The Comparative Guide to American Hospitals

Volume 3

Fourth Edition

The Comparative Guide to American Hospitals

Volume 3: Central Region

4,834 Hospitals with Key Personnel and
67 Quality Measures Relating to Heart Attack, Heart Failure, Pneumonia, Stroke, Blood Clots, Childhood Asthma, Emergency Room Care, Surgical Care, Preventative Care, Medical Imaging and Patient Experience

A SEDGWICK PRESS Book

Grey House Publishing

PUBLISHER: Leslie Mackenzie
SENIOR EDITOR: David Garoogian
EDITORIAL DIRECTOR: Laura Mars
PRODUCTION MANAGER: Kristen Thatcher
MARKETING DIRECTOR: Jessica Moody

A Sedgewick Press Book
Grey House Publishing, Inc.
4919 Route 22
Amenia, NY 12501
518.789.8700
FAX 845.373.6390
www.greyhouse.com
e-mail: books @greyhouse.com

Fourth Edition

Printed in the Canada

Comparative guide to American hospitals. Vol. 3, Central region; [ed. David Garoogian]. — 4th ed. (2014)

4 v. ; cm.

Includes index.
"4,834 Hospitals with Key Personnel and 67 Quality Measures Relating to Heart Attack, Heart Failure, Pneumonia, Stroke, Blood Clots, Childhood Asthma, Emergency Room Care, Surgical Care, Preventative Care, Medical Imaging and Patient Experience."

1. Hospitals—United States—Directories. 2. Hospitals—United States—Periodicals. 3. Hospitals—Ratings—United States—Statistics—Periodicals. 4. Myocardial infarction—Hospitals—United States—Directories. 5. Heart failure—Hospitals—United States—Directories. 6. Pneumonia—Hospitals—United States—Directories. I. Garoogian, David.

RA977 .C66
610/.025

4-Volume Set	ISBN: 978-1-61925-457-2
Volume 1	ISBN: 978-1-61925-458-9
Volume 2	ISBN: 978-1-61925-459-6
Volume 3	**ISBN: 978-1-61925-460-2**
Volume 4	ISBN: 978-1-61925-461-9

Table of Contents

Introduction

This is the fourth edition of *The Comparative Guide to American Hospitals*. It reports on how 4,834 hospitals—**141 more than last edition**—in America measure up when caring for patients with a number of specific conditions. The third edition reported on **Heart Attacks, Heart Failure, Pneumonia, Childhood Asthma, Surgical Care, Use of Medical Imaging**, and **Patients' Hospital Experiences**. This fourth edition includes new data on **Blood Clot Prevention and Treatment, Emergency Room Care, Preventative Care, Stroke,** and **Medicare Spending**. Also new are appendices on **Surgical Complication Rates** and **Best Hospitals by Category**.

This work is based on a Federal study (Hospital Compare) in which short-term acute care and critical access hospitals around the country voluntarily report on quality measures to receive an incentive payment established by the Medicare Prescription Drug, Improvement and Modernization Act of 2003. Each hospital in this edition is rated on 67 recognized quality measures—**18 more than last edition**—and is compared to both state and national averages.

In *The Comparative Guide to American Hospitals,* the data is organized, sorted and ranked by our editors. It is this organization and ranking that makes *The Comparative Guide to American Hospitals* a unique and valuable tool to the health care consumer. Data is presented in such a way as to inform and educate the user, who can then put the facts into a meaningful context as hospitals are evaluated state by state.

Due to the increased data, and the regional use of such data, this edition is again comprised of four regional volumes—**Eastern, Southern, Central** and **Western**. In addition to comprehensive **hospital rankings and profiles** for all states in the region, each volume includes four Appendices with additional information.

In addition to the data from Hospital Compare, each hospital profile in *The Comparative Guide to American Hospitals* is comprised of value-added data from Grey House's *Directory of Hospital Personnel*. This critical contact data includes fax numbers, web sites, email addresses, and number of beds plus 24,458 key contact names—**783 more names than last edition**. In addition, each state chapter includes **State Hospital Rankings**.

Section One: State Hospital Rankings & State Profiles

The first section of each regional volume of *The Comparative Guide to American Hospitals* is arranged alphabetically by state. Each state chapter starts with a ranking section, unique to Grey House, that ranks hospitals in that state on how often they meet each of the 67 accepted quality protocols. The quality measures ranked in *The Comparative Guide to American Hospitals* are based on accepted, effective treatments supported by the Centers for Medicare & Medical Services of the US Department of Health & Human Services and the Hospital Quality Alliance (HQA)—a public/private collaboration established to promote on hospital quality of care. HQA represents consumers, hospitals, doctors, employers, accrediting organizations and Federal agencies.

Following the ranking section, hospital profiles are listed first by city, then alpha within city. Profiles include name, address, phone, fax, web site, hospital type and ownership, number of beds, and whether the hospital provides emergency services. Further, each profile includes an average of five key medical contacts—representing not only the facility's top administration but also the physicians specifically responsible for the care of heart, pneumonia, and asthma patients, as well as surgical care. Again, these data points are unique to *The Comparative Guide to American Hospitals*, and complete the picture for health care consumers searching for quality care.

The remainder of each hospital profile examines the 67 quality measures in detail, comparing the hospital's score with both the state and national average: These measures include:

- **Timely and Effective Care:**
  - **Blood Clot Prevention and Treatment** ***(NEW)*** measures include anticoagulation overlap therapy, ICU venous thromboembolism prophylaxis, incidence of potentially preventable VTE, UFH with dosages/platelet count monitoring, venous thromboembolism prophylaxis, and warfarin therapy discharge instructions
  - **Chest Pain/Possible Heart Attack Care** measures include aspirin at arrival, median time to ECG, median time to transfer, and fibrinolytic medication timing
  - **Children's Asthma Care** measures include receiving systemic corticosteroids, receiving home management plan, and receiving reliever medication
  - **Emergency Department** ***(NEW)*** measures include admittance decision time, head CT results within 45 minutes of arrival, patients who left ER before being seen, time from ER arrival to admittance, time from ER arrival to discharge, time spent in ER before being evaluated, and time to pain medications for long-bone fractures
  - **Heart Attack Care** measures include aspirin given at discharge, statin prescribed at discharge, fibrinolytic medication timing, and percutaneous coronary intervention within 90 minutes of arrival
  - **Heart Failure Care** measures include angiotensin converting enzyme inhibitor or angiotensin receptor blocker for left ventricular systolic dysfunction, discharge instructions given, and evaluation of left ventricular systolic function
  - **Pneumonia Care** measures include appropriate initial antibiotic, and blood culture timing
  - **Pregnancy and Delivery Care** ***(NEW)*** measures include newborn deliveries scheduled early
  - **Preventive Care** ***(NEW)*** measures include immunization for influenza and immunization for pneumonia
  - **Stroke Care** ***(NEW)*** measures include anticoagulation therapy for atrial fibrillation, antithrombotic therapy timing, assessed for rehabilitation, discharged on antithrombotic therapy, discharged on statin medication, thrombolytic therapy timing, venous thromboembolism prophylaxis, and written stroke educational materials given
  - **Surgical Care** measures include appropriate venous thromboembolism prophylaxis within 24 hours, appropriate beta blocker usage, controlled postoperative blood glucose, perioperative temperature management ***(NEW)***, prophylactic antibiotic timing, prophylactic antibiotic selection, prophylactic antibiotic stopped, and urinary catheter removal
- **Medicare Spending** ***(NEW)*** measures include Medicare spending per beneficiary
- **Use of Medical Imaging** measures include MRI for low back pain, cardiac imaging stress test before surgery ***(NEW)***, follow-up mammogram/ultrasound, combination brain/sinus CT scan ***(NEW)***, combination abdominal CT scan, and combination chest CT scan.
- **Survey of Patients' Hospital Experiences**
  HCAHPS (Hospital Consumer Assessment of Healthcare Providers and Systems) is a national, standardized survey of hospital patients. HCAHPS (pronounced "H-caps") was created to publicly report the patient's perspective of hospital care. The survey asks a random sample of recently discharged patients about important aspects of their hospital experience. The HCAHPS results allow consumers to make fair and objective comparisons between hospitals, and of individual hospitals to state and national benchmarks, on ten important measures of patients' perspectives of care:
  - How do patients rate the hospital overall?
  - How often did doctors communicate well with patients?
  - How often did nurses communicate well with patients?
  - How often did patients receive help quickly from hospital staff?
  - How often did staff explain about medicines before giving them to patients?
  - How often was patients' pain well controlled?
  - How often was the area around patients' rooms kept quiet at night?
  - How often were the patients' rooms and bathrooms kept clean?
  - Were patients given information about what to do during their recovery at home?
  - Would patients recommend the hospital to friends and family?

Section Two: Appendixes & Index

The second section of *The Comparative Guide to American Hospitals* includes:

- **Appendix A: 30-Day Death (Mortality) Rates** Unique to Grey House, this section takes data and organize it in a helpful, informative way for the reader. It lists hospitals nationwide that are "better" or "worse" than the national average, plus a State and National Summary of Hospital Mortality Rates.
- **Appendix B: 30-Day Readmission Rates** lists hospitals nationwide that are "better" or "worse" than the national average, plus a State and National Summary of Hospital Readmission Rates.
- **Appendix C: Surgical Complication Rates** lists hospitals nationwide that are "better" or "worse" than the national average, plus a State and National Summary of Hospital Readmission Rates. Surgical complications covered include:
    - A Wound That Splits Open After Surgery on the Abdomen or Pelvis
    - Accidental Cuts and Tears From Medical Treatment
    - Collapsed Lung Due to Medical Treatment
    - Deaths Among Patients With Serious Treatable Complications After Surgery
    - Rate of Complications for Hip/Knee Replacement Patients
    - Serious Blood Clots After Surgery
    - Serious Complications
- **Appendix D: Best Hospitals by Selected Category** lists best hospitals nationwide based on their average scores in 11 categories. The categories are:
    - Blood Clot Prevention and Treatment
    - Children's Asthma Care
    - Emergency Department Care
    - Heart Care
    - Pneumonia Care
    - Preventative Care
    - Stroke Care
    - Surgical Care
    - Patient's Hospital Experiences
    - Use of Medical Imaging
    - Lowest Medicare Spending per Beneficiary
- **Appendix E: Glossary** provides a list of 87 medical terms to make the best use possible of the data in this edition.
- **Regional Hospital Profile Index** lists hospitals included in each regional volume alphabetically, including city and state.
- **National Hospital Profile Index** lists all hospitals nationwide alphabetically, including volume number, city and state. Appears in Volume 4 only.

This completely revised fourth edition of *The Comparative Guide to American Hospitals* is a valuable guide for the entire medical community, with more hospitals, more criteria measures and more key executives than the last edition. It offers an indispensable snapshot of how hospitals measure up, not only to established "best practices," but also to each other.

We welcome your comments to this edition.

User's Guide

What is the *Comparative Guide to American Hospitals*?

The *Comparative Guide to American Hospitals* (CGAH) is based on a Federal study (Hospital Compare) in which short-term acute care and critical access hospitals around the country voluntarily report on quality measures to receive an incentive payment established by the Medicare Prescription Drug, Improvement and Modernization Act of 2003. Each hospital in this edition is rated on 67 recognized quality measures and is compared to both state and national averages. The measures are grouped into four major categories: Timely and Effective Care; Survey of Patients' Experiences; Use of Medical Imaging; and Medicare Spending Per Beneficiary.

Timely and Effective Care Measures (aka "Process of Care" Measures)

Process of care measures reported under the Hospital Inpatient Quality Reporting (IQR) and Outpatient Quality Reporting (OQR) programs show: 1) The percentage of hospital patients who receive treatments known to get the best results for certain common, serious medical conditions or surgical procedures; 2) How quickly hospitals treat patients who come to the hospital with certain medical emergencies. The measures only apply to patients for whom the recommended treatment would be appropriate. By law, any measures reported on the Hospital Compare website must reflect accepted standards of care, based on current scientific evidence. The measures are regularly reviewed and revised to ensure that they are up-to-date, and new measures and types of conditions and treatments are added over time. Process of care measures include:

- Blood Clot Prevention and Treatment
- Chest Pain/Possible Heart Attack Care
- Children's Asthma Care
- Emergency Department Care
- Heart Attack Care
- Heart Failure Care
- Pneumonia Care
- Pregnancy and Delivery Care
- Preventative Care
- Stroke Care
- Surgical Care Improvment Project

Where the Information Comes From

Measures of timely and effective care come from the data that hospitals get from medical records of their eligible patients, following standards for abstracting and reporting the information. Data submissions include auditing procedures and edit checks to assess whether data submitted are consistent with CMS's defined specifications. In addition, CMS validates the data submitted to provide assurance that the hospital, or its designated agent, can accurately abstract patient medical records and accurately submit data.

What Patients the Measures Apply To

The measures of timely and effective care apply to any adult patients treated at hospitals participating in the IQR and OQR programs for whom the recommended treatments would be appropriate, including Medicare patients, Medicare managed care patients, and non-Medicare patients. Hospitals with a large number of discharges may provide data from a sample of eligible Medicare and non-Medicare patients, based CMS sampling rules.

Risk Adjustment

The measures of timely and effective care do not require risk adjustment, because patients for whom the recommended treatment would not be appropriate are not included in the calculations.

Significance Testing

CMS does not perform tests of statistical significance in reporting the measures of timely and effective care. However, the smaller the sample size, the greater the difference in rates must be in order for that difference to be statistically meaningful. Large differences between individual hospitals' rates may be significant, but small differences between hospitals are usually not significant.

Reporting Period

These 50 measures are based on a reporting period of October 1, 2012 through September 30, 2013 except for the following: Emergency Department Care—Percentage of Patients Who Left the Emergency Department Before Being Seen—January 1, 2012 through December 31, 2012; Preventative Care—Patients Assessed and Given Influenza Vaccination—October 1, 2012 through March 31, 2013; All eight Stroke Care measures—January 1, 2013 through September 30, 2013; All six Blood Clot Prevention and Treatment measures—January 1, 2013 through September 30, 2013.

Survey of Patients' Experiences

The Centers for Medicare & Medicaid Services (CMS), along with the Agency for Healthcare Research and Quality (AHRQ), developed the HCAHPS (Hospital Consumer Assessment of Healthcare Providers and Systems) Survey, also known as Hospital CAHPS®, to provide a standardized survey instrument and data collection methodology for measuring patients' perspectives on hospital care. The HCAHPS Survey is administered to a random sample of patients continuously throughout the year. CMS cleans, adjusts and analyzes the data, then publicly reports the results.

Which Patients are Included
The HCAHPS survey is administered to a random sample of adult patients across medical conditions between 48 hours and six weeks after discharge; the survey is not restricted to Medicare beneficiaries.

Where the Information Comes From
All short-term, acute care, non-specialty hospitals are invited to participate in the HCAHPS Survey. Over 4,000 hospitals participate in HCAHPS. The goal is for each hospital to get at least 300 completed patient surveys per year. In general, the more patients that respond to the survey, the more the results shown on this website will reflect the experiences of all the patients who used that hospital. HCAHPS survey data must be collected by organizations that are trained by the federal government in HCAHPS data collection procedures. Data submitted to the HCAHPS data warehouse is cleaned, adjusted and analyzed by CMS, which calculates hospitals' HCAHPS scores and publicly reports them on the Hospital Compare website.

Adjusting Rates
Preparing the data for public reporting includes taking certain factors into account to ensure fair comparisons among hospitals. For example, the mix of patients can differ from one hospital to the next, and these differences in the patient mix can affect a hospital's HCAHPS results. Patient-mix adjustment takes these differences into account so that the survey results reported on this website are what would be expected for each hospital if all hospitals had a similar mix of patients.

Reporting Period
These 10 measures are based on a reporting period of October 1, 2012 through September 30, 2013.

Use of Medical Imaging

The six measures on the use of medical imaging show how often a hospital provides specific imaging tests for Medicare beneficiaries under circumstances where they may not be medically appropriate. Lower percentages suggest more efficient use of medical imaging. The purpose of reporting these measures is to reduce unnecessary exposure to contrast materials and/or radiation, to ensure adherence to evidence-based medicine and practice guidelines, and to prevent wasteful use of Medicare resources. The measures only apply to Medicare patients treated in hospital outpatient departments. It does not include tests performed in other ambulatory care settings or hospital inpatient settings.

What Patients are Included
Outpatient imaging efficiency measures apply only to Medicare beneficiaries enrolled in Original Medicare who were treated as outpatients in hospital facilities reimbursed through the Outpatient Prospective Payment System (OPPS). They do not include Medicare managed care patients, non-Medicare patients, or patients who were admitted to the hospital as inpatients.

Where the Information Comes From
CMS calculates imaging efficiency measures using data from claims that hospitals and physicians submit for Medicare beneficiaries enrolled in Original Medicare. The data are calculated only for hospitals paid through the Outpatient Prospective Payment System (OPPS). The measures are part of the Hospital Outpatient Quality Reporting Program (OQR).

Risk Adjustment
Outpatient imaging efficiency measures are not risk adjusted. However, measures specifications do not include cases where there were clear medical reasons for performing the tests.

Significance Testing
CMS does not perform tests of statistical significance in reporting the outpatient imaging efficiency measures. Large differences between hospitals' percentages may be significant, but small differences usually are not.

Reporting Period
These six measures are based on a reporting period of July 1, 2012 through June 30, 2013.

Medicare Spending per Beneficiary

The Medicare Spending per Beneficiary (MSPB) measure assesses Medicare Part A and Part B payments for services provided to a Medicare beneficiary during a spending-per-beneficiary episode that spans from three days prior to an inpatient hospital admission through 30 days after discharge. The payments included in this measure are price-standardized and risk-adjusted. Price standardization removes sources of variation that are due to geographic payment differences such as wage index and geographic practice cost differences, as well as indirect medical education (IME) or disproportionate share hospital (DSH) payments. Risk adjustment accounts for variation due to patient health status.

By measuring cost of care through this measure, CMS hopes to increase the transparency of care for consumers and recognize hospitals that are involved in the provision of high-quality care at lower cost to Medicare.

Reporting Period
This measure is based on a reporting period of January 1, 2012 through December 31, 2012.

Sample Entry

The listing below illustrates the kind of information that is or might be included in a Hospital Profile. Each numbered item of information is described in the paragraphs following the example.

1 ▶ **Cleveland Clinic**
9500 Euclid Avenue
Cleveland, OH 44195
Phone: 216-444-2200
Fax: 216-445-7758
URL: www.clevelandclinic.org
Type: Acute Care Hospitals
Emergency Services: Yes
Ownership: Voluntary non-profit - Private
Beds: 1,113

2 ▶ **Key Personnel:**
CEO/President. . . . . Delos M Cosgrove, MD
Chief of Medical Staff. . . . . Marc Harrison, MD
Infection Control. . . . . David L Longworth, MD
Operating Room. . . . . Allan Siperstein, MD
Pediatric Ambulatory Care . . . . . . Robert Wyllie, MD
Quality Assurance . . . . J Michael Henderson, MD
Radiology. . . . . Gregory P Borkowski, MD

	Measure	Cases	This Hosp.	State Avg.	U.S. Avg.
3 ▶					
4 ▶	**Blood Clot Prevention and Treatment**				
	Anticoagulation Overlap Therapy[2]	400	98%	93%	93%
	ICU Venous Thromboembolism Prophylaxis[2]	84	98%	93%	92%
	Incidence of Potentially Preventable VTE[2]	168	2%	6%	10%
	UFH with Dosages/Platelet Monitoring[2]	444	100%	98%	97%
	Venous Thromboembolism Prophylaxis[2]	347	96%	88%	85%
	Warfarin Therapy Discharge Instructions[2]	237	89%	79%	75%
5 ▶	**Chest Pain/Possible Heart Attack Care**				
	Aspirin Given Within 24 Hours of Arrival	190	96%	97%	96%
	Fibrinolytic Meds Within 30 Min. of Arrival[7]	-	-	44%	58%
	Median Time to ECG (minutes)	197	6	6	7
	Median Time to Transfer (minutes)[1]	-	-	58	60
6 ▶	**Children's Asthma Care**				
	Received Home Management Plan of Care	74	99%	85%	88%
	Received Reliever Medication	75	100%	100%	100%
	Received Systemic Corticosteroids	74	100%	100%	100%
7 ▶	**Emergency Department**				
	Admittance Decision Time (minutes)[2]	227	102	90	98%
	Head CT Results Within 45 Min. of Arrival	11	91%	63%	57%
	Patients Who Left ER Before Being Seen	82,229	2%	2%	2%
	Time from ER Arrival to Admit. (minutes)[2]	228	304	265	274
	Time from ER Arrival to Discharge (minutes)	294	131	128	134
	Time in ER Before Being Evaluated (minutes)	417	11	22	26
	Time to Pain Meds for Fractures (minutes)	194	46	54	57
8 ▶	**Heart Attack Care**				
	Aspirin Given at Discharge	868	100%	99%	99%
	Fibrinolytic Meds Within 30 Min. of Arrival[7]	-	-	80%	54%
	PCI Within 90 Minutes of Arrival	13	92%	97%	96%
	Statin Prescribed at Discharge	834	100%	98%	98%
9 ▶	**Heart Failure Care**				
	ACE Inhibitor or ARB for LVSD[2]	287	99%	97%	97%
	Discharge Instructions Given[2]	712	94%	96%	94%
	Evaluation of LVS Function[2]	858	100%	100%	99%
10 ▶	**Medicare Spending**				
	Medicare Hospital Spending per Patient	-	0.99	1.01	0.98
11 ▶	**Pneumonia Care**				
	Appropriate Initial Antibiotic Given	84	94%	96%	95%
	Blood Culture Timing	176	95%	98%	98%
12 ▶	**Pregnancy and Delivery Care**				
	Newborn Deliveries Scheduled Early[1]	-	-	5%	6%
13 ▶	**Preventive Care**				
	Immunization for Influenza[2]	577	96%	93%	90%
	Immunization for Pneumonia[2]	747	95%	94%	92%
14 ▶	**Stroke Care**				
	Anticoagulation Therapy for Atrial Fibrillation[2]	34	100%	95%	95%
	Antithrombotic Therapy Timing[2]	180	96%	98%	98%
	Assessed for Rehabilitation[2]	333	98%	98%	97%
	Discharged on Antithrombotic Therapy[2]	221	100%	99%	99%
	Discharged on Statin Medication[2]	152	99%	95%	94%
	Thrombolytic Therapy Timing[1,2]	-	-	65%	66%
	Venous Thromboembolism Prophylaxis[2]	349	100%	95%	94%
	Written Stroke Educational Materials Given[2]	125	98%	92%	88%
15 ▶	**Surgical Care Improvement Project**				
	Appropriate Beta Blocker Usage[2]	356	99%	98%	98%
	Appropriate VTP Within 24 Hours[2]	447	99%	98%	98%
	Controlled Postoperative Blood Glucose[2]	253	96%	97%	97%
	Perioperative Temperature Management[2]	625	100%	100%	100%
	Prophylactic Antibiotic Selection[2]	570	99%	99%	99%
	Prophylactic Antibiotic Selection (Outpatient)	1,080	100%	98%	98%
	Prophylactic Antibiotic Stopped[2]	554	97%	98%	98%
	Prophylactic Antibiotic Timing[2]	570	99%	99%	99%
	Prophylactic Antibiotic Timing (Outpatient)	563	97%	97%	98%
	Urinary Catheter Removal[2]	381	98%	97%	97%
16 ▶	**Survey of Patients' Hospital Experiences**				
	Area Around Room 'Always' Quiet at Night	300+	57%	58%	61%
	Doctors 'Always' Communicated Well	300+	82%	80%	82%
	Home Recovery Information Given	300+	90%	87%	85%
	Hospital Given 9 or 10 on 10 Point Scale	300+	84%	72%	71%
	Meds 'Always' Explained Before Given	300+	66%	64%	64%
	Nurses 'Always' Communicated Well	300+	83%	81%	79%
	Pain 'Always' Well Controlled	300+	72%	71%	71%
	Room and Bathroom 'Always' Clean	300+	78%	75%	73%
	Timely Help 'Always' Received	300+	68%	70%	68%
	Would Definitely Recommend Hospital	300+	87%	71%	71%
17 ▶	**Use of Medical Imaging**				
	Cardiac Imaging Stress Test before Surgery	4,179	6.7%	5.4%	5.3%
	Combination Abdominal CT Scan	5,813	13.0%	7.1%	10.5%
	Combination Brain/Sinus CT Scan	2,131	1.7%	2.8%	2.7%
	Combination Chest CT Scan	6,539	0.1%	1.7%	2.7%
	Follow-up Mammogram/Ultrasound	9,962	9.3%	8.7%	8.8%
	Lumbar Spine MRI for Low Back Pain	661	31.9%	34.7%	37.2%

1▶ **Hospital Name and Record Header:** hospital name; street address; phone; fax; e-mail; URL; hospital type; ownership; emergency services (Yes/No); and number of beds.

2▶ **Key Personnel:** includes the names of key personnel primarily related to the conditions covered in this publication.

3▶ **Hospital Compare Data:** each profile contains data covering 67 measures contained in the Centers for Medicare & Medicaid Services Hospital Compare database. There are five columns:

Measure: the 67 quality measures reported.

There are 14 possible footnotes:

(1) The number of cases/patients is too few to report
This footnote is applied: when the number of cases/patients does not meet the required minimum amount for public reporting; when the number of cases/patients is too small to reliably tell how well a hospital is performing; and/or to protect personal health information.

(2) Data submitted were based on a sample of cases/patients
This footnote indicates that a hospital chose to submit data for a random sample of its cases/patients while following specific rules for how to select the patients.

(3) Results are based on a shorter time period than required
This footnote indicates that the hospital's results were based on data from less than the maximum possible time period generally used to collect data for a measure. See Reporting Periods for more information.

(4) Data suppressed by CMS (Centers for Medicare and Medicaid Services) for one or more quarters
The results for these measures were excluded for various reasons, such as data inaccuracies.

(5) Results are not available for this reporting period
This footnote is applied when the hospital does not have data to report.

(6) Fewer than 100 patients completed the HCAHPS survey.
This footnote is applied when the number of completed surveys the hospital or its vendor provided to CMS is less than 100. Use these scores with caution, as the number of surveys may be too low to reliably assess hospital performance.

(7) No cases met the criteria for this measure
This footnote is applied when a hospital did not have any cases meet the inclusion criteria for a measure.

(8) The lower limit of the confidence interval cannot be calculated
The lower limit of the confidence interval cannot be calculated if the number of observed infections equals zero.

(9) No data are available from the state/territory for this reporting period
This footnote is applied when: too few hospitals in a state/territory had data available; or no data was reported for this state/territory.

(10) The scores shown reflect fewer than 50 completed surveys.
This footnote is applied when the number of completed surveys the hospital or its vendor provided to CMS is less than 50. Use these scores with caution, as the number of surveys may be too low to reliably assess hospital performance.

(11) There were discrepancies in the data collection process
This footnote is applied when there have been deviations from data collection protocols. CMS is working to correct this situation.

(12) This measure does not apply to this hospital for this reporting period
This footnote is applied when: there were zero device days or procedures; the hospital does not have ICU locations; the hospital is a new member of the registry and didn't have an opportunity to submit any cases; or the hospital does not report this voluntary measure.

(13) Results cannot be calculated for this reporting period
This footnote is applied when: the number of predicted infections is less than 1; the number of observed MRSA or Clostridium difficile infections present on admission (community-onset prevalence) was above a pre-determined cut-point.

(14) The results for this state are combined with nearby states to protect confidentiality
This footnote is applied when a state has fewer than 10 hospitals in order to protect confidentiality. Results are combined as follows: 1) the District of Columbia and Delaware are combined; 2) Alaska and Washington are combined; 3) North Dakota and South Dakota are combined; and 4) New Hampshire and Vermont are combined. Hospitals located in Maryland and U.S. territories are excluded from the measure calculation.

Cases: the size of the data sample (number of patients) for each hospital and quality measure. In addition, the notation "0" is applied when a hospital provided care to patients with a condition, such as pneumonia, but the cases that the hospital submitted did not meet the specific criteria for being included in the calculation of the measure.

This Hospital: the performance rate that the hospital achieved for each quality measure. This value is expressed as a percentage of the sample size that was measured. The performance rate is calculated by dividing the numerator by the denominator. The denominator is the sum of all eligible cases (as defined in the measure specifications) submitted to the QIO Clinical Data Warehouse for the reporting period. The numerator is the sum of all eligible cases submitted for the same reporting period where the recommended care was provided.

State Average: the average rate for all hospitals reporting data in the state the hospital is located in.

U.S. Average: the average rate for all hospitals reporting nationwide.

Note: Beginning in December 2010, state and national averages for the process of care measures are calculated by summing the cases in the state or nation that "passed" the measure (Numerator) and dividing that sum by the number of cases in the state or national Denominator. For the national and state averages, a simple average was constructed where the numerator was the sum of all non-excluded hospitals' scores and the denominator was the total number of hospitals, each calculated at either the national or individual state level. For the process and survey measures, the national and state averages are calculated before excluding suppressed rates and are not recalculated using only published rates as was done prior to September 2009. Acute Care-VA Medical Centers are not included in the calculation of the national and state comparison rates.

The children's asthma care national and state averages are calculated differently. The average rate for all healthcare organizations in the nation that provide results for a measure. The average rate is calculated by dividing the total number of patients who had the recommended care provided for a measure by the total number of patients who met the inclusion and exclusion criteria for that measure in the nation for the timeframe being reported.

4▸ Blood Clot Prevention and Treatment

The measures listed below show how well hospitals are providing recommended care known to prevent or treat blood clots and how often blood clots occur that could have been prevented.

Anticoagulation Overlap Therapy

Patients with blood clots who got the recommended treatment, which includes using two different blood thinner medicines at the same time.
Patients who develop blood clots in their veins (also called venous thromboembolism, or VTE) need to get treatment that can break up the clots quickly and prevent others from forming. The recommended treatment is to first give a blood thinner that can get into the bloodstream quickly through an IV or injection (heparin), then give a slower-acting oral blood thinner medicine (warfarin), and continue giving both blood thinners for 5 days or until it is safe for the patient to transition off of the IV blood thinner and use only the oral blood thinner medicine. This measure shows the percentage of hospital patients who had a confirmed diagnosis of blood clot at hospital admission or during their hospital stay, and received both medicines for at least 5 days, or were discharged from the hospital on both kinds of medicine, unless their blood work showed they no longer needed it. *Higher percentages are better.*

ICU Venous Thromboembolism Prophylaxis

Patients who got treatment to prevent blood clots on the day of or day after being admitted to the intensive care unit (ICU).
Patients in the Intensive Care Unit (ICU) are at increased risk for developing blood clots in their veins (venous thromboembolism, or VTE), because they are in bed for a long period of time. These clots can break off and travel to other parts of the body, causing serious harm. Hospitals can prevent blood clots by routinely evaluating all patients for their risk of developing blood clots and using appropriate prevention and treatment procedures. Prevention can include compression stockings, blood thinners, and/or other medicines. This measure shows the percentage of ICU patients who received treatment to prevent blood clots: on the day of or day after arrival at the hospital; or on the day of or day after transfer to the ICU; or on the day of or day after having surgery. Patients who did not receive treatment may also be included in this measure, if they had paperwork in their chart to explain why. Reasons for not receiving treatment may include having a massive wound, actively bleeding, or having an allergy to blood thinners. *Higher percentages are better.*

Incidence of Potentially Preventable VTE
Patients who developed a blood clot while in the hospital who did not get treatment that could have prevented it. Because hospital patients often have to stay in bed for long periods of time, all patients admitted to the hospital are at increased risk of developing blood clots in their veins (also called venous thromboembolism or VTE) that can break off and travel to other parts of the body, like the heart, brain, or lung. Hospitals can prevent blood clots by routinely evaluating patients for their risk of developing blood clots and using appropriate prevention and treatment procedures. Prevention can include compression stockings, blood thinners, and/or other medicines. This measure shows the percentage of patients who developed blood clots while in the hospital who did not receive preventative treatment beforehand. *Lower percentages are better.*

UFH with Dosages/Platelet Monitoring
Patients with blood clots who were treated with an intravenous blood thinner, and then were checked to determine if the blood thinner was putting the patient at an increased risk of bleeding.
Patients who have been diagnosed with a blood clot (also called venous thromboembolism, or VTE) are usually treated with a blood thinner such as IV heparin. Some patients may be prescribed a type of IV heparin called unfractionated heparin (UFH). Unfractionated heparin carries a higher risk of increased bleeding than a different type of IV heparin (called low molecular weight heparin). Risk for bleeding increases because blood thinners increase the time it takes your blood to clot. The most common signs of increased bleeding include unusual bruising, nosebleeds, and bleeding gums. Because of their higher risk of bleeding, patients getting unfractionated heparin should be given regular blood tests to determine if they are at an increased risk of bleeding from getting the medication. This measure shows the percentage of patients who developed a blood clot at admission or during their hospital stay, treated with unfractionated IV heparin who had their blood checked using recommended procedures. *Higher percentages are better.*

Venous Thromboembolism Prophylaxis
Patients who got treatment to prevent blood clots on the day of or day after hospital admission or surgery.
Because hospital patients often have to stay in bed for long periods of time, all patients admitted to the hospital are at increased risk of developing blood clots in their veins (also called venous thromboembolism, or VTE) that can break off and travel to other parts of the body, like the heart, brain, or lung. Hospitals can prevent blood clots by routinely evaluating patients for their risk of developing blood clots and using appropriate prevention and treatment procedures. Prevention can include compression stockings, blood thinners, and/or other medicines. This measure shows the percentage of patients who received treatment to prevent blood clots: on the day of or day after arrival at the hospital; or on the day of or day after having surgery. Patients who did not receive treatment may also be included in this measure, if they had paperwork in their chart to explain why. Reasons for not receiving treatment may include having a massive wound, actively bleeding, or having an allergy to blood thinners. *Higher percentages are better.*

Warfarin Therapy Discharge Instructions
Patients with blood clots who were discharged on a blood thinner medicine and received written instructions about that medicine.
Patients who develop blood clots (also called venous thromboembolism or VTE) will usually be given blood thinner medicines to take when they leave the hospital. Educating patients about how to take the medicine and its possible side effects can help prevent problems that could bring them back to the hospital. Before leaving the hospital, patients with a blood clot, who are taking a blood thinner medicine, and their caregiver should receive information about the following topics: Compliance (how to follow medication instructions); Diet (how to eat a healthy diet and avoid foods that interfere with blood thinners); Monitoring their blood thinner medicine; Adverse drug reactions (difficulty breathing, vomiting, nausea); When to call your health care provider (dizziness or weakness, a fall, bright red bleeding). This measure shows the percentage of patients diagnosed with a blood clot (either at admission or during their hospital stay) discharged from the hospital on blood thinners (anticoagulants or anticoagulant therapy or warfarin therapy) who received written educational instructions at hospital discharge. *Higher percentages are better.*

5▶ Chest Pain/Possible Heart Attack Care

Scientific evidence shows that the following measures represent the best practices for the treatment of chest pain/possible heart attack.

Aspirin Given Within 24 Hours of Arrival
Outpatients with chest pain or possible heart attack who got aspirin within 24 hours of arrival.
Blood clots can cause heart attacks. For many patients having a heart attack, taking aspirin soon after symptoms of a heart attack begin may help break up a clot and make the heart attack less severe. If patients have not taken aspirin themselves before going to the hospital, they should get aspirin when they arrive. Standards for care say that patients should get aspirin within 24 hours of arriving at the hospital. This measure tells what percent of patients got aspirin within this time period. *Higher percentages are better.*

Fibrinolytic Meds Within 30 Minutes of Arrival
Outpatients with chest pain or possible heart attack who got drugs to break up blood clots within 30 minutes of arrival.
Blood clots can cause heart attacks. Certain patients having a heart attack should get a "clot busting" drug to help break up the blood clots and improve blood flow to the heart. Standards for care say that a clot busting drug should be given within 30 minutes of arrival at the hospital. This measure tells the percent of patients who were given a clot busting drug within this time period. *Higher percentages are better.*

Average Time to ECG (minutes)
Average number of minutes before outpatients with chest pain or possible heart attack got an ECG.
"ECG" (sometimes called EKG) stands for electrocardiogram. An ECG is a test that can help doctors know whether patients are having a heart attack. Standards of care say that patients with chest pain or a possible heart attack should have an ECG upon arrival, preferably within 10 minutes. This measure shows the average number of minutes it takes before patients had an ECG (calculated as an arithmetic median). Sometimes patients get an ECG done before they get to the hospital (for example, by the ambulance staff). This is counted as "0 minutes." *Lower numbers are better.*

Average Time to Transfer (minutes)
Average number of minutes before outpatients with chest pain or possible heart attack who needed specialized care were transferred to another hospital.
If a hospital does not have the facilities to provide specialized heart attack care, it transfers patients with possible heart attack to another hospital that can give them this care. This measure shows how long it takes, on average, for hospitals to identify patients who need specialized heart attack care the hospital cannot provide and begin their transfer to another hospital. Specifically, it shows the average (arithmetic median) number of minutes it takes from the time patients arrive in the emergency department until they are transported to a different hospital. *Lower numbers are better.*

6 ▸ Children's Asthma Care

Scientific evidence shows that the following measures represent best practices for treating children with asthma.

Received Home Management Plan of Care
Children and their caregivers who received a home management plan of care document while hospitalized for asthma.
This measure shows the percentage of children with asthma and their caregivers who were given a home management plan of care document while hospitalized. Because asthma is a chronic condition, controlling a child's asthma symptoms at home will help reduce the risk of further attacks. Knowledge about the disease and its treatment is the key to good asthma control. Asthma that is not managed effectively may lead to more visits to the hospital. Medications can help prevent asthma symptoms and attacks from starting in the first place and can reduce how often attacks happen and severity of the attacks. It is important for children with asthma and their caregivers to know how to prevent asthma symptoms and attacks before they happen. The home management plan of care helps children with asthma and their caregivers develop a plan to manage the child's asthma symptoms and to know when to take action. It should address all of the following: arrangements for follow-up care; environmental control and control of other triggers; method and timing of rescue actions; use of controller medications; use of reliever medications. *Higher percentages are better.*

Received Reliever Medication
Children who received reliever medication while hospitalized for asthma.
National guidelines for treating children with asthma recommend using relievers in the severe phase and gradually cutting down the dosage of medications to provide control of asthma symptoms. Although there are guidelines for medication therapy for children with asthma, there is evidence that these guidelines are not being consistently followed. Using the appropriate medications will lower the risk of severe illness and/or death. This measure shows the percentage of children with asthma who were given reliever medication (like albuterol) while hospitalized. Relievers are medications that relax the bands of muscle surrounding the airways and make breathing easier. *Higher percentages are better.*

Received Systemic Corticosteroids
Children who received systemic corticosteroid medication (oral and IV medication that reduces inflammation and controls symptoms) while hospitalized for asthma.
Oral or IV steroid medications control severe asthma well. That is why they are important for hospital care. Unfortunately, they can cause serious side effects when used long-term. That is why they are mainly used for severe episodes or chronic severe asthma, which cannot be controlled with other medications (like inhaled or oral bronchodilators and anti-inflammatory medications). This measure shows the percentage of children with asthma who were given oral or IV steroid medications while hospitalized. These medications work in the body as a whole,

rather than just on the lungs. They help reduce inflammation and control allergic reactions. *Higher percentages are better.*

7▶ Emergency Department Care

Timely and effective care in hospital emergency departments is essential for good patient outcomes. Delays before receiving care in the emergency department can reduce the quality of care and increase risks and discomfort for patients with serious illnesses or injuries. Waiting times at different hospitals can vary widely, depending on the number of patients seen, staffing levels, efficiency, admitting procedures, or the availability of inpatient beds.

Admittance Decision Time (minutes)

For patients who had to be admitted to the hospital as an inpatient, average time patients spent in the emergency department, after the doctor decided to admit them as an inpatient before leaving the emergency department for their inpatient room.

Delays in transferring emergency department patients to an inpatient unit may be a sign that there's not enough staff or there's poor coordination among hospital departments. Long delays can also create more stress for patients and families. This measure shows the average (arithmetic median) time patients spent in the emergency department—from the time the doctor decided to admit them to the time they left the emergency department for an inpatient bed. *Lower numbers are better.*

Head CT Results Within 45 Minutes of Arrival

Percentage of patients who came to the emergency department with stroke symptoms who received brain scan results within 45 minutes of arrival.

People who suffer from strokes need to receive treatment immediately to lessen the amount of brain damage that occurs with any stroke. A scan of the brain must be taken to determine the type and severity of the stroke before treatment can be provided. Long waits may be a sign that the emergency department is understaffed or overcrowded and can lead to delayed diagnosis and treatment and may lead to further brain damage. Standards of care say that patients with stroke symptoms should receive brain scan results (to diagnose whether and how severely a stroke occurred) within 45 minutes of arriving at the emergency department. This measure shows the percentage of emergency department patients with stroke symptoms who received brain scan results within that time period. *Lower numbers are better.*

Patients Who Left ER Before Being Seen

Percentage of patients who left the emergency department before being seen.

Hospital emergency departments that have high percentages of patients who leave without being seen may not have the staff or resources to provide timely and effective emergency room care. Patients who leave the emergency department without being seen may be seriously ill, putting themselves at higher risk for poor health outcomes. This measure shows the percentage of all individuals who signed into an emergency department but left before being evaluated by a healthcare professional. *Lower numbers are better.*

Time from ER Arrival to Admittance (minutes)

For patients who had to be admitted to the hospital as an inpatient, average time patients spent in the emergency department, before they were admitted to the hospital as an inpatient.

Long stays in an emergency department before a patient is admitted may be a sign that the emergency department is understaffed or overcrowded. This may result in delays in treatment or lower quality care. This measure shows the average (arithmetic median) time patients spent in the emergency department—from the time they arrived to the time they left the emergency department for an inpatient bed. This number only includes patients who were admitted to the hospital as an inpatient. It does not include those people who went home. *Lower numbers are better.*

Time from ER Arrival to Discharge (minutes)

Average time patients spent in the emergency department before being sent home.

Long stays in the emergency department before a patient is sent home may be a sign that the emergency department is understaffed or overcrowded. This may result in delays in treatment, increased suffering for those who wait, and unpleasant treatment environments. This measure shows the average (arithmetic median) time in minutes that patients spent in the emergency department—from the time they arrived to the time they were sent home. It does not include patients who were later admitted to the hospital as inpatients, admitted for observation, transferred to another acute care hospital, or who left without being seen by a licensed provider. *Lower numbers are better.*

Time in ER Before Being Evaluated (minutes)

Average time patients spent in the emergency department before they were seen by a healthcare professional.

Delays in being seen by a healthcare provider may be a sign that the emergency department is understaffed or overcrowded. This may result in delays in treatment, lower quality care, and more stress for patients and families. For patients who were later sent home, this measure shows the average (arithmetic median) time in minutes spent in the emergency department—from the time they arrived until the time they were seen by a healthcare professional. It does not include patients who were admitted to the hospital, who died in the emergency department, or who left without being seen. *Lower numbers are better.*

Time to Pain Meds for Fractures (minutes)
Average time patients who came to the emergency department with broken bones had to wait before receiving pain medication.
Long waits before a patient is treated may be a sign that the emergency department is understaffed or overcrowded. For patients with broken bones, long waits without pain medication cause unnecessary suffering. For all patients 2 years and older who came to the emergency department with a broken arm or leg, this shows the average (arithmetic median) time they waited before receiving pain medication. *Lower numbers are better.*

8▶ Heart Attack Care

Scientific evidence shows that the following measures represent the best practices for the treatment of heart attack.

Aspirin Given at Discharge
Heart attack patients given aspirin at discharge.
Blood clots can block blood vessels. Aspirin can help prevent blood clots from forming or help dissolve blood clots that have formed. Following a heart attack, continued use of aspirin may help reduce the risk of another heart attack. Aspirin can have side effects like stomach inflammation, bleeding, or allergic reactions. Talk to your health care provider before using aspirin on a regular basis to make sure it's safe for you. This measure shows what percentage of patients were given aspirin upon leaving the hospital. *Higher percentages are better.*

Fibrinolytic Meds Within 30 Minutes of Arrival
Heart attack patients given fibrinolytic medication within 30 minutes of arrival.
The heart is a muscle that gets oxygen through blood vessels. Sometimes blood clots can block these blood vessels and the heart can't get enough oxygen. This can cause a heart attack. Fibrinolytic drugs are medicines that can help dissolve blood clots in blood vessels and improve blood flow to your heart. Standards for care say that patients should get them within 30 minutes of arrival at the hospital. This measure shows what percentage of patients got fibrinolytic drugs within this time period. *Higher percentages are better.*

PCI Within 90 Minutes of Arrival
Heart attack patients given PCI within 90 minutes of arrival.
The heart is a muscle that gets oxygen through blood vessels. Sometimes blood clots can block these blood vessels, and the heart cannot get enough oxygen. This can cause a heart attack. Percutaneous coronary interventions (PCI) are procedures that are among the most effective ways to open blocked blood vessels and help prevent further heart muscle damage. A PCI is performed by a doctor to open the blockage and increase blood flow in blocked blood vessels. Improving blood flow to your heart as quickly as possible lessens the damage to your heart muscle, and it also can increase your chances of surviving a heart attack. There are three procedures commonly described by the term PCI. These procedures all involve a catheter (a flexible tube) that is inserted, often through your leg, and guided through the blood vessels to the blockage. The three procedures are: angioplasty—a balloon is inflated to open the blood vessel; stenting—a small wire tube called a stent is placed in the blood vessel to hold it open; atherectomy—a blade or laser cuts through and removes the blockage. Standards for care say that patients should receive a PCI within 90 minutes of arriving at the hospital. This measure shows what percentage of patients got a PCI within this time period. *Higher percentages are better.*

Statin Prescribed at Discharge
Heart attack patients given a prescription for a statin at discharge.
Statins are drugs used to lower cholesterol. Cholesterol is a fat (also called a lipid) that your body needs to work properly. Cholesterol levels that are too high can increase your chance of getting heart disease, stroke, and other problems. For patients who have had one or more heart attacks and have high cholesterol, taking statins can lower the chance that they'll have another heart attack or die. This measure shows the percent of patients who had a heart attack who got a prescription for a statin upon leaving the hospital. Patients who shouldn't take statins aren't included in this measure. *Higher numbers are better.*

9▶ Heart Failure Care

Scientific evidence shows that the following measures represent the best practices for the treatment of heart failure.

ACE Inhibitor or ARB for LVSD
Heart failure patients given ACE inhibitor or ARB for left ventricular systolic dysfunction (LVSD).
ACE (angiotensin converting enzyme) inhibitors and ARBs (angiotensin receptor blockers) are medicines used to treat patients with heart failure and are particularly beneficial in those patients with decreased function of the left side of the heart. Early treatment with ACE inhibitors and ARBs in patients who have heart failure symptoms or decreased heart function after a heart attack can also reduce their risk of death from future heart attacks. ACE

inhibitors and ARBs work by limiting the effects of a hormone that narrows blood vessels, and may thus lower blood pressure and reduce the work the heart has to perform. Since the ways in which these two kinds of drugs work are different, your doctor will decide which drug is most appropriate for you. Standards for care say that if patients have a heart attack and/or heart failure, they should get a prescription for ACE inhibitors or ARBs if they have decreased heart function before leaving the hospital. *Higher percentages are better.*

Discharge Instructions Given
Heart failure patients given discharge instructions.
Heart failure is a chronic condition. It results in symptoms such as shortness of breath, dizziness, and fatigue. Before you leave the hospital, the staff at the hospital should provide you with information to help you manage the symptoms after you get home. The information should include your information about: activity level (what you can and can't do); diet (what you should, and shouldn't eat or drink); medications; your follow-up appointment; watching your daily weight; and what to do if your symptoms get worse. *Higher percentages are better.*

Evaluation of LVS Function
Heart failure patients given an evaluation of left ventricular systolic (LVS) function.
The proper treatment for heart failure depends on what area of your heart is affected. An important test is to check how your heart is pumping, called an "evaluation of the left ventricular systolic function." It can tell your health care provider whether the left side of your heart is pumping properly. Other ways to check on how your heart is pumping include: your medical history; a physical examination; listening to your heart sounds; and other tests as ordered by a physician (like an ECG (electrocardiogram), chest x-ray, blood work, and an echocardiogram) *Higher percentages are better.*

10 ▶ Medicare Spending

The Medicare Hospital Spending per Patient measure shows whether Medicare spends more, less, or about the same on an episode of care for a Medicare patient treated in a specific hospital compared to how much Medicare spends on an episode of care across all hospitals nationally. This measure includes any Medicare Part A and Part B payments made for services provided to a patient during an episode of care, which includes the 3 days prior to the hospital stay, during the stay, and during the 30 days after discharge from the hospital. This result is a ratio calculated by dividing the amount Medicare spends per patient for an episode of care initiated at this hospital by the median (or middle) amount Medicare spent per episode of care nationally.

- A ratio equal to the national average means that Medicare spends ABOUT THE SAME per patient for an episode of care initiated at this hospital as it does per episode of care across all hospitals nationally.
- A ratio that is more than the national average means that Medicare spends MORE per patient for an episode of care initiated at this hospital than it does per episode of care across all hospitals nationally.
- A ratio that is less than the national average means that Medicare spends LESS per patient for an episode of care initiated at this hospital than it does per episode of care across all hospitals nationally.

11 ▶ Pneumonia Care

Scientific evidence shows that the following measures represent the best practices for the treatment of community-acquired pneumonia.

Appropriate Initial Antibiotic Given
Pneumonia patients given the most appropriate initial antibiotic(s).
Pneumonia is a lung infection that is usually caused by bacteria or a virus. If pneumonia is caused by bacteria, hospitals will treat the infection with antibiotics. Different bacteria are treated with different antibiotics. *Higher percentages are better.*

Blood Culture Timing
Pneumonia patients whose initial emergency room blood culture was performed prior to the administration of the first hospital dose of antibiotics.
Different types of bacteria can cause pneumonia. A blood culture is a test that can help your health care provider identify which bacteria may have caused your pneumonia, and which antibiotic should be prescribed. A blood culture is not always needed, but for patients who are first seen in the hospital emergency department, it is important for the accuracy of the test that a blood culture be conducted before any antibiotics are started. It is also important to start antibiotics as soon as possible. *Higher percentages are better.*

12▶ Pregnancy and Delivery Care

Newborn Deliveries Scheduled Early
Percent of newborns whose deliveries were scheduled too early (1-3 weeks early), when a scheduled delivery was not medically necessary.
Guidelines developed by doctors and researchers say it's best to wait until the 39th completed week of pregnancy to deliver your baby because important fetal development takes place in your baby's brain and lungs during the last few weeks of pregnancy. Sometimes women go into early labor on their own, and early deliveries can't be prevented. Sometimes, doctors decide that inducing labor or delivering a baby early by C-section (called "elective delivery") is in the best interest of the mother and the baby. In these cases, early deliveries are medically necessary. However, doctors may also decide to induce labor or deliver babies by C-section early as a convenience to themselves or their patient. This practice is not recommended. Hospitals should work with doctors and patients to avoid early elective deliveries when they are not medically necessary. This measure shows the percent of pregnancy women who had elective deliveries 1-3 weeks early (either vaginally or by C-section) who early deliveries were not medically necessary. Higher numbers may indicate that hospitals aren't doing enough to discourage this unsafe practice. *Lower percentages are better.*

13▶ Preventive Care

Hospitals and other healthcare providers play a crucial role in promoting, providing and educating patients about preventive services and screenings and maintaining the health of their communities. Many diseases are preventable through immunizations, screenings, treatment, and lifestyle changes. The information below shows how well the hospitals you selected are providing preventive services.

Immunization for Influenza
Patients assessed and given influenza vaccination.
Influenza, or the "flu," is a respiratory illness that is caused by flu viruses and easily spread from person to person. There are over 200,000 hospitalizations from the flu on average every year. An average of 36,000 Americans die annually due to the flu and its complications. The best way to prevent the flu is to get a flu shot each year during the fall season. Because flu viruses change from year to year, it is important to get a flu shot each year. *Higher percentages are better.*

Immunization for Pneumonia
Patients assessed and given pneumonia vaccination.
Pneumonia is an infection of the lungs that is caused by bacteria or a virus and can spread from person to person. A cold or flu that gets worse can turn into pneumonia. Although antibiotics such as penicillin were once very effective at treating pneumonia, the disease has mutated (changed) so these treatments are not as effective. The best way to prevent pneumonia is to get a flu shot each year (as flu often leads to pneumonia) and frequently washing your hands. Those who are more at risk of getting pneumonia, such as young children, people over the age of 65, people with a chronic illness (such as heart or lung disease or diabetes), or people who have had pneumonia before, should get the pneumonia vaccine. Ask your doctor when the best time to be vaccinated is for you. *Higher percentages are better.*

14▶ Stroke Care

Scientific evidence shows that the following measures show some of the standards of stroke care that hospitals should follow, for adults who have had a stroke.

Anticoagulation Therapy for Atrial Fibrillation
Ischemic stroke patients with a type of irregular heartbeat who were given a prescription for a blood thinner at discharge.
Patients admitted with an ischemic stroke who have an irregular heartbeat (also called atrial fibrillation or atrial flutter) are at greater risk of having another stroke. Research suggests that medicine that thins the blood (called an anticoagulant) reduces the chance of another stroke in these patients. This measure shows the percentage of patients admitted with ischemic stroke and an irregular heartbeat (atrial fibrillation/atrial flutter) who were prescribed an anticoagulant before they were discharged from the hospital. *Higher percentages are better.*

Antithrombotic Therapy Timing
Ischemic stroke patients who received medicine known to prevent complications caused by blood clots within 2 days of arriving at the hospital.
Ischemic stroke patients should get medicine known to reduce death, disability and the risk of another stroke (known as Antithrombotic Therapy) while in the hospital. Research shows that hospitals should start this medicine within 2 days of arriving at the hospital to prevent and treat clots and reduce the risk of complications from the stroke. Serious complications caused by strokes include changes in thinking and memory; muscle, joint, and nerve problems; or difficulty swallowing or eating; or blood clots. This measure shows the percentage of patients

admitted with an ischemic stroke who got antithrombotic therapy started within 2 days of arriving at the hospital. *Higher percentages are better.*

Assessed for Rehabilitation

Ischemic or hemorrhagic stroke patients who were evaluated for rehabilitation services.

Many ischemic stroke or hemorrhagic stroke patients will experience moderate or severe disability, including problems with physical, speech and mental functions. Stroke rehabilitation can help patients relearn those lost skills and regain independence. Once the stroke symptoms and related problems are under control, the hospital appropriate health care professionals should review the status of the patient and begin rehabilitation as soon as possible. Appropriate health care professionals include physicians, physical therapists, occupational therapists, speech and language therapists, and/or neuropsychologist. The earlier the patient starts rehabilitation, the better the recovery process. Patients who need stroke rehabilitation may begin while they are still at the hospital and continue in a rehabilitation setting that is right for the patient. These options include inpatient rehabilitation units (either stand-alone or part of a hospital/clinic), outpatient units (usually part of a hospital/clinic), nursing home, or home-based programs. This measure shows the percentage of patients admitted with an ischemic stroke or a hemorrhagic stroke who were evaluated for their need for rehabilitation services. *Higher percentages are better.*

Discharged on Antithrombotic Therapy

Ischemic stroke patients who received a prescription for medicine known to prevent complications caused by blood clots before discharge.

Patients admitted with an ischemic stroke are at risk for developing complications like another stroke even after discharge. These patients should get a prescription at discharge for a blood thinner that prevents complications like another stroke (called Antithrombotic Therapy.) Serious complications caused by strokes include changes in thinking and memory; muscle, joint, and nerve problems; or difficulty swallowing or eating; or blood clots. This measure shows the percentage of patients who were admitted with an ischemic stroke who were given a prescription for an antithrombotic before they were discharged from the hospital. *Higher percentages are better.*

Discharged on Statin Medication

Ischemic stroke patients needing medicine to lower cholesterol, who were given a prescription for this medicine before discharge.

Cholesterol is a fat (also called a lipid) that the body needs to work properly. Levels of bad cholesterol (LDL) that are too high can increase the chance of stroke, heart disease, and other problems. Medicines called statins can help lower LDL cholesterol levels. In patients with ischemic stroke who have high cholesterol, taking statins can help lower the chance of another stroke. This measure shows the percentage of patients admitted with an ischemic stroke who got a prescription for a statin before they were discharged from the hospital. Patients who shouldn't take statins are not included in this measure. *Higher percentages are better.*

Thrombolytic Therapy Timing

Ischemic stroke patients who got medicine to break up a blood clot within 3 hours after symptoms started.

Patients with ischemic stroke should get medicine called tissue plasminogen activator, or t-PA, to break up a blood clot within 3 hours after their symptoms start. T-PA is a kind of thrombolytic therapy. Research shows that hospitals that give t-PA within 3 hours after symptoms start can limit the damage and disability caused by an ischemic stroke. This measure shows the percentage of patients admitted with ischemic stroke who arrived in the emergency department (ED) within 2 hours of the onset of their symptoms and who got t-PA within three hours after the onset of their symptoms. *Higher percentages are better.*

Venous Thromboembolism Prophylaxis

Ischemic or hemorrhagic stroke patients who received treatment to keep blood clots from forming anywhere in the body within 2 days of arriving at the hospital.

Patients admitted to the hospital with ischemic stroke or hemorrhagic stroke are at increased risk of developing new blood clots in their veins that break off and travel to other parts of the body, like the brain or lung (also called venous thromboembolism). Research shows that hospitals should begin treatment to prevent new blood clots on the day of or day after these patients are arrived at the hospital. Treatment can include medicine, medical devices, or tightly fitting stockings designed to keep blood from clotting. This measure shows the percentage of patients admitted with an ischemic stroke or hemorrhagic stroke who either received treatment to prevent blood clots on the day of or day after arrival at the hospital or had paperwork in their chart to explain why they had not received this treatment. *Higher percentages are better.*

Written Stroke Educational Materials Given

Ischemic or hemorrhagic stroke patients or caregivers who received written educational materials about stroke care and prevention during the hospital stay.

Educating patients with ischemic stroke and hemorrhagic stroke and their caregivers about stroke care and prevention helps patients live healthier lives and reduces health care costs. During the hospital stay, hospital staff should give stroke patients and caregivers written information on: how to activate the hospital emergency system; the importance of doing follow-up after being released from the hospital; medicines prescribed at discharge;

what increases the chance of stroke; warning signs and symptoms of stroke. This measure shows the percentage of patients with an ischemic stroke or a hemorrhagic stroke or their caregivers who received written information about these topics during their hospital stay. *Higher percentages are better.*

15▶ Surgical Care Improvement Project

Scientific evidence shows that the following measures represent the best practices for preventing complications after certain surgeries: colon surgery, hip replacement, knee replacement, abdominal and vaginal hysterectomy, cardiac surgery- including coronary artery bypass grafts (CABG), and vascular surgery.

Appropriate Beta Blocker Usage

Surgery patients who were taking heart drugs called beta blockers before coming to the hospital, who were kept on the beta blockers during the period just before and after their surgery.

It is often standard procedure to stop taking usual medications for a while before and after surgery. But if patients who have been taking beta blockers suddenly stop taking them, they can have heart problems such as a fast heartbeat. For these patients, staying on beta blockers before and after surgery makes it less likely that they will have heart problems. This measure shows the percentage of patients who remained on beta blockers within this time period. *Higher percentages are better.*

Appropriate VTP Within 24 Hours

Patients who got treatment (venous thromboembolism prevention) at the right time (within 24 hours before or after their surgery) to help prevent blood clots after certain types of surgery.

Many factors influence a surgery patient's risk of developing a blood clot, including the type of surgery. When patients stay still for a long time after some types of surgery, they are more likely to develop a blood clot in the veins of the legs, thighs, or pelvis. A blood clot slows down the flow of blood, causing swelling, redness, and pain. A blood clot can also break off and travel to other parts of the body. If the blood clot gets into the lung, it is a serious problem that can sometimes cause death. Doctors can order treatments including blood-thinning medications, elastic support stockings, or mechanical air stockings that help with blood flow in the legs. These treatments need to be started at the right time, which is typically during the period that begins 24 hours before surgery and ends 24 hours after surgery. This measure shows the percentage of patients who received these treatments this time period. *Higher percentages are better.*

Controlled Postoperative Blood Glucose

Heart surgery patients whose blood sugar (blood glucose) is kept under good control in the days right after surgery.

Even if heart surgery patients do not have diabetes, keeping blood sugar under good control (200 mg/dL or less) after surgery lowers the risk of infection and other problems. This measure shows the percentage of patients who had their blood sugar kept under good control in the days right after surgery. *Higher percentages are better.*

Perioperative Temperature Management

Patients having surgery who were actively warmed in the operating room or whose body temperature was near normal by the end of surgery.

Hospitals can prevent surgical wound infections and other complications by keeping the patient's body temperature near normal during surgery. Medical research has shown that patients whose body temperatures drop during surgery have a greater risk of infection and their wounds may not heal as quickly. Standards of care say that patients should have their body temperature normal or near normal during the time period 30 minutes before the end of surgery to 15 minutes after anesthesia ended. This measure shows the percent of patients whose body temperature was normal or near normal within this time period. *Higher percentages are better.*

Prophylactic Antibiotic Selection

Surgery patients who were given the right kind of antibiotic to help prevent infection.

Surgical wound infections can be prevented. Medical research has shown that certain antibiotics work better to prevent wound infections for certain types of surgery. This measure shows the percentage of surgery patients who were given the right antibiotic during surgery. *Higher percentages are better.*

Prophylactic Antibiotic Selection (Outpatient)

Outpatients having surgery who got the right kind of antibiotic.

Hospitals can prevent surgical wound infections. Medical research has shown that certain antibiotics work better to prevent wound infections for certain types of surgery. Hospital staff should make sure patients get the antibiotic that works best for their type of surgery. This measure shows the percentage of patients who got the right antibiotic during surgery. *Higher percentages are better.*

Prophylactic Antibiotic Stopped

Surgery patients whose preventive antibiotics were stopped at the right time (within 24 hours after surgery).

Antibiotics are often given to patients before surgery to prevent infection. Taking these antibiotics for more than 24 hours after routine surgery is usually not necessary. Continuing the medication longer than necessary can increase the risk of side effects such as stomach aches and serious types of diarrhea. Also, when antibiotics are used for too long, patients can develop resistance to them and the antibiotics won't work as well. This measure shows the percentage of patients who stopped getting preventive antibiotics within this time period. *Higher percentages are better.*

Prophylactic Antibiotic Timing
Surgery patients who were given an antibiotic at the right time (within one hour before surgery) to help prevent infection.
Surgical wound infections can be prevented. Medical research shows that surgery patients who get antibiotics within the hour before their surgery are less likely to get wound infections. Getting an antibiotic earlier, or after surgery begins, is not as effective. Hospital staff should make sure surgery patients get antibiotics at the right time. This measure shows the percentage of patients who got an antibiotic to prevent infection in this time period. *Higher percentages are better.*

Prophylactic Antibiotic Timing (Outpatient)
Outpatients having surgery who got an antibiotic at the right time (within one hour before surgery).
Hospitals can prevent surgical wound infections. Standards for care say that surgery patients who get antibiotics within an hour of their surgery are less likely to get wound infections. Getting an antibiotic earlier, or after surgery begins, is not as effective. This measure shows the percentage of patients who got an antibiotic in this time period. *Higher percentages are better.*

Urinary Catheter Removal
Surgery patients whose urinary catheters were removed on the first or second day after surgery.
Sometimes surgical patients need to have a urinary catheter, or thin tube, inserted into their bladder to help drain the urine. Catheters are usually attached to a bag that collects the urine. Surgery patients can develop infections when urinary catheters are left in place too long after surgery. Standards of care say that most surgery patients should have their urinary catheters removed within 2 days after surgery to help prevent infection. This measure shows the percent of surgery patients whose urinary catheters were removed on the first or second day after surgery. *Higher percentages are better.*

16 ▶ Survey of Patients' Hospital Experiences

The HCAHPS (Hospital Consumer Assessment of Healthcare Providers and Systems) Survey, also known as the CAHPS® Hospital Survey or Hospital CAHPS®, is a standardized survey instrument and data collection methodology that has been in use since 2006 to measure patients' perspectives of hospital care. A partnership of public and private organizations led by the Federal government, specifically the Centers for Medicare & Medicaid Services (CMS) and the Agency for Healthcare Research and Quality (AHRQ), created HCAHPS (pronounced "H-caps") to publicly report the patient's perspective of hospital care. The HCAHPS results posted on Hospital Compare allow consumers to make fair and objective comparisons between hospitals and with state and national averages, on important measures of patients' perspectives of care. For more on HCAHPS information, please visit the official HCAHPS website: www.hcahpsonline.org

The HCAHPS survey asks patients to give feedback about topics for which they are the best source of information. The survey asks patients to answer questions about their experiences in the hospital. To make sure the HCAHPS survey data is meaningful; patients only answer questions about topics with which they have experience. The HCAHPS survey asks patients to answer questions related to ten topics. The topics and questions are listed in the table below. Answers shown in italics are included in this publication.

Measure as it Appears in CGAH	HCAHPS Topic Text	HCAHPS Answer Description
Would Definitely Recommend Hospital	How do patients rate the hospital overall?	*Patients who gave a rating of 9 or 10 (high)*
		Patients who gave a rating of 7 or 8 (medium)
		Patients who gave a rating of 6 or lower (low)
Doctors 'Always' Communicated Well	How often did doctors communicate well with patients?	*Doctors always communicated well*
		Doctors usually communicated well
		Doctors sometimes or never communicated well
Nurses 'Always' Communicated Well	How often did nurses communicate well with patients?	*Nurses always communicated well*
		Nurses usually communicated well
		Nurses sometimes or never communicated well
Timely Help 'Always' Received	How often did patients receive help quickly from hospital staff?	*Patients always received help as soon as they wanted*
		Patients usually received help as soon as they wanted
		Patients sometimes or never received help as soon as they wanted

Measure as it Appears in CGAH	HCAHPS Topic Text	HCAHPS Answer Description
Meds 'Always' Explained Before Given	How often did staff explain about medicines before giving them to patients?	*Staff always explained*
		Staff usually explained
		Staff sometimes or never explained
Pain 'Always' Well Controlled	How often was patients' pain well controlled?	*Pain was always well controlled*
		Pain was usually well controlled
		Pain was sometimes or never well controlled
Area Around Room 'Always' Quiet at Night	How often was the area around patients' rooms kept quiet at night?	*Always quiet at night*
		Usually quiet at night
		Sometimes or never quiet at night
Room and Bathroom 'Always' Clean	How often were the patients' rooms and bathrooms kept clean?	*Room was always clean*
		Room was usually clean
		Room was sometimes or never clean
Home Recovery Information Given	Were patients given information about what to do during their recovery at home?	*YES, staff did give patients this information*
		NO, staff did not give patients this information
Would Definitely Recommend Hospital	Would patients recommend the hospital to friends and family?	*YES, patients would definitely recommend the hospital*
		YES, patients would probably recommend the hospital
		NO, patients would not recommend the hospital (they probably would not or definitely would not recommend it)

17▶ Use of Medical Imaging

"Medical imaging" tests create images of various parts of the body to screen for or diagnose medical conditions. Examples of medical imaging include CT scans, MRIs, and mammograms.

Cardiac Imaging Stress Test before Surgery

Outpatients who got cardiac imaging stress tests before low-risk outpatient surgery.
A cardiac stress test measures the heart's ability to respond when it is stressed, and can be useful in evaluating a patient's surgical risk. Experts agree, however, that these tests are not necessary before most low-risk outpatient surgical procedures, such as colonoscopies, cataract surgery, biopsies, or endoscopies (using an instrument to look inside the body) because these procedures put very little stress on the heart. Patients with certain risk factors that increase the likelihood of having complications are not included in the measure. This measure shows the percentage of all cardiac stress tests done in a hospital outpatient imaging department (using echocardiograms, CT scans, and MRIs) for Medicare patients who were going to have certain low-risk outpatient surgical procedures. Hospital outpatient imaging departments that have higher percentages on this measure may be giving people more tests than they need. *Hospitals that are rated well will have lower percentages.* If a percentage is high, it may mean that the facility is doing unnecessary cardiac imaging before some low-risk surgeries.

Combination Abdominal CT Scan

Outpatient CT scans of the abdomen that were "combination" (double) scans.
A CT scan (also called a CAT scan) uses multiple X-rays to produce detailed pictures of the inside of the body (bones, organs, and other body parts). For some, a substance called "contrast" is put into the patient's body before the scan begins, which help make parts of the body stand out more clearly. Contrast can be either swallowed or injected into a vein. Risks of contrast include possible harm to the kidneys or allergic reactions. Contrast shouldn't be used if it isn't needed. "Combination" CT scan means that the patient gets two CT scans—one scan without contrast, followed by a second scan with contrast. Standards of quality care say that most patients who are getting a CT scan of the chest should be given a single CT scan rather than a "combination" CT scan. Although combination CT scans are appropriate for some parts of the body and for some medical conditions, combination scans are usually not appropriate for the chest. The range for these measures is from 0% to 100%. For hospitals with higher percentages, it may mean that the facility is routinely giving patients combination CT scans of the chest or abdomen when a single scan is all they need. Giving patients two scans when they only need one needlessly doubles their exposure to radiation: Radiation exposure from a single CT scan of the chest is about 350 times higher than for an ordinary chest X-ray. For combination CT scans, radiation exposure is 700 times higher than for a chest X-ray because the patient is given two scans. For a combination CT scan, radiation exposure is 22 times higher than for an X-ray of the abdomen because the patient is given two scans. Radiation exposure from a single CT scan of the abdomen is about 11 times higher than for an ordinary X-ray of the abdomen. When contrast is used, there are risks that can include possible harm to the kidneys or allergic reactions (especially if the contrast is injected). To avoid unnecessary risk, contrast should be used only when it is needed. If you need to have a CT scan of the chest or abdomen, feel free to ask your doctor these questions to determine

what's best for your medical condition: Do you need a single scan—either with or without contrast—or is a combination scan necessary? Is using contrast appropriate for your medical condition? *Hospitals that are rated well will have lower percentages.* If a percentage is high, it may mean that the facility is doing unnecessary double/combination scans.

Combination Brain/Sinus CT Scan

Outpatients with brain CT scans who got a sinus CT scan at the same time.

Brain CTs and sinus CTs can be important tools for diagnosing problems that may be causing severe headaches or chronic sinus infections, but they also expose patients to high levels of radiation. Brain CT scans cover large parts of the sinuses, so ordering both tests may be unnecessary. For patients with chronic sinusitis, a sinus CT is usually done first before deciding if a brain CT is also needed. Experts do not recommend doing both tests at once, unless patients have head injuries or tumors. Hospital outpatient imaging departments that have higher percentages on this measure may be giving people more tests than they need, exposing them to too much radiation. This measure shows the percentage of brain CT scans done in a hospital outpatient imaging department where a sinus CT scan was done at the same time on the same Medicare patient. It does not count cases where doctors had questions about complications due to injuries, cancer, or serious infections. *Hospitals that are rated well will have lower percentages.* If a percentage is high, it may mean that the facility is doing unnecessary scans.

Combination Chest CT Scan

Outpatient CT scans of the chest that were "combination" (double) scans.

A CT scan (also called a CAT scan) uses multiple X-rays to produce detailed pictures of the inside of the body (bones, organs, and other body parts). For some, a substance called "contrast" is put into the patient's body before the scan begins, which help make parts of the body stand out more clearly. Contrast can be either swallowed or injected into a vein. Risks of contrast include possible harm to the kidneys or allergic reactions. Contrast shouldn't be used if it isn't needed. "Combination" CT scan means that the patient gets two CT scans—one scan without contrast, followed by a second scan with contrast. Standards of quality care say that most patients who are getting a CT scan of the chest should be given a single CT scan rather than a "combination" CT scan. Although combination CT scans are appropriate for some parts of the body and for some medical conditions, combination scans are usually not appropriate for the chest. The range for these measures is from 0% to 100%. For hospitals with higher percentages, it may mean that the facility is routinely giving patients combination CT scans of the chest or abdomen when a single scan is all they need. Giving patients two scans when they only need one needlessly doubles their exposure to radiation. Radiation exposure from a single CT scan of the chest is about 350 times higher than for an ordinary chest X-ray. For combination CT scans, radiation exposure is 700 times higher than for a chest X-ray because the patient is given two scans. For a combination CT scan, radiation exposure is 22 times higher than for an X-ray of the abdomen because the patient is given two scans. Radiation exposure from a single CT scan of the abdomen is about 11 times higher than for an ordinary X-ray of the abdomen. When contrast is used, there are risks that can include possible harm to the kidneys or allergic reactions (especially if the contrast is injected). To avoid unnecessary risk, contrast should be used only when it is needed. If you need to have a CT scan of the chest or abdomen, feel free to ask your doctor these questions to determine what's best for your medical condition: Do you need a single scan - either with or without contrast - or is a combination scan necessary? Is using contrast appropriate for your medical condition? *Hospitals that are rated well will have lower percentages.* If a percentage is high, it may mean that the facility is doing unnecessary double/combination scans.

Follow-up Mammogram/Ultrasound

Outpatients who had a follow-up mammogram, ultrasound, or MRI of the breast within 45 days after a screening mammogram.

A screening mammogram is an X-ray of the breast to check for possible breast cancer before it can be detected by women or health care professionals. Although mammography is a good test, it is not perfect. Some women who do not have breast cancer will have an abnormal mammogram (even though they are cancer free), and some women with breast cancer will have a normal screening mammogram (their cancer is missed). Some women may be asked to come back for follow-up testing if there are signs of possible breast cancer. A follow-up visit usually means having more tests (mammograms, an ultrasound, and/or an MRI of the breast). The numbers of women asked to follow-up varies widely among mammography facilities in the United States. There are many reasons for differences in follow-up rates including poor technique (blurry X-rays that need to be repeated), a lack of skill or experience interpreting the screening mammograms, medical history of the woman undergoing screening, and whether a woman is being screened for the first time or has previously undergone mammography screening. The follow-up rates reported here for mammography facilities include follow-up exams performed on the same day as screening mammograms, as well as those performed up to 45 days later. Medical evidence suggests that there may be a problem if a facility has either a very low or very high rate of follow-ups. *Although values for a very low follow-up rate have not been established, a follow-up rate near zero may indicate a facility that misses signs of cancer. Follow-up rates around 9% are typical. Research has established that a follow-up rate above 14% is not appropriate, and may indicate a facility doing unnecessary follow up.* If you have a screening mammogram and you are called back for additional testing, ask your doctor why and what this additional testing means in your case for how he or she makes an accurate diagnosis.

Lumbar Spine MRI for Low Back Pain

Outpatients with low back pain who had an MRI without trying recommended treatments first, such as physical therapy.

An MRI (magnetic resonance imaging) is a test that uses a powerful magnetic field and a computer to produce detailed pictures of the inside of the body (bones, organs, and other body parts). Although MRI scans can be helpful for diagnosing low back pain, they can also be used too much. Low back pain can improve or go away within six weeks and an MRI may not be needed. Standards of care say that most patients with low back pain should start with treatment such as physical therapy or chiropractic care, and have an MRI only if the treatment doesn't help. Finding out whether treatment helps or not before having an MRI can be a safe and effective way to avoid unnecessary stress, risk, or cost of doing an MRI. For patients with certain conditions, getting an MRI right away is appropriate care. Patients with these conditions are not included in this measure. If you have low back pain, you, your doctor, and the medical imaging facility staff can talk about the best time to do an MRI if you need one. Since MRIs use magnets rather than x-rays, there is no radiation risk. However, because the magnets attract some kinds of metal, it's important for the technician to know if there are any metal objects or implants inside your body, such as pacemakers, artificial joints, screws, stents, plates, or staples. Metal objects can pose serious risk to you during the MRI and interfere with the test. For some MRIs, a substance called "contrast" is injected before the test to make parts of the body stand out more clearly on the images. Risks of contrast include possible harm to the kidneys or allergic reactions. Contrast shouldn't be used if it isn't needed. Having the test can be stressful for some people. Patients must hold still for about 15 to 45 minutes while lying on a table that moves inside a large scanning machine. While images are being taken, the machine makes loud noises. *Hospitals that are rated well will have lower percentages.* If a percentage is high, it may mean that the facility is doing unnecessary MRIs for low back pain.

Blood Clot Prevention and Treatment

Anticoagulation Overlap Therapy

Hospital Name	City	Rate	Cases
Adventist Bolingbrook Hospital[2]	Bolingbrook	100%	38
Genesis Health System[2]	Silvis	100%	26
Good Samaritan Regional Health Center[2]	Mount Vernon	100%	35
Heartland Regional Medical Center[2]	Marion	100%	33
Herrin Hospital[2]	Herrin	100%	27
Katherine Shaw Bethea Hospital[2]	Dixon	100%	30
Kishwaukee Community Hospital[2]	Dekalb	100%	45
Memorial Hospital[2]	Belleville	100%	98
Metrosouth Medical Center[2]	Blue Island	100%	106
Northwest Community Hospital[2]	Arlington Hgts	100%	142
Presence Saint Francis Hospital[2]	Evanston	100%	53
Saint Anthony's Health Center[2]	Alton	100%	27
Sherman Hospital[2]	Elgin	100%	119
Advocate Good Samaritan Hospital[2]	Downers Grove	99%	149
Lake Forest Hospital[2]	Lake Forest	99%	90
Louis A Weiss Memorial Hospital[2]	Chicago	99%	77
Memorial Hospital of Carbondale[2]	Carbondale	99%	70
Riverside Medical Center[2]	Kankakee	99%	87
Blessing Hospital[2]	Quincy	98%	64
Loyola University Medical Center[2]	Maywood	98%	127
Methodist Medical Center of Illinois[2]	Peoria	98%	55
Presence Mercy Medical Center[2]	Aurora	98%	63
Presence Our Lady of the Res Med Ctr[2]	Chicago	98%	58
Rush Oak Park Hospital[2]	Oak Park	98%	50
Trinity Rock Island[2]	Rock Island	98%	65
The University of Chicago Medical Center[2]	Chicago	98%	155
Advocate Illinois Masonic Medical Center[2]	Chicago	97%	94
Decatur Memorial Hospital[2]	Decatur	97%	115
Passavant Area Hospital[2]	Jacksonville	97%	30
Presence United Samaritans Medical Center[2]	Danville	97%	62
Saint Marys Hospital[2]	Centralia	97%	30
Alton Memorial Hospital[2]	Alton	96%	67
Edward Hospital[2]	Naperville	96%	191
Hinsdale Hospital[2]	Hinsdale	96%	74
Ingalls Memorial Hospital[2]	Harvey	96%	137
Presence Sts Mary & Elizabeth Med Ctr[2]	Chicago	96%	67
Vista Medical Center East[2]	Waukegan	96%	79
Alexian Brothers Medical Center[2]	Elk Grove Vlg	95%	156
Carle Foundation Hospital[2]	Urbana	95%	164
Copley Memorial Hospital[2]	Aurora	95%	79
Evanston Hospital[2]	Evanston	95%	264
Memorial Medical Center[2]	Springfield	95%	178
Northwestern Memorial Hospital[2]	Chicago	95%	282
Saint Francis Medical Center[2]	Peoria	95%	169
Saint Joseph Medical Center[2]	Bloomington	95%	42
Advocate Lutheran General Hospital[2]	Park Ridge	94%	122
Central Dupage Hospital[2]	Winfield	94%	163
Rockford Memorial Hospital[2]	Rockford	94%	97
Saint Alexius Medical Center[2]	Hoffman Estates	94%	129
Saint Anthony Medical Center[2]	Rockford	94%	114
Saint Elizabeth Hospital[2]	Belleville	94%	52
University of Illinois Hospital[2]	Chicago	94%	112
Advocate Bromenn Medical Center	Normal	93%	42
Advocate Good Shepherd Hospital[2]	Barrington	93%	82
Galesburg Cottage Hospital[2]	Galesburg	93%	29
Presence Resurrection Medical Center[2]	Chicago	93%	67
Saint Anthonys Memorial Hospital[2]	Effingham	93%	43
Advocate Trinity Hospital[2]	Chicago	92%	136
CGH Medical Center[2]	Sterling	92%	38
Delnor Community Hospital[2]	Geneva	92%	51
Macneal Hospital[2]	Berwyn	92%	88
Presence Covenant Medical Center[2]	Urbana	92%	51
Advocate Christ Hospital & Medical Center[2]	Oak Lawn	91%	270
Proctor Hospital[2]	Peoria	91%	34
Saint Johns Hospital[2]	Springfield	91%	87
Advocate Condell Medical Center[2]	Libertyville	90%	124
John H Stroger Jr Hospital[2]	Chicago	90%	129
Little Company of Mary Hospital[2]	Evergreen Park	90%	175
Palos Community Hospital[2]	Palos Heights	90%	168
Morris Hospital & Healthcare Centers[2]	Morris	89%	35
Centegra Health Sys-Mc Henry Hosp[2]	Mchenry	88%	77
Mount Sinai Hospital Medical Center[2]	Chicago	88%	56
Presence Saint Marys Hospital[2]	Kankakee	88%	42
Advocate South Suburban Hospital[2]	Hazel Crest	86%	121
Mercy Hospital & Medical Center[2]	Chicago	86%	87
Saint Bernard Hospital[2]	Chicago	86%	29
Saint Mary Medical Center[2]	Galesburg	86%	35
Elmhurst Memorial Hospital[2]	Elmhurst	85%	143
Sarah Bush Lincoln Health Center[2]	Mattoon	85%	40
Adventist La Grange Memorial Hospital[2]	La Grange	84%	62
Franciscan Saint James Health[2]	Olympia Fields	84%	161
Swedish American Hospital[2]	Rockford	83%	103
West Suburban Medical Center[2]	Oak Park	83%	47
Anderson Hospital[2]	Maryville	82%	40
Rush University Medical Center[2]	Chicago	82%	163
Fhn Memorial Hospital[2]	Freeport	80%	49
Presence Saint Joseph Hospital - Elgin[2]	Elgin	80%	66
Presence Saint Joseph Medical Center[2]	Joliet	77%	162
Centegra Health Sys-Woodstock Hosp[2]	Woodstock	76%	49
Silver Cross Hospital & Medical Centers[2]	New Lenox	76%	107
Roseland Community Hospital[2]	Chicago	68%	28
Holy Cross Hospital[2]	Chicago	66%	86
Norwegian - American Hospital[2]	Chicago	65%	34
Swedish Covenant Hospital[2]	Chicago	59%	74
Loyola Gottlieb Memorial Hospital[2]	Melrose Park	48%	33
Saint Marys Hospital[2]	Decatur	27%	37

ICU Venous Thromboembolism Prophylaxis

Hospital Name	City	Rate	Cases
Adventist Bolingbrook Hospital[2]	Bolingbrook	100%	87
Alton Memorial Hospital[2]	Alton	100%	62
Copley Memorial Hospital[2]	Aurora	100%	85
Crossroads Community Hospital[2]	Mount Vernon	100%	71
Galesburg Cottage Hospital[2]	Galesburg	100%	106
Louis A Weiss Memorial Hospital[2]	Chicago	100%	77
Memorial Hospital of Carbondale[2]	Carbondale	100%	69
Northwestern Memorial Hospital[2]	Chicago	100%	111
Presence Saint Joseph Hospital - Chicago[2]	Chicago	100%	83
Riverside Medical Center[2]	Kankakee	100%	78
Saint Alexius Medical Center[2]	Hoffman Estates	100%	70
Saint Anthony's Health Center[2]	Alton	100%	76
Saint Mary Medical Center[2]	Galesburg	100%	85
Touchette Regional Hospital[2]	Centreville	100%	25
Vista Medical Center East[2]	Waukegan	100%	107
Ingalls Memorial Hospital[2]	Harvey	99%	91
Kishwaukee Community Hospital[2]	Dekalb	99%	73
Methodist Medical Center of Illinois[2]	Peoria	99%	67
Metrosouth Medical Center[2]	Blue Island	99%	116
Presence Mercy Medical Center[2]	Aurora	99%	101
Presence Our Lady of the Res Med Ctr[2]	Chicago	99%	116
Saint Anthony Hospital[2]	Chicago	99%	100
Saint Elizabeth Hospital[2]	Belleville	99%	78
Sherman Hospital[2]	Elgin	99%	77
Advocate Illinois Masonic Medical Center[2]	Chicago	98%	50
Carle Foundation Hospital[2]	Urbana	98%	41
Centegra Health Sys-Woodstock Hosp[2]	Woodstock	98%	81
Genesis Health System[2]	Silvis	98%	61
Herrin Hospital[2]	Herrin	98%	80
Hinsdale Hospital[2]	Hinsdale	98%	65
Mount Sinai Hospital Medical Center[2]	Chicago	98%	63
Passavant Area Hospital[2]	Jacksonville	98%	53
Presence Resurrection Medical Center[2]	Chicago	98%	147
Presence Saint Joseph Hospital - Elgin[2]	Elgin	98%	102
Presence Sts Mary & Elizabeth Med Ctr[2]	Chicago	98%	58
Saint Bernard Hospital[2]	Chicago	98%	41
Alexian Brothers Medical Center[2]	Elk Grove Vlg	97%	96
Decatur Memorial Hospital[2]	Decatur	97%	58
Good Samaritan Regional Health Center[2]	Mount Vernon	97%	79
Memorial Medical Center[2]	Springfield	97%	61
Rockford Memorial Hospital[2]	Rockford	97%	92
Rush Oak Park Hospital[2]	Oak Park	97%	116
Saint James Hospital[2]	Pontiac	97%	33
Advocate Bromenn Medical Center	Normal	96%	355
Gateway Regional Medical Center[2]	Granite City	96%	208
Heartland Regional Medical Center[2]	Marion	96%	136
Memorial Hospital[2]	Belleville	96%	57
Mercy Hospital & Medical Center[2]	Chicago	96%	91
Saint Anthony Medical Center[2]	Rockford	96%	125
Saint Margarets Hospital[2]	Spring Valley	96%	28
Thorek Memorial Hospital[2]	Chicago	96%	56
Advocate Good Shepherd Hospital[2]	Barrington	95%	116
Palos Community Hospital[2]	Palos Heights	95%	86
Pekin Memorial Hospital[2]	Pekin	95%	65
Rush University Medical Center[2]	Chicago	95%	113
Saint Joseph Medical Center[2]	Bloomington	95%	41
Saint Marys Hospital[2]	Centralia	95%	75
The University of Chicago Medical Center[2]	Chicago	95%	79
University of Illinois Hospital[2]	Chicago	95%	88
Adventist Glenoaks[2]	Glendale Hghts	94%	97
Advocate Christ Hospital & Medical Center[2]	Oak Lawn	94%	124
Advocate Trinity Hospital[2]	Chicago	94%	33
Katherine Shaw Bethea Hospital[2]	Dixon	94%	107
Lake Forest Hospital[2]	Lake Forest	94%	65
Presence United Samaritans Medical Center[2]	Danville	94%	79
Proctor Hospital[2]	Peoria	94%	78
Saint Johns Hospital[2]	Springfield	94%	80
Advocate Good Samaritan Hospital[2]	Downers Grove	93%	91
Delnor Community Hospital[2]	Geneva	93%	61
Macneal Hospital[2]	Berwyn	93%	58
Northwest Community Hospital[2]	Arlington Hgts	93%	85
Saint Marys Hospital[2]	Streator	93%	27
Advocate Lutheran General Hospital[2]	Park Ridge	92%	87
Blessing Hospital[2]	Quincy	92%	71
Central Dupage Hospital[2]	Winfield	92%	61
Holy Cross Hospital[2]	Chicago	92%	113
Presence Saint Marys Hospital[2]	Kankakee	92%	157
Sarah Bush Lincoln Health Center[2]	Mattoon	92%	53
Swedish American Hospital[2]	Rockford	92%	83
Swedish Covenant Hospital[2]	Chicago	92%	53
Advocate Condell Medical Center[2]	Libertyville	91%	67
Centegra Health Sys-Mc Henry Hosp[2]	Mchenry	91%	80
Franciscan Saint James Health[2]	Olympia Fields	91%	118
Ottawa Reg Hosp & Healthcare Ctr[2]	Ottawa	91%	32
Presence Saint Francis Hospital[2]	Evanston	91%	141
West Suburban Medical Center[2]	Oak Park	91%	81
Westlake Community Hospital[2]	Melrose Park	91%	64
Loyola University Medical Center[2]	Maywood	90%	107
Roseland Community Hospital[2]	Chicago	90%	60
Elmhurst Memorial Hospital[2]	Elmhurst	89%	111
Evanston Hospital[2]	Evanston	89%	75
Saint Marys Hospital[2]	Decatur	89%	55
Midwestern Region Medical Center[2]	Zion	88%	26
Saint Anthonys Memorial Hospital[2]	Effingham	88%	56
CGH Medical Center[2]	Sterling	86%	92
John H Stroger Jr Hospital[2]	Chicago	86%	59
Saint Francis Medical Center[2]	Peoria	86%	44
Adventist La Grange Memorial Hospital[2]	La Grange	85%	39
Iroquois Memorial Hospital[2]	Watseka	85%	27
Little Company of Mary Hospital[2]	Evergreen Park	85%	87
Loretto Hospital[2]	Chicago	85%	89
Fhn Memorial Hospital[2]	Freeport	84%	109
Silver Cross Hospital & Medical Centers[2]	New Lenox	84%	56
Advocate South Suburban Hospital[2]	Hazel Crest	83%	116
Loyola Gottlieb Memorial Hospital[2]	Melrose Park	82%	88
Morris Hospital & Healthcare Centers[2]	Morris	81%	119
Edward Hospital[2]	Naperville	79%	92
Presence Covenant Medical Center[2]	Urbana	78%	83
Presence Saint Joseph Medical Center[2]	Joliet	78%	59
Trinity Rock Island[2]	Rock Island	78%	65
McDonough District Hospital[2]	Macomb	74%	35
Anderson Hospital[2]	Maryville	73%	48
South Shore Hospital[2]	Chicago	67%	46
Graham Hospital Association[2]	Canton	62%	47
Norwegian - American Hospital[2]	Chicago	57%	61

Incidence of Potentially Preventable VTE

Hospital Name	City	Rate	Cases
Advocate Illinois Masonic Medical Center[2]	Chicago	0%	25
Rush University Medical Center[2]	Chicago	2%	56
University of Illinois Hospital[2]	Chicago	2%	90
Advocate Christ Hospital & Medical Center[2]	Oak Lawn	5%	81
Memorial Medical Center[2]	Springfield	5%	37
Advocate Good Samaritan Hospital[2]	Downers Grove	6%	33
Evanston Hospital[2]	Evanston	6%	34
Loyola University Medical Center[2]	Maywood	6%	35
Carle Foundation Hospital[2]	Urbana	7%	30
Mercy Hospital & Medical Center[2]	Chicago	7%	30
Northwestern Memorial Hospital[2]	Chicago	7%	156
Advocate Lutheran General Hospital[2]	Park Ridge	8%	53
Louis A Weiss Memorial Hospital[2]	Chicago	8%	38
Northwest Community Hospital[2]	Arlington Hgts	8%	39
Saint Francis Medical Center[2]	Peoria	8%	39
Central Dupage Hospital[2]	Winfield	9%	53
Alexian Brothers Medical Center[2]	Elk Grove Vlg	10%	39
Advocate Trinity Hospital[2]	Chicago	11%	28
Palos Community Hospital[2]	Palos Heights	11%	37
Presence Saint Joseph Medical Center[2]	Joliet	11%	28
The University of Chicago Medical Center[2]	Chicago	14%	85
Edward Hospital[2]	Naperville	16%	51
John H Stroger Jr Hospital[2]	Chicago	19%	31
Little Company of Mary Hospital[2]	Evergreen Park	20%	41
Franciscan Saint James Health[2]	Olympia Fields	24%	41
Holy Cross Hospital[2]	Chicago	35%	31

UFH with Dosages/Platelet Count Monitoring

Hospital Name	City	Rate	Cases
Advocate Good Shepherd Hospital[2]	Barrington	100%	68
Advocate Trinity Hospital[2]	Chicago	100%	95
Blessing Hospital[2]	Quincy	100%	36
Centegra Health Sys-Mc Henry Hosp[2]	Mchenry	100%	66
Centegra Health Sys-Woodstock Hosp[2]	Woodstock	100%	35
Copley Memorial Hospital[2]	Aurora	100%	41
Decatur Memorial Hospital[2]	Decatur	100%	58
Elmhurst Memorial Hospital[2]	Elmhurst	100%	114
Evanston Hospital[2]	Evanston	100%	142
Franciscan Saint James Health[2]	Olympia Fields	100%	92
Galesburg Cottage Hospital[2]	Galesburg	100%	27
Ingalls Memorial Hospital[2]	Harvey	100%	119
Lake Forest Hospital[2]	Lake Forest	100%	31
Little Company of Mary Hospital[2]	Evergreen Park	100%	159
Louis A Weiss Memorial Hospital[2]	Chicago	100%	29
Loyola University Medical Center[2]	Maywood	100%	109
Macneal Hospital[2]	Berwyn	100%	55
Memorial Hospital[2]	Belleville	100%	120
Metrosouth Medical Center[2]	Blue Island	100%	75
Morris Hospital & Healthcare Centers[2]	Morris	100%	28
Northwest Community Hospital[2]	Arlington Hgts	100%	118

NOTE: Hospital profiles are in alphabetical order by state, then city, then hospital within the city; Rankings exclude hospitals with less than 25 cases except for patient surveys which excludes hospitals with less than 100 cases; (a) 100-299 cases; (1) The number of cases/patients is too few to report; (2) Data submitted were based on a sample of cases/patients; (3) Results are based on a shorter time period than required; (4) Data suppressed by CMS for one or more quarters; (5) Results are not available for this reporting period; (6) Fewer than 100 patients completed the HCAHPS survey; (7) No cases met the criteria for this measure; (8) The lower limit of the confidence interval cannot be calculated if the number of observed infections equals zero; (9) No data are available from the state/territory for this reporting period; (10) The scores shown reflect fewer than 50 completed surveys; (11) There were discrepancies in the data collection process; (12) This measure does not apply to this hospital for this reporting period; (13) Results cannot be calculated for this reporting period; (14) The results for this state are combined with nearby states to protect confidentiality; Please refer to the User's Guide for a full explanation of data.

Palos Community Hospital[2]	Palos Heights	100%	179
Presence Mercy Medical Center[2]	Aurora	100%	25
Presence Saint Francis Hospital[2]	Evanston	100%	28
Presence Saint Joseph Hospital - Elgin[2]	Elgin	100%	42
Presence Saint Joseph Medical Center[2]	Joliet	100%	48
Presence Sts Mary & Elizabeth Med Ctr[2]	Chicago	100%	39
Riverside Medical Center[2]	Kankakee	100%	72
Saint Elizabeth Hospital[2]	Belleville	100%	35
Saint Francis Medical Center[2]	Peoria	100%	103
Saint Johns Hospital[2]	Springfield	100%	68
Saint Mary Medical Center[2]	Galesburg	100%	28
Sherman Hospital[2]	Elgin	100%	97
Silver Cross Hospital & Medical Centers[2]	New Lenox	100%	54
Swedish Covenant Hospital[2]	Chicago	100%	64
Vista Medical Center East[2]	Waukegan	100%	37
Advocate Christ Hospital & Medical Center[2]	Oak Lawn	99%	201
Edward Hospital[2]	Naperville	99%	205
University of Illinois Hospital[2]	Chicago	99%	129
Alexian Brothers Medical Center[2]	Elk Grove Vlg	98%	150
Hinsdale Hospital[2]	Hinsdale	98%	42
Methodist Medical Center of Illinois[2]	Peoria	98%	40
Advocate Condell Medical Center[2]	Libertyville	97%	33
Advocate Illinois Masonic Medical Center[2]	Chicago	97%	61
Advocate Lutheran General Hospital[2]	Park Ridge	97%	32
The University of Chicago Medical Center[2]	Chicago	97%	153
Advocate Good Samaritan Hospital[2]	Downers Grove	96%	109
Saint Alexius Medical Center[2]	Hoffman Estates	96%	105
Advocate South Suburban Hospital[2]	Hazel Crest	94%	52
Swedish American Hospital[2]	Rockford	94%	32
Memorial Medical Center[2]	Springfield	93%	143
Adventist La Grange Memorial Hospital[2]	La Grange	91%	58
Carle Foundation Hospital[2]	Urbana	88%	147
Mercy Hospital & Medical Center[2]	Chicago	86%	65
Northwestern Memorial Hospital[2]	Chicago	75%	226
Rush University Medical Center[2]	Chicago	74%	145
Central Dupage Hospital[2]	Winfield	62%	101
Holy Cross Hospital[2]	Chicago	34%	44
John H Stroger Jr Hospital[2]	Chicago	15%	48

Venous Thromboembolism Prophylaxis

Hospital Name	City	Rate	Cases
Genesis Health System[2]	Silvis	100%	289
Presence Mercy Medical Center[2]	Aurora	100%	303
Saint Joseph's Hospital[2]	Breese	100%	116
Vista Medical Center East[2]	Waukegan	100%	395
Galesburg Cottage Hospital[2]	Galesburg	99%	189
Red Bud Regional Hospital[2]	Red Bud	99%	371
Riverside Medical Center[2]	Kankakee	99%	300
Saint Anthony Hospital[2]	Chicago	99%	213
Valley West Community Hospital[2]	Sandwich	99%	87
Adventist Bolingbrook Hospital[2]	Bolingbrook	98%	322
Alton Memorial Hospital[2]	Alton	98%	345
Ingalls Memorial Hospital[2]	Harvey	98%	432
Kishwaukee Community Hospital[2]	Dekalb	98%	324
Methodist Hospital of Chicago[2]	Chicago	98%	148
Saint Anthony's Health Center[2]	Alton	98%	250
Union County Hospital[2]	Anna	98%	324
Copley Memorial Hospital[2]	Aurora	97%	290
Memorial Hospital of Carbondale[2]	Carbondale	97%	336
Presence Saint Joseph Hospital - Elgin[2]	Elgin	97%	320
Saint James Hospital[2]	Pontiac	97%	60
Saint Joseph Memorial Hospital	Murphysboro	97%	353
Saint Margarets Hospital[2]	Spring Valley	97%	147
Crossroads Community Hospital[2]	Mount Vernon	96%	294
Heartland Regional Medical Center[2]	Marion	96%	278
Richland Memorial Hospital[2]	Olney	96%	175
Roseland Community Hospital[2]	Chicago	96%	174
Advocate Bromenn Medical Center	Normal	95%	2329
Carle Foundation Hospital[2]	Urbana	95%	362
Evanston Hospital[2]	Evanston	95%	320
Metrosouth Medical Center[2]	Blue Island	95%	335
Saint Bernard Hospital[2]	Chicago	95%	307
Saint Elizabeth Hospital[2]	Belleville	95%	259
Advocate Eureka Hospital	Eureka	94%	125
Good Samaritan Regional Health Center[2]	Mount Vernon	94%	339
Herrin Hospital[2]	Herrin	94%	365
Louis A Weiss Memorial Hospital[2]	Chicago	94%	343
Rush Oak Park Hospital[2]	Oak Park	94%	331
Advocate Illinois Masonic Medical Center[2]	Chicago	93%	314
Advocate Trinity Hospital[2]	Chicago	93%	395
Gateway Regional Medical Center[2]	Granite City	93%	1090
Illini Community Hospital[3]	Pittsfield	93%	43
Katherine Shaw Bethea Hospital[2]	Dixon	93%	252
Memorial Hospital[2]	Belleville	93%	388
Morris Hospital & Healthcare Centers[2]	Morris	93%	231
Rush University Medical Center[2]	Chicago	93%	274
Jackson Park Hospital[2]	Chicago	92%	216
Mercy Harvard Hospital[2]	Harvard	92%	124
Northwest Community Hospital[2]	Arlington Hgts	92%	355
Presence Sts Mary & Elizabeth Med Ctr[2]	Chicago	92%	321
Abraham Lincoln Memorial Hospital[2]	Lincoln	91%	216
Ottawa Reg Hosp & Healthcare Ctr[2]	Ottawa	91%	185
Fhn Memorial Hospital[2]	Freeport	90%	334
Loyola University Medical Center[2]	Maywood	90%	261
Presence Saint Joseph Hospital - Chicago[2]	Chicago	90%	354
Saint Mary Medical Center[2]	Galesburg	90%	229
Saint Marys Hospital[2]	Streator	90%	175
Swedish American Hospital[2]	Rockford	90%	368
Advocate Christ Hospital & Medical Center[2]	Oak Lawn	89%	341
Holy Cross Hospital[2]	Chicago	89%	337
Presence Our Lady of the Res Med Ctr[2]	Chicago	89%	348
Saint Alexius Medical Center[2]	Hoffman Estates	89%	335
University of Illinois Hospital[2]	Chicago	89%	348
Advocate Good Samaritan Hospital[2]	Downers Grove	88%	336
Franciscan Saint James Health[2]	Olympia Fields	88%	708
Little Company of Mary Hospital[2]	Evergreen Park	88%	378
Mercy Hospital & Medical Center[2]	Chicago	88%	324
Presence United Samaritans Medical Center[2]	Danville	88%	346
Proctor Hospital[2]	Peoria	88%	360
Saint Marys Hospital[2]	Centralia	88%	388
Greenville Regional Hospital[2]	Greenville	87%	126
Harrisburg Medical Center[2]	Harrisburg	87%	110
Presence Saint Francis Hospital[2]	Evanston	87%	280
Westlake Community Hospital[2]	Melrose Park	87%	247
Centegra Health Sys-Woodstock Hosp[2]	Woodstock	86%	311
Illinois Valley Community Hospital[2]	Peru	86%	194
Mount Sinai Hospital Medical Center[2]	Chicago	86%	303
Northwestern Memorial Hospital[2]	Chicago	86%	297
Presence Resurrection Medical Center[2]	Chicago	86%	306
West Suburban Medical Center[2]	Oak Park	86%	352
Alexian Brothers Medical Center[2]	Elk Grove Vlg	85%	333
CGH Medical Center[2]	Sterling	85%	304
Delnor Community Hospital[2]	Geneva	85%	299
Rockford Memorial Hospital[2]	Rockford	85%	476
Swedish Covenant Hospital[2]	Chicago	85%	407
Advocate Good Shepherd Hospital[2]	Barrington	84%	315
Central Dupage Hospital[2]	Winfield	84%	258
Paris Community Hospital[2]	Paris	84%	90
Saint Anthonys Memorial Hospital[2]	Effingham	84%	291
Saint Joseph Medical Center[2]	Bloomington	84%	341
Advocate Lutheran General Hospital[2]	Park Ridge	83%	323
Centegra Health Sys-Mc Henry Hosp[2]	Mchenry	83%	333
Elmhurst Memorial Hospital[2]	Elmhurst	83%	301
Methodist Medical Center of Illinois[2]	Peoria	83%	293
Saint Johns Hospital[2]	Springfield	83%	305
Touchette Regional Hospital[2]	Centreville	83%	103
Adventist Glenoaks[2]	Glendale Hghts	82%	149
Adventist La Grange Memorial Hospital[2]	La Grange	81%	363
Hinsdale Hospital[2]	Hinsdale	81%	295
Palos Community Hospital[2]	Palos Heights	81%	355
Pekin Memorial Hospital[2]	Pekin	81%	234
Macneal Hospital[2]	Berwyn	80%	352
Presence Saint Marys Hospital[2]	Kankakee	80%	295
Saint Anthony Medical Center[2]	Rockford	80%	307
Saint Francis Medical Center[2]	Peoria	80%	347
Advocate South Suburban Hospital[2]	Hazel Crest	79%	356
Decatur Memorial Hospital[2]	Decatur	79%	323
Edward Hospital[2]	Naperville	79%	304
Thorek Memorial Hospital[2]	Chicago	79%	213
John H Stroger Jr Hospital[2]	Chicago	78%	424
Lake Forest Hospital[2]	Lake Forest	78%	290
Sarah Bush Lincoln Health Center[2]	Mattoon	78%	345
Trinity Rock Island[2]	Rock Island	78%	330
McDonough District Hospital[2]	Macomb	77%	155
Blessing Hospital[2]	Quincy	76%	297
Presence Covenant Medical Center[2]	Urbana	75%	329
The University of Chicago Medical Center[2]	Chicago	75%	354
Memorial Medical Center[2]	Springfield	74%	334
Midwestern Region Medical Center[2]	Zion	74%	179
Shelby Memorial Hospital	Shelbyville	74%	233
Sherman Hospital[2]	Elgin	74%	330
Advocate Condell Medical Center[2]	Libertyville	73%	352
Anderson Hospital[2]	Maryville	73%	328
Passavant Area Hospital[2]	Jacksonville	73%	282
Iroquois Memorial Hospital[2]	Watseka	72%	92
Presence Saint Joseph Medical Center[2]	Joliet	71%	378
Loretto Hospital[2]	Chicago	69%	155
Provident Hospital of Chicago[2]	Chicago	69%	186
Loyola Gottlieb Memorial Hospital[2]	Melrose Park	66%	358
Silver Cross Hospital & Medical Centers[2]	New Lenox	61%	343
Norwegian - American Hospital[2]	Chicago	54%	191
Saint Marys Hospital[2]	Decatur	54%	261
South Shore Hospital[2]	Chicago	54%	283
Graham Hospital Association[2]	Canton	52%	171
Jersey Community Hospital[2]	Jerseyville	49%	239
Mendota Community Hospital[2,3]	Mendota	29%	98
Taylorville Memorial Hospital[2]	Taylorville	26%	167

Warfarin Therapy Discharge Instructions

Hospital Name	City	Rate	Cases
Copley Memorial Hospital[2]	Aurora	100%	68
Decatur Memorial Hospital[2]	Decatur	100%	85
Memorial Hospital of Carbondale[2]	Carbondale	100%	59
Northwest Community Hospital[2]	Arlington Hgts	100%	83
Presence Sts Mary & Elizabeth Med Ctr[2]	Chicago	100%	44
Riverside Medical Center[2]	Kankakee	100%	61
Saint Elizabeth Hospital[2]	Belleville	100%	36
Vista Medical Center East[2]	Waukegan	100%	54
Ingalls Memorial Hospital[2]	Harvey	99%	103
Alton Memorial Hospital[2]	Alton	98%	53
Sherman Hospital[2]	Elgin	98%	102
Kishwaukee Community Hospital[2]	Dekalb	97%	34
Metrosouth Medical Center[2]	Blue Island	97%	67
Advocate Bromenn Medical Center	Normal	96%	28
Katherine Shaw Bethea Hospital[2]	Dixon	96%	28
Morris Hospital & Healthcare Centers[2]	Morris	96%	25
Presence Saint Joseph Hospital - Elgin[2]	Elgin	96%	52
Saint Anthonys Memorial Hospital[2]	Effingham	96%	28
Silver Cross Hospital & Medical Centers[2]	New Lenox	96%	68
Palos Community Hospital[2]	Palos Heights	94%	120
Presence Mercy Medical Center[2]	Aurora	94%	47
Adventist Bolingbrook Hospital[2]	Bolingbrook	93%	27
Methodist Medical Center of Illinois[2]	Peoria	93%	41
Fhn Memorial Hospital[2]	Freeport	92%	38
Lake Forest Hospital[2]	Lake Forest	92%	71
Mercy Hospital & Medical Center[2]	Chicago	91%	58
Presence United Samaritans Medical Center[2]	Danville	91%	45
Swedish Covenant Hospital[2]	Chicago	91%	43
Evanston Hospital[2]	Evanston	90%	168
Good Samaritan Regional Health Center[2]	Mount Vernon	89%	28
Little Company of Mary Hospital[2]	Evergreen Park	89%	124
Saint Alexius Medical Center[2]	Hoffman Estates	89%	81
Blessing Hospital[2]	Quincy	87%	39
Memorial Hospital[2]	Belleville	86%	59
Presence Saint Joseph Medical Center[2]	Joliet	85%	124
Saint Mary Medical Center[2]	Galesburg	85%	27
Advocate Lutheran General Hospital[2]	Park Ridge	84%	69
Saint Marys Hospital[2]	Centralia	84%	25
Saint Marys Hospital[2]	Decatur	84%	31
Alexian Brothers Medical Center[2]	Elk Grove Vlg	83%	101
Presence Our Lady of the Res Med Ctr[2]	Chicago	83%	29
Louis A Weiss Memorial Hospital[2]	Chicago	81%	36
Proctor Hospital[2]	Peoria	78%	27
Swedish American Hospital[2]	Rockford	77%	77
Rush Oak Park Hospital[2]	Oak Park	76%	41
Rush University Medical Center[2]	Chicago	75%	114
Advocate Good Samaritan Hospital[2]	Downers Grove	73%	84
Norwegian - American Hospital[2]	Chicago	73%	26
Advocate Good Shepherd Hospital[2]	Barrington	72%	60
Advocate Trinity Hospital[2]	Chicago	71%	89
Carle Foundation Hospital[2]	Urbana	71%	120
Advocate Illinois Masonic Medical Center[2]	Chicago	70%	60
Presence Covenant Medical Center[2]	Urbana	70%	33
Saint Francis Medical Center[2]	Peoria	69%	122
Hinsdale Hospital[2]	Hinsdale	68%	44
Macneal Hospital[2]	Berwyn	68%	57
Saint Joseph Medical Center[2]	Bloomington	68%	38
Edward Hospital[2]	Naperville	67%	144
Adventist La Grange Memorial Hospital[2]	La Grange	65%	37
University of Illinois Hospital[2]	Chicago	65%	77
Trinity Rock Island[2]	Rock Island	64%	50
Centegra Health Sys-Mc Henry Hosp[2]	Mchenry	62%	56
Centegra Health Sys-Woodstock Hosp[2]	Woodstock	62%	37
John H Stroger Jr Hospital[2]	Chicago	62%	112
Presence Saint Marys Hospital[2]	Kankakee	61%	33
Sarah Bush Lincoln Health Center[2]	Mattoon	60%	30
Elmhurst Memorial Hospital[2]	Elmhurst	59%	111
The University of Chicago Medical Center[2]	Chicago	57%	106
Memorial Medical Center[2]	Springfield	53%	132
Presence Saint Francis Hospital[2]	Evanston	53%	34
Franciscan Saint James Health[2]	Olympia Fields	44%	115
Saint Anthony Medical Center[2]	Rockford	41%	80
Advocate Christ Hospital & Medical Center[2]	Oak Lawn	39%	163
Northwestern Memorial Hospital[2]	Chicago	34%	205
CGH Medical Center[2]	Sterling	30%	30
Loyola University Medical Center[2]	Maywood	30%	93
Advocate South Suburban Hospital[2]	Hazel Crest	29%	85
Central Dupage Hospital[2]	Winfield	29%	118
West Suburban Medical Center[2]	Oak Park	29%	38
Saint Johns Hospital[2]	Springfield	28%	60
Advocate Condell Medical Center[2]	Libertyville	26%	73
Rockford Memorial Hospital[2]	Rockford	22%	74
Presence Resurrection Medical Center[2]	Chicago	18%	40
Holy Cross Hospital[2]	Chicago	16%	44
Delnor Community Hospital[2]	Geneva	14%	36
Mount Sinai Hospital Medical Center[2]	Chicago	0%	32

Chest Pain/Possible Heart Attack Care

Aspirin Given Within 24 Hours of Arrival

Hospital Name	City	Rate	Cases
Alton Memorial Hospital	Alton	100%	46

NOTE: Hospital profiles are in alphabetical order by state, then city, then hospital within the city; Rankings exclude hospitals with less than 25 cases except for patient surveys which excludes hospitals with less than 100 cases; (a) 100-299 cases; (1) The number of cases/patients is too few to report; (2) Data submitted were based on a sample of cases/patients; (3) Results are based on a shorter time period than required; (4) Data suppressed by CMS for one or more quarters; (5) Results are not available for this reporting period; (6) Fewer than 100 patients completed the HCAHPS survey; (7) No cases met the criteria for this measure; (8) The lower limit of the confidence interval cannot be calculated if the number of observed infections equals zero; (9) No data are available from the state/territory for this reporting period; (10) The scores shown reflect fewer than 50 completed surveys; (11) There were discrepancies in the data collection process; (12) This measure does not apply to this hospital for this reporting period; (13) Results cannot be calculated for this reporting period; (14) The results for this state are combined with nearby states to protect confidentiality; Please refer to the User's Guide for a full explanation of data.

Hospital Name	City	Rate	Cases
Carlinville Area Hospital	Carlinville	100%	30
Graham Hospital Association	Canton	100%	59
Illinois Valley Community Hospital	Peru	100%	44
Memorial Hospital	Chester	100%	39
Richland Memorial Hospital	Olney	100%	36
Saint James Hospital	Pontiac	100%	54
Saint Joseph's Hospital	Breese	100%	48
Saint Marys Hospital	Streator	100%	77
Herrin Hospital	Herrin	99%	160
McDonough District Hospital	Macomb	99%	82
Clay County Hospital	Flora	98%	98
Fhn Memorial Hospital	Freeport	98%	41
Galesburg Cottage Hospital	Galesburg	98%	49
Harrisburg Medical Center	Harrisburg	98%	48
Saint Anthonys Memorial Hospital	Effingham	98%	106
Saint Margarets Hospital	Spring Valley	98%	49
Union County Hospital	Anna	98%	64
Abraham Lincoln Memorial Hospital	Lincoln	97%	79
Hardin County General Hospital	Rosiclare	97%	38
Saint Mary Medical Center	Galesburg	97%	77
Saint Marys Hospital	Centralia	97%	61
Sarah Bush Lincoln Health Center	Mattoon	97%	108
Valley West Community Hospital	Sandwich	97%	31
Jersey Community Hospital	Jerseyville	96%	53
Red Bud Regional Hospital	Red Bud	96%	74
Centegra Health Sys-Woodstock Hosp	Woodstock	95%	42
Fairfield Memorial Hospital	Fairfield	95%	39
Ottawa Reg Hosp & Healthcare Ctr	Ottawa	95%	65
Taylorville Memorial Hospital	Taylorville	95%	74
Shelby Memorial Hospital	Shelbyville	94%	36
Anderson Hospital	Maryville	93%	29
CGH Medical Center	Sterling	93%	29
Greenville Regional Hospital[3]	Greenville	93%	29
Passavant Area Hospital	Jacksonville	93%	135
Presence United Samaritans Medical Center	Danville	93%	132
Saint Bernard Hospital	Chicago	91%	53
Provident Hospital of Chicago	Chicago	89%	54
Holy Cross Hospital	Chicago	86%	35
Massac Memorial Hospital[3]	Metropolis	74%	43

Average Time to ECG (minutes)

Hospital Name	City	Min.	Cases
Illinois Valley Community Hospital	Peru	2	43
Sarah Bush Lincoln Health Center	Mattoon	2	111
Abraham Lincoln Memorial Hospital	Lincoln	3	80
Fairfield Memorial Hospital	Fairfield	3	41
Fhn Memorial Hospital	Freeport	3	46
Saint Bernard Hospital	Chicago	3	54
Taylorville Memorial Hospital	Taylorville	3	80
Anderson Hospital	Maryville	4	29
Centegra Health Sys-Woodstock Hosp	Woodstock	4	44
Hardin County General Hospital	Rosiclare	4	40
Herrin Hospital	Herrin	4	163
Memorial Hospital	Chester	4	39
Red Bud Regional Hospital	Red Bud	4	76
Union County Hospital	Anna	4	68
Valley West Community Hospital	Sandwich	4	32
CGH Medical Center	Sterling	5	29
Saint James Hospital	Pontiac	5	58
Saint Margarets Hospital	Spring Valley	5	49
Saint Marys Hospital	Streator	5	81
Wabash General Hospital	Mount Carmel	5	31
Carlinville Area Hospital	Carlinville	6	31
Harrisburg Medical Center	Harrisburg	6	50
Jersey Community Hospital	Jerseyville	6	51
McDonough District Hospital	Macomb	6	82
Ottawa Reg Hosp & Healthcare Ctr	Ottawa	6	65
Saint Mary Medical Center	Galesburg	6	79
Saint Marys Hospital	Centralia	6	62
Clay County Hospital	Flora	7	97
Richland Memorial Hospital	Olney	7	37
Alton Memorial Hospital	Alton	8	44
Galesburg Cottage Hospital	Galesburg	8	50
Shelby Memorial Hospital	Shelbyville	8	37
Presence United Samaritans Medical Center	Danville	9	137
Saint Joseph's Hospital	Breese	9	49
Graham Hospital Association	Canton	10	60
Passavant Area Hospital	Jacksonville	10	141
Swedish Covenant Hospital	Chicago	10	25
Massac Memorial Hospital[3]	Metropolis	12	44
Greenville Regional Hospital[3]	Greenville	13	30
Saint Anthonys Memorial Hospital	Effingham	13	104
Holy Cross Hospital	Chicago	14	35
Provident Hospital of Chicago	Chicago	80	62

Average Time to Transfer (minutes)

Hospital Name	City	Min.	Cases
Herrin Hospital	Herrin	29	29
Passavant Area Hospital	Jacksonville	38	25
Presence United Samaritans Medical Center	Danville	60	27

Children's Asthma Care

Received Home Management Plan of Care

Hospital Name	City	Rate	Cases
Little Company of Mary Hospital	Evergreen Park	96%	26
Loyola University Medical Center	Maywood	90%	167
Saint Johns Hospital	Springfield	88%	96
The University of Chicago Medical Center[2]	Chicago	84%	275

Received Reliever Medication

Hospital Name	City	Rate	Cases
Little Company of Mary Hospital	Evergreen Park	100%	27
Loyola University Medical Center	Maywood	100%	169
Saint Johns Hospital	Springfield	100%	97
The University of Chicago Medical Center[2]	Chicago	100%	280

Received Systemic Corticosteroids

Hospital Name	City	Rate	Cases
Little Company of Mary Hospital	Evergreen Park	100%	27
Loyola University Medical Center	Maywood	100%	167
Saint Johns Hospital	Springfield	100%	97
The University of Chicago Medical Center[2]	Chicago	100%	279

Emergency Department

Admittance Decision Time (minutes)

Hospital Name	City	Min.	Cases
Jackson Park Hospital[2]	Chicago	0	180
Harrisburg Medical Center[2]	Harrisburg	3	162
Shelby Memorial Hospital	Shelbyville	37	220
Mendota Community Hospital[3]	Mendota	40	118
Mercy Harvard Hospital	Harvard	40	276
Saint Margarets Hospital[2]	Spring Valley	43	224
Illinois Valley Community Hospital[2]	Peru	45	325
Massac Memorial Hospital[2]	Metropolis	45	160
Saint Joseph's Hospital[2]	Breese	45	239
Graham Hospital Association[2]	Canton	49	339
Morris Hospital & Healthcare Centers[2]	Morris	49	581
Mason District Hospital[2,3]	Havana	50	79
OSF Holy Family Medical Center[2]	Monmouth	50	112
Valley West Community Hospital[2]	Sandwich	52	312
CGH Medical Center[2]	Sterling	53	648
Advocate Eureka Hospital	Eureka	54	175
Richland Memorial Hospital[2]	Olney	54	273
Greenville Regional Hospital	Greenville	55	377
Pinckneyville Community Hospital[2]	Pinckneyville	55	186
Crossroads Community Hospital[2]	Mount Vernon	56	463
Fairfield Memorial Hospital[2]	Fairfield	58	158
Fhn Memorial Hospital[2]	Freeport	58	424
Ottawa Reg Hosp & Healthcare Ctr[2]	Ottawa	58	351
Rush Oak Park Hospital[2]	Oak Park	58	695
Saint James Hospital[2]	Pontiac	58	420
Swedish American Hospital[2]	Rockford	58	564
Saint Anthony's Health Center[2]	Alton	59	347
Abraham Lincoln Memorial Hospital[2]	Lincoln	61	285
Proctor Hospital[2]	Peoria	61	370
Red Bud Regional Hospital[2]	Red Bud	62	459
Gateway Regional Medical Center[2]	Granite City	64	1775
McDonough District Hospital[2]	Macomb	64	312
Northwest Community Hospital[2]	Arlington Hgts	64	484
Alton Memorial Hospital[2]	Alton	65	303
Saint Anthonys Memorial Hospital[2]	Effingham	65	437
Galesburg Cottage Hospital[2]	Galesburg	67	331
Katherine Shaw Bethea Hospital[2]	Dixon	68	406
Presence Resurrection Medical Center[2]	Chicago	68	753
Saint Joseph Memorial Hospital	Murphysboro	68	363
Union County Hospital[2]	Anna	69	295
Elmhurst Memorial Hospital[2]	Elmhurst	70	688
Herrin Hospital[2]	Herrin	70	690
Passavant Area Hospital[2]	Jacksonville	70	494
Taylorville Memorial Hospital[2]	Taylorville	70	331
Advocate Lutheran General Hospital[2]	Park Ridge	72	442
Blessing Hospital[2]	Quincy	72	395
Clay County Hospital[2]	Flora	72	567
Trinity Rock Island[2]	Rock Island	72	433
Genesis Health System[2]	Silvis	74	439
Good Samaritan Regional Health Center[2]	Mount Vernon	75	445
Pekin Memorial Hospital[2]	Pekin	75	324
Presence United Samaritans Medical Center[2]	Danville	75	671
Saint Marys Hospital[2]	Centralia	75	632
Rockford Memorial Hospital[2]	Rockford	76	616
Methodist Hospital of Chicago[2]	Chicago	77	226
Evanston Hospital[2]	Evanston	78	393
Kishwaukee Community Hospital[2]	Dekalb	78	466
Sarah Bush Lincoln Health Center[2]	Mattoon	78	577
Saint Alexius Medical Center[2]	Hoffman Estates	79	594
Saint Mary Medical Center[2]	Galesburg	79	331
Centegra Health Sys-Woodstock Hosp[2]	Woodstock	80	500
Iroquois Memorial Hospital[2]	Watseka	80	274
Anderson Hospital[2]	Maryville	81	453
Saint Joseph Medical Center[2]	Bloomington	81	352
Carle Foundation Hospital[2]	Urbana	82	543
Palos Community Hospital[2]	Palos Heights	83	612
Saint Elizabeth Hospital[2]	Belleville	84	516
Silver Cross Hospital & Medical Centers[2]	New Lenox	84	424
Ingalls Memorial Hospital[2]	Harvey	85	464
Presence Saint Marys Hospital[2]	Kankakee	85	700
Saint Anthony Medical Center[2]	Rockford	86	618
Louis A Weiss Memorial Hospital[2]	Chicago	87	690
Sherman Hospital[2]	Elgin	87	515
Methodist Medical Center of Illinois[2]	Peoria	88	455
Advocate Good Samaritan Hospital[2]	Downers Grove	90	542
Jersey Community Hospital[2]	Jerseyville	90	393
Saint Marys Hospital[2]	Decatur	91	540
Loyola Gottlieb Memorial Hospital[2]	Melrose Park	92	412
Adventist Glenoaks[2]	Glendale Hghts	93	266
Little Company of Mary Hospital[2]	Evergreen Park	93	824
Presence Saint Joseph Hospital - Elgin[2]	Elgin	93	653
Advocate Illinois Masonic Medical Center[2]	Chicago	94	460
Central Dupage Hospital[2]	Winfield	94	408
Memorial Medical Center[2]	Springfield	94	485
Adventist Bolingbrook Hospital[2]	Bolingbrook	95	515
Alexian Brothers Medical Center[2]	Elk Grove Vlg	95	687
Heartland Regional Medical Center[2]	Marion	95	430
Lake Forest Hospital[2]	Lake Forest	95	454
Presence Mercy Medical Center[2]	Aurora	95	648
Presence Saint Joseph Medical Center[2]	Joliet	95	555
Edward Hospital[2]	Naperville	96	485
Riverside Medical Center[2]	Kankakee	97	529
Adventist La Grange Memorial Hospital[2]	La Grange	98	376
Touchette Regional Hospital[2]	Centreville	98	197
Delnor Community Hospital[2]	Geneva	100	397
Memorial Hospital of Carbondale[2]	Carbondale	100	314
Swedish Covenant Hospital[2]	Chicago	100	429
Advocate Bromenn Medical Center[2]	Normal	102	460
Hinsdale Hospital[2]	Hinsdale	103	310
Memorial Hospital[2]	Belleville	103	797
Saint Anthony Hospital[2]	Chicago	103	529
Copley Memorial Hospital[2]	Aurora	104	393
Advocate Good Shepherd Hospital[2]	Barrington	105	457
Franciscan Saint James Health[2]	Olympia Fields	105	1520
Presence Saint Joseph Hospital - Chicago[2]	Chicago	105	364
Advocate South Suburban Hospital[2]	Hazel Crest	108	609
Centegra Health Sys-Mc Henry Hosp[2]	Mchenry	111	577
Presence Covenant Medical Center[2]	Urbana	115	493
Vista Medical Center East[2]	Waukegan	115	777
Westlake Community Hospital[2]	Melrose Park	115	365
Saint Johns Hospital[2]	Springfield	116	370
West Suburban Medical Center[2]	Oak Park	120	622
Advocate Trinity Hospital[2]	Chicago	122	664
Norwegian - American Hospital[2]	Chicago	124	239
Decatur Memorial Hospital[2]	Decatur	125	519
Thorek Memorial Hospital[2]	Chicago	125	207
Presence Saint Francis Hospital[2]	Evanston	130	632
Loretto Hospital[2]	Chicago	132	322
Northwestern Memorial Hospital[2]	Chicago	132	246
Advocate Condell Medical Center[2]	Libertyville	135	521
Presence Sts Mary & Elizabeth Med Ctr[2]	Chicago	136	561
Saint Marys Hospital[2]	Streator	137	331
University of Illinois Hospital[2]	Chicago	137	500
Mercy Hospital & Medical Center[2]	Chicago	138	584
Saint Francis Medical Center[2]	Peoria	142	520
Presence Our Lady of the Res Med Ctr[2]	Chicago	150	856
Metrosouth Medical Center[2]	Blue Island	156	605
South Shore Hospital[2]	Chicago	164	443
Loyola University Medical Center[2]	Maywood	170	383
Rush University Medical Center[2]	Chicago	170	406
Mount Sinai Hospital Medical Center[2]	Chicago	174	537
Macneal Hospital[2]	Berwyn	178	694
Roseland Community Hospital[2]	Chicago	185	459
Advocate Christ Hospital & Medical Center[2]	Oak Lawn	210	557
John H Stroger Jr Hospital[2]	Chicago	210	811
Holy Cross Hospital[2]	Chicago	229	943
Provident Hospital of Chicago[2]	Chicago	242	512
The University of Chicago Medical Center[2]	Chicago	277	447
Saint Bernard Hospital[2]	Chicago	305	616

Head CT Results Within 45 Minutes of Arrival

Hospital Name	City	Rate	Cases
Sherman Hospital	Elgin	98%	49
Alton Memorial Hospital	Alton	91%	32
Franciscan Saint James Health	Olympia Fields	78%	36
Palos Community Hospital	Palos Heights	71%	35
Anderson Hospital	Maryville	70%	37
Advocate Trinity Hospital	Chicago	59%	27
Passavant Area Hospital	Jacksonville	34%	41

NOTE: Hospital profiles are in alphabetical order by state, then city, then hospital within the city; Rankings exclude hospitals with less than 25 cases except for patient surveys which excludes hospitals with less than 100 cases; (a) 100-299 cases; (1) The number of cases/patients is too few to report; (2) Data submitted were based on a sample of cases/patients; (3) Results are based on a shorter time period than required; (4) Data suppressed by CMS for one or more quarters; (5) Results are not available for this reporting period; (6) Fewer than 100 patients completed the HCAHPS survey; (7) No cases met the criteria for this measure; (8) The lower limit of the confidence interval cannot be calculated if the number of observed infections equals zero; (9) No data are available from the state/territory for this reporting period; (10) The scores shown reflect fewer than 50 completed surveys; (11) There were discrepancies in the data collection process; (12) This measure does not apply to this hospital for this reporting period; (13) Results cannot be calculated for this reporting period; (14) The results for this state are combined with nearby states to protect confidentiality; Please refer to the User's Guide for a full explanation of data.

Patients Who Left ER Before Being Seen

Hospital Name	City	Rate	Cases
Adventist Glenoaks	Glendale Hghts	0%	19899
Advocate Condell Medical Center	Libertyville	0%	56924
Carle Foundation Hospital	Urbana	0%	70356
Edward Hospital	Naperville	0%	93106
Gibson Community Hospital	Gibson City	0%	6262
Illini Community Hospital	Pittsfield	0%	7025
Iroquois Memorial Hospital	Watseka	0%	10739
Jackson Park Hospital	Chicago	0%	15989
Memorial Hospital	Chester	0%	6046
Methodist Hospital of Chicago	Chicago	0%	3989
Ottawa Reg Hosp & Healthcare Ctr	Ottawa	0%	15895
Presence Resurrection Medical Center	Chicago	0%	40201
Presence Saint Francis Hospital	Evanston	0%	36849
Presence Saint Joseph Hospital - Chicago	Chicago	0%	20222
Saint James Hospital	Pontiac	0%	14647
Saint Marys Hospital	Centralia	0%	24005
Saint Marys Hospital	Streator	0%	12518
Taylorville Memorial Hospital	Taylorville	0%	15562
Thorek Memorial Hospital	Chicago	0%	8202
Abraham Lincoln Memorial Hospital	Lincoln	1%	17464
Adventist Bolingbrook Hospital	Bolingbrook	1%	33434
Adventist La Grange Memorial Hospital	La Grange	1%	27023
Advocate Good Samaritan Hospital	Downers Grove	1%	44589
Advocate Good Shepherd Hospital	Barrington	1%	34092
Advocate Lutheran General Hospital	Park Ridge	1%	63801
Alexian Brothers Medical Center	Elk Grove Vlg	1%	49973
Blessing Hospital	Quincy	1%	53703
Central Dupage Hospital	Winfield	1%	72326
CGH Medical Center	Sterling	1%	29271
Crossroads Community Hospital	Mount Vernon	1%	9993
Decatur Memorial Hospital	Decatur	1%	50727
Elmhurst Memorial Hospital	Elmhurst	1%	50406
Evanston Hospital	Evanston	1%	103257
Fhn Memorial Hospital	Freeport	1%	26996
Galesburg Cottage Hospital	Galesburg	1%	14435
Genesis Health System	Silvis	1%	25496
Graham Hospital Association	Canton	1%	16234
Greenville Regional Hospital	Greenville	1%	9336
Harrisburg Medical Center	Harrisburg	1%	12964
Hinsdale Hospital	Hinsdale	1%	27525
Illinois Valley Community Hospital	Peru	1%	14941
Jersey Community Hospital	Jerseyville	1%	12536
Katherine Shaw Bethea Hospital	Dixon	1%	18719
Lake Forest Hospital	Lake Forest	1%	52625
McDonough District Hospital	Macomb	1%	14500
Memorial Hospital	Belleville	1%	66977
Memorial Hospital of Carbondale	Carbondale	1%	33166
Mendota Community Hospital	Mendota	1%	6558
Morris Hospital & Healthcare Centers	Morris	1%	26797
Morrison Community Hospital	Morrison	1%	1489
Mount Sinai Hospital Medical Center	Chicago	1%	54714
Northwest Community Hospital	Arlington Hgts	1%	74955
Passavant Area Hospital	Jacksonville	1%	16564
Pekin Memorial Hospital	Pekin	1%	41588
Presence Our Lady of the Res Med Ctr	Chicago	1%	45754
Presence Saint Joseph Hospital - Elgin	Elgin	1%	30773
Presence United Samaritans Medical Center	Danville	1%	39914
Proctor Hospital	Peoria	1%	20575
Red Bud Regional Hospital	Red Bud	1%	6304
Richland Memorial Hospital	Olney	1%	9572
Rush Oak Park Hospital	Oak Park	1%	23872
Saint Alexius Medical Center	Hoffman Estates	1%	57021
Saint Anthony Hospital	Chicago	1%	37920
Saint Anthony's Health Center	Alton	1%	23367
Saint Anthonys Memorial Hospital	Effingham	1%	25786
Saint Francis Medical Center	Peoria	1%	87429
Saint Joseph's Hospital	Breese	1%	8565
Saint Joseph's Hospital	Highland	1%	6370
Saint Margarets Hospital	Spring Valley	1%	9879
Shelby Memorial Hospital	Shelbyville	1%	5668
Sherman Hospital	Elgin	1%	60739
Trinity Rock Island	Rock Island	1%	63265
Union County Hospital	Anna	1%	8470
Valley West Community Hospital	Sandwich	1%	9327
Vista Medical Center East	Waukegan	1%	42973
Vista Medical Center West	Waukegan	1%	12494
West Suburban Medical Center	Oak Park	1%	60134
Advocate Illinois Masonic Medical Center	Chicago	2%	44204
Anderson Hospital	Maryville	2%	34962
Centegra Health Sys-Mc Henry Hosp	Mchenry	2%	37712
Centegra Health Sys-Woodstock Hosp	Woodstock	2%	27577
Delnor Community Hospital	Geneva	2%	33714
Franciscan Saint James Health	Olympia Fields	2%	81419
Heartland Regional Medical Center	Marion	2%	17954
Ingalls Memorial Hospital	Harvey	2%	50435
Kishwaukee Community Hospital	Dekalb	2%	27181
Louis A Weiss Memorial Hospital	Chicago	2%	24215
Macneal Hospital	Berwyn	2%	61619
Metrosouth Medical Center	Blue Island	2%	49919
Palos Community Hospital	Palos Heights	2%	47408
Pana Community Hospital	Pana	2%	8847
Presence Saint Marys Hospital	Kankakee	2%	33735
Presence Sts Mary & Elizabeth Med Ctr	Chicago	2%	69677
Riverside Medical Center	Kankakee	2%	40912
Saint Mary Medical Center	Galesburg	2%	21156
Saint Marys Hospital	Decatur	2%	33535
Sarah Bush Lincoln Health Center	Mattoon	2%	38559
Silver Cross Hospital & Medical Centers	New Lenox	2%	70182
Advocate Bromenn Medical Center	Normal	3%	36944
Advocate Christ Hospital & Medical Center	Oak Lawn	3%	98236
Alton Memorial Hospital	Alton	3%	42943
Copley Memorial Hospital	Aurora	3%	73392
Ferrell Hospital Community Foundations	Eldorado	3%	7375
Gateway Regional Medical Center	Granite City	3%	26367
Good Samaritan Regional Health Center	Mount Vernon	3%	23844
Herrin Hospital	Herrin	3%	25843
Methodist Medical Center of Illinois	Peoria	3%	56545
Midwestern Region Medical Center	Zion	3%	2219
Presence Covenant Medical Center	Urbana	3%	29333
Presence Mercy Medical Center	Aurora	3%	41265
Rockford Memorial Hospital	Rockford	3%	52600
Saint Anthony Medical Center	Rockford	3%	38266
Saint Elizabeth Hospital	Belleville	3%	17742
Saint Johns Hospital	Springfield	3%	55941
Saint Joseph Medical Center	Bloomington	3%	31023
Swedish American Hospital	Rockford	3%	64657
Advocate South Suburban Hospital	Hazel Crest	4%	46788
Loyola University Medical Center	Maywood	4%	48828
Memorial Medical Center	Springfield	4%	69792
Northwestern Memorial Hospital	Chicago	4%	88850
Norwegian - American Hospital	Chicago	4%	26589
Presence Saint Joseph Medical Center	Joliet	4%	74004
South Shore Hospital	Chicago	4%	14980
Swedish Covenant Hospital	Chicago	4%	49834
Touchette Regional Hospital	Centreville	4%	18798
University of Illinois Hospital	Chicago	4%	51565
Westlake Community Hospital	Melrose Park	4%	21558
Advocate Trinity Hospital	Chicago	5%	44936
Mercy Hospital & Medical Center	Chicago	5%	61812
Little Company of Mary Hospital	Evergreen Park	6%	48369
Loretto Hospital	Chicago	6%	15576
Roseland Community Hospital	Chicago	6%	27188
Rush University Medical Center	Chicago	6%	63360
Holy Cross Hospital	Chicago	7%	49182
Loyola Gottlieb Memorial Hospital	Melrose Park	7%	25040
John H Stroger Jr Hospital	Chicago	10%	140701
Provident Hospital of Chicago	Chicago	10%	36921
The University of Chicago Medical Center	Chicago	10%	78857
Saint Bernard Hospital	Chicago	12%	43452

Time from ER Arrival to Being Admitted (minutes)

Hospital Name	City	Min.	Cases
Harrisburg Medical Center[2]	Harrisburg	125	163
Shelby Memorial Hospital	Shelbyville	153	230
Illinois Valley Community Hospital[2]	Peru	171	330
Graham Hospital Association[2]	Canton	174	339
Saint Margarets Hospital[2]	Spring Valley	174	246
Saint Marys Hospital[2]	Streator	179	331
Pinckneyville Community Hospital[2]	Pinckneyville	180	188
Katherine Shaw Bethea Hospital[2]	Dixon	181	430
Crossroads Community Hospital[2]	Mount Vernon	185	463
Massac Memorial Hospital[2]	Metropolis	186	165
Saint James Hospital[2]	Pontiac	189	420
Fairfield Memorial Hospital[2]	Fairfield	191	160
OSF Holy Family Medical Center[2]	Monmouth	192	167
Proctor Hospital[2]	Peoria	192	507
Ottawa Reg Hosp & Healthcare Ctr[2]	Ottawa	193	351
McDonough District Hospital[2]	Macomb	194	328
Mason District Hospital[2,3]	Havana	195	79
Blessing Hospital[2]	Quincy	196	405
CGH Medical Center[2]	Sterling	198	650
Mercy Harvard Hospital	Harvard	200	281
Morris Hospital & Healthcare Centers[2]	Morris	200	582
Rush Oak Park Hospital[2]	Oak Park	201	699
Advocate Eureka Hospital	Eureka	205	181
Mendota Community Hospital[3]	Mendota	206	118
Taylorville Memorial Hospital[2]	Taylorville	209	335
Saint Anthonys Memorial Hospital[2]	Effingham	210	454
Saint Joseph's Hospital[2]	Breese	211	244
Presence Saint Joseph Hospital - Chicago[2]	Chicago	212	364
Saint Anthony's Health Center[2]	Alton	213	385
Gateway Regional Medical Center[2]	Granite City	216	1786
Abraham Lincoln Memorial Hospital[2]	Lincoln	218	290
Genesis Health System[2]	Silvis	218	459
Sarah Bush Lincoln Health Center[2]	Mattoon	218	598
Red Bud Regional Hospital[2]	Red Bud	219	460
Iroquois Memorial Hospital[2]	Watseka	220	313
Presence Resurrection Medical Center[2]	Chicago	220	755
Trinity Rock Island[2]	Rock Island	221	437
Galesburg Cottage Hospital[2]	Galesburg	223	335
Richland Memorial Hospital[2]	Olney	224	274
Valley West Community Hospital[2]	Sandwich	224	332
Greenville Regional Hospital	Greenville	228	381
Heartland Regional Medical Center[2]	Marion	228	587
Presence United Samaritans Medical Center[2]	Danville	228	706
Union County Hospital[2]	Anna	229	447
Evanston Hospital[2]	Evanston	232	394
Pekin Memorial Hospital[2]	Pekin	232	328
Fhn Memorial Hospital[2]	Freeport	233	424
Lake Forest Hospital[2]	Lake Forest	233	462
Sherman Hospital[2]	Elgin	234	531
Saint Joseph Memorial Hospital	Murphysboro	237	424
Central Dupage Hospital[2]	Winfield	238	412
Elmhurst Memorial Hospital[2]	Elmhurst	238	694
Saint Anthony Medical Center[2]	Rockford	238	632
Alton Memorial Hospital[2]	Alton	242	410
Methodist Hospital of Chicago[2]	Chicago	242	226
Presence Saint Marys Hospital[2]	Kankakee	242	715
Jersey Community Hospital[2]	Jerseyville	243	399
Silver Cross Hospital & Medical Centers[2]	New Lenox	243	425
Rockford Memorial Hospital[2]	Rockford	244	617
Alexian Brothers Medical Center[2]	Elk Grove Vlg	245	687
Saint Mary Medical Center[2]	Galesburg	245	359
Edward Hospital[2]	Naperville	246	499
Kishwaukee Community Hospital[2]	Dekalb	246	467
Northwest Community Hospital[2]	Arlington Hgts	248	538
Advocate Lutheran General Hospital[2]	Park Ridge	249	448
Centegra Health Sys-Woodstock Hosp[2]	Woodstock	249	535
Swedish American Hospital[2]	Rockford	249	564
Passavant Area Hospital[2]	Jacksonville	250	563
Adventist La Grange Memorial Hospital[2]	La Grange	251	701
Methodist Medical Center of Illinois[2]	Peoria	251	487
Adventist Glenoaks[2]	Glendale Hghts	252	289
Palos Community Hospital[2]	Palos Heights	252	688
Delnor Community Hospital[2]	Geneva	253	454
Anderson Hospital[2]	Maryville	254	477
Saint Joseph Medical Center[2]	Bloomington	254	401
Carle Foundation Hospital[2]	Urbana	255	549
Thorek Memorial Hospital[2]	Chicago	256	248
Saint Elizabeth Hospital[2]	Belleville	257	518
Louis A Weiss Memorial Hospital[2]	Chicago	258	775
Clay County Hospital[2]	Flora	259	569
Saint Marys Hospital[2]	Centralia	260	650
Hinsdale Hospital[2]	Hinsdale	261	450
Saint Alexius Medical Center[2]	Hoffman Estates	261	595
Adventist Bolingbrook Hospital[2]	Bolingbrook	263	557
Presence Saint Joseph Hospital - Elgin[2]	Elgin	264	667
Herrin Hospital[2]	Herrin	265	737
Presence Covenant Medical Center[2]	Urbana	265	527
Memorial Hospital of Carbondale[2]	Carbondale	266	367
Advocate Bromenn Medical Center[2]	Normal	267	479
Swedish Covenant Hospital[2]	Chicago	269	437
Copley Memorial Hospital[2]	Aurora	270	401
Presence Saint Francis Hospital[2]	Evanston	273	647
Riverside Medical Center[2]	Kankakee	274	532
Saint Marys Hospital[2]	Decatur	276	559
Vista Medical Center East[2]	Waukegan	276	778
Presence Our Lady of the Res Med Ctr[2]	Chicago	277	893
Advocate Condell Medical Center[2]	Libertyville	280	558
Saint Anthony Hospital[2]	Chicago	280	534
Decatur Memorial Hospital[2]	Decatur	281	519
Advocate Good Shepherd Hospital[2]	Barrington	283	511
West Suburban Medical Center[2]	Oak Park	284	633
Loyola Gottlieb Memorial Hospital[2]	Melrose Park	285	449
Little Company of Mary Hospital[2]	Evergreen Park	286	824
Saint Francis Medical Center[2]	Peoria	286	527
Ingalls Memorial Hospital[2]	Harvey	287	465
Advocate Good Samaritan Hospital[2]	Downers Grove	288	567
Presence Mercy Medical Center[2]	Aurora	288	702
Memorial Medical Center[2]	Springfield	290	537
Good Samaritan Regional Health Center[2]	Mount Vernon	292	471
Touchette Regional Hospital[2]	Centreville	292	197
Presence Saint Joseph Medical Center[2]	Joliet	294	566
Advocate Illinois Masonic Medical Center[2]	Chicago	295	522
Centegra Health Sys-Mc Henry Hosp[2]	Mchenry	295	616
Franciscan Saint James Health[2]	Olympia Fields	295	1532
Saint Johns Hospital[2]	Springfield	304	384
Memorial Hospital[2]	Belleville	307	798
Norwegian - American Hospital[2]	Chicago	309	302
Presence Sts Mary & Elizabeth Med Ctr[2]	Chicago	314	570
Metrosouth Medical Center[2]	Blue Island	316	606
Advocate South Suburban Hospital[2]	Hazel Crest	320	616
Jackson Park Hospital[2]	Chicago	331	180
Westlake Community Hospital[2]	Melrose Park	336	367
Northwestern Memorial Hospital[2]	Chicago	351	251
Rush University Medical Center[2]	Chicago	358	410
Advocate Christ Hospital & Medical Center[2]	Oak Lawn	360	599
Advocate Trinity Hospital[2]	Chicago	374	664
Macneal Hospital[2]	Berwyn	378	701
Loretto Hospital[2]	Chicago	385	351

NOTE: Hospital profiles are in alphabetical order by state, then city, then hospital within the city; Rankings exclude hospitals with less than 25 cases except for patient surveys which excludes hospitals with less than 100 cases; (a) 100-299 cases; (1) The number of cases/patients is too few to report; (2) Data submitted were based on a sample of cases/patients; (3) Results are based on a shorter time period than required; (4) Data suppressed by CMS for one or more quarters; (5) Results are not available for this reporting period; (6) Fewer than 100 patients completed the HCAHPS survey; (7) No cases met the criteria for this measure; (8) The lower limit of the confidence interval cannot be calculated if the number of observed infections equals zero; (9) No data are available from the state/territory for this reporting period; (10) The scores shown reflect fewer than 50 completed surveys; (11) There were discrepancies in the data collection process; (12) This measure does not apply to this hospital for this reporting period; (13) Results cannot be calculated for this reporting period; (14) The results for this state are combined with nearby states to protect confidentiality; Please refer to the User's Guide for a full explanation of data.

Loyola University Medical Center[2]	Maywood	385	388
South Shore Hospital[2]	Chicago	387	443
Mercy Hospital & Medical Center[2]	Chicago	389	603
University of Illinois Hospital[2]	Chicago	406	502
Mount Sinai Hospital Medical Center[2]	Chicago	426	539
Holy Cross Hospital[2]	Chicago	428	948
Saint Bernard Hospital[2]	Chicago	442	616
Roseland Community Hospital[2]	Chicago	480	460
The University of Chicago Medical Center[2]	Chicago	504	447
John H Stroger Jr Hospital[2]	Chicago	578	816
Provident Hospital of Chicago[2]	Chicago	647	513

Time from ER Arrival to Discharge (minutes)

Hospital Name	City	Min.	Cases
Illinois Valley Community Hospital	Peru	76	522
Harrisburg Medical Center	Harrisburg	80	293
Crossroads Community Hospital	Mount Vernon	83	404
Graham Hospital Association	Canton	85	362
Taylorville Memorial Hospital	Taylorville	85	343
Saint Marys Hospital	Streator	87	347
Iroquois Memorial Hospital	Watseka	88	379
Mercy Harvard Hospital	Harvard	90	389
Abraham Lincoln Memorial Hospital	Lincoln	91	356
McDonough District Hospital	Macomb	91	383
Ottawa Reg Hosp & Healthcare Ctr	Ottawa	92	416
Saint James Hospital	Pontiac	94	360
Jersey Community Hospital	Jerseyville	95	212
Carle Foundation Hospital	Urbana	96	344
Advocate Eureka Hospital	Eureka	97	343
Midwestern Region Medical Center	Zion	98	238
Shelby Memorial Hospital	Shelbyville	98	366
Red Bud Regional Hospital	Red Bud	100	365
Katherine Shaw Bethea Hospital	Dixon	101	343
Pekin Memorial Hospital	Pekin	101	354
Vista Medical Center West	Waukegan	101	335
Saint Margarets Hospital	Spring Valley	102	324
Greenville Regional Hospital	Greenville	103	331
Proctor Hospital	Peoria	104	470
Valley West Community Hospital	Sandwich	104	396
Saint Anthony's Health Center	Alton	106	342
Thorek Memorial Hospital	Chicago	107	311
Galesburg Cottage Hospital	Galesburg	108	374
Rush Oak Park Hospital	Oak Park	108	379
Saint Anthonys Memorial Hospital	Effingham	108	370
Morris Hospital & Healthcare Centers	Morris	109	407
Adventist Glenoaks	Glendale Hghts	110	342
Edward Hospital	Naperville	110	373
Vista Medical Center East	Waukegan	111	390
Presence Saint Joseph Hospital - Chicago	Chicago	112	368
Richland Memorial Hospital	Olney	114	372
Union County Hospital	Anna	114	333
Alton Memorial Hospital	Alton	115	774
Fairfield Memorial Hospital	Fairfield	115	692
OSF Holy Family Medical Center[3]	Monmouth	115	133
Presence Saint Marys Hospital	Kankakee	115	384
Trinity Rock Island	Rock Island	115	374
Gateway Regional Medical Center	Granite City	116	378
Heartland Regional Medical Center	Marion	116	369
Touchette Regional Hospital	Centreville	116	401
Ingalls Memorial Hospital	Harvey	118	360
Saint Joseph's Hospital	Breese	120	420
Presence Covenant Medical Center	Urbana	121	328
Fhn Memorial Hospital	Freeport	122	429
Riverside Medical Center	Kankakee	122	360
Sarah Bush Lincoln Health Center	Mattoon	123	311
Sherman Hospital	Elgin	123	408
Presence Resurrection Medical Center	Chicago	128	357
CGH Medical Center	Sterling	131	370
Saint Mary Medical Center	Galesburg	132	385
West Suburban Medical Center	Oak Park	133	355
Centegra Health Sys-Woodstock Hosp	Woodstock	134	391
Memorial Hospital of Carbondale	Carbondale	134	386
Passavant Area Hospital	Jacksonville	134	376
Anderson Hospital	Maryville	135	373
Elmhurst Memorial Hospital	Elmhurst	135	357
Metrosouth Medical Center	Blue Island	135	383
Kishwaukee Community Hospital	Dekalb	136	364
Lake Forest Hospital	Lake Forest	137	404
Genesis Health System	Silvis	138	374
Louis A Weiss Memorial Hospital	Chicago	139	333
Saint Marys Hospital	Centralia	139	356
Macneal Hospital	Berwyn	141	374
Saint Elizabeth Hospital	Belleville	142	374
Copley Memorial Hospital	Aurora	143	384
Presence Saint Francis Hospital	Evanston	143	362
Presence Saint Joseph Hospital - Elgin	Elgin	143	349
Presence Our Lady of the Res Med Ctr	Chicago	144	398
Silver Cross Hospital & Medical Centers	New Lenox	144	374
Swedish American Hospital	Rockford	146	391
Adventist Bolingbrook Hospital	Bolingbrook	148	337
Blessing Hospital	Quincy	148	346
Saint Johns Hospital	Springfield	149	382
Advocate Condell Medical Center	Libertyville	150	353
Decatur Memorial Hospital	Decatur	150	368
Hinsdale Hospital	Hinsdale	150	334
Norwegian - American Hospital	Chicago	150	360
Saint Anthony Medical Center	Rockford	150	361
Alexian Brothers Medical Center	Elk Grove Vlg	152	393
Delnor Community Hospital	Geneva	153	354
Central Dupage Hospital	Winfield	154	378
Presence Sts Mary & Elizabeth Med Ctr	Chicago	155	403
Presence United Samaritans Medical Center	Danville	155	345
Franciscan Saint James Health	Olympia Fields	156	687
Rockford Memorial Hospital	Rockford	156	753
Adventist La Grange Memorial Hospital	La Grange	157	340
Herrin Hospital	Herrin	157	368
Good Samaritan Regional Health Center	Mount Vernon	158	364
Memorial Hospital	Belleville	158	374
Saint Marys Hospital	Decatur	158	360
Advocate Bromenn Medical Center	Normal	159	382
Little Company of Mary Hospital	Evergreen Park	160	1391
Northwest Community Hospital	Arlington Hgts	160	371
Loyola University Medical Center	Maywood	161	308
Saint Anthony Hospital	Chicago	163	351
Advocate Good Samaritan Hospital	Downers Grove	164	376
Evanston Hospital	Evanston	164	750
Saint Joseph Medical Center	Bloomington	164	370
Loretto Hospital	Chicago	167	320
Palos Community Hospital	Palos Heights	167	332
Centegra Health Sys-Mc Henry Hosp	Mchenry	168	373
Saint Alexius Medical Center	Hoffman Estates	168	370
Westlake Community Hospital	Melrose Park	168	360
Advocate Good Shepherd Hospital	Barrington	169	385
Advocate South Suburban Hospital	Hazel Crest	169	367
Memorial Medical Center	Springfield	172	371
Methodist Hospital of Chicago	Chicago	178	226
Swedish Covenant Hospital	Chicago	178	410
Methodist Medical Center of Illinois	Peoria	179	351
Advocate Lutheran General Hospital	Park Ridge	180	384
Roseland Community Hospital	Chicago	180	417
Saint Francis Medical Center	Peoria	182	398
Advocate Trinity Hospital	Chicago	186	382
Presence Mercy Medical Center	Aurora	188	390
Presence Saint Joseph Medical Center	Joliet	190	370
Advocate Christ Hospital & Medical Center	Oak Lawn	195	383
Saint Bernard Hospital	Chicago	198	327
Advocate Illinois Masonic Medical Center	Chicago	200	346
Jackson Park Hospital	Chicago	201	49
Mercy Hospital & Medical Center	Chicago	201	333
Holy Cross Hospital	Chicago	214	311
Loyola Gottlieb Memorial Hospital	Melrose Park	219	294
Mount Sinai Hospital Medical Center	Chicago	220	318
University of Illinois Hospital	Chicago	220	384
South Shore Hospital	Chicago	224	236
Northwestern Memorial Hospital	Chicago	225	316
Provident Hospital of Chicago	Chicago	230	370
Rush University Medical Center	Chicago	239	336
The University of Chicago Medical Center	Chicago	259	359
John H Stroger Jr Hospital	Chicago	292	374

Time in ER Before Being Evaluated (minutes)

Hospital Name	City	Min.	Cases
Jackson Park Hospital	Chicago	0	400
Methodist Hospital of Chicago	Chicago	6	276
Presence Saint Joseph Hospital - Chicago	Chicago	8	406
Saint James Hospital	Pontiac	9	408
South Shore Hospital	Chicago	9	283
Edward Hospital	Naperville	10	387
Illinois Valley Community Hospital	Peru	10	544
Ingalls Memorial Hospital	Harvey	10	398
Memorial Hospital	Belleville	10	417
Vista Medical Center West	Waukegan	12	421
Iroquois Memorial Hospital	Watseka	13	420
Saint Anthony's Health Center	Alton	13	267
Graham Hospital Association	Canton	14	407
Presence Resurrection Medical Center	Chicago	14	213
Red Bud Regional Hospital	Red Bud	14	421
Saint Marys Hospital	Streator	14	402
Sarah Bush Lincoln Health Center	Mattoon	14	342
Advocate Eureka Hospital	Eureka	15	370
Crossroads Community Hospital	Mount Vernon	15	445
McDonough District Hospital	Macomb	15	423
OSF Holy Family Medical Center[3]	Monmouth	15	151
Saint Mary Medical Center	Galesburg	15	416
Norwegian - American Hospital	Chicago	16	436
Valley West Community Hospital	Sandwich	16	350
Adventist Glenoaks	Glendale Hghts	17	358
Gateway Regional Medical Center	Granite City	17	497
Shelby Memorial Hospital	Shelbyville	17	481
Vista Medical Center East	Waukegan	17	416
Abraham Lincoln Memorial Hospital	Lincoln	18	372
Carle Foundation Hospital	Urbana	18	254
Galesburg Cottage Hospital	Galesburg	18	417
Heartland Regional Medical Center	Marion	18	414
Presence Saint Joseph Hospital - Elgin	Elgin	18	399
Saint Joseph's Hospital	Breese	18	479
Saint Margarets Hospital	Spring Valley	18	316
Taylorville Memorial Hospital	Taylorville	18	276
Elmhurst Memorial Hospital	Elmhurst	19	397
Mercy Harvard Hospital	Harvard	19	448
Proctor Hospital	Peoria	19	474
Sherman Hospital	Elgin	19	442
Morris Hospital & Healthcare Centers	Morris	20	353
Presence Saint Francis Hospital	Evanston	20	209
Rush Oak Park Hospital	Oak Park	20	318
Saint Anthonys Memorial Hospital	Effingham	20	405
Methodist Medical Center of Illinois	Peoria	21	384
Metrosouth Medical Center	Blue Island	21	421
Ottawa Reg Hosp & Healthcare Ctr	Ottawa	21	446
Saint Anthony Medical Center	Rockford	21	402
Trinity Rock Island	Rock Island	21	380
Alexian Brothers Medical Center	Elk Grove Vlg	22	428
Jersey Community Hospital	Jerseyville	22	331
CGH Medical Center	Sterling	23	409
Fairfield Memorial Hospital	Fairfield	23	689
Saint Elizabeth Hospital	Belleville	23	418
Blessing Hospital	Quincy	24	305
Memorial Medical Center	Springfield	24	400
Pekin Memorial Hospital	Pekin	24	318
Union County Hospital	Anna	24	396
Adventist La Grange Memorial Hospital	La Grange	25	313
Mercy Hospital & Medical Center	Chicago	25	371
Richland Memorial Hospital	Olney	25	419
Saint Francis Medical Center	Peoria	25	437
Swedish American Hospital	Rockford	25	430
Saint Alexius Medical Center	Hoffman Estates	26	426
Saint Joseph Medical Center	Bloomington	26	405
Fhn Memorial Hospital	Freeport	27	476
Riverside Medical Center	Kankakee	27	392
Central Dupage Hospital	Winfield	28	328
Kishwaukee Community Hospital	Dekalb	28	407
Lake Forest Hospital	Lake Forest	28	350
Louis A Weiss Memorial Hospital	Chicago	28	401
Saint Johns Hospital	Springfield	28	402
Alton Memorial Hospital	Alton	29	785
Greenville Regional Hospital	Greenville	29	382
Memorial Hospital of Carbondale	Carbondale	29	443
Advocate Condell Medical Center	Libertyville	30	409
Genesis Health System	Silvis	30	403
Presence Covenant Medical Center	Urbana	30	398
Presence Saint Marys Hospital	Kankakee	30	405
Thorek Memorial Hospital	Chicago	30	320
Delnor Community Hospital	Geneva	31	352
Franciscan Saint James Health	Olympia Fields	31	745
Adventist Bolingbrook Hospital	Bolingbrook	32	268
Advocate Bromenn Medical Center	Normal	32	419
Northwest Community Hospital	Arlington Hgts	32	434
Hinsdale Hospital	Hinsdale	33	294
Presence United Samaritans Medical Center	Danville	33	408
Macneal Hospital	Berwyn	34	411
Presence Our Lady of the Res Med Ctr	Chicago	34	423
Herrin Hospital	Herrin	35	433
Passavant Area Hospital	Jacksonville	35	275
Advocate Good Samaritan Hospital	Downers Grove	36	396
Little Company of Mary Hospital	Evergreen Park	36	1208
Presence Mercy Medical Center	Aurora	36	399
Presence Saint Joseph Medical Center	Joliet	36	383
Presence Sts Mary & Elizabeth Med Ctr	Chicago	36	464
Saint Marys Hospital	Centralia	36	399
Copley Memorial Hospital	Aurora	37	402
West Suburban Medical Center	Oak Park	37	363
Centegra Health Sys-Woodstock Hosp	Woodstock	38	429
Decatur Memorial Hospital	Decatur	39	407
Harrisburg Medical Center	Harrisburg	39	361
Midwestern Region Medical Center	Zion	39	163
Anderson Hospital	Maryville	40	408
Good Samaritan Regional Health Center	Mount Vernon	41	395
Katherine Shaw Bethea Hospital	Dixon	41	347
Saint Bernard Hospital	Chicago	42	390
Advocate Lutheran General Hospital	Park Ridge	43	332
Centegra Health Sys-Mc Henry Hosp	Mchenry	45	405
Westlake Community Hospital	Melrose Park	47	400
Evanston Hospital	Evanston	48	860
Advocate Good Shepherd Hospital	Barrington	49	376
Advocate Illinois Masonic Medical Center	Chicago	49	387
Saint Marys Hospital	Decatur	50	404
Northwestern Memorial Hospital	Chicago	51	282
Palos Community Hospital	Palos Heights	52	398
Loyola University Medical Center	Maywood	53	356
Touchette Regional Hospital	Centreville	53	449
Loretto Hospital	Chicago	54	347
Silver Cross Hospital & Medical Centers	New Lenox	60	327
University of Illinois Hospital	Chicago	62	392

NOTE: Hospital profiles are in alphabetical order by state, then city, then hospital within the city; Rankings exclude hospitals with less than 25 cases except for patient surveys which excludes hospitals with less than 100 cases; (a) 100-299 cases; (1) The number of cases/patients is too few to report; (2) Data submitted were based on a sample of cases/patients; (3) Results are based on a shorter time period than required; (4) Data suppressed by CMS for one or more quarters; (5) Results are not available for this reporting period; (6) Fewer than 100 patients completed the HCAHPS survey; (7) No cases met the criteria for this measure; (8) The lower limit of the confidence interval cannot be calculated if the number of observed infections equals zero; (9) No data are available from the state/territory for this reporting period; (10) The scores shown reflect fewer than 50 completed surveys; (11) There were discrepancies in the data collection process; (12) This measure does not apply to this hospital for this reporting period; (13) Results cannot be calculated for this reporting period; (14) The results for this state are combined with nearby states to protect confidentiality; Please refer to the User's Guide for a full explanation of data.

Advocate South Suburban Hospital	Hazel Crest	64	387
Holy Cross Hospital	Chicago	65	354
Advocate Trinity Hospital	Chicago	66	409
Mount Sinai Hospital Medical Center	Chicago	66	349
Rockford Memorial Hospital	Rockford	67	761
Roseland Community Hospital	Chicago	75	434
Swedish Covenant Hospital	Chicago	75	494
The University of Chicago Medical Center	Chicago	79	335
Advocate Christ Hospital & Medical Center	Oak Lawn	81	255
Loyola Gottlieb Memorial Hospital	Melrose Park	85	170
Saint Anthony Hospital	Chicago	86	370
Rush University Medical Center	Chicago	107	331
Provident Hospital of Chicago	Chicago	109	417
John H Stroger Jr Hospital	Chicago	153	379

Time to Pain Meds for Bone Fractures (minutes)

Hospital Name	City	Min.	Cases
Advocate Christ Hospital & Medical Center	Oak Lawn	19	294
Northwest Community Hospital	Arlington Hgts	23	219
Shelby Memorial Hospital	Shelbyville	24	30
Iroquois Memorial Hospital	Watseka	25	25
Abraham Lincoln Memorial Hospital	Lincoln	26	80
Edward Hospital	Naperville	26	346
The University of Chicago Medical Center	Chicago	27	133
Valley West Community Hospital	Sandwich	28	65
Proctor Hospital	Peoria	29	69
Saint James Hospital	Pontiac	29	66
Graham Hospital Association	Canton	30	62
Saint Margarets Hospital	Spring Valley	30	36
Alexian Brothers Medical Center	Elk Grove Vlg	31	171
McDonough District Hospital	Macomb	31	73
Sarah Bush Lincoln Health Center	Mattoon	31	117
Crossroads Community Hospital	Mount Vernon	32	35
Saint Joseph's Hospital	Breese	32	36
Ottawa Reg Hosp & Healthcare Ctr	Ottawa	33	75
Advocate Condell Medical Center	Libertyville	36	221
CGH Medical Center	Sterling	36	89
Saint Alexius Medical Center	Hoffman Estates	36	200
Taylorville Memorial Hospital	Taylorville	36	45
Central Dupage Hospital	Winfield	37	264
Memorial Hospital	Belleville	37	229
Ingalls Memorial Hospital	Harvey	38	183
Riverside Medical Center	Kankakee	38	137
Westlake Community Hospital	Melrose Park	38	46
Pekin Memorial Hospital	Pekin	39	112
Saint Anthony's Health Center	Alton	40	48
Thorek Memorial Hospital	Chicago	40	27
Galesburg Cottage Hospital	Galesburg	41	60
Lake Forest Hospital	Lake Forest	41	189
Trinity Rock Island	Rock Island	41	188
Adventist Glenoaks	Glendale Hghts	42	76
Red Bud Regional Hospital	Red Bud	42	34
Vista Medical Center East	Waukegan	42	194
Macneal Hospital	Berwyn	43	180
Adventist Bolingbrook Hospital	Bolingbrook	44	111
Alton Memorial Hospital	Alton	44	129
Elmhurst Memorial Hospital	Elmhurst	44	152
Norwegian - American Hospital[3]	Chicago	44	47
Sherman Hospital	Elgin	44	300
Delnor Community Hospital	Geneva	45	164
Presence Our Lady of the Res Med Ctr	Chicago	45	151
Rush Oak Park Hospital	Oak Park	46	76
Greenville Regional Hospital	Greenville	47	33
Saint Anthony Hospital	Chicago	47	179
Saint Marys Hospital	Streator	47	41
Fairfield Memorial Hospital	Fairfield	48	53
Genesis Health System	Silvis	48	88
Morris Hospital & Healthcare Centers	Morris	48	164
Passavant Area Hospital	Jacksonville	48	112
Presence Resurrection Medical Center	Chicago	48	291
Saint Anthonys Memorial Hospital	Effingham	48	108
Katherine Shaw Bethea Hospital	Dixon	49	44
Kishwaukee Community Hospital	Dekalb	49	90
Blessing Hospital	Quincy	50	105
Centegra Health Sys-Woodstock Hosp	Woodstock	50	88
Copley Memorial Hospital	Aurora	50	299
Illini Community Hospital[3]	Pittsfield	50	26
Jersey Community Hospital	Jerseyville	50	71
Louis A Weiss Memorial Hospital	Chicago	50	56
Presence Saint Joseph Hospital - Chicago	Chicago	50	38
Presence Saint Joseph Medical Center	Joliet	50	173
Methodist Medical Center of Illinois	Peoria	51	68
Saint Marys Hospital	Centralia	51	85
Illinois Valley Community Hospital	Peru	52	61
Presence Saint Marys Hospital	Kankakee	52	98
Clay County Hospital	Flora	53	32
Memorial Hospital of Carbondale	Carbondale	53	96
Adventist La Grange Memorial Hospital	La Grange	54	88
Advocate Illinois Masonic Medical Center	Chicago	54	118
Harrisburg Medical Center	Harrisburg	54	59
Advocate Good Samaritan Hospital	Downers Grove	56	137
Evanston Hospital	Evanston	56	228
Franciscan Saint James Health	Olympia Fields	56	164
Hinsdale Hospital	Hinsdale	56	131
Mercy Hospital & Medical Center	Chicago	56	69
Saint Mary Medical Center	Galesburg	56	50
West Suburban Medical Center	Oak Park	56	69
Presence Saint Joseph Hospital - Elgin	Elgin	57	95
Advocate Lutheran General Hospital	Park Ridge	58	224
Anderson Hospital	Maryville	58	190
Carle Foundation Hospital	Urbana	58	154
Fhn Memorial Hospital	Freeport	58	70
Richland Memorial Hospital	Olney	58	33
Swedish American Hospital	Rockford	58	249
Metrosouth Medical Center	Blue Island	59	193
Saint Joseph Medical Center	Bloomington	59	95
Herrin Hospital	Herrin	61	73
Presence Covenant Medical Center	Urbana	61	68
Northwestern Memorial Hospital	Chicago	62	90
Saint Anthony Medical Center	Rockford	62	174
Advocate Good Shepherd Hospital	Barrington	63	131
Gateway Regional Medical Center	Granite City	63	80
Heartland Regional Medical Center	Marion	63	65
Presence Sts Mary & Elizabeth Med Ctr	Chicago	63	285
Saint Francis Medical Center	Peoria	63	138
Presence Mercy Medical Center	Aurora	64	164
Silver Cross Hospital & Medical Centers	New Lenox	64	270
Good Samaritan Regional Health Center	Mount Vernon	65	116
Saint Bernard Hospital	Chicago	65	26
Advocate Bromenn Medical Center	Normal	66	112
Advocate South Suburban Hospital	Hazel Crest	67	71
Union County Hospital	Anna	67	43
Touchette Regional Hospital	Centreville	68	28
Presence Saint Francis Hospital	Evanston	70	127
Rockford Memorial Hospital	Rockford	70	128
Decatur Memorial Hospital	Decatur	72	187
Memorial Medical Center	Springfield	72	234
Presence United Samaritans Medical Center	Danville	72	129
Palos Community Hospital	Palos Heights	74	187
Holy Cross Hospital	Chicago	75	103
Centegra Health Sys-Mc Henry Hosp	Mchenry	78	143
Saint Elizabeth Hospital	Belleville	78	116
Saint Marys Hospital	Decatur	78	81
Saint Johns Hospital	Springfield	79	211
Swedish Covenant Hospital	Chicago	80	252
Little Company of Mary Hospital	Evergreen Park	83	71
Loyola Gottlieb Memorial Hospital	Melrose Park	85	81
Loyola University Medical Center	Maywood	88	101
Mount Sinai Hospital Medical Center	Chicago	89	137
University of Illinois Hospital	Chicago	90	76
Rush University Medical Center	Chicago	92	104
Advocate Trinity Hospital	Chicago	114	108
Provident Hospital of Chicago	Chicago	126	45
John H Stroger Jr Hospital	Chicago	171	331

Heart Attack Care

Aspirin Given at Discharge

Hospital Name	City	Rate	Cases
Adventist Bolingbrook Hospital	Bolingbrook	100%	74
Adventist Glenoaks[2]	Glendale Hghts	100%	42
Adventist La Grange Memorial Hospital	La Grange	100%	77
Advocate Bromenn Medical Center	Normal	100%	135
Advocate Christ Hospital & Medical Center[2]	Oak Lawn	100%	304
Advocate Condell Medical Center	Libertyville	100%	323
Advocate Good Samaritan Hospital	Downers Grove	100%	209
Advocate Good Shepherd Hospital	Barrington	100%	202
Advocate Illinois Masonic Medical Center	Chicago	100%	156
Advocate Lutheran General Hospital	Park Ridge	100%	243
Advocate South Suburban Hospital[2]	Hazel Crest	100%	183
Advocate Trinity Hospital	Chicago	100%	119
Alexian Brothers Medical Center	Elk Grove Vlg	100%	242
Blessing Hospital	Quincy	100%	235
Central Dupage Hospital	Winfield	100%	191
Decatur Memorial Hospital	Decatur	100%	124
Edward Hospital	Naperville	100%	233
Elmhurst Memorial Hospital	Elmhurst	100%	195
Evanston Hospital	Evanston	100%	428
Fhn Memorial Hospital	Freeport	100%	29
Gateway Regional Medical Center	Granite City	100%	110
Genesis Health System	Silvis	100%	109
Good Samaritan Regional Health Center	Mount Vernon	100%	275
Heartland Regional Medical Center	Marion	100%	85
Hines VA Medical Center	Hines	100%	63
Hinsdale Hospital	Hinsdale	100%	97
Ingalls Memorial Hospital[2]	Harvey	100%	248
Katherine Shaw Bethea Hospital	Dixon	100%	49
Kishwaukee Community Hospital	Dekalb	100%	65
Lake Forest Hospital	Lake Forest	100%	51
Little Company of Mary Hospital	Evergreen Park	100%	94
Louis A Weiss Memorial Hospital	Chicago	100%	98
Loyola University Medical Center	Maywood	100%	224
Macneal Hospital	Berwyn	100%	228
Memorial Hospital of Carbondale	Carbondale	100%	447
Memorial Medical Center[2]	Springfield	100%	301
Methodist Medical Center of Illinois	Peoria	100%	216
Mount Sinai Hospital Medical Center	Chicago	100%	118
Northwest Community Hospital[2]	Arlington Hgts	100%	312
Northwestern Memorial Hospital	Chicago	100%	258
Palos Community Hospital[2]	Palos Heights	100%	264
Presence Our Lady of the Res Med Ctr	Chicago	100%	150
Presence Resurrection Medical Center	Chicago	100%	331
Presence Saint Joseph Hospital - Chicago	Chicago	100%	82
Presence Saint Marys Hospital	Kankakee	100%	36
Presence Sts Mary & Elizabeth Med Ctr	Chicago	100%	147
Riverside Medical Center	Kankakee	100%	128
Rockford Memorial Hospital	Rockford	100%	243
Saint Alexius Medical Center	Hoffman Estates	100%	147
Saint Anthony's Health Center	Alton	100%	80
Saint Elizabeth Hospital	Belleville	100%	278
Saint Johns Hospital	Springfield	100%	647
Saint Marys Hospital	Centralia	100%	33
Saint Marys Hospital	Decatur	100%	158
Sarah Bush Lincoln Health Center	Mattoon	100%	46
Sherman Hospital	Elgin	100%	222
Swedish American Hospital	Rockford	100%	249
The University of Chicago Medical Center	Chicago	100%	159
Vista Medical Center East	Waukegan	100%	127
Alton Memorial Hospital	Alton	99%	79
Anderson Hospital	Maryville	99%	105
Centegra Health Sys-Mc Henry Hosp	Mchenry	99%	310
Delnor Community Hospital	Geneva	99%	86
Franciscan Saint James Health	Olympia Fields	99%	250
John H Stroger Jr Hospital[2]	Chicago	99%	188
Memorial Hospital	Belleville	99%	316
Metrosouth Medical Center	Blue Island	99%	126
Presence Covenant Medical Center	Urbana	99%	186
Presence Mercy Medical Center	Aurora	99%	140
Presence Saint Francis Hospital	Evanston	99%	123
Presence Saint Joseph Medical Center[2]	Joliet	99%	293
Rush University Medical Center	Chicago	99%	167
Saint Anthony Medical Center	Rockford	99%	268
Saint Francis Medical Center	Peoria	99%	665
Silver Cross Hospital & Medical Centers	New Lenox	99%	254
Swedish Covenant Hospital	Chicago	99%	224
West Suburban Medical Center	Oak Park	99%	112
Carle Foundation Hospital[2]	Urbana	98%	304
Copley Memorial Hospital	Aurora	98%	149
Holy Cross Hospital[2]	Chicago	98%	53
Jesse Brown VA Med Ctr-VA Chicago	Chicago	98%	65
Loyola Gottlieb Memorial Hospital	Melrose Park	98%	136
Morris Hospital & Healthcare Centers	Morris	98%	57
Presence Saint Joseph Hospital - Elgin	Elgin	98%	85
Proctor Hospital	Peoria	98%	87
Saint Joseph Medical Center	Bloomington	98%	180
Trinity Rock Island	Rock Island	98%	508
CGH Medical Center	Sterling	97%	59
Mercy Hospital & Medical Center	Chicago	97%	219
University of Illinois Hospital	Chicago	96%	112
Westlake Community Hospital	Melrose Park	96%	48
Rush Oak Park Hospital	Oak Park	95%	44
Presence United Samaritans Medical Center	Danville	94%	32
Norwegian - American Hospital	Chicago	88%	26

PCI Within 90 Minutes of Arrival

Hospital Name	City	Rate	Cases
Advocate Bromenn Medical Center	Normal	100%	33
Advocate Christ Hospital & Medical Center[2]	Oak Lawn	100%	32
Advocate Condell Medical Center	Libertyville	100%	50
Advocate Good Shepherd Hospital	Barrington	100%	27
Alexian Brothers Medical Center	Elk Grove Vlg	100%	58
Carle Foundation Hospital[2]	Urbana	100%	25
Central Dupage Hospital	Winfield	100%	61
Copley Memorial Hospital	Aurora	100%	30
Edward Hospital	Naperville	100%	46
Franciscan Saint James Health	Olympia Fields	100%	32
Memorial Hospital of Carbondale	Carbondale	100%	34
Methodist Medical Center of Illinois	Peoria	100%	26
Northwest Community Hospital[2]	Arlington Hgts	100%	76
Northwestern Memorial Hospital	Chicago	100%	57
Presence Resurrection Medical Center	Chicago	100%	65
Rockford Memorial Hospital	Rockford	100%	32
Saint Alexius Medical Center	Hoffman Estates	100%	39
Saint Elizabeth Hospital	Belleville	100%	32
Saint Francis Medical Center	Peoria	100%	79
Saint Johns Hospital	Springfield	100%	47
Silver Cross Hospital & Medical Centers	New Lenox	100%	55
Trinity Rock Island	Rock Island	100%	32
The University of Chicago Medical Center	Chicago	100%	31
Vista Medical Center East	Waukegan	100%	31
Evanston Hospital	Evanston	99%	79
Blessing Hospital	Quincy	98%	50

NOTE: Hospital profiles are in alphabetical order by state, then city, then hospital within the city; Rankings exclude hospitals with less than 25 cases except for patient surveys which excludes hospitals with less than 100 cases; (a) 100-299 cases; (1) The number of cases/patients is too few to report; (2) Data submitted were based on a sample of cases/patients; (3) Results are based on a shorter time period than required; (4) Data suppressed by CMS for one or more quarters; (5) Results are not available for this reporting period; (6) Fewer than 100 patients completed the HCAHPS survey; (7) No cases met the criteria for this measure; (8) The lower limit of the confidence interval cannot be calculated if the number of observed infections equals zero; (9) No data are available from the state/territory for this reporting period; (10) The scores shown reflect fewer than 50 completed surveys; (11) There were discrepancies in the data collection process; (12) This measure does not apply to this hospital for this reporting period; (13) Results cannot be calculated for this reporting period; (14) The results for this state are combined with nearby states to protect confidentiality; Please refer to the User's Guide for a full explanation of data.

Hospital Name	City	Rate	Cases
Elmhurst Memorial Hospital	Elmhurst	98%	45
Presence Saint Joseph Medical Center[2]	Joliet	98%	47
Saint Anthony Medical Center	Rockford	98%	42
Sherman Hospital	Elgin	98%	57
Adventist Bolingbrook Hospital	Bolingbrook	96%	25
Advocate Good Samaritan Hospital	Downers Grove	96%	57
Advocate Lutheran General Hospital	Park Ridge	96%	55
Genesis Health System	Silvis	96%	26
Memorial Hospital	Belleville	96%	28
Swedish American Hospital	Rockford	96%	51
Macneal Hospital	Berwyn	95%	61
Saint Joseph Medical Center	Bloomington	95%	43
Centegra Health Sys-Mc Henry Hosp	Mchenry	94%	51
Palos Community Hospital[2]	Palos Heights	94%	69
Delnor Community Hospital	Geneva	93%	30
Presence Sts Mary & Elizabeth Med Ctr	Chicago	93%	29
Anderson Hospital	Maryville	91%	33
Memorial Medical Center[2]	Springfield	90%	29
Swedish Covenant Hospital	Chicago	84%	32
Mercy Hospital & Medical Center	Chicago	81%	31

Statin Prescribed at Discharge

Hospital Name	City	Rate	Cases
Adventist Bolingbrook Hospital	Bolingbrook	100%	73
Adventist La Grange Memorial Hospital	La Grange	100%	77
Advocate Christ Hospital & Medical Center[2]	Oak Lawn	100%	290
Advocate Condell Medical Center	Libertyville	100%	302
Advocate Good Samaritan Hospital	Downers Grove	100%	201
Advocate Good Shepherd Hospital	Barrington	100%	194
Advocate Illinois Masonic Medical Center	Chicago	100%	155
Advocate Lutheran General Hospital	Park Ridge	100%	240
Advocate South Suburban Hospital[2]	Hazel Crest	100%	185
Alexian Brothers Medical Center	Elk Grove Vlg	100%	236
Alton Memorial Hospital	Alton	100%	80
Copley Memorial Hospital	Aurora	100%	147
Decatur Memorial Hospital	Decatur	100%	132
Elmhurst Memorial Hospital	Elmhurst	100%	191
Fhn Memorial Hospital	Freeport	100%	30
Gateway Regional Medical Center	Granite City	100%	98
Genesis Health System	Silvis	100%	102
Good Samaritan Regional Health Center	Mount Vernon	100%	254
Ingalls Memorial Hospital[2]	Harvey	100%	222
Kishwaukee Community Hospital	Dekalb	100%	57
Lake Forest Hospital	Lake Forest	100%	50
Little Company of Mary Hospital	Evergreen Park	100%	93
Loyola University Medical Center	Maywood	100%	231
Macneal Hospital	Berwyn	100%	225
Memorial Hospital of Carbondale	Carbondale	100%	434
Mount Sinai Hospital Medical Center	Chicago	100%	108
Northwest Community Hospital[2]	Arlington Hgts	100%	302
Northwestern Memorial Hospital	Chicago	100%	254
Palos Community Hospital[2]	Palos Heights	100%	266
Presence Covenant Medical Center	Urbana	100%	186
Presence Saint Marys Hospital	Kankakee	100%	36
Presence Sts Mary & Elizabeth Med Ctr	Chicago	100%	141
Riverside Medical Center	Kankakee	100%	121
Rush Oak Park Hospital	Oak Park	100%	39
Saint Anthony's Health Center	Alton	100%	66
Saint Elizabeth Hospital	Belleville	100%	268
Saint Francis Medical Center	Peoria	100%	644
Sarah Bush Lincoln Health Center	Mattoon	100%	46
Sherman Hospital	Elgin	100%	214
Swedish American Hospital	Rockford	100%	245
The University of Chicago Medical Center	Chicago	100%	148
Vista Medical Center East	Waukegan	100%	132
Advocate Bromenn Medical Center	Normal	99%	130
Advocate Trinity Hospital	Chicago	99%	123
Carle Foundation Hospital[2]	Urbana	99%	296
Centegra Health Sys-Mc Henry Hosp	Mchenry	99%	295
Central Dupage Hospital	Winfield	99%	187
Delnor Community Hospital	Geneva	99%	84
Evanston Hospital	Evanston	99%	425
John H Stroger Jr Hospital[2]	Chicago	99%	188
Louis A Weiss Memorial Hospital	Chicago	99%	100
Presence Our Lady of the Res Med Ctr	Chicago	99%	146
Presence Resurrection Medical Center	Chicago	99%	330
Presence Saint Joseph Hospital - Chicago	Chicago	99%	74
Presence Saint Joseph Hospital - Elgin	Elgin	99%	84
Rockford Memorial Hospital	Rockford	99%	242
Rush University Medical Center	Chicago	99%	163
Saint Alexius Medical Center	Hoffman Estates	99%	145
Saint Johns Hospital	Springfield	99%	631
Swedish Covenant Hospital	Chicago	99%	222
West Suburban Medical Center	Oak Park	99%	106
Blessing Hospital	Quincy	98%	215
Edward Hospital	Naperville	98%	218
Franciscan Saint James Health	Olympia Fields	98%	249
Heartland Regional Medical Center	Marion	98%	82
Hines VA Medical Center	Hines	98%	65
Hinsdale Hospital	Hinsdale	98%	97
Katherine Shaw Bethea Hospital	Dixon	98%	47
Memorial Medical Center[2]	Springfield	98%	291
Mercy Hospital & Medical Center	Chicago	98%	220
Methodist Medical Center of Illinois	Peoria	98%	199
Morris Hospital & Healthcare Centers	Morris	98%	51
Presence Mercy Medical Center	Aurora	98%	140
Presence Saint Joseph Medical Center[2]	Joliet	98%	265
Saint Anthony Medical Center	Rockford	98%	253
Saint Joseph Medical Center	Bloomington	98%	177
Westlake Community Hospital	Melrose Park	98%	47
Adventist Glenoaks[2]	Glendale Hghts	97%	39
Jesse Brown VA Med Ctr-VA Chicago	Chicago	97%	63
Loyola Gottlieb Memorial Hospital	Melrose Park	97%	136
Saint Marys Hospital	Decatur	97%	145
Silver Cross Hospital & Medical Centers	New Lenox	97%	237
CGH Medical Center	Sterling	96%	57
Memorial Hospital	Belleville	96%	289
Proctor Hospital	Peoria	96%	81
Metrosouth Medical Center	Blue Island	94%	120
Presence Saint Francis Hospital	Evanston	94%	123
University of Illinois Hospital	Chicago	94%	112
Anderson Hospital	Maryville	93%	106
Saint Marys Hospital	Centralia	93%	29
Presence United Samaritans Medical Center	Danville	92%	38
Trinity Rock Island	Rock Island	90%	477
Holy Cross Hospital[2]	Chicago	89%	53

Heart Failure Care

ACE Inhibitor or ARB for LVSD

Hospital Name	City	Rate	Cases
Adventist Bolingbrook Hospital	Bolingbrook	100%	45
Adventist La Grange Memorial Hospital	La Grange	100%	61
Advocate Christ Hospital & Medical Center[2]	Oak Lawn	100%	106
Advocate Condell Medical Center[2]	Libertyville	100%	86
Advocate Good Samaritan Hospital[2]	Downers Grove	100%	105
Advocate Good Shepherd Hospital	Barrington	100%	45
Advocate Illinois Masonic Medical Center[2]	Chicago	100%	95
Advocate Lutheran General Hospital[2]	Park Ridge	100%	77
Advocate South Suburban Hospital[2]	Hazel Crest	100%	128
Alexian Brothers Medical Center	Elk Grove Vlg	100%	92
Blessing Hospital	Quincy	100%	70
Centegra Health Sys-Mc Henry Hosp	Mchenry	100%	82
Decatur Memorial Hospital	Decatur	100%	71
Elmhurst Memorial Hospital[2]	Elmhurst	100%	92
Fhn Memorial Hospital	Freeport	100%	48
Gateway Regional Medical Center	Granite City	100%	40
Genesis Health System	Silvis	100%	44
Good Samaritan Regional Health Center	Mount Vernon	100%	53
Heartland Regional Medical Center	Marion	100%	38
Herrin Hospital	Herrin	100%	25
Hinsdale Hospital	Hinsdale	100%	39
Illinois Valley Community Hospital[2]	Peru	100%	31
Ingalls Memorial Hospital[2]	Harvey	100%	107
John H Stroger Jr Hospital[2]	Chicago	100%	156
Kishwaukee Community Hospital	Dekalb	100%	40
Lake Forest Hospital	Lake Forest	100%	43
Louis A Weiss Memorial Hospital	Chicago	100%	64
Loyola University Medical Center	Maywood	100%	212
Macneal Hospital	Berwyn	100%	97
Memorial Hospital of Carbondale	Carbondale	100%	67
North Chicago VA Medical Center	North Chicago	100%	32
Northwest Community Hospital[2]	Arlington Hgts	100%	36
Northwestern Memorial Hospital	Chicago	100%	282
Palos Community Hospital[2]	Palos Heights	100%	54
Presence Covenant Medical Center	Urbana	100%	59
Presence Our Lady of the Res Med Ctr	Chicago	100%	82
Presence Saint Joseph Medical Center[2]	Joliet	100%	85
Presence Sts Mary & Elizabeth Med Ctr	Chicago	100%	100
Proctor Hospital	Peoria	100%	38
Riverside Medical Center	Kankakee	100%	105
Saint Alexius Medical Center	Hoffman Estates	100%	73
Saint Anthony Hospital	Chicago	100%	43
Saint Anthonys Memorial Hospital	Effingham	100%	41
Saint Mary Medical Center	Galesburg	100%	46
Saint Marys Hospital	Centralia	100%	29
Saint Marys Hospital	Decatur	100%	56
Sarah Bush Lincoln Health Center	Mattoon	100%	58
Swedish Covenant Hospital	Chicago	100%	130
Vista Medical Center East	Waukegan	100%	141
Alton Memorial Hospital[2]	Alton	99%	68
Central Dupage Hospital	Winfield	99%	111
Hines VA Medical Center	Hines	99%	127
Jackson Park Hospital	Chicago	99%	95
Jesse Brown VA Med Ctr-VA Chicago	Chicago	99%	154
Metrosouth Medical Center	Blue Island	99%	153
Presence United Samaritans Medical Center	Danville	99%	87
Provident Hospital of Chicago[2]	Chicago	99%	86
Rush Oak Park Hospital	Oak Park	99%	79
Saint Elizabeth Hospital	Belleville	99%	88
Saint Francis Medical Center	Peoria	99%	182
Saint Johns Hospital[2]	Springfield	99%	88
Sherman Hospital	Elgin	99%	93
Silver Cross Hospital & Medical Centers	New Lenox	99%	140
Advocate Bromenn Medical Center	Normal	98%	62
Carle Foundation Hospital[2]	Urbana	98%	123
Edward Hospital[2]	Naperville	98%	141
Loyola Gottlieb Memorial Hospital	Melrose Park	98%	64
Mount Sinai Hospital Medical Center	Chicago	98%	183
Presence Saint Joseph Hospital - Chicago	Chicago	98%	49
Presence Saint Marys Hospital	Kankakee	98%	52
Rush University Medical Center[2]	Chicago	98%	138
West Suburban Medical Center	Oak Park	98%	160
Advocate Trinity Hospital[2]	Chicago	97%	146
Evanston Hospital[2]	Evanston	97%	115
Katherine Shaw Bethea Hospital	Dixon	97%	30
Little Company of Mary Hospital[2]	Evergreen Park	97%	104
Memorial Hospital	Belleville	97%	220
Memorial Medical Center[2]	Springfield	97%	87
Presence Resurrection Medical Center	Chicago	97%	116
Saint Joseph Medical Center	Bloomington	97%	59
Swedish American Hospital	Rockford	97%	142
The University of Chicago Medical Center[2]	Chicago	97%	133
Copley Memorial Hospital	Aurora	96%	55
Galesburg Cottage Hospital	Galesburg	96%	25
Methodist Medical Center of Illinois	Peoria	96%	105
Rockford Memorial Hospital	Rockford	96%	85
Saint Anthony Medical Center	Rockford	96%	101
University of Illinois Hospital[2]	Chicago	96%	140
Presence Mercy Medical Center	Aurora	95%	44
Presence Saint Francis Hospital	Evanston	95%	73
Delnor Community Hospital	Geneva	94%	49
Franciscan Saint James Health[2]	Olympia Fields	94%	202
Holy Cross Hospital[2]	Chicago	94%	142
Saint Bernard Hospital	Chicago	94%	101
Touchette Regional Hospital	Centreville	94%	35
Norwegian - American Hospital	Chicago	93%	43
Trinity Rock Island[2]	Rock Island	93%	81
Anderson Hospital[2]	Maryville	92%	72
Mercy Hospital & Medical Center[2]	Chicago	92%	144
Roseland Community Hospital[2]	Chicago	92%	39
Pekin Memorial Hospital	Pekin	90%	31
CGH Medical Center	Sterling	89%	55
Presence Saint Joseph Hospital - Elgin	Elgin	88%	25
Richland Memorial Hospital[2]	Olney	88%	25
South Shore Hospital	Chicago	85%	54
Westlake Community Hospital	Melrose Park	85%	53
Loretto Hospital	Chicago	82%	33

Discharge Instructions Given

Hospital Name	City	Rate	Cases
Abraham Lincoln Memorial Hospital	Lincoln	100%	28
Advocate Good Samaritan Hospital[2]	Downers Grove	100%	221
Advocate Good Shepherd Hospital	Barrington	100%	203
Advocate Illinois Masonic Medical Center[2]	Chicago	100%	193
Advocate Lutheran General Hospital[2]	Park Ridge	100%	246
Carle Foundation Hospital[2]	Urbana	100%	216
Central Dupage Hospital	Winfield	100%	418
CGH Medical Center	Sterling	100%	163
Clay County Hospital	Flora	100%	32
Decatur Memorial Hospital	Decatur	100%	200
Elmhurst Memorial Hospital[2]	Elmhurst	100%	235
Fayette County Hospital	Vandalia	100%	32
Gateway Regional Medical Center	Granite City	100%	133
Harrisburg Medical Center	Harrisburg	100%	32
Hines VA Medical Center	Hines	100%	272
Ingalls Memorial Hospital[2]	Harvey	100%	253
Jesse Brown VA Med Ctr-VA Chicago	Chicago	100%	362
Kewanee Hospital[2]	Kewanee	100%	26
Loyola University Medical Center	Maywood	100%	435
Metrosouth Medical Center	Blue Island	100%	369
Mount Sinai Hospital Medical Center	Chicago	100%	272
Perry Memorial Hospital	Princeton	100%	37
Presence Our Lady of the Res Med Ctr	Chicago	100%	195
Presence Resurrection Medical Center	Chicago	100%	387
Presence Saint Francis Hospital	Evanston	100%	165
Presence Saint Joseph Hospital - Chicago	Chicago	100%	202
Presence Sts Mary & Elizabeth Med Ctr	Chicago	100%	199
Rush University Medical Center[2]	Chicago	100%	262
Saint Anthony Hospital	Chicago	100%	93
Saint Anthony Medical Center	Rockford	100%	281
Saint Anthony's Health Center	Alton	100%	120
Saint James Hospital	Pontiac	100%	37
Saint Joseph Medical Center	Bloomington	100%	153
Saint Joseph's Hospital	Breese	100%	25
Saint Mary Medical Center	Galesburg	100%	92
Saint Marys Hospital	Centralia	100%	110
Sarah Bush Lincoln Health Center	Mattoon	100%	174
South Shore Hospital	Chicago	100%	113
Swedish Covenant Hospital	Chicago	100%	315
Valley West Community Hospital	Sandwich	100%	26
Vista Medical Center East	Waukegan	100%	286

NOTE: Hospital profiles are in alphabetical order by state, then city, then hospital within the city; Rankings exclude hospitals with less than 25 cases except for patient surveys which excludes hospitals with less than 100 cases; (a) 100-299 cases; (1) The number of cases/patients is too few to report; (2) Data submitted were based on a sample of cases/patients; (3) Results are based on a shorter time period than required; (4) Data suppressed by CMS for one or more quarters; (5) Results are not available for this reporting period; (6) Fewer than 100 patients completed the HCAHPS survey; (7) No cases met the criteria for this measure; (8) The lower limit of the confidence interval cannot be calculated if the number of observed infections equals zero; (9) No data are available from the state/territory for this reporting period; (10) The scores shown reflect fewer than 50 completed surveys; (11) There were discrepancies in the data collection process; (12) This measure does not apply to this hospital for this reporting period; (13) Results cannot be calculated for this reporting period; (14) The results for this state are combined with nearby states to protect confidentiality; Please refer to the User's Guide for a full explanation of data.

Adventist La Grange Memorial Hospital	La Grange	99%	194
Alexian Brothers Medical Center	Elk Grove Vlg	99%	344
Alton Memorial Hospital[2]	Alton	99%	183
Evanston Hospital[2]	Evanston	99%	346
Genesis Health System	Silvis	99%	94
Good Samaritan Regional Health Center	Mount Vernon	99%	158
Jackson Park Hospital	Chicago	99%	143
Kishwaukee Community Hospital	Dekalb	99%	93
Loretto Hospital	Chicago	99%	72
Presence Covenant Medical Center	Urbana	99%	180
Presence Mercy Medical Center	Aurora	99%	152
Proctor Hospital	Peoria	99%	93
Saint Elizabeth Hospital	Belleville	99%	306
Saint Marys Hospital	Streator	99%	74
Sherman Hospital	Elgin	99%	277
Swedish American Hospital	Rockford	99%	331
West Suburban Medical Center	Oak Park	99%	330
Adventist Bolingbrook Hospital	Bolingbrook	98%	125
Advocate Christ Hospital & Medical Center[2]	Oak Lawn	98%	280
Advocate South Suburban Hospital[2]	Hazel Crest	98%	263
Advocate Trinity Hospital[2]	Chicago	98%	318
Louis A Weiss Memorial Hospital	Chicago	98%	135
Memorial Medical Center[2]	Springfield	98%	236
Morris Hospital & Healthcare Centers	Morris	98%	83
North Chicago VA Medical Center	North Chicago	98%	58
Northwest Community Hospital[2]	Arlington Hgts	98%	160
Norwegian - American Hospital	Chicago	98%	83
Saint Alexius Medical Center	Hoffman Estates	98%	224
Saint Johns Hospital[2]	Springfield	98%	241
Thorek Memorial Hospital	Chicago	98%	60
Delnor Community Hospital	Geneva	97%	170
Fhn Memorial Hospital	Freeport	97%	126
Jersey Community Hospital	Jerseyville	97%	34
Loyola Gottlieb Memorial Hospital	Melrose Park	97%	198
Marion Il VA Medical Center	Marion	97%	72
Mercy Hospital & Medical Center[2]	Chicago	97%	260
Northwestern Memorial Hospital	Chicago	97%	759
Pekin Memorial Hospital	Pekin	97%	79
Riverside Medical Center	Kankakee	97%	168
Saint Francis Medical Center	Peoria	97%	514
Trinity Rock Island[2]	Rock Island	97%	232
Advocate Condell Medical Center[2]	Libertyville	96%	210
Heartland Regional Medical Center	Marion	96%	75
Little Company of Mary Hospital[2]	Evergreen Park	96%	245
Saint Anthonys Memorial Hospital	Effingham	96%	126
Saint Bernard Hospital	Chicago	96%	259
Silver Cross Hospital & Medical Centers	New Lenox	96%	477
University of Illinois Hospital[2]	Chicago	96%	294
Advocate Bromenn Medical Center	Normal	95%	156
Centegra Health Sys-Woodstock Hosp	Woodstock	95%	62
Herrin Hospital	Herrin	95%	94
Macneal Hospital	Berwyn	95%	270
Presence Saint Marys Hospital	Kankakee	95%	115
Saint Marys Hospital	Decatur	95%	191
Adventist Glenoaks[2]	Glendale Hghts	94%	49
Centegra Health Sys-Mc Henry Hosp	Mchenry	94%	191
Copley Memorial Hospital	Aurora	94%	166
Graham Hospital Association	Canton	94%	63
Hinsdale Hospital	Hinsdale	94%	141
Lake Forest Hospital	Lake Forest	94%	101
McDonough District Hospital	Macomb	94%	50
Memorial Hospital	Belleville	94%	576
Methodist Medical Center of Illinois	Peoria	94%	215
Palos Community Hospital[2]	Palos Heights	94%	236
Taylorville Memorial Hospital	Taylorville	94%	50
Anderson Hospital[2]	Maryville	93%	183
Blessing Hospital	Quincy	93%	238
Memorial Hospital of Carbondale	Carbondale	93%	195
Touchette Regional Hospital	Centreville	93%	102
VA Illiana Healthcare System - Danville	Danville	93%	28
John H Stroger Jr Hospital[2]	Chicago	92%	325
Ottawa Reg Hosp & Healthcare Ctr	Ottawa	92%	60
Presence Saint Joseph Hospital - Elgin	Elgin	92%	100
Saint Margarets Hospital	Spring Valley	92%	38
Franciscan Saint James Health[2]	Olympia Fields	91%	437
Katherine Shaw Bethea Hospital	Dixon	91%	80
Presence United Samaritans Medical Center	Danville	91%	185
Provident Hospital of Chicago[2]	Chicago	91%	175
Rush Oak Park Hospital	Oak Park	91%	165
The University of Chicago Medical Center[2]	Chicago	91%	264
Westlake Community Hospital	Melrose Park	91%	116
Mendota Community Hospital[2]	Mendota	89%	35
Richland Memorial Hospital[2]	Olney	89%	61
Edward Hospital[2]	Naperville	86%	376
Galesburg Cottage Hospital	Galesburg	85%	47
Rockford Memorial Hospital	Rockford	84%	230
Presence Saint Joseph Medical Center[2]	Joliet	83%	246
Holy Cross Hospital[2]	Chicago	79%	272
Roseland Community Hospital[2]	Chicago	78%	148
Illinois Valley Community Hospital[2]	Peru	75%	110
Saint Francis Hospital	Litchfield	72%	32
Passavant Area Hospital	Jacksonville	61%	46

Evaluation of LVS Function

Hospital Name	City	Rate	Cases
Adventist Bolingbrook Hospital	Bolingbrook	100%	159
Adventist Glenoaks[2]	Glendale Hghts	100%	69
Adventist La Grange Memorial Hospital	La Grange	100%	288
Advocate Bromenn Medical Center	Normal	100%	198
Advocate Christ Hospital & Medical Center[2]	Oak Lawn	100%	329
Advocate Condell Medical Center[2]	Libertyville	100%	292
Advocate Good Samaritan Hospital[2]	Downers Grove	100%	314
Advocate Good Shepherd Hospital	Barrington	100%	262
Advocate Illinois Masonic Medical Center[2]	Chicago	100%	244
Advocate Lutheran General Hospital[2]	Park Ridge	100%	348
Advocate South Suburban Hospital[2]	Hazel Crest	100%	333
Alexian Brothers Medical Center	Elk Grove Vlg	100%	434
Anderson Hospital[2]	Maryville	100%	264
Blessing Hospital	Quincy	100%	370
Carle Foundation Hospital[2]	Urbana	100%	281
Centegra Health Sys-Mc Henry Hosp	Mchenry	100%	249
Centegra Health Sys-Woodstock Hosp	Woodstock	100%	94
Central Dupage Hospital	Winfield	100%	523
CGH Medical Center	Sterling	100%	204
Clay County Hospital	Flora	100%	49
Copley Memorial Hospital	Aurora	100%	219
Crawford Memorial Hospital[3]	Robinson	100%	25
Crossroads Community Hospital	Mount Vernon	100%	29
Decatur Memorial Hospital	Decatur	100%	269
Delnor Community Hospital	Geneva	100%	215
Edward Hospital[2]	Naperville	100%	453
Elmhurst Memorial Hospital[2]	Elmhurst	100%	305
Evanston Hospital[2]	Evanston	100%	508
Fayette County Hospital	Vandalia	100%	49
Fhn Memorial Hospital	Freeport	100%	171
Galesburg Cottage Hospital	Galesburg	100%	96
Gateway Regional Medical Center	Granite City	100%	157
Genesis Health System	Silvis	100%	140
Good Samaritan Regional Health Center	Mount Vernon	100%	188
Hammond Henry Hospital	Geneseo	100%	38
Hardin County General Hospital[3]	Rosiclare	100%	29
Heartland Regional Medical Center	Marion	100%	98
Herrin Hospital	Herrin	100%	127
Hillsboro Area Hospital	Hillsboro	100%	31
Hines VA Medical Center	Hines	100%	288
Hinsdale Hospital	Hinsdale	100%	210
Ingalls Memorial Hospital[2]	Harvey	100%	299
Jesse Brown VA Med Ctr-VA Chicago	Chicago	100%	386
Katherine Shaw Bethea Hospital	Dixon	100%	109
Kishwaukee Community Hospital	Dekalb	100%	129
Lake Forest Hospital	Lake Forest	100%	141
Little Company of Mary Hospital[2]	Evergreen Park	100%	312
Louis A Weiss Memorial Hospital	Chicago	100%	183
Loyola Gottlieb Memorial Hospital	Melrose Park	100%	253
Loyola University Medical Center	Maywood	100%	485
Macneal Hospital	Berwyn	100%	347
McDonough District Hospital	Macomb	100%	71
Memorial Hospital	Belleville	100%	690
Memorial Hospital of Carbondale	Carbondale	100%	225
Memorial Medical Center[2]	Springfield	100%	307
Methodist Hospital of Chicago	Chicago	100%	42
Methodist Medical Center of Illinois	Peoria	100%	273
Metrosouth Medical Center	Blue Island	100%	418
Morris Hospital & Healthcare Centers	Morris	100%	94
Mount Sinai Hospital Medical Center	Chicago	100%	305
North Chicago VA Medical Center	North Chicago	100%	65
Northwest Community Hospital[2]	Arlington Hgts	100%	265
Northwestern Memorial Hospital	Chicago	100%	853
Palos Community Hospital[2]	Palos Heights	100%	312
Presence Covenant Medical Center	Urbana	100%	244
Presence Our Lady of the Res Med Ctr	Chicago	100%	330
Presence Resurrection Medical Center	Chicago	100%	608
Presence Saint Francis Hospital	Evanston	100%	231
Presence Saint Joseph Hospital - Chicago	Chicago	100%	277
Presence Saint Joseph Medical Center[2]	Joliet	100%	335
Presence Saint Marys Hospital	Kankakee	100%	146
Presence Sts Mary & Elizabeth Med Ctr	Chicago	100%	236
Presence United Samaritans Medical Center	Danville	100%	254
Red Bud Regional Hospital	Red Bud	100%	28
Riverside Medical Center	Kankakee	100%	249
Rush Oak Park Hospital	Oak Park	100%	201
Rush University Medical Center[2]	Chicago	100%	294
Saint Alexius Medical Center	Hoffman Estates	100%	299
Saint Anthony Hospital	Chicago	100%	108
Saint Anthony Medical Center	Rockford	100%	384
Saint Anthony's Health Center	Alton	100%	152
Saint Anthonys Memorial Hospital	Effingham	100%	178
Saint Elizabeth Hospital	Belleville	100%	371
Saint Francis Medical Center	Peoria	100%	632
Saint James Hospital	Pontiac	100%	47
Saint Johns Hospital[2]	Springfield	100%	308
Saint Joseph Medical Center	Bloomington	100%	196
Saint Joseph's Hospital	Breese	100%	32
Saint Margarets Hospital	Spring Valley	100%	63
Saint Marys Hospital	Centralia	100%	156
Saint Marys Hospital	Decatur	100%	257
Saint Marys Hospital	Streator	100%	94
Sarah Bush Lincoln Health Center	Mattoon	100%	249
Sherman Hospital	Elgin	100%	363
Silver Cross Hospital & Medical Centers	New Lenox	100%	582
Swedish American Hospital	Rockford	100%	403
Swedish Covenant Hospital	Chicago	100%	414
Thorek Memorial Hospital	Chicago	100%	77
Union County Hospital	Anna	100%	30
The University of Chicago Medical Center[2]	Chicago	100%	298
University of Illinois Hospital[2]	Chicago	100%	306
VA Illiana Healthcare System - Danville	Danville	100%	37
Valley West Community Hospital	Sandwich	100%	36
Vista Medical Center East	Waukegan	100%	375
Wabash General Hospital	Mount Carmel	100%	29
West Suburban Medical Center	Oak Park	100%	374
Westlake Community Hospital	Melrose Park	100%	147
Advocate Trinity Hospital[2]	Chicago	99%	364
Alton Memorial Hospital[2]	Alton	99%	232
Franciscan Saint James Health[2]	Olympia Fields	99%	521
Illinois Valley Community Hospital[2]	Peru	99%	142
Jackson Park Hospital	Chicago	99%	184
John H Stroger Jr Hospital[2]	Chicago	99%	326
Mercy Hospital & Medical Center[2]	Chicago	99%	292
Ottawa Reg Hosp & Healthcare Ctr	Ottawa	99%	92
Pekin Memorial Hospital	Pekin	99%	109
Perry Memorial Hospital	Princeton	99%	73
Presence Mercy Medical Center	Aurora	99%	192
Proctor Hospital	Peoria	99%	151
Rockford Memorial Hospital	Rockford	99%	293
Roseland Community Hospital[2]	Chicago	99%	139
Saint Bernard Hospital	Chicago	99%	286
Saint Mary Medical Center	Galesburg	99%	130
Taylorville Memorial Hospital	Taylorville	99%	70
Trinity Rock Island[2]	Rock Island	99%	286
Graham Hospital Association	Canton	98%	91
Harrisburg Medical Center	Harrisburg	98%	50
Loretto Hospital	Chicago	98%	83
Marion Il VA Medical Center	Marion	98%	80
Shelby Memorial Hospital	Shelbyville	98%	49
Holy Cross Hospital[2]	Chicago	97%	316
Norwegian - American Hospital	Chicago	97%	96
Passavant Area Hospital	Jacksonville	97%	88
Presence Saint Joseph Hospital - Elgin	Elgin	97%	143
Richland Memorial Hospital[2]	Olney	97%	105
Touchette Regional Hospital	Centreville	97%	107
Hamilton Memorial Hospital District	Mcleansboro	96%	25
Rochelle Community Hospital	Rochelle	96%	27
South Shore Hospital	Chicago	96%	146
Abraham Lincoln Memorial Hospital	Lincoln	95%	41
Provident Hospital of Chicago[2]	Chicago	95%	175
Kewanee Hospital[2]	Kewanee	94%	34
Pinckneyville Community Hospital	Pinckneyville	92%	25
Jersey Community Hospital	Jerseyville	90%	49
Paris Community Hospital	Paris	88%	26
Saint Francis Hospital	Litchfield	87%	39
Mendota Community Hospital[2]	Mendota	86%	44
Greenville Regional Hospital	Greenville	77%	35
Lawrence County Memorial Hospital	Lawrenceville	65%	43

Medicare Spending

Medicare Spending per Patient (ratio)

Hospital Name	City	Ratio	Cases
Provident Hospital of Chicago	Chicago	0.73	-
John H Stroger Jr Hospital	Chicago	0.81	-
Saint Anthonys Memorial Hospital	Effingham	0.88	-
Graham Hospital Association	Canton	0.89	-
McDonough District Hospital	Macomb	0.89	-
Alton Memorial Hospital	Alton	0.90	-
Harrisburg Medical Center	Harrisburg	0.90	-
Iroquois Memorial Hospital	Watseka	0.90	-
Saint James Hospital	Pontiac	0.90	-
Touchette Regional Hospital	Centreville	0.90	-
Saint Marys Hospital	Streator	0.91	-
Fhn Memorial Hospital	Freeport	0.92	-
Greenville Regional Hospital	Greenville	0.92	-
Katherine Shaw Bethea Hospital	Dixon	0.92	-
Saint Elizabeth Hospital	Belleville	0.92	-
Good Samaritan Regional Health Center	Mount Vernon	0.93	-
Proctor Hospital	Peoria	0.93	-
Saint Johns Hospital	Springfield	0.93	-
Carle Foundation Hospital	Urbana	0.94	-
Memorial Hospital	Belleville	0.94	-
Saint Francis Medical Center	Peoria	0.94	-
Saint Joseph Medical Center	Bloomington	0.94	-
Sarah Bush Lincoln Health Center	Mattoon	0.94	-

NOTE: Hospital profiles are in alphabetical order by state, then city, then hospital within the city; Rankings exclude hospitals with less than 25 cases except for patient surveys which excludes hospitals with less than 100 cases; (a) 100-299 cases; (1) The number of cases/patients is too few to report; (2) Data submitted were based on a sample of cases/patients; (3) Results are based on a shorter time period than required; (4) Data suppressed by CMS for one or more quarters; (5) Results are not available for this reporting period; (6) Fewer than 100 patients completed the HCAHPS survey; (7) No cases met the criteria for this measure; (8) The lower limit of the confidence interval cannot be calculated if the number of observed infections equals zero; (9) No data are available from the state/territory for this reporting period; (10) The scores shown reflect fewer than 50 completed surveys; (11) There were discrepancies in the data collection process; (12) This measure does not apply to this hospital for this reporting period; (13) Results cannot be calculated for this reporting period; (14) The results for this state are combined with nearby states to protect confidentiality; Please refer to the User's Guide for a full explanation of data.

Anderson Hospital	Maryville	0.95	-
CGH Medical Center	Sterling	0.95	-
Crossroads Community Hospital	Mount Vernon	0.95	-
Gateway Regional Medical Center	Granite City	0.95	-
Genesis Health System	Silvis	0.95	-
Presence Saint Marys Hospital	Kankakee	0.95	-
Saint Anthony's Health Center	Alton	0.95	-
Blessing Hospital	Quincy	0.96	-
Decatur Memorial Hospital	Decatur	0.96	-
Illinois Valley Community Hospital	Peru	0.96	-
Memorial Medical Center	Springfield	0.96	-
Passavant Area Hospital	Jacksonville	0.96	-
Pekin Memorial Hospital	Pekin	0.96	-
Rush University Medical Center	Chicago	0.96	-
Saint Joseph's Hospital	Breese	0.96	-
Saint Marys Hospital	Centralia	0.96	-
Saint Marys Hospital	Decatur	0.96	-
Presence Covenant Medical Center	Urbana	0.97	-
Presence United Samaritans Medical Center	Danville	0.97	-
Richland Memorial Hospital	Olney	0.97	-
University of Illinois Hospital	Chicago	0.97	-
Advocate South Suburban Hospital	Hazel Crest	0.98	-
Loyola University Medical Center	Maywood	0.98	-
Memorial Hospital of Carbondale	Carbondale	0.98	-
Mercy Hospital & Medical Center	Chicago	0.98	-
Saint Margarets Hospital	Spring Valley	0.98	-
Trinity Rock Island	Rock Island	0.98	-
Advocate Bromenn Medical Center	Normal	0.99	-
Franciscan Saint James Health	Olympia Fields	0.99	-
Galesburg Cottage Hospital	Galesburg	0.99	-
Kishwaukee Community Hospital	Dekalb	0.99	-
Lake Forest Hospital	Lake Forest	0.99	-
Methodist Medical Center of Illinois	Peoria	0.99	-
Presence Mercy Medical Center	Aurora	0.99	-
Saint Mary Medical Center	Galesburg	0.99	-
Shelby Memorial Hospital	Shelbyville	0.99	-
Swedish American Hospital	Rockford	0.99	-
West Suburban Medical Center	Oak Park	0.99	-
Centegra Health Sys-Woodstock Hosp	Woodstock	1.00	-
Loyola Gottlieb Memorial Hospital	Melrose Park	1.00	-
Macneal Hospital	Berwyn	1.00	-
Riverside Medical Center	Kankakee	1.00	-
Rockford Memorial Hospital	Rockford	1.00	-
Advocate Trinity Hospital	Chicago	1.01	-
Little Company of Mary Hospital	Evergreen Park	1.01	-
Metrosouth Medical Center	Blue Island	1.01	-
Mount Sinai Hospital Medical Center	Chicago	1.01	-
Northwestern Memorial Hospital	Chicago	1.01	-
Roseland Community Hospital	Chicago	1.01	-
Centegra Health Sys-Mc Henry Hosp	Mchenry	1.02	-
Central Dupage Hospital	Winfield	1.02	-
Evanston Hospital	Evanston	1.02	-
Heartland Regional Medical Center	Marion	1.02	-
Presence Sts Mary & Elizabeth Med Ctr	Chicago	1.02	-
Saint Anthony Medical Center	Rockford	1.02	-
Silver Cross Hospital & Medical Centers	New Lenox	1.02	-
The University of Chicago Medical Center	Chicago	1.02	-
Advocate Good Shepherd Hospital	Barrington	1.03	-
Advocate Illinois Masonic Medical Center	Chicago	1.03	-
Copley Memorial Hospital	Aurora	1.03	-
Delnor Community Hospital	Geneva	1.03	-
Edward Hospital	Naperville	1.03	-
Herrin Hospital	Herrin	1.03	-
Jackson Park Hospital	Chicago	1.03	-
Morris Hospital & Healthcare Centers	Morris	1.03	-
Ottawa Reg Hosp & Healthcare Ctr	Ottawa	1.03	-
Palos Community Hospital	Palos Heights	1.03	-
Rush Oak Park Hospital	Oak Park	1.03	-
Saint Anthony Hospital	Chicago	1.03	-
Thorek Memorial Hospital	Chicago	1.03	-
Adventist La Grange Memorial Hospital	La Grange	1.04	-
Advocate Christ Hospital & Medical Center	Oak Lawn	1.04	-
Ingalls Memorial Hospital	Harvey	1.04	-
Jersey Community Hospital	Jerseyville	1.04	-
Methodist Hospital of Chicago	Chicago	1.04	-
Presence Saint Joseph Hospital - Chicago	Chicago	1.04	-
Swedish Covenant Hospital	Chicago	1.04	-
Vista Medical Center East	Waukegan	1.04	-
Advocate Condell Medical Center	Libertyville	1.05	-
Presence Saint Joseph Medical Center	Joliet	1.05	-
Sherman Hospital	Elgin	1.05	-
Adventist Bolingbrook Hospital	Bolingbrook	1.06	-
Advocate Lutheran General Hospital	Park Ridge	1.06	-
Elmhurst Memorial Hospital	Elmhurst	1.06	-
Alexian Brothers Medical Center	Elk Grove Vlg	1.07	-
Norwegian - American Hospital	Chicago	1.07	-
Saint Bernard Hospital	Chicago	1.07	-
South Shore Hospital	Chicago	1.07	-
Hinsdale Hospital	Hinsdale	1.08	-
Loretto Hospital	Chicago	1.08	-
Northwest Community Hospital	Arlington Hgts	1.08	-
Saint Alexius Medical Center	Hoffman Estates	1.08	-
Advocate Good Samaritan Hospital	Downers Grove	1.09	-
Presence Our Lady of the Res Med Ctr	Chicago	1.09	-
Presence Saint Francis Hospital	Evanston	1.09	-
Westlake Community Hospital	Melrose Park	1.09	-
Adventist Glenoaks	Glendale Hghts	1.11	-
Presence Saint Joseph Hospital - Elgin	Elgin	1.11	-
Louis A Weiss Memorial Hospital	Chicago	1.12	-
Holy Cross Hospital	Chicago	1.13	-
Presence Resurrection Medical Center	Chicago	1.13	-
Midwestern Region Medical Center	Zion	1.36	-

Pneumonia Care

Appropriate Initial Antibiotic Given

Hospital Name	City	Rate	Cases
Advocate Christ Hospital & Medical Center[2]	Oak Lawn	100%	46
Advocate Illinois Masonic Medical Center[2]	Chicago	100%	56
Clay County Hospital	Flora	100%	63
Hammond Henry Hospital	Geneseo	100%	60
Hillsboro Area Hospital	Hillsboro	100%	44
Hines VA Medical Center	Hines	100%	44
Ingalls Memorial Hospital[2]	Harvey	100%	59
Kishwaukee Community Hospital	Dekalb	100%	114
Lake Forest Hospital	Lake Forest	100%	78
Little Company of Mary Hospital[2]	Evergreen Park	100%	90
Louis A Weiss Memorial Hospital	Chicago	100%	34
Mason District Hospital	Havana	100%	29
Ottawa Reg Hosp & Healthcare Ctr	Ottawa	100%	75
Palos Community Hospital[2]	Palos Heights	100%	91
Presence Saint Joseph Hospital - Chicago	Chicago	100%	69
Rockford Memorial Hospital	Rockford	100%	160
Saint Anthony Hospital	Chicago	100%	62
Saint Anthony's Health Center	Alton	100%	118
Saint James Hospital	Pontiac	100%	25
Saint Joseph's Hospital	Breese	100%	27
Saint Margarets Hospital	Spring Valley	100%	34
Saint Marys Hospital	Streator	100%	49
Sparta Community Hospital	Sparta	100%	28
Thorek Memorial Hospital	Chicago	100%	31
VA Illiana Healthcare System - Danville	Danville	100%	36
Valley West Community Hospital	Sandwich	100%	26
Adventist Bolingbrook Hospital	Bolingbrook	99%	77
Advocate Good Samaritan Hospital[2]	Downers Grove	99%	103
Alton Memorial Hospital[2]	Alton	99%	140
Carle Foundation Hospital[2]	Urbana	99%	68
Fhn Memorial Hospital	Freeport	99%	86
Harrisburg Medical Center[2]	Harrisburg	99%	67
Herrin Hospital	Herrin	99%	141
Macneal Hospital	Berwyn	99%	146
Memorial Hospital of Carbondale	Carbondale	99%	88
Presence Resurrection Medical Center	Chicago	99%	151
Presence Saint Joseph Medical Center[2]	Joliet	99%	85
Presence Sts Mary & Elizabeth Med Ctr	Chicago	99%	154
Saint Elizabeth Hospital	Belleville	99%	163
Swedish Covenant Hospital[2]	Chicago	99%	160
Vista Medical Center East	Waukegan	99%	150
Advocate Lutheran General Hospital[2]	Park Ridge	98%	97
Advocate Trinity Hospital[2]	Chicago	98%	99
Blessing Hospital	Quincy	98%	154
Centegra Health Sys-Mc Henry Hosp[2]	Mchenry	98%	103
Central Dupage Hospital	Winfield	98%	201
Crossroads Community Hospital	Mount Vernon	98%	60
Delnor Community Hospital[2]	Geneva	98%	136
Evanston Hospital[2]	Evanston	98%	64
Genesis Health System	Silvis	98%	114
Good Samaritan Regional Health Center	Mount Vernon	98%	89
Graham Hospital Association[2]	Canton	98%	53
Hinsdale Hospital	Hinsdale	98%	114
McDonough District Hospital	Macomb	98%	48
Metrosouth Medical Center	Blue Island	98%	126
North Chicago VA Medical Center	North Chicago	98%	66
Presence Mercy Medical Center[2]	Aurora	98%	81
Presence Our Lady of the Res Med Ctr	Chicago	98%	115
Provident Hospital of Chicago[2]	Chicago	98%	50
Saint Anthony Medical Center	Rockford	98%	173
Saint Francis Hospital	Litchfield	98%	44
Saint Joseph Memorial Hospital	Murphysboro	98%	42
Saint Joseph's Hospital	Highland	98%	42
Sherman Hospital	Elgin	98%	206
Trinity Rock Island[2]	Rock Island	98%	101
Westlake Community Hospital	Melrose Park	98%	45
Alexian Brothers Medical Center	Elk Grove Vlg	97%	185
Copley Memorial Hospital	Aurora	97%	113
Edward Hospital[2]	Naperville	97%	140
Fayette County Hospital	Vandalia	97%	34
Galesburg Cottage Hospital	Galesburg	97%	38
Katherine Shaw Bethea Hospital	Dixon	97%	65
Memorial Hospital	Belleville	97%	354
Methodist Medical Center of Illinois	Peoria	97%	175
Morris Hospital & Healthcare Centers[2]	Morris	97%	86
Passavant Area Hospital[2]	Jacksonville	97%	86
Red Bud Regional Hospital	Red Bud	97%	37
Riverside Medical Center	Kankakee	97%	115
Rush Oak Park Hospital	Oak Park	97%	58
Saint Alexius Medical Center	Hoffman Estates	97%	155
Saint Francis Medical Center	Peoria	97%	226
Saint Johns Hospital[2]	Springfield	97%	67
Saint Mary Medical Center	Galesburg	97%	92
Sarah Bush Lincoln Health Center	Mattoon	97%	126
Silver Cross Hospital & Medical Centers	New Lenox	97%	199
Adventist La Grange Memorial Hospital	La Grange	96%	140
Advocate Condell Medical Center[2]	Libertyville	96%	74
Advocate South Suburban Hospital[2]	Hazel Crest	96%	69
Centegra Health Sys-Woodstock Hosp	Woodstock	96%	71
Franciscan Saint James Health[2]	Olympia Fields	96%	102
Loyola University Medical Center	Maywood	96%	97
Marion Il VA Medical Center	Marion	96%	25
Northwest Community Hospital[2]	Arlington Hgts	96%	102
Presence Saint Francis Hospital	Evanston	96%	90
Saint Bernard Hospital	Chicago	96%	84
Saint Marys Hospital	Centralia	96%	77
Swedish American Hospital	Rockford	96%	210
University of Illinois Hospital[2]	Chicago	96%	53
West Suburban Medical Center	Oak Park	96%	106
Advocate Good Shepherd Hospital[2]	Barrington	95%	87
Anderson Hospital[2]	Maryville	95%	104
Northwestern Memorial Hospital	Chicago	95%	161
Proctor Hospital	Peoria	95%	109
Richland Memorial Hospital[2]	Olney	95%	60
CGH Medical Center	Sterling	94%	109
Greenville Regional Hospital	Greenville	94%	36
Mount Sinai Hospital Medical Center	Chicago	94%	72
Presence United Samaritans Medical Center	Danville	94%	107
Saint Anthonys Memorial Hospital	Effingham	94%	84
Union County Hospital	Anna	94%	32
Decatur Memorial Hospital	Decatur	93%	152
Jesse Brown VA Med Ctr-VA Chicago	Chicago	93%	44
Pekin Memorial Hospital	Pekin	93%	123
Presence Covenant Medical Center	Urbana	93%	92
Presence Saint Joseph Hospital - Elgin[2]	Elgin	93%	92
Saint Joseph Medical Center	Bloomington	93%	90
Shelby Memorial Hospital	Shelbyville	93%	30
Elmhurst Memorial Hospital[2]	Elmhurst	92%	98
Presence Saint Marys Hospital[2]	Kankakee	92%	60
Rush University Medical Center[2]	Chicago	92%	39
Advocate Bromenn Medical Center	Normal	91%	68
Loyola Gottlieb Memorial Hospital	Melrose Park	91%	91
Touchette Regional Hospital	Centreville	91%	57
Heartland Regional Medical Center	Marion	90%	49
Holy Cross Hospital[2]	Chicago	90%	70
Illinois Valley Community Hospital	Peru	90%	41
Kewanee Hospital[2]	Kewanee	90%	31
Loretto Hospital	Chicago	90%	60
Memorial Medical Center[2]	Springfield	89%	62
Mercy Hospital & Medical Center[2]	Chicago	89%	76
Norwegian - American Hospital	Chicago	89%	57
Jersey Community Hospital	Jerseyville	88%	81
Mendota Community Hospital	Mendota	88%	26
Saint Marys Hospital	Decatur	88%	115
South Shore Hospital	Chicago	87%	47
Wabash General Hospital	Mount Carmel	87%	46
Abraham Lincoln Memorial Hospital	Lincoln	86%	50
Iroquois Memorial Hospital	Watseka	84%	37
Taylorville Memorial Hospital	Taylorville	84%	57
John H Stroger Jr Hospital[2]	Chicago	83%	107
Roseland Community Hospital[2]	Chicago	82%	94
Pinckneyville Community Hospital	Pinckneyville	81%	31
Ferrell Hospital Community Foundations	Eldorado	80%	44
Massac Memorial Hospital[2]	Metropolis	75%	40
Perry Memorial Hospital	Princeton	75%	32
Jackson Park Hospital[2]	Chicago	72%	121
Rochelle Community Hospital[2]	Rochelle	72%	32
Salem Township Hospital[3]	Salem	70%	27
Lawrence County Memorial Hospital	Lawrenceville	44%	32

Blood Culture Timing

Hospital Name	City	Rate	Cases
Abraham Lincoln Memorial Hospital	Lincoln	100%	61
Adventist Glenoaks[2]	Glendale Hghts	100%	81
Adventist La Grange Memorial Hospital	La Grange	100%	253
Advocate Christ Hospital & Medical Center[2]	Oak Lawn	100%	90
Advocate Good Samaritan Hospital[2]	Downers Grove	100%	190
Advocate Good Shepherd Hospital[2]	Barrington	100%	141
Advocate Illinois Masonic Medical Center[2]	Chicago	100%	148
Blessing Hospital	Quincy	100%	325
Carlinville Area Hospital[3]	Carlinville	100%	25
CGH Medical Center	Sterling	100%	222
Copley Memorial Hospital	Aurora	100%	232
Edward Hospital[2]	Naperville	100%	277
Evanston Hospital[2]	Evanston	100%	151

NOTE: Hospital profiles are in alphabetical order by state, then city, then hospital within the city; Rankings exclude hospitals with less than 25 cases except for patient surveys which excludes hospitals with less than 100 cases; (a) 100-299 cases; (1) The number of cases/patients is too few to report; (2) Data submitted were based on a sample of cases/patients; (3) Results are based on a shorter time period than required; (4) Data suppressed by CMS for one or more quarters; (5) Results are not available for this reporting period; (6) Fewer than 100 patients completed the HCAHPS survey; (7) No cases met the criteria for this measure; (8) The lower limit of the confidence interval cannot be calculated if the number of observed infections equals zero; (9) No data are available from the state/territory for this reporting period; (10) The scores shown reflect fewer than 50 completed surveys; (11) There were discrepancies in the data collection process; (12) This measure does not apply to this hospital for this reporting period; (13) Results cannot be calculated for this reporting period; (14) The results for this state are combined with nearby states to protect confidentiality; Please refer to the User's Guide for a full explanation of data.

Fairfield Memorial Hospital	Fairfield	100%	31
Fhn Memorial Hospital	Freeport	100%	195
Genesis Health System	Silvis	100%	151
Greenville Regional Hospital	Greenville	100%	54
Hammond Henry Hospital	Geneseo	100%	70
Heartland Regional Medical Center	Marion	100%	152
Illini Community Hospital	Pittsfield	100%	34
Ingalls Memorial Hospital[2]	Harvey	100%	86
Kewanee Hospital[2]	Kewanee	100%	55
Lake Forest Hospital	Lake Forest	100%	187
Little Company of Mary Hospital[2]	Evergreen Park	100%	171
Loyola University Medical Center	Maywood	100%	223
Macneal Hospital	Berwyn	100%	276
Marion Il VA Medical Center	Marion	100%	49
Memorial Hospital	Chester	100%	39
Memorial Hospital of Carbondale	Carbondale	100%	206
Metrosouth Medical Center	Blue Island	100%	241
Mount Sinai Hospital Medical Center	Chicago	100%	167
Presence Resurrection Medical Center	Chicago	100%	342
Red Bud Regional Hospital	Red Bud	100%	45
Riverside Medical Center	Kankakee	100%	247
Rockford Memorial Hospital	Rockford	100%	278
Saint Alexius Medical Center	Hoffman Estates	100%	342
Saint Anthony Hospital	Chicago	100%	112
Saint Anthony's Health Center	Alton	100%	195
Saint Elizabeth Hospital	Belleville	100%	299
Saint James Hospital	Pontiac	100%	70
Saint Joseph's Hospital	Breese	100%	52
Saint Joseph's Hospital	Highland	100%	56
Saint Margarets Hospital	Spring Valley	100%	82
Sherman Hospital	Elgin	100%	377
Taylorville Memorial Hospital	Taylorville	100%	65
Thorek Memorial Hospital	Chicago	100%	44
Valley West Community Hospital	Sandwich	100%	59
Vista Medical Center East	Waukegan	100%	281
Advocate Condell Medical Center[2]	Libertyville	99%	178
Advocate Lutheran General Hospital[2]	Park Ridge	99%	189
Alexian Brothers Medical Center	Elk Grove Vlg	99%	418
Centegra Health Sys-Mc Henry Hosp[2]	Mchenry	99%	165
Centegra Health Sys-Woodstock Hosp	Woodstock	99%	120
Clay County Hospital	Flora	99%	90
Crossroads Community Hospital	Mount Vernon	99%	106
Galesburg Cottage Hospital	Galesburg	99%	130
Graham Hospital Association[2]	Canton	99%	106
Herrin Hospital	Herrin	99%	387
Hines VA Medical Center	Hines	99%	96
Hinsdale Hospital	Hinsdale	99%	282
Iroquois Memorial Hospital	Watseka	99%	76
Jersey Community Hospital	Jerseyville	99%	122
Katherine Shaw Bethea Hospital	Dixon	99%	90
Kishwaukee Community Hospital	Dekalb	99%	139
Loretto Hospital	Chicago	99%	104
Louis A Weiss Memorial Hospital	Chicago	99%	112
Memorial Hospital	Belleville	99%	500
Methodist Medical Center of Illinois	Peoria	99%	263
Northwest Community Hospital[2]	Arlington Hgts	99%	204
Ottawa Reg Hosp & Healthcare Ctr	Ottawa	99%	106
Palos Community Hospital[2]	Palos Heights	99%	168
Pekin Memorial Hospital	Pekin	99%	184
Presence Our Lady of the Res Med Ctr	Chicago	99%	169
Presence Saint Francis Hospital	Evanston	99%	355
Presence Saint Joseph Hospital - Chicago	Chicago	99%	181
Presence Saint Marys Hospital[2]	Kankakee	99%	162
Presence Sts Mary & Elizabeth Med Ctr	Chicago	99%	325
Rush University Medical Center[2]	Chicago	99%	94
Saint Anthony Medical Center	Rockford	99%	309
Saint Anthonys Memorial Hospital	Effingham	99%	148
Saint Francis Medical Center	Peoria	99%	549
Saint Johns Hospital[2]	Springfield	99%	108
Saint Joseph Medical Center	Bloomington	99%	117
Saint Joseph Memorial Hospital	Murphysboro	99%	78
Saint Marys Hospital	Centralia	99%	149
Saint Marys Hospital	Streator	99%	100
Trinity Rock Island[2]	Rock Island	99%	160
University of Illinois Hospital[2]	Chicago	99%	163
West Suburban Medical Center	Oak Park	99%	185
Adventist Bolingbrook Hospital	Bolingbrook	98%	160
Advocate South Suburban Hospital[2]	Hazel Crest	98%	86
Advocate Trinity Hospital[2]	Chicago	98%	154
Alton Memorial Hospital[2]	Alton	98%	257
Anderson Hospital[2]	Maryville	98%	170
Decatur Memorial Hospital	Decatur	98%	281
Delnor Community Hospital[2]	Geneva	98%	215
Elmhurst Memorial Hospital[2]	Elmhurst	98%	144
Fayette County Hospital	Vandalia	98%	56
Franciscan Saint James Health[2]	Olympia Fields	98%	249
Good Samaritan Regional Health Center	Mount Vernon	98%	144
Holy Cross Hospital[2]	Chicago	98%	120
Illinois Valley Community Hospital	Peru	98%	63
Jackson Park Hospital[2]	Chicago	98%	132
Jesse Brown VA Med Ctr-VA Chicago	Chicago	98%	84
McDonough District Hospital	Macomb	98%	66
Mendota Community Hospital	Mendota	98%	40
Morris Hospital & Healthcare Centers[2]	Morris	98%	186
North Chicago VA Medical Center	North Chicago	98%	100
Northwestern Memorial Hospital	Chicago	98%	491
Norwegian - American Hospital	Chicago	98%	98
Presence Mercy Medical Center[2]	Aurora	98%	173
Presence Saint Joseph Hospital - Elgin[2]	Elgin	98%	172
Proctor Hospital	Peoria	98%	139
Saint Francis Hospital	Litchfield	98%	62
Saint Mary Medical Center	Galesburg	98%	128
Saint Marys Hospital	Decatur	98%	189
Sarah Bush Lincoln Health Center	Mattoon	98%	171
Shelby Memorial Hospital	Shelbyville	98%	46
Swedish Covenant Hospital[2]	Chicago	98%	317
Union County Hospital	Anna	98%	49
Wabash General Hospital	Mount Carmel	98%	43
Westlake Community Hospital	Melrose Park	98%	81
Advocate Bromenn Medical Center	Normal	97%	113
Carle Foundation Hospital[2]	Urbana	97%	109
Central Dupage Hospital	Winfield	97%	300
Hardin County General Hospital[2,3]	Rosiclare	97%	37
Hillsboro Area Hospital	Hillsboro	97%	67
Loyola Gottlieb Memorial Hospital	Melrose Park	97%	155
Presence Covenant Medical Center	Urbana	97%	136
Roseland Community Hospital[2]	Chicago	97%	111
Silver Cross Hospital & Medical Centers	New Lenox	97%	145
Sparta Community Hospital	Sparta	97%	32
VA Illiana Healthcare System - Danville	Danville	97%	33
John H Stroger Jr Hospital[2]	Chicago	96%	127
Methodist Hospital of Chicago	Chicago	96%	84
Passavant Area Hospital[2]	Jacksonville	96%	138
Presence United Samaritans Medical Center	Danville	96%	203
Richland Memorial Hospital[2]	Olney	96%	73
Rush Oak Park Hospital	Oak Park	96%	97
Swedish American Hospital	Rockford	96%	303
The University of Chicago Medical Center[2]	Chicago	96%	77
Gateway Regional Medical Center	Granite City	95%	102
Gibson Community Hospital	Gibson City	95%	39
Memorial Medical Center[2]	Springfield	95%	116
Presence Saint Joseph Medical Center[2]	Joliet	95%	167
Mason District Hospital	Havana	94%	33
Harrisburg Medical Center[2]	Harrisburg	93%	126
Mercy Hospital & Medical Center[2]	Chicago	93%	148
Pana Community Hospital	Pana	93%	27
Salem Township Hospital[3]	Salem	93%	28
South Shore Hospital	Chicago	93%	102
Pinckneyville Community Hospital	Pinckneyville	92%	37
Rochelle Community Hospital[2]	Rochelle	91%	45
John & Mary Kirby Hospital[2]	Monticello	89%	27
Touchette Regional Hospital	Centreville	89%	91
Massac Memorial Hospital[2]	Metropolis	88%	41
Perry Memorial Hospital	Princeton	87%	39
Provident Hospital of Chicago[2]	Chicago	83%	54
Lawrence County Memorial Hospital	Lawrenceville	76%	41

Pregnancy and Delivery Care

Newborns whose Deliveries were Scheduled Early

Hospital Name	City	Rate	Cases
Advocate Condell Medical Center	Libertyville	0%	249
Advocate South Suburban Hospital	Hazel Crest	0%	101
Alexian Brothers Medical Center[2]	Elk Grove Vlg	0%	53
Blessing Hospital[2]	Quincy	0%	26
Carle Foundation Hospital[2]	Urbana	0%	432
Decatur Memorial Hospital[2]	Decatur	0%	35
Delnor Community Hospital[2]	Geneva	0%	31
Elmhurst Memorial Hospital[2]	Elmhurst	0%	26
Evanston Hospital[2]	Evanston	0%	45
Fhn Memorial Hospital	Freeport	0%	26
Franciscan Saint James Health[2]	Olympia Fields	0%	31
Galesburg Cottage Hospital[2]	Galesburg	0%	29
Illinois Valley Community Hospital	Peru	0%	39
Loyola University Medical Center	Maywood	0%	55
Mercy Hospital & Medical Center	Chicago	0%	176
Metrosouth Medical Center[2]	Blue Island	0%	47
Morris Hospital & Healthcare Centers	Morris	0%	54
Northwestern Memorial Hospital[2]	Chicago	0%	109
Norwegian - American Hospital[2]	Chicago	0%	32
Palos Community Hospital[2]	Palos Heights	0%	28
Presence Covenant Medical Center	Urbana	0%	48
Presence Mercy Medical Center	Aurora	0%	26
Richland Memorial Hospital	Olney	0%	28
Riverside Medical Center[2]	Kankakee	0%	31
Roseland Community Hospital	Chicago	0%	47
Saint Alexius Medical Center[2]	Hoffman Estates	0%	75
Saint Anthony Hospital[2]	Chicago	0%	37
Saint Anthony Medical Center	Rockford	0%	48
Saint Anthony's Health Center[2]	Alton	0%	29
Saint Bernard Hospital[2]	Chicago	0%	29
Saint Elizabeth Hospital[2]	Belleville	0%	32
Saint Joseph Medical Center	Bloomington	0%	78
Saint Joseph's Hospital[2]	Breese	0%	29
Saint Mary Medical Center	Galesburg	0%	32
Saint Marys Hospital	Centralia	0%	33
Sherman Hospital[2]	Elgin	0%	64
Advocate Bromenn Medical Center	Normal	1%	158
Advocate Good Samaritan Hospital	Downers Grove	1%	150
Advocate Illinois Masonic Medical Center	Chicago	1%	162
Advocate Lutheran General Hospital	Park Ridge	1%	387
Advocate Trinity Hospital	Chicago	1%	95
Good Samaritan Regional Health Center[2]	Mount Vernon	1%	111
Ingalls Memorial Hospital[2]	Harvey	1%	70
Memorial Hospital	Belleville	1%	184
Presence Resurrection Medical Center	Chicago	1%	100
Presence United Samaritans Medical Center	Danville	1%	70
Sarah Bush Lincoln Health Center	Mattoon	1%	120
Adventist Glenoaks[2]	Glendale Hghts	2%	43
Advocate Christ Hospital & Medical Center	Oak Lawn	2%	274
Copley Memorial Hospital	Aurora	2%	343
Heartland Regional Medical Center[2]	Marion	2%	45
Memorial Hospital of Carbondale[2]	Carbondale	2%	42
Memorial Medical Center	Springfield	2%	43
Presence Saint Joseph Medical Center	Joliet	2%	124
Saint Anthonys Memorial Hospital[2]	Effingham	2%	52
Advocate Good Shepherd Hospital	Barrington	3%	150
Central Dupage Hospital[2]	Winfield	3%	243
Edward Hospital[2]	Naperville	3%	37
Graham Hospital Association[2]	Canton	3%	29
Katherine Shaw Bethea Hospital	Dixon	3%	29
Kishwaukee Community Hospital	Dekalb	3%	39
Macneal Hospital[2]	Berwyn	3%	29
Mount Sinai Hospital Medical Center[2]	Chicago	3%	34
Presence Sts Mary & Elizabeth Med Ctr[2]	Chicago	3%	33
Centegra Health Sys-Mc Henry Hosp	Mchenry	4%	75
Centegra Health Sys-Woodstock Hosp	Woodstock	4%	97
Genesis Health System	Silvis	4%	48
Swedish American Hospital[2]	Rockford	4%	50
Anderson Hospital[2]	Maryville	5%	39
Holy Cross Hospital[2]	Chicago	5%	43
Saint Francis Medical Center	Peoria	5%	158
Saint Marys Hospital	Decatur	5%	38
Swedish Covenant Hospital[2]	Chicago	5%	43
Westlake Community Hospital[2]	Melrose Park	5%	40
Methodist Medical Center of Illinois[2]	Peoria	6%	36
Lake Forest Hospital[2]	Lake Forest	7%	30
University of Illinois Hospital[2]	Chicago	7%	30
Northwest Community Hospital[2]	Arlington Hgts	8%	39
Pekin Memorial Hospital[2]	Pekin	8%	37
Valley West Community Hospital	Sandwich	9%	32
Adventist La Grange Memorial Hospital[2]	La Grange	10%	30
John H Stroger Jr Hospital[2]	Chicago	10%	135
Silver Cross Hospital & Medical Centers[2]	New Lenox	11%	35
Proctor Hospital	Peoria	14%	42
Hinsdale Hospital[2]	Hinsdale	15%	34
Passavant Area Hospital[2]	Jacksonville	15%	33
Adventist Bolingbrook Hospital	Bolingbrook	20%	94
Little Company of Mary Hospital[2]	Evergreen Park	21%	39

Preventive Care

Immunization for Influenza

Hospital Name	City	Rate	Cases
Abraham Lincoln Memorial Hospital[2]	Lincoln	100%	251
Alton Memorial Hospital[2]	Alton	100%	527
Clay County Hospital[2]	Flora	100%	331
Ingalls Memorial Hospital[2]	Harvey	100%	564
Jackson Park Hospital[2]	Chicago	100%	585
Mercy Harvard Hospital	Harvard	100%	201
Roseland Community Hospital[2]	Chicago	100%	471
Rush University Medical Center[2]	Chicago	100%	538
Saint Joseph's Hospital[2]	Breese	100%	271
Valley West Community Hospital[2]	Sandwich	100%	273
Vista Medical Center East[2]	Waukegan	100%	642
Crossroads Community Hospital[2]	Mount Vernon	99%	352
Galesburg Cottage Hospital[2]	Galesburg	99%	319
Good Samaritan Regional Health Center[2]	Mount Vernon	99%	521
Heartland Regional Medical Center[2]	Marion	99%	502
Katherine Shaw Bethea Hospital[2]	Dixon	99%	413
Kishwaukee Community Hospital[2]	Dekalb	99%	483
Methodist Hospital of Chicago[2]	Chicago	99%	381
Metrosouth Medical Center[2]	Blue Island	99%	622
Palos Community Hospital[2]	Palos Heights	99%	578
Rush Oak Park Hospital[2]	Oak Park	99%	441
Saint Alexius Medical Center[2]	Hoffman Estates	99%	600
Saint Anthony's Health Center[2]	Alton	99%	374
Shelby Memorial Hospital	Shelbyville	99%	194
Sherman Hospital[2]	Elgin	99%	485
Union County Hospital[2]	Anna	99%	301
Advocate Good Shepherd Hospital[2]	Barrington	98%	569

NOTE: Hospital profiles are in alphabetical order by state, then city, then hospital within the city; Rankings exclude hospitals with less than 25 cases except for patient surveys which excludes hospitals with less than 100 cases; (a) 100-299 cases; (1) The number of cases/patients is too few to report; (2) Data submitted were based on a sample of cases/patients; (3) Results are based on a shorter time period than required; (4) Data suppressed by CMS for one or more quarters; (5) Results are not available for this reporting period; (6) Fewer than 100 patients completed the HCAHPS survey; (7) No cases met the criteria for this measure; (8) The lower limit of the confidence interval cannot be calculated if the number of observed infections equals zero; (9) No data are available from the state/territory for this reporting period; (10) The scores shown reflect fewer than 50 completed surveys; (11) There were discrepancies in the data collection process; (12) This measure does not apply to this hospital for this reporting period; (13) Results cannot be calculated for this reporting period; (14) The results for this state are combined with nearby states to protect confidentiality; Please refer to the User's Guide for a full explanation of data.

Hospital Name	City	Rate	Cases
Franciscan Saint James Health[2]	Olympia Fields	98%	1120
Kewanee Hospital[3]	Kewanee	98%	120
Lake Forest Hospital[2]	Lake Forest	98%	519
Louis A Weiss Memorial Hospital[2]	Chicago	98%	533
Ottawa Reg Hosp & Healthcare Ctr[2]	Ottawa	98%	265
Red Bud Regional Hospital[2]	Red Bud	98%	327
Saint Anthony Hospital[2]	Chicago	98%	463
Saint Elizabeth Hospital[2]	Belleville	98%	548
Saint Marys Hospital[2]	Centralia	98%	541
Silver Cross Hospital & Medical Centers[2]	New Lenox	98%	522
The University of Chicago Medical Center[2]	Chicago	98%	610
Vista Medical Center West[2]	Waukegan	98%	262
Advocate Bromenn Medical Center[2]	Normal	97%	562
Advocate Condell Medical Center[2]	Libertyville	97%	563
Centegra Health Sys-Woodstock Hosp[2]	Woodstock	97%	543
Edward Hospital[2]	Naperville	97%	539
Genesis Health System[2]	Silvis	97%	404
Memorial Hospital of Carbondale[2]	Carbondale	97%	552
Northwestern Memorial Hospital[2]	Chicago	97%	456
Presence Our Lady of the Res Med Ctr[2]	Chicago	97%	635
Richland Memorial Hospital[2]	Olney	97%	243
Saint Marys Hospital[2]	Streator	97%	277
Adventist Bolingbrook Hospital[2]	Bolingbrook	96%	497
Advocate Eureka Hospital	Eureka	96%	117
Advocate Illinois Masonic Medical Center[2]	Chicago	96%	540
Advocate Lutheran General Hospital[2]	Park Ridge	96%	551
Centegra Health Sys-Mc Henry Hosp[2]	Mchenry	96%	588
Evanston Hospital[2]	Evanston	96%	640
Fairfield Memorial Hospital	Fairfield	96%	216
Iroquois Memorial Hospital[2]	Watseka	96%	260
Memorial Hospital[2]	Chester	96%	214
Morris Hospital & Healthcare Centers[2]	Morris	96%	400
Pinckneyville Community Hospital[2]	Pinckneyville	96%	27
Saint James Hospital[2]	Pontiac	96%	531
Taylorville Memorial Hospital[2]	Taylorville	96%	314
Advocate South Suburban Hospital[2]	Hazel Crest	95%	599
Delnor Community Hospital[2]	Geneva	95%	501
Gateway Regional Medical Center[2]	Granite City	95%	1309
Holy Cross Hospital[2]	Chicago	95%	564
McDonough District Hospital[2]	Macomb	95%	267
Pekin Memorial Hospital[2]	Pekin	95%	347
Presence United Samaritans Medical Center[2]	Danville	95%	557
Riverside Medical Center[2]	Kankakee	95%	547
Saint Joseph Memorial Hospital	Murphysboro	95%	334
Thorek Memorial Hospital[2]	Chicago	95%	466
University of Illinois Hospital[2]	Chicago	95%	644
Alexian Brothers Medical Center[2]	Elk Grove Vlg	94%	633
Anderson Hospital[2]	Maryville	94%	467
Elmhurst Memorial Hospital[2]	Elmhurst	94%	567
Herrin Hospital[2]	Herrin	94%	519
Hinsdale Hospital[2]	Hinsdale	94%	487
Macneal Hospital[2]	Berwyn	94%	548
Memorial Hospital[2]	Belleville	94%	555
Memorial Medical Center[2]	Springfield	94%	591
Presence Sts Mary & Elizabeth Med Ctr[2]	Chicago	94%	714
Saint Joseph Medical Center[2]	Bloomington	94%	515
Fhn Memorial Hospital[2]	Freeport	93%	468
Little Company of Mary Hospital[2]	Evergreen Park	93%	657
Loyola Gottlieb Memorial Hospital[2]	Melrose Park	93%	568
Saint Johns Hospital[2]	Springfield	93%	574
Saint Margarets Hospital[2]	Spring Valley	93%	248
West Suburban Medical Center[2]	Oak Park	93%	496
Methodist Medical Center of Illinois[2]	Peoria	92%	519
Presence Mercy Medical Center[2]	Aurora	92%	583
Saint Anthonys Memorial Hospital[2]	Effingham	92%	502
Saint Mary Medical Center[2]	Galesburg	92%	341
Advocate Good Samaritan Hospital[2]	Downers Grove	91%	587
Central Dupage Hospital[2]	Winfield	91%	581
CGH Medical Center[2]	Sterling	91%	539
Adventist La Grange Memorial Hospital[2]	La Grange	90%	556
Advocate Christ Hospital & Medical Center[2]	Oak Lawn	90%	575
Greenville Regional Hospital	Greenville	90%	236
Loyola University Medical Center[2]	Maywood	90%	521
Swedish American Hospital[2]	Rockford	90%	519
Swedish Covenant Hospital[2]	Chicago	90%	555
Graham Hospital Association[2]	Canton	89%	269
Mercy Hospital & Medical Center[2]	Chicago	89%	489
Carle Foundation Hospital[2]	Urbana	88%	516
Massac Memorial Hospital[2]	Metropolis	88%	122
OSF Holy Family Medical Center[2]	Monmouth	88%	118
Passavant Area Hospital[2]	Jacksonville	88%	554
Proctor Hospital[2]	Peoria	88%	594
Rockford Memorial Hospital[2]	Rockford	88%	617
Saint Francis Medical Center[2]	Peoria	88%	541
Presence Saint Francis Hospital[2]	Evanston	87%	553
Saint Marys Hospital[2]	Decatur	87%	542
Saint Anthony Medical Center[2]	Rockford	86%	582
Sarah D Culbertson Memorial Hospital[2]	Rushville	86%	49
South Shore Hospital[2]	Chicago	86%	320
Advocate Trinity Hospital[2]	Chicago	85%	581
Blessing Hospital[2]	Quincy	85%	574
Midwestern Region Medical Center[2]	Zion	85%	291
Northwest Community Hospital[2]	Arlington Hgts	85%	530
Presence Saint Marys Hospital[2]	Kankakee	85%	531
Sarah Bush Lincoln Health Center[2]	Mattoon	85%	509
Westlake Community Hospital[2]	Melrose Park	85%	415
Presence Saint Joseph Hospital - Elgin[2]	Elgin	84%	472
Adventist Glenoaks[2]	Glendale Hghts	83%	287
Harrisburg Medical Center[2]	Harrisburg	83%	314
Provident Hospital of Chicago[2]	Chicago	83%	311
Copley Memorial Hospital[2]	Aurora	81%	486
Decatur Memorial Hospital[2]	Decatur	81%	559
Illinois Valley Community Hospital[2]	Peru	80%	341
Marion Il VA Medical Center[2,3]	Marion	80%	134
Touchette Regional Hospital[2]	Centreville	80%	258
John & Mary Kirby Hospital	Monticello	79%	118
Presence Covenant Medical Center[2]	Urbana	76%	563
John H Stroger Jr Hospital[2]	Chicago	75%	599
Loretto Hospital[2]	Chicago	70%	391
Saint Bernard Hospital[2]	Chicago	70%	522
Trinity Rock Island[2]	Rock Island	69%	496
Norwegian - American Hospital[2]	Chicago	67%	501
Jersey Community Hospital[2]	Jerseyville	66%	270
Presence Resurrection Medical Center[2]	Chicago	65%	571
Presence Saint Joseph Hospital - Chicago[2]	Chicago	64%	533
Presence Saint Joseph Medical Center[2]	Joliet	64%	594
Mount Sinai Hospital Medical Center[2]	Chicago	62%	506

Immunization for Pneumonia

Hospital Name	City	Rate	Cases
Alton Memorial Hospital[2]	Alton	100%	717
Clay County Hospital[2]	Flora	100%	520
Crossroads Community Hospital[2]	Mount Vernon	100%	506
Galesburg Cottage Hospital[2]	Galesburg	100%	414
Heartland Regional Medical Center[2]	Marion	100%	605
Ingalls Memorial Hospital[2]	Harvey	100%	735
Kishwaukee Community Hospital[2]	Dekalb	100%	609
Metrosouth Medical Center[2]	Blue Island	100%	819
Palos Community Hospital[2]	Palos Heights	100%	865
Red Bud Regional Hospital[2]	Red Bud	100%	508
Rush University Medical Center[2]	Chicago	100%	582
Saint Anthony Hospital[2]	Chicago	100%	466
Shelby Memorial Hospital	Shelbyville	100%	314
Valley West Community Hospital[2]	Sandwich	100%	273
Vista Medical Center East[2]	Waukegan	100%	700
Fhn Memorial Hospital[2]	Freeport	99%	610
Kewanee Hospital[3]	Kewanee	99%	258
Mercy Harvard Hospital	Harvard	99%	277
Methodist Hospital of Chicago[2]	Chicago	99%	486
Morris Hospital & Healthcare Centers[2]	Morris	99%	459
Riverside Medical Center[2]	Kankakee	99%	653
Rush Oak Park Hospital[2]	Oak Park	99%	609
Saint Anthony's Health Center[2]	Alton	99%	510
Saint Joseph's Hospital[2]	Breese	99%	232
Saint Marys Hospital[2]	Centralia	99%	696
Union County Hospital[2]	Anna	99%	449
Abraham Lincoln Memorial Hospital[2]	Lincoln	98%	327
Advocate Bromenn Medical Center[2]	Normal	98%	583
Good Samaritan Regional Health Center[2]	Mount Vernon	98%	663
Katherine Shaw Bethea Hospital[2]	Dixon	98%	565
Louis A Weiss Memorial Hospital[2]	Chicago	98%	812
Midwestern Region Medical Center[2]	Zion	98%	155
Presence Mercy Medical Center[2]	Aurora	98%	802
Presence United Samaritans Medical Center[2]	Danville	98%	757
Richland Memorial Hospital[2]	Olney	98%	299
Roseland Community Hospital[2]	Chicago	98%	523
Saint James Hospital[2]	Pontiac	98%	536
Saint Margarets Hospital[2]	Spring Valley	98%	343
Saint Marys Hospital[2]	Streator	98%	384
Sherman Hospital[2]	Elgin	98%	556
Taylorville Memorial Hospital[2]	Taylorville	98%	523
Adventist Bolingbrook Hospital[2]	Bolingbrook	97%	525
Centegra Health Sys-Mc Henry Hosp[2]	Mchenry	97%	773
Gateway Regional Medical Center[2]	Granite City	97%	1687
Genesis Health System[2]	Silvis	97%	488
Mason District Hospital[2,3]	Havana	97%	79
Memorial Hospital[2]	Chester	97%	336
Memorial Hospital of Carbondale[2]	Carbondale	97%	617
Pekin Memorial Hospital[2]	Pekin	97%	406
Saint Alexius Medical Center[2]	Hoffman Estates	97%	615
The University of Chicago Medical Center[2]	Chicago	97%	538
University of Illinois Hospital[2]	Chicago	97%	542
West Suburban Medical Center[2]	Oak Park	97%	556
Advocate Condell Medical Center[2]	Libertyville	96%	635
Centegra Health Sys-Woodstock Hosp[2]	Woodstock	96%	603
Delnor Community Hospital[2]	Geneva	96%	573
Evanston Hospital[2]	Evanston	96%	721
Pinckneyville Community Hospital[2]	Pinckneyville	96%	57
Saint Elizabeth Hospital[2]	Belleville	96%	647
Saint Joseph Memorial Hospital	Murphysboro	96%	501
Swedish American Hospital[2]	Rockford	96%	574
Adventist Glenoaks[2]	Glendale Hghts	95%	306
Advocate Eureka Hospital	Eureka	95%	183
Advocate Good Shepherd Hospital[2]	Barrington	95%	635
Alexian Brothers Medical Center[2]	Elk Grove Vlg	95%	836
CGH Medical Center[2]	Sterling	95%	662
Fairfield Memorial Hospital	Fairfield	95%	321
Franciscan Saint James Health[2]	Olympia Fields	95%	1589
Graham Hospital Association[2]	Canton	95%	363
Herrin Hospital[2]	Herrin	95%	820
Holy Cross Hospital[2]	Chicago	95%	862
Iroquois Memorial Hospital[2]	Watseka	95%	390
Macneal Hospital[2]	Berwyn	95%	647
Ottawa Reg Hosp & Healthcare Ctr[2]	Ottawa	95%	343
Presence Our Lady of the Res Med Ctr[2]	Chicago	95%	946
Adventist La Grange Memorial Hospital[2]	La Grange	94%	809
Advocate Christ Hospital & Medical Center[2]	Oak Lawn	94%	694
Advocate Lutheran General Hospital[2]	Park Ridge	94%	543
Advocate South Suburban Hospital[2]	Hazel Crest	94%	769
Anderson Hospital[2]	Maryville	94%	517
Elmhurst Memorial Hospital[2]	Elmhurst	94%	713
Greenville Regional Hospital	Greenville	94%	423
Lake Forest Hospital[2]	Lake Forest	94%	468
Methodist Medical Center of Illinois[2]	Peoria	94%	654
Saint Anthonys Memorial Hospital[2]	Effingham	94%	643
Saint Joseph Medical Center[2]	Bloomington	94%	701
McDonough District Hospital[2]	Macomb	93%	328
Presence Saint Marys Hospital[2]	Kankakee	93%	638
Saint Johns Hospital[2]	Springfield	93%	659
Saint Mary Medical Center[2]	Galesburg	93%	448
Sarah Bush Lincoln Health Center[2]	Mattoon	93%	659
Silver Cross Hospital & Medical Centers[2]	New Lenox	93%	593
Advocate Illinois Masonic Medical Center[2]	Chicago	92%	556
Carle Foundation Hospital[2]	Urbana	92%	592
Hinsdale Hospital[2]	Hinsdale	92%	500
Marion Il VA Medical Center[2,3]	Marion	92%	330
Memorial Hospital[2]	Belleville	92%	737
Northwest Community Hospital[2]	Arlington Hgts	92%	659
Presence Saint Francis Hospital[2]	Evanston	92%	750
Presence Sts Mary & Elizabeth Med Ctr[2]	Chicago	92%	709
Swedish Covenant Hospital[2]	Chicago	92%	678
Westlake Community Hospital[2]	Melrose Park	92%	407
Memorial Medical Center[2]	Springfield	91%	766
Passavant Area Hospital[2]	Jacksonville	91%	692
Thorek Memorial Hospital[2]	Chicago	91%	558
Little Company of Mary Hospital[2]	Evergreen Park	90%	863
Northwestern Memorial Hospital[2]	Chicago	90%	403
Saint Marys Hospital[2]	Decatur	90%	651
Advocate Good Samaritan Hospital[2]	Downers Grove	89%	707
Loyola University Medical Center[2]	Maywood	89%	520
Mercy Hospital & Medical Center[2]	Chicago	89%	575
South Shore Hospital[2]	Chicago	89%	488
Presence Saint Joseph Hospital - Elgin[2]	Elgin	88%	725
Central Dupage Hospital[2]	Winfield	87%	581
OSF Holy Family Medical Center[2]	Monmouth	87%	203
Touchette Regional Hospital[2]	Centreville	87%	189
Blessing Hospital[2]	Quincy	86%	601
Harrisburg Medical Center[2]	Harrisburg	86%	362
Loyola Gottlieb Memorial Hospital[2]	Melrose Park	86%	727
Massac Memorial Hospital[2]	Metropolis	86%	221
Jackson Park Hospital[2]	Chicago	85%	629
Sarah D Culbertson Memorial Hospital[2]	Rushville	85%	92
Illinois Valley Community Hospital[2]	Peru	84%	447
Saint Anthony Medical Center[2]	Rockford	84%	832
Advocate Trinity Hospital[2]	Chicago	83%	825
Decatur Memorial Hospital[2]	Decatur	83%	755
John & Mary Kirby Hospital	Monticello	83%	181
Saint Francis Medical Center[2]	Peoria	83%	569
Proctor Hospital[2]	Peoria	82%	764
Rockford Memorial Hospital[2]	Rockford	82%	754
Edward Hospital[2]	Naperville	81%	603
Saint Bernard Hospital[2]	Chicago	81%	568
Copley Memorial Hospital[2]	Aurora	79%	453
Norwegian - American Hospital[2]	Chicago	78%	437
Provident Hospital of Chicago[2]	Chicago	78%	412
Mount Sinai Hospital Medical Center[2]	Chicago	77%	419
Presence Covenant Medical Center[2]	Urbana	77%	708
Loretto Hospital[2]	Chicago	76%	455
Trinity Rock Island[2]	Rock Island	76%	637
Presence Saint Joseph Hospital - Chicago[2]	Chicago	72%	524
Jersey Community Hospital[2]	Jerseyville	71%	455
Presence Saint Joseph Medical Center[2]	Joliet	68%	780
Presence Resurrection Medical Center[2]	Chicago	67%	808
John H Stroger Jr Hospital[2]	Chicago	49%	677

Stroke Care

Anticoagulation Therapy for Atrial Fibrillation

Hospital Name	City	Rate	Cases
Advocate Christ Hospital & Medical Center	Oak Lawn	100%	53
Edward Hospital	Naperville	100%	36
Evanston Hospital	Evanston	100%	51

NOTE: Hospital profiles are in alphabetical order by state, then city, then hospital within the city; Rankings exclude hospitals with less than 25 cases except for patient surveys which excludes hospitals with less than 100 cases; (a) 100-299 cases; (1) The number of cases/patients is too few to report; (2) Data submitted were based on a sample of cases/patients; (3) Results are based on a shorter time period than required; (4) Data suppressed by CMS for one or more quarters; (5) Results are not available for this reporting period; (6) Fewer than 100 patients completed the HCAHPS survey; (7) No cases met the criteria for this measure; (8) The lower limit of the confidence interval cannot be calculated if the number of observed infections equals zero; (9) No data are available from the state/territory for this reporting period; (10) The scores shown reflect fewer than 50 completed surveys; (11) There were discrepancies in the data collection process; (12) This measure does not apply to this hospital for this reporting period; (13) Results cannot be calculated for this reporting period; (14) The results for this state are combined with nearby states to protect confidentiality; Please refer to the User's Guide for a full explanation of data.

Hospital Name	City	Rate	Cases
Northwest Community Hospital	Arlington Hgts	100%	41
Rush University Medical Center	Chicago	100%	33
Saint Johns Hospital	Springfield	100%	48
Advocate Lutheran General Hospital	Park Ridge	98%	42
Northwestern Memorial Hospital	Chicago	98%	45
Advocate Condell Medical Center	Libertyville	97%	30
Little Company of Mary Hospital	Evergreen Park	96%	25
Silver Cross Hospital & Medical Centers	New Lenox	96%	25
Alexian Brothers Medical Center	Elk Grove Vlg	94%	36
Saint Francis Medical Center	Peoria	90%	70
Blessing Hospital	Quincy	88%	25

Antithrombotic Therapy Timing

Hospital Name	City	Rate	Cases
Adventist La Grange Memorial Hospital	La Grange	100%	74
Advocate Bromenn Medical Center	Normal	100%	59
Advocate Christ Hospital & Medical Center	Oak Lawn	100%	306
Advocate Good Shepherd Hospital	Barrington	100%	71
Advocate Illinois Masonic Medical Center	Chicago	100%	64
Blessing Hospital	Quincy	100%	133
CGH Medical Center	Sterling	100%	33
Copley Memorial Hospital	Aurora	100%	90
Delnor Community Hospital[2]	Geneva	100%	62
Fhn Memorial Hospital	Freeport	100%	52
Good Samaritan Regional Health Center	Mount Vernon	100%	69
Herrin Hospital	Herrin	100%	48
Hinsdale Hospital	Hinsdale	100%	68
Ingalls Memorial Hospital[2]	Harvey	100%	107
Jackson Park Hospital	Chicago	100%	35
Katherine Shaw Bethea Hospital	Dixon	100%	26
Kishwaukee Community Hospital	Dekalb	100%	33
Lake Forest Hospital	Lake Forest	100%	51
Macneal Hospital[2]	Berwyn	100%	95
Metrosouth Medical Center	Blue Island	100%	98
Morris Hospital & Healthcare Centers	Morris	100%	43
Northwest Community Hospital	Arlington Hgts	100%	192
Presence Covenant Medical Center	Urbana	100%	89
Presence Mercy Medical Center	Aurora	100%	57
Presence Our Lady of the Res Med Ctr[2]	Chicago	100%	103
Presence Saint Francis Hospital	Evanston	100%	73
Presence Saint Joseph Hospital - Elgin	Elgin	100%	56
Presence Saint Marys Hospital	Kankakee	100%	42
Presence Sts Mary & Elizabeth Med Ctr[2]	Chicago	100%	126
Proctor Hospital	Peoria	100%	60
Rockford Memorial Hospital	Rockford	100%	95
Rush Oak Park Hospital	Oak Park	100%	36
Saint Anthony Medical Center	Rockford	100%	131
Saint Anthony's Health Center	Alton	100%	32
Saint Elizabeth Hospital	Belleville	100%	96
Saint Johns Hospital	Springfield	100%	204
Sherman Hospital	Elgin	100%	73
Vista Medical Center East	Waukegan	100%	96
Westlake Community Hospital	Melrose Park	100%	34
Advocate Condell Medical Center	Libertyville	99%	150
Advocate Lutheran General Hospital	Park Ridge	99%	181
Advocate Trinity Hospital	Chicago	99%	172
Alexian Brothers Medical Center	Elk Grove Vlg	99%	148
Decatur Memorial Hospital[2]	Decatur	99%	98
Evanston Hospital	Evanston	99%	250
Memorial Hospital	Belleville	99%	140
Memorial Medical Center[2]	Springfield	99%	74
Presence Resurrection Medical Center	Chicago	99%	193
Saint Joseph Medical Center	Bloomington	99%	80
Advocate Good Samaritan Hospital	Downers Grove	98%	124
Alton Memorial Hospital[2]	Alton	98%	64
Anderson Hospital	Maryville	98%	54
Carle Foundation Hospital	Urbana	98%	179
Centegra Health Sys-Woodstock Hosp	Woodstock	98%	50
Central Dupage Hospital[2]	Winfield	98%	66
Edward Hospital	Naperville	98%	185
John H Stroger Jr Hospital[2]	Chicago	98%	200
Little Company of Mary Hospital	Evergreen Park	98%	170
Loyola University Medical Center[2]	Maywood	98%	63
Mercy Hospital & Medical Center	Chicago	98%	146
Northwestern Memorial Hospital	Chicago	98%	273
Presence Saint Joseph Hospital - Chicago	Chicago	98%	54
Presence United Samaritans Medical Center	Danville	98%	52
Rush University Medical Center	Chicago	98%	195
Saint Alexius Medical Center	Hoffman Estates	98%	107
Silver Cross Hospital & Medical Centers	New Lenox	98%	169
Trinity Rock Island[2]	Rock Island	98%	66
The University of Chicago Medical Center[2]	Chicago	98%	92
Adventist Bolingbrook Hospital	Bolingbrook	97%	33
Advocate South Suburban Hospital	Hazel Crest	97%	116
Elmhurst Memorial Hospital	Elmhurst	97%	127
Heartland Regional Medical Center	Marion	97%	35
Memorial Hospital of Carbondale	Carbondale	97%	74
Methodist Medical Center of Illinois	Peoria	97%	90
Mount Sinai Hospital Medical Center[2]	Chicago	97%	74
Riverside Medical Center	Kankakee	97%	89
Saint Anthonys Memorial Hospital	Effingham	97%	30
Swedish American Hospital	Rockford	97%	121
Centegra Health Sys-Mc Henry Hosp	Mchenry	96%	78
Franciscan Saint James Health[2]	Olympia Fields	96%	138
University of Illinois Hospital	Chicago	96%	97
West Suburban Medical Center	Oak Park	96%	101
Palos Community Hospital[2]	Palos Heights	95%	110
Saint Marys Hospital	Centralia	95%	41
Swedish Covenant Hospital[2]	Chicago	95%	81
Presence Saint Joseph Medical Center[2]	Joliet	94%	81
Holy Cross Hospital[2]	Chicago	93%	147
Loyola Gottlieb Memorial Hospital	Melrose Park	93%	55
Saint Marys Hospital	Decatur	93%	29
Saint Mary Medical Center	Galesburg	90%	30
Saint Francis Medical Center	Peoria	89%	332
Sarah Bush Lincoln Health Center	Mattoon	86%	36

Assessed for Rehabilitation

Hospital Name	City	Rate	Cases
Adventist Bolingbrook Hospital	Bolingbrook	100%	31
Adventist La Grange Memorial Hospital	La Grange	100%	95
Advocate Good Shepherd Hospital	Barrington	100%	89
Alexian Brothers Medical Center	Elk Grove Vlg	100%	232
Alton Memorial Hospital[2]	Alton	100%	63
Blessing Hospital	Quincy	100%	158
CGH Medical Center	Sterling	100%	34
Decatur Memorial Hospital[2]	Decatur	100%	132
Genesis Health System	Silvis	100%	25
Good Samaritan Regional Health Center	Mount Vernon	100%	67
Heartland Regional Medical Center	Marion	100%	34
Lake Forest Hospital	Lake Forest	100%	50
Louis A Weiss Memorial Hospital	Chicago	100%	27
Northwest Community Hospital	Arlington Hgts	100%	239
Presence Covenant Medical Center	Urbana	100%	90
Presence Mercy Medical Center	Aurora	100%	58
Presence Our Lady of the Res Med Ctr[2]	Chicago	100%	133
Presence Saint Joseph Medical Center[2]	Joliet	100%	106
Riverside Medical Center	Kankakee	100%	110
Rush Oak Park Hospital	Oak Park	100%	35
Rush University Medical Center	Chicago	100%	470
Saint Alexius Medical Center	Hoffman Estates	100%	117
Saint Anthony's Health Center	Alton	100%	40
Saint Johns Hospital	Springfield	100%	269
Sherman Hospital	Elgin	100%	101
Vista Medical Center East	Waukegan	100%	133
Advocate Condell Medical Center	Libertyville	99%	179
Advocate Lutheran General Hospital	Park Ridge	99%	245
Advocate South Suburban Hospital	Hazel Crest	99%	134
Centegra Health Sys-Mc Henry Hosp	Mchenry	99%	92
Central Dupage Hospital[2]	Winfield	99%	116
Copley Memorial Hospital	Aurora	99%	104
Elmhurst Memorial Hospital	Elmhurst	99%	148
Evanston Hospital	Evanston	99%	347
Ingalls Memorial Hospital[2]	Harvey	99%	108
Little Company of Mary Hospital	Evergreen Park	99%	179
Mercy Hospital & Medical Center	Chicago	99%	148
Metrosouth Medical Center	Blue Island	99%	113
Mount Sinai Hospital Medical Center[2]	Chicago	99%	103
Northwestern Memorial Hospital	Chicago	99%	389
Presence Resurrection Medical Center	Chicago	99%	205
Presence Sts Mary & Elizabeth Med Ctr[2]	Chicago	99%	140
Saint Joseph Medical Center	Bloomington	99%	126
Advocate Bromenn Medical Center	Normal	98%	85
Carle Foundation Hospital	Urbana	98%	292
Centegra Health Sys-Woodstock Hosp	Woodstock	98%	61
Herrin Hospital	Herrin	98%	54
Hinsdale Hospital	Hinsdale	98%	101
Macneal Hospital[2]	Berwyn	98%	104
Memorial Medical Center[2]	Springfield	98%	100
Methodist Medical Center of Illinois	Peoria	98%	125
Presence Saint Joseph Hospital - Chicago	Chicago	98%	53
Presence Saint Joseph Hospital - Elgin	Elgin	98%	59
Saint Francis Medical Center	Peoria	98%	581
Swedish American Hospital	Rockford	98%	158
Swedish Covenant Hospital[2]	Chicago	98%	114
University of Illinois Hospital	Chicago	98%	248
Advocate Good Samaritan Hospital	Downers Grove	97%	145
Advocate Illinois Masonic Medical Center	Chicago	97%	86
Advocate Trinity Hospital	Chicago	97%	175
Delnor Community Hospital[2]	Geneva	97%	73
Jackson Park Hospital	Chicago	97%	39
Katherine Shaw Bethea Hospital	Dixon	97%	29
Kishwaukee Community Hospital	Dekalb	97%	35
Loyola University Medical Center[2]	Maywood	97%	104
Saint Anthony Medical Center	Rockford	97%	187
Saint Anthonys Memorial Hospital	Effingham	97%	31
Saint Marys Hospital	Centralia	97%	39
The University of Chicago Medical Center[2]	Chicago	97%	118
Edward Hospital	Naperville	96%	223
Fhn Memorial Hospital	Freeport	96%	55
Presence Saint Marys Hospital	Kankakee	96%	48
Presence United Samaritans Medical Center	Danville	96%	51
Saint Elizabeth Hospital	Belleville	96%	115
Silver Cross Hospital & Medical Centers	New Lenox	96%	193
Advocate Christ Hospital & Medical Center	Oak Lawn	95%	446
Memorial Hospital	Belleville	95%	144
Memorial Hospital of Carbondale	Carbondale	95%	126
Presence Saint Francis Hospital	Evanston	95%	94
West Suburban Medical Center	Oak Park	95%	97
Saint Marys Hospital	Decatur	94%	52
Anderson Hospital	Maryville	92%	59
Franciscan Saint James Health[2]	Olympia Fields	92%	157
Holy Cross Hospital[2]	Chicago	91%	148
Palos Community Hospital[2]	Palos Heights	91%	101
Rockford Memorial Hospital	Rockford	91%	125
John H Stroger Jr Hospital[2]	Chicago	90%	208
Saint Mary Medical Center	Galesburg	90%	29
Trinity Rock Island[2]	Rock Island	90%	79
Proctor Hospital	Peoria	85%	60
Westlake Community Hospital	Melrose Park	85%	39
Loyola Gottlieb Memorial Hospital	Melrose Park	82%	61
Morris Hospital & Healthcare Centers	Morris	78%	40
Sarah Bush Lincoln Health Center	Mattoon	77%	47

Discharged on Antithrombotic Therapy

Hospital Name	City	Rate	Cases
Adventist Bolingbrook Hospital	Bolingbrook	100%	30
Adventist La Grange Memorial Hospital	La Grange	100%	90
Advocate Christ Hospital & Medical Center	Oak Lawn	100%	339
Advocate Good Shepherd Hospital	Barrington	100%	77
Advocate Lutheran General Hospital	Park Ridge	100%	218
Alton Memorial Hospital[2]	Alton	100%	60
Anderson Hospital	Maryville	100%	59
Blessing Hospital	Quincy	100%	146
Carle Foundation Hospital	Urbana	100%	221
Centegra Health Sys-Mc Henry Hosp	Mchenry	100%	79
Centegra Health Sys-Woodstock Hosp	Woodstock	100%	57
Central Dupage Hospital[2]	Winfield	100%	92
Delnor Community Hospital[2]	Geneva	100%	64
Elmhurst Memorial Hospital	Elmhurst	100%	138
Evanston Hospital	Evanston	100%	286
Fhn Memorial Hospital	Freeport	100%	55
Good Samaritan Regional Health Center	Mount Vernon	100%	67
Heartland Regional Medical Center	Marion	100%	34
Herrin Hospital	Herrin	100%	53
Katherine Shaw Bethea Hospital	Dixon	100%	28
Kishwaukee Community Hospital	Dekalb	100%	34
Loyola University Medical Center[2]	Maywood	100%	81
Macneal Hospital[2]	Berwyn	100%	91
Memorial Hospital of Carbondale	Carbondale	100%	115
Methodist Medical Center of Illinois	Peoria	100%	109
Morris Hospital & Healthcare Centers	Morris	100%	40
Mount Sinai Hospital Medical Center[2]	Chicago	100%	80
Northwest Community Hospital	Arlington Hgts	100%	213
Palos Community Hospital[2]	Palos Heights	100%	99
Presence Covenant Medical Center	Urbana	100%	89
Presence Mercy Medical Center	Aurora	100%	56
Presence Our Lady of the Res Med Ctr[2]	Chicago	100%	112
Presence Sts Mary & Elizabeth Med Ctr[2]	Chicago	100%	126
Presence United Samaritans Medical Center	Danville	100%	44
Proctor Hospital	Peoria	100%	59
Riverside Medical Center	Kankakee	100%	96
Rockford Memorial Hospital	Rockford	100%	103
Rush University Medical Center	Chicago	100%	257
Saint Alexius Medical Center	Hoffman Estates	100%	101
Saint Anthony's Health Center	Alton	100%	40
Saint Elizabeth Hospital	Belleville	100%	110
Saint Johns Hospital	Springfield	100%	243
Saint Joseph Medical Center	Bloomington	100%	113
Saint Mary Medical Center	Galesburg	100%	28
Sarah Bush Lincoln Health Center	Mattoon	100%	43
Sherman Hospital	Elgin	100%	88
Vista Medical Center East	Waukegan	100%	100
Advocate Condell Medical Center	Libertyville	99%	163
Advocate Good Samaritan Hospital	Downers Grove	99%	132
Advocate Trinity Hospital	Chicago	99%	169
Alexian Brothers Medical Center	Elk Grove Vlg	99%	186
Copley Memorial Hospital	Aurora	99%	88
Decatur Memorial Hospital[2]	Decatur	99%	121
Hinsdale Hospital	Hinsdale	99%	84
Ingalls Memorial Hospital[2]	Harvey	99%	98
John H Stroger Jr Hospital[2]	Chicago	99%	196
Memorial Hospital	Belleville	99%	138
Memorial Medical Center[2]	Springfield	99%	89
Mercy Hospital & Medical Center	Chicago	99%	141
Northwestern Memorial Hospital	Chicago	99%	313
Presence Resurrection Medical Center	Chicago	99%	179
Saint Anthony Medical Center	Rockford	99%	150
Saint Francis Medical Center	Peoria	99%	463
Silver Cross Hospital & Medical Centers	New Lenox	99%	166
The University of Chicago Medical Center[2]	Chicago	99%	96
University of Illinois Hospital	Chicago	99%	106
Advocate South Suburban Hospital	Hazel Crest	98%	124

NOTE: Hospital profiles are in alphabetical order by state, then city, then hospital within the city; Rankings exclude hospitals with less than 25 cases except for patient surveys which excludes hospitals with less than 100 cases; (a) 100-299 cases; (1) The number of cases/patients is too few to report; (2) Data submitted were based on a sample of cases/patients; (3) Results are based on a shorter time period than required; (4) Data suppressed by CMS for one or more quarters; (5) Results are not available for this reporting period; (6) Fewer than 100 patients completed the HCAHPS survey; (7) No cases met the criteria for this measure; (8) The lower limit of the confidence interval cannot be calculated if the number of observed infections equals zero; (9) No data are available from the state/territory for this reporting period; (10) The scores shown reflect fewer than 50 completed surveys; (11) There were discrepancies in the data collection process; (12) This measure does not apply to this hospital for this reporting period; (13) Results cannot be calculated for this reporting period; (14) The results for this state are combined with nearby states to protect confidentiality; Please refer to the User's Guide for a full explanation of data.

Hospital Name	City	Rate	Cases
Lake Forest Hospital	Lake Forest	98%	49
Little Company of Mary Hospital	Evergreen Park	98%	169
Metrosouth Medical Center	Blue Island	98%	109
Presence Saint Marys Hospital	Kankakee	98%	46
Swedish American Hospital	Rockford	98%	139
Advocate Bromenn Medical Center	Normal	97%	73
Jackson Park Hospital	Chicago	97%	38
Presence Saint Francis Hospital	Evanston	97%	76
Rush Oak Park Hospital	Oak Park	97%	34
Saint Marys Hospital	Centralia	97%	38
Presence Saint Joseph Hospital - Elgin	Elgin	96%	51
Saint Anthonys Memorial Hospital	Effingham	96%	28
Saint Marys Hospital	Decatur	96%	45
Edward Hospital	Naperville	95%	199
Loyola Gottlieb Memorial Hospital	Melrose Park	95%	56
Presence Saint Joseph Medical Center[2]	Joliet	95%	82
Swedish Covenant Hospital[2]	Chicago	95%	92
Westlake Community Hospital	Melrose Park	95%	38
Advocate Illinois Masonic Medical Center	Chicago	94%	69
CGH Medical Center	Sterling	94%	32
Presence Saint Joseph Hospital - Chicago	Chicago	94%	48
Franciscan Saint James Health[2]	Olympia Fields	93%	142
Trinity Rock Island[2]	Rock Island	93%	73
Holy Cross Hospital[2]	Chicago	85%	144
West Suburban Medical Center	Oak Park	85%	94

Discharged on Statin Medication

Hospital Name	City	Rate	Cases
Centegra Health Sys-Mc Henry Hosp	Mchenry	100%	62
Centegra Health Sys-Woodstock Hosp	Woodstock	100%	47
Fhn Memorial Hospital	Freeport	100%	37
Herrin Hospital	Herrin	100%	41
Hinsdale Hospital	Hinsdale	100%	60
Macneal Hospital[2]	Berwyn	100%	68
Mount Sinai Hospital Medical Center[2]	Chicago	100%	56
Presence Our Lady of the Res Med Ctr[2]	Chicago	100%	91
Presence Sts Mary & Elizabeth Med Ctr[2]	Chicago	100%	106
Riverside Medical Center	Kankakee	100%	57
Rush University Medical Center	Chicago	100%	195
Saint Anthony's Health Center	Alton	100%	26
Sherman Hospital	Elgin	100%	63
The University of Chicago Medical Center[2]	Chicago	100%	69
University of Illinois Hospital	Chicago	100%	91
Vista Medical Center East	Waukegan	100%	78
Loyola University Medical Center[2]	Maywood	99%	67
Metrosouth Medical Center	Blue Island	99%	85
Northwest Community Hospital	Arlington Hgts	99%	157
Saint Alexius Medical Center	Hoffman Estates	99%	82
Saint Johns Hospital	Springfield	99%	197
Advocate Lutheran General Hospital	Park Ridge	98%	178
Advocate South Suburban Hospital	Hazel Crest	98%	105
Decatur Memorial Hospital[2]	Decatur	98%	89
Evanston Hospital	Evanston	98%	226
Good Samaritan Regional Health Center	Mount Vernon	98%	49
Ingalls Memorial Hospital[2]	Harvey	98%	81
Little Company of Mary Hospital	Evergreen Park	98%	125
Memorial Hospital of Carbondale	Carbondale	98%	99
Memorial Medical Center[2]	Springfield	98%	81
Presence Mercy Medical Center	Aurora	98%	42
Presence Saint Francis Hospital	Evanston	98%	54
Adventist La Grange Memorial Hospital	La Grange	97%	72
Alexian Brothers Medical Center	Elk Grove Vlg	97%	143
Elmhurst Memorial Hospital	Elmhurst	97%	116
Lake Forest Hospital	Lake Forest	97%	35
Mercy Hospital & Medical Center	Chicago	97%	96
Methodist Medical Center of Illinois	Peoria	97%	90
Northwestern Memorial Hospital	Chicago	97%	245
Palos Community Hospital[2]	Palos Heights	97%	66
Presence Saint Marys Hospital	Kankakee	97%	36
Saint Joseph Medical Center	Bloomington	97%	78
Saint Marys Hospital	Centralia	97%	30
Advocate Good Samaritan Hospital	Downers Grove	96%	107
Copley Memorial Hospital	Aurora	96%	74
John H Stroger Jr Hospital[2]	Chicago	96%	158
Saint Anthony Medical Center	Rockford	96%	102
Saint Elizabeth Hospital	Belleville	96%	75
Advocate Good Shepherd Hospital	Barrington	95%	66
Blessing Hospital	Quincy	95%	100
Carle Foundation Hospital	Urbana	95%	177
Central Dupage Hospital[2]	Winfield	95%	65
Jackson Park Hospital	Chicago	95%	38
Presence Saint Joseph Hospital - Elgin	Elgin	95%	38
Saint Francis Medical Center	Peoria	95%	363
Swedish American Hospital	Rockford	95%	107
Advocate Christ Hospital & Medical Center	Oak Lawn	94%	272
Advocate Condell Medical Center	Libertyville	94%	122
Alton Memorial Hospital[2]	Alton	94%	52
Delnor Community Hospital[2]	Geneva	94%	53
Presence Covenant Medical Center	Urbana	94%	72
Rockford Memorial Hospital	Rockford	94%	87
Advocate Bromenn Medical Center	Normal	93%	55
Edward Hospital	Naperville	93%	151
Presence Saint Joseph Hospital - Chicago	Chicago	93%	43
Swedish Covenant Hospital[2]	Chicago	93%	81
Advocate Illinois Masonic Medical Center	Chicago	92%	62
Silver Cross Hospital & Medical Centers	New Lenox	92%	129
Memorial Hospital	Belleville	91%	115
Westlake Community Hospital	Melrose Park	91%	34
Presence Resurrection Medical Center	Chicago	90%	134
Rush Oak Park Hospital	Oak Park	90%	29
Advocate Trinity Hospital	Chicago	88%	143
Franciscan Saint James Health[2]	Olympia Fields	85%	122
Morris Hospital & Healthcare Centers	Morris	83%	30
Presence Saint Joseph Medical Center[2]	Joliet	80%	64
Presence United Samaritans Medical Center	Danville	78%	40
Proctor Hospital	Peoria	77%	44
West Suburban Medical Center	Oak Park	76%	83
Saint Marys Hospital	Decatur	74%	35
Loyola Gottlieb Memorial Hospital	Melrose Park	73%	48
Sarah Bush Lincoln Health Center	Mattoon	71%	42
Holy Cross Hospital[2]	Chicago	69%	121
Saint Mary Medical Center	Galesburg	69%	26
Trinity Rock Island[2]	Rock Island	69%	59
Anderson Hospital	Maryville	67%	49

Thrombolytic Therapy Timing

Hospital Name	City	Rate	Cases
Alexian Brothers Medical Center	Elk Grove Vlg	100%	26
Evanston Hospital	Evanston	100%	32
Advocate Lutheran General Hospital	Park Ridge	96%	27
Saint Francis Medical Center	Peoria	95%	38
Presence Resurrection Medical Center	Chicago	38%	56
Presence Saint Francis Hospital	Evanston	19%	26

Venous Thromboembolism (VTE) Prophylaxis

Hospital Name	City	Rate	Cases
Adventist Bolingbrook Hospital	Bolingbrook	100%	32
Centegra Health Sys-Woodstock Hosp	Woodstock	100%	58
Decatur Memorial Hospital[2]	Decatur	100%	112
Delnor Community Hospital[2]	Geneva	100%	67
Genesis Health System	Silvis	100%	26
Heartland Regional Medical Center	Marion	100%	35
Northwest Community Hospital	Arlington Hgts	100%	247
Presence Sts Mary & Elizabeth Med Ctr[2]	Chicago	100%	144
Rush University Medical Center	Chicago	100%	521
Saint Anthony's Health Center	Alton	100%	36
University of Illinois Hospital	Chicago	100%	270
Vista Medical Center East	Waukegan	100%	142
Alexian Brothers Medical Center	Elk Grove Vlg	99%	245
Carle Foundation Hospital	Urbana	99%	307
Copley Memorial Hospital	Aurora	99%	103
Good Samaritan Regional Health Center	Mount Vernon	99%	69
Memorial Hospital of Carbondale	Carbondale	99%	120
Northwestern Memorial Hospital	Chicago	99%	393
Riverside Medical Center	Kankakee	99%	116
Saint Alexius Medical Center	Hoffman Estates	99%	123
Saint Johns Hospital	Springfield	99%	268
Sherman Hospital	Elgin	99%	90
Swedish American Hospital	Rockford	99%	153
Advocate Good Shepherd Hospital	Barrington	98%	84
Centegra Health Sys-Mc Henry Hosp	Mchenry	98%	97
Central Dupage Hospital[2]	Winfield	98%	114
Herrin Hospital	Herrin	98%	48
Ingalls Memorial Hospital[2]	Harvey	98%	116
Little Company of Mary Hospital	Evergreen Park	98%	197
Memorial Medical Center[2]	Springfield	98%	98
Metrosouth Medical Center	Blue Island	98%	119
Presence Mercy Medical Center	Aurora	98%	56
Presence Saint Joseph Hospital - Elgin	Elgin	98%	64
Adventist La Grange Memorial Hospital	La Grange	97%	87
Advocate Lutheran General Hospital	Park Ridge	97%	247
Alton Memorial Hospital[2]	Alton	97%	68
Kishwaukee Community Hospital	Dekalb	97%	31
Loyola University Medical Center[2]	Maywood	97%	99
Macneal Hospital[2]	Berwyn	97%	115
Proctor Hospital	Peoria	97%	65
Saint Mary Medical Center	Galesburg	97%	31
Blessing Hospital	Quincy	96%	150
Evanston Hospital	Evanston	96%	373
Katherine Shaw Bethea Hospital	Dixon	96%	27
Methodist Medical Center of Illinois	Peoria	96%	121
Mount Sinai Hospital Medical Center[2]	Chicago	96%	112
Presence Our Lady of the Res Med Ctr[2]	Chicago	96%	140
Saint Bernard Hospital	Chicago	96%	28
Advocate Illinois Masonic Medical Center	Chicago	95%	85
Hinsdale Hospital	Hinsdale	95%	92
Jackson Park Hospital	Chicago	95%	38
Memorial Hospital	Belleville	95%	149
Presence Saint Joseph Hospital - Chicago	Chicago	95%	56
Saint Anthony Medical Center	Rockford	95%	199
Advocate Christ Hospital & Medical Center	Oak Lawn	94%	472
Advocate South Suburban Hospital	Hazel Crest	94%	135
Fhn Memorial Hospital	Freeport	94%	50
Mercy Hospital & Medical Center	Chicago	94%	155
Presence Saint Francis Hospital	Evanston	94%	104
Elmhurst Memorial Hospital	Elmhurst	93%	149
Gateway Regional Medical Center	Granite City	93%	27
Presence Saint Marys Hospital	Kankakee	93%	46
Saint Elizabeth Hospital	Belleville	93%	109
Saint Francis Medical Center	Peoria	93%	570
Saint Joseph Medical Center	Bloomington	93%	108
Advocate Bromenn Medical Center	Normal	92%	79
CGH Medical Center	Sterling	92%	36
Franciscan Saint James Health[2]	Olympia Fields	92%	164
John H Stroger Jr Hospital[2]	Chicago	92%	209
Presence Resurrection Medical Center	Chicago	92%	228
Rush Oak Park Hospital	Oak Park	92%	40
Presence United Samaritans Medical Center	Danville	91%	47
Saint Marys Hospital	Decatur	91%	47
Swedish Covenant Hospital[2]	Chicago	91%	114
The University of Chicago Medical Center[2]	Chicago	91%	124
Advocate Condell Medical Center	Libertyville	90%	179
Advocate Good Samaritan Hospital	Downers Grove	90%	140
Edward Hospital	Naperville	90%	230
Holy Cross Hospital[2]	Chicago	90%	158
Presence Covenant Medical Center	Urbana	90%	86
Saint Marys Hospital	Centralia	90%	41
Advocate Trinity Hospital	Chicago	89%	183
West Suburban Medical Center	Oak Park	89%	106
Louis A Weiss Memorial Hospital	Chicago	88%	26
Trinity Rock Island[2]	Rock Island	87%	83
Palos Community Hospital[2]	Palos Heights	86%	114
Morris Hospital & Healthcare Centers	Morris	84%	38
Saint Anthonys Memorial Hospital	Effingham	84%	32
Sarah Bush Lincoln Health Center	Mattoon	84%	38
Lake Forest Hospital	Lake Forest	83%	47
Westlake Community Hospital	Melrose Park	83%	35
Presence Saint Joseph Medical Center[2]	Joliet	82%	115
Silver Cross Hospital & Medical Centers	New Lenox	80%	211
Rockford Memorial Hospital	Rockford	79%	136
Loyola Gottlieb Memorial Hospital	Melrose Park	70%	61
Anderson Hospital	Maryville	67%	52

Written Stroke Educational Materials Given

Hospital Name	City	Rate	Cases
Advocate Good Shepherd Hospital	Barrington	100%	46
Advocate South Suburban Hospital	Hazel Crest	100%	72
Alton Memorial Hospital[2]	Alton	100%	41
Decatur Memorial Hospital[2]	Decatur	100%	93
Delnor Community Hospital[2]	Geneva	100%	37
Ingalls Memorial Hospital[2]	Harvey	100%	59
Lake Forest Hospital	Lake Forest	100%	36
Macneal Hospital[2]	Berwyn	100%	54
Northwest Community Hospital	Arlington Hgts	100%	119
Presence Sts Mary & Elizabeth Med Ctr[2]	Chicago	100%	73
Riverside Medical Center	Kankakee	100%	35
Sherman Hospital	Elgin	100%	54
Advocate Lutheran General Hospital	Park Ridge	99%	108
Adventist La Grange Memorial Hospital	La Grange	98%	49
Advocate Bromenn Medical Center	Normal	98%	41
Advocate Good Samaritan Hospital	Downers Grove	98%	61
Central Dupage Hospital[2]	Winfield	98%	60
Good Samaritan Regional Health Center	Mount Vernon	98%	44
Metrosouth Medical Center	Blue Island	98%	59
Presence Covenant Medical Center	Urbana	98%	57
Saint Johns Hospital	Springfield	98%	151
Vista Medical Center East	Waukegan	98%	59
Centegra Health Sys-Woodstock Hosp	Woodstock	97%	32
Herrin Hospital	Herrin	97%	37
Presence Mercy Medical Center	Aurora	97%	34
Elmhurst Memorial Hospital	Elmhurst	96%	77
Fhn Memorial Hospital	Freeport	96%	28
Copley Memorial Hospital	Aurora	95%	55
Mercy Hospital & Medical Center	Chicago	95%	73
Methodist Medical Center of Illinois	Peoria	95%	64
Mount Sinai Hospital Medical Center[2]	Chicago	95%	44
Rush University Medical Center	Chicago	95%	219
Advocate Condell Medical Center	Libertyville	94%	87
Centegra Health Sys-Mc Henry Hosp	Mchenry	94%	54
Holy Cross Hospital[2]	Chicago	94%	72
Loyola University Medical Center[2]	Maywood	94%	69
Advocate Christ Hospital & Medical Center	Oak Lawn	93%	212
Evanston Hospital	Evanston	93%	170
Presence Our Lady of the Res Med Ctr[2]	Chicago	93%	55
Presence Resurrection Medical Center	Chicago	93%	70
Saint Anthony Medical Center	Rockford	93%	92
Saint Elizabeth Hospital	Belleville	93%	61
Saint Marys Hospital	Decatur	93%	27
Alexian Brothers Medical Center	Elk Grove Vlg	92%	116
Memorial Medical Center[2]	Springfield	92%	60
University of Illinois Hospital	Chicago	92%	140
Hinsdale Hospital	Hinsdale	91%	55

NOTE: Hospital profiles are in alphabetical order by state, then city, then hospital within the city; Rankings exclude hospitals with less than 25 cases except for patient surveys which excludes hospitals with less than 100 cases; (a) 100-299 cases; (1) The number of cases/patients is too few to report; (2) Data submitted were based on a sample of cases/patients; (3) Results are based on a shorter time period than required; (4) Data suppressed by CMS for one or more quarters; (5) Results are not available for this reporting period; (6) Fewer than 100 patients completed the HCAHPS survey; (7) No cases met the criteria for this measure; (8) The lower limit of the confidence interval cannot be calculated if the number of observed infections equals zero; (9) No data are available from the state/territory for this reporting period; (10) The scores shown reflect fewer than 50 completed surveys; (11) There were discrepancies in the data collection process; (12) This measure does not apply to this hospital for this reporting period; (13) Results cannot be calculated for this reporting period; (14) The results for this state are combined with nearby states to protect confidentiality; Please refer to the User's Guide for a full explanation of data.

Hospital Name	City	Rate	Cases
Swedish American Hospital	Rockford	91%	90
Swedish Covenant Hospital[2]	Chicago	91%	57
Carle Foundation Hospital	Urbana	90%	146
Advocate Illinois Masonic Medical Center	Chicago	89%	36
John H Stroger Jr Hospital[2]	Chicago	89%	180
Saint Francis Medical Center	Peoria	89%	354
Little Company of Mary Hospital	Evergreen Park	88%	96
Blessing Hospital	Quincy	87%	77
Advocate Trinity Hospital	Chicago	85%	80
Memorial Hospital of Carbondale	Carbondale	84%	89
Presence Saint Joseph Hospital - Elgin	Elgin	84%	25
Edward Hospital	Naperville	83%	121
Saint Alexius Medical Center	Hoffman Estates	79%	61
Northwestern Memorial Hospital	Chicago	78%	244
Silver Cross Hospital & Medical Centers	New Lenox	77%	105
Morris Hospital & Healthcare Centers	Morris	76%	29
Saint Joseph Medical Center	Bloomington	73%	85
Memorial Hospital	Belleville	72%	76
Presence Saint Francis Hospital	Evanston	72%	43
West Suburban Medical Center	Oak Park	71%	48
The University of Chicago Medical Center[2]	Chicago	68%	47
Franciscan Saint James Health[2]	Olympia Fields	66%	85
Trinity Rock Island[2]	Rock Island	62%	29
Rockford Memorial Hospital	Rockford	53%	68
Proctor Hospital	Peoria	45%	29
Palos Community Hospital[2]	Palos Heights	44%	50
Presence Saint Joseph Medical Center[2]	Joliet	37%	57
Sarah Bush Lincoln Health Center	Mattoon	32%	31
Anderson Hospital	Maryville	22%	27
Loyola Gottlieb Memorial Hospital	Melrose Park	9%	34

Surgical Care Improvement Project

Appropriate Beta Blocker Usage

Hospital Name	City	Rate	Cases
Abraham Lincoln Memorial Hospital	Lincoln	100%	34
Adventist Bolingbrook Hospital	Bolingbrook	100%	50
Adventist La Grange Memorial Hospital[2]	La Grange	100%	126
Advocate Bromenn Medical Center[2]	Normal	100%	220
Advocate Good Shepherd Hospital[2]	Barrington	100%	307
Advocate South Suburban Hospital[2]	Hazel Crest	100%	155
Copley Memorial Hospital[2]	Aurora	100%	295
Edward Hospital[2]	Naperville	100%	245
Franciscan Saint James Health[2]	Olympia Fields	100%	217
Gateway Regional Medical Center	Granite City	100%	84
Genesis Health System[2]	Silvis	100%	76
Good Samaritan Regional Health Center	Mount Vernon	100%	188
Hammond Henry Hospital	Geneseo	100%	59
Illinois Valley Community Hospital	Peru	100%	89
Ingalls Memorial Hospital[2]	Harvey	100%	139
John H Stroger Jr Hospital[2]	Chicago	100%	138
Kishwaukee Community Hospital	Dekalb	100%	132
Louis A Weiss Memorial Hospital[2]	Chicago	100%	150
Loyola Gottlieb Memorial Hospital[2]	Melrose Park	100%	106
Loyola University Medical Center[2]	Maywood	100%	246
Macneal Hospital[2]	Berwyn	100%	227
Methodist Medical Center of Illinois[2]	Peoria	100%	266
Morris Hospital & Healthcare Centers	Morris	100%	53
Presence Saint Joseph Hospital - Chicago[2]	Chicago	100%	111
Presence Saint Joseph Medical Center[2]	Joliet	100%	237
Presence Sts Mary & Elizabeth Med Ctr[2]	Chicago	100%	113
Riverside Medical Center[2]	Kankakee	100%	230
Saint Anthony's Health Center	Alton	100%	48
Saint Elizabeth Hospital	Belleville	100%	202
Saint James Hospital	Pontiac	100%	49
Saint Joseph's Hospital	Highland	100%	25
Saint Marys Hospital	Streator	100%	26
Sarah Bush Lincoln Health Center	Mattoon	100%	137
The University of Chicago Medical Center[2]	Chicago	100%	221
Advocate Condell Medical Center[2]	Libertyville	99%	294
Advocate Good Samaritan Hospital[2]	Downers Grove	99%	189
Alexian Brothers Medical Center[2]	Elk Grove Vlg	99%	249
Alton Memorial Hospital[2]	Alton	99%	82
Centegra Health Sys-Woodstock Hosp[2]	Woodstock	99%	158
Central Dupage Hospital[2]	Winfield	99%	163
Delnor Community Hospital[2]	Geneva	99%	120
Evanston Hospital[2]	Evanston	99%	276
Fhn Memorial Hospital	Freeport	99%	136
Hines VA Medical Center[2]	Hines	99%	136
Katherine Shaw Bethea Hospital	Dixon	99%	76
Little Company of Mary Hospital[2]	Evergreen Park	99%	131
Memorial Medical Center[2]	Springfield	99%	282
Metrosouth Medical Center	Blue Island	99%	108
Northwest Community Hospital[2]	Arlington Hgts	99%	220
Palos Community Hospital[2]	Palos Heights	99%	233
Pekin Memorial Hospital	Pekin	99%	80
Presence Covenant Medical Center[2]	Urbana	99%	188
Presence Mercy Medical Center[2]	Aurora	99%	180
Presence Resurrection Medical Center[2]	Chicago	99%	219
Presence Saint Joseph Hospital - Elgin[2]	Elgin	99%	155
Presence Saint Marys Hospital	Kankakee	99%	94
Rockford Memorial Hospital	Rockford	99%	328
Rush Oak Park Hospital	Oak Park	99%	84
Rush University Medical Center[2]	Chicago	99%	188
Saint Anthonys Memorial Hospital	Effingham	99%	303
Saint Francis Medical Center[2]	Peoria	99%	524
Saint Johns Hospital[2]	Springfield	99%	353
Saint Joseph Medical Center	Bloomington	99%	275
Sherman Hospital	Elgin	99%	436
Advocate Christ Hospital & Medical Center[2]	Oak Lawn	98%	385
Advocate Illinois Masonic Medical Center[2]	Chicago	98%	194
Blessing Hospital	Quincy	98%	242
Carle Foundation Hospital[2]	Urbana	98%	199
Centegra Health Sys-Mc Henry Hosp[2]	Mchenry	98%	267
CGH Medical Center[2]	Sterling	98%	165
Decatur Memorial Hospital[2]	Decatur	98%	222
Galesburg Cottage Hospital	Galesburg	98%	61
Gibson Community Hospital	Gibson City	98%	48
Heartland Regional Medical Center	Marion	98%	84
Herrin Hospital	Herrin	98%	139
Memorial Hospital[2]	Belleville	98%	249
Memorial Hospital of Carbondale	Carbondale	98%	376
Saint Alexius Medical Center[2]	Hoffman Estates	98%	132
Saint Anthony Medical Center[2]	Rockford	98%	365
Saint Margarets Hospital	Spring Valley	98%	110
Saint Marys Hospital	Centralia	98%	42
Silver Cross Hospital & Medical Centers[2]	New Lenox	98%	184
Swedish American Hospital[2]	Rockford	98%	371
Trinity Rock Island[2]	Rock Island	98%	153
Vista Medical Center East	Waukegan	98%	125
Adventist Glenoaks[2]	Glendale Hghts	97%	32
Advocate Lutheran General Hospital[2]	Park Ridge	97%	302
Elmhurst Memorial Hospital[2]	Elmhurst	97%	160
Graham Hospital Association[2]	Canton	97%	71
Hinsdale Hospital[2]	Hinsdale	97%	134
McDonough District Hospital	Macomb	97%	30
Mount Sinai Hospital Medical Center[2]	Chicago	97%	78
Northwestern Memorial Hospital[2]	Chicago	97%	236
Ottawa Reg Hosp & Healthcare Ctr	Ottawa	97%	36
Presence Our Lady of the Res Med Ctr	Chicago	97%	76
Saint Mary Medical Center	Galesburg	97%	102
Westlake Community Hospital[2]	Melrose Park	97%	37
Mercy Hospital & Medical Center	Chicago	96%	157
Passavant Area Hospital[2]	Jacksonville	96%	82
University of Illinois Hospital[2]	Chicago	95%	168
Anderson Hospital[2]	Maryville	94%	125
Lake Forest Hospital	Lake Forest	94%	177
Presence United Samaritans Medical Center	Danville	94%	70
Proctor Hospital[2]	Peoria	94%	104
Saint Marys Hospital	Decatur	94%	104
Swedish Covenant Hospital[2]	Chicago	94%	199
Jesse Brown VA Med Ctr-VA Chicago[2]	Chicago	93%	42
Presence Saint Francis Hospital[2]	Evanston	93%	103
West Suburban Medical Center[2]	Oak Park	93%	122
Advocate Trinity Hospital[2]	Chicago	92%	120
Crossroads Community Hospital	Mount Vernon	92%	40
Paris Community Hospital	Paris	92%	25
Holy Cross Hospital[2]	Chicago	85%	47
North Chicago VA Medical Center[2]	North Chicago	73%	30

Appropriate VTP Within 24 Hours

Hospital Name	City	Rate	Cases
Adventist Glenoaks[2]	Glendale Hghts	100%	94
Adventist La Grange Memorial Hospital[2]	La Grange	100%	272
Advocate Condell Medical Center[2]	Libertyville	100%	455
Advocate Good Shepherd Hospital[2]	Barrington	100%	418
Advocate South Suburban Hospital[2]	Hazel Crest	100%	407
Advocate Trinity Hospital[2]	Chicago	100%	307
Alexian Brothers Medical Center[2]	Elk Grove Vlg	100%	460
Centegra Health Sys-Woodstock Hosp[2]	Woodstock	100%	446
Fhn Memorial Hospital	Freeport	100%	374
Gateway Regional Medical Center	Granite City	100%	239
Genesis Health System[2]	Silvis	100%	269
Good Samaritan Regional Health Center	Mount Vernon	100%	325
Hammond Henry Hospital	Geneseo	100%	95
Heartland Regional Medical Center	Marion	100%	241
Hines VA Medical Center[2]	Hines	100%	169
Loretto Hospital	Chicago	100%	35
Louis A Weiss Memorial Hospital[2]	Chicago	100%	430
Loyola University Medical Center[2]	Maywood	100%	337
Macneal Hospital[2]	Berwyn	100%	516
Mercy Harvard Hospital	Harvard	100%	31
Northwestern Memorial Hospital[2]	Chicago	100%	406
Perry Memorial Hospital	Princeton	100%	25
Presence Resurrection Medical Center[2]	Chicago	100%	412
Presence Saint Joseph Hospital - Chicago[2]	Chicago	100%	302
Presence Saint Joseph Medical Center[2]	Joliet	100%	461
Provident Hospital of Chicago[2]	Chicago	100%	70
Richland Memorial Hospital[2]	Olney	100%	49
Riverside Medical Center[2]	Kankakee	100%	419
Roseland Community Hospital[2]	Chicago	100%	34
Saint Anthony Hospital	Chicago	100%	98
Saint Anthony's Health Center	Alton	100%	133
Saint Bernard Hospital	Chicago	100%	64
Saint Joseph's Hospital	Breese	100%	54
Saint Joseph's Hospital	Highland	100%	68
Saint Margarets Hospital	Spring Valley	100%	321
Saint Marys Hospital	Centralia	100%	122
Silver Cross Hospital & Medical Centers[2]	New Lenox	100%	654
Vista Medical Center East	Waukegan	100%	300
Abraham Lincoln Memorial Hospital	Lincoln	99%	104
Advocate Bromenn Medical Center[2]	Normal	99%	586
Advocate Good Samaritan Hospital[2]	Downers Grove	99%	439
Advocate Lutheran General Hospital[2]	Park Ridge	99%	467
Carle Foundation Hospital[2]	Urbana	99%	289
CGH Medical Center[2]	Sterling	99%	355
Crossroads Community Hospital	Mount Vernon	99%	135
Decatur Memorial Hospital[2]	Decatur	99%	431
Franciscan Saint James Health[2]	Olympia Fields	99%	447
Herrin Hospital	Herrin	99%	396
Illinois Valley Community Hospital	Peru	99%	222
Kishwaukee Community Hospital	Dekalb	99%	393
Little Company of Mary Hospital[2]	Evergreen Park	99%	404
Memorial Hospital[2]	Belleville	99%	412
Memorial Hospital of Carbondale	Carbondale	99%	673
Methodist Medical Center of Illinois[2]	Peoria	99%	574
Metrosouth Medical Center	Blue Island	99%	295
Midwestern Region Medical Center[2]	Zion	99%	151
Morris Hospital & Healthcare Centers	Morris	99%	225
Palos Community Hospital[2]	Palos Heights	99%	447
Pekin Memorial Hospital	Pekin	99%	293
Presence Sts Mary & Elizabeth Med Ctr[2]	Chicago	99%	392
Rush University Medical Center[2]	Chicago	99%	371
Saint Anthonys Memorial Hospital	Effingham	99%	769
Saint Elizabeth Hospital	Belleville	99%	282
Saint Joseph Medical Center	Bloomington	99%	489
Saint Mary Medical Center	Galesburg	99%	285
Sherman Hospital	Elgin	99%	937
The University of Chicago Medical Center[2]	Chicago	99%	350
Adventist Bolingbrook Hospital	Bolingbrook	98%	173
Advocate Christ Hospital & Medical Center[2]	Oak Lawn	98%	464
Advocate Illinois Masonic Medical Center[2]	Chicago	98%	441
Blessing Hospital	Quincy	98%	364
Centegra Health Sys-Mc Henry Hosp[2]	Mchenry	98%	506
Central Dupage Hospital[2]	Winfield	98%	367
Copley Memorial Hospital[2]	Aurora	98%	619
Delnor Community Hospital[2]	Geneva	98%	308
Edward Hospital[2]	Naperville	98%	420
Galesburg Cottage Hospital	Galesburg	98%	178
Hinsdale Hospital[2]	Hinsdale	98%	280
Ingalls Memorial Hospital[2]	Harvey	98%	308
John H Stroger Jr Hospital[2]	Chicago	98%	304
Lake Forest Hospital	Lake Forest	98%	813
Loyola Gottlieb Memorial Hospital[2]	Melrose Park	98%	283
Mercy Hospital & Medical Center	Chicago	98%	403
Mount Sinai Hospital Medical Center[2]	Chicago	98%	223
Presence Covenant Medical Center[2]	Urbana	98%	388
Presence Our Lady of the Res Med Ctr	Chicago	98%	245
Presence Saint Joseph Hospital - Elgin[2]	Elgin	98%	341
Rush Oak Park Hospital	Oak Park	98%	246
Saint Alexius Medical Center[2]	Hoffman Estates	98%	428
Saint Anthony Medical Center[2]	Rockford	98%	662
Saint Francis Medical Center[2]	Peoria	98%	960
Saint James Hospital	Pontiac	98%	117
Saint Marys Hospital	Decatur	98%	262
Sarah Bush Lincoln Health Center	Mattoon	98%	500
Swedish American Hospital[2]	Rockford	98%	787
Swedish Covenant Hospital[2]	Chicago	98%	427
Evanston Hospital[2]	Evanston	97%	489
Graham Hospital Association[2]	Canton	97%	151
Iroquois Memorial Hospital	Watseka	97%	29
Jesse Brown VA Med Ctr-VA Chicago[2]	Chicago	97%	141
Memorial Hospital	Chester	97%	33
Northwest Community Hospital[2]	Arlington Hgts	97%	406
Presence Saint Marys Hospital	Kankakee	97%	313
Saint Johns Hospital[2]	Springfield	97%	323
Saint Marys Hospital	Streator	97%	92
University of Illinois Hospital[2]	Chicago	97%	421
Valley West Community Hospital	Sandwich	97%	39
West Suburban Medical Center[2]	Oak Park	97%	337
Westlake Community Hospital[2]	Melrose Park	97%	94
Alton Memorial Hospital[2]	Alton	96%	248
Elmhurst Memorial Hospital[2]	Elmhurst	96%	352
Gibson Community Hospital	Gibson City	96%	180
McDonough District Hospital	Macomb	96%	98
Red Bud Regional Hospital	Red Bud	96%	25
South Shore Hospital	Chicago	96%	50
Thorek Memorial Hospital	Chicago	96%	80
Trinity Rock Island[2]	Rock Island	96%	300
Memorial Medical Center[2]	Springfield	95%	342
Ottawa Reg Hosp & Healthcare Ctr	Ottawa	95%	125
Presence Mercy Medical Center[2]	Aurora	95%	304

NOTE: Hospital profiles are in alphabetical order by state, then city, then hospital within the city; Rankings exclude hospitals with less than 25 cases except for patient surveys which excludes hospitals with less than 100 cases; (a) 100-299 cases; (1) The number of cases/patients is too few to report; (2) Data submitted were based on a sample of cases/patients; (3) Results are based on a shorter time period than required; (4) Data suppressed by CMS for one or more quarters; (5) Results are not available for this reporting period; (6) Fewer than 100 patients completed the HCAHPS survey; (7) No cases met the criteria for this measure; (8) The lower limit of the confidence interval cannot be calculated if the number of observed infections equals zero; (9) No data are available from the state/territory for this reporting period; (10) The scores shown reflect fewer than 50 completed surveys; (11) There were discrepancies in the data collection process; (12) This measure does not apply to this hospital for this reporting period; (13) Results cannot be calculated for this reporting period; (14) The results for this state are combined with nearby states to protect confidentiality; Please refer to the User's Guide for a full explanation of data.

Hospital Name	City	Rate	Cases
Presence Saint Francis Hospital[2]	Evanston	95%	379
Rockford Memorial Hospital	Rockford	95%	699
Touchette Regional Hospital	Centreville	95%	41
Anderson Hospital[2]	Maryville	94%	364
Katherine Shaw Bethea Hospital	Dixon	94%	177
Presence United Samaritans Medical Center	Danville	94%	171
Proctor Hospital[2]	Peoria	94%	230
Wabash General Hospital	Mount Carmel	94%	120
Paris Community Hospital	Paris	93%	58
North Chicago VA Medical Center[2]	North Chicago	91%	96
Passavant Area Hospital[2]	Jacksonville	90%	245
Holy Cross Hospital[2]	Chicago	88%	146
Norwegian - American Hospital	Chicago	85%	48
Jersey Community Hospital	Jerseyville	77%	26
Mendota Community Hospital[3]	Mendota	76%	29

Controlled Postoperative Blood Glucose

Hospital Name	City	Rate	Cases
Adventist La Grange Memorial Hospital[2]	La Grange	100%	42
Central Dupage Hospital[2]	Winfield	100%	117
Ingalls Memorial Hospital[2]	Harvey	100%	41
Loyola Gottlieb Memorial Hospital[2]	Melrose Park	100%	50
Memorial Hospital[2]	Belleville	100%	107
Mount Sinai Hospital Medical Center[2]	Chicago	100%	39
Rush University Medical Center[2]	Chicago	100%	107
Saint Anthony Medical Center[2]	Rockford	100%	138
Advocate Condell Medical Center[2]	Libertyville	99%	117
Advocate Good Shepherd Hospital[2]	Barrington	99%	110
Alexian Brothers Medical Center[2]	Elk Grove Vlg	99%	135
Evanston Hospital[2]	Evanston	99%	221
Franciscan Saint James Health[2]	Olympia Fields	99%	74
Memorial Hospital of Carbondale	Carbondale	99%	156
Northwest Community Hospital[2]	Arlington Hgts	99%	128
Presence Mercy Medical Center[2]	Aurora	99%	131
Saint Francis Medical Center[2]	Peoria	99%	260
Swedish Covenant Hospital[2]	Chicago	99%	76
Advocate Bromenn Medical Center[2]	Normal	98%	42
Advocate Christ Hospital & Medical Center[2]	Oak Lawn	98%	157
Advocate Good Samaritan Hospital[2]	Downers Grove	98%	119
Advocate Illinois Masonic Medical Center[2]	Chicago	98%	89
Advocate Lutheran General Hospital[2]	Park Ridge	98%	113
Blessing Hospital	Quincy	98%	66
Copley Memorial Hospital[2]	Aurora	98%	105
Hinsdale Hospital[2]	Hinsdale	98%	51
Macneal Hospital[2]	Berwyn	98%	66
Methodist Medical Center of Illinois[2]	Peoria	98%	114
Saint Johns Hospital[2]	Springfield	98%	205
Sherman Hospital	Elgin	98%	158
Trinity Rock Island[2]	Rock Island	98%	114
The University of Chicago Medical Center[2]	Chicago	98%	133
University of Illinois Hospital[2]	Chicago	98%	48
Carle Foundation Hospital[2]	Urbana	97%	122
Decatur Memorial Hospital[2]	Decatur	97%	64
Elmhurst Memorial Hospital[2]	Elmhurst	97%	110
Presence Saint Joseph Hospital - Chicago[2]	Chicago	97%	65
Presence Saint Joseph Hospital - Elgin[2]	Elgin	97%	38
Riverside Medical Center[2]	Kankakee	97%	125
Saint Elizabeth Hospital	Belleville	97%	119
Swedish American Hospital[2]	Rockford	97%	153
Edward Hospital[2]	Naperville	96%	161
Good Samaritan Regional Health Center	Mount Vernon	96%	74
Mercy Hospital & Medical Center	Chicago	96%	49
Metrosouth Medical Center	Blue Island	96%	26
Northwestern Memorial Hospital[2]	Chicago	96%	145
Presence Resurrection Medical Center[2]	Chicago	96%	115
Rockford Memorial Hospital	Rockford	96%	78
Saint Joseph Medical Center	Bloomington	96%	54
Palos Community Hospital[2]	Palos Heights	95%	152
Presence Saint Francis Hospital[2]	Evanston	95%	41
Vista Medical Center East	Waukegan	95%	65
Centegra Health Sys-Mc Henry Hosp[2]	Mchenry	94%	96
Presence Saint Joseph Medical Center[2]	Joliet	94%	141
Hines VA Medical Center[2]	Hines	93%	105
Presence Sts Mary & Elizabeth Med Ctr[2]	Chicago	93%	43
Memorial Medical Center[2]	Springfield	92%	139
John H Stroger Jr Hospital[2]	Chicago	91%	99
Presence Covenant Medical Center[2]	Urbana	91%	77
Loyola University Medical Center[2]	Maywood	86%	132
West Suburban Medical Center[2]	Oak Park	86%	35

Perioperative Temperature Management

Hospital Name	City	Rate	Cases
Adventist Bolingbrook Hospital	Bolingbrook	100%	191
Adventist La Grange Memorial Hospital[2]	La Grange	100%	334
Advocate Bromenn Medical Center[2]	Normal	100%	758
Advocate Christ Hospital & Medical Center[2]	Oak Lawn	100%	652
Advocate Condell Medical Center[2]	Libertyville	100%	564
Advocate Good Samaritan Hospital[2]	Downers Grove	100%	518
Advocate Good Shepherd Hospital[2]	Barrington	100%	513
Advocate Illinois Masonic Medical Center[2]	Chicago	100%	530
Advocate Lutheran General Hospital[2]	Park Ridge	100%	580
Advocate South Suburban Hospital[2]	Hazel Crest	100%	498
Advocate Trinity Hospital[2]	Chicago	100%	419
Alexian Brothers Medical Center[2]	Elk Grove Vlg	100%	523
Alton Memorial Hospital[2]	Alton	100%	270
Anderson Hospital[2]	Maryville	100%	410
Blessing Hospital	Quincy	100%	477
Centegra Health Sys-Mc Henry Hosp[2]	Mchenry	100%	617
Centegra Health Sys-Woodstock Hosp[2]	Woodstock	100%	514
Central Dupage Hospital[2]	Winfield	100%	445
CGH Medical Center[2]	Sterling	100%	424
Crawford Memorial Hospital[3]	Robinson	100%	41
Crossroads Community Hospital	Mount Vernon	100%	143
Decatur Memorial Hospital[2]	Decatur	100%	562
Edward Hospital[2]	Naperville	100%	512
Elmhurst Memorial Hospital[2]	Elmhurst	100%	408
Evanston Hospital[2]	Evanston	100%	591
Fairfield Memorial Hospital	Fairfield	100%	26
Fhn Memorial Hospital	Freeport	100%	417
Franciscan Saint James Health[2]	Olympia Fields	100%	522
Galesburg Cottage Hospital	Galesburg	100%	206
Gateway Regional Medical Center	Granite City	100%	255
Genesis Health System[2]	Silvis	100%	299
Gibson Community Hospital	Gibson City	100%	194
Good Samaritan Regional Health Center	Mount Vernon	100%	382
Graham Hospital Association[2]	Canton	100%	186
Hammond Henry Hospital	Geneseo	100%	153
Heartland Regional Medical Center	Marion	100%	304
Herrin Hospital	Herrin	100%	428
Hinsdale Hospital[2]	Hinsdale	100%	338
Ingalls Memorial Hospital[2]	Harvey	100%	378
Jackson Park Hospital	Chicago	100%	48
Katherine Shaw Bethea Hospital	Dixon	100%	245
Kishwaukee Community Hospital	Dekalb	100%	434
Lake Forest Hospital	Lake Forest	100%	850
Little Company of Mary Hospital[2]	Evergreen Park	100%	499
Loretto Hospital	Chicago	100%	45
Louis A Weiss Memorial Hospital[2]	Chicago	100%	455
Loyola Gottlieb Memorial Hospital[2]	Melrose Park	100%	316
Loyola University Medical Center[2]	Maywood	100%	438
Macneal Hospital[2]	Berwyn	100%	631
McDonough District Hospital	Macomb	100%	113
Memorial Hospital[2]	Belleville	100%	503
Memorial Hospital	Chester	100%	37
Memorial Hospital of Carbondale	Carbondale	100%	788
Memorial Medical Center[2]	Springfield	100%	503
Methodist Hospital of Chicago	Chicago	100%	38
Methodist Medical Center of Illinois[2]	Peoria	100%	682
Metrosouth Medical Center	Blue Island	100%	346
Midwestern Region Medical Center[2]	Zion	100%	153
Morris Hospital & Healthcare Centers	Morris	100%	251
Mount Sinai Hospital Medical Center[2]	Chicago	100%	290
Northwest Community Hospital[2]	Arlington Hgts	100%	491
Ottawa Reg Hosp & Healthcare Ctr	Ottawa	100%	141
Palos Community Hospital[2]	Palos Heights	100%	537
Paris Community Hospital	Paris	100%	68
Passavant Area Hospital[2]	Jacksonville	100%	265
Pekin Memorial Hospital	Pekin	100%	320
Perry Memorial Hospital	Princeton	100%	28
Presence Covenant Medical Center[2]	Urbana	100%	454
Presence Mercy Medical Center[2]	Aurora	100%	336
Presence Our Lady of the Res Med Ctr	Chicago	100%	284
Presence Resurrection Medical Center[2]	Chicago	100%	522
Presence Saint Francis Hospital[2]	Evanston	100%	421
Presence Saint Joseph Hospital - Chicago[2]	Chicago	100%	336
Presence Saint Joseph Medical Center[2]	Joliet	100%	546
Presence Saint Marys Hospital	Kankakee	100%	347
Presence Sts Mary & Elizabeth Med Ctr[2]	Chicago	100%	455
Presence United Samaritans Medical Center	Danville	100%	213
Proctor Hospital[2]	Peoria	100%	347
Red Bud Regional Hospital	Red Bud	100%	33
Richland Memorial Hospital[2]	Olney	100%	96
Riverside Medical Center[2]	Kankakee	100%	472
Rockford Memorial Hospital	Rockford	100%	867
Roseland Community Hospital[2]	Chicago	100%	44
Rush Oak Park Hospital	Oak Park	100%	282
Rush University Medical Center[2]	Chicago	100%	502
Saint Alexius Medical Center[2]	Hoffman Estates	100%	473
Saint Anthony Hospital	Chicago	100%	122
Saint Anthony Medical Center[2]	Rockford	100%	803
Saint Anthony's Health Center	Alton	100%	143
Saint Anthonys Memorial Hospital	Effingham	100%	834
Saint Elizabeth Hospital	Belleville	100%	400
Saint Francis Medical Center[2]	Peoria	100%	1214
Saint James Hospital	Pontiac	100%	140
Saint Johns Hospital[2]	Springfield	100%	532
Saint Joseph Medical Center	Bloomington	100%	688
Saint Joseph's Hospital	Breese	100%	78
Saint Joseph's Hospital	Highland	100%	70
Saint Margarets Hospital	Spring Valley	100%	380
Saint Mary Medical Center	Galesburg	100%	311
Saint Marys Hospital	Decatur	100%	291
Saint Marys Hospital	Streator	100%	98
Sarah Bush Lincoln Health Center	Mattoon	100%	576
Sherman Hospital	Elgin	100%	1094
Silver Cross Hospital & Medical Centers[2]	New Lenox	100%	724
Swedish American Hospital[2]	Rockford	100%	992
Swedish Covenant Hospital[2]	Chicago	100%	589
Taylorville Memorial Hospital	Taylorville	100%	33
Thorek Memorial Hospital	Chicago	100%	90
Touchette Regional Hospital	Centreville	100%	41
Trinity Rock Island[2]	Rock Island	100%	368
The University of Chicago Medical Center[2]	Chicago	100%	576
University of Illinois Hospital[2]	Chicago	100%	528
Valley West Community Hospital	Sandwich	100%	50
Vista Medical Center East	Waukegan	100%	344
Wabash General Hospital	Mount Carmel	100%	136
West Suburban Medical Center[2]	Oak Park	100%	392
Westlake Community Hospital[2]	Melrose Park	100%	114
Abraham Lincoln Memorial Hospital	Lincoln	99%	111
Carle Foundation Hospital[2]	Urbana	99%	422
Copley Memorial Hospital[2]	Aurora	99%	771
Delnor Community Hospital[2]	Geneva	99%	414
Hines VA Medical Center[2]	Hines	99%	268
Holy Cross Hospital[2]	Chicago	99%	172
Illinois Valley Community Hospital	Peru	99%	275
John H Stroger Jr Hospital[2]	Chicago	99%	385
Mercy Hospital & Medical Center	Chicago	99%	462
Northwestern Memorial Hospital[2]	Chicago	99%	580
Presence Saint Joseph Hospital - Elgin[2]	Elgin	99%	397
Saint Marys Hospital	Centralia	99%	138
Adventist Glenoaks[2]	Glendale Hghts	98%	108
Iroquois Memorial Hospital	Watseka	98%	49
Jesse Brown VA Med Ctr-VA Chicago[2]	Chicago	98%	177
Mercy Harvard Hospital	Harvard	98%	44
Norwegian - American Hospital	Chicago	98%	63
Provident Hospital of Chicago[2]	Chicago	98%	80
Mendota Community Hospital[3]	Mendota	97%	30
Saint Bernard Hospital	Chicago	97%	71
North Chicago VA Medical Center[2]	North Chicago	95%	101
Jersey Community Hospital	Jerseyville	90%	31

Prophylactic Antibiotic Selection

Hospital Name	City	Rate	Cases
Adventist Glenoaks[2]	Glendale Hghts	100%	66
Advocate Bromenn Medical Center[2]	Normal	100%	581
Advocate Condell Medical Center[2]	Libertyville	100%	475
Advocate Illinois Masonic Medical Center[2]	Chicago	100%	439
Advocate Lutheran General Hospital[2]	Park Ridge	100%	466
Alton Memorial Hospital[2]	Alton	100%	187
Copley Memorial Hospital[2]	Aurora	100%	715
Elmhurst Memorial Hospital[2]	Elmhurst	100%	356
Evanston Hospital[2]	Evanston	100%	587
Franciscan Saint James Health[2]	Olympia Fields	100%	383
Gateway Regional Medical Center	Granite City	100%	177
Genesis Health System[2]	Silvis	100%	214
Good Samaritan Regional Health Center	Mount Vernon	100%	312
Heartland Regional Medical Center	Marion	100%	200
Herrin Hospital	Herrin	100%	330
Hines VA Medical Center	Hines	100%	187
Hinsdale Hospital[2]	Hinsdale	100%	270
Illinois Valley Community Hospital	Peru	100%	223
Ingalls Memorial Hospital[2]	Harvey	100%	303
Jesse Brown VA Med Ctr-VA Chicago	Chicago	100%	74
Kishwaukee Community Hospital	Dekalb	100%	321
Louis A Weiss Memorial Hospital[2]	Chicago	100%	313
Loyola University Medical Center[2]	Maywood	100%	372
Macneal Hospital[2]	Berwyn	100%	469
Memorial Hospital of Carbondale	Carbondale	100%	659
Methodist Hospital of Chicago	Chicago	100%	28
Methodist Medical Center of Illinois[2]	Peoria	100%	614
Metrosouth Medical Center	Blue Island	100%	258
Morris Hospital & Healthcare Centers	Morris	100%	178
North Chicago VA Medical Center	North Chicago	100%	60
Ottawa Reg Hosp & Healthcare Ctr	Ottawa	100%	61
Paris Community Hospital	Paris	100%	51
Presence Covenant Medical Center[2]	Urbana	100%	350
Presence Resurrection Medical Center[2]	Chicago	100%	464
Presence Saint Joseph Hospital - Chicago[2]	Chicago	100%	281
Presence Saint Joseph Hospital - Elgin[2]	Elgin	100%	279
Presence Sts Mary & Elizabeth Med Ctr[2]	Chicago	100%	341
Richland Memorial Hospital[2]	Olney	100%	56
Riverside Medical Center[2]	Kankakee	100%	441
Rush University Medical Center[2]	Chicago	100%	423
Saint Anthony Medical Center[2]	Rockford	100%	723
Saint Anthony's Health Center	Alton	100%	95
Saint James Hospital	Pontiac	100%	109
Saint Joseph Medical Center	Bloomington	100%	491
Saint Joseph's Hospital	Breese	100%	48
Saint Joseph's Hospital	Highland	100%	56
Saint Margarets Hospital	Spring Valley	100%	249
Saint Mary Medical Center	Galesburg	100%	222

NOTE: Hospital profiles are in alphabetical order by state, then city, then hospital within the city; Rankings exclude hospitals with less than 25 cases except for patient surveys which excludes hospitals with less than 100 cases; (a) 100-299 cases; (1) The number of cases/patients is too few to report; (2) Data submitted were based on a sample of cases/patients; (3) Results are based on a shorter time period than required; (4) Data suppressed by CMS for one or more quarters; (5) Results are not available for this reporting period; (6) Fewer than 100 patients completed the HCAHPS survey; (7) No cases met the criteria for this measure; (8) The lower limit of the confidence interval cannot be calculated if the number of observed infections equals zero; (9) No data are available from the state/territory for this reporting period; (10) The scores shown reflect fewer than 50 completed surveys; (11) There were discrepancies in the data collection process; (12) This measure does not apply to this hospital for this reporting period; (13) Results cannot be calculated for this reporting period; (14) The results for this state are combined with nearby states to protect confidentiality; Please refer to the User's Guide for a full explanation of data.

Hospital Name	City	Rate	Cases
Saint Marys Hospital	Streator	100%	63
Sarah Bush Lincoln Health Center	Mattoon	100%	420
Sherman Hospital	Elgin	100%	812
The University of Chicago Medical Center[2]	Chicago	100%	394
Vista Medical Center East	Waukegan	100%	272
Wabash General Hospital	Mount Carmel	100%	121
Abraham Lincoln Memorial Hospital	Lincoln	99%	95
Adventist La Grange Memorial Hospital[2]	La Grange	99%	248
Advocate Christ Hospital & Medical Center[2]	Oak Lawn	99%	538
Advocate Good Samaritan Hospital[2]	Downers Grove	99%	455
Advocate Good Shepherd Hospital[2]	Barrington	99%	420
Advocate South Suburban Hospital[2]	Hazel Crest	99%	336
Advocate Trinity Hospital[2]	Chicago	99%	217
Alexian Brothers Medical Center[2]	Elk Grove Vlg	99%	468
Anderson Hospital[2]	Maryville	99%	272
Blessing Hospital	Quincy	99%	352
Carle Foundation Hospital[2]	Urbana	99%	410
Centegra Health Sys-Mc Henry Hosp[2]	Mchenry	99%	542
Centegra Health Sys-Woodstock Hosp[2]	Woodstock	99%	390
Central Dupage Hospital[2]	Winfield	99%	418
CGH Medical Center[2]	Sterling	99%	304
Crossroads Community Hospital	Mount Vernon	99%	106
Decatur Memorial Hospital[2]	Decatur	99%	428
Delnor Community Hospital[2]	Geneva	99%	278
Edward Hospital[2]	Naperville	99%	459
Fhn Memorial Hospital	Freeport	99%	299
Gibson Community Hospital	Gibson City	99%	148
Holy Cross Hospital[2]	Chicago	99%	95
Katherine Shaw Bethea Hospital	Dixon	99%	184
Little Company of Mary Hospital[2]	Evergreen Park	99%	251
Memorial Hospital[2]	Belleville	99%	406
Memorial Medical Center[2]	Springfield	99%	453
Mercy Hospital & Medical Center	Chicago	99%	325
Midwestern Region Medical Center[2]	Zion	99%	71
Northwest Community Hospital[2]	Arlington Hgts	99%	438
Northwestern Memorial Hospital[2]	Chicago	99%	468
Palos Community Hospital[2]	Palos Heights	99%	483
Presence Mercy Medical Center[2]	Aurora	99%	346
Presence Our Lady of the Res Med Ctr	Chicago	99%	120
Presence Saint Francis Hospital[2]	Evanston	99%	310
Presence Saint Marys Hospital	Kankakee	99%	227
Presence United Samaritans Medical Center	Danville	99%	163
Rockford Memorial Hospital	Rockford	99%	575
Saint Alexius Medical Center[2]	Hoffman Estates	99%	320
Saint Anthonys Memorial Hospital	Effingham	99%	654
Saint Elizabeth Hospital	Belleville	99%	373
Saint Francis Medical Center[2]	Peoria	99%	1103
Saint Johns Hospital[2]	Springfield	99%	492
Saint Marys Hospital	Centralia	99%	86
Silver Cross Hospital & Medical Centers[2]	New Lenox	99%	550
Swedish American Hospital[2]	Rockford	99%	925
Swedish Covenant Hospital[2]	Chicago	99%	356
Trinity Rock Island[2]	Rock Island	99%	347
West Suburban Medical Center[2]	Oak Park	99%	296
Westlake Community Hospital[2]	Melrose Park	99%	67
Galesburg Cottage Hospital	Galesburg	98%	119
Graham Hospital Association[2]	Canton	98%	146
Lake Forest Hospital	Lake Forest	98%	702
Mount Sinai Hospital Medical Center[2]	Chicago	98%	207
Passavant Area Hospital[2]	Jacksonville	98%	170
Pekin Memorial Hospital	Pekin	98%	211
Presence Saint Joseph Medical Center[2]	Joliet	98%	508
Proctor Hospital[2]	Peoria	98%	256
Rush Oak Park Hospital	Oak Park	98%	163
Saint Anthony Hospital	Chicago	98%	45
Adventist Bolingbrook Hospital	Bolingbrook	97%	92
Hammond Henry Hospital	Geneseo	97%	118
John H Stroger Jr Hospital[2]	Chicago	97%	310
McDonough District Hospital	Macomb	97%	64
Memorial Hospital	Chester	97%	30
Provident Hospital of Chicago[2]	Chicago	97%	76
Saint Marys Hospital	Decatur	97%	221
Iroquois Memorial Hospital	Watseka	96%	25
Norwegian - American Hospital	Chicago	96%	27
University of Illinois Hospital[2]	Chicago	96%	393
Loyola Gottlieb Memorial Hospital[2]	Melrose Park	95%	262
Thorek Memorial Hospital	Chicago	95%	38
Touchette Regional Hospital	Centreville	94%	35
Crawford Memorial Hospital[3]	Robinson	92%	37
South Shore Hospital	Chicago	92%	39

Prophylactic Antibiotic Selection (Outpatient)

Hospital Name	City	Rate	Cases
Adventist La Grange Memorial Hospital	La Grange	100%	94
Advocate Good Shepherd Hospital	Barrington	100%	368
Alton Memorial Hospital	Alton	100%	133
Copley Memorial Hospital	Aurora	100%	435
Crossroads Community Hospital	Mount Vernon	100%	108
Decatur Memorial Hospital	Decatur	100%	334
Elmhurst Memorial Hospital	Elmhurst	100%	351
Gateway Regional Medical Center	Granite City	100%	133
Hinsdale Hospital	Hinsdale	100%	370
Illinois Valley Community Hospital	Peru	100%	57
Ingalls Memorial Hospital	Harvey	100%	164
Jersey Community Hospital	Jerseyville	100%	26
Katherine Shaw Bethea Hospital	Dixon	100%	145
Kishwaukee Community Hospital	Dekalb	100%	112
Metrosouth Medical Center	Blue Island	100%	135
Mount Sinai Hospital Medical Center	Chicago	100%	181
Ottawa Reg Hosp & Healthcare Ctr	Ottawa	100%	43
Palos Community Hospital	Palos Heights	100%	220
Pekin Memorial Hospital	Pekin	100%	47
Presence United Samaritans Medical Center	Danville	100%	43
Saint Marys Hospital	Centralia	100%	46
Saint Marys Hospital	Streator	100%	37
Advocate Condell Medical Center	Libertyville	99%	456
Advocate Good Samaritan Hospital	Downers Grove	99%	354
Advocate Illinois Masonic Medical Center	Chicago	99%	470
Advocate Lutheran General Hospital	Park Ridge	99%	683
Advocate Trinity Hospital	Chicago	99%	80
Anderson Hospital	Maryville	99%	319
Centegra Health Sys-Mc Henry Hosp	Mchenry	99%	125
Evanston Hospital	Evanston	99%	857
Fhn Memorial Hospital	Freeport	99%	140
Heartland Regional Medical Center	Marion	99%	78
Lake Forest Hospital	Lake Forest	99%	190
Memorial Hospital	Belleville	99%	394
Memorial Hospital of Carbondale	Carbondale	99%	444
Methodist Medical Center of Illinois	Peoria	99%	383
Morris Hospital & Healthcare Centers	Morris	99%	148
Northwest Community Hospital	Arlington Hgts	99%	483
Passavant Area Hospital	Jacksonville	99%	82
Presence Covenant Medical Center	Urbana	99%	323
Presence Our Lady of the Res Med Ctr	Chicago	99%	106
Presence Sts Mary & Elizabeth Med Ctr	Chicago	99%	137
Rush University Medical Center	Chicago	99%	420
Saint Alexius Medical Center	Hoffman Estates	99%	429
Saint Anthony's Health Center	Alton	99%	105
Saint Elizabeth Hospital	Belleville	99%	205
Saint Francis Medical Center	Peoria	99%	565
Saint Marys Hospital	Decatur	99%	155
Sherman Hospital	Elgin	99%	269
Swedish American Hospital	Rockford	99%	439
The University of Chicago Medical Center	Chicago	99%	517
Vista Medical Center East	Waukegan	99%	210
Advocate Bromenn Medical Center	Normal	98%	379
Advocate South Suburban Hospital	Hazel Crest	98%	178
Blessing Hospital	Quincy	98%	268
Carle Foundation Hospital	Urbana	98%	400
Central Dupage Hospital	Winfield	98%	423
Edward Hospital	Naperville	98%	588
Louis A Weiss Memorial Hospital	Chicago	98%	196
Loyola University Medical Center	Maywood	98%	523
Memorial Medical Center	Springfield	98%	696
Presence Mercy Medical Center	Aurora	98%	122
Riverside Medical Center	Kankakee	98%	330
Saint Johns Hospital	Springfield	98%	578
Silver Cross Hospital & Medical Centers	New Lenox	98%	556
Swedish Covenant Hospital	Chicago	98%	168
CGH Medical Center	Sterling	97%	123
Good Samaritan Regional Health Center	Mount Vernon	97%	355
Little Company of Mary Hospital	Evergreen Park	97%	218
Loyola Gottlieb Memorial Hospital	Melrose Park	97%	94
Mercy Hospital & Medical Center	Chicago	97%	112
Northwestern Memorial Hospital	Chicago	97%	571
Presence Saint Joseph Hospital - Chicago	Chicago	97%	192
Presence Saint Joseph Hospital - Elgin	Elgin	97%	104
Presence Saint Marys Hospital	Kankakee	97%	126
Rockford Memorial Hospital	Rockford	97%	267
Saint Anthony Hospital	Chicago	97%	63
Saint Joseph Medical Center	Bloomington	97%	188
Touchette Regional Hospital	Centreville	97%	33
Advocate Christ Hospital & Medical Center	Oak Lawn	96%	583
Alexian Brothers Medical Center	Elk Grove Vlg	96%	425
Franciscan Saint James Health	Olympia Fields	96%	232
Galesburg Cottage Hospital	Galesburg	96%	76
Genesis Health System	Silvis	96%	83
Graham Hospital Association	Canton	96%	46
Iroquois Memorial Hospital	Watseka	96%	56
McDonough District Hospital	Macomb	96%	68
Presence Resurrection Medical Center	Chicago	96%	254
Presence Saint Joseph Medical Center	Joliet	96%	367
Saint Anthony Medical Center	Rockford	96%	427
Saint Mary Medical Center	Galesburg	96%	53
Centegra Health Sys-Woodstock Hosp	Woodstock	95%	44
Proctor Hospital	Peoria	95%	128
Sarah Bush Lincoln Health Center	Mattoon	95%	74
Trinity Rock Island	Rock Island	95%	440
University of Illinois Hospital	Chicago	95%	251
Adventist Bolingbrook Hospital	Bolingbrook	94%	79
Westlake Community Hospital	Melrose Park	94%	68
Fairfield Memorial Hospital	Fairfield	92%	37
Rush Oak Park Hospital	Oak Park	92%	25
Holy Cross Hospital	Chicago	91%	44
John H Stroger Jr Hospital	Chicago	90%	188
Macneal Hospital	Berwyn	90%	357
Presence Saint Francis Hospital	Evanston	89%	62
Delnor Community Hospital	Geneva	87%	159
Adventist Glenoaks	Glendale Hghts	85%	26
Saint Anthonys Memorial Hospital	Effingham	85%	85
West Suburban Medical Center	Oak Park	84%	152
Midwestern Region Medical Center	Zion	75%	55

Prophylactic Antibiotic Stopped

Hospital Name	City	Rate	Cases
Abraham Lincoln Memorial Hospital	Lincoln	100%	94
Adventist Glenoaks[2]	Glendale Hghts	100%	61
Advocate Condell Medical Center[2]	Libertyville	100%	451
Advocate Good Shepherd Hospital[2]	Barrington	100%	410
Advocate Illinois Masonic Medical Center[2]	Chicago	100%	418
Advocate South Suburban Hospital[2]	Hazel Crest	100%	326
Blessing Hospital	Quincy	100%	324
Crawford Memorial Hospital[3]	Robinson	100%	36
Evanston Hospital[2]	Evanston	100%	575
Fhn Memorial Hospital	Freeport	100%	285
Genesis Health System[2]	Silvis	100%	211
Herrin Hospital	Herrin	100%	319
Illinois Valley Community Hospital	Peru	100%	222
Ingalls Memorial Hospital[2]	Harvey	100%	285
Jesse Brown VA Med Ctr-VA Chicago	Chicago	100%	74
Little Company of Mary Hospital[2]	Evergreen Park	100%	237
Memorial Hospital	Chester	100%	29
Methodist Hospital of Chicago	Chicago	100%	28
Morris Hospital & Healthcare Centers	Morris	100%	176
North Chicago VA Medical Center	North Chicago	100%	59
Norwegian - American Hospital	Chicago	100%	27
Presence Sts Mary & Elizabeth Med Ctr[2]	Chicago	100%	318
Rush Oak Park Hospital	Oak Park	100%	158
Saint Anthony Hospital	Chicago	100%	37
Saint James Hospital	Pontiac	100%	107
Saint Joseph's Hospital	Breese	100%	48
Saint Joseph's Hospital	Highland	100%	54
Saint Margarets Hospital	Spring Valley	100%	242
Sherman Hospital	Elgin	100%	789
Swedish Covenant Hospital[2]	Chicago	100%	336
Vista Medical Center East	Waukegan	100%	272
Adventist Bolingbrook Hospital	Bolingbrook	99%	90
Adventist La Grange Memorial Hospital[2]	La Grange	99%	234
Advocate Bromenn Medical Center[2]	Normal	99%	577
Advocate Christ Hospital & Medical Center[2]	Oak Lawn	99%	521
Advocate Good Samaritan Hospital[2]	Downers Grove	99%	438
Advocate Lutheran General Hospital[2]	Park Ridge	99%	453
CGH Medical Center[2]	Sterling	99%	298
Copley Memorial Hospital[2]	Aurora	99%	695
Decatur Memorial Hospital[2]	Decatur	99%	423
Delnor Community Hospital[2]	Geneva	99%	277
Franciscan Saint James Health[2]	Olympia Fields	99%	346
Gateway Regional Medical Center	Granite City	99%	175
Hines VA Medical Center	Hines	99%	182
Hinsdale Hospital[2]	Hinsdale	99%	261
Kishwaukee Community Hospital	Dekalb	99%	314
Lake Forest Hospital	Lake Forest	99%	700
Louis A Weiss Memorial Hospital[2]	Chicago	99%	292
Macneal Hospital[2]	Berwyn	99%	449
Methodist Medical Center of Illinois[2]	Peoria	99%	602
Metrosouth Medical Center	Blue Island	99%	251
Presence Saint Joseph Hospital - Chicago[2]	Chicago	99%	279
Presence Saint Joseph Hospital - Elgin[2]	Elgin	99%	268
Provident Hospital of Chicago[2]	Chicago	99%	76
Saint Anthony Medical Center[2]	Rockford	99%	710
Saint Anthony's Health Center	Alton	99%	89
Saint Anthonys Memorial Hospital	Effingham	99%	649
Saint Elizabeth Hospital	Belleville	99%	359
Saint Francis Medical Center[2]	Peoria	99%	1075
Saint Joseph Medical Center	Bloomington	99%	473
Saint Mary Medical Center	Galesburg	99%	209
Silver Cross Hospital & Medical Centers[2]	New Lenox	99%	534
West Suburban Medical Center[2]	Oak Park	99%	289
Alexian Brothers Medical Center[2]	Elk Grove Vlg	98%	445
Alton Memorial Hospital[2]	Alton	98%	173
Carle Foundation Hospital[2]	Urbana	98%	406
Centegra Health Sys-Mc Henry Hosp[2]	Mchenry	98%	532
Centegra Health Sys-Woodstock Hosp[2]	Woodstock	98%	387
Crossroads Community Hospital	Mount Vernon	98%	104
Elmhurst Memorial Hospital[2]	Elmhurst	98%	348
Gibson Community Hospital	Gibson City	98%	145
Good Samaritan Regional Health Center	Mount Vernon	98%	294
Hammond Henry Hospital	Geneseo	98%	116
Katherine Shaw Bethea Hospital	Dixon	98%	160
Loyola Gottlieb Memorial Hospital[2]	Melrose Park	98%	258
Loyola University Medical Center[2]	Maywood	98%	364
Memorial Medical Center[2]	Springfield	98%	443
Midwestern Region Medical Center[2]	Zion	98%	65

NOTE: Hospital profiles are in alphabetical order by state, then city, then hospital within the city; Rankings exclude hospitals with less than 25 cases except for patient surveys which excludes hospitals with less than 100 cases; (a) 100-299 cases; (1) The number of cases/patients is too few to report; (2) Data submitted were based on a sample of cases/patients; (3) Results are based on a shorter time period than required; (4) Data suppressed by CMS for one or more quarters; (5) Results are not available for this reporting period; (6) Fewer than 100 patients completed the HCAHPS survey; (7) No cases met the criteria for this measure; (8) The lower limit of the confidence interval cannot be calculated if the number of observed infections equals zero; (9) No data are available from the state/territory for this reporting period; (10) The scores shown reflect fewer than 50 completed surveys; (11) There were discrepancies in the data collection process; (12) This measure does not apply to this hospital for this reporting period; (13) Results cannot be calculated for this reporting period; (14) The results for this state are combined with nearby states to protect confidentiality; Please refer to the User's Guide for a full explanation of data.

Hospital Name	City	Rate	Cases
Northwestern Memorial Hospital[2]	Chicago	98%	449
Ottawa Reg Hosp & Healthcare Ctr	Ottawa	98%	54
Palos Community Hospital[2]	Palos Heights	98%	472
Pekin Memorial Hospital	Pekin	98%	207
Presence Covenant Medical Center[2]	Urbana	98%	339
Presence Mercy Medical Center[2]	Aurora	98%	331
Presence Resurrection Medical Center[2]	Chicago	98%	449
Presence United Samaritans Medical Center	Danville	98%	162
Richland Memorial Hospital[2]	Olney	98%	56
Riverside Medical Center[2]	Kankakee	98%	430
Rush University Medical Center[2]	Chicago	98%	410
Saint Alexius Medical Center[2]	Hoffman Estates	98%	310
Saint Johns Hospital[2]	Springfield	98%	483
Saint Marys Hospital	Centralia	98%	80
Saint Marys Hospital	Decatur	98%	219
Sarah Bush Lincoln Health Center	Mattoon	98%	398
Swedish American Hospital[2]	Rockford	98%	916
The University of Chicago Medical Center[2]	Chicago	98%	372
University of Illinois Hospital[2]	Chicago	98%	374
Anderson Hospital[2]	Maryville	97%	268
Edward Hospital[2]	Naperville	97%	449
Graham Hospital Association[2]	Canton	97%	145
John H Stroger Jr Hospital[2]	Chicago	97%	304
McDonough District Hospital	Macomb	97%	63
Memorial Hospital[2]	Belleville	97%	391
Memorial Hospital of Carbondale	Carbondale	97%	641
Presence Our Lady of the Res Med Ctr	Chicago	97%	108
Presence Saint Francis Hospital[2]	Evanston	97%	304
Presence Saint Joseph Medical Center[2]	Joliet	97%	485
Rockford Memorial Hospital	Rockford	97%	555
South Shore Hospital	Chicago	97%	38
Thorek Memorial Hospital	Chicago	97%	37
Advocate Trinity Hospital[2]	Chicago	96%	207
Central Dupage Hospital[2]	Winfield	96%	413
Heartland Regional Medical Center	Marion	96%	186
Mercy Hospital & Medical Center	Chicago	96%	311
Mount Sinai Hospital Medical Center[2]	Chicago	96%	198
Northwest Community Hospital[2]	Arlington Hgts	96%	409
Passavant Area Hospital[2]	Jacksonville	96%	156
Trinity Rock Island[2]	Rock Island	96%	341
Holy Cross Hospital[2]	Chicago	95%	93
Proctor Hospital[2]	Peoria	95%	254
Westlake Community Hospital[2]	Melrose Park	95%	62
Paris Community Hospital	Paris	94%	50
Presence Saint Marys Hospital	Kankakee	94%	216
Saint Marys Hospital	Streator	94%	62
Touchette Regional Hospital	Centreville	94%	33
Wabash General Hospital	Mount Carmel	94%	120
Galesburg Cottage Hospital	Galesburg	93%	115

Prophylactic Antibiotic Timing

Hospital Name	City	Rate	Cases
Adventist Bolingbrook Hospital	Bolingbrook	100%	92
Adventist Glenoaks[2]	Glendale Hghts	100%	66
Advocate Bromenn Medical Center[2]	Normal	100%	580
Advocate Christ Hospital & Medical Center[2]	Oak Lawn	100%	538
Advocate Good Samaritan Hospital[2]	Downers Grove	100%	456
Advocate Illinois Masonic Medical Center[2]	Chicago	100%	439
Advocate Lutheran General Hospital[2]	Park Ridge	100%	466
Advocate South Suburban Hospital[2]	Hazel Crest	100%	337
Advocate Trinity Hospital[2]	Chicago	100%	218
Alexian Brothers Medical Center[2]	Elk Grove Vlg	100%	468
Blessing Hospital	Quincy	100%	355
Centegra Health Sys-Mc Henry Hosp[2]	Mchenry	100%	542
Copley Memorial Hospital[2]	Aurora	100%	715
Crossroads Community Hospital	Mount Vernon	100%	106
Fhn Memorial Hospital	Freeport	100%	300
Genesis Health System[2]	Silvis	100%	215
Heartland Regional Medical Center	Marion	100%	200
Hinsdale Hospital[2]	Hinsdale	100%	270
Ingalls Memorial Hospital[2]	Harvey	100%	304
Iroquois Memorial Hospital	Watseka	100%	25
Little Company of Mary Hospital[2]	Evergreen Park	100%	251
Louis A Weiss Memorial Hospital[2]	Chicago	100%	313
Macneal Hospital[2]	Berwyn	100%	469
Methodist Medical Center of Illinois[2]	Peoria	100%	615
Metrosouth Medical Center	Blue Island	100%	258
Morris Hospital & Healthcare Centers	Morris	100%	178
North Chicago VA Medical Center	North Chicago	100%	60
Ottawa Reg Hosp & Healthcare Ctr	Ottawa	100%	61
Palos Community Hospital[2]	Palos Heights	100%	483
Pekin Memorial Hospital	Pekin	100%	211
Presence Covenant Medical Center[2]	Urbana	100%	350
Presence Resurrection Medical Center[2]	Chicago	100%	464
Presence Saint Francis Hospital[2]	Evanston	100%	310
Presence Saint Joseph Medical Center[2]	Joliet	100%	509
Presence Sts Mary & Elizabeth Med Ctr[2]	Chicago	100%	341
Presence United Samaritans Medical Center	Danville	100%	163
Provident Hospital of Chicago[2]	Chicago	100%	76
Riverside Medical Center[2]	Kankakee	100%	443
Rush University Medical Center[2]	Chicago	100%	426
Saint Alexius Medical Center[2]	Hoffman Estates	100%	320
Saint Anthony Hospital	Chicago	100%	46
Saint Anthony's Health Center	Alton	100%	95
Saint Anthonys Memorial Hospital	Effingham	100%	654
Saint Elizabeth Hospital	Belleville	100%	373
Saint James Hospital	Pontiac	100%	109
Saint Joseph Medical Center	Bloomington	100%	491
Saint Joseph's Hospital	Highland	100%	56
Saint Margarets Hospital	Spring Valley	100%	249
Saint Marys Hospital	Streator	100%	63
Sherman Hospital	Elgin	100%	812
Swedish American Hospital[2]	Rockford	100%	925
Vista Medical Center East	Waukegan	100%	273
Westlake Community Hospital[2]	Melrose Park	100%	67
Advocate Condell Medical Center[2]	Libertyville	99%	476
Advocate Good Shepherd Hospital[2]	Barrington	99%	420
Carle Foundation Hospital[2]	Urbana	99%	410
Centegra Health Sys-Woodstock Hosp[2]	Woodstock	99%	390
CGH Medical Center[2]	Sterling	99%	304
Decatur Memorial Hospital[2]	Decatur	99%	428
Edward Hospital[2]	Naperville	99%	460
Elmhurst Memorial Hospital[2]	Elmhurst	99%	356
Evanston Hospital[2]	Evanston	99%	586
Franciscan Saint James Health[2]	Olympia Fields	99%	385
Galesburg Cottage Hospital	Galesburg	99%	119
Good Samaritan Regional Health Center	Mount Vernon	99%	313
Hammond Henry Hospital	Geneseo	99%	119
Herrin Hospital	Herrin	99%	330
Katherine Shaw Bethea Hospital	Dixon	99%	184
Kishwaukee Community Hospital	Dekalb	99%	321
Loyola University Medical Center[2]	Maywood	99%	372
Memorial Hospital[2]	Belleville	99%	406
Memorial Hospital of Carbondale	Carbondale	99%	659
Mercy Hospital & Medical Center	Chicago	99%	325
Mount Sinai Hospital Medical Center[2]	Chicago	99%	208
Presence Mercy Medical Center[2]	Aurora	99%	348
Presence Our Lady of the Res Med Ctr	Chicago	99%	120
Presence Saint Joseph Hospital - Chicago[2]	Chicago	99%	281
Presence Saint Joseph Hospital - Elgin[2]	Elgin	99%	279
Presence Saint Marys Hospital	Kankakee	99%	226
Rockford Memorial Hospital	Rockford	99%	575
Saint Anthony Medical Center[2]	Rockford	99%	724
Saint Francis Medical Center[2]	Peoria	99%	1103
Saint Johns Hospital[2]	Springfield	99%	493
Saint Marys Hospital	Centralia	99%	86
Saint Marys Hospital	Decatur	99%	223
Sarah Bush Lincoln Health Center	Mattoon	99%	420
Silver Cross Hospital & Medical Centers[2]	New Lenox	99%	551
Swedish Covenant Hospital[2]	Chicago	99%	356
Trinity Rock Island[2]	Rock Island	99%	347
The University of Chicago Medical Center[2]	Chicago	99%	395
University of Illinois Hospital[2]	Chicago	99%	394
Wabash General Hospital	Mount Carmel	99%	121
West Suburban Medical Center[2]	Oak Park	99%	296
Adventist La Grange Memorial Hospital[2]	La Grange	98%	248
Alton Memorial Hospital[2]	Alton	98%	187
Anderson Hospital[2]	Maryville	98%	272
Gateway Regional Medical Center	Granite City	98%	177
Hines VA Medical Center	Hines	98%	188
Illinois Valley Community Hospital	Peru	98%	223
Lake Forest Hospital	Lake Forest	98%	703
Loyola Gottlieb Memorial Hospital[2]	Melrose Park	98%	265
Memorial Medical Center[2]	Springfield	98%	453
Northwest Community Hospital[2]	Arlington Hgts	98%	439
Rush Oak Park Hospital	Oak Park	98%	163
Saint Mary Medical Center	Galesburg	98%	222
Abraham Lincoln Memorial Hospital	Lincoln	97%	95
Crawford Memorial Hospital[3]	Robinson	97%	37
Delnor Community Hospital[2]	Geneva	97%	279
Graham Hospital Association[2]	Canton	97%	146
Methodist Hospital of Chicago	Chicago	97%	29
Midwestern Region Medical Center[2]	Zion	97%	71
Passavant Area Hospital[2]	Jacksonville	97%	170
Proctor Hospital[2]	Peoria	97%	256
Thorek Memorial Hospital	Chicago	97%	38
Gibson Community Hospital	Gibson City	96%	148
Jesse Brown VA Med Ctr-VA Chicago	Chicago	96%	76
John H Stroger Jr Hospital[2]	Chicago	96%	313
Northwestern Memorial Hospital[2]	Chicago	96%	470
Richland Memorial Hospital[2]	Olney	96%	56
Saint Joseph's Hospital	Breese	96%	48
Central Dupage Hospital[2]	Winfield	95%	420
Paris Community Hospital	Paris	94%	51
Holy Cross Hospital[2]	Chicago	93%	95
Memorial Hospital	Chester	93%	30
McDonough District Hospital	Macomb	92%	64
Touchette Regional Hospital	Centreville	89%	35
South Shore Hospital	Chicago	87%	39
Norwegian - American Hospital	Chicago	85%	27

Prophylactic Antibiotic Timing (Outpatient)

Hospital Name	City	Rate	Cases
Advocate Good Samaritan Hospital	Downers Grove	100%	355
Advocate Good Shepherd Hospital	Barrington	100%	368
Advocate Lutheran General Hospital	Park Ridge	100%	683
Alton Memorial Hospital	Alton	100%	133
Crossroads Community Hospital	Mount Vernon	100%	81
Fairfield Memorial Hospital	Fairfield	100%	36
Galesburg Cottage Hospital	Galesburg	100%	76
Gateway Regional Medical Center	Granite City	100%	133
Genesis Health System	Silvis	100%	83
Graham Hospital Association	Canton	100%	46
Heartland Regional Medical Center	Marion	100%	78
Hinsdale Hospital	Hinsdale	100%	370
Louis A Weiss Memorial Hospital	Chicago	100%	182
Methodist Medical Center of Illinois	Peoria	100%	381
Metrosouth Medical Center	Blue Island	100%	135
Mount Sinai Hospital Medical Center	Chicago	100%	71
Riverside Medical Center	Kankakee	100%	331
Saint Alexius Medical Center	Hoffman Estates	100%	423
Saint Anthony's Health Center	Alton	100%	105
Saint Mary Medical Center	Galesburg	100%	53
Saint Marys Hospital	Streator	100%	37
Sherman Hospital	Elgin	100%	184
Vista Medical Center East	Waukegan	100%	208
Adventist La Grange Memorial Hospital	La Grange	99%	95
Advocate Condell Medical Center	Libertyville	99%	457
Advocate Illinois Masonic Medical Center	Chicago	99%	428
Anderson Hospital	Maryville	99%	321
Blessing Hospital	Quincy	99%	269
Centegra Health Sys-Mc Henry Hosp	Mchenry	99%	122
Decatur Memorial Hospital	Decatur	99%	334
Elmhurst Memorial Hospital	Elmhurst	99%	251
Fhn Memorial Hospital	Freeport	99%	79
Ingalls Memorial Hospital	Harvey	99%	165
Kishwaukee Community Hospital	Dekalb	99%	112
Memorial Hospital	Belleville	99%	394
Northwest Community Hospital	Arlington Hgts	99%	471
Palos Community Hospital	Palos Heights	99%	220
Passavant Area Hospital	Jacksonville	99%	81
Presence Our Lady of the Res Med Ctr	Chicago	99%	104
Presence Saint Joseph Hospital - Chicago	Chicago	99%	192
Presence Saint Joseph Medical Center	Joliet	99%	370
Rockford Memorial Hospital	Rockford	99%	269
Saint Anthony Medical Center	Rockford	99%	428
Saint Joseph Medical Center	Bloomington	99%	190
Saint Marys Hospital	Decatur	99%	156
Swedish American Hospital	Rockford	99%	440
Swedish Covenant Hospital	Chicago	99%	168
Adventist Bolingbrook Hospital	Bolingbrook	98%	81
Advocate Bromenn Medical Center	Normal	98%	379
Advocate South Suburban Hospital	Hazel Crest	98%	178
Alexian Brothers Medical Center	Elk Grove Vlg	98%	424
Centegra Health Sys-Woodstock Hosp	Woodstock	98%	44
Copley Memorial Hospital	Aurora	98%	437
Evanston Hospital	Evanston	98%	778
Franciscan Saint James Health	Olympia Fields	98%	202
Good Samaritan Regional Health Center	Mount Vernon	98%	358
Loyola Gottlieb Memorial Hospital	Melrose Park	98%	94
Loyola University Medical Center	Maywood	98%	400
Midwestern Region Medical Center	Zion	98%	56
Morris Hospital & Healthcare Centers	Morris	98%	142
Ottawa Reg Hosp & Healthcare Ctr	Ottawa	98%	43
Presence Covenant Medical Center	Urbana	98%	326
Presence Mercy Medical Center	Aurora	98%	123
Presence Saint Marys Hospital	Kankakee	98%	124
Rush University Medical Center	Chicago	98%	421
Saint Francis Medical Center	Peoria	98%	565
Saint Marys Hospital	Centralia	98%	45
Trinity Rock Island	Rock Island	98%	445
The University of Chicago Medical Center	Chicago	98%	287
Edward Hospital	Naperville	97%	589
Iroquois Memorial Hospital	Watseka	97%	58
Little Company of Mary Hospital	Evergreen Park	97%	218
Memorial Hospital of Carbondale	Carbondale	97%	453
Memorial Medical Center	Springfield	97%	705
Proctor Hospital	Peoria	97%	130
Saint Elizabeth Hospital	Belleville	97%	211
Saint Johns Hospital	Springfield	97%	585
Silver Cross Hospital & Medical Centers	New Lenox	97%	559
Adventist Glenoaks	Glendale Hghts	96%	26
Mercy Hospital & Medical Center	Chicago	96%	114
Pekin Memorial Hospital	Pekin	96%	46
Presence United Samaritans Medical Center	Danville	96%	45
Westlake Community Hospital	Melrose Park	96%	70
Advocate Trinity Hospital	Chicago	95%	82
Carle Foundation Hospital	Urbana	95%	363
John H Stroger Jr Hospital	Chicago	95%	193
Lake Forest Hospital	Lake Forest	95%	188
Presence Resurrection Medical Center	Chicago	95%	259

NOTE: Hospital profiles are in alphabetical order by state, then city, then hospital within the city; Rankings exclude hospitals with less than 25 cases except for patient surveys which excludes hospitals with less than 100 cases; (a) 100-299 cases; (1) The number of cases/patients is too few to report; (2) Data submitted were based on a sample of cases/patients; (3) Results are based on a shorter time period than required; (4) Data suppressed by CMS for one or more quarters; (5) Results are not available for this reporting period; (6) Fewer than 100 patients completed the HCAHPS survey; (7) No cases met the criteria for this measure; (8) The lower limit of the confidence interval cannot be calculated if the number of observed infections equals zero; (9) No data are available from the state/territory for this reporting period; (10) The scores shown reflect fewer than 50 completed surveys; (11) There were discrepancies in the data collection process; (12) This measure does not apply to this hospital for this reporting period; (13) Results cannot be calculated for this reporting period; (14) The results for this state are combined with nearby states to protect confidentiality; Please refer to the User's Guide for a full explanation of data.

Hospital Name	City	Rate	Cases
Saint Anthony Hospital	Chicago	95%	65
Saint Anthonys Memorial Hospital	Effingham	95%	87
Sarah Bush Lincoln Health Center	Mattoon	95%	75
Advocate Christ Hospital & Medical Center	Oak Lawn	94%	586
Katherine Shaw Bethea Hospital	Dixon	94%	80
Northwestern Memorial Hospital	Chicago	94%	591
Presence Sts Mary & Elizabeth Med Ctr	Chicago	94%	145
University of Illinois Hospital	Chicago	94%	196
Central Dupage Hospital	Winfield	93%	439
Illinois Valley Community Hospital	Peru	93%	58
Holy Cross Hospital	Chicago	91%	46
McDonough District Hospital	Macomb	89%	72
CGH Medical Center	Sterling	88%	92
Macneal Hospital	Berwyn	88%	380
Presence Saint Joseph Hospital - Elgin	Elgin	88%	74
Rush Oak Park Hospital	Oak Park	88%	26
Delnor Community Hospital	Geneva	86%	165
Presence Saint Francis Hospital	Evanston	73%	66
Norwegian - American Hospital	Chicago	72%	29
West Suburban Medical Center	Oak Park	71%	176

Urinary Catheter Removal

Hospital Name	City	Rate	Cases
Abraham Lincoln Memorial Hospital	Lincoln	100%	67
Advocate Condell Medical Center[2]	Libertyville	100%	406
Advocate Illinois Masonic Medical Center[2]	Chicago	100%	223
Advocate Lutheran General Hospital[2]	Park Ridge	100%	304
Advocate South Suburban Hospital[2]	Hazel Crest	100%	263
Centegra Health Sys-Woodstock Hosp[2]	Woodstock	100%	374
Galesburg Cottage Hospital	Galesburg	100%	152
Gateway Regional Medical Center	Granite City	100%	111
Herrin Hospital	Herrin	100%	386
Hines VA Medical Center[2]	Hines	100%	233
Ingalls Memorial Hospital[2]	Harvey	100%	138
John H Stroger Jr Hospital[2]	Chicago	100%	208
Kishwaukee Community Hospital	Dekalb	100%	338
Louis A Weiss Memorial Hospital[2]	Chicago	100%	384
Macneal Hospital[2]	Berwyn	100%	457
Methodist Hospital of Chicago	Chicago	100%	34
Methodist Medical Center of Illinois[2]	Peoria	100%	537
Metrosouth Medical Center	Blue Island	100%	232
Midwestern Region Medical Center[2]	Zion	100%	40
Morris Hospital & Healthcare Centers	Morris	100%	200
Northwestern Memorial Hospital[2]	Chicago	100%	413
Ottawa Reg Hosp & Healthcare Ctr	Ottawa	100%	87
Presence Saint Joseph Hospital - Chicago[2]	Chicago	100%	92
Presence Saint Joseph Medical Center[2]	Joliet	100%	321
Presence Saint Marys Hospital	Kankakee	100%	219
Presence Sts Mary & Elizabeth Med Ctr[2]	Chicago	100%	189
Presence United Samaritans Medical Center	Danville	100%	111
Riverside Medical Center[2]	Kankakee	100%	353
Rush Oak Park Hospital	Oak Park	100%	211
Rush University Medical Center[2]	Chicago	100%	345
Saint Anthony Hospital	Chicago	100%	39
Saint Anthony's Health Center	Alton	100%	104
Saint Elizabeth Hospital	Belleville	100%	309
Saint James Hospital	Pontiac	100%	99
Saint Joseph's Hospital	Breese	100%	37
Saint Joseph's Hospital	Highland	100%	59
Saint Margarets Hospital	Spring Valley	100%	294
Saint Marys Hospital	Decatur	100%	211
Sherman Hospital	Elgin	100%	270
Trinity Rock Island[2]	Rock Island	100%	128
Valley West Community Hospital	Sandwich	100%	25
Vista Medical Center East	Waukegan	100%	199
Adventist La Grange Memorial Hospital[2]	La Grange	99%	225
Advocate Good Samaritan Hospital[2]	Downers Grove	99%	275
Advocate Good Shepherd Hospital[2]	Barrington	99%	386
Alexian Brothers Medical Center[2]	Elk Grove Vlg	99%	377
Alton Memorial Hospital[2]	Alton	99%	183
Blessing Hospital	Quincy	99%	270
Centegra Health Sys-Mc Henry Hosp[2]	Mchenry	99%	500
CGH Medical Center[2]	Sterling	99%	310
Copley Memorial Hospital[2]	Aurora	99%	556
Elmhurst Memorial Hospital[2]	Elmhurst	99%	318
Fhn Memorial Hospital	Freeport	99%	87
Franciscan Saint James Health[2]	Olympia Fields	99%	186
Illinois Valley Community Hospital	Peru	99%	206
Katherine Shaw Bethea Hospital	Dixon	99%	126
Little Company of Mary Hospital[2]	Evergreen Park	99%	194
Memorial Medical Center[2]	Springfield	99%	426
Mount Sinai Hospital Medical Center[2]	Chicago	99%	127
Pekin Memorial Hospital	Pekin	99%	184
Presence Covenant Medical Center[2]	Urbana	99%	372
Presence Resurrection Medical Center[2]	Chicago	99%	292
Presence Saint Joseph Hospital - Elgin[2]	Elgin	99%	205
Saint Marys Hospital	Centralia	99%	87
Sarah Bush Lincoln Health Center	Mattoon	99%	259
Swedish American Hospital[2]	Rockford	99%	367
Adventist Bolingbrook Hospital	Bolingbrook	98%	87
Adventist Glenoaks[2]	Glendale Hghts	98%	66
Advocate Bromenn Medical Center[2]	Normal	98%	162
Advocate Christ Hospital & Medical Center[2]	Oak Lawn	98%	314
Genesis Health System[2]	Silvis	98%	45
Gibson Community Hospital	Gibson City	98%	163
Good Samaritan Regional Health Center	Mount Vernon	98%	160
Jesse Brown VA Med Ctr-VA Chicago[2]	Chicago	98%	107
Lake Forest Hospital	Lake Forest	98%	676
Loyola Gottlieb Memorial Hospital[2]	Melrose Park	98%	207
Loyola University Medical Center[2]	Maywood	98%	303
North Chicago VA Medical Center[2]	North Chicago	98%	51
Northwest Community Hospital[2]	Arlington Hgts	98%	358
Proctor Hospital[2]	Peoria	98%	237
Saint Anthony Medical Center[2]	Rockford	98%	195
Saint Francis Medical Center[2]	Peoria	98%	949
Saint Johns Hospital[2]	Springfield	98%	458
Saint Joseph Medical Center	Bloomington	98%	347
Saint Mary Medical Center	Galesburg	98%	247
Silver Cross Hospital & Medical Centers[2]	New Lenox	98%	476
The University of Chicago Medical Center[2]	Chicago	98%	315
Wabash General Hospital	Mount Carmel	98%	125
Evanston Hospital[2]	Evanston	97%	514
Memorial Hospital[2]	Belleville	97%	407
Memorial Hospital of Carbondale	Carbondale	97%	558
Mercy Harvard Hospital	Harvard	97%	32
Palos Community Hospital[2]	Palos Heights	97%	298
Presence Mercy Medical Center[2]	Aurora	97%	321
Presence Our Lady of the Res Med Ctr	Chicago	97%	110
Presence Saint Francis Hospital[2]	Evanston	97%	191
Saint Alexius Medical Center[2]	Hoffman Estates	97%	246
Swedish Covenant Hospital[2]	Chicago	97%	301
Carle Foundation Hospital[2]	Urbana	96%	260
Central Dupage Hospital[2]	Winfield	96%	286
Edward Hospital[2]	Naperville	96%	443
Heartland Regional Medical Center	Marion	96%	138
Hinsdale Hospital[2]	Hinsdale	96%	157
Memorial Hospital	Chester	96%	27
Saint Anthonys Memorial Hospital	Effingham	96%	283
University of Illinois Hospital[2]	Chicago	96%	287
Crossroads Community Hospital	Mount Vernon	95%	65
Decatur Memorial Hospital[2]	Decatur	95%	389
Mercy Hospital & Medical Center	Chicago	95%	254
Saint Marys Hospital	Streator	95%	60
Anderson Hospital[2]	Maryville	94%	154
West Suburban Medical Center[2]	Oak Park	93%	168
Iroquois Memorial Hospital	Watseka	92%	39
McDonough District Hospital	Macomb	92%	53
Paris Community Hospital	Paris	92%	48
Graham Hospital Association[2]	Canton	89%	129
Passavant Area Hospital[2]	Jacksonville	89%	76
Crawford Memorial Hospital[3]	Robinson	88%	25
Thorek Memorial Hospital	Chicago	87%	39
Delnor Community Hospital[2]	Geneva	86%	95
Rockford Memorial Hospital	Rockford	86%	290
Advocate Trinity Hospital[2]	Chicago	85%	79
Holy Cross Hospital[2]	Chicago	78%	72
Norwegian - American Hospital	Chicago	77%	26

Survey of Patients' Hospital Experiences

Area Around Room 'Always' Quiet at Night

Hospital Name	City	Rate	Cases
OSF Holy Family Medical Center	Monmouth	78%	(a)
Provident Hospital of Chicago	Chicago	78%	(a)
Saint Joseph's Hospital	Breese	77%	300+
Valley West Community Hospital	Sandwich	77%	(a)
Crossroads Community Hospital	Mount Vernon	73%	300+
Saint Joseph Memorial Hospital	Murphysboro	73%	(a)
Touchette Regional Hospital	Centreville	73%	(a)
Kewanee Hospital	Kewanee	72%	(a)
Massac Memorial Hospital	Metropolis	71%	(a)
Sparta Community Hospital	Sparta	71%	(a)
Rush University Medical Center	Chicago	70%	300+
Union County Hospital	Anna	70%	(a)
Adventist Bolingbrook Hospital[11]	Bolingbrook	69%	300+
Elmhurst Memorial Hospital	Elmhurst	69%	300+
Presence United Samaritans Medical Center	Danville	69%	300+
Gibson Community Hospital	Gibson City	68%	300+
Mendota Community Hospital	Mendota	68%	(a)
Sherman Hospital	Elgin	68%	300+
Central Dupage Hospital	Winfield	67%	300+
Presence Mercy Medical Center	Aurora	67%	300+
Presence Saint Marys Hospital	Kankakee	67%	300+
Rochelle Community Hospital	Rochelle	67%	(a)
Saint Francis Hospital	Litchfield	67%	300+
Saint Joseph's Hospital	Highland	67%	(a)
Saint Marys Hospital	Centralia	67%	300+
Silver Cross Hospital & Medical Centers	New Lenox	67%	300+
Wabash General Hospital	Mount Carmel	67%	(a)
Alton Memorial Hospital[11]	Alton	66%	300+
Richland Memorial Hospital	Olney	66%	300+
Rush Oak Park Hospital	Oak Park	66%	300+
Saint James Hospital	Pontiac	66%	(a)
Abraham Lincoln Memorial Hospital	Lincoln	65%	(a)
McDonough District Hospital	Macomb	65%	300+
Metrosouth Medical Center	Blue Island	65%	300+
Northwestern Memorial Hospital	Chicago	65%	300+
Saint Joseph Medical Center	Bloomington	65%	300+
Advocate Trinity Hospital	Chicago	64%	300+
Good Samaritan Regional Health Center	Mount Vernon	64%	300+
Hammond Henry Hospital	Geneseo	64%	300+
Hillsboro Area Hospital	Hillsboro	64%	(a)
Midwestern Region Medical Center	Zion	64%	300+
Red Bud Regional Hospital	Red Bud	64%	(a)
Saint Marys Hospital	Streator	64%	300+
Adventist La Grange Memorial Hospital[11]	La Grange	63%	300+
Jersey Community Hospital	Jerseyville	63%	(a)
Perry Memorial Hospital	Princeton	63%	(a)
Riverside Medical Center	Kankakee	63%	300+
Decatur Memorial Hospital	Decatur	62%	300+
Gateway Regional Medical Center	Granite City	62%	300+
Saint Anthony's Health Center	Alton	62%	300+
Saint Mary Medical Center	Galesburg	62%	300+
South Shore Hospital	Chicago	62%	(a)
Advocate Bromenn Medical Center	Normal	61%	300+
Anderson Hospital	Maryville	61%	300+
CGH Medical Center	Sterling	61%	300+
Little Company of Mary Hospital	Evergreen Park	61%	300+
Loretto Hospital	Chicago	61%	(a)
Memorial Hospital of Carbondale	Carbondale	61%	300+
Mercy Hospital & Medical Center	Chicago	61%	300+
Methodist Medical Center of Illinois	Peoria	61%	300+
Northwest Community Hospital	Arlington Hgts	61%	300+
Presence Saint Joseph Medical Center	Joliet	61%	300+
Proctor Hospital	Peoria	61%	300+
Saint Bernard Hospital	Chicago	61%	300+
Advocate Condell Medical Center	Libertyville	60%	300+
Fhn Memorial Hospital	Freeport	60%	300+
Harrisburg Medical Center	Harrisburg	60%	(a)
Kishwaukee Community Hospital	Dekalb	60%	300+
Morris Hospital & Healthcare Centers[11]	Morris	60%	(a)
Presence Covenant Medical Center	Urbana	60%	300+
Presence Saint Joseph Hospital - Elgin	Elgin	60%	300+
Roseland Community Hospital[3]	Chicago	60%	(a)
Saint Margarets Hospital	Spring Valley	60%	300+
Saint Marys Hospital	Decatur	60%	300+
Salem Township Hospital	Salem	60%	(a)
Advocate Lutheran General Hospital	Park Ridge	59%	300+
Galesburg Cottage Hospital	Galesburg	59%	300+
Herrin Hospital	Herrin	59%	300+
Hinsdale Hospital[11]	Hinsdale	59%	300+
Memorial Hospital	Belleville	59%	300+
Mount Sinai Hospital Medical Center	Chicago	59%	300+
Ottawa Reg Hosp & Healthcare Ctr	Ottawa	59%	300+
Saint Elizabeth Hospital	Belleville	59%	300+
Sarah Bush Lincoln Health Center	Mattoon	59%	300+
West Suburban Medical Center[11]	Oak Park	59%	300+
Greenville Regional Hospital	Greenville	58%	(a)
Holy Cross Hospital	Chicago	58%	300+
Katherine Shaw Bethea Hospital	Dixon	58%	300+
Presence Sts Mary & Elizabeth Med Ctr	Chicago	58%	300+
Thorek Memorial Hospital	Chicago	58%	(a)
University of Illinois Hospital	Chicago	58%	300+
Advocate Illinois Masonic Medical Center	Chicago	57%	300+
Alexian Brothers Medical Center	Elk Grove Vlg	57%	300+
Delnor Community Hospital	Geneva	57%	300+
Edward Hospital	Naperville	57%	300+
Ingalls Memorial Hospital	Harvey	57%	300+
Pinckneyville Community Hospital	Pinckneyville	57%	(a)
Presence Resurrection Medical Center	Chicago	57%	300+
Presence Saint Joseph Hospital - Chicago	Chicago	57%	300+
Rockford Memorial Hospital	Rockford	57%	300+
Advocate South Suburban Hospital	Hazel Crest	56%	300+
Crawford Memorial Hospital	Robinson	56%	(a)
Presence Saint Francis Hospital	Evanston	56%	300+
Saint Anthony Hospital	Chicago	56%	300+
Illinois Valley Community Hospital[11]	Peru	55%	300+
Passavant Area Hospital	Jacksonville	55%	300+
Saint Anthonys Memorial Hospital	Effingham	55%	300+
Advocate Christ Hospital & Medical Center	Oak Lawn	54%	300+
Copley Memorial Hospital	Aurora	54%	300+
Genesis Health System	Silvis	54%	300+
Iroquois Memorial Hospital	Watseka	54%	(a)
Louis A Weiss Memorial Hospital[11]	Chicago	54%	300+
Memorial Medical Center	Springfield	54%	300+
Swedish American Hospital	Rockford	54%	300+
Taylorville Memorial Hospital	Taylorville	54%	300+
Trinity Rock Island	Rock Island	54%	300+
The University of Chicago Medical Center	Chicago	54%	300+
Vista Medical Center East	Waukegan	54%	300+
Advocate Good Samaritan Hospital	Downers Grove	53%	300+
Blessing Hospital[11]	Quincy	53%	300+

NOTE: Hospital profiles are in alphabetical order by state, then city, then hospital within the city; Rankings exclude hospitals with less than 25 cases except for patient surveys which excludes hospitals with less than 100 cases; (a) 100-299 cases; (1) The number of cases/patients is too few to report; (2) Data submitted were based on a sample of cases/patients; (3) Results are based on a shorter time period than required; (4) Data suppressed by CMS for one or more quarters; (5) Results are not available for this reporting period; (6) Fewer than 100 patients completed the HCAHPS survey; (7) No cases met the criteria for this measure; (8) The lower limit of the confidence interval cannot be calculated if the number of observed infections equals zero; (9) No data are available from the state/territory for this reporting period; (10) The scores shown reflect fewer than 50 completed surveys; (11) There were discrepancies in the data collection process; (12) This measure does not apply to this hospital for this reporting period; (13) Results cannot be calculated for this reporting period; (14) The results for this state are combined with nearby states to protect confidentiality; Please refer to the User's Guide for a full explanation of data.

Carle Foundation Hospital[11]	Urbana	53%	300+
Evanston Hospital[11]	Evanston	53%	300+
Franciscan Saint James Health	Olympia Fields	53%	300+
Heartland Regional Medical Center	Marion	53%	300+
Saint Francis Medical Center	Peoria	53%	300+
Adventist Glenoaks[11]	Glendale Hghts	52%	300+
Centegra Health Sys-Woodstock Hosp	Woodstock	52%	300+
Graham Hospital Association	Canton	52%	300+
Lake Forest Hospital	Lake Forest	52%	300+
Norwegian - American Hospital	Chicago	52%	300+
Saint Alexius Medical Center	Hoffman Estates	52%	300+
Saint Johns Hospital	Springfield	52%	300+
John H Stroger Jr Hospital	Chicago	51%	300+
Loyola University Medical Center	Maywood	51%	300+
Macneal Hospital[11]	Berwyn	51%	300+
Advocate Good Shepherd Hospital	Barrington	50%	300+
Jackson Park Hospital	Chicago	50%	300+
Pekin Memorial Hospital	Pekin	50%	300+
Loyola Gottlieb Memorial Hospital	Melrose Park	49%	300+
Palos Community Hospital	Palos Heights	48%	300+
Swedish Covenant Hospital	Chicago	48%	300+
Centegra Health Sys-Mc Henry Hosp	Mchenry	47%	300+
Clay County Hospital	Flora	47%	(a)
Presence Our Lady of the Res Med Ctr	Chicago	47%	300+
Westlake Community Hospital[11]	Melrose Park	47%	300+
Saint Anthony Medical Center	Rockford	45%	300+

Doctors 'Always' Communicated Well

Hospital Name	City	Rate	Cases
OSF Holy Family Medical Center	Monmouth	93%	(a)
Hillsboro Area Hospital	Hillsboro	92%	(a)
Union County Hospital	Anna	91%	(a)
Abraham Lincoln Memorial Hospital	Lincoln	90%	(a)
Hammond Henry Hospital	Geneseo	90%	300+
Salem Township Hospital	Salem	90%	(a)
Rochelle Community Hospital	Rochelle	89%	(a)
Saint Joseph's Hospital	Highland	89%	(a)
Taylorville Memorial Hospital	Taylorville	89%	300+
Gibson Community Hospital	Gibson City	88%	300+
Massac Memorial Hospital	Metropolis	88%	(a)
Pinckneyville Community Hospital	Pinckneyville	88%	(a)
Saint Francis Hospital	Litchfield	88%	300+
Saint Joseph's Hospital	Breese	88%	300+
Saint Marys Hospital	Centralia	88%	300+
Wabash General Hospital	Mount Carmel	88%	(a)
Crawford Memorial Hospital	Robinson	87%	(a)
Richland Memorial Hospital	Olney	87%	300+
Saint Mary Medical Center	Galesburg	87%	300+
Sarah Bush Lincoln Health Center	Mattoon	87%	300+
Valley West Community Hospital	Sandwich	87%	(a)
Graham Hospital Association	Canton	86%	300+
Presence Saint Marys Hospital	Kankakee	86%	300+
Red Bud Regional Hospital	Red Bud	86%	(a)
Saint Joseph Memorial Hospital	Murphysboro	86%	(a)
Saint Margarets Hospital	Spring Valley	86%	300+
Saint Marys Hospital	Streator	86%	300+
Anderson Hospital	Maryville	85%	300+
Illinois Valley Community Hospital[11]	Peru	85%	300+
Kewanee Hospital	Kewanee	85%	(a)
Provident Hospital of Chicago	Chicago	85%	(a)
Saint Joseph Medical Center	Bloomington	85%	300+
Crossroads Community Hospital	Mount Vernon	84%	300+
Galesburg Cottage Hospital	Galesburg	84%	300+
Midwestern Region Medical Center	Zion	84%	300+
Perry Memorial Hospital	Princeton	84%	(a)
Rush Oak Park Hospital	Oak Park	84%	300+
Saint James Hospital	Pontiac	84%	(a)
Adventist La Grange Memorial Hospital[11]	La Grange	83%	300+
Advocate Bromenn Medical Center	Normal	83%	300+
CGH Medical Center	Sterling	83%	300+
Clay County Hospital	Flora	83%	(a)
Decatur Memorial Hospital	Decatur	83%	300+
Hinsdale Hospital[11]	Hinsdale	83%	300+
Kishwaukee Community Hospital	Dekalb	83%	300+
McDonough District Hospital	Macomb	83%	300+
Mendota Community Hospital	Mendota	83%	(a)
Morris Hospital & Healthcare Centers[11]	Morris	83%	(a)
Pekin Memorial Hospital	Pekin	83%	300+
Presence United Samaritans Medical Center	Danville	83%	300+
Touchette Regional Hospital	Centreville	83%	(a)
Copley Memorial Hospital	Aurora	82%	300+
Good Samaritan Regional Health Center	Mount Vernon	82%	300+
Greenville Regional Hospital	Greenville	82%	(a)
Iroquois Memorial Hospital	Watseka	82%	(a)
Little Company of Mary Hospital	Evergreen Park	82%	300+
Memorial Hospital of Carbondale	Carbondale	82%	300+
Metrosouth Medical Center	Blue Island	82%	300+
Ottawa Reg Hosp & Healthcare Ctr	Ottawa	82%	300+
Rush University Medical Center	Chicago	82%	300+
Saint Anthonys Memorial Hospital	Effingham	82%	300+
West Suburban Medical Center[11]	Oak Park	82%	300+
Advocate Good Samaritan Hospital	Downers Grove	81%	300+
Advocate Good Shepherd Hospital	Barrington	81%	300+
Advocate South Suburban Hospital	Hazel Crest	81%	300+
Alexian Brothers Medical Center	Elk Grove Vlg	81%	300+
Alton Memorial Hospital[11]	Alton	81%	300+
Carle Foundation Hospital[11]	Urbana	81%	300+
Centegra Health Sys-Woodstock Hosp	Woodstock	81%	300+
Central Dupage Hospital	Winfield	81%	300+
Edward Hospital	Naperville	81%	300+
Harrisburg Medical Center	Harrisburg	81%	(a)
Heartland Regional Medical Center	Marion	81%	300+
Jersey Community Hospital	Jerseyville	81%	(a)
Katherine Shaw Bethea Hospital	Dixon	81%	300+
Memorial Medical Center	Springfield	81%	300+
Mercy Hospital & Medical Center	Chicago	81%	300+
Methodist Medical Center of Illinois	Peoria	81%	300+
Palos Community Hospital	Palos Heights	81%	300+
Presence Saint Francis Hospital	Evanston	81%	300+
Saint Elizabeth Hospital	Belleville	81%	300+
Adventist Bolingbrook Hospital[11]	Bolingbrook	80%	300+
Advocate Christ Hospital & Medical Center	Oak Lawn	80%	300+
Advocate Lutheran General Hospital	Park Ridge	80%	300+
Advocate Trinity Hospital	Chicago	80%	300+
Blessing Hospital[11]	Quincy	80%	300+
Elmhurst Memorial Hospital	Elmhurst	80%	300+
Genesis Health System	Silvis	80%	300+
Herrin Hospital	Herrin	80%	300+
Lake Forest Hospital	Lake Forest	80%	300+
Macneal Hospital[11]	Berwyn	80%	300+
Memorial Hospital	Belleville	80%	300+
Northwestern Memorial Hospital	Chicago	80%	300+
Passavant Area Hospital	Jacksonville	80%	300+
Presence Saint Joseph Hospital - Elgin	Elgin	80%	300+
Riverside Medical Center	Kankakee	80%	300+
Saint Alexius Medical Center	Hoffman Estates	80%	300+
Saint Anthony Hospital	Chicago	80%	300+
Saint Anthony Medical Center	Rockford	80%	300+
Saint Francis Medical Center	Peoria	80%	300+
The University of Chicago Medical Center	Chicago	80%	300+
Advocate Illinois Masonic Medical Center	Chicago	79%	300+
Centegra Health Sys-Mc Henry Hosp	Mchenry	79%	300+
Evanston Hospital[11]	Evanston	79%	300+
Fhn Memorial Hospital	Freeport	79%	300+
John H Stroger Jr Hospital	Chicago	79%	300+
Louis A Weiss Memorial Hospital[11]	Chicago	79%	300+
Loyola Gottlieb Memorial Hospital	Melrose Park	79%	300+
Loyola University Medical Center	Maywood	79%	300+
Presence Mercy Medical Center	Aurora	79%	300+
Presence Our Lady of the Res Med Ctr	Chicago	79%	300+
Presence Resurrection Medical Center	Chicago	79%	300+
Saint Anthony's Health Center	Alton	79%	300+
Saint Johns Hospital	Springfield	79%	300+
Saint Marys Hospital	Decatur	79%	300+
Silver Cross Hospital & Medical Centers	New Lenox	79%	300+
Swedish American Hospital	Rockford	79%	300+
Vista Medical Center East	Waukegan	79%	300+
Westlake Community Hospital[11]	Melrose Park	79%	300+
Advocate Condell Medical Center	Libertyville	78%	300+
Delnor Community Hospital	Geneva	78%	300+
Gateway Regional Medical Center	Granite City	78%	300+
Mount Sinai Hospital Medical Center	Chicago	78%	300+
Presence Covenant Medical Center	Urbana	78%	300+
Presence Saint Joseph Medical Center	Joliet	78%	300+
Presence Sts Mary & Elizabeth Med Ctr	Chicago	78%	300+
Proctor Hospital	Peoria	78%	300+
Sherman Hospital	Elgin	78%	300+
Swedish Covenant Hospital	Chicago	78%	300+
Trinity Rock Island	Rock Island	78%	300+
Ingalls Memorial Hospital	Harvey	77%	300+
Rockford Memorial Hospital	Rockford	77%	300+
Franciscan Saint James Health	Olympia Fields	76%	300+
Northwest Community Hospital	Arlington Hgts	76%	300+
Presence Saint Joseph Hospital - Chicago	Chicago	76%	300+
University of Illinois Hospital	Chicago	76%	300+
Adventist Glenoaks[11]	Glendale Hghts	75%	300+
Holy Cross Hospital	Chicago	75%	300+
Sparta Community Hospital	Sparta	75%	(a)
Thorek Memorial Hospital	Chicago	75%	(a)
Norwegian - American Hospital	Chicago	74%	300+
Loretto Hospital	Chicago	73%	(a)
Saint Bernard Hospital	Chicago	72%	300+
South Shore Hospital	Chicago	72%	(a)
Jackson Park Hospital	Chicago	71%	300+
Roseland Community Hospital[3]	Chicago	70%	(a)

Home Recovery Information Given

Hospital Name	City	Rate	Cases
Blessing Hospital[11]	Quincy	94%	300+
Pinckneyville Community Hospital	Pinckneyville	93%	(a)
Richland Memorial Hospital	Olney	93%	300+
Rochelle Community Hospital	Rochelle	93%	(a)
Abraham Lincoln Memorial Hospital	Lincoln	92%	(a)
Gibson Community Hospital	Gibson City	92%	300+
Hillsboro Area Hospital	Hillsboro	92%	(a)
Mendota Community Hospital	Mendota	92%	(a)
Midwestern Region Medical Center	Zion	92%	300+
Red Bud Regional Hospital	Red Bud	92%	(a)
Saint James Hospital	Pontiac	92%	(a)
Saint Joseph's Hospital	Breese	92%	300+
Kewanee Hospital	Kewanee	91%	(a)
McDonough District Hospital	Macomb	91%	300+
OSF Holy Family Medical Center	Monmouth	91%	(a)
Presence Saint Marys Hospital	Kankakee	91%	300+
Sparta Community Hospital	Sparta	91%	(a)
Clay County Hospital	Flora	90%	(a)
Crawford Memorial Hospital	Robinson	90%	(a)
Delnor Community Hospital	Geneva	90%	300+
Iroquois Memorial Hospital	Watseka	90%	(a)
Morris Hospital & Healthcare Centers[11]	Morris	90%	(a)
Saint Marys Hospital	Centralia	90%	300+
Sarah Bush Lincoln Health Center	Mattoon	90%	300+
Valley West Community Hospital	Sandwich	90%	(a)
Wabash General Hospital	Mount Carmel	90%	(a)
Advocate Good Shepherd Hospital	Barrington	89%	300+
Alton Memorial Hospital[11]	Alton	89%	300+
Anderson Hospital	Maryville	89%	300+
Centegra Health Sys-Mc Henry Hosp	Mchenry	89%	300+
Galesburg Cottage Hospital	Galesburg	89%	300+
Kishwaukee Community Hospital	Dekalb	89%	300+
Presence United Samaritans Medical Center	Danville	89%	300+
Saint Francis Medical Center	Peoria	89%	300+
Saint Margarets Hospital	Spring Valley	89%	300+
Saint Mary Medical Center	Galesburg	89%	300+
Advocate Christ Hospital & Medical Center	Oak Lawn	88%	300+
Centegra Health Sys-Woodstock Hosp	Woodstock	88%	300+
Central Dupage Hospital	Winfield	88%	300+
CGH Medical Center	Sterling	88%	300+
Copley Memorial Hospital	Aurora	88%	300+
Decatur Memorial Hospital	Decatur	88%	300+
Good Samaritan Regional Health Center	Mount Vernon	88%	300+
Greenville Regional Hospital	Greenville	88%	(a)
Hammond Henry Hospital	Geneseo	88%	300+
Herrin Hospital	Herrin	88%	300+
Illinois Valley Community Hospital[11]	Peru	88%	300+
Ingalls Memorial Hospital	Harvey	88%	300+
Katherine Shaw Bethea Hospital	Dixon	88%	300+
Presence Mercy Medical Center	Aurora	88%	300+
Presence Saint Joseph Hospital - Elgin	Elgin	88%	300+
Riverside Medical Center	Kankakee	88%	300+
Saint Alexius Medical Center	Hoffman Estates	88%	300+
Saint Joseph Medical Center	Bloomington	88%	300+
Swedish American Hospital	Rockford	88%	300+
Union County Hospital	Anna	88%	(a)
Adventist La Grange Memorial Hospital[11]	La Grange	87%	300+
Advocate Bromenn Medical Center	Normal	87%	300+
Advocate Good Samaritan Hospital	Downers Grove	87%	300+
Advocate Lutheran General Hospital	Park Ridge	87%	300+
Alexian Brothers Medical Center	Elk Grove Vlg	87%	300+
Crossroads Community Hospital	Mount Vernon	87%	300+
Memorial Hospital of Carbondale	Carbondale	87%	300+
Methodist Medical Center of Illinois	Peoria	87%	300+
Ottawa Reg Hosp & Healthcare Ctr	Ottawa	87%	300+
Pekin Memorial Hospital	Pekin	87%	300+
Presence Covenant Medical Center	Urbana	87%	300+
Proctor Hospital	Peoria	87%	300+
Rush University Medical Center	Chicago	87%	300+
Saint Anthony's Health Center	Alton	87%	300+
Saint Joseph's Hospital	Highland	87%	(a)
Salem Township Hospital	Salem	87%	(a)
Sherman Hospital	Elgin	87%	300+
Trinity Rock Island	Rock Island	87%	300+
Advocate Illinois Masonic Medical Center	Chicago	86%	300+
Elmhurst Memorial Hospital	Elmhurst	86%	300+
Evanston Hospital[11]	Evanston	86%	300+
Fhn Memorial Hospital	Freeport	86%	300+
Genesis Health System	Silvis	86%	300+
Hinsdale Hospital[11]	Hinsdale	86%	300+
Loyola University Medical Center	Maywood	86%	300+
Massac Memorial Hospital	Metropolis	86%	(a)
Memorial Hospital	Belleville	86%	300+
Metrosouth Medical Center	Blue Island	86%	300+
Passavant Area Hospital	Jacksonville	86%	300+
Presence Resurrection Medical Center	Chicago	86%	300+
Presence Saint Joseph Hospital - Chicago	Chicago	86%	300+
Saint Anthony Medical Center	Rockford	86%	300+
Saint Anthonys Memorial Hospital	Effingham	86%	300+
Saint Elizabeth Hospital	Belleville	86%	300+
Saint Francis Hospital	Litchfield	86%	300+
Saint Marys Hospital	Streator	86%	300+
Advocate Condell Medical Center	Libertyville	85%	300+
Carle Foundation Hospital[11]	Urbana	85%	300+
Heartland Regional Medical Center	Marion	85%	300+

NOTE: Hospital profiles are in alphabetical order by state, then city, then hospital within the city; Rankings exclude hospitals with less than 25 cases except for patient surveys which excludes hospitals with less than 100 cases; (a) 100-299 cases; (1) The number of cases/patients is too few to report; (2) Data submitted were based on a sample of cases/patients; (3) Results are based on a shorter time period than required; (4) Data suppressed by CMS for one or more quarters; (5) Results are not available for this reporting period; (6) Fewer than 100 patients completed the HCAHPS survey; (7) No cases met the criteria for this measure; (8) The lower limit of the confidence interval cannot be calculated if the number of observed infections equals zero; (9) No data are available from the state/territory for this reporting period; (10) The scores shown reflect fewer than 50 completed surveys; (11) There were discrepancies in the data collection process; (12) This measure does not apply to this hospital for this reporting period; (13) Results cannot be calculated for this reporting period; (14) The results for this state are combined with nearby states to protect confidentiality; Please refer to the User's Guide for a full explanation of data.

Hospital Name	City	Rate	Cases
Macneal Hospital[11]	Berwyn	85%	300+
Memorial Medical Center	Springfield	85%	300+
Northwest Community Hospital	Arlington Hgts	85%	300+
Perry Memorial Hospital	Princeton	85%	(a)
Saint Johns Hospital	Springfield	85%	300+
Vista Medical Center East	Waukegan	85%	300+
West Suburban Medical Center[11]	Oak Park	85%	300+
Advocate South Suburban Hospital	Hazel Crest	84%	300+
Gateway Regional Medical Center	Granite City	84%	300+
Graham Hospital Association	Canton	84%	300+
Little Company of Mary Hospital	Evergreen Park	84%	300+
Presence Saint Joseph Medical Center	Joliet	84%	300+
Adventist Bolingbrook Hospital[11]	Bolingbrook	83%	300+
Adventist Glenoaks[11]	Glendale Hghts	83%	300+
Edward Hospital	Naperville	83%	300+
Louis A Weiss Memorial Hospital[11]	Chicago	83%	300+
Mount Sinai Hospital Medical Center	Chicago	83%	300+
Rockford Memorial Hospital	Rockford	83%	300+
Rush Oak Park Hospital	Oak Park	83%	300+
The University of Chicago Medical Center	Chicago	83%	300+
Westlake Community Hospital[11]	Melrose Park	83%	300+
Franciscan Saint James Health	Olympia Fields	82%	300+
Mercy Hospital & Medical Center	Chicago	82%	300+
Palos Community Hospital	Palos Heights	82%	300+
Presence Our Lady of the Res Med Ctr	Chicago	82%	300+
Presence Saint Francis Hospital	Evanston	82%	300+
Presence Sts Mary & Elizabeth Med Ctr	Chicago	82%	300+
Saint Joseph Memorial Hospital	Murphysboro	82%	(a)
Saint Marys Hospital	Decatur	82%	300+
Silver Cross Hospital & Medical Centers	New Lenox	82%	300+
Taylorville Memorial Hospital	Taylorville	82%	300+
Thorek Memorial Hospital	Chicago	82%	(a)
Advocate Trinity Hospital	Chicago	81%	300+
Holy Cross Hospital	Chicago	81%	300+
Jersey Community Hospital	Jerseyville	81%	300+
Saint Anthony Hospital	Chicago	81%	300+
Touchette Regional Hospital	Centreville	81%	(a)
Harrisburg Medical Center	Harrisburg	80%	(a)
Lake Forest Hospital	Lake Forest	80%	300+
Loyola Gottlieb Memorial Hospital	Melrose Park	80%	300+
Northwestern Memorial Hospital	Chicago	80%	300+
Swedish Covenant Hospital	Chicago	80%	300+
University of Illinois Hospital	Chicago	80%	300+
Provident Hospital of Chicago	Chicago	77%	(a)
John H Stroger Jr Hospital	Chicago	76%	300+
Norwegian - American Hospital	Chicago	76%	300+
Saint Bernard Hospital	Chicago	73%	300+
South Shore Hospital	Chicago	71%	(a)
Loretto Hospital	Chicago	67%	(a)
Roseland Community Hospital[3]	Chicago	65%	(a)
Jackson Park Hospital	Chicago	64%	300+

Hospital Given 9 or 10 on 10 Point Scale

Hospital Name	City	Rate	Cases
Midwestern Region Medical Center	Zion	88%	300+
Gibson Community Hospital	Gibson City	87%	300+
Saint Joseph Memorial Hospital	Murphysboro	87%	(a)
Saint Joseph's Hospital	Breese	86%	300+
OSF Holy Family Medical Center	Monmouth	85%	(a)
Abraham Lincoln Memorial Hospital	Lincoln	84%	(a)
Central Dupage Hospital	Winfield	83%	300+
Hillsboro Area Hospital	Hillsboro	83%	(a)
Mendota Community Hospital	Mendota	82%	(a)
Taylorville Memorial Hospital	Taylorville	81%	300+
Valley West Community Hospital	Sandwich	81%	(a)
Hammond Henry Hospital	Geneseo	80%	300+
Massac Memorial Hospital	Metropolis	80%	(a)
Morris Hospital & Healthcare Centers[11]	Morris	80%	(a)
Rush University Medical Center	Chicago	80%	300+
Saint Joseph Medical Center	Bloomington	80%	300+
Wabash General Hospital	Mount Carmel	80%	(a)
Saint Marys Hospital	Centralia	79%	300+
Salem Township Hospital	Salem	79%	(a)
Adventist La Grange Memorial Hospital[11]	La Grange	78%	300+
Advocate Bromenn Medical Center	Normal	78%	300+
Advocate Lutheran General Hospital	Park Ridge	78%	300+
Hinsdale Hospital[11]	Hinsdale	78%	300+
Saint Mary Medical Center	Galesburg	78%	300+
Edward Hospital	Naperville	77%	300+
Sarah Bush Lincoln Health Center	Mattoon	77%	300+
CGH Medical Center	Sterling	76%	300+
Clay County Hospital	Flora	76%	(a)
Crawford Memorial Hospital	Robinson	76%	(a)
Illinois Valley Community Hospital[11]	Peru	76%	300+
Little Company of Mary Hospital	Evergreen Park	76%	300+
Memorial Medical Center	Springfield	76%	300+
Presence Saint Marys Hospital	Kankakee	76%	300+
Presence United Samaritans Medical Center	Danville	76%	300+
Rochelle Community Hospital	Rochelle	76%	(a)
Saint Francis Hospital	Litchfield	76%	300+
Silver Cross Hospital & Medical Centers	New Lenox	76%	300+
Delnor Community Hospital	Geneva	75%	300+
Elmhurst Memorial Hospital	Elmhurst	75%	300+
Greenville Regional Hospital	Greenville	75%	(a)
Memorial Hospital	Belleville	75%	300+
Northwestern Memorial Hospital	Chicago	75%	300+
Richland Memorial Hospital	Olney	75%	300+
Riverside Medical Center	Kankakee	75%	300+
Saint Francis Medical Center	Peoria	75%	300+
Alexian Brothers Medical Center	Elk Grove Vlg	74%	300+
Anderson Hospital	Maryville	74%	300+
Good Samaritan Regional Health Center	Mount Vernon	74%	300+
Herrin Hospital	Herrin	74%	300+
Kewanee Hospital	Kewanee	74%	(a)
Methodist Medical Center of Illinois	Peoria	74%	300+
Northwest Community Hospital	Arlington Hgts	74%	300+
Presence Saint Francis Hospital	Evanston	74%	300+
Saint Anthony's Health Center	Alton	74%	300+
Sherman Hospital	Elgin	74%	300+
Advocate Christ Hospital & Medical Center	Oak Lawn	73%	300+
Advocate Condell Medical Center	Libertyville	73%	300+
Advocate Good Samaritan Hospital	Downers Grove	73%	300+
Alton Memorial Hospital[11]	Alton	73%	300+
Carle Foundation Hospital[11]	Urbana	73%	300+
Genesis Health System	Silvis	73%	300+
Memorial Hospital of Carbondale	Carbondale	73%	300+
Rush Oak Park Hospital	Oak Park	73%	300+
Saint James Hospital	Pontiac	73%	(a)
Saint Joseph's Hospital	Highland	73%	(a)
Saint Margarets Hospital	Spring Valley	73%	300+
Swedish American Hospital	Rockford	73%	300+
Adventist Bolingbrook Hospital[11]	Bolingbrook	72%	300+
Advocate Good Shepherd Hospital	Barrington	72%	300+
Crossroads Community Hospital	Mount Vernon	72%	300+
Evanston Hospital[11]	Evanston	72%	300+
Kishwaukee Community Hospital	Dekalb	72%	300+
Perry Memorial Hospital	Princeton	72%	(a)
Red Bud Regional Hospital	Red Bud	72%	(a)
Saint Marys Hospital	Decatur	72%	300+
Advocate Illinois Masonic Medical Center	Chicago	71%	300+
Copley Memorial Hospital	Aurora	71%	300+
Passavant Area Hospital	Jacksonville	71%	300+
Presence Saint Joseph Hospital - Chicago	Chicago	71%	300+
Saint Anthony Medical Center	Rockford	71%	300+
Saint Johns Hospital	Springfield	71%	300+
Katherine Shaw Bethea Hospital	Dixon	70%	300+
Presence Covenant Medical Center	Urbana	70%	300+
Presence Saint Joseph Hospital - Elgin	Elgin	70%	300+
Saint Alexius Medical Center	Hoffman Estates	70%	300+
Saint Marys Hospital	Streator	70%	300+
Union County Hospital	Anna	70%	(a)
Blessing Hospital[11]	Quincy	69%	300+
Decatur Memorial Hospital	Decatur	69%	300+
Galesburg Cottage Hospital	Galesburg	69%	300+
Loyola University Medical Center	Maywood	69%	300+
Macneal Hospital[11]	Berwyn	69%	300+
Mercy Hospital & Medical Center	Chicago	69%	300+
Ottawa Reg Hosp & Healthcare Ctr	Ottawa	69%	300+
Rockford Memorial Hospital	Rockford	69%	300+
Saint Elizabeth Hospital	Belleville	69%	300+
Advocate South Suburban Hospital	Hazel Crest	68%	300+
Fhn Memorial Hospital	Freeport	68%	300+
Graham Hospital Association	Canton	68%	300+
Iroquois Memorial Hospital	Watseka	68%	(a)
Jersey Community Hospital	Jerseyville	68%	(a)
McDonough District Hospital	Macomb	68%	300+
Saint Anthonys Memorial Hospital	Effingham	68%	300+
Trinity Rock Island	Rock Island	68%	300+
Centegra Health Sys-Mc Henry Hosp	Mchenry	67%	300+
Centegra Health Sys-Woodstock Hosp	Woodstock	67%	300+
Metrosouth Medical Center	Blue Island	67%	300+
Pinckneyville Community Hospital	Pinckneyville	67%	(a)
Presence Mercy Medical Center	Aurora	67%	300+
The University of Chicago Medical Center	Chicago	67%	300+
Advocate Trinity Hospital	Chicago	66%	300+
Heartland Regional Medical Center	Marion	66%	300+
Presence Sts Mary & Elizabeth Med Ctr	Chicago	66%	300+
Proctor Hospital	Peoria	66%	300+
Sparta Community Hospital	Sparta	66%	(a)
Palos Community Hospital	Palos Heights	65%	300+
Presence Resurrection Medical Center	Chicago	65%	300+
Presence Saint Joseph Medical Center	Joliet	65%	300+
Ingalls Memorial Hospital	Harvey	64%	300+
Lake Forest Hospital	Lake Forest	64%	300+
Saint Anthony Hospital	Chicago	64%	300+
Gateway Regional Medical Center	Granite City	63%	300+
Harrisburg Medical Center	Harrisburg	63%	(a)
Pekin Memorial Hospital	Pekin	63%	300+
Swedish Covenant Hospital	Chicago	63%	300+
Touchette Regional Hospital	Centreville	63%	(a)
Presence Our Lady of the Res Med Ctr	Chicago	62%	300+
Provident Hospital of Chicago	Chicago	62%	(a)
Vista Medical Center East	Waukegan	61%	300+
Westlake Community Hospital[11]	Melrose Park	61%	300+
Louis A Weiss Memorial Hospital[11]	Chicago	60%	300+
West Suburban Medical Center[11]	Oak Park	60%	300+
Loyola Gottlieb Memorial Hospital	Melrose Park	59%	300+
Mount Sinai Hospital Medical Center	Chicago	59%	300+
University of Illinois Hospital	Chicago	59%	300+
Adventist Glenoaks[11]	Glendale Hghts	58%	300+
Franciscan Saint James Health	Olympia Fields	58%	300+
John H Stroger Jr Hospital	Chicago	54%	300+
Holy Cross Hospital	Chicago	53%	300+
Thorek Memorial Hospital	Chicago	52%	(a)
Norwegian - American Hospital	Chicago	50%	300+
South Shore Hospital	Chicago	48%	(a)
Saint Bernard Hospital	Chicago	46%	300+
Loretto Hospital	Chicago	43%	(a)
Roseland Community Hospital[3]	Chicago	41%	(a)
Jackson Park Hospital	Chicago	35%	300+

Meds 'Always' Explained Before Given

Hospital Name	City	Rate	Cases
Saint Joseph's Hospital	Breese	82%	300+
OSF Holy Family Medical Center	Monmouth	78%	(a)
Hillsboro Area Hospital	Hillsboro	76%	(a)
Pinckneyville Community Hospital	Pinckneyville	73%	(a)
Red Bud Regional Hospital	Red Bud	73%	(a)
Saint Marys Hospital	Centralia	73%	300+
Crawford Memorial Hospital	Robinson	72%	(a)
Gibson Community Hospital	Gibson City	72%	300+
Hammond Henry Hospital	Geneseo	72%	300+
Morris Hospital & Healthcare Centers[11]	Morris	72%	(a)
Ottawa Reg Hosp & Healthcare Ctr	Ottawa	72%	300+
Rochelle Community Hospital	Rochelle	72%	(a)
Saint James Hospital	Pontiac	72%	(a)
Saint Mary Medical Center	Galesburg	72%	300+
Sparta Community Hospital	Sparta	71%	(a)
Salem Township Hospital	Salem	70%	(a)
Sarah Bush Lincoln Health Center	Mattoon	70%	300+
Taylorville Memorial Hospital	Taylorville	70%	300+
Abraham Lincoln Memorial Hospital	Lincoln	69%	(a)
Illinois Valley Community Hospital[11]	Peru	69%	300+
Midwestern Region Medical Center	Zion	69%	300+
Saint Joseph Memorial Hospital	Murphysboro	69%	(a)
Saint Margarets Hospital	Spring Valley	69%	300+
Union County Hospital	Anna	69%	(a)
Blessing Hospital[11]	Quincy	68%	300+
Herrin Hospital	Herrin	68%	300+
Mendota Community Hospital	Mendota	68%	(a)
Rush Oak Park Hospital	Oak Park	68%	300+
Valley West Community Hospital	Sandwich	68%	(a)
Central Dupage Hospital	Winfield	67%	300+
CGH Medical Center	Sterling	67%	300+
Clay County Hospital	Flora	67%	(a)
Decatur Memorial Hospital	Decatur	67%	300+
Graham Hospital Association	Canton	67%	300+
Presence United Samaritans Medical Center	Danville	67%	300+
Saint Alexius Medical Center	Hoffman Estates	67%	300+
Saint Joseph Medical Center	Bloomington	67%	300+
Adventist La Grange Memorial Hospital[11]	La Grange	66%	300+
Advocate Trinity Hospital	Chicago	66%	300+
Crossroads Community Hospital	Mount Vernon	66%	300+
Galesburg Cottage Hospital	Galesburg	66%	300+
Harrisburg Medical Center	Harrisburg	66%	(a)
Iroquois Memorial Hospital	Watseka	66%	(a)
Jersey Community Hospital	Jerseyville	66%	(a)
McDonough District Hospital	Macomb	66%	300+
Rush University Medical Center	Chicago	66%	300+
Saint Francis Hospital	Litchfield	66%	300+
Saint Marys Hospital	Streator	66%	300+
Wabash General Hospital	Mount Carmel	66%	(a)
Advocate Bromenn Medical Center	Normal	65%	300+
Advocate Christ Hospital & Medical Center	Oak Lawn	65%	300+
Advocate Good Samaritan Hospital	Downers Grove	65%	300+
Advocate Illinois Masonic Medical Center	Chicago	65%	300+
Advocate Lutheran General Hospital	Park Ridge	65%	300+
Anderson Hospital	Maryville	65%	300+
Centegra Health Sys-Woodstock Hosp	Woodstock	65%	300+
Good Samaritan Regional Health Center	Mount Vernon	65%	300+
Katherine Shaw Bethea Hospital	Dixon	65%	300+
Memorial Hospital	Belleville	65%	300+
Passavant Area Hospital	Jacksonville	65%	300+
Perry Memorial Hospital	Princeton	65%	(a)
Presence Saint Marys Hospital	Kankakee	65%	300+
Richland Memorial Hospital	Olney	65%	300+
Riverside Medical Center	Kankakee	65%	300+
Saint Anthony's Health Center	Alton	65%	300+
Saint Joseph's Hospital	Highland	65%	(a)
Adventist Bolingbrook Hospital[11]	Bolingbrook	64%	300+
Advocate Good Shepherd Hospital	Barrington	64%	300+
Advocate South Suburban Hospital	Hazel Crest	64%	300+
Copley Memorial Hospital	Aurora	64%	300+

NOTE: Hospital profiles are in alphabetical order by state, then city, then hospital within the city; Rankings exclude hospitals with less than 25 cases except for patient surveys which excludes hospitals with less than 100 cases; (a) 100-299 cases; (1) The number of cases/patients is too few to report; (2) Data submitted were based on a sample of cases/patients; (3) Results are based on a shorter time period than required; (4) Data suppressed by CMS for one or more quarters; (5) Results are not available for this reporting period; (6) Fewer than 100 patients completed the HCAHPS survey; (7) No cases met the criteria for this measure; (8) The lower limit of the confidence interval cannot be calculated if the number of observed infections equals zero; (9) No data are available from the state/territory for this reporting period; (10) The scores shown reflect fewer than 50 completed surveys; (11) There were discrepancies in the data collection process; (12) This measure does not apply to this hospital for this reporting period; (13) Results cannot be calculated for this reporting period; (14) The results for this state are combined with nearby states to protect confidentiality; Please refer to the User's Guide for a full explanation of data.

Hospital Name	City	Rate	Cases
Elmhurst Memorial Hospital	Elmhurst	64%	300+
Genesis Health System	Silvis	64%	300+
Memorial Medical Center	Springfield	64%	300+
Metrosouth Medical Center	Blue Island	64%	300+
Provident Hospital of Chicago	Chicago	64%	(a)
Saint Anthony Medical Center	Rockford	64%	300+
Saint Elizabeth Hospital	Belleville	64%	300+
Saint Francis Medical Center	Peoria	64%	300+
Silver Cross Hospital & Medical Centers	New Lenox	64%	300+
Swedish American Hospital	Rockford	64%	300+
Carle Foundation Hospital[11]	Urbana	63%	300+
Edward Hospital	Naperville	63%	300+
Greenville Regional Hospital	Greenville	63%	(a)
Kewanee Hospital	Kewanee	63%	(a)
Little Company of Mary Hospital	Evergreen Park	63%	300+
Memorial Hospital of Carbondale	Carbondale	63%	300+
Methodist Medical Center of Illinois	Peoria	63%	300+
Northwest Community Hospital	Arlington Hgts	63%	300+
Saint Anthonys Memorial Hospital	Effingham	63%	300+
Sherman Hospital	Elgin	63%	300+
Touchette Regional Hospital	Centreville	63%	(a)
Advocate Condell Medical Center	Libertyville	62%	300+
Fhn Memorial Hospital	Freeport	62%	300+
Gateway Regional Medical Center	Granite City	62%	300+
Kishwaukee Community Hospital	Dekalb	62%	300+
Presence Mercy Medical Center	Aurora	62%	300+
Presence Resurrection Medical Center	Chicago	62%	300+
Presence Saint Joseph Medical Center	Joliet	62%	300+
Saint Johns Hospital	Springfield	62%	300+
Adventist Glenoaks[11]	Glendale Hghts	61%	300+
Alexian Brothers Medical Center	Elk Grove Vlg	61%	300+
Centegra Health Sys-Mc Henry Hosp	Mchenry	61%	300+
Delnor Community Hospital	Geneva	61%	300+
Evanston Hospital[11]	Evanston	61%	300+
Hinsdale Hospital[11]	Hinsdale	61%	300+
Ingalls Memorial Hospital	Harvey	61%	300+
Northwestern Memorial Hospital	Chicago	61%	300+
Alton Memorial Hospital[11]	Alton	60%	300+
Heartland Regional Medical Center	Marion	60%	300+
Loyola University Medical Center	Maywood	60%	300+
Mount Sinai Hospital Medical Center	Chicago	60%	300+
Pekin Memorial Hospital	Pekin	60%	300+
Presence Saint Joseph Hospital - Elgin	Elgin	60%	300+
Rockford Memorial Hospital	Rockford	60%	300+
West Suburban Medical Center[11]	Oak Park	60%	300+
Franciscan Saint James Health	Olympia Fields	59%	300+
Macneal Hospital[11]	Berwyn	59%	300+
Massac Memorial Hospital	Metropolis	59%	(a)
Palos Community Hospital	Palos Heights	59%	300+
Presence Covenant Medical Center	Urbana	59%	300+
Presence Saint Francis Hospital	Evanston	59%	300+
Presence Sts Mary & Elizabeth Med Ctr	Chicago	59%	300+
Saint Marys Hospital	Decatur	59%	300+
Trinity Rock Island	Rock Island	59%	300+
Holy Cross Hospital	Chicago	58%	300+
Presence Saint Joseph Hospital - Chicago	Chicago	58%	300+
The University of Chicago Medical Center	Chicago	58%	300+
Vista Medical Center East	Waukegan	58%	300+
Westlake Community Hospital[11]	Melrose Park	58%	300+
Lake Forest Hospital	Lake Forest	57%	300+
Thorek Memorial Hospital	Chicago	57%	(a)
Louis A Weiss Memorial Hospital[11]	Chicago	56%	300+
Loyola Gottlieb Memorial Hospital	Melrose Park	56%	300+
Presence Our Lady of the Res Med Ctr	Chicago	56%	300+
Proctor Hospital	Peoria	56%	300+
Mercy Hospital & Medical Center	Chicago	55%	300+
Swedish Covenant Hospital	Chicago	55%	300+
University of Illinois Hospital	Chicago	55%	300+
South Shore Hospital	Chicago	53%	(a)
John H Stroger Jr Hospital	Chicago	50%	300+
Saint Anthony Hospital	Chicago	50%	300+
Saint Bernard Hospital	Chicago	50%	300+
Roseland Community Hospital[3]	Chicago	49%	(a)
Loretto Hospital	Chicago	48%	(a)
Norwegian - American Hospital	Chicago	48%	300+
Jackson Park Hospital	Chicago	45%	300+

Nurses 'Always' Communicated Well

Hospital Name	City	Rate	Cases
OSF Holy Family Medical Center	Monmouth	94%	(a)
Hillsboro Area Hospital	Hillsboro	92%	(a)
Saint Joseph's Hospital	Breese	91%	300+
Rochelle Community Hospital	Rochelle	90%	(a)
Salem Township Hospital	Salem	88%	(a)
Pinckneyville Community Hospital	Pinckneyville	87%	(a)
Saint Marys Hospital	Centralia	87%	300+
Wabash General Hospital	Mount Carmel	87%	(a)
McDonough District Hospital	Macomb	86%	300+
Mendota Community Hospital	Mendota	86%	(a)
Saint Joseph Memorial Hospital	Murphysboro	86%	(a)
Abraham Lincoln Memorial Hospital	Lincoln	85%	(a)
Crawford Memorial Hospital	Robinson	85%	(a)
Illinois Valley Community Hospital[11]	Peru	85%	300+
Sarah Bush Lincoln Health Center	Mattoon	85%	300+
Taylorville Memorial Hospital	Taylorville	85%	300+
Gibson Community Hospital	Gibson City	84%	300+
Hammond Henry Hospital	Geneseo	84%	300+
Massac Memorial Hospital	Metropolis	84%	(a)
Morris Hospital & Healthcare Centers[11]	Morris	84%	(a)
Ottawa Reg Hosp & Healthcare Ctr	Ottawa	84%	300+
Red Bud Regional Hospital	Red Bud	84%	(a)
Adventist La Grange Memorial Hospital[11]	La Grange	83%	300+
Advocate Bromenn Medical Center	Normal	83%	300+
Harrisburg Medical Center	Harrisburg	83%	(a)
Memorial Hospital	Belleville	83%	300+
Midwestern Region Medical Center	Zion	83%	300+
Presence United Samaritans Medical Center	Danville	83%	300+
Rush Oak Park Hospital	Oak Park	83%	300+
Rush University Medical Center	Chicago	83%	300+
Saint Francis Hospital	Litchfield	83%	300+
Saint James Hospital	Pontiac	83%	(a)
Saint Joseph Medical Center	Bloomington	83%	300+
Saint Joseph's Hospital	Highland	83%	(a)
Saint Mary Medical Center	Galesburg	83%	300+
Sparta Community Hospital	Sparta	83%	(a)
Advocate Christ Hospital & Medical Center	Oak Lawn	82%	300+
Advocate Good Samaritan Hospital	Downers Grove	82%	300+
Advocate Trinity Hospital	Chicago	82%	300+
Blessing Hospital[11]	Quincy	82%	300+
Carle Foundation Hospital[11]	Urbana	82%	300+
CGH Medical Center	Sterling	82%	300+
Clay County Hospital	Flora	82%	(a)
Good Samaritan Regional Health Center	Mount Vernon	82%	300+
Kewanee Hospital	Kewanee	82%	(a)
Presence Saint Marys Hospital	Kankakee	82%	300+
Richland Memorial Hospital	Olney	82%	300+
Saint Francis Medical Center	Peoria	82%	300+
Saint Margarets Hospital	Spring Valley	82%	300+
Saint Marys Hospital	Streator	82%	300+
Union County Hospital	Anna	82%	(a)
Valley West Community Hospital	Sandwich	82%	(a)
Advocate Good Shepherd Hospital	Barrington	81%	300+
Advocate South Suburban Hospital	Hazel Crest	81%	300+
Anderson Hospital	Maryville	81%	300+
Central Dupage Hospital	Winfield	81%	300+
Graham Hospital Association	Canton	81%	300+
Greenville Regional Hospital	Greenville	81%	(a)
Hinsdale Hospital[11]	Hinsdale	81%	300+
Memorial Hospital of Carbondale	Carbondale	81%	300+
Methodist Medical Center of Illinois	Peoria	81%	300+
Passavant Area Hospital	Jacksonville	81%	300+
Perry Memorial Hospital	Princeton	81%	(a)
Adventist Glenoaks[11]	Glendale Hghts	80%	300+
Advocate Illinois Masonic Medical Center	Chicago	80%	300+
Advocate Lutheran General Hospital	Park Ridge	80%	300+
Delnor Community Hospital	Geneva	80%	300+
Galesburg Cottage Hospital	Galesburg	80%	300+
Genesis Health System	Silvis	80%	300+
Herrin Hospital	Herrin	80%	300+
Jersey Community Hospital	Jerseyville	80%	(a)
Katherine Shaw Bethea Hospital	Dixon	80%	300+
Little Company of Mary Hospital	Evergreen Park	80%	300+
Memorial Medical Center	Springfield	80%	300+
Presence Resurrection Medical Center	Chicago	80%	300+
Provident Hospital of Chicago	Chicago	80%	(a)
Riverside Medical Center	Kankakee	80%	300+
Saint Alexius Medical Center	Hoffman Estates	80%	300+
Saint Anthony Medical Center	Rockford	80%	300+
Saint Elizabeth Hospital	Belleville	80%	300+
Sherman Hospital	Elgin	80%	300+
Adventist Bolingbrook Hospital[11]	Bolingbrook	79%	300+
Alexian Brothers Medical Center	Elk Grove Vlg	79%	300+
Alton Memorial Hospital[11]	Alton	79%	300+
Centegra Health Sys-Mc Henry Hosp	Mchenry	79%	300+
Centegra Health Sys-Woodstock Hosp	Woodstock	79%	300+
Copley Memorial Hospital	Aurora	79%	300+
Crossroads Community Hospital	Mount Vernon	79%	300+
Presence Mercy Medical Center	Aurora	79%	300+
Saint Anthony's Health Center	Alton	79%	300+
Saint Anthonys Memorial Hospital	Effingham	79%	300+
Swedish American Hospital	Rockford	79%	300+
Advocate Condell Medical Center	Libertyville	78%	300+
Edward Hospital	Naperville	78%	300+
Elmhurst Memorial Hospital	Elmhurst	78%	300+
Evanston Hospital[11]	Evanston	78%	300+
Gateway Regional Medical Center	Granite City	78%	300+
Kishwaukee Community Hospital	Dekalb	78%	300+
Palos Community Hospital	Palos Heights	78%	300+
Presence Covenant Medical Center	Urbana	78%	300+
Presence Saint Joseph Hospital - Elgin	Elgin	78%	300+
Saint Johns Hospital	Springfield	78%	300+
Saint Marys Hospital	Decatur	78%	300+
Silver Cross Hospital & Medical Centers	New Lenox	78%	300+
Touchette Regional Hospital	Centreville	78%	(a)
Trinity Rock Island	Rock Island	78%	300+
Decatur Memorial Hospital	Decatur	77%	300+
Fhn Memorial Hospital	Freeport	77%	300+
Iroquois Memorial Hospital	Watseka	77%	(a)
Macneal Hospital[11]	Berwyn	77%	300+
Metrosouth Medical Center	Blue Island	77%	300+
Presence Saint Francis Hospital	Evanston	77%	300+
Presence Sts Mary & Elizabeth Med Ctr	Chicago	77%	300+
Rockford Memorial Hospital	Rockford	77%	300+
Loyola Gottlieb Memorial Hospital	Melrose Park	76%	300+
Loyola University Medical Center	Maywood	76%	300+
Northwest Community Hospital	Arlington Hgts	76%	300+
Northwestern Memorial Hospital	Chicago	76%	300+
Pekin Memorial Hospital	Pekin	76%	300+
Presence Saint Joseph Hospital - Chicago	Chicago	76%	300+
Heartland Regional Medical Center	Marion	75%	300+
Ingalls Memorial Hospital	Harvey	75%	300+
Presence Our Lady of the Res Med Ctr	Chicago	75%	300+
Proctor Hospital	Peoria	75%	300+
Mercy Hospital & Medical Center	Chicago	74%	300+
Presence Saint Joseph Medical Center	Joliet	74%	300+
West Suburban Medical Center[11]	Oak Park	74%	300+
Franciscan Saint James Health	Olympia Fields	73%	300+
Saint Anthony Hospital	Chicago	73%	300+
Swedish Covenant Hospital	Chicago	72%	300+
Vista Medical Center East	Waukegan	72%	300+
Louis A Weiss Memorial Hospital[11]	Chicago	71%	300+
Mount Sinai Hospital Medical Center	Chicago	71%	300+
The University of Chicago Medical Center	Chicago	71%	300+
University of Illinois Hospital	Chicago	71%	300+
Holy Cross Hospital	Chicago	70%	300+
Lake Forest Hospital	Lake Forest	70%	300+
Westlake Community Hospital[11]	Melrose Park	70%	300+
Thorek Memorial Hospital	Chicago	69%	(a)
South Shore Hospital	Chicago	65%	(a)
John H Stroger Jr Hospital	Chicago	64%	300+
Loretto Hospital	Chicago	64%	(a)
Roseland Community Hospital[3]	Chicago	64%	(a)
Saint Bernard Hospital	Chicago	63%	300+
Norwegian - American Hospital	Chicago	60%	300+
Jackson Park Hospital	Chicago	59%	300+

Pain 'Always' Well Controlled

Hospital Name	City	Rate	Cases
Hillsboro Area Hospital	Hillsboro	87%	(a)
Rochelle Community Hospital	Rochelle	84%	(a)
Saint Joseph Memorial Hospital	Murphysboro	82%	(a)
Crawford Memorial Hospital	Robinson	81%	(a)
Saint Joseph's Hospital	Breese	81%	300+
OSF Holy Family Medical Center	Monmouth	80%	(a)
Presence Saint Marys Hospital	Kankakee	79%	300+
Pinckneyville Community Hospital	Pinckneyville	77%	(a)
Adventist La Grange Memorial Hospital[11]	La Grange	76%	300+
Central Dupage Hospital	Winfield	76%	300+
Clay County Hospital	Flora	76%	(a)
Gibson Community Hospital	Gibson City	76%	300+
Good Samaritan Regional Health Center	Mount Vernon	76%	300+
Massac Memorial Hospital	Metropolis	76%	(a)
Midwestern Region Medical Center	Zion	76%	300+
Saint Francis Hospital	Litchfield	76%	300+
Saint Mary Medical Center	Galesburg	76%	300+
Anderson Hospital	Maryville	75%	300+
Hammond Henry Hospital	Geneseo	75%	300+
Memorial Hospital	Belleville	75%	300+
Mendota Community Hospital	Mendota	75%	(a)
Red Bud Regional Hospital	Red Bud	75%	(a)
Richland Memorial Hospital	Olney	75%	300+
Union County Hospital	Anna	75%	(a)
Genesis Health System	Silvis	74%	300+
Illinois Valley Community Hospital[11]	Peru	74%	300+
Katherine Shaw Bethea Hospital	Dixon	74%	300+
Little Company of Mary Hospital	Evergreen Park	74%	300+
Morris Hospital & Healthcare Centers[11]	Morris	74%	(a)
Presence United Samaritans Medical Center	Danville	74%	300+
Saint James Hospital	Pontiac	74%	(a)
Saint Marys Hospital	Centralia	74%	300+
Salem Township Hospital	Salem	74%	(a)
Sparta Community Hospital	Sparta	74%	(a)
Touchette Regional Hospital	Centreville	74%	(a)
Valley West Community Hospital	Sandwich	74%	(a)
Advocate Good Samaritan Hospital	Downers Grove	73%	300+
Advocate Lutheran General Hospital	Park Ridge	73%	300+
Advocate South Suburban Hospital	Hazel Crest	73%	300+
Carle Foundation Hospital[11]	Urbana	73%	300+
Galesburg Cottage Hospital	Galesburg	73%	300+
Hinsdale Hospital[11]	Hinsdale	73%	300+
Ottawa Reg Hosp & Healthcare Ctr	Ottawa	73%	300+
Presence Mercy Medical Center	Aurora	73%	300+
Presence Resurrection Medical Center	Chicago	73%	300+

NOTE: Hospital profiles are in alphabetical order by state, then city, then hospital within the city; Rankings exclude hospitals with less than 25 cases except for patient surveys which excludes hospitals with less than 100 cases; (a) 100-299 cases; (1) The number of cases/patients is too few to report; (2) Data submitted were based on a sample of cases/patients; (3) Results are based on a shorter time period than required; (4) Data suppressed by CMS for one or more quarters; (5) Results are not available for this reporting period; (6) Fewer than 100 patients completed the HCAHPS survey; (7) No cases met the criteria for this measure; (8) The lower limit of the confidence interval cannot be calculated if the number of observed infections equals zero; (9) No data are available from the state/territory for this reporting period; (10) The scores shown reflect fewer than 50 completed surveys; (11) There were discrepancies in the data collection process; (12) This measure does not apply to this hospital for this reporting period; (13) Results cannot be calculated for this reporting period; (14) The results for this state are combined with nearby states to protect confidentiality; Please refer to the User's Guide for a full explanation of data.

Hospital Name	City	Rate	Cases
Provident Hospital of Chicago	Chicago	73%	(a)
Rush Oak Park Hospital	Oak Park	73%	300+
Saint Elizabeth Hospital	Belleville	73%	300+
Saint Joseph Medical Center	Bloomington	73%	300+
Swedish American Hospital	Rockford	73%	300+
Advocate Bromenn Medical Center	Normal	72%	300+
Advocate Christ Hospital & Medical Center	Oak Lawn	72%	300+
Advocate Trinity Hospital	Chicago	72%	300+
Alexian Brothers Medical Center	Elk Grove Vlg	72%	300+
Blessing Hospital[11]	Quincy	72%	300+
Copley Memorial Hospital	Aurora	72%	300+
Crossroads Community Hospital	Mount Vernon	72%	300+
Edward Hospital	Naperville	72%	300+
Kishwaukee Community Hospital	Dekalb	72%	300+
Methodist Medical Center of Illinois	Peoria	72%	300+
Northwest Community Hospital	Arlington Hgts	72%	300+
Rush University Medical Center	Chicago	72%	300+
Saint Anthony Medical Center	Rockford	72%	300+
Saint Anthony's Health Center	Alton	72%	300+
Saint Francis Medical Center	Peoria	72%	300+
Saint Margarets Hospital	Spring Valley	72%	300+
Sarah Bush Lincoln Health Center	Mattoon	72%	300+
Taylorville Memorial Hospital	Taylorville	72%	300+
Adventist Bolingbrook Hospital[11]	Bolingbrook	71%	300+
Advocate Good Shepherd Hospital	Barrington	71%	300+
Advocate Illinois Masonic Medical Center	Chicago	71%	300+
Centegra Health Sys-Woodstock Hosp	Woodstock	71%	300+
Graham Hospital Association	Canton	71%	300+
Herrin Hospital	Herrin	71%	300+
McDonough District Hospital	Macomb	71%	300+
Memorial Medical Center	Springfield	71%	300+
Metrosouth Medical Center	Blue Island	71%	300+
Palos Community Hospital	Palos Heights	71%	300+
Passavant Area Hospital	Jacksonville	71%	300+
Presence Saint Joseph Hospital - Elgin	Elgin	71%	300+
Riverside Medical Center	Kankakee	71%	300+
Saint Alexius Medical Center	Hoffman Estates	71%	300+
Sherman Hospital	Elgin	71%	300+
Advocate Condell Medical Center	Libertyville	70%	300+
Alton Memorial Hospital[11]	Alton	70%	300+
Centegra Health Sys-Mc Henry Hosp	Mchenry	70%	300+
CGH Medical Center	Sterling	70%	300+
Greenville Regional Hospital	Greenville	70%	(a)
Harrisburg Medical Center	Harrisburg	70%	(a)
Macneal Hospital[11]	Berwyn	70%	300+
Memorial Hospital of Carbondale	Carbondale	70%	300+
Northwestern Memorial Hospital	Chicago	70%	300+
Silver Cross Hospital & Medical Centers	New Lenox	70%	300+
Swedish Covenant Hospital	Chicago	70%	300+
Trinity Rock Island	Rock Island	70%	300+
Abraham Lincoln Memorial Hospital	Lincoln	69%	(a)
Adventist Glenoaks[11]	Glendale Hghts	69%	300+
Decatur Memorial Hospital	Decatur	69%	300+
Delnor Community Hospital	Geneva	69%	300+
Fhn Memorial Hospital	Freeport	69%	300+
Gateway Regional Medical Center	Granite City	69%	300+
Jersey Community Hospital	Jerseyville	69%	(a)
Loyola University Medical Center	Maywood	69%	300+
Mercy Hospital & Medical Center	Chicago	69%	300+
Presence Our Lady of the Res Med Ctr	Chicago	69%	300+
Rockford Memorial Hospital	Rockford	69%	300+
Saint Anthonys Memorial Hospital	Effingham	69%	300+
Saint Johns Hospital	Springfield	69%	300+
Elmhurst Memorial Hospital	Elmhurst	68%	300+
Evanston Hospital[11]	Evanston	68%	300+
Iroquois Memorial Hospital	Watseka	68%	(a)
Perry Memorial Hospital	Princeton	68%	(a)
Presence Saint Francis Hospital	Evanston	68%	300+
Saint Joseph's Hospital	Highland	68%	(a)
West Suburban Medical Center[11]	Oak Park	68%	300+
Kewanee Hospital	Kewanee	67%	(a)
Loyola Gottlieb Memorial Hospital	Melrose Park	67%	300+
Pekin Memorial Hospital	Pekin	67%	300+
Presence Covenant Medical Center	Urbana	67%	300+
Saint Marys Hospital	Streator	67%	300+
Wabash General Hospital	Mount Carmel	67%	(a)
Westlake Community Hospital[11]	Melrose Park	67%	300+
Franciscan Saint James Health	Olympia Fields	66%	300+
Heartland Regional Medical Center	Marion	66%	300+
Presence Sts Mary & Elizabeth Med Ctr	Chicago	66%	300+
Vista Medical Center East	Waukegan	66%	300+
Ingalls Memorial Hospital	Harvey	65%	300+
Lake Forest Hospital	Lake Forest	65%	300+
Saint Marys Hospital	Decatur	65%	300+
The University of Chicago Medical Center	Chicago	65%	300+
Holy Cross Hospital	Chicago	64%	300+
Louis A Weiss Memorial Hospital[11]	Chicago	64%	300+
Mount Sinai Hospital Medical Center	Chicago	64%	300+
Presence Saint Joseph Medical Center	Joliet	64%	300+
Presence Saint Joseph Hospital - Chicago	Chicago	63%	300+
Saint Anthony Hospital	Chicago	63%	300+
John H Stroger Jr Hospital	Chicago	62%	300+
Proctor Hospital	Peoria	62%	300+
University of Illinois Hospital	Chicago	62%	300+
Saint Bernard Hospital	Chicago	59%	300+
South Shore Hospital	Chicago	58%	(a)
Roseland Community Hospital[3]	Chicago	57%	(a)
Thorek Memorial Hospital	Chicago	57%	(a)
Jackson Park Hospital	Chicago	55%	300+
Norwegian - American Hospital	Chicago	55%	300+
Loretto Hospital	Chicago	54%	(a)

Room and Bathroom 'Always' Clean

Hospital Name	City	Rate	Cases
OSF Holy Family Medical Center	Monmouth	97%	(a)
Saint Joseph's Hospital	Breese	92%	300+
Saint Marys Hospital	Centralia	91%	300+
Hillsboro Area Hospital	Hillsboro	90%	(a)
Rochelle Community Hospital	Rochelle	90%	(a)
Massac Memorial Hospital	Metropolis	87%	(a)
Crawford Memorial Hospital	Robinson	86%	(a)
Mendota Community Hospital	Mendota	86%	(a)
Saint Francis Hospital	Litchfield	86%	300+
Wabash General Hospital	Mount Carmel	85%	(a)
Good Samaritan Regional Health Center	Mount Vernon	84%	300+
Jersey Community Hospital	Jerseyville	84%	(a)
McDonough District Hospital	Macomb	84%	300+
Salem Township Hospital	Salem	84%	(a)
Sparta Community Hospital	Sparta	84%	(a)
Abraham Lincoln Memorial Hospital	Lincoln	83%	(a)
CGH Medical Center	Sterling	83%	300+
Saint Marys Hospital	Streator	83%	300+
Saint Joseph Memorial Hospital	Murphysboro	82%	(a)
Advocate Condell Medical Center	Libertyville	81%	300+
Harrisburg Medical Center	Harrisburg	81%	(a)
Ottawa Reg Hosp & Healthcare Ctr	Ottawa	81%	300+
Perry Memorial Hospital	Princeton	81%	(a)
Pinckneyville Community Hospital	Pinckneyville	81%	(a)
Taylorville Memorial Hospital	Taylorville	81%	300+
Illinois Valley Community Hospital[11]	Peru	80%	300+
Saint Joseph Medical Center	Bloomington	80%	300+
Centegra Health Sys-Woodstock Hosp	Woodstock	79%	300+
Clay County Hospital	Flora	79%	(a)
Iroquois Memorial Hospital	Watseka	79%	(a)
Kewanee Hospital	Kewanee	79%	(a)
Passavant Area Hospital	Jacksonville	79%	300+
Saint Margarets Hospital	Spring Valley	79%	300+
Saint Mary Medical Center	Galesburg	79%	300+
Silver Cross Hospital & Medical Centers	New Lenox	79%	300+
Advocate Bromenn Medical Center	Normal	78%	300+
Blessing Hospital[11]	Quincy	78%	300+
Gibson Community Hospital	Gibson City	78%	300+
Northwest Community Hospital	Arlington Hgts	78%	300+
Adventist Bolingbrook Hospital[11]	Bolingbrook	77%	300+
Adventist La Grange Memorial Hospital[11]	La Grange	77%	300+
Advocate Illinois Masonic Medical Center	Chicago	77%	300+
Advocate Lutheran General Hospital	Park Ridge	77%	300+
Greenville Regional Hospital	Greenville	77%	(a)
Hinsdale Hospital[11]	Hinsdale	77%	300+
Methodist Medical Center of Illinois	Peoria	77%	300+
Midwestern Region Medical Center	Zion	77%	300+
Morris Hospital & Healthcare Centers[11]	Morris	77%	(a)
Saint James Hospital	Pontiac	77%	(a)
Saint Joseph's Hospital	Highland	77%	(a)
Advocate Trinity Hospital	Chicago	76%	300+
Anderson Hospital	Maryville	76%	300+
Copley Memorial Hospital	Aurora	76%	300+
Presence Saint Marys Hospital	Kankakee	76%	300+
Presence United Samaritans Medical Center	Danville	76%	300+
Central Dupage Hospital	Winfield	75%	300+
Crossroads Community Hospital	Mount Vernon	75%	300+
Memorial Hospital	Belleville	75%	300+
Provident Hospital of Chicago	Chicago	75%	(a)
Rush University Medical Center	Chicago	75%	300+
Saint Anthony's Health Center	Alton	75%	300+
Sarah Bush Lincoln Health Center	Mattoon	75%	300+
Sherman Hospital	Elgin	75%	300+
Adventist Glenoaks[11]	Glendale Hghts	74%	300+
Advocate Good Samaritan Hospital	Downers Grove	74%	300+
Alexian Brothers Medical Center	Elk Grove Vlg	74%	300+
Centegra Health Sys-Mc Henry Hosp	Mchenry	74%	300+
Graham Hospital Association	Canton	74%	300+
Memorial Hospital of Carbondale	Carbondale	74%	300+
Presence Resurrection Medical Center	Chicago	74%	300+
Rush Oak Park Hospital	Oak Park	74%	300+
Saint Anthony Medical Center	Rockford	74%	300+
Saint Francis Medical Center	Peoria	74%	300+
Genesis Health System	Silvis	73%	300+
Hammond Henry Hospital	Geneseo	73%	300+
Katherine Shaw Bethea Hospital	Dixon	73%	300+
Presence Saint Joseph Hospital - Elgin	Elgin	73%	300+
Richland Memorial Hospital	Olney	73%	300+
Saint Anthonys Memorial Hospital	Effingham	73%	300+
Saint Johns Hospital	Springfield	73%	300+
Saint Marys Hospital	Decatur	73%	300+
Valley West Community Hospital	Sandwich	73%	(a)
Alton Memorial Hospital[11]	Alton	72%	300+
Edward Hospital	Naperville	72%	300+
Elmhurst Memorial Hospital	Elmhurst	72%	300+
Herrin Hospital	Herrin	72%	300+
Metrosouth Medical Center	Blue Island	72%	300+
Presence Mercy Medical Center	Aurora	72%	300+
Presence Saint Francis Hospital	Evanston	72%	300+
Saint Anthony Hospital	Chicago	72%	300+
Kishwaukee Community Hospital	Dekalb	71%	300+
Lake Forest Hospital	Lake Forest	71%	300+
Loyola Gottlieb Memorial Hospital	Melrose Park	71%	300+
Pekin Memorial Hospital	Pekin	71%	300+
Presence Our Lady of the Res Med Ctr	Chicago	71%	300+
Red Bud Regional Hospital	Red Bud	71%	(a)
Riverside Medical Center	Kankakee	71%	300+
Saint Elizabeth Hospital	Belleville	71%	300+
Swedish American Hospital	Rockford	71%	300+
Swedish Covenant Hospital	Chicago	71%	300+
Touchette Regional Hospital	Centreville	71%	(a)
Advocate Christ Hospital & Medical Center	Oak Lawn	70%	300+
Advocate Good Shepherd Hospital	Barrington	70%	300+
Carle Foundation Hospital[11]	Urbana	70%	300+
Delnor Community Hospital	Geneva	70%	300+
Evanston Hospital[11]	Evanston	70%	300+
Fhn Memorial Hospital	Freeport	70%	300+
Little Company of Mary Hospital	Evergreen Park	70%	300+
Memorial Medical Center	Springfield	70%	300+
Mercy Hospital & Medical Center	Chicago	70%	300+
Rockford Memorial Hospital	Rockford	70%	300+
Trinity Rock Island	Rock Island	70%	300+
Decatur Memorial Hospital	Decatur	69%	300+
Franciscan Saint James Health	Olympia Fields	69%	300+
Advocate South Suburban Hospital	Hazel Crest	68%	300+
Galesburg Cottage Hospital	Galesburg	68%	300+
Presence Saint Joseph Medical Center	Joliet	68%	300+
Saint Alexius Medical Center	Hoffman Estates	68%	300+
Gateway Regional Medical Center	Granite City	67%	300+
Heartland Regional Medical Center	Marion	67%	300+
Holy Cross Hospital	Chicago	67%	300+
Presence Covenant Medical Center	Urbana	67%	300+
Presence Saint Joseph Hospital - Chicago	Chicago	67%	300+
Vista Medical Center East	Waukegan	67%	300+
Ingalls Memorial Hospital	Harvey	66%	300+
Macneal Hospital[11]	Berwyn	66%	300+
Palos Community Hospital	Palos Heights	66%	300+
Proctor Hospital	Peoria	65%	300+
Saint Bernard Hospital	Chicago	65%	300+
Union County Hospital	Anna	65%	(a)
South Shore Hospital	Chicago	64%	(a)
University of Illinois Hospital	Chicago	64%	300+
Roseland Community Hospital[3]	Chicago	63%	(a)
Thorek Memorial Hospital	Chicago	63%	(a)
Loretto Hospital	Chicago	62%	(a)
Louis A Weiss Memorial Hospital[11]	Chicago	62%	300+
Loyola University Medical Center	Maywood	62%	300+
Northwestern Memorial Hospital	Chicago	62%	300+
The University of Chicago Medical Center	Chicago	62%	300+
Westlake Community Hospital[11]	Melrose Park	62%	300+
West Suburban Medical Center[11]	Oak Park	61%	300+
Presence Sts Mary & Elizabeth Med Ctr	Chicago	60%	300+
Norwegian - American Hospital	Chicago	59%	300+
Mount Sinai Hospital Medical Center	Chicago	58%	300+
Jackson Park Hospital	Chicago	54%	300+
John H Stroger Jr Hospital	Chicago	48%	300+

Timely Help 'Always' Received

Hospital Name	City	Rate	Cases
OSF Holy Family Medical Center	Monmouth	91%	(a)
Hillsboro Area Hospital	Hillsboro	85%	(a)
Saint Joseph's Hospital	Breese	85%	300+
Saint Joseph Memorial Hospital	Murphysboro	84%	(a)
Salem Township Hospital	Salem	83%	(a)
Rochelle Community Hospital	Rochelle	82%	(a)
Saint Marys Hospital	Centralia	82%	300+
Massac Memorial Hospital	Metropolis	81%	(a)
Wabash General Hospital	Mount Carmel	81%	(a)
Mendota Community Hospital	Mendota	80%	(a)
Gibson Community Hospital	Gibson City	78%	300+
Harrisburg Medical Center	Harrisburg	78%	(a)
Jersey Community Hospital	Jerseyville	78%	(a)
Sparta Community Hospital	Sparta	78%	(a)
Hammond Henry Hospital	Geneseo	77%	300+
Ottawa Reg Hosp & Healthcare Ctr	Ottawa	77%	300+
Pinckneyville Community Hospital	Pinckneyville	77%	(a)
Union County Hospital	Anna	76%	(a)
Adventist La Grange Memorial Hospital[11]	La Grange	75%	300+
Clay County Hospital	Flora	75%	(a)

NOTE: Hospital profiles are in alphabetical order by state, then city, then hospital within the city; Rankings exclude hospitals with less than 25 cases except for patient surveys which excludes hospitals with less than 100 cases; (a) 100-299 cases; (1) The number of cases/patients is too few to report; (2) Data submitted were based on a sample of cases/patients; (3) Results are based on a shorter time period than required; (4) Data suppressed by CMS for one or more quarters; (5) Results are not available for this reporting period; (6) Fewer than 100 patients completed the HCAHPS survey; (7) No cases met the criteria for this measure; (8) The lower limit of the confidence interval cannot be calculated if the number of observed infections equals zero; (9) No data are available from the state/territory for this reporting period; (10) The scores shown reflect fewer than 50 completed surveys; (11) There were discrepancies in the data collection process; (12) This measure does not apply to this hospital for this reporting period; (13) Results cannot be calculated for this reporting period; (14) The results for this state are combined with nearby states to protect confidentiality; Please refer to the User's Guide for a full explanation of data.

Illinois Valley Community Hospital[11]	Peru	75%	300+
Morris Hospital & Healthcare Centers[11]	Morris	75%	(a)
Saint Francis Hospital	Litchfield	75%	300+
Saint James Hospital	Pontiac	75%	(a)
McDonough District Hospital	Macomb	74%	300+
Saint Joseph's Hospital	Highland	74%	(a)
Saint Mary Medical Center	Galesburg	74%	300+
Anderson Hospital	Maryville	73%	300+
Crawford Memorial Hospital	Robinson	73%	(a)
Kewanee Hospital	Kewanee	73%	(a)
Richland Memorial Hospital	Olney	73%	300+
Taylorville Memorial Hospital	Taylorville	73%	300+
Valley West Community Hospital	Sandwich	73%	(a)
Advocate Good Samaritan Hospital	Downers Grove	72%	300+
CGH Medical Center	Sterling	72%	300+
Good Samaritan Regional Health Center	Mount Vernon	72%	300+
Midwestern Region Medical Center	Zion	72%	300+
Rush Oak Park Hospital	Oak Park	72%	300+
Blessing Hospital[11]	Quincy	70%	300+
Centegra Health Sys-Mc Henry Hosp	Mchenry	70%	300+
Crossroads Community Hospital	Mount Vernon	70%	300+
Genesis Health System	Silvis	70%	300+
Iroquois Memorial Hospital	Watseka	70%	(a)
Memorial Hospital	Belleville	70%	300+
Methodist Medical Center of Illinois	Peoria	70%	300+
Saint Margarets Hospital	Spring Valley	70%	300+
Saint Marys Hospital	Streator	70%	300+
Sarah Bush Lincoln Health Center	Mattoon	70%	300+
Abraham Lincoln Memorial Hospital	Lincoln	69%	(a)
Advocate Christ Hospital & Medical Center	Oak Lawn	69%	300+
Advocate Illinois Masonic Medical Center	Chicago	69%	300+
Centegra Health Sys-Woodstock Hosp	Woodstock	69%	300+
Delnor Community Hospital	Geneva	69%	300+
Hinsdale Hospital[11]	Hinsdale	69%	300+
Passavant Area Hospital	Jacksonville	69%	300+
Presence Saint Marys Hospital	Kankakee	69%	300+
Swedish American Hospital	Rockford	69%	300+
Advocate Bromenn Medical Center	Normal	68%	300+
Little Company of Mary Hospital	Evergreen Park	68%	300+
Presence United Samaritans Medical Center	Danville	68%	300+
Riverside Medical Center	Kankakee	68%	300+
Saint Alexius Medical Center	Hoffman Estates	68%	300+
Saint Joseph Medical Center	Bloomington	68%	300+
Adventist Glenoaks[11]	Glendale Hghts	67%	300+
Central Dupage Hospital	Winfield	67%	300+
Graham Hospital Association	Canton	67%	300+
Katherine Shaw Bethea Hospital	Dixon	67%	300+
Saint Elizabeth Hospital	Belleville	67%	300+
Saint Johns Hospital	Springfield	67%	300+
Sherman Hospital	Elgin	67%	300+
Silver Cross Hospital & Medical Centers	New Lenox	67%	300+
Greenville Regional Hospital	Greenville	66%	(a)
Memorial Hospital of Carbondale	Carbondale	66%	300+
Memorial Medical Center	Springfield	66%	300+
Perry Memorial Hospital	Princeton	66%	(a)
Rush University Medical Center	Chicago	66%	300+
Saint Anthonys Memorial Hospital	Effingham	66%	300+
Advocate Condell Medical Center	Libertyville	65%	300+
Advocate Lutheran General Hospital	Park Ridge	65%	300+
Advocate South Suburban Hospital	Hazel Crest	65%	300+
Advocate Trinity Hospital	Chicago	65%	300+
Herrin Hospital	Herrin	65%	300+
Metrosouth Medical Center	Blue Island	65%	300+
Northwest Community Hospital	Arlington Hgts	65%	300+
Provident Hospital of Chicago	Chicago	65%	(a)
Red Bud Regional Hospital	Red Bud	65%	(a)
Saint Francis Medical Center	Peoria	65%	300+
Advocate Good Shepherd Hospital	Barrington	64%	300+
Alexian Brothers Medical Center	Elk Grove Vlg	64%	300+
Alton Memorial Hospital[11]	Alton	64%	300+
Heartland Regional Medical Center	Marion	64%	300+
Macneal Hospital[11]	Berwyn	64%	300+
Saint Anthony Medical Center	Rockford	64%	300+
Adventist Bolingbrook Hospital[11]	Bolingbrook	63%	300+
Carle Foundation Hospital[11]	Urbana	63%	300+
Galesburg Cottage Hospital	Galesburg	63%	300+
Pekin Memorial Hospital	Pekin	63%	300+
Presence Resurrection Medical Center	Chicago	63%	300+
Proctor Hospital	Peoria	63%	300+
Swedish Covenant Hospital	Chicago	63%	300+
Touchette Regional Hospital	Centreville	63%	(a)
Edward Hospital	Naperville	62%	300+
Fhn Memorial Hospital	Freeport	62%	300+
Gateway Regional Medical Center	Granite City	62%	300+
Loyola Gottlieb Memorial Hospital	Melrose Park	62%	300+
Loyola University Medical Center	Maywood	62%	300+
Palos Community Hospital	Palos Heights	62%	300+
Copley Memorial Hospital	Aurora	61%	300+
Decatur Memorial Hospital	Decatur	61%	300+
Elmhurst Memorial Hospital	Elmhurst	61%	300+
Kishwaukee Community Hospital	Dekalb	61%	300+
Presence Our Lady of the Res Med Ctr	Chicago	61%	300+
Rockford Memorial Hospital	Rockford	61%	300+
Evanston Hospital[11]	Evanston	60%	300+
Northwestern Memorial Hospital	Chicago	60%	300+
Presence Covenant Medical Center	Urbana	60%	300+
Presence Mercy Medical Center	Aurora	60%	300+
Presence Saint Francis Hospital	Evanston	60%	300+
Presence Sts Mary & Elizabeth Med Ctr	Chicago	60%	300+
Saint Anthony's Health Center	Alton	60%	300+
Mercy Hospital & Medical Center	Chicago	59%	300+
Presence Saint Joseph Hospital - Chicago	Chicago	59%	300+
Presence Saint Joseph Medical Center	Joliet	59%	300+
Saint Marys Hospital	Decatur	59%	300+
Holy Cross Hospital	Chicago	58%	300+
Presence Saint Joseph Hospital - Elgin	Elgin	58%	300+
Saint Anthony Hospital	Chicago	58%	300+
Trinity Rock Island	Rock Island	58%	300+
West Suburban Medical Center[11]	Oak Park	58%	300+
Mount Sinai Hospital Medical Center	Chicago	56%	300+
Vista Medical Center East	Waukegan	56%	300+
Ingalls Memorial Hospital	Harvey	55%	300+
Lake Forest Hospital	Lake Forest	55%	300+
The University of Chicago Medical Center	Chicago	55%	300+
Franciscan Saint James Health	Olympia Fields	54%	300+
Louis A Weiss Memorial Hospital[11]	Chicago	54%	300+
University of Illinois Hospital	Chicago	54%	300+
John H Stroger Jr Hospital	Chicago	53%	300+
Norwegian - American Hospital	Chicago	53%	300+
Westlake Community Hospital[11]	Melrose Park	52%	300+
Loretto Hospital	Chicago	51%	(a)
Thorek Memorial Hospital	Chicago	50%	(a)
Jackson Park Hospital	Chicago	44%	300+
Saint Bernard Hospital	Chicago	44%	300+
South Shore Hospital	Chicago	44%	(a)
Roseland Community Hospital[3]	Chicago	41%	(a)

Would Definitely Recommend Hospital

Hospital Name	City	Rate	Cases
Midwestern Region Medical Center	Zion	90%	300+
Saint Joseph's Hospital	Breese	86%	300+
Gibson Community Hospital	Gibson City	85%	300+
Abraham Lincoln Memorial Hospital	Lincoln	84%	(a)
Saint Mary Medical Center	Galesburg	84%	300+
Central Dupage Hospital	Winfield	83%	300+
Rush University Medical Center	Chicago	83%	300+
Saint Joseph Memorial Hospital	Murphysboro	83%	(a)
Saint Joseph Medical Center	Bloomington	82%	300+
Edward Hospital	Naperville	81%	300+
OSF Holy Family Medical Center	Monmouth	81%	(a)
Presence Saint Marys Hospital	Kankakee	81%	300+
Adventist La Grange Memorial Hospital[11]	La Grange	80%	300+
Advocate Lutheran General Hospital	Park Ridge	80%	300+
Hammond Henry Hospital	Geneseo	80%	300+
Illinois Valley Community Hospital[11]	Peru	80%	300+
Northwestern Memorial Hospital	Chicago	80%	300+
Taylorville Memorial Hospital	Taylorville	80%	300+
Advocate Bromenn Medical Center	Normal	79%	300+
Herrin Hospital	Herrin	79%	300+
Hillsboro Area Hospital	Hillsboro	79%	(a)
Hinsdale Hospital[11]	Hinsdale	79%	300+
Memorial Medical Center	Springfield	79%	300+
Morris Hospital & Healthcare Centers[11]	Morris	79%	(a)
Silver Cross Hospital & Medical Centers	New Lenox	79%	300+
Evanston Hospital[11]	Evanston	78%	300+
Memorial Hospital	Belleville	78%	300+
Memorial Hospital of Carbondale	Carbondale	78%	300+
Methodist Medical Center of Illinois	Peoria	78%	300+
Northwest Community Hospital	Arlington Hgts	78%	300+
Swedish American Hospital	Rockford	78%	300+
Carle Foundation Hospital[11]	Urbana	77%	300+
Riverside Medical Center	Kankakee	77%	300+
Saint Francis Medical Center	Peoria	77%	300+
Saint Marys Hospital	Centralia	77%	300+
Advocate Good Samaritan Hospital	Downers Grove	76%	300+
Advocate Good Shepherd Hospital	Barrington	76%	300+
Alexian Brothers Medical Center	Elk Grove Vlg	76%	300+
Elmhurst Memorial Hospital	Elmhurst	76%	300+
Little Company of Mary Hospital	Evergreen Park	76%	300+
Advocate Condell Medical Center	Libertyville	75%	300+
Alton Memorial Hospital[11]	Alton	75%	300+
Anderson Hospital	Maryville	75%	300+
Massac Memorial Hospital	Metropolis	75%	(a)
Mendota Community Hospital	Mendota	75%	(a)
Rochelle Community Hospital	Rochelle	75%	(a)
Sherman Hospital	Elgin	75%	300+
Valley West Community Hospital	Sandwich	75%	(a)
Wabash General Hospital	Mount Carmel	75%	(a)
Advocate Christ Hospital & Medical Center	Oak Lawn	74%	300+
Blessing Hospital[11]	Quincy	74%	300+
Copley Memorial Hospital	Aurora	74%	300+
Delnor Community Hospital	Geneva	74%	300+
Presence Saint Joseph Hospital - Chicago	Chicago	74%	300+
Richland Memorial Hospital	Olney	74%	300+
Saint Alexius Medical Center	Hoffman Estates	74%	300+
Saint Anthony Medical Center	Rockford	74%	300+
Saint Johns Hospital	Springfield	74%	300+
Saint Marys Hospital	Decatur	74%	300+
Advocate Illinois Masonic Medical Center	Chicago	73%	300+
Good Samaritan Regional Health Center	Mount Vernon	73%	300+
Katherine Shaw Bethea Hospital	Dixon	73%	300+
Presence Covenant Medical Center	Urbana	73%	300+
Saint Anthony's Health Center	Alton	73%	300+
Sarah Bush Lincoln Health Center	Mattoon	73%	300+
Crawford Memorial Hospital	Robinson	72%	(a)
Loyola University Medical Center	Maywood	72%	300+
Proctor Hospital	Peoria	72%	300+
Rush Oak Park Hospital	Oak Park	72%	300+
Saint Margarets Hospital	Spring Valley	72%	300+
Adventist Bolingbrook Hospital[11]	Bolingbrook	71%	300+
CGH Medical Center	Sterling	71%	300+
Decatur Memorial Hospital	Decatur	71%	300+
Genesis Health System	Silvis	71%	300+
Saint Francis Hospital	Litchfield	71%	300+
Salem Township Hospital	Salem	71%	(a)
The University of Chicago Medical Center	Chicago	71%	300+
Clay County Hospital	Flora	70%	(a)
Crossroads Community Hospital	Mount Vernon	70%	300+
Presence Resurrection Medical Center	Chicago	70%	300+
Rockford Memorial Hospital	Rockford	70%	300+
Saint Joseph's Hospital	Highland	70%	(a)
Trinity Rock Island	Rock Island	70%	300+
Centegra Health Sys-Woodstock Hosp	Woodstock	69%	300+
Kishwaukee Community Hospital	Dekalb	69%	300+
Pinckneyville Community Hospital	Pinckneyville	69%	(a)
Presence Saint Francis Hospital	Evanston	69%	300+
Presence Sts Mary & Elizabeth Med Ctr	Chicago	69%	300+
Presence United Samaritans Medical Center	Danville	69%	300+
McDonough District Hospital	Macomb	68%	300+
Metrosouth Medical Center	Blue Island	68%	300+
Palos Community Hospital	Palos Heights	68%	300+
Red Bud Regional Hospital	Red Bud	68%	(a)
Saint Elizabeth Hospital	Belleville	68%	300+
Centegra Health Sys-Mc Henry Hosp	Mchenry	67%	300+
Greenville Regional Hospital	Greenville	67%	(a)
Macneal Hospital[11]	Berwyn	67%	300+
Perry Memorial Hospital	Princeton	67%	(a)
Presence Mercy Medical Center	Aurora	67%	300+
Presence Saint Joseph Hospital - Elgin	Elgin	67%	300+
Advocate South Suburban Hospital	Hazel Crest	66%	300+
Galesburg Cottage Hospital	Galesburg	66%	300+
Ingalls Memorial Hospital	Harvey	66%	300+
Lake Forest Hospital	Lake Forest	66%	300+
Mercy Hospital & Medical Center	Chicago	66%	300+
Passavant Area Hospital	Jacksonville	66%	300+
Presence Saint Joseph Medical Center	Joliet	66%	300+
Saint Anthony Hospital	Chicago	66%	300+
Saint Anthonys Memorial Hospital	Effingham	66%	300+
Swedish Covenant Hospital	Chicago	66%	300+
Iroquois Memorial Hospital	Watseka	65%	(a)
Ottawa Reg Hosp & Healthcare Ctr	Ottawa	65%	300+
Saint James Hospital	Pontiac	65%	(a)
University of Illinois Hospital	Chicago	65%	300+
Graham Hospital Association	Canton	64%	300+
Advocate Trinity Hospital	Chicago	63%	300+
Fhn Memorial Hospital	Freeport	63%	300+
Pekin Memorial Hospital	Pekin	63%	300+
Saint Marys Hospital	Streator	63%	300+
Union County Hospital	Anna	63%	(a)
Harrisburg Medical Center	Harrisburg	62%	(a)
Jersey Community Hospital	Jerseyville	62%	(a)
Kewanee Hospital	Kewanee	62%	(a)
Louis A Weiss Memorial Hospital[11]	Chicago	62%	300+
Presence Our Lady of the Res Med Ctr	Chicago	62%	300+
Provident Hospital of Chicago	Chicago	62%	(a)
Heartland Regional Medical Center	Marion	61%	300+
John H Stroger Jr Hospital	Chicago	61%	300+
Loyola Gottlieb Memorial Hospital	Melrose Park	61%	300+
Mount Sinai Hospital Medical Center	Chicago	61%	300+
Franciscan Saint James Health	Olympia Fields	60%	300+
Touchette Regional Hospital	Centreville	59%	(a)
West Suburban Medical Center[11]	Oak Park	59%	300+
Vista Medical Center East	Waukegan	58%	300+
Adventist Glenoaks[11]	Glendale Hghts	57%	300+
Gateway Regional Medical Center	Granite City	57%	300+
Westlake Community Hospital[11]	Melrose Park	57%	300+
Thorek Memorial Hospital	Chicago	55%	(a)
Holy Cross Hospital	Chicago	54%	300+
Sparta Community Hospital	Sparta	53%	(a)
Norwegian - American Hospital	Chicago	47%	300+
South Shore Hospital	Chicago	43%	(a)
Roseland Community Hospital[3]	Chicago	37%	(a)
Saint Bernard Hospital	Chicago	37%	300+

NOTE: Hospital profiles are in alphabetical order by state, then city, then hospital within the city; Rankings exclude hospitals with less than 25 cases except for patient surveys which excludes hospitals with less than 100 cases; (a) 100-299 cases; (1) The number of cases/patients is too few to report; (2) Data submitted were based on a sample of cases/patients; (3) Results are based on a shorter time period than required; (4) Data suppressed by CMS for one or more quarters; (5) Results are not available for this reporting period; (6) Fewer than 100 patients completed the HCAHPS survey; (7) No cases met the criteria for this measure; (8) The lower limit of the confidence interval cannot be calculated if the number of observed infections equals zero; (9) No data are available from the state/territory for this reporting period; (10) The scores shown reflect fewer than 50 completed surveys; (11) There were discrepancies in the data collection process; (12) This measure does not apply to this hospital for this reporting period; (13) Results cannot be calculated for this reporting period; (14) The results for this state are combined with nearby states to protect confidentiality; Please refer to the User's Guide for a full explanation of data.

Jackson Park Hospital	Chicago	36%	300+
Loretto Hospital	Chicago	36%	(a)

Use of Medical Imaging

Cardiac Imaging Stress Test before OP Surgery

Hospital Name	City	Rate	Cases
Abraham Lincoln Memorial Hospital	Lincoln	0.0%	62
Ferrell Hospital Community Foundations	Eldorado	0.0%	49
Iroquois Memorial Hospital	Watseka	0.0%	61
Memorial Hospital	Chester	0.0%	131
Hammond Henry Hospital	Geneseo	0.9%	108
Paris Community Hospital	Paris	1.1%	92
Trinity Rock Island	Rock Island	1.3%	153
Taylorville Memorial Hospital	Taylorville	1.5%	136
Advocate Trinity Hospital	Chicago	1.6%	254
Graham Hospital Association	Canton	2.0%	152
South Shore Hospital	Chicago	2.0%	49
McDonough District Hospital	Macomb	2.1%	97
Presence Covenant Medical Center	Urbana	2.3%	213
Proctor Hospital	Peoria	2.5%	282
Mercy Hospital & Medical Center	Chicago	2.6%	533
John H Stroger Jr Hospital	Chicago	2.9%	171
Doctor John Warner Hospital	Clinton	3.1%	65
Mendota Community Hospital	Mendota	3.1%	130
Saint Marys Hospital	Streator	3.1%	225
Galesburg Cottage Hospital	Galesburg	3.2%	186
Westlake Community Hospital	Melrose Park	3.2%	158
Clay County Hospital	Flora	3.3%	61
Crossroads Community Hospital	Mount Vernon	3.3%	91
Red Bud Regional Hospital	Red Bud	3.3%	123
Advocate Eureka Hospital	Eureka	3.4%	59
Saint Anthony Medical Center	Rockford	3.5%	1646
Pekin Memorial Hospital	Pekin	3.7%	219
Illini Community Hospital	Pittsfield	3.8%	79
Saint Anthonys Memorial Hospital	Effingham	3.8%	771
Saint James Hospital	Pontiac	3.8%	240
University of Illinois Hospital	Chicago	3.8%	366
Presence Sts Mary & Elizabeth Med Ctr	Chicago	3.9%	517
Edward Hospital	Naperville	4.0%	2044
Ottawa Reg Hosp & Healthcare Ctr	Ottawa	4.0%	198
Good Samaritan Regional Health Center	Mount Vernon	4.1%	344
Saint Mary Medical Center	Galesburg	4.1%	268
Katherine Shaw Bethea Hospital	Dixon	4.2%	381
Delnor Community Hospital	Geneva	4.3%	552
The University of Chicago Medical Center	Chicago	4.3%	790
Advocate Bromenn Medical Center	Normal	4.4%	339
Adventist Bolingbrook Hospital	Bolingbrook	4.5%	178
Saint Francis Hospital	Litchfield	4.5%	202
Alexian Brothers Medical Center	Elk Grove Vlg	4.6%	1554
Fairfield Memorial Hospital	Fairfield	4.6%	151
Hinsdale Hospital	Hinsdale	4.6%	1253
Riverside Medical Center	Kankakee	4.6%	395
Saint Johns Hospital	Springfield	4.6%	2450
Loyola Gottlieb Memorial Hospital	Melrose Park	4.7%	493
Little Company of Mary Hospital	Evergreen Park	4.8%	606
Methodist Medical Center of Illinois	Peoria	4.8%	537
Mount Sinai Hospital Medical Center	Chicago	4.8%	228
Saint Anthony's Health Center	Alton	4.9%	244
Swedish American Hospital	Rockford	4.9%	965
Memorial Hospital of Carbondale	Carbondale	5.0%	1518
Advocate Good Shepherd Hospital	Barrington	5.2%	756
Decatur Memorial Hospital	Decatur	5.2%	677
Louis A Weiss Memorial Hospital	Chicago	5.2%	309
Memorial Hospital	Belleville	5.2%	698
Memorial Medical Center	Springfield	5.2%	344
Saint Anthony Hospital	Chicago	5.2%	134
Saint Marys Hospital	Decatur	5.2%	845
Sarah Bush Lincoln Health Center	Mattoon	5.2%	610
Central Dupage Hospital	Winfield	5.3%	737
CGH Medical Center	Sterling	5.3%	787
Kishwaukee Community Hospital	Dekalb	5.3%	281
Presence Saint Joseph Hospital - Chicago	Chicago	5.3%	395
Saint Francis Medical Center	Peoria	5.3%	1628
Blessing Hospital	Quincy	5.4%	569
Metrosouth Medical Center	Blue Island	5.4%	186
Advocate Christ Hospital & Medical Center	Oak Lawn	5.5%	963
Morris Hospital & Healthcare Centers	Morris	5.5%	329
Rockford Memorial Hospital	Rockford	5.5%	924
Gibson Community Hospital	Gibson City	5.6%	71
Saint Joseph Medical Center	Bloomington	5.6%	571
Franciscan Saint James Health	Olympia Fields	5.7%	969
Loyola University Medical Center	Maywood	5.7%	1626
Rush Oak Park Hospital	Oak Park	5.7%	247
Harrisburg Medical Center	Harrisburg	5.8%	121
Presence Resurrection Medical Center	Chicago	5.8%	741
Saint Elizabeth Hospital	Belleville	5.8%	607
Advocate South Suburban Hospital	Hazel Crest	5.9%	459
Fhn Memorial Hospital	Freeport	5.9%	404
Illinois Valley Community Hospital	Peru	6.0%	284
Ingalls Memorial Hospital	Harvey	6.0%	737
Presence Our Lady of the Res Med Ctr	Chicago	6.0%	383
Valley West Community Hospital	Sandwich	6.0%	83
Thorek Memorial Hospital	Chicago	6.1%	115
Genesis Health System	Silvis	6.2%	130
Macneal Hospital	Berwyn	6.2%	307
Presence Mercy Medical Center	Aurora	6.2%	291
Saint Alexius Medical Center	Hoffman Estates	6.2%	534
Massac Memorial Hospital	Metropolis	6.3%	96
Rush University Medical Center	Chicago	6.3%	1292
Sherman Hospital	Elgin	6.3%	863
Silver Cross Hospital & Medical Centers	New Lenox	6.3%	448
Evanston Hospital	Evanston	6.4%	4048
Swedish Covenant Hospital	Chicago	6.4%	849
Advocate Lutheran General Hospital	Park Ridge	6.5%	664
Anderson Hospital	Maryville	6.6%	151
Elmhurst Memorial Hospital	Elmhurst	6.6%	792
Palos Community Hospital	Palos Heights	6.6%	1141
Saint Margarets Hospital	Spring Valley	6.6%	151
West Suburban Medical Center	Oak Park	6.6%	211
Advocate Illinois Masonic Medical Center	Chicago	6.7%	342
Centegra Health Sys-Mc Henry Hosp	Mchenry	6.7%	675
Saint Joseph's Hospital	Breese	6.7%	224
Northwestern Memorial Hospital	Chicago	6.8%	2217
Presence United Samaritans Medical Center	Danville	6.8%	117
Centegra Health Sys-Woodstock Hosp	Woodstock	6.9%	361
Norwegian - American Hospital	Chicago	6.9%	72
Passavant Area Hospital	Jacksonville	7.0%	114
Presence Saint Marys Hospital	Kankakee	7.0%	214
Carlinville Area Hospital	Carlinville	7.1%	85
Herrin Hospital	Herrin	7.2%	765
Presence Saint Francis Hospital	Evanston	7.2%	445
Northwest Community Hospital	Arlington Hgts	7.3%	1126
Adventist La Grange Memorial Hospital	La Grange	7.4%	282
Carle Foundation Hospital	Urbana	7.4%	472
Greenville Regional Hospital	Greenville	7.4%	81
Holy Cross Hospital	Chicago	7.4%	162
Adventist Glenoaks	Glendale Hghts	7.5%	120
Advocate Condell Medical Center	Libertyville	7.5%	523
Presence Saint Joseph Hospital - Elgin	Elgin	7.5%	413
Heartland Regional Medical Center	Marion	7.6%	291
Copley Memorial Hospital	Aurora	7.7%	855
Lake Forest Hospital	Lake Forest	7.7%	413
Alton Memorial Hospital	Alton	8.0%	237
Presence Saint Joseph Medical Center	Joliet	8.4%	789
Shelby Memorial Hospital	Shelbyville	8.4%	83
Richland Memorial Hospital	Olney	8.5%	177
Advocate Good Samaritan Hospital	Downers Grove	9.4%	488
Vista Medical Center East	Waukegan	9.4%	159
Mercy Harvard Hospital	Harvard	10.4%	106
Saint Joseph's Hospital	Highland	10.5%	86
Saint Marys Hospital	Centralia	12.3%	195

Combination Abdominal CT Scan

Hospital Name	City	Rate	Cases
Jackson Park Hospital	Chicago	0.0%	130
CGH Medical Center	Sterling	1.1%	749
Saint Anthony Hospital	Chicago	1.4%	218
Clay County Hospital	Flora	1.5%	333
Fhn Memorial Hospital	Freeport	1.5%	593
Presence Covenant Medical Center	Urbana	1.5%	272
Holy Cross Hospital	Chicago	1.6%	425
Kishwaukee Community Hospital	Dekalb	1.9%	474
Hopedale Medical Complex	Hopedale	2.2%	136
Advocate Condell Medical Center	Libertyville	2.3%	1449
Advocate Trinity Hospital	Chicago	2.3%	522
Genesis Health System	Silvis	2.3%	308
Memorial Hospital	Chester	2.3%	177
Advocate Illinois Masonic Medical Center	Chicago	2.7%	729
Passavant Area Hospital	Jacksonville	2.7%	752
Valley West Community Hospital	Sandwich	2.7%	333
Metrosouth Medical Center	Blue Island	2.8%	392
Alton Memorial Hospital	Alton	2.9%	842
Anderson Hospital	Maryville	3.0%	770
Mercy Harvard Hospital	Harvard	3.0%	101
OSF Holy Family Medical Center	Monmouth	3.1%	127
Mercy Hospital & Medical Center	Chicago	3.2%	820
Blessing Hospital	Quincy	3.3%	769
Illini Community Hospital	Pittsfield	3.3%	242
Palos Community Hospital	Palos Heights	3.4%	1889
Galesburg Cottage Hospital	Galesburg	3.5%	254
Trinity Rock Island	Rock Island	3.5%	1025
Advocate Good Shepherd Hospital	Barrington	3.8%	1051
Hoopeston Community Memorial Hospital	Hoopeston	3.8%	104
Swedish American Hospital	Rockford	3.8%	1669
Decatur Memorial Hospital	Decatur	3.9%	1301
Macneal Hospital	Berwyn	4.0%	730
Presence Mercy Medical Center	Aurora	4.0%	803
Sarah Bush Lincoln Health Center	Mattoon	4.3%	1035
Advocate Lutheran General Hospital	Park Ridge	4.4%	2083
Advocate South Suburban Hospital	Hazel Crest	4.4%	850
Memorial Medical Center	Springfield	4.5%	2577
Katherine Shaw Bethea Hospital	Dixon	4.6%	411
Copley Memorial Hospital	Aurora	4.7%	1193
Adventist La Grange Memorial Hospital	La Grange	4.9%	933
Advocate Christ Hospital & Medical Center	Oak Lawn	5.0%	1517
Pekin Memorial Hospital	Pekin	5.1%	511
Presence Saint Joseph Hospital - Elgin	Elgin	5.1%	622
Riverside Medical Center	Kankakee	5.1%	1060
Rush University Medical Center	Chicago	5.1%	534
Saint Anthony Medical Center	Rockford	5.1%	1537
Westlake Community Hospital	Melrose Park	5.3%	208
Central Dupage Hospital	Winfield	5.4%	1701
Mount Sinai Hospital Medical Center	Chicago	5.5%	455
Hammond Henry Hospital	Geneseo	5.6%	306
Silver Cross Hospital & Medical Centers	New Lenox	5.6%	933
Graham Hospital Association	Canton	5.7%	336
Saint James Hospital	Pontiac	5.7%	422
Presence Saint Joseph Hospital - Chicago	Chicago	5.8%	431
Northwest Community Hospital	Arlington Hgts	5.9%	3853
Shelby Memorial Hospital	Shelbyville	5.9%	220
Saint Anthonys Memorial Hospital	Effingham	6.0%	998
Thorek Memorial Hospital	Chicago	6.0%	182
Loretto Hospital	Chicago	6.2%	65
Heartland Regional Medical Center	Marion	6.4%	422
Little Company of Mary Hospital	Evergreen Park	6.4%	903
Abraham Lincoln Memorial Hospital	Lincoln	6.6%	501
Carle Foundation Hospital	Urbana	6.6%	918
Proctor Hospital	Peoria	6.7%	416
Adventist Bolingbrook Hospital	Bolingbrook	6.9%	447
Saint Joseph's Hospital	Highland	6.9%	291
Advocate Good Samaritan Hospital	Downers Grove	7.1%	939
Ingalls Memorial Hospital	Harvey	7.1%	1917
Saint Marys Hospital	Decatur	7.1%	660
Saint Bernard Hospital	Chicago	7.2%	138
Doctor John Warner Hospital	Clinton	7.3%	124
Memorial Hospital	Belleville	7.3%	1650
Rush Oak Park Hospital	Oak Park	7.3%	449
Elmhurst Memorial Hospital	Elmhurst	7.5%	1643
Presence Sts Mary & Elizabeth Med Ctr	Chicago	7.5%	831
Mendota Community Hospital	Mendota	7.6%	275
The University of Chicago Medical Center	Chicago	7.6%	3514
Centegra Health Sys-Mc Henry Hosp	Mchenry	7.7%	987
Presence Our Lady of the Res Med Ctr	Chicago	7.7%	610
Edward Hospital	Naperville	7.8%	1980
Pana Community Hospital	Pana	7.9%	331
Saint Mary Medical Center	Galesburg	7.9%	580
Presence Saint Francis Hospital	Evanston	8.1%	582
Taylorville Memorial Hospital	Taylorville	8.1%	541
Saint Alexius Medical Center	Hoffman Estates	8.2%	1265
University of Illinois Hospital	Chicago	8.2%	635
Carlinville Area Hospital	Carlinville	8.3%	206
Centegra Health Sys-Woodstock Hosp	Woodstock	8.3%	639
Sherman Hospital	Elgin	8.3%	1517
Rockford Memorial Hospital	Rockford	8.4%	666
Illinois Valley Community Hospital	Peru	8.6%	406
Evanston Hospital	Evanston	8.9%	5153
Adventist Glenoaks	Glendale Hghts	9.5%	147
Alexian Brothers Medical Center	Elk Grove Vlg	9.5%	1763
Crossroads Community Hospital	Mount Vernon	9.7%	237
Morris Hospital & Healthcare Centers	Morris	9.9%	776
Saint Joseph Medical Center	Bloomington	10.4%	655
Massac Memorial Hospital	Metropolis	10.7%	373
Franciscan Saint James Health	Olympia Fields	11.0%	948
Mason District Hospital	Havana	11.0%	172
Memorial Hospital of Carbondale	Carbondale	11.0%	976
Louis A Weiss Memorial Hospital	Chicago	11.2%	492
Norwegian - American Hospital	Chicago	11.5%	191
Saint Joseph's Hospital	Breese	11.5%	304
Hinsdale Hospital	Hinsdale	11.7%	844
Swedish Covenant Hospital	Chicago	11.8%	1124
Saint Francis Medical Center	Peoria	12.0%	1488
Greenville Regional Hospital	Greenville	12.3%	269
Saint Anthony's Health Center	Alton	12.3%	506
Herrin Hospital	Herrin	12.6%	1396
Presence Resurrection Medical Center	Chicago	12.9%	1296
Red Bud Regional Hospital	Red Bud	13.0%	207
Loyola University Medical Center	Maywood	13.1%	2739
Loyola Gottlieb Memorial Hospital	Melrose Park	13.3%	677
Union County Hospital	Anna	13.4%	247
Ottawa Reg Hosp & Healthcare Ctr	Ottawa	14.1%	474
Northwestern Memorial Hospital	Chicago	14.8%	4510
Saint Margarets Hospital	Spring Valley	15.2%	302
Hardin County General Hospital	Rosiclare	15.4%	104
Saint Johns Hospital	Springfield	15.5%	975
Gateway Regional Medical Center	Granite City	16.0%	332
John H Stroger Jr Hospital	Chicago	16.3%	650
Touchette Regional Hospital	Centreville	16.3%	92
Presence United Samaritans Medical Center	Danville	16.4%	451
Vista Medical Center East	Waukegan	17.1%	858
Methodist Medical Center of Illinois	Peoria	17.3%	969
Presence Saint Joseph Medical Center	Joliet	17.7%	1072

NOTE: Hospital profiles are in alphabetical order by state, then city, then hospital within the city; Rankings exclude hospitals with less than 25 cases except for patient surveys which excludes hospitals with less than 100 cases; (a) 100-299 cases; (1) The number of cases/patients is too few to report; (2) Data submitted were based on a sample of cases/patients; (3) Results are based on a shorter time period than required; (4) Data suppressed by CMS for one or more quarters; (5) Results are not available for this reporting period; (6) Fewer than 100 patients completed the HCAHPS survey; (7) No cases met the criteria for this measure; (8) The lower limit of the confidence interval cannot be calculated if the number of observed infections equals zero; (9) No data are available from the state/territory for this reporting period; (10) The scores shown reflect fewer than 50 completed surveys; (11) There were discrepancies in the data collection process; (12) This measure does not apply to this hospital for this reporting period; (13) Results cannot be calculated for this reporting period; (14) The results for this state are combined with nearby states to protect confidentiality; Please refer to the User's Guide for a full explanation of data.

Hospital Name	City	Rate	Cases
Gibson Community Hospital	Gibson City	18.6%	194
West Suburban Medical Center	Oak Park	18.6%	506
Good Samaritan Regional Health Center	Mount Vernon	18.7%	713
Lake Forest Hospital	Lake Forest	19.5%	1204
Saint Joseph Memorial Hospital	Murphysboro	20.0%	480
Presence Saint Marys Hospital	Kankakee	20.1%	583
Richland Memorial Hospital	Olney	20.1%	294
Paris Community Hospital	Paris	20.5%	249
Saint Elizabeth Hospital	Belleville	21.0%	632
Franklin Hospital	Benton	21.2%	165
Saint Marys Hospital	Streator	21.6%	352
Ferrell Hospital Community Foundations	Eldorado	23.0%	213
Harrisburg Medical Center	Harrisburg	23.2%	569
Saint Marys Hospital	Centralia	23.2%	689
Delnor Community Hospital	Geneva	23.3%	1090
Jersey Community Hospital	Jerseyville	23.8%	223
Methodist Hospital of Chicago	Chicago	24.7%	89
Advocate Bromenn Medical Center	Normal	24.8%	540
Wabash General Hospital	Mount Carmel	28.4%	194
Advocate Eureka Hospital	Eureka	30.2%	86
Provident Hospital of Chicago	Chicago	34.4%	96
Saint Francis Hospital	Litchfield	38.9%	568
Fairfield Memorial Hospital	Fairfield	40.8%	395
Iroquois Memorial Hospital	Watseka	42.2%	249
Salem Township Hospital	Salem	47.4%	323
Roseland Community Hospital	Chicago	53.9%	76
South Shore Hospital	Chicago	54.3%	105
McDonough District Hospital	Macomb	60.6%	360
Midwestern Region Medical Center	Zion	96.4%	949

Combination Brain/Sinus CT Scan

Hospital Name	City	Rate	Cases
Loretto Hospital	Chicago	0.0%	136
Saint Joseph Medical Center	Bloomington	0.0%	472
Genesis Health System	Silvis	0.3%	352
Delnor Community Hospital	Geneva	0.4%	734
Advocate Trinity Hospital	Chicago	0.5%	579
Hoopeston Community Memorial Hospital	Hoopeston	0.6%	181
Union County Hospital	Anna	0.6%	309
John H Stroger Jr Hospital	Chicago	0.7%	291
Edward Hospital	Naperville	0.8%	1449
Advocate Christ Hospital & Medical Center	Oak Lawn	1.0%	1275
Central Dupage Hospital	Winfield	1.0%	1342
Mount Sinai Hospital Medical Center	Chicago	1.0%	387
Paris Community Hospital	Paris	1.0%	299
Rockford Memorial Hospital	Rockford	1.0%	735
Riverside Medical Center	Kankakee	1.1%	984
Northwestern Memorial Hospital	Chicago	1.2%	1599
Presence Mercy Medical Center	Aurora	1.2%	642
West Suburban Medical Center	Oak Park	1.2%	505
Iroquois Memorial Hospital	Watseka	1.3%	378
Ottawa Reg Hosp & Healthcare Ctr	Ottawa	1.3%	311
Presence Saint Joseph Hospital - Chicago	Chicago	1.3%	459
Carle Foundation Hospital	Urbana	1.4%	797
Hammond Henry Hospital	Geneseo	1.4%	351
Presence Sts Mary & Elizabeth Med Ctr	Chicago	1.4%	733
Saint Marys Hospital	Streator	1.4%	346
Swedish American Hospital	Rockford	1.4%	1332
University of Illinois Hospital	Chicago	1.4%	640
Advocate South Suburban Hospital	Hazel Crest	1.5%	819
CGH Medical Center	Sterling	1.5%	740
Metrosouth Medical Center	Blue Island	1.5%	593
Elmhurst Memorial Hospital	Elmhurst	1.6%	1223
Harrisburg Medical Center	Harrisburg	1.6%	577
Little Company of Mary Hospital	Evergreen Park	1.6%	1031
Advocate Illinois Masonic Medical Center	Chicago	1.7%	576
Copley Memorial Hospital	Aurora	1.7%	1205
Galesburg Cottage Hospital	Galesburg	1.7%	405
Kishwaukee Community Hospital	Dekalb	1.7%	697
Saint Mary Medical Center	Galesburg	1.7%	478
Holy Cross Hospital	Chicago	1.8%	704
Loyola University Medical Center	Maywood	1.8%	963
Advocate Bromenn Medical Center	Normal	1.9%	622
Gateway Regional Medical Center	Granite City	1.9%	463
The University of Chicago Medical Center	Chicago	2.0%	856
Advocate Good Samaritan Hospital	Downers Grove	2.1%	1197
Alexian Brothers Medical Center	Elk Grove Vlg	2.1%	1191
Proctor Hospital	Peoria	2.1%	433
Silver Cross Hospital & Medical Centers	New Lenox	2.1%	963
Trinity Rock Island	Rock Island	2.1%	960
Advocate Condell Medical Center	Libertyville	2.2%	1292
Jersey Community Hospital	Jerseyville	2.2%	415
Pekin Memorial Hospital	Pekin	2.2%	448
Sarah Bush Lincoln Health Center	Mattoon	2.2%	915
Evanston Hospital	Evanston	2.3%	3192
Palos Community Hospital	Palos Heights	2.3%	1606
Advocate Good Shepherd Hospital	Barrington	2.4%	904
Fhn Memorial Hospital	Freeport	2.4%	547
Mercy Hospital & Medical Center	Chicago	2.4%	1021
Saint Alexius Medical Center	Hoffman Estates	2.5%	1114
Saint Anthony Medical Center	Rockford	2.5%	1382
Blessing Hospital	Quincy	2.6%	913
Presence Our Lady of the Res Med Ctr	Chicago	2.6%	874
Presence Resurrection Medical Center	Chicago	2.6%	1372
Sherman Hospital	Elgin	2.6%	1176
Presence Saint Joseph Medical Center	Joliet	2.7%	1467
Adventist La Grange Memorial Hospital	La Grange	2.8%	751
Advocate Lutheran General Hospital	Park Ridge	2.8%	1526
Methodist Medical Center of Illinois	Peoria	2.8%	968
Rush University Medical Center	Chicago	2.8%	751
Saint Anthonys Memorial Hospital	Effingham	2.9%	688
Ingalls Memorial Hospital	Harvey	3.0%	1152
Presence Saint Francis Hospital	Evanston	3.1%	703
Decatur Memorial Hospital	Decatur	3.2%	971
Memorial Hospital	Belleville	3.2%	1522
Swedish Covenant Hospital	Chicago	3.2%	988
Northwest Community Hospital	Arlington Hgts	3.4%	2143
Saint Francis Medical Center	Peoria	3.4%	1017
Centegra Health Sys-Mc Henry Hosp	Mchenry	3.5%	849
Franciscan Saint James Health	Olympia Fields	3.6%	828
Passavant Area Hospital	Jacksonville	3.6%	750
Herrin Hospital	Herrin	3.9%	1099
Saint Johns Hospital	Springfield	4.0%	845
Pana Community Hospital	Pana	4.2%	425
Centegra Health Sys-Woodstock Hosp	Woodstock	4.3%	602
Saint Joseph's Hospital	Breese	4.4%	339
Adventist Bolingbrook Hospital	Bolingbrook	4.5%	425
Macneal Hospital	Berwyn	4.5%	793
Memorial Medical Center	Springfield	4.6%	1879
Saint Elizabeth Hospital	Belleville	4.7%	559
Saint Marys Hospital	Decatur	4.7%	662
Heartland Regional Medical Center	Marion	4.8%	418
Anderson Hospital	Maryville	4.9%	760
Westlake Community Hospital	Melrose Park	5.1%	197
Gibson Community Hospital	Gibson City	5.2%	192
Jackson Park Hospital	Chicago	5.2%	230
Alton Memorial Hospital	Alton	5.3%	842
Mason District Hospital	Havana	5.3%	151
Touchette Regional Hospital	Centreville	5.3%	169
Vista Medical Center East	Waukegan	5.3%	912
Massac Memorial Hospital	Metropolis	5.5%	309
Memorial Hospital of Carbondale	Carbondale	5.7%	770
Good Samaritan Regional Health Center	Mount Vernon	6.0%	620
Roseland Community Hospital	Chicago	6.1%	279
South Shore Hospital	Chicago	6.6%	166
Memorial Hospital	Chester	7.7%	207

Combination Chest CT Scan

Hospital Name	City	Rate	Cases
Abraham Lincoln Memorial Hospital	Lincoln	0.0%	387
Anderson Hospital	Maryville	0.0%	580
Blessing Hospital	Quincy	0.0%	573
Fairfield Memorial Hospital	Fairfield	0.0%	253
Fhn Memorial Hospital	Freeport	0.0%	303
Illini Community Hospital	Pittsfield	0.0%	201
Kishwaukee Community Hospital	Dekalb	0.0%	367
Memorial Hospital	Chester	0.0%	79
Mendota Community Hospital	Mendota	0.0%	123
Midwestern Region Medical Center	Zion	0.0%	1060
Northwestern Memorial Hospital	Chicago	0.0%	5326
OSF Holy Family Medical Center	Monmouth	0.0%	89
Pekin Memorial Hospital	Pekin	0.0%	417
Rockford Memorial Hospital	Rockford	0.0%	518
Rush Oak Park Hospital	Oak Park	0.0%	363
Saint Anthony Hospital	Chicago	0.0%	86
Sarah Bush Lincoln Health Center	Mattoon	0.0%	486
Thorek Memorial Hospital	Chicago	0.0%	109
Trinity Rock Island	Rock Island	0.0%	709
Union County Hospital	Anna	0.0%	104
The University of Chicago Medical Center	Chicago	0.0%	4373
University of Illinois Hospital	Chicago	0.0%	661
Swedish American Hospital	Rockford	0.1%	1094
Advocate Illinois Masonic Medical Center	Chicago	0.2%	493
Alton Memorial Hospital	Alton	0.2%	643
Saint Francis Medical Center	Peoria	0.2%	1350
Saint Marys Hospital	Centralia	0.2%	414
Graham Hospital Association	Canton	0.3%	308
Presence Saint Joseph Hospital - Chicago	Chicago	0.3%	302
Saint James Hospital	Pontiac	0.3%	342
Advocate Condell Medical Center	Libertyville	0.4%	793
Carle Foundation Hospital	Urbana	0.4%	779
Katherine Shaw Bethea Hospital	Dixon	0.4%	235
Palos Community Hospital	Palos Heights	0.4%	1912
Advocate Good Samaritan Hospital	Downers Grove	0.5%	802
CGH Medical Center	Sterling	0.5%	437
Macneal Hospital	Berwyn	0.5%	585
Northwest Community Hospital	Arlington Hgts	0.5%	2438
Presence Saint Joseph Hospital - Elgin	Elgin	0.5%	423
Saint Mary Medical Center	Galesburg	0.5%	379
Loyola University Medical Center	Maywood	0.6%	2786
Morris Hospital & Healthcare Centers	Morris	0.6%	511
Passavant Area Hospital	Jacksonville	0.6%	522
Good Samaritan Regional Health Center	Mount Vernon	0.7%	401
Hinsdale Hospital	Hinsdale	0.7%	543
Presence Covenant Medical Center	Urbana	0.7%	145
Riverside Medical Center	Kankakee	0.7%	610
Copley Memorial Hospital	Aurora	0.8%	641
Hopedale Medical Complex	Hopedale	0.8%	124
Illinois Valley Community Hospital	Peru	0.8%	242
Presence Resurrection Medical Center	Chicago	0.8%	783
Carlinville Area Hospital	Carlinville	0.9%	115
Central Dupage Hospital	Winfield	0.9%	1288
Heartland Regional Medical Center	Marion	0.9%	325
Saint Anthony Medical Center	Rockford	0.9%	1100
Shelby Memorial Hospital	Shelbyville	0.9%	108
Adventist Glenoaks	Glendale Hghts	1.0%	104
Hoopeston Community Memorial Hospital	Hoopeston	1.0%	98
Metrosouth Medical Center	Blue Island	1.0%	205
Saint Margarets Hospital	Spring Valley	1.0%	293
Clay County Hospital	Flora	1.1%	280
Louis A Weiss Memorial Hospital	Chicago	1.1%	369
Elmhurst Memorial Hospital	Elmhurst	1.2%	1403
Ingalls Memorial Hospital	Harvey	1.2%	1443
Presence Sts Mary & Elizabeth Med Ctr	Chicago	1.2%	164
Silver Cross Hospital & Medical Centers	New Lenox	1.2%	936
Little Company of Mary Hospital	Evergreen Park	1.4%	917
Mercy Hospital & Medical Center	Chicago	1.4%	369
Presence Mercy Medical Center	Aurora	1.4%	784
Decatur Memorial Hospital	Decatur	1.5%	672
Edward Hospital	Naperville	1.5%	1696
Jackson Park Hospital	Chicago	1.5%	133
Advocate Christ Hospital & Medical Center	Oak Lawn	1.6%	1756
Holy Cross Hospital	Chicago	1.6%	246
Memorial Hospital	Belleville	1.6%	1152
Mount Sinai Hospital Medical Center	Chicago	1.6%	245
Saint Joseph Medical Center	Bloomington	1.6%	696
Advocate Good Shepherd Hospital	Barrington	1.7%	947
Galesburg Cottage Hospital	Galesburg	1.7%	240
Presence Our Lady of the Res Med Ctr	Chicago	1.7%	287
Valley West Community Hospital	Sandwich	1.8%	171
Sherman Hospital	Elgin	1.9%	979
Crossroads Community Hospital	Mount Vernon	2.0%	98
Taylorville Memorial Hospital	Taylorville	2.1%	427
Saint Anthonys Memorial Hospital	Effingham	2.2%	603
Red Bud Regional Hospital	Red Bud	2.3%	87
Saint Alexius Medical Center	Hoffman Estates	2.3%	948
Swedish Covenant Hospital	Chicago	2.3%	622
Advocate Lutheran General Hospital	Park Ridge	2.4%	1647
Evanston Hospital	Evanston	2.6%	6195
Advocate Trinity Hospital	Chicago	2.7%	226
Norwegian - American Hospital	Chicago	2.7%	75
Memorial Medical Center	Springfield	2.8%	2382
Advocate South Suburban Hospital	Hazel Crest	2.9%	583
Greenville Regional Hospital	Greenville	2.9%	210
Salem Township Hospital	Salem	2.9%	174
Pana Community Hospital	Pana	3.0%	100
Genesis Health System	Silvis	3.1%	162
Methodist Medical Center of Illinois	Peoria	3.1%	809
Presence Saint Joseph Medical Center	Joliet	3.3%	635
Saint Anthony's Health Center	Alton	3.3%	273
Loyola Gottlieb Memorial Hospital	Melrose Park	3.5%	405
Saint Joseph's Hospital	Highland	3.6%	165
Saint Joseph's Hospital	Breese	3.7%	217
Centegra Health Sys-Mc Henry Hosp	Mchenry	3.8%	744
Ottawa Reg Hosp & Healthcare Ctr	Ottawa	3.8%	367
Presence Saint Francis Hospital	Evanston	4.0%	403
Vista Medical Center East	Waukegan	4.0%	495
Touchette Regional Hospital	Centreville	4.3%	70
Westlake Community Hospital	Melrose Park	4.3%	93
Centegra Health Sys-Woodstock Hosp	Woodstock	4.6%	391
Saint Johns Hospital	Springfield	4.6%	675
Proctor Hospital	Peoria	5.0%	241
Hammond Henry Hospital	Geneseo	5.1%	118
Saint Bernard Hospital	Chicago	5.2%	77
Saint Marys Hospital	Decatur	5.5%	307
John H Stroger Jr Hospital	Chicago	5.8%	550
Mercy Harvard Hospital	Harvard	6.0%	83
Saint Marys Hospital	Streator	6.1%	231
Jersey Community Hospital	Jerseyville	6.3%	143
Gateway Regional Medical Center	Granite City	6.5%	186
Rush University Medical Center	Chicago	6.8%	323
Alexian Brothers Medical Center	Elk Grove Vlg	7.1%	1377
Franciscan Saint James Health	Olympia Fields	7.7%	712
Saint Francis Hospital	Litchfield	8.0%	338
West Suburban Medical Center	Oak Park	8.4%	287
Doctor John Warner Hospital	Clinton	8.7%	104
Adventist La Grange Memorial Hospital	La Grange	8.8%	740
Lake Forest Hospital	Lake Forest	9.4%	819
Massac Memorial Hospital	Metropolis	9.4%	171
Saint Joseph Memorial Hospital	Murphysboro	9.5%	200
Mason District Hospital	Havana	9.8%	132
Memorial Hospital of Carbondale	Carbondale	10.0%	691
Presence Saint Marys Hospital	Kankakee	11.3%	248

NOTE: Hospital profiles are in alphabetical order by state, then city, then hospital within the city; Rankings exclude hospitals with less than 25 cases except for patient surveys which excludes hospitals with less than 100 cases; (a) 100-299 cases; (1) The number of cases/patients is too few to report; (2) Data submitted were based on a sample of cases/patients; (3) Results are based on a shorter time period than required; (4) Data suppressed by CMS for one or more quarters; (5) Results are not available for this reporting period; (6) Fewer than 100 patients completed the HCAHPS survey; (7) No cases met the criteria for this measure; (8) The lower limit of the confidence interval cannot be calculated if the number of observed infections equals zero; (9) No data are available from the state/territory for this reporting period; (10) The scores shown reflect fewer than 50 completed surveys; (11) There were discrepancies in the data collection process; (12) This measure does not apply to this hospital for this reporting period; (13) Results cannot be calculated for this reporting period; (14) The results for this state are combined with nearby states to protect confidentiality; Please refer to the User's Guide for a full explanation of data.

Hospital Name	City	Rate	Cases
Roseland Community Hospital	Chicago	11.4%	88
Gibson Community Hospital	Gibson City	11.9%	135
McDonough District Hospital	Macomb	12.3%	365
Paris Community Hospital	Paris	12.4%	161
Herrin Hospital	Herrin	12.7%	1098
Presence United Samaritans Medical Center	Danville	12.9%	371
Saint Elizabeth Hospital	Belleville	13.6%	381
Advocate Bromenn Medical Center	Normal	13.9%	540
Delnor Community Hospital	Geneva	15.6%	789
Methodist Hospital of Chicago	Chicago	15.6%	96
Adventist Bolingbrook Hospital	Bolingbrook	18.4%	272
Richland Memorial Hospital	Olney	20.8%	221
Advocate Eureka Hospital	Eureka	24.5%	106
Provident Hospital of Chicago	Chicago	27.9%	68
Wabash General Hospital	Mount Carmel	28.4%	102
Iroquois Memorial Hospital	Watseka	34.2%	117
Harrisburg Medical Center	Harrisburg	41.3%	286
Ferrell Hospital Community Foundations	Eldorado	48.6%	109
South Shore Hospital	Chicago	50.0%	34
Hardin County General Hospital	Rosiclare	53.3%	45

Follow-up Mammogram/Ultrasound

A follow-up rate near zero may indicate missed cancer; a rate higher than 14% may mean there is unnecessary follow up.

Hospital Name	City	Rate	Cases
Provident Hospital of Chicago	Chicago	1.9%	526
Hopedale Medical Complex	Hopedale	2.6%	193
Sarah Bush Lincoln Health Center	Mattoon	3.0%	1510
Holy Cross Hospital	Chicago	3.2%	408
Fairfield Memorial Hospital	Fairfield	3.3%	365
Riverside Medical Center	Kankakee	3.3%	2524
Mercy Hospital & Medical Center	Chicago	3.9%	2241
Gateway Regional Medical Center	Granite City	4.2%	687
Presence Sts Mary & Elizabeth Med Ctr	Chicago	4.3%	1115
Vista Medical Center East	Waukegan	4.3%	2256
Mercy Harvard Hospital	Harvard	4.4%	91
Alton Memorial Hospital	Alton	4.5%	1850
Mason District Hospital	Havana	4.6%	195
Saint Marys Hospital	Decatur	4.6%	1141
Evanston Hospital	Evanston	4.7%	13333
Saint Bernard Hospital	Chicago	4.8%	187
Carle Foundation Hospital	Urbana	5.2%	1448
Hoopeston Community Memorial Hospital	Hoopeston	5.3%	114
Memorial Medical Center	Springfield	5.3%	3562
University of Illinois Hospital	Chicago	5.3%	1175
Metrosouth Medical Center	Blue Island	5.4%	836
Presence Saint Joseph Medical Center	Joliet	5.4%	2512
Saint Marys Hospital	Streator	5.4%	924
Advocate Lutheran General Hospital	Park Ridge	5.7%	4903
Franklin Hospital	Benton	5.8%	139
Morris Hospital & Healthcare Centers	Morris	5.8%	988
Silver Cross Hospital & Medical Centers	New Lenox	5.8%	1760
Copley Memorial Hospital	Aurora	5.9%	1416
Presence Saint Marys Hospital	Kankakee	5.9%	768
Centegra Health Sys-Woodstock Hosp	Woodstock	6.0%	1558
Roseland Community Hospital	Chicago	6.0%	100
Presence Saint Joseph Hospital - Chicago	Chicago	6.1%	1386
Advocate Condell Medical Center	Libertyville	6.3%	1888
Taylorville Memorial Hospital	Taylorville	6.3%	728
Union County Hospital	Anna	6.3%	303
Midwestern Region Medical Center	Zion	6.4%	173
Sherman Hospital	Elgin	6.4%	2079
Advocate Bromenn Medical Center	Normal	6.5%	1352
Clay County Hospital	Flora	6.5%	398
Good Samaritan Regional Health Center	Mount Vernon	6.5%	1233
Mount Sinai Hospital Medical Center	Chicago	6.5%	831
Saint Alexius Medical Center	Hoffman Estates	6.5%	2630
Central Dupage Hospital	Winfield	6.6%	3183
Richland Memorial Hospital	Olney	6.6%	516
Loyola University Medical Center	Maywood	6.7%	3118
Alexian Brothers Medical Center	Elk Grove Vlg	6.8%	2918
Northwest Community Hospital	Arlington Hgts	6.8%	6511
Hardin County General Hospital	Rosiclare	6.9%	102
South Shore Hospital	Chicago	6.9%	202
Jersey Community Hospital	Jerseyville	7.0%	369
Proctor Hospital	Peoria	7.0%	342
Saint Joseph's Hospital	Breese	7.0%	839
Salem Township Hospital	Salem	7.0%	387
Passavant Area Hospital	Jacksonville	7.1%	1105
Rush Oak Park Hospital	Oak Park	7.2%	923
Blessing Hospital	Quincy	7.3%	1868
McDonough District Hospital	Macomb	7.3%	600
Saint Anthony Medical Center	Rockford	7.3%	2473
Fhn Memorial Hospital	Freeport	7.4%	1140
Illini Community Hospital	Pittsfield	7.4%	244
Ferrell Hospital Community Foundations	Eldorado	7.5%	268
Ingalls Memorial Hospital	Harvey	7.5%	3291
Saint Margarets Hospital	Spring Valley	7.5%	616
Carlinville Area Hospital	Carlinville	7.8%	270
Franciscan Saint James Health	Olympia Fields	7.9%	2421
Morrison Community Hospital	Morrison	7.9%	63
Presence Our Lady of the Res Med Ctr	Chicago	7.9%	1057
Abraham Lincoln Memorial Hospital	Lincoln	8.0%	540
Advocate Eureka Hospital	Eureka	8.0%	176
Advocate Christ Hospital & Medical Center	Oak Lawn	8.1%	3361
Centegra Health Sys-Mc Henry Hosp	Mchenry	8.1%	2156
Galesburg Cottage Hospital	Galesburg	8.1%	669
Loyola Gottlieb Memorial Hospital	Melrose Park	8.2%	1275
Saint Joseph's Hospital	Highland	8.2%	390
Wabash General Hospital	Mount Carmel	8.3%	253
Westlake Community Hospital	Melrose Park	8.4%	407
Genesis Health System	Silvis	8.5%	730
Saint Anthony Hospital	Chicago	8.5%	375
Swedish American Hospital	Rockford	8.5%	3617
Advocate Good Shepherd Hospital	Barrington	8.6%	2177
Macneal Hospital	Berwyn	8.6%	1651
Saint Anthony's Health Center	Alton	8.6%	966
Doctor John Warner Hospital	Clinton	8.7%	150
The University of Chicago Medical Center	Chicago	8.7%	2290
Louis A Weiss Memorial Hospital	Chicago	8.8%	296
Gibson Community Hospital	Gibson City	8.9%	563
John H Stroger Jr Hospital	Chicago	8.9%	257
Delnor Community Hospital	Geneva	9.0%	1646
Illinois Valley Community Hospital	Peru	9.0%	787
Northwestern Memorial Hospital	Chicago	9.0%	6582
Methodist Medical Center of Illinois	Peoria	9.1%	2520
Saint Marys Hospital	Centralia	9.1%	1076
Heartland Regional Medical Center	Marion	9.3%	616
Hammond Henry Hospital	Geneseo	9.4%	468
Advocate Illinois Masonic Medical Center	Chicago	9.5%	1173
Elmhurst Memorial Hospital	Elmhurst	9.5%	2756
Trinity Rock Island	Rock Island	9.7%	2303
Palos Community Hospital	Palos Heights	9.8%	2900
Saint Anthonys Memorial Hospital	Effingham	9.8%	1752
Little Company of Mary Hospital	Evergreen Park	9.9%	1770
Norwegian - American Hospital	Chicago	9.9%	262
Presence Saint Francis Hospital	Evanston	9.9%	1318
Memorial Hospital of Carbondale	Carbondale	10.0%	2837
Red Bud Regional Hospital	Red Bud	10.1%	358
Saint James Hospital	Pontiac	10.1%	872
Crossroads Community Hospital	Mount Vernon	10.2%	521
Katherine Shaw Bethea Hospital	Dixon	10.4%	906
OSF Holy Family Medical Center	Monmouth	10.4%	299
Swedish Covenant Hospital	Chicago	10.5%	1625
Advocate Trinity Hospital	Chicago	10.7%	974
CGH Medical Center	Sterling	10.7%	1552
Herrin Hospital	Herrin	10.8%	1302
Saint Joseph Medical Center	Bloomington	10.8%	1443
Hinsdale Hospital	Hinsdale	10.9%	3530
Paris Community Hospital	Paris	10.9%	265
Decatur Memorial Hospital	Decatur	11.1%	3427
Edward Hospital	Naperville	11.2%	2939
Memorial Hospital	Belleville	11.2%	2433
Saint Mary Medical Center	Galesburg	11.2%	1529
Graham Hospital Association	Canton	11.5%	477
Rush University Medical Center	Chicago	11.5%	3001
Presence Saint Joseph Hospital - Elgin	Elgin	11.6%	805
Iroquois Memorial Hospital	Watseka	11.7%	429
Jackson Park Hospital	Chicago	11.7%	111
Advocate Good Samaritan Hospital	Downers Grove	11.8%	2580
Harrisburg Medical Center	Harrisburg	11.8%	729
Saint Elizabeth Hospital	Belleville	11.8%	1638
West Suburban Medical Center	Oak Park	11.8%	849
Presence Resurrection Medical Center	Chicago	11.9%	2762
Greenville Regional Hospital	Greenville	12.0%	498
Anderson Hospital	Maryville	12.1%	978
Saint Francis Medical Center	Peoria	12.2%	5128
Adventist La Grange Memorial Hospital	La Grange	12.3%	1942
Advocate South Suburban Hospital	Hazel Crest	12.3%	1639
Touchette Regional Hospital	Centreville	12.4%	267
Massac Memorial Hospital	Metropolis	12.9%	263
Valley West Community Hospital	Sandwich	13.1%	374
Saint Francis Hospital	Litchfield	13.5%	809
Pekin Memorial Hospital	Pekin	13.6%	843
Pana Community Hospital	Pana	14.2%	225
Adventist Bolingbrook Hospital	Bolingbrook	14.3%	545
Presence Mercy Medical Center	Aurora	14.4%	445
Thorek Memorial Hospital	Chicago	14.4%	243
Presence Covenant Medical Center	Urbana	14.5%	296
Ottawa Reg Hosp & Healthcare Ctr	Ottawa	14.8%	824
Shelby Memorial Hospital	Shelbyville	14.9%	248
Saint Johns Hospital	Springfield	15.0%	1837
Kishwaukee Community Hospital	Dekalb	16.0%	720
Mendota Community Hospital	Mendota	16.1%	392
Memorial Hospital	Chester	17.1%	240
Lake Forest Hospital	Lake Forest	18.1%	3247
Loretto Hospital	Chicago	18.1%	83
Presence United Samaritans Medical Center	Danville	18.6%	474
Adventist Glenoaks	Glendale Hghts	19.4%	134
Methodist Hospital of Chicago	Chicago	22.0%	91

Lumbar Spine MRI for Low Back Pain

Hospital Name	City	Rate	Cases
Sherman Hospital	Elgin	26.5%	151
Louis A Weiss Memorial Hospital	Chicago	26.7%	90
Franciscan Saint James Health	Olympia Fields	27.3%	154
Alexian Brothers Medical Center	Elk Grove Vlg	27.6%	228
Advocate Good Shepherd Hospital	Barrington	27.8%	115
Centegra Health Sys-Woodstock Hosp	Woodstock	28.0%	161
University of Illinois Hospital	Chicago	28.0%	100
Advocate Trinity Hospital	Chicago	28.6%	70
Katherine Shaw Bethea Hospital	Dixon	29.2%	65
Saint Alexius Medical Center	Hoffman Estates	29.5%	224
Sarah Bush Lincoln Health Center	Mattoon	29.5%	227
Saint Joseph Medical Center	Bloomington	30.0%	90
Pekin Memorial Hospital	Pekin	30.2%	53
Morris Hospital & Healthcare Centers	Morris	30.4%	102
Memorial Hospital of Carbondale	Carbondale	30.6%	111
Saint Marys Hospital	Centralia	31.0%	58
Advocate Condell Medical Center	Libertyville	31.1%	190
Saint Francis Hospital	Litchfield	31.4%	86
Presence Saint Joseph Medical Center	Joliet	31.9%	323
Advocate Bromenn Medical Center	Normal	32.1%	81
Delnor Community Hospital	Geneva	32.1%	109
West Suburban Medical Center	Oak Park	32.1%	56
Lake Forest Hospital	Lake Forest	32.2%	245
Memorial Medical Center	Springfield	32.5%	231
Silver Cross Hospital & Medical Centers	New Lenox	32.9%	246
Edward Hospital	Naperville	33.5%	212
Anderson Hospital	Maryville	33.9%	127
Methodist Medical Center of Illinois	Peoria	34.3%	137
The University of Chicago Medical Center	Chicago	34.4%	209
Kishwaukee Community Hospital	Dekalb	34.6%	81
CGH Medical Center	Sterling	34.8%	141
Northwest Community Hospital	Arlington Hgts	34.8%	597
Central Dupage Hospital	Winfield	35.2%	216
Evanston Hospital	Evanston	35.3%	976
Mercy Hospital & Medical Center	Chicago	35.3%	136
Saint Anthonys Memorial Hospital	Effingham	35.3%	295
Saint Francis Medical Center	Peoria	35.4%	302
Gibson Community Hospital	Gibson City	35.5%	62
Hinsdale Hospital	Hinsdale	35.5%	110
Ottawa Reg Hosp & Healthcare Ctr	Ottawa	35.5%	76
Northwestern Memorial Hospital	Chicago	35.6%	390
Galesburg Cottage Hospital	Galesburg	35.7%	56
Presence United Samaritans Medical Center	Danville	36.0%	50
Fhn Memorial Hospital	Freeport	36.1%	119
Advocate South Suburban Hospital	Hazel Crest	36.4%	99
Advocate Good Samaritan Hospital	Downers Grove	36.8%	125
Riverside Medical Center	Kankakee	36.8%	337
Swedish American Hospital	Rockford	36.8%	193
Swedish Covenant Hospital	Chicago	36.9%	287
Elmhurst Memorial Hospital	Elmhurst	37.0%	319
Presence Saint Francis Hospital	Evanston	37.1%	70
Vista Medical Center East	Waukegan	37.1%	224
Advocate Lutheran General Hospital	Park Ridge	37.2%	290
Herrin Hospital	Herrin	37.3%	153
Advocate Christ Hospital & Medical Center	Oak Lawn	37.4%	147
Loyola University Medical Center	Maywood	37.6%	258
Memorial Hospital	Belleville	37.8%	233
Ingalls Memorial Hospital	Harvey	37.9%	385
Saint Johns Hospital	Springfield	38.0%	92
Rockford Memorial Hospital	Rockford	38.1%	160
Little Company of Mary Hospital	Evergreen Park	38.8%	85
Presence Mercy Medical Center	Aurora	39.6%	53
Copley Memorial Hospital	Aurora	40.0%	160
Graham Hospital Association	Canton	40.0%	50
Presence Saint Joseph Hospital - Chicago	Chicago	40.0%	85
Saint Joseph's Hospital	Breese	40.0%	45
Adventist Bolingbrook Hospital	Bolingbrook	40.3%	62
Presence Saint Joseph Hospital - Elgin	Elgin	40.4%	57
Adventist La Grange Memorial Hospital	La Grange	40.5%	111
McDonough District Hospital	Macomb	40.6%	64
Saint Marys Hospital	Decatur	40.9%	127
Blessing Hospital	Quincy	41.0%	122
Saint Marys Hospital	Streator	41.0%	39
Decatur Memorial Hospital	Decatur	41.2%	335
Saint Margarets Hospital	Spring Valley	41.5%	65
Saint Mary Medical Center	Galesburg	41.6%	113
Centegra Health Sys-Mc Henry Hosp	Mchenry	41.9%	198
Presence Resurrection Medical Center	Chicago	42.0%	176
Presence Sts Mary & Elizabeth Med Ctr	Chicago	42.1%	107
Saint Anthony Medical Center	Rockford	42.2%	206
Taylorville Memorial Hospital	Taylorville	42.3%	78
Palos Community Hospital	Palos Heights	42.4%	99
Loyola Gottlieb Memorial Hospital	Melrose Park	42.7%	110
Proctor Hospital	Peoria	43.1%	58
Good Samaritan Regional Health Center	Mount Vernon	43.6%	55
Abraham Lincoln Memorial Hospital	Lincoln	43.9%	66
Carle Foundation Hospital	Urbana	44.4%	99
Macneal Hospital	Berwyn	44.8%	203

NOTE: Hospital profiles are in alphabetical order by state, then city, then hospital within the city; Rankings exclude hospitals with less than 25 cases except for patient surveys which excludes hospitals with less than 100 cases; (a) 100-299 cases; (1) The number of cases/patients is too few to report; (2) Data submitted were based on a sample of cases/patients; (3) Results are based on a shorter time period than required; (4) Data suppressed by CMS for one or more quarters; (5) Results are not available for this reporting period; (6) Fewer than 100 patients completed the HCAHPS survey; (7) No cases met the criteria for this measure; (8) The lower limit of the confidence interval cannot be calculated if the number of observed infections equals zero; (9) No data are available from the state/territory for this reporting period; (10) The scores shown reflect fewer than 50 completed surveys; (11) There were discrepancies in the data collection process; (12) This measure does not apply to this hospital for this reporting period; (13) Results cannot be calculated for this reporting period; (14) The results for this state are combined with nearby states to protect confidentiality; Please refer to the User's Guide for a full explanation of data.

Illinois Valley Community Hospital	Peru	45.0%	131
Advocate Illinois Masonic Medical Center	Chicago	45.7%	116
Presence Saint Marys Hospital	Kankakee	45.8%	59
Saint Anthony's Health Center	Alton	46.9%	64
Gateway Regional Medical Center	Granite City	48.0%	98
Presence Our Lady of the Res Med Ctr	Chicago	48.7%	76
Massac Memorial Hospital	Metropolis	48.8%	43
Holy Cross Hospital	Chicago	50.0%	32
Iroquois Memorial Hospital	Watseka	50.0%	34
Saint James Hospital	Pontiac	50.0%	66
Passavant Area Hospital	Jacksonville	50.8%	126
Memorial Hospital	Chester	52.6%	38
Jersey Community Hospital	Jerseyville	60.3%	58

NOTE: Hospital profiles are in alphabetical order by state, then city, then hospital within the city; Rankings exclude hospitals with less than 25 cases except for patient surveys which excludes hospitals with less than 100 cases; (a) 100-299 cases; (1) The number of cases/patients is too few to report; (2) Data submitted were based on a sample of cases/patients; (3) Results are based on a shorter time period than required; (4) Data suppressed by CMS for one or more quarters; (5) Results are not available for this reporting period; (6) Fewer than 100 patients completed the HCAHPS survey; (7) No cases met the criteria for this measure; (8) The lower limit of the confidence interval cannot be calculated if the number of observed infections equals zero; (9) No data are available from the state/territory for this reporting period; (10) The scores shown reflect fewer than 50 completed surveys; (11) There were discrepancies in the data collection process; (12) This measure does not apply to this hospital for this reporting period; (13) Results cannot be calculated for this reporting period; (14) The results for this state are combined with nearby states to protect confidentiality; Please refer to the User's Guide for a full explanation of data.

Genesis Medical Center - Aledo

409 Nw 9th Avenue Phone: 309-582-5301
Aledo, IL 61231
URL: www.mercerhospital.org
Type: Critical Access Hospitals Emergency Services: Yes
Ownership: Voluntary non-profit - Private Beds: 22
Key Personnel:
Administrator . . . . Ted Rogalski

Measure	Cases	This Hosp.	State Avg.	U.S. Avg.
Blood Clot Prevention and Treatment				
Anticoagulation Overlap Therapy[5]	-	-	91%	93%
ICU Venous Thromboembolism Prophylaxis[5]	-	-	93%	92%
Incidence of Potentially Preventable VTE[5]	-	-	11%	10%
UFH with Dosages/Platelet Monitoring[5]	-	-	94%	97%
Venous Thromboembolism Prophylaxis[5]	-	-	86%	85%
Warfarin Therapy Discharge Instructions[5]	-	-	71%	75%
Chest Pain/Possible Heart Attack Care				
Aspirin Given Within 24 Hours of Arrival	-	-	96%	96%
Fibrinolytic Meds Within 30 Min. of Arrival	-	-	65%	58%
Average Time to ECG (minutes)	-	-	6	7
Average Time to Transfer (minutes)	-	-	63	60
Children's Asthma Care				
Received Home Management Plan of Care	-	-	-	88%
Received Reliever Medication	-	-	-	100%
Received Systemic Corticosteroids	-	-	-	100%
Emergency Department				
Admittance Decision Time (minutes)[5]	-	-	89	98
Head CT Results Within 45 Min. of Arrival	-	-	64%	57%
Patients Who Left ER Before Being Seen	-	-	3%	2%
Time from ER Arrival to Admit. (minutes)[5]	-	-	260	274
Time from ER Arrival to Discharge (minutes)	-	-	138	134
Time in ER Before Being Evaluated (minutes)	-	-	28	26
Time to Pain Meds for Fractures (minutes)	-	-	52	57
Heart Attack Care				
Aspirin Given at Discharge[5]	-	-	99%	99%
Fibrinolytic Meds Within 30 Min. of Arrival[5]	-	-	33%	54%
PCI Within 90 Minutes of Arrival[5]	-	-	97%	96%
Statin Prescribed at Discharge[5]	-	-	98%	98%
Heart Failure Care				
ACE Inhibitor or ARB for LVSD[5]	-	-	98%	97%
Discharge Instructions Given[5]	-	-	96%	94%
Evaluation of LVS Function[5]	-	-	99%	99%
Medicare Spending				
Medicare Spending per Patient (ratio)	-	-	1	0.98
Pneumonia Care				
Appropriate Initial Antibiotic Given[5]	-	-	95%	95%
Blood Culture Timing[5]	-	-	98%	98%
Pregnancy and Delivery Care				
Newborn Deliveries Scheduled Early[5]	-	-	2%	6%
Preventive Care				
Immunization for Influenza[5]	-	-	92%	90%
Immunization for Pneumonia[5]	-	-	92%	92%
Stroke Care				
Anticoagulation Therapy for Atrial Fibrillation[5]	-	-	94%	95%
Antithrombotic Therapy Timing[5]	-	-	98%	98%
Assessed for Rehabilitation[5]	-	-	97%	97%
Discharged on Antithrombotic Therapy[5]	-	-	99%	99%
Discharged on Statin Medication[5]	-	-	94%	94%
Thrombolytic Therapy Timing[5]	-	-	66%	66%
Venous Thromboembolism Prophylaxis[5]	-	-	94%	94%
Written Stroke Educational Materials Given[5]	-	-	87%	88%
Surgical Care Improvement Project				
Appropriate Beta Blocker Usage[5]	-	-	98%	98%
Appropriate VTP Within 24 Hours[5]	-	-	98%	98%
Controlled Postoperative Blood Glucose[5]	-	-	97%	97%
Perioperative Temperature Management[5]	-	-	100%	100%
Prophylactic Antibiotic Selection[5]	-	-	99%	99%
Prophylactic Antibiotic Selection (Outpatient)	-	-	98%	98%
Prophylactic Antibiotic Stopped[5]	-	-	98%	98%
Prophylactic Antibiotic Timing[5]	-	-	99%	99%
Prophylactic Antibiotic Timing (Outpatient)	-	-	97%	98%
Urinary Catheter Removal[5]	-	-	98%	97%
Survey of Patients' Hospital Experiences				
Area Around Room 'Always' Quiet at Night[5]	-	-	60%	61%
Doctors 'Always' Communicated Well[5]	-	-	81%	82%
Home Recovery Information Given[5]	-	-	86%	85%
Hospital Given 9 or 10 on 10 Point Scale[5]	-	-	70%	71%
Meds 'Always' Explained Before Given[5]	-	-	64%	64%
Nurses 'Always' Communicated Well[5]	-	-	79%	79%
Pain 'Always' Well Controlled[5]	-	-	71%	71%
Room and Bathroom 'Always' Clean[5]	-	-	74%	73%
Timely Help 'Always' Received[5]	-	-	67%	68%
Would Definitely Recommend Hospital[5]	-	-	70%	71%
Use of Medical Imaging				
Cardiac Imaging Stress Test before Surgery	-	-	5.5%	5.3%
Combination Abdominal CT Scan	-	-	10.1%	10.5%
Combination Brain/Sinus CT Scan	-	-	2.6%	2.7%
Combination Chest CT Scan	-	-	2.8%	2.7%
Follow-up Mammogram/Ultrasound	-	-	8.4%	8.8%
Lumbar Spine MRI for Low Back Pain	-	-	36.6%	37.2%

Alton Memorial Hospital

One Memorial Drive Phone: 618-463-7300
Alton, IL 62002 Fax: 618-463-7850
URL: www.altonmemorialhospital.org
Type: Acute Care Hospitals Emergency Services: Yes
Ownership: Voluntary non-profit - Private Beds: 222
Key Personnel:
President . . . . Dave Braasch

Measure	Cases	This Hosp.	State Avg.	U.S. Avg.
Blood Clot Prevention and Treatment				
Anticoagulation Overlap Therapy[2]	67	96%	91%	93%
ICU Venous Thromboembolism Prophylaxis[2]	62	100%	93%	92%
Incidence of Potentially Preventable VTE[1,2]	-	-	11%	10%
UFH with Dosages/Platelet Monitoring[2]	11	73%	94%	97%
Venous Thromboembolism Prophylaxis[2]	345	98%	86%	85%
Warfarin Therapy Discharge Instructions[2]	53	98%	71%	75%
Chest Pain/Possible Heart Attack Care				
Aspirin Given Within 24 Hours of Arrival	46	100%	96%	96%
Fibrinolytic Meds Within 30 Min. of Arrival[7]	-	-	65%	58%
Average Time to ECG (minutes)	44	8	6	7
Average Time to Transfer (minutes)[1]	-	-	63	60
Children's Asthma Care				
Received Home Management Plan of Care	-	-	-	88%
Received Reliever Medication	-	-	-	100%
Received Systemic Corticosteroids	-	-	-	100%
Emergency Department				
Admittance Decision Time (minutes)[2]	303	65	89	98
Head CT Results Within 45 Min. of Arrival	32	91%	64%	57%
Patients Who Left ER Before Being Seen	42,943	3%	3%	2%
Time from ER Arrival to Admit. (minutes)[2]	410	242	260	274
Time from ER Arrival to Discharge (minutes)	774	115	138	134
Time in ER Before Being Evaluated (minutes)	785	29	28	26
Time to Pain Meds for Fractures (minutes)	129	44	52	57
Heart Attack Care				
Aspirin Given at Discharge	79	99%	99%	99%
Fibrinolytic Meds Within 30 Min. of Arrival[7]	-	-	33%	54%
PCI Within 90 Minutes of Arrival[1]	-	-	97%	96%
Statin Prescribed at Discharge	80	100%	98%	98%
Heart Failure Care				
ACE Inhibitor or ARB for LVSD[2]	68	99%	98%	97%
Discharge Instructions Given[2]	183	99%	96%	94%
Evaluation of LVS Function[2]	232	99%	99%	99%
Medicare Spending				
Medicare Spending per Patient (ratio)	-	0.90	1	0.98
Pneumonia Care				
Appropriate Initial Antibiotic Given[2]	140	99%	95%	95%
Blood Culture Timing[2]	257	98%	98%	98%
Pregnancy and Delivery Care				
Newborn Deliveries Scheduled Early[2]	20	0%	2%	6%
Preventive Care				
Immunization for Influenza[2]	527	100%	92%	90%
Immunization for Pneumonia[2]	717	100%	92%	92%
Stroke Care				
Anticoagulation Therapy for Atrial Fibrillation[2]	11	91%	94%	95%
Antithrombotic Therapy Timing[2]	64	98%	98%	98%
Assessed for Rehabilitation[2]	63	100%	97%	97%
Discharged on Antithrombotic Therapy[2]	60	100%	99%	99%
Discharged on Statin Medication[2]	52	94%	94%	94%
Thrombolytic Therapy Timing[1,2]	-	-	66%	66%
Venous Thromboembolism Prophylaxis[2]	68	97%	94%	94%
Written Stroke Educational Materials Given[2]	41	100%	87%	88%
Surgical Care Improvement Project				
Appropriate Beta Blocker Usage[2]	82	99%	98%	98%
Appropriate VTP Within 24 Hours[2]	248	96%	98%	98%
Controlled Postoperative Blood Glucose[2,7]	-	-	97%	97%
Perioperative Temperature Management[2]	270	100%	100%	100%
Prophylactic Antibiotic Selection[2]	187	100%	99%	99%
Prophylactic Antibiotic Selection (Outpatient)	133	100%	98%	98%
Prophylactic Antibiotic Stopped[2]	173	98%	98%	98%
Prophylactic Antibiotic Timing[2]	187	98%	99%	99%
Prophylactic Antibiotic Timing (Outpatient)	133	100%	97%	98%
Urinary Catheter Removal[2]	183	99%	98%	97%
Survey of Patients' Hospital Experiences				
Area Around Room 'Always' Quiet at Night[11]	300+	66%	60%	61%
Doctors 'Always' Communicated Well[11]	300+	81%	81%	82%
Home Recovery Information Given[11]	300+	89%	86%	85%
Hospital Given 9 or 10 on 10 Point Scale[11]	300+	73%	70%	71%
Meds 'Always' Explained Before Given[11]	300+	60%	64%	64%
Nurses 'Always' Communicated Well[11]	300+	79%	79%	79%
Pain 'Always' Well Controlled[11]	300+	70%	71%	71%
Room and Bathroom 'Always' Clean[11]	300+	72%	74%	73%
Timely Help 'Always' Received[11]	300+	64%	67%	68%
Would Definitely Recommend Hospital[11]	300+	75%	70%	71%
Use of Medical Imaging				
Cardiac Imaging Stress Test before Surgery	237	8.0%	5.5%	5.3%
Combination Abdominal CT Scan	842	2.9%	10.1%	10.5%
Combination Brain/Sinus CT Scan	842	5.3%	2.6%	2.7%
Combination Chest CT Scan	643	0.2%	2.8%	2.7%
Follow-up Mammogram/Ultrasound	1,850	4.5%	8.4%	8.8%
Lumbar Spine MRI for Low Back Pain[1]	-	-	36.6%	37.2%

Saint Anthony's Health Center

Saint Anthony's Way Phone: 618-465-2571
Alton, IL 62002 Fax: 618-474-4860
URL: www.sahc.org
Type: Acute Care Hospitals Emergency Services: Yes
Ownership: Voluntary non-profit - Church Beds: 192
Key Personnel:
Quality Assurance . . . . Susan Hornsey
Cardiac Laboratory. . . . . Pamela Kratovil
CEO/President. . . . . E J Kuiper
Chief of Medical Staff . . . . Salvador LoBianco, MD
Emergency Room . . . . Karen Marzluf

Measure	Cases	This Hosp.	State Avg.	U.S. Avg.
Blood Clot Prevention and Treatment				
Anticoagulation Overlap Therapy[2]	27	100%	91%	93%
ICU Venous Thromboembolism Prophylaxis[2]	76	100%	93%	92%
Incidence of Potentially Preventable VTE[1,2]	-	-	11%	10%
UFH with Dosages/Platelet Monitoring[1,2]	-	-	94%	97%
Venous Thromboembolism Prophylaxis[2]	250	98%	86%	85%
Warfarin Therapy Discharge Instructions[2]	21	100%	71%	75%
Chest Pain/Possible Heart Attack Care				
Aspirin Given Within 24 Hours of Arrival	14	100%	96%	96%
Fibrinolytic Meds Within 30 Min. of Arrival[7]	-	-	65%	58%
Average Time to ECG (minutes)	15	2	6	7
Average Time to Transfer (minutes)[1]	-	-	63	60
Children's Asthma Care				
Received Home Management Plan of Care	-	-	-	88%
Received Reliever Medication	-	-	-	100%
Received Systemic Corticosteroids	-	-	-	100%
Emergency Department				
Admittance Decision Time (minutes)[2]	347	59	89	98
Head CT Results Within 45 Min. of Arrival	13	100%	64%	57%
Patients Who Left ER Before Being Seen	23,367	1%	3%	2%
Time from ER Arrival to Admit. (minutes)[2]	385	213	260	274
Time from ER Arrival to Discharge (minutes)	342	106	138	134
Time in ER Before Being Evaluated (minutes)	267	13	28	26
Time to Pain Meds for Fractures (minutes)	48	40	52	57

NOTE: Hospital profiles are in alphabetical order by state, then city, then hospital within the city; Rankings exclude hospitals with less than 25 cases except for patient surveys which excludes hospitals with less than 100 cases; (a) 100-299 cases; (1) The number of cases/patients is too few to report; (2) Data submitted were based on a sample of cases/patients; (3) Results are based on a shorter time period than required; (4) Data suppressed by CMS for one or more quarters; (5) Results are not available for this reporting period; (6) Fewer than 100 patients completed the HCAHPS survey; (7) No cases met the criteria for this measure; (8) The lower limit of the confidence interval cannot be calculated if the number of observed infections equals zero; (9) No data are available from the state/territory for this reporting period; (10) The scores shown reflect fewer than 50 completed surveys; (11) There were discrepancies in the data collection process; (12) This measure does not apply to this hospital for this reporting period; (13) Results cannot be calculated for this reporting period; (14) The results for this state are combined with nearby states to protect confidentiality; Please refer to the User's Guide for a full explanation of data.

Measure	Cases	This Hosp.	State Avg.	U.S. Avg.
Heart Attack Care				
Aspirin Given at Discharge	80	100%	99%	99%
Fibrinolytic Meds Within 30 Min. of Arrival[7]	-	-	33%	54%
PCI Within 90 Minutes of Arrival[1]	-	-	97%	96%
Statin Prescribed at Discharge	66	100%	98%	98%
Heart Failure Care				
ACE Inhibitor or ARB for LVSD	24	100%	98%	97%
Discharge Instructions Given	120	100%	96%	94%
Evaluation of LVS Function	152	100%	99%	99%
Medicare Spending				
Medicare Spending per Patient (ratio)	-	0.95	1	0.98
Pneumonia Care				
Appropriate Initial Antibiotic Given	118	100%	95%	95%
Blood Culture Timing	195	100%	98%	98%
Pregnancy and Delivery Care				
Newborn Deliveries Scheduled Early[2]	29	0%	2%	6%
Preventive Care				
Immunization for Influenza[2]	374	99%	92%	90%
Immunization for Pneumonia[2]	510	99%	92%	92%
Stroke Care				
Anticoagulation Therapy for Atrial Fibrillation[1]	-	-	94%	95%
Antithrombotic Therapy Timing	32	100%	98%	98%
Assessed for Rehabilitation	40	100%	97%	97%
Discharged on Antithrombotic Therapy	40	100%	99%	99%
Discharged on Statin Medication	26	100%	94%	94%
Thrombolytic Therapy Timing[1]	-	-	66%	66%
Venous Thromboembolism Prophylaxis	36	100%	94%	94%
Written Stroke Educational Materials Given	24	96%	87%	88%
Surgical Care Improvement Project				
Appropriate Beta Blocker Usage	48	100%	98%	98%
Appropriate VTP Within 24 Hours	133	100%	98%	98%
Controlled Postoperative Blood Glucose[7]	-	-	97%	97%
Perioperative Temperature Management	143	100%	100%	100%
Prophylactic Antibiotic Selection	95	100%	99%	99%
Prophylactic Antibiotic Selection (Outpatient)	105	99%	98%	98%
Prophylactic Antibiotic Stopped	89	99%	98%	98%
Prophylactic Antibiotic Timing	95	100%	99%	99%
Prophylactic Antibiotic Timing (Outpatient)	105	100%	97%	98%
Urinary Catheter Removal	104	100%	98%	97%
Survey of Patients' Hospital Experiences				
Area Around Room 'Always' Quiet at Night	300+	62%	60%	61%
Doctors 'Always' Communicated Well	300+	79%	81%	82%
Home Recovery Information Given	300+	87%	86%	85%
Hospital Given 9 or 10 on 10 Point Scale	300+	74%	70%	71%
Meds 'Always' Explained Before Given	300+	65%	64%	64%
Nurses 'Always' Communicated Well	300+	79%	79%	79%
Pain 'Always' Well Controlled	300+	72%	71%	71%
Room and Bathroom 'Always' Clean	300+	75%	74%	73%
Timely Help 'Always' Received	300+	60%	67%	68%
Would Definitely Recommend Hospital	300+	73%	70%	71%
Use of Medical Imaging				
Cardiac Imaging Stress Test before Surgery	244	4.9%	5.5%	5.3%
Combination Abdominal CT Scan	506	12.3%	10.1%	10.5%
Combination Brain/Sinus CT Scan[1]	-	-	2.6%	2.7%
Combination Chest CT Scan	273	3.3%	2.8%	2.7%
Follow-up Mammogram/Ultrasound	966	8.6%	8.4%	8.8%
Lumbar Spine MRI for Low Back Pain	64	46.9%	36.6%	37.2%

Union County Hospital

517 North Main Street
Anna, IL 62906
Phone: 618-833-4511
Fax: 618-833-4183
Type: Critical Access Hospitals
Emergency Services: Yes
Ownership: Proprietary
Beds: 58

Key Personnel:
Quality Assurance . . . . Tonia Capel, RN
CEO/President. . . . . James R Farris
Emergency Room . . . . Judy Lewis, RN
Operating Room. . . . . Paula Parr, RN
Chief of Medical Staff . . . . Deanna St Germain, DO
Radiology. . . . . Peter Wories

Measure	Cases	This Hosp.	State Avg.	U.S. Avg.
Blood Clot Prevention and Treatment				
Anticoagulation Overlap Therapy[1,2]	-	-	91%	93%
ICU Venous Thromboembolism Prophylaxis[2,7]	-	-	93%	92%
Incidence of Potentially Preventable VTE[1,2]	-	-	11%	10%
UFH with Dosages/Platelet Monitoring[1,2]	-	-	94%	97%
Venous Thromboembolism Prophylaxis[2]	324	98%	86%	85%
Warfarin Therapy Discharge Instructions[1,2]	-	-	71%	75%
Chest Pain/Possible Heart Attack Care				
Aspirin Given Within 24 Hours of Arrival	64	98%	96%	96%
Fibrinolytic Meds Within 30 Min. of Arrival[1]	-	-	65%	58%
Average Time to ECG (minutes)	68	4	6	7
Average Time to Transfer (minutes)[1]	-	-	63	60
Children's Asthma Care				
Received Home Management Plan of Care	-	-	-	88%
Received Reliever Medication	-	-	-	100%
Received Systemic Corticosteroids	-	-	-	100%
Emergency Department				
Admittance Decision Time (minutes)[2]	295	69	89	98
Head CT Results Within 45 Min. of Arrival[1]	-	-	64%	57%
Patients Who Left ER Before Being Seen	8,470	1%	3%	2%
Time from ER Arrival to Admit. (minutes)[2]	447	229	260	274
Time from ER Arrival to Discharge (minutes)	333	114	138	134
Time in ER Before Being Evaluated (minutes)	396	24	28	26
Time to Pain Meds for Fractures (minutes)	43	67	52	57
Heart Attack Care				
Aspirin Given at Discharge[1,3]	-	-	99%	99%
Fibrinolytic Meds Within 30 Min. of Arrival[3,7]	-	-	33%	54%
PCI Within 90 Minutes of Arrival[3,7]	-	-	97%	96%
Statin Prescribed at Discharge[1,3]	-	-	98%	98%
Heart Failure Care				
ACE Inhibitor or ARB for LVSD[1]	-	-	98%	97%
Discharge Instructions Given	18	94%	96%	94%
Evaluation of LVS Function	30	100%	99%	99%
Medicare Spending				
Medicare Spending per Patient (ratio)	-	-	1	0.98
Pneumonia Care				
Appropriate Initial Antibiotic Given	32	94%	95%	95%
Blood Culture Timing	49	98%	98%	98%
Pregnancy and Delivery Care				
Newborn Deliveries Scheduled Early[5]	-	-	2%	6%
Preventive Care				
Immunization for Influenza[2]	301	99%	92%	90%
Immunization for Pneumonia[2]	449	99%	92%	92%
Stroke Care				
Anticoagulation Therapy for Atrial Fibrillation[3,7]	-	-	94%	95%
Antithrombotic Therapy Timing[1,3]	-	-	98%	98%
Assessed for Rehabilitation[1,3]	-	-	97%	97%
Discharged on Antithrombotic Therapy[1,3]	-	-	99%	99%
Discharged on Statin Medication[1,3]	-	-	94%	94%
Thrombolytic Therapy Timing[3,7]	-	-	66%	66%
Venous Thromboembolism Prophylaxis[1,3]	-	-	94%	94%
Written Stroke Educational Materials Given[1,3]	-	-	87%	88%
Surgical Care Improvement Project				
Appropriate Beta Blocker Usage[5]	-	-	98%	98%
Appropriate VTP Within 24 Hours[5]	-	-	98%	98%
Controlled Postoperative Blood Glucose[5]	-	-	97%	97%
Perioperative Temperature Management[5]	-	-	100%	100%
Prophylactic Antibiotic Selection[5]	-	-	99%	99%
Prophylactic Antibiotic Selection (Outpatient)[5]	-	-	98%	98%
Prophylactic Antibiotic Stopped[5]	-	-	98%	98%
Prophylactic Antibiotic Timing[5]	-	-	99%	99%
Prophylactic Antibiotic Timing (Outpatient)[5]	-	-	97%	98%
Urinary Catheter Removal[5]	-	-	98%	97%
Survey of Patients' Hospital Experiences				
Area Around Room 'Always' Quiet at Night	(a)	70%	60%	61%
Doctors 'Always' Communicated Well	(a)	91%	81%	82%
Home Recovery Information Given	(a)	88%	86%	85%
Hospital Given 9 or 10 on 10 Point Scale	(a)	70%	70%	71%
Meds 'Always' Explained Before Given	(a)	69%	64%	64%
Nurses 'Always' Communicated Well	(a)	82%	79%	79%
Pain 'Always' Well Controlled	(a)	75%	71%	71%
Room and Bathroom 'Always' Clean	(a)	65%	74%	73%
Timely Help 'Always' Received	(a)	76%	67%	68%
Would Definitely Recommend Hospital	(a)	63%	70%	71%
Use of Medical Imaging				
Cardiac Imaging Stress Test before Surgery[1]	-	-	5.5%	5.3%
Combination Abdominal CT Scan	247	13.4%	10.1%	10.5%
Combination Brain/Sinus CT Scan	309	0.6%	2.6%	2.7%
Combination Chest CT Scan	104	0.0%	2.8%	2.7%
Follow-up Mammogram/Ultrasound	303	6.3%	8.4%	8.8%
Lumbar Spine MRI for Low Back Pain[1]	-	-	36.6%	37.2%

Northwest Community Hospital

800 W Central Road
Arlington Heights, IL 60005
Phone: 847-618-1000
Fax: 847-618-5509
URL: www.nch.org
Type: Acute Care Hospitals
Emergency Services: Yes
Ownership: Voluntary non-profit - Other
Beds: 488

Key Personnel:
CEO/President. . . . . Bruce K Crowther
Pediatric In-Patient Care . . . . Timothy Geleske, MD
Infection Control. . . . . Karen Gormen
Operating Room. . . . . Mark Levin, MD
Quality Assurance . . . . Joyce McComb
Chief of Medical Staff . . . . Donald E Pochly
Cardiac Laboratory. . . . . Gilbert Sita, MD
Radiology. . . . . Clifford Wolf, MD

Measure	Cases	This Hosp.	State Avg.	U.S. Avg.
Blood Clot Prevention and Treatment				
Anticoagulation Overlap Therapy[2]	142	100%	91%	93%
ICU Venous Thromboembolism Prophylaxis[2]	85	93%	93%	92%
Incidence of Potentially Preventable VTE[2]	39	8%	11%	10%
UFH with Dosages/Platelet Monitoring[2]	118	100%	94%	97%
Venous Thromboembolism Prophylaxis[2]	355	92%	86%	85%
Warfarin Therapy Discharge Instructions[2]	83	100%	71%	75%
Chest Pain/Possible Heart Attack Care				
Aspirin Given Within 24 Hours of Arrival[1,3]	-	-	96%	96%
Fibrinolytic Meds Within 30 Min. of Arrival[5]	-	-	65%	58%
Average Time to ECG (minutes)[3,7]	-	-	6	7
Average Time to Transfer (minutes)[5]	-	-	63	60
Children's Asthma Care				
Received Home Management Plan of Care	-	-	-	88%
Received Reliever Medication	-	-	-	100%
Received Systemic Corticosteroids	-	-	-	100%
Emergency Department				
Admittance Decision Time (minutes)[2]	484	64	89	98
Head CT Results Within 45 Min. of Arrival[1]	-	-	64%	57%
Patients Who Left ER Before Being Seen	74,955	1%	3%	2%
Time from ER Arrival to Admit. (minutes)[2]	538	248	260	274
Time from ER Arrival to Discharge (minutes)	371	160	138	134
Time in ER Before Being Evaluated (minutes)	434	32	28	26
Time to Pain Meds for Fractures (minutes)	219	23	52	57
Heart Attack Care				
Aspirin Given at Discharge[2]	312	100%	99%	99%
Fibrinolytic Meds Within 30 Min. of Arrival[2,7]	-	-	33%	54%
PCI Within 90 Minutes of Arrival[2]	76	100%	97%	96%
Statin Prescribed at Discharge[2]	302	100%	98%	98%
Heart Failure Care				
ACE Inhibitor or ARB for LVSD[2]	36	100%	98%	97%
Discharge Instructions Given[2]	160	98%	96%	94%
Evaluation of LVS Function[2]	265	100%	99%	99%
Medicare Spending				
Medicare Spending per Patient (ratio)	-	1.08	1	0.98
Pneumonia Care				
Appropriate Initial Antibiotic Given[2]	102	96%	95%	95%
Blood Culture Timing[2]	204	99%	98%	98%
Pregnancy and Delivery Care				
Newborn Deliveries Scheduled Early[2]	39	8%	2%	6%
Preventive Care				
Immunization for Influenza[2]	530	85%	92%	90%
Immunization for Pneumonia[2]	659	92%	92%	92%
Stroke Care				
Anticoagulation Therapy for Atrial Fibrillation	41	100%	94%	95%
Antithrombotic Therapy Timing	192	100%	98%	98%
Assessed for Rehabilitation	239	100%	97%	97%
Discharged on Antithrombotic Therapy	213	100%	99%	99%
Discharged on Statin Medication	157	99%	94%	94%
Thrombolytic Therapy Timing	15	100%	66%	66%
Venous Thromboembolism Prophylaxis	247	100%	94%	94%

NOTE: Hospital profiles are in alphabetical order by state, then city, then hospital within the city; Rankings exclude hospitals with less than 25 cases except for patient surveys which excludes hospitals with less than 100 cases; (a) 100-299 cases; (1) The number of cases/patients is too few to report; (2) Data submitted were based on a sample of cases/patients; (3) Results are based on a shorter time period than required; (4) Data suppressed by CMS for one or more quarters; (5) Results are not available for this reporting period; (6) Fewer than 100 patients completed the HCAHPS survey; (7) No cases met the criteria for this measure; (8) The lower limit of the confidence interval cannot be calculated if the number of observed infections equals zero; (9) No data are available from the state/territory for this reporting period; (10) The scores shown reflect fewer than 50 completed surveys; (11) There were discrepancies in the data collection process; (12) This measure does not apply to this hospital for this reporting period; (13) Results cannot be calculated for this reporting period; (14) The results for this state are combined with nearby states to protect confidentiality; Please refer to the User's Guide for a full explanation of data.

Measure	Cases	This Hosp.	State Avg.	U.S. Avg.
Written Stroke Educational Materials Given	119	100%	87%	88%
Surgical Care Improvement Project				
Appropriate Beta Blocker Usage[2]	220	99%	98%	98%
Appropriate VTP Within 24 Hours[2]	406	97%	98%	98%
Controlled Postoperative Blood Glucose[2]	128	99%	97%	97%
Perioperative Temperature Management[2]	491	100%	100%	100%
Prophylactic Antibiotic Selection[2]	438	99%	99%	99%
Prophylactic Antibiotic Selection (Outpatient)	483	99%	98%	98%
Prophylactic Antibiotic Stopped[2]	409	96%	98%	98%
Prophylactic Antibiotic Timing[2]	439	98%	99%	99%
Prophylactic Antibiotic Timing (Outpatient)	471	99%	97%	98%
Urinary Catheter Removal[2]	358	98%	98%	97%
Survey of Patients' Hospital Experiences				
Area Around Room 'Always' Quiet at Night	300+	61%	60%	61%
Doctors 'Always' Communicated Well	300+	76%	81%	82%
Home Recovery Information Given	300+	85%	86%	85%
Hospital Given 9 or 10 on 10 Point Scale	300+	74%	70%	71%
Meds 'Always' Explained Before Given	300+	63%	64%	64%
Nurses 'Always' Communicated Well	300+	76%	79%	79%
Pain 'Always' Well Controlled	300+	72%	71%	71%
Room and Bathroom 'Always' Clean	300+	78%	74%	73%
Timely Help 'Always' Received	300+	65%	67%	68%
Would Definitely Recommend Hospital	300+	78%	70%	71%
Use of Medical Imaging				
Cardiac Imaging Stress Test before Surgery	1,126	7.3%	5.5%	5.3%
Combination Abdominal CT Scan	3,853	5.9%	10.1%	10.5%
Combination Brain/Sinus CT Scan	2,143	3.4%	2.6%	2.7%
Combination Chest CT Scan	2,438	0.5%	2.8%	2.7%
Follow-up Mammogram/Ultrasound	6,511	6.8%	8.4%	8.8%
Lumbar Spine MRI for Low Back Pain	597	34.8%	36.6%	37.2%

Copley Memorial Hospital

2000 Ogden Avenue
Aurora, IL 60504
Phone: 630-978-6200
Fax: 630-978-6888
E-mail: clord@rsh.net
URL: www.rushcopley.com
Type: Acute Care Hospitals
Emergency Services: Yes
Ownership: Voluntary non-profit - Private
Beds: 183

Key Personnel:
Radiology. . . . . Syed A Akbar
Quality Assurance . . . . Lisa Brady, MS
CEO/President. . . . . Barry C Finn, MBA CPA
Chief of Medical Staff. . . . . Steven B Lowenthal, MD
Infection Control. . . . . Maria Montero
Operating Room. . . . . David Reinhaft
Pediatric In-Patient Care . . . . Janet Smith, RN

Measure	Cases	This Hosp.	State Avg.	U.S. Avg.
Blood Clot Prevention and Treatment				
Anticoagulation Overlap Therapy[2]	79	95%	91%	93%
ICU Venous Thromboembolism Prophylaxis[2]	85	100%	93%	92%
Incidence of Potentially Preventable VTE[2]	11	0%	11%	10%
UFH with Dosages/Platelet Monitoring[2]	41	100%	94%	97%
Venous Thromboembolism Prophylaxis[2]	290	97%	86%	85%
Warfarin Therapy Discharge Instructions[2]	68	100%	71%	75%
Chest Pain/Possible Heart Attack Care				
Aspirin Given Within 24 Hours of Arrival[5]	-	-	96%	96%
Fibrinolytic Meds Within 30 Min. of Arrival[5]	-	-	65%	58%
Average Time to ECG (minutes)[5]	-	-	6	7
Average Time to Transfer (minutes)[5]	-	-	63	60
Children's Asthma Care				
Received Home Management Plan of Care	-	-	-	88%
Received Reliever Medication	-	-	-	100%
Received Systemic Corticosteroids	-	-	-	100%
Emergency Department				
Admittance Decision Time (minutes)[2]	393	104	89	98
Head CT Results Within 45 Min. of Arrival[1]	-	-	64%	57%
Patients Who Left ER Before Being Seen	73,392	3%	3%	2%
Time from ER Arrival to Admit. (minutes)[2]	401	270	260	274
Time from ER Arrival to Discharge (minutes)	384	143	138	134
Time in ER Before Being Evaluated (minutes)	402	37	28	26
Time to Pain Meds for Fractures (minutes)	299	50	52	57
Heart Attack Care				
Aspirin Given at Discharge	149	98%	99%	99%
Fibrinolytic Meds Within 30 Min. of Arrival[7]	-	-	33%	54%
PCI Within 90 Minutes of Arrival	30	100%	97%	96%
Statin Prescribed at Discharge	147	100%	98%	98%
Heart Failure Care				
ACE Inhibitor or ARB for LVSD	55	96%	98%	97%
Discharge Instructions Given	166	94%	96%	94%
Evaluation of LVS Function	219	100%	99%	99%
Medicare Spending				
Medicare Spending per Patient (ratio)	-	1.03	1	0.98
Pneumonia Care				
Appropriate Initial Antibiotic Given	113	97%	95%	95%
Blood Culture Timing	232	100%	98%	98%
Pregnancy and Delivery Care				
Newborn Deliveries Scheduled Early	343	2%	2%	6%
Preventive Care				
Immunization for Influenza[2]	486	81%	92%	90%
Immunization for Pneumonia[2]	453	79%	92%	92%
Stroke Care				
Anticoagulation Therapy for Atrial Fibrillation	14	100%	94%	95%
Antithrombotic Therapy Timing	90	100%	98%	98%
Assessed for Rehabilitation	104	99%	97%	97%
Discharged on Antithrombotic Therapy	88	99%	99%	99%
Discharged on Statin Medication	74	96%	94%	94%
Thrombolytic Therapy Timing[1]	-	-	66%	66%
Venous Thromboembolism Prophylaxis	103	99%	94%	94%
Written Stroke Educational Materials Given	55	95%	87%	88%
Surgical Care Improvement Project				
Appropriate Beta Blocker Usage[2]	295	100%	98%	98%
Appropriate VTP Within 24 Hours[2]	619	98%	98%	98%
Controlled Postoperative Blood Glucose[2]	105	98%	97%	97%
Perioperative Temperature Management[2]	771	99%	100%	100%
Prophylactic Antibiotic Selection[2]	715	100%	99%	99%
Prophylactic Antibiotic Selection (Outpatient)	435	100%	98%	98%
Prophylactic Antibiotic Stopped[2]	695	99%	98%	98%
Prophylactic Antibiotic Timing[2]	715	100%	99%	99%
Prophylactic Antibiotic Timing (Outpatient)	437	98%	97%	98%
Urinary Catheter Removal[2]	556	99%	98%	97%
Survey of Patients' Hospital Experiences				
Area Around Room 'Always' Quiet at Night	300+	54%	60%	61%
Doctors 'Always' Communicated Well	300+	82%	81%	82%
Home Recovery Information Given	300+	88%	86%	85%
Hospital Given 9 or 10 on 10 Point Scale	300+	71%	70%	71%
Meds 'Always' Explained Before Given	300+	64%	64%	64%
Nurses 'Always' Communicated Well	300+	79%	79%	79%
Pain 'Always' Well Controlled	300+	72%	71%	71%
Room and Bathroom 'Always' Clean	300+	76%	74%	73%
Timely Help 'Always' Received	300+	61%	67%	68%
Would Definitely Recommend Hospital	300+	74%	70%	71%
Use of Medical Imaging				
Cardiac Imaging Stress Test before Surgery	855	7.7%	5.5%	5.3%
Combination Abdominal CT Scan	1,193	4.7%	10.1%	10.5%
Combination Brain/Sinus CT Scan	1,205	1.7%	2.6%	2.7%
Combination Chest CT Scan	641	0.8%	2.8%	2.7%
Follow-up Mammogram/Ultrasound	1,416	5.9%	8.4%	8.8%
Lumbar Spine MRI for Low Back Pain	160	40.0%	36.6%	37.2%

Presence Mercy Medical Center

1325 N Highland Avenue
Aurora, IL 60506
Phone: 630-859-2222
Fax: 630-801-2608
URL: www.provena.org/mercy
Type: Acute Care Hospitals
Emergency Services: Yes
Ownership: Voluntary non-profit - Church
Beds: 293

Key Personnel:
Radiology. . . . . EH Dolin, MD
Infection Control. . . . . Kathy Hettinger
Emergency Room . . . . James Kolka, MD
Chief of Medical Staff. . . . . Michael Loebach, MD
Operating Room. . . . . Kathleen Satchel, RN
CEO/President. . . . . Teresa Stokes
Anesthesiology. . . . . HF Tsang, MD

Measure	Cases	This Hosp.	State Avg.	U.S. Avg.
Blood Clot Prevention and Treatment				
Anticoagulation Overlap Therapy[2]	63	98%	91%	93%
ICU Venous Thromboembolism Prophylaxis[2]	101	99%	93%	92%
Incidence of Potentially Preventable VTE[2]	18	0%	11%	10%
UFH with Dosages/Platelet Monitoring[2]	25	100%	94%	97%
Venous Thromboembolism Prophylaxis[2]	303	100%	86%	85%
Warfarin Therapy Discharge Instructions[2]	47	94%	71%	75%
Chest Pain/Possible Heart Attack Care				
Aspirin Given Within 24 Hours of Arrival[1,3]	-	-	96%	96%
Fibrinolytic Meds Within 30 Min. of Arrival[5]	-	-	65%	58%
Average Time to ECG (minutes)[1,3]	-	-	6	7
Average Time to Transfer (minutes)[5]	-	-	63	60
Children's Asthma Care				
Received Home Management Plan of Care	-	-	-	88%
Received Reliever Medication	-	-	-	100%
Received Systemic Corticosteroids	-	-	-	100%
Emergency Department				
Admittance Decision Time (minutes)[2]	648	95	89	98
Head CT Results Within 45 Min. of Arrival	11	73%	64%	57%
Patients Who Left ER Before Being Seen	41,265	3%	3%	2%
Time from ER Arrival to Admit. (minutes)[2]	702	288	260	274
Time from ER Arrival to Discharge (minutes)	390	188	138	134
Time in ER Before Being Evaluated (minutes)	399	36	28	26
Time to Pain Meds for Fractures (minutes)	164	64	52	57
Heart Attack Care				
Aspirin Given at Discharge	140	99%	99%	99%
Fibrinolytic Meds Within 30 Min. of Arrival[7]	-	-	33%	54%
PCI Within 90 Minutes of Arrival	22	82%	97%	96%
Statin Prescribed at Discharge	140	98%	98%	98%
Heart Failure Care				
ACE Inhibitor or ARB for LVSD	44	95%	98%	97%
Discharge Instructions Given	152	99%	96%	94%
Evaluation of LVS Function	192	99%	99%	99%
Medicare Spending				
Medicare Spending per Patient (ratio)	-	0.99	1	0.98
Pneumonia Care				
Appropriate Initial Antibiotic Given[2]	81	98%	95%	95%
Blood Culture Timing[2]	173	98%	98%	98%
Pregnancy and Delivery Care				
Newborn Deliveries Scheduled Early	26	0%	2%	6%
Preventive Care				
Immunization for Influenza[2]	583	92%	92%	90%
Immunization for Pneumonia[2]	802	98%	92%	92%
Stroke Care				
Anticoagulation Therapy for Atrial Fibrillation[1]	-	-	94%	95%
Antithrombotic Therapy Timing	57	100%	98%	98%
Assessed for Rehabilitation	58	100%	97%	97%
Discharged on Antithrombotic Therapy	56	100%	99%	99%
Discharged on Statin Medication	42	98%	94%	94%
Thrombolytic Therapy Timing[1]	-	-	66%	66%
Venous Thromboembolism Prophylaxis	56	98%	94%	94%
Written Stroke Educational Materials Given	34	97%	87%	88%
Surgical Care Improvement Project				
Appropriate Beta Blocker Usage[2]	180	99%	98%	98%
Appropriate VTP Within 24 Hours[2]	304	95%	98%	98%
Controlled Postoperative Blood Glucose[2]	131	99%	97%	97%
Perioperative Temperature Management[2]	336	100%	100%	100%
Prophylactic Antibiotic Selection[2]	346	99%	99%	99%
Prophylactic Antibiotic Selection (Outpatient)	122	98%	98%	98%
Prophylactic Antibiotic Stopped[2]	331	98%	98%	98%
Prophylactic Antibiotic Timing[2]	348	99%	99%	99%
Prophylactic Antibiotic Timing (Outpatient)	123	98%	97%	98%
Urinary Catheter Removal[2]	321	97%	98%	97%
Survey of Patients' Hospital Experiences				
Area Around Room 'Always' Quiet at Night	300+	67%	60%	61%
Doctors 'Always' Communicated Well	300+	79%	81%	82%
Home Recovery Information Given	300+	88%	86%	85%
Hospital Given 9 or 10 on 10 Point Scale	300+	67%	70%	71%
Meds 'Always' Explained Before Given	300+	62%	64%	64%
Nurses 'Always' Communicated Well	300+	79%	79%	79%
Pain 'Always' Well Controlled	300+	73%	71%	71%
Room and Bathroom 'Always' Clean	300+	72%	74%	73%
Timely Help 'Always' Received	300+	60%	67%	68%
Would Definitely Recommend Hospital	300+	67%	70%	71%
Use of Medical Imaging				
Cardiac Imaging Stress Test before Surgery	291	6.2%	5.5%	5.3%

NOTE: Hospital profiles are in alphabetical order by state, then city, then hospital within the city; Rankings exclude hospitals with less than 25 cases except for patient surveys which excludes hospitals with less than 100 cases; (a) 100-299 cases; (1) The number of cases/patients is too few to report; (2) Data submitted were based on a sample of cases/patients; (3) Results are based on a shorter time period than required; (4) Data suppressed by CMS for one or more quarters; (5) Results are not available for this reporting period; (6) Fewer than 100 patients completed the HCAHPS survey; (7) No cases met the criteria for this measure; (8) The lower limit of the confidence interval cannot be calculated if the number of observed infections equals zero; (9) No data are available from the state/territory for this reporting period; (10) The scores shown reflect fewer than 50 completed surveys; (11) There were discrepancies in the data collection process; (12) This measure does not apply to this hospital for this reporting period; (13) Results cannot be calculated for this reporting period; (14) The results for this state are combined with nearby states to protect confidentiality; Please refer to the User's Guide for a full explanation of data.

Measure	Cases	This Hosp.	State Avg.	U.S. Avg.
Combination Abdominal CT Scan	803	4.0%	10.1%	10.5%
Combination Brain/Sinus CT Scan	642	1.2%	2.6%	2.7%
Combination Chest CT Scan	784	1.4%	2.8%	2.7%
Follow-up Mammogram/Ultrasound	445	14.4%	8.4%	8.8%
Lumbar Spine MRI for Low Back Pain	53	39.6%	36.6%	37.2%

Advocate Good Shepherd Hospital

450 West Highway 22 Phone: 847-381-9600
Barrington, IL 60010 Fax: 847-842-4060
URL: www.advocatehealth.com
Type: Acute Care Hospitals Emergency Services: Yes
Ownership: Voluntary non-profit - Church Beds: 154
Key Personnel:
Radiology. . . . . Sebouh Guevikia, MD
CEO/President. . . . . Karen Lambert
Quality Assurance . . . . Mike Wiegel

Measure	Cases	This Hosp.	State Avg.	U.S. Avg.
Blood Clot Prevention and Treatment				
Anticoagulation Overlap Therapy[2]	82	93%	91%	93%
ICU Venous Thromboembolism Prophylaxis[2]	116	95%	93%	92%
Incidence of Potentially Preventable VTE[1,2]	-	-	11%	10%
UFH with Dosages/Platelet Monitoring[2]	68	100%	94%	97%
Venous Thromboembolism Prophylaxis[2]	315	84%	86%	85%
Warfarin Therapy Discharge Instructions[2]	60	72%	71%	75%
Chest Pain/Possible Heart Attack Care				
Aspirin Given Within 24 Hours of Arrival[1]	-	-	96%	96%
Fibrinolytic Meds Within 30 Min. of Arrival[5]	-	-	65%	58%
Average Time to ECG (minutes)[1]	-	-	6	7
Average Time to Transfer (minutes)[5]	-	-	63	60
Children's Asthma Care				
Received Home Management Plan of Care	-	-	-	88%
Received Reliever Medication	-	-	-	100%
Received Systemic Corticosteroids	-	-	-	100%
Emergency Department				
Admittance Decision Time (minutes)[2]	457	105	89	98
Head CT Results Within 45 Min. of Arrival[1]	-	-	64%	57%
Patients Who Left ER Before Being Seen	34,092	1%	3%	2%
Time from ER Arrival to Admit. (minutes)[2]	511	283	260	274
Time from ER Arrival to Discharge (minutes)	385	169	138	134
Time in ER Before Being Evaluated (minutes)	376	49	28	26
Time to Pain Meds for Fractures (minutes)	131	63	52	57
Heart Attack Care				
Aspirin Given at Discharge	202	100%	99%	99%
Fibrinolytic Meds Within 30 Min. of Arrival[7]	-	-	33%	54%
PCI Within 90 Minutes of Arrival	27	100%	97%	96%
Statin Prescribed at Discharge	194	100%	98%	98%
Heart Failure Care				
ACE Inhibitor or ARB for LVSD	45	100%	98%	97%
Discharge Instructions Given	203	100%	96%	94%
Evaluation of LVS Function	262	100%	99%	99%
Medicare Spending				
Medicare Spending per Patient (ratio)	-	1.03	1	0.98
Pneumonia Care				
Appropriate Initial Antibiotic Given[2]	87	95%	95%	95%
Blood Culture Timing[2]	141	100%	98%	98%
Pregnancy and Delivery Care				
Newborn Deliveries Scheduled Early	150	3%	2%	6%
Preventive Care				
Immunization for Influenza[2]	569	98%	92%	90%
Immunization for Pneumonia[2]	635	95%	92%	92%
Stroke Care				
Anticoagulation Therapy for Atrial Fibrillation	12	100%	94%	95%
Antithrombotic Therapy Timing	71	100%	98%	98%
Assessed for Rehabilitation	89	100%	97%	97%
Discharged on Antithrombotic Therapy	77	100%	99%	99%
Discharged on Statin Medication	66	95%	94%	94%
Thrombolytic Therapy Timing[1]	-	-	66%	66%
Venous Thromboembolism Prophylaxis	84	98%	94%	94%
Written Stroke Educational Materials Given	46	100%	87%	88%
Surgical Care Improvement Project				
Appropriate Beta Blocker Usage[2]	307	100%	98%	98%
Appropriate VTP Within 24 Hours[2]	418	100%	98%	98%
Controlled Postoperative Blood Glucose[2]	110	99%	97%	97%
Perioperative Temperature Management[2]	513	100%	100%	100%
Prophylactic Antibiotic Selection[2]	420	99%	99%	99%
Prophylactic Antibiotic Selection (Outpatient)	368	100%	98%	98%
Prophylactic Antibiotic Stopped[2]	410	100%	98%	98%
Prophylactic Antibiotic Timing[2]	420	99%	99%	99%
Prophylactic Antibiotic Timing (Outpatient)	368	100%	97%	98%
Urinary Catheter Removal[2]	386	99%	98%	97%
Survey of Patients' Hospital Experiences				
Area Around Room 'Always' Quiet at Night	300+	50%	60%	61%
Doctors 'Always' Communicated Well	300+	81%	81%	82%
Home Recovery Information Given	300+	89%	86%	85%
Hospital Given 9 or 10 on 10 Point Scale	300+	72%	70%	71%
Meds 'Always' Explained Before Given	300+	64%	64%	64%
Nurses 'Always' Communicated Well	300+	81%	79%	79%
Pain 'Always' Well Controlled	300+	71%	71%	71%
Room and Bathroom 'Always' Clean	300+	70%	74%	73%
Timely Help 'Always' Received	300+	64%	67%	68%
Would Definitely Recommend Hospital	300+	76%	70%	71%
Use of Medical Imaging				
Cardiac Imaging Stress Test before Surgery	756	5.2%	5.5%	5.3%
Combination Abdominal CT Scan	1,051	3.8%	10.1%	10.5%
Combination Brain/Sinus CT Scan	904	2.4%	2.6%	2.7%
Combination Chest CT Scan	947	1.7%	2.8%	2.7%
Follow-up Mammogram/Ultrasound	2,177	8.6%	8.4%	8.8%
Lumbar Spine MRI for Low Back Pain	115	27.8%	36.6%	37.2%

Memorial Hospital

4500 Memorial Drive Phone: 618-233-7750
Belleville, IL 62226 Fax: 618-257-6911
E-mail: info@memhosp.com
URL: www.memhosp.com
Type: Acute Care Hospitals Emergency Services: Yes
Ownership: Voluntary non-profit - Private Beds: 316
Key Personnel:
Emergency Room . . . . Thomas Byrne, MD
Chief of Medical Staff. . . . . William Casperson, MD
Infection Control. . . . . Kathy Harms
Intensive Care Unit. . . . . Kim Howell
Operating Room. . . . . Brian Johnson, RN
Anesthesiology. . . . . Paul Sander, MD
CEO/President. . . . . Mark J Turner
Quality Assurance . . . . Kerry Wrigley

Measure	Cases	This Hosp.	State Avg.	U.S. Avg.
Blood Clot Prevention and Treatment				
Anticoagulation Overlap Therapy[2]	98	100%	91%	93%
ICU Venous Thromboembolism Prophylaxis[2]	57	96%	93%	92%
Incidence of Potentially Preventable VTE[2]	14	7%	11%	10%
UFH with Dosages/Platelet Monitoring[2]	120	100%	94%	97%
Venous Thromboembolism Prophylaxis[2]	388	93%	86%	85%
Warfarin Therapy Discharge Instructions[2]	59	86%	71%	75%
Chest Pain/Possible Heart Attack Care				
Aspirin Given Within 24 Hours of Arrival	12	100%	96%	96%
Fibrinolytic Meds Within 30 Min. of Arrival[3,7]	-	-	65%	58%
Average Time to ECG (minutes)	13	6	6	7
Average Time to Transfer (minutes)[3,7]	-	-	63	60
Children's Asthma Care				
Received Home Management Plan of Care	-	-	-	88%
Received Reliever Medication	-	-	-	100%
Received Systemic Corticosteroids	-	-	-	100%
Emergency Department				
Admittance Decision Time (minutes)[2]	797	103	89	98
Head CT Results Within 45 Min. of Arrival	24	75%	64%	57%
Patients Who Left ER Before Being Seen	66,977	1%	3%	2%
Time from ER Arrival to Admit. (minutes)[2]	798	307	260	274
Time from ER Arrival to Discharge (minutes)	374	158	138	134
Time in ER Before Being Evaluated (minutes)	417	10	28	26
Time to Pain Meds for Fractures (minutes)	229	37	52	57
Heart Attack Care				
Aspirin Given at Discharge	316	99%	99%	99%
Fibrinolytic Meds Within 30 Min. of Arrival[7]	-	-	33%	54%
PCI Within 90 Minutes of Arrival	28	96%	97%	96%
Statin Prescribed at Discharge	289	96%	98%	98%
Heart Failure Care				
ACE Inhibitor or ARB for LVSD	220	97%	98%	97%
Discharge Instructions Given	576	94%	96%	94%
Evaluation of LVS Function	690	100%	99%	99%
Medicare Spending				
Medicare Spending per Patient (ratio)	-	0.94	1	0.98
Pneumonia Care				
Appropriate Initial Antibiotic Given	354	97%	95%	95%
Blood Culture Timing	500	99%	98%	98%
Pregnancy and Delivery Care				
Newborn Deliveries Scheduled Early	184	1%	2%	6%
Preventive Care				
Immunization for Influenza[2]	555	94%	92%	90%
Immunization for Pneumonia[2]	737	92%	92%	92%
Stroke Care				
Anticoagulation Therapy for Atrial Fibrillation	20	85%	94%	95%
Antithrombotic Therapy Timing	140	99%	98%	98%
Assessed for Rehabilitation	144	95%	97%	97%
Discharged on Antithrombotic Therapy	138	99%	99%	99%
Discharged on Statin Medication	115	91%	94%	94%
Thrombolytic Therapy Timing[1]	-	-	66%	66%
Venous Thromboembolism Prophylaxis	149	95%	94%	94%
Written Stroke Educational Materials Given	76	72%	87%	88%
Surgical Care Improvement Project				
Appropriate Beta Blocker Usage[2]	249	98%	98%	98%
Appropriate VTP Within 24 Hours[2]	412	99%	98%	98%
Controlled Postoperative Blood Glucose[2]	107	100%	97%	97%
Perioperative Temperature Management[2]	503	100%	100%	100%
Prophylactic Antibiotic Selection[2]	406	99%	99%	99%
Prophylactic Antibiotic Selection (Outpatient)	394	99%	98%	98%
Prophylactic Antibiotic Stopped[2]	391	97%	98%	98%
Prophylactic Antibiotic Timing[2]	406	99%	99%	99%
Prophylactic Antibiotic Timing (Outpatient)	394	99%	97%	98%
Urinary Catheter Removal[2]	407	97%	98%	97%
Survey of Patients' Hospital Experiences				
Area Around Room 'Always' Quiet at Night	300+	59%	60%	61%
Doctors 'Always' Communicated Well	300+	80%	81%	82%
Home Recovery Information Given	300+	86%	86%	85%
Hospital Given 9 or 10 on 10 Point Scale	300+	75%	70%	71%
Meds 'Always' Explained Before Given	300+	65%	64%	64%
Nurses 'Always' Communicated Well	300+	83%	79%	79%
Pain 'Always' Well Controlled	300+	75%	71%	71%
Room and Bathroom 'Always' Clean	300+	75%	74%	73%
Timely Help 'Always' Received	300+	70%	67%	68%
Would Definitely Recommend Hospital	300+	78%	70%	71%
Use of Medical Imaging				
Cardiac Imaging Stress Test before Surgery	698	5.2%	5.5%	5.3%
Combination Abdominal CT Scan	1,650	7.3%	10.1%	10.5%
Combination Brain/Sinus CT Scan	1,522	3.2%	2.6%	2.7%
Combination Chest CT Scan	1,152	1.6%	2.8%	2.7%
Follow-up Mammogram/Ultrasound	2,433	11.2%	8.4%	8.8%
Lumbar Spine MRI for Low Back Pain	233	37.8%	36.6%	37.2%

Saint Elizabeth Hospital

211 S Third St Phone: 618-234-2120
Belleville, IL 62220 Fax: 618-222-4650
URL: www.steliz.org
Type: Acute Care Hospitals Emergency Services: Yes
Ownership: Voluntary non-profit - Church Beds: 498
Key Personnel:
Intensive Care Unit. . . . . Terry Brown
Pediatric In-Patient Care . . . . Salil Gupta, MD
Chief of Medical Staff. . . . . Shelly Harkins, MD
Quality Assurance . . . . Lana Peters
Emergency Room . . . . Paul Saba
Radiology. . . . . Paul Schroeder, MD
Operating Room. . . . . Andrea Spalter
Infection Control. . . . . Laura Stollard

Measure	Cases	This Hosp.	State Avg.	U.S. Avg.
Blood Clot Prevention and Treatment				
Anticoagulation Overlap Therapy[2]	52	94%	91%	93%
ICU Venous Thromboembolism Prophylaxis[2]	78	99%	93%	92%
Incidence of Potentially Preventable VTE[1,2]	-	-	11%	10%
UFH with Dosages/Platelet Monitoring[2]	35	100%	94%	97%
Venous Thromboembolism Prophylaxis[2]	259	95%	86%	85%
Warfarin Therapy Discharge Instructions[2]	36	100%	71%	75%

NOTE: Hospital profiles are in alphabetical order by state, then city, then hospital within the city; Rankings exclude hospitals with less than 25 cases except for patient surveys which excludes hospitals with less than 100 cases; (a) 100-299 cases; (1) The number of cases/patients is too few to report; (2) Data submitted were based on a sample of cases/patients; (3) Results are based on a shorter time period than required; (4) Data suppressed by CMS for one or more quarters; (5) Results are not available for this reporting period; (6) Fewer than 100 patients completed the HCAHPS survey; (7) No cases met the criteria for this measure; (8) The lower limit of the confidence interval cannot be calculated if the number of observed infections equals zero; (9) No data are available from the state/territory for this reporting period; (10) The scores shown reflect fewer than 50 completed surveys; (11) There were discrepancies in the data collection process; (12) This measure does not apply to this hospital for this reporting period; (13) Results cannot be calculated for this reporting period; (14) The results for this state are combined with nearby states to protect confidentiality; Please refer to the User's Guide for a full explanation of data.

Measure	Cases	This Hosp.	State Avg.	U.S. Avg.
Chest Pain/Possible Heart Attack Care				
Aspirin Given Within 24 Hours of Arrival[1,3]	-	-	96%	96%
Fibrinolytic Meds Within 30 Min. of Arrival[5]	-	-	65%	58%
Average Time to ECG (minutes)[1,3]	-	-	6	7
Average Time to Transfer (minutes)[5]	-	-	63	60
Children's Asthma Care				
Received Home Management Plan of Care	-	-	-	88%
Received Reliever Medication	-	-	-	100%
Received Systemic Corticosteroids	-	-	-	100%
Emergency Department				
Admittance Decision Time (minutes)[2]	516	84	89	98
Head CT Results Within 45 Min. of Arrival[1]	-	-	64%	57%
Patients Who Left ER Before Being Seen	17,742	3%	3%	2%
Time from ER Arrival to Admit. (minutes)[2]	518	257	260	274
Time from ER Arrival to Discharge (minutes)	374	142	138	134
Time in ER Before Being Evaluated (minutes)	418	23	28	26
Time to Pain Meds for Fractures (minutes)	116	78	52	57
Heart Attack Care				
Aspirin Given at Discharge	278	100%	99%	99%
Fibrinolytic Meds Within 30 Min. of Arrival[7]	-	-	33%	54%
PCI Within 90 Minutes of Arrival	32	100%	97%	96%
Statin Prescribed at Discharge	268	100%	98%	98%
Heart Failure Care				
ACE Inhibitor or ARB for LVSD	88	99%	98%	97%
Discharge Instructions Given	306	99%	96%	94%
Evaluation of LVS Function	371	100%	99%	99%
Medicare Spending				
Medicare Spending per Patient (ratio)	-	0.92	1	0.98
Pneumonia Care				
Appropriate Initial Antibiotic Given	163	99%	95%	95%
Blood Culture Timing	299	100%	98%	98%
Pregnancy and Delivery Care				
Newborn Deliveries Scheduled Early[2]	32	0%	2%	6%
Preventive Care				
Immunization for Influenza[2]	548	98%	92%	90%
Immunization for Pneumonia[2]	647	96%	92%	92%
Stroke Care				
Anticoagulation Therapy for Atrial Fibrillation[1]	-	-	94%	95%
Antithrombotic Therapy Timing	96	100%	98%	98%
Assessed for Rehabilitation	115	96%	97%	97%
Discharged on Antithrombotic Therapy	110	100%	99%	99%
Discharged on Statin Medication	75	96%	94%	94%
Thrombolytic Therapy Timing[1]	-	-	66%	66%
Venous Thromboembolism Prophylaxis	109	93%	94%	94%
Written Stroke Educational Materials Given	61	93%	87%	88%
Surgical Care Improvement Project				
Appropriate Beta Blocker Usage	202	100%	98%	98%
Appropriate VTP Within 24 Hours	282	99%	98%	98%
Controlled Postoperative Blood Glucose	119	97%	97%	97%
Perioperative Temperature Management	400	100%	100%	100%
Prophylactic Antibiotic Selection	373	99%	99%	99%
Prophylactic Antibiotic Selection (Outpatient)	205	99%	98%	98%
Prophylactic Antibiotic Stopped	359	99%	98%	98%
Prophylactic Antibiotic Timing	373	100%	99%	99%
Prophylactic Antibiotic Timing (Outpatient)	211	97%	97%	98%
Urinary Catheter Removal	309	100%	98%	97%
Survey of Patients' Hospital Experiences				
Area Around Room 'Always' Quiet at Night	300+	59%	60%	61%
Doctors 'Always' Communicated Well	300+	81%	81%	82%
Home Recovery Information Given	300+	86%	86%	85%
Hospital Given 9 or 10 on 10 Point Scale	300+	69%	70%	71%
Meds 'Always' Explained Before Given	300+	64%	64%	64%
Nurses 'Always' Communicated Well	300+	80%	79%	79%
Pain 'Always' Well Controlled	300+	73%	71%	71%
Room and Bathroom 'Always' Clean	300+	71%	74%	73%
Timely Help 'Always' Received	300+	67%	67%	68%
Would Definitely Recommend Hospital	300+	68%	70%	71%
Use of Medical Imaging				
Cardiac Imaging Stress Test before Surgery	607	5.8%	5.5%	5.3%
Combination Abdominal CT Scan	632	21.0%	10.1%	10.5%
Combination Brain/Sinus CT Scan	559	4.7%	2.6%	2.7%
Combination Chest CT Scan	381	13.6%	2.8%	2.7%
Follow-up Mammogram/Ultrasound	1,638	11.8%	8.4%	8.8%
Lumbar Spine MRI for Low Back Pain[1]	-	-	36.6%	37.2%

Franklin Hospital

201 Bailey Lane
Benton, IL 62812
Phone: 618-439-3761
Type: Critical Access Hospitals
Emergency Services: Yes
Ownership: Govt - Hospital Dist/Auth

Measure	Cases	This Hosp.	State Avg.	U.S. Avg.
Blood Clot Prevention and Treatment				
Anticoagulation Overlap Therapy	-	-	91%	93%
ICU Venous Thromboembolism Prophylaxis	-	-	93%	92%
Incidence of Potentially Preventable VTE	-	-	11%	10%
UFH with Dosages/Platelet Monitoring	-	-	94%	97%
Venous Thromboembolism Prophylaxis	-	-	86%	85%
Warfarin Therapy Discharge Instructions	-	-	71%	75%
Chest Pain/Possible Heart Attack Care				
Aspirin Given Within 24 Hours of Arrival[5]	-	-	96%	96%
Fibrinolytic Meds Within 30 Min. of Arrival[5]	-	-	65%	58%
Average Time to ECG (minutes)[5]	-	-	6	7
Average Time to Transfer (minutes)[5]	-	-	63	60
Children's Asthma Care				
Received Home Management Plan of Care	-	-	-	88%
Received Reliever Medication	-	-	-	100%
Received Systemic Corticosteroids	-	-	-	100%
Emergency Department				
Admittance Decision Time (minutes)	-	-	89	98
Head CT Results Within 45 Min. of Arrival[5]	-	-	64%	57%
Patients Who Left ER Before Being Seen[5]	-	-	3%	2%
Time from ER Arrival to Admit. (minutes)	-	-	260	274
Time from ER Arrival to Discharge (minutes)[5]	-	-	138	134
Time in ER Before Being Evaluated (minutes)[5]	-	-	28	26
Time to Pain Meds for Fractures (minutes)[5]	-	-	52	57
Heart Attack Care				
Aspirin Given at Discharge	-	-	99%	99%
Fibrinolytic Meds Within 30 Min. of Arrival	-	-	33%	54%
PCI Within 90 Minutes of Arrival	-	-	97%	96%
Statin Prescribed at Discharge	-	-	98%	98%
Heart Failure Care				
ACE Inhibitor or ARB for LVSD	-	-	98%	97%
Discharge Instructions Given	-	-	96%	94%
Evaluation of LVS Function	-	-	99%	99%
Medicare Spending				
Medicare Spending per Patient (ratio)	-	-	1	0.98
Pneumonia Care				
Appropriate Initial Antibiotic Given	-	-	95%	95%
Blood Culture Timing	-	-	98%	98%
Pregnancy and Delivery Care				
Newborn Deliveries Scheduled Early	-	-	2%	6%
Preventive Care				
Immunization for Influenza	-	-	92%	90%
Immunization for Pneumonia	-	-	92%	92%
Stroke Care				
Anticoagulation Therapy for Atrial Fibrillation	-	-	94%	95%
Antithrombotic Therapy Timing	-	-	98%	98%
Assessed for Rehabilitation	-	-	97%	97%
Discharged on Antithrombotic Therapy	-	-	99%	99%
Discharged on Statin Medication	-	-	94%	94%
Thrombolytic Therapy Timing	-	-	66%	66%
Venous Thromboembolism Prophylaxis	-	-	94%	94%
Written Stroke Educational Materials Given	-	-	87%	88%
Surgical Care Improvement Project				
Appropriate Beta Blocker Usage	-	-	98%	98%
Appropriate VTP Within 24 Hours	-	-	98%	98%
Controlled Postoperative Blood Glucose	-	-	97%	97%
Perioperative Temperature Management	-	-	100%	100%
Prophylactic Antibiotic Selection	-	-	99%	99%
Prophylactic Antibiotic Selection (Outpatient)[5]	-	-	98%	98%
Prophylactic Antibiotic Stopped	-	-	98%	98%
Prophylactic Antibiotic Timing	-	-	99%	99%
Prophylactic Antibiotic Timing (Outpatient)[5]	-	-	97%	98%
Urinary Catheter Removal	-	-	98%	97%
Survey of Patients' Hospital Experiences				
Area Around Room 'Always' Quiet at Night	-	-	60%	61%
Doctors 'Always' Communicated Well	-	-	81%	82%
Home Recovery Information Given	-	-	86%	85%
Hospital Given 9 or 10 on 10 Point Scale	-	-	70%	71%
Meds 'Always' Explained Before Given	-	-	64%	64%
Nurses 'Always' Communicated Well	-	-	79%	79%
Pain 'Always' Well Controlled	-	-	71%	71%
Room and Bathroom 'Always' Clean	-	-	74%	73%
Timely Help 'Always' Received	-	-	67%	68%
Would Definitely Recommend Hospital	-	-	70%	71%
Use of Medical Imaging				
Cardiac Imaging Stress Test before Surgery[1]	-	-	5.5%	5.3%
Combination Abdominal CT Scan	165	21.2%	10.1%	10.5%
Combination Brain/Sinus CT Scan[1]	-	-	2.6%	2.7%
Combination Chest CT Scan[1]	-	-	2.8%	2.7%
Follow-up Mammogram/Ultrasound	139	5.8%	8.4%	8.8%
Lumbar Spine MRI for Low Back Pain[1]	-	-	36.6%	37.2%

Macneal Hospital

3249 South Oak Park Avenue
Berwyn, IL 60402
Phone: 708-783-9100
Fax: 708-783-3489
URL: www.macneal.com
Type: Acute Care Hospitals
Emergency Services: Yes
Ownership: Proprietary
Beds: 400

Key Personnel:
Cardiac Laboratory............ Donald Dickson
Emergency Room.......... Brian Fchurgin
CEO/President............... Brian Lemon
Chief of Medical Staff.......... Gary Wainer

Measure	Cases	This Hosp.	State Avg.	U.S. Avg.
Blood Clot Prevention and Treatment				
Anticoagulation Overlap Therapy[2]	88	92%	91%	93%
ICU Venous Thromboembolism Prophylaxis[2]	58	93%	93%	92%
Incidence of Potentially Preventable VTE[2]	16	12%	11%	10%
UFH with Dosages/Platelet Monitoring[2]	55	100%	94%	97%
Venous Thromboembolism Prophylaxis[2]	352	80%	86%	85%
Warfarin Therapy Discharge Instructions[2]	57	68%	71%	75%
Chest Pain/Possible Heart Attack Care				
Aspirin Given Within 24 Hours of Arrival[1,3]	-	-	96%	96%
Fibrinolytic Meds Within 30 Min. of Arrival[5]	-	-	65%	58%
Average Time to ECG (minutes)[1,3]	-	-	6	7
Average Time to Transfer (minutes)[5]	-	-	63	60
Children's Asthma Care				
Received Home Management Plan of Care	-	-	-	88%
Received Reliever Medication	-	-	-	100%
Received Systemic Corticosteroids	-	-	-	100%
Emergency Department				
Admittance Decision Time (minutes)[2]	694	178	89	98
Head CT Results Within 45 Min. of Arrival	13	38%	64%	57%
Patients Who Left ER Before Being Seen	61,619	2%	3%	2%
Time from ER Arrival to Admit. (minutes)[2]	701	378	260	274
Time from ER Arrival to Discharge (minutes)	374	141	138	134
Time in ER Before Being Evaluated (minutes)	411	34	28	26
Time to Pain Meds for Fractures (minutes)	180	43	52	57
Heart Attack Care				
Aspirin Given at Discharge	228	100%	99%	99%
Fibrinolytic Meds Within 30 Min. of Arrival[7]	-	-	33%	54%
PCI Within 90 Minutes of Arrival	61	95%	97%	96%
Statin Prescribed at Discharge	225	100%	98%	98%
Heart Failure Care				
ACE Inhibitor or ARB for LVSD	97	100%	98%	97%
Discharge Instructions Given	270	95%	96%	94%
Evaluation of LVS Function	347	100%	99%	99%
Medicare Spending				
Medicare Spending per Patient (ratio)	-	1.00	1	0.98
Pneumonia Care				
Appropriate Initial Antibiotic Given	146	99%	95%	95%
Blood Culture Timing	276	100%	98%	98%
Pregnancy and Delivery Care				
Newborn Deliveries Scheduled Early[2]	29	3%	2%	6%
Preventive Care				
Immunization for Influenza[2]	548	94%	92%	90%

NOTE: Hospital profiles are in alphabetical order by state, then city, then hospital within the city; Rankings exclude hospitals with less than 25 cases except for patient surveys which excludes hospitals with less than 100 cases; (a) 100-299 cases; (1) The number of cases/patients is too few to report; (2) Data submitted were based on a sample of cases/patients; (3) Results are based on a shorter time period than required; (4) Data suppressed by CMS for one or more quarters; (5) Results are not available for this reporting period; (6) Fewer than 100 patients completed the HCAHPS survey; (7) No cases met the criteria for this measure; (8) The lower limit of the confidence interval cannot be calculated if the number of observed infections equals zero; (9) No data are available from the state/territory for this reporting period; (10) The scores shown reflect fewer than 50 completed surveys; (11) There were discrepancies in the data collection process; (12) This measure does not apply to this hospital for this reporting period; (13) Results cannot be calculated for this reporting period; (14) The results for this state are combined with nearby states to protect confidentiality; Please refer to the User's Guide for a full explanation of data.

Immunization for Pneumonia[2]	647	95%	92%	92%
Stroke Care				
Anticoagulation Therapy for Atrial Fibrillation[2]	14	100%	94%	95%
Antithrombotic Therapy Timing[2]	95	100%	98%	98%
Assessed for Rehabilitation[2]	104	98%	97%	97%
Discharged on Antithrombotic Therapy[2]	91	100%	99%	99%
Discharged on Statin Medication[2]	68	100%	94%	94%
Thrombolytic Therapy Timing[1,2]	-	-	66%	66%
Venous Thromboembolism Prophylaxis[2]	115	97%	94%	94%
Written Stroke Educational Materials Given[2]	54	100%	87%	88%
Surgical Care Improvement Project				
Appropriate Beta Blocker Usage[2]	227	100%	98%	98%
Appropriate VTP Within 24 Hours[2]	516	100%	98%	98%
Controlled Postoperative Blood Glucose[2]	66	98%	97%	97%
Perioperative Temperature Management[2]	631	100%	100%	100%
Prophylactic Antibiotic Selection[2]	469	100%	99%	99%
Prophylactic Antibiotic Selection (Outpatient)	357	90%	98%	98%
Prophylactic Antibiotic Stopped[2]	449	99%	98%	98%
Prophylactic Antibiotic Timing[2]	469	100%	99%	99%
Prophylactic Antibiotic Timing (Outpatient)	380	88%	97%	98%
Urinary Catheter Removal[2]	457	100%	98%	97%
Survey of Patients' Hospital Experiences				
Area Around Room 'Always' Quiet at Night[11]	300+	51%	60%	61%
Doctors 'Always' Communicated Well[11]	300+	80%	81%	82%
Home Recovery Information Given[11]	300+	85%	86%	85%
Hospital Given 9 or 10 on 10 Point Scale[11]	300+	69%	70%	71%
Meds 'Always' Explained Before Given[11]	300+	59%	64%	64%
Nurses 'Always' Communicated Well[11]	300+	77%	79%	79%
Pain 'Always' Well Controlled[11]	300+	70%	71%	71%
Room and Bathroom 'Always' Clean[11]	300+	66%	74%	73%
Timely Help 'Always' Received[11]	300+	64%	67%	68%
Would Definitely Recommend Hospital[11]	300+	67%	70%	71%
Use of Medical Imaging				
Cardiac Imaging Stress Test before Surgery	307	6.2%	5.5%	5.3%
Combination Abdominal CT Scan	730	4.0%	10.1%	10.5%
Combination Brain/Sinus CT Scan	793	4.5%	2.6%	2.7%
Combination Chest CT Scan	585	0.5%	2.8%	2.7%
Follow-up Mammogram/Ultrasound	1,651	8.6%	8.4%	8.8%
Lumbar Spine MRI for Low Back Pain	203	44.8%	36.6%	37.2%

Saint Joseph Medical Center

2200 E Washington
Bloomington, IL 61701
Phone: 309-662-3311
Fax: 309-662-7665
Type: Acute Care Hospitals
Emergency Services: Yes
Ownership: Voluntary non-profit - Church
Beds: 182

Key Personnel:

Quality Assurance . . . . Kathy Haig
Radiology. . . . . James McGee, MD
CEO/President. . . . . Kenneth Natzke
Operating Room. . . . . Marsha Reeves
Pediatric Ambulatory Care . . . . . . Mark Ulbrich, MD
Pediatric In-Patient Care . . . . Mark Ulbrich, MD
Chief of Medical Staff. . . . . Herbert Weiser, MD

Measure	Cases	This Hosp.	State Avg.	U.S. Avg.
Blood Clot Prevention and Treatment				
Anticoagulation Overlap Therapy[2]	42	95%	91%	93%
ICU Venous Thromboembolism Prophylaxis[2]	41	95%	93%	92%
Incidence of Potentially Preventable VTE[1,2]	-	-	11%	10%
UFH with Dosages/Platelet Monitoring[2]	19	100%	94%	97%
Venous Thromboembolism Prophylaxis[2]	341	84%	86%	85%
Warfarin Therapy Discharge Instructions[2]	38	68%	71%	75%
Chest Pain/Possible Heart Attack Care				
Aspirin Given Within 24 Hours of Arrival[5]	-	-	96%	96%
Fibrinolytic Meds Within 30 Min. of Arrival[5]	-	-	65%	58%
Average Time to ECG (minutes)[5]	-	-	6	7
Average Time to Transfer (minutes)[5]	-	-	63	60
Children's Asthma Care				
Received Home Management Plan of Care	-	-	-	88%
Received Reliever Medication	-	-	-	100%
Received Systemic Corticosteroids	-	-	-	100%
Emergency Department				
Admittance Decision Time (minutes)[2]	352	81	89	98
Head CT Results Within 45 Min. of Arrival[1]	-	-	64%	57%
Patients Who Left ER Before Being Seen	31,023	3%	3%	2%
Time from ER Arrival to Admit. (minutes)[2]	401	254	260	274
Time from ER Arrival to Discharge (minutes)	370	164	138	134
Time in ER Before Being Evaluated (minutes)	405	26	28	26
Time to Pain Meds for Fractures (minutes)	95	59	52	57
Heart Attack Care				
Aspirin Given at Discharge	180	98%	99%	99%
Fibrinolytic Meds Within 30 Min. of Arrival[7]	-	-	33%	54%
PCI Within 90 Minutes of Arrival	43	95%	97%	96%
Statin Prescribed at Discharge	177	98%	98%	98%
Heart Failure Care				
ACE Inhibitor or ARB for LVSD	59	97%	98%	97%
Discharge Instructions Given	153	100%	96%	94%
Evaluation of LVS Function	196	100%	99%	99%
Medicare Spending				
Medicare Spending per Patient (ratio)	-	0.94	1	0.98
Pneumonia Care				
Appropriate Initial Antibiotic Given	90	93%	95%	95%
Blood Culture Timing	117	99%	98%	98%
Pregnancy and Delivery Care				
Newborn Deliveries Scheduled Early	78	0%	2%	6%
Preventive Care				
Immunization for Influenza[2]	515	94%	92%	90%
Immunization for Pneumonia[2]	701	94%	92%	92%
Stroke Care				
Anticoagulation Therapy for Atrial Fibrillation	12	100%	94%	95%
Antithrombotic Therapy Timing	80	99%	98%	98%
Assessed for Rehabilitation	126	99%	97%	97%
Discharged on Antithrombotic Therapy	113	100%	99%	99%
Discharged on Statin Medication	78	97%	94%	94%
Thrombolytic Therapy Timing	12	100%	66%	66%
Venous Thromboembolism Prophylaxis	108	93%	94%	94%
Written Stroke Educational Materials Given	85	73%	87%	88%
Surgical Care Improvement Project				
Appropriate Beta Blocker Usage	275	99%	98%	98%
Appropriate VTP Within 24 Hours	489	99%	98%	98%
Controlled Postoperative Blood Glucose	54	96%	97%	97%
Perioperative Temperature Management	688	100%	100%	100%
Prophylactic Antibiotic Selection	491	100%	99%	99%
Prophylactic Antibiotic Selection (Outpatient)	188	97%	98%	98%
Prophylactic Antibiotic Stopped	473	99%	98%	98%
Prophylactic Antibiotic Timing	491	100%	99%	99%
Prophylactic Antibiotic Timing (Outpatient)	190	99%	97%	98%
Urinary Catheter Removal	347	98%	98%	97%
Survey of Patients' Hospital Experiences				
Area Around Room 'Always' Quiet at Night	300+	65%	60%	61%
Doctors 'Always' Communicated Well	300+	85%	81%	82%
Home Recovery Information Given	300+	88%	86%	85%
Hospital Given 9 or 10 on 10 Point Scale	300+	80%	70%	71%
Meds 'Always' Explained Before Given	300+	67%	64%	64%
Nurses 'Always' Communicated Well	300+	83%	79%	79%
Pain 'Always' Well Controlled	300+	73%	71%	71%
Room and Bathroom 'Always' Clean	300+	80%	74%	73%
Timely Help 'Always' Received	300+	68%	67%	68%
Would Definitely Recommend Hospital	300+	82%	70%	71%
Use of Medical Imaging				
Cardiac Imaging Stress Test before Surgery	571	5.6%	5.5%	5.3%
Combination Abdominal CT Scan	655	10.4%	10.1%	10.5%
Combination Brain/Sinus CT Scan	472	0.0%	2.6%	2.7%
Combination Chest CT Scan	696	1.6%	2.8%	2.7%
Follow-up Mammogram/Ultrasound	1,443	10.8%	8.4%	8.8%
Lumbar Spine MRI for Low Back Pain	90	30.0%	36.6%	37.2%

Metrosouth Medical Center

12935 S Gregory
Blue Island, IL 60406
Phone: 708-597-2000
Fax: 708-389-9480
URL: www.stfrancisblueisland.com
Type: Acute Care Hospitals
Emergency Services: Yes
Ownership: Proprietary
Beds: 410

Key Personnel:

Chief of Medical Staff. . . . . Kurt Erickson, MD
Infection Control. . . . . Robert Fliegelman, MD
CEO/President. . . . . Colleen Kannaday
Operating Room. . . . . Nancy Kasper, RN
Emergency Room . . . . Daniel Kowalzyk, MD
Radiology. . . . . Vicki McFarlane

Measure	Cases	This Hosp.	State Avg.	U.S. Avg.
Blood Clot Prevention and Treatment				
Anticoagulation Overlap Therapy[2]	106	100%	91%	93%
ICU Venous Thromboembolism Prophylaxis[2]	116	99%	93%	92%
Incidence of Potentially Preventable VTE[2]	15	0%	11%	10%
UFH with Dosages/Platelet Monitoring[2]	75	100%	94%	97%
Venous Thromboembolism Prophylaxis[2]	335	95%	86%	85%
Warfarin Therapy Discharge Instructions[2]	67	97%	71%	75%
Chest Pain/Possible Heart Attack Care				
Aspirin Given Within 24 Hours of Arrival[5]	-	-	96%	96%
Fibrinolytic Meds Within 30 Min. of Arrival[5]	-	-	65%	58%
Average Time to ECG (minutes)[5]	-	-	6	7
Average Time to Transfer (minutes)[5]	-	-	63	60
Children's Asthma Care				
Received Home Management Plan of Care	-	-	-	88%
Received Reliever Medication	-	-	-	100%
Received Systemic Corticosteroids	-	-	-	100%
Emergency Department				
Admittance Decision Time (minutes)[2]	605	156	89	98
Head CT Results Within 45 Min. of Arrival	15	87%	64%	57%
Patients Who Left ER Before Being Seen	49,919	2%	3%	2%
Time from ER Arrival to Admit. (minutes)[2]	606	316	260	274
Time from ER Arrival to Discharge (minutes)	383	135	138	134
Time in ER Before Being Evaluated (minutes)	421	21	28	26
Time to Pain Meds for Fractures (minutes)	193	59	52	57
Heart Attack Care				
Aspirin Given at Discharge	126	99%	99%	99%
Fibrinolytic Meds Within 30 Min. of Arrival[7]	-	-	33%	54%
PCI Within 90 Minutes of Arrival	20	100%	97%	96%
Statin Prescribed at Discharge	120	94%	98%	98%
Heart Failure Care				
ACE Inhibitor or ARB for LVSD	153	99%	98%	97%
Discharge Instructions Given	369	100%	96%	94%
Evaluation of LVS Function	418	100%	99%	99%
Medicare Spending				
Medicare Spending per Patient (ratio)	-	1.01	1	0.98
Pneumonia Care				
Appropriate Initial Antibiotic Given	126	98%	95%	95%
Blood Culture Timing	241	100%	98%	98%
Pregnancy and Delivery Care				
Newborn Deliveries Scheduled Early[2]	47	0%	2%	6%
Preventive Care				
Immunization for Influenza[2]	622	99%	92%	90%
Immunization for Pneumonia[2]	819	100%	92%	92%
Stroke Care				
Anticoagulation Therapy for Atrial Fibrillation[1]	-	-	94%	95%
Antithrombotic Therapy Timing	98	100%	98%	98%
Assessed for Rehabilitation	113	99%	97%	97%
Discharged on Antithrombotic Therapy	109	98%	99%	99%
Discharged on Statin Medication	85	99%	94%	94%
Thrombolytic Therapy Timing	13	100%	66%	66%
Venous Thromboembolism Prophylaxis	119	98%	94%	94%
Written Stroke Educational Materials Given	59	98%	87%	88%
Surgical Care Improvement Project				
Appropriate Beta Blocker Usage	108	99%	98%	98%
Appropriate VTP Within 24 Hours	295	99%	98%	98%
Controlled Postoperative Blood Glucose	26	96%	97%	97%
Perioperative Temperature Management	346	100%	100%	100%
Prophylactic Antibiotic Selection	258	100%	99%	99%
Prophylactic Antibiotic Selection (Outpatient)	135	100%	98%	98%
Prophylactic Antibiotic Stopped	251	99%	98%	98%
Prophylactic Antibiotic Timing	258	100%	99%	99%
Prophylactic Antibiotic Timing (Outpatient)	135	100%	97%	98%
Urinary Catheter Removal	232	100%	98%	97%
Survey of Patients' Hospital Experiences				
Area Around Room 'Always' Quiet at Night	300+	65%	60%	61%
Doctors 'Always' Communicated Well	300+	82%	81%	82%
Home Recovery Information Given	300+	86%	86%	85%
Hospital Given 9 or 10 on 10 Point Scale	300+	67%	70%	71%
Meds 'Always' Explained Before Given	300+	64%	64%	64%
Nurses 'Always' Communicated Well	300+	77%	79%	79%
Pain 'Always' Well Controlled	300+	71%	71%	71%

NOTE: Hospital profiles are in alphabetical order by state, then city, then hospital within the city; Rankings exclude hospitals with less than 25 cases except for patient surveys which excludes hospitals with less than 100 cases; (a) 100-299 cases; (1) The number of cases/patients is too few to report; (2) Data submitted were based on a sample of cases/patients; (3) Results are based on a shorter time period than required; (4) Data suppressed by CMS for one or more quarters; (5) Results are not available for this reporting period; (6) Fewer than 100 patients completed the HCAHPS survey; (7) No cases met the criteria for this measure; (8) The lower limit of the confidence interval cannot be calculated if the number of observed infections equals zero; (9) No data are available from the state/territory for this reporting period; (10) The scores shown reflect fewer than 50 completed surveys; (11) There were discrepancies in the data collection process; (12) This measure does not apply to this hospital for this reporting period; (13) Results cannot be calculated for this reporting period; (14) The results for this state are combined with nearby states to protect confidentiality; Please refer to the User's Guide for a full explanation of data.

Measure	Cases	This Hosp.	State Avg.	U.S. Avg.
Room and Bathroom 'Always' Clean	300+	72%	74%	73%
Timely Help 'Always' Received	300+	65%	67%	68%
Would Definitely Recommend Hospital	300+	68%	70%	71%
Use of Medical Imaging				
Cardiac Imaging Stress Test before Surgery	186	5.4%	5.5%	5.3%
Combination Abdominal CT Scan	392	2.8%	10.1%	10.5%
Combination Brain/Sinus CT Scan	593	1.5%	2.6%	2.7%
Combination Chest CT Scan	205	1.0%	2.8%	2.7%
Follow-up Mammogram/Ultrasound	836	5.4%	8.4%	8.8%
Lumbar Spine MRI for Low Back Pain[1]	-	-	36.6%	37.2%

Adventist Bolingbrook Hospital

500 Remington Boulevard
Bolingbrook, IL 60440
Phone: 630-226-8100
URL: www.keepingyouwell.com
Type: Acute Care Hospitals
Emergency Services: Yes
Ownership: Voluntary non-profit - Private

Measure	Cases	This Hosp.	State Avg.	U.S. Avg.
Blood Clot Prevention and Treatment				
Anticoagulation Overlap Therapy[2]	38	100%	91%	93%
ICU Venous Thromboembolism Prophylaxis[2]	87	100%	93%	92%
Incidence of Potentially Preventable VTE[1,2]	-	-	11%	10%
UFH with Dosages/Platelet Monitoring[2]	16	100%	94%	97%
Venous Thromboembolism Prophylaxis[2]	322	98%	86%	85%
Warfarin Therapy Discharge Instructions[2]	27	93%	71%	75%
Chest Pain/Possible Heart Attack Care				
Aspirin Given Within 24 Hours of Arrival[1,3]	-	-	96%	96%
Fibrinolytic Meds Within 30 Min. of Arrival[5]	-	-	65%	58%
Average Time to ECG (minutes)[1,3]	-	-	6	7
Average Time to Transfer (minutes)[5]	-	-	63	60
Children's Asthma Care				
Received Home Management Plan of Care	-	-	-	88%
Received Reliever Medication	-	-	-	100%
Received Systemic Corticosteroids	-	-	-	100%
Emergency Department				
Admittance Decision Time (minutes)[2]	515	95	89	98
Head CT Results Within 45 Min. of Arrival[1]	-	-	64%	57%
Patients Who Left ER Before Being Seen	33,434	1%	3%	2%
Time from ER Arrival to Admit. (minutes)[2]	557	263	260	274
Time from ER Arrival to Discharge (minutes)	337	148	138	134
Time in ER Before Being Evaluated (minutes)	268	32	28	26
Time to Pain Meds for Fractures (minutes)	111	44	52	57
Heart Attack Care				
Aspirin Given at Discharge	74	100%	99%	99%
Fibrinolytic Meds Within 30 Min. of Arrival[7]	-	-	33%	54%
PCI Within 90 Minutes of Arrival	25	96%	97%	96%
Statin Prescribed at Discharge	73	100%	98%	98%
Heart Failure Care				
ACE Inhibitor or ARB for LVSD	45	100%	98%	97%
Discharge Instructions Given	125	98%	96%	94%
Evaluation of LVS Function	159	100%	99%	99%
Medicare Spending				
Medicare Spending per Patient (ratio)	-	1.06	1	0.98
Pneumonia Care				
Appropriate Initial Antibiotic Given	77	99%	95%	95%
Blood Culture Timing	160	98%	98%	98%
Pregnancy and Delivery Care				
Newborn Deliveries Scheduled Early	94	20%	2%	6%
Preventive Care				
Immunization for Influenza[2]	497	96%	92%	90%
Immunization for Pneumonia[2]	525	97%	92%	92%
Stroke Care				
Anticoagulation Therapy for Atrial Fibrillation[1]	-	-	94%	95%
Antithrombotic Therapy Timing	33	97%	98%	98%
Assessed for Rehabilitation	31	100%	97%	97%
Discharged on Antithrombotic Therapy	30	100%	99%	99%
Discharged on Statin Medication	17	100%	94%	94%
Thrombolytic Therapy Timing[1]	-	-	66%	66%
Venous Thromboembolism Prophylaxis	32	100%	94%	94%
Written Stroke Educational Materials Given	18	83%	87%	88%
Surgical Care Improvement Project				
Appropriate Beta Blocker Usage	50	100%	98%	98%
Appropriate VTP Within 24 Hours	173	98%	98%	98%
Controlled Postoperative Blood Glucose[7]	-	-	97%	97%
Perioperative Temperature Management	191	100%	100%	100%
Prophylactic Antibiotic Selection	92	97%	99%	99%
Prophylactic Antibiotic Selection (Outpatient)	79	94%	98%	98%
Prophylactic Antibiotic Stopped	90	99%	98%	98%
Prophylactic Antibiotic Timing	92	100%	99%	99%
Prophylactic Antibiotic Timing (Outpatient)	81	98%	97%	98%
Urinary Catheter Removal	87	98%	98%	97%
Survey of Patients' Hospital Experiences				
Area Around Room 'Always' Quiet at Night[11]	300+	69%	60%	61%
Doctors 'Always' Communicated Well[11]	300+	80%	81%	82%
Home Recovery Information Given[11]	300+	83%	86%	85%
Hospital Given 9 or 10 on 10 Point Scale[11]	300+	72%	70%	71%
Meds 'Always' Explained Before Given[11]	300+	64%	64%	64%
Nurses 'Always' Communicated Well[11]	300+	79%	79%	79%
Pain 'Always' Well Controlled[11]	300+	71%	71%	71%
Room and Bathroom 'Always' Clean[11]	300+	77%	74%	73%
Timely Help 'Always' Received[11]	300+	63%	67%	68%
Would Definitely Recommend Hospital[11]	300+	71%	70%	71%
Use of Medical Imaging				
Cardiac Imaging Stress Test before Surgery	178	4.5%	5.5%	5.3%
Combination Abdominal CT Scan	447	6.9%	10.1%	10.5%
Combination Brain/Sinus CT Scan	425	4.5%	2.6%	2.7%
Combination Chest CT Scan	272	18.4%	2.8%	2.7%
Follow-up Mammogram/Ultrasound	545	14.3%	8.4%	8.8%
Lumbar Spine MRI for Low Back Pain	62	40.3%	36.6%	37.2%

Saint Joseph's Hospital

9515 Holy Cross Ln
Breese, IL 62230
Phone: 618-526-4511
Fax: 618-526-8022
E-mail: phinton@sjh.hshs.org
URL: www.stjoebreese.com
Type: Acute Care Hospitals
Emergency Services: Yes
Ownership: Voluntary non-profit - Church
Beds: 85

Key Personnel:
Radiology. . . . . Thomas Doyle
Operating Room. . . . . Renato Rivera, RN
Quality Assurance . . . . Jan Robert, RN
CEO/President. . . . . Jacolyn Schlautman

Measure	Cases	This Hosp.	State Avg.	U.S. Avg.
Blood Clot Prevention and Treatment				
Anticoagulation Overlap Therapy[2]	12	100%	91%	93%
ICU Venous Thromboembolism Prophylaxis[2,7]	-	-	93%	92%
Incidence of Potentially Preventable VTE[1,2]	-	-	11%	10%
UFH with Dosages/Platelet Monitoring[1,2]	-	-	94%	97%
Venous Thromboembolism Prophylaxis[2]	116	100%	86%	85%
Warfarin Therapy Discharge Instructions[1,2]	-	-	71%	75%
Chest Pain/Possible Heart Attack Care				
Aspirin Given Within 24 Hours of Arrival	48	100%	96%	96%
Fibrinolytic Meds Within 30 Min. of Arrival[7]	-	-	65%	58%
Average Time to ECG (minutes)	49	9	6	7
Average Time to Transfer (minutes)	11	68	63	60
Children's Asthma Care				
Received Home Management Plan of Care	-	-	-	88%
Received Reliever Medication	-	-	-	100%
Received Systemic Corticosteroids	-	-	-	100%
Emergency Department				
Admittance Decision Time (minutes)[2]	239	45	89	98
Head CT Results Within 45 Min. of Arrival	14	71%	64%	57%
Patients Who Left ER Before Being Seen	8,565	1%	3%	2%
Time from ER Arrival to Admit. (minutes)[2]	244	211	260	274
Time from ER Arrival to Discharge (minutes)	420	120	138	134
Time in ER Before Being Evaluated (minutes)	479	18	28	26
Time to Pain Meds for Fractures (minutes)	36	32	52	57
Heart Attack Care				
Aspirin Given at Discharge[7]	-	-	99%	99%
Fibrinolytic Meds Within 30 Min. of Arrival[7]	-	-	33%	54%
PCI Within 90 Minutes of Arrival[7]	-	-	97%	96%
Statin Prescribed at Discharge[7]	-	-	98%	98%
Heart Failure Care				
ACE Inhibitor or ARB for LVSD[1]	-	-	98%	97%
Discharge Instructions Given	25	100%	96%	94%
Evaluation of LVS Function	32	100%	99%	99%
Medicare Spending				
Medicare Spending per Patient (ratio)	-	0.96	1	0.98
Pneumonia Care				
Appropriate Initial Antibiotic Given	27	100%	95%	95%
Blood Culture Timing	52	100%	98%	98%
Pregnancy and Delivery Care				
Newborn Deliveries Scheduled Early[2]	29	0%	2%	6%
Preventive Care				
Immunization for Influenza[2]	271	100%	92%	90%
Immunization for Pneumonia[2]	232	99%	92%	92%
Stroke Care				
Anticoagulation Therapy for Atrial Fibrillation[7]	-	-	94%	95%
Antithrombotic Therapy Timing[1]	-	-	98%	98%
Assessed for Rehabilitation[1]	-	-	97%	97%
Discharged on Antithrombotic Therapy[1]	-	-	99%	99%
Discharged on Statin Medication[1]	-	-	94%	94%
Thrombolytic Therapy Timing[7]	-	-	66%	66%
Venous Thromboembolism Prophylaxis[1]	-	-	94%	94%
Written Stroke Educational Materials Given[1]	-	-	87%	88%
Surgical Care Improvement Project				
Appropriate Beta Blocker Usage	17	100%	98%	98%
Appropriate VTP Within 24 Hours	54	100%	98%	98%
Controlled Postoperative Blood Glucose[7]	-	-	97%	97%
Perioperative Temperature Management	78	100%	100%	100%
Prophylactic Antibiotic Selection	48	100%	99%	99%
Prophylactic Antibiotic Selection (Outpatient)[3]	13	100%	98%	98%
Prophylactic Antibiotic Stopped	48	100%	98%	98%
Prophylactic Antibiotic Timing	48	96%	99%	99%
Prophylactic Antibiotic Timing (Outpatient)[3]	12	100%	97%	98%
Urinary Catheter Removal	37	100%	98%	97%
Survey of Patients' Hospital Experiences				
Area Around Room 'Always' Quiet at Night	300+	77%	60%	61%
Doctors 'Always' Communicated Well	300+	88%	81%	82%
Home Recovery Information Given	300+	92%	86%	85%
Hospital Given 9 or 10 on 10 Point Scale	300+	86%	70%	71%
Meds 'Always' Explained Before Given	300+	82%	64%	64%
Nurses 'Always' Communicated Well	300+	91%	79%	79%
Pain 'Always' Well Controlled	300+	81%	71%	71%
Room and Bathroom 'Always' Clean	300+	92%	74%	73%
Timely Help 'Always' Received	300+	85%	67%	68%
Would Definitely Recommend Hospital	300+	86%	70%	71%
Use of Medical Imaging				
Cardiac Imaging Stress Test before Surgery	224	6.7%	5.5%	5.3%
Combination Abdominal CT Scan	304	11.5%	10.1%	10.5%
Combination Brain/Sinus CT Scan	339	4.4%	2.6%	2.7%
Combination Chest CT Scan	217	3.7%	2.8%	2.7%
Follow-up Mammogram/Ultrasound	839	7.0%	8.4%	8.8%
Lumbar Spine MRI for Low Back Pain	45	40.0%	36.6%	37.2%

Graham Hospital Association

210 West Walnut Street
Canton, IL 61520
Phone: 309-647-5240
Fax: 309-649-5197
URL: www.grahamhospital.org
Type: Acute Care Hospitals
Emergency Services: Yes
Ownership: Voluntary non-profit - Other
Beds: 124

Key Personnel:
Operating Room. . . . . Mary Ahn
Chief of Medical Staff. . . . . Shirley Frantz, MD
CEO/President. . . . . Robert Senneff
Chairman/CEO . . . . Michael Walters
Quality Assurance . . . . Carol Welch

Measure	Cases	This Hosp.	State Avg.	U.S. Avg.
Blood Clot Prevention and Treatment				
Anticoagulation Overlap Therapy[2]	11	82%	91%	93%
ICU Venous Thromboembolism Prophylaxis[2]	47	62%	93%	92%
Incidence of Potentially Preventable VTE[1,2]	-	-	11%	10%
UFH with Dosages/Platelet Monitoring[2,7]	-	-	94%	97%
Venous Thromboembolism Prophylaxis[2]	171	52%	86%	85%
Warfarin Therapy Discharge Instructions[1,2]	-	-	71%	75%
Chest Pain/Possible Heart Attack Care				
Aspirin Given Within 24 Hours of Arrival	59	100%	96%	96%
Fibrinolytic Meds Within 30 Min. of Arrival[7]	-	-	65%	58%

NOTE: Hospital profiles are in alphabetical order by state, then city, then hospital within the city; Rankings exclude hospitals with less than 25 cases except for patient surveys which excludes hospitals with less than 100 cases; (a) 100-299 cases; (1) The number of cases/patients is too few to report; (2) Data submitted were based on a sample of cases/patients; (3) Results are based on a shorter time period than required; (4) Data suppressed by CMS for one or more quarters; (5) Results are not available for this reporting period; (6) Fewer than 100 patients completed the HCAHPS survey; (7) No cases met the criteria for this measure; (8) The lower limit of the confidence interval cannot be calculated if the number of observed infections equals zero; (9) No data are available from the state/territory for this reporting period; (10) The scores shown reflect fewer than 50 completed surveys; (11) There were discrepancies in the data collection process; (12) This measure does not apply to this hospital for this reporting period; (13) Results cannot be calculated for this reporting period; (14) The results for this state are combined with nearby states to protect confidentiality; Please refer to the User's Guide for a full explanation of data.

Measure	Cases	This Hosp.	State Avg.	U.S. Avg.
Average Time to ECG (minutes)	60	10	6	7
Average Time to Transfer (minutes)[1]	-	-	63	60
Children's Asthma Care				
Received Home Management Plan of Care	-	-	-	88%
Received Reliever Medication	-	-	-	100%
Received Systemic Corticosteroids	-	-	-	100%
Emergency Department				
Admittance Decision Time (minutes)[2]	339	49	89	98
Head CT Results Within 45 Min. of Arrival	12	92%	64%	57%
Patients Who Left ER Before Being Seen	16,234	1%	3%	2%
Time from ER Arrival to Admit. (minutes)[2]	339	174	260	274
Time from ER Arrival to Discharge (minutes)	362	85	138	134
Time in ER Before Being Evaluated (minutes)	407	14	28	26
Time to Pain Meds for Fractures (minutes)	62	30	52	57
Heart Attack Care				
Aspirin Given at Discharge[1]	-	-	99%	99%
Fibrinolytic Meds Within 30 Min. of Arrival[7]	-	-	33%	54%
PCI Within 90 Minutes of Arrival[7]	-	-	97%	96%
Statin Prescribed at Discharge[1]	-	-	98%	98%
Heart Failure Care				
ACE Inhibitor or ARB for LVSD	22	95%	98%	97%
Discharge Instructions Given	63	94%	96%	94%
Evaluation of LVS Function	91	98%	99%	99%
Medicare Spending				
Medicare Spending per Patient (ratio)	-	0.89	1	0.98
Pneumonia Care				
Appropriate Initial Antibiotic Given[2]	53	98%	95%	95%
Blood Culture Timing[2]	106	99%	98%	98%
Pregnancy and Delivery Care				
Newborn Deliveries Scheduled Early[2]	29	3%	2%	6%
Preventive Care				
Immunization for Influenza[2]	269	89%	92%	90%
Immunization for Pneumonia[2]	363	95%	92%	92%
Stroke Care				
Anticoagulation Therapy for Atrial Fibrillation[1]	-	-	94%	95%
Antithrombotic Therapy Timing	19	100%	98%	98%
Assessed for Rehabilitation	19	95%	97%	97%
Discharged on Antithrombotic Therapy	19	100%	99%	99%
Discharged on Statin Medication	18	39%	94%	94%
Thrombolytic Therapy Timing[7]	-	-	66%	66%
Venous Thromboembolism Prophylaxis	18	83%	94%	94%
Written Stroke Educational Materials Given[1]	-	-	87%	88%
Surgical Care Improvement Project				
Appropriate Beta Blocker Usage[2]	71	97%	98%	98%
Appropriate VTP Within 24 Hours[2]	151	97%	98%	98%
Controlled Postoperative Blood Glucose[2,7]	-	-	97%	97%
Perioperative Temperature Management[2]	186	100%	100%	100%
Prophylactic Antibiotic Selection[2]	146	98%	99%	99%
Prophylactic Antibiotic Selection (Outpatient)	46	96%	98%	98%
Prophylactic Antibiotic Stopped[2]	145	97%	98%	98%
Prophylactic Antibiotic Timing[2]	146	97%	99%	99%
Prophylactic Antibiotic Timing (Outpatient)	46	100%	97%	98%
Urinary Catheter Removal[2]	129	89%	98%	97%
Survey of Patients' Hospital Experiences				
Area Around Room 'Always' Quiet at Night	300+	52%	60%	61%
Doctors 'Always' Communicated Well	300+	86%	81%	82%
Home Recovery Information Given	300+	84%	86%	85%
Hospital Given 9 or 10 on 10 Point Scale	300+	68%	70%	71%
Meds 'Always' Explained Before Given	300+	67%	64%	64%
Nurses 'Always' Communicated Well	300+	81%	79%	79%
Pain 'Always' Well Controlled	300+	71%	71%	71%
Room and Bathroom 'Always' Clean	300+	74%	74%	73%
Timely Help 'Always' Received	300+	67%	67%	68%
Would Definitely Recommend Hospital	300+	64%	70%	71%
Use of Medical Imaging				
Cardiac Imaging Stress Test before Surgery	152	2.0%	5.5%	5.3%
Combination Abdominal CT Scan	336	5.7%	10.1%	10.5%
Combination Brain/Sinus CT Scan[1]	-	-	2.6%	2.7%
Combination Chest CT Scan	308	0.3%	2.8%	2.7%
Follow-up Mammogram/Ultrasound	477	11.5%	8.4%	8.8%
Lumbar Spine MRI for Low Back Pain	50	40.0%	36.6%	37.2%

Memorial Hospital of Carbondale

405 W Jackson
Carbondale, IL 62902
URL: www.sih.net
Phone: 618-549-0721
Fax: 618-529-0449
Type: Acute Care Hospitals
Emergency Services: Yes
Ownership: Voluntary non-profit - Private
Beds: 150

Key Personnel:

Emergency Room . . . . Kent Arnold
Operating Room. . . . . R Judson Brewer
CEO/President. . . . . Rex Budde
Administrator . . . . Bart Millstead
Chief of Medical Staff . . . . Marci Moore-Connelley, MD
Chair/CEO . . . . Steve Sabens

Measure	Cases	This Hosp.	State Avg.	U.S. Avg.
Blood Clot Prevention and Treatment				
Anticoagulation Overlap Therapy[2]	70	99%	91%	93%
ICU Venous Thromboembolism Prophylaxis[2]	69	100%	93%	92%
Incidence of Potentially Preventable VTE[1,2]	-	-	11%	10%
UFH with Dosages/Platelet Monitoring[2]	16	88%	94%	97%
Venous Thromboembolism Prophylaxis[2]	336	97%	86%	85%
Warfarin Therapy Discharge Instructions[2]	59	100%	71%	75%
Chest Pain/Possible Heart Attack Care				
Aspirin Given Within 24 Hours of Arrival[5]	-	-	96%	96%
Fibrinolytic Meds Within 30 Min. of Arrival[5]	-	-	65%	58%
Average Time to ECG (minutes)[5]	-	-	6	7
Average Time to Transfer (minutes)[5]	-	-	63	60
Children's Asthma Care				
Received Home Management Plan of Care	-	-	-	88%
Received Reliever Medication	-	-	-	100%
Received Systemic Corticosteroids	-	-	-	100%
Emergency Department				
Admittance Decision Time (minutes)[2]	314	100	89	98
Head CT Results Within 45 Min. of Arrival[1]	-	-	64%	57%
Patients Who Left ER Before Being Seen	33,166	1%	3%	2%
Time from ER Arrival to Admit. (minutes)[2]	367	266	260	274
Time from ER Arrival to Discharge (minutes)	386	134	138	134
Time in ER Before Being Evaluated (minutes)	443	29	28	26
Time to Pain Meds for Fractures (minutes)	96	53	52	57
Heart Attack Care				
Aspirin Given at Discharge	447	100%	99%	99%
Fibrinolytic Meds Within 30 Min. of Arrival[7]	-	-	33%	54%
PCI Within 90 Minutes of Arrival	34	100%	97%	96%
Statin Prescribed at Discharge	434	100%	98%	98%
Heart Failure Care				
ACE Inhibitor or ARB for LVSD	67	100%	98%	97%
Discharge Instructions Given	195	93%	96%	94%
Evaluation of LVS Function	225	100%	99%	99%
Medicare Spending				
Medicare Spending per Patient (ratio)	-	0.98	1	0.98
Pneumonia Care				
Appropriate Initial Antibiotic Given	88	99%	95%	95%
Blood Culture Timing	206	100%	98%	98%
Pregnancy and Delivery Care				
Newborn Deliveries Scheduled Early[2]	42	2%	2%	6%
Preventive Care				
Immunization for Influenza[2]	552	97%	92%	90%
Immunization for Pneumonia[2]	617	97%	92%	92%
Stroke Care				
Anticoagulation Therapy for Atrial Fibrillation	18	100%	94%	95%
Antithrombotic Therapy Timing	74	97%	98%	98%
Assessed for Rehabilitation	126	95%	97%	97%
Discharged on Antithrombotic Therapy	115	100%	99%	99%
Discharged on Statin Medication	99	98%	94%	94%
Thrombolytic Therapy Timing[1]	-	-	66%	66%
Venous Thromboembolism Prophylaxis	120	99%	94%	94%
Written Stroke Educational Materials Given	89	84%	87%	88%
Surgical Care Improvement Project				
Appropriate Beta Blocker Usage	376	98%	98%	98%
Appropriate VTP Within 24 Hours	673	99%	98%	98%
Controlled Postoperative Blood Glucose	156	99%	97%	97%
Perioperative Temperature Management	788	100%	100%	100%
Prophylactic Antibiotic Selection	659	100%	99%	99%
Prophylactic Antibiotic Selection (Outpatient)	444	99%	98%	98%
Prophylactic Antibiotic Stopped	641	97%	98%	98%
Prophylactic Antibiotic Timing	659	99%	99%	99%
Prophylactic Antibiotic Timing (Outpatient)	453	97%	97%	98%
Urinary Catheter Removal	558	97%	98%	97%
Survey of Patients' Hospital Experiences				
Area Around Room 'Always' Quiet at Night	300+	61%	60%	61%
Doctors 'Always' Communicated Well	300+	82%	81%	82%
Home Recovery Information Given	300+	87%	86%	85%
Hospital Given 9 or 10 on 10 Point Scale	300+	73%	70%	71%
Meds 'Always' Explained Before Given	300+	63%	64%	64%
Nurses 'Always' Communicated Well	300+	81%	79%	79%
Pain 'Always' Well Controlled	300+	70%	71%	71%
Room and Bathroom 'Always' Clean	300+	74%	74%	73%
Timely Help 'Always' Received	300+	66%	67%	68%
Would Definitely Recommend Hospital	300+	78%	70%	71%
Use of Medical Imaging				
Cardiac Imaging Stress Test before Surgery	1,518	5.0%	5.5%	5.3%
Combination Abdominal CT Scan	976	11.0%	10.1%	10.5%
Combination Brain/Sinus CT Scan	770	5.7%	2.6%	2.7%
Combination Chest CT Scan	691	10.0%	2.8%	2.7%
Follow-up Mammogram/Ultrasound	2,837	10.0%	8.4%	8.8%
Lumbar Spine MRI for Low Back Pain	111	30.6%	36.6%	37.2%

Carlinville Area Hospital

20733 N Broad Street
Carlinville, IL 62626
Phone: 217-854-3141
Fax: 217-854-7861
Type: Critical Access Hospitals
Emergency Services: Yes
Ownership: Voluntary non-profit - Private
Beds: 33

Key Personnel:

Surgery . . . . Jon E. Andersen, D.O.
Operating Room. . . . . Rosie Arnett
Emergency Room . . . . Robert England, MD
CEO/President. . . . . Steve Hannah
Quality Assurance . . . . Nick Tex

Measure	Cases	This Hosp.	State Avg.	U.S. Avg.
Blood Clot Prevention and Treatment				
Anticoagulation Overlap Therapy[5]	-	-	91%	93%
ICU Venous Thromboembolism Prophylaxis[5]	-	-	93%	92%
Incidence of Potentially Preventable VTE[5]	-	-	11%	10%
UFH with Dosages/Platelet Monitoring[5]	-	-	94%	97%
Venous Thromboembolism Prophylaxis[5]	-	-	86%	85%
Warfarin Therapy Discharge Instructions[5]	-	-	71%	75%
Chest Pain/Possible Heart Attack Care				
Aspirin Given Within 24 Hours of Arrival	30	100%	96%	96%
Fibrinolytic Meds Within 30 Min. of Arrival[3,7]	-	-	65%	58%
Average Time to ECG (minutes)	31	6	6	7
Average Time to Transfer (minutes)[1,3]	-	-	63	60
Children's Asthma Care				
Received Home Management Plan of Care	-	-	-	88%
Received Reliever Medication	-	-	-	100%
Received Systemic Corticosteroids	-	-	-	100%
Emergency Department				
Admittance Decision Time (minutes)[5]	-	-	89	98
Head CT Results Within 45 Min. of Arrival[5]	-	-	64%	57%
Patients Who Left ER Before Being Seen[5]	-	-	3%	2%
Time from ER Arrival to Admit. (minutes)[5]	-	-	260	274
Time from ER Arrival to Discharge (minutes)[5]	-	-	138	134
Time in ER Before Being Evaluated (minutes)[5]	-	-	28	26
Time to Pain Meds for Fractures (minutes)[5]	-	-	52	57
Heart Attack Care				
Aspirin Given at Discharge[1,3]	-	-	99%	99%
Fibrinolytic Meds Within 30 Min. of Arrival[5]	-	-	33%	54%
PCI Within 90 Minutes of Arrival[5]	-	-	97%	96%
Statin Prescribed at Discharge[1,3]	-	-	98%	98%
Heart Failure Care				
ACE Inhibitor or ARB for LVSD[1,3]	-	-	98%	97%
Discharge Instructions Given[1,3]	-	-	96%	94%
Evaluation of LVS Function[3]	19	100%	99%	99%
Medicare Spending				
Medicare Spending per Patient (ratio)	-	-	1	0.98
Pneumonia Care				
Appropriate Initial Antibiotic Given[3]	16	94%	95%	95%
Blood Culture Timing[3]	25	100%	98%	98%
Pregnancy and Delivery Care				

NOTE: Hospital profiles are in alphabetical order by state, then city, then hospital within the city; Rankings exclude hospitals with less than 25 cases except for patient surveys which excludes hospitals with less than 100 cases; (a) 100-299 cases; (1) The number of cases/patients is too few to report; (2) Data submitted were based on a sample of cases/patients; (3) Results are based on a shorter time period than required; (4) Data suppressed by CMS for one or more quarters; (5) Results are not available for this reporting period; (6) Fewer than 100 patients completed the HCAHPS survey; (7) No cases met the criteria for this measure; (8) The lower limit of the confidence interval cannot be calculated if the number of observed infections equals zero; (9) No data are available from the state/territory for this reporting period; (10) The scores shown reflect fewer than 50 completed surveys; (11) There were discrepancies in the data collection process; (12) This measure does not apply to this hospital for this reporting period; (13) Results cannot be calculated for this reporting period; (14) The results for this state are combined with nearby states to protect confidentiality; Please refer to the User's Guide for a full explanation of data.

Measure	Cases	This Hosp.	State Avg.	U.S. Avg.
Newborn Deliveries Scheduled Early[5]	-	-	2%	6%
Preventive Care				
Immunization for Influenza[5]	-	-	92%	90%
Immunization for Pneumonia[5]	-	-	92%	92%
Stroke Care				
Anticoagulation Therapy for Atrial Fibrillation[5]	-	-	94%	95%
Antithrombotic Therapy Timing[5]	-	-	98%	98%
Assessed for Rehabilitation[5]	-	-	97%	97%
Discharged on Antithrombotic Therapy[5]	-	-	99%	99%
Discharged on Statin Medication[5]	-	-	94%	94%
Thrombolytic Therapy Timing[5]	-	-	66%	66%
Venous Thromboembolism Prophylaxis[5]	-	-	94%	94%
Written Stroke Educational Materials Given[5]	-	-	87%	88%
Surgical Care Improvement Project				
Appropriate Beta Blocker Usage[5]	-	-	98%	98%
Appropriate VTP Within 24 Hours[5]	-	-	98%	98%
Controlled Postoperative Blood Glucose[5]	-	-	97%	97%
Perioperative Temperature Management[5]	-	-	100%	100%
Prophylactic Antibiotic Selection[5]	-	-	99%	99%
Prophylactic Antibiotic Selection (Outpatient)[5]	-	-	98%	98%
Prophylactic Antibiotic Stopped[5]	-	-	98%	98%
Prophylactic Antibiotic Timing[5]	-	-	99%	99%
Prophylactic Antibiotic Timing (Outpatient)[5]	-	-	97%	98%
Urinary Catheter Removal[5]	-	-	98%	97%
Survey of Patients' Hospital Experiences				
Area Around Room 'Always' Quiet at Night[6]	<100	65%	60%	61%
Doctors 'Always' Communicated Well[6]	<100	78%	81%	82%
Home Recovery Information Given[6]	<100	84%	86%	85%
Hospital Given 9 or 10 on 10 Point Scale[6]	<100	84%	70%	71%
Meds 'Always' Explained Before Given[6]	<100	66%	64%	64%
Nurses 'Always' Communicated Well[6]	<100	84%	79%	79%
Pain 'Always' Well Controlled[6]	<100	71%	71%	71%
Room and Bathroom 'Always' Clean[6]	<100	94%	74%	73%
Timely Help 'Always' Received[6]	<100	70%	67%	68%
Would Definitely Recommend Hospital[6]	<100	77%	70%	71%
Use of Medical Imaging				
Cardiac Imaging Stress Test before Surgery	85	7.1%	5.5%	5.3%
Combination Abdominal CT Scan	206	8.3%	10.1%	10.5%
Combination Brain/Sinus CT Scan[1]	-	-	2.6%	2.7%
Combination Chest CT Scan	115	0.9%	2.8%	2.7%
Follow-up Mammogram/Ultrasound	270	7.8%	8.4%	8.8%
Lumbar Spine MRI for Low Back Pain[1]	-	-	36.6%	37.2%

Thomas H Boyd Memorial Hospital

800 School St — Phone: 217-942-6946
Carrollton, IL 62016 — Fax: 217-942-6091
Type: Critical Access Hospitals — Emergency Services: Yes
Ownership: Voluntary non-profit - Private — Beds: 65

Key Personnel:

Chief of Medical Staff.......... August Adams
Operating Room.............. Judy Brannan
CEO/President.............. Deborah Campbell
Quality Assurance .... Jenny Clough
Cardiac Laboratory............ Terry Grooms
Radiology.................. Cathy Handlin
Emergency Room .... Kris Templin

Measure	Cases	This Hosp.	State Avg.	U.S. Avg.
Blood Clot Prevention and Treatment				
Anticoagulation Overlap Therapy[5]	-	-	91%	93%
ICU Venous Thromboembolism Prophylaxis[5]	-	-	93%	92%
Incidence of Potentially Preventable VTE[5]	-	-	11%	10%
UFH with Dosages/Platelet Monitoring[5]	-	-	94%	97%
Venous Thromboembolism Prophylaxis[5]	-	-	86%	85%
Warfarin Therapy Discharge Instructions[5]	-	-	71%	75%
Chest Pain/Possible Heart Attack Care				
Aspirin Given Within 24 Hours of Arrival	-	-	96%	96%
Fibrinolytic Meds Within 30 Min. of Arrival	-	-	65%	58%
Average Time to ECG (minutes)	-	-	6	7
Average Time to Transfer (minutes)	-	-	63	60
Children's Asthma Care				
Received Home Management Plan of Care	-	-	-	88%
Received Reliever Medication	-	-	-	100%
Received Systemic Corticosteroids	-	-	-	100%
Emergency Department				
Admittance Decision Time (minutes)[5]	-	-	89	98
Head CT Results Within 45 Min. of Arrival	-	-	64%	57%
Patients Who Left ER Before Being Seen	-	-	3%	2%
Time from ER Arrival to Admit. (minutes)[5]	-	-	260	274
Time from ER Arrival to Discharge (minutes)	-	-	138	134
Time in ER Before Being Evaluated (minutes)	-	-	28	26
Time to Pain Meds for Fractures (minutes)	-	-	52	57
Heart Attack Care				
Aspirin Given at Discharge[3,7]	-	-	99%	99%
Fibrinolytic Meds Within 30 Min. of Arrival[3,7]	-	-	33%	54%
PCI Within 90 Minutes of Arrival[3,7]	-	-	97%	96%
Statin Prescribed at Discharge[1,3]	-	-	98%	98%
Heart Failure Care				
ACE Inhibitor or ARB for LVSD[3,7]	-	-	98%	97%
Discharge Instructions Given[1,3]	-	-	96%	94%
Evaluation of LVS Function[1,3]	-	-	99%	99%
Medicare Spending				
Medicare Spending per Patient (ratio)	-	-	1	0.98
Pneumonia Care				
Appropriate Initial Antibiotic Given[3]	11	64%	95%	95%
Blood Culture Timing[3]	12	83%	98%	98%
Pregnancy and Delivery Care				
Newborn Deliveries Scheduled Early[5]	-	-	2%	6%
Preventive Care				
Immunization for Influenza[5]	-	-	92%	90%
Immunization for Pneumonia[5]	-	-	92%	92%
Stroke Care				
Anticoagulation Therapy for Atrial Fibrillation[5]	-	-	94%	95%
Antithrombotic Therapy Timing[5]	-	-	98%	98%
Assessed for Rehabilitation[5]	-	-	97%	97%
Discharged on Antithrombotic Therapy[5]	-	-	99%	99%
Discharged on Statin Medication[5]	-	-	94%	94%
Thrombolytic Therapy Timing[5]	-	-	66%	66%
Venous Thromboembolism Prophylaxis[5]	-	-	94%	94%
Written Stroke Educational Materials Given[5]	-	-	87%	88%
Surgical Care Improvement Project				
Appropriate Beta Blocker Usage[5]	-	-	98%	98%
Appropriate VTP Within 24 Hours[5]	-	-	98%	98%
Controlled Postoperative Blood Glucose[5]	-	-	97%	97%
Perioperative Temperature Management[5]	-	-	100%	100%
Prophylactic Antibiotic Selection[5]	-	-	99%	99%
Prophylactic Antibiotic Selection (Outpatient)	-	-	98%	98%
Prophylactic Antibiotic Stopped[5]	-	-	98%	98%
Prophylactic Antibiotic Timing[5]	-	-	99%	99%
Prophylactic Antibiotic Timing (Outpatient)	-	-	97%	98%
Urinary Catheter Removal[5]	-	-	98%	97%
Survey of Patients' Hospital Experiences				
Area Around Room 'Always' Quiet at Night[5]	-	-	60%	61%
Doctors 'Always' Communicated Well[5]	-	-	81%	82%
Home Recovery Information Given[5]	-	-	86%	85%
Hospital Given 9 or 10 on 10 Point Scale[5]	-	-	70%	71%
Meds 'Always' Explained Before Given[5]	-	-	64%	64%
Nurses 'Always' Communicated Well[5]	-	-	79%	79%
Pain 'Always' Well Controlled[5]	-	-	71%	71%
Room and Bathroom 'Always' Clean[5]	-	-	74%	73%
Timely Help 'Always' Received[5]	-	-	67%	68%
Would Definitely Recommend Hospital[5]	-	-	70%	71%
Use of Medical Imaging				
Cardiac Imaging Stress Test before Surgery	-	-	5.5%	5.3%
Combination Abdominal CT Scan	-	-	10.1%	10.5%
Combination Brain/Sinus CT Scan	-	-	2.6%	2.7%
Combination Chest CT Scan	-	-	2.8%	2.7%
Follow-up Mammogram/Ultrasound	-	-	8.4%	8.8%
Lumbar Spine MRI for Low Back Pain	-	-	36.6%	37.2%

Memorial Hospital

South Adams St, PO Box 160 — Phone: 217-357-3131
Carthage, IL 62321
Type: Critical Access Hospitals — Emergency Services: Yes
Ownership: Voluntary non-profit - Private

Measure	Cases	This Hosp.	State Avg.	U.S. Avg.
Blood Clot Prevention and Treatment				
Anticoagulation Overlap Therapy[5]	-	-	91%	93%
ICU Venous Thromboembolism Prophylaxis[5]	-	-	93%	92%
Incidence of Potentially Preventable VTE[5]	-	-	11%	10%
UFH with Dosages/Platelet Monitoring[5]	-	-	94%	97%
Venous Thromboembolism Prophylaxis[5]	-	-	86%	85%
Warfarin Therapy Discharge Instructions[5]	-	-	71%	75%
Chest Pain/Possible Heart Attack Care				
Aspirin Given Within 24 Hours of Arrival[5]	-	-	96%	96%
Fibrinolytic Meds Within 30 Min. of Arrival[5]	-	-	65%	58%
Average Time to ECG (minutes)[5]	-	-	6	7
Average Time to Transfer (minutes)[5]	-	-	63	60
Children's Asthma Care				
Received Home Management Plan of Care	-	-	-	88%
Received Reliever Medication	-	-	-	100%
Received Systemic Corticosteroids	-	-	-	100%
Emergency Department				
Admittance Decision Time (minutes)[5]	-	-	89	98
Head CT Results Within 45 Min. of Arrival[5]	-	-	64%	57%
Patients Who Left ER Before Being Seen[5]	-	-	3%	2%
Time from ER Arrival to Admit. (minutes)[5]	-	-	260	274
Time from ER Arrival to Discharge (minutes)[5]	-	-	138	134
Time in ER Before Being Evaluated (minutes)[5]	-	-	28	26
Time to Pain Meds for Fractures (minutes)[5]	-	-	52	57
Heart Attack Care				
Aspirin Given at Discharge[5]	-	-	99%	99%
Fibrinolytic Meds Within 30 Min. of Arrival[5]	-	-	33%	54%
PCI Within 90 Minutes of Arrival[5]	-	-	97%	96%
Statin Prescribed at Discharge[5]	-	-	98%	98%
Heart Failure Care				
ACE Inhibitor or ARB for LVSD[7]	-	-	98%	97%
Discharge Instructions Given[1]	-	-	96%	94%
Evaluation of LVS Function[1]	-	-	99%	99%
Medicare Spending				
Medicare Spending per Patient (ratio)	-	-	1	0.98
Pneumonia Care				
Appropriate Initial Antibiotic Given[7]	-	-	95%	95%
Blood Culture Timing[7]	-	-	98%	98%
Pregnancy and Delivery Care				
Newborn Deliveries Scheduled Early[5]	-	-	2%	6%
Preventive Care				
Immunization for Influenza[5]	-	-	92%	90%
Immunization for Pneumonia[5]	-	-	92%	92%
Stroke Care				
Anticoagulation Therapy for Atrial Fibrillation[5]	-	-	94%	95%
Antithrombotic Therapy Timing[5]	-	-	98%	98%
Assessed for Rehabilitation[5]	-	-	97%	97%
Discharged on Antithrombotic Therapy[5]	-	-	99%	99%
Discharged on Statin Medication[5]	-	-	94%	94%
Thrombolytic Therapy Timing[5]	-	-	66%	66%
Venous Thromboembolism Prophylaxis[5]	-	-	94%	94%
Written Stroke Educational Materials Given[5]	-	-	87%	88%
Surgical Care Improvement Project				
Appropriate Beta Blocker Usage[1]	-	-	98%	98%
Appropriate VTP Within 24 Hours	21	100%	98%	98%
Controlled Postoperative Blood Glucose[7]	-	-	97%	97%
Perioperative Temperature Management	24	46%	100%	100%
Prophylactic Antibiotic Selection	24	96%	99%	99%
Prophylactic Antibiotic Selection (Outpatient)[5]	-	-	98%	98%
Prophylactic Antibiotic Stopped	23	100%	98%	98%
Prophylactic Antibiotic Timing	24	92%	99%	99%
Prophylactic Antibiotic Timing (Outpatient)[5]	-	-	97%	98%
Urinary Catheter Removal[1]	-	-	98%	97%
Survey of Patients' Hospital Experiences				
Area Around Room 'Always' Quiet at Night[5]	-	-	60%	61%
Doctors 'Always' Communicated Well[5]	-	-	81%	82%
Home Recovery Information Given[5]	-	-	86%	85%
Hospital Given 9 or 10 on 10 Point Scale[5]	-	-	70%	71%
Meds 'Always' Explained Before Given[5]	-	-	64%	64%
Nurses 'Always' Communicated Well[5]	-	-	79%	79%
Pain 'Always' Well Controlled[5]	-	-	71%	71%
Room and Bathroom 'Always' Clean[5]	-	-	74%	73%
Timely Help 'Always' Received[5]	-	-	67%	68%

NOTE: Hospital profiles are in alphabetical order by state, then city, then hospital within the city; Rankings exclude hospitals with less than 25 cases except for patient surveys which excludes hospitals with less than 100 cases; (a) 100-299 cases; (1) The number of cases/patients is too few to report; (2) Data submitted were based on a sample of cases/patients; (3) Results are based on a shorter time period than required; (4) Data suppressed by CMS for one or more quarters; (5) Results are not available for this reporting period; (6) Fewer than 100 patients completed the HCAHPS survey; (7) No cases met the criteria for this measure; (8) The lower limit of the confidence interval cannot be calculated if the number of observed infections equals zero; (9) No data are available from the state/territory for this reporting period; (10) The scores shown reflect fewer than 50 completed surveys; (11) There were discrepancies in the data collection process; (12) This measure does not apply to this hospital for this reporting period; (13) Results cannot be calculated for this reporting period; (14) The results for this state are combined with nearby states to protect confidentiality; Please refer to the User's Guide for a full explanation of data.

Would Definitely Recommend Hospital[5]	-	-	70%	71%
Use of Medical Imaging				
Cardiac Imaging Stress Test before Surgery[5]	-	-	5.5%	5.3%
Combination Abdominal CT Scan[5]	-	-	10.1%	10.5%
Combination Brain/Sinus CT Scan[5]	-	-	2.6%	2.7%
Combination Chest CT Scan[5]	-	-	2.8%	2.7%
Follow-up Mammogram/Ultrasound[5]	-	-	8.4%	8.8%
Lumbar Spine MRI for Low Back Pain[5]	-	-	36.6%	37.2%

Saint Marys Hospital

400 North Pleasant Avenue
Centralia, IL 62801
Phone: 618-436-6519
Fax: 618-436-8046
URL: www.stmarys-goodsamaritan.com
Type: Acute Care Hospitals
Emergency Services: Yes
Ownership: Voluntary non-profit - Church
Beds: 276

Key Personnel:
Pediatric Ambulatory Care . . . . . . Nazir Ahmad, MD
Pediatric In-Patient Care . . . . Nazir Ahmad, MD
Operating Room. . . . . James Jeffers, RN
Chief of Medical Staff . . . . Tom Martin, MD
Radiology. . . . . Richard Rudman, MD
CEO/President. . . . . James W Sanger
Cardiac Laboratory. . . . . Trecy Siscus
Quality Assurance . . . . Mary Lynn Szperra

Measure	Cases	This Hosp.	State Avg.	U.S. Avg.
Blood Clot Prevention and Treatment				
Anticoagulation Overlap Therapy[2]	30	97%	91%	93%
ICU Venous Thromboembolism Prophylaxis[2]	75	95%	93%	92%
Incidence of Potentially Preventable VTE[1,2]	-	-	11%	10%
UFH with Dosages/Platelet Monitoring[2]	18	100%	94%	97%
Venous Thromboembolism Prophylaxis[2]	388	88%	86%	85%
Warfarin Therapy Discharge Instructions[2]	25	84%	71%	75%
Chest Pain/Possible Heart Attack Care				
Aspirin Given Within 24 Hours of Arrival	61	97%	96%	96%
Fibrinolytic Meds Within 30 Min. of Arrival[7]	-	-	65%	58%
Average Time to ECG (minutes)	62	6	6	7
Average Time to Transfer (minutes)[1]	-	-	63	60
Children's Asthma Care				
Received Home Management Plan of Care	-	-	-	88%
Received Reliever Medication	-	-	-	100%
Received Systemic Corticosteroids	-	-	-	100%
Emergency Department				
Admittance Decision Time (minutes)[2]	632	75	89	98
Head CT Results Within 45 Min. of Arrival[1]	-	-	64%	57%
Patients Who Left ER Before Being Seen	24,005	0%	3%	2%
Time from ER Arrival to Admit. (minutes)[2]	650	260	260	274
Time from ER Arrival to Discharge (minutes)	356	139	138	134
Time in ER Before Being Evaluated (minutes)	399	36	28	26
Time to Pain Meds for Fractures (minutes)	85	51	52	57
Heart Attack Care				
Aspirin Given at Discharge	33	100%	99%	99%
Fibrinolytic Meds Within 30 Min. of Arrival[7]	-	-	33%	54%
PCI Within 90 Minutes of Arrival[7]	-	-	97%	96%
Statin Prescribed at Discharge	29	93%	98%	98%
Heart Failure Care				
ACE Inhibitor or ARB for LVSD	29	100%	98%	97%
Discharge Instructions Given	110	100%	96%	94%
Evaluation of LVS Function	156	100%	99%	99%
Medicare Spending				
Medicare Spending per Patient (ratio)	-	0.96	1	0.98
Pneumonia Care				
Appropriate Initial Antibiotic Given	77	96%	95%	95%
Blood Culture Timing	149	99%	98%	98%
Pregnancy and Delivery Care				
Newborn Deliveries Scheduled Early	33	0%	2%	6%
Preventive Care				
Immunization for Influenza[2]	541	98%	92%	90%
Immunization for Pneumonia[2]	696	99%	92%	92%
Stroke Care				
Anticoagulation Therapy for Atrial Fibrillation[1]	-	-	94%	95%
Antithrombotic Therapy Timing	41	95%	98%	98%
Assessed for Rehabilitation	39	97%	97%	97%
Discharged on Antithrombotic Therapy	38	97%	99%	99%
Discharged on Statin Medication	30	97%	94%	94%
Thrombolytic Therapy Timing[1]	-	-	66%	66%
Venous Thromboembolism Prophylaxis	41	90%	94%	94%
Written Stroke Educational Materials Given	23	96%	87%	88%
Surgical Care Improvement Project				
Appropriate Beta Blocker Usage	42	98%	98%	98%
Appropriate VTP Within 24 Hours	122	100%	98%	98%
Controlled Postoperative Blood Glucose[7]	-	-	97%	97%
Perioperative Temperature Management	138	99%	100%	100%
Prophylactic Antibiotic Selection	86	99%	99%	99%
Prophylactic Antibiotic Selection (Outpatient)	46	100%	98%	98%
Prophylactic Antibiotic Stopped	80	98%	98%	98%
Prophylactic Antibiotic Timing	86	99%	99%	99%
Prophylactic Antibiotic Timing (Outpatient)	45	98%	97%	98%
Urinary Catheter Removal	87	99%	98%	97%
Survey of Patients' Hospital Experiences				
Area Around Room 'Always' Quiet at Night	300+	67%	60%	61%
Doctors 'Always' Communicated Well	300+	88%	81%	82%
Home Recovery Information Given	300+	90%	86%	85%
Hospital Given 9 or 10 on 10 Point Scale	300+	79%	70%	71%
Meds 'Always' Explained Before Given	300+	73%	64%	64%
Nurses 'Always' Communicated Well	300+	87%	79%	79%
Pain 'Always' Well Controlled	300+	74%	71%	71%
Room and Bathroom 'Always' Clean	300+	91%	74%	73%
Timely Help 'Always' Received	300+	82%	67%	68%
Would Definitely Recommend Hospital	300+	77%	70%	71%
Use of Medical Imaging				
Cardiac Imaging Stress Test before Surgery	195	12.3%	5.5%	5.3%
Combination Abdominal CT Scan	689	23.2%	10.1%	10.5%
Combination Brain/Sinus CT Scan[1]	-	-	2.6%	2.7%
Combination Chest CT Scan	414	0.2%	2.8%	2.7%
Follow-up Mammogram/Ultrasound	1,076	9.1%	8.4%	8.8%
Lumbar Spine MRI for Low Back Pain	58	31.0%	36.6%	37.2%

Touchette Regional Hospital

5900 Bond Avenue
Centreville, IL 62207
Phone: 618-332-3060
Fax: 618-332-5256
URL: www.touchette.org
Type: Acute Care Hospitals
Emergency Services: Yes
Ownership: Voluntary non-profit - Private
Beds: 114

Key Personnel:
Anesthesiology. . . . . Brad Bernstein
Operating Room. . . . . Patricia Clark
Emergency Room . . . . Louis Gary
Infection Control. . . . . Pat Giacin
Quality Assurance . . . . Rich Hampson
Radiology. . . . . David Hunter
CEO/President. . . . . Robert Klutts
Chief of Medical Staff. . . . . Jose Ramon

Measure	Cases	This Hosp.	State Avg.	U.S. Avg.
Blood Clot Prevention and Treatment				
Anticoagulation Overlap Therapy[1,2]	-	-	91%	93%
ICU Venous Thromboembolism Prophylaxis[2]	25	100%	93%	92%
Incidence of Potentially Preventable VTE[2,7]	-	-	11%	10%
UFH with Dosages/Platelet Monitoring[1,2]	-	-	94%	97%
Venous Thromboembolism Prophylaxis[2]	103	83%	86%	85%
Warfarin Therapy Discharge Instructions[1,2]	-	-	71%	75%
Chest Pain/Possible Heart Attack Care				
Aspirin Given Within 24 Hours of Arrival[1,3]	-	-	96%	96%
Fibrinolytic Meds Within 30 Min. of Arrival[5]	-	-	65%	58%
Average Time to ECG (minutes)[1,3]	-	-	6	7
Average Time to Transfer (minutes)[5]	-	-	63	60
Children's Asthma Care				
Received Home Management Plan of Care	-	-	-	88%
Received Reliever Medication	-	-	-	100%
Received Systemic Corticosteroids	-	-	-	100%
Emergency Department				
Admittance Decision Time (minutes)[2]	197	98	89	98
Head CT Results Within 45 Min. of Arrival[1]	-	-	64%	57%
Patients Who Left ER Before Being Seen	18,798	4%	3%	2%
Time from ER Arrival to Admit. (minutes)[2]	197	292	260	274
Time from ER Arrival to Discharge (minutes)	401	116	138	134
Time in ER Before Being Evaluated (minutes)	449	53	28	26
Time to Pain Meds for Fractures (minutes)	28	68	52	57
Heart Attack Care				
Aspirin Given at Discharge[1]	-	-	99%	99%
Fibrinolytic Meds Within 30 Min. of Arrival[7]	-	-	33%	54%
PCI Within 90 Minutes of Arrival[7]	-	-	97%	96%
Statin Prescribed at Discharge[1]	-	-	98%	98%
Heart Failure Care				
ACE Inhibitor or ARB for LVSD	35	94%	98%	97%
Discharge Instructions Given	102	93%	96%	94%
Evaluation of LVS Function	107	97%	99%	99%
Medicare Spending				
Medicare Spending per Patient (ratio)	-	0.90	1	0.98
Pneumonia Care				
Appropriate Initial Antibiotic Given	57	91%	95%	95%
Blood Culture Timing	91	89%	98%	98%
Pregnancy and Delivery Care				
Newborn Deliveries Scheduled Early[2]	22	5%	2%	6%
Preventive Care				
Immunization for Influenza[2]	258	80%	92%	90%
Immunization for Pneumonia[2]	189	87%	92%	92%
Stroke Care				
Anticoagulation Therapy for Atrial Fibrillation[3,7]	-	-	94%	95%
Antithrombotic Therapy Timing[1,3]	-	-	98%	98%
Assessed for Rehabilitation[1,3]	-	-	97%	97%
Discharged on Antithrombotic Therapy[1,3]	-	-	99%	99%
Discharged on Statin Medication[1,3]	-	-	94%	94%
Thrombolytic Therapy Timing[3,7]	-	-	66%	66%
Venous Thromboembolism Prophylaxis[1,3]	-	-	94%	94%
Written Stroke Educational Materials Given[1,3]	-	-	87%	88%
Surgical Care Improvement Project				
Appropriate Beta Blocker Usage[1]	-	-	98%	98%
Appropriate VTP Within 24 Hours	41	95%	98%	98%
Controlled Postoperative Blood Glucose[7]	-	-	97%	97%
Perioperative Temperature Management	41	100%	100%	100%
Prophylactic Antibiotic Selection	35	94%	99%	99%
Prophylactic Antibiotic Selection (Outpatient)	33	97%	98%	98%
Prophylactic Antibiotic Stopped	33	94%	98%	98%
Prophylactic Antibiotic Timing	35	89%	99%	99%
Prophylactic Antibiotic Timing (Outpatient)[1]	-	-	97%	98%
Urinary Catheter Removal	15	87%	98%	97%
Survey of Patients' Hospital Experiences				
Area Around Room 'Always' Quiet at Night	(a)	73%	60%	61%
Doctors 'Always' Communicated Well	(a)	83%	81%	82%
Home Recovery Information Given	(a)	81%	86%	85%
Hospital Given 9 or 10 on 10 Point Scale	(a)	63%	70%	71%
Meds 'Always' Explained Before Given	(a)	63%	64%	64%
Nurses 'Always' Communicated Well	(a)	78%	79%	79%
Pain 'Always' Well Controlled	(a)	74%	71%	71%
Room and Bathroom 'Always' Clean	(a)	71%	74%	73%
Timely Help 'Always' Received	(a)	63%	67%	68%
Would Definitely Recommend Hospital	(a)	59%	70%	71%
Use of Medical Imaging				
Cardiac Imaging Stress Test before Surgery[1]	-	-	5.5%	5.3%
Combination Abdominal CT Scan	92	16.3%	10.1%	10.5%
Combination Brain/Sinus CT Scan	169	5.3%	2.6%	2.7%
Combination Chest CT Scan	70	4.3%	2.8%	2.7%
Follow-up Mammogram/Ultrasound	267	12.4%	8.4%	8.8%
Lumbar Spine MRI for Low Back Pain[1]	-	-	36.6%	37.2%

Memorial Hospital

1900 State Street
Chester, IL 62233
Phone: 618-826-4581
Fax: 618-826-4813
URL: www.mhchester.com
Type: Critical Access Hospitals
Emergency Services: Yes
Ownership: Govt - Hospital Dist/Auth
Beds: 25

Key Personnel:
CEO . . . . Brett Bollmann
Radiology. . . . . Joseph Dugan
Infection Control. . . . . Machelle Kureker
Chief of Medical Staff . . . . Allen Liefer, MD
Operating Room. . . . . Patricia Nanney, RN
Emergency Room . . . . Mary Rosendohl, RN
Intensive Care Unit. . . . . Karen Wolf

Measure	Cases	This Hosp.	State Avg.	U.S. Avg.
Blood Clot Prevention and Treatment				
Anticoagulation Overlap Therapy[5]	-	-	91%	93%

NOTE: Hospital profiles are in alphabetical order by state, then city, then hospital within the city; Rankings exclude hospitals with less than 25 cases except for patient surveys which excludes hospitals with less than 100 cases; (a) 100-299 cases; (1) The number of cases/patients is too few to report; (2) Data submitted were based on a sample of cases/patients; (3) Results are based on a shorter time period than required; (4) Data suppressed by CMS for one or more quarters; (5) Results are not available for this reporting period; (6) Fewer than 100 patients completed the HCAHPS survey; (7) No cases met the criteria for this measure; (8) The lower limit of the confidence interval cannot be calculated if the number of observed infections equals zero; (9) No data are available from the state/territory for this reporting period; (10) The scores shown reflect fewer than 50 completed surveys; (11) There were discrepancies in the data collection process; (12) This measure does not apply to this hospital for this reporting period; (13) Results cannot be calculated for this reporting period; (14) The results for this state are combined with nearby states to protect confidentiality; Please refer to the User's Guide for a full explanation of data.

Measure	Cases	This Hosp.	State Avg.	U.S. Avg.
ICU Venous Thromboembolism Prophylaxis[5]	-	-	93%	92%
Incidence of Potentially Preventable VTE[5]	-	-	11%	10%
UFH with Dosages/Platelet Monitoring[5]	-	-	94%	97%
Venous Thromboembolism Prophylaxis[5]	-	-	86%	85%
Warfarin Therapy Discharge Instructions[5]	-	-	71%	75%
Chest Pain/Possible Heart Attack Care				
Aspirin Given Within 24 Hours of Arrival	39	100%	96%	96%
Fibrinolytic Meds Within 30 Min. of Arrival[7]	-	-	65%	58%
Average Time to ECG (minutes)	39	4	6	7
Average Time to Transfer (minutes)[1]	-	-	63	60
Children's Asthma Care				
Received Home Management Plan of Care	-	-	-	88%
Received Reliever Medication	-	-	-	100%
Received Systemic Corticosteroids	-	-	-	100%
Emergency Department				
Admittance Decision Time (minutes)[5]	-	-	89	98
Head CT Results Within 45 Min. of Arrival[5]	-	-	64%	57%
Patients Who Left ER Before Being Seen	6,046	0%	3%	2%
Time from ER Arrival to Admit. (minutes)[5]	-	-	260	274
Time from ER Arrival to Discharge (minutes)[5]	-	-	138	134
Time in ER Before Being Evaluated (minutes)[5]	-	-	28	26
Time to Pain Meds for Fractures (minutes)[5]	-	-	52	57
Heart Attack Care				
Aspirin Given at Discharge[1,3]	-	-	99%	99%
Fibrinolytic Meds Within 30 Min. of Arrival[3,7]	-	-	33%	54%
PCI Within 90 Minutes of Arrival[3,7]	-	-	97%	96%
Statin Prescribed at Discharge[3,7]	-	-	98%	98%
Heart Failure Care				
ACE Inhibitor or ARB for LVSD[1]	-	-	98%	97%
Discharge Instructions Given	21	86%	96%	94%
Evaluation of LVS Function	23	100%	99%	99%
Medicare Spending				
Medicare Spending per Patient (ratio)	-	-	1	0.98
Pneumonia Care				
Appropriate Initial Antibiotic Given	22	100%	95%	95%
Blood Culture Timing	39	100%	98%	98%
Pregnancy and Delivery Care				
Newborn Deliveries Scheduled Early[5]	-	-	2%	6%
Preventive Care				
Immunization for Influenza[2]	214	96%	92%	90%
Immunization for Pneumonia[2]	336	97%	92%	92%
Stroke Care				
Anticoagulation Therapy for Atrial Fibrillation[5]	-	-	94%	95%
Antithrombotic Therapy Timing[5]	-	-	98%	98%
Assessed for Rehabilitation[5]	-	-	97%	97%
Discharged on Antithrombotic Therapy[5]	-	-	99%	99%
Discharged on Statin Medication[5]	-	-	94%	94%
Thrombolytic Therapy Timing[5]	-	-	66%	66%
Venous Thromboembolism Prophylaxis[5]	-	-	94%	94%
Written Stroke Educational Materials Given[5]	-	-	87%	88%
Surgical Care Improvement Project				
Appropriate Beta Blocker Usage	12	92%	98%	98%
Appropriate VTP Within 24 Hours	33	97%	98%	98%
Controlled Postoperative Blood Glucose[3,7]	-	-	97%	97%
Perioperative Temperature Management	37	100%	100%	100%
Prophylactic Antibiotic Selection	30	97%	99%	99%
Prophylactic Antibiotic Selection (Outpatient)	14	93%	98%	98%
Prophylactic Antibiotic Stopped	29	100%	98%	98%
Prophylactic Antibiotic Timing	30	93%	99%	99%
Prophylactic Antibiotic Timing (Outpatient)	16	81%	97%	98%
Urinary Catheter Removal	27	96%	98%	97%
Survey of Patients' Hospital Experiences				
Area Around Room 'Always' Quiet at Night[5]	-	-	60%	61%
Doctors 'Always' Communicated Well[5]	-	-	81%	82%
Home Recovery Information Given[5]	-	-	86%	85%
Hospital Given 9 or 10 on 10 Point Scale[5]	-	-	70%	71%
Meds 'Always' Explained Before Given[5]	-	-	64%	64%
Nurses 'Always' Communicated Well[5]	-	-	79%	79%
Pain 'Always' Well Controlled[5]	-	-	71%	71%
Room and Bathroom 'Always' Clean[5]	-	-	74%	73%
Timely Help 'Always' Received[5]	-	-	67%	68%
Would Definitely Recommend Hospital[5]	-	-	70%	71%
Use of Medical Imaging				
Cardiac Imaging Stress Test before Surgery	131	0.0%	5.5%	5.3%
Combination Abdominal CT Scan	177	2.3%	10.1%	10.5%
Combination Brain/Sinus CT Scan	207	7.7%	2.6%	2.7%
Combination Chest CT Scan	79	0.0%	2.8%	2.7%
Follow-up Mammogram/Ultrasound	240	17.1%	8.4%	8.8%
Lumbar Spine MRI for Low Back Pain	38	52.6%	36.6%	37.2%

Advocate Illinois Masonic Medical Center

836 West Wellington Avenue
Chicago, IL 60657
Phone: 773-975-1600
Fax: 773-296-8119
URL: www.advocatehealth.com/immc
Type: Acute Care Hospitals
Emergency Services: Yes
Ownership: Voluntary non-profit - Church
Beds: 370
Key Personnel:
Patient Relations . . . . Ellen Donovan
CEO/President . . . . Susan Nordstrom Lopez

Measure	Cases	This Hosp.	State Avg.	U.S. Avg.
Blood Clot Prevention and Treatment				
Anticoagulation Overlap Therapy[2]	94	97%	91%	93%
ICU Venous Thromboembolism Prophylaxis[2]	50	98%	93%	92%
Incidence of Potentially Preventable VTE[2]	25	0%	11%	10%
UFH with Dosages/Platelet Monitoring[2]	61	97%	94%	97%
Venous Thromboembolism Prophylaxis[2]	314	93%	86%	85%
Warfarin Therapy Discharge Instructions[2]	60	70%	71%	75%
Chest Pain/Possible Heart Attack Care				
Aspirin Given Within 24 Hours of Arrival[3,7]	-	-	96%	96%
Fibrinolytic Meds Within 30 Min. of Arrival[5]	-	-	65%	58%
Average Time to ECG (minutes)[3,7]	-	-	6	7
Average Time to Transfer (minutes)[5]	-	-	63	60
Children's Asthma Care				
Received Home Management Plan of Care	-	-	-	88%
Received Reliever Medication	-	-	-	100%
Received Systemic Corticosteroids	-	-	-	100%
Emergency Department				
Admittance Decision Time (minutes)[2]	460	94	89	98
Head CT Results Within 45 Min. of Arrival[1,3]	-	-	64%	57%
Patients Who Left ER Before Being Seen	44,204	2%	3%	2%
Time from ER Arrival to Admit. (minutes)[2]	522	295	260	274
Time from ER Arrival to Discharge (minutes)	346	200	138	134
Time in ER Before Being Evaluated (minutes)	387	49	28	26
Time to Pain Meds for Fractures (minutes)	118	54	52	57
Heart Attack Care				
Aspirin Given at Discharge	156	100%	99%	99%
Fibrinolytic Meds Within 30 Min. of Arrival[7]	-	-	33%	54%
PCI Within 90 Minutes of Arrival	13	100%	97%	96%
Statin Prescribed at Discharge	155	100%	98%	98%
Heart Failure Care				
ACE Inhibitor or ARB for LVSD[2]	95	100%	98%	97%
Discharge Instructions Given[2]	193	100%	96%	94%
Evaluation of LVS Function[2]	244	100%	99%	99%
Medicare Spending				
Medicare Spending per Patient (ratio)	-	1.03	1	0.98
Pneumonia Care				
Appropriate Initial Antibiotic Given[2]	56	100%	95%	95%
Blood Culture Timing[2]	148	100%	98%	98%
Pregnancy and Delivery Care				
Newborn Deliveries Scheduled Early	162	1%	2%	6%
Preventive Care				
Immunization for Influenza[2]	540	96%	92%	90%
Immunization for Pneumonia[2]	556	92%	92%	92%
Stroke Care				
Anticoagulation Therapy for Atrial Fibrillation[1]	-	-	94%	95%
Antithrombotic Therapy Timing	64	100%	98%	98%
Assessed for Rehabilitation	86	97%	97%	97%
Discharged on Antithrombotic Therapy	69	94%	99%	99%
Discharged on Statin Medication	62	92%	94%	94%
Thrombolytic Therapy Timing[1]	-	-	66%	66%
Venous Thromboembolism Prophylaxis	85	95%	94%	94%
Written Stroke Educational Materials Given	36	89%	87%	88%
Surgical Care Improvement Project				
Appropriate Beta Blocker Usage[2]	194	98%	98%	98%
Appropriate VTP Within 24 Hours[2]	441	98%	98%	98%
Controlled Postoperative Blood Glucose[2]	89	98%	97%	97%
Perioperative Temperature Management[2]	530	100%	100%	100%
Prophylactic Antibiotic Selection[2]	439	100%	99%	99%
Prophylactic Antibiotic Selection (Outpatient)	470	99%	98%	98%
Prophylactic Antibiotic Stopped[2]	418	100%	98%	98%
Prophylactic Antibiotic Timing[2]	439	100%	99%	99%
Prophylactic Antibiotic Timing (Outpatient)	428	99%	97%	98%
Urinary Catheter Removal[2]	223	100%	98%	97%
Survey of Patients' Hospital Experiences				
Area Around Room 'Always' Quiet at Night	300+	57%	60%	61%
Doctors 'Always' Communicated Well	300+	79%	81%	82%
Home Recovery Information Given	300+	86%	86%	85%
Hospital Given 9 or 10 on 10 Point Scale	300+	71%	70%	71%
Meds 'Always' Explained Before Given	300+	65%	64%	64%
Nurses 'Always' Communicated Well	300+	80%	79%	79%
Pain 'Always' Well Controlled	300+	71%	71%	71%
Room and Bathroom 'Always' Clean	300+	77%	74%	73%
Timely Help 'Always' Received	300+	69%	67%	68%
Would Definitely Recommend Hospital	300+	73%	70%	71%
Use of Medical Imaging				
Cardiac Imaging Stress Test before Surgery	342	6.7%	5.5%	5.3%
Combination Abdominal CT Scan	729	2.7%	10.1%	10.5%
Combination Brain/Sinus CT Scan	576	1.7%	2.6%	2.7%
Combination Chest CT Scan	493	0.2%	2.8%	2.7%
Follow-up Mammogram/Ultrasound	1,173	9.5%	8.4%	8.8%
Lumbar Spine MRI for Low Back Pain	116	45.7%	36.6%	37.2%

Advocate Trinity Hospital

2320 E 93rd St
Chicago, IL 60617
Phone: 773-967-2000
Fax: 773-967-4209
URL: www.advocatehealth.com/trin
Type: Acute Care Hospitals
Emergency Services: Yes
Ownership: Voluntary non-profit - Other
Key Personnel:
Radiology . . . . Ari Mintz
CEO/President . . . . Anthony Munroe

Measure	Cases	This Hosp.	State Avg.	U.S. Avg.
Blood Clot Prevention and Treatment				
Anticoagulation Overlap Therapy[2]	136	92%	91%	93%
ICU Venous Thromboembolism Prophylaxis[2]	33	94%	93%	92%
Incidence of Potentially Preventable VTE[2]	28	11%	11%	10%
UFH with Dosages/Platelet Monitoring[2]	95	100%	94%	97%
Venous Thromboembolism Prophylaxis[2]	395	93%	86%	85%
Warfarin Therapy Discharge Instructions[2]	89	71%	71%	75%
Chest Pain/Possible Heart Attack Care				
Aspirin Given Within 24 Hours of Arrival[1,3]	-	-	96%	96%
Fibrinolytic Meds Within 30 Min. of Arrival[5]	-	-	65%	58%
Average Time to ECG (minutes)[1,3]	-	-	6	7
Average Time to Transfer (minutes)[5]	-	-	63	60
Children's Asthma Care				
Received Home Management Plan of Care	-	-	-	88%
Received Reliever Medication	-	-	-	100%
Received Systemic Corticosteroids	-	-	-	100%
Emergency Department				
Admittance Decision Time (minutes)[2]	664	122	89	98
Head CT Results Within 45 Min. of Arrival	27	59%	64%	57%
Patients Who Left ER Before Being Seen	44,936	5%	3%	2%
Time from ER Arrival to Admit. (minutes)[2]	664	374	260	274
Time from ER Arrival to Discharge (minutes)	382	186	138	134
Time in ER Before Being Evaluated (minutes)	409	66	28	26
Time to Pain Meds for Fractures (minutes)	108	114	52	57
Heart Attack Care				
Aspirin Given at Discharge	119	100%	99%	99%
Fibrinolytic Meds Within 30 Min. of Arrival[7]	-	-	33%	54%
PCI Within 90 Minutes of Arrival	17	88%	97%	96%
Statin Prescribed at Discharge	123	99%	98%	98%
Heart Failure Care				
ACE Inhibitor or ARB for LVSD[2]	146	97%	98%	97%
Discharge Instructions Given[2]	318	98%	96%	94%
Evaluation of LVS Function[2]	364	99%	99%	99%
Medicare Spending				
Medicare Spending per Patient (ratio)	-	1.01	1	0.98
Pneumonia Care				

NOTE: Hospital profiles are in alphabetical order by state, then city, then hospital within the city; Rankings exclude hospitals with less than 25 cases except for patient surveys which excludes hospitals with less than 100 cases; (a) 100-299 cases; (1) The number of cases/patients is too few to report; (2) Data submitted were based on a sample of cases/patients; (3) Results are based on a shorter time period than required; (4) Data suppressed by CMS for one or more quarters; (5) Results are not available for this reporting period; (6) Fewer than 100 patients completed the HCAHPS survey; (7) No cases met the criteria for this measure; (8) The lower limit of the confidence interval cannot be calculated if the number of observed infections equals zero; (9) No data are available from the state/territory for this reporting period; (10) The scores shown reflect fewer than 50 completed surveys; (11) There were discrepancies in the data collection process; (12) This measure does not apply to this hospital for this reporting period; (13) Results cannot be calculated for this reporting period; (14) The results for this state are combined with nearby states to protect confidentiality; Please refer to the User's Guide for a full explanation of data.

Measure	Cases	This Hosp.	State Avg.	U.S. Avg.
Appropriate Initial Antibiotic Given[2]	99	98%	95%	95%
Blood Culture Timing[2]	154	98%	98%	98%
Pregnancy and Delivery Care				
Newborn Deliveries Scheduled Early	95	1%	2%	6%
Preventive Care				
Immunization for Influenza[2]	581	85%	92%	90%
Immunization for Pneumonia[2]	825	83%	92%	92%
Stroke Care				
Anticoagulation Therapy for Atrial Fibrillation	19	84%	94%	95%
Antithrombotic Therapy Timing	172	99%	98%	98%
Assessed for Rehabilitation	175	97%	97%	97%
Discharged on Antithrombotic Therapy	169	99%	99%	99%
Discharged on Statin Medication	143	88%	94%	94%
Thrombolytic Therapy Timing	24	42%	66%	66%
Venous Thromboembolism Prophylaxis	183	89%	94%	94%
Written Stroke Educational Materials Given	80	85%	87%	88%
Surgical Care Improvement Project				
Appropriate Beta Blocker Usage[2]	120	92%	98%	98%
Appropriate VTP Within 24 Hours[2]	307	100%	98%	98%
Controlled Postoperative Blood Glucose[2,7]	-	-	97%	97%
Perioperative Temperature Management[2]	419	100%	100%	100%
Prophylactic Antibiotic Selection[2]	217	99%	99%	99%
Prophylactic Antibiotic Selection (Outpatient)	80	99%	98%	98%
Prophylactic Antibiotic Stopped[2]	207	96%	98%	98%
Prophylactic Antibiotic Timing[2]	218	100%	99%	99%
Prophylactic Antibiotic Timing (Outpatient)	82	95%	97%	98%
Urinary Catheter Removal[2]	79	85%	98%	97%
Survey of Patients' Hospital Experiences				
Area Around Room 'Always' Quiet at Night	300+	64%	60%	61%
Doctors 'Always' Communicated Well	300+	80%	81%	82%
Home Recovery Information Given	300+	81%	86%	85%
Hospital Given 9 or 10 on 10 Point Scale	300+	66%	70%	71%
Meds 'Always' Explained Before Given	300+	66%	64%	64%
Nurses 'Always' Communicated Well	300+	82%	79%	79%
Pain 'Always' Well Controlled	300+	72%	71%	71%
Room and Bathroom 'Always' Clean	300+	76%	74%	73%
Timely Help 'Always' Received	300+	65%	67%	68%
Would Definitely Recommend Hospital	300+	63%	70%	71%
Use of Medical Imaging				
Cardiac Imaging Stress Test before Surgery	254	1.6%	5.5%	5.3%
Combination Abdominal CT Scan	522	2.3%	10.1%	10.5%
Combination Brain/Sinus CT Scan	579	0.5%	2.6%	2.7%
Combination Chest CT Scan	226	2.7%	2.8%	2.7%
Follow-up Mammogram/Ultrasound	974	10.7%	8.4%	8.8%
Lumbar Spine MRI for Low Back Pain	70	28.6%	36.6%	37.2%

Holy Cross Hospital

2701 W 68th Street
Chicago, IL 60629
Phone: 773-471-8000
Fax: 773-884-8013
URL: www.holycrosshospital.org
Type: Acute Care Hospitals
Emergency Services: Yes
Ownership: Voluntary non-profit - Private
Beds: 244

Key Personnel:

Quality Assurance .... Michael Jucius
CEO/President................ Brian Lemon
Emergency Room .... Ann Reninger, RN
Operating Room.............. Suzanne Rich
Chief of Medical Staff .... Chin Waung

Measure	Cases	This Hosp.	State Avg.	U.S. Avg.
Blood Clot Prevention and Treatment				
Anticoagulation Overlap Therapy[2]	86	66%	91%	93%
ICU Venous Thromboembolism Prophylaxis[2]	113	92%	93%	92%
Incidence of Potentially Preventable VTE[2]	31	35%	11%	10%
UFH with Dosages/Platelet Monitoring[2]	44	34%	94%	97%
Venous Thromboembolism Prophylaxis[2]	337	89%	86%	85%
Warfarin Therapy Discharge Instructions[2]	44	16%	71%	75%
Chest Pain/Possible Heart Attack Care				
Aspirin Given Within 24 Hours of Arrival	35	86%	96%	96%
Fibrinolytic Meds Within 30 Min. of Arrival[7]	-	-	65%	58%
Average Time to ECG (minutes)	35	14	6	7
Average Time to Transfer (minutes)	19	137	63	60
Children's Asthma Care				
Received Home Management Plan of Care	-	-	-	88%
Received Reliever Medication	-	-	-	100%
Received Systemic Corticosteroids	-	-	-	100%
Emergency Department				
Admittance Decision Time (minutes)[2]	943	229	89	98
Head CT Results Within 45 Min. of Arrival	22	45%	64%	57%
Patients Who Left ER Before Being Seen	49,182	7%	3%	2%
Time from ER Arrival to Admit. (minutes)[2]	948	428	260	274
Time from ER Arrival to Discharge (minutes)	311	214	138	134
Time in ER Before Being Evaluated (minutes)	354	65	28	26
Time to Pain Meds for Fractures (minutes)	103	75	52	57
Heart Attack Care				
Aspirin Given at Discharge[2]	53	98%	99%	99%
Fibrinolytic Meds Within 30 Min. of Arrival[2,7]	-	-	33%	54%
PCI Within 90 Minutes of Arrival[2,7]	-	-	97%	96%
Statin Prescribed at Discharge[2]	53	89%	98%	98%
Heart Failure Care				
ACE Inhibitor or ARB for LVSD[2]	142	94%	98%	97%
Discharge Instructions Given[2]	272	79%	96%	94%
Evaluation of LVS Function[2]	316	97%	99%	99%
Medicare Spending				
Medicare Spending per Patient (ratio)	-	1.13	1	0.98
Pneumonia Care				
Appropriate Initial Antibiotic Given[2]	70	90%	95%	95%
Blood Culture Timing[2]	120	98%	98%	98%
Pregnancy and Delivery Care				
Newborn Deliveries Scheduled Early[2]	43	5%	2%	6%
Preventive Care				
Immunization for Influenza[2]	564	95%	92%	90%
Immunization for Pneumonia[2]	862	95%	92%	92%
Stroke Care				
Anticoagulation Therapy for Atrial Fibrillation[2]	11	64%	94%	95%
Antithrombotic Therapy Timing[2]	147	93%	98%	98%
Assessed for Rehabilitation[2]	148	91%	97%	97%
Discharged on Antithrombotic Therapy[2]	144	85%	99%	99%
Discharged on Statin Medication[2]	121	69%	94%	94%
Thrombolytic Therapy Timing[2]	13	46%	66%	66%
Venous Thromboembolism Prophylaxis[2]	158	90%	94%	94%
Written Stroke Educational Materials Given[2]	72	94%	87%	88%
Surgical Care Improvement Project				
Appropriate Beta Blocker Usage[2]	47	85%	98%	98%
Appropriate VTP Within 24 Hours[2]	146	88%	98%	98%
Controlled Postoperative Blood Glucose[2,7]	-	-	97%	97%
Perioperative Temperature Management[2]	172	99%	100%	100%
Prophylactic Antibiotic Selection[2]	95	99%	99%	99%
Prophylactic Antibiotic Selection (Outpatient)	44	91%	98%	98%
Prophylactic Antibiotic Stopped[2]	93	95%	98%	98%
Prophylactic Antibiotic Timing[2]	95	93%	99%	99%
Prophylactic Antibiotic Timing (Outpatient)	46	91%	97%	98%
Urinary Catheter Removal[2]	72	78%	98%	97%
Survey of Patients' Hospital Experiences				
Area Around Room 'Always' Quiet at Night	300+	58%	60%	61%
Doctors 'Always' Communicated Well	300+	75%	81%	82%
Home Recovery Information Given	300+	81%	86%	85%
Hospital Given 9 or 10 on 10 Point Scale	300+	53%	70%	71%
Meds 'Always' Explained Before Given	300+	58%	64%	64%
Nurses 'Always' Communicated Well	300+	70%	79%	79%
Pain 'Always' Well Controlled	300+	64%	71%	71%
Room and Bathroom 'Always' Clean	300+	67%	74%	73%
Timely Help 'Always' Received	300+	58%	67%	68%
Would Definitely Recommend Hospital	300+	54%	70%	71%
Use of Medical Imaging				
Cardiac Imaging Stress Test before Surgery	162	7.4%	5.5%	5.3%
Combination Abdominal CT Scan	425	1.6%	10.1%	10.5%
Combination Brain/Sinus CT Scan	704	1.8%	2.6%	2.7%
Combination Chest CT Scan	246	1.6%	2.8%	2.7%
Follow-up Mammogram/Ultrasound	408	3.2%	8.4%	8.8%
Lumbar Spine MRI for Low Back Pain	32	50.0%	36.6%	37.2%

Jackson Park Hospital

7531 S Stony Island Ave
Chicago, IL 60649
Phone: 773-947-7500
Fax: 773-947-7791
URL: www.jacksonparkhospital.org
Type: Acute Care Hospitals
Emergency Services: Yes
Ownership: Voluntary non-profit - Private
Beds: 336

Key Personnel:

Quality Assurance .... Rosemary Albright
Patient Relations .... Magdalene Armstead, MSN RN
Intensive Care Unit........... Produb David, RN
CEO/President.............. Merritt J. Hasbrouck
Cardiac Laboratory............. D Kumar, MD
Infection Control............. Martha Lyons, RN
Chief of Medical Staff.......... Michael A Wilczynski, MD

Measure	Cases	This Hosp.	State Avg.	U.S. Avg.
Blood Clot Prevention and Treatment				
Anticoagulation Overlap Therapy[2]	22	86%	91%	93%
ICU Venous Thromboembolism Prophylaxis[2]	11	82%	93%	92%
Incidence of Potentially Preventable VTE[1,2]	-	-	11%	10%
UFH with Dosages/Platelet Monitoring[2]	24	100%	94%	97%
Venous Thromboembolism Prophylaxis[2]	216	92%	86%	85%
Warfarin Therapy Discharge Instructions[2,7]	-	-	71%	75%
Chest Pain/Possible Heart Attack Care				
Aspirin Given Within 24 Hours of Arrival[5]	-	-	96%	96%
Fibrinolytic Meds Within 30 Min. of Arrival[5]	-	-	65%	58%
Average Time to ECG (minutes)[5]	-	-	6	7
Average Time to Transfer (minutes)[5]	-	-	63	60
Children's Asthma Care				
Received Home Management Plan of Care	-	-	-	88%
Received Reliever Medication	-	-	-	100%
Received Systemic Corticosteroids	-	-	-	100%
Emergency Department				
Admittance Decision Time (minutes)[2]	180	0	89	98
Head CT Results Within 45 Min. of Arrival[7]	-	-	64%	57%
Patients Who Left ER Before Being Seen	15,989	0%	3%	2%
Time from ER Arrival to Admit. (minutes)[2]	180	331	260	274
Time from ER Arrival to Discharge (minutes)	49	201	138	134
Time in ER Before Being Evaluated (minutes)	400	0	28	26
Time to Pain Meds for Fractures (minutes)[1]	-	-	52	57
Heart Attack Care				
Aspirin Given at Discharge	19	100%	99%	99%
Fibrinolytic Meds Within 30 Min. of Arrival[1]	-	-	33%	54%
PCI Within 90 Minutes of Arrival[7]	-	-	97%	96%
Statin Prescribed at Discharge	19	100%	98%	98%
Heart Failure Care				
ACE Inhibitor or ARB for LVSD	95	99%	98%	97%
Discharge Instructions Given	143	99%	96%	94%
Evaluation of LVS Function	184	99%	99%	99%
Medicare Spending				
Medicare Spending per Patient (ratio)	-	1.03	1	0.98
Pneumonia Care				
Appropriate Initial Antibiotic Given[2]	121	72%	95%	95%
Blood Culture Timing[2]	132	98%	98%	98%
Pregnancy and Delivery Care				
Newborn Deliveries Scheduled Early	16	0%	2%	6%
Preventive Care				
Immunization for Influenza[2]	585	100%	92%	90%
Immunization for Pneumonia[2]	629	85%	92%	92%
Stroke Care				
Anticoagulation Therapy for Atrial Fibrillation[1]	-	-	94%	95%
Antithrombotic Therapy Timing	35	100%	98%	98%
Assessed for Rehabilitation	39	97%	97%	97%
Discharged on Antithrombotic Therapy	38	97%	99%	99%
Discharged on Statin Medication	38	95%	94%	94%
Thrombolytic Therapy Timing[1]	-	-	66%	66%
Venous Thromboembolism Prophylaxis	38	95%	94%	94%
Written Stroke Educational Materials Given	17	100%	87%	88%
Surgical Care Improvement Project				
Appropriate Beta Blocker Usage[1]	-	-	98%	98%
Appropriate VTP Within 24 Hours	12	92%	98%	98%
Controlled Postoperative Blood Glucose[7]	-	-	97%	97%
Perioperative Temperature Management	48	100%	100%	100%
Prophylactic Antibiotic Selection	23	70%	99%	99%
Prophylactic Antibiotic Selection (Outpatient)[1]	-	-	98%	98%

NOTE: Hospital profiles are in alphabetical order by state, then city, then hospital within the city; Rankings exclude hospitals with less than 25 cases except for patient surveys which excludes hospitals with less than 100 cases; (a) 100-299 cases; (1) The number of cases/patients is too few to report; (2) Data submitted were based on a sample of cases/patients; (3) Results are based on a shorter time period than required; (4) Data suppressed by CMS for one or more quarters; (5) Results are not available for this reporting period; (6) Fewer than 100 patients completed the HCAHPS survey; (7) No cases met the criteria for this measure; (8) The lower limit of the confidence interval cannot be calculated if the number of observed infections equals zero; (9) No data are available from the state/territory for this reporting period; (10) The scores shown reflect fewer than 50 completed surveys; (11) There were discrepancies in the data collection process; (12) This measure does not apply to this hospital for this reporting period; (13) Results cannot be calculated for this reporting period; (14) The results for this state are combined with nearby states to protect confidentiality; Please refer to the User's Guide for a full explanation of data.

Measure	Cases	This Hosp.	State Avg.	U.S. Avg.
Prophylactic Antibiotic Stopped	23	100%	98%	98%
Prophylactic Antibiotic Timing	23	61%	99%	99%
Prophylactic Antibiotic Timing (Outpatient)[1]	-	-	97%	98%
Urinary Catheter Removal	14	93%	98%	97%
Survey of Patients' Hospital Experiences				
Area Around Room 'Always' Quiet at Night	300+	50%	60%	61%
Doctors 'Always' Communicated Well	300+	71%	81%	82%
Home Recovery Information Given	300+	64%	86%	85%
Hospital Given 9 or 10 on 10 Point Scale	300+	35%	70%	71%
Meds 'Always' Explained Before Given	300+	45%	64%	64%
Nurses 'Always' Communicated Well	300+	59%	79%	79%
Pain 'Always' Well Controlled	300+	55%	71%	71%
Room and Bathroom 'Always' Clean	300+	54%	74%	73%
Timely Help 'Always' Received	300+	44%	67%	68%
Would Definitely Recommend Hospital	300+	36%	70%	71%
Use of Medical Imaging				
Cardiac Imaging Stress Test before Surgery[1]	-	-	5.5%	5.3%
Combination Abdominal CT Scan	130	0.0%	10.1%	10.5%
Combination Brain/Sinus CT Scan	230	5.2%	2.6%	2.7%
Combination Chest CT Scan	133	1.5%	2.8%	2.7%
Follow-up Mammogram/Ultrasound	111	11.7%	8.4%	8.8%
Lumbar Spine MRI for Low Back Pain[7]	-	-	36.6%	37.2%

Jesse Brown VA Medical Center - VA Chicago

820 S Damen Street
Chicago, IL 60612
URL: www.va.gov
Phone: 312-569-8387
Fax: 312-569-6188
Type: Acute Care - VA
Ownership: Government Federal
Emergency Services: No
Beds: 337

Key Personnel:
Radiology. . . . . Edwin April, MD
CEO/President. . . . . Richard Centron
Quality Assurance . . . . James Curry
Operating Room. . . . . Darlene Rzepka, RN
Chief of Medical Staff. . . . . Wendy Weinstock Brown, MD, MPH

Measure	Cases	This Hosp.	State Avg.	U.S. Avg.
Blood Clot Prevention and Treatment				
Anticoagulation Overlap Therapy	-	-	91%	93%
ICU Venous Thromboembolism Prophylaxis	-	-	93%	92%
Incidence of Potentially Preventable VTE	-	-	11%	10%
UFH with Dosages/Platelet Monitoring	-	-	94%	97%
Venous Thromboembolism Prophylaxis	-	-	86%	85%
Warfarin Therapy Discharge Instructions	-	-	71%	75%
Chest Pain/Possible Heart Attack Care				
Aspirin Given Within 24 Hours of Arrival	-	-	96%	96%
Fibrinolytic Meds Within 30 Min. of Arrival	-	-	65%	58%
Average Time to ECG (minutes)	-	-	6	7
Average Time to Transfer (minutes)	-	-	63	60
Children's Asthma Care				
Received Home Management Plan of Care	-	-	-	88%
Received Reliever Medication	-	-	-	100%
Received Systemic Corticosteroids	-	-	-	100%
Emergency Department				
Admittance Decision Time (minutes)	-	-	89	98
Head CT Results Within 45 Min. of Arrival	-	-	64%	57%
Patients Who Left ER Before Being Seen	-	-	3%	2%
Time from ER Arrival to Admit. (minutes)	-	-	260	274
Time from ER Arrival to Discharge (minutes)	-	-	138	134
Time in ER Before Being Evaluated (minutes)	-	-	28	26
Time to Pain Meds for Fractures (minutes)	-	-	52	57
Heart Attack Care				
Aspirin Given at Discharge	65	98%	99%	99%
Fibrinolytic Meds Within 30 Min. of Arrival[5]	-	-	33%	54%
PCI Within 90 Minutes of Arrival[1]	-	-	97%	96%
Statin Prescribed at Discharge	63	97%	98%	98%
Heart Failure Care				
ACE Inhibitor or ARB for LVSD	154	99%	98%	97%
Discharge Instructions Given	362	100%	96%	94%
Evaluation of LVS Function	386	100%	99%	99%
Medicare Spending				
Medicare Spending per Patient (ratio)	-	-	1	0.98
Pneumonia Care				
Appropriate Initial Antibiotic Given	44	93%	95%	95%
Blood Culture Timing	84	98%	98%	98%
Pregnancy and Delivery Care				
Newborn Deliveries Scheduled Early	-	-	2%	6%
Preventive Care				
Immunization for Influenza[5]	-	-	92%	90%
Immunization for Pneumonia[5]	-	-	92%	92%
Stroke Care				
Anticoagulation Therapy for Atrial Fibrillation	-	-	94%	95%
Antithrombotic Therapy Timing	-	-	98%	98%
Assessed for Rehabilitation	-	-	97%	97%
Discharged on Antithrombotic Therapy	-	-	99%	99%
Discharged on Statin Medication	-	-	94%	94%
Thrombolytic Therapy Timing	-	-	66%	66%
Venous Thromboembolism Prophylaxis	-	-	94%	94%
Written Stroke Educational Materials Given	-	-	87%	88%
Surgical Care Improvement Project				
Appropriate Beta Blocker Usage[2]	42	93%	98%	98%
Appropriate VTP Within 24 Hours[2]	141	97%	98%	98%
Controlled Postoperative Blood Glucose[5]	-	-	97%	97%
Perioperative Temperature Management[2]	177	98%	100%	100%
Prophylactic Antibiotic Selection	74	100%	99%	99%
Prophylactic Antibiotic Selection (Outpatient)	-	-	98%	98%
Prophylactic Antibiotic Stopped	74	100%	98%	98%
Prophylactic Antibiotic Timing	76	96%	99%	99%
Prophylactic Antibiotic Timing (Outpatient)	-	-	97%	98%
Urinary Catheter Removal[2]	107	98%	98%	97%
Survey of Patients' Hospital Experiences				
Area Around Room 'Always' Quiet at Night	-	-	60%	61%
Doctors 'Always' Communicated Well	-	-	81%	82%
Home Recovery Information Given	-	-	86%	85%
Hospital Given 9 or 10 on 10 Point Scale	-	-	70%	71%
Meds 'Always' Explained Before Given	-	-	64%	64%
Nurses 'Always' Communicated Well	-	-	79%	79%
Pain 'Always' Well Controlled	-	-	71%	71%
Room and Bathroom 'Always' Clean	-	-	74%	73%
Timely Help 'Always' Received	-	-	67%	68%
Would Definitely Recommend Hospital	-	-	70%	71%
Use of Medical Imaging				
Cardiac Imaging Stress Test before Surgery	-	-	5.5%	5.3%
Combination Abdominal CT Scan	-	-	10.1%	10.5%
Combination Brain/Sinus CT Scan	-	-	2.6%	2.7%
Combination Chest CT Scan	-	-	2.8%	2.7%
Follow-up Mammogram/Ultrasound	-	-	8.4%	8.8%
Lumbar Spine MRI for Low Back Pain	-	-	36.6%	37.2%

John H Stroger Jr Hospital

1901 W Harrison St
Chicago, IL 60612
URL: www.cookcountygov.com
Phone: 312-864-6000
Fax: 312-864-9725
Type: Acute Care Hospitals
Ownership: Government - Local
Emergency Services: Yes
Beds: 464

Key Personnel:
Chief of Medical Staff. . . . . Stephen Hamburger, MD
Quality Assurance . . . . Margaret Martin
Intensive Care Unit. . . . . Mary O'Flaherty
CEO/President. . . . . Lacy L Thomas
Infection Control. . . . . Robert Weinstein, MD
Operating Room. . . . . Brenda White

Measure	Cases	This Hosp.	State Avg.	U.S. Avg.
Blood Clot Prevention and Treatment				
Anticoagulation Overlap Therapy[2]	129	90%	91%	93%
ICU Venous Thromboembolism Prophylaxis[2]	59	86%	93%	92%
Incidence of Potentially Preventable VTE[2]	31	19%	11%	10%
UFH with Dosages/Platelet Monitoring[2]	48	15%	94%	97%
Venous Thromboembolism Prophylaxis[2]	424	78%	86%	85%
Warfarin Therapy Discharge Instructions[2]	112	62%	71%	75%
Chest Pain/Possible Heart Attack Care				
Aspirin Given Within 24 Hours of Arrival[5]	-	-	96%	96%
Fibrinolytic Meds Within 30 Min. of Arrival[5]	-	-	65%	58%
Average Time to ECG (minutes)[5]	-	-	6	7
Average Time to Transfer (minutes)[5]	-	-	63	60
Children's Asthma Care				
Received Home Management Plan of Care	-	-	-	88%
Received Reliever Medication	-	-	-	100%
Received Systemic Corticosteroids	-	-	-	100%
Emergency Department				
Admittance Decision Time (minutes)[2]	811	210	89	98
Head CT Results Within 45 Min. of Arrival[3,7]	-	-	64%	57%
Patients Who Left ER Before Being Seen	>100k	10%	3%	2%
Time from ER Arrival to Admit. (minutes)[2]	816	578	260	274
Time from ER Arrival to Discharge (minutes)	374	292	138	134
Time in ER Before Being Evaluated (minutes)	379	153	28	26
Time to Pain Meds for Fractures (minutes)	331	171	52	57
Heart Attack Care				
Aspirin Given at Discharge[2]	188	99%	99%	99%
Fibrinolytic Meds Within 30 Min. of Arrival[2,7]	-	-	33%	54%
PCI Within 90 Minutes of Arrival[2]	14	79%	97%	96%
Statin Prescribed at Discharge[2]	188	99%	98%	98%
Heart Failure Care				
ACE Inhibitor or ARB for LVSD[2]	156	100%	98%	97%
Discharge Instructions Given[2]	325	92%	96%	94%
Evaluation of LVS Function[2]	326	99%	99%	99%
Medicare Spending				
Medicare Spending per Patient (ratio)	-	0.81	1	0.98
Pneumonia Care				
Appropriate Initial Antibiotic Given[2]	107	83%	95%	95%
Blood Culture Timing[2]	127	96%	98%	98%
Pregnancy and Delivery Care				
Newborn Deliveries Scheduled Early[2]	135	10%	2%	6%
Preventive Care				
Immunization for Influenza[2]	599	75%	92%	90%
Immunization for Pneumonia[2]	677	49%	92%	92%
Stroke Care				
Anticoagulation Therapy for Atrial Fibrillation[1,2]	-	-	94%	95%
Antithrombotic Therapy Timing[2]	200	98%	98%	98%
Assessed for Rehabilitation[2]	208	90%	97%	97%
Discharged on Antithrombotic Therapy[2]	196	99%	99%	99%
Discharged on Statin Medication[2]	158	96%	94%	94%
Thrombolytic Therapy Timing[1,2]	-	-	66%	66%
Venous Thromboembolism Prophylaxis[2]	209	92%	94%	94%
Written Stroke Educational Materials Given[2]	180	89%	87%	88%
Surgical Care Improvement Project				
Appropriate Beta Blocker Usage[2]	138	100%	98%	98%
Appropriate VTP Within 24 Hours[2]	304	98%	98%	98%
Controlled Postoperative Blood Glucose[2]	99	91%	97%	97%
Perioperative Temperature Management[2]	385	99%	100%	100%
Prophylactic Antibiotic Selection[2]	310	97%	99%	99%
Prophylactic Antibiotic Selection (Outpatient)	188	90%	98%	98%
Prophylactic Antibiotic Stopped[2]	304	97%	98%	98%
Prophylactic Antibiotic Timing[2]	313	96%	99%	99%
Prophylactic Antibiotic Timing (Outpatient)	193	95%	97%	98%
Urinary Catheter Removal[2]	208	100%	98%	97%
Survey of Patients' Hospital Experiences				
Area Around Room 'Always' Quiet at Night	300+	51%	60%	61%
Doctors 'Always' Communicated Well	300+	79%	81%	82%
Home Recovery Information Given	300+	76%	86%	85%
Hospital Given 9 or 10 on 10 Point Scale	300+	54%	70%	71%
Meds 'Always' Explained Before Given	300+	50%	64%	64%
Nurses 'Always' Communicated Well	300+	64%	79%	79%
Pain 'Always' Well Controlled	300+	62%	71%	71%
Room and Bathroom 'Always' Clean	300+	48%	74%	73%
Timely Help 'Always' Received	300+	53%	67%	68%
Would Definitely Recommend Hospital	300+	61%	70%	71%
Use of Medical Imaging				
Cardiac Imaging Stress Test before Surgery	171	2.9%	5.5%	5.3%
Combination Abdominal CT Scan	650	16.3%	10.1%	10.5%
Combination Brain/Sinus CT Scan	291	0.7%	2.6%	2.7%
Combination Chest CT Scan	550	5.8%	2.8%	2.7%
Follow-up Mammogram/Ultrasound	257	8.9%	8.4%	8.8%
Lumbar Spine MRI for Low Back Pain[1]	-	-	36.6%	37.2%

NOTE: Hospital profiles are in alphabetical order by state, then city, then hospital within the city; Rankings exclude hospitals with less than 25 cases except for patient surveys which excludes hospitals with less than 100 cases; (a) 100-299 cases; (1) The number of cases/patients is too few to report; (2) Data submitted were based on a sample of cases/patients; (3) Results are based on a shorter time period than required; (4) Data suppressed by CMS for one or more quarters; (5) Results are not available for this reporting period; (6) Fewer than 100 patients completed the HCAHPS survey; (7) No cases met the criteria for this measure; (8) The lower limit of the confidence interval cannot be calculated if the number of observed infections equals zero; (9) No data are available from the state/territory for this reporting period; (10) The scores shown reflect fewer than 50 completed surveys; (11) There were discrepancies in the data collection process; (12) This measure does not apply to this hospital for this reporting period; (13) Results cannot be calculated for this reporting period; (14) The results for this state are combined with nearby states to protect confidentiality; Please refer to the User's Guide for a full explanation of data.

Loretto Hospital

645 South Central Ave
Chicago, IL 60644
URL: www.lorettohospital.org
Type: Acute Care Hospitals
Ownership: Proprietary

Phone: 773-626-4300
Fax: 773-626-2613
Emergency Services: Yes
Beds: 189

Key Personnel:
Operating Room. . . . . Mary Frolik
Ambulatory Care . . . . Deen Gaddam, MD
President . . . . Eliyazar Gaddam, MD
Chief of Medical Staff. . . . . Humid M Humayum, MD
Infection Control. . . . . Omar Jrab
Emergency Room . . . . Patricia Lindeman

Measure	Cases	This Hosp.	State Avg.	U.S. Avg.
Blood Clot Prevention and Treatment				
Anticoagulation Overlap Therapy[2]	15	73%	91%	93%
ICU Venous Thromboembolism Prophylaxis[2]	89	85%	93%	92%
Incidence of Potentially Preventable VTE[1,2]	-	-	11%	10%
UFH with Dosages/Platelet Monitoring[1,2]	-	-	94%	97%
Venous Thromboembolism Prophylaxis[2]	155	69%	86%	85%
Warfarin Therapy Discharge Instructions[1,2]	-	-	71%	75%
Chest Pain/Possible Heart Attack Care				
Aspirin Given Within 24 Hours of Arrival[1]	-	-	96%	96%
Fibrinolytic Meds Within 30 Min. of Arrival[3,7]	-	-	65%	58%
Average Time to ECG (minutes)[1]	-	-	6	7
Average Time to Transfer (minutes)[1,3]	-	-	63	60
Children's Asthma Care				
Received Home Management Plan of Care	-	-	-	88%
Received Reliever Medication	-	-	-	100%
Received Systemic Corticosteroids	-	-	-	100%
Emergency Department				
Admittance Decision Time (minutes)[2]	322	132	89	98
Head CT Results Within 45 Min. of Arrival[1]	-	-	64%	57%
Patients Who Left ER Before Being Seen	15,576	6%	3%	2%
Time from ER Arrival to Admit. (minutes)[2]	351	385	260	274
Time from ER Arrival to Discharge (minutes)	320	167	138	134
Time in ER Before Being Evaluated (minutes)	347	54	28	26
Time to Pain Meds for Fractures (minutes)	13	51	52	57
Heart Attack Care				
Aspirin Given at Discharge[1]	-	-	99%	99%
Fibrinolytic Meds Within 30 Min. of Arrival[7]	-	-	33%	54%
PCI Within 90 Minutes of Arrival[7]	-	-	97%	96%
Statin Prescribed at Discharge[1]	-	-	98%	98%
Heart Failure Care				
ACE Inhibitor or ARB for LVSD	33	82%	98%	97%
Discharge Instructions Given	72	99%	96%	94%
Evaluation of LVS Function	83	98%	99%	99%
Medicare Spending				
Medicare Spending per Patient (ratio)	-	1.08	1	0.98
Pneumonia Care				
Appropriate Initial Antibiotic Given	60	90%	95%	95%
Blood Culture Timing	104	99%	98%	98%
Pregnancy and Delivery Care				
Newborn Deliveries Scheduled Early[2,7]	-	-	2%	6%
Preventive Care				
Immunization for Influenza[2]	391	70%	92%	90%
Immunization for Pneumonia[2]	455	76%	92%	92%
Stroke Care				
Anticoagulation Therapy for Atrial Fibrillation[7]	-	-	94%	95%
Antithrombotic Therapy Timing	16	100%	98%	98%
Assessed for Rehabilitation	13	92%	97%	97%
Discharged on Antithrombotic Therapy	13	92%	99%	99%
Discharged on Statin Medication	12	75%	94%	94%
Thrombolytic Therapy Timing[7]	-	-	66%	66%
Venous Thromboembolism Prophylaxis	16	75%	94%	94%
Written Stroke Educational Materials Given[1]	-	-	87%	88%
Surgical Care Improvement Project				
Appropriate Beta Blocker Usage	13	85%	98%	98%
Appropriate VTP Within 24 Hours	35	100%	98%	98%
Controlled Postoperative Blood Glucose[7]	-	-	97%	97%
Perioperative Temperature Management	45	100%	100%	100%
Prophylactic Antibiotic Selection	13	69%	99%	99%
Prophylactic Antibiotic Selection (Outpatient)	17	100%	98%	98%
Prophylactic Antibiotic Stopped[1]	-	-	98%	98%
Prophylactic Antibiotic Timing	13	100%	99%	99%
Prophylactic Antibiotic Timing (Outpatient)	17	100%	97%	98%
Urinary Catheter Removal	24	67%	98%	97%
Survey of Patients' Hospital Experiences				
Area Around Room 'Always' Quiet at Night	(a)	61%	60%	61%
Doctors 'Always' Communicated Well	(a)	73%	81%	82%
Home Recovery Information Given	(a)	67%	86%	85%
Hospital Given 9 or 10 on 10 Point Scale	(a)	43%	70%	71%
Meds 'Always' Explained Before Given	(a)	48%	64%	64%
Nurses 'Always' Communicated Well	(a)	64%	79%	79%
Pain 'Always' Well Controlled	(a)	54%	71%	71%
Room and Bathroom 'Always' Clean	(a)	62%	74%	73%
Timely Help 'Always' Received	(a)	51%	67%	68%
Would Definitely Recommend Hospital	(a)	36%	70%	71%
Use of Medical Imaging				
Cardiac Imaging Stress Test before Surgery[1]	-	-	5.5%	5.3%
Combination Abdominal CT Scan	65	6.2%	10.1%	10.5%
Combination Brain/Sinus CT Scan	136	0.0%	2.6%	2.7%
Combination Chest CT Scan[1]	-	-	2.8%	2.7%
Follow-up Mammogram/Ultrasound	83	18.1%	8.4%	8.8%
Lumbar Spine MRI for Low Back Pain[7]	-	-	36.6%	37.2%

Louis A Weiss Memorial Hospital

4646 N Marine Drive
Chicago, IL 60640
E-mail: cboykin@weisshospital.org
URL: www.weisshospital.org
Type: Acute Care Hospitals
Ownership: Proprietary

Phone: 773-878-8700
Fax: 773-564-5359
Emergency Services: Yes
Beds: 357

Key Personnel:
Radiology. . . . . Hiroyuki Abe, MD
Operating Room. . . . . Marc Adajar
Infection Control. . . . . David Balling, MD
Quality Assurance . . . . Chris Brady, RN
Emergency Room . . . . Leo Dilan, MD
Chief of Medical Staff. . . . . Stuart Kraussn, MD
Anesthesiology. . . . . Kenneth Rodino, MD
CEO/President. . . . . Tracey Rogers

Measure	Cases	This Hosp.	State Avg.	U.S. Avg.
Blood Clot Prevention and Treatment				
Anticoagulation Overlap Therapy[2]	77	99%	91%	93%
ICU Venous Thromboembolism Prophylaxis[2]	77	100%	93%	92%
Incidence of Potentially Preventable VTE[2]	38	8%	11%	10%
UFH with Dosages/Platelet Monitoring[2]	29	100%	94%	97%
Venous Thromboembolism Prophylaxis[2]	343	94%	86%	85%
Warfarin Therapy Discharge Instructions[2]	36	81%	71%	75%
Chest Pain/Possible Heart Attack Care				
Aspirin Given Within 24 Hours of Arrival[5]	-	-	96%	96%
Fibrinolytic Meds Within 30 Min. of Arrival[5]	-	-	65%	58%
Average Time to ECG (minutes)[5]	-	-	6	7
Average Time to Transfer (minutes)[5]	-	-	63	60
Children's Asthma Care				
Received Home Management Plan of Care	-	-	-	88%
Received Reliever Medication	-	-	-	100%
Received Systemic Corticosteroids	-	-	-	100%
Emergency Department				
Admittance Decision Time (minutes)[2]	690	87	89	98
Head CT Results Within 45 Min. of Arrival[5]	-	-	64%	57%
Patients Who Left ER Before Being Seen	24,215	2%	3%	2%
Time from ER Arrival to Admit. (minutes)[2]	775	258	260	274
Time from ER Arrival to Discharge (minutes)	333	139	138	134
Time in ER Before Being Evaluated (minutes)	401	28	28	26
Time to Pain Meds for Fractures (minutes)	56	50	52	57
Heart Attack Care				
Aspirin Given at Discharge	98	100%	99%	99%
Fibrinolytic Meds Within 30 Min. of Arrival[1]	-	-	33%	54%
PCI Within 90 Minutes of Arrival	17	88%	97%	96%
Statin Prescribed at Discharge	100	99%	98%	98%
Heart Failure Care				
ACE Inhibitor or ARB for LVSD	64	100%	98%	97%
Discharge Instructions Given	135	98%	96%	94%
Evaluation of LVS Function	183	100%	99%	99%
Medicare Spending				
Medicare Spending per Patient (ratio)	-	1.12	1	0.98
Pneumonia Care				
Appropriate Initial Antibiotic Given	34	100%	95%	95%
Blood Culture Timing	112	99%	98%	98%
Pregnancy and Delivery Care				
Newborn Deliveries Scheduled Early[7]	-	-	2%	6%
Preventive Care				
Immunization for Influenza[2]	533	98%	92%	90%
Immunization for Pneumonia[2]	812	98%	92%	92%
Stroke Care				
Anticoagulation Therapy for Atrial Fibrillation[1]	-	-	94%	95%
Antithrombotic Therapy Timing	22	100%	98%	98%
Assessed for Rehabilitation	27	100%	97%	97%
Discharged on Antithrombotic Therapy	24	100%	99%	99%
Discharged on Statin Medication	19	100%	94%	94%
Thrombolytic Therapy Timing[7]	-	-	66%	66%
Venous Thromboembolism Prophylaxis	26	88%	94%	94%
Written Stroke Educational Materials Given	13	69%	87%	88%
Surgical Care Improvement Project				
Appropriate Beta Blocker Usage[2]	150	100%	98%	98%
Appropriate VTP Within 24 Hours[2]	430	100%	98%	98%
Controlled Postoperative Blood Glucose[2]	16	81%	97%	97%
Perioperative Temperature Management[2]	455	100%	100%	100%
Prophylactic Antibiotic Selection[2]	313	100%	99%	99%
Prophylactic Antibiotic Selection (Outpatient)	196	98%	98%	98%
Prophylactic Antibiotic Stopped[2]	292	99%	98%	98%
Prophylactic Antibiotic Timing[2]	313	100%	99%	99%
Prophylactic Antibiotic Timing (Outpatient)	182	100%	97%	98%
Urinary Catheter Removal[2]	384	100%	98%	97%
Survey of Patients' Hospital Experiences				
Area Around Room 'Always' Quiet at Night[11]	300+	54%	60%	61%
Doctors 'Always' Communicated Well[11]	300+	79%	81%	82%
Home Recovery Information Given[11]	300+	83%	86%	85%
Hospital Given 9 or 10 on 10 Point Scale[11]	300+	60%	70%	71%
Meds 'Always' Explained Before Given[11]	300+	56%	64%	64%
Nurses 'Always' Communicated Well[11]	300+	71%	79%	79%
Pain 'Always' Well Controlled[11]	300+	64%	71%	71%
Room and Bathroom 'Always' Clean[11]	300+	62%	74%	73%
Timely Help 'Always' Received[11]	300+	54%	67%	68%
Would Definitely Recommend Hospital[11]	300+	62%	70%	71%
Use of Medical Imaging				
Cardiac Imaging Stress Test before Surgery	309	5.2%	5.5%	5.3%
Combination Abdominal CT Scan	492	11.2%	10.1%	10.5%
Combination Brain/Sinus CT Scan[1]	-	-	2.6%	2.7%
Combination Chest CT Scan	369	1.1%	2.8%	2.7%
Follow-up Mammogram/Ultrasound	296	8.8%	8.4%	8.8%
Lumbar Spine MRI for Low Back Pain	90	26.7%	36.6%	37.2%

Mercy Hospital & Medical Center

2525 S Michigan Ave
Chicago, IL 60616
E-mail: mercy@mercy-chicago.org
URL: www.mercy-chicago.org
Type: Acute Care Hospitals
Ownership: Voluntary non-profit - Private

Phone: 312-567-2000
Emergency Services: Yes
Beds: 507

Key Personnel:
Anesthesiology. . . . . Milorad Cupic, MD
Pediatric Ambulatory Care . . . . . . Jere E. Freidheim, MD
CEO/President. . . . . Carol L. Garikes Schneid
Quality Assurance . . . . Nancy Hill Davis
Infection Control. . . . . Jean Kirk, RN
Operating Room. . . . . Mary Alice Ledenmeyer
Radiology. . . . . Shahrooz Sepahdari, MD
Cardiac Laboratory. . . . . Karen Walker

Measure	Cases	This Hosp.	State Avg.	U.S. Avg.
Blood Clot Prevention and Treatment				
Anticoagulation Overlap Therapy[2]	87	86%	91%	93%
ICU Venous Thromboembolism Prophylaxis[2]	91	96%	93%	92%
Incidence of Potentially Preventable VTE[2]	30	7%	11%	10%
UFH with Dosages/Platelet Monitoring[2]	65	86%	94%	97%
Venous Thromboembolism Prophylaxis[2]	324	88%	86%	85%
Warfarin Therapy Discharge Instructions[2]	58	91%	71%	75%
Chest Pain/Possible Heart Attack Care				
Aspirin Given Within 24 Hours of Arrival[5]	-	-	96%	96%
Fibrinolytic Meds Within 30 Min. of Arrival[5]	-	-	65%	58%

NOTE: Hospital profiles are in alphabetical order by state, then city, then hospital within the city; Rankings exclude hospitals with less than 25 cases except for patient surveys which excludes hospitals with less than 100 cases; (a) 100-299 cases; (1) The number of cases/patients is too few to report; (2) Data submitted were based on a sample of cases/patients; (3) Results are based on a shorter time period than required; (4) Data suppressed by CMS for one or more quarters; (5) Results are not available for this reporting period; (6) Fewer than 100 patients completed the HCAHPS survey; (7) No cases met the criteria for this measure; (8) The lower limit of the confidence interval cannot be calculated if the number of observed infections equals zero; (9) No data are available from the state/territory for this reporting period; (10) The scores shown reflect fewer than 50 completed surveys; (11) There were discrepancies in the data collection process; (12) This measure does not apply to this hospital for this reporting period; (13) Results cannot be calculated for this reporting period; (14) The results for this state are combined with nearby states to protect confidentiality; Please refer to the User's Guide for a full explanation of data.

Measure	Cases	This Hosp.	State Avg.	U.S. Avg.
Average Time to ECG (minutes)[5]	-	-	6	7
Average Time to Transfer (minutes)[5]	-	-	63	60
Children's Asthma Care				
Received Home Management Plan of Care	-	-	-	88%
Received Reliever Medication	-	-	-	100%
Received Systemic Corticosteroids	-	-	-	100%
Emergency Department				
Admittance Decision Time (minutes)[2]	584	138	89	98
Head CT Results Within 45 Min. of Arrival	12	83%	64%	57%
Patients Who Left ER Before Being Seen	61,812	5%	3%	2%
Time from ER Arrival to Admit. (minutes)[2]	603	389	260	274
Time from ER Arrival to Discharge (minutes)	333	201	138	134
Time in ER Before Being Evaluated (minutes)	371	25	28	26
Time to Pain Meds for Fractures (minutes)	69	56	52	57
Heart Attack Care				
Aspirin Given at Discharge	219	97%	99%	99%
Fibrinolytic Meds Within 30 Min. of Arrival[7]	-	-	33%	54%
PCI Within 90 Minutes of Arrival	31	81%	97%	96%
Statin Prescribed at Discharge	220	98%	98%	98%
Heart Failure Care				
ACE Inhibitor or ARB for LVSD[2]	144	92%	98%	97%
Discharge Instructions Given[2]	260	97%	96%	94%
Evaluation of LVS Function[2]	292	99%	99%	99%
Medicare Spending				
Medicare Spending per Patient (ratio)	-	0.98	1	0.98
Pneumonia Care				
Appropriate Initial Antibiotic Given[2]	76	89%	95%	95%
Blood Culture Timing[2]	148	93%	98%	98%
Pregnancy and Delivery Care				
Newborn Deliveries Scheduled Early	176	0%	2%	6%
Preventive Care				
Immunization for Influenza[2]	489	89%	92%	90%
Immunization for Pneumonia[2]	575	89%	92%	92%
Stroke Care				
Anticoagulation Therapy for Atrial Fibrillation[1]	-	-	94%	95%
Antithrombotic Therapy Timing	146	98%	98%	98%
Assessed for Rehabilitation	148	99%	97%	97%
Discharged on Antithrombotic Therapy	141	99%	99%	99%
Discharged on Statin Medication	96	97%	94%	94%
Thrombolytic Therapy Timing[1]	-	-	66%	66%
Venous Thromboembolism Prophylaxis	155	94%	94%	94%
Written Stroke Educational Materials Given	73	95%	87%	88%
Surgical Care Improvement Project				
Appropriate Beta Blocker Usage	157	96%	98%	98%
Appropriate VTP Within 24 Hours	403	98%	98%	98%
Controlled Postoperative Blood Glucose	49	96%	97%	97%
Perioperative Temperature Management	462	99%	100%	100%
Prophylactic Antibiotic Selection	325	99%	99%	99%
Prophylactic Antibiotic Selection (Outpatient)	112	97%	98%	98%
Prophylactic Antibiotic Stopped	311	96%	98%	98%
Prophylactic Antibiotic Timing	325	99%	99%	99%
Prophylactic Antibiotic Timing (Outpatient)	114	96%	97%	98%
Urinary Catheter Removal	254	95%	98%	97%
Survey of Patients' Hospital Experiences				
Area Around Room 'Always' Quiet at Night	300+	61%	60%	61%
Doctors 'Always' Communicated Well	300+	81%	81%	82%
Home Recovery Information Given	300+	82%	86%	85%
Hospital Given 9 or 10 on 10 Point Scale	300+	69%	70%	71%
Meds 'Always' Explained Before Given	300+	55%	64%	64%
Nurses 'Always' Communicated Well	300+	74%	79%	79%
Pain 'Always' Well Controlled	300+	69%	71%	71%
Room and Bathroom 'Always' Clean	300+	70%	74%	73%
Timely Help 'Always' Received	300+	59%	67%	68%
Would Definitely Recommend Hospital	300+	66%	70%	71%
Use of Medical Imaging				
Cardiac Imaging Stress Test before Surgery	533	2.6%	5.5%	5.3%
Combination Abdominal CT Scan	820	3.2%	10.1%	10.5%
Combination Brain/Sinus CT Scan	1,021	2.4%	2.6%	2.7%
Combination Chest CT Scan	369	1.4%	2.8%	2.7%
Follow-up Mammogram/Ultrasound	2,241	3.9%	8.4%	8.8%
Lumbar Spine MRI for Low Back Pain	136	35.3%	36.6%	37.2%

Methodist Hospital of Chicago

5025 N Paulina Street
Chicago, IL 60640
URL: www.methodistchicago.org
Type: Acute Care Hospitals
Ownership: Voluntary non-profit - Private
Phone: 773-271-9040
Fax: 773-989-1348
Emergency Services: Yes
Beds: 198

Key Personnel:
CEO/President. . . . . Steven Dahl
Chief of Medical Staff . . . . Irzing Tracer, MD
Quality Assurance . . . . Eleanor Wolrfram

Measure	Cases	This Hosp.	State Avg.	U.S. Avg.
Blood Clot Prevention and Treatment				
Anticoagulation Overlap Therapy[1,2]	-	-	91%	93%
ICU Venous Thromboembolism Prophylaxis[1,2]	-	-	93%	92%
Incidence of Potentially Preventable VTE[2,7]	-	-	11%	10%
UFH with Dosages/Platelet Monitoring[1,2]	-	-	94%	97%
Venous Thromboembolism Prophylaxis[2]	148	98%	86%	85%
Warfarin Therapy Discharge Instructions[1,2]	-	-	71%	75%
Chest Pain/Possible Heart Attack Care				
Aspirin Given Within 24 Hours of Arrival[1,3]	-	-	96%	96%
Fibrinolytic Meds Within 30 Min. of Arrival[5]	-	-	65%	58%
Average Time to ECG (minutes)[1,3]	-	-	6	7
Average Time to Transfer (minutes)[5]	-	-	63	60
Children's Asthma Care				
Received Home Management Plan of Care	-	-	-	88%
Received Reliever Medication	-	-	-	100%
Received Systemic Corticosteroids	-	-	-	100%
Emergency Department				
Admittance Decision Time (minutes)[2]	226	77	89	98
Head CT Results Within 45 Min. of Arrival[5]	-	-	64%	57%
Patients Who Left ER Before Being Seen	3,989	0%	3%	2%
Time from ER Arrival to Admit. (minutes)[2]	226	242	260	274
Time from ER Arrival to Discharge (minutes)	226	178	138	134
Time in ER Before Being Evaluated (minutes)	276	6	28	26
Time to Pain Meds for Fractures (minutes)[1]	-	-	52	57
Heart Attack Care				
Aspirin Given at Discharge[1,3]	-	-	99%	99%
Fibrinolytic Meds Within 30 Min. of Arrival[3,7]	-	-	33%	54%
PCI Within 90 Minutes of Arrival[3,7]	-	-	97%	96%
Statin Prescribed at Discharge[1,3]	-	-	98%	98%
Heart Failure Care				
ACE Inhibitor or ARB for LVSD[1]	-	-	98%	97%
Discharge Instructions Given	15	100%	96%	94%
Evaluation of LVS Function	42	100%	99%	99%
Medicare Spending				
Medicare Spending per Patient (ratio)	-	1.04	1	0.98
Pneumonia Care				
Appropriate Initial Antibiotic Given	17	88%	95%	95%
Blood Culture Timing	84	96%	98%	98%
Pregnancy and Delivery Care				
Newborn Deliveries Scheduled Early[7]	-	-	2%	6%
Preventive Care				
Immunization for Influenza[2]	381	99%	92%	90%
Immunization for Pneumonia[2]	486	99%	92%	92%
Stroke Care				
Anticoagulation Therapy for Atrial Fibrillation[3,7]	-	-	94%	95%
Antithrombotic Therapy Timing[1,3]	-	-	98%	98%
Assessed for Rehabilitation[1,3]	-	-	97%	97%
Discharged on Antithrombotic Therapy[1,3]	-	-	99%	99%
Discharged on Statin Medication[1,3]	-	-	94%	94%
Thrombolytic Therapy Timing[3,7]	-	-	66%	66%
Venous Thromboembolism Prophylaxis[1,3]	-	-	94%	94%
Written Stroke Educational Materials Given[3,7]	-	-	87%	88%
Surgical Care Improvement Project				
Appropriate Beta Blocker Usage	19	100%	98%	98%
Appropriate VTP Within 24 Hours	21	90%	98%	98%
Controlled Postoperative Blood Glucose[7]	-	-	97%	97%
Perioperative Temperature Management	38	100%	100%	100%
Prophylactic Antibiotic Selection	28	100%	99%	99%
Prophylactic Antibiotic Selection (Outpatient)	19	84%	98%	98%
Prophylactic Antibiotic Stopped	28	100%	98%	98%
Prophylactic Antibiotic Timing	29	97%	99%	99%
Prophylactic Antibiotic Timing (Outpatient)	17	100%	97%	98%
Urinary Catheter Removal	34	100%	98%	97%
Survey of Patients' Hospital Experiences				
Area Around Room 'Always' Quiet at Night[6,11]	<100	59%	60%	61%
Doctors 'Always' Communicated Well[6,11]	<100	74%	81%	82%
Home Recovery Information Given[6,11]	<100	79%	86%	85%
Hospital Given 9 or 10 on 10 Point Scale[6,11]	<100	62%	70%	71%
Meds 'Always' Explained Before Given[6,11]	<100	60%	64%	64%
Nurses 'Always' Communicated Well[6,11]	<100	72%	79%	79%
Pain 'Always' Well Controlled[6,11]	<100	74%	71%	71%
Room and Bathroom 'Always' Clean[6,11]	<100	69%	74%	73%
Timely Help 'Always' Received[6,11]	<100	73%	67%	68%
Would Definitely Recommend Hospital[6,11]	<100	55%	70%	71%
Use of Medical Imaging				
Cardiac Imaging Stress Test before Surgery[1]	-	-	5.5%	5.3%
Combination Abdominal CT Scan	89	24.7%	10.1%	10.5%
Combination Brain/Sinus CT Scan[1]	-	-	2.6%	2.7%
Combination Chest CT Scan	96	15.6%	2.8%	2.7%
Follow-up Mammogram/Ultrasound	91	22.0%	8.4%	8.8%
Lumbar Spine MRI for Low Back Pain[1]	-	-	36.6%	37.2%

Mount Sinai Hospital Medical Center

15th Street at California
Chicago, IL 60608
URL: www.sinai.org
Type: Acute Care Hospitals
Ownership: Voluntary non-profit - Private
Phone: 773-257-6751
Fax: 773-257-6208
Emergency Services: Yes
Beds: 432

Key Personnel:
Radiology. . . . . Randy Boberg
Infection Control. . . . . Jan Lepenski
Operating Room. . . . . Sue McKenna
Intensive Care Unit. . . . . Barbara Shields-Johnson
Quality Assurance . . . . Robert Tarver
Anesthesiology. . . . . John Vazquez, MD
Chief of Medical Staff. . . . . John Vazquez, MD
Emergency Room . . . . Leslie Zun, MD

Measure	Cases	This Hosp.	State Avg.	U.S. Avg.
Blood Clot Prevention and Treatment				
Anticoagulation Overlap Therapy[2]	56	88%	91%	93%
ICU Venous Thromboembolism Prophylaxis[2]	63	98%	93%	92%
Incidence of Potentially Preventable VTE[2]	11	9%	11%	10%
UFH with Dosages/Platelet Monitoring[2]	17	100%	94%	97%
Venous Thromboembolism Prophylaxis[2]	303	86%	86%	85%
Warfarin Therapy Discharge Instructions[2]	32	0%	71%	75%
Chest Pain/Possible Heart Attack Care				
Aspirin Given Within 24 Hours of Arrival[1,3]	-	-	96%	96%
Fibrinolytic Meds Within 30 Min. of Arrival[5]	-	-	65%	58%
Average Time to ECG (minutes)[1,3]	-	-	6	7
Average Time to Transfer (minutes)[5]	-	-	63	60
Children's Asthma Care				
Received Home Management Plan of Care	-	-	-	88%
Received Reliever Medication	-	-	-	100%
Received Systemic Corticosteroids	-	-	-	100%
Emergency Department				
Admittance Decision Time (minutes)[2]	537	174	89	98
Head CT Results Within 45 Min. of Arrival[1]	-	-	64%	57%
Patients Who Left ER Before Being Seen	54,714	1%	3%	2%
Time from ER Arrival to Admit. (minutes)[2]	539	426	260	274
Time from ER Arrival to Discharge (minutes)	318	220	138	134
Time in ER Before Being Evaluated (minutes)	349	66	28	26
Time to Pain Meds for Fractures (minutes)	137	89	52	57
Heart Attack Care				
Aspirin Given at Discharge	118	100%	99%	99%
Fibrinolytic Meds Within 30 Min. of Arrival[7]	-	-	33%	54%
PCI Within 90 Minutes of Arrival	12	92%	97%	96%
Statin Prescribed at Discharge	108	100%	98%	98%
Heart Failure Care				
ACE Inhibitor or ARB for LVSD	183	98%	98%	97%
Discharge Instructions Given	272	100%	96%	94%
Evaluation of LVS Function	305	100%	99%	99%
Medicare Spending				
Medicare Spending per Patient (ratio)	-	1.01	1	0.98
Pneumonia Care				
Appropriate Initial Antibiotic Given	72	94%	95%	95%
Blood Culture Timing	167	100%	98%	98%

NOTE: Hospital profiles are in alphabetical order by state, then city, then hospital within the city; Rankings exclude hospitals with less than 25 cases except for patient surveys which excludes hospitals with less than 100 cases; (a) 100-299 cases; (1) The number of cases/patients is too few to report; (2) Data submitted were based on a sample of cases/patients; (3) Results are based on a shorter time period than required; (4) Data suppressed by CMS for one or more quarters; (5) Results are not available for this reporting period; (6) Fewer than 100 patients completed the HCAHPS survey; (7) No cases met the criteria for this measure; (8) The lower limit of the confidence interval cannot be calculated if the number of observed infections equals zero; (9) No data are available from the state/territory for this reporting period; (10) The scores shown reflect fewer than 50 completed surveys; (11) There were discrepancies in the data collection process; (12) This measure does not apply to this hospital for this reporting period; (13) Results cannot be calculated for this reporting period; (14) The results for this state are combined with nearby states to protect confidentiality; Please refer to the User's Guide for a full explanation of data.

Measure	Cases	This Hosp.	State Avg.	U.S. Avg.
Pregnancy and Delivery Care				
Newborn Deliveries Scheduled Early[2]	34	3%	2%	6%
Preventive Care				
Immunization for Influenza[2]	506	62%	92%	90%
Immunization for Pneumonia[2]	419	77%	92%	92%
Stroke Care				
Anticoagulation Therapy for Atrial Fibrillation[1,2]	-	-	94%	95%
Antithrombotic Therapy Timing[2]	74	97%	98%	98%
Assessed for Rehabilitation[2]	103	99%	97%	97%
Discharged on Antithrombotic Therapy[2]	80	100%	99%	99%
Discharged on Statin Medication[2]	56	100%	94%	94%
Thrombolytic Therapy Timing[1,2]	-	-	66%	66%
Venous Thromboembolism Prophylaxis[2]	112	96%	94%	94%
Written Stroke Educational Materials Given[2]	44	95%	87%	88%
Surgical Care Improvement Project				
Appropriate Beta Blocker Usage[2]	78	97%	98%	98%
Appropriate VTP Within 24 Hours[2]	223	98%	98%	98%
Controlled Postoperative Blood Glucose[2]	39	100%	97%	97%
Perioperative Temperature Management[2]	290	100%	100%	100%
Prophylactic Antibiotic Selection[2]	207	98%	99%	99%
Prophylactic Antibiotic Selection (Outpatient)	181	100%	98%	98%
Prophylactic Antibiotic Stopped[2]	198	96%	98%	98%
Prophylactic Antibiotic Timing[2]	208	99%	99%	99%
Prophylactic Antibiotic Timing (Outpatient)	71	100%	97%	98%
Urinary Catheter Removal[2]	127	99%	98%	97%
Survey of Patients' Hospital Experiences				
Area Around Room 'Always' Quiet at Night	300+	59%	60%	61%
Doctors 'Always' Communicated Well	300+	78%	81%	82%
Home Recovery Information Given	300+	83%	86%	85%
Hospital Given 9 or 10 on 10 Point Scale	300+	59%	70%	71%
Meds 'Always' Explained Before Given	300+	60%	64%	64%
Nurses 'Always' Communicated Well	300+	71%	79%	79%
Pain 'Always' Well Controlled	300+	64%	71%	71%
Room and Bathroom 'Always' Clean	300+	58%	74%	73%
Timely Help 'Always' Received	300+	56%	67%	68%
Would Definitely Recommend Hospital	300+	61%	70%	71%
Use of Medical Imaging				
Cardiac Imaging Stress Test before Surgery	228	4.8%	5.5%	5.3%
Combination Abdominal CT Scan	455	5.5%	10.1%	10.5%
Combination Brain/Sinus CT Scan	387	1.0%	2.6%	2.7%
Combination Chest CT Scan	245	1.6%	2.8%	2.7%
Follow-up Mammogram/Ultrasound	831	6.5%	8.4%	8.8%
Lumbar Spine MRI for Low Back Pain[1]	-	-	36.6%	37.2%

Northwestern Memorial Hospital

251 E Huron St
Chicago, IL 60611
URL: www.nmh.org
Type: Acute Care Hospitals
Ownership: Voluntary non-profit - Private
Phone: 312-926-2000
Fax: 312-926-3858
Emergency Services: Yes
Beds: 744

Key Personnel:
Chief of Medical Staff.......... John Clarke, MD
CEO/President............... Dean M Harrison
Cardiac Laboratory............ Alan Kadish, MD
Operating Room............. Michael Langerfeld
Quality Assurance .... Laura Lingl
Pediatric Ambulatory Care ...... Martin Myers, MD
Radiology.................... Eric Russell, MD
Infection Control.............. Steve Wolinsky, MD

Measure	Cases	This Hosp.	State Avg.	U.S. Avg.
Blood Clot Prevention and Treatment				
Anticoagulation Overlap Therapy[2]	282	95%	91%	93%
ICU Venous Thromboembolism Prophylaxis[2]	111	100%	93%	92%
Incidence of Potentially Preventable VTE[2]	156	7%	11%	10%
UFH with Dosages/Platelet Monitoring[2]	226	75%	94%	97%
Venous Thromboembolism Prophylaxis[2]	297	86%	86%	85%
Warfarin Therapy Discharge Instructions[2]	205	34%	71%	75%
Chest Pain/Possible Heart Attack Care				
Aspirin Given Within 24 Hours of Arrival[3,7]	-	-	96%	96%
Fibrinolytic Meds Within 30 Min. of Arrival[5]	-	-	65%	58%
Average Time to ECG (minutes)[3,7]	-	-	6	7
Average Time to Transfer (minutes)[5]	-	-	63	60
Children's Asthma Care				
Received Home Management Plan of Care	-	-	-	88%
Received Reliever Medication	-	-	-	100%
Received Systemic Corticosteroids	-	-	-	100%
Emergency Department				
Admittance Decision Time (minutes)[2]	246	132	89	98
Head CT Results Within 45 Min. of Arrival[7]	-	-	64%	57%
Patients Who Left ER Before Being Seen	88,850	4%	3%	2%
Time from ER Arrival to Admit. (minutes)[2]	251	351	260	274
Time from ER Arrival to Discharge (minutes)	316	225	138	134
Time in ER Before Being Evaluated (minutes)	282	51	28	26
Time to Pain Meds for Fractures (minutes)	90	62	52	57
Heart Attack Care				
Aspirin Given at Discharge	258	100%	99%	99%
Fibrinolytic Meds Within 30 Min. of Arrival[7]	-	-	33%	54%
PCI Within 90 Minutes of Arrival	57	100%	97%	96%
Statin Prescribed at Discharge	254	100%	98%	98%
Heart Failure Care				
ACE Inhibitor or ARB for LVSD	282	100%	98%	97%
Discharge Instructions Given	759	97%	96%	94%
Evaluation of LVS Function	853	100%	99%	99%
Medicare Spending				
Medicare Spending per Patient (ratio)	-	1.01	1	0.98
Pneumonia Care				
Appropriate Initial Antibiotic Given	161	95%	95%	95%
Blood Culture Timing	491	98%	98%	98%
Pregnancy and Delivery Care				
Newborn Deliveries Scheduled Early[2]	109	0%	2%	6%
Preventive Care				
Immunization for Influenza[2]	456	97%	92%	90%
Immunization for Pneumonia[2]	403	90%	92%	92%
Stroke Care				
Anticoagulation Therapy for Atrial Fibrillation	45	98%	94%	95%
Antithrombotic Therapy Timing	273	98%	98%	98%
Assessed for Rehabilitation	389	99%	97%	97%
Discharged on Antithrombotic Therapy	313	99%	99%	99%
Discharged on Statin Medication	245	97%	94%	94%
Thrombolytic Therapy Timing	18	94%	66%	66%
Venous Thromboembolism Prophylaxis	393	99%	94%	94%
Written Stroke Educational Materials Given	244	78%	87%	88%
Surgical Care Improvement Project				
Appropriate Beta Blocker Usage[2]	236	97%	98%	98%
Appropriate VTP Within 24 Hours[2]	406	100%	98%	98%
Controlled Postoperative Blood Glucose[2]	145	96%	97%	97%
Perioperative Temperature Management[2]	580	99%	100%	100%
Prophylactic Antibiotic Selection[2]	468	99%	99%	99%
Prophylactic Antibiotic Selection (Outpatient)	571	97%	98%	98%
Prophylactic Antibiotic Stopped[2]	449	98%	98%	98%
Prophylactic Antibiotic Timing[2]	470	96%	99%	99%
Prophylactic Antibiotic Timing (Outpatient)	591	94%	97%	98%
Urinary Catheter Removal[2]	413	100%	98%	97%
Survey of Patients' Hospital Experiences				
Area Around Room 'Always' Quiet at Night	300+	65%	60%	61%
Doctors 'Always' Communicated Well	300+	80%	81%	82%
Home Recovery Information Given	300+	80%	86%	85%
Hospital Given 9 or 10 on 10 Point Scale	300+	75%	70%	71%
Meds 'Always' Explained Before Given	300+	61%	64%	64%
Nurses 'Always' Communicated Well	300+	76%	79%	79%
Pain 'Always' Well Controlled	300+	70%	71%	71%
Room and Bathroom 'Always' Clean	300+	62%	74%	73%
Timely Help 'Always' Received	300+	60%	67%	68%
Would Definitely Recommend Hospital	300+	80%	70%	71%
Use of Medical Imaging				
Cardiac Imaging Stress Test before Surgery	2,217	6.8%	5.5%	5.3%
Combination Abdominal CT Scan	4,510	14.8%	10.1%	10.5%
Combination Brain/Sinus CT Scan	1,599	1.2%	2.6%	2.7%
Combination Chest CT Scan	5,326	0.0%	2.8%	2.7%
Follow-up Mammogram/Ultrasound	6,582	9.0%	8.4%	8.8%
Lumbar Spine MRI for Low Back Pain	390	35.6%	36.6%	37.2%

Norwegian - American Hospital

1044 N Francisco Ave
Chicago, IL 60622
URL: www.nahospital.org
Type: Acute Care Hospitals
Ownership: Voluntary non-profit - Private
Phone: 773-292-8200
Fax: 773-278-3531
Emergency Services: Yes
Beds: 200

Key Personnel:
Emergency Room .... Lilia Charpe, RN
Chief of Medical Staff.......... Jose De Leon, MD
Operating Room............. Rose Garcia, RN
President................... Manuel Martinez, MD
Quality Assurance .... James McCracken
Pediatric In-Patient Care .... Henry Munez, MD

Measure	Cases	This Hosp.	State Avg.	U.S. Avg.
Blood Clot Prevention and Treatment				
Anticoagulation Overlap Therapy[2]	34	65%	91%	93%
ICU Venous Thromboembolism Prophylaxis[2]	61	57%	93%	92%
Incidence of Potentially Preventable VTE[1,2]	-	-	11%	10%
UFH with Dosages/Platelet Monitoring[2]	18	100%	94%	97%
Venous Thromboembolism Prophylaxis[2]	191	54%	86%	85%
Warfarin Therapy Discharge Instructions[2]	26	73%	71%	75%
Chest Pain/Possible Heart Attack Care				
Aspirin Given Within 24 Hours of Arrival[5]	-	-	96%	96%
Fibrinolytic Meds Within 30 Min. of Arrival[5]	-	-	65%	58%
Average Time to ECG (minutes)[5]	-	-	6	7
Average Time to Transfer (minutes)[5]	-	-	63	60
Children's Asthma Care				
Received Home Management Plan of Care	-	-	-	88%
Received Reliever Medication	-	-	-	100%
Received Systemic Corticosteroids	-	-	-	100%
Emergency Department				
Admittance Decision Time (minutes)[2]	239	124	89	98
Head CT Results Within 45 Min. of Arrival[3,7]	-	-	64%	57%
Patients Who Left ER Before Being Seen	26,589	4%	3%	2%
Time from ER Arrival to Admit. (minutes)[2]	302	309	260	274
Time from ER Arrival to Discharge (minutes)	360	150	138	134
Time in ER Before Being Evaluated (minutes)	436	16	28	26
Time to Pain Meds for Fractures (minutes)[3]	47	44	52	57
Heart Attack Care				
Aspirin Given at Discharge	26	88%	99%	99%
Fibrinolytic Meds Within 30 Min. of Arrival[7]	-	-	33%	54%
PCI Within 90 Minutes of Arrival[1]	-	-	97%	96%
Statin Prescribed at Discharge	20	90%	98%	98%
Heart Failure Care				
ACE Inhibitor or ARB for LVSD	43	93%	98%	97%
Discharge Instructions Given	83	98%	96%	94%
Evaluation of LVS Function	96	97%	99%	99%
Medicare Spending				
Medicare Spending per Patient (ratio)	-	1.07	1	0.98
Pneumonia Care				
Appropriate Initial Antibiotic Given	57	89%	95%	95%
Blood Culture Timing	98	98%	98%	98%
Pregnancy and Delivery Care				
Newborn Deliveries Scheduled Early[2]	32	0%	2%	6%
Preventive Care				
Immunization for Influenza[2]	501	67%	92%	90%
Immunization for Pneumonia[2]	437	78%	92%	92%
Stroke Care				
Anticoagulation Therapy for Atrial Fibrillation[7]	-	-	94%	95%
Antithrombotic Therapy Timing[1]	-	-	98%	98%
Assessed for Rehabilitation[1]	-	-	97%	97%
Discharged on Antithrombotic Therapy[1]	-	-	99%	99%
Discharged on Statin Medication[1]	-	-	94%	94%
Thrombolytic Therapy Timing[1]	-	-	66%	66%
Venous Thromboembolism Prophylaxis	12	100%	94%	94%
Written Stroke Educational Materials Given[1]	-	-	87%	88%
Surgical Care Improvement Project				
Appropriate Beta Blocker Usage[1]	-	-	98%	98%
Appropriate VTP Within 24 Hours	48	85%	98%	98%
Controlled Postoperative Blood Glucose[7]	-	-	97%	97%
Perioperative Temperature Management	63	98%	100%	100%
Prophylactic Antibiotic Selection	27	96%	99%	99%
Prophylactic Antibiotic Selection (Outpatient)	23	100%	98%	98%
Prophylactic Antibiotic Stopped	27	100%	98%	98%

NOTE: Hospital profiles are in alphabetical order by state, then city, then hospital within the city; Rankings exclude hospitals with less than 25 cases except for patient surveys which excludes hospitals with less than 100 cases; (a) 100-299 cases; (1) The number of cases/patients is too few to report; (2) Data submitted were based on a sample of cases/patients; (3) Results are based on a shorter time period than required; (4) Data suppressed by CMS for one or more quarters; (5) Results are not available for this reporting period; (6) Fewer than 100 patients completed the HCAHPS survey; (7) No cases met the criteria for this measure; (8) The lower limit of the confidence interval cannot be calculated if the number of observed infections equals zero; (9) No data are available from the state/territory for this reporting period; (10) The scores shown reflect fewer than 50 completed surveys; (11) There were discrepancies in the data collection process; (12) This measure does not apply to this hospital for this reporting period; (13) Results cannot be calculated for this reporting period; (14) The results for this state are combined with nearby states to protect confidentiality; Please refer to the User's Guide for a full explanation of data.

Measure	Cases	This Hosp.	State Avg.	U.S. Avg.
Prophylactic Antibiotic Timing	27	85%	99%	99%
Prophylactic Antibiotic Timing (Outpatient)	29	72%	97%	98%
Urinary Catheter Removal	26	77%	98%	97%
Survey of Patients' Hospital Experiences				
Area Around Room 'Always' Quiet at Night	300+	52%	60%	61%
Doctors 'Always' Communicated Well	300+	74%	81%	82%
Home Recovery Information Given	300+	76%	86%	85%
Hospital Given 9 or 10 on 10 Point Scale	300+	50%	70%	71%
Meds 'Always' Explained Before Given	300+	48%	64%	64%
Nurses 'Always' Communicated Well	300+	60%	79%	79%
Pain 'Always' Well Controlled	300+	55%	71%	71%
Room and Bathroom 'Always' Clean	300+	59%	74%	73%
Timely Help 'Always' Received	300+	53%	67%	68%
Would Definitely Recommend Hospital	300+	47%	70%	71%
Use of Medical Imaging				
Cardiac Imaging Stress Test before Surgery	72	6.9%	5.5%	5.3%
Combination Abdominal CT Scan	191	11.5%	10.1%	10.5%
Combination Brain/Sinus CT Scan[1]	-	-	2.6%	2.7%
Combination Chest CT Scan	75	2.7%	2.8%	2.7%
Follow-up Mammogram/Ultrasound	262	9.9%	8.4%	8.8%
Lumbar Spine MRI for Low Back Pain[1]	-	-	36.6%	37.2%

Presence Our Lady of the Resurrection Medical Center

5645 W Addison
Chicago, IL 60634
Phone: 773-282-7000
Fax: 773-794-8353
URL: www.reshealth.org
Type: Acute Care Hospitals
Emergency Services: Yes
Ownership: Voluntary non-profit - Private
Beds: 264

Key Personnel:

Quality Assurance . . . . George Einhorn
Operating Room. . . . . Crystal Mobley, RN
Infection Control. . . . . Ann Marie Ogle, RN
Cardiac Laboratory. . . . . Sue Schaub
Chief of Medical Staff . . . . Shirish Shah, MD
CEO/President. . . . . John Short

Measure	Cases	This Hosp.	State Avg.	U.S. Avg.
Blood Clot Prevention and Treatment				
Anticoagulation Overlap Therapy[2]	58	98%	91%	93%
ICU Venous Thromboembolism Prophylaxis[2]	116	99%	93%	92%
Incidence of Potentially Preventable VTE[2]	15	7%	11%	10%
UFH with Dosages/Platelet Monitoring[2]	13	100%	94%	97%
Venous Thromboembolism Prophylaxis[2]	348	89%	86%	85%
Warfarin Therapy Discharge Instructions[2]	29	83%	71%	75%
Chest Pain/Possible Heart Attack Care				
Aspirin Given Within 24 Hours of Arrival[1,3]	-	-	96%	96%
Fibrinolytic Meds Within 30 Min. of Arrival[3,7]	-	-	65%	58%
Average Time to ECG (minutes)[1,3]	-	-	6	7
Average Time to Transfer (minutes)[3,7]	-	-	63	60
Children's Asthma Care				
Received Home Management Plan of Care	-	-	-	88%
Received Reliever Medication	-	-	-	100%
Received Systemic Corticosteroids	-	-	-	100%
Emergency Department				
Admittance Decision Time (minutes)[2]	856	150	89	98
Head CT Results Within 45 Min. of Arrival[1]	-	-	64%	57%
Patients Who Left ER Before Being Seen	45,754	1%	3%	2%
Time from ER Arrival to Admit. (minutes)[2]	893	277	260	274
Time from ER Arrival to Discharge (minutes)	398	144	138	134
Time in ER Before Being Evaluated (minutes)	423	34	28	26
Time to Pain Meds for Fractures (minutes)	151	45	52	57
Heart Attack Care				
Aspirin Given at Discharge	150	100%	99%	99%
Fibrinolytic Meds Within 30 Min. of Arrival[7]	-	-	33%	54%
PCI Within 90 Minutes of Arrival	20	100%	97%	96%
Statin Prescribed at Discharge	146	99%	98%	98%
Heart Failure Care				
ACE Inhibitor or ARB for LVSD	82	100%	98%	97%
Discharge Instructions Given	195	100%	96%	94%
Evaluation of LVS Function	330	100%	99%	99%
Medicare Spending				
Medicare Spending per Patient (ratio)	-	1.09	1	0.98
Pneumonia Care				
Appropriate Initial Antibiotic Given	115	98%	95%	95%
Blood Culture Timing	169	99%	98%	98%
Pregnancy and Delivery Care				
Newborn Deliveries Scheduled Early[7]	-	-	2%	6%
Preventive Care				
Immunization for Influenza[2]	635	97%	92%	90%
Immunization for Pneumonia[2]	946	95%	92%	92%
Stroke Care				
Anticoagulation Therapy for Atrial Fibrillation[2]	16	100%	94%	95%
Antithrombotic Therapy Timing[2]	103	100%	98%	98%
Assessed for Rehabilitation[2]	133	100%	97%	97%
Discharged on Antithrombotic Therapy[2]	112	100%	99%	99%
Discharged on Statin Medication[2]	91	100%	94%	94%
Thrombolytic Therapy Timing[2]	13	85%	66%	66%
Venous Thromboembolism Prophylaxis[2]	140	96%	94%	94%
Written Stroke Educational Materials Given[2]	55	93%	87%	88%
Surgical Care Improvement Project				
Appropriate Beta Blocker Usage	76	97%	98%	98%
Appropriate VTP Within 24 Hours	245	98%	98%	98%
Controlled Postoperative Blood Glucose[7]	-	-	97%	97%
Perioperative Temperature Management	284	100%	100%	100%
Prophylactic Antibiotic Selection	120	99%	99%	99%
Prophylactic Antibiotic Selection (Outpatient)	106	99%	98%	98%
Prophylactic Antibiotic Stopped	108	97%	98%	98%
Prophylactic Antibiotic Timing	120	99%	99%	99%
Prophylactic Antibiotic Timing (Outpatient)	104	99%	97%	98%
Urinary Catheter Removal	110	97%	98%	97%
Survey of Patients' Hospital Experiences				
Area Around Room 'Always' Quiet at Night	300+	47%	60%	61%
Doctors 'Always' Communicated Well	300+	79%	81%	82%
Home Recovery Information Given	300+	82%	86%	85%
Hospital Given 9 or 10 on 10 Point Scale	300+	62%	70%	71%
Meds 'Always' Explained Before Given	300+	56%	64%	64%
Nurses 'Always' Communicated Well	300+	75%	79%	79%
Pain 'Always' Well Controlled	300+	69%	71%	71%
Room and Bathroom 'Always' Clean	300+	71%	74%	73%
Timely Help 'Always' Received	300+	61%	67%	68%
Would Definitely Recommend Hospital	300+	62%	70%	71%
Use of Medical Imaging				
Cardiac Imaging Stress Test before Surgery	383	6.0%	5.5%	5.3%
Combination Abdominal CT Scan	610	7.7%	10.1%	10.5%
Combination Brain/Sinus CT Scan	874	2.6%	2.6%	2.7%
Combination Chest CT Scan	287	1.7%	2.8%	2.7%
Follow-up Mammogram/Ultrasound	1,057	7.9%	8.4%	8.8%
Lumbar Spine MRI for Low Back Pain	76	48.7%	36.6%	37.2%

Presence Resurrection Medical Center

7435 W Talcott Avenue
Chicago, IL 60631
Phone: 773-774-8000
Fax: 773-792-9926
URL: www.reshealthcare.org
Type: Acute Care Hospitals
Emergency Services: Yes
Ownership: Voluntary non-profit - Church
Beds: 434

Key Personnel:

Infection Control. . . . . Marcia Beckerdite
CEO/President. . . . . Sandra Brue
Chief of Medical Staff. . . . . Rosa Cubria
Quality Assurance . . . . Vicky Malone
Radiology. . . . . John McGreevy
Pediatric Ambulatory Care . . . . . . Kathy Nierzwicki, RN
Operating Room. . . . . Debbie Serwa

Measure	Cases	This Hosp.	State Avg.	U.S. Avg.
Blood Clot Prevention and Treatment				
Anticoagulation Overlap Therapy[2]	67	93%	91%	93%
ICU Venous Thromboembolism Prophylaxis[2]	147	98%	93%	92%
Incidence of Potentially Preventable VTE[1,2]	-	-	11%	10%
UFH with Dosages/Platelet Monitoring[1,2]	-	-	94%	97%
Venous Thromboembolism Prophylaxis[2]	306	86%	86%	85%
Warfarin Therapy Discharge Instructions[2]	40	18%	71%	75%
Chest Pain/Possible Heart Attack Care				
Aspirin Given Within 24 Hours of Arrival[1,3]	-	-	96%	96%
Fibrinolytic Meds Within 30 Min. of Arrival[5]	-	-	65%	58%
Average Time to ECG (minutes)[1,3]	-	-	6	7
Average Time to Transfer (minutes)[5]	-	-	63	60
Children's Asthma Care				
Received Home Management Plan of Care	-	-	-	88%
Received Reliever Medication	-	-	-	100%
Received Systemic Corticosteroids	-	-	-	100%
Emergency Department				
Admittance Decision Time (minutes)[2]	753	68	89	98
Head CT Results Within 45 Min. of Arrival	12	58%	64%	57%
Patients Who Left ER Before Being Seen	40,201	0%	3%	2%
Time from ER Arrival to Admit. (minutes)[2]	755	220	260	274
Time from ER Arrival to Discharge (minutes)	357	128	138	134
Time in ER Before Being Evaluated (minutes)	213	14	28	26
Time to Pain Meds for Fractures (minutes)	291	48	52	57
Heart Attack Care				
Aspirin Given at Discharge	331	100%	99%	99%
Fibrinolytic Meds Within 30 Min. of Arrival[7]	-	-	33%	54%
PCI Within 90 Minutes of Arrival	65	100%	97%	96%
Statin Prescribed at Discharge	330	99%	98%	98%
Heart Failure Care				
ACE Inhibitor or ARB for LVSD	116	97%	98%	97%
Discharge Instructions Given	387	100%	96%	94%
Evaluation of LVS Function	608	100%	99%	99%
Medicare Spending				
Medicare Spending per Patient (ratio)	-	1.13	1	0.98
Pneumonia Care				
Appropriate Initial Antibiotic Given	151	99%	95%	95%
Blood Culture Timing	342	100%	98%	98%
Pregnancy and Delivery Care				
Newborn Deliveries Scheduled Early	100	1%	2%	6%
Preventive Care				
Immunization for Influenza[2]	571	65%	92%	90%
Immunization for Pneumonia[2]	808	67%	92%	92%
Stroke Care				
Anticoagulation Therapy for Atrial Fibrillation	24	96%	94%	95%
Antithrombotic Therapy Timing	193	99%	98%	98%
Assessed for Rehabilitation	205	99%	97%	97%
Discharged on Antithrombotic Therapy	179	99%	99%	99%
Discharged on Statin Medication	134	90%	94%	94%
Thrombolytic Therapy Timing	56	38%	66%	66%
Venous Thromboembolism Prophylaxis	228	92%	94%	94%
Written Stroke Educational Materials Given	70	93%	87%	88%
Surgical Care Improvement Project				
Appropriate Beta Blocker Usage[2]	219	99%	98%	98%
Appropriate VTP Within 24 Hours[2]	412	100%	98%	98%
Controlled Postoperative Blood Glucose[2]	115	96%	97%	97%
Perioperative Temperature Management[2]	522	100%	100%	100%
Prophylactic Antibiotic Selection[2]	464	100%	99%	99%
Prophylactic Antibiotic Selection (Outpatient)	254	96%	98%	98%
Prophylactic Antibiotic Stopped[2]	449	98%	98%	98%
Prophylactic Antibiotic Timing[2]	464	100%	99%	99%
Prophylactic Antibiotic Timing (Outpatient)	259	95%	97%	98%
Urinary Catheter Removal[2]	292	99%	98%	97%
Survey of Patients' Hospital Experiences				
Area Around Room 'Always' Quiet at Night	300+	57%	60%	61%
Doctors 'Always' Communicated Well	300+	79%	81%	82%
Home Recovery Information Given	300+	86%	86%	85%
Hospital Given 9 or 10 on 10 Point Scale	300+	65%	70%	71%
Meds 'Always' Explained Before Given	300+	62%	64%	64%
Nurses 'Always' Communicated Well	300+	80%	79%	79%
Pain 'Always' Well Controlled	300+	73%	71%	71%
Room and Bathroom 'Always' Clean	300+	74%	74%	73%
Timely Help 'Always' Received	300+	63%	67%	68%
Would Definitely Recommend Hospital	300+	70%	70%	71%
Use of Medical Imaging				
Cardiac Imaging Stress Test before Surgery	741	5.8%	5.5%	5.3%
Combination Abdominal CT Scan	1,296	12.9%	10.1%	10.5%
Combination Brain/Sinus CT Scan	1,372	2.6%	2.6%	2.7%
Combination Chest CT Scan	783	0.8%	2.8%	2.7%
Follow-up Mammogram/Ultrasound	2,762	11.9%	8.4%	8.8%
Lumbar Spine MRI for Low Back Pain	176	42.0%	36.6%	37.2%

NOTE: Hospital profiles are in alphabetical order by state, then city, then hospital within the city; Rankings exclude hospitals with less than 25 cases except for patient surveys which excludes hospitals with less than 100 cases; (a) 100-299 cases; (1) The number of cases/patients is too few to report; (2) Data submitted were based on a sample of cases/patients; (3) Results are based on a shorter time period than required; (4) Data suppressed by CMS for one or more quarters; (5) Results are not available for this reporting period; (6) Fewer than 100 patients completed the HCAHPS survey; (7) No cases met the criteria for this measure; (8) The lower limit of the confidence interval cannot be calculated if the number of observed infections equals zero; (9) No data are available from the state/territory for this reporting period; (10) The scores shown reflect fewer than 50 completed surveys; (11) There were discrepancies in the data collection process; (12) This measure does not apply to this hospital for this reporting period; (13) Results cannot be calculated for this reporting period; (14) The results for this state are combined with nearby states to protect confidentiality; Please refer to the User's Guide for a full explanation of data.

Presence Saint Joseph Hospital - Chicago

2900 North Lake Shore Drive
Chicago, IL 60657
Phone: 773-665-3000
Fax: 773-665-6502
URL: www.res-health.org
Type: Acute Care Hospitals
Emergency Services: Yes
Ownership: Voluntary non-profit - Church
Beds: 492

Key Personnel:

CEO/President............... Sandra Bruce
Hemotology Center........... Leon Dragon
Radiology................... Howard Gerard, MD
Chief of Medical Staff.......... Andrew Gorchynky
Emergency Room............ Geoffery Grassle
Quality Assurance.......... Margaret Heinrich
Cardiac Laboratory........... Kathy Pyme
Anesthesiology.............. Cathy Watt, MD

Measure	Cases	This Hosp.	State Avg.	U.S. Avg.
Blood Clot Prevention and Treatment				
Anticoagulation Overlap Therapy[2]	20	100%	91%	93%
ICU Venous Thromboembolism Prophylaxis[2]	83	100%	93%	92%
Incidence of Potentially Preventable VTE[1,2]	-	-	11%	10%
UFH with Dosages/Platelet Monitoring[1,2]	-	-	94%	97%
Venous Thromboembolism Prophylaxis[2]	354	90%	86%	85%
Warfarin Therapy Discharge Instructions[2]	11	64%	71%	75%
Chest Pain/Possible Heart Attack Care				
Aspirin Given Within 24 Hours of Arrival[5]	-	-	96%	96%
Fibrinolytic Meds Within 30 Min. of Arrival[5]	-	-	65%	58%
Average Time to ECG (minutes)[5]	-	-	6	7
Average Time to Transfer (minutes)[5]	-	-	63	60
Children's Asthma Care				
Received Home Management Plan of Care	-	-	-	88%
Received Reliever Medication	-	-	-	100%
Received Systemic Corticosteroids	-	-	-	100%
Emergency Department				
Admittance Decision Time (minutes)[2]	364	105	89	98
Head CT Results Within 45 Min. of Arrival[1]	-	-	64%	57%
Patients Who Left ER Before Being Seen	20,222	0%	3%	2%
Time from ER Arrival to Admit. (minutes)[2]	364	212	260	274
Time from ER Arrival to Discharge (minutes)	368	112	138	134
Time in ER Before Being Evaluated (minutes)	406	8	28	26
Time to Pain Meds for Fractures (minutes)	38	50	52	57
Heart Attack Care				
Aspirin Given at Discharge	82	100%	99%	99%
Fibrinolytic Meds Within 30 Min. of Arrival[7]	-	-	33%	54%
PCI Within 90 Minutes of Arrival[1]	-	-	97%	96%
Statin Prescribed at Discharge	74	99%	98%	98%
Heart Failure Care				
ACE Inhibitor or ARB for LVSD	49	98%	98%	97%
Discharge Instructions Given	202	100%	96%	94%
Evaluation of LVS Function	277	100%	99%	99%
Medicare Spending				
Medicare Spending per Patient (ratio)	-	1.04	1	0.98
Pneumonia Care				
Appropriate Initial Antibiotic Given	69	100%	95%	95%
Blood Culture Timing	181	99%	98%	98%
Pregnancy and Delivery Care				
Newborn Deliveries Scheduled Early[2]	22	5%	2%	6%
Preventive Care				
Immunization for Influenza[2]	533	64%	92%	90%
Immunization for Pneumonia[2]	524	72%	92%	92%
Stroke Care				
Anticoagulation Therapy for Atrial Fibrillation[1]	-	-	94%	95%
Antithrombotic Therapy Timing	54	98%	98%	98%
Assessed for Rehabilitation	53	98%	97%	97%
Discharged on Antithrombotic Therapy	48	94%	99%	99%
Discharged on Statin Medication	43	93%	94%	94%
Thrombolytic Therapy Timing	12	8%	66%	66%
Venous Thromboembolism Prophylaxis	56	95%	94%	94%
Written Stroke Educational Materials Given	22	86%	87%	88%
Surgical Care Improvement Project				
Appropriate Beta Blocker Usage[2]	111	100%	98%	98%
Appropriate VTP Within 24 Hours[2]	302	100%	98%	98%
Controlled Postoperative Blood Glucose[2]	65	97%	97%	97%
Perioperative Temperature Management[2]	336	100%	100%	100%
Prophylactic Antibiotic Selection[2]	281	100%	99%	99%
Prophylactic Antibiotic Selection (Outpatient)	192	97%	98%	98%
Prophylactic Antibiotic Stopped[2]	279	99%	98%	98%
Prophylactic Antibiotic Timing[2]	281	99%	99%	99%
Prophylactic Antibiotic Timing (Outpatient)	192	99%	97%	98%
Urinary Catheter Removal[2]	92	100%	98%	97%
Survey of Patients' Hospital Experiences				
Area Around Room 'Always' Quiet at Night	300+	57%	60%	61%
Doctors 'Always' Communicated Well	300+	76%	81%	82%
Home Recovery Information Given	300+	86%	86%	85%
Hospital Given 9 or 10 on 10 Point Scale	300+	71%	70%	71%
Meds 'Always' Explained Before Given	300+	58%	64%	64%
Nurses 'Always' Communicated Well	300+	76%	79%	79%
Pain 'Always' Well Controlled	300+	63%	71%	71%
Room and Bathroom 'Always' Clean	300+	67%	74%	73%
Timely Help 'Always' Received	300+	59%	67%	68%
Would Definitely Recommend Hospital	300+	74%	70%	71%
Use of Medical Imaging				
Cardiac Imaging Stress Test before Surgery	395	5.3%	5.5%	5.3%
Combination Abdominal CT Scan	431	5.8%	10.1%	10.5%
Combination Brain/Sinus CT Scan	459	1.3%	2.6%	2.7%
Combination Chest CT Scan	302	0.3%	2.8%	2.7%
Follow-up Mammogram/Ultrasound	1,386	6.1%	8.4%	8.8%
Lumbar Spine MRI for Low Back Pain	85	40.0%	36.6%	37.2%

Presence Saints Mary & Elizabeth Medical Center

2233 W Division St
Chicago, IL 60622
Phone: 312-770-2000
Fax: 312-770-2392
URL: www.reshealth.org
Type: Acute Care Hospitals
Emergency Services: Yes
Ownership: Voluntary non-profit - Church
Beds: 387

Key Personnel:

Infection Control.............. Pat Alexander, RN
Operating Room............... Gail Alkovich
Quality Assurance............. Patti Graham, RN
CEO/President................ Margaret McDermott
Radiology.................... William Plos
Cardiac Laboratory............ John Sedivy
Chief of Medical Staff.......... Hugo Velrade, MD

Measure	Cases	This Hosp.	State Avg.	U.S. Avg.
Blood Clot Prevention and Treatment				
Anticoagulation Overlap Therapy[2]	67	96%	91%	93%
ICU Venous Thromboembolism Prophylaxis[2]	58	98%	93%	92%
Incidence of Potentially Preventable VTE[1,2]	-	-	11%	10%
UFH with Dosages/Platelet Monitoring[2]	39	100%	94%	97%
Venous Thromboembolism Prophylaxis[2]	321	92%	86%	85%
Warfarin Therapy Discharge Instructions[2]	44	100%	71%	75%
Chest Pain/Possible Heart Attack Care				
Aspirin Given Within 24 Hours of Arrival[1]	-	-	96%	96%
Fibrinolytic Meds Within 30 Min. of Arrival[5]	-	-	65%	58%
Average Time to ECG (minutes)[1]	-	-	6	7
Average Time to Transfer (minutes)[5]	-	-	63	60
Children's Asthma Care				
Received Home Management Plan of Care	-	-	-	88%
Received Reliever Medication	-	-	-	100%
Received Systemic Corticosteroids	-	-	-	100%
Emergency Department				
Admittance Decision Time (minutes)[2]	561	136	89	98
Head CT Results Within 45 Min. of Arrival	15	7%	64%	57%
Patients Who Left ER Before Being Seen	69,677	2%	3%	2%
Time from ER Arrival to Admit. (minutes)[2]	570	314	260	274
Time from ER Arrival to Discharge (minutes)	403	155	138	134
Time in ER Before Being Evaluated (minutes)	464	36	28	26
Time to Pain Meds for Fractures (minutes)	285	63	52	57
Heart Attack Care				
Aspirin Given at Discharge	147	100%	99%	99%
Fibrinolytic Meds Within 30 Min. of Arrival[7]	-	-	33%	54%
PCI Within 90 Minutes of Arrival	29	93%	97%	96%
Statin Prescribed at Discharge	141	100%	98%	98%
Heart Failure Care				
ACE Inhibitor or ARB for LVSD	100	100%	98%	97%
Discharge Instructions Given	199	100%	96%	94%
Evaluation of LVS Function	236	100%	99%	99%
Medicare Spending				
Medicare Spending per Patient (ratio)	-	1.02	1	0.98
Pneumonia Care				
Appropriate Initial Antibiotic Given	154	99%	95%	95%
Blood Culture Timing	325	99%	98%	98%
Pregnancy and Delivery Care				
Newborn Deliveries Scheduled Early[2]	33	3%	2%	6%
Preventive Care				
Immunization for Influenza[2]	714	94%	92%	90%
Immunization for Pneumonia[2]	709	92%	92%	92%
Stroke Care				
Anticoagulation Therapy for Atrial Fibrillation[1,2]	-	-	94%	95%
Antithrombotic Therapy Timing[2]	126	100%	98%	98%
Assessed for Rehabilitation[2]	140	99%	97%	97%
Discharged on Antithrombotic Therapy[2]	126	100%	99%	99%
Discharged on Statin Medication[2]	106	100%	94%	94%
Thrombolytic Therapy Timing[2]	12	83%	66%	66%
Venous Thromboembolism Prophylaxis[2]	144	100%	94%	94%
Written Stroke Educational Materials Given[2]	73	100%	87%	88%
Surgical Care Improvement Project				
Appropriate Beta Blocker Usage[2]	113	100%	98%	98%
Appropriate VTP Within 24 Hours[2]	392	99%	98%	98%
Controlled Postoperative Blood Glucose[2]	43	93%	97%	97%
Perioperative Temperature Management[2]	455	100%	100%	100%
Prophylactic Antibiotic Selection[2]	341	100%	99%	99%
Prophylactic Antibiotic Selection (Outpatient)	137	99%	98%	98%
Prophylactic Antibiotic Stopped[2]	318	100%	98%	98%
Prophylactic Antibiotic Timing[2]	341	100%	99%	99%
Prophylactic Antibiotic Timing (Outpatient)	145	94%	97%	98%
Urinary Catheter Removal[2]	189	100%	98%	97%
Survey of Patients' Hospital Experiences				
Area Around Room 'Always' Quiet at Night	300+	58%	60%	61%
Doctors 'Always' Communicated Well	300+	78%	81%	82%
Home Recovery Information Given	300+	82%	86%	85%
Hospital Given 9 or 10 on 10 Point Scale	300+	66%	70%	71%
Meds 'Always' Explained Before Given	300+	59%	64%	64%
Nurses 'Always' Communicated Well	300+	77%	79%	79%
Pain 'Always' Well Controlled	300+	66%	71%	71%
Room and Bathroom 'Always' Clean	300+	60%	74%	73%
Timely Help 'Always' Received	300+	60%	67%	68%
Would Definitely Recommend Hospital	300+	69%	70%	71%
Use of Medical Imaging				
Cardiac Imaging Stress Test before Surgery	517	3.9%	5.5%	5.3%
Combination Abdominal CT Scan	831	7.5%	10.1%	10.5%
Combination Brain/Sinus CT Scan	733	1.4%	2.6%	2.7%
Combination Chest CT Scan	164	1.2%	2.8%	2.7%
Follow-up Mammogram/Ultrasound	1,115	4.3%	8.4%	8.8%
Lumbar Spine MRI for Low Back Pain	107	42.1%	36.6%	37.2%

Provident Hospital of Chicago

500 E 51st St
Chicago, IL 60615
Phone: 312-572-2000
Fax: 312-572-2796
URL: www.providentfoundation.org
Type: Acute Care Hospitals
Emergency Services: Yes
Ownership: Government - Local
Beds: 243

Key Personnel:

Quality Assurance............ Joseph Coty
Chief of Medical Staff.......... James Myles

Measure	Cases	This Hosp.	State Avg.	U.S. Avg.
Blood Clot Prevention and Treatment				
Anticoagulation Overlap Therapy[2]	17	94%	91%	93%
ICU Venous Thromboembolism Prophylaxis[2,7]	-	-	93%	92%
Incidence of Potentially Preventable VTE[1,2]	-	-	11%	10%
UFH with Dosages/Platelet Monitoring[1,2]	-	-	94%	97%
Venous Thromboembolism Prophylaxis[2]	186	69%	86%	85%
Warfarin Therapy Discharge Instructions[2]	15	100%	71%	75%
Chest Pain/Possible Heart Attack Care				
Aspirin Given Within 24 Hours of Arrival	54	89%	96%	96%
Fibrinolytic Meds Within 30 Min. of Arrival[7]	-	-	65%	58%
Average Time to ECG (minutes)	62	80	6	7
Average Time to Transfer (minutes)[1]	-	-	63	60
Children's Asthma Care				
Received Home Management Plan of Care	-	-	-	88%
Received Reliever Medication	-	-	-	100%
Received Systemic Corticosteroids	-	-	-	100%

NOTE: Hospital profiles are in alphabetical order by state, then city, then hospital within the city; Rankings exclude hospitals with less than 25 cases except for patient surveys which excludes hospitals with less than 100 cases; (a) 100-299 cases; (1) The number of cases/patients is too few to report; (2) Data submitted were based on a sample of cases/patients; (3) Results are based on a shorter time period than required; (4) Data suppressed by CMS for one or more quarters; (5) Results are not available for this reporting period; (6) Fewer than 100 patients completed the HCAHPS survey; (7) No cases met the criteria for this measure; (8) The lower limit of the confidence interval cannot be calculated if the number of observed infections equals zero; (9) No data are available from the state/territory for this reporting period; (10) The scores shown reflect fewer than 50 completed surveys; (11) There were discrepancies in the data collection process; (12) This measure does not apply to this hospital for this reporting period; (13) Results cannot be calculated for this reporting period; (14) The results for this state are combined with nearby states to protect confidentiality; Please refer to the User's Guide for a full explanation of data.

Measure	Cases	This Hosp.	State Avg.	U.S. Avg.
Emergency Department				
Admittance Decision Time (minutes)[2]	512	242	89	98
Head CT Results Within 45 Min. of Arrival[1,3]	-	-	64%	57%
Patients Who Left ER Before Being Seen	36,921	10%	3%	2%
Time from ER Arrival to Admit. (minutes)[2]	513	647	260	274
Time from ER Arrival to Discharge (minutes)	370	230	138	134
Time in ER Before Being Evaluated (minutes)	417	109	28	26
Time to Pain Meds for Fractures (minutes)	45	126	52	57
Heart Attack Care				
Aspirin Given at Discharge[5]	-	-	99%	99%
Fibrinolytic Meds Within 30 Min. of Arrival[5]	-	-	33%	54%
PCI Within 90 Minutes of Arrival[5]	-	-	97%	96%
Statin Prescribed at Discharge[5]	-	-	98%	98%
Heart Failure Care				
ACE Inhibitor or ARB for LVSD[2]	86	99%	98%	97%
Discharge Instructions Given[2]	175	91%	96%	94%
Evaluation of LVS Function[2]	175	95%	99%	99%
Medicare Spending				
Medicare Spending per Patient (ratio)	-	0.73	1	0.98
Pneumonia Care				
Appropriate Initial Antibiotic Given[2]	50	98%	95%	95%
Blood Culture Timing[2]	54	83%	98%	98%
Pregnancy and Delivery Care				
Newborn Deliveries Scheduled Early[7]	-	-	2%	6%
Preventive Care				
Immunization for Influenza[2]	311	83%	92%	90%
Immunization for Pneumonia[2]	412	78%	92%	92%
Stroke Care				
Anticoagulation Therapy for Atrial Fibrillation[5]	-	-	94%	95%
Antithrombotic Therapy Timing[5]	-	-	98%	98%
Assessed for Rehabilitation[5]	-	-	97%	97%
Discharged on Antithrombotic Therapy[5]	-	-	99%	99%
Discharged on Statin Medication[5]	-	-	94%	94%
Thrombolytic Therapy Timing[5]	-	-	66%	66%
Venous Thromboembolism Prophylaxis[5]	-	-	94%	94%
Written Stroke Educational Materials Given[5]	-	-	87%	88%
Surgical Care Improvement Project				
Appropriate Beta Blocker Usage[1,2]	-	-	98%	98%
Appropriate VTP Within 24 Hours[2]	70	100%	98%	98%
Controlled Postoperative Blood Glucose[2,7]	-	-	97%	97%
Perioperative Temperature Management[2]	80	98%	100%	100%
Prophylactic Antibiotic Selection[2]	76	97%	99%	99%
Prophylactic Antibiotic Selection (Outpatient)	20	85%	98%	98%
Prophylactic Antibiotic Stopped[2]	76	99%	98%	98%
Prophylactic Antibiotic Timing[2]	76	100%	99%	99%
Prophylactic Antibiotic Timing (Outpatient)	18	50%	97%	98%
Urinary Catheter Removal[2,7]	-	-	98%	97%
Survey of Patients' Hospital Experiences				
Area Around Room 'Always' Quiet at Night	(a)	78%	60%	61%
Doctors 'Always' Communicated Well	(a)	85%	81%	82%
Home Recovery Information Given	(a)	77%	86%	85%
Hospital Given 9 or 10 on 10 Point Scale	(a)	62%	70%	71%
Meds 'Always' Explained Before Given	(a)	64%	64%	64%
Nurses 'Always' Communicated Well	(a)	80%	79%	79%
Pain 'Always' Well Controlled	(a)	73%	71%	71%
Room and Bathroom 'Always' Clean	(a)	75%	74%	73%
Timely Help 'Always' Received	(a)	65%	67%	68%
Would Definitely Recommend Hospital	(a)	62%	70%	71%
Use of Medical Imaging				
Cardiac Imaging Stress Test before Surgery[1]	-	-	5.5%	5.3%
Combination Abdominal CT Scan	96	34.4%	10.1%	10.5%
Combination Brain/Sinus CT Scan[1]	-	-	2.6%	2.7%
Combination Chest CT Scan	68	27.9%	2.8%	2.7%
Follow-up Mammogram/Ultrasound	526	1.9%	8.4%	8.8%
Lumbar Spine MRI for Low Back Pain[7]	-	-	36.6%	37.2%

Roseland Community Hospital

45 W 111th Street
Chicago, IL 60628
URL: www.roselandhospital.org
Phone: 773-995-3000
Fax: 773-995-1052
Type: Acute Care Hospitals
Emergency Services: Yes
Ownership: Voluntary non-profit - Other
Beds: 162

Key Personnel:

Radiology.................. Conrad Brown
CEO/President.............. Tim Egan
Administrator................ Kathleen Kinsella
Quality Assurance........... Mary Walker
Operating Room.............. Gladys Williams

Measure	Cases	This Hosp.	State Avg.	U.S. Avg.
Blood Clot Prevention and Treatment				
Anticoagulation Overlap Therapy[2]	28	68%	91%	93%
ICU Venous Thromboembolism Prophylaxis[2]	60	90%	93%	92%
Incidence of Potentially Preventable VTE[1,2]	-	-	11%	10%
UFH with Dosages/Platelet Monitoring[2]	23	96%	94%	97%
Venous Thromboembolism Prophylaxis[2]	174	96%	86%	85%
Warfarin Therapy Discharge Instructions[2]	23	74%	71%	75%
Chest Pain/Possible Heart Attack Care				
Aspirin Given Within 24 Hours of Arrival[1,3]	-	-	96%	96%
Fibrinolytic Meds Within 30 Min. of Arrival[3,7]	-	-	65%	58%
Average Time to ECG (minutes)[3]	12	17	6	7
Average Time to Transfer (minutes)[1,3]	-	-	63	60
Children's Asthma Care				
Received Home Management Plan of Care	-	-	-	88%
Received Reliever Medication	-	-	-	100%
Received Systemic Corticosteroids	-	-	-	100%
Emergency Department				
Admittance Decision Time (minutes)[2]	459	185	89	98
Head CT Results Within 45 Min. of Arrival[1,3]	-	-	64%	57%
Patients Who Left ER Before Being Seen	27,188	6%	3%	2%
Time from ER Arrival to Admit. (minutes)[2]	460	480	260	274
Time from ER Arrival to Discharge (minutes)	417	180	138	134
Time in ER Before Being Evaluated (minutes)	434	75	28	26
Time to Pain Meds for Fractures (minutes)[3]	11	98	52	57
Heart Attack Care				
Aspirin Given at Discharge[2]	12	83%	99%	99%
Fibrinolytic Meds Within 30 Min. of Arrival[2,7]	-	-	33%	54%
PCI Within 90 Minutes of Arrival[2,7]	-	-	97%	96%
Statin Prescribed at Discharge[1,2]	-	-	98%	98%
Heart Failure Care				
ACE Inhibitor or ARB for LVSD[2]	39	92%	98%	97%
Discharge Instructions Given[2]	148	78%	96%	94%
Evaluation of LVS Function[2]	139	99%	99%	99%
Medicare Spending				
Medicare Spending per Patient (ratio)	-	1.01	1	0.98
Pneumonia Care				
Appropriate Initial Antibiotic Given[2]	94	82%	95%	95%
Blood Culture Timing[2]	111	97%	98%	98%
Pregnancy and Delivery Care				
Newborn Deliveries Scheduled Early	47	0%	2%	6%
Preventive Care				
Immunization for Influenza[2]	471	100%	92%	90%
Immunization for Pneumonia[2]	523	98%	92%	92%
Stroke Care				
Anticoagulation Therapy for Atrial Fibrillation[3,7]	-	-	94%	95%
Antithrombotic Therapy Timing[1,3]	-	-	98%	98%
Assessed for Rehabilitation[1,3]	-	-	97%	97%
Discharged on Antithrombotic Therapy[1,3]	-	-	99%	99%
Discharged on Statin Medication[1,3]	-	-	94%	94%
Thrombolytic Therapy Timing[1,3]	-	-	66%	66%
Venous Thromboembolism Prophylaxis[1,3]	-	-	94%	94%
Written Stroke Educational Materials Given[1,3]	-	-	87%	88%
Surgical Care Improvement Project				
Appropriate Beta Blocker Usage[1,2]	-	-	98%	98%
Appropriate VTP Within 24 Hours[2]	34	100%	98%	98%
Controlled Postoperative Blood Glucose[2,7]	-	-	97%	97%
Perioperative Temperature Management[2]	44	100%	100%	100%
Prophylactic Antibiotic Selection[1,2]	-	-	99%	99%
Prophylactic Antibiotic Selection (Outpatient)[5]	-	-	98%	98%
Prophylactic Antibiotic Stopped[1,2]	-	-	98%	98%
Prophylactic Antibiotic Timing[1,2]	-	-	99%	99%
Prophylactic Antibiotic Timing (Outpatient)[5]	-	-	97%	98%
Urinary Catheter Removal[2]	11	91%	98%	97%
Survey of Patients' Hospital Experiences				
Area Around Room 'Always' Quiet at Night[3]	(a)	60%	60%	61%
Doctors 'Always' Communicated Well[3]	(a)	70%	81%	82%
Home Recovery Information Given[3]	(a)	65%	86%	85%
Hospital Given 9 or 10 on 10 Point Scale[3]	(a)	41%	70%	71%
Meds 'Always' Explained Before Given[3]	(a)	49%	64%	64%
Nurses 'Always' Communicated Well[3]	(a)	64%	79%	79%
Pain 'Always' Well Controlled[3]	(a)	57%	71%	71%
Room and Bathroom 'Always' Clean[3]	(a)	63%	74%	73%
Timely Help 'Always' Received[3]	(a)	41%	67%	68%
Would Definitely Recommend Hospital[3]	(a)	37%	70%	71%
Use of Medical Imaging				
Cardiac Imaging Stress Test before Surgery[1]	-	-	5.5%	5.3%
Combination Abdominal CT Scan	76	53.9%	10.1%	10.5%
Combination Brain/Sinus CT Scan	279	6.1%	2.6%	2.7%
Combination Chest CT Scan	88	11.4%	2.8%	2.7%
Follow-up Mammogram/Ultrasound	100	6.0%	8.4%	8.8%
Lumbar Spine MRI for Low Back Pain[7]	-	-	36.6%	37.2%

Rush University Medical Center

1653 West Congress Parkway
Chicago, IL 60612
URL: www.ruch.edu
Phone: 312-942-5000
Fax: 312-942-8021
Type: Acute Care Hospitals
Emergency Services: No
Ownership: Voluntary non-profit - Private
Beds: 618

Key Personnel:

Chief of Medical Staff.......... David A Ansell, MD
CEO/President.................. Larry M Goodman, MD
Pediatric In-Patient Care....... Samuel P Gotoff, MD
Emergency Room................ Paul K Hanashiro, MD
Intensive Care Unit............. Joan Mathien, RN
Quality Assurance.............. Susan O'Leary
Radiology...................... Jerry Petasnick, MD
Infection Control............... Gorden Trenholme, MD

Measure	Cases	This Hosp.	State Avg.	U.S. Avg.
Blood Clot Prevention and Treatment				
Anticoagulation Overlap Therapy[2]	163	82%	91%	93%
ICU Venous Thromboembolism Prophylaxis[2]	113	95%	93%	92%
Incidence of Potentially Preventable VTE[2]	56	2%	11%	10%
UFH with Dosages/Platelet Monitoring[2]	145	74%	94%	97%
Venous Thromboembolism Prophylaxis[2]	274	93%	86%	85%
Warfarin Therapy Discharge Instructions[2]	114	75%	71%	75%
Chest Pain/Possible Heart Attack Care				
Aspirin Given Within 24 Hours of Arrival[5]	-	-	96%	96%
Fibrinolytic Meds Within 30 Min. of Arrival[5]	-	-	65%	58%
Average Time to ECG (minutes)[5]	-	-	6	7
Average Time to Transfer (minutes)[5]	-	-	63	60
Children's Asthma Care				
Received Home Management Plan of Care	-	-	-	88%
Received Reliever Medication	-	-	-	100%
Received Systemic Corticosteroids	-	-	-	100%
Emergency Department				
Admittance Decision Time (minutes)[2]	406	170	89	98
Head CT Results Within 45 Min. of Arrival[1,3]	-	-	64%	57%
Patients Who Left ER Before Being Seen	63,360	6%	3%	2%
Time from ER Arrival to Admit. (minutes)[2]	410	358	260	274
Time from ER Arrival to Discharge (minutes)	336	239	138	134
Time in ER Before Being Evaluated (minutes)	331	107	28	26
Time to Pain Meds for Fractures (minutes)	104	92	52	57
Heart Attack Care				
Aspirin Given at Discharge	167	99%	99%	99%
Fibrinolytic Meds Within 30 Min. of Arrival[7]	-	-	33%	54%
PCI Within 90 Minutes of Arrival	19	95%	97%	96%
Statin Prescribed at Discharge	163	99%	98%	98%
Heart Failure Care				
ACE Inhibitor or ARB for LVSD[2]	138	98%	98%	97%
Discharge Instructions Given[2]	262	100%	96%	94%
Evaluation of LVS Function[2]	294	100%	99%	99%
Medicare Spending				
Medicare Spending per Patient (ratio)	-	0.96	1	0.98
Pneumonia Care				
Appropriate Initial Antibiotic Given[2]	39	92%	95%	95%
Blood Culture Timing[2]	94	99%	98%	98%
Pregnancy and Delivery Care				
Newborn Deliveries Scheduled Early[2]	21	10%	2%	6%
Preventive Care				
Immunization for Influenza[2]	538	100%	92%	90%
Immunization for Pneumonia[2]	582	100%	92%	92%

NOTE: Hospital profiles are in alphabetical order by state, then city, then hospital within the city; Rankings exclude hospitals with less than 25 cases except for patient surveys which excludes hospitals with less than 100 cases; (a) 100-299 cases; (1) The number of cases/patients is too few to report; (2) Data submitted were based on a sample of cases/patients; (3) Results are based on a shorter time period than required; (4) Data suppressed by CMS for one or more quarters; (5) Results are not available for this reporting period; (6) Fewer than 100 patients completed the HCAHPS survey; (7) No cases met the criteria for this measure; (8) The lower limit of the confidence interval cannot be calculated if the number of observed infections equals zero; (9) No data are available from the state/territory for this reporting period; (10) The scores shown reflect fewer than 50 completed surveys; (11) There were discrepancies in the data collection process; (12) This measure does not apply to this hospital for this reporting period; (13) Results cannot be calculated for this reporting period; (14) The results for this state are combined with nearby states to protect confidentiality; Please refer to the User's Guide for a full explanation of data.

Stroke Care				
Anticoagulation Therapy for Atrial Fibrillation	33	100%	94%	95%
Antithrombotic Therapy Timing	195	98%	98%	98%
Assessed for Rehabilitation	470	100%	97%	97%
Discharged on Antithrombotic Therapy	257	100%	99%	99%
Discharged on Statin Medication	195	100%	94%	94%
Thrombolytic Therapy Timing	12	92%	66%	66%
Venous Thromboembolism Prophylaxis	521	100%	94%	94%
Written Stroke Educational Materials Given	219	95%	87%	88%
Surgical Care Improvement Project				
Appropriate Beta Blocker Usage[2]	188	99%	98%	98%
Appropriate VTP Within 24 Hours[2]	371	99%	98%	98%
Controlled Postoperative Blood Glucose[2]	107	100%	97%	97%
Perioperative Temperature Management[2]	502	100%	100%	100%
Prophylactic Antibiotic Selection[2]	423	100%	99%	99%
Prophylactic Antibiotic Selection (Outpatient)	420	99%	98%	98%
Prophylactic Antibiotic Stopped[2]	410	98%	98%	98%
Prophylactic Antibiotic Timing[2]	426	100%	99%	99%
Prophylactic Antibiotic Timing (Outpatient)	421	98%	97%	98%
Urinary Catheter Removal[2]	345	100%	98%	97%
Survey of Patients' Hospital Experiences				
Area Around Room 'Always' Quiet at Night	300+	70%	60%	61%
Doctors 'Always' Communicated Well	300+	82%	81%	82%
Home Recovery Information Given	300+	87%	86%	85%
Hospital Given 9 or 10 on 10 Point Scale	300+	80%	70%	71%
Meds 'Always' Explained Before Given	300+	66%	64%	64%
Nurses 'Always' Communicated Well	300+	83%	79%	79%
Pain 'Always' Well Controlled	300+	72%	71%	71%
Room and Bathroom 'Always' Clean	300+	75%	74%	73%
Timely Help 'Always' Received	300+	66%	67%	68%
Would Definitely Recommend Hospital	300+	83%	70%	71%
Use of Medical Imaging				
Cardiac Imaging Stress Test before Surgery	1,292	6.3%	5.5%	5.3%
Combination Abdominal CT Scan	534	5.1%	10.1%	10.5%
Combination Brain/Sinus CT Scan	751	2.8%	2.6%	2.7%
Combination Chest CT Scan	323	6.8%	2.8%	2.7%
Follow-up Mammogram/Ultrasound	3,001	11.5%	8.4%	8.8%
Lumbar Spine MRI for Low Back Pain[1]	-	-	36.6%	37.2%

Saint Anthony Hospital

2875 West 19th Street
Chicago, IL 60623
Phone: 773-521-1710
Fax: 773-521-7902
URL: www.cath-health.org
Type: Acute Care Hospitals
Emergency Services: Yes
Ownership: Voluntary non-profit - Church
Beds: 183

Key Personnel:
CEO/President. . . . . Kathleen K DeVine
Quality Assurance . . . . Tom Forbes
Operating Room. . . . . Oscar Herbas
Chief of Medical Staff. . . . . Rolando Lara, MD
Pediatric In-Patient Care . . . . Denisse Roque-Leon
Infection Control. . . . . Julie Sammarco
Cardiac Laboratory. . . . . Fran Washington

Measure	Cases	This Hosp.	State Avg.	U.S. Avg.
Blood Clot Prevention and Treatment				
Anticoagulation Overlap Therapy[2]	19	100%	91%	93%
ICU Venous Thromboembolism Prophylaxis[2]	100	99%	93%	92%
Incidence of Potentially Preventable VTE[1,2]	-	-	11%	10%
UFH with Dosages/Platelet Monitoring[1,2]	-	-	94%	97%
Venous Thromboembolism Prophylaxis[2]	213	99%	86%	85%
Warfarin Therapy Discharge Instructions[2]	17	100%	71%	75%
Chest Pain/Possible Heart Attack Care				
Aspirin Given Within 24 Hours of Arrival[1]	-	-	96%	96%
Fibrinolytic Meds Within 30 Min. of Arrival[7]	-	-	65%	58%
Average Time to ECG (minutes)[1]	-	-	6	7
Average Time to Transfer (minutes)[1]	-	-	63	60
Children's Asthma Care				
Received Home Management Plan of Care	-	-		88%
Received Reliever Medication	-	-	-	100%
Received Systemic Corticosteroids	-	-	-	100%
Emergency Department				
Admittance Decision Time (minutes)[2]	529	103	89	98
Head CT Results Within 45 Min. of Arrival[1]	-	-	64%	57%
Patients Who Left ER Before Being Seen	37,920	1%	3%	2%
Time from ER Arrival to Admit. (minutes)[2]	534	280	260	274
Time from ER Arrival to Discharge (minutes)	351	163	138	134
Time in ER Before Being Evaluated (minutes)	370	86	28	26
Time to Pain Meds for Fractures (minutes)	179	47	52	57
Heart Attack Care				
Aspirin Given at Discharge	11	100%	99%	99%
Fibrinolytic Meds Within 30 Min. of Arrival[7]	-	-	33%	54%
PCI Within 90 Minutes of Arrival[7]	-	-	97%	96%
Statin Prescribed at Discharge[1]	-	-	98%	98%
Heart Failure Care				
ACE Inhibitor or ARB for LVSD	43	100%	98%	97%
Discharge Instructions Given	93	100%	96%	94%
Evaluation of LVS Function	108	100%	99%	99%
Medicare Spending				
Medicare Spending per Patient (ratio)	-	1.03	1	0.98
Pneumonia Care				
Appropriate Initial Antibiotic Given	62	100%	95%	95%
Blood Culture Timing	112	100%	98%	98%
Pregnancy and Delivery Care				
Newborn Deliveries Scheduled Early[2]	37	0%	2%	6%
Preventive Care				
Immunization for Influenza[2]	463	98%	92%	90%
Immunization for Pneumonia[2]	466	100%	92%	92%
Stroke Care				
Anticoagulation Therapy for Atrial Fibrillation[7]	-	-	94%	95%
Antithrombotic Therapy Timing	16	100%	98%	98%
Assessed for Rehabilitation	21	100%	97%	97%
Discharged on Antithrombotic Therapy	20	100%	99%	99%
Discharged on Statin Medication	13	100%	94%	94%
Thrombolytic Therapy Timing[7]	-	-	66%	66%
Venous Thromboembolism Prophylaxis	22	100%	94%	94%
Written Stroke Educational Materials Given	14	100%	87%	88%
Surgical Care Improvement Project				
Appropriate Beta Blocker Usage[1]	-	-	98%	98%
Appropriate VTP Within 24 Hours	98	100%	98%	98%
Controlled Postoperative Blood Glucose[7]	-	-	97%	97%
Perioperative Temperature Management	122	100%	100%	100%
Prophylactic Antibiotic Selection	45	98%	99%	99%
Prophylactic Antibiotic Selection (Outpatient)	63	97%	98%	98%
Prophylactic Antibiotic Stopped	37	100%	98%	98%
Prophylactic Antibiotic Timing	46	100%	99%	99%
Prophylactic Antibiotic Timing (Outpatient)	65	95%	97%	98%
Urinary Catheter Removal	39	100%	98%	97%
Survey of Patients' Hospital Experiences				
Area Around Room 'Always' Quiet at Night	300+	56%	60%	61%
Doctors 'Always' Communicated Well	300+	80%	81%	82%
Home Recovery Information Given	300+	81%	86%	85%
Hospital Given 9 or 10 on 10 Point Scale	300+	64%	70%	71%
Meds 'Always' Explained Before Given	300+	50%	64%	64%
Nurses 'Always' Communicated Well	300+	73%	79%	79%
Pain 'Always' Well Controlled	300+	63%	71%	71%
Room and Bathroom 'Always' Clean	300+	72%	74%	73%
Timely Help 'Always' Received	300+	58%	67%	68%
Would Definitely Recommend Hospital	300+	66%	70%	71%
Use of Medical Imaging				
Cardiac Imaging Stress Test before Surgery	134	5.2%	5.5%	5.3%
Combination Abdominal CT Scan	218	1.4%	10.1%	10.5%
Combination Brain/Sinus CT Scan[1]	-	-	2.6%	2.7%
Combination Chest CT Scan	86	0.0%	2.8%	2.7%
Follow-up Mammogram/Ultrasound	375	8.5%	8.4%	8.8%
Lumbar Spine MRI for Low Back Pain[1]	-	-	36.6%	37.2%

Saint Bernard Hospital

326 W 64th St
Chicago, IL 60621
Phone: 773-962-3900
Fax: 773-962-0034
E-mail: info@stbh.org
URL: www.stbernardhospital.com
Type: Acute Care Hospitals
Emergency Services: Yes
Ownership: Voluntary non-profit - Private
Beds: 183

Key Personnel:
Quality Assurance . . . . Roland Abellera
Radiology. . . . . James Beckett
Patient Relations . . . . Roland Campbell
Chief of Medical Staff. . . . . Rogelio Cave
CEO/President. . . . . Charles Holland

Measure	Cases	This Hosp.	State Avg.	U.S. Avg.
Blood Clot Prevention and Treatment				
Anticoagulation Overlap Therapy[2]	29	86%	91%	93%
ICU Venous Thromboembolism Prophylaxis[2]	41	98%	93%	92%
Incidence of Potentially Preventable VTE[1,2]	-	-	11%	10%
UFH with Dosages/Platelet Monitoring[1,2]	-	-	94%	97%
Venous Thromboembolism Prophylaxis[2]	307	95%	86%	85%
Warfarin Therapy Discharge Instructions[2]	23	100%	71%	75%
Chest Pain/Possible Heart Attack Care				
Aspirin Given Within 24 Hours of Arrival	53	91%	96%	96%
Fibrinolytic Meds Within 30 Min. of Arrival[7]	-	-	65%	58%
Average Time to ECG (minutes)	54	3	6	7
Average Time to Transfer (minutes)[1]	-	-	63	60
Children's Asthma Care				
Received Home Management Plan of Care	-	-		88%
Received Reliever Medication	-	-	-	100%
Received Systemic Corticosteroids	-	-	-	100%
Emergency Department				
Admittance Decision Time (minutes)[2]	616	305	89	98
Head CT Results Within 45 Min. of Arrival[1]	-	-	64%	57%
Patients Who Left ER Before Being Seen	43,452	12%	3%	2%
Time from ER Arrival to Admit. (minutes)[2]	616	442	260	274
Time from ER Arrival to Discharge (minutes)	327	198	138	134
Time in ER Before Being Evaluated (minutes)	390	42	28	26
Time to Pain Meds for Fractures (minutes)	26	65	52	57
Heart Attack Care				
Aspirin Given at Discharge[1]	-	-	99%	99%
Fibrinolytic Meds Within 30 Min. of Arrival[7]	-	-	33%	54%
PCI Within 90 Minutes of Arrival[7]	-	-	97%	96%
Statin Prescribed at Discharge[1]	-	-	98%	98%
Heart Failure Care				
ACE Inhibitor or ARB for LVSD	101	94%	98%	97%
Discharge Instructions Given	259	96%	96%	94%
Evaluation of LVS Function	286	99%	99%	99%
Medicare Spending				
Medicare Spending per Patient (ratio)	-	1.07	1	0.98
Pneumonia Care				
Appropriate Initial Antibiotic Given	84	96%	95%	95%
Blood Culture Timing	24	100%	98%	98%
Pregnancy and Delivery Care				
Newborn Deliveries Scheduled Early[2]	29	0%	2%	6%
Preventive Care				
Immunization for Influenza[2]	522	70%	92%	90%
Immunization for Pneumonia[2]	568	81%	92%	92%
Stroke Care				
Anticoagulation Therapy for Atrial Fibrillation[1]	-	-	94%	95%
Antithrombotic Therapy Timing	24	100%	98%	98%
Assessed for Rehabilitation	23	96%	97%	97%
Discharged on Antithrombotic Therapy	15	100%	99%	99%
Discharged on Statin Medication	17	53%	94%	94%
Thrombolytic Therapy Timing[7]	-	-	66%	66%
Venous Thromboembolism Prophylaxis	28	96%	94%	94%
Written Stroke Educational Materials Given[1]	-	-	87%	88%
Surgical Care Improvement Project				
Appropriate Beta Blocker Usage[1]	-	-	98%	98%
Appropriate VTP Within 24 Hours	64	100%	98%	98%
Controlled Postoperative Blood Glucose[7]	-	-	97%	97%
Perioperative Temperature Management	71	97%	100%	100%
Prophylactic Antibiotic Selection[1]	-	-	99%	99%
Prophylactic Antibiotic Selection (Outpatient)[1]	-	-	98%	98%
Prophylactic Antibiotic Stopped[1]	-	-	98%	98%
Prophylactic Antibiotic Timing[1]	-	-	99%	99%
Prophylactic Antibiotic Timing (Outpatient)[1]	-	-	97%	98%
Urinary Catheter Removal[1]	-	-	98%	97%
Survey of Patients' Hospital Experiences				
Area Around Room 'Always' Quiet at Night	300+	61%	60%	61%
Doctors 'Always' Communicated Well	300+	72%	81%	82%
Home Recovery Information Given	300+	73%	86%	85%
Hospital Given 9 or 10 on 10 Point Scale	300+	46%	70%	71%
Meds 'Always' Explained Before Given	300+	50%	64%	64%
Nurses 'Always' Communicated Well	300+	63%	79%	79%
Pain 'Always' Well Controlled	300+	59%	71%	71%

NOTE: Hospital profiles are in alphabetical order by state, then city, then hospital within the city; Rankings exclude hospitals with less than 25 cases except for patient surveys which excludes hospitals with less than 100 cases; (a) 100-299 cases; (1) The number of cases/patients is too few to report; (2) Data submitted were based on a sample of cases/patients; (3) Results are based on a shorter time period than required; (4) Data suppressed by CMS for one or more quarters; (5) Results are not available for this reporting period; (6) Fewer than 100 patients completed the HCAHPS survey; (7) No cases met the criteria for this measure; (8) The lower limit of the confidence interval cannot be calculated if the number of observed infections equals zero; (9) No data are available from the state/territory for this reporting period; (10) The scores shown reflect fewer than 50 completed surveys; (11) There were discrepancies in the data collection process; (12) This measure does not apply to this hospital for this reporting period; (13) Results cannot be calculated for this reporting period; (14) The results for this state are combined with nearby states to protect confidentiality; Please refer to the User's Guide for a full explanation of data.

Measure	Cases	This Hosp.	State Avg.	U.S. Avg.
Room and Bathroom 'Always' Clean	300+	65%	74%	73%
Timely Help 'Always' Received	300+	44%	67%	68%
Would Definitely Recommend Hospital	300+	37%	70%	71%
Use of Medical Imaging				
Cardiac Imaging Stress Test before Surgery[1]	-	-	5.5%	5.3%
Combination Abdominal CT Scan	138	7.2%	10.1%	10.5%
Combination Brain/Sinus CT Scan[1]	-	-	2.6%	2.7%
Combination Chest CT Scan	77	5.2%	2.8%	2.7%
Follow-up Mammogram/Ultrasound	187	4.8%	8.4%	8.8%
Lumbar Spine MRI for Low Back Pain[7]	-	-	36.6%	37.2%

South Shore Hospital

8012 South Crandon Avenue
Chicago, IL 60617
Phone: 773-768-0810
Fax: 773-768-8154
URL: www.southshorehospital.com
Type: Acute Care Hospitals
Emergency Services: Yes
Ownership: Voluntary non-profit - Private
Beds: 170

Key Personnel:

CEO/President. . . . . Richard Aubut
Chair/CEO . . . . Kenneth Kirkland
Emergency Room . . . . Jackie Levandowski, RN
Operating Room. . . . . Flortina McCoo, RN
Quality Assurance . . . . Marisel Pineda
Patient Relations . . . . Leslie M Rogers
Chief of Medical Staff. . . . . John Stevenson, MD
Radiology. . . . . Tim Williams

Measure	Cases	This Hosp.	State Avg.	U.S. Avg.
Blood Clot Prevention and Treatment				
Anticoagulation Overlap Therapy[1,2]	-	-	91%	93%
ICU Venous Thromboembolism Prophylaxis[2]	46	67%	93%	92%
Incidence of Potentially Preventable VTE[1,2]	-	-	11%	10%
UFH with Dosages/Platelet Monitoring[1,2]	-	-	94%	97%
Venous Thromboembolism Prophylaxis[2]	283	54%	86%	85%
Warfarin Therapy Discharge Instructions[1,2]	-	-	71%	75%
Chest Pain/Possible Heart Attack Care				
Aspirin Given Within 24 Hours of Arrival[1,3]	-	-	96%	96%
Fibrinolytic Meds Within 30 Min. of Arrival[3,7]	-	-	65%	58%
Average Time to ECG (minutes)[3]	11	33	6	7
Average Time to Transfer (minutes)[1,3]	-	-	63	60
Children's Asthma Care				
Received Home Management Plan of Care	-	-	-	88%
Received Reliever Medication	-	-	-	100%
Received Systemic Corticosteroids	-	-	-	100%
Emergency Department				
Admittance Decision Time (minutes)[2]	443	164	89	98
Head CT Results Within 45 Min. of Arrival[1,3]	-	-	64%	57%
Patients Who Left ER Before Being Seen	14,980	4%	3%	2%
Time from ER Arrival to Admit. (minutes)[2]	443	387	260	274
Time from ER Arrival to Discharge (minutes)	236	224	138	134
Time in ER Before Being Evaluated (minutes)	283	9	28	26
Time to Pain Meds for Fractures (minutes)[1,3]	-	-	52	57
Heart Attack Care				
Aspirin Given at Discharge	13	92%	99%	99%
Fibrinolytic Meds Within 30 Min. of Arrival[7]	-	-	33%	54%
PCI Within 90 Minutes of Arrival[7]	-	-	97%	96%
Statin Prescribed at Discharge	13	77%	98%	98%
Heart Failure Care				
ACE Inhibitor or ARB for LVSD	54	85%	98%	97%
Discharge Instructions Given	113	100%	96%	94%
Evaluation of LVS Function	146	96%	99%	99%
Medicare Spending				
Medicare Spending per Patient (ratio)	-	1.07	1	0.98
Pneumonia Care				
Appropriate Initial Antibiotic Given	47	87%	95%	95%
Blood Culture Timing	102	93%	98%	98%
Pregnancy and Delivery Care				
Newborn Deliveries Scheduled Early[2,7]	-	-	2%	6%
Preventive Care				
Immunization for Influenza[2]	320	86%	92%	90%
Immunization for Pneumonia[2]	488	89%	92%	92%
Stroke Care				
Anticoagulation Therapy for Atrial Fibrillation[1]	-	-	94%	95%
Antithrombotic Therapy Timing	20	95%	98%	98%
Assessed for Rehabilitation	16	81%	97%	97%
Discharged on Antithrombotic Therapy	16	94%	99%	99%
Discharged on Statin Medication[1]	-	-	94%	94%
Thrombolytic Therapy Timing[1]	-	-	66%	66%
Venous Thromboembolism Prophylaxis	21	57%	94%	94%
Written Stroke Educational Materials Given[1]	-	-	87%	88%
Surgical Care Improvement Project				
Appropriate Beta Blocker Usage[1]	-	-	98%	98%
Appropriate VTP Within 24 Hours	50	96%	98%	98%
Controlled Postoperative Blood Glucose[7]	-	-	97%	97%
Perioperative Temperature Management	18	100%	100%	100%
Prophylactic Antibiotic Selection	39	92%	99%	99%
Prophylactic Antibiotic Selection (Outpatient)[1]	-	-	98%	98%
Prophylactic Antibiotic Stopped	38	97%	98%	98%
Prophylactic Antibiotic Timing	39	87%	99%	99%
Prophylactic Antibiotic Timing (Outpatient)[1]	-	-	97%	98%
Urinary Catheter Removal[1]	-	-	98%	97%
Survey of Patients' Hospital Experiences				
Area Around Room 'Always' Quiet at Night	(a)	62%	60%	61%
Doctors 'Always' Communicated Well	(a)	72%	81%	82%
Home Recovery Information Given	(a)	71%	86%	85%
Hospital Given 9 or 10 on 10 Point Scale	(a)	48%	70%	71%
Meds 'Always' Explained Before Given	(a)	53%	64%	64%
Nurses 'Always' Communicated Well	(a)	65%	79%	79%
Pain 'Always' Well Controlled	(a)	58%	71%	71%
Room and Bathroom 'Always' Clean	(a)	64%	74%	73%
Timely Help 'Always' Received	(a)	44%	67%	68%
Would Definitely Recommend Hospital	(a)	43%	70%	71%
Use of Medical Imaging				
Cardiac Imaging Stress Test before Surgery	49	2.0%	5.5%	5.3%
Combination Abdominal CT Scan	105	54.3%	10.1%	10.5%
Combination Brain/Sinus CT Scan	166	6.6%	2.6%	2.7%
Combination Chest CT Scan	34	50.0%	2.8%	2.7%
Follow-up Mammogram/Ultrasound	202	6.9%	8.4%	8.8%
Lumbar Spine MRI for Low Back Pain[1]	-	-	36.6%	37.2%

Swedish Covenant Hospital

5145 N California Ave
Chicago, IL 60625
Phone: 773-878-8200
Fax: 773-878-6152
URL: www.swedishcovenant.org
Type: Acute Care Hospitals
Emergency Services: Yes
Ownership: Voluntary non-profit - Church
Beds: 330

Key Personnel:

Pediatric Ambulatory Care . . . . . . Roberto Espinosa, MD
Pediatric In-Patient Care . . . . Roberto Espinosa, MD
CEO/President. . . . . Mark Newton
Quality Assurance . . . . Janis Rueping
Chief of Medical Staff. . . . . Albert Saporta, MD
Cardiac Laboratory. . . . . Jerrad Shapiro
Operating Room. . . . . Mary Shehan
Radiology. . . . . Bruce Silver, MD

Measure	Cases	This Hosp.	State Avg.	U.S. Avg.
Blood Clot Prevention and Treatment				
Anticoagulation Overlap Therapy[2]	74	59%	91%	93%
ICU Venous Thromboembolism Prophylaxis[2]	53	92%	93%	92%
Incidence of Potentially Preventable VTE[2]	13	23%	11%	10%
UFH with Dosages/Platelet Monitoring[2]	64	100%	94%	97%
Venous Thromboembolism Prophylaxis[2]	407	85%	86%	85%
Warfarin Therapy Discharge Instructions[2]	43	91%	71%	75%
Chest Pain/Possible Heart Attack Care				
Aspirin Given Within 24 Hours of Arrival	22	100%	96%	96%
Fibrinolytic Meds Within 30 Min. of Arrival[3,7]	-	-	65%	58%
Average Time to ECG (minutes)	25	10	6	7
Average Time to Transfer (minutes)[3,7]	-	-	63	60
Children's Asthma Care				
Received Home Management Plan of Care	-	-	-	88%
Received Reliever Medication	-	-	-	100%
Received Systemic Corticosteroids	-	-	-	100%
Emergency Department				
Admittance Decision Time (minutes)[2]	429	100	89	98
Head CT Results Within 45 Min. of Arrival[1]	-	-	64%	57%
Patients Who Left ER Before Being Seen	49,834	4%	3%	2%
Time from ER Arrival to Admit. (minutes)[2]	437	269	260	274
Time from ER Arrival to Discharge (minutes)	410	178	138	134
Time in ER Before Being Evaluated (minutes)	494	75	28	26
Time to Pain Meds for Fractures (minutes)	252	80	52	57
Heart Attack Care				
Aspirin Given at Discharge	224	99%	99%	99%
Fibrinolytic Meds Within 30 Min. of Arrival[7]	-	-	33%	54%
PCI Within 90 Minutes of Arrival	32	84%	97%	96%
Statin Prescribed at Discharge	222	99%	98%	98%
Heart Failure Care				
ACE Inhibitor or ARB for LVSD	130	100%	98%	97%
Discharge Instructions Given	315	100%	96%	94%
Evaluation of LVS Function	414	100%	99%	99%
Medicare Spending				
Medicare Spending per Patient (ratio)	-	1.04	1	0.98
Pneumonia Care				
Appropriate Initial Antibiotic Given[2]	160	99%	95%	95%
Blood Culture Timing[2]	317	98%	98%	98%
Pregnancy and Delivery Care				
Newborn Deliveries Scheduled Early[2]	43	5%	2%	6%
Preventive Care				
Immunization for Influenza[2]	555	90%	92%	90%
Immunization for Pneumonia[2]	678	92%	92%	92%
Stroke Care				
Anticoagulation Therapy for Atrial Fibrillation[2]	20	50%	94%	95%
Antithrombotic Therapy Timing[2]	81	95%	98%	98%
Assessed for Rehabilitation[2]	114	98%	97%	97%
Discharged on Antithrombotic Therapy[2]	92	95%	99%	99%
Discharged on Statin Medication[2]	81	93%	94%	94%
Thrombolytic Therapy Timing[2]	14	29%	66%	66%
Venous Thromboembolism Prophylaxis[2]	114	91%	94%	94%
Written Stroke Educational Materials Given[2]	57	91%	87%	88%
Surgical Care Improvement Project				
Appropriate Beta Blocker Usage[2]	199	94%	98%	98%
Appropriate VTP Within 24 Hours[2]	427	98%	98%	98%
Controlled Postoperative Blood Glucose[2]	76	99%	97%	97%
Perioperative Temperature Management[2]	589	100%	100%	100%
Prophylactic Antibiotic Selection[2]	356	99%	99%	99%
Prophylactic Antibiotic Selection (Outpatient)	168	98%	98%	98%
Prophylactic Antibiotic Stopped[2]	336	100%	98%	98%
Prophylactic Antibiotic Timing[2]	356	99%	99%	99%
Prophylactic Antibiotic Timing (Outpatient)	168	99%	97%	98%
Urinary Catheter Removal[2]	301	97%	98%	97%
Survey of Patients' Hospital Experiences				
Area Around Room 'Always' Quiet at Night	300+	48%	60%	61%
Doctors 'Always' Communicated Well	300+	78%	81%	82%
Home Recovery Information Given	300+	80%	86%	85%
Hospital Given 9 or 10 on 10 Point Scale	300+	63%	70%	71%
Meds 'Always' Explained Before Given	300+	55%	64%	64%
Nurses 'Always' Communicated Well	300+	72%	79%	79%
Pain 'Always' Well Controlled	300+	70%	71%	71%
Room and Bathroom 'Always' Clean	300+	71%	74%	73%
Timely Help 'Always' Received	300+	63%	67%	68%
Would Definitely Recommend Hospital	300+	66%	70%	71%
Use of Medical Imaging				
Cardiac Imaging Stress Test before Surgery	849	6.4%	5.5%	5.3%
Combination Abdominal CT Scan	1,124	11.8%	10.1%	10.5%
Combination Brain/Sinus CT Scan	988	3.2%	2.6%	2.7%
Combination Chest CT Scan	622	2.3%	2.8%	2.7%
Follow-up Mammogram/Ultrasound	1,625	10.5%	8.4%	8.8%
Lumbar Spine MRI for Low Back Pain	287	36.9%	36.6%	37.2%

Thorek Memorial Hospital

850 W Irving Park Rd
Chicago, IL 60613
Phone: 312-525-6780
Fax: 773-975-6703
URL: www.thorek.org
Type: Acute Care Hospitals
Emergency Services: Yes
Ownership: Voluntary non-profit - Private
Beds: 218

Key Personnel:

Radiology. . . . . Peter Berger, MD
Quality Assurance . . . . John Danielson
Emergency Room . . . . Effie Heale
Chief of Medical Staff. . . . . Jagan Mohan, MD
Operating Room. . . . . Gregory Nacopoulos

Measure	Cases	This Hosp.	State Avg.	U.S. Avg.
Blood Clot Prevention and Treatment				
Anticoagulation Overlap Therapy[2]	16	62%	91%	93%

NOTE: Hospital profiles are in alphabetical order by state, then city, then hospital within the city; Rankings exclude hospitals with less than 25 cases except for patient surveys which excludes hospitals with less than 100 cases; (a) 100-299 cases; (1) The number of cases/patients is too few to report; (2) Data submitted were based on a sample of cases/patients; (3) Results are based on a shorter time period than required; (4) Data suppressed by CMS for one or more quarters; (5) Results are not available for this reporting period; (6) Fewer than 100 patients completed the HCAHPS survey; (7) No cases met the criteria for this measure; (8) The lower limit of the confidence interval cannot be calculated if the number of observed infections equals zero; (9) No data are available from the state/territory for this reporting period; (10) The scores shown reflect fewer than 50 completed surveys; (11) There were discrepancies in the data collection process; (12) This measure does not apply to this hospital for this reporting period; (13) Results cannot be calculated for this reporting period; (14) The results for this state are combined with nearby states to protect confidentiality; Please refer to the User's Guide for a full explanation of data.

Measure	Cases	This Hosp.	State Avg.	U.S. Avg.
ICU Venous Thromboembolism Prophylaxis[2]	56	96%	93%	92%
Incidence of Potentially Preventable VTE[1,2]	-	-	11%	10%
UFH with Dosages/Platelet Monitoring[1,2]	-	-	94%	97%
Venous Thromboembolism Prophylaxis[2]	213	79%	86%	85%
Warfarin Therapy Discharge Instructions[1,2]	-	-	71%	75%
Chest Pain/Possible Heart Attack Care				
Aspirin Given Within 24 Hours of Arrival[5]	-	-	96%	96%
Fibrinolytic Meds Within 30 Min. of Arrival[5]	-	-	65%	58%
Average Time to ECG (minutes)[5]	-	-	6	7
Average Time to Transfer (minutes)[5]	-	-	63	60
Children's Asthma Care				
Received Home Management Plan of Care	-	-	-	88%
Received Reliever Medication	-	-	-	100%
Received Systemic Corticosteroids	-	-	-	100%
Emergency Department				
Admittance Decision Time (minutes)[2]	207	125	89	98
Head CT Results Within 45 Min. of Arrival[5]	-	-	64%	57%
Patients Who Left ER Before Being Seen	8,202	0%	3%	2%
Time from ER Arrival to Admit. (minutes)[2]	248	256	260	274
Time from ER Arrival to Discharge (minutes)	311	107	138	134
Time in ER Before Being Evaluated (minutes)	320	30	28	26
Time to Pain Meds for Fractures (minutes)	27	40	52	57
Heart Attack Care				
Aspirin Given at Discharge	11	100%	99%	99%
Fibrinolytic Meds Within 30 Min. of Arrival[7]	-	-	33%	54%
PCI Within 90 Minutes of Arrival[7]	-	-	97%	96%
Statin Prescribed at Discharge[1]	-	-	98%	98%
Heart Failure Care				
ACE Inhibitor or ARB for LVSD	19	100%	98%	97%
Discharge Instructions Given	60	98%	96%	94%
Evaluation of LVS Function	77	100%	99%	99%
Medicare Spending				
Medicare Spending per Patient (ratio)	-	1.03	1	0.98
Pneumonia Care				
Appropriate Initial Antibiotic Given	31	100%	95%	95%
Blood Culture Timing	44	100%	98%	98%
Pregnancy and Delivery Care				
Newborn Deliveries Scheduled Early[7]	-	-	2%	6%
Preventive Care				
Immunization for Influenza[2]	466	95%	92%	90%
Immunization for Pneumonia[2]	558	91%	92%	92%
Stroke Care				
Anticoagulation Therapy for Atrial Fibrillation[1]	-	-	94%	95%
Antithrombotic Therapy Timing	17	76%	98%	98%
Assessed for Rehabilitation	17	82%	97%	97%
Discharged on Antithrombotic Therapy	16	75%	99%	99%
Discharged on Statin Medication	14	57%	94%	94%
Thrombolytic Therapy Timing[7]	-	-	66%	66%
Venous Thromboembolism Prophylaxis	17	76%	94%	94%
Written Stroke Educational Materials Given	12	42%	87%	88%
Surgical Care Improvement Project				
Appropriate Beta Blocker Usage	21	86%	98%	98%
Appropriate VTP Within 24 Hours	80	96%	98%	98%
Controlled Postoperative Blood Glucose[7]	-	-	97%	97%
Perioperative Temperature Management	90	100%	100%	100%
Prophylactic Antibiotic Selection	38	95%	99%	99%
Prophylactic Antibiotic Selection (Outpatient)[5]	-	-	98%	98%
Prophylactic Antibiotic Stopped	37	97%	98%	98%
Prophylactic Antibiotic Timing	38	97%	99%	99%
Prophylactic Antibiotic Timing (Outpatient)[5]	-	-	97%	98%
Urinary Catheter Removal	39	87%	98%	97%
Survey of Patients' Hospital Experiences				
Area Around Room 'Always' Quiet at Night	(a)	58%	60%	61%
Doctors 'Always' Communicated Well	(a)	75%	81%	82%
Home Recovery Information Given	(a)	82%	86%	85%
Hospital Given 9 or 10 on 10 Point Scale	(a)	52%	70%	71%
Meds 'Always' Explained Before Given	(a)	57%	64%	64%
Nurses 'Always' Communicated Well	(a)	69%	79%	79%
Pain 'Always' Well Controlled	(a)	57%	71%	71%
Room and Bathroom 'Always' Clean	(a)	63%	74%	73%
Timely Help 'Always' Received	(a)	50%	67%	68%
Would Definitely Recommend Hospital	(a)	55%	70%	71%
Use of Medical Imaging				
Cardiac Imaging Stress Test before Surgery	115	6.1%	5.5%	5.3%
Combination Abdominal CT Scan	182	6.0%	10.1%	10.5%
Combination Brain/Sinus CT Scan[1]	-	-	2.6%	2.7%
Combination Chest CT Scan	109	0.0%	2.8%	2.7%
Follow-up Mammogram/Ultrasound	243	14.4%	8.4%	8.8%
Lumbar Spine MRI for Low Back Pain[1]	-	-	36.6%	37.2%

The University of Chicago Medical Center

5841 South Maryland
Chicago, IL 60637
Phone: 773-702-1000
Fax: 773-702-9005
URL: www.uchospitals.edu
Type: Acute Care Hospitals
Emergency Services: Yes
Ownership: Voluntary non-profit - Private
Beds: 662

Key Personnel:

Radiology. . . . . Richard Baron, MD
Quality Assurance . . . . Krista Curell
Ambulatory Care . . . . Laurence Dry
Anesthesiology. . . . . David Glick
Pediatric In-Patient Care . . . . Kim Taaca, MD

Measure	Cases	This Hosp.	State Avg.	U.S. Avg.
Blood Clot Prevention and Treatment				
Anticoagulation Overlap Therapy[2]	155	98%	91%	93%
ICU Venous Thromboembolism Prophylaxis[2]	79	95%	93%	92%
Incidence of Potentially Preventable VTE[2]	85	14%	11%	10%
UFH with Dosages/Platelet Monitoring[2]	153	97%	94%	97%
Venous Thromboembolism Prophylaxis[2]	354	75%	86%	85%
Warfarin Therapy Discharge Instructions[2]	106	57%	71%	75%
Chest Pain/Possible Heart Attack Care				
Aspirin Given Within 24 Hours of Arrival[5]	-	-	96%	96%
Fibrinolytic Meds Within 30 Min. of Arrival[5]	-	-	65%	58%
Average Time to ECG (minutes)[5]	-	-	6	7
Average Time to Transfer (minutes)[5]	-	-	63	60
Children's Asthma Care				
Received Home Management Plan of Care[2]	275	84%	-	88%
Received Reliever Medication[2]	280	100%	-	100%
Received Systemic Corticosteroids[2]	279	100%	-	100%
Emergency Department				
Admittance Decision Time (minutes)[2]	447	277	89	98
Head CT Results Within 45 Min. of Arrival[5]	-	-	64%	57%
Patients Who Left ER Before Being Seen	78,857	10%	3%	2%
Time from ER Arrival to Admit. (minutes)[2]	447	504	260	274
Time from ER Arrival to Discharge (minutes)	359	259	138	134
Time in ER Before Being Evaluated (minutes)	335	79	28	26
Time to Pain Meds for Fractures (minutes)	133	27	52	57
Heart Attack Care				
Aspirin Given at Discharge	159	100%	99%	99%
Fibrinolytic Meds Within 30 Min. of Arrival[7]	-	-	33%	54%
PCI Within 90 Minutes of Arrival	31	100%	97%	96%
Statin Prescribed at Discharge	148	100%	98%	98%
Heart Failure Care				
ACE Inhibitor or ARB for LVSD[2]	133	97%	98%	97%
Discharge Instructions Given[2]	264	91%	96%	94%
Evaluation of LVS Function[2]	298	100%	99%	99%
Medicare Spending				
Medicare Spending per Patient (ratio)	-	1.02	1	0.98
Pneumonia Care				
Appropriate Initial Antibiotic Given[2]	24	92%	95%	95%
Blood Culture Timing[2]	77	96%	98%	98%
Pregnancy and Delivery Care				
Newborn Deliveries Scheduled Early[2]	21	0%	2%	6%
Preventive Care				
Immunization for Influenza[2]	610	98%	92%	90%
Immunization for Pneumonia[2]	538	97%	92%	92%
Stroke Care				
Anticoagulation Therapy for Atrial Fibrillation[1,2]	-	-	94%	95%
Antithrombotic Therapy Timing[2]	92	98%	98%	98%
Assessed for Rehabilitation[2]	118	97%	97%	97%
Discharged on Antithrombotic Therapy[2]	96	99%	99%	99%
Discharged on Statin Medication[2]	69	100%	94%	94%
Thrombolytic Therapy Timing[1,2]	-	-	66%	66%
Venous Thromboembolism Prophylaxis[2]	124	91%	94%	94%
Written Stroke Educational Materials Given[2]	47	68%	87%	88%
Surgical Care Improvement Project				
Appropriate Beta Blocker Usage[2]	221	100%	98%	98%
Appropriate VTP Within 24 Hours[2]	350	99%	98%	98%
Controlled Postoperative Blood Glucose[2]	133	98%	97%	97%
Perioperative Temperature Management[2]	576	100%	100%	100%
Prophylactic Antibiotic Selection[2]	394	100%	99%	99%
Prophylactic Antibiotic Selection (Outpatient)	517	99%	98%	98%
Prophylactic Antibiotic Stopped[2]	372	98%	98%	98%
Prophylactic Antibiotic Timing[2]	395	99%	99%	99%
Prophylactic Antibiotic Timing (Outpatient)	287	98%	97%	98%
Urinary Catheter Removal[2]	315	98%	98%	97%
Survey of Patients' Hospital Experiences				
Area Around Room 'Always' Quiet at Night	300+	54%	60%	61%
Doctors 'Always' Communicated Well	300+	80%	81%	82%
Home Recovery Information Given	300+	83%	86%	85%
Hospital Given 9 or 10 on 10 Point Scale	300+	67%	70%	71%
Meds 'Always' Explained Before Given	300+	58%	64%	64%
Nurses 'Always' Communicated Well	300+	71%	79%	79%
Pain 'Always' Well Controlled	300+	65%	71%	71%
Room and Bathroom 'Always' Clean	300+	62%	74%	73%
Timely Help 'Always' Received	300+	55%	67%	68%
Would Definitely Recommend Hospital	300+	71%	70%	71%
Use of Medical Imaging				
Cardiac Imaging Stress Test before Surgery	790	4.3%	5.5%	5.3%
Combination Abdominal CT Scan	3,514	7.6%	10.1%	10.5%
Combination Brain/Sinus CT Scan	856	2.0%	2.6%	2.7%
Combination Chest CT Scan	4,373	0.0%	2.8%	2.7%
Follow-up Mammogram/Ultrasound	2,290	8.7%	8.4%	8.8%
Lumbar Spine MRI for Low Back Pain	209	34.4%	36.6%	37.2%

University of Illinois Hospital

1740 West Taylor Saint Suite 1400
Chicago, IL 60612
Phone: 312-996-3900
Fax: 312-996-7049
URL: www.uic.edu
Type: Acute Care Hospitals
Emergency Services: Yes
Ownership: Government - State
Beds: 570

Key Personnel:

Infection Control. . . . . James L Cook, MD
CEO/President. . . . . John DeNardo
Chief of Medical Staff . . . . Lawrence Frohman, MD
Pediatric Ambulatory Care . . . . . . George R Honig, MD
Pediatric In-Patient Care . . . . George R Honig, MD
Quality Assurance . . . . Debra Krause
Radiology. . . . . Mahmood Mafee, MD
Operating Room. . . . . Barbara Vela

Measure	Cases	This Hosp.	State Avg.	U.S. Avg.
Blood Clot Prevention and Treatment				
Anticoagulation Overlap Therapy[2]	112	94%	91%	93%
ICU Venous Thromboembolism Prophylaxis[2]	88	95%	93%	92%
Incidence of Potentially Preventable VTE[2]	90	2%	11%	10%
UFH with Dosages/Platelet Monitoring[2]	129	99%	94%	97%
Venous Thromboembolism Prophylaxis[2]	348	89%	86%	85%
Warfarin Therapy Discharge Instructions[2]	77	65%	71%	75%
Chest Pain/Possible Heart Attack Care				
Aspirin Given Within 24 Hours of Arrival[5]	-	-	96%	96%
Fibrinolytic Meds Within 30 Min. of Arrival[5]	-	-	65%	58%
Average Time to ECG (minutes)[5]	-	-	6	7
Average Time to Transfer (minutes)[5]	-	-	63	60
Children's Asthma Care				
Received Home Management Plan of Care	-	-	-	88%
Received Reliever Medication	-	-	-	100%
Received Systemic Corticosteroids	-	-	-	100%
Emergency Department				
Admittance Decision Time (minutes)[2]	500	137	89	98
Head CT Results Within 45 Min. of Arrival[5]	-	-	64%	57%
Patients Who Left ER Before Being Seen	51,565	4%	3%	2%
Time from ER Arrival to Admit. (minutes)[2]	502	406	260	274
Time from ER Arrival to Discharge (minutes)	384	220	138	134
Time in ER Before Being Evaluated (minutes)	392	62	28	26
Time to Pain Meds for Fractures (minutes)	76	90	52	57
Heart Attack Care				
Aspirin Given at Discharge	112	96%	99%	99%
Fibrinolytic Meds Within 30 Min. of Arrival[7]	-	-	33%	54%
PCI Within 90 Minutes of Arrival	12	83%	97%	96%
Statin Prescribed at Discharge	112	94%	98%	98%

NOTE: Hospital profiles are in alphabetical order by state, then city, then hospital within the city; Rankings exclude hospitals with less than 25 cases except for patient surveys which excludes hospitals with less than 100 cases; (a) 100-299 cases; (1) The number of cases/patients is too few to report; (2) Data submitted were based on a sample of cases/patients; (3) Results are based on a shorter time period than required; (4) Data suppressed by CMS for one or more quarters; (5) Results are not available for this reporting period; (6) Fewer than 100 patients completed the HCAHPS survey; (7) No cases met the criteria for this measure; (8) The lower limit of the confidence interval cannot be calculated if the number of observed infections equals zero; (9) No data are available from the state/territory for this reporting period; (10) The scores shown reflect fewer than 50 completed surveys; (11) There were discrepancies in the data collection process; (12) This measure does not apply to this hospital for this reporting period; (13) Results cannot be calculated for this reporting period; (14) The results for this state are combined with nearby states to protect confidentiality; Please refer to the User's Guide for a full explanation of data.

Measure	Cases	This Hosp.	State Avg.	U.S. Avg.
Heart Failure Care				
ACE Inhibitor or ARB for LVSD[2]	140	96%	98%	97%
Discharge Instructions Given[2]	294	96%	96%	94%
Evaluation of LVS Function[2]	306	100%	99%	99%
Medicare Spending				
Medicare Spending per Patient (ratio)	-	0.97	1	0.98
Pneumonia Care				
Appropriate Initial Antibiotic Given[2]	53	96%	95%	95%
Blood Culture Timing[2]	163	99%	98%	98%
Pregnancy and Delivery Care				
Newborn Deliveries Scheduled Early[2]	30	7%	2%	6%
Preventive Care				
Immunization for Influenza[2]	644	95%	92%	90%
Immunization for Pneumonia[2]	542	97%	92%	92%
Stroke Care				
Anticoagulation Therapy for Atrial Fibrillation	11	100%	94%	95%
Antithrombotic Therapy Timing	97	96%	98%	98%
Assessed for Rehabilitation	248	98%	97%	97%
Discharged on Antithrombotic Therapy	106	99%	99%	99%
Discharged on Statin Medication	91	100%	94%	94%
Thrombolytic Therapy Timing[1]	-	-	66%	66%
Venous Thromboembolism Prophylaxis	270	100%	94%	94%
Written Stroke Educational Materials Given	140	92%	87%	88%
Surgical Care Improvement Project				
Appropriate Beta Blocker Usage[2]	168	95%	98%	98%
Appropriate VTP Within 24 Hours[2]	421	97%	98%	98%
Controlled Postoperative Blood Glucose[2]	48	98%	97%	97%
Perioperative Temperature Management[2]	528	100%	100%	100%
Prophylactic Antibiotic Selection[2]	393	96%	99%	99%
Prophylactic Antibiotic Selection (Outpatient)	251	95%	98%	98%
Prophylactic Antibiotic Stopped[2]	374	98%	98%	98%
Prophylactic Antibiotic Timing[2]	394	99%	99%	99%
Prophylactic Antibiotic Timing (Outpatient)	196	94%	97%	98%
Urinary Catheter Removal[2]	287	96%	98%	97%
Survey of Patients' Hospital Experiences				
Area Around Room 'Always' Quiet at Night	300+	58%	60%	61%
Doctors 'Always' Communicated Well	300+	76%	81%	82%
Home Recovery Information Given	300+	80%	86%	85%
Hospital Given 9 or 10 on 10 Point Scale	300+	59%	70%	71%
Meds 'Always' Explained Before Given	300+	55%	64%	64%
Nurses 'Always' Communicated Well	300+	71%	79%	79%
Pain 'Always' Well Controlled	300+	62%	71%	71%
Room and Bathroom 'Always' Clean	300+	64%	74%	73%
Timely Help 'Always' Received	300+	54%	67%	68%
Would Definitely Recommend Hospital	300+	65%	70%	71%
Use of Medical Imaging				
Cardiac Imaging Stress Test before Surgery	366	3.8%	5.5%	5.3%
Combination Abdominal CT Scan	635	8.2%	10.1%	10.5%
Combination Brain/Sinus CT Scan	640	1.4%	2.6%	2.7%
Combination Chest CT Scan	661	0.0%	2.8%	2.7%
Follow-up Mammogram/Ultrasound	1,175	5.3%	8.4%	8.8%
Lumbar Spine MRI for Low Back Pain	100	28.0%	36.6%	37.2%

Doctor John Warner Hospital

422 W White St
Clinton, IL 61727
Phone: 217-935-9571
Fax: 217-937-5244
URL: www.djwhospital.org
Type: Critical Access Hospitals
Emergency Services: Yes
Ownership: Government - Local
Beds: 25

Key Personnel:

Emergency Room . . . . Heidi Cook
Infection Control. . . . . Heidi Coook
Quality Assurance . . . . Kathy Isaac
Intensive Care Unit. . . . . Brenda Lehman
Operating Room. . . . . Brenda Saubert
Chief of Medical Staff . . . . Dr Tricia Scerba
CEO/President. . . . . Earl N Sheehy
Ambulatory Care . . . . Karen Welch

Measure	Cases	This Hosp.	State Avg.	U.S. Avg.
Blood Clot Prevention and Treatment				
Anticoagulation Overlap Therapy[5]	-	-	91%	93%
ICU Venous Thromboembolism Prophylaxis[5]	-	-	93%	92%
Incidence of Potentially Preventable VTE[5]	-	-	11%	10%
UFH with Dosages/Platelet Monitoring[5]	-	-	94%	97%
Venous Thromboembolism Prophylaxis[5]	-	-	86%	85%
Warfarin Therapy Discharge Instructions[5]	-	-	71%	75%
Chest Pain/Possible Heart Attack Care				
Aspirin Given Within 24 Hours of Arrival[5]	-	-	96%	96%
Fibrinolytic Meds Within 30 Min. of Arrival[5]	-	-	65%	58%
Average Time to ECG (minutes)[5]	-	-	6	7
Average Time to Transfer (minutes)[5]	-	-	63	60
Children's Asthma Care				
Received Home Management Plan of Care	-	-	-	88%
Received Reliever Medication	-	-	-	100%
Received Systemic Corticosteroids	-	-	-	100%
Emergency Department				
Admittance Decision Time (minutes)[5]	-	-	89	98
Head CT Results Within 45 Min. of Arrival[5]	-	-	64%	57%
Patients Who Left ER Before Being Seen[5]	-	-	3%	2%
Time from ER Arrival to Admit. (minutes)[5]	-	-	260	274
Time from ER Arrival to Discharge (minutes)[5]	-	-	138	134
Time in ER Before Being Evaluated (minutes)[5]	-	-	28	26
Time to Pain Meds for Fractures (minutes)[5]	-	-	52	57
Heart Attack Care				
Aspirin Given at Discharge[1,3]	-	-	99%	99%
Fibrinolytic Meds Within 30 Min. of Arrival[3,7]	-	-	33%	54%
PCI Within 90 Minutes of Arrival[3,7]	-	-	97%	96%
Statin Prescribed at Discharge[1,3]	-	-	98%	98%
Heart Failure Care				
ACE Inhibitor or ARB for LVSD[1,3]	-	-	98%	97%
Discharge Instructions Given[1,3]	-	-	96%	94%
Evaluation of LVS Function[1,3]	-	-	99%	99%
Medicare Spending				
Medicare Spending per Patient (ratio)	-	-	1	0.98
Pneumonia Care				
Appropriate Initial Antibiotic Given[1,3]	-	-	95%	95%
Blood Culture Timing[3]	13	77%	98%	98%
Pregnancy and Delivery Care				
Newborn Deliveries Scheduled Early[5]	-	-	2%	6%
Preventive Care				
Immunization for Influenza[5]	-	-	92%	90%
Immunization for Pneumonia[5]	-	-	92%	92%
Stroke Care				
Anticoagulation Therapy for Atrial Fibrillation[5]	-	-	94%	95%
Antithrombotic Therapy Timing[5]	-	-	98%	98%
Assessed for Rehabilitation[5]	-	-	97%	97%
Discharged on Antithrombotic Therapy[5]	-	-	99%	99%
Discharged on Statin Medication[5]	-	-	94%	94%
Thrombolytic Therapy Timing[5]	-	-	66%	66%
Venous Thromboembolism Prophylaxis[5]	-	-	94%	94%
Written Stroke Educational Materials Given[5]	-	-	87%	88%
Surgical Care Improvement Project				
Appropriate Beta Blocker Usage[1,3]	-	-	98%	98%
Appropriate VTP Within 24 Hours[1,3]	-	-	98%	98%
Controlled Postoperative Blood Glucose[3,7]	-	-	97%	97%
Perioperative Temperature Management[1,3]	-	-	100%	100%
Prophylactic Antibiotic Selection[1,3]	-	-	99%	99%
Prophylactic Antibiotic Selection (Outpatient)[5]	-	-	98%	98%
Prophylactic Antibiotic Stopped[1,3]	-	-	98%	98%
Prophylactic Antibiotic Timing[1,3]	-	-	99%	99%
Prophylactic Antibiotic Timing (Outpatient)[5]	-	-	97%	98%
Urinary Catheter Removal[1,3]	-	-	98%	97%
Survey of Patients' Hospital Experiences				
Area Around Room 'Always' Quiet at Night[5]	-	-	60%	61%
Doctors 'Always' Communicated Well[5]	-	-	81%	82%
Home Recovery Information Given[5]	-	-	86%	85%
Hospital Given 9 or 10 on 10 Point Scale[5]	-	-	70%	71%
Meds 'Always' Explained Before Given[5]	-	-	64%	64%
Nurses 'Always' Communicated Well[5]	-	-	79%	79%
Pain 'Always' Well Controlled[5]	-	-	71%	71%
Room and Bathroom 'Always' Clean[5]	-	-	74%	73%
Timely Help 'Always' Received[5]	-	-	67%	68%
Would Definitely Recommend Hospital[5]	-	-	70%	71%
Use of Medical Imaging				
Cardiac Imaging Stress Test before Surgery	65	3.1%	5.5%	5.3%
Combination Abdominal CT Scan	124	7.3%	10.1%	10.5%
Combination Brain/Sinus CT Scan[1]	-	-	2.6%	2.7%
Combination Chest CT Scan	104	8.7%	2.8%	2.7%
Follow-up Mammogram/Ultrasound	150	8.7%	8.4%	8.8%
Lumbar Spine MRI for Low Back Pain[1]	-	-	36.6%	37.2%

Presence United Samaritans Medical Center

812 N Logan
Danville, IL 61832
Phone: 217-443-5000
Fax: 217-443-1965
URL: www.provena.org/usmc
Type: Acute Care Hospitals
Emergency Services: Yes
Ownership: Voluntary non-profit - Church
Beds: 210

Key Personnel:

Radiology. . . . . Prasad Devabhak
Infection Control. . . . . JoAnne Guyman, RN
President/CEO. . . . . Joseph Hugar
Hemotology Center . . . . J Labyog, MD
Pediatric In-Patient Care . . . . Ray Maciejewski, MD
Emergency Room . . . . Mary Miller, RN
Chief of Medical Staff. . . . . Charanjit Rakalla, MD
Intensive Care Unit. . . . . Sharon Tuggle

Measure	Cases	This Hosp.	State Avg.	U.S. Avg.
Blood Clot Prevention and Treatment				
Anticoagulation Overlap Therapy[2]	62	97%	91%	93%
ICU Venous Thromboembolism Prophylaxis[2]	79	94%	93%	92%
Incidence of Potentially Preventable VTE[1,2]	-	-	11%	10%
UFH with Dosages/Platelet Monitoring[1,2]	-	-	94%	97%
Venous Thromboembolism Prophylaxis[2]	346	88%	86%	85%
Warfarin Therapy Discharge Instructions[2]	45	91%	71%	75%
Chest Pain/Possible Heart Attack Care				
Aspirin Given Within 24 Hours of Arrival	132	93%	96%	96%
Fibrinolytic Meds Within 30 Min. of Arrival[7]	-	-	65%	58%
Average Time to ECG (minutes)	137	9	6	7
Average Time to Transfer (minutes)	27	60	63	60
Children's Asthma Care				
Received Home Management Plan of Care	-	-	-	88%
Received Reliever Medication	-	-	-	100%
Received Systemic Corticosteroids	-	-	-	100%
Emergency Department				
Admittance Decision Time (minutes)[2]	671	75	89	98
Head CT Results Within 45 Min. of Arrival	23	65%	64%	57%
Patients Who Left ER Before Being Seen	39,914	1%	3%	2%
Time from ER Arrival to Admit. (minutes)[2]	706	228	260	274
Time from ER Arrival to Discharge (minutes)	345	155	138	134
Time in ER Before Being Evaluated (minutes)	408	33	28	26
Time to Pain Meds for Fractures (minutes)	129	72	52	57
Heart Attack Care				
Aspirin Given at Discharge	32	94%	99%	99%
Fibrinolytic Meds Within 30 Min. of Arrival[7]	-	-	33%	54%
PCI Within 90 Minutes of Arrival[7]	-	-	97%	96%
Statin Prescribed at Discharge	38	92%	98%	98%
Heart Failure Care				
ACE Inhibitor or ARB for LVSD	87	99%	98%	97%
Discharge Instructions Given	185	91%	96%	94%
Evaluation of LVS Function	254	100%	99%	99%
Medicare Spending				
Medicare Spending per Patient (ratio)	-	0.97	1	0.98
Pneumonia Care				
Appropriate Initial Antibiotic Given	107	94%	95%	95%
Blood Culture Timing	203	96%	98%	98%
Pregnancy and Delivery Care				
Newborn Deliveries Scheduled Early	70	1%	2%	6%
Preventive Care				
Immunization for Influenza[2]	557	95%	92%	90%
Immunization for Pneumonia[2]	757	98%	92%	92%
Stroke Care				
Anticoagulation Therapy for Atrial Fibrillation[1]	-	-	94%	95%
Antithrombotic Therapy Timing	52	98%	98%	98%
Assessed for Rehabilitation	51	96%	97%	97%
Discharged on Antithrombotic Therapy	44	100%	99%	99%
Discharged on Statin Medication	40	78%	94%	94%
Thrombolytic Therapy Timing[7]	-	-	66%	66%
Venous Thromboembolism Prophylaxis	47	91%	94%	94%
Written Stroke Educational Materials Given	24	79%	87%	88%
Surgical Care Improvement Project				

NOTE: Hospital profiles are in alphabetical order by state, then city, then hospital within the city; Rankings exclude hospitals with less than 25 cases except for patient surveys which excludes hospitals with less than 100 cases; (a) 100-299 cases; (1) The number of cases/patients is too few to report; (2) Data submitted were based on a sample of cases/patients; (3) Results are based on a shorter time period than required; (4) Data suppressed by CMS for one or more quarters; (5) Results are not available for this reporting period; (6) Fewer than 100 patients completed the HCAHPS survey; (7) No cases met the criteria for this measure; (8) The lower limit of the confidence interval cannot be calculated if the number of observed infections equals zero; (9) No data are available from the state/territory for this reporting period; (10) The scores shown reflect fewer than 50 completed surveys; (11) There were discrepancies in the data collection process; (12) This measure does not apply to this hospital for this reporting period; (13) Results cannot be calculated for this reporting period; (14) The results for this state are combined with nearby states to protect confidentiality; Please refer to the User's Guide for a full explanation of data.

Measure	Cases	This Hosp.	State Avg.	U.S. Avg.
Appropriate Beta Blocker Usage	70	94%	98%	98%
Appropriate VTP Within 24 Hours	171	94%	98%	98%
Controlled Postoperative Blood Glucose[7]	-	-	97%	97%
Perioperative Temperature Management	213	100%	100%	100%
Prophylactic Antibiotic Selection	163	99%	99%	99%
Prophylactic Antibiotic Selection (Outpatient)	43	100%	98%	98%
Prophylactic Antibiotic Stopped	162	98%	98%	98%
Prophylactic Antibiotic Timing	163	100%	99%	99%
Prophylactic Antibiotic Timing (Outpatient)	45	96%	97%	98%
Urinary Catheter Removal	111	100%	98%	97%
Survey of Patients' Hospital Experiences				
Area Around Room 'Always' Quiet at Night	300+	69%	60%	61%
Doctors 'Always' Communicated Well	300+	83%	81%	82%
Home Recovery Information Given	300+	89%	86%	85%
Hospital Given 9 or 10 on 10 Point Scale	300+	76%	70%	71%
Meds 'Always' Explained Before Given	300+	67%	64%	64%
Nurses 'Always' Communicated Well	300+	83%	79%	79%
Pain 'Always' Well Controlled	300+	74%	71%	71%
Room and Bathroom 'Always' Clean	300+	76%	74%	73%
Timely Help 'Always' Received	300+	68%	67%	68%
Would Definitely Recommend Hospital	300+	69%	70%	71%
Use of Medical Imaging				
Cardiac Imaging Stress Test before Surgery	117	6.8%	5.5%	5.3%
Combination Abdominal CT Scan	451	16.4%	10.1%	10.5%
Combination Brain/Sinus CT Scan[1]	-	-	2.6%	2.7%
Combination Chest CT Scan	371	12.9%	2.8%	2.7%
Follow-up Mammogram/Ultrasound	474	18.6%	8.4%	8.8%
Lumbar Spine MRI for Low Back Pain	50	36.0%	36.6%	37.2%

VA Illiana Healthcare System - Danville

1900 E. Main
Danville, IL 61832
URL: www.va.gov
Type: Acute Care - VA
Ownership: Government Federal

Phone: 217-554-3000
Fax: 217-554-4552

Emergency Services: No
Beds: 361

Key Personnel:
Radiology. M Gai, MD
Quality Assurance . . . . Kim Gibson
Patient Relations . . . . Kim Grossman
Chief of Medical Staff . . . . Nirmala Rozario, MD
CEO/President. . . . . Romero Zamberletti

Measure	Cases	This Hosp.	State Avg.	U.S. Avg.
Blood Clot Prevention and Treatment				
Anticoagulation Overlap Therapy	-	-	91%	93%
ICU Venous Thromboembolism Prophylaxis	-	-	93%	92%
Incidence of Potentially Preventable VTE	-	-	11%	10%
UFH with Dosages/Platelet Monitoring	-	-	94%	97%
Venous Thromboembolism Prophylaxis	-	-	86%	85%
Warfarin Therapy Discharge Instructions	-	-	71%	75%
Chest Pain/Possible Heart Attack Care				
Aspirin Given Within 24 Hours of Arrival	-	-	96%	96%
Fibrinolytic Meds Within 30 Min. of Arrival	-	-	65%	58%
Average Time to ECG (minutes)	-	-	6	7
Average Time to Transfer (minutes)	-	-	63	60
Children's Asthma Care				
Received Home Management Plan of Care	-	-	-	88%
Received Reliever Medication	-	-	-	100%
Received Systemic Corticosteroids	-	-	-	100%
Emergency Department				
Admittance Decision Time (minutes)	-	-	89	98
Head CT Results Within 45 Min. of Arrival	-	-	64%	57%
Patients Who Left ER Before Being Seen	-	-	3%	2%
Time from ER Arrival to Admit. (minutes)	-	-	260	274
Time from ER Arrival to Discharge (minutes)	-	-	138	134
Time in ER Before Being Evaluated (minutes)	-	-	28	26
Time to Pain Meds for Fractures (minutes)	-	-	52	57
Heart Attack Care				
Aspirin Given at Discharge[5]	-	-	99%	99%
Fibrinolytic Meds Within 30 Min. of Arrival[5]	-	-	33%	54%
PCI Within 90 Minutes of Arrival[5]	-	-	97%	96%
Statin Prescribed at Discharge[5]	-	-	98%	98%
Heart Failure Care				
ACE Inhibitor or ARB for LVSD[1]	15	100%	98%	97%
Discharge Instructions Given	28	93%	96%	94%
Evaluation of LVS Function	37	100%	99%	99%
Medicare Spending				
Medicare Spending per Patient (ratio)	-	-	1	0.98
Pneumonia Care				
Appropriate Initial Antibiotic Given	36	100%	95%	95%
Blood Culture Timing	33	97%	98%	98%
Pregnancy and Delivery Care				
Newborn Deliveries Scheduled Early	-	-	2%	6%
Preventive Care				
Immunization for Influenza[5]	-	-	92%	90%
Immunization for Pneumonia[5]	-	-	92%	92%
Stroke Care				
Anticoagulation Therapy for Atrial Fibrillation	-	-	94%	95%
Antithrombotic Therapy Timing	-	-	98%	98%
Assessed for Rehabilitation	-	-	97%	97%
Discharged on Antithrombotic Therapy	-	-	99%	99%
Discharged on Statin Medication	-	-	94%	94%
Thrombolytic Therapy Timing	-	-	66%	66%
Venous Thromboembolism Prophylaxis	-	-	94%	94%
Written Stroke Educational Materials Given	-	-	87%	88%
Surgical Care Improvement Project				
Appropriate Beta Blocker Usage[5]	-	-	98%	98%
Appropriate VTP Within 24 Hours[5]	-	-	98%	98%
Controlled Postoperative Blood Glucose[5]	-	-	97%	97%
Perioperative Temperature Management[5]	-	-	100%	100%
Prophylactic Antibiotic Selection[5]	-	-	99%	99%
Prophylactic Antibiotic Selection (Outpatient)	-	-	98%	98%
Prophylactic Antibiotic Stopped[5]	-	-	98%	98%
Prophylactic Antibiotic Timing[5]	-	-	99%	99%
Prophylactic Antibiotic Timing (Outpatient)	-	-	97%	98%
Urinary Catheter Removal[5]	-	-	98%	97%
Survey of Patients' Hospital Experiences				
Area Around Room 'Always' Quiet at Night	-	-	60%	61%
Doctors 'Always' Communicated Well	-	-	81%	82%
Home Recovery Information Given	-	-	86%	85%
Hospital Given 9 or 10 on 10 Point Scale	-	-	70%	71%
Meds 'Always' Explained Before Given	-	-	64%	64%
Nurses 'Always' Communicated Well	-	-	79%	79%
Pain 'Always' Well Controlled	-	-	71%	71%
Room and Bathroom 'Always' Clean	-	-	74%	73%
Timely Help 'Always' Received	-	-	67%	68%
Would Definitely Recommend Hospital	-	-	70%	71%
Use of Medical Imaging				
Cardiac Imaging Stress Test before Surgery	-	-	5.5%	5.3%
Combination Abdominal CT Scan	-	-	10.1%	10.5%
Combination Brain/Sinus CT Scan	-	-	2.6%	2.7%
Combination Chest CT Scan	-	-	2.8%	2.7%
Follow-up Mammogram/Ultrasound	-	-	8.4%	8.8%
Lumbar Spine MRI for Low Back Pain	-	-	36.6%	37.2%

Decatur Memorial Hospital

2300 North Edward Street
Decatur, IL 62526
URL: www.dmhcares.org
Type: Acute Care Hospitals
Ownership: Voluntary non-profit - Other

Phone: 217-877-8121
Fax: 217-876-6118

Emergency Services: Yes
Beds: 314

Key Personnel:
Pediatric In-Patient Care . . . . MA Arzon, MD
Operating Room. . . . . Sally Hodges
Radiology. . . . . G Richard Locke, MD
Infection Control. . . . . Alma Miller, RN
Quality Assurance . . . . Beth Paul, RN
CEO/President. . . . . Kenneth Smithmier
Chief of Medical Staff. . . . . Jame L Wade, MD
Intensive Care Unit. . . . . Michael Zia, MD

Measure	Cases	This Hosp.	State Avg.	U.S. Avg.
Blood Clot Prevention and Treatment				
Anticoagulation Overlap Therapy[2]	115	97%	91%	93%
ICU Venous Thromboembolism Prophylaxis[2]	58	97%	93%	92%
Incidence of Potentially Preventable VTE[2]	15	0%	11%	10%
UFH with Dosages/Platelet Monitoring[2]	58	100%	94%	97%
Venous Thromboembolism Prophylaxis[2]	323	79%	86%	85%
Warfarin Therapy Discharge Instructions[2]	85	100%	71%	75%
Chest Pain/Possible Heart Attack Care				
Aspirin Given Within 24 Hours of Arrival[5]	-	-	96%	96%
Fibrinolytic Meds Within 30 Min. of Arrival[5]	-	-	65%	58%
Average Time to ECG (minutes)[5]	-	-	6	7
Average Time to Transfer (minutes)[5]	-	-	63	60
Children's Asthma Care				
Received Home Management Plan of Care	-	-	-	88%
Received Reliever Medication	-	-	-	100%
Received Systemic Corticosteroids	-	-	-	100%
Emergency Department				
Admittance Decision Time (minutes)[2]	519	125	89	98
Head CT Results Within 45 Min. of Arrival[1,3]	-	-	64%	57%
Patients Who Left ER Before Being Seen	50,727	1%	3%	2%
Time from ER Arrival to Admit. (minutes)[2]	519	281	260	274
Time from ER Arrival to Discharge (minutes)	368	150	138	134
Time in ER Before Being Evaluated (minutes)	407	39	28	26
Time to Pain Meds for Fractures (minutes)	187	72	52	57
Heart Attack Care				
Aspirin Given at Discharge	124	100%	99%	99%
Fibrinolytic Meds Within 30 Min. of Arrival[7]	-	-	33%	54%
PCI Within 90 Minutes of Arrival	23	96%	97%	96%
Statin Prescribed at Discharge	132	100%	98%	98%
Heart Failure Care				
ACE Inhibitor or ARB for LVSD	71	100%	98%	97%
Discharge Instructions Given	200	100%	96%	94%
Evaluation of LVS Function	269	100%	99%	99%
Medicare Spending				
Medicare Spending per Patient (ratio)	-	0.96	1	0.98
Pneumonia Care				
Appropriate Initial Antibiotic Given	152	93%	95%	95%
Blood Culture Timing	281	98%	98%	98%
Pregnancy and Delivery Care				
Newborn Deliveries Scheduled Early[2]	35	0%	2%	6%
Preventive Care				
Immunization for Influenza[2]	559	81%	92%	90%
Immunization for Pneumonia[2]	755	83%	92%	92%
Stroke Care				
Anticoagulation Therapy for Atrial Fibrillation[2]	16	100%	94%	95%
Antithrombotic Therapy Timing[2]	98	99%	98%	98%
Assessed for Rehabilitation[2]	132	100%	97%	97%
Discharged on Antithrombotic Therapy[2]	121	99%	99%	99%
Discharged on Statin Medication[2]	89	98%	94%	94%
Thrombolytic Therapy Timing[1,2]	-	-	66%	66%
Venous Thromboembolism Prophylaxis[2]	112	100%	94%	94%
Written Stroke Educational Materials Given[2]	93	100%	87%	88%
Surgical Care Improvement Project				
Appropriate Beta Blocker Usage[2]	222	98%	98%	98%
Appropriate VTP Within 24 Hours[2]	431	99%	98%	98%
Controlled Postoperative Blood Glucose[2]	64	97%	97%	97%
Perioperative Temperature Management[2]	562	100%	100%	100%
Prophylactic Antibiotic Selection[2]	428	99%	99%	99%
Prophylactic Antibiotic Selection (Outpatient)	334	100%	98%	98%
Prophylactic Antibiotic Stopped[2]	423	99%	98%	98%
Prophylactic Antibiotic Timing[2]	428	99%	99%	99%
Prophylactic Antibiotic Timing (Outpatient)	334	99%	97%	98%
Urinary Catheter Removal[2]	389	95%	98%	97%
Survey of Patients' Hospital Experiences				
Area Around Room 'Always' Quiet at Night	300+	62%	60%	61%
Doctors 'Always' Communicated Well	300+	83%	81%	82%
Home Recovery Information Given	300+	88%	86%	85%
Hospital Given 9 or 10 on 10 Point Scale	300+	69%	70%	71%
Meds 'Always' Explained Before Given	300+	67%	64%	64%
Nurses 'Always' Communicated Well	300+	77%	79%	79%
Pain 'Always' Well Controlled	300+	69%	71%	71%
Room and Bathroom 'Always' Clean	300+	69%	74%	73%
Timely Help 'Always' Received	300+	61%	67%	68%
Would Definitely Recommend Hospital	300+	71%	70%	71%
Use of Medical Imaging				
Cardiac Imaging Stress Test before Surgery	677	5.2%	5.5%	5.3%
Combination Abdominal CT Scan	1,301	3.9%	10.1%	10.5%
Combination Brain/Sinus CT Scan	971	3.2%	2.6%	2.7%
Combination Chest CT Scan	672	1.5%	2.8%	2.7%

NOTE: Hospital profiles are in alphabetical order by state, then city, then hospital within the city; Rankings exclude hospitals with less than 25 cases except for patient surveys which excludes hospitals with less than 100 cases; (a) 100-299 cases; (1) The number of cases/patients is too few to report; (2) Data submitted were based on a sample of cases/patients; (3) Results are based on a shorter time period than required; (4) Data suppressed by CMS for one or more quarters; (5) Results are not available for this reporting period; (6) Fewer than 100 patients completed the HCAHPS survey; (7) No cases met the criteria for this measure; (8) The lower limit of the confidence interval cannot be calculated if the number of observed infections equals zero; (9) No data are available from the state/territory for this reporting period; (10) The scores shown reflect fewer than 50 completed surveys; (11) There were discrepancies in the data collection process; (12) This measure does not apply to this hospital for this reporting period; (13) Results cannot be calculated for this reporting period; (14) The results for this state are combined with nearby states to protect confidentiality; Please refer to the User's Guide for a full explanation of data.

Follow-up Mammogram/Ultrasound	3,427	11.1%	8.4%	8.8%
Lumbar Spine MRI for Low Back Pain	335	41.2%	36.6%	37.2%

Saint Marys Hospital

1800 E Lake Shore Dr
Decatur, IL 62521
Phone: 217-464-7000
Fax: 217-464-1616
URL: www.stmarys-hospital.com
Type: Acute Care Hospitals
Emergency Services: Yes
Ownership: Voluntary non-profit - Private
Beds: 371

Key Personnel:
Intensive Care Unit. . . . . Steven Arnold, MD
Chief of Medical Staff. . . . . Phillip Barnell, MD
Emergency Room . . . . Phillip Barnell, MD
Pediatric Ambulatory Care . . . . . . G Chiligiris, MD
Anesthesiology. . . . . John Furry, MD
Coronary Care . . . . Glen Griesheim, RN
Quality Assurance . . . . Gayla Hislope
CEO/President. . . . . Dan Perryman

Measure	Cases	This Hosp.	State Avg.	U.S. Avg.
Blood Clot Prevention and Treatment				
Anticoagulation Overlap Therapy[2]	37	27%	91%	93%
ICU Venous Thromboembolism Prophylaxis[2]	55	89%	93%	92%
Incidence of Potentially Preventable VTE[1,2]	-	-	11%	10%
UFH with Dosages/Platelet Monitoring[2]	24	96%	94%	97%
Venous Thromboembolism Prophylaxis[2]	261	54%	86%	85%
Warfarin Therapy Discharge Instructions[2]	31	84%	71%	75%
Chest Pain/Possible Heart Attack Care				
Aspirin Given Within 24 Hours of Arrival[1,3]	-	-	96%	96%
Fibrinolytic Meds Within 30 Min. of Arrival[5]	-	-	65%	58%
Average Time to ECG (minutes)[1,3]	-	-	6	7
Average Time to Transfer (minutes)[5]	-	-	63	60
Children's Asthma Care				
Received Home Management Plan of Care	-	-	-	88%
Received Reliever Medication	-	-	-	100%
Received Systemic Corticosteroids	-	-	-	100%
Emergency Department				
Admittance Decision Time (minutes)[2]	540	91	89	98
Head CT Results Within 45 Min. of Arrival	18	17%	64%	57%
Patients Who Left ER Before Being Seen	33,535	2%	3%	2%
Time from ER Arrival to Admit. (minutes)[2]	559	276	260	274
Time from ER Arrival to Discharge (minutes)	360	158	138	134
Time in ER Before Being Evaluated (minutes)	404	50	28	26
Time to Pain Meds for Fractures (minutes)	81	78	52	57
Heart Attack Care				
Aspirin Given at Discharge	158	100%	99%	99%
Fibrinolytic Meds Within 30 Min. of Arrival[1]	-	-	33%	54%
PCI Within 90 Minutes of Arrival	19	100%	97%	96%
Statin Prescribed at Discharge	145	97%	98%	98%
Heart Failure Care				
ACE Inhibitor or ARB for LVSD	56	100%	98%	97%
Discharge Instructions Given	191	95%	96%	94%
Evaluation of LVS Function	257	100%	99%	99%
Medicare Spending				
Medicare Spending per Patient (ratio)	-	0.96	1	0.98
Pneumonia Care				
Appropriate Initial Antibiotic Given	115	88%	95%	95%
Blood Culture Timing	189	98%	98%	98%
Pregnancy and Delivery Care				
Newborn Deliveries Scheduled Early	38	5%	2%	6%
Preventive Care				
Immunization for Influenza[2]	542	87%	92%	90%
Immunization for Pneumonia[2]	651	90%	92%	92%
Stroke Care				
Anticoagulation Therapy for Atrial Fibrillation[1]	-	-	94%	95%
Antithrombotic Therapy Timing	29	93%	98%	98%
Assessed for Rehabilitation	52	94%	97%	97%
Discharged on Antithrombotic Therapy	45	96%	99%	99%
Discharged on Statin Medication	35	74%	94%	94%
Thrombolytic Therapy Timing	11	27%	66%	66%
Venous Thromboembolism Prophylaxis	47	91%	94%	94%
Written Stroke Educational Materials Given	27	93%	87%	88%
Surgical Care Improvement Project				
Appropriate Beta Blocker Usage	104	94%	98%	98%
Appropriate VTP Within 24 Hours	262	98%	98%	98%
Controlled Postoperative Blood Glucose[7]	-	-	97%	97%
Perioperative Temperature Management	291	100%	100%	100%
Prophylactic Antibiotic Selection	221	97%	99%	99%
Prophylactic Antibiotic Selection (Outpatient)	155	99%	98%	98%
Prophylactic Antibiotic Stopped	219	98%	98%	98%
Prophylactic Antibiotic Timing	223	99%	99%	99%
Prophylactic Antibiotic Timing (Outpatient)	156	99%	97%	98%
Urinary Catheter Removal	211	100%	98%	97%
Survey of Patients' Hospital Experiences				
Area Around Room 'Always' Quiet at Night	300+	60%	60%	61%
Doctors 'Always' Communicated Well	300+	79%	81%	82%
Home Recovery Information Given	300+	82%	86%	85%
Hospital Given 9 or 10 on 10 Point Scale	300+	72%	70%	71%
Meds 'Always' Explained Before Given	300+	59%	64%	64%
Nurses 'Always' Communicated Well	300+	78%	79%	79%
Pain 'Always' Well Controlled	300+	65%	71%	71%
Room and Bathroom 'Always' Clean	300+	73%	74%	73%
Timely Help 'Always' Received	300+	59%	67%	68%
Would Definitely Recommend Hospital	300+	74%	70%	71%
Use of Medical Imaging				
Cardiac Imaging Stress Test before Surgery	845	5.2%	5.5%	5.3%
Combination Abdominal CT Scan	660	7.1%	10.1%	10.5%
Combination Brain/Sinus CT Scan	662	4.7%	2.6%	2.7%
Combination Chest CT Scan	307	5.5%	2.8%	2.7%
Follow-up Mammogram/Ultrasound	1,141	4.6%	8.4%	8.8%
Lumbar Spine MRI for Low Back Pain	127	40.9%	36.6%	37.2%

Kishwaukee Community Hospital

One Kish Hospital Drive
Dekalb, IL 60115
Phone: 815-756-1521
Fax: 815-756-7665
URL: www.kishhospital.org
Type: Acute Care Hospitals
Emergency Services: Yes
Ownership: Voluntary non-profit - Private
Beds: 172

Key Personnel:
Radiology. . . . . Thomas R Cain, MD
Pediatric Ambulatory Care . . . . . . Suzanne Cook, MD
Pediatric In-Patient Care . . . . Suzanne Cook, MD
Quality Assurance . . . . Brad Copple
Chief of Medical Staff. . . . . Pamela Duffy
Patient Relations . . . . Pamela Duffy
Operating Room. . . . . Stephen R Goldman
CEO/President. . . . . Kevin Poorten

Measure	Cases	This Hosp.	State Avg.	U.S. Avg.
Blood Clot Prevention and Treatment				
Anticoagulation Overlap Therapy[2]	45	100%	91%	93%
ICU Venous Thromboembolism Prophylaxis[2]	73	99%	93%	92%
Incidence of Potentially Preventable VTE[1,2]	-	-	11%	10%
UFH with Dosages/Platelet Monitoring[2]	19	100%	94%	97%
Venous Thromboembolism Prophylaxis[2]	324	98%	86%	85%
Warfarin Therapy Discharge Instructions[2]	34	97%	71%	75%
Chest Pain/Possible Heart Attack Care				
Aspirin Given Within 24 Hours of Arrival[1]	-	-	96%	96%
Fibrinolytic Meds Within 30 Min. of Arrival[3,7]	-	-	65%	58%
Average Time to ECG (minutes)[1]	-	-	6	7
Average Time to Transfer (minutes)[3,7]	-	-	63	60
Children's Asthma Care				
Received Home Management Plan of Care	-	-	-	88%
Received Reliever Medication	-	-	-	100%
Received Systemic Corticosteroids	-	-	-	100%
Emergency Department				
Admittance Decision Time (minutes)[2]	466	78	89	98
Head CT Results Within 45 Min. of Arrival	15	60%	64%	57%
Patients Who Left ER Before Being Seen	27,181	2%	3%	2%
Time from ER Arrival to Admit. (minutes)[2]	467	246	260	274
Time from ER Arrival to Discharge (minutes)	364	136	138	134
Time in ER Before Being Evaluated (minutes)	407	28	28	26
Time to Pain Meds for Fractures (minutes)	90	49	52	57
Heart Attack Care				
Aspirin Given at Discharge	65	100%	99%	99%
Fibrinolytic Meds Within 30 Min. of Arrival[7]	-	-	33%	54%
PCI Within 90 Minutes of Arrival	19	95%	97%	96%
Statin Prescribed at Discharge	57	100%	98%	98%
Heart Failure Care				
ACE Inhibitor or ARB for LVSD	40	100%	98%	97%
Discharge Instructions Given	93	99%	96%	94%
Evaluation of LVS Function	129	100%	99%	99%
Medicare Spending				
Medicare Spending per Patient (ratio)	-	0.99	1	0.98
Pneumonia Care				
Appropriate Initial Antibiotic Given	114	100%	95%	95%
Blood Culture Timing	139	99%	98%	98%
Pregnancy and Delivery Care				
Newborn Deliveries Scheduled Early	39	3%	2%	6%
Preventive Care				
Immunization for Influenza[2]	483	99%	92%	90%
Immunization for Pneumonia[2]	609	100%	92%	92%
Stroke Care				
Anticoagulation Therapy for Atrial Fibrillation[1]	-	-	94%	95%
Antithrombotic Therapy Timing	33	100%	98%	98%
Assessed for Rehabilitation	35	97%	97%	97%
Discharged on Antithrombotic Therapy	34	100%	99%	99%
Discharged on Statin Medication	23	96%	94%	94%
Thrombolytic Therapy Timing[7]	-	-	66%	66%
Venous Thromboembolism Prophylaxis	31	97%	94%	94%
Written Stroke Educational Materials Given	15	93%	87%	88%
Surgical Care Improvement Project				
Appropriate Beta Blocker Usage	132	100%	98%	98%
Appropriate VTP Within 24 Hours	393	99%	98%	98%
Controlled Postoperative Blood Glucose[7]	-	-	97%	97%
Perioperative Temperature Management	434	100%	100%	100%
Prophylactic Antibiotic Selection	321	100%	99%	99%
Prophylactic Antibiotic Selection (Outpatient)	112	100%	98%	98%
Prophylactic Antibiotic Stopped	314	99%	98%	98%
Prophylactic Antibiotic Timing	321	99%	99%	99%
Prophylactic Antibiotic Timing (Outpatient)	112	99%	97%	98%
Urinary Catheter Removal	338	100%	98%	97%
Survey of Patients' Hospital Experiences				
Area Around Room 'Always' Quiet at Night	300+	60%	60%	61%
Doctors 'Always' Communicated Well	300+	83%	81%	82%
Home Recovery Information Given	300+	89%	86%	85%
Hospital Given 9 or 10 on 10 Point Scale	300+	72%	70%	71%
Meds 'Always' Explained Before Given	300+	62%	64%	64%
Nurses 'Always' Communicated Well	300+	78%	79%	79%
Pain 'Always' Well Controlled	300+	72%	71%	71%
Room and Bathroom 'Always' Clean	300+	71%	74%	73%
Timely Help 'Always' Received	300+	61%	67%	68%
Would Definitely Recommend Hospital	300+	69%	70%	71%
Use of Medical Imaging				
Cardiac Imaging Stress Test before Surgery	281	5.3%	5.5%	5.3%
Combination Abdominal CT Scan	474	1.9%	10.1%	10.5%
Combination Brain/Sinus CT Scan	697	1.7%	2.6%	2.7%
Combination Chest CT Scan	367	0.0%	2.8%	2.7%
Follow-up Mammogram/Ultrasound	720	16.0%	8.4%	8.8%
Lumbar Spine MRI for Low Back Pain	81	34.6%	36.6%	37.2%

Katherine Shaw Bethea Hospital

403 E 1st St
Dixon, IL 61021
Phone: 815-288-5531
Type: Acute Care Hospitals
Emergency Services: Yes
Ownership: Voluntary non-profit - Private

Key Personnel:
Radiology. . . . . Imre Almassy, MD
Anesthesiology. . . . . Yolanda P. Dela Cruz, MD
CEO/President. . . . . David Schreiner

Measure	Cases	This Hosp.	State Avg.	U.S. Avg.
Blood Clot Prevention and Treatment				
Anticoagulation Overlap Therapy[2]	30	100%	91%	93%
ICU Venous Thromboembolism Prophylaxis[2]	107	94%	93%	92%
Incidence of Potentially Preventable VTE[2,7]	-	-	11%	10%
UFH with Dosages/Platelet Monitoring[1,2]	-	-	94%	97%
Venous Thromboembolism Prophylaxis[2]	252	93%	86%	85%
Warfarin Therapy Discharge Instructions[2]	28	96%	71%	75%
Chest Pain/Possible Heart Attack Care				
Aspirin Given Within 24 Hours of Arrival[1,3]	-	-	96%	96%
Fibrinolytic Meds Within 30 Min. of Arrival[3,7]	-	-	65%	58%
Average Time to ECG (minutes)[1,3]	-	-	6	7
Average Time to Transfer (minutes)[1,3]	-	-	63	60

NOTE: Hospital profiles are in alphabetical order by state, then city, then hospital within the city; Rankings exclude hospitals with less than 25 cases except for patient surveys which excludes hospitals with less than 100 cases; (a) 100-299 cases; (1) The number of cases/patients is too few to report; (2) Data submitted were based on a sample of cases/patients; (3) Results are based on a shorter time period than required; (4) Data suppressed by CMS for one or more quarters; (5) Results are not available for this reporting period; (6) Fewer than 100 patients completed the HCAHPS survey; (7) No cases met the criteria for this measure; (8) The lower limit of the confidence interval cannot be calculated if the number of observed infections equals zero; (9) No data are available from the state/territory for this reporting period; (10) The scores shown reflect fewer than 50 completed surveys; (11) There were discrepancies in the data collection process; (12) This measure does not apply to this hospital for this reporting period; (13) Results cannot be calculated for this reporting period; (14) The results for this state are combined with nearby states to protect confidentiality; Please refer to the User's Guide for a full explanation of data.

Measure	Cases	This Hosp.	State Avg.	U.S. Avg.
Children's Asthma Care				
Received Home Management Plan of Care	-	-	-	88%
Received Reliever Medication	-	-	-	100%
Received Systemic Corticosteroids	-	-	-	100%
Emergency Department				
Admittance Decision Time (minutes)[2]	406	68	89	98
Head CT Results Within 45 Min. of Arrival[1]	-	-	64%	57%
Patients Who Left ER Before Being Seen	18,719	1%	3%	2%
Time from ER Arrival to Admit. (minutes)[2]	430	181	260	274
Time from ER Arrival to Discharge (minutes)	343	101	138	134
Time in ER Before Being Evaluated (minutes)	347	41	28	26
Time to Pain Meds for Fractures (minutes)	44	49	52	57
Heart Attack Care				
Aspirin Given at Discharge	49	100%	99%	99%
Fibrinolytic Meds Within 30 Min. of Arrival[7]	-	-	33%	54%
PCI Within 90 Minutes of Arrival[1]	-	-	97%	96%
Statin Prescribed at Discharge	47	98%	98%	98%
Heart Failure Care				
ACE Inhibitor or ARB for LVSD	30	97%	98%	97%
Discharge Instructions Given	80	91%	96%	94%
Evaluation of LVS Function	109	100%	99%	99%
Medicare Spending				
Medicare Spending per Patient (ratio)	-	0.92	1	0.98
Pneumonia Care				
Appropriate Initial Antibiotic Given	65	97%	95%	95%
Blood Culture Timing	90	99%	98%	98%
Pregnancy and Delivery Care				
Newborn Deliveries Scheduled Early	29	3%	2%	6%
Preventive Care				
Immunization for Influenza[2]	413	99%	92%	90%
Immunization for Pneumonia[2]	565	98%	92%	92%
Stroke Care				
Anticoagulation Therapy for Atrial Fibrillation[1]	-	-	94%	95%
Antithrombotic Therapy Timing	26	100%	98%	98%
Assessed for Rehabilitation	29	97%	97%	97%
Discharged on Antithrombotic Therapy	28	100%	99%	99%
Discharged on Statin Medication	21	90%	94%	94%
Thrombolytic Therapy Timing[1]	-	-	66%	66%
Venous Thromboembolism Prophylaxis	27	96%	94%	94%
Written Stroke Educational Materials Given	15	67%	87%	88%
Surgical Care Improvement Project				
Appropriate Beta Blocker Usage	76	99%	98%	98%
Appropriate VTP Within 24 Hours	177	94%	98%	98%
Controlled Postoperative Blood Glucose[7]	-	-	97%	97%
Perioperative Temperature Management	245	100%	100%	100%
Prophylactic Antibiotic Selection	184	99%	99%	99%
Prophylactic Antibiotic Selection (Outpatient)	145	100%	98%	98%
Prophylactic Antibiotic Stopped	160	98%	98%	98%
Prophylactic Antibiotic Timing	184	99%	99%	99%
Prophylactic Antibiotic Timing (Outpatient)	80	94%	97%	98%
Urinary Catheter Removal	126	99%	98%	97%
Survey of Patients' Hospital Experiences				
Area Around Room 'Always' Quiet at Night	300+	58%	60%	61%
Doctors 'Always' Communicated Well	300+	81%	81%	82%
Home Recovery Information Given	300+	88%	86%	85%
Hospital Given 9 or 10 on 10 Point Scale	300+	70%	70%	71%
Meds 'Always' Explained Before Given	300+	65%	64%	64%
Nurses 'Always' Communicated Well	300+	80%	79%	79%
Pain 'Always' Well Controlled	300+	74%	71%	71%
Room and Bathroom 'Always' Clean	300+	73%	74%	73%
Timely Help 'Always' Received	300+	67%	67%	68%
Would Definitely Recommend Hospital	300+	73%	70%	71%
Use of Medical Imaging				
Cardiac Imaging Stress Test before Surgery	381	4.2%	5.5%	5.3%
Combination Abdominal CT Scan	411	4.6%	10.1%	10.5%
Combination Brain/Sinus CT Scan[1]	-	-	2.6%	2.7%
Combination Chest CT Scan	235	0.4%	2.8%	2.7%
Follow-up Mammogram/Ultrasound	906	10.4%	8.4%	8.8%
Lumbar Spine MRI for Low Back Pain	65	29.2%	36.6%	37.2%

Advocate Good Samaritan Hospital

3815 Highland Avenue Phone: 630-275-5900
Downers Grove, IL 60515 Fax: 630-963-8605
URL: www.advocatehealth.com/gsam
Type: Acute Care Hospitals Emergency Services: Yes
Ownership: Voluntary non-profit - Church Beds: 327

Key Personnel:
CEO/President. . . . . Jon Bruss
Chief of Medical Staff. . . . . Timothy Payne
Pediatric In-Patient Care . . . . Gus Rousonebs, MD
Radiology. . . . . R William Wayne, LVN

Measure	Cases	This Hosp.	State Avg.	U.S. Avg.
Blood Clot Prevention and Treatment				
Anticoagulation Overlap Therapy[2]	149	99%	91%	93%
ICU Venous Thromboembolism Prophylaxis[2]	91	93%	93%	92%
Incidence of Potentially Preventable VTE[2]	33	6%	11%	10%
UFH with Dosages/Platelet Monitoring[2]	109	96%	94%	97%
Venous Thromboembolism Prophylaxis[2]	336	88%	86%	85%
Warfarin Therapy Discharge Instructions[2]	84	73%	71%	75%
Chest Pain/Possible Heart Attack Care				
Aspirin Given Within 24 Hours of Arrival[3,7]	-	-	96%	96%
Fibrinolytic Meds Within 30 Min. of Arrival[5]	-	-	65%	58%
Average Time to ECG (minutes)[1,3]	-	-	6	7
Average Time to Transfer (minutes)[5]	-	-	63	60
Children's Asthma Care				
Received Home Management Plan of Care	-	-	-	88%
Received Reliever Medication	-	-	-	100%
Received Systemic Corticosteroids	-	-	-	100%
Emergency Department				
Admittance Decision Time (minutes)[2]	542	90	89	98
Head CT Results Within 45 Min. of Arrival	13	62%	64%	57%
Patients Who Left ER Before Being Seen	44,589	1%	3%	2%
Time from ER Arrival to Admit. (minutes)[2]	567	288	260	274
Time from ER Arrival to Discharge (minutes)	376	164	138	134
Time in ER Before Being Evaluated (minutes)	396	36	28	26
Time to Pain Meds for Fractures (minutes)	137	56	52	57
Heart Attack Care				
Aspirin Given at Discharge	209	100%	99%	99%
Fibrinolytic Meds Within 30 Min. of Arrival[7]	-	-	33%	54%
PCI Within 90 Minutes of Arrival	57	96%	97%	96%
Statin Prescribed at Discharge	201	100%	98%	98%
Heart Failure Care				
ACE Inhibitor or ARB for LVSD[2]	105	100%	98%	97%
Discharge Instructions Given[2]	221	100%	96%	94%
Evaluation of LVS Function[2]	314	100%	99%	99%
Medicare Spending				
Medicare Spending per Patient (ratio)	-	1.09	1	0.98
Pneumonia Care				
Appropriate Initial Antibiotic Given[2]	103	99%	95%	95%
Blood Culture Timing[2]	190	100%	98%	98%
Pregnancy and Delivery Care				
Newborn Deliveries Scheduled Early	150	1%	2%	6%
Preventive Care				
Immunization for Influenza[2]	587	91%	92%	90%
Immunization for Pneumonia[2]	707	89%	92%	92%
Stroke Care				
Anticoagulation Therapy for Atrial Fibrillation	17	94%	94%	95%
Antithrombotic Therapy Timing	124	98%	98%	98%
Assessed for Rehabilitation	145	97%	97%	97%
Discharged on Antithrombotic Therapy	132	99%	99%	99%
Discharged on Statin Medication	107	96%	94%	94%
Thrombolytic Therapy Timing[1]	-	-	66%	66%
Venous Thromboembolism Prophylaxis	140	90%	94%	94%
Written Stroke Educational Materials Given	61	98%	87%	88%
Surgical Care Improvement Project				
Appropriate Beta Blocker Usage[2]	189	99%	98%	98%
Appropriate VTP Within 24 Hours[2]	439	99%	98%	98%
Controlled Postoperative Blood Glucose[2]	119	98%	97%	97%
Perioperative Temperature Management[2]	518	100%	100%	100%
Prophylactic Antibiotic Selection[2]	455	99%	99%	99%
Prophylactic Antibiotic Selection (Outpatient)	354	99%	98%	98%
Prophylactic Antibiotic Stopped[2]	438	99%	98%	98%
Prophylactic Antibiotic Timing[2]	456	100%	99%	99%
Prophylactic Antibiotic Timing (Outpatient)	355	100%	97%	98%
Urinary Catheter Removal[2]	275	99%	98%	97%
Survey of Patients' Hospital Experiences				
Area Around Room 'Always' Quiet at Night	300+	53%	60%	61%
Doctors 'Always' Communicated Well	300+	81%	81%	82%
Home Recovery Information Given	300+	87%	86%	85%
Hospital Given 9 or 10 on 10 Point Scale	300+	73%	70%	71%
Meds 'Always' Explained Before Given	300+	65%	64%	64%
Nurses 'Always' Communicated Well	300+	82%	79%	79%
Pain 'Always' Well Controlled	300+	73%	71%	71%
Room and Bathroom 'Always' Clean	300+	74%	74%	73%
Timely Help 'Always' Received	300+	72%	67%	68%
Would Definitely Recommend Hospital	300+	76%	70%	71%
Use of Medical Imaging				
Cardiac Imaging Stress Test before Surgery	488	9.4%	5.5%	5.3%
Combination Abdominal CT Scan	939	7.1%	10.1%	10.5%
Combination Brain/Sinus CT Scan	1,197	2.1%	2.6%	2.7%
Combination Chest CT Scan	802	0.5%	2.8%	2.7%
Follow-up Mammogram/Ultrasound	2,580	11.8%	8.4%	8.8%
Lumbar Spine MRI for Low Back Pain	125	36.8%	36.6%	37.2%

Marshall Browning Hospital

900 North Washington Street Phone: 618-542-2146
Du Quoin, IL 62832 Fax: 618-542-4756
URL: www.marshallbrowninghospital.com
Type: Critical Access Hospitals Emergency Services: Yes
Ownership: Voluntary non-profit - Private Beds: 25

Key Personnel:
CEO . . . . Edwin A. Gast

Measure	Cases	This Hosp.	State Avg.	U.S. Avg.
Blood Clot Prevention and Treatment				
Anticoagulation Overlap Therapy[5]	-	-	91%	93%
ICU Venous Thromboembolism Prophylaxis[5]	-	-	93%	92%
Incidence of Potentially Preventable VTE[5]	-	-	11%	10%
UFH with Dosages/Platelet Monitoring[5]	-	-	94%	97%
Venous Thromboembolism Prophylaxis[5]	-	-	86%	85%
Warfarin Therapy Discharge Instructions[5]	-	-	71%	75%
Chest Pain/Possible Heart Attack Care				
Aspirin Given Within 24 Hours of Arrival	-	-	96%	96%
Fibrinolytic Meds Within 30 Min. of Arrival	-	-	65%	58%
Average Time to ECG (minutes)	-	-	6	7
Average Time to Transfer (minutes)	-	-	63	60
Children's Asthma Care				
Received Home Management Plan of Care	-	-	-	88%
Received Reliever Medication	-	-	-	100%
Received Systemic Corticosteroids	-	-	-	100%
Emergency Department				
Admittance Decision Time (minutes)[5]	-	-	89	98
Head CT Results Within 45 Min. of Arrival	-	-	64%	57%
Patients Who Left ER Before Being Seen	-	-	3%	2%
Time from ER Arrival to Admit. (minutes)[5]	-	-	260	274
Time from ER Arrival to Discharge (minutes)	-	-	138	134
Time in ER Before Being Evaluated (minutes)	-	-	28	26
Time to Pain Meds for Fractures (minutes)	-	-	52	57
Heart Attack Care				
Aspirin Given at Discharge[1,3]	-	-	99%	99%
Fibrinolytic Meds Within 30 Min. of Arrival[3,7]	-	-	33%	54%
PCI Within 90 Minutes of Arrival[3,7]	-	-	97%	96%
Statin Prescribed at Discharge[1,3]	-	-	98%	98%
Heart Failure Care				
ACE Inhibitor or ARB for LVSD[1,3]	-	-	98%	97%
Discharge Instructions Given[1,3]	-	-	96%	94%
Evaluation of LVS Function[3]	12	67%	99%	99%
Medicare Spending				
Medicare Spending per Patient (ratio)	-	-	1	0.98
Pneumonia Care				
Appropriate Initial Antibiotic Given[3]	12	92%	95%	95%
Blood Culture Timing[3]	22	100%	98%	98%
Pregnancy and Delivery Care				
Newborn Deliveries Scheduled Early[5]	-	-	2%	6%
Preventive Care				
Immunization for Influenza[5]	-	-	92%	90%
Immunization for Pneumonia[5]	-	-	92%	92%

NOTE: Hospital profiles are in alphabetical order by state, then city, then hospital within the city; Rankings exclude hospitals with less than 25 cases except for patient surveys which excludes hospitals with less than 100 cases; (a) 100-299 cases; (1) The number of cases/patients is too few to report; (2) Data submitted were based on a sample of cases/patients; (3) Results are based on a shorter time period than required; (4) Data suppressed by CMS for one or more quarters; (5) Results are not available for this reporting period; (6) Fewer than 100 patients completed the HCAHPS survey; (7) No cases met the criteria for this measure; (8) The lower limit of the confidence interval cannot be calculated if the number of observed infections equals zero; (9) No data are available from the state/territory for this reporting period; (10) The scores shown reflect fewer than 50 completed surveys; (11) There were discrepancies in the data collection process; (12) This measure does not apply to this hospital for this reporting period; (13) Results cannot be calculated for this reporting period; (14) The results for this state are combined with nearby states to protect confidentiality; Please refer to the User's Guide for a full explanation of data.

Stroke Care				
Anticoagulation Therapy for Atrial Fibrillation[5]	-	-	94%	95%
Antithrombotic Therapy Timing[5]	-	-	98%	98%
Assessed for Rehabilitation[5]	-	-	97%	97%
Discharged on Antithrombotic Therapy[5]	-	-	99%	99%
Discharged on Statin Medication[5]	-	-	94%	94%
Thrombolytic Therapy Timing[5]	-	-	66%	66%
Venous Thromboembolism Prophylaxis[5]	-	-	94%	94%
Written Stroke Educational Materials Given[5]	-	-	87%	88%
Surgical Care Improvement Project				
Appropriate Beta Blocker Usage[5]	-	-	98%	98%
Appropriate VTP Within 24 Hours[5]	-	-	98%	98%
Controlled Postoperative Blood Glucose[5]	-	-	97%	97%
Perioperative Temperature Management[5]	-	-	100%	100%
Prophylactic Antibiotic Selection[5]	-	-	99%	99%
Prophylactic Antibiotic Selection (Outpatient)	-	-	98%	98%
Prophylactic Antibiotic Stopped[5]	-	-	98%	98%
Prophylactic Antibiotic Timing[5]	-	-	99%	99%
Prophylactic Antibiotic Timing (Outpatient)	-	-	97%	98%
Urinary Catheter Removal[5]	-	-	98%	97%
Survey of Patients' Hospital Experiences				
Area Around Room 'Always' Quiet at Night[5]	-	-	60%	61%
Doctors 'Always' Communicated Well[5]	-	-	81%	82%
Home Recovery Information Given[5]	-	-	86%	85%
Hospital Given 9 or 10 on 10 Point Scale[5]	-	-	70%	71%
Meds 'Always' Explained Before Given[5]	-	-	64%	64%
Nurses 'Always' Communicated Well[5]	-	-	79%	79%
Pain 'Always' Well Controlled[5]	-	-	71%	71%
Room and Bathroom 'Always' Clean[5]	-	-	74%	73%
Timely Help 'Always' Received[5]	-	-	67%	68%
Would Definitely Recommend Hospital[5]	-	-	70%	71%
Use of Medical Imaging				
Cardiac Imaging Stress Test before Surgery	-	-	5.5%	5.3%
Combination Abdominal CT Scan	-	-	10.1%	10.5%
Combination Brain/Sinus CT Scan	-	-	2.6%	2.7%
Combination Chest CT Scan	-	-	2.8%	2.7%
Follow-up Mammogram/Ultrasound	-	-	8.4%	8.8%
Lumbar Spine MRI for Low Back Pain	-	-	36.6%	37.2%

Saint Anthonys Memorial Hospital

503 N Maple Street
Effingham, IL 62401
Phone: 217-342-2121
Fax: 217-347-1563
E-mail: hospital@effingham.net
URL: www.stanthonyshospital.org
Type: Acute Care Hospitals
Emergency Services: Yes
Ownership: Voluntary non-profit - Church
Beds: 146

Key Personnel:
Radiology. Marily Boone
Operating Room. . . . . Ruben Boyajian
Quality Assurance . . . . Mary Finley
Infection Control. . . . . Kim Howell
Chief of Medical Staff. . . . . Dr. Ryan Jennings
Coronary Care . . . . Sharyn Phillips
Pediatric In-Patient Care . . . . Sharyn Phillips
CEO/President. . . . . Theresa Rutherford

Measure	Cases	This Hosp.	State Avg.	U.S. Avg.
Blood Clot Prevention and Treatment				
Anticoagulation Overlap Therapy[2]	43	93%	91%	93%
ICU Venous Thromboembolism Prophylaxis[2]	56	88%	93%	92%
Incidence of Potentially Preventable VTE[1,2]	-	-	11%	10%
UFH with Dosages/Platelet Monitoring[2]	20	100%	94%	97%
Venous Thromboembolism Prophylaxis[2]	291	84%	86%	85%
Warfarin Therapy Discharge Instructions[2]	28	96%	71%	75%
Chest Pain/Possible Heart Attack Care				
Aspirin Given Within 24 Hours of Arrival	106	98%	96%	96%
Fibrinolytic Meds Within 30 Min. of Arrival[7]	-	-	65%	58%
Average Time to ECG (minutes)	104	13	6	7
Average Time to Transfer (minutes)[7]	-	-	63	60
Children's Asthma Care				
Received Home Management Plan of Care	-	-	-	88%
Received Reliever Medication	-	-	-	100%
Received Systemic Corticosteroids	-	-	-	100%
Emergency Department				
Admittance Decision Time (minutes)[2]	437	65	89	98
Head CT Results Within 45 Min. of Arrival	12	67%	64%	57%
Patients Who Left ER Before Being Seen	25,786	1%	3%	2%
Time from ER Arrival to Admit. (minutes)[2]	454	210	260	274
Time from ER Arrival to Discharge (minutes)	370	108	138	134
Time in ER Before Being Evaluated (minutes)	405	20	28	26
Time to Pain Meds for Fractures (minutes)	108	48	52	57
Heart Attack Care				
Aspirin Given at Discharge	23	100%	99%	99%
Fibrinolytic Meds Within 30 Min. of Arrival[7]	-	-	33%	54%
PCI Within 90 Minutes of Arrival[7]	-	-	97%	96%
Statin Prescribed at Discharge	19	100%	98%	98%
Heart Failure Care				
ACE Inhibitor or ARB for LVSD	41	100%	98%	97%
Discharge Instructions Given	126	96%	96%	94%
Evaluation of LVS Function	178	100%	99%	99%
Medicare Spending				
Medicare Spending per Patient (ratio)	-	0.88	1	0.98
Pneumonia Care				
Appropriate Initial Antibiotic Given	84	94%	95%	95%
Blood Culture Timing	148	99%	98%	98%
Pregnancy and Delivery Care				
Newborn Deliveries Scheduled Early[2]	52	2%	2%	6%
Preventive Care				
Immunization for Influenza[2]	502	92%	92%	90%
Immunization for Pneumonia[2]	643	94%	92%	92%
Stroke Care				
Anticoagulation Therapy for Atrial Fibrillation[1]	-	-	94%	95%
Antithrombotic Therapy Timing	30	97%	98%	98%
Assessed for Rehabilitation	31	97%	97%	97%
Discharged on Antithrombotic Therapy	28	96%	99%	99%
Discharged on Statin Medication	21	90%	94%	94%
Thrombolytic Therapy Timing[1]	-	-	66%	66%
Venous Thromboembolism Prophylaxis	32	84%	94%	94%
Written Stroke Educational Materials Given	14	57%	87%	88%
Surgical Care Improvement Project				
Appropriate Beta Blocker Usage	303	99%	98%	98%
Appropriate VTP Within 24 Hours	769	99%	98%	98%
Controlled Postoperative Blood Glucose[7]	-	-	97%	97%
Perioperative Temperature Management	834	100%	100%	100%
Prophylactic Antibiotic Selection	654	99%	99%	99%
Prophylactic Antibiotic Selection (Outpatient)	85	85%	98%	98%
Prophylactic Antibiotic Stopped	649	99%	98%	98%
Prophylactic Antibiotic Timing	654	100%	99%	99%
Prophylactic Antibiotic Timing (Outpatient)	87	95%	97%	98%
Urinary Catheter Removal	283	96%	98%	97%
Survey of Patients' Hospital Experiences				
Area Around Room 'Always' Quiet at Night	300+	55%	60%	61%
Doctors 'Always' Communicated Well	300+	82%	81%	82%
Home Recovery Information Given	300+	86%	86%	85%
Hospital Given 9 or 10 on 10 Point Scale	300+	68%	70%	71%
Meds 'Always' Explained Before Given	300+	63%	64%	64%
Nurses 'Always' Communicated Well	300+	79%	79%	79%
Pain 'Always' Well Controlled	300+	69%	71%	71%
Room and Bathroom 'Always' Clean	300+	73%	74%	73%
Timely Help 'Always' Received	300+	66%	67%	68%
Would Definitely Recommend Hospital	300+	66%	70%	71%
Use of Medical Imaging				
Cardiac Imaging Stress Test before Surgery	771	3.8%	5.5%	5.3%
Combination Abdominal CT Scan	998	6.0%	10.1%	10.5%
Combination Brain/Sinus CT Scan	688	2.9%	2.6%	2.7%
Combination Chest CT Scan	603	2.2%	2.8%	2.7%
Follow-up Mammogram/Ultrasound	1,752	9.8%	8.4%	8.8%
Lumbar Spine MRI for Low Back Pain	295	35.3%	36.6%	37.2%

Ferrell Hospital Community Foundations

1201 Pine Street
Eldorado, IL 62930
Phone: 618-273-3361
Fax: 618-273-2571
Type: Critical Access Hospitals
Emergency Services: Yes
Ownership: Voluntary non-profit - Private
Beds: 51

Key Personnel:
Operating Room. . . . . Samir F Abdo
Cardiology . . . . Sridhar Banuru
CEO/President. . . . . Donald Brown
Chairman/CEO . . . . Gene Morris
Chief of Medical Staff . . . . Eliott Partirdge
Radiology. Bill Scroggins
Emergency Room . . . . Jackie Tripp

Measure	Cases	This Hosp.	State Avg.	U.S. Avg.
Blood Clot Prevention and Treatment				
Anticoagulation Overlap Therapy[5]	-	-	91%	93%
ICU Venous Thromboembolism Prophylaxis[5]	-	-	93%	92%
Incidence of Potentially Preventable VTE[5]	-	-	11%	10%
UFH with Dosages/Platelet Monitoring[5]	-	-	94%	97%
Venous Thromboembolism Prophylaxis[5]	-	-	86%	85%
Warfarin Therapy Discharge Instructions[5]	-	-	71%	75%
Chest Pain/Possible Heart Attack Care				
Aspirin Given Within 24 Hours of Arrival[5]	-	-	96%	96%
Fibrinolytic Meds Within 30 Min. of Arrival[5]	-	-	65%	58%
Average Time to ECG (minutes)[5]	-	-	6	7
Average Time to Transfer (minutes)[5]	-	-	63	60
Children's Asthma Care				
Received Home Management Plan of Care	-	-	-	88%
Received Reliever Medication	-	-	-	100%
Received Systemic Corticosteroids	-	-	-	100%
Emergency Department				
Admittance Decision Time (minutes)[5]	-	-	89	98
Head CT Results Within 45 Min. of Arrival[5]	-	-	64%	57%
Patients Who Left ER Before Being Seen	7,375	3%	3%	2%
Time from ER Arrival to Admit. (minutes)[5]	-	-	260	274
Time from ER Arrival to Discharge (minutes)[5]	-	-	138	134
Time in ER Before Being Evaluated (minutes)[5]	-	-	28	26
Time to Pain Meds for Fractures (minutes)[5]	-	-	52	57
Heart Attack Care				
Aspirin Given at Discharge[1]	-	-	99%	99%
Fibrinolytic Meds Within 30 Min. of Arrival[7]	-	-	33%	54%
PCI Within 90 Minutes of Arrival[7]	-	-	97%	96%
Statin Prescribed at Discharge[1]	-	-	98%	98%
Heart Failure Care				
ACE Inhibitor or ARB for LVSD[1]	-	-	98%	97%
Discharge Instructions Given	15	53%	96%	94%
Evaluation of LVS Function	18	39%	99%	99%
Medicare Spending				
Medicare Spending per Patient (ratio)	-	-	1	0.98
Pneumonia Care				
Appropriate Initial Antibiotic Given	44	80%	95%	95%
Blood Culture Timing	22	100%	98%	98%
Pregnancy and Delivery Care				
Newborn Deliveries Scheduled Early[5]	-	-	2%	6%
Preventive Care				
Immunization for Influenza[5]	-	-	92%	90%
Immunization for Pneumonia[5]	-	-	92%	92%
Stroke Care				
Anticoagulation Therapy for Atrial Fibrillation[5]	-	-	94%	95%
Antithrombotic Therapy Timing[5]	-	-	98%	98%
Assessed for Rehabilitation[5]	-	-	97%	97%
Discharged on Antithrombotic Therapy[5]	-	-	99%	99%
Discharged on Statin Medication[5]	-	-	94%	94%
Thrombolytic Therapy Timing[5]	-	-	66%	66%
Venous Thromboembolism Prophylaxis[5]	-	-	94%	94%
Written Stroke Educational Materials Given[5]	-	-	87%	88%
Surgical Care Improvement Project				
Appropriate Beta Blocker Usage[5]	-	-	98%	98%
Appropriate VTP Within 24 Hours[5]	-	-	98%	98%
Controlled Postoperative Blood Glucose[5]	-	-	97%	97%
Perioperative Temperature Management[5]	-	-	100%	100%
Prophylactic Antibiotic Selection[5]	-	-	99%	99%
Prophylactic Antibiotic Selection (Outpatient)[5]	-	-	98%	98%
Prophylactic Antibiotic Stopped[5]	-	-	98%	98%
Prophylactic Antibiotic Timing[5]	-	-	99%	99%
Prophylactic Antibiotic Timing (Outpatient)[5]	-	-	97%	98%
Urinary Catheter Removal[5]	-	-	98%	97%
Survey of Patients' Hospital Experiences				
Area Around Room 'Always' Quiet at Night[5]	-	-	60%	61%
Doctors 'Always' Communicated Well[5]	-	-	81%	82%
Home Recovery Information Given[5]	-	-	86%	85%
Hospital Given 9 or 10 on 10 Point Scale[5]	-	-	70%	71%

NOTE: Hospital profiles are in alphabetical order by state, then city, then hospital within the city; Rankings exclude hospitals with less than 25 cases except for patient surveys which excludes hospitals with less than 100 cases; (a) 100-299 cases; (1) The number of cases/patients is too few to report; (2) Data submitted were based on a sample of cases/patients; (3) Results are based on a shorter time period than required; (4) Data suppressed by CMS for one or more quarters; (5) Results are not available for this reporting period; (6) Fewer than 100 patients completed the HCAHPS survey; (7) No cases met the criteria for this measure; (8) The lower limit of the confidence interval cannot be calculated if the number of observed infections equals zero; (9) No data are available from the state/territory for this reporting period; (10) The scores shown reflect fewer than 50 completed surveys; (11) There were discrepancies in the data collection process; (12) This measure does not apply to this hospital for this reporting period; (13) Results cannot be calculated for this reporting period; (14) The results for this state are combined with nearby states to protect confidentiality; Please refer to the User's Guide for a full explanation of data.

Measure	Cases	This Hosp.	State Avg.	U.S. Avg.
Meds 'Always' Explained Before Given[5]	-	-	64%	64%
Nurses 'Always' Communicated Well[5]	-	-	79%	79%
Pain 'Always' Well Controlled[5]	-	-	71%	71%
Room and Bathroom 'Always' Clean[5]	-	-	74%	73%
Timely Help 'Always' Received[5]	-	-	67%	68%
Would Definitely Recommend Hospital[5]	-	-	70%	71%
Use of Medical Imaging				
Cardiac Imaging Stress Test before Surgery	49	0.0%	5.5%	5.3%
Combination Abdominal CT Scan	213	23.0%	10.1%	10.5%
Combination Brain/Sinus CT Scan[1]	-	-	2.6%	2.7%
Combination Chest CT Scan	109	48.6%	2.8%	2.7%
Follow-up Mammogram/Ultrasound	268	7.5%	8.4%	8.8%
Lumbar Spine MRI for Low Back Pain[1]	-	-	36.6%	37.2%

Presence Saint Joseph Hospital - Elgin

77 N Airlite Street
Elgin, IL 60123
Phone: 847-695-3200
Fax: 847-622-2070
URL: www.provenasaintjoeph.com
Type: Acute Care Hospitals
Emergency Services: Yes
Ownership: Voluntary non-profit - Church
Beds: 260

Key Personnel:
Operating Room. . . . . Feli Bayani
Cardiac Laboratory. . . . . Jeff Berchner
CEO/President. . . . . Sandra Bruce
Chief of Medical Staff . . . . Charles Carallo, MD
Quality Assurance . . . . Carol Fodge
Infection Control. . . . . Kathy Hogan
Radiology. . . . . Laurie Schachtner

Measure	Cases	This Hosp.	State Avg.	U.S. Avg.
Blood Clot Prevention and Treatment				
Anticoagulation Overlap Therapy[2]	66	80%	91%	93%
ICU Venous Thromboembolism Prophylaxis[2]	102	98%	93%	92%
Incidence of Potentially Preventable VTE[2]	12	0%	11%	10%
UFH with Dosages/Platelet Monitoring[2]	42	100%	94%	97%
Venous Thromboembolism Prophylaxis[2]	320	97%	86%	85%
Warfarin Therapy Discharge Instructions[2]	52	96%	71%	75%
Chest Pain/Possible Heart Attack Care				
Aspirin Given Within 24 Hours of Arrival[1,3]	-	-	96%	96%
Fibrinolytic Meds Within 30 Min. of Arrival[3,7]	-	-	65%	58%
Average Time to ECG (minutes)[1,3]	-	-	6	7
Average Time to Transfer (minutes)[1,3]	-	-	63	60
Children's Asthma Care				
Received Home Management Plan of Care	-	-	-	88%
Received Reliever Medication	-	-	-	100%
Received Systemic Corticosteroids	-	-	-	100%
Emergency Department				
Admittance Decision Time (minutes)[2]	653	93	89	98
Head CT Results Within 45 Min. of Arrival	13	62%	64%	57%
Patients Who Left ER Before Being Seen	30,773	1%	3%	2%
Time from ER Arrival to Admit. (minutes)[2]	667	264	260	274
Time from ER Arrival to Discharge (minutes)	349	143	138	134
Time in ER Before Being Evaluated (minutes)	399	18	28	26
Time to Pain Meds for Fractures (minutes)	95	57	52	57
Heart Attack Care				
Aspirin Given at Discharge	85	98%	99%	99%
Fibrinolytic Meds Within 30 Min. of Arrival[7]	-	-	33%	54%
PCI Within 90 Minutes of Arrival	20	90%	97%	96%
Statin Prescribed at Discharge	84	99%	98%	98%
Heart Failure Care				
ACE Inhibitor or ARB for LVSD	25	88%	98%	97%
Discharge Instructions Given	100	92%	96%	94%
Evaluation of LVS Function	143	97%	99%	99%
Medicare Spending				
Medicare Spending per Patient (ratio)	-	1.11	1	0.98
Pneumonia Care				
Appropriate Initial Antibiotic Given[2]	92	93%	95%	95%
Blood Culture Timing[2]	172	98%	98%	98%
Pregnancy and Delivery Care				
Newborn Deliveries Scheduled Early[7]	-	-	2%	6%
Preventive Care				
Immunization for Influenza[2]	472	84%	92%	90%
Immunization for Pneumonia[2]	725	88%	92%	92%
Stroke Care				
Anticoagulation Therapy for Atrial Fibrillation[1]	-	-	94%	95%
Antithrombotic Therapy Timing	56	100%	98%	98%
Assessed for Rehabilitation	59	98%	97%	97%
Discharged on Antithrombotic Therapy	51	96%	99%	99%
Discharged on Statin Medication	38	95%	94%	94%
Thrombolytic Therapy Timing[1]	-	-	66%	66%
Venous Thromboembolism Prophylaxis	64	98%	94%	94%
Written Stroke Educational Materials Given	25	84%	87%	88%
Surgical Care Improvement Project				
Appropriate Beta Blocker Usage[2]	155	99%	98%	98%
Appropriate VTP Within 24 Hours[2]	341	98%	98%	98%
Controlled Postoperative Blood Glucose[2]	38	97%	97%	97%
Perioperative Temperature Management[2]	397	99%	100%	100%
Prophylactic Antibiotic Selection[2]	279	100%	99%	99%
Prophylactic Antibiotic Selection (Outpatient)	104	97%	98%	98%
Prophylactic Antibiotic Stopped[2]	268	99%	98%	98%
Prophylactic Antibiotic Timing[2]	279	99%	99%	99%
Prophylactic Antibiotic Timing (Outpatient)	74	88%	97%	98%
Urinary Catheter Removal[2]	205	99%	98%	97%
Survey of Patients' Hospital Experiences				
Area Around Room 'Always' Quiet at Night	300+	60%	60%	61%
Doctors 'Always' Communicated Well	300+	80%	81%	82%
Home Recovery Information Given	300+	88%	86%	85%
Hospital Given 9 or 10 on 10 Point Scale	300+	70%	70%	71%
Meds 'Always' Explained Before Given	300+	60%	64%	64%
Nurses 'Always' Communicated Well	300+	78%	79%	79%
Pain 'Always' Well Controlled	300+	71%	71%	71%
Room and Bathroom 'Always' Clean	300+	73%	74%	73%
Timely Help 'Always' Received	300+	58%	67%	68%
Would Definitely Recommend Hospital	300+	67%	70%	71%
Use of Medical Imaging				
Cardiac Imaging Stress Test before Surgery	413	7.5%	5.5%	5.3%
Combination Abdominal CT Scan	622	5.1%	10.1%	10.5%
Combination Brain/Sinus CT Scan[1]	-	-	2.6%	2.7%
Combination Chest CT Scan	423	0.5%	2.8%	2.7%
Follow-up Mammogram/Ultrasound	805	11.6%	8.4%	8.8%
Lumbar Spine MRI for Low Back Pain	57	40.4%	36.6%	37.2%

Sherman Hospital

1425 North Randall Road
Elgin, IL 60123
Phone: 847-742-9800
Fax: 847-429-2035
URL: www.shermanhealth.com
Type: Acute Care Hospitals
Emergency Services: Yes
Ownership: Voluntary non-profit - Private
Beds: 353

Key Personnel:
Operating Room. . . . . Paula Bergschneider
CEO/President. . . . . Linda Deering
Pediatric Ambulatory Care . . . . . . Patrick Esposito, MD
Pediatric In-Patient Care . . . . Patrick Esposito, MD
Chief of Medical Staff. . . . . Edgar Feldman, MD, FACS
Quality Assurance . . . . Barbara Giardino
Radiology. . . . . Debbie Petges
Infection Control. . . . . Sallie Rivera, RN

Measure	Cases	This Hosp.	State Avg.	U.S. Avg.
Blood Clot Prevention and Treatment				
Anticoagulation Overlap Therapy[2]	119	100%	91%	93%
ICU Venous Thromboembolism Prophylaxis[2]	77	99%	93%	92%
Incidence of Potentially Preventable VTE[2]	14	14%	11%	10%
UFH with Dosages/Platelet Monitoring[2]	97	100%	94%	97%
Venous Thromboembolism Prophylaxis[2]	330	74%	86%	85%
Warfarin Therapy Discharge Instructions[2]	102	98%	71%	75%
Chest Pain/Possible Heart Attack Care				
Aspirin Given Within 24 Hours of Arrival[1,3]	-	-	96%	96%
Fibrinolytic Meds Within 30 Min. of Arrival[5]	-	-	65%	58%
Average Time to ECG (minutes)[1,3]	-	-	6	7
Average Time to Transfer (minutes)[5]	-	-	63	60
Children's Asthma Care				
Received Home Management Plan of Care	-	-	-	88%
Received Reliever Medication	-	-	-	100%
Received Systemic Corticosteroids	-	-	-	100%
Emergency Department				
Admittance Decision Time (minutes)[2]	515	87	89	98
Head CT Results Within 45 Min. of Arrival	49	98%	64%	57%
Patients Who Left ER Before Being Seen	60,739	1%	3%	2%
Time from ER Arrival to Admit. (minutes)[2]	531	234	260	274
Time from ER Arrival to Discharge (minutes)	408	123	138	134
Time in ER Before Being Evaluated (minutes)	442	19	28	26
Time to Pain Meds for Fractures (minutes)	300	44	52	57
Heart Attack Care				
Aspirin Given at Discharge	222	100%	99%	99%
Fibrinolytic Meds Within 30 Min. of Arrival[7]	-	-	33%	54%
PCI Within 90 Minutes of Arrival	57	98%	97%	96%
Statin Prescribed at Discharge	214	100%	98%	98%
Heart Failure Care				
ACE Inhibitor or ARB for LVSD	93	99%	98%	97%
Discharge Instructions Given	277	99%	96%	94%
Evaluation of LVS Function	363	100%	99%	99%
Medicare Spending				
Medicare Spending per Patient (ratio)	-	1.05	1	0.98
Pneumonia Care				
Appropriate Initial Antibiotic Given	206	98%	95%	95%
Blood Culture Timing	377	100%	98%	98%
Pregnancy and Delivery Care				
Newborn Deliveries Scheduled Early[2]	64	0%	2%	6%
Preventive Care				
Immunization for Influenza[2]	485	99%	92%	90%
Immunization for Pneumonia[2]	556	98%	92%	92%
Stroke Care				
Anticoagulation Therapy for Atrial Fibrillation	14	100%	94%	95%
Antithrombotic Therapy Timing	73	100%	98%	98%
Assessed for Rehabilitation	101	100%	97%	97%
Discharged on Antithrombotic Therapy	88	100%	99%	99%
Discharged on Statin Medication	63	100%	94%	94%
Thrombolytic Therapy Timing[7]	-	-	66%	66%
Venous Thromboembolism Prophylaxis	90	99%	94%	94%
Written Stroke Educational Materials Given	54	100%	87%	88%
Surgical Care Improvement Project				
Appropriate Beta Blocker Usage	436	99%	98%	98%
Appropriate VTP Within 24 Hours	937	99%	98%	98%
Controlled Postoperative Blood Glucose	158	98%	97%	97%
Perioperative Temperature Management	1,094	100%	100%	100%
Prophylactic Antibiotic Selection	812	100%	99%	99%
Prophylactic Antibiotic Selection (Outpatient)	269	99%	98%	98%
Prophylactic Antibiotic Stopped	789	100%	98%	98%
Prophylactic Antibiotic Timing	812	100%	99%	99%
Prophylactic Antibiotic Timing (Outpatient)	184	100%	97%	98%
Urinary Catheter Removal	270	100%	98%	97%
Survey of Patients' Hospital Experiences				
Area Around Room 'Always' Quiet at Night	300+	68%	60%	61%
Doctors 'Always' Communicated Well	300+	78%	81%	82%
Home Recovery Information Given	300+	87%	86%	85%
Hospital Given 9 or 10 on 10 Point Scale	300+	74%	70%	71%
Meds 'Always' Explained Before Given	300+	63%	64%	64%
Nurses 'Always' Communicated Well	300+	80%	79%	79%
Pain 'Always' Well Controlled	300+	71%	71%	71%
Room and Bathroom 'Always' Clean	300+	75%	74%	73%
Timely Help 'Always' Received	300+	67%	67%	68%
Would Definitely Recommend Hospital	300+	75%	70%	71%
Use of Medical Imaging				
Cardiac Imaging Stress Test before Surgery	863	6.3%	5.5%	5.3%
Combination Abdominal CT Scan	1,517	8.3%	10.1%	10.5%
Combination Brain/Sinus CT Scan	1,176	2.6%	2.6%	2.7%
Combination Chest CT Scan	979	1.9%	2.8%	2.7%
Follow-up Mammogram/Ultrasound	2,079	6.4%	8.4%	8.8%
Lumbar Spine MRI for Low Back Pain	151	26.5%	36.6%	37.2%

Alexian Brothers Medical Center

800 W Biesterfield Rd
Elk Grove Village, IL 60007
Phone: 847-437-5500
Fax: 847-981-5766
URL: www.alexian.org
Type: Acute Care Hospitals
Emergency Services: Yes
Ownership: Voluntary non-profit - Church
Beds: 483

Key Personnel:
Pediatric In-Patient Care . . . . Patsy Buckberg
CEO/President. . . . . Mark Frey
Chief of Medical Staff . . . . Barry Glick, MD
Cardiac Laboratory. . . . . Paul J Grunenwald
Radiology. . . . . Steve Jung
Infection Control. . . . . Laura Marconnet
Intensive Care Unit. . . . . Debra Perrin-Davis

NOTE: Hospital profiles are in alphabetical order by state, then city, then hospital within the city; Rankings exclude hospitals with less than 25 cases except for patient surveys which excludes hospitals with less than 100 cases; (a) 100-299 cases; (1) The number of cases/patients is too few to report; (2) Data submitted were based on a sample of cases/patients; (3) Results are based on a shorter time period than required; (4) Data suppressed by CMS for one or more quarters; (5) Results are not available for this reporting period; (6) Fewer than 100 patients completed the HCAHPS survey; (7) No cases met the criteria for this measure; (8) The lower limit of the confidence interval cannot be calculated if the number of observed infections equals zero; (9) No data are available from the state/territory for this reporting period; (10) The scores shown reflect fewer than 50 completed surveys; (11) There were discrepancies in the data collection process; (12) This measure does not apply to this hospital for this reporting period; (13) Results cannot be calculated for this reporting period; (14) The results for this state are combined with nearby states to protect confidentiality; Please refer to the User's Guide for a full explanation of data.

Emergency Room . . . . Rick Stephani, CHRM

Measure	Cases	This Hosp.	State Avg.	U.S. Avg.
Blood Clot Prevention and Treatment				
Anticoagulation Overlap Therapy[2]	156	95%	91%	93%
ICU Venous Thromboembolism Prophylaxis[2]	96	97%	93%	92%
Incidence of Potentially Preventable VTE[2]	39	10%	11%	10%
UFH with Dosages/Platelet Monitoring[2]	150	98%	94%	97%
Venous Thromboembolism Prophylaxis[2]	333	85%	86%	85%
Warfarin Therapy Discharge Instructions[2]	101	83%	71%	75%
Chest Pain/Possible Heart Attack Care				
Aspirin Given Within 24 Hours of Arrival[5]	-	-	96%	96%
Fibrinolytic Meds Within 30 Min. of Arrival[5]	-	-	65%	58%
Average Time to ECG (minutes)[5]	-	-	6	7
Average Time to Transfer (minutes)[5]	-	-	63	60
Children's Asthma Care				
Received Home Management Plan of Care	-	-	-	88%
Received Reliever Medication	-	-	-	100%
Received Systemic Corticosteroids	-	-	-	100%
Emergency Department				
Admittance Decision Time (minutes)[2]	687	95	89	98
Head CT Results Within 45 Min. of Arrival[5]	-	64%	57%	
Patients Who Left ER Before Being Seen	49,973	1%	3%	2%
Time from ER Arrival to Admit. (minutes)[2]	687	245	260	274
Time from ER Arrival to Discharge (minutes)	393	152	138	134
Time in ER Before Being Evaluated (minutes)	428	22	28	26
Time to Pain Meds for Fractures (minutes)	171	31	52	57
Heart Attack Care				
Aspirin Given at Discharge	242	100%	99%	99%
Fibrinolytic Meds Within 30 Min. of Arrival[7]	-	-	33%	54%
PCI Within 90 Minutes of Arrival	58	100%	97%	96%
Statin Prescribed at Discharge	236	100%	98%	98%
Heart Failure Care				
ACE Inhibitor or ARB for LVSD	92	100%	98%	97%
Discharge Instructions Given	344	99%	96%	94%
Evaluation of LVS Function	434	100%	99%	99%
Medicare Spending				
Medicare Spending per Patient (ratio)	-	1.07	1	0.98
Pneumonia Care				
Appropriate Initial Antibiotic Given	185	97%	95%	95%
Blood Culture Timing	418	99%	98%	98%
Pregnancy and Delivery Care				
Newborn Deliveries Scheduled Early[2]	53	0%	2%	6%
Preventive Care				
Immunization for Influenza[2]	633	94%	92%	90%
Immunization for Pneumonia[2]	836	95%	92%	92%
Stroke Care				
Anticoagulation Therapy for Atrial Fibrillation	36	94%	94%	95%
Antithrombotic Therapy Timing	148	99%	98%	98%
Assessed for Rehabilitation	232	100%	97%	97%
Discharged on Antithrombotic Therapy	186	99%	99%	99%
Discharged on Statin Medication	143	97%	94%	94%
Thrombolytic Therapy Timing	26	100%	66%	66%
Venous Thromboembolism Prophylaxis	245	99%	94%	94%
Written Stroke Educational Materials Given	116	92%	87%	88%
Surgical Care Improvement Project				
Appropriate Beta Blocker Usage[2]	249	99%	98%	98%
Appropriate VTP Within 24 Hours[2]	460	100%	98%	98%
Controlled Postoperative Blood Glucose[2]	135	99%	97%	97%
Perioperative Temperature Management[2]	523	100%	100%	100%
Prophylactic Antibiotic Selection[2]	468	99%	99%	99%
Prophylactic Antibiotic Selection (Outpatient)	425	96%	98%	98%
Prophylactic Antibiotic Stopped[2]	445	98%	98%	98%
Prophylactic Antibiotic Timing[2]	468	100%	99%	99%
Prophylactic Antibiotic Timing (Outpatient)	424	98%	97%	98%
Urinary Catheter Removal[2]	377	99%	98%	97%
Survey of Patients' Hospital Experiences				
Area Around Room 'Always' Quiet at Night	300+	57%	60%	61%
Doctors 'Always' Communicated Well	300+	81%	81%	82%
Home Recovery Information Given	300+	87%	86%	85%
Hospital Given 9 or 10 on 10 Point Scale	300+	74%	70%	71%
Meds 'Always' Explained Before Given	300+	61%	64%	64%
Nurses 'Always' Communicated Well	300+	79%	79%	79%
Pain 'Always' Well Controlled	300+	72%	71%	71%
Room and Bathroom 'Always' Clean	300+	74%	74%	73%
Timely Help 'Always' Received	300+	64%	67%	68%
Would Definitely Recommend Hospital	300+	76%	70%	71%
Use of Medical Imaging				
Cardiac Imaging Stress Test before Surgery	1,554	4.6%	5.5%	5.3%
Combination Abdominal CT Scan	1,763	9.5%	10.1%	10.5%
Combination Brain/Sinus CT Scan	1,191	2.1%	2.6%	2.7%
Combination Chest CT Scan	1,377	7.1%	2.8%	2.7%
Follow-up Mammogram/Ultrasound	2,918	6.8%	8.4%	8.8%
Lumbar Spine MRI for Low Back Pain	228	27.6%	36.6%	37.2%

Elmhurst Memorial Hospital

155 East Brush Hill Road
Elmhurst, IL 60126
URL: www.emhc.org
Type: Acute Care Hospitals
Ownership: Proprietary

Phone: 630-833-1400
Fax: 630-782-7844
Emergency Services: Yes
Beds: 427

Key Personnel:
Operating Room. . . . . Diane Drugas, MD
Infection Control. . . . . Patricia Funderburk
Quality Assurance . . . . Craig Grothaus
Emergency Room . . . . Fred Jacobs, MD
CEO/President. . . . . Mary Lou Mastro
Radiology. . . . . Aloyzas Pakalniskis, MD
Pediatric In-Patient Care . . . . . . Victoria Uribe, MD
Chief of Medical Staff . . . . Karl L. Vos, MD

Measure	Cases	This Hosp.	State Avg.	U.S. Avg.
Blood Clot Prevention and Treatment				
Anticoagulation Overlap Therapy[2]	143	85%	91%	93%
ICU Venous Thromboembolism Prophylaxis[2]	111	89%	93%	92%
Incidence of Potentially Preventable VTE[1,2]	-	-	11%	10%
UFH with Dosages/Platelet Monitoring[2]	114	100%	94%	97%
Venous Thromboembolism Prophylaxis[2]	301	83%	86%	85%
Warfarin Therapy Discharge Instructions[2]	111	59%	71%	75%
Chest Pain/Possible Heart Attack Care				
Aspirin Given Within 24 Hours of Arrival[5]	-	-	96%	96%
Fibrinolytic Meds Within 30 Min. of Arrival[5]	-	-	65%	58%
Average Time to ECG (minutes)[5]	-	-	6	7
Average Time to Transfer (minutes)[5]	-	-	63	60
Children's Asthma Care				
Received Home Management Plan of Care	-	-	-	88%
Received Reliever Medication	-	-	-	100%
Received Systemic Corticosteroids	-	-	-	100%
Emergency Department				
Admittance Decision Time (minutes)[2]	688	70	89	98
Head CT Results Within 45 Min. of Arrival	11	55%	64%	57%
Patients Who Left ER Before Being Seen	50,406	1%	3%	2%
Time from ER Arrival to Admit. (minutes)[2]	694	238	260	274
Time from ER Arrival to Discharge (minutes)	357	135	138	134
Time in ER Before Being Evaluated (minutes)	397	19	28	26
Time to Pain Meds for Fractures (minutes)	152	44	52	57
Heart Attack Care				
Aspirin Given at Discharge	195	100%	99%	99%
Fibrinolytic Meds Within 30 Min. of Arrival[7]	-	-	33%	54%
PCI Within 90 Minutes of Arrival	45	98%	97%	96%
Statin Prescribed at Discharge	191	100%	98%	98%
Heart Failure Care				
ACE Inhibitor or ARB for LVSD[2]	92	100%	98%	97%
Discharge Instructions Given[2]	235	100%	96%	94%
Evaluation of LVS Function[2]	305	100%	99%	99%
Medicare Spending				
Medicare Spending per Patient (ratio)	-	1.06	1	0.98
Pneumonia Care				
Appropriate Initial Antibiotic Given[2]	98	92%	95%	95%
Blood Culture Timing[2]	144	98%	98%	98%
Pregnancy and Delivery Care				
Newborn Deliveries Scheduled Early[2]	26	0%	2%	6%
Preventive Care				
Immunization for Influenza[2]	567	94%	92%	90%
Immunization for Pneumonia[2]	713	94%	92%	92%
Stroke Care				
Anticoagulation Therapy for Atrial Fibrillation	15	87%	94%	95%
Antithrombotic Therapy Timing	127	97%	98%	98%
Assessed for Rehabilitation	148	99%	97%	97%
Discharged on Antithrombotic Therapy	138	100%	99%	99%
Discharged on Statin Medication	116	97%	94%	94%
Thrombolytic Therapy Timing	16	62%	66%	66%
Venous Thromboembolism Prophylaxis	149	93%	94%	94%
Written Stroke Educational Materials Given	77	96%	87%	88%
Surgical Care Improvement Project				
Appropriate Beta Blocker Usage[2]	160	97%	98%	98%
Appropriate VTP Within 24 Hours[2]	352	96%	98%	98%
Controlled Postoperative Blood Glucose[2]	110	97%	97%	97%
Perioperative Temperature Management[2]	408	100%	100%	100%
Prophylactic Antibiotic Selection[2]	356	100%	99%	99%
Prophylactic Antibiotic Selection (Outpatient)	351	100%	98%	98%
Prophylactic Antibiotic Stopped[2]	348	98%	98%	98%
Prophylactic Antibiotic Timing[2]	356	99%	99%	99%
Prophylactic Antibiotic Timing (Outpatient)	251	99%	97%	98%
Urinary Catheter Removal[2]	318	99%	98%	97%
Survey of Patients' Hospital Experiences				
Area Around Room 'Always' Quiet at Night	300+	69%	60%	61%
Doctors 'Always' Communicated Well	300+	80%	81%	82%
Home Recovery Information Given	300+	86%	86%	85%
Hospital Given 9 or 10 on 10 Point Scale	300+	75%	70%	71%
Meds 'Always' Explained Before Given	300+	64%	64%	64%
Nurses 'Always' Communicated Well	300+	78%	79%	79%
Pain 'Always' Well Controlled	300+	68%	71%	71%
Room and Bathroom 'Always' Clean	300+	72%	74%	73%
Timely Help 'Always' Received	300+	61%	67%	68%
Would Definitely Recommend Hospital	300+	76%	70%	71%
Use of Medical Imaging				
Cardiac Imaging Stress Test before Surgery	792	6.6%	5.5%	5.3%
Combination Abdominal CT Scan	1,643	7.5%	10.1%	10.5%
Combination Brain/Sinus CT Scan	1,223	1.6%	2.6%	2.7%
Combination Chest CT Scan	1,403	1.2%	2.8%	2.7%
Follow-up Mammogram/Ultrasound	2,756	9.5%	8.4%	8.8%
Lumbar Spine MRI for Low Back Pain	319	37.0%	36.6%	37.2%

Advocate Eureka Hospital

101 S Major St
Eureka, IL 61530
E-mail: webmaster@bromenn.org
URL: www.eurekahospital.org
Type: Critical Access Hospitals
Ownership: Voluntary non-profit - Private

Phone: 309-467-2371
Fax: 309-467-2880
Emergency Services: Yes
Beds: 25

Key Personnel:
Operating Room. . . . . Steve Holman
CEO/President. . . . . Roger S Hunt
Infection Control. . . . . Henrietta Iwema, RN
Chief of Medical Staff . . . . Steven K Jones, DO
Anesthesiology. . . . . Rodney T McCalla, MD
Quality Assurance . . . . Jane Ulrich
Coronary Care . . . . Jeff Williams
Emergency Room . . . . Jeff Williams

Measure	Cases	This Hosp.	State Avg.	U.S. Avg.
Blood Clot Prevention and Treatment				
Anticoagulation Overlap Therapy[1]	-	-	91%	93%
ICU Venous Thromboembolism Prophylaxis[7]	-	-	93%	92%
Incidence of Potentially Preventable VTE[7]	-	-	11%	10%
UFH with Dosages/Platelet Monitoring[7]	-	-	94%	97%
Venous Thromboembolism Prophylaxis	125	94%	86%	85%
Warfarin Therapy Discharge Instructions[1]	-	-	71%	75%
Chest Pain/Possible Heart Attack Care				
Aspirin Given Within 24 Hours of Arrival[1,3]	-	-	96%	96%
Fibrinolytic Meds Within 30 Min. of Arrival[3,7]	-	-	65%	58%
Average Time to ECG (minutes)[1,3]	-	-	6	7
Average Time to Transfer (minutes)[1,3]	-	-	63	60
Children's Asthma Care				
Received Home Management Plan of Care	-	-	-	88%
Received Reliever Medication	-	-	-	100%
Received Systemic Corticosteroids	-	-	-	100%
Emergency Department				
Admittance Decision Time (minutes)	175	54	89	98
Head CT Results Within 45 Min. of Arrival[5]	-	-	64%	57%
Patients Who Left ER Before Being Seen[5]	-	-	3%	2%

NOTE: Hospital profiles are in alphabetical order by state, then city, then hospital within the city; Rankings exclude hospitals with less than 25 cases except for patient surveys which excludes hospitals with less than 100 cases; (a) 100-299 cases; (1) The number of cases/patients is too few to report; (2) Data submitted were based on a sample of cases/patients; (3) Results are based on a shorter time period than required; (4) Data suppressed by CMS for one or more quarters; (5) Results are not available for this reporting period; (6) Fewer than 100 patients completed the HCAHPS survey; (7) No cases met the criteria for this measure; (8) The lower limit of the confidence interval cannot be calculated if the number of observed infections equals zero; (9) No data are available from the state/territory for this reporting period; (10) The scores shown reflect fewer than 50 completed surveys; (11) There were discrepancies in the data collection process; (12) This measure does not apply to this hospital for this reporting period; (13) Results cannot be calculated for this reporting period; (14) The results for this state are combined with nearby states to protect confidentiality; Please refer to the User's Guide for a full explanation of data.

Measure	Cases	This Hosp.	State Avg.	U.S. Avg.
Time from ER Arrival to Admit. (minutes)	181	205	260	274
Time from ER Arrival to Discharge (minutes)	343	97	138	134
Time in ER Before Being Evaluated (minutes)	370	15	28	26
Time to Pain Meds for Fractures (minutes)	23	53	52	57
Heart Attack Care				
Aspirin Given at Discharge[5]	-	-	99%	99%
Fibrinolytic Meds Within 30 Min. of Arrival[5]	-	-	33%	54%
PCI Within 90 Minutes of Arrival[5]	-	-	97%	96%
Statin Prescribed at Discharge[5]	-	-	98%	98%
Heart Failure Care				
ACE Inhibitor or ARB for LVSD[1]	-	-	98%	97%
Discharge Instructions Given[1]	-	-	96%	94%
Evaluation of LVS Function	20	100%	99%	99%
Medicare Spending				
Medicare Spending per Patient (ratio)	-	-	1	0.98
Pneumonia Care				
Appropriate Initial Antibiotic Given	15	100%	95%	95%
Blood Culture Timing	17	94%	98%	98%
Pregnancy and Delivery Care				
Newborn Deliveries Scheduled Early[5]	-	-	2%	6%
Preventive Care				
Immunization for Influenza	117	96%	92%	90%
Immunization for Pneumonia	183	95%	92%	92%
Stroke Care				
Anticoagulation Therapy for Atrial Fibrillation[5]	-	-	94%	95%
Antithrombotic Therapy Timing[5]	-	-	98%	98%
Assessed for Rehabilitation[5]	-	-	97%	97%
Discharged on Antithrombotic Therapy[5]	-	-	99%	99%
Discharged on Statin Medication[5]	-	-	94%	94%
Thrombolytic Therapy Timing[5]	-	-	66%	66%
Venous Thromboembolism Prophylaxis[5]	-	-	94%	94%
Written Stroke Educational Materials Given[5]	-	-	87%	88%
Surgical Care Improvement Project				
Appropriate Beta Blocker Usage[3,7]	-	-	98%	98%
Appropriate VTP Within 24 Hours[1,3]	-	-	98%	98%
Controlled Postoperative Blood Glucose[5]	-	-	97%	97%
Perioperative Temperature Management[1,3]	-	-	100%	100%
Prophylactic Antibiotic Selection[1,3]	-	-	99%	99%
Prophylactic Antibiotic Selection (Outpatient)[5]	-	-	98%	98%
Prophylactic Antibiotic Stopped[1,3]	-	-	98%	98%
Prophylactic Antibiotic Timing[1,3]	-	-	99%	99%
Prophylactic Antibiotic Timing (Outpatient)[5]	-	-	97%	98%
Urinary Catheter Removal[1,3]	-	-	98%	97%
Survey of Patients' Hospital Experiences				
Area Around Room 'Always' Quiet at Night[5]	-	-	60%	61%
Doctors 'Always' Communicated Well[5]	-	-	81%	82%
Home Recovery Information Given[5]	-	-	86%	85%
Hospital Given 9 or 10 on 10 Point Scale[5]	-	-	70%	71%
Meds 'Always' Explained Before Given[5]	-	-	64%	64%
Nurses 'Always' Communicated Well[5]	-	-	79%	79%
Pain 'Always' Well Controlled[5]	-	-	71%	71%
Room and Bathroom 'Always' Clean[5]	-	-	74%	73%
Timely Help 'Always' Received[5]	-	-	67%	68%
Would Definitely Recommend Hospital[5]	-	-	70%	71%
Use of Medical Imaging				
Cardiac Imaging Stress Test before Surgery	59	3.4%	5.5%	5.3%
Combination Abdominal CT Scan	86	30.2%	10.1%	10.5%
Combination Brain/Sinus CT Scan[1]	-	-	2.6%	2.7%
Combination Chest CT Scan	106	24.5%	2.8%	2.7%
Follow-up Mammogram/Ultrasound	176	8.0%	8.4%	8.8%
Lumbar Spine MRI for Low Back Pain[1]	-	-	36.6%	37.2%

Evanston Hospital

2650 Ridge Ave
Evanston, IL 60201
URL: www.enh.org
Phone: 847-432-8000
Fax: 847-570-5243
Type: Acute Care Hospitals
Emergency Services: Yes
Ownership: Voluntary non-profit - Other
Beds: 635

Key Personnel:
Operating Room. . . . . Bill Duffy
Quality Assurance . . . . Emma Hooks
CEO/President. . . . . Mark Neaman
Infection Control. . . . . Kay O'Connor, RN
Chief of Medical Staff. . . . . Arnold Wagner
Radiology. . . . . Russell Zage

Measure	Cases	This Hosp.	State Avg.	U.S. Avg.
Blood Clot Prevention and Treatment				
Anticoagulation Overlap Therapy[2]	264	95%	91%	93%
ICU Venous Thromboembolism Prophylaxis[2]	75	89%	93%	92%
Incidence of Potentially Preventable VTE[2]	34	6%	11%	10%
UFH with Dosages/Platelet Monitoring[2]	142	100%	94%	97%
Venous Thromboembolism Prophylaxis[2]	320	95%	86%	85%
Warfarin Therapy Discharge Instructions[2]	168	90%	71%	75%
Chest Pain/Possible Heart Attack Care				
Aspirin Given Within 24 Hours of Arrival[1,3]	-	-	96%	96%
Fibrinolytic Meds Within 30 Min. of Arrival[5]	-	-	65%	58%
Average Time to ECG (minutes)[1,3]	-	-	6	7
Average Time to Transfer (minutes)[5]	-	-	63	60
Children's Asthma Care				
Received Home Management Plan of Care	-	-	-	88%
Received Reliever Medication	-	-	-	100%
Received Systemic Corticosteroids	-	-	-	100%
Emergency Department				
Admittance Decision Time (minutes)[2]	393	78	89	98
Head CT Results Within 45 Min. of Arrival[1]	-	-	64%	57%
Patients Who Left ER Before Being Seen	>100k	1%	3%	2%
Time from ER Arrival to Admit. (minutes)[2]	394	232	260	274
Time from ER Arrival to Discharge (minutes)	750	164	138	134
Time in ER Before Being Evaluated (minutes)	860	48	28	26
Time to Pain Meds for Fractures (minutes)	228	56	52	57
Heart Attack Care				
Aspirin Given at Discharge	428	100%	99%	99%
Fibrinolytic Meds Within 30 Min. of Arrival[7]	-	-	33%	54%
PCI Within 90 Minutes of Arrival	79	99%	97%	96%
Statin Prescribed at Discharge	425	99%	98%	98%
Heart Failure Care				
ACE Inhibitor or ARB for LVSD[2]	115	97%	98%	97%
Discharge Instructions Given[2]	346	99%	96%	94%
Evaluation of LVS Function[2]	508	100%	99%	99%
Medicare Spending				
Medicare Spending per Patient (ratio)	-	1.02	1	0.98
Pneumonia Care				
Appropriate Initial Antibiotic Given[2]	64	98%	95%	95%
Blood Culture Timing[2]	151	100%	98%	98%
Pregnancy and Delivery Care				
Newborn Deliveries Scheduled Early[2]	45	0%	2%	6%
Preventive Care				
Immunization for Influenza[2]	640	96%	92%	90%
Immunization for Pneumonia[2]	721	96%	92%	92%
Stroke Care				
Anticoagulation Therapy for Atrial Fibrillation	51	100%	94%	95%
Antithrombotic Therapy Timing	250	99%	98%	98%
Assessed for Rehabilitation	347	99%	97%	97%
Discharged on Antithrombotic Therapy	286	100%	99%	99%
Discharged on Statin Medication	226	98%	94%	94%
Thrombolytic Therapy Timing	32	100%	66%	66%
Venous Thromboembolism Prophylaxis	373	96%	94%	94%
Written Stroke Educational Materials Given	170	93%	87%	88%
Surgical Care Improvement Project				
Appropriate Beta Blocker Usage[2]	276	99%	98%	98%
Appropriate VTP Within 24 Hours[2]	489	97%	98%	98%
Controlled Postoperative Blood Glucose[2]	221	99%	97%	97%
Perioperative Temperature Management[2]	591	100%	100%	100%
Prophylactic Antibiotic Selection[2]	587	100%	99%	99%
Prophylactic Antibiotic Selection (Outpatient)	857	99%	98%	98%
Prophylactic Antibiotic Stopped[2]	575	100%	98%	98%
Prophylactic Antibiotic Timing[2]	586	99%	99%	99%
Prophylactic Antibiotic Timing (Outpatient)	778	98%	97%	98%
Urinary Catheter Removal[2]	514	97%	98%	97%
Survey of Patients' Hospital Experiences				
Area Around Room 'Always' Quiet at Night[11]	300+	53%	60%	61%
Doctors 'Always' Communicated Well[11]	300+	79%	81%	82%
Home Recovery Information Given[11]	300+	86%	86%	85%
Hospital Given 9 or 10 on 10 Point Scale[11]	300+	72%	70%	71%
Meds 'Always' Explained Before Given[11]	300+	61%	64%	64%
Nurses 'Always' Communicated Well[11]	300+	78%	79%	79%
Pain 'Always' Well Controlled[11]	300+	68%	71%	71%
Room and Bathroom 'Always' Clean[11]	300+	70%	74%	73%
Timely Help 'Always' Received[11]	300+	60%	67%	68%
Would Definitely Recommend Hospital[11]	300+	78%	70%	71%
Use of Medical Imaging				
Cardiac Imaging Stress Test before Surgery	4,048	6.4%	5.5%	5.3%
Combination Abdominal CT Scan	5,153	8.9%	10.1%	10.5%
Combination Brain/Sinus CT Scan	3,192	2.3%	2.6%	2.7%
Combination Chest CT Scan	6,195	2.6%	2.8%	2.7%
Follow-up Mammogram/Ultrasound	13,333	4.7%	8.4%	8.8%
Lumbar Spine MRI for Low Back Pain	976	35.3%	36.6%	37.2%

Presence Saint Francis Hospital

355 Ridge Ave
Evanston, IL 60202
URL: www.reshealth.org
Phone: 847-316-4000
Fax: 847-316-4500
Type: Acute Care Hospitals
Emergency Services: Yes
Ownership: Voluntary non-profit - Church
Beds: 445

Key Personnel:
Operating Room. . . . . Pamela Bemaung, RN
Quality Assurance . . . . Lori Biala-Smith
Infection Control. . . . . Chris Costas, MD
Pediatric Ambulatory Care . . . . . . Chris Costas, MD
Pediatric In-Patient Care . . . . Chris Costas, MD
Radiology. . . . . Thomas Cronin, MD
Chief of Medical Staff . . . . Ann Kinnealey, MD
CEO/President. . . . . Jeffrey Murphy

Measure	Cases	This Hosp.	State Avg.	U.S. Avg.
Blood Clot Prevention and Treatment				
Anticoagulation Overlap Therapy[2]	53	100%	91%	93%
ICU Venous Thromboembolism Prophylaxis[2]	141	91%	93%	92%
Incidence of Potentially Preventable VTE[2]	12	17%	11%	10%
UFH with Dosages/Platelet Monitoring[2]	28	100%	94%	97%
Venous Thromboembolism Prophylaxis[2]	280	87%	86%	85%
Warfarin Therapy Discharge Instructions[2]	34	53%	71%	75%
Chest Pain/Possible Heart Attack Care				
Aspirin Given Within 24 Hours of Arrival[1,3]	-	-	96%	96%
Fibrinolytic Meds Within 30 Min. of Arrival[5]	-	-	65%	58%
Average Time to ECG (minutes)[1,3]	-	-	6	7
Average Time to Transfer (minutes)[5]	-	-	63	60
Children's Asthma Care				
Received Home Management Plan of Care	-	-	-	88%
Received Reliever Medication	-	-	-	100%
Received Systemic Corticosteroids	-	-	-	100%
Emergency Department				
Admittance Decision Time (minutes)[2]	632	130	89	98
Head CT Results Within 45 Min. of Arrival[1]	-	-	64%	57%
Patients Who Left ER Before Being Seen	36,849	0%	3%	2%
Time from ER Arrival to Admit. (minutes)[2]	647	273	260	274
Time from ER Arrival to Discharge (minutes)	362	143	138	134
Time in ER Before Being Evaluated (minutes)	209	20	28	26
Time to Pain Meds for Fractures (minutes)	127	70	52	57
Heart Attack Care				
Aspirin Given at Discharge	123	99%	99%	99%
Fibrinolytic Meds Within 30 Min. of Arrival[7]	-	-	33%	54%
PCI Within 90 Minutes of Arrival	16	94%	97%	96%
Statin Prescribed at Discharge	123	94%	98%	98%
Heart Failure Care				
ACE Inhibitor or ARB for LVSD	73	95%	98%	97%
Discharge Instructions Given	165	100%	96%	94%
Evaluation of LVS Function	231	100%	99%	99%
Medicare Spending				
Medicare Spending per Patient (ratio)	-	1.09	1	0.98
Pneumonia Care				
Appropriate Initial Antibiotic Given	90	96%	95%	95%
Blood Culture Timing	355	99%	98%	98%
Pregnancy and Delivery Care				
Newborn Deliveries Scheduled Early[2]	21	0%	2%	6%
Preventive Care				
Immunization for Influenza[2]	553	87%	92%	90%
Immunization for Pneumonia[2]	750	92%	92%	92%
Stroke Care				
Anticoagulation Therapy for Atrial Fibrillation	13	100%	94%	95%
Antithrombotic Therapy Timing	73	100%	98%	98%
Assessed for Rehabilitation	94	95%	97%	97%

NOTE: Hospital profiles are in alphabetical order by state, then city, then hospital within the city; Rankings exclude hospitals with less than 25 cases except for patient surveys which excludes hospitals with less than 100 cases; (a) 100-299 cases; (1) The number of cases/patients is too few to report; (2) Data submitted were based on a sample of cases/patients; (3) Results are based on a shorter time period than required; (4) Data suppressed by CMS for one or more quarters; (5) Results are not available for this reporting period; (6) Fewer than 100 patients completed the HCAHPS survey; (7) No cases met the criteria for this measure; (8) The lower limit of the confidence interval cannot be calculated if the number of observed infections equals zero; (9) No data are available from the state/territory for this reporting period; (10) The scores shown reflect fewer than 50 completed surveys; (11) There were discrepancies in the data collection process; (12) This measure does not apply to this hospital for this reporting period; (13) Results cannot be calculated for this reporting period; (14) The results for this state are combined with nearby states to protect confidentiality; Please refer to the User's Guide for a full explanation of data.

Measure	Cases	This Hosp.	State Avg.	U.S. Avg.
Discharged on Antithrombotic Therapy	76	97%	99%	99%
Discharged on Statin Medication	54	98%	94%	94%
Thrombolytic Therapy Timing	26	19%	66%	66%
Venous Thromboembolism Prophylaxis	104	94%	94%	94%
Written Stroke Educational Materials Given	43	72%	87%	88%
Surgical Care Improvement Project				
Appropriate Beta Blocker Usage[2]	103	93%	98%	98%
Appropriate VTP Within 24 Hours[2]	379	95%	98%	98%
Controlled Postoperative Blood Glucose[2]	41	95%	97%	97%
Perioperative Temperature Management[2]	421	100%	100%	100%
Prophylactic Antibiotic Selection[2]	310	99%	99%	99%
Prophylactic Antibiotic Selection (Outpatient)	62	89%	98%	98%
Prophylactic Antibiotic Stopped[2]	304	97%	98%	98%
Prophylactic Antibiotic Timing[2]	310	100%	99%	99%
Prophylactic Antibiotic Timing (Outpatient)	66	73%	97%	98%
Urinary Catheter Removal[2]	191	97%	98%	97%
Survey of Patients' Hospital Experiences				
Area Around Room 'Always' Quiet at Night	300+	56%	60%	61%
Doctors 'Always' Communicated Well	300+	81%	81%	82%
Home Recovery Information Given	300+	82%	86%	85%
Hospital Given 9 or 10 on 10 Point Scale	300+	74%	70%	71%
Meds 'Always' Explained Before Given	300+	59%	64%	64%
Nurses 'Always' Communicated Well	300+	77%	79%	79%
Pain 'Always' Well Controlled	300+	68%	71%	71%
Room and Bathroom 'Always' Clean	300+	72%	74%	73%
Timely Help 'Always' Received	300+	60%	67%	68%
Would Definitely Recommend Hospital	300+	69%	70%	71%
Use of Medical Imaging				
Cardiac Imaging Stress Test before Surgery	445	7.2%	5.5%	5.3%
Combination Abdominal CT Scan	582	8.1%	10.1%	10.5%
Combination Brain/Sinus CT Scan	703	3.1%	2.6%	2.7%
Combination Chest CT Scan	403	4.0%	2.8%	2.7%
Follow-up Mammogram/Ultrasound	1,318	9.9%	8.4%	8.8%
Lumbar Spine MRI for Low Back Pain	70	37.1%	36.6%	37.2%

Little Company of Mary Hospital

2800 W 95th St
Evergreen Park, IL 60805
Phone: 708-422-6200
Fax: 708-229-6733
URL: www.lcmh.org
Type: Acute Care Hospitals
Emergency Services: Yes
Ownership: Voluntary non-profit - Church
Beds: 487

Key Personnel:

Pediatric Ambulatory Care . . . . . . Hassan Alzan, MD
Chief of Medical Staff. . . . . Kent Armruster, MD
Intensive Care Unit. . . . . Jim Boyle
Operating Room. . . . . Marilyn Coonin
Infection Control. . . . . Carol Hoffman
Emergency Room . . . . Michael O'Mara DO
Cardiac Laboratory. . . . . Kathy Paul
Radiology. . . . . George Saprenza

Measure	Cases	This Hosp.	State Avg.	U.S. Avg.
Blood Clot Prevention and Treatment				
Anticoagulation Overlap Therapy[2]	175	90%	91%	93%
ICU Venous Thromboembolism Prophylaxis[2]	87	85%	93%	92%
Incidence of Potentially Preventable VTE[2]	41	20%	11%	10%
UFH with Dosages/Platelet Monitoring[2]	159	100%	94%	97%
Venous Thromboembolism Prophylaxis[2]	378	88%	86%	85%
Warfarin Therapy Discharge Instructions[2]	124	89%	71%	75%
Chest Pain/Possible Heart Attack Care				
Aspirin Given Within 24 Hours of Arrival[1,3]	-	-	96%	96%
Fibrinolytic Meds Within 30 Min. of Arrival[5]	-	-	65%	58%
Average Time to ECG (minutes)[1,3]	-	-	6	7
Average Time to Transfer (minutes)[5]	-	-	63	60
Children's Asthma Care				
Received Home Management Plan of Care	26	96%	-	88%
Received Reliever Medication	27	100%	-	100%
Received Systemic Corticosteroids	27	100%	-	100%
Emergency Department				
Admittance Decision Time (minutes)[2]	824	93	89	98
Head CT Results Within 45 Min. of Arrival	19	63%	64%	57%
Patients Who Left ER Before Being Seen	48,369	6%	3%	2%
Time from ER Arrival to Admit. (minutes)[2]	824	286	260	274
Time from ER Arrival to Discharge (minutes)	1,391	160	138	134
Time in ER Before Being Evaluated (minutes)	1,208	36	28	26
Time to Pain Meds for Fractures (minutes)	71	83	52	57
Heart Attack Care				
Aspirin Given at Discharge	94	100%	99%	99%
Fibrinolytic Meds Within 30 Min. of Arrival[7]	-	-	33%	54%
PCI Within 90 Minutes of Arrival	19	100%	97%	96%
Statin Prescribed at Discharge	93	100%	98%	98%
Heart Failure Care				
ACE Inhibitor or ARB for LVSD[2]	104	97%	98%	97%
Discharge Instructions Given[2]	245	96%	96%	94%
Evaluation of LVS Function[2]	312	100%	99%	99%
Medicare Spending				
Medicare Spending per Patient (ratio)	-	1.01	1	0.98
Pneumonia Care				
Appropriate Initial Antibiotic Given[2]	90	100%	95%	95%
Blood Culture Timing[2]	171	100%	98%	98%
Pregnancy and Delivery Care				
Newborn Deliveries Scheduled Early[2]	39	21%	2%	6%
Preventive Care				
Immunization for Influenza[2]	657	93%	92%	90%
Immunization for Pneumonia[2]	863	90%	92%	92%
Stroke Care				
Anticoagulation Therapy for Atrial Fibrillation	25	96%	94%	95%
Antithrombotic Therapy Timing	170	98%	98%	98%
Assessed for Rehabilitation	179	99%	97%	97%
Discharged on Antithrombotic Therapy	169	98%	99%	99%
Discharged on Statin Medication	125	98%	94%	94%
Thrombolytic Therapy Timing	11	100%	66%	66%
Venous Thromboembolism Prophylaxis	197	98%	94%	94%
Written Stroke Educational Materials Given	96	88%	87%	88%
Surgical Care Improvement Project				
Appropriate Beta Blocker Usage[2]	131	99%	98%	98%
Appropriate VTP Within 24 Hours[2]	404	99%	98%	98%
Controlled Postoperative Blood Glucose[2,7]	-	-	97%	97%
Perioperative Temperature Management[2]	499	100%	100%	100%
Prophylactic Antibiotic Selection[2]	251	99%	99%	99%
Prophylactic Antibiotic Selection (Outpatient)	218	97%	98%	98%
Prophylactic Antibiotic Stopped[2]	237	100%	98%	98%
Prophylactic Antibiotic Timing[2]	251	100%	99%	99%
Prophylactic Antibiotic Timing (Outpatient)	218	97%	97%	98%
Urinary Catheter Removal[2]	194	99%	98%	97%
Survey of Patients' Hospital Experiences				
Area Around Room 'Always' Quiet at Night	300+	61%	60%	61%
Doctors 'Always' Communicated Well	300+	82%	81%	82%
Home Recovery Information Given	300+	84%	86%	85%
Hospital Given 9 or 10 on 10 Point Scale	300+	76%	70%	71%
Meds 'Always' Explained Before Given	300+	63%	64%	64%
Nurses 'Always' Communicated Well	300+	80%	79%	79%
Pain 'Always' Well Controlled	300+	74%	71%	71%
Room and Bathroom 'Always' Clean	300+	70%	74%	73%
Timely Help 'Always' Received	300+	68%	67%	68%
Would Definitely Recommend Hospital	300+	76%	70%	71%
Use of Medical Imaging				
Cardiac Imaging Stress Test before Surgery	606	4.8%	5.5%	5.3%
Combination Abdominal CT Scan	903	6.4%	10.1%	10.5%
Combination Brain/Sinus CT Scan	1,031	1.6%	2.6%	2.7%
Combination Chest CT Scan	917	1.4%	2.8%	2.7%
Follow-up Mammogram/Ultrasound	1,770	9.9%	8.4%	8.8%
Lumbar Spine MRI for Low Back Pain	85	38.8%	36.6%	37.2%

Fairfield Memorial Hospital

303 N W 11th Street
Fairfield, IL 62837
Phone: 618-842-2611
Fax: 618-842-2011
URL: www.fairfieldob.com
Type: Critical Access Hospitals
Emergency Services: Yes
Ownership: Voluntary non-profit - Private
Beds: 80

Key Personnel:

Infection Control. . . . . Hazel Best, RN
Radiology. . . . . Enrique Bouffar, III
CEO/President. . . . . Michale Brown
Chief of Medical Staff . . . . Patrick Molt
Emergency Room . . . . Bo Schneider, MD
Quality Assurance . . . . Frances Strange

Measure	Cases	This Hosp.	State Avg.	U.S. Avg.
Blood Clot Prevention and Treatment				
Anticoagulation Overlap Therapy[1,3]	-	-	91%	93%
ICU Venous Thromboembolism Prophylaxis[3,7]	-	-	93%	92%
Incidence of Potentially Preventable VTE[3,7]	-	-	11%	10%
UFH with Dosages/Platelet Monitoring[1,3]	-	-	94%	97%
Venous Thromboembolism Prophylaxis[3,7]	-	-	86%	85%
Warfarin Therapy Discharge Instructions[1,3]	-	-	71%	75%
Chest Pain/Possible Heart Attack Care				
Aspirin Given Within 24 Hours of Arrival	39	95%	96%	96%
Fibrinolytic Meds Within 30 Min. of Arrival[1]	-	-	65%	58%
Average Time to ECG (minutes)	41	3	6	7
Average Time to Transfer (minutes)[1]	-	-	63	60
Children's Asthma Care				
Received Home Management Plan of Care	-	-	-	88%
Received Reliever Medication	-	-	-	100%
Received Systemic Corticosteroids	-	-	-	100%
Emergency Department				
Admittance Decision Time (minutes)[2]	158	58	89	98
Head CT Results Within 45 Min. of Arrival[1]	-	-	64%	57%
Patients Who Left ER Before Being Seen[5]	-	-	3%	2%
Time from ER Arrival to Admit. (minutes)[2]	160	191	260	274
Time from ER Arrival to Discharge (minutes)	692	115	138	134
Time in ER Before Being Evaluated (minutes)	689	23	28	26
Time to Pain Meds for Fractures (minutes)	53	48	52	57
Heart Attack Care				
Aspirin Given at Discharge[1]	-	-	99%	99%
Fibrinolytic Meds Within 30 Min. of Arrival[7]	-	-	33%	54%
PCI Within 90 Minutes of Arrival[7]	-	-	97%	96%
Statin Prescribed at Discharge[1]	-	-	98%	98%
Heart Failure Care				
ACE Inhibitor or ARB for LVSD[1]	-	-	98%	97%
Discharge Instructions Given	12	75%	96%	94%
Evaluation of LVS Function	20	90%	99%	99%
Medicare Spending				
Medicare Spending per Patient (ratio)	-	-	1	0.98
Pneumonia Care				
Appropriate Initial Antibiotic Given	18	83%	95%	95%
Blood Culture Timing	31	100%	98%	98%
Pregnancy and Delivery Care				
Newborn Deliveries Scheduled Early[5]	-	-	2%	6%
Preventive Care				
Immunization for Influenza	216	96%	92%	90%
Immunization for Pneumonia	321	95%	92%	92%
Stroke Care				
Anticoagulation Therapy for Atrial Fibrillation[1]	-	-	94%	95%
Antithrombotic Therapy Timing	13	92%	98%	98%
Assessed for Rehabilitation	15	100%	97%	97%
Discharged on Antithrombotic Therapy	13	92%	99%	99%
Discharged on Statin Medication[1]	-	-	94%	94%
Thrombolytic Therapy Timing[1]	-	-	66%	66%
Venous Thromboembolism Prophylaxis	17	94%	94%	94%
Written Stroke Educational Materials Given[1]	-	-	87%	88%
Surgical Care Improvement Project				
Appropriate Beta Blocker Usage[1]	-	-	98%	98%
Appropriate VTP Within 24 Hours	22	100%	98%	98%
Controlled Postoperative Blood Glucose[7]	-	-	97%	97%
Perioperative Temperature Management	26	100%	100%	100%
Prophylactic Antibiotic Selection[1]	-	-	99%	99%
Prophylactic Antibiotic Selection (Outpatient)	37	92%	98%	98%
Prophylactic Antibiotic Stopped[1]	-	-	98%	98%
Prophylactic Antibiotic Timing[1]	-	-	99%	99%
Prophylactic Antibiotic Timing (Outpatient)	36	100%	97%	98%
Urinary Catheter Removal[1]	-	-	98%	97%
Survey of Patients' Hospital Experiences				
Area Around Room 'Always' Quiet at Night[5]	-	-	60%	61%
Doctors 'Always' Communicated Well[5]	-	-	81%	82%
Home Recovery Information Given[5]	-	-	86%	85%
Hospital Given 9 or 10 on 10 Point Scale[5]	-	-	70%	71%
Meds 'Always' Explained Before Given[5]	-	-	64%	64%
Nurses 'Always' Communicated Well[5]	-	-	79%	79%
Pain 'Always' Well Controlled[5]	-	-	71%	71%
Room and Bathroom 'Always' Clean[5]	-	-	74%	73%
Timely Help 'Always' Received[5]	-	-	67%	68%

NOTE: Hospital profiles are in alphabetical order by state, then city, then hospital within the city; Rankings exclude hospitals with less than 25 cases except for patient surveys which excludes hospitals with less than 100 cases; (a) 100-299 cases; (1) The number of cases/patients is too few to report; (2) Data submitted were based on a sample of cases/patients; (3) Results are based on a shorter time period than required; (4) Data suppressed by CMS for one or more quarters; (5) Results are not available for this reporting period; (6) Fewer than 100 patients completed the HCAHPS survey; (7) No cases met the criteria for this measure; (8) The lower limit of the confidence interval cannot be calculated if the number of observed infections equals zero; (9) No data are available from the state/territory for this reporting period; (10) The scores shown reflect fewer than 50 completed surveys; (11) There were discrepancies in the data collection process; (12) This measure does not apply to this hospital for this reporting period; (13) Results cannot be calculated for this reporting period; (14) The results for this state are combined with nearby states to protect confidentiality; Please refer to the User's Guide for a full explanation of data.

Measure	Cases	This Hosp.	State Avg.	U.S. Avg.
Would Definitely Recommend Hospital[5]	-	-	70%	71%
Use of Medical Imaging				
Cardiac Imaging Stress Test before Surgery	151	4.6%	5.5%	5.3%
Combination Abdominal CT Scan	395	40.8%	10.1%	10.5%
Combination Brain/Sinus CT Scan[1]	-	-	2.6%	2.7%
Combination Chest CT Scan	253	0.0%	2.8%	2.7%
Follow-up Mammogram/Ultrasound	365	3.3%	8.4%	8.8%
Lumbar Spine MRI for Low Back Pain[1]	-	-	36.6%	37.2%

Clay County Hospital

911 Stacy Burk Drive
Flora, IL 62839
Phone: 618-662-2131
Fax: 618-662-1486
E-mail: cchdas@wabash.net
URL: www.claycountyhospital.org
Type: Critical Access Hospitals
Emergency Services: Yes
Ownership: Government - Local
Beds: 18

Key Personnel:
Quality Assurance .... Mike Anderson
Emergency Room .... Eileen Enlow, RN
CEO/President............... Steven H Lipstein
Chief of Medical Staff.......... Jennifer Maneja
Radiology................... Preecha Tawjareon

Measure	Cases	This Hosp.	State Avg.	U.S. Avg.
Blood Clot Prevention and Treatment				
Anticoagulation Overlap Therapy[5]	-	-	91%	93%
ICU Venous Thromboembolism Prophylaxis[5]	-	-	93%	92%
Incidence of Potentially Preventable VTE[5]	-	-	11%	10%
UFH with Dosages/Platelet Monitoring[5]	-	-	94%	97%
Venous Thromboembolism Prophylaxis[5]	-	-	86%	85%
Warfarin Therapy Discharge Instructions[5]	-	-	71%	75%
Chest Pain/Possible Heart Attack Care				
Aspirin Given Within 24 Hours of Arrival	98	98%	96%	96%
Fibrinolytic Meds Within 30 Min. of Arrival[7]	-	-	65%	58%
Average Time to ECG (minutes)	97	7	6	7
Average Time to Transfer (minutes)[1]	-	-	63	60
Children's Asthma Care				
Received Home Management Plan of Care	-	-	-	88%
Received Reliever Medication	-	-	-	100%
Received Systemic Corticosteroids	-	-	-	100%
Emergency Department				
Admittance Decision Time (minutes)[2]	567	72	89	98
Head CT Results Within 45 Min. of Arrival[1]	-	-	64%	57%
Patients Who Left ER Before Being Seen[5]	-	-	3%	2%
Time from ER Arrival to Admit. (minutes)[2]	569	259	260	274
Time from ER Arrival to Discharge (minutes)[5]	-	-	138	134
Time in ER Before Being Evaluated (minutes)[5]	-	-	28	26
Time to Pain Meds for Fractures (minutes)	32	53	52	57
Heart Attack Care				
Aspirin Given at Discharge[1]	-	-	99%	99%
Fibrinolytic Meds Within 30 Min. of Arrival[7]	-	-	33%	54%
PCI Within 90 Minutes of Arrival[7]	-	-	97%	96%
Statin Prescribed at Discharge[1]	-	-	98%	98%
Heart Failure Care				
ACE Inhibitor or ARB for LVSD[1]	-	-	98%	97%
Discharge Instructions Given	32	100%	96%	94%
Evaluation of LVS Function	49	100%	99%	99%
Medicare Spending				
Medicare Spending per Patient (ratio)	-	-	1	0.98
Pneumonia Care				
Appropriate Initial Antibiotic Given	63	100%	95%	95%
Blood Culture Timing	90	99%	98%	98%
Pregnancy and Delivery Care				
Newborn Deliveries Scheduled Early[3,7]	-	-	2%	6%
Preventive Care				
Immunization for Influenza[2]	331	100%	92%	90%
Immunization for Pneumonia[2]	520	100%	92%	92%
Stroke Care				
Anticoagulation Therapy for Atrial Fibrillation[5]	-	-	94%	95%
Antithrombotic Therapy Timing[5]	-	-	98%	98%
Assessed for Rehabilitation[5]	-	-	97%	97%
Discharged on Antithrombotic Therapy[5]	-	-	99%	99%
Discharged on Statin Medication[5]	-	-	94%	94%
Thrombolytic Therapy Timing[5]	-	-	66%	66%
Venous Thromboembolism Prophylaxis[5]	-	-	94%	94%
Written Stroke Educational Materials Given[5]	-	-	87%	88%
Surgical Care Improvement Project				
Appropriate Beta Blocker Usage[1]	-	-	98%	98%
Appropriate VTP Within 24 Hours	12	100%	98%	98%
Controlled Postoperative Blood Glucose[7]	-	-	97%	97%
Perioperative Temperature Management	12	100%	100%	100%
Prophylactic Antibiotic Selection[1]	-	-	99%	99%
Prophylactic Antibiotic Selection (Outpatient)[1]	-	-	98%	98%
Prophylactic Antibiotic Stopped[1]	-	-	98%	98%
Prophylactic Antibiotic Timing[1]	-	-	99%	99%
Prophylactic Antibiotic Timing (Outpatient)[1]	-	-	97%	98%
Urinary Catheter Removal	12	100%	98%	97%
Survey of Patients' Hospital Experiences				
Area Around Room 'Always' Quiet at Night	(a)	47%	60%	61%
Doctors 'Always' Communicated Well	(a)	83%	81%	82%
Home Recovery Information Given	(a)	90%	86%	85%
Hospital Given 9 or 10 on 10 Point Scale	(a)	76%	70%	71%
Meds 'Always' Explained Before Given	(a)	67%	64%	64%
Nurses 'Always' Communicated Well	(a)	82%	79%	79%
Pain 'Always' Well Controlled	(a)	76%	71%	71%
Room and Bathroom 'Always' Clean	(a)	79%	74%	73%
Timely Help 'Always' Received	(a)	75%	67%	68%
Would Definitely Recommend Hospital	(a)	70%	70%	71%
Use of Medical Imaging				
Cardiac Imaging Stress Test before Surgery	61	3.3%	5.5%	5.3%
Combination Abdominal CT Scan	333	1.5%	10.1%	10.5%
Combination Brain/Sinus CT Scan[1]	-	-	2.6%	2.7%
Combination Chest CT Scan	280	1.1%	2.8%	2.7%
Follow-up Mammogram/Ultrasound	398	6.5%	8.4%	8.8%
Lumbar Spine MRI for Low Back Pain[1]	-	-	36.6%	37.2%

Fhn Memorial Hospital

1045 West Stephenson Street
Freeport, IL 61032
Phone: 815-235-4131
Fax: 815-599-6417
E-mail: wecare@fhn.org
URL: www.fhn.org
Type: Acute Care Hospitals
Emergency Services: Yes
Ownership: Voluntary non-profit - Private
Beds: 194

Key Personnel:
Operating Room............. Barry Barnes
Chief of Medical Staff.......... Alan Esker
Radiology................... Gustavo Espinosa
CEO/President............... Michael Perry

Measure	Cases	This Hosp.	State Avg.	U.S. Avg.
Blood Clot Prevention and Treatment				
Anticoagulation Overlap Therapy[2]	49	80%	91%	93%
ICU Venous Thromboembolism Prophylaxis[2]	109	84%	93%	92%
Incidence of Potentially Preventable VTE[2]	12	0%	11%	10%
UFH with Dosages/Platelet Monitoring[1,2]	-	-	94%	97%
Venous Thromboembolism Prophylaxis[2]	334	90%	86%	85%
Warfarin Therapy Discharge Instructions[2]	38	92%	71%	75%
Chest Pain/Possible Heart Attack Care				
Aspirin Given Within 24 Hours of Arrival	41	98%	96%	96%
Fibrinolytic Meds Within 30 Min. of Arrival[7]	-	-	65%	58%
Average Time to ECG (minutes)	46	3	6	7
Average Time to Transfer (minutes)	12	74	63	60
Children's Asthma Care				
Received Home Management Plan of Care	-	-	-	88%
Received Reliever Medication	-	-	-	100%
Received Systemic Corticosteroids	-	-	-	100%
Emergency Department				
Admittance Decision Time (minutes)[2]	424	58	89	98
Head CT Results Within 45 Min. of Arrival	22	73%	64%	57%
Patients Who Left ER Before Being Seen	26,996	1%	3%	2%
Time from ER Arrival to Admit. (minutes)[2]	424	233	260	274
Time from ER Arrival to Discharge (minutes)	429	122	138	134
Time in ER Before Being Evaluated (minutes)	476	27	28	26
Time to Pain Meds for Fractures (minutes)	70	58	52	57
Heart Attack Care				
Aspirin Given at Discharge	29	100%	99%	99%
Fibrinolytic Meds Within 30 Min. of Arrival[7]	-	-	33%	54%
PCI Within 90 Minutes of Arrival[1]	-	-	97%	96%
Statin Prescribed at Discharge	30	100%	98%	98%
Heart Failure Care				
ACE Inhibitor or ARB for LVSD	48	100%	98%	97%
Discharge Instructions Given	126	97%	96%	94%
Evaluation of LVS Function	171	100%	99%	99%
Medicare Spending				
Medicare Spending per Patient (ratio)	-	0.92	1	0.98
Pneumonia Care				
Appropriate Initial Antibiotic Given	86	99%	95%	95%
Blood Culture Timing	195	100%	98%	98%
Pregnancy and Delivery Care				
Newborn Deliveries Scheduled Early	26	0%	2%	6%
Preventive Care				
Immunization for Influenza[2]	468	93%	92%	90%
Immunization for Pneumonia[2]	610	99%	92%	92%
Stroke Care				
Anticoagulation Therapy for Atrial Fibrillation	12	100%	94%	95%
Antithrombotic Therapy Timing	52	100%	98%	98%
Assessed for Rehabilitation	55	96%	97%	97%
Discharged on Antithrombotic Therapy	55	100%	99%	99%
Discharged on Statin Medication	37	100%	94%	94%
Thrombolytic Therapy Timing[1]	-	-	66%	66%
Venous Thromboembolism Prophylaxis	50	94%	94%	94%
Written Stroke Educational Materials Given	28	96%	87%	88%
Surgical Care Improvement Project				
Appropriate Beta Blocker Usage	136	99%	98%	98%
Appropriate VTP Within 24 Hours	374	100%	98%	98%
Controlled Postoperative Blood Glucose[7]	-	-	97%	97%
Perioperative Temperature Management	417	100%	100%	100%
Prophylactic Antibiotic Selection	299	99%	99%	99%
Prophylactic Antibiotic Selection (Outpatient)	140	99%	98%	98%
Prophylactic Antibiotic Stopped	285	100%	98%	98%
Prophylactic Antibiotic Timing	300	100%	99%	99%
Prophylactic Antibiotic Timing (Outpatient)	79	99%	97%	98%
Urinary Catheter Removal	87	99%	98%	97%
Survey of Patients' Hospital Experiences				
Area Around Room 'Always' Quiet at Night	300+	60%	60%	61%
Doctors 'Always' Communicated Well	300+	79%	81%	82%
Home Recovery Information Given	300+	86%	86%	85%
Hospital Given 9 or 10 on 10 Point Scale	300+	68%	70%	71%
Meds 'Always' Explained Before Given	300+	62%	64%	64%
Nurses 'Always' Communicated Well	300+	77%	79%	79%
Pain 'Always' Well Controlled	300+	69%	71%	71%
Room and Bathroom 'Always' Clean	300+	70%	74%	73%
Timely Help 'Always' Received	300+	62%	67%	68%
Would Definitely Recommend Hospital	300+	63%	70%	71%
Use of Medical Imaging				
Cardiac Imaging Stress Test before Surgery	404	5.9%	5.5%	5.3%
Combination Abdominal CT Scan	593	1.5%	10.1%	10.5%
Combination Brain/Sinus CT Scan	547	2.4%	2.6%	2.7%
Combination Chest CT Scan	303	0.0%	2.8%	2.7%
Follow-up Mammogram/Ultrasound	1,140	7.4%	8.4%	8.8%
Lumbar Spine MRI for Low Back Pain	119	36.1%	36.6%	37.2%

Midwest Medical Center

One Medical Center Drive
Galena, IL 61036
Phone: 815-777-1340
Type: Critical Access Hospitals
Emergency Services: Yes
Ownership: Voluntary non-profit - Private

Measure	Cases	This Hosp.	State Avg.	U.S. Avg.
Blood Clot Prevention and Treatment				
Anticoagulation Overlap Therapy[5]	-	-	91%	93%
ICU Venous Thromboembolism Prophylaxis[5]	-	-	93%	92%
Incidence of Potentially Preventable VTE[5]	-	-	11%	10%
UFH with Dosages/Platelet Monitoring[5]	-	-	94%	97%
Venous Thromboembolism Prophylaxis[5]	-	-	86%	85%
Warfarin Therapy Discharge Instructions[5]	-	-	71%	75%
Chest Pain/Possible Heart Attack Care				
Aspirin Given Within 24 Hours of Arrival	-	-	96%	96%
Fibrinolytic Meds Within 30 Min. of Arrival	-	-	65%	58%
Average Time to ECG (minutes)	-	-	6	7
Average Time to Transfer (minutes)	-	-	63	60
Children's Asthma Care				

NOTE: Hospital profiles are in alphabetical order by state, then city, then hospital within the city; Rankings exclude hospitals with less than 25 cases except for patient surveys which excludes hospitals with less than 100 cases; (a) 100-299 cases; (1) The number of cases/patients is too few to report; (2) Data submitted were based on a sample of cases/patients; (3) Results are based on a shorter time period than required; (4) Data suppressed by CMS for one or more quarters; (5) Results are not available for this reporting period; (6) Fewer than 100 patients completed the HCAHPS survey; (7) No cases met the criteria for this measure; (8) The lower limit of the confidence interval cannot be calculated if the number of observed infections equals zero; (9) No data are available from the state/territory for this reporting period; (10) The scores shown reflect fewer than 50 completed surveys; (11) There were discrepancies in the data collection process; (12) This measure does not apply to this hospital for this reporting period; (13) Results cannot be calculated for this reporting period; (14) The results for this state are combined with nearby states to protect confidentiality; Please refer to the User's Guide for a full explanation of data.

Measure	Cases	This Hosp.	State Avg.	U.S. Avg.
Received Home Management Plan of Care	-	-	-	88%
Received Reliever Medication	-	-	-	100%
Received Systemic Corticosteroids	-	-	-	100%
Emergency Department				
Admittance Decision Time (minutes)[5]	-	-	89	98
Head CT Results Within 45 Min. of Arrival	-	-	64%	57%
Patients Who Left ER Before Being Seen	-	-	3%	2%
Time from ER Arrival to Admit. (minutes)[5]	-	-	260	274
Time from ER Arrival to Discharge (minutes)	-	-	138	134
Time in ER Before Being Evaluated (minutes)	-	-	28	26
Time to Pain Meds for Fractures (minutes)	-	-	52	57
Heart Attack Care				
Aspirin Given at Discharge[5]	-	-	99%	99%
Fibrinolytic Meds Within 30 Min. of Arrival[5]	-	-	33%	54%
PCI Within 90 Minutes of Arrival[5]	-	-	97%	96%
Statin Prescribed at Discharge[5]	-	-	98%	98%
Heart Failure Care				
ACE Inhibitor or ARB for LVSD[1]	-	-	98%	97%
Discharge Instructions Given[1]	-	-	96%	94%
Evaluation of LVS Function[1]	-	-	99%	99%
Medicare Spending				
Medicare Spending per Patient (ratio)	-	-	1	0.98
Pneumonia Care				
Appropriate Initial Antibiotic Given	11	91%	95%	95%
Blood Culture Timing[1]	-	-	98%	98%
Pregnancy and Delivery Care				
Newborn Deliveries Scheduled Early[5]	-	-	2%	6%
Preventive Care				
Immunization for Influenza[5]	-	-	92%	90%
Immunization for Pneumonia[5]	-	-	92%	92%
Stroke Care				
Anticoagulation Therapy for Atrial Fibrillation[5]	-	-	94%	95%
Antithrombotic Therapy Timing[5]	-	-	98%	98%
Assessed for Rehabilitation[5]	-	-	97%	97%
Discharged on Antithrombotic Therapy[5]	-	-	99%	99%
Discharged on Statin Medication[5]	-	-	94%	94%
Thrombolytic Therapy Timing[5]	-	-	66%	66%
Venous Thromboembolism Prophylaxis[5]	-	-	94%	94%
Written Stroke Educational Materials Given[5]	-	-	87%	88%
Surgical Care Improvement Project				
Appropriate Beta Blocker Usage[3,7]	-	-	98%	98%
Appropriate VTP Within 24 Hours[1,3]	-	-	98%	98%
Controlled Postoperative Blood Glucose[3,7]	-	-	97%	97%
Perioperative Temperature Management[1,3]	-	-	100%	100%
Prophylactic Antibiotic Selection[1,3]	-	-	99%	99%
Prophylactic Antibiotic Selection (Outpatient)	-	-	98%	98%
Prophylactic Antibiotic Stopped[1,3]	-	-	98%	98%
Prophylactic Antibiotic Timing[1,3]	-	-	99%	99%
Prophylactic Antibiotic Timing (Outpatient)	-	-	97%	98%
Urinary Catheter Removal[1,3]	-	-	98%	97%
Survey of Patients' Hospital Experiences				
Area Around Room 'Always' Quiet at Night[5]	-	-	60%	61%
Doctors 'Always' Communicated Well[5]	-	-	81%	82%
Home Recovery Information Given[5]	-	-	86%	85%
Hospital Given 9 or 10 on 10 Point Scale[5]	-	-	70%	71%
Meds 'Always' Explained Before Given[5]	-	-	64%	64%
Nurses 'Always' Communicated Well[5]	-	-	79%	79%
Pain 'Always' Well Controlled[5]	-	-	71%	71%
Room and Bathroom 'Always' Clean[5]	-	-	74%	73%
Timely Help 'Always' Received[5]	-	-	67%	68%
Would Definitely Recommend Hospital[5]	-	-	70%	71%
Use of Medical Imaging				
Cardiac Imaging Stress Test before Surgery	-	-	5.5%	5.3%
Combination Abdominal CT Scan	-	-	10.1%	10.5%
Combination Brain/Sinus CT Scan	-	-	2.6%	2.7%
Combination Chest CT Scan	-	-	2.8%	2.7%
Follow-up Mammogram/Ultrasound	-	-	8.4%	8.8%
Lumbar Spine MRI for Low Back Pain	-	-	36.6%	37.2%

Galesburg Cottage Hospital

695 N Kellogg St
Galesburg, IL 61401
URL: www.cottagehospital.com
Type: Acute Care Hospitals
Ownership: Proprietary
Phone: 309-345-4555
Fax: 309-343-2393
Emergency Services: Yes
Beds: 170

Key Personnel:

Radiology. . . . . Jared Browning
Chief of Medical Staff . . . . Mark Daus, MD
CEO/President. . . . . Kenneth Hutchennider
Infection Control. . . . . Linda Newcomb
Coronary Care . . . . Deb Rickard
Cardiac Laboratory. . . . . Johanna Steller
Operating Room. . . . . Alan Willis

Measure	Cases	This Hosp.	State Avg.	U.S. Avg.
Blood Clot Prevention and Treatment				
Anticoagulation Overlap Therapy[2]	29	93%	91%	93%
ICU Venous Thromboembolism Prophylaxis[2]	106	100%	93%	92%
Incidence of Potentially Preventable VTE[1,2]	-	-	11%	10%
UFH with Dosages/Platelet Monitoring[2]	27	100%	94%	97%
Venous Thromboembolism Prophylaxis[2]	189	99%	86%	85%
Warfarin Therapy Discharge Instructions[2]	12	100%	71%	75%
Chest Pain/Possible Heart Attack Care				
Aspirin Given Within 24 Hours of Arrival	49	98%	96%	96%
Fibrinolytic Meds Within 30 Min. of Arrival[1]	-	-	65%	58%
Average Time to ECG (minutes)	50	8	6	7
Average Time to Transfer (minutes)[1]	-	-	63	60
Children's Asthma Care				
Received Home Management Plan of Care	-	-	-	88%
Received Reliever Medication	-	-	-	100%
Received Systemic Corticosteroids	-	-	-	100%
Emergency Department				
Admittance Decision Time (minutes)[2]	331	67	89	98
Head CT Results Within 45 Min. of Arrival[1]	-	-	64%	57%
Patients Who Left ER Before Being Seen	14,435	1%	3%	2%
Time from ER Arrival to Admit. (minutes)[2]	335	223	260	274
Time from ER Arrival to Discharge (minutes)	374	108	138	134
Time in ER Before Being Evaluated (minutes)	417	18	28	26
Time to Pain Meds for Fractures (minutes)	60	41	52	57
Heart Attack Care				
Aspirin Given at Discharge	11	100%	99%	99%
Fibrinolytic Meds Within 30 Min. of Arrival[7]	-	-	33%	54%
PCI Within 90 Minutes of Arrival[7]	-	-	97%	96%
Statin Prescribed at Discharge	11	100%	98%	98%
Heart Failure Care				
ACE Inhibitor or ARB for LVSD	25	96%	98%	97%
Discharge Instructions Given	47	85%	96%	94%
Evaluation of LVS Function	96	100%	99%	99%
Medicare Spending				
Medicare Spending per Patient (ratio)	-	0.99	1	0.98
Pneumonia Care				
Appropriate Initial Antibiotic Given	38	97%	95%	95%
Blood Culture Timing	130	99%	98%	98%
Pregnancy and Delivery Care				
Newborn Deliveries Scheduled Early[2]	29	0%	2%	6%
Preventive Care				
Immunization for Influenza[2]	319	99%	92%	90%
Immunization for Pneumonia[2]	414	100%	92%	92%
Stroke Care				
Anticoagulation Therapy for Atrial Fibrillation[1]	-	-	94%	95%
Antithrombotic Therapy Timing	22	100%	98%	98%
Assessed for Rehabilitation	23	96%	97%	97%
Discharged on Antithrombotic Therapy	22	100%	99%	99%
Discharged on Statin Medication	14	100%	94%	94%
Thrombolytic Therapy Timing[1]	-	-	66%	66%
Venous Thromboembolism Prophylaxis	22	95%	94%	94%
Written Stroke Educational Materials Given[1]	-	-	87%	88%
Surgical Care Improvement Project				
Appropriate Beta Blocker Usage	61	98%	98%	98%
Appropriate VTP Within 24 Hours	178	98%	98%	98%
Controlled Postoperative Blood Glucose[7]	-	-	97%	97%
Perioperative Temperature Management	206	100%	100%	100%
Prophylactic Antibiotic Selection	119	98%	99%	99%
Prophylactic Antibiotic Selection (Outpatient)	76	96%	98%	98%
Prophylactic Antibiotic Stopped	115	93%	98%	98%
Prophylactic Antibiotic Timing	119	99%	99%	99%
Prophylactic Antibiotic Timing (Outpatient)	76	100%	97%	98%
Urinary Catheter Removal	152	100%	98%	97%
Survey of Patients' Hospital Experiences				
Area Around Room 'Always' Quiet at Night	300+	59%	60%	61%
Doctors 'Always' Communicated Well	300+	84%	81%	82%
Home Recovery Information Given	300+	89%	86%	85%
Hospital Given 9 or 10 on 10 Point Scale	300+	69%	70%	71%
Meds 'Always' Explained Before Given	300+	66%	64%	64%
Nurses 'Always' Communicated Well	300+	80%	79%	79%
Pain 'Always' Well Controlled	300+	73%	71%	71%
Room and Bathroom 'Always' Clean	300+	68%	74%	73%
Timely Help 'Always' Received	300+	63%	67%	68%
Would Definitely Recommend Hospital	300+	66%	70%	71%
Use of Medical Imaging				
Cardiac Imaging Stress Test before Surgery	186	3.2%	5.5%	5.3%
Combination Abdominal CT Scan	254	3.5%	10.1%	10.5%
Combination Brain/Sinus CT Scan	405	1.7%	2.6%	2.7%
Combination Chest CT Scan	240	1.7%	2.8%	2.7%
Follow-up Mammogram/Ultrasound	669	8.1%	8.4%	8.8%
Lumbar Spine MRI for Low Back Pain	56	35.7%	36.6%	37.2%

Saint Mary Medical Center

3333 North Seminary
Galesburg, IL 61401
URL: www.osfhealthcare.org
Type: Acute Care Hospitals
Ownership: Voluntary non-profit - Church
Phone: 309-344-3161
Fax: 309-344-9494
Emergency Services: No
Beds: 156

Key Personnel:

Emergency Room . . . . Cathy Anderson
Anesthesiology. . . . . Gary Daligowski
Infection Control. . . . . Bonnie Fransene
Coronary Care . . . . Rosie Friend
Intensive Care Unit. . . . . Rosie Friend
Pediatric In-Patient Care . . . . Carrie Hagen
CEO/President. . . . . Richard Kowalski
Operating Room. . . . . Julia Nielsen

Measure	Cases	This Hosp.	State Avg.	U.S. Avg.
Blood Clot Prevention and Treatment				
Anticoagulation Overlap Therapy[2]	35	86%	91%	93%
ICU Venous Thromboembolism Prophylaxis[2]	85	100%	93%	92%
Incidence of Potentially Preventable VTE[1,2]	-	-	11%	10%
UFH with Dosages/Platelet Monitoring[2]	28	100%	94%	97%
Venous Thromboembolism Prophylaxis[2]	229	90%	86%	85%
Warfarin Therapy Discharge Instructions[2]	27	85%	71%	75%
Chest Pain/Possible Heart Attack Care				
Aspirin Given Within 24 Hours of Arrival	77	97%	96%	96%
Fibrinolytic Meds Within 30 Min. of Arrival[7]	-	-	65%	58%
Average Time to ECG (minutes)	79	6	6	7
Average Time to Transfer (minutes)	14	66	63	60
Children's Asthma Care				
Received Home Management Plan of Care	-	-	-	88%
Received Reliever Medication	-	-	-	100%
Received Systemic Corticosteroids	-	-	-	100%
Emergency Department				
Admittance Decision Time (minutes)[2]	331	79	89	98
Head CT Results Within 45 Min. of Arrival	18	44%	64%	57%
Patients Who Left ER Before Being Seen	21,156	2%	3%	2%
Time from ER Arrival to Admit. (minutes)[2]	359	245	260	274
Time from ER Arrival to Discharge (minutes)	385	132	138	134
Time in ER Before Being Evaluated (minutes)	416	15	28	26
Time to Pain Meds for Fractures (minutes)	50	56	52	57
Heart Attack Care				
Aspirin Given at Discharge	15	93%	99%	99%
Fibrinolytic Meds Within 30 Min. of Arrival[1]	-	-	33%	54%
PCI Within 90 Minutes of Arrival[7]	-	-	97%	96%
Statin Prescribed at Discharge	16	81%	98%	98%
Heart Failure Care				
ACE Inhibitor or ARB for LVSD	46	100%	98%	97%
Discharge Instructions Given	92	100%	96%	94%
Evaluation of LVS Function	130	99%	99%	99%
Medicare Spending				
Medicare Spending per Patient (ratio)	-	0.99	1	0.98

NOTE: Hospital profiles are in alphabetical order by state, then city, then hospital within the city; Rankings exclude hospitals with less than 25 cases except for patient surveys which excludes hospitals with less than 100 cases; (a) 100-299 cases; (1) The number of cases/patients is too few to report; (2) Data submitted were based on a sample of cases/patients; (3) Results are based on a shorter time period than required; (4) Data suppressed by CMS for one or more quarters; (5) Results are not available for this reporting period; (6) Fewer than 100 patients completed the HCAHPS survey; (7) No cases met the criteria for this measure; (8) The lower limit of the confidence interval cannot be calculated if the number of observed infections equals zero; (9) No data are available from the state/territory for this reporting period; (10) The scores shown reflect fewer than 50 completed surveys; (11) There were discrepancies in the data collection process; (12) This measure does not apply to this hospital for this reporting period; (13) Results cannot be calculated for this reporting period; (14) The results for this state are combined with nearby states to protect confidentiality; Please refer to the User's Guide for a full explanation of data.

Measure	Cases	This Hosp.	State Avg.	U.S. Avg.
Pneumonia Care				
Appropriate Initial Antibiotic Given	92	97%	95%	95%
Blood Culture Timing	128	98%	98%	98%
Pregnancy and Delivery Care				
Newborn Deliveries Scheduled Early	32	0%	2%	6%
Preventive Care				
Immunization for Influenza[2]	341	92%	92%	90%
Immunization for Pneumonia[2]	448	93%	92%	92%
Stroke Care				
Anticoagulation Therapy for Atrial Fibrillation[1]	-	-	94%	95%
Antithrombotic Therapy Timing	30	90%	98%	98%
Assessed for Rehabilitation	29	90%	97%	97%
Discharged on Antithrombotic Therapy	28	100%	99%	99%
Discharged on Statin Medication	26	69%	94%	94%
Thrombolytic Therapy Timing[1]	-	-	66%	66%
Venous Thromboembolism Prophylaxis	31	97%	94%	94%
Written Stroke Educational Materials Given	11	18%	87%	88%
Surgical Care Improvement Project				
Appropriate Beta Blocker Usage	102	97%	98%	98%
Appropriate VTP Within 24 Hours	285	99%	98%	98%
Controlled Postoperative Blood Glucose[7]	-	-	97%	97%
Perioperative Temperature Management	311	100%	100%	100%
Prophylactic Antibiotic Selection	222	100%	99%	99%
Prophylactic Antibiotic Selection (Outpatient)	53	96%	98%	98%
Prophylactic Antibiotic Stopped	209	99%	98%	98%
Prophylactic Antibiotic Timing	222	98%	99%	99%
Prophylactic Antibiotic Timing (Outpatient)	53	100%	97%	98%
Urinary Catheter Removal	247	98%	98%	97%
Survey of Patients' Hospital Experiences				
Area Around Room 'Always' Quiet at Night	300+	62%	60%	61%
Doctors 'Always' Communicated Well	300+	87%	81%	82%
Home Recovery Information Given	300+	89%	86%	85%
Hospital Given 9 or 10 on 10 Point Scale	300+	78%	70%	71%
Meds 'Always' Explained Before Given	300+	72%	64%	64%
Nurses 'Always' Communicated Well	300+	83%	79%	79%
Pain 'Always' Well Controlled	300+	76%	71%	71%
Room and Bathroom 'Always' Clean	300+	79%	74%	73%
Timely Help 'Always' Received	300+	74%	67%	68%
Would Definitely Recommend Hospital	300+	84%	70%	71%
Use of Medical Imaging				
Cardiac Imaging Stress Test before Surgery	268	4.1%	5.5%	5.3%
Combination Abdominal CT Scan	580	7.9%	10.1%	10.5%
Combination Brain/Sinus CT Scan	478	1.7%	2.6%	2.7%
Combination Chest CT Scan	379	0.5%	2.8%	2.7%
Follow-up Mammogram/Ultrasound	1,529	11.2%	8.4%	8.8%
Lumbar Spine MRI for Low Back Pain	113	41.6%	36.6%	37.2%

Hammond Henry Hospital

600 N College Avenue
Geneseo, IL 61254
E-mail: hhh@hammondhenry.com
URL: www.hammondhenry.com
Phone: 309-944-6431
Fax: 309-944-5299
Type: Critical Access Hospitals
Ownership: Govt - Hospital Dist/Auth
Emergency Services: No
Beds: 105

Key Personnel:
Intensive Care Unit. . . . . Karen Crossman
Infection Control. . . . . Geri Egert
Quality Assurance . . . . Geri Egert
Emergency Room . . . . Lokanathum Gumadyala, MD
Chief of Medical Staff. . . . . L Gumidyala
Operating Room. . . . . Yogin Parikh
CEO/President. . . . . Bradley Solberg
Patient Relations . . . . Diane Swaggen

Measure	Cases	This Hosp.	State Avg.	U.S. Avg.
Blood Clot Prevention and Treatment				
Anticoagulation Overlap Therapy[5]	-	-	91%	93%
ICU Venous Thromboembolism Prophylaxis[5]	-	-	93%	92%
Incidence of Potentially Preventable VTE[5]	-	-	11%	10%
UFH with Dosages/Platelet Monitoring[5]	-	-	94%	97%
Venous Thromboembolism Prophylaxis[5]	-	-	86%	85%
Warfarin Therapy Discharge Instructions[5]	-	-	71%	75%
Chest Pain/Possible Heart Attack Care				
Aspirin Given Within 24 Hours of Arrival[5]	-	-	96%	96%
Fibrinolytic Meds Within 30 Min. of Arrival[5]	-	-	65%	58%
Average Time to ECG (minutes)[5]	-	-	6	7
Average Time to Transfer (minutes)[5]	-	-	63	60
Children's Asthma Care				
Received Home Management Plan of Care	-	-	-	88%
Received Reliever Medication	-	-	-	100%
Received Systemic Corticosteroids	-	-	-	100%
Emergency Department				
Admittance Decision Time (minutes)[5]	-	-	89	98
Head CT Results Within 45 Min. of Arrival[5]	-	-	64%	57%
Patients Who Left ER Before Being Seen[5]	-	-	3%	2%
Time from ER Arrival to Admit. (minutes)[5]	-	-	260	274
Time from ER Arrival to Discharge (minutes)[5]	-	-	138	134
Time in ER Before Being Evaluated (minutes)[5]	-	-	28	26
Time to Pain Meds for Fractures (minutes)[5]	-	-	52	57
Heart Attack Care				
Aspirin Given at Discharge[5]	-	-	99%	99%
Fibrinolytic Meds Within 30 Min. of Arrival[5]	-	-	33%	54%
PCI Within 90 Minutes of Arrival[5]	-	-	97%	96%
Statin Prescribed at Discharge[5]	-	-	98%	98%
Heart Failure Care				
ACE Inhibitor or ARB for LVSD[1]	-	-	98%	97%
Discharge Instructions Given	23	100%	96%	94%
Evaluation of LVS Function	38	100%	99%	99%
Medicare Spending				
Medicare Spending per Patient (ratio)	-	-	1	0.98
Pneumonia Care				
Appropriate Initial Antibiotic Given	60	100%	95%	95%
Blood Culture Timing	70	100%	98%	98%
Pregnancy and Delivery Care				
Newborn Deliveries Scheduled Early[5]	-	-	2%	6%
Preventive Care				
Immunization for Influenza[5]	-	-	92%	90%
Immunization for Pneumonia[5]	-	-	92%	92%
Stroke Care				
Anticoagulation Therapy for Atrial Fibrillation[5]	-	-	94%	95%
Antithrombotic Therapy Timing[5]	-	-	98%	98%
Assessed for Rehabilitation[5]	-	-	97%	97%
Discharged on Antithrombotic Therapy[5]	-	-	99%	99%
Discharged on Statin Medication[5]	-	-	94%	94%
Thrombolytic Therapy Timing[5]	-	-	66%	66%
Venous Thromboembolism Prophylaxis[5]	-	-	94%	94%
Written Stroke Educational Materials Given[5]	-	-	87%	88%
Surgical Care Improvement Project				
Appropriate Beta Blocker Usage	59	100%	98%	98%
Appropriate VTP Within 24 Hours	95	100%	98%	98%
Controlled Postoperative Blood Glucose[7]	-	-	97%	97%
Perioperative Temperature Management	153	100%	100%	100%
Prophylactic Antibiotic Selection	118	97%	99%	99%
Prophylactic Antibiotic Selection (Outpatient)[5]	-	-	98%	98%
Prophylactic Antibiotic Stopped	116	98%	98%	98%
Prophylactic Antibiotic Timing	119	99%	99%	99%
Prophylactic Antibiotic Timing (Outpatient)[5]	-	-	97%	98%
Urinary Catheter Removal	24	100%	98%	97%
Survey of Patients' Hospital Experiences				
Area Around Room 'Always' Quiet at Night	300+	64%	60%	61%
Doctors 'Always' Communicated Well	300+	90%	81%	82%
Home Recovery Information Given	300+	88%	86%	85%
Hospital Given 9 or 10 on 10 Point Scale	300+	80%	70%	71%
Meds 'Always' Explained Before Given	300+	72%	64%	64%
Nurses 'Always' Communicated Well	300+	84%	79%	79%
Pain 'Always' Well Controlled	300+	75%	71%	71%
Room and Bathroom 'Always' Clean	300+	73%	74%	73%
Timely Help 'Always' Received	300+	77%	67%	68%
Would Definitely Recommend Hospital	300+	80%	70%	71%
Use of Medical Imaging				
Cardiac Imaging Stress Test before Surgery	108	0.9%	5.5%	5.3%
Combination Abdominal CT Scan	306	5.6%	10.1%	10.5%
Combination Brain/Sinus CT Scan	351	1.4%	2.6%	2.7%
Combination Chest CT Scan	118	5.1%	2.8%	2.7%
Follow-up Mammogram/Ultrasound	468	9.4%	8.4%	8.8%
Lumbar Spine MRI for Low Back Pain[1]	-	-	36.6%	37.2%

Delnor Community Hospital

300 Randall Rd
Geneva, IL 60134
E-mail: info@delnor.com
URL: www.delnor.com
Phone: 630-208-3000
Fax: 630-208-3478
Type: Acute Care Hospitals
Ownership: Voluntary non-profit - Other
Emergency Services: Yes
Beds: 118

Key Personnel:
Quality Assurance . . . . Linda Adams
Operating Room. . . . . Paul Batty
Pediatric Ambulatory Care . . . . . . Cathy Brill
Pediatric In-Patient Care . . . . Cathy Brill
Radiology. . . . . Sidney Jain
CEO/President. . . . . Craig A Livermore

Measure	Cases	This Hosp.	State Avg.	U.S. Avg.
Blood Clot Prevention and Treatment				
Anticoagulation Overlap Therapy[2]	51	92%	91%	93%
ICU Venous Thromboembolism Prophylaxis[2]	61	93%	93%	92%
Incidence of Potentially Preventable VTE[1,2]	-	-	11%	10%
UFH with Dosages/Platelet Monitoring[1,2]	-	-	94%	97%
Venous Thromboembolism Prophylaxis[2]	299	85%	86%	85%
Warfarin Therapy Discharge Instructions[2]	36	14%	71%	75%
Chest Pain/Possible Heart Attack Care				
Aspirin Given Within 24 Hours of Arrival[3,7]	-	-	96%	96%
Fibrinolytic Meds Within 30 Min. of Arrival[5]	-	-	65%	58%
Average Time to ECG (minutes)[3,7]	-	-	6	7
Average Time to Transfer (minutes)[5]	-	-	63	60
Children's Asthma Care				
Received Home Management Plan of Care	-	-	-	88%
Received Reliever Medication	-	-	-	100%
Received Systemic Corticosteroids	-	-	-	100%
Emergency Department				
Admittance Decision Time (minutes)[2]	397	100	89	98
Head CT Results Within 45 Min. of Arrival	22	73%	64%	57%
Patients Who Left ER Before Being Seen	33,714	2%	3%	2%
Time from ER Arrival to Admit. (minutes)[2]	454	253	260	274
Time from ER Arrival to Discharge (minutes)	354	153	138	134
Time in ER Before Being Evaluated (minutes)	352	31	28	26
Time to Pain Meds for Fractures (minutes)	164	45	52	57
Heart Attack Care				
Aspirin Given at Discharge	86	99%	99%	99%
Fibrinolytic Meds Within 30 Min. of Arrival[7]	-	-	33%	54%
PCI Within 90 Minutes of Arrival	30	93%	97%	96%
Statin Prescribed at Discharge	84	99%	98%	98%
Heart Failure Care				
ACE Inhibitor or ARB for LVSD	49	94%	98%	97%
Discharge Instructions Given	170	97%	96%	94%
Evaluation of LVS Function	215	100%	99%	99%
Medicare Spending				
Medicare Spending per Patient (ratio)	-	1.03	1	0.98
Pneumonia Care				
Appropriate Initial Antibiotic Given[2]	136	98%	95%	95%
Blood Culture Timing[2]	215	98%	98%	98%
Pregnancy and Delivery Care				
Newborn Deliveries Scheduled Early[2]	31	0%	2%	6%
Preventive Care				
Immunization for Influenza[2]	501	95%	92%	90%
Immunization for Pneumonia[2]	573	96%	92%	92%
Stroke Care				
Anticoagulation Therapy for Atrial Fibrillation[2]	12	83%	94%	95%
Antithrombotic Therapy Timing[2]	62	100%	98%	98%
Assessed for Rehabilitation[2]	73	97%	97%	97%
Discharged on Antithrombotic Therapy[2]	64	100%	99%	99%
Discharged on Statin Medication[2]	53	94%	94%	94%
Thrombolytic Therapy Timing[1,2]	-	-	66%	66%
Venous Thromboembolism Prophylaxis[2]	67	100%	94%	94%
Written Stroke Educational Materials Given[2]	37	100%	87%	88%
Surgical Care Improvement Project				
Appropriate Beta Blocker Usage[2]	120	99%	98%	98%
Appropriate VTP Within 24 Hours[2]	308	98%	98%	98%
Controlled Postoperative Blood Glucose[2,7]	-	-	97%	97%
Perioperative Temperature Management[2]	414	99%	100%	100%
Prophylactic Antibiotic Selection[2]	278	99%	99%	99%
Prophylactic Antibiotic Selection (Outpatient)	159	87%	98%	98%

NOTE: Hospital profiles are in alphabetical order by state, then city, then hospital within the city; Rankings exclude hospitals with less than 25 cases except for patient surveys which excludes hospitals with less than 100 cases; (a) 100-299 cases; (1) The number of cases/patients is too few to report; (2) Data submitted were based on a sample of cases/patients; (3) Results are based on a shorter time period than required; (4) Data suppressed by CMS for one or more quarters; (5) Results are not available for this reporting period; (6) Fewer than 100 patients completed the HCAHPS survey; (7) No cases met the criteria for this measure; (8) The lower limit of the confidence interval cannot be calculated if the number of observed infections equals zero; (9) No data are available from the state/territory for this reporting period; (10) The scores shown reflect fewer than 50 completed surveys; (11) There were discrepancies in the data collection process; (12) This measure does not apply to this hospital for this reporting period; (13) Results cannot be calculated for this reporting period; (14) The results for this state are combined with nearby states to protect confidentiality; Please refer to the User's Guide for a full explanation of data.

Prophylactic Antibiotic Stopped[2]	277	99%	98%	98%
Prophylactic Antibiotic Timing[2]	279	97%	99%	99%
Prophylactic Antibiotic Timing (Outpatient)	165	86%	97%	98%
Urinary Catheter Removal[2]	95	86%	98%	97%
Survey of Patients' Hospital Experiences				
Area Around Room 'Always' Quiet at Night	300+	57%	60%	61%
Doctors 'Always' Communicated Well	300+	78%	81%	82%
Home Recovery Information Given	300+	90%	86%	85%
Hospital Given 9 or 10 on 10 Point Scale	300+	75%	70%	71%
Meds 'Always' Explained Before Given	300+	61%	64%	64%
Nurses 'Always' Communicated Well	300+	80%	79%	79%
Pain 'Always' Well Controlled	300+	69%	71%	71%
Room and Bathroom 'Always' Clean	300+	70%	74%	73%
Timely Help 'Always' Received	300+	69%	67%	68%
Would Definitely Recommend Hospital	300+	74%	70%	71%
Use of Medical Imaging				
Cardiac Imaging Stress Test before Surgery	552	4.3%	5.5%	5.3%
Combination Abdominal CT Scan	1,090	23.3%	10.1%	10.5%
Combination Brain/Sinus CT Scan	734	0.4%	2.6%	2.7%
Combination Chest CT Scan	789	15.6%	2.8%	2.7%
Follow-up Mammogram/Ultrasound	1,646	9.0%	8.4%	8.8%
Lumbar Spine MRI for Low Back Pain	109	32.1%	36.6%	37.2%

Gibson Community Hospital

1120 N Melvin Street
Gibson City, IL 60936
URL: www.gibsonhospital.org
Type: Critical Access Hospitals
Ownership: Voluntary non-profit - Private
Phone: 217-784-4251
Fax: 217-784-2610
Emergency Services: Yes
Beds: 82

Key Personnel:
Emergency Room . . . . Almuhannad Alfrhan
Anesthesiology. . . . . Roger Birky
Quality Assurance . . . . Sylvia Day
Infection Control. . . . . Becki Garard
Radiology. . . . . Daniel Ha
Operating Room. . . . . Eric Kivisto
CEO/President. . . . . Rob Schmitt
Intensive Care Unit. . . . . Brenda Standerfer

Measure	Cases	This Hosp.	State Avg.	U.S. Avg.
Blood Clot Prevention and Treatment				
Anticoagulation Overlap Therapy[5]	-	-	91%	93%
ICU Venous Thromboembolism Prophylaxis[5]	-	-	93%	92%
Incidence of Potentially Preventable VTE[5]	-	-	11%	10%
UFH with Dosages/Platelet Monitoring[5]	-	-	94%	97%
Venous Thromboembolism Prophylaxis[5]	-	-	86%	85%
Warfarin Therapy Discharge Instructions[5]	-	-	71%	75%
Chest Pain/Possible Heart Attack Care				
Aspirin Given Within 24 Hours of Arrival[5]	-	-	96%	96%
Fibrinolytic Meds Within 30 Min. of Arrival[5]	-	-	65%	58%
Average Time to ECG (minutes)[5]	-	-	6	7
Average Time to Transfer (minutes)[5]	-	-	63	60
Children's Asthma Care				
Received Home Management Plan of Care	-	-	-	88%
Received Reliever Medication	-	-	-	100%
Received Systemic Corticosteroids	-	-	-	100%
Emergency Department				
Admittance Decision Time (minutes)[5]	-	-	89	98
Head CT Results Within 45 Min. of Arrival[5]	-	-	64%	57%
Patients Who Left ER Before Being Seen	6,262	0%	3%	2%
Time from ER Arrival to Admit. (minutes)[5]	-	-	260	274
Time from ER Arrival to Discharge (minutes)[5]	-	-	138	134
Time in ER Before Being Evaluated (minutes)[5]	-	-	28	26
Time to Pain Meds for Fractures (minutes)[5]	-	-	52	57
Heart Attack Care				
Aspirin Given at Discharge[3,7]	-	-	99%	99%
Fibrinolytic Meds Within 30 Min. of Arrival[3,7]	-	-	33%	54%
PCI Within 90 Minutes of Arrival[3,7]	-	-	97%	96%
Statin Prescribed at Discharge[3,7]	-	-	98%	98%
Heart Failure Care				
ACE Inhibitor or ARB for LVSD[1]	-	-	98%	97%
Discharge Instructions Given[1]	-	-	96%	94%
Evaluation of LVS Function	13	100%	99%	99%
Medicare Spending				
Medicare Spending per Patient (ratio)	-	-	1	0.98
Pneumonia Care				
Appropriate Initial Antibiotic Given	22	86%	95%	95%
Blood Culture Timing	39	95%	98%	98%
Pregnancy and Delivery Care				
Newborn Deliveries Scheduled Early[5]	-	-	2%	6%
Preventive Care				
Immunization for Influenza[5]	-	-	92%	90%
Immunization for Pneumonia[5]	-	-	92%	92%
Stroke Care				
Anticoagulation Therapy for Atrial Fibrillation[5]	-	-	94%	95%
Antithrombotic Therapy Timing[5]	-	-	98%	98%
Assessed for Rehabilitation[5]	-	-	97%	97%
Discharged on Antithrombotic Therapy[5]	-	-	99%	99%
Discharged on Statin Medication[5]	-	-	94%	94%
Thrombolytic Therapy Timing[5]	-	-	66%	66%
Venous Thromboembolism Prophylaxis[5]	-	-	94%	94%
Written Stroke Educational Materials Given[5]	-	-	87%	88%
Surgical Care Improvement Project				
Appropriate Beta Blocker Usage	48	98%	98%	98%
Appropriate VTP Within 24 Hours	180	96%	98%	98%
Controlled Postoperative Blood Glucose[7]	-	-	97%	97%
Perioperative Temperature Management	194	100%	100%	100%
Prophylactic Antibiotic Selection	148	99%	99%	99%
Prophylactic Antibiotic Selection (Outpatient)[5]	-	-	98%	98%
Prophylactic Antibiotic Stopped	145	98%	98%	98%
Prophylactic Antibiotic Timing	148	96%	99%	99%
Prophylactic Antibiotic Timing (Outpatient)[5]	-	-	97%	98%
Urinary Catheter Removal	163	98%	98%	97%
Survey of Patients' Hospital Experiences				
Area Around Room 'Always' Quiet at Night	300+	68%	60%	61%
Doctors 'Always' Communicated Well	300+	88%	81%	82%
Home Recovery Information Given	300+	92%	86%	85%
Hospital Given 9 or 10 on 10 Point Scale	300+	87%	70%	71%
Meds 'Always' Explained Before Given	300+	72%	64%	64%
Nurses 'Always' Communicated Well	300+	84%	79%	79%
Pain 'Always' Well Controlled	300+	76%	71%	71%
Room and Bathroom 'Always' Clean	300+	78%	74%	73%
Timely Help 'Always' Received	300+	78%	67%	68%
Would Definitely Recommend Hospital	300+	85%	70%	71%
Use of Medical Imaging				
Cardiac Imaging Stress Test before Surgery	71	5.6%	5.5%	5.3%
Combination Abdominal CT Scan	194	18.6%	10.1%	10.5%
Combination Brain/Sinus CT Scan	192	5.2%	2.6%	2.7%
Combination Chest CT Scan	135	11.9%	2.8%	2.7%
Follow-up Mammogram/Ultrasound	563	8.9%	8.4%	8.8%
Lumbar Spine MRI for Low Back Pain	62	35.5%	36.6%	37.2%

Adventist Glenoaks

701 Winthrop Avenue
Glendale Heights, IL 60139
URL: www.keepingyouwell.com
Type: Acute Care Hospitals
Ownership: Voluntary non-profit - Other
Phone: 630-545-6160
Fax: 630-545-3920
Emergency Services: Yes
Beds: 186

Key Personnel:
Infection Control. . . . . Darlene Gallagher
Cardiac Laboratory. . . . . Richard Kenney
Radiology. . . . . Patricia Lee
CEO/President. . . . . Brinsley Lewis
Operating Room. . . . . Judy Papendorf
Quality Assurance . . . . Chris Rendl
Chief of Medical Staff. . . . . Lisa Wohl, MD

Measure	Cases	This Hosp.	State Avg.	U.S. Avg.
Blood Clot Prevention and Treatment				
Anticoagulation Overlap Therapy[2]	14	100%	91%	93%
ICU Venous Thromboembolism Prophylaxis[2]	97	94%	93%	92%
Incidence of Potentially Preventable VTE[1,2]	-	-	11%	10%
UFH with Dosages/Platelet Monitoring[1,2]	-	-	94%	97%
Venous Thromboembolism Prophylaxis[2]	149	82%	86%	85%
Warfarin Therapy Discharge Instructions[2]	11	73%	71%	75%
Chest Pain/Possible Heart Attack Care				
Aspirin Given Within 24 Hours of Arrival[1,3]	-	-	96%	96%
Fibrinolytic Meds Within 30 Min. of Arrival[3,7]	-	-	65%	58%
Average Time to ECG (minutes)[1,3]	-	-	6	7
Average Time to Transfer (minutes)[3,7]	-	-	63	60
Children's Asthma Care				
Received Home Management Plan of Care	-	-	-	88%
Received Reliever Medication	-	-	-	100%
Received Systemic Corticosteroids	-	-	-	100%
Emergency Department				
Admittance Decision Time (minutes)[2]	266	93	89	98
Head CT Results Within 45 Min. of Arrival[1]	-	-	64%	57%
Patients Who Left ER Before Being Seen	19,899	0%	3%	2%
Time from ER Arrival to Admit. (minutes)[2]	289	252	260	274
Time from ER Arrival to Discharge (minutes)	342	110	138	134
Time in ER Before Being Evaluated (minutes)	358	17	28	26
Time to Pain Meds for Fractures (minutes)	76	42	52	57
Heart Attack Care				
Aspirin Given at Discharge[2]	42	100%	99%	99%
Fibrinolytic Meds Within 30 Min. of Arrival[2,7]	-	-	33%	54%
PCI Within 90 Minutes of Arrival[2]	11	100%	97%	96%
Statin Prescribed at Discharge[2]	39	97%	98%	98%
Heart Failure Care				
ACE Inhibitor or ARB for LVSD[2]	22	100%	98%	97%
Discharge Instructions Given[2]	49	94%	96%	94%
Evaluation of LVS Function[2]	69	100%	99%	99%
Medicare Spending				
Medicare Spending per Patient (ratio)	-	1.11	1	0.98
Pneumonia Care				
Appropriate Initial Antibiotic Given[2]	24	100%	95%	95%
Blood Culture Timing[2]	81	100%	98%	98%
Pregnancy and Delivery Care				
Newborn Deliveries Scheduled Early[2]	43	2%	2%	6%
Preventive Care				
Immunization for Influenza[2]	287	83%	92%	90%
Immunization for Pneumonia[2]	306	95%	92%	92%
Stroke Care				
Anticoagulation Therapy for Atrial Fibrillation[1,2]	-	-	94%	95%
Antithrombotic Therapy Timing[2]	20	100%	98%	98%
Assessed for Rehabilitation[2]	24	96%	97%	97%
Discharged on Antithrombotic Therapy[2]	22	100%	99%	99%
Discharged on Statin Medication[2]	20	85%	94%	94%
Thrombolytic Therapy Timing[1,2]	-	-	66%	66%
Venous Thromboembolism Prophylaxis[2]	24	67%	94%	94%
Written Stroke Educational Materials Given[2]	11	82%	87%	88%
Surgical Care Improvement Project				
Appropriate Beta Blocker Usage[2]	32	97%	98%	98%
Appropriate VTP Within 24 Hours[2]	94	100%	98%	98%
Controlled Postoperative Blood Glucose[2,7]	-	-	97%	97%
Perioperative Temperature Management[2]	108	98%	100%	100%
Prophylactic Antibiotic Selection[2]	66	100%	99%	99%
Prophylactic Antibiotic Selection (Outpatient)	26	85%	98%	98%
Prophylactic Antibiotic Stopped[2]	61	100%	98%	98%
Prophylactic Antibiotic Timing[2]	66	100%	99%	99%
Prophylactic Antibiotic Timing (Outpatient)	26	96%	97%	98%
Urinary Catheter Removal[2]	66	98%	98%	97%
Survey of Patients' Hospital Experiences				
Area Around Room 'Always' Quiet at Night[11]	300+	52%	60%	61%
Doctors 'Always' Communicated Well[11]	300+	75%	81%	82%
Home Recovery Information Given[11]	300+	83%	86%	85%
Hospital Given 9 or 10 on 10 Point Scale[11]	300+	58%	70%	71%
Meds 'Always' Explained Before Given[11]	300+	61%	64%	64%
Nurses 'Always' Communicated Well[11]	300+	80%	79%	79%
Pain 'Always' Well Controlled[11]	300+	69%	71%	71%
Room and Bathroom 'Always' Clean[11]	300+	74%	74%	73%
Timely Help 'Always' Received[11]	300+	67%	67%	68%
Would Definitely Recommend Hospital[11]	300+	57%	70%	71%
Use of Medical Imaging				
Cardiac Imaging Stress Test before Surgery	120	7.5%	5.5%	5.3%
Combination Abdominal CT Scan	147	9.5%	10.1%	10.5%
Combination Brain/Sinus CT Scan[1]	-	-	2.6%	2.7%
Combination Chest CT Scan	104	1.0%	2.8%	2.7%
Follow-up Mammogram/Ultrasound	134	19.4%	8.4%	8.8%
Lumbar Spine MRI for Low Back Pain[1]	-	-	36.6%	37.2%

NOTE: Hospital profiles are in alphabetical order by state, then city, then hospital within the city; Rankings exclude hospitals with less than 25 cases except for patient surveys which excludes hospitals with less than 100 cases; (a) 100-299 cases; (1) The number of cases/patients is too few to report; (2) Data submitted were based on a sample of cases/patients; (3) Results are based on a shorter time period than required; (4) Data suppressed by CMS for one or more quarters; (5) Results are not available for this reporting period; (6) Fewer than 100 patients completed the HCAHPS survey; (7) No cases met the criteria for this measure; (8) The lower limit of the confidence interval cannot be calculated if the number of observed infections equals zero; (9) No data are available from the state/territory for this reporting period; (10) The scores shown reflect fewer than 50 completed surveys; (11) There were discrepancies in the data collection process; (12) This measure does not apply to this hospital for this reporting period; (13) Results cannot be calculated for this reporting period; (14) The results for this state are combined with nearby states to protect confidentiality; Please refer to the User's Guide for a full explanation of data.

Gateway Regional Medical Center

2100 Madison Avenue
Granite City, IL 62040
URL: www.sehs.com
Phone: 618-798-3175
Fax: 618-798-3853
Type: Acute Care Hospitals
Ownership: Proprietary
Emergency Services: Yes
Beds: 393

Key Personnel:
Radiology. . . . . Karen Aderholdt, MD
Pediatric Ambulatory Care . . . . . . S Ahmad, MD
Pediatric In-Patient Care . . . . S Ahmad, MD
Infection Control. . . . . Ruth Ann Gabriel
Operating Room. . . . . Wesley Harris
Chief of Medical Staff. . . . . K Konzen, MD
Quality Assurance . . . . Marcia Walker

Measure	Cases	This Hosp.	State Avg.	U.S. Avg.
Blood Clot Prevention and Treatment				
Anticoagulation Overlap Therapy[2]	21	100%	91%	93%
ICU Venous Thromboembolism Prophylaxis[2]	208	96%	93%	92%
Incidence of Potentially Preventable VTE[1,2]	-	-	11%	10%
UFH with Dosages/Platelet Monitoring[1,2]	-	-	94%	97%
Venous Thromboembolism Prophylaxis[2]	1,090	93%	86%	85%
Warfarin Therapy Discharge Instructions[2]	15	93%	71%	75%
Chest Pain/Possible Heart Attack Care				
Aspirin Given Within 24 Hours of Arrival[1,3]	-	-	96%	96%
Fibrinolytic Meds Within 30 Min. of Arrival[3,7]	-	-	65%	58%
Average Time to ECG (minutes)[3]	11	4	6	7
Average Time to Transfer (minutes)[3,7]	-	-	63	60
Children's Asthma Care				
Received Home Management Plan of Care	-	-	-	88%
Received Reliever Medication	-	-	-	100%
Received Systemic Corticosteroids	-	-	-	100%
Emergency Department				
Admittance Decision Time (minutes)[2]	1,775	64	89	98
Head CT Results Within 45 Min. of Arrival[1]	-	-	64%	57%
Patients Who Left ER Before Being Seen	26,367	3%	3%	2%
Time from ER Arrival to Admit. (minutes)[2]	1,786	216	260	274
Time from ER Arrival to Discharge (minutes)	378	116	138	134
Time in ER Before Being Evaluated (minutes)	497	17	28	26
Time to Pain Meds for Fractures (minutes)	80	63	52	57
Heart Attack Care				
Aspirin Given at Discharge	110	100%	99%	99%
Fibrinolytic Meds Within 30 Min. of Arrival[7]	-	-	33%	54%
PCI Within 90 Minutes of Arrival[1]	-	-	97%	96%
Statin Prescribed at Discharge	98	100%	98%	98%
Heart Failure Care				
ACE Inhibitor or ARB for LVSD	40	100%	98%	97%
Discharge Instructions Given	133	100%	96%	94%
Evaluation of LVS Function	157	100%	99%	99%
Medicare Spending				
Medicare Spending per Patient (ratio)	-	0.95	1	0.98
Pneumonia Care				
Appropriate Initial Antibiotic Given	16	94%	95%	95%
Blood Culture Timing	102	95%	98%	98%
Pregnancy and Delivery Care				
Newborn Deliveries Scheduled Early[2]	19	0%	2%	6%
Preventive Care				
Immunization for Influenza[2]	1,309	95%	92%	90%
Immunization for Pneumonia[2]	1,687	97%	92%	92%
Stroke Care				
Anticoagulation Therapy for Atrial Fibrillation[1]	-	-	94%	95%
Antithrombotic Therapy Timing	12	83%	98%	98%
Assessed for Rehabilitation	24	96%	97%	97%
Discharged on Antithrombotic Therapy	15	93%	99%	99%
Discharged on Statin Medication	16	94%	94%	94%
Thrombolytic Therapy Timing[7]	-	-	66%	66%
Venous Thromboembolism Prophylaxis	27	93%	94%	94%
Written Stroke Educational Materials Given	14	86%	87%	88%
Surgical Care Improvement Project				
Appropriate Beta Blocker Usage	84	100%	98%	98%
Appropriate VTP Within 24 Hours	239	100%	98%	98%
Controlled Postoperative Blood Glucose[7]	-	-	97%	97%
Perioperative Temperature Management	255	100%	100%	100%
Prophylactic Antibiotic Selection	177	100%	99%	99%
Prophylactic Antibiotic Selection (Outpatient)	133	100%	98%	98%
Prophylactic Antibiotic Stopped	175	99%	98%	98%
Prophylactic Antibiotic Timing	177	98%	99%	99%
Prophylactic Antibiotic Timing (Outpatient)	133	100%	97%	98%
Urinary Catheter Removal	111	100%	98%	97%
Survey of Patients' Hospital Experiences				
Area Around Room 'Always' Quiet at Night	300+	62%	60%	61%
Doctors 'Always' Communicated Well	300+	78%	81%	82%
Home Recovery Information Given	300+	84%	86%	85%
Hospital Given 9 or 10 on 10 Point Scale	300+	63%	70%	71%
Meds 'Always' Explained Before Given	300+	62%	64%	64%
Nurses 'Always' Communicated Well	300+	78%	79%	79%
Pain 'Always' Well Controlled	300+	69%	71%	71%
Room and Bathroom 'Always' Clean	300+	67%	74%	73%
Timely Help 'Always' Received	300+	62%	67%	68%
Would Definitely Recommend Hospital	300+	57%	70%	71%
Use of Medical Imaging				
Cardiac Imaging Stress Test before Surgery[1]	-	-	5.5%	5.3%
Combination Abdominal CT Scan	332	16.0%	10.1%	10.5%
Combination Brain/Sinus CT Scan	463	1.9%	2.6%	2.7%
Combination Chest CT Scan	186	6.5%	2.8%	2.7%
Follow-up Mammogram/Ultrasound	687	4.2%	8.4%	8.8%
Lumbar Spine MRI for Low Back Pain	98	48.0%	36.6%	37.2%

Greenville Regional Hospital

200 Healthcare Dr
Greenville, IL 62246
Phone: 618-664-1230
Fax: 618-664-9750
Type: Acute Care Hospitals
Ownership: Voluntary non-profit - Other
Emergency Services: Yes
Beds: 50

Key Personnel:
Quality Assurance . . . . Alisa Beck
Emergency Room . . . . Sara McPeak
CEO/President. . . . . Brian Nall

Measure	Cases	This Hosp.	State Avg.	U.S. Avg.
Blood Clot Prevention and Treatment				
Anticoagulation Overlap Therapy[1,2]	-	-	91%	93%
ICU Venous Thromboembolism Prophylaxis[2,7]	-	-	93%	92%
Incidence of Potentially Preventable VTE[2,7]	-	-	11%	10%
UFH with Dosages/Platelet Monitoring[1,2]	-	-	94%	97%
Venous Thromboembolism Prophylaxis[2]	126	87%	86%	85%
Warfarin Therapy Discharge Instructions[1,2]	-	-	71%	75%
Chest Pain/Possible Heart Attack Care				
Aspirin Given Within 24 Hours of Arrival[3]	29	93%	96%	96%
Fibrinolytic Meds Within 30 Min. of Arrival[1,3]	-	-	65%	58%
Average Time to ECG (minutes)[3]	30	13	6	7
Average Time to Transfer (minutes)[1,3]	-	-	63	60
Children's Asthma Care				
Received Home Management Plan of Care	-	-	-	88%
Received Reliever Medication	-	-	-	100%
Received Systemic Corticosteroids	-	-	-	100%
Emergency Department				
Admittance Decision Time (minutes)	377	55	89	98
Head CT Results Within 45 Min. of Arrival[1,3]	-	-	64%	57%
Patients Who Left ER Before Being Seen	9,336	1%	3%	2%
Time from ER Arrival to Admit. (minutes)	381	228	260	274
Time from ER Arrival to Discharge (minutes)	331	103	138	134
Time in ER Before Being Evaluated (minutes)	382	29	28	26
Time to Pain Meds for Fractures (minutes)	33	47	52	57
Heart Attack Care				
Aspirin Given at Discharge[1]	-	-	99%	99%
Fibrinolytic Meds Within 30 Min. of Arrival[7]	-	-	33%	54%
PCI Within 90 Minutes of Arrival[7]	-	-	97%	96%
Statin Prescribed at Discharge[1]	-	-	98%	98%
Heart Failure Care				
ACE Inhibitor or ARB for LVSD[1]	-	-	98%	97%
Discharge Instructions Given	23	91%	96%	94%
Evaluation of LVS Function	35	77%	99%	99%
Medicare Spending				
Medicare Spending per Patient (ratio)	-	0.92	1	0.98
Pneumonia Care				
Appropriate Initial Antibiotic Given	36	94%	95%	95%
Blood Culture Timing	54	100%	98%	98%
Pregnancy and Delivery Care				
Newborn Deliveries Scheduled Early	22	0%	2%	6%
Preventive Care				
Immunization for Influenza	236	90%	92%	90%
Immunization for Pneumonia	423	94%	92%	92%
Stroke Care				
Anticoagulation Therapy for Atrial Fibrillation[3,7]	-	-	94%	95%
Antithrombotic Therapy Timing[1,3]	-	-	98%	98%
Assessed for Rehabilitation[1,3]	-	-	97%	97%
Discharged on Antithrombotic Therapy[1,3]	-	-	99%	99%
Discharged on Statin Medication[3,7]	-	-	94%	94%
Thrombolytic Therapy Timing[3,7]	-	-	66%	66%
Venous Thromboembolism Prophylaxis[1,3]	-	-	94%	94%
Written Stroke Educational Materials Given[1,3]	-	-	87%	88%
Surgical Care Improvement Project				
Appropriate Beta Blocker Usage[1,3]	-	-	98%	98%
Appropriate VTP Within 24 Hours[1,3]	-	-	98%	98%
Controlled Postoperative Blood Glucose[3,7]	-	-	97%	97%
Perioperative Temperature Management[1,3]	-	-	100%	100%
Prophylactic Antibiotic Selection[1,3]	-	-	99%	99%
Prophylactic Antibiotic Selection (Outpatient)	12	83%	98%	98%
Prophylactic Antibiotic Stopped[1,3]	-	-	98%	98%
Prophylactic Antibiotic Timing[1,3]	-	-	99%	99%
Prophylactic Antibiotic Timing (Outpatient)	12	100%	97%	98%
Urinary Catheter Removal[3,7]	-	-	98%	97%
Survey of Patients' Hospital Experiences				
Area Around Room 'Always' Quiet at Night	(a)	58%	60%	61%
Doctors 'Always' Communicated Well	(a)	82%	81%	82%
Home Recovery Information Given	(a)	88%	86%	85%
Hospital Given 9 or 10 on 10 Point Scale	(a)	75%	70%	71%
Meds 'Always' Explained Before Given	(a)	63%	64%	64%
Nurses 'Always' Communicated Well	(a)	81%	79%	79%
Pain 'Always' Well Controlled	(a)	70%	71%	71%
Room and Bathroom 'Always' Clean	(a)	77%	74%	73%
Timely Help 'Always' Received	(a)	66%	67%	68%
Would Definitely Recommend Hospital	(a)	67%	70%	71%
Use of Medical Imaging				
Cardiac Imaging Stress Test before Surgery	81	7.4%	5.5%	5.3%
Combination Abdominal CT Scan	269	12.3%	10.1%	10.5%
Combination Brain/Sinus CT Scan[1]	-	-	2.6%	2.7%
Combination Chest CT Scan	210	2.9%	2.8%	2.7%
Follow-up Mammogram/Ultrasound	498	12.0%	8.4%	8.8%
Lumbar Spine MRI for Low Back Pain[1]	-	-	36.6%	37.2%

Harrisburg Medical Center

100 Doctor Warren Tuttle Dr
Harrisburg, IL 62946
Phone: 618-253-7671
Fax: 618-252-7274
E-mail: cchatterton@harrisburgmed.org
Type: Acute Care Hospitals
Ownership: Voluntary non-profit - Other
Emergency Services: Yes
Beds: 86

Key Personnel:
CEO/President. . . . . Vince Ashley
Infection Control. . . . . Brenda Duckworth, RN
Quality Assurance . . . . Danny Lampley
Chief of Medical Staff . . . . Vinay Mehta, MD
Operating Room. . . . . Linda Murphy, RN
Radiology. . . . . H T Youssef, MD

Measure	Cases	This Hosp.	State Avg.	U.S. Avg.
Blood Clot Prevention and Treatment				
Anticoagulation Overlap Therapy[2]	13	100%	91%	93%
ICU Venous Thromboembolism Prophylaxis[2,7]	-	-	93%	92%
Incidence of Potentially Preventable VTE[2,7]	-	-	11%	10%
UFH with Dosages/Platelet Monitoring[2,7]	-	-	94%	97%
Venous Thromboembolism Prophylaxis[2]	110	87%	86%	85%
Warfarin Therapy Discharge Instructions[1,2]	-	-	71%	75%
Chest Pain/Possible Heart Attack Care				
Aspirin Given Within 24 Hours of Arrival	48	98%	96%	96%
Fibrinolytic Meds Within 30 Min. of Arrival[7]	-	-	65%	58%
Average Time to ECG (minutes)	50	6	6	7
Average Time to Transfer (minutes)[1]	-	-	63	60
Children's Asthma Care				
Received Home Management Plan of Care	-	-	-	88%
Received Reliever Medication	-	-	-	100%
Received Systemic Corticosteroids	-	-	-	100%
Emergency Department				
Admittance Decision Time (minutes)[2]	162	3	89	98

NOTE: *Hospital profiles are in alphabetical order by state, then city, then hospital within the city; Rankings exclude hospitals with less than 25 cases except for patient surveys which excludes hospitals with less than 100 cases; (a) 100-299 cases; (1) The number of cases/patients is too few to report; (2) Data submitted were based on a sample of cases/patients; (3) Results are based on a shorter time period than required; (4) Data suppressed by CMS for one or more quarters; (5) Results are not available for this reporting period; (6) Fewer than 100 patients completed the HCAHPS survey; (7) No cases met the criteria for this measure; (8) The lower limit of the confidence interval cannot be calculated if the number of observed infections equals zero; (9) No data are available from the state/territory for this reporting period; (10) The scores shown reflect fewer than 50 completed surveys; (11) There were discrepancies in the data collection process; (12) This measure does not apply to this hospital for this reporting period; (13) Results cannot be calculated for this reporting period; (14) The results for this state are combined with nearby states to protect confidentiality; Please refer to the User's Guide for a full explanation of data.*

Measure	Cases	This Hosp.	State Avg.	U.S. Avg.
Head CT Results Within 45 Min. of Arrival[1]	-	-	64%	57%
Patients Who Left ER Before Being Seen	12,964	1%	3%	2%
Time from ER Arrival to Admit. (minutes)[2]	163	125	260	274
Time from ER Arrival to Discharge (minutes)	293	80	138	134
Time in ER Before Being Evaluated (minutes)	361	39	28	26
Time to Pain Meds for Fractures (minutes)	59	54	52	57
Heart Attack Care				
Aspirin Given at Discharge[1]	-	-	99%	99%
Fibrinolytic Meds Within 30 Min. of Arrival[7]	-	-	33%	54%
PCI Within 90 Minutes of Arrival[7]	-	-	97%	96%
Statin Prescribed at Discharge[1]	-	-	98%	98%
Heart Failure Care				
ACE Inhibitor or ARB for LVSD[1]	-	-	98%	97%
Discharge Instructions Given	32	100%	96%	94%
Evaluation of LVS Function	50	98%	99%	99%
Medicare Spending				
Medicare Spending per Patient (ratio)	-	0.90	1	0.98
Pneumonia Care				
Appropriate Initial Antibiotic Given[2]	67	99%	95%	95%
Blood Culture Timing[2]	126	93%	98%	98%
Pregnancy and Delivery Care				
Newborn Deliveries Scheduled Early[7]	-	-	2%	6%
Preventive Care				
Immunization for Influenza[2]	314	83%	92%	90%
Immunization for Pneumonia[2]	362	86%	92%	92%
Stroke Care				
Anticoagulation Therapy for Atrial Fibrillation[1]	-	-	94%	95%
Antithrombotic Therapy Timing[1]	-	-	98%	98%
Assessed for Rehabilitation[1]	-	-	97%	97%
Discharged on Antithrombotic Therapy[1]	-	-	99%	99%
Discharged on Statin Medication[1]	-	-	94%	94%
Thrombolytic Therapy Timing[7]	-	-	66%	66%
Venous Thromboembolism Prophylaxis[1]	-	-	94%	94%
Written Stroke Educational Materials Given[1]	-	-	87%	88%
Surgical Care Improvement Project				
Appropriate Beta Blocker Usage[1]	-	-	98%	98%
Appropriate VTP Within 24 Hours	18	89%	98%	98%
Controlled Postoperative Blood Glucose[7]	-	-	97%	97%
Perioperative Temperature Management	22	100%	100%	100%
Prophylactic Antibiotic Selection[1]	-	-	99%	99%
Prophylactic Antibiotic Selection (Outpatient)[3,7]	-	-	98%	98%
Prophylactic Antibiotic Stopped[1]	-	-	98%	98%
Prophylactic Antibiotic Timing[1]	-	-	99%	99%
Prophylactic Antibiotic Timing (Outpatient)[1,3]	-	-	97%	98%
Urinary Catheter Removal	14	93%	98%	97%
Survey of Patients' Hospital Experiences				
Area Around Room 'Always' Quiet at Night	(a)	60%	60%	61%
Doctors 'Always' Communicated Well	(a)	81%	81%	82%
Home Recovery Information Given	(a)	80%	86%	85%
Hospital Given 9 or 10 on 10 Point Scale	(a)	63%	70%	71%
Meds 'Always' Explained Before Given	(a)	66%	64%	64%
Nurses 'Always' Communicated Well	(a)	83%	79%	79%
Pain 'Always' Well Controlled	(a)	70%	71%	71%
Room and Bathroom 'Always' Clean	(a)	81%	74%	73%
Timely Help 'Always' Received	(a)	78%	67%	68%
Would Definitely Recommend Hospital	(a)	62%	70%	71%
Use of Medical Imaging				
Cardiac Imaging Stress Test before Surgery	121	5.8%	5.5%	5.3%
Combination Abdominal CT Scan	569	23.2%	10.1%	10.5%
Combination Brain/Sinus CT Scan	577	1.6%	2.6%	2.7%
Combination Chest CT Scan	286	41.3%	2.8%	2.7%
Follow-up Mammogram/Ultrasound	729	11.8%	8.4%	8.8%
Lumbar Spine MRI for Low Back Pain[7]	-	-	36.6%	37.2%

Mercy Harvard Hospital

901 Grant Street
Harvard, IL 60033
E-mail: custserv@mhsjvl.org
URL: www.mercyhealthsystem.org
Type: Critical Access Hospitals
Ownership: Voluntary non-profit - Private
Phone: 815-943-5431
Fax: 815-943-2493
Emergency Services: Yes
Beds: 46

Key Personnel:

Emergency Room . . . . Brian Aldred, MD
CEO/President. . . . . Javon R. Bea
Radiology. Leon F DeJongh
Chief of Medical Staff . . . . Joseph Levenstein, MD
Patient Relations . . . . Connie Secor, RN

Measure	Cases	This Hosp.	State Avg.	U.S. Avg.
Blood Clot Prevention and Treatment				
Anticoagulation Overlap Therapy[1,2]	-	-	91%	93%
ICU Venous Thromboembolism Prophylaxis[2]	21	76%	93%	92%
Incidence of Potentially Preventable VTE[2,7]	-	-	11%	10%
UFH with Dosages/Platelet Monitoring[2,7]	-	-	94%	97%
Venous Thromboembolism Prophylaxis[2]	124	92%	86%	85%
Warfarin Therapy Discharge Instructions[1,2]	-	-	71%	75%
Chest Pain/Possible Heart Attack Care				
Aspirin Given Within 24 Hours of Arrival	15	100%	96%	96%
Fibrinolytic Meds Within 30 Min. of Arrival[3,7]	-	-	65%	58%
Average Time to ECG (minutes)	16	6	6	7
Average Time to Transfer (minutes)[1,3]	-	-	63	60
Children's Asthma Care				
Received Home Management Plan of Care	-	-	-	88%
Received Reliever Medication	-	-	-	100%
Received Systemic Corticosteroids	-	-	-	100%
Emergency Department				
Admittance Decision Time (minutes)	276	40	89	98
Head CT Results Within 45 Min. of Arrival[1]	-	-	64%	57%
Patients Who Left ER Before Being Seen[5]	-	-	3%	2%
Time from ER Arrival to Admit. (minutes)	281	200	260	274
Time from ER Arrival to Discharge (minutes)	389	90	138	134
Time in ER Before Being Evaluated (minutes)	448	19	28	26
Time to Pain Meds for Fractures (minutes)	24	46	52	57
Heart Attack Care				
Aspirin Given at Discharge[5]	-	-	99%	99%
Fibrinolytic Meds Within 30 Min. of Arrival[5]	-	-	33%	54%
PCI Within 90 Minutes of Arrival[5]	-	-	97%	96%
Statin Prescribed at Discharge[5]	-	-	98%	98%
Heart Failure Care				
ACE Inhibitor or ARB for LVSD[1]	-	-	98%	97%
Discharge Instructions Given[1]	-	-	96%	94%
Evaluation of LVS Function[1]	-	-	99%	99%
Medicare Spending				
Medicare Spending per Patient (ratio)	-	-	1	0.98
Pneumonia Care				
Appropriate Initial Antibiotic Given[1]	-	-	95%	95%
Blood Culture Timing	11	100%	98%	98%
Pregnancy and Delivery Care				
Newborn Deliveries Scheduled Early[5]	-	-	2%	6%
Preventive Care				
Immunization for Influenza	201	100%	92%	90%
Immunization for Pneumonia	277	99%	92%	92%
Stroke Care				
Anticoagulation Therapy for Atrial Fibrillation[3,7]	-	-	94%	95%
Antithrombotic Therapy Timing[1,3]	-	-	98%	98%
Assessed for Rehabilitation[1,3]	-	-	97%	97%
Discharged on Antithrombotic Therapy[1,3]	-	-	99%	99%
Discharged on Statin Medication[1,3]	-	-	94%	94%
Thrombolytic Therapy Timing[3,7]	-	-	66%	66%
Venous Thromboembolism Prophylaxis[1,3]	-	-	94%	94%
Written Stroke Educational Materials Given[3,7]	-	-	87%	88%
Surgical Care Improvement Project				
Appropriate Beta Blocker Usage	11	100%	98%	98%
Appropriate VTP Within 24 Hours	31	100%	98%	98%
Controlled Postoperative Blood Glucose[7]	-	-	97%	97%
Perioperative Temperature Management	44	98%	100%	100%
Prophylactic Antibiotic Selection	20	100%	99%	99%
Prophylactic Antibiotic Selection (Outpatient)[1,3]	-	-	98%	98%
Prophylactic Antibiotic Stopped	18	94%	98%	98%
Prophylactic Antibiotic Timing	20	100%	99%	99%
Prophylactic Antibiotic Timing (Outpatient)[1,3]	-	-	97%	98%
Urinary Catheter Removal	32	97%	98%	97%
Survey of Patients' Hospital Experiences				
Area Around Room 'Always' Quiet at Night[5]	-	-	60%	61%
Doctors 'Always' Communicated Well[5]	-	-	81%	82%
Home Recovery Information Given[5]	-	-	86%	85%
Hospital Given 9 or 10 on 10 Point Scale[5]	-	-	70%	71%
Meds 'Always' Explained Before Given[5]	-	-	64%	64%
Nurses 'Always' Communicated Well[5]	-	-	79%	79%
Pain 'Always' Well Controlled[5]	-	-	71%	71%
Room and Bathroom 'Always' Clean[5]	-	-	74%	73%
Timely Help 'Always' Received[5]	-	-	67%	68%
Would Definitely Recommend Hospital[5]	-	-	70%	71%
Use of Medical Imaging				
Cardiac Imaging Stress Test before Surgery	106	10.4%	5.5%	5.3%
Combination Abdominal CT Scan	101	3.0%	10.1%	10.5%
Combination Brain/Sinus CT Scan[1]	-	-	2.6%	2.7%
Combination Chest CT Scan	83	6.0%	2.8%	2.7%
Follow-up Mammogram/Ultrasound	91	4.4%	8.4%	8.8%
Lumbar Spine MRI for Low Back Pain[1]	-	-	36.6%	37.2%

Ingalls Memorial Hospital

One Ingalls Drive
Harvey, IL 60426
URL: www.ingalls.org
Type: Acute Care Hospitals
Ownership: Voluntary non-profit - Private
Phone: 708-333-2300
Fax: 708-915-2707
Emergency Services: Yes
Beds: 326

Key Personnel:

Cardiology . . . . Tahir Abbasi, MD
Anesthesiology. . . . . Suresh Agarwal, MD
Pediatrics. . . . . Yahya Ahmadian, MD
Hemotology Center . . . . Vasia Ahmed, MD
Radiology. . . . . Lavanya Chekuri, MD
Surgery . . . . Bohdan Iwanetz, MD
CEO/President. . . . . Kurt Johnson
Infection Control. . . . . Bazgha Siddiqui, MD

Measure	Cases	This Hosp.	State Avg.	U.S. Avg.
Blood Clot Prevention and Treatment				
Anticoagulation Overlap Therapy[2]	137	96%	91%	93%
ICU Venous Thromboembolism Prophylaxis[2]	91	99%	93%	92%
Incidence of Potentially Preventable VTE[2]	14	21%	11%	10%
UFH with Dosages/Platelet Monitoring[2]	119	100%	94%	97%
Venous Thromboembolism Prophylaxis[2]	432	98%	86%	85%
Warfarin Therapy Discharge Instructions[2]	103	99%	71%	75%
Chest Pain/Possible Heart Attack Care				
Aspirin Given Within 24 Hours of Arrival[1,3]	-	-	96%	96%
Fibrinolytic Meds Within 30 Min. of Arrival[3,7]	-	-	65%	58%
Average Time to ECG (minutes)[1,3]	-	-	6	7
Average Time to Transfer (minutes)[3,7]	-	-	63	60
Children's Asthma Care				
Received Home Management Plan of Care	-	-	-	88%
Received Reliever Medication	-	-	-	100%
Received Systemic Corticosteroids	-	-	-	100%
Emergency Department				
Admittance Decision Time (minutes)[2]	464	85	89	98
Head CT Results Within 45 Min. of Arrival[1]	-	-	64%	57%
Patients Who Left ER Before Being Seen	50,435	2%	3%	2%
Time from ER Arrival to Admit. (minutes)[2]	465	287	260	274
Time from ER Arrival to Discharge (minutes)	360	118	138	134
Time in ER Before Being Evaluated (minutes)	398	10	28	26
Time to Pain Meds for Fractures (minutes)	183	38	52	57
Heart Attack Care				
Aspirin Given at Discharge[2]	248	100%	99%	99%
Fibrinolytic Meds Within 30 Min. of Arrival[2,7]	-	-	33%	54%
PCI Within 90 Minutes of Arrival[2]	13	92%	97%	96%
Statin Prescribed at Discharge[2]	222	100%	98%	98%
Heart Failure Care				
ACE Inhibitor or ARB for LVSD[2]	107	100%	98%	97%
Discharge Instructions Given[2]	253	100%	96%	94%
Evaluation of LVS Function[2]	299	100%	99%	99%
Medicare Spending				
Medicare Spending per Patient (ratio)	-	1.04	1	0.98
Pneumonia Care				
Appropriate Initial Antibiotic Given[2]	59	100%	95%	95%
Blood Culture Timing[2]	86	100%	98%	98%
Pregnancy and Delivery Care				
Newborn Deliveries Scheduled Early[2]	70	1%	2%	6%
Preventive Care				
Immunization for Influenza[2]	564	100%	92%	90%
Immunization for Pneumonia[2]	735	100%	92%	92%
Stroke Care				

NOTE: Hospital profiles are in alphabetical order by state, then city, then hospital within the city; Rankings exclude hospitals with less than 25 cases except for patient surveys which excludes hospitals with less than 100 cases; (a) 100-299 cases; (1) The number of cases/patients is too few to report; (2) Data submitted were based on a sample of cases/patients; (3) Results are based on a shorter time period than required; (4) Data suppressed by CMS for one or more quarters; (5) Results are not available for this reporting period; (6) Fewer than 100 patients completed the HCAHPS survey; (7) No cases met the criteria for this measure; (8) The lower limit of the confidence interval cannot be calculated if the number of observed infections equals zero; (9) No data are available from the state/territory for this reporting period; (10) The scores shown reflect fewer than 50 completed surveys; (11) There were discrepancies in the data collection process; (12) This measure does not apply to this hospital for this reporting period; (13) Results cannot be calculated for this reporting period; (14) The results for this state are combined with nearby states to protect confidentiality; Please refer to the User's Guide for a full explanation of data.

Measure	Cases	This Hosp.	State Avg.	U.S. Avg.
Anticoagulation Therapy for Atrial Fibrillation[1,2]	-	-	94%	95%
Antithrombotic Therapy Timing[2]	107	100%	98%	98%
Assessed for Rehabilitation[2]	108	99%	97%	97%
Discharged on Antithrombotic Therapy[2]	98	99%	99%	99%
Discharged on Statin Medication[2]	81	98%	94%	94%
Thrombolytic Therapy Timing[1,2]	-	-	66%	66%
Venous Thromboembolism Prophylaxis[2]	116	98%	94%	94%
Written Stroke Educational Materials Given[2]	59	100%	87%	88%
Surgical Care Improvement Project				
Appropriate Beta Blocker Usage[2]	139	100%	98%	98%
Appropriate VTP Within 24 Hours[2]	308	98%	98%	98%
Controlled Postoperative Blood Glucose[2]	41	100%	97%	97%
Perioperative Temperature Management[2]	378	100%	100%	100%
Prophylactic Antibiotic Selection[2]	303	100%	99%	99%
Prophylactic Antibiotic Selection (Outpatient)	164	100%	98%	98%
Prophylactic Antibiotic Stopped[2]	285	100%	98%	98%
Prophylactic Antibiotic Timing[2]	304	100%	99%	99%
Prophylactic Antibiotic Timing (Outpatient)	165	99%	97%	98%
Urinary Catheter Removal[2]	138	100%	98%	97%
Survey of Patients' Hospital Experiences				
Area Around Room 'Always' Quiet at Night	300+	57%	60%	61%
Doctors 'Always' Communicated Well	300+	77%	81%	82%
Home Recovery Information Given	300+	88%	86%	85%
Hospital Given 9 or 10 on 10 Point Scale	300+	64%	70%	71%
Meds 'Always' Explained Before Given	300+	61%	64%	64%
Nurses 'Always' Communicated Well	300+	75%	79%	79%
Pain 'Always' Well Controlled	300+	65%	71%	71%
Room and Bathroom 'Always' Clean	300+	66%	74%	73%
Timely Help 'Always' Received	300+	55%	67%	68%
Would Definitely Recommend Hospital	300+	66%	70%	71%
Use of Medical Imaging				
Cardiac Imaging Stress Test before Surgery	737	6.0%	5.5%	5.3%
Combination Abdominal CT Scan	1,917	7.1%	10.1%	10.5%
Combination Brain/Sinus CT Scan	1,152	3.0%	2.6%	2.7%
Combination Chest CT Scan	1,443	1.2%	2.8%	2.7%
Follow-up Mammogram/Ultrasound	3,291	7.5%	8.4%	8.8%
Lumbar Spine MRI for Low Back Pain	385	37.9%	36.6%	37.2%

Mason District Hospital

615 North Promenade Street,p O Box 530 Phone: 309-543-4431
Havana, IL 62644 Fax: 309-543-8523
E-mail: hwolin@fgi.net
URL: www.masondistricthospital.org
Type: Critical Access Hospitals Emergency Services: Yes
Ownership: Govt - Hospital Dist/Auth Beds: 48

Key Personnel:
Quality Assurance . . . . Gail Behrends
Operating Room. . . . . Darci Bull, RN
Infection Control . . . . Lori Canada
Emergency Room . . . . Rhonda Hine, RN
Chairman/CEO . . . . Daniel Houghton
Chief of Medical Staff. . . . . Tad A Yetter

Measure	Cases	This Hosp.	State Avg.	U.S. Avg.
Blood Clot Prevention and Treatment				
Anticoagulation Overlap Therapy[5]	-	-	91%	93%
ICU Venous Thromboembolism Prophylaxis[5]	-	-	93%	92%
Incidence of Potentially Preventable VTE[5]	-	-	11%	10%
UFH with Dosages/Platelet Monitoring[5]	-	-	94%	97%
Venous Thromboembolism Prophylaxis[5]	-	-	86%	85%
Warfarin Therapy Discharge Instructions[5]	-	-	71%	75%
Chest Pain/Possible Heart Attack Care				
Aspirin Given Within 24 Hours of Arrival[5]	-	-	96%	96%
Fibrinolytic Meds Within 30 Min. of Arrival[5]	-	-	65%	58%
Average Time to ECG (minutes)[5]	-	-	6	7
Average Time to Transfer (minutes)[5]	-	-	63	60
Children's Asthma Care				
Received Home Management Plan of Care	-	-	-	88%
Received Reliever Medication	-	-	-	100%
Received Systemic Corticosteroids	-	-	-	100%
Emergency Department				
Admittance Decision Time (minutes)[2,3]	79	50	89	98
Head CT Results Within 45 Min. of Arrival[5]	-	-	64%	57%
Patients Who Left ER Before Being Seen[5]	-	-	3%	2%
Time from ER Arrival to Admit. (minutes)[2,3]	79	195	260	274
Time from ER Arrival to Discharge (minutes)[5]	-	-	138	134
Time in ER Before Being Evaluated (minutes)[5]	-	-	28	26
Time to Pain Meds for Fractures (minutes)[5]	-	-	52	57
Heart Attack Care				
Aspirin Given at Discharge[1,3]	-	-	99%	99%
Fibrinolytic Meds Within 30 Min. of Arrival[3,7]	-	-	33%	54%
PCI Within 90 Minutes of Arrival[3,7]	-	-	97%	96%
Statin Prescribed at Discharge[1,3]	-	-	98%	98%
Heart Failure Care				
ACE Inhibitor or ARB for LVSD[7]	-	-	98%	97%
Discharge Instructions Given[1]	-	-	96%	94%
Evaluation of LVS Function	14	100%	99%	99%
Medicare Spending				
Medicare Spending per Patient (ratio)	-	-	1	0.98
Pneumonia Care				
Appropriate Initial Antibiotic Given	29	100%	95%	95%
Blood Culture Timing	33	94%	98%	98%
Pregnancy and Delivery Care				
Newborn Deliveries Scheduled Early[5]	-	-	2%	6%
Preventive Care				
Immunization for Influenza[5]	-	-	92%	90%
Immunization for Pneumonia[2,3]	79	97%	92%	92%
Stroke Care				
Anticoagulation Therapy for Atrial Fibrillation[5]	-	-	94%	95%
Antithrombotic Therapy Timing[5]	-	-	98%	98%
Assessed for Rehabilitation[5]	-	-	97%	97%
Discharged on Antithrombotic Therapy[5]	-	-	99%	99%
Discharged on Statin Medication[5]	-	-	94%	94%
Thrombolytic Therapy Timing[5]	-	-	66%	66%
Venous Thromboembolism Prophylaxis[5]	-	-	94%	94%
Written Stroke Educational Materials Given[5]	-	-	87%	88%
Surgical Care Improvement Project				
Appropriate Beta Blocker Usage[3,7]	-	-	98%	98%
Appropriate VTP Within 24 Hours[1,3]	-	-	98%	98%
Controlled Postoperative Blood Glucose[3,7]	-	-	97%	97%
Perioperative Temperature Management[1,3]	-	-	100%	100%
Prophylactic Antibiotic Selection[1,3]	-	-	99%	99%
Prophylactic Antibiotic Selection (Outpatient)[5]	-	-	98%	98%
Prophylactic Antibiotic Stopped[1,3]	-	-	98%	98%
Prophylactic Antibiotic Timing[1,3]	-	-	99%	99%
Prophylactic Antibiotic Timing (Outpatient)[5]	-	-	97%	98%
Urinary Catheter Removal[1,3]	-	-	98%	97%
Survey of Patients' Hospital Experiences				
Area Around Room 'Always' Quiet at Night[6]	<100	67%	60%	61%
Doctors 'Always' Communicated Well[6]	<100	89%	81%	82%
Home Recovery Information Given[6]	<100	94%	86%	85%
Hospital Given 9 or 10 on 10 Point Scale[6]	<100	91%	70%	71%
Meds 'Always' Explained Before Given[6]	<100	78%	64%	64%
Nurses 'Always' Communicated Well[6]	<100	88%	79%	79%
Pain 'Always' Well Controlled[6]	<100	76%	71%	71%
Room and Bathroom 'Always' Clean[6]	<100	77%	74%	73%
Timely Help 'Always' Received[6]	<100	86%	67%	68%
Would Definitely Recommend Hospital[6]	<100	82%	70%	71%
Use of Medical Imaging				
Cardiac Imaging Stress Test before Surgery[1]	-	-	5.5%	5.3%
Combination Abdominal CT Scan	172	11.0%	10.1%	10.5%
Combination Brain/Sinus CT Scan	151	5.3%	2.6%	2.7%
Combination Chest CT Scan	132	9.8%	2.8%	2.7%
Follow-up Mammogram/Ultrasound	195	4.6%	8.4%	8.8%
Lumbar Spine MRI for Low Back Pain[1]	-	-	36.6%	37.2%

Advocate South Suburban Hospital

17800 S Kedzie Ave Phone: 708-799-8000
Hazel Crest, IL 60429 Fax: 773-967-4217
E-mail: maureen.daugherty@advocatehealth.com
URL: www.advocatehealth.com
Type: Acute Care Hospitals Emergency Services: Yes
Ownership: Voluntary non-profit - Church Beds: 291

Key Personnel:
Intensive Care Unit. . . . . Donna Gurley
Chief of Medical Staff . . . . Asta Kelly, MD
Quality Assurance . . . . Mary Lange
CEO/President. . . . . Pat Martin
Radiology. . . . . J Nayden, MD
Operating Room. . . . . Cynthia Newell
Emergency Room . . . . Diane Warbuton

Measure	Cases	This Hosp.	State Avg.	U.S. Avg.
Blood Clot Prevention and Treatment				
Anticoagulation Overlap Therapy[2]	121	86%	91%	93%
ICU Venous Thromboembolism Prophylaxis[2]	116	83%	93%	92%
Incidence of Potentially Preventable VTE[2]	18	11%	11%	10%
UFH with Dosages/Platelet Monitoring[2]	52	94%	94%	97%
Venous Thromboembolism Prophylaxis[2]	356	79%	86%	85%
Warfarin Therapy Discharge Instructions[2]	85	29%	71%	75%
Chest Pain/Possible Heart Attack Care				
Aspirin Given Within 24 Hours of Arrival[1]	-	-	96%	96%
Fibrinolytic Meds Within 30 Min. of Arrival[5]	-	-	65%	58%
Average Time to ECG (minutes)[1]	-	-	6	7
Average Time to Transfer (minutes)[5]	-	-	63	60
Children's Asthma Care				
Received Home Management Plan of Care	-	-	-	88%
Received Reliever Medication	-	-	-	100%
Received Systemic Corticosteroids	-	-	-	100%
Emergency Department				
Admittance Decision Time (minutes)[2]	609	108	89	98
Head CT Results Within 45 Min. of Arrival	12	92%	64%	57%
Patients Who Left ER Before Being Seen	46,788	4%	3%	2%
Time from ER Arrival to Admit. (minutes)[2]	616	320	260	274
Time from ER Arrival to Discharge (minutes)	367	169	138	134
Time in ER Before Being Evaluated (minutes)	387	64	28	26
Time to Pain Meds for Fractures (minutes)	71	67	52	57
Heart Attack Care				
Aspirin Given at Discharge[2]	183	100%	99%	99%
Fibrinolytic Meds Within 30 Min. of Arrival[2,7]	-	-	33%	54%
PCI Within 90 Minutes of Arrival[2]	24	96%	97%	96%
Statin Prescribed at Discharge[2]	185	100%	98%	98%
Heart Failure Care				
ACE Inhibitor or ARB for LVSD[2]	128	100%	98%	97%
Discharge Instructions Given[2]	263	98%	96%	94%
Evaluation of LVS Function[2]	333	100%	99%	99%
Medicare Spending				
Medicare Spending per Patient (ratio)	-	0.98	1	0.98
Pneumonia Care				
Appropriate Initial Antibiotic Given[2]	69	96%	95%	95%
Blood Culture Timing[2]	86	98%	98%	98%
Pregnancy and Delivery Care				
Newborn Deliveries Scheduled Early	101	0%	2%	6%
Preventive Care				
Immunization for Influenza[2]	599	95%	92%	90%
Immunization for Pneumonia[2]	769	94%	92%	92%
Stroke Care				
Anticoagulation Therapy for Atrial Fibrillation	15	87%	94%	95%
Antithrombotic Therapy Timing	116	97%	98%	98%
Assessed for Rehabilitation	134	99%	97%	97%
Discharged on Antithrombotic Therapy	124	98%	99%	99%
Discharged on Statin Medication	105	98%	94%	94%
Thrombolytic Therapy Timing	14	93%	66%	66%
Venous Thromboembolism Prophylaxis	135	94%	94%	94%
Written Stroke Educational Materials Given	72	100%	87%	88%
Surgical Care Improvement Project				
Appropriate Beta Blocker Usage[2]	155	100%	98%	98%
Appropriate VTP Within 24 Hours[2]	407	100%	98%	98%
Controlled Postoperative Blood Glucose[2,7]	-	-	97%	97%
Perioperative Temperature Management[2]	498	100%	100%	100%
Prophylactic Antibiotic Selection[2]	336	99%	99%	99%
Prophylactic Antibiotic Selection (Outpatient)	178	98%	98%	98%
Prophylactic Antibiotic Stopped[2]	326	100%	98%	98%
Prophylactic Antibiotic Timing[2]	337	100%	99%	99%
Prophylactic Antibiotic Timing (Outpatient)	178	98%	97%	98%
Urinary Catheter Removal[2]	263	100%	98%	97%
Survey of Patients' Hospital Experiences				
Area Around Room 'Always' Quiet at Night	300+	56%	60%	61%
Doctors 'Always' Communicated Well	300+	81%	81%	82%
Home Recovery Information Given	300+	84%	86%	85%
Hospital Given 9 or 10 on 10 Point Scale	300+	68%	70%	71%
Meds 'Always' Explained Before Given	300+	64%	64%	64%

NOTE: Hospital profiles are in alphabetical order by state, then city, then hospital within the city; Rankings exclude hospitals with less than 25 cases except for patient surveys which excludes hospitals with less than 100 cases; (a) 100-299 cases; (1) The number of cases/patients is too few to report; (2) Data submitted were based on a sample of cases/patients; (3) Results are based on a shorter time period than required; (4) Data suppressed by CMS for one or more quarters; (5) Results are not available for this reporting period; (6) Fewer than 100 patients completed the HCAHPS survey; (7) No cases met the criteria for this measure; (8) The lower limit of the confidence interval cannot be calculated if the number of observed infections equals zero; (9) No data are available from the state/territory for this reporting period; (10) The scores shown reflect fewer than 50 completed surveys; (11) There were discrepancies in the data collection process; (12) This measure does not apply to this hospital for this reporting period; (13) Results cannot be calculated for this reporting period; (14) The results for this state are combined with nearby states to protect confidentiality; Please refer to the User's Guide for a full explanation of data.

Measure	Cases	This Hosp.	State Avg.	U.S. Avg.
Nurses 'Always' Communicated Well	300+	81%	79%	79%
Pain 'Always' Well Controlled	300+	73%	71%	71%
Room and Bathroom 'Always' Clean	300+	68%	74%	73%
Timely Help 'Always' Received	300+	65%	67%	68%
Would Definitely Recommend Hospital	300+	66%	70%	71%
Use of Medical Imaging				
Cardiac Imaging Stress Test before Surgery	459	5.9%	5.5%	5.3%
Combination Abdominal CT Scan	850	4.4%	10.1%	10.5%
Combination Brain/Sinus CT Scan	819	1.5%	2.6%	2.7%
Combination Chest CT Scan	583	2.9%	2.8%	2.7%
Follow-up Mammogram/Ultrasound	1,639	12.3%	8.4%	8.8%
Lumbar Spine MRI for Low Back Pain	99	36.4%	36.6%	37.2%

Herrin Hospital

201 S 14th St
Herrin, IL 62948
URL: www.sih.net
Phone: 618-942-2171
Fax: 618-351-4929
Type: Acute Care Hospitals
Emergency Services: Yes
Ownership: Voluntary non-profit - Private
Beds: 102

Key Personnel:

Quality Assurance . . . . Paula Alters
Chief of Medical Staff . . . . Pramote Anantachai, MD
Emergency Room . . . . Daniel Bercu, MD
Radiology. . . . . James Borders
President/CEO. . . . . Rex Budde
Operating Room. . . . . Antoni Kos, RN
Infection Control. . . . . Dottie Throgmorton, RN
Intensive Care Unit. . . . . Dottie Throgmorton, RN

Measure	Cases	This Hosp.	State Avg.	U.S. Avg.
Blood Clot Prevention and Treatment				
Anticoagulation Overlap Therapy[2]	27	100%	91%	93%
ICU Venous Thromboembolism Prophylaxis[2]	80	98%	93%	92%
Incidence of Potentially Preventable VTE[1,2]	-	-	11%	10%
UFH with Dosages/Platelet Monitoring[1,2]	-	-	94%	97%
Venous Thromboembolism Prophylaxis[2]	365	94%	86%	85%
Warfarin Therapy Discharge Instructions[2]	18	94%	71%	75%
Chest Pain/Possible Heart Attack Care				
Aspirin Given Within 24 Hours of Arrival	160	99%	96%	96%
Fibrinolytic Meds Within 30 Min. of Arrival[7]	-	-	65%	58%
Average Time to ECG (minutes)	163	4	6	7
Average Time to Transfer (minutes)	29	29	63	60
Children's Asthma Care				
Received Home Management Plan of Care	-	-	-	88%
Received Reliever Medication	-	-	-	100%
Received Systemic Corticosteroids	-	-	-	100%
Emergency Department				
Admittance Decision Time (minutes)[2]	690	70	89	98
Head CT Results Within 45 Min. of Arrival	22	82%	64%	57%
Patients Who Left ER Before Being Seen	25,843	3%	3%	2%
Time from ER Arrival to Admit. (minutes)[2]	737	265	260	274
Time from ER Arrival to Discharge (minutes)	368	157	138	134
Time in ER Before Being Evaluated (minutes)	433	35	28	26
Time to Pain Meds for Fractures (minutes)	73	61	52	57
Heart Attack Care				
Aspirin Given at Discharge	18	100%	99%	99%
Fibrinolytic Meds Within 30 Min. of Arrival[7]	-	-	33%	54%
PCI Within 90 Minutes of Arrival[7]	-	-	97%	96%
Statin Prescribed at Discharge	18	89%	98%	98%
Heart Failure Care				
ACE Inhibitor or ARB for LVSD	25	100%	98%	97%
Discharge Instructions Given	94	95%	96%	94%
Evaluation of LVS Function	127	100%	99%	99%
Medicare Spending				
Medicare Spending per Patient (ratio)	-	1.03	1	0.98
Pneumonia Care				
Appropriate Initial Antibiotic Given	141	99%	95%	95%
Blood Culture Timing	387	99%	98%	98%
Pregnancy and Delivery Care				
Newborn Deliveries Scheduled Early[7]	-	-	2%	6%
Preventive Care				
Immunization for Influenza[2]	519	94%	92%	90%
Immunization for Pneumonia[2]	820	95%	92%	92%
Stroke Care				
Anticoagulation Therapy for Atrial Fibrillation[1]	-	-	94%	95%
Antithrombotic Therapy Timing	48	100%	98%	98%
Assessed for Rehabilitation	54	98%	97%	97%
Discharged on Antithrombotic Therapy	53	100%	99%	99%
Discharged on Statin Medication	41	100%	94%	94%
Thrombolytic Therapy Timing[7]	-	-	66%	66%
Venous Thromboembolism Prophylaxis	48	98%	94%	94%
Written Stroke Educational Materials Given	37	97%	87%	88%
Surgical Care Improvement Project				
Appropriate Beta Blocker Usage	139	98%	98%	98%
Appropriate VTP Within 24 Hours	396	99%	98%	98%
Controlled Postoperative Blood Glucose[7]	-	-	97%	97%
Perioperative Temperature Management	428	100%	100%	100%
Prophylactic Antibiotic Selection	330	100%	99%	99%
Prophylactic Antibiotic Selection (Outpatient)	14	100%	98%	98%
Prophylactic Antibiotic Stopped	319	100%	98%	98%
Prophylactic Antibiotic Timing	330	99%	99%	99%
Prophylactic Antibiotic Timing (Outpatient)	14	93%	97%	98%
Urinary Catheter Removal	386	100%	98%	97%
Survey of Patients' Hospital Experiences				
Area Around Room 'Always' Quiet at Night	300+	59%	60%	61%
Doctors 'Always' Communicated Well	300+	80%	81%	82%
Home Recovery Information Given	300+	88%	86%	85%
Hospital Given 9 or 10 on 10 Point Scale	300+	74%	70%	71%
Meds 'Always' Explained Before Given	300+	68%	64%	64%
Nurses 'Always' Communicated Well	300+	80%	79%	79%
Pain 'Always' Well Controlled	300+	71%	71%	71%
Room and Bathroom 'Always' Clean	300+	72%	74%	73%
Timely Help 'Always' Received	300+	65%	67%	68%
Would Definitely Recommend Hospital	300+	79%	70%	71%
Use of Medical Imaging				
Cardiac Imaging Stress Test before Surgery	765	7.2%	5.5%	5.3%
Combination Abdominal CT Scan	1,396	12.6%	10.1%	10.5%
Combination Brain/Sinus CT Scan	1,099	3.9%	2.6%	2.7%
Combination Chest CT Scan	1,098	12.7%	2.8%	2.7%
Follow-up Mammogram/Ultrasound	1,302	10.8%	8.4%	8.8%
Lumbar Spine MRI for Low Back Pain	153	37.3%	36.6%	37.2%

Saint Joseph's Hospital

12866 Troxler Avenue
Highland, IL 62249
Phone: 618-651-2600
Fax: 618-654-2012
Type: Critical Access Hospitals
Emergency Services: Yes
Ownership: Voluntary non-profit - Church
Beds: 106

Key Personnel:

Anesthesiology. . . . . Brad Bernstein
Radiology. . . . . Robert Killian
Emergency Room . . . . Armand Miranda, MD
Chief of Medical Staff . . . . Greg Mirianda
President . . . . Kathryn H. Ruscitto

Measure	Cases	This Hosp.	State Avg.	U.S. Avg.
Blood Clot Prevention and Treatment				
Anticoagulation Overlap Therapy[5]	-	-	91%	93%
ICU Venous Thromboembolism Prophylaxis[5]	-	-	93%	92%
Incidence of Potentially Preventable VTE[5]	-	-	11%	10%
UFH with Dosages/Platelet Monitoring[5]	-	-	94%	97%
Venous Thromboembolism Prophylaxis[5]	-	-	86%	85%
Warfarin Therapy Discharge Instructions[5]	-	-	71%	75%
Chest Pain/Possible Heart Attack Care				
Aspirin Given Within 24 Hours of Arrival[5]	-	-	96%	96%
Fibrinolytic Meds Within 30 Min. of Arrival[5]	-	-	65%	58%
Average Time to ECG (minutes)[5]	-	-	6	7
Average Time to Transfer (minutes)[5]	-	-	63	60
Children's Asthma Care				
Received Home Management Plan of Care	-	-	-	88%
Received Reliever Medication	-	-	-	100%
Received Systemic Corticosteroids	-	-	-	100%
Emergency Department				
Admittance Decision Time (minutes)[5]	-	-	89	98
Head CT Results Within 45 Min. of Arrival[5]	-	-	64%	57%
Patients Who Left ER Before Being Seen	6,370	1%	3%	2%
Time from ER Arrival to Admit. (minutes)[5]	-	-	260	274
Time from ER Arrival to Discharge (minutes)[5]	-	-	138	134
Time in ER Before Being Evaluated (minutes)[5]	-	-	28	26
Time to Pain Meds for Fractures (minutes)[5]	-	-	52	57
Heart Attack Care				
Aspirin Given at Discharge[1]	-	-	99%	99%
Fibrinolytic Meds Within 30 Min. of Arrival[7]	-	-	33%	54%
PCI Within 90 Minutes of Arrival[3,7]	-	-	97%	96%
Statin Prescribed at Discharge[1]	-	-	98%	98%
Heart Failure Care				
ACE Inhibitor or ARB for LVSD[1]	-	-	98%	97%
Discharge Instructions Given	11	100%	96%	94%
Evaluation of LVS Function	21	100%	99%	99%
Medicare Spending				
Medicare Spending per Patient (ratio)	-	-	1	0.98
Pneumonia Care				
Appropriate Initial Antibiotic Given	42	98%	95%	95%
Blood Culture Timing	56	100%	98%	98%
Pregnancy and Delivery Care				
Newborn Deliveries Scheduled Early[5]	-	-	2%	6%
Preventive Care				
Immunization for Influenza[5]	-	-	92%	90%
Immunization for Pneumonia[5]	-	-	92%	92%
Stroke Care				
Anticoagulation Therapy for Atrial Fibrillation[5]	-	-	94%	95%
Antithrombotic Therapy Timing[5]	-	-	98%	98%
Assessed for Rehabilitation[5]	-	-	97%	97%
Discharged on Antithrombotic Therapy[5]	-	-	99%	99%
Discharged on Statin Medication[5]	-	-	94%	94%
Thrombolytic Therapy Timing[5]	-	-	66%	66%
Venous Thromboembolism Prophylaxis[5]	-	-	94%	94%
Written Stroke Educational Materials Given[5]	-	-	87%	88%
Surgical Care Improvement Project				
Appropriate Beta Blocker Usage	25	100%	98%	98%
Appropriate VTP Within 24 Hours	68	100%	98%	98%
Controlled Postoperative Blood Glucose[3,7]	-	-	97%	97%
Perioperative Temperature Management	70	100%	100%	100%
Prophylactic Antibiotic Selection	56	100%	99%	99%
Prophylactic Antibiotic Selection (Outpatient)[5]	-	-	98%	98%
Prophylactic Antibiotic Stopped	54	100%	98%	98%
Prophylactic Antibiotic Timing	56	100%	99%	99%
Prophylactic Antibiotic Timing (Outpatient)[5]	-	-	97%	98%
Urinary Catheter Removal	59	100%	98%	97%
Survey of Patients' Hospital Experiences				
Area Around Room 'Always' Quiet at Night	(a)	67%	60%	61%
Doctors 'Always' Communicated Well	(a)	89%	81%	82%
Home Recovery Information Given	(a)	87%	86%	85%
Hospital Given 9 or 10 on 10 Point Scale	(a)	73%	70%	71%
Meds 'Always' Explained Before Given	(a)	65%	64%	64%
Nurses 'Always' Communicated Well	(a)	83%	79%	79%
Pain 'Always' Well Controlled	(a)	68%	71%	71%
Room and Bathroom 'Always' Clean	(a)	77%	74%	73%
Timely Help 'Always' Received	(a)	74%	67%	68%
Would Definitely Recommend Hospital	(a)	70%	70%	71%
Use of Medical Imaging				
Cardiac Imaging Stress Test before Surgery	86	10.5%	5.5%	5.3%
Combination Abdominal CT Scan	291	6.9%	10.1%	10.5%
Combination Brain/Sinus CT Scan[1]	-	-	2.6%	2.7%
Combination Chest CT Scan	165	3.6%	2.8%	2.7%
Follow-up Mammogram/Ultrasound	390	8.2%	8.4%	8.8%
Lumbar Spine MRI for Low Back Pain[1]	-	-	36.6%	37.2%

Hillsboro Area Hospital

1200 E Tremont Street
Hillsboro, IL 62049
URL: www.hillsboroareahospital.org
Phone: 217-532-6111
Fax: 217-532-2726
Type: Critical Access Hospitals
Emergency Services: Yes
Ownership: Voluntary non-profit - Private
Beds: 100

Key Personnel:

President/CEO. . . . . Rex Brown, MD
Quality Assurance . . . . Angie Dugan
Quality Assurance . . . . Theresa Rapp
Surgery . . . . Theresa Rapp
Pediatric In-Patient Care . . . . Deehan Rives
Infection Control. . . . . Deehon Rives
Infection Control. . . . . Kathy Sullivan, RN
Radiology. . . . . Patricia Weaver

Measure	Cases	This Hosp.	State Avg.	U.S. Avg.

NOTE: Hospital profiles are in alphabetical order by state, then city, then hospital within the city; Rankings exclude hospitals with less than 25 cases except for patient surveys which excludes hospitals with less than 100 cases; (a) 100-299 cases; (1) The number of cases/patients is too few to report; (2) Data submitted were based on a sample of cases/patients; (3) Results are based on a shorter time period than required; (4) Data suppressed by CMS for one or more quarters; (5) Results are not available for this reporting period; (6) Fewer than 100 patients completed the HCAHPS survey; (7) No cases met the criteria for this measure; (8) The lower limit of the confidence interval cannot be calculated if the number of observed infections equals zero; (9) No data are available from the state/territory for this reporting period; (10) The scores shown reflect fewer than 50 completed surveys; (11) There were discrepancies in the data collection process; (12) This measure does not apply to this hospital for this reporting period; (13) Results cannot be calculated for this reporting period; (14) The results for this state are combined with nearby states to protect confidentiality; Please refer to the User's Guide for a full explanation of data.

Blood Clot Prevention and Treatment				
Anticoagulation Overlap Therapy[5]	-	-	91%	93%
ICU Venous Thromboembolism Prophylaxis[5]	-	-	93%	92%
Incidence of Potentially Preventable VTE[5]	-	-	11%	10%
UFH with Dosages/Platelet Monitoring[5]	-	-	94%	97%
Venous Thromboembolism Prophylaxis[5]	-	-	86%	85%
Warfarin Therapy Discharge Instructions[5]	-	-	71%	75%
Chest Pain/Possible Heart Attack Care				
Aspirin Given Within 24 Hours of Arrival	-	-	96%	96%
Fibrinolytic Meds Within 30 Min. of Arrival	-	-	65%	58%
Average Time to ECG (minutes)	-	-	6	7
Average Time to Transfer (minutes)	-	-	63	60
Children's Asthma Care				
Received Home Management Plan of Care	-	-	-	88%
Received Reliever Medication	-	-	-	100%
Received Systemic Corticosteroids	-	-	-	100%
Emergency Department				
Admittance Decision Time (minutes)[5]	-	-	89	98
Head CT Results Within 45 Min. of Arrival	-	-	64%	57%
Patients Who Left ER Before Being Seen	-	-	3%	2%
Time from ER Arrival to Admit. (minutes)[5]	-	-	260	274
Time from ER Arrival to Discharge (minutes)	-	-	138	134
Time in ER Before Being Evaluated (minutes)	-	-	28	26
Time to Pain Meds for Fractures (minutes)	-	-	52	57
Heart Attack Care				
Aspirin Given at Discharge[1]	-	-	99%	99%
Fibrinolytic Meds Within 30 Min. of Arrival[7]	-	-	33%	54%
PCI Within 90 Minutes of Arrival[5]	-	-	97%	96%
Statin Prescribed at Discharge[1]	-	-	98%	98%
Heart Failure Care				
ACE Inhibitor or ARB for LVSD[1]	-	-	98%	97%
Discharge Instructions Given	18	100%	96%	94%
Evaluation of LVS Function	31	100%	99%	99%
Medicare Spending				
Medicare Spending per Patient (ratio)	-	-	1	0.98
Pneumonia Care				
Appropriate Initial Antibiotic Given	44	100%	95%	95%
Blood Culture Timing	67	97%	98%	98%
Pregnancy and Delivery Care				
Newborn Deliveries Scheduled Early[5]	-	-	2%	6%
Preventive Care				
Immunization for Influenza[5]	-	-	92%	90%
Immunization for Pneumonia[5]	-	-	92%	92%
Stroke Care				
Anticoagulation Therapy for Atrial Fibrillation[5]	-	-	94%	95%
Antithrombotic Therapy Timing[5]	-	-	98%	98%
Assessed for Rehabilitation[5]	-	-	97%	97%
Discharged on Antithrombotic Therapy[5]	-	-	99%	99%
Discharged on Statin Medication[5]	-	-	94%	94%
Thrombolytic Therapy Timing[5]	-	-	66%	66%
Venous Thromboembolism Prophylaxis[5]	-	-	94%	94%
Written Stroke Educational Materials Given[5]	-	-	87%	88%
Surgical Care Improvement Project				
Appropriate Beta Blocker Usage[3,7]	-	-	98%	98%
Appropriate VTP Within 24 Hours[1,3]	-	-	98%	98%
Controlled Postoperative Blood Glucose[5]	-	-	97%	97%
Perioperative Temperature Management[1,3]	-	-	100%	100%
Prophylactic Antibiotic Selection[3,7]	-	-	99%	99%
Prophylactic Antibiotic Selection (Outpatient)	-	-	98%	98%
Prophylactic Antibiotic Stopped[3,7]	-	-	98%	98%
Prophylactic Antibiotic Timing[3,7]	-	-	99%	99%
Prophylactic Antibiotic Timing (Outpatient)	-	-	97%	98%
Urinary Catheter Removal[1,3]	-	-	98%	97%
Survey of Patients' Hospital Experiences				
Area Around Room 'Always' Quiet at Night	(a)	64%	60%	61%
Doctors 'Always' Communicated Well	(a)	92%	81%	82%
Home Recovery Information Given	(a)	92%	86%	85%
Hospital Given 9 or 10 on 10 Point Scale	(a)	83%	70%	71%
Meds 'Always' Explained Before Given	(a)	76%	64%	64%
Nurses 'Always' Communicated Well	(a)	92%	79%	79%
Pain 'Always' Well Controlled	(a)	87%	71%	71%
Room and Bathroom 'Always' Clean	(a)	90%	74%	73%
Timely Help 'Always' Received	(a)	85%	67%	68%
Would Definitely Recommend Hospital	(a)	79%	70%	71%
Use of Medical Imaging				
Cardiac Imaging Stress Test before Surgery	-	-	5.5%	5.3%
Combination Abdominal CT Scan	-	-	10.1%	10.5%
Combination Brain/Sinus CT Scan	-	-	2.6%	2.7%
Combination Chest CT Scan	-	-	2.8%	2.7%
Follow-up Mammogram/Ultrasound	-	-	8.4%	8.8%
Lumbar Spine MRI for Low Back Pain	-	-	36.6%	37.2%

Hines VA Medical Center

5th Street & Roosevelt Avenue
Hines, IL 60141
URL: www.visn12.med.va.gov/hines
Type: Acute Care - VA
Ownership: Government Federal

Phone: 708-202-8387
Fax: 708-202-2725
Emergency Services: No
Beds: 472

Key Personnel:
Quality Assurance . . . . L Beverly
Chief of Medical Staff . . . . Jack Bulmash, MD
Anesthesiology. . . . . B Kleinmann, MD
Emergency Room . . . . P Murdoch, MD
Operating Room. . . . . E Pierce, RN
Intensive Care Unit. . . . . L Rutledge, RN
Infection Control. . . . . D Schaaff, MD
Radiology. . . . . Mark VanDrunen, MD

Measure	Cases	This Hosp.	State Avg.	U.S. Avg.
Blood Clot Prevention and Treatment				
Anticoagulation Overlap Therapy	-	-	91%	93%
ICU Venous Thromboembolism Prophylaxis	-	-	93%	92%
Incidence of Potentially Preventable VTE	-	-	11%	10%
UFH with Dosages/Platelet Monitoring	-	-	94%	97%
Venous Thromboembolism Prophylaxis	-	-	86%	85%
Warfarin Therapy Discharge Instructions	-	-	71%	75%
Chest Pain/Possible Heart Attack Care				
Aspirin Given Within 24 Hours of Arrival	-	-	96%	96%
Fibrinolytic Meds Within 30 Min. of Arrival	-	-	65%	58%
Average Time to ECG (minutes)	-	-	6	7
Average Time to Transfer (minutes)	-	-	63	60
Children's Asthma Care				
Received Home Management Plan of Care	-	-	-	88%
Received Reliever Medication	-	-	-	100%
Received Systemic Corticosteroids	-	-	-	100%
Emergency Department				
Admittance Decision Time (minutes)	-	-	89	98
Head CT Results Within 45 Min. of Arrival	-	-	64%	57%
Patients Who Left ER Before Being Seen	-	-	3%	2%
Time from ER Arrival to Admit. (minutes)	-	-	260	274
Time from ER Arrival to Discharge (minutes)	-	-	138	134
Time in ER Before Being Evaluated (minutes)	-	-	28	26
Time to Pain Meds for Fractures (minutes)	-	-	52	57
Heart Attack Care				
Aspirin Given at Discharge	63	100%	99%	99%
Fibrinolytic Meds Within 30 Min. of Arrival[5]	-	-	33%	54%
PCI Within 90 Minutes of Arrival[5]	-	-	97%	96%
Statin Prescribed at Discharge	65	98%	98%	98%
Heart Failure Care				
ACE Inhibitor or ARB for LVSD	127	99%	98%	97%
Discharge Instructions Given	272	100%	96%	94%
Evaluation of LVS Function	288	100%	99%	99%
Medicare Spending				
Medicare Spending per Patient (ratio)	-	-	1	0.98
Pneumonia Care				
Appropriate Initial Antibiotic Given	44	100%	95%	95%
Blood Culture Timing	96	99%	98%	98%
Pregnancy and Delivery Care				
Newborn Deliveries Scheduled Early	-	-	2%	6%
Preventive Care				
Immunization for Influenza[5]	-	-	92%	90%
Immunization for Pneumonia[5]	-	-	92%	92%
Stroke Care				
Anticoagulation Therapy for Atrial Fibrillation	-	-	94%	95%
Antithrombotic Therapy Timing	-	-	98%	98%
Assessed for Rehabilitation	-	-	97%	97%
Discharged on Antithrombotic Therapy	-	-	99%	99%
Discharged on Statin Medication	-	-	94%	94%
Thrombolytic Therapy Timing	-	-	66%	66%
Venous Thromboembolism Prophylaxis	-	-	94%	94%
Written Stroke Educational Materials Given	-	-	87%	88%
Surgical Care Improvement Project				
Appropriate Beta Blocker Usage[2]	136	99%	98%	98%
Appropriate VTP Within 24 Hours[2]	169	100%	98%	98%
Controlled Postoperative Blood Glucose[2]	105	93%	97%	97%
Perioperative Temperature Management[2]	268	99%	100%	100%
Prophylactic Antibiotic Selection	187	100%	99%	99%
Prophylactic Antibiotic Selection (Outpatient)	-	-	98%	98%
Prophylactic Antibiotic Stopped	182	99%	98%	98%
Prophylactic Antibiotic Timing	188	98%	99%	99%
Prophylactic Antibiotic Timing (Outpatient)	-	-	97%	98%
Urinary Catheter Removal[2]	233	100%	98%	97%
Survey of Patients' Hospital Experiences				
Area Around Room 'Always' Quiet at Night	-	-	60%	61%
Doctors 'Always' Communicated Well	-	-	81%	82%
Home Recovery Information Given	-	-	86%	85%
Hospital Given 9 or 10 on 10 Point Scale	-	-	70%	71%
Meds 'Always' Explained Before Given	-	-	64%	64%
Nurses 'Always' Communicated Well	-	-	79%	79%
Pain 'Always' Well Controlled	-	-	71%	71%
Room and Bathroom 'Always' Clean	-	-	74%	73%
Timely Help 'Always' Received	-	-	67%	68%
Would Definitely Recommend Hospital	-	-	70%	71%
Use of Medical Imaging				
Cardiac Imaging Stress Test before Surgery	-	-	5.5%	5.3%
Combination Abdominal CT Scan	-	-	10.1%	10.5%
Combination Brain/Sinus CT Scan	-	-	2.6%	2.7%
Combination Chest CT Scan	-	-	2.8%	2.7%
Follow-up Mammogram/Ultrasound	-	-	8.4%	8.8%
Lumbar Spine MRI for Low Back Pain	-	-	36.6%	37.2%

Hinsdale Hospital

120 North Oak St
Hinsdale, IL 60521
URL: www.keepingyouwell.com
Type: Acute Care Hospitals
Ownership: Voluntary non-profit - Church

Phone: 630-856-9000
Fax: 630-856-7560
Emergency Services: Yes
Beds: 426

Key Personnel:
Radiology. . . . . Val Lavezzi
Quality Assurance . . . . Donita Phillips
CEO/President. . . . . Ernie Sadau
Ambulatory Care . . . . Sue Smith
Emergency Room . . . . Sue Smith
Chief of Medical Staff . . . . Robert Zeck, MD

Measure	Cases	This Hosp.	State Avg.	U.S. Avg.
Blood Clot Prevention and Treatment				
Anticoagulation Overlap Therapy[2]	74	96%	91%	93%
ICU Venous Thromboembolism Prophylaxis[2]	65	98%	93%	92%
Incidence of Potentially Preventable VTE[2]	12	0%	11%	10%
UFH with Dosages/Platelet Monitoring[2]	42	98%	94%	97%
Venous Thromboembolism Prophylaxis[2]	295	81%	86%	85%
Warfarin Therapy Discharge Instructions[2]	44	68%	71%	75%
Chest Pain/Possible Heart Attack Care				
Aspirin Given Within 24 Hours of Arrival[5]	-	-	96%	96%
Fibrinolytic Meds Within 30 Min. of Arrival[5]	-	-	65%	58%
Average Time to ECG (minutes)[5]	-	-	6	7
Average Time to Transfer (minutes)[5]	-	-	63	60
Children's Asthma Care				
Received Home Management Plan of Care	-	-	-	88%
Received Reliever Medication	-	-	-	100%
Received Systemic Corticosteroids	-	-	-	100%
Emergency Department				
Admittance Decision Time (minutes)[2]	310	103	89	98
Head CT Results Within 45 Min. of Arrival[3,7]	-	-	64%	57%
Patients Who Left ER Before Being Seen	27,525	1%	3%	2%
Time from ER Arrival to Admit. (minutes)[2]	450	261	260	274
Time from ER Arrival to Discharge (minutes)	334	150	138	134
Time in ER Before Being Evaluated (minutes)	294	33	28	26
Time to Pain Meds for Fractures (minutes)	131	56	52	57
Heart Attack Care				
Aspirin Given at Discharge	97	100%	99%	99%

NOTE: Hospital profiles are in alphabetical order by state, then city, then hospital within the city; Rankings exclude hospitals with less than 25 cases except for patient surveys which excludes hospitals with less than 100 cases; (a) 100-299 cases; (1) The number of cases/patients is too few to report; (2) Data submitted were based on a sample of cases/patients; (3) Results are based on a shorter time period than required; (4) Data suppressed by CMS for one or more quarters; (5) Results are not available for this reporting period; (6) Fewer than 100 patients completed the HCAHPS survey; (7) No cases met the criteria for this measure; (8) The lower limit of the confidence interval cannot be calculated if the number of observed infections equals zero; (9) No data are available from the state/territory for this reporting period; (10) The scores shown reflect fewer than 50 completed surveys; (11) There were discrepancies in the data collection process; (12) This measure does not apply to this hospital for this reporting period; (13) Results cannot be calculated for this reporting period; (14) The results for this state are combined with nearby states to protect confidentiality; Please refer to the User's Guide for a full explanation of data.

Measure	Cases	This Hosp.	State Avg.	U.S. Avg.
Fibrinolytic Meds Within 30 Min. of Arrival[7]	-	-	33%	54%
PCI Within 90 Minutes of Arrival	24	100%	97%	96%
Statin Prescribed at Discharge	97	98%	98%	98%
Heart Failure Care				
ACE Inhibitor or ARB for LVSD	39	100%	98%	97%
Discharge Instructions Given	141	94%	96%	94%
Evaluation of LVS Function	210	100%	99%	99%
Medicare Spending				
Medicare Spending per Patient (ratio)	-	1.08	1	0.98
Pneumonia Care				
Appropriate Initial Antibiotic Given	114	98%	95%	95%
Blood Culture Timing	282	99%	98%	98%
Pregnancy and Delivery Care				
Newborn Deliveries Scheduled Early[2]	34	15%	2%	6%
Preventive Care				
Immunization for Influenza[2]	487	94%	92%	90%
Immunization for Pneumonia[2]	500	92%	92%	92%
Stroke Care				
Anticoagulation Therapy for Atrial Fibrillation	12	100%	94%	95%
Antithrombotic Therapy Timing	68	100%	98%	98%
Assessed for Rehabilitation	101	98%	97%	97%
Discharged on Antithrombotic Therapy	84	99%	99%	99%
Discharged on Statin Medication	60	100%	94%	94%
Thrombolytic Therapy Timing[1]	-	-	66%	66%
Venous Thromboembolism Prophylaxis	92	95%	94%	94%
Written Stroke Educational Materials Given	55	91%	87%	88%
Surgical Care Improvement Project				
Appropriate Beta Blocker Usage[2]	134	97%	98%	98%
Appropriate VTP Within 24 Hours[2]	280	98%	98%	98%
Controlled Postoperative Blood Glucose[2]	51	98%	97%	97%
Perioperative Temperature Management[2]	338	100%	100%	100%
Prophylactic Antibiotic Selection[2]	270	100%	99%	99%
Prophylactic Antibiotic Selection (Outpatient)	370	100%	98%	98%
Prophylactic Antibiotic Stopped[2]	261	99%	98%	98%
Prophylactic Antibiotic Timing[2]	270	100%	99%	99%
Prophylactic Antibiotic Timing (Outpatient)	370	100%	97%	98%
Urinary Catheter Removal[2]	157	96%	98%	97%
Survey of Patients' Hospital Experiences				
Area Around Room 'Always' Quiet at Night[11]	300+	59%	60%	61%
Doctors 'Always' Communicated Well[11]	300+	83%	81%	82%
Home Recovery Information Given[11]	300+	86%	86%	85%
Hospital Given 9 or 10 on 10 Point Scale[11]	300+	78%	70%	71%
Meds 'Always' Explained Before Given[11]	300+	61%	64%	64%
Nurses 'Always' Communicated Well[11]	300+	81%	79%	79%
Pain 'Always' Well Controlled[11]	300+	73%	71%	71%
Room and Bathroom 'Always' Clean[11]	300+	77%	74%	73%
Timely Help 'Always' Received[11]	300+	69%	67%	68%
Would Definitely Recommend Hospital[11]	300+	79%	70%	71%
Use of Medical Imaging				
Cardiac Imaging Stress Test before Surgery	1,253	4.6%	5.5%	5.3%
Combination Abdominal CT Scan	844	11.7%	10.1%	10.5%
Combination Brain/Sinus CT Scan[1]	-	-	2.6%	2.7%
Combination Chest CT Scan	543	0.7%	2.8%	2.7%
Follow-up Mammogram/Ultrasound	3,530	10.9%	8.4%	8.8%
Lumbar Spine MRI for Low Back Pain	110	35.5%	36.6%	37.2%

Saint Alexius Medical Center

1555 N Barrington Rd
Hoffman Estates, IL 60194
Phone: 847-843-2000
Fax: 847-781-3914
E-mail: linda.baker@stalexius.net
URL: www.alexianbrothershealth.org
Type: Acute Care Hospitals
Emergency Services: Yes
Ownership: Voluntary non-profit - Church
Beds: 331

Key Personnel:

Radiology. . . . . Scott Baker
Operating Room. . . . . Barb Cerwin
Cardiac Laboratory. . . . . Laura Fiaccato
Emergency Room . . . . Keith Hill, RN
Pediatric In-Patient Care . . . . Laurie Miller, RN
Hemotology Center . . . . Carol Pfeifer, RN
Intensive Care Unit. . . . . Barb Wallace
CEO/President. . . . . Len Wilk

Measure	Cases	This Hosp.	State Avg.	U.S. Avg.
Blood Clot Prevention and Treatment				
Anticoagulation Overlap Therapy[2]	129	94%	91%	93%
ICU Venous Thromboembolism Prophylaxis[2]	70	100%	93%	92%
Incidence of Potentially Preventable VTE[2]	23	13%	11%	10%
UFH with Dosages/Platelet Monitoring[2]	105	96%	94%	97%
Venous Thromboembolism Prophylaxis[2]	335	89%	86%	85%
Warfarin Therapy Discharge Instructions[2]	81	89%	71%	75%
Chest Pain/Possible Heart Attack Care				
Aspirin Given Within 24 Hours of Arrival[5]	-	-	96%	96%
Fibrinolytic Meds Within 30 Min. of Arrival[5]	-	-	65%	58%
Average Time to ECG (minutes)[5]	-	-	6	7
Average Time to Transfer (minutes)[5]	-	-	63	60
Children's Asthma Care				
Received Home Management Plan of Care	-	-	-	88%
Received Reliever Medication	-	-	-	100%
Received Systemic Corticosteroids	-	-	-	100%
Emergency Department				
Admittance Decision Time (minutes)[2]	594	79	89	98
Head CT Results Within 45 Min. of Arrival[1,3]	-	-	64%	57%
Patients Who Left ER Before Being Seen	57,021	1%	3%	2%
Time from ER Arrival to Admit. (minutes)[2]	595	261	260	274
Time from ER Arrival to Discharge (minutes)	370	168	138	134
Time in ER Before Being Evaluated (minutes)	426	26	28	26
Time to Pain Meds for Fractures (minutes)	200	36	52	57
Heart Attack Care				
Aspirin Given at Discharge	147	100%	99%	99%
Fibrinolytic Meds Within 30 Min. of Arrival[7]	-	-	33%	54%
PCI Within 90 Minutes of Arrival	39	100%	97%	96%
Statin Prescribed at Discharge	145	99%	98%	98%
Heart Failure Care				
ACE Inhibitor or ARB for LVSD	73	100%	98%	97%
Discharge Instructions Given	224	98%	96%	94%
Evaluation of LVS Function	299	100%	99%	99%
Medicare Spending				
Medicare Spending per Patient (ratio)	-	1.08	1	0.98
Pneumonia Care				
Appropriate Initial Antibiotic Given	155	97%	95%	95%
Blood Culture Timing	342	100%	98%	98%
Pregnancy and Delivery Care				
Newborn Deliveries Scheduled Early[2]	75	0%	2%	6%
Preventive Care				
Immunization for Influenza[2]	600	99%	92%	90%
Immunization for Pneumonia[2]	615	97%	92%	92%
Stroke Care				
Anticoagulation Therapy for Atrial Fibrillation	11	91%	94%	95%
Antithrombotic Therapy Timing	107	98%	98%	98%
Assessed for Rehabilitation	117	100%	97%	97%
Discharged on Antithrombotic Therapy	101	100%	99%	99%
Discharged on Statin Medication	82	99%	94%	94%
Thrombolytic Therapy Timing[1]	-	-	66%	66%
Venous Thromboembolism Prophylaxis	123	99%	94%	94%
Written Stroke Educational Materials Given	61	79%	87%	88%
Surgical Care Improvement Project				
Appropriate Beta Blocker Usage[2]	132	98%	98%	98%
Appropriate VTP Within 24 Hours[2]	428	98%	98%	98%
Controlled Postoperative Blood Glucose[2,7]	-	-	97%	97%
Perioperative Temperature Management[2]	473	100%	100%	100%
Prophylactic Antibiotic Selection[2]	320	99%	99%	99%
Prophylactic Antibiotic Selection (Outpatient)	429	99%	98%	98%
Prophylactic Antibiotic Stopped[2]	310	98%	98%	98%
Prophylactic Antibiotic Timing[2]	320	100%	99%	99%
Prophylactic Antibiotic Timing (Outpatient)	423	100%	97%	98%
Urinary Catheter Removal[2]	246	97%	98%	97%
Survey of Patients' Hospital Experiences				
Area Around Room 'Always' Quiet at Night	300+	52%	60%	61%
Doctors 'Always' Communicated Well	300+	80%	81%	82%
Home Recovery Information Given	300+	88%	86%	85%
Hospital Given 9 or 10 on 10 Point Scale	300+	70%	70%	71%
Meds 'Always' Explained Before Given	300+	67%	64%	64%
Nurses 'Always' Communicated Well	300+	80%	79%	79%
Pain 'Always' Well Controlled	300+	71%	71%	71%
Room and Bathroom 'Always' Clean	300+	68%	74%	73%
Timely Help 'Always' Received	300+	68%	67%	68%
Would Definitely Recommend Hospital	300+	74%	70%	71%
Use of Medical Imaging				
Cardiac Imaging Stress Test before Surgery	534	6.2%	5.5%	5.3%
Combination Abdominal CT Scan	1,265	8.2%	10.1%	10.5%
Combination Brain/Sinus CT Scan	1,114	2.5%	2.6%	2.7%
Combination Chest CT Scan	948	2.3%	2.8%	2.7%
Follow-up Mammogram/Ultrasound	2,630	6.5%	8.4%	8.8%
Lumbar Spine MRI for Low Back Pain	224	29.5%	36.6%	37.2%

Hoopeston Community Memorial Hospital

701 East Orange Street
Hoopeston, IL 60942
Phone: 217-283-5531
Fax: 217-283-7991
Type: Critical Access Hospitals
Emergency Services: Yes
Ownership: Voluntary non-profit - Private
Beds: 25

Key Personnel:

Anesthesiology. . . . . Dennis Birkey, CRNA
Infection Control. . . . . Carole Bond
CEO/President. . . . . Frank T Caruso
Operating Room. . . . . Dr San Diego, RN
Chief of Medical Staff. . . . . Daesun Oh, MD
Quality Assurance . . . . Dianne Vance, LPN

Measure	Cases	This Hosp.	State Avg.	U.S. Avg.
Blood Clot Prevention and Treatment				
Anticoagulation Overlap Therapy[5]	-	-	91%	93%
ICU Venous Thromboembolism Prophylaxis[5]	-	-	93%	92%
Incidence of Potentially Preventable VTE[5]	-	-	11%	10%
UFH with Dosages/Platelet Monitoring[5]	-	-	94%	97%
Venous Thromboembolism Prophylaxis[5]	-	-	86%	85%
Warfarin Therapy Discharge Instructions[5]	-	-	71%	75%
Chest Pain/Possible Heart Attack Care				
Aspirin Given Within 24 Hours of Arrival[5]	-	-	96%	96%
Fibrinolytic Meds Within 30 Min. of Arrival[5]	-	-	65%	58%
Average Time to ECG (minutes)[5]	-	-	6	7
Average Time to Transfer (minutes)[5]	-	-	63	60
Children's Asthma Care				
Received Home Management Plan of Care	-	-	-	88%
Received Reliever Medication	-	-	-	100%
Received Systemic Corticosteroids	-	-	-	100%
Emergency Department				
Admittance Decision Time (minutes)[5]	-	-	89	98
Head CT Results Within 45 Min. of Arrival[5]	-	-	64%	57%
Patients Who Left ER Before Being Seen[5]	-	-	3%	2%
Time from ER Arrival to Admit. (minutes)[5]	-	-	260	274
Time from ER Arrival to Discharge (minutes)[5]	-	-	138	134
Time in ER Before Being Evaluated (minutes)[5]	-	-	28	26
Time to Pain Meds for Fractures (minutes)[5]	-	-	52	57
Heart Attack Care				
Aspirin Given at Discharge[1,3]	-	-	99%	99%
Fibrinolytic Meds Within 30 Min. of Arrival[3,7]	-	-	33%	54%
PCI Within 90 Minutes of Arrival[3,7]	-	-	97%	96%
Statin Prescribed at Discharge[3,7]	-	-	98%	98%
Heart Failure Care				
ACE Inhibitor or ARB for LVSD[1]	-	-	98%	97%
Discharge Instructions Given	12	42%	96%	94%
Evaluation of LVS Function	19	53%	99%	99%
Medicare Spending				
Medicare Spending per Patient (ratio)	-	-	1	0.98
Pneumonia Care				
Appropriate Initial Antibiotic Given	11	73%	95%	95%
Blood Culture Timing[1]	-	-	98%	98%
Pregnancy and Delivery Care				
Newborn Deliveries Scheduled Early[5]	-	-	2%	6%
Preventive Care				
Immunization for Influenza[5]	-	-	92%	90%
Immunization for Pneumonia[5]	-	-	92%	92%
Stroke Care				
Anticoagulation Therapy for Atrial Fibrillation[5]	-	-	94%	95%
Antithrombotic Therapy Timing[5]	-	-	98%	98%
Assessed for Rehabilitation[5]	-	-	97%	97%
Discharged on Antithrombotic Therapy[5]	-	-	99%	99%
Discharged on Statin Medication[5]	-	-	94%	94%
Thrombolytic Therapy Timing[5]	-	-	66%	66%
Venous Thromboembolism Prophylaxis[5]	-	-	94%	94%
Written Stroke Educational Materials Given[5]	-	-	87%	88%

NOTE: Hospital profiles are in alphabetical order by state, then city, then hospital within the city; Rankings exclude hospitals with less than 25 cases except for patient surveys which excludes hospitals with less than 100 cases; (a) 100-299 cases; (1) The number of cases/patients is too few to report; (2) Data submitted were based on a sample of cases/patients; (3) Results are based on a shorter time period than required; (4) Data suppressed by CMS for one or more quarters; (5) Results are not available for this reporting period; (6) Fewer than 100 patients completed the HCAHPS survey; (7) No cases met the criteria for this measure; (8) The lower limit of the confidence interval cannot be calculated if the number of observed infections equals zero; (9) No data are available from the state/territory for this reporting period; (10) The scores shown reflect fewer than 50 completed surveys; (11) There were discrepancies in the data collection process; (12) This measure does not apply to this hospital for this reporting period; (13) Results cannot be calculated for this reporting period; (14) The results for this state are combined with nearby states to protect confidentiality; Please refer to the User's Guide for a full explanation of data.

Measure	Cases	This Hosp.	State Avg.	U.S. Avg.
Surgical Care Improvement Project				
Appropriate Beta Blocker Usage[1]	-	-	98%	98%
Appropriate VTP Within 24 Hours	16	100%	98%	98%
Controlled Postoperative Blood Glucose[7]	-	-	97%	97%
Perioperative Temperature Management	17	94%	100%	100%
Prophylactic Antibiotic Selection	17	100%	99%	99%
Prophylactic Antibiotic Selection (Outpatient)[5]	-	-	98%	98%
Prophylactic Antibiotic Stopped	15	100%	98%	98%
Prophylactic Antibiotic Timing	17	94%	99%	99%
Prophylactic Antibiotic Timing (Outpatient)[5]	-	-	97%	98%
Urinary Catheter Removal	16	69%	98%	97%
Survey of Patients' Hospital Experiences				
Area Around Room 'Always' Quiet at Night[5]	-	-	60%	61%
Doctors 'Always' Communicated Well[5]	-	-	81%	82%
Home Recovery Information Given[5]	-	-	86%	85%
Hospital Given 9 or 10 on 10 Point Scale[5]	-	-	70%	71%
Meds 'Always' Explained Before Given[5]	-	-	64%	64%
Nurses 'Always' Communicated Well[5]	-	-	79%	79%
Pain 'Always' Well Controlled[5]	-	-	71%	71%
Room and Bathroom 'Always' Clean[5]	-	-	74%	73%
Timely Help 'Always' Received[5]	-	-	67%	68%
Would Definitely Recommend Hospital[5]	-	-	70%	71%
Use of Medical Imaging				
Cardiac Imaging Stress Test before Surgery[1]	-	-	5.5%	5.3%
Combination Abdominal CT Scan	104	3.8%	10.1%	10.5%
Combination Brain/Sinus CT Scan	181	0.6%	2.6%	2.7%
Combination Chest CT Scan	98	1.0%	2.8%	2.7%
Follow-up Mammogram/Ultrasound	114	5.3%	8.4%	8.8%
Lumbar Spine MRI for Low Back Pain[1]	-	-	36.6%	37.2%

Hopedale Medical Complex

107 Tremont Street Phone: 309-449-3321
Hopedale, IL 61747
Type: Critical Access Hospitals Emergency Services: Yes
Ownership: Voluntary non-profit - Private

Measure	Cases	This Hosp.	State Avg.	U.S. Avg.
Blood Clot Prevention and Treatment				
Anticoagulation Overlap Therapy[5]	-	-	91%	93%
ICU Venous Thromboembolism Prophylaxis[5]	-	-	93%	92%
Incidence of Potentially Preventable VTE[5]	-	-	11%	10%
UFH with Dosages/Platelet Monitoring[5]	-	-	94%	97%
Venous Thromboembolism Prophylaxis[5]	-	-	86%	85%
Warfarin Therapy Discharge Instructions[5]	-	-	71%	75%
Chest Pain/Possible Heart Attack Care				
Aspirin Given Within 24 Hours of Arrival[5]	-	-	96%	96%
Fibrinolytic Meds Within 30 Min. of Arrival[5]	-	-	65%	58%
Average Time to ECG (minutes)[5]	-	-	6	7
Average Time to Transfer (minutes)[5]	-	-	63	60
Children's Asthma Care				
Received Home Management Plan of Care	-	-	-	88%
Received Reliever Medication	-	-	-	100%
Received Systemic Corticosteroids	-	-	-	100%
Emergency Department				
Admittance Decision Time (minutes)[5]	-	-	89	98
Head CT Results Within 45 Min. of Arrival[5]	-	-	64%	57%
Patients Who Left ER Before Being Seen[5]	-	-	3%	2%
Time from ER Arrival to Admit. (minutes)[5]	-	-	260	274
Time from ER Arrival to Discharge (minutes)[5]	-	-	138	134
Time in ER Before Being Evaluated (minutes)[5]	-	-	28	26
Time to Pain Meds for Fractures (minutes)[5]	-	-	52	57
Heart Attack Care				
Aspirin Given at Discharge[5]	-	-	99%	99%
Fibrinolytic Meds Within 30 Min. of Arrival[5]	-	-	33%	54%
PCI Within 90 Minutes of Arrival[5]	-	-	97%	96%
Statin Prescribed at Discharge[5]	-	-	98%	98%
Heart Failure Care				
ACE Inhibitor or ARB for LVSD[5]	-	-	98%	97%
Discharge Instructions Given[5]	-	-	96%	94%
Evaluation of LVS Function[5]	-	-	99%	99%
Medicare Spending				
Medicare Spending per Patient (ratio)	-	-	1	0.98
Pneumonia Care				
Appropriate Initial Antibiotic Given[5]	-	-	95%	95%
Blood Culture Timing[5]	-	-	98%	98%
Pregnancy and Delivery Care				
Newborn Deliveries Scheduled Early[5]	-	-	2%	6%
Preventive Care				
Immunization for Influenza[5]	-	-	92%	90%
Immunization for Pneumonia[5]	-	-	92%	92%
Stroke Care				
Anticoagulation Therapy for Atrial Fibrillation[5]	-	-	94%	95%
Antithrombotic Therapy Timing[5]	-	-	98%	98%
Assessed for Rehabilitation[5]	-	-	97%	97%
Discharged on Antithrombotic Therapy[5]	-	-	99%	99%
Discharged on Statin Medication[5]	-	-	94%	94%
Thrombolytic Therapy Timing[5]	-	-	66%	66%
Venous Thromboembolism Prophylaxis[5]	-	-	94%	94%
Written Stroke Educational Materials Given[5]	-	-	87%	88%
Surgical Care Improvement Project				
Appropriate Beta Blocker Usage[5]	-	-	98%	98%
Appropriate VTP Within 24 Hours[5]	-	-	98%	98%
Controlled Postoperative Blood Glucose[5]	-	-	97%	97%
Perioperative Temperature Management[5]	-	-	100%	100%
Prophylactic Antibiotic Selection[5]	-	-	99%	99%
Prophylactic Antibiotic Selection (Outpatient)[5]	-	-	98%	98%
Prophylactic Antibiotic Stopped[5]	-	-	98%	98%
Prophylactic Antibiotic Timing[5]	-	-	99%	99%
Prophylactic Antibiotic Timing (Outpatient)[5]	-	-	97%	98%
Urinary Catheter Removal[5]	-	-	98%	97%
Survey of Patients' Hospital Experiences				
Area Around Room 'Always' Quiet at Night[5]	-	-	60%	61%
Doctors 'Always' Communicated Well[5]	-	-	81%	82%
Home Recovery Information Given[5]	-	-	86%	85%
Hospital Given 9 or 10 on 10 Point Scale[5]	-	-	70%	71%
Meds 'Always' Explained Before Given[5]	-	-	64%	64%
Nurses 'Always' Communicated Well[5]	-	-	79%	79%
Pain 'Always' Well Controlled[5]	-	-	71%	71%
Room and Bathroom 'Always' Clean[5]	-	-	74%	73%
Timely Help 'Always' Received[5]	-	-	67%	68%
Would Definitely Recommend Hospital[5]	-	-	70%	71%
Use of Medical Imaging				
Cardiac Imaging Stress Test before Surgery[1]	-	-	5.5%	5.3%
Combination Abdominal CT Scan	136	2.2%	10.1%	10.5%
Combination Brain/Sinus CT Scan[1]	-	-	2.6%	2.7%
Combination Chest CT Scan	124	0.8%	2.8%	2.7%
Follow-up Mammogram/Ultrasound	193	2.6%	8.4%	8.8%
Lumbar Spine MRI for Low Back Pain[1]	-	-	36.6%	37.2%

Passavant Area Hospital

1600 W Walnut St Phone: 217-245-9551
Jacksonville, IL 62650 Fax: 217-479-5637
E-mail: info@passavanthospital.com
URL: www.passavanthospital.com
Type: Acute Care Hospitals Emergency Services: Yes
Ownership: Voluntary non-profit - Private Beds: 173

Key Personnel:

Intensive Care Unit. . . . . Terry Beachamp
Infection Control. . . . . Anne Beck
Operating Room. . . . . Tracy Mills, RN
Quality Assurance . . . . Connie Mudd
CEO/President. . . . . Doug Rahn, DBA
Chief of Medical Staff. . . . . Tara Ramsey, MD
Radiology. . . . . Robert Stallworth, MD
Emergency Room . . . . Michael Whitmore, MD

Measure	Cases	This Hosp.	State Avg.	U.S. Avg.
Blood Clot Prevention and Treatment				
Anticoagulation Overlap Therapy[2]	30	97%	91%	93%
ICU Venous Thromboembolism Prophylaxis[2]	53	98%	93%	92%
Incidence of Potentially Preventable VTE[1,2]	-	-	11%	10%
UFH with Dosages/Platelet Monitoring[2]	21	100%	94%	97%
Venous Thromboembolism Prophylaxis[2]	282	73%	86%	85%
Warfarin Therapy Discharge Instructions[2]	21	100%	71%	75%
Chest Pain/Possible Heart Attack Care				
Aspirin Given Within 24 Hours of Arrival	135	93%	96%	96%
Fibrinolytic Meds Within 30 Min. of Arrival[7]	-	-	65%	58%
Average Time to ECG (minutes)	141	10	6	7
Average Time to Transfer (minutes)	25	38	63	60
Children's Asthma Care				
Received Home Management Plan of Care	-	-	-	88%
Received Reliever Medication	-	-	-	100%
Received Systemic Corticosteroids	-	-	-	100%
Emergency Department				
Admittance Decision Time (minutes)[2]	494	70	89	98
Head CT Results Within 45 Min. of Arrival	41	34%	64%	57%
Patients Who Left ER Before Being Seen	16,564	1%	3%	2%
Time from ER Arrival to Admit. (minutes)[2]	563	250	260	274
Time from ER Arrival to Discharge (minutes)	376	134	138	134
Time in ER Before Being Evaluated (minutes)	275	35	28	26
Time to Pain Meds for Fractures (minutes)	112	48	52	57
Heart Attack Care				
Aspirin Given at Discharge[1]	-	-	99%	99%
Fibrinolytic Meds Within 30 Min. of Arrival[7]	-	-	33%	54%
PCI Within 90 Minutes of Arrival[7]	-	-	97%	96%
Statin Prescribed at Discharge[1]	-	-	98%	98%
Heart Failure Care				
ACE Inhibitor or ARB for LVSD	19	84%	98%	97%
Discharge Instructions Given	46	61%	96%	94%
Evaluation of LVS Function	88	97%	99%	99%
Medicare Spending				
Medicare Spending per Patient (ratio)	-	0.96	1	0.98
Pneumonia Care				
Appropriate Initial Antibiotic Given[2]	86	97%	95%	95%
Blood Culture Timing[2]	138	96%	98%	98%
Pregnancy and Delivery Care				
Newborn Deliveries Scheduled Early[2]	33	15%	2%	6%
Preventive Care				
Immunization for Influenza[2]	554	88%	92%	90%
Immunization for Pneumonia[2]	692	91%	92%	92%
Stroke Care				
Anticoagulation Therapy for Atrial Fibrillation[1]	-	-	94%	95%
Antithrombotic Therapy Timing	20	100%	98%	98%
Assessed for Rehabilitation	20	95%	97%	97%
Discharged on Antithrombotic Therapy	20	90%	99%	99%
Discharged on Statin Medication	17	53%	94%	94%
Thrombolytic Therapy Timing[1]	-	-	66%	66%
Venous Thromboembolism Prophylaxis	18	72%	94%	94%
Written Stroke Educational Materials Given[1]	-	-	87%	88%
Surgical Care Improvement Project				
Appropriate Beta Blocker Usage[2]	82	96%	98%	98%
Appropriate VTP Within 24 Hours[2]	245	90%	98%	98%
Controlled Postoperative Blood Glucose[2,7]	-	-	97%	97%
Perioperative Temperature Management[2]	265	100%	100%	100%
Prophylactic Antibiotic Selection[2]	170	98%	99%	99%
Prophylactic Antibiotic Selection (Outpatient)	82	99%	98%	98%
Prophylactic Antibiotic Stopped[2]	156	96%	98%	98%
Prophylactic Antibiotic Timing[2]	170	97%	99%	99%
Prophylactic Antibiotic Timing (Outpatient)	81	99%	97%	98%
Urinary Catheter Removal[2]	76	89%	98%	97%
Survey of Patients' Hospital Experiences				
Area Around Room 'Always' Quiet at Night	300+	55%	60%	61%
Doctors 'Always' Communicated Well	300+	80%	81%	82%
Home Recovery Information Given	300+	86%	86%	85%
Hospital Given 9 or 10 on 10 Point Scale	300+	71%	70%	71%
Meds 'Always' Explained Before Given	300+	65%	64%	64%
Nurses 'Always' Communicated Well	300+	81%	79%	79%
Pain 'Always' Well Controlled	300+	71%	71%	71%
Room and Bathroom 'Always' Clean	300+	79%	74%	73%
Timely Help 'Always' Received	300+	69%	67%	68%
Would Definitely Recommend Hospital	300+	66%	70%	71%
Use of Medical Imaging				
Cardiac Imaging Stress Test before Surgery	114	7.0%	5.5%	5.3%
Combination Abdominal CT Scan	752	2.7%	10.1%	10.5%
Combination Brain/Sinus CT Scan	750	3.6%	2.6%	2.7%
Combination Chest CT Scan	522	0.6%	2.8%	2.7%
Follow-up Mammogram/Ultrasound	1,105	7.1%	8.4%	8.8%
Lumbar Spine MRI for Low Back Pain	126	50.8%	36.6%	37.2%

NOTE: Hospital profiles are in alphabetical order by state, then city, then hospital within the city; Rankings exclude hospitals with less than 25 cases except for patient surveys which excludes hospitals with less than 100 cases; (a) 100-299 cases; (1) The number of cases/patients is too few to report; (2) Data submitted were based on a sample of cases/patients; (3) Results are based on a shorter time period than required; (4) Data suppressed by CMS for one or more quarters; (5) Results are not available for this reporting period; (6) Fewer than 100 patients completed the HCAHPS survey; (7) No cases met the criteria for this measure; (8) The lower limit of the confidence interval cannot be calculated if the number of observed infections equals zero; (9) No data are available from the state/territory for this reporting period; (10) The scores shown reflect fewer than 50 completed surveys; (11) There were discrepancies in the data collection process; (12) This measure does not apply to this hospital for this reporting period; (13) Results cannot be calculated for this reporting period; (14) The results for this state are combined with nearby states to protect confidentiality; Please refer to the User's Guide for a full explanation of data.

Jersey Community Hospital

400 Maple Summit Road
Jerseyville, IL 62052
Phone: 618-498-6402
Fax: 618-498-8492
Type: Acute Care Hospitals
Emergency Services: Yes
Ownership: Government - Local
Beds: 67

Key Personnel:
CEO/President . . . . Larry Bear
Emergency Room . . . . Alvina Isringhausen
Chief of Medical Staff. . . . . Susan Vritweiser
Quality Assurance . . . . Nancy Wollenwebber

Measure	Cases	This Hosp.	State Avg.	U.S. Avg.
Blood Clot Prevention and Treatment				
Anticoagulation Overlap Therapy[1,2]	-	-	91%	93%
ICU Venous Thromboembolism Prophylaxis[2]	21	48%	93%	92%
Incidence of Potentially Preventable VTE[2,7]	-	-	11%	10%
UFH with Dosages/Platelet Monitoring[1,2]	-	-	94%	97%
Venous Thromboembolism Prophylaxis[2]	239	49%	86%	85%
Warfarin Therapy Discharge Instructions[1,2]	-	-	71%	75%
Chest Pain/Possible Heart Attack Care				
Aspirin Given Within 24 Hours of Arrival	53	96%	96%	96%
Fibrinolytic Meds Within 30 Min. of Arrival[1]	-	-	65%	58%
Average Time to ECG (minutes)	51	6	6	7
Average Time to Transfer (minutes)[1]	-	-	63	60
Children's Asthma Care				
Received Home Management Plan of Care	-	-	-	88%
Received Reliever Medication	-	-	-	100%
Received Systemic Corticosteroids	-	-	-	100%
Emergency Department				
Admittance Decision Time (minutes)[2]	393	90	89	98
Head CT Results Within 45 Min. of Arrival	18	11%	64%	57%
Patients Who Left ER Before Being Seen	12,536	1%	3%	2%
Time from ER Arrival to Admit. (minutes)[2]	399	243	260	274
Time from ER Arrival to Discharge (minutes)	212	95	138	134
Time in ER Before Being Evaluated (minutes)	331	22	28	26
Time to Pain Meds for Fractures (minutes)	71	50	52	57
Heart Attack Care				
Aspirin Given at Discharge[1]	-	-	99%	99%
Fibrinolytic Meds Within 30 Min. of Arrival[7]	-	-	33%	54%
PCI Within 90 Minutes of Arrival[7]	-	-	97%	96%
Statin Prescribed at Discharge[1]	-	-	98%	98%
Heart Failure Care				
ACE Inhibitor or ARB for LVSD[1]	-	-	98%	97%
Discharge Instructions Given	34	97%	96%	94%
Evaluation of LVS Function	49	90%	99%	99%
Medicare Spending				
Medicare Spending per Patient (ratio)	-	1.04	1	0.98
Pneumonia Care				
Appropriate Initial Antibiotic Given	81	88%	95%	95%
Blood Culture Timing	122	99%	98%	98%
Pregnancy and Delivery Care				
Newborn Deliveries Scheduled Early	12	8%	2%	6%
Preventive Care				
Immunization for Influenza[2]	270	66%	92%	90%
Immunization for Pneumonia[2]	455	71%	92%	92%
Stroke Care				
Anticoagulation Therapy for Atrial Fibrillation[1]	-	-	94%	95%
Antithrombotic Therapy Timing[1]	-	-	98%	98%
Assessed for Rehabilitation[1]	-	-	97%	97%
Discharged on Antithrombotic Therapy[1]	-	-	99%	99%
Discharged on Statin Medication[1]	-	-	94%	94%
Thrombolytic Therapy Timing[1]	-	-	66%	66%
Venous Thromboembolism Prophylaxis[1]	-	-	94%	94%
Written Stroke Educational Materials Given[1]	-	-	87%	88%
Surgical Care Improvement Project				
Appropriate Beta Blocker Usage[1]	-	-	98%	98%
Appropriate VTP Within 24 Hours	26	77%	98%	98%
Controlled Postoperative Blood Glucose[7]	-	-	97%	97%
Perioperative Temperature Management	31	90%	100%	100%
Prophylactic Antibiotic Selection	14	93%	99%	99%
Prophylactic Antibiotic Selection (Outpatient)	26	100%	98%	98%
Prophylactic Antibiotic Stopped	14	71%	98%	98%
Prophylactic Antibiotic Timing	15	93%	99%	99%
Prophylactic Antibiotic Timing (Outpatient)[1]	-	-	97%	98%
Urinary Catheter Removal[1]	-	-	98%	97%
Survey of Patients' Hospital Experiences				
Area Around Room 'Always' Quiet at Night	(a)	63%	60%	61%
Doctors 'Always' Communicated Well	(a)	81%	81%	82%
Home Recovery Information Given	(a)	81%	86%	85%
Hospital Given 9 or 10 on 10 Point Scale	(a)	68%	70%	71%
Meds 'Always' Explained Before Given	(a)	66%	64%	64%
Nurses 'Always' Communicated Well	(a)	80%	79%	79%
Pain 'Always' Well Controlled	(a)	69%	71%	71%
Room and Bathroom 'Always' Clean	(a)	84%	74%	73%
Timely Help 'Always' Received	(a)	78%	67%	68%
Would Definitely Recommend Hospital	(a)	62%	70%	71%
Use of Medical Imaging				
Cardiac Imaging Stress Test before Surgery[1]	-	-	5.5%	5.3%
Combination Abdominal CT Scan	223	23.8%	10.1%	10.5%
Combination Brain/Sinus CT Scan	415	2.2%	2.6%	2.7%
Combination Chest CT Scan	143	6.3%	2.8%	2.7%
Follow-up Mammogram/Ultrasound	369	7.0%	8.4%	8.8%
Lumbar Spine MRI for Low Back Pain	58	60.3%	36.6%	37.2%

Presence Saint Joseph Medical Center

333 N Madison
Joliet, IL 60435
Phone: 815-725-7133
Fax: 815-741-7121
URL: www.provena.org/stjoes
Type: Acute Care Hospitals
Emergency Services: Yes
Ownership: Voluntary non-profit - Church
Beds: 452

Key Personnel:
Chief of Medical Staff. . . . . David Franzblau, MD
CEO/President. . . . . Beth Hughes
Emergency Room . . . . Rao Kilaru, MD
Quality Assurance . . . . Lon McPherson, MD
Patient Relations . . . . Kathleen Mikos
Infection Control. . . . . Peg Sheehan
Pediatric Ambulatory Care . . . . . . Rhea Simons, MD
Pediatric In-Patient Care . . . . Rhea Simons, MD

Measure	Cases	This Hosp.	State Avg.	U.S. Avg.
Blood Clot Prevention and Treatment				
Anticoagulation Overlap Therapy[2]	162	77%	91%	93%
ICU Venous Thromboembolism Prophylaxis[2]	59	78%	93%	92%
Incidence of Potentially Preventable VTE[2]	28	11%	11%	10%
UFH with Dosages/Platelet Monitoring[2]	48	100%	94%	97%
Venous Thromboembolism Prophylaxis[2]	378	71%	86%	85%
Warfarin Therapy Discharge Instructions[2]	124	85%	71%	75%
Chest Pain/Possible Heart Attack Care				
Aspirin Given Within 24 Hours of Arrival[5]	-	-	96%	96%
Fibrinolytic Meds Within 30 Min. of Arrival[5]	-	-	65%	58%
Average Time to ECG (minutes)[5]	-	-	6	7
Average Time to Transfer (minutes)[5]	-	-	63	60
Children's Asthma Care				
Received Home Management Plan of Care	-	-	-	88%
Received Reliever Medication	-	-	-	100%
Received Systemic Corticosteroids	-	-	-	100%
Emergency Department				
Admittance Decision Time (minutes)[2]	555	95	89	98
Head CT Results Within 45 Min. of Arrival[5]	-	-	64%	57%
Patients Who Left ER Before Being Seen	74,004	4%	3%	2%
Time from ER Arrival to Admit. (minutes)[2]	566	294	260	274
Time from ER Arrival to Discharge (minutes)	370	190	138	134
Time in ER Before Being Evaluated (minutes)	383	36	28	26
Time to Pain Meds for Fractures (minutes)	173	50	52	57
Heart Attack Care				
Aspirin Given at Discharge[2]	293	99%	99%	99%
Fibrinolytic Meds Within 30 Min. of Arrival[2,7]	-	-	33%	54%
PCI Within 90 Minutes of Arrival[2]	47	98%	97%	96%
Statin Prescribed at Discharge[2]	265	98%	98%	98%
Heart Failure Care				
ACE Inhibitor or ARB for LVSD[2]	85	100%	98%	97%
Discharge Instructions Given[2]	246	83%	96%	94%
Evaluation of LVS Function[2]	335	100%	99%	99%
Medicare Spending				
Medicare Spending per Patient (ratio)	-	1.05	1	0.98
Pneumonia Care				
Appropriate Initial Antibiotic Given[2]	85	99%	95%	95%
Blood Culture Timing[2]	167	95%	98%	98%
Pregnancy and Delivery Care				
Newborn Deliveries Scheduled Early	124	2%	2%	6%
Preventive Care				
Immunization for Influenza[2]	594	64%	92%	90%
Immunization for Pneumonia[2]	780	68%	92%	92%
Stroke Care				
Anticoagulation Therapy for Atrial Fibrillation[2]	13	100%	94%	95%
Antithrombotic Therapy Timing[2]	81	94%	98%	98%
Assessed for Rehabilitation[2]	106	100%	97%	97%
Discharged on Antithrombotic Therapy[2]	82	95%	99%	99%
Discharged on Statin Medication[2]	64	80%	94%	94%
Thrombolytic Therapy Timing[1,2]	-	-	66%	66%
Venous Thromboembolism Prophylaxis[2]	115	82%	94%	94%
Written Stroke Educational Materials Given[2]	57	37%	87%	88%
Surgical Care Improvement Project				
Appropriate Beta Blocker Usage[2]	237	100%	98%	98%
Appropriate VTP Within 24 Hours[2]	461	100%	98%	98%
Controlled Postoperative Blood Glucose[2]	141	94%	97%	97%
Perioperative Temperature Management[2]	546	100%	100%	100%
Prophylactic Antibiotic Selection[2]	508	98%	99%	99%
Prophylactic Antibiotic Selection (Outpatient)	367	96%	98%	98%
Prophylactic Antibiotic Stopped[2]	485	97%	98%	98%
Prophylactic Antibiotic Timing[2]	509	100%	99%	99%
Prophylactic Antibiotic Timing (Outpatient)	370	99%	97%	98%
Urinary Catheter Removal[2]	321	100%	98%	97%
Survey of Patients' Hospital Experiences				
Area Around Room 'Always' Quiet at Night	300+	61%	60%	61%
Doctors 'Always' Communicated Well	300+	78%	81%	82%
Home Recovery Information Given	300+	84%	86%	85%
Hospital Given 9 or 10 on 10 Point Scale	300+	65%	70%	71%
Meds 'Always' Explained Before Given	300+	62%	64%	64%
Nurses 'Always' Communicated Well	300+	74%	79%	79%
Pain 'Always' Well Controlled	300+	64%	71%	71%
Room and Bathroom 'Always' Clean	300+	68%	74%	73%
Timely Help 'Always' Received	300+	59%	67%	68%
Would Definitely Recommend Hospital	300+	66%	70%	71%
Use of Medical Imaging				
Cardiac Imaging Stress Test before Surgery	789	8.4%	5.5%	5.3%
Combination Abdominal CT Scan	1,072	17.7%	10.1%	10.5%
Combination Brain/Sinus CT Scan	1,467	2.7%	2.6%	2.7%
Combination Chest CT Scan	635	3.3%	2.8%	2.7%
Follow-up Mammogram/Ultrasound	2,512	5.4%	8.4%	8.8%
Lumbar Spine MRI for Low Back Pain	323	31.9%	36.6%	37.2%

Presence Saint Marys Hospital

500 W Court St
Kankakee, IL 60901
Phone: 815-937-2490
Fax: 815-937-8772
URL: www.provenastmarys.com
Type: Acute Care Hospitals
Emergency Services: Yes
Ownership: Voluntary non-profit - Other
Beds: 210

Key Personnel:
Operating Room. . . . . Robert E Brockman, RN
Emergency Room . . . . Tony Brunello
Chief of Medical Staff. . . . . Hippen Hammer
Cardiac Laboratory. . . . . Michelle Hardesty
President/CEO. . . . . Joseph Hugar
Infection Control. . . . . Julie Nehls
Quality Assurance . . . . Len Winnicki

Measure	Cases	This Hosp.	State Avg.	U.S. Avg.
Blood Clot Prevention and Treatment				
Anticoagulation Overlap Therapy[2]	42	88%	91%	93%
ICU Venous Thromboembolism Prophylaxis[2]	157	92%	93%	92%
Incidence of Potentially Preventable VTE[1,2]	-	-	11%	10%
UFH with Dosages/Platelet Monitoring[2]	21	95%	94%	97%
Venous Thromboembolism Prophylaxis[2]	295	80%	86%	85%
Warfarin Therapy Discharge Instructions[2]	33	61%	71%	75%
Chest Pain/Possible Heart Attack Care				
Aspirin Given Within 24 Hours of Arrival[1,3]	-	-	96%	96%
Fibrinolytic Meds Within 30 Min. of Arrival[5]	-	-	65%	58%
Average Time to ECG (minutes)[1,3]	-	-	6	7
Average Time to Transfer (minutes)[5]	-	-	63	60
Children's Asthma Care				
Received Home Management Plan of Care	-	-	-	88%
Received Reliever Medication	-	-	-	100%

NOTE: Hospital profiles are in alphabetical order by state, then city, then hospital within the city; Rankings exclude hospitals with less than 25 cases except for patient surveys which excludes hospitals with less than 100 cases; (a) 100-299 cases; (1) The number of cases/patients is too few to report; (2) Data submitted were based on a sample of cases/patients; (3) Results are based on a shorter time period than required; (4) Data suppressed by CMS for one or more quarters; (5) Results are not available for this reporting period; (6) Fewer than 100 patients completed the HCAHPS survey; (7) No cases met the criteria for this measure; (8) The lower limit of the confidence interval cannot be calculated if the number of observed infections equals zero; (9) No data are available from the state/territory for this reporting period; (10) The scores shown reflect fewer than 50 completed surveys; (11) There were discrepancies in the data collection process; (12) This measure does not apply to this hospital for this reporting period; (13) Results cannot be calculated for this reporting period; (14) The results for this state are combined with nearby states to protect confidentiality; Please refer to the User's Guide for a full explanation of data.

Received Systemic Corticosteroids	-	-	-	100%
Emergency Department				
Admittance Decision Time (minutes)[2]	700	85	89	98
Head CT Results Within 45 Min. of Arrival[7]	-	-	64%	57%
Patients Who Left ER Before Being Seen	33,735	2%	3%	2%
Time from ER Arrival to Admit. (minutes)[2]	715	242	260	274
Time from ER Arrival to Discharge (minutes)	384	115	138	134
Time in ER Before Being Evaluated (minutes)	405	30	28	26
Time to Pain Meds for Fractures (minutes)	98	52	52	57
Heart Attack Care				
Aspirin Given at Discharge	36	100%	99%	99%
Fibrinolytic Meds Within 30 Min. of Arrival[7]	-	-	33%	54%
PCI Within 90 Minutes of Arrival	11	100%	97%	96%
Statin Prescribed at Discharge	36	100%	98%	98%
Heart Failure Care				
ACE Inhibitor or ARB for LVSD	52	98%	98%	97%
Discharge Instructions Given	115	95%	96%	94%
Evaluation of LVS Function	146	100%	99%	99%
Medicare Spending				
Medicare Spending per Patient (ratio)	-	0.95	1	0.98
Pneumonia Care				
Appropriate Initial Antibiotic Given[2]	60	92%	95%	95%
Blood Culture Timing[2]	162	99%	98%	98%
Pregnancy and Delivery Care				
Newborn Deliveries Scheduled Early[2]	16	6%	2%	6%
Preventive Care				
Immunization for Influenza[2]	531	85%	92%	90%
Immunization for Pneumonia[2]	638	93%	92%	92%
Stroke Care				
Anticoagulation Therapy for Atrial Fibrillation[1]	-	-	94%	95%
Antithrombotic Therapy Timing	42	100%	98%	98%
Assessed for Rehabilitation	48	96%	97%	97%
Discharged on Antithrombotic Therapy	46	98%	99%	99%
Discharged on Statin Medication	36	97%	94%	94%
Thrombolytic Therapy Timing[1]	-	-	66%	66%
Venous Thromboembolism Prophylaxis	46	93%	94%	94%
Written Stroke Educational Materials Given	24	100%	87%	88%
Surgical Care Improvement Project				
Appropriate Beta Blocker Usage	94	99%	98%	98%
Appropriate VTP Within 24 Hours	313	97%	98%	98%
Controlled Postoperative Blood Glucose[7]	-	-	97%	97%
Perioperative Temperature Management	347	100%	100%	100%
Prophylactic Antibiotic Selection	227	99%	99%	99%
Prophylactic Antibiotic Selection (Outpatient)	126	97%	98%	98%
Prophylactic Antibiotic Stopped	216	94%	98%	98%
Prophylactic Antibiotic Timing	226	99%	99%	99%
Prophylactic Antibiotic Timing (Outpatient)	124	98%	97%	98%
Urinary Catheter Removal	219	100%	98%	97%
Survey of Patients' Hospital Experiences				
Area Around Room 'Always' Quiet at Night	300+	67%	60%	61%
Doctors 'Always' Communicated Well	300+	86%	81%	82%
Home Recovery Information Given	300+	91%	86%	85%
Hospital Given 9 or 10 on 10 Point Scale	300+	76%	70%	71%
Meds 'Always' Explained Before Given	300+	65%	64%	64%
Nurses 'Always' Communicated Well	300+	82%	79%	79%
Pain 'Always' Well Controlled	300+	79%	71%	71%
Room and Bathroom 'Always' Clean	300+	76%	74%	73%
Timely Help 'Always' Received	300+	69%	67%	68%
Would Definitely Recommend Hospital	300+	81%	70%	71%
Use of Medical Imaging				
Cardiac Imaging Stress Test before Surgery	214	7.0%	5.5%	5.3%
Combination Abdominal CT Scan	583	20.1%	10.1%	10.5%
Combination Brain/Sinus CT Scan[1]	-	-	2.6%	2.7%
Combination Chest CT Scan	248	11.3%	2.8%	2.7%
Follow-up Mammogram/Ultrasound	768	5.9%	8.4%	8.8%
Lumbar Spine MRI for Low Back Pain	59	45.8%	36.6%	37.2%

Riverside Medical Center

350 N Wall St
Kankakee, IL 60901
URL: www.riversidehealthcare.org
Type: Acute Care Hospitals
Ownership: Voluntary non-profit - Private

Phone: 815-933-1671
Fax: 815-935-7823

Emergency Services: Yes
Beds: 336

Key Personnel:

Emergency Room . . . . Crystal Allen
Chief of Medical Staff . . . . John V. Jurica
CEO/President . . . . Phillip M. Kambic
Operating Room . . . . Sandra Kegg, RN
Coronary Care . . . . Allen Kelly
Quality Assurance . . . . Mary Schore
Radiology . . . . Nicholas Slimuck, MD

Measure	Cases	This Hosp.	State Avg.	U.S. Avg.
Blood Clot Prevention and Treatment				
Anticoagulation Overlap Therapy[2]	87	99%	91%	93%
ICU Venous Thromboembolism Prophylaxis[2]	78	100%	93%	92%
Incidence of Potentially Preventable VTE[1,2]	-	-	11%	10%
UFH with Dosages/Platelet Monitoring[2]	72	100%	94%	97%
Venous Thromboembolism Prophylaxis[2]	300	99%	86%	85%
Warfarin Therapy Discharge Instructions[2]	61	100%	71%	75%
Chest Pain/Possible Heart Attack Care				
Aspirin Given Within 24 Hours of Arrival[1,3]	-	-	96%	96%
Fibrinolytic Meds Within 30 Min. of Arrival[5]	-	-	65%	58%
Average Time to ECG (minutes)[1,3]	-	-	6	7
Average Time to Transfer (minutes)[5]	-	-	63	60
Children's Asthma Care				
Received Home Management Plan of Care	-	-	-	88%
Received Reliever Medication	-	-	-	100%
Received Systemic Corticosteroids	-	-	-	100%
Emergency Department				
Admittance Decision Time (minutes)[2]	529	97	89	98
Head CT Results Within 45 Min. of Arrival[1]	-	-	64%	57%
Patients Who Left ER Before Being Seen	40,912	2%	3%	2%
Time from ER Arrival to Admit. (minutes)[2]	532	274	260	274
Time from ER Arrival to Discharge (minutes)	360	122	138	134
Time in ER Before Being Evaluated (minutes)	392	27	28	26
Time to Pain Meds for Fractures (minutes)	137	38	52	57
Heart Attack Care				
Aspirin Given at Discharge	128	100%	99%	99%
Fibrinolytic Meds Within 30 Min. of Arrival[7]	-	-	33%	54%
PCI Within 90 Minutes of Arrival	22	100%	97%	96%
Statin Prescribed at Discharge	121	100%	98%	98%
Heart Failure Care				
ACE Inhibitor or ARB for LVSD	105	100%	98%	97%
Discharge Instructions Given	168	97%	96%	94%
Evaluation of LVS Function	249	100%	99%	99%
Medicare Spending				
Medicare Spending per Patient (ratio)	-	1.00	1	0.98
Pneumonia Care				
Appropriate Initial Antibiotic Given	115	97%	95%	95%
Blood Culture Timing	247	100%	98%	98%
Pregnancy and Delivery Care				
Newborn Deliveries Scheduled Early[2]	31	0%	2%	6%
Preventive Care				
Immunization for Influenza[2]	547	95%	92%	90%
Immunization for Pneumonia[2]	653	99%	92%	92%
Stroke Care				
Anticoagulation Therapy for Atrial Fibrillation[1]	-	-	94%	95%
Antithrombotic Therapy Timing	89	97%	98%	98%
Assessed for Rehabilitation	110	100%	97%	97%
Discharged on Antithrombotic Therapy	96	100%	99%	99%
Discharged on Statin Medication	57	100%	94%	94%
Thrombolytic Therapy Timing[1]	-	-	66%	66%
Venous Thromboembolism Prophylaxis	116	99%	94%	94%
Written Stroke Educational Materials Given	35	100%	87%	88%
Surgical Care Improvement Project				
Appropriate Beta Blocker Usage[2]	230	100%	98%	98%
Appropriate VTP Within 24 Hours[2]	419	100%	98%	98%
Controlled Postoperative Blood Glucose[2]	125	97%	97%	97%
Perioperative Temperature Management[2]	472	100%	100%	100%
Prophylactic Antibiotic Selection[2]	441	100%	99%	99%
Prophylactic Antibiotic Selection (Outpatient)	330	98%	98%	98%
Prophylactic Antibiotic Stopped[2]	430	98%	98%	98%
Prophylactic Antibiotic Timing[2]	443	100%	99%	99%
Prophylactic Antibiotic Timing (Outpatient)	331	100%	97%	98%
Urinary Catheter Removal[2]	353	100%	98%	97%
Survey of Patients' Hospital Experiences				
Area Around Room 'Always' Quiet at Night	300+	63%	60%	61%
Doctors 'Always' Communicated Well	300+	80%	81%	82%
Home Recovery Information Given	300+	88%	86%	85%
Hospital Given 9 or 10 on 10 Point Scale	300+	75%	70%	71%
Meds 'Always' Explained Before Given	300+	65%	64%	64%
Nurses 'Always' Communicated Well	300+	80%	79%	79%
Pain 'Always' Well Controlled	300+	71%	71%	71%
Room and Bathroom 'Always' Clean	300+	71%	74%	73%
Timely Help 'Always' Received	300+	68%	67%	68%
Would Definitely Recommend Hospital	300+	77%	70%	71%
Use of Medical Imaging				
Cardiac Imaging Stress Test before Surgery	395	4.6%	5.5%	5.3%
Combination Abdominal CT Scan	1,060	5.1%	10.1%	10.5%
Combination Brain/Sinus CT Scan	984	1.1%	2.6%	2.7%
Combination Chest CT Scan	610	0.7%	2.8%	2.7%
Follow-up Mammogram/Ultrasound	2,524	3.3%	8.4%	8.8%
Lumbar Spine MRI for Low Back Pain	337	36.8%	36.6%	37.2%

Kewanee Hospital

1051 West South Street
Kewanee, IL 61443
E-mail: rlindner@kewaneehospital.com
URL: www.kewaneehospital.com
Type: Critical Access Hospitals
Ownership: Voluntary non-profit - Private

Phone: 309-853-3361
Fax: 309-854-5209

Emergency Services: Yes
Beds: 82

Key Personnel:

Anesthesiology . . . . Keith Barnhill
Chief of Medical Staff . . . . Rick Cernovich, MD
CEO/President . . . . Margaret Gustafson
Quality Assurance . . . . Colleen Lewis
Emergency Room . . . . Adam Reading
Hemotology Center . . . . Jan Sams
Operating Room . . . . Karen Swan
Infection Control . . . . Brenda Wager

Measure	Cases	This Hosp.	State Avg.	U.S. Avg.
Blood Clot Prevention and Treatment				
Anticoagulation Overlap Therapy[5]	-	-	91%	93%
ICU Venous Thromboembolism Prophylaxis[5]	-	-	93%	92%
Incidence of Potentially Preventable VTE[5]	-	-	11%	10%
UFH with Dosages/Platelet Monitoring[5]	-	-	94%	97%
Venous Thromboembolism Prophylaxis[5]	-	-	86%	85%
Warfarin Therapy Discharge Instructions[5]	-	-	71%	75%
Chest Pain/Possible Heart Attack Care				
Aspirin Given Within 24 Hours of Arrival	-	-	96%	96%
Fibrinolytic Meds Within 30 Min. of Arrival	-	-	65%	58%
Average Time to ECG (minutes)	-	-	6	7
Average Time to Transfer (minutes)	-	-	63	60
Children's Asthma Care				
Received Home Management Plan of Care	-	-	-	88%
Received Reliever Medication	-	-	-	100%
Received Systemic Corticosteroids	-	-	-	100%
Emergency Department				
Admittance Decision Time (minutes)[5]	-	-	89	98
Head CT Results Within 45 Min. of Arrival	-	-	64%	57%
Patients Who Left ER Before Being Seen	-	-	3%	2%
Time from ER Arrival to Admit. (minutes)[5]	-	-	260	274
Time from ER Arrival to Discharge (minutes)	-	-	138	134
Time in ER Before Being Evaluated (minutes)	-	-	28	26
Time to Pain Meds for Fractures (minutes)	-	-	52	57
Heart Attack Care				
Aspirin Given at Discharge[1,3]	-	-	99%	99%
Fibrinolytic Meds Within 30 Min. of Arrival[3,7]	-	-	33%	54%
PCI Within 90 Minutes of Arrival[5]	-	-	97%	96%
Statin Prescribed at Discharge[3,7]	-	-	98%	98%
Heart Failure Care				
ACE Inhibitor or ARB for LVSD[1,2]	-	-	98%	97%
Discharge Instructions Given[2]	26	100%	96%	94%
Evaluation of LVS Function[2]	34	94%	99%	99%
Medicare Spending				

NOTE: Hospital profiles are in alphabetical order by state, then city, then hospital within the city; Rankings exclude hospitals with less than 25 cases except for patient surveys which excludes hospitals with less than 100 cases; (a) 100-299 cases; (1) The number of cases/patients is too few to report; (2) Data submitted were based on a sample of cases/patients; (3) Results are based on a shorter time period than required; (4) Data suppressed by CMS for one or more quarters; (5) Results are not available for this reporting period; (6) Fewer than 100 patients completed the HCAHPS survey; (7) No cases met the criteria for this measure; (8) The lower limit of the confidence interval cannot be calculated if the number of observed infections equals zero; (9) No data are available from the state/territory for this reporting period; (10) The scores shown reflect fewer than 50 completed surveys; (11) There were discrepancies in the data collection process; (12) This measure does not apply to this hospital for this reporting period; (13) Results cannot be calculated for this reporting period; (14) The results for this state are combined with nearby states to protect confidentiality; Please refer to the User's Guide for a full explanation of data.

Medicare Spending per Patient (ratio)	-	-	1	0.98
Pneumonia Care				
Appropriate Initial Antibiotic Given[2]	31	90%	95%	95%
Blood Culture Timing[2]	55	100%	98%	98%
Pregnancy and Delivery Care				
Newborn Deliveries Scheduled Early[5]	-	-	2%	6%
Preventive Care				
Immunization for Influenza[3]	120	98%	92%	90%
Immunization for Pneumonia[3]	258	99%	92%	92%
Stroke Care				
Anticoagulation Therapy for Atrial Fibrillation[5]	-	-	94%	95%
Antithrombotic Therapy Timing[5]	-	-	98%	98%
Assessed for Rehabilitation[5]	-	-	97%	97%
Discharged on Antithrombotic Therapy[5]	-	-	99%	99%
Discharged on Statin Medication[5]	-	-	94%	94%
Thrombolytic Therapy Timing[5]	-	-	66%	66%
Venous Thromboembolism Prophylaxis[5]	-	-	94%	94%
Written Stroke Educational Materials Given[5]	-	-	87%	88%
Surgical Care Improvement Project				
Appropriate Beta Blocker Usage[1]	-	-	98%	98%
Appropriate VTP Within 24 Hours[1]	-	-	98%	98%
Controlled Postoperative Blood Glucose[5]	-	-	97%	97%
Perioperative Temperature Management[1]	-	-	100%	100%
Prophylactic Antibiotic Selection[1]	-	-	99%	99%
Prophylactic Antibiotic Selection (Outpatient)	-	-	98%	98%
Prophylactic Antibiotic Stopped[1]	-	-	98%	98%
Prophylactic Antibiotic Timing[1]	-	-	99%	99%
Prophylactic Antibiotic Timing (Outpatient)	-	-	97%	98%
Urinary Catheter Removal[1]	-	-	98%	97%
Survey of Patients' Hospital Experiences				
Area Around Room 'Always' Quiet at Night	(a)	72%	60%	61%
Doctors 'Always' Communicated Well	(a)	85%	81%	82%
Home Recovery Information Given	(a)	91%	86%	85%
Hospital Given 9 or 10 on 10 Point Scale	(a)	74%	70%	71%
Meds 'Always' Explained Before Given	(a)	63%	64%	64%
Nurses 'Always' Communicated Well	(a)	82%	79%	79%
Pain 'Always' Well Controlled	(a)	67%	71%	71%
Room and Bathroom 'Always' Clean	(a)	79%	74%	73%
Timely Help 'Always' Received	(a)	73%	67%	68%
Would Definitely Recommend Hospital	(a)	62%	70%	71%
Use of Medical Imaging				
Cardiac Imaging Stress Test before Surgery	-	-	5.5%	5.3%
Combination Abdominal CT Scan	-	-	10.1%	10.5%
Combination Brain/Sinus CT Scan	-	-	2.6%	2.7%
Combination Chest CT Scan	-	-	2.8%	2.7%
Follow-up Mammogram/Ultrasound	-	-	8.4%	8.8%
Lumbar Spine MRI for Low Back Pain	-	-	36.6%	37.2%

Adventist La Grange Memorial Hospital

5101 S Willow Springs Rd Phone: 708-352-1200
La Grange, IL 60525 Fax: 708-245-5627
E-mail: egervain@ahss.org
URL: www.keepingyouwell.com
Type: Acute Care Hospitals Emergency Services: Yes
Ownership: Voluntary non-profit - Church Beds: 274

Key Personnel:
Quality Assurance . . . . Sue Cunningham
Pediatric In-Patient Care . . . . Marc Freed, DO
Operating Room. . . . . Lori Kaspar, RN
Radiology. . . . . Timothy N Merrill, MD
Chief of Medical Staff . . . . Patrick Quirke, MD
Emergency Room . . . . Gail Weimer, RN
CEO/President. . . . . Rick Wright

Measure	Cases	This Hosp.	State Avg.	U.S. Avg.
Blood Clot Prevention and Treatment				
Anticoagulation Overlap Therapy[2]	62	84%	91%	93%
ICU Venous Thromboembolism Prophylaxis[2]	39	85%	93%	92%
Incidence of Potentially Preventable VTE[2]	12	25%	11%	10%
UFH with Dosages/Platelet Monitoring[2]	58	91%	94%	97%
Venous Thromboembolism Prophylaxis[2]	363	81%	86%	85%
Warfarin Therapy Discharge Instructions[2]	37	65%	71%	75%
Chest Pain/Possible Heart Attack Care				
Aspirin Given Within 24 Hours of Arrival[5]	-	-	96%	96%
Fibrinolytic Meds Within 30 Min. of Arrival[5]	-	-	65%	58%
Average Time to ECG (minutes)[5]	-	-	6	7
Average Time to Transfer (minutes)[5]	-	-	63	60
Children's Asthma Care				
Received Home Management Plan of Care	-	-	-	88%
Received Reliever Medication	-	-	-	100%
Received Systemic Corticosteroids	-	-	-	100%
Emergency Department				
Admittance Decision Time (minutes)[2]	376	98	89	98
Head CT Results Within 45 Min. of Arrival[1,3]	-	-	64%	57%
Patients Who Left ER Before Being Seen	27,023	1%	3%	2%
Time from ER Arrival to Admit. (minutes)[2]	701	251	260	274
Time from ER Arrival to Discharge (minutes)	340	157	138	134
Time in ER Before Being Evaluated (minutes)	313	25	28	26
Time to Pain Meds for Fractures (minutes)	88	54	52	57
Heart Attack Care				
Aspirin Given at Discharge	77	100%	99%	99%
Fibrinolytic Meds Within 30 Min. of Arrival[7]	-	-	33%	54%
PCI Within 90 Minutes of Arrival	21	95%	97%	96%
Statin Prescribed at Discharge	77	100%	98%	98%
Heart Failure Care				
ACE Inhibitor or ARB for LVSD	61	100%	98%	97%
Discharge Instructions Given	194	99%	96%	94%
Evaluation of LVS Function	288	100%	99%	99%
Medicare Spending				
Medicare Spending per Patient (ratio)	-	1.04	1	0.98
Pneumonia Care				
Appropriate Initial Antibiotic Given	140	96%	95%	95%
Blood Culture Timing	253	100%	98%	98%
Pregnancy and Delivery Care				
Newborn Deliveries Scheduled Early[2]	30	10%	2%	6%
Preventive Care				
Immunization for Influenza[2]	556	90%	92%	90%
Immunization for Pneumonia[2]	809	94%	92%	92%
Stroke Care				
Anticoagulation Therapy for Atrial Fibrillation[1]	-	-	94%	95%
Antithrombotic Therapy Timing	74	100%	98%	98%
Assessed for Rehabilitation	95	100%	97%	97%
Discharged on Antithrombotic Therapy	90	100%	99%	99%
Discharged on Statin Medication	72	97%	94%	94%
Thrombolytic Therapy Timing[1]	-	-	66%	66%
Venous Thromboembolism Prophylaxis	87	97%	94%	94%
Written Stroke Educational Materials Given	49	98%	87%	88%
Surgical Care Improvement Project				
Appropriate Beta Blocker Usage[2]	126	100%	98%	98%
Appropriate VTP Within 24 Hours[2]	272	100%	98%	98%
Controlled Postoperative Blood Glucose[2]	42	100%	97%	97%
Perioperative Temperature Management[2]	334	100%	100%	100%
Prophylactic Antibiotic Selection[2]	248	99%	99%	99%
Prophylactic Antibiotic Selection (Outpatient)	94	100%	98%	98%
Prophylactic Antibiotic Stopped[2]	234	99%	98%	98%
Prophylactic Antibiotic Timing[2]	248	98%	99%	99%
Prophylactic Antibiotic Timing (Outpatient)	95	99%	97%	98%
Urinary Catheter Removal[2]	225	99%	98%	97%
Survey of Patients' Hospital Experiences				
Area Around Room 'Always' Quiet at Night[11]	300+	63%	60%	61%
Doctors 'Always' Communicated Well[11]	300+	83%	81%	82%
Home Recovery Information Given[11]	300+	87%	86%	85%
Hospital Given 9 or 10 on 10 Point Scale[11]	300+	78%	70%	71%
Meds 'Always' Explained Before Given[11]	300+	66%	64%	64%
Nurses 'Always' Communicated Well[11]	300+	83%	79%	79%
Pain 'Always' Well Controlled[11]	300+	76%	71%	71%
Room and Bathroom 'Always' Clean[11]	300+	77%	74%	73%
Timely Help 'Always' Received[11]	300+	75%	67%	68%
Would Definitely Recommend Hospital[11]	300+	80%	70%	71%
Use of Medical Imaging				
Cardiac Imaging Stress Test before Surgery	282	7.4%	5.5%	5.3%
Combination Abdominal CT Scan	933	4.9%	10.1%	10.5%
Combination Brain/Sinus CT Scan	751	2.8%	2.6%	2.7%
Combination Chest CT Scan	740	8.8%	2.8%	2.7%
Follow-up Mammogram/Ultrasound	1,942	12.3%	8.4%	8.8%
Lumbar Spine MRI for Low Back Pain	111	40.5%	36.6%	37.2%

Lake Forest Hospital

660 N Westmoreland Road Phone: 847-234-5600
Lake Forest, IL 60045 Fax: 847-535-7846
URL: www.lakeforesthospital.com
Type: Acute Care Hospitals Emergency Services: Yes
Ownership: Voluntary non-profit - Other Beds: 261

Key Personnel:
Chief of Medical Staff . . . . Michael G. Ankin, MD
CEO/President. . . . . Thomas J. McAfee

Measure	Cases	This Hosp.	State Avg.	U.S. Avg.
Blood Clot Prevention and Treatment				
Anticoagulation Overlap Therapy[2]	90	99%	91%	93%
ICU Venous Thromboembolism Prophylaxis[2]	65	94%	93%	92%
Incidence of Potentially Preventable VTE[1,2]	-	-	11%	10%
UFH with Dosages/Platelet Monitoring[2]	31	100%	94%	97%
Venous Thromboembolism Prophylaxis[2]	290	78%	86%	85%
Warfarin Therapy Discharge Instructions[2]	71	92%	71%	75%
Chest Pain/Possible Heart Attack Care				
Aspirin Given Within 24 Hours of Arrival[1]	-	-	96%	96%
Fibrinolytic Meds Within 30 Min. of Arrival[3,7]	-	-	65%	58%
Average Time to ECG (minutes)	11	6	6	7
Average Time to Transfer (minutes)[3,7]	-	-	63	60
Children's Asthma Care				
Received Home Management Plan of Care	-	-	-	88%
Received Reliever Medication	-	-	-	100%
Received Systemic Corticosteroids	-	-	-	100%
Emergency Department				
Admittance Decision Time (minutes)[2]	454	95	89	98
Head CT Results Within 45 Min. of Arrival[1]	-	-	64%	57%
Patients Who Left ER Before Being Seen	52,625	1%	3%	2%
Time from ER Arrival to Admit. (minutes)[2]	462	233	260	274
Time from ER Arrival to Discharge (minutes)	404	137	138	134
Time in ER Before Being Evaluated (minutes)	350	28	28	26
Time to Pain Meds for Fractures (minutes)	189	41	52	57
Heart Attack Care				
Aspirin Given at Discharge	51	100%	99%	99%
Fibrinolytic Meds Within 30 Min. of Arrival[7]	-	-	33%	54%
PCI Within 90 Minutes of Arrival	13	100%	97%	96%
Statin Prescribed at Discharge	50	100%	98%	98%
Heart Failure Care				
ACE Inhibitor or ARB for LVSD	43	100%	98%	97%
Discharge Instructions Given	101	94%	96%	94%
Evaluation of LVS Function	141	100%	99%	99%
Medicare Spending				
Medicare Spending per Patient (ratio)	-	0.99	1	0.98
Pneumonia Care				
Appropriate Initial Antibiotic Given	78	100%	95%	95%
Blood Culture Timing	187	100%	98%	98%
Pregnancy and Delivery Care				
Newborn Deliveries Scheduled Early[2]	30	7%	2%	6%
Preventive Care				
Immunization for Influenza[2]	519	98%	92%	90%
Immunization for Pneumonia[2]	468	94%	92%	92%
Stroke Care				
Anticoagulation Therapy for Atrial Fibrillation[1]	-	-	94%	95%
Antithrombotic Therapy Timing	51	100%	98%	98%
Assessed for Rehabilitation	50	100%	97%	97%
Discharged on Antithrombotic Therapy	49	98%	99%	99%
Discharged on Statin Medication	35	97%	94%	94%
Thrombolytic Therapy Timing[1]	-	-	66%	66%
Venous Thromboembolism Prophylaxis	47	83%	94%	94%
Written Stroke Educational Materials Given	36	100%	87%	88%
Surgical Care Improvement Project				
Appropriate Beta Blocker Usage	177	94%	98%	98%
Appropriate VTP Within 24 Hours	813	98%	98%	98%
Controlled Postoperative Blood Glucose[7]	-	-	97%	97%
Perioperative Temperature Management	850	100%	100%	100%
Prophylactic Antibiotic Selection	702	98%	99%	99%
Prophylactic Antibiotic Selection (Outpatient)	190	99%	98%	98%
Prophylactic Antibiotic Stopped	700	99%	98%	98%
Prophylactic Antibiotic Timing	703	98%	99%	99%
Prophylactic Antibiotic Timing (Outpatient)	188	95%	97%	98%
Urinary Catheter Removal	676	98%	98%	97%

NOTE: Hospital profiles are in alphabetical order by state, then city, then hospital within the city; Rankings exclude hospitals with less than 25 cases except for patient surveys which excludes hospitals with less than 100 cases; (a) 100-299 cases; (1) The number of cases/patients is too few to report; (2) Data submitted were based on a sample of cases/patients; (3) Results are based on a shorter time period than required; (4) Data suppressed by CMS for one or more quarters; (5) Results are not available for this reporting period; (6) Fewer than 100 patients completed the HCAHPS survey; (7) No cases met the criteria for this measure; (8) The lower limit of the confidence interval cannot be calculated if the number of observed infections equals zero; (9) No data are available from the state/territory for this reporting period; (10) The scores shown reflect fewer than 50 completed surveys; (11) There were discrepancies in the data collection process; (12) This measure does not apply to this hospital for this reporting period; (13) Results cannot be calculated for this reporting period; (14) The results for this state are combined with nearby states to protect confidentiality; Please refer to the User's Guide for a full explanation of data.

Measure	Cases	This Hosp.	State Avg.	U.S. Avg.
Survey of Patients' Hospital Experiences				
Area Around Room 'Always' Quiet at Night	300+	52%	60%	61%
Doctors 'Always' Communicated Well	300+	80%	81%	82%
Home Recovery Information Given	300+	80%	86%	85%
Hospital Given 9 or 10 on 10 Point Scale	300+	64%	70%	71%
Meds 'Always' Explained Before Given	300+	57%	64%	64%
Nurses 'Always' Communicated Well	300+	70%	79%	79%
Pain 'Always' Well Controlled	300+	65%	71%	71%
Room and Bathroom 'Always' Clean	300+	71%	74%	73%
Timely Help 'Always' Received	300+	55%	67%	68%
Would Definitely Recommend Hospital	300+	66%	70%	71%
Use of Medical Imaging				
Cardiac Imaging Stress Test before Surgery	413	7.7%	5.5%	5.3%
Combination Abdominal CT Scan	1,204	19.5%	10.1%	10.5%
Combination Brain/Sinus CT Scan[1]	-	-	2.6%	2.7%
Combination Chest CT Scan	819	9.4%	2.8%	2.7%
Follow-up Mammogram/Ultrasound	3,247	18.1%	8.4%	8.8%
Lumbar Spine MRI for Low Back Pain	245	32.2%	36.6%	37.2%

Lawrence County Memorial Hospital

2200 W State St
Lawrenceville, IL 62439
Phone: 618-943-1000
Fax: 618-943-7230
Type: Critical Access Hospitals
Emergency Services: Yes
Ownership: Voluntary non-profit - Other
Beds: 25

Key Personnel:
Chief of Medical Staff.......... Gary Carr, MD
CEO .... Doug Florkowski
Emergency Room .... Rita Garvey
Quality Assurance .... Debbie Gregory
Infection Control.............. Deborah Lemeroa, RN
Radiology.................... Debbie Miller
Anesthesiology............... Tim Williams, DO

Measure	Cases	This Hosp.	State Avg.	U.S. Avg.
Blood Clot Prevention and Treatment				
Anticoagulation Overlap Therapy[1,3]	-	-	91%	93%
ICU Venous Thromboembolism Prophylaxis[3,7]	-	-	93%	92%
Incidence of Potentially Preventable VTE[3,7]	-	-	11%	10%
UFH with Dosages/Platelet Monitoring[3,7]	-	-	94%	97%
Venous Thromboembolism Prophylaxis[3,7]	-	-	86%	85%
Warfarin Therapy Discharge Instructions[1,3]	-	-	71%	75%
Chest Pain/Possible Heart Attack Care				
Aspirin Given Within 24 Hours of Arrival	-	-	96%	96%
Fibrinolytic Meds Within 30 Min. of Arrival	-	-	65%	58%
Average Time to ECG (minutes)	-	-	6	7
Average Time to Transfer (minutes)	-	-	63	60
Children's Asthma Care				
Received Home Management Plan of Care	-	-	-	88%
Received Reliever Medication	-	-	-	100%
Received Systemic Corticosteroids	-	-	-	100%
Emergency Department				
Admittance Decision Time (minutes)[5]	-	-	89	98
Head CT Results Within 45 Min. of Arrival	-	-	64%	57%
Patients Who Left ER Before Being Seen	-	-	3%	2%
Time from ER Arrival to Admit. (minutes)[5]	-	-	260	274
Time from ER Arrival to Discharge (minutes)	-	-	138	134
Time in ER Before Being Evaluated (minutes)	-	-	28	26
Time to Pain Meds for Fractures (minutes)	-	-	52	57
Heart Attack Care				
Aspirin Given at Discharge[5]	-	-	99%	99%
Fibrinolytic Meds Within 30 Min. of Arrival[5]	-	-	33%	54%
PCI Within 90 Minutes of Arrival[5]	-	-	97%	96%
Statin Prescribed at Discharge[5]	-	-	98%	98%
Heart Failure Care				
ACE Inhibitor or ARB for LVSD[1]	-	-	98%	97%
Discharge Instructions Given	21	33%	96%	94%
Evaluation of LVS Function	43	65%	99%	99%
Medicare Spending				
Medicare Spending per Patient (ratio)	-	-	1	0.98
Pneumonia Care				
Appropriate Initial Antibiotic Given	32	44%	95%	95%
Blood Culture Timing	41	76%	98%	98%
Pregnancy and Delivery Care				
Newborn Deliveries Scheduled Early[5]	-	-	2%	6%
Preventive Care				
Immunization for Influenza[5]	-	-	92%	90%
Immunization for Pneumonia[5]	-	-	92%	92%
Stroke Care				
Anticoagulation Therapy for Atrial Fibrillation[5]	-	-	94%	95%
Antithrombotic Therapy Timing[5]	-	-	98%	98%
Assessed for Rehabilitation[5]	-	-	97%	97%
Discharged on Antithrombotic Therapy[5]	-	-	99%	99%
Discharged on Statin Medication[5]	-	-	94%	94%
Thrombolytic Therapy Timing[5]	-	-	66%	66%
Venous Thromboembolism Prophylaxis[5]	-	-	94%	94%
Written Stroke Educational Materials Given[5]	-	-	87%	88%
Surgical Care Improvement Project				
Appropriate Beta Blocker Usage[5]	-	-	98%	98%
Appropriate VTP Within 24 Hours[5]	-	-	98%	98%
Controlled Postoperative Blood Glucose[5]	-	-	97%	97%
Perioperative Temperature Management[5]	-	-	100%	100%
Prophylactic Antibiotic Selection[5]	-	-	99%	99%
Prophylactic Antibiotic Selection (Outpatient)	-	-	98%	98%
Prophylactic Antibiotic Stopped[5]	-	-	98%	98%
Prophylactic Antibiotic Timing[5]	-	-	99%	99%
Prophylactic Antibiotic Timing (Outpatient)	-	-	97%	98%
Urinary Catheter Removal[5]	-	-	98%	97%
Survey of Patients' Hospital Experiences				
Area Around Room 'Always' Quiet at Night[5]	-	-	60%	61%
Doctors 'Always' Communicated Well[5]	-	-	81%	82%
Home Recovery Information Given[5]	-	-	86%	85%
Hospital Given 9 or 10 on 10 Point Scale[5]	-	-	70%	71%
Meds 'Always' Explained Before Given[5]	-	-	64%	64%
Nurses 'Always' Communicated Well[5]	-	-	79%	79%
Pain 'Always' Well Controlled[5]	-	-	71%	71%
Room and Bathroom 'Always' Clean[5]	-	-	74%	73%
Timely Help 'Always' Received[5]	-	-	67%	68%
Would Definitely Recommend Hospital[5]	-	-	70%	71%
Use of Medical Imaging				
Cardiac Imaging Stress Test before Surgery	-	-	5.5%	5.3%
Combination Abdominal CT Scan	-	-	10.1%	10.5%
Combination Brain/Sinus CT Scan	-	-	2.6%	2.7%
Combination Chest CT Scan	-	-	2.8%	2.7%
Follow-up Mammogram/Ultrasound	-	-	8.4%	8.8%
Lumbar Spine MRI for Low Back Pain	-	-	36.6%	37.2%

Advocate Condell Medical Center

801 S Milwaukee Ave
Libertyville, IL 60048
Phone: 847-990-5200
Fax: 847-362-1721
URL: www.condell.org
Type: Acute Care Hospitals
Emergency Services: Yes
Ownership: Voluntary non-profit - Private
Beds: 305

Key Personnel:
Infection Control.............. Emily Bergman
Radiology................... Daniel Y Kim
Emergency Room .... William E Maloney
Quality Assurance .... Kathleen Mika
CEO/President............... Eugene Pritchard
Intensive Care Unit........... Sharon Reich
Cardiac Laboratory............ Vinda Russo

Measure	Cases	This Hosp.	State Avg.	U.S. Avg.
Blood Clot Prevention and Treatment				
Anticoagulation Overlap Therapy[2]	124	90%	91%	93%
ICU Venous Thromboembolism Prophylaxis[2]	67	91%	93%	92%
Incidence of Potentially Preventable VTE[2]	22	5%	11%	10%
UFH with Dosages/Platelet Monitoring[2]	33	97%	94%	97%
Venous Thromboembolism Prophylaxis[2]	352	73%	86%	85%
Warfarin Therapy Discharge Instructions[2]	73	26%	71%	75%
Chest Pain/Possible Heart Attack Care				
Aspirin Given Within 24 Hours of Arrival[1,3]	-	-	96%	96%
Fibrinolytic Meds Within 30 Min. of Arrival[5]	-	-	65%	58%
Average Time to ECG (minutes)[1,3]	-	-	6	7
Average Time to Transfer (minutes)[5]	-	-	63	60
Children's Asthma Care				
Received Home Management Plan of Care	-	-	-	88%
Received Reliever Medication	-	-	-	100%
Received Systemic Corticosteroids	-	-	-	100%
Emergency Department				
Admittance Decision Time (minutes)[2]	521	135	89	98
Head CT Results Within 45 Min. of Arrival	12	92%	64%	57%
Patients Who Left ER Before Being Seen	56,924	0%	3%	2%
Time from ER Arrival to Admit. (minutes)[2]	558	280	260	274
Time from ER Arrival to Discharge (minutes)	353	150	138	134
Time in ER Before Being Evaluated (minutes)	409	30	28	26
Time to Pain Meds for Fractures (minutes)	221	36	52	57
Heart Attack Care				
Aspirin Given at Discharge	323	100%	99%	99%
Fibrinolytic Meds Within 30 Min. of Arrival[7]	-	-	33%	54%
PCI Within 90 Minutes of Arrival	50	100%	97%	96%
Statin Prescribed at Discharge	302	100%	98%	98%
Heart Failure Care				
ACE Inhibitor or ARB for LVSD[2]	86	100%	98%	97%
Discharge Instructions Given[2]	210	96%	96%	94%
Evaluation of LVS Function[2]	292	100%	99%	99%
Medicare Spending				
Medicare Spending per Patient (ratio)	-	1.05	1	0.98
Pneumonia Care				
Appropriate Initial Antibiotic Given[2]	74	96%	95%	95%
Blood Culture Timing[2]	178	99%	98%	98%
Pregnancy and Delivery Care				
Newborn Deliveries Scheduled Early	249	0%	2%	6%
Preventive Care				
Immunization for Influenza[2]	563	97%	92%	90%
Immunization for Pneumonia[2]	635	96%	92%	92%
Stroke Care				
Anticoagulation Therapy for Atrial Fibrillation	30	97%	94%	95%
Antithrombotic Therapy Timing	150	99%	98%	98%
Assessed for Rehabilitation	179	99%	97%	97%
Discharged on Antithrombotic Therapy	163	99%	99%	99%
Discharged on Statin Medication	122	94%	94%	94%
Thrombolytic Therapy Timing	19	79%	66%	66%
Venous Thromboembolism Prophylaxis	179	90%	94%	94%
Written Stroke Educational Materials Given	87	94%	87%	88%
Surgical Care Improvement Project				
Appropriate Beta Blocker Usage[2]	294	99%	98%	98%
Appropriate VTP Within 24 Hours[2]	455	100%	98%	98%
Controlled Postoperative Blood Glucose[2]	117	99%	97%	97%
Perioperative Temperature Management[2]	564	100%	100%	100%
Prophylactic Antibiotic Selection[2]	475	100%	99%	99%
Prophylactic Antibiotic Selection (Outpatient)	456	99%	98%	98%
Prophylactic Antibiotic Stopped[2]	451	100%	98%	98%
Prophylactic Antibiotic Timing[2]	476	99%	99%	99%
Prophylactic Antibiotic Timing (Outpatient)	457	99%	97%	98%
Urinary Catheter Removal[2]	406	100%	98%	97%
Survey of Patients' Hospital Experiences				
Area Around Room 'Always' Quiet at Night	300+	60%	60%	61%
Doctors 'Always' Communicated Well	300+	78%	81%	82%
Home Recovery Information Given	300+	85%	86%	85%
Hospital Given 9 or 10 on 10 Point Scale	300+	73%	70%	71%
Meds 'Always' Explained Before Given	300+	62%	64%	64%
Nurses 'Always' Communicated Well	300+	78%	79%	79%
Pain 'Always' Well Controlled	300+	70%	71%	71%
Room and Bathroom 'Always' Clean	300+	81%	74%	73%
Timely Help 'Always' Received	300+	65%	67%	68%
Would Definitely Recommend Hospital	300+	75%	70%	71%
Use of Medical Imaging				
Cardiac Imaging Stress Test before Surgery	523	7.5%	5.5%	5.3%
Combination Abdominal CT Scan	1,449	2.3%	10.1%	10.5%
Combination Brain/Sinus CT Scan	1,292	2.2%	2.6%	2.7%
Combination Chest CT Scan	793	0.4%	2.8%	2.7%
Follow-up Mammogram/Ultrasound	1,888	6.3%	8.4%	8.8%
Lumbar Spine MRI for Low Back Pain	190	31.1%	36.6%	37.2%

Abraham Lincoln Memorial Hospital

200 Stahlhut Drive
Lincoln, IL 62656
Phone: 217-732-2161
Fax: 217-732-7481
URL: www.almh.org
Type: Critical Access Hospitals
Emergency Services: Yes
Ownership: Voluntary non-profit - Private
Beds: 66

Key Personnel:
Intensive Care Unit............. Judy Evans
Infection Control............... Margaret Evers, RN
Operating Room............... Debbie Morrow, RN

NOTE: Hospital profiles are in alphabetical order by state, then city, then hospital within the city; Rankings exclude hospitals with less than 25 cases except for patient surveys which excludes hospitals with less than 100 cases; (a) 100-299 cases; (1) The number of cases/patients is too few to report; (2) Data submitted were based on a sample of cases/patients; (3) Results are based on a shorter time period than required; (4) Data suppressed by CMS for one or more quarters; (5) Results are not available for this reporting period; (6) Fewer than 100 patients completed the HCAHPS survey; (7) No cases met the criteria for this measure; (8) The lower limit of the confidence interval cannot be calculated if the number of observed infections equals zero; (9) No data are available from the state/territory for this reporting period; (10) The scores shown reflect fewer than 50 completed surveys; (11) There were discrepancies in the data collection process; (12) This measure does not apply to this hospital for this reporting period; (13) Results cannot be calculated for this reporting period; (14) The results for this state are combined with nearby states to protect confidentiality; Please refer to the User's Guide for a full explanation of data.

Radiology. . . . . Charles Neal
Emergency Room . . . . Larry Pinter, MD
Anesthesiology. . . . . Gene Quint
Quality Assurance . . . . Kathleen Vipond
Chief of Medical Staff. . . . . Amir John Wahab, MD

Measure	Cases	This Hosp.	State Avg.	U.S. Avg.
Blood Clot Prevention and Treatment				
Anticoagulation Overlap Therapy[1,2]	-	-	91%	93%
ICU Venous Thromboembolism Prophylaxis[2,7]	-	-	93%	92%
Incidence of Potentially Preventable VTE[2,7]	-	-	11%	10%
UFH with Dosages/Platelet Monitoring[1,2]	-	-	94%	97%
Venous Thromboembolism Prophylaxis[2]	100	91%	86%	85%
Warfarin Therapy Discharge Instructions[1,2]	-	-	71%	75%
Chest Pain/Possible Heart Attack Care				
Aspirin Given Within 24 Hours of Arrival	79	97%	96%	96%
Fibrinolytic Meds Within 30 Min. of Arrival[7]	-	-	65%	58%
Average Time to ECG (minutes)	80	3	6	7
Average Time to Transfer (minutes)[1]	-	-	63	60
Children's Asthma Care				
Received Home Management Plan of Care	-	-	-	88%
Received Reliever Medication	-	-	-	100%
Received Systemic Corticosteroids	-	-	-	100%
Emergency Department				
Admittance Decision Time (minutes)[2]	285	61	89	98
Head CT Results Within 45 Min. of Arrival	13	62%	64%	57%
Patients Who Left ER Before Being Seen	17,464	1%	3%	2%
Time from ER Arrival to Admit. (minutes)[2]	290	218	260	274
Time from ER Arrival to Discharge (minutes)	356	91	138	134
Time in ER Before Being Evaluated (minutes)	372	18	28	26
Time to Pain Meds for Fractures (minutes)	80	26	52	57
Heart Attack Care				
Aspirin Given at Discharge[1]	-	-	99%	99%
Fibrinolytic Meds Within 30 Min. of Arrival[7]	-	-	33%	54%
PCI Within 90 Minutes of Arrival[7]	-	-	97%	96%
Statin Prescribed at Discharge[1]	-	-	98%	98%
Heart Failure Care				
ACE Inhibitor or ARB for LVSD[1]	-	-	98%	97%
Discharge Instructions Given	28	100%	96%	94%
Evaluation of LVS Function	41	95%	99%	99%
Medicare Spending				
Medicare Spending per Patient (ratio)	-	-	1	0.98
Pneumonia Care				
Appropriate Initial Antibiotic Given	50	86%	95%	95%
Blood Culture Timing	61	100%	98%	98%
Pregnancy and Delivery Care				
Newborn Deliveries Scheduled Early[5]	-	-	2%	6%
Preventive Care				
Immunization for Influenza[2]	251	100%	92%	90%
Immunization for Pneumonia[2]	327	98%	92%	92%
Stroke Care				
Anticoagulation Therapy for Atrial Fibrillation[5]	-	-	94%	95%
Antithrombotic Therapy Timing[5]	-	-	98%	98%
Assessed for Rehabilitation[5]	-	-	97%	97%
Discharged on Antithrombotic Therapy[5]	-	-	99%	99%
Discharged on Statin Medication[5]	-	-	94%	94%
Thrombolytic Therapy Timing[5]	-	-	66%	66%
Venous Thromboembolism Prophylaxis[5]	-	-	94%	94%
Written Stroke Educational Materials Given[5]	-	-	87%	88%
Surgical Care Improvement Project				
Appropriate Beta Blocker Usage	34	100%	98%	98%
Appropriate VTP Within 24 Hours	104	99%	98%	98%
Controlled Postoperative Blood Glucose[7]	-	-	97%	97%
Perioperative Temperature Management	111	99%	100%	100%
Prophylactic Antibiotic Selection	95	99%	99%	99%
Prophylactic Antibiotic Selection (Outpatient)[5]	-	-	98%	98%
Prophylactic Antibiotic Stopped	94	100%	98%	98%
Prophylactic Antibiotic Timing	95	97%	99%	99%
Prophylactic Antibiotic Timing (Outpatient)[5]	-	-	97%	98%
Urinary Catheter Removal	67	100%	98%	97%
Survey of Patients' Hospital Experiences				
Area Around Room 'Always' Quiet at Night	(a)	65%	60%	61%
Doctors 'Always' Communicated Well	(a)	90%	81%	82%
Home Recovery Information Given	(a)	92%	86%	85%
Hospital Given 9 or 10 on 10 Point Scale	(a)	84%	70%	71%
Meds 'Always' Explained Before Given	(a)	69%	64%	64%
Nurses 'Always' Communicated Well	(a)	85%	79%	79%
Pain 'Always' Well Controlled	(a)	69%	71%	71%
Room and Bathroom 'Always' Clean	(a)	83%	74%	73%
Timely Help 'Always' Received	(a)	69%	67%	68%
Would Definitely Recommend Hospital	(a)	84%	70%	71%
Use of Medical Imaging				
Cardiac Imaging Stress Test before Surgery	62	0.0%	5.5%	5.3%
Combination Abdominal CT Scan	501	6.6%	10.1%	10.5%
Combination Brain/Sinus CT Scan[1]	-	-	2.6%	2.7%
Combination Chest CT Scan	387	0.0%	2.8%	2.7%
Follow-up Mammogram/Ultrasound	540	8.0%	8.4%	8.8%
Lumbar Spine MRI for Low Back Pain	66	43.9%	36.6%	37.2%

Saint Francis Hospital

1215 Franciscan Dr
Litchfield, IL 62056
URL: www.stfrancis-litchfield.org
Phone: 217-324-2191
Fax: 217-324-3081
Type: Critical Access Hospitals
Emergency Services: Yes
Ownership: Voluntary non-profit - Church
Beds: 25

Key Personnel:
Operating Room. . . . . D Billiter
Quality Assurance . . . . Bev Deaton
Emergency Room . . . . Vicky Fuller, RN
Chief of Medical Staff. . . . . Timothy Ishmael, MD
Radiology. . . . . Laura Smalley
Infection Control. . . . . Angie Tefteller, RN
Intensive Care Unit. . . . . Pat Wernsing, RN

Measure	Cases	This Hosp.	State Avg.	U.S. Avg.
Blood Clot Prevention and Treatment				
Anticoagulation Overlap Therapy[5]	-	-	91%	93%
ICU Venous Thromboembolism Prophylaxis[5]	-	-	93%	92%
Incidence of Potentially Preventable VTE[5]	-	-	11%	10%
UFH with Dosages/Platelet Monitoring[5]	-	-	94%	97%
Venous Thromboembolism Prophylaxis[5]	-	-	86%	85%
Warfarin Therapy Discharge Instructions[5]	-	-	71%	75%
Chest Pain/Possible Heart Attack Care				
Aspirin Given Within 24 Hours of Arrival[5]	-	-	96%	96%
Fibrinolytic Meds Within 30 Min. of Arrival[5]	-	-	65%	58%
Average Time to ECG (minutes)[5]	-	-	6	7
Average Time to Transfer (minutes)[5]	-	-	63	60
Children's Asthma Care				
Received Home Management Plan of Care	-	-	-	88%
Received Reliever Medication	-	-	-	100%
Received Systemic Corticosteroids	-	-	-	100%
Emergency Department				
Admittance Decision Time (minutes)[5]	-	-	89	98
Head CT Results Within 45 Min. of Arrival[5]	-	-	64%	57%
Patients Who Left ER Before Being Seen[5]	-	-	3%	2%
Time from ER Arrival to Admit. (minutes)[5]	-	-	260	274
Time from ER Arrival to Discharge (minutes)[5]	-	-	138	134
Time in ER Before Being Evaluated (minutes)[5]	-	-	28	26
Time to Pain Meds for Fractures (minutes)[5]	-	-	52	57
Heart Attack Care				
Aspirin Given at Discharge[5]	-	-	99%	99%
Fibrinolytic Meds Within 30 Min. of Arrival[5]	-	-	33%	54%
PCI Within 90 Minutes of Arrival[5]	-	-	97%	96%
Statin Prescribed at Discharge[5]	-	-	98%	98%
Heart Failure Care				
ACE Inhibitor or ARB for LVSD	13	85%	98%	97%
Discharge Instructions Given	32	72%	96%	94%
Evaluation of LVS Function	39	87%	99%	99%
Medicare Spending				
Medicare Spending per Patient (ratio)	-	-	1	0.98
Pneumonia Care				
Appropriate Initial Antibiotic Given	44	98%	95%	95%
Blood Culture Timing	62	98%	98%	98%
Pregnancy and Delivery Care				
Newborn Deliveries Scheduled Early[5]	-	-	2%	6%
Preventive Care				
Immunization for Influenza[5]	-	-	92%	90%
Immunization for Pneumonia[5]	-	-	92%	92%
Stroke Care				
Anticoagulation Therapy for Atrial Fibrillation[5]	-	-	94%	95%
Antithrombotic Therapy Timing[5]	-	-	98%	98%
Assessed for Rehabilitation[5]	-	-	97%	97%
Discharged on Antithrombotic Therapy[5]	-	-	99%	99%
Discharged on Statin Medication[5]	-	-	94%	94%
Thrombolytic Therapy Timing[5]	-	-	66%	66%
Venous Thromboembolism Prophylaxis[5]	-	-	94%	94%
Written Stroke Educational Materials Given[5]	-	-	87%	88%
Surgical Care Improvement Project				
Appropriate Beta Blocker Usage[1]	-	-	98%	98%
Appropriate VTP Within 24 Hours	20	90%	98%	98%
Controlled Postoperative Blood Glucose[3,7]	-	-	97%	97%
Perioperative Temperature Management	22	100%	100%	100%
Prophylactic Antibiotic Selection	15	100%	99%	99%
Prophylactic Antibiotic Selection (Outpatient)[5]	-	-	98%	98%
Prophylactic Antibiotic Stopped	12	92%	98%	98%
Prophylactic Antibiotic Timing	15	100%	99%	99%
Prophylactic Antibiotic Timing (Outpatient)[5]	-	-	97%	98%
Urinary Catheter Removal	20	95%	98%	97%
Survey of Patients' Hospital Experiences				
Area Around Room 'Always' Quiet at Night	300+	67%	60%	61%
Doctors 'Always' Communicated Well	300+	88%	81%	82%
Home Recovery Information Given	300+	86%	86%	85%
Hospital Given 9 or 10 on 10 Point Scale	300+	76%	70%	71%
Meds 'Always' Explained Before Given	300+	66%	64%	64%
Nurses 'Always' Communicated Well	300+	83%	79%	79%
Pain 'Always' Well Controlled	300+	76%	71%	71%
Room and Bathroom 'Always' Clean	300+	86%	74%	73%
Timely Help 'Always' Received	300+	75%	67%	68%
Would Definitely Recommend Hospital	300+	71%	70%	71%
Use of Medical Imaging				
Cardiac Imaging Stress Test before Surgery	202	4.5%	5.5%	5.3%
Combination Abdominal CT Scan	568	38.9%	10.1%	10.5%
Combination Brain/Sinus CT Scan[1]	-	-	2.6%	2.7%
Combination Chest CT Scan	338	8.0%	2.8%	2.7%
Follow-up Mammogram/Ultrasound	809	13.5%	8.4%	8.8%
Lumbar Spine MRI for Low Back Pain	86	31.4%	36.6%	37.2%

McDonough District Hospital

525 East Grant Street
Macomb, IL 61455
URL: www.mdh.org
Phone: 309-833-4101
Fax: 309-836-1507
Type: Acute Care Hospitals
Emergency Services: Yes
Ownership: Govt - Hospital Dist/Auth
Beds: 113

Key Personnel:
President/CEO. . . . . Kenny Boyd, MS
Quality Assurance . . . . Linda Dace
Chief of Medical Staff. . . . . Dr Charles O'Neill
Radiology. . . . . Ronald Rigdon, MD
Infection Control. . . . . Carol Rowland-Maguire, RN
Operating Room. . . . . Linda Sampson

Measure	Cases	This Hosp.	State Avg.	U.S. Avg.
Blood Clot Prevention and Treatment				
Anticoagulation Overlap Therapy[2]	21	100%	91%	93%
ICU Venous Thromboembolism Prophylaxis[2]	35	74%	93%	92%
Incidence of Potentially Preventable VTE[2,7]	-	-	11%	10%
UFH with Dosages/Platelet Monitoring[2]	13	100%	94%	97%
Venous Thromboembolism Prophylaxis[2]	155	77%	86%	85%
Warfarin Therapy Discharge Instructions[2]	14	100%	71%	75%
Chest Pain/Possible Heart Attack Care				
Aspirin Given Within 24 Hours of Arrival	82	99%	96%	96%
Fibrinolytic Meds Within 30 Min. of Arrival[7]	-	-	65%	58%
Average Time to ECG (minutes)	82	6	6	7
Average Time to Transfer (minutes)[1]	-	-	63	60
Children's Asthma Care				
Received Home Management Plan of Care	-	-	-	88%
Received Reliever Medication	-	-	-	100%
Received Systemic Corticosteroids	-	-	-	100%
Emergency Department				
Admittance Decision Time (minutes)[2]	312	64	89	98
Head CT Results Within 45 Min. of Arrival	16	75%	64%	57%
Patients Who Left ER Before Being Seen	14,500	1%	3%	2%
Time from ER Arrival to Admit. (minutes)[2]	328	194	260	274

NOTE: Hospital profiles are in alphabetical order by state, then city, then hospital within the city; Rankings exclude hospitals with less than 25 cases except for patient surveys which excludes hospitals with less than 100 cases; (a) 100-299 cases; (1) The number of cases/patients is too few to report; (2) Data submitted were based on a sample of cases/patients; (3) Results are based on a shorter time period than required; (4) Data suppressed by CMS for one or more quarters; (5) Results are not available for this reporting period; (6) Fewer than 100 patients completed the HCAHPS survey; (7) No cases met the criteria for this measure; (8) The lower limit of the confidence interval cannot be calculated if the number of observed infections equals zero; (9) No data are available from the state/territory for this reporting period; (10) The scores shown reflect fewer than 50 completed surveys; (11) There were discrepancies in the data collection process; (12) This measure does not apply to this hospital for this reporting period; (13) Results cannot be calculated for this reporting period; (14) The results for this state are combined with nearby states to protect confidentiality; Please refer to the User's Guide for a full explanation of data.

Time from ER Arrival to Discharge (minutes)	383	91	138	134
Time in ER Before Being Evaluated (minutes)	423	15	28	26
Time to Pain Meds for Fractures (minutes)	73	31	52	57
Heart Attack Care				
Aspirin Given at Discharge[1,3]	-	-	99%	99%
Fibrinolytic Meds Within 30 Min. of Arrival[3,7]	-	-	33%	54%
PCI Within 90 Minutes of Arrival[3,7]	-	-	97%	96%
Statin Prescribed at Discharge[1,3]	-	-	98%	98%
Heart Failure Care				
ACE Inhibitor or ARB for LVSD	20	95%	98%	97%
Discharge Instructions Given	50	94%	96%	94%
Evaluation of LVS Function	71	100%	99%	99%
Medicare Spending				
Medicare Spending per Patient (ratio)	-	0.89	1	0.98
Pneumonia Care				
Appropriate Initial Antibiotic Given	48	98%	95%	95%
Blood Culture Timing	66	98%	98%	98%
Pregnancy and Delivery Care				
Newborn Deliveries Scheduled Early	24	0%	2%	6%
Preventive Care				
Immunization for Influenza[2]	267	95%	92%	90%
Immunization for Pneumonia[2]	328	93%	92%	92%
Stroke Care				
Anticoagulation Therapy for Atrial Fibrillation[1]	-	-	94%	95%
Antithrombotic Therapy Timing	11	100%	98%	98%
Assessed for Rehabilitation	15	100%	97%	97%
Discharged on Antithrombotic Therapy	13	100%	99%	99%
Discharged on Statin Medication[1]	-	-	94%	94%
Thrombolytic Therapy Timing[7]	-	-	66%	66%
Venous Thromboembolism Prophylaxis	13	92%	94%	94%
Written Stroke Educational Materials Given[1]	-	-	87%	88%
Surgical Care Improvement Project				
Appropriate Beta Blocker Usage	30	97%	98%	98%
Appropriate VTP Within 24 Hours	98	96%	98%	98%
Controlled Postoperative Blood Glucose[7]	-	-	97%	97%
Perioperative Temperature Management	113	100%	100%	100%
Prophylactic Antibiotic Selection	64	97%	99%	99%
Prophylactic Antibiotic Selection (Outpatient)	68	96%	98%	98%
Prophylactic Antibiotic Stopped	63	97%	98%	98%
Prophylactic Antibiotic Timing	64	92%	99%	99%
Prophylactic Antibiotic Timing (Outpatient)	72	89%	97%	98%
Urinary Catheter Removal	53	92%	98%	97%
Survey of Patients' Hospital Experiences				
Area Around Room 'Always' Quiet at Night	300+	65%	60%	61%
Doctors 'Always' Communicated Well	300+	83%	81%	82%
Home Recovery Information Given	300+	91%	86%	85%
Hospital Given 9 or 10 on 10 Point Scale	300+	68%	70%	71%
Meds 'Always' Explained Before Given	300+	66%	64%	64%
Nurses 'Always' Communicated Well	300+	86%	79%	79%
Pain 'Always' Well Controlled	300+	71%	71%	71%
Room and Bathroom 'Always' Clean	300+	84%	74%	73%
Timely Help 'Always' Received	300+	74%	67%	68%
Would Definitely Recommend Hospital	300+	68%	70%	71%
Use of Medical Imaging				
Cardiac Imaging Stress Test before Surgery	97	2.1%	5.5%	5.3%
Combination Abdominal CT Scan	360	60.6%	10.1%	10.5%
Combination Brain/Sinus CT Scan[1]	-	-	2.6%	2.7%
Combination Chest CT Scan	365	12.3%	2.8%	2.7%
Follow-up Mammogram/Ultrasound	600	7.3%	8.4%	8.8%
Lumbar Spine MRI for Low Back Pain	64	40.6%	36.6%	37.2%

Heartland Regional Medical Center

3333 W De Young
Marion, IL 62959
URL: www.heartlandregional.com
Type: Acute Care Hospitals
Ownership: Proprietary

Phone: 618-998-7000
Emergency Services: Yes
Beds: 92

Measure	Cases	This Hosp.	State Avg.	U.S. Avg.
Blood Clot Prevention and Treatment				
Anticoagulation Overlap Therapy[2]	33	100%	91%	93%
ICU Venous Thromboembolism Prophylaxis[2]	136	96%	93%	92%
Incidence of Potentially Preventable VTE[1,2]	-	-	11%	10%
UFH with Dosages/Platelet Monitoring[1,2]	-	-	94%	97%
Venous Thromboembolism Prophylaxis[2]	278	96%	86%	85%
Warfarin Therapy Discharge Instructions[2]	21	95%	71%	75%
Chest Pain/Possible Heart Attack Care				
Aspirin Given Within 24 Hours of Arrival[1,3]	-	-	96%	96%
Fibrinolytic Meds Within 30 Min. of Arrival[5]	-	-	65%	58%
Average Time to ECG (minutes)[1,3]	-	-	6	7
Average Time to Transfer (minutes)[5]	-	-	63	60
Children's Asthma Care				
Received Home Management Plan of Care	-	-	-	88%
Received Reliever Medication	-	-	-	100%
Received Systemic Corticosteroids	-	-	-	100%
Emergency Department				
Admittance Decision Time (minutes)[2]	430	95	89	98
Head CT Results Within 45 Min. of Arrival[1]	-	-	64%	57%
Patients Who Left ER Before Being Seen	17,954	2%	3%	2%
Time from ER Arrival to Admit. (minutes)[2]	587	228	260	274
Time from ER Arrival to Discharge (minutes)	369	116	138	134
Time in ER Before Being Evaluated (minutes)	414	18	28	26
Time to Pain Meds for Fractures (minutes)	65	63	52	57
Heart Attack Care				
Aspirin Given at Discharge	85	100%	99%	99%
Fibrinolytic Meds Within 30 Min. of Arrival[7]	-	-	33%	54%
PCI Within 90 Minutes of Arrival	16	94%	97%	96%
Statin Prescribed at Discharge	82	98%	98%	98%
Heart Failure Care				
ACE Inhibitor or ARB for LVSD	38	100%	98%	97%
Discharge Instructions Given	75	96%	96%	94%
Evaluation of LVS Function	98	100%	99%	99%
Medicare Spending				
Medicare Spending per Patient (ratio)	-	1.02	1	0.98
Pneumonia Care				
Appropriate Initial Antibiotic Given	49	90%	95%	95%
Blood Culture Timing	152	100%	98%	98%
Pregnancy and Delivery Care				
Newborn Deliveries Scheduled Early[2]	45	2%	2%	6%
Preventive Care				
Immunization for Influenza[2]	502	99%	92%	90%
Immunization for Pneumonia[2]	605	100%	92%	92%
Stroke Care				
Anticoagulation Therapy for Atrial Fibrillation[1]	-	-	94%	95%
Antithrombotic Therapy Timing	35	97%	98%	98%
Assessed for Rehabilitation	34	100%	97%	97%
Discharged on Antithrombotic Therapy	34	100%	99%	99%
Discharged on Statin Medication	24	96%	94%	94%
Thrombolytic Therapy Timing[1]	-	-	66%	66%
Venous Thromboembolism Prophylaxis	35	100%	94%	94%
Written Stroke Educational Materials Given	22	91%	87%	88%
Surgical Care Improvement Project				
Appropriate Beta Blocker Usage	84	98%	98%	98%
Appropriate VTP Within 24 Hours	241	100%	98%	98%
Controlled Postoperative Blood Glucose[1]	-	-	97%	97%
Perioperative Temperature Management	304	100%	100%	100%
Prophylactic Antibiotic Selection	200	100%	99%	99%
Prophylactic Antibiotic Selection (Outpatient)	78	99%	98%	98%
Prophylactic Antibiotic Stopped	186	96%	98%	98%
Prophylactic Antibiotic Timing	200	100%	99%	99%
Prophylactic Antibiotic Timing (Outpatient)	78	100%	97%	98%
Urinary Catheter Removal	138	96%	98%	97%
Survey of Patients' Hospital Experiences				
Area Around Room 'Always' Quiet at Night	300+	53%	60%	61%
Doctors 'Always' Communicated Well	300+	81%	81%	82%
Home Recovery Information Given	300+	85%	86%	85%
Hospital Given 9 or 10 on 10 Point Scale	300+	66%	70%	71%
Meds 'Always' Explained Before Given	300+	60%	64%	64%
Nurses 'Always' Communicated Well	300+	75%	79%	79%
Pain 'Always' Well Controlled	300+	66%	71%	71%
Room and Bathroom 'Always' Clean	300+	67%	74%	73%
Timely Help 'Always' Received	300+	64%	67%	68%
Would Definitely Recommend Hospital	300+	61%	70%	71%
Use of Medical Imaging				
Cardiac Imaging Stress Test before Surgery	291	7.6%	5.5%	5.3%
Combination Abdominal CT Scan	422	6.4%	10.1%	10.5%
Combination Brain/Sinus CT Scan	418	4.8%	2.6%	2.7%
Combination Chest CT Scan	325	0.9%	2.8%	2.7%
Follow-up Mammogram/Ultrasound	616	9.3%	8.4%	8.8%
Lumbar Spine MRI for Low Back Pain[1]	-	-	36.6%	37.2%

Marion II VA Medical Center

2401 West Main
Marion, IL 62959
Type: Acute Care - VA
Ownership: Government Federal

Phone: 618-997-5311
Fax: 618-998-5667
Emergency Services: No
Beds: 39

Key Personnel:
Operating Room. . . . . Debbie Bertramd
Infection Control. . . . . Jan Collins
Emergency Room . . . . Betty Dunbar
CEO/President. . . . . Arpakorn Kantatan, MD
Chief of Medical Staff . . . . Michael R. Ladwig
Intensive Care Unit. . . . . Cheryl Sherrill

Measure	Cases	This Hosp.	State Avg.	U.S. Avg.
Blood Clot Prevention and Treatment				
Anticoagulation Overlap Therapy	-	-	91%	93%
ICU Venous Thromboembolism Prophylaxis	-	-	93%	92%
Incidence of Potentially Preventable VTE	-	-	11%	10%
UFH with Dosages/Platelet Monitoring	-	-	94%	97%
Venous Thromboembolism Prophylaxis	-	-	86%	85%
Warfarin Therapy Discharge Instructions	-	-	71%	75%
Chest Pain/Possible Heart Attack Care				
Aspirin Given Within 24 Hours of Arrival	-	-	96%	96%
Fibrinolytic Meds Within 30 Min. of Arrival	-	-	65%	58%
Average Time to ECG (minutes)	-	-	6	7
Average Time to Transfer (minutes)	-	-	63	60
Children's Asthma Care				
Received Home Management Plan of Care	-	-	-	88%
Received Reliever Medication	-	-	-	100%
Received Systemic Corticosteroids	-	-	-	100%
Emergency Department				
Admittance Decision Time (minutes)	-	-	89	98
Head CT Results Within 45 Min. of Arrival	-	-	64%	57%
Patients Who Left ER Before Being Seen	-	-	3%	2%
Time from ER Arrival to Admit. (minutes)	-	-	260	274
Time from ER Arrival to Discharge (minutes)	-	-	138	134
Time in ER Before Being Evaluated (minutes)	-	-	28	26
Time to Pain Meds for Fractures (minutes)	-	-	52	57
Heart Attack Care				
Aspirin Given at Discharge[5]	-	-	99%	99%
Fibrinolytic Meds Within 30 Min. of Arrival[5]	-	-	33%	54%
PCI Within 90 Minutes of Arrival[5]	-	-	97%	96%
Statin Prescribed at Discharge[5]	-	-	98%	98%
Heart Failure Care				
ACE Inhibitor or ARB for LVSD[1]	24	79%	98%	97%
Discharge Instructions Given	72	97%	96%	94%
Evaluation of LVS Function	80	98%	99%	99%
Medicare Spending				
Medicare Spending per Patient (ratio)	-	-	1	0.98
Pneumonia Care				
Appropriate Initial Antibiotic Given	25	96%	95%	95%
Blood Culture Timing	49	100%	98%	98%
Pregnancy and Delivery Care				
Newborn Deliveries Scheduled Early	-	-	2%	6%
Preventive Care				
Immunization for Influenza[2,3]	134	80%	92%	90%
Immunization for Pneumonia[2,3]	330	92%	92%	92%
Stroke Care				
Anticoagulation Therapy for Atrial Fibrillation	-	-	94%	95%
Antithrombotic Therapy Timing	-	-	98%	98%
Assessed for Rehabilitation	-	-	97%	97%
Discharged on Antithrombotic Therapy	-	-	99%	99%
Discharged on Statin Medication	-	-	94%	94%
Thrombolytic Therapy Timing	-	-	66%	66%
Venous Thromboembolism Prophylaxis	-	-	94%	94%
Written Stroke Educational Materials Given	-	-	87%	88%
Surgical Care Improvement Project				
Appropriate Beta Blocker Usage[5]	-	-	98%	98%
Appropriate VTP Within 24 Hours[5]	-	-	98%	98%

NOTE: Hospital profiles are in alphabetical order by state, then city, then hospital within the city; Rankings exclude hospitals with less than 25 cases except for patient surveys which excludes hospitals with less than 100 cases; (a) 100-299 cases; (1) The number of cases/patients is too few to report; (2) Data submitted were based on a sample of cases/patients; (3) Results are based on a shorter time period than required; (4) Data suppressed by CMS for one or more quarters; (5) Results are not available for this reporting period; (6) Fewer than 100 patients completed the HCAHPS survey; (7) No cases met the criteria for this measure; (8) The lower limit of the confidence interval cannot be calculated if the number of observed infections equals zero; (9) No data are available from the state/territory for this reporting period; (10) The scores shown reflect fewer than 50 completed surveys; (11) There were discrepancies in the data collection process; (12) This measure does not apply to this hospital for this reporting period; (13) Results cannot be calculated for this reporting period; (14) The results for this state are combined with nearby states to protect confidentiality; Please refer to the User's Guide for a full explanation of data.

Controlled Postoperative Blood Glucose[5]	-	-	97%	97%
Perioperative Temperature Management[5]	-	-	100%	100%
Prophylactic Antibiotic Selection[5]	-	-	99%	99%
Prophylactic Antibiotic Selection (Outpatient)	-	-	98%	98%
Prophylactic Antibiotic Stopped[5]	-	-	98%	98%
Prophylactic Antibiotic Timing[5]	-	-	99%	99%
Prophylactic Antibiotic Timing (Outpatient)	-	-	97%	98%
Urinary Catheter Removal[5]	-	-	98%	97%
Survey of Patients' Hospital Experiences				
Area Around Room 'Always' Quiet at Night	-	-	60%	61%
Doctors 'Always' Communicated Well	-	-	81%	82%
Home Recovery Information Given	-	-	86%	85%
Hospital Given 9 or 10 on 10 Point Scale	-	-	70%	71%
Meds 'Always' Explained Before Given	-	-	64%	64%
Nurses 'Always' Communicated Well	-	-	79%	79%
Pain 'Always' Well Controlled	-	-	71%	71%
Room and Bathroom 'Always' Clean	-	-	74%	73%
Timely Help 'Always' Received	-	-	67%	68%
Would Definitely Recommend Hospital	-	-	70%	71%
Use of Medical Imaging				
Cardiac Imaging Stress Test before Surgery	-	-	5.5%	5.3%
Combination Abdominal CT Scan	-	-	10.1%	10.5%
Combination Brain/Sinus CT Scan	-	-	2.6%	2.7%
Combination Chest CT Scan	-	-	2.8%	2.7%
Follow-up Mammogram/Ultrasound	-	-	8.4%	8.8%
Lumbar Spine MRI for Low Back Pain	-	-	36.6%	37.2%

Anderson Hospital

6800 State Route 162
Maryville, IL 62062
Phone: 618-288-5711
Fax: 618-288-4088
URL: www.andersonhospital.org
Type: Acute Care Hospitals
Emergency Services: Yes
Ownership: Voluntary non-profit - Private
Beds: 130

Key Personnel:
Pediatric Ambulatory Care ...... Lizabeth Didriksen, MD
Pediatric In-Patient Care ...... Lizabeth Didriksen, MD
Infection Control.............. Doris Driscoll, RN
Chief of Medical Staff........... Rod Greeling, MD
CEO/President............... Keith Page
Quality Assurance .... Dolores Phelps
Operating Room.............. Scott A Wong, RN

Measure	Cases	This Hosp.	State Avg.	U.S. Avg.
Blood Clot Prevention and Treatment				
Anticoagulation Overlap Therapy[2]	40	82%	91%	93%
ICU Venous Thromboembolism Prophylaxis[2]	48	73%	93%	92%
Incidence of Potentially Preventable VTE[2]	11	27%	11%	10%
UFH with Dosages/Platelet Monitoring[2]	18	94%	94%	97%
Venous Thromboembolism Prophylaxis[2]	328	73%	86%	85%
Warfarin Therapy Discharge Instructions[2]	24	25%	71%	75%
Chest Pain/Possible Heart Attack Care				
Aspirin Given Within 24 Hours of Arrival	29	93%	96%	96%
Fibrinolytic Meds Within 30 Min. of Arrival[3,7]	-	-	65%	58%
Average Time to ECG (minutes)	29	4	6	7
Average Time to Transfer (minutes)[1,3]	-	-	63	60
Children's Asthma Care				
Received Home Management Plan of Care	-	-	-	88%
Received Reliever Medication	-	-	-	100%
Received Systemic Corticosteroids	-	-	-	100%
Emergency Department				
Admittance Decision Time (minutes)[2]	453	81	89	98
Head CT Results Within 45 Min. of Arrival	37	70%	64%	57%
Patients Who Left ER Before Being Seen	34,962	2%	3%	2%
Time from ER Arrival to Admit. (minutes)[2]	477	254	260	274
Time from ER Arrival to Discharge (minutes)	373	135	138	134
Time in ER Before Being Evaluated (minutes)	408	40	28	26
Time to Pain Meds for Fractures (minutes)	190	58	52	57
Heart Attack Care				
Aspirin Given at Discharge	105	99%	99%	99%
Fibrinolytic Meds Within 30 Min. of Arrival[7]	-	-	33%	54%
PCI Within 90 Minutes of Arrival	33	91%	97%	96%
Statin Prescribed at Discharge	106	93%	98%	98%
Heart Failure Care				
ACE Inhibitor or ARB for LVSD[2]	72	92%	98%	97%
Discharge Instructions Given[2]	183	93%	96%	94%
Evaluation of LVS Function[2]	264	100%	99%	99%
Medicare Spending				
Medicare Spending per Patient (ratio)	-	0.95	1	0.98
Pneumonia Care				
Appropriate Initial Antibiotic Given[2]	104	95%	95%	95%
Blood Culture Timing[2]	170	98%	98%	98%
Pregnancy and Delivery Care				
Newborn Deliveries Scheduled Early[2]	39	5%	2%	6%
Preventive Care				
Immunization for Influenza[2]	467	94%	92%	90%
Immunization for Pneumonia[2]	517	94%	92%	92%
Stroke Care				
Anticoagulation Therapy for Atrial Fibrillation[1]	-	-	94%	95%
Antithrombotic Therapy Timing	54	98%	98%	98%
Assessed for Rehabilitation	59	92%	97%	97%
Discharged on Antithrombotic Therapy	59	100%	99%	99%
Discharged on Statin Medication	49	67%	94%	94%
Thrombolytic Therapy Timing[1]	-	-	66%	66%
Venous Thromboembolism Prophylaxis	52	67%	94%	94%
Written Stroke Educational Materials Given	27	22%	87%	88%
Surgical Care Improvement Project				
Appropriate Beta Blocker Usage[2]	125	94%	98%	98%
Appropriate VTP Within 24 Hours[2]	364	94%	98%	98%
Controlled Postoperative Blood Glucose[2,7]	-	-	97%	97%
Perioperative Temperature Management[2]	410	100%	100%	100%
Prophylactic Antibiotic Selection[2]	272	99%	99%	99%
Prophylactic Antibiotic Selection (Outpatient)	319	99%	98%	98%
Prophylactic Antibiotic Stopped[2]	268	97%	98%	98%
Prophylactic Antibiotic Timing[2]	272	98%	99%	99%
Prophylactic Antibiotic Timing (Outpatient)	321	99%	97%	98%
Urinary Catheter Removal[2]	154	94%	98%	97%
Survey of Patients' Hospital Experiences				
Area Around Room 'Always' Quiet at Night	300+	61%	60%	61%
Doctors 'Always' Communicated Well	300+	85%	81%	82%
Home Recovery Information Given	300+	89%	86%	85%
Hospital Given 9 or 10 on 10 Point Scale	300+	74%	70%	71%
Meds 'Always' Explained Before Given	300+	65%	64%	64%
Nurses 'Always' Communicated Well	300+	81%	79%	79%
Pain 'Always' Well Controlled	300+	75%	71%	71%
Room and Bathroom 'Always' Clean	300+	76%	74%	73%
Timely Help 'Always' Received	300+	73%	67%	68%
Would Definitely Recommend Hospital	300+	75%	70%	71%
Use of Medical Imaging				
Cardiac Imaging Stress Test before Surgery	151	6.6%	5.5%	5.3%
Combination Abdominal CT Scan	770	3.0%	10.1%	10.5%
Combination Brain/Sinus CT Scan	760	4.9%	2.6%	2.7%
Combination Chest CT Scan	580	0.0%	2.8%	2.7%
Follow-up Mammogram/Ultrasound	978	12.1%	8.4%	8.8%
Lumbar Spine MRI for Low Back Pain	127	33.9%	36.6%	37.2%

Sarah Bush Lincoln Health Center

1000 Health Center Drive PO Box 372
Mattoon, IL 61938
Phone: 217-258-2572
Fax: 217-258-2111
E-mail: jpierce@sblhs.org
Type: Acute Care Hospitals
Emergency Services: Yes
Ownership: Voluntary non-profit - Private
Beds: 202

Key Personnel:
Radiology..................... Jon Banas, DO
CEO/President................. Gary L Barnett
Chief of Medical Staff.......... Dr Joseph Burton
Quality Assurance .... Cheryl Creasy, RN
Operating Room.............. Carol Ray
Pediatric Ambulatory Care .... Thomas Snowden, MD
Pediatric In-Patient Care .... Thomas Snowden, MD
Infection Control............... Ramona Tomshack

Measure	Cases	This Hosp.	State Avg.	U.S. Avg.
Blood Clot Prevention and Treatment				
Anticoagulation Overlap Therapy[2]	40	85%	91%	93%
ICU Venous Thromboembolism Prophylaxis[2]	53	92%	93%	92%
Incidence of Potentially Preventable VTE[1,2]	-	-	11%	10%
UFH with Dosages/Platelet Monitoring[1,2]	-	-	94%	97%
Venous Thromboembolism Prophylaxis[2]	345	78%	86%	85%
Warfarin Therapy Discharge Instructions[2]	30	60%	71%	75%
Chest Pain/Possible Heart Attack Care				
Aspirin Given Within 24 Hours of Arrival	108	97%	96%	96%
Fibrinolytic Meds Within 30 Min. of Arrival[1]	-	-	65%	58%
Average Time to ECG (minutes)	111	2	6	7
Average Time to Transfer (minutes)	23	65	63	60
Children's Asthma Care				
Received Home Management Plan of Care	-	-	-	88%
Received Reliever Medication	-	-	-	100%
Received Systemic Corticosteroids	-	-	-	100%
Emergency Department				
Admittance Decision Time (minutes)[2]	577	78	89	98
Head CT Results Within 45 Min. of Arrival	21	24%	64%	57%
Patients Who Left ER Before Being Seen	38,559	2%	3%	2%
Time from ER Arrival to Admit. (minutes)[2]	598	218	260	274
Time from ER Arrival to Discharge (minutes)	311	123	138	134
Time in ER Before Being Evaluated (minutes)	342	14	28	26
Time to Pain Meds for Fractures (minutes)	117	31	52	57
Heart Attack Care				
Aspirin Given at Discharge	46	100%	99%	99%
Fibrinolytic Meds Within 30 Min. of Arrival[7]	-	-	33%	54%
PCI Within 90 Minutes of Arrival[7]	-	-	97%	96%
Statin Prescribed at Discharge	46	100%	98%	98%
Heart Failure Care				
ACE Inhibitor or ARB for LVSD	58	100%	98%	97%
Discharge Instructions Given	174	100%	96%	94%
Evaluation of LVS Function	249	100%	99%	99%
Medicare Spending				
Medicare Spending per Patient (ratio)	-	0.94	1	0.98
Pneumonia Care				
Appropriate Initial Antibiotic Given	126	97%	95%	95%
Blood Culture Timing	171	98%	98%	98%
Pregnancy and Delivery Care				
Newborn Deliveries Scheduled Early	120	1%	2%	6%
Preventive Care				
Immunization for Influenza[2]	509	85%	92%	90%
Immunization for Pneumonia[2]	659	93%	92%	92%
Stroke Care				
Anticoagulation Therapy for Atrial Fibrillation[1]	-	-	94%	95%
Antithrombotic Therapy Timing	36	86%	98%	98%
Assessed for Rehabilitation	47	77%	97%	97%
Discharged on Antithrombotic Therapy	43	100%	99%	99%
Discharged on Statin Medication	42	71%	94%	94%
Thrombolytic Therapy Timing[1]	-	-	66%	66%
Venous Thromboembolism Prophylaxis	38	84%	94%	94%
Written Stroke Educational Materials Given	31	32%	87%	88%
Surgical Care Improvement Project				
Appropriate Beta Blocker Usage	137	100%	98%	98%
Appropriate VTP Within 24 Hours	500	98%	98%	98%
Controlled Postoperative Blood Glucose[7]	-	-	97%	97%
Perioperative Temperature Management	576	100%	100%	100%
Prophylactic Antibiotic Selection	420	100%	99%	99%
Prophylactic Antibiotic Selection (Outpatient)	74	95%	98%	98%
Prophylactic Antibiotic Stopped	398	98%	98%	98%
Prophylactic Antibiotic Timing	420	99%	99%	99%
Prophylactic Antibiotic Timing (Outpatient)	75	95%	97%	98%
Urinary Catheter Removal	259	99%	98%	97%
Survey of Patients' Hospital Experiences				
Area Around Room 'Always' Quiet at Night	300+	59%	60%	61%
Doctors 'Always' Communicated Well	300+	87%	81%	82%
Home Recovery Information Given	300+	90%	86%	85%
Hospital Given 9 or 10 on 10 Point Scale	300+	77%	70%	71%
Meds 'Always' Explained Before Given	300+	70%	64%	64%
Nurses 'Always' Communicated Well	300+	85%	79%	79%
Pain 'Always' Well Controlled	300+	72%	71%	71%
Room and Bathroom 'Always' Clean	300+	75%	74%	73%
Timely Help 'Always' Received	300+	70%	67%	68%
Would Definitely Recommend Hospital	300+	73%	70%	71%
Use of Medical Imaging				
Cardiac Imaging Stress Test before Surgery	610	5.2%	5.5%	5.3%
Combination Abdominal CT Scan	1,035	4.3%	10.1%	10.5%
Combination Brain/Sinus CT Scan	915	2.2%	2.6%	2.7%
Combination Chest CT Scan	486	0.0%	2.8%	2.7%
Follow-up Mammogram/Ultrasound	1,510	3.0%	8.4%	8.8%

NOTE: Hospital profiles are in alphabetical order by state, then city, then hospital within the city; Rankings exclude hospitals with less than 25 cases except for patient surveys which excludes hospitals with less than 100 cases; (a) 100-299 cases; (1) The number of cases/patients is too few to report; (2) Data submitted were based on a sample of cases/patients; (3) Results are based on a shorter time period than required; (4) Data suppressed by CMS for one or more quarters; (5) Results are not available for this reporting period; (6) Fewer than 100 patients completed the HCAHPS survey; (7) No cases met the criteria for this measure; (8) The lower limit of the confidence interval cannot be calculated if the number of observed infections equals zero; (9) No data are available from the state/territory for this reporting period; (10) The scores shown reflect fewer than 50 completed surveys; (11) There were discrepancies in the data collection process; (12) This measure does not apply to this hospital for this reporting period; (13) Results cannot be calculated for this reporting period; (14) The results for this state are combined with nearby states to protect confidentiality; Please refer to the User's Guide for a full explanation of data.

Measure	Cases	This Hosp.	State Avg.	U.S. Avg.
Lumbar Spine MRI for Low Back Pain	227	29.5%	36.6%	37.2%

Loyola University Medical Center

2160 S 1st Avenue
Maywood, IL 60153
URL: www.lumc.edu
Phone: 708-216-9000
Fax: 708-216-5690
Type: Acute Care Hospitals
Emergency Services: Yes
Ownership: Voluntary non-profit - Private
Beds: 589

Key Personnel:
CEO/President. . . . . Anthony L Barbato, MD
Quality Assurance . . . . Paul C. Kuo, MD, MBA, FACS
Radiology. . . . . Scott A. Mirowitz, MD, MMM, FACR,
Infection Control. . . . . Paul O'Keefe, MD
Pediatric Ambulatory Care . . . . . . Jerold M. Stirling, MD, FAAP
Chief of Medical Staff. . . . . Leonard L Vertuno, MD
Operating Room. . . . . Margaret Vorrier
Cardiac Laboratory. . . . . David Wilber

Measure	Cases	This Hosp.	State Avg.	U.S. Avg.
Blood Clot Prevention and Treatment				
Anticoagulation Overlap Therapy[2]	127	98%	91%	93%
ICU Venous Thromboembolism Prophylaxis[2]	107	90%	93%	92%
Incidence of Potentially Preventable VTE[2]	35	6%	11%	10%
UFH with Dosages/Platelet Monitoring[2]	109	100%	94%	97%
Venous Thromboembolism Prophylaxis[2]	261	90%	86%	85%
Warfarin Therapy Discharge Instructions[2]	93	30%	71%	75%
Chest Pain/Possible Heart Attack Care				
Aspirin Given Within 24 Hours of Arrival[5]	-	-	96%	96%
Fibrinolytic Meds Within 30 Min. of Arrival[5]	-	-	65%	58%
Average Time to ECG (minutes)[5]	-	-	6	7
Average Time to Transfer (minutes)[5]	-	-	63	60
Children's Asthma Care				
Received Home Management Plan of Care	167	90%	-	88%
Received Reliever Medication	169	100%	-	100%
Received Systemic Corticosteroids	167	100%	-	100%
Emergency Department				
Admittance Decision Time (minutes)[2]	383	170	89	98
Head CT Results Within 45 Min. of Arrival[5]	-	-	64%	57%
Patients Who Left ER Before Being Seen	48,828	4%	3%	2%
Time from ER Arrival to Admit. (minutes)[2]	388	385	260	274
Time from ER Arrival to Discharge (minutes)	308	161	138	134
Time in ER Before Being Evaluated (minutes)	356	53	28	26
Time to Pain Meds for Fractures (minutes)	101	88	52	57
Heart Attack Care				
Aspirin Given at Discharge	224	100%	99%	99%
Fibrinolytic Meds Within 30 Min. of Arrival[7]	-	-	33%	54%
PCI Within 90 Minutes of Arrival	24	96%	97%	96%
Statin Prescribed at Discharge	231	100%	98%	98%
Heart Failure Care				
ACE Inhibitor or ARB for LVSD	212	100%	98%	97%
Discharge Instructions Given	435	100%	96%	94%
Evaluation of LVS Function	485	100%	99%	99%
Medicare Spending				
Medicare Spending per Patient (ratio)	-	0.98	1	0.98
Pneumonia Care				
Appropriate Initial Antibiotic Given	97	96%	95%	95%
Blood Culture Timing	223	100%	98%	98%
Pregnancy and Delivery Care				
Newborn Deliveries Scheduled Early	55	0%	2%	6%
Preventive Care				
Immunization for Influenza[2]	521	90%	92%	90%
Immunization for Pneumonia[2]	520	89%	92%	92%
Stroke Care				
Anticoagulation Therapy for Atrial Fibrillation[2]	23	91%	94%	95%
Antithrombotic Therapy Timing[2]	63	98%	98%	98%
Assessed for Rehabilitation[2]	104	97%	97%	97%
Discharged on Antithrombotic Therapy[2]	81	100%	99%	99%
Discharged on Statin Medication[2]	67	99%	94%	94%
Thrombolytic Therapy Timing[1,2]	-	-	66%	66%
Venous Thromboembolism Prophylaxis[2]	99	97%	94%	94%
Written Stroke Educational Materials Given[2]	69	94%	87%	88%
Surgical Care Improvement Project				
Appropriate Beta Blocker Usage[2]	246	100%	98%	98%
Appropriate VTP Within 24 Hours[2]	337	100%	98%	98%
Controlled Postoperative Blood Glucose[2]	132	86%	97%	97%
Perioperative Temperature Management[2]	438	100%	100%	100%
Prophylactic Antibiotic Selection[2]	372	100%	99%	99%
Prophylactic Antibiotic Selection (Outpatient)	523	98%	98%	98%
Prophylactic Antibiotic Stopped[2]	364	98%	98%	98%
Prophylactic Antibiotic Timing[2]	372	99%	99%	99%
Prophylactic Antibiotic Timing (Outpatient)	400	98%	97%	98%
Urinary Catheter Removal[2]	303	98%	98%	97%
Survey of Patients' Hospital Experiences				
Area Around Room 'Always' Quiet at Night	300+	51%	60%	61%
Doctors 'Always' Communicated Well	300+	79%	81%	82%
Home Recovery Information Given	300+	86%	86%	85%
Hospital Given 9 or 10 on 10 Point Scale	300+	69%	70%	71%
Meds 'Always' Explained Before Given	300+	60%	64%	64%
Nurses 'Always' Communicated Well	300+	76%	79%	79%
Pain 'Always' Well Controlled	300+	69%	71%	71%
Room and Bathroom 'Always' Clean	300+	62%	74%	73%
Timely Help 'Always' Received	300+	62%	67%	68%
Would Definitely Recommend Hospital	300+	72%	70%	71%
Use of Medical Imaging				
Cardiac Imaging Stress Test before Surgery	1,626	5.7%	5.5%	5.3%
Combination Abdominal CT Scan	2,739	13.1%	10.1%	10.5%
Combination Brain/Sinus CT Scan	963	1.8%	2.6%	2.7%
Combination Chest CT Scan	2,786	0.6%	2.8%	2.7%
Follow-up Mammogram/Ultrasound	3,118	6.7%	8.4%	8.8%
Lumbar Spine MRI for Low Back Pain	258	37.6%	36.6%	37.2%

Centegra Health System - Mc Henry Hospital

4201 Medical Center Drive
Mchenry, IL 60050
URL: www.centegra.org
Phone: 815-344-5000
Fax: 815-759-8094
Type: Acute Care Hospitals
Emergency Services: Yes
Ownership: Voluntary non-profit - Other
Beds: 196

Key Personnel:
CEO . . . . Michael S Eesley
Infection Control. . . . . Pat Kinney
Chief of Medical Staff . . . . Z Thaddeus Lorenc, MD
Emergency Room . . . . Amy Moerschbaecher
President. . . . . Jason Sciarro
Quality Assurance . . . . Aaron Shepley

Measure	Cases	This Hosp.	State Avg.	U.S. Avg.
Blood Clot Prevention and Treatment				
Anticoagulation Overlap Therapy[2]	77	88%	91%	93%
ICU Venous Thromboembolism Prophylaxis[2]	80	91%	93%	92%
Incidence of Potentially Preventable VTE[1,2]	-	-	11%	10%
UFH with Dosages/Platelet Monitoring[2]	66	100%	94%	97%
Venous Thromboembolism Prophylaxis[2]	333	83%	86%	85%
Warfarin Therapy Discharge Instructions[2]	56	62%	71%	75%
Chest Pain/Possible Heart Attack Care				
Aspirin Given Within 24 Hours of Arrival[5]	-	-	96%	96%
Fibrinolytic Meds Within 30 Min. of Arrival[5]	-	-	65%	58%
Average Time to ECG (minutes)[5]	-	-	6	7
Average Time to Transfer (minutes)[5]	-	-	63	60
Children's Asthma Care				
Received Home Management Plan of Care	-	-	-	88%
Received Reliever Medication	-	-	-	100%
Received Systemic Corticosteroids	-	-	-	100%
Emergency Department				
Admittance Decision Time (minutes)[2]	577	111	89	98
Head CT Results Within 45 Min. of Arrival	12	42%	64%	57%
Patients Who Left ER Before Being Seen	37,712	2%	3%	2%
Time from ER Arrival to Admit. (minutes)[2]	616	295	260	274
Time from ER Arrival to Discharge (minutes)	373	168	138	134
Time in ER Before Being Evaluated (minutes)	405	45	28	26
Time to Pain Meds for Fractures (minutes)	143	78	52	57
Heart Attack Care				
Aspirin Given at Discharge	310	99%	99%	99%
Fibrinolytic Meds Within 30 Min. of Arrival[7]	-	-	33%	54%
PCI Within 90 Minutes of Arrival	51	94%	97%	96%
Statin Prescribed at Discharge	295	99%	98%	98%
Heart Failure Care				
ACE Inhibitor or ARB for LVSD	82	100%	98%	97%
Discharge Instructions Given	191	94%	96%	94%
Evaluation of LVS Function	249	100%	99%	99%
Medicare Spending				
Medicare Spending per Patient (ratio)	-	1.02	1	0.98
Pneumonia Care				
Appropriate Initial Antibiotic Given[2]	103	98%	95%	95%
Blood Culture Timing[2]	165	99%	98%	98%
Pregnancy and Delivery Care				
Newborn Deliveries Scheduled Early	75	4%	2%	6%
Preventive Care				
Immunization for Influenza[2]	588	96%	92%	90%
Immunization for Pneumonia[2]	773	97%	92%	92%
Stroke Care				
Anticoagulation Therapy for Atrial Fibrillation	13	100%	94%	95%
Antithrombotic Therapy Timing	78	96%	98%	98%
Assessed for Rehabilitation	92	99%	97%	97%
Discharged on Antithrombotic Therapy	79	100%	99%	99%
Discharged on Statin Medication	62	100%	94%	94%
Thrombolytic Therapy Timing[1]	-	-	66%	66%
Venous Thromboembolism Prophylaxis	97	98%	94%	94%
Written Stroke Educational Materials Given	54	94%	87%	88%
Surgical Care Improvement Project				
Appropriate Beta Blocker Usage[2]	267	98%	98%	98%
Appropriate VTP Within 24 Hours[2]	506	98%	98%	98%
Controlled Postoperative Blood Glucose[2]	96	94%	97%	97%
Perioperative Temperature Management[2]	617	100%	100%	100%
Prophylactic Antibiotic Selection[2]	542	99%	99%	99%
Prophylactic Antibiotic Selection (Outpatient)	125	99%	98%	98%
Prophylactic Antibiotic Stopped[2]	532	98%	98%	98%
Prophylactic Antibiotic Timing[2]	542	100%	99%	99%
Prophylactic Antibiotic Timing (Outpatient)	122	99%	97%	98%
Urinary Catheter Removal[2]	500	99%	98%	97%
Survey of Patients' Hospital Experiences				
Area Around Room 'Always' Quiet at Night	300+	47%	60%	61%
Doctors 'Always' Communicated Well	300+	79%	81%	82%
Home Recovery Information Given	300+	89%	86%	85%
Hospital Given 9 or 10 on 10 Point Scale	300+	67%	70%	71%
Meds 'Always' Explained Before Given	300+	61%	64%	64%
Nurses 'Always' Communicated Well	300+	79%	79%	79%
Pain 'Always' Well Controlled	300+	70%	71%	71%
Room and Bathroom 'Always' Clean	300+	74%	74%	73%
Timely Help 'Always' Received	300+	70%	67%	68%
Would Definitely Recommend Hospital	300+	67%	70%	71%
Use of Medical Imaging				
Cardiac Imaging Stress Test before Surgery	675	6.7%	5.5%	5.3%
Combination Abdominal CT Scan	987	7.7%	10.1%	10.5%
Combination Brain/Sinus CT Scan	849	3.5%	2.6%	2.7%
Combination Chest CT Scan	744	3.8%	2.8%	2.7%
Follow-up Mammogram/Ultrasound	2,156	8.1%	8.4%	8.8%
Lumbar Spine MRI for Low Back Pain	198	41.9%	36.6%	37.2%

Hamilton Memorial Hospital District

611 S Marshall Avenue
Mcleansboro, IL 62859
URL: www.mcleansboro.com
Phone: 618-643-2361
Fax: 618-643-2875
Type: Critical Access Hospitals
Emergency Services: Yes
Ownership: Govt - Hospital Dist/Auth
Beds: 85

Key Personnel:
CEO/President. . . . . Randall W Dauby

Measure	Cases	This Hosp.	State Avg.	U.S. Avg.
Blood Clot Prevention and Treatment				
Anticoagulation Overlap Therapy[5]	-	-	91%	93%
ICU Venous Thromboembolism Prophylaxis[5]	-	-	93%	92%
Incidence of Potentially Preventable VTE[5]	-	-	11%	10%
UFH with Dosages/Platelet Monitoring[5]	-	-	94%	97%
Venous Thromboembolism Prophylaxis[5]	-	-	86%	85%
Warfarin Therapy Discharge Instructions[5]	-	-	71%	75%
Chest Pain/Possible Heart Attack Care				
Aspirin Given Within 24 Hours of Arrival	-	-	96%	96%
Fibrinolytic Meds Within 30 Min. of Arrival	-	-	65%	58%
Average Time to ECG (minutes)	-	-	6	7
Average Time to Transfer (minutes)	-	-	63	60
Children's Asthma Care				
Received Home Management Plan of Care	-	-	-	88%
Received Reliever Medication	-	-	-	100%

NOTE: Hospital profiles are in alphabetical order by state, then city, then hospital within the city; Rankings exclude hospitals with less than 25 cases except for patient surveys which excludes hospitals with less than 100 cases; (a) 100-299 cases; (1) The number of cases/patients is too few to report; (2) Data submitted were based on a sample of cases/patients; (3) Results are based on a shorter time period than required; (4) Data suppressed by CMS for one or more quarters; (5) Results are not available for this reporting period; (6) Fewer than 100 patients completed the HCAHPS survey; (7) No cases met the criteria for this measure; (8) The lower limit of the confidence interval cannot be calculated if the number of observed infections equals zero; (9) No data are available from the state/territory for this reporting period; (10) The scores shown reflect fewer than 50 completed surveys; (11) There were discrepancies in the data collection process; (12) This measure does not apply to this hospital for this reporting period; (13) Results cannot be calculated for this reporting period; (14) The results for this state are combined with nearby states to protect confidentiality; Please refer to the User's Guide for a full explanation of data.

Measure	Cases	This Hosp.	State Avg.	U.S. Avg.
Received Systemic Corticosteroids	-	-	-	100%
Emergency Department				
Admittance Decision Time (minutes)[5]	-	-	89	98
Head CT Results Within 45 Min. of Arrival	-	-	64%	57%
Patients Who Left ER Before Being Seen	-	-	3%	2%
Time from ER Arrival to Admit. (minutes)[5]	-	-	260	274
Time from ER Arrival to Discharge (minutes)	-	-	138	134
Time in ER Before Being Evaluated (minutes)	-	-	28	26
Time to Pain Meds for Fractures (minutes)	-	-	52	57
Heart Attack Care				
Aspirin Given at Discharge[5]	-	-	99%	99%
Fibrinolytic Meds Within 30 Min. of Arrival[5]	-	-	33%	54%
PCI Within 90 Minutes of Arrival[5]	-	-	97%	96%
Statin Prescribed at Discharge[5]	-	-	98%	98%
Heart Failure Care				
ACE Inhibitor or ARB for LVSD[1]	-	-	98%	97%
Discharge Instructions Given	19	100%	96%	94%
Evaluation of LVS Function	25	96%	99%	99%
Medicare Spending				
Medicare Spending per Patient (ratio)	-	-	1	0.98
Pneumonia Care				
Appropriate Initial Antibiotic Given	16	75%	95%	95%
Blood Culture Timing	23	100%	98%	98%
Pregnancy and Delivery Care				
Newborn Deliveries Scheduled Early[5]	-	-	2%	6%
Preventive Care				
Immunization for Influenza[5]	-	-	92%	90%
Immunization for Pneumonia[5]	-	-	92%	92%
Stroke Care				
Anticoagulation Therapy for Atrial Fibrillation[5]	-	-	94%	95%
Antithrombotic Therapy Timing[5]	-	-	98%	98%
Assessed for Rehabilitation[5]	-	-	97%	97%
Discharged on Antithrombotic Therapy[5]	-	-	99%	99%
Discharged on Statin Medication[5]	-	-	94%	94%
Thrombolytic Therapy Timing[5]	-	-	66%	66%
Venous Thromboembolism Prophylaxis[5]	-	-	94%	94%
Written Stroke Educational Materials Given[5]	-	-	87%	88%
Surgical Care Improvement Project				
Appropriate Beta Blocker Usage[3,7]	-	-	98%	98%
Appropriate VTP Within 24 Hours[1,3]	-	-	98%	98%
Controlled Postoperative Blood Glucose[3,7]	-	-	97%	97%
Perioperative Temperature Management[1,3]	-	-	100%	100%
Prophylactic Antibiotic Selection[1,3]	-	-	99%	99%
Prophylactic Antibiotic Selection (Outpatient)	-	-	98%	98%
Prophylactic Antibiotic Stopped[1,3]	-	-	98%	98%
Prophylactic Antibiotic Timing[1,3]	-	-	99%	99%
Prophylactic Antibiotic Timing (Outpatient)	-	-	97%	98%
Urinary Catheter Removal[1,3]	-	-	98%	97%
Survey of Patients' Hospital Experiences				
Area Around Room 'Always' Quiet at Night[5]	-	-	60%	61%
Doctors 'Always' Communicated Well[5]	-	-	81%	82%
Home Recovery Information Given[5]	-	-	86%	85%
Hospital Given 9 or 10 on 10 Point Scale[5]	-	-	70%	71%
Meds 'Always' Explained Before Given[5]	-	-	64%	64%
Nurses 'Always' Communicated Well[5]	-	-	79%	79%
Pain 'Always' Well Controlled[5]	-	-	71%	71%
Room and Bathroom 'Always' Clean[5]	-	-	74%	73%
Timely Help 'Always' Received[5]	-	-	67%	68%
Would Definitely Recommend Hospital[5]	-	-	70%	71%
Use of Medical Imaging				
Cardiac Imaging Stress Test before Surgery	-	-	5.5%	5.3%
Combination Abdominal CT Scan	-	-	10.1%	10.5%
Combination Brain/Sinus CT Scan	-	-	2.6%	2.7%
Combination Chest CT Scan	-	-	2.8%	2.7%
Follow-up Mammogram/Ultrasound	-	-	8.4%	8.8%
Lumbar Spine MRI for Low Back Pain	-	-	36.6%	37.2%

Loyola Gottlieb Memorial Hospital

701 West North Ave
Melrose Park, IL 60160
URL: www.gottliebhospital.org
Type: Acute Care Hospitals
Ownership: Voluntary non-profit - Private
Phone: 708-450-4924
Fax: 708-681-0078
Emergency Services: Yes
Beds: 250

Key Personnel:
CEO/President. . . . . Pat Cassidy
Emergency Room . . . . Mark E. Cichon, DO, FACEP, FACO
Anesthesiology. . . . . W. Scott Jellish, MD, PHD
Operating Room. . . . . Kathy Kozerski, RN
Chief of Medical Staff . . . . Anand Lal, MD
Quality Assurance . . . . Bev McAdam
Infection Control. . . . . Cathy Paulas
Radiology. . . . . Ron Shimonis

Measure	Cases	This Hosp.	State Avg.	U.S. Avg.
Blood Clot Prevention and Treatment				
Anticoagulation Overlap Therapy[2]	33	48%	91%	93%
ICU Venous Thromboembolism Prophylaxis[2]	88	82%	93%	92%
Incidence of Potentially Preventable VTE[1,2]	-	-	11%	10%
UFH with Dosages/Platelet Monitoring[2]	19	68%	94%	97%
Venous Thromboembolism Prophylaxis[2]	358	66%	86%	85%
Warfarin Therapy Discharge Instructions[2]	23	70%	71%	75%
Chest Pain/Possible Heart Attack Care				
Aspirin Given Within 24 Hours of Arrival[1]	-	-	96%	96%
Fibrinolytic Meds Within 30 Min. of Arrival[5]	-	-	65%	58%
Average Time to ECG (minutes)[1]	-	-	6	7
Average Time to Transfer (minutes)[5]	-	-	63	60
Children's Asthma Care				
Received Home Management Plan of Care	-	-	-	88%
Received Reliever Medication	-	-	-	100%
Received Systemic Corticosteroids	-	-	-	100%
Emergency Department				
Admittance Decision Time (minutes)[2]	412	92	89	98
Head CT Results Within 45 Min. of Arrival[1]	-	-	64%	57%
Patients Who Left ER Before Being Seen	25,040	7%	3%	2%
Time from ER Arrival to Admit. (minutes)[2]	449	285	260	274
Time from ER Arrival to Discharge (minutes)	294	219	138	134
Time in ER Before Being Evaluated (minutes)	170	85	28	26
Time to Pain Meds for Fractures (minutes)	81	85	52	57
Heart Attack Care				
Aspirin Given at Discharge	136	98%	99%	99%
Fibrinolytic Meds Within 30 Min. of Arrival[7]	-	-	33%	54%
PCI Within 90 Minutes of Arrival	23	83%	97%	96%
Statin Prescribed at Discharge	136	97%	98%	98%
Heart Failure Care				
ACE Inhibitor or ARB for LVSD	64	98%	98%	97%
Discharge Instructions Given	198	97%	96%	94%
Evaluation of LVS Function	253	100%	99%	99%
Medicare Spending				
Medicare Spending per Patient (ratio)	-	1.00	1	0.98
Pneumonia Care				
Appropriate Initial Antibiotic Given	91	91%	95%	95%
Blood Culture Timing	155	97%	98%	98%
Pregnancy and Delivery Care				
Newborn Deliveries Scheduled Early[2]	24	0%	2%	6%
Preventive Care				
Immunization for Influenza[2]	568	93%	92%	90%
Immunization for Pneumonia[2]	727	86%	92%	92%
Stroke Care				
Anticoagulation Therapy for Atrial Fibrillation[1]	-	-	94%	95%
Antithrombotic Therapy Timing	55	93%	98%	98%
Assessed for Rehabilitation	61	82%	97%	97%
Discharged on Antithrombotic Therapy	56	95%	99%	99%
Discharged on Statin Medication	48	73%	94%	94%
Thrombolytic Therapy Timing[1]	-	-	66%	66%
Venous Thromboembolism Prophylaxis	61	70%	94%	94%
Written Stroke Educational Materials Given	34	9%	87%	88%
Surgical Care Improvement Project				
Appropriate Beta Blocker Usage[2]	106	100%	98%	98%
Appropriate VTP Within 24 Hours[2]	283	98%	98%	98%
Controlled Postoperative Blood Glucose[2]	50	100%	97%	97%
Perioperative Temperature Management[2]	316	100%	100%	100%
Prophylactic Antibiotic Selection[2]	262	95%	99%	99%
Prophylactic Antibiotic Selection (Outpatient)	94	97%	98%	98%
Prophylactic Antibiotic Stopped[2]	258	98%	98%	98%
Prophylactic Antibiotic Timing[2]	265	98%	99%	99%
Prophylactic Antibiotic Timing (Outpatient)	94	98%	97%	98%
Urinary Catheter Removal[2]	207	98%	98%	97%
Survey of Patients' Hospital Experiences				
Area Around Room 'Always' Quiet at Night	300+	49%	60%	61%
Doctors 'Always' Communicated Well	300+	79%	81%	82%
Home Recovery Information Given	300+	80%	86%	85%
Hospital Given 9 or 10 on 10 Point Scale	300+	59%	70%	71%
Meds 'Always' Explained Before Given	300+	56%	64%	64%
Nurses 'Always' Communicated Well	300+	76%	79%	79%
Pain 'Always' Well Controlled	300+	67%	71%	71%
Room and Bathroom 'Always' Clean	300+	71%	74%	73%
Timely Help 'Always' Received	300+	62%	67%	68%
Would Definitely Recommend Hospital	300+	61%	70%	71%
Use of Medical Imaging				
Cardiac Imaging Stress Test before Surgery	493	4.7%	5.5%	5.3%
Combination Abdominal CT Scan	677	13.3%	10.1%	10.5%
Combination Brain/Sinus CT Scan[1]	-	-	2.6%	2.7%
Combination Chest CT Scan	405	3.5%	2.8%	2.7%
Follow-up Mammogram/Ultrasound	1,275	8.2%	8.4%	8.8%
Lumbar Spine MRI for Low Back Pain	110	42.7%	36.6%	37.2%

Westlake Community Hospital

1225 Lake St
Melrose Park, IL 60160
URL: www.reshealth.org
Type: Acute Care Hospitals
Ownership: Voluntary non-profit - Other
Phone: 708-938-4000
Fax: 708-938-7905
Emergency Services: Yes
Beds: 326

Key Personnel:
Pediatric Ambulatory Care . . . . . . Kundankumar Giri, MD
Pediatric In-Patient Care . . . . Kundankumar Giri, MD
Operating Room. . . . . Julio Jiminez
Radiology. . . . . Robert Liebman, MD
Emergency Room . . . . Steve Meeks
Chief of Medical Staff . . . . Nabil Saleh
CEO/President. . . . . Pat Shehorn
Quality Assurance . . . . Paulette Thomas

Measure	Cases	This Hosp.	State Avg.	U.S. Avg.
Blood Clot Prevention and Treatment				
Anticoagulation Overlap Therapy[2]	24	83%	91%	93%
ICU Venous Thromboembolism Prophylaxis[2]	64	91%	93%	92%
Incidence of Potentially Preventable VTE[1,2]	-	-	11%	10%
UFH with Dosages/Platelet Monitoring[1,2]	-	-	94%	97%
Venous Thromboembolism Prophylaxis[2]	247	87%	86%	85%
Warfarin Therapy Discharge Instructions[2]	15	73%	71%	75%
Chest Pain/Possible Heart Attack Care				
Aspirin Given Within 24 Hours of Arrival[1,3]	-	-	96%	96%
Fibrinolytic Meds Within 30 Min. of Arrival[3,7]	-	-	65%	58%
Average Time to ECG (minutes)[1,3]	-	-	6	7
Average Time to Transfer (minutes)[1,3]	-	-	63	60
Children's Asthma Care				
Received Home Management Plan of Care	-	-	-	88%
Received Reliever Medication	-	-	-	100%
Received Systemic Corticosteroids	-	-	-	100%
Emergency Department				
Admittance Decision Time (minutes)[2]	365	115	89	98
Head CT Results Within 45 Min. of Arrival[1]	-	-	64%	57%
Patients Who Left ER Before Being Seen	21,558	4%	3%	2%
Time from ER Arrival to Admit. (minutes)[2]	367	336	260	274
Time from ER Arrival to Discharge (minutes)	360	168	138	134
Time in ER Before Being Evaluated (minutes)	400	47	28	26
Time to Pain Meds for Fractures (minutes)	46	38	52	57
Heart Attack Care				
Aspirin Given at Discharge	48	96%	99%	99%
Fibrinolytic Meds Within 30 Min. of Arrival[7]	-	-	33%	54%
PCI Within 90 Minutes of Arrival[1]	-	-	97%	96%
Statin Prescribed at Discharge	47	98%	98%	98%
Heart Failure Care				
ACE Inhibitor or ARB for LVSD	53	85%	98%	97%
Discharge Instructions Given	116	91%	96%	94%
Evaluation of LVS Function	147	100%	99%	99%

NOTE: Hospital profiles are in alphabetical order by state, then city, then hospital within the city; Rankings exclude hospitals with less than 25 cases except for patient surveys which excludes hospitals with less than 100 cases; (a) 100-299 cases; (1) The number of cases/patients is too few to report; (2) Data submitted were based on a sample of cases/patients; (3) Results are based on a shorter time period than required; (4) Data suppressed by CMS for one or more quarters; (5) Results are not available for this reporting period; (6) Fewer than 100 patients completed the HCAHPS survey; (7) No cases met the criteria for this measure; (8) The lower limit of the confidence interval cannot be calculated if the number of observed infections equals zero; (9) No data are available from the state/territory for this reporting period; (10) The scores shown reflect fewer than 50 completed surveys; (11) There were discrepancies in the data collection process; (12) This measure does not apply to this hospital for this reporting period; (13) Results cannot be calculated for this reporting period; (14) The results for this state are combined with nearby states to protect confidentiality; Please refer to the User's Guide for a full explanation of data.

Medicare Spending				
Medicare Spending per Patient (ratio)	-	1.09	1	0.98
Pneumonia Care				
Appropriate Initial Antibiotic Given	45	98%	95%	95%
Blood Culture Timing	81	98%	98%	98%
Pregnancy and Delivery Care				
Newborn Deliveries Scheduled Early[2]	40	5%	2%	6%
Preventive Care				
Immunization for Influenza[2]	415	85%	92%	90%
Immunization for Pneumonia[2]	407	92%	92%	92%
Stroke Care				
Anticoagulation Therapy for Atrial Fibrillation[1]	-	-	94%	95%
Antithrombotic Therapy Timing	34	100%	98%	98%
Assessed for Rehabilitation	39	85%	97%	97%
Discharged on Antithrombotic Therapy	38	95%	99%	99%
Discharged on Statin Medication	34	91%	94%	94%
Thrombolytic Therapy Timing[1]	-	-	66%	66%
Venous Thromboembolism Prophylaxis	35	83%	94%	94%
Written Stroke Educational Materials Given	22	50%	87%	88%
Surgical Care Improvement Project				
Appropriate Beta Blocker Usage[2]	37	97%	98%	98%
Appropriate VTP Within 24 Hours[2]	94	97%	98%	98%
Controlled Postoperative Blood Glucose[2,7]	-	-	97%	97%
Perioperative Temperature Management[2]	114	100%	100%	100%
Prophylactic Antibiotic Selection[2]	67	99%	99%	99%
Prophylactic Antibiotic Selection (Outpatient)	68	94%	98%	98%
Prophylactic Antibiotic Stopped[2]	62	95%	98%	98%
Prophylactic Antibiotic Timing[2]	67	100%	99%	99%
Prophylactic Antibiotic Timing (Outpatient)	70	96%	97%	98%
Urinary Catheter Removal[2]	19	84%	98%	97%
Survey of Patients' Hospital Experiences				
Area Around Room 'Always' Quiet at Night[11]	300+	47%	60%	61%
Doctors 'Always' Communicated Well[11]	300+	79%	81%	82%
Home Recovery Information Given[11]	300+	83%	86%	85%
Hospital Given 9 or 10 on 10 Point Scale[11]	300+	61%	70%	71%
Meds 'Always' Explained Before Given[11]	300+	58%	64%	64%
Nurses 'Always' Communicated Well[11]	300+	70%	79%	79%
Pain 'Always' Well Controlled[11]	300+	67%	71%	71%
Room and Bathroom 'Always' Clean[11]	300+	62%	74%	73%
Timely Help 'Always' Received[11]	300+	52%	67%	68%
Would Definitely Recommend Hospital[11]	300+	57%	70%	71%
Use of Medical Imaging				
Cardiac Imaging Stress Test before Surgery	158	3.2%	5.5%	5.3%
Combination Abdominal CT Scan	208	5.3%	10.1%	10.5%
Combination Brain/Sinus CT Scan	197	5.1%	2.6%	2.7%
Combination Chest CT Scan	93	4.3%	2.8%	2.7%
Follow-up Mammogram/Ultrasound	407	8.4%	8.4%	8.8%
Lumbar Spine MRI for Low Back Pain[1]	-	-	36.6%	37.2%

Mendota Community Hospital

1401 E 12th Street
Mendota, IL 61342
URL: www.mendotahospital.org
Type: Critical Access Hospitals
Ownership: Voluntary non-profit - Private

Phone: 815-539-7461
Fax: 815-538-5516
Emergency Services: Yes
Beds: 32

Key Personnel:

Chief of Medical Staff . . . . Mary Chin
President . . . . Margo Gallagher Schmi
Operating Room. . . . . Jason Goliath
Quality Assurance . . . . Janet Lane
Pediatric Ambulatory Care . . . . . . Deepak Nathani, MD
Pediatric In-Patient Care . . . . Deepak Nathani, MD

Measure	Cases	This Hosp.	State Avg.	U.S. Avg.
Blood Clot Prevention and Treatment				
Anticoagulation Overlap Therapy[1,2]	-	-	91%	93%
ICU Venous Thromboembolism Prophylaxis[2,3]	17	59%	93%	92%
Incidence of Potentially Preventable VTE[2,3]	-	-	11%	10%
UFH with Dosages/Platelet Monitoring[1,2]	-	-	94%	97%
Venous Thromboembolism Prophylaxis[2,3]	98	29%	86%	85%
Warfarin Therapy Discharge Instructions[1,2]	-	-	71%	75%
Chest Pain/Possible Heart Attack Care				
Aspirin Given Within 24 Hours of Arrival[3]	13	100%	96%	96%
Fibrinolytic Meds Within 30 Min. of Arrival[1,3]	-	-	65%	58%
Average Time to ECG (minutes)[3]	13	9	6	7
Average Time to Transfer (minutes)[3,7]	-	-	63	60
Children's Asthma Care				
Received Home Management Plan of Care	-	-	-	88%
Received Reliever Medication	-	-	-	100%
Received Systemic Corticosteroids	-	-	-	100%
Emergency Department				
Admittance Decision Time (minutes)[3]	118	40	89	98
Head CT Results Within 45 Min. of Arrival[1,3]	-	-	64%	57%
Patients Who Left ER Before Being Seen	6,558	1%	3%	2%
Time from ER Arrival to Admit. (minutes)[3]	118	206	260	274
Time from ER Arrival to Discharge (minutes)[5]	-	-	138	134
Time in ER Before Being Evaluated (minutes)[5]	-	-	28	26
Time to Pain Meds for Fractures (minutes)[3]	15	50	52	57
Heart Attack Care				
Aspirin Given at Discharge[1,3]	-	-	99%	99%
Fibrinolytic Meds Within 30 Min. of Arrival[3,7]	-	-	33%	54%
PCI Within 90 Minutes of Arrival[3,7]	-	-	97%	96%
Statin Prescribed at Discharge[1,3]	-	-	98%	98%
Heart Failure Care				
ACE Inhibitor or ARB for LVSD[1,2]	-	-	98%	97%
Discharge Instructions Given[2]	35	89%	96%	94%
Evaluation of LVS Function[2]	44	86%	99%	99%
Medicare Spending				
Medicare Spending per Patient (ratio)	-	-	1	0.98
Pneumonia Care				
Appropriate Initial Antibiotic Given	26	88%	95%	95%
Blood Culture Timing	40	98%	98%	98%
Pregnancy and Delivery Care				
Newborn Deliveries Scheduled Early[3,7]	-	-	2%	6%
Preventive Care				
Immunization for Influenza[5]	-	-	92%	90%
Immunization for Pneumonia[5]	-	-	92%	92%
Stroke Care				
Anticoagulation Therapy for Atrial Fibrillation[5]	-	-	94%	95%
Antithrombotic Therapy Timing[5]	-	-	98%	98%
Assessed for Rehabilitation[5]	-	-	97%	97%
Discharged on Antithrombotic Therapy[5]	-	-	99%	99%
Discharged on Statin Medication[5]	-	-	94%	94%
Thrombolytic Therapy Timing[5]	-	-	66%	66%
Venous Thromboembolism Prophylaxis[5]	-	-	94%	94%
Written Stroke Educational Materials Given[5]	-	-	87%	88%
Surgical Care Improvement Project				
Appropriate Beta Blocker Usage[1,3]	-	-	98%	98%
Appropriate VTP Within 24 Hours[3]	29	76%	98%	98%
Controlled Postoperative Blood Glucose[3,7]	-	-	97%	97%
Perioperative Temperature Management[3]	30	97%	100%	100%
Prophylactic Antibiotic Selection[3]	12	75%	99%	99%
Prophylactic Antibiotic Selection (Outpatient)[1,3]	-	-	98%	98%
Prophylactic Antibiotic Stopped[3]	12	92%	98%	98%
Prophylactic Antibiotic Timing[3]	12	100%	99%	99%
Prophylactic Antibiotic Timing (Outpatient)[1,3]	-	-	97%	98%
Urinary Catheter Removal[3]	12	83%	98%	97%
Survey of Patients' Hospital Experiences				
Area Around Room 'Always' Quiet at Night	(a)	68%	60%	61%
Doctors 'Always' Communicated Well	(a)	83%	81%	82%
Home Recovery Information Given	(a)	92%	86%	85%
Hospital Given 9 or 10 on 10 Point Scale	(a)	82%	70%	71%
Meds 'Always' Explained Before Given	(a)	68%	64%	64%
Nurses 'Always' Communicated Well	(a)	86%	79%	79%
Pain 'Always' Well Controlled	(a)	75%	71%	71%
Room and Bathroom 'Always' Clean	(a)	86%	74%	73%
Timely Help 'Always' Received	(a)	80%	67%	68%
Would Definitely Recommend Hospital	(a)	75%	70%	71%
Use of Medical Imaging				
Cardiac Imaging Stress Test before Surgery	130	3.1%	5.5%	5.3%
Combination Abdominal CT Scan	275	7.6%	10.1%	10.5%
Combination Brain/Sinus CT Scan[1]	-	-	2.6%	2.7%
Combination Chest CT Scan	123	0.0%	2.8%	2.7%
Follow-up Mammogram/Ultrasound	392	16.1%	8.4%	8.8%
Lumbar Spine MRI for Low Back Pain[1]	-	-	36.6%	37.2%

Massac Memorial Hospital

28 Chick Street, PO Box 850
Metropolis, IL 62960
Type: Critical Access Hospitals
Ownership: Govt - Hospital Dist/Auth

Phone: 618-524-2176
Emergency Services: Yes

Measure	Cases	This Hosp.	State Avg.	U.S. Avg.
Blood Clot Prevention and Treatment				
Anticoagulation Overlap Therapy[5]	-	-	91%	93%
ICU Venous Thromboembolism Prophylaxis[5]	-	-	93%	92%
Incidence of Potentially Preventable VTE[5]	-	-	11%	10%
UFH with Dosages/Platelet Monitoring[5]	-	-	94%	97%
Venous Thromboembolism Prophylaxis[5]	-	-	86%	85%
Warfarin Therapy Discharge Instructions[5]	-	-	71%	75%
Chest Pain/Possible Heart Attack Care				
Aspirin Given Within 24 Hours of Arrival[3]	43	74%	96%	96%
Fibrinolytic Meds Within 30 Min. of Arrival[3,7]	-	-	65%	58%
Average Time to ECG (minutes)[3]	44	12	6	7
Average Time to Transfer (minutes)[1,3]	-	-	63	60
Children's Asthma Care				
Received Home Management Plan of Care	-	-	-	88%
Received Reliever Medication	-	-	-	100%
Received Systemic Corticosteroids	-	-	-	100%
Emergency Department				
Admittance Decision Time (minutes)[2]	160	45	89	98
Head CT Results Within 45 Min. of Arrival[5]	-	-	64%	57%
Patients Who Left ER Before Being Seen[5]	-	-	3%	2%
Time from ER Arrival to Admit. (minutes)[2]	165	186	260	274
Time from ER Arrival to Discharge (minutes)[5]	-	-	138	134
Time in ER Before Being Evaluated (minutes)[5]	-	-	28	26
Time to Pain Meds for Fractures (minutes)[5]	-	-	52	57
Heart Attack Care				
Aspirin Given at Discharge[3,7]	-	-	99%	99%
Fibrinolytic Meds Within 30 Min. of Arrival[3,7]	-	-	33%	54%
PCI Within 90 Minutes of Arrival[3,7]	-	-	97%	96%
Statin Prescribed at Discharge[1,3]	-	-	98%	98%
Heart Failure Care				
ACE Inhibitor or ARB for LVSD[1]	-	-	98%	97%
Discharge Instructions Given	21	86%	96%	94%
Evaluation of LVS Function	24	88%	99%	99%
Medicare Spending				
Medicare Spending per Patient (ratio)	-	-	1	0.98
Pneumonia Care				
Appropriate Initial Antibiotic Given[2]	40	75%	95%	95%
Blood Culture Timing[2]	41	88%	98%	98%
Pregnancy and Delivery Care				
Newborn Deliveries Scheduled Early[5]	-	-	2%	6%
Preventive Care				
Immunization for Influenza[2]	122	88%	92%	90%
Immunization for Pneumonia[2]	221	86%	92%	92%
Stroke Care				
Anticoagulation Therapy for Atrial Fibrillation[5]	-	-	94%	95%
Antithrombotic Therapy Timing[5]	-	-	98%	98%
Assessed for Rehabilitation[5]	-	-	97%	97%
Discharged on Antithrombotic Therapy[5]	-	-	99%	99%
Discharged on Statin Medication[5]	-	-	94%	94%
Thrombolytic Therapy Timing[5]	-	-	66%	66%
Venous Thromboembolism Prophylaxis[5]	-	-	94%	94%
Written Stroke Educational Materials Given[5]	-	-	87%	88%
Surgical Care Improvement Project				
Appropriate Beta Blocker Usage[5]	-	-	98%	98%
Appropriate VTP Within 24 Hours[5]	-	-	98%	98%
Controlled Postoperative Blood Glucose[5]	-	-	97%	97%
Perioperative Temperature Management[5]	-	-	100%	100%
Prophylactic Antibiotic Selection[5]	-	-	99%	99%
Prophylactic Antibiotic Selection (Outpatient)[1,3]	-	-	98%	98%
Prophylactic Antibiotic Stopped[5]	-	-	98%	98%
Prophylactic Antibiotic Timing[5]	-	-	99%	99%
Prophylactic Antibiotic Timing (Outpatient)[1,3]	-	-	97%	98%
Urinary Catheter Removal[5]	-	-	98%	97%
Survey of Patients' Hospital Experiences				
Area Around Room 'Always' Quiet at Night	(a)	71%	60%	61%
Doctors 'Always' Communicated Well	(a)	88%	81%	82%

NOTE: Hospital profiles are in alphabetical order by state, then city, then hospital within the city; Rankings exclude hospitals with less than 25 cases except for patient surveys which excludes hospitals with less than 100 cases; (a) 100-299 cases; (1) The number of cases/patients is too few to report; (2) Data submitted were based on a sample of cases/patients; (3) Results are based on a shorter time period than required; (4) Data suppressed by CMS for one or more quarters; (5) Results are not available for this reporting period; (6) Fewer than 100 patients completed the HCAHPS survey; (7) No cases met the criteria for this measure; (8) The lower limit of the confidence interval cannot be calculated if the number of observed infections equals zero; (9) No data are available from the state/territory for this reporting period; (10) The scores shown reflect fewer than 50 completed surveys; (11) There were discrepancies in the data collection process; (12) This measure does not apply to this hospital for this reporting period; (13) Results cannot be calculated for this reporting period; (14) The results for this state are combined with nearby states to protect confidentiality; Please refer to the User's Guide for a full explanation of data.

Measure	Cases	This Hosp.	State Avg.	U.S. Avg.
Home Recovery Information Given	(a)	86%	86%	85%
Hospital Given 9 or 10 on 10 Point Scale	(a)	80%	70%	71%
Meds 'Always' Explained Before Given	(a)	59%	64%	64%
Nurses 'Always' Communicated Well	(a)	84%	79%	79%
Pain 'Always' Well Controlled	(a)	76%	71%	71%
Room and Bathroom 'Always' Clean	(a)	87%	74%	73%
Timely Help 'Always' Received	(a)	81%	67%	68%
Would Definitely Recommend Hospital	(a)	75%	70%	71%
Use of Medical Imaging				
Cardiac Imaging Stress Test before Surgery	96	6.3%	5.5%	5.3%
Combination Abdominal CT Scan	373	10.7%	10.1%	10.5%
Combination Brain/Sinus CT Scan	309	5.5%	2.6%	2.7%
Combination Chest CT Scan	171	9.4%	2.8%	2.7%
Follow-up Mammogram/Ultrasound	263	12.9%	8.4%	8.8%
Lumbar Spine MRI for Low Back Pain	43	48.8%	36.6%	37.2%

OSF Holy Family Medical Center

1000 W Harlem Avenue | Phone: 309-734-3141
Monmouth, IL 61462 | Fax: 309-734-3029
URL: www.cmchospital.com
Type: Critical Access Hospitals | Emergency Services: Yes
Ownership: Voluntary non-profit - Private | Beds: 68

Key Personnel:
CEO/President. . . . . Donald G Brown
Quality Assurance . . . . Mary Craig, RN
Emergency Room . . . . Laura Elliott
Cardiac Laboratory. . . . . Sara Glasnovich
Radiology. . . . . Byung Hyun
Chief of Medical Staff . . . . Ruben Medrano
Operating Room. . . . . Lisa Morris

Measure	Cases	This Hosp.	State Avg.	U.S. Avg.
Blood Clot Prevention and Treatment				
Anticoagulation Overlap Therapy[3,7]	-	-	91%	93%
ICU Venous Thromboembolism Prophylaxis[3,7]	-	-	93%	92%
Incidence of Potentially Preventable VTE[3,7]	-	-	11%	10%
UFH with Dosages/Platelet Monitoring[3,7]	-	-	94%	97%
Venous Thromboembolism Prophylaxis[3,7]	-	-	86%	85%
Warfarin Therapy Discharge Instructions[3,7]	-	-	71%	75%
Chest Pain/Possible Heart Attack Care				
Aspirin Given Within 24 Hours of Arrival[3]	11	100%	96%	96%
Fibrinolytic Meds Within 30 Min. of Arrival[3,7]	-	-	65%	58%
Average Time to ECG (minutes)[3]	11	6	6	7
Average Time to Transfer (minutes)[1,3]	-	-	63	60
Children's Asthma Care				
Received Home Management Plan of Care	-	-	-	88%
Received Reliever Medication	-	-	-	100%
Received Systemic Corticosteroids	-	-	-	100%
Emergency Department				
Admittance Decision Time (minutes)[2]	112	50	89	98
Head CT Results Within 45 Min. of Arrival[1,3]	-	-	64%	57%
Patients Who Left ER Before Being Seen[5]	-	-	3%	2%
Time from ER Arrival to Admit. (minutes)[2]	167	192	260	274
Time from ER Arrival to Discharge (minutes)[3]	133	115	138	134
Time in ER Before Being Evaluated (minutes)[3]	151	15	28	26
Time to Pain Meds for Fractures (minutes)[1,3]	-	-	52	57
Heart Attack Care				
Aspirin Given at Discharge[3,7]	-	-	99%	99%
Fibrinolytic Meds Within 30 Min. of Arrival[3,7]	-	-	33%	54%
PCI Within 90 Minutes of Arrival[3,7]	-	-	97%	96%
Statin Prescribed at Discharge[3,7]	-	-	98%	98%
Heart Failure Care				
ACE Inhibitor or ARB for LVSD[1,2]	-	-	98%	97%
Discharge Instructions Given[2]	13	100%	96%	94%
Evaluation of LVS Function[2]	23	100%	99%	99%
Medicare Spending				
Medicare Spending per Patient (ratio)	-	-	1	0.98
Pneumonia Care				
Appropriate Initial Antibiotic Given[7]	-	-	95%	95%
Blood Culture Timing	21	100%	98%	98%
Pregnancy and Delivery Care				
Newborn Deliveries Scheduled Early[5]	-	-	2%	6%
Preventive Care				
Immunization for Influenza[2]	118	88%	92%	90%
Immunization for Pneumonia[2]	203	87%	92%	92%
Stroke Care				
Anticoagulation Therapy for Atrial Fibrillation[3,7]	-	-	94%	95%
Antithrombotic Therapy Timing[1,3]	-	-	98%	98%
Assessed for Rehabilitation[1,3]	-	-	97%	97%
Discharged on Antithrombotic Therapy[1,3]	-	-	99%	99%
Discharged on Statin Medication[1,3]	-	-	94%	94%
Thrombolytic Therapy Timing[3,7]	-	-	66%	66%
Venous Thromboembolism Prophylaxis[1,3]	-	-	94%	94%
Written Stroke Educational Materials Given[1,3]	-	-	87%	88%
Surgical Care Improvement Project				
Appropriate Beta Blocker Usage[1]	-	-	98%	98%
Appropriate VTP Within 24 Hours	12	100%	98%	98%
Controlled Postoperative Blood Glucose[7]	-	-	97%	97%
Perioperative Temperature Management	13	100%	100%	100%
Prophylactic Antibiotic Selection[1]	-	-	99%	99%
Prophylactic Antibiotic Selection (Outpatient)[5]	-	-	98%	98%
Prophylactic Antibiotic Stopped[1]	-	-	98%	98%
Prophylactic Antibiotic Timing[1]	-	-	99%	99%
Prophylactic Antibiotic Timing (Outpatient)[5]	-	-	97%	98%
Urinary Catheter Removal[1]	-	-	98%	97%
Survey of Patients' Hospital Experiences				
Area Around Room 'Always' Quiet at Night	(a)	78%	60%	61%
Doctors 'Always' Communicated Well	(a)	93%	81%	82%
Home Recovery Information Given	(a)	91%	86%	85%
Hospital Given 9 or 10 on 10 Point Scale	(a)	85%	70%	71%
Meds 'Always' Explained Before Given	(a)	78%	64%	64%
Nurses 'Always' Communicated Well	(a)	94%	79%	79%
Pain 'Always' Well Controlled	(a)	80%	71%	71%
Room and Bathroom 'Always' Clean	(a)	97%	74%	73%
Timely Help 'Always' Received	(a)	91%	67%	68%
Would Definitely Recommend Hospital	(a)	81%	70%	71%
Use of Medical Imaging				
Cardiac Imaging Stress Test before Surgery[1]	-	-	5.5%	5.3%
Combination Abdominal CT Scan	127	3.1%	10.1%	10.5%
Combination Brain/Sinus CT Scan[1]	-	-	2.6%	2.7%
Combination Chest CT Scan	89	0.0%	2.8%	2.7%
Follow-up Mammogram/Ultrasound	299	10.4%	8.4%	8.8%
Lumbar Spine MRI for Low Back Pain[1]	-	-	36.6%	37.2%

John & Mary Kirby Hospital

1111 N State St | Phone: 217-762-2115
Monticello, IL 61856 | Fax: 217-762-6267
Type: Critical Access Hospitals | Emergency Services: Yes
Ownership: Voluntary non-profit - Private | Beds: 17

Measure	Cases	This Hosp.	State Avg.	U.S. Avg.
Blood Clot Prevention and Treatment				
Anticoagulation Overlap Therapy[3,7]	-	-	91%	93%
ICU Venous Thromboembolism Prophylaxis[3,7]	-	-	93%	92%
Incidence of Potentially Preventable VTE[3,7]	-	-	11%	10%
UFH with Dosages/Platelet Monitoring[3,7]	-	-	94%	97%
Venous Thromboembolism Prophylaxis[3,7]	-	-	86%	85%
Warfarin Therapy Discharge Instructions[3,7]	-	-	71%	75%
Chest Pain/Possible Heart Attack Care				
Aspirin Given Within 24 Hours of Arrival	-	-	96%	96%
Fibrinolytic Meds Within 30 Min. of Arrival	-	-	65%	58%
Average Time to ECG (minutes)	-	-	6	7
Average Time to Transfer (minutes)	-	-	63	60
Children's Asthma Care				
Received Home Management Plan of Care	-	-	-	88%
Received Reliever Medication	-	-	-	100%
Received Systemic Corticosteroids	-	-	-	100%
Emergency Department				
Admittance Decision Time (minutes)[1,3]	-	-	89	98
Head CT Results Within 45 Min. of Arrival	-	-	64%	57%
Patients Who Left ER Before Being Seen	-	-	3%	2%
Time from ER Arrival to Admit. (minutes)[3]	15	209	260	274
Time from ER Arrival to Discharge (minutes)	-	-	138	134
Time in ER Before Being Evaluated (minutes)	-	-	28	26
Time to Pain Meds for Fractures (minutes)	-	-	52	57
Heart Attack Care				
Aspirin Given at Discharge[5]	-	-	99%	99%
Fibrinolytic Meds Within 30 Min. of Arrival[5]	-	-	33%	54%
PCI Within 90 Minutes of Arrival[5]	-	-	97%	96%
Statin Prescribed at Discharge[5]	-	-	98%	98%
Heart Failure Care				
ACE Inhibitor or ARB for LVSD[1]	-	-	98%	97%
Discharge Instructions Given[1]	-	-	96%	94%
Evaluation of LVS Function	20	75%	99%	99%
Medicare Spending				
Medicare Spending per Patient (ratio)	-	-	1	0.98
Pneumonia Care				
Appropriate Initial Antibiotic Given[2]	22	50%	95%	95%
Blood Culture Timing[2]	27	89%	98%	98%
Pregnancy and Delivery Care				
Newborn Deliveries Scheduled Early[5]	-	-	2%	6%
Preventive Care				
Immunization for Influenza	118	79%	92%	90%
Immunization for Pneumonia	181	83%	92%	92%
Stroke Care				
Anticoagulation Therapy for Atrial Fibrillation[5]	-	-	94%	95%
Antithrombotic Therapy Timing[5]	-	-	98%	98%
Assessed for Rehabilitation[5]	-	-	97%	97%
Discharged on Antithrombotic Therapy[5]	-	-	99%	99%
Discharged on Statin Medication[5]	-	-	94%	94%
Thrombolytic Therapy Timing[5]	-	-	66%	66%
Venous Thromboembolism Prophylaxis[5]	-	-	94%	94%
Written Stroke Educational Materials Given[5]	-	-	87%	88%
Surgical Care Improvement Project				
Appropriate Beta Blocker Usage[5]	-	-	98%	98%
Appropriate VTP Within 24 Hours[5]	-	-	98%	98%
Controlled Postoperative Blood Glucose[5]	-	-	97%	97%
Perioperative Temperature Management[5]	-	-	100%	100%
Prophylactic Antibiotic Selection[5]	-	-	99%	99%
Prophylactic Antibiotic Selection (Outpatient)	-	-	98%	98%
Prophylactic Antibiotic Stopped[5]	-	-	98%	98%
Prophylactic Antibiotic Timing[5]	-	-	99%	99%
Prophylactic Antibiotic Timing (Outpatient)	-	-	97%	98%
Urinary Catheter Removal[5]	-	-	98%	97%
Survey of Patients' Hospital Experiences				
Area Around Room 'Always' Quiet at Night[5]	-	-	60%	61%
Doctors 'Always' Communicated Well[5]	-	-	81%	82%
Home Recovery Information Given[5]	-	-	86%	85%
Hospital Given 9 or 10 on 10 Point Scale[5]	-	-	70%	71%
Meds 'Always' Explained Before Given[5]	-	-	64%	64%
Nurses 'Always' Communicated Well[5]	-	-	79%	79%
Pain 'Always' Well Controlled[5]	-	-	71%	71%
Room and Bathroom 'Always' Clean[5]	-	-	74%	73%
Timely Help 'Always' Received[5]	-	-	67%	68%
Would Definitely Recommend Hospital[5]	-	-	70%	71%
Use of Medical Imaging				
Cardiac Imaging Stress Test before Surgery	-	-	5.5%	5.3%
Combination Abdominal CT Scan	-	-	10.1%	10.5%
Combination Brain/Sinus CT Scan	-	-	2.6%	2.7%
Combination Chest CT Scan	-	-	2.8%	2.7%
Follow-up Mammogram/Ultrasound	-	-	8.4%	8.8%
Lumbar Spine MRI for Low Back Pain	-	-	36.6%	37.2%

Morris Hospital & Healthcare Centers

150 W High St | Phone: 815-942-2932
Morris, IL 60450 | Fax: 815-942-3154
URL: www.morrishospital.org
Type: Acute Care Hospitals | Emergency Services: Yes
Ownership: Voluntary non-profit - Private | Beds: 82

Key Personnel:
Emergency Room . . . . Sean C Atchison
CEO/President. . . . . Bill Bruce
Radiology. . . . . Jeffrey E Chung
Chief of Medical Staff . . . . Sherwin Ritz, MD

Measure	Cases	This Hosp.	State Avg.	U.S. Avg.
Blood Clot Prevention and Treatment				
Anticoagulation Overlap Therapy[2]	35	89%	91%	93%
ICU Venous Thromboembolism Prophylaxis[2]	119	81%	93%	92%
Incidence of Potentially Preventable VTE[1,2]	-	-	11%	10%
UFH with Dosages/Platelet Monitoring[2]	28	100%	94%	97%
Venous Thromboembolism Prophylaxis[2]	231	93%	86%	85%

NOTE: Hospital profiles are in alphabetical order by state, then city, then hospital within the city; Rankings exclude hospitals with less than 25 cases except for patient surveys which excludes hospitals with less than 100 cases; (a) 100-299 cases; (1) The number of cases/patients is too few to report; (2) Data submitted were based on a sample of cases/patients; (3) Results are based on a shorter time period than required; (4) Data suppressed by CMS for one or more quarters; (5) Results are not available for this reporting period; (6) Fewer than 100 patients completed the HCAHPS survey; (7) No cases met the criteria for this measure; (8) The lower limit of the confidence interval cannot be calculated if the number of observed infections equals zero; (9) No data are available from the state/territory for this reporting period; (10) The scores shown reflect fewer than 50 completed surveys; (11) There were discrepancies in the data collection process; (12) This measure does not apply to this hospital for this reporting period; (13) Results cannot be calculated for this reporting period; (14) The results for this state are combined with nearby states to protect confidentiality; Please refer to the User's Guide for a full explanation of data.

Measure	Cases	This Hosp.	State Avg.	U.S. Avg.
Warfarin Therapy Discharge Instructions[2]	25	96%	71%	75%
Chest Pain/Possible Heart Attack Care				
Aspirin Given Within 24 Hours of Arrival	13	100%	96%	96%
Fibrinolytic Meds Within 30 Min. of Arrival[3,7]	-	-	65%	58%
Average Time to ECG (minutes)	19	3	6	7
Average Time to Transfer (minutes)[1,3]	-	-	63	60
Children's Asthma Care				
Received Home Management Plan of Care	-	-	-	88%
Received Reliever Medication	-	-	-	100%
Received Systemic Corticosteroids	-	-	-	100%
Emergency Department				
Admittance Decision Time (minutes)[2]	581	49	89	98
Head CT Results Within 45 Min. of Arrival	21	76%	64%	57%
Patients Who Left ER Before Being Seen	26,797	1%	3%	2%
Time from ER Arrival to Admit. (minutes)[2]	582	200	260	274
Time from ER Arrival to Discharge (minutes)	407	109	138	134
Time in ER Before Being Evaluated (minutes)	353	20	28	26
Time to Pain Meds for Fractures (minutes)	164	48	52	57
Heart Attack Care				
Aspirin Given at Discharge	57	98%	99%	99%
Fibrinolytic Meds Within 30 Min. of Arrival[7]	-	-	33%	54%
PCI Within 90 Minutes of Arrival	23	100%	97%	96%
Statin Prescribed at Discharge	51	98%	98%	98%
Heart Failure Care				
ACE Inhibitor or ARB for LVSD	24	96%	98%	97%
Discharge Instructions Given	83	98%	96%	94%
Evaluation of LVS Function	94	100%	99%	99%
Medicare Spending				
Medicare Spending per Patient (ratio)	-	1.03	1	0.98
Pneumonia Care				
Appropriate Initial Antibiotic Given[2]	86	97%	95%	95%
Blood Culture Timing[2]	186	98%	98%	98%
Pregnancy and Delivery Care				
Newborn Deliveries Scheduled Early	54	0%	2%	6%
Preventive Care				
Immunization for Influenza[2]	400	96%	92%	90%
Immunization for Pneumonia[2]	459	99%	92%	92%
Stroke Care				
Anticoagulation Therapy for Atrial Fibrillation[1]	-	-	94%	95%
Antithrombotic Therapy Timing	43	100%	98%	98%
Assessed for Rehabilitation	40	78%	97%	97%
Discharged on Antithrombotic Therapy	40	100%	99%	99%
Discharged on Statin Medication	30	83%	94%	94%
Thrombolytic Therapy Timing[1]	-	-	66%	66%
Venous Thromboembolism Prophylaxis	38	84%	94%	94%
Written Stroke Educational Materials Given	29	76%	87%	88%
Surgical Care Improvement Project				
Appropriate Beta Blocker Usage	53	100%	98%	98%
Appropriate VTP Within 24 Hours	225	99%	98%	98%
Controlled Postoperative Blood Glucose[7]	-	-	97%	97%
Perioperative Temperature Management	251	100%	100%	100%
Prophylactic Antibiotic Selection	178	100%	99%	99%
Prophylactic Antibiotic Selection (Outpatient)	148	99%	98%	98%
Prophylactic Antibiotic Stopped	176	100%	98%	98%
Prophylactic Antibiotic Timing	178	100%	99%	99%
Prophylactic Antibiotic Timing (Outpatient)	142	98%	97%	98%
Urinary Catheter Removal	200	100%	98%	97%
Survey of Patients' Hospital Experiences				
Area Around Room 'Always' Quiet at Night[11]	(a)	60%	60%	61%
Doctors 'Always' Communicated Well[11]	(a)	83%	81%	82%
Home Recovery Information Given[11]	(a)	90%	86%	85%
Hospital Given 9 or 10 on 10 Point Scale[11]	(a)	80%	70%	71%
Meds 'Always' Explained Before Given[11]	(a)	72%	64%	64%
Nurses 'Always' Communicated Well[11]	(a)	84%	79%	79%
Pain 'Always' Well Controlled[11]	(a)	74%	71%	71%
Room and Bathroom 'Always' Clean[11]	(a)	77%	74%	73%
Timely Help 'Always' Received[11]	(a)	75%	67%	68%
Would Definitely Recommend Hospital[11]	(a)	79%	70%	71%
Use of Medical Imaging				
Cardiac Imaging Stress Test before Surgery	329	5.5%	5.5%	5.3%
Combination Abdominal CT Scan	776	9.9%	10.1%	10.5%
Combination Brain/Sinus CT Scan[1]	-	-	2.6%	2.7%
Combination Chest CT Scan	511	0.6%	2.8%	2.7%
Follow-up Mammogram/Ultrasound	988	5.8%	8.4%	8.8%
Lumbar Spine MRI for Low Back Pain	102	30.4%	36.6%	37.2%

Morrison Community Hospital

303 N Jackson Street Phone: 815-772-4003
Morrison, IL 61270
Type: Critical Access Hospitals Emergency Services: Yes
Ownership: Govt - Hospital Dist/Auth

Measure	Cases	This Hosp.	State Avg.	U.S. Avg.
Blood Clot Prevention and Treatment				
Anticoagulation Overlap Therapy[5]	-	-	91%	93%
ICU Venous Thromboembolism Prophylaxis[5]	-	-	93%	92%
Incidence of Potentially Preventable VTE[5]	-	-	11%	10%
UFH with Dosages/Platelet Monitoring[5]	-	-	94%	97%
Venous Thromboembolism Prophylaxis[5]	-	-	86%	85%
Warfarin Therapy Discharge Instructions[5]	-	-	71%	75%
Chest Pain/Possible Heart Attack Care				
Aspirin Given Within 24 Hours of Arrival[5]	-	-	96%	96%
Fibrinolytic Meds Within 30 Min. of Arrival[5]	-	-	65%	58%
Average Time to ECG (minutes)[5]	-	-	6	7
Average Time to Transfer (minutes)[5]	-	-	63	60
Children's Asthma Care				
Received Home Management Plan of Care	-	-	-	88%
Received Reliever Medication	-	-	-	100%
Received Systemic Corticosteroids	-	-	-	100%
Emergency Department				
Admittance Decision Time (minutes)[5]	-	-	89	98
Head CT Results Within 45 Min. of Arrival[5]	-	-	64%	57%
Patients Who Left ER Before Being Seen	1,489	1%	3%	2%
Time from ER Arrival to Admit. (minutes)[5]	-	-	260	274
Time from ER Arrival to Discharge (minutes)[5]	-	-	138	134
Time in ER Before Being Evaluated (minutes)[5]	-	-	28	26
Time to Pain Meds for Fractures (minutes)[5]	-	-	52	57
Heart Attack Care				
Aspirin Given at Discharge[5]	-	-	99%	99%
Fibrinolytic Meds Within 30 Min. of Arrival[5]	-	-	33%	54%
PCI Within 90 Minutes of Arrival[5]	-	-	97%	96%
Statin Prescribed at Discharge[5]	-	-	98%	98%
Heart Failure Care				
ACE Inhibitor or ARB for LVSD[5]	-	-	98%	97%
Discharge Instructions Given[5]	-	-	96%	94%
Evaluation of LVS Function[5]	-	-	99%	99%
Medicare Spending				
Medicare Spending per Patient (ratio)	-	-	1	0.98
Pneumonia Care				
Appropriate Initial Antibiotic Given[5]	-	-	95%	95%
Blood Culture Timing[5]	-	-	98%	98%
Pregnancy and Delivery Care				
Newborn Deliveries Scheduled Early[5]	-	-	2%	6%
Preventive Care				
Immunization for Influenza[5]	-	-	92%	90%
Immunization for Pneumonia[5]	-	-	92%	92%
Stroke Care				
Anticoagulation Therapy for Atrial Fibrillation[5]	-	-	94%	95%
Antithrombotic Therapy Timing[5]	-	-	98%	98%
Assessed for Rehabilitation[5]	-	-	97%	97%
Discharged on Antithrombotic Therapy[5]	-	-	99%	99%
Discharged on Statin Medication[5]	-	-	94%	94%
Thrombolytic Therapy Timing[5]	-	-	66%	66%
Venous Thromboembolism Prophylaxis[5]	-	-	94%	94%
Written Stroke Educational Materials Given[5]	-	-	87%	88%
Surgical Care Improvement Project				
Appropriate Beta Blocker Usage[5]	-	-	98%	98%
Appropriate VTP Within 24 Hours[5]	-	-	98%	98%
Controlled Postoperative Blood Glucose[5]	-	-	97%	97%
Perioperative Temperature Management[5]	-	-	100%	100%
Prophylactic Antibiotic Selection[5]	-	-	99%	99%
Prophylactic Antibiotic Selection (Outpatient)[5]	-	-	98%	98%
Prophylactic Antibiotic Stopped[5]	-	-	98%	98%
Prophylactic Antibiotic Timing[5]	-	-	99%	99%
Prophylactic Antibiotic Timing (Outpatient)[5]	-	-	97%	98%
Urinary Catheter Removal[5]	-	-	98%	97%
Survey of Patients' Hospital Experiences				
Area Around Room 'Always' Quiet at Night[6]	<100	74%	60%	61%
Doctors 'Always' Communicated Well[6]	<100	71%	81%	82%
Home Recovery Information Given[6]	<100	88%	86%	85%
Hospital Given 9 or 10 on 10 Point Scale[6]	<100	65%	70%	71%
Meds 'Always' Explained Before Given[6]	<100	51%	64%	64%
Nurses 'Always' Communicated Well[6]	<100	70%	79%	79%
Pain 'Always' Well Controlled[6]	<100	79%	71%	71%
Room and Bathroom 'Always' Clean[6]	<100	81%	74%	73%
Timely Help 'Always' Received[6]	<100	78%	67%	68%
Would Definitely Recommend Hospital[6]	<100	68%	70%	71%
Use of Medical Imaging				
Cardiac Imaging Stress Test before Surgery[7]	-	-	5.5%	5.3%
Combination Abdominal CT Scan[1]	-	-	10.1%	10.5%
Combination Brain/Sinus CT Scan[1]	-	-	2.6%	2.7%
Combination Chest CT Scan[1]	-	-	2.8%	2.7%
Follow-up Mammogram/Ultrasound	63	7.9%	8.4%	8.8%
Lumbar Spine MRI for Low Back Pain[7]	-	-	36.6%	37.2%

Wabash General Hospital

1418 College Drive Phone: 618-262-8621
Mount Carmel, IL 62863 Fax: 618-263-6461
URL: www.wabashgeneral.com
Type: Critical Access Hospitals Emergency Services: Yes
Ownership: Govt - Hospital Dist/Auth Beds: 56
Key Personnel:
CEO/President. . . . . Jay Purvis
Radiology. . . . . H Youssef

Measure	Cases	This Hosp.	State Avg.	U.S. Avg.
Blood Clot Prevention and Treatment				
Anticoagulation Overlap Therapy[5]	-	-	91%	93%
ICU Venous Thromboembolism Prophylaxis[5]	-	-	93%	92%
Incidence of Potentially Preventable VTE[5]	-	-	11%	10%
UFH with Dosages/Platelet Monitoring[5]	-	-	94%	97%
Venous Thromboembolism Prophylaxis[5]	-	-	86%	85%
Warfarin Therapy Discharge Instructions[5]	-	-	71%	75%
Chest Pain/Possible Heart Attack Care				
Aspirin Given Within 24 Hours of Arrival	24	100%	96%	96%
Fibrinolytic Meds Within 30 Min. of Arrival[7]	-	-	65%	58%
Average Time to ECG (minutes)	31	5	6	7
Average Time to Transfer (minutes)[7]	-	-	63	60
Children's Asthma Care				
Received Home Management Plan of Care	-	-	-	88%
Received Reliever Medication	-	-	-	100%
Received Systemic Corticosteroids	-	-	-	100%
Emergency Department				
Admittance Decision Time (minutes)[5]	-	-	89	98
Head CT Results Within 45 Min. of Arrival[5]	-	-	64%	57%
Patients Who Left ER Before Being Seen[5]	-	-	3%	2%
Time from ER Arrival to Admit. (minutes)[5]	-	-	260	274
Time from ER Arrival to Discharge (minutes)[5]	-	-	138	134
Time in ER Before Being Evaluated (minutes)[5]	-	-	28	26
Time to Pain Meds for Fractures (minutes)[5]	-	-	52	57
Heart Attack Care				
Aspirin Given at Discharge[1,3]	-	-	99%	99%
Fibrinolytic Meds Within 30 Min. of Arrival[3,7]	-	-	33%	54%
PCI Within 90 Minutes of Arrival[5]	-	-	97%	96%
Statin Prescribed at Discharge[1,3]	-	-	98%	98%
Heart Failure Care				
ACE Inhibitor or ARB for LVSD[1]	-	-	98%	97%
Discharge Instructions Given	20	100%	96%	94%
Evaluation of LVS Function	29	100%	99%	99%
Medicare Spending				
Medicare Spending per Patient (ratio)	-	-	1	0.98
Pneumonia Care				
Appropriate Initial Antibiotic Given	46	87%	95%	95%
Blood Culture Timing	43	98%	98%	98%
Pregnancy and Delivery Care				
Newborn Deliveries Scheduled Early[5]	-	-	2%	6%
Preventive Care				
Immunization for Influenza[5]	-	-	92%	90%
Immunization for Pneumonia[5]	-	-	92%	92%

NOTE: Hospital profiles are in alphabetical order by state, then city, then hospital within the city; Rankings exclude hospitals with less than 25 cases except for patient surveys which excludes hospitals with less than 100 cases; (a) 100-299 cases; (1) The number of cases/patients is too few to report; (2) Data submitted were based on a sample of cases/patients; (3) Results are based on a shorter time period than required; (4) Data suppressed by CMS for one or more quarters; (5) Results are not available for this reporting period; (6) Fewer than 100 patients completed the HCAHPS survey; (7) No cases met the criteria for this measure; (8) The lower limit of the confidence interval cannot be calculated if the number of observed infections equals zero; (9) No data are available from the state/territory for this reporting period; (10) The scores shown reflect fewer than 50 completed surveys; (11) There were discrepancies in the data collection process; (12) This measure does not apply to this hospital for this reporting period; (13) Results cannot be calculated for this reporting period; (14) The results for this state are combined with nearby states to protect confidentiality; Please refer to the User's Guide for a full explanation of data.

Measure	Cases	This Hosp.	State Avg.	U.S. Avg.
Stroke Care				
Anticoagulation Therapy for Atrial Fibrillation[5]	-	-	94%	95%
Antithrombotic Therapy Timing[5]	-	-	98%	98%
Assessed for Rehabilitation[5]	-	-	97%	97%
Discharged on Antithrombotic Therapy[5]	-	-	99%	99%
Discharged on Statin Medication[5]	-	-	94%	94%
Thrombolytic Therapy Timing[5]	-	-	66%	66%
Venous Thromboembolism Prophylaxis[5]	-	-	94%	94%
Written Stroke Educational Materials Given[5]	-	-	87%	88%
Surgical Care Improvement Project				
Appropriate Beta Blocker Usage	18	100%	98%	98%
Appropriate VTP Within 24 Hours	120	94%	98%	98%
Controlled Postoperative Blood Glucose[7]	-	-	97%	97%
Perioperative Temperature Management	136	100%	100%	100%
Prophylactic Antibiotic Selection	121	100%	99%	99%
Prophylactic Antibiotic Selection (Outpatient)[1,3]	-	-	98%	98%
Prophylactic Antibiotic Stopped	120	94%	98%	98%
Prophylactic Antibiotic Timing	121	99%	99%	99%
Prophylactic Antibiotic Timing (Outpatient)[1,3]	-	-	97%	98%
Urinary Catheter Removal	125	98%	98%	97%
Survey of Patients' Hospital Experiences				
Area Around Room 'Always' Quiet at Night	(a)	67%	60%	61%
Doctors 'Always' Communicated Well	(a)	88%	81%	82%
Home Recovery Information Given	(a)	90%	86%	85%
Hospital Given 9 or 10 on 10 Point Scale	(a)	80%	70%	71%
Meds 'Always' Explained Before Given	(a)	66%	64%	64%
Nurses 'Always' Communicated Well	(a)	87%	79%	79%
Pain 'Always' Well Controlled	(a)	67%	71%	71%
Room and Bathroom 'Always' Clean	(a)	85%	74%	73%
Timely Help 'Always' Received	(a)	81%	67%	68%
Would Definitely Recommend Hospital	(a)	75%	70%	71%
Use of Medical Imaging				
Cardiac Imaging Stress Test before Surgery[1]	-	-	5.5%	5.3%
Combination Abdominal CT Scan	194	28.4%	10.1%	10.5%
Combination Brain/Sinus CT Scan[1]	-	-	2.6%	2.7%
Combination Chest CT Scan	102	28.4%	2.8%	2.7%
Follow-up Mammogram/Ultrasound	253	8.3%	8.4%	8.8%
Lumbar Spine MRI for Low Back Pain[1]	-	-	36.6%	37.2%

Crossroads Community Hospital

8 Doctors Park Road
Mount Vernon, IL 62864
Phone: 618-244-5500
Fax: 618-244-5566
URL: www.crossroadscommnityhospital.com
Type: Acute Care Hospitals
Emergency Services: Yes
Ownership: Proprietary
Beds: 55

Key Personnel:
Infection Control. . . . . Mike Beirman, RN
Radiology. . . . . Andrew Holz
Quality Assurance . . . . Karen Salamone
Operating Room. . . . . Doris Shields, RN
CEO/President. . . . . Gregory F Simsniel, RN
Chief of Medical Staff. . . . . Alan Sroehling

Measure	Cases	This Hosp.	State Avg.	U.S. Avg.
Blood Clot Prevention and Treatment				
Anticoagulation Overlap Therapy[1,2]	-	-	91%	93%
ICU Venous Thromboembolism Prophylaxis[2]	71	100%	93%	92%
Incidence of Potentially Preventable VTE[2,7]	-	-	11%	10%
UFH with Dosages/Platelet Monitoring[1,2]	-	-	94%	97%
Venous Thromboembolism Prophylaxis[2]	294	96%	86%	85%
Warfarin Therapy Discharge Instructions[1,2]	-	-	71%	75%
Chest Pain/Possible Heart Attack Care				
Aspirin Given Within 24 Hours of Arrival	23	96%	96%	96%
Fibrinolytic Meds Within 30 Min. of Arrival[7]	-	-	65%	58%
Average Time to ECG (minutes)	23	1	6	7
Average Time to Transfer (minutes)[1]	-	-	63	60
Children's Asthma Care				
Received Home Management Plan of Care	-	-	-	88%
Received Reliever Medication	-	-	-	100%
Received Systemic Corticosteroids	-	-	-	100%
Emergency Department				
Admittance Decision Time (minutes)[2]	463	56	89	98
Head CT Results Within 45 Min. of Arrival[1]	-	-	64%	57%
Patients Who Left ER Before Being Seen	9,993	1%	3%	2%
Time from ER Arrival to Admit. (minutes)[2]	463	185	260	274
Time from ER Arrival to Discharge (minutes)	404	83	138	134
Time in ER Before Being Evaluated (minutes)	445	15	28	26
Time to Pain Meds for Fractures (minutes)	35	32	52	57
Heart Attack Care				
Aspirin Given at Discharge[1]	-	-	99%	99%
Fibrinolytic Meds Within 30 Min. of Arrival[7]	-	-	33%	54%
PCI Within 90 Minutes of Arrival[7]	-	-	97%	96%
Statin Prescribed at Discharge[1]	-	-	98%	98%
Heart Failure Care				
ACE Inhibitor or ARB for LVSD[1]	-	-	98%	97%
Discharge Instructions Given	18	67%	96%	94%
Evaluation of LVS Function	29	100%	99%	99%
Medicare Spending				
Medicare Spending per Patient (ratio)	-	0.95	1	0.98
Pneumonia Care				
Appropriate Initial Antibiotic Given	60	98%	95%	95%
Blood Culture Timing	106	99%	98%	98%
Pregnancy and Delivery Care				
Newborn Deliveries Scheduled Early[2,7]	-	-	2%	6%
Preventive Care				
Immunization for Influenza[2]	352	99%	92%	90%
Immunization for Pneumonia[2]	506	100%	92%	92%
Stroke Care				
Anticoagulation Therapy for Atrial Fibrillation[1]	-	-	94%	95%
Antithrombotic Therapy Timing[1]	-	-	98%	98%
Assessed for Rehabilitation[1]	-	-	97%	97%
Discharged on Antithrombotic Therapy[1]	-	-	99%	99%
Discharged on Statin Medication[1]	-	-	94%	94%
Thrombolytic Therapy Timing[1]	-	-	66%	66%
Venous Thromboembolism Prophylaxis[1]	-	-	94%	94%
Written Stroke Educational Materials Given[1]	-	-	87%	88%
Surgical Care Improvement Project				
Appropriate Beta Blocker Usage	40	92%	98%	98%
Appropriate VTP Within 24 Hours	135	99%	98%	98%
Controlled Postoperative Blood Glucose[7]	-	-	97%	97%
Perioperative Temperature Management	143	100%	100%	100%
Prophylactic Antibiotic Selection	106	99%	99%	99%
Prophylactic Antibiotic Selection (Outpatient)	108	100%	98%	98%
Prophylactic Antibiotic Stopped	104	98%	98%	98%
Prophylactic Antibiotic Timing	106	100%	99%	99%
Prophylactic Antibiotic Timing (Outpatient)	81	100%	97%	98%
Urinary Catheter Removal	65	95%	98%	97%
Survey of Patients' Hospital Experiences				
Area Around Room 'Always' Quiet at Night	300+	73%	60%	61%
Doctors 'Always' Communicated Well	300+	84%	81%	82%
Home Recovery Information Given	300+	87%	86%	85%
Hospital Given 9 or 10 on 10 Point Scale	300+	72%	70%	71%
Meds 'Always' Explained Before Given	300+	66%	64%	64%
Nurses 'Always' Communicated Well	300+	79%	79%	79%
Pain 'Always' Well Controlled	300+	72%	71%	71%
Room and Bathroom 'Always' Clean	300+	75%	74%	73%
Timely Help 'Always' Received	300+	70%	67%	68%
Would Definitely Recommend Hospital	300+	70%	70%	71%
Use of Medical Imaging				
Cardiac Imaging Stress Test before Surgery	91	3.3%	5.5%	5.3%
Combination Abdominal CT Scan	237	9.7%	10.1%	10.5%
Combination Brain/Sinus CT Scan[1]	-	-	2.6%	2.7%
Combination Chest CT Scan	98	2.0%	2.8%	2.7%
Follow-up Mammogram/Ultrasound	521	10.2%	8.4%	8.8%
Lumbar Spine MRI for Low Back Pain[1]	-	-	36.6%	37.2%

Good Samaritan Regional Health Center

1 Good Samaritan Way
Mount Vernon, IL 62864
Phone: 618-899-1469
Fax: 618-242-3196
URL: www.smgsi.com
Type: Acute Care Hospitals
Emergency Services: Yes
Ownership: Voluntary non-profit - Church
Beds: 175

Key Personnel:
Intensive Care Unit. . . . . Darren Bock
Radiology. . . . . Henry Chen, MD
CEO/President. . . . . Leo F Childers, Jr
Operating Room. . . . . Kevin Claffey, RN
Quality Assurance . . . . Joby Glenn
Emergency Room . . . . Scott Roustio, MD
Infection Control. . . . . Jeralee Sargent, RN
Chief of Medical Staff. . . . . Jitendra Trivedi, MD

Measure	Cases	This Hosp.	State Avg.	U.S. Avg.
Blood Clot Prevention and Treatment				
Anticoagulation Overlap Therapy[2]	35	100%	91%	93%
ICU Venous Thromboembolism Prophylaxis[2]	79	97%	93%	92%
Incidence of Potentially Preventable VTE[1,2]	-	-	11%	10%
UFH with Dosages/Platelet Monitoring[2]	24	100%	94%	97%
Venous Thromboembolism Prophylaxis[2]	339	94%	86%	85%
Warfarin Therapy Discharge Instructions[2]	28	89%	71%	75%
Chest Pain/Possible Heart Attack Care				
Aspirin Given Within 24 Hours of Arrival	11	91%	96%	96%
Fibrinolytic Meds Within 30 Min. of Arrival[3,7]	-	-	65%	58%
Average Time to ECG (minutes)	11	9	6	7
Average Time to Transfer (minutes)[3,7]	-	-	63	60
Children's Asthma Care				
Received Home Management Plan of Care	-	-	-	88%
Received Reliever Medication	-	-	-	100%
Received Systemic Corticosteroids	-	-	-	100%
Emergency Department				
Admittance Decision Time (minutes)[2]	445	75	89	98
Head CT Results Within 45 Min. of Arrival[1]	-	-	64%	57%
Patients Who Left ER Before Being Seen	23,844	3%	3%	2%
Time from ER Arrival to Admit. (minutes)[2]	471	292	260	274
Time from ER Arrival to Discharge (minutes)	364	158	138	134
Time in ER Before Being Evaluated (minutes)	395	41	28	26
Time to Pain Meds for Fractures (minutes)	116	65	52	57
Heart Attack Care				
Aspirin Given at Discharge	275	100%	99%	99%
Fibrinolytic Meds Within 30 Min. of Arrival[7]	-	-	33%	54%
PCI Within 90 Minutes of Arrival	19	84%	97%	96%
Statin Prescribed at Discharge	254	100%	98%	98%
Heart Failure Care				
ACE Inhibitor or ARB for LVSD	53	100%	98%	97%
Discharge Instructions Given	158	99%	96%	94%
Evaluation of LVS Function	188	100%	99%	99%
Medicare Spending				
Medicare Spending per Patient (ratio)	-	0.93	1	0.98
Pneumonia Care				
Appropriate Initial Antibiotic Given	89	98%	95%	95%
Blood Culture Timing	144	98%	98%	98%
Pregnancy and Delivery Care				
Newborn Deliveries Scheduled Early[2]	111	1%	2%	6%
Preventive Care				
Immunization for Influenza[2]	521	99%	92%	90%
Immunization for Pneumonia[2]	663	98%	92%	92%
Stroke Care				
Anticoagulation Therapy for Atrial Fibrillation	16	100%	94%	95%
Antithrombotic Therapy Timing	69	100%	98%	98%
Assessed for Rehabilitation	67	100%	97%	97%
Discharged on Antithrombotic Therapy	67	100%	99%	99%
Discharged on Statin Medication	49	98%	94%	94%
Thrombolytic Therapy Timing[1]	-	-	66%	66%
Venous Thromboembolism Prophylaxis	69	99%	94%	94%
Written Stroke Educational Materials Given	44	98%	87%	88%
Surgical Care Improvement Project				
Appropriate Beta Blocker Usage	188	100%	98%	98%
Appropriate VTP Within 24 Hours	325	100%	98%	98%
Controlled Postoperative Blood Glucose	74	96%	97%	97%
Perioperative Temperature Management	382	100%	100%	100%
Prophylactic Antibiotic Selection	312	100%	99%	99%
Prophylactic Antibiotic Selection (Outpatient)	355	97%	98%	98%
Prophylactic Antibiotic Stopped	294	98%	98%	98%
Prophylactic Antibiotic Timing	313	99%	99%	99%
Prophylactic Antibiotic Timing (Outpatient)	358	98%	97%	98%
Urinary Catheter Removal	160	98%	98%	97%
Survey of Patients' Hospital Experiences				
Area Around Room 'Always' Quiet at Night	300+	64%	60%	61%
Doctors 'Always' Communicated Well	300+	82%	81%	82%
Home Recovery Information Given	300+	88%	86%	85%
Hospital Given 9 or 10 on 10 Point Scale	300+	74%	70%	71%
Meds 'Always' Explained Before Given	300+	65%	64%	64%

NOTE: Hospital profiles are in alphabetical order by state, then city, then hospital within the city; Rankings exclude hospitals with less than 25 cases except for patient surveys which excludes hospitals with less than 100 cases; (a) 100-299 cases; (1) The number of cases/patients is too few to report; (2) Data submitted were based on a sample of cases/patients; (3) Results are based on a shorter time period than required; (4) Data suppressed by CMS for one or more quarters; (5) Results are not available for this reporting period; (6) Fewer than 100 patients completed the HCAHPS survey; (7) No cases met the criteria for this measure; (8) The lower limit of the confidence interval cannot be calculated if the number of observed infections equals zero; (9) No data are available from the state/territory for this reporting period; (10) The scores shown reflect fewer than 50 completed surveys; (11) There were discrepancies in the data collection process; (12) This measure does not apply to this hospital for this reporting period; (13) Results cannot be calculated for this reporting period; (14) The results for this state are combined with nearby states to protect confidentiality; Please refer to the User's Guide for a full explanation of data.

Measure	Cases	This Hosp.	State Avg.	U.S. Avg.
Nurses 'Always' Communicated Well	300+	82%	79%	79%
Pain 'Always' Well Controlled	300+	76%	71%	71%
Room and Bathroom 'Always' Clean	300+	84%	74%	73%
Timely Help 'Always' Received	300+	72%	67%	68%
Would Definitely Recommend Hospital	300+	73%	70%	71%
Use of Medical Imaging				
Cardiac Imaging Stress Test before Surgery	344	4.1%	5.5%	5.3%
Combination Abdominal CT Scan	713	18.7%	10.1%	10.5%
Combination Brain/Sinus CT Scan	620	6.0%	2.6%	2.7%
Combination Chest CT Scan	401	0.7%	2.8%	2.7%
Follow-up Mammogram/Ultrasound	1,233	6.5%	8.4%	8.8%
Lumbar Spine MRI for Low Back Pain	55	43.6%	36.6%	37.2%

Saint Joseph Memorial Hospital

2 South Hospital Drive
Murphysboro, IL 62966
E-mail: info@sih.net
URL: www.sih.net
Phone: 618-684-3156
Fax: 618-529-0535

Type: Critical Access Hospitals
Ownership: Voluntary non-profit - Private
Emergency Services: Yes
Beds: 59

Key Personnel:

Chief of Medical Staff.......... Dale Blaise, MD
Administrator................ John Brothers
Operating Room.............. David Clutts
Infection Control............. Tammy Jurgens
Quality Assurance .... Tammy Jurgens
Emergency Room .... Karen Robert
Intensive Care Unit........... Ann Smith, RN
Anesthesiology............... Louise Vaughn

Measure	Cases	This Hosp.	State Avg.	U.S. Avg.
Blood Clot Prevention and Treatment				
Anticoagulation Overlap Therapy[1]	-	-	91%	93%
ICU Venous Thromboembolism Prophylaxis[7]	-	-	93%	92%
Incidence of Potentially Preventable VTE[7]	-	-	11%	10%
UFH with Dosages/Platelet Monitoring[7]	-	-	94%	97%
Venous Thromboembolism Prophylaxis	353	97%	86%	85%
Warfarin Therapy Discharge Instructions[1]	-	-	71%	75%
Chest Pain/Possible Heart Attack Care				
Aspirin Given Within 24 Hours of Arrival[5]	-	-	96%	96%
Fibrinolytic Meds Within 30 Min. of Arrival[5]	-	-	65%	58%
Average Time to ECG (minutes)[5]	-	-	6	7
Average Time to Transfer (minutes)[5]	-	-	63	60
Children's Asthma Care				
Received Home Management Plan of Care	-	-	-	88%
Received Reliever Medication	-	-	-	100%
Received Systemic Corticosteroids	-	-	-	100%
Emergency Department				
Admittance Decision Time (minutes)	363	68	89	98
Head CT Results Within 45 Min. of Arrival[5]	-	-	64%	57%
Patients Who Left ER Before Being Seen[5]	-	-	3%	2%
Time from ER Arrival to Admit. (minutes)	424	237	260	274
Time from ER Arrival to Discharge (minutes)[5]	-	-	138	134
Time in ER Before Being Evaluated (minutes)[5]	-	-	28	26
Time to Pain Meds for Fractures (minutes)[5]	-	-	52	57
Heart Attack Care				
Aspirin Given at Discharge[1,3]	-	-	99%	99%
Fibrinolytic Meds Within 30 Min. of Arrival[3,7]	-	-	33%	54%
PCI Within 90 Minutes of Arrival[3,7]	-	-	97%	96%
Statin Prescribed at Discharge[1,3]	-	-	98%	98%
Heart Failure Care				
ACE Inhibitor or ARB for LVSD[1]	-	-	98%	97%
Discharge Instructions Given[1]	-	-	96%	94%
Evaluation of LVS Function	15	100%	99%	99%
Medicare Spending				
Medicare Spending per Patient (ratio)	-	-	1	0.98
Pneumonia Care				
Appropriate Initial Antibiotic Given	42	98%	95%	95%
Blood Culture Timing	78	99%	98%	98%
Pregnancy and Delivery Care				
Newborn Deliveries Scheduled Early[7]	-	-	2%	6%
Preventive Care				
Immunization for Influenza	334	95%	92%	90%
Immunization for Pneumonia	501	96%	92%	92%
Stroke Care				
Anticoagulation Therapy for Atrial Fibrillation[5]	-	-	94%	95%
Antithrombotic Therapy Timing[5]	-	-	98%	98%
Assessed for Rehabilitation[5]	-	-	97%	97%
Discharged on Antithrombotic Therapy[5]	-	-	99%	99%
Discharged on Statin Medication[5]	-	-	94%	94%
Thrombolytic Therapy Timing[5]	-	-	66%	66%
Venous Thromboembolism Prophylaxis[5]	-	-	94%	94%
Written Stroke Educational Materials Given[5]	-	-	87%	88%
Surgical Care Improvement Project				
Appropriate Beta Blocker Usage[5]	-	-	98%	98%
Appropriate VTP Within 24 Hours[5]	-	-	98%	98%
Controlled Postoperative Blood Glucose[5]	-	-	97%	97%
Perioperative Temperature Management[5]	-	-	100%	100%
Prophylactic Antibiotic Selection[5]	-	-	99%	99%
Prophylactic Antibiotic Selection (Outpatient)[5]	-	-	98%	98%
Prophylactic Antibiotic Stopped[5]	-	-	98%	98%
Prophylactic Antibiotic Timing[5]	-	-	99%	99%
Prophylactic Antibiotic Timing (Outpatient)[5]	-	-	97%	98%
Urinary Catheter Removal[5]	-	-	98%	97%
Survey of Patients' Hospital Experiences				
Area Around Room 'Always' Quiet at Night	(a)	73%	60%	61%
Doctors 'Always' Communicated Well	(a)	86%	81%	82%
Home Recovery Information Given	(a)	82%	86%	85%
Hospital Given 9 or 10 on 10 Point Scale	(a)	87%	70%	71%
Meds 'Always' Explained Before Given	(a)	69%	64%	64%
Nurses 'Always' Communicated Well	(a)	86%	79%	79%
Pain 'Always' Well Controlled	(a)	82%	71%	71%
Room and Bathroom 'Always' Clean	(a)	82%	74%	73%
Timely Help 'Always' Received	(a)	84%	67%	68%
Would Definitely Recommend Hospital	(a)	83%	70%	71%
Use of Medical Imaging				
Cardiac Imaging Stress Test before Surgery[1]	-	-	5.5%	5.3%
Combination Abdominal CT Scan	480	20.0%	10.1%	10.5%
Combination Brain/Sinus CT Scan[1]	-	-	2.6%	2.7%
Combination Chest CT Scan	200	9.5%	2.8%	2.7%
Follow-up Mammogram/Ultrasound[7]	-	-	8.4%	8.8%
Lumbar Spine MRI for Low Back Pain[1]	-	-	36.6%	37.2%

Edward Hospital

801 South Washington
Naperville, IL 60540
URL: www.edward.org
Phone: 630-527-3000
Fax: 630-961-4910

Type: Acute Care Hospitals
Ownership: Voluntary non-profit - Private
Emergency Services: Yes
Beds: 179

Key Personnel:

Operating Room.............. Mohan Airan
Infection Control.............. Robert Chase, MD
Chief of Medical Staff.......... Glenn Grobe
Radiology.................... Yuk-Pui Li, MD
CEO/President................ Pamela Meyer-Davis
Quality Assurance .... Jane Mitchell
Pediatric Ambulatory Care ...... Timothy Wall
Pediatric In-Patient Care .... Timothy Wall

Measure	Cases	This Hosp.	State Avg.	U.S. Avg.
Blood Clot Prevention and Treatment				
Anticoagulation Overlap Therapy[2]	191	96%	91%	93%
ICU Venous Thromboembolism Prophylaxis[2]	92	79%	93%	92%
Incidence of Potentially Preventable VTE[2]	51	16%	11%	10%
UFH with Dosages/Platelet Monitoring[2]	205	99%	94%	97%
Venous Thromboembolism Prophylaxis[2]	304	79%	86%	85%
Warfarin Therapy Discharge Instructions[2]	144	67%	71%	75%
Chest Pain/Possible Heart Attack Care				
Aspirin Given Within 24 Hours of Arrival[1,3]	-	-	96%	96%
Fibrinolytic Meds Within 30 Min. of Arrival[5]	-	-	65%	58%
Average Time to ECG (minutes)[1,3]	-	-	6	7
Average Time to Transfer (minutes)[5]	-	-	63	60
Children's Asthma Care				
Received Home Management Plan of Care	-	-	-	88%
Received Reliever Medication	-	-	-	100%
Received Systemic Corticosteroids	-	-	-	100%
Emergency Department				
Admittance Decision Time (minutes)[2]	485	96	89	98
Head CT Results Within 45 Min. of Arrival[1]	-	-	64%	57%
Patients Who Left ER Before Being Seen	93,106	0%	3%	2%
Time from ER Arrival to Admit. (minutes)[2]	499	246	260	274
Time from ER Arrival to Discharge (minutes)	373	110	138	134
Time in ER Before Being Evaluated (minutes)	387	10	28	26
Time to Pain Meds for Fractures (minutes)	346	26	52	57
Heart Attack Care				
Aspirin Given at Discharge	233	100%	99%	99%
Fibrinolytic Meds Within 30 Min. of Arrival[7]	-	-	33%	54%
PCI Within 90 Minutes of Arrival	46	100%	97%	96%
Statin Prescribed at Discharge	218	98%	98%	98%
Heart Failure Care				
ACE Inhibitor or ARB for LVSD[2]	141	98%	98%	97%
Discharge Instructions Given[2]	376	86%	96%	94%
Evaluation of LVS Function[2]	453	100%	99%	99%
Medicare Spending				
Medicare Spending per Patient (ratio)	-	1.03	1	0.98
Pneumonia Care				
Appropriate Initial Antibiotic Given[2]	140	97%	95%	95%
Blood Culture Timing[2]	277	100%	98%	98%
Pregnancy and Delivery Care				
Newborn Deliveries Scheduled Early[2]	37	3%	2%	6%
Preventive Care				
Immunization for Influenza[2]	539	97%	92%	90%
Immunization for Pneumonia[2]	603	81%	92%	92%
Stroke Care				
Anticoagulation Therapy for Atrial Fibrillation	36	100%	94%	95%
Antithrombotic Therapy Timing	185	98%	98%	98%
Assessed for Rehabilitation	223	96%	97%	97%
Discharged on Antithrombotic Therapy	199	95%	99%	99%
Discharged on Statin Medication	151	93%	94%	94%
Thrombolytic Therapy Timing	23	57%	66%	66%
Venous Thromboembolism Prophylaxis	230	90%	94%	94%
Written Stroke Educational Materials Given	121	83%	87%	88%
Surgical Care Improvement Project				
Appropriate Beta Blocker Usage[2]	245	100%	98%	98%
Appropriate VTP Within 24 Hours[2]	420	98%	98%	98%
Controlled Postoperative Blood Glucose[2]	161	96%	97%	97%
Perioperative Temperature Management[2]	512	100%	100%	100%
Prophylactic Antibiotic Selection[2]	459	99%	99%	99%
Prophylactic Antibiotic Selection (Outpatient)	588	98%	98%	98%
Prophylactic Antibiotic Stopped[2]	449	97%	98%	98%
Prophylactic Antibiotic Timing[2]	460	99%	99%	99%
Prophylactic Antibiotic Timing (Outpatient)	589	97%	97%	98%
Urinary Catheter Removal[2]	443	96%	98%	97%
Survey of Patients' Hospital Experiences				
Area Around Room 'Always' Quiet at Night	300+	57%	60%	61%
Doctors 'Always' Communicated Well	300+	81%	81%	82%
Home Recovery Information Given	300+	83%	86%	85%
Hospital Given 9 or 10 on 10 Point Scale	300+	77%	70%	71%
Meds 'Always' Explained Before Given	300+	63%	64%	64%
Nurses 'Always' Communicated Well	300+	78%	79%	79%
Pain 'Always' Well Controlled	300+	72%	71%	71%
Room and Bathroom 'Always' Clean	300+	72%	74%	73%
Timely Help 'Always' Received	300+	62%	67%	68%
Would Definitely Recommend Hospital	300+	81%	70%	71%
Use of Medical Imaging				
Cardiac Imaging Stress Test before Surgery	2,044	4.0%	5.5%	5.3%
Combination Abdominal CT Scan	1,980	7.8%	10.1%	10.5%
Combination Brain/Sinus CT Scan	1,449	0.8%	2.6%	2.7%
Combination Chest CT Scan	1,696	1.5%	2.8%	2.7%
Follow-up Mammogram/Ultrasound	2,939	11.2%	8.4%	8.8%
Lumbar Spine MRI for Low Back Pain	212	33.5%	36.6%	37.2%

Silver Cross Hospital & Medical Centers

1900 Silver Cross Blvd
New Lenox, IL 60451
E-mail: tsimons@silvercross.org
URL: www.silvercross.org
Phone: 815-300-1100
Fax: 815-740-3561

Type: Acute Care Hospitals
Ownership: Voluntary non-profit - Private
Emergency Services: Yes
Beds: 297

Key Personnel:

Chief of Medical Staff.......... Kishor Ajmere
Radiology.................... Salwa Asaad
Pediatric In-Patient Care .... Peggy Gricus
CEO/President................ Paul Pawlak
Infection Control.............. Margaret Rodegher

NOTE: Hospital profiles are in alphabetical order by state, then city, then hospital within the city; Rankings exclude hospitals with less than 25 cases except for patient surveys which excludes hospitals with less than 100 cases; (a) 100-299 cases; (1) The number of cases/patients is too few to report; (2) Data submitted were based on a sample of cases/patients; (3) Results are based on a shorter time period than required; (4) Data suppressed by CMS for one or more quarters; (5) Results are not available for this reporting period; (6) Fewer than 100 patients completed the HCAHPS survey; (7) No cases met the criteria for this measure; (8) The lower limit of the confidence interval cannot be calculated if the number of observed infections equals zero; (9) No data are available from the state/territory for this reporting period; (10) The scores shown reflect fewer than 50 completed surveys; (11) There were discrepancies in the data collection process; (12) This measure does not apply to this hospital for this reporting period; (13) Results cannot be calculated for this reporting period; (14) The results for this state are combined with nearby states to protect confidentiality; Please refer to the User's Guide for a full explanation of data.

Quality Assurance .... Billie Schimanski
Cardiac Laboratory............ Paula Simpson

Measure	Cases	This Hosp.	State Avg.	U.S. Avg.
Blood Clot Prevention and Treatment				
Anticoagulation Overlap Therapy[2]	107	76%	91%	93%
ICU Venous Thromboembolism Prophylaxis[2]	56	84%	93%	92%
Incidence of Potentially Preventable VTE[2]	19	53%	11%	10%
UFH with Dosages/Platelet Monitoring[2]	54	100%	94%	97%
Venous Thromboembolism Prophylaxis[2]	343	61%	86%	85%
Warfarin Therapy Discharge Instructions[2]	68	96%	71%	75%
Chest Pain/Possible Heart Attack Care				
Aspirin Given Within 24 Hours of Arrival[1]	-	-	96%	96%
Fibrinolytic Meds Within 30 Min. of Arrival[3,7]	-	-	65%	58%
Average Time to ECG (minutes)[1]	-	-	6	7
Average Time to Transfer (minutes)[3,7]	-	-	63	60
Children's Asthma Care				
Received Home Management Plan of Care	-	-	-	88%
Received Reliever Medication	-	-	-	100%
Received Systemic Corticosteroids	-	-	-	100%
Emergency Department				
Admittance Decision Time (minutes)[2]	424	84	89	98
Head CT Results Within 45 Min. of Arrival[1,3]	-	-	64%	57%
Patients Who Left ER Before Being Seen	70,182	2%	3%	2%
Time from ER Arrival to Admit. (minutes)[2]	425	243	260	274
Time from ER Arrival to Discharge (minutes)	374	144	138	134
Time in ER Before Being Evaluated (minutes)	327	60	28	26
Time to Pain Meds for Fractures (minutes)	270	64	52	57
Heart Attack Care				
Aspirin Given at Discharge	254	99%	99%	99%
Fibrinolytic Meds Within 30 Min. of Arrival[7]	-	-	33%	54%
PCI Within 90 Minutes of Arrival	55	100%	97%	96%
Statin Prescribed at Discharge	237	97%	98%	98%
Heart Failure Care				
ACE Inhibitor or ARB for LVSD	140	99%	98%	97%
Discharge Instructions Given	477	96%	96%	94%
Evaluation of LVS Function	582	100%	99%	99%
Medicare Spending				
Medicare Spending per Patient (ratio)	-	1.02	1	0.98
Pneumonia Care				
Appropriate Initial Antibiotic Given	199	97%	95%	95%
Blood Culture Timing	145	97%	98%	98%
Pregnancy and Delivery Care				
Newborn Deliveries Scheduled Early[2]	35	11%	2%	6%
Preventive Care				
Immunization for Influenza[2]	522	98%	92%	90%
Immunization for Pneumonia[2]	593	93%	92%	92%
Stroke Care				
Anticoagulation Therapy for Atrial Fibrillation	25	96%	94%	95%
Antithrombotic Therapy Timing	169	98%	98%	98%
Assessed for Rehabilitation	193	96%	97%	97%
Discharged on Antithrombotic Therapy	166	99%	99%	99%
Discharged on Statin Medication	129	92%	94%	94%
Thrombolytic Therapy Timing	13	100%	66%	66%
Venous Thromboembolism Prophylaxis	211	80%	94%	94%
Written Stroke Educational Materials Given	105	77%	87%	88%
Surgical Care Improvement Project				
Appropriate Beta Blocker Usage[2]	184	98%	98%	98%
Appropriate VTP Within 24 Hours[2]	654	100%	98%	98%
Controlled Postoperative Blood Glucose[2,7]	-	-	97%	97%
Perioperative Temperature Management[2]	724	100%	100%	100%
Prophylactic Antibiotic Selection[2]	550	99%	99%	99%
Prophylactic Antibiotic Selection (Outpatient)	556	98%	98%	98%
Prophylactic Antibiotic Stopped[2]	534	99%	98%	98%
Prophylactic Antibiotic Timing[2]	551	99%	99%	99%
Prophylactic Antibiotic Timing (Outpatient)	559	97%	97%	98%
Urinary Catheter Removal[2]	476	98%	98%	97%
Survey of Patients' Hospital Experiences				
Area Around Room 'Always' Quiet at Night	300+	67%	60%	61%
Doctors 'Always' Communicated Well	300+	79%	81%	82%
Home Recovery Information Given	300+	82%	86%	85%
Hospital Given 9 or 10 on 10 Point Scale	300+	76%	70%	71%
Meds 'Always' Explained Before Given	300+	64%	64%	64%
Nurses 'Always' Communicated Well	300+	78%	79%	79%
Pain 'Always' Well Controlled	300+	70%	71%	71%
Room and Bathroom 'Always' Clean	300+	79%	74%	73%
Timely Help 'Always' Received	300+	67%	67%	68%
Would Definitely Recommend Hospital	300+	79%	70%	71%
Use of Medical Imaging				
Cardiac Imaging Stress Test before Surgery	448	6.3%	5.5%	5.3%
Combination Abdominal CT Scan	933	5.6%	10.1%	10.5%
Combination Brain/Sinus CT Scan	963	2.1%	2.6%	2.7%
Combination Chest CT Scan	936	1.2%	2.8%	2.7%
Follow-up Mammogram/Ultrasound	1,760	5.8%	8.4%	8.8%
Lumbar Spine MRI for Low Back Pain	246	32.9%	36.6%	37.2%

Advocate Bromenn Medical Center

1304 Franklin Avenue
Normal, IL 61761
Phone: 309-454-1400
Type: Acute Care Hospitals
Emergency Services: Yes
Ownership: Voluntary non-profit - Church

Key Personnel:
CEO/President............... Roger S Hunt

Measure	Cases	This Hosp.	State Avg.	U.S. Avg.
Blood Clot Prevention and Treatment				
Anticoagulation Overlap Therapy	42	93%	91%	93%
ICU Venous Thromboembolism Prophylaxis	355	96%	93%	92%
Incidence of Potentially Preventable VTE[1]	-	-	11%	10%
UFH with Dosages/Platelet Monitoring	19	100%	94%	97%
Venous Thromboembolism Prophylaxis	2,329	95%	86%	85%
Warfarin Therapy Discharge Instructions	28	96%	71%	75%
Chest Pain/Possible Heart Attack Care				
Aspirin Given Within 24 Hours of Arrival[5]	-	-	96%	96%
Fibrinolytic Meds Within 30 Min. of Arrival[5]	-	-	65%	58%
Average Time to ECG (minutes)[5]	-	-	6	7
Average Time to Transfer (minutes)[5]	-	-	63	60
Children's Asthma Care				
Received Home Management Plan of Care	-	-	-	88%
Received Reliever Medication	-	-	-	100%
Received Systemic Corticosteroids	-	-	-	100%
Emergency Department				
Admittance Decision Time (minutes)[2]	460	102	89	98
Head CT Results Within 45 Min. of Arrival[5]	-	-	64%	57%
Patients Who Left ER Before Being Seen	36,944	3%	3%	2%
Time from ER Arrival to Admit. (minutes)[2]	479	267	260	274
Time from ER Arrival to Discharge (minutes)	382	159	138	134
Time in ER Before Being Evaluated (minutes)	419	32	28	26
Time to Pain Meds for Fractures (minutes)	112	66	52	57
Heart Attack Care				
Aspirin Given at Discharge	135	100%	99%	99%
Fibrinolytic Meds Within 30 Min. of Arrival[7]	-	-	33%	54%
PCI Within 90 Minutes of Arrival	33	100%	97%	96%
Statin Prescribed at Discharge	130	99%	98%	98%
Heart Failure Care				
ACE Inhibitor or ARB for LVSD	62	98%	98%	97%
Discharge Instructions Given	156	95%	96%	94%
Evaluation of LVS Function	198	100%	99%	99%
Medicare Spending				
Medicare Spending per Patient (ratio)	-	0.99	1	0.98
Pneumonia Care				
Appropriate Initial Antibiotic Given	68	91%	95%	95%
Blood Culture Timing	113	97%	98%	98%
Pregnancy and Delivery Care				
Newborn Deliveries Scheduled Early	158	1%	2%	6%
Preventive Care				
Immunization for Influenza[2]	562	97%	92%	90%
Immunization for Pneumonia[2]	583	98%	92%	92%
Stroke Care				
Anticoagulation Therapy for Atrial Fibrillation	12	100%	94%	95%
Antithrombotic Therapy Timing	59	100%	98%	98%
Assessed for Rehabilitation	85	98%	97%	97%
Discharged on Antithrombotic Therapy	73	97%	99%	99%
Discharged on Statin Medication	55	93%	94%	94%
Thrombolytic Therapy Timing	13	62%	66%	66%
Venous Thromboembolism Prophylaxis	79	92%	94%	94%
Written Stroke Educational Materials Given	41	98%	87%	88%
Surgical Care Improvement Project				
Appropriate Beta Blocker Usage[2]	220	100%	98%	98%
Appropriate VTP Within 24 Hours[2]	586	99%	98%	98%
Controlled Postoperative Blood Glucose[2]	42	98%	97%	97%
Perioperative Temperature Management[2]	758	100%	100%	100%
Prophylactic Antibiotic Selection[2]	581	100%	99%	99%
Prophylactic Antibiotic Selection (Outpatient)	379	98%	98%	98%
Prophylactic Antibiotic Stopped[2]	577	99%	98%	98%
Prophylactic Antibiotic Timing[2]	580	100%	99%	99%
Prophylactic Antibiotic Timing (Outpatient)	379	98%	97%	98%
Urinary Catheter Removal[2]	162	98%	98%	97%
Survey of Patients' Hospital Experiences				
Area Around Room 'Always' Quiet at Night	300+	61%	60%	61%
Doctors 'Always' Communicated Well	300+	83%	81%	82%
Home Recovery Information Given	300+	87%	86%	85%
Hospital Given 9 or 10 on 10 Point Scale	300+	78%	70%	71%
Meds 'Always' Explained Before Given	300+	65%	64%	64%
Nurses 'Always' Communicated Well	300+	83%	79%	79%
Pain 'Always' Well Controlled	300+	72%	71%	71%
Room and Bathroom 'Always' Clean	300+	78%	74%	73%
Timely Help 'Always' Received	300+	68%	67%	68%
Would Definitely Recommend Hospital	300+	79%	70%	71%
Use of Medical Imaging				
Cardiac Imaging Stress Test before Surgery	339	4.4%	5.5%	5.3%
Combination Abdominal CT Scan	540	24.8%	10.1%	10.5%
Combination Brain/Sinus CT Scan	622	1.9%	2.6%	2.7%
Combination Chest CT Scan	540	13.9%	2.8%	2.7%
Follow-up Mammogram/Ultrasound	1,352	6.5%	8.4%	8.8%
Lumbar Spine MRI for Low Back Pain	81	32.1%	36.6%	37.2%

North Chicago VA Medical Center

3001 Greenbay Road
North Chicago, IL 60064
Phone: 847-688-1900
Fax: 224-610-3806
URL: www.northchicago.va.gov
Type: Acute Care - VA
Emergency Services: No
Ownership: Government Federal

Key Personnel:
Intensive Care Unit............ Celestina Bobadilla, RN
Radiology.................... Wonsang Chun, MD
Chief of Medical Staff.......... Tariq Hassan, MD
Emergency Room .... Frank Maldonado, MD
Quality Assurance .... Sharon Pusateri
CEO/President................ Patrick L Sullivan, FACHE

Measure	Cases	This Hosp.	State Avg.	U.S. Avg.
Blood Clot Prevention and Treatment				
Anticoagulation Overlap Therapy	-	-	91%	93%
ICU Venous Thromboembolism Prophylaxis	-	-	93%	92%
Incidence of Potentially Preventable VTE	-	-	11%	10%
UFH with Dosages/Platelet Monitoring	-	-	94%	97%
Venous Thromboembolism Prophylaxis	-	-	86%	85%
Warfarin Therapy Discharge Instructions	-	-	71%	75%
Chest Pain/Possible Heart Attack Care				
Aspirin Given Within 24 Hours of Arrival	-	-	96%	96%
Fibrinolytic Meds Within 30 Min. of Arrival	-	-	65%	58%
Average Time to ECG (minutes)	-	-	6	7
Average Time to Transfer (minutes)	-	-	63	60
Children's Asthma Care				
Received Home Management Plan of Care	-	-	-	88%
Received Reliever Medication	-	-	-	100%
Received Systemic Corticosteroids	-	-	-	100%
Emergency Department				
Admittance Decision Time (minutes)	-	-	89	98
Head CT Results Within 45 Min. of Arrival	-	-	64%	57%
Patients Who Left ER Before Being Seen	-	-	3%	2%
Time from ER Arrival to Admit. (minutes)	-	-	260	274
Time from ER Arrival to Discharge (minutes)	-	-	138	134
Time in ER Before Being Evaluated (minutes)	-	-	28	26
Time to Pain Meds for Fractures (minutes)	-	-	52	57
Heart Attack Care				
Aspirin Given at Discharge[1]	-	-	99%	99%
Fibrinolytic Meds Within 30 Min. of Arrival[5]	-	-	33%	54%
PCI Within 90 Minutes of Arrival[5]	-	-	97%	96%
Statin Prescribed at Discharge[1]	-	-	98%	98%
Heart Failure Care				

NOTE: Hospital profiles are in alphabetical order by state, then city, then hospital within the city; Rankings exclude hospitals with less than 25 cases except for patient surveys which excludes hospitals with less than 100 cases; (a) 100-299 cases; (1) The number of cases/patients is too few to report; (2) Data submitted were based on a sample of cases/patients; (3) Results are based on a shorter time period than required; (4) Data suppressed by CMS for one or more quarters; (5) Results are not available for this reporting period; (6) Fewer than 100 patients completed the HCAHPS survey; (7) No cases met the criteria for this measure; (8) The lower limit of the confidence interval cannot be calculated if the number of observed infections equals zero; (9) No data are available from the state/territory for this reporting period; (10) The scores shown reflect fewer than 50 completed surveys; (11) There were discrepancies in the data collection process; (12) This measure does not apply to this hospital for this reporting period; (13) Results cannot be calculated for this reporting period; (14) The results for this state are combined with nearby states to protect confidentiality; Please refer to the User's Guide for a full explanation of data.

Measure	Cases	This Hosp.	State Avg.	U.S. Avg.
ACE Inhibitor or ARB for LVSD	32	100%	98%	97%
Discharge Instructions Given	58	98%	96%	94%
Evaluation of LVS Function	65	100%	99%	99%
Medicare Spending				
Medicare Spending per Patient (ratio)	-	-	1	0.98
Pneumonia Care				
Appropriate Initial Antibiotic Given	66	98%	95%	95%
Blood Culture Timing	100	98%	98%	98%
Pregnancy and Delivery Care				
Newborn Deliveries Scheduled Early	-	-	2%	6%
Preventive Care				
Immunization for Influenza[5]	-	-	92%	90%
Immunization for Pneumonia[5]	-	-	92%	92%
Stroke Care				
Anticoagulation Therapy for Atrial Fibrillation	-	-	94%	95%
Antithrombotic Therapy Timing	-	-	98%	98%
Assessed for Rehabilitation	-	-	97%	97%
Discharged on Antithrombotic Therapy	-	-	99%	99%
Discharged on Statin Medication	-	-	94%	94%
Thrombolytic Therapy Timing	-	-	66%	66%
Venous Thromboembolism Prophylaxis	-	-	94%	94%
Written Stroke Educational Materials Given	-	-	87%	88%
Surgical Care Improvement Project				
Appropriate Beta Blocker Usage[2]	30	73%	98%	98%
Appropriate VTP Within 24 Hours[2]	96	91%	98%	98%
Controlled Postoperative Blood Glucose[5]	-	-	97%	97%
Perioperative Temperature Management[2]	101	95%	100%	100%
Prophylactic Antibiotic Selection	60	100%	99%	99%
Prophylactic Antibiotic Selection (Outpatient)	-	-	98%	98%
Prophylactic Antibiotic Stopped	59	100%	98%	98%
Prophylactic Antibiotic Timing	60	100%	99%	99%
Prophylactic Antibiotic Timing (Outpatient)	-	-	97%	98%
Urinary Catheter Removal[2]	51	98%	98%	97%
Survey of Patients' Hospital Experiences				
Area Around Room 'Always' Quiet at Night	-	-	60%	61%
Doctors 'Always' Communicated Well	-	-	81%	82%
Home Recovery Information Given	-	-	86%	85%
Hospital Given 9 or 10 on 10 Point Scale	-	-	70%	71%
Meds 'Always' Explained Before Given	-	-	64%	64%
Nurses 'Always' Communicated Well	-	-	79%	79%
Pain 'Always' Well Controlled	-	-	71%	71%
Room and Bathroom 'Always' Clean	-	-	74%	73%
Timely Help 'Always' Received	-	-	67%	68%
Would Definitely Recommend Hospital	-	-	70%	71%
Use of Medical Imaging				
Cardiac Imaging Stress Test before Surgery	-	-	5.5%	5.3%
Combination Abdominal CT Scan	-	-	10.1%	10.5%
Combination Brain/Sinus CT Scan	-	-	2.6%	2.7%
Combination Chest CT Scan	-	-	2.8%	2.7%
Follow-up Mammogram/Ultrasound	-	-	8.4%	8.8%
Lumbar Spine MRI for Low Back Pain	-	-	36.6%	37.2%

Advocate Christ Hospital & Medical Center

4440 W 95th Street
Oak Lawn, IL 60453
URL: www.advocatehealth.com
Type: Acute Care Hospitals
Ownership: Voluntary non-profit - Church
Phone: 708-684-8000
Fax: 708-864-4440
Emergency Services: Yes
Beds: 64

Key Personnel:
Radiology. . . . . Sangarappillai Asoka
CEO/President. . . . . James H. Skogsbergh

Measure	Cases	This Hosp.	State Avg.	U.S. Avg.
Blood Clot Prevention and Treatment				
Anticoagulation Overlap Therapy[2]	270	91%	91%	93%
ICU Venous Thromboembolism Prophylaxis[2]	124	94%	93%	92%
Incidence of Potentially Preventable VTE[2]	81	5%	11%	10%
UFH with Dosages/Platelet Monitoring[2]	201	99%	94%	97%
Venous Thromboembolism Prophylaxis[2]	341	89%	86%	85%
Warfarin Therapy Discharge Instructions[2]	163	39%	71%	75%
Chest Pain/Possible Heart Attack Care				
Aspirin Given Within 24 Hours of Arrival[1,3]	-	-	96%	96%
Fibrinolytic Meds Within 30 Min. of Arrival[5]	-	-	65%	58%
Average Time to ECG (minutes)[1,3]	-	-	6	7
Average Time to Transfer (minutes)[5]	-	-	63	60
Children's Asthma Care				
Received Home Management Plan of Care	-	-	-	88%
Received Reliever Medication	-	-	-	100%
Received Systemic Corticosteroids	-	-	-	100%
Emergency Department				
Admittance Decision Time (minutes)[2]	557	210	89	98
Head CT Results Within 45 Min. of Arrival[1]	-	-	64%	57%
Patients Who Left ER Before Being Seen	98,236	3%	3%	2%
Time from ER Arrival to Admit. (minutes)[2]	599	360	260	274
Time from ER Arrival to Discharge (minutes)	383	195	138	134
Time in ER Before Being Evaluated (minutes)	255	81	28	26
Time to Pain Meds for Fractures (minutes)	294	19	52	57
Heart Attack Care				
Aspirin Given at Discharge[2]	304	100%	99%	99%
Fibrinolytic Meds Within 30 Min. of Arrival[2,7]	-	-	33%	54%
PCI Within 90 Minutes of Arrival[2]	32	100%	97%	96%
Statin Prescribed at Discharge[2]	290	100%	98%	98%
Heart Failure Care				
ACE Inhibitor or ARB for LVSD[2]	106	100%	98%	97%
Discharge Instructions Given[2]	280	98%	96%	94%
Evaluation of LVS Function[2]	329	100%	99%	99%
Medicare Spending				
Medicare Spending per Patient (ratio)	-	1.04	1	0.98
Pneumonia Care				
Appropriate Initial Antibiotic Given[2]	46	100%	95%	95%
Blood Culture Timing[2]	90	100%	98%	98%
Pregnancy and Delivery Care				
Newborn Deliveries Scheduled Early	274	2%	2%	6%
Preventive Care				
Immunization for Influenza[2]	575	90%	92%	90%
Immunization for Pneumonia[2]	694	94%	92%	92%
Stroke Care				
Anticoagulation Therapy for Atrial Fibrillation	53	100%	94%	95%
Antithrombotic Therapy Timing	306	100%	98%	98%
Assessed for Rehabilitation	446	95%	97%	97%
Discharged on Antithrombotic Therapy	339	100%	99%	99%
Discharged on Statin Medication	272	94%	94%	94%
Thrombolytic Therapy Timing	23	91%	66%	66%
Venous Thromboembolism Prophylaxis	472	94%	94%	94%
Written Stroke Educational Materials Given	212	93%	87%	88%
Surgical Care Improvement Project				
Appropriate Beta Blocker Usage[2]	385	98%	98%	98%
Appropriate VTP Within 24 Hours[2]	464	98%	98%	98%
Controlled Postoperative Blood Glucose[2]	157	98%	97%	97%
Perioperative Temperature Management[2]	652	100%	100%	100%
Prophylactic Antibiotic Selection[2]	538	99%	99%	99%
Prophylactic Antibiotic Selection (Outpatient)	583	96%	98%	98%
Prophylactic Antibiotic Stopped[2]	521	99%	98%	98%
Prophylactic Antibiotic Timing[2]	538	100%	99%	99%
Prophylactic Antibiotic Timing (Outpatient)	586	94%	97%	98%
Urinary Catheter Removal[2]	314	98%	98%	97%
Survey of Patients' Hospital Experiences				
Area Around Room 'Always' Quiet at Night	300+	54%	60%	61%
Doctors 'Always' Communicated Well	300+	80%	81%	82%
Home Recovery Information Given	300+	88%	86%	85%
Hospital Given 9 or 10 on 10 Point Scale	300+	73%	70%	71%
Meds 'Always' Explained Before Given	300+	65%	64%	64%
Nurses 'Always' Communicated Well	300+	82%	79%	79%
Pain 'Always' Well Controlled	300+	72%	71%	71%
Room and Bathroom 'Always' Clean	300+	70%	74%	73%
Timely Help 'Always' Received	300+	69%	67%	68%
Would Definitely Recommend Hospital	300+	74%	70%	71%
Use of Medical Imaging				
Cardiac Imaging Stress Test before Surgery	963	5.5%	5.5%	5.3%
Combination Abdominal CT Scan	1,517	5.0%	10.1%	10.5%
Combination Brain/Sinus CT Scan	1,275	1.0%	2.6%	2.7%
Combination Chest CT Scan	1,756	1.6%	2.8%	2.7%
Follow-up Mammogram/Ultrasound	3,361	8.1%	8.4%	8.8%
Lumbar Spine MRI for Low Back Pain	147	37.4%	36.6%	37.2%

Rush Oak Park Hospital

520 S Maple Ave
Oak Park, IL 60304
URL: www.oakparkhospital.org
Type: Acute Care Hospitals
Ownership: Voluntary non-profit - Church
Phone: 708-383-9300
Fax: 708-660-6658
Emergency Services: No
Beds: 296

Key Personnel:
Chief of Medical Staff. . . . . David Ansell, MD
Quality Assurance . . . . Mary Barrie, RN
CEO/President. . . . . Bruce M Elegant, MPH, FACHE
Radiology. . . . . William Mollihan, MD
Emergency Room . . . . Daniel Noonan, MD
Operating Room. . . . . Diane Vendola

Measure	Cases	This Hosp.	State Avg.	U.S. Avg.
Blood Clot Prevention and Treatment				
Anticoagulation Overlap Therapy[2]	50	98%	91%	93%
ICU Venous Thromboembolism Prophylaxis[2]	116	97%	93%	92%
Incidence of Potentially Preventable VTE[1,2]	-	-	11%	10%
UFH with Dosages/Platelet Monitoring[2]	21	100%	94%	97%
Venous Thromboembolism Prophylaxis[2]	331	94%	86%	85%
Warfarin Therapy Discharge Instructions[2]	41	76%	71%	75%
Chest Pain/Possible Heart Attack Care				
Aspirin Given Within 24 Hours of Arrival[1,3]	-	-	96%	96%
Fibrinolytic Meds Within 30 Min. of Arrival[3,7]	-	-	65%	58%
Average Time to ECG (minutes)[1,3]	-	-	6	7
Average Time to Transfer (minutes)[3,7]	-	-	63	60
Children's Asthma Care				
Received Home Management Plan of Care	-	-	-	88%
Received Reliever Medication	-	-	-	100%
Received Systemic Corticosteroids	-	-	-	100%
Emergency Department				
Admittance Decision Time (minutes)[2]	695	58	89	98
Head CT Results Within 45 Min. of Arrival[1]	-	-	64%	57%
Patients Who Left ER Before Being Seen	23,872	1%	3%	2%
Time from ER Arrival to Admit. (minutes)[2]	699	201	260	274
Time from ER Arrival to Discharge (minutes)	379	108	138	134
Time in ER Before Being Evaluated (minutes)	318	20	28	26
Time to Pain Meds for Fractures (minutes)	76	46	52	57
Heart Attack Care				
Aspirin Given at Discharge	44	95%	99%	99%
Fibrinolytic Meds Within 30 Min. of Arrival[7]	-	-	33%	54%
PCI Within 90 Minutes of Arrival[1]	-	-	97%	96%
Statin Prescribed at Discharge	39	100%	98%	98%
Heart Failure Care				
ACE Inhibitor or ARB for LVSD	79	99%	98%	97%
Discharge Instructions Given	165	91%	96%	94%
Evaluation of LVS Function	201	100%	99%	99%
Medicare Spending				
Medicare Spending per Patient (ratio)	-	1.03	1	0.98
Pneumonia Care				
Appropriate Initial Antibiotic Given	58	97%	95%	95%
Blood Culture Timing	97	96%	98%	98%
Pregnancy and Delivery Care				
Newborn Deliveries Scheduled Early[7]	-	-	2%	6%
Preventive Care				
Immunization for Influenza[2]	441	99%	92%	90%
Immunization for Pneumonia[2]	609	99%	92%	92%
Stroke Care				
Anticoagulation Therapy for Atrial Fibrillation[1]	-	-	94%	95%
Antithrombotic Therapy Timing	36	100%	98%	98%
Assessed for Rehabilitation	35	100%	97%	97%
Discharged on Antithrombotic Therapy	34	97%	99%	99%
Discharged on Statin Medication	29	90%	94%	94%
Thrombolytic Therapy Timing[1]	-	-	66%	66%
Venous Thromboembolism Prophylaxis	40	92%	94%	94%
Written Stroke Educational Materials Given	19	89%	87%	88%
Surgical Care Improvement Project				
Appropriate Beta Blocker Usage	84	99%	98%	98%
Appropriate VTP Within 24 Hours	246	98%	98%	98%
Controlled Postoperative Blood Glucose[7]	-	-	97%	97%
Perioperative Temperature Management	282	100%	100%	100%
Prophylactic Antibiotic Selection	163	98%	99%	99%
Prophylactic Antibiotic Selection (Outpatient)	25	92%	98%	98%
Prophylactic Antibiotic Stopped	158	100%	98%	98%

NOTE: Hospital profiles are in alphabetical order by state, then city, then hospital within the city; Rankings exclude hospitals with less than 25 cases except for patient surveys which excludes hospitals with less than 100 cases; (a) 100-299 cases; (1) The number of cases/patients is too few to report; (2) Data submitted were based on a sample of cases/patients; (3) Results are based on a shorter time period than required; (4) Data suppressed by CMS for one or more quarters; (5) Results are not available for this reporting period; (6) Fewer than 100 patients completed the HCAHPS survey; (7) No cases met the criteria for this measure; (8) The lower limit of the confidence interval cannot be calculated if the number of observed infections equals zero; (9) No data are available from the state/territory for this reporting period; (10) The scores shown reflect fewer than 50 completed surveys; (11) There were discrepancies in the data collection process; (12) This measure does not apply to this hospital for this reporting period; (13) Results cannot be calculated for this reporting period; (14) The results for this state are combined with nearby states to protect confidentiality; Please refer to the User's Guide for a full explanation of data.

Measure	Cases	This Hosp.	State Avg.	U.S. Avg.
Prophylactic Antibiotic Timing	163	98%	99%	99%
Prophylactic Antibiotic Timing (Outpatient)	26	88%	97%	98%
Urinary Catheter Removal	211	100%	98%	97%
Survey of Patients' Hospital Experiences				
Area Around Room 'Always' Quiet at Night	300+	66%	60%	61%
Doctors 'Always' Communicated Well	300+	84%	81%	82%
Home Recovery Information Given	300+	83%	86%	85%
Hospital Given 9 or 10 on 10 Point Scale	300+	73%	70%	71%
Meds 'Always' Explained Before Given	300+	68%	64%	64%
Nurses 'Always' Communicated Well	300+	83%	79%	79%
Pain 'Always' Well Controlled	300+	73%	71%	71%
Room and Bathroom 'Always' Clean	300+	74%	74%	73%
Timely Help 'Always' Received	300+	72%	67%	68%
Would Definitely Recommend Hospital	300+	72%	70%	71%
Use of Medical Imaging				
Cardiac Imaging Stress Test before Surgery	247	5.7%	5.5%	5.3%
Combination Abdominal CT Scan	449	7.3%	10.1%	10.5%
Combination Brain/Sinus CT Scan[1]	-	-	2.6%	2.7%
Combination Chest CT Scan	363	0.0%	2.8%	2.7%
Follow-up Mammogram/Ultrasound	923	7.2%	8.4%	8.8%
Lumbar Spine MRI for Low Back Pain[1]	-	-	36.6%	37.2%

West Suburban Medical Center

3 Erie Court
Oak Park, IL 60302
Phone: 708-383-6200
Fax: 708-386-9246
URL: www.wshmc.org
Type: Acute Care Hospitals
Emergency Services: Yes
Ownership: Voluntary non-profit - Other
Beds: 258

Key Personnel:

Quality Assurance . . . . Christine Clark
Patient Relations . . . . Deborah Davisson
Chief of Medical Staff . . . . Roy Horras, MD
CEO/President . . . . Jay Kreuzer
Anesthesiology . . . . Vermeri Murthy, MD
Radiology . . . . Gayle Payonk
Emergency Room . . . . Sandra Watkins
Operating Room . . . . Margaret Zeinthiewicz

Measure	Cases	This Hosp.	State Avg.	U.S. Avg.
Blood Clot Prevention and Treatment				
Anticoagulation Overlap Therapy[2]	47	83%	91%	93%
ICU Venous Thromboembolism Prophylaxis[2]	81	91%	93%	92%
Incidence of Potentially Preventable VTE[1,2]	-	-	11%	10%
UFH with Dosages/Platelet Monitoring[2]	18	78%	94%	97%
Venous Thromboembolism Prophylaxis[2]	352	86%	86%	85%
Warfarin Therapy Discharge Instructions[2]	38	29%	71%	75%
Chest Pain/Possible Heart Attack Care				
Aspirin Given Within 24 Hours of Arrival[5]	-	-	96%	96%
Fibrinolytic Meds Within 30 Min. of Arrival[5]	-	-	65%	58%
Average Time to ECG (minutes)[5]	-	-	6	7
Average Time to Transfer (minutes)[5]	-	-	63	60
Children's Asthma Care				
Received Home Management Plan of Care	-	-	-	88%
Received Reliever Medication	-	-	-	100%
Received Systemic Corticosteroids	-	-	-	100%
Emergency Department				
Admittance Decision Time (minutes)[2]	622	120	89	98
Head CT Results Within 45 Min. of Arrival	20	20%	64%	57%
Patients Who Left ER Before Being Seen	60,134	1%	3%	2%
Time from ER Arrival to Admit. (minutes)[2]	633	284	260	274
Time from ER Arrival to Discharge (minutes)	355	133	138	134
Time in ER Before Being Evaluated (minutes)	363	37	28	26
Time to Pain Meds for Fractures (minutes)	69	56	52	57
Heart Attack Care				
Aspirin Given at Discharge	112	99%	99%	99%
Fibrinolytic Meds Within 30 Min. of Arrival[7]	-	-	33%	54%
PCI Within 90 Minutes of Arrival[1]	-	-	97%	96%
Statin Prescribed at Discharge	106	99%	98%	98%
Heart Failure Care				
ACE Inhibitor or ARB for LVSD	160	98%	98%	97%
Discharge Instructions Given	330	99%	96%	94%
Evaluation of LVS Function	374	100%	99%	99%
Medicare Spending				
Medicare Spending per Patient (ratio)	-	0.99	1	0.98
Pneumonia Care				
Appropriate Initial Antibiotic Given	106	96%	95%	95%
Blood Culture Timing	185	99%	98%	98%
Pregnancy and Delivery Care				
Newborn Deliveries Scheduled Early[2]	18	0%	2%	6%
Preventive Care				
Immunization for Influenza[2]	496	93%	92%	90%
Immunization for Pneumonia[2]	556	97%	92%	92%
Stroke Care				
Anticoagulation Therapy for Atrial Fibrillation[1]	-	-	94%	95%
Antithrombotic Therapy Timing	101	96%	98%	98%
Assessed for Rehabilitation	97	95%	97%	97%
Discharged on Antithrombotic Therapy	94	85%	99%	99%
Discharged on Statin Medication	83	76%	94%	94%
Thrombolytic Therapy Timing	24	0%	66%	66%
Venous Thromboembolism Prophylaxis	106	89%	94%	94%
Written Stroke Educational Materials Given	48	71%	87%	88%
Surgical Care Improvement Project				
Appropriate Beta Blocker Usage[2]	122	93%	98%	98%
Appropriate VTP Within 24 Hours[2]	337	97%	98%	98%
Controlled Postoperative Blood Glucose[2]	35	86%	97%	97%
Perioperative Temperature Management[2]	392	100%	100%	100%
Prophylactic Antibiotic Selection[2]	296	99%	99%	99%
Prophylactic Antibiotic Selection (Outpatient)	152	84%	98%	98%
Prophylactic Antibiotic Stopped[2]	289	99%	98%	98%
Prophylactic Antibiotic Timing[2]	296	99%	99%	99%
Prophylactic Antibiotic Timing (Outpatient)	176	71%	97%	98%
Urinary Catheter Removal[2]	168	93%	98%	97%
Survey of Patients' Hospital Experiences				
Area Around Room 'Always' Quiet at Night[11]	300+	59%	60%	61%
Doctors 'Always' Communicated Well[11]	300+	82%	81%	82%
Home Recovery Information Given[11]	300+	85%	86%	85%
Hospital Given 9 or 10 on 10 Point Scale[11]	300+	60%	70%	71%
Meds 'Always' Explained Before Given[11]	300+	60%	64%	64%
Nurses 'Always' Communicated Well[11]	300+	74%	79%	79%
Pain 'Always' Well Controlled[11]	300+	68%	71%	71%
Room and Bathroom 'Always' Clean[11]	300+	61%	74%	73%
Timely Help 'Always' Received[11]	300+	58%	67%	68%
Would Definitely Recommend Hospital[11]	300+	59%	70%	71%
Use of Medical Imaging				
Cardiac Imaging Stress Test before Surgery	211	6.6%	5.5%	5.3%
Combination Abdominal CT Scan	506	18.6%	10.1%	10.5%
Combination Brain/Sinus CT Scan	505	1.2%	2.6%	2.7%
Combination Chest CT Scan	287	8.4%	2.8%	2.7%
Follow-up Mammogram/Ultrasound	849	11.8%	8.4%	8.8%
Lumbar Spine MRI for Low Back Pain	56	32.1%	36.6%	37.2%

Richland Memorial Hospital

800 East Locust
Olney, IL 62450
Phone: 618-395-2131
Fax: 618-392-3228
URL: www.richlandmemorial.com
Type: Acute Care Hospitals
Emergency Services: Yes
Ownership: Voluntary non-profit - Private
Beds: 135

Key Personnel:

CEO . . . . David Allen
Radiology . . . . Randy Bishop
Emergency Room . . . . Donna Brown
Operating Room . . . . Kathy Cowman
Infection Control . . . . Penni Kuenstler
Chief of Medical Staff . . . . Robert Nash, MD
Quality Assurance . . . . Lana Royse
Intensive Care Unit . . . . Joan Sager

Measure	Cases	This Hosp.	State Avg.	U.S. Avg.
Blood Clot Prevention and Treatment				
Anticoagulation Overlap Therapy[1,2]	-	-	91%	93%
ICU Venous Thromboembolism Prophylaxis[1,2]	-	-	93%	92%
Incidence of Potentially Preventable VTE[2,7]	-	-	11%	10%
UFH with Dosages/Platelet Monitoring[1,2]	-	-	94%	97%
Venous Thromboembolism Prophylaxis[2]	175	96%	86%	85%
Warfarin Therapy Discharge Instructions[1,2]	-	-	71%	75%
Chest Pain/Possible Heart Attack Care				
Aspirin Given Within 24 Hours of Arrival	36	100%	96%	96%
Fibrinolytic Meds Within 30 Min. of Arrival[1]	-	-	65%	58%
Average Time to ECG (minutes)	37	7	6	7
Average Time to Transfer (minutes)[1]	-	-	63	60
Children's Asthma Care				
Received Home Management Plan of Care	-	-	-	88%
Received Reliever Medication	-	-	-	100%
Received Systemic Corticosteroids	-	-	-	100%
Emergency Department				
Admittance Decision Time (minutes)[2]	273	54	89	98
Head CT Results Within 45 Min. of Arrival[1]	-	-	64%	57%
Patients Who Left ER Before Being Seen	9,572	1%	3%	2%
Time from ER Arrival to Admit. (minutes)[2]	274	224	260	274
Time from ER Arrival to Discharge (minutes)	372	114	138	134
Time in ER Before Being Evaluated (minutes)	419	25	28	26
Time to Pain Meds for Fractures (minutes)	33	58	52	57
Heart Attack Care				
Aspirin Given at Discharge[1]	-	-	99%	99%
Fibrinolytic Meds Within 30 Min. of Arrival[7]	-	-	33%	54%
PCI Within 90 Minutes of Arrival[7]	-	-	97%	96%
Statin Prescribed at Discharge[1]	-	-	98%	98%
Heart Failure Care				
ACE Inhibitor or ARB for LVSD[2]	25	88%	98%	97%
Discharge Instructions Given[2]	61	89%	96%	94%
Evaluation of LVS Function[2]	105	97%	99%	99%
Medicare Spending				
Medicare Spending per Patient (ratio)	-	0.97	1	0.98
Pneumonia Care				
Appropriate Initial Antibiotic Given[2]	60	95%	95%	95%
Blood Culture Timing[2]	73	96%	98%	98%
Pregnancy and Delivery Care				
Newborn Deliveries Scheduled Early	28	0%	2%	6%
Preventive Care				
Immunization for Influenza[2]	243	97%	92%	90%
Immunization for Pneumonia[2]	299	98%	92%	92%
Stroke Care				
Anticoagulation Therapy for Atrial Fibrillation[1]	-	-	94%	95%
Antithrombotic Therapy Timing	12	100%	98%	98%
Assessed for Rehabilitation	11	100%	97%	97%
Discharged on Antithrombotic Therapy	11	100%	99%	99%
Discharged on Statin Medication[1]	-	-	94%	94%
Thrombolytic Therapy Timing[7]	-	-	66%	66%
Venous Thromboembolism Prophylaxis	12	100%	94%	94%
Written Stroke Educational Materials Given[1]	-	-	87%	88%
Surgical Care Improvement Project				
Appropriate Beta Blocker Usage[1,2]	-	-	98%	98%
Appropriate VTP Within 24 Hours[2]	49	100%	98%	98%
Controlled Postoperative Blood Glucose[2,7]	-	-	97%	97%
Perioperative Temperature Management[2]	96	100%	100%	100%
Prophylactic Antibiotic Selection[2]	56	100%	99%	99%
Prophylactic Antibiotic Selection (Outpatient)[1,3]	-	-	98%	98%
Prophylactic Antibiotic Stopped[2]	56	98%	98%	98%
Prophylactic Antibiotic Timing[2]	56	96%	99%	99%
Prophylactic Antibiotic Timing (Outpatient)[1,3]	-	-	97%	98%
Urinary Catheter Removal[1,2]	-	-	98%	97%
Survey of Patients' Hospital Experiences				
Area Around Room 'Always' Quiet at Night	300+	66%	60%	61%
Doctors 'Always' Communicated Well	300+	87%	81%	82%
Home Recovery Information Given	300+	93%	86%	85%
Hospital Given 9 or 10 on 10 Point Scale	300+	75%	70%	71%
Meds 'Always' Explained Before Given	300+	65%	64%	64%
Nurses 'Always' Communicated Well	300+	82%	79%	79%
Pain 'Always' Well Controlled	300+	75%	71%	71%
Room and Bathroom 'Always' Clean	300+	73%	74%	73%
Timely Help 'Always' Received	300+	73%	67%	68%
Would Definitely Recommend Hospital	300+	74%	70%	71%
Use of Medical Imaging				
Cardiac Imaging Stress Test before Surgery	177	8.5%	5.5%	5.3%
Combination Abdominal CT Scan	294	20.1%	10.1%	10.5%
Combination Brain/Sinus CT Scan[1]	-	-	2.6%	2.7%
Combination Chest CT Scan	221	20.8%	2.8%	2.7%
Follow-up Mammogram/Ultrasound	516	6.6%	8.4%	8.8%
Lumbar Spine MRI for Low Back Pain[1]	-	-	36.6%	37.2%

NOTE: Hospital profiles are in alphabetical order by state, then city, then hospital within the city; Rankings exclude hospitals with less than 25 cases except for patient surveys which excludes hospitals with less than 100 cases; (a) 100-299 cases; (1) The number of cases/patients is too few to report; (2) Data submitted were based on a sample of cases/patients; (3) Results are based on a shorter time period than required; (4) Data suppressed by CMS for one or more quarters; (5) Results are not available for this reporting period; (6) Fewer than 100 patients completed the HCAHPS survey; (7) No cases met the criteria for this measure; (8) The lower limit of the confidence interval cannot be calculated if the number of observed infections equals zero; (9) No data are available from the state/territory for this reporting period; (10) The scores shown reflect fewer than 50 completed surveys; (11) There were discrepancies in the data collection process; (12) This measure does not apply to this hospital for this reporting period; (13) Results cannot be calculated for this reporting period; (14) The results for this state are combined with nearby states to protect confidentiality; Please refer to the User's Guide for a full explanation of data.

Franciscan Saint James Health

20201 S Crawford Avenue
Olympia Fields, IL 60461
URL: www.franciscanalliance.org
Type: Acute Care Hospitals
Ownership: Proprietary

Phone: 708-747-4000
Fax: 708-756-6763
Emergency Services: Yes
Beds: 201

Key Personnel:
CEO/President. . . . . Arnie Kimmel
Chief of Medical Staff. . . . . Aswatch Subram, MD

Measure	Cases	This Hosp.	State Avg.	U.S. Avg.
Blood Clot Prevention and Treatment				
Anticoagulation Overlap Therapy[2]	161	84%	91%	93%
ICU Venous Thromboembolism Prophylaxis[2]	118	91%	93%	92%
Incidence of Potentially Preventable VTE[2]	41	24%	11%	10%
UFH with Dosages/Platelet Monitoring[2]	92	100%	94%	97%
Venous Thromboembolism Prophylaxis[2]	708	88%	86%	85%
Warfarin Therapy Discharge Instructions[2]	115	44%	71%	75%
Chest Pain/Possible Heart Attack Care				
Aspirin Given Within 24 Hours of Arrival[1]	-	-	96%	96%
Fibrinolytic Meds Within 30 Min. of Arrival[3,7]	-	-	65%	58%
Average Time to ECG (minutes)[1]	-	-	6	7
Average Time to Transfer (minutes)[3,7]	-	-	63	60
Children's Asthma Care				
Received Home Management Plan of Care	-	-	-	88%
Received Reliever Medication	-	-	-	100%
Received Systemic Corticosteroids	-	-	-	100%
Emergency Department				
Admittance Decision Time (minutes)[2]	1,520	105	89	98
Head CT Results Within 45 Min. of Arrival	36	78%	64%	57%
Patients Who Left ER Before Being Seen	81,419	2%	3%	2%
Time from ER Arrival to Admit. (minutes)[2]	1,532	295	260	274
Time from ER Arrival to Discharge (minutes)	687	156	138	134
Time in ER Before Being Evaluated (minutes)	745	31	28	26
Time to Pain Meds for Fractures (minutes)	164	56	52	57
Heart Attack Care				
Aspirin Given at Discharge	250	99%	99%	99%
Fibrinolytic Meds Within 30 Min. of Arrival[7]	-	-	33%	54%
PCI Within 90 Minutes of Arrival	32	100%	97%	96%
Statin Prescribed at Discharge	249	98%	98%	98%
Heart Failure Care				
ACE Inhibitor or ARB for LVSD[2]	202	94%	98%	97%
Discharge Instructions Given[2]	437	91%	96%	94%
Evaluation of LVS Function[2]	521	99%	99%	99%
Medicare Spending				
Medicare Spending per Patient (ratio)	-	0.99	1	0.98
Pneumonia Care				
Appropriate Initial Antibiotic Given[2]	102	96%	95%	95%
Blood Culture Timing[2]	249	98%	98%	98%
Pregnancy and Delivery Care				
Newborn Deliveries Scheduled Early[2]	31	0%	2%	6%
Preventive Care				
Immunization for Influenza[2]	1,120	98%	92%	90%
Immunization for Pneumonia[2]	1,589	95%	92%	92%
Stroke Care				
Anticoagulation Therapy for Atrial Fibrillation[2]	16	75%	94%	95%
Antithrombotic Therapy Timing[2]	138	96%	98%	98%
Assessed for Rehabilitation[2]	157	92%	97%	97%
Discharged on Antithrombotic Therapy[2]	142	93%	99%	99%
Discharged on Statin Medication[2]	122	85%	94%	94%
Thrombolytic Therapy Timing[1,2]	-	-	66%	66%
Venous Thromboembolism Prophylaxis[2]	164	92%	94%	94%
Written Stroke Educational Materials Given[2]	85	66%	87%	88%
Surgical Care Improvement Project				
Appropriate Beta Blocker Usage[2]	217	100%	98%	98%
Appropriate VTP Within 24 Hours[2]	447	99%	98%	98%
Controlled Postoperative Blood Glucose[2]	74	99%	97%	97%
Perioperative Temperature Management[2]	522	100%	100%	100%
Prophylactic Antibiotic Selection[2]	383	100%	99%	99%
Prophylactic Antibiotic Selection (Outpatient)	232	96%	98%	98%
Prophylactic Antibiotic Stopped[2]	346	99%	98%	98%
Prophylactic Antibiotic Timing[2]	385	99%	99%	99%
Prophylactic Antibiotic Timing (Outpatient)	202	98%	97%	98%
Urinary Catheter Removal[2]	186	99%	98%	97%
Survey of Patients' Hospital Experiences				
Area Around Room 'Always' Quiet at Night	300+	53%	60%	61%
Doctors 'Always' Communicated Well	300+	76%	81%	82%
Home Recovery Information Given	300+	82%	86%	85%
Hospital Given 9 or 10 on 10 Point Scale	300+	58%	70%	71%
Meds 'Always' Explained Before Given	300+	59%	64%	64%
Nurses 'Always' Communicated Well	300+	73%	79%	79%
Pain 'Always' Well Controlled	300+	66%	71%	71%
Room and Bathroom 'Always' Clean	300+	69%	74%	73%
Timely Help 'Always' Received	300+	54%	67%	68%
Would Definitely Recommend Hospital	300+	60%	70%	71%
Use of Medical Imaging				
Cardiac Imaging Stress Test before Surgery	969	5.7%	5.5%	5.3%
Combination Abdominal CT Scan	948	11.0%	10.1%	10.5%
Combination Brain/Sinus CT Scan	828	3.6%	2.6%	2.7%
Combination Chest CT Scan	712	7.7%	2.8%	2.7%
Follow-up Mammogram/Ultrasound	2,421	7.9%	8.4%	8.8%
Lumbar Spine MRI for Low Back Pain	154	27.3%	36.6%	37.2%

Ottawa Regional Hospital & Healthcare Center

1100 East Norris Drive
Ottawa, IL 61350
URL: www.community-hospital.org
Type: Acute Care Hospitals
Ownership: Voluntary non-profit - Private

Phone: 815-433-3100
Fax: 815-431-5500
Emergency Services: Yes
Beds: 124

Key Personnel:
Operating Room. . . . . Caner Celeboglu
Infection Control. . . . . Kerry Gerding
Emergency Room . . . . Linda Grey, RN
Intensive Care Unit. . . . . Kathy Jakubek, RN
Radiology. . . . . Byron Johnson, MD
Chief of Medical Staff. . . . . Joseph S Kokoszka, MD
Quality Assurance . . . . Marcy Perkunas
CEO/President. . . . . Robert I Schmelter

Measure	Cases	This Hosp.	State Avg.	U.S. Avg.
Blood Clot Prevention and Treatment				
Anticoagulation Overlap Therapy[2]	12	100%	91%	93%
ICU Venous Thromboembolism Prophylaxis[2]	32	91%	93%	92%
Incidence of Potentially Preventable VTE[2,7]	-	-	11%	10%
UFH with Dosages/Platelet Monitoring[2,7]	-	-	94%	97%
Venous Thromboembolism Prophylaxis[2]	185	91%	86%	85%
Warfarin Therapy Discharge Instructions[2]	11	100%	71%	75%
Chest Pain/Possible Heart Attack Care				
Aspirin Given Within 24 Hours of Arrival	65	95%	96%	96%
Fibrinolytic Meds Within 30 Min. of Arrival[7]	-	-	65%	58%
Average Time to ECG (minutes)	65	6	6	7
Average Time to Transfer (minutes)[1]	-	-	63	60
Children's Asthma Care				
Received Home Management Plan of Care	-	-	-	88%
Received Reliever Medication	-	-	-	100%
Received Systemic Corticosteroids	-	-	-	100%
Emergency Department				
Admittance Decision Time (minutes)[2]	351	58	89	98
Head CT Results Within 45 Min. of Arrival	14	36%	64%	57%
Patients Who Left ER Before Being Seen	15,895	0%	3%	2%
Time from ER Arrival to Admit. (minutes)[2]	351	193	260	274
Time from ER Arrival to Discharge (minutes)	416	92	138	134
Time in ER Before Being Evaluated (minutes)	446	21	28	26
Time to Pain Meds for Fractures (minutes)	75	33	52	57
Heart Attack Care				
Aspirin Given at Discharge[1,3]	-	-	99%	99%
Fibrinolytic Meds Within 30 Min. of Arrival[3,7]	-	-	33%	54%
PCI Within 90 Minutes of Arrival[3,7]	-	-	97%	96%
Statin Prescribed at Discharge[1,3]	-	-	98%	98%
Heart Failure Care				
ACE Inhibitor or ARB for LVSD	17	100%	98%	97%
Discharge Instructions Given	60	92%	96%	94%
Evaluation of LVS Function	92	99%	99%	99%
Medicare Spending				
Medicare Spending per Patient (ratio)	-	1.03	1	0.98
Pneumonia Care				
Appropriate Initial Antibiotic Given	75	100%	95%	95%
Blood Culture Timing	106	99%	98%	98%
Pregnancy and Delivery Care				
Newborn Deliveries Scheduled Early[2]	21	5%	2%	6%
Preventive Care				
Immunization for Influenza[2]	265	98%	92%	90%
Immunization for Pneumonia[2]	343	95%	92%	92%
Stroke Care				
Anticoagulation Therapy for Atrial Fibrillation[1]	-	-	94%	95%
Antithrombotic Therapy Timing	23	100%	98%	98%
Assessed for Rehabilitation	16	94%	97%	97%
Discharged on Antithrombotic Therapy	16	100%	99%	99%
Discharged on Statin Medication	15	73%	94%	94%
Thrombolytic Therapy Timing[7]	-	-	66%	66%
Venous Thromboembolism Prophylaxis	23	91%	94%	94%
Written Stroke Educational Materials Given[1]	-	-	87%	88%
Surgical Care Improvement Project				
Appropriate Beta Blocker Usage	36	97%	98%	98%
Appropriate VTP Within 24 Hours	125	95%	98%	98%
Controlled Postoperative Blood Glucose[7]	-	-	97%	97%
Perioperative Temperature Management	141	100%	100%	100%
Prophylactic Antibiotic Selection	61	100%	99%	99%
Prophylactic Antibiotic Selection (Outpatient)	43	100%	98%	98%
Prophylactic Antibiotic Stopped	54	98%	98%	98%
Prophylactic Antibiotic Timing	61	100%	99%	99%
Prophylactic Antibiotic Timing (Outpatient)	43	98%	97%	98%
Urinary Catheter Removal	87	100%	98%	97%
Survey of Patients' Hospital Experiences				
Area Around Room 'Always' Quiet at Night	300+	59%	60%	61%
Doctors 'Always' Communicated Well	300+	82%	81%	82%
Home Recovery Information Given	300+	87%	86%	85%
Hospital Given 9 or 10 on 10 Point Scale	300+	69%	70%	71%
Meds 'Always' Explained Before Given	300+	72%	64%	64%
Nurses 'Always' Communicated Well	300+	84%	79%	79%
Pain 'Always' Well Controlled	300+	73%	71%	71%
Room and Bathroom 'Always' Clean	300+	81%	74%	73%
Timely Help 'Always' Received	300+	77%	67%	68%
Would Definitely Recommend Hospital	300+	65%	70%	71%
Use of Medical Imaging				
Cardiac Imaging Stress Test before Surgery	198	4.0%	5.5%	5.3%
Combination Abdominal CT Scan	474	14.1%	10.1%	10.5%
Combination Brain/Sinus CT Scan	311	1.3%	2.6%	2.7%
Combination Chest CT Scan	367	3.8%	2.8%	2.7%
Follow-up Mammogram/Ultrasound	824	14.8%	8.4%	8.8%
Lumbar Spine MRI for Low Back Pain	76	35.5%	36.6%	37.2%

Palos Community Hospital

12251 South 80th Avenue
Palos Heights, IL 60463
URL: www.paloshospital.org
Type: Acute Care Hospitals
Ownership: Voluntary non-profit - Private

Phone: 708-923-4000
Fax: 708-923-4620
Emergency Services: Yes
Beds: 436

Key Personnel:
Cardiac Laboratory. . . . . Julie Callahan
Quality Assurance . . . . Nancy Kayse
Chief of Medical Staff. . . . . Thomas Lavery
Emergency Room . . . . Lori Stott
CEO/President. . . . . Sr Margaret Wright

Measure	Cases	This Hosp.	State Avg.	U.S. Avg.
Blood Clot Prevention and Treatment				
Anticoagulation Overlap Therapy[2]	168	90%	91%	93%
ICU Venous Thromboembolism Prophylaxis[2]	86	95%	93%	92%
Incidence of Potentially Preventable VTE[2]	37	11%	11%	10%
UFH with Dosages/Platelet Monitoring[2]	179	100%	94%	97%
Venous Thromboembolism Prophylaxis[2]	355	81%	86%	85%
Warfarin Therapy Discharge Instructions[2]	120	94%	71%	75%
Chest Pain/Possible Heart Attack Care				
Aspirin Given Within 24 Hours of Arrival[1,3]	-	-	96%	96%
Fibrinolytic Meds Within 30 Min. of Arrival[3,7]	-	-	65%	58%
Average Time to ECG (minutes)[1,3]	-	-	6	7
Average Time to Transfer (minutes)[3,7]	-	-	63	60
Children's Asthma Care				
Received Home Management Plan of Care	-	-	-	88%
Received Reliever Medication	-	-	-	100%
Received Systemic Corticosteroids	-	-	-	100%
Emergency Department				

NOTE: Hospital profiles are in alphabetical order by state, then city, then hospital within the city; Rankings exclude hospitals with less than 25 cases except for patient surveys which excludes hospitals with less than 100 cases; (a) 100-299 cases; (1) The number of cases/patients is too few to report; (2) Data submitted were based on a sample of cases/patients; (3) Results are based on a shorter time period than required; (4) Data suppressed by CMS for one or more quarters; (5) Results are not available for this reporting period; (6) Fewer than 100 patients completed the HCAHPS survey; (7) No cases met the criteria for this measure; (8) The lower limit of the confidence interval cannot be calculated if the number of observed infections equals zero; (9) No data are available from the state/territory for this reporting period; (10) The scores shown reflect fewer than 50 completed surveys; (11) There were discrepancies in the data collection process; (12) This measure does not apply to this hospital for this reporting period; (13) Results cannot be calculated for this reporting period; (14) The results for this state are combined with nearby states to protect confidentiality; Please refer to the User's Guide for a full explanation of data.

Measure	Cases	This Hosp.	State Avg.	U.S. Avg.
Admittance Decision Time (minutes)[2]	612	83	89	98
Head CT Results Within 45 Min. of Arrival	35	71%	64%	57%
Patients Who Left ER Before Being Seen	47,408	2%	3%	2%
Time from ER Arrival to Admit. (minutes)[2]	688	252	260	274
Time from ER Arrival to Discharge (minutes)	332	167	138	134
Time in ER Before Being Evaluated (minutes)	398	52	28	26
Time to Pain Meds for Fractures (minutes)	187	74	52	57
Heart Attack Care				
Aspirin Given at Discharge[2]	264	100%	99%	99%
Fibrinolytic Meds Within 30 Min. of Arrival[2,7]	-	-	33%	54%
PCI Within 90 Minutes of Arrival[2]	69	94%	97%	96%
Statin Prescribed at Discharge[2]	266	100%	98%	98%
Heart Failure Care				
ACE Inhibitor or ARB for LVSD[2]	54	100%	98%	97%
Discharge Instructions Given[2]	236	94%	96%	94%
Evaluation of LVS Function[2]	312	100%	99%	99%
Medicare Spending				
Medicare Spending per Patient (ratio)	-	1.03	1	0.98
Pneumonia Care				
Appropriate Initial Antibiotic Given[2]	91	100%	95%	95%
Blood Culture Timing[2]	168	99%	98%	98%
Pregnancy and Delivery Care				
Newborn Deliveries Scheduled Early[2]	28	0%	2%	6%
Preventive Care				
Immunization for Influenza[2]	578	99%	92%	90%
Immunization for Pneumonia[2]	865	100%	92%	92%
Stroke Care				
Anticoagulation Therapy for Atrial Fibrillation[2]	21	86%	94%	95%
Antithrombotic Therapy Timing[2]	110	95%	98%	98%
Assessed for Rehabilitation[2]	101	91%	97%	97%
Discharged on Antithrombotic Therapy[2]	99	100%	99%	99%
Discharged on Statin Medication[2]	66	97%	94%	94%
Thrombolytic Therapy Timing[1,2]	-	-	66%	66%
Venous Thromboembolism Prophylaxis[2]	114	86%	94%	94%
Written Stroke Educational Materials Given[2]	50	44%	87%	88%
Surgical Care Improvement Project				
Appropriate Beta Blocker Usage[2]	233	99%	98%	98%
Appropriate VTP Within 24 Hours[2]	447	99%	98%	98%
Controlled Postoperative Blood Glucose[2]	152	95%	97%	97%
Perioperative Temperature Management[2]	537	100%	100%	100%
Prophylactic Antibiotic Selection[2]	483	99%	99%	99%
Prophylactic Antibiotic Selection (Outpatient)	220	100%	98%	98%
Prophylactic Antibiotic Stopped[2]	472	98%	98%	98%
Prophylactic Antibiotic Timing[2]	483	100%	99%	99%
Prophylactic Antibiotic Timing (Outpatient)	220	99%	97%	98%
Urinary Catheter Removal[2]	298	97%	98%	97%
Survey of Patients' Hospital Experiences				
Area Around Room 'Always' Quiet at Night	300+	48%	60%	61%
Doctors 'Always' Communicated Well	300+	81%	81%	82%
Home Recovery Information Given	300+	82%	86%	85%
Hospital Given 9 or 10 on 10 Point Scale	300+	65%	70%	71%
Meds 'Always' Explained Before Given	300+	59%	64%	64%
Nurses 'Always' Communicated Well	300+	78%	79%	79%
Pain 'Always' Well Controlled	300+	71%	71%	71%
Room and Bathroom 'Always' Clean	300+	66%	74%	73%
Timely Help 'Always' Received	300+	62%	67%	68%
Would Definitely Recommend Hospital	300+	68%	70%	71%
Use of Medical Imaging				
Cardiac Imaging Stress Test before Surgery	1,141	6.6%	5.5%	5.3%
Combination Abdominal CT Scan	1,889	3.4%	10.1%	10.5%
Combination Brain/Sinus CT Scan	1,606	2.3%	2.6%	2.7%
Combination Chest CT Scan	1,912	0.4%	2.8%	2.7%
Follow-up Mammogram/Ultrasound	2,900	9.8%	8.4%	8.8%
Lumbar Spine MRI for Low Back Pain	99	42.4%	36.6%	37.2%

Pana Community Hospital

101 E Ninth Street
Pana, IL 62557
Phone: 217-562-2131
Fax: 217-562-6270
Type: Critical Access Hospitals
Emergency Services: Yes
Ownership: Voluntary non-profit - Private
Beds: 44

Key Personnel:

CEO/President. . . . . Roland Carlson
Chief of Medical Staff . . . . Allen Frigy, MD
Infection Control. . . . . Sheri Trexler
Operating Room. . . . . Nora Washburn, RN

Measure	Cases	This Hosp.	State Avg.	U.S. Avg.
Blood Clot Prevention and Treatment				
Anticoagulation Overlap Therapy[5]	-	-	91%	93%
ICU Venous Thromboembolism Prophylaxis[5]	-	-	93%	92%
Incidence of Potentially Preventable VTE[5]	-	-	11%	10%
UFH with Dosages/Platelet Monitoring[5]	-	-	94%	97%
Venous Thromboembolism Prophylaxis[5]	-	-	86%	85%
Warfarin Therapy Discharge Instructions[5]	-	-	71%	75%
Chest Pain/Possible Heart Attack Care				
Aspirin Given Within 24 Hours of Arrival[5]	-	-	96%	96%
Fibrinolytic Meds Within 30 Min. of Arrival[5]	-	-	65%	58%
Average Time to ECG (minutes)[5]	-	-	6	7
Average Time to Transfer (minutes)[5]	-	-	63	60
Children's Asthma Care				
Received Home Management Plan of Care	-	-	-	88%
Received Reliever Medication	-	-	-	100%
Received Systemic Corticosteroids	-	-	-	100%
Emergency Department				
Admittance Decision Time (minutes)[5]	-	-	89	98
Head CT Results Within 45 Min. of Arrival[5]	-	-	64%	57%
Patients Who Left ER Before Being Seen	8,847	2%	3%	2%
Time from ER Arrival to Admit. (minutes)[5]	-	-	260	274
Time from ER Arrival to Discharge (minutes)[5]	-	-	138	134
Time in ER Before Being Evaluated (minutes)[5]	-	-	28	26
Time to Pain Meds for Fractures (minutes)[5]	-	-	52	57
Heart Attack Care				
Aspirin Given at Discharge[5]	-	-	99%	99%
Fibrinolytic Meds Within 30 Min. of Arrival[5]	-	-	33%	54%
PCI Within 90 Minutes of Arrival[5]	-	-	97%	96%
Statin Prescribed at Discharge[5]	-	-	98%	98%
Heart Failure Care				
ACE Inhibitor or ARB for LVSD[1,3]	-	-	98%	97%
Discharge Instructions Given[1,3]	-	-	96%	94%
Evaluation of LVS Function[3]	12	75%	99%	99%
Medicare Spending				
Medicare Spending per Patient (ratio)	-	-	1	0.98
Pneumonia Care				
Appropriate Initial Antibiotic Given	15	67%	95%	95%
Blood Culture Timing	27	93%	98%	98%
Pregnancy and Delivery Care				
Newborn Deliveries Scheduled Early[5]	-	-	2%	6%
Preventive Care				
Immunization for Influenza[5]	-	-	92%	90%
Immunization for Pneumonia[5]	-	-	92%	92%
Stroke Care				
Anticoagulation Therapy for Atrial Fibrillation[5]	-	-	94%	95%
Antithrombotic Therapy Timing[5]	-	-	98%	98%
Assessed for Rehabilitation[5]	-	-	97%	97%
Discharged on Antithrombotic Therapy[5]	-	-	99%	99%
Discharged on Statin Medication[5]	-	-	94%	94%
Thrombolytic Therapy Timing[5]	-	-	66%	66%
Venous Thromboembolism Prophylaxis[5]	-	-	94%	94%
Written Stroke Educational Materials Given[5]	-	-	87%	88%
Surgical Care Improvement Project				
Appropriate Beta Blocker Usage[5]	-	-	98%	98%
Appropriate VTP Within 24 Hours[5]	-	-	98%	98%
Controlled Postoperative Blood Glucose[5]	-	-	97%	97%
Perioperative Temperature Management[5]	-	-	100%	100%
Prophylactic Antibiotic Selection[5]	-	-	99%	99%
Prophylactic Antibiotic Selection (Outpatient)[5]	-	-	98%	98%
Prophylactic Antibiotic Stopped[5]	-	-	98%	98%
Prophylactic Antibiotic Timing[5]	-	-	99%	99%
Prophylactic Antibiotic Timing (Outpatient)[5]	-	-	97%	98%
Urinary Catheter Removal[5]	-	-	98%	97%
Survey of Patients' Hospital Experiences				
Area Around Room 'Always' Quiet at Night[5]	-	-	60%	61%
Doctors 'Always' Communicated Well[5]	-	-	81%	82%
Home Recovery Information Given[5]	-	-	86%	85%
Hospital Given 9 or 10 on 10 Point Scale[5]	-	-	70%	71%
Meds 'Always' Explained Before Given[5]	-	-	64%	64%
Nurses 'Always' Communicated Well[5]	-	-	79%	79%
Pain 'Always' Well Controlled[5]	-	-	71%	71%
Room and Bathroom 'Always' Clean[5]	-	-	74%	73%
Timely Help 'Always' Received[5]	-	-	67%	68%
Would Definitely Recommend Hospital[5]	-	-	70%	71%
Use of Medical Imaging				
Cardiac Imaging Stress Test before Surgery[1]	-	-	5.5%	5.3%
Combination Abdominal CT Scan	331	7.9%	10.1%	10.5%
Combination Brain/Sinus CT Scan	425	4.2%	2.6%	2.7%
Combination Chest CT Scan	100	3.0%	2.8%	2.7%
Follow-up Mammogram/Ultrasound	225	14.2%	8.4%	8.8%
Lumbar Spine MRI for Low Back Pain[1]	-	-	36.6%	37.2%

Paris Community Hospital

721 E Court Street
Paris, IL 61944
Phone: 217-465-4141
Fax: 217-463-2096
URL: www.pariscommunityhospital.com
Type: Critical Access Hospitals
Emergency Services: Yes
Ownership: Voluntary non-profit - Other
Beds: 49

Key Personnel:

Operating Room. . . . . Katrina Conine, RN
Chief of Medical Staff . . . . Daniel R Gilbert, DO
Quality Assurance . . . . Robin Gordon
Infection Control. . . . . Tammy Hewitt, RN
Radiology. . . . . Bruce Houle
CEO/President. . . . . Oliver Smith, RPh
Emergency Room . . . . Rachel Woltman, DO
Intensive Care Unit. . . . . Rachel Young, RN

Measure	Cases	This Hosp.	State Avg.	U.S. Avg.
Blood Clot Prevention and Treatment				
Anticoagulation Overlap Therapy[1,2]	-	-	91%	93%
ICU Venous Thromboembolism Prophylaxis[2,7]	-	-	93%	92%
Incidence of Potentially Preventable VTE[2,7]	-	-	11%	10%
UFH with Dosages/Platelet Monitoring[2,7]	-	-	94%	97%
Venous Thromboembolism Prophylaxis[2]	90	84%	86%	85%
Warfarin Therapy Discharge Instructions[1,2]	-	-	71%	75%
Chest Pain/Possible Heart Attack Care				
Aspirin Given Within 24 Hours of Arrival[5]	-	-	96%	96%
Fibrinolytic Meds Within 30 Min. of Arrival[5]	-	-	65%	58%
Average Time to ECG (minutes)[5]	-	-	6	7
Average Time to Transfer (minutes)[5]	-	-	63	60
Children's Asthma Care				
Received Home Management Plan of Care	-	-	-	88%
Received Reliever Medication	-	-	-	100%
Received Systemic Corticosteroids	-	-	-	100%
Emergency Department				
Admittance Decision Time (minutes)[5]	-	-	89	98
Head CT Results Within 45 Min. of Arrival[5]	-	-	64%	57%
Patients Who Left ER Before Being Seen[5]	-	-	3%	2%
Time from ER Arrival to Admit. (minutes)[5]	-	-	260	274
Time from ER Arrival to Discharge (minutes)[5]	-	-	138	134
Time in ER Before Being Evaluated (minutes)[5]	-	-	28	26
Time to Pain Meds for Fractures (minutes)[5]	-	-	52	57
Heart Attack Care				
Aspirin Given at Discharge[1,3]	-	-	99%	99%
Fibrinolytic Meds Within 30 Min. of Arrival[3,7]	-	-	33%	54%
PCI Within 90 Minutes of Arrival[3,7]	-	-	97%	96%
Statin Prescribed at Discharge[1,3]	-	-	98%	98%
Heart Failure Care				
ACE Inhibitor or ARB for LVSD[1]	-	-	98%	97%
Discharge Instructions Given	17	100%	96%	94%
Evaluation of LVS Function	26	88%	99%	99%
Medicare Spending				
Medicare Spending per Patient (ratio)	-	-	1	0.98
Pneumonia Care				
Appropriate Initial Antibiotic Given	22	95%	95%	95%
Blood Culture Timing	20	100%	98%	98%
Pregnancy and Delivery Care				
Newborn Deliveries Scheduled Early[5]	-	-	2%	6%
Preventive Care				
Immunization for Influenza[5]	-	-	92%	90%
Immunization for Pneumonia[5]	-	-	92%	92%
Stroke Care				
Anticoagulation Therapy for Atrial Fibrillation[7]	-	-	94%	95%

NOTE: Hospital profiles are in alphabetical order by state, then city, then hospital within the city; Rankings exclude hospitals with less than 25 cases except for patient surveys which excludes hospitals with less than 100 cases; (a) 100-299 cases; (1) The number of cases/patients is too few to report; (2) Data submitted were based on a sample of cases/patients; (3) Results are based on a shorter time period than required; (4) Data suppressed by CMS for one or more quarters; (5) Results are not available for this reporting period; (6) Fewer than 100 patients completed the HCAHPS survey; (7) No cases met the criteria for this measure; (8) The lower limit of the confidence interval cannot be calculated if the number of observed infections equals zero; (9) No data are available from the state/territory for this reporting period; (10) The scores shown reflect fewer than 50 completed surveys; (11) There were discrepancies in the data collection process; (12) This measure does not apply to this hospital for this reporting period; (13) Results cannot be calculated for this reporting period; (14) The results for this state are combined with nearby states to protect confidentiality; Please refer to the User's Guide for a full explanation of data.

Measure	Cases	This Hosp.	State Avg.	U.S. Avg.
Antithrombotic Therapy Timing[1]	-	-	98%	98%
Assessed for Rehabilitation[1]	-	-	97%	97%
Discharged on Antithrombotic Therapy[1]	-	-	99%	99%
Discharged on Statin Medication[1]	-	-	94%	94%
Thrombolytic Therapy Timing[7]	-	-	66%	66%
Venous Thromboembolism Prophylaxis[1]	-	-	94%	94%
Written Stroke Educational Materials Given[1]	-	-	87%	88%
Surgical Care Improvement Project				
Appropriate Beta Blocker Usage	25	92%	98%	98%
Appropriate VTP Within 24 Hours	58	93%	98%	98%
Controlled Postoperative Blood Glucose[7]	-	-	97%	97%
Perioperative Temperature Management	68	100%	100%	100%
Prophylactic Antibiotic Selection	51	100%	99%	99%
Prophylactic Antibiotic Selection (Outpatient)[5]	-	-	98%	98%
Prophylactic Antibiotic Stopped	50	94%	98%	98%
Prophylactic Antibiotic Timing	51	94%	99%	99%
Prophylactic Antibiotic Timing (Outpatient)[5]	-	-	97%	98%
Urinary Catheter Removal	48	92%	98%	97%
Survey of Patients' Hospital Experiences				
Area Around Room 'Always' Quiet at Night[6]	<100	67%	60%	61%
Doctors 'Always' Communicated Well[6]	<100	85%	81%	82%
Home Recovery Information Given[6]	<100	85%	86%	85%
Hospital Given 9 or 10 on 10 Point Scale[6]	<100	71%	70%	71%
Meds 'Always' Explained Before Given[6]	<100	72%	64%	64%
Nurses 'Always' Communicated Well[6]	<100	81%	79%	79%
Pain 'Always' Well Controlled[6]	<100	72%	71%	71%
Room and Bathroom 'Always' Clean[6]	<100	78%	74%	73%
Timely Help 'Always' Received[6]	<100	65%	67%	68%
Would Definitely Recommend Hospital[6]	<100	65%	70%	71%
Use of Medical Imaging				
Cardiac Imaging Stress Test before Surgery	92	1.1%	5.5%	5.3%
Combination Abdominal CT Scan	249	20.5%	10.1%	10.5%
Combination Brain/Sinus CT Scan	299	1.0%	2.6%	2.7%
Combination Chest CT Scan	161	12.4%	2.8%	2.7%
Follow-up Mammogram/Ultrasound	265	10.9%	8.4%	8.8%
Lumbar Spine MRI for Low Back Pain[1]	-	-	36.6%	37.2%

Advocate Lutheran General Hospital

1775 Dempster St
Park Ridge, IL 60068
URL: www.advocatehealth.com
Type: Acute Care Hospitals
Ownership: Voluntary non-profit - Church
Phone: 847-723-2210
Fax: 847-696-2612
Emergency Services: Yes

Key Personnel:
CEO/President. . . . . Bruce C Campbell
Radiology. . . . . John McFadden
Chief of Medical Staff. . . . . John Sage

Measure	Cases	This Hosp.	State Avg.	U.S. Avg.
Blood Clot Prevention and Treatment				
Anticoagulation Overlap Therapy[2]	122	94%	91%	93%
ICU Venous Thromboembolism Prophylaxis[2]	87	92%	93%	92%
Incidence of Potentially Preventable VTE[2]	53	8%	11%	10%
UFH with Dosages/Platelet Monitoring[2]	32	97%	94%	97%
Venous Thromboembolism Prophylaxis[2]	323	83%	86%	85%
Warfarin Therapy Discharge Instructions[2]	69	84%	71%	75%
Chest Pain/Possible Heart Attack Care				
Aspirin Given Within 24 Hours of Arrival[1,3]	-	-	96%	96%
Fibrinolytic Meds Within 30 Min. of Arrival[5]	-	-	65%	58%
Average Time to ECG (minutes)[1,3]	-	-	6	7
Average Time to Transfer (minutes)[5]	-	-	63	60
Children's Asthma Care				
Received Home Management Plan of Care	-	-	-	88%
Received Reliever Medication	-	-	-	100%
Received Systemic Corticosteroids	-	-	-	100%
Emergency Department				
Admittance Decision Time (minutes)[2]	442	72	89	98
Head CT Results Within 45 Min. of Arrival[1]	-	-	64%	57%
Patients Who Left ER Before Being Seen	63,801	1%	3%	2%
Time from ER Arrival to Admit. (minutes)[2]	448	249	260	274
Time from ER Arrival to Discharge (minutes)	384	180	138	134
Time in ER Before Being Evaluated (minutes)	332	43	28	26
Time to Pain Meds for Fractures (minutes)	224	58	52	57
Heart Attack Care				
Aspirin Given at Discharge	243	100%	99%	99%
Fibrinolytic Meds Within 30 Min. of Arrival[7]	-	-	33%	54%
PCI Within 90 Minutes of Arrival	55	96%	97%	96%
Statin Prescribed at Discharge	240	100%	98%	98%
Heart Failure Care				
ACE Inhibitor or ARB for LVSD[2]	77	100%	98%	97%
Discharge Instructions Given[2]	246	100%	96%	94%
Evaluation of LVS Function[2]	348	100%	99%	99%
Medicare Spending				
Medicare Spending per Patient (ratio)	-	1.06	1	0.98
Pneumonia Care				
Appropriate Initial Antibiotic Given[2]	97	98%	95%	95%
Blood Culture Timing[2]	189	99%	98%	98%
Pregnancy and Delivery Care				
Newborn Deliveries Scheduled Early	387	1%	2%	6%
Preventive Care				
Immunization for Influenza[2]	551	96%	92%	90%
Immunization for Pneumonia[2]	543	94%	92%	92%
Stroke Care				
Anticoagulation Therapy for Atrial Fibrillation	42	98%	94%	95%
Antithrombotic Therapy Timing	181	99%	98%	98%
Assessed for Rehabilitation	245	99%	97%	97%
Discharged on Antithrombotic Therapy	218	100%	99%	99%
Discharged on Statin Medication	178	98%	94%	94%
Thrombolytic Therapy Timing	27	96%	66%	66%
Venous Thromboembolism Prophylaxis	247	97%	94%	94%
Written Stroke Educational Materials Given	108	99%	87%	88%
Surgical Care Improvement Project				
Appropriate Beta Blocker Usage[2]	302	97%	98%	98%
Appropriate VTP Within 24 Hours[2]	467	99%	98%	98%
Controlled Postoperative Blood Glucose[2]	113	98%	97%	97%
Perioperative Temperature Management[2]	580	100%	100%	100%
Prophylactic Antibiotic Selection[2]	466	100%	99%	99%
Prophylactic Antibiotic Selection (Outpatient)	683	99%	98%	98%
Prophylactic Antibiotic Stopped[2]	453	99%	98%	98%
Prophylactic Antibiotic Timing[2]	466	100%	99%	99%
Prophylactic Antibiotic Timing (Outpatient)	683	100%	97%	98%
Urinary Catheter Removal[2]	304	100%	98%	97%
Survey of Patients' Hospital Experiences				
Area Around Room 'Always' Quiet at Night	300+	59%	60%	61%
Doctors 'Always' Communicated Well	300+	80%	81%	82%
Home Recovery Information Given	300+	87%	86%	85%
Hospital Given 9 or 10 on 10 Point Scale	300+	78%	70%	71%
Meds 'Always' Explained Before Given	300+	65%	64%	64%
Nurses 'Always' Communicated Well	300+	80%	79%	79%
Pain 'Always' Well Controlled	300+	73%	71%	71%
Room and Bathroom 'Always' Clean	300+	77%	74%	73%
Timely Help 'Always' Received	300+	65%	67%	68%
Would Definitely Recommend Hospital	300+	80%	70%	71%
Use of Medical Imaging				
Cardiac Imaging Stress Test before Surgery	664	6.5%	5.5%	5.3%
Combination Abdominal CT Scan	2,083	4.4%	10.1%	10.5%
Combination Brain/Sinus CT Scan	1,526	2.8%	2.6%	2.7%
Combination Chest CT Scan	1,647	2.4%	2.8%	2.7%
Follow-up Mammogram/Ultrasound	4,903	5.7%	8.4%	8.8%
Lumbar Spine MRI for Low Back Pain	290	37.2%	36.6%	37.2%

Pekin Memorial Hospital

600 South 13th Street
Pekin, IL 61554
URL: www.pekinhospital.org
Type: Acute Care Hospitals
Ownership: Voluntary non-profit - Private
Phone: 309-347-1151
Fax: 309-347-5453
Emergency Services: Yes
Beds: 125

Key Personnel:
Quality Assurance . . . . Sandy Brooks
CEO . . . . Bob J. Haley
CEO/President. . . . . Robert Moore
Chairman/CEO . . . . Andrew J. Sparks

Measure	Cases	This Hosp.	State Avg.	U.S. Avg.
Blood Clot Prevention and Treatment				
Anticoagulation Overlap Therapy[2]	19	100%	91%	93%
ICU Venous Thromboembolism Prophylaxis[2]	65	95%	93%	92%
Incidence of Potentially Preventable VTE[1,2]	-	-	11%	10%
UFH with Dosages/Platelet Monitoring[2]	16	100%	94%	97%
Venous Thromboembolism Prophylaxis[2]	234	81%	86%	85%
Warfarin Therapy Discharge Instructions[2]	15	80%	71%	75%
Chest Pain/Possible Heart Attack Care				
Aspirin Given Within 24 Hours of Arrival	16	100%	96%	96%
Fibrinolytic Meds Within 30 Min. of Arrival[7]	-	-	65%	58%
Average Time to ECG (minutes)	16	6	6	7
Average Time to Transfer (minutes)[1]	-	-	63	60
Children's Asthma Care				
Received Home Management Plan of Care	-	-	-	88%
Received Reliever Medication	-	-	-	100%
Received Systemic Corticosteroids	-	-	-	100%
Emergency Department				
Admittance Decision Time (minutes)[2]	324	75	89	98
Head CT Results Within 45 Min. of Arrival	14	36%	64%	57%
Patients Who Left ER Before Being Seen	41,588	1%	3%	2%
Time from ER Arrival to Admit. (minutes)[2]	328	232	260	274
Time from ER Arrival to Discharge (minutes)	354	101	138	134
Time in ER Before Being Evaluated (minutes)	318	24	28	26
Time to Pain Meds for Fractures (minutes)	112	39	52	57
Heart Attack Care				
Aspirin Given at Discharge	21	100%	99%	99%
Fibrinolytic Meds Within 30 Min. of Arrival[7]	-	-	33%	54%
PCI Within 90 Minutes of Arrival[7]	-	-	97%	96%
Statin Prescribed at Discharge	18	94%	98%	98%
Heart Failure Care				
ACE Inhibitor or ARB for LVSD	31	90%	98%	97%
Discharge Instructions Given	79	97%	96%	94%
Evaluation of LVS Function	109	99%	99%	99%
Medicare Spending				
Medicare Spending per Patient (ratio)	-	0.96	1	0.98
Pneumonia Care				
Appropriate Initial Antibiotic Given	123	93%	95%	95%
Blood Culture Timing	184	99%	98%	98%
Pregnancy and Delivery Care				
Newborn Deliveries Scheduled Early[2]	37	8%	2%	6%
Preventive Care				
Immunization for Influenza[2]	347	95%	92%	90%
Immunization for Pneumonia[2]	406	97%	92%	92%
Stroke Care				
Anticoagulation Therapy for Atrial Fibrillation[1]	-	-	94%	95%
Antithrombotic Therapy Timing	16	100%	98%	98%
Assessed for Rehabilitation	14	100%	97%	97%
Discharged on Antithrombotic Therapy	13	100%	99%	99%
Discharged on Statin Medication	12	83%	94%	94%
Thrombolytic Therapy Timing[7]	-	-	66%	66%
Venous Thromboembolism Prophylaxis	17	88%	94%	94%
Written Stroke Educational Materials Given[1]	-	-	87%	88%
Surgical Care Improvement Project				
Appropriate Beta Blocker Usage	80	99%	98%	98%
Appropriate VTP Within 24 Hours	293	99%	98%	98%
Controlled Postoperative Blood Glucose[7]	-	-	97%	97%
Perioperative Temperature Management	320	100%	100%	100%
Prophylactic Antibiotic Selection	211	98%	99%	99%
Prophylactic Antibiotic Selection (Outpatient)	47	100%	98%	98%
Prophylactic Antibiotic Stopped	207	98%	98%	98%
Prophylactic Antibiotic Timing	211	100%	99%	99%
Prophylactic Antibiotic Timing (Outpatient)	46	96%	97%	98%
Urinary Catheter Removal	184	99%	98%	97%
Survey of Patients' Hospital Experiences				
Area Around Room 'Always' Quiet at Night	300+	50%	60%	61%
Doctors 'Always' Communicated Well	300+	83%	81%	82%
Home Recovery Information Given	300+	87%	86%	85%
Hospital Given 9 or 10 on 10 Point Scale	300+	63%	70%	71%
Meds 'Always' Explained Before Given	300+	60%	64%	64%
Nurses 'Always' Communicated Well	300+	76%	79%	79%
Pain 'Always' Well Controlled	300+	67%	71%	71%
Room and Bathroom 'Always' Clean	300+	71%	74%	73%
Timely Help 'Always' Received	300+	63%	67%	68%
Would Definitely Recommend Hospital	300+	63%	70%	71%
Use of Medical Imaging				
Cardiac Imaging Stress Test before Surgery	219	3.7%	5.5%	5.3%

NOTE: Hospital profiles are in alphabetical order by state, then city, then hospital within the city; Rankings exclude hospitals with less than 25 cases except for patient surveys which excludes hospitals with less than 100 cases; (a) 100-299 cases; (1) The number of cases/patients is too few to report; (2) Data submitted were based on a sample of cases/patients; (3) Results are based on a shorter time period than required; (4) Data suppressed by CMS for one or more quarters; (5) Results are not available for this reporting period; (6) Fewer than 100 patients completed the HCAHPS survey; (7) No cases met the criteria for this measure; (8) The lower limit of the confidence interval cannot be calculated if the number of observed infections equals zero; (9) No data are available from the state/territory for this reporting period; (10) The scores shown reflect fewer than 50 completed surveys; (11) There were discrepancies in the data collection process; (12) This measure does not apply to this hospital for this reporting period; (13) Results cannot be calculated for this reporting period; (14) The results for this state are combined with nearby states to protect confidentiality; Please refer to the User's Guide for a full explanation of data.

Combination Abdominal CT Scan	511	5.1%	10.1%	10.5%
Combination Brain/Sinus CT Scan	448	2.2%	2.6%	2.7%
Combination Chest CT Scan	417	0.0%	2.8%	2.7%
Follow-up Mammogram/Ultrasound	843	13.6%	8.4%	8.8%
Lumbar Spine MRI for Low Back Pain	53	30.2%	36.6%	37.2%

Methodist Medical Center of Illinois

221 N E Glen Oak Ave
Peoria, IL 61636
URL: www.mmci.org
Phone: 309-672-5522
Fax: 309-671-8303
Type: Acute Care Hospitals
Emergency Services: Yes
Ownership: Voluntary non-profit - Other
Beds: 330

Key Personnel:

Infection Control.............. Linda Barton
Chief of Medical Staff.......... Gary Knepp, DO
Quality Assurance .... Sandy Pryor
CEO/President................ Debbie Simon
Cardiac Laboratory............ Jeanine Spain, RN
Operating Room............... Jeanine Spain
Patient Relations .... Shelley Wilkes
Radiology.................... Carter Young, DO

Measure	Cases	This Hosp.	State Avg.	U.S. Avg.
Blood Clot Prevention and Treatment				
Anticoagulation Overlap Therapy[2]	55	98%	91%	93%
ICU Venous Thromboembolism Prophylaxis[2]	67	99%	93%	92%
Incidence of Potentially Preventable VTE[1,2]	-	-	11%	10%
UFH with Dosages/Platelet Monitoring[2]	40	98%	94%	97%
Venous Thromboembolism Prophylaxis[2]	293	83%	86%	85%
Warfarin Therapy Discharge Instructions[2]	41	93%	71%	75%
Chest Pain/Possible Heart Attack Care				
Aspirin Given Within 24 Hours of Arrival[5]	-	-	96%	96%
Fibrinolytic Meds Within 30 Min. of Arrival[5]	-	-	65%	58%
Average Time to ECG (minutes)[5]	-	-	6	7
Average Time to Transfer (minutes)[5]	-	-	63	60
Children's Asthma Care				
Received Home Management Plan of Care	-	-	-	88%
Received Reliever Medication	-	-	-	100%
Received Systemic Corticosteroids	-	-	-	100%
Emergency Department				
Admittance Decision Time (minutes)[2]	455	88	89	98
Head CT Results Within 45 Min. of Arrival[5]	-	-	64%	57%
Patients Who Left ER Before Being Seen	56,545	3%	3%	2%
Time from ER Arrival to Admit. (minutes)[2]	487	251	260	274
Time from ER Arrival to Discharge (minutes)	351	179	138	134
Time in ER Before Being Evaluated (minutes)	384	21	28	26
Time to Pain Meds for Fractures (minutes)	68	51	52	57
Heart Attack Care				
Aspirin Given at Discharge	216	100%	99%	99%
Fibrinolytic Meds Within 30 Min. of Arrival[7]	-	-	33%	54%
PCI Within 90 Minutes of Arrival	26	100%	97%	96%
Statin Prescribed at Discharge	199	98%	98%	98%
Heart Failure Care				
ACE Inhibitor or ARB for LVSD	105	96%	98%	97%
Discharge Instructions Given	215	94%	96%	94%
Evaluation of LVS Function	273	100%	99%	99%
Medicare Spending				
Medicare Spending per Patient (ratio)	-	0.99	1	0.98
Pneumonia Care				
Appropriate Initial Antibiotic Given	175	97%	95%	95%
Blood Culture Timing	263	99%	98%	98%
Pregnancy and Delivery Care				
Newborn Deliveries Scheduled Early[2]	36	6%	2%	6%
Preventive Care				
Immunization for Influenza[2]	519	92%	92%	90%
Immunization for Pneumonia[2]	654	94%	92%	92%
Stroke Care				
Anticoagulation Therapy for Atrial Fibrillation	18	94%	94%	95%
Antithrombotic Therapy Timing	90	97%	98%	98%
Assessed for Rehabilitation	125	98%	97%	97%
Discharged on Antithrombotic Therapy	109	100%	99%	99%
Discharged on Statin Medication	90	97%	94%	94%
Thrombolytic Therapy Timing[1]	-	-	66%	66%
Venous Thromboembolism Prophylaxis	121	96%	94%	94%
Written Stroke Educational Materials Given	64	95%	87%	88%
Surgical Care Improvement Project				
Appropriate Beta Blocker Usage[2]	266	100%	98%	98%
Appropriate VTP Within 24 Hours[2]	574	99%	98%	98%
Controlled Postoperative Blood Glucose[2]	114	98%	97%	97%
Perioperative Temperature Management[2]	682	100%	100%	100%
Prophylactic Antibiotic Selection[2]	614	100%	99%	99%
Prophylactic Antibiotic Selection (Outpatient)	383	99%	98%	98%
Prophylactic Antibiotic Stopped[2]	602	99%	98%	98%
Prophylactic Antibiotic Timing[2]	615	100%	99%	99%
Prophylactic Antibiotic Timing (Outpatient)	381	100%	97%	98%
Urinary Catheter Removal[2]	537	100%	98%	97%
Survey of Patients' Hospital Experiences				
Area Around Room 'Always' Quiet at Night	300+	61%	60%	61%
Doctors 'Always' Communicated Well	300+	81%	81%	82%
Home Recovery Information Given	300+	87%	86%	85%
Hospital Given 9 or 10 on 10 Point Scale	300+	74%	70%	71%
Meds 'Always' Explained Before Given	300+	63%	64%	64%
Nurses 'Always' Communicated Well	300+	81%	79%	79%
Pain 'Always' Well Controlled	300+	72%	71%	71%
Room and Bathroom 'Always' Clean	300+	77%	74%	73%
Timely Help 'Always' Received	300+	70%	67%	68%
Would Definitely Recommend Hospital	300+	78%	70%	71%
Use of Medical Imaging				
Cardiac Imaging Stress Test before Surgery	537	4.8%	5.5%	5.3%
Combination Abdominal CT Scan	969	17.3%	10.1%	10.5%
Combination Brain/Sinus CT Scan	968	2.8%	2.6%	2.7%
Combination Chest CT Scan	809	3.1%	2.8%	2.7%
Follow-up Mammogram/Ultrasound	2,520	9.1%	8.4%	8.8%
Lumbar Spine MRI for Low Back Pain	137	34.3%	36.6%	37.2%

Proctor Hospital

5409 N Knoxville Ave
Peoria, IL 61614
E-mail: information@proctor.org
URL: www.proctor.org
Phone: 309-691-1000
Fax: 309-689-6062
Type: Acute Care Hospitals
Emergency Services: Yes
Ownership: Voluntary non-profit - Private
Beds: 175

Key Personnel:

Pediatrics.................... Amy Christison, MD
Quality Assurance .... Marty Dorgan
CEO/President................ Debbie Simon
Anesthesiology................ Kenneth Strum, MD
Radiology.................... Carter Young, DO

Measure	Cases	This Hosp.	State Avg.	U.S. Avg.
Blood Clot Prevention and Treatment				
Anticoagulation Overlap Therapy[2]	34	91%	91%	93%
ICU Venous Thromboembolism Prophylaxis[2]	78	94%	93%	92%
Incidence of Potentially Preventable VTE[1,2]	-	-	11%	10%
UFH with Dosages/Platelet Monitoring[2]	15	87%	94%	97%
Venous Thromboembolism Prophylaxis[2]	360	88%	86%	85%
Warfarin Therapy Discharge Instructions[2]	27	78%	71%	75%
Chest Pain/Possible Heart Attack Care				
Aspirin Given Within 24 Hours of Arrival[5]	-	-	96%	96%
Fibrinolytic Meds Within 30 Min. of Arrival[5]	-	-	65%	58%
Average Time to ECG (minutes)[5]	-	-	6	7
Average Time to Transfer (minutes)[5]	-	-	63	60
Children's Asthma Care				
Received Home Management Plan of Care	-	-	-	88%
Received Reliever Medication	-	-	-	100%
Received Systemic Corticosteroids	-	-	-	100%
Emergency Department				
Admittance Decision Time (minutes)[2]	370	61	89	98
Head CT Results Within 45 Min. of Arrival[1]	-	-	64%	57%
Patients Who Left ER Before Being Seen	20,575	1%	3%	2%
Time from ER Arrival to Admit. (minutes)[2]	507	192	260	274
Time from ER Arrival to Discharge (minutes)	470	104	138	134
Time in ER Before Being Evaluated (minutes)	474	19	28	26
Time to Pain Meds for Fractures (minutes)	69	29	52	57
Heart Attack Care				
Aspirin Given at Discharge	87	98%	99%	99%
Fibrinolytic Meds Within 30 Min. of Arrival[7]	-	-	33%	54%
PCI Within 90 Minutes of Arrival	19	100%	97%	96%
Statin Prescribed at Discharge	81	96%	98%	98%
Heart Failure Care				
ACE Inhibitor or ARB for LVSD	38	100%	98%	97%
Discharge Instructions Given	93	99%	96%	94%
Evaluation of LVS Function	151	99%	99%	99%
Medicare Spending				
Medicare Spending per Patient (ratio)	-	0.93	1	0.98
Pneumonia Care				
Appropriate Initial Antibiotic Given	109	95%	95%	95%
Blood Culture Timing	139	98%	98%	98%
Pregnancy and Delivery Care				
Newborn Deliveries Scheduled Early	42	14%	2%	6%
Preventive Care				
Immunization for Influenza[2]	594	88%	92%	90%
Immunization for Pneumonia[2]	764	82%	92%	92%
Stroke Care				
Anticoagulation Therapy for Atrial Fibrillation[1]	-	-	94%	95%
Antithrombotic Therapy Timing	60	100%	98%	98%
Assessed for Rehabilitation	60	85%	97%	97%
Discharged on Antithrombotic Therapy	59	100%	99%	99%
Discharged on Statin Medication	44	77%	94%	94%
Thrombolytic Therapy Timing[1]	-	-	66%	66%
Venous Thromboembolism Prophylaxis	65	97%	94%	94%
Written Stroke Educational Materials Given	29	45%	87%	88%
Surgical Care Improvement Project				
Appropriate Beta Blocker Usage[2]	104	94%	98%	98%
Appropriate VTP Within 24 Hours[2]	230	94%	98%	98%
Controlled Postoperative Blood Glucose[2]	17	94%	97%	97%
Perioperative Temperature Management[2]	347	100%	100%	100%
Prophylactic Antibiotic Selection[2]	256	98%	99%	99%
Prophylactic Antibiotic Selection (Outpatient)	128	95%	98%	98%
Prophylactic Antibiotic Stopped[2]	254	95%	98%	98%
Prophylactic Antibiotic Timing[2]	256	97%	99%	99%
Prophylactic Antibiotic Timing (Outpatient)	130	97%	97%	98%
Urinary Catheter Removal[2]	237	98%	98%	97%
Survey of Patients' Hospital Experiences				
Area Around Room 'Always' Quiet at Night	300+	61%	60%	61%
Doctors 'Always' Communicated Well	300+	78%	81%	82%
Home Recovery Information Given	300+	87%	86%	85%
Hospital Given 9 or 10 on 10 Point Scale	300+	66%	70%	71%
Meds 'Always' Explained Before Given	300+	56%	64%	64%
Nurses 'Always' Communicated Well	300+	75%	79%	79%
Pain 'Always' Well Controlled	300+	62%	71%	71%
Room and Bathroom 'Always' Clean	300+	65%	74%	73%
Timely Help 'Always' Received	300+	63%	67%	68%
Would Definitely Recommend Hospital	300+	72%	70%	71%
Use of Medical Imaging				
Cardiac Imaging Stress Test before Surgery	282	2.5%	5.5%	5.3%
Combination Abdominal CT Scan	416	6.7%	10.1%	10.5%
Combination Brain/Sinus CT Scan	433	2.1%	2.6%	2.7%
Combination Chest CT Scan	241	5.0%	2.8%	2.7%
Follow-up Mammogram/Ultrasound	342	7.0%	8.4%	8.8%
Lumbar Spine MRI for Low Back Pain	58	43.1%	36.6%	37.2%

Saint Francis Medical Center

530 Ne Glen Oak Ave
Peoria, IL 61637
URL: www.osfsaintfrancis.org
Phone: 309-655-2000
Fax: 309-671-8996
Type: Acute Care Hospitals
Emergency Services: Yes
Ownership: Voluntary non-profit - Church
Beds: 731

Key Personnel:

Infection Control.............. Patricia Ham
Chief of Medical Staff.......... Tim Miller, MD
Pediatric Ambulatory Care .... Kay Saving, MD
Cardiac Laboratory............ Delmar Smith
Quality Assurance .... Gail Strunk
Operating Room............... Judy Winkler, MD
Radiology.................... Gary Zwicky, MD

Measure	Cases	This Hosp.	State Avg.	U.S. Avg.
Blood Clot Prevention and Treatment				
Anticoagulation Overlap Therapy[2]	169	95%	91%	93%
ICU Venous Thromboembolism Prophylaxis[2]	44	86%	93%	92%
Incidence of Potentially Preventable VTE[2]	39	8%	11%	10%
UFH with Dosages/Platelet Monitoring[2]	103	100%	94%	97%
Venous Thromboembolism Prophylaxis[2]	347	80%	86%	85%
Warfarin Therapy Discharge Instructions[2]	122	69%	71%	75%

NOTE: Hospital profiles are in alphabetical order by state, then city, then hospital within the city; Rankings exclude hospitals with less than 25 cases except for patient surveys which excludes hospitals with less than 100 cases; (a) 100-299 cases; (1) The number of cases/patients is too few to report; (2) Data submitted were based on a sample of cases/patients; (3) Results are based on a shorter time period than required; (4) Data suppressed by CMS for one or more quarters; (5) Results are not available for this reporting period; (6) Fewer than 100 patients completed the HCAHPS survey; (7) No cases met the criteria for this measure; (8) The lower limit of the confidence interval cannot be calculated if the number of observed infections equals zero; (9) No data are available from the state/territory for this reporting period; (10) The scores shown reflect fewer than 50 completed surveys; (11) There were discrepancies in the data collection process; (12) This measure does not apply to this hospital for this reporting period; (13) Results cannot be calculated for this reporting period; (14) The results for this state are combined with nearby states to protect confidentiality; Please refer to the User's Guide for a full explanation of data.

Measure	Cases	This Hosp.	State Avg.	U.S. Avg.
Chest Pain/Possible Heart Attack Care				
Aspirin Given Within 24 Hours of Arrival[5]	-	-	96%	96%
Fibrinolytic Meds Within 30 Min. of Arrival[5]	-	-	65%	58%
Average Time to ECG (minutes)[5]	-	-	6	7
Average Time to Transfer (minutes)[5]	-	-	63	60
Children's Asthma Care				
Received Home Management Plan of Care	-	-	-	88%
Received Reliever Medication	-	-	-	100%
Received Systemic Corticosteroids	-	-	-	100%
Emergency Department				
Admittance Decision Time (minutes)[2]	520	142	89	98
Head CT Results Within 45 Min. of Arrival[1]	-	-	64%	57%
Patients Who Left ER Before Being Seen	87,429	1%	3%	2%
Time from ER Arrival to Admit. (minutes)[2]	527	286	260	274
Time from ER Arrival to Discharge (minutes)	398	182	138	134
Time in ER Before Being Evaluated (minutes)	437	25	28	26
Time to Pain Meds for Fractures (minutes)	138	63	52	57
Heart Attack Care				
Aspirin Given at Discharge	665	99%	99%	99%
Fibrinolytic Meds Within 30 Min. of Arrival[7]	-	-	33%	54%
PCI Within 90 Minutes of Arrival	79	100%	97%	96%
Statin Prescribed at Discharge	644	100%	98%	98%
Heart Failure Care				
ACE Inhibitor or ARB for LVSD	182	99%	98%	97%
Discharge Instructions Given	514	97%	96%	94%
Evaluation of LVS Function	632	100%	99%	99%
Medicare Spending				
Medicare Spending per Patient (ratio)	-	0.94	1	0.98
Pneumonia Care				
Appropriate Initial Antibiotic Given	226	97%	95%	95%
Blood Culture Timing	549	99%	98%	98%
Pregnancy and Delivery Care				
Newborn Deliveries Scheduled Early	158	5%	2%	6%
Preventive Care				
Immunization for Influenza[2]	541	88%	92%	90%
Immunization for Pneumonia[2]	569	83%	92%	92%
Stroke Care				
Anticoagulation Therapy for Atrial Fibrillation	70	90%	94%	95%
Antithrombotic Therapy Timing	332	89%	98%	98%
Assessed for Rehabilitation	581	98%	97%	97%
Discharged on Antithrombotic Therapy	463	99%	99%	99%
Discharged on Statin Medication	363	95%	94%	94%
Thrombolytic Therapy Timing	38	95%	66%	66%
Venous Thromboembolism Prophylaxis	570	93%	94%	94%
Written Stroke Educational Materials Given	354	89%	87%	88%
Surgical Care Improvement Project				
Appropriate Beta Blocker Usage[2]	524	99%	98%	98%
Appropriate VTP Within 24 Hours[2]	960	98%	98%	98%
Controlled Postoperative Blood Glucose[2]	260	99%	97%	97%
Perioperative Temperature Management[2]	1,214	100%	100%	100%
Prophylactic Antibiotic Selection[2]	1,103	99%	99%	99%
Prophylactic Antibiotic Selection (Outpatient)	565	99%	98%	98%
Prophylactic Antibiotic Stopped[2]	1,075	99%	98%	98%
Prophylactic Antibiotic Timing[2]	1,103	99%	99%	99%
Prophylactic Antibiotic Timing (Outpatient)	565	98%	97%	98%
Urinary Catheter Removal[2]	949	98%	98%	97%
Survey of Patients' Hospital Experiences				
Area Around Room 'Always' Quiet at Night	300+	53%	60%	61%
Doctors 'Always' Communicated Well	300+	80%	81%	82%
Home Recovery Information Given	300+	89%	86%	85%
Hospital Given 9 or 10 on 10 Point Scale	300+	75%	70%	71%
Meds 'Always' Explained Before Given	300+	64%	64%	64%
Nurses 'Always' Communicated Well	300+	82%	79%	79%
Pain 'Always' Well Controlled	300+	72%	71%	71%
Room and Bathroom 'Always' Clean	300+	74%	74%	73%
Timely Help 'Always' Received	300+	65%	67%	68%
Would Definitely Recommend Hospital	300+	77%	70%	71%
Use of Medical Imaging				
Cardiac Imaging Stress Test before Surgery	1,628	5.3%	5.5%	5.3%
Combination Abdominal CT Scan	1,488	12.0%	10.1%	10.5%
Combination Brain/Sinus CT Scan	1,017	3.4%	2.6%	2.7%
Combination Chest CT Scan	1,350	0.2%	2.8%	2.7%
Follow-up Mammogram/Ultrasound	5,128	12.2%	8.4%	8.8%
Lumbar Spine MRI for Low Back Pain	302	35.4%	36.6%	37.2%

Illinois Valley Community Hospital

925 West St
Peru, IL 61354
Phone: 815-223-3300
Fax: 815-223-3394
E-mail: prelate@ivch.org
URL: www.ivch.org
Type: Acute Care Hospitals
Emergency Services: Yes
Ownership: Voluntary non-profit - Private
Beds: 172

Key Personnel:

Chief of Medical Staff.......... Mario Cote, MD
Radiology.................... Steven Coventry, MD
Emergency Room .... Greg Guard, MD
Quality Assurance .... Carol Myer
Anesthesiology............... Deofil Orteza, MD
Infection Control............. Deb Patyk
President .... Kris Paul
Operating Room.............. Elizabeth Soeder

Measure	Cases	This Hosp.	State Avg.	U.S. Avg.
Blood Clot Prevention and Treatment				
Anticoagulation Overlap Therapy[1,2]	-	-	91%	93%
ICU Venous Thromboembolism Prophylaxis[2]	18	100%	93%	92%
Incidence of Potentially Preventable VTE[2,7]	-	-	11%	10%
UFH with Dosages/Platelet Monitoring[1,2]	-	-	94%	97%
Venous Thromboembolism Prophylaxis[2]	194	86%	86%	85%
Warfarin Therapy Discharge Instructions[1,2]	-	-	71%	75%
Chest Pain/Possible Heart Attack Care				
Aspirin Given Within 24 Hours of Arrival	44	100%	96%	96%
Fibrinolytic Meds Within 30 Min. of Arrival[1]	-	-	65%	58%
Average Time to ECG (minutes)	43	2	6	7
Average Time to Transfer (minutes)[1]	-	-	63	60
Children's Asthma Care				
Received Home Management Plan of Care	-	-	-	88%
Received Reliever Medication	-	-	-	100%
Received Systemic Corticosteroids	-	-	-	100%
Emergency Department				
Admittance Decision Time (minutes)[2]	325	45	89	98
Head CT Results Within 45 Min. of Arrival	15	67%	64%	57%
Patients Who Left ER Before Being Seen	14,941	1%	3%	2%
Time from ER Arrival to Admit. (minutes)[2]	330	171	260	274
Time from ER Arrival to Discharge (minutes)	522	76	138	134
Time in ER Before Being Evaluated (minutes)	544	10	28	26
Time to Pain Meds for Fractures (minutes)	61	52	52	57
Heart Attack Care				
Aspirin Given at Discharge[1]	-	-	99%	99%
Fibrinolytic Meds Within 30 Min. of Arrival[7]	-	-	33%	54%
PCI Within 90 Minutes of Arrival[7]	-	-	97%	96%
Statin Prescribed at Discharge[1]	-	-	98%	98%
Heart Failure Care				
ACE Inhibitor or ARB for LVSD[2]	31	100%	98%	97%
Discharge Instructions Given[2]	110	75%	96%	94%
Evaluation of LVS Function[2]	142	99%	99%	99%
Medicare Spending				
Medicare Spending per Patient (ratio)	-	0.96	1	0.98
Pneumonia Care				
Appropriate Initial Antibiotic Given	41	90%	95%	95%
Blood Culture Timing	63	98%	98%	98%
Pregnancy and Delivery Care				
Newborn Deliveries Scheduled Early	39	0%	2%	6%
Preventive Care				
Immunization for Influenza[2]	341	80%	92%	90%
Immunization for Pneumonia[2]	447	84%	92%	92%
Stroke Care				
Anticoagulation Therapy for Atrial Fibrillation[1]	-	-	94%	95%
Antithrombotic Therapy Timing[1]	-	-	98%	98%
Assessed for Rehabilitation	18	89%	97%	97%
Discharged on Antithrombotic Therapy	16	81%	99%	99%
Discharged on Statin Medication	16	81%	94%	94%
Thrombolytic Therapy Timing[1]	-	-	66%	66%
Venous Thromboembolism Prophylaxis	21	86%	94%	94%
Written Stroke Educational Materials Given[1]	-	-	87%	88%
Surgical Care Improvement Project				
Appropriate Beta Blocker Usage	89	100%	98%	98%
Appropriate VTP Within 24 Hours	222	99%	98%	98%
Controlled Postoperative Blood Glucose[7]	-	-	97%	97%
Perioperative Temperature Management	275	99%	100%	100%
Prophylactic Antibiotic Selection	223	100%	99%	99%
Prophylactic Antibiotic Selection (Outpatient)	57	100%	98%	98%
Prophylactic Antibiotic Stopped	222	100%	98%	98%
Prophylactic Antibiotic Timing	223	98%	99%	99%
Prophylactic Antibiotic Timing (Outpatient)	58	93%	97%	98%
Urinary Catheter Removal	206	99%	98%	97%
Survey of Patients' Hospital Experiences				
Area Around Room 'Always' Quiet at Night[11]	300+	55%	60%	61%
Doctors 'Always' Communicated Well[11]	300+	85%	81%	82%
Home Recovery Information Given[11]	300+	88%	86%	85%
Hospital Given 9 or 10 on 10 Point Scale[11]	300+	76%	70%	71%
Meds 'Always' Explained Before Given[11]	300+	69%	64%	64%
Nurses 'Always' Communicated Well[11]	300+	85%	79%	79%
Pain 'Always' Well Controlled[11]	300+	74%	71%	71%
Room and Bathroom 'Always' Clean[11]	300+	80%	74%	73%
Timely Help 'Always' Received[11]	300+	75%	67%	68%
Would Definitely Recommend Hospital[11]	300+	80%	70%	71%
Use of Medical Imaging				
Cardiac Imaging Stress Test before Surgery	284	6.0%	5.5%	5.3%
Combination Abdominal CT Scan	406	8.6%	10.1%	10.5%
Combination Brain/Sinus CT Scan[1]	-	-	2.6%	2.7%
Combination Chest CT Scan	242	0.8%	2.8%	2.7%
Follow-up Mammogram/Ultrasound	787	9.0%	8.4%	8.8%
Lumbar Spine MRI for Low Back Pain	131	45.0%	36.6%	37.2%

Pinckneyville Community Hospital

101 N Walnut
Pinckneyville, IL 62274
Phone: 618-357-2187
Fax: 618-357-6740
Type: Critical Access Hospitals
Emergency Services: Yes
Ownership: Govt - Hospital Dist/Auth
Beds: 85

Key Personnel:

Chief of Medical Staff.......... Craig Fovard

Measure	Cases	This Hosp.	State Avg.	U.S. Avg.
Blood Clot Prevention and Treatment				
Anticoagulation Overlap Therapy[1,3]	-	-	91%	93%
ICU Venous Thromboembolism Prophylaxis[3,7]	-	-	93%	92%
Incidence of Potentially Preventable VTE[3,7]	-	-	11%	10%
UFH with Dosages/Platelet Monitoring[3,7]	-	-	94%	97%
Venous Thromboembolism Prophylaxis[3,7]	-	-	86%	85%
Warfarin Therapy Discharge Instructions[1,3]	-	-	71%	75%
Chest Pain/Possible Heart Attack Care				
Aspirin Given Within 24 Hours of Arrival	-	-	96%	96%
Fibrinolytic Meds Within 30 Min. of Arrival	-	-	65%	58%
Average Time to ECG (minutes)	-	-	6	7
Average Time to Transfer (minutes)	-	-	63	60
Children's Asthma Care				
Received Home Management Plan of Care	-	-	-	88%
Received Reliever Medication	-	-	-	100%
Received Systemic Corticosteroids	-	-	-	100%
Emergency Department				
Admittance Decision Time (minutes)[2]	186	55	89	98
Head CT Results Within 45 Min. of Arrival	-	-	64%	57%
Patients Who Left ER Before Being Seen	-	-	3%	2%
Time from ER Arrival to Admit. (minutes)[2]	188	180	260	274
Time from ER Arrival to Discharge (minutes)	-	-	138	134
Time in ER Before Being Evaluated (minutes)	-	-	28	26
Time to Pain Meds for Fractures (minutes)	-	-	52	57
Heart Attack Care				
Aspirin Given at Discharge[1,3]	-	-	99%	99%
Fibrinolytic Meds Within 30 Min. of Arrival[3,7]	-	-	33%	54%
PCI Within 90 Minutes of Arrival[3,7]	-	-	97%	96%
Statin Prescribed at Discharge[1,3]	-	-	98%	98%
Heart Failure Care				
ACE Inhibitor or ARB for LVSD[1]	-	-	98%	97%
Discharge Instructions Given	17	100%	96%	94%
Evaluation of LVS Function	25	92%	99%	99%
Medicare Spending				
Medicare Spending per Patient (ratio)	-	-	1	0.98
Pneumonia Care				

NOTE: Hospital profiles are in alphabetical order by state, then city, then hospital within the city; Rankings exclude hospitals with less than 25 cases except for patient surveys which excludes hospitals with less than 100 cases; (a) 100-299 cases; (1) The number of cases/patients is too few to report; (2) Data submitted were based on a sample of cases/patients; (3) Results are based on a shorter time period than required; (4) Data suppressed by CMS for one or more quarters; (5) Results are not available for this reporting period; (6) Fewer than 100 patients completed the HCAHPS survey; (7) No cases met the criteria for this measure; (8) The lower limit of the confidence interval cannot be calculated if the number of observed infections equals zero; (9) No data are available from the state/territory for this reporting period; (10) The scores shown reflect fewer than 50 completed surveys; (11) There were discrepancies in the data collection process; (12) This measure does not apply to this hospital for this reporting period; (13) Results cannot be calculated for this reporting period; (14) The results for this state are combined with nearby states to protect confidentiality; Please refer to the User's Guide for a full explanation of data.

Measure	Cases	This Hosp.	State Avg.	U.S. Avg.
Appropriate Initial Antibiotic Given	31	81%	95%	95%
Blood Culture Timing	37	92%	98%	98%
Pregnancy and Delivery Care				
Newborn Deliveries Scheduled Early[5]	-	-	2%	6%
Preventive Care				
Immunization for Influenza[2]	27	96%	92%	90%
Immunization for Pneumonia[2]	57	96%	92%	92%
Stroke Care				
Anticoagulation Therapy for Atrial Fibrillation[7]	-	-	94%	95%
Antithrombotic Therapy Timing[1]	-	-	98%	98%
Assessed for Rehabilitation[1]	-	-	97%	97%
Discharged on Antithrombotic Therapy[1]	-	-	99%	99%
Discharged on Statin Medication[1]	-	-	94%	94%
Thrombolytic Therapy Timing[1]	-	-	66%	66%
Venous Thromboembolism Prophylaxis[1]	-	-	94%	94%
Written Stroke Educational Materials Given[1]	-	-	87%	88%
Surgical Care Improvement Project				
Appropriate Beta Blocker Usage[5]	-	-	98%	98%
Appropriate VTP Within 24 Hours[5]	-	-	98%	98%
Controlled Postoperative Blood Glucose[5]	-	-	97%	97%
Perioperative Temperature Management[5]	-	-	100%	100%
Prophylactic Antibiotic Selection[5]	-	-	99%	99%
Prophylactic Antibiotic Selection (Outpatient)	-	-	98%	98%
Prophylactic Antibiotic Stopped[5]	-	-	98%	98%
Prophylactic Antibiotic Timing[5]	-	-	99%	99%
Prophylactic Antibiotic Timing (Outpatient)	-	-	97%	98%
Urinary Catheter Removal[5]	-	-	98%	97%
Survey of Patients' Hospital Experiences				
Area Around Room 'Always' Quiet at Night	(a)	57%	60%	61%
Doctors 'Always' Communicated Well	(a)	88%	81%	82%
Home Recovery Information Given	(a)	93%	86%	85%
Hospital Given 9 or 10 on 10 Point Scale	(a)	67%	70%	71%
Meds 'Always' Explained Before Given	(a)	73%	64%	64%
Nurses 'Always' Communicated Well	(a)	87%	79%	79%
Pain 'Always' Well Controlled	(a)	77%	71%	71%
Room and Bathroom 'Always' Clean	(a)	81%	74%	73%
Timely Help 'Always' Received	(a)	77%	67%	68%
Would Definitely Recommend Hospital	(a)	69%	70%	71%
Use of Medical Imaging				
Cardiac Imaging Stress Test before Surgery	-	-	5.5%	5.3%
Combination Abdominal CT Scan	-	-	10.1%	10.5%
Combination Brain/Sinus CT Scan	-	-	2.6%	2.7%
Combination Chest CT Scan	-	-	2.8%	2.7%
Follow-up Mammogram/Ultrasound	-	-	8.4%	8.8%
Lumbar Spine MRI for Low Back Pain	-	-	36.6%	37.2%

Illini Community Hospital

640 W Washington
Pittsfield, IL 62363
Phone: 217-285-2113
Fax: 217-285-5090
Type: Critical Access Hospitals
Emergency Services: Yes
Ownership: Voluntary non-profit - Private
Beds: 37

Measure	Cases	This Hosp.	State Avg.	U.S. Avg.
Blood Clot Prevention and Treatment				
Anticoagulation Overlap Therapy[3,7]	-	-	91%	93%
ICU Venous Thromboembolism Prophylaxis[3,7]	-	-	93%	92%
Incidence of Potentially Preventable VTE[3,7]	-	-	11%	10%
UFH with Dosages/Platelet Monitoring[3,7]	-	-	94%	97%
Venous Thromboembolism Prophylaxis[3]	43	93%	86%	85%
Warfarin Therapy Discharge Instructions[3,7]	-	-	71%	75%
Chest Pain/Possible Heart Attack Care				
Aspirin Given Within 24 Hours of Arrival[3]	24	92%	96%	96%
Fibrinolytic Meds Within 30 Min. of Arrival[3,7]	-	-	65%	58%
Average Time to ECG (minutes)[3]	24	10	6	7
Average Time to Transfer (minutes)[3,7]	-	-	63	60
Children's Asthma Care				
Received Home Management Plan of Care	-	-	-	88%
Received Reliever Medication	-	-	-	100%
Received Systemic Corticosteroids	-	-	-	100%
Emergency Department				
Admittance Decision Time (minutes)[5]	-	-	89	98
Head CT Results Within 45 Min. of Arrival[5]	-	-	64%	57%
Patients Who Left ER Before Being Seen	7,025	0%	3%	2%
Time from ER Arrival to Admit. (minutes)[5]	-	-	260	274
Time from ER Arrival to Discharge (minutes)[5]	-	-	138	134
Time in ER Before Being Evaluated (minutes)[5]	-	-	28	26
Time to Pain Meds for Fractures (minutes)[3]	26	50	52	57
Heart Attack Care				
Aspirin Given at Discharge[5]	-	-	99%	99%
Fibrinolytic Meds Within 30 Min. of Arrival[5]	-	-	33%	54%
PCI Within 90 Minutes of Arrival[5]	-	-	97%	96%
Statin Prescribed at Discharge[5]	-	-	98%	98%
Heart Failure Care				
ACE Inhibitor or ARB for LVSD[1]	-	-	98%	97%
Discharge Instructions Given	15	93%	96%	94%
Evaluation of LVS Function	21	100%	99%	99%
Medicare Spending				
Medicare Spending per Patient (ratio)	-	-	1	0.98
Pneumonia Care				
Appropriate Initial Antibiotic Given	19	95%	95%	95%
Blood Culture Timing	34	100%	98%	98%
Pregnancy and Delivery Care				
Newborn Deliveries Scheduled Early[5]	-	-	2%	6%
Preventive Care				
Immunization for Influenza[5]	-	-	92%	90%
Immunization for Pneumonia[5]	-	-	92%	92%
Stroke Care				
Anticoagulation Therapy for Atrial Fibrillation[5]	-	-	94%	95%
Antithrombotic Therapy Timing[5]	-	-	98%	98%
Assessed for Rehabilitation[5]	-	-	97%	97%
Discharged on Antithrombotic Therapy[5]	-	-	99%	99%
Discharged on Statin Medication[5]	-	-	94%	94%
Thrombolytic Therapy Timing[5]	-	-	66%	66%
Venous Thromboembolism Prophylaxis[5]	-	-	94%	94%
Written Stroke Educational Materials Given[5]	-	-	87%	88%
Surgical Care Improvement Project				
Appropriate Beta Blocker Usage[5]	-	-	98%	98%
Appropriate VTP Within 24 Hours[5]	-	-	98%	98%
Controlled Postoperative Blood Glucose[5]	-	-	97%	97%
Perioperative Temperature Management[5]	-	-	100%	100%
Prophylactic Antibiotic Selection[5]	-	-	99%	99%
Prophylactic Antibiotic Selection (Outpatient)[5]	-	-	98%	98%
Prophylactic Antibiotic Stopped[5]	-	-	98%	98%
Prophylactic Antibiotic Timing[5]	-	-	99%	99%
Prophylactic Antibiotic Timing (Outpatient)[5]	-	-	97%	98%
Urinary Catheter Removal[5]	-	-	98%	97%
Survey of Patients' Hospital Experiences				
Area Around Room 'Always' Quiet at Night[6]	<100	75%	60%	61%
Doctors 'Always' Communicated Well[6]	<100	80%	81%	82%
Home Recovery Information Given[6]	<100	93%	86%	85%
Hospital Given 9 or 10 on 10 Point Scale[6]	<100	74%	70%	71%
Meds 'Always' Explained Before Given[6]	<100	71%	64%	64%
Nurses 'Always' Communicated Well[6]	<100	91%	79%	79%
Pain 'Always' Well Controlled[6]	<100	84%	71%	71%
Room and Bathroom 'Always' Clean[6]	<100	89%	74%	73%
Timely Help 'Always' Received[6]	<100	91%	67%	68%
Would Definitely Recommend Hospital[6]	<100	75%	70%	71%
Use of Medical Imaging				
Cardiac Imaging Stress Test before Surgery	79	3.8%	5.5%	5.3%
Combination Abdominal CT Scan	242	3.3%	10.1%	10.5%
Combination Brain/Sinus CT Scan[1]	-	-	2.6%	2.7%
Combination Chest CT Scan	201	0.0%	2.8%	2.7%
Follow-up Mammogram/Ultrasound	244	7.4%	8.4%	8.8%
Lumbar Spine MRI for Low Back Pain[1]	-	-	36.6%	37.2%

Saint James Hospital

2500 West Reynolds Street
Pontiac, IL 61764
URL: www.osfsaintjames.org
Phone: 815-842-2828
Fax: 815-842-4912
Type: Acute Care Hospitals
Emergency Services: Yes
Ownership: Voluntary non-profit - Church
Beds: 89

Key Personnel:
Emergency Room . . . . Nan Marx
Operating Room. . . . . Rajendra Shrivastav

Measure	Cases	This Hosp.	State Avg.	U.S. Avg.
Blood Clot Prevention and Treatment				
Anticoagulation Overlap Therapy[1,2]	-	-	91%	93%
ICU Venous Thromboembolism Prophylaxis[2]	33	97%	93%	92%
Incidence of Potentially Preventable VTE[1,2]	-	-	11%	10%
UFH with Dosages/Platelet Monitoring[1,2]	-	-	94%	97%
Venous Thromboembolism Prophylaxis[2]	60	97%	86%	85%
Warfarin Therapy Discharge Instructions[1,2]	-	-	71%	75%
Chest Pain/Possible Heart Attack Care				
Aspirin Given Within 24 Hours of Arrival	54	100%	96%	96%
Fibrinolytic Meds Within 30 Min. of Arrival[7]	-	-	65%	58%
Average Time to ECG (minutes)	58	5	6	7
Average Time to Transfer (minutes)[1]	-	-	63	60
Children's Asthma Care				
Received Home Management Plan of Care	-	-	-	88%
Received Reliever Medication	-	-	-	100%
Received Systemic Corticosteroids	-	-	-	100%
Emergency Department				
Admittance Decision Time (minutes)[2]	420	58	89	98
Head CT Results Within 45 Min. of Arrival	23	74%	64%	57%
Patients Who Left ER Before Being Seen	14,647	0%	3%	2%
Time from ER Arrival to Admit. (minutes)[2]	420	189	260	274
Time from ER Arrival to Discharge (minutes)	360	94	138	134
Time in ER Before Being Evaluated (minutes)	408	9	28	26
Time to Pain Meds for Fractures (minutes)	66	29	52	57
Heart Attack Care				
Aspirin Given at Discharge[1]	-	-	99%	99%
Fibrinolytic Meds Within 30 Min. of Arrival[7]	-	-	33%	54%
PCI Within 90 Minutes of Arrival[7]	-	-	97%	96%
Statin Prescribed at Discharge[1]	-	-	98%	98%
Heart Failure Care				
ACE Inhibitor or ARB for LVSD	19	100%	98%	97%
Discharge Instructions Given	37	100%	96%	94%
Evaluation of LVS Function	47	100%	99%	99%
Medicare Spending				
Medicare Spending per Patient (ratio)	-	0.90	1	0.98
Pneumonia Care				
Appropriate Initial Antibiotic Given	25	100%	95%	95%
Blood Culture Timing	70	100%	98%	98%
Pregnancy and Delivery Care				
Newborn Deliveries Scheduled Early	14	0%	2%	6%
Preventive Care				
Immunization for Influenza[2]	531	96%	92%	90%
Immunization for Pneumonia[2]	536	98%	92%	92%
Stroke Care				
Anticoagulation Therapy for Atrial Fibrillation[7]	-	-	94%	95%
Antithrombotic Therapy Timing[1]	-	-	98%	98%
Assessed for Rehabilitation[1]	-	-	97%	97%
Discharged on Antithrombotic Therapy[1]	-	-	99%	99%
Discharged on Statin Medication[1]	-	-	94%	94%
Thrombolytic Therapy Timing[7]	-	-	66%	66%
Venous Thromboembolism Prophylaxis[1]	-	-	94%	94%
Written Stroke Educational Materials Given[1]	-	-	87%	88%
Surgical Care Improvement Project				
Appropriate Beta Blocker Usage	49	100%	98%	98%
Appropriate VTP Within 24 Hours	117	98%	98%	98%
Controlled Postoperative Blood Glucose[7]	-	-	97%	97%
Perioperative Temperature Management	140	100%	100%	100%
Prophylactic Antibiotic Selection	109	100%	99%	99%
Prophylactic Antibiotic Selection (Outpatient)[1,3]	-	-	98%	98%
Prophylactic Antibiotic Stopped	107	100%	98%	98%
Prophylactic Antibiotic Timing	109	100%	99%	99%
Prophylactic Antibiotic Timing (Outpatient)[1,3]	-	-	97%	98%
Urinary Catheter Removal	99	100%	98%	97%
Survey of Patients' Hospital Experiences				
Area Around Room 'Always' Quiet at Night	(a)	66%	60%	61%
Doctors 'Always' Communicated Well	(a)	84%	81%	82%
Home Recovery Information Given	(a)	92%	86%	85%
Hospital Given 9 or 10 on 10 Point Scale	(a)	73%	70%	71%
Meds 'Always' Explained Before Given	(a)	72%	64%	64%
Nurses 'Always' Communicated Well	(a)	83%	79%	79%
Pain 'Always' Well Controlled	(a)	74%	71%	71%
Room and Bathroom 'Always' Clean	(a)	77%	74%	73%
Timely Help 'Always' Received	(a)	75%	67%	68%

NOTE: Hospital profiles are in alphabetical order by state, then city, then hospital within the city; Rankings exclude hospitals with less than 25 cases except for patient surveys which excludes hospitals with less than 100 cases; (a) 100-299 cases; (1) The number of cases/patients is too few to report; (2) Data submitted were based on a sample of cases/patients; (3) Results are based on a shorter time period than required; (4) Data suppressed by CMS for one or more quarters; (5) Results are not available for this reporting period; (6) Fewer than 100 patients completed the HCAHPS survey; (7) No cases met the criteria for this measure; (8) The lower limit of the confidence interval cannot be calculated if the number of observed infections equals zero; (9) No data are available from the state/territory for this reporting period; (10) The scores shown reflect fewer than 50 completed surveys; (11) There were discrepancies in the data collection process; (12) This measure does not apply to this hospital for this reporting period; (13) Results cannot be calculated for this reporting period; (14) The results for this state are combined with nearby states to protect confidentiality; Please refer to the User's Guide for a full explanation of data.

Measure	Cases	This Hosp.	State Avg.	U.S. Avg.
Would Definitely Recommend Hospital	(a)	65%	70%	71%
Use of Medical Imaging				
Cardiac Imaging Stress Test before Surgery	240	3.8%	5.5%	5.3%
Combination Abdominal CT Scan	422	5.7%	10.1%	10.5%
Combination Brain/Sinus CT Scan[1]	-	-	2.6%	2.7%
Combination Chest CT Scan	342	0.3%	2.8%	2.7%
Follow-up Mammogram/Ultrasound	872	10.1%	8.4%	8.8%
Lumbar Spine MRI for Low Back Pain	66	50.0%	36.6%	37.2%

Perry Memorial Hospital

530 Park Avenue East
Princeton, IL 61356
Phone: 815-875-2811
Fax: 815-872-6006
URL: www.perry-memorial.org
Type: Critical Access Hospitals
Emergency Services: Yes
Ownership: Government - Local
Beds: 98

Key Personnel:
Emergency Room . . . . Earel Belford, MD
Chief of Medical Staff . . . . E Doran, MD
Patient Relations . . . . Jeanine Dressler
Quality Assurance . . . . Denise Jackson
CEO/President . . . . Robert Senneff

Measure	Cases	This Hosp.	State Avg.	U.S. Avg.
Blood Clot Prevention and Treatment				
Anticoagulation Overlap Therapy[5]	-	-	91%	93%
ICU Venous Thromboembolism Prophylaxis[5]	-	-	93%	92%
Incidence of Potentially Preventable VTE[5]	-	-	11%	10%
UFH with Dosages/Platelet Monitoring[5]	-	-	94%	97%
Venous Thromboembolism Prophylaxis[5]	-	-	86%	85%
Warfarin Therapy Discharge Instructions[5]	-	-	71%	75%
Chest Pain/Possible Heart Attack Care				
Aspirin Given Within 24 Hours of Arrival	-	-	96%	96%
Fibrinolytic Meds Within 30 Min. of Arrival	-	-	65%	58%
Average Time to ECG (minutes)	-	-	6	7
Average Time to Transfer (minutes)	-	-	63	60
Children's Asthma Care				
Received Home Management Plan of Care	-	-	-	88%
Received Reliever Medication	-	-	-	100%
Received Systemic Corticosteroids	-	-	-	100%
Emergency Department				
Admittance Decision Time (minutes)[5]	-	-	89	98
Head CT Results Within 45 Min. of Arrival	-	-	64%	57%
Patients Who Left ER Before Being Seen	-	-	3%	2%
Time from ER Arrival to Admit. (minutes)[5]	-	-	260	274
Time from ER Arrival to Discharge (minutes)	-	-	138	134
Time in ER Before Being Evaluated (minutes)	-	-	28	26
Time to Pain Meds for Fractures (minutes)	-	-	52	57
Heart Attack Care				
Aspirin Given at Discharge[1]	-	-	99%	99%
Fibrinolytic Meds Within 30 Min. of Arrival[7]	-	-	33%	54%
PCI Within 90 Minutes of Arrival[7]	-	-	97%	96%
Statin Prescribed at Discharge[1]	-	-	98%	98%
Heart Failure Care				
ACE Inhibitor or ARB for LVSD[1]	-	-	98%	97%
Discharge Instructions Given	37	100%	96%	94%
Evaluation of LVS Function	73	99%	99%	99%
Medicare Spending				
Medicare Spending per Patient (ratio)	-	-	1	0.98
Pneumonia Care				
Appropriate Initial Antibiotic Given	32	75%	95%	95%
Blood Culture Timing	39	87%	98%	98%
Pregnancy and Delivery Care				
Newborn Deliveries Scheduled Early[5]	-	-	2%	6%
Preventive Care				
Immunization for Influenza[5]	-	-	92%	90%
Immunization for Pneumonia[5]	-	-	92%	92%
Stroke Care				
Anticoagulation Therapy for Atrial Fibrillation[5]	-	-	94%	95%
Antithrombotic Therapy Timing[5]	-	-	98%	98%
Assessed for Rehabilitation[5]	-	-	97%	97%
Discharged on Antithrombotic Therapy[5]	-	-	99%	99%
Discharged on Statin Medication[5]	-	-	94%	94%
Thrombolytic Therapy Timing[5]	-	-	66%	66%
Venous Thromboembolism Prophylaxis[5]	-	-	94%	94%
Written Stroke Educational Materials Given[5]	-	-	87%	88%
Surgical Care Improvement Project				
Appropriate Beta Blocker Usage[1]	-	-	98%	98%
Appropriate VTP Within 24 Hours	25	100%	98%	98%
Controlled Postoperative Blood Glucose[7]	-	-	97%	97%
Perioperative Temperature Management	28	100%	100%	100%
Prophylactic Antibiotic Selection	18	100%	99%	99%
Prophylactic Antibiotic Selection (Outpatient)	-	-	98%	98%
Prophylactic Antibiotic Stopped	13	100%	98%	98%
Prophylactic Antibiotic Timing	18	94%	99%	99%
Prophylactic Antibiotic Timing (Outpatient)	-	-	97%	98%
Urinary Catheter Removal	18	100%	98%	97%
Survey of Patients' Hospital Experiences				
Area Around Room 'Always' Quiet at Night	(a)	63%	60%	61%
Doctors 'Always' Communicated Well	(a)	84%	81%	82%
Home Recovery Information Given	(a)	85%	86%	85%
Hospital Given 9 or 10 on 10 Point Scale	(a)	72%	70%	71%
Meds 'Always' Explained Before Given	(a)	65%	64%	64%
Nurses 'Always' Communicated Well	(a)	81%	79%	79%
Pain 'Always' Well Controlled	(a)	68%	71%	71%
Room and Bathroom 'Always' Clean	(a)	81%	74%	73%
Timely Help 'Always' Received	(a)	66%	67%	68%
Would Definitely Recommend Hospital	(a)	67%	70%	71%
Use of Medical Imaging				
Cardiac Imaging Stress Test before Surgery	-	-	5.5%	5.3%
Combination Abdominal CT Scan	-	-	10.1%	10.5%
Combination Brain/Sinus CT Scan	-	-	2.6%	2.7%
Combination Chest CT Scan	-	-	2.8%	2.7%
Follow-up Mammogram/Ultrasound	-	-	8.4%	8.8%
Lumbar Spine MRI for Low Back Pain	-	-	36.6%	37.2%

Blessing Hospital

Broadway at 11th Street
Quincy, IL 62301
Phone: 217-223-5811
Fax: 217-223-1200
E-mail: sfelde@blessinghospital.com
URL: www.blessinghealthsystem.org
Type: Acute Care Hospitals
Emergency Services: Yes
Ownership: Voluntary non-profit - Private
Beds: 426

Key Personnel:
CEO/President . . . . Brad Billings
Operating Room . . . . William Birsic, RN
Pediatric In-Patient Care . . . . Joan Hynek, RN
Quality Assurance . . . . Tena Jones
Cardiac Laboratory . . . . James Kase
Radiology . . . . Bonnie Kleissle
Infection Control . . . . Carleen Orton, RN
Chief of Medical Staff . . . . Steve Sanders, DO

Measure	Cases	This Hosp.	State Avg.	U.S. Avg.
Blood Clot Prevention and Treatment				
Anticoagulation Overlap Therapy[2]	64	98%	91%	93%
ICU Venous Thromboembolism Prophylaxis[2]	71	92%	93%	92%
Incidence of Potentially Preventable VTE[1,2]	-	-	11%	10%
UFH with Dosages/Platelet Monitoring[2]	36	100%	94%	97%
Venous Thromboembolism Prophylaxis[2]	297	76%	86%	85%
Warfarin Therapy Discharge Instructions[2]	39	87%	71%	75%
Chest Pain/Possible Heart Attack Care				
Aspirin Given Within 24 Hours of Arrival[1,3]	-	-	96%	96%
Fibrinolytic Meds Within 30 Min. of Arrival[5]	-	-	65%	58%
Average Time to ECG (minutes)[1,3]	-	-	6	7
Average Time to Transfer (minutes)[5]	-	-	63	60
Children's Asthma Care				
Received Home Management Plan of Care	-	-	-	88%
Received Reliever Medication	-	-	-	100%
Received Systemic Corticosteroids	-	-	-	100%
Emergency Department				
Admittance Decision Time (minutes)[2]	395	72	89	98
Head CT Results Within 45 Min. of Arrival[1]	-	-	64%	57%
Patients Who Left ER Before Being Seen	53,703	1%	3%	2%
Time from ER Arrival to Admit. (minutes)[2]	405	196	260	274
Time from ER Arrival to Discharge (minutes)	346	148	138	134
Time in ER Before Being Evaluated (minutes)	305	24	28	26
Time to Pain Meds for Fractures (minutes)	105	50	52	57
Heart Attack Care				
Aspirin Given at Discharge	235	100%	99%	99%
Fibrinolytic Meds Within 30 Min. of Arrival[7]	-	-	33%	54%
PCI Within 90 Minutes of Arrival	50	98%	97%	96%
Statin Prescribed at Discharge	215	98%	98%	98%
Heart Failure Care				
ACE Inhibitor or ARB for LVSD	70	100%	98%	97%
Discharge Instructions Given	238	93%	96%	94%
Evaluation of LVS Function	370	100%	99%	99%
Medicare Spending				
Medicare Spending per Patient (ratio)	-	0.96	1	0.98
Pneumonia Care				
Appropriate Initial Antibiotic Given	154	98%	95%	95%
Blood Culture Timing	325	100%	98%	98%
Pregnancy and Delivery Care				
Newborn Deliveries Scheduled Early[2]	26	0%	2%	6%
Preventive Care				
Immunization for Influenza[2]	574	85%	92%	90%
Immunization for Pneumonia[2]	601	86%	92%	92%
Stroke Care				
Anticoagulation Therapy for Atrial Fibrillation	25	88%	94%	95%
Antithrombotic Therapy Timing	133	100%	98%	98%
Assessed for Rehabilitation	158	100%	97%	97%
Discharged on Antithrombotic Therapy	146	100%	99%	99%
Discharged on Statin Medication	100	95%	94%	94%
Thrombolytic Therapy Timing[1]	-	-	66%	66%
Venous Thromboembolism Prophylaxis	150	96%	94%	94%
Written Stroke Educational Materials Given	77	87%	87%	88%
Surgical Care Improvement Project				
Appropriate Beta Blocker Usage	242	98%	98%	98%
Appropriate VTP Within 24 Hours	364	98%	98%	98%
Controlled Postoperative Blood Glucose	66	98%	97%	97%
Perioperative Temperature Management	477	100%	100%	100%
Prophylactic Antibiotic Selection	352	99%	99%	99%
Prophylactic Antibiotic Selection (Outpatient)	268	98%	98%	98%
Prophylactic Antibiotic Stopped	324	100%	98%	98%
Prophylactic Antibiotic Timing	355	100%	99%	99%
Prophylactic Antibiotic Timing (Outpatient)	269	99%	97%	98%
Urinary Catheter Removal	270	99%	98%	97%
Survey of Patients' Hospital Experiences				
Area Around Room 'Always' Quiet at Night[11]	300+	53%	60%	61%
Doctors 'Always' Communicated Well[11]	300+	80%	81%	82%
Home Recovery Information Given[11]	300+	94%	86%	85%
Hospital Given 9 or 10 on 10 Point Scale[11]	300+	69%	70%	71%
Meds 'Always' Explained Before Given[11]	300+	68%	64%	64%
Nurses 'Always' Communicated Well[11]	300+	82%	79%	79%
Pain 'Always' Well Controlled[11]	300+	72%	71%	71%
Room and Bathroom 'Always' Clean[11]	300+	78%	74%	73%
Timely Help 'Always' Received[11]	300+	70%	67%	68%
Would Definitely Recommend Hospital[11]	300+	74%	70%	71%
Use of Medical Imaging				
Cardiac Imaging Stress Test before Surgery	569	5.4%	5.5%	5.3%
Combination Abdominal CT Scan	769	3.3%	10.1%	10.5%
Combination Brain/Sinus CT Scan	913	2.6%	2.6%	2.7%
Combination Chest CT Scan	573	0.0%	2.8%	2.7%
Follow-up Mammogram/Ultrasound	1,868	7.3%	8.4%	8.8%
Lumbar Spine MRI for Low Back Pain	122	41.0%	36.6%	37.2%

Red Bud Regional Hospital

325 Spring Street
Red Bud, IL 62278
Phone: 618-282-3831
Fax: 618-282-6101
Type: Critical Access Hospitals
Emergency Services: Yes
Ownership: Proprietary
Beds: 202

Key Personnel:
Emergency Room . . . . Steven Elster
Chief of Medical Staff . . . . Chung Khan
CEO . . . . Shane Watson

Measure	Cases	This Hosp.	State Avg.	U.S. Avg.
Blood Clot Prevention and Treatment				
Anticoagulation Overlap Therapy[1,2]	-	-	91%	93%
ICU Venous Thromboembolism Prophylaxis[2,7]	-	-	93%	92%
Incidence of Potentially Preventable VTE[1,2]	-	-	11%	10%
UFH with Dosages/Platelet Monitoring[2,7]	-	-	94%	97%
Venous Thromboembolism Prophylaxis[2]	371	99%	86%	85%
Warfarin Therapy Discharge Instructions[1,2]	-	-	71%	75%
Chest Pain/Possible Heart Attack Care				

NOTE: Hospital profiles are in alphabetical order by state, then city, then hospital within the city; Rankings exclude hospitals with less than 25 cases except for patient surveys which excludes hospitals with less than 100 cases; (a) 100-299 cases; (1) The number of cases/patients is too few to report; (2) Data submitted were based on a sample of cases/patients; (3) Results are based on a shorter time period than required; (4) Data suppressed by CMS for one or more quarters; (5) Results are not available for this reporting period; (6) Fewer than 100 patients completed the HCAHPS survey; (7) No cases met the criteria for this measure; (8) The lower limit of the confidence interval cannot be calculated if the number of observed infections equals zero; (9) No data are available from the state/territory for this reporting period; (10) The scores shown reflect fewer than 50 completed surveys; (11) There were discrepancies in the data collection process; (12) This measure does not apply to this hospital for this reporting period; (13) Results cannot be calculated for this reporting period; (14) The results for this state are combined with nearby states to protect confidentiality; Please refer to the User's Guide for a full explanation of data.

Measure	Cases	This Hosp.	State Avg.	U.S. Avg.
Aspirin Given Within 24 Hours of Arrival	74	96%	96%	96%
Fibrinolytic Meds Within 30 Min. of Arrival[1]	-	-	65%	58%
Average Time to ECG (minutes)	76	4	6	7
Average Time to Transfer (minutes)[1]	-	-	63	60
Children's Asthma Care				
Received Home Management Plan of Care	-	-	-	88%
Received Reliever Medication	-	-	-	100%
Received Systemic Corticosteroids	-	-	-	100%
Emergency Department				
Admittance Decision Time (minutes)[2]	459	62	89	98
Head CT Results Within 45 Min. of Arrival[1]	-	-	64%	57%
Patients Who Left ER Before Being Seen	6,304	1%	3%	2%
Time from ER Arrival to Admit. (minutes)[2]	460	219	260	274
Time from ER Arrival to Discharge (minutes)	365	100	138	134
Time in ER Before Being Evaluated (minutes)	421	14	28	26
Time to Pain Meds for Fractures (minutes)	34	42	52	57
Heart Attack Care				
Aspirin Given at Discharge[1]	-	-	99%	99%
Fibrinolytic Meds Within 30 Min. of Arrival[7]	-	-	33%	54%
PCI Within 90 Minutes of Arrival[7]	-	-	97%	96%
Statin Prescribed at Discharge[1]	-	-	98%	98%
Heart Failure Care				
ACE Inhibitor or ARB for LVSD[1]	-	-	98%	97%
Discharge Instructions Given[1]	-	-	96%	94%
Evaluation of LVS Function	28	100%	99%	99%
Medicare Spending				
Medicare Spending per Patient (ratio)	-	-	1	0.98
Pneumonia Care				
Appropriate Initial Antibiotic Given	37	97%	95%	95%
Blood Culture Timing	45	100%	98%	98%
Pregnancy and Delivery Care				
Newborn Deliveries Scheduled Early[2,3]	-	-	2%	6%
Preventive Care				
Immunization for Influenza[2]	327	98%	92%	90%
Immunization for Pneumonia[2]	508	100%	92%	92%
Stroke Care				
Anticoagulation Therapy for Atrial Fibrillation[1]	-	-	94%	95%
Antithrombotic Therapy Timing[1]	-	-	98%	98%
Assessed for Rehabilitation[1]	-	-	97%	97%
Discharged on Antithrombotic Therapy[1]	-	-	99%	99%
Discharged on Statin Medication[1]	-	-	94%	94%
Thrombolytic Therapy Timing[7]	-	-	66%	66%
Venous Thromboembolism Prophylaxis[1]	-	-	94%	94%
Written Stroke Educational Materials Given[1]	-	-	87%	88%
Surgical Care Improvement Project				
Appropriate Beta Blocker Usage[1]	-	-	98%	98%
Appropriate VTP Within 24 Hours	25	96%	98%	98%
Controlled Postoperative Blood Glucose[7]	-	-	97%	97%
Perioperative Temperature Management	33	100%	100%	100%
Prophylactic Antibiotic Selection	17	100%	99%	99%
Prophylactic Antibiotic Selection (Outpatient)	19	100%	98%	98%
Prophylactic Antibiotic Stopped	16	100%	98%	98%
Prophylactic Antibiotic Timing	17	100%	99%	99%
Prophylactic Antibiotic Timing (Outpatient)	19	100%	97%	98%
Urinary Catheter Removal[1]	-	-	98%	97%
Survey of Patients' Hospital Experiences				
Area Around Room 'Always' Quiet at Night	(a)	64%	60%	61%
Doctors 'Always' Communicated Well	(a)	86%	81%	82%
Home Recovery Information Given	(a)	92%	86%	85%
Hospital Given 9 or 10 on 10 Point Scale	(a)	72%	70%	71%
Meds 'Always' Explained Before Given	(a)	73%	64%	64%
Nurses 'Always' Communicated Well	(a)	84%	79%	79%
Pain 'Always' Well Controlled	(a)	75%	71%	71%
Room and Bathroom 'Always' Clean	(a)	71%	74%	73%
Timely Help 'Always' Received	(a)	65%	67%	68%
Would Definitely Recommend Hospital	(a)	68%	70%	71%
Use of Medical Imaging				
Cardiac Imaging Stress Test before Surgery	123	3.3%	5.5%	5.3%
Combination Abdominal CT Scan	207	13.0%	10.1%	10.5%
Combination Brain/Sinus CT Scan[1]	-	-	2.6%	2.7%
Combination Chest CT Scan	87	2.3%	2.8%	2.7%
Follow-up Mammogram/Ultrasound	358	10.1%	8.4%	8.8%
Lumbar Spine MRI for Low Back Pain[1]	-	-	36.6%	37.2%

Crawford Memorial Hospital

1000 North Allen Street
Robinson, IL 62454
Phone: 618-546-2514
Fax: 618-546-2600
E-mail: debbie.robinson@crawfordmh.org
URL: www.crawfordmh.com
Type: Critical Access Hospitals
Emergency Services: Yes
Ownership: Govt - Hospital Dist/Auth
Beds: 93

Key Personnel:
Quality Assurance . . . . Darra Beard
Chief of Medical Staff . . . . Michael Elliott, MD
CEO/President . . . . Randy Simmons, MHA

Measure	Cases	This Hosp.	State Avg.	U.S. Avg.
Blood Clot Prevention and Treatment				
Anticoagulation Overlap Therapy[5]	-	-	91%	93%
ICU Venous Thromboembolism Prophylaxis[5]	-	-	93%	92%
Incidence of Potentially Preventable VTE[5]	-	-	11%	10%
UFH with Dosages/Platelet Monitoring[5]	-	-	94%	97%
Venous Thromboembolism Prophylaxis[5]	-	-	86%	85%
Warfarin Therapy Discharge Instructions[5]	-	-	71%	75%
Chest Pain/Possible Heart Attack Care				
Aspirin Given Within 24 Hours of Arrival	-	-	96%	96%
Fibrinolytic Meds Within 30 Min. of Arrival	-	-	65%	58%
Average Time to ECG (minutes)	-	-	6	7
Average Time to Transfer (minutes)	-	-	63	60
Children's Asthma Care				
Received Home Management Plan of Care	-	-	-	88%
Received Reliever Medication	-	-	-	100%
Received Systemic Corticosteroids	-	-	-	100%
Emergency Department				
Admittance Decision Time (minutes)[5]	-	-	89	98
Head CT Results Within 45 Min. of Arrival	-	-	64%	57%
Patients Who Left ER Before Being Seen	-	-	3%	2%
Time from ER Arrival to Admit. (minutes)[5]	-	-	260	274
Time from ER Arrival to Discharge (minutes)	-	-	138	134
Time in ER Before Being Evaluated (minutes)	-	-	28	26
Time to Pain Meds for Fractures (minutes)	-	-	52	57
Heart Attack Care				
Aspirin Given at Discharge[1,3]	-	-	99%	99%
Fibrinolytic Meds Within 30 Min. of Arrival[3,7]	-	-	33%	54%
PCI Within 90 Minutes of Arrival[3,7]	-	-	97%	96%
Statin Prescribed at Discharge[1,3]	-	-	98%	98%
Heart Failure Care				
ACE Inhibitor or ARB for LVSD[1,3]	-	-	98%	97%
Discharge Instructions Given[3]	20	95%	96%	94%
Evaluation of LVS Function[3]	25	100%	99%	99%
Medicare Spending				
Medicare Spending per Patient (ratio)	-	-	1	0.98
Pneumonia Care				
Appropriate Initial Antibiotic Given[3]	21	100%	95%	95%
Blood Culture Timing[3]	24	100%	98%	98%
Pregnancy and Delivery Care				
Newborn Deliveries Scheduled Early[5]	-	-	2%	6%
Preventive Care				
Immunization for Influenza[5]	-	-	92%	90%
Immunization for Pneumonia[5]	-	-	92%	92%
Stroke Care				
Anticoagulation Therapy for Atrial Fibrillation[5]	-	-	94%	95%
Antithrombotic Therapy Timing[5]	-	-	98%	98%
Assessed for Rehabilitation[5]	-	-	97%	97%
Discharged on Antithrombotic Therapy[5]	-	-	99%	99%
Discharged on Statin Medication[5]	-	-	94%	94%
Thrombolytic Therapy Timing[5]	-	-	66%	66%
Venous Thromboembolism Prophylaxis[5]	-	-	94%	94%
Written Stroke Educational Materials Given[5]	-	-	87%	88%
Surgical Care Improvement Project				
Appropriate Beta Blocker Usage[1,3]	-	-	98%	98%
Appropriate VTP Within 24 Hours[1,3]	-	-	98%	98%
Controlled Postoperative Blood Glucose[3,7]	-	-	97%	97%
Perioperative Temperature Management[3]	41	100%	100%	100%
Prophylactic Antibiotic Selection[3]	37	92%	99%	99%
Prophylactic Antibiotic Selection (Outpatient)	-	-	98%	98%
Prophylactic Antibiotic Stopped[3]	36	100%	98%	98%
Prophylactic Antibiotic Timing[3]	37	97%	99%	99%
Prophylactic Antibiotic Timing (Outpatient)	-	-	97%	98%
Urinary Catheter Removal[3]	25	88%	98%	97%
Survey of Patients' Hospital Experiences				
Area Around Room 'Always' Quiet at Night	(a)	56%	60%	61%
Doctors 'Always' Communicated Well	(a)	87%	81%	82%
Home Recovery Information Given	(a)	90%	86%	85%
Hospital Given 9 or 10 on 10 Point Scale	(a)	76%	70%	71%
Meds 'Always' Explained Before Given	(a)	72%	64%	64%
Nurses 'Always' Communicated Well	(a)	85%	79%	79%
Pain 'Always' Well Controlled	(a)	81%	71%	71%
Room and Bathroom 'Always' Clean	(a)	86%	74%	73%
Timely Help 'Always' Received	(a)	73%	67%	68%
Would Definitely Recommend Hospital	(a)	72%	70%	71%
Use of Medical Imaging				
Cardiac Imaging Stress Test before Surgery	-	-	5.5%	5.3%
Combination Abdominal CT Scan	-	-	10.1%	10.5%
Combination Brain/Sinus CT Scan	-	-	2.6%	2.7%
Combination Chest CT Scan	-	-	2.8%	2.7%
Follow-up Mammogram/Ultrasound	-	-	8.4%	8.8%
Lumbar Spine MRI for Low Back Pain	-	-	36.6%	37.2%

Rochelle Community Hospital

900 N 2nd St
Rochelle, IL 61068
Phone: 815-562-2181
Fax: 815-562-5474
URL: www.rcha.net
Type: Critical Access Hospitals
Emergency Services: Yes
Ownership: Voluntary non-profit - Private
Beds: 42

Key Personnel:
CEO/President . . . . Mark J. Batty
Radiology . . . . Nester S Cuasay
Infection Control . . . . Dorrie Kasman
Emergency Room . . . . Janet Lodico, RN
Chief of Medical Staff . . . . John Prabbaker, MD
Quality Assurance . . . . Karen Tracey, RN

Measure	Cases	This Hosp.	State Avg.	U.S. Avg.
Blood Clot Prevention and Treatment				
Anticoagulation Overlap Therapy[5]	-	-	91%	93%
ICU Venous Thromboembolism Prophylaxis[5]	-	-	93%	92%
Incidence of Potentially Preventable VTE[5]	-	-	11%	10%
UFH with Dosages/Platelet Monitoring[5]	-	-	94%	97%
Venous Thromboembolism Prophylaxis[5]	-	-	86%	85%
Warfarin Therapy Discharge Instructions[5]	-	-	71%	75%
Chest Pain/Possible Heart Attack Care				
Aspirin Given Within 24 Hours of Arrival	-	-	96%	96%
Fibrinolytic Meds Within 30 Min. of Arrival	-	-	65%	58%
Average Time to ECG (minutes)	-	-	6	7
Average Time to Transfer (minutes)	-	-	63	60
Children's Asthma Care				
Received Home Management Plan of Care	-	-	-	88%
Received Reliever Medication	-	-	-	100%
Received Systemic Corticosteroids	-	-	-	100%
Emergency Department				
Admittance Decision Time (minutes)[5]	-	-	89	98
Head CT Results Within 45 Min. of Arrival	-	-	64%	57%
Patients Who Left ER Before Being Seen	-	-	3%	2%
Time from ER Arrival to Admit. (minutes)[5]	-	-	260	274
Time from ER Arrival to Discharge (minutes)	-	-	138	134
Time in ER Before Being Evaluated (minutes)	-	-	28	26
Time to Pain Meds for Fractures (minutes)	-	-	52	57
Heart Attack Care				
Aspirin Given at Discharge[1,3]	-	-	99%	99%
Fibrinolytic Meds Within 30 Min. of Arrival[3,7]	-	-	33%	54%
PCI Within 90 Minutes of Arrival[3,7]	-	-	97%	96%
Statin Prescribed at Discharge[1,3]	-	-	98%	98%
Heart Failure Care				
ACE Inhibitor or ARB for LVSD	11	45%	98%	97%
Discharge Instructions Given	22	77%	96%	94%
Evaluation of LVS Function	27	96%	99%	99%
Medicare Spending				
Medicare Spending per Patient (ratio)	-	-	1	0.98
Pneumonia Care				
Appropriate Initial Antibiotic Given[2]	32	72%	95%	95%

NOTE: Hospital profiles are in alphabetical order by state, then city, then hospital within the city; Rankings exclude hospitals with less than 25 cases except for patient surveys which excludes hospitals with less than 100 cases; (a) 100-299 cases; (1) The number of cases/patients is too few to report; (2) Data submitted were based on a sample of cases/patients; (3) Results are based on a shorter time period than required; (4) Data suppressed by CMS for one or more quarters; (5) Results are not available for this reporting period; (6) Fewer than 100 patients completed the HCAHPS survey; (7) No cases met the criteria for this measure; (8) The lower limit of the confidence interval cannot be calculated if the number of observed infections equals zero; (9) No data are available from the state/territory for this reporting period; (10) The scores shown reflect fewer than 50 completed surveys; (11) There were discrepancies in the data collection process; (12) This measure does not apply to this hospital for this reporting period; (13) Results cannot be calculated for this reporting period; (14) The results for this state are combined with nearby states to protect confidentiality; Please refer to the User's Guide for a full explanation of data.

Measure	Cases	This Hosp.	State Avg.	U.S. Avg.
Blood Culture Timing[2]	45	91%	98%	98%
Pregnancy and Delivery Care				
Newborn Deliveries Scheduled Early[5]	-	-	2%	6%
Preventive Care				
Immunization for Influenza[5]	-	-	92%	90%
Immunization for Pneumonia[5]	-	-	92%	92%
Stroke Care				
Anticoagulation Therapy for Atrial Fibrillation[5]	-	-	94%	95%
Antithrombotic Therapy Timing[5]	-	-	98%	98%
Assessed for Rehabilitation[5]	-	-	97%	97%
Discharged on Antithrombotic Therapy[5]	-	-	99%	99%
Discharged on Statin Medication[5]	-	-	94%	94%
Thrombolytic Therapy Timing[5]	-	-	66%	66%
Venous Thromboembolism Prophylaxis[5]	-	-	94%	94%
Written Stroke Educational Materials Given[5]	-	-	87%	88%
Surgical Care Improvement Project				
Appropriate Beta Blocker Usage[1]	-	-	98%	98%
Appropriate VTP Within 24 Hours	23	100%	98%	98%
Controlled Postoperative Blood Glucose[7]	-	-	97%	97%
Perioperative Temperature Management	23	100%	100%	100%
Prophylactic Antibiotic Selection	21	100%	99%	99%
Prophylactic Antibiotic Selection (Outpatient)	-	-	98%	98%
Prophylactic Antibiotic Stopped	21	81%	98%	98%
Prophylactic Antibiotic Timing	21	90%	99%	99%
Prophylactic Antibiotic Timing (Outpatient)	-	-	97%	98%
Urinary Catheter Removal	20	90%	98%	97%
Survey of Patients' Hospital Experiences				
Area Around Room 'Always' Quiet at Night	(a)	67%	60%	61%
Doctors 'Always' Communicated Well	(a)	89%	81%	82%
Home Recovery Information Given	(a)	93%	86%	85%
Hospital Given 9 or 10 on 10 Point Scale	(a)	76%	70%	71%
Meds 'Always' Explained Before Given	(a)	72%	64%	64%
Nurses 'Always' Communicated Well	(a)	90%	79%	79%
Pain 'Always' Well Controlled	(a)	84%	71%	71%
Room and Bathroom 'Always' Clean	(a)	90%	74%	73%
Timely Help 'Always' Received	(a)	82%	67%	68%
Would Definitely Recommend Hospital	(a)	75%	70%	71%
Use of Medical Imaging				
Cardiac Imaging Stress Test before Surgery	-	-	5.5%	5.3%
Combination Abdominal CT Scan	-	-	10.1%	10.5%
Combination Brain/Sinus CT Scan	-	-	2.6%	2.7%
Combination Chest CT Scan	-	-	2.8%	2.7%
Follow-up Mammogram/Ultrasound	-	-	8.4%	8.8%
Lumbar Spine MRI for Low Back Pain	-	-	36.6%	37.2%

Trinity Rock Island

2701 17th St
Rock Island, IL 61201
URL: www.trinityqc.com
Phone: 309-779-5000
Fax: 309-779-2695
Type: Acute Care Hospitals
Emergency Services: Yes
Ownership: Voluntary non-profit - Other
Beds: 349

Key Personnel:

Operating Room. . . . . Cherie Fulks
Quality Assurance . . . . Cheryl Jackson
Pediatric Ambulatory Care . . . . . . Paulito Juazon, MD
Pediatric In-Patient Care . . . . Paulito Juazon, MD
CEO/President. . . . . Rick Seidler
Radiology. . . . . Craig Tillman, MD
Infection Control. . . . . Marilynn Van Vliete, RN
Chief of Medical Staff. . . . . Harry Wallner, MD

Measure	Cases	This Hosp.	State Avg.	U.S. Avg.
Blood Clot Prevention and Treatment				
Anticoagulation Overlap Therapy[2]	65	98%	91%	93%
ICU Venous Thromboembolism Prophylaxis[2]	65	78%	93%	92%
Incidence of Potentially Preventable VTE[2]	17	12%	11%	10%
UFH with Dosages/Platelet Monitoring[1,2]	-	-	94%	97%
Venous Thromboembolism Prophylaxis[2]	330	78%	86%	85%
Warfarin Therapy Discharge Instructions[2]	50	64%	71%	75%
Chest Pain/Possible Heart Attack Care				
Aspirin Given Within 24 Hours of Arrival[1,3]	-	-	96%	96%
Fibrinolytic Meds Within 30 Min. of Arrival[5]	-	-	65%	58%
Average Time to ECG (minutes)[1,3]	-	-	6	7
Average Time to Transfer (minutes)[5]	-	-	63	60
Children's Asthma Care				
Received Home Management Plan of Care	-	-	-	88%
Received Reliever Medication	-	-	-	100%
Received Systemic Corticosteroids	-	-	-	100%
Emergency Department				
Admittance Decision Time (minutes)[2]	433	72	89	98
Head CT Results Within 45 Min. of Arrival	17	94%	64%	57%
Patients Who Left ER Before Being Seen	63,265	1%	3%	2%
Time from ER Arrival to Admit. (minutes)[2]	437	221	260	274
Time from ER Arrival to Discharge (minutes)	374	115	138	134
Time in ER Before Being Evaluated (minutes)	380	21	28	26
Time to Pain Meds for Fractures (minutes)	188	41	52	57
Heart Attack Care				
Aspirin Given at Discharge	508	98%	99%	99%
Fibrinolytic Meds Within 30 Min. of Arrival[7]	-	-	33%	54%
PCI Within 90 Minutes of Arrival	32	100%	97%	96%
Statin Prescribed at Discharge	477	90%	98%	98%
Heart Failure Care				
ACE Inhibitor or ARB for LVSD[2]	81	93%	98%	97%
Discharge Instructions Given[2]	232	97%	96%	94%
Evaluation of LVS Function[2]	286	99%	99%	99%
Medicare Spending				
Medicare Spending per Patient (ratio)	-	0.98	1	0.98
Pneumonia Care				
Appropriate Initial Antibiotic Given[2]	101	98%	95%	95%
Blood Culture Timing[2]	160	99%	98%	98%
Pregnancy and Delivery Care				
Newborn Deliveries Scheduled Early[2]	23	0%	2%	6%
Preventive Care				
Immunization for Influenza[2]	496	69%	92%	90%
Immunization for Pneumonia[2]	637	76%	92%	92%
Stroke Care				
Anticoagulation Therapy for Atrial Fibrillation[1,2]	-	-	94%	95%
Antithrombotic Therapy Timing[2]	66	98%	98%	98%
Assessed for Rehabilitation[2]	79	90%	97%	97%
Discharged on Antithrombotic Therapy[2]	73	93%	99%	99%
Discharged on Statin Medication[2]	59	69%	94%	94%
Thrombolytic Therapy Timing[1,2]	-	-	66%	66%
Venous Thromboembolism Prophylaxis[2]	83	87%	94%	94%
Written Stroke Educational Materials Given[2]	29	62%	87%	88%
Surgical Care Improvement Project				
Appropriate Beta Blocker Usage[2]	153	98%	98%	98%
Appropriate VTP Within 24 Hours[2]	300	96%	98%	98%
Controlled Postoperative Blood Glucose[2]	114	98%	97%	97%
Perioperative Temperature Management[2]	368	100%	100%	100%
Prophylactic Antibiotic Selection[2]	347	99%	99%	99%
Prophylactic Antibiotic Selection (Outpatient)	440	95%	98%	98%
Prophylactic Antibiotic Stopped[2]	341	96%	98%	98%
Prophylactic Antibiotic Timing[2]	347	99%	99%	99%
Prophylactic Antibiotic Timing (Outpatient)	445	98%	97%	98%
Urinary Catheter Removal[2]	128	100%	98%	97%
Survey of Patients' Hospital Experiences				
Area Around Room 'Always' Quiet at Night	300+	54%	60%	61%
Doctors 'Always' Communicated Well	300+	78%	81%	82%
Home Recovery Information Given	300+	87%	86%	85%
Hospital Given 9 or 10 on 10 Point Scale	300+	68%	70%	71%
Meds 'Always' Explained Before Given	300+	59%	64%	64%
Nurses 'Always' Communicated Well	300+	78%	79%	79%
Pain 'Always' Well Controlled	300+	70%	71%	71%
Room and Bathroom 'Always' Clean	300+	70%	74%	73%
Timely Help 'Always' Received	300+	58%	67%	68%
Would Definitely Recommend Hospital	300+	70%	70%	71%
Use of Medical Imaging				
Cardiac Imaging Stress Test before Surgery	153	1.3%	5.5%	5.3%
Combination Abdominal CT Scan	1,025	3.5%	10.1%	10.5%
Combination Brain/Sinus CT Scan	960	2.1%	2.6%	2.7%
Combination Chest CT Scan	709	0.0%	2.8%	2.7%
Follow-up Mammogram/Ultrasound	2,303	9.7%	8.4%	8.8%
Lumbar Spine MRI for Low Back Pain[1]	-	-	36.6%	37.2%

Rockford Memorial Hospital

2400 North Rockton Avenue
Rockford, IL 61103
URL: www.rhsnet.org
Phone: 815-968-6861
Fax: 815-971-6167
Type: Acute Care Hospitals
Emergency Services: Yes
Ownership: Voluntary non-profit - Private
Beds: 396

Key Personnel:

CEO/President. . . . . Gary E. Kaatz
Chief of Medical Staff. . . . . Milton Schmitt, MD
Emergency Room . . . . Dennis Veharra, MD

Measure	Cases	This Hosp.	State Avg.	U.S. Avg.
Blood Clot Prevention and Treatment				
Anticoagulation Overlap Therapy[2]	97	94%	91%	93%
ICU Venous Thromboembolism Prophylaxis[2]	92	97%	93%	92%
Incidence of Potentially Preventable VTE[2]	19	5%	11%	10%
UFH with Dosages/Platelet Monitoring[1,2]	-	-	94%	97%
Venous Thromboembolism Prophylaxis[2]	476	85%	86%	85%
Warfarin Therapy Discharge Instructions[2]	74	22%	71%	75%
Chest Pain/Possible Heart Attack Care				
Aspirin Given Within 24 Hours of Arrival[5]	-	-	96%	96%
Fibrinolytic Meds Within 30 Min. of Arrival[5]	-	-	65%	58%
Average Time to ECG (minutes)[5]	-	-	6	7
Average Time to Transfer (minutes)[5]	-	-	63	60
Children's Asthma Care				
Received Home Management Plan of Care	-	-	-	88%
Received Reliever Medication	-	-	-	100%
Received Systemic Corticosteroids	-	-	-	100%
Emergency Department				
Admittance Decision Time (minutes)[2]	616	76	89	98
Head CT Results Within 45 Min. of Arrival[1,3]	-	-	64%	57%
Patients Who Left ER Before Being Seen	52,600	3%	3%	2%
Time from ER Arrival to Admit. (minutes)[2]	617	244	260	274
Time from ER Arrival to Discharge (minutes)	753	156	138	134
Time in ER Before Being Evaluated (minutes)	761	67	28	26
Time to Pain Meds for Fractures (minutes)	128	70	52	57
Heart Attack Care				
Aspirin Given at Discharge	243	100%	99%	99%
Fibrinolytic Meds Within 30 Min. of Arrival[7]	-	-	33%	54%
PCI Within 90 Minutes of Arrival	32	100%	97%	96%
Statin Prescribed at Discharge	242	99%	98%	98%
Heart Failure Care				
ACE Inhibitor or ARB for LVSD	85	96%	98%	97%
Discharge Instructions Given	230	84%	96%	94%
Evaluation of LVS Function	293	99%	99%	99%
Medicare Spending				
Medicare Spending per Patient (ratio)	-	1.00	1	0.98
Pneumonia Care				
Appropriate Initial Antibiotic Given	160	100%	95%	95%
Blood Culture Timing	278	100%	98%	98%
Pregnancy and Delivery Care				
Newborn Deliveries Scheduled Early[2]	24	0%	2%	6%
Preventive Care				
Immunization for Influenza[2]	617	88%	92%	90%
Immunization for Pneumonia[2]	754	82%	92%	92%
Stroke Care				
Anticoagulation Therapy for Atrial Fibrillation	15	87%	94%	95%
Antithrombotic Therapy Timing	95	100%	98%	98%
Assessed for Rehabilitation	125	91%	97%	97%
Discharged on Antithrombotic Therapy	103	100%	99%	99%
Discharged on Statin Medication	87	94%	94%	94%
Thrombolytic Therapy Timing	12	67%	66%	66%
Venous Thromboembolism Prophylaxis	136	79%	94%	94%
Written Stroke Educational Materials Given	68	53%	87%	88%
Surgical Care Improvement Project				
Appropriate Beta Blocker Usage	328	99%	98%	98%
Appropriate VTP Within 24 Hours	699	95%	98%	98%
Controlled Postoperative Blood Glucose	78	96%	97%	97%
Perioperative Temperature Management	867	100%	100%	100%
Prophylactic Antibiotic Selection	575	99%	99%	99%
Prophylactic Antibiotic Selection (Outpatient)	267	97%	98%	98%
Prophylactic Antibiotic Stopped	555	97%	98%	98%
Prophylactic Antibiotic Timing	575	99%	99%	99%
Prophylactic Antibiotic Timing (Outpatient)	269	99%	97%	98%

NOTE: Hospital profiles are in alphabetical order by state, then city, then hospital within the city; Rankings exclude hospitals with less than 25 cases except for patient surveys which excludes hospitals with less than 100 cases; (a) 100-299 cases; (1) The number of cases/patients is too few to report; (2) Data submitted were based on a sample of cases/patients; (3) Results are based on a shorter time period than required; (4) Data suppressed by CMS for one or more quarters; (5) Results are not available for this reporting period; (6) Fewer than 100 patients completed the HCAHPS survey; (7) No cases met the criteria for this measure; (8) The lower limit of the confidence interval cannot be calculated if the number of observed infections equals zero; (9) No data are available from the state/territory for this reporting period; (10) The scores shown reflect fewer than 50 completed surveys; (11) There were discrepancies in the data collection process; (12) This measure does not apply to this hospital for this reporting period; (13) Results cannot be calculated for this reporting period; (14) The results for this state are combined with nearby states to protect confidentiality; Please refer to the User's Guide for a full explanation of data.

Measure	Cases	This Hosp.	State Avg.	U.S. Avg.
Urinary Catheter Removal	290	86%	98%	97%
Survey of Patients' Hospital Experiences				
Area Around Room 'Always' Quiet at Night	300+	57%	60%	61%
Doctors 'Always' Communicated Well	300+	77%	81%	82%
Home Recovery Information Given	300+	83%	86%	85%
Hospital Given 9 or 10 on 10 Point Scale	300+	69%	70%	71%
Meds 'Always' Explained Before Given	300+	60%	64%	64%
Nurses 'Always' Communicated Well	300+	77%	79%	79%
Pain 'Always' Well Controlled	300+	69%	71%	71%
Room and Bathroom 'Always' Clean	300+	70%	74%	73%
Timely Help 'Always' Received	300+	61%	67%	68%
Would Definitely Recommend Hospital	300+	70%	70%	71%
Use of Medical Imaging				
Cardiac Imaging Stress Test before Surgery	924	5.5%	5.5%	5.3%
Combination Abdominal CT Scan	666	8.4%	10.1%	10.5%
Combination Brain/Sinus CT Scan	735	1.0%	2.6%	2.7%
Combination Chest CT Scan	518	0.0%	2.8%	2.7%
Follow-up Mammogram/Ultrasound[7]	-	-	8.4%	8.8%
Lumbar Spine MRI for Low Back Pain	160	38.1%	36.6%	37.2%

Saint Anthony Medical Center

5666 East State Street
Rockford, IL 61108
URL: www.osfhealth.com
Type: Acute Care Hospitals
Ownership: Voluntary non-profit - Church
Phone: 815-226-2000
Fax: 815-395-5449
Emergency Services: Yes
Beds: 254

Key Personnel:
Pediatric Ambulatory Care . . . . Errol C Baptist, MD
Infection Control . . . . Larry Brown, RN
Radiology . . . . David Childers
CEO/President . . . . David A Schertz
Coronary Care . . . . Brenda Schroeder, RN
Quality Assurance . . . . Susan Taphorn, RN
Operating Room . . . . Sarah Walder, RN
Chief of Medical Staff . . . . Robert White, MD

Measure	Cases	This Hosp.	State Avg.	U.S. Avg.
Blood Clot Prevention and Treatment				
Anticoagulation Overlap Therapy[2]	114	94%	91%	93%
ICU Venous Thromboembolism Prophylaxis[2]	125	96%	93%	92%
Incidence of Potentially Preventable VTE[2]	11	18%	11%	10%
UFH with Dosages/Platelet Monitoring[2]	17	0%	94%	97%
Venous Thromboembolism Prophylaxis[2]	307	80%	86%	85%
Warfarin Therapy Discharge Instructions[2]	80	41%	71%	75%
Chest Pain/Possible Heart Attack Care				
Aspirin Given Within 24 Hours of Arrival[1,3]	-	-	96%	96%
Fibrinolytic Meds Within 30 Min. of Arrival[3,7]	-	-	65%	58%
Average Time to ECG (minutes)[1,3]	-	-	6	7
Average Time to Transfer (minutes)[3,7]	-	-	63	60
Children's Asthma Care				
Received Home Management Plan of Care	-	-	-	88%
Received Reliever Medication	-	-	-	100%
Received Systemic Corticosteroids	-	-	-	100%
Emergency Department				
Admittance Decision Time (minutes)[2]	618	86	89	98
Head CT Results Within 45 Min. of Arrival[1]	-	-	64%	57%
Patients Who Left ER Before Being Seen	38,266	3%	3%	2%
Time from ER Arrival to Admit. (minutes)[2]	632	238	260	274
Time from ER Arrival to Discharge (minutes)	361	150	138	134
Time in ER Before Being Evaluated (minutes)	402	21	28	26
Time to Pain Meds for Fractures (minutes)	174	62	52	57
Heart Attack Care				
Aspirin Given at Discharge	268	99%	99%	99%
Fibrinolytic Meds Within 30 Min. of Arrival[7]	-	-	33%	54%
PCI Within 90 Minutes of Arrival	42	98%	97%	96%
Statin Prescribed at Discharge	253	98%	98%	98%
Heart Failure Care				
ACE Inhibitor or ARB for LVSD	101	96%	98%	97%
Discharge Instructions Given	281	100%	96%	94%
Evaluation of LVS Function	384	100%	99%	99%
Medicare Spending				
Medicare Spending per Patient (ratio)	-	1.02	1	0.98
Pneumonia Care				
Appropriate Initial Antibiotic Given	173	98%	95%	95%
Blood Culture Timing	309	99%	98%	98%
Pregnancy and Delivery Care				
Newborn Deliveries Scheduled Early	48	0%	2%	6%
Preventive Care				
Immunization for Influenza[2]	582	86%	92%	90%
Immunization for Pneumonia[2]	832	84%	92%	92%
Stroke Care				
Anticoagulation Therapy for Atrial Fibrillation	14	100%	94%	95%
Antithrombotic Therapy Timing	131	100%	98%	98%
Assessed for Rehabilitation	187	97%	97%	97%
Discharged on Antithrombotic Therapy	150	99%	99%	99%
Discharged on Statin Medication	102	96%	94%	94%
Thrombolytic Therapy Timing	16	81%	66%	66%
Venous Thromboembolism Prophylaxis	199	95%	94%	94%
Written Stroke Educational Materials Given	92	93%	87%	88%
Surgical Care Improvement Project				
Appropriate Beta Blocker Usage[2]	365	98%	98%	98%
Appropriate VTP Within 24 Hours[2]	662	98%	98%	98%
Controlled Postoperative Blood Glucose[2]	138	100%	97%	97%
Perioperative Temperature Management[2]	803	100%	100%	100%
Prophylactic Antibiotic Selection[2]	723	100%	99%	99%
Prophylactic Antibiotic Selection (Outpatient)	427	96%	98%	98%
Prophylactic Antibiotic Stopped[2]	710	99%	98%	98%
Prophylactic Antibiotic Timing[2]	724	99%	99%	99%
Prophylactic Antibiotic Timing (Outpatient)	428	99%	97%	98%
Urinary Catheter Removal[2]	195	98%	98%	97%
Survey of Patients' Hospital Experiences				
Area Around Room 'Always' Quiet at Night	300+	45%	60%	61%
Doctors 'Always' Communicated Well	300+	80%	81%	82%
Home Recovery Information Given	300+	86%	86%	85%
Hospital Given 9 or 10 on 10 Point Scale	300+	71%	70%	71%
Meds 'Always' Explained Before Given	300+	64%	64%	64%
Nurses 'Always' Communicated Well	300+	80%	79%	79%
Pain 'Always' Well Controlled	300+	72%	71%	71%
Room and Bathroom 'Always' Clean	300+	74%	74%	73%
Timely Help 'Always' Received	300+	64%	67%	68%
Would Definitely Recommend Hospital	300+	74%	70%	71%
Use of Medical Imaging				
Cardiac Imaging Stress Test before Surgery	1,646	3.5%	5.5%	5.3%
Combination Abdominal CT Scan	1,537	5.1%	10.1%	10.5%
Combination Brain/Sinus CT Scan	1,382	2.5%	2.6%	2.7%
Combination Chest CT Scan	1,100	0.9%	2.8%	2.7%
Follow-up Mammogram/Ultrasound	2,473	7.3%	8.4%	8.8%
Lumbar Spine MRI for Low Back Pain	206	42.2%	36.6%	37.2%

Swedish American Hospital

1401 East State Street
Rockford, IL 61104
URL: www.swedishamerican.org
Type: Acute Care Hospitals
Ownership: Voluntary non-profit - Other
Phone: 815-968-4400
Fax: 815-961-2445
Emergency Services: Yes
Beds: 357

Key Personnel:
Intensive Care Unit . . . . Kathy Arnold
Radiology . . . . Dr Marc Bernstein
Pediatric Ambulatory Care . . . . . . Dr Glen Burress
Chief of Medical Staff . . . . Dr Kathleen Kelly
Quality Assurance . . . . Beverly Merfeld
Infection Control . . . . Gary Rifkin, MD
Anesthesiology . . . . Dr Timothy Starck
Emergency Room . . . . Dr John Underwood

Measure	Cases	This Hosp.	State Avg.	U.S. Avg.
Blood Clot Prevention and Treatment				
Anticoagulation Overlap Therapy[2]	103	83%	91%	93%
ICU Venous Thromboembolism Prophylaxis[2]	83	92%	93%	92%
Incidence of Potentially Preventable VTE[2]	11	0%	11%	10%
UFH with Dosages/Platelet Monitoring[2]	32	94%	94%	97%
Venous Thromboembolism Prophylaxis[2]	368	90%	86%	85%
Warfarin Therapy Discharge Instructions[2]	77	77%	71%	75%
Chest Pain/Possible Heart Attack Care				
Aspirin Given Within 24 Hours of Arrival	16	100%	96%	96%
Fibrinolytic Meds Within 30 Min. of Arrival[3,7]	-	-	65%	58%
Average Time to ECG (minutes)	16	0	6	7
Average Time to Transfer (minutes)[3,7]	-	-	63	60
Children's Asthma Care				
Received Home Management Plan of Care	-	-	-	88%
Received Reliever Medication	-	-	-	100%
Received Systemic Corticosteroids	-	-	-	100%
Emergency Department				
Admittance Decision Time (minutes)[2]	564	58	89	98
Head CT Results Within 45 Min. of Arrival[1]	-	-	64%	57%
Patients Who Left ER Before Being Seen	64,657	3%	3%	2%
Time from ER Arrival to Admit. (minutes)[2]	564	249	260	274
Time from ER Arrival to Discharge (minutes)	391	146	138	134
Time in ER Before Being Evaluated (minutes)	430	25	28	26
Time to Pain Meds for Fractures (minutes)	249	58	52	57
Heart Attack Care				
Aspirin Given at Discharge	249	100%	99%	99%
Fibrinolytic Meds Within 30 Min. of Arrival[7]	-	-	33%	54%
PCI Within 90 Minutes of Arrival	51	96%	97%	96%
Statin Prescribed at Discharge	245	100%	98%	98%
Heart Failure Care				
ACE Inhibitor or ARB for LVSD	142	97%	98%	97%
Discharge Instructions Given	331	99%	96%	94%
Evaluation of LVS Function	403	100%	99%	99%
Medicare Spending				
Medicare Spending per Patient (ratio)	-	0.99	1	0.98
Pneumonia Care				
Appropriate Initial Antibiotic Given	210	96%	95%	95%
Blood Culture Timing	303	96%	98%	98%
Pregnancy and Delivery Care				
Newborn Deliveries Scheduled Early[2]	50	4%	2%	6%
Preventive Care				
Immunization for Influenza[2]	519	90%	92%	90%
Immunization for Pneumonia[2]	574	96%	92%	92%
Stroke Care				
Anticoagulation Therapy for Atrial Fibrillation	13	92%	94%	95%
Antithrombotic Therapy Timing	121	97%	98%	98%
Assessed for Rehabilitation	158	98%	97%	97%
Discharged on Antithrombotic Therapy	139	98%	99%	99%
Discharged on Statin Medication	107	95%	94%	94%
Thrombolytic Therapy Timing[1]	-	-	66%	66%
Venous Thromboembolism Prophylaxis	153	99%	94%	94%
Written Stroke Educational Materials Given	90	91%	87%	88%
Surgical Care Improvement Project				
Appropriate Beta Blocker Usage[2]	371	98%	98%	98%
Appropriate VTP Within 24 Hours[2]	787	98%	98%	98%
Controlled Postoperative Blood Glucose[2]	153	97%	97%	97%
Perioperative Temperature Management[2]	992	100%	100%	100%
Prophylactic Antibiotic Selection[2]	925	99%	99%	99%
Prophylactic Antibiotic Selection (Outpatient)	439	99%	98%	98%
Prophylactic Antibiotic Stopped[2]	916	98%	98%	98%
Prophylactic Antibiotic Timing[2]	925	100%	99%	99%
Prophylactic Antibiotic Timing (Outpatient)	440	99%	97%	98%
Urinary Catheter Removal[2]	367	99%	98%	97%
Survey of Patients' Hospital Experiences				
Area Around Room 'Always' Quiet at Night	300+	54%	60%	61%
Doctors 'Always' Communicated Well	300+	79%	81%	82%
Home Recovery Information Given	300+	88%	86%	85%
Hospital Given 9 or 10 on 10 Point Scale	300+	73%	70%	71%
Meds 'Always' Explained Before Given	300+	64%	64%	64%
Nurses 'Always' Communicated Well	300+	79%	79%	79%
Pain 'Always' Well Controlled	300+	73%	71%	71%
Room and Bathroom 'Always' Clean	300+	71%	74%	73%
Timely Help 'Always' Received	300+	69%	67%	68%
Would Definitely Recommend Hospital	300+	78%	70%	71%
Use of Medical Imaging				
Cardiac Imaging Stress Test before Surgery	965	4.9%	5.5%	5.3%
Combination Abdominal CT Scan	1,669	3.8%	10.1%	10.5%
Combination Brain/Sinus CT Scan	1,332	1.4%	2.6%	2.7%
Combination Chest CT Scan	1,094	0.1%	2.8%	2.7%
Follow-up Mammogram/Ultrasound	3,617	8.5%	8.4%	8.8%
Lumbar Spine MRI for Low Back Pain	193	36.8%	36.6%	37.2%

NOTE: Hospital profiles are in alphabetical order by state, then city, then hospital within the city; Rankings exclude hospitals with less than 25 cases except for patient surveys which excludes hospitals with less than 100 cases; (a) 100-299 cases; (1) The number of cases/patients is too few to report; (2) Data submitted were based on a sample of cases/patients; (3) Results are based on a shorter time period than required; (4) Data suppressed by CMS for one or more quarters; (5) Results are not available for this reporting period; (6) Fewer than 100 patients completed the HCAHPS survey; (7) No cases met the criteria for this measure; (8) The lower limit of the confidence interval cannot be calculated if the number of observed infections equals zero; (9) No data are available from the state/territory for this reporting period; (10) The scores shown reflect fewer than 50 completed surveys; (11) There were discrepancies in the data collection process; (12) This measure does not apply to this hospital for this reporting period; (13) Results cannot be calculated for this reporting period; (14) The results for this state are combined with nearby states to protect confidentiality; Please refer to the User's Guide for a full explanation of data.

Hardin County General Hospital

Ferrell Road
Rosiclare, IL 62982
Phone: 618-285-6634
Fax: 618-285-3564
Type: Critical Access Hospitals
Emergency Services: Yes
Ownership: Voluntary non-profit - Private
Beds: 25

Key Personnel:
Emergency Room . . . . Marsha Broadway, RN
Quality Assurance . . . . Jan Donbrow, RN
Radiology. . . . . Alice Kayler
Chief of Medical Staff. . . . . Marcos Sunga, MD
CEO/President. . . . . Roby Williams

Measure	Cases	This Hosp.	State Avg.	U.S. Avg.
Blood Clot Prevention and Treatment				
Anticoagulation Overlap Therapy[5]	-	-	91%	93%
ICU Venous Thromboembolism Prophylaxis[5]	-	-	93%	92%
Incidence of Potentially Preventable VTE[5]	-	-	11%	10%
UFH with Dosages/Platelet Monitoring[5]	-	-	94%	97%
Venous Thromboembolism Prophylaxis[5]	-	-	86%	85%
Warfarin Therapy Discharge Instructions[5]	-	-	71%	75%
Chest Pain/Possible Heart Attack Care				
Aspirin Given Within 24 Hours of Arrival	38	97%	96%	96%
Fibrinolytic Meds Within 30 Min. of Arrival[1]	-	-	65%	58%
Average Time to ECG (minutes)	40	4	6	7
Average Time to Transfer (minutes)[1]	-	-	63	60
Children's Asthma Care				
Received Home Management Plan of Care	-	-	-	88%
Received Reliever Medication	-	-	-	100%
Received Systemic Corticosteroids	-	-	-	100%
Emergency Department				
Admittance Decision Time (minutes)[5]	-	-	89	98
Head CT Results Within 45 Min. of Arrival[1,3]	-	-	64%	57%
Patients Who Left ER Before Being Seen[5]	-	-	3%	2%
Time from ER Arrival to Admit. (minutes)[5]	-	-	260	274
Time from ER Arrival to Discharge (minutes)[5]	-	-	138	134
Time in ER Before Being Evaluated (minutes)[5]	-	-	28	26
Time to Pain Meds for Fractures (minutes)[5]	-	-	52	57
Heart Attack Care				
Aspirin Given at Discharge[5]	-	-	99%	99%
Fibrinolytic Meds Within 30 Min. of Arrival[5]	-	-	33%	54%
PCI Within 90 Minutes of Arrival[5]	-	-	97%	96%
Statin Prescribed at Discharge[5]	-	-	98%	98%
Heart Failure Care				
ACE Inhibitor or ARB for LVSD[1,3]	-	-	98%	97%
Discharge Instructions Given[3]	22	95%	96%	94%
Evaluation of LVS Function[3]	29	100%	99%	99%
Medicare Spending				
Medicare Spending per Patient (ratio)	-	-	1	0.98
Pneumonia Care				
Appropriate Initial Antibiotic Given[2,3]	18	100%	95%	95%
Blood Culture Timing[2,3]	37	97%	98%	98%
Pregnancy and Delivery Care				
Newborn Deliveries Scheduled Early[5]	-	-	2%	6%
Preventive Care				
Immunization for Influenza[5]	-	-	92%	90%
Immunization for Pneumonia[5]	-	-	92%	92%
Stroke Care				
Anticoagulation Therapy for Atrial Fibrillation[5]	-	-	94%	95%
Antithrombotic Therapy Timing[5]	-	-	98%	98%
Assessed for Rehabilitation[5]	-	-	97%	97%
Discharged on Antithrombotic Therapy[5]	-	-	99%	99%
Discharged on Statin Medication[5]	-	-	94%	94%
Thrombolytic Therapy Timing[5]	-	-	66%	66%
Venous Thromboembolism Prophylaxis[5]	-	-	94%	94%
Written Stroke Educational Materials Given[5]	-	-	87%	88%
Surgical Care Improvement Project				
Appropriate Beta Blocker Usage[5]	-	-	98%	98%
Appropriate VTP Within 24 Hours[5]	-	-	98%	98%
Controlled Postoperative Blood Glucose[5]	-	-	97%	97%
Perioperative Temperature Management[5]	-	-	100%	100%
Prophylactic Antibiotic Selection[5]	-	-	99%	99%
Prophylactic Antibiotic Selection (Outpatient)[5]	-	-	98%	98%
Prophylactic Antibiotic Stopped[5]	-	-	98%	98%
Prophylactic Antibiotic Timing[5]	-	-	99%	99%
Prophylactic Antibiotic Timing (Outpatient)[5]	-	-	97%	98%
Urinary Catheter Removal[5]	-	-	98%	97%
Survey of Patients' Hospital Experiences				
Area Around Room 'Always' Quiet at Night[5]	-	-	60%	61%
Doctors 'Always' Communicated Well[5]	-	-	81%	82%
Home Recovery Information Given[5]	-	-	86%	85%
Hospital Given 9 or 10 on 10 Point Scale[5]	-	-	70%	71%
Meds 'Always' Explained Before Given[5]	-	-	64%	64%
Nurses 'Always' Communicated Well[5]	-	-	79%	79%
Pain 'Always' Well Controlled[5]	-	-	71%	71%
Room and Bathroom 'Always' Clean[5]	-	-	74%	73%
Timely Help 'Always' Received[5]	-	-	67%	68%
Would Definitely Recommend Hospital[5]	-	-	70%	71%
Use of Medical Imaging				
Cardiac Imaging Stress Test before Surgery[7]	-	-	5.5%	5.3%
Combination Abdominal CT Scan	104	15.4%	10.1%	10.5%
Combination Brain/Sinus CT Scan[1]	-	-	2.6%	2.7%
Combination Chest CT Scan	45	53.3%	2.8%	2.7%
Follow-up Mammogram/Ultrasound	102	6.9%	8.4%	8.8%
Lumbar Spine MRI for Low Back Pain[1]	-	-	36.6%	37.2%

Sarah D Culbertson Memorial Hospital

238 South Congress Street
Rushville, IL 62681
Phone: 217-322-4321
Fax: 217-322-6425
E-mail: cmh@cmhospital.com
URL: www.cmhospital.com
Type: Critical Access Hospitals
Emergency Services: Yes
Ownership: Govt - Hospital Dist/Auth
Beds: 64

Key Personnel:
Chief of Medical Staff. . . . . Lisa Downs, RN
Emergency Room . . . . Lisa Downs, RN
Chairman/CEO . . . . David Hester
Quality Assurance . . . . Judy Richy
CEO/President. . . . . David Sniff

Measure	Cases	This Hosp.	State Avg.	U.S. Avg.
Blood Clot Prevention and Treatment				
Anticoagulation Overlap Therapy[5]	-	-	91%	93%
ICU Venous Thromboembolism Prophylaxis[5]	-	-	93%	92%
Incidence of Potentially Preventable VTE[5]	-	-	11%	10%
UFH with Dosages/Platelet Monitoring[5]	-	-	94%	97%
Venous Thromboembolism Prophylaxis[5]	-	-	86%	85%
Warfarin Therapy Discharge Instructions[5]	-	-	71%	75%
Chest Pain/Possible Heart Attack Care				
Aspirin Given Within 24 Hours of Arrival	-	-	96%	96%
Fibrinolytic Meds Within 30 Min. of Arrival	-	-	65%	58%
Average Time to ECG (minutes)	-	-	6	7
Average Time to Transfer (minutes)	-	-	63	60
Children's Asthma Care				
Received Home Management Plan of Care	-	-	-	88%
Received Reliever Medication	-	-	-	100%
Received Systemic Corticosteroids	-	-	-	100%
Emergency Department				
Admittance Decision Time (minutes)[5]	-	-	89	98
Head CT Results Within 45 Min. of Arrival	-	-	64%	57%
Patients Who Left ER Before Being Seen	-	-	3%	2%
Time from ER Arrival to Admit. (minutes)[5]	-	-	260	274
Time from ER Arrival to Discharge (minutes)	-	-	138	134
Time in ER Before Being Evaluated (minutes)	-	-	28	26
Time to Pain Meds for Fractures (minutes)	-	-	52	57
Heart Attack Care				
Aspirin Given at Discharge[5]	-	-	99%	99%
Fibrinolytic Meds Within 30 Min. of Arrival[5]	-	-	33%	54%
PCI Within 90 Minutes of Arrival[5]	-	-	97%	96%
Statin Prescribed at Discharge[5]	-	-	98%	98%
Heart Failure Care				
ACE Inhibitor or ARB for LVSD[1,3]	-	-	98%	97%
Discharge Instructions Given[1,3]	-	-	96%	94%
Evaluation of LVS Function[1,3]	-	-	99%	99%
Medicare Spending				
Medicare Spending per Patient (ratio)	-	-	1	0.98
Pneumonia Care				
Appropriate Initial Antibiotic Given[1]	-	-	95%	95%
Blood Culture Timing[1]	-	-	98%	98%
Pregnancy and Delivery Care				
Newborn Deliveries Scheduled Early[5]	-	-	2%	6%
Preventive Care				
Immunization for Influenza[2]	49	86%	92%	90%
Immunization for Pneumonia[2]	92	85%	92%	92%
Stroke Care				
Anticoagulation Therapy for Atrial Fibrillation[5]	-	-	94%	95%
Antithrombotic Therapy Timing[5]	-	-	98%	98%
Assessed for Rehabilitation[5]	-	-	97%	97%
Discharged on Antithrombotic Therapy[6]	-	-	99%	99%
Discharged on Statin Medication[5]	-	-	94%	94%
Thrombolytic Therapy Timing[5]	-	-	66%	66%
Venous Thromboembolism Prophylaxis[5]	-	-	94%	94%
Written Stroke Educational Materials Given[5]	-	-	87%	88%
Surgical Care Improvement Project				
Appropriate Beta Blocker Usage[3,7]	-	-	98%	98%
Appropriate VTP Within 24 Hours[1,3]	-	-	98%	98%
Controlled Postoperative Blood Glucose[3,7]	-	-	97%	97%
Perioperative Temperature Management[1,3]	-	-	100%	100%
Prophylactic Antibiotic Selection[1,3]	-	-	99%	99%
Prophylactic Antibiotic Selection (Outpatient)	-	-	98%	98%
Prophylactic Antibiotic Stopped[1,3]	-	-	98%	98%
Prophylactic Antibiotic Timing[1,3]	-	-	99%	99%
Prophylactic Antibiotic Timing (Outpatient)	-	-	97%	98%
Urinary Catheter Removal[3,7]	-	-	98%	97%
Survey of Patients' Hospital Experiences				
Area Around Room 'Always' Quiet at Night[5]	-	-	60%	61%
Doctors 'Always' Communicated Well[5]	-	-	81%	82%
Home Recovery Information Given[5]	-	-	86%	85%
Hospital Given 9 or 10 on 10 Point Scale[5]	-	-	70%	71%
Meds 'Always' Explained Before Given[5]	-	-	64%	64%
Nurses 'Always' Communicated Well[5]	-	-	79%	79%
Pain 'Always' Well Controlled[5]	-	-	71%	71%
Room and Bathroom 'Always' Clean[5]	-	-	74%	73%
Timely Help 'Always' Received[5]	-	-	67%	68%
Would Definitely Recommend Hospital[5]	-	-	70%	71%
Use of Medical Imaging				
Cardiac Imaging Stress Test before Surgery	-	-	5.5%	5.3%
Combination Abdominal CT Scan	-	-	10.1%	10.5%
Combination Brain/Sinus CT Scan	-	-	2.6%	2.7%
Combination Chest CT Scan	-	-	2.8%	2.7%
Follow-up Mammogram/Ultrasound	-	-	8.4%	8.8%
Lumbar Spine MRI for Low Back Pain	-	-	36.6%	37.2%

Salem Township Hospital

1201 Ricker Drive
Salem, IL 62881
Phone: 618-548-3194
Fax: 618-548-6831
Type: Critical Access Hospitals
Emergency Services: Yes
Ownership: Government - Local
Beds: 46

Key Personnel:
Emergency Room . . . . Roberto Garcia
Infection Control. . . . . Wilma Gott, RN, B
Operating Room. . . . . S Lakshmanan, RN
CEO/President. . . . . Rithilll Rennegarve
Quality Assurance . . . . Sheri Schultz
Chief of Medical Staff. . . . . Hyet Settlemoir, DO
Intensive Care Unit. . . . . P Suppiah, MD
Radiology. . . . . Preecha Tawjare, MD

Measure	Cases	This Hosp.	State Avg.	U.S. Avg.
Blood Clot Prevention and Treatment				
Anticoagulation Overlap Therapy[5]	-	-	91%	93%
ICU Venous Thromboembolism Prophylaxis[5]	-	-	93%	92%
Incidence of Potentially Preventable VTE[5]	-	-	11%	10%
UFH with Dosages/Platelet Monitoring[5]	-	-	94%	97%
Venous Thromboembolism Prophylaxis[5]	-	-	86%	85%
Warfarin Therapy Discharge Instructions[5]	-	-	71%	75%
Chest Pain/Possible Heart Attack Care				
Aspirin Given Within 24 Hours of Arrival[5]	-	-	96%	96%
Fibrinolytic Meds Within 30 Min. of Arrival[5]	-	-	65%	58%
Average Time to ECG (minutes)[5]	-	-	6	7
Average Time to Transfer (minutes)[5]	-	-	63	60
Children's Asthma Care				
Received Home Management Plan of Care	-	-	-	88%
Received Reliever Medication	-	-	-	100%
Received Systemic Corticosteroids	-	-	-	100%

NOTE: Hospital profiles are in alphabetical order by state, then city, then hospital within the city; Rankings exclude hospitals with less than 25 cases except for patient surveys which excludes hospitals with less than 100 cases; (a) 100-299 cases; (1) The number of cases/patients is too few to report; (2) Data submitted were based on a sample of cases/patients; (3) Results are based on a shorter time period than required; (4) Data suppressed by CMS for one or more quarters; (5) Results are not available for this reporting period; (6) Fewer than 100 patients completed the HCAHPS survey; (7) No cases met the criteria for this measure; (8) The lower limit of the confidence interval cannot be calculated if the number of observed infections equals zero; (9) No data are available from the state/territory for this reporting period; (10) The scores shown reflect fewer than 50 completed surveys; (11) There were discrepancies in the data collection process; (12) This measure does not apply to this hospital for this reporting period; (13) Results cannot be calculated for this reporting period; (14) The results for this state are combined with nearby states to protect confidentiality; Please refer to the User's Guide for a full explanation of data.

Measure	Cases	This Hosp.	State Avg.	U.S. Avg.
Emergency Department				
Admittance Decision Time (minutes)[5]	-	-	89	98
Head CT Results Within 45 Min. of Arrival[5]	-	-	64%	57%
Patients Who Left ER Before Being Seen[5]	-	-	3%	2%
Time from ER Arrival to Admit. (minutes)[5]	-	-	260	274
Time from ER Arrival to Discharge (minutes)[5]	-	-	138	134
Time in ER Before Being Evaluated (minutes)[5]	-	-	28	26
Time to Pain Meds for Fractures (minutes)[5]	-	-	52	57
Heart Attack Care				
Aspirin Given at Discharge[5]	-	-	99%	99%
Fibrinolytic Meds Within 30 Min. of Arrival[5]	-	-	33%	54%
PCI Within 90 Minutes of Arrival[5]	-	-	97%	96%
Statin Prescribed at Discharge[5]	-	-	98%	98%
Heart Failure Care				
ACE Inhibitor or ARB for LVSD[1,3]	-	-	98%	97%
Discharge Instructions Given[3]	14	93%	96%	94%
Evaluation of LVS Function[3]	23	96%	99%	99%
Medicare Spending				
Medicare Spending per Patient (ratio)	-	-	1	0.98
Pneumonia Care				
Appropriate Initial Antibiotic Given[3]	27	70%	95%	95%
Blood Culture Timing[3]	28	93%	98%	98%
Pregnancy and Delivery Care				
Newborn Deliveries Scheduled Early[5]	-	-	2%	6%
Preventive Care				
Immunization for Influenza[5]	-	-	92%	90%
Immunization for Pneumonia[5]	-	-	92%	92%
Stroke Care				
Anticoagulation Therapy for Atrial Fibrillation[5]	-	-	94%	95%
Antithrombotic Therapy Timing[5]	-	-	98%	98%
Assessed for Rehabilitation[5]	-	-	97%	97%
Discharged on Antithrombotic Therapy[5]	-	-	99%	99%
Discharged on Statin Medication[5]	-	-	94%	94%
Thrombolytic Therapy Timing[5]	-	-	66%	66%
Venous Thromboembolism Prophylaxis[5]	-	-	94%	94%
Written Stroke Educational Materials Given[5]	-	-	87%	88%
Surgical Care Improvement Project				
Appropriate Beta Blocker Usage[1,3]	-	-	98%	98%
Appropriate VTP Within 24 Hours[3]	13	100%	98%	98%
Controlled Postoperative Blood Glucose[3,7]	-	-	97%	97%
Perioperative Temperature Management[3]	15	100%	100%	100%
Prophylactic Antibiotic Selection[1,3]	-	-	99%	99%
Prophylactic Antibiotic Selection (Outpatient)[5]	-	-	98%	98%
Prophylactic Antibiotic Stopped[1,3]	-	-	98%	98%
Prophylactic Antibiotic Timing[1,3]	-	-	99%	99%
Prophylactic Antibiotic Timing (Outpatient)[5]	-	-	97%	98%
Urinary Catheter Removal[1,3]	-	-	98%	97%
Survey of Patients' Hospital Experiences				
Area Around Room 'Always' Quiet at Night	(a)	60%	60%	61%
Doctors 'Always' Communicated Well	(a)	90%	81%	82%
Home Recovery Information Given	(a)	87%	86%	85%
Hospital Given 9 or 10 on 10 Point Scale	(a)	79%	70%	71%
Meds 'Always' Explained Before Given	(a)	70%	64%	64%
Nurses 'Always' Communicated Well	(a)	88%	79%	79%
Pain 'Always' Well Controlled	(a)	74%	71%	71%
Room and Bathroom 'Always' Clean	(a)	84%	74%	73%
Timely Help 'Always' Received	(a)	83%	67%	68%
Would Definitely Recommend Hospital	(a)	71%	70%	71%
Use of Medical Imaging				
Cardiac Imaging Stress Test before Surgery[1]	-	-	5.5%	5.3%
Combination Abdominal CT Scan	323	47.4%	10.1%	10.5%
Combination Brain/Sinus CT Scan[1]	-	-	2.6%	2.7%
Combination Chest CT Scan	174	2.9%	2.8%	2.7%
Follow-up Mammogram/Ultrasound	387	7.0%	8.4%	8.8%
Lumbar Spine MRI for Low Back Pain[1]	-	-	36.6%	37.2%

Valley West Community Hospital

1301 North Main Street
Sandwich, IL 60548
Phone: 815-786-8484
Fax: 815-786-3705
E-mail: sandhosp@snd.softfarm.com/sandhosp
URL: www.snd.softfarm.com/sandhosp
Type: Critical Access Hospitals
Emergency Services: Yes
Ownership: Voluntary non-profit - Private
Beds: 84

Key Personnel:
Chief of Medical Staff. . . . . Martin Brauweiler
Radiology. . . . . Thomas R Cain, MD
Emergency Room . . . . Victor Garber, MD
Operating Room. . . . . Richard W Mason
CEO/President. . . . . Brad Topple
Infection Control. . . . . Carol Vignali
Intensive Care Unit. . . . . Kris Wyant, RN

Measure	Cases	This Hosp.	State Avg.	U.S. Avg.
Blood Clot Prevention and Treatment				
Anticoagulation Overlap Therapy[2]	13	100%	91%	93%
ICU Venous Thromboembolism Prophylaxis[2]	12	100%	93%	92%
Incidence of Potentially Preventable VTE[1,2]	-	-	11%	10%
UFH with Dosages/Platelet Monitoring[1,2]	-	-	94%	97%
Venous Thromboembolism Prophylaxis[2]	87	99%	86%	85%
Warfarin Therapy Discharge Instructions[1,2]	-	-	71%	75%
Chest Pain/Possible Heart Attack Care				
Aspirin Given Within 24 Hours of Arrival	31	97%	96%	96%
Fibrinolytic Meds Within 30 Min. of Arrival[1]	-	-	65%	58%
Average Time to ECG (minutes)	32	4	6	7
Average Time to Transfer (minutes)[1]	-	-	63	60
Children's Asthma Care				
Received Home Management Plan of Care	-	-	-	88%
Received Reliever Medication	-	-	-	100%
Received Systemic Corticosteroids	-	-	-	100%
Emergency Department				
Admittance Decision Time (minutes)[2]	312	52	89	98
Head CT Results Within 45 Min. of Arrival[1]	-	-	64%	57%
Patients Who Left ER Before Being Seen	9,327	1%	3%	2%
Time from ER Arrival to Admit. (minutes)[2]	332	224	260	274
Time from ER Arrival to Discharge (minutes)	396	104	138	134
Time in ER Before Being Evaluated (minutes)	350	16	28	26
Time to Pain Meds for Fractures (minutes)	65	28	52	57
Heart Attack Care				
Aspirin Given at Discharge[1,3]	-	-	99%	99%
Fibrinolytic Meds Within 30 Min. of Arrival[3,7]	-	-	33%	54%
PCI Within 90 Minutes of Arrival[3,7]	-	-	97%	96%
Statin Prescribed at Discharge[3,7]	-	-	98%	98%
Heart Failure Care				
ACE Inhibitor or ARB for LVSD	12	100%	98%	97%
Discharge Instructions Given	26	100%	96%	94%
Evaluation of LVS Function	36	100%	99%	99%
Medicare Spending				
Medicare Spending per Patient (ratio)	-	-	1	0.98
Pneumonia Care				
Appropriate Initial Antibiotic Given	26	100%	95%	95%
Blood Culture Timing	59	100%	98%	98%
Pregnancy and Delivery Care				
Newborn Deliveries Scheduled Early	32	9%	2%	6%
Preventive Care				
Immunization for Influenza[2]	273	100%	92%	90%
Immunization for Pneumonia[2]	273	100%	92%	92%
Stroke Care				
Anticoagulation Therapy for Atrial Fibrillation[1]	-	-	94%	95%
Antithrombotic Therapy Timing[1]	-	-	98%	98%
Assessed for Rehabilitation[1]	-	-	97%	97%
Discharged on Antithrombotic Therapy[1]	-	-	99%	99%
Discharged on Statin Medication[1]	-	-	94%	94%
Thrombolytic Therapy Timing[7]	-	-	66%	66%
Venous Thromboembolism Prophylaxis[1]	-	-	94%	94%
Written Stroke Educational Materials Given[7]	-	-	87%	88%
Surgical Care Improvement Project				
Appropriate Beta Blocker Usage[1]	-	-	98%	98%
Appropriate VTP Within 24 Hours	39	97%	98%	98%
Controlled Postoperative Blood Glucose[7]	-	-	97%	97%
Perioperative Temperature Management	50	100%	100%	100%
Prophylactic Antibiotic Selection	18	100%	99%	99%
Prophylactic Antibiotic Selection (Outpatient)	16	88%	98%	98%
Prophylactic Antibiotic Stopped	18	100%	98%	98%
Prophylactic Antibiotic Timing	18	100%	99%	99%
Prophylactic Antibiotic Timing (Outpatient)	16	100%	97%	98%
Urinary Catheter Removal	25	100%	98%	97%
Survey of Patients' Hospital Experiences				
Area Around Room 'Always' Quiet at Night	(a)	77%	60%	61%
Doctors 'Always' Communicated Well	(a)	87%	81%	82%
Home Recovery Information Given	(a)	90%	86%	85%
Hospital Given 9 or 10 on 10 Point Scale	(a)	81%	70%	71%
Meds 'Always' Explained Before Given	(a)	68%	64%	64%
Nurses 'Always' Communicated Well	(a)	82%	79%	79%
Pain 'Always' Well Controlled	(a)	74%	71%	71%
Room and Bathroom 'Always' Clean	(a)	73%	74%	73%
Timely Help 'Always' Received	(a)	73%	67%	68%
Would Definitely Recommend Hospital	(a)	75%	70%	71%
Use of Medical Imaging				
Cardiac Imaging Stress Test before Surgery	83	6.0%	5.5%	5.3%
Combination Abdominal CT Scan	333	2.7%	10.1%	10.5%
Combination Brain/Sinus CT Scan[1]	-	-	2.6%	2.7%
Combination Chest CT Scan	171	1.8%	2.8%	2.7%
Follow-up Mammogram/Ultrasound	374	13.1%	8.4%	8.8%
Lumbar Spine MRI for Low Back Pain[1]	-	-	36.6%	37.2%

Shelby Memorial Hospital

200 S Cedar St
Shelbyville, IL 62565
Phone: 217-774-3961
Fax: 217-774-5100
URL: www.mysmh.org
Type: Acute Care Hospitals
Emergency Services: Yes
Ownership: Voluntary non-profit - Private
Beds: 54

Key Personnel:
Chief of Medical Staff. . . . . Arnold V Agapito
Quality Assurance . . . . Donna Bales, RN
Infection Control. . . . . Meredith Barnes
Operating Room. . . . . Meredith Barnes
Emergency Room . . . . U Dauz, MD
Intensive Care Unit. . . . . Das Gurujal, MD
Radiology. . . . . Caroline Rodman, MD
CEO . . . . Marilyn Sears

Measure	Cases	This Hosp.	State Avg.	U.S. Avg.
Blood Clot Prevention and Treatment				
Anticoagulation Overlap Therapy[1]	-	-	91%	93%
ICU Venous Thromboembolism Prophylaxis[7]	-	-	93%	92%
Incidence of Potentially Preventable VTE[1]	-	-	11%	10%
UFH with Dosages/Platelet Monitoring[1]	-	-	94%	97%
Venous Thromboembolism Prophylaxis	233	74%	86%	85%
Warfarin Therapy Discharge Instructions[1]	-	-	71%	75%
Chest Pain/Possible Heart Attack Care				
Aspirin Given Within 24 Hours of Arrival	36	94%	96%	96%
Fibrinolytic Meds Within 30 Min. of Arrival[3,7]	-	-	65%	58%
Average Time to ECG (minutes)	37	8	6	7
Average Time to Transfer (minutes)[1,3]	-	-	63	60
Children's Asthma Care				
Received Home Management Plan of Care	-	-	-	88%
Received Reliever Medication	-	-	-	100%
Received Systemic Corticosteroids	-	-	-	100%
Emergency Department				
Admittance Decision Time (minutes)	220	37	89	98
Head CT Results Within 45 Min. of Arrival[1]	-	-	64%	57%
Patients Who Left ER Before Being Seen	5,668	1%	3%	2%
Time from ER Arrival to Admit. (minutes)	230	153	260	274
Time from ER Arrival to Discharge (minutes)	366	98	138	134
Time in ER Before Being Evaluated (minutes)	481	17	28	26
Time to Pain Meds for Fractures (minutes)	30	24	52	57
Heart Attack Care				
Aspirin Given at Discharge[1,3]	-	-	99%	99%
Fibrinolytic Meds Within 30 Min. of Arrival[3,7]	-	-	33%	54%
PCI Within 90 Minutes of Arrival[3,7]	-	-	97%	96%
Statin Prescribed at Discharge[3,7]	-	-	98%	98%
Heart Failure Care				
ACE Inhibitor or ARB for LVSD	11	91%	98%	97%
Discharge Instructions Given	11	100%	96%	94%
Evaluation of LVS Function	49	98%	99%	99%
Medicare Spending				

NOTE: Hospital profiles are in alphabetical order by state, then city, then hospital within the city; Rankings exclude hospitals with less than 25 cases except for patient surveys which excludes hospitals with less than 100 cases; (a) 100-299 cases; (1) The number of cases/patients is too few to report; (2) Data submitted were based on a sample of cases/patients; (3) Results are based on a shorter time period than required; (4) Data suppressed by CMS for one or more quarters; (5) Results are not available for this reporting period; (6) Fewer than 100 patients completed the HCAHPS survey; (7) No cases met the criteria for this measure; (8) The lower limit of the confidence interval cannot be calculated if the number of observed infections equals zero; (9) No data are available from the state/territory for this reporting period; (10) The scores shown reflect fewer than 50 completed surveys; (11) There were discrepancies in the data collection process; (12) This measure does not apply to this hospital for this reporting period; (13) Results cannot be calculated for this reporting period; (14) The results for this state are combined with nearby states to protect confidentiality; Please refer to the User's Guide for a full explanation of data.

Measure	Cases	This Hosp.	State Avg.	U.S. Avg.
Medicare Spending per Patient (ratio)	-	0.99	1	0.98
Pneumonia Care				
Appropriate Initial Antibiotic Given	30	93%	95%	95%
Blood Culture Timing	46	98%	98%	98%
Pregnancy and Delivery Care				
Newborn Deliveries Scheduled Early[7]	-	-	2%	6%
Preventive Care				
Immunization for Influenza	194	99%	92%	90%
Immunization for Pneumonia	314	100%	92%	92%
Stroke Care				
Anticoagulation Therapy for Atrial Fibrillation[1,3]	-	-	94%	95%
Antithrombotic Therapy Timing[1,3]	-	-	98%	98%
Assessed for Rehabilitation[1,3]	-	-	97%	97%
Discharged on Antithrombotic Therapy[1,3]	-	-	99%	99%
Discharged on Statin Medication[1,3]	-	-	94%	94%
Thrombolytic Therapy Timing[3,7]	-	-	66%	66%
Venous Thromboembolism Prophylaxis[1,3]	-	-	94%	94%
Written Stroke Educational Materials Given[3,7]	-	-	87%	88%
Surgical Care Improvement Project				
Appropriate Beta Blocker Usage[5]	-	-	98%	98%
Appropriate VTP Within 24 Hours[5]	-	-	98%	98%
Controlled Postoperative Blood Glucose[5]	-	-	97%	97%
Perioperative Temperature Management[5]	-	-	100%	100%
Prophylactic Antibiotic Selection[5]	-	-	99%	99%
Prophylactic Antibiotic Selection (Outpatient)[5]	-	-	98%	98%
Prophylactic Antibiotic Stopped[5]	-	-	98%	98%
Prophylactic Antibiotic Timing[5]	-	-	99%	99%
Prophylactic Antibiotic Timing (Outpatient)[5]	-	-	97%	98%
Urinary Catheter Removal[5]	-	-	98%	97%
Survey of Patients' Hospital Experiences				
Area Around Room 'Always' Quiet at Night[6]	<100	61%	60%	61%
Doctors 'Always' Communicated Well[6]	<100	84%	81%	82%
Home Recovery Information Given[6]	<100	85%	86%	85%
Hospital Given 9 or 10 on 10 Point Scale[6]	<100	68%	70%	71%
Meds 'Always' Explained Before Given[6]	<100	63%	64%	64%
Nurses 'Always' Communicated Well[6]	<100	82%	79%	79%
Pain 'Always' Well Controlled[6]	<100	71%	71%	71%
Room and Bathroom 'Always' Clean[6]	<100	81%	74%	73%
Timely Help 'Always' Received[6]	<100	73%	67%	68%
Would Definitely Recommend Hospital[6]	<100	57%	70%	71%
Use of Medical Imaging				
Cardiac Imaging Stress Test before Surgery	83	8.4%	5.5%	5.3%
Combination Abdominal CT Scan	220	5.9%	10.1%	10.5%
Combination Brain/Sinus CT Scan[1]	-	-	2.6%	2.7%
Combination Chest CT Scan	108	0.9%	2.8%	2.7%
Follow-up Mammogram/Ultrasound	248	14.9%	8.4%	8.8%
Lumbar Spine MRI for Low Back Pain[1]	-	-	36.6%	37.2%

Genesis Health System

801 Illini Drive
Silvis, IL 61282
Phone: 309-792-9363
Fax: 309-792-4274
Type: Acute Care Hospitals
Emergency Services: Yes
Ownership: Government - Local
Beds: 150

Key Personnel:
Anesthesiology. . . . . Iwona Bobela, MD
CEO/President. . . . . Douglas P. Cropper
Emergency Room . . . . Janet Eckhart, RN
Operating Room. . . . . Sandy Freddy
Infection Control. . . . . Anne Lewis
Cardiac Laboratory. . . . . Andy Nelson
Chief of Medical Staff . . . . Thomas VonGilliern, MD
Cardiology . . . . Jessica A. Witter

Measure	Cases	This Hosp.	State Avg.	U.S. Avg.
Blood Clot Prevention and Treatment				
Anticoagulation Overlap Therapy[2]	26	100%	91%	93%
ICU Venous Thromboembolism Prophylaxis[2]	61	98%	93%	92%
Incidence of Potentially Preventable VTE[1,2]	-	-	11%	10%
UFH with Dosages/Platelet Monitoring[1,2]	-	-	94%	97%
Venous Thromboembolism Prophylaxis[2]	289	100%	86%	85%
Warfarin Therapy Discharge Instructions[2]	17	100%	71%	75%
Chest Pain/Possible Heart Attack Care				
Aspirin Given Within 24 Hours of Arrival	21	100%	96%	96%
Fibrinolytic Meds Within 30 Min. of Arrival[3,7]	-	-	65%	58%
Average Time to ECG (minutes)	24	9	6	7
Average Time to Transfer (minutes)[3,7]	-	-	63	60
Children's Asthma Care				
Received Home Management Plan of Care	-	-	-	88%
Received Reliever Medication	-	-	-	100%
Received Systemic Corticosteroids	-	-	-	100%
Emergency Department				
Admittance Decision Time (minutes)[2]	439	74	89	98
Head CT Results Within 45 Min. of Arrival	19	79%	64%	57%
Patients Who Left ER Before Being Seen	25,496	1%	3%	2%
Time from ER Arrival to Admit. (minutes)[2]	459	218	260	274
Time from ER Arrival to Discharge (minutes)	374	138	138	134
Time in ER Before Being Evaluated (minutes)	403	30	28	26
Time to Pain Meds for Fractures (minutes)	88	48	52	57
Heart Attack Care				
Aspirin Given at Discharge	109	100%	99%	99%
Fibrinolytic Meds Within 30 Min. of Arrival[7]	-	-	33%	54%
PCI Within 90 Minutes of Arrival	26	96%	97%	96%
Statin Prescribed at Discharge	102	100%	98%	98%
Heart Failure Care				
ACE Inhibitor or ARB for LVSD	44	100%	98%	97%
Discharge Instructions Given	94	99%	96%	94%
Evaluation of LVS Function	140	100%	99%	99%
Medicare Spending				
Medicare Spending per Patient (ratio)	-	0.95	1	0.98
Pneumonia Care				
Appropriate Initial Antibiotic Given	114	98%	95%	95%
Blood Culture Timing	151	100%	98%	98%
Pregnancy and Delivery Care				
Newborn Deliveries Scheduled Early	48	4%	2%	6%
Preventive Care				
Immunization for Influenza[2]	404	97%	92%	90%
Immunization for Pneumonia[2]	488	97%	92%	92%
Stroke Care				
Anticoagulation Therapy for Atrial Fibrillation[1]	-	-	94%	95%
Antithrombotic Therapy Timing	24	100%	98%	98%
Assessed for Rehabilitation	25	100%	97%	97%
Discharged on Antithrombotic Therapy	24	100%	99%	99%
Discharged on Statin Medication	19	100%	94%	94%
Thrombolytic Therapy Timing[1]	-	-	66%	66%
Venous Thromboembolism Prophylaxis	26	100%	94%	94%
Written Stroke Educational Materials Given	13	100%	87%	88%
Surgical Care Improvement Project				
Appropriate Beta Blocker Usage[2]	76	100%	98%	98%
Appropriate VTP Within 24 Hours[2]	269	100%	98%	98%
Controlled Postoperative Blood Glucose[2,7]	-	-	97%	97%
Perioperative Temperature Management[2]	299	100%	100%	100%
Prophylactic Antibiotic Selection[2]	214	100%	99%	99%
Prophylactic Antibiotic Selection (Outpatient)	83	96%	98%	98%
Prophylactic Antibiotic Stopped[2]	211	100%	98%	98%
Prophylactic Antibiotic Timing[2]	215	100%	99%	99%
Prophylactic Antibiotic Timing (Outpatient)	83	100%	97%	98%
Urinary Catheter Removal[2]	45	98%	98%	97%
Survey of Patients' Hospital Experiences				
Area Around Room 'Always' Quiet at Night	300+	54%	60%	61%
Doctors 'Always' Communicated Well	300+	80%	81%	82%
Home Recovery Information Given	300+	86%	86%	85%
Hospital Given 9 or 10 on 10 Point Scale	300+	73%	70%	71%
Meds 'Always' Explained Before Given	300+	64%	64%	64%
Nurses 'Always' Communicated Well	300+	80%	79%	79%
Pain 'Always' Well Controlled	300+	74%	71%	71%
Room and Bathroom 'Always' Clean	300+	73%	74%	73%
Timely Help 'Always' Received	300+	70%	67%	68%
Would Definitely Recommend Hospital	300+	71%	70%	71%
Use of Medical Imaging				
Cardiac Imaging Stress Test before Surgery	130	6.2%	5.5%	5.3%
Combination Abdominal CT Scan	308	2.3%	10.1%	10.5%
Combination Brain/Sinus CT Scan	352	0.3%	2.6%	2.7%
Combination Chest CT Scan	162	3.1%	2.8%	2.7%
Follow-up Mammogram/Ultrasound	730	8.5%	8.4%	8.8%
Lumbar Spine MRI for Low Back Pain[1]	-	-	36.6%	37.2%

Sparta Community Hospital

818 E Broadway
Sparta, IL 62286
Phone: 618-443-2177
Fax: 618-443-1383
E-mail: hertzingp@spartahospital.com
URL: www.spartahospital.com
Type: Critical Access Hospitals
Emergency Services: Yes
Ownership: Govt - Hospital Dist/Auth
Beds: 39

Key Personnel:
Infection Control. . . . . Donna Chappell, RN
Emergency Room . . . . Sharon Hall, MD
Quality Assurance . . . . Ruth Holloway
Chief of Medical Staff . . . . Wim Sippo, MD
Anesthesiology. . . . . Debbie Weatherspoon
Operating Room. . . . . Janet Zeidler, RN

Measure	Cases	This Hosp.	State Avg.	U.S. Avg.
Blood Clot Prevention and Treatment				
Anticoagulation Overlap Therapy[5]	-	-	91%	93%
ICU Venous Thromboembolism Prophylaxis[5]	-	-	93%	92%
Incidence of Potentially Preventable VTE[5]	-	-	11%	10%
UFH with Dosages/Platelet Monitoring[5]	-	-	94%	97%
Venous Thromboembolism Prophylaxis[5]	-	-	86%	85%
Warfarin Therapy Discharge Instructions[5]	-	-	71%	75%
Chest Pain/Possible Heart Attack Care				
Aspirin Given Within 24 Hours of Arrival	-	-	96%	96%
Fibrinolytic Meds Within 30 Min. of Arrival	-	-	65%	58%
Average Time to ECG (minutes)	-	-	6	7
Average Time to Transfer (minutes)	-	-	63	60
Children's Asthma Care				
Received Home Management Plan of Care	-	-	-	88%
Received Reliever Medication	-	-	-	100%
Received Systemic Corticosteroids	-	-	-	100%
Emergency Department				
Admittance Decision Time (minutes)[5]	-	-	89	98
Head CT Results Within 45 Min. of Arrival	-	-	64%	57%
Patients Who Left ER Before Being Seen	-	-	3%	2%
Time from ER Arrival to Admit. (minutes)[5]	-	-	260	274
Time from ER Arrival to Discharge (minutes)	-	-	138	134
Time in ER Before Being Evaluated (minutes)	-	-	28	26
Time to Pain Meds for Fractures (minutes)	-	-	52	57
Heart Attack Care				
Aspirin Given at Discharge[1,3]	-	-	99%	99%
Fibrinolytic Meds Within 30 Min. of Arrival[3,7]	-	-	33%	54%
PCI Within 90 Minutes of Arrival[3,7]	-	-	97%	96%
Statin Prescribed at Discharge[1,3]	-	-	98%	98%
Heart Failure Care				
ACE Inhibitor or ARB for LVSD[1]	-	-	98%	97%
Discharge Instructions Given[1]	-	-	96%	94%
Evaluation of LVS Function	17	100%	99%	99%
Medicare Spending				
Medicare Spending per Patient (ratio)	-	-	1	0.98
Pneumonia Care				
Appropriate Initial Antibiotic Given	28	100%	95%	95%
Blood Culture Timing	32	97%	98%	98%
Pregnancy and Delivery Care				
Newborn Deliveries Scheduled Early[5]	-	-	2%	6%
Preventive Care				
Immunization for Influenza[5]	-	-	92%	90%
Immunization for Pneumonia[5]	-	-	92%	92%
Stroke Care				
Anticoagulation Therapy for Atrial Fibrillation[5]	-	-	94%	95%
Antithrombotic Therapy Timing[5]	-	-	98%	98%
Assessed for Rehabilitation[5]	-	-	97%	97%
Discharged on Antithrombotic Therapy[5]	-	-	99%	99%
Discharged on Statin Medication[5]	-	-	94%	94%
Thrombolytic Therapy Timing[5]	-	-	66%	66%
Venous Thromboembolism Prophylaxis[5]	-	-	94%	94%
Written Stroke Educational Materials Given[5]	-	-	87%	88%
Surgical Care Improvement Project				
Appropriate Beta Blocker Usage[1]	-	-	98%	98%
Appropriate VTP Within 24 Hours	16	100%	98%	98%
Controlled Postoperative Blood Glucose[7]	-	-	97%	97%
Perioperative Temperature Management	19	100%	100%	100%
Prophylactic Antibiotic Selection	17	100%	99%	99%
Prophylactic Antibiotic Selection (Outpatient)	-	-	98%	98%

NOTE: Hospital profiles are in alphabetical order by state, then city, then hospital within the city; Rankings exclude hospitals with less than 25 cases except for patient surveys which excludes hospitals with less than 100 cases; (a) 100-299 cases; (1) The number of cases/patients is too few to report; (2) Data submitted were based on a sample of cases/patients; (3) Results are based on a shorter time period than required; (4) Data suppressed by CMS for one or more quarters; (5) Results are not available for this reporting period; (6) Fewer than 100 patients completed the HCAHPS survey; (7) No cases met the criteria for this measure; (8) The lower limit of the confidence interval cannot be calculated if the number of observed infections equals zero; (9) No data are available from the state/territory for this reporting period; (10) The scores shown reflect fewer than 50 completed surveys; (11) There were discrepancies in the data collection process; (12) This measure does not apply to this hospital for this reporting period; (13) Results cannot be calculated for this reporting period; (14) The results for this state are combined with nearby states to protect confidentiality; Please refer to the User's Guide for a full explanation of data.

Measure	Cases	This Hosp.	State Avg.	U.S. Avg.
Prophylactic Antibiotic Stopped	17	88%	98%	98%
Prophylactic Antibiotic Timing	17	100%	99%	99%
Prophylactic Antibiotic Timing (Outpatient)	-	-	97%	98%
Urinary Catheter Removal	18	94%	98%	97%
Survey of Patients' Hospital Experiences				
Area Around Room 'Always' Quiet at Night	(a)	71%	60%	61%
Doctors 'Always' Communicated Well	(a)	75%	81%	82%
Home Recovery Information Given	(a)	91%	86%	85%
Hospital Given 9 or 10 on 10 Point Scale	(a)	66%	70%	71%
Meds 'Always' Explained Before Given	(a)	71%	64%	64%
Nurses 'Always' Communicated Well	(a)	83%	79%	79%
Pain 'Always' Well Controlled	(a)	74%	71%	71%
Room and Bathroom 'Always' Clean	(a)	84%	74%	73%
Timely Help 'Always' Received	(a)	78%	67%	68%
Would Definitely Recommend Hospital	(a)	53%	70%	71%
Use of Medical Imaging				
Cardiac Imaging Stress Test before Surgery	-	-	5.5%	5.3%
Combination Abdominal CT Scan	-	-	10.1%	10.5%
Combination Brain/Sinus CT Scan	-	-	2.6%	2.7%
Combination Chest CT Scan	-	-	2.8%	2.7%
Follow-up Mammogram/Ultrasound	-	-	8.4%	8.8%
Lumbar Spine MRI for Low Back Pain	-	-	36.6%	37.2%

Saint Margarets Hospital

600 E 1st St
Spring Valley, IL 61362
Phone: 815-664-1176
Fax: 815-664-1608
E-mail: hrdir@st-margarets.com
URL: www.aboutsmh.org
Type: Acute Care Hospitals
Emergency Services: Yes
Ownership: Voluntary non-profit - Church
Beds: 155

Key Personnel:
Chief of Medical Staff.......... Marshal Cummings
CEO/President............... Tim Muntz
Chairman/CEO .... Dr. Frank Zeller

Measure	Cases	This Hosp.	State Avg.	U.S. Avg.
Blood Clot Prevention and Treatment				
Anticoagulation Overlap Therapy[1,2]	-	-	91%	93%
ICU Venous Thromboembolism Prophylaxis[2]	28	96%	93%	92%
Incidence of Potentially Preventable VTE[1,2]	-	-	11%	10%
UFH with Dosages/Platelet Monitoring[1,2]	-	-	94%	97%
Venous Thromboembolism Prophylaxis[2]	147	97%	86%	85%
Warfarin Therapy Discharge Instructions[1,2]	-	-	71%	75%
Chest Pain/Possible Heart Attack Care				
Aspirin Given Within 24 Hours of Arrival	49	98%	96%	96%
Fibrinolytic Meds Within 30 Min. of Arrival[1]	-	-	65%	58%
Average Time to ECG (minutes)	49	5	6	7
Average Time to Transfer (minutes)[1]	-	-	63	60
Children's Asthma Care				
Received Home Management Plan of Care	-	-	-	88%
Received Reliever Medication	-	-	-	100%
Received Systemic Corticosteroids	-	-	-	100%
Emergency Department				
Admittance Decision Time (minutes)[2]	224	43	89	98
Head CT Results Within 45 Min. of Arrival[1,3]	-	-	64%	57%
Patients Who Left ER Before Being Seen	9,879	1%	3%	2%
Time from ER Arrival to Admit. (minutes)[2]	246	174	260	274
Time from ER Arrival to Discharge (minutes)	324	102	138	134
Time in ER Before Being Evaluated (minutes)	316	18	28	26
Time to Pain Meds for Fractures (minutes)	36	30	52	57
Heart Attack Care				
Aspirin Given at Discharge[5]	-	-	99%	99%
Fibrinolytic Meds Within 30 Min. of Arrival[5]	-	-	33%	54%
PCI Within 90 Minutes of Arrival[5]	-	-	97%	96%
Statin Prescribed at Discharge[5]	-	-	98%	98%
Heart Failure Care				
ACE Inhibitor or ARB for LVSD[1]	-	-	98%	97%
Discharge Instructions Given	38	92%	96%	94%
Evaluation of LVS Function	63	100%	99%	99%
Medicare Spending				
Medicare Spending per Patient (ratio)	-	0.98	1	0.98
Pneumonia Care				
Appropriate Initial Antibiotic Given	34	100%	95%	95%
Blood Culture Timing	82	100%	98%	98%
Pregnancy and Delivery Care				
Newborn Deliveries Scheduled Early	20	10%	2%	6%
Preventive Care				
Immunization for Influenza[2]	248	93%	92%	90%
Immunization for Pneumonia[2]	343	98%	92%	92%
Stroke Care				
Anticoagulation Therapy for Atrial Fibrillation[1,2]	-	-	94%	95%
Antithrombotic Therapy Timing[1,2]	-	-	98%	98%
Assessed for Rehabilitation[1,2]	-	-	97%	97%
Discharged on Antithrombotic Therapy[1,2]	-	-	99%	99%
Discharged on Statin Medication[1,2]	-	-	94%	94%
Thrombolytic Therapy Timing[2,3]	-	-	66%	66%
Venous Thromboembolism Prophylaxis[1,2]	-	-	94%	94%
Written Stroke Educational Materials Given[1,2]	-	-	87%	88%
Surgical Care Improvement Project				
Appropriate Beta Blocker Usage	110	98%	98%	98%
Appropriate VTP Within 24 Hours	321	100%	98%	98%
Controlled Postoperative Blood Glucose[7]	-	-	97%	97%
Perioperative Temperature Management	380	100%	100%	100%
Prophylactic Antibiotic Selection	249	100%	99%	99%
Prophylactic Antibiotic Selection (Outpatient)	23	96%	98%	98%
Prophylactic Antibiotic Stopped	242	100%	98%	98%
Prophylactic Antibiotic Timing	249	100%	99%	99%
Prophylactic Antibiotic Timing (Outpatient)	22	100%	97%	98%
Urinary Catheter Removal	294	100%	98%	97%
Survey of Patients' Hospital Experiences				
Area Around Room 'Always' Quiet at Night	300+	60%	60%	61%
Doctors 'Always' Communicated Well	300+	86%	81%	82%
Home Recovery Information Given	300+	89%	86%	85%
Hospital Given 9 or 10 on 10 Point Scale	300+	73%	70%	71%
Meds 'Always' Explained Before Given	300+	69%	64%	64%
Nurses 'Always' Communicated Well	300+	82%	79%	79%
Pain 'Always' Well Controlled	300+	72%	71%	71%
Room and Bathroom 'Always' Clean	300+	79%	74%	73%
Timely Help 'Always' Received	300+	70%	67%	68%
Would Definitely Recommend Hospital	300+	72%	70%	71%
Use of Medical Imaging				
Cardiac Imaging Stress Test before Surgery	151	6.6%	5.5%	5.3%
Combination Abdominal CT Scan	302	15.2%	10.1%	10.5%
Combination Brain/Sinus CT Scan[1]	-	-	2.6%	2.7%
Combination Chest CT Scan	293	1.0%	2.8%	2.7%
Follow-up Mammogram/Ultrasound	616	7.5%	8.4%	8.8%
Lumbar Spine MRI for Low Back Pain	65	41.5%	36.6%	37.2%

Memorial Medical Center

701 N First St
Springfield, IL 62781
Phone: 217-788-3000
Fax: 217-788-5594
URL: www.memorialmedical.com
Type: Acute Care Hospitals
Emergency Services: Yes
Ownership: Voluntary non-profit - Private
Beds: 444

Key Personnel:
Radiology.................... Kathy Ambs
Coronary Care............... Donna Crompton, RN
CEO/President............... Edgar J Curtis, FACHE
Operating Room.............. Sandy Flattery, RN
Chief of Medical Staff.......... Rajesh G. Govindaiah, MD
Patient Relations .... Marsha Prater, PhD RN
Quality Assurance .... Todd Riplinger
Infection Control.............. Margaret Roth, RN

Measure	Cases	This Hosp.	State Avg.	U.S. Avg.
Blood Clot Prevention and Treatment				
Anticoagulation Overlap Therapy[2]	178	95%	91%	93%
ICU Venous Thromboembolism Prophylaxis[2]	61	97%	93%	92%
Incidence of Potentially Preventable VTE[2]	37	5%	11%	10%
UFH with Dosages/Platelet Monitoring[2]	143	93%	94%	97%
Venous Thromboembolism Prophylaxis[2]	334	74%	86%	85%
Warfarin Therapy Discharge Instructions[2]	132	53%	71%	75%
Chest Pain/Possible Heart Attack Care				
Aspirin Given Within 24 Hours of Arrival[1,3]	-	-	96%	96%
Fibrinolytic Meds Within 30 Min. of Arrival[3,7]	-	-	65%	58%
Average Time to ECG (minutes)[1,3]	-	-	6	7
Average Time to Transfer (minutes)[3,7]	-	-	63	60
Children's Asthma Care				
Received Home Management Plan of Care	-	-	-	88%
Received Reliever Medication	-	-	-	100%
Received Systemic Corticosteroids	-	-	-	100%
Emergency Department				
Admittance Decision Time (minutes)[2]	485	94	89	98
Head CT Results Within 45 Min. of Arrival[1]	-	-	64%	57%
Patients Who Left ER Before Being Seen	69,792	4%	3%	2%
Time from ER Arrival to Admit. (minutes)[2]	537	290	260	274
Time from ER Arrival to Discharge (minutes)	371	172	138	134
Time in ER Before Being Evaluated (minutes)	400	24	28	26
Time to Pain Meds for Fractures (minutes)	234	72	52	57
Heart Attack Care				
Aspirin Given at Discharge[2]	301	100%	99%	99%
Fibrinolytic Meds Within 30 Min. of Arrival[2,7]	-	-	33%	54%
PCI Within 90 Minutes of Arrival[2]	29	90%	97%	96%
Statin Prescribed at Discharge[2]	291	98%	98%	98%
Heart Failure Care				
ACE Inhibitor or ARB for LVSD[2]	87	97%	98%	97%
Discharge Instructions Given[2]	236	98%	96%	94%
Evaluation of LVS Function[2]	307	100%	99%	99%
Medicare Spending				
Medicare Spending per Patient (ratio)	-	0.96	1	0.98
Pneumonia Care				
Appropriate Initial Antibiotic Given[2]	62	89%	95%	95%
Blood Culture Timing[2]	116	95%	98%	98%
Pregnancy and Delivery Care				
Newborn Deliveries Scheduled Early	43	2%	2%	6%
Preventive Care				
Immunization for Influenza[2]	591	94%	92%	90%
Immunization for Pneumonia[2]	766	91%	92%	92%
Stroke Care				
Anticoagulation Therapy for Atrial Fibrillation[2]	14	100%	94%	95%
Antithrombotic Therapy Timing[2]	74	99%	98%	98%
Assessed for Rehabilitation[2]	100	98%	97%	97%
Discharged on Antithrombotic Therapy[2]	89	99%	99%	99%
Discharged on Statin Medication[2]	81	98%	94%	94%
Thrombolytic Therapy Timing[1,2]	-	-	66%	66%
Venous Thromboembolism Prophylaxis[2]	98	98%	94%	94%
Written Stroke Educational Materials Given[2]	60	92%	87%	88%
Surgical Care Improvement Project				
Appropriate Beta Blocker Usage[2]	282	99%	98%	98%
Appropriate VTP Within 24 Hours[2]	342	95%	98%	98%
Controlled Postoperative Blood Glucose[2]	139	92%	97%	97%
Perioperative Temperature Management[2]	503	100%	100%	100%
Prophylactic Antibiotic Selection[2]	453	99%	99%	99%
Prophylactic Antibiotic Selection (Outpatient)	696	98%	98%	98%
Prophylactic Antibiotic Stopped[2]	443	98%	98%	98%
Prophylactic Antibiotic Timing[2]	453	98%	99%	99%
Prophylactic Antibiotic Timing (Outpatient)	705	97%	97%	98%
Urinary Catheter Removal[2]	426	99%	98%	97%
Survey of Patients' Hospital Experiences				
Area Around Room 'Always' Quiet at Night	300+	54%	60%	61%
Doctors 'Always' Communicated Well	300+	81%	81%	82%
Home Recovery Information Given	300+	85%	86%	85%
Hospital Given 9 or 10 on 10 Point Scale	300+	76%	70%	71%
Meds 'Always' Explained Before Given	300+	64%	64%	64%
Nurses 'Always' Communicated Well	300+	80%	79%	79%
Pain 'Always' Well Controlled	300+	71%	71%	71%
Room and Bathroom 'Always' Clean	300+	70%	74%	73%
Timely Help 'Always' Received	300+	66%	67%	68%
Would Definitely Recommend Hospital	300+	79%	70%	71%
Use of Medical Imaging				
Cardiac Imaging Stress Test before Surgery	344	5.2%	5.5%	5.3%
Combination Abdominal CT Scan	2,577	4.5%	10.1%	10.5%
Combination Brain/Sinus CT Scan	1,879	4.6%	2.6%	2.7%
Combination Chest CT Scan	2,382	2.8%	2.8%	2.7%
Follow-up Mammogram/Ultrasound	3,562	5.3%	8.4%	8.8%
Lumbar Spine MRI for Low Back Pain	231	32.5%	36.6%	37.2%

NOTE: Hospital profiles are in alphabetical order by state, then city, then hospital within the city; Rankings exclude hospitals with less than 25 cases except for patient surveys which excludes hospitals with less than 100 cases; (a) 100-299 cases; (1) The number of cases/patients is too few to report; (2) Data submitted were based on a sample of cases/patients; (3) Results are based on a shorter time period than required; (4) Data suppressed by CMS for one or more quarters; (5) Results are not available for this reporting period; (6) Fewer than 100 patients completed the HCAHPS survey; (7) No cases met the criteria for this measure; (8) The lower limit of the confidence interval cannot be calculated if the number of observed infections equals zero; (9) No data are available from the state/territory for this reporting period; (10) The scores shown reflect fewer than 50 completed surveys; (11) There were discrepancies in the data collection process; (12) This measure does not apply to this hospital for this reporting period; (13) Results cannot be calculated for this reporting period; (14) The results for this state are combined with nearby states to protect confidentiality; Please refer to the User's Guide for a full explanation of data.

Saint Johns Hospital

800 E Carpenter St
Springfield, IL 62769
URL: www.st-johns.org
Phone: 217-544-6464
Fax: 217-535-3989
Type: Acute Care Hospitals
Emergency Services: Yes
Ownership: Voluntary non-profit - Church
Beds: 742

Key Personnel:
Chief of Medical Staff. . . . . Craig Backs, MD
Infection Control. . . . . Carol Coleman, RN
Radiology. . . . . Pat Hynes
Emergency Room . . . . Amy Jones
CEO/President. . . . . Charles Lucore, MD
Intensive Care Unit. . . . . Betty Meisser
Chair/CEO . . . . John Slayton

Measure	Cases	This Hosp.	State Avg.	U.S. Avg.
Blood Clot Prevention and Treatment				
Anticoagulation Overlap Therapy[2]	87	91%	91%	93%
ICU Venous Thromboembolism Prophylaxis[2]	80	94%	93%	92%
Incidence of Potentially Preventable VTE[2]	23	4%	11%	10%
UFH with Dosages/Platelet Monitoring[2]	68	100%	94%	97%
Venous Thromboembolism Prophylaxis[2]	305	83%	86%	85%
Warfarin Therapy Discharge Instructions[2]	60	28%	71%	75%
Chest Pain/Possible Heart Attack Care				
Aspirin Given Within 24 Hours of Arrival[5]	-	-	96%	96%
Fibrinolytic Meds Within 30 Min. of Arrival[5]	-	-	65%	58%
Average Time to ECG (minutes)[5]	-	-	6	7
Average Time to Transfer (minutes)[5]	-	-	63	60
Children's Asthma Care				
Received Home Management Plan of Care	96	88%	-	88%
Received Reliever Medication	97	100%	-	100%
Received Systemic Corticosteroids	97	100%	-	100%
Emergency Department				
Admittance Decision Time (minutes)[2]	370	116	89	98
Head CT Results Within 45 Min. of Arrival[1]	-	-	64%	57%
Patients Who Left ER Before Being Seen	55,941	3%	3%	2%
Time from ER Arrival to Admit. (minutes)[2]	384	304	260	274
Time from ER Arrival to Discharge (minutes)	382	149	138	134
Time in ER Before Being Evaluated (minutes)	402	28	28	26
Time to Pain Meds for Fractures (minutes)	211	79	52	57
Heart Attack Care				
Aspirin Given at Discharge	647	100%	99%	99%
Fibrinolytic Meds Within 30 Min. of Arrival[7]	-	-	33%	54%
PCI Within 90 Minutes of Arrival	47	100%	97%	96%
Statin Prescribed at Discharge	631	99%	98%	98%
Heart Failure Care				
ACE Inhibitor or ARB for LVSD[2]	88	99%	98%	97%
Discharge Instructions Given[2]	241	98%	96%	94%
Evaluation of LVS Function[2]	308	100%	99%	99%
Medicare Spending				
Medicare Spending per Patient (ratio)	-	0.93	1	0.98
Pneumonia Care				
Appropriate Initial Antibiotic Given[2]	67	97%	95%	95%
Blood Culture Timing[2]	108	99%	98%	98%
Pregnancy and Delivery Care				
Newborn Deliveries Scheduled Early[2]	23	4%	2%	6%
Preventive Care				
Immunization for Influenza[2]	574	93%	92%	90%
Immunization for Pneumonia[2]	659	93%	92%	92%
Stroke Care				
Anticoagulation Therapy for Atrial Fibrillation	48	100%	94%	95%
Antithrombotic Therapy Timing	204	100%	98%	98%
Assessed for Rehabilitation	269	100%	97%	97%
Discharged on Antithrombotic Therapy	243	100%	99%	99%
Discharged on Statin Medication	197	99%	94%	94%
Thrombolytic Therapy Timing	11	91%	66%	66%
Venous Thromboembolism Prophylaxis	268	99%	94%	94%
Written Stroke Educational Materials Given	151	98%	87%	88%
Surgical Care Improvement Project				
Appropriate Beta Blocker Usage[2]	353	99%	98%	98%
Appropriate VTP Within 24 Hours[2]	323	97%	98%	98%
Controlled Postoperative Blood Glucose[2]	205	98%	97%	97%
Perioperative Temperature Management[2]	532	100%	100%	100%
Prophylactic Antibiotic Selection[2]	492	99%	99%	99%
Prophylactic Antibiotic Selection (Outpatient)	578	98%	98%	98%
Prophylactic Antibiotic Stopped[2]	483	98%	98%	98%
Prophylactic Antibiotic Timing[2]	493	99%	99%	99%
Prophylactic Antibiotic Timing (Outpatient)	585	97%	97%	98%
Urinary Catheter Removal[2]	458	98%	98%	97%
Survey of Patients' Hospital Experiences				
Area Around Room 'Always' Quiet at Night	300+	52%	60%	61%
Doctors 'Always' Communicated Well	300+	79%	81%	82%
Home Recovery Information Given	300+	85%	86%	85%
Hospital Given 9 or 10 on 10 Point Scale	300+	71%	70%	71%
Meds 'Always' Explained Before Given	300+	62%	64%	64%
Nurses 'Always' Communicated Well	300+	78%	79%	79%
Pain 'Always' Well Controlled	300+	69%	71%	71%
Room and Bathroom 'Always' Clean	300+	73%	74%	73%
Timely Help 'Always' Received	300+	67%	67%	68%
Would Definitely Recommend Hospital	300+	74%	70%	71%
Use of Medical Imaging				
Cardiac Imaging Stress Test before Surgery	2,450	4.6%	5.5%	5.3%
Combination Abdominal CT Scan	975	15.5%	10.1%	10.5%
Combination Brain/Sinus CT Scan	845	4.0%	2.6%	2.7%
Combination Chest CT Scan	675	4.6%	2.8%	2.7%
Follow-up Mammogram/Ultrasound	1,837	15.0%	8.4%	8.8%
Lumbar Spine MRI for Low Back Pain	92	38.0%	36.6%	37.2%

Community Memorial Hospital

400 Caldwell
Staunton, IL 62088
Phone: 618-635-2200
Fax: 618-635-3400
E-mail: mbellovich@stauntonhospital.org
URL: www.stauntonhospital.org
Type: Critical Access Hospitals
Emergency Services: Yes
Ownership: Voluntary non-profit - Private
Beds: 49

Key Personnel:
Operating Room. . . . . Joseph Blazer, RN
CEO/President. . . . . Patrick B Heise
Chief of Medical Staff . . . . Manish Mathur
Infection Control. . . . . Judy Matteson, RN
Quality Assurance . . . . Judy Matteson, RN
Emergency Room . . . . Roberta Monsholt, RN

Measure	Cases	This Hosp.	State Avg.	U.S. Avg.
Blood Clot Prevention and Treatment				
Anticoagulation Overlap Therapy[5]	-	-	91%	93%
ICU Venous Thromboembolism Prophylaxis[5]	-	-	93%	92%
Incidence of Potentially Preventable VTE[5]	-	-	11%	10%
UFH with Dosages/Platelet Monitoring[5]	-	-	94%	97%
Venous Thromboembolism Prophylaxis[5]	-	-	86%	85%
Warfarin Therapy Discharge Instructions[5]	-	-	71%	75%
Chest Pain/Possible Heart Attack Care				
Aspirin Given Within 24 Hours of Arrival	-	-	96%	96%
Fibrinolytic Meds Within 30 Min. of Arrival	-	-	65%	58%
Average Time to ECG (minutes)	-	-	6	7
Average Time to Transfer (minutes)	-	-	63	60
Children's Asthma Care				
Received Home Management Plan of Care	-	-	-	88%
Received Reliever Medication	-	-	-	100%
Received Systemic Corticosteroids	-	-	-	100%
Emergency Department				
Admittance Decision Time (minutes)[5]	-	-	89	98
Head CT Results Within 45 Min. of Arrival	-	-	64%	57%
Patients Who Left ER Before Being Seen	-	-	3%	2%
Time from ER Arrival to Admit. (minutes)[5]	-	-	260	274
Time from ER Arrival to Discharge (minutes)	-	-	138	134
Time in ER Before Being Evaluated (minutes)	-	-	28	26
Time to Pain Meds for Fractures (minutes)	-	-	52	57
Heart Attack Care				
Aspirin Given at Discharge[1]	-	-	99%	99%
Fibrinolytic Meds Within 30 Min. of Arrival[7]	-	-	33%	54%
PCI Within 90 Minutes of Arrival[7]	-	-	97%	96%
Statin Prescribed at Discharge[1]	-	-	98%	98%
Heart Failure Care				
ACE Inhibitor or ARB for LVSD[1]	-	-	98%	97%
Discharge Instructions Given[1]	-	-	96%	94%
Evaluation of LVS Function[1]	-	-	99%	99%
Medicare Spending				
Medicare Spending per Patient (ratio)	-	-	1	0.98
Pneumonia Care				
Appropriate Initial Antibiotic Given	19	89%	95%	95%
Blood Culture Timing	17	100%	98%	98%
Pregnancy and Delivery Care				
Newborn Deliveries Scheduled Early[5]	-	-	2%	6%
Preventive Care				
Immunization for Influenza[5]	-	-	92%	90%
Immunization for Pneumonia[5]	-	-	92%	92%
Stroke Care				
Anticoagulation Therapy for Atrial Fibrillation[5]	-	-	94%	95%
Antithrombotic Therapy Timing[5]	-	-	98%	98%
Assessed for Rehabilitation[5]	-	-	97%	97%
Discharged on Antithrombotic Therapy[5]	-	-	99%	99%
Discharged on Statin Medication[5]	-	-	94%	94%
Thrombolytic Therapy Timing[5]	-	-	66%	66%
Venous Thromboembolism Prophylaxis[5]	-	-	94%	94%
Written Stroke Educational Materials Given[5]	-	-	87%	88%
Surgical Care Improvement Project				
Appropriate Beta Blocker Usage[3,7]	-	-	98%	98%
Appropriate VTP Within 24 Hours[1,3]	-	-	98%	98%
Controlled Postoperative Blood Glucose[3,7]	-	-	97%	97%
Perioperative Temperature Management[1,3]	-	-	100%	100%
Prophylactic Antibiotic Selection[1,3]	-	-	99%	99%
Prophylactic Antibiotic Selection (Outpatient)	-	-	98%	98%
Prophylactic Antibiotic Stopped[1,3]	-	-	98%	98%
Prophylactic Antibiotic Timing[1,3]	-	-	99%	99%
Prophylactic Antibiotic Timing (Outpatient)	-	-	97%	98%
Urinary Catheter Removal[1,3]	-	-	98%	97%
Survey of Patients' Hospital Experiences				
Area Around Room 'Always' Quiet at Night[5]	-	-	60%	61%
Doctors 'Always' Communicated Well[5]	-	-	81%	82%
Home Recovery Information Given[5]	-	-	86%	85%
Hospital Given 9 or 10 on 10 Point Scale[5]	-	-	70%	71%
Meds 'Always' Explained Before Given[5]	-	-	64%	64%
Nurses 'Always' Communicated Well[5]	-	-	79%	79%
Pain 'Always' Well Controlled[5]	-	-	71%	71%
Room and Bathroom 'Always' Clean[5]	-	-	74%	73%
Timely Help 'Always' Received[5]	-	-	67%	68%
Would Definitely Recommend Hospital[5]	-	-	70%	71%
Use of Medical Imaging				
Cardiac Imaging Stress Test before Surgery	-	-	5.5%	5.3%
Combination Abdominal CT Scan	-	-	10.1%	10.5%
Combination Brain/Sinus CT Scan	-	-	2.6%	2.7%
Combination Chest CT Scan	-	-	2.8%	2.7%
Follow-up Mammogram/Ultrasound	-	-	8.4%	8.8%
Lumbar Spine MRI for Low Back Pain	-	-	36.6%	37.2%

CGH Medical Center

100 East Lefevre Road
Sterling, IL 61081
Phone: 815-625-0400
Fax: 815-625-4825
URL: www.cghmc.com
Type: Acute Care Hospitals
Emergency Services: Yes
Ownership: Government - Local
Beds: 139

Key Personnel:
CEO/President. . . . . Ed Andersen
Chief of Medical Staff . . . . Angel Biazquez, MD
Radiology. . . . . Eugene W Brown, MD
Quality Assurance . . . . Theresa Friel-Draper, RN
Pediatric Ambulatory Care . . . . . . Mandrama Herman, MD
Pediatric In-Patient Care . . . . Mandrama Herman, MD
Operating Room. . . . . Thomas P McGlone
Infection Control. . . . . Sandra Westbo, RN

Measure	Cases	This Hosp.	State Avg.	U.S. Avg.
Blood Clot Prevention and Treatment				
Anticoagulation Overlap Therapy[2]	38	92%	91%	93%
ICU Venous Thromboembolism Prophylaxis[2]	92	86%	93%	92%
Incidence of Potentially Preventable VTE[1,2]	-	-	11%	10%
UFH with Dosages/Platelet Monitoring[1,2]	-	-	94%	97%
Venous Thromboembolism Prophylaxis[2]	304	85%	86%	85%
Warfarin Therapy Discharge Instructions[2]	30	30%	71%	75%
Chest Pain/Possible Heart Attack Care				
Aspirin Given Within 24 Hours of Arrival	29	93%	96%	96%
Fibrinolytic Meds Within 30 Min. of Arrival[3,7]	-	-	65%	58%
Average Time to ECG (minutes)	29	5	6	7
Average Time to Transfer (minutes)[3,7]	-	-	63	60

NOTE: Hospital profiles are in alphabetical order by state, then city, then hospital within the city; Rankings exclude hospitals with less than 25 cases except for patient surveys which excludes hospitals with less than 100 cases; (a) 100-299 cases; (1) The number of cases/patients is too few to report; (2) Data submitted were based on a sample of cases/patients; (3) Results are based on a shorter time period than required; (4) Data suppressed by CMS for one or more quarters; (5) Results are not available for this reporting period; (6) Fewer than 100 patients completed the HCAHPS survey; (7) No cases met the criteria for this measure; (8) The lower limit of the confidence interval cannot be calculated if the number of observed infections equals zero; (9) No data are available from the state/territory for this reporting period; (10) The scores shown reflect fewer than 50 completed surveys; (11) There were discrepancies in the data collection process; (12) This measure does not apply to this hospital for this reporting period; (13) Results cannot be calculated for this reporting period; (14) The results for this state are combined with nearby states to protect confidentiality; Please refer to the User's Guide for a full explanation of data.

Measure	Cases	This Hosp.	State Avg.	U.S. Avg.
Children's Asthma Care				
Received Home Management Plan of Care	-	-	-	88%
Received Reliever Medication	-	-	-	100%
Received Systemic Corticosteroids	-	-	-	100%
Emergency Department				
Admittance Decision Time (minutes)[2]	648	53	89	98
Head CT Results Within 45 Min. of Arrival	21	81%	64%	57%
Patients Who Left ER Before Being Seen	29,271	1%	3%	2%
Time from ER Arrival to Admit. (minutes)[2]	650	198	260	274
Time from ER Arrival to Discharge (minutes)	370	131	138	134
Time in ER Before Being Evaluated (minutes)	409	23	28	26
Time to Pain Meds for Fractures (minutes)	89	36	52	57
Heart Attack Care				
Aspirin Given at Discharge	59	97%	99%	99%
Fibrinolytic Meds Within 30 Min. of Arrival[7]	-	-	33%	54%
PCI Within 90 Minutes of Arrival[1]	-	-	97%	96%
Statin Prescribed at Discharge	57	96%	98%	98%
Heart Failure Care				
ACE Inhibitor or ARB for LVSD	55	89%	98%	97%
Discharge Instructions Given	163	100%	96%	94%
Evaluation of LVS Function	204	100%	99%	99%
Medicare Spending				
Medicare Spending per Patient (ratio)	-	0.95	1	0.98
Pneumonia Care				
Appropriate Initial Antibiotic Given	109	94%	95%	95%
Blood Culture Timing	222	100%	98%	98%
Pregnancy and Delivery Care				
Newborn Deliveries Scheduled Early[2]	20	5%	2%	6%
Preventive Care				
Immunization for Influenza[2]	539	91%	92%	90%
Immunization for Pneumonia[2]	662	95%	92%	92%
Stroke Care				
Anticoagulation Therapy for Atrial Fibrillation[1]	-	-	94%	95%
Antithrombotic Therapy Timing	33	100%	98%	98%
Assessed for Rehabilitation	34	100%	97%	97%
Discharged on Antithrombotic Therapy	32	94%	99%	99%
Discharged on Statin Medication	20	95%	94%	94%
Thrombolytic Therapy Timing[1]	-	-	66%	66%
Venous Thromboembolism Prophylaxis	36	92%	94%	94%
Written Stroke Educational Materials Given	22	64%	87%	88%
Surgical Care Improvement Project				
Appropriate Beta Blocker Usage[2]	165	98%	98%	98%
Appropriate VTP Within 24 Hours[2]	355	99%	98%	98%
Controlled Postoperative Blood Glucose[2,7]	-	-	97%	97%
Perioperative Temperature Management[2]	424	100%	100%	100%
Prophylactic Antibiotic Selection[2]	304	99%	99%	99%
Prophylactic Antibiotic Selection (Outpatient)	123	97%	98%	98%
Prophylactic Antibiotic Stopped[2]	298	99%	98%	98%
Prophylactic Antibiotic Timing[2]	304	99%	99%	99%
Prophylactic Antibiotic Timing (Outpatient)	92	88%	97%	98%
Urinary Catheter Removal[2]	310	99%	98%	97%
Survey of Patients' Hospital Experiences				
Area Around Room 'Always' Quiet at Night	300+	61%	60%	61%
Doctors 'Always' Communicated Well	300+	83%	81%	82%
Home Recovery Information Given	300+	88%	86%	85%
Hospital Given 9 or 10 on 10 Point Scale	300+	76%	70%	71%
Meds 'Always' Explained Before Given	300+	67%	64%	64%
Nurses 'Always' Communicated Well	300+	82%	79%	79%
Pain 'Always' Well Controlled	300+	70%	71%	71%
Room and Bathroom 'Always' Clean	300+	83%	74%	73%
Timely Help 'Always' Received	300+	72%	67%	68%
Would Definitely Recommend Hospital	300+	71%	70%	71%
Use of Medical Imaging				
Cardiac Imaging Stress Test before Surgery	787	5.3%	5.5%	5.3%
Combination Abdominal CT Scan	749	1.1%	10.1%	10.5%
Combination Brain/Sinus CT Scan	740	1.5%	2.6%	2.7%
Combination Chest CT Scan	437	0.5%	2.8%	2.7%
Follow-up Mammogram/Ultrasound	1,552	10.7%	8.4%	8.8%
Lumbar Spine MRI for Low Back Pain	141	34.8%	36.6%	37.2%

Saint Marys Hospital

111 Spring Street
Streator, IL 61364
Phone: 815-673-2311
Fax: 815-673-4592
URL: www.stmaryshospital.org
Type: Acute Care Hospitals
Emergency Services: No
Ownership: Voluntary non-profit - Church
Beds: 251

Key Personnel:
Pediatric Ambulatory Care . . . . . . Bella Baz, MD
Pediatric In-Patient Care . . . . Bella Baz, MD
CEO/President. . . . . Marker Heller
Radiology. . . . . Mark Hilborn, MD
Operating Room. . . . . Bonnie Ostrem, RN
Chief of Medical Staff . . . . Glen Ricca
Emergency Room . . . . Susan Taylor, RN
Quality Assurance . . . . Walter Wahl

Measure	Cases	This Hosp.	State Avg.	U.S. Avg.
Blood Clot Prevention and Treatment				
Anticoagulation Overlap Therapy[1,2]	-	-	91%	93%
ICU Venous Thromboembolism Prophylaxis[2]	27	93%	93%	92%
Incidence of Potentially Preventable VTE[2,7]	-	-	11%	10%
UFH with Dosages/Platelet Monitoring[1,2]	-	-	94%	97%
Venous Thromboembolism Prophylaxis[2]	175	90%	86%	85%
Warfarin Therapy Discharge Instructions[1,2]	-	-	71%	75%
Chest Pain/Possible Heart Attack Care				
Aspirin Given Within 24 Hours of Arrival	77	100%	96%	96%
Fibrinolytic Meds Within 30 Min. of Arrival[1]	-	-	65%	58%
Average Time to ECG (minutes)	81	5	6	7
Average Time to Transfer (minutes)[1]	-	-	63	60
Children's Asthma Care				
Received Home Management Plan of Care	-	-	-	88%
Received Reliever Medication	-	-	-	100%
Received Systemic Corticosteroids	-	-	-	100%
Emergency Department				
Admittance Decision Time (minutes)[2]	331	137	89	98
Head CT Results Within 45 Min. of Arrival[1]	-	-	64%	57%
Patients Who Left ER Before Being Seen	12,518	0%	3%	2%
Time from ER Arrival to Admit. (minutes)[2]	331	179	260	274
Time from ER Arrival to Discharge (minutes)	347	87	138	134
Time in ER Before Being Evaluated (minutes)	402	14	28	26
Time to Pain Meds for Fractures (minutes)	41	47	52	57
Heart Attack Care				
Aspirin Given at Discharge	11	100%	99%	99%
Fibrinolytic Meds Within 30 Min. of Arrival[7]	-	-	33%	54%
PCI Within 90 Minutes of Arrival[7]	-	-	97%	96%
Statin Prescribed at Discharge	14	100%	98%	98%
Heart Failure Care				
ACE Inhibitor or ARB for LVSD	24	100%	98%	97%
Discharge Instructions Given	74	99%	96%	94%
Evaluation of LVS Function	94	100%	99%	99%
Medicare Spending				
Medicare Spending per Patient (ratio)	-	0.91	1	0.98
Pneumonia Care				
Appropriate Initial Antibiotic Given	49	100%	95%	95%
Blood Culture Timing	100	99%	98%	98%
Pregnancy and Delivery Care				
Newborn Deliveries Scheduled Early	21	10%	2%	6%
Preventive Care				
Immunization for Influenza[2]	277	97%	92%	90%
Immunization for Pneumonia[2]	384	98%	92%	92%
Stroke Care				
Anticoagulation Therapy for Atrial Fibrillation[1]	-	-	94%	95%
Antithrombotic Therapy Timing[1]	-	-	98%	98%
Assessed for Rehabilitation	11	100%	97%	97%
Discharged on Antithrombotic Therapy[1]	-	-	99%	99%
Discharged on Statin Medication[1]	-	-	94%	94%
Thrombolytic Therapy Timing[7]	-	-	66%	66%
Venous Thromboembolism Prophylaxis	12	83%	94%	94%
Written Stroke Educational Materials Given[1]	-	-	87%	88%
Surgical Care Improvement Project				
Appropriate Beta Blocker Usage	26	100%	98%	98%
Appropriate VTP Within 24 Hours	92	97%	98%	98%
Controlled Postoperative Blood Glucose[7]	-	-	97%	97%
Perioperative Temperature Management	98	100%	100%	100%
Prophylactic Antibiotic Selection	63	100%	99%	99%
Prophylactic Antibiotic Selection (Outpatient)	37	100%	98%	98%
Prophylactic Antibiotic Stopped	62	94%	98%	98%
Prophylactic Antibiotic Timing	63	100%	99%	99%
Prophylactic Antibiotic Timing (Outpatient)	37	100%	97%	98%
Urinary Catheter Removal	60	95%	98%	97%
Survey of Patients' Hospital Experiences				
Area Around Room 'Always' Quiet at Night	300+	64%	60%	61%
Doctors 'Always' Communicated Well	300+	86%	81%	82%
Home Recovery Information Given	300+	86%	86%	85%
Hospital Given 9 or 10 on 10 Point Scale	300+	70%	70%	71%
Meds 'Always' Explained Before Given	300+	66%	64%	64%
Nurses 'Always' Communicated Well	300+	82%	79%	79%
Pain 'Always' Well Controlled	300+	67%	71%	71%
Room and Bathroom 'Always' Clean	300+	83%	74%	73%
Timely Help 'Always' Received	300+	70%	67%	68%
Would Definitely Recommend Hospital	300+	63%	70%	71%
Use of Medical Imaging				
Cardiac Imaging Stress Test before Surgery	225	3.1%	5.5%	5.3%
Combination Abdominal CT Scan	352	21.6%	10.1%	10.5%
Combination Brain/Sinus CT Scan	346	1.4%	2.6%	2.7%
Combination Chest CT Scan	231	6.1%	2.8%	2.7%
Follow-up Mammogram/Ultrasound	924	5.4%	8.4%	8.8%
Lumbar Spine MRI for Low Back Pain	39	41.0%	36.6%	37.2%

Taylorville Memorial Hospital

201 East Pleasant Street
Taylorville, IL 62568
Phone: 217-824-3331
Fax: 217-824-1638
URL: www.svmh.org
Type: Critical Access Hospitals
Emergency Services: Yes
Ownership: Voluntary non-profit - Private
Beds: 74

Key Personnel:
Chief of Medical Staff . . . . Richard K DelValle
CEO/President. . . . . Dan Raab
Emergency Room . . . . Matthew Yociss, MD

Measure	Cases	This Hosp.	State Avg.	U.S. Avg.
Blood Clot Prevention and Treatment				
Anticoagulation Overlap Therapy[1,2]	-	-	91%	93%
ICU Venous Thromboembolism Prophylaxis[2,7]	-	-	93%	92%
Incidence of Potentially Preventable VTE[1,2]	-	-	11%	10%
UFH with Dosages/Platelet Monitoring[1,2]	-	-	94%	97%
Venous Thromboembolism Prophylaxis[2]	167	26%	86%	85%
Warfarin Therapy Discharge Instructions[1,2]	-	-	71%	75%
Chest Pain/Possible Heart Attack Care				
Aspirin Given Within 24 Hours of Arrival	74	95%	96%	96%
Fibrinolytic Meds Within 30 Min. of Arrival[1]	-	-	65%	58%
Average Time to ECG (minutes)	80	3	6	7
Average Time to Transfer (minutes)[7]	-	-	63	60
Children's Asthma Care				
Received Home Management Plan of Care	-	-	-	88%
Received Reliever Medication	-	-	-	100%
Received Systemic Corticosteroids	-	-	-	100%
Emergency Department				
Admittance Decision Time (minutes)[2]	331	70	89	98
Head CT Results Within 45 Min. of Arrival	11	82%	64%	57%
Patients Who Left ER Before Being Seen	15,562	0%	3%	2%
Time from ER Arrival to Admit. (minutes)[2]	335	209	260	274
Time from ER Arrival to Discharge (minutes)	343	85	138	134
Time in ER Before Being Evaluated (minutes)	276	18	28	26
Time to Pain Meds for Fractures (minutes)	45	36	52	57
Heart Attack Care				
Aspirin Given at Discharge[1]	-	-	99%	99%
Fibrinolytic Meds Within 30 Min. of Arrival[7]	-	-	33%	54%
PCI Within 90 Minutes of Arrival[3,7]	-	-	97%	96%
Statin Prescribed at Discharge[1]	-	-	98%	98%
Heart Failure Care				
ACE Inhibitor or ARB for LVSD	15	100%	98%	97%
Discharge Instructions Given	50	94%	96%	94%
Evaluation of LVS Function	70	99%	99%	99%
Medicare Spending				
Medicare Spending per Patient (ratio)	-	-	1	0.98
Pneumonia Care				
Appropriate Initial Antibiotic Given	57	84%	95%	95%
Blood Culture Timing	65	100%	98%	98%

NOTE: Hospital profiles are in alphabetical order by state, then city, then hospital within the city; Rankings exclude hospitals with less than 25 cases except for patient surveys which excludes hospitals with less than 100 cases; (a) 100-299 cases; (1) The number of cases/patients is too few to report; (2) Data submitted were based on a sample of cases/patients; (3) Results are based on a shorter time period than required; (4) Data suppressed by CMS for one or more quarters; (5) Results are not available for this reporting period; (6) Fewer than 100 patients completed the HCAHPS survey; (7) No cases met the criteria for this measure; (8) The lower limit of the confidence interval cannot be calculated if the number of observed infections equals zero; (9) No data are available from the state/territory for this reporting period; (10) The scores shown reflect fewer than 50 completed surveys; (11) There were discrepancies in the data collection process; (12) This measure does not apply to this hospital for this reporting period; (13) Results cannot be calculated for this reporting period; (14) The results for this state are combined with nearby states to protect confidentiality; Please refer to the User's Guide for a full explanation of data.

Measure	Cases	This Hosp.	State Avg.	U.S. Avg.
Pregnancy and Delivery Care				
Newborn Deliveries Scheduled Early[5]	-	-	2%	6%
Preventive Care				
Immunization for Influenza[2]	314	96%	92%	90%
Immunization for Pneumonia[2]	523	98%	92%	92%
Stroke Care				
Anticoagulation Therapy for Atrial Fibrillation[5]	-	-	94%	95%
Antithrombotic Therapy Timing[5]	-	-	98%	98%
Assessed for Rehabilitation[5]	-	-	97%	97%
Discharged on Antithrombotic Therapy[5]	-	-	99%	99%
Discharged on Statin Medication[5]	-	-	94%	94%
Thrombolytic Therapy Timing[5]	-	-	66%	66%
Venous Thromboembolism Prophylaxis[5]	-	-	94%	94%
Written Stroke Educational Materials Given[5]	-	-	87%	88%
Surgical Care Improvement Project				
Appropriate Beta Blocker Usage[1]	-	-	98%	98%
Appropriate VTP Within 24 Hours	23	100%	98%	98%
Controlled Postoperative Blood Glucose[7]	-	-	97%	97%
Perioperative Temperature Management	33	100%	100%	100%
Prophylactic Antibiotic Selection	23	100%	99%	99%
Prophylactic Antibiotic Selection (Outpatient)[5]	-	-	98%	98%
Prophylactic Antibiotic Stopped	22	95%	98%	98%
Prophylactic Antibiotic Timing	23	96%	99%	99%
Prophylactic Antibiotic Timing (Outpatient)[5]	-	-	97%	98%
Urinary Catheter Removal[1]	-	-	98%	97%
Survey of Patients' Hospital Experiences				
Area Around Room 'Always' Quiet at Night	300+	54%	60%	61%
Doctors 'Always' Communicated Well	300+	89%	81%	82%
Home Recovery Information Given	300+	82%	86%	85%
Hospital Given 9 or 10 on 10 Point Scale	300+	81%	70%	71%
Meds 'Always' Explained Before Given	300+	70%	64%	64%
Nurses 'Always' Communicated Well	300+	85%	79%	79%
Pain 'Always' Well Controlled	300+	72%	71%	71%
Room and Bathroom 'Always' Clean	300+	81%	74%	73%
Timely Help 'Always' Received	300+	73%	67%	68%
Would Definitely Recommend Hospital	300+	80%	70%	71%
Use of Medical Imaging				
Cardiac Imaging Stress Test before Surgery	136	1.5%	5.5%	5.3%
Combination Abdominal CT Scan	541	8.1%	10.1%	10.5%
Combination Brain/Sinus CT Scan[1]	-	-	2.6%	2.7%
Combination Chest CT Scan	427	2.1%	2.8%	2.7%
Follow-up Mammogram/Ultrasound	728	6.3%	8.4%	8.8%
Lumbar Spine MRI for Low Back Pain	78	42.3%	36.6%	37.2%

Carle Foundation Hospital

611 West Park Street
Urbana, IL 61801
Phone: 217-383-3311
Fax: 217-383-3373
URL: www.carle.com
Type: Acute Care Hospitals
Emergency Services: Yes
Ownership: Voluntary non-profit - Private
Beds: 345

Key Personnel:

Operating Room. . . . . Sue Cook
Quality Assurance . . . . LJ Fallon
Chief of Medical Staff. . . . . David Graham, MD
Radiology. . . . . Jon Hendrickson, MD
Pediatric In-Patient Care . . . . Malcolm Hill, MD
CEO/President. . . . . James C Leanard
Emergency Room . . . . Jay Yambert

Measure	Cases	This Hosp.	State Avg.	U.S. Avg.
Blood Clot Prevention and Treatment				
Anticoagulation Overlap Therapy[2]	164	95%	91%	93%
ICU Venous Thromboembolism Prophylaxis[2]	41	98%	93%	92%
Incidence of Potentially Preventable VTE[2]	30	7%	11%	10%
UFH with Dosages/Platelet Monitoring[2]	147	88%	94%	97%
Venous Thromboembolism Prophylaxis[2]	362	95%	86%	85%
Warfarin Therapy Discharge Instructions[2]	120	71%	71%	75%
Chest Pain/Possible Heart Attack Care				
Aspirin Given Within 24 Hours of Arrival[1,3]	-	-	96%	96%
Fibrinolytic Meds Within 30 Min. of Arrival[5]	-	-	65%	58%
Average Time to ECG (minutes)[1,3]	-	-	6	7
Average Time to Transfer (minutes)[5]	-	-	63	60
Children's Asthma Care				
Received Home Management Plan of Care	-	-	-	88%
Received Reliever Medication	-	-	-	100%
Received Systemic Corticosteroids	-	-	-	100%
Emergency Department				
Admittance Decision Time (minutes)[2]	543	82	89	98
Head CT Results Within 45 Min. of Arrival[1]	-	-	64%	57%
Patients Who Left ER Before Being Seen	70,356	0%	3%	2%
Time from ER Arrival to Admit. (minutes)[2]	549	255	260	274
Time from ER Arrival to Discharge (minutes)	344	96	138	134
Time in ER Before Being Evaluated (minutes)	254	18	28	26
Time to Pain Meds for Fractures (minutes)	154	58	52	57
Heart Attack Care				
Aspirin Given at Discharge[2]	304	98%	99%	99%
Fibrinolytic Meds Within 30 Min. of Arrival[2,7]	-	-	33%	54%
PCI Within 90 Minutes of Arrival[2]	25	100%	97%	96%
Statin Prescribed at Discharge[2]	296	99%	98%	98%
Heart Failure Care				
ACE Inhibitor or ARB for LVSD[2]	123	98%	98%	97%
Discharge Instructions Given[2]	216	100%	96%	94%
Evaluation of LVS Function[2]	281	100%	99%	99%
Medicare Spending				
Medicare Spending per Patient (ratio)	-	0.94	1	0.98
Pneumonia Care				
Appropriate Initial Antibiotic Given[2]	68	99%	95%	95%
Blood Culture Timing[2]	109	97%	98%	98%
Pregnancy and Delivery Care				
Newborn Deliveries Scheduled Early[2]	432	0%	2%	6%
Preventive Care				
Immunization for Influenza[2]	516	88%	92%	90%
Immunization for Pneumonia[2]	592	92%	92%	92%
Stroke Care				
Anticoagulation Therapy for Atrial Fibrillation	18	100%	94%	95%
Antithrombotic Therapy Timing	179	98%	98%	98%
Assessed for Rehabilitation	292	98%	97%	97%
Discharged on Antithrombotic Therapy	221	100%	99%	99%
Discharged on Statin Medication	177	95%	94%	94%
Thrombolytic Therapy Timing	11	91%	66%	66%
Venous Thromboembolism Prophylaxis	307	99%	94%	94%
Written Stroke Educational Materials Given	146	90%	87%	88%
Surgical Care Improvement Project				
Appropriate Beta Blocker Usage[2]	199	98%	98%	98%
Appropriate VTP Within 24 Hours[2]	289	99%	98%	98%
Controlled Postoperative Blood Glucose[2]	122	97%	97%	97%
Perioperative Temperature Management[2]	422	99%	100%	100%
Prophylactic Antibiotic Selection[2]	410	99%	99%	99%
Prophylactic Antibiotic Selection (Outpatient)	400	98%	98%	98%
Prophylactic Antibiotic Stopped[2]	406	98%	98%	98%
Prophylactic Antibiotic Timing[2]	410	99%	99%	99%
Prophylactic Antibiotic Timing (Outpatient)	363	95%	97%	98%
Urinary Catheter Removal[2]	260	96%	98%	97%
Survey of Patients' Hospital Experiences				
Area Around Room 'Always' Quiet at Night[11]	300+	53%	60%	61%
Doctors 'Always' Communicated Well[11]	300+	81%	81%	82%
Home Recovery Information Given[11]	300+	85%	86%	85%
Hospital Given 9 or 10 on 10 Point Scale[11]	300+	73%	70%	71%
Meds 'Always' Explained Before Given[11]	300+	63%	64%	64%
Nurses 'Always' Communicated Well[11]	300+	82%	79%	79%
Pain 'Always' Well Controlled[11]	300+	73%	71%	71%
Room and Bathroom 'Always' Clean[11]	300+	70%	74%	73%
Timely Help 'Always' Received[11]	300+	63%	67%	68%
Would Definitely Recommend Hospital[11]	300+	77%	70%	71%
Use of Medical Imaging				
Cardiac Imaging Stress Test before Surgery	472	7.4%	5.5%	5.3%
Combination Abdominal CT Scan	918	6.6%	10.1%	10.5%
Combination Brain/Sinus CT Scan	797	1.4%	2.6%	2.7%
Combination Chest CT Scan	779	0.4%	2.8%	2.7%
Follow-up Mammogram/Ultrasound	1,448	5.2%	8.4%	8.8%
Lumbar Spine MRI for Low Back Pain	99	44.4%	36.6%	37.2%

Presence Covenant Medical Center

1400 West Park Avenue
Urbana, IL 61801
Phone: 217-337-2000
Fax: 217-337-2619
URL: www.provena.org/covenant
Type: Acute Care Hospitals
Emergency Services: Yes
Ownership: Voluntary non-profit - Church
Beds: 210

Key Personnel:

Chief of Medical Staff. . . . . Kathy Collins, MD
Radiology. . . . . Ed Mabry
Pediatric In-Patient Care . . . . Barbara Michell, MD
CEO/President. . . . . Jared C. Rogers
Chair/CEO . . . . Steve Thomas

Measure	Cases	This Hosp.	State Avg.	U.S. Avg.
Blood Clot Prevention and Treatment				
Anticoagulation Overlap Therapy[2]	51	92%	91%	93%
ICU Venous Thromboembolism Prophylaxis[2]	83	78%	93%	92%
Incidence of Potentially Preventable VTE[1,2]	-	-	11%	10%
UFH with Dosages/Platelet Monitoring[2]	24	100%	94%	97%
Venous Thromboembolism Prophylaxis[2]	329	75%	86%	85%
Warfarin Therapy Discharge Instructions[2]	33	70%	71%	75%
Chest Pain/Possible Heart Attack Care				
Aspirin Given Within 24 Hours of Arrival[1,3]	-	-	96%	96%
Fibrinolytic Meds Within 30 Min. of Arrival[5]	-	-	65%	58%
Average Time to ECG (minutes)[1,3]	-	-	6	7
Average Time to Transfer (minutes)[5]	-	-	63	60
Children's Asthma Care				
Received Home Management Plan of Care	-	-	-	88%
Received Reliever Medication	-	-	-	100%
Received Systemic Corticosteroids	-	-	-	100%
Emergency Department				
Admittance Decision Time (minutes)[2]	493	115	89	98
Head CT Results Within 45 Min. of Arrival	13	69%	64%	57%
Patients Who Left ER Before Being Seen	29,333	3%	3%	2%
Time from ER Arrival to Admit. (minutes)[2]	527	265	260	274
Time from ER Arrival to Discharge (minutes)	328	121	138	134
Time in ER Before Being Evaluated (minutes)	398	30	28	26
Time to Pain Meds for Fractures (minutes)	68	61	52	57
Heart Attack Care				
Aspirin Given at Discharge	186	99%	99%	99%
Fibrinolytic Meds Within 30 Min. of Arrival[7]	-	-	33%	54%
PCI Within 90 Minutes of Arrival	16	94%	97%	96%
Statin Prescribed at Discharge	186	100%	98%	98%
Heart Failure Care				
ACE Inhibitor or ARB for LVSD	59	100%	98%	97%
Discharge Instructions Given	180	99%	96%	94%
Evaluation of LVS Function	244	100%	99%	99%
Medicare Spending				
Medicare Spending per Patient (ratio)	-	0.97	1	0.98
Pneumonia Care				
Appropriate Initial Antibiotic Given	92	93%	95%	95%
Blood Culture Timing	136	97%	98%	98%
Pregnancy and Delivery Care				
Newborn Deliveries Scheduled Early	48	0%	2%	6%
Preventive Care				
Immunization for Influenza[2]	563	76%	92%	90%
Immunization for Pneumonia[2]	708	77%	92%	92%
Stroke Care				
Anticoagulation Therapy for Atrial Fibrillation[1]	-	-	94%	95%
Antithrombotic Therapy Timing	89	100%	98%	98%
Assessed for Rehabilitation	90	100%	97%	97%
Discharged on Antithrombotic Therapy	89	100%	99%	99%
Discharged on Statin Medication	72	94%	94%	94%
Thrombolytic Therapy Timing[1]	-	-	66%	66%
Venous Thromboembolism Prophylaxis	86	90%	94%	94%
Written Stroke Educational Materials Given	57	98%	87%	88%
Surgical Care Improvement Project				
Appropriate Beta Blocker Usage[2]	188	99%	98%	98%
Appropriate VTP Within 24 Hours[2]	388	98%	98%	98%
Controlled Postoperative Blood Glucose[2]	77	91%	97%	97%
Perioperative Temperature Management[2]	454	100%	100%	100%
Prophylactic Antibiotic Selection[2]	350	100%	99%	99%
Prophylactic Antibiotic Selection (Outpatient)	323	99%	98%	98%
Prophylactic Antibiotic Stopped[2]	339	98%	98%	98%

NOTE: Hospital profiles are in alphabetical order by state, then city, then hospital within the city; Rankings exclude hospitals with less than 25 cases except for patient surveys which excludes hospitals with less than 100 cases; (a) 100-299 cases; (1) The number of cases/patients is too few to report; (2) Data submitted were based on a sample of cases/patients; (3) Results are based on a shorter time period than required; (4) Data suppressed by CMS for one or more quarters; (5) Results are not available for this reporting period; (6) Fewer than 100 patients completed the HCAHPS survey; (7) No cases met the criteria for this measure; (8) The lower limit of the confidence interval cannot be calculated if the number of observed infections equals zero; (9) No data are available from the state/territory for this reporting period; (10) The scores shown reflect fewer than 50 completed surveys; (11) There were discrepancies in the data collection process; (12) This measure does not apply to this hospital for this reporting period; (13) Results cannot be calculated for this reporting period; (14) The results for this state are combined with nearby states to protect confidentiality; Please refer to the User's Guide for a full explanation of data.

Measure	Cases	This Hosp.	State Avg.	U.S. Avg.
Prophylactic Antibiotic Timing[2]	350	100%	99%	99%
Prophylactic Antibiotic Timing (Outpatient)	326	98%	97%	98%
Urinary Catheter Removal[2]	372	99%	98%	97%
Survey of Patients' Hospital Experiences				
Area Around Room 'Always' Quiet at Night	300+	60%	60%	61%
Doctors 'Always' Communicated Well	300+	78%	81%	82%
Home Recovery Information Given	300+	87%	86%	85%
Hospital Given 9 or 10 on 10 Point Scale	300+	70%	70%	71%
Meds 'Always' Explained Before Given	300+	59%	64%	64%
Nurses 'Always' Communicated Well	300+	78%	79%	79%
Pain 'Always' Well Controlled	300+	67%	71%	71%
Room and Bathroom 'Always' Clean	300+	67%	74%	73%
Timely Help 'Always' Received	300+	60%	67%	68%
Would Definitely Recommend Hospital	300+	73%	70%	71%
Use of Medical Imaging				
Cardiac Imaging Stress Test before Surgery	213	2.3%	5.5%	5.3%
Combination Abdominal CT Scan	272	1.5%	10.1%	10.5%
Combination Brain/Sinus CT Scan[1]		-	2.6%	2.7%
Combination Chest CT Scan	145	0.7%	2.8%	2.7%
Follow-up Mammogram/Ultrasound	296	14.5%	8.4%	8.8%
Lumbar Spine MRI for Low Back Pain[1]		-	36.6%	37.2%

Fayette County Hospital

7th & Taylor
Vandalia, IL 62471
Phone: 618-283-1231
Fax: 618-283-4652
URL: www.fayettecountyhospital.org
Type: Critical Access Hospitals
Emergency Services: Yes
Ownership: Voluntary non-profit - Other
Beds: 160

Key Personnel:
Cardiac Laboratory. . . . . John Cowinjano
CEO/President. . . . . Denich Hucchison
Chief of Medical Staff. . . . . Brunch Schwarm

Measure	Cases	This Hosp.	State Avg.	U.S. Avg.
Blood Clot Prevention and Treatment				
Anticoagulation Overlap Therapy[5]	-	-	91%	93%
ICU Venous Thromboembolism Prophylaxis[5]	-	-	93%	92%
Incidence of Potentially Preventable VTE[5]	-	-	11%	10%
UFH with Dosages/Platelet Monitoring[5]	-	-	94%	97%
Venous Thromboembolism Prophylaxis[5]	-	-	86%	85%
Warfarin Therapy Discharge Instructions[5]	-	-	71%	75%
Chest Pain/Possible Heart Attack Care				
Aspirin Given Within 24 Hours of Arrival	-	-	96%	96%
Fibrinolytic Meds Within 30 Min. of Arrival	-	-	65%	58%
Average Time to ECG (minutes)	-	-	6	7
Average Time to Transfer (minutes)	-	-	63	60
Children's Asthma Care				
Received Home Management Plan of Care	-	-	-	88%
Received Reliever Medication	-	-	-	100%
Received Systemic Corticosteroids	-	-	-	100%
Emergency Department				
Admittance Decision Time (minutes)[5]	-	-	89	98
Head CT Results Within 45 Min. of Arrival	-	-	64%	57%
Patients Who Left ER Before Being Seen	-	-	3%	2%
Time from ER Arrival to Admit. (minutes)[5]	-	-	260	274
Time from ER Arrival to Discharge (minutes)	-	-	138	134
Time in ER Before Being Evaluated (minutes)	-	-	28	26
Time to Pain Meds for Fractures (minutes)	-	-	52	57
Heart Attack Care				
Aspirin Given at Discharge[5]	-	-	99%	99%
Fibrinolytic Meds Within 30 Min. of Arrival[5]	-	-	33%	54%
PCI Within 90 Minutes of Arrival[5]	-	-	97%	96%
Statin Prescribed at Discharge[5]	-	-	98%	98%
Heart Failure Care				
ACE Inhibitor or ARB for LVSD[1]	-	-	98%	97%
Discharge Instructions Given	32	100%	96%	94%
Evaluation of LVS Function	49	100%	99%	99%
Medicare Spending				
Medicare Spending per Patient (ratio)	-	-	1	0.98
Pneumonia Care				
Appropriate Initial Antibiotic Given	34	97%	95%	95%
Blood Culture Timing	56	98%	98%	98%
Pregnancy and Delivery Care				
Newborn Deliveries Scheduled Early[5]	-	-	2%	6%
Preventive Care				
Immunization for Influenza[5]	-	-	92%	90%
Immunization for Pneumonia[5]	-	-	92%	92%
Stroke Care				
Anticoagulation Therapy for Atrial Fibrillation[5]	-	-	94%	95%
Antithrombotic Therapy Timing[5]	-	-	98%	98%
Assessed for Rehabilitation[5]	-	-	97%	97%
Discharged on Antithrombotic Therapy[5]	-	-	99%	99%
Discharged on Statin Medication[5]	-	-	94%	94%
Thrombolytic Therapy Timing[5]	-	-	66%	66%
Venous Thromboembolism Prophylaxis[5]	-	-	94%	94%
Written Stroke Educational Materials Given[5]	-	-	87%	88%
Surgical Care Improvement Project				
Appropriate Beta Blocker Usage[1]	-	-	98%	98%
Appropriate VTP Within 24 Hours[1]	-	-	98%	98%
Controlled Postoperative Blood Glucose[7]	-	-	97%	97%
Perioperative Temperature Management[1]	-	-	100%	100%
Prophylactic Antibiotic Selection[1]	-	-	99%	99%
Prophylactic Antibiotic Selection (Outpatient)	-	-	98%	98%
Prophylactic Antibiotic Stopped[1]	-	-	98%	98%
Prophylactic Antibiotic Timing[1]	-	-	99%	99%
Prophylactic Antibiotic Timing (Outpatient)	-	-	97%	98%
Urinary Catheter Removal[1]	-	-	98%	97%
Survey of Patients' Hospital Experiences				
Area Around Room 'Always' Quiet at Night[5]	-	-	60%	61%
Doctors 'Always' Communicated Well[5]	-	-	81%	82%
Home Recovery Information Given[5]	-	-	86%	85%
Hospital Given 9 or 10 on 10 Point Scale[5]	-	-	70%	71%
Meds 'Always' Explained Before Given[5]	-	-	64%	64%
Nurses 'Always' Communicated Well[5]	-	-	79%	79%
Pain 'Always' Well Controlled[5]	-	-	71%	71%
Room and Bathroom 'Always' Clean[5]	-	-	74%	73%
Timely Help 'Always' Received[5]	-	-	67%	68%
Would Definitely Recommend Hospital[5]	-	-	70%	71%
Use of Medical Imaging				
Cardiac Imaging Stress Test before Surgery	-	-	5.5%	5.3%
Combination Abdominal CT Scan	-	-	10.1%	10.5%
Combination Brain/Sinus CT Scan	-	-	2.6%	2.7%
Combination Chest CT Scan	-	-	2.8%	2.7%
Follow-up Mammogram/Ultrasound	-	-	8.4%	8.8%
Lumbar Spine MRI for Low Back Pain	-	-	36.6%	37.2%

Iroquois Memorial Hospital

200 Fairman Street
Watseka, IL 60970
Phone: 815-432-5201
Fax: 815-432-7821
E-mail: info@iroquoimemorial.com
URL: www.iroquoismemorial.com
Type: Acute Care Hospitals
Emergency Services: Yes
Ownership: Voluntary non-profit - Private
Beds: 94

Key Personnel:
Infection Control. . . . . Lou Wonna Bell
Patient Relations . . . . Terri Fanning
Operating Room. . . . . Sharon Hilgendorf
Radiology. . . . . Kenneth Hurst
Coronary Care . . . . Peggy Jaskula
Intensive Care Unit. . . . . Peggy Jaskula, RN
CEO/President. . . . . Steve Leurck
Quality Assurance . . . . Tom McCann

Measure	Cases	This Hosp.	State Avg.	U.S. Avg.
Blood Clot Prevention and Treatment				
Anticoagulation Overlap Therapy[1,2]	-	-	91%	93%
ICU Venous Thromboembolism Prophylaxis[2]	27	85%	93%	92%
Incidence of Potentially Preventable VTE[1,2]	-	-	11%	10%
UFH with Dosages/Platelet Monitoring[1,2]	-	-	94%	97%
Venous Thromboembolism Prophylaxis[2]	92	72%	86%	85%
Warfarin Therapy Discharge Instructions[1,2]	-	-	71%	75%
Chest Pain/Possible Heart Attack Care				
Aspirin Given Within 24 Hours of Arrival[3]	15	93%	96%	96%
Fibrinolytic Meds Within 30 Min. of Arrival[1,3]	-	-	65%	58%
Average Time to ECG (minutes)[3]	15	13	6	7
Average Time to Transfer (minutes)[1,3]	-	-	63	60
Children's Asthma Care				
Received Home Management Plan of Care	-	-	-	88%
Received Reliever Medication	-	-	-	100%
Received Systemic Corticosteroids	-	-	-	100%
Emergency Department				
Admittance Decision Time (minutes)[2]	274	80	89	98
Head CT Results Within 45 Min. of Arrival[1]	-	-	64%	57%
Patients Who Left ER Before Being Seen	10,739	0%	3%	2%
Time from ER Arrival to Admit. (minutes)[2]	313	220	260	274
Time from ER Arrival to Discharge (minutes)	379	88	138	134
Time in ER Before Being Evaluated (minutes)	420	13	28	26
Time to Pain Meds for Fractures (minutes)	25	25	52	57
Heart Attack Care				
Aspirin Given at Discharge	16	88%	99%	99%
Fibrinolytic Meds Within 30 Min. of Arrival[1]	-	-	33%	54%
PCI Within 90 Minutes of Arrival[7]	-	-	97%	96%
Statin Prescribed at Discharge	17	76%	98%	98%
Heart Failure Care				
ACE Inhibitor or ARB for LVSD[1]	-	-	98%	97%
Discharge Instructions Given	12	83%	96%	94%
Evaluation of LVS Function	19	100%	99%	99%
Medicare Spending				
Medicare Spending per Patient (ratio)	-	0.90	1	0.98
Pneumonia Care				
Appropriate Initial Antibiotic Given	37	84%	95%	95%
Blood Culture Timing	76	99%	98%	98%
Pregnancy and Delivery Care				
Newborn Deliveries Scheduled Early[1,2]	-	-	2%	6%
Preventive Care				
Immunization for Influenza[2]	260	96%	92%	90%
Immunization for Pneumonia[2]	390	95%	92%	92%
Stroke Care				
Anticoagulation Therapy for Atrial Fibrillation[1]	-	-	94%	95%
Antithrombotic Therapy Timing[1]	-	-	98%	98%
Assessed for Rehabilitation[1]	-	-	97%	97%
Discharged on Antithrombotic Therapy[1]	-	-	99%	99%
Discharged on Statin Medication[1]	-	-	94%	94%
Thrombolytic Therapy Timing[7]	-	-	66%	66%
Venous Thromboembolism Prophylaxis[1]	-	-	94%	94%
Written Stroke Educational Materials Given[1]	-	-	87%	88%
Surgical Care Improvement Project				
Appropriate Beta Blocker Usage	18	94%	98%	98%
Appropriate VTP Within 24 Hours	29	97%	98%	98%
Controlled Postoperative Blood Glucose[7]	-	-	97%	97%
Perioperative Temperature Management	49	98%	100%	100%
Prophylactic Antibiotic Selection	25	96%	99%	99%
Prophylactic Antibiotic Selection (Outpatient)	56	96%	98%	98%
Prophylactic Antibiotic Stopped	23	91%	98%	98%
Prophylactic Antibiotic Timing	25	100%	99%	99%
Prophylactic Antibiotic Timing (Outpatient)	58	97%	97%	98%
Urinary Catheter Removal	39	92%	98%	97%
Survey of Patients' Hospital Experiences				
Area Around Room 'Always' Quiet at Night	(a)	54%	60%	61%
Doctors 'Always' Communicated Well	(a)	82%	81%	82%
Home Recovery Information Given	(a)	90%	86%	85%
Hospital Given 9 or 10 on 10 Point Scale	(a)	68%	70%	71%
Meds 'Always' Explained Before Given	(a)	66%	64%	64%
Nurses 'Always' Communicated Well	(a)	77%	79%	79%
Pain 'Always' Well Controlled	(a)	68%	71%	71%
Room and Bathroom 'Always' Clean	(a)	79%	74%	73%
Timely Help 'Always' Received	(a)	70%	67%	68%
Would Definitely Recommend Hospital	(a)	65%	70%	71%
Use of Medical Imaging				
Cardiac Imaging Stress Test before Surgery	61	0.0%	5.5%	5.3%
Combination Abdominal CT Scan	249	42.2%	10.1%	10.5%
Combination Brain/Sinus CT Scan	378	1.3%	2.6%	2.7%
Combination Chest CT Scan	117	34.2%	2.8%	2.7%
Follow-up Mammogram/Ultrasound	429	11.7%	8.4%	8.8%
Lumbar Spine MRI for Low Back Pain	34	50.0%	36.6%	37.2%

NOTE: Hospital profiles are in alphabetical order by state, then city, then hospital within the city; Rankings exclude hospitals with less than 25 cases except for patient surveys which excludes hospitals with less than 100 cases; (a) 100-299 cases; (1) The number of cases/patients is too few to report; (2) Data submitted were based on a sample of cases/patients; (3) Results are based on a shorter time period than required; (4) Data suppressed by CMS for one or more quarters; (5) Results are not available for this reporting period; (6) Fewer than 100 patients completed the HCAHPS survey; (7) No cases met the criteria for this measure; (8) The lower limit of the confidence interval cannot be calculated if the number of observed infections equals zero; (9) No data are available from the state/territory for this reporting period; (10) The scores shown reflect fewer than 50 completed surveys; (11) There were discrepancies in the data collection process; (12) This measure does not apply to this hospital for this reporting period; (13) Results cannot be calculated for this reporting period; (14) The results for this state are combined with nearby states to protect confidentiality; Please refer to the User's Guide for a full explanation of data.

Vista Medical Center East

1324 North Sheridan Road
Waukegan, IL 60085
URL: www.vistahealth.com
Type: Acute Care Hospitals
Ownership: Voluntary non-profit - Other
Phone: 847-360-4000
Fax: 847-360-4230
Emergency Services: Yes
Beds: 299

Key Personnel:
CEO/President. . . . . Timothy Harrington
Quality Assurance . . . . Lora Johnas

Measure	Cases	This Hosp.	State Avg.	U.S. Avg.
Blood Clot Prevention and Treatment				
Anticoagulation Overlap Therapy[2]	79	96%	91%	93%
ICU Venous Thromboembolism Prophylaxis[2]	107	100%	93%	92%
Incidence of Potentially Preventable VTE[2]	13	23%	11%	10%
UFH with Dosages/Platelet Monitoring[2]	37	100%	94%	97%
Venous Thromboembolism Prophylaxis[2]	395	100%	86%	85%
Warfarin Therapy Discharge Instructions[2]	54	100%	71%	75%
Chest Pain/Possible Heart Attack Care				
Aspirin Given Within 24 Hours of Arrival[1,3]	-	-	96%	96%
Fibrinolytic Meds Within 30 Min. of Arrival[5]	-	-	65%	58%
Average Time to ECG (minutes)[1,3]	-	-	6	7
Average Time to Transfer (minutes)[5]	-	-	63	60
Children's Asthma Care				
Received Home Management Plan of Care	-	-	-	88%
Received Reliever Medication	-	-	-	100%
Received Systemic Corticosteroids	-	-	-	100%
Emergency Department				
Admittance Decision Time (minutes)[2]	777	115	89	98
Head CT Results Within 45 Min. of Arrival[1]	-	-	64%	57%
Patients Who Left ER Before Being Seen	42,973	1%	3%	2%
Time from ER Arrival to Admit. (minutes)[2]	778	276	260	274
Time from ER Arrival to Discharge (minutes)	390	111	138	134
Time in ER Before Being Evaluated (minutes)	416	17	28	26
Time to Pain Meds for Fractures (minutes)	194	42	52	57
Heart Attack Care				
Aspirin Given at Discharge	127	100%	99%	99%
Fibrinolytic Meds Within 30 Min. of Arrival[7]	-	-	33%	54%
PCI Within 90 Minutes of Arrival	31	100%	97%	96%
Statin Prescribed at Discharge	132	100%	98%	98%
Heart Failure Care				
ACE Inhibitor or ARB for LVSD	141	100%	98%	97%
Discharge Instructions Given	286	100%	96%	94%
Evaluation of LVS Function	375	100%	99%	99%
Medicare Spending				
Medicare Spending per Patient (ratio)	-	1.04	1	0.98
Pneumonia Care				
Appropriate Initial Antibiotic Given	150	99%	95%	95%
Blood Culture Timing	281	100%	98%	98%
Pregnancy and Delivery Care				
Newborn Deliveries Scheduled Early[2]	23	0%	2%	6%
Preventive Care				
Immunization for Influenza[2]	642	100%	92%	90%
Immunization for Pneumonia[2]	700	100%	92%	92%
Stroke Care				
Anticoagulation Therapy for Atrial Fibrillation	15	93%	94%	95%
Antithrombotic Therapy Timing	96	100%	98%	98%
Assessed for Rehabilitation	133	100%	97%	97%
Discharged on Antithrombotic Therapy	100	100%	99%	99%
Discharged on Statin Medication	78	100%	94%	94%
Thrombolytic Therapy Timing[1]	-	-	66%	66%
Venous Thromboembolism Prophylaxis	142	100%	94%	94%
Written Stroke Educational Materials Given	59	98%	87%	88%
Surgical Care Improvement Project				
Appropriate Beta Blocker Usage	125	98%	98%	98%
Appropriate VTP Within 24 Hours	300	100%	98%	98%
Controlled Postoperative Blood Glucose	65	95%	97%	97%
Perioperative Temperature Management	344	100%	100%	100%
Prophylactic Antibiotic Selection	272	100%	99%	99%
Prophylactic Antibiotic Selection (Outpatient)	210	99%	98%	98%
Prophylactic Antibiotic Stopped	272	100%	98%	98%
Prophylactic Antibiotic Timing	273	100%	99%	99%
Prophylactic Antibiotic Timing (Outpatient)	208	100%	97%	98%
Urinary Catheter Removal	199	100%	98%	97%
Survey of Patients' Hospital Experiences				
Area Around Room 'Always' Quiet at Night	300+	54%	60%	61%
Doctors 'Always' Communicated Well	300+	79%	81%	82%
Home Recovery Information Given	300+	85%	86%	85%
Hospital Given 9 or 10 on 10 Point Scale	300+	61%	70%	71%
Meds 'Always' Explained Before Given	300+	58%	64%	64%
Nurses 'Always' Communicated Well	300+	72%	79%	79%
Pain 'Always' Well Controlled	300+	66%	71%	71%
Room and Bathroom 'Always' Clean	300+	67%	74%	73%
Timely Help 'Always' Received	300+	56%	67%	68%
Would Definitely Recommend Hospital	300+	58%	70%	71%
Use of Medical Imaging				
Cardiac Imaging Stress Test before Surgery	159	9.4%	5.5%	5.3%
Combination Abdominal CT Scan	858	17.1%	10.1%	10.5%
Combination Brain/Sinus CT Scan	912	5.3%	2.6%	2.7%
Combination Chest CT Scan	495	4.0%	2.8%	2.7%
Follow-up Mammogram/Ultrasound	2,256	4.3%	8.4%	8.8%
Lumbar Spine MRI for Low Back Pain	224	37.1%	36.6%	37.2%

Vista Medical Center West

2615 Washington St
Waukegan, IL 60085
URL: www.vistahealth.com
Type: Acute Care Hospitals
Ownership: Voluntary non-profit - Church
Phone: 847-249-3900
Fax: 847-360-4230
Emergency Services: Yes
Beds: 388

Key Personnel:
Intensive Care Unit. . . . . Kathy Dumalski
Operating Room. . . . . Marianne Finlay
CEO/President. . . . . Timothy J Harrington
Quality Assurance . . . . Lora Johnas
Radiology. . . . . Elaine Pape, MD
Emergency Room . . . . Denise Tucker, RN
Infection Control. . . . . Karen VanBuren
Patient Relations . . . . Mary Anne Yuknay

Measure	Cases	This Hosp.	State Avg.	U.S. Avg.
Blood Clot Prevention and Treatment				
Anticoagulation Overlap Therapy[2,7]	-	-	91%	93%
ICU Venous Thromboembolism Prophylaxis[2,7]	-	-	93%	92%
Incidence of Potentially Preventable VTE[2,7]	-	-	11%	10%
UFH with Dosages/Platelet Monitoring[2,7]	-	-	94%	97%
Venous Thromboembolism Prophylaxis[2,7]	-	-	86%	85%
Warfarin Therapy Discharge Instructions[2,7]	-	-	71%	75%
Chest Pain/Possible Heart Attack Care				
Aspirin Given Within 24 Hours of Arrival	16	100%	96%	96%
Fibrinolytic Meds Within 30 Min. of Arrival[3,7]	-	-	65%	58%
Average Time to ECG (minutes)	16	5	6	7
Average Time to Transfer (minutes)[1,3]	-	-	63	60
Children's Asthma Care				
Received Home Management Plan of Care	-	-	-	88%
Received Reliever Medication	-	-	-	100%
Received Systemic Corticosteroids	-	-	-	100%
Emergency Department				
Admittance Decision Time (minutes)[2,7]	-	-	89	98
Head CT Results Within 45 Min. of Arrival[1]	-	-	64%	57%
Patients Who Left ER Before Being Seen	12,494	1%	3%	2%
Time from ER Arrival to Admit. (minutes)[2,7]	-	-	260	274
Time from ER Arrival to Discharge (minutes)	335	101	138	134
Time in ER Before Being Evaluated (minutes)	421	12	28	26
Time to Pain Meds for Fractures (minutes)	21	48	52	57
Heart Attack Care				
Aspirin Given at Discharge[5]	-	-	99%	99%
Fibrinolytic Meds Within 30 Min. of Arrival[5]	-	-	33%	54%
PCI Within 90 Minutes of Arrival[5]	-	-	97%	96%
Statin Prescribed at Discharge[5]	-	-	98%	98%
Heart Failure Care				
ACE Inhibitor or ARB for LVSD[5]	-	-	98%	97%
Discharge Instructions Given[5]	-	-	96%	94%
Evaluation of LVS Function[5]	-	-	99%	99%
Medicare Spending				
Medicare Spending per Patient (ratio)	-	-	1	0.98
Pneumonia Care				
Appropriate Initial Antibiotic Given[5]	-	-	95%	95%
Blood Culture Timing[5]	-	-	98%	98%
Pregnancy and Delivery Care				
Newborn Deliveries Scheduled Early[2,7]	-	-	2%	6%
Preventive Care				
Immunization for Influenza[2]	262	98%	92%	90%
Immunization for Pneumonia[1,2]	-	-	92%	92%
Stroke Care				
Anticoagulation Therapy for Atrial Fibrillation[5]	-	-	94%	95%
Antithrombotic Therapy Timing[5]	-	-	98%	98%
Assessed for Rehabilitation[5]	-	-	97%	97%
Discharged on Antithrombotic Therapy[5]	-	-	99%	99%
Discharged on Statin Medication[5]	-	-	94%	94%
Thrombolytic Therapy Timing[5]	-	-	66%	66%
Venous Thromboembolism Prophylaxis[5]	-	-	94%	94%
Written Stroke Educational Materials Given[5]	-	-	87%	88%
Surgical Care Improvement Project				
Appropriate Beta Blocker Usage[5]	-	-	98%	98%
Appropriate VTP Within 24 Hours[5]	-	-	98%	98%
Controlled Postoperative Blood Glucose[5]	-	-	97%	97%
Perioperative Temperature Management[5]	-	-	100%	100%
Prophylactic Antibiotic Selection[5]	-	-	99%	99%
Prophylactic Antibiotic Selection (Outpatient)[5]	-	-	98%	98%
Prophylactic Antibiotic Stopped[5]	-	-	98%	98%
Prophylactic Antibiotic Timing[5]	-	-	99%	99%
Prophylactic Antibiotic Timing (Outpatient)[5]	-	-	97%	98%
Urinary Catheter Removal[5]	-	-	98%	97%
Survey of Patients' Hospital Experiences				
Area Around Room 'Always' Quiet at Night[1]	-	-	60%	61%
Doctors 'Always' Communicated Well[1]	-	-	81%	82%
Home Recovery Information Given[1]	-	-	86%	85%
Hospital Given 9 or 10 on 10 Point Scale[1]	-	-	70%	71%
Meds 'Always' Explained Before Given[1]	-	-	64%	64%
Nurses 'Always' Communicated Well[1]	-	-	79%	79%
Pain 'Always' Well Controlled[1]	-	-	71%	71%
Room and Bathroom 'Always' Clean[1]	-	-	74%	73%
Timely Help 'Always' Received[1]	-	-	67%	68%
Would Definitely Recommend Hospital[1]	-	-	70%	71%
Use of Medical Imaging				
Cardiac Imaging Stress Test before Surgery[7]	-	-	5.5%	5.3%
Combination Abdominal CT Scan[1]	-	-	10.1%	10.5%
Combination Brain/Sinus CT Scan[1]	-	-	2.6%	2.7%
Combination Chest CT Scan[1]	-	-	2.8%	2.7%
Follow-up Mammogram/Ultrasound[7]	-	-	8.4%	8.8%
Lumbar Spine MRI for Low Back Pain[7]	-	-	36.6%	37.2%

Central Dupage Hospital

25 North Winfield Road
Winfield, IL 60190
E-mail: cdh_information@cdh.org
URL: www.cdh.org
Type: Acute Care Hospitals
Ownership: Voluntary non-profit - Private
Phone: 630-682-1600
Fax: 630-933-1300
Emergency Services: Yes
Beds: 20

Key Personnel:
Chief of Medical Staff . . . . Kevin Most
CEO/President. . . . . Michael Vivoda

Measure	Cases	This Hosp.	State Avg.	U.S. Avg.
Blood Clot Prevention and Treatment				
Anticoagulation Overlap Therapy[2]	163	94%	91%	93%
ICU Venous Thromboembolism Prophylaxis[2]	61	92%	93%	92%
Incidence of Potentially Preventable VTE[2]	53	9%	11%	10%
UFH with Dosages/Platelet Monitoring[2]	101	62%	94%	97%
Venous Thromboembolism Prophylaxis[2]	258	84%	86%	85%
Warfarin Therapy Discharge Instructions[2]	118	29%	71%	75%
Chest Pain/Possible Heart Attack Care				
Aspirin Given Within 24 Hours of Arrival[5]	-	-	96%	96%
Fibrinolytic Meds Within 30 Min. of Arrival[5]	-	-	65%	58%
Average Time to ECG (minutes)[5]	-	-	6	7
Average Time to Transfer (minutes)[5]	-	-	63	60
Children's Asthma Care				
Received Home Management Plan of Care	-	-	-	88%
Received Reliever Medication	-	-	-	100%
Received Systemic Corticosteroids	-	-	-	100%
Emergency Department				
Admittance Decision Time (minutes)[2]	408	94	89	98
Head CT Results Within 45 Min. of Arrival[5]	-	-	64%	57%

NOTE: Hospital profiles are in alphabetical order by state, then city, then hospital within the city; Rankings exclude hospitals with less than 25 cases except for patient surveys which excludes hospitals with less than 100 cases; (a) 100-299 cases; (1) The number of cases/patients is too few to report; (2) Data submitted were based on a sample of cases/patients; (3) Results are based on a shorter time period than required; (4) Data suppressed by CMS for one or more quarters; (5) Results are not available for this reporting period; (6) Fewer than 100 patients completed the HCAHPS survey; (7) No cases met the criteria for this measure; (8) The lower limit of the confidence interval cannot be calculated if the number of observed infections equals zero; (9) No data are available from the state/territory for this reporting period; (10) The scores shown reflect fewer than 50 completed surveys; (11) There were discrepancies in the data collection process; (12) This measure does not apply to this hospital for this reporting period; (13) Results cannot be calculated for this reporting period; (14) The results for this state are combined with nearby states to protect confidentiality; Please refer to the User's Guide for a full explanation of data.

Measure	Cases	This Hosp.	State Avg.	U.S. Avg.
Patients Who Left ER Before Being Seen	72,326	1%	3%	2%
Time from ER Arrival to Admit. (minutes)[2]	412	238	260	274
Time from ER Arrival to Discharge (minutes)	378	154	138	134
Time in ER Before Being Evaluated (minutes)	328	28	28	26
Time to Pain Meds for Fractures (minutes)	264	37	52	57
Heart Attack Care				
Aspirin Given at Discharge	191	100%	99%	99%
Fibrinolytic Meds Within 30 Min. of Arrival[7]	-	-	33%	54%
PCI Within 90 Minutes of Arrival	61	100%	97%	96%
Statin Prescribed at Discharge	187	99%	98%	98%
Heart Failure Care				
ACE Inhibitor or ARB for LVSD	111	99%	98%	97%
Discharge Instructions Given	418	100%	96%	94%
Evaluation of LVS Function	523	100%	99%	99%
Medicare Spending				
Medicare Spending per Patient (ratio)	-	1.02	1	0.98
Pneumonia Care				
Appropriate Initial Antibiotic Given	201	98%	95%	95%
Blood Culture Timing	300	97%	98%	98%
Pregnancy and Delivery Care				
Newborn Deliveries Scheduled Early[2]	243	3%	2%	6%
Preventive Care				
Immunization for Influenza[2]	581	91%	92%	90%
Immunization for Pneumonia[2]	581	87%	92%	92%
Stroke Care				
Anticoagulation Therapy for Atrial Fibrillation[1,2]	-	-	94%	95%
Antithrombotic Therapy Timing[2]	66	98%	98%	98%
Assessed for Rehabilitation[2]	116	99%	97%	97%
Discharged on Antithrombotic Therapy[2]	92	100%	99%	99%
Discharged on Statin Medication[2]	65	95%	94%	94%
Thrombolytic Therapy Timing[1,2]	-	-	66%	66%
Venous Thromboembolism Prophylaxis[2]	114	98%	94%	94%
Written Stroke Educational Materials Given[2]	60	98%	87%	88%
Surgical Care Improvement Project				
Appropriate Beta Blocker Usage[2]	163	99%	98%	98%
Appropriate VTP Within 24 Hours[2]	367	98%	98%	98%
Controlled Postoperative Blood Glucose[2]	117	100%	97%	97%
Perioperative Temperature Management[2]	445	100%	100%	100%
Prophylactic Antibiotic Selection[2]	418	99%	99%	99%
Prophylactic Antibiotic Selection (Outpatient)	423	98%	98%	98%
Prophylactic Antibiotic Stopped[2]	413	96%	98%	98%
Prophylactic Antibiotic Timing[2]	420	95%	99%	99%
Prophylactic Antibiotic Timing (Outpatient)	439	93%	97%	98%
Urinary Catheter Removal[2]	286	96%	98%	97%
Survey of Patients' Hospital Experiences				
Area Around Room 'Always' Quiet at Night	300+	67%	60%	61%
Doctors 'Always' Communicated Well	300+	81%	81%	82%
Home Recovery Information Given	300+	88%	86%	85%
Hospital Given 9 or 10 on 10 Point Scale	300+	83%	70%	71%
Meds 'Always' Explained Before Given	300+	67%	64%	64%
Nurses 'Always' Communicated Well	300+	81%	79%	79%
Pain 'Always' Well Controlled	300+	76%	71%	71%
Room and Bathroom 'Always' Clean	300+	75%	74%	73%
Timely Help 'Always' Received	300+	67%	67%	68%
Would Definitely Recommend Hospital	300+	83%	70%	71%
Use of Medical Imaging				
Cardiac Imaging Stress Test before Surgery	737	5.3%	5.5%	5.3%
Combination Abdominal CT Scan	1,701	5.4%	10.1%	10.5%
Combination Brain/Sinus CT Scan	1,342	1.0%	2.6%	2.7%
Combination Chest CT Scan	1,288	0.9%	2.8%	2.7%
Follow-up Mammogram/Ultrasound	3,183	6.6%	8.4%	8.8%
Lumbar Spine MRI for Low Back Pain	216	35.2%	36.6%	37.2%

Centegra Health System - Woodstock Hospital

3701 Doty Road
Woodstock, IL 60098
Phone: 815-788-5823
Fax: 815-334-3948
URL: www.centegra.org
Type: Acute Care Hospitals
Emergency Services: Yes
Ownership: Voluntary non-profit - Private
Beds: 154

Key Personnel:
CEO . . . . Michael S. Eesley
CEO/President. . . . . Paul Laubick

Measure	Cases	This Hosp.	State Avg.	U.S. Avg.
Blood Clot Prevention and Treatment				
Anticoagulation Overlap Therapy[2]	49	76%	91%	93%
ICU Venous Thromboembolism Prophylaxis[2]	81	98%	93%	92%
Incidence of Potentially Preventable VTE[1,2]	-	-	11%	10%
UFH with Dosages/Platelet Monitoring[2]	35	100%	94%	97%
Venous Thromboembolism Prophylaxis[2]	311	86%	86%	85%
Warfarin Therapy Discharge Instructions[2]	37	62%	71%	75%
Chest Pain/Possible Heart Attack Care				
Aspirin Given Within 24 Hours of Arrival	42	95%	96%	96%
Fibrinolytic Meds Within 30 Min. of Arrival[7]	-	-	65%	58%
Average Time to ECG (minutes)	44	4	6	7
Average Time to Transfer (minutes)	18	49	63	60
Children's Asthma Care				
Received Home Management Plan of Care	-	-	-	88%
Received Reliever Medication	-	-	-	100%
Received Systemic Corticosteroids	-	-	-	100%
Emergency Department				
Admittance Decision Time (minutes)[2]	500	80	89	98
Head CT Results Within 45 Min. of Arrival[1]	-	-	64%	57%
Patients Who Left ER Before Being Seen	27,577	2%	3%	2%
Time from ER Arrival to Admit. (minutes)[2]	535	249	260	274
Time from ER Arrival to Discharge (minutes)	391	134	138	134
Time in ER Before Being Evaluated (minutes)	429	38	28	26
Time to Pain Meds for Fractures (minutes)	88	50	52	57
Heart Attack Care				
Aspirin Given at Discharge[1]	-	-	99%	99%
Fibrinolytic Meds Within 30 Min. of Arrival[7]	-	-	33%	54%
PCI Within 90 Minutes of Arrival[7]	-	-	97%	96%
Statin Prescribed at Discharge[1]	-	-	98%	98%
Heart Failure Care				
ACE Inhibitor or ARB for LVSD	15	93%	98%	97%
Discharge Instructions Given	62	95%	96%	94%
Evaluation of LVS Function	94	100%	99%	99%
Medicare Spending				
Medicare Spending per Patient (ratio)	-	1.00	1	0.98
Pneumonia Care				
Appropriate Initial Antibiotic Given	71	96%	95%	95%
Blood Culture Timing	120	99%	98%	98%
Pregnancy and Delivery Care				
Newborn Deliveries Scheduled Early	97	4%	2%	6%
Preventive Care				
Immunization for Influenza[2]	543	97%	92%	90%
Immunization for Pneumonia[2]	603	96%	92%	92%
Stroke Care				
Anticoagulation Therapy for Atrial Fibrillation[1]	-	-	94%	95%
Antithrombotic Therapy Timing	50	98%	98%	98%
Assessed for Rehabilitation	61	98%	97%	97%
Discharged on Antithrombotic Therapy	57	100%	99%	99%
Discharged on Statin Medication	47	100%	94%	94%
Thrombolytic Therapy Timing[1]	-	-	66%	66%
Venous Thromboembolism Prophylaxis	58	100%	94%	94%
Written Stroke Educational Materials Given	32	97%	87%	88%
Surgical Care Improvement Project				
Appropriate Beta Blocker Usage[2]	158	99%	98%	98%
Appropriate VTP Within 24 Hours[2]	446	100%	98%	98%
Controlled Postoperative Blood Glucose[2,7]	-	-	97%	97%
Perioperative Temperature Management[2]	514	100%	100%	100%
Prophylactic Antibiotic Selection[2]	390	99%	99%	99%
Prophylactic Antibiotic Selection (Outpatient)	44	95%	98%	98%
Prophylactic Antibiotic Stopped[2]	387	98%	98%	98%
Prophylactic Antibiotic Timing[2]	390	99%	99%	99%
Prophylactic Antibiotic Timing (Outpatient)	44	98%	97%	98%
Urinary Catheter Removal[2]	374	100%	98%	97%
Survey of Patients' Hospital Experiences				
Area Around Room 'Always' Quiet at Night	300+	52%	60%	61%
Doctors 'Always' Communicated Well	300+	81%	81%	82%
Home Recovery Information Given	300+	88%	86%	85%
Hospital Given 9 or 10 on 10 Point Scale	300+	67%	70%	71%
Meds 'Always' Explained Before Given	300+	65%	64%	64%
Nurses 'Always' Communicated Well	300+	79%	79%	79%
Pain 'Always' Well Controlled	300+	71%	71%	71%
Room and Bathroom 'Always' Clean	300+	79%	74%	73%
Timely Help 'Always' Received	300+	69%	67%	68%
Would Definitely Recommend Hospital	300+	69%	70%	71%
Use of Medical Imaging				
Cardiac Imaging Stress Test before Surgery	361	6.9%	5.5%	5.3%
Combination Abdominal CT Scan	639	8.3%	10.1%	10.5%
Combination Brain/Sinus CT Scan	602	4.3%	2.6%	2.7%
Combination Chest CT Scan	391	4.6%	2.8%	2.7%
Follow-up Mammogram/Ultrasound	1,558	6.0%	8.4%	8.8%
Lumbar Spine MRI for Low Back Pain	161	28.0%	36.6%	37.2%

Midwestern Region Medical Center

2520 Elisha Avenue
Zion, IL 60099
Phone: 847-872-4561
Fax: 847-872-6222
E-mail: susan.thomas@mrmc-ctca.com
URL: www.cancercare.com
Type: Acute Care Hospitals
Emergency Services: Yes
Ownership: Proprietary
Beds: 95

Key Personnel:
CEO/President. . . . . Roger Cary
Operating Room. . . . . Sharon Dimitrijevich
Chief of Medical Staff . . . . Joel Granitk
Infection Control. . . . . Debra Horton
Quality Assurance . . . . Carol Lepper
Radiology. . . . . Pakorn Sirijintakarn, MD

Measure	Cases	This Hosp.	State Avg.	U.S. Avg.
Blood Clot Prevention and Treatment				
Anticoagulation Overlap Therapy[2,7]	-	-	91%	93%
ICU Venous Thromboembolism Prophylaxis[2]	26	88%	93%	92%
Incidence of Potentially Preventable VTE[1,2]	-	-	11%	10%
UFH with Dosages/Platelet Monitoring[1,2]	-	-	94%	97%
Venous Thromboembolism Prophylaxis[2]	179	74%	86%	85%
Warfarin Therapy Discharge Instructions[2,7]	-	-	71%	75%
Chest Pain/Possible Heart Attack Care				
Aspirin Given Within 24 Hours of Arrival[1,3]	-	-	96%	96%
Fibrinolytic Meds Within 30 Min. of Arrival[3,7]	-	-	65%	58%
Average Time to ECG (minutes)[1,3]	-	-	6	7
Average Time to Transfer (minutes)[3,7]	-	-	63	60
Children's Asthma Care				
Received Home Management Plan of Care	-	-	-	88%
Received Reliever Medication	-	-	-	100%
Received Systemic Corticosteroids	-	-	-	100%
Emergency Department				
Admittance Decision Time (minutes)[2]	20	146	89	98
Head CT Results Within 45 Min. of Arrival[5]	-	-	64%	57%
Patients Who Left ER Before Being Seen	2,219	3%	3%	2%
Time from ER Arrival to Admit. (minutes)[2]	22	306	260	274
Time from ER Arrival to Discharge (minutes)	238	98	138	134
Time in ER Before Being Evaluated (minutes)	163	39	28	26
Time to Pain Meds for Fractures (minutes)[1]	-	-	52	57
Heart Attack Care				
Aspirin Given at Discharge[1,3]	-	-	99%	99%
Fibrinolytic Meds Within 30 Min. of Arrival[3,7]	-	-	33%	54%
PCI Within 90 Minutes of Arrival[3,7]	-	-	97%	96%
Statin Prescribed at Discharge[3,7]	-	-	98%	98%
Heart Failure Care				
ACE Inhibitor or ARB for LVSD[1]	-	-	98%	97%
Discharge Instructions Given[1]	-	-	96%	94%
Evaluation of LVS Function[1]	-	-	99%	99%
Medicare Spending				
Medicare Spending per Patient (ratio)	-	1.36	1	0.98
Pneumonia Care				
Appropriate Initial Antibiotic Given[1]	-	-	95%	95%
Blood Culture Timing[1]	-	-	98%	98%
Pregnancy and Delivery Care				
Newborn Deliveries Scheduled Early[7]	-	-	2%	6%
Preventive Care				
Immunization for Influenza[2]	291	85%	92%	90%
Immunization for Pneumonia[2]	155	98%	92%	92%
Stroke Care				
Anticoagulation Therapy for Atrial Fibrillation[3,7]	-	-	94%	95%
Antithrombotic Therapy Timing[1,3]	-	-	98%	98%
Assessed for Rehabilitation[1,3]	-	-	97%	97%
Discharged on Antithrombotic Therapy[1,3]	-	-	99%	99%
Discharged on Statin Medication[1,3]	-	-	94%	94%

NOTE: Hospital profiles are in alphabetical order by state, then city, then hospital within the city; Rankings exclude hospitals with less than 25 cases except for patient surveys which excludes hospitals with less than 100 cases; (a) 100-299 cases; (1) The number of cases/patients is too few to report; (2) Data submitted were based on a sample of cases/patients; (3) Results are based on a shorter time period than required; (4) Data suppressed by CMS for one or more quarters; (5) Results are not available for this reporting period; (6) Fewer than 100 patients completed the HCAHPS survey; (7) No cases met the criteria for this measure; (8) The lower limit of the confidence interval cannot be calculated if the number of observed infections equals zero; (9) No data are available from the state/territory for this reporting period; (10) The scores shown reflect fewer than 50 completed surveys; (11) There were discrepancies in the data collection process; (12) This measure does not apply to this hospital for this reporting period; (13) Results cannot be calculated for this reporting period; (14) The results for this state are combined with nearby states to protect confidentiality; Please refer to the User's Guide for a full explanation of data.

Thrombolytic Therapy Timing[3,7]	-	-	66%	66%
Venous Thromboembolism Prophylaxis[1,3]	-	-	94%	94%
Written Stroke Educational Materials Given[1,3]	-	-	87%	88%
Surgical Care Improvement Project				
Appropriate Beta Blocker Usage[2]	19	100%	98%	98%
Appropriate VTP Within 24 Hours[2]	151	99%	98%	98%
Controlled Postoperative Blood Glucose[2,7]	-	-	97%	97%
Perioperative Temperature Management[2]	153	100%	100%	100%
Prophylactic Antibiotic Selection[2]	71	99%	99%	99%
Prophylactic Antibiotic Selection (Outpatient)	55	75%	98%	98%
Prophylactic Antibiotic Stopped[2]	65	98%	98%	98%
Prophylactic Antibiotic Timing[2]	71	97%	99%	99%
Prophylactic Antibiotic Timing (Outpatient)	56	98%	97%	98%
Urinary Catheter Removal[2]	40	100%	98%	97%
Survey of Patients' Hospital Experiences				
Area Around Room 'Always' Quiet at Night	300+	64%	60%	61%
Doctors 'Always' Communicated Well	300+	84%	81%	82%
Home Recovery Information Given	300+	92%	86%	85%
Hospital Given 9 or 10 on 10 Point Scale	300+	88%	70%	71%
Meds 'Always' Explained Before Given	300+	69%	64%	64%
Nurses 'Always' Communicated Well	300+	83%	79%	79%
Pain 'Always' Well Controlled	300+	76%	71%	71%
Room and Bathroom 'Always' Clean	300+	77%	74%	73%
Timely Help 'Always' Received	300+	72%	67%	68%
Would Definitely Recommend Hospital	300+	90%	70%	71%
Use of Medical Imaging				
Cardiac Imaging Stress Test before Surgery[1]	-	-	5.5%	5.3%
Combination Abdominal CT Scan	949	96.4%	10.1%	10.5%
Combination Brain/Sinus CT Scan[1]	-	-	2.6%	2.7%
Combination Chest CT Scan	1,060	0.0%	2.8%	2.7%
Follow-up Mammogram/Ultrasound	173	6.4%	8.4%	8.8%
Lumbar Spine MRI for Low Back Pain[1]	-	-	36.6%	37.2%

NOTE: Hospital profiles are in alphabetical order by state, then city, then hospital within the city; Rankings exclude hospitals with less than 25 cases except for patient surveys which excludes hospitals with less than 100 cases; (a) 100-299 cases; (1) The number of cases/patients is too few to report; (2) Data submitted were based on a sample of cases/patients; (3) Results are based on a shorter time period than required; (4) Data suppressed by CMS for one or more quarters; (5) Results are not available for this reporting period; (6) Fewer than 100 patients completed the HCAHPS survey; (7) No cases met the criteria for this measure; (8) The lower limit of the confidence interval cannot be calculated if the number of observed infections equals zero; (9) No data are available from the state/territory for this reporting period; (10) The scores shown reflect fewer than 50 completed surveys; (11) There were discrepancies in the data collection process; (12) This measure does not apply to this hospital for this reporting period; (13) Results cannot be calculated for this reporting period; (14) The results for this state are combined with nearby states to protect confidentiality; Please refer to the User's Guide for a full explanation of data.

Blood Clot Prevention and Treatment

Anticoagulation Overlap Therapy

Hospital Name	City	Rate	Cases
Eskenazi Health[2]	Indianapolis	100%	39
Hendricks Regional Health[2]	Danville	100%	32
Saint Catherine Hospital[2]	East Chicago	100%	29
Saint Joseph Regional Medical Center[2]	Mishawaka	100%	117
Saint Mary Medical Center[2]	Hobart	100%	62
Terre Haute Regional Hospital[2]	Terre Haute	100%	25
Floyd Memorial Hospital & Health Services[2]	New Albany	99%	105
Indiana Univ Health Bloomington Hosp[2]	Bloomington	99%	87
Reid Hospital & Health Care Services[2]	Richmond	99%	67
Saint Vincent Hospital & Health Services[2]	Indianapolis	99%	164
Columbus Regional Hospital[2]	Columbus	98%	55
Indiana University Health[2]	Indianapolis	98%	226
Lutheran Hospital of Indiana[2]	Fort Wayne	98%	167
Union Hospital[2]	Terre Haute	98%	112
Elkhart General Hospital[2]	Elkhart	97%	139
Kosciusko Community Hospital[2]	Warsaw	97%	32
Riverview Hospital[2]	Noblesville	97%	29
Community Hospital[2]	Munster	96%	124
Community Howard Regional Health[2]	Kokomo	96%	28
Saint Mary's Medical Center of Evansville[2]	Evansville	96%	128
Franciscan St Anthony Health-Crown Pt[2]	Crown Point	95%	77
Franciscan Saint Margaret Health - Dyer[2]	Dyer	95%	42
Franciscan St Margaret Health-Hammond[2]	Hammond	95%	100
Indiana Univ Health Ball Mem Hosp[2]	Muncie	95%	133
Franciscan St Francis Hlth-Indianapolis[2]	Indianapolis	94%	107
Indiana University Health North Hospital[2]	Carmel	94%	33
IU Health West Hospital[2]	Avon	94%	54
Henry County Memorial Hospital[2]	New Castle	93%	27
Deaconess Hospital[2]	Evansville	92%	149
Saint Vincent Anderson Regional Hospital[2]	Anderson	92%	48
Community Hospital East[2]	Indianapolis	91%	74
Comm Hosp of Anderson/Madison Co[2]	Anderson	91%	32
Memorial Hospital & Health Care Center[2]	Jasper	91%	32
Parkview Regional Medical Center[2]	Fort Wayne	90%	195
Indiana University Health Arnett Hospital[2]	Lafayette	89%	81
Johnson Memorial Hospital[2]	Franklin	88%	32
Community Hospital South[2]	Indianapolis	86%	50
Franciscan St Elizabeth Health[2]	Lafayette	85%	27
Memorial Hospital of South Bend[2]	South Bend	85%	131
Clark Memorial Hospital[2]	Jeffersonville	84%	73
Community Hospital North[2]	Indianapolis	82%	93
Dearborn County Hospital[2]	Lawrenceburg	82%	40
Methodist Hospitals[2]	Gary	82%	131
Indiana Univ Health La Porte Hosp[2]	La Porte	79%	38
IU Health Goshen Hospital[2]	Goshen	79%	57
Franciscan St Elizabeth Health[2]	Lafayette	78%	40
King's Daughters' Health[2]	Madison	76%	25
Franciscan St Anthony Health[2]	Michigan City	74%	42
Porter Regional Hospital[2]	Valparaiso	73%	84
Marion General Hospital[2]	Marion	70%	30
Good Samaritan Hospital[2]	Vincennes	66%	44

ICU Venous Thromboembolism Prophylaxis

Hospital Name	City	Rate	Cases
Bluffton Regional Medical Center[2]	Bluffton	100%	61
Dukes Memorial Hospital[2]	Peru	100%	45
Dupont Hospital[2]	Fort Wayne	100%	27
Franciscan St Francis Health[2]	Mooresville	100%	36
Hancock Regional Hospital[2]	Greenfield	100%	52
Indiana University Health Arnett Hospital[2]	Lafayette	100%	35
Kosciusko Community Hospital[2]	Warsaw	100%	52
Riverview Hospital[2]	Noblesville	100%	126
Saint Catherine Hospital[2]	East Chicago	100%	72
Saint Joseph Hospital & Health Center[2]	Kokomo	100%	51
Schneck Medical Center[2]	Seymour	100%	54
Terre Haute Regional Hospital[2]	Terre Haute	100%	88
Union Hospital[2]	Terre Haute	100%	145
Union Hospital Clinton	Clinton	100%	87
Hendricks Regional Health[2]	Danville	99%	88
Henry County Memorial Hospital[2]	New Castle	99%	70
Deaconess Hospital[2]	Evansville	98%	128
Eskenazi Health[2]	Indianapolis	98%	48
Floyd Memorial Hospital & Health Services[2]	New Albany	98%	53
Indiana Univ Health Bloomington Hosp[2]	Bloomington	98%	87
Saint Joseph Hospital[2]	Fort Wayne	98%	99
Saint Mary Medical Center[2]	Hobart	98%	56
Dekalb Health[2]	Auburn	97%	194
Elkhart General Hospital[2]	Elkhart	97%	158
Lutheran Hospital of Indiana[2]	Fort Wayne	97%	225
Major Hospital[2]	Shelbyville	97%	65
Franciscan St Francis Hlth-Indianapolis[2]	Indianapolis	96%	112
IU Health Goshen Hospital[2]	Goshen	96%	76
Parkview Regional Medical Center[2]	Fort Wayne	96%	78
Saint Vincent Carmel Hospital[2]	Carmel	96%	26
Community Howard Regional Health[2]	Kokomo	95%	94
Community Westview Hospital[2]	Indianapolis	95%	39
Memorial Hospital	Logansport	95%	143
Memorial Hospital of South Bend[2]	South Bend	95%	38
Reid Hospital & Health Care Services[2]	Richmond	95%	97
Franciscan St Anthony Health-Crown Pt[2]	Crown Point	94%	35
Indiana Univ Health Ball Mem Hosp[2]	Muncie	94%	77
Saint Joseph Regional Medical Center[2]	Mishawaka	94%	71
Scott Memorial Hospital[2]	Scottsburg	94%	35
Columbus Regional Hospital[2]	Columbus	93%	91
Community Hospital[2]	Munster	93%	71
Community Hospital East[2]	Indianapolis	93%	27
Franciscan St Margaret Health-Hammond[2]	Hammond	93%	72
Methodist Hospitals[2]	Gary	93%	75
Saint Mary's Medical Center of Evansville[2]	Evansville	93%	101
Franciscan Healthcare - Munster	Munster	92%	64
Johnson Memorial Hospital[2]	Franklin	92%	84
Marion General Hospital[2]	Marion	91%	92
Saint Vincent Hospital & Health Services[2]	Indianapolis	91%	76
Memorial Hospital & Health Care Center[2]	Jasper	90%	72
Witham Health Services[2]	Lebanon	90%	42
Franciscan Saint Margaret Health - Dyer[2]	Dyer	89%	66
The Heart Hospital at Deaconess Gateway[2]	Newburgh	89%	70
Indiana University Health Tipton Hospital	Tipton	89%	103
Indiana University Health North Hospital[2]	Carmel	87%	30
Parkview Noble Hospital[2]	Kendallville	87%	30
Indiana University Health[2]	Indianapolis	86%	73
Clark Memorial Hospital[2]	Jeffersonville	85%	52
Comm Hosp of Anderson/Madison Co[2]	Anderson	85%	61
Franciscan St Elizabeth Health[2]	Lafayette	85%	47
Good Samaritan Hospital[2]	Vincennes	85%	67
Franciscan St Elizabeth Health[2]	Lafayette	82%	50
Indiana Univ Health La Porte Hosp[2]	La Porte	82%	97
Porter Regional Hospital[2]	Valparaiso	82%	97
St Joseph Reg Med Ctr-Plymouth[2]	Plymouth	82%	61
Franciscan St Anthony Health[2]	Michigan City	81%	91
Franciscan St Elizabeth Health[2]	Crawfordsville	81%	26
Saint Vincent Heart Center of Indiana[2]	Indianapolis	81%	93
Daviess Community Hospital[2]	Washington	77%	70
Indiana University Health Morgan Hospital[2]	Martinsville	77%	56
Community Hospital North[2]	Indianapolis	75%	32
Community Hospital South[2]	Indianapolis	74%	46
Dearborn County Hospital[2]	Lawrenceburg	74%	133
The Indiana Heart Hospital[2]	Indianapolis	74%	165
Saint Vincent Anderson Regional Hospital[2]	Anderson	72%	116
Kentuckiana Medical Center[2]	Clarksville	70%	71
King's Daughters' Health[2]	Madison	55%	65

Incidence of Potentially Preventable VTE

Hospital Name	City	Rate	Cases
Lutheran Hospital of Indiana[2]	Fort Wayne	0%	33
Memorial Hospital of South Bend[2]	South Bend	0%	27
Saint Mary's Medical Center of Evansville[2]	Evansville	0%	25
Indiana University Health[2]	Indianapolis	5%	85
Indiana Univ Health Ball Mem Hosp[2]	Muncie	7%	28
Saint Vincent Hospital & Health Services[2]	Indianapolis	11%	53
Porter Regional Hospital[2]	Valparaiso	14%	29

UFH with Dosages/Platelet Count Monitoring

Hospital Name	City	Rate	Cases
Community Hospital[2]	Munster	100%	68
Deaconess Hospital[2]	Evansville	100%	30
Floyd Memorial Hospital & Health Services[2]	New Albany	100%	28
Franciscan St Francis Hlth-Indianapolis[2]	Indianapolis	100%	60
Good Samaritan Hospital[2]	Vincennes	100%	31
Indiana University Health[2]	Indianapolis	100%	135
Indiana Univ Health Ball Mem Hosp[2]	Muncie	100%	96
IU Health Goshen Hospital[2]	Goshen	100%	28
Lutheran Hospital of Indiana[2]	Fort Wayne	100%	163
Porter Regional Hospital[2]	Valparaiso	100%	65
Saint Joseph Regional Medical Center[2]	Mishawaka	100%	60
Saint Mary Medical Center[2]	Hobart	100%	30
Saint Mary's Medical Center of Evansville[2]	Evansville	100%	47
Parkview Regional Medical Center[2]	Fort Wayne	99%	176
Elkhart General Hospital[2]	Elkhart	95%	152
Methodist Hospitals[2]	Gary	89%	64
Franciscan St Margaret Health-Hammond[2]	Hammond	84%	44
Saint Vincent Hospital & Health Services[2]	Indianapolis	81%	54
Memorial Hospital of South Bend[2]	South Bend	73%	74
Clark Memorial Hospital[2]	Jeffersonville	6%	36

Venous Thromboembolism Prophylaxis

Hospital Name	City	Rate	Cases
Dupont Hospital[2]	Fort Wayne	100%	135
Orthopaedic Hospital at Parkview North[2]	Fort Wayne	100%	48
Riverview Hospital[2]	Noblesville	100%	242
Saint Joseph Hospital & Health Center[2]	Kokomo	100%	278
Union Hospital Clinton	Clinton	100%	332
Unity Medical & Surgical Hospital[2]	Mishawaka	100%	103
Bluffton Regional Medical Center[2]	Bluffton	99%	328
Hancock Regional Hospital[2]	Greenfield	99%	190
Saint Catherine Hospital[2]	East Chicago	99%	380
Saint Mary Medical Center[2]	Hobart	99%	375
Terre Haute Regional Hospital[2]	Terre Haute	99%	302
Hendricks Regional Health[2]	Danville	97%	337
Kosciusko Community Hospital[2]	Warsaw	97%	303
The Ortho Hosp/Lutheran Health Network[2]	Fort Wayne	97%	145
Schneck Medical Center[2]	Seymour	97%	219
Dukes Memorial Hospital[2]	Peru	96%	206
Franciscan St Anthony Health-Crown Pt[2]	Crown Point	96%	380
Jay County Hospital	Portland	96%	295
Saint Vincent Carmel Hospital[2]	Carmel	96%	287
Wabash County Hospital[2]	Wabash	96%	52
Community Westview Hospital[2]	Indianapolis	95%	115
Dekalb Health[2]	Auburn	95%	86
Indiana Orthopaedic Hospital[2]	Indianapolis	95%	77
Reid Hospital & Health Care Services[2]	Richmond	95%	329
Eskenazi Health[2]	Indianapolis	94%	302
Franciscan St Francis Hlth-Indianapolis[2]	Indianapolis	94%	496
Henry County Memorial Hospital[2]	New Castle	94%	140
Fayette Regional Health System[2]	Connersville	93%	122
IU Health West Hospital[2]	Avon	93%	402
Lutheran Hospital of Indiana[2]	Fort Wayne	93%	359
Major Hospital[2]	Shelbyville	93%	249
Pulaski Memorial Hospital	Winamac	93%	227
Saint Joseph Hospital[2]	Fort Wayne	92%	319
Franciscan Healthcare - Munster	Munster	91%	382
Franciscan St Francis Health[2]	Mooresville	91%	140
Indiana University Health Arnett Hospital[2]	Lafayette	91%	383
Indiana University Health Morgan Hospital[2]	Martinsville	91%	82
Saint Vincent Mercy Hospital	Elwood	91%	297
Saint Vincent Williamsport Hospital	Williamsport	91%	387
Deaconess Hospital[2]	Evansville	90%	313
Elkhart General Hospital[2]	Elkhart	90%	401
Indiana Univ Health Bloomington Hosp[2]	Bloomington	90%	263
IU Health Goshen Hospital[2]	Goshen	89%	324
Memorial Hospital of South Bend[2]	South Bend	89%	306
Saint Vincent Frankfort Hospital[2]	Frankfort	89%	108
Witham Health Services[2]	Lebanon	89%	152
Community Howard Regional Health[2]	Kokomo	88%	298
Indiana Univ Health Ball Mem Hosp[2]	Muncie	88%	318
Parkview Regional Medical Center[2]	Fort Wayne	88%	389
Columbus Regional Hospital[2]	Columbus	87%	315
Community Hospital[2]	Munster	87%	340
Indiana University Health Starke Hospital[2]	Knox	87%	103
Marion General Hospital[2]	Marion	87%	356
Scott Memorial Hospital[2]	Scottsburg	87%	92
Union Hospital[2]	Terre Haute	87%	561
Cameron Memorial Community Hospital[2]	Angola	86%	103
Methodist Hospitals[2]	Gary	86%	393
Indiana University Health Tipton Hospital	Tipton	85%	389
Memorial Hospital	Logansport	85%	511
Parkview Huntington Hospital[2]	Huntington	85%	160
Franciscan St Elizabeth Health[2]	Lafayette	84%	319
Indiana University Health North Hospital[2]	Carmel	84%	300
Parkview Whitley Hospital[2]	Columbia City	83%	126
Saint Joseph Regional Medical Center[2]	Mishawaka	83%	334
Good Samaritan Hospital[2]	Vincennes	82%	348
Indiana University Health[2]	Indianapolis	82%	352
Franciscan St Margaret Health-Hammond[2]	Hammond	81%	361
Porter Regional Hospital[2]	Valparaiso	81%	438
Community Hospital South[2]	Indianapolis	80%	326
The Heart Hospital at Deaconess Gateway[2]	Newburgh	80%	130
Memorial Hospital & Health Care Center[2]	Jasper	80%	288
Saint Mary's Medical Center of Evansville[2]	Evansville	80%	325
The Women's Hospital	Newburgh	80%	25
Indiana Univ Health La Porte Hosp[2]	La Porte	79%	251
Pinnacle Hospital[2]	Crown Point	79%	332
Community Hospital East[2]	Indianapolis	78%	255
Community Hospital North[2]	Indianapolis	77%	390
Franciscan St Elizabeth Health[2]	Lafayette	76%	298
Johnson Memorial Hospital[2]	Franklin	76%	221
Parkview Lagrange Hospital[2]	Lagrange	76%	91
Saint Vincent Heart Center of Indiana[2]	Indianapolis	76%	359
Daviess Community Hospital[2]	Washington	75%	176
Saint Vincent Hospital & Health Services[2]	Indianapolis	74%	344
Franciscan Saint Margaret Health - Dyer[2]	Dyer	73%	343
Floyd Memorial Hospital & Health Services[2]	New Albany	72%	393
Monroe Hospital[2]	Bloomington	72%	126
Comm Hosp of Anderson/Madison Co[2]	Anderson	71%	329
Franciscan St Anthony Health[2]	Michigan City	70%	358
Parkview Noble Hospital[2]	Kendallville	70%	145
St Joseph Reg Med Ctr-Plymouth[2]	Plymouth	70%	117
Kentuckiana Medical Center[2]	Clarksville	69%	112
Saint Vincent Anderson Regional Hospital[2]	Anderson	68%	1058
Franciscan St Elizabeth Health[2]	Crawfordsville	65%	130
Saint Mary's Warrick Hospital[2]	Boonville	63%	180
Saint Vincent Randolph Hospital	Winchester	59%	321
King's Daughters' Health[2]	Madison	56%	338
Dearborn County Hospital[2]	Lawrenceburg	55%	295
The Indiana Heart Hospital[2]	Indianapolis	55%	212
Clark Memorial Hospital[2]	Jeffersonville	50%	345
Saint Catherine Regional Hospital[2]	Charlestown	21%	150

NOTE: Hospital profiles are in alphabetical order by state, then city, then hospital within the city; Rankings exclude hospitals with less than 25 cases except for patient surveys which excludes hospitals with less than 100 cases; (a) 100-299 cases; (1) The number of cases/patients is too few to report; (2) Data submitted were based on a sample of cases/patients; (3) Results are based on a shorter time period than required; (4) Data suppressed by CMS for one or more quarters; (5) Results are not available for this reporting period; (6) Fewer than 100 patients completed the HCAHPS survey; (7) No cases met the criteria for this measure; (8) The lower limit of the confidence interval cannot be calculated if the number of observed infections equals zero; (9) No data are available from the state/territory for this reporting period; (10) The scores shown reflect fewer than 50 completed surveys; (11) There were discrepancies in the data collection process; (12) This measure does not apply to this hospital for this reporting period; (13) Results cannot be calculated for this reporting period; (14) The results for this state are combined with nearby states to protect confidentiality; Please refer to the User's Guide for a full explanation of data.

Hospital Name	City	Rate	Cases
Rush Memorial Hospital	Rushville	12%	240

Warfarin Therapy Discharge Instructions

Hospital Name	City	Rate	Cases
Eskenazi Health[2]	Indianapolis	100%	34
Floyd Memorial Hospital & Health Services[2]	New Albany	100%	73
Saint Mary Medical Center[2]	Hobart	100%	48
Saint Mary's Medical Center of Evansville[2]	Evansville	100%	77
Methodist Hospitals[2]	Gary	99%	89
Union Hospital[2]	Terre Haute	97%	72
Lutheran Hospital of Indiana[2]	Fort Wayne	95%	132
Community Hospital[2]	Munster	94%	83
Reid Hospital & Health Care Services[2]	Richmond	93%	44
Franciscan St Anthony Health[2]	Michigan City	89%	35
Indiana University Health Arnett Hospital[2]	Lafayette	88%	57
Parkview Regional Medical Center[2]	Fort Wayne	87%	135
Deaconess Hospital[2]	Evansville	86%	105
Dearborn County Hospital[2]	Lawrenceburg	85%	27
Franciscan St Anthony Health-Crown Pt[2]	Crown Point	85%	60
Saint Vincent Anderson Regional Hospital[2]	Anderson	85%	27
Franciscan St Francis Hlth-Indianapolis[2]	Indianapolis	81%	85
Good Samaritan Hospital[2]	Vincennes	81%	37
Johnson Memorial Hospital[2]	Franklin	80%	25
Franciscan St Margaret Health-Hammond[2]	Hammond	76%	66
Indiana Univ Health Ball Mem Hosp[2]	Muncie	75%	102
IU Health Goshen Hospital[2]	Goshen	75%	51
Saint Joseph Regional Medical Center[2]	Mishawaka	69%	86
Elkhart General Hospital[2]	Elkhart	68%	115
Indiana Univ Health Bloomington Hosp[2]	Bloomington	68%	66
Hendricks Regional Health[2]	Danville	64%	25
Franciscan St Elizabeth Health[2]	Lafayette	57%	30
Clark Memorial Hospital[2]	Jeffersonville	47%	49
Franciscan Saint Margaret Health - Dyer[2]	Dyer	47%	36
Memorial Hospital of South Bend[2]	South Bend	46%	109
IU Health West Hospital[2]	Avon	45%	47
Indiana University Health North Hospital[2]	Carmel	41%	27
Indiana University Health[2]	Indianapolis	38%	169
Indiana Univ Health La Porte Hosp[2]	La Porte	33%	27
Columbus Regional Hospital[2]	Columbus	26%	42
Porter Regional Hospital[2]	Valparaiso	26%	68
Saint Vincent Hospital & Health Services[2]	Indianapolis	25%	115
Community Hospital North[2]	Indianapolis	22%	68
Community Hospital South[2]	Indianapolis	18%	28
Community Hospital East[2]	Indianapolis	12%	60

Chest Pain/Possible Heart Attack Care

Aspirin Given Within 24 Hours of Arrival

Hospital Name	City	Rate	Cases
Bluffton Regional Medical Center	Bluffton	100%	54
Comm Hosp of Anderson/Madison Co	Anderson	100%	64
Dekalb Health	Auburn	100%	45
Dupont Hospital	Fort Wayne	100%	35
Hancock Regional Hospital	Greenfield	100%	60
Hendricks Regional Health	Danville	100%	159
Indiana Univ Health Blackford Hosp	Hartford City	100%	55
Indiana University Health Morgan Hospital	Martinsville	100%	42
Indiana University Health Tipton Hospital	Tipton	100%	30
IU Health West Hospital	Avon	100%	35
Johnson Memorial Hospital	Franklin	100%	30
Kosciusko Community Hospital	Warsaw	100%	76
Margaret Mary Community Hospital	Batesville	100%	109
Parkview Noble Hospital	Kendallville	100%	40
Parkview Whitley Hospital	Columbia City	100%	44
Rush Memorial Hospital	Rushville	100%	50
St Joseph Reg Med Ctr-Plymouth	Plymouth	100%	41
Saint Vincent Carmel Hospital	Carmel	100%	70
Saint Vincent Frankfort Hospital[3]	Frankfort	100%	28
Wabash County Hospital[3]	Wabash	100%	31
Witham Health Services	Lebanon	100%	47
Deaconess Hospital	Evansville	99%	178
Decatur County Memorial Hospital	Greensburg	99%	67
Saint Vincent Anderson Regional Hospital	Anderson	99%	103
Cameron Memorial Community Hospital	Angola	98%	92
Dukes Memorial Hospital	Peru	98%	63
Indiana University Health Starke Hospital	Knox	98%	43
King's Daughters' Health	Madison	98%	206
Saint Vincent Williamsport Hospital	Williamsport	98%	43
Memorial Hospital	Logansport	97%	67
Parkview Lagrange Hospital	Lagrange	97%	39
Schneck Medical Center	Seymour	97%	170
Daviess Community Hospital	Washington	96%	53
Franciscan St Elizabeth Health	Crawfordsville	96%	81
Franciscan St Francis Health	Mooresville	96%	93
Jasper County Hospital	Rensselaer	96%	55
Saint Vincent Dunn Hospital	Bedford	96%	28
Sullivan County Community Hospital	Sullivan	96%	54
Dearborn County Hospital	Lawrenceburg	95%	88
Henry County Memorial Hospital	New Castle	95%	124
Marion General Hospital	Marion	95%	189
Saint Vincent Hospital & Health Services[3]	Indianapolis	95%	39
Union Hospital Clinton	Clinton	95%	43
Harrison County Hospital	Corydon	94%	34
Indiana Univ Health Bedford Hosp	Bedford	94%	54
IU Health Goshen Hospital	Goshen	94%	36
Jay County Hospital	Portland	94%	53
Parkview Huntington Hospital	Huntington	94%	54
Saint Joseph Hospital & Health Center	Kokomo	94%	71
Major Hospital	Shelbyville	93%	44
Perry County Memorial Hospital	Tell City	92%	50
Putnam County Hospital	Greencastle	92%	36
Fayette Regional Health System	Connersville	91%	75
Saint Vincent Randolph Hospital	Winchester	91%	57
Saint Vincent Mercy Hospital	Elwood	89%	53
Saint Vincent Clay Hospital	Brazil	88%	25
Community Hospital North	Indianapolis	87%	109
The Indiana Heart Hospital	Indianapolis	86%	29
Pulaski Memorial Hospital	Winamac	82%	51

Average Time to ECG (minutes)

Hospital Name	City	Min.	Cases
Henry County Memorial Hospital	New Castle	2	132
Jay County Hospital	Portland	2	57
Franciscan St Francis Health	Mooresville	3	100
Hancock Regional Hospital	Greenfield	3	60
The Indiana Heart Hospital	Indianapolis	3	31
Johnson Memorial Hospital	Franklin	3	31
Kosciusko Community Hospital	Warsaw	3	78
Bluffton Regional Medical Center	Bluffton	4	55
Dupont Hospital	Fort Wayne	4	36
Hendricks Regional Health	Danville	4	162
Indiana University Health Morgan Hospital	Martinsville	4	43
Major Hospital	Shelbyville	4	46
Margaret Mary Community Hospital	Batesville	4	114
Parkview Lagrange Hospital	Lagrange	4	41
Saint Vincent Dunn Hospital	Bedford	4	30
Community Hospital East	Indianapolis	5	27
Comm Hosp of Anderson/Madison Co	Anderson	5	66
Fayette Regional Health System	Connersville	5	83
Parkview Noble Hospital	Kendallville	5	39
Saint Vincent Anderson Regional Hospital	Anderson	5	103
Saint Vincent Carmel Hospital	Carmel	5	78
Saint Vincent Frankfort Hospital[3]	Frankfort	5	30
Saint Vincent Hospital & Health Services[3]	Indianapolis	5	41
Schneck Medical Center	Seymour	5	177
Sullivan County Community Hospital	Sullivan	5	57
Daviess Community Hospital	Washington	6	56
Dearborn County Hospital	Lawrenceburg	6	92
Decatur County Memorial Hospital	Greensburg	6	75
Indiana Univ Health Blackford Hosp	Hartford City	6	56
Indiana University Health Starke Hospital	Knox	6	48
Indiana University Health Tipton Hospital	Tipton	6	30
IU Health Goshen Hospital	Goshen	6	37
IU Health West Hospital	Avon	6	36
Jasper County Hospital	Rensselaer	6	56
King's Daughters' Health	Madison	6	208
Pulaski Memorial Hospital	Winamac	6	55
Putnam County Hospital	Greencastle	6	40
Witham Health Services	Lebanon	6	48
Dekalb Health	Auburn	7	47
Dukes Memorial Hospital	Peru	7	65
Indiana Univ Health Bedford Hosp	Bedford	7	55
Marion General Hospital	Marion	7	193
Memorial Hospital	Logansport	7	72
Parkview Whitley Hospital	Columbia City	7	47
Saint Vincent Mercy Hospital	Elwood	7	57
Saint Vincent Randolph Hospital	Winchester	7	57
Union Hospital Clinton	Clinton	7	45
Wabash County Hospital[3]	Wabash	7	42
Deaconess Hospital	Evansville	8	184
Franciscan St Elizabeth Health	Crawfordsville	8	83
Perry County Memorial Hospital	Tell City	8	56
Saint Vincent Williamsport Hospital	Williamsport	8	46
Cameron Memorial Community Hospital	Angola	9	100
Saint Vincent Clay Hospital	Brazil	9	26
Harrison County Hospital	Corydon	10	36
Parkview Huntington Hospital	Huntington	10	52
Saint Joseph Hospital & Health Center	Kokomo	10	79
Rush Memorial Hospital	Rushville	12	51
Community Hospital North	Indianapolis	13	111
St Joseph Reg Med Ctr-Plymouth	Plymouth	14	41

Average Time to Transfer (minutes)

Hospital Name	City	Min.	Cases
Saint Vincent Anderson Regional Hospital	Anderson	27	29
Deaconess Hospital	Evansville	34	43
Hendricks Regional Health	Danville	43	33
Marion General Hospital	Marion	50	53
Saint Joseph Hospital & Health Center	Kokomo	54	32
Hancock Regional Hospital	Greenfield	76	26

Children's Asthma Care

Received Home Management Plan of Care

Hospital Name	City	Rate	Cases
Indiana University Health North Hospital[2]	Carmel	76%	50

Received Reliever Medication

Hospital Name	City	Rate	Cases
Indiana University Health North Hospital	Carmel	100%	51

Received Systemic Corticosteroids

Hospital Name	City	Rate	Cases
Indiana University Health North Hospital	Carmel	100%	51

Emergency Department

Admittance Decision Time (minutes)

Hospital Name	City	Min.	Cases
Saint Vincent Salem Hospital[2,3]	Salem	15	50
Saint Catherine Regional Hospital	Charlestown	27	247
The Women's Hospital[2]	Newburgh	32	120
Major Hospital[2]	Shelbyville	37	467
Indiana University Health Starke Hospital[2]	Knox	41	393
St Joseph Reg Med Ctr-Plymouth[2]	Plymouth	42	328
Adams Memorial Hospital[2]	Decatur	44	525
Schneck Medical Center[2]	Seymour	44	315
Rush Memorial Hospital[2]	Rushville	45	220
Bluffton Regional Medical Center[2]	Bluffton	48	374
Decatur County Memorial Hospital[2]	Greensburg	48	279
The Indiana Heart Hospital[2]	Indianapolis	48	179
Comm Hosp of Anderson/Madison Co[2]	Anderson	49	591
Deaconess Hospital[2]	Evansville	49	448
Saint Mary's Warrick Hospital[2]	Boonville	50	318
Saint Vincent Frankfort Hospital[2]	Frankfort	50	257
Cameron Memorial Community Hospital[2]	Angola	51	407
Saint Vincent Anderson Regional Hospital[2]	Anderson	54	631
Jay County Hospital	Portland	55	528
Harrison County Hospital[2]	Corydon	58	440
Indiana Univ Health Blackford Hosp	Hartford City	58	212
Daviess Community Hospital[2]	Washington	59	351
Saint Joseph Hospital & Health Center[2]	Kokomo	59	475
Henry County Memorial Hospital[2]	New Castle	60	374
Indiana Univ Health La Porte Hosp[2]	La Porte	60	527
Parkview Lagrange Hospital[2]	Lagrange	60	154
Terre Haute Regional Hospital[2]	Terre Haute	60	458
Pulaski Memorial Hospital	Winamac	61	333
Columbus Regional Hospital[2]	Columbus	62	447
Fayette Regional Health System[2]	Connersville	64	400
Marion General Hospital[2]	Marion	64	515
Dupont Hospital[2]	Fort Wayne	65	235
Memorial Hospital	Logansport	65	811
Saint Vincent Clay Hospital	Brazil	65	254
Good Samaritan Hospital[2]	Vincennes	66	685
Riverview Hospital[2]	Noblesville	66	742
Union Hospital Clinton	Clinton	66	463
Monroe Hospital[2]	Bloomington	67	231
Parkview Noble Hospital[2]	Kendallville	67	298
Franciscan St Elizabeth Health[2]	Crawfordsville	68	448
Memorial Hospital & Health Care Center[2]	Jasper	69	551
Reid Hospital & Health Care Services[2]	Richmond	69	676
Clark Memorial Hospital[2]	Jeffersonville	70	584
Kosciusko Community Hospital[2]	Warsaw	70	580
Indiana Univ Health Bedford Hosp[2,3]	Bedford	72	294
Indiana Univ Health Bloomington Hosp[2]	Bloomington	74	460
Saint Vincent Williamsport Hospital	Williamsport	74	395
Indiana University Health Tipton Hospital	Tipton	75	543
Jasper County Hospital[3]	Rensselaer	75	47
Parkview Huntington Hospital[2]	Huntington	76	274
Porter Regional Hospital[2]	Valparaiso	76	829
Saint Vincent Carmel Hospital[2]	Carmel	76	240
Dukes Memorial Hospital[2]	Peru	77	317
Indiana University Health Morgan Hospital[2]	Martinsville	77	536
King's Daughters' Health[2]	Madison	78	384
Saint Joseph Regional Medical Center[2]	Mishawaka	81	620
Dearborn County Hospital[2]	Lawrenceburg	82	493
Parkview Whitley Hospital[2]	Columbia City	82	277
Saint Vincent Hospital & Health Services[2]	Indianapolis	82	425
Witham Health Services[2]	Lebanon	82	352
Floyd Memorial Hospital & Health Services[2]	New Albany	83	577
Union Hospital[2]	Terre Haute	83	686
Saint Vincent Dunn Hospital[2]	Bedford	85	183
Hendricks Regional Health[2]	Danville	90	542
Memorial Hospital of South Bend[2]	South Bend	91	373
Saint Mary's Medical Center of Evansville[2]	Evansville	93	506
Johnson Memorial Hospital[2]	Franklin	94	408
Lutheran Hospital of Indiana[2]	Fort Wayne	94	662
Dekalb Health[2]	Auburn	96	231
Franciscan Saint Margaret Health - Dyer[2]	Dyer	96	658
Indiana University Health Arnett Hospital[2]	Lafayette	96	676

NOTE: Hospital profiles are in alphabetical order by state, then city, then hospital within the city; Rankings exclude hospitals with less than 25 cases except for patient surveys which excludes hospitals with less than 100 cases; (a) 100-299 cases; (1) The number of cases/patients is too few to report; (2) Data submitted were based on a sample of cases/patients; (3) Results are based on a shorter time period than required; (4) Data suppressed by CMS for one or more quarters; (5) Results are not available for this reporting period; (6) Fewer than 100 patients completed the HCAHPS survey; (7) No cases met the criteria for this measure; (8) The lower limit of the confidence interval cannot be calculated if the number of observed infections equals zero; (9) No data are available from the state/territory for this reporting period; (10) The scores shown reflect fewer than 50 completed surveys; (11) There were discrepancies in the data collection process; (12) This measure does not apply to this hospital for this reporting period; (13) Results cannot be calculated for this reporting period; (14) The results for this state are combined with nearby states to protect confidentiality; Please refer to the User's Guide for a full explanation of data.

Franciscan St Anthony Health[2]	Michigan City	97	795
Franciscan St Elizabeth Health[2]	Lafayette	98	228
Community Westview Hospital[2]	Indianapolis	100	469
Saint Vincent Randolph Hospital[2]	Winchester	100	278
Franciscan St Elizabeth Health[2]	Lafayette	101	253
Elkhart General Hospital[2]	Elkhart	103	637
Franciscan St Margaret Health-Hammond[2]	Hammond	107	919
Indiana Univ Health Ball Mem Hosp[2]	Muncie	109	569
Community Hospital South[2]	Indianapolis	110	589
Saint Catherine Hospital[2]	East Chicago	111	708
Saint Joseph Hospital[2]	Fort Wayne	118	468
Community Howard Regional Health[2]	Kokomo	119	452
Parkview Regional Medical Center[2]	Fort Wayne	122	542
IU Health Goshen Hospital[2]	Goshen	124	455
Indiana University Health North Hospital[2]	Carmel	130	250
Franciscan St Anthony Health-Crown Pt[2]	Crown Point	135	395
IU Health West Hospital[2]	Avon	138	716
Community Hospital[2]	Munster	146	649
Methodist Hospitals[2]	Gary	146	754
Hancock Regional Hospital[2]	Greenfield	148	456
Saint Vincent Heart Center of Indiana[2]	Indianapolis	150	74
Indiana University Health[2]	Indianapolis	154	382
Saint Mary Medical Center[2]	Hobart	166	805
Community Hospital East[2]	Indianapolis	180	679
Franciscan St Francis Health[2]	Mooresville	191	370
Eskenazi Health[2]	Indianapolis	249	382
Franciscan St Francis Hlth-Indianapolis[2]	Indianapolis	281	601

Head CT Results Within 45 Minutes of Arrival

Hospital Name	City	Rate	Cases
Franciscan St Margaret Health-Hammond	Hammond	48%	29

Patients Who Left ER Before Being Seen

Hospital Name	City	Rate	Cases
Adams Memorial Hospital	Decatur	0%	11725
Bluffton Regional Medical Center	Bluffton	0%	9669
Comm Hosp of Anderson/Madison Co	Anderson	0%	30714
Community Westview Hospital	Indianapolis	0%	8793
Decatur County Memorial Hospital	Greensburg	0%	16099
Franciscan St Francis Health	Mooresville	0%	29628
Good Samaritan Hospital	Vincennes	0%	35950
Hendricks Regional Health	Danville	0%	30396
The Indiana Heart Hospital	Indianapolis	0%	4832
Indiana Univ Health La Porte Hosp	La Porte	0%	19169
Indiana University Health North Hospital	Carmel	0%	17465
Indiana University Health Starke Hospital	Knox	0%	7331
Indiana University Health Tipton Hospital	Tipton	0%	5899
Indiana Univ Health White Mem Hosp	Monticello	0%	14187
Lutheran Hospital of Indiana	Fort Wayne	0%	43522
Margaret Mary Community Hospital	Batesville	0%	16093
Parkview Lagrange Hospital	Lagrange	0%	8065
Parkview Noble Hospital	Kendallville	0%	18065
Porter Regional Hospital	Valparaiso	0%	54995
Pulaski Memorial Hospital	Winamac	0%	4986
Reid Hospital & Health Care Services	Richmond	0%	46877
Riverview Hospital	Noblesville	0%	22679
Saint Catherine Regional Hospital	Charlestown	0%	4914
Saint Joseph Hospital	Fort Wayne	0%	29189
Saint Vincent Carmel Hospital	Carmel	0%	17043
Saint Vincent Heart Center of Indiana	Indianapolis	0%	3021
Saint Vincent Randolph Hospital	Winchester	0%	11797
Saint Vincent Williamsport Hospital	Williamsport	0%	11563
Terre Haute Regional Hospital	Terre Haute	0%	21385
Union Hospital	Terre Haute	0%	54263
Union Hospital Clinton	Clinton	0%	11537
Witham Health Services	Lebanon	0%	21163
The Women's Hospital	Newburgh	0%	4117
Woodlawn Hospital	Rochester	0%	7519
Community Hospital	Munster	1%	65403
Community Hospital North	Indianapolis	1%	52254
Daviess Community Hospital	Washington	1%	13650
Deaconess Hospital	Evansville	1%	91032
Dekalb Health	Auburn	1%	18185
Dupont Hospital	Fort Wayne	1%	21037
Elkhart General Hospital	Elkhart	1%	63114
Fayette Regional Health System	Connersville	1%	15801
Franciscan St Anthony Health-Crown Pt	Crown Point	1%	32704
Franciscan St Anthony Health	Michigan City	1%	41228
Franciscan St Elizabeth Health	Crawfordsville	1%	20458
Franciscan St Elizabeth Health	Lafayette	1%	27779
Franciscan St Elizabeth Health	Lafayette	1%	37490
Franciscan St Francis Hlth-Indianapolis	Indianapolis	1%	83211
Franciscan Saint Margaret Health - Dyer	Dyer	1%	11484
Gibson General Hospital	Princeton	1%	12643
Greene County General Hospital	Linton	1%	9028
Harrison County Hospital	Corydon	1%	15730
Indiana University Health	Indianapolis	1%	166864
Indiana Univ Health Blackford Hosp	Hartford City	1%	10165
Indiana University Health Paoli Hospital	Paoli	1%	10793
IU Health Goshen Hospital	Goshen	1%	33469
Jasper County Hospital	Rensselaer	1%	9903
Jay County Hospital	Portland	1%	10233
Johnson Memorial Hospital	Franklin	1%	22822
Kosciusko Community Hospital	Warsaw	1%	24296
Marion General Hospital	Marion	1%	44733
Memorial Hospital & Health Care Center	Jasper	1%	25921
Memorial Hospital of South Bend	South Bend	1%	56583
Monroe Hospital	Bloomington	1%	13316
Parkview Huntington Hospital	Huntington	1%	14790
Parkview Regional Medical Center	Fort Wayne	1%	76591
Parkview Whitley Hospital	Columbia City	1%	12823
Perry County Memorial Hospital	Tell City	1%	13120
Putnam County Hospital	Greencastle	1%	11532
Rush Memorial Hospital	Rushville	1%	9992
Saint Joseph Regional Medical Center	Mishawaka	1%	58352
St Joseph Reg Med Ctr-Plymouth	Plymouth	1%	15767
Saint Mary's Medical Center of Evansville	Evansville	1%	64264
Saint Vincent Anderson Regional Hospital	Anderson	1%	46722
Saint Vincent Clay Hospital	Brazil	1%	10647
Saint Vincent Dunn Hospital	Bedford	1%	9188
Saint Vincent Jennings Hospital	North Vernon	1%	9254
Saint Vincent Mercy Hospital	Elwood	1%	9927
Saint Vincent Salem Hospital	Salem	1%	8285
Sullivan County Community Hospital	Sullivan	1%	8839
Wabash County Hospital	Wabash	1%	10724
Clark Memorial Hospital	Jeffersonville	2%	31528
Community Hospital South	Indianapolis	2%	41425
Eskenazi Health	Indianapolis	2%	108396
Floyd Memorial Hospital & Health Services	New Albany	2%	45882
Hancock Regional Hospital	Greenfield	2%	33279
Henry County Memorial Hospital	New Castle	2%	18058
Indiana University Health Arnett Hospital	Lafayette	2%	33398
Indiana Univ Health Bedford Hosp	Bedford	2%	12357
Indiana University Health Morgan Hospital	Martinsville	2%	15937
IU Health West Hospital	Avon	2%	48060
Major Hospital	Shelbyville	2%	23279
Saint Catherine Hospital	East Chicago	2%	33458
Schneck Medical Center	Seymour	2%	29743
Columbus Regional Hospital	Columbus	3%	41675
Dearborn County Hospital	Lawrenceburg	3%	19050
Dukes Memorial Hospital	Peru	3%	11250
Franciscan St Margaret Health-Hammond	Hammond	3%	43121
King's Daughters' Health	Madison	3%	18068
Memorial Hospital	Logansport	3%	14514
Saint Mary's Warrick Hospital	Boonville	3%	8364
Saint Vincent Hospital & Health Services	Indianapolis	3%	64788
Community Hospital East	Indianapolis	4%	67445
Community Howard Regional Health	Kokomo	4%	21853
Indiana Univ Health Ball Mem Hosp	Muncie	4%	61367
Methodist Hospitals	Gary	4%	61080
Indiana Univ Health Bloomington Hosp	Bloomington	5%	52475
Saint Mary Medical Center	Hobart	5%	37699
Saint Joseph Hospital & Health Center	Kokomo	8%	23413

Time from ER Arrival to Being Admitted (minutes)

Hospital Name	City	Min.	Cases
The Women's Hospital[2]	Newburgh	97	127
The Indiana Heart Hospital[2]	Indianapolis	149	184
Saint Mary's Warrick Hospital[2]	Boonville	149	334
Adams Memorial Hospital[2]	Decatur	170	548
Saint Catherine Regional Hospital	Charlestown	172	247
Deaconess Hospital[2]	Evansville	177	488
Decatur County Memorial Hospital[2]	Greensburg	180	279
Saint Vincent Salem Hospital[2,3]	Salem	182	50
Bluffton Regional Medical Center[2]	Bluffton	184	391
Jasper County Hospital[3]	Rensselaer	184	47
Columbus Regional Hospital[2]	Columbus	185	497
Comm Hosp of Anderson/Madison Co[2]	Anderson	185	712
Indiana University Health Starke Hospital[2]	Knox	190	490
Daviess Community Hospital[2]	Washington	191	363
Dupont Hospital[2]	Fort Wayne	193	236
Parkview Lagrange Hospital[2]	Lagrange	193	174
Good Samaritan Hospital[2]	Vincennes	194	705
Schneck Medical Center[2]	Seymour	195	350
Union Hospital Clinton	Clinton	195	532
Saint Vincent Williamsport Hospital	Williamsport	196	395
Riverview Hospital[2]	Noblesville	197	749
St Joseph Reg Med Ctr-Plymouth[2]	Plymouth	197	329
Rush Memorial Hospital[2]	Rushville	198	242
Memorial Hospital & Health Care Center[2]	Jasper	203	576
Indiana Univ Health La Porte Hosp[2]	La Porte	204	544
Saint Vincent Frankfort Hospital[2]	Frankfort	207	274
Parkview Noble Hospital[2]	Kendallville	209	351
Franciscan St Elizabeth Health[2]	Crawfordsville	210	457
Terre Haute Regional Hospital[2]	Terre Haute	210	460
Major Hospital[2]	Shelbyville	212	470
Henry County Memorial Hospital[2]	New Castle	213	385
Indiana University Health Tipton Hospital	Tipton	215	553
Jay County Hospital	Portland	220	562
Cameron Memorial Community Hospital[2]	Angola	223	415
Fayette Regional Health System[2]	Connersville	224	400
Pulaski Memorial Hospital	Winamac	224	336
Saint Vincent Anderson Regional Hospital[2]	Anderson	226	646
Hendricks Regional Health[2]	Danville	227	586
Marion General Hospital[2]	Marion	228	607
Saint Mary's Medical Center of Evansville[2]	Evansville	228	550
Dekalb Health[2]	Auburn	229	251
Parkview Whitley Hospital[2]	Columbia City	230	333
Memorial Hospital	Logansport	232	882
Union Hospital[2]	Terre Haute	232	745
Harrison County Hospital[2]	Corydon	234	461
Indiana Univ Health Bedford Hosp[2,3]	Bedford	234	294
Saint Vincent Heart Center of Indiana[2]	Indianapolis	236	93
Reid Hospital & Health Care Services[2]	Richmond	237	747
Monroe Hospital[2]	Bloomington	238	232
Porter Regional Hospital[2]	Valparaiso	239	863
Indiana Univ Health Bloomington Hosp[2]	Bloomington	240	472
Indiana University Health Morgan Hospital[2]	Martinsville	240	545
Dukes Memorial Hospital[2]	Peru	242	334
Johnson Memorial Hospital[2]	Franklin	242	453
Saint Vincent Carmel Hospital[2]	Carmel	242	242
Franciscan St Elizabeth Health[2]	Lafayette	244	262
Franciscan St Elizabeth Health[2]	Lafayette	246	228
Community Westview Hospital[2]	Indianapolis	247	505
Franciscan St Francis Health[2]	Mooresville	247	380
Franciscan Saint Margaret Health - Dyer[2]	Dyer	247	658
Indiana Univ Health Blackford Hosp	Hartford City	247	223
Saint Vincent Hospital & Health Services[2]	Indianapolis	247	435
Witham Health Services[2]	Lebanon	247	410
Parkview Huntington Hospital[2]	Huntington	249	302
Franciscan St Anthony Health[2]	Michigan City	250	799
Saint Vincent Clay Hospital	Brazil	250	329
Floyd Memorial Hospital & Health Services[2]	New Albany	252	791
Lutheran Hospital of Indiana[2]	Fort Wayne	252	682
Memorial Hospital of South Bend[2]	South Bend	252	398
Elkhart General Hospital[2]	Elkhart	254	637
Dearborn County Hospital[2]	Lawrenceburg	260	508
Kosciusko Community Hospital[2]	Warsaw	262	580
Community Hospital South[2]	Indianapolis	263	609
Saint Joseph Regional Medical Center[2]	Mishawaka	263	625
IU Health Goshen Hospital[2]	Goshen	264	474
Saint Catherine Hospital[2]	East Chicago	264	708
Saint Joseph Hospital[2]	Fort Wayne	270	473
Saint Vincent Randolph Hospital[2]	Winchester	270	298
Community Hospital[2]	Munster	274	649
Indiana University Health North Hospital[2]	Carmel	274	253
Saint Vincent Dunn Hospital[2]	Bedford	274	211
King's Daughters' Health[2]	Madison	275	387
Saint Joseph Hospital & Health Center[2]	Kokomo	276	500
Hancock Regional Hospital[2]	Greenfield	280	456
Indiana University Health Arnett Hospital[2]	Lafayette	281	689
Franciscan St Anthony Health-Crown Pt[2]	Crown Point	285	463
Franciscan St Margaret Health-Hammond[2]	Hammond	286	919
Indiana Univ Health Ball Mem Hosp[2]	Muncie	300	573
Clark Memorial Hospital[2]	Jeffersonville	302	591
Community Howard Regional Health[2]	Kokomo	307	474
Community Hospital East[2]	Indianapolis	308	700
Parkview Regional Medical Center[2]	Fort Wayne	309	605
Indiana University Health[2]	Indianapolis	318	386
IU Health West Hospital[2]	Avon	334	721
Franciscan St Francis Hlth-Indianapolis[2]	Indianapolis	348	613
Methodist Hospitals[2]	Gary	361	754
Saint Mary Medical Center[2]	Hobart	364	806
Eskenazi Health[2]	Indianapolis	498	392

Time from ER Arrival to Discharge (minutes)

Hospital Name	City	Min.	Cases
Saint Catherine Regional Hospital	Charlestown	68	441
Margaret Mary Community Hospital	Batesville	78	350
Parkview Lagrange Hospital	Lagrange	84	380
Parkview Noble Hospital	Kendallville	85	395
Schneck Medical Center	Seymour	87	351
Monroe Hospital	Bloomington	90	354
Dekalb Health	Auburn	94	430
Saint Vincent Frankfort Hospital[3]	Frankfort	94	245
Parkview Whitley Hospital	Columbia City	95	385
Decatur County Memorial Hospital	Greensburg	97	518
Fayette Regional Health System	Connersville	97	359
Dupont Hospital	Fort Wayne	98	405
Daviess Community Hospital	Washington	100	423
Johnson Memorial Hospital	Franklin	100	516
Franciscan St Elizabeth Health	Crawfordsville	101	404
Jasper County Hospital	Rensselaer	101	8320
Riverview Hospital	Noblesville	101	385
Community Westview Hospital	Indianapolis	104	432
Franciscan St Elizabeth Health	Lafayette	104	387
Witham Health Services	Lebanon	105	370
Indiana University Health Tipton Hospital	Tipton	106	430
Cameron Memorial Community Hospital	Angola	108	341
St Joseph Reg Med Ctr-Plymouth	Plymouth	108	397
Bluffton Regional Medical Center	Bluffton	110	377
Indiana University Health Starke Hospital	Knox	110	385

NOTE: Hospital profiles are in alphabetical order by state, then city, then hospital within the city; Rankings exclude hospitals with less than 25 cases except for patient surveys which excludes hospitals with less than 100 cases; (a) 100-299 cases; (1) The number of cases/patients is too few to report; (2) Data submitted were based on a sample of cases/patients; (3) Results are based on a shorter time period than required; (4) Data suppressed by CMS for one or more quarters; (5) Results are not available for this reporting period; (6) Fewer than 100 patients completed the HCAHPS survey; (7) No cases met the criteria for this measure; (8) The lower limit of the confidence interval cannot be calculated if the number of observed infections equals zero; (9) No data are available from the state/territory for this reporting period; (10) The scores shown reflect fewer than 50 completed surveys; (11) There were discrepancies in the data collection process; (12) This measure does not apply to this hospital for this reporting period; (13) Results cannot be calculated for this reporting period; (14) The results for this state are combined with nearby states to protect confidentiality; Please refer to the User's Guide for a full explanation of data.

Hospital Name	City	Min.	Cases
Elkhart General Hospital	Elkhart	111	563
Good Samaritan Hospital	Vincennes	112	373
Union Hospital Clinton	Clinton	113	522
Franciscan St Anthony Health	Michigan City	114	482
Franciscan St Francis Health	Mooresville	114	416
Saint Joseph Hospital	Fort Wayne	114	391
Indiana Univ Health Blackford Hosp	Hartford City	116	366
Saint Vincent Salem Hospital[3]	Salem	117	257
Comm Hosp of Anderson/Madison Co	Anderson	118	385
Franciscan St Elizabeth Health	Lafayette	120	404
Franciscan Saint Margaret Health - Dyer	Dyer	120	477
Indiana University Health Morgan Hospital	Martinsville	121	470
Jay County Hospital[3]	Portland	121	642
Parkview Huntington Hospital	Huntington	122	371
Saint Vincent Dunn Hospital[3]	Bedford	122	270
Terre Haute Regional Hospital	Terre Haute	123	404
Saint Vincent Anderson Regional Hospital	Anderson	124	386
Dukes Memorial Hospital	Peru	126	363
Memorial Hospital & Health Care Center	Jasper	126	361
Saint Mary's Medical Center of Evansville	Evansville	126	365
Deaconess Hospital	Evansville	127	329
Hendricks Regional Health	Danville	127	754
Harrison County Hospital	Corydon	128	343
Community Hospital	Munster	129	381
Memorial Hospital	Logansport	129	523
Franciscan St Anthony Health-Crown Pt	Crown Point	130	372
Porter Regional Hospital	Valparaiso	130	392
Columbus Regional Hospital	Columbus	131	460
Marion General Hospital	Marion	131	375
Reid Hospital & Health Care Services	Richmond	133	367
IU Health Goshen Hospital	Goshen	134	377
Saint Vincent Clay Hospital	Brazil	134	320
Henry County Memorial Hospital	New Castle	136	274
Saint Vincent Randolph Hospital	Winchester	137	343
Union Hospital	Terre Haute	137	526
Major Hospital	Shelbyville	138	460
Parkview Regional Medical Center	Fort Wayne	139	535
Floyd Memorial Hospital & Health Services	New Albany	141	414
Saint Joseph Regional Medical Center	Mishawaka	141	398
Kosciusko Community Hospital	Warsaw	142	395
The Women's Hospital	Newburgh	143	434
Community Hospital South	Indianapolis	144	406
Indiana Univ Health La Porte Hosp	La Porte	146	437
Indiana University Health North Hospital	Carmel	146	387
Saint Catherine Hospital	East Chicago	146	389
Saint Vincent Carmel Hospital	Carmel	146	355
Community Hospital East	Indianapolis	147	397
Dearborn County Hospital	Lawrenceburg	147	353
Franciscan St Francis Hlth-Indianapolis	Indianapolis	148	423
Lutheran Hospital of Indiana	Fort Wayne	148	390
The Indiana Heart Hospital	Indianapolis	149	341
Franciscan St Margaret Health-Hammond	Hammond	150	461
Saint Vincent Hospital & Health Services	Indianapolis	150	374
Community Howard Regional Health	Kokomo	167	523
Indiana Univ Health Bloomington Hosp	Bloomington	167	385
Hancock Regional Hospital	Greenfield	168	457
Indiana University Health	Indianapolis	168	373
Clark Memorial Hospital	Jeffersonville	171	370
Indiana University Health Arnett Hospital	Lafayette	173	371
Methodist Hospitals	Gary	173	328
Indiana Univ Health Ball Mem Hosp	Muncie	174	403
King's Daughters' Health	Madison	175	357
IU Health West Hospital	Avon	181	375
Saint Mary Medical Center	Hobart	182	382
Eskenazi Health	Indianapolis	185	364
Saint Joseph Hospital & Health Center	Kokomo	191	367
Saint Vincent Heart Center of Indiana	Indianapolis	192	124
Memorial Hospital of South Bend	South Bend	197	441

Time in ER Before Being Evaluated (minutes)

Hospital Name	City	Min.	Cases
Major Hospital	Shelbyville	5	477
Saint Catherine Regional Hospital	Charlestown	6	488
Witham Health Services	Lebanon	7	376
Decatur County Memorial Hospital	Greensburg	10	810
St Joseph Reg Med Ctr-Plymouth	Plymouth	10	430
Saint Vincent Heart Center of Indiana	Indianapolis	10	259
The Women's Hospital	Newburgh	10	452
The Indiana Heart Hospital	Indianapolis	11	275
Johnson Memorial Hospital	Franklin	11	600
Union Hospital	Terre Haute	11	469
Saint Vincent Frankfort Hospital[3]	Frankfort	12	276
Indiana University Health Morgan Hospital	Martinsville	13	496
Union Hospital Clinton	Clinton	13	583
Deaconess Hospital	Evansville	15	416
Indiana University Health Tipton Hospital	Tipton	15	399
Bluffton Regional Medical Center	Bluffton	16	409
Daviess Community Hospital	Washington	16	517
Dupont Hospital	Fort Wayne	16	423
Jay County Hospital[3]	Portland	16	700
Lutheran Hospital of Indiana	Fort Wayne	16	410
Margaret Mary Community Hospital	Batesville	17	375
Memorial Hospital & Health Care Center	Jasper	17	328
Porter Regional Hospital	Valparaiso	17	403
Saint Joseph Regional Medical Center	Mishawaka	17	425
Terre Haute Regional Hospital	Terre Haute	17	460
Fayette Regional Health System	Connersville	18	408
Franciscan St Elizabeth Health	Crawfordsville	18	285
IU Health Goshen Hospital	Goshen	18	400
Saint Vincent Dunn Hospital[3]	Bedford	18	296
Cameron Memorial Community Hospital	Angola	19	357
Community Hospital North	Indianapolis	19	409
Franciscan St Elizabeth Health	Lafayette	19	281
Franciscan St Elizabeth Health	Lafayette	19	281
Indiana University Health North Hospital	Carmel	19	404
Elkhart General Hospital	Elkhart	20	579
Saint Joseph Hospital	Fort Wayne	20	411
Saint Vincent Salem Hospital[3]	Salem	20	214
Schneck Medical Center	Seymour	20	358
Community Hospital South	Indianapolis	21	283
Dekalb Health	Auburn	21	449
Dukes Memorial Hospital	Peru	21	401
Franciscan St Anthony Health-Crown Pt	Crown Point	21	415
Jasper County Hospital	Rensselaer	21	8983
Riverview Hospital	Noblesville	21	398
Harrison County Hospital	Corydon	22	409
Henry County Memorial Hospital	New Castle	22	353
IU Health West Hospital	Avon	22	370
Monroe Hospital	Bloomington	22	370
Saint Mary's Medical Center of Evansville	Evansville	22	380
Comm Hosp of Anderson/Madison Co	Anderson	23	384
Franciscan St Francis Hlth-Indianapolis	Indianapolis	23	445
Indiana University Health Starke Hospital	Knox	23	385
Saint Mary Medical Center	Hobart	23	416
Franciscan St Anthony Health	Michigan City	24	428
Franciscan St Francis Health	Mooresville	24	438
Good Samaritan Hospital	Vincennes	24	391
Hendricks Regional Health	Danville	24	840
Memorial Hospital	Logansport	24	571
Parkview Whitley Hospital	Columbia City	24	381
Saint Vincent Carmel Hospital	Carmel	24	348
Community Hospital East	Indianapolis	26	294
Hancock Regional Hospital	Greenfield	26	500
Indiana Univ Health Blackford Hosp	Hartford City	26	407
Indiana Univ Health Bloomington Hosp	Bloomington	26	412
Kosciusko Community Hospital	Warsaw	26	401
Parkview Noble Hospital	Kendallville	26	372
Saint Catherine Hospital	East Chicago	26	418
Community Westview Hospital	Indianapolis	27	453
Franciscan Saint Margaret Health - Dyer	Dyer	28	503
Indiana University Health	Indianapolis	28	374
Indiana University Health Arnett Hospital	Lafayette	28	395
Parkview Lagrange Hospital	Lagrange	28	318
Community Hospital	Munster	29	425
Saint Vincent Clay Hospital	Brazil	29	368
Marion General Hospital	Marion	30	390
Parkview Regional Medical Center	Fort Wayne	31	547
Indiana Univ Health Ball Mem Hosp	Muncie	32	453
Saint Vincent Hospital & Health Services	Indianapolis	33	322
Columbus Regional Hospital	Columbus	34	468
Franciscan St Margaret Health-Hammond	Hammond	34	502
Saint Vincent Anderson Regional Hospital	Anderson	34	390
Floyd Memorial Hospital & Health Services	New Albany	35	354
Saint Vincent Randolph Hospital	Winchester	35	373
Indiana Univ Health La Porte Hosp	La Porte	37	479
Reid Hospital & Health Care Services	Richmond	37	369
Clark Memorial Hospital	Jeffersonville	38	390
King's Daughters' Health	Madison	38	417
Dearborn County Hospital	Lawrenceburg	40	423
Parkview Huntington Hospital	Huntington	40	348
Community Howard Regional Health	Kokomo	45	556
Eskenazi Health	Indianapolis	52	370
Memorial Hospital of South Bend	South Bend	68	467
Methodist Hospitals	Gary	74	272
Saint Joseph Hospital & Health Center	Kokomo	100	401

Time to Pain Meds for Bone Fractures (minutes)

Hospital Name	City	Min.	Cases
Parkview Lagrange Hospital	Lagrange	21	43
Cameron Memorial Community Hospital	Angola	25	83
Decatur County Memorial Hospital	Greensburg	26	41
Dupont Hospital	Fort Wayne	26	71
Parkview Whitley Hospital	Columbia City	30	42
Parkview Noble Hospital	Kendallville	31	61
Daviess Community Hospital	Washington	32	46
Terre Haute Regional Hospital	Terre Haute	33	59
Indiana University Health Starke Hospital	Knox	34	39
Johnson Memorial Hospital	Franklin	34	60
Rush Memorial Hospital	Rushville	34	31
Margaret Mary Community Hospital	Batesville	37	38
Union Hospital Clinton	Clinton	37	62
Franciscan St Francis Hlth-Indianapolis	Indianapolis	38	182
Franciscan St Elizabeth Health	Crawfordsville	39	91
Franciscan St Francis Health	Mooresville	40	64
Saint Joseph Hospital	Fort Wayne	40	92
Memorial Hospital	Logansport	41	63
Dekalb Health	Auburn	42	62
Henry County Memorial Hospital	New Castle	42	93
Schneck Medical Center	Seymour	42	65
Saint Vincent Carmel Hospital	Carmel	43	135
Bluffton Regional Medical Center	Bluffton	44	53
Elkhart General Hospital	Elkhart	44	155
Franciscan St Anthony Health	Michigan City	44	130
Indiana Univ Health Bedford Hosp	Bedford	44	38
Indiana University Health North Hospital	Carmel	44	98
Lutheran Hospital of Indiana	Fort Wayne	44	256
Parkview Huntington Hospital	Huntington	44	60
Witham Health Services	Lebanon	44	106
Community Hospital	Munster	45	164
Dukes Memorial Hospital	Peru	45	53
Sullivan County Community Hospital	Sullivan	45	42
Franciscan St Anthony Health-Crown Pt	Crown Point	46	124
Franciscan Saint Margaret Health - Dyer	Dyer	46	80
Franciscan St Elizabeth Health	Lafayette	47	135
Clark Memorial Hospital	Jeffersonville	48	94
Franciscan St Elizabeth Health	Lafayette	48	57
St Joseph Reg Med Ctr-Plymouth	Plymouth	48	81
Saint Vincent Hospital & Health Services	Indianapolis	48	349
Union Hospital	Terre Haute	49	170
Good Samaritan Hospital	Vincennes	51	127
Major Hospital	Shelbyville	51	78
Columbus Regional Hospital	Columbus	52	177
Community Hospital North	Indianapolis	52	253
Community Howard Regional Health	Kokomo	53	95
Hancock Regional Hospital	Greenfield	53	123
Hendricks Regional Health	Danville	53	112
Harrison County Hospital	Corydon	54	53
Porter Regional Hospital	Valparaiso	54	304
Riverview Hospital	Noblesville	54	105
Saint Vincent Salem Hospital[3]	Salem	54	39
Community Hospital South	Indianapolis	55	161
Fayette Regional Health System	Connersville	55	60
Deaconess Hospital	Evansville	56	193
Franciscan St Margaret Health-Hammond	Hammond	56	96
Indiana University Health Morgan Hospital	Martinsville	56	84
IU Health Goshen Hospital	Goshen	56	162
Kosciusko Community Hospital	Warsaw	56	90
Monroe Hospital	Bloomington	56	42
Comm Hosp of Anderson/Madison Co	Anderson	57	75
Memorial Hospital & Health Care Center	Jasper	58	129
Parkview Regional Medical Center	Fort Wayne	58	344
Saint Catherine Hospital	East Chicago	58	113
Saint Joseph Regional Medical Center	Mishawaka	58	154
Indiana Univ Health Bloomington Hosp	Bloomington	59	196
Reid Hospital & Health Care Services	Richmond	59	117
Community Hospital East	Indianapolis	60	168
Indiana University Health Arnett Hospital	Lafayette	61	120
Indiana Univ Health Ball Mem Hosp	Muncie	61	170
Dearborn County Hospital	Lawrenceburg	63	93
Marion General Hospital	Marion	63	118
Saint Vincent Anderson Regional Hospital	Anderson	63	107
IU Health West Hospital	Avon	64	197
Saint Mary's Medical Center of Evansville	Evansville	65	142
Saint Mary Medical Center	Hobart	66	119
Indiana University Health	Indianapolis	68	182
Jasper County Hospital	Rensselaer	68	40
Floyd Memorial Hospital & Health Services	New Albany	70	173
Indiana Univ Health Blackford Hosp	Hartford City	72	43
King's Daughters' Health	Madison	72	71
Eskenazi Health	Indianapolis	75	95
Indiana Univ Health La Porte Hosp	La Porte	75	93
Methodist Hospitals	Gary	78	124
Saint Joseph Hospital & Health Center	Kokomo	84	80
Memorial Hospital of South Bend	South Bend	86	182

Heart Attack Care

Aspirin Given at Discharge

Hospital Name	City	Rate	Cases
Columbus Regional Hospital	Columbus	100%	259
Community Hospital South	Indianapolis	100%	170
Eskenazi Health	Indianapolis	100%	244
Floyd Memorial Hospital & Health Services	New Albany	100%	338
Franciscan St Francis Hlth-Indianapolis	Indianapolis	100%	417
Franciscan Saint Margaret Health - Dyer	Dyer	100%	89
Good Samaritan Hospital	Vincennes	100%	115
Hancock Regional Hospital	Greenfield	100%	38
The Heart Hospital at Deaconess Gateway	Newburgh	100%	294
Indiana University Health	Indianapolis	100%	610
Indiana Univ Health Bloomington Hosp[2]	Bloomington	100%	323
Indiana University Health North Hospital	Carmel	100%	41
IU Health West Hospital	Avon	100%	82

NOTE: Hospital profiles are in alphabetical order by state, then city, then hospital within the city; Rankings exclude hospitals with less than 25 cases except for patient surveys which excludes hospitals with less than 100 cases; (a) 100-299 cases; (1) The number of cases/patients is too few to report; (2) Data submitted were based on a sample of cases/patients; (3) Results are based on a shorter time period than required; (4) Data suppressed by CMS for one or more quarters; (5) Results are not available for this reporting period; (6) Fewer than 100 patients completed the HCAHPS survey; (7) No cases met the criteria for this measure; (8) The lower limit of the confidence interval cannot be calculated if the number of observed infections equals zero; (9) No data are available from the state/territory for this reporting period; (10) The scores shown reflect fewer than 50 completed surveys; (11) There were discrepancies in the data collection process; (12) This measure does not apply to this hospital for this reporting period; (13) Results cannot be calculated for this reporting period; (14) The results for this state are combined with nearby states to protect confidentiality; Please refer to the User's Guide for a full explanation of data.

Hospital Name	City	Rate	Cases
Lutheran Hospital of Indiana	Fort Wayne	100%	544
Memorial Hospital & Health Care Center	Jasper	100%	212
Parkview Regional Medical Center	Fort Wayne	100%	675
Porter Regional Hospital	Valparaiso	100%	287
Riverview Hospital	Noblesville	100%	80
Saint Catherine Hospital	East Chicago	100%	65
Saint Joseph Regional Medical Center	Mishawaka	100%	242
St Joseph Reg Med Ctr-Plymouth	Plymouth	100%	39
Saint Mary Medical Center	Hobart	100%	97
Saint Mary's Medical Center of Evansville	Evansville	100%	307
Saint Vincent Heart Center of Indiana	Indianapolis	100%	955
Saint Vincent Hospital & Health Services	Indianapolis	100%	302
Terre Haute Regional Hospital	Terre Haute	100%	172
Union Hospital	Terre Haute	100%	535
Witham Health Services	Lebanon	100%	31
Community Hospital	Munster	99%	170
Community Hospital East	Indianapolis	99%	159
Community Howard Regional Health	Kokomo	99%	126
Deaconess Hospital	Evansville	99%	313
Elkhart General Hospital[2]	Elkhart	99%	285
Franciscan St Anthony Health-Crown Pt	Crown Point	99%	158
Franciscan St Anthony Health	Michigan City	99%	105
Franciscan St Margaret Health-Hammond	Hammond	99%	139
The Indiana Heart Hospital	Indianapolis	99%	264
Indiana University Health Arnett Hospital	Lafayette	99%	215
Indianapolis VA Medical Center	Indianapolis	99%	125
IU Health Goshen Hospital	Goshen	99%	89
Memorial Hospital of South Bend	South Bend	99%	301
Reid Hospital & Health Care Services	Richmond	99%	386
Saint Joseph Hospital	Fort Wayne	99%	129
Comm Hosp of Anderson/Madison Co	Anderson	98%	48
Franciscan St Elizabeth Health	Lafayette	98%	200
Indiana Univ Health Ball Mem Hosp	Muncie	98%	381
Methodist Hospitals[2]	Gary	98%	126
Clark Memorial Hospital	Jeffersonville	97%	193
Indiana Univ Health La Porte Hosp	La Porte	97%	115
Saint Vincent Anderson Regional Hospital	Anderson	97%	32
Marion General Hospital	Marion	96%	26
Hendricks Regional Health	Danville	94%	50
Dearborn County Hospital	Lawrenceburg	91%	35

PCI Within 90 Minutes of Arrival

Hospital Name	City	Rate	Cases
Community Hospital	Munster	100%	32
Community Hospital East	Indianapolis	100%	46
Community Howard Regional Health	Kokomo	100%	29
Franciscan St Anthony Health-Crown Pt	Crown Point	100%	35
Franciscan St Francis Hlth-Indianapolis	Indianapolis	100%	86
Franciscan St Margaret Health-Hammond	Hammond	100%	29
The Indiana Heart Hospital	Indianapolis	100%	54
Indiana Univ Health Bloomington Hosp[2]	Bloomington	100%	63
Porter Regional Hospital	Valparaiso	100%	49
Saint Vincent Hospital & Health Services	Indianapolis	100%	27
Indiana Univ Health Ball Mem Hosp	Muncie	99%	70
Memorial Hospital of South Bend	South Bend	99%	68
Columbus Regional Hospital	Columbus	98%	62
Elkhart General Hospital[2]	Elkhart	98%	65
Indiana University Health	Indianapolis	98%	109
Reid Hospital & Health Care Services	Richmond	98%	52
Saint Mary's Medical Center of Evansville	Evansville	98%	49
Lutheran Hospital of Indiana	Fort Wayne	97%	59
Deaconess Hospital	Evansville	96%	54
Saint Joseph Hospital	Fort Wayne	96%	27
Saint Joseph Regional Medical Center	Mishawaka	96%	56
Indiana University Health Arnett Hospital	Lafayette	95%	39
Union Hospital	Terre Haute	95%	61
Community Hospital South	Indianapolis	94%	49
Franciscan St Elizabeth Health	Lafayette	94%	36
Indiana Univ Health La Porte Hosp	La Porte	93%	29
Parkview Regional Medical Center	Fort Wayne	93%	54
Methodist Hospitals[2]	Gary	89%	35
Clark Memorial Hospital	Jeffersonville	86%	37
Floyd Memorial Hospital & Health Services	New Albany	81%	53

Statin Prescribed at Discharge

Hospital Name	City	Rate	Cases
Columbus Regional Hospital	Columbus	100%	254
Elkhart General Hospital[2]	Elkhart	100%	282
Eskenazi Health	Indianapolis	100%	242
Franciscan St Francis Hlth-Indianapolis	Indianapolis	100%	406
Indiana University Health	Indianapolis	100%	625
Indiana Univ Health Ball Mem Hosp	Muncie	100%	373
Indiana Univ Health Bloomington Hosp[2]	Bloomington	100%	322
Indiana Univ Health La Porte Hosp	La Porte	100%	116
Indianapolis VA Medical Center	Indianapolis	100%	119
IU Health Goshen Hospital	Goshen	100%	88
Lutheran Hospital of Indiana	Fort Wayne	100%	526
Marion General Hospital	Marion	100%	28
Porter Regional Hospital	Valparaiso	100%	279
Riverview Hospital	Noblesville	100%	77
Saint Catherine Hospital	East Chicago	100%	65
St Joseph Reg Med Ctr-Plymouth	Plymouth	100%	39
Saint Mary Medical Center	Hobart	100%	92
Saint Vincent Anderson Regional Hospital	Anderson	100%	31
Saint Vincent Heart Center of Indiana	Indianapolis	100%	936
Saint Vincent Hospital & Health Services	Indianapolis	100%	297
Terre Haute Regional Hospital	Terre Haute	100%	168
Community Hospital South	Indianapolis	99%	161
Deaconess Hospital	Evansville	99%	306
Franciscan St Anthony Health	Michigan City	99%	100
Franciscan St Elizabeth Health	Lafayette	99%	190
The Heart Hospital at Deaconess Gateway	Newburgh	99%	286
The Indiana Heart Hospital	Indianapolis	99%	250
IU Health West Hospital	Avon	99%	81
Parkview Regional Medical Center	Fort Wayne	99%	650
Reid Hospital & Health Care Services	Richmond	99%	387
Saint Joseph Hospital	Fort Wayne	99%	118
Saint Joseph Regional Medical Center	Mishawaka	99%	237
Union Hospital	Terre Haute	99%	499
Community Hospital	Munster	98%	169
Community Hospital East	Indianapolis	98%	158
Comm Hosp of Anderson/Madison Co	Anderson	98%	49
Floyd Memorial Hospital & Health Services	New Albany	98%	314
Franciscan Saint Margaret Health - Dyer	Dyer	98%	87
Indiana University Health Arnett Hospital	Lafayette	98%	212
Memorial Hospital & Health Care Center	Jasper	98%	208
Memorial Hospital of South Bend	South Bend	98%	304
Saint Mary's Medical Center of Evansville	Evansville	98%	298
Community Howard Regional Health	Kokomo	97%	127
Hancock Regional Hospital	Greenfield	97%	37
Indiana University Health North Hospital	Carmel	97%	34
Franciscan St Margaret Health-Hammond	Hammond	96%	133
Franciscan St Anthony Health-Crown Pt	Crown Point	95%	153
Good Samaritan Hospital	Vincennes	95%	111
Methodist Hospitals[2]	Gary	95%	125
Clark Memorial Hospital	Jeffersonville	94%	171
Dearborn County Hospital	Lawrenceburg	94%	33
Witham Health Services	Lebanon	94%	32
Hendricks Regional Health	Danville	87%	46

Heart Failure Care

ACE Inhibitor or ARB for LVSD

Hospital Name	City	Rate	Cases
Community Hospital East	Indianapolis	100%	108
Community Hospital South	Indianapolis	100%	70
Franciscan St Anthony Health	Michigan City	100%	90
Franciscan St Francis Hlth-Indianapolis	Indianapolis	100%	101
The Indiana Heart Hospital	Indianapolis	100%	94
Indiana University Health Arnett Hospital[2]	Lafayette	100%	44
Indiana Univ Health Bloomington Hosp	Bloomington	100%	70
IU Health Goshen Hospital	Goshen	100%	25
IU Health West Hospital	Avon	100%	37
Major Hospital	Shelbyville	100%	26
Memorial Hospital of South Bend	South Bend	100%	104
Porter Regional Hospital	Valparaiso	100%	116
Saint Joseph Hospital	Fort Wayne	100%	51
Saint Joseph Hospital & Health Center	Kokomo	100%	50
Saint Joseph Regional Medical Center	Mishawaka	100%	68
Saint Mary Medical Center[2]	Hobart	100%	118
Saint Vincent Anderson Regional Hospital	Anderson	100%	71
Saint Vincent Heart Center of Indiana	Indianapolis	100%	112
Terre Haute Regional Hospital	Terre Haute	100%	48
Columbus Regional Hospital	Columbus	99%	93
Franciscan St Elizabeth Health	Lafayette	99%	68
Indiana University Health[2]	Indianapolis	99%	208
Lutheran Hospital of Indiana	Fort Wayne	99%	117
Saint Mary's Medical Center of Evansville	Evansville	99%	138
Saint Vincent Hospital & Health Services	Indianapolis	99%	196
Union Hospital	Terre Haute	99%	159
Comm Hosp of Anderson/Madison Co	Anderson	98%	64
Eskenazi Health	Indianapolis	98%	185
Hendricks Regional Health	Danville	98%	46
Indiana Univ Health La Porte Hosp	La Porte	98%	53
Indianapolis VA Medical Center	Indianapolis	98%	103
Marion General Hospital	Marion	98%	40
Methodist Hospitals[2]	Gary	98%	145
Parkview Regional Medical Center[2]	Fort Wayne	98%	81
Saint Catherine Hospital	East Chicago	98%	93
Floyd Memorial Hospital & Health Services	New Albany	97%	104
Franciscan St Anthony Health-Crown Pt[2]	Crown Point	97%	65
Franciscan Saint Margaret Health - Dyer	Dyer	97%	63
Franciscan St Margaret Health-Hammond[2]	Hammond	97%	102
The Heart Hospital at Deaconess Gateway	Newburgh	97%	31
Bluffton Regional Medical Center	Bluffton	96%	26
Community Howard Regional Health	Kokomo	96%	45
Kentuckiana Medical Center[2]	Clarksville	96%	28
Memorial Hospital & Health Care Center	Jasper	96%	54
Reid Hospital & Health Care Services	Richmond	96%	75
Deaconess Hospital	Evansville	95%	193
Elkhart General Hospital[2]	Elkhart	95%	146
Good Samaritan Hospital	Vincennes	95%	80
Clark Memorial Hospital	Jeffersonville	94%	83
Community Hospital North	Indianapolis	91%	33
Indiana Univ Health Ball Mem Hosp[2]	Muncie	91%	74
Community Hospital[2]	Munster	89%	81
Dearborn County Hospital	Lawrenceburg	84%	25
King's Daughters' Health	Madison	65%	37

Discharge Instructions Given

Hospital Name	City	Rate	Cases
Decatur County Memorial Hospital	Greensburg	100%	39
Dupont Hospital	Fort Wayne	100%	28
Eskenazi Health	Indianapolis	100%	362
Franciscan St Elizabeth Health	Crawfordsville	100%	51
Indiana Univ Health Ball Mem Hosp[2]	Muncie	100%	218
Indiana Univ Health Bloomington Hosp	Bloomington	100%	146
Indiana University Health Morgan Hospital	Martinsville	100%	47
Indiana University Health North Hospital	Carmel	100%	50
Indiana University Health Starke Hospital	Knox	100%	40
Indiana Univ Health White Mem Hosp	Monticello	100%	29
Indianapolis VA Medical Center	Indianapolis	100%	232
Margaret Mary Community Hospital	Batesville	100%	27
Memorial Hospital	Logansport	100%	41
Porter Regional Hospital	Valparaiso	100%	294
Saint Mary Medical Center[2]	Hobart	100%	240
Saint Mary's Medical Center of Evansville	Evansville	100%	338
Saint Vincent Dunn Hospital	Bedford	100%	33
Saint Vincent Williamsport Hospital	Williamsport	100%	28
Schneck Medical Center	Seymour	100%	37
Witham Health Services	Lebanon	100%	61
Woodlawn Hospital	Rochester	100%	30
Franciscan St Anthony Health	Michigan City	99%	199
IU Health West Hospital	Avon	99%	145
Memorial Hospital of South Bend	South Bend	99%	314
Saint Catherine Hospital	East Chicago	99%	222
Saint Joseph Hospital	Fort Wayne	99%	154
Saint Vincent Anderson Regional Hospital	Anderson	99%	138
Bluffton Regional Medical Center	Bluffton	98%	41
Community Hospital[2]	Munster	98%	266
Comm Hosp of Anderson/Madison Co	Anderson	98%	158
Community Hospital South	Indianapolis	98%	175
Dekalb Health	Auburn	98%	47
Franciscan St Francis Hlth-Indianapolis	Indianapolis	98%	344
Indiana Univ Health La Porte Hosp	La Porte	98%	129
IU Health Goshen Hospital	Goshen	98%	88
Saint Joseph Regional Medical Center	Mishawaka	98%	277
St Joseph Reg Med Ctr-Plymouth	Plymouth	98%	43
Saint Vincent Heart Center of Indiana	Indianapolis	98%	268
Terre Haute Regional Hospital	Terre Haute	98%	146
Cameron Memorial Community Hospital	Angola	97%	33
Fayette Regional Health System	Connersville	97%	34
King's Daughters' Health	Madison	97%	77
Major Hospital	Shelbyville	97%	72
Memorial Hospital & Health Care Center	Jasper	97%	128
Parkview Whitley Hospital	Columbia City	97%	31
Community Hospital East	Indianapolis	96%	256
Franciscan Saint Margaret Health - Dyer	Dyer	96%	188
The Indiana Heart Hospital	Indianapolis	96%	205
Lutheran Hospital of Indiana	Fort Wayne	96%	387
Marion General Hospital	Marion	96%	158
Parkview Noble Hospital	Kendallville	96%	51
Riverview Hospital	Noblesville	96%	73
Adams Memorial Hospital	Decatur	95%	41
Franciscan St Margaret Health-Hammond[2]	Hammond	95%	267
Hendricks Regional Health	Danville	95%	86
Henry County Memorial Hospital	New Castle	95%	39
Indiana University Health[2]	Indianapolis	95%	584
Parkview Regional Medical Center[2]	Fort Wayne	95%	242
Saint Joseph Hospital & Health Center	Kokomo	95%	109
Saint Vincent Hospital & Health Services	Indianapolis	95%	587
Indiana University Health Arnett Hospital[2]	Lafayette	94%	148
Reid Hospital & Health Care Services	Richmond	94%	276
Franciscan St Anthony Health-Crown Pt[2]	Crown Point	93%	198
Franciscan St Elizabeth Health	Lafayette	93%	147
Kosciusko Community Hospital	Warsaw	93%	87
Community Hospital North	Indianapolis	92%	113
Dearborn County Hospital	Lawrenceburg	92%	64
Floyd Memorial Hospital & Health Services	New Albany	92%	298
Union Hospital	Terre Haute	92%	391
Clark Memorial Hospital	Jeffersonville	91%	215
Parkview Huntington Hospital	Huntington	91%	46
Union Hospital Clinton	Clinton	91%	32
Elkhart General Hospital[2]	Elkhart	89%	398
Franciscan Healthcare - Munster	Munster	89%	38
Franciscan St Elizabeth Health	Lafayette	89%	46
Kentuckiana Medical Center[2]	Clarksville	89%	45
Methodist Hospitals[2]	Gary	88%	254
Columbus Regional Hospital	Columbus	87%	211
Hancock Regional Hospital	Greenfield	87%	54
Deaconess Hospital	Evansville	86%	511

NOTE: Hospital profiles are in alphabetical order by state, then city, then hospital within the city; Rankings exclude hospitals with less than 25 cases except for patient surveys which excludes hospitals with less than 100 cases; (a) 100-299 cases; (1) The number of cases/patients is too few to report; (2) Data submitted were based on a sample of cases/patients; (3) Results are based on a shorter time period than required; (4) Data suppressed by CMS for one or more quarters; (5) Results are not available for this reporting period; (6) Fewer than 100 patients completed the HCAHPS survey; (7) No cases met the criteria for this measure; (8) The lower limit of the confidence interval cannot be calculated if the number of observed infections equals zero; (9) No data are available from the state/territory for this reporting period; (10) The scores shown reflect fewer than 50 completed surveys; (11) There were discrepancies in the data collection process; (12) This measure does not apply to this hospital for this reporting period; (13) Results cannot be calculated for this reporting period; (14) The results for this state are combined with nearby states to protect confidentiality; Please refer to the User's Guide for a full explanation of data.

Community Westview Hospital[2]	Indianapolis	85%	48
Johnson Memorial Hospital	Franklin	85%	54
Sullivan County Community Hospital	Sullivan	85%	26
Community Howard Regional Health	Kokomo	83%	87
Good Samaritan Hospital	Vincennes	83%	170
The Heart Hospital at Deaconess Gateway	Newburgh	83%	54
Daviess Community Hospital	Washington	80%	30
Greene County General Hospital	Linton	79%	39
Jasper County Hospital	Rensselaer	78%	36
Scott Memorial Hospital	Scottsburg	76%	25
Perry County Memorial Hospital	Tell City	73%	37

Evaluation of LVS Function

Hospital Name	City	Rate	Cases
Adams Memorial Hospital	Decatur	100%	60
Bluffton Regional Medical Center	Bluffton	100%	61
Cameron Memorial Community Hospital	Angola	100%	46
Clark Memorial Hospital	Jeffersonville	100%	294
Columbus Regional Hospital	Columbus	100%	288
Community Hospital[2]	Munster	100%	322
Community Hospital North	Indianapolis	100%	172
Comm Hosp of Anderson/Madison Co	Anderson	100%	205
Community Hospital South	Indianapolis	100%	252
Community Westview Hospital[2]	Indianapolis	100%	56
Deaconess Hospital	Evansville	100%	686
Dearborn County Hospital	Lawrenceburg	100%	94
Decatur County Memorial Hospital	Greensburg	100%	64
Dekalb Health	Auburn	100%	72
Dupont Hospital	Fort Wayne	100%	37
Elkhart General Hospital[2]	Elkhart	100%	483
Eskenazi Health	Indianapolis	100%	400
Fayette Regional Health System	Connersville	100%	43
Franciscan Healthcare - Munster	Munster	100%	42
Franciscan St Anthony Health-Crown Pt[2]	Crown Point	100%	274
Franciscan St Anthony Health	Michigan City	100%	244
Franciscan St Francis Hlth-Indianapolis	Indianapolis	100%	455
Franciscan St Francis Health	Mooresville	100%	25
Franciscan Saint Margaret Health - Dyer	Dyer	100%	240
Hancock Regional Hospital	Greenfield	100%	78
The Heart Hospital at Deaconess Gateway	Newburgh	100%	61
Henry County Memorial Hospital	New Castle	100%	55
The Indiana Heart Hospital	Indianapolis	100%	269
Indiana University Health[2]	Indianapolis	100%	722
Indiana University Health Arnett Hospital[2]	Lafayette	100%	205
Indiana Univ Health Ball Mem Hosp[2]	Muncie	100%	275
Indiana Univ Health Bloomington Hosp	Bloomington	100%	216
Indiana Univ Health La Porte Hosp	La Porte	100%	164
Indiana University Health Starke Hospital	Knox	100%	41
Indiana University Health Tipton Hospital	Tipton	100%	31
Indianapolis VA Medical Center	Indianapolis	100%	246
IU Health Goshen Hospital	Goshen	100%	114
IU Health West Hospital	Avon	100%	190
Johnson Memorial Hospital	Franklin	100%	81
Kosciusko Community Hospital	Warsaw	100%	118
Lutheran Hospital of Indiana	Fort Wayne	100%	466
Major Hospital	Shelbyville	100%	87
Marion General Hospital	Marion	100%	200
Memorial Hospital	Logansport	100%	63
Memorial Hospital & Health Care Center	Jasper	100%	169
Memorial Hospital of South Bend	South Bend	100%	399
Methodist Hospitals[2]	Gary	100%	310
Parkview Noble Hospital	Kendallville	100%	74
Parkview Regional Medical Center[2]	Fort Wayne	100%	311
Parkview Whitley Hospital	Columbia City	100%	40
Porter Regional Hospital	Valparaiso	100%	369
Reid Hospital & Health Care Services	Richmond	100%	387
Saint Joseph Hospital	Fort Wayne	100%	185
Saint Joseph Hospital & Health Center	Kokomo	100%	145
Saint Joseph Regional Medical Center	Mishawaka	100%	364
St Joseph Reg Med Ctr-Plymouth	Plymouth	100%	59
Saint Mary Medical Center[2]	Hobart	100%	301
Saint Mary's Medical Center of Evansville	Evansville	100%	424
Saint Vincent Anderson Regional Hospital	Anderson	100%	192
Saint Vincent Carmel Hospital	Carmel	100%	31
Saint Vincent Dunn Hospital	Bedford	100%	54
Saint Vincent Hospital & Health Services	Indianapolis	100%	749
Saint Vincent Randolph Hospital	Winchester	100%	28
Schneck Medical Center	Seymour	100%	62
Terre Haute Regional Hospital	Terre Haute	100%	190
Union Hospital	Terre Haute	100%	511
Union Hospital Clinton	Clinton	100%	41
Wabash County Hospital	Wabash	100%	26
Community Hospital East	Indianapolis	99%	328
Floyd Memorial Hospital & Health Services	New Albany	99%	402
Franciscan St Elizabeth Health	Lafayette	99%	178
Good Samaritan Hospital	Vincennes	99%	231
Hendricks Regional Health	Danville	99%	117
King's Daughters' Health	Madison	99%	117
Parkview Huntington Hospital	Huntington	99%	70
Riverview Hospital	Noblesville	99%	93
Saint Catherine Hospital	East Chicago	99%	281
Community Howard Regional Health	Kokomo	98%	123
Indiana University Health Morgan Hospital	Martinsville	98%	66
Indiana University Health North Hospital	Carmel	98%	64
Margaret Mary Community Hospital	Batesville	98%	45
Saint Vincent Williamsport Hospital	Williamsport	98%	45
Franciscan St Elizabeth Health	Crawfordsville	97%	64
Franciscan St Elizabeth Health	Lafayette	97%	68
Franciscan St Margaret Health-Hammond[2]	Hammond	97%	313
Jasper County Hospital	Rensselaer	97%	67
Scott Memorial Hospital	Scottsburg	97%	36
Indiana Univ Health White Mem Hosp	Monticello	96%	45
Pulaski Memorial Hospital	Winamac	96%	26
Saint Vincent Heart Center of Indiana	Indianapolis	96%	316
Witham Health Services	Lebanon	96%	81
Sullivan County Community Hospital	Sullivan	95%	41
Gibson General Hospital	Princeton	93%	28
Kentuckiana Medical Center[2]	Clarksville	90%	41
Daviess Community Hospital	Washington	88%	40
Saint Vincent Mercy Hospital	Elwood	83%	30
Greene County General Hospital	Linton	77%	61
Woodlawn Hospital	Rochester	69%	36

Medicare Spending

Medicare Spending per Patient (ratio)

Hospital Name	City	Ratio	Cases
Fairbanks	Indianapolis	0.85	-
Physicians' Medical Center	New Albany	0.86	-
The Ortho Hosp/Lutheran Health Network	Fort Wayne	0.90	-
Parkview Whitley Hospital	Columbia City	0.90	-
Indiana Orthopaedic Hospital	Indianapolis	0.91	-
Schneck Medical Center	Seymour	0.91	-
Franciscan St Elizabeth Health	Crawfordsville	0.92	-
Franciscan St Francis Health	Mooresville	0.94	-
Bluffton Regional Medical Center	Bluffton	0.96	-
Columbus Regional Hospital	Columbus	0.96	-
Dupont Hospital	Fort Wayne	0.96	-
Eskenazi Health	Indianapolis	0.96	-
Memorial Hospital & Health Care Center	Jasper	0.96	-
Pinnacle Hospital	Crown Point	0.96	-
Dearborn County Hospital	Lawrenceburg	0.97	-
Fayette Regional Health System	Connersville	0.97	-
Kosciusko Community Hospital	Warsaw	0.97	-
Elkhart General Hospital	Elkhart	0.98	-
Memorial Hospital of South Bend	South Bend	0.98	-
Orthopaedic Hospital at Parkview North	Fort Wayne	0.98	-
St Joseph Reg Med Ctr-Plymouth	Plymouth	0.98	-
Saint Vincent Carmel Hospital	Carmel	0.98	-
Comm Hosp of Anderson/Madison Co	Anderson	0.99	-
Franciscan Healthcare - Munster	Munster	0.99	-
Franciscan St Anthony Health-Crown Pt	Crown Point	0.99	-
Franciscan St Elizabeth Health	Lafayette	0.99	-
Good Samaritan Hospital	Vincennes	0.99	-
Hendricks Regional Health	Danville	0.99	-
Indiana Univ Health La Porte Hosp	La Porte	0.99	-
Indiana University Health Starke Hospital	Knox	0.99	-
IU Health West Hospital	Avon	0.99	-
King's Daughters' Health	Madison	0.99	-
Parkview Noble Hospital	Kendallville	0.99	-
Saint Mary Medical Center	Hobart	0.99	-
Saint Vincent Heart Center of Indiana	Indianapolis	0.99	-
The Women's Hospital	Newburgh	0.99	-
Franciscan St Elizabeth Health	Lafayette	1.00	-
The Heart Hospital at Deaconess Gateway	Newburgh	1.00	-
Lutheran Hospital of Indiana	Fort Wayne	1.00	-
Parkview Huntington Hospital	Huntington	1.00	-
Parkview Regional Medical Center	Fort Wayne	1.00	-
Witham Health Services	Lebanon	1.00	-
Clark Memorial Hospital	Jeffersonville	1.01	-
Community Hospital East	Indianapolis	1.01	-
Floyd Memorial Hospital & Health Services	New Albany	1.01	-
Franciscan St Anthony Health	Michigan City	1.01	-
Indiana University Health	Indianapolis	1.01	-
Indiana Univ Health Ball Mem Hosp	Muncie	1.01	-
Reid Hospital & Health Care Services	Richmond	1.01	-
Saint Catherine Regional Hospital	Charlestown	1.01	-
Saint Joseph Regional Medical Center	Mishawaka	1.01	-
Saint Mary's Medical Center of Evansville	Evansville	1.01	-
Community Hospital North	Indianapolis	1.02	-
Community Hospital South	Indianapolis	1.02	-
Dekalb Health	Auburn	1.02	-
The Indiana Heart Hospital	Indianapolis	1.02	-
Major Hospital	Shelbyville	1.02	-
Marion General Hospital	Marion	1.02	-
Saint Vincent Hospital & Health Services	Indianapolis	1.02	-
Terre Haute Regional Hospital	Terre Haute	1.02	-
Community Westview Hospital	Indianapolis	1.03	-
Deaconess Hospital	Evansville	1.03	-
Henry County Memorial Hospital	New Castle	1.03	-
IU Health Goshen Hospital	Goshen	1.03	-
Johnson Memorial Hospital	Franklin	1.03	-
Porter Regional Hospital	Valparaiso	1.03	-
Riverview Hospital	Noblesville	1.03	-
Saint Vincent Anderson Regional Hospital	Anderson	1.03	-
Union Hospital	Terre Haute	1.03	-
Community Howard Regional Health	Kokomo	1.04	-
Franciscan St Francis Hlth-Indianapolis	Indianapolis	1.04	-
Hancock Regional Hospital	Greenfield	1.04	-
Indiana Univ Health Bloomington Hosp	Bloomington	1.04	-
Monroe Hospital	Bloomington	1.04	-
Saint Joseph Hospital	Fort Wayne	1.04	-
Franciscan Saint Margaret Health - Dyer	Dyer	1.05	-
Franciscan St Margaret Health-Hammond	Hammond	1.05	-
Indiana University Health Arnett Hospital	Lafayette	1.05	-
Indiana University Health Morgan Hospital	Martinsville	1.05	-
Kentuckiana Medical Center	Clarksville	1.05	-
Community Hospital	Munster	1.06	-
Saint Joseph Hospital & Health Center	Kokomo	1.06	-
Indiana University Health North Hospital	Carmel	1.07	-
Memorial Hospital	Logansport	1.07	-
Methodist Hospitals	Gary	1.07	-
Saint Catherine Hospital	East Chicago	1.14	-
Daviess Community Hospital	Washington	1.22	-
Unity Medical & Surgical Hospital	Mishawaka	1.49	-

Pneumonia Care

Appropriate Initial Antibiotic Given

Hospital Name	City	Rate	Cases
Decatur County Memorial Hospital	Greensburg	100%	43
Dupont Hospital	Fort Wayne	100%	33
Franciscan St Anthony Health	Michigan City	100%	97
Franciscan St Elizabeth Health[2]	Lafayette	100%	34
Franciscan St Elizabeth Health[2]	Lafayette	100%	30
Franciscan Saint Margaret Health - Dyer	Dyer	100%	57
Memorial Hospital	Logansport	100%	92
Methodist Hospitals[2]	Gary	100%	59
Putnam County Hospital	Greencastle	100%	44
Saint Catherine Hospital	East Chicago	100%	68
Saint Joseph Hospital	Fort Wayne	100%	59
Saint Joseph Hospital & Health Center	Kokomo	100%	86
St Joseph Reg Med Ctr-Plymouth	Plymouth	100%	57
Saint Mary Medical Center[2]	Hobart	100%	72
Saint Vincent Anderson Regional Hospital	Anderson	100%	114
Union Hospital Clinton	Clinton	100%	45
Bluffton Regional Medical Center	Bluffton	99%	72
Dekalb Health	Auburn	99%	71
Elkhart General Hospital[2]	Elkhart	99%	85
Indiana Univ Health Ball Mem Hosp[2]	Muncie	99%	70
Kosciusko Community Hospital	Warsaw	99%	79
Marion General Hospital	Marion	99%	136
Parkview Huntington Hospital	Huntington	99%	80
Parkview Noble Hospital	Kendallville	99%	83
Saint Joseph Regional Medical Center	Mishawaka	99%	211
Columbus Regional Hospital	Columbus	98%	161
Comm Hosp of Anderson/Madison Co[2]	Anderson	98%	58
Eskenazi Health[2]	Indianapolis	98%	65
Franciscan St Margaret Health-Hammond[2]	Hammond	98%	65
Good Samaritan Hospital	Vincennes	98%	137
Henry County Memorial Hospital	New Castle	98%	97
Indiana University Health[2]	Indianapolis	98%	58
Memorial Hospital & Health Care Center[2]	Jasper	98%	94
Reid Hospital & Health Care Services	Richmond	98%	239
Saint Vincent Hospital & Health Services	Indianapolis	98%	170
Community Hospital North[2]	Indianapolis	97%	96
Floyd Memorial Hospital & Health Services	New Albany	97%	230
Hancock Regional Hospital[2]	Greenfield	97%	73
IU Health Goshen Hospital	Goshen	97%	149
Saint Mary's Warrick Hospital	Boonville	97%	31
Saint Vincent Dunn Hospital	Bedford	97%	33
Saint Vincent Randolph Hospital	Winchester	97%	32
Sullivan County Community Hospital	Sullivan	97%	33
Terre Haute Regional Hospital	Terre Haute	97%	64
Clark Memorial Hospital	Jeffersonville	96%	211
Community Hospital[2]	Munster	96%	76
Deaconess Hospital[2]	Evansville	96%	68
Fayette Regional Health System	Connersville	96%	73
Indiana Univ Health Bedford Hosp	Bedford	96%	55
Indiana Univ Health Blackford Hosp	Hartford City	96%	26
Indiana University Health Tipton Hospital	Tipton	96%	53
King's Daughters' Health[2]	Madison	96%	77
Margaret Mary Community Hospital	Batesville	96%	53
Parkview Lagrange Hospital	Lagrange	96%	47
Porter Regional Hospital	Valparaiso	96%	163
Pulaski Memorial Hospital	Winamac	96%	26
Saint Mary's Medical Center of Evansville	Evansville	96%	200
Schneck Medical Center	Seymour	96%	81
Union Hospital	Terre Haute	96%	320
Witham Health Services	Lebanon	96%	69
Community Hospital East[2]	Indianapolis	95%	124

NOTE: Hospital profiles are in alphabetical order by state, then city, then hospital within the city; Rankings exclude hospitals with less than 25 cases except for patient surveys which excludes hospitals with less than 100 cases; (a) 100-299 cases; (1) The number of cases/patients is too few to report; (2) Data submitted were based on a sample of cases/patients; (3) Results are based on a shorter time period than required; (4) Data suppressed by CMS for one or more quarters; (5) Results are not available for this reporting period; (6) Fewer than 100 patients completed the HCAHPS survey; (7) No cases met the criteria for this measure; (8) The lower limit of the confidence interval cannot be calculated if the number of observed infections equals zero; (9) No data are available from the state/territory for this reporting period; (10) The scores shown reflect fewer than 50 completed surveys; (11) There were discrepancies in the data collection process; (12) This measure does not apply to this hospital for this reporting period; (13) Results cannot be calculated for this reporting period; (14) The results for this state are combined with nearby states to protect confidentiality; Please refer to the User's Guide for a full explanation of data.

Hospital Name	City	Rate	Cases
Community Howard Regional Health	Kokomo	95%	123
Franciscan St Anthony Health-Crown Pt[2]	Crown Point	95%	78
Franciscan St Elizabeth Health	Crawfordsville	95%	38
Hendricks Regional Health	Danville	95%	115
Indiana Univ Health Bloomington Hosp[2]	Bloomington	95%	97
Indianapolis VA Medical Center	Indianapolis	95%	100
Jay County Hospital	Portland	95%	44
Major Hospital	Shelbyville	95%	58
Memorial Hospital of South Bend	South Bend	95%	188
Parkview Whitley Hospital	Columbia City	95%	55
Perry County Memorial Hospital	Tell City	95%	43
Saint Vincent Frankfort Hospital	Frankfort	95%	44
Cameron Memorial Community Hospital	Angola	94%	72
Indiana University Health Arnett Hospital[2]	Lafayette	94%	64
Indiana Univ Health La Porte Hosp	La Porte	94%	108
Indiana University Health Morgan Hospital	Martinsville	94%	31
Parkview Regional Medical Center[2]	Fort Wayne	94%	80
Saint Vincent Salem Hospital	Salem	94%	31
Dearborn County Hospital	Lawrenceburg	93%	76
Franciscan St Francis Hlth-Indianapolis	Indianapolis	93%	349
Saint Vincent Carmel Hospital	Carmel	93%	55
Scott Memorial Hospital	Scottsburg	93%	74
Daviess Community Hospital	Washington	92%	53
Indiana University Health Starke Hospital	Knox	92%	49
Lutheran Hospital of Indiana	Fort Wayne	92%	102
Riverview Hospital	Noblesville	92%	106
Jasper County Hospital	Rensselaer	91%	32
Dukes Memorial Hospital	Peru	90%	29
Indiana Univ Health White Mem Hosp	Monticello	90%	41
IU Health West Hospital[2]	Avon	90%	81
Franciscan St Francis Health	Mooresville	89%	92
Adams Memorial Hospital	Decatur	88%	64
Community Hospital South[2]	Indianapolis	88%	91
Indiana University Health North Hospital[2]	Carmel	88%	42
Saint Vincent Mercy Hospital	Elwood	87%	46
Saint Vincent Williamsport Hospital	Williamsport	85%	39
Johnson Memorial Hospital	Franklin	84%	82
Woodlawn Hospital	Rochester	81%	48
Saint Vincent Jennings Hospital	North Vernon	80%	35
Monroe Hospital	Bloomington	73%	30
Saint Catherine Regional Hospital	Charlestown	61%	31
Harrison County Hospital	Corydon	49%	59

Blood Culture Timing

Hospital Name	City	Rate	Cases
Bluffton Regional Medical Center	Bluffton	100%	85
Cameron Memorial Community Hospital	Angola	100%	77
Clark Memorial Hospital	Jeffersonville	100%	346
Columbus Regional Hospital	Columbus	100%	266
Comm Hosp of Anderson/Madison Co[2]	Anderson	100%	88
Dukes Memorial Hospital	Peru	100%	31
Dupont Hospital	Fort Wayne	100%	50
Elkhart General Hospital[2]	Elkhart	100%	149
Franciscan St Anthony Health	Michigan City	100%	81
Franciscan St Elizabeth Health[2]	Lafayette	100%	55
Hancock Regional Hospital[2]	Greenfield	100%	106
Henry County Memorial Hospital	New Castle	100%	123
Indiana University Health Morgan Hospital	Martinsville	100%	57
Indiana University Health North Hospital[2]	Carmel	100%	77
Indiana University Health Paoli Hospital	Paoli	100%	36
Indiana University Health Tipton Hospital	Tipton	100%	65
Indiana Univ Health White Mem Hosp	Monticello	100%	53
IU Health Goshen Hospital	Goshen	100%	229
Jasper County Hospital	Rensselaer	100%	40
Memorial Hospital of South Bend	South Bend	100%	311
Parkview Lagrange Hospital	Lagrange	100%	56
Parkview Noble Hospital	Kendallville	100%	123
Parkview Regional Medical Center[2]	Fort Wayne	100%	100
Parkview Whitley Hospital	Columbia City	100%	78
Reid Hospital & Health Care Services	Richmond	100%	435
Saint Catherine Hospital	East Chicago	100%	103
Saint Joseph Hospital	Fort Wayne	100%	60
Saint Joseph Hospital & Health Center	Kokomo	100%	162
St Joseph Reg Med Ctr-Plymouth	Plymouth	100%	101
Saint Mary Medical Center[2]	Hobart	100%	135
Saint Vincent Anderson Regional Hospital	Anderson	100%	239
Saint Vincent Dunn Hospital	Bedford	100%	50
Saint Vincent Salem Hospital	Salem	100%	28
Saint Vincent Williamsport Hospital	Williamsport	100%	44
Terre Haute Regional Hospital	Terre Haute	100%	98
Community Hospital[2]	Munster	99%	158
Community Hospital East[2]	Indianapolis	99%	164
Community Hospital North[2]	Indianapolis	99%	171
Community Howard Regional Health	Kokomo	99%	149
Dekalb Health	Auburn	99%	105
Franciscan St Anthony Health-Crown Pt[2]	Crown Point	99%	127
Franciscan St Margaret Health-Hammond[2]	Hammond	99%	155
Good Samaritan Hospital	Vincennes	99%	248
Indiana Univ Health Bedford Hosp	Bedford	99%	95
IU Health West Hospital[2]	Avon	99%	164
Kosciusko Community Hospital	Warsaw	99%	135
Lutheran Hospital of Indiana	Fort Wayne	99%	186
Major Hospital	Shelbyville	99%	115
Margaret Mary Community Hospital	Batesville	99%	106
Memorial Hospital	Logansport	99%	99
Methodist Hospitals[2]	Gary	99%	117
Porter Regional Hospital	Valparaiso	99%	364
Riverview Hospital	Noblesville	99%	161
Saint Joseph Regional Medical Center	Mishawaka	99%	344
Saint Vincent Frankfort Hospital	Frankfort	99%	68
Adams Memorial Hospital	Decatur	98%	82
Community Hospital South[2]	Indianapolis	98%	153
Eskenazi Health[2]	Indianapolis	98%	114
Fayette Regional Health System	Connersville	98%	99
Franciscan St Francis Hlth-Indianapolis	Indianapolis	98%	780
Franciscan St Francis Health	Mooresville	98%	127
Indiana University Health[2]	Indianapolis	98%	139
Indianapolis VA Medical Center	Indianapolis	98%	185
Parkview Huntington Hospital	Huntington	98%	109
Saint Mary's Medical Center of Evansville	Evansville	98%	298
Saint Vincent Hospital & Health Services	Indianapolis	98%	337
Schneck Medical Center	Seymour	98%	94
Union Hospital	Terre Haute	98%	358
Witham Health Services	Lebanon	98%	121
Community Westview Hospital[2]	Indianapolis	97%	35
Daviess Community Hospital	Washington	97%	79
Franciscan St Elizabeth Health[2]	Lafayette	97%	61
Indiana University Health Arnett Hospital[2]	Lafayette	97%	157
Indiana Univ Health Blackford Hosp	Hartford City	97%	39
Johnson Memorial Hospital	Franklin	97%	109
King's Daughters' Health[2]	Madison	97%	112
Marion General Hospital	Marion	97%	158
Memorial Hospital & Health Care Center[2]	Jasper	97%	112
Pulaski Memorial Hospital	Winamac	97%	34
Wabash County Hospital	Wabash	97%	34
Dearborn County Hospital	Lawrenceburg	96%	113
Decatur County Memorial Hospital	Greensburg	96%	50
Floyd Memorial Hospital & Health Services	New Albany	96%	410
Franciscan Saint Margaret Health - Dyer	Dyer	96%	146
Indiana Univ Health Ball Mem Hosp[2]	Muncie	96%	131
Indiana Univ Health Bloomington Hosp[2]	Bloomington	96%	150
Putnam County Hospital	Greencastle	96%	77
Deaconess Hospital[2]	Evansville	95%	132
Hendricks Regional Health	Danville	95%	174
Perry County Memorial Hospital	Tell City	95%	66
Franciscan St Elizabeth Health	Crawfordsville	94%	53
Gibson General Hospital	Princeton	94%	34
Indiana Univ Health La Porte Hosp	La Porte	94%	166
Saint Mary's Warrick Hospital	Boonville	94%	32
Saint Vincent Mercy Hospital	Elwood	94%	50
Harrison County Hospital	Corydon	93%	69
Jay County Hospital	Portland	93%	43
Scott Memorial Hospital	Scottsburg	93%	83
Sullivan County Community Hospital	Sullivan	93%	58
Greene County General Hospital	Linton	92%	37
Saint Vincent Jennings Hospital	North Vernon	91%	43
Saint Vincent Randolph Hospital	Winchester	91%	44
Indiana University Health Starke Hospital	Knox	90%	63
Saint Vincent Carmel Hospital	Carmel	88%	90
Woodlawn Hospital	Rochester	76%	45

Pregnancy and Delivery Care

Newborns whose Deliveries were Scheduled Early

Hospital Name	City	Rate	Cases
Columbus Regional Hospital[2]	Columbus	0%	77
Dearborn County Hospital	Lawrenceburg	0%	33
Dekalb Health	Auburn	0%	37
Eskenazi Health[2]	Indianapolis	0%	35
Fayette Regional Health System	Connersville	0%	25
Hancock Regional Hospital[2]	Greenfield	0%	28
Indiana Univ Health Bloomington Hosp[2]	Bloomington	0%	30
Indiana Univ Health La Porte Hosp[2]	La Porte	0%	34
IU Health West Hospital[2]	Avon	0%	26
King's Daughters' Health[2]	Madison	0%	32
Methodist Hospitals[2]	Gary	0%	32
Saint Catherine Hospital[2]	East Chicago	0%	39
Saint Joseph Hospital[2]	Fort Wayne	0%	35
Saint Joseph Regional Medical Center[2]	Mishawaka	0%	27
Saint Mary Medical Center[2]	Hobart	0%	28
Saint Vincent Hospital & Health Services[2]	Indianapolis	0%	665
Saint Vincent Randolph Hospital[2,3]	Winchester	0%	26
Terre Haute Regional Hospital[2]	Terre Haute	0%	49
Witham Health Services[2]	Lebanon	0%	37
IU Health Goshen Hospital	Goshen	1%	82
Dupont Hospital[2]	Fort Wayne	2%	56
Elkhart General Hospital	Elkhart	2%	163
Hendricks Regional Health	Danville	2%	198
Indiana University Health	Indianapolis	2%	206
Franciscan St Francis Hlth-Indianapolis[2]	Indianapolis	3%	108
Franciscan Saint Margaret Health - Dyer[2]	Dyer	3%	29
Saint Mary's Medical Center of Evansville	Evansville	3%	127
Community Hospital North[2]	Indianapolis	4%	72
Community Hospital South[2]	Indianapolis	4%	25
Lutheran Hospital of Indiana[2]	Fort Wayne	4%	46
Memorial Hospital	Logansport	4%	48
Memorial Hospital & Health Care Center	Jasper	4%	136
Memorial Hospital of South Bend	South Bend	4%	184
St Joseph Reg Med Ctr-Plymouth[2]	Plymouth	4%	25
Indiana University Health Arnett Hospital[2]	Lafayette	5%	38
Franciscan St Elizabeth Health[2]	Lafayette	6%	35
Clark Memorial Hospital	Jeffersonville	7%	118
Franciscan St Margaret Health-Hammond[2]	Hammond	7%	45
Parkview Regional Medical Center[2]	Fort Wayne	7%	54
Saint Vincent Carmel Hospital[2]	Carmel	7%	29
Indiana University Health North Hospital[2]	Carmel	8%	49
Union Hospital	Terre Haute	8%	178
Good Samaritan Hospital	Vincennes	9%	44
Community Hospital[2]	Munster	10%	41
Harrison County Hospital[2]	Corydon	10%	62
Indiana Univ Health Ball Mem Hosp[2]	Muncie	10%	31
Kosciusko Community Hospital[2]	Warsaw	11%	28
Floyd Memorial Hospital & Health Services	New Albany	12%	66
Marion General Hospital[2]	Marion	12%	51
Schneck Medical Center[2]	Seymour	12%	76
Johnson Memorial Hospital	Franklin	13%	30
Reid Hospital & Health Care Services	Richmond	13%	62
Saint Vincent Anderson Regional Hospital	Anderson	16%	64
Community Hospital East[2]	Indianapolis	17%	29
The Women's Hospital[2]	Newburgh	24%	62
Daviess Community Hospital	Washington	32%	76
Franciscan St Francis Health[2]	Mooresville	58%	36

Preventive Care

Immunization for Influenza

Hospital Name	City	Rate	Cases
Bluffton Regional Medical Center[2]	Bluffton	100%	337
Community Westview Hospital[2]	Indianapolis	100%	347
Dupont Hospital[2]	Fort Wayne	100%	446
Henry County Memorial Hospital[2]	New Castle	100%	289
Indiana Univ Health Blackford Hosp	Hartford City	100%	176
The Ortho Hosp/Lutheran Health Network[2]	Fort Wayne	100%	340
Parkview Huntington Hospital[2]	Huntington	100%	251
Parkview Whitley Hospital[2]	Columbia City	100%	263
Saint Joseph Hospital & Health Center[2]	Kokomo	100%	508
Saint Mary Medical Center[2]	Hobart	100%	602
Terre Haute Regional Hospital[2]	Terre Haute	100%	531
Dekalb Health[2]	Auburn	99%	228
Franciscan Healthcare - Munster	Munster	99%	447
Franciscan St Anthony Health-Crown Pt[2]	Crown Point	99%	520
Franciscan St Francis Health[2]	Mooresville	99%	737
Good Samaritan Hospital[2]	Vincennes	99%	561
Indiana Univ Health Bedford Hosp[2,3]	Bedford	99%	134
Lutheran Hospital of Indiana[2]	Fort Wayne	99%	789
Memorial Hospital of South Bend[2]	South Bend	99%	517
Parkview Lagrange Hospital[2]	Lagrange	99%	226
Saint Mary's Warrick Hospital[2]	Boonville	99%	247
Schneck Medical Center[2]	Seymour	99%	361
Clark Memorial Hospital[2]	Jeffersonville	98%	546
Deaconess Hospital[2]	Evansville	98%	610
Elkhart General Hospital[2]	Elkhart	98%	534
Fairbanks[2]	Indianapolis	98%	288
Fayette Regional Health System[2]	Connersville	98%	269
Franciscan St Elizabeth Health[2]	Lafayette	98%	317
Franciscan St Elizabeth Health[2]	Lafayette	98%	491
Franciscan St Francis Hlth-Indianapolis[2]	Indianapolis	98%	596
Hancock Regional Hospital[2]	Greenfield	98%	322
Major Hospital[2]	Shelbyville	98%	334
Saint Vincent Dunn Hospital[2]	Bedford	98%	265
Saint Vincent Williamsport Hospital	Williamsport	98%	333
Union Hospital Clinton	Clinton	98%	455
The Women's Hospital[2]	Newburgh	98%	390
Community Hospital[2]	Munster	97%	565
Dearborn County Hospital[2]	Lawrenceburg	97%	440
The Heart Hospital at Deaconess Gateway[2]	Newburgh	97%	308
Indiana University Health Starke Hospital[2]	Knox	97%	300
IU Health Goshen Hospital[2]	Goshen	97%	515
Kosciusko Community Hospital[2]	Warsaw	97%	442
Memorial Hospital & Health Care Center[2]	Jasper	97%	489
Riverview Hospital[2]	Noblesville	97%	471
Columbus Regional Hospital[2]	Columbus	96%	850
Comm Hosp of Anderson/Madison Co[2]	Anderson	96%	713
Dukes Memorial Hospital[2]	Peru	96%	283
Franciscan St Anthony Health[2]	Michigan City	96%	567
Indiana University Health North Hospital[2]	Carmel	96%	452
King's Daughters' Health[2]	Madison	96%	376
Marion General Hospital[2]	Marion	96%	548
Parkview Noble Hospital[2]	Kendallville	96%	253
Pulaski Memorial Hospital	Winamac	96%	246
St Joseph Reg Med Ctr-Plymouth[2]	Plymouth	96%	256

NOTE: Hospital profiles are in alphabetical order by state, then city, then hospital within the city; Rankings exclude hospitals with less than 25 cases except for patient surveys which excludes hospitals with less than 100 cases; (a) 100-299 cases; (1) The number of cases/patients is too few to report; (2) Data submitted were based on a sample of cases/patients; (3) Results are based on a shorter time period than required; (4) Data suppressed by CMS for one or more quarters; (5) Results are not available for this reporting period; (6) Fewer than 100 patients completed the HCAHPS survey; (7) No cases met the criteria for this measure; (8) The lower limit of the confidence interval cannot be calculated if the number of observed infections equals zero; (9) No data are available from the state/territory for this reporting period; (10) The scores shown reflect fewer than 50 completed surveys; (11) There were discrepancies in the data collection process; (12) This measure does not apply to this hospital for this reporting period; (13) Results cannot be calculated for this reporting period; (14) The results for this state are combined with nearby states to protect confidentiality; Please refer to the User's Guide for a full explanation of data.

Hospital Name	City	Rate	Cases
Hendricks Regional Health[2]	Danville	95%	487
Indiana Univ Health Ball Mem Hosp[2]	Muncie	95%	560
IU Health West Hospital[2]	Avon	95%	505
Jay County Hospital	Portland	95%	582
Memorial Hospital	Logansport	95%	919
Orthopaedic Hospital at Parkview North[2]	Fort Wayne	95%	325
Saint Catherine Hospital[2]	East Chicago	95%	585
Saint Joseph Hospital[2]	Fort Wayne	95%	454
Saint Mary's Medical Center of Evansville[2]	Evansville	95%	536
Saint Vincent Carmel Hospital[2]	Carmel	95%	469
Saint Vincent Frankfort Hospital[2]	Frankfort	95%	219
Witham Health Services[2]	Lebanon	95%	268
Cameron Memorial Community Hospital[2]	Angola	94%	373
Decatur County Memorial Hospital[2]	Greensburg	94%	372
Indiana University Health Arnett Hospital[2]	Lafayette	94%	505
Indiana Univ Health Bloomington Hosp[2]	Bloomington	94%	577
Porter Regional Hospital[2]	Valparaiso	93%	696
Franciscan St Elizabeth Health[2]	Crawfordsville	92%	318
Saint Vincent Randolph Hospital[2]	Winchester	92%	336
Indiana University Health[2]	Indianapolis	91%	515
Indiana University Health Morgan Hospital[2]	Martinsville	91%	286
Unity Medical & Surgical Hospital[2]	Mishawaka	91%	212
Parkview Regional Medical Center[2]	Fort Wayne	90%	558
Saint Joseph Regional Medical Center[2]	Mishawaka	90%	550
Johnson Memorial Hospital[2]	Franklin	88%	378
Indiana University Health Tipton Hospital	Tipton	87%	434
Saint Vincent Heart Center of Indiana[2]	Indianapolis	87%	534
Community Howard Regional Health[2]	Kokomo	86%	578
Indiana Univ Health La Porte Hosp[2]	La Porte	86%	627
Kentuckiana Medical Center[2]	Clarksville	86%	307
Saint Vincent Anderson Regional Hospital[2]	Anderson	86%	600
Saint Vincent Hospital & Health Services[2]	Indianapolis	86%	545
Saint Vincent Salem Hospital[2,3]	Salem	86%	78
Franciscan Saint Margaret Health - Dyer[2]	Dyer	85%	533
Physicians' Medical Center[2]	New Albany	85%	128
Floyd Memorial Hospital & Health Services[2]	New Albany	83%	617
Reid Hospital & Health Care Services[2]	Richmond	83%	569
Adams Memorial Hospital[2]	Decatur	81%	282
Franciscan St Margaret Health-Hammond[2]	Hammond	81%	544
Saint Vincent Clay Hospital	Brazil	81%	283
VA N Indiana Healthcare Sys-Marion[2,3]	Marion	81%	136
Methodist Hospitals[2]	Gary	79%	549
Pinnacle Hospital[2]	Crown Point	79%	312
Rush Memorial Hospital[2]	Rushville	78%	207
Union Hospital[2]	Terre Haute	77%	695
Community Hospital South[2]	Indianapolis	72%	566
Harrison County Hospital[2]	Corydon	71%	360
Daviess Community Hospital[2]	Washington	69%	432
Community Hospital East[2]	Indianapolis	66%	896
The Indiana Heart Hospital[2]	Indianapolis	66%	317
Monroe Hospital[2]	Bloomington	66%	345
Community Hospital North[2]	Indianapolis	64%	505
Eskenazi Health[2]	Indianapolis	49%	495
Indiana Orthopaedic Hospital[2]	Indianapolis	49%	318
Saint Catherine Regional Hospital	Charlestown	2%	228

Immunization for Pneumonia

Hospital Name	City	Rate	Cases
Dekalb Health[2]	Auburn	100%	255
Doctors NeuroMed Hosp & Brain Inst[2,3]	Bremen	100%	132
Henry County Memorial Hospital[2]	New Castle	100%	459
Indiana Univ Health Blackford Hosp	Hartford City	100%	268
Saint Joseph Hospital & Health Center[2]	Kokomo	100%	562
Terre Haute Regional Hospital[2]	Terre Haute	100%	763
Bluffton Regional Medical Center[2]	Bluffton	99%	530
Community Hospital[2]	Munster	99%	774
Community Westview Hospital[2]	Indianapolis	99%	578
Dukes Memorial Hospital[2]	Peru	99%	341
Dupont Hospital[2]	Fort Wayne	99%	272
Fayette Regional Health System[2]	Connersville	99%	363
Franciscan Healthcare - Munster	Munster	99%	625
Franciscan St Anthony Health-Crown Pt[2]	Crown Point	99%	641
Franciscan St Francis Hlth-Indianapolis[2]	Indianapolis	99%	823
Franciscan St Francis Health[2]	Mooresville	99%	989
Good Samaritan Hospital[2]	Vincennes	99%	802
Hancock Regional Hospital[2]	Greenfield	99%	428
Lutheran Hospital of Indiana[2]	Fort Wayne	99%	1058
Major Hospital[2]	Shelbyville	99%	405
Memorial Hospital	Logansport	99%	896
Parkview Lagrange Hospital[2]	Lagrange	99%	189
Parkview Noble Hospital[2]	Kendallville	99%	321
Saint Mary's Warrick Hospital[2]	Boonville	99%	356
Elkhart General Hospital[2]	Elkhart	98%	669
Indiana University Health Starke Hospital[2]	Knox	98%	420
Kosciusko Community Hospital[2]	Warsaw	98%	489
Memorial Hospital & Health Care Center[2]	Jasper	98%	596
Parkview Huntington Hospital[2]	Huntington	98%	299
Parkview Whitley Hospital[2]	Columbia City	98%	292
Riverview Hospital[2]	Noblesville	98%	782
Saint Catherine Hospital[2]	East Chicago	98%	772
Saint Mary Medical Center[2]	Hobart	98%	901
Saint Vincent Frankfort Hospital[2]	Frankfort	98%	243
Saint Vincent Williamsport Hospital	Williamsport	98%	546
Clark Memorial Hospital[2]	Jeffersonville	97%	699
Dearborn County Hospital[2]	Lawrenceburg	97%	545
Franciscan St Anthony Health[2]	Michigan City	97%	734
Hendricks Regional Health[2]	Danville	97%	578
Jay County Hospital	Portland	97%	752
The Ortho Hosp/Lutheran Health Network[2]	Fort Wayne	97%	458
Pulaski Memorial Hospital	Winamac	97%	311
Saint Vincent Dunn Hospital[2]	Bedford	97%	252
Schneck Medical Center[2]	Seymour	97%	381
Union Hospital Clinton	Clinton	97%	711
Comm Hosp of Anderson/Madison Co[2]	Anderson	96%	813
Indiana Univ Health Bedford Hosp[2,3]	Bedford	96%	306
IU Health Goshen Hospital[2]	Goshen	96%	579
Johnson Memorial Hospital[2]	Franklin	96%	475
King's Daughters' Health[2]	Madison	96%	512
Marion General Hospital[2]	Marion	96%	670
Memorial Hospital of South Bend[2]	South Bend	96%	509
Saint Vincent Carmel Hospital[2]	Carmel	96%	410
Saint Vincent Randolph Hospital[2]	Winchester	96%	341
Columbus Regional Hospital[2]	Columbus	95%	1091
Deaconess Hospital[2]	Evansville	95%	908
Franciscan St Elizabeth Health[2]	Lafayette	95%	511
The Heart Hospital at Deaconess Gateway[2]	Newburgh	95%	503
Orthopaedic Hospital at Parkview North[2]	Fort Wayne	95%	435
Porter Regional Hospital[2]	Valparaiso	95%	875
Reid Hospital & Health Care Services[2]	Richmond	95%	846
Saint Joseph Hospital[2]	Fort Wayne	95%	645
Saint Mary's Medical Center of Evansville[2]	Evansville	95%	703
Cameron Memorial Community Hospital[2]	Angola	94%	449
Indiana University Health Arnett Hospital[2]	Lafayette	94%	658
IU Health West Hospital[2]	Avon	94%	639
Parkview Regional Medical Center[2]	Fort Wayne	94%	698
VA N Indiana Healthcare Sys-Marion[2,3]	Marion	94%	202
Witham Health Services[2]	Lebanon	94%	399
Saint Vincent Salem Hospital[2,3]	Salem	93%	141
Franciscan St Elizabeth Health[2]	Lafayette	92%	539
Indiana Univ Health Ball Mem Hosp[2]	Muncie	92%	670
Indiana University Health Morgan Hospital[2]	Martinsville	92%	486
St Joseph Reg Med Ctr-Plymouth[2]	Plymouth	92%	329
Franciscan St Elizabeth Health[2]	Crawfordsville	91%	522
Indiana University Health Tipton Hospital	Tipton	91%	702
Floyd Memorial Hospital & Health Services[2]	New Albany	90%	864
Indiana Univ Health Bloomington Hosp[2]	Bloomington	90%	609
Kentuckiana Medical Center[2]	Clarksville	89%	390
Community Howard Regional Health[2]	Kokomo	88%	683
Indiana University Health[2]	Indianapolis	88%	502
Franciscan St Margaret Health-Hammond[2]	Hammond	87%	818
Indiana Univ Health La Porte Hosp[2]	La Porte	87%	717
Physicians' Medical Center[2]	New Albany	87%	60
Saint Vincent Clay Hospital	Brazil	87%	412
Unity Medical & Surgical Hospital[2]	Mishawaka	87%	119
Daviess Community Hospital[2]	Washington	86%	352
Franciscan Saint Margaret Health - Dyer[2]	Dyer	86%	696
Saint Vincent Hospital & Health Services[2]	Indianapolis	86%	596
Indiana University Health North Hospital[2]	Carmel	85%	350
Union Hospital[2]	Terre Haute	84%	900
Decatur County Memorial Hospital[2]	Greensburg	83%	421
Pinnacle Hospital[2]	Crown Point	83%	239
Rush Memorial Hospital[2]	Rushville	83%	301
Saint Joseph Regional Medical Center[2]	Mishawaka	82%	704
Community Hospital South[2]	Indianapolis	81%	647
Saint Vincent Anderson Regional Hospital[2]	Anderson	81%	684
Saint Vincent Heart Center of Indiana[2]	Indianapolis	80%	874
Adams Memorial Hospital[2]	Decatur	79%	482
Community Hospital East[2]	Indianapolis	73%	840
Methodist Hospitals[2]	Gary	73%	716
Community Hospital North[2]	Indianapolis	70%	511
The Indiana Heart Hospital[2]	Indianapolis	70%	523
Monroe Hospital[2]	Bloomington	67%	458
Indiana Orthopaedic Hospital[2]	Indianapolis	60%	367
Harrison County Hospital[2]	Corydon	58%	465
Eskenazi Health[2]	Indianapolis	56%	535
Fairbanks[2]	Indianapolis	38%	40
Saint Catherine Regional Hospital	Charlestown	2%	290

Stroke Care

Anticoagulation Therapy for Atrial Fibrillation

Hospital Name	City	Rate	Cases
Franciscan St Francis Hlth-Indianapolis	Indianapolis	100%	35
Lutheran Hospital of Indiana	Fort Wayne	100%	26
Parkview Regional Medical Center	Fort Wayne	100%	48
Saint Vincent Hospital & Health Services	Indianapolis	97%	64
Community Hospital North	Indianapolis	93%	41
Saint Mary's Medical Center of Evansville	Evansville	92%	26
Deaconess Hospital	Evansville	88%	51

Antithrombotic Therapy Timing

Hospital Name	City	Rate	Cases
Comm Hosp of Anderson/Madison Co	Anderson	100%	67
Community Howard Regional Health	Kokomo	100%	44
Dearborn County Hospital	Lawrenceburg	100%	34
Floyd Memorial Hospital & Health Services	New Albany	100%	147
Franciscan St Elizabeth Health	Lafayette	100%	65
Good Samaritan Hospital	Vincennes	100%	104
Hancock Regional Hospital[2]	Greenfield	100%	38
Hendricks Regional Health	Danville	100%	44
Indiana Univ Health Bloomington Hosp	Bloomington	100%	154
Indiana Univ Health La Porte Hosp[2]	La Porte	100%	57
Indiana University Health North Hospital	Carmel	100%	31
IU Health Goshen Hospital	Goshen	100%	57
IU Health West Hospital	Avon	100%	75
Kosciusko Community Hospital	Warsaw	100%	34
Major Hospital	Shelbyville	100%	35
Memorial Hospital & Health Care Center	Jasper	100%	67
Parkview Regional Medical Center	Fort Wayne	100%	323
Riverview Hospital	Noblesville	100%	41
Saint Joseph Hospital	Fort Wayne	100%	31
Saint Joseph Hospital & Health Center	Kokomo	100%	64
Saint Mary Medical Center[2]	Hobart	100%	99
Schneck Medical Center	Seymour	100%	39
Union Hospital	Terre Haute	100%	146
Columbus Regional Hospital	Columbus	99%	93
Community Hospital	Munster	99%	177
Franciscan St Francis Hlth-Indianapolis	Indianapolis	99%	199
Franciscan St Margaret Health-Hammond[2]	Hammond	99%	89
Indiana University Health Arnett Hospital[2]	Lafayette	99%	88
Indiana Univ Health Ball Mem Hosp[2]	Muncie	98%	84
Johnson Memorial Hospital	Franklin	98%	42
Saint Joseph Regional Medical Center	Mishawaka	98%	138
Saint Vincent Anderson Regional Hospital	Anderson	98%	63
Saint Vincent Hospital & Health Services	Indianapolis	98%	324
Deaconess Hospital	Evansville	97%	325
Elkhart General Hospital[2]	Elkhart	97%	125
Franciscan St Anthony Health-Crown Pt[2]	Crown Point	97%	72
Franciscan St Elizabeth Health	Lafayette	97%	31
Franciscan Saint Margaret Health - Dyer	Dyer	97%	67
Indiana University Health[2]	Indianapolis	97%	65
Lutheran Hospital of Indiana	Fort Wayne	97%	166
Memorial Hospital of South Bend	South Bend	97%	146
Methodist Hospitals[2]	Gary	97%	92
Reid Hospital & Health Care Services	Richmond	97%	138
Porter Regional Hospital	Valparaiso	96%	121
Community Hospital North	Indianapolis	95%	181
Community Hospital South	Indianapolis	95%	66
Eskenazi Health[2]	Indianapolis	95%	80
Saint Catherine Hospital	East Chicago	95%	75
Saint Mary's Medical Center of Evansville	Evansville	95%	133
Clark Memorial Hospital	Jeffersonville	94%	72
Franciscan St Anthony Health	Michigan City	94%	52
Marion General Hospital	Marion	94%	33
Community Hospital East	Indianapolis	93%	136
King's Daughters' Health	Madison	89%	27
Doctors NeuroMed Hosp & Brain Inst[2,3]	Bremen	12%	26

Assessed for Rehabilitation

Hospital Name	City	Rate	Cases
Columbus Regional Hospital	Columbus	100%	106
Comm Hosp of Anderson/Madison Co	Anderson	100%	77
Community Hospital South	Indianapolis	100%	91
Hancock Regional Hospital[2]	Greenfield	100%	53
Hendricks Regional Health	Danville	100%	62
Indiana Univ Health Ball Mem Hosp[2]	Muncie	100%	101
Indiana Univ Health La Porte Hosp[2]	La Porte	100%	69
IU Health Goshen Hospital	Goshen	100%	63
Johnson Memorial Hospital	Franklin	100%	47
Kosciusko Community Hospital	Warsaw	100%	40
Memorial Hospital & Health Care Center	Jasper	100%	82
Parkview Regional Medical Center	Fort Wayne	100%	420
Riverview Hospital	Noblesville	100%	40
Saint Joseph Regional Medical Center	Mishawaka	100%	179
Saint Mary Medical Center[2]	Hobart	100%	111
Saint Vincent Anderson Regional Hospital	Anderson	100%	89
Deaconess Hospital	Evansville	99%	411
Memorial Hospital of South Bend	South Bend	99%	194
Methodist Hospitals[2]	Gary	99%	116
Reid Hospital & Health Care Services	Richmond	99%	142
Saint Catherine Hospital	East Chicago	99%	85
Union Hospital	Terre Haute	99%	171
Franciscan St Francis Hlth-Indianapolis	Indianapolis	98%	239
Indiana Univ Health Bloomington Hosp	Bloomington	98%	225
Saint Mary's Medical Center of Evansville	Evansville	98%	176
Schneck Medical Center	Seymour	98%	40
Good Samaritan Hospital	Vincennes	97%	107
Saint Joseph Hospital	Fort Wayne	97%	29
Saint Joseph Hospital & Health Center	Kokomo	97%	77
Elkhart General Hospital[2]	Elkhart	96%	148

NOTE: Hospital profiles are in alphabetical order by state, then city, then hospital within the city; Rankings exclude hospitals with less than 25 cases except for patient surveys which excludes hospitals with less than 100 cases; (a) 100-299 cases; (1) The number of cases/patients is too few to report; (2) Data submitted were based on a sample of cases/patients; (3) Results are based on a shorter time period than required; (4) Data suppressed by CMS for one or more quarters; (5) Results are not available for this reporting period; (6) Fewer than 100 patients completed the HCAHPS survey; (7) No cases met the criteria for this measure; (8) The lower limit of the confidence interval cannot be calculated if the number of observed infections equals zero; (9) No data are available from the state/territory for this reporting period; (10) The scores shown reflect fewer than 50 completed surveys; (11) There were discrepancies in the data collection process; (12) This measure does not apply to this hospital for this reporting period; (13) Results cannot be calculated for this reporting period; (14) The results for this state are combined with nearby states to protect confidentiality; Please refer to the User's Guide for a full explanation of data.

Hospital Name	City	Rate	Cases
Floyd Memorial Hospital & Health Services	New Albany	96%	172
Franciscan St Anthony Health	Michigan City	96%	68
Franciscan St Elizabeth Health	Lafayette	96%	28
Franciscan Saint Margaret Health - Dyer	Dyer	96%	84
Lutheran Hospital of Indiana	Fort Wayne	96%	224
Community Hospital North	Indianapolis	95%	209
Indiana University Health[2]	Indianapolis	95%	105
IU Health West Hospital	Avon	95%	73
Saint Vincent Hospital & Health Services	Indianapolis	95%	422
Dearborn County Hospital	Lawrenceburg	94%	36
Franciscan St Anthony Health-Crown Pt[2]	Crown Point	94%	85
Community Howard Regional Health	Kokomo	93%	56
Indiana University Health Arnett Hospital[2]	Lafayette	93%	85
Community Hospital East	Indianapolis	92%	166
Franciscan St Elizabeth Health	Lafayette	92%	87
Marion General Hospital	Marion	92%	36
Franciscan St Margaret Health-Hammond[2]	Hammond	91%	95
Major Hospital	Shelbyville	91%	35
Indiana University Health North Hospital	Carmel	88%	42
Eskenazi Health[2]	Indianapolis	87%	107
Porter Regional Hospital	Valparaiso	83%	127
Community Hospital	Munster	82%	205
Clark Memorial Hospital	Jeffersonville	80%	69
Doctors NeuroMed Hosp & Brain Inst[2,3]	Bremen	19%	31

Discharged on Antithrombotic Therapy

Hospital Name	City	Rate	Cases
Columbus Regional Hospital	Columbus	100%	105
Comm Hosp of Anderson/Madison Co	Anderson	100%	75
Eskenazi Health[2]	Indianapolis	100%	95
Floyd Memorial Hospital & Health Services	New Albany	100%	158
Franciscan St Elizabeth Health	Lafayette	100%	28
Good Samaritan Hospital	Vincennes	100%	102
Hancock Regional Hospital[2]	Greenfield	100%	51
Indiana University Health[2]	Indianapolis	100%	74
Indiana University Health Arnett Hospital[2]	Lafayette	100%	79
Indiana Univ Health Ball Mem Hosp[2]	Muncie	100%	89
Indiana Univ Health La Porte Hosp[2]	La Porte	100%	62
IU Health Goshen Hospital	Goshen	100%	58
Kosciusko Community Hospital	Warsaw	100%	40
Lutheran Hospital of Indiana	Fort Wayne	100%	187
Major Hospital	Shelbyville	100%	33
Marion General Hospital	Marion	100%	34
Memorial Hospital & Health Care Center	Jasper	100%	82
Parkview Regional Medical Center	Fort Wayne	100%	350
Riverview Hospital	Noblesville	100%	40
Saint Joseph Hospital	Fort Wayne	100%	29
Saint Joseph Hospital & Health Center	Kokomo	100%	71
Saint Mary Medical Center[2]	Hobart	100%	97
Saint Mary's Medical Center of Evansville	Evansville	100%	153
Saint Vincent Anderson Regional Hospital	Anderson	100%	85
Union Hospital	Terre Haute	100%	152
Community Hospital North	Indianapolis	99%	193
Franciscan St Francis Hlth-Indianapolis	Indianapolis	99%	212
IU Health West Hospital	Avon	99%	73
Saint Joseph Regional Medical Center	Mishawaka	99%	159
Saint Vincent Hospital & Health Services	Indianapolis	99%	340
Deaconess Hospital	Evansville	98%	346
Elkhart General Hospital[2]	Elkhart	98%	133
Franciscan St Anthony Health	Michigan City	98%	66
Franciscan St Margaret Health-Hammond[2]	Hammond	98%	88
Hendricks Regional Health	Danville	98%	53
Indiana Univ Health Bloomington Hosp	Bloomington	98%	198
Indiana University Health North Hospital	Carmel	98%	40
Johnson Memorial Hospital	Franklin	98%	47
Porter Regional Hospital	Valparaiso	98%	120
Reid Hospital & Health Care Services	Richmond	98%	133
Saint Catherine Hospital	East Chicago	98%	81
Clark Memorial Hospital	Jeffersonville	97%	69
Community Hospital East	Indianapolis	97%	139
Community Hospital South	Indianapolis	97%	75
Dearborn County Hospital	Lawrenceburg	97%	34
Franciscan Saint Margaret Health - Dyer	Dyer	97%	73
Memorial Hospital of South Bend	South Bend	97%	163
Methodist Hospitals[2]	Gary	97%	92
Community Howard Regional Health	Kokomo	96%	53
Franciscan St Anthony Health-Crown Pt[2]	Crown Point	95%	76
Schneck Medical Center	Seymour	95%	39
Franciscan St Elizabeth Health	Lafayette	93%	76
Community Hospital	Munster	92%	180
Doctors NeuroMed Hosp & Brain Inst[2,3]	Bremen	30%	27

Discharged on Statin Medication

Hospital Name	City	Rate	Cases
Comm Hosp of Anderson/Madison Co	Anderson	100%	61
Hendricks Regional Health	Danville	100%	40
Kosciusko Community Hospital	Warsaw	100%	29
Saint Mary Medical Center[2]	Hobart	100%	67
Saint Vincent Anderson Regional Hospital	Anderson	100%	76
Lutheran Hospital of Indiana	Fort Wayne	99%	140
Saint Joseph Regional Medical Center	Mishawaka	99%	134
Franciscan Saint Margaret Health - Dyer	Dyer	98%	60
Indiana University Health[2]	Indianapolis	98%	60
Indiana Univ Health Bloomington Hosp	Bloomington	98%	161
Saint Joseph Hospital & Health Center	Kokomo	98%	51
Deaconess Hospital	Evansville	97%	287
IU Health West Hospital	Avon	97%	65
Hancock Regional Hospital[2]	Greenfield	96%	45
Franciscan St Francis Hlth-Indianapolis	Indianapolis	95%	168
Indiana Univ Health Ball Mem Hosp[2]	Muncie	95%	61
Porter Regional Hospital	Valparaiso	95%	99
Saint Mary's Medical Center of Evansville	Evansville	95%	123
Eskenazi Health[2]	Indianapolis	94%	79
Memorial Hospital & Health Care Center	Jasper	94%	63
Good Samaritan Hospital	Vincennes	93%	85
Indiana University Health Arnett Hospital[2]	Lafayette	93%	67
IU Health Goshen Hospital	Goshen	93%	44
Union Hospital	Terre Haute	93%	113
Elkhart General Hospital[2]	Elkhart	92%	91
Johnson Memorial Hospital	Franklin	92%	37
Parkview Regional Medical Center	Fort Wayne	92%	280
Community Hospital North	Indianapolis	91%	162
Memorial Hospital of South Bend	South Bend	91%	133
Saint Catherine Hospital	East Chicago	91%	67
Indiana Univ Health La Porte Hosp[2]	La Porte	90%	49
Saint Vincent Hospital & Health Services	Indianapolis	90%	276
Community Hospital South	Indianapolis	89%	65
Reid Hospital & Health Care Services	Richmond	89%	98
Franciscan St Anthony Health-Crown Pt[2]	Crown Point	88%	59
Franciscan St Anthony Health	Michigan City	88%	43
Marion General Hospital	Marion	88%	33
Schneck Medical Center	Seymour	88%	33
Methodist Hospitals[2]	Gary	87%	71
Franciscan St Margaret Health-Hammond[2]	Hammond	86%	66
Franciscan St Elizabeth Health	Lafayette	85%	62
Clark Memorial Hospital	Jeffersonville	84%	63
Columbus Regional Hospital	Columbus	84%	76
Floyd Memorial Hospital & Health Services	New Albany	83%	130
Riverview Hospital	Noblesville	81%	36
Community Howard Regional Health	Kokomo	80%	46
Community Hospital	Munster	78%	126
Community Hospital East	Indianapolis	76%	110
Indiana University Health North Hospital	Carmel	74%	31
Dearborn County Hospital	Lawrenceburg	71%	31
Doctors NeuroMed Hosp & Brain Inst[2,3]	Bremen	19%	31

Thrombolytic Therapy Timing

Hospital Name	City	Rate	Cases
Porter Regional Hospital	Valparaiso	50%	26
Eskenazi Health[2]	Indianapolis	16%	43
Indiana University Health Arnett Hospital[2]	Lafayette	7%	30

Venous Thromboembolism (VTE) Prophylaxis

Hospital Name	City	Rate	Cases
Hancock Regional Hospital[2]	Greenfield	100%	34
Hendricks Regional Health	Danville	100%	52
Major Hospital	Shelbyville	100%	40
Riverview Hospital	Noblesville	100%	45
Saint Joseph Hospital & Health Center	Kokomo	100%	72
Saint Mary Medical Center[2]	Hobart	100%	115
Schneck Medical Center	Seymour	100%	40
Terre Haute Regional Hospital	Terre Haute	100%	26
Comm Hosp of Anderson/Madison Co	Anderson	99%	75
Good Samaritan Hospital	Vincennes	99%	107
Indiana Univ Health Ball Mem Hosp[2]	Muncie	98%	107
Parkview Regional Medical Center	Fort Wayne	98%	443
Reid Hospital & Health Care Services	Richmond	98%	150
Saint Joseph Regional Medical Center	Mishawaka	98%	175
Indiana Univ Health Bloomington Hosp	Bloomington	97%	203
Lutheran Hospital of Indiana	Fort Wayne	97%	242
Memorial Hospital of South Bend	South Bend	97%	203
Saint Vincent Anderson Regional Hospital	Anderson	97%	78
Union Hospital	Terre Haute	97%	170
Franciscan St Francis Hlth-Indianapolis	Indianapolis	96%	221
Indiana University Health[2]	Indianapolis	96%	113
IU Health Goshen Hospital	Goshen	96%	57
Saint Mary's Medical Center of Evansville	Evansville	96%	187
Indiana University Health Arnett Hospital[2]	Lafayette	95%	98
Memorial Hospital & Health Care Center	Jasper	94%	77
Saint Joseph Hospital	Fort Wayne	94%	33
Deaconess Hospital	Evansville	93%	391
Franciscan St Anthony Health-Crown Pt[2]	Crown Point	92%	87
IU Health West Hospital	Avon	92%	79
Community Hospital South	Indianapolis	91%	92
Elkhart General Hospital[2]	Elkhart	91%	151
Indiana Univ Health La Porte Hosp[2]	La Porte	91%	75
Kosciusko Community Hospital	Warsaw	91%	35
Columbus Regional Hospital	Columbus	90%	101
Franciscan Saint Margaret Health - Dyer	Dyer	90%	88
Floyd Memorial Hospital & Health Services	New Albany	89%	170
Methodist Hospitals[2]	Gary	88%	127
Porter Regional Hospital	Valparaiso	88%	142
Franciscan St Elizabeth Health	Lafayette	87%	31
Saint Vincent Hospital & Health Services	Indianapolis	87%	445
Franciscan St Elizabeth Health	Lafayette	86%	83
Franciscan St Margaret Health-Hammond[2]	Hammond	86%	94
Marion General Hospital	Marion	86%	35
Saint Catherine Hospital	East Chicago	86%	84
Community Howard Regional Health	Kokomo	85%	53
Community Hospital	Munster	84%	212
Indiana University Health North Hospital	Carmel	82%	34
Community Hospital North	Indianapolis	79%	209
Community Hospital East	Indianapolis	77%	179
Eskenazi Health[2]	Indianapolis	76%	97
Franciscan St Anthony Health	Michigan City	76%	71
Johnson Memorial Hospital	Franklin	73%	44
Clark Memorial Hospital	Jeffersonville	58%	71
Dearborn County Hospital	Lawrenceburg	58%	33
Doctors NeuroMed Hosp & Brain Inst[2,3]	Bremen	39%	31
King's Daughters' Health	Madison	38%	26

Written Stroke Educational Materials Given

Hospital Name	City	Rate	Cases
Columbus Regional Hospital	Columbus	100%	45
Community Hospital	Munster	100%	114
Indiana Univ Health La Porte Hosp[2]	La Porte	100%	39
Saint Mary's Medical Center of Evansville	Evansville	99%	82
Community Hospital South	Indianapolis	98%	41
Saint Vincent Anderson Regional Hospital	Anderson	98%	45
Franciscan St Anthony Health	Michigan City	97%	39
Methodist Hospitals[2]	Gary	97%	61
Porter Regional Hospital	Valparaiso	97%	73
Saint Joseph Hospital & Health Center	Kokomo	97%	37
Hancock Regional Hospital[2]	Greenfield	96%	25
IU Health Goshen Hospital	Goshen	94%	32
Saint Mary Medical Center[2]	Hobart	94%	66
Comm Hosp of Anderson/Madison Co	Anderson	93%	41
Parkview Regional Medical Center	Fort Wayne	93%	210
Lutheran Hospital of Indiana	Fort Wayne	92%	101
Memorial Hospital of South Bend	South Bend	92%	89
Franciscan St Anthony Health-Crown Pt[2]	Crown Point	91%	45
Indiana Univ Health Bloomington Hosp	Bloomington	91%	99
Saint Catherine Hospital	East Chicago	91%	43
Franciscan Saint Margaret Health - Dyer	Dyer	90%	50
Union Hospital	Terre Haute	90%	83
Good Samaritan Hospital	Vincennes	89%	53
Reid Hospital & Health Care Services	Richmond	89%	63
Saint Joseph Regional Medical Center	Mishawaka	88%	92
Franciscan St Francis Hlth-Indianapolis	Indianapolis	87%	121
Community Hospital North	Indianapolis	85%	116
Franciscan St Elizabeth Health	Lafayette	85%	41
Indiana University Health[2]	Indianapolis	85%	52
Deaconess Hospital	Evansville	84%	192
Elkhart General Hospital[2]	Elkhart	84%	74
Indiana Univ Health Ball Mem Hosp[2]	Muncie	84%	56
Community Hospital East	Indianapolis	78%	78
Hendricks Regional Health	Danville	77%	35
Indiana University Health Arnett Hospital[2]	Lafayette	71%	52
Saint Vincent Hospital & Health Services	Indianapolis	69%	223
IU Health West Hospital	Avon	65%	49
Memorial Hospital & Health Care Center	Jasper	62%	32
Franciscan St Margaret Health-Hammond[2]	Hammond	61%	41
Indiana University Health North Hospital	Carmel	56%	27
Floyd Memorial Hospital & Health Services	New Albany	53%	108
Clark Memorial Hospital	Jeffersonville	22%	41
Eskenazi Health[2]	Indianapolis	1%	86

Surgical Care Improvement Project

Appropriate Beta Blocker Usage

Hospital Name	City	Rate	Cases
Community Westview Hospital	Indianapolis	100%	35
Decatur County Memorial Hospital	Greensburg	100%	27
Dekalb Health	Auburn	100%	28
Dupont Hospital	Fort Wayne	100%	69
Eskenazi Health[2]	Indianapolis	100%	58
Floyd Memorial Hospital & Health Services	New Albany	100%	398
Franciscan St Anthony Health	Michigan City	100%	138
Good Samaritan Hospital	Vincennes	100%	158
The Heart Hospital at Deaconess Gateway[2]	Newburgh	100%	191
Indiana Univ Health Bloomington Hosp[2]	Bloomington	100%	243
Kosciusko Community Hospital	Warsaw	100%	77
Margaret Mary Community Hospital	Batesville	100%	32
Memorial Hospital	Logansport	100%	25
Methodist Hospitals[2]	Gary	100%	125
Parkview Huntington Hospital	Huntington	100%	26
Reid Hospital & Health Care Services	Richmond	100%	338
Saint Catherine Hospital	East Chicago	100%	67
Saint Joseph Hospital	Fort Wayne	100%	39
Saint Joseph Hospital & Health Center	Kokomo	100%	115

NOTE: Hospital profiles are in alphabetical order by state, then city, then hospital within the city; Rankings exclude hospitals with less than 25 cases except for patient surveys which excludes hospitals with less than 100 cases; (a) 100-299 cases; (1) The number of cases/patients is too few to report; (2) Data submitted were based on a sample of cases/patients; (3) Results are based on a shorter time period than required; (4) Data suppressed by CMS for one or more quarters; (5) Results are not available for this reporting period; (6) Fewer than 100 patients completed the HCAHPS survey; (7) No cases met the criteria for this measure; (8) The lower limit of the confidence interval cannot be calculated if the number of observed infections equals zero; (9) No data are available from the state/territory for this reporting period; (10) The scores shown reflect fewer than 50 completed surveys; (11) There were discrepancies in the data collection process; (12) This measure does not apply to this hospital for this reporting period; (13) Results cannot be calculated for this reporting period; (14) The results for this state are combined with nearby states to protect confidentiality; Please refer to the User's Guide for a full explanation of data.

Saint Joseph Regional Medical Center	Mishawaka	100%	362
St Joseph Reg Med Ctr-Plymouth	Plymouth	100%	37
Saint Mary Medical Center[2]	Hobart	100%	174
Saint Vincent Anderson Regional Hospital	Anderson	100%	140
Terre Haute Regional Hospital	Terre Haute	100%	118
Unity Medical & Surgical Hospital[2]	Mishawaka	100%	25
Witham Health Services	Lebanon	100%	35
Community Hospital North[2]	Indianapolis	99%	140
Deaconess Hospital[2]	Evansville	99%	180
Dearborn County Hospital	Lawrenceburg	99%	81
Franciscan St Francis Hlth-Indianapolis	Indianapolis	99%	668
Franciscan St Francis Health[2]	Mooresville	99%	414
Franciscan Saint Margaret Health - Dyer	Dyer	99%	134
Hancock Regional Hospital	Greenfield	99%	70
Hendricks Regional Health	Danville	99%	175
Indiana University Health[2]	Indianapolis	99%	339
Indiana Univ Health Ball Mem Hosp[2]	Muncie	99%	388
Indianapolis VA Medical Center[2]	Indianapolis	99%	272
IU Health Goshen Hospital	Goshen	99%	158
The Ortho Hosp/Lutheran Health Network	Fort Wayne	99%	476
Saint Mary's Medical Center of Evansville[2]	Evansville	99%	514
Saint Vincent Carmel Hospital[2]	Carmel	99%	77
Saint Vincent Heart Center of Indiana	Indianapolis	99%	424
Saint Vincent Hospital & Health Services[2]	Indianapolis	99%	706
Clark Memorial Hospital[2]	Jeffersonville	98%	225
Community Hospital[2]	Munster	98%	278
Comm Hosp of Anderson/Madison Co	Anderson	98%	127
Elkhart General Hospital[2]	Elkhart	98%	421
Henry County Memorial Hospital	New Castle	98%	128
The Indiana Heart Hospital[2]	Indianapolis	98%	266
Indiana Orthopaedic Hospital[2]	Indianapolis	98%	122
Indiana University Health Arnett Hospital[2]	Lafayette	98%	163
Indiana Univ Health La Porte Hosp	La Porte	98%	127
IU Health West Hospital[2]	Avon	98%	110
King's Daughters' Health[2]	Madison	98%	54
Lutheran Hospital of Indiana	Fort Wayne	98%	599
Major Hospital	Shelbyville	98%	65
Memorial Hospital of South Bend[2]	South Bend	98%	231
Orthopaedic Hospital at Parkview North[2]	Fort Wayne	98%	164
Parkview Regional Medical Center[2]	Fort Wayne	98%	263
Community Hospital South[2]	Indianapolis	97%	156
Franciscan Healthcare - Munster	Munster	97%	39
Franciscan St Elizabeth Health	Crawfordsville	97%	29
Indiana University Health North Hospital[2]	Carmel	97%	79
Indiana University Health Tipton Hospital	Tipton	97%	38
Memorial Hospital & Health Care Center[2]	Jasper	97%	172
Porter Regional Hospital	Valparaiso	97%	413
Union Hospital	Terre Haute	97%	453
Columbus Regional Hospital	Columbus	96%	225
Community Howard Regional Health	Kokomo	96%	52
Franciscan St Elizabeth Health[2]	Lafayette	96%	209
Franciscan St Margaret Health-Hammond	Hammond	96%	79
Marion General Hospital[2]	Marion	96%	96
Schneck Medical Center	Seymour	96%	84
Community Hospital East[2]	Indianapolis	95%	95
Franciscan St Anthony Health-Crown Pt[2]	Crown Point	94%	115
Kentuckiana Medical Center[2]	Clarksville	93%	70
Riverview Hospital	Noblesville	93%	156
Monroe Hospital	Bloomington	84%	79

Appropriate VTP Within 24 Hours

Hospital Name	City	Rate	Cases
Bluffton Regional Medical Center	Bluffton	100%	65
Community Westview Hospital	Indianapolis	100%	82
Decatur County Memorial Hospital	Greensburg	100%	76
Dukes Memorial Hospital	Peru	100%	35
Dupont Hospital	Fort Wayne	100%	260
Franciscan St Francis Health[2]	Mooresville	100%	1063
Good Samaritan Hospital	Vincennes	100%	389
Henry County Memorial Hospital	New Castle	100%	323
Indiana Univ Health Bedford Hosp	Bedford	100%	38
Indiana Univ Health Bloomington Hosp[2]	Bloomington	100%	366
Indiana Univ Health La Porte Hosp	La Porte	100%	289
Indiana University Health North Hospital[2]	Carmel	100%	248
Indiana University Health Tipton Hospital	Tipton	100%	138
Kosciusko Community Hospital	Warsaw	100%	230
Major Hospital	Shelbyville	100%	167
Memorial Hospital	Logansport	100%	91
Methodist Hospitals[2]	Gary	100%	329
Orthopaedic Hospital at Parkview North[2]	Fort Wayne	100%	499
The Ortho Hosp/Lutheran Health Network	Fort Wayne	100%	981
Parkview Huntington Hospital	Huntington	100%	92
Parkview Noble Hospital	Kendallville	100%	62
Parkview Whitley Hospital	Columbia City	100%	34
Pulaski Memorial Hospital	Winamac	100%	25
Saint Catherine Hospital	East Chicago	100%	132
Saint Joseph Hospital & Health Center	Kokomo	100%	275
Saint Joseph Regional Medical Center	Mishawaka	100%	1055
Saint Mary Medical Center[2]	Hobart	100%	255
Saint Vincent Anderson Regional Hospital	Anderson	100%	339
Saint Vincent Carmel Hospital[2]	Carmel	100%	295
Terre Haute Regional Hospital	Terre Haute	100%	200
Unity Medical & Surgical Hospital[2]	Mishawaka	100%	39
Clark Memorial Hospital[2]	Jeffersonville	99%	610
Community Hospital North[2]	Indianapolis	99%	473
Comm Hosp of Anderson/Madison Co	Anderson	99%	368
Dearborn County Hospital	Lawrenceburg	99%	259
Elkhart General Hospital[2]	Elkhart	99%	782
Floyd Memorial Hospital & Health Services	New Albany	99%	596
Franciscan Healthcare - Munster	Munster	99%	96
Franciscan St Anthony Health-Crown Pt[2]	Crown Point	99%	282
Franciscan St Anthony Health	Michigan City	99%	274
Franciscan St Francis Hlth-Indianapolis	Indianapolis	99%	1035
Franciscan Saint Margaret Health - Dyer	Dyer	99%	452
Hendricks Regional Health	Danville	99%	482
Indiana Orthopaedic Hospital[2]	Indianapolis	99%	246
Indiana University Health[2]	Indianapolis	99%	709
Indiana Univ Health Ball Mem Hosp[2]	Muncie	99%	755
Lutheran Hospital of Indiana	Fort Wayne	99%	654
Margaret Mary Community Hospital	Batesville	99%	127
Reid Hospital & Health Care Services	Richmond	99%	662
Schneck Medical Center	Seymour	99%	251
Columbus Regional Hospital	Columbus	98%	458
Community Hospital South[2]	Indianapolis	98%	399
Dekalb Health	Auburn	98%	88
Fayette Regional Health System	Connersville	98%	50
Hancock Regional Hospital	Greenfield	98%	200
Indianapolis VA Medical Center[2]	Indianapolis	98%	376
IU Health West Hospital[2]	Avon	98%	322
Johnson Memorial Hospital	Franklin	98%	106
Parkview Lagrange Hospital	Lagrange	98%	42
Physicians' Medical Center[2]	New Albany	98%	55
Porter Regional Hospital	Valparaiso	98%	353
Saint Mary's Medical Center of Evansville[2]	Evansville	98%	1238
Union Hospital	Terre Haute	98%	765
Cameron Memorial Community Hospital	Angola	97%	59
Deaconess Hospital[2]	Evansville	97%	345
Eskenazi Health[2]	Indianapolis	97%	277
IU Health Goshen Hospital	Goshen	97%	442
Memorial Hospital of South Bend[2]	South Bend	97%	405
Riverview Hospital	Noblesville	97%	518
St Joseph Reg Med Ctr-Plymouth	Plymouth	97%	78
Saint Vincent Hospital & Health Services[2]	Indianapolis	97%	1112
Wabash County Hospital	Wabash	97%	66
Witham Health Services	Lebanon	97%	114
Marion General Hospital[2]	Marion	96%	308
Memorial Hospital & Health Care Center[2]	Jasper	96%	489
Parkview Regional Medical Center[2]	Fort Wayne	96%	365
Pinnacle Hospital[2]	Crown Point	96%	27
Community Howard Regional Health	Kokomo	95%	143
Franciscan St Elizabeth Health[2]	Lafayette	95%	371
Franciscan St Margaret Health-Hammond	Hammond	95%	157
Indiana University Health Arnett Hospital[2]	Lafayette	95%	273
Saint Joseph Hospital	Fort Wayne	95%	63
Adams Memorial Hospital	Decatur	94%	63
Community Hospital[2]	Munster	94%	446
Community Hospital East[2]	Indianapolis	94%	340
Franciscan St Elizabeth Health	Crawfordsville	94%	90
King's Daughters' Health[2]	Madison	94%	106
The Women's Hospital	Newburgh	94%	89
Monroe Hospital	Bloomington	91%	281
Daviess Community Hospital	Washington	88%	42
Jay County Hospital	Portland	69%	35
Harrison County Hospital	Corydon	54%	28

Controlled Postoperative Blood Glucose

Hospital Name	City	Rate	Cases
Columbus Regional Hospital	Columbus	100%	57
Elkhart General Hospital[2]	Elkhart	100%	203
Franciscan St Anthony Health	Michigan City	100%	31
Franciscan Saint Margaret Health - Dyer	Dyer	100%	25
Indiana University Health Arnett Hospital[2]	Lafayette	100%	83
Saint Catherine Hospital	East Chicago	100%	39
Terre Haute Regional Hospital	Terre Haute	100%	38
Floyd Memorial Hospital & Health Services	New Albany	99%	216
Indiana Univ Health Ball Mem Hosp[2]	Muncie	99%	116
Indiana Univ Health Bloomington Hosp[2]	Bloomington	99%	129
Memorial Hospital of South Bend[2]	South Bend	99%	156
Porter Regional Hospital	Valparaiso	99%	98
Saint Mary Medical Center[2]	Hobart	99%	88
Community Hospital[2]	Munster	98%	161
Franciscan St Anthony Health-Crown Pt[2]	Crown Point	98%	53
Franciscan St Francis Hlth-Indianapolis	Indianapolis	98%	354
Franciscan St Margaret Health-Hammond	Hammond	98%	43
The Heart Hospital at Deaconess Gateway[2]	Newburgh	98%	280
Methodist Hospitals[2]	Gary	98%	57
Parkview Regional Medical Center[2]	Fort Wayne	98%	182
Reid Hospital & Health Care Services	Richmond	98%	162
Saint Joseph Regional Medical Center	Mishawaka	98%	124
Saint Vincent Heart Center of Indiana	Indianapolis	98%	764
Union Hospital	Terre Haute	98%	175
Indianapolis VA Medical Center[2]	Indianapolis	97%	71
Lutheran Hospital of Indiana	Fort Wayne	97%	300
Saint Joseph Hospital	Fort Wayne	97%	31
Franciscan St Elizabeth Health[2]	Lafayette	95%	62
Saint Vincent Hospital & Health Services[2]	Indianapolis	95%	307
The Indiana Heart Hospital[2]	Indianapolis	94%	244
Indiana Univ Health La Porte Hosp	La Porte	94%	64
Saint Mary's Medical Center of Evansville[2]	Evansville	94%	140
Indiana University Health[2]	Indianapolis	92%	139
Deaconess Hospital[2]	Evansville	85%	48
Kentuckiana Medical Center[2]	Clarksville	84%	122

Perioperative Temperature Management

Hospital Name	City	Rate	Cases
Adams Memorial Hospital	Decatur	100%	65
Bluffton Regional Medical Center	Bluffton	100%	76
Cameron Memorial Community Hospital	Angola	100%	65
Clark Memorial Hospital[2]	Jeffersonville	100%	650
Columbus Regional Hospital	Columbus	100%	536
Community Hospital[2]	Munster	100%	556
Community Hospital East[2]	Indianapolis	100%	356
Community Hospital North[2]	Indianapolis	100%	509
Comm Hosp of Anderson/Madison Co	Anderson	100%	461
Community Hospital South[2]	Indianapolis	100%	445
Community Westview Hospital	Indianapolis	100%	102
Daviess Community Hospital	Washington	100%	56
Deaconess Hospital[2]	Evansville	100%	478
Dearborn County Hospital	Lawrenceburg	100%	281
Decatur County Memorial Hospital	Greensburg	100%	88
Dekalb Health	Auburn	100%	98
Dukes Memorial Hospital	Peru	100%	39
Dupont Hospital	Fort Wayne	100%	306
Elkhart General Hospital[2]	Elkhart	100%	1016
Eskenazi Health[2]	Indianapolis	100%	334
Fayette Regional Health System	Connersville	100%	58
Floyd Memorial Hospital & Health Services	New Albany	100%	739
Franciscan Healthcare - Munster	Munster	100%	102
Franciscan St Anthony Health-Crown Pt[2]	Crown Point	100%	328
Franciscan St Elizabeth Health	Crawfordsville	100%	104
Franciscan St Francis Health[2]	Mooresville	100%	1200
Franciscan Saint Margaret Health - Dyer	Dyer	100%	508
Franciscan St Margaret Health-Hammond	Hammond	100%	190
Good Samaritan Hospital	Vincennes	100%	461
Hancock Regional Hospital	Greenfield	100%	226
Hendricks Regional Health	Danville	100%	523
Henry County Memorial Hospital	New Castle	100%	350
Indiana Orthopaedic Hospital[2]	Indianapolis	100%	265
Indiana University Health[2]	Indianapolis	100%	935
Indiana University Health Arnett Hospital[2]	Lafayette	100%	314
Indiana Univ Health Ball Mem Hosp[2]	Muncie	100%	838
Indiana Univ Health Bedford Hosp	Bedford	100%	56
Indiana Univ Health Bloomington Hosp[2]	Bloomington	100%	502
Indiana Univ Health La Porte Hosp	La Porte	100%	380
Indiana University Health North Hospital[2]	Carmel	100%	314
Indiana University Health Tipton Hospital	Tipton	100%	145
Indianapolis VA Medical Center[2]	Indianapolis	100%	572
IU Health Goshen Hospital	Goshen	100%	567
IU Health West Hospital[2]	Avon	100%	340
Johnson Memorial Hospital	Franklin	100%	115
Kosciusko Community Hospital	Warsaw	100%	267
Lutheran Hospital of Indiana	Fort Wayne	100%	1015
Margaret Mary Community Hospital	Batesville	100%	144
Marion General Hospital[2]	Marion	100%	342
Memorial Hospital	Logansport	100%	99
Memorial Hospital & Health Care Center[2]	Jasper	100%	522
Memorial Hospital of South Bend[2]	South Bend	100%	600
Methodist Hospitals[2]	Gary	100%	377
Monroe Hospital	Bloomington	100%	302
Orthopaedic Hospital at Parkview North[2]	Fort Wayne	100%	527
The Ortho Hosp/Lutheran Health Network	Fort Wayne	100%	1470
Parkview Huntington Hospital	Huntington	100%	96
Parkview Lagrange Hospital	Lagrange	100%	46
Parkview Noble Hospital	Kendallville	100%	77
Parkview Regional Medical Center[2]	Fort Wayne	100%	561
Parkview Whitley Hospital	Columbia City	100%	41
Pinnacle Hospital[2]	Crown Point	100%	30
Porter Regional Hospital	Valparaiso	100%	1061
Pulaski Memorial Hospital	Winamac	100%	34
Putnam County Hospital	Greencastle	100%	32
Reid Hospital & Health Care Services	Richmond	100%	775
Riverview Hospital	Noblesville	100%	607
Saint Catherine Hospital	East Chicago	100%	189
Saint Joseph Hospital	Fort Wayne	100%	75
Saint Joseph Hospital & Health Center	Kokomo	100%	358
Saint Joseph Regional Medical Center	Mishawaka	100%	1814
St Joseph Reg Med Ctr-Plymouth	Plymouth	100%	144
Saint Mary Medical Center[2]	Hobart	100%	450
Saint Mary's Medical Center of Evansville[2]	Evansville	100%	1366
Saint Vincent Anderson Regional Hospital	Anderson	100%	432
Saint Vincent Carmel Hospital[2]	Carmel	100%	318
Saint Vincent Hospital & Health Services[2]	Indianapolis	100%	1596
Schneck Medical Center	Seymour	100%	267

NOTE: Hospital profiles are in alphabetical order by state, then city, then hospital within the city; Rankings exclude hospitals with less than 25 cases except for patient surveys which excludes hospitals with less than 100 cases; (a) 100-299 cases; (1) The number of cases/patients is too few to report; (2) Data submitted were based on a sample of cases/patients; (3) Results are based on a shorter time period than required; (4) Data suppressed by CMS for one or more quarters; (5) Results are not available for this reporting period; (6) Fewer than 100 patients completed the HCAHPS survey; (7) No cases met the criteria for this measure; (8) The lower limit of the confidence interval cannot be calculated if the number of observed infections equals zero; (9) No data are available from the state/territory for this reporting period; (10) The scores shown reflect fewer than 50 completed surveys; (11) There were discrepancies in the data collection process; (12) This measure does not apply to this hospital for this reporting period; (13) Results cannot be calculated for this reporting period; (14) The results for this state are combined with nearby states to protect confidentiality; Please refer to the User's Guide for a full explanation of data.

Hospital Name	City	Rate	Cases
Terre Haute Regional Hospital	Terre Haute	100%	247
Union Hospital	Terre Haute	100%	886
Unity Medical & Surgical Hospital[2]	Mishawaka	100%	130
Wabash County Hospital	Wabash	100%	70
Witham Health Services	Lebanon	100%	124
The Women's Hospital	Newburgh	100%	92
Community Howard Regional Health	Kokomo	99%	156
Franciscan St Anthony Health	Michigan City	99%	357
Franciscan St Elizabeth Health[2]	Lafayette	99%	521
Franciscan St Francis Hlth-Indianapolis	Indianapolis	99%	1196
King's Daughters' Health[2]	Madison	99%	176
Major Hospital	Shelbyville	99%	197
The Indiana Heart Hospital[2]	Indianapolis	98%	200
Jay County Hospital	Portland	98%	42
Saint Vincent Heart Center of Indiana	Indianapolis	98%	65
Harrison County Hospital	Corydon	94%	32
Physicians' Medical Center[2]	New Albany	89%	97

Prophylactic Antibiotic Selection

Hospital Name	City	Rate	Cases
Bluffton Regional Medical Center	Bluffton	100%	60
Clark Memorial Hospital[2]	Jeffersonville	100%	518
Comm Hosp of Anderson/Madison Co	Anderson	100%	328
Community Westview Hospital	Indianapolis	100%	81
Decatur County Memorial Hospital	Greensburg	100%	63
Dekalb Health	Auburn	100%	62
Dupont Hospital	Fort Wayne	100%	207
Elkhart General Hospital[2]	Elkhart	100%	797
Eskenazi Health[2]	Indianapolis	100%	238
Fayette Regional Health System	Connersville	100%	35
Franciscan St Anthony Health	Michigan City	100%	258
Franciscan St Francis Hlth-Indianapolis	Indianapolis	100%	939
Franciscan St Francis Health[2]	Mooresville	100%	892
Good Samaritan Hospital	Vincennes	100%	332
The Heart Hospital at Deaconess Gateway[2]	Newburgh	100%	205
Henry County Memorial Hospital	New Castle	100%	283
The Indiana Heart Hospital[2]	Indianapolis	100%	338
Indiana Orthopaedic Hospital[2]	Indianapolis	100%	211
Indiana Univ Health Ball Mem Hosp[2]	Muncie	100%	790
Indiana Univ Health Bloomington Hosp[2]	Bloomington	100%	432
Indiana University Health North Hospital[2]	Carmel	100%	218
IU Health West Hospital[2]	Avon	100%	220
Kentuckiana Medical Center[2]	Clarksville	100%	87
Kosciusko Community Hospital	Warsaw	100%	207
Lutheran Hospital of Indiana	Fort Wayne	100%	568
Major Hospital	Shelbyville	100%	143
Memorial Hospital of South Bend[2]	South Bend	100%	573
Orthopaedic Hospital at Parkview North[2]	Fort Wayne	100%	441
The Ortho Hosp/Lutheran Health Network	Fort Wayne	100%	1202
Parkview Huntington Hospital	Huntington	100%	88
Parkview Lagrange Hospital	Lagrange	100%	37
Parkview Noble Hospital	Kendallville	100%	61
Reid Hospital & Health Care Services	Richmond	100%	693
Riverview Hospital	Noblesville	100%	482
Saint Joseph Hospital	Fort Wayne	100%	65
Saint Joseph Hospital & Health Center	Kokomo	100%	270
St Joseph Reg Med Ctr-Plymouth	Plymouth	100%	110
Saint Mary Medical Center[2]	Hobart	100%	354
Saint Mary's Medical Center of Evansville[2]	Evansville	100%	1214
Saint Vincent Anderson Regional Hospital	Anderson	100%	295
Saint Vincent Heart Center of Indiana	Indianapolis	100%	721
Union Hospital	Terre Haute	100%	718
Unity Medical & Surgical Hospital[2]	Mishawaka	100%	108
Witham Health Services	Lebanon	100%	95
The Women's Hospital	Newburgh	100%	54
Columbus Regional Hospital	Columbus	99%	418
Community Hospital[2]	Munster	99%	527
Community Hospital East[2]	Indianapolis	99%	243
Community Hospital North[2]	Indianapolis	99%	349
Deaconess Hospital[2]	Evansville	99%	347
Dearborn County Hospital	Lawrenceburg	99%	211
Floyd Memorial Hospital & Health Services	New Albany	99%	594
Franciscan St Elizabeth Health[2]	Lafayette	99%	402
Franciscan Saint Margaret Health - Dyer	Dyer	99%	389
Hancock Regional Hospital	Greenfield	99%	153
Hendricks Regional Health	Danville	99%	402
Indiana University Health[2]	Indianapolis	99%	688
Indiana Univ Health La Porte Hosp	La Porte	99%	276
Indiana University Health Tipton Hospital	Tipton	99%	111
Indianapolis VA Medical Center	Indianapolis	99%	428
IU Health Goshen Hospital	Goshen	99%	368
Johnson Memorial Hospital	Franklin	99%	75
King's Daughters' Health[2]	Madison	99%	123
Margaret Mary Community Hospital	Batesville	99%	109
Methodist Hospitals[2]	Gary	99%	290
Parkview Regional Medical Center[2]	Fort Wayne	99%	539
Porter Regional Hospital	Valparaiso	99%	779
Saint Catherine Hospital	East Chicago	99%	143
Saint Joseph Regional Medical Center	Mishawaka	99%	1545
Saint Vincent Hospital & Health Services[2]	Indianapolis	99%	1234
Schneck Medical Center	Seymour	99%	178
Terre Haute Regional Hospital	Terre Haute	99%	196
Community Hospital South[2]	Indianapolis	98%	317
Franciscan St Anthony Health-Crown Pt[2]	Crown Point	98%	273
Franciscan St Margaret Health-Hammond	Hammond	98%	124
Indiana University Health Arnett Hospital[2]	Lafayette	98%	281
Monroe Hospital	Bloomington	98%	245
Saint Vincent Carmel Hospital[2]	Carmel	98%	198
Wabash County Hospital	Wabash	98%	60
Daviess Community Hospital	Washington	97%	36
Franciscan Healthcare - Munster	Munster	97%	79
Franciscan St Elizabeth Health	Crawfordsville	97%	95
Jay County Hospital	Portland	97%	31
Parkview Whitley Hospital	Columbia City	97%	31
Community Howard Regional Health	Kokomo	96%	114
Cameron Memorial Community Hospital	Angola	95%	44
Memorial Hospital	Logansport	94%	54
Memorial Hospital & Health Care Center[2]	Jasper	94%	408
Marion General Hospital[2]	Marion	93%	246
Indiana Univ Health Bedford Hosp	Bedford	91%	32
Physicians' Medical Center[2]	New Albany	88%	77

Prophylactic Antibiotic Selection (Outpatient)

Hospital Name	City	Rate	Cases
Columbus Regional Hospital	Columbus	100%	417
Dukes Memorial Hospital	Peru	100%	33
Dupont Hospital	Fort Wayne	100%	586
Eskenazi Health	Indianapolis	100%	66
Franciscan St Francis Health	Mooresville	100%	58
The Indiana Heart Hospital	Indianapolis	100%	393
Indiana Orthopaedic Hospital	Indianapolis	100%	529
Kosciusko Community Hospital	Warsaw	100%	59
Margaret Mary Community Hospital	Batesville	100%	104
Orthopaedic Hospital at Parkview North	Fort Wayne	100%	206
The Ortho Hosp/Lutheran Health Network	Fort Wayne	100%	622
Parkview Lagrange Hospital[3]	Lagrange	100%	28
Parkview Noble Hospital	Kendallville	100%	32
Parkview Whitley Hospital	Columbia City	100%	59
Porter Regional Hospital	Valparaiso	100%	407
Reid Hospital & Health Care Services	Richmond	100%	417
Riverview Hospital	Noblesville	100%	101
Saint Joseph Hospital	Fort Wayne	100%	62
St Joseph Reg Med Ctr-Plymouth	Plymouth	100%	26
Saint Vincent Heart Center of Indiana	Indianapolis	100%	411
The Women's Hospital	Newburgh	100%	476
Community Hospital	Munster	99%	496
Community Howard Regional Health	Kokomo	99%	99
Community Westview Hospital	Indianapolis	99%	68
Dekalb Health	Auburn	99%	71
Franciscan Healthcare - Munster	Munster	99%	88
Franciscan St Anthony Health	Michigan City	99%	300
Franciscan St Elizabeth Health	Lafayette	99%	593
Franciscan St Francis Hlth-Indianapolis	Indianapolis	99%	832
Franciscan Saint Margaret Health - Dyer	Dyer	99%	211
The Heart Hospital at Deaconess Gateway	Newburgh	99%	420
Henry County Memorial Hospital	New Castle	99%	100
Indiana University Health Arnett Hospital	Lafayette	99%	428
Indiana Univ Health Ball Mem Hosp	Muncie	99%	419
Indiana Univ Health La Porte Hosp	La Porte	99%	304
IU Health West Hospital	Avon	99%	256
Johnson Memorial Hospital	Franklin	99%	152
Lutheran Hospital of Indiana	Fort Wayne	99%	1055
Methodist Hospitals	Gary	99%	241
Parkview Regional Medical Center	Fort Wayne	99%	623
Saint Mary Medical Center	Hobart	99%	294
Saint Mary's Medical Center of Evansville	Evansville	99%	1076
Saint Vincent Anderson Regional Hospital	Anderson	99%	168
Clark Memorial Hospital	Jeffersonville	98%	386
Community Hospital East	Indianapolis	98%	249
Community Hospital North	Indianapolis	98%	439
Comm Hosp of Anderson/Madison Co	Anderson	98%	163
Community Hospital South	Indianapolis	98%	372
Dearborn County Hospital	Lawrenceburg	98%	84
Elkhart General Hospital	Elkhart	98%	357
Good Samaritan Hospital	Vincennes	98%	152
Hancock Regional Hospital	Greenfield	98%	42
Hendricks Regional Health	Danville	98%	216
Indiana Univ Health Bloomington Hosp	Bloomington	98%	681
Indiana University Health North Hospital	Carmel	98%	352
IU Health Goshen Hospital	Goshen	98%	159
King's Daughters' Health	Madison	98%	89
Memorial Hospital of South Bend	South Bend	98%	530
Monroe Hospital	Bloomington	98%	127
Parkview Huntington Hospital	Huntington	98%	52
Terre Haute Regional Hospital	Terre Haute	98%	121
Cameron Memorial Community Hospital	Angola	97%	29
Deaconess Hospital	Evansville	97%	653
Marion General Hospital	Marion	97%	232
Memorial Hospital	Logansport	97%	128
Memorial Hospital & Health Care Center	Jasper	97%	248
Saint Catherine Hospital	East Chicago	97%	66
Saint Joseph Hospital & Health Center	Kokomo	97%	128
Saint Vincent Carmel Hospital	Carmel	97%	138
Saint Vincent Hospital & Health Services	Indianapolis	97%	758
Schneck Medical Center	Seymour	97%	141
Union Hospital	Terre Haute	97%	675
Saint Joseph Regional Medical Center	Mishawaka	96%	326
Franciscan St Anthony Health-Crown Pt	Crown Point	95%	292
Franciscan St Margaret Health-Hammond	Hammond	95%	85
Indiana University Health Morgan Hospital	Martinsville	95%	41
Indiana University Health	Indianapolis	93%	771
Kentuckiana Medical Center[3]	Clarksville	89%	27
Daviess Community Hospital	Washington	88%	77
Indiana Univ Health Bedford Hosp	Bedford	88%	26
Floyd Memorial Hospital & Health Services	New Albany	84%	311
Franciscan St Elizabeth Health	Crawfordsville	84%	63
Physicians' Medical Center	New Albany	83%	182

Prophylactic Antibiotic Stopped

Hospital Name	City	Rate	Cases
Cameron Memorial Community Hospital	Angola	100%	44
Community Hospital East[2]	Indianapolis	100%	243
Community Westview Hospital	Indianapolis	100%	74
Elkhart General Hospital[2]	Elkhart	100%	763
Fayette Regional Health System	Connersville	100%	34
Franciscan Healthcare - Munster	Munster	100%	74
Franciscan St Anthony Health	Michigan City	100%	246
Indiana Orthopaedic Hospital[2]	Indianapolis	100%	210
Indiana Univ Health Bloomington Hosp[2]	Bloomington	100%	409
Indiana University Health Tipton Hospital	Tipton	100%	111
Jay County Hospital	Portland	100%	31
Kentuckiana Medical Center[2]	Clarksville	100%	82
Methodist Hospitals[2]	Gary	100%	263
The Ortho Hosp/Lutheran Health Network	Fort Wayne	100%	1199
Parkview Lagrange Hospital	Lagrange	100%	35
Saint Catherine Hospital	East Chicago	100%	137
Saint Joseph Hospital & Health Center	Kokomo	100%	256
Saint Joseph Regional Medical Center	Mishawaka	100%	1545
St Joseph Reg Med Ctr-Plymouth	Plymouth	100%	108
Saint Mary Medical Center[2]	Hobart	100%	344
Saint Vincent Anderson Regional Hospital	Anderson	100%	292
Wabash County Hospital	Wabash	100%	60
Community Hospital North[2]	Indianapolis	99%	346
Comm Hosp of Anderson/Madison Co	Anderson	99%	319
Community Hospital South[2]	Indianapolis	99%	314
Dupont Hospital	Fort Wayne	99%	202
Franciscan St Elizabeth Health[2]	Lafayette	99%	387
Franciscan St Francis Hlth-Indianapolis	Indianapolis	99%	893
Franciscan Saint Margaret Health - Dyer	Dyer	99%	378
Franciscan St Margaret Health-Hammond	Hammond	99%	121
Good Samaritan Hospital	Vincennes	99%	316
Hancock Regional Hospital	Greenfield	99%	152
Hendricks Regional Health	Danville	99%	399
Henry County Memorial Hospital	New Castle	99%	279
The Indiana Heart Hospital[2]	Indianapolis	99%	323
Indiana Univ Health Ball Mem Hosp[2]	Muncie	99%	778
Indiana University Health North Hospital[2]	Carmel	99%	216
Indianapolis VA Medical Center	Indianapolis	99%	420
IU Health Goshen Hospital	Goshen	99%	363
Major Hospital	Shelbyville	99%	139
Margaret Mary Community Hospital	Batesville	99%	108
Parkview Huntington Hospital	Huntington	99%	87
Porter Regional Hospital	Valparaiso	99%	765
Reid Hospital & Health Care Services	Richmond	99%	652
Saint Mary's Medical Center of Evansville[2]	Evansville	99%	1198
Saint Vincent Heart Center of Indiana	Indianapolis	99%	708
Terre Haute Regional Hospital	Terre Haute	99%	153
Bluffton Regional Medical Center	Bluffton	98%	56
Clark Memorial Hospital[2]	Jeffersonville	98%	511
Columbus Regional Hospital	Columbus	98%	390
Community Hospital[2]	Munster	98%	506
Deaconess Hospital[2]	Evansville	98%	338
Decatur County Memorial Hospital	Greensburg	98%	62
Dekalb Health	Auburn	98%	61
Eskenazi Health[2]	Indianapolis	98%	237
Floyd Memorial Hospital & Health Services	New Albany	98%	582
Franciscan St Francis Health[2]	Mooresville	98%	878
Indiana University Health[2]	Indianapolis	98%	667
Indiana University Health Arnett Hospital[2]	Lafayette	98%	272
Indiana Univ Health La Porte Hosp	La Porte	98%	270
IU Health West Hospital[2]	Avon	98%	207
Kosciusko Community Hospital	Warsaw	98%	207
Memorial Hospital	Logansport	98%	48
Memorial Hospital of South Bend[2]	South Bend	98%	557
Riverview Hospital	Noblesville	98%	475
Saint Joseph Hospital	Fort Wayne	98%	63
Saint Vincent Hospital & Health Services[2]	Indianapolis	98%	1214
Schneck Medical Center	Seymour	98%	167
Union Hospital	Terre Haute	98%	676
Community Howard Regional Health	Kokomo	97%	109
Franciscan St Elizabeth Health	Crawfordsville	97%	93
The Heart Hospital at Deaconess Gateway[2]	Newburgh	97%	199
Indiana Univ Health Bedford Hosp	Bedford	97%	32

NOTE: Hospital profiles are in alphabetical order by state, then city, then hospital within the city; Rankings exclude hospitals with less than 25 cases except for patient surveys which excludes hospitals with less than 100 cases; (a) 100-299 cases; (1) The number of cases/patients is too few to report; (2) Data submitted were based on a sample of cases/patients; (3) Results are based on a shorter time period than required; (4) Data suppressed by CMS for one or more quarters; (5) Results are not available for this reporting period; (6) Fewer than 100 patients completed the HCAHPS survey; (7) No cases met the criteria for this measure; (8) The lower limit of the confidence interval cannot be calculated if the number of observed infections equals zero; (9) No data are available from the state/territory for this reporting period; (10) The scores shown reflect fewer than 50 completed surveys; (11) There were discrepancies in the data collection process; (12) This measure does not apply to this hospital for this reporting period; (13) Results cannot be calculated for this reporting period; (14) The results for this state are combined with nearby states to protect confidentiality; Please refer to the User's Guide for a full explanation of data.

Hospital Name	City	Rate	Cases
King's Daughters' Health[2]	Madison	97%	119
Lutheran Hospital of Indiana	Fort Wayne	97%	537
Marion General Hospital[2]	Marion	97%	236
Orthopaedic Hospital at Parkview North[2]	Fort Wayne	97%	440
Saint Vincent Carmel Hospital[2]	Carmel	97%	197
Johnson Memorial Hospital	Franklin	96%	74
Memorial Hospital & Health Care Center[2]	Jasper	96%	399
Parkview Regional Medical Center[2]	Fort Wayne	96%	525
Witham Health Services	Lebanon	96%	94
Franciscan St Anthony Health-Crown Pt[2]	Crown Point	95%	261
Dearborn County Hospital	Lawrenceburg	94%	198
Parkview Whitley Hospital	Columbia City	94%	31
The Women's Hospital	Newburgh	94%	52
Parkview Noble Hospital	Kendallville	92%	60
Physicians' Medical Center[2]	New Albany	91%	76
Unity Medical & Surgical Hospital[2]	Mishawaka	90%	103
Monroe Hospital	Bloomington	88%	241
Daviess Community Hospital	Washington	84%	31

Prophylactic Antibiotic Timing

Hospital Name	City	Rate	Cases
Bluffton Regional Medical Center	Bluffton	100%	60
Cameron Memorial Community Hospital	Angola	100%	44
Clark Memorial Hospital[2]	Jeffersonville	100%	518
Community Westview Hospital	Indianapolis	100%	81
Dupont Hospital	Fort Wayne	100%	207
Elkhart General Hospital[2]	Elkhart	100%	797
Franciscan St Elizabeth Health	Crawfordsville	100%	95
Franciscan St Francis Hlth-Indianapolis	Indianapolis	100%	940
Franciscan Saint Margaret Health - Dyer	Dyer	100%	389
Franciscan St Margaret Health-Hammond	Hammond	100%	124
Good Samaritan Hospital	Vincennes	100%	332
Hancock Regional Hospital	Greenfield	100%	153
The Heart Hospital at Deaconess Gateway[2]	Newburgh	100%	205
Henry County Memorial Hospital	New Castle	100%	283
The Indiana Heart Hospital[2]	Indianapolis	100%	339
Indiana Orthopaedic Hospital[2]	Indianapolis	100%	211
Indiana University Health[2]	Indianapolis	100%	692
Indiana University Health Arnett Hospital[2]	Lafayette	100%	280
Indiana Univ Health Bedford Hosp	Bedford	100%	32
Indiana University Health North Hospital[2]	Carmel	100%	218
Indiana University Health Tipton Hospital	Tipton	100%	111
IU Health West Hospital[2]	Avon	100%	222
Jay County Hospital	Portland	100%	31
King's Daughters' Health[2]	Madison	100%	123
Kosciusko Community Hospital	Warsaw	100%	207
Major Hospital	Shelbyville	100%	143
Memorial Hospital	Logansport	100%	54
Memorial Hospital of South Bend[2]	South Bend	100%	575
Methodist Hospitals[2]	Gary	100%	291
Orthopaedic Hospital at Parkview North[2]	Fort Wayne	100%	441
The Ortho Hosp/Lutheran Health Network	Fort Wayne	100%	1202
Parkview Noble Hospital	Kendallville	100%	61
Parkview Whitley Hospital	Columbia City	100%	31
Reid Hospital & Health Care Services	Richmond	100%	693
Saint Catherine Hospital	East Chicago	100%	144
Saint Joseph Hospital & Health Center	Kokomo	100%	270
Saint Joseph Regional Medical Center	Mishawaka	100%	1547
Saint Mary Medical Center[2]	Hobart	100%	355
Saint Mary's Medical Center of Evansville[2]	Evansville	100%	1214
Saint Vincent Anderson Regional Hospital	Anderson	100%	295
Saint Vincent Heart Center of Indiana	Indianapolis	100%	724
Terre Haute Regional Hospital	Terre Haute	100%	196
Columbus Regional Hospital	Columbus	99%	420
Community Hospital[2]	Munster	99%	528
Comm Hosp of Anderson/Madison Co	Anderson	99%	328
Eskenazi Health[2]	Indianapolis	99%	238
Franciscan St Anthony Health-Crown Pt[2]	Crown Point	99%	273
Franciscan St Anthony Health	Michigan City	99%	259
Franciscan St Francis Health[2]	Mooresville	99%	892
Hendricks Regional Health	Danville	99%	402
Indiana Univ Health Ball Mem Hosp[2]	Muncie	99%	790
Indiana Univ Health Bloomington Hosp[2]	Bloomington	99%	433
Indiana Univ Health La Porte Hosp	La Porte	99%	276
Indianapolis VA Medical Center	Indianapolis	99%	428
IU Health Goshen Hospital	Goshen	99%	369
Lutheran Hospital of Indiana	Fort Wayne	99%	569
Parkview Huntington Hospital	Huntington	99%	88
Porter Regional Hospital	Valparaiso	99%	779
Riverview Hospital	Noblesville	99%	482
St Joseph Reg Med Ctr-Plymouth	Plymouth	99%	110
Saint Vincent Hospital & Health Services[2]	Indianapolis	99%	1237
Union Hospital	Terre Haute	99%	724
Witham Health Services	Lebanon	99%	96
Community Hospital North[2]	Indianapolis	98%	349
Decatur County Memorial Hospital	Greensburg	98%	64
Dekalb Health	Auburn	98%	62
Floyd Memorial Hospital & Health Services	New Albany	98%	594
Franciscan St Elizabeth Health[2]	Lafayette	98%	403
Margaret Mary Community Hospital	Batesville	98%	109
Parkview Regional Medical Center[2]	Fort Wayne	98%	542
Saint Joseph Hospital	Fort Wayne	98%	65
Schneck Medical Center	Seymour	98%	179
Unity Medical & Surgical Hospital[2]	Mishawaka	98%	108
The Women's Hospital	Newburgh	98%	54
Fayette Regional Health System	Connersville	97%	35
Franciscan Healthcare - Munster	Munster	97%	79
Johnson Memorial Hospital	Franklin	97%	75
Memorial Hospital & Health Care Center[2]	Jasper	97%	408
Saint Vincent Carmel Hospital[2]	Carmel	97%	199
Deaconess Hospital[2]	Evansville	96%	347
Marion General Hospital[2]	Marion	96%	248
Community Hospital East[2]	Indianapolis	95%	244
Community Howard Regional Health	Kokomo	95%	115
Kentuckiana Medical Center[2]	Clarksville	95%	87
Parkview Lagrange Hospital	Lagrange	95%	37
Wabash County Hospital	Wabash	95%	60
Community Hospital South[2]	Indianapolis	94%	317
Monroe Hospital	Bloomington	94%	245
Dearborn County Hospital	Lawrenceburg	92%	212
Daviess Community Hospital	Washington	89%	36
Physicians' Medical Center[2]	New Albany	88%	78

Prophylactic Antibiotic Timing (Outpatient)

Hospital Name	City	Rate	Cases
Clark Memorial Hospital	Jeffersonville	100%	386
Comm Hosp of Anderson/Madison Co	Anderson	100%	163
Dekalb Health	Auburn	100%	71
Dukes Memorial Hospital	Peru	100%	33
Eskenazi Health	Indianapolis	100%	66
Franciscan St Francis Health	Mooresville	100%	57
Henry County Memorial Hospital	New Castle	100%	100
Indiana Orthopaedic Hospital	Indianapolis	100%	529
Indiana Univ Health Ball Mem Hosp	Muncie	100%	420
Indiana Univ Health Bedford Hosp	Bedford	100%	26
Indiana University Health North Hospital	Carmel	100%	352
IU Health West Hospital	Avon	100%	256
Kentuckiana Medical Center[3]	Clarksville	100%	26
Kosciusko Community Hospital	Warsaw	100%	59
Margaret Mary Community Hospital	Batesville	100%	88
Orthopaedic Hospital at Parkview North	Fort Wayne	100%	206
The Ortho Hosp/Lutheran Health Network	Fort Wayne	100%	622
Riverview Hospital	Noblesville	100%	101
Saint Catherine Hospital	East Chicago	100%	58
St Joseph Reg Med Ctr-Plymouth	Plymouth	100%	26
Saint Mary Medical Center	Hobart	100%	286
Saint Mary's Medical Center of Evansville	Evansville	100%	1076
Community Hospital East	Indianapolis	99%	250
Dupont Hospital	Fort Wayne	99%	586
Franciscan Healthcare - Munster	Munster	99%	89
Franciscan St Anthony Health-Crown Pt	Crown Point	99%	293
Franciscan St Francis Hlth-Indianapolis	Indianapolis	99%	834
The Heart Hospital at Deaconess Gateway	Newburgh	99%	420
Indiana University Health	Indianapolis	99%	653
Indiana University Health Arnett Hospital	Lafayette	99%	427
Indiana Univ Health Bloomington Hosp	Bloomington	99%	681
Lutheran Hospital of Indiana	Fort Wayne	99%	1055
Memorial Hospital of South Bend	South Bend	99%	531
Parkview Regional Medical Center	Fort Wayne	99%	627
Reid Hospital & Health Care Services	Richmond	99%	418
Saint Joseph Regional Medical Center	Mishawaka	99%	326
Schneck Medical Center	Seymour	99%	140
Terre Haute Regional Hospital	Terre Haute	99%	121
Union Hospital	Terre Haute	99%	673
Community Hospital North	Indianapolis	98%	440
Deaconess Hospital	Evansville	98%	621
Elkhart General Hospital	Elkhart	98%	360
Hendricks Regional Health	Danville	98%	216
Methodist Hospitals	Gary	98%	242
Parkview Huntington Hospital	Huntington	98%	53
Porter Regional Hospital	Valparaiso	98%	411
Saint Joseph Hospital	Fort Wayne	98%	62
Saint Vincent Heart Center of Indiana	Indianapolis	98%	411
The Women's Hospital	Newburgh	98%	476
Cameron Memorial Community Hospital	Angola	97%	30
Columbus Regional Hospital	Columbus	97%	420
Community Hospital	Munster	97%	497
Community Westview Hospital	Indianapolis	97%	68
Floyd Memorial Hospital & Health Services	New Albany	97%	319
Franciscan St Anthony Health	Michigan City	97%	226
Franciscan St Elizabeth Health	Lafayette	97%	602
Franciscan St Margaret Health-Hammond	Hammond	97%	77
Good Samaritan Hospital	Vincennes	97%	153
The Indiana Heart Hospital	Indianapolis	97%	396
King's Daughters' Health	Madison	97%	88
Marion General Hospital	Marion	97%	236
Memorial Hospital	Logansport	97%	95
Parkview Noble Hospital	Kendallville	97%	33
Parkview Whitley Hospital	Columbia City	97%	60
Physicians' Medical Center	New Albany	97%	171
Saint Joseph Hospital & Health Center	Kokomo	97%	129
Saint Vincent Carmel Hospital	Carmel	97%	140
Indiana Univ Health La Porte Hosp	La Porte	96%	253
IU Health Goshen Hospital	Goshen	96%	161
Johnson Memorial Hospital	Franklin	96%	153
Monroe Hospital	Bloomington	96%	129
Saint Vincent Anderson Regional Hospital	Anderson	96%	164
Daviess Community Hospital	Washington	95%	77
Franciscan Saint Margaret Health - Dyer	Dyer	95%	194
Hancock Regional Hospital	Greenfield	95%	43
Community Hospital South	Indianapolis	94%	379
Saint Vincent Hospital & Health Services	Indianapolis	94%	770
Parkview Lagrange Hospital[3]	Lagrange	93%	29
Franciscan St Elizabeth Health	Crawfordsville	91%	66
Community Howard Regional Health	Kokomo	87%	105
Dearborn County Hospital	Lawrenceburg	82%	60
Jasper County Hospital	Rensselaer	78%	27
Memorial Hospital & Health Care Center	Jasper	77%	310

Urinary Catheter Removal

Hospital Name	City	Rate	Cases
Bluffton Regional Medical Center	Bluffton	100%	51
Community Westview Hospital	Indianapolis	100%	60
Decatur County Memorial Hospital	Greensburg	100%	65
Dekalb Health	Auburn	100%	28
Dupont Hospital	Fort Wayne	100%	91
Elkhart General Hospital[2]	Elkhart	100%	834
Floyd Memorial Hospital & Health Services	New Albany	100%	569
Franciscan St Anthony Health	Michigan City	100%	204
Franciscan St Francis Health[2]	Mooresville	100%	1074
Hancock Regional Hospital	Greenfield	100%	45
The Heart Hospital at Deaconess Gateway[2]	Newburgh	100%	259
Indiana Univ Health Bloomington Hosp[2]	Bloomington	100%	418
Indiana Univ Health La Porte Hosp	La Porte	100%	240
Indiana University Health Tipton Hospital	Tipton	100%	128
Major Hospital	Shelbyville	100%	139
Memorial Hospital	Logansport	100%	30
Orthopaedic Hospital at Parkview North[2]	Fort Wayne	100%	422
Parkview Huntington Hospital	Huntington	100%	85
Parkview Lagrange Hospital	Lagrange	100%	26
Physicians' Medical Center[2]	New Albany	100%	32
Riverview Hospital	Noblesville	100%	445
Saint Catherine Hospital	East Chicago	100%	85
Saint Joseph Hospital & Health Center	Kokomo	100%	274
Saint Joseph Regional Medical Center	Mishawaka	100%	212
Saint Mary Medical Center[2]	Hobart	100%	172
Clark Memorial Hospital[2]	Jeffersonville	99%	502
Columbus Regional Hospital	Columbus	99%	447
Deaconess Hospital[2]	Evansville	99%	253
Eskenazi Health[2]	Indianapolis	99%	199
Franciscan St Francis Hlth-Indianapolis	Indianapolis	99%	757
Franciscan Saint Margaret Health - Dyer	Dyer	99%	134
Hendricks Regional Health	Danville	99%	380
Henry County Memorial Hospital	New Castle	99%	91
The Indiana Heart Hospital[2]	Indianapolis	99%	370
Indiana University Health Arnett Hospital[2]	Lafayette	99%	281
Indiana Univ Health Ball Mem Hosp[2]	Muncie	99%	764
IU Health Goshen Hospital	Goshen	99%	311
IU Health West Hospital[2]	Avon	99%	271
Lutheran Hospital of Indiana	Fort Wayne	99%	617
Methodist Hospitals[2]	Gary	99%	213
The Ortho Hosp/Lutheran Health Network	Fort Wayne	99%	356
Saint Mary's Medical Center of Evansville[2]	Evansville	99%	933
Saint Vincent Anderson Regional Hospital	Anderson	99%	310
Saint Vincent Carmel Hospital[2]	Carmel	99%	87
Saint Vincent Heart Center of Indiana	Indianapolis	99%	470
Terre Haute Regional Hospital	Terre Haute	99%	128
Cameron Memorial Community Hospital	Angola	98%	52
Franciscan Healthcare - Munster	Munster	98%	59
Indiana Orthopaedic Hospital[2]	Indianapolis	98%	50
Indiana University Health[2]	Indianapolis	98%	702
Indiana University Health North Hospital[2]	Carmel	98%	196
Indianapolis VA Medical Center[2]	Indianapolis	98%	413
Memorial Hospital & Health Care Center[2]	Jasper	98%	208
Parkview Noble Hospital	Kendallville	98%	44
Parkview Regional Medical Center[2]	Fort Wayne	98%	348
Porter Regional Hospital	Valparaiso	98%	296
Reid Hospital & Health Care Services	Richmond	98%	518
Schneck Medical Center	Seymour	98%	46
Wabash County Hospital	Wabash	98%	42
Witham Health Services	Lebanon	98%	94
Comm Hosp of Anderson/Madison Co	Anderson	97%	322
Community Hospital South[2]	Indianapolis	97%	125
Kosciusko Community Hospital	Warsaw	97%	38
Saint Vincent Hospital & Health Services[2]	Indianapolis	97%	847
Community Howard Regional Health	Kokomo	96%	113
Dearborn County Hospital	Lawrenceburg	96%	185
Franciscan St Elizabeth Health[2]	Lafayette	96%	164
Good Samaritan Hospital	Vincennes	96%	114
Johnson Memorial Hospital	Franklin	96%	82
Margaret Mary Community Hospital	Batesville	96%	67
Union Hospital	Terre Haute	96%	677
Adams Memorial Hospital	Decatur	95%	43

NOTE: Hospital profiles are in alphabetical order by state, then city, then hospital within the city; Rankings exclude hospitals with less than 25 cases except for patient surveys which excludes hospitals with less than 100 cases; (a) 100-299 cases; (1) The number of cases/patients is too few to report; (2) Data submitted were based on a sample of cases/patients; (3) Results are based on a shorter time period than required; (4) Data suppressed by CMS for one or more quarters; (5) Results are not available for this reporting period; (6) Fewer than 100 patients completed the HCAHPS survey; (7) No cases met the criteria for this measure; (8) The lower limit of the confidence interval cannot be calculated if the number of observed infections equals zero; (9) No data are available from the state/territory for this reporting period; (10) The scores shown reflect fewer than 50 completed surveys; (11) There were discrepancies in the data collection process; (12) This measure does not apply to this hospital for this reporting period; (13) Results cannot be calculated for this reporting period; (14) The results for this state are combined with nearby states to protect confidentiality; Please refer to the User's Guide for a full explanation of data.

Daviess Community Hospital	Washington	95%	37
Franciscan St Anthony Health-Crown Pt[2]	Crown Point	95%	209
Community Hospital East[2]	Indianapolis	94%	107
Kentuckiana Medical Center[2]	Clarksville	94%	69
Monroe Hospital	Bloomington	94%	248
Franciscan St Margaret Health-Hammond	Hammond	93%	75
Marion General Hospital[2]	Marion	93%	81
Community Hospital[2]	Munster	92%	317
Community Hospital North[2]	Indianapolis	91%	117
King's Daughters' Health[2]	Madison	91%	70
Memorial Hospital of South Bend[2]	South Bend	91%	227
Saint Joseph Hospital	Fort Wayne	89%	38

Survey of Patients' Hospital Experiences

Area Around Room 'Always' Quiet at Night

Hospital Name	City	Rate	Cases
Physicians' Medical Center	New Albany	87%	(a)
Indiana Orthopaedic Hospital	Indianapolis	81%	300+
Kentuckiana Medical Center	Clarksville	77%	300+
Unity Medical & Surgical Hospital	Mishawaka	76%	(a)
Franciscan St Elizabeth Health	Crawfordsville	73%	(a)
Gibson General Hospital	Princeton	72%	(a)
Jay County Hospital	Portland	72%	300+
Monroe Hospital	Bloomington	72%	300+
Franciscan Healthcare - Munster	Munster	71%	300+
The Women's Hospital	Newburgh	71%	300+
The Heart Hospital at Deaconess Gateway	Newburgh	70%	300+
The Indiana Heart Hospital	Indianapolis	69%	300+
Orthopaedic Hospital at Parkview North	Fort Wayne	69%	300+
The Ortho Hosp/Lutheran Health Network	Fort Wayne	69%	300+
Pinnacle Hospital	Crown Point	69%	(a)
Fayette Regional Health System	Connersville	68%	300+
Memorial Hospital & Health Care Center	Jasper	68%	300+
Schneck Medical Center	Seymour	68%	300+
Indiana University Health North Hospital	Carmel	67%	300+
Parkview Regional Medical Center	Fort Wayne	67%	300+
Saint Vincent Dunn Hospital	Bedford	67%	(a)
Saint Vincent Frankfort Hospital	Frankfort	66%	(a)
Community Hospital South	Indianapolis	65%	300+
IU Health West Hospital	Avon	65%	300+
Parkview Lagrange Hospital	Lagrange	65%	(a)
Pulaski Memorial Hospital	Winamac	65%	(a)
Saint Catherine Hospital	East Chicago	65%	300+
Woodlawn Hospital	Rochester	65%	(a)
Hendricks Regional Health	Danville	64%	300+
Kosciusko Community Hospital	Warsaw	64%	300+
Margaret Mary Community Hospital	Batesville	64%	300+
Parkview Huntington Hospital	Huntington	64%	300+
Perry County Memorial Hospital	Tell City	64%	(a)
Saint Joseph Regional Medical Center	Mishawaka	64%	300+
Saint Vincent Mercy Hospital	Elwood	64%	(a)
Wabash County Hospital	Wabash	64%	(a)
Hancock Regional Hospital	Greenfield	63%	300+
Indiana University Health Arnett Hospital	Lafayette	63%	300+
Indiana University Health Tipton Hospital	Tipton	63%	(a)
Saint Mary's Medical Center of Evansville	Evansville	63%	300+
Eskenazi Health	Indianapolis	62%	300+
Floyd Memorial Hospital & Health Services	New Albany	62%	(a)
Franciscan St Elizabeth Health	Lafayette	62%	300+
Parkview Noble Hospital	Kendallville	62%	300+
Rush Memorial Hospital	Rushville	62%	(a)
Saint Vincent Randolph Hospital	Winchester	62%	(a)
Adams Memorial Hospital	Decatur	61%	300+
Bluffton Regional Medical Center	Bluffton	61%	300+
Community Howard Regional Health	Kokomo	61%	300+
Harrison County Hospital	Corydon	61%	(a)
King's Daughters' Health	Madison	61%	300+
Saint Vincent Clay Hospital	Brazil	61%	(a)
Union Hospital	Terre Haute	61%	300+
Witham Health Services	Lebanon	61%	300+
Deaconess Hospital	Evansville	60%	300+
Dearborn County Hospital	Lawrenceburg	60%	300+
Franciscan St Francis Health	Mooresville	60%	300+
Porter Regional Hospital	Valparaiso	60%	300+
Reid Hospital & Health Care Services	Richmond	60%	300+
Scott Memorial Hospital	Scottsburg	60%	(a)
Community Hospital North	Indianapolis	59%	300+
Henry County Memorial Hospital	New Castle	59%	300+
Indiana Univ Health Ball Mem Hosp	Muncie	59%	300+
Methodist Hospitals	Gary	59%	300+
Parkview Whitley Hospital	Columbia City	59%	300+
Riverview Hospital	Noblesville	59%	300+
Saint Joseph Hospital	Fort Wayne	59%	300+
Saint Vincent Anderson Regional Hospital	Anderson	59%	300+
Saint Vincent Heart Center of Indiana	Indianapolis	59%	300+
Sullivan County Community Hospital	Sullivan	59%	(a)
Cameron Memorial Community Hospital	Angola	58%	300+
Columbus Regional Hospital	Columbus	58%	300+
Indiana Univ Health White Mem Hosp	Monticello	58%	(a)
Major Hospital	Shelbyville	58%	300+
Saint Vincent Carmel Hospital	Carmel	58%	300+
Daviess Community Hospital	Washington	57%	300+
Dukes Memorial Hospital	Peru	57%	(a)
Dupont Hospital	Fort Wayne	57%	300+
Franciscan St Anthony Health-Crown Pt	Crown Point	57%	300+
Franciscan St Anthony Health	Michigan City	57%	300+
Franciscan St Margaret Health-Hammond	Hammond	57%	300+
Good Samaritan Hospital	Vincennes	57%	300+
Indiana University Health Morgan Hospital	Martinsville	57%	(a)
Johnson Memorial Hospital	Franklin	57%	300+
Lutheran Hospital of Indiana	Fort Wayne	57%	300+
Marion General Hospital[11]	Marion	57%	300+
St Joseph Reg Med Ctr-Plymouth	Plymouth	57%	300+
Saint Mary Medical Center	Hobart	57%	300+
Saint Vincent Hospital & Health Services[11]	Indianapolis	57%	300+
Saint Vincent Williamsport Hospital	Williamsport	57%	(a)
Indiana University Health	Indianapolis	56%	300+
Union Hospital Clinton	Clinton	56%	(a)
Community Hospital	Munster	55%	300+
Community Hospital East	Indianapolis	55%	300+
Elkhart General Hospital	Elkhart	55%	300+
Memorial Hospital	Logansport	55%	300+
Terre Haute Regional Hospital	Terre Haute	55%	300+
Franciscan Saint Margaret Health - Dyer	Dyer	54%	300+
Indiana Univ Health Bloomington Hosp	Bloomington	54%	300+
Indiana University Health Starke Hospital	Knox	54%	(a)
IU Health Goshen Hospital	Goshen	54%	300+
Saint Joseph Hospital & Health Center	Kokomo	54%	300+
Community Westview Hospital	Indianapolis	53%	(a)
Decatur County Memorial Hospital	Greensburg	53%	(a)
Franciscan St Francis Hlth-Indianapolis	Indianapolis	53%	300+
Indiana Univ Health La Porte Hosp	La Porte	53%	300+
Clark Memorial Hospital	Jeffersonville	52%	300+
Comm Hosp of Anderson/Madison Co	Anderson	52%	300+
Indiana Univ Health Bedford Hosp	Bedford	52%	(a)
Putnam County Hospital	Greencastle	50%	(a)
Dekalb Health	Auburn	49%	(a)
Franciscan St Elizabeth Health	Lafayette	49%	300+
Memorial Hospital of South Bend	South Bend	47%	300+
Jasper County Hospital	Rensselaer	45%	(a)

Doctors 'Always' Communicated Well

Hospital Name	City	Rate	Cases
Saint Vincent Clay Hospital	Brazil	90%	(a)
Gibson General Hospital	Princeton	89%	(a)
Indiana University Health Tipton Hospital	Tipton	89%	(a)
Margaret Mary Community Hospital	Batesville	89%	300+
Indiana Univ Health Bedford Hosp	Bedford	88%	(a)
Johnson Memorial Hospital	Franklin	88%	300+
Kentuckiana Medical Center	Clarksville	88%	300+
Union Hospital Clinton	Clinton	88%	(a)
Harrison County Hospital	Corydon	87%	(a)
Indiana Orthopaedic Hospital	Indianapolis	87%	300+
Orthopaedic Hospital at Parkview North	Fort Wayne	87%	300+
Parkview Noble Hospital	Kendallville	87%	300+
Saint Vincent Heart Center of Indiana	Indianapolis	87%	300+
Saint Vincent Williamsport Hospital	Williamsport	87%	(a)
Woodlawn Hospital	Rochester	87%	(a)
Dekalb Health	Auburn	86%	300+
Franciscan St Francis Health	Mooresville	86%	300+
Good Samaritan Hospital	Vincennes	86%	300+
Hendricks Regional Health	Danville	86%	300+
Rush Memorial Hospital	Rushville	86%	(a)
Saint Vincent Frankfort Hospital	Frankfort	86%	(a)
Schneck Medical Center	Seymour	86%	300+
Dukes Memorial Hospital	Peru	85%	(a)
Floyd Memorial Hospital & Health Services	New Albany	85%	(a)
The Heart Hospital at Deaconess Gateway	Newburgh	85%	300+
Indiana University Health Morgan Hospital	Martinsville	85%	(a)
Jay County Hospital	Portland	85%	300+
King's Daughters' Health	Madison	85%	300+
Memorial Hospital & Health Care Center	Jasper	85%	300+
The Ortho Hosp/Lutheran Health Network	Fort Wayne	85%	300+
Parkview Huntington Hospital	Huntington	85%	300+
Parkview Whitley Hospital	Columbia City	85%	300+
Putnam County Hospital	Greencastle	85%	(a)
Saint Joseph Hospital & Health Center	Kokomo	85%	300+
Saint Vincent Carmel Hospital	Carmel	85%	300+
Saint Vincent Dunn Hospital	Bedford	85%	(a)
Saint Vincent Randolph Hospital	Winchester	85%	(a)
Sullivan County Community Hospital	Sullivan	85%	(a)
Wabash County Hospital	Wabash	85%	(a)
Decatur County Memorial Hospital	Greensburg	84%	(a)
Hancock Regional Hospital	Greenfield	84%	300+
Indiana University Health North Hospital	Carmel	84%	300+
Major Hospital	Shelbyville	84%	300+
Monroe Hospital	Bloomington	84%	300+
Perry County Memorial Hospital	Tell City	84%	(a)
Pinnacle Hospital	Crown Point	84%	(a)
Pulaski Memorial Hospital	Winamac	84%	(a)
Saint Vincent Mercy Hospital	Elwood	84%	(a)
Witham Health Services	Lebanon	84%	300+
Columbus Regional Hospital	Columbus	83%	300+
Dearborn County Hospital	Lawrenceburg	83%	300+
Dupont Hospital	Fort Wayne	83%	300+
Franciscan Healthcare - Munster	Munster	83%	300+
Franciscan St Elizabeth Health	Crawfordsville	83%	(a)
Henry County Memorial Hospital	New Castle	83%	300+
The Indiana Heart Hospital	Indianapolis	83%	300+
Marion General Hospital[11]	Marion	83%	300+
Memorial Hospital	Logansport	83%	300+
Riverview Hospital	Noblesville	83%	300+
Saint Vincent Anderson Regional Hospital	Anderson	83%	300+
Adams Memorial Hospital	Decatur	82%	300+
Cameron Memorial Community Hospital	Angola	82%	300+
Comm Hosp of Anderson/Madison Co	Anderson	82%	300+
Community Westview Hospital	Indianapolis	82%	(a)
Franciscan Saint Margaret Health - Dyer	Dyer	82%	300+
IU Health West Hospital	Avon	82%	300+
Parkview Lagrange Hospital	Lagrange	82%	(a)
Physicians' Medical Center	New Albany	82%	(a)
Saint Vincent Hospital & Health Services[11]	Indianapolis	82%	300+
Scott Memorial Hospital	Scottsburg	82%	(a)
Community Howard Regional Health	Kokomo	81%	300+
Deaconess Hospital	Evansville	81%	300+
Fayette Regional Health System	Connersville	81%	300+
Indiana Univ Health Bloomington Hosp	Bloomington	81%	300+
Indiana Univ Health White Mem Hosp	Monticello	81%	(a)
Kosciusko Community Hospital	Warsaw	81%	300+
Reid Hospital & Health Care Services	Richmond	81%	300+
Saint Mary Medical Center	Hobart	81%	300+
Unity Medical & Surgical Hospital	Mishawaka	81%	(a)
The Women's Hospital	Newburgh	81%	300+
Bluffton Regional Medical Center	Bluffton	80%	300+
Community Hospital	Munster	80%	300+
Eskenazi Health	Indianapolis	80%	300+
Franciscan St Anthony Health	Michigan City	80%	300+
Franciscan St Elizabeth Health	Lafayette	80%	300+
Franciscan St Francis Hlth-Indianapolis	Indianapolis	80%	300+
Indiana University Health	Indianapolis	80%	300+
Jasper County Hospital	Rensselaer	80%	(a)
Memorial Hospital of South Bend	South Bend	80%	300+
Saint Catherine Hospital	East Chicago	80%	300+
Saint Joseph Hospital	Fort Wayne	80%	300+
Saint Mary's Medical Center of Evansville	Evansville	80%	300+
Terre Haute Regional Hospital	Terre Haute	80%	300+
Clark Memorial Hospital	Jeffersonville	79%	300+
Daviess Community Hospital	Washington	79%	300+
Franciscan St Anthony Health-Crown Pt	Crown Point	79%	300+
IU Health Goshen Hospital	Goshen	79%	300+
Porter Regional Hospital	Valparaiso	79%	300+
St Joseph Reg Med Ctr-Plymouth	Plymouth	79%	300+
Community Hospital South	Indianapolis	78%	300+
Indiana Univ Health Ball Mem Hosp	Muncie	78%	300+
Lutheran Hospital of Indiana	Fort Wayne	78%	300+
Methodist Hospitals	Gary	78%	300+
Saint Joseph Regional Medical Center	Mishawaka	78%	300+
Community Hospital North	Indianapolis	77%	300+
Elkhart General Hospital	Elkhart	77%	300+
Parkview Regional Medical Center	Fort Wayne	77%	300+
Indiana University Health Arnett Hospital	Lafayette	76%	300+
Community Hospital East	Indianapolis	75%	300+
Union Hospital	Terre Haute	75%	300+
Franciscan St Margaret Health-Hammond	Hammond	74%	300+
Franciscan St Elizabeth Health	Lafayette	73%	300+
Indiana Univ Health La Porte Hosp	La Porte	73%	300+
Indiana University Health Starke Hospital	Knox	71%	(a)

Home Recovery Information Given

Hospital Name	City	Rate	Cases
Indiana Orthopaedic Hospital	Indianapolis	93%	300+
Woodlawn Hospital	Rochester	93%	(a)
Orthopaedic Hospital at Parkview North	Fort Wayne	92%	300+
Franciscan St Francis Health	Mooresville	91%	300+
Indiana Univ Health Bedford Hosp	Bedford	91%	(a)
The Ortho Hosp/Lutheran Health Network	Fort Wayne	91%	300+
Parkview Huntington Hospital	Huntington	91%	300+
Pulaski Memorial Hospital	Winamac	91%	(a)
Putnam County Hospital	Greencastle	91%	(a)
Saint Vincent Anderson Regional Hospital	Anderson	91%	300+
Union Hospital Clinton	Clinton	91%	(a)
Unity Medical & Surgical Hospital	Mishawaka	91%	(a)
Decatur County Memorial Hospital	Greensburg	90%	(a)
Franciscan St Elizabeth Health	Crawfordsville	90%	(a)
Good Samaritan Hospital	Vincennes	90%	300+
Parkview Noble Hospital	Kendallville	90%	300+
Saint Mary's Medical Center of Evansville	Evansville	90%	300+
Union Hospital	Terre Haute	90%	300+
Dupont Hospital	Fort Wayne	89%	300+
Hancock Regional Hospital	Greenfield	89%	300+
Hendricks Regional Health	Danville	89%	300+

NOTE: Hospital profiles are in alphabetical order by state, then city, then hospital within the city; Rankings exclude hospitals with less than 25 cases except for patient surveys which excludes hospitals with less than 100 cases; (a) 100-299 cases; (1) The number of cases/patients is too few to report; (2) Data submitted were based on a sample of cases/patients; (3) Results are based on a shorter time period than required; (4) Data suppressed by CMS for one or more quarters; (5) Results are not available for this reporting period; (6) Fewer than 100 patients completed the HCAHPS survey; (7) No cases met the criteria for this measure; (8) The lower limit of the confidence interval cannot be calculated if the number of observed infections equals zero; (9) No data are available from the state/territory for this reporting period; (10) The scores shown reflect fewer than 50 completed surveys; (11) There were discrepancies in the data collection process; (12) This measure does not apply to this hospital for this reporting period; (13) Results cannot be calculated for this reporting period; (14) The results for this state are combined with nearby states to protect confidentiality; Please refer to the User's Guide for a full explanation of data.

Henry County Memorial Hospital	New Castle	89%	300+
Johnson Memorial Hospital	Franklin	89%	300+
Major Hospital	Shelbyville	89%	300+
Reid Hospital & Health Care Services	Richmond	89%	300+
Saint Vincent Frankfort Hospital	Frankfort	89%	(a)
Bluffton Regional Medical Center	Bluffton	88%	300+
Cameron Memorial Community Hospital	Angola	88%	300+
Columbus Regional Hospital	Columbus	88%	300+
Daviess Community Hospital	Washington	88%	300+
Dearborn County Hospital	Lawrenceburg	88%	300+
Dekalb Health	Auburn	88%	300+
Fayette Regional Health System	Connersville	88%	300+
Franciscan St Elizabeth Health	Lafayette	88%	300+
Gibson General Hospital	Princeton	88%	(a)
The Heart Hospital at Deaconess Gateway	Newburgh	88%	300+
Indiana Univ Health Bloomington Hosp	Bloomington	88%	300+
IU Health Goshen Hospital	Goshen	88%	300+
Memorial Hospital & Health Care Center	Jasper	88%	300+
Memorial Hospital of South Bend	South Bend	88%	300+
Parkview Lagrange Hospital	Lagrange	88%	(a)
Parkview Whitley Hospital	Columbia City	88%	300+
Saint Joseph Hospital & Health Center	Kokomo	88%	300+
St Joseph Reg Med Ctr-Plymouth	Plymouth	88%	300+
The Women's Hospital	Newburgh	88%	300+
The Indiana Heart Hospital	Indianapolis	87%	300+
Indiana University Health	Indianapolis	87%	300+
Indiana University Health North Hospital	Carmel	87%	300+
Kosciusko Community Hospital	Warsaw	87%	300+
Margaret Mary Community Hospital	Batesville	87%	300+
Parkview Regional Medical Center	Fort Wayne	87%	300+
Riverview Hospital	Noblesville	87%	300+
Saint Vincent Heart Center of Indiana	Indianapolis	87%	300+
Saint Vincent Randolph Hospital	Winchester	87%	(a)
Sullivan County Community Hospital	Sullivan	87%	(a)
Terre Haute Regional Hospital	Terre Haute	87%	300+
Adams Memorial Hospital	Decatur	86%	300+
Community Hospital North	Indianapolis	86%	300+
Dukes Memorial Hospital	Peru	86%	(a)
Elkhart General Hospital	Elkhart	86%	300+
Harrison County Hospital	Corydon	86%	(a)
Indiana University Health Morgan Hospital	Martinsville	86%	(a)
IU Health West Hospital	Avon	86%	300+
King's Daughters' Health	Madison	86%	300+
Lutheran Hospital of Indiana	Fort Wayne	86%	300+
Marion General Hospital[11]	Marion	86%	300+
Perry County Memorial Hospital	Tell City	86%	(a)
Porter Regional Hospital	Valparaiso	86%	300+
Saint Joseph Regional Medical Center	Mishawaka	86%	300+
Saint Mary Medical Center	Hobart	86%	300+
Saint Vincent Dunn Hospital	Bedford	86%	(a)
Community Hospital	Munster	85%	300+
Community Hospital South	Indianapolis	85%	300+
Community Howard Regional Health	Kokomo	85%	300+
Community Westview Hospital	Indianapolis	85%	(a)
Deaconess Hospital	Evansville	85%	300+
Floyd Memorial Hospital & Health Services	New Albany	85%	(a)
Franciscan St Anthony Health	Michigan City	85%	300+
Indiana University Health Arnett Hospital	Lafayette	85%	300+
Indiana Univ Health La Porte Hosp	La Porte	85%	300+
Indiana University Health Tipton Hospital	Tipton	85%	(a)
Jay County Hospital	Portland	85%	300+
Saint Joseph Hospital	Fort Wayne	85%	300+
Saint Vincent Clay Hospital	Brazil	85%	(a)
Saint Vincent Williamsport Hospital	Williamsport	85%	(a)
Schneck Medical Center	Seymour	85%	300+
Scott Memorial Hospital	Scottsburg	85%	(a)
Comm Hosp of Anderson/Madison Co	Anderson	84%	300+
Franciscan Healthcare - Munster	Munster	84%	300+
Franciscan St Francis Hlth-Indianapolis	Indianapolis	84%	300+
Kentuckiana Medical Center	Clarksville	84%	300+
Physicians' Medical Center	New Albany	84%	(a)
Pinnacle Hospital	Crown Point	84%	(a)
Saint Catherine Hospital	East Chicago	84%	300+
Saint Vincent Hospital & Health Services[11]	Indianapolis	84%	300+
Saint Vincent Mercy Hospital	Elwood	84%	(a)
Witham Health Services	Lebanon	84%	300+
Eskenazi Health	Indianapolis	83%	300+
Franciscan St Anthony Health-Crown Pt	Crown Point	83%	300+
Indiana Univ Health Ball Mem Hosp	Muncie	83%	300+
Indiana University Health Starke Hospital	Knox	83%	(a)
Indiana Univ Health White Mem Hosp	Monticello	83%	(a)
Saint Vincent Carmel Hospital	Carmel	83%	300+
Community Hospital East	Indianapolis	82%	300+
Franciscan St Elizabeth Health	Lafayette	82%	300+
Franciscan Saint Margaret Health - Dyer	Dyer	82%	300+
Memorial Hospital	Logansport	82%	300+
Methodist Hospitals	Gary	82%	300+
Monroe Hospital	Bloomington	82%	300+
Wabash County Hospital	Wabash	82%	(a)
Clark Memorial Hospital	Jeffersonville	80%	300+
Franciscan St Margaret Health-Hammond	Hammond	80%	300+
Jasper County Hospital	Rensselaer	80%	(a)
Rush Memorial Hospital	Rushville	80%	(a)

Hospital Given 9 or 10 on 10 Point Scale

Hospital Name	City	Rate	Cases
Indiana Orthopaedic Hospital	Indianapolis	90%	300+
The Heart Hospital at Deaconess Gateway	Newburgh	88%	300+
Indiana University Health North Hospital	Carmel	86%	300+
Saint Vincent Heart Center of Indiana	Indianapolis	85%	300+
Franciscan St Francis Health	Mooresville	84%	300+
The Indiana Heart Hospital	Indianapolis	84%	300+
Kentuckiana Medical Center	Clarksville	84%	300+
Hendricks Regional Health	Danville	83%	300+
Physicians' Medical Center	New Albany	83%	(a)
The Women's Hospital	Newburgh	83%	300+
Indiana University Health Tipton Hospital	Tipton	82%	(a)
Orthopaedic Hospital at Parkview North	Fort Wayne	82%	300+
Parkview Noble Hospital	Kendallville	82%	300+
Pulaski Memorial Hospital	Winamac	82%	(a)
Union Hospital Clinton	Clinton	82%	(a)
Floyd Memorial Hospital & Health Services	New Albany	81%	(a)
IU Health West Hospital	Avon	81%	300+
Margaret Mary Community Hospital	Batesville	81%	300+
Memorial Hospital & Health Care Center	Jasper	81%	300+
Parkview Whitley Hospital	Columbia City	81%	300+
Dupont Hospital	Fort Wayne	80%	300+
Hancock Regional Hospital	Greenfield	80%	300+
Indiana Univ Health Bedford Hosp	Bedford	80%	(a)
Johnson Memorial Hospital	Franklin	79%	300+
The Ortho Hosp/Lutheran Health Network	Fort Wayne	79%	300+
Community Hospital	Munster	78%	300+
Community Hospital North	Indianapolis	78%	300+
Good Samaritan Hospital	Vincennes	78%	300+
Jay County Hospital	Portland	78%	300+
Parkview Huntington Hospital	Huntington	78%	300+
Parkview Lagrange Hospital	Lagrange	78%	(a)
Saint Joseph Hospital & Health Center	Kokomo	78%	300+
Saint Mary Medical Center	Hobart	78%	300+
Saint Vincent Carmel Hospital	Carmel	78%	300+
Saint Vincent Hospital & Health Services[11]	Indianapolis	78%	300+
Unity Medical & Surgical Hospital	Mishawaka	78%	(a)
Henry County Memorial Hospital	New Castle	77%	300+
Parkview Regional Medical Center	Fort Wayne	77%	300+
Schneck Medical Center	Seymour	77%	300+
Community Hospital South	Indianapolis	76%	300+
Deaconess Hospital	Evansville	76%	300+
Franciscan St Francis Hlth-Indianapolis	Indianapolis	76%	300+
Harrison County Hospital	Corydon	76%	(a)
Monroe Hospital	Bloomington	76%	300+
Pinnacle Hospital	Crown Point	76%	(a)
Saint Joseph Regional Medical Center	Mishawaka	76%	300+
Saint Mary's Medical Center of Evansville	Evansville	76%	300+
Saint Vincent Dunn Hospital	Bedford	76%	(a)
Witham Health Services	Lebanon	76%	300+
Bluffton Regional Medical Center	Bluffton	75%	300+
Franciscan St Elizabeth Health	Lafayette	75%	300+
Lutheran Hospital of Indiana	Fort Wayne	75%	300+
Major Hospital	Shelbyville	75%	300+
Memorial Hospital of South Bend	South Bend	75%	300+
Saint Vincent Frankfort Hospital	Frankfort	75%	(a)
Scott Memorial Hospital	Scottsburg	75%	(a)
Union Hospital	Terre Haute	75%	300+
Woodlawn Hospital	Rochester	75%	(a)
Adams Memorial Hospital	Decatur	74%	300+
Comm Hosp of Anderson/Madison Co	Anderson	74%	300+
Decatur County Memorial Hospital	Greensburg	74%	(a)
Gibson General Hospital	Princeton	74%	(a)
Indiana University Health	Indianapolis	74%	300+
Indiana University Health Arnett Hospital	Lafayette	74%	300+
St Joseph Reg Med Ctr-Plymouth	Plymouth	74%	300+
Wabash County Hospital	Wabash	74%	(a)
Dekalb Health	Auburn	73%	300+
Reid Hospital & Health Care Services	Richmond	73%	300+
Riverview Hospital	Noblesville	73%	300+
Saint Catherine Hospital	East Chicago	73%	300+
Saint Vincent Anderson Regional Hospital	Anderson	73%	300+
Saint Vincent Williamsport Hospital	Williamsport	73%	(a)
Terre Haute Regional Hospital	Terre Haute	73%	300+
Cameron Memorial Community Hospital	Angola	72%	300+
Eskenazi Health	Indianapolis	72%	300+
Fayette Regional Health System	Connersville	72%	300+
Franciscan Healthcare - Munster	Munster	72%	300+
Indiana Univ Health Bloomington Hosp	Bloomington	72%	300+
Indiana Univ Health White Mem Hosp	Monticello	72%	(a)
IU Health Goshen Hospital	Goshen	72%	300+
Perry County Memorial Hospital	Tell City	72%	(a)
Porter Regional Hospital	Valparaiso	72%	300+
Sullivan County Community Hospital	Sullivan	72%	(a)
Columbus Regional Hospital	Columbus	71%	300+
Dearborn County Hospital	Lawrenceburg	71%	300+
Franciscan St Anthony Health-Crown Pt	Crown Point	71%	300+
Franciscan St Anthony Health	Michigan City	71%	300+
Marion General Hospital[11]	Marion	71%	300+
Franciscan St Elizabeth Health	Crawfordsville	70%	(a)
Methodist Hospitals	Gary	70%	300+
Saint Vincent Randolph Hospital	Winchester	70%	(a)
Clark Memorial Hospital	Jeffersonville	69%	300+
Community Hospital East	Indianapolis	69%	300+
Community Howard Regional Health	Kokomo	69%	300+
Elkhart General Hospital	Elkhart	69%	300+
Saint Vincent Mercy Hospital	Elwood	69%	(a)
Franciscan Saint Margaret Health - Dyer	Dyer	68%	300+
Indiana University Health Morgan Hospital	Martinsville	68%	(a)
Kosciusko Community Hospital	Warsaw	68%	300+
Saint Vincent Clay Hospital	Brazil	68%	(a)
Indiana Univ Health Ball Mem Hosp	Muncie	67%	300+
Indiana Univ Health La Porte Hosp	La Porte	67%	300+
Community Westview Hospital	Indianapolis	66%	(a)
Dukes Memorial Hospital	Peru	66%	(a)
King's Daughters' Health	Madison	66%	300+
Rush Memorial Hospital	Rushville	66%	(a)
Saint Joseph Hospital	Fort Wayne	66%	300+
Franciscan St Margaret Health-Hammond	Hammond	65%	300+
Daviess Community Hospital	Washington	64%	300+
Franciscan St Elizabeth Health	Lafayette	63%	300+
Memorial Hospital	Logansport	62%	300+
Indiana University Health Starke Hospital	Knox	61%	(a)
Putnam County Hospital	Greencastle	61%	(a)
Jasper County Hospital	Rensselaer	59%	(a)

Meds 'Always' Explained Before Given

Hospital Name	City	Rate	Cases
Indiana Orthopaedic Hospital	Indianapolis	77%	300+
Scott Memorial Hospital	Scottsburg	77%	(a)
Gibson General Hospital	Princeton	72%	(a)
Memorial Hospital & Health Care Center	Jasper	72%	300+
Perry County Memorial Hospital	Tell City	72%	(a)
Physicians' Medical Center	New Albany	72%	(a)
Decatur County Memorial Hospital	Greensburg	71%	(a)
Henry County Memorial Hospital	New Castle	71%	300+
The Indiana Heart Hospital	Indianapolis	71%	300+
Johnson Memorial Hospital	Franklin	70%	300+
Sullivan County Community Hospital	Sullivan	70%	(a)
Woodlawn Hospital	Rochester	70%	(a)
Franciscan St Elizabeth Health	Crawfordsville	69%	(a)
Franciscan St Francis Health	Mooresville	69%	300+
Hancock Regional Hospital	Greenfield	69%	300+
Saint Vincent Clay Hospital	Brazil	69%	(a)
Union Hospital Clinton	Clinton	69%	(a)
Wabash County Hospital	Wabash	69%	(a)
Eskenazi Health	Indianapolis	68%	300+
Indiana University Health Tipton Hospital	Tipton	68%	(a)
Kentuckiana Medical Center	Clarksville	68%	300+
Marion General Hospital[11]	Marion	68%	300+
Saint Vincent Frankfort Hospital	Frankfort	68%	(a)
Schneck Medical Center	Seymour	68%	300+
Good Samaritan Hospital	Vincennes	67%	300+
Harrison County Hospital	Corydon	67%	(a)
Jay County Hospital	Portland	67%	300+
Major Hospital	Shelbyville	67%	300+
Parkview Huntington Hospital	Huntington	67%	300+
Pulaski Memorial Hospital	Winamac	67%	(a)
Unity Medical & Surgical Hospital	Mishawaka	67%	(a)
Community Hospital	Munster	66%	300+
Fayette Regional Health System	Connersville	66%	300+
Floyd Memorial Hospital & Health Services	New Albany	66%	(a)
Franciscan Saint Margaret Health - Dyer	Dyer	66%	300+
Indiana Univ Health Bedford Hosp	Bedford	66%	(a)
Margaret Mary Community Hospital	Batesville	66%	300+
Reid Hospital & Health Care Services	Richmond	66%	300+
Saint Catherine Hospital	East Chicago	66%	300+
Saint Vincent Dunn Hospital	Bedford	66%	(a)
Saint Vincent Randolph Hospital	Winchester	66%	(a)
Bluffton Regional Medical Center	Bluffton	65%	300+
Dearborn County Hospital	Lawrenceburg	65%	300+
Franciscan St Elizabeth Health	Lafayette	65%	300+
The Heart Hospital at Deaconess Gateway	Newburgh	65%	300+
Hendricks Regional Health	Danville	65%	300+
Indiana University Health Starke Hospital	Knox	65%	(a)
Kosciusko Community Hospital	Warsaw	65%	300+
Orthopaedic Hospital at Parkview North	Fort Wayne	65%	300+
Parkview Noble Hospital	Kendallville	65%	300+
Parkview Whitley Hospital	Columbia City	65%	300+
Rush Memorial Hospital	Rushville	65%	(a)
Saint Joseph Hospital & Health Center	Kokomo	65%	300+
Saint Vincent Heart Center of Indiana	Indianapolis	65%	300+
Witham Health Services	Lebanon	65%	300+
Cameron Memorial Community Hospital	Angola	64%	300+
Columbus Regional Hospital	Columbus	64%	300+
Daviess Community Hospital	Washington	64%	300+
Franciscan Healthcare - Munster	Munster	64%	300+
Indiana University Health	Indianapolis	64%	300+

NOTE: Hospital profiles are in alphabetical order by state, then city, then hospital within the city; Rankings exclude hospitals with less than 25 cases except for patient surveys which excludes hospitals with less than 100 cases; (a) 100-299 cases; (1) The number of cases/patients is too few to report; (2) Data submitted were based on a sample of cases/patients; (3) Results are based on a shorter time period than required; (4) Data suppressed by CMS for one or more quarters; (5) Results are not available for this reporting period; (6) Fewer than 100 patients completed the HCAHPS survey; (7) No cases met the criteria for this measure; (8) The lower limit of the confidence interval cannot be calculated if the number of observed infections equals zero; (9) No data are available from the state/territory for this reporting period; (10) The scores shown reflect fewer than 50 completed surveys; (11) There were discrepancies in the data collection process; (12) This measure does not apply to this hospital for this reporting period; (13) Results cannot be calculated for this reporting period; (14) The results for this state are combined with nearby states to protect confidentiality; Please refer to the User's Guide for a full explanation of data.

Indiana University Health North Hospital	Carmel	64%	300+
IU Health Goshen Hospital	Goshen	64%	300+
IU Health West Hospital	Avon	64%	300+
Methodist Hospitals	Gary	64%	300+
Riverview Hospital	Noblesville	64%	300+
Saint Mary Medical Center	Hobart	64%	300+
Community Howard Regional Health	Kokomo	63%	300+
Deaconess Hospital	Evansville	63%	300+
Dekalb Health	Auburn	63%	300+
Dukes Memorial Hospital	Peru	63%	(a)
Indiana Univ Health White Mem Hosp	Monticello	63%	(a)
The Ortho Hosp/Lutheran Health Network	Fort Wayne	63%	300+
Saint Vincent Mercy Hospital	Elwood	63%	(a)
The Women's Hospital	Newburgh	63%	300+
Adams Memorial Hospital	Decatur	62%	300+
Franciscan St Anthony Health	Michigan City	62%	300+
Indiana Univ Health Ball Mem Hosp	Muncie	62%	300+
Indiana Univ Health Bloomington Hosp	Bloomington	62%	300+
Indiana Univ Health La Porte Hosp	La Porte	62%	300+
King's Daughters' Health	Madison	62%	300+
Parkview Lagrange Hospital	Lagrange	62%	(a)
Saint Joseph Hospital	Fort Wayne	62%	300+
Saint Vincent Carmel Hospital	Carmel	62%	300+
Clark Memorial Hospital	Jeffersonville	61%	300+
Community Hospital North	Indianapolis	61%	300+
Comm Hosp of Anderson/Madison Co	Anderson	61%	300+
Dupont Hospital	Fort Wayne	61%	300+
Franciscan St Anthony Health-Crown Pt	Crown Point	61%	300+
Monroe Hospital	Bloomington	61%	300+
Saint Mary's Medical Center of Evansville	Evansville	61%	300+
Terre Haute Regional Hospital	Terre Haute	61%	300+
Community Hospital South	Indianapolis	60%	300+
Franciscan St Elizabeth Health	Lafayette	60%	300+
Franciscan St Margaret Health-Hammond	Hammond	60%	300+
Indiana University Health Morgan Hospital	Martinsville	60%	(a)
Lutheran Hospital of Indiana	Fort Wayne	60%	300+
Memorial Hospital of South Bend	South Bend	60%	300+
Pinnacle Hospital	Crown Point	60%	(a)
St Joseph Reg Med Ctr-Plymouth	Plymouth	60%	300+
Community Hospital East	Indianapolis	59%	300+
Community Westview Hospital	Indianapolis	59%	(a)
Elkhart General Hospital	Elkhart	59%	300+
Franciscan St Francis Hlth-Indianapolis	Indianapolis	59%	300+
Jasper County Hospital	Rensselaer	59%	(a)
Parkview Regional Medical Center	Fort Wayne	59%	300+
Saint Vincent Hospital & Health Services[11]	Indianapolis	59%	300+
Saint Vincent Williamsport Hospital	Williamsport	59%	(a)
Union Hospital	Terre Haute	59%	300+
Putnam County Hospital	Greencastle	58%	(a)
Saint Joseph Regional Medical Center	Mishawaka	58%	300+
Saint Vincent Anderson Regional Hospital	Anderson	57%	300+
Indiana University Health Arnett Hospital	Lafayette	56%	300+
Porter Regional Hospital	Valparaiso	56%	300+
Memorial Hospital	Logansport	53%	300+

Nurses 'Always' Communicated Well

Hospital Name	City	Rate	Cases
Indiana Orthopaedic Hospital	Indianapolis	91%	300+
Gibson General Hospital	Princeton	89%	(a)
Union Hospital Clinton	Clinton	89%	(a)
Good Samaritan Hospital	Vincennes	87%	300+
Kentuckiana Medical Center	Clarksville	87%	300+
Margaret Mary Community Hospital	Batesville	87%	300+
Franciscan St Elizabeth Health	Crawfordsville	86%	(a)
Perry County Memorial Hospital	Tell City	86%	(a)
Unity Medical & Surgical Hospital	Mishawaka	86%	(a)
The Heart Hospital at Deaconess Gateway	Newburgh	85%	300+
Henry County Memorial Hospital	New Castle	85%	300+
The Indiana Heart Hospital	Indianapolis	85%	300+
Indiana University Health North Hospital	Carmel	85%	300+
Physicians' Medical Center	New Albany	85%	(a)
Schneck Medical Center	Seymour	85%	300+
Adams Memorial Hospital	Decatur	84%	300+
Cameron Memorial Community Hospital	Angola	84%	300+
Community Hospital	Munster	84%	300+
Floyd Memorial Hospital & Health Services	New Albany	84%	(a)
Franciscan Healthcare - Munster	Munster	84%	300+
Hancock Regional Hospital	Greenfield	84%	300+
Indiana Univ Health Bedford Hosp	Bedford	84%	(a)
Parkview Huntington Hospital	Huntington	84%	300+
Pulaski Memorial Hospital	Winamac	84%	(a)
Putnam County Hospital	Greencastle	84%	(a)
Saint Vincent Clay Hospital	Brazil	84%	(a)
Saint Vincent Heart Center of Indiana	Indianapolis	84%	300+
Scott Memorial Hospital	Scottsburg	84%	(a)
Wabash County Hospital	Wabash	84%	(a)
Bluffton Regional Medical Center	Bluffton	83%	300+
Decatur County Memorial Hospital	Greensburg	83%	(a)
Fayette Regional Health System	Connersville	83%	300+
Franciscan St Francis Health	Mooresville	83%	300+
Hendricks Regional Health	Danville	83%	300+
Indiana University Health Morgan Hospital	Martinsville	83%	(a)
Jay County Hospital	Portland	83%	300+
Major Hospital	Shelbyville	83%	300+
Memorial Hospital & Health Care Center	Jasper	83%	300+
Orthopaedic Hospital at Parkview North	Fort Wayne	83%	300+
Parkview Whitley Hospital	Columbia City	83%	300+
Saint Mary Medical Center	Hobart	83%	300+
The Women's Hospital	Newburgh	83%	300+
Woodlawn Hospital	Rochester	83%	(a)
Community Howard Regional Health	Kokomo	82%	300+
Harrison County Hospital	Corydon	82%	(a)
Indiana University Health Tipton Hospital	Tipton	82%	(a)
Johnson Memorial Hospital	Franklin	82%	300+
Methodist Hospitals	Gary	82%	300+
Parkview Lagrange Hospital	Lagrange	82%	(a)
Parkview Noble Hospital	Kendallville	82%	300+
Rush Memorial Hospital	Rushville	82%	(a)
Saint Catherine Hospital	East Chicago	82%	300+
Saint Vincent Dunn Hospital	Bedford	82%	(a)
Comm Hosp of Anderson/Madison Co	Anderson	81%	300+
Deaconess Hospital	Evansville	81%	300+
Dearborn County Hospital	Lawrenceburg	81%	300+
Franciscan St Elizabeth Health	Lafayette	81%	300+
Franciscan St Francis Hlth-Indianapolis	Indianapolis	81%	300+
Franciscan Saint Margaret Health - Dyer	Dyer	81%	300+
Marion General Hospital[11]	Marion	81%	300+
Saint Vincent Mercy Hospital	Elwood	81%	(a)
Saint Vincent Randolph Hospital	Winchester	81%	(a)
Saint Vincent Williamsport Hospital	Williamsport	81%	(a)
Sullivan County Community Hospital	Sullivan	81%	(a)
Clark Memorial Hospital	Jeffersonville	80%	300+
Columbus Regional Hospital	Columbus	80%	300+
Dukes Memorial Hospital	Peru	80%	(a)
Franciscan St Anthony Health	Michigan City	80%	300+
Memorial Hospital of South Bend	South Bend	80%	300+
Monroe Hospital	Bloomington	80%	300+
St Joseph Reg Med Ctr-Plymouth	Plymouth	80%	300+
Saint Vincent Anderson Regional Hospital	Anderson	80%	300+
Witham Health Services	Lebanon	80%	300+
Community Hospital South	Indianapolis	79%	300+
Daviess Community Hospital	Washington	79%	300+
Dekalb Health	Auburn	79%	300+
Dupont Hospital	Fort Wayne	79%	300+
Franciscan St Elizabeth Health	Lafayette	79%	300+
Indiana Univ Health Ball Mem Hosp	Muncie	79%	300+
Indiana Univ Health Bloomington Hosp	Bloomington	79%	300+
Indiana Univ Health La Porte Hosp	La Porte	79%	300+
IU Health Goshen Hospital	Goshen	79%	300+
IU Health West Hospital	Avon	79%	300+
Lutheran Hospital of Indiana	Fort Wayne	79%	300+
The Ortho Hosp/Lutheran Health Network	Fort Wayne	79%	300+
Parkview Regional Medical Center	Fort Wayne	79%	300+
Reid Hospital & Health Care Services	Richmond	79%	300+
Saint Joseph Hospital & Health Center	Kokomo	79%	300+
Saint Vincent Frankfort Hospital	Frankfort	79%	(a)
Franciscan St Anthony Health-Crown Pt	Crown Point	78%	300+
Indiana University Health	Indianapolis	78%	300+
King's Daughters' Health	Madison	78%	300+
Porter Regional Hospital	Valparaiso	78%	300+
Saint Mary's Medical Center of Evansville	Evansville	78%	300+
Saint Vincent Hospital & Health Services[11]	Indianapolis	78%	300+
Terre Haute Regional Hospital	Terre Haute	78%	300+
Indiana University Health Arnett Hospital	Lafayette	77%	300+
Indiana Univ Health White Mem Hosp	Monticello	77%	(a)
Memorial Hospital	Logansport	77%	300+
Pinnacle Hospital	Crown Point	77%	(a)
Riverview Hospital	Noblesville	77%	300+
Saint Joseph Hospital	Fort Wayne	77%	300+
Union Hospital	Terre Haute	77%	300+
Community Hospital North	Indianapolis	76%	300+
Elkhart General Hospital	Elkhart	76%	300+
Eskenazi Health	Indianapolis	76%	300+
Franciscan St Margaret Health-Hammond	Hammond	76%	300+
Indiana University Health Starke Hospital	Knox	76%	(a)
Kosciusko Community Hospital	Warsaw	76%	300+
Saint Joseph Regional Medical Center	Mishawaka	76%	300+
Saint Vincent Carmel Hospital	Carmel	76%	300+
Community Hospital East	Indianapolis	75%	300+
Jasper County Hospital	Rensselaer	75%	(a)
Community Westview Hospital	Indianapolis	72%	(a)

Pain 'Always' Well Controlled

Hospital Name	City	Rate	Cases
Saint Vincent Mercy Hospital	Elwood	84%	(a)
Gibson General Hospital	Princeton	81%	(a)
Indiana Orthopaedic Hospital	Indianapolis	80%	300+
Perry County Memorial Hospital	Tell City	80%	(a)
Union Hospital Clinton	Clinton	80%	(a)
Indiana University Health Morgan Hospital	Martinsville	79%	(a)
Margaret Mary Community Hospital	Batesville	79%	300+
Saint Vincent Heart Center of Indiana	Indianapolis	79%	300+
Decatur County Memorial Hospital	Greensburg	78%	(a)
Kentuckiana Medical Center	Clarksville	78%	300+
Pulaski Memorial Hospital	Winamac	78%	(a)
Schneck Medical Center	Seymour	78%	300+
Unity Medical & Surgical Hospital	Mishawaka	78%	(a)
Cameron Memorial Community Hospital	Angola	77%	300+
Floyd Memorial Hospital & Health Services	New Albany	77%	(a)
Franciscan St Elizabeth Health	Crawfordsville	77%	(a)
Franciscan St Francis Health	Mooresville	77%	300+
Good Samaritan Hospital	Vincennes	77%	300+
The Heart Hospital at Deaconess Gateway	Newburgh	77%	300+
The Indiana Heart Hospital	Indianapolis	77%	300+
Indiana University Health North Hospital	Carmel	77%	300+
Parkview Huntington Hospital	Huntington	77%	300+
Physicians' Medical Center	New Albany	77%	(a)
Jay County Hospital	Portland	76%	300+
Marion General Hospital[11]	Marion	76%	300+
Methodist Hospitals	Gary	76%	300+
Parkview Lagrange Hospital	Lagrange	76%	(a)
Rush Memorial Hospital	Rushville	76%	(a)
Community Hospital	Munster	75%	300+
Indiana University Health Tipton Hospital	Tipton	75%	(a)
Memorial Hospital & Health Care Center	Jasper	75%	300+
St Joseph Reg Med Ctr-Plymouth	Plymouth	75%	300+
Saint Vincent Carmel Hospital	Carmel	75%	300+
Saint Vincent Dunn Hospital	Bedford	75%	(a)
Sullivan County Community Hospital	Sullivan	75%	(a)
Woodlawn Hospital	Rochester	75%	(a)
Fayette Regional Health System	Connersville	74%	300+
Franciscan St Anthony Health	Michigan City	74%	300+
Hancock Regional Hospital	Greenfield	74%	300+
Major Hospital	Shelbyville	74%	300+
Monroe Hospital	Bloomington	74%	300+
Parkview Noble Hospital	Kendallville	74%	300+
Parkview Whitley Hospital	Columbia City	74%	300+
Saint Catherine Hospital	East Chicago	74%	300+
Saint Mary Medical Center	Hobart	74%	300+
Comm Hosp of Anderson/Madison Co	Anderson	73%	300+
Dupont Hospital	Fort Wayne	73%	300+
Franciscan St Elizabeth Health	Lafayette	73%	300+
Franciscan St Francis Hlth-Indianapolis	Indianapolis	73%	300+
Hendricks Regional Health	Danville	73%	300+
Henry County Memorial Hospital	New Castle	73%	300+
Indiana Univ Health Bloomington Hosp	Bloomington	73%	300+
Johnson Memorial Hospital	Franklin	73%	300+
Lutheran Hospital of Indiana	Fort Wayne	73%	300+
Orthopaedic Hospital at Parkview North	Fort Wayne	73%	300+
Saint Vincent Anderson Regional Hospital	Anderson	73%	300+
Saint Vincent Clay Hospital	Brazil	73%	(a)
Columbus Regional Hospital	Columbus	72%	300+
Dearborn County Hospital	Lawrenceburg	72%	300+
Indiana Univ Health Ball Mem Hosp	Muncie	72%	300+
Indiana Univ Health Bedford Hosp	Bedford	72%	(a)
IU Health Goshen Hospital	Goshen	72%	300+
Parkview Regional Medical Center	Fort Wayne	72%	300+
Bluffton Regional Medical Center	Bluffton	71%	300+
Community Hospital East	Indianapolis	71%	300+
Community Hospital North	Indianapolis	71%	300+
Deaconess Hospital	Evansville	71%	300+
Dekalb Health	Auburn	71%	300+
Dukes Memorial Hospital	Peru	71%	(a)
Eskenazi Health	Indianapolis	71%	300+
Franciscan Healthcare - Munster	Munster	71%	300+
Franciscan St Anthony Health-Crown Pt	Crown Point	71%	300+
Franciscan St Margaret Health-Hammond	Hammond	71%	300+
Indiana University Health Arnett Hospital	Lafayette	71%	300+
Kosciusko Community Hospital	Warsaw	71%	300+
Memorial Hospital	Logansport	71%	300+
The Ortho Hosp/Lutheran Health Network	Fort Wayne	71%	300+
Saint Joseph Hospital	Fort Wayne	71%	300+
Saint Joseph Hospital & Health Center	Kokomo	71%	300+
Saint Mary's Medical Center of Evansville	Evansville	71%	300+
Saint Vincent Frankfort Hospital	Frankfort	71%	(a)
Saint Vincent Randolph Hospital	Winchester	71%	(a)
Terre Haute Regional Hospital	Terre Haute	71%	300+
Wabash County Hospital	Wabash	71%	(a)
Witham Health Services	Lebanon	71%	300+
The Women's Hospital	Newburgh	71%	300+
Adams Memorial Hospital	Decatur	70%	300+
Community Howard Regional Health	Kokomo	70%	300+
Community Westview Hospital	Indianapolis	70%	(a)
Daviess Community Hospital	Washington	70%	300+
Indiana University Health	Indianapolis	70%	300+
IU Health West Hospital	Avon	70%	300+
Memorial Hospital of South Bend	South Bend	70%	300+
Porter Regional Hospital	Valparaiso	70%	300+
Riverview Hospital	Noblesville	70%	300+
Scott Memorial Hospital	Scottsburg	70%	(a)
Clark Memorial Hospital	Jeffersonville	69%	300+
Community Hospital South	Indianapolis	69%	300+
Elkhart General Hospital	Elkhart	69%	300+

NOTE: Hospital profiles are in alphabetical order by state, then city, then hospital within the city; Rankings exclude hospitals with less than 25 cases except for patient surveys which excludes hospitals with less than 100 cases; (a) 100-299 cases; (1) The number of cases/patients is too few to report; (2) Data submitted were based on a sample of cases/patients; (3) Results are based on a shorter time period than required; (4) Data suppressed by CMS for one or more quarters; (5) Results are not available for this reporting period; (6) Fewer than 100 patients completed the HCAHPS survey; (7) No cases met the criteria for this measure; (8) The lower limit of the confidence interval cannot be calculated if the number of observed infections equals zero; (9) No data are available from the state/territory for this reporting period; (10) The scores shown reflect fewer than 50 completed surveys; (11) There were discrepancies in the data collection process; (12) This measure does not apply to this hospital for this reporting period; (13) Results cannot be calculated for this reporting period; (14) The results for this state are combined with nearby states to protect confidentiality; Please refer to the User's Guide for a full explanation of data.

Hospital Name	City	Rate	Cases
Franciscan Saint Margaret Health - Dyer	Dyer	69%	300+
Harrison County Hospital	Corydon	69%	(a)
Indiana Univ Health La Porte Hosp	La Porte	69%	300+
Jasper County Hospital	Rensselaer	69%	(a)
Putnam County Hospital	Greencastle	69%	(a)
Reid Hospital & Health Care Services	Richmond	69%	300+
Saint Joseph Regional Medical Center	Mishawaka	69%	300+
Saint Vincent Hospital & Health Services[11]	Indianapolis	69%	300+
Saint Vincent Williamsport Hospital	Williamsport	69%	(a)
King's Daughters' Health	Madison	68%	300+
Franciscan St Elizabeth Health	Lafayette	67%	300+
Indiana University Health Starke Hospital	Knox	67%	(a)
Pinnacle Hospital	Crown Point	67%	(a)
Union Hospital	Terre Haute	67%	300+
Indiana Univ Health White Mem Hosp	Monticello	63%	(a)

Room and Bathroom 'Always' Clean

Hospital Name	City	Rate	Cases
Indiana Orthopaedic Hospital	Indianapolis	89%	300+
Good Samaritan Hospital	Vincennes	88%	300+
Saint Vincent Dunn Hospital	Bedford	88%	(a)
Adams Memorial Hospital	Decatur	87%	300+
Dearborn County Hospital	Lawrenceburg	85%	300+
Memorial Hospital & Health Care Center	Jasper	85%	300+
Perry County Memorial Hospital	Tell City	84%	(a)
Wabash County Hospital	Wabash	84%	(a)
Indiana Univ Health Bedford Hosp	Bedford	83%	(a)
Indiana University Health Tipton Hospital	Tipton	83%	(a)
Franciscan St Elizabeth Health	Crawfordsville	82%	(a)
Major Hospital	Shelbyville	82%	300+
Margaret Mary Community Hospital	Batesville	82%	300+
Monroe Hospital	Bloomington	82%	300+
Parkview Lagrange Hospital	Lagrange	82%	(a)
Parkview Noble Hospital	Kendallville	82%	300+
Rush Memorial Hospital	Rushville	82%	(a)
The Women's Hospital	Newburgh	82%	300+
Bluffton Regional Medical Center	Bluffton	81%	300+
Franciscan St Francis Health	Mooresville	81%	300+
Harrison County Hospital	Corydon	81%	(a)
Indiana University Health North Hospital	Carmel	81%	300+
Kentuckiana Medical Center	Clarksville	81%	300+
Schneck Medical Center	Seymour	81%	300+
Cameron Memorial Community Hospital	Angola	80%	300+
Fayette Regional Health System	Connersville	80%	300+
Gibson General Hospital	Princeton	80%	(a)
Henry County Memorial Hospital	New Castle	80%	300+
The Indiana Heart Hospital	Indianapolis	80%	300+
Johnson Memorial Hospital	Franklin	80%	300+
Reid Hospital & Health Care Services	Richmond	80%	300+
Unity Medical & Surgical Hospital	Mishawaka	80%	(a)
Decatur County Memorial Hospital	Greensburg	79%	(a)
Orthopaedic Hospital at Parkview North	Fort Wayne	79%	300+
Parkview Whitley Hospital	Columbia City	79%	300+
Physicians' Medical Center	New Albany	79%	(a)
Scott Memorial Hospital	Scottsburg	79%	(a)
Witham Health Services	Lebanon	79%	300+
Columbus Regional Hospital	Columbus	78%	300+
Community Hospital	Munster	78%	300+
Community Howard Regional Health	Kokomo	78%	300+
Hancock Regional Hospital	Greenfield	78%	300+
Indiana University Health Morgan Hospital	Martinsville	78%	(a)
Indiana University Health Starke Hospital	Knox	78%	(a)
Terre Haute Regional Hospital	Terre Haute	78%	300+
Union Hospital Clinton	Clinton	78%	(a)
Franciscan St Elizabeth Health	Lafayette	77%	300+
Franciscan St Margaret Health-Hammond	Hammond	77%	300+
Hendricks Regional Health	Danville	77%	300+
Indiana Univ Health White Mem Hosp	Monticello	77%	(a)
King's Daughters' Health	Madison	77%	300+
Saint Mary Medical Center	Hobart	77%	300+
Union Hospital	Terre Haute	77%	300+
Woodlawn Hospital	Rochester	77%	(a)
Community Hospital North	Indianapolis	76%	300+
Floyd Memorial Hospital & Health Services	New Albany	76%	(a)
Franciscan St Anthony Health	Michigan City	76%	300+
Franciscan Saint Margaret Health - Dyer	Dyer	76%	300+
Pulaski Memorial Hospital	Winamac	76%	(a)
Saint Vincent Clay Hospital	Brazil	76%	(a)
Sullivan County Community Hospital	Sullivan	76%	(a)
Clark Memorial Hospital	Jeffersonville	75%	300+
Parkview Huntington Hospital	Huntington	75%	300+
Saint Vincent Williamsport Hospital	Williamsport	75%	(a)
Community Hospital South	Indianapolis	74%	300+
Elkhart General Hospital	Elkhart	74%	300+
Franciscan St Anthony Health-Crown Pt	Crown Point	74%	300+
Jay County Hospital	Portland	74%	300+
Parkview Regional Medical Center	Fort Wayne	74%	300+
Saint Catherine Hospital	East Chicago	74%	300+
Saint Mary's Medical Center of Evansville	Evansville	74%	300+
Saint Vincent Anderson Regional Hospital	Anderson	74%	300+
Community Hospital East	Indianapolis	73%	300+
Dukes Memorial Hospital	Peru	73%	(a)
IU Health Goshen Hospital	Goshen	73%	300+
Jasper County Hospital	Rensselaer	73%	(a)
Porter Regional Hospital	Valparaiso	73%	300+
Saint Joseph Hospital & Health Center	Kokomo	73%	300+
Franciscan Healthcare - Munster	Munster	72%	300+
Indiana Univ Health Ball Mem Hosp	Muncie	72%	300+
Kosciusko Community Hospital	Warsaw	72%	300+
Marion General Hospital[11]	Marion	72%	300+
Memorial Hospital of South Bend	South Bend	72%	300+
Methodist Hospitals	Gary	72%	300+
Saint Vincent Heart Center of Indiana	Indianapolis	72%	300+
Comm Hosp of Anderson/Madison Co	Anderson	71%	300+
Deaconess Hospital	Evansville	71%	300+
Dekalb Health	Auburn	71%	300+
Franciscan St Elizabeth Health	Lafayette	71%	300+
Franciscan St Francis Hlth-Indianapolis	Indianapolis	71%	300+
The Heart Hospital at Deaconess Gateway	Newburgh	71%	300+
IU Health West Hospital	Avon	71%	300+
Memorial Hospital	Logansport	71%	300+
Pinnacle Hospital	Crown Point	71%	(a)
Saint Joseph Regional Medical Center	Mishawaka	71%	300+
St Joseph Reg Med Ctr-Plymouth	Plymouth	71%	300+
Saint Vincent Mercy Hospital	Elwood	71%	(a)
Indiana University Health	Indianapolis	70%	300+
The Ortho Hosp/Lutheran Health Network	Fort Wayne	70%	300+
Riverview Hospital	Noblesville	70%	300+
Saint Vincent Frankfort Hospital	Frankfort	70%	(a)
Saint Vincent Randolph Hospital	Winchester	70%	(a)
Eskenazi Health	Indianapolis	69%	300+
Lutheran Hospital of Indiana	Fort Wayne	69%	300+
Saint Joseph Hospital	Fort Wayne	69%	300+
Indiana Univ Health Bloomington Hosp	Bloomington	68%	300+
Putnam County Hospital	Greencastle	68%	(a)
Daviess Community Hospital	Washington	67%	300+
Indiana Univ Health La Porte Hosp	La Porte	67%	300+
Community Westview Hospital	Indianapolis	64%	(a)
Dupont Hospital	Fort Wayne	64%	300+
Indiana University Health Arnett Hospital	Lafayette	64%	300+
Saint Vincent Carmel Hospital	Carmel	63%	300+
Saint Vincent Hospital & Health Services[11]	Indianapolis	60%	300+

Timely Help 'Always' Received

Hospital Name	City	Rate	Cases
Perry County Memorial Hospital	Tell City	85%	(a)
Physicians' Medical Center	New Albany	85%	(a)
Indiana Orthopaedic Hospital	Indianapolis	84%	300+
Gibson General Hospital	Princeton	82%	(a)
Indiana University Health Starke Hospital	Knox	82%	(a)
Pulaski Memorial Hospital	Winamac	82%	(a)
Saint Vincent Williamsport Hospital	Williamsport	82%	(a)
Cameron Memorial Community Hospital	Angola	81%	300+
Wabash County Hospital	Wabash	81%	(a)
Franciscan St Elizabeth Health	Crawfordsville	80%	(a)
Scott Memorial Hospital	Scottsburg	79%	(a)
Unity Medical & Surgical Hospital	Mishawaka	79%	(a)
The Heart Hospital at Deaconess Gateway	Newburgh	78%	300+
Kentuckiana Medical Center	Clarksville	78%	300+
Floyd Memorial Hospital & Health Services	New Albany	77%	(a)
Indiana Univ Health Bedford Hosp	Bedford	77%	(a)
Jay County Hospital	Portland	77%	300+
Parkview Lagrange Hospital	Lagrange	77%	(a)
Rush Memorial Hospital	Rushville	77%	(a)
Fayette Regional Health System	Connersville	76%	300+
Good Samaritan Hospital	Vincennes	76%	300+
Parkview Noble Hospital	Kendallville	76%	300+
Parkview Whitley Hospital	Columbia City	76%	300+
Saint Vincent Heart Center of Indiana	Indianapolis	76%	300+
Sullivan County Community Hospital	Sullivan	76%	(a)
The Indiana Heart Hospital	Indianapolis	75%	300+
Major Hospital	Shelbyville	75%	300+
Parkview Huntington Hospital	Huntington	75%	300+
Union Hospital Clinton	Clinton	75%	(a)
Adams Memorial Hospital	Decatur	74%	300+
Decatur County Memorial Hospital	Greensburg	74%	(a)
Franciscan Healthcare - Munster	Munster	74%	300+
Harrison County Hospital	Corydon	74%	(a)
Johnson Memorial Hospital	Franklin	74%	300+
Marion General Hospital[11]	Marion	74%	300+
Memorial Hospital & Health Care Center	Jasper	74%	300+
Putnam County Hospital	Greencastle	74%	(a)
Schneck Medical Center	Seymour	74%	300+
Community Hospital	Munster	73%	300+
Franciscan Saint Margaret Health - Dyer	Dyer	73%	300+
Orthopaedic Hospital at Parkview North	Fort Wayne	73%	300+
Saint Vincent Frankfort Hospital	Frankfort	73%	(a)
Saint Vincent Mercy Hospital	Elwood	73%	(a)
Daviess Community Hospital	Washington	72%	300+
Indiana University Health Morgan Hospital	Martinsville	72%	(a)
Margaret Mary Community Hospital	Batesville	72%	300+
Memorial Hospital of South Bend	South Bend	72%	300+
Pinnacle Hospital	Crown Point	72%	(a)
Saint Vincent Dunn Hospital	Bedford	72%	(a)
Woodlawn Hospital	Rochester	72%	(a)
Columbus Regional Hospital	Columbus	71%	300+
Dupont Hospital	Fort Wayne	71%	300+
Franciscan St Anthony Health	Michigan City	71%	300+
Henry County Memorial Hospital	New Castle	71%	300+
Clark Memorial Hospital	Jeffersonville	70%	300+
Dearborn County Hospital	Lawrenceburg	70%	300+
Dekalb Health	Auburn	70%	300+
Franciscan St Francis Hlth-Indianapolis	Indianapolis	70%	300+
Franciscan St Francis Health	Mooresville	70%	300+
Indiana Univ Health Bloomington Hosp	Bloomington	70%	300+
Indiana Univ Health White Mem Hosp	Monticello	70%	(a)
Methodist Hospitals	Gary	70%	300+
The Ortho Hosp/Lutheran Health Network	Fort Wayne	70%	300+
Saint Vincent Randolph Hospital	Winchester	70%	(a)
Bluffton Regional Medical Center	Bluffton	69%	300+
Community Howard Regional Health	Kokomo	69%	300+
Hancock Regional Hospital	Greenfield	69%	300+
Indiana Univ Health La Porte Hosp	La Porte	69%	300+
Indiana University Health North Hospital	Carmel	69%	300+
King's Daughters' Health	Madison	69%	300+
Saint Catherine Hospital	East Chicago	69%	300+
St Joseph Reg Med Ctr-Plymouth	Plymouth	69%	300+
Saint Mary Medical Center	Hobart	69%	300+
Dukes Memorial Hospital	Peru	68%	(a)
Franciscan St Elizabeth Health	Lafayette	68%	300+
Hendricks Regional Health	Danville	68%	300+
Indiana University Health Tipton Hospital	Tipton	68%	(a)
IU Health Goshen Hospital	Goshen	68%	300+
Monroe Hospital	Bloomington	68%	300+
Community Hospital East	Indianapolis	67%	300+
Lutheran Hospital of Indiana	Fort Wayne	67%	300+
Parkview Regional Medical Center	Fort Wayne	67%	300+
The Women's Hospital	Newburgh	67%	300+
Comm Hosp of Anderson/Madison Co	Anderson	66%	300+
Deaconess Hospital	Evansville	66%	300+
Reid Hospital & Health Care Services	Richmond	66%	300+
Saint Joseph Hospital	Fort Wayne	66%	300+
Saint Vincent Clay Hospital	Brazil	66%	(a)
Terre Haute Regional Hospital	Terre Haute	66%	300+
Union Hospital	Terre Haute	66%	300+
Community Hospital South	Indianapolis	65%	300+
Franciscan St Elizabeth Health	Lafayette	65%	300+
Witham Health Services	Lebanon	65%	300+
Saint Mary's Medical Center of Evansville	Evansville	64%	300+
Elkhart General Hospital	Elkhart	63%	300+
Indiana Univ Health Ball Mem Hosp	Muncie	63%	300+
IU Health West Hospital	Avon	63%	300+
Kosciusko Community Hospital	Warsaw	63%	300+
Memorial Hospital	Logansport	63%	300+
Saint Vincent Anderson Regional Hospital	Anderson	63%	300+
Eskenazi Health	Indianapolis	62%	300+
Riverview Hospital	Noblesville	62%	300+
Saint Joseph Hospital & Health Center	Kokomo	62%	300+
Saint Joseph Regional Medical Center	Mishawaka	62%	300+
Saint Vincent Carmel Hospital	Carmel	62%	300+
Saint Vincent Hospital & Health Services[11]	Indianapolis	61%	300+
Franciscan St Anthony Health-Crown Pt	Crown Point	60%	300+
Franciscan St Margaret Health-Hammond	Hammond	60%	300+
Indiana University Health	Indianapolis	60%	300+
Indiana University Health Arnett Hospital	Lafayette	60%	300+
Community Westview Hospital	Indianapolis	59%	(a)
Jasper County Hospital	Rensselaer	58%	(a)
Porter Regional Hospital	Valparaiso	58%	300+
Community Hospital North	Indianapolis	56%	300+

Would Definitely Recommend Hospital

Hospital Name	City	Rate	Cases
Indiana Orthopaedic Hospital	Indianapolis	92%	300+
The Heart Hospital at Deaconess Gateway	Newburgh	89%	300+
Indiana University Health North Hospital	Carmel	88%	300+
Saint Vincent Heart Center of Indiana	Indianapolis	88%	300+
Franciscan St Francis Health	Mooresville	86%	300+
The Indiana Heart Hospital	Indianapolis	86%	300+
Kentuckiana Medical Center	Clarksville	85%	300+
Orthopaedic Hospital at Parkview North	Fort Wayne	85%	300+
Hendricks Regional Health	Danville	84%	300+
The Women's Hospital	Newburgh	83%	300+
IU Health West Hospital	Avon	82%	300+
Margaret Mary Community Hospital	Batesville	82%	300+
The Ortho Hosp/Lutheran Health Network	Fort Wayne	82%	300+
Saint Joseph Hospital & Health Center	Kokomo	82%	300+
Saint Vincent Dunn Hospital	Bedford	82%	(a)
Unity Medical & Surgical Hospital	Mishawaka	82%	(a)
Franciscan St Francis Hlth-Indianapolis	Indianapolis	81%	300+
Union Hospital Clinton	Clinton	81%	(a)
Community Hospital	Munster	80%	300+
Community Hospital North	Indianapolis	80%	300+
Floyd Memorial Hospital & Health Services	New Albany	80%	(a)

NOTE: Hospital profiles are in alphabetical order by state, then city, then hospital within the city; Rankings exclude hospitals with less than 25 cases except for patient surveys which excludes hospitals with less than 100 cases; (a) 100-299 cases; (1) The number of cases/patients is too few to report; (2) Data submitted were based on a sample of cases/patients; (3) Results are based on a shorter time period than required; (4) Data suppressed by CMS for one or more quarters; (5) Results are not available for this reporting period; (6) Fewer than 100 patients completed the HCAHPS survey; (7) No cases met the criteria for this measure; (8) The lower limit of the confidence interval cannot be calculated if the number of observed infections equals zero; (9) No data are available from the state/territory for this reporting period; (10) The scores shown reflect fewer than 50 completed surveys; (11) There were discrepancies in the data collection process; (12) This measure does not apply to this hospital for this reporting period; (13) Results cannot be calculated for this reporting period; (14) The results for this state are combined with nearby states to protect confidentiality; Please refer to the User's Guide for a full explanation of data.

Hospital Name	City	Rate	Cases
Memorial Hospital of South Bend	South Bend	80%	300+
Saint Mary Medical Center	Hobart	80%	300+
Deaconess Hospital	Evansville	79%	300+
Dupont Hospital	Fort Wayne	79%	300+
Hancock Regional Hospital	Greenfield	79%	300+
Physicians' Medical Center	New Albany	79%	(a)
Saint Vincent Carmel Hospital	Carmel	79%	300+
Saint Vincent Hospital & Health Services[11]	Indianapolis	79%	300+
Good Samaritan Hospital	Vincennes	78%	300+
Indiana University Health	Indianapolis	78%	300+
Indiana Univ Health Bedford Hosp	Bedford	78%	(a)
Lutheran Hospital of Indiana	Fort Wayne	78%	300+
Parkview Huntington Hospital	Huntington	78%	300+
Parkview Regional Medical Center	Fort Wayne	78%	300+
Parkview Whitley Hospital	Columbia City	78%	300+
Pinnacle Hospital	Crown Point	78%	(a)
Union Hospital	Terre Haute	78%	300+
Comm Hosp of Anderson/Madison Co	Anderson	77%	300+
Franciscan St Elizabeth Health	Lafayette	77%	300+
Parkview Lagrange Hospital	Lagrange	77%	(a)
Saint Joseph Regional Medical Center	Mishawaka	77%	300+
Saint Mary's Medical Center of Evansville	Evansville	77%	300+
Woodlawn Hospital	Rochester	77%	(a)
Bluffton Regional Medical Center	Bluffton	76%	300+
Eskenazi Health	Indianapolis	76%	300+
Memorial Hospital & Health Care Center	Jasper	76%	300+
Monroe Hospital	Bloomington	76%	300+
Parkview Noble Hospital	Kendallville	76%	300+
Pulaski Memorial Hospital	Winamac	76%	(a)
Community Hospital South	Indianapolis	75%	300+
Franciscan Healthcare - Munster	Munster	75%	300+
Henry County Memorial Hospital	New Castle	75%	300+
Indiana Univ Health Bloomington Hosp	Bloomington	75%	300+
IU Health Goshen Hospital	Goshen	75%	300+
Johnson Memorial Hospital	Franklin	75%	300+
Schneck Medical Center	Seymour	75%	300+
Terre Haute Regional Hospital	Terre Haute	75%	300+
Witham Health Services	Lebanon	75%	300+
Harrison County Hospital	Corydon	74%	(a)
Indiana University Health Arnett Hospital	Lafayette	74%	300+
Indiana University Health Tipton Hospital	Tipton	74%	(a)
Saint Catherine Hospital	East Chicago	74%	300+
Riverview Hospital	Noblesville	73%	300+
Saint Vincent Anderson Regional Hospital	Anderson	73%	300+
Clark Memorial Hospital	Jeffersonville	72%	300+
Gibson General Hospital	Princeton	72%	(a)
Jay County Hospital	Portland	72%	300+
Porter Regional Hospital	Valparaiso	72%	300+
Elkhart General Hospital	Elkhart	71%	300+
Franciscan St Anthony Health-Crown Pt	Crown Point	71%	300+
Major Hospital	Shelbyville	71%	300+
Franciscan St Elizabeth Health	Lafayette	70%	300+
Franciscan Saint Margaret Health - Dyer	Dyer	70%	300+
Methodist Hospitals	Gary	70%	300+
Reid Hospital & Health Care Services	Richmond	70%	300+
St Joseph Reg Med Ctr-Plymouth	Plymouth	70%	300+
Adams Memorial Hospital	Decatur	69%	300+
Columbus Regional Hospital	Columbus	69%	300+
Community Hospital East	Indianapolis	69%	300+
Community Howard Regional Health	Kokomo	69%	300+
Decatur County Memorial Hospital	Greensburg	69%	(a)
Dearborn County Hospital	Lawrenceburg	68%	300+
Dekalb Health	Auburn	68%	300+
Franciscan St Anthony Health	Michigan City	68%	300+
King's Daughters' Health	Madison	68%	300+
Saint Vincent Frankfort Hospital	Frankfort	68%	(a)
Saint Vincent Mercy Hospital	Elwood	68%	(a)
Saint Vincent Randolph Hospital	Winchester	68%	(a)
Scott Memorial Hospital	Scottsburg	68%	(a)
Sullivan County Community Hospital	Sullivan	68%	(a)
Cameron Memorial Community Hospital	Angola	67%	300+
Rush Memorial Hospital	Rushville	67%	(a)
Saint Joseph Hospital	Fort Wayne	67%	300+
Indiana Univ Health White Mem Hosp	Monticello	66%	(a)
Kosciusko Community Hospital	Warsaw	66%	300+
Perry County Memorial Hospital	Tell City	66%	(a)
Dukes Memorial Hospital	Peru	65%	(a)
Fayette Regional Health System	Connersville	65%	300+
Franciscan St Elizabeth Health	Crawfordsville	65%	(a)
Saint Vincent Clay Hospital	Brazil	65%	(a)
Community Westview Hospital	Indianapolis	64%	(a)
Saint Vincent Williamsport Hospital	Williamsport	64%	(a)
Wabash County Hospital	Wabash	64%	(a)
Franciscan St Margaret Health-Hammond	Hammond	63%	300+
Indiana Univ Health La Porte Hosp	La Porte	63%	300+
Marion General Hospital[11]	Marion	63%	300+
Indiana Univ Health Ball Mem Hosp	Muncie	61%	300+
Indiana University Health Morgan Hospital	Martinsville	59%	(a)
Indiana University Health Starke Hospital	Knox	59%	(a)
Daviess Community Hospital	Washington	58%	300+
Memorial Hospital	Logansport	56%	300+
Putnam County Hospital	Greencastle	54%	(a)
Jasper County Hospital	Rensselaer	47%	(a)

Use of Medical Imaging

Cardiac Imaging Stress Test before OP Surgery

Hospital Name	City	Rate	Cases
Indiana Univ Health White Mem Hosp	Monticello	0.0%	76
Union Hospital	Terre Haute	1.2%	81
Fayette Regional Health System	Connersville	1.3%	160
Parkview Huntington Hospital	Huntington	1.8%	57
Dekalb Health	Auburn	2.1%	48
Union Hospital Clinton	Clinton	2.1%	48
Indiana University Health Starke Hospital	Knox	2.2%	91
Daviess Community Hospital	Washington	2.3%	129
Franciscan St Anthony Health	Michigan City	2.4%	340
St Joseph Reg Med Ctr-Plymouth	Plymouth	2.6%	196
Adams Memorial Hospital	Decatur	3.2%	62
Comm Hosp of Anderson/Madison Co	Anderson	3.4%	495
Dearborn County Hospital	Lawrenceburg	3.4%	266
Kosciusko Community Hospital	Warsaw	3.5%	113
Saint Vincent Jennings Hospital	North Vernon	3.6%	55
Schneck Medical Center	Seymour	3.6%	220
Franciscan Healthcare - Munster	Munster	3.7%	82
Community Hospital South	Indianapolis	3.8%	341
Elkhart General Hospital	Elkhart	3.8%	1049
Methodist Hospitals	Gary	3.8%	238
Eskenazi Health	Indianapolis	4.0%	347
Saint Joseph Hospital	Fort Wayne	4.0%	99
Community Hospital East	Indianapolis	4.1%	317
Decatur County Memorial Hospital	Greensburg	4.1%	195
Harrison County Hospital	Corydon	4.2%	119
Porter Regional Hospital	Valparaiso	4.2%	239
Indiana University Health Morgan Hospital	Martinsville	4.4%	68
Lutheran Hospital of Indiana	Fort Wayne	4.4%	834
Memorial Hospital	Logansport	4.4%	206
Wabash County Hospital	Wabash	4.4%	114
The Indiana Heart Hospital	Indianapolis	4.6%	1115
Saint Joseph Hospital & Health Center	Kokomo	4.6%	672
Saint Vincent Hospital & Health Services	Indianapolis	4.6%	3254
Indiana Univ Health Bedford Hosp	Bedford	4.7%	214
Reid Hospital & Health Care Services	Richmond	4.7%	1023
Saint Vincent Anderson Regional Hospital	Anderson	4.7%	551
Memorial Hospital of South Bend	South Bend	4.8%	583
Franciscan St Francis Health	Mooresville	5.0%	341
Major Hospital	Shelbyville	5.1%	253
Franciscan St Francis Hlth-Indianapolis	Indianapolis	5.2%	1411
Saint Vincent Heart Center of Indiana	Indianapolis	5.2%	174
IU Health West Hospital	Avon	5.3%	284
Saint Mary Medical Center	Hobart	5.3%	244
Saint Vincent Mercy Hospital	Elwood	5.4%	56
Franciscan St Elizabeth Health	Lafayette	5.5%	361
Good Samaritan Hospital	Vincennes	5.5%	506
Witham Health Services	Lebanon	5.5%	164
Franciscan Saint Margaret Health - Dyer	Dyer	5.6%	252
The Heart Hospital at Deaconess Gateway	Newburgh	5.7%	123
Indiana Univ Health Ball Mem Hosp	Muncie	5.7%	419
Indiana University Health Tipton Hospital	Tipton	5.7%	122
Indiana Univ Health La Porte Hosp	La Porte	5.8%	814
Indiana University Health	Indianapolis	5.9%	1083
Clark Memorial Hospital	Jeffersonville	6.0%	416
Franciscan St Elizabeth Health	Crawfordsville	6.1%	196
Greene County General Hospital	Linton	6.1%	98
Parkview Regional Medical Center	Fort Wayne	6.1%	1107
Saint Catherine Hospital	East Chicago	6.1%	375
Saint Joseph Regional Medical Center	Mishawaka	6.1%	375
IU Health Goshen Hospital	Goshen	6.2%	241
Hendricks Regional Health	Danville	6.3%	191
Parkview Noble Hospital	Kendallville	6.3%	79
Terre Haute Regional Hospital	Terre Haute	6.3%	142
Indiana University Health Arnett Hospital	Lafayette	6.4%	543
Dukes Memorial Hospital	Peru	6.5%	153
King's Daughters' Health	Madison	6.5%	354
Community Howard Regional Health	Kokomo	6.6%	411
Margaret Mary Community Hospital	Batesville	6.6%	151
Franciscan St Margaret Health-Hammond	Hammond	6.7%	193
Saint Vincent Salem Hospital	Salem	6.7%	105
Riverview Hospital	Noblesville	6.8%	177
Rush Memorial Hospital	Rushville	6.8%	74
Johnson Memorial Hospital	Franklin	6.9%	291
Memorial Hospital & Health Care Center	Jasper	6.9%	621
Saint Mary's Medical Center of Evansville	Evansville	6.9%	793
Hancock Regional Hospital	Greenfield	7.0%	157
Community Westview Hospital	Indianapolis	7.2%	83
Indiana Univ Health Bloomington Hosp	Bloomington	7.8%	463
Monroe Hospital	Bloomington	7.8%	90
Perry County Memorial Hospital	Tell City	7.8%	103
Floyd Memorial Hospital & Health Services	New Albany	7.9%	529
Deaconess Hospital	Evansville	8.2%	754
Franciscan St Anthony Health-Crown Pt	Crown Point	8.5%	82
Columbus Regional Hospital	Columbus	8.9%	124
Community Hospital	Munster	8.9%	503
Indiana University Health North Hospital	Carmel	9.9%	91
Henry County Memorial Hospital	New Castle	10.1%	308

Combination Abdominal CT Scan

Hospital Name	City	Rate	Cases
Dekalb Health	Auburn	0.0%	229
Saint Mary's Warrick Hospital	Boonville	0.0%	129
Community Westview Hospital	Indianapolis	0.5%	189
Jay County Hospital	Portland	1.3%	305
Indiana University Health Paoli Hospital	Paoli	1.5%	336
Indiana Univ Health Blackford Hosp	Hartford City	1.6%	243
Dukes Memorial Hospital	Peru	1.8%	225
Adams Memorial Hospital	Decatur	1.9%	209
Dupont Hospital	Fort Wayne	2.0%	303
Franciscan St Elizabeth Health	Lafayette	2.2%	225
Indiana Univ Health Ball Mem Hosp	Muncie	2.2%	1302
Saint Mary's Medical Center of Evansville	Evansville	2.3%	1221
IU Health Goshen Hospital	Goshen	2.6%	892
Parkview Lagrange Hospital	Lagrange	2.7%	187
Community Hospital South	Indianapolis	2.8%	651
Fayette Regional Health System	Connersville	2.8%	285
Saint Vincent Dunn Hospital	Bedford	2.8%	250
Saint Vincent Frankfort Hospital	Frankfort	2.8%	179
Comm Hosp of Anderson/Madison Co	Anderson	2.9%	687
Lutheran Hospital of Indiana	Fort Wayne	2.9%	853
Saint Joseph Hospital	Fort Wayne	2.9%	209
Indiana University Health Arnett Hospital	Lafayette	3.0%	731
Kosciusko Community Hospital	Warsaw	3.0%	573
Saint Joseph Regional Medical Center	Mishawaka	3.0%	922
Schneck Medical Center	Seymour	3.0%	593
Indiana University Health Starke Hospital	Knox	3.1%	291
Union Hospital Clinton	Clinton	3.1%	360
Community Hospital of Bremen	Bremen	3.3%	122
Elkhart General Hospital	Elkhart	3.3%	1047
Monroe Hospital	Bloomington	3.4%	383
Saint Catherine Hospital	East Chicago	3.4%	590
Woodlawn Hospital	Rochester	3.6%	196
Parkview Noble Hospital	Kendallville	3.8%	314
Saint Vincent Williamsport Hospital	Williamsport	3.8%	236
Terre Haute Regional Hospital	Terre Haute	4.0%	453
Cameron Memorial Community Hospital	Angola	4.1%	267
Daviess Community Hospital	Washington	4.1%	271
Indiana University Health	Indianapolis	4.3%	4148
Saint Joseph Hospital & Health Center	Kokomo	4.3%	743
Memorial Hospital & Health Care Center	Jasper	4.4%	1201
Saint Vincent Salem Hospital	Salem	4.4%	182
Saint Vincent Jennings Hospital	North Vernon	4.5%	243
Franciscan St Elizabeth Health	Crawfordsville	4.6%	549
Indiana Univ Health White Mem Hosp	Monticello	4.6%	417
St Joseph Reg Med Ctr-Plymouth	Plymouth	4.7%	404
Bluffton Regional Medical Center	Bluffton	4.8%	249
Clark Memorial Hospital	Jeffersonville	4.9%	886
Saint Vincent Anderson Regional Hospital	Anderson	4.9%	923
IU Health West Hospital	Avon	5.1%	1001
Jasper County Hospital	Rensselaer	5.1%	257
Indiana University Health North Hospital	Carmel	5.2%	687
Saint Vincent Hospital & Health Services	Indianapolis	5.2%	1779
Saint Vincent Randolph Hospital	Winchester	5.2%	268
Franciscan St Francis Hlth-Indianapolis	Indianapolis	5.3%	1817
Memorial Hospital	Logansport	5.3%	452
Saint Vincent Carmel Hospital	Carmel	5.3%	454
Indiana Univ Health La Porte Hosp	La Porte	5.5%	669
Eskenazi Health	Indianapolis	5.6%	754
Memorial Hospital of South Bend	South Bend	5.9%	863
Community Hospital	Munster	6.0%	2212
Parkview Huntington Hospital	Huntington	6.1%	163
Saint Mary Medical Center	Hobart	6.1%	1141
Wabash County Hospital	Wabash	6.2%	260
Deaconess Hospital	Evansville	6.3%	2797
Columbus Regional Hospital	Columbus	6.4%	1005
Reid Hospital & Health Care Services	Richmond	6.5%	1707
Johnson Memorial Hospital	Franklin	6.8%	457
Indiana Univ Health Bedford Hosp	Bedford	7.0%	485
Riverview Hospital	Noblesville	7.0%	661
Rush Memorial Hospital	Rushville	7.3%	192
Franciscan St Francis Health	Mooresville	7.4%	706
Indiana Univ Health Bloomington Hosp	Bloomington	7.4%	1020
King's Daughters' Health	Madison	7.7%	607
Indiana University Health Tipton Hospital	Tipton	7.8%	193
Witham Health Services	Lebanon	8.0%	512
Community Howard Regional Health	Kokomo	8.3%	747
Franciscan St Elizabeth Health	Lafayette	8.3%	735
Gibson General Hospital	Princeton	8.8%	205
Indiana University Health Morgan Hospital	Martinsville	8.9%	270
Henry County Memorial Hospital	New Castle	9.0%	687
Community Hospital East	Indianapolis	9.1%	1063
Hancock Regional Hospital	Greenfield	9.1%	671
Marion General Hospital	Marion	9.1%	1105
Putnam County Hospital	Greencastle	9.1%	318

NOTE: Hospital profiles are in alphabetical order by state, then city, then hospital within the city; Rankings exclude hospitals with less than 25 cases except for patient surveys which excludes hospitals with less than 100 cases; (a) 100-299 cases; (1) The number of cases/patients is too few to report; (2) Data submitted were based on a sample of cases/patients; (3) Results are based on a shorter time period than required; (4) Data suppressed by CMS for one or more quarters; (5) Results are not available for this reporting period; (6) Fewer than 100 patients completed the HCAHPS survey; (7) No cases met the criteria for this measure; (8) The lower limit of the confidence interval cannot be calculated if the number of observed infections equals zero; (9) No data are available from the state/territory for this reporting period; (10) The scores shown reflect fewer than 50 completed surveys; (11) There were discrepancies in the data collection process; (12) This measure does not apply to this hospital for this reporting period; (13) Results cannot be calculated for this reporting period; (14) The results for this state are combined with nearby states to protect confidentiality; Please refer to the User's Guide for a full explanation of data.

Parkview Whitley Hospital	Columbia City	9.2%	218
Saint Catherine Regional Hospital	Charlestown	10.1%	69
Saint Vincent Mercy Hospital	Elwood	10.6%	199
Community Hospital North	Indianapolis	11.0%	1111
Parkview Regional Medical Center	Fort Wayne	11.8%	1081
Major Hospital	Shelbyville	13.7%	461
Franciscan St Anthony Health-Crown Pt	Crown Point	15.7%	1149
Margaret Mary Community Hospital	Batesville	15.8%	385
Harrison County Hospital	Corydon	17.2%	424
Porter Regional Hospital	Valparaiso	17.3%	1295
Sullivan County Community Hospital	Sullivan	18.5%	324
Union Hospital	Terre Haute	18.8%	1953
Floyd Memorial Hospital & Health Services	New Albany	20.7%	1145
Greene County General Hospital	Linton	25.8%	322
Franciscan St Anthony Health	Michigan City	26.4%	785
Hendricks Regional Health	Danville	27.0%	930
Franciscan St Margaret Health-Hammond	Hammond	27.1%	554
Methodist Hospitals	Gary	28.5%	1211
Pinnacle Hospital	Crown Point	30.6%	108
Good Samaritan Hospital	Vincennes	31.4%	1049
Franciscan Saint Margaret Health - Dyer	Dyer	32.0%	541
Perry County Memorial Hospital	Tell City	32.4%	318
Pulaski Memorial Hospital	Winamac	32.9%	173
Dearborn County Hospital	Lawrenceburg	39.7%	466
Decatur County Memorial Hospital	Greensburg	41.1%	236
Franciscan Healthcare - Munster	Munster	42.6%	451
Saint Vincent Clay Hospital	Brazil	45.3%	256

Combination Brain/Sinus CT Scan

Hospital Name	City	Rate	Cases
Community Hospital of Bremen	Bremen	0.0%	123
Pulaski Memorial Hospital	Winamac	0.0%	144
Rush Memorial Hospital	Rushville	0.0%	180
Saint Vincent Heart Center of Indiana	Indianapolis	0.0%	63
Adams Memorial Hospital	Decatur	0.4%	240
Parkview Huntington Hospital	Huntington	0.4%	229
Indiana University Health Morgan Hospital	Martinsville	0.6%	174
Parkview Lagrange Hospital	Lagrange	0.6%	176
Cameron Memorial Community Hospital	Angola	0.7%	283
Saint Joseph Hospital	Fort Wayne	0.8%	262
Saint Vincent Anderson Regional Hospital	Anderson	0.8%	724
Indiana Univ Health Blackford Hosp	Hartford City	0.9%	329
Memorial Hospital & Health Care Center	Jasper	0.9%	805
Decatur County Memorial Hospital	Greensburg	1.0%	384
Woodlawn Hospital	Rochester	1.0%	202
Franciscan St Francis Health	Mooresville	1.1%	450
Saint Vincent Williamsport Hospital	Williamsport	1.1%	272
Elkhart General Hospital	Elkhart	1.2%	1041
Saint Vincent Jennings Hospital	North Vernon	1.2%	259
IU Health Goshen Hospital	Goshen	1.3%	615
IU Health West Hospital	Avon	1.4%	644
Comm Hosp of Anderson/Madison Co	Anderson	1.5%	478
Franciscan St Francis Hlth-Indianapolis	Indianapolis	1.5%	1309
Hendricks Regional Health	Danville	1.5%	595
Memorial Hospital	Logansport	1.5%	404
Fayette Regional Health System	Connersville	1.6%	377
Memorial Hospital of South Bend	South Bend	1.6%	861
Saint Joseph Hospital & Health Center	Kokomo	1.6%	555
Dearborn County Hospital	Lawrenceburg	1.7%	481
Franciscan St Anthony Health-Crown Pt	Crown Point	1.7%	811
Henry County Memorial Hospital	New Castle	1.7%	591
Hancock Regional Hospital	Greenfield	1.8%	562
Floyd Memorial Hospital & Health Services	New Albany	1.9%	837
Johnson Memorial Hospital	Franklin	1.9%	520
Witham Health Services	Lebanon	1.9%	430
Indiana Univ Health Bloomington Hosp	Bloomington	2.0%	1128
Good Samaritan Hospital	Vincennes	2.3%	820
Indiana University Health Arnett Hospital	Lafayette	2.3%	724
Lutheran Hospital of Indiana	Fort Wayne	2.3%	858
Reid Hospital & Health Care Services	Richmond	2.3%	991
Clark Memorial Hospital	Jeffersonville	2.4%	752
Community Hospital	Munster	2.4%	1608
Franciscan St Elizabeth Health	Lafayette	2.4%	743
Indiana Univ Health White Mem Hosp	Monticello	2.4%	507
Marion General Hospital	Marion	2.4%	931
Columbus Regional Hospital	Columbus	2.5%	948
Indiana Univ Health Ball Mem Hosp	Muncie	2.5%	1175
Saint Vincent Hospital & Health Services	Indianapolis	2.6%	1175
Indiana University Health	Indianapolis	2.7%	1374
Saint Joseph Regional Medical Center	Mishawaka	2.7%	857
Community Hospital South	Indianapolis	2.8%	611
Community Hospital North	Indianapolis	2.9%	917
Porter Regional Hospital	Valparaiso	3.0%	1045
Community Hospital East	Indianapolis	3.1%	867
Franciscan St Margaret Health-Hammond	Hammond	3.3%	723
Union Hospital	Terre Haute	3.3%	1474
Saint Mary Medical Center	Hobart	3.4%	709
Parkview Regional Medical Center	Fort Wayne	3.5%	967
Saint Mary's Medical Center of Evansville	Evansville	3.5%	961
Methodist Hospitals	Gary	3.6%	1231
Community Howard Regional Health	Kokomo	4.1%	631
Union Hospital Clinton	Clinton	4.2%	427
Franciscan St Anthony Health	Michigan City	4.4%	729
Saint Vincent Mercy Hospital	Elwood	5.0%	221
Eskenazi Health	Indianapolis	5.1%	508
Daviess Community Hospital	Washington	5.3%	301
Deaconess Hospital	Evansville	5.8%	2051
Dupont Hospital	Fort Wayne	5.9%	270
Indiana University Health North Hospital	Carmel	6.0%	301
Perry County Memorial Hospital	Tell City	6.5%	308
Saint Mary's Warrick Hospital	Boonville	7.1%	127
Saint Catherine Regional Hospital	Charlestown	10.4%	96

Combination Chest CT Scan

Hospital Name	City	Rate	Cases
Bluffton Regional Medical Center	Bluffton	0.0%	108
Cameron Memorial Community Hospital	Angola	0.0%	170
Clark Memorial Hospital	Jeffersonville	0.0%	843
Community Hospital of Bremen	Bremen	0.0%	50
Community Westview Hospital	Indianapolis	0.0%	53
Dekalb Health	Auburn	0.0%	111
Jasper County Hospital	Rensselaer	0.0%	148
Jay County Hospital	Portland	0.0%	170
Parkview Huntington Hospital	Huntington	0.0%	110
St Joseph Reg Med Ctr-Plymouth	Plymouth	0.0%	246
Saint Vincent Carmel Hospital	Carmel	0.0%	226
Saint Vincent Clay Hospital	Brazil	0.0%	165
Saint Vincent Dunn Hospital	Bedford	0.0%	99
Saint Vincent Frankfort Hospital	Frankfort	0.0%	87
Saint Vincent Mercy Hospital	Elwood	0.0%	79
Saint Vincent Williamsport Hospital	Williamsport	0.0%	88
Columbus Regional Hospital	Columbus	0.1%	862
Deaconess Hospital	Evansville	0.1%	1763
Indiana University Health	Indianapolis	0.1%	3296
Saint Mary Medical Center	Hobart	0.1%	818
Elkhart General Hospital	Elkhart	0.2%	474
Lutheran Hospital of Indiana	Fort Wayne	0.2%	609
Saint Joseph Hospital & Health Center	Kokomo	0.2%	544
IU Health Goshen Hospital	Goshen	0.3%	736
King's Daughters' Health	Madison	0.3%	372
Parkview Regional Medical Center	Fort Wayne	0.3%	724
Saint Vincent Hospital & Health Services	Indianapolis	0.3%	1480
Schneck Medical Center	Seymour	0.3%	359
Saint Vincent Anderson Regional Hospital	Anderson	0.4%	744
Riverview Hospital	Noblesville	0.5%	595
Saint Catherine Hospital	East Chicago	0.5%	216
Community Hospital	Munster	0.6%	1243
Fayette Regional Health System	Connersville	0.7%	141
Reid Hospital & Health Care Services	Richmond	0.7%	985
Terre Haute Regional Hospital	Terre Haute	0.7%	441
Dupont Hospital	Fort Wayne	0.8%	125
Indiana University Health North Hospital	Carmel	0.8%	483
Monroe Hospital	Bloomington	0.8%	264
Saint Joseph Regional Medical Center	Mishawaka	0.8%	369
Wabash County Hospital	Wabash	0.8%	129
Indiana Univ Health Blackford Hosp	Hartford City	0.9%	116
IU Health West Hospital	Avon	0.9%	793
Kosciusko Community Hospital	Warsaw	0.9%	326
Community Hospital South	Indianapolis	1.0%	391
Franciscan St Elizabeth Health	Lafayette	1.0%	104
Indiana Univ Health Ball Mem Hosp	Muncie	1.0%	1034
Adams Memorial Hospital	Decatur	1.1%	93
Johnson Memorial Hospital	Franklin	1.1%	186
Parkview Noble Hospital	Kendallville	1.1%	185
Dukes Memorial Hospital	Peru	1.2%	167
Franciscan St Elizabeth Health	Crawfordsville	1.3%	235
Memorial Hospital	Logansport	1.3%	224
Memorial Hospital & Health Care Center	Jasper	1.3%	850
Indiana University Health Paoli Hospital	Paoli	1.4%	142
Parkview Lagrange Hospital	Lagrange	1.4%	73
Saint Joseph Hospital	Fort Wayne	1.6%	125
Union Hospital Clinton	Clinton	1.6%	184
Franciscan St Elizabeth Health	Lafayette	1.7%	472
Franciscan St Francis Health	Mooresville	1.7%	346
Franciscan Healthcare - Munster	Munster	1.8%	602
Greene County General Hospital	Linton	1.8%	111
Indiana Univ Health Bloomington Hosp	Bloomington	1.8%	340
Witham Health Services	Lebanon	1.8%	328
Indiana University Health Arnett Hospital	Lafayette	1.9%	376
Woodlawn Hospital	Rochester	2.1%	146
Franciscan St Francis Hlth-Indianapolis	Indianapolis	2.2%	1325
Comm Hosp of Anderson/Madison Co	Anderson	2.5%	519
Saint Vincent Jennings Hospital	North Vernon	2.7%	74
Indiana Univ Health White Mem Hosp	Monticello	2.8%	177
Eskenazi Health	Indianapolis	2.9%	552
Indiana University Health Tipton Hospital	Tipton	3.1%	128
Memorial Hospital of South Bend	South Bend	3.2%	505
Sullivan County Community Hospital	Sullivan	3.4%	145
Daviess Community Hospital	Washington	3.5%	141
Indiana Univ Health La Porte Hosp	La Porte	3.6%	276
Hancock Regional Hospital	Greenfield	3.9%	636
Parkview Whitley Hospital	Columbia City	3.9%	127
Saint Vincent Salem Hospital	Salem	4.0%	99
Marion General Hospital	Marion	4.1%	491
Indiana Univ Health Bedford Hosp	Bedford	4.7%	275
Community Howard Regional Health	Kokomo	4.8%	861
Floyd Memorial Hospital & Health Services	New Albany	5.8%	914
Rush Memorial Hospital	Rushville	6.2%	81
Putnam County Hospital	Greencastle	6.6%	244
Indiana University Health Starke Hospital	Knox	7.1%	126
Indiana University Health Morgan Hospital	Martinsville	7.3%	164
Community Hospital East	Indianapolis	7.8%	529
Saint Vincent Randolph Hospital	Winchester	8.4%	178
Harrison County Hospital	Corydon	9.2%	228
Community Hospital North	Indianapolis	9.3%	722
Henry County Memorial Hospital	New Castle	9.7%	217
Porter Regional Hospital	Valparaiso	10.1%	883
Major Hospital	Shelbyville	12.7%	308
Margaret Mary Community Hospital	Batesville	13.3%	256
Union Hospital	Terre Haute	15.0%	1322
Franciscan Saint Margaret Health - Dyer	Dyer	15.5%	265
Dearborn County Hospital	Lawrenceburg	15.6%	430
Franciscan St Anthony Health-Crown Pt	Crown Point	16.4%	688
Saint Mary's Medical Center of Evansville	Evansville	16.8%	951
Gibson General Hospital	Princeton	17.4%	69
Perry County Memorial Hospital	Tell City	20.6%	107
Hendricks Regional Health	Danville	23.2%	495
Franciscan St Margaret Health-Hammond	Hammond	25.2%	234
Methodist Hospitals	Gary	27.1%	597
Pulaski Memorial Hospital	Winamac	29.1%	86
Franciscan St Anthony Health	Michigan City	31.2%	311
Good Samaritan Hospital	Vincennes	34.9%	501
Decatur County Memorial Hospital	Greensburg	54.3%	105

Follow-up Mammogram/Ultrasound

A follow-up rate near zero may indicate missed cancer; a rate higher than 14% may mean there is unnecessary follow up.

Hospital Name	City	Rate	Cases
Rush Memorial Hospital	Rushville	2.8%	218
Franciscan St Anthony Health	Michigan City	3.3%	1466
Sullivan County Community Hospital	Sullivan	3.4%	232
Saint Vincent Clay Hospital	Brazil	3.6%	252
Major Hospital	Shelbyville	3.7%	676
Decatur County Memorial Hospital	Greensburg	4.3%	530
Franciscan St Elizabeth Health	Crawfordsville	4.3%	820
Saint Mary's Warrick Hospital	Boonville	4.4%	68
Kosciusko Community Hospital	Warsaw	4.5%	669
Saint Joseph Hospital	Fort Wayne	4.5%	890
Lutheran Hospital of Indiana	Fort Wayne	4.8%	932
Henry County Memorial Hospital	New Castle	5.2%	916
Good Samaritan Hospital	Vincennes	5.4%	1729
Johnson Memorial Hospital	Franklin	5.5%	671
Deaconess Hospital	Evansville	5.6%	3952
Jasper County Hospital	Rensselaer	5.6%	252
Woodlawn Hospital	Rochester	5.6%	180
Indiana Univ Health Bedford Hosp	Bedford	5.8%	843
Saint Vincent Randolph Hospital	Winchester	6.0%	315
Bluffton Regional Medical Center	Bluffton	6.1%	587
Reid Hospital & Health Care Services	Richmond	6.1%	2102
Porter Regional Hospital	Valparaiso	6.2%	1780
Greene County General Hospital	Linton	6.4%	283
Dukes Memorial Hospital	Peru	6.5%	201
Eskenazi Health	Indianapolis	6.5%	1427
Parkview Noble Hospital	Kendallville	6.5%	355
IU Health Goshen Hospital	Goshen	6.6%	1396
Memorial Hospital of South Bend	South Bend	6.6%	2166
Perry County Memorial Hospital	Tell City	6.6%	317
Elkhart General Hospital	Elkhart	6.8%	2333
Putnam County Hospital	Greencastle	6.8%	411
Franciscan St Francis Health	Mooresville	6.9%	1259
Pulaski Memorial Hospital	Winamac	6.9%	203
Community Westview Hospital	Indianapolis	7.0%	286
Saint Vincent Dunn Hospital	Bedford	7.0%	301
Wabash County Hospital	Wabash	7.0%	387
Hendricks Regional Health	Danville	7.1%	1381
Dupont Hospital	Fort Wayne	7.2%	389
Indiana University Health	Indianapolis	7.3%	2375
Indiana University Health North Hospital	Carmel	7.3%	522
Indiana Univ Health White Mem Hosp	Monticello	7.3%	427
St Joseph Reg Med Ctr-Plymouth	Plymouth	7.3%	508
King's Daughters' Health	Madison	7.4%	176
Community Howard Regional Health	Kokomo	7.5%	824
Columbus Regional Hospital	Columbus	7.6%	1957
Parkview Lagrange Hospital	Lagrange	7.6%	342
Franciscan St Elizabeth Health	Lafayette	7.7%	1694
Franciscan St Francis Hlth-Indianapolis	Indianapolis	7.8%	3019
Saint Vincent Carmel Hospital	Carmel	7.8%	768
Saint Mary Medical Center	Hobart	7.9%	1224
Franciscan St Anthony Health-Crown Pt	Crown Point	8.1%	1923
Hancock Regional Hospital	Greenfield	8.1%	1464
Indiana Univ Health Ball Mem Hosp	Muncie	8.2%	2414
Union Hospital	Terre Haute	8.2%	2668
Franciscan St Elizabeth Health	Lafayette	8.4%	275

NOTE: Hospital profiles are in alphabetical order by state, then city, then hospital within the city; Rankings exclude hospitals with less than 25 cases except for patient surveys which excludes hospitals with less than 100 cases; (a) 100-299 cases; (1) The number of cases/patients is too few to report; (2) Data submitted were based on a sample of cases/patients; (3) Results are based on a shorter time period than required; (4) Data suppressed by CMS for one or more quarters; (5) Results are not available for this reporting period; (6) Fewer than 100 patients completed the HCAHPS survey; (7) No cases met the criteria for this measure; (8) The lower limit of the confidence interval cannot be calculated if the number of observed infections equals zero; (9) No data are available from the state/territory for this reporting period; (10) The scores shown reflect fewer than 50 completed surveys; (11) There were discrepancies in the data collection process; (12) This measure does not apply to this hospital for this reporting period; (13) Results cannot be calculated for this reporting period; (14) The results for this state are combined with nearby states to protect confidentiality; Please refer to the User's Guide for a full explanation of data.

Saint Joseph Hospital & Health Center	Kokomo	8.4%	848
Saint Vincent Williamsport Hospital	Williamsport	8.4%	143
Clark Memorial Hospital	Jeffersonville	8.6%	1866
Memorial Hospital & Health Care Center	Jasper	8.7%	1513
Community Hospital	Munster	8.8%	3447
Franciscan Healthcare - Munster	Munster	8.8%	856
Marion General Hospital	Marion	8.8%	1763
Adams Memorial Hospital	Decatur	8.9%	359
Community Hospital of Bremen	Bremen	8.9%	192
IU Health West Hospital	Avon	8.9%	728
Methodist Hospitals	Gary	8.9%	1880
Saint Vincent Hospital & Health Services	Indianapolis	8.9%	3574
Saint Catherine Hospital	East Chicago	9.1%	778
Floyd Memorial Hospital & Health Services	New Albany	9.2%	1849
Indiana Univ Health La Porte Hosp	La Porte	9.2%	1287
Memorial Hospital	Logansport	9.2%	976
Indiana Univ Health Blackford Hosp	Hartford City	9.3%	236
Dekalb Health	Auburn	9.4%	385
Saint Vincent Salem Hospital	Salem	9.4%	180
Margaret Mary Community Hospital	Batesville	9.5%	603
Community Hospital South	Indianapolis	9.8%	1743
Indiana University Health Paoli Hospital	Paoli	9.8%	244
Union Hospital Clinton	Clinton	9.9%	302
Dearborn County Hospital	Lawrenceburg	10.1%	752
Franciscan St Margaret Health-Hammond	Hammond	10.4%	618
Terre Haute Regional Hospital	Terre Haute	10.4%	511
Parkview Whitley Hospital	Columbia City	10.7%	270
Saint Vincent Frankfort Hospital	Frankfort	10.7%	382
Riverview Hospital	Noblesville	10.8%	1076
Saint Joseph Regional Medical Center	Mishawaka	10.9%	1564
Fayette Regional Health System	Connersville	11.0%	456
Harrison County Hospital	Corydon	11.2%	401
Indiana University Health Starke Hospital	Knox	11.2%	278
Witham Health Services	Lebanon	11.2%	599
Schneck Medical Center	Seymour	11.4%	657
Indiana University Health Morgan Hospital	Martinsville	11.9%	328
Parkview Huntington Hospital	Huntington	12.6%	326
Community Hospital East	Indianapolis	13.0%	1663
Franciscan Saint Margaret Health - Dyer	Dyer	13.3%	585
Monroe Hospital	Bloomington	13.6%	132
Daviess Community Hospital	Washington	13.8%	455
Community Hospital North	Indianapolis	14.0%	1789
Saint Vincent Anderson Regional Hospital	Anderson	14.2%	1747
Comm Hosp of Anderson/Madison Co	Anderson	14.3%	1364
Jay County Hospital	Portland	15.2%	343
Saint Vincent Jennings Hospital	North Vernon	15.4%	285
Gibson General Hospital	Princeton	16.3%	227
Indiana University Health Tipton Hospital	Tipton	17.0%	341
Cameron Memorial Community Hospital	Angola	17.5%	366
Saint Vincent Mercy Hospital	Elwood	21.1%	261

Lumbar Spine MRI for Low Back Pain

Hospital Name	City	Rate	Cases
Columbus Regional Hospital	Columbus	26.2%	107
Wabash County Hospital	Wabash	27.1%	59
Dekalb Health	Auburn	28.6%	56
Indiana University Health Starke Hospital	Knox	32.2%	87
Community Hospital South	Indianapolis	32.5%	80
Indiana Univ Health La Porte Hosp	La Porte	32.9%	231
Indiana Univ Health Bloomington Hosp	Bloomington	33.3%	93
King's Daughters' Health	Madison	33.7%	92
Marion General Hospital	Marion	33.8%	219
Elkhart General Hospital	Elkhart	34.6%	156
Major Hospital	Shelbyville	34.7%	95
Eskenazi Health	Indianapolis	34.8%	138
Porter Regional Hospital	Valparaiso	34.8%	227
Saint Vincent Anderson Regional Hospital	Anderson	35.1%	228
Hancock Regional Hospital	Greenfield	35.2%	128
Kosciusko Community Hospital	Warsaw	35.2%	108
Community Howard Regional Health	Kokomo	35.3%	133
Saint Joseph Hospital	Fort Wayne	35.4%	48
Unity Medical & Surgical Hospital	Mishawaka	35.5%	62
Fayette Regional Health System	Connersville	35.7%	70
Indiana University Health	Indianapolis	35.8%	313
Community Hospital North	Indianapolis	36.0%	286
Franciscan St Anthony Health	Michigan City	36.1%	155
Adams Memorial Hospital	Decatur	36.2%	47
Johnson Memorial Hospital	Franklin	36.2%	58
Reid Hospital & Health Care Services	Richmond	36.3%	311
IU Health West Hospital	Avon	36.4%	132
Parkview Regional Medical Center	Fort Wayne	36.4%	151
Indiana Orthopaedic Hospital	Indianapolis	36.6%	295
Parkview Noble Hospital	Kendallville	36.6%	82
Saint Vincent Williamsport Hospital	Williamsport	36.7%	49
Saint Catherine Hospital	East Chicago	36.8%	57
Community Hospital	Munster	37.3%	354
Cameron Memorial Community Hospital	Angola	37.5%	72
Saint Vincent Carmel Hospital	Carmel	37.6%	165
Dupont Hospital	Fort Wayne	37.7%	61
Floyd Memorial Hospital & Health Services	New Albany	37.7%	223
Monroe Hospital	Bloomington	37.9%	174
Lutheran Hospital of Indiana	Fort Wayne	38.3%	149
Saint Mary's Medical Center of Evansville	Evansville	38.3%	316
Franciscan St Francis Hlth-Indianapolis	Indianapolis	38.6%	303
Community Hospital East	Indianapolis	39.0%	277
Deaconess Hospital	Evansville	39.3%	397
Saint Joseph Hospital & Health Center	Kokomo	39.3%	112
Indiana Univ Health Ball Mem Hosp	Muncie	39.5%	86
Clark Memorial Hospital	Jeffersonville	40.2%	179
Dearborn County Hospital	Lawrenceburg	40.2%	92
Union Hospital	Terre Haute	40.4%	230
Franciscan St Francis Health	Mooresville	40.7%	123
Memorial Hospital	Logansport	41.2%	51
Saint Vincent Hospital & Health Services	Indianapolis	41.2%	272
Riverview Hospital	Noblesville	41.3%	143
Methodist Hospitals	Gary	41.5%	135
IU Health Goshen Hospital	Goshen	41.6%	125
Putnam County Hospital	Greencastle	42.1%	38
Franciscan St Anthony Health-Crown Pt	Crown Point	42.2%	249
Harrison County Hospital	Corydon	42.3%	78
Franciscan Healthcare - Munster	Munster	42.5%	134
Franciscan St Elizabeth Health	Lafayette	42.9%	63
The Ortho Hosp/Lutheran Health Network	Fort Wayne	43.1%	65
Good Samaritan Hospital	Vincennes	43.2%	176
Henry County Memorial Hospital	New Castle	43.3%	60
Witham Health Services	Lebanon	43.5%	85
Memorial Hospital & Health Care Center	Jasper	43.8%	130
Saint Mary Medical Center	Hobart	43.8%	162
Comm Hosp of Anderson/Madison Co	Anderson	44.2%	147
Daviess Community Hospital	Washington	44.2%	52
Indiana University Health Arnett Hospital	Lafayette	44.2%	77
Jay County Hospital	Portland	44.2%	43
Indiana Univ Health Bedford Hosp	Bedford	44.6%	56
Parkview Huntington Hospital	Huntington	44.7%	38
Franciscan Saint Margaret Health - Dyer	Dyer	45.2%	73
Hendricks Regional Health	Danville	46.3%	123
Schneck Medical Center	Seymour	47.6%	103
Parkview Whitley Hospital	Columbia City	47.9%	48
Franciscan St Elizabeth Health	Crawfordsville	50.0%	52
Jasper County Hospital	Rensselaer	53.2%	47
Parkview Lagrange Hospital	Lagrange	53.5%	43
Saint Vincent Salem Hospital	Salem	54.1%	37
Pinnacle Hospital	Crown Point	61.4%	70

NOTE: Hospital profiles are in alphabetical order by state, then city, then hospital within the city; Rankings exclude hospitals with less than 25 cases except for patient surveys which excludes hospitals with less than 100 cases; (a) 100-299 cases; (1) The number of cases/patients is too few to report; (2) Data submitted were based on a sample of cases/patients; (3) Results are based on a shorter time period than required; (4) Data suppressed by CMS for one or more quarters; (5) Results are not available for this reporting period; (6) Fewer than 100 patients completed the HCAHPS survey; (7) No cases met the criteria for this measure; (8) The lower limit of the confidence interval cannot be calculated if the number of observed infections equals zero; (9) No data are available from the state/territory for this reporting period; (10) The scores shown reflect fewer than 50 completed surveys; (11) There were discrepancies in the data collection process; (12) This measure does not apply to this hospital for this reporting period; (13) Results cannot be calculated for this reporting period; (14) The results for this state are combined with nearby states to protect confidentiality; Please refer to the User's Guide for a full explanation of data.

Community Hospital of Anderson & Madison County

1515 N Madison Ave
Phone: 765-298-4242
Anderson, IN 46011
URL: www.communityanderson.com
Type: Acute Care Hospitals
Emergency Services: Yes
Ownership: Voluntary non-profit - Private

Measure	Cases	This Hosp.	State Avg.	U.S. Avg.
Blood Clot Prevention and Treatment				
Anticoagulation Overlap Therapy[2]	32	91%	92%	93%
ICU Venous Thromboembolism Prophylaxis[2]	61	85%	91%	92%
Incidence of Potentially Preventable VTE[1,2]	-	-	10%	10%
UFH with Dosages/Platelet Monitoring[2]	11	100%	95%	97%
Venous Thromboembolism Prophylaxis[2]	329	71%	83%	85%
Warfarin Therapy Discharge Instructions[2]	23	100%	71%	75%
Chest Pain/Possible Heart Attack Care				
Aspirin Given Within 24 Hours of Arrival	64	100%	96%	96%
Fibrinolytic Meds Within 30 Min. of Arrival[7]	-	-	48%	58%
Average Time to ECG (minutes)	66	5	6	7
Average Time to Transfer (minutes)	19	36	46	60
Children's Asthma Care				
Received Home Management Plan of Care	-	-	-	88%
Received Reliever Medication	-	-	-	100%
Received Systemic Corticosteroids	-	-	-	100%
Emergency Department				
Admittance Decision Time (minutes)[2]	591	49	80	98
Head CT Results Within 45 Min. of Arrival[1,3]	-	-	60%	57%
Patients Who Left ER Before Being Seen	30,714	0%	2%	2%
Time from ER Arrival to Admit. (minutes)[2]	712	185	241	274
Time from ER Arrival to Discharge (minutes)	385	118	122	134
Time in ER Before Being Evaluated (minutes)	384	23	22	26
Time to Pain Meds for Fractures (minutes)	75	57	52	57
Heart Attack Care				
Aspirin Given at Discharge	48	98%	99%	99%
Fibrinolytic Meds Within 30 Min. of Arrival[7]	-	-	67%	54%
PCI Within 90 Minutes of Arrival[1]	-	-	97%	96%
Statin Prescribed at Discharge	49	98%	99%	98%
Heart Failure Care				
ACE Inhibitor or ARB for LVSD	64	98%	97%	97%
Discharge Instructions Given	158	98%	95%	94%
Evaluation of LVS Function	205	100%	99%	99%
Medicare Spending				
Medicare Spending per Patient (ratio)	-	0.99	1.01	0.98
Pneumonia Care				
Appropriate Initial Antibiotic Given[2]	58	98%	95%	95%
Blood Culture Timing[2]	88	100%	98%	98%
Pregnancy and Delivery Care				
Newborn Deliveries Scheduled Early[2]	15	7%	5%	6%
Preventive Care				
Immunization for Influenza[2]	713	96%	91%	90%
Immunization for Pneumonia[2]	813	96%	92%	92%
Stroke Care				
Anticoagulation Therapy for Atrial Fibrillation[1]	-	-	94%	95%
Antithrombotic Therapy Timing	67	100%	97%	98%
Assessed for Rehabilitation	77	100%	96%	97%
Discharged on Antithrombotic Therapy	75	100%	98%	99%
Discharged on Statin Medication	61	100%	91%	94%
Thrombolytic Therapy Timing[1]	-	-	54%	66%
Venous Thromboembolism Prophylaxis	75	99%	91%	94%
Written Stroke Educational Materials Given	41	93%	82%	88%
Surgical Care Improvement Project				
Appropriate Beta Blocker Usage	127	98%	98%	98%
Appropriate VTP Within 24 Hours	368	99%	98%	98%
Controlled Postoperative Blood Glucose[7]	-	-	97%	97%
Perioperative Temperature Management	461	100%	100%	100%
Prophylactic Antibiotic Selection	328	100%	99%	99%
Prophylactic Antibiotic Selection (Outpatient)	163	98%	98%	98%
Prophylactic Antibiotic Stopped	319	99%	98%	98%
Prophylactic Antibiotic Timing	328	99%	99%	99%
Prophylactic Antibiotic Timing (Outpatient)	163	100%	98%	98%
Urinary Catheter Removal	322	97%	98%	97%
Survey of Patients' Hospital Experiences				
Area Around Room 'Always' Quiet at Night	300+	52%	61%	61%
Doctors 'Always' Communicated Well	300+	82%	83%	82%
Home Recovery Information Given	300+	84%	86%	85%
Hospital Given 9 or 10 on 10 Point Scale	300+	74%	74%	71%
Meds 'Always' Explained Before Given	300+	61%	64%	64%
Nurses 'Always' Communicated Well	300+	81%	81%	79%
Pain 'Always' Well Controlled	300+	73%	73%	71%
Room and Bathroom 'Always' Clean	300+	71%	76%	73%
Timely Help 'Always' Received	300+	66%	71%	68%
Would Definitely Recommend Hospital	300+	77%	73%	71%
Use of Medical Imaging				
Cardiac Imaging Stress Test before Surgery	495	3.4%	5.4%	5.3%
Combination Abdominal CT Scan	687	2.9%	9.3%	10.5%
Combination Brain/Sinus CT Scan	478	1.5%	2.6%	2.7%
Combination Chest CT Scan	519	2.5%	4.6%	2.7%
Follow-up Mammogram/Ultrasound	1,364	14.3%	8.4%	8.8%
Lumbar Spine MRI for Low Back Pain	147	44.2%	38.7%	37.2%

Saint Vincent Anderson Regional Hospital

2015 Jackson St
Phone: 765-646-8373
Anderson, IN 46016
Fax: 765-646-8504
URL: www.stjohnshealthsystem.org
Type: Acute Care Hospitals
Emergency Services: Yes
Ownership: Voluntary non-profit - Private
Beds: 225

Key Personnel:
Pediatric In-Patient Care .... David Beahm, MD
Quality Assurance .... Ross Brodhead
Radiology.................. Henry Jones, MD
Intensive Care Unit........... Tracy MCallister
Emergency Room .... Robert Steele
President.................. Richard Tofel
Anesthesiology.............. John Vu, MD

Measure	Cases	This Hosp.	State Avg.	U.S. Avg.
Blood Clot Prevention and Treatment				
Anticoagulation Overlap Therapy[2]	48	92%	92%	93%
ICU Venous Thromboembolism Prophylaxis[2]	116	72%	91%	92%
Incidence of Potentially Preventable VTE[1,2]	-	-	10%	10%
UFH with Dosages/Platelet Monitoring[1,2]	-	-	95%	97%
Venous Thromboembolism Prophylaxis[2]	1,058	68%	83%	85%
Warfarin Therapy Discharge Instructions[2]	27	85%	71%	75%
Chest Pain/Possible Heart Attack Care				
Aspirin Given Within 24 Hours of Arrival	103	99%	96%	96%
Fibrinolytic Meds Within 30 Min. of Arrival[7]	-	-	48%	58%
Average Time to ECG (minutes)	103	5	6	7
Average Time to Transfer (minutes)	29	27	46	60
Children's Asthma Care				
Received Home Management Plan of Care	-	-	-	88%
Received Reliever Medication	-	-	-	100%
Received Systemic Corticosteroids	-	-	-	100%
Emergency Department				
Admittance Decision Time (minutes)[2]	631	54	80	98
Head CT Results Within 45 Min. of Arrival[1]	-	-	60%	57%
Patients Who Left ER Before Being Seen	46,722	1%	2%	2%
Time from ER Arrival to Admit. (minutes)[2]	646	226	241	274
Time from ER Arrival to Discharge (minutes)	386	124	122	134
Time in ER Before Being Evaluated (minutes)	390	34	22	26
Time to Pain Meds for Fractures (minutes)	107	63	52	57
Heart Attack Care				
Aspirin Given at Discharge	32	97%	99%	99%
Fibrinolytic Meds Within 30 Min. of Arrival[1]	-	-	67%	54%
PCI Within 90 Minutes of Arrival[7]	-	-	97%	96%
Statin Prescribed at Discharge	31	100%	99%	98%
Heart Failure Care				
ACE Inhibitor or ARB for LVSD	71	100%	97%	97%
Discharge Instructions Given	138	99%	95%	94%
Evaluation of LVS Function	192	100%	99%	99%
Medicare Spending				
Medicare Spending per Patient (ratio)	-	1.03	1.01	0.98
Pneumonia Care				
Appropriate Initial Antibiotic Given	114	100%	95%	95%
Blood Culture Timing	239	100%	98%	98%
Pregnancy and Delivery Care				
Newborn Deliveries Scheduled Early	64	16%	5%	6%
Preventive Care				
Immunization for Influenza[2]	600	86%	91%	90%
Immunization for Pneumonia[2]	684	81%	92%	92%
Stroke Care				
Anticoagulation Therapy for Atrial Fibrillation	12	100%	94%	95%
Antithrombotic Therapy Timing	63	98%	97%	98%
Assessed for Rehabilitation	89	100%	96%	97%
Discharged on Antithrombotic Therapy	85	100%	98%	99%
Discharged on Statin Medication	76	100%	91%	94%
Thrombolytic Therapy Timing	12	92%	54%	66%
Venous Thromboembolism Prophylaxis	78	97%	91%	94%
Written Stroke Educational Materials Given	45	98%	82%	88%
Surgical Care Improvement Project				
Appropriate Beta Blocker Usage	140	100%	98%	98%
Appropriate VTP Within 24 Hours	339	100%	98%	98%
Controlled Postoperative Blood Glucose[7]	-	-	97%	97%
Perioperative Temperature Management	432	100%	100%	100%
Prophylactic Antibiotic Selection	295	100%	99%	99%
Prophylactic Antibiotic Selection (Outpatient)	168	99%	98%	98%
Prophylactic Antibiotic Stopped	292	100%	98%	98%
Prophylactic Antibiotic Timing	295	100%	99%	99%
Prophylactic Antibiotic Timing (Outpatient)	164	96%	98%	98%
Urinary Catheter Removal	310	99%	98%	97%
Survey of Patients' Hospital Experiences				
Area Around Room 'Always' Quiet at Night	300+	59%	61%	61%
Doctors 'Always' Communicated Well	300+	83%	83%	82%
Home Recovery Information Given	300+	91%	86%	85%
Hospital Given 9 or 10 on 10 Point Scale	300+	73%	74%	71%
Meds 'Always' Explained Before Given	300+	57%	64%	64%
Nurses 'Always' Communicated Well	300+	80%	81%	79%
Pain 'Always' Well Controlled	300+	73%	73%	71%
Room and Bathroom 'Always' Clean	300+	74%	76%	73%
Timely Help 'Always' Received	300+	63%	71%	68%
Would Definitely Recommend Hospital	300+	73%	73%	71%
Use of Medical Imaging				
Cardiac Imaging Stress Test before Surgery	551	4.7%	5.4%	5.3%
Combination Abdominal CT Scan	923	4.9%	9.3%	10.5%
Combination Brain/Sinus CT Scan	724	0.8%	2.6%	2.7%
Combination Chest CT Scan	744	0.4%	4.6%	2.7%
Follow-up Mammogram/Ultrasound	1,747	14.2%	8.4%	8.8%
Lumbar Spine MRI for Low Back Pain	228	35.1%	38.7%	37.2%

Cameron Memorial Community Hospital

416 E Maumee St
Phone: 260-665-2141
Angola, IN 46703
Fax: 260-665-2879
URL: www.cameronmch.com
Type: Critical Access Hospitals
Emergency Services: Yes
Ownership: Voluntary non-profit - Private
Beds: 25

Key Personnel:
President/CEO............... Gregory T. Burns
Chief of Medical Staff.......... Michael E Holton

Measure	Cases	This Hosp.	State Avg.	U.S. Avg.
Blood Clot Prevention and Treatment				
Anticoagulation Overlap Therapy[1,2]	-	-	92%	93%
ICU Venous Thromboembolism Prophylaxis[1,2]	-	-	91%	92%
Incidence of Potentially Preventable VTE[2,7]	-	-	10%	10%
UFH with Dosages/Platelet Monitoring[1,2]	-	-	95%	97%
Venous Thromboembolism Prophylaxis[2]	103	86%	83%	85%
Warfarin Therapy Discharge Instructions[1,2]	-	-	71%	75%
Chest Pain/Possible Heart Attack Care				
Aspirin Given Within 24 Hours of Arrival	92	98%	96%	96%
Fibrinolytic Meds Within 30 Min. of Arrival[7]	-	-	48%	58%
Average Time to ECG (minutes)	100	9	6	7
Average Time to Transfer (minutes)	12	51	46	60
Children's Asthma Care				
Received Home Management Plan of Care	-	-	-	88%
Received Reliever Medication	-	-	-	100%
Received Systemic Corticosteroids	-	-	-	100%
Emergency Department				
Admittance Decision Time (minutes)[2]	407	51	80	98
Head CT Results Within 45 Min. of Arrival[1]	-	-	60%	57%
Patients Who Left ER Before Being Seen[5]	-	-	2%	2%
Time from ER Arrival to Admit. (minutes)[2]	415	223	241	274
Time from ER Arrival to Discharge (minutes)	341	108	122	134

NOTE: Hospital profiles are in alphabetical order by state, then city, then hospital within the city; Rankings exclude hospitals with less than 25 cases except for patient surveys which excludes hospitals with less than 100 cases; (a) 100-299 cases; (1) The number of cases/patients is too few to report; (2) Data submitted were based on a sample of cases/patients; (3) Results are based on a shorter time period than required; (4) Data suppressed by CMS for one or more quarters; (5) Results are not available for this reporting period; (6) Fewer than 100 patients completed the HCAHPS survey; (7) No cases met the criteria for this measure; (8) The lower limit of the confidence interval cannot be calculated if the number of observed infections equals zero; (9) No data are available from the state/territory for this reporting period; (10) The scores shown reflect fewer than 50 completed surveys; (11) There were discrepancies in the data collection process; (12) This measure does not apply to this hospital for this reporting period; (13) Results cannot be calculated for this reporting period; (14) The results for this state are combined with nearby states to protect confidentiality; Please refer to the User's Guide for a full explanation of data.

Measure	Cases	This Hosp.	State Avg.	U.S. Avg.
Time in ER Before Being Evaluated (minutes)	357	19	22	26
Time to Pain Meds for Fractures (minutes)	83	25	52	57
Heart Attack Care				
Aspirin Given at Discharge[1]	-	-	99%	99%
Fibrinolytic Meds Within 30 Min. of Arrival[7]	-	-	67%	54%
PCI Within 90 Minutes of Arrival[7]	-	-	97%	96%
Statin Prescribed at Discharge[1]	-	-	99%	98%
Heart Failure Care				
ACE Inhibitor or ARB for LVSD	11	91%	97%	97%
Discharge Instructions Given	33	97%	95%	94%
Evaluation of LVS Function	46	100%	99%	99%
Medicare Spending				
Medicare Spending per Patient (ratio)	-	-	1.01	0.98
Pneumonia Care				
Appropriate Initial Antibiotic Given	72	94%	95%	95%
Blood Culture Timing	77	100%	98%	98%
Pregnancy and Delivery Care				
Newborn Deliveries Scheduled Early[5]	-	-	5%	6%
Preventive Care				
Immunization for Influenza[2]	373	94%	91%	90%
Immunization for Pneumonia[2]	449	94%	92%	92%
Stroke Care				
Anticoagulation Therapy for Atrial Fibrillation[1]	-	-	94%	95%
Antithrombotic Therapy Timing	21	100%	97%	98%
Assessed for Rehabilitation	19	100%	96%	97%
Discharged on Antithrombotic Therapy	19	100%	98%	99%
Discharged on Statin Medication	12	100%	91%	94%
Thrombolytic Therapy Timing[7]	-	-	54%	66%
Venous Thromboembolism Prophylaxis	21	95%	91%	94%
Written Stroke Educational Materials Given	15	93%	82%	88%
Surgical Care Improvement Project				
Appropriate Beta Blocker Usage	14	100%	98%	98%
Appropriate VTP Within 24 Hours	59	97%	98%	98%
Controlled Postoperative Blood Glucose[7]	-	-	97%	97%
Perioperative Temperature Management	65	100%	100%	100%
Prophylactic Antibiotic Selection	44	95%	99%	99%
Prophylactic Antibiotic Selection (Outpatient)	29	97%	98%	98%
Prophylactic Antibiotic Stopped	44	100%	98%	98%
Prophylactic Antibiotic Timing	44	100%	99%	99%
Prophylactic Antibiotic Timing (Outpatient)	30	97%	98%	98%
Urinary Catheter Removal	52	98%	98%	97%
Survey of Patients' Hospital Experiences				
Area Around Room 'Always' Quiet at Night	300+	58%	61%	61%
Doctors 'Always' Communicated Well	300+	82%	83%	82%
Home Recovery Information Given	300+	88%	86%	85%
Hospital Given 9 or 10 on 10 Point Scale	300+	72%	74%	71%
Meds 'Always' Explained Before Given	300+	64%	64%	64%
Nurses 'Always' Communicated Well	300+	84%	81%	79%
Pain 'Always' Well Controlled	300+	77%	73%	71%
Room and Bathroom 'Always' Clean	300+	80%	76%	73%
Timely Help 'Always' Received	300+	81%	71%	68%
Would Definitely Recommend Hospital	300+	67%	73%	71%
Use of Medical Imaging				
Cardiac Imaging Stress Test before Surgery[7]	-	-	5.4%	5.3%
Combination Abdominal CT Scan	267	4.1%	9.3%	10.5%
Combination Brain/Sinus CT Scan	283	0.7%	2.6%	2.7%
Combination Chest CT Scan	170	0.0%	4.6%	2.7%
Follow-up Mammogram/Ultrasound	366	17.5%	8.4%	8.8%
Lumbar Spine MRI for Low Back Pain	72	37.5%	38.7%	37.2%

Dekalb Health

1316 E Seventh St
Auburn, IN 46706
Phone: 260-925-4600
Fax: 260-925-4733
E-mail: info@dekalbmemorial.com
URL: www.dekalbmemorial.com
Type: Acute Care Hospitals
Emergency Services: Yes
Ownership: Voluntary non-profit - Private
Beds: 47

Key Personnel:

Infection Control. . . . . Mary Bigelow, RN
CEO/President. . . . . JM Corey
Operating Room. . . . . Jeffrey Justice, RN
Quality Assurance . . . . Cheryl Markiton, RN
Pediatric Ambulatory Care . . . . . . David Marquis, MD
Pediatric In-Patient Care . . . . David Marquis, MD
CEO . . . . Fred Price
Chief of Medical Staff . . . . Emilio Vazquez, MD

Measure	Cases	This Hosp.	State Avg.	U.S. Avg.
Blood Clot Prevention and Treatment				
Anticoagulation Overlap Therapy[2]	19	100%	92%	93%
ICU Venous Thromboembolism Prophylaxis[2]	194	97%	91%	92%
Incidence of Potentially Preventable VTE[1,2]	-	-	10%	10%
UFH with Dosages/Platelet Monitoring[2]	14	100%	95%	97%
Venous Thromboembolism Prophylaxis[2]	86	95%	83%	85%
Warfarin Therapy Discharge Instructions[2]	14	93%	71%	75%
Chest Pain/Possible Heart Attack Care				
Aspirin Given Within 24 Hours of Arrival	45	100%	96%	96%
Fibrinolytic Meds Within 30 Min. of Arrival[7]	-	-	48%	58%
Average Time to ECG (minutes)	47	7	6	7
Average Time to Transfer (minutes)[1]	-	-	46	60
Children's Asthma Care				
Received Home Management Plan of Care	-	-	-	88%
Received Reliever Medication	-	-	-	100%
Received Systemic Corticosteroids	-	-	-	100%
Emergency Department				
Admittance Decision Time (minutes)[2]	231	96	80	98
Head CT Results Within 45 Min. of Arrival[1]	-	-	60%	57%
Patients Who Left ER Before Being Seen	18,185	1%	2%	2%
Time from ER Arrival to Admit. (minutes)[2]	251	229	241	274
Time from ER Arrival to Discharge (minutes)	430	94	122	134
Time in ER Before Being Evaluated (minutes)	449	21	22	26
Time to Pain Meds for Fractures (minutes)	62	42	52	57
Heart Attack Care				
Aspirin Given at Discharge	12	100%	99%	99%
Fibrinolytic Meds Within 30 Min. of Arrival[7]	-	-	67%	54%
PCI Within 90 Minutes of Arrival[7]	-	-	97%	96%
Statin Prescribed at Discharge[1]	-	-	99%	98%
Heart Failure Care				
ACE Inhibitor or ARB for LVSD	13	100%	97%	97%
Discharge Instructions Given	47	98%	95%	94%
Evaluation of LVS Function	72	100%	99%	99%
Medicare Spending				
Medicare Spending per Patient (ratio)	-	1.02	1.01	0.98
Pneumonia Care				
Appropriate Initial Antibiotic Given	71	99%	95%	95%
Blood Culture Timing	105	99%	98%	98%
Pregnancy and Delivery Care				
Newborn Deliveries Scheduled Early	37	0%	5%	6%
Preventive Care				
Immunization for Influenza[2]	228	99%	91%	90%
Immunization for Pneumonia[2]	255	100%	92%	92%
Stroke Care				
Anticoagulation Therapy for Atrial Fibrillation[1]	-	-	94%	95%
Antithrombotic Therapy Timing	15	100%	97%	98%
Assessed for Rehabilitation	18	100%	96%	97%
Discharged on Antithrombotic Therapy	18	100%	98%	99%
Discharged on Statin Medication	14	100%	91%	94%
Thrombolytic Therapy Timing[7]	-	-	54%	66%
Venous Thromboembolism Prophylaxis	16	100%	91%	94%
Written Stroke Educational Materials Given[1]	-	-	82%	88%
Surgical Care Improvement Project				
Appropriate Beta Blocker Usage	28	100%	98%	98%
Appropriate VTP Within 24 Hours	88	98%	98%	98%
Controlled Postoperative Blood Glucose[7]	-	-	97%	97%
Perioperative Temperature Management	98	100%	100%	100%
Prophylactic Antibiotic Selection	62	100%	99%	99%
Prophylactic Antibiotic Selection (Outpatient)	71	99%	98%	98%
Prophylactic Antibiotic Stopped	61	98%	98%	98%
Prophylactic Antibiotic Timing	62	98%	99%	99%
Prophylactic Antibiotic Timing (Outpatient)	71	100%	98%	98%
Urinary Catheter Removal	28	100%	98%	97%
Survey of Patients' Hospital Experiences				
Area Around Room 'Always' Quiet at Night	300+	49%	61%	61%
Doctors 'Always' Communicated Well	300+	86%	83%	82%
Home Recovery Information Given	300+	88%	86%	85%
Hospital Given 9 or 10 on 10 Point Scale	300+	73%	74%	71%
Meds 'Always' Explained Before Given	300+	63%	64%	64%
Nurses 'Always' Communicated Well	300+	79%	81%	79%
Pain 'Always' Well Controlled	300+	71%	73%	71%
Room and Bathroom 'Always' Clean	300+	71%	76%	73%
Timely Help 'Always' Received	300+	70%	71%	68%
Would Definitely Recommend Hospital	300+	68%	73%	71%
Use of Medical Imaging				
Cardiac Imaging Stress Test before Surgery	48	2.1%	5.4%	5.3%
Combination Abdominal CT Scan	229	0.0%	9.3%	10.5%
Combination Brain/Sinus CT Scan[1]	-	-	2.6%	2.7%
Combination Chest CT Scan	111	0.0%	4.6%	2.7%
Follow-up Mammogram/Ultrasound	385	9.4%	8.4%	8.8%
Lumbar Spine MRI for Low Back Pain	56	28.6%	38.7%	37.2%

IU Health West Hospital

1111 N Ronald Reagan Pkwy
Avon, IN 46123
Phone: 317-217-3000
URL: www.iuhealth.org/west
Type: Acute Care Hospitals
Emergency Services: Yes
Ownership: Proprietary

Key Personnel:

CEO/President. . . . . Matt Bailey, FACHE
Chief of Medical Staff . . . . Andrew Nigh, MD

Measure	Cases	This Hosp.	State Avg.	U.S. Avg.
Blood Clot Prevention and Treatment				
Anticoagulation Overlap Therapy[2]	54	94%	92%	93%
ICU Venous Thromboembolism Prophylaxis[2]	17	100%	91%	92%
Incidence of Potentially Preventable VTE[2]	16	25%	10%	10%
UFH with Dosages/Platelet Monitoring[2]	14	100%	95%	97%
Venous Thromboembolism Prophylaxis[2]	402	93%	83%	85%
Warfarin Therapy Discharge Instructions[2]	47	45%	71%	75%
Chest Pain/Possible Heart Attack Care				
Aspirin Given Within 24 Hours of Arrival	35	100%	96%	96%
Fibrinolytic Meds Within 30 Min. of Arrival[7]	-	-	48%	58%
Average Time to ECG (minutes)	36	6	6	7
Average Time to Transfer (minutes)	13	38	46	60
Children's Asthma Care				
Received Home Management Plan of Care	-	-	-	88%
Received Reliever Medication	-	-	-	100%
Received Systemic Corticosteroids	-	-	-	100%
Emergency Department				
Admittance Decision Time (minutes)[2]	716	138	80	98
Head CT Results Within 45 Min. of Arrival[1]	-	-	60%	57%
Patients Who Left ER Before Being Seen	48,060	2%	2%	2%
Time from ER Arrival to Admit. (minutes)[2]	721	334	241	274
Time from ER Arrival to Discharge (minutes)	375	181	122	134
Time in ER Before Being Evaluated (minutes)	370	22	22	26
Time to Pain Meds for Fractures (minutes)	197	64	52	57
Heart Attack Care				
Aspirin Given at Discharge	82	100%	99%	99%
Fibrinolytic Meds Within 30 Min. of Arrival[7]	-	-	67%	54%
PCI Within 90 Minutes of Arrival	13	92%	97%	96%
Statin Prescribed at Discharge	81	99%	99%	98%
Heart Failure Care				
ACE Inhibitor or ARB for LVSD	37	100%	97%	97%
Discharge Instructions Given	145	99%	95%	94%
Evaluation of LVS Function	190	100%	99%	99%
Medicare Spending				
Medicare Spending per Patient (ratio)	-	0.99	1.01	0.98
Pneumonia Care				
Appropriate Initial Antibiotic Given[2]	81	90%	95%	95%
Blood Culture Timing[2]	164	99%	98%	98%
Pregnancy and Delivery Care				
Newborn Deliveries Scheduled Early[2]	26	0%	5%	6%
Preventive Care				
Immunization for Influenza[2]	505	95%	91%	90%
Immunization for Pneumonia[2]	639	94%	92%	92%
Stroke Care				
Anticoagulation Therapy for Atrial Fibrillation	13	85%	94%	95%
Antithrombotic Therapy Timing	75	100%	97%	98%
Assessed for Rehabilitation	73	95%	96%	97%
Discharged on Antithrombotic Therapy	73	99%	98%	99%
Discharged on Statin Medication	65	97%	91%	94%
Thrombolytic Therapy Timing[1]	-	-	54%	66%
Venous Thromboembolism Prophylaxis	79	92%	91%	94%
Written Stroke Educational Materials Given	49	65%	82%	88%

NOTE: Hospital profiles are in alphabetical order by state, then city, then hospital within the city; Rankings exclude hospitals with less than 25 cases except for patient surveys which excludes hospitals with less than 100 cases; (a) 100-299 cases; (1) The number of cases/patients is too few to report; (2) Data submitted were based on a sample of cases/patients; (3) Results are based on a shorter time period than required; (4) Data suppressed by CMS for one or more quarters; (5) Results are not available for this reporting period; (6) Fewer than 100 patients completed the HCAHPS survey; (7) No cases met the criteria for this measure; (8) The lower limit of the confidence interval cannot be calculated if the number of observed infections equals zero; (9) No data are available from the state/territory for this reporting period; (10) The scores shown reflect fewer than 50 completed surveys; (11) There were discrepancies in the data collection process; (12) This measure does not apply to this hospital for this reporting period; (13) Results cannot be calculated for this reporting period; (14) The results for this state are combined with nearby states to protect confidentiality; Please refer to the User's Guide for a full explanation of data.

Measure	Cases	This Hosp.	State Avg.	U.S. Avg.
Surgical Care Improvement Project				
Appropriate Beta Blocker Usage[2]	110	98%	98%	98%
Appropriate VTP Within 24 Hours[2]	322	98%	98%	98%
Controlled Postoperative Blood Glucose[2,7]	-	-	97%	97%
Perioperative Temperature Management[2]	340	100%	100%	100%
Prophylactic Antibiotic Selection[2]	220	100%	99%	99%
Prophylactic Antibiotic Selection (Outpatient)	256	99%	98%	98%
Prophylactic Antibiotic Stopped[2]	207	98%	98%	98%
Prophylactic Antibiotic Timing[2]	222	100%	99%	99%
Prophylactic Antibiotic Timing (Outpatient)	256	100%	98%	98%
Urinary Catheter Removal[2]	271	99%	98%	97%
Survey of Patients' Hospital Experiences				
Area Around Room 'Always' Quiet at Night	300+	65%	61%	61%
Doctors 'Always' Communicated Well	300+	82%	83%	82%
Home Recovery Information Given	300+	86%	86%	85%
Hospital Given 9 or 10 on 10 Point Scale	300+	81%	74%	71%
Meds 'Always' Explained Before Given	300+	64%	64%	64%
Nurses 'Always' Communicated Well	300+	79%	81%	79%
Pain 'Always' Well Controlled	300+	70%	73%	71%
Room and Bathroom 'Always' Clean	300+	71%	76%	73%
Timely Help 'Always' Received	300+	63%	71%	68%
Would Definitely Recommend Hospital	300+	82%	73%	71%
Use of Medical Imaging				
Cardiac Imaging Stress Test before Surgery	284	5.3%	5.4%	5.3%
Combination Abdominal CT Scan	1,001	5.1%	9.3%	10.5%
Combination Brain/Sinus CT Scan	644	1.4%	2.6%	2.7%
Combination Chest CT Scan	793	0.9%	4.6%	2.7%
Follow-up Mammogram/Ultrasound	728	8.9%	8.4%	8.8%
Lumbar Spine MRI for Low Back Pain	132	36.4%	38.7%	37.2%

Margaret Mary Community Hospital

321 Mitchell Ave
Batesville, IN 47006
Phone: 812-934-6624
Fax: 812-934-5373
E-mail: mmch@venus.net
URL: www.mmch.org

Type: Critical Access Hospitals
Emergency Services: Yes
Ownership: Voluntary non-profit - Private
Beds: 79

Key Personnel:
Operating Room. . . . . Brian Albers
Infection Control. . . . . Lisa Banks
Quality Assurance . . . . Lisa Banks
Radiology. . . . . James Browne
Chief of Medical Staff. . . . . Janet Ford, MD
CEO/President. . . . . Timothy L Putnam

Measure	Cases	This Hosp.	State Avg.	U.S. Avg.
Blood Clot Prevention and Treatment				
Anticoagulation Overlap Therapy[5]	-	-	92%	93%
ICU Venous Thromboembolism Prophylaxis[5]	-	-	91%	92%
Incidence of Potentially Preventable VTE[5]	-	-	10%	10%
UFH with Dosages/Platelet Monitoring[5]	-	-	95%	97%
Venous Thromboembolism Prophylaxis[5]	-	-	83%	85%
Warfarin Therapy Discharge Instructions[5]	-	-	71%	75%
Chest Pain/Possible Heart Attack Care				
Aspirin Given Within 24 Hours of Arrival	109	100%	96%	96%
Fibrinolytic Meds Within 30 Min. of Arrival[7]	-	-	48%	58%
Average Time to ECG (minutes)	114	4	6	7
Average Time to Transfer (minutes)	17	43	46	60
Children's Asthma Care				
Received Home Management Plan of Care	-	-	-	88%
Received Reliever Medication	-	-	-	100%
Received Systemic Corticosteroids	-	-	-	100%
Emergency Department				
Admittance Decision Time (minutes)[5]	-	-	80	98
Head CT Results Within 45 Min. of Arrival[1]	-	-	60%	57%
Patients Who Left ER Before Being Seen	16,093	0%	2%	2%
Time from ER Arrival to Admit. (minutes)[5]	-	-	241	274
Time from ER Arrival to Discharge (minutes)	350	78	122	134
Time in ER Before Being Evaluated (minutes)	375	17	22	26
Time to Pain Meds for Fractures (minutes)	38	37	52	57
Heart Attack Care				
Aspirin Given at Discharge[1]	-	-	99%	99%
Fibrinolytic Meds Within 30 Min. of Arrival[7]	-	-	67%	54%
PCI Within 90 Minutes of Arrival[5]	-	-	97%	96%
Statin Prescribed at Discharge[1]	-	-	99%	98%
Heart Failure Care				
ACE Inhibitor or ARB for LVSD[1]	-	-	97%	97%
Discharge Instructions Given	27	100%	95%	94%
Evaluation of LVS Function	45	98%	99%	99%
Medicare Spending				
Medicare Spending per Patient (ratio)	-	-	1.01	0.98
Pneumonia Care				
Appropriate Initial Antibiotic Given	53	96%	95%	95%
Blood Culture Timing	106	99%	98%	98%
Pregnancy and Delivery Care				
Newborn Deliveries Scheduled Early[5]	-	-	5%	6%
Preventive Care				
Immunization for Influenza[5]	-	-	91%	90%
Immunization for Pneumonia[5]	-	-	92%	92%
Stroke Care				
Anticoagulation Therapy for Atrial Fibrillation[5]	-	-	94%	95%
Antithrombotic Therapy Timing[5]	-	-	97%	98%
Assessed for Rehabilitation[5]	-	-	96%	97%
Discharged on Antithrombotic Therapy[5]	-	-	98%	99%
Discharged on Statin Medication[5]	-	-	91%	94%
Thrombolytic Therapy Timing[5]	-	-	54%	66%
Venous Thromboembolism Prophylaxis[5]	-	-	91%	94%
Written Stroke Educational Materials Given[5]	-	-	82%	88%
Surgical Care Improvement Project				
Appropriate Beta Blocker Usage	32	100%	98%	98%
Appropriate VTP Within 24 Hours	127	99%	98%	98%
Controlled Postoperative Blood Glucose[5]	-	-	97%	97%
Perioperative Temperature Management	144	100%	100%	100%
Prophylactic Antibiotic Selection	109	99%	99%	99%
Prophylactic Antibiotic Selection (Outpatient)	104	100%	98%	98%
Prophylactic Antibiotic Stopped	108	99%	98%	98%
Prophylactic Antibiotic Timing	109	98%	99%	99%
Prophylactic Antibiotic Timing (Outpatient)	88	100%	98%	98%
Urinary Catheter Removal	67	96%	98%	97%
Survey of Patients' Hospital Experiences				
Area Around Room 'Always' Quiet at Night	300+	64%	61%	61%
Doctors 'Always' Communicated Well	300+	89%	83%	82%
Home Recovery Information Given	300+	87%	86%	85%
Hospital Given 9 or 10 on 10 Point Scale	300+	81%	74%	71%
Meds 'Always' Explained Before Given	300+	66%	64%	64%
Nurses 'Always' Communicated Well	300+	87%	81%	79%
Pain 'Always' Well Controlled	300+	79%	73%	71%
Room and Bathroom 'Always' Clean	300+	82%	76%	73%
Timely Help 'Always' Received	300+	72%	71%	68%
Would Definitely Recommend Hospital	300+	82%	73%	71%
Use of Medical Imaging				
Cardiac Imaging Stress Test before Surgery	151	6.6%	5.4%	5.3%
Combination Abdominal CT Scan	385	15.8%	9.3%	10.5%
Combination Brain/Sinus CT Scan[1]	-	-	2.6%	2.7%
Combination Chest CT Scan	256	13.3%	4.6%	2.7%
Follow-up Mammogram/Ultrasound	603	9.5%	8.4%	8.8%
Lumbar Spine MRI for Low Back Pain[1]	-	-	38.7%	37.2%

Indiana University Health Bedford Hospital

2900 W 16th St
Bedford, IN 47421
Phone: 812-275-1200
Fax: 812-275-1450
E-mail: kellis@kiva.net
URL: www.brmchealthcare.com

Type: Critical Access Hospitals
Emergency Services: Yes
Ownership: Voluntary non-profit - Private
Beds: 49

Key Personnel:
Radiology. . . . . Steven A Archibald
Chief of Medical Staff. . . . . Cristina Bickford
CEO/President. . . . . Bradford W Dykes

Measure	Cases	This Hosp.	State Avg.	U.S. Avg.
Blood Clot Prevention and Treatment				
Anticoagulation Overlap Therapy[5]	-	-	92%	93%
ICU Venous Thromboembolism Prophylaxis[5]	-	-	91%	92%
Incidence of Potentially Preventable VTE[5]	-	-	10%	10%
UFH with Dosages/Platelet Monitoring[5]	-	-	95%	97%
Venous Thromboembolism Prophylaxis[5]	-	-	83%	85%
Warfarin Therapy Discharge Instructions[5]	-	-	71%	75%
Chest Pain/Possible Heart Attack Care				
Aspirin Given Within 24 Hours of Arrival	54	94%	96%	96%
Fibrinolytic Meds Within 30 Min. of Arrival[7]	-	-	48%	58%
Average Time to ECG (minutes)	55	7	6	7
Average Time to Transfer (minutes)	16	38	46	60
Children's Asthma Care				
Received Home Management Plan of Care	-	-	-	88%
Received Reliever Medication	-	-	-	100%
Received Systemic Corticosteroids	-	-	-	100%
Emergency Department				
Admittance Decision Time (minutes)[2,3]	294	72	80	98
Head CT Results Within 45 Min. of Arrival[1]	-	-	60%	57%
Patients Who Left ER Before Being Seen	12,357	2%	2%	2%
Time from ER Arrival to Admit. (minutes)[2,3]	294	234	241	274
Time from ER Arrival to Discharge (minutes)[5]	-	-	122	134
Time in ER Before Being Evaluated (minutes)[5]	-	-	22	26
Time to Pain Meds for Fractures (minutes)	38	44	52	57
Heart Attack Care				
Aspirin Given at Discharge[1]	-	-	99%	99%
Fibrinolytic Meds Within 30 Min. of Arrival[7]	-	-	67%	54%
PCI Within 90 Minutes of Arrival[3,7]	-	-	97%	96%
Statin Prescribed at Discharge[1]	-	-	99%	98%
Heart Failure Care				
ACE Inhibitor or ARB for LVSD[1]	-	-	97%	97%
Discharge Instructions Given	12	100%	95%	94%
Evaluation of LVS Function	17	100%	99%	99%
Medicare Spending				
Medicare Spending per Patient (ratio)	-	-	1.01	0.98
Pneumonia Care				
Appropriate Initial Antibiotic Given	55	96%	95%	95%
Blood Culture Timing	95	99%	98%	98%
Pregnancy and Delivery Care				
Newborn Deliveries Scheduled Early[5]	-	-	5%	6%
Preventive Care				
Immunization for Influenza[2,3]	134	99%	91%	90%
Immunization for Pneumonia[2,3]	306	96%	92%	92%
Stroke Care				
Anticoagulation Therapy for Atrial Fibrillation[5]	-	-	94%	95%
Antithrombotic Therapy Timing[5]	-	-	97%	98%
Assessed for Rehabilitation[5]	-	-	96%	97%
Discharged on Antithrombotic Therapy[5]	-	-	98%	99%
Discharged on Statin Medication[5]	-	-	91%	94%
Thrombolytic Therapy Timing[5]	-	-	54%	66%
Venous Thromboembolism Prophylaxis[5]	-	-	91%	94%
Written Stroke Educational Materials Given[5]	-	-	82%	88%
Surgical Care Improvement Project				
Appropriate Beta Blocker Usage[1]	-	-	98%	98%
Appropriate VTP Within 24 Hours	38	100%	98%	98%
Controlled Postoperative Blood Glucose[3,7]	-	-	97%	97%
Perioperative Temperature Management	56	100%	100%	100%
Prophylactic Antibiotic Selection	32	91%	99%	99%
Prophylactic Antibiotic Selection (Outpatient)	26	88%	98%	98%
Prophylactic Antibiotic Stopped	32	97%	98%	98%
Prophylactic Antibiotic Timing	32	100%	99%	99%
Prophylactic Antibiotic Timing (Outpatient)	26	100%	98%	98%
Urinary Catheter Removal	24	100%	98%	97%
Survey of Patients' Hospital Experiences				
Area Around Room 'Always' Quiet at Night	(a)	52%	61%	61%
Doctors 'Always' Communicated Well	(a)	88%	83%	82%
Home Recovery Information Given	(a)	91%	86%	85%
Hospital Given 9 or 10 on 10 Point Scale	(a)	80%	74%	71%
Meds 'Always' Explained Before Given	(a)	66%	64%	64%
Nurses 'Always' Communicated Well	(a)	84%	81%	79%
Pain 'Always' Well Controlled	(a)	72%	73%	71%
Room and Bathroom 'Always' Clean	(a)	83%	76%	73%
Timely Help 'Always' Received	(a)	77%	71%	68%
Would Definitely Recommend Hospital	(a)	78%	73%	71%
Use of Medical Imaging				
Cardiac Imaging Stress Test before Surgery	214	4.7%	5.4%	5.3%
Combination Abdominal CT Scan	485	7.0%	9.3%	10.5%
Combination Brain/Sinus CT Scan[1]	-	-	2.6%	2.7%
Combination Chest CT Scan	275	4.7%	4.6%	2.7%
Follow-up Mammogram/Ultrasound	843	5.8%	8.4%	8.8%

NOTE: Hospital profiles are in alphabetical order by state, then city, then hospital within the city; Rankings exclude hospitals with less than 25 cases except for patient surveys which excludes hospitals with less than 100 cases; (a) 100-299 cases; (1) The number of cases/patients is too few to report; (2) Data submitted were based on a sample of cases/patients; (3) Results are based on a shorter time period than required; (4) Data suppressed by CMS for one or more quarters; (5) Results are not available for this reporting period; (6) Fewer than 100 patients completed the HCAHPS survey; (7) No cases met the criteria for this measure; (8) The lower limit of the confidence interval cannot be calculated if the number of observed infections equals zero; (9) No data are available from the state/territory for this reporting period; (10) The scores shown reflect fewer than 50 completed surveys; (11) There were discrepancies in the data collection process; (12) This measure does not apply to this hospital for this reporting period; (13) Results cannot be calculated for this reporting period; (14) The results for this state are combined with nearby states to protect confidentiality; Please refer to the User's Guide for a full explanation of data.

Measure	Cases	This Hosp.	State Avg.	U.S. Avg.
Lumbar Spine MRI for Low Back Pain	56	44.6%	38.7%	37.2%

Saint Vincent Dunn Hospital

1600 23rd St
Bedford, IN 47421
Phone: 812-275-3331
Fax: 812-276-1211
URL: www.stvincent.org/St-Vincent-Dunn
Type: Critical Access Hospitals
Emergency Services: Yes
Ownership: Voluntary non-profit - Other
Beds: 137

Key Personnel:
Cardiac Laboratory. . . . . Audi Baer
Emergency Room . . . . Rodney Beeler
CEO/President. . . . . D Bruner
Chief of Medical Staff. . . . . RB Kalari

Measure	Cases	This Hosp.	State Avg.	U.S. Avg.
Blood Clot Prevention and Treatment				
Anticoagulation Overlap Therapy[5]	-	-	92%	93%
ICU Venous Thromboembolism Prophylaxis[5]	-	-	91%	92%
Incidence of Potentially Preventable VTE[5]	-	-	10%	10%
UFH with Dosages/Platelet Monitoring[5]	-	-	95%	97%
Venous Thromboembolism Prophylaxis[5]	-	-	83%	85%
Warfarin Therapy Discharge Instructions[5]	-	-	71%	75%
Chest Pain/Possible Heart Attack Care				
Aspirin Given Within 24 Hours of Arrival	28	96%	96%	96%
Fibrinolytic Meds Within 30 Min. of Arrival[7]	-	-	48%	58%
Average Time to ECG (minutes)	30	4	6	7
Average Time to Transfer (minutes)[1]	-	-	46	60
Children's Asthma Care				
Received Home Management Plan of Care	-	-	-	88%
Received Reliever Medication	-	-	-	100%
Received Systemic Corticosteroids	-	-	-	100%
Emergency Department				
Admittance Decision Time (minutes)[2]	183	85	80	98
Head CT Results Within 45 Min. of Arrival[1,3]	-	-	60%	57%
Patients Who Left ER Before Being Seen	9,188	1%	2%	2%
Time from ER Arrival to Admit. (minutes)[2]	211	274	241	274
Time from ER Arrival to Discharge (minutes)[3]	270	122	122	134
Time in ER Before Being Evaluated (minutes)[3]	296	18	22	26
Time to Pain Meds for Fractures (minutes)[3]	24	38	52	57
Heart Attack Care				
Aspirin Given at Discharge	24	100%	99%	99%
Fibrinolytic Meds Within 30 Min. of Arrival[7]	-	-	67%	54%
PCI Within 90 Minutes of Arrival[7]	-	-	97%	96%
Statin Prescribed at Discharge	21	100%	99%	98%
Heart Failure Care				
ACE Inhibitor or ARB for LVSD	13	100%	97%	97%
Discharge Instructions Given	33	100%	95%	94%
Evaluation of LVS Function	54	100%	99%	99%
Medicare Spending				
Medicare Spending per Patient (ratio)	-	-	1.01	0.98
Pneumonia Care				
Appropriate Initial Antibiotic Given	33	97%	95%	95%
Blood Culture Timing	50	100%	98%	98%
Pregnancy and Delivery Care				
Newborn Deliveries Scheduled Early[5]	-	-	5%	6%
Preventive Care				
Immunization for Influenza[2]	265	98%	91%	90%
Immunization for Pneumonia[2]	252	97%	92%	92%
Stroke Care				
Anticoagulation Therapy for Atrial Fibrillation[1,3]	-	-	94%	95%
Antithrombotic Therapy Timing[1,3]	-	-	97%	98%
Assessed for Rehabilitation[1,3]	-	-	96%	97%
Discharged on Antithrombotic Therapy[1,3]	-	-	98%	99%
Discharged on Statin Medication[1,3]	-	-	91%	94%
Thrombolytic Therapy Timing[1,3]	-	-	54%	66%
Venous Thromboembolism Prophylaxis[1,3]	-	-	91%	94%
Written Stroke Educational Materials Given[1,3]	-	-	82%	88%
Surgical Care Improvement Project				
Appropriate Beta Blocker Usage[1,3]	-	-	98%	98%
Appropriate VTP Within 24 Hours[3]	23	100%	98%	98%
Controlled Postoperative Blood Glucose[3,7]	-	-	97%	97%
Perioperative Temperature Management[3]	23	100%	100%	100%
Prophylactic Antibiotic Selection[3]	11	100%	99%	99%
Prophylactic Antibiotic Selection (Outpatient)[3,7]	-	-	98%	98%
Prophylactic Antibiotic Stopped[3]	11	91%	98%	98%
Prophylactic Antibiotic Timing[3]	11	82%	99%	99%
Prophylactic Antibiotic Timing (Outpatient)[3,7]	-	-	98%	98%
Urinary Catheter Removal[3]	14	93%	98%	97%
Survey of Patients' Hospital Experiences				
Area Around Room 'Always' Quiet at Night	(a)	67%	61%	61%
Doctors 'Always' Communicated Well	(a)	85%	83%	82%
Home Recovery Information Given	(a)	86%	86%	85%
Hospital Given 9 or 10 on 10 Point Scale	(a)	76%	74%	71%
Meds 'Always' Explained Before Given	(a)	66%	64%	64%
Nurses 'Always' Communicated Well	(a)	82%	81%	79%
Pain 'Always' Well Controlled	(a)	75%	73%	71%
Room and Bathroom 'Always' Clean	(a)	88%	76%	73%
Timely Help 'Always' Received	(a)	72%	71%	68%
Would Definitely Recommend Hospital	(a)	82%	73%	71%
Use of Medical Imaging				
Cardiac Imaging Stress Test before Surgery[1]	-	-	5.4%	5.3%
Combination Abdominal CT Scan	250	2.8%	9.3%	10.5%
Combination Brain/Sinus CT Scan[1]	-	-	2.6%	2.7%
Combination Chest CT Scan	99	0.0%	4.6%	2.7%
Follow-up Mammogram/Ultrasound	301	7.0%	8.4%	8.8%
Lumbar Spine MRI for Low Back Pain[1]	-	-	38.7%	37.2%

Indiana University Health Bloomington Hospital

601 W Second St
Bloomington, IN 47403
Phone: 812-353-9555
Fax: 812-353-9321
E-mail: info@bloomingtonhospital.org
URL: www.bloomingtonhospital.org
Type: Acute Care Hospitals
Emergency Services: Yes
Ownership: Voluntary non-profit - Private
Beds: 355

Key Personnel:
Chief of Medical Staff. . . . . Ken Marshall, MD
CEO/President. . . . . Mark E Moore
Radiology. . . . . Bruce Riley

Measure	Cases	This Hosp.	State Avg.	U.S. Avg.
Blood Clot Prevention and Treatment				
Anticoagulation Overlap Therapy[2]	87	99%	92%	93%
ICU Venous Thromboembolism Prophylaxis[2]	87	98%	91%	92%
Incidence of Potentially Preventable VTE[1,2]	-	-	10%	10%
UFH with Dosages/Platelet Monitoring[2]	24	100%	95%	97%
Venous Thromboembolism Prophylaxis[2]	263	90%	83%	85%
Warfarin Therapy Discharge Instructions[2]	66	68%	71%	75%
Chest Pain/Possible Heart Attack Care				
Aspirin Given Within 24 Hours of Arrival[1,3]	-	-	96%	96%
Fibrinolytic Meds Within 30 Min. of Arrival[3,7]	-	-	48%	58%
Average Time to ECG (minutes)[1,3]	-	-	6	7
Average Time to Transfer (minutes)[3,7]	-	-	46	60
Children's Asthma Care				
Received Home Management Plan of Care	-	-	-	88%
Received Reliever Medication	-	-	-	100%
Received Systemic Corticosteroids	-	-	-	100%
Emergency Department				
Admittance Decision Time (minutes)[2]	460	74	80	98
Head CT Results Within 45 Min. of Arrival[1]	-	-	60%	57%
Patients Who Left ER Before Being Seen	52,475	5%	2%	2%
Time from ER Arrival to Admit. (minutes)[2]	472	240	241	274
Time from ER Arrival to Discharge (minutes)	385	167	122	134
Time in ER Before Being Evaluated (minutes)	412	26	22	26
Time to Pain Meds for Fractures (minutes)	196	59	52	57
Heart Attack Care				
Aspirin Given at Discharge[2]	323	100%	99%	99%
Fibrinolytic Meds Within 30 Min. of Arrival[2,7]	-	-	67%	54%
PCI Within 90 Minutes of Arrival[2]	63	100%	97%	96%
Statin Prescribed at Discharge[2]	322	100%	99%	98%
Heart Failure Care				
ACE Inhibitor or ARB for LVSD	70	100%	97%	97%
Discharge Instructions Given	146	100%	95%	94%
Evaluation of LVS Function	216	100%	99%	99%
Medicare Spending				
Medicare Spending per Patient (ratio)	-	1.04	1.01	0.98
Pneumonia Care				
Appropriate Initial Antibiotic Given[2]	97	95%	95%	95%
Blood Culture Timing[2]	150	96%	98%	98%
Pregnancy and Delivery Care				
Newborn Deliveries Scheduled Early[2]	30	0%	5%	6%
Preventive Care				
Immunization for Influenza[2]	577	94%	91%	90%
Immunization for Pneumonia[2]	609	90%	92%	92%
Stroke Care				
Anticoagulation Therapy for Atrial Fibrillation	22	95%	94%	95%
Antithrombotic Therapy Timing	154	100%	97%	98%
Assessed for Rehabilitation	225	98%	96%	97%
Discharged on Antithrombotic Therapy	198	98%	98%	99%
Discharged on Statin Medication	161	98%	91%	94%
Thrombolytic Therapy Timing	15	93%	54%	66%
Venous Thromboembolism Prophylaxis	203	97%	91%	94%
Written Stroke Educational Materials Given	99	91%	82%	88%
Surgical Care Improvement Project				
Appropriate Beta Blocker Usage[2]	243	100%	98%	98%
Appropriate VTP Within 24 Hours[2]	366	100%	98%	98%
Controlled Postoperative Blood Glucose[2]	129	99%	97%	97%
Perioperative Temperature Management[2]	502	100%	100%	100%
Prophylactic Antibiotic Selection[2]	432	100%	99%	99%
Prophylactic Antibiotic Selection (Outpatient)	681	98%	98%	98%
Prophylactic Antibiotic Stopped[2]	409	100%	98%	98%
Prophylactic Antibiotic Timing[2]	433	99%	99%	99%
Prophylactic Antibiotic Timing (Outpatient)	681	99%	98%	98%
Urinary Catheter Removal[2]	418	100%	98%	97%
Survey of Patients' Hospital Experiences				
Area Around Room 'Always' Quiet at Night	300+	54%	61%	61%
Doctors 'Always' Communicated Well	300+	81%	83%	82%
Home Recovery Information Given	300+	88%	86%	85%
Hospital Given 9 or 10 on 10 Point Scale	300+	72%	74%	71%
Meds 'Always' Explained Before Given	300+	62%	64%	64%
Nurses 'Always' Communicated Well	300+	79%	81%	79%
Pain 'Always' Well Controlled	300+	73%	73%	71%
Room and Bathroom 'Always' Clean	300+	68%	76%	73%
Timely Help 'Always' Received	300+	70%	71%	68%
Would Definitely Recommend Hospital	300+	75%	73%	71%
Use of Medical Imaging				
Cardiac Imaging Stress Test before Surgery	463	7.8%	5.4%	5.3%
Combination Abdominal CT Scan	1,020	7.4%	9.3%	10.5%
Combination Brain/Sinus CT Scan	1,128	2.0%	2.6%	2.7%
Combination Chest CT Scan	340	1.8%	4.6%	2.7%
Follow-up Mammogram/Ultrasound[7]	-	-	8.4%	8.8%
Lumbar Spine MRI for Low Back Pain	93	33.3%	38.7%	37.2%

Monroe Hospital

4011 S Monroe Medical Park Blvd
Bloomington, IN 47403
Phone: 812-825-1111
URL: www.monroehospital.com
Type: Acute Care Hospitals
Emergency Services: Yes
Ownership: Proprietary

Measure	Cases	This Hosp.	State Avg.	U.S. Avg.
Blood Clot Prevention and Treatment				
Anticoagulation Overlap Therapy[2]	11	64%	92%	93%
ICU Venous Thromboembolism Prophylaxis[2]	21	81%	91%	92%
Incidence of Potentially Preventable VTE[1,2]	-	-	10%	10%
UFH with Dosages/Platelet Monitoring[1,2]	-	-	95%	97%
Venous Thromboembolism Prophylaxis[2]	126	72%	83%	85%
Warfarin Therapy Discharge Instructions[1,2]	-	-	71%	75%
Chest Pain/Possible Heart Attack Care				
Aspirin Given Within 24 Hours of Arrival	21	90%	96%	96%
Fibrinolytic Meds Within 30 Min. of Arrival[7]	-	-	48%	58%
Average Time to ECG (minutes)	23	9	6	7
Average Time to Transfer (minutes)	14	124	46	60
Children's Asthma Care				
Received Home Management Plan of Care	-	-	-	88%
Received Reliever Medication	-	-	-	100%
Received Systemic Corticosteroids	-	-	-	100%
Emergency Department				
Admittance Decision Time (minutes)[2]	231	67	80	98
Head CT Results Within 45 Min. of Arrival[1]	-	-	60%	57%
Patients Who Left ER Before Being Seen	13,316	1%	2%	2%
Time from ER Arrival to Admit. (minutes)[2]	232	238	241	274

NOTE: Hospital profiles are in alphabetical order by state, then city, then hospital within the city; Rankings exclude hospitals with less than 25 cases except for patient surveys which excludes hospitals with less than 100 cases; (a) 100-299 cases; (1) The number of cases/patients is too few to report; (2) Data submitted were based on a sample of cases/patients; (3) Results are based on a shorter time period than required; (4) Data suppressed by CMS for one or more quarters; (5) Results are not available for this reporting period; (6) Fewer than 100 patients completed the HCAHPS survey; (7) No cases met the criteria for this measure; (8) The lower limit of the confidence interval cannot be calculated if the number of observed infections equals zero; (9) No data are available from the state/territory for this reporting period; (10) The scores shown reflect fewer than 50 completed surveys; (11) There were discrepancies in the data collection process; (12) This measure does not apply to this hospital for this reporting period; (13) Results cannot be calculated for this reporting period; (14) The results for this state are combined with nearby states to protect confidentiality; Please refer to the User's Guide for a full explanation of data.

Measure	Cases	This Hosp.	State Avg.	U.S. Avg.
Time from ER Arrival to Discharge (minutes)	354	90	122	134
Time in ER Before Being Evaluated (minutes)	370	22	22	26
Time to Pain Meds for Fractures (minutes)	42	56	52	57
Heart Attack Care				
Aspirin Given at Discharge[3,7]	-	-	99%	99%
Fibrinolytic Meds Within 30 Min. of Arrival[3,7]	-	-	67%	54%
PCI Within 90 Minutes of Arrival[3,7]	-	-	97%	96%
Statin Prescribed at Discharge[3,7]	-	-	99%	98%
Heart Failure Care				
ACE Inhibitor or ARB for LVSD[1]	-	-	97%	97%
Discharge Instructions Given	12	42%	95%	94%
Evaluation of LVS Function	16	75%	99%	99%
Medicare Spending				
Medicare Spending per Patient (ratio)	-	1.04	1.01	0.98
Pneumonia Care				
Appropriate Initial Antibiotic Given	30	73%	95%	95%
Blood Culture Timing	22	100%	98%	98%
Pregnancy and Delivery Care				
Newborn Deliveries Scheduled Early[7]	-	-	5%	6%
Preventive Care				
Immunization for Influenza[2]	345	66%	91%	90%
Immunization for Pneumonia[2]	458	67%	92%	92%
Stroke Care				
Anticoagulation Therapy for Atrial Fibrillation[1]	-	-	94%	95%
Antithrombotic Therapy Timing[1]	-	-	97%	98%
Assessed for Rehabilitation[1]	-	-	96%	97%
Discharged on Antithrombotic Therapy[1]	-	-	98%	99%
Discharged on Statin Medication[1]	-	-	91%	94%
Thrombolytic Therapy Timing[7]	-	-	54%	66%
Venous Thromboembolism Prophylaxis[1]	-	-	91%	94%
Written Stroke Educational Materials Given[1]	-	-	82%	88%
Surgical Care Improvement Project				
Appropriate Beta Blocker Usage	79	84%	98%	98%
Appropriate VTP Within 24 Hours	281	91%	98%	98%
Controlled Postoperative Blood Glucose[7]	-	-	97%	97%
Perioperative Temperature Management	302	100%	100%	100%
Prophylactic Antibiotic Selection	245	98%	99%	99%
Prophylactic Antibiotic Selection (Outpatient)	127	98%	98%	98%
Prophylactic Antibiotic Stopped	241	88%	98%	98%
Prophylactic Antibiotic Timing	245	94%	99%	99%
Prophylactic Antibiotic Timing (Outpatient)	129	96%	98%	98%
Urinary Catheter Removal	248	94%	98%	97%
Survey of Patients' Hospital Experiences				
Area Around Room 'Always' Quiet at Night	300+	72%	61%	61%
Doctors 'Always' Communicated Well	300+	84%	83%	82%
Home Recovery Information Given	300+	82%	86%	85%
Hospital Given 9 or 10 on 10 Point Scale	300+	76%	74%	71%
Meds 'Always' Explained Before Given	300+	61%	64%	64%
Nurses 'Always' Communicated Well	300+	80%	81%	79%
Pain 'Always' Well Controlled	300+	74%	73%	71%
Room and Bathroom 'Always' Clean	300+	82%	76%	73%
Timely Help 'Always' Received	300+	68%	71%	68%
Would Definitely Recommend Hospital	300+	76%	73%	71%
Use of Medical Imaging				
Cardiac Imaging Stress Test before Surgery	90	7.8%	5.4%	5.3%
Combination Abdominal CT Scan	383	3.4%	9.3%	10.5%
Combination Brain/Sinus CT Scan[1]	-	-	2.6%	2.7%
Combination Chest CT Scan	264	0.8%	4.6%	2.7%
Follow-up Mammogram/Ultrasound	132	13.6%	8.4%	8.8%
Lumbar Spine MRI for Low Back Pain	174	37.9%	38.7%	37.2%

Bluffton Regional Medical Center

303 S Main St
Bluffton, IN 46714
Phone: 260-824-3210
Fax: 260-919-3851
URL: www.blufftonregional.com
Type: Acute Care Hospitals
Emergency Services: Yes
Ownership: Proprietary
Beds: 79

Key Personnel:
CEO/President. . . . . Thomas Clark
Radiology. . . . . Brett Hagedorn
Emergency Room . . . . Derrick Williams

Measure	Cases	This Hosp.	State Avg.	U.S. Avg.
Blood Clot Prevention and Treatment				
Anticoagulation Overlap Therapy[2]	18	100%	92%	93%
ICU Venous Thromboembolism Prophylaxis[2]	61	100%	91%	92%
Incidence of Potentially Preventable VTE[1,2]	-	-	10%	10%
UFH with Dosages/Platelet Monitoring[1,2]	-	-	95%	97%
Venous Thromboembolism Prophylaxis[2]	328	99%	83%	85%
Warfarin Therapy Discharge Instructions[2]	14	100%	71%	75%
Chest Pain/Possible Heart Attack Care				
Aspirin Given Within 24 Hours of Arrival	54	100%	96%	96%
Fibrinolytic Meds Within 30 Min. of Arrival[7]	-	-	48%	58%
Average Time to ECG (minutes)	55	4	6	7
Average Time to Transfer (minutes)[1]	-	-	46	60
Children's Asthma Care				
Received Home Management Plan of Care	-	-	-	88%
Received Reliever Medication	-	-	-	100%
Received Systemic Corticosteroids	-	-	-	100%
Emergency Department				
Admittance Decision Time (minutes)[2]	374	48	80	98
Head CT Results Within 45 Min. of Arrival[1]	-	-	60%	57%
Patients Who Left ER Before Being Seen	9,669	0%	2%	2%
Time from ER Arrival to Admit. (minutes)[2]	391	184	241	274
Time from ER Arrival to Discharge (minutes)	377	110	122	134
Time in ER Before Being Evaluated (minutes)	409	16	22	26
Time to Pain Meds for Fractures (minutes)	53	44	52	57
Heart Attack Care				
Aspirin Given at Discharge[1]	-	-	99%	99%
Fibrinolytic Meds Within 30 Min. of Arrival[7]	-	-	67%	54%
PCI Within 90 Minutes of Arrival[7]	-	-	97%	96%
Statin Prescribed at Discharge[1]	-	-	99%	98%
Heart Failure Care				
ACE Inhibitor or ARB for LVSD	26	96%	97%	97%
Discharge Instructions Given	41	98%	95%	94%
Evaluation of LVS Function	61	100%	99%	99%
Medicare Spending				
Medicare Spending per Patient (ratio)	-	0.96	1.01	0.98
Pneumonia Care				
Appropriate Initial Antibiotic Given	72	99%	95%	95%
Blood Culture Timing	85	100%	98%	98%
Pregnancy and Delivery Care				
Newborn Deliveries Scheduled Early	20	0%	5%	6%
Preventive Care				
Immunization for Influenza[2]	337	100%	91%	90%
Immunization for Pneumonia[2]	530	99%	92%	92%
Stroke Care				
Anticoagulation Therapy for Atrial Fibrillation[1]	-	-	94%	95%
Antithrombotic Therapy Timing	14	100%	97%	98%
Assessed for Rehabilitation	16	100%	96%	97%
Discharged on Antithrombotic Therapy	13	100%	98%	99%
Discharged on Statin Medication	12	100%	91%	94%
Thrombolytic Therapy Timing[7]	-	-	54%	66%
Venous Thromboembolism Prophylaxis	14	93%	91%	94%
Written Stroke Educational Materials Given[1]	-	-	82%	88%
Surgical Care Improvement Project				
Appropriate Beta Blocker Usage	23	100%	98%	98%
Appropriate VTP Within 24 Hours	65	100%	98%	98%
Controlled Postoperative Blood Glucose[7]	-	-	97%	97%
Perioperative Temperature Management	76	100%	100%	100%
Prophylactic Antibiotic Selection	60	100%	99%	99%
Prophylactic Antibiotic Selection (Outpatient)[3]	14	93%	98%	98%
Prophylactic Antibiotic Stopped	56	98%	98%	98%
Prophylactic Antibiotic Timing	60	100%	99%	99%
Prophylactic Antibiotic Timing (Outpatient)[3]	14	100%	98%	98%
Urinary Catheter Removal	51	100%	98%	97%
Survey of Patients' Hospital Experiences				
Area Around Room 'Always' Quiet at Night	300+	61%	61%	61%
Doctors 'Always' Communicated Well	300+	80%	83%	82%
Home Recovery Information Given	300+	88%	86%	85%
Hospital Given 9 or 10 on 10 Point Scale	300+	75%	74%	71%
Meds 'Always' Explained Before Given	300+	65%	64%	64%
Nurses 'Always' Communicated Well	300+	83%	81%	79%
Pain 'Always' Well Controlled	300+	71%	73%	71%
Room and Bathroom 'Always' Clean	300+	81%	76%	73%
Timely Help 'Always' Received	300+	69%	71%	68%
Would Definitely Recommend Hospital	300+	76%	73%	71%
Use of Medical Imaging				
Cardiac Imaging Stress Test before Surgery[1]	-	-	5.4%	5.3%
Combination Abdominal CT Scan	249	4.8%	9.3%	10.5%
Combination Brain/Sinus CT Scan[1]	-	-	2.6%	2.7%
Combination Chest CT Scan	108	0.0%	4.6%	2.7%
Follow-up Mammogram/Ultrasound	587	6.1%	8.4%	8.8%
Lumbar Spine MRI for Low Back Pain[1]	-	-	38.7%	37.2%

Saint Mary's Warrick Hospital

1116 Millis Ave
Boonville, IN 47601
Phone: 812-897-4800
Fax: 812-897-7375
URL: www.stmarys.org
Type: Critical Access Hospitals
Emergency Services: Yes
Ownership: Voluntary non-profit - Private
Beds: 25

Key Personnel:
Emergency Room . . . . David Baughn
CEO/President. . . . . Marc Dooley
Chief of Medical Staff . . . . David Vaughn

Measure	Cases	This Hosp.	State Avg.	U.S. Avg.
Blood Clot Prevention and Treatment				
Anticoagulation Overlap Therapy[2,7]	-	-	92%	93%
ICU Venous Thromboembolism Prophylaxis[2,7]	-	-	91%	92%
Incidence of Potentially Preventable VTE[2,7]	-	-	10%	10%
UFH with Dosages/Platelet Monitoring[2,7]	-	-	95%	97%
Venous Thromboembolism Prophylaxis[2]	180	63%	83%	85%
Warfarin Therapy Discharge Instructions[2,7]	-	-	71%	75%
Chest Pain/Possible Heart Attack Care				
Aspirin Given Within 24 Hours of Arrival[5]	-	-	96%	96%
Fibrinolytic Meds Within 30 Min. of Arrival[5]	-	-	48%	58%
Average Time to ECG (minutes)[5]	-	-	6	7
Average Time to Transfer (minutes)[5]	-	-	46	60
Children's Asthma Care				
Received Home Management Plan of Care	-	-	-	88%
Received Reliever Medication	-	-	-	100%
Received Systemic Corticosteroids	-	-	-	100%
Emergency Department				
Admittance Decision Time (minutes)[2]	318	50	80	98
Head CT Results Within 45 Min. of Arrival[5]	-	-	60%	57%
Patients Who Left ER Before Being Seen	8,364	3%	2%	2%
Time from ER Arrival to Admit. (minutes)[2]	334	149	241	274
Time from ER Arrival to Discharge (minutes)[5]	-	-	122	134
Time in ER Before Being Evaluated (minutes)[5]	-	-	22	26
Time to Pain Meds for Fractures (minutes)[5]	-	-	52	57
Heart Attack Care				
Aspirin Given at Discharge[3,7]	-	-	99%	99%
Fibrinolytic Meds Within 30 Min. of Arrival[3,7]	-	-	67%	54%
PCI Within 90 Minutes of Arrival[3,7]	-	-	97%	96%
Statin Prescribed at Discharge[3,7]	-	-	99%	98%
Heart Failure Care				
ACE Inhibitor or ARB for LVSD[1]	-	-	97%	97%
Discharge Instructions Given[1]	-	-	95%	94%
Evaluation of LVS Function[1]	-	-	99%	99%
Medicare Spending				
Medicare Spending per Patient (ratio)	-	-	1.01	0.98
Pneumonia Care				
Appropriate Initial Antibiotic Given	31	97%	95%	95%
Blood Culture Timing	32	94%	98%	98%
Pregnancy and Delivery Care				
Newborn Deliveries Scheduled Early[3,7]	-	-	5%	6%
Preventive Care				
Immunization for Influenza[2]	247	99%	91%	90%
Immunization for Pneumonia[2]	356	99%	92%	92%
Stroke Care				
Anticoagulation Therapy for Atrial Fibrillation[5]	-	-	94%	95%
Antithrombotic Therapy Timing[5]	-	-	97%	98%
Assessed for Rehabilitation[5]	-	-	96%	97%
Discharged on Antithrombotic Therapy[5]	-	-	98%	99%
Discharged on Statin Medication[5]	-	-	91%	94%
Thrombolytic Therapy Timing[5]	-	-	54%	66%
Venous Thromboembolism Prophylaxis[5]	-	-	91%	94%
Written Stroke Educational Materials Given[5]	-	-	82%	88%
Surgical Care Improvement Project				

NOTE: Hospital profiles are in alphabetical order by state, then city, then hospital within the city; Rankings exclude hospitals with less than 25 cases except for patient surveys which excludes hospitals with less than 100 cases; (a) 100-299 cases; (1) The number of cases/patients is too few to report; (2) Data submitted were based on a sample of cases/patients; (3) Results are based on a shorter time period than required; (4) Data suppressed by CMS for one or more quarters; (5) Results are not available for this reporting period; (6) Fewer than 100 patients completed the HCAHPS survey; (7) No cases met the criteria for this measure; (8) The lower limit of the confidence interval cannot be calculated if the number of observed infections equals zero; (9) No data are available from the state/territory for this reporting period; (10) The scores shown reflect fewer than 50 completed surveys; (11) There were discrepancies in the data collection process; (12) This measure does not apply to this hospital for this reporting period; (13) Results cannot be calculated for this reporting period; (14) The results for this state are combined with nearby states to protect confidentiality; Please refer to the User's Guide for a full explanation of data.

Appropriate Beta Blocker Usage[5]	-	-	98%	98%
Appropriate VTP Within 24 Hours[5]	-	-	98%	98%
Controlled Postoperative Blood Glucose[5]	-	-	97%	97%
Perioperative Temperature Management[5]	-	-	100%	100%
Prophylactic Antibiotic Selection[5]	-	-	99%	99%
Prophylactic Antibiotic Selection (Outpatient)[5]	-	-	98%	98%
Prophylactic Antibiotic Stopped[5]	-	-	98%	98%
Prophylactic Antibiotic Timing[5]	-	-	99%	99%
Prophylactic Antibiotic Timing (Outpatient)[5]	-	-	98%	98%
Urinary Catheter Removal[5]	-	-	98%	97%
Survey of Patients' Hospital Experiences				
Area Around Room 'Always' Quiet at Night[5]	-	-	61%	61%
Doctors 'Always' Communicated Well[5]	-	-	83%	82%
Home Recovery Information Given[5]	-	-	86%	85%
Hospital Given 9 or 10 on 10 Point Scale[5]	-	-	74%	71%
Meds 'Always' Explained Before Given[5]	-	-	64%	64%
Nurses 'Always' Communicated Well[5]	-	-	81%	79%
Pain 'Always' Well Controlled[5]	-	-	73%	71%
Room and Bathroom 'Always' Clean[5]	-	-	76%	73%
Timely Help 'Always' Received[5]	-	-	71%	68%
Would Definitely Recommend Hospital[5]	-	-	73%	71%
Use of Medical Imaging				
Cardiac Imaging Stress Test before Surgery[1]	-	-	5.4%	5.3%
Combination Abdominal CT Scan	129	0.0%	9.3%	10.5%
Combination Brain/Sinus CT Scan	127	7.1%	2.6%	2.7%
Combination Chest CT Scan[1]	-	-	4.6%	2.7%
Follow-up Mammogram/Ultrasound	68	4.4%	8.4%	8.8%
Lumbar Spine MRI for Low Back Pain[1]	-	-	38.7%	37.2%

Saint Vincent Clay Hospital

1206 E National Ave
Brazil, IN 47834
URL: www.stvincent.org/faccen/clay
Phone: 812-442-2500
Fax: 812-442-2605
Type: Critical Access Hospitals
Ownership: Voluntary non-profit - Private
Emergency Services: Yes
Beds: 58

Key Personnel:
Chief of Medical Staff.......... Catherine Brush
Quality Assurance .... Thomas Falen, RN
CEO/President................ Jonathan Nalli
Emergency Room .... R Curtis Oehler, MD
Operating Room............... Jamie J Webster

Measure	Cases	This Hosp.	State Avg.	U.S. Avg.
Blood Clot Prevention and Treatment				
Anticoagulation Overlap Therapy[5]	-	-	92%	93%
ICU Venous Thromboembolism Prophylaxis[5]	-	-	91%	92%
Incidence of Potentially Preventable VTE[5]	-	-	10%	10%
UFH with Dosages/Platelet Monitoring[5]	-	-	95%	97%
Venous Thromboembolism Prophylaxis[5]	-	-	83%	85%
Warfarin Therapy Discharge Instructions[5]	-	-	71%	75%
Chest Pain/Possible Heart Attack Care				
Aspirin Given Within 24 Hours of Arrival	25	88%	96%	96%
Fibrinolytic Meds Within 30 Min. of Arrival[7]	-	-	48%	58%
Average Time to ECG (minutes)	26	9	6	7
Average Time to Transfer (minutes)[1]	-	-	46	60
Children's Asthma Care				
Received Home Management Plan of Care	-	-	-	88%
Received Reliever Medication	-	-	-	100%
Received Systemic Corticosteroids	-	-	-	100%
Emergency Department				
Admittance Decision Time (minutes)	254	65	80	98
Head CT Results Within 45 Min. of Arrival[1]	-	-	60%	57%
Patients Who Left ER Before Being Seen	10,647	1%	2%	2%
Time from ER Arrival to Admit. (minutes)	329	250	241	274
Time from ER Arrival to Discharge (minutes)	320	134	122	134
Time in ER Before Being Evaluated (minutes)	368	29	22	26
Time to Pain Meds for Fractures (minutes)[5]	-	-	52	57
Heart Attack Care				
Aspirin Given at Discharge[3,7]	-	-	99%	99%
Fibrinolytic Meds Within 30 Min. of Arrival[3,7]	-	-	67%	54%
PCI Within 90 Minutes of Arrival[3,7]	-	-	97%	96%
Statin Prescribed at Discharge[3,7]	-	-	99%	98%
Heart Failure Care				
ACE Inhibitor or ARB for LVSD[1]	-	-	97%	97%
Discharge Instructions Given	17	76%	95%	94%
Evaluation of LVS Function	21	86%	99%	99%
Medicare Spending				
Medicare Spending per Patient (ratio)	-	-	1.01	0.98
Pneumonia Care				
Appropriate Initial Antibiotic Given	16	94%	95%	95%
Blood Culture Timing	14	100%	98%	98%
Pregnancy and Delivery Care				
Newborn Deliveries Scheduled Early[5]	-	-	5%	6%
Preventive Care				
Immunization for Influenza	283	81%	91%	90%
Immunization for Pneumonia	412	87%	92%	92%
Stroke Care				
Anticoagulation Therapy for Atrial Fibrillation[3,7]	-	-	94%	95%
Antithrombotic Therapy Timing[1,3]	-	-	97%	98%
Assessed for Rehabilitation[1,3]	-	-	96%	97%
Discharged on Antithrombotic Therapy[1,3]	-	-	98%	99%
Discharged on Statin Medication[1,3]	-	-	91%	94%
Thrombolytic Therapy Timing[1,3]	-	-	54%	66%
Venous Thromboembolism Prophylaxis[1,3]	-	-	91%	94%
Written Stroke Educational Materials Given[1,3]	-	-	82%	88%
Surgical Care Improvement Project				
Appropriate Beta Blocker Usage[1]	-	-	98%	98%
Appropriate VTP Within 24 Hours	12	100%	98%	98%
Controlled Postoperative Blood Glucose[3,7]	-	-	97%	97%
Perioperative Temperature Management	13	100%	100%	100%
Prophylactic Antibiotic Selection[1]	-	-	99%	99%
Prophylactic Antibiotic Selection (Outpatient)[5]	-	-	98%	98%
Prophylactic Antibiotic Stopped[1]	-	-	98%	98%
Prophylactic Antibiotic Timing[1]	-	-	99%	99%
Prophylactic Antibiotic Timing (Outpatient)[5]	-	-	98%	98%
Urinary Catheter Removal[1]	-	-	98%	97%
Survey of Patients' Hospital Experiences				
Area Around Room 'Always' Quiet at Night	(a)	61%	61%	61%
Doctors 'Always' Communicated Well	(a)	90%	83%	82%
Home Recovery Information Given	(a)	85%	86%	85%
Hospital Given 9 or 10 on 10 Point Scale	(a)	68%	74%	71%
Meds 'Always' Explained Before Given	(a)	69%	64%	64%
Nurses 'Always' Communicated Well	(a)	84%	81%	79%
Pain 'Always' Well Controlled	(a)	73%	73%	71%
Room and Bathroom 'Always' Clean	(a)	76%	76%	73%
Timely Help 'Always' Received	(a)	66%	71%	68%
Would Definitely Recommend Hospital	(a)	65%	73%	71%
Use of Medical Imaging				
Cardiac Imaging Stress Test before Surgery[1]	-	-	5.4%	5.3%
Combination Abdominal CT Scan	256	45.3%	9.3%	10.5%
Combination Brain/Sinus CT Scan[1]	-	-	2.6%	2.7%
Combination Chest CT Scan	165	0.0%	4.6%	2.7%
Follow-up Mammogram/Ultrasound	252	3.6%	8.4%	8.8%
Lumbar Spine MRI for Low Back Pain[1]	-	-	38.7%	37.2%

Community Hospital of Bremen

1020 High Rd
Bremen, IN 46506
E-mail: pboard@bremenhospital.com
URL: www.bremenhospital.com
Phone: 574-546-2211
Fax: 574-546-4312
Type: Critical Access Hospitals
Ownership: Voluntary non-profit - Private
Emergency Services: Yes
Beds: 24

Key Personnel:
Quality Assurance .... Dick Balmer
Infection Control.............. Teresa Brown, RN
Chief of Medical Staff.......... Carey Gear, MD
Emergency Room .... Carey Gear, MD
CEO/President................ Scott Graybill
Cardiology .... John Katsaropoulos, M.D.
Anesthesiology................ Great Lakes

Measure	Cases	This Hosp.	State Avg.	U.S. Avg.
Blood Clot Prevention and Treatment				
Anticoagulation Overlap Therapy[1]	-	-	92%	93%
ICU Venous Thromboembolism Prophylaxis[7]	-	-	91%	92%
Incidence of Potentially Preventable VTE[7]	-	-	10%	10%
UFH with Dosages/Platelet Monitoring[7]	-	-	95%	97%
Venous Thromboembolism Prophylaxis[7]	-	-	83%	85%
Warfarin Therapy Discharge Instructions[1]	-	-	71%	75%
Chest Pain/Possible Heart Attack Care				
Aspirin Given Within 24 Hours of Arrival[3]	11	100%	96%	96%
Fibrinolytic Meds Within 30 Min. of Arrival[3,7]	-	-	48%	58%
Average Time to ECG (minutes)[3]	12	12	6	7
Average Time to Transfer (minutes)[1,3]	-	-	46	60
Children's Asthma Care				
Received Home Management Plan of Care	-	-	-	88%
Received Reliever Medication	-	-	-	100%
Received Systemic Corticosteroids	-	-	-	100%
Emergency Department				
Admittance Decision Time (minutes)[5]	-	-	80	98
Head CT Results Within 45 Min. of Arrival[5]	-	-	60%	57%
Patients Who Left ER Before Being Seen	24	33%	2%	2%
Time from ER Arrival to Admit. (minutes)[5]	-	-	241	274
Time from ER Arrival to Discharge (minutes)[5]	-	-	122	134
Time in ER Before Being Evaluated (minutes)[5]	-	-	22	26
Time to Pain Meds for Fractures (minutes)[5]	-	-	52	57
Heart Attack Care				
Aspirin Given at Discharge[1,3]	-	-	99%	99%
Fibrinolytic Meds Within 30 Min. of Arrival[3,7]	-	-	67%	54%
PCI Within 90 Minutes of Arrival[3,7]	-	-	97%	96%
Statin Prescribed at Discharge[1,3]	-	-	99%	98%
Heart Failure Care				
ACE Inhibitor or ARB for LVSD[1]	-	-	97%	97%
Discharge Instructions Given	18	61%	95%	94%
Evaluation of LVS Function	21	90%	99%	99%
Medicare Spending				
Medicare Spending per Patient (ratio)	-	-	1.01	0.98
Pneumonia Care				
Appropriate Initial Antibiotic Given[1,2]	-	-	95%	95%
Blood Culture Timing[1,2]	-	-	98%	98%
Pregnancy and Delivery Care				
Newborn Deliveries Scheduled Early[5]	-	-	5%	6%
Preventive Care				
Immunization for Influenza[5]	-	-	91%	90%
Immunization for Pneumonia[5]	-	-	92%	92%
Stroke Care				
Anticoagulation Therapy for Atrial Fibrillation[7]	-	-	94%	95%
Antithrombotic Therapy Timing[1]	-	-	97%	98%
Assessed for Rehabilitation[1]	-	-	96%	97%
Discharged on Antithrombotic Therapy[1]	-	-	98%	99%
Discharged on Statin Medication[1]	-	-	91%	94%
Thrombolytic Therapy Timing[1]	-	-	54%	66%
Venous Thromboembolism Prophylaxis[1]	-	-	91%	94%
Written Stroke Educational Materials Given[1]	-	-	82%	88%
Surgical Care Improvement Project				
Appropriate Beta Blocker Usage[1]	-	-	98%	98%
Appropriate VTP Within 24 Hours	19	95%	98%	98%
Controlled Postoperative Blood Glucose[7]	-	-	97%	97%
Perioperative Temperature Management	22	95%	100%	100%
Prophylactic Antibiotic Selection	17	94%	99%	99%
Prophylactic Antibiotic Selection (Outpatient)[1,3]	-	-	98%	98%
Prophylactic Antibiotic Stopped	17	88%	98%	98%
Prophylactic Antibiotic Timing	17	88%	99%	99%
Prophylactic Antibiotic Timing (Outpatient)[1,3]	-	-	98%	98%
Urinary Catheter Removal	13	100%	98%	97%
Survey of Patients' Hospital Experiences				
Area Around Room 'Always' Quiet at Night[5]	-	-	61%	61%
Doctors 'Always' Communicated Well[5]	-	-	83%	82%
Home Recovery Information Given[5]	-	-	86%	85%
Hospital Given 9 or 10 on 10 Point Scale[5]	-	-	74%	71%
Meds 'Always' Explained Before Given[5]	-	-	64%	64%
Nurses 'Always' Communicated Well[5]	-	-	81%	79%
Pain 'Always' Well Controlled[5]	-	-	73%	71%
Room and Bathroom 'Always' Clean[5]	-	-	76%	73%
Timely Help 'Always' Received[5]	-	-	71%	68%
Would Definitely Recommend Hospital[5]	-	-	73%	71%
Use of Medical Imaging				
Cardiac Imaging Stress Test before Surgery[7]	-	-	5.4%	5.3%
Combination Abdominal CT Scan	122	3.3%	9.3%	10.5%
Combination Brain/Sinus CT Scan	123	0.0%	2.6%	2.7%
Combination Chest CT Scan	50	0.0%	4.6%	2.7%

NOTE: Hospital profiles are in alphabetical order by state, then city, then hospital within the city; Rankings exclude hospitals with less than 25 cases except for patient surveys which excludes hospitals with less than 100 cases; (a) 100-299 cases; (1) The number of cases/patients is too few to report; (2) Data submitted were based on a sample of cases/patients; (3) Results are based on a shorter time period than required; (4) Data suppressed by CMS for one or more quarters; (5) Results are not available for this reporting period; (6) Fewer than 100 patients completed the HCAHPS survey; (7) No cases met the criteria for this measure; (8) The lower limit of the confidence interval cannot be calculated if the number of observed infections equals zero; (9) No data are available from the state/territory for this reporting period; (10) The scores shown reflect fewer than 50 completed surveys; (11) There were discrepancies in the data collection process; (12) This measure does not apply to this hospital for this reporting period; (13) Results cannot be calculated for this reporting period; (14) The results for this state are combined with nearby states to protect confidentiality; Please refer to the User's Guide for a full explanation of data.

Follow-up Mammogram/Ultrasound	192	8.9%	8.4%	8.8%
Lumbar Spine MRI for Low Back Pain[1]	-	-	38.7%	37.2%

Doctors Neuromedical Hospital & Brain Institute

411 S Whitlock St Phone: 574-546-3830
Bremen, IN 46506
Type: Acute Care Hospitals Emergency Services: No
Ownership: Proprietary

Measure	Cases	This Hosp.	State Avg.	U.S. Avg.
Blood Clot Prevention and Treatment				
Anticoagulation Overlap Therapy[1,2]	-	-	92%	93%
ICU Venous Thromboembolism Prophylaxis[2,3]	-	-	91%	92%
Incidence of Potentially Preventable VTE[2,3]	-	-	10%	10%
UFH with Dosages/Platelet Monitoring[2,3]	-	-	95%	97%
Venous Thromboembolism Prophylaxis[2,3]	23	0%	83%	85%
Warfarin Therapy Discharge Instructions[2,3]	-	-	71%	75%
Chest Pain/Possible Heart Attack Care				
Aspirin Given Within 24 Hours of Arrival[5]	-	-	96%	96%
Fibrinolytic Meds Within 30 Min. of Arrival[5]	-	-	48%	58%
Average Time to ECG (minutes)[5]	-	-	6	7
Average Time to Transfer (minutes)[5]	-	-	46	60
Children's Asthma Care				
Received Home Management Plan of Care	-	-	-	88%
Received Reliever Medication	-	-	-	100%
Received Systemic Corticosteroids	-	-	-	100%
Emergency Department				
Admittance Decision Time (minutes)[2,3]	-	-	80	98
Head CT Results Within 45 Min. of Arrival[5]	-	-	60%	57%
Patients Who Left ER Before Being Seen[5]	-	-	2%	2%
Time from ER Arrival to Admit. (minutes)[2,3]	-	-	241	274
Time from ER Arrival to Discharge (minutes)[5]	-	-	122	134
Time in ER Before Being Evaluated (minutes)[5]	-	-	22	26
Time to Pain Meds for Fractures (minutes)[5]	-	-	52	57
Heart Attack Care				
Aspirin Given at Discharge[5]	-	-	99%	99%
Fibrinolytic Meds Within 30 Min. of Arrival[5]	-	-	67%	54%
PCI Within 90 Minutes of Arrival[5]	-	-	97%	96%
Statin Prescribed at Discharge[5]	-	-	99%	98%
Heart Failure Care				
ACE Inhibitor or ARB for LVSD[2,3]	-	-	97%	97%
Discharge Instructions Given[1,2]	-	-	95%	94%
Evaluation of LVS Function[1,2]	-	-	99%	99%
Medicare Spending				
Medicare Spending per Patient (ratio)	-	-	1.01	0.98
Pneumonia Care				
Appropriate Initial Antibiotic Given[2,3]	-	-	95%	95%
Blood Culture Timing[2,3]	-	-	98%	98%
Pregnancy and Delivery Care				
Newborn Deliveries Scheduled Early[3,7]	-	-	5%	6%
Preventive Care				
Immunization for Influenza[5]	-	-	91%	90%
Immunization for Pneumonia[2,3]	132	100%	92%	92%
Stroke Care				
Anticoagulation Therapy for Atrial Fibrillation[1,2]	-	-	94%	95%
Antithrombotic Therapy Timing[2,3]	26	12%	97%	98%
Assessed for Rehabilitation[2,3]	31	19%	96%	97%
Discharged on Antithrombotic Therapy[2,3]	27	30%	98%	99%
Discharged on Statin Medication[2,3]	31	19%	91%	94%
Thrombolytic Therapy Timing[2,3]	-	-	54%	66%
Venous Thromboembolism Prophylaxis[2,3]	31	39%	91%	94%
Written Stroke Educational Materials Given[1,2]	-	-	82%	88%
Surgical Care Improvement Project				
Appropriate Beta Blocker Usage[5]	-	-	98%	98%
Appropriate VTP Within 24 Hours[5]	-	-	98%	98%
Controlled Postoperative Blood Glucose[5]	-	-	97%	97%
Perioperative Temperature Management[5]	-	-	100%	100%
Prophylactic Antibiotic Selection[5]	-	-	99%	99%
Prophylactic Antibiotic Selection (Outpatient)[5]	-	-	98%	98%
Prophylactic Antibiotic Stopped[5]	-	-	98%	98%
Prophylactic Antibiotic Timing[5]	-	-	99%	99%
Prophylactic Antibiotic Timing (Outpatient)[5]	-	-	98%	98%
Urinary Catheter Removal[5]	-	-	98%	97%
Survey of Patients' Hospital Experiences				
Area Around Room 'Always' Quiet at Night[5]	-	-	61%	61%
Doctors 'Always' Communicated Well[5]	-	-	83%	82%
Home Recovery Information Given[5]	-	-	86%	85%
Hospital Given 9 or 10 on 10 Point Scale[5]	-	-	74%	71%
Meds 'Always' Explained Before Given[5]	-	-	64%	64%
Nurses 'Always' Communicated Well[5]	-	-	81%	79%
Pain 'Always' Well Controlled[5]	-	-	73%	71%
Room and Bathroom 'Always' Clean[5]	-	-	76%	73%
Timely Help 'Always' Received[5]	-	-	71%	68%
Would Definitely Recommend Hospital[5]	-	-	73%	71%
Use of Medical Imaging				
Cardiac Imaging Stress Test before Surgery[7]	-	-	5.4%	5.3%
Combination Abdominal CT Scan[7]	-	-	9.3%	10.5%
Combination Brain/Sinus CT Scan[7]	-	-	2.6%	2.7%
Combination Chest CT Scan[7]	-	-	4.6%	2.7%
Follow-up Mammogram/Ultrasound[7]	-	-	8.4%	8.8%
Lumbar Spine MRI for Low Back Pain[7]	-	-	38.7%	37.2%

Franciscan Saint Francis Health - Carmel

12188 B North Meridian Street Phone: 317-705-4500
Carmel, IN 46032
Type: Acute Care Hospitals Emergency Services: No
Ownership: Voluntary non-profit - Church

Measure	Cases	This Hosp.	State Avg.	U.S. Avg.
Blood Clot Prevention and Treatment				
Anticoagulation Overlap Therapy[5]	-	-	92%	93%
ICU Venous Thromboembolism Prophylaxis[5]	-	-	91%	92%
Incidence of Potentially Preventable VTE[5]	-	-	10%	10%
UFH with Dosages/Platelet Monitoring[5]	-	-	95%	97%
Venous Thromboembolism Prophylaxis[5]	-	-	83%	85%
Warfarin Therapy Discharge Instructions[5]	-	-	71%	75%
Chest Pain/Possible Heart Attack Care				
Aspirin Given Within 24 Hours of Arrival[5]	-	-	96%	96%
Fibrinolytic Meds Within 30 Min. of Arrival[5]	-	-	48%	58%
Average Time to ECG (minutes)[5]	-	-	6	7
Average Time to Transfer (minutes)[5]	-	-	46	60
Children's Asthma Care				
Received Home Management Plan of Care	-	-	-	88%
Received Reliever Medication	-	-	-	100%
Received Systemic Corticosteroids	-	-	-	100%
Emergency Department				
Admittance Decision Time (minutes)[5]	-	-	80	98
Head CT Results Within 45 Min. of Arrival[5]	-	-	60%	57%
Patients Who Left ER Before Being Seen[5]	-	-	2%	2%
Time from ER Arrival to Admit. (minutes)[5]	-	-	241	274
Time from ER Arrival to Discharge (minutes)[5]	-	-	122	134
Time in ER Before Being Evaluated (minutes)[5]	-	-	22	26
Time to Pain Meds for Fractures (minutes)[5]	-	-	52	57
Heart Attack Care				
Aspirin Given at Discharge[5]	-	-	99%	99%
Fibrinolytic Meds Within 30 Min. of Arrival[5]	-	-	67%	54%
PCI Within 90 Minutes of Arrival[5]	-	-	97%	96%
Statin Prescribed at Discharge[5]	-	-	99%	98%
Heart Failure Care				
ACE Inhibitor or ARB for LVSD[5]	-	-	97%	97%
Discharge Instructions Given[5]	-	-	95%	94%
Evaluation of LVS Function[5]	-	-	99%	99%
Medicare Spending				
Medicare Spending per Patient (ratio)	-	-	1.01	0.98
Pneumonia Care				
Appropriate Initial Antibiotic Given[5]	-	-	95%	95%
Blood Culture Timing[5]	-	-	98%	98%
Pregnancy and Delivery Care				
Newborn Deliveries Scheduled Early[5]	-	-	5%	6%
Preventive Care				
Immunization for Influenza[5]	-	-	91%	90%
Immunization for Pneumonia[5]	-	-	92%	92%
Stroke Care				
Anticoagulation Therapy for Atrial Fibrillation[5]	-	-	94%	95%
Antithrombotic Therapy Timing[5]	-	-	97%	98%
Assessed for Rehabilitation[5]	-	-	96%	97%
Discharged on Antithrombotic Therapy[5]	-	-	98%	99%
Discharged on Statin Medication[5]	-	-	91%	94%
Thrombolytic Therapy Timing[5]	-	-	54%	66%
Venous Thromboembolism Prophylaxis[5]	-	-	91%	94%
Written Stroke Educational Materials Given[5]	-	-	82%	88%
Surgical Care Improvement Project				
Appropriate Beta Blocker Usage[5]	-	-	98%	98%
Appropriate VTP Within 24 Hours[5]	-	-	98%	98%
Controlled Postoperative Blood Glucose[5]	-	-	97%	97%
Perioperative Temperature Management[5]	-	-	100%	100%
Prophylactic Antibiotic Selection[5]	-	-	99%	99%
Prophylactic Antibiotic Selection (Outpatient)[5]	-	-	98%	98%
Prophylactic Antibiotic Stopped[5]	-	-	98%	98%
Prophylactic Antibiotic Timing[5]	-	-	99%	99%
Prophylactic Antibiotic Timing (Outpatient)[5]	-	-	98%	98%
Urinary Catheter Removal[5]	-	-	98%	97%
Survey of Patients' Hospital Experiences				
Area Around Room 'Always' Quiet at Night[5]	-	-	61%	61%
Doctors 'Always' Communicated Well[5]	-	-	83%	82%
Home Recovery Information Given[5]	-	-	86%	85%
Hospital Given 9 or 10 on 10 Point Scale[5]	-	-	74%	71%
Meds 'Always' Explained Before Given[5]	-	-	64%	64%
Nurses 'Always' Communicated Well[5]	-	-	81%	79%
Pain 'Always' Well Controlled[5]	-	-	73%	71%
Room and Bathroom 'Always' Clean[5]	-	-	76%	73%
Timely Help 'Always' Received[5]	-	-	71%	68%
Would Definitely Recommend Hospital[5]	-	-	73%	71%
Use of Medical Imaging				
Cardiac Imaging Stress Test before Surgery[7]	-	-	5.4%	5.3%
Combination Abdominal CT Scan[7]	-	-	9.3%	10.5%
Combination Brain/Sinus CT Scan[7]	-	-	2.6%	2.7%
Combination Chest CT Scan[7]	-	-	4.6%	2.7%
Follow-up Mammogram/Ultrasound[7]	-	-	8.4%	8.8%
Lumbar Spine MRI for Low Back Pain[7]	-	-	38.7%	37.2%

Indiana University Health North Hospital

11700 N Meridian St Phone: 317-688-2000
Carmel, IN 46032
URL: www.iuhealth.org/north
Type: Acute Care Hospitals Emergency Services: Yes
Ownership: Proprietary
Key Personnel:
Chief of Medical Staff . . . . Paul Calkins
CEO/President. . . . . Jonathan R Goble

Measure	Cases	This Hosp.	State Avg.	U.S. Avg.
Blood Clot Prevention and Treatment				
Anticoagulation Overlap Therapy[2]	33	94%	92%	93%
ICU Venous Thromboembolism Prophylaxis[2]	30	87%	91%	92%
Incidence of Potentially Preventable VTE[1,2]	-	-	10%	10%
UFH with Dosages/Platelet Monitoring[2]	18	89%	95%	97%
Venous Thromboembolism Prophylaxis[2]	300	84%	83%	85%
Warfarin Therapy Discharge Instructions[2]	27	41%	71%	75%
Chest Pain/Possible Heart Attack Care				
Aspirin Given Within 24 Hours of Arrival[5]	-	-	96%	96%
Fibrinolytic Meds Within 30 Min. of Arrival[5]	-	-	48%	58%
Average Time to ECG (minutes)[5]	-	-	6	7
Average Time to Transfer (minutes)[5]	-	-	46	60
Children's Asthma Care				
Received Home Management Plan of Care[2]	50	76%	-	88%
Received Reliever Medication	51	100%	-	100%
Received Systemic Corticosteroids	51	100%	-	100%
Emergency Department				
Admittance Decision Time (minutes)[2]	250	130	80	98
Head CT Results Within 45 Min. of Arrival[1]	-	-	60%	57%
Patients Who Left ER Before Being Seen	17,465	0%	2%	2%
Time from ER Arrival to Admit. (minutes)[2]	253	274	241	274
Time from ER Arrival to Discharge (minutes)	387	146	122	134
Time in ER Before Being Evaluated (minutes)	404	19	22	26
Time to Pain Meds for Fractures (minutes)	98	44	52	57
Heart Attack Care				
Aspirin Given at Discharge	41	100%	99%	99%
Fibrinolytic Meds Within 30 Min. of Arrival[7]	-	-	67%	54%
PCI Within 90 Minutes of Arrival[1]	-	-	97%	96%

NOTE: Hospital profiles are in alphabetical order by state, then city, then hospital within the city; Rankings exclude hospitals with less than 25 cases except for patient surveys which excludes hospitals with less than 100 cases; (a) 100-299 cases; (1) The number of cases/patients is too few to report; (2) Data submitted were based on a sample of cases/patients; (3) Results are based on a shorter time period than required; (4) Data suppressed by CMS for one or more quarters; (5) Results are not available for this reporting period; (6) Fewer than 100 patients completed the HCAHPS survey; (7) No cases met the criteria for this measure; (8) The lower limit of the confidence interval cannot be calculated if the number of observed infections equals zero; (9) No data are available from the state/territory for this reporting period; (10) The scores shown reflect fewer than 50 completed surveys; (11) There were discrepancies in the data collection process; (12) This measure does not apply to this hospital for this reporting period; (13) Results cannot be calculated for this reporting period; (14) The results for this state are combined with nearby states to protect confidentiality; Please refer to the User's Guide for a full explanation of data.

Statin Prescribed at Discharge	34	97%	99%	98%
Heart Failure Care				
ACE Inhibitor or ARB for LVSD	20	95%	97%	97%
Discharge Instructions Given	50	100%	95%	94%
Evaluation of LVS Function	64	98%	99%	99%
Medicare Spending				
Medicare Spending per Patient (ratio)	-	1.07	1.01	0.98
Pneumonia Care				
Appropriate Initial Antibiotic Given[2]	42	88%	95%	95%
Blood Culture Timing[2]	77	100%	98%	98%
Pregnancy and Delivery Care				
Newborn Deliveries Scheduled Early[2]	49	8%	5%	6%
Preventive Care				
Immunization for Influenza[2]	452	96%	91%	90%
Immunization for Pneumonia[2]	350	85%	92%	92%
Stroke Care				
Anticoagulation Therapy for Atrial Fibrillation[1]	-	-	94%	95%
Antithrombotic Therapy Timing	31	100%	97%	98%
Assessed for Rehabilitation	42	88%	96%	97%
Discharged on Antithrombotic Therapy	40	98%	98%	99%
Discharged on Statin Medication	31	74%	91%	94%
Thrombolytic Therapy Timing	12	0%	54%	66%
Venous Thromboembolism Prophylaxis	34	82%	91%	94%
Written Stroke Educational Materials Given	27	56%	82%	88%
Surgical Care Improvement Project				
Appropriate Beta Blocker Usage[2]	79	97%	98%	98%
Appropriate VTP Within 24 Hours[2]	248	100%	98%	98%
Controlled Postoperative Blood Glucose[2,7]	-	-	97%	97%
Perioperative Temperature Management[2]	314	100%	100%	100%
Prophylactic Antibiotic Selection[2]	218	100%	99%	99%
Prophylactic Antibiotic Selection (Outpatient)	352	98%	98%	98%
Prophylactic Antibiotic Stopped[2]	216	99%	98%	98%
Prophylactic Antibiotic Timing[2]	218	100%	99%	99%
Prophylactic Antibiotic Timing (Outpatient)	352	100%	98%	98%
Urinary Catheter Removal[2]	196	98%	98%	97%
Survey of Patients' Hospital Experiences				
Area Around Room 'Always' Quiet at Night	300+	67%	61%	61%
Doctors 'Always' Communicated Well	300+	84%	83%	82%
Home Recovery Information Given	300+	87%	86%	85%
Hospital Given 9 or 10 on 10 Point Scale	300+	86%	74%	71%
Meds 'Always' Explained Before Given	300+	64%	64%	64%
Nurses 'Always' Communicated Well	300+	85%	81%	79%
Pain 'Always' Well Controlled	300+	77%	73%	71%
Room and Bathroom 'Always' Clean	300+	81%	76%	73%
Timely Help 'Always' Received	300+	69%	71%	68%
Would Definitely Recommend Hospital	300+	88%	73%	71%
Use of Medical Imaging				
Cardiac Imaging Stress Test before Surgery	91	9.9%	5.4%	5.3%
Combination Abdominal CT Scan	687	5.2%	9.3%	10.5%
Combination Brain/Sinus CT Scan	301	6.0%	2.6%	2.7%
Combination Chest CT Scan	483	0.8%	4.6%	2.7%
Follow-up Mammogram/Ultrasound	522	7.3%	8.4%	8.8%
Lumbar Spine MRI for Low Back Pain[1]	-	-	38.7%	37.2%

Saint Vincent Carmel Hospital

13500 N Meridian St
Carmel, IN 46032
Phone: 317-582-7000
URL: www.carmel.stvincent.org
Type: Acute Care Hospitals
Emergency Services: Yes
Ownership: Voluntary non-profit - Church
Beds: 100

Key Personnel:
Emergency Room . . . . Kay Darnell
Operating Room. . . . . Carrie Drummond
Intensive Care Unit. . . . . Ted Eads
Anesthesiology. . . . . Steve Priddy, MD
Chief of Medical Staff. . . . . Steve Priddy, MD
Quality Assurance . . . . Cindy Ransford

Measure	Cases	This Hosp.	State Avg.	U.S. Avg.
Blood Clot Prevention and Treatment				
Anticoagulation Overlap Therapy[2]	14	100%	92%	93%
ICU Venous Thromboembolism Prophylaxis[2]	26	96%	91%	92%
Incidence of Potentially Preventable VTE[1,2]	-	-	10%	10%
UFH with Dosages/Platelet Monitoring[2,7]	-	-	95%	97%
Venous Thromboembolism Prophylaxis[2]	287	96%	83%	85%
Warfarin Therapy Discharge Instructions[1,2]	-	-	71%	75%
Chest Pain/Possible Heart Attack Care				
Aspirin Given Within 24 Hours of Arrival	70	100%	96%	96%
Fibrinolytic Meds Within 30 Min. of Arrival[7]	-	-	48%	58%
Average Time to ECG (minutes)	78	5	6	7
Average Time to Transfer (minutes)[1]	-	-	46	60
Children's Asthma Care				
Received Home Management Plan of Care	-	-	-	88%
Received Reliever Medication	-	-	-	100%
Received Systemic Corticosteroids	-	-	-	100%
Emergency Department				
Admittance Decision Time (minutes)[2]	240	76	80	98
Head CT Results Within 45 Min. of Arrival[1]	-	-	60%	57%
Patients Who Left ER Before Being Seen	17,043	0%	2%	2%
Time from ER Arrival to Admit. (minutes)[2]	242	242	241	274
Time from ER Arrival to Discharge (minutes)	355	146	122	134
Time in ER Before Being Evaluated (minutes)	348	24	22	26
Time to Pain Meds for Fractures (minutes)	135	43	52	57
Heart Attack Care				
Aspirin Given at Discharge[1,3]	-	-	99%	99%
Fibrinolytic Meds Within 30 Min. of Arrival[3,7]	-	-	67%	54%
PCI Within 90 Minutes of Arrival[3,7]	-	-	97%	96%
Statin Prescribed at Discharge[3,7]	-	-	99%	98%
Heart Failure Care				
ACE Inhibitor or ARB for LVSD[1]	-	-	97%	97%
Discharge Instructions Given	21	100%	95%	94%
Evaluation of LVS Function	31	100%	99%	99%
Medicare Spending				
Medicare Spending per Patient (ratio)	-	0.98	1.01	0.98
Pneumonia Care				
Appropriate Initial Antibiotic Given	55	93%	95%	95%
Blood Culture Timing	90	88%	98%	98%
Pregnancy and Delivery Care				
Newborn Deliveries Scheduled Early[2]	29	7%	5%	6%
Preventive Care				
Immunization for Influenza[2]	469	95%	91%	90%
Immunization for Pneumonia[2]	410	96%	92%	92%
Stroke Care				
Anticoagulation Therapy for Atrial Fibrillation[1]	-	-	94%	95%
Antithrombotic Therapy Timing	11	100%	97%	98%
Assessed for Rehabilitation	13	77%	96%	97%
Discharged on Antithrombotic Therapy	12	100%	98%	99%
Discharged on Statin Medication	12	75%	91%	94%
Thrombolytic Therapy Timing[1]	-	-	54%	66%
Venous Thromboembolism Prophylaxis	11	91%	91%	94%
Written Stroke Educational Materials Given[1]	-	-	82%	88%
Surgical Care Improvement Project				
Appropriate Beta Blocker Usage[2]	77	99%	98%	98%
Appropriate VTP Within 24 Hours[2]	295	100%	98%	98%
Controlled Postoperative Blood Glucose[2,7]	-	-	97%	97%
Perioperative Temperature Management[2]	318	100%	100%	100%
Prophylactic Antibiotic Selection[2]	198	98%	99%	99%
Prophylactic Antibiotic Selection (Outpatient)	138	97%	98%	98%
Prophylactic Antibiotic Stopped[2]	197	97%	98%	98%
Prophylactic Antibiotic Timing[2]	199	97%	99%	99%
Prophylactic Antibiotic Timing (Outpatient)	140	97%	98%	98%
Urinary Catheter Removal[2]	87	99%	98%	97%
Survey of Patients' Hospital Experiences				
Area Around Room 'Always' Quiet at Night	300+	58%	61%	61%
Doctors 'Always' Communicated Well	300+	85%	83%	82%
Home Recovery Information Given	300+	83%	86%	85%
Hospital Given 9 or 10 on 10 Point Scale	300+	78%	74%	71%
Meds 'Always' Explained Before Given	300+	62%	64%	64%
Nurses 'Always' Communicated Well	300+	76%	81%	79%
Pain 'Always' Well Controlled	300+	75%	73%	71%
Room and Bathroom 'Always' Clean	300+	63%	76%	73%
Timely Help 'Always' Received	300+	62%	71%	68%
Would Definitely Recommend Hospital	300+	79%	73%	71%
Use of Medical Imaging				
Cardiac Imaging Stress Test before Surgery[1]	-	-	5.4%	5.3%
Combination Abdominal CT Scan	454	5.3%	9.3%	10.5%
Combination Brain/Sinus CT Scan[1]	-	-	2.6%	2.7%
Combination Chest CT Scan	226	0.0%	4.6%	2.7%
Follow-up Mammogram/Ultrasound	768	7.8%	8.4%	8.8%
Lumbar Spine MRI for Low Back Pain	165	37.6%	38.7%	37.2%

Saint Catherine Regional Hospital

2200 Market St
Charlestown, IN 47111
Phone: 812-256-3301
Fax: 812-256-0201
E-mail: wobertate@altavista.net
Type: Acute Care Hospitals
Emergency Services: Yes
Ownership: Proprietary
Beds: 96

Measure	Cases	This Hosp.	State Avg.	U.S. Avg.
Blood Clot Prevention and Treatment				
Anticoagulation Overlap Therapy[2,7]	-	-	92%	93%
ICU Venous Thromboembolism Prophylaxis[2,7]	-	-	91%	92%
Incidence of Potentially Preventable VTE[2,7]	-	-	10%	10%
UFH with Dosages/Platelet Monitoring[2,7]	-	-	95%	97%
Venous Thromboembolism Prophylaxis[2]	150	21%	83%	85%
Warfarin Therapy Discharge Instructions[2,7]	-	-	71%	75%
Chest Pain/Possible Heart Attack Care				
Aspirin Given Within 24 Hours of Arrival[1,3]	-	-	96%	96%
Fibrinolytic Meds Within 30 Min. of Arrival[1,3]	-	-	48%	58%
Average Time to ECG (minutes)[1,3]	-	-	6	7
Average Time to Transfer (minutes)[1,3]	-	-	46	60
Children's Asthma Care				
Received Home Management Plan of Care	-	-	-	88%
Received Reliever Medication	-	-	-	100%
Received Systemic Corticosteroids	-	-	-	100%
Emergency Department				
Admittance Decision Time (minutes)	247	27	80	98
Head CT Results Within 45 Min. of Arrival[1,3]	-	-	60%	57%
Patients Who Left ER Before Being Seen	4,914	0%	2%	2%
Time from ER Arrival to Admit. (minutes)	247	172	241	274
Time from ER Arrival to Discharge (minutes)	441	68	122	134
Time in ER Before Being Evaluated (minutes)	488	6	22	26
Time to Pain Meds for Fractures (minutes)[3]	12	37	52	57
Heart Attack Care				
Aspirin Given at Discharge[3,7]	-	-	99%	99%
Fibrinolytic Meds Within 30 Min. of Arrival[3,7]	-	-	67%	54%
PCI Within 90 Minutes of Arrival[3,7]	-	-	97%	96%
Statin Prescribed at Discharge[3,7]	-	-	99%	98%
Heart Failure Care				
ACE Inhibitor or ARB for LVSD[3,7]	-	-	97%	97%
Discharge Instructions Given[1,3]	-	-	95%	94%
Evaluation of LVS Function[1,3]	-	-	99%	99%
Medicare Spending				
Medicare Spending per Patient (ratio)	-	1.01	1.01	0.98
Pneumonia Care				
Appropriate Initial Antibiotic Given	31	61%	95%	95%
Blood Culture Timing	22	95%	98%	98%
Pregnancy and Delivery Care				
Newborn Deliveries Scheduled Early[7]	-	-	5%	6%
Preventive Care				
Immunization for Influenza	228	2%	91%	90%
Immunization for Pneumonia	290	2%	92%	92%
Stroke Care				
Anticoagulation Therapy for Atrial Fibrillation[3,7]	-	-	94%	95%
Antithrombotic Therapy Timing[1,3]	-	-	97%	98%
Assessed for Rehabilitation[1,3]	-	-	96%	97%
Discharged on Antithrombotic Therapy[1,3]	-	-	98%	99%
Discharged on Statin Medication[1,3]	-	-	91%	94%
Thrombolytic Therapy Timing[1,3]	-	-	54%	66%
Venous Thromboembolism Prophylaxis[1,3]	-	-	91%	94%
Written Stroke Educational Materials Given[3,7]	-	-	82%	88%
Surgical Care Improvement Project				
Appropriate Beta Blocker Usage[5]	-	-	98%	98%
Appropriate VTP Within 24 Hours[5]	-	-	98%	98%
Controlled Postoperative Blood Glucose[5]	-	-	97%	97%
Perioperative Temperature Management[5]	-	-	100%	100%
Prophylactic Antibiotic Selection[5]	-	-	99%	99%
Prophylactic Antibiotic Selection (Outpatient)[5]	-	-	98%	98%
Prophylactic Antibiotic Stopped[5]	-	-	98%	98%
Prophylactic Antibiotic Timing[5]	-	-	99%	99%

NOTE: Hospital profiles are in alphabetical order by state, then city, then hospital within the city; Rankings exclude hospitals with less than 25 cases except for patient surveys which excludes hospitals with less than 100 cases; (a) 100-299 cases; (1) The number of cases/patients is too few to report; (2) Data submitted were based on a sample of cases/patients; (3) Results are based on a shorter time period than required; (4) Data suppressed by CMS for one or more quarters; (5) Results are not available for this reporting period; (6) Fewer than 100 patients completed the HCAHPS survey; (7) No cases met the criteria for this measure; (8) The lower limit of the confidence interval cannot be calculated if the number of observed infections equals zero; (9) No data are available from the state/territory for this reporting period; (10) The scores shown reflect fewer than 50 completed surveys; (11) There were discrepancies in the data collection process; (12) This measure does not apply to this hospital for this reporting period; (13) Results cannot be calculated for this reporting period; (14) The results for this state are combined with nearby states to protect confidentiality; Please refer to the User's Guide for a full explanation of data.

Prophylactic Antibiotic Timing (Outpatient)[5]	-	-	98%	98%
Urinary Catheter Removal[5]	-	-	98%	97%
Survey of Patients' Hospital Experiences				
Area Around Room 'Always' Quiet at Night[6]	<100	58%	61%	61%
Doctors 'Always' Communicated Well[6]	<100	80%	83%	82%
Home Recovery Information Given[6]	<100	73%	86%	85%
Hospital Given 9 or 10 on 10 Point Scale[6]	<100	44%	74%	71%
Meds 'Always' Explained Before Given[6]	<100	43%	64%	64%
Nurses 'Always' Communicated Well[6]	<100	71%	81%	79%
Pain 'Always' Well Controlled[6]	<100	64%	73%	71%
Room and Bathroom 'Always' Clean[6]	<100	68%	76%	73%
Timely Help 'Always' Received[6]	<100	56%	71%	68%
Would Definitely Recommend Hospital[6]	<100	44%	73%	71%
Use of Medical Imaging				
Cardiac Imaging Stress Test before Surgery[1]	-	-	5.4%	5.3%
Combination Abdominal CT Scan	69	10.1%	9.3%	10.5%
Combination Brain/Sinus CT Scan	96	10.4%	2.6%	2.7%
Combination Chest CT Scan[1]	-	-	4.6%	2.7%
Follow-up Mammogram/Ultrasound[1]	-	-	8.4%	8.8%
Lumbar Spine MRI for Low Back Pain[1]	-	-	38.7%	37.2%

Kentuckiana Medical Center

4601 Medical Plaza Way
Clarksville, IN 47129
Phone: 812-280-3300
URL: www.kentuckianamedcen.com
Type: Acute Care Hospitals
Emergency Services: No
Ownership: Proprietary
Beds: 34
Key Personnel:
CEO . . . . Chris Staves

Measure	Cases	This Hosp.	State Avg.	U.S. Avg.
Blood Clot Prevention and Treatment				
Anticoagulation Overlap Therapy[1,2]	-	-	92%	93%
ICU Venous Thromboembolism Prophylaxis[2]	71	70%	91%	92%
Incidence of Potentially Preventable VTE[1,2]	-	-	10%	10%
UFH with Dosages/Platelet Monitoring[1,2]	-	-	95%	97%
Venous Thromboembolism Prophylaxis[2]	112	69%	83%	85%
Warfarin Therapy Discharge Instructions[1,2]	-	-	71%	75%
Chest Pain/Possible Heart Attack Care				
Aspirin Given Within 24 Hours of Arrival[5]	-	-	96%	96%
Fibrinolytic Meds Within 30 Min. of Arrival[5]	-	-	48%	58%
Average Time to ECG (minutes)[5]	-	-	6	7
Average Time to Transfer (minutes)[5]	-	-	46	60
Children's Asthma Care				
Received Home Management Plan of Care	-	-	-	88%
Received Reliever Medication	-	-	-	100%
Received Systemic Corticosteroids	-	-	-	100%
Emergency Department				
Admittance Decision Time (minutes)[2,7]	-	-	80	98
Head CT Results Within 45 Min. of Arrival[5]	-	-	60%	57%
Patients Who Left ER Before Being Seen[5]	-	-	2%	2%
Time from ER Arrival to Admit. (minutes)[2,7]	-	-	241	274
Time from ER Arrival to Discharge (minutes)[5]	-	-	122	134
Time in ER Before Being Evaluated (minutes)[5]	-	-	22	26
Time to Pain Meds for Fractures (minutes)[5]	-	-	52	57
Heart Attack Care				
Aspirin Given at Discharge[2]	21	100%	99%	99%
Fibrinolytic Meds Within 30 Min. of Arrival[1,2]	-	-	67%	54%
PCI Within 90 Minutes of Arrival[2,7]	-	-	97%	96%
Statin Prescribed at Discharge[2]	23	96%	99%	98%
Heart Failure Care				
ACE Inhibitor or ARB for LVSD[2]	28	96%	97%	97%
Discharge Instructions Given[2]	45	89%	95%	94%
Evaluation of LVS Function[2]	41	90%	99%	99%
Medicare Spending				
Medicare Spending per Patient (ratio)	-	1.05	1.01	0.98
Pneumonia Care				
Appropriate Initial Antibiotic Given[2]	16	31%	95%	95%
Blood Culture Timing[1,2]	-	-	98%	98%
Pregnancy and Delivery Care				
Newborn Deliveries Scheduled Early[7]	-	-	5%	6%
Preventive Care				
Immunization for Influenza[2]	307	86%	91%	90%
Immunization for Pneumonia[2]	390	89%	92%	92%
Stroke Care				
Anticoagulation Therapy for Atrial Fibrillation[2,7]	-	-	94%	95%
Antithrombotic Therapy Timing[1,2]	-	-	97%	98%
Assessed for Rehabilitation[1,2]	-	-	96%	97%
Discharged on Antithrombotic Therapy[1,2]	-	-	98%	99%
Discharged on Statin Medication[1,2]	-	-	91%	94%
Thrombolytic Therapy Timing[2,7]	-	-	54%	66%
Venous Thromboembolism Prophylaxis[1,2]	-	-	91%	94%
Written Stroke Educational Materials Given[1,2]	-	-	82%	88%
Surgical Care Improvement Project				
Appropriate Beta Blocker Usage[2]	70	93%	98%	98%
Appropriate VTP Within 24 Hours[2,7]	-	-	98%	98%
Controlled Postoperative Blood Glucose[2]	122	84%	97%	97%
Perioperative Temperature Management[1,2]	-	-	100%	100%
Prophylactic Antibiotic Selection[2]	87	100%	99%	99%
Prophylactic Antibiotic Selection (Outpatient)[3]	27	89%	98%	98%
Prophylactic Antibiotic Stopped[2]	82	100%	98%	98%
Prophylactic Antibiotic Timing[2]	87	95%	99%	99%
Prophylactic Antibiotic Timing (Outpatient)[3]	26	100%	98%	98%
Urinary Catheter Removal[2]	69	94%	98%	97%
Survey of Patients' Hospital Experiences				
Area Around Room 'Always' Quiet at Night	300+	77%	61%	61%
Doctors 'Always' Communicated Well	300+	88%	83%	82%
Home Recovery Information Given	300+	84%	86%	85%
Hospital Given 9 or 10 on 10 Point Scale	300+	84%	74%	71%
Meds 'Always' Explained Before Given	300+	68%	64%	64%
Nurses 'Always' Communicated Well	300+	87%	81%	79%
Pain 'Always' Well Controlled	300+	78%	73%	71%
Room and Bathroom 'Always' Clean	300+	81%	76%	73%
Timely Help 'Always' Received	300+	78%	71%	68%
Would Definitely Recommend Hospital	300+	85%	73%	71%
Use of Medical Imaging				
Cardiac Imaging Stress Test before Surgery[1]	-	-	5.4%	5.3%
Combination Abdominal CT Scan[1]	-	-	9.3%	10.5%
Combination Brain/Sinus CT Scan[1]	-	-	2.6%	2.7%
Combination Chest CT Scan[1]	-	-	4.6%	2.7%
Follow-up Mammogram/Ultrasound[7]	-	-	8.4%	8.8%
Lumbar Spine MRI for Low Back Pain[7]	-	-	38.7%	37.2%

Union Hospital Clinton

801 S Main St
Clinton, IN 47842
Phone: 765-832-1234
E-mail: prpublic@uhhg.org
URL: www.unionhospitalhealthgroup.org/wcch
Type: Critical Access Hospitals
Emergency Services: Yes
Ownership: Voluntary non-profit - Private
Key Personnel:
CEO/President. . . . . Steven M. Holman, FACHE
Quality Assurance . . . . Jeanette Spradlin

Measure	Cases	This Hosp.	State Avg.	U.S. Avg.
Blood Clot Prevention and Treatment				
Anticoagulation Overlap Therapy[1]	-	-	92%	93%
ICU Venous Thromboembolism Prophylaxis	87	100%	91%	92%
Incidence of Potentially Preventable VTE[7]	-	-	10%	10%
UFH with Dosages/Platelet Monitoring[1]	-	-	95%	97%
Venous Thromboembolism Prophylaxis	332	100%	83%	85%
Warfarin Therapy Discharge Instructions[1]	-	-	71%	75%
Chest Pain/Possible Heart Attack Care				
Aspirin Given Within 24 Hours of Arrival	43	95%	96%	96%
Fibrinolytic Meds Within 30 Min. of Arrival[7]	-	-	48%	58%
Average Time to ECG (minutes)	45	7	6	7
Average Time to Transfer (minutes)	11	32	46	60
Children's Asthma Care				
Received Home Management Plan of Care	-	-	-	88%
Received Reliever Medication	-	-	-	100%
Received Systemic Corticosteroids	-	-	-	100%
Emergency Department				
Admittance Decision Time (minutes)	463	66	80	98
Head CT Results Within 45 Min. of Arrival[1]	-	-	60%	57%
Patients Who Left ER Before Being Seen	11,537	0%	2%	2%
Time from ER Arrival to Admit. (minutes)	532	195	241	274
Time from ER Arrival to Discharge (minutes)	522	113	122	134
Time in ER Before Being Evaluated (minutes)	583	13	22	26
Time to Pain Meds for Fractures (minutes)	62	37	52	57
Heart Attack Care				
Aspirin Given at Discharge[1]	-	-	99%	99%
Fibrinolytic Meds Within 30 Min. of Arrival[7]	-	-	67%	54%
PCI Within 90 Minutes of Arrival[7]	-	-	97%	96%
Statin Prescribed at Discharge[1]	-	-	99%	98%
Heart Failure Care				
ACE Inhibitor or ARB for LVSD[1]	-	-	97%	97%
Discharge Instructions Given	32	91%	95%	94%
Evaluation of LVS Function	41	100%	99%	99%
Medicare Spending				
Medicare Spending per Patient (ratio)	-	-	1.01	0.98
Pneumonia Care				
Appropriate Initial Antibiotic Given	45	100%	95%	95%
Blood Culture Timing	24	100%	98%	98%
Pregnancy and Delivery Care				
Newborn Deliveries Scheduled Early[5]	-	-	5%	6%
Preventive Care				
Immunization for Influenza	455	98%	91%	90%
Immunization for Pneumonia	711	97%	92%	92%
Stroke Care				
Anticoagulation Therapy for Atrial Fibrillation[1]	-	-	94%	95%
Antithrombotic Therapy Timing[1]	-	-	97%	98%
Assessed for Rehabilitation[1]	-	-	96%	97%
Discharged on Antithrombotic Therapy[1]	-	-	98%	99%
Discharged on Statin Medication[1]	-	-	91%	94%
Thrombolytic Therapy Timing[7]	-	-	54%	66%
Venous Thromboembolism Prophylaxis[1]	-	-	91%	94%
Written Stroke Educational Materials Given[1]	-	-	82%	88%
Surgical Care Improvement Project				
Appropriate Beta Blocker Usage[1]	-	-	98%	98%
Appropriate VTP Within 24 Hours	16	100%	98%	98%
Controlled Postoperative Blood Glucose[7]	-	-	97%	97%
Perioperative Temperature Management	17	100%	100%	100%
Prophylactic Antibiotic Selection[1]	-	-	99%	99%
Prophylactic Antibiotic Selection (Outpatient)[1,3]	-	-	98%	98%
Prophylactic Antibiotic Stopped[1]	-	-	98%	98%
Prophylactic Antibiotic Timing[1]	-	-	99%	99%
Prophylactic Antibiotic Timing (Outpatient)[1,3]	-	-	98%	98%
Urinary Catheter Removal	11	100%	98%	97%
Survey of Patients' Hospital Experiences				
Area Around Room 'Always' Quiet at Night	(a)	56%	61%	61%
Doctors 'Always' Communicated Well	(a)	88%	83%	82%
Home Recovery Information Given	(a)	91%	86%	85%
Hospital Given 9 or 10 on 10 Point Scale	(a)	82%	74%	71%
Meds 'Always' Explained Before Given	(a)	69%	64%	64%
Nurses 'Always' Communicated Well	(a)	89%	81%	79%
Pain 'Always' Well Controlled	(a)	80%	73%	71%
Room and Bathroom 'Always' Clean	(a)	78%	76%	73%
Timely Help 'Always' Received	(a)	75%	71%	68%
Would Definitely Recommend Hospital	(a)	81%	73%	71%
Use of Medical Imaging				
Cardiac Imaging Stress Test before Surgery	48	2.1%	5.4%	5.3%
Combination Abdominal CT Scan	360	3.1%	9.3%	10.5%
Combination Brain/Sinus CT Scan	427	4.2%	2.6%	2.7%
Combination Chest CT Scan	184	1.6%	4.6%	2.7%
Follow-up Mammogram/Ultrasound	302	9.9%	8.4%	8.8%
Lumbar Spine MRI for Low Back Pain[7]	-	-	38.7%	37.2%

Parkview Whitley Hospital

1260 E Sr 205
Columbia City, IN 46725
Phone: 260-248-9301
Fax: 260-248-9107
URL: www.parkview.com
Type: Acute Care Hospitals
Emergency Services: Yes
Ownership: Voluntary non-profit - Private
Beds: 45
Key Personnel:
Chief of Medical Staff . . . . Greg Johnson
CEO/President. . . . . Mike Packnett
President . . . . Mitchell B. Stucky

Measure	Cases	This Hosp.	State Avg.	U.S. Avg.
Blood Clot Prevention and Treatment				
Anticoagulation Overlap Therapy[2]	14	93%	92%	93%
ICU Venous Thromboembolism Prophylaxis[2]	21	76%	91%	92%

NOTE: Hospital profiles are in alphabetical order by state, then city, then hospital within the city; Rankings exclude hospitals with less than 25 cases except for patient surveys which excludes hospitals with less than 100 cases; (a) 100-299 cases; (1) The number of cases/patients is too few to report; (2) Data submitted were based on a sample of cases/patients; (3) Results are based on a shorter time period than required; (4) Data suppressed by CMS for one or more quarters; (5) Results are not available for this reporting period; (6) Fewer than 100 patients completed the HCAHPS survey; (7) No cases met the criteria for this measure; (8) The lower limit of the confidence interval cannot be calculated if the number of observed infections equals zero; (9) No data are available from the state/territory for this reporting period; (10) The scores shown reflect fewer than 50 completed surveys; (11) There were discrepancies in the data collection process; (12) This measure does not apply to this hospital for this reporting period; (13) Results cannot be calculated for this reporting period; (14) The results for this state are combined with nearby states to protect confidentiality; Please refer to the User's Guide for a full explanation of data.

Measure	Cases	This Hosp.	State Avg.	U.S. Avg.
Incidence of Potentially Preventable VTE[1,2]	-	-	10%	10%
UFH with Dosages/Platelet Monitoring[1,2]	-	-	95%	97%
Venous Thromboembolism Prophylaxis[2]	126	83%	83%	85%
Warfarin Therapy Discharge Instructions[2]	12	83%	71%	75%
Chest Pain/Possible Heart Attack Care				
Aspirin Given Within 24 Hours of Arrival	44	100%	96%	96%
Fibrinolytic Meds Within 30 Min. of Arrival[7]	-	-	48%	58%
Average Time to ECG (minutes)	47	7	6	7
Average Time to Transfer (minutes)[1]	-	-	46	60
Children's Asthma Care				
Received Home Management Plan of Care	-	-	-	88%
Received Reliever Medication	-	-	-	100%
Received Systemic Corticosteroids	-	-	-	100%
Emergency Department				
Admittance Decision Time (minutes)[2]	277	82	80	98
Head CT Results Within 45 Min. of Arrival[1]	-	-	60%	57%
Patients Who Left ER Before Being Seen	12,823	1%	2%	2%
Time from ER Arrival to Admit. (minutes)[2]	333	230	241	274
Time from ER Arrival to Discharge (minutes)	385	95	122	134
Time in ER Before Being Evaluated (minutes)	381	24	22	26
Time to Pain Meds for Fractures (minutes)	42	30	52	57
Heart Attack Care				
Aspirin Given at Discharge[1,3]	-	-	99%	99%
Fibrinolytic Meds Within 30 Min. of Arrival[3,7]	-	-	67%	54%
PCI Within 90 Minutes of Arrival[3,7]	-	-	97%	96%
Statin Prescribed at Discharge[1,3]	-	-	99%	98%
Heart Failure Care				
ACE Inhibitor or ARB for LVSD[1]	-	-	97%	97%
Discharge Instructions Given	31	97%	95%	94%
Evaluation of LVS Function	40	100%	99%	99%
Medicare Spending				
Medicare Spending per Patient (ratio)	-	0.90	1.01	0.98
Pneumonia Care				
Appropriate Initial Antibiotic Given	55	95%	95%	95%
Blood Culture Timing	78	100%	98%	98%
Pregnancy and Delivery Care				
Newborn Deliveries Scheduled Early	24	0%	5%	6%
Preventive Care				
Immunization for Influenza[2]	263	100%	91%	90%
Immunization for Pneumonia[2]	292	98%	92%	92%
Stroke Care				
Anticoagulation Therapy for Atrial Fibrillation[1]	-	-	94%	95%
Antithrombotic Therapy Timing[1]	-	-	97%	98%
Assessed for Rehabilitation[1]	-	-	96%	97%
Discharged on Antithrombotic Therapy[1]	-	-	98%	99%
Discharged on Statin Medication[1]	-	-	91%	94%
Thrombolytic Therapy Timing[7]	-	-	54%	66%
Venous Thromboembolism Prophylaxis	11	64%	91%	94%
Written Stroke Educational Materials Given[1]	-	-	82%	88%
Surgical Care Improvement Project				
Appropriate Beta Blocker Usage[1]	-	-	98%	98%
Appropriate VTP Within 24 Hours	34	100%	98%	98%
Controlled Postoperative Blood Glucose[7]	-	-	97%	97%
Perioperative Temperature Management	41	100%	100%	100%
Prophylactic Antibiotic Selection	31	97%	99%	99%
Prophylactic Antibiotic Selection (Outpatient)	59	100%	98%	98%
Prophylactic Antibiotic Stopped	31	94%	98%	98%
Prophylactic Antibiotic Timing	31	100%	99%	99%
Prophylactic Antibiotic Timing (Outpatient)	60	97%	98%	98%
Urinary Catheter Removal	21	100%	98%	97%
Survey of Patients' Hospital Experiences				
Area Around Room 'Always' Quiet at Night	300+	59%	61%	61%
Doctors 'Always' Communicated Well	300+	85%	83%	82%
Home Recovery Information Given	300+	88%	86%	85%
Hospital Given 9 or 10 on 10 Point Scale	300+	81%	74%	71%
Meds 'Always' Explained Before Given	300+	65%	64%	64%
Nurses 'Always' Communicated Well	300+	83%	81%	79%
Pain 'Always' Well Controlled	300+	74%	73%	71%
Room and Bathroom 'Always' Clean	300+	79%	76%	73%
Timely Help 'Always' Received	300+	76%	71%	68%
Would Definitely Recommend Hospital	300+	78%	73%	71%
Use of Medical Imaging				
Cardiac Imaging Stress Test before Surgery[1]	-	-	5.4%	5.3%
Combination Abdominal CT Scan	218	9.2%	9.3%	10.5%
Combination Brain/Sinus CT Scan[1]	-	-	2.6%	2.7%
Combination Chest CT Scan	127	3.9%	4.6%	2.7%
Follow-up Mammogram/Ultrasound	270	10.7%	8.4%	8.8%
Lumbar Spine MRI for Low Back Pain	48	47.9%	38.7%	37.2%

Columbus Regional Hospital

2400 E 17th St
Columbus, IN 47201
URL: www.crh.org
Type: Acute Care Hospitals
Ownership: Government - Local
Phone: 812-379-4441
Fax: 812-376-5001
Emergency Services: Yes
Beds: 225

Key Personnel:
President/CEO. . . . . Jim Bickel
Radiology. . . . . Martha J Dwenger
Infection Control. . . . . Cindy Fields
Quality Assurance . . . . Martha Myers
Chief of Medical Staff. . . . . Thomas Sauderman, MD

Measure	Cases	This Hosp.	State Avg.	U.S. Avg.
Blood Clot Prevention and Treatment				
Anticoagulation Overlap Therapy[2]	55	98%	92%	93%
ICU Venous Thromboembolism Prophylaxis[2]	91	93%	91%	92%
Incidence of Potentially Preventable VTE[1,2]	-	-	10%	10%
UFH with Dosages/Platelet Monitoring[1,2]	-	-	95%	97%
Venous Thromboembolism Prophylaxis[2]	315	87%	83%	85%
Warfarin Therapy Discharge Instructions[2]	42	26%	71%	75%
Chest Pain/Possible Heart Attack Care				
Aspirin Given Within 24 Hours of Arrival[1]	-	-	96%	96%
Fibrinolytic Meds Within 30 Min. of Arrival[3,7]	-	-	48%	58%
Average Time to ECG (minutes)[1]	-	-	6	7
Average Time to Transfer (minutes)[3,7]	-	-	46	60
Children's Asthma Care				
Received Home Management Plan of Care	-	-	-	88%
Received Reliever Medication	-	-	-	100%
Received Systemic Corticosteroids	-	-	-	100%
Emergency Department				
Admittance Decision Time (minutes)[2]	447	62	80	98
Head CT Results Within 45 Min. of Arrival[1]	-	-	60%	57%
Patients Who Left ER Before Being Seen	41,675	3%	2%	2%
Time from ER Arrival to Admit. (minutes)[2]	497	185	241	274
Time from ER Arrival to Discharge (minutes)	460	131	122	134
Time in ER Before Being Evaluated (minutes)	468	34	22	26
Time to Pain Meds for Fractures (minutes)	177	52	52	57
Heart Attack Care				
Aspirin Given at Discharge	259	100%	99%	99%
Fibrinolytic Meds Within 30 Min. of Arrival[7]	-	-	67%	54%
PCI Within 90 Minutes of Arrival	62	98%	97%	96%
Statin Prescribed at Discharge	254	100%	99%	98%
Heart Failure Care				
ACE Inhibitor or ARB for LVSD	93	99%	97%	97%
Discharge Instructions Given	211	87%	95%	94%
Evaluation of LVS Function	288	100%	99%	99%
Medicare Spending				
Medicare Spending per Patient (ratio)	-	0.96	1.01	0.98
Pneumonia Care				
Appropriate Initial Antibiotic Given	161	98%	95%	95%
Blood Culture Timing	266	100%	98%	98%
Pregnancy and Delivery Care				
Newborn Deliveries Scheduled Early[2]	77	0%	5%	6%
Preventive Care				
Immunization for Influenza[2]	850	96%	91%	90%
Immunization for Pneumonia[2]	1,091	95%	92%	92%
Stroke Care				
Anticoagulation Therapy for Atrial Fibrillation	12	92%	94%	95%
Antithrombotic Therapy Timing	93	99%	97%	98%
Assessed for Rehabilitation	106	100%	96%	97%
Discharged on Antithrombotic Therapy	105	100%	98%	99%
Discharged on Statin Medication	76	84%	91%	94%
Thrombolytic Therapy Timing[1]	-	-	54%	66%
Venous Thromboembolism Prophylaxis	101	90%	91%	94%
Written Stroke Educational Materials Given	45	100%	82%	88%
Surgical Care Improvement Project				
Appropriate Beta Blocker Usage	225	96%	98%	98%
Appropriate VTP Within 24 Hours	458	98%	98%	98%
Controlled Postoperative Blood Glucose	57	100%	97%	97%
Perioperative Temperature Management	536	100%	100%	100%
Prophylactic Antibiotic Selection	418	99%	99%	99%
Prophylactic Antibiotic Selection (Outpatient)	417	100%	98%	98%
Prophylactic Antibiotic Stopped	390	98%	98%	98%
Prophylactic Antibiotic Timing	420	99%	99%	99%
Prophylactic Antibiotic Timing (Outpatient)	420	97%	98%	98%
Urinary Catheter Removal	447	99%	98%	97%
Survey of Patients' Hospital Experiences				
Area Around Room 'Always' Quiet at Night	300+	58%	61%	61%
Doctors 'Always' Communicated Well	300+	83%	83%	82%
Home Recovery Information Given	300+	88%	86%	85%
Hospital Given 9 or 10 on 10 Point Scale	300+	71%	74%	71%
Meds 'Always' Explained Before Given	300+	64%	64%	64%
Nurses 'Always' Communicated Well	300+	80%	81%	79%
Pain 'Always' Well Controlled	300+	72%	73%	71%
Room and Bathroom 'Always' Clean	300+	78%	76%	73%
Timely Help 'Always' Received	300+	71%	71%	68%
Would Definitely Recommend Hospital	300+	69%	73%	71%
Use of Medical Imaging				
Cardiac Imaging Stress Test before Surgery	124	8.9%	5.4%	5.3%
Combination Abdominal CT Scan	1,005	6.4%	9.3%	10.5%
Combination Brain/Sinus CT Scan	948	2.5%	2.6%	2.7%
Combination Chest CT Scan	862	0.1%	4.6%	2.7%
Follow-up Mammogram/Ultrasound	1,957	7.6%	8.4%	8.8%
Lumbar Spine MRI for Low Back Pain	107	26.2%	38.7%	37.2%

Fayette Regional Health System

1941 Virginia Ave
Connersville, IN 47331
URL: www.fayettememorial.org
Type: Acute Care Hospitals
Ownership: Proprietary
Phone: 765-825-5131
Fax: 765-827-7775
Emergency Services: Yes
Beds: 140

Key Personnel:
Intensive Care Unit. . . . . Paula Anderson
Cardiac Laboratory. . . . . Joan Baum, DO
Anesthesiology. . . . . Abdul Khan, MD
Quality Assurance . . . . Betty Klein
Emergency Room . . . . Shelley Millor
Chief of Medical Staff. . . . . Michael Rowe, MD
Operating Room. . . . . Peggy Stang
CEO/President. . . . . Randy White, MBA, MS, FACHE

Measure	Cases	This Hosp.	State Avg.	U.S. Avg.
Blood Clot Prevention and Treatment				
Anticoagulation Overlap Therapy[1,2]	-	-	92%	93%
ICU Venous Thromboembolism Prophylaxis[1,2]	-	-	91%	92%
Incidence of Potentially Preventable VTE[1,2]	-	-	10%	10%
UFH with Dosages/Platelet Monitoring[1,2]	-	-	95%	97%
Venous Thromboembolism Prophylaxis[2]	122	93%	83%	85%
Warfarin Therapy Discharge Instructions[1,2]	-	-	71%	75%
Chest Pain/Possible Heart Attack Care				
Aspirin Given Within 24 Hours of Arrival	75	91%	96%	96%
Fibrinolytic Meds Within 30 Min. of Arrival[7]	-	-	48%	58%
Average Time to ECG (minutes)	83	5	6	7
Average Time to Transfer (minutes)	15	47	46	60
Children's Asthma Care				
Received Home Management Plan of Care	-	-	-	88%
Received Reliever Medication	-	-	-	100%
Received Systemic Corticosteroids	-	-	-	100%
Emergency Department				
Admittance Decision Time (minutes)[2]	400	64	80	98
Head CT Results Within 45 Min. of Arrival[1]	-	-	60%	57%
Patients Who Left ER Before Being Seen	15,801	1%	2%	2%
Time from ER Arrival to Admit. (minutes)[2]	400	224	241	274
Time from ER Arrival to Discharge (minutes)	359	97	122	134
Time in ER Before Being Evaluated (minutes)	408	18	22	26
Time to Pain Meds for Fractures (minutes)	60	55	52	57
Heart Attack Care				
Aspirin Given at Discharge[1]	-	-	99%	99%
Fibrinolytic Meds Within 30 Min. of Arrival[7]	-	-	67%	54%
PCI Within 90 Minutes of Arrival[7]	-	-	97%	96%
Statin Prescribed at Discharge[1]	-	-	99%	98%
Heart Failure Care				

NOTE: Hospital profiles are in alphabetical order by state, then city, then hospital within the city; Rankings exclude hospitals with less than 25 cases except for patient surveys which excludes hospitals with less than 100 cases; (a) 100-299 cases; (1) The number of cases/patients is too few to report; (2) Data submitted were based on a sample of cases/patients; (3) Results are based on a shorter time period than required; (4) Data suppressed by CMS for one or more quarters; (5) Results are not available for this reporting period; (6) Fewer than 100 patients completed the HCAHPS survey; (7) No cases met the criteria for this measure; (8) The lower limit of the confidence interval cannot be calculated if the number of observed infections equals zero; (9) No data are available from the state/territory for this reporting period; (10) The scores shown reflect fewer than 50 completed surveys; (11) There were discrepancies in the data collection process; (12) This measure does not apply to this hospital for this reporting period; (13) Results cannot be calculated for this reporting period; (14) The results for this state are combined with nearby states to protect confidentiality; Please refer to the User's Guide for a full explanation of data.

Measure	Cases	This Hosp.	State Avg.	U.S. Avg.
ACE Inhibitor or ARB for LVSD	12	100%	97%	97%
Discharge Instructions Given	34	97%	95%	94%
Evaluation of LVS Function	43	100%	99%	99%
Medicare Spending				
Medicare Spending per Patient (ratio)	-	0.97	1.01	0.98
Pneumonia Care				
Appropriate Initial Antibiotic Given	73	96%	95%	95%
Blood Culture Timing	99	98%	98%	98%
Pregnancy and Delivery Care				
Newborn Deliveries Scheduled Early	25	0%	5%	6%
Preventive Care				
Immunization for Influenza[2]	269	98%	91%	90%
Immunization for Pneumonia[2]	363	99%	92%	92%
Stroke Care				
Anticoagulation Therapy for Atrial Fibrillation[1]	-	-	94%	95%
Antithrombotic Therapy Timing	19	89%	97%	98%
Assessed for Rehabilitation	22	86%	96%	97%
Discharged on Antithrombotic Therapy	21	95%	98%	99%
Discharged on Statin Medication	13	85%	91%	94%
Thrombolytic Therapy Timing[1]	-	-	54%	66%
Venous Thromboembolism Prophylaxis	21	95%	91%	94%
Written Stroke Educational Materials Given	12	42%	82%	88%
Surgical Care Improvement Project				
Appropriate Beta Blocker Usage	12	92%	98%	98%
Appropriate VTP Within 24 Hours	50	98%	98%	98%
Controlled Postoperative Blood Glucose[7]	-	-	97%	97%
Perioperative Temperature Management	58	100%	100%	100%
Prophylactic Antibiotic Selection	35	100%	99%	99%
Prophylactic Antibiotic Selection (Outpatient)	22	91%	98%	98%
Prophylactic Antibiotic Stopped	34	100%	98%	98%
Prophylactic Antibiotic Timing	35	97%	99%	99%
Prophylactic Antibiotic Timing (Outpatient)	24	92%	98%	98%
Urinary Catheter Removal	24	88%	98%	97%
Survey of Patients' Hospital Experiences				
Area Around Room 'Always' Quiet at Night	300+	68%	61%	61%
Doctors 'Always' Communicated Well	300+	81%	83%	82%
Home Recovery Information Given	300+	88%	86%	85%
Hospital Given 9 or 10 on 10 Point Scale	300+	72%	74%	71%
Meds 'Always' Explained Before Given	300+	66%	64%	64%
Nurses 'Always' Communicated Well	300+	83%	81%	79%
Pain 'Always' Well Controlled	300+	74%	73%	71%
Room and Bathroom 'Always' Clean	300+	80%	76%	73%
Timely Help 'Always' Received	300+	76%	71%	68%
Would Definitely Recommend Hospital	300+	65%	73%	71%
Use of Medical Imaging				
Cardiac Imaging Stress Test before Surgery	160	1.3%	5.4%	5.3%
Combination Abdominal CT Scan	285	2.8%	9.3%	10.5%
Combination Brain/Sinus CT Scan	377	1.6%	2.6%	2.7%
Combination Chest CT Scan	141	0.7%	4.6%	2.7%
Follow-up Mammogram/Ultrasound	456	11.0%	8.4%	8.8%
Lumbar Spine MRI for Low Back Pain	70	35.7%	38.7%	37.2%

Harrison County Hospital

1141 Hospital Dr Nw
Corydon, IN 47112
URL: www.hchin.org
Phone: 812-738-4251
Fax: 812-738-7829
Type: Critical Access Hospitals
Ownership: Government - Local
Emergency Services: Yes
Beds: 68

Key Personnel:
Quality Assurance . . . . Jonell Dailey
Radiology. . . . . Christopher J Day
Infection Control. . . . . Debra Gibson
Operating Room. . . . . Rashidul Islam, RN
Chief of Medical Staff . . . . Reggie Lyell, MD
Pediatric Ambulatory Care . . . . . . John Norton, MD
Pediatric In-Patient Care . . . . John Norton, MD
CEO/President. . . . . Steve Taylor

Measure	Cases	This Hosp.	State Avg.	U.S. Avg.
Blood Clot Prevention and Treatment				
Anticoagulation Overlap Therapy[5]	-	-	92%	93%
ICU Venous Thromboembolism Prophylaxis[5]	-	-	91%	92%
Incidence of Potentially Preventable VTE[5]	-	-	10%	10%
UFH with Dosages/Platelet Monitoring[5]	-	-	95%	97%
Venous Thromboembolism Prophylaxis[5]	-	-	83%	85%
Warfarin Therapy Discharge Instructions[5]	-	-	71%	75%
Chest Pain/Possible Heart Attack Care				
Aspirin Given Within 24 Hours of Arrival	34	94%	96%	96%
Fibrinolytic Meds Within 30 Min. of Arrival[1,3]	-	-	48%	58%
Average Time to ECG (minutes)	36	10	6	7
Average Time to Transfer (minutes)[3]	13	144	46	60
Children's Asthma Care				
Received Home Management Plan of Care	-	-	-	88%
Received Reliever Medication	-	-	-	100%
Received Systemic Corticosteroids	-	-	-	100%
Emergency Department				
Admittance Decision Time (minutes)[2]	440	58	80	98
Head CT Results Within 45 Min. of Arrival[1,3]	-	-	60%	57%
Patients Who Left ER Before Being Seen	15,730	1%	2%	2%
Time from ER Arrival to Admit. (minutes)[2]	461	234	241	274
Time from ER Arrival to Discharge (minutes)	343	128	122	134
Time in ER Before Being Evaluated (minutes)	409	22	22	26
Time to Pain Meds for Fractures (minutes)	53	54	52	57
Heart Attack Care				
Aspirin Given at Discharge[1,3]	-	-	99%	99%
Fibrinolytic Meds Within 30 Min. of Arrival[3,7]	-	-	67%	54%
PCI Within 90 Minutes of Arrival[3,7]	-	-	97%	96%
Statin Prescribed at Discharge[1,3]	-	-	99%	98%
Heart Failure Care				
ACE Inhibitor or ARB for LVSD[1]	-	-	97%	97%
Discharge Instructions Given	11	91%	95%	94%
Evaluation of LVS Function	15	93%	99%	99%
Medicare Spending				
Medicare Spending per Patient (ratio)	-	-	1.01	0.98
Pneumonia Care				
Appropriate Initial Antibiotic Given	59	49%	95%	95%
Blood Culture Timing	69	93%	98%	98%
Pregnancy and Delivery Care				
Newborn Deliveries Scheduled Early[2]	62	10%	5%	6%
Preventive Care				
Immunization for Influenza[2]	360	71%	91%	90%
Immunization for Pneumonia[2]	465	58%	92%	92%
Stroke Care				
Anticoagulation Therapy for Atrial Fibrillation[1]	-	-	94%	95%
Antithrombotic Therapy Timing[1]	-	-	97%	98%
Assessed for Rehabilitation	12	83%	96%	97%
Discharged on Antithrombotic Therapy[1]	-	-	98%	99%
Discharged on Statin Medication[1]	-	-	91%	94%
Thrombolytic Therapy Timing[1]	-	-	54%	66%
Venous Thromboembolism Prophylaxis	12	83%	91%	94%
Written Stroke Educational Materials Given[1]	-	-	82%	88%
Surgical Care Improvement Project				
Appropriate Beta Blocker Usage[1]	-	-	98%	98%
Appropriate VTP Within 24 Hours	28	54%	98%	98%
Controlled Postoperative Blood Glucose[7]	-	-	97%	97%
Perioperative Temperature Management	32	94%	100%	100%
Prophylactic Antibiotic Selection[1]	-	-	99%	99%
Prophylactic Antibiotic Selection (Outpatient)[1,3]	-	-	98%	98%
Prophylactic Antibiotic Stopped[1]	-	-	98%	98%
Prophylactic Antibiotic Timing[1]	-	-	99%	99%
Prophylactic Antibiotic Timing (Outpatient)[1,3]	-	-	98%	98%
Urinary Catheter Removal	22	68%	98%	97%
Survey of Patients' Hospital Experiences				
Area Around Room 'Always' Quiet at Night	(a)	61%	61%	61%
Doctors 'Always' Communicated Well	(a)	87%	83%	82%
Home Recovery Information Given	(a)	86%	86%	85%
Hospital Given 9 or 10 on 10 Point Scale	(a)	76%	74%	71%
Meds 'Always' Explained Before Given	(a)	67%	64%	64%
Nurses 'Always' Communicated Well	(a)	82%	81%	79%
Pain 'Always' Well Controlled	(a)	69%	73%	71%
Room and Bathroom 'Always' Clean	(a)	81%	76%	73%
Timely Help 'Always' Received	(a)	74%	71%	68%
Would Definitely Recommend Hospital	(a)	74%	73%	71%
Use of Medical Imaging				
Cardiac Imaging Stress Test before Surgery	119	4.2%	5.4%	5.3%
Combination Abdominal CT Scan	424	17.2%	9.3%	10.5%
Combination Brain/Sinus CT Scan[1]	-	-	2.6%	2.7%
Combination Chest CT Scan	228	9.2%	4.6%	2.7%
Follow-up Mammogram/Ultrasound	401	11.2%	8.4%	8.8%
Lumbar Spine MRI for Low Back Pain	78	42.3%	38.7%	37.2%

Franciscan Saint Elizabeth Health - Crawfordsville

1710 Lafayette Rd
Crawfordsville, IN 47933
URL: www.stclaremedical.org
Phone: 765-362-2800
Fax: 765-364-9010
Type: Acute Care Hospitals
Ownership: Voluntary non-profit - Church
Emergency Services: Yes
Beds: 120

Key Personnel:
Radiology. . . . . Barry E Allen
Chief of Medical Staff . . . . Jude Momodu
CEO . . . . Terry Wilson

Measure	Cases	This Hosp.	State Avg.	U.S. Avg.
Blood Clot Prevention and Treatment				
Anticoagulation Overlap Therapy[1,2]	-	-	92%	93%
ICU Venous Thromboembolism Prophylaxis[2]	26	81%	91%	92%
Incidence of Potentially Preventable VTE[2,7]	-	-	10%	10%
UFH with Dosages/Platelet Monitoring[1,2]	-	-	95%	97%
Venous Thromboembolism Prophylaxis[2]	130	65%	83%	85%
Warfarin Therapy Discharge Instructions[1,2]	-	-	71%	75%
Chest Pain/Possible Heart Attack Care				
Aspirin Given Within 24 Hours of Arrival	81	96%	96%	96%
Fibrinolytic Meds Within 30 Min. of Arrival[7]	-	-	48%	58%
Average Time to ECG (minutes)	83	8	6	7
Average Time to Transfer (minutes)[1]	-	-	46	60
Children's Asthma Care				
Received Home Management Plan of Care	-	-	-	88%
Received Reliever Medication	-	-	-	100%
Received Systemic Corticosteroids	-	-	-	100%
Emergency Department				
Admittance Decision Time (minutes)[2]	448	68	80	98
Head CT Results Within 45 Min. of Arrival	17	65%	60%	57%
Patients Who Left ER Before Being Seen	20,458	1%	2%	2%
Time from ER Arrival to Admit. (minutes)[2]	457	210	241	274
Time from ER Arrival to Discharge (minutes)	404	101	122	134
Time in ER Before Being Evaluated (minutes)	285	18	22	26
Time to Pain Meds for Fractures (minutes)	91	39	52	57
Heart Attack Care				
Aspirin Given at Discharge[1,3]	-	-	99%	99%
Fibrinolytic Meds Within 30 Min. of Arrival[3,7]	-	-	67%	54%
PCI Within 90 Minutes of Arrival[3,7]	-	-	97%	96%
Statin Prescribed at Discharge[1,3]	-	-	99%	98%
Heart Failure Care				
ACE Inhibitor or ARB for LVSD	17	94%	97%	97%
Discharge Instructions Given	51	100%	95%	94%
Evaluation of LVS Function	64	97%	99%	99%
Medicare Spending				
Medicare Spending per Patient (ratio)	-	0.92	1.01	0.98
Pneumonia Care				
Appropriate Initial Antibiotic Given	38	95%	95%	95%
Blood Culture Timing	53	94%	98%	98%
Pregnancy and Delivery Care				
Newborn Deliveries Scheduled Early[7]	-	-	5%	6%
Preventive Care				
Immunization for Influenza[2]	318	92%	91%	90%
Immunization for Pneumonia[2]	522	91%	92%	92%
Stroke Care				
Anticoagulation Therapy for Atrial Fibrillation[1]	-	-	94%	95%
Antithrombotic Therapy Timing	13	100%	97%	98%
Assessed for Rehabilitation	12	100%	96%	97%
Discharged on Antithrombotic Therapy	12	100%	98%	99%
Discharged on Statin Medication[1]	-	-	91%	94%
Thrombolytic Therapy Timing[1]	-	-	54%	66%
Venous Thromboembolism Prophylaxis	11	91%	91%	94%
Written Stroke Educational Materials Given[1]	-	-	82%	88%
Surgical Care Improvement Project				
Appropriate Beta Blocker Usage	29	97%	98%	98%
Appropriate VTP Within 24 Hours	90	94%	98%	98%
Controlled Postoperative Blood Glucose[7]	-	-	97%	97%
Perioperative Temperature Management	104	100%	100%	100%
Prophylactic Antibiotic Selection	95	97%	99%	99%

NOTE: Hospital profiles are in alphabetical order by state, then city, then hospital within the city; Rankings exclude hospitals with less than 25 cases except for patient surveys which excludes hospitals with less than 100 cases; (a) 100-299 cases; (1) The number of cases/patients is too few to report; (2) Data submitted were based on a sample of cases/patients; (3) Results are based on a shorter time period than required; (4) Data suppressed by CMS for one or more quarters; (5) Results are not available for this reporting period; (6) Fewer than 100 patients completed the HCAHPS survey; (7) No cases met the criteria for this measure; (8) The lower limit of the confidence interval cannot be calculated if the number of observed infections equals zero; (9) No data are available from the state/territory for this reporting period; (10) The scores shown reflect fewer than 50 completed surveys; (11) There were discrepancies in the data collection process; (12) This measure does not apply to this hospital for this reporting period; (13) Results cannot be calculated for this reporting period; (14) The results for this state are combined with nearby states to protect confidentiality; Please refer to the User's Guide for a full explanation of data.

Measure	Cases	This Hosp.	State Avg.	U.S. Avg.
Prophylactic Antibiotic Selection (Outpatient)	63	84%	98%	98%
Prophylactic Antibiotic Stopped	93	97%	98%	98%
Prophylactic Antibiotic Timing	95	100%	99%	99%
Prophylactic Antibiotic Timing (Outpatient)	66	91%	98%	98%
Urinary Catheter Removal	17	88%	98%	97%
Survey of Patients' Hospital Experiences				
Area Around Room 'Always' Quiet at Night	(a)	73%	61%	61%
Doctors 'Always' Communicated Well	(a)	83%	83%	82%
Home Recovery Information Given	(a)	90%	86%	85%
Hospital Given 9 or 10 on 10 Point Scale	(a)	70%	74%	71%
Meds 'Always' Explained Before Given	(a)	69%	64%	64%
Nurses 'Always' Communicated Well	(a)	86%	81%	79%
Pain 'Always' Well Controlled	(a)	77%	73%	71%
Room and Bathroom 'Always' Clean	(a)	82%	76%	73%
Timely Help 'Always' Received	(a)	80%	71%	68%
Would Definitely Recommend Hospital	(a)	65%	73%	71%
Use of Medical Imaging				
Cardiac Imaging Stress Test before Surgery	196	6.1%	5.4%	5.3%
Combination Abdominal CT Scan	549	4.6%	9.3%	10.5%
Combination Brain/Sinus CT Scan[1]	-		2.6%	2.7%
Combination Chest CT Scan	235	1.3%	4.6%	2.7%
Follow-up Mammogram/Ultrasound	820	4.3%	8.4%	8.8%
Lumbar Spine MRI for Low Back Pain	52	50.0%	38.7%	37.2%

Franciscan Saint Anthony Health - Crown Point

1201 S Main St
Crown Point, IN 46307
Phone: 219-757-6100
Fax: 219-757-6242
URL: www.stanthonymedicalcenter.com
Type: Acute Care Hospitals
Emergency Services: Yes
Ownership: Voluntary non-profit - Church
Beds: 411

Key Personnel:
Radiology. . . . . Mohammed Abbas, MD
Operating Room. . . . . Carla McArdle
CEO/President. . . . . David F Ruskowski
Pediatric Ambulatory Care . . . . . . Darlene Sekerez, MD
Pediatric In-Patient Care . . . . Darlene Sekerez, MD
Infection Control. . . . . Chris Shakula
Cardiac Laboratory. . . . . Susan Slivka
Quality Assurance . . . . Sharon Werner

Measure	Cases	This Hosp.	State Avg.	U.S. Avg.
Blood Clot Prevention and Treatment				
Anticoagulation Overlap Therapy[2]	77	95%	92%	93%
ICU Venous Thromboembolism Prophylaxis[2]	35	94%	91%	92%
Incidence of Potentially Preventable VTE[1,2]	-	-	10%	10%
UFH with Dosages/Platelet Monitoring[2]	14	100%	95%	97%
Venous Thromboembolism Prophylaxis[2]	380	96%	83%	85%
Warfarin Therapy Discharge Instructions[2]	60	85%	71%	75%
Chest Pain/Possible Heart Attack Care				
Aspirin Given Within 24 Hours of Arrival[5]	-	-	96%	96%
Fibrinolytic Meds Within 30 Min. of Arrival[5]	-	-	48%	58%
Average Time to ECG (minutes)[5]	-	-	6	7
Average Time to Transfer (minutes)[5]	-	-	46	60
Children's Asthma Care				
Received Home Management Plan of Care	-	-	-	88%
Received Reliever Medication	-	-	-	100%
Received Systemic Corticosteroids	-	-	-	100%
Emergency Department				
Admittance Decision Time (minutes)[2]	395	135	80	98
Head CT Results Within 45 Min. of Arrival[1]	-	-	60%	57%
Patients Who Left ER Before Being Seen	32,704	1%	2%	2%
Time from ER Arrival to Admit. (minutes)[2]	463	285	241	274
Time from ER Arrival to Discharge (minutes)	372	130	122	134
Time in ER Before Being Evaluated (minutes)	415	21	22	26
Time to Pain Meds for Fractures (minutes)	124	46	52	57
Heart Attack Care				
Aspirin Given at Discharge	158	99%	99%	99%
Fibrinolytic Meds Within 30 Min. of Arrival[7]	-	-	67%	54%
PCI Within 90 Minutes of Arrival	35	100%	97%	96%
Statin Prescribed at Discharge	153	95%	99%	98%
Heart Failure Care				
ACE Inhibitor or ARB for LVSD[2]	65	97%	97%	97%
Discharge Instructions Given[2]	198	93%	95%	94%
Evaluation of LVS Function[2]	274	100%	99%	99%
Medicare Spending				
Medicare Spending per Patient (ratio)	-	0.99	1.01	0.98
Pneumonia Care				
Appropriate Initial Antibiotic Given[2]	78	95%	95%	95%
Blood Culture Timing[2]	127	99%	98%	98%
Pregnancy and Delivery Care				
Newborn Deliveries Scheduled Early[2]	24	4%	5%	6%
Preventive Care				
Immunization for Influenza[2]	520	99%	91%	90%
Immunization for Pneumonia[2]	641	99%	92%	92%
Stroke Care				
Anticoagulation Therapy for Atrial Fibrillation[2]	12	100%	94%	95%
Antithrombotic Therapy Timing[2]	72	97%	97%	98%
Assessed for Rehabilitation[2]	85	94%	96%	97%
Discharged on Antithrombotic Therapy[2]	76	95%	98%	99%
Discharged on Statin Medication[2]	59	88%	91%	94%
Thrombolytic Therapy Timing[1,2]	-	-	54%	66%
Venous Thromboembolism Prophylaxis[2]	87	92%	91%	94%
Written Stroke Educational Materials Given[2]	45	91%	82%	88%
Surgical Care Improvement Project				
Appropriate Beta Blocker Usage[2]	115	94%	98%	98%
Appropriate VTP Within 24 Hours[2]	282	99%	98%	98%
Controlled Postoperative Blood Glucose[2]	53	98%	97%	97%
Perioperative Temperature Management[2]	328	100%	100%	100%
Prophylactic Antibiotic Selection[2]	273	98%	99%	99%
Prophylactic Antibiotic Selection (Outpatient)	292	95%	98%	98%
Prophylactic Antibiotic Stopped[2]	261	95%	98%	98%
Prophylactic Antibiotic Timing[2]	273	99%	99%	99%
Prophylactic Antibiotic Timing (Outpatient)	293	99%	98%	98%
Urinary Catheter Removal[2]	209	95%	98%	97%
Survey of Patients' Hospital Experiences				
Area Around Room 'Always' Quiet at Night	300+	57%	61%	61%
Doctors 'Always' Communicated Well	300+	79%	83%	82%
Home Recovery Information Given	300+	83%	86%	85%
Hospital Given 9 or 10 on 10 Point Scale	300+	71%	74%	71%
Meds 'Always' Explained Before Given	300+	61%	64%	64%
Nurses 'Always' Communicated Well	300+	78%	81%	79%
Pain 'Always' Well Controlled	300+	71%	73%	71%
Room and Bathroom 'Always' Clean	300+	74%	76%	73%
Timely Help 'Always' Received	300+	60%	71%	68%
Would Definitely Recommend Hospital	300+	71%	73%	71%
Use of Medical Imaging				
Cardiac Imaging Stress Test before Surgery	82	8.5%	5.4%	5.3%
Combination Abdominal CT Scan	1,149	15.7%	9.3%	10.5%
Combination Brain/Sinus CT Scan	811	1.7%	2.6%	2.7%
Combination Chest CT Scan	688	16.4%	4.6%	2.7%
Follow-up Mammogram/Ultrasound	1,923	8.1%	8.4%	8.8%
Lumbar Spine MRI for Low Back Pain	249	42.2%	38.7%	37.2%

Pinnacle Hospital

9301 Connecticut Dr
Crown Point, IN 46307
Phone: 219-756-2100
URL: www.pinnaclehealthcare.net
Type: Acute Care Hospitals
Emergency Services: No
Ownership: Physician
Beds: 18

Measure	Cases	This Hosp.	State Avg.	U.S. Avg.
Blood Clot Prevention and Treatment				
Anticoagulation Overlap Therapy[1,2]	-	-	92%	93%
ICU Venous Thromboembolism Prophylaxis[2,7]	-	-	91%	92%
Incidence of Potentially Preventable VTE[2,7]	-	-	10%	10%
UFH with Dosages/Platelet Monitoring[1,2]	-	-	95%	97%
Venous Thromboembolism Prophylaxis[2]	332	79%	83%	85%
Warfarin Therapy Discharge Instructions[1,2]	-	-	71%	75%
Chest Pain/Possible Heart Attack Care				
Aspirin Given Within 24 Hours of Arrival[5]	-	-	96%	96%
Fibrinolytic Meds Within 30 Min. of Arrival[5]	-	-	48%	58%
Average Time to ECG (minutes)[5]	-	-	6	7
Average Time to Transfer (minutes)[5]	-	-	46	60
Children's Asthma Care				
Received Home Management Plan of Care	-	-	-	88%
Received Reliever Medication	-	-	-	100%
Received Systemic Corticosteroids	-	-	-	100%
Emergency Department				
Admittance Decision Time (minutes)[2,7]	-	-	80	98
Head CT Results Within 45 Min. of Arrival[5]	-	-	60%	57%
Patients Who Left ER Before Being Seen[5]	-	-	2%	2%
Time from ER Arrival to Admit. (minutes)[2,7]	-	-	241	274
Time from ER Arrival to Discharge (minutes)[5]	-	-	122	134
Time in ER Before Being Evaluated (minutes)[5]	-	-	22	26
Time to Pain Meds for Fractures (minutes)[5]	-	-	52	57
Heart Attack Care				
Aspirin Given at Discharge[5]	-	-	99%	99%
Fibrinolytic Meds Within 30 Min. of Arrival[5]	-	-	67%	54%
PCI Within 90 Minutes of Arrival[5]	-	-	97%	96%
Statin Prescribed at Discharge[5]	-	-	99%	98%
Heart Failure Care				
ACE Inhibitor or ARB for LVSD[1,2]	-	-	97%	97%
Discharge Instructions Given[1,2]	-	-	95%	94%
Evaluation of LVS Function[1,2]	-	-	99%	99%
Medicare Spending				
Medicare Spending per Patient (ratio)	-	0.96	1.01	0.98
Pneumonia Care				
Appropriate Initial Antibiotic Given[1,2]	-	-	95%	95%
Blood Culture Timing[1,2]	-	-	98%	98%
Pregnancy and Delivery Care				
Newborn Deliveries Scheduled Early[2,7]	-	-	5%	6%
Preventive Care				
Immunization for Influenza[2]	312	79%	91%	90%
Immunization for Pneumonia[2]	239	83%	92%	92%
Stroke Care				
Anticoagulation Therapy for Atrial Fibrillation[2,3]	-	-	94%	95%
Antithrombotic Therapy Timing[1,2]	-	-	97%	98%
Assessed for Rehabilitation[1,2]	-	-	96%	97%
Discharged on Antithrombotic Therapy[1,2]	-	-	98%	99%
Discharged on Statin Medication[1,2]	-	-	91%	94%
Thrombolytic Therapy Timing[2,3]	-	-	54%	66%
Venous Thromboembolism Prophylaxis[1,2]	-	-	91%	94%
Written Stroke Educational Materials Given[1,2]	-	-	82%	88%
Surgical Care Improvement Project				
Appropriate Beta Blocker Usage[1,2]	-	-	98%	98%
Appropriate VTP Within 24 Hours[2]	27	96%	98%	98%
Controlled Postoperative Blood Glucose[2,7]	-	-	97%	97%
Perioperative Temperature Management[2]	30	100%	100%	100%
Prophylactic Antibiotic Selection[2]	21	90%	99%	99%
Prophylactic Antibiotic Selection (Outpatient)[5]	-	-	98%	98%
Prophylactic Antibiotic Stopped[2]	21	86%	98%	98%
Prophylactic Antibiotic Timing[2]	21	100%	99%	99%
Prophylactic Antibiotic Timing (Outpatient)[5]	-	-	98%	98%
Urinary Catheter Removal[1,2]	-	-	98%	97%
Survey of Patients' Hospital Experiences				
Area Around Room 'Always' Quiet at Night	(a)	69%	61%	61%
Doctors 'Always' Communicated Well	(a)	84%	83%	82%
Home Recovery Information Given	(a)	84%	86%	85%
Hospital Given 9 or 10 on 10 Point Scale	(a)	76%	74%	71%
Meds 'Always' Explained Before Given	(a)	60%	64%	64%
Nurses 'Always' Communicated Well	(a)	77%	81%	79%
Pain 'Always' Well Controlled	(a)	67%	73%	71%
Room and Bathroom 'Always' Clean	(a)	71%	76%	73%
Timely Help 'Always' Received	(a)	72%	71%	68%
Would Definitely Recommend Hospital	(a)	78%	73%	71%
Use of Medical Imaging				
Cardiac Imaging Stress Test before Surgery[7]	-	-	5.4%	5.3%
Combination Abdominal CT Scan	108	30.6%	9.3%	10.5%
Combination Brain/Sinus CT Scan[1]	-	-	2.6%	2.7%
Combination Chest CT Scan[1]	-	-	4.6%	2.7%
Follow-up Mammogram/Ultrasound[7]	-	-	8.4%	8.8%
Lumbar Spine MRI for Low Back Pain	70	61.4%	38.7%	37.2%

Hendricks Regional Health

1000 E Main St
Danville, IN 46122
Phone: 317-745-4451
Fax: 317-745-8325
URL: www.hendricksregional.org
Type: Acute Care Hospitals
Emergency Services: Yes
Ownership: Government - Local
Beds: 141

Key Personnel:
Pediatric In-Patient Care . . . . Deb Case
Operating Room. . . . . Christopher M Evanson

NOTE: Hospital profiles are in alphabetical order by state, then city, then hospital within the city; Rankings exclude hospitals with less than 25 cases except for patient surveys which excludes hospitals with less than 100 cases; (a) 100-299 cases; (1) The number of cases/patients is too few to report; (2) Data submitted were based on a sample of cases/patients; (3) Results are based on a shorter time period than required; (4) Data suppressed by CMS for one or more quarters; (5) Results are not available for this reporting period; (6) Fewer than 100 patients completed the HCAHPS survey; (7) No cases met the criteria for this measure; (8) The lower limit of the confidence interval cannot be calculated if the number of observed infections equals zero; (9) No data are available from the state/territory for this reporting period; (10) The scores shown reflect fewer than 50 completed surveys; (11) There were discrepancies in the data collection process; (12) This measure does not apply to this hospital for this reporting period; (13) Results cannot be calculated for this reporting period; (14) The results for this state are combined with nearby states to protect confidentiality; Please refer to the User's Guide for a full explanation of data.

Radiology. . . . . Mark G Ferrara
Coronary Care . . . . Jo Morton
Intensive Care Unit. . . . . Jo Morton
Chief of Medical Staff . . . . Gordon Reed, MD
CEO/President. . . . . Kevin P. Speer, JD
Patient Relations . . . . Trudy Tharp

Measure	Cases	This Hosp.	State Avg.	U.S. Avg.
Blood Clot Prevention and Treatment				
Anticoagulation Overlap Therapy[2]	32	100%	92%	93%
ICU Venous Thromboembolism Prophylaxis[2]	88	99%	91%	92%
Incidence of Potentially Preventable VTE[1,2]	-	-	10%	10%
UFH with Dosages/Platelet Monitoring[1,2]	-	-	95%	97%
Venous Thromboembolism Prophylaxis[2]	337	97%	83%	85%
Warfarin Therapy Discharge Instructions[2]	25	64%	71%	75%
Chest Pain/Possible Heart Attack Care				
Aspirin Given Within 24 Hours of Arrival	159	100%	96%	96%
Fibrinolytic Meds Within 30 Min. of Arrival[7]	-	-	48%	58%
Average Time to ECG (minutes)	162	4	6	7
Average Time to Transfer (minutes)	33	43	46	60
Children's Asthma Care				
Received Home Management Plan of Care	-	-	-	88%
Received Reliever Medication	-	-	-	100%
Received Systemic Corticosteroids	-	-	-	100%
Emergency Department				
Admittance Decision Time (minutes)[2]	542	90	80	98
Head CT Results Within 45 Min. of Arrival[1]	-	-	60%	57%
Patients Who Left ER Before Being Seen	30,396	0%	2%	2%
Time from ER Arrival to Admit. (minutes)[2]	586	227	241	274
Time from ER Arrival to Discharge (minutes)	754	127	122	134
Time in ER Before Being Evaluated (minutes)	840	24	22	26
Time to Pain Meds for Fractures (minutes)	112	53	52	57
Heart Attack Care				
Aspirin Given at Discharge	50	94%	99%	99%
Fibrinolytic Meds Within 30 Min. of Arrival[7]	-	-	67%	54%
PCI Within 90 Minutes of Arrival[1]	-	-	97%	96%
Statin Prescribed at Discharge	46	87%	99%	98%
Heart Failure Care				
ACE Inhibitor or ARB for LVSD	46	98%	97%	97%
Discharge Instructions Given	86	95%	95%	94%
Evaluation of LVS Function	117	99%	99%	99%
Medicare Spending				
Medicare Spending per Patient (ratio)	-	0.99	1.01	0.98
Pneumonia Care				
Appropriate Initial Antibiotic Given	115	95%	95%	95%
Blood Culture Timing	174	95%	98%	98%
Pregnancy and Delivery Care				
Newborn Deliveries Scheduled Early	198	2%	5%	6%
Preventive Care				
Immunization for Influenza[2]	487	95%	91%	90%
Immunization for Pneumonia[2]	578	97%	92%	92%
Stroke Care				
Anticoagulation Therapy for Atrial Fibrillation[1]	-	-	94%	95%
Antithrombotic Therapy Timing	44	100%	97%	98%
Assessed for Rehabilitation	62	100%	96%	97%
Discharged on Antithrombotic Therapy	53	98%	98%	99%
Discharged on Statin Medication	40	100%	91%	94%
Thrombolytic Therapy Timing[1]	-	-	54%	66%
Venous Thromboembolism Prophylaxis	52	100%	91%	94%
Written Stroke Educational Materials Given	35	77%	82%	88%
Surgical Care Improvement Project				
Appropriate Beta Blocker Usage	175	99%	98%	98%
Appropriate VTP Within 24 Hours	482	99%	98%	98%
Controlled Postoperative Blood Glucose[7]	-	-	97%	97%
Perioperative Temperature Management	523	100%	100%	100%
Prophylactic Antibiotic Selection	402	99%	99%	99%
Prophylactic Antibiotic Selection (Outpatient)	216	98%	98%	98%
Prophylactic Antibiotic Stopped	399	99%	98%	98%
Prophylactic Antibiotic Timing	402	99%	99%	99%
Prophylactic Antibiotic Timing (Outpatient)	216	98%	98%	98%
Urinary Catheter Removal	380	99%	98%	97%
Survey of Patients' Hospital Experiences				
Area Around Room 'Always' Quiet at Night	300+	64%	61%	61%
Doctors 'Always' Communicated Well	300+	86%	83%	82%
Home Recovery Information Given	300+	89%	86%	85%
Hospital Given 9 or 10 on 10 Point Scale	300+	83%	74%	71%
Meds 'Always' Explained Before Given	300+	65%	64%	64%
Nurses 'Always' Communicated Well	300+	83%	81%	79%
Pain 'Always' Well Controlled	300+	73%	73%	71%
Room and Bathroom 'Always' Clean	300+	77%	76%	73%
Timely Help 'Always' Received	300+	68%	71%	68%
Would Definitely Recommend Hospital	300+	84%	73%	71%
Use of Medical Imaging				
Cardiac Imaging Stress Test before Surgery	191	6.3%	5.4%	5.3%
Combination Abdominal CT Scan	930	27.0%	9.3%	10.5%
Combination Brain/Sinus CT Scan	595	1.5%	2.6%	2.7%
Combination Chest CT Scan	495	23.2%	4.6%	2.7%
Follow-up Mammogram/Ultrasound	1,381	7.1%	8.4%	8.8%
Lumbar Spine MRI for Low Back Pain	123	46.3%	38.7%	37.2%

Adams Memorial Hospital

1100 Mercer Ave
Decatur, IN 46733
Phone: 260-724-2145
Fax: 260-728-3865
URL: www.adamshospital.com
Type: Critical Access Hospitals
Emergency Services: Yes
Ownership: Government - Local
Beds: 87

Key Personnel:
Anesthesiology. . . . . Donald Advent, MD
Cardiac Laboratory. . . . . Ronda Brune
Infection Control . . . . Peggy LaFountaine
Emergency Room . . . . Lesley Scholl, MD
Chief of Medical Staff . . . . Brian Zurcher, MD

Measure	Cases	This Hosp.	State Avg.	U.S. Avg.
Blood Clot Prevention and Treatment				
Anticoagulation Overlap Therapy[5]	-	-	92%	93%
ICU Venous Thromboembolism Prophylaxis[5]	-	-	91%	92%
Incidence of Potentially Preventable VTE[5]	-	-	10%	10%
UFH with Dosages/Platelet Monitoring[5]	-	-	95%	97%
Venous Thromboembolism Prophylaxis[5]	-	-	83%	85%
Warfarin Therapy Discharge Instructions[5]	-	-	71%	75%
Chest Pain/Possible Heart Attack Care				
Aspirin Given Within 24 Hours of Arrival[5]	-	-	96%	96%
Fibrinolytic Meds Within 30 Min. of Arrival[5]	-	-	48%	58%
Average Time to ECG (minutes)[5]	-	-	6	7
Average Time to Transfer (minutes)[5]	-	-	46	60
Children's Asthma Care				
Received Home Management Plan of Care	-	-	-	88%
Received Reliever Medication	-	-	-	100%
Received Systemic Corticosteroids	-	-	-	100%
Emergency Department				
Admittance Decision Time (minutes)[2]	525	44	80	98
Head CT Results Within 45 Min. of Arrival[5]	-	-	60%	57%
Patients Who Left ER Before Being Seen	11,725	0%	2%	2%
Time from ER Arrival to Admit. (minutes)[2]	548	170	241	274
Time from ER Arrival to Discharge (minutes)[5]	-	-	122	134
Time in ER Before Being Evaluated (minutes)[5]	-	-	22	26
Time to Pain Meds for Fractures (minutes)[5]	-	-	52	57
Heart Attack Care				
Aspirin Given at Discharge[1]	-	-	99%	99%
Fibrinolytic Meds Within 30 Min. of Arrival[7]	-	-	67%	54%
PCI Within 90 Minutes of Arrival[7]	-	-	97%	96%
Statin Prescribed at Discharge[1]	-	-	99%	98%
Heart Failure Care				
ACE Inhibitor or ARB for LVSD	11	91%	97%	97%
Discharge Instructions Given	41	95%	95%	94%
Evaluation of LVS Function	60	100%	99%	99%
Medicare Spending				
Medicare Spending per Patient (ratio)	-	-	1.01	0.98
Pneumonia Care				
Appropriate Initial Antibiotic Given	64	88%	95%	95%
Blood Culture Timing	82	98%	98%	98%
Pregnancy and Delivery Care				
Newborn Deliveries Scheduled Early[1,3]	-	-	5%	6%
Preventive Care				
Immunization for Influenza[2]	282	81%	91%	90%
Immunization for Pneumonia[2]	482	79%	92%	92%
Stroke Care				
Anticoagulation Therapy for Atrial Fibrillation[5]	-	-	94%	95%
Antithrombotic Therapy Timing[5]	-	-	97%	98%
Assessed for Rehabilitation[5]	-	-	96%	97%
Discharged on Antithrombotic Therapy[5]	-	-	98%	99%
Discharged on Statin Medication[5]	-	-	91%	94%
Thrombolytic Therapy Timing[5]	-	-	54%	66%
Venous Thromboembolism Prophylaxis[5]	-	-	91%	94%
Written Stroke Educational Materials Given[5]	-	-	82%	88%
Surgical Care Improvement Project				
Appropriate Beta Blocker Usage	15	93%	98%	98%
Appropriate VTP Within 24 Hours	63	94%	98%	98%
Controlled Postoperative Blood Glucose[3,7]	-	-	97%	97%
Perioperative Temperature Management	65	100%	100%	100%
Prophylactic Antibiotic Selection	12	100%	99%	99%
Prophylactic Antibiotic Selection (Outpatient)[5]	-	-	98%	98%
Prophylactic Antibiotic Stopped	12	83%	98%	98%
Prophylactic Antibiotic Timing	12	92%	99%	99%
Prophylactic Antibiotic Timing (Outpatient)[5]	-	-	98%	98%
Urinary Catheter Removal	43	95%	98%	97%
Survey of Patients' Hospital Experiences				
Area Around Room 'Always' Quiet at Night	300+	61%	61%	61%
Doctors 'Always' Communicated Well	300+	82%	83%	82%
Home Recovery Information Given	300+	86%	86%	85%
Hospital Given 9 or 10 on 10 Point Scale	300+	74%	74%	71%
Meds 'Always' Explained Before Given	300+	62%	64%	64%
Nurses 'Always' Communicated Well	300+	84%	81%	79%
Pain 'Always' Well Controlled	300+	70%	73%	71%
Room and Bathroom 'Always' Clean	300+	87%	76%	73%
Timely Help 'Always' Received	300+	74%	71%	68%
Would Definitely Recommend Hospital	300+	69%	73%	71%
Use of Medical Imaging				
Cardiac Imaging Stress Test before Surgery	62	3.2%	5.4%	5.3%
Combination Abdominal CT Scan	209	1.9%	9.3%	10.5%
Combination Brain/Sinus CT Scan	240	0.4%	2.6%	2.7%
Combination Chest CT Scan	93	1.1%	4.6%	2.7%
Follow-up Mammogram/Ultrasound	359	8.9%	8.4%	8.8%
Lumbar Spine MRI for Low Back Pain	47	36.2%	38.7%	37.2%

Franciscan Saint Margaret Health - Dyer

24 Joliet St
Dyer, IN 46311
Phone: 219-865-2141
Fax: 219-864-2585
URL: www.smmhc.com
Type: Acute Care Hospitals
Emergency Services: Yes
Ownership: Voluntary non-profit - Private
Beds: 794

Key Personnel:
CEO/President. . . . . Eugene Diamond
Radiology. . . . . Wally Grzych
Chief of Medical Staff . . . . R Kanuru, MD
Pediatric In-Patient Care . . . . Anne Leus
Quality Assurance . . . . Joanne O'Malley
Cardiac Laboratory. . . . . Dora Slupsizi

Measure	Cases	This Hosp.	State Avg.	U.S. Avg.
Blood Clot Prevention and Treatment				
Anticoagulation Overlap Therapy[2]	42	95%	92%	93%
ICU Venous Thromboembolism Prophylaxis[2]	66	89%	91%	92%
Incidence of Potentially Preventable VTE[1,2]	-	-	10%	10%
UFH with Dosages/Platelet Monitoring[2]	21	90%	95%	97%
Venous Thromboembolism Prophylaxis[2]	343	73%	83%	85%
Warfarin Therapy Discharge Instructions[2]	36	47%	71%	75%
Chest Pain/Possible Heart Attack Care				
Aspirin Given Within 24 Hours of Arrival[1,3]	-	-	96%	96%
Fibrinolytic Meds Within 30 Min. of Arrival[5]	-	-	48%	58%
Average Time to ECG (minutes)[1,3]	-	-	6	7
Average Time to Transfer (minutes)[5]	-	-	46	60
Children's Asthma Care				
Received Home Management Plan of Care	-	-	-	88%
Received Reliever Medication	-	-	-	100%
Received Systemic Corticosteroids	-	-	-	100%
Emergency Department				
Admittance Decision Time (minutes)[2]	658	96	80	98
Head CT Results Within 45 Min. of Arrival	11	73%	60%	57%
Patients Who Left ER Before Being Seen	11,484	1%	2%	2%
Time from ER Arrival to Admit. (minutes)[2]	658	247	241	274
Time from ER Arrival to Discharge (minutes)	477	120	122	134
Time in ER Before Being Evaluated (minutes)	503	28	22	26

NOTE: Hospital profiles are in alphabetical order by state, then city, then hospital within the city; Rankings exclude hospitals with less than 25 cases except for patient surveys which excludes hospitals with less than 100 cases; (a) 100-299 cases; (1) The number of cases/patients is too few to report; (2) Data submitted were based on a sample of cases/patients; (3) Results are based on a shorter time period than required; (4) Data suppressed by CMS for one or more quarters; (5) Results are not available for this reporting period; (6) Fewer than 100 patients completed the HCAHPS survey; (7) No cases met the criteria for this measure; (8) The lower limit of the confidence interval cannot be calculated if the number of observed infections equals zero; (9) No data are available from the state/territory for this reporting period; (10) The scores shown reflect fewer than 50 completed surveys; (11) There were discrepancies in the data collection process; (12) This measure does not apply to this hospital for this reporting period; (13) Results cannot be calculated for this reporting period; (14) The results for this state are combined with nearby states to protect confidentiality; Please refer to the User's Guide for a full explanation of data.

Measure	Cases	This Hosp.	State Avg.	U.S. Avg.
Time to Pain Meds for Fractures (minutes)	80	46	52	57
Heart Attack Care				
Aspirin Given at Discharge	89	100%	99%	99%
Fibrinolytic Meds Within 30 Min. of Arrival[7]	-	-	67%	54%
PCI Within 90 Minutes of Arrival	18	94%	97%	96%
Statin Prescribed at Discharge	87	98%	99%	98%
Heart Failure Care				
ACE Inhibitor or ARB for LVSD	63	97%	97%	97%
Discharge Instructions Given	188	96%	95%	94%
Evaluation of LVS Function	240	100%	99%	99%
Medicare Spending				
Medicare Spending per Patient (ratio)	-	1.05	1.01	0.98
Pneumonia Care				
Appropriate Initial Antibiotic Given	57	100%	95%	95%
Blood Culture Timing	146	96%	98%	98%
Pregnancy and Delivery Care				
Newborn Deliveries Scheduled Early[2]	29	3%	5%	6%
Preventive Care				
Immunization for Influenza[2]	533	85%	91%	90%
Immunization for Pneumonia[2]	696	86%	92%	92%
Stroke Care				
Anticoagulation Therapy for Atrial Fibrillation	12	83%	94%	95%
Antithrombotic Therapy Timing	67	97%	97%	98%
Assessed for Rehabilitation	84	96%	96%	97%
Discharged on Antithrombotic Therapy	73	97%	98%	99%
Discharged on Statin Medication	60	98%	91%	94%
Thrombolytic Therapy Timing[1]	-	-	54%	66%
Venous Thromboembolism Prophylaxis	88	90%	91%	94%
Written Stroke Educational Materials Given	50	90%	82%	88%
Surgical Care Improvement Project				
Appropriate Beta Blocker Usage	134	99%	98%	98%
Appropriate VTP Within 24 Hours	452	99%	98%	98%
Controlled Postoperative Blood Glucose	25	100%	97%	97%
Perioperative Temperature Management	508	100%	100%	100%
Prophylactic Antibiotic Selection	389	99%	99%	99%
Prophylactic Antibiotic Selection (Outpatient)	211	99%	98%	98%
Prophylactic Antibiotic Stopped	378	99%	98%	98%
Prophylactic Antibiotic Timing	389	100%	99%	99%
Prophylactic Antibiotic Timing (Outpatient)	194	95%	98%	98%
Urinary Catheter Removal	134	99%	98%	97%
Survey of Patients' Hospital Experiences				
Area Around Room 'Always' Quiet at Night	300+	54%	61%	61%
Doctors 'Always' Communicated Well	300+	82%	83%	82%
Home Recovery Information Given	300+	82%	86%	85%
Hospital Given 9 or 10 on 10 Point Scale	300+	68%	74%	71%
Meds 'Always' Explained Before Given	300+	66%	64%	64%
Nurses 'Always' Communicated Well	300+	81%	81%	79%
Pain 'Always' Well Controlled	300+	69%	73%	71%
Room and Bathroom 'Always' Clean	300+	76%	76%	73%
Timely Help 'Always' Received	300+	73%	71%	68%
Would Definitely Recommend Hospital	300+	70%	73%	71%
Use of Medical Imaging				
Cardiac Imaging Stress Test before Surgery	252	5.6%	5.4%	5.3%
Combination Abdominal CT Scan	541	32.0%	9.3%	10.5%
Combination Brain/Sinus CT Scan[1]	-	-	2.6%	2.7%
Combination Chest CT Scan	265	15.5%	4.6%	2.7%
Follow-up Mammogram/Ultrasound	585	13.3%	8.4%	8.8%
Lumbar Spine MRI for Low Back Pain	73	45.2%	38.7%	37.2%

Saint Catherine Hospital

4321 Fir St
East Chicago, IN 46312
URL: www.comhs.org/stcatherine
Type: Acute Care Hospitals
Ownership: Voluntary non-profit - Private

Phone: 219-392-7004
Fax: 219-392-7622
Emergency Services: Yes
Beds: 290

Key Personnel:

CEO . . . . JoAnn Birdzell
Emergency Room . . . . Jeffery Dubnow
Cardiac Laboratory. . . . . Miguel Gambette
Chief of Medical Staff. . . . . John Griep
Operating Room. . . . . Lori McBride, RN

Measure	Cases	This Hosp.	State Avg.	U.S. Avg.
Blood Clot Prevention and Treatment				
Anticoagulation Overlap Therapy[2]	29	100%	92%	93%
ICU Venous Thromboembolism Prophylaxis[2]	72	100%	91%	92%
Incidence of Potentially Preventable VTE[1,2]	-	-	10%	10%
UFH with Dosages/Platelet Monitoring[1,2]	-	-	95%	97%
Venous Thromboembolism Prophylaxis[2]	380	99%	83%	85%
Warfarin Therapy Discharge Instructions[2]	21	100%	71%	75%
Chest Pain/Possible Heart Attack Care				
Aspirin Given Within 24 Hours of Arrival[5]	-	-	96%	96%
Fibrinolytic Meds Within 30 Min. of Arrival[5]	-	-	48%	58%
Average Time to ECG (minutes)[5]	-	-	6	7
Average Time to Transfer (minutes)[5]	-	-	46	60
Children's Asthma Care				
Received Home Management Plan of Care	-	-	-	88%
Received Reliever Medication	-	-	-	100%
Received Systemic Corticosteroids	-	-	-	100%
Emergency Department				
Admittance Decision Time (minutes)[2]	708	111	80	98
Head CT Results Within 45 Min. of Arrival[1]	-	-	60%	57%
Patients Who Left ER Before Being Seen	33,458	2%	2%	2%
Time from ER Arrival to Admit. (minutes)[2]	708	264	241	274
Time from ER Arrival to Discharge (minutes)	389	146	122	134
Time in ER Before Being Evaluated (minutes)	418	26	22	26
Time to Pain Meds for Fractures (minutes)	113	58	52	57
Heart Attack Care				
Aspirin Given at Discharge	65	100%	99%	99%
Fibrinolytic Meds Within 30 Min. of Arrival[7]	-	-	67%	54%
PCI Within 90 Minutes of Arrival	15	100%	97%	96%
Statin Prescribed at Discharge	65	100%	99%	98%
Heart Failure Care				
ACE Inhibitor or ARB for LVSD	93	98%	97%	97%
Discharge Instructions Given	222	99%	95%	94%
Evaluation of LVS Function	281	99%	99%	99%
Medicare Spending				
Medicare Spending per Patient (ratio)	-	1.14	1.01	0.98
Pneumonia Care				
Appropriate Initial Antibiotic Given	68	100%	95%	95%
Blood Culture Timing	103	100%	98%	98%
Pregnancy and Delivery Care				
Newborn Deliveries Scheduled Early[2]	39	0%	5%	6%
Preventive Care				
Immunization for Influenza[2]	585	95%	91%	90%
Immunization for Pneumonia[2]	772	98%	92%	92%
Stroke Care				
Anticoagulation Therapy for Atrial Fibrillation	11	82%	94%	95%
Antithrombotic Therapy Timing	75	95%	97%	98%
Assessed for Rehabilitation	85	99%	96%	97%
Discharged on Antithrombotic Therapy	81	98%	98%	99%
Discharged on Statin Medication	67	91%	91%	94%
Thrombolytic Therapy Timing[1]	-	-	54%	66%
Venous Thromboembolism Prophylaxis	84	86%	91%	94%
Written Stroke Educational Materials Given	43	91%	82%	88%
Surgical Care Improvement Project				
Appropriate Beta Blocker Usage	67	100%	98%	98%
Appropriate VTP Within 24 Hours	132	100%	98%	98%
Controlled Postoperative Blood Glucose	39	100%	97%	97%
Perioperative Temperature Management	189	100%	100%	100%
Prophylactic Antibiotic Selection	143	99%	99%	99%
Prophylactic Antibiotic Selection (Outpatient)	66	97%	98%	98%
Prophylactic Antibiotic Stopped	137	100%	98%	98%
Prophylactic Antibiotic Timing	144	100%	99%	99%
Prophylactic Antibiotic Timing (Outpatient)	58	100%	98%	98%
Urinary Catheter Removal	85	100%	98%	97%
Survey of Patients' Hospital Experiences				
Area Around Room 'Always' Quiet at Night	300+	65%	61%	61%
Doctors 'Always' Communicated Well	300+	80%	83%	82%
Home Recovery Information Given	300+	84%	86%	85%
Hospital Given 9 or 10 on 10 Point Scale	300+	73%	74%	71%
Meds 'Always' Explained Before Given	300+	66%	64%	64%
Nurses 'Always' Communicated Well	300+	82%	81%	79%
Pain 'Always' Well Controlled	300+	74%	73%	71%
Room and Bathroom 'Always' Clean	300+	74%	76%	73%
Timely Help 'Always' Received	300+	69%	71%	68%
Would Definitely Recommend Hospital	300+	74%	73%	71%
Use of Medical Imaging				
Cardiac Imaging Stress Test before Surgery	375	6.1%	5.4%	5.3%
Combination Abdominal CT Scan	590	3.4%	9.3%	10.5%
Combination Brain/Sinus CT Scan[1]	-	-	2.6%	2.7%
Combination Chest CT Scan	216	0.5%	4.6%	2.7%
Follow-up Mammogram/Ultrasound	778	9.1%	8.4%	8.8%
Lumbar Spine MRI for Low Back Pain	57	36.8%	38.7%	37.2%

Elkhart General Hospital

600 E Blvd
Elkhart, IN 46514
URL: www.egh.org
Type: Acute Care Hospitals
Ownership: Government - Local

Phone: 574-294-2621
Fax: 574-523-3495
Emergency Services: Yes
Beds: 365

Key Personnel:

Emergency Room . . . . Colleen Nowlin
Chairman/CEO . . . . Matthew Pletcher
Quality Assurance . . . . Jean Putnam
CEO/President. . . . . Mary Thornton

Measure	Cases	This Hosp.	State Avg.	U.S. Avg.
Blood Clot Prevention and Treatment				
Anticoagulation Overlap Therapy[2]	139	97%	92%	93%
ICU Venous Thromboembolism Prophylaxis[2]	158	97%	91%	92%
Incidence of Potentially Preventable VTE[2]	20	10%	10%	10%
UFH with Dosages/Platelet Monitoring[2]	152	95%	95%	97%
Venous Thromboembolism Prophylaxis[2]	401	90%	83%	85%
Warfarin Therapy Discharge Instructions[2]	115	68%	71%	75%
Chest Pain/Possible Heart Attack Care				
Aspirin Given Within 24 Hours of Arrival[5]	-	-	96%	96%
Fibrinolytic Meds Within 30 Min. of Arrival[5]	-	-	48%	58%
Average Time to ECG (minutes)[5]	-	-	6	7
Average Time to Transfer (minutes)[5]	-	-	46	60
Children's Asthma Care				
Received Home Management Plan of Care	-	-	-	88%
Received Reliever Medication	-	-	-	100%
Received Systemic Corticosteroids	-	-	-	100%
Emergency Department				
Admittance Decision Time (minutes)[2]	637	103	80	98
Head CT Results Within 45 Min. of Arrival[1,3]	-	-	60%	57%
Patients Who Left ER Before Being Seen	63,114	1%	2%	2%
Time from ER Arrival to Admit. (minutes)[2]	637	254	241	274
Time from ER Arrival to Discharge (minutes)	563	111	122	134
Time in ER Before Being Evaluated (minutes)	579	20	22	26
Time to Pain Meds for Fractures (minutes)	155	44	52	57
Heart Attack Care				
Aspirin Given at Discharge[2]	285	99%	99%	99%
Fibrinolytic Meds Within 30 Min. of Arrival[1,2]	-	-	67%	54%
PCI Within 90 Minutes of Arrival[2]	65	98%	97%	96%
Statin Prescribed at Discharge[2]	282	100%	99%	98%
Heart Failure Care				
ACE Inhibitor or ARB for LVSD[2]	146	95%	97%	97%
Discharge Instructions Given[2]	398	89%	95%	94%
Evaluation of LVS Function[2]	483	100%	99%	99%
Medicare Spending				
Medicare Spending per Patient (ratio)	-	0.98	1.01	0.98
Pneumonia Care				
Appropriate Initial Antibiotic Given[2]	85	99%	95%	95%
Blood Culture Timing[2]	149	100%	98%	98%
Pregnancy and Delivery Care				
Newborn Deliveries Scheduled Early	163	2%	5%	6%
Preventive Care				
Immunization for Influenza[2]	534	98%	91%	90%
Immunization for Pneumonia[2]	669	98%	92%	92%
Stroke Care				
Anticoagulation Therapy for Atrial Fibrillation[2]	23	100%	94%	95%
Antithrombotic Therapy Timing[2]	125	97%	97%	98%
Assessed for Rehabilitation[2]	148	96%	96%	97%
Discharged on Antithrombotic Therapy[2]	133	98%	98%	99%
Discharged on Statin Medication[2]	91	92%	91%	94%
Thrombolytic Therapy Timing[1,2]	-	-	54%	66%
Venous Thromboembolism Prophylaxis[2]	151	91%	91%	94%
Written Stroke Educational Materials Given[2]	74	84%	82%	88%
Surgical Care Improvement Project				

NOTE: Hospital profiles are in alphabetical order by state, then city, then hospital within the city; Rankings exclude hospitals with less than 25 cases except for patient surveys which excludes hospitals with less than 100 cases; (a) 100-299 cases; (1) The number of cases/patients is too few to report; (2) Data submitted were based on a sample of cases/patients; (3) Results are based on a shorter time period than required; (4) Data suppressed by CMS for one or more quarters; (5) Results are not available for this reporting period; (6) Fewer than 100 patients completed the HCAHPS survey; (7) No cases met the criteria for this measure; (8) The lower limit of the confidence interval cannot be calculated if the number of observed infections equals zero; (9) No data are available from the state/territory for this reporting period; (10) The scores shown reflect fewer than 50 completed surveys; (11) There were discrepancies in the data collection process; (12) This measure does not apply to this hospital for this reporting period; (13) Results cannot be calculated for this reporting period; (14) The results for this state are combined with nearby states to protect confidentiality; Please refer to the User's Guide for a full explanation of data.

Appropriate Beta Blocker Usage[2]	421	98%	98%	98%
Appropriate VTP Within 24 Hours[2]	782	99%	98%	98%
Controlled Postoperative Blood Glucose[2]	203	100%	97%	97%
Perioperative Temperature Management[2]	1,016	100%	100%	100%
Prophylactic Antibiotic Selection[2]	797	100%	99%	99%
Prophylactic Antibiotic Selection (Outpatient)	357	98%	98%	98%
Prophylactic Antibiotic Stopped[2]	763	100%	98%	98%
Prophylactic Antibiotic Timing[2]	797	100%	99%	99%
Prophylactic Antibiotic Timing (Outpatient)	360	98%	98%	98%
Urinary Catheter Removal[2]	834	100%	98%	97%
Survey of Patients' Hospital Experiences				
Area Around Room 'Always' Quiet at Night	300+	55%	61%	61%
Doctors 'Always' Communicated Well	300+	77%	83%	82%
Home Recovery Information Given	300+	86%	86%	85%
Hospital Given 9 or 10 on 10 Point Scale	300+	69%	74%	71%
Meds 'Always' Explained Before Given	300+	59%	64%	64%
Nurses 'Always' Communicated Well	300+	76%	81%	79%
Pain 'Always' Well Controlled	300+	69%	73%	71%
Room and Bathroom 'Always' Clean	300+	74%	76%	73%
Timely Help 'Always' Received	300+	63%	71%	68%
Would Definitely Recommend Hospital	300+	71%	73%	71%
Use of Medical Imaging				
Cardiac Imaging Stress Test before Surgery	1,049	3.8%	5.4%	5.3%
Combination Abdominal CT Scan	1,047	3.3%	9.3%	10.5%
Combination Brain/Sinus CT Scan	1,041	1.2%	2.6%	2.7%
Combination Chest CT Scan	474	0.2%	4.6%	2.7%
Follow-up Mammogram/Ultrasound	2,333	6.8%	8.4%	8.8%
Lumbar Spine MRI for Low Back Pain	156	34.6%	38.7%	37.2%

Saint Vincent Mercy Hospital

1331 S A St
Elwood, IN 46036
URL: www.stvincent.org
Phone: 765-552-4743
Fax: 765-552-4700
Type: Critical Access Hospitals
Emergency Services: Yes
Ownership: Voluntary non-profit - Church
Beds: 25

Key Personnel:

Radiology . . . . Maria S Coutz
Quality Assurance . . . . John D Doyle
Emergency Room . . . . Brad Hayes
Chief of Medical Staff . . . . Robert Helm, MD
Intensive Care Unit . . . . Tamala Hobbs
Operating Room . . . . Sheryl Miller, RN
CEO . . . . Jonathan Nalli
Infection Control . . . . Candy Robinson

Measure	Cases	This Hosp.	State Avg.	U.S. Avg.
Blood Clot Prevention and Treatment				
Anticoagulation Overlap Therapy[1]	-	-	92%	93%
ICU Venous Thromboembolism Prophylaxis[7]	-	-	91%	92%
Incidence of Potentially Preventable VTE[7]	-	-	10%	10%
UFH with Dosages/Platelet Monitoring[1]	-	-	95%	97%
Venous Thromboembolism Prophylaxis	297	91%	83%	85%
Warfarin Therapy Discharge Instructions[1]	-	-	71%	75%
Chest Pain/Possible Heart Attack Care				
Aspirin Given Within 24 Hours of Arrival	53	89%	96%	96%
Fibrinolytic Meds Within 30 Min. of Arrival[1]	-	-	48%	58%
Average Time to ECG (minutes)	57	7	6	7
Average Time to Transfer (minutes)	14	106	46	60
Children's Asthma Care				
Received Home Management Plan of Care	-	-	-	88%
Received Reliever Medication	-	-	-	100%
Received Systemic Corticosteroids	-	-	-	100%
Emergency Department				
Admittance Decision Time (minutes)[5]	-	-	80	98
Head CT Results Within 45 Min. of Arrival[5]	-	-	60%	57%
Patients Who Left ER Before Being Seen	9,927	1%	2%	2%
Time from ER Arrival to Admit. (minutes)[5]	-	-	241	274
Time from ER Arrival to Discharge (minutes)[5]	-	-	122	134
Time in ER Before Being Evaluated (minutes)[5]	-	-	22	26
Time to Pain Meds for Fractures (minutes)[5]	-	-	52	57
Heart Attack Care				
Aspirin Given at Discharge[1,3]	-	-	99%	99%
Fibrinolytic Meds Within 30 Min. of Arrival[3,7]	-	-	67%	54%
PCI Within 90 Minutes of Arrival[3,7]	-	-	97%	96%
Statin Prescribed at Discharge[1,3]	-	-	99%	98%
Heart Failure Care				
ACE Inhibitor or ARB for LVSD[1]	-	-	97%	97%
Discharge Instructions Given	17	100%	95%	94%
Evaluation of LVS Function	30	83%	99%	99%
Medicare Spending				
Medicare Spending per Patient (ratio)	-	-	1.01	0.98
Pneumonia Care				
Appropriate Initial Antibiotic Given	46	87%	95%	95%
Blood Culture Timing	50	94%	98%	98%
Pregnancy and Delivery Care				
Newborn Deliveries Scheduled Early[5]	-	-	5%	6%
Preventive Care				
Immunization for Influenza[5]	-	-	91%	90%
Immunization for Pneumonia[5]	-	-	92%	92%
Stroke Care				
Anticoagulation Therapy for Atrial Fibrillation[1]	-	-	94%	95%
Antithrombotic Therapy Timing	11	73%	97%	98%
Assessed for Rehabilitation	12	100%	96%	97%
Discharged on Antithrombotic Therapy	12	83%	98%	99%
Discharged on Statin Medication	12	58%	91%	94%
Thrombolytic Therapy Timing[1]	-	-	54%	66%
Venous Thromboembolism Prophylaxis	12	83%	91%	94%
Written Stroke Educational Materials Given[1]	-	-	82%	88%
Surgical Care Improvement Project				
Appropriate Beta Blocker Usage[1]	-	-	98%	98%
Appropriate VTP Within 24 Hours	17	88%	98%	98%
Controlled Postoperative Blood Glucose[7]	-	-	97%	97%
Perioperative Temperature Management	18	100%	100%	100%
Prophylactic Antibiotic Selection[1]	-	-	99%	99%
Prophylactic Antibiotic Selection (Outpatient)[3,7]	-	-	98%	98%
Prophylactic Antibiotic Stopped[1]	-	-	98%	98%
Prophylactic Antibiotic Timing[1]	-	-	99%	99%
Prophylactic Antibiotic Timing (Outpatient)[1,3]	-	-	98%	98%
Urinary Catheter Removal	17	94%	98%	97%
Survey of Patients' Hospital Experiences				
Area Around Room 'Always' Quiet at Night	(a)	64%	61%	61%
Doctors 'Always' Communicated Well	(a)	84%	83%	82%
Home Recovery Information Given	(a)	84%	86%	85%
Hospital Given 9 or 10 on 10 Point Scale	(a)	69%	74%	71%
Meds 'Always' Explained Before Given	(a)	63%	64%	64%
Nurses 'Always' Communicated Well	(a)	81%	81%	79%
Pain 'Always' Well Controlled	(a)	84%	73%	71%
Room and Bathroom 'Always' Clean	(a)	71%	76%	73%
Timely Help 'Always' Received	(a)	73%	71%	68%
Would Definitely Recommend Hospital	(a)	68%	73%	71%
Use of Medical Imaging				
Cardiac Imaging Stress Test before Surgery	56	5.4%	5.4%	5.3%
Combination Abdominal CT Scan	199	10.6%	9.3%	10.5%
Combination Brain/Sinus CT Scan	221	5.0%	2.6%	2.7%
Combination Chest CT Scan	79	0.0%	4.6%	2.7%
Follow-up Mammogram/Ultrasound	261	21.1%	8.4%	8.8%
Lumbar Spine MRI for Low Back Pain[1]	-	-	38.7%	37.2%

Deaconess Hospital

600 Mary St
Evansville, IN 47747
URL: www.deaconess.com
Phone: 812-450-5000
Fax: 812-450-6051
Type: Acute Care Hospitals
Emergency Services: Yes
Ownership: Voluntary non-profit - Private
Beds: 400

Key Personnel:

Quality Assurance . . . . Tom Alvey
Cardiac Laboratory . . . . Joan Fedor-Bassemier
Coronary Care . . . . Joana Fedor-Bessemier
Operating Room . . . . Lynn Lingafelter
Infection Control . . . . Mellodee Montgomery
Chief of Medical Staff . . . . James R. Porter, MD, FAAP, FACHE
Radiology . . . . Ray Poston
CEO/President . . . . Linda E. White

Measure	Cases	This Hosp.	State Avg.	U.S. Avg.
Blood Clot Prevention and Treatment				
Anticoagulation Overlap Therapy[2]	149	92%	92%	93%
ICU Venous Thromboembolism Prophylaxis[2]	128	98%	91%	92%
Incidence of Potentially Preventable VTE[2]	23	0%	10%	10%
UFH with Dosages/Platelet Monitoring[2]	30	100%	95%	97%
Venous Thromboembolism Prophylaxis[2]	313	90%	83%	85%
Warfarin Therapy Discharge Instructions[2]	105	86%	71%	75%
Chest Pain/Possible Heart Attack Care				
Aspirin Given Within 24 Hours of Arrival	178	99%	96%	96%
Fibrinolytic Meds Within 30 Min. of Arrival[7]	-	-	48%	58%
Average Time to ECG (minutes)	184	8	6	7
Average Time to Transfer (minutes)	43	34	46	60
Children's Asthma Care				
Received Home Management Plan of Care	-	-	-	88%
Received Reliever Medication	-	-	-	100%
Received Systemic Corticosteroids	-	-	-	100%
Emergency Department				
Admittance Decision Time (minutes)[2]	448	49	80	98
Head CT Results Within 45 Min. of Arrival	12	75%	60%	57%
Patients Who Left ER Before Being Seen	91,032	1%	2%	2%
Time from ER Arrival to Admit. (minutes)[2]	488	177	241	274
Time from ER Arrival to Discharge (minutes)	329	127	122	134
Time in ER Before Being Evaluated (minutes)	416	15	22	26
Time to Pain Meds for Fractures (minutes)	193	56	52	57
Heart Attack Care				
Aspirin Given at Discharge	313	99%	99%	99%
Fibrinolytic Meds Within 30 Min. of Arrival[7]	-	-	67%	54%
PCI Within 90 Minutes of Arrival	54	96%	97%	96%
Statin Prescribed at Discharge	306	99%	99%	98%
Heart Failure Care				
ACE Inhibitor or ARB for LVSD	193	95%	97%	97%
Discharge Instructions Given	511	86%	95%	94%
Evaluation of LVS Function	686	100%	99%	99%
Medicare Spending				
Medicare Spending per Patient (ratio)	-	1.03	1.01	0.98
Pneumonia Care				
Appropriate Initial Antibiotic Given[2]	68	96%	95%	95%
Blood Culture Timing[2]	132	95%	98%	98%
Pregnancy and Delivery Care				
Newborn Deliveries Scheduled Early[7]	-	-	5%	6%
Preventive Care				
Immunization for Influenza[2]	610	98%	91%	90%
Immunization for Pneumonia[2]	908	95%	92%	92%
Stroke Care				
Anticoagulation Therapy for Atrial Fibrillation	51	88%	94%	95%
Antithrombotic Therapy Timing	325	97%	97%	98%
Assessed for Rehabilitation	411	99%	96%	97%
Discharged on Antithrombotic Therapy	346	98%	98%	99%
Discharged on Statin Medication	287	97%	91%	94%
Thrombolytic Therapy Timing	15	93%	54%	66%
Venous Thromboembolism Prophylaxis	391	93%	91%	94%
Written Stroke Educational Materials Given	192	84%	82%	88%
Surgical Care Improvement Project				
Appropriate Beta Blocker Usage[2]	180	99%	98%	98%
Appropriate VTP Within 24 Hours[2]	345	97%	98%	98%
Controlled Postoperative Blood Glucose[2]	48	85%	97%	97%
Perioperative Temperature Management[2]	478	100%	100%	100%
Prophylactic Antibiotic Selection[2]	347	99%	99%	99%
Prophylactic Antibiotic Selection (Outpatient)	653	97%	98%	98%
Prophylactic Antibiotic Stopped[2]	338	98%	98%	98%
Prophylactic Antibiotic Timing[2]	347	96%	99%	99%
Prophylactic Antibiotic Timing (Outpatient)	621	98%	98%	98%
Urinary Catheter Removal[2]	253	99%	98%	97%
Survey of Patients' Hospital Experiences				
Area Around Room 'Always' Quiet at Night	300+	60%	61%	61%
Doctors 'Always' Communicated Well	300+	81%	83%	82%
Home Recovery Information Given	300+	85%	86%	85%
Hospital Given 9 or 10 on 10 Point Scale	300+	76%	74%	71%
Meds 'Always' Explained Before Given	300+	63%	64%	64%
Nurses 'Always' Communicated Well	300+	81%	81%	79%
Pain 'Always' Well Controlled	300+	71%	73%	71%
Room and Bathroom 'Always' Clean	300+	71%	76%	73%
Timely Help 'Always' Received	300+	66%	71%	68%
Would Definitely Recommend Hospital	300+	79%	73%	71%
Use of Medical Imaging				
Cardiac Imaging Stress Test before Surgery	754	8.2%	5.4%	5.3%

NOTE: Hospital profiles are in alphabetical order by state, then city, then hospital within the city; Rankings exclude hospitals with less than 25 cases except for patient surveys which excludes hospitals with less than 100 cases; (a) 100-299 cases; (1) The number of cases/patients is too few to report; (2) Data submitted were based on a sample of cases/patients; (3) Results are based on a shorter time period than required; (4) Data suppressed by CMS for one or more quarters; (5) Results are not available for this reporting period; (6) Fewer than 100 patients completed the HCAHPS survey; (7) No cases met the criteria for this measure; (8) The lower limit of the confidence interval cannot be calculated if the number of observed infections equals zero; (9) No data are available from the state/territory for this reporting period; (10) The scores shown reflect fewer than 50 completed surveys; (11) There were discrepancies in the data collection process; (12) This measure does not apply to this hospital for this reporting period; (13) Results cannot be calculated for this reporting period; (14) The results for this state are combined with nearby states to protect confidentiality; Please refer to the User's Guide for a full explanation of data.

Combination Abdominal CT Scan	2,797	6.3%	9.3%	10.5%
Combination Brain/Sinus CT Scan	2,051	5.8%	2.6%	2.7%
Combination Chest CT Scan	1,763	0.1%	4.6%	2.7%
Follow-up Mammogram/Ultrasound	3,952	5.6%	8.4%	8.8%
Lumbar Spine MRI for Low Back Pain	397	39.3%	38.7%	37.2%

Saint Mary's Medical Center of Evansville

3700 Washington Ave
Evansville, IN 47750
Phone: 812-485-4000
Fax: 812-485-7800
URL: www.stmarys.org
Type: Acute Care Hospitals
Emergency Services: Yes
Ownership: Voluntary non-profit - Private
Beds: 508

Key Personnel:
Pediatric Ambulatory Care . . . . . . Kishor Bhatt, MD
Pediatric In-Patient Care . . . . Kishor Bhatt, MD
Emergency Room . . . . Connie Brandes
Infection Control . . . . Donna Bratt
Radiology . . . . Paul Hargan, MD
CEO/President . . . . Keith Jewell, MD
Operating Room . . . . Lisa McGuire
Quality Assurance . . . . Marty Runge

Measure	Cases	This Hosp.	State Avg.	U.S. Avg.
Blood Clot Prevention and Treatment				
Anticoagulation Overlap Therapy[2]	128	96%	92%	93%
ICU Venous Thromboembolism Prophylaxis[2]	101	93%	91%	92%
Incidence of Potentially Preventable VTE[2]	25	0%	10%	10%
UFH with Dosages/Platelet Monitoring[2]	47	100%	95%	97%
Venous Thromboembolism Prophylaxis[2]	325	80%	83%	85%
Warfarin Therapy Discharge Instructions[2]	77	100%	71%	75%
Chest Pain/Possible Heart Attack Care				
Aspirin Given Within 24 Hours of Arrival[1,3]	-	-	96%	96%
Fibrinolytic Meds Within 30 Min. of Arrival[5]	-	-	48%	58%
Average Time to ECG (minutes)[1,3]	-	-	6	7
Average Time to Transfer (minutes)[5]	-	-	46	60
Children's Asthma Care				
Received Home Management Plan of Care	-	-	-	88%
Received Reliever Medication	-	-	-	100%
Received Systemic Corticosteroids	-	-	-	100%
Emergency Department				
Admittance Decision Time (minutes)[2]	506	93	80	98
Head CT Results Within 45 Min. of Arrival[1]	-	-	60%	57%
Patients Who Left ER Before Being Seen	64,264	1%	2%	2%
Time from ER Arrival to Admit. (minutes)[2]	550	228	241	274
Time from ER Arrival to Discharge (minutes)	365	126	122	134
Time in ER Before Being Evaluated (minutes)	380	22	22	26
Time to Pain Meds for Fractures (minutes)	142	65	52	57
Heart Attack Care				
Aspirin Given at Discharge	307	100%	99%	99%
Fibrinolytic Meds Within 30 Min. of Arrival[7]	-	-	67%	54%
PCI Within 90 Minutes of Arrival	49	98%	97%	96%
Statin Prescribed at Discharge	298	98%	99%	98%
Heart Failure Care				
ACE Inhibitor or ARB for LVSD	138	99%	97%	97%
Discharge Instructions Given	338	100%	95%	94%
Evaluation of LVS Function	424	100%	99%	99%
Medicare Spending				
Medicare Spending per Patient (ratio)	-	1.01	1.01	0.98
Pneumonia Care				
Appropriate Initial Antibiotic Given	200	96%	95%	95%
Blood Culture Timing	298	98%	98%	98%
Pregnancy and Delivery Care				
Newborn Deliveries Scheduled Early	127	3%	5%	6%
Preventive Care				
Immunization for Influenza[2]	536	95%	91%	90%
Immunization for Pneumonia[2]	703	95%	92%	92%
Stroke Care				
Anticoagulation Therapy for Atrial Fibrillation	26	92%	94%	95%
Antithrombotic Therapy Timing	133	95%	97%	98%
Assessed for Rehabilitation	176	98%	96%	97%
Discharged on Antithrombotic Therapy	153	100%	98%	99%
Discharged on Statin Medication	123	95%	91%	94%
Thrombolytic Therapy Timing	17	29%	54%	66%
Venous Thromboembolism Prophylaxis	187	96%	91%	94%
Written Stroke Educational Materials Given	82	99%	82%	88%
Surgical Care Improvement Project				
Appropriate Beta Blocker Usage[2]	514	99%	98%	98%
Appropriate VTP Within 24 Hours[2]	1,238	98%	98%	98%
Controlled Postoperative Blood Glucose[2]	140	94%	97%	97%
Perioperative Temperature Management[2]	1,366	100%	100%	100%
Prophylactic Antibiotic Selection[2]	1,214	100%	99%	99%
Prophylactic Antibiotic Selection (Outpatient)	1,076	99%	98%	98%
Prophylactic Antibiotic Stopped[2]	1,198	99%	98%	98%
Prophylactic Antibiotic Timing[2]	1,214	100%	99%	99%
Prophylactic Antibiotic Timing (Outpatient)	1,076	100%	98%	98%
Urinary Catheter Removal[2]	933	99%	98%	97%
Survey of Patients' Hospital Experiences				
Area Around Room 'Always' Quiet at Night	300+	63%	61%	61%
Doctors 'Always' Communicated Well	300+	80%	83%	82%
Home Recovery Information Given	300+	90%	86%	85%
Hospital Given 9 or 10 on 10 Point Scale	300+	76%	74%	71%
Meds 'Always' Explained Before Given	300+	61%	64%	64%
Nurses 'Always' Communicated Well	300+	78%	81%	79%
Pain 'Always' Well Controlled	300+	71%	73%	71%
Room and Bathroom 'Always' Clean	300+	74%	76%	73%
Timely Help 'Always' Received	300+	64%	71%	68%
Would Definitely Recommend Hospital	300+	77%	73%	71%
Use of Medical Imaging				
Cardiac Imaging Stress Test before Surgery	793	6.9%	5.4%	5.3%
Combination Abdominal CT Scan	1,221	2.3%	9.3%	10.5%
Combination Brain/Sinus CT Scan	961	3.5%	2.6%	2.7%
Combination Chest CT Scan	951	16.8%	4.6%	2.7%
Follow-up Mammogram/Ultrasound[7]	-	-	8.4%	8.8%
Lumbar Spine MRI for Low Back Pain	316	38.3%	38.7%	37.2%

Saint Vincent Fishers Hospital

13861 Olio Road
Fishers, IN 46037
Phone: 317-415-9000
Type: Acute Care Hospitals
Emergency Services: Yes
Ownership: Voluntary non-profit - Private

Measure	Cases	This Hosp.	State Avg.	U.S. Avg.
Blood Clot Prevention and Treatment				
Anticoagulation Overlap Therapy[5]	-	-	92%	93%
ICU Venous Thromboembolism Prophylaxis[5]	-	-	91%	92%
Incidence of Potentially Preventable VTE[5]	-	-	10%	10%
UFH with Dosages/Platelet Monitoring[5]	-	-	95%	97%
Venous Thromboembolism Prophylaxis[5]	-	-	83%	85%
Warfarin Therapy Discharge Instructions[5]	-	-	71%	75%
Chest Pain/Possible Heart Attack Care				
Aspirin Given Within 24 Hours of Arrival[5]	-	-	96%	96%
Fibrinolytic Meds Within 30 Min. of Arrival[5]	-	-	48%	58%
Average Time to ECG (minutes)[5]	-	-	6	7
Average Time to Transfer (minutes)[5]	-	-	46	60
Children's Asthma Care				
Received Home Management Plan of Care	-	-	-	88%
Received Reliever Medication	-	-	-	100%
Received Systemic Corticosteroids	-	-	-	100%
Emergency Department				
Admittance Decision Time (minutes)[5]	-	-	80	98
Head CT Results Within 45 Min. of Arrival[5]	-	-	60%	57%
Patients Who Left ER Before Being Seen[5]	-	-	2%	2%
Time from ER Arrival to Admit. (minutes)[5]	-	-	241	274
Time from ER Arrival to Discharge (minutes)[5]	-	-	122	134
Time in ER Before Being Evaluated (minutes)[5]	-	-	22	26
Time to Pain Meds for Fractures (minutes)[5]	-	-	52	57
Heart Attack Care				
Aspirin Given at Discharge[5]	-	-	99%	99%
Fibrinolytic Meds Within 30 Min. of Arrival[5]	-	-	67%	54%
PCI Within 90 Minutes of Arrival[5]	-	-	97%	96%
Statin Prescribed at Discharge[5]	-	-	99%	98%
Heart Failure Care				
ACE Inhibitor or ARB for LVSD[5]	-	-	97%	97%
Discharge Instructions Given[5]	-	-	95%	94%
Evaluation of LVS Function[5]	-	-	99%	99%
Medicare Spending				
Medicare Spending per Patient (ratio)	-	-	1.01	0.98
Pneumonia Care				
Appropriate Initial Antibiotic Given[5]	-	-	95%	95%
Blood Culture Timing[5]	-	-	98%	98%
Pregnancy and Delivery Care				
Newborn Deliveries Scheduled Early[5]	-	-	5%	6%
Preventive Care				
Immunization for Influenza[5]	-	-	91%	90%
Immunization for Pneumonia[5]	-	-	92%	92%
Stroke Care				
Anticoagulation Therapy for Atrial Fibrillation[5]	-	-	94%	95%
Antithrombotic Therapy Timing[5]	-	-	97%	98%
Assessed for Rehabilitation[5]	-	-	96%	97%
Discharged on Antithrombotic Therapy[5]	-	-	98%	99%
Discharged on Statin Medication[5]	-	-	91%	94%
Thrombolytic Therapy Timing[5]	-	-	54%	66%
Venous Thromboembolism Prophylaxis[5]	-	-	91%	94%
Written Stroke Educational Materials Given[5]	-	-	82%	88%
Surgical Care Improvement Project				
Appropriate Beta Blocker Usage[5]	-	-	98%	98%
Appropriate VTP Within 24 Hours[5]	-	-	98%	98%
Controlled Postoperative Blood Glucose[5]	-	-	97%	97%
Perioperative Temperature Management[5]	-	-	100%	100%
Prophylactic Antibiotic Selection[5]	-	-	99%	99%
Prophylactic Antibiotic Selection (Outpatient)[5]	-	-	98%	98%
Prophylactic Antibiotic Stopped[5]	-	-	98%	98%
Prophylactic Antibiotic Timing[5]	-	-	99%	99%
Prophylactic Antibiotic Timing (Outpatient)[5]	-	-	98%	98%
Urinary Catheter Removal[5]	-	-	98%	97%
Survey of Patients' Hospital Experiences				
Area Around Room 'Always' Quiet at Night[5]	-	-	61%	61%
Doctors 'Always' Communicated Well[5]	-	-	83%	82%
Home Recovery Information Given[5]	-	-	86%	85%
Hospital Given 9 or 10 on 10 Point Scale[5]	-	-	74%	71%
Meds 'Always' Explained Before Given[5]	-	-	64%	64%
Nurses 'Always' Communicated Well[5]	-	-	81%	79%
Pain 'Always' Well Controlled[5]	-	-	73%	71%
Room and Bathroom 'Always' Clean[5]	-	-	76%	73%
Timely Help 'Always' Received[5]	-	-	71%	68%
Would Definitely Recommend Hospital[5]	-	-	73%	71%
Use of Medical Imaging				
Cardiac Imaging Stress Test before Surgery[1]	-	-	5.4%	5.3%
Combination Abdominal CT Scan[1]	-	-	9.3%	10.5%
Combination Brain/Sinus CT Scan[1]	-	-	2.6%	2.7%
Combination Chest CT Scan[1]	-	-	4.6%	2.7%
Follow-up Mammogram/Ultrasound[7]	-	-	8.4%	8.8%
Lumbar Spine MRI for Low Back Pain[1]	-	-	38.7%	37.2%

Dupont Hospital

2520 E Dupont Rd
Fort Wayne, IN 46825
Phone: 260-416-3000
URL: www.theduponthospital.com
Type: Acute Care Hospitals
Emergency Services: Yes
Ownership: Proprietary
Beds: 131

Key Personnel:
Quality Assurance . . . . Diana S. Hupe, MSN, RN
CEO/President . . . . Mike Schatzlein
CEO . . . . Chad Towner, BS, MBA

Measure	Cases	This Hosp.	State Avg.	U.S. Avg.
Blood Clot Prevention and Treatment				
Anticoagulation Overlap Therapy[2]	18	100%	92%	93%
ICU Venous Thromboembolism Prophylaxis[2]	27	100%	91%	92%
Incidence of Potentially Preventable VTE[2,7]	-	-	10%	10%
UFH with Dosages/Platelet Monitoring[2]	16	100%	95%	97%
Venous Thromboembolism Prophylaxis[2]	135	100%	83%	85%
Warfarin Therapy Discharge Instructions[2]	15	100%	71%	75%
Chest Pain/Possible Heart Attack Care				
Aspirin Given Within 24 Hours of Arrival	35	100%	96%	96%
Fibrinolytic Meds Within 30 Min. of Arrival[7]	-	-	48%	58%
Average Time to ECG (minutes)	36	4	6	7
Average Time to Transfer (minutes)	13	41	46	60
Children's Asthma Care				
Received Home Management Plan of Care	-	-	-	88%
Received Reliever Medication	-	-	-	100%
Received Systemic Corticosteroids	-	-	-	100%

NOTE: Hospital profiles are in alphabetical order by state, then city, then hospital within the city; Rankings exclude hospitals with less than 25 cases except for patient surveys which excludes hospitals with less than 100 cases; (a) 100-299 cases; (1) The number of cases/patients is too few to report; (2) Data submitted were based on a sample of cases/patients; (3) Results are based on a shorter time period than required; (4) Data suppressed by CMS for one or more quarters; (5) Results are not available for this reporting period; (6) Fewer than 100 patients completed the HCAHPS survey; (7) No cases met the criteria for this measure; (8) The lower limit of the confidence interval cannot be calculated if the number of observed infections equals zero; (9) No data are available from the state/territory for this reporting period; (10) The scores shown reflect fewer than 50 completed surveys; (11) There were discrepancies in the data collection process; (12) This measure does not apply to this hospital for this reporting period; (13) Results cannot be calculated for this reporting period; (14) The results for this state are combined with nearby states to protect confidentiality; Please refer to the User's Guide for a full explanation of data.

Measure	Cases	This Hosp.	State Avg.	U.S. Avg.
Emergency Department				
Admittance Decision Time (minutes)[2]	235	65	80	98
Head CT Results Within 45 Min. of Arrival[1]	-	-	60%	57%
Patients Who Left ER Before Being Seen	21,037	1%	2%	2%
Time from ER Arrival to Admit. (minutes)[2]	236	193	241	274
Time from ER Arrival to Discharge (minutes)	405	98	122	134
Time in ER Before Being Evaluated (minutes)	423	16	22	26
Time to Pain Meds for Fractures (minutes)	71	26	52	57
Heart Attack Care				
Aspirin Given at Discharge[1]	-	-	99%	99%
Fibrinolytic Meds Within 30 Min. of Arrival[7]	-	-	67%	54%
PCI Within 90 Minutes of Arrival[7]	-	-	97%	96%
Statin Prescribed at Discharge[1]	-	-	99%	98%
Heart Failure Care				
ACE Inhibitor or ARB for LVSD[1]	-	-	97%	97%
Discharge Instructions Given	28	100%	95%	94%
Evaluation of LVS Function	37	100%	99%	99%
Medicare Spending				
Medicare Spending per Patient (ratio)	-	0.96	1.01	0.98
Pneumonia Care				
Appropriate Initial Antibiotic Given	33	100%	95%	95%
Blood Culture Timing	50	100%	98%	98%
Pregnancy and Delivery Care				
Newborn Deliveries Scheduled Early[2]	56	2%	5%	6%
Preventive Care				
Immunization for Influenza[2]	446	100%	91%	90%
Immunization for Pneumonia[2]	272	99%	92%	92%
Stroke Care				
Anticoagulation Therapy for Atrial Fibrillation[1]	-	-	94%	95%
Antithrombotic Therapy Timing	11	100%	97%	98%
Assessed for Rehabilitation[1]	-	-	96%	97%
Discharged on Antithrombotic Therapy[1]	-	-	98%	99%
Discharged on Statin Medication[1]	-	-	91%	94%
Thrombolytic Therapy Timing[7]	-	-	54%	66%
Venous Thromboembolism Prophylaxis	11	100%	91%	94%
Written Stroke Educational Materials Given[1]	-	-	82%	88%
Surgical Care Improvement Project				
Appropriate Beta Blocker Usage	69	100%	98%	98%
Appropriate VTP Within 24 Hours	260	100%	98%	98%
Controlled Postoperative Blood Glucose[7]	-	-	97%	97%
Perioperative Temperature Management	306	100%	100%	100%
Prophylactic Antibiotic Selection	207	100%	99%	99%
Prophylactic Antibiotic Selection (Outpatient)	586	100%	98%	98%
Prophylactic Antibiotic Stopped	202	99%	98%	98%
Prophylactic Antibiotic Timing	207	100%	99%	99%
Prophylactic Antibiotic Timing (Outpatient)	586	99%	98%	98%
Urinary Catheter Removal	91	100%	98%	97%
Survey of Patients' Hospital Experiences				
Area Around Room 'Always' Quiet at Night	300+	57%	61%	61%
Doctors 'Always' Communicated Well	300+	83%	83%	82%
Home Recovery Information Given	300+	89%	86%	85%
Hospital Given 9 or 10 on 10 Point Scale	300+	80%	74%	71%
Meds 'Always' Explained Before Given	300+	61%	64%	64%
Nurses 'Always' Communicated Well	300+	79%	81%	79%
Pain 'Always' Well Controlled	300+	73%	73%	71%
Room and Bathroom 'Always' Clean	300+	64%	76%	73%
Timely Help 'Always' Received	300+	71%	71%	68%
Would Definitely Recommend Hospital	300+	79%	73%	71%
Use of Medical Imaging				
Cardiac Imaging Stress Test before Surgery[1]	-	-	5.4%	5.3%
Combination Abdominal CT Scan	303	2.0%	9.3%	10.5%
Combination Brain/Sinus CT Scan	270	5.9%	2.6%	2.7%
Combination Chest CT Scan	125	0.8%	4.6%	2.7%
Follow-up Mammogram/Ultrasound	389	7.2%	8.4%	8.8%
Lumbar Spine MRI for Low Back Pain	61	37.7%	38.7%	37.2%

Lutheran Hospital of Indiana

7950 W Jefferson Blvd
Fort Wayne, IN 46804
Phone: 260-435-7001
Fax: 260-435-7640
URL: www.lutheranhospital.com
Type: Acute Care Hospitals
Emergency Services: Yes
Ownership: Proprietary
Beds: 435
Key Personnel:
Chief of Medical Staff. . . . . B V House, MD
CEO/President. . . . . Thomas D Miller

Measure	Cases	This Hosp.	State Avg.	U.S. Avg.
Blood Clot Prevention and Treatment				
Anticoagulation Overlap Therapy[2]	167	98%	92%	93%
ICU Venous Thromboembolism Prophylaxis[2]	225	97%	91%	92%
Incidence of Potentially Preventable VTE[2]	33	0%	10%	10%
UFH with Dosages/Platelet Monitoring[2]	163	100%	95%	97%
Venous Thromboembolism Prophylaxis[2]	359	93%	83%	85%
Warfarin Therapy Discharge Instructions[2]	132	95%	71%	75%
Chest Pain/Possible Heart Attack Care				
Aspirin Given Within 24 Hours of Arrival[5]	-	-	96%	96%
Fibrinolytic Meds Within 30 Min. of Arrival[5]	-	-	48%	58%
Average Time to ECG (minutes)[5]	-	-	6	7
Average Time to Transfer (minutes)[5]	-	-	46	60
Children's Asthma Care				
Received Home Management Plan of Care	-	-	-	88%
Received Reliever Medication	-	-	-	100%
Received Systemic Corticosteroids	-	-	-	100%
Emergency Department				
Admittance Decision Time (minutes)[2]	662	94	80	98
Head CT Results Within 45 Min. of Arrival[1,3]	-	-	60%	57%
Patients Who Left ER Before Being Seen	43,522	0%	2%	2%
Time from ER Arrival to Admit. (minutes)[2]	682	252	241	274
Time from ER Arrival to Discharge (minutes)	390	148	122	134
Time in ER Before Being Evaluated (minutes)	410	16	22	26
Time to Pain Meds for Fractures (minutes)	256	44	52	57
Heart Attack Care				
Aspirin Given at Discharge	544	100%	99%	99%
Fibrinolytic Meds Within 30 Min. of Arrival[7]	-	-	67%	54%
PCI Within 90 Minutes of Arrival	59	97%	97%	96%
Statin Prescribed at Discharge	526	100%	99%	98%
Heart Failure Care				
ACE Inhibitor or ARB for LVSD	117	99%	97%	97%
Discharge Instructions Given	387	96%	95%	94%
Evaluation of LVS Function	466	100%	99%	99%
Medicare Spending				
Medicare Spending per Patient (ratio)	-	1.00	1.01	0.98
Pneumonia Care				
Appropriate Initial Antibiotic Given	102	92%	95%	95%
Blood Culture Timing	186	99%	98%	98%
Pregnancy and Delivery Care				
Newborn Deliveries Scheduled Early[2]	46	4%	5%	6%
Preventive Care				
Immunization for Influenza[2]	789	99%	91%	90%
Immunization for Pneumonia[2]	1,058	99%	92%	92%
Stroke Care				
Anticoagulation Therapy for Atrial Fibrillation	26	100%	94%	95%
Antithrombotic Therapy Timing	166	97%	97%	98%
Assessed for Rehabilitation	224	96%	96%	97%
Discharged on Antithrombotic Therapy	187	100%	98%	99%
Discharged on Statin Medication	140	99%	91%	94%
Thrombolytic Therapy Timing[1]	-	-	54%	66%
Venous Thromboembolism Prophylaxis	242	97%	91%	94%
Written Stroke Educational Materials Given	101	92%	82%	88%
Surgical Care Improvement Project				
Appropriate Beta Blocker Usage	599	98%	98%	98%
Appropriate VTP Within 24 Hours	654	99%	98%	98%
Controlled Postoperative Blood Glucose	300	97%	97%	97%
Perioperative Temperature Management	1,015	100%	100%	100%
Prophylactic Antibiotic Selection	568	100%	99%	99%
Prophylactic Antibiotic Selection (Outpatient)	1,055	99%	98%	98%
Prophylactic Antibiotic Stopped	537	97%	98%	98%
Prophylactic Antibiotic Timing	569	99%	99%	99%
Prophylactic Antibiotic Timing (Outpatient)	1,055	99%	98%	98%
Urinary Catheter Removal	617	99%	98%	97%
Survey of Patients' Hospital Experiences				
Area Around Room 'Always' Quiet at Night	300+	57%	61%	61%
Doctors 'Always' Communicated Well	300+	78%	83%	82%
Home Recovery Information Given	300+	86%	86%	85%
Hospital Given 9 or 10 on 10 Point Scale	300+	75%	74%	71%
Meds 'Always' Explained Before Given	300+	60%	64%	64%
Nurses 'Always' Communicated Well	300+	79%	81%	79%
Pain 'Always' Well Controlled	300+	73%	73%	71%
Room and Bathroom 'Always' Clean	300+	69%	76%	73%
Timely Help 'Always' Received	300+	67%	71%	68%
Would Definitely Recommend Hospital	300+	78%	73%	71%
Use of Medical Imaging				
Cardiac Imaging Stress Test before Surgery	834	4.4%	5.4%	5.3%
Combination Abdominal CT Scan	853	2.9%	9.3%	10.5%
Combination Brain/Sinus CT Scan	858	2.3%	2.6%	2.7%
Combination Chest CT Scan	609	0.2%	4.6%	2.7%
Follow-up Mammogram/Ultrasound	932	4.8%	8.4%	8.8%
Lumbar Spine MRI for Low Back Pain	149	38.3%	38.7%	37.2%

Orthopaedic Hospital at Parkview North

11130 Parkview Circle Dr
Fort Wayne, IN 46845
Phone: 260-672-4050
URL: www.parkview.com
Type: Acute Care Hospitals
Emergency Services: Yes
Ownership: Voluntary non-profit - Private
Beds: 37
Key Personnel:
President/CEO. . . . . Michael Packnett

Measure	Cases	This Hosp.	State Avg.	U.S. Avg.
Blood Clot Prevention and Treatment				
Anticoagulation Overlap Therapy[1,2]	-	-	92%	93%
ICU Venous Thromboembolism Prophylaxis[2,7]	-	-	91%	92%
Incidence of Potentially Preventable VTE[1,2]	-	-	10%	10%
UFH with Dosages/Platelet Monitoring[2,7]	-	-	95%	97%
Venous Thromboembolism Prophylaxis[2]	48	100%	83%	85%
Warfarin Therapy Discharge Instructions[2,7]	-	-	71%	75%
Chest Pain/Possible Heart Attack Care				
Aspirin Given Within 24 Hours of Arrival[5]	-	-	96%	96%
Fibrinolytic Meds Within 30 Min. of Arrival[5]	-	-	48%	58%
Average Time to ECG (minutes)[5]	-	-	6	7
Average Time to Transfer (minutes)[5]	-	-	46	60
Children's Asthma Care				
Received Home Management Plan of Care	-	-	-	88%
Received Reliever Medication	-	-	-	100%
Received Systemic Corticosteroids	-	-	-	100%
Emergency Department				
Admittance Decision Time (minutes)[2,7]	-	-	80	98
Head CT Results Within 45 Min. of Arrival[5]	-	-	60%	57%
Patients Who Left ER Before Being Seen[5]	-	-	2%	2%
Time from ER Arrival to Admit. (minutes)[2,7]	-	-	241	274
Time from ER Arrival to Discharge (minutes)[5]	-	-	122	134
Time in ER Before Being Evaluated (minutes)[5]	-	-	22	26
Time to Pain Meds for Fractures (minutes)[5]	-	-	52	57
Heart Attack Care				
Aspirin Given at Discharge[5]	-	-	99%	99%
Fibrinolytic Meds Within 30 Min. of Arrival[5]	-	-	67%	54%
PCI Within 90 Minutes of Arrival[5]	-	-	97%	96%
Statin Prescribed at Discharge[5]	-	-	99%	98%
Heart Failure Care				
ACE Inhibitor or ARB for LVSD[5]	-	-	97%	97%
Discharge Instructions Given[5]	-	-	95%	94%
Evaluation of LVS Function[5]	-	-	99%	99%
Medicare Spending				
Medicare Spending per Patient (ratio)	-	0.98	1.01	0.98
Pneumonia Care				
Appropriate Initial Antibiotic Given[5]	-	-	95%	95%
Blood Culture Timing[5]	-	-	98%	98%
Pregnancy and Delivery Care				
Newborn Deliveries Scheduled Early[7]	-	-	5%	6%
Preventive Care				
Immunization for Influenza[2]	325	95%	91%	90%
Immunization for Pneumonia[2]	435	95%	92%	92%
Stroke Care				
Anticoagulation Therapy for Atrial Fibrillation[5]	-	-	94%	95%
Antithrombotic Therapy Timing[5]	-	-	97%	98%
Assessed for Rehabilitation[5]	-	-	96%	97%
Discharged on Antithrombotic Therapy[5]	-	-	98%	99%
Discharged on Statin Medication[5]	-	-	91%	94%
Thrombolytic Therapy Timing[5]	-	-	54%	66%
Venous Thromboembolism Prophylaxis[5]	-	-	91%	94%

NOTE: Hospital profiles are in alphabetical order by state, then city, then hospital within the city; Rankings exclude hospitals with less than 25 cases except for patient surveys which excludes hospitals with less than 100 cases; (a) 100-299 cases; (1) The number of cases/patients is too few to report; (2) Data submitted were based on a sample of cases/patients; (3) Results are based on a shorter time period than required; (4) Data suppressed by CMS for one or more quarters; (5) Results are not available for this reporting period; (6) Fewer than 100 patients completed the HCAHPS survey; (7) No cases met the criteria for this measure; (8) The lower limit of the confidence interval cannot be calculated if the number of observed infections equals zero; (9) No data are available from the state/territory for this reporting period; (10) The scores shown reflect fewer than 50 completed surveys; (11) There were discrepancies in the data collection process; (12) This measure does not apply to this hospital for this reporting period; (13) Results cannot be calculated for this reporting period; (14) The results for this state are combined with nearby states to protect confidentiality; Please refer to the User's Guide for a full explanation of data.

Measure	Cases	This Hosp.	State Avg.	U.S. Avg.
Written Stroke Educational Materials Given[5]	-	-	82%	88%
Surgical Care Improvement Project				
Appropriate Beta Blocker Usage[2]	164	98%	98%	98%
Appropriate VTP Within 24 Hours[2]	499	100%	98%	98%
Controlled Postoperative Blood Glucose[2,7]	-	-	97%	97%
Perioperative Temperature Management[2]	527	100%	100%	100%
Prophylactic Antibiotic Selection[2]	441	100%	99%	99%
Prophylactic Antibiotic Selection (Outpatient)	206	100%	98%	98%
Prophylactic Antibiotic Stopped[2]	440	97%	98%	98%
Prophylactic Antibiotic Timing[2]	441	100%	99%	99%
Prophylactic Antibiotic Timing (Outpatient)	206	100%	98%	98%
Urinary Catheter Removal[2]	422	100%	98%	97%
Survey of Patients' Hospital Experiences				
Area Around Room 'Always' Quiet at Night	300+	69%	61%	61%
Doctors 'Always' Communicated Well	300+	87%	83%	82%
Home Recovery Information Given	300+	92%	86%	85%
Hospital Given 9 or 10 on 10 Point Scale	300+	82%	74%	71%
Meds 'Always' Explained Before Given	300+	65%	64%	64%
Nurses 'Always' Communicated Well	300+	83%	81%	79%
Pain 'Always' Well Controlled	300+	73%	73%	71%
Room and Bathroom 'Always' Clean	300+	79%	76%	73%
Timely Help 'Always' Received	300+	73%	71%	68%
Would Definitely Recommend Hospital	300+	85%	73%	71%
Use of Medical Imaging				
Cardiac Imaging Stress Test before Surgery[7]	-	-	5.4%	5.3%
Combination Abdominal CT Scan[7]	-	-	9.3%	10.5%
Combination Brain/Sinus CT Scan[7]	-	-	2.6%	2.7%
Combination Chest CT Scan[7]	-	-	4.6%	2.7%
Follow-up Mammogram/Ultrasound[7]	-	-	8.4%	8.8%
Lumbar Spine MRI for Low Back Pain[7]	-	-	38.7%	37.2%

The Orthopaedic Hospital of Lutheran Health Network

7952 W Jefferson Blvd
Fort Wayne, IN 46804
Phone: 260-435-2999
URL: www.lutheranhealth.net
Type: Acute Care Hospitals
Ownership: Proprietary
Emergency Services: No
Beds: 39
Key Personnel:
CEO . . . . Shelly Miller

Measure	Cases	This Hosp.	State Avg.	U.S. Avg.
Blood Clot Prevention and Treatment				
Anticoagulation Overlap Therapy[1,2]	-	-	92%	93%
ICU Venous Thromboembolism Prophylaxis[2,7]	-	-	91%	92%
Incidence of Potentially Preventable VTE[1,2]	-	-	10%	10%
UFH with Dosages/Platelet Monitoring[1,2]	-	-	95%	97%
Venous Thromboembolism Prophylaxis[2]	145	97%	83%	85%
Warfarin Therapy Discharge Instructions[1,2]	-	-	71%	75%
Chest Pain/Possible Heart Attack Care				
Aspirin Given Within 24 Hours of Arrival[5]	-	-	96%	96%
Fibrinolytic Meds Within 30 Min. of Arrival[5]	-	-	48%	58%
Average Time to ECG (minutes)[5]	-	-	6	7
Average Time to Transfer (minutes)[5]	-	-	46	60
Children's Asthma Care				
Received Home Management Plan of Care	-	-	-	88%
Received Reliever Medication	-	-	-	100%
Received Systemic Corticosteroids	-	-	-	100%
Emergency Department				
Admittance Decision Time (minutes)[2,7]	-	-	80	98
Head CT Results Within 45 Min. of Arrival[5]	-	-	60%	57%
Patients Who Left ER Before Being Seen[5]	-	-	2%	2%
Time from ER Arrival to Admit. (minutes)[2,7]	-	-	241	274
Time from ER Arrival to Discharge (minutes)[5]	-	-	122	134
Time in ER Before Being Evaluated (minutes)[5]	-	-	22	26
Time to Pain Meds for Fractures (minutes)[5]	-	-	52	57
Heart Attack Care				
Aspirin Given at Discharge[5]	-	-	99%	99%
Fibrinolytic Meds Within 30 Min. of Arrival[5]	-	-	67%	54%
PCI Within 90 Minutes of Arrival[5]	-	-	97%	96%
Statin Prescribed at Discharge[5]	-	-	99%	98%
Heart Failure Care				
ACE Inhibitor or ARB for LVSD[5]	-	-	97%	97%
Discharge Instructions Given[5]	-	-	95%	94%
Evaluation of LVS Function[5]	-	-	99%	99%
Medicare Spending				
Medicare Spending per Patient (ratio)	-	0.90	1.01	0.98
Pneumonia Care				
Appropriate Initial Antibiotic Given[5]	-	-	95%	95%
Blood Culture Timing[5]	-	-	98%	98%
Pregnancy and Delivery Care				
Newborn Deliveries Scheduled Early[2,7]	-	-	5%	6%
Preventive Care				
Immunization for Influenza[2]	340	100%	91%	90%
Immunization for Pneumonia[2]	458	97%	92%	92%
Stroke Care				
Anticoagulation Therapy for Atrial Fibrillation[5]	-	-	94%	95%
Antithrombotic Therapy Timing[5]	-	-	97%	98%
Assessed for Rehabilitation[5]	-	-	96%	97%
Discharged on Antithrombotic Therapy[5]	-	-	98%	99%
Discharged on Statin Medication[5]	-	-	91%	94%
Thrombolytic Therapy Timing[5]	-	-	54%	66%
Venous Thromboembolism Prophylaxis[5]	-	-	91%	94%
Written Stroke Educational Materials Given[5]	-	-	82%	88%
Surgical Care Improvement Project				
Appropriate Beta Blocker Usage	476	99%	98%	98%
Appropriate VTP Within 24 Hours	981	100%	98%	98%
Controlled Postoperative Blood Glucose[7]	-	-	97%	97%
Perioperative Temperature Management	1,470	100%	100%	100%
Prophylactic Antibiotic Selection	1,202	100%	99%	99%
Prophylactic Antibiotic Selection (Outpatient)	622	100%	98%	98%
Prophylactic Antibiotic Stopped	1,199	100%	98%	98%
Prophylactic Antibiotic Timing	1,202	100%	99%	99%
Prophylactic Antibiotic Timing (Outpatient)	622	100%	98%	98%
Urinary Catheter Removal	356	99%	98%	97%
Survey of Patients' Hospital Experiences				
Area Around Room 'Always' Quiet at Night	300+	69%	61%	61%
Doctors 'Always' Communicated Well	300+	85%	83%	82%
Home Recovery Information Given	300+	91%	86%	85%
Hospital Given 9 or 10 on 10 Point Scale	300+	79%	74%	71%
Meds 'Always' Explained Before Given	300+	63%	64%	64%
Nurses 'Always' Communicated Well	300+	79%	81%	79%
Pain 'Always' Well Controlled	300+	71%	73%	71%
Room and Bathroom 'Always' Clean	300+	70%	76%	73%
Timely Help 'Always' Received	300+	70%	71%	68%
Would Definitely Recommend Hospital	300+	82%	73%	71%
Use of Medical Imaging				
Cardiac Imaging Stress Test before Surgery[7]	-	-	5.4%	5.3%
Combination Abdominal CT Scan[7]	-	-	9.3%	10.5%
Combination Brain/Sinus CT Scan[7]	-	-	2.6%	2.7%
Combination Chest CT Scan[7]	-	-	4.6%	2.7%
Follow-up Mammogram/Ultrasound[7]	-	-	8.4%	8.8%
Lumbar Spine MRI for Low Back Pain	65	43.1%	38.7%	37.2%

Parkview Regional Medical Center

11109 Parkview Plaza Drive
Fort Wayne, IN 46845
Phone: 260-266-1000
Fax: 260-483-1373
E-mail: fdb@parkview.com
URL: www.parkview.com
Type: Acute Care Hospitals
Ownership: Voluntary non-profit - Private
Emergency Services: Yes
Beds: 656
Key Personnel:
Radiology. Claudia Bergdoll
Pediatric Ambulatory Care . . . . . . Michael Dick, MD
Pediatric In-Patient Care . . . . Michael Dick, MD
Quality Assurance . . . . Sue Ehinger
Infection Control. . . . . Joan Kennedy, RN
Chief of Medical Staff . . . . Richard Neilsen, MD
CEO/President. . . . . Mike Packnett, MD
Operating Room. . . . . Katie Smith

Measure	Cases	This Hosp.	State Avg.	U.S. Avg.
Blood Clot Prevention and Treatment				
Anticoagulation Overlap Therapy[2]	195	90%	92%	93%
ICU Venous Thromboembolism Prophylaxis[2]	78	96%	91%	92%
Incidence of Potentially Preventable VTE[2]	21	0%	10%	10%
UFH with Dosages/Platelet Monitoring[2]	176	99%	95%	97%
Venous Thromboembolism Prophylaxis[2]	389	88%	83%	85%
Warfarin Therapy Discharge Instructions[2]	135	87%	71%	75%
Chest Pain/Possible Heart Attack Care				
Aspirin Given Within 24 Hours of Arrival[5]	-	-	96%	96%
Fibrinolytic Meds Within 30 Min. of Arrival[5]	-	-	48%	58%
Average Time to ECG (minutes)[5]	-	-	6	7
Average Time to Transfer (minutes)[5]	-	-	46	60
Children's Asthma Care				
Received Home Management Plan of Care	-	-	-	88%
Received Reliever Medication	-	-	-	100%
Received Systemic Corticosteroids	-	-	-	100%
Emergency Department				
Admittance Decision Time (minutes)[2]	542	122	80	98
Head CT Results Within 45 Min. of Arrival[1,3]	-	-	60%	57%
Patients Who Left ER Before Being Seen	76,591	1%	2%	2%
Time from ER Arrival to Admit. (minutes)[2]	605	309	241	274
Time from ER Arrival to Discharge (minutes)	535	139	122	134
Time in ER Before Being Evaluated (minutes)	547	31	22	26
Time to Pain Meds for Fractures (minutes)	344	58	52	57
Heart Attack Care				
Aspirin Given at Discharge	675	100%	99%	99%
Fibrinolytic Meds Within 30 Min. of Arrival[7]	-	-	67%	54%
PCI Within 90 Minutes of Arrival	54	93%	97%	96%
Statin Prescribed at Discharge	650	99%	99%	98%
Heart Failure Care				
ACE Inhibitor or ARB for LVSD[2]	81	98%	97%	97%
Discharge Instructions Given[2]	242	95%	95%	94%
Evaluation of LVS Function[2]	311	100%	99%	99%
Medicare Spending				
Medicare Spending per Patient (ratio)	-	1.00	1.01	0.98
Pneumonia Care				
Appropriate Initial Antibiotic Given[2]	80	94%	95%	95%
Blood Culture Timing[2]	100	100%	98%	98%
Pregnancy and Delivery Care				
Newborn Deliveries Scheduled Early[2]	54	7%	5%	6%
Preventive Care				
Immunization for Influenza[2]	558	90%	91%	90%
Immunization for Pneumonia[2]	698	94%	92%	92%
Stroke Care				
Anticoagulation Therapy for Atrial Fibrillation	48	100%	94%	95%
Antithrombotic Therapy Timing	323	100%	97%	98%
Assessed for Rehabilitation	420	100%	96%	97%
Discharged on Antithrombotic Therapy	350	100%	98%	99%
Discharged on Statin Medication	280	92%	91%	94%
Thrombolytic Therapy Timing	20	100%	54%	66%
Venous Thromboembolism Prophylaxis	443	98%	91%	94%
Written Stroke Educational Materials Given	210	93%	82%	88%
Surgical Care Improvement Project				
Appropriate Beta Blocker Usage[2]	263	98%	98%	98%
Appropriate VTP Within 24 Hours[2]	365	96%	98%	98%
Controlled Postoperative Blood Glucose[2]	182	98%	97%	97%
Perioperative Temperature Management[2]	561	100%	100%	100%
Prophylactic Antibiotic Selection[2]	539	99%	99%	99%
Prophylactic Antibiotic Selection (Outpatient)	623	99%	98%	98%
Prophylactic Antibiotic Stopped[2]	525	96%	98%	98%
Prophylactic Antibiotic Timing[2]	542	98%	99%	99%
Prophylactic Antibiotic Timing (Outpatient)	627	99%	98%	98%
Urinary Catheter Removal[2]	348	98%	98%	97%
Survey of Patients' Hospital Experiences				
Area Around Room 'Always' Quiet at Night	300+	67%	61%	61%
Doctors 'Always' Communicated Well	300+	77%	83%	82%
Home Recovery Information Given	300+	87%	86%	85%
Hospital Given 9 or 10 on 10 Point Scale	300+	77%	74%	71%
Meds 'Always' Explained Before Given	300+	59%	64%	64%
Nurses 'Always' Communicated Well	300+	79%	81%	79%
Pain 'Always' Well Controlled	300+	72%	73%	71%
Room and Bathroom 'Always' Clean	300+	74%	76%	73%
Timely Help 'Always' Received	300+	67%	71%	68%
Would Definitely Recommend Hospital	300+	78%	73%	71%
Use of Medical Imaging				
Cardiac Imaging Stress Test before Surgery	1,107	6.1%	5.4%	5.3%
Combination Abdominal CT Scan	1,081	11.8%	9.3%	10.5%
Combination Brain/Sinus CT Scan	967	3.5%	2.6%	2.7%
Combination Chest CT Scan	724	0.3%	4.6%	2.7%

NOTE: Hospital profiles are in alphabetical order by state, then city, then hospital within the city; Rankings exclude hospitals with less than 25 cases except for patient surveys which excludes hospitals with less than 100 cases; (a) 100-299 cases; (1) The number of cases/patients is too few to report; (2) Data submitted were based on a sample of cases/patients; (3) Results are based on a shorter time period than required; (4) Data suppressed by CMS for one or more quarters; (5) Results are not available for this reporting period; (6) Fewer than 100 patients completed the HCAHPS survey; (7) No cases met the criteria for this measure; (8) The lower limit of the confidence interval cannot be calculated if the number of observed infections equals zero; (9) No data are available from the state/territory for this reporting period; (10) The scores shown reflect fewer than 50 completed surveys; (11) There were discrepancies in the data collection process; (12) This measure does not apply to this hospital for this reporting period; (13) Results cannot be calculated for this reporting period; (14) The results for this state are combined with nearby states to protect confidentiality; Please refer to the User's Guide for a full explanation of data.

Measure	Cases	This Hosp.	State Avg.	U.S. Avg.
Follow-up Mammogram/Ultrasound[7]	-	-	8.4%	8.8%
Lumbar Spine MRI for Low Back Pain	151	36.4%	38.7%	37.2%

Saint Joseph Hospital

700 Broadway
Fort Wayne, IN 46802
URL: www.stjoehospital.com
Type: Acute Care Hospitals
Ownership: Proprietary

Phone: 260-425-3000
Fax: 260-425-3013
Emergency Services: Yes
Beds: 191

Key Personnel:

CEO/President. . . . . Kirk Bay
Operating Room. . . . . Bernice Ewing
Chief of Medical Staff . . . . Bryan E Flueckiger
Quality Assurance . . . . Cheryl Rieves
Emergency Room . . . . Jernice Watson, RN

Measure	Cases	This Hosp.	State Avg.	U.S. Avg.
Blood Clot Prevention and Treatment				
Anticoagulation Overlap Therapy[2]	18	94%	92%	93%
ICU Venous Thromboembolism Prophylaxis[2]	99	98%	91%	92%
Incidence of Potentially Preventable VTE[1,2]	-	-	10%	10%
UFH with Dosages/Platelet Monitoring[2]	20	100%	95%	97%
Venous Thromboembolism Prophylaxis[2]	319	92%	83%	85%
Warfarin Therapy Discharge Instructions[2]	16	81%	71%	75%
Chest Pain/Possible Heart Attack Care				
Aspirin Given Within 24 Hours of Arrival[5]	-	-	96%	96%
Fibrinolytic Meds Within 30 Min. of Arrival[5]	-	-	48%	58%
Average Time to ECG (minutes)[5]	-	-	6	7
Average Time to Transfer (minutes)[5]	-	-	46	60
Children's Asthma Care				
Received Home Management Plan of Care	-	-	-	88%
Received Reliever Medication	-	-	-	100%
Received Systemic Corticosteroids	-	-	-	100%
Emergency Department				
Admittance Decision Time (minutes)[2]	468	118	80	98
Head CT Results Within 45 Min. of Arrival[1]	-	-	60%	57%
Patients Who Left ER Before Being Seen	29,189	0%	2%	2%
Time from ER Arrival to Admit. (minutes)[2]	473	270	241	274
Time from ER Arrival to Discharge (minutes)	391	114	122	134
Time in ER Before Being Evaluated (minutes)	411	20	22	26
Time to Pain Meds for Fractures (minutes)	92	40	52	57
Heart Attack Care				
Aspirin Given at Discharge	129	99%	99%	99%
Fibrinolytic Meds Within 30 Min. of Arrival[7]	-	-	67%	54%
PCI Within 90 Minutes of Arrival	27	96%	97%	96%
Statin Prescribed at Discharge	118	99%	99%	98%
Heart Failure Care				
ACE Inhibitor or ARB for LVSD	51	100%	97%	97%
Discharge Instructions Given	154	99%	95%	94%
Evaluation of LVS Function	185	100%	99%	99%
Medicare Spending				
Medicare Spending per Patient (ratio)	-	1.04	1.01	0.98
Pneumonia Care				
Appropriate Initial Antibiotic Given	59	100%	95%	95%
Blood Culture Timing	60	100%	98%	98%
Pregnancy and Delivery Care				
Newborn Deliveries Scheduled Early[2]	35	0%	5%	6%
Preventive Care				
Immunization for Influenza[2]	454	95%	91%	90%
Immunization for Pneumonia[2]	645	95%	92%	92%
Stroke Care				
Anticoagulation Therapy for Atrial Fibrillation[1]	-	-	94%	95%
Antithrombotic Therapy Timing	31	100%	97%	98%
Assessed for Rehabilitation	29	97%	96%	97%
Discharged on Antithrombotic Therapy	29	100%	98%	99%
Discharged on Statin Medication	23	96%	91%	94%
Thrombolytic Therapy Timing[1]	-	-	54%	66%
Venous Thromboembolism Prophylaxis	33	94%	91%	94%
Written Stroke Educational Materials Given	15	93%	82%	88%
Surgical Care Improvement Project				
Appropriate Beta Blocker Usage	39	100%	98%	98%
Appropriate VTP Within 24 Hours	63	95%	98%	98%
Controlled Postoperative Blood Glucose	31	97%	97%	97%
Perioperative Temperature Management	75	100%	100%	100%
Prophylactic Antibiotic Selection	65	100%	99%	99%
Prophylactic Antibiotic Selection (Outpatient)	62	100%	98%	98%
Prophylactic Antibiotic Stopped	63	98%	98%	98%
Prophylactic Antibiotic Timing	65	98%	99%	99%
Prophylactic Antibiotic Timing (Outpatient)	62	98%	98%	98%
Urinary Catheter Removal	38	89%	98%	97%
Survey of Patients' Hospital Experiences				
Area Around Room 'Always' Quiet at Night	300+	59%	61%	61%
Doctors 'Always' Communicated Well	300+	80%	83%	82%
Home Recovery Information Given	300+	85%	86%	85%
Hospital Given 9 or 10 on 10 Point Scale	300+	66%	74%	71%
Meds 'Always' Explained Before Given	300+	62%	64%	64%
Nurses 'Always' Communicated Well	300+	77%	81%	79%
Pain 'Always' Well Controlled	300+	71%	73%	71%
Room and Bathroom 'Always' Clean	300+	69%	76%	73%
Timely Help 'Always' Received	300+	66%	71%	68%
Would Definitely Recommend Hospital	300+	67%	73%	71%
Use of Medical Imaging				
Cardiac Imaging Stress Test before Surgery	99	4.0%	5.4%	5.3%
Combination Abdominal CT Scan	209	2.9%	9.3%	10.5%
Combination Brain/Sinus CT Scan	262	0.8%	2.6%	2.7%
Combination Chest CT Scan	125	1.6%	4.6%	2.7%
Follow-up Mammogram/Ultrasound	890	4.5%	8.4%	8.8%
Lumbar Spine MRI for Low Back Pain	48	35.4%	38.7%	37.2%

Saint Vincent Frankfort Hospital

1300 S Jackson St
Frankfort, IN 46041
URL: www.stvincent.org
Type: Critical Access Hospitals
Ownership: Voluntary non-profit - Church

Phone: 765-656-3000
Fax: 765-654-6881
Emergency Services: Yes
Beds: 25

Key Personnel:

Anesthesiology. . . . . Alexandra Dominik, MD
Quality Assurance . . . . John D Doyle
Radiology. . . . . Stevan A Fritsch, MD
Intensive Care Unit. . . . . Debbie Lineback, RN
Operating Room. . . . . Cindi Mattingly, RN
CEO . . . . Jonathan Nalli
Emergency Room . . . . James Rudolph, MD
Chief of Medical Staff . . . . Stephen D Thorp, MD

Measure	Cases	This Hosp.	State Avg.	U.S. Avg.
Blood Clot Prevention and Treatment				
Anticoagulation Overlap Therapy[1,2]	-	-	92%	93%
ICU Venous Thromboembolism Prophylaxis[2,7]	-	-	91%	92%
Incidence of Potentially Preventable VTE[2,7]	-	-	10%	10%
UFH with Dosages/Platelet Monitoring[2,7]	-	-	95%	97%
Venous Thromboembolism Prophylaxis[2]	108	89%	83%	85%
Warfarin Therapy Discharge Instructions[1,2]	-	-	71%	75%
Chest Pain/Possible Heart Attack Care				
Aspirin Given Within 24 Hours of Arrival[3]	28	100%	96%	96%
Fibrinolytic Meds Within 30 Min. of Arrival[3,7]	-	-	48%	58%
Average Time to ECG (minutes)[3]	30	5	6	7
Average Time to Transfer (minutes)[1,3]	-	-	46	60
Children's Asthma Care				
Received Home Management Plan of Care	-	-	-	88%
Received Reliever Medication	-	-	-	100%
Received Systemic Corticosteroids	-	-	-	100%
Emergency Department				
Admittance Decision Time (minutes)[2]	257	50	80	98
Head CT Results Within 45 Min. of Arrival[5]	-	-	60%	57%
Patients Who Left ER Before Being Seen[5]	-	-	2%	2%
Time from ER Arrival to Admit. (minutes)[2]	274	207	241	274
Time from ER Arrival to Discharge (minutes)[3]	245	94	122	134
Time in ER Before Being Evaluated (minutes)[3]	276	12	22	26
Time to Pain Meds for Fractures (minutes)[5]	-	-	52	57
Heart Attack Care				
Aspirin Given at Discharge[3,7]	-	-	99%	99%
Fibrinolytic Meds Within 30 Min. of Arrival[3,7]	-	-	67%	54%
PCI Within 90 Minutes of Arrival[3,7]	-	-	97%	96%
Statin Prescribed at Discharge[3,7]	-	-	99%	98%
Heart Failure Care				
ACE Inhibitor or ARB for LVSD[1]	-	-	97%	97%
Discharge Instructions Given[1]	-	-	95%	94%
Evaluation of LVS Function	14	93%	99%	99%
Medicare Spending				
Medicare Spending per Patient (ratio)	-	-	1.01	0.98
Pneumonia Care				
Appropriate Initial Antibiotic Given	44	95%	95%	95%
Blood Culture Timing	68	99%	98%	98%
Pregnancy and Delivery Care				
Newborn Deliveries Scheduled Early[5]	-	-	5%	6%
Preventive Care				
Immunization for Influenza[2]	219	95%	91%	90%
Immunization for Pneumonia[2]	243	98%	92%	92%
Stroke Care				
Anticoagulation Therapy for Atrial Fibrillation[5]	-	-	94%	95%
Antithrombotic Therapy Timing[5]	-	-	97%	98%
Assessed for Rehabilitation[5]	-	-	96%	97%
Discharged on Antithrombotic Therapy[5]	-	-	98%	99%
Discharged on Statin Medication[5]	-	-	91%	94%
Thrombolytic Therapy Timing[5]	-	-	54%	66%
Venous Thromboembolism Prophylaxis[5]	-	-	91%	94%
Written Stroke Educational Materials Given[5]	-	-	82%	88%
Surgical Care Improvement Project				
Appropriate Beta Blocker Usage[1]	-	-	98%	98%
Appropriate VTP Within 24 Hours	17	100%	98%	98%
Controlled Postoperative Blood Glucose[3,7]	-	-	97%	97%
Perioperative Temperature Management	19	100%	100%	100%
Prophylactic Antibiotic Selection	15	93%	99%	99%
Prophylactic Antibiotic Selection (Outpatient)[3]	19	100%	98%	98%
Prophylactic Antibiotic Stopped	15	100%	98%	98%
Prophylactic Antibiotic Timing	15	93%	99%	99%
Prophylactic Antibiotic Timing (Outpatient)[3]	19	95%	98%	98%
Urinary Catheter Removal[1]	-	-	98%	97%
Survey of Patients' Hospital Experiences				
Area Around Room 'Always' Quiet at Night	(a)	66%	61%	61%
Doctors 'Always' Communicated Well	(a)	86%	83%	82%
Home Recovery Information Given	(a)	89%	86%	85%
Hospital Given 9 or 10 on 10 Point Scale	(a)	75%	74%	71%
Meds 'Always' Explained Before Given	(a)	68%	64%	64%
Nurses 'Always' Communicated Well	(a)	79%	81%	79%
Pain 'Always' Well Controlled	(a)	71%	73%	71%
Room and Bathroom 'Always' Clean	(a)	70%	76%	73%
Timely Help 'Always' Received	(a)	73%	71%	68%
Would Definitely Recommend Hospital	(a)	68%	73%	71%
Use of Medical Imaging				
Cardiac Imaging Stress Test before Surgery[1]	-	-	5.4%	5.3%
Combination Abdominal CT Scan	179	2.8%	9.3%	10.5%
Combination Brain/Sinus CT Scan[1]	-	-	2.6%	2.7%
Combination Chest CT Scan	87	0.0%	4.6%	2.7%
Follow-up Mammogram/Ultrasound	382	10.7%	8.4%	8.8%
Lumbar Spine MRI for Low Back Pain[1]	-	-	38.7%	37.2%

Johnson Memorial Hospital

1125 W Jefferson St
Franklin, IN 46131
URL: www.johnsonmemorial.org
Type: Acute Care Hospitals
Ownership: Government - Local

Phone: 317-736-3300
Fax: 317-738-7894
Emergency Services: Yes
Beds: 161

Key Personnel:

Anesthesiology. . . . . D Buch, MD
Radiology. . . . . Richard Buck
CEO/President. . . . . Larry R. Heydon, MBA
Quality Assurance . . . . Cindy Lewis
Operating Room. . . . . Vickie McCullough
Chief of Medical Staff . . . . John Norris, MD
Intensive Care Unit. . . . . Karen Robards
Emergency Room . . . . Carla M Taylor

Measure	Cases	This Hosp.	State Avg.	U.S. Avg.
Blood Clot Prevention and Treatment				
Anticoagulation Overlap Therapy[2]	32	88%	92%	93%
ICU Venous Thromboembolism Prophylaxis[2]	84	92%	91%	92%
Incidence of Potentially Preventable VTE[1,2]	-	-	10%	10%
UFH with Dosages/Platelet Monitoring[1,2]	-	-	95%	97%
Venous Thromboembolism Prophylaxis[2]	221	76%	83%	85%
Warfarin Therapy Discharge Instructions[2]	25	80%	71%	75%
Chest Pain/Possible Heart Attack Care				
Aspirin Given Within 24 Hours of Arrival	30	100%	96%	96%
Fibrinolytic Meds Within 30 Min. of Arrival[7]	-	-	48%	58%

NOTE: Hospital profiles are in alphabetical order by state, then city, then hospital within the city; Rankings exclude hospitals with less than 25 cases except for patient surveys which excludes hospitals with less than 100 cases; (a) 100-299 cases; (1) The number of cases/patients is too few to report; (2) Data submitted were based on a sample of cases/patients; (3) Results are based on a shorter time period than required; (4) Data suppressed by CMS for one or more quarters; (5) Results are not available for this reporting period; (6) Fewer than 100 patients completed the HCAHPS survey; (7) No cases met the criteria for this measure; (8) The lower limit of the confidence interval cannot be calculated if the number of observed infections equals zero; (9) No data are available from the state/territory for this reporting period; (10) The scores shown reflect fewer than 50 completed surveys; (11) There were discrepancies in the data collection process; (12) This measure does not apply to this hospital for this reporting period; (13) Results cannot be calculated for this reporting period; (14) The results for this state are combined with nearby states to protect confidentiality; Please refer to the User's Guide for a full explanation of data.

Average Time to ECG (minutes)	31	3	6	7
Average Time to Transfer (minutes)	17	32	46	60
Children's Asthma Care				
Received Home Management Plan of Care	-	-	-	88%
Received Reliever Medication	-	-	-	100%
Received Systemic Corticosteroids	-	-	-	100%
Emergency Department				
Admittance Decision Time (minutes)[2]	408	94	80	98
Head CT Results Within 45 Min. of Arrival[1]	-	-	60%	57%
Patients Who Left ER Before Being Seen	22,822	1%	2%	2%
Time from ER Arrival to Admit. (minutes)[2]	453	242	241	274
Time from ER Arrival to Discharge (minutes)	516	100	122	134
Time in ER Before Being Evaluated (minutes)	600	11	22	26
Time to Pain Meds for Fractures (minutes)	60	34	52	57
Heart Attack Care				
Aspirin Given at Discharge	13	92%	99%	99%
Fibrinolytic Meds Within 30 Min. of Arrival[7]	-	-	67%	54%
PCI Within 90 Minutes of Arrival[7]	-	-	97%	96%
Statin Prescribed at Discharge	13	92%	99%	98%
Heart Failure Care				
ACE Inhibitor or ARB for LVSD	18	94%	97%	97%
Discharge Instructions Given	54	85%	95%	94%
Evaluation of LVS Function	81	100%	99%	99%
Medicare Spending				
Medicare Spending per Patient (ratio)	-	1.03	1.01	0.98
Pneumonia Care				
Appropriate Initial Antibiotic Given	82	84%	95%	95%
Blood Culture Timing	109	97%	98%	98%
Pregnancy and Delivery Care				
Newborn Deliveries Scheduled Early	30	13%	5%	6%
Preventive Care				
Immunization for Influenza[2]	378	88%	91%	90%
Immunization for Pneumonia[2]	475	96%	92%	92%
Stroke Care				
Anticoagulation Therapy for Atrial Fibrillation[1]	-	-	94%	95%
Antithrombotic Therapy Timing	42	98%	97%	98%
Assessed for Rehabilitation	47	100%	96%	97%
Discharged on Antithrombotic Therapy	47	98%	98%	99%
Discharged on Statin Medication	37	92%	91%	94%
Thrombolytic Therapy Timing[1]	-	-	54%	66%
Venous Thromboembolism Prophylaxis	44	73%	91%	94%
Written Stroke Educational Materials Given	18	100%	82%	88%
Surgical Care Improvement Project				
Appropriate Beta Blocker Usage	23	100%	98%	98%
Appropriate VTP Within 24 Hours	106	98%	98%	98%
Controlled Postoperative Blood Glucose[7]	-	-	97%	97%
Perioperative Temperature Management	115	100%	100%	100%
Prophylactic Antibiotic Selection	75	99%	99%	99%
Prophylactic Antibiotic Selection (Outpatient)	152	99%	98%	98%
Prophylactic Antibiotic Stopped	74	96%	98%	98%
Prophylactic Antibiotic Timing	75	97%	99%	99%
Prophylactic Antibiotic Timing (Outpatient)	153	96%	98%	98%
Urinary Catheter Removal	82	96%	98%	97%
Survey of Patients' Hospital Experiences				
Area Around Room 'Always' Quiet at Night	300+	57%	61%	61%
Doctors 'Always' Communicated Well	300+	88%	83%	82%
Home Recovery Information Given	300+	89%	86%	85%
Hospital Given 9 or 10 on 10 Point Scale	300+	79%	74%	71%
Meds 'Always' Explained Before Given	300+	70%	64%	64%
Nurses 'Always' Communicated Well	300+	82%	81%	79%
Pain 'Always' Well Controlled	300+	73%	73%	71%
Room and Bathroom 'Always' Clean	300+	80%	76%	73%
Timely Help 'Always' Received	300+	74%	71%	68%
Would Definitely Recommend Hospital	300+	75%	73%	71%
Use of Medical Imaging				
Cardiac Imaging Stress Test before Surgery	291	6.9%	5.4%	5.3%
Combination Abdominal CT Scan	457	6.8%	9.3%	10.5%
Combination Brain/Sinus CT Scan	520	1.9%	2.6%	2.7%
Combination Chest CT Scan	186	1.1%	4.6%	2.7%
Follow-up Mammogram/Ultrasound	671	5.5%	8.4%	8.8%
Lumbar Spine MRI for Low Back Pain	58	36.2%	38.7%	37.2%

Methodist Hospitals

600 Grant St
Gary, IN 46402
URL: www.methodisthospital.org
Type: Acute Care Hospitals
Ownership: Voluntary non-profit - Private
Phone: 219-886-4642
Fax: 219-886-4592
Emergency Services: Yes
Beds: 469

Key Personnel:

CEO/President. . . . . Michael Davenport, MD
Anesthesiology. . . . . Ronald Hayes, MD
Emergency Room . . . . Michael McGee, MD
Cardiac Laboratory. . . . . Nazzal Obaid, MD
Surgery . . . . Ray Sawaqed, MD
Radiology. . . . . Tulsi Sawlani, MD
Pediatric Ambulatory Care . . . . . . Steve Simpson, MD
Chief of Medical Staff . . . . Katrina Wright, MD

Measure	Cases	This Hosp.	State Avg.	U.S. Avg.
Blood Clot Prevention and Treatment				
Anticoagulation Overlap Therapy[2]	131	82%	92%	93%
ICU Venous Thromboembolism Prophylaxis[2]	75	93%	91%	92%
Incidence of Potentially Preventable VTE[2]	21	14%	10%	10%
UFH with Dosages/Platelet Monitoring[2]	64	89%	95%	97%
Venous Thromboembolism Prophylaxis[2]	393	86%	83%	85%
Warfarin Therapy Discharge Instructions[2]	89	99%	71%	75%
Chest Pain/Possible Heart Attack Care				
Aspirin Given Within 24 Hours of Arrival[1]	-	-	96%	96%
Fibrinolytic Meds Within 30 Min. of Arrival[5]	-	-	48%	58%
Average Time to ECG (minutes)[1]	-	-	6	7
Average Time to Transfer (minutes)[5]	-	-	46	60
Children's Asthma Care				
Received Home Management Plan of Care	-	-	-	88%
Received Reliever Medication	-	-	-	100%
Received Systemic Corticosteroids	-	-	-	100%
Emergency Department				
Admittance Decision Time (minutes)[2]	754	146	80	98
Head CT Results Within 45 Min. of Arrival[1]	-	-	60%	57%
Patients Who Left ER Before Being Seen	61,080	4%	2%	2%
Time from ER Arrival to Admit. (minutes)[2]	754	361	241	274
Time from ER Arrival to Discharge (minutes)	328	173	122	134
Time in ER Before Being Evaluated (minutes)	272	74	22	26
Time to Pain Meds for Fractures (minutes)	124	78	52	57
Heart Attack Care				
Aspirin Given at Discharge[2]	126	98%	99%	99%
Fibrinolytic Meds Within 30 Min. of Arrival[2,7]	-	-	67%	54%
PCI Within 90 Minutes of Arrival[2]	35	89%	97%	96%
Statin Prescribed at Discharge[2]	125	95%	99%	98%
Heart Failure Care				
ACE Inhibitor or ARB for LVSD[2]	145	98%	97%	97%
Discharge Instructions Given[2]	254	88%	95%	94%
Evaluation of LVS Function[2]	310	100%	99%	99%
Medicare Spending				
Medicare Spending per Patient (ratio)	-	1.07	1.01	0.98
Pneumonia Care				
Appropriate Initial Antibiotic Given[2]	59	100%	95%	95%
Blood Culture Timing[2]	117	99%	98%	98%
Pregnancy and Delivery Care				
Newborn Deliveries Scheduled Early[2]	32	0%	5%	6%
Preventive Care				
Immunization for Influenza[2]	549	79%	91%	90%
Immunization for Pneumonia[2]	716	73%	92%	92%
Stroke Care				
Anticoagulation Therapy for Atrial Fibrillation[2]	11	91%	94%	95%
Antithrombotic Therapy Timing[2]	92	97%	97%	98%
Assessed for Rehabilitation[2]	116	99%	96%	97%
Discharged on Antithrombotic Therapy[2]	92	97%	98%	99%
Discharged on Statin Medication[2]	71	87%	91%	94%
Thrombolytic Therapy Timing[1,2]	-	-	54%	66%
Venous Thromboembolism Prophylaxis[2]	127	88%	91%	94%
Written Stroke Educational Materials Given[2]	61	97%	82%	88%
Surgical Care Improvement Project				
Appropriate Beta Blocker Usage[2]	125	100%	98%	98%
Appropriate VTP Within 24 Hours[2]	329	100%	98%	98%
Controlled Postoperative Blood Glucose[2]	57	98%	97%	97%
Perioperative Temperature Management[2]	377	100%	100%	100%
Prophylactic Antibiotic Selection[2]	290	99%	99%	99%
Prophylactic Antibiotic Selection (Outpatient)	241	99%	98%	98%
Prophylactic Antibiotic Stopped[2]	263	100%	98%	98%
Prophylactic Antibiotic Timing[2]	291	100%	99%	99%
Prophylactic Antibiotic Timing (Outpatient)	242	98%	98%	98%
Urinary Catheter Removal[2]	213	99%	98%	97%
Survey of Patients' Hospital Experiences				
Area Around Room 'Always' Quiet at Night	300+	59%	61%	61%
Doctors 'Always' Communicated Well	300+	78%	83%	82%
Home Recovery Information Given	300+	82%	86%	85%
Hospital Given 9 or 10 on 10 Point Scale	300+	70%	74%	71%
Meds 'Always' Explained Before Given	300+	64%	64%	64%
Nurses 'Always' Communicated Well	300+	82%	81%	79%
Pain 'Always' Well Controlled	300+	76%	73%	71%
Room and Bathroom 'Always' Clean	300+	72%	76%	73%
Timely Help 'Always' Received	300+	70%	71%	68%
Would Definitely Recommend Hospital	300+	70%	73%	71%
Use of Medical Imaging				
Cardiac Imaging Stress Test before Surgery	238	3.8%	5.4%	5.3%
Combination Abdominal CT Scan	1,211	28.5%	9.3%	10.5%
Combination Brain/Sinus CT Scan	1,231	3.6%	2.6%	2.7%
Combination Chest CT Scan	597	27.1%	4.6%	2.7%
Follow-up Mammogram/Ultrasound	1,880	8.9%	8.4%	8.8%
Lumbar Spine MRI for Low Back Pain	135	41.5%	38.7%	37.2%

IU Health Goshen Hospital

200 High Park Ave
Goshen, IN 46526
E-mail: ksearcy@goshenhealth.com
URL: www.goshenhosp.com
Type: Acute Care Hospitals
Ownership: Voluntary non-profit - Private
Phone: 574-364-1000
Fax: 574-535-2859
Emergency Services: Yes
Beds: 115

Key Personnel:

Emergency Room . . . . Candes Andersen
Radiology. . . . . Jody Barber
Operating Room. . . . . Wil Beachy
Chief of Medical Staff . . . . Randy Cammengade
Cardiac Laboratory. . . . . Scott Ereksen
CEO/President. . . . . Dan Evans

Measure	Cases	This Hosp.	State Avg.	U.S. Avg.
Blood Clot Prevention and Treatment				
Anticoagulation Overlap Therapy[2]	57	79%	92%	93%
ICU Venous Thromboembolism Prophylaxis[2]	76	96%	91%	92%
Incidence of Potentially Preventable VTE[1,2]	-	-	10%	10%
UFH with Dosages/Platelet Monitoring[2]	28	100%	95%	97%
Venous Thromboembolism Prophylaxis[2]	324	89%	83%	85%
Warfarin Therapy Discharge Instructions[2]	51	75%	71%	75%
Chest Pain/Possible Heart Attack Care				
Aspirin Given Within 24 Hours of Arrival	36	94%	96%	96%
Fibrinolytic Meds Within 30 Min. of Arrival[7]	-	-	48%	58%
Average Time to ECG (minutes)	37	6	6	7
Average Time to Transfer (minutes)[1]	-	-	46	60
Children's Asthma Care				
Received Home Management Plan of Care	-	-	-	88%
Received Reliever Medication	-	-	-	100%
Received Systemic Corticosteroids	-	-	-	100%
Emergency Department				
Admittance Decision Time (minutes)[2]	455	124	80	98
Head CT Results Within 45 Min. of Arrival	14	43%	60%	57%
Patients Who Left ER Before Being Seen	33,469	1%	2%	2%
Time from ER Arrival to Admit. (minutes)[2]	474	264	241	274
Time from ER Arrival to Discharge (minutes)	377	134	122	134
Time in ER Before Being Evaluated (minutes)	400	18	22	26
Time to Pain Meds for Fractures (minutes)	162	56	52	57
Heart Attack Care				
Aspirin Given at Discharge	89	99%	99%	99%
Fibrinolytic Meds Within 30 Min. of Arrival[7]	-	-	67%	54%
PCI Within 90 Minutes of Arrival	19	100%	97%	96%
Statin Prescribed at Discharge	88	100%	99%	98%
Heart Failure Care				
ACE Inhibitor or ARB for LVSD	25	100%	97%	97%
Discharge Instructions Given	88	98%	95%	94%
Evaluation of LVS Function	114	100%	99%	99%
Medicare Spending				
Medicare Spending per Patient (ratio)	-	1.03	1.01	0.98

NOTE: Hospital profiles are in alphabetical order by state, then city, then hospital within the city; Rankings exclude hospitals with less than 25 cases except for patient surveys which excludes hospitals with less than 100 cases; (a) 100-299 cases; (1) The number of cases/patients is too few to report; (2) Data submitted were based on a sample of cases/patients; (3) Results are based on a shorter time period than required; (4) Data suppressed by CMS for one or more quarters; (5) Results are not available for this reporting period; (6) Fewer than 100 patients completed the HCAHPS survey; (7) No cases met the criteria for this measure; (8) The lower limit of the confidence interval cannot be calculated if the number of observed infections equals zero; (9) No data are available from the state/territory for this reporting period; (10) The scores shown reflect fewer than 50 completed surveys; (11) There were discrepancies in the data collection process; (12) This measure does not apply to this hospital for this reporting period; (13) Results cannot be calculated for this reporting period; (14) The results for this state are combined with nearby states to protect confidentiality; Please refer to the User's Guide for a full explanation of data.

Measure	Cases	This Hosp.	State Avg.	U.S. Avg.
Pneumonia Care				
Appropriate Initial Antibiotic Given	149	97%	95%	95%
Blood Culture Timing	229	100%	98%	98%
Pregnancy and Delivery Care				
Newborn Deliveries Scheduled Early	82	1%	5%	6%
Preventive Care				
Immunization for Influenza[2]	515	97%	91%	90%
Immunization for Pneumonia[2]	579	96%	92%	92%
Stroke Care				
Anticoagulation Therapy for Atrial Fibrillation[1]	-	-	94%	95%
Antithrombotic Therapy Timing	57	100%	97%	98%
Assessed for Rehabilitation	63	100%	96%	97%
Discharged on Antithrombotic Therapy	58	100%	98%	99%
Discharged on Statin Medication	44	93%	91%	94%
Thrombolytic Therapy Timing[1]	-	-	54%	66%
Venous Thromboembolism Prophylaxis	57	96%	91%	94%
Written Stroke Educational Materials Given	32	94%	82%	88%
Surgical Care Improvement Project				
Appropriate Beta Blocker Usage	158	99%	98%	98%
Appropriate VTP Within 24 Hours	442	97%	98%	98%
Controlled Postoperative Blood Glucose[7]	-	-	97%	97%
Perioperative Temperature Management	567	100%	100%	100%
Prophylactic Antibiotic Selection	368	99%	99%	99%
Prophylactic Antibiotic Selection (Outpatient)	159	98%	98%	98%
Prophylactic Antibiotic Stopped	363	99%	98%	98%
Prophylactic Antibiotic Timing	369	99%	99%	99%
Prophylactic Antibiotic Timing (Outpatient)	161	96%	98%	98%
Urinary Catheter Removal	311	99%	98%	97%
Survey of Patients' Hospital Experiences				
Area Around Room 'Always' Quiet at Night	300+	54%	61%	61%
Doctors 'Always' Communicated Well	300+	79%	83%	82%
Home Recovery Information Given	300+	88%	86%	85%
Hospital Given 9 or 10 on 10 Point Scale	300+	72%	74%	71%
Meds 'Always' Explained Before Given	300+	64%	64%	64%
Nurses 'Always' Communicated Well	300+	79%	81%	79%
Pain 'Always' Well Controlled	300+	72%	73%	71%
Room and Bathroom 'Always' Clean	300+	73%	76%	73%
Timely Help 'Always' Received	300+	68%	71%	68%
Would Definitely Recommend Hospital	300+	75%	73%	71%
Use of Medical Imaging				
Cardiac Imaging Stress Test before Surgery	241	6.2%	5.4%	5.3%
Combination Abdominal CT Scan	892	2.6%	9.3%	10.5%
Combination Brain/Sinus CT Scan	615	1.3%	2.6%	2.7%
Combination Chest CT Scan	736	0.3%	4.6%	2.7%
Follow-up Mammogram/Ultrasound	1,396	6.6%	8.4%	8.8%
Lumbar Spine MRI for Low Back Pain	125	41.6%	38.7%	37.2%

Putnam County Hospital

1542 S Bloomington St
Greencastle, IN 46135
Phone: 765-655-2620
Fax: 765-655-2625
Type: Critical Access Hospitals
Emergency Services: Yes
Ownership: Government - Local
Beds: 85

Key Personnel:

Intensive Care Unit............ Jackie Eitel
Cardiac Laboratory............ Douglas Eley
Chief of Medical Staff.......... Donna Gennaway
Radiology.................... Paul Sanders
Infection Control.............. Suzanne Tucker
CEO/President............... Dennis Weatherford
Quality Assurance .... Dennis Weatherford
Operating Room.............. Jodie Wyndham

Measure	Cases	This Hosp.	State Avg.	U.S. Avg.
Blood Clot Prevention and Treatment				
Anticoagulation Overlap Therapy[5]	-	-	92%	93%
ICU Venous Thromboembolism Prophylaxis[5]	-	-	91%	92%
Incidence of Potentially Preventable VTE[5]	-	-	10%	10%
UFH with Dosages/Platelet Monitoring[5]	-	-	95%	97%
Venous Thromboembolism Prophylaxis[5]	-	-	83%	85%
Warfarin Therapy Discharge Instructions[5]	-	-	71%	75%
Chest Pain/Possible Heart Attack Care				
Aspirin Given Within 24 Hours of Arrival	36	92%	96%	96%
Fibrinolytic Meds Within 30 Min. of Arrival[7]	-	-	48%	58%
Average Time to ECG (minutes)	40	6	6	7
Average Time to Transfer (minutes)[1]	-	-	46	60
Children's Asthma Care				
Received Home Management Plan of Care	-	-	-	88%
Received Reliever Medication	-	-	-	100%
Received Systemic Corticosteroids	-	-	-	100%
Emergency Department				
Admittance Decision Time (minutes)[5]	-	-	80	98
Head CT Results Within 45 Min. of Arrival[5]	-	-	60%	57%
Patients Who Left ER Before Being Seen	11,532	1%	2%	2%
Time from ER Arrival to Admit. (minutes)[5]	-	-	241	274
Time from ER Arrival to Discharge (minutes)[5]	-	-	122	134
Time in ER Before Being Evaluated (minutes)[5]	-	-	22	26
Time to Pain Meds for Fractures (minutes)[5]	-	-	52	57
Heart Attack Care				
Aspirin Given at Discharge[3,7]	-	-	99%	99%
Fibrinolytic Meds Within 30 Min. of Arrival[3,7]	-	-	67%	54%
PCI Within 90 Minutes of Arrival[3,7]	-	-	97%	96%
Statin Prescribed at Discharge[3,7]	-	-	99%	98%
Heart Failure Care				
ACE Inhibitor or ARB for LVSD[1]	-	-	97%	97%
Discharge Instructions Given	17	100%	95%	94%
Evaluation of LVS Function	24	100%	99%	99%
Medicare Spending				
Medicare Spending per Patient (ratio)	-	-	1.01	0.98
Pneumonia Care				
Appropriate Initial Antibiotic Given	44	100%	95%	95%
Blood Culture Timing	77	96%	98%	98%
Pregnancy and Delivery Care				
Newborn Deliveries Scheduled Early[5]	-	-	5%	6%
Preventive Care				
Immunization for Influenza[5]	-	-	91%	90%
Immunization for Pneumonia[5]	-	-	92%	92%
Stroke Care				
Anticoagulation Therapy for Atrial Fibrillation[5]	-	-	94%	95%
Antithrombotic Therapy Timing[5]	-	-	97%	98%
Assessed for Rehabilitation[5]	-	-	96%	97%
Discharged on Antithrombotic Therapy[5]	-	-	98%	99%
Discharged on Statin Medication[5]	-	-	91%	94%
Thrombolytic Therapy Timing[5]	-	-	54%	66%
Venous Thromboembolism Prophylaxis[5]	-	-	91%	94%
Written Stroke Educational Materials Given[5]	-	-	82%	88%
Surgical Care Improvement Project				
Appropriate Beta Blocker Usage	13	85%	98%	98%
Appropriate VTP Within 24 Hours	24	96%	98%	98%
Controlled Postoperative Blood Glucose[3,7]	-	-	97%	97%
Perioperative Temperature Management	32	100%	100%	100%
Prophylactic Antibiotic Selection	22	100%	99%	99%
Prophylactic Antibiotic Selection (Outpatient)[1,3]	-	-	98%	98%
Prophylactic Antibiotic Stopped	20	90%	98%	98%
Prophylactic Antibiotic Timing	22	95%	99%	99%
Prophylactic Antibiotic Timing (Outpatient)[1,3]	-	-	98%	98%
Urinary Catheter Removal	17	100%	98%	97%
Survey of Patients' Hospital Experiences				
Area Around Room 'Always' Quiet at Night	(a)	50%	61%	61%
Doctors 'Always' Communicated Well	(a)	85%	83%	82%
Home Recovery Information Given	(a)	91%	86%	85%
Hospital Given 9 or 10 on 10 Point Scale	(a)	61%	74%	71%
Meds 'Always' Explained Before Given	(a)	58%	64%	64%
Nurses 'Always' Communicated Well	(a)	84%	81%	79%
Pain 'Always' Well Controlled	(a)	69%	73%	71%
Room and Bathroom 'Always' Clean	(a)	68%	76%	73%
Timely Help 'Always' Received	(a)	74%	71%	68%
Would Definitely Recommend Hospital	(a)	54%	73%	71%
Use of Medical Imaging				
Cardiac Imaging Stress Test before Surgery[1]	-	-	5.4%	5.3%
Combination Abdominal CT Scan	318	9.1%	9.3%	10.5%
Combination Brain/Sinus CT Scan[1]	-	-	2.6%	2.7%
Combination Chest CT Scan	244	6.6%	4.6%	2.7%
Follow-up Mammogram/Ultrasound	411	6.8%	8.4%	8.8%
Lumbar Spine MRI for Low Back Pain	38	42.1%	38.7%	37.2%

Hancock Regional Hospital

801 N State St
Greenfield, IN 46140
Phone: 317-468-4410
URL: www.hancockregional.org
Type: Acute Care Hospitals
Emergency Services: Yes
Ownership: Government - Local
Beds: 94

Key Personnel:

Operating Room............... Brenda Cole
Chief of Medical Staff.......... Michael Fletcher, MD
Emergency Room .... Judy Hall
CEO/President............... Bobby Keen, MD
Coronary Care............... Tammy Strunk, RN
Radiology.................... Lisa Wood

Measure	Cases	This Hosp.	State Avg.	U.S. Avg.
Blood Clot Prevention and Treatment				
Anticoagulation Overlap Therapy[2]	15	100%	92%	93%
ICU Venous Thromboembolism Prophylaxis[2]	52	100%	91%	92%
Incidence of Potentially Preventable VTE[1,2]	-	-	10%	10%
UFH with Dosages/Platelet Monitoring[1,2]	-	-	95%	97%
Venous Thromboembolism Prophylaxis[2]	190	99%	83%	85%
Warfarin Therapy Discharge Instructions[2]	11	82%	71%	75%
Chest Pain/Possible Heart Attack Care				
Aspirin Given Within 24 Hours of Arrival	60	100%	96%	96%
Fibrinolytic Meds Within 30 Min. of Arrival[7]	-	-	48%	58%
Average Time to ECG (minutes)	60	3	6	7
Average Time to Transfer (minutes)	26	76	46	60
Children's Asthma Care				
Received Home Management Plan of Care	-	-	-	88%
Received Reliever Medication	-	-	-	100%
Received Systemic Corticosteroids	-	-	-	100%
Emergency Department				
Admittance Decision Time (minutes)[2]	456	148	80	98
Head CT Results Within 45 Min. of Arrival	15	47%	60%	57%
Patients Who Left ER Before Being Seen	33,279	2%	2%	2%
Time from ER Arrival to Admit. (minutes)[2]	456	280	241	274
Time from ER Arrival to Discharge (minutes)	457	168	122	134
Time in ER Before Being Evaluated (minutes)	500	26	22	26
Time to Pain Meds for Fractures (minutes)	123	53	52	57
Heart Attack Care				
Aspirin Given at Discharge	38	100%	99%	99%
Fibrinolytic Meds Within 30 Min. of Arrival[7]	-	-	67%	54%
PCI Within 90 Minutes of Arrival[1]	-	-	97%	96%
Statin Prescribed at Discharge	37	97%	99%	98%
Heart Failure Care				
ACE Inhibitor or ARB for LVSD	17	100%	97%	97%
Discharge Instructions Given	54	87%	95%	94%
Evaluation of LVS Function	78	100%	99%	99%
Medicare Spending				
Medicare Spending per Patient (ratio)	-	1.04	1.01	0.98
Pneumonia Care				
Appropriate Initial Antibiotic Given[2]	73	97%	95%	95%
Blood Culture Timing[2]	106	100%	98%	98%
Pregnancy and Delivery Care				
Newborn Deliveries Scheduled Early[2]	28	0%	5%	6%
Preventive Care				
Immunization for Influenza[2]	322	98%	91%	90%
Immunization for Pneumonia[2]	428	99%	92%	92%
Stroke Care				
Anticoagulation Therapy for Atrial Fibrillation[1,2]	-	-	94%	95%
Antithrombotic Therapy Timing[2]	38	100%	97%	98%
Assessed for Rehabilitation[2]	53	100%	96%	97%
Discharged on Antithrombotic Therapy[2]	51	100%	98%	99%
Discharged on Statin Medication[2]	45	96%	91%	94%
Thrombolytic Therapy Timing[1,2]	-	-	54%	66%
Venous Thromboembolism Prophylaxis[2]	34	100%	91%	94%
Written Stroke Educational Materials Given[2]	25	96%	82%	88%
Surgical Care Improvement Project				
Appropriate Beta Blocker Usage	70	99%	98%	98%
Appropriate VTP Within 24 Hours	200	98%	98%	98%
Controlled Postoperative Blood Glucose[7]	-	-	97%	97%
Perioperative Temperature Management	226	100%	100%	100%
Prophylactic Antibiotic Selection	153	99%	99%	99%
Prophylactic Antibiotic Selection (Outpatient)	42	98%	98%	98%
Prophylactic Antibiotic Stopped	152	99%	98%	98%

NOTE: Hospital profiles are in alphabetical order by state, then city, then hospital within the city; Rankings exclude hospitals with less than 25 cases except for patient surveys which excludes hospitals with less than 100 cases; (a) 100-299 cases; (1) The number of cases/patients is too few to report; (2) Data submitted were based on a sample of cases/patients; (3) Results are based on a shorter time period than required; (4) Data suppressed by CMS for one or more quarters; (5) Results are not available for this reporting period; (6) Fewer than 100 patients completed the HCAHPS survey; (7) No cases met the criteria for this measure; (8) The lower limit of the confidence interval cannot be calculated if the number of observed infections equals zero; (9) No data are available from the state/territory for this reporting period; (10) The scores shown reflect fewer than 50 completed surveys; (11) There were discrepancies in the data collection process; (12) This measure does not apply to this hospital for this reporting period; (13) Results cannot be calculated for this reporting period; (14) The results for this state are combined with nearby states to protect confidentiality; Please refer to the User's Guide for a full explanation of data.

Measure	Cases	This Hosp.	State Avg.	U.S. Avg.
Prophylactic Antibiotic Timing	153	100%	99%	99%
Prophylactic Antibiotic Timing (Outpatient)	43	95%	98%	98%
Urinary Catheter Removal	45	100%	98%	97%
Survey of Patients' Hospital Experiences				
Area Around Room 'Always' Quiet at Night	300+	63%	61%	61%
Doctors 'Always' Communicated Well	300+	84%	83%	82%
Home Recovery Information Given	300+	89%	86%	85%
Hospital Given 9 or 10 on 10 Point Scale	300+	80%	74%	71%
Meds 'Always' Explained Before Given	300+	69%	64%	64%
Nurses 'Always' Communicated Well	300+	84%	81%	79%
Pain 'Always' Well Controlled	300+	74%	73%	71%
Room and Bathroom 'Always' Clean	300+	78%	76%	73%
Timely Help 'Always' Received	300+	69%	71%	68%
Would Definitely Recommend Hospital	300+	79%	73%	71%
Use of Medical Imaging				
Cardiac Imaging Stress Test before Surgery	157	7.0%	5.4%	5.3%
Combination Abdominal CT Scan	671	9.1%	9.3%	10.5%
Combination Brain/Sinus CT Scan	562	1.8%	2.6%	2.7%
Combination Chest CT Scan	636	3.9%	4.6%	2.7%
Follow-up Mammogram/Ultrasound	1,464	8.1%	8.4%	8.8%
Lumbar Spine MRI for Low Back Pain	128	35.2%	38.7%	37.2%

Decatur County Memorial Hospital

720 N Lincoln St
Greensburg, IN 47240
URL: www.dcmh.net
Type: Critical Access Hospitals
Ownership: Government - Local

Phone: 812-663-4331
Fax: 812-663-9738

Emergency Services: Yes
Beds: 115

Key Personnel:

Infection Control. . . . . Pat Barnes, RN
Anesthesiology. . . . . Sergio Bisono, MD
Chief of Medical Staff. . . . . Dr. Jennifer Fletcher
Intensive Care Unit. . . . . Cindy Grote, RN
Emergency Room . . . . Michael McCarthy, MD
Operating Room. . . . . Jae Riedeman
CEO/President. . . . . Linda Simmons
Radiology. . . . . Barbara Taylor

Measure	Cases	This Hosp.	State Avg.	U.S. Avg.
Blood Clot Prevention and Treatment				
Anticoagulation Overlap Therapy[5]	-	-	92%	93%
ICU Venous Thromboembolism Prophylaxis[5]	-	-	91%	92%
Incidence of Potentially Preventable VTE[5]	-	-	10%	10%
UFH with Dosages/Platelet Monitoring[5]	-	-	95%	97%
Venous Thromboembolism Prophylaxis[5]	-	-	83%	85%
Warfarin Therapy Discharge Instructions[5]	-	-	71%	75%
Chest Pain/Possible Heart Attack Care				
Aspirin Given Within 24 Hours of Arrival	67	99%	96%	96%
Fibrinolytic Meds Within 30 Min. of Arrival[7]	-	-	48%	58%
Average Time to ECG (minutes)	75	6	6	7
Average Time to Transfer (minutes)[1]	-	-	46	60
Children's Asthma Care				
Received Home Management Plan of Care	-	-	-	88%
Received Reliever Medication	-	-	-	100%
Received Systemic Corticosteroids	-	-	-	100%
Emergency Department				
Admittance Decision Time (minutes)[2]	279	48	80	98
Head CT Results Within 45 Min. of Arrival[1,3]	-	-	60%	57%
Patients Who Left ER Before Being Seen	16,099	0%	2%	2%
Time from ER Arrival to Admit. (minutes)[2]	279	180	241	274
Time from ER Arrival to Discharge (minutes)	518	97	122	134
Time in ER Before Being Evaluated (minutes)	810	10	22	26
Time to Pain Meds for Fractures (minutes)	41	26	52	57
Heart Attack Care				
Aspirin Given at Discharge[5]	-	-	99%	99%
Fibrinolytic Meds Within 30 Min. of Arrival[5]	-	-	67%	54%
PCI Within 90 Minutes of Arrival[5]	-	-	97%	96%
Statin Prescribed at Discharge[5]	-	-	99%	98%
Heart Failure Care				
ACE Inhibitor or ARB for LVSD[1]	-	-	97%	97%
Discharge Instructions Given	39	100%	95%	94%
Evaluation of LVS Function	64	100%	99%	99%
Medicare Spending				
Medicare Spending per Patient (ratio)	-	-	1.01	0.98
Pneumonia Care				
Appropriate Initial Antibiotic Given	43	100%	95%	95%
Blood Culture Timing	50	96%	98%	98%
Pregnancy and Delivery Care				
Newborn Deliveries Scheduled Early[3]	16	0%	5%	6%
Preventive Care				
Immunization for Influenza[2]	372	94%	91%	90%
Immunization for Pneumonia[2]	421	83%	92%	92%
Stroke Care				
Anticoagulation Therapy for Atrial Fibrillation[5]	-	-	94%	95%
Antithrombotic Therapy Timing[5]	-	-	97%	98%
Assessed for Rehabilitation[5]	-	-	96%	97%
Discharged on Antithrombotic Therapy[5]	-	-	98%	99%
Discharged on Statin Medication[5]	-	-	91%	94%
Thrombolytic Therapy Timing[5]	-	-	54%	66%
Venous Thromboembolism Prophylaxis[5]	-	-	91%	94%
Written Stroke Educational Materials Given[5]	-	-	82%	88%
Surgical Care Improvement Project				
Appropriate Beta Blocker Usage	27	100%	98%	98%
Appropriate VTP Within 24 Hours	76	100%	98%	98%
Controlled Postoperative Blood Glucose[3,7]	-	-	97%	97%
Perioperative Temperature Management	88	100%	100%	100%
Prophylactic Antibiotic Selection	63	100%	99%	99%
Prophylactic Antibiotic Selection (Outpatient)	11	100%	98%	98%
Prophylactic Antibiotic Stopped	62	98%	98%	98%
Prophylactic Antibiotic Timing	64	98%	99%	99%
Prophylactic Antibiotic Timing (Outpatient)	11	100%	98%	98%
Urinary Catheter Removal	65	100%	98%	97%
Survey of Patients' Hospital Experiences				
Area Around Room 'Always' Quiet at Night	(a)	53%	61%	61%
Doctors 'Always' Communicated Well	(a)	84%	83%	82%
Home Recovery Information Given	(a)	90%	86%	85%
Hospital Given 9 or 10 on 10 Point Scale	(a)	74%	74%	71%
Meds 'Always' Explained Before Given	(a)	71%	64%	64%
Nurses 'Always' Communicated Well	(a)	83%	81%	79%
Pain 'Always' Well Controlled	(a)	78%	73%	71%
Room and Bathroom 'Always' Clean	(a)	79%	76%	73%
Timely Help 'Always' Received	(a)	74%	71%	68%
Would Definitely Recommend Hospital	(a)	69%	73%	71%
Use of Medical Imaging				
Cardiac Imaging Stress Test before Surgery	195	4.1%	5.4%	5.3%
Combination Abdominal CT Scan	236	41.1%	9.3%	10.5%
Combination Brain/Sinus CT Scan	384	1.0%	2.6%	2.7%
Combination Chest CT Scan	105	54.3%	4.6%	2.7%
Follow-up Mammogram/Ultrasound	530	4.3%	8.4%	8.8%
Lumbar Spine MRI for Low Back Pain[1]	-	-	38.7%	37.2%

Franciscan Saint Margaret Health - Hammond

5454 Hohman Ave
Hammond, IN 46320
URL: www.smmhc.com
Type: Acute Care Hospitals
Ownership: Voluntary non-profit - Church

Phone: 219-932-2300
Fax: 219-933-2585

Emergency Services: Yes
Beds: 475

Key Personnel:

Infection Control. . . . . Sally Bola
CEO/President. . . . . Jean Diamond
Radiology. . . . . J Marcus Lee
Operating Room. . . . . Harvey J Levin, RN
Quality Assurance . . . . Jess McHenry
Chief of Medical Staff . . . . J Patel
Pediatric Ambulatory Care . . . . . . S Paul
Pediatric In-Patient Care . . . . S Paul

Measure	Cases	This Hosp.	State Avg.	U.S. Avg.
Blood Clot Prevention and Treatment				
Anticoagulation Overlap Therapy[2]	100	95%	92%	93%
ICU Venous Thromboembolism Prophylaxis[2]	72	93%	91%	92%
Incidence of Potentially Preventable VTE[2]	24	12%	10%	10%
UFH with Dosages/Platelet Monitoring[2]	44	84%	95%	97%
Venous Thromboembolism Prophylaxis[2]	361	81%	83%	85%
Warfarin Therapy Discharge Instructions[2]	66	76%	71%	75%
Chest Pain/Possible Heart Attack Care				
Aspirin Given Within 24 Hours of Arrival[1,3]	-	-	96%	96%
Fibrinolytic Meds Within 30 Min. of Arrival[5]	-	-	48%	58%
Average Time to ECG (minutes)[1,3]	-	-	6	7
Average Time to Transfer (minutes)[5]	-	-	46	60
Children's Asthma Care				
Received Home Management Plan of Care	-	-	-	88%
Received Reliever Medication	-	-	-	100%
Received Systemic Corticosteroids	-	-	-	100%
Emergency Department				
Admittance Decision Time (minutes)[2]	919	107	80	98
Head CT Results Within 45 Min. of Arrival	29	48%	60%	57%
Patients Who Left ER Before Being Seen	43,121	3%	2%	2%
Time from ER Arrival to Admit. (minutes)[2]	919	286	241	274
Time from ER Arrival to Discharge (minutes)	461	150	122	134
Time in ER Before Being Evaluated (minutes)	502	34	22	26
Time to Pain Meds for Fractures (minutes)	96	56	52	57
Heart Attack Care				
Aspirin Given at Discharge	139	99%	99%	99%
Fibrinolytic Meds Within 30 Min. of Arrival[7]	-	-	67%	54%
PCI Within 90 Minutes of Arrival	29	100%	97%	96%
Statin Prescribed at Discharge	133	96%	99%	98%
Heart Failure Care				
ACE Inhibitor or ARB for LVSD[2]	102	97%	97%	97%
Discharge Instructions Given[2]	267	95%	95%	94%
Evaluation of LVS Function[2]	313	97%	99%	99%
Medicare Spending				
Medicare Spending per Patient (ratio)	-	1.05	1.01	0.98
Pneumonia Care				
Appropriate Initial Antibiotic Given[2]	65	98%	95%	95%
Blood Culture Timing[2]	155	99%	98%	98%
Pregnancy and Delivery Care				
Newborn Deliveries Scheduled Early[2]	45	7%	5%	6%
Preventive Care				
Immunization for Influenza[2]	544	81%	91%	90%
Immunization for Pneumonia[2]	818	87%	92%	92%
Stroke Care				
Anticoagulation Therapy for Atrial Fibrillation[1,2]	-	-	94%	95%
Antithrombotic Therapy Timing[2]	89	99%	97%	98%
Assessed for Rehabilitation[2]	95	91%	96%	97%
Discharged on Antithrombotic Therapy[2]	88	98%	98%	99%
Discharged on Statin Medication[2]	66	86%	91%	94%
Thrombolytic Therapy Timing[1,2]	-	-	54%	66%
Venous Thromboembolism Prophylaxis[2]	94	86%	91%	94%
Written Stroke Educational Materials Given[2]	41	61%	82%	88%
Surgical Care Improvement Project				
Appropriate Beta Blocker Usage	79	96%	98%	98%
Appropriate VTP Within 24 Hours	157	95%	98%	98%
Controlled Postoperative Blood Glucose	43	98%	97%	97%
Perioperative Temperature Management	190	100%	100%	100%
Prophylactic Antibiotic Selection	124	98%	99%	99%
Prophylactic Antibiotic Selection (Outpatient)	85	95%	98%	98%
Prophylactic Antibiotic Stopped	121	99%	98%	98%
Prophylactic Antibiotic Timing	124	100%	99%	99%
Prophylactic Antibiotic Timing (Outpatient)	77	97%	98%	98%
Urinary Catheter Removal	75	93%	98%	97%
Survey of Patients' Hospital Experiences				
Area Around Room 'Always' Quiet at Night	300+	57%	61%	61%
Doctors 'Always' Communicated Well	300+	74%	83%	82%
Home Recovery Information Given	300+	80%	86%	85%
Hospital Given 9 or 10 on 10 Point Scale	300+	65%	74%	71%
Meds 'Always' Explained Before Given	300+	60%	64%	64%
Nurses 'Always' Communicated Well	300+	76%	81%	79%
Pain 'Always' Well Controlled	300+	71%	73%	71%
Room and Bathroom 'Always' Clean	300+	77%	76%	73%
Timely Help 'Always' Received	300+	60%	71%	68%
Would Definitely Recommend Hospital	300+	63%	73%	71%
Use of Medical Imaging				
Cardiac Imaging Stress Test before Surgery	193	6.7%	5.4%	5.3%
Combination Abdominal CT Scan	554	27.1%	9.3%	10.5%
Combination Brain/Sinus CT Scan	723	3.3%	2.6%	2.7%
Combination Chest CT Scan	234	25.2%	4.6%	2.7%
Follow-up Mammogram/Ultrasound	618	10.4%	8.4%	8.8%
Lumbar Spine MRI for Low Back Pain[1]	-	-	38.7%	37.2%

NOTE: Hospital profiles are in alphabetical order by state, then city, then hospital within the city; Rankings exclude hospitals with less than 25 cases except for patient surveys which excludes hospitals with less than 100 cases; (a) 100-299 cases; (1) The number of cases/patients is too few to report; (2) Data submitted were based on a sample of cases/patients; (3) Results are based on a shorter time period than required; (4) Data suppressed by CMS for one or more quarters; (5) Results are not available for this reporting period; (6) Fewer than 100 patients completed the HCAHPS survey; (7) No cases met the criteria for this measure; (8) The lower limit of the confidence interval cannot be calculated if the number of observed infections equals zero; (9) No data are available from the state/territory for this reporting period; (10) The scores shown reflect fewer than 50 completed surveys; (11) There were discrepancies in the data collection process; (12) This measure does not apply to this hospital for this reporting period; (13) Results cannot be calculated for this reporting period; (14) The results for this state are combined with nearby states to protect confidentiality; Please refer to the User's Guide for a full explanation of data.

Indiana University Health Blackford Hospital

410 Pilgrim Blvd
Hartford City, IN 47348
Phone: 765-348-0300
Fax: 765-348-0574
URL: www.accesschs.org
Type: Critical Access Hospitals
Emergency Services: Yes
Ownership: Voluntary non-profit - Private
Beds: 15

Key Personnel:
CEO/President. . . . . Dan Evans
Quality Assurance . . . . Nancy Hedden
Infection Control. . . . . Jennifer Horsley
Chief of Medical Staff. . . . . John C. Kohne, MD
Emergency Room . . . . Thomas Lee
Operating Room. . . . . Gail Lewis

Measure	Cases	This Hosp.	State Avg.	U.S. Avg.
Blood Clot Prevention and Treatment				
Anticoagulation Overlap Therapy[5]	-	-	92%	93%
ICU Venous Thromboembolism Prophylaxis[5]	-	-	91%	92%
Incidence of Potentially Preventable VTE[5]	-	-	10%	10%
UFH with Dosages/Platelet Monitoring[5]	-	-	95%	97%
Venous Thromboembolism Prophylaxis[5]	-	-	83%	85%
Warfarin Therapy Discharge Instructions[5]	-	-	71%	75%
Chest Pain/Possible Heart Attack Care				
Aspirin Given Within 24 Hours of Arrival	55	100%	96%	96%
Fibrinolytic Meds Within 30 Min. of Arrival[7]	-	-	48%	58%
Average Time to ECG (minutes)	56	6	6	7
Average Time to Transfer (minutes)[7]	-	-	46	60
Children's Asthma Care				
Received Home Management Plan of Care	-	-	-	88%
Received Reliever Medication	-	-	-	100%
Received Systemic Corticosteroids	-	-	-	100%
Emergency Department				
Admittance Decision Time (minutes)	212	58	80	98
Head CT Results Within 45 Min. of Arrival[1]	-	-	60%	57%
Patients Who Left ER Before Being Seen	10,165	1%	2%	2%
Time from ER Arrival to Admit. (minutes)	223	247	241	274
Time from ER Arrival to Discharge (minutes)	366	116	122	134
Time in ER Before Being Evaluated (minutes)	407	26	22	26
Time to Pain Meds for Fractures (minutes)	43	72	52	57
Heart Attack Care				
Aspirin Given at Discharge[5]	-	-	99%	99%
Fibrinolytic Meds Within 30 Min. of Arrival[5]	-	-	67%	54%
PCI Within 90 Minutes of Arrival[5]	-	-	97%	96%
Statin Prescribed at Discharge[5]	-	-	99%	98%
Heart Failure Care				
ACE Inhibitor or ARB for LVSD[1]	-	-	97%	97%
Discharge Instructions Given[1]	-	-	95%	94%
Evaluation of LVS Function[1]	-	-	99%	99%
Medicare Spending				
Medicare Spending per Patient (ratio)	-	-	1.01	0.98
Pneumonia Care				
Appropriate Initial Antibiotic Given	26	96%	95%	95%
Blood Culture Timing	39	97%	98%	98%
Pregnancy and Delivery Care				
Newborn Deliveries Scheduled Early[5]	-	-	5%	6%
Preventive Care				
Immunization for Influenza	176	100%	91%	90%
Immunization for Pneumonia	268	100%	92%	92%
Stroke Care				
Anticoagulation Therapy for Atrial Fibrillation[5]	-	-	94%	95%
Antithrombotic Therapy Timing[5]	-	-	97%	98%
Assessed for Rehabilitation[5]	-	-	96%	97%
Discharged on Antithrombotic Therapy[5]	-	-	98%	99%
Discharged on Statin Medication[5]	-	-	91%	94%
Thrombolytic Therapy Timing[5]	-	-	54%	66%
Venous Thromboembolism Prophylaxis[5]	-	-	91%	94%
Written Stroke Educational Materials Given[5]	-	-	82%	88%
Surgical Care Improvement Project				
Appropriate Beta Blocker Usage[3,7]	-	-	98%	98%
Appropriate VTP Within 24 Hours[1]	-	-	98%	98%
Controlled Postoperative Blood Glucose[7]	-	-	97%	97%
Perioperative Temperature Management[1,3]	-	-	100%	100%
Prophylactic Antibiotic Selection[1]	-	-	99%	99%
Prophylactic Antibiotic Selection (Outpatient)[5]	-	-	98%	98%
Prophylactic Antibiotic Stopped[1]	-	-	98%	98%
Prophylactic Antibiotic Timing[1]	-	-	99%	99%
Prophylactic Antibiotic Timing (Outpatient)[5]	-	-	98%	98%
Urinary Catheter Removal[1,3]	-	-	98%	97%
Survey of Patients' Hospital Experiences				
Area Around Room 'Always' Quiet at Night[6]	<100	54%	61%	61%
Doctors 'Always' Communicated Well[6]	<100	90%	83%	82%
Home Recovery Information Given[6]	<100	94%	86%	85%
Hospital Given 9 or 10 on 10 Point Scale[6]	<100	79%	74%	71%
Meds 'Always' Explained Before Given[6]	<100	63%	64%	64%
Nurses 'Always' Communicated Well[6]	<100	84%	81%	79%
Pain 'Always' Well Controlled[6]	<100	72%	73%	71%
Room and Bathroom 'Always' Clean[6]	<100	86%	76%	73%
Timely Help 'Always' Received[6]	<100	66%	71%	68%
Would Definitely Recommend Hospital[6]	<100	70%	73%	71%
Use of Medical Imaging				
Cardiac Imaging Stress Test before Surgery[7]	-	-	5.4%	5.3%
Combination Abdominal CT Scan	243	1.6%	9.3%	10.5%
Combination Brain/Sinus CT Scan	329	0.9%	2.6%	2.7%
Combination Chest CT Scan	116	0.9%	4.6%	2.7%
Follow-up Mammogram/Ultrasound	236	9.3%	8.4%	8.8%
Lumbar Spine MRI for Low Back Pain[1]	-	-	38.7%	37.2%

Saint Mary Medical Center

1500 S Lake Park Ave
Hobart, IN 46342
Phone: 219-942-0551
URL: www.comhs.org/stmary
Type: Acute Care Hospitals
Emergency Services: Yes
Ownership: Voluntary non-profit - Private
Beds: 190

Key Personnel:
CEO/President. . . . . Janice Ryba

Measure	Cases	This Hosp.	State Avg.	U.S. Avg.
Blood Clot Prevention and Treatment				
Anticoagulation Overlap Therapy[2]	62	100%	92%	93%
ICU Venous Thromboembolism Prophylaxis[2]	56	98%	91%	92%
Incidence of Potentially Preventable VTE[1,2]	-	-	10%	10%
UFH with Dosages/Platelet Monitoring[2]	30	100%	95%	97%
Venous Thromboembolism Prophylaxis[2]	375	99%	83%	85%
Warfarin Therapy Discharge Instructions[2]	48	100%	71%	75%
Chest Pain/Possible Heart Attack Care				
Aspirin Given Within 24 Hours of Arrival[5]	-	-	96%	96%
Fibrinolytic Meds Within 30 Min. of Arrival[5]	-	-	48%	58%
Average Time to ECG (minutes)[5]	-	-	6	7
Average Time to Transfer (minutes)[5]	-	-	46	60
Children's Asthma Care				
Received Home Management Plan of Care	-	-	-	88%
Received Reliever Medication	-	-	-	100%
Received Systemic Corticosteroids	-	-	-	100%
Emergency Department				
Admittance Decision Time (minutes)[2]	805	166	80	98
Head CT Results Within 45 Min. of Arrival[3,7]	-	-	60%	57%
Patients Who Left ER Before Being Seen	37,699	5%	2%	2%
Time from ER Arrival to Admit. (minutes)[2]	806	364	241	274
Time from ER Arrival to Discharge (minutes)	382	182	122	134
Time in ER Before Being Evaluated (minutes)	416	23	22	26
Time to Pain Meds for Fractures (minutes)	119	66	52	57
Heart Attack Care				
Aspirin Given at Discharge	97	100%	99%	99%
Fibrinolytic Meds Within 30 Min. of Arrival[7]	-	-	67%	54%
PCI Within 90 Minutes of Arrival	24	100%	97%	96%
Statin Prescribed at Discharge	92	100%	99%	98%
Heart Failure Care				
ACE Inhibitor or ARB for LVSD[2]	118	100%	97%	97%
Discharge Instructions Given[2]	240	100%	95%	94%
Evaluation of LVS Function[2]	301	100%	99%	99%
Medicare Spending				
Medicare Spending per Patient (ratio)	-	0.99	1.01	0.98
Pneumonia Care				
Appropriate Initial Antibiotic Given[2]	72	100%	95%	95%
Blood Culture Timing[2]	135	100%	98%	98%
Pregnancy and Delivery Care				
Newborn Deliveries Scheduled Early[2]	28	0%	5%	6%
Preventive Care				
Immunization for Influenza[2]	602	100%	91%	90%
Immunization for Pneumonia[2]	901	98%	92%	92%
Stroke Care				
Anticoagulation Therapy for Atrial Fibrillation[2]	13	100%	94%	95%
Antithrombotic Therapy Timing[2]	99	100%	97%	98%
Assessed for Rehabilitation[2]	111	100%	96%	97%
Discharged on Antithrombotic Therapy[2]	97	100%	98%	99%
Discharged on Statin Medication[2]	67	100%	91%	94%
Thrombolytic Therapy Timing[1,2]	-	-	54%	66%
Venous Thromboembolism Prophylaxis[2]	115	100%	91%	94%
Written Stroke Educational Materials Given[2]	66	94%	82%	88%
Surgical Care Improvement Project				
Appropriate Beta Blocker Usage[2]	174	100%	98%	98%
Appropriate VTP Within 24 Hours[2]	255	100%	98%	98%
Controlled Postoperative Blood Glucose[2]	88	99%	97%	97%
Perioperative Temperature Management[2]	450	100%	100%	100%
Prophylactic Antibiotic Selection[2]	354	100%	99%	99%
Prophylactic Antibiotic Selection (Outpatient)	294	99%	98%	98%
Prophylactic Antibiotic Stopped[2]	344	100%	98%	98%
Prophylactic Antibiotic Timing[2]	355	100%	99%	99%
Prophylactic Antibiotic Timing (Outpatient)	286	100%	98%	98%
Urinary Catheter Removal[2]	172	100%	98%	97%
Survey of Patients' Hospital Experiences				
Area Around Room 'Always' Quiet at Night	300+	57%	61%	61%
Doctors 'Always' Communicated Well	300+	81%	83%	82%
Home Recovery Information Given	300+	86%	86%	85%
Hospital Given 9 or 10 on 10 Point Scale	300+	78%	74%	71%
Meds 'Always' Explained Before Given	300+	64%	64%	64%
Nurses 'Always' Communicated Well	300+	83%	81%	79%
Pain 'Always' Well Controlled	300+	74%	73%	71%
Room and Bathroom 'Always' Clean	300+	77%	76%	73%
Timely Help 'Always' Received	300+	69%	71%	68%
Would Definitely Recommend Hospital	300+	80%	73%	71%
Use of Medical Imaging				
Cardiac Imaging Stress Test before Surgery	244	5.3%	5.4%	5.3%
Combination Abdominal CT Scan	1,141	6.1%	9.3%	10.5%
Combination Brain/Sinus CT Scan	709	3.4%	2.6%	2.7%
Combination Chest CT Scan	818	0.1%	4.6%	2.7%
Follow-up Mammogram/Ultrasound	1,224	7.9%	8.4%	8.8%
Lumbar Spine MRI for Low Back Pain	162	43.8%	38.7%	37.2%

Parkview Huntington Hospital

2001 Stults Rd
Huntington, IN 46750
Phone: 260-355-3000
Fax: 260-355-3346
URL: www.parkview.com
Type: Acute Care Hospitals
Emergency Services: Yes
Ownership: Voluntary non-profit - Private
Beds: 36

Key Personnel:
Chief of Medical Staff. . . . . Jeffrey Brookes
Emergency Room . . . . Mary Johnson, RN
Quality Assurance . . . . Mary Johnson, RN

Measure	Cases	This Hosp.	State Avg.	U.S. Avg.
Blood Clot Prevention and Treatment				
Anticoagulation Overlap Therapy[2]	18	100%	92%	93%
ICU Venous Thromboembolism Prophylaxis[2]	18	78%	91%	92%
Incidence of Potentially Preventable VTE[1,2]	-	-	10%	10%
UFH with Dosages/Platelet Monitoring[1,2]	-	-	95%	97%
Venous Thromboembolism Prophylaxis[2]	160	85%	83%	85%
Warfarin Therapy Discharge Instructions[2]	14	64%	71%	75%
Chest Pain/Possible Heart Attack Care				
Aspirin Given Within 24 Hours of Arrival	54	94%	96%	96%
Fibrinolytic Meds Within 30 Min. of Arrival[7]	-	-	48%	58%
Average Time to ECG (minutes)	52	10	6	7
Average Time to Transfer (minutes)[1]	-	-	46	60
Children's Asthma Care				
Received Home Management Plan of Care	-	-	-	88%
Received Reliever Medication	-	-	-	100%
Received Systemic Corticosteroids	-	-	-	100%
Emergency Department				
Admittance Decision Time (minutes)[2]	274	76	80	98
Head CT Results Within 45 Min. of Arrival[1]	-	-	60%	57%
Patients Who Left ER Before Being Seen	14,790	1%	2%	2%
Time from ER Arrival to Admit. (minutes)[2]	302	249	241	274
Time from ER Arrival to Discharge (minutes)	371	122	122	134

NOTE: Hospital profiles are in alphabetical order by state, then city, then hospital within the city; Rankings exclude hospitals with less than 25 cases except for patient surveys which excludes hospitals with less than 100 cases; (a) 100-299 cases; (1) The number of cases/patients is too few to report; (2) Data submitted were based on a sample of cases/patients; (3) Results are based on a shorter time period than required; (4) Data suppressed by CMS for one or more quarters; (5) Results are not available for this reporting period; (6) Fewer than 100 patients completed the HCAHPS survey; (7) No cases met the criteria for this measure; (8) The lower limit of the confidence interval cannot be calculated if the number of observed infections equals zero; (9) No data are available from the state/territory for this reporting period; (10) The scores shown reflect fewer than 50 completed surveys; (11) There were discrepancies in the data collection process; (12) This measure does not apply to this hospital for this reporting period; (13) Results cannot be calculated for this reporting period; (14) The results for this state are combined with nearby states to protect confidentiality; Please refer to the User's Guide for a full explanation of data.

Measure	Cases	This Hosp.	State Avg.	U.S. Avg.
Time in ER Before Being Evaluated (minutes)	348	40	22	26
Time to Pain Meds for Fractures (minutes)	60	44	52	57
Heart Attack Care				
Aspirin Given at Discharge[1,3]	-	-	99%	99%
Fibrinolytic Meds Within 30 Min. of Arrival[3,7]	-	-	67%	54%
PCI Within 90 Minutes of Arrival[3,7]	-	-	97%	96%
Statin Prescribed at Discharge[1,3]	-	-	99%	98%
Heart Failure Care				
ACE Inhibitor or ARB for LVSD	17	94%	97%	97%
Discharge Instructions Given	46	91%	95%	94%
Evaluation of LVS Function	70	99%	99%	99%
Medicare Spending				
Medicare Spending per Patient (ratio)	-	1.00	1.01	0.98
Pneumonia Care				
Appropriate Initial Antibiotic Given	80	99%	95%	95%
Blood Culture Timing	109	98%	98%	98%
Pregnancy and Delivery Care				
Newborn Deliveries Scheduled Early	17	0%	5%	6%
Preventive Care				
Immunization for Influenza[2]	251	100%	91%	90%
Immunization for Pneumonia[2]	299	98%	92%	92%
Stroke Care				
Anticoagulation Therapy for Atrial Fibrillation[7]	-	-	94%	95%
Antithrombotic Therapy Timing[1]	-	-	97%	98%
Assessed for Rehabilitation	12	100%	96%	97%
Discharged on Antithrombotic Therapy	11	100%	98%	99%
Discharged on Statin Medication	11	73%	91%	94%
Thrombolytic Therapy Timing[7]	-	-	54%	66%
Venous Thromboembolism Prophylaxis	11	82%	91%	94%
Written Stroke Educational Materials Given[1]	-	-	82%	88%
Surgical Care Improvement Project				
Appropriate Beta Blocker Usage	26	100%	98%	98%
Appropriate VTP Within 24 Hours	92	100%	98%	98%
Controlled Postoperative Blood Glucose[7]	-	-	97%	97%
Perioperative Temperature Management	96	100%	100%	100%
Prophylactic Antibiotic Selection	88	100%	99%	99%
Prophylactic Antibiotic Selection (Outpatient)	52	98%	98%	98%
Prophylactic Antibiotic Stopped	87	99%	98%	98%
Prophylactic Antibiotic Timing	88	99%	99%	99%
Prophylactic Antibiotic Timing (Outpatient)	53	98%	98%	98%
Urinary Catheter Removal	85	100%	98%	97%
Survey of Patients' Hospital Experiences				
Area Around Room 'Always' Quiet at Night	300+	64%	61%	61%
Doctors 'Always' Communicated Well	300+	85%	83%	82%
Home Recovery Information Given	300+	91%	86%	85%
Hospital Given 9 or 10 on 10 Point Scale	300+	78%	74%	71%
Meds 'Always' Explained Before Given	300+	67%	64%	64%
Nurses 'Always' Communicated Well	300+	84%	81%	79%
Pain 'Always' Well Controlled	300+	77%	73%	71%
Room and Bathroom 'Always' Clean	300+	75%	76%	73%
Timely Help 'Always' Received	300+	75%	71%	68%
Would Definitely Recommend Hospital	300+	78%	73%	71%
Use of Medical Imaging				
Cardiac Imaging Stress Test before Surgery	57	1.8%	5.4%	5.3%
Combination Abdominal CT Scan	163	6.1%	9.3%	10.5%
Combination Brain/Sinus CT Scan	229	0.4%	2.6%	2.7%
Combination Chest CT Scan	110	0.0%	4.6%	2.7%
Follow-up Mammogram/Ultrasound	326	12.6%	8.4%	8.8%
Lumbar Spine MRI for Low Back Pain	38	44.7%	38.7%	37.2%

Community Hospital East

1500 N Ritter Ave
Indianapolis, IN 46219
Phone: 317-355-5411
Fax: 317-351-7726
URL: www.ecommunity.com
Type: Acute Care Hospitals
Emergency Services: Yes
Ownership: Voluntary non-profit - Private
Beds: 1,025

Key Personnel:
Quality Assurance . . . . Ruth Adams
Infection Control. . . . . Robert Baker, MD
Chief of Medical Staff . . . . Clif Knight, MD
CEO/President. . . . . Bryan A Mills
Radiology. . . . . Michael Mullinix, MD
Pediatric Ambulatory Care . . . . . . Jerrald Smith
Pediatric In-Patient Care . . . . Jerrald Smith

Measure	Cases	This Hosp.	State Avg.	U.S. Avg.
Blood Clot Prevention and Treatment				
Anticoagulation Overlap Therapy[2]	74	91%	92%	93%
ICU Venous Thromboembolism Prophylaxis[2]	27	93%	91%	92%
Incidence of Potentially Preventable VTE[1,2]	-	-	10%	10%
UFH with Dosages/Platelet Monitoring[1,2]	-	-	95%	97%
Venous Thromboembolism Prophylaxis[2]	255	78%	83%	85%
Warfarin Therapy Discharge Instructions[2]	60	12%	71%	75%
Chest Pain/Possible Heart Attack Care				
Aspirin Given Within 24 Hours of Arrival	24	88%	96%	96%
Fibrinolytic Meds Within 30 Min. of Arrival[3,7]	-	-	48%	58%
Average Time to ECG (minutes)	27	5	6	7
Average Time to Transfer (minutes)[1,3]	-	-	46	60
Children's Asthma Care				
Received Home Management Plan of Care	-	-	-	88%
Received Reliever Medication	-	-	-	100%
Received Systemic Corticosteroids	-	-	-	100%
Emergency Department				
Admittance Decision Time (minutes)[2]	679	180	80	98
Head CT Results Within 45 Min. of Arrival[1,3]	-	-	60%	57%
Patients Who Left ER Before Being Seen	67,445	4%	2%	2%
Time from ER Arrival to Admit. (minutes)[2]	700	308	241	274
Time from ER Arrival to Discharge (minutes)	397	147	122	134
Time in ER Before Being Evaluated (minutes)	294	26	22	26
Time to Pain Meds for Fractures (minutes)	168	60	52	57
Heart Attack Care				
Aspirin Given at Discharge	159	99%	99%	99%
Fibrinolytic Meds Within 30 Min. of Arrival[7]	-	-	67%	54%
PCI Within 90 Minutes of Arrival	46	100%	97%	96%
Statin Prescribed at Discharge	158	98%	99%	98%
Heart Failure Care				
ACE Inhibitor or ARB for LVSD	108	100%	97%	97%
Discharge Instructions Given	256	96%	95%	94%
Evaluation of LVS Function	328	99%	99%	99%
Medicare Spending				
Medicare Spending per Patient (ratio)	-	1.01	1.01	0.98
Pneumonia Care				
Appropriate Initial Antibiotic Given[2]	124	95%	95%	95%
Blood Culture Timing[2]	164	99%	98%	98%
Pregnancy and Delivery Care				
Newborn Deliveries Scheduled Early[2]	29	17%	5%	6%
Preventive Care				
Immunization for Influenza[2]	896	66%	91%	90%
Immunization for Pneumonia[2]	840	73%	92%	92%
Stroke Care				
Anticoagulation Therapy for Atrial Fibrillation	19	68%	94%	95%
Antithrombotic Therapy Timing	136	93%	97%	98%
Assessed for Rehabilitation	166	92%	96%	97%
Discharged on Antithrombotic Therapy	139	97%	98%	99%
Discharged on Statin Medication	110	76%	91%	94%
Thrombolytic Therapy Timing	20	40%	54%	66%
Venous Thromboembolism Prophylaxis	179	77%	91%	94%
Written Stroke Educational Materials Given	78	78%	82%	88%
Surgical Care Improvement Project				
Appropriate Beta Blocker Usage[2]	95	95%	98%	98%
Appropriate VTP Within 24 Hours[2]	340	94%	98%	98%
Controlled Postoperative Blood Glucose[2,7]	-	-	97%	97%
Perioperative Temperature Management[2]	356	100%	100%	100%
Prophylactic Antibiotic Selection[2]	243	99%	99%	99%
Prophylactic Antibiotic Selection (Outpatient)	249	98%	98%	98%
Prophylactic Antibiotic Stopped[2]	243	100%	98%	98%
Prophylactic Antibiotic Timing[2]	244	95%	99%	99%
Prophylactic Antibiotic Timing (Outpatient)	250	99%	98%	98%
Urinary Catheter Removal[2]	107	94%	98%	97%
Survey of Patients' Hospital Experiences				
Area Around Room 'Always' Quiet at Night	300+	55%	61%	61%
Doctors 'Always' Communicated Well	300+	75%	83%	82%
Home Recovery Information Given	300+	82%	86%	85%
Hospital Given 9 or 10 on 10 Point Scale	300+	69%	74%	71%
Meds 'Always' Explained Before Given	300+	59%	64%	64%
Nurses 'Always' Communicated Well	300+	75%	81%	79%
Pain 'Always' Well Controlled	300+	71%	73%	71%
Room and Bathroom 'Always' Clean	300+	73%	76%	73%
Timely Help 'Always' Received	300+	67%	71%	68%
Would Definitely Recommend Hospital	300+	69%	73%	71%
Use of Medical Imaging				
Cardiac Imaging Stress Test before Surgery	317	4.1%	5.4%	5.3%
Combination Abdominal CT Scan	1,063	9.1%	9.3%	10.5%
Combination Brain/Sinus CT Scan	867	3.1%	2.6%	2.7%
Combination Chest CT Scan	529	7.8%	4.6%	2.7%
Follow-up Mammogram/Ultrasound	1,663	13.0%	8.4%	8.8%
Lumbar Spine MRI for Low Back Pain	277	39.0%	38.7%	37.2%

Community Hospital North

7150 Clearvista Dr
Indianapolis, IN 46256
Phone: 317-621-5335
Fax: 317-621-3627
URL: www.ecommunity.com/north
Type: Acute Care Hospitals
Emergency Services: Yes
Ownership: Voluntary non-profit - Private
Beds: 282

Key Personnel:
CEO/President. . . . . William Corley
Chief of Medical Staff . . . . Mark Dixon
Radiology. . . . . Jeff Jackson

Measure	Cases	This Hosp.	State Avg.	U.S. Avg.
Blood Clot Prevention and Treatment				
Anticoagulation Overlap Therapy[2]	93	82%	92%	93%
ICU Venous Thromboembolism Prophylaxis[2]	32	75%	91%	92%
Incidence of Potentially Preventable VTE[2]	14	36%	10%	10%
UFH with Dosages/Platelet Monitoring[2]	21	100%	95%	97%
Venous Thromboembolism Prophylaxis[2]	390	77%	83%	85%
Warfarin Therapy Discharge Instructions[2]	68	22%	71%	75%
Chest Pain/Possible Heart Attack Care				
Aspirin Given Within 24 Hours of Arrival	109	87%	96%	96%
Fibrinolytic Meds Within 30 Min. of Arrival[7]	-	-	48%	58%
Average Time to ECG (minutes)	111	13	6	7
Average Time to Transfer (minutes)	14	41	46	60
Children's Asthma Care				
Received Home Management Plan of Care	-	-	-	88%
Received Reliever Medication	-	-	-	100%
Received Systemic Corticosteroids	-	-	-	100%
Emergency Department				
Admittance Decision Time (minutes)[2,7]	-	-	80	98
Head CT Results Within 45 Min. of Arrival[1]	-	-	60%	57%
Patients Who Left ER Before Being Seen	52,254	1%	2%	2%
Time from ER Arrival to Admit. (minutes)[2,7]	-	-	241	274
Time from ER Arrival to Discharge (minutes)[7]	-	-	122	134
Time in ER Before Being Evaluated (minutes)	409	19	22	26
Time to Pain Meds for Fractures (minutes)	253	52	52	57
Heart Attack Care				
Aspirin Given at Discharge	13	85%	99%	99%
Fibrinolytic Meds Within 30 Min. of Arrival[7]	-	-	67%	54%
PCI Within 90 Minutes of Arrival[7]	-	-	97%	96%
Statin Prescribed at Discharge	11	91%	99%	98%
Heart Failure Care				
ACE Inhibitor or ARB for LVSD	33	91%	97%	97%
Discharge Instructions Given	113	92%	95%	94%
Evaluation of LVS Function	172	100%	99%	99%
Medicare Spending				
Medicare Spending per Patient (ratio)	-	1.02	1.01	0.98
Pneumonia Care				
Appropriate Initial Antibiotic Given[2]	96	97%	95%	95%
Blood Culture Timing[2]	171	99%	98%	98%
Pregnancy and Delivery Care				
Newborn Deliveries Scheduled Early[2]	72	4%	5%	6%
Preventive Care				
Immunization for Influenza[2]	505	64%	91%	90%
Immunization for Pneumonia[2]	511	70%	92%	92%
Stroke Care				
Anticoagulation Therapy for Atrial Fibrillation	41	93%	94%	95%
Antithrombotic Therapy Timing	181	95%	97%	98%
Assessed for Rehabilitation	209	95%	96%	97%
Discharged on Antithrombotic Therapy	193	99%	98%	99%
Discharged on Statin Medication	162	91%	91%	94%
Thrombolytic Therapy Timing	20	55%	54%	66%
Venous Thromboembolism Prophylaxis	209	79%	91%	94%

NOTE: Hospital profiles are in alphabetical order by state, then city, then hospital within the city; Rankings exclude hospitals with less than 25 cases except for patient surveys which excludes hospitals with less than 100 cases; (a) 100-299 cases; (1) The number of cases/patients is too few to report; (2) Data submitted were based on a sample of cases/patients; (3) Results are based on a shorter time period than required; (4) Data suppressed by CMS for one or more quarters; (5) Results are not available for this reporting period; (6) Fewer than 100 patients completed the HCAHPS survey; (7) No cases met the criteria for this measure; (8) The lower limit of the confidence interval cannot be calculated if the number of observed infections equals zero; (9) No data are available from the state/territory for this reporting period; (10) The scores shown reflect fewer than 50 completed surveys; (11) There were discrepancies in the data collection process; (12) This measure does not apply to this hospital for this reporting period; (13) Results cannot be calculated for this reporting period; (14) The results for this state are combined with nearby states to protect confidentiality; Please refer to the User's Guide for a full explanation of data.

Measure	Cases	This Hosp.	State Avg.	U.S. Avg.
Written Stroke Educational Materials Given	116	85%	82%	88%
Surgical Care Improvement Project				
Appropriate Beta Blocker Usage[2]	140	99%	98%	98%
Appropriate VTP Within 24 Hours[2]	473	99%	98%	98%
Controlled Postoperative Blood Glucose[2,7]	-	-	97%	97%
Perioperative Temperature Management[2]	509	100%	100%	100%
Prophylactic Antibiotic Selection[2]	349	99%	99%	99%
Prophylactic Antibiotic Selection (Outpatient)	439	98%	98%	98%
Prophylactic Antibiotic Stopped[2]	346	99%	98%	98%
Prophylactic Antibiotic Timing[2]	349	98%	99%	99%
Prophylactic Antibiotic Timing (Outpatient)	440	98%	98%	98%
Urinary Catheter Removal[2]	117	91%	98%	97%
Survey of Patients' Hospital Experiences				
Area Around Room 'Always' Quiet at Night	300+	59%	61%	61%
Doctors 'Always' Communicated Well	300+	77%	83%	82%
Home Recovery Information Given	300+	86%	86%	85%
Hospital Given 9 or 10 on 10 Point Scale	300+	78%	74%	71%
Meds 'Always' Explained Before Given	300+	61%	64%	64%
Nurses 'Always' Communicated Well	300+	76%	81%	79%
Pain 'Always' Well Controlled	300+	71%	73%	71%
Room and Bathroom 'Always' Clean	300+	76%	76%	73%
Timely Help 'Always' Received	300+	56%	71%	68%
Would Definitely Recommend Hospital	300+	80%	73%	71%
Use of Medical Imaging				
Cardiac Imaging Stress Test before Surgery[1]	-	-	5.4%	5.3%
Combination Abdominal CT Scan	1,111	11.0%	9.3%	10.5%
Combination Brain/Sinus CT Scan	917	2.9%	2.6%	2.7%
Combination Chest CT Scan	722	9.3%	4.6%	2.7%
Follow-up Mammogram/Ultrasound	1,789	14.0%	8.4%	8.8%
Lumbar Spine MRI for Low Back Pain	286	36.0%	38.7%	37.2%

Community Hospital South

1402 E County Line Rd S
Indianapolis, IN 46227
URL: www.ecommunity.com/south
Type: Acute Care Hospitals
Ownership: Voluntary non-profit - Private
Phone: 317-887-7112
Fax: 317-887-4670
Emergency Services: Yes

Key Personnel:
Radiology. . . . . Thomas Belt
Quality Assurance . . . . Cleo Burgard
CEO/President. . . . . William Corley
Pediatric Ambulatory Care . . . . . . Sue Sandberg
Coronary Care . . . . Kerry Sawin
Operating Room. . . . . Mark Walke
Infection Control. . . . . Gayle Walsh
Chief of Medical Staff . . . . Carolyn Waymire

Measure	Cases	This Hosp.	State Avg.	U.S. Avg.
Blood Clot Prevention and Treatment				
Anticoagulation Overlap Therapy[2]	50	86%	92%	93%
ICU Venous Thromboembolism Prophylaxis[2]	46	74%	91%	92%
Incidence of Potentially Preventable VTE[1,2]	-	-	10%	10%
UFH with Dosages/Platelet Monitoring[2]	12	100%	95%	97%
Venous Thromboembolism Prophylaxis[2]	326	80%	83%	85%
Warfarin Therapy Discharge Instructions[2]	28	18%	71%	75%
Chest Pain/Possible Heart Attack Care				
Aspirin Given Within 24 Hours of Arrival[1]	-	-	96%	96%
Fibrinolytic Meds Within 30 Min. of Arrival[3,7]	-	-	48%	58%
Average Time to ECG (minutes)[1]	-	-	6	7
Average Time to Transfer (minutes)[1,3]	-	-	46	60
Children's Asthma Care				
Received Home Management Plan of Care	-	-	-	88%
Received Reliever Medication	-	-	-	100%
Received Systemic Corticosteroids	-	-	-	100%
Emergency Department				
Admittance Decision Time (minutes)[2]	589	110	80	98
Head CT Results Within 45 Min. of Arrival[1]	-	-	60%	57%
Patients Who Left ER Before Being Seen	41,425	2%	2%	2%
Time from ER Arrival to Admit. (minutes)[2]	609	263	241	274
Time from ER Arrival to Discharge (minutes)	406	144	122	134
Time in ER Before Being Evaluated (minutes)	283	21	22	26
Time to Pain Meds for Fractures (minutes)	161	55	52	57
Heart Attack Care				
Aspirin Given at Discharge	170	100%	99%	99%
Fibrinolytic Meds Within 30 Min. of Arrival[7]	-	-	67%	54%
PCI Within 90 Minutes of Arrival	49	94%	97%	96%
Statin Prescribed at Discharge	161	99%	99%	98%
Heart Failure Care				
ACE Inhibitor or ARB for LVSD	70	100%	97%	97%
Discharge Instructions Given	175	98%	95%	94%
Evaluation of LVS Function	252	100%	99%	99%
Medicare Spending				
Medicare Spending per Patient (ratio)	-	1.02	1.01	0.98
Pneumonia Care				
Appropriate Initial Antibiotic Given[2]	91	88%	95%	95%
Blood Culture Timing[2]	153	98%	98%	98%
Pregnancy and Delivery Care				
Newborn Deliveries Scheduled Early[2]	25	4%	5%	6%
Preventive Care				
Immunization for Influenza[2]	566	72%	91%	90%
Immunization for Pneumonia[2]	647	81%	92%	92%
Stroke Care				
Anticoagulation Therapy for Atrial Fibrillation	12	83%	94%	95%
Antithrombotic Therapy Timing	66	95%	97%	98%
Assessed for Rehabilitation	91	100%	96%	97%
Discharged on Antithrombotic Therapy	75	97%	98%	99%
Discharged on Statin Medication	65	89%	91%	94%
Thrombolytic Therapy Timing	11	64%	54%	66%
Venous Thromboembolism Prophylaxis	92	91%	91%	94%
Written Stroke Educational Materials Given	41	98%	82%	88%
Surgical Care Improvement Project				
Appropriate Beta Blocker Usage[2]	156	97%	98%	98%
Appropriate VTP Within 24 Hours[2]	399	98%	98%	98%
Controlled Postoperative Blood Glucose[2,7]	-	-	97%	97%
Perioperative Temperature Management[2]	445	100%	100%	100%
Prophylactic Antibiotic Selection[2]	317	98%	99%	99%
Prophylactic Antibiotic Selection (Outpatient)	372	98%	98%	98%
Prophylactic Antibiotic Stopped[2]	314	99%	98%	98%
Prophylactic Antibiotic Timing[2]	317	94%	99%	99%
Prophylactic Antibiotic Timing (Outpatient)	379	94%	98%	98%
Urinary Catheter Removal[2]	125	97%	98%	97%
Survey of Patients' Hospital Experiences				
Area Around Room 'Always' Quiet at Night	300+	65%	61%	61%
Doctors 'Always' Communicated Well	300+	78%	83%	82%
Home Recovery Information Given	300+	85%	86%	85%
Hospital Given 9 or 10 on 10 Point Scale	300+	76%	74%	71%
Meds 'Always' Explained Before Given	300+	60%	64%	64%
Nurses 'Always' Communicated Well	300+	79%	81%	79%
Pain 'Always' Well Controlled	300+	69%	73%	71%
Room and Bathroom 'Always' Clean	300+	74%	76%	73%
Timely Help 'Always' Received	300+	65%	71%	68%
Would Definitely Recommend Hospital	300+	75%	73%	71%
Use of Medical Imaging				
Cardiac Imaging Stress Test before Surgery	341	3.8%	5.4%	5.3%
Combination Abdominal CT Scan	651	2.8%	9.3%	10.5%
Combination Brain/Sinus CT Scan	611	2.8%	2.6%	2.7%
Combination Chest CT Scan	391	1.0%	4.6%	2.7%
Follow-up Mammogram/Ultrasound	1,743	9.8%	8.4%	8.8%
Lumbar Spine MRI for Low Back Pain	80	32.5%	38.7%	37.2%

Community Westview Hospital

3630 Guion Rd
Indianapolis, IN 46222
E-mail: info@westviewhospital.org
URL: www.westviewhospital.org
Type: Acute Care Hospitals
Ownership: Voluntary non-profit - Private
Phone: 317-920-7288
Fax: 317-920-7551
Emergency Services: Yes
Beds: 116

Key Personnel:
Quality Assurance . . . . Michele Borten
CEO/President. . . . . Jerry Porter

Measure	Cases	This Hosp.	State Avg.	U.S. Avg.
Blood Clot Prevention and Treatment				
Anticoagulation Overlap Therapy[2]	17	94%	92%	93%
ICU Venous Thromboembolism Prophylaxis[2]	39	95%	91%	92%
Incidence of Potentially Preventable VTE[1,2]	-	-	10%	10%
UFH with Dosages/Platelet Monitoring[1,2]	-	-	95%	97%
Venous Thromboembolism Prophylaxis[2]	115	95%	83%	85%
Warfarin Therapy Discharge Instructions[2]	15	73%	71%	75%
Chest Pain/Possible Heart Attack Care				
Aspirin Given Within 24 Hours of Arrival	12	100%	96%	96%
Fibrinolytic Meds Within 30 Min. of Arrival[7]	-	-	48%	58%
Average Time to ECG (minutes)	14	6	6	7
Average Time to Transfer (minutes)[1]	-	-	46	60
Children's Asthma Care				
Received Home Management Plan of Care	-	-	-	88%
Received Reliever Medication	-	-	-	100%
Received Systemic Corticosteroids	-	-	-	100%
Emergency Department				
Admittance Decision Time (minutes)[2]	469	100	80	98
Head CT Results Within 45 Min. of Arrival[1]	-	-	60%	57%
Patients Who Left ER Before Being Seen	8,793	0%	2%	2%
Time from ER Arrival to Admit. (minutes)[2]	505	247	241	274
Time from ER Arrival to Discharge (minutes)	432	104	122	134
Time in ER Before Being Evaluated (minutes)	453	27	22	26
Time to Pain Meds for Fractures (minutes)	20	47	52	57
Heart Attack Care				
Aspirin Given at Discharge[1,3]	-	-	99%	99%
Fibrinolytic Meds Within 30 Min. of Arrival[3,7]	-	-	67%	54%
PCI Within 90 Minutes of Arrival[3,7]	-	-	97%	96%
Statin Prescribed at Discharge[1,3]	-	-	99%	98%
Heart Failure Care				
ACE Inhibitor or ARB for LVSD[1,2]	-	-	97%	97%
Discharge Instructions Given[2]	48	85%	95%	94%
Evaluation of LVS Function[2]	56	100%	99%	99%
Medicare Spending				
Medicare Spending per Patient (ratio)	-	1.03	1.01	0.98
Pneumonia Care				
Appropriate Initial Antibiotic Given[2]	20	100%	95%	95%
Blood Culture Timing[2]	35	97%	98%	98%
Pregnancy and Delivery Care				
Newborn Deliveries Scheduled Early[7]	-	-	5%	6%
Preventive Care				
Immunization for Influenza[2]	347	100%	91%	90%
Immunization for Pneumonia[2]	578	99%	92%	92%
Stroke Care				
Anticoagulation Therapy for Atrial Fibrillation[7]	-	-	94%	95%
Antithrombotic Therapy Timing[1]	-	-	97%	98%
Assessed for Rehabilitation[1]	-	-	96%	97%
Discharged on Antithrombotic Therapy[1]	-	-	98%	99%
Discharged on Statin Medication[1]	-	-	91%	94%
Thrombolytic Therapy Timing[7]	-	-	54%	66%
Venous Thromboembolism Prophylaxis[1]	-	-	91%	94%
Written Stroke Educational Materials Given[1]	-	-	82%	88%
Surgical Care Improvement Project				
Appropriate Beta Blocker Usage	35	100%	98%	98%
Appropriate VTP Within 24 Hours	82	100%	98%	98%
Controlled Postoperative Blood Glucose[7]	-	-	97%	97%
Perioperative Temperature Management	102	100%	100%	100%
Prophylactic Antibiotic Selection	81	100%	99%	99%
Prophylactic Antibiotic Selection (Outpatient)	68	99%	98%	98%
Prophylactic Antibiotic Stopped	74	100%	98%	98%
Prophylactic Antibiotic Timing	81	100%	99%	99%
Prophylactic Antibiotic Timing (Outpatient)	68	97%	98%	98%
Urinary Catheter Removal	60	100%	98%	97%
Survey of Patients' Hospital Experiences				
Area Around Room 'Always' Quiet at Night	(a)	53%	61%	61%
Doctors 'Always' Communicated Well	(a)	82%	83%	82%
Home Recovery Information Given	(a)	85%	86%	85%
Hospital Given 9 or 10 on 10 Point Scale	(a)	66%	74%	71%
Meds 'Always' Explained Before Given	(a)	59%	64%	64%
Nurses 'Always' Communicated Well	(a)	72%	81%	79%
Pain 'Always' Well Controlled	(a)	70%	73%	71%
Room and Bathroom 'Always' Clean	(a)	64%	76%	73%
Timely Help 'Always' Received	(a)	59%	71%	68%
Would Definitely Recommend Hospital	(a)	64%	73%	71%
Use of Medical Imaging				
Cardiac Imaging Stress Test before Surgery	83	7.2%	5.4%	5.3%
Combination Abdominal CT Scan	189	0.5%	9.3%	10.5%
Combination Brain/Sinus CT Scan[1]	-	-	2.6%	2.7%
Combination Chest CT Scan	53	0.0%	4.6%	2.7%

NOTE: Hospital profiles are in alphabetical order by state, then city, then hospital within the city; Rankings exclude hospitals with less than 25 cases except for patient surveys which excludes hospitals with less than 100 cases; (a) 100-299 cases; (1) The number of cases/patients is too few to report; (2) Data submitted were based on a sample of cases/patients; (3) Results are based on a shorter time period than required; (4) Data suppressed by CMS for one or more quarters; (5) Results are not available for this reporting period; (6) Fewer than 100 patients completed the HCAHPS survey; (7) No cases met the criteria for this measure; (8) The lower limit of the confidence interval cannot be calculated if the number of observed infections equals zero; (9) No data are available from the state/territory for this reporting period; (10) The scores shown reflect fewer than 50 completed surveys; (11) There were discrepancies in the data collection process; (12) This measure does not apply to this hospital for this reporting period; (13) Results cannot be calculated for this reporting period; (14) The results for this state are combined with nearby states to protect confidentiality; Please refer to the User's Guide for a full explanation of data.

Measure	Cases	This Hosp.	State Avg.	U.S. Avg.
Follow-up Mammogram/Ultrasound	286	7.0%	8.4%	8.8%
Lumbar Spine MRI for Low Back Pain[1]	-	-	38.7%	37.2%

Eskenazi Health

720 Eskenazi Avenue
Indianapolis, IN 46254
URL: www.wishard.edu
Type: Acute Care Hospitals
Ownership: Government - Local
Phone: 317-880-4818
Fax: 317-630-7678
Emergency Services: Yes
Beds: 354

Key Personnel:
CEO/President . . . . Lisa E Harris, MD
Chair/CEO . . . . James D. Miner, MD

Measure	Cases	This Hosp.	State Avg.	U.S. Avg.
Blood Clot Prevention and Treatment				
Anticoagulation Overlap Therapy[2]	39	100%	92%	93%
ICU Venous Thromboembolism Prophylaxis[2]	48	98%	91%	92%
Incidence of Potentially Preventable VTE[2]	14	0%	10%	10%
UFH with Dosages/Platelet Monitoring[2]	21	100%	95%	97%
Venous Thromboembolism Prophylaxis[2]	302	94%	83%	85%
Warfarin Therapy Discharge Instructions[2]	34	100%	71%	75%
Chest Pain/Possible Heart Attack Care				
Aspirin Given Within 24 Hours of Arrival[5]	-	-	96%	96%
Fibrinolytic Meds Within 30 Min. of Arrival[5]	-	-	48%	58%
Average Time to ECG (minutes)[5]	-	-	6	7
Average Time to Transfer (minutes)[5]	-	-	46	60
Children's Asthma Care				
Received Home Management Plan of Care	-	-	-	88%
Received Reliever Medication	-	-	-	100%
Received Systemic Corticosteroids	-	-	-	100%
Emergency Department				
Admittance Decision Time (minutes)[2]	382	249	80	98
Head CT Results Within 45 Min. of Arrival[1,3]	-	-	60%	57%
Patients Who Left ER Before Being Seen	>100k	2%	2%	2%
Time from ER Arrival to Admit. (minutes)[2]	392	498	241	274
Time from ER Arrival to Discharge (minutes)	364	185	122	134
Time in ER Before Being Evaluated (minutes)	370	52	22	26
Time to Pain Meds for Fractures (minutes)	95	75	52	57
Heart Attack Care				
Aspirin Given at Discharge	244	100%	99%	99%
Fibrinolytic Meds Within 30 Min. of Arrival[7]	-	-	67%	54%
PCI Within 90 Minutes of Arrival	11	100%	97%	96%
Statin Prescribed at Discharge	242	100%	99%	98%
Heart Failure Care				
ACE Inhibitor or ARB for LVSD	185	98%	97%	97%
Discharge Instructions Given	362	100%	95%	94%
Evaluation of LVS Function	400	100%	99%	99%
Medicare Spending				
Medicare Spending per Patient (ratio)	-	0.96	1.01	0.98
Pneumonia Care				
Appropriate Initial Antibiotic Given[2]	65	98%	95%	95%
Blood Culture Timing[2]	114	98%	98%	98%
Pregnancy and Delivery Care				
Newborn Deliveries Scheduled Early[2]	35	0%	5%	6%
Preventive Care				
Immunization for Influenza[2]	495	49%	91%	90%
Immunization for Pneumonia[2]	535	56%	92%	92%
Stroke Care				
Anticoagulation Therapy for Atrial Fibrillation[1,2]	-	-	94%	95%
Antithrombotic Therapy Timing[2]	80	95%	97%	98%
Assessed for Rehabilitation[2]	107	87%	96%	97%
Discharged on Antithrombotic Therapy[2]	95	100%	98%	99%
Discharged on Statin Medication[2]	79	94%	91%	94%
Thrombolytic Therapy Timing[2]	43	16%	54%	66%
Venous Thromboembolism Prophylaxis[2]	97	76%	91%	94%
Written Stroke Educational Materials Given[2]	86	1%	82%	88%
Surgical Care Improvement Project				
Appropriate Beta Blocker Usage[2]	58	100%	98%	98%
Appropriate VTP Within 24 Hours[2]	277	97%	98%	98%
Controlled Postoperative Blood Glucose[2,7]	-	-	97%	97%
Perioperative Temperature Management[2]	334	100%	100%	100%
Prophylactic Antibiotic Selection[2]	238	100%	99%	99%
Prophylactic Antibiotic Selection (Outpatient)	66	100%	98%	98%
Prophylactic Antibiotic Stopped[2]	237	98%	98%	98%
Prophylactic Antibiotic Timing[2]	238	99%	99%	99%
Prophylactic Antibiotic Timing (Outpatient)	66	100%	98%	98%
Urinary Catheter Removal[2]	199	99%	98%	97%
Survey of Patients' Hospital Experiences				
Area Around Room 'Always' Quiet at Night	300+	62%	61%	61%
Doctors 'Always' Communicated Well	300+	80%	83%	82%
Home Recovery Information Given	300+	83%	86%	85%
Hospital Given 9 or 10 on 10 Point Scale	300+	72%	74%	71%
Meds 'Always' Explained Before Given	300+	68%	64%	64%
Nurses 'Always' Communicated Well	300+	76%	81%	79%
Pain 'Always' Well Controlled	300+	71%	73%	71%
Room and Bathroom 'Always' Clean	300+	69%	76%	73%
Timely Help 'Always' Received	300+	62%	71%	68%
Would Definitely Recommend Hospital	300+	76%	73%	71%
Use of Medical Imaging				
Cardiac Imaging Stress Test before Surgery	347	4.0%	5.4%	5.3%
Combination Abdominal CT Scan	754	5.6%	9.3%	10.5%
Combination Brain/Sinus CT Scan	508	5.1%	2.6%	2.7%
Combination Chest CT Scan	552	2.9%	4.6%	2.7%
Follow-up Mammogram/Ultrasound	1,427	6.5%	8.4%	8.8%
Lumbar Spine MRI for Low Back Pain	138	34.8%	38.7%	37.2%

Fairbanks

8102 Clearvista Parkway
Indianapolis, IN 46256
Type: Acute Care Hospitals
Ownership: Voluntary non-profit - Private
Phone: 317-849-8222
Emergency Services: No

Measure	Cases	This Hosp.	State Avg.	U.S. Avg.
Blood Clot Prevention and Treatment				
Anticoagulation Overlap Therapy[2,7]	-	-	92%	93%
ICU Venous Thromboembolism Prophylaxis[2,7]	-	-	91%	92%
Incidence of Potentially Preventable VTE[2,7]	-	-	10%	10%
UFH with Dosages/Platelet Monitoring[2,7]	-	-	95%	97%
Venous Thromboembolism Prophylaxis[1,2]	-	-	83%	85%
Warfarin Therapy Discharge Instructions[2,7]	-	-	71%	75%
Chest Pain/Possible Heart Attack Care				
Aspirin Given Within 24 Hours of Arrival[5]	-	-	96%	96%
Fibrinolytic Meds Within 30 Min. of Arrival[5]	-	-	48%	58%
Average Time to ECG (minutes)[5]	-	-	6	7
Average Time to Transfer (minutes)[5]	-	-	46	60
Children's Asthma Care				
Received Home Management Plan of Care	-	-	-	88%
Received Reliever Medication	-	-	-	100%
Received Systemic Corticosteroids	-	-	-	100%
Emergency Department				
Admittance Decision Time (minutes)[2,7]	-	-	80	98
Head CT Results Within 45 Min. of Arrival[5]	-	-	60%	57%
Patients Who Left ER Before Being Seen[5]	-	-	2%	2%
Time from ER Arrival to Admit. (minutes)[2,7]	-	-	241	274
Time from ER Arrival to Discharge (minutes)[5]	-	-	122	134
Time in ER Before Being Evaluated (minutes)[5]	-	-	22	26
Time to Pain Meds for Fractures (minutes)[5]	-	-	52	57
Heart Attack Care				
Aspirin Given at Discharge[5]	-	-	99%	99%
Fibrinolytic Meds Within 30 Min. of Arrival[5]	-	-	67%	54%
PCI Within 90 Minutes of Arrival[5]	-	-	97%	96%
Statin Prescribed at Discharge[5]	-	-	99%	98%
Heart Failure Care				
ACE Inhibitor or ARB for LVSD[5]	-	-	97%	97%
Discharge Instructions Given[5]	-	-	95%	94%
Evaluation of LVS Function[5]	-	-	99%	99%
Medicare Spending				
Medicare Spending per Patient (ratio)	-	0.85	1.01	0.98
Pneumonia Care				
Appropriate Initial Antibiotic Given[5]	-	-	95%	95%
Blood Culture Timing[5]	-	-	98%	98%
Pregnancy and Delivery Care				
Newborn Deliveries Scheduled Early[7]	-	-	5%	6%
Preventive Care				
Immunization for Influenza[2]	288	98%	91%	90%
Immunization for Pneumonia[2]	40	38%	92%	92%
Stroke Care				
Anticoagulation Therapy for Atrial Fibrillation[5]	-	-	94%	95%
Antithrombotic Therapy Timing[5]	-	-	97%	98%
Assessed for Rehabilitation[5]	-	-	96%	97%
Discharged on Antithrombotic Therapy[5]	-	-	98%	99%
Discharged on Statin Medication[5]	-	-	91%	94%
Thrombolytic Therapy Timing[5]	-	-	54%	66%
Venous Thromboembolism Prophylaxis[5]	-	-	91%	94%
Written Stroke Educational Materials Given[5]	-	-	82%	88%
Surgical Care Improvement Project				
Appropriate Beta Blocker Usage[5]	-	-	98%	98%
Appropriate VTP Within 24 Hours[5]	-	-	98%	98%
Controlled Postoperative Blood Glucose[5]	-	-	97%	97%
Perioperative Temperature Management[5]	-	-	100%	100%
Prophylactic Antibiotic Selection[5]	-	-	99%	99%
Prophylactic Antibiotic Selection (Outpatient)[5]	-	-	98%	98%
Prophylactic Antibiotic Stopped[5]	-	-	98%	98%
Prophylactic Antibiotic Timing[5]	-	-	99%	99%
Prophylactic Antibiotic Timing (Outpatient)[5]	-	-	98%	98%
Urinary Catheter Removal[5]	-	-	98%	97%
Survey of Patients' Hospital Experiences				
Area Around Room 'Always' Quiet at Night[1]	-	-	61%	61%
Doctors 'Always' Communicated Well[1]	-	-	83%	82%
Home Recovery Information Given[1]	-	-	86%	85%
Hospital Given 9 or 10 on 10 Point Scale[1]	-	-	74%	71%
Meds 'Always' Explained Before Given[1]	-	-	64%	64%
Nurses 'Always' Communicated Well[1]	-	-	81%	79%
Pain 'Always' Well Controlled[1]	-	-	73%	71%
Room and Bathroom 'Always' Clean[1]	-	-	76%	73%
Timely Help 'Always' Received[1]	-	-	71%	68%
Would Definitely Recommend Hospital[1]	-	-	73%	71%
Use of Medical Imaging				
Cardiac Imaging Stress Test before Surgery[7]	-	-	5.4%	5.3%
Combination Abdominal CT Scan[7]	-	-	9.3%	10.5%
Combination Brain/Sinus CT Scan[7]	-	-	2.6%	2.7%
Combination Chest CT Scan[7]	-	-	4.6%	2.7%
Follow-up Mammogram/Ultrasound[7]	-	-	8.4%	8.8%
Lumbar Spine MRI for Low Back Pain[7]	-	-	38.7%	37.2%

Franciscan Saint Francis Health - Indianapolis

8111 S Emerson Ave
Indianapolis, IN 46237
URL: www.stfrancishospitals.org
Type: Acute Care Hospitals
Ownership: Voluntary non-profit - Church
Phone: 317-865-5001
Fax: 317-783-8152
Emergency Services: Yes

Key Personnel:
CEO/President . . . . Robert Brody
Chief of Medical Staff . . . . Alan Gillespie

Measure	Cases	This Hosp.	State Avg.	U.S. Avg.
Blood Clot Prevention and Treatment				
Anticoagulation Overlap Therapy[2]	107	94%	92%	93%
ICU Venous Thromboembolism Prophylaxis[2]	112	96%	91%	92%
Incidence of Potentially Preventable VTE[2]	15	7%	10%	10%
UFH with Dosages/Platelet Monitoring[2]	60	100%	95%	97%
Venous Thromboembolism Prophylaxis[2]	496	94%	83%	85%
Warfarin Therapy Discharge Instructions[2]	85	81%	71%	75%
Chest Pain/Possible Heart Attack Care				
Aspirin Given Within 24 Hours of Arrival[1,3]	-	-	96%	96%
Fibrinolytic Meds Within 30 Min. of Arrival[3,7]	-	-	48%	58%
Average Time to ECG (minutes)[1,3]	-	-	6	7
Average Time to Transfer (minutes)[3,7]	-	-	46	60
Children's Asthma Care				
Received Home Management Plan of Care	-	-	-	88%
Received Reliever Medication	-	-	-	100%
Received Systemic Corticosteroids	-	-	-	100%
Emergency Department				
Admittance Decision Time (minutes)[2]	601	281	80	98
Head CT Results Within 45 Min. of Arrival[1]	-	-	60%	57%
Patients Who Left ER Before Being Seen	83,211	1%	2%	2%
Time from ER Arrival to Admit. (minutes)[2]	613	348	241	274
Time from ER Arrival to Discharge (minutes)	423	148	122	134
Time in ER Before Being Evaluated (minutes)	445	23	22	26
Time to Pain Meds for Fractures (minutes)	182	38	52	57
Heart Attack Care				

NOTE: Hospital profiles are in alphabetical order by state, then city, then hospital within the city; Rankings exclude hospitals with less than 25 cases except for patient surveys which excludes hospitals with less than 100 cases; (a) 100-299 cases; (1) The number of cases/patients is too few to report; (2) Data submitted were based on a sample of cases/patients; (3) Results are based on a shorter time period than required; (4) Data suppressed by CMS for one or more quarters; (5) Results are not available for this reporting period; (6) Fewer than 100 patients completed the HCAHPS survey; (7) No cases met the criteria for this measure; (8) The lower limit of the confidence interval cannot be calculated if the number of observed infections equals zero; (9) No data are available from the state/territory for this reporting period; (10) The scores shown reflect fewer than 50 completed surveys; (11) There were discrepancies in the data collection process; (12) This measure does not apply to this hospital for this reporting period; (13) Results cannot be calculated for this reporting period; (14) The results for this state are combined with nearby states to protect confidentiality; Please refer to the User's Guide for a full explanation of data.

Measure	Cases	This Hosp.	State Avg.	U.S. Avg.
Aspirin Given at Discharge	417	100%	99%	99%
Fibrinolytic Meds Within 30 Min. of Arrival[7]	-	-	67%	54%
PCI Within 90 Minutes of Arrival	86	100%	97%	96%
Statin Prescribed at Discharge	406	100%	99%	98%
Heart Failure Care				
ACE Inhibitor or ARB for LVSD	101	100%	97%	97%
Discharge Instructions Given	344	98%	95%	94%
Evaluation of LVS Function	455	100%	99%	99%
Medicare Spending				
Medicare Spending per Patient (ratio)	-	1.04	1.01	0.98
Pneumonia Care				
Appropriate Initial Antibiotic Given	349	93%	95%	95%
Blood Culture Timing	780	98%	98%	98%
Pregnancy and Delivery Care				
Newborn Deliveries Scheduled Early[2]	108	3%	5%	6%
Preventive Care				
Immunization for Influenza[2]	596	98%	91%	90%
Immunization for Pneumonia[2]	823	99%	92%	92%
Stroke Care				
Anticoagulation Therapy for Atrial Fibrillation	35	100%	94%	95%
Antithrombotic Therapy Timing	199	99%	97%	98%
Assessed for Rehabilitation	239	98%	96%	97%
Discharged on Antithrombotic Therapy	212	99%	98%	99%
Discharged on Statin Medication	168	95%	91%	94%
Thrombolytic Therapy Timing[1]	-	-	54%	66%
Venous Thromboembolism Prophylaxis	221	96%	91%	94%
Written Stroke Educational Materials Given	121	87%	82%	88%
Surgical Care Improvement Project				
Appropriate Beta Blocker Usage	668	99%	98%	98%
Appropriate VTP Within 24 Hours	1,035	99%	98%	98%
Controlled Postoperative Blood Glucose	354	98%	97%	97%
Perioperative Temperature Management	1,196	99%	100%	100%
Prophylactic Antibiotic Selection	939	100%	99%	99%
Prophylactic Antibiotic Selection (Outpatient)	832	99%	98%	98%
Prophylactic Antibiotic Stopped	893	99%	98%	98%
Prophylactic Antibiotic Timing	940	100%	99%	99%
Prophylactic Antibiotic Timing (Outpatient)	834	99%	98%	98%
Urinary Catheter Removal	757	99%	98%	97%
Survey of Patients' Hospital Experiences				
Area Around Room 'Always' Quiet at Night	300+	53%	61%	61%
Doctors 'Always' Communicated Well	300+	80%	83%	82%
Home Recovery Information Given	300+	84%	86%	85%
Hospital Given 9 or 10 on 10 Point Scale	300+	76%	74%	71%
Meds 'Always' Explained Before Given	300+	59%	64%	64%
Nurses 'Always' Communicated Well	300+	81%	81%	79%
Pain 'Always' Well Controlled	300+	73%	73%	71%
Room and Bathroom 'Always' Clean	300+	71%	76%	73%
Timely Help 'Always' Received	300+	70%	71%	68%
Would Definitely Recommend Hospital	300+	81%	73%	71%
Use of Medical Imaging				
Cardiac Imaging Stress Test before Surgery	1,411	5.2%	5.4%	5.3%
Combination Abdominal CT Scan	1,817	5.3%	9.3%	10.5%
Combination Brain/Sinus CT Scan	1,309	1.5%	2.6%	2.7%
Combination Chest CT Scan	1,325	2.2%	4.6%	2.7%
Follow-up Mammogram/Ultrasound	3,019	7.8%	8.4%	8.8%
Lumbar Spine MRI for Low Back Pain	303	38.6%	38.7%	37.2%

The Indiana Heart Hospital

8075 N Shadeland Ave
Indianapolis, IN 46250
URL: www.hearthospital.com
Type: Acute Care Hospitals
Ownership: Voluntary non-profit - Other
Phone: 317-621-8063
Fax: 317-621-8111
Emergency Services: Yes
Beds: 72

Key Personnel:
CEO/President. . . . . Thomas A Malasto

Measure	Cases	This Hosp.	State Avg.	U.S. Avg.
Blood Clot Prevention and Treatment				
Anticoagulation Overlap Therapy[2]	12	83%	92%	93%
ICU Venous Thromboembolism Prophylaxis[2]	165	74%	91%	92%
Incidence of Potentially Preventable VTE[1,2]	-	-	10%	10%
UFH with Dosages/Platelet Monitoring[1,2]	-	-	95%	97%
Venous Thromboembolism Prophylaxis[2]	212	55%	83%	85%
Warfarin Therapy Discharge Instructions[1,2]	-	-	71%	75%
Chest Pain/Possible Heart Attack Care				
Aspirin Given Within 24 Hours of Arrival	29	86%	96%	96%
Fibrinolytic Meds Within 30 Min. of Arrival[5]	-	-	48%	58%
Average Time to ECG (minutes)	31	3	6	7
Average Time to Transfer (minutes)[5]	-	-	46	60
Children's Asthma Care				
Received Home Management Plan of Care	-	-	-	88%
Received Reliever Medication	-	-	-	100%
Received Systemic Corticosteroids	-	-	-	100%
Emergency Department				
Admittance Decision Time (minutes)[2]	179	48	80	98
Head CT Results Within 45 Min. of Arrival[1]	-	-	60%	57%
Patients Who Left ER Before Being Seen	4,832	0%	2%	2%
Time from ER Arrival to Admit. (minutes)[2]	184	149	241	274
Time from ER Arrival to Discharge (minutes)	341	149	122	134
Time in ER Before Being Evaluated (minutes)	275	11	22	26
Time to Pain Meds for Fractures (minutes)[5]	-	-	52	57
Heart Attack Care				
Aspirin Given at Discharge	264	99%	99%	99%
Fibrinolytic Meds Within 30 Min. of Arrival[7]	-	-	67%	54%
PCI Within 90 Minutes of Arrival	54	100%	97%	96%
Statin Prescribed at Discharge	250	99%	99%	98%
Heart Failure Care				
ACE Inhibitor or ARB for LVSD	94	100%	97%	97%
Discharge Instructions Given	205	96%	95%	94%
Evaluation of LVS Function	269	100%	99%	99%
Medicare Spending				
Medicare Spending per Patient (ratio)	-	1.02	1.01	0.98
Pneumonia Care				
Appropriate Initial Antibiotic Given[1]	-	-	95%	95%
Blood Culture Timing[1]	-	-	98%	98%
Pregnancy and Delivery Care				
Newborn Deliveries Scheduled Early[7]	-	-	5%	6%
Preventive Care				
Immunization for Influenza[2]	317	66%	91%	90%
Immunization for Pneumonia[2]	523	70%	92%	92%
Stroke Care				
Anticoagulation Therapy for Atrial Fibrillation[7]	-	-	94%	95%
Antithrombotic Therapy Timing[1]	-	-	97%	98%
Assessed for Rehabilitation[1]	-	-	96%	97%
Discharged on Antithrombotic Therapy[1]	-	-	98%	99%
Discharged on Statin Medication[1]	-	-	91%	94%
Thrombolytic Therapy Timing[7]	-	-	54%	66%
Venous Thromboembolism Prophylaxis[1]	-	-	91%	94%
Written Stroke Educational Materials Given[1]	-	-	82%	88%
Surgical Care Improvement Project				
Appropriate Beta Blocker Usage[2]	266	98%	98%	98%
Appropriate VTP Within 24 Hours[1,2]	-	-	98%	98%
Controlled Postoperative Blood Glucose[2]	244	94%	97%	97%
Perioperative Temperature Management[2]	200	98%	100%	100%
Prophylactic Antibiotic Selection[2]	338	100%	99%	99%
Prophylactic Antibiotic Selection (Outpatient)	393	100%	98%	98%
Prophylactic Antibiotic Stopped[2]	323	99%	98%	98%
Prophylactic Antibiotic Timing[2]	339	100%	99%	99%
Prophylactic Antibiotic Timing (Outpatient)	396	97%	98%	98%
Urinary Catheter Removal[2]	370	99%	98%	97%
Survey of Patients' Hospital Experiences				
Area Around Room 'Always' Quiet at Night	300+	69%	61%	61%
Doctors 'Always' Communicated Well	300+	83%	83%	82%
Home Recovery Information Given	300+	87%	86%	85%
Hospital Given 9 or 10 on 10 Point Scale	300+	84%	74%	71%
Meds 'Always' Explained Before Given	300+	71%	64%	64%
Nurses 'Always' Communicated Well	300+	85%	81%	79%
Pain 'Always' Well Controlled	300+	77%	73%	71%
Room and Bathroom 'Always' Clean	300+	80%	76%	73%
Timely Help 'Always' Received	300+	75%	71%	68%
Would Definitely Recommend Hospital	300+	86%	73%	71%
Use of Medical Imaging				
Cardiac Imaging Stress Test before Surgery	1,115	4.6%	5.4%	5.3%
Combination Abdominal CT Scan[1]	-	-	9.3%	10.5%
Combination Brain/Sinus CT Scan[1]	-	-	2.6%	2.7%
Combination Chest CT Scan[1]	-	-	4.6%	2.7%
Follow-up Mammogram/Ultrasound[7]	-	-	8.4%	8.8%
Lumbar Spine MRI for Low Back Pain[7]	-	-	38.7%	37.2%

Indiana Orthopaedic Hospital

8400 Northwest Blvd
Indianapolis, IN 46278
URL: www.indianaorthopaedichospital.com
Type: Acute Care Hospitals
Ownership: Physician
Phone: 317-956-1000
Emergency Services: No

Measure	Cases	This Hosp.	State Avg.	U.S. Avg.
Blood Clot Prevention and Treatment				
Anticoagulation Overlap Therapy[1,2]	-	-	92%	93%
ICU Venous Thromboembolism Prophylaxis[2,7]	-	-	91%	92%
Incidence of Potentially Preventable VTE[2,7]	-	-	10%	10%
UFH with Dosages/Platelet Monitoring[2,7]	-	-	95%	97%
Venous Thromboembolism Prophylaxis[2]	77	95%	83%	85%
Warfarin Therapy Discharge Instructions[1,2]	-	-	71%	75%
Chest Pain/Possible Heart Attack Care				
Aspirin Given Within 24 Hours of Arrival[5]	-	-	96%	96%
Fibrinolytic Meds Within 30 Min. of Arrival[5]	-	-	48%	58%
Average Time to ECG (minutes)[5]	-	-	6	7
Average Time to Transfer (minutes)[5]	-	-	46	60
Children's Asthma Care				
Received Home Management Plan of Care	-	-	-	88%
Received Reliever Medication	-	-	-	100%
Received Systemic Corticosteroids	-	-	-	100%
Emergency Department				
Admittance Decision Time (minutes)[2,7]	-	-	80	98
Head CT Results Within 45 Min. of Arrival[5]	-	-	60%	57%
Patients Who Left ER Before Being Seen[5]	-	-	2%	2%
Time from ER Arrival to Admit. (minutes)[2,7]	-	-	241	274
Time from ER Arrival to Discharge (minutes)[5]	-	-	122	134
Time in ER Before Being Evaluated (minutes)[5]	-	-	22	26
Time to Pain Meds for Fractures (minutes)[5]	-	-	52	57
Heart Attack Care				
Aspirin Given at Discharge[5]	-	-	99%	99%
Fibrinolytic Meds Within 30 Min. of Arrival[5]	-	-	67%	54%
PCI Within 90 Minutes of Arrival[5]	-	-	97%	96%
Statin Prescribed at Discharge[5]	-	-	99%	98%
Heart Failure Care				
ACE Inhibitor or ARB for LVSD[5]	-	-	97%	97%
Discharge Instructions Given[5]	-	-	95%	94%
Evaluation of LVS Function[5]	-	-	99%	99%
Medicare Spending				
Medicare Spending per Patient (ratio)	-	0.91	1.01	0.98
Pneumonia Care				
Appropriate Initial Antibiotic Given[5]	-	-	95%	95%
Blood Culture Timing[5]	-	-	98%	98%
Pregnancy and Delivery Care				
Newborn Deliveries Scheduled Early[7]	-	-	5%	6%
Preventive Care				
Immunization for Influenza[2]	318	49%	91%	90%
Immunization for Pneumonia[2]	367	60%	92%	92%
Stroke Care				
Anticoagulation Therapy for Atrial Fibrillation[5]	-	-	94%	95%
Antithrombotic Therapy Timing[5]	-	-	97%	98%
Assessed for Rehabilitation[5]	-	-	96%	97%
Discharged on Antithrombotic Therapy[5]	-	-	98%	99%
Discharged on Statin Medication[5]	-	-	91%	94%
Thrombolytic Therapy Timing[5]	-	-	54%	66%
Venous Thromboembolism Prophylaxis[5]	-	-	91%	94%
Written Stroke Educational Materials Given[5]	-	-	82%	88%
Surgical Care Improvement Project				
Appropriate Beta Blocker Usage[2]	122	98%	98%	98%
Appropriate VTP Within 24 Hours[2]	246	99%	98%	98%
Controlled Postoperative Blood Glucose[2,7]	-	-	97%	97%
Perioperative Temperature Management[2]	265	100%	100%	100%
Prophylactic Antibiotic Selection[2]	211	100%	99%	99%
Prophylactic Antibiotic Selection (Outpatient)	529	100%	98%	98%
Prophylactic Antibiotic Stopped[2]	210	100%	98%	98%
Prophylactic Antibiotic Timing[2]	211	100%	99%	99%
Prophylactic Antibiotic Timing (Outpatient)	529	100%	98%	98%

NOTE: Hospital profiles are in alphabetical order by state, then city, then hospital within the city; Rankings exclude hospitals with less than 25 cases except for patient surveys which excludes hospitals with less than 100 cases; (a) 100-299 cases; (1) The number of cases/patients is too few to report; (2) Data submitted were based on a sample of cases/patients; (3) Results are based on a shorter time period than required; (4) Data suppressed by CMS for one or more quarters; (5) Results are not available for this reporting period; (6) Fewer than 100 patients completed the HCAHPS survey; (7) No cases met the criteria for this measure; (8) The lower limit of the confidence interval cannot be calculated if the number of observed infections equals zero; (9) No data are available from the state/territory for this reporting period; (10) The scores shown reflect fewer than 50 completed surveys; (11) There were discrepancies in the data collection process; (12) This measure does not apply to this hospital for this reporting period; (13) Results cannot be calculated for this reporting period; (14) The results for this state are combined with nearby states to protect confidentiality; Please refer to the User's Guide for a full explanation of data.

Measure	Cases	This Hosp.	State Avg.	U.S. Avg.
Urinary Catheter Removal[2]	50	98%	98%	97%
Survey of Patients' Hospital Experiences				
Area Around Room 'Always' Quiet at Night	300+	81%	61%	61%
Doctors 'Always' Communicated Well	300+	87%	83%	82%
Home Recovery Information Given	300+	93%	86%	85%
Hospital Given 9 or 10 on 10 Point Scale	300+	90%	74%	71%
Meds 'Always' Explained Before Given	300+	77%	64%	64%
Nurses 'Always' Communicated Well	300+	91%	81%	79%
Pain 'Always' Well Controlled	300+	80%	73%	71%
Room and Bathroom 'Always' Clean	300+	89%	76%	73%
Timely Help 'Always' Received	300+	84%	71%	68%
Would Definitely Recommend Hospital	300+	92%	73%	71%
Use of Medical Imaging				
Cardiac Imaging Stress Test before Surgery[7]	-	-	5.4%	5.3%
Combination Abdominal CT Scan[1]	-	-	9.3%	10.5%
Combination Brain/Sinus CT Scan[1]	-	-	2.6%	2.7%
Combination Chest CT Scan[1]	-	-	4.6%	2.7%
Follow-up Mammogram/Ultrasound[7]	-	-	8.4%	8.8%
Lumbar Spine MRI for Low Back Pain	295	36.6%	38.7%	37.2%

Indiana University Health

1701 N Senate Blvd
Indianapolis, IN 46202
URL: www.iuhealth.org
Type: Acute Care Hospitals
Ownership: Voluntary non-profit - Private

Phone: 317-962-5900
Fax: 317-962-1867
Emergency Services: Yes
Beds: 1,120

Measure	Cases	This Hosp.	State Avg.	U.S. Avg.
Blood Clot Prevention and Treatment				
Anticoagulation Overlap Therapy[2]	226	98%	92%	93%
ICU Venous Thromboembolism Prophylaxis[2]	73	86%	91%	92%
Incidence of Potentially Preventable VTE[2]	85	5%	10%	10%
UFH with Dosages/Platelet Monitoring[2]	135	100%	95%	97%
Venous Thromboembolism Prophylaxis[2]	352	82%	83%	85%
Warfarin Therapy Discharge Instructions[2]	169	38%	71%	75%
Chest Pain/Possible Heart Attack Care				
Aspirin Given Within 24 Hours of Arrival[5]	-	-	96%	96%
Fibrinolytic Meds Within 30 Min. of Arrival[5]	-	-	48%	58%
Average Time to ECG (minutes)[5]	-	-	6	7
Average Time to Transfer (minutes)[5]	-	-	46	60
Children's Asthma Care				
Received Home Management Plan of Care	-	-	-	88%
Received Reliever Medication	-	-	-	100%
Received Systemic Corticosteroids	-	-	-	100%
Emergency Department				
Admittance Decision Time (minutes)[2]	382	154	80	98
Head CT Results Within 45 Min. of Arrival[1]	-	-	60%	57%
Patients Who Left ER Before Being Seen	>100k	1%	2%	2%
Time from ER Arrival to Admit. (minutes)[2]	386	318	241	274
Time from ER Arrival to Discharge (minutes)	373	168	122	134
Time in ER Before Being Evaluated (minutes)	374	28	22	26
Time to Pain Meds for Fractures (minutes)	182	68	52	57
Heart Attack Care				
Aspirin Given at Discharge	610	100%	99%	99%
Fibrinolytic Meds Within 30 Min. of Arrival[7]	-	-	67%	54%
PCI Within 90 Minutes of Arrival	109	98%	97%	96%
Statin Prescribed at Discharge	625	100%	99%	98%
Heart Failure Care				
ACE Inhibitor or ARB for LVSD[2]	208	99%	97%	97%
Discharge Instructions Given[2]	584	95%	95%	94%
Evaluation of LVS Function[2]	722	100%	99%	99%
Medicare Spending				
Medicare Spending per Patient (ratio)	-	1.01	1.01	0.98
Pneumonia Care				
Appropriate Initial Antibiotic Given[2]	58	98%	95%	95%
Blood Culture Timing[2]	139	98%	98%	98%
Pregnancy and Delivery Care				
Newborn Deliveries Scheduled Early	206	2%	5%	6%
Preventive Care				
Immunization for Influenza[2]	515	91%	91%	90%
Immunization for Pneumonia[2]	502	88%	92%	92%
Stroke Care				
Anticoagulation Therapy for Atrial Fibrillation[2]	12	100%	94%	95%
Antithrombotic Therapy Timing[2]	65	97%	97%	98%
Assessed for Rehabilitation[2]	105	95%	96%	97%
Discharged on Antithrombotic Therapy[2]	74	100%	98%	99%
Discharged on Statin Medication[2]	60	98%	91%	94%
Thrombolytic Therapy Timing[1,2]	-	-	54%	66%
Venous Thromboembolism Prophylaxis[2]	113	96%	91%	94%
Written Stroke Educational Materials Given[2]	52	85%	82%	88%
Surgical Care Improvement Project				
Appropriate Beta Blocker Usage[2]	339	99%	98%	98%
Appropriate VTP Within 24 Hours[2]	709	99%	98%	98%
Controlled Postoperative Blood Glucose[2]	139	92%	97%	97%
Perioperative Temperature Management[2]	935	100%	100%	100%
Prophylactic Antibiotic Selection[2]	688	99%	99%	99%
Prophylactic Antibiotic Selection (Outpatient)	771	93%	98%	98%
Prophylactic Antibiotic Stopped[2]	667	98%	98%	98%
Prophylactic Antibiotic Timing[2]	692	100%	99%	99%
Prophylactic Antibiotic Timing (Outpatient)	653	99%	98%	98%
Urinary Catheter Removal[2]	702	98%	98%	97%
Survey of Patients' Hospital Experiences				
Area Around Room 'Always' Quiet at Night	300+	56%	61%	61%
Doctors 'Always' Communicated Well	300+	80%	83%	82%
Home Recovery Information Given	300+	87%	86%	85%
Hospital Given 9 or 10 on 10 Point Scale	300+	74%	74%	71%
Meds 'Always' Explained Before Given	300+	64%	64%	64%
Nurses 'Always' Communicated Well	300+	78%	81%	79%
Pain 'Always' Well Controlled	300+	70%	73%	71%
Room and Bathroom 'Always' Clean	300+	70%	76%	73%
Timely Help 'Always' Received	300+	60%	71%	68%
Would Definitely Recommend Hospital	300+	78%	73%	71%
Use of Medical Imaging				
Cardiac Imaging Stress Test before Surgery	1,083	5.9%	5.4%	5.3%
Combination Abdominal CT Scan	4,148	4.3%	9.3%	10.5%
Combination Brain/Sinus CT Scan	1,374	2.7%	2.6%	2.7%
Combination Chest CT Scan	3,296	0.1%	4.6%	2.7%
Follow-up Mammogram/Ultrasound	2,375	7.3%	8.4%	8.8%
Lumbar Spine MRI for Low Back Pain	313	35.8%	38.7%	37.2%

Indianapolis VA Medical Center

1481 W. Tenth Street
Indianapolis, IN 46202
URL: www.indianapolis.va.gov
Type: Acute Care - VA
Ownership: Government Federal

Phone: 317-554-0000
Fax: 317-988-2701
Emergency Services: No
Beds: 170

Key Personnel:
Patient Relations . . . . Ann Barrett
Chief of Medical Staff . . . . Chowdry-Mujahid Bashir, MD
Operating Room. . . . . Delores Cikrit, MD
CEO/President. . . . . Thomas Mattice
Anesthesiology. . . . . SS Moorthy, MD
Quality Assurance . . . . Mary Ann Payne
Ambulatory Care . . . . Peter Woodbridge, MD

Measure	Cases	This Hosp.	State Avg.	U.S. Avg.
Blood Clot Prevention and Treatment				
Anticoagulation Overlap Therapy	-	-	92%	93%
ICU Venous Thromboembolism Prophylaxis	-	-	91%	92%
Incidence of Potentially Preventable VTE	-	-	10%	10%
UFH with Dosages/Platelet Monitoring	-	-	95%	97%
Venous Thromboembolism Prophylaxis	-	-	83%	85%
Warfarin Therapy Discharge Instructions	-	-	71%	75%
Chest Pain/Possible Heart Attack Care				
Aspirin Given Within 24 Hours of Arrival	-	-	96%	96%
Fibrinolytic Meds Within 30 Min. of Arrival	-	-	48%	58%
Average Time to ECG (minutes)	-	-	6	7
Average Time to Transfer (minutes)	-	-	46	60
Children's Asthma Care				
Received Home Management Plan of Care	-	-	-	88%
Received Reliever Medication	-	-	-	100%
Received Systemic Corticosteroids	-	-	-	100%
Emergency Department				
Admittance Decision Time (minutes)	-	-	80	98
Head CT Results Within 45 Min. of Arrival	-	-	60%	57%
Patients Who Left ER Before Being Seen	-	-	2%	2%
Time from ER Arrival to Admit. (minutes)	-	-	241	274
Time from ER Arrival to Discharge (minutes)	-	-	122	134
Time in ER Before Being Evaluated (minutes)	-	-	22	26
Time to Pain Meds for Fractures (minutes)	-	-	52	57
Heart Attack Care				
Aspirin Given at Discharge	125	99%	99%	99%
Fibrinolytic Meds Within 30 Min. of Arrival[5]	-	-	67%	54%
PCI Within 90 Minutes of Arrival[1]	19	95%	97%	96%
Statin Prescribed at Discharge	119	100%	99%	98%
Heart Failure Care				
ACE Inhibitor or ARB for LVSD	103	98%	97%	97%
Discharge Instructions Given	232	100%	95%	94%
Evaluation of LVS Function	246	100%	99%	99%
Medicare Spending				
Medicare Spending per Patient (ratio)	-	-	1.01	0.98
Pneumonia Care				
Appropriate Initial Antibiotic Given	100	95%	95%	95%
Blood Culture Timing	185	98%	98%	98%
Pregnancy and Delivery Care				
Newborn Deliveries Scheduled Early	-	-	5%	6%
Preventive Care				
Immunization for Influenza[5]	-	-	91%	90%
Immunization for Pneumonia[5]	-	-	92%	92%
Stroke Care				
Anticoagulation Therapy for Atrial Fibrillation	-	-	94%	95%
Antithrombotic Therapy Timing	-	-	97%	98%
Assessed for Rehabilitation	-	-	96%	97%
Discharged on Antithrombotic Therapy	-	-	98%	99%
Discharged on Statin Medication	-	-	91%	94%
Thrombolytic Therapy Timing	-	-	54%	66%
Venous Thromboembolism Prophylaxis	-	-	91%	94%
Written Stroke Educational Materials Given	-	-	82%	88%
Surgical Care Improvement Project				
Appropriate Beta Blocker Usage[2]	272	99%	98%	98%
Appropriate VTP Within 24 Hours[2]	376	98%	98%	98%
Controlled Postoperative Blood Glucose[2]	71	97%	97%	97%
Perioperative Temperature Management[2]	572	100%	100%	100%
Prophylactic Antibiotic Selection	428	99%	99%	99%
Prophylactic Antibiotic Selection (Outpatient)	-	-	98%	98%
Prophylactic Antibiotic Stopped	420	99%	98%	98%
Prophylactic Antibiotic Timing	428	99%	99%	99%
Prophylactic Antibiotic Timing (Outpatient)	-	-	98%	98%
Urinary Catheter Removal[2]	413	98%	98%	97%
Survey of Patients' Hospital Experiences				
Area Around Room 'Always' Quiet at Night	-	-	61%	61%
Doctors 'Always' Communicated Well	-	-	83%	82%
Home Recovery Information Given	-	-	86%	85%
Hospital Given 9 or 10 on 10 Point Scale	-	-	74%	71%
Meds 'Always' Explained Before Given	-	-	64%	64%
Nurses 'Always' Communicated Well	-	-	81%	79%
Pain 'Always' Well Controlled	-	-	73%	71%
Room and Bathroom 'Always' Clean	-	-	76%	73%
Timely Help 'Always' Received	-	-	71%	68%
Would Definitely Recommend Hospital	-	-	73%	71%
Use of Medical Imaging				
Cardiac Imaging Stress Test before Surgery	-	-	5.4%	5.3%
Combination Abdominal CT Scan	-	-	9.3%	10.5%
Combination Brain/Sinus CT Scan	-	-	2.6%	2.7%
Combination Chest CT Scan	-	-	4.6%	2.7%
Follow-up Mammogram/Ultrasound	-	-	8.4%	8.8%
Lumbar Spine MRI for Low Back Pain	-	-	38.7%	37.2%

Saint Vincent Heart Center of Indiana

10580 N Meridian St
Indianapolis, IN 46290
E-mail: marketing@theheathcenter.com
URL: www.theheartcenter.com
Type: Acute Care Hospitals
Ownership: Proprietary

Phone: 317-583-5000
Fax: 317-583-5002
Emergency Services: Yes
Beds: 80

Key Personnel:
Cardiac Laboratory. . . . . Gregg Elsener
CEO/President. . . . . John Stewart
Chief of Medical Staff . . . . William Store

Measure	Cases	This Hosp.	State Avg.	U.S. Avg.
Blood Clot Prevention and Treatment				

NOTE: Hospital profiles are in alphabetical order by state, then city, then hospital within the city; Rankings exclude hospitals with less than 25 cases except for patient surveys which excludes hospitals with less than 100 cases; (a) 100-299 cases; (1) The number of cases/patients is too few to report; (2) Data submitted were based on a sample of cases/patients; (3) Results are based on a shorter time period than required; (4) Data suppressed by CMS for one or more quarters; (5) Results are not available for this reporting period; (6) Fewer than 100 patients completed the HCAHPS survey; (7) No cases met the criteria for this measure; (8) The lower limit of the confidence interval cannot be calculated if the number of observed infections equals zero; (9) No data are available from the state/territory for this reporting period; (10) The scores shown reflect fewer than 50 completed surveys; (11) There were discrepancies in the data collection process; (12) This measure does not apply to this hospital for this reporting period; (13) Results cannot be calculated for this reporting period; (14) The results for this state are combined with nearby states to protect confidentiality; Please refer to the User's Guide for a full explanation of data.

Measure	Cases	This Hosp.	State Avg.	U.S. Avg.
Anticoagulation Overlap Therapy[1,2]	-	-	92%	93%
ICU Venous Thromboembolism Prophylaxis[2]	93	81%	91%	92%
Incidence of Potentially Preventable VTE[1,2]	-	-	10%	10%
UFH with Dosages/Platelet Monitoring[1,2]	-	-	95%	97%
Venous Thromboembolism Prophylaxis[2]	359	76%	83%	85%
Warfarin Therapy Discharge Instructions[1,2]	-	-	71%	75%
Chest Pain/Possible Heart Attack Care				
Aspirin Given Within 24 Hours of Arrival	13	77%	96%	96%
Fibrinolytic Meds Within 30 Min. of Arrival[5]	-	-	48%	58%
Average Time to ECG (minutes)	18	6	6	7
Average Time to Transfer (minutes)[5]	-	-	46	60
Children's Asthma Care				
Received Home Management Plan of Care	-	-	-	88%
Received Reliever Medication	-	-	-	100%
Received Systemic Corticosteroids	-	-	-	100%
Emergency Department				
Admittance Decision Time (minutes)[2]	74	150	80	98
Head CT Results Within 45 Min. of Arrival[1]	-	-	60%	57%
Patients Who Left ER Before Being Seen	3,021	0%	2%	2%
Time from ER Arrival to Admit. (minutes)[2]	93	236	241	274
Time from ER Arrival to Discharge (minutes)	124	192	122	134
Time in ER Before Being Evaluated (minutes)	259	10	22	26
Time to Pain Meds for Fractures (minutes)[3,7]	-	-	52	57
Heart Attack Care				
Aspirin Given at Discharge	955	100%	99%	99%
Fibrinolytic Meds Within 30 Min. of Arrival[7]	-	-	67%	54%
PCI Within 90 Minutes of Arrival	21	95%	97%	96%
Statin Prescribed at Discharge	936	100%	99%	98%
Heart Failure Care				
ACE Inhibitor or ARB for LVSD	112	100%	97%	97%
Discharge Instructions Given	268	98%	95%	94%
Evaluation of LVS Function	316	96%	99%	99%
Medicare Spending				
Medicare Spending per Patient (ratio)	-	0.99	1.01	0.98
Pneumonia Care				
Appropriate Initial Antibiotic Given[1]	-	-	95%	95%
Blood Culture Timing[1]	-	-	98%	98%
Pregnancy and Delivery Care				
Newborn Deliveries Scheduled Early[7]	-	-	5%	6%
Preventive Care				
Immunization for Influenza[2]	534	87%	91%	90%
Immunization for Pneumonia[2]	874	80%	92%	92%
Stroke Care				
Anticoagulation Therapy for Atrial Fibrillation[1]	-	-	94%	95%
Antithrombotic Therapy Timing[1]	-	-	97%	98%
Assessed for Rehabilitation[1]	-	-	96%	97%
Discharged on Antithrombotic Therapy[1]	-	-	98%	99%
Discharged on Statin Medication[1]	-	-	91%	94%
Thrombolytic Therapy Timing[7]	-	-	54%	66%
Venous Thromboembolism Prophylaxis[1]	-	-	91%	94%
Written Stroke Educational Materials Given[1]	-	-	82%	88%
Surgical Care Improvement Project				
Appropriate Beta Blocker Usage	424	99%	98%	98%
Appropriate VTP Within 24 Hours[7]	-	-	98%	98%
Controlled Postoperative Blood Glucose	764	98%	97%	97%
Perioperative Temperature Management	65	98%	100%	100%
Prophylactic Antibiotic Selection	721	100%	99%	99%
Prophylactic Antibiotic Selection (Outpatient)	411	100%	98%	98%
Prophylactic Antibiotic Stopped	708	99%	98%	98%
Prophylactic Antibiotic Timing	724	100%	99%	99%
Prophylactic Antibiotic Timing (Outpatient)	411	98%	98%	98%
Urinary Catheter Removal	470	99%	98%	97%
Survey of Patients' Hospital Experiences				
Area Around Room 'Always' Quiet at Night	300+	59%	61%	61%
Doctors 'Always' Communicated Well	300+	87%	83%	82%
Home Recovery Information Given	300+	87%	86%	85%
Hospital Given 9 or 10 on 10 Point Scale	300+	85%	74%	71%
Meds 'Always' Explained Before Given	300+	65%	64%	64%
Nurses 'Always' Communicated Well	300+	84%	81%	79%
Pain 'Always' Well Controlled	300+	79%	73%	71%
Room and Bathroom 'Always' Clean	300+	72%	76%	73%
Timely Help 'Always' Received	300+	76%	71%	68%
Would Definitely Recommend Hospital	300+	88%	73%	71%
Use of Medical Imaging				
Cardiac Imaging Stress Test before Surgery	174	5.2%	5.4%	5.3%
Combination Abdominal CT Scan[1]	-	-	9.3%	10.5%
Combination Brain/Sinus CT Scan	63	0.0%	2.6%	2.7%
Combination Chest CT Scan[1]	-	-	4.6%	2.7%
Follow-up Mammogram/Ultrasound[7]	-	-	8.4%	8.8%
Lumbar Spine MRI for Low Back Pain[1]	-	-	38.7%	37.2%

Saint Vincent Hospital & Health Services

2001 W 86th St
Indianapolis, IN 46260
Phone: 317-338-7000
Fax: 317-338-7005
URL: www.indianapolis.stvincent.org
Type: Acute Care Hospitals
Emergency Services: Yes
Ownership: Voluntary non-profit - Church
Beds: 650

Key Personnel:
Coronary Care . . . . Andrew Allen
Radiology. . . . . Peter D Arfken, MD
Pediatric In-Patient Care . . . . Edward Aull, MD
CEO/President. . . . . Sr Bernice Coreil, DC
Infection Control. . . . . Carolyn Davee
Quality Assurance . . . . John D Doyle
CEO . . . . Jonathan Nalli
Anesthesiology. . . . . Steven R Young, MD

Measure	Cases	This Hosp.	State Avg.	U.S. Avg.
Blood Clot Prevention and Treatment				
Anticoagulation Overlap Therapy[2]	164	99%	92%	93%
ICU Venous Thromboembolism Prophylaxis[2]	76	91%	91%	92%
Incidence of Potentially Preventable VTE[2]	53	11%	10%	10%
UFH with Dosages/Platelet Monitoring[2]	54	81%	95%	97%
Venous Thromboembolism Prophylaxis[2]	344	74%	83%	85%
Warfarin Therapy Discharge Instructions[2]	115	25%	71%	75%
Chest Pain/Possible Heart Attack Care				
Aspirin Given Within 24 Hours of Arrival[3]	39	95%	96%	96%
Fibrinolytic Meds Within 30 Min. of Arrival[3,7]	-	-	48%	58%
Average Time to ECG (minutes)[3]	41	5	6	7
Average Time to Transfer (minutes)[1,3]	-	-	46	60
Children's Asthma Care				
Received Home Management Plan of Care	-	-	-	88%
Received Reliever Medication	-	-	-	100%
Received Systemic Corticosteroids	-	-	-	100%
Emergency Department				
Admittance Decision Time (minutes)[2]	425	82	80	98
Head CT Results Within 45 Min. of Arrival[1]	-	-	60%	57%
Patients Who Left ER Before Being Seen	64,788	3%	2%	2%
Time from ER Arrival to Admit. (minutes)[2]	435	247	241	274
Time from ER Arrival to Discharge (minutes)	374	150	122	134
Time in ER Before Being Evaluated (minutes)	322	33	22	26
Time to Pain Meds for Fractures (minutes)	349	48	52	57
Heart Attack Care				
Aspirin Given at Discharge	302	100%	99%	99%
Fibrinolytic Meds Within 30 Min. of Arrival[7]	-	-	67%	54%
PCI Within 90 Minutes of Arrival	27	100%	97%	96%
Statin Prescribed at Discharge	297	100%	99%	98%
Heart Failure Care				
ACE Inhibitor or ARB for LVSD	196	99%	97%	97%
Discharge Instructions Given	587	95%	95%	94%
Evaluation of LVS Function	749	100%	99%	99%
Medicare Spending				
Medicare Spending per Patient (ratio)	-	1.02	1.01	0.98
Pneumonia Care				
Appropriate Initial Antibiotic Given	170	98%	95%	95%
Blood Culture Timing	337	98%	98%	98%
Pregnancy and Delivery Care				
Newborn Deliveries Scheduled Early[2]	665	0%	5%	6%
Preventive Care				
Immunization for Influenza[2]	545	86%	91%	90%
Immunization for Pneumonia[2]	596	86%	92%	92%
Stroke Care				
Anticoagulation Therapy for Atrial Fibrillation	64	97%	94%	95%
Antithrombotic Therapy Timing	324	98%	97%	98%
Assessed for Rehabilitation	422	95%	96%	97%
Discharged on Antithrombotic Therapy	340	99%	98%	99%
Discharged on Statin Medication	276	90%	91%	94%
Thrombolytic Therapy Timing	20	50%	54%	66%
Venous Thromboembolism Prophylaxis	445	87%	91%	94%
Written Stroke Educational Materials Given	223	69%	82%	88%
Surgical Care Improvement Project				
Appropriate Beta Blocker Usage[2]	706	99%	98%	98%
Appropriate VTP Within 24 Hours[2]	1,112	97%	98%	98%
Controlled Postoperative Blood Glucose[2]	307	95%	97%	97%
Perioperative Temperature Management[2]	1,596	100%	100%	100%
Prophylactic Antibiotic Selection[2]	1,234	99%	99%	99%
Prophylactic Antibiotic Selection (Outpatient)	758	97%	98%	98%
Prophylactic Antibiotic Stopped[2]	1,214	98%	98%	98%
Prophylactic Antibiotic Timing[2]	1,237	99%	99%	99%
Prophylactic Antibiotic Timing (Outpatient)	770	94%	98%	98%
Urinary Catheter Removal[2]	847	97%	98%	97%
Survey of Patients' Hospital Experiences				
Area Around Room 'Always' Quiet at Night[11]	300+	57%	61%	61%
Doctors 'Always' Communicated Well[11]	300+	82%	83%	82%
Home Recovery Information Given[11]	300+	84%	86%	85%
Hospital Given 9 or 10 on 10 Point Scale[11]	300+	78%	74%	71%
Meds 'Always' Explained Before Given[11]	300+	59%	64%	64%
Nurses 'Always' Communicated Well[11]	300+	78%	81%	79%
Pain 'Always' Well Controlled[11]	300+	69%	73%	71%
Room and Bathroom 'Always' Clean[11]	300+	60%	76%	73%
Timely Help 'Always' Received[11]	300+	61%	71%	68%
Would Definitely Recommend Hospital[11]	300+	79%	73%	71%
Use of Medical Imaging				
Cardiac Imaging Stress Test before Surgery	3,254	4.6%	5.4%	5.3%
Combination Abdominal CT Scan	1,779	5.2%	9.3%	10.5%
Combination Brain/Sinus CT Scan	1,175	2.6%	2.6%	2.7%
Combination Chest CT Scan	1,480	0.3%	4.6%	2.7%
Follow-up Mammogram/Ultrasound	3,574	8.9%	8.4%	8.8%
Lumbar Spine MRI for Low Back Pain	272	41.2%	38.7%	37.2%

Memorial Hospital & Health Care Center

800 W 9th St
Jasper, IN 47546
Phone: 812-996-2345
Fax: 812-482-0302
URL: www.mhhcc.org
Type: Acute Care Hospitals
Emergency Services: Yes
Ownership: Voluntary non-profit - Church
Beds: 131

Key Personnel:
Pediatric Ambulatory Care . . . . . . Suzanne Burgess, RN
Pediatric In-Patient Care . . . . Suzanne Burgess, RN
Chief of Medical Staff. . . . . Robert Earhard, MD
Coronary Care . . . . Kathy Howell
Quality Assurance . . . . Denise Kaatzal, RN
Radiology. . . . . Elaine Schitter
CEO/President. . . . . Ray Snowden
Infection Control. . . . . Sue Willis, RN

Measure	Cases	This Hosp.	State Avg.	U.S. Avg.
Blood Clot Prevention and Treatment				
Anticoagulation Overlap Therapy[2]	32	91%	92%	93%
ICU Venous Thromboembolism Prophylaxis[2]	72	90%	91%	92%
Incidence of Potentially Preventable VTE[1,2]	-	-	10%	10%
UFH with Dosages/Platelet Monitoring[2]	14	100%	95%	97%
Venous Thromboembolism Prophylaxis[2]	288	80%	83%	85%
Warfarin Therapy Discharge Instructions[2]	20	95%	71%	75%
Chest Pain/Possible Heart Attack Care				
Aspirin Given Within 24 Hours of Arrival[1]	-	-	96%	96%
Fibrinolytic Meds Within 30 Min. of Arrival[3,7]	-	-	48%	58%
Average Time to ECG (minutes)[1]	-	-	6	7
Average Time to Transfer (minutes)[3,7]	-	-	46	60
Children's Asthma Care				
Received Home Management Plan of Care	-	-	-	88%
Received Reliever Medication	-	-	-	100%
Received Systemic Corticosteroids	-	-	-	100%
Emergency Department				
Admittance Decision Time (minutes)[2]	551	69	80	98
Head CT Results Within 45 Min. of Arrival[1]	-	-	60%	57%
Patients Who Left ER Before Being Seen	25,921	1%	2%	2%
Time from ER Arrival to Admit. (minutes)[2]	576	203	241	274
Time from ER Arrival to Discharge (minutes)	361	126	122	134
Time in ER Before Being Evaluated (minutes)	328	17	22	26
Time to Pain Meds for Fractures (minutes)	129	58	52	57
Heart Attack Care				

NOTE: Hospital profiles are in alphabetical order by state, then city, then hospital within the city; Rankings exclude hospitals with less than 25 cases except for patient surveys which excludes hospitals with less than 100 cases; (a) 100-299 cases; (1) The number of cases/patients is too few to report; (2) Data submitted were based on a sample of cases/patients; (3) Results are based on a shorter time period than required; (4) Data suppressed by CMS for one or more quarters; (5) Results are not available for this reporting period; (6) Fewer than 100 patients completed the HCAHPS survey; (7) No cases met the criteria for this measure; (8) The lower limit of the confidence interval cannot be calculated if the number of observed infections equals zero; (9) No data are available from the state/territory for this reporting period; (10) The scores shown reflect fewer than 50 completed surveys; (11) There were discrepancies in the data collection process; (12) This measure does not apply to this hospital for this reporting period; (13) Results cannot be calculated for this reporting period; (14) The results for this state are combined with nearby states to protect confidentiality; Please refer to the User's Guide for a full explanation of data.

Aspirin Given at Discharge	212	100%	99%	99%
Fibrinolytic Meds Within 30 Min. of Arrival[7]	-	-	67%	54%
PCI Within 90 Minutes of Arrival	19	100%	97%	96%
Statin Prescribed at Discharge	208	98%	99%	98%
Heart Failure Care				
ACE Inhibitor or ARB for LVSD	54	96%	97%	97%
Discharge Instructions Given	128	97%	95%	94%
Evaluation of LVS Function	169	100%	99%	99%
Medicare Spending				
Medicare Spending per Patient (ratio)	-	0.96	1.01	0.98
Pneumonia Care				
Appropriate Initial Antibiotic Given[2]	94	98%	95%	95%
Blood Culture Timing[2]	112	97%	98%	98%
Pregnancy and Delivery Care				
Newborn Deliveries Scheduled Early	136	4%	5%	6%
Preventive Care				
Immunization for Influenza[2]	489	97%	91%	90%
Immunization for Pneumonia[2]	596	98%	92%	92%
Stroke Care				
Anticoagulation Therapy for Atrial Fibrillation	14	93%	94%	95%
Antithrombotic Therapy Timing	67	100%	97%	98%
Assessed for Rehabilitation	82	100%	96%	97%
Discharged on Antithrombotic Therapy	82	100%	98%	99%
Discharged on Statin Medication	63	94%	91%	94%
Thrombolytic Therapy Timing[1]	-	-	54%	66%
Venous Thromboembolism Prophylaxis	77	94%	91%	94%
Written Stroke Educational Materials Given	32	62%	82%	88%
Surgical Care Improvement Project				
Appropriate Beta Blocker Usage[2]	172	97%	98%	98%
Appropriate VTP Within 24 Hours[2]	489	96%	98%	98%
Controlled Postoperative Blood Glucose[2,7]	-	-	97%	97%
Perioperative Temperature Management[2]	522	100%	100%	100%
Prophylactic Antibiotic Selection[2]	408	94%	99%	99%
Prophylactic Antibiotic Selection (Outpatient)	248	97%	98%	98%
Prophylactic Antibiotic Stopped[2]	399	96%	98%	98%
Prophylactic Antibiotic Timing[2]	408	97%	99%	99%
Prophylactic Antibiotic Timing (Outpatient)	310	77%	98%	98%
Urinary Catheter Removal[2]	208	98%	98%	97%
Survey of Patients' Hospital Experiences				
Area Around Room 'Always' Quiet at Night	300+	68%	61%	61%
Doctors 'Always' Communicated Well	300+	85%	83%	82%
Home Recovery Information Given	300+	88%	86%	85%
Hospital Given 9 or 10 on 10 Point Scale	300+	81%	74%	71%
Meds 'Always' Explained Before Given	300+	72%	64%	64%
Nurses 'Always' Communicated Well	300+	83%	81%	79%
Pain 'Always' Well Controlled	300+	75%	73%	71%
Room and Bathroom 'Always' Clean	300+	85%	76%	73%
Timely Help 'Always' Received	300+	74%	71%	68%
Would Definitely Recommend Hospital	300+	76%	73%	71%
Use of Medical Imaging				
Cardiac Imaging Stress Test before Surgery	621	6.9%	5.4%	5.3%
Combination Abdominal CT Scan	1,201	4.4%	9.3%	10.5%
Combination Brain/Sinus CT Scan	805	0.9%	2.6%	2.7%
Combination Chest CT Scan	850	1.3%	4.6%	2.7%
Follow-up Mammogram/Ultrasound	1,513	8.7%	8.4%	8.8%
Lumbar Spine MRI for Low Back Pain	130	43.8%	38.7%	37.2%

Clark Memorial Hospital

1220 Missouri Ave
Jeffersonville, IN 47130
Phone: 812-283-2142
Fax: 812-283-2688
E-mail: paula.lamb@clarkmemorial.org
URL: www.clarkmemorial.org
Type: Acute Care Hospitals
Emergency Services: Yes
Ownership: Voluntary non-profit - Other
Beds: 241

Key Personnel:

Radiology. . . . . Asma Ahmad, MD
Chief of Medical Staff . . . . Warlito A Bautista
Quality Assurance . . . . Chad Brough
Emergency Room . . . . Lynn Meuer
CEO/President. . . . . Martin Padgett
Operating Room. . . . . Ruth Schmidt

Measure	Cases	This Hosp.	State Avg.	U.S. Avg.
Blood Clot Prevention and Treatment				
Anticoagulation Overlap Therapy[2]	73	84%	92%	93%
ICU Venous Thromboembolism Prophylaxis[2]	52	85%	91%	92%
Incidence of Potentially Preventable VTE[2]	13	38%	10%	10%
UFH with Dosages/Platelet Monitoring[2]	36	6%	95%	97%
Venous Thromboembolism Prophylaxis[2]	345	50%	83%	85%
Warfarin Therapy Discharge Instructions[2]	49	47%	71%	75%
Chest Pain/Possible Heart Attack Care				
Aspirin Given Within 24 Hours of Arrival[1,3]	-	-	96%	96%
Fibrinolytic Meds Within 30 Min. of Arrival[3,7]	-	-	48%	58%
Average Time to ECG (minutes)[1,3]	-	-	6	7
Average Time to Transfer (minutes)[3,7]	-	-	46	60
Children's Asthma Care				
Received Home Management Plan of Care	-	-	-	88%
Received Reliever Medication	-	-	-	100%
Received Systemic Corticosteroids	-	-	-	100%
Emergency Department				
Admittance Decision Time (minutes)[2]	584	70	80	98
Head CT Results Within 45 Min. of Arrival[1]	-	-	60%	57%
Patients Who Left ER Before Being Seen	31,528	2%	2%	2%
Time from ER Arrival to Admit. (minutes)[2]	591	302	241	274
Time from ER Arrival to Discharge (minutes)	370	171	122	134
Time in ER Before Being Evaluated (minutes)	390	38	22	26
Time to Pain Meds for Fractures (minutes)	94	48	52	57
Heart Attack Care				
Aspirin Given at Discharge	193	97%	99%	99%
Fibrinolytic Meds Within 30 Min. of Arrival[7]	-	-	67%	54%
PCI Within 90 Minutes of Arrival	37	86%	97%	96%
Statin Prescribed at Discharge	171	94%	99%	98%
Heart Failure Care				
ACE Inhibitor or ARB for LVSD	83	94%	97%	97%
Discharge Instructions Given	215	91%	95%	94%
Evaluation of LVS Function	294	100%	99%	99%
Medicare Spending				
Medicare Spending per Patient (ratio)	-	1.01	1.01	0.98
Pneumonia Care				
Appropriate Initial Antibiotic Given	211	96%	95%	95%
Blood Culture Timing	346	100%	98%	98%
Pregnancy and Delivery Care				
Newborn Deliveries Scheduled Early	118	7%	5%	6%
Preventive Care				
Immunization for Influenza[2]	546	98%	91%	90%
Immunization for Pneumonia[2]	699	97%	92%	92%
Stroke Care				
Anticoagulation Therapy for Atrial Fibrillation	11	73%	94%	95%
Antithrombotic Therapy Timing	72	94%	97%	98%
Assessed for Rehabilitation	69	80%	96%	97%
Discharged on Antithrombotic Therapy	69	97%	98%	99%
Discharged on Statin Medication	63	84%	91%	94%
Thrombolytic Therapy Timing[1]	-	-	54%	66%
Venous Thromboembolism Prophylaxis	71	58%	91%	94%
Written Stroke Educational Materials Given	41	22%	82%	88%
Surgical Care Improvement Project				
Appropriate Beta Blocker Usage[2]	225	98%	98%	98%
Appropriate VTP Within 24 Hours[2]	610	99%	98%	98%
Controlled Postoperative Blood Glucose[2,7]	-	-	97%	97%
Perioperative Temperature Management[2]	650	100%	100%	100%
Prophylactic Antibiotic Selection[2]	518	100%	99%	99%
Prophylactic Antibiotic Selection (Outpatient)	386	98%	98%	98%
Prophylactic Antibiotic Stopped[2]	511	98%	98%	98%
Prophylactic Antibiotic Timing[2]	518	100%	99%	99%
Prophylactic Antibiotic Timing (Outpatient)	386	100%	98%	98%
Urinary Catheter Removal[2]	502	99%	98%	97%
Survey of Patients' Hospital Experiences				
Area Around Room 'Always' Quiet at Night	300+	52%	61%	61%
Doctors 'Always' Communicated Well	300+	79%	83%	82%
Home Recovery Information Given	300+	80%	86%	85%
Hospital Given 9 or 10 on 10 Point Scale	300+	69%	74%	71%
Meds 'Always' Explained Before Given	300+	61%	64%	64%
Nurses 'Always' Communicated Well	300+	80%	81%	79%
Pain 'Always' Well Controlled	300+	69%	73%	71%
Room and Bathroom 'Always' Clean	300+	75%	76%	73%
Timely Help 'Always' Received	300+	70%	71%	68%
Would Definitely Recommend Hospital	300+	72%	73%	71%
Use of Medical Imaging				
Cardiac Imaging Stress Test before Surgery	416	6.0%	5.4%	5.3%
Combination Abdominal CT Scan	886	4.9%	9.3%	10.5%
Combination Brain/Sinus CT Scan	752	2.4%	2.6%	2.7%
Combination Chest CT Scan	843	0.0%	4.6%	2.7%
Follow-up Mammogram/Ultrasound	1,866	8.6%	8.4%	8.8%
Lumbar Spine MRI for Low Back Pain	179	40.2%	38.7%	37.2%

Parkview Noble Hospital

401 Sawyer Rd
Kendallville, IN 46755
Phone: 260-347-8700
E-mail: mashek4126@aol.com
URL: www.parkview.com
Type: Acute Care Hospitals
Emergency Services: Yes
Ownership: Voluntary non-profit - Private
Beds: 66

Key Personnel:

CEO/President. . . . . John Berhow
Infection Control. . . . . Karen Denny
Operating Room. . . . . Holly Goe
Quality Assurance . . . . Mary Hageman
Emergency Room . . . . Kim Horan
Chief of Medical Staff . . . . Abdali Jan, MD
Intensive Care Unit. . . . . Mindy Kurtz
Hemotology Center . . . . Karen Stroman

Measure	Cases	This Hosp.	State Avg.	U.S. Avg.
Blood Clot Prevention and Treatment				
Anticoagulation Overlap Therapy[1,2]	-	-	92%	93%
ICU Venous Thromboembolism Prophylaxis[2]	30	87%	91%	92%
Incidence of Potentially Preventable VTE[2,7]	-	-	10%	10%
UFH with Dosages/Platelet Monitoring[1,2]	-	-	95%	97%
Venous Thromboembolism Prophylaxis[2]	145	70%	83%	85%
Warfarin Therapy Discharge Instructions[1,2]	-	-	71%	75%
Chest Pain/Possible Heart Attack Care				
Aspirin Given Within 24 Hours of Arrival	40	100%	96%	96%
Fibrinolytic Meds Within 30 Min. of Arrival[3,7]	-	-	48%	58%
Average Time to ECG (minutes)	39	5	6	7
Average Time to Transfer (minutes)[1,3]	-	-	46	60
Children's Asthma Care				
Received Home Management Plan of Care	-	-	-	88%
Received Reliever Medication	-	-	-	100%
Received Systemic Corticosteroids	-	-	-	100%
Emergency Department				
Admittance Decision Time (minutes)[2]	298	67	80	98
Head CT Results Within 45 Min. of Arrival	12	83%	60%	57%
Patients Who Left ER Before Being Seen	18,065	0%	2%	2%
Time from ER Arrival to Admit. (minutes)[2]	351	209	241	274
Time from ER Arrival to Discharge (minutes)	395	85	122	134
Time in ER Before Being Evaluated (minutes)	372	26	22	26
Time to Pain Meds for Fractures (minutes)	61	31	52	57
Heart Attack Care				
Aspirin Given at Discharge[1]	-	-	99%	99%
Fibrinolytic Meds Within 30 Min. of Arrival[7]	-	-	67%	54%
PCI Within 90 Minutes of Arrival[7]	-	-	97%	96%
Statin Prescribed at Discharge[1]	-	-	99%	98%
Heart Failure Care				
ACE Inhibitor or ARB for LVSD	13	100%	97%	97%
Discharge Instructions Given	51	96%	95%	94%
Evaluation of LVS Function	74	100%	99%	99%
Medicare Spending				
Medicare Spending per Patient (ratio)	-	0.99	1.01	0.98
Pneumonia Care				
Appropriate Initial Antibiotic Given	83	99%	95%	95%
Blood Culture Timing	123	100%	98%	98%
Pregnancy and Delivery Care				
Newborn Deliveries Scheduled Early	15	0%	5%	6%
Preventive Care				
Immunization for Influenza[2]	253	96%	91%	90%
Immunization for Pneumonia[2]	321	99%	92%	92%
Stroke Care				
Anticoagulation Therapy for Atrial Fibrillation[1]	-	-	94%	95%
Antithrombotic Therapy Timing	12	83%	97%	98%
Assessed for Rehabilitation[1]	-	-	96%	97%
Discharged on Antithrombotic Therapy[1]	-	-	98%	99%
Discharged on Statin Medication[1]	-	-	91%	94%

NOTE: Hospital profiles are in alphabetical order by state, then city, then hospital within the city; Rankings exclude hospitals with less than 25 cases except for patient surveys which excludes hospitals with less than 100 cases; (a) 100-299 cases; (1) The number of cases/patients is too few to report; (2) Data submitted were based on a sample of cases/patients; (3) Results are based on a shorter time period than required; (4) Data suppressed by CMS for one or more quarters; (5) Results are not available for this reporting period; (6) Fewer than 100 patients completed the HCAHPS survey; (7) No cases met the criteria for this measure; (8) The lower limit of the confidence interval cannot be calculated if the number of observed infections equals zero; (9) No data are available from the state/territory for this reporting period; (10) The scores shown reflect fewer than 50 completed surveys; (11) There were discrepancies in the data collection process; (12) This measure does not apply to this hospital for this reporting period; (13) Results cannot be calculated for this reporting period; (14) The results for this state are combined with nearby states to protect confidentiality; Please refer to the User's Guide for a full explanation of data.

Measure	Cases	This Hosp.	State Avg.	U.S. Avg.
Thrombolytic Therapy Timing[7]	-	-	54%	66%
Venous Thromboembolism Prophylaxis	13	54%	91%	94%
Written Stroke Educational Materials Given[1]	-	-	82%	88%
Surgical Care Improvement Project				
Appropriate Beta Blocker Usage	21	95%	98%	98%
Appropriate VTP Within 24 Hours	62	100%	98%	98%
Controlled Postoperative Blood Glucose[7]	-	-	97%	97%
Perioperative Temperature Management	77	100%	100%	100%
Prophylactic Antibiotic Selection	61	100%	99%	99%
Prophylactic Antibiotic Selection (Outpatient)	32	100%	98%	98%
Prophylactic Antibiotic Stopped	60	92%	98%	98%
Prophylactic Antibiotic Timing	61	100%	99%	99%
Prophylactic Antibiotic Timing (Outpatient)	33	97%	98%	98%
Urinary Catheter Removal	44	98%	98%	97%
Survey of Patients' Hospital Experiences				
Area Around Room 'Always' Quiet at Night	300+	62%	61%	61%
Doctors 'Always' Communicated Well	300+	87%	83%	82%
Home Recovery Information Given	300+	90%	86%	85%
Hospital Given 9 or 10 on 10 Point Scale	300+	82%	74%	71%
Meds 'Always' Explained Before Given	300+	65%	64%	64%
Nurses 'Always' Communicated Well	300+	82%	81%	79%
Pain 'Always' Well Controlled	300+	74%	73%	71%
Room and Bathroom 'Always' Clean	300+	82%	76%	73%
Timely Help 'Always' Received	300+	76%	71%	68%
Would Definitely Recommend Hospital	300+	76%	73%	71%
Use of Medical Imaging				
Cardiac Imaging Stress Test before Surgery	79	6.3%	5.4%	5.3%
Combination Abdominal CT Scan	314	3.8%	9.3%	10.5%
Combination Brain/Sinus CT Scan[1]	-	-	2.6%	2.7%
Combination Chest CT Scan	185	1.1%	4.6%	2.7%
Follow-up Mammogram/Ultrasound	355	6.5%	8.4%	8.8%
Lumbar Spine MRI for Low Back Pain	82	36.6%	38.7%	37.2%

Indiana University Health Starke Hospital

102 E Culver Rd
Knox, IN 46534
Phone: 574-772-1102
Fax: 574-772-1144
E-mail: info@starkememorial.com
URL: www.starkememorial.com
Type: Acute Care Hospitals
Emergency Services: Yes
Ownership: Proprietary
Beds: 53

Key Personnel:
Chief of Medical Staff.......... Patricia Alexander
Coronary Care............... Tanya Emory
President.................... Craig Felty, RN, BSN, MBA, C
Emergency Room .... Kathie Jones, RN
Quality Assurance .... Peggy Madsen
CEO/President............... Michael Meadows

Measure	Cases	This Hosp.	State Avg.	U.S. Avg.
Blood Clot Prevention and Treatment				
Anticoagulation Overlap Therapy[1,2]	-	-	92%	93%
ICU Venous Thromboembolism Prophylaxis[2]	12	50%	91%	92%
Incidence of Potentially Preventable VTE[1,2]	-	-	10%	10%
UFH with Dosages/Platelet Monitoring[1,2]	-	-	95%	97%
Venous Thromboembolism Prophylaxis[2]	103	87%	83%	85%
Warfarin Therapy Discharge Instructions[1,2]	-	-	71%	75%
Chest Pain/Possible Heart Attack Care				
Aspirin Given Within 24 Hours of Arrival	43	98%	96%	96%
Fibrinolytic Meds Within 30 Min. of Arrival[1]	-	-	48%	58%
Average Time to ECG (minutes)	48	6	6	7
Average Time to Transfer (minutes)[1]	-	-	46	60
Children's Asthma Care				
Received Home Management Plan of Care	-	-	-	88%
Received Reliever Medication	-	-	-	100%
Received Systemic Corticosteroids	-	-	-	100%
Emergency Department				
Admittance Decision Time (minutes)[2]	393	41	80	98
Head CT Results Within 45 Min. of Arrival[1]	-	-	60%	57%
Patients Who Left ER Before Being Seen	7,331	0%	2%	2%
Time from ER Arrival to Admit. (minutes)[2]	490	190	241	274
Time from ER Arrival to Discharge (minutes)	385	110	122	134
Time in ER Before Being Evaluated (minutes)	385	23	22	26
Time to Pain Meds for Fractures (minutes)	39	34	52	57
Heart Attack Care				
Aspirin Given at Discharge[1]	-	-	99%	99%
Fibrinolytic Meds Within 30 Min. of Arrival[7]	-	-	67%	54%
PCI Within 90 Minutes of Arrival[7]	-	-	97%	96%
Statin Prescribed at Discharge[1]	-	-	99%	98%
Heart Failure Care				
ACE Inhibitor or ARB for LVSD[1]	-	-	97%	97%
Discharge Instructions Given	40	100%	95%	94%
Evaluation of LVS Function	41	100%	99%	99%
Medicare Spending				
Medicare Spending per Patient (ratio)	-	0.99	1.01	0.98
Pneumonia Care				
Appropriate Initial Antibiotic Given	49	92%	95%	95%
Blood Culture Timing	63	90%	98%	98%
Pregnancy and Delivery Care				
Newborn Deliveries Scheduled Early[7]	-	-	5%	6%
Preventive Care				
Immunization for Influenza[2]	300	97%	91%	90%
Immunization for Pneumonia[2]	420	98%	92%	92%
Stroke Care				
Anticoagulation Therapy for Atrial Fibrillation[3,7]	-	-	94%	95%
Antithrombotic Therapy Timing[1,3]	-	-	97%	98%
Assessed for Rehabilitation[1,3]	-	-	96%	97%
Discharged on Antithrombotic Therapy[1,3]	-	-	98%	99%
Discharged on Statin Medication[1,3]	-	-	91%	94%
Thrombolytic Therapy Timing[1,3]	-	-	54%	66%
Venous Thromboembolism Prophylaxis[1,3]	-	-	91%	94%
Written Stroke Educational Materials Given[1,3]	-	-	82%	88%
Surgical Care Improvement Project				
Appropriate Beta Blocker Usage[1]	-	-	98%	98%
Appropriate VTP Within 24 Hours	13	100%	98%	98%
Controlled Postoperative Blood Glucose[7]	-	-	97%	97%
Perioperative Temperature Management	13	100%	100%	100%
Prophylactic Antibiotic Selection[1]	-	-	99%	99%
Prophylactic Antibiotic Selection (Outpatient)[1,3]	-	-	98%	98%
Prophylactic Antibiotic Stopped[1]	-	-	98%	98%
Prophylactic Antibiotic Timing[1]	-	-	99%	99%
Prophylactic Antibiotic Timing (Outpatient)[1,3]	-	-	98%	98%
Urinary Catheter Removal[1]	-	-	98%	97%
Survey of Patients' Hospital Experiences				
Area Around Room 'Always' Quiet at Night	(a)	54%	61%	61%
Doctors 'Always' Communicated Well	(a)	71%	83%	82%
Home Recovery Information Given	(a)	83%	86%	85%
Hospital Given 9 or 10 on 10 Point Scale	(a)	61%	74%	71%
Meds 'Always' Explained Before Given	(a)	65%	64%	64%
Nurses 'Always' Communicated Well	(a)	76%	81%	79%
Pain 'Always' Well Controlled	(a)	67%	73%	71%
Room and Bathroom 'Always' Clean	(a)	78%	76%	73%
Timely Help 'Always' Received	(a)	82%	71%	68%
Would Definitely Recommend Hospital	(a)	59%	73%	71%
Use of Medical Imaging				
Cardiac Imaging Stress Test before Surgery	91	2.2%	5.4%	5.3%
Combination Abdominal CT Scan	291	3.1%	9.3%	10.5%
Combination Brain/Sinus CT Scan[1]	-	-	2.6%	2.7%
Combination Chest CT Scan	126	7.1%	4.6%	2.7%
Follow-up Mammogram/Ultrasound	278	11.2%	8.4%	8.8%
Lumbar Spine MRI for Low Back Pain	87	32.2%	38.7%	37.2%

Community Howard Regional Health

3500 S Lafountain St
Kokomo, IN 46902
Phone: 765-453-8371
Fax: 765-453-8087
URL: www.howardcommunity.org
Type: Acute Care Hospitals
Emergency Services: Yes
Ownership: Voluntary non-profit - Private
Beds: 150

Key Personnel:
CEO/President................ James P Alender
Radiology..................... William I Babchuk, MD
Chief of Medical Staff.......... Bruce Hughes, MD
Anesthesiology................ Marvin Lodde, MD
Infection Control.............. Danel Peterson

Measure	Cases	This Hosp.	State Avg.	U.S. Avg.
Blood Clot Prevention and Treatment				
Anticoagulation Overlap Therapy[2]	28	96%	92%	93%
ICU Venous Thromboembolism Prophylaxis[2]	94	95%	91%	92%
Incidence of Potentially Preventable VTE[1,2]	-	-	10%	10%
UFH with Dosages/Platelet Monitoring[1,2]	-	-	95%	97%
Venous Thromboembolism Prophylaxis[2]	298	88%	83%	85%
Warfarin Therapy Discharge Instructions[2]	21	67%	71%	75%
Chest Pain/Possible Heart Attack Care				
Aspirin Given Within 24 Hours of Arrival[1,3]	-	-	96%	96%
Fibrinolytic Meds Within 30 Min. of Arrival[3,7]	-	-	48%	58%
Average Time to ECG (minutes)[1,3]	-	-	6	7
Average Time to Transfer (minutes)[1,3]	-	-	46	60
Children's Asthma Care				
Received Home Management Plan of Care	-	-	-	88%
Received Reliever Medication	-	-	-	100%
Received Systemic Corticosteroids	-	-	-	100%
Emergency Department				
Admittance Decision Time (minutes)[2]	452	119	80	98
Head CT Results Within 45 Min. of Arrival	13	62%	60%	57%
Patients Who Left ER Before Being Seen	21,853	4%	2%	2%
Time from ER Arrival to Admit. (minutes)[2]	474	307	241	274
Time from ER Arrival to Discharge (minutes)	523	167	122	134
Time in ER Before Being Evaluated (minutes)	556	45	22	26
Time to Pain Meds for Fractures (minutes)	95	53	52	57
Heart Attack Care				
Aspirin Given at Discharge	126	99%	99%	99%
Fibrinolytic Meds Within 30 Min. of Arrival[7]	-	-	67%	54%
PCI Within 90 Minutes of Arrival	29	100%	97%	96%
Statin Prescribed at Discharge	127	97%	99%	98%
Heart Failure Care				
ACE Inhibitor or ARB for LVSD	45	96%	97%	97%
Discharge Instructions Given	87	83%	95%	94%
Evaluation of LVS Function	123	98%	99%	99%
Medicare Spending				
Medicare Spending per Patient (ratio)	-	1.04	1.01	0.98
Pneumonia Care				
Appropriate Initial Antibiotic Given	123	95%	95%	95%
Blood Culture Timing	149	99%	98%	98%
Pregnancy and Delivery Care				
Newborn Deliveries Scheduled Early	19	0%	5%	6%
Preventive Care				
Immunization for Influenza[2]	578	86%	91%	90%
Immunization for Pneumonia[2]	683	88%	92%	92%
Stroke Care				
Anticoagulation Therapy for Atrial Fibrillation	14	100%	94%	95%
Antithrombotic Therapy Timing	44	100%	97%	98%
Assessed for Rehabilitation	56	93%	96%	97%
Discharged on Antithrombotic Therapy	53	96%	98%	99%
Discharged on Statin Medication	46	80%	91%	94%
Thrombolytic Therapy Timing[1]	-	-	54%	66%
Venous Thromboembolism Prophylaxis	53	85%	91%	94%
Written Stroke Educational Materials Given	21	38%	82%	88%
Surgical Care Improvement Project				
Appropriate Beta Blocker Usage	52	96%	98%	98%
Appropriate VTP Within 24 Hours	143	95%	98%	98%
Controlled Postoperative Blood Glucose	13	100%	97%	97%
Perioperative Temperature Management	156	99%	100%	100%
Prophylactic Antibiotic Selection	114	96%	99%	99%
Prophylactic Antibiotic Selection (Outpatient)	99	99%	98%	98%
Prophylactic Antibiotic Stopped	109	97%	98%	98%
Prophylactic Antibiotic Timing	115	95%	99%	99%
Prophylactic Antibiotic Timing (Outpatient)	105	87%	98%	98%
Urinary Catheter Removal	113	96%	98%	97%
Survey of Patients' Hospital Experiences				
Area Around Room 'Always' Quiet at Night	300+	61%	61%	61%
Doctors 'Always' Communicated Well	300+	81%	83%	82%
Home Recovery Information Given	300+	85%	86%	85%
Hospital Given 9 or 10 on 10 Point Scale	300+	69%	74%	71%
Meds 'Always' Explained Before Given	300+	63%	64%	64%
Nurses 'Always' Communicated Well	300+	82%	81%	79%
Pain 'Always' Well Controlled	300+	70%	73%	71%
Room and Bathroom 'Always' Clean	300+	78%	76%	73%
Timely Help 'Always' Received	300+	69%	71%	68%
Would Definitely Recommend Hospital	300+	69%	73%	71%
Use of Medical Imaging				
Cardiac Imaging Stress Test before Surgery	411	6.6%	5.4%	5.3%

NOTE: Hospital profiles are in alphabetical order by state, then city, then hospital within the city; Rankings exclude hospitals with less than 25 cases except for patient surveys which excludes hospitals with less than 100 cases; (a) 100-299 cases; (1) The number of cases/patients is too few to report; (2) Data submitted were based on a sample of cases/patients; (3) Results are based on a shorter time period than required; (4) Data suppressed by CMS for one or more quarters; (5) Results are not available for this reporting period; (6) Fewer than 100 patients completed the HCAHPS survey; (7) No cases met the criteria for this measure; (8) The lower limit of the confidence interval cannot be calculated if the number of observed infections equals zero; (9) No data are available from the state/territory for this reporting period; (10) The scores shown reflect fewer than 50 completed surveys; (11) There were discrepancies in the data collection process; (12) This measure does not apply to this hospital for this reporting period; (13) Results cannot be calculated for this reporting period; (14) The results for this state are combined with nearby states to protect confidentiality; Please refer to the User's Guide for a full explanation of data.

Combination Abdominal CT Scan	747	8.3%	9.3%	10.5%
Combination Brain/Sinus CT Scan	631	4.1%	2.6%	2.7%
Combination Chest CT Scan	861	4.8%	4.6%	2.7%
Follow-up Mammogram/Ultrasound	824	7.5%	8.4%	8.8%
Lumbar Spine MRI for Low Back Pain	133	35.3%	38.7%	37.2%

Saint Joseph Hospital & Health Center

1907 W Sycamore St
Kokomo, IN 46904
Phone: 765-456-5300
Fax: 765-456-5779
URL: www.stvincent.org
Type: Acute Care Hospitals
Emergency Services: Yes
Ownership: Voluntary non-profit - Church
Beds: 156

Key Personnel:
Radiology. Peter D Arfken, MD
Emergency Room . . . . John Ayers
CEO/President. . . . . Darcy Burghay
Quality Assurance . . . . Polly Jones
Cardiac Laboratory. . . . . Shapor Khosravipour
Ambulatory Care . . . . Mark E. Murphy, RN,NP
Chief of Medical Staff. . . . . RJ Steele, MD
Operating Room. . . . . Michael B Tempel, RN

Measure	Cases	This Hosp.	State Avg.	U.S. Avg.
Blood Clot Prevention and Treatment				
Anticoagulation Overlap Therapy[2]	24	100%	92%	93%
ICU Venous Thromboembolism Prophylaxis[2]	51	100%	91%	92%
Incidence of Potentially Preventable VTE[1,2]	-	-	10%	10%
UFH with Dosages/Platelet Monitoring[1,2]	-	-	95%	97%
Venous Thromboembolism Prophylaxis[2]	278	100%	83%	85%
Warfarin Therapy Discharge Instructions[2]	19	95%	71%	75%
Chest Pain/Possible Heart Attack Care				
Aspirin Given Within 24 Hours of Arrival	71	94%	96%	96%
Fibrinolytic Meds Within 30 Min. of Arrival[7]	-	-	48%	58%
Average Time to ECG (minutes)	79	10	6	7
Average Time to Transfer (minutes)	32	54	46	60
Children's Asthma Care				
Received Home Management Plan of Care	-	-	-	88%
Received Reliever Medication	-	-	-	100%
Received Systemic Corticosteroids	-	-	-	100%
Emergency Department				
Admittance Decision Time (minutes)[2]	475	59	80	98
Head CT Results Within 45 Min. of Arrival[1]	-	-	60%	57%
Patients Who Left ER Before Being Seen	23,413	8%	2%	2%
Time from ER Arrival to Admit. (minutes)[2]	500	276	241	274
Time from ER Arrival to Discharge (minutes)	367	191	122	134
Time in ER Before Being Evaluated (minutes)	401	100	22	26
Time to Pain Meds for Fractures (minutes)	80	84	52	57
Heart Attack Care				
Aspirin Given at Discharge[1]	-	-	99%	99%
Fibrinolytic Meds Within 30 Min. of Arrival[7]	-	-	67%	54%
PCI Within 90 Minutes of Arrival[7]	-	-	97%	96%
Statin Prescribed at Discharge[1]	-	-	99%	98%
Heart Failure Care				
ACE Inhibitor or ARB for LVSD	50	100%	97%	97%
Discharge Instructions Given	109	95%	95%	94%
Evaluation of LVS Function	145	100%	99%	99%
Medicare Spending				
Medicare Spending per Patient (ratio)	-	1.06	1.01	0.98
Pneumonia Care				
Appropriate Initial Antibiotic Given	86	100%	95%	95%
Blood Culture Timing	162	100%	98%	98%
Pregnancy and Delivery Care				
Newborn Deliveries Scheduled Early[2]	19	0%	5%	6%
Preventive Care				
Immunization for Influenza[2]	508	100%	91%	90%
Immunization for Pneumonia[2]	562	100%	92%	92%
Stroke Care				
Anticoagulation Therapy for Atrial Fibrillation[1]	-	-	94%	95%
Antithrombotic Therapy Timing	64	100%	97%	98%
Assessed for Rehabilitation	77	97%	96%	97%
Discharged on Antithrombotic Therapy	71	100%	98%	99%
Discharged on Statin Medication	51	98%	91%	94%
Thrombolytic Therapy Timing[1]	-	-	54%	66%
Venous Thromboembolism Prophylaxis	72	100%	91%	94%
Written Stroke Educational Materials Given	37	97%	82%	88%
Surgical Care Improvement Project				
Appropriate Beta Blocker Usage	115	100%	98%	98%
Appropriate VTP Within 24 Hours	275	100%	98%	98%
Controlled Postoperative Blood Glucose[7]	-	-	97%	97%
Perioperative Temperature Management	358	100%	100%	100%
Prophylactic Antibiotic Selection	270	100%	99%	99%
Prophylactic Antibiotic Selection (Outpatient)	128	97%	98%	98%
Prophylactic Antibiotic Stopped	256	100%	98%	98%
Prophylactic Antibiotic Timing	270	100%	99%	99%
Prophylactic Antibiotic Timing (Outpatient)	129	97%	98%	98%
Urinary Catheter Removal	274	100%	98%	97%
Survey of Patients' Hospital Experiences				
Area Around Room 'Always' Quiet at Night	300+	54%	61%	61%
Doctors 'Always' Communicated Well	300+	85%	83%	82%
Home Recovery Information Given	300+	88%	86%	85%
Hospital Given 9 or 10 on 10 Point Scale	300+	78%	74%	71%
Meds 'Always' Explained Before Given	300+	65%	64%	64%
Nurses 'Always' Communicated Well	300+	79%	81%	79%
Pain 'Always' Well Controlled	300+	71%	73%	71%
Room and Bathroom 'Always' Clean	300+	73%	76%	73%
Timely Help 'Always' Received	300+	62%	71%	68%
Would Definitely Recommend Hospital	300+	82%	73%	71%
Use of Medical Imaging				
Cardiac Imaging Stress Test before Surgery	672	4.6%	5.4%	5.3%
Combination Abdominal CT Scan	743	4.3%	9.3%	10.5%
Combination Brain/Sinus CT Scan	555	1.6%	2.6%	2.7%
Combination Chest CT Scan	544	0.2%	4.6%	2.7%
Follow-up Mammogram/Ultrasound	848	8.4%	8.4%	8.8%
Lumbar Spine MRI for Low Back Pain	112	39.3%	38.7%	37.2%

Indiana University Health La Porte Hospital

1007 Lincolnway
La Porte, IN 46350
Phone: 219-326-1234
Fax: 219-326-2509
URL: www.laportehealth.org
Type: Acute Care Hospitals
Emergency Services: Yes
Ownership: Voluntary non-profit - Private
Beds: 227

Key Personnel:
Cardiology. Abul Basher, MD
Chief of Medical Staff. . . . . Dabi Baughman
Operating Room. . . . . James Cornwell, RN
CEO/President. . . . . Michael Haley
Quality Assurance . . . . Leigh E Morris
Radiology. Edward Neyman
Pediatric In-Patient Care . . . . Marwan Saman, MD

Measure	Cases	This Hosp.	State Avg.	U.S. Avg.
Blood Clot Prevention and Treatment				
Anticoagulation Overlap Therapy[2]	38	79%	92%	93%
ICU Venous Thromboembolism Prophylaxis[2]	97	82%	91%	92%
Incidence of Potentially Preventable VTE[1,2]	-	-	10%	10%
UFH with Dosages/Platelet Monitoring[2]	16	100%	95%	97%
Venous Thromboembolism Prophylaxis[2]	251	79%	83%	85%
Warfarin Therapy Discharge Instructions[2]	27	33%	71%	75%
Chest Pain/Possible Heart Attack Care				
Aspirin Given Within 24 Hours of Arrival[1,3]	-	-	96%	96%
Fibrinolytic Meds Within 30 Min. of Arrival[3,7]	-	-	48%	58%
Average Time to ECG (minutes)[1,3]	-	-	6	7
Average Time to Transfer (minutes)[3,7]	-	-	46	60
Children's Asthma Care				
Received Home Management Plan of Care	-	-	-	88%
Received Reliever Medication	-	-	-	100%
Received Systemic Corticosteroids	-	-	-	100%
Emergency Department				
Admittance Decision Time (minutes)[2]	527	60	80	98
Head CT Results Within 45 Min. of Arrival[1,3]	-	-	60%	57%
Patients Who Left ER Before Being Seen	19,169	0%	2%	2%
Time from ER Arrival to Admit. (minutes)[2]	544	204	241	274
Time from ER Arrival to Discharge (minutes)	437	146	122	134
Time in ER Before Being Evaluated (minutes)	479	37	22	26
Time to Pain Meds for Fractures (minutes)	93	75	52	57
Heart Attack Care				
Aspirin Given at Discharge	115	97%	99%	99%
Fibrinolytic Meds Within 30 Min. of Arrival[7]	-	-	67%	54%
PCI Within 90 Minutes of Arrival	29	93%	97%	96%
Statin Prescribed at Discharge	116	100%	99%	98%
Heart Failure Care				
ACE Inhibitor or ARB for LVSD	53	98%	97%	97%
Discharge Instructions Given	129	98%	95%	94%
Evaluation of LVS Function	164	100%	99%	99%
Medicare Spending				
Medicare Spending per Patient (ratio)	-	0.99	1.01	0.98
Pneumonia Care				
Appropriate Initial Antibiotic Given	108	94%	95%	95%
Blood Culture Timing	166	94%	98%	98%
Pregnancy and Delivery Care				
Newborn Deliveries Scheduled Early[2]	34	0%	5%	6%
Preventive Care				
Immunization for Influenza[2]	627	86%	91%	90%
Immunization for Pneumonia[2]	717	87%	92%	92%
Stroke Care				
Anticoagulation Therapy for Atrial Fibrillation[1,2]	-	-	94%	95%
Antithrombotic Therapy Timing[2]	57	100%	97%	98%
Assessed for Rehabilitation[2]	69	100%	96%	97%
Discharged on Antithrombotic Therapy[2]	62	100%	98%	99%
Discharged on Statin Medication[2]	49	90%	91%	94%
Thrombolytic Therapy Timing[1,2]	-	-	54%	66%
Venous Thromboembolism Prophylaxis[2]	75	91%	91%	94%
Written Stroke Educational Materials Given[2]	39	100%	82%	88%
Surgical Care Improvement Project				
Appropriate Beta Blocker Usage	127	98%	98%	98%
Appropriate VTP Within 24 Hours	289	100%	98%	98%
Controlled Postoperative Blood Glucose	64	94%	97%	97%
Perioperative Temperature Management	380	100%	100%	100%
Prophylactic Antibiotic Selection	276	99%	99%	99%
Prophylactic Antibiotic Selection (Outpatient)	304	99%	98%	98%
Prophylactic Antibiotic Stopped	270	98%	98%	98%
Prophylactic Antibiotic Timing	276	99%	99%	99%
Prophylactic Antibiotic Timing (Outpatient)	253	96%	98%	98%
Urinary Catheter Removal	240	100%	98%	97%
Survey of Patients' Hospital Experiences				
Area Around Room 'Always' Quiet at Night	300+	53%	61%	61%
Doctors 'Always' Communicated Well	300+	73%	83%	82%
Home Recovery Information Given	300+	85%	86%	85%
Hospital Given 9 or 10 on 10 Point Scale	300+	67%	74%	71%
Meds 'Always' Explained Before Given	300+	62%	64%	64%
Nurses 'Always' Communicated Well	300+	79%	81%	79%
Pain 'Always' Well Controlled	300+	69%	73%	71%
Room and Bathroom 'Always' Clean	300+	67%	76%	73%
Timely Help 'Always' Received	300+	69%	71%	68%
Would Definitely Recommend Hospital	300+	63%	73%	71%
Use of Medical Imaging				
Cardiac Imaging Stress Test before Surgery	814	5.8%	5.4%	5.3%
Combination Abdominal CT Scan	669	5.5%	9.3%	10.5%
Combination Brain/Sinus CT Scan[1]	-	-	2.6%	2.7%
Combination Chest CT Scan	276	3.6%	4.6%	2.7%
Follow-up Mammogram/Ultrasound	1,287	9.2%	8.4%	8.8%
Lumbar Spine MRI for Low Back Pain	231	32.9%	38.7%	37.2%

Franciscan Saint Elizabeth Health - Lafayette Central

1501 Hartford St
Lafayette, IN 47904
Phone: 765-502-4334
Fax: 765-423-6925
URL: www.glhsi.org
Type: Acute Care Hospitals
Emergency Services: Yes
Ownership: Voluntary non-profit - Church
Beds: 375

Key Personnel:
Infection Control. . . . . Patricia Boardman, RN
Cardiac Laboratory. . . . . Larry Drummond
Chief of Medical Staff. . . . . Donald Edelen, MD
Quality Assurance . . . . Donald Edelen, MD
Radiology. Steve Good, MD
Operating Room. . . . . Joan Miller, RN
Pediatric In-Patient Care . . . . Marcia Sukits, RN
CEO/President. . . . . Terrence Wilson

Measure	Cases	This Hosp.	State Avg.	U.S. Avg.
Blood Clot Prevention and Treatment				
Anticoagulation Overlap Therapy[2]	27	85%	92%	93%
ICU Venous Thromboembolism Prophylaxis[2]	50	82%	91%	92%
Incidence of Potentially Preventable VTE[2,7]	-	-	10%	10%
UFH with Dosages/Platelet Monitoring[1,2]	-	-	95%	97%

NOTE: Hospital profiles are in alphabetical order by state, then city, then hospital within the city; Rankings exclude hospitals with less than 25 cases except for patient surveys which excludes hospitals with less than 100 cases; (a) 100-299 cases; (1) The number of cases/patients is too few to report; (2) Data submitted were based on a sample of cases/patients; (3) Results are based on a shorter time period than required; (4) Data suppressed by CMS for one or more quarters; (5) Results are not available for this reporting period; (6) Fewer than 100 patients completed the HCAHPS survey; (7) No cases met the criteria for this measure; (8) The lower limit of the confidence interval cannot be calculated if the number of observed infections equals zero; (9) No data are available from the state/territory for this reporting period; (10) The scores shown reflect fewer than 50 completed surveys; (11) There were discrepancies in the data collection process; (12) This measure does not apply to this hospital for this reporting period; (13) Results cannot be calculated for this reporting period; (14) The results for this state are combined with nearby states to protect confidentiality; Please refer to the User's Guide for a full explanation of data.

Measure	Cases	This Hosp.	State Avg.	U.S. Avg.
Venous Thromboembolism Prophylaxis[2]	319	84%	83%	85%
Warfarin Therapy Discharge Instructions[2]	21	76%	71%	75%
Chest Pain/Possible Heart Attack Care				
Aspirin Given Within 24 Hours of Arrival	21	95%	96%	96%
Fibrinolytic Meds Within 30 Min. of Arrival[3,7]	-	-	48%	58%
Average Time to ECG (minutes)	21	5	6	7
Average Time to Transfer (minutes)[1,3]	-	-	46	60
Children's Asthma Care				
Received Home Management Plan of Care	-	-	-	88%
Received Reliever Medication	-	-	-	100%
Received Systemic Corticosteroids	-	-	-	100%
Emergency Department				
Admittance Decision Time (minutes)[2]	228	98	80	98
Head CT Results Within 45 Min. of Arrival[1,3]	-	-	60%	57%
Patients Who Left ER Before Being Seen	27,779	1%	2%	2%
Time from ER Arrival to Admit. (minutes)[2]	228	246	241	274
Time from ER Arrival to Discharge (minutes)	387	104	122	134
Time in ER Before Being Evaluated (minutes)	281	19	22	26
Time to Pain Meds for Fractures (minutes)	57	48	52	57
Heart Attack Care				
Aspirin Given at Discharge[1,3]	-	-	99%	99%
Fibrinolytic Meds Within 30 Min. of Arrival[3,7]	-	-	67%	54%
PCI Within 90 Minutes of Arrival[3,7]	-	-	97%	96%
Statin Prescribed at Discharge[1,3]	-	-	99%	98%
Heart Failure Care				
ACE Inhibitor or ARB for LVSD[1]	-	-	97%	97%
Discharge Instructions Given	46	89%	95%	94%
Evaluation of LVS Function	68	97%	99%	99%
Medicare Spending				
Medicare Spending per Patient (ratio)	-	1.00	1.01	0.98
Pneumonia Care				
Appropriate Initial Antibiotic Given[2]	34	100%	95%	95%
Blood Culture Timing[2]	61	97%	98%	98%
Pregnancy and Delivery Care				
Newborn Deliveries Scheduled Early[7]	-	-	5%	6%
Preventive Care				
Immunization for Influenza[2]	317	98%	91%	90%
Immunization for Pneumonia[2]	511	95%	92%	92%
Stroke Care				
Anticoagulation Therapy for Atrial Fibrillation[1]	-	-	94%	95%
Antithrombotic Therapy Timing	31	97%	97%	98%
Assessed for Rehabilitation	28	96%	96%	97%
Discharged on Antithrombotic Therapy	28	100%	98%	99%
Discharged on Statin Medication	18	94%	91%	94%
Thrombolytic Therapy Timing[1]	-	-	54%	66%
Venous Thromboembolism Prophylaxis	31	87%	91%	94%
Written Stroke Educational Materials Given	16	69%	82%	88%
Surgical Care Improvement Project				
Appropriate Beta Blocker Usage[5]	-	-	98%	98%
Appropriate VTP Within 24 Hours[5]	-	-	98%	98%
Controlled Postoperative Blood Glucose[5]	-	-	97%	97%
Perioperative Temperature Management[5]	-	-	100%	100%
Prophylactic Antibiotic Selection[5]	-	-	99%	99%
Prophylactic Antibiotic Selection (Outpatient)[5]	-	-	98%	98%
Prophylactic Antibiotic Stopped[5]	-	-	98%	98%
Prophylactic Antibiotic Timing[5]	-	-	99%	99%
Prophylactic Antibiotic Timing (Outpatient)[5]	-	-	98%	98%
Urinary Catheter Removal[5]	-	-	98%	97%
Survey of Patients' Hospital Experiences				
Area Around Room 'Always' Quiet at Night	300+	49%	61%	61%
Doctors 'Always' Communicated Well	300+	73%	83%	82%
Home Recovery Information Given	300+	82%	86%	85%
Hospital Given 9 or 10 on 10 Point Scale	300+	63%	74%	71%
Meds 'Always' Explained Before Given	300+	60%	64%	64%
Nurses 'Always' Communicated Well	300+	79%	81%	79%
Pain 'Always' Well Controlled	300+	67%	73%	71%
Room and Bathroom 'Always' Clean	300+	71%	76%	73%
Timely Help 'Always' Received	300+	65%	71%	68%
Would Definitely Recommend Hospital	300+	70%	73%	71%
Use of Medical Imaging				
Cardiac Imaging Stress Test before Surgery[1]	-	-	5.4%	5.3%
Combination Abdominal CT Scan	225	2.2%	9.3%	10.5%
Combination Brain/Sinus CT Scan[1]	-	-	2.6%	2.7%
Combination Chest CT Scan	104	1.0%	4.6%	2.7%
Follow-up Mammogram/Ultrasound	1,694	7.7%	8.4%	8.8%
Lumbar Spine MRI for Low Back Pain[1]	-	-	38.7%	37.2%

Franciscan Saint Elizabeth Health - Lafayette East

1701 S Creasy Ln
Lafayette, IN 47905
URL: www.ste.org
Type: Acute Care Hospitals
Ownership: Voluntary non-profit - Church

Phone: 765-502-4334
Fax: 765-423-6475
Emergency Services: Yes
Beds: 263

Key Personnel:
Infection Control.............. Laura Aschenberg
Intensive Care Unit............ Carol Bailey
Pediatric In-Patient Care .... Marcia Cherry
Cardiac Laboratory............ Sam Haskett
Quality Assurance .... Terry Janssen
Emergency Room .... Wayne O'Connor
Radiology.................. Carlos Vasquez
CEO/President............... Terry Wilson

Measure	Cases	This Hosp.	State Avg.	U.S. Avg.
Blood Clot Prevention and Treatment				
Anticoagulation Overlap Therapy[2]	40	78%	92%	93%
ICU Venous Thromboembolism Prophylaxis[2]	47	85%	91%	92%
Incidence of Potentially Preventable VTE[1,2]	-	-	10%	10%
UFH with Dosages/Platelet Monitoring[2]	16	100%	95%	97%
Venous Thromboembolism Prophylaxis[2]	298	76%	83%	85%
Warfarin Therapy Discharge Instructions[2]	30	57%	71%	75%
Chest Pain/Possible Heart Attack Care				
Aspirin Given Within 24 Hours of Arrival[1]	-	-	96%	96%
Fibrinolytic Meds Within 30 Min. of Arrival[3,7]	-	-	48%	58%
Average Time to ECG (minutes)[1]	-	-	6	7
Average Time to Transfer (minutes)[3,7]	-	-	46	60
Children's Asthma Care				
Received Home Management Plan of Care	-	-	-	88%
Received Reliever Medication	-	-	-	100%
Received Systemic Corticosteroids	-	-	-	100%
Emergency Department				
Admittance Decision Time (minutes)[2]	253	101	80	98
Head CT Results Within 45 Min. of Arrival[1]	-	-	60%	57%
Patients Who Left ER Before Being Seen	37,490	1%	2%	2%
Time from ER Arrival to Admit. (minutes)[2]	262	244	241	274
Time from ER Arrival to Discharge (minutes)	404	120	122	134
Time in ER Before Being Evaluated (minutes)	281	19	22	26
Time to Pain Meds for Fractures (minutes)	135	47	52	57
Heart Attack Care				
Aspirin Given at Discharge	200	98%	99%	99%
Fibrinolytic Meds Within 30 Min. of Arrival[7]	-	-	67%	54%
PCI Within 90 Minutes of Arrival	36	94%	97%	96%
Statin Prescribed at Discharge	190	99%	99%	98%
Heart Failure Care				
ACE Inhibitor or ARB for LVSD	68	99%	97%	97%
Discharge Instructions Given	147	93%	95%	94%
Evaluation of LVS Function	178	99%	99%	99%
Medicare Spending				
Medicare Spending per Patient (ratio)	-	0.99	1.01	0.98
Pneumonia Care				
Appropriate Initial Antibiotic Given[2]	30	100%	95%	95%
Blood Culture Timing[2]	55	100%	98%	98%
Pregnancy and Delivery Care				
Newborn Deliveries Scheduled Early[2]	35	6%	5%	6%
Preventive Care				
Immunization for Influenza[2]	491	98%	91%	90%
Immunization for Pneumonia[2]	539	92%	92%	92%
Stroke Care				
Anticoagulation Therapy for Atrial Fibrillation	13	85%	94%	95%
Antithrombotic Therapy Timing	65	100%	97%	98%
Assessed for Rehabilitation	87	92%	96%	97%
Discharged on Antithrombotic Therapy	76	93%	98%	99%
Discharged on Statin Medication	62	85%	91%	94%
Thrombolytic Therapy Timing[1]	-	-	54%	66%
Venous Thromboembolism Prophylaxis	83	86%	91%	94%
Written Stroke Educational Materials Given	41	85%	82%	88%
Surgical Care Improvement Project				
Appropriate Beta Blocker Usage[2]	209	96%	98%	98%
Appropriate VTP Within 24 Hours[2]	371	95%	98%	98%
Controlled Postoperative Blood Glucose[2]	62	95%	97%	97%
Perioperative Temperature Management[2]	521	99%	100%	100%
Prophylactic Antibiotic Selection[2]	402	99%	99%	99%
Prophylactic Antibiotic Selection (Outpatient)	593	99%	98%	98%
Prophylactic Antibiotic Stopped[2]	387	99%	98%	98%
Prophylactic Antibiotic Timing[2]	403	98%	99%	99%
Prophylactic Antibiotic Timing (Outpatient)	602	97%	98%	98%
Urinary Catheter Removal[2]	164	96%	98%	97%
Survey of Patients' Hospital Experiences				
Area Around Room 'Always' Quiet at Night	300+	62%	61%	61%
Doctors 'Always' Communicated Well	300+	80%	83%	82%
Home Recovery Information Given	300+	88%	86%	85%
Hospital Given 9 or 10 on 10 Point Scale	300+	75%	74%	71%
Meds 'Always' Explained Before Given	300+	65%	64%	64%
Nurses 'Always' Communicated Well	300+	81%	81%	79%
Pain 'Always' Well Controlled	300+	73%	73%	71%
Room and Bathroom 'Always' Clean	300+	77%	76%	73%
Timely Help 'Always' Received	300+	68%	71%	68%
Would Definitely Recommend Hospital	300+	77%	73%	71%
Use of Medical Imaging				
Cardiac Imaging Stress Test before Surgery	361	5.5%	5.4%	5.3%
Combination Abdominal CT Scan	735	8.3%	9.3%	10.5%
Combination Brain/Sinus CT Scan	743	2.4%	2.6%	2.7%
Combination Chest CT Scan	472	1.7%	4.6%	2.7%
Follow-up Mammogram/Ultrasound	275	8.4%	8.4%	8.8%
Lumbar Spine MRI for Low Back Pain	63	42.9%	38.7%	37.2%

Indiana University Health Arnett Hospital

5165 Mccarty Ln
Lafayette, IN 47905
URL: www.iuhealth.org/arnett
Type: Acute Care Hospitals
Ownership: Voluntary non-profit - Private

Phone: 765-448-8000
Emergency Services: Yes

Key Personnel:
CEO .... Al Gatmaitan

Measure	Cases	This Hosp.	State Avg.	U.S. Avg.
Blood Clot Prevention and Treatment				
Anticoagulation Overlap Therapy[2]	81	89%	92%	93%
ICU Venous Thromboembolism Prophylaxis[2]	35	100%	91%	92%
Incidence of Potentially Preventable VTE[1,2]	-	-	10%	10%
UFH with Dosages/Platelet Monitoring[1,2]	-	-	95%	97%
Venous Thromboembolism Prophylaxis[2]	383	91%	83%	85%
Warfarin Therapy Discharge Instructions[2]	57	88%	71%	75%
Chest Pain/Possible Heart Attack Care				
Aspirin Given Within 24 Hours of Arrival[5]	-	-	96%	96%
Fibrinolytic Meds Within 30 Min. of Arrival[5]	-	-	48%	58%
Average Time to ECG (minutes)[5]	-	-	6	7
Average Time to Transfer (minutes)[5]	-	-	46	60
Children's Asthma Care				
Received Home Management Plan of Care	-	-	-	88%
Received Reliever Medication	-	-	-	100%
Received Systemic Corticosteroids	-	-	-	100%
Emergency Department				
Admittance Decision Time (minutes)[2]	676	96	80	98
Head CT Results Within 45 Min. of Arrival[1,3]	-	-	60%	57%
Patients Who Left ER Before Being Seen	33,398	2%	2%	2%
Time from ER Arrival to Admit. (minutes)[2]	689	281	241	274
Time from ER Arrival to Discharge (minutes)	371	173	122	134
Time in ER Before Being Evaluated (minutes)	395	28	22	26
Time to Pain Meds for Fractures (minutes)	120	61	52	57
Heart Attack Care				
Aspirin Given at Discharge	215	99%	99%	99%
Fibrinolytic Meds Within 30 Min. of Arrival[7]	-	-	67%	54%
PCI Within 90 Minutes of Arrival	39	95%	97%	96%
Statin Prescribed at Discharge	212	98%	99%	98%
Heart Failure Care				
ACE Inhibitor or ARB for LVSD[2]	44	100%	97%	97%
Discharge Instructions Given[2]	148	94%	95%	94%
Evaluation of LVS Function[2]	205	100%	99%	99%
Medicare Spending				
Medicare Spending per Patient (ratio)	-	1.05	1.01	0.98

NOTE: Hospital profiles are in alphabetical order by state, then city, then hospital within the city; Rankings exclude hospitals with less than 25 cases except for patient surveys which excludes hospitals with less than 100 cases; (a) 100-299 cases; (1) The number of cases/patients is too few to report; (2) Data submitted were based on a sample of cases/patients; (3) Results are based on a shorter time period than required; (4) Data suppressed by CMS for one or more quarters; (5) Results are not available for this reporting period; (6) Fewer than 100 patients completed the HCAHPS survey; (7) No cases met the criteria for this measure; (8) The lower limit of the confidence interval cannot be calculated if the number of observed infections equals zero; (9) No data are available from the state/territory for this reporting period; (10) The scores shown reflect fewer than 50 completed surveys; (11) There were discrepancies in the data collection process; (12) This measure does not apply to this hospital for this reporting period; (13) Results cannot be calculated for this reporting period; (14) The results for this state are combined with nearby states to protect confidentiality; Please refer to the User's Guide for a full explanation of data.

Measure	Cases	This Hosp.	State Avg.	U.S. Avg.
Pneumonia Care				
Appropriate Initial Antibiotic Given[2]	64	94%	95%	95%
Blood Culture Timing[2]	157	97%	98%	98%
Pregnancy and Delivery Care				
Newborn Deliveries Scheduled Early[2]	38	5%	5%	6%
Preventive Care				
Immunization for Influenza[2]	505	94%	91%	90%
Immunization for Pneumonia[2]	658	94%	92%	92%
Stroke Care				
Anticoagulation Therapy for Atrial Fibrillation[2]	16	94%	94%	95%
Antithrombotic Therapy Timing[2]	88	99%	97%	98%
Assessed for Rehabilitation[2]	85	93%	96%	97%
Discharged on Antithrombotic Therapy[2]	79	100%	98%	99%
Discharged on Statin Medication[2]	67	93%	91%	94%
Thrombolytic Therapy Timing[2]	30	7%	54%	66%
Venous Thromboembolism Prophylaxis[2]	98	95%	91%	94%
Written Stroke Educational Materials Given[2]	52	71%	82%	88%
Surgical Care Improvement Project				
Appropriate Beta Blocker Usage[2]	163	98%	98%	98%
Appropriate VTP Within 24 Hours[2]	273	95%	98%	98%
Controlled Postoperative Blood Glucose[2]	83	100%	97%	97%
Perioperative Temperature Management[2]	314	100%	100%	100%
Prophylactic Antibiotic Selection[2]	281	98%	99%	99%
Prophylactic Antibiotic Selection (Outpatient)	428	99%	98%	98%
Prophylactic Antibiotic Stopped[2]	272	98%	98%	98%
Prophylactic Antibiotic Timing[2]	280	100%	99%	99%
Prophylactic Antibiotic Timing (Outpatient)	427	99%	98%	98%
Urinary Catheter Removal[2]	281	99%	98%	97%
Survey of Patients' Hospital Experiences				
Area Around Room 'Always' Quiet at Night	300+	63%	61%	61%
Doctors 'Always' Communicated Well	300+	76%	83%	82%
Home Recovery Information Given	300+	85%	86%	85%
Hospital Given 9 or 10 on 10 Point Scale	300+	74%	74%	71%
Meds 'Always' Explained Before Given	300+	56%	64%	64%
Nurses 'Always' Communicated Well	300+	77%	81%	79%
Pain 'Always' Well Controlled	300+	71%	73%	71%
Room and Bathroom 'Always' Clean	300+	64%	76%	73%
Timely Help 'Always' Received	300+	60%	71%	68%
Would Definitely Recommend Hospital	300+	74%	73%	71%
Use of Medical Imaging				
Cardiac Imaging Stress Test before Surgery	543	6.4%	5.4%	5.3%
Combination Abdominal CT Scan	731	3.0%	9.3%	10.5%
Combination Brain/Sinus CT Scan	724	2.3%	2.6%	2.7%
Combination Chest CT Scan	376	1.9%	4.6%	2.7%
Follow-up Mammogram/Ultrasound[7]	-	-	8.4%	8.8%
Lumbar Spine MRI for Low Back Pain	77	44.2%	38.7%	37.2%

Parkview Lagrange Hospital

207 N Townline Rd
Lagrange, IN 46761
URL: www.parkview.com
Phone: 260-463-9000
Fax: 260-463-3190
Type: Critical Access Hospitals
Ownership: Voluntary non-profit - Private
Emergency Services: Yes
Beds: 62

Key Personnel:
Quality Assurance . . . . Diane Barnes
Infection Control. . . . . Jane Case
Chief of Medical Staff . . . . Shashank Kashyap, MD
Emergency Room . . . . Scott Smith, MD
Anesthesiology. . . . . Evan Thompson, MD
Radiology. . . . . James Wehrenberg, MD

Measure	Cases	This Hosp.	State Avg.	U.S. Avg.
Blood Clot Prevention and Treatment				
Anticoagulation Overlap Therapy[1,2]	-	-	92%	93%
ICU Venous Thromboembolism Prophylaxis[2]	21	76%	91%	92%
Incidence of Potentially Preventable VTE[2,7]	-	-	10%	10%
UFH with Dosages/Platelet Monitoring[1,2]	-	-	95%	97%
Venous Thromboembolism Prophylaxis[2]	91	76%	83%	85%
Warfarin Therapy Discharge Instructions[1,2]	-	-	71%	75%
Chest Pain/Possible Heart Attack Care				
Aspirin Given Within 24 Hours of Arrival	39	97%	96%	96%
Fibrinolytic Meds Within 30 Min. of Arrival[7]	-	-	48%	58%
Average Time to ECG (minutes)	41	4	6	7
Average Time to Transfer (minutes)[1]	-	-	46	60
Children's Asthma Care				
Received Home Management Plan of Care	-	-	-	88%
Received Reliever Medication	-	-	-	100%
Received Systemic Corticosteroids	-	-	-	100%
Emergency Department				
Admittance Decision Time (minutes)[2]	154	60	80	98
Head CT Results Within 45 Min. of Arrival[1]	-	-	60%	57%
Patients Who Left ER Before Being Seen	8,065	0%	2%	2%
Time from ER Arrival to Admit. (minutes)[2]	174	193	241	274
Time from ER Arrival to Discharge (minutes)	380	84	122	134
Time in ER Before Being Evaluated (minutes)	318	28	22	26
Time to Pain Meds for Fractures (minutes)	43	21	52	57
Heart Attack Care				
Aspirin Given at Discharge[1,3]	-	-	99%	99%
Fibrinolytic Meds Within 30 Min. of Arrival[3,7]	-	-	67%	54%
PCI Within 90 Minutes of Arrival[3,7]	-	-	97%	96%
Statin Prescribed at Discharge[1,3]	-	-	99%	98%
Heart Failure Care				
ACE Inhibitor or ARB for LVSD[1]	-	-	97%	97%
Discharge Instructions Given	19	95%	95%	94%
Evaluation of LVS Function	21	100%	99%	99%
Medicare Spending				
Medicare Spending per Patient (ratio)	-	-	1.01	0.98
Pneumonia Care				
Appropriate Initial Antibiotic Given	47	96%	95%	95%
Blood Culture Timing	56	100%	98%	98%
Pregnancy and Delivery Care				
Newborn Deliveries Scheduled Early[3]	17	0%	5%	6%
Preventive Care				
Immunization for Influenza[2]	226	99%	91%	90%
Immunization for Pneumonia[2]	189	99%	92%	92%
Stroke Care				
Anticoagulation Therapy for Atrial Fibrillation[7]	-	-	94%	95%
Antithrombotic Therapy Timing[1]	-	-	97%	98%
Assessed for Rehabilitation[1]	-	-	96%	97%
Discharged on Antithrombotic Therapy[1]	-	-	98%	99%
Discharged on Statin Medication[1]	-	-	91%	94%
Thrombolytic Therapy Timing[7]	-	-	54%	66%
Venous Thromboembolism Prophylaxis[1]	-	-	91%	94%
Written Stroke Educational Materials Given[1]	-	-	82%	88%
Surgical Care Improvement Project				
Appropriate Beta Blocker Usage	12	100%	98%	98%
Appropriate VTP Within 24 Hours	42	98%	98%	98%
Controlled Postoperative Blood Glucose[7]	-	-	97%	97%
Perioperative Temperature Management	46	100%	100%	100%
Prophylactic Antibiotic Selection	37	100%	99%	99%
Prophylactic Antibiotic Selection (Outpatient)[3]	28	100%	98%	98%
Prophylactic Antibiotic Stopped	35	100%	98%	98%
Prophylactic Antibiotic Timing	37	95%	99%	99%
Prophylactic Antibiotic Timing (Outpatient)[3]	29	93%	98%	98%
Urinary Catheter Removal	26	100%	98%	97%
Survey of Patients' Hospital Experiences				
Area Around Room 'Always' Quiet at Night	(a)	65%	61%	61%
Doctors 'Always' Communicated Well	(a)	82%	83%	82%
Home Recovery Information Given	(a)	88%	86%	85%
Hospital Given 9 or 10 on 10 Point Scale	(a)	78%	74%	71%
Meds 'Always' Explained Before Given	(a)	62%	64%	64%
Nurses 'Always' Communicated Well	(a)	82%	81%	79%
Pain 'Always' Well Controlled	(a)	76%	73%	71%
Room and Bathroom 'Always' Clean	(a)	82%	76%	73%
Timely Help 'Always' Received	(a)	77%	71%	68%
Would Definitely Recommend Hospital	(a)	77%	73%	71%
Use of Medical Imaging				
Cardiac Imaging Stress Test before Surgery[1]	-	-	5.4%	5.3%
Combination Abdominal CT Scan	187	2.7%	9.3%	10.5%
Combination Brain/Sinus CT Scan	176	0.6%	2.6%	2.7%
Combination Chest CT Scan	73	1.4%	4.6%	2.7%
Follow-up Mammogram/Ultrasound	342	7.6%	8.4%	8.8%
Lumbar Spine MRI for Low Back Pain	43	53.5%	38.7%	37.2%

Dearborn County Hospital

600 Wilson Creek Rd
Lawrenceburg, IN 47025
E-mail: hhinds@dch.org
URL: www.dhc.org
Phone: 812-537-1010
Fax: 812-537-2897
Type: Acute Care Hospitals
Ownership: Government - Local
Emergency Services: Yes
Beds: 144

Key Personnel:
Intensive Care Unit. . . . . Keri Amberger, RN
Radiology. . . . . John A Botsford
Pediatric Ambulatory Care . . . . . . Michael Caudy, MD
Operating Room. . . . . Connie Cecil
Quality Assurance . . . . Stephanie Craig, RN
Chief of Medical Staff . . . . Stephen Eliason, MD
Emergency Room . . . . Ellen McCracken
Anesthesiology. . . . . Joseph Uehlein, MD

Measure	Cases	This Hosp.	State Avg.	U.S. Avg.
Blood Clot Prevention and Treatment				
Anticoagulation Overlap Therapy[2]	40	82%	92%	93%
ICU Venous Thromboembolism Prophylaxis[2]	133	74%	91%	92%
Incidence of Potentially Preventable VTE[1,2]	-	-	10%	10%
UFH with Dosages/Platelet Monitoring[2]	18	100%	95%	97%
Venous Thromboembolism Prophylaxis[2]	295	55%	83%	85%
Warfarin Therapy Discharge Instructions[2]	27	85%	71%	75%
Chest Pain/Possible Heart Attack Care				
Aspirin Given Within 24 Hours of Arrival	88	95%	96%	96%
Fibrinolytic Meds Within 30 Min. of Arrival[1]	-	-	48%	58%
Average Time to ECG (minutes)	92	6	6	7
Average Time to Transfer (minutes)	23	64	46	60
Children's Asthma Care				
Received Home Management Plan of Care	-	-	-	88%
Received Reliever Medication	-	-	-	100%
Received Systemic Corticosteroids	-	-	-	100%
Emergency Department				
Admittance Decision Time (minutes)[2]	493	82	80	98
Head CT Results Within 45 Min. of Arrival	15	87%	60%	57%
Patients Who Left ER Before Being Seen	19,050	3%	2%	2%
Time from ER Arrival to Admit. (minutes)[2]	508	260	241	274
Time from ER Arrival to Discharge (minutes)	353	147	122	134
Time in ER Before Being Evaluated (minutes)	423	40	22	26
Time to Pain Meds for Fractures (minutes)	93	63	52	57
Heart Attack Care				
Aspirin Given at Discharge	35	91%	99%	99%
Fibrinolytic Meds Within 30 Min. of Arrival[7]	-	-	67%	54%
PCI Within 90 Minutes of Arrival[7]	-	-	97%	96%
Statin Prescribed at Discharge	33	94%	99%	98%
Heart Failure Care				
ACE Inhibitor or ARB for LVSD	25	84%	97%	97%
Discharge Instructions Given	64	92%	95%	94%
Evaluation of LVS Function	94	100%	99%	99%
Medicare Spending				
Medicare Spending per Patient (ratio)	-	0.97	1.01	0.98
Pneumonia Care				
Appropriate Initial Antibiotic Given	76	93%	95%	95%
Blood Culture Timing	113	96%	98%	98%
Pregnancy and Delivery Care				
Newborn Deliveries Scheduled Early	33	0%	5%	6%
Preventive Care				
Immunization for Influenza[2]	440	97%	91%	90%
Immunization for Pneumonia[2]	545	97%	92%	92%
Stroke Care				
Anticoagulation Therapy for Atrial Fibrillation[1]	-	-	94%	95%
Antithrombotic Therapy Timing	34	100%	97%	98%
Assessed for Rehabilitation	36	94%	96%	97%
Discharged on Antithrombotic Therapy	34	97%	98%	99%
Discharged on Statin Medication	31	71%	91%	94%
Thrombolytic Therapy Timing[1]	-	-	54%	66%
Venous Thromboembolism Prophylaxis	33	58%	91%	94%
Written Stroke Educational Materials Given	18	100%	82%	88%
Surgical Care Improvement Project				
Appropriate Beta Blocker Usage	81	99%	98%	98%
Appropriate VTP Within 24 Hours	259	99%	98%	98%
Controlled Postoperative Blood Glucose[7]	-	-	97%	97%
Perioperative Temperature Management	281	100%	100%	100%

NOTE: Hospital profiles are in alphabetical order by state, then city, then hospital within the city; Rankings exclude hospitals with less than 25 cases except for patient surveys which excludes hospitals with less than 100 cases; (a) 100-299 cases; (1) The number of cases/patients is too few to report; (2) Data submitted were based on a sample of cases/patients; (3) Results are based on a shorter time period than required; (4) Data suppressed by CMS for one or more quarters; (5) Results are not available for this reporting period; (6) Fewer than 100 patients completed the HCAHPS survey; (7) No cases met the criteria for this measure; (8) The lower limit of the confidence interval cannot be calculated if the number of observed infections equals zero; (9) No data are available from the state/territory for this reporting period; (10) The scores shown reflect fewer than 50 completed surveys; (11) There were discrepancies in the data collection process; (12) This measure does not apply to this hospital for this reporting period; (13) Results cannot be calculated for this reporting period; (14) The results for this state are combined with nearby states to protect confidentiality; Please refer to the User's Guide for a full explanation of data.

Prophylactic Antibiotic Selection	211	99%	99%	99%
Prophylactic Antibiotic Selection (Outpatient)	84	98%	98%	98%
Prophylactic Antibiotic Stopped	198	94%	98%	98%
Prophylactic Antibiotic Timing	212	92%	99%	99%
Prophylactic Antibiotic Timing (Outpatient)	60	82%	98%	98%
Urinary Catheter Removal	185	96%	98%	97%
Survey of Patients' Hospital Experiences				
Area Around Room 'Always' Quiet at Night	300+	60%	61%	61%
Doctors 'Always' Communicated Well	300+	83%	83%	82%
Home Recovery Information Given	300+	88%	86%	85%
Hospital Given 9 or 10 on 10 Point Scale	300+	71%	74%	71%
Meds 'Always' Explained Before Given	300+	65%	64%	64%
Nurses 'Always' Communicated Well	300+	81%	81%	79%
Pain 'Always' Well Controlled	300+	72%	73%	71%
Room and Bathroom 'Always' Clean	300+	85%	76%	73%
Timely Help 'Always' Received	300+	70%	71%	68%
Would Definitely Recommend Hospital	300+	68%	73%	71%
Use of Medical Imaging				
Cardiac Imaging Stress Test before Surgery	266	3.4%	5.4%	5.3%
Combination Abdominal CT Scan	466	39.7%	9.3%	10.5%
Combination Brain/Sinus CT Scan	481	1.7%	2.6%	2.7%
Combination Chest CT Scan	430	15.6%	4.6%	2.7%
Follow-up Mammogram/Ultrasound	752	10.1%	8.4%	8.8%
Lumbar Spine MRI for Low Back Pain	92	40.2%	38.7%	37.2%

Witham Health Services

2605 N Lebanon St
Lebanon, IN 46052
Phone: 765-485-8000
Fax: 765-482-8688
URL: www.witham.org
Type: Acute Care Hospitals
Emergency Services: Yes
Ownership: Government - Local
Beds: 80

Key Personnel:
Radiology. . . . . Homer Beltz
Patient Relations . . . . Diane Feder, RN, MSN
CEO/President. . . . . Raymond Ingham
Coronary Care . . . . Cindy Line
Chief of Medical Staff. . . . . Robert Watt, PhD, MD

Measure	Cases	This Hosp.	State Avg.	U.S. Avg.
Blood Clot Prevention and Treatment				
Anticoagulation Overlap Therapy[1,2]	-	-	92%	93%
ICU Venous Thromboembolism Prophylaxis[2]	42	90%	91%	92%
Incidence of Potentially Preventable VTE[2,7]	-	-	10%	10%
UFH with Dosages/Platelet Monitoring[2,7]	-	-	95%	97%
Venous Thromboembolism Prophylaxis[2]	152	89%	83%	85%
Warfarin Therapy Discharge Instructions[1,2]	-	-	71%	75%
Chest Pain/Possible Heart Attack Care				
Aspirin Given Within 24 Hours of Arrival	47	100%	96%	96%
Fibrinolytic Meds Within 30 Min. of Arrival[7]	-	-	48%	58%
Average Time to ECG (minutes)	48	6	6	7
Average Time to Transfer (minutes)[1]	-	-	46	60
Children's Asthma Care				
Received Home Management Plan of Care	-	-	-	88%
Received Reliever Medication	-	-	-	100%
Received Systemic Corticosteroids	-	-	-	100%
Emergency Department				
Admittance Decision Time (minutes)[2]	352	82	80	98
Head CT Results Within 45 Min. of Arrival[1]	-	-	60%	57%
Patients Who Left ER Before Being Seen	21,163	0%	2%	2%
Time from ER Arrival to Admit. (minutes)[2]	410	247	241	274
Time from ER Arrival to Discharge (minutes)	370	105	122	134
Time in ER Before Being Evaluated (minutes)	376	7	22	26
Time to Pain Meds for Fractures (minutes)	106	44	52	57
Heart Attack Care				
Aspirin Given at Discharge	31	100%	99%	99%
Fibrinolytic Meds Within 30 Min. of Arrival[7]	-	-	67%	54%
PCI Within 90 Minutes of Arrival[1]	-	-	97%	96%
Statin Prescribed at Discharge	32	94%	99%	98%
Heart Failure Care				
ACE Inhibitor or ARB for LVSD	15	93%	97%	97%
Discharge Instructions Given	61	100%	95%	94%
Evaluation of LVS Function	81	96%	99%	99%
Medicare Spending				
Medicare Spending per Patient (ratio)	-	1.00	1.01	0.98
Pneumonia Care				
Appropriate Initial Antibiotic Given	69	96%	95%	95%
Blood Culture Timing	121	98%	98%	98%
Pregnancy and Delivery Care				
Newborn Deliveries Scheduled Early[2]	37	0%	5%	6%
Preventive Care				
Immunization for Influenza[2]	268	95%	91%	90%
Immunization for Pneumonia[2]	399	94%	92%	92%
Stroke Care				
Anticoagulation Therapy for Atrial Fibrillation[1]	-	-	94%	95%
Antithrombotic Therapy Timing[1]	-	-	97%	98%
Assessed for Rehabilitation	12	100%	96%	97%
Discharged on Antithrombotic Therapy	12	100%	98%	99%
Discharged on Statin Medication	11	91%	91%	94%
Thrombolytic Therapy Timing[7]	-	-	54%	66%
Venous Thromboembolism Prophylaxis[1]	-	-	91%	94%
Written Stroke Educational Materials Given[1]	-	-	82%	88%
Surgical Care Improvement Project				
Appropriate Beta Blocker Usage	35	100%	98%	98%
Appropriate VTP Within 24 Hours	114	97%	98%	98%
Controlled Postoperative Blood Glucose[7]	-	-	97%	97%
Perioperative Temperature Management	124	100%	100%	100%
Prophylactic Antibiotic Selection	95	100%	99%	99%
Prophylactic Antibiotic Selection (Outpatient)	20	85%	98%	98%
Prophylactic Antibiotic Stopped	94	96%	98%	98%
Prophylactic Antibiotic Timing	96	99%	99%	99%
Prophylactic Antibiotic Timing (Outpatient)	20	100%	98%	98%
Urinary Catheter Removal	94	98%	98%	97%
Survey of Patients' Hospital Experiences				
Area Around Room 'Always' Quiet at Night	300+	61%	61%	61%
Doctors 'Always' Communicated Well	300+	84%	83%	82%
Home Recovery Information Given	300+	84%	86%	85%
Hospital Given 9 or 10 on 10 Point Scale	300+	76%	74%	71%
Meds 'Always' Explained Before Given	300+	65%	64%	64%
Nurses 'Always' Communicated Well	300+	80%	81%	79%
Pain 'Always' Well Controlled	300+	71%	73%	71%
Room and Bathroom 'Always' Clean	300+	79%	76%	73%
Timely Help 'Always' Received	300+	65%	71%	68%
Would Definitely Recommend Hospital	300+	75%	73%	71%
Use of Medical Imaging				
Cardiac Imaging Stress Test before Surgery	164	5.5%	5.4%	5.3%
Combination Abdominal CT Scan	512	8.0%	9.3%	10.5%
Combination Brain/Sinus CT Scan	430	1.9%	2.6%	2.7%
Combination Chest CT Scan	328	1.8%	4.6%	2.7%
Follow-up Mammogram/Ultrasound	599	11.2%	8.4%	8.8%
Lumbar Spine MRI for Low Back Pain	85	43.5%	38.7%	37.2%

Greene County General Hospital

1185 N 1000 W
Linton, IN 47441
Phone: 812-847-2281
Fax: 812-847-6166
URL: www.greenecountyhospital.com
Type: Critical Access Hospitals
Emergency Services: Yes
Ownership: Government - Local
Beds: 76

Key Personnel:
Chief of Medical Staff. . . . . Jitender Bhandari
Infection Control. . . . . Cheryl Corbin
Emergency Room . . . . Tim Hale
Intensive Care Unit. . . . . Amy Miller
Radiology. . . . . Martina Swaby-Steele, MD
Quality Assurance . . . . Janet Sweet
CEO/President. . . . . Jonas Uland

Measure	Cases	This Hosp.	State Avg.	U.S. Avg.
Blood Clot Prevention and Treatment				
Anticoagulation Overlap Therapy[5]	-	-	92%	93%
ICU Venous Thromboembolism Prophylaxis[5]	-	-	91%	92%
Incidence of Potentially Preventable VTE[5]	-	-	10%	10%
UFH with Dosages/Platelet Monitoring[5]	-	-	95%	97%
Venous Thromboembolism Prophylaxis[5]	-	-	83%	85%
Warfarin Therapy Discharge Instructions[5]	-	-	71%	75%
Chest Pain/Possible Heart Attack Care				
Aspirin Given Within 24 Hours of Arrival[5]	-	-	96%	96%
Fibrinolytic Meds Within 30 Min. of Arrival[5]	-	-	48%	58%
Average Time to ECG (minutes)[5]	-	-	6	7
Average Time to Transfer (minutes)[5]	-	-	46	60
Children's Asthma Care				
Received Home Management Plan of Care	-	-	-	88%
Received Reliever Medication	-	-	-	100%
Received Systemic Corticosteroids	-	-	-	100%
Emergency Department				
Admittance Decision Time (minutes)[5]	-	-	80	98
Head CT Results Within 45 Min. of Arrival[5]	-	-	60%	57%
Patients Who Left ER Before Being Seen	9,028	1%	2%	2%
Time from ER Arrival to Admit. (minutes)[5]	-	-	241	274
Time from ER Arrival to Discharge (minutes)[5]	-	-	122	134
Time in ER Before Being Evaluated (minutes)[5]	-	-	22	26
Time to Pain Meds for Fractures (minutes)[5]	-	-	52	57
Heart Attack Care				
Aspirin Given at Discharge[1,3]	-	-	99%	99%
Fibrinolytic Meds Within 30 Min. of Arrival[3,7]	-	-	67%	54%
PCI Within 90 Minutes of Arrival[5]	-	-	97%	96%
Statin Prescribed at Discharge[1,3]	-	-	99%	98%
Heart Failure Care				
ACE Inhibitor or ARB for LVSD	12	92%	97%	97%
Discharge Instructions Given	39	79%	95%	94%
Evaluation of LVS Function	61	77%	99%	99%
Medicare Spending				
Medicare Spending per Patient (ratio)	-	-	1.01	0.98
Pneumonia Care				
Appropriate Initial Antibiotic Given	22	95%	95%	95%
Blood Culture Timing	37	92%	98%	98%
Pregnancy and Delivery Care				
Newborn Deliveries Scheduled Early[5]	-	-	5%	6%
Preventive Care				
Immunization for Influenza[5]	-	-	91%	90%
Immunization for Pneumonia[5]	-	-	92%	92%
Stroke Care				
Anticoagulation Therapy for Atrial Fibrillation[5]	-	-	94%	95%
Antithrombotic Therapy Timing[5]	-	-	97%	98%
Assessed for Rehabilitation[5]	-	-	96%	97%
Discharged on Antithrombotic Therapy[5]	-	-	98%	99%
Discharged on Statin Medication[5]	-	-	91%	94%
Thrombolytic Therapy Timing[5]	-	-	54%	66%
Venous Thromboembolism Prophylaxis[5]	-	-	91%	94%
Written Stroke Educational Materials Given[5]	-	-	82%	88%
Surgical Care Improvement Project				
Appropriate Beta Blocker Usage[5]	-	-	98%	98%
Appropriate VTP Within 24 Hours[5]	-	-	98%	98%
Controlled Postoperative Blood Glucose[5]	-	-	97%	97%
Perioperative Temperature Management[5]	-	-	100%	100%
Prophylactic Antibiotic Selection[5]	-	-	99%	99%
Prophylactic Antibiotic Selection (Outpatient)[5]	-	-	98%	98%
Prophylactic Antibiotic Stopped[5]	-	-	98%	98%
Prophylactic Antibiotic Timing[5]	-	-	99%	99%
Prophylactic Antibiotic Timing (Outpatient)[5]	-	-	98%	98%
Urinary Catheter Removal[5]	-	-	98%	97%
Survey of Patients' Hospital Experiences				
Area Around Room 'Always' Quiet at Night[5]	-	-	61%	61%
Doctors 'Always' Communicated Well[5]	-	-	83%	82%
Home Recovery Information Given[5]	-	-	86%	85%
Hospital Given 9 or 10 on 10 Point Scale[5]	-	-	74%	71%
Meds 'Always' Explained Before Given[5]	-	-	64%	64%
Nurses 'Always' Communicated Well[5]	-	-	81%	79%
Pain 'Always' Well Controlled[5]	-	-	73%	71%
Room and Bathroom 'Always' Clean[5]	-	-	76%	73%
Timely Help 'Always' Received[5]	-	-	71%	68%
Would Definitely Recommend Hospital[5]	-	-	73%	71%
Use of Medical Imaging				
Cardiac Imaging Stress Test before Surgery	98	6.1%	5.4%	5.3%
Combination Abdominal CT Scan	322	25.8%	9.3%	10.5%
Combination Brain/Sinus CT Scan[1]	-	-	2.6%	2.7%
Combination Chest CT Scan	111	1.8%	4.6%	2.7%
Follow-up Mammogram/Ultrasound	283	6.4%	8.4%	8.8%
Lumbar Spine MRI for Low Back Pain[7]	-	-	38.7%	37.2%

NOTE: Hospital profiles are in alphabetical order by state, then city, then hospital within the city; Rankings exclude hospitals with less than 25 cases except for patient surveys which excludes hospitals with less than 100 cases; (a) 100-299 cases; (1) The number of cases/patients is too few to report; (2) Data submitted were based on a sample of cases/patients; (3) Results are based on a shorter time period than required; (4) Data suppressed by CMS for one or more quarters; (5) Results are not available for this reporting period; (6) Fewer than 100 patients completed the HCAHPS survey; (7) No cases met the criteria for this measure; (8) The lower limit of the confidence interval cannot be calculated if the number of observed infections equals zero; (9) No data are available from the state/territory for this reporting period; (10) The scores shown reflect fewer than 50 completed surveys; (11) There were discrepancies in the data collection process; (12) This measure does not apply to this hospital for this reporting period; (13) Results cannot be calculated for this reporting period; (14) The results for this state are combined with nearby states to protect confidentiality; Please refer to the User's Guide for a full explanation of data.

Memorial Hospital

1101 Michigan Ave
Logansport, IN 46947
Phone: 574-753-7541
E-mail: info@mhlogan.org
URL: www.mhlogan.org
Type: Acute Care Hospitals
Emergency Services: Yes
Ownership: Government - Local
Beds: 104

Key Personnel:
Intensive Care Unit. . . . . Angela Cleland, RN
Radiology. . . . . William Harvey
Infection Control. . . . . Sebrena Ide, RN
Chief of Medical Staff . . . . Charles Montgomery, MD
Quality Assurance . . . . Kathy Pattee, RN
Patient Relations . . . . Alice Rothermel
CEO/President. . . . . Brian Shockney
Operating Room. . . . . Todd Weinstein, RN

Measure	Cases	This Hosp.	State Avg.	U.S. Avg.
Blood Clot Prevention and Treatment				
Anticoagulation Overlap Therapy	16	75%	92%	93%
ICU Venous Thromboembolism Prophylaxis	143	95%	91%	92%
Incidence of Potentially Preventable VTE[7]	-	-	10%	10%
UFH with Dosages/Platelet Monitoring[1]	-	-	95%	97%
Venous Thromboembolism Prophylaxis	511	85%	83%	85%
Warfarin Therapy Discharge Instructions	13	100%	71%	75%
Chest Pain/Possible Heart Attack Care				
Aspirin Given Within 24 Hours of Arrival	67	97%	96%	96%
Fibrinolytic Meds Within 30 Min. of Arrival[1]	-	-	48%	58%
Average Time to ECG (minutes)	72	7	6	7
Average Time to Transfer (minutes)[1]	-	-	46	60
Children's Asthma Care				
Received Home Management Plan of Care	-	-	-	88%
Received Reliever Medication	-	-	-	100%
Received Systemic Corticosteroids	-	-	-	100%
Emergency Department				
Admittance Decision Time (minutes)	811	65	80	98
Head CT Results Within 45 Min. of Arrival	14	50%	60%	57%
Patients Who Left ER Before Being Seen	14,514	3%	2%	2%
Time from ER Arrival to Admit. (minutes)	882	232	241	274
Time from ER Arrival to Discharge (minutes)	523	129	122	134
Time in ER Before Being Evaluated (minutes)	571	24	22	26
Time to Pain Meds for Fractures (minutes)	63	41	52	57
Heart Attack Care				
Aspirin Given at Discharge[1]	-	-	99%	99%
Fibrinolytic Meds Within 30 Min. of Arrival[7]	-	-	67%	54%
PCI Within 90 Minutes of Arrival[7]	-	-	97%	96%
Statin Prescribed at Discharge[1]	-	-	99%	98%
Heart Failure Care				
ACE Inhibitor or ARB for LVSD	20	100%	97%	97%
Discharge Instructions Given	41	100%	95%	94%
Evaluation of LVS Function	63	100%	99%	99%
Medicare Spending				
Medicare Spending per Patient (ratio)	-	1.07	1.01	0.98
Pneumonia Care				
Appropriate Initial Antibiotic Given	92	100%	95%	95%
Blood Culture Timing	99	99%	98%	98%
Pregnancy and Delivery Care				
Newborn Deliveries Scheduled Early	48	4%	5%	6%
Preventive Care				
Immunization for Influenza	919	95%	91%	90%
Immunization for Pneumonia	896	99%	92%	92%
Stroke Care				
Anticoagulation Therapy for Atrial Fibrillation[1]	-	-	94%	95%
Antithrombotic Therapy Timing	20	100%	97%	98%
Assessed for Rehabilitation	17	100%	96%	97%
Discharged on Antithrombotic Therapy	16	100%	98%	99%
Discharged on Statin Medication	13	92%	91%	94%
Thrombolytic Therapy Timing[1]	-	-	54%	66%
Venous Thromboembolism Prophylaxis	21	76%	91%	94%
Written Stroke Educational Materials Given[1]	-	-	82%	88%
Surgical Care Improvement Project				
Appropriate Beta Blocker Usage	25	100%	98%	98%
Appropriate VTP Within 24 Hours	91	100%	98%	98%
Controlled Postoperative Blood Glucose[7]	-	-	97%	97%
Perioperative Temperature Management	99	100%	100%	100%
Prophylactic Antibiotic Selection	54	94%	99%	99%
Prophylactic Antibiotic Selection (Outpatient)	128	97%	98%	98%
Prophylactic Antibiotic Stopped	48	98%	98%	98%
Prophylactic Antibiotic Timing	54	100%	99%	99%
Prophylactic Antibiotic Timing (Outpatient)	95	97%	98%	98%
Urinary Catheter Removal	30	100%	98%	97%
Survey of Patients' Hospital Experiences				
Area Around Room 'Always' Quiet at Night	300+	55%	61%	61%
Doctors 'Always' Communicated Well	300+	83%	83%	82%
Home Recovery Information Given	300+	82%	86%	85%
Hospital Given 9 or 10 on 10 Point Scale	300+	62%	74%	71%
Meds 'Always' Explained Before Given	300+	53%	64%	64%
Nurses 'Always' Communicated Well	300+	77%	81%	79%
Pain 'Always' Well Controlled	300+	71%	73%	71%
Room and Bathroom 'Always' Clean	300+	71%	76%	73%
Timely Help 'Always' Received	300+	63%	71%	68%
Would Definitely Recommend Hospital	300+	56%	73%	71%
Use of Medical Imaging				
Cardiac Imaging Stress Test before Surgery	206	4.4%	5.4%	5.3%
Combination Abdominal CT Scan	452	5.3%	9.3%	10.5%
Combination Brain/Sinus CT Scan	404	1.5%	2.6%	2.7%
Combination Chest CT Scan	224	1.3%	4.6%	2.7%
Follow-up Mammogram/Ultrasound	976	9.2%	8.4%	8.8%
Lumbar Spine MRI for Low Back Pain	51	41.2%	38.7%	37.2%

King's Daughters' Health

1373 East Sr 62
Madison, IN 47250
Phone: 812-801-0105
Fax: 812-265-0680
E-mail: kdh@seida.com
URL: www.kdhhs.org
Type: Acute Care Hospitals
Emergency Services: Yes
Ownership: Voluntary non-profit - Private
Beds: 142

Key Personnel:
Emergency Room . . . . L Bernard
Operating Room. . . . . Kathy Brown
Infection Control. . . . . Vikki Conners, RN
Chief of Medical Staff . . . . William Estes, MD
Quality Assurance . . . . Judy Gill
Intensive Care Unit. . . . . Nick James, RN
Radiology. . . . . Robert Leatherm, MD
Hemotology Center . . . . Judy Tingle

Measure	Cases	This Hosp.	State Avg.	U.S. Avg.
Blood Clot Prevention and Treatment				
Anticoagulation Overlap Therapy[2]	25	76%	92%	93%
ICU Venous Thromboembolism Prophylaxis[2]	65	55%	91%	92%
Incidence of Potentially Preventable VTE[1,2]	-	-	10%	10%
UFH with Dosages/Platelet Monitoring[1,2]	-	-	95%	97%
Venous Thromboembolism Prophylaxis[2]	338	56%	83%	85%
Warfarin Therapy Discharge Instructions[2]	23	96%	71%	75%
Chest Pain/Possible Heart Attack Care				
Aspirin Given Within 24 Hours of Arrival	206	98%	96%	96%
Fibrinolytic Meds Within 30 Min. of Arrival[1]	-	-	48%	58%
Average Time to ECG (minutes)	208	6	6	7
Average Time to Transfer (minutes)	12	64	46	60
Children's Asthma Care				
Received Home Management Plan of Care	-	-	-	88%
Received Reliever Medication	-	-	-	100%
Received Systemic Corticosteroids	-	-	-	100%
Emergency Department				
Admittance Decision Time (minutes)[2]	384	78	80	98
Head CT Results Within 45 Min. of Arrival	20	60%	60%	57%
Patients Who Left ER Before Being Seen	18,068	3%	2%	2%
Time from ER Arrival to Admit. (minutes)[2]	387	275	241	274
Time from ER Arrival to Discharge (minutes)	357	175	122	134
Time in ER Before Being Evaluated (minutes)	417	38	22	26
Time to Pain Meds for Fractures (minutes)	71	72	52	57
Heart Attack Care				
Aspirin Given at Discharge[1]	-	-	99%	99%
Fibrinolytic Meds Within 30 Min. of Arrival[7]	-	-	67%	54%
PCI Within 90 Minutes of Arrival[7]	-	-	97%	96%
Statin Prescribed at Discharge[1]	-	-	99%	98%
Heart Failure Care				
ACE Inhibitor or ARB for LVSD	37	65%	97%	97%
Discharge Instructions Given	77	97%	95%	94%
Evaluation of LVS Function	117	99%	99%	99%
Medicare Spending				
Medicare Spending per Patient (ratio)	-	0.99	1.01	0.98
Pneumonia Care				
Appropriate Initial Antibiotic Given[2]	77	96%	95%	95%
Blood Culture Timing[2]	112	97%	98%	98%
Pregnancy and Delivery Care				
Newborn Deliveries Scheduled Early[2]	32	0%	5%	6%
Preventive Care				
Immunization for Influenza[2]	376	96%	91%	90%
Immunization for Pneumonia[2]	512	96%	92%	92%
Stroke Care				
Anticoagulation Therapy for Atrial Fibrillation[1]	-	-	94%	95%
Antithrombotic Therapy Timing	27	89%	97%	98%
Assessed for Rehabilitation	24	79%	96%	97%
Discharged on Antithrombotic Therapy	24	100%	98%	99%
Discharged on Statin Medication	22	77%	91%	94%
Thrombolytic Therapy Timing[7]	-	-	54%	66%
Venous Thromboembolism Prophylaxis	26	38%	91%	94%
Written Stroke Educational Materials Given	12	50%	82%	88%
Surgical Care Improvement Project				
Appropriate Beta Blocker Usage[2]	54	98%	98%	98%
Appropriate VTP Within 24 Hours[2]	106	94%	98%	98%
Controlled Postoperative Blood Glucose[2,7]	-	-	97%	97%
Perioperative Temperature Management[2]	176	99%	100%	100%
Prophylactic Antibiotic Selection[2]	123	99%	99%	99%
Prophylactic Antibiotic Selection (Outpatient)	89	98%	98%	98%
Prophylactic Antibiotic Stopped[2]	119	97%	98%	98%
Prophylactic Antibiotic Timing[2]	123	100%	99%	99%
Prophylactic Antibiotic Timing (Outpatient)	88	97%	98%	98%
Urinary Catheter Removal[2]	70	91%	98%	97%
Survey of Patients' Hospital Experiences				
Area Around Room 'Always' Quiet at Night	300+	61%	61%	61%
Doctors 'Always' Communicated Well	300+	85%	83%	82%
Home Recovery Information Given	300+	86%	86%	85%
Hospital Given 9 or 10 on 10 Point Scale	300+	66%	74%	71%
Meds 'Always' Explained Before Given	300+	62%	64%	64%
Nurses 'Always' Communicated Well	300+	78%	81%	79%
Pain 'Always' Well Controlled	300+	68%	73%	71%
Room and Bathroom 'Always' Clean	300+	77%	76%	73%
Timely Help 'Always' Received	300+	69%	71%	68%
Would Definitely Recommend Hospital	300+	68%	73%	71%
Use of Medical Imaging				
Cardiac Imaging Stress Test before Surgery	354	6.5%	5.4%	5.3%
Combination Abdominal CT Scan	607	7.7%	9.3%	10.5%
Combination Brain/Sinus CT Scan[1]	-	-	2.6%	2.7%
Combination Chest CT Scan	372	0.3%	4.6%	2.7%
Follow-up Mammogram/Ultrasound	176	7.4%	8.4%	8.8%
Lumbar Spine MRI for Low Back Pain	92	33.7%	38.7%	37.2%

Marion General Hospital

441 N Wabash Ave
Marion, IN 46952
Phone: 765-660-6000
Fax: 765-662-4842
URL: www.mgh.net
Type: Acute Care Hospitals
Emergency Services: Yes
Ownership: Voluntary non-profit - Private
Beds: 191

Key Personnel:
Radiology. . . . . Sheri L Brinker
Operating Room. . . . . Robert Crowell
Infection Control. . . . . B Eppler, RN
Chief of Medical Staff . . . . Aaron M Fritz
Quality Assurance . . . . Ruth Masiongale
President/CEO. . . . . Paul L. Usher, FACHE

Measure	Cases	This Hosp.	State Avg.	U.S. Avg.
Blood Clot Prevention and Treatment				
Anticoagulation Overlap Therapy[2]	30	70%	92%	93%
ICU Venous Thromboembolism Prophylaxis[2]	92	91%	91%	92%
Incidence of Potentially Preventable VTE[1,2]	-	-	10%	10%
UFH with Dosages/Platelet Monitoring[1,2]	-	-	95%	97%
Venous Thromboembolism Prophylaxis[2]	356	87%	83%	85%
Warfarin Therapy Discharge Instructions[2]	23	100%	71%	75%
Chest Pain/Possible Heart Attack Care				
Aspirin Given Within 24 Hours of Arrival	189	95%	96%	96%
Fibrinolytic Meds Within 30 Min. of Arrival[7]	-	-	48%	58%

NOTE: Hospital profiles are in alphabetical order by state, then city, then hospital within the city; Rankings exclude hospitals with less than 25 cases except for patient surveys which excludes hospitals with less than 100 cases; (a) 100-299 cases; (1) The number of cases/patients is too few to report; (2) Data submitted were based on a sample of cases/patients; (3) Results are based on a shorter time period than required; (4) Data suppressed by CMS for one or more quarters; (5) Results are not available for this reporting period; (6) Fewer than 100 patients completed the HCAHPS survey; (7) No cases met the criteria for this measure; (8) The lower limit of the confidence interval cannot be calculated if the number of observed infections equals zero; (9) No data are available from the state/territory for this reporting period; (10) The scores shown reflect fewer than 50 completed surveys; (11) There were discrepancies in the data collection process; (12) This measure does not apply to this hospital for this reporting period; (13) Results cannot be calculated for this reporting period; (14) The results for this state are combined with nearby states to protect confidentiality; Please refer to the User's Guide for a full explanation of data.

Measure	Cases	This Hosp.	State Avg.	U.S. Avg.
Average Time to ECG (minutes)	193	7	6	7
Average Time to Transfer (minutes)	53	50	46	60
Children's Asthma Care				
Received Home Management Plan of Care	-	-	-	88%
Received Reliever Medication	-	-	-	100%
Received Systemic Corticosteroids	-	-	-	100%
Emergency Department				
Admittance Decision Time (minutes)[2]	515	64	80	98
Head CT Results Within 45 Min. of Arrival	19	47%	60%	57%
Patients Who Left ER Before Being Seen	44,733	1%	2%	2%
Time from ER Arrival to Admit. (minutes)[2]	607	228	241	274
Time from ER Arrival to Discharge (minutes)	375	131	122	134
Time in ER Before Being Evaluated (minutes)	390	30	22	26
Time to Pain Meds for Fractures (minutes)	118	63	52	57
Heart Attack Care				
Aspirin Given at Discharge	26	96%	99%	99%
Fibrinolytic Meds Within 30 Min. of Arrival[7]	-	-	67%	54%
PCI Within 90 Minutes of Arrival[7]	-	-	97%	96%
Statin Prescribed at Discharge	28	100%	99%	98%
Heart Failure Care				
ACE Inhibitor or ARB for LVSD	40	98%	97%	97%
Discharge Instructions Given	158	96%	95%	94%
Evaluation of LVS Function	200	100%	99%	99%
Medicare Spending				
Medicare Spending per Patient (ratio)	-	1.02	1.01	0.98
Pneumonia Care				
Appropriate Initial Antibiotic Given	136	99%	95%	95%
Blood Culture Timing	158	97%	98%	98%
Pregnancy and Delivery Care				
Newborn Deliveries Scheduled Early[2]	51	12%	5%	6%
Preventive Care				
Immunization for Influenza[2]	548	96%	91%	90%
Immunization for Pneumonia[2]	670	96%	92%	92%
Stroke Care				
Anticoagulation Therapy for Atrial Fibrillation[1]	-	-	94%	95%
Antithrombotic Therapy Timing	33	94%	97%	98%
Assessed for Rehabilitation	36	92%	96%	97%
Discharged on Antithrombotic Therapy	34	100%	98%	99%
Discharged on Statin Medication	33	88%	91%	94%
Thrombolytic Therapy Timing[1]	-	-	54%	66%
Venous Thromboembolism Prophylaxis	35	86%	91%	94%
Written Stroke Educational Materials Given	15	67%	82%	88%
Surgical Care Improvement Project				
Appropriate Beta Blocker Usage[2]	96	96%	98%	98%
Appropriate VTP Within 24 Hours[2]	308	96%	98%	98%
Controlled Postoperative Blood Glucose[2,7]	-	-	97%	97%
Perioperative Temperature Management[2]	342	100%	100%	100%
Prophylactic Antibiotic Selection[2]	246	93%	99%	99%
Prophylactic Antibiotic Selection (Outpatient)	232	97%	98%	98%
Prophylactic Antibiotic Stopped[2]	236	97%	98%	98%
Prophylactic Antibiotic Timing[2]	248	96%	99%	99%
Prophylactic Antibiotic Timing (Outpatient)	236	97%	98%	98%
Urinary Catheter Removal[2]	81	93%	98%	97%
Survey of Patients' Hospital Experiences				
Area Around Room 'Always' Quiet at Night[11]	300+	57%	61%	61%
Doctors 'Always' Communicated Well[11]	300+	83%	83%	82%
Home Recovery Information Given[11]	300+	86%	86%	85%
Hospital Given 9 or 10 on 10 Point Scale[11]	300+	71%	74%	71%
Meds 'Always' Explained Before Given[11]	300+	68%	64%	64%
Nurses 'Always' Communicated Well[11]	300+	81%	81%	79%
Pain 'Always' Well Controlled[11]	300+	76%	73%	71%
Room and Bathroom 'Always' Clean[11]	300+	72%	76%	73%
Timely Help 'Always' Received[11]	300+	74%	71%	68%
Would Definitely Recommend Hospital[11]	300+	63%	73%	71%
Use of Medical Imaging				
Cardiac Imaging Stress Test before Surgery[1]	-	-	5.4%	5.3%
Combination Abdominal CT Scan	1,105	9.1%	9.3%	10.5%
Combination Brain/Sinus CT Scan	931	2.4%	2.6%	2.7%
Combination Chest CT Scan	491	4.1%	4.6%	2.7%
Follow-up Mammogram/Ultrasound	1,763	8.8%	8.4%	8.8%
Lumbar Spine MRI for Low Back Pain	219	33.8%	38.7%	37.2%

VA Northern Indiana Healthcare System - Marion

1700 E. 38th Street
Marion, IN 46953
Phone: 765-674-3321
URL: www.northernindiana.va.gov
Type: Acute Care - VA
Emergency Services: No
Ownership: Government Federal

Measure	Cases	This Hosp.	State Avg.	U.S. Avg.
Blood Clot Prevention and Treatment				
Anticoagulation Overlap Therapy	-	-	92%	93%
ICU Venous Thromboembolism Prophylaxis	-	-	91%	92%
Incidence of Potentially Preventable VTE	-	-	10%	10%
UFH with Dosages/Platelet Monitoring	-	-	95%	97%
Venous Thromboembolism Prophylaxis	-	-	83%	85%
Warfarin Therapy Discharge Instructions	-	-	71%	75%
Chest Pain/Possible Heart Attack Care				
Aspirin Given Within 24 Hours of Arrival	-	-	96%	96%
Fibrinolytic Meds Within 30 Min. of Arrival	-	-	48%	58%
Average Time to ECG (minutes)	-	-	6	7
Average Time to Transfer (minutes)	-	-	46	60
Children's Asthma Care				
Received Home Management Plan of Care	-	-	-	88%
Received Reliever Medication	-	-	-	100%
Received Systemic Corticosteroids	-	-	-	100%
Emergency Department				
Admittance Decision Time (minutes)	-	-	80	98
Head CT Results Within 45 Min. of Arrival	-	-	60%	57%
Patients Who Left ER Before Being Seen	-	-	2%	2%
Time from ER Arrival to Admit. (minutes)	-	-	241	274
Time from ER Arrival to Discharge (minutes)	-	-	122	134
Time in ER Before Being Evaluated (minutes)	-	-	22	26
Time to Pain Meds for Fractures (minutes)	-	-	52	57
Heart Attack Care				
Aspirin Given at Discharge[5]	-	-	99%	99%
Fibrinolytic Meds Within 30 Min. of Arrival[5]	-	-	67%	54%
PCI Within 90 Minutes of Arrival[5]	-	-	97%	96%
Statin Prescribed at Discharge[5]	-	-	99%	98%
Heart Failure Care				
ACE Inhibitor or ARB for LVSD[1]	-	-	97%	97%
Discharge Instructions Given[1]	13	100%	95%	94%
Evaluation of LVS Function[1]	14	100%	99%	99%
Medicare Spending				
Medicare Spending per Patient (ratio)	-	-	1.01	0.98
Pneumonia Care				
Appropriate Initial Antibiotic Given[1]	11	91%	95%	95%
Blood Culture Timing[1]	11	100%	98%	98%
Pregnancy and Delivery Care				
Newborn Deliveries Scheduled Early	-	-	5%	6%
Preventive Care				
Immunization for Influenza[2,3]	136	81%	91%	90%
Immunization for Pneumonia[2,3]	202	94%	92%	92%
Stroke Care				
Anticoagulation Therapy for Atrial Fibrillation	-	-	94%	95%
Antithrombotic Therapy Timing	-	-	97%	98%
Assessed for Rehabilitation	-	-	96%	97%
Discharged on Antithrombotic Therapy	-	-	98%	99%
Discharged on Statin Medication	-	-	91%	94%
Thrombolytic Therapy Timing	-	-	54%	66%
Venous Thromboembolism Prophylaxis	-	-	91%	94%
Written Stroke Educational Materials Given	-	-	82%	88%
Surgical Care Improvement Project				
Appropriate Beta Blocker Usage[5]	-	-	98%	98%
Appropriate VTP Within 24 Hours[5]	-	-	98%	98%
Controlled Postoperative Blood Glucose[5]	-	-	97%	97%
Perioperative Temperature Management[5]	-	-	100%	100%
Prophylactic Antibiotic Selection[5]	-	-	99%	99%
Prophylactic Antibiotic Selection (Outpatient)	-	-	98%	98%
Prophylactic Antibiotic Stopped[5]	-	-	98%	98%
Prophylactic Antibiotic Timing[5]	-	-	99%	99%
Prophylactic Antibiotic Timing (Outpatient)	-	-	98%	98%
Urinary Catheter Removal[5]	-	-	98%	97%
Survey of Patients' Hospital Experiences				
Area Around Room 'Always' Quiet at Night	-	-	61%	61%
Doctors 'Always' Communicated Well	-	-	83%	82%
Home Recovery Information Given	-	-	86%	85%
Hospital Given 9 or 10 on 10 Point Scale	-	-	74%	71%
Meds 'Always' Explained Before Given	-	-	64%	64%
Nurses 'Always' Communicated Well	-	-	81%	79%
Pain 'Always' Well Controlled	-	-	73%	71%
Room and Bathroom 'Always' Clean	-	-	76%	73%
Timely Help 'Always' Received	-	-	71%	68%
Would Definitely Recommend Hospital	-	-	73%	71%
Use of Medical Imaging				
Cardiac Imaging Stress Test before Surgery	-	-	5.4%	5.3%
Combination Abdominal CT Scan	-	-	9.3%	10.5%
Combination Brain/Sinus CT Scan	-	-	2.6%	2.7%
Combination Chest CT Scan	-	-	4.6%	2.7%
Follow-up Mammogram/Ultrasound	-	-	8.4%	8.8%
Lumbar Spine MRI for Low Back Pain	-	-	38.7%	37.2%

Indiana University Health Morgan Hospital

2209 John R Wooden Dr
Martinsville, IN 46151
Phone: 765-349-6938
Fax: 765-349-5411
Type: Acute Care Hospitals
Emergency Services: Yes
Ownership: Voluntary non-profit - Private
Beds: 106

Key Personnel:

Radiology.............. Caryn C Anderson
Operating Room.............. Michael D Boyer
Hemotology Center.............. Vicki Elliff
Patient Relations.............. Debra Frenn
Chief of Medical Staff.............. Warren L Gray
CEO/President.............. Tom Laux
Infection Control.............. Deanna Skaggs

Measure	Cases	This Hosp.	State Avg.	U.S. Avg.
Blood Clot Prevention and Treatment				
Anticoagulation Overlap Therapy[2]	11	91%	92%	93%
ICU Venous Thromboembolism Prophylaxis[2]	56	77%	91%	92%
Incidence of Potentially Preventable VTE[2,7]	-	-	10%	10%
UFH with Dosages/Platelet Monitoring[1,2]	-	-	95%	97%
Venous Thromboembolism Prophylaxis[2]	82	91%	83%	85%
Warfarin Therapy Discharge Instructions[2]	11	91%	71%	75%
Chest Pain/Possible Heart Attack Care				
Aspirin Given Within 24 Hours of Arrival	42	100%	96%	96%
Fibrinolytic Meds Within 30 Min. of Arrival[7]	-	-	48%	58%
Average Time to ECG (minutes)	43	4	6	7
Average Time to Transfer (minutes)	13	50	46	60
Children's Asthma Care				
Received Home Management Plan of Care	-	-	-	88%
Received Reliever Medication	-	-	-	100%
Received Systemic Corticosteroids	-	-	-	100%
Emergency Department				
Admittance Decision Time (minutes)[2]	536	77	80	98
Head CT Results Within 45 Min. of Arrival[1]	-	-	60%	57%
Patients Who Left ER Before Being Seen	15,937	2%	2%	2%
Time from ER Arrival to Admit. (minutes)[2]	545	240	241	274
Time from ER Arrival to Discharge (minutes)	470	121	122	134
Time in ER Before Being Evaluated (minutes)	496	13	22	26
Time to Pain Meds for Fractures (minutes)	84	56	52	57
Heart Attack Care				
Aspirin Given at Discharge[1]	-	-	99%	99%
Fibrinolytic Meds Within 30 Min. of Arrival[7]	-	-	67%	54%
PCI Within 90 Minutes of Arrival[7]	-	-	97%	96%
Statin Prescribed at Discharge[1]	-	-	99%	98%
Heart Failure Care				
ACE Inhibitor or ARB for LVSD	22	95%	97%	97%
Discharge Instructions Given	47	100%	95%	94%
Evaluation of LVS Function	66	98%	99%	99%
Medicare Spending				
Medicare Spending per Patient (ratio)	-	1.05	1.01	0.98
Pneumonia Care				
Appropriate Initial Antibiotic Given	31	94%	95%	95%
Blood Culture Timing	57	100%	98%	98%
Pregnancy and Delivery Care				
Newborn Deliveries Scheduled Early[1]	-	-	5%	6%
Preventive Care				
Immunization for Influenza[2]	286	91%	91%	90%
Immunization for Pneumonia[2]	486	92%	92%	92%

NOTE: Hospital profiles are in alphabetical order by state, then city, then hospital within the city; Rankings exclude hospitals with less than 25 cases except for patient surveys which excludes hospitals with less than 100 cases; (a) 100-299 cases; (1) The number of cases/patients is too few to report; (2) Data submitted were based on a sample of cases/patients; (3) Results are based on a shorter time period than required; (4) Data suppressed by CMS for one or more quarters; (5) Results are not available for this reporting period; (6) Fewer than 100 patients completed the HCAHPS survey; (7) No cases met the criteria for this measure; (8) The lower limit of the confidence interval cannot be calculated if the number of observed infections equals zero; (9) No data are available from the state/territory for this reporting period; (10) The scores shown reflect fewer than 50 completed surveys; (11) There were discrepancies in the data collection process; (12) This measure does not apply to this hospital for this reporting period; (13) Results cannot be calculated for this reporting period; (14) The results for this state are combined with nearby states to protect confidentiality; Please refer to the User's Guide for a full explanation of data.

Measure	Cases	This Hosp.	State Avg.	U.S. Avg.
Stroke Care				
Anticoagulation Therapy for Atrial Fibrillation[1]	-	-	94%	95%
Antithrombotic Therapy Timing[1]	-	-	97%	98%
Assessed for Rehabilitation[1]	-	-	96%	97%
Discharged on Antithrombotic Therapy[1]	-	-	98%	99%
Discharged on Statin Medication[1]	-	-	91%	94%
Thrombolytic Therapy Timing[7]	-	-	54%	66%
Venous Thromboembolism Prophylaxis[1]	-	-	91%	94%
Written Stroke Educational Materials Given[1]	-	-	82%	88%
Surgical Care Improvement Project				
Appropriate Beta Blocker Usage[1,3]	-	-	98%	98%
Appropriate VTP Within 24 Hours[1,3]	-	-	98%	98%
Controlled Postoperative Blood Glucose[3,7]	-	-	97%	97%
Perioperative Temperature Management[1,3]	-	-	100%	100%
Prophylactic Antibiotic Selection[1,3]	-	-	99%	99%
Prophylactic Antibiotic Selection (Outpatient)	41	95%	98%	98%
Prophylactic Antibiotic Stopped[1,3]	-	-	98%	98%
Prophylactic Antibiotic Timing[1,3]	-	-	99%	99%
Prophylactic Antibiotic Timing (Outpatient)	24	92%	98%	98%
Urinary Catheter Removal[1,3]	-	-	98%	97%
Survey of Patients' Hospital Experiences				
Area Around Room 'Always' Quiet at Night	(a)	57%	61%	61%
Doctors 'Always' Communicated Well	(a)	85%	83%	82%
Home Recovery Information Given	(a)	86%	86%	85%
Hospital Given 9 or 10 on 10 Point Scale	(a)	68%	74%	71%
Meds 'Always' Explained Before Given	(a)	60%	64%	64%
Nurses 'Always' Communicated Well	(a)	83%	81%	79%
Pain 'Always' Well Controlled	(a)	79%	73%	71%
Room and Bathroom 'Always' Clean	(a)	78%	76%	73%
Timely Help 'Always' Received	(a)	72%	71%	68%
Would Definitely Recommend Hospital	(a)	59%	73%	71%
Use of Medical Imaging				
Cardiac Imaging Stress Test before Surgery	68	4.4%	5.4%	5.3%
Combination Abdominal CT Scan	270	8.9%	9.3%	10.5%
Combination Brain/Sinus CT Scan	174	0.6%	2.6%	2.7%
Combination Chest CT Scan	164	7.3%	4.6%	2.7%
Follow-up Mammogram/Ultrasound	328	11.9%	8.4%	8.8%
Lumbar Spine MRI for Low Back Pain[1]	-	-	38.7%	37.2%

Franciscan Saint Anthony Health - Michigan City

301 W Homer St
Michigan City, IN 46360
Phone: 219-879-8511
Fax: 219-877-1684
URL: www.samhc.org
Type: Acute Care Hospitals
Emergency Services: Yes
Ownership: Voluntary non-profit - Church
Beds: 310

Key Personnel:
Chief of Medical Staff. . . . . James Callaghan, MD
Quality Assurance . . . . Gloria Covert
Infection Control. . . . . Janene Gumz-Pulaski
Radiology. . . . . Cheryl Hoas
Operating Room. . . . . Maria Petti
CEO/President. . . . . Bruce Rampage
Cardiac Laboratory. . . . . Linda Rempala

Measure	Cases	This Hosp.	State Avg.	U.S. Avg.
Blood Clot Prevention and Treatment				
Anticoagulation Overlap Therapy[2]	42	74%	92%	93%
ICU Venous Thromboembolism Prophylaxis[2]	91	81%	91%	92%
Incidence of Potentially Preventable VTE[1,2]	-	-	10%	10%
UFH with Dosages/Platelet Monitoring[2]	22	100%	95%	97%
Venous Thromboembolism Prophylaxis[2]	358	70%	83%	85%
Warfarin Therapy Discharge Instructions[2]	35	89%	71%	75%
Chest Pain/Possible Heart Attack Care				
Aspirin Given Within 24 Hours of Arrival[1,3]	-	-	96%	96%
Fibrinolytic Meds Within 30 Min. of Arrival[5]	-	-	48%	58%
Average Time to ECG (minutes)[1,3]	-	-	6	7
Average Time to Transfer (minutes)[5]	-	-	46	60
Children's Asthma Care				
Received Home Management Plan of Care	-	-	-	88%
Received Reliever Medication	-	-	-	100%
Received Systemic Corticosteroids	-	-	-	100%
Emergency Department				
Admittance Decision Time (minutes)[2]	795	97	80	98
Head CT Results Within 45 Min. of Arrival[1]	-	-	60%	57%
Patients Who Left ER Before Being Seen	41,228	1%	2%	2%
Time from ER Arrival to Admit. (minutes)[2]	799	250	241	274
Time from ER Arrival to Discharge (minutes)	482	114	122	134
Time in ER Before Being Evaluated (minutes)	428	24	22	26
Time to Pain Meds for Fractures (minutes)	130	44	52	57
Heart Attack Care				
Aspirin Given at Discharge	105	99%	99%	99%
Fibrinolytic Meds Within 30 Min. of Arrival[7]	-	-	67%	54%
PCI Within 90 Minutes of Arrival	19	100%	97%	96%
Statin Prescribed at Discharge	100	99%	99%	98%
Heart Failure Care				
ACE Inhibitor or ARB for LVSD	90	100%	97%	97%
Discharge Instructions Given	199	99%	95%	94%
Evaluation of LVS Function	244	100%	99%	99%
Medicare Spending				
Medicare Spending per Patient (ratio)	-	1.01	1.01	0.98
Pneumonia Care				
Appropriate Initial Antibiotic Given	97	100%	95%	95%
Blood Culture Timing	81	100%	98%	98%
Pregnancy and Delivery Care				
Newborn Deliveries Scheduled Early[2]	24	0%	5%	6%
Preventive Care				
Immunization for Influenza[2]	567	96%	91%	90%
Immunization for Pneumonia[2]	734	97%	92%	92%
Stroke Care				
Anticoagulation Therapy for Atrial Fibrillation[1]	-	-	94%	95%
Antithrombotic Therapy Timing	52	94%	97%	98%
Assessed for Rehabilitation	68	96%	96%	97%
Discharged on Antithrombotic Therapy	66	98%	98%	99%
Discharged on Statin Medication	43	88%	91%	94%
Thrombolytic Therapy Timing[1]	-	-	54%	66%
Venous Thromboembolism Prophylaxis	71	76%	91%	94%
Written Stroke Educational Materials Given	39	97%	82%	88%
Surgical Care Improvement Project				
Appropriate Beta Blocker Usage	138	100%	98%	98%
Appropriate VTP Within 24 Hours	274	99%	98%	98%
Controlled Postoperative Blood Glucose	31	100%	97%	97%
Perioperative Temperature Management	357	99%	100%	100%
Prophylactic Antibiotic Selection	258	100%	99%	99%
Prophylactic Antibiotic Selection (Outpatient)	300	99%	98%	98%
Prophylactic Antibiotic Stopped	246	100%	98%	98%
Prophylactic Antibiotic Timing	259	99%	99%	99%
Prophylactic Antibiotic Timing (Outpatient)	226	97%	98%	98%
Urinary Catheter Removal	204	100%	98%	97%
Survey of Patients' Hospital Experiences				
Area Around Room 'Always' Quiet at Night	300+	57%	61%	61%
Doctors 'Always' Communicated Well	300+	80%	83%	82%
Home Recovery Information Given	300+	85%	86%	85%
Hospital Given 9 or 10 on 10 Point Scale	300+	71%	74%	71%
Meds 'Always' Explained Before Given	300+	62%	64%	64%
Nurses 'Always' Communicated Well	300+	80%	81%	79%
Pain 'Always' Well Controlled	300+	74%	73%	71%
Room and Bathroom 'Always' Clean	300+	76%	76%	73%
Timely Help 'Always' Received	300+	71%	71%	68%
Would Definitely Recommend Hospital	300+	68%	73%	71%
Use of Medical Imaging				
Cardiac Imaging Stress Test before Surgery	340	2.4%	5.4%	5.3%
Combination Abdominal CT Scan	785	26.4%	9.3%	10.5%
Combination Brain/Sinus CT Scan	729	4.4%	2.6%	2.7%
Combination Chest CT Scan	311	31.2%	4.6%	2.7%
Follow-up Mammogram/Ultrasound	1,466	3.3%	8.4%	8.8%
Lumbar Spine MRI for Low Back Pain	155	36.1%	38.7%	37.2%

Saint Joseph Regional Medical Center

5215 Holy Cross Pkwy
Mishawaka, IN 46545
Phone: 574-335-5000
Fax: 574-247-5401
URL: www.sjmed.com
Type: Acute Care Hospitals
Emergency Services: Yes
Ownership: Voluntary non-profit - Private
Beds: 125

Key Personnel:
Chief of Medical Staff. . . . . Stephen Anderson, MD, MMM
CEO/President. . . . . Albert Gutierrez
Emergency Room . . . . Bruce Harley
Chair/CEO. . . . . Abraham Marcus

Measure	Cases	This Hosp.	State Avg.	U.S. Avg.
Blood Clot Prevention and Treatment				
Anticoagulation Overlap Therapy[2]	117	100%	92%	93%
ICU Venous Thromboembolism Prophylaxis[2]	71	94%	91%	92%
Incidence of Potentially Preventable VTE[2]	20	0%	10%	10%
UFH with Dosages/Platelet Monitoring[2]	60	100%	95%	97%
Venous Thromboembolism Prophylaxis[2]	334	83%	83%	85%
Warfarin Therapy Discharge Instructions[2]	86	69%	71%	75%
Chest Pain/Possible Heart Attack Care				
Aspirin Given Within 24 Hours of Arrival[5]	-	-	96%	96%
Fibrinolytic Meds Within 30 Min. of Arrival[5]	-	-	48%	58%
Average Time to ECG (minutes)[5]	-	-	6	7
Average Time to Transfer (minutes)[5]	-	-	46	60
Children's Asthma Care				
Received Home Management Plan of Care	-	-	-	88%
Received Reliever Medication	-	-	-	100%
Received Systemic Corticosteroids	-	-	-	100%
Emergency Department				
Admittance Decision Time (minutes)[2]	620	81	80	98
Head CT Results Within 45 Min. of Arrival[1,3]	-	-	60%	57%
Patients Who Left ER Before Being Seen	58,352	1%	2%	2%
Time from ER Arrival to Admit. (minutes)[2]	625	263	241	274
Time from ER Arrival to Discharge (minutes)	398	141	122	134
Time in ER Before Being Evaluated (minutes)	425	17	22	26
Time to Pain Meds for Fractures (minutes)	154	58	52	57
Heart Attack Care				
Aspirin Given at Discharge	242	100%	99%	99%
Fibrinolytic Meds Within 30 Min. of Arrival[7]	-	-	67%	54%
PCI Within 90 Minutes of Arrival	56	96%	97%	96%
Statin Prescribed at Discharge	237	99%	99%	98%
Heart Failure Care				
ACE Inhibitor or ARB for LVSD	68	100%	97%	97%
Discharge Instructions Given	277	98%	95%	94%
Evaluation of LVS Function	364	100%	99%	99%
Medicare Spending				
Medicare Spending per Patient (ratio)	-	1.01	1.01	0.98
Pneumonia Care				
Appropriate Initial Antibiotic Given	211	99%	95%	95%
Blood Culture Timing	344	99%	98%	98%
Pregnancy and Delivery Care				
Newborn Deliveries Scheduled Early[2]	27	0%	5%	6%
Preventive Care				
Immunization for Influenza[2]	550	90%	91%	90%
Immunization for Pneumonia[2]	704	82%	92%	92%
Stroke Care				
Anticoagulation Therapy for Atrial Fibrillation	21	100%	94%	95%
Antithrombotic Therapy Timing	138	98%	97%	98%
Assessed for Rehabilitation	179	100%	96%	97%
Discharged on Antithrombotic Therapy	159	99%	98%	99%
Discharged on Statin Medication	134	99%	91%	94%
Thrombolytic Therapy Timing	11	100%	54%	66%
Venous Thromboembolism Prophylaxis	175	98%	91%	94%
Written Stroke Educational Materials Given	92	88%	82%	88%
Surgical Care Improvement Project				
Appropriate Beta Blocker Usage	362	100%	98%	98%
Appropriate VTP Within 24 Hours	1,055	100%	98%	98%
Controlled Postoperative Blood Glucose	124	98%	97%	97%
Perioperative Temperature Management	1,814	100%	100%	100%
Prophylactic Antibiotic Selection	1,545	99%	99%	99%
Prophylactic Antibiotic Selection (Outpatient)	326	96%	98%	98%
Prophylactic Antibiotic Stopped	1,545	100%	98%	98%
Prophylactic Antibiotic Timing	1,547	100%	99%	99%
Prophylactic Antibiotic Timing (Outpatient)	326	99%	98%	98%
Urinary Catheter Removal	212	100%	98%	97%
Survey of Patients' Hospital Experiences				
Area Around Room 'Always' Quiet at Night	300+	64%	61%	61%
Doctors 'Always' Communicated Well	300+	78%	83%	82%
Home Recovery Information Given	300+	86%	86%	85%
Hospital Given 9 or 10 on 10 Point Scale	300+	76%	74%	71%
Meds 'Always' Explained Before Given	300+	58%	64%	64%
Nurses 'Always' Communicated Well	300+	76%	81%	79%
Pain 'Always' Well Controlled	300+	69%	73%	71%

NOTE: Hospital profiles are in alphabetical order by state, then city, then hospital within the city; Rankings exclude hospitals with less than 25 cases except for patient surveys which excludes hospitals with less than 100 cases; (a) 100-299 cases; (1) The number of cases/patients is too few to report; (2) Data submitted were based on a sample of cases/patients; (3) Results are based on a shorter time period than required; (4) Data suppressed by CMS for one or more quarters; (5) Results are not available for this reporting period; (6) Fewer than 100 patients completed the HCAHPS survey; (7) No cases met the criteria for this measure; (8) The lower limit of the confidence interval cannot be calculated if the number of observed infections equals zero; (9) No data are available from the state/territory for this reporting period; (10) The scores shown reflect fewer than 50 completed surveys; (11) There were discrepancies in the data collection process; (12) This measure does not apply to this hospital for this reporting period; (13) Results cannot be calculated for this reporting period; (14) The results for this state are combined with nearby states to protect confidentiality; Please refer to the User's Guide for a full explanation of data.

Room and Bathroom 'Always' Clean	300+	71%	76%	73%
Timely Help 'Always' Received	300+	62%	71%	68%
Would Definitely Recommend Hospital	300+	77%	73%	71%
Use of Medical Imaging				
Cardiac Imaging Stress Test before Surgery	375	6.1%	5.4%	5.3%
Combination Abdominal CT Scan	922	3.0%	9.3%	10.5%
Combination Brain/Sinus CT Scan	857	2.7%	2.6%	2.7%
Combination Chest CT Scan	369	0.8%	4.6%	2.7%
Follow-up Mammogram/Ultrasound	1,564	10.9%	8.4%	8.8%
Lumbar Spine MRI for Low Back Pain[1]	-	-	38.7%	37.2%

Unity Medical & Surgical Hospital

4455 Edison Lakes Pkwy Phone: 574-231-6800
Mishawaka, IN 46545
URL: www.physicianshospitalsystem.net
Type: Acute Care Hospitals Emergency Services: No
Ownership: Proprietary
Key Personnel:
President/CEO . . . . Cameron Gilbert, PhD

Measure	Cases	This Hosp.	State Avg.	U.S. Avg.
Blood Clot Prevention and Treatment				
Anticoagulation Overlap Therapy[2,7]	-	-	92%	93%
ICU Venous Thromboembolism Prophylaxis[2,7]	-	-	91%	92%
Incidence of Potentially Preventable VTE[2,7]	-	-	10%	10%
UFH with Dosages/Platelet Monitoring[2,7]	-	-	95%	97%
Venous Thromboembolism Prophylaxis[2]	103	100%	83%	85%
Warfarin Therapy Discharge Instructions[2,7]	-	-	71%	75%
Chest Pain/Possible Heart Attack Care				
Aspirin Given Within 24 Hours of Arrival[5]	-	-	96%	96%
Fibrinolytic Meds Within 30 Min. of Arrival[5]	-	-	48%	58%
Average Time to ECG (minutes)[5]	-	-	6	7
Average Time to Transfer (minutes)[5]	-	-	46	60
Children's Asthma Care				
Received Home Management Plan of Care	-	-	-	88%
Received Reliever Medication	-	-	-	100%
Received Systemic Corticosteroids	-	-	-	100%
Emergency Department				
Admittance Decision Time (minutes)[2,7]	-	-	80	98
Head CT Results Within 45 Min. of Arrival[5]	-	-	60%	57%
Patients Who Left ER Before Being Seen[5]	-	-	2%	2%
Time from ER Arrival to Admit. (minutes)[2,7]	-	-	241	274
Time from ER Arrival to Discharge (minutes)[5]	-	-	122	134
Time in ER Before Being Evaluated (minutes)[5]	-	-	22	26
Time to Pain Meds for Fractures (minutes)[5]	-	-	52	57
Heart Attack Care				
Aspirin Given at Discharge[3,7]	-	-	99%	99%
Fibrinolytic Meds Within 30 Min. of Arrival[3,7]	-	-	67%	54%
PCI Within 90 Minutes of Arrival[3,7]	-	-	97%	96%
Statin Prescribed at Discharge[3,7]	-	-	99%	98%
Heart Failure Care				
ACE Inhibitor or ARB for LVSD[5]	-	-	97%	97%
Discharge Instructions Given[5]	-	-	95%	94%
Evaluation of LVS Function[5]	-	-	99%	99%
Medicare Spending				
Medicare Spending per Patient (ratio)	-	1.49	1.01	0.98
Pneumonia Care				
Appropriate Initial Antibiotic Given[3,7]	-	-	95%	95%
Blood Culture Timing[3,7]	-	-	98%	98%
Pregnancy and Delivery Care				
Newborn Deliveries Scheduled Early[7]	-	-	5%	6%
Preventive Care				
Immunization for Influenza[2]	212	91%	91%	90%
Immunization for Pneumonia[2]	119	87%	92%	92%
Stroke Care				
Anticoagulation Therapy for Atrial Fibrillation[5]	-	-	94%	95%
Antithrombotic Therapy Timing[5]	-	-	97%	98%
Assessed for Rehabilitation[5]	-	-	96%	97%
Discharged on Antithrombotic Therapy[5]	-	-	98%	99%
Discharged on Statin Medication[5]	-	-	91%	94%
Thrombolytic Therapy Timing[5]	-	-	54%	66%
Venous Thromboembolism Prophylaxis[5]	-	-	91%	94%
Written Stroke Educational Materials Given[5]	-	-	82%	88%
Surgical Care Improvement Project				
Appropriate Beta Blocker Usage[2]	25	100%	98%	98%
Appropriate VTP Within 24 Hours[2]	39	100%	98%	98%
Controlled Postoperative Blood Glucose[2,7]	-	-	97%	97%
Perioperative Temperature Management[2]	130	100%	100%	100%
Prophylactic Antibiotic Selection[2]	108	100%	99%	99%
Prophylactic Antibiotic Selection (Outpatient)[5]	-	-	98%	98%
Prophylactic Antibiotic Stopped[2]	103	90%	98%	98%
Prophylactic Antibiotic Timing[2]	108	98%	99%	99%
Prophylactic Antibiotic Timing (Outpatient)[5]	-	-	98%	98%
Urinary Catheter Removal[1,2]	-	-	98%	97%
Survey of Patients' Hospital Experiences				
Area Around Room 'Always' Quiet at Night	(a)	76%	61%	61%
Doctors 'Always' Communicated Well	(a)	81%	83%	82%
Home Recovery Information Given	(a)	91%	86%	85%
Hospital Given 9 or 10 on 10 Point Scale	(a)	78%	74%	71%
Meds 'Always' Explained Before Given	(a)	67%	64%	64%
Nurses 'Always' Communicated Well	(a)	86%	81%	79%
Pain 'Always' Well Controlled	(a)	78%	73%	71%
Room and Bathroom 'Always' Clean	(a)	80%	76%	73%
Timely Help 'Always' Received	(a)	79%	71%	68%
Would Definitely Recommend Hospital	(a)	82%	73%	71%
Use of Medical Imaging				
Cardiac Imaging Stress Test before Surgery[7]	-	-	5.4%	5.3%
Combination Abdominal CT Scan[1]	-	-	9.3%	10.5%
Combination Brain/Sinus CT Scan[1]	-	-	2.6%	2.7%
Combination Chest CT Scan[1]	-	-	4.6%	2.7%
Follow-up Mammogram/Ultrasound[7]	-	-	8.4%	8.8%
Lumbar Spine MRI for Low Back Pain	62	35.5%	38.7%	37.2%

Indiana University Health White Memorial Hospital

720 South Sixth St Phone: 574-583-7111
Monticello, IN 47960
E-mail: tcreamer@whitecmh.org
URL: www.whitecmh.org
Type: Critical Access Hospitals Emergency Services: Yes
Ownership: Voluntary non-profit - Private Beds: 25
Key Personnel:
Chief of Medical Staff . . . . David Bailey
Operating Room. . . . . Joni Diener
Quality Assurance . . . . Dave Ley
Infection Control. . . . . Robin Smith
President . . . . Dorothy Snowberger
Emergency Room . . . . Denise Voetz

Measure	Cases	This Hosp.	State Avg.	U.S. Avg.
Blood Clot Prevention and Treatment				
Anticoagulation Overlap Therapy[5]	-	-	92%	93%
ICU Venous Thromboembolism Prophylaxis[5]	-	-	91%	92%
Incidence of Potentially Preventable VTE[5]	-	-	10%	10%
UFH with Dosages/Platelet Monitoring[5]	-	-	95%	97%
Venous Thromboembolism Prophylaxis[5]	-	-	83%	85%
Warfarin Therapy Discharge Instructions[5]	-	-	71%	75%
Chest Pain/Possible Heart Attack Care				
Aspirin Given Within 24 Hours of Arrival[5]	-	-	96%	96%
Fibrinolytic Meds Within 30 Min. of Arrival[5]	-	-	48%	58%
Average Time to ECG (minutes)[5]	-	-	6	7
Average Time to Transfer (minutes)[5]	-	-	46	60
Children's Asthma Care				
Received Home Management Plan of Care	-	-	-	88%
Received Reliever Medication	-	-	-	100%
Received Systemic Corticosteroids	-	-	-	100%
Emergency Department				
Admittance Decision Time (minutes)[5]	-	-	80	98
Head CT Results Within 45 Min. of Arrival[5]	-	-	60%	57%
Patients Who Left ER Before Being Seen	14,187	0%	2%	2%
Time from ER Arrival to Admit. (minutes)[5]	-	-	241	274
Time from ER Arrival to Discharge (minutes)[5]	-	-	122	134
Time in ER Before Being Evaluated (minutes)[5]	-	-	22	26
Time to Pain Meds for Fractures (minutes)[5]	-	-	52	57
Heart Attack Care				
Aspirin Given at Discharge[3,7]	-	-	99%	99%
Fibrinolytic Meds Within 30 Min. of Arrival[5]	-	-	67%	54%
PCI Within 90 Minutes of Arrival[5]	-	-	97%	96%
Statin Prescribed at Discharge[1,3]	-	-	99%	98%
Heart Failure Care				
ACE Inhibitor or ARB for LVSD[1]	-	-	97%	97%
Discharge Instructions Given	29	100%	95%	94%
Evaluation of LVS Function	45	96%	99%	99%
Medicare Spending				
Medicare Spending per Patient (ratio)	-	-	1.01	0.98
Pneumonia Care				
Appropriate Initial Antibiotic Given	41	90%	95%	95%
Blood Culture Timing	53	100%	98%	98%
Pregnancy and Delivery Care				
Newborn Deliveries Scheduled Early[5]	-	-	5%	6%
Preventive Care				
Immunization for Influenza[5]	-	-	91%	90%
Immunization for Pneumonia[5]	-	-	92%	92%
Stroke Care				
Anticoagulation Therapy for Atrial Fibrillation[5]	-	-	94%	95%
Antithrombotic Therapy Timing[5]	-	-	97%	98%
Assessed for Rehabilitation[5]	-	-	96%	97%
Discharged on Antithrombotic Therapy[5]	-	-	98%	99%
Discharged on Statin Medication[5]	-	-	91%	94%
Thrombolytic Therapy Timing[5]	-	-	54%	66%
Venous Thromboembolism Prophylaxis[5]	-	-	91%	94%
Written Stroke Educational Materials Given[5]	-	-	82%	88%
Surgical Care Improvement Project				
Appropriate Beta Blocker Usage[5]	-	-	98%	98%
Appropriate VTP Within 24 Hours[5]	-	-	98%	98%
Controlled Postoperative Blood Glucose[5]	-	-	97%	97%
Perioperative Temperature Management[1,3]	-	-	100%	100%
Prophylactic Antibiotic Selection[1,3]	-	-	99%	99%
Prophylactic Antibiotic Selection (Outpatient)[5]	-	-	98%	98%
Prophylactic Antibiotic Stopped[1,3]	-	-	98%	98%
Prophylactic Antibiotic Timing[1,3]	-	-	99%	99%
Prophylactic Antibiotic Timing (Outpatient)[5]	-	-	98%	98%
Urinary Catheter Removal[1,3]	-	-	98%	97%
Survey of Patients' Hospital Experiences				
Area Around Room 'Always' Quiet at Night	(a)	58%	61%	61%
Doctors 'Always' Communicated Well	(a)	81%	83%	82%
Home Recovery Information Given	(a)	83%	86%	85%
Hospital Given 9 or 10 on 10 Point Scale	(a)	72%	74%	71%
Meds 'Always' Explained Before Given	(a)	63%	64%	64%
Nurses 'Always' Communicated Well	(a)	77%	81%	79%
Pain 'Always' Well Controlled	(a)	63%	73%	71%
Room and Bathroom 'Always' Clean	(a)	77%	76%	73%
Timely Help 'Always' Received	(a)	70%	71%	68%
Would Definitely Recommend Hospital	(a)	66%	73%	71%
Use of Medical Imaging				
Cardiac Imaging Stress Test before Surgery	76	0.0%	5.4%	5.3%
Combination Abdominal CT Scan	417	4.6%	9.3%	10.5%
Combination Brain/Sinus CT Scan	507	2.4%	2.6%	2.7%
Combination Chest CT Scan	177	2.8%	4.6%	2.7%
Follow-up Mammogram/Ultrasound	427	7.3%	8.4%	8.8%
Lumbar Spine MRI for Low Back Pain[1]	-	-	38.7%	37.2%

Franciscan Saint Francis Health - Mooresville

1201 Hadley Rd Phone: 317-831-1160
Mooresville, IN 46158 Fax: 317-831-9315
URL: www.stfrancishospitals.org
Type: Acute Care Hospitals Emergency Services: Yes
Ownership: Voluntary non-profit - Church Beds: 64
Key Personnel:
CEO/President. . . . . Robert J Brody
Chief of Medical Staff . . . . Alan Gillespie
Radiology. . . . . Katie Lee, RT(T)

Measure	Cases	This Hosp.	State Avg.	U.S. Avg.
Blood Clot Prevention and Treatment				
Anticoagulation Overlap Therapy[2]	17	82%	92%	93%
ICU Venous Thromboembolism Prophylaxis[2]	36	100%	91%	92%
Incidence of Potentially Preventable VTE[1,2]	-	-	10%	10%
UFH with Dosages/Platelet Monitoring[1,2]	-	-	95%	97%
Venous Thromboembolism Prophylaxis[2]	140	91%	83%	85%
Warfarin Therapy Discharge Instructions[2]	12	75%	71%	75%
Chest Pain/Possible Heart Attack Care				
Aspirin Given Within 24 Hours of Arrival	93	96%	96%	96%
Fibrinolytic Meds Within 30 Min. of Arrival[7]	-	-	48%	58%

NOTE: *Hospital profiles are in alphabetical order by state, then city, then hospital within the city; Rankings exclude hospitals with less than 25 cases except for patient surveys which excludes hospitals with less than 100 cases; (a) 100-299 cases; (1) The number of cases/patients is too few to report; (2) Data submitted were based on a sample of cases/patients; (3) Results are based on a shorter time period than required; (4) Data suppressed by CMS for one or more quarters; (5) Results are not available for this reporting period; (6) Fewer than 100 patients completed the HCAHPS survey; (7) No cases met the criteria for this measure; (8) The lower limit of the confidence interval cannot be calculated if the number of observed infections equals zero; (9) No data are available from the state/territory for this reporting period; (10) The scores shown reflect fewer than 50 completed surveys; (11) There were discrepancies in the data collection process; (12) This measure does not apply to this hospital for this reporting period; (13) Results cannot be calculated for this reporting period; (14) The results for this state are combined with nearby states to protect confidentiality; Please refer to the User's Guide for a full explanation of data.*

Average Time to ECG (minutes)	100	3	6	7
Average Time to Transfer (minutes)	18	42	46	60
Children's Asthma Care				
Received Home Management Plan of Care	-	-	-	88%
Received Reliever Medication	-	-	-	100%
Received Systemic Corticosteroids	-	-	-	100%
Emergency Department				
Admittance Decision Time (minutes)[2]	370	191	80	98
Head CT Results Within 45 Min. of Arrival[1]	-	-	60%	57%
Patients Who Left ER Before Being Seen	29,628	0%	2%	2%
Time from ER Arrival to Admit. (minutes)[2]	380	247	241	274
Time from ER Arrival to Discharge (minutes)	416	114	122	134
Time in ER Before Being Evaluated (minutes)	438	24	22	26
Time to Pain Meds for Fractures (minutes)	64	40	52	57
Heart Attack Care				
Aspirin Given at Discharge[5]	-	-	99%	99%
Fibrinolytic Meds Within 30 Min. of Arrival[5]	-	-	67%	54%
PCI Within 90 Minutes of Arrival[5]	-	-	97%	96%
Statin Prescribed at Discharge[5]	-	-	99%	98%
Heart Failure Care				
ACE Inhibitor or ARB for LVSD[1]	-	-	97%	97%
Discharge Instructions Given	17	94%	95%	94%
Evaluation of LVS Function	25	100%	99%	99%
Medicare Spending				
Medicare Spending per Patient (ratio)	-	0.94	1.01	0.98
Pneumonia Care				
Appropriate Initial Antibiotic Given	92	89%	95%	95%
Blood Culture Timing	127	98%	98%	98%
Pregnancy and Delivery Care				
Newborn Deliveries Scheduled Early[2]	36	58%	5%	6%
Preventive Care				
Immunization for Influenza[2]	737	99%	91%	90%
Immunization for Pneumonia[2]	989	99%	92%	92%
Stroke Care				
Anticoagulation Therapy for Atrial Fibrillation[3,7]	-	-	94%	95%
Antithrombotic Therapy Timing[1,3]	-	-	97%	98%
Assessed for Rehabilitation[3,7]	-	-	96%	97%
Discharged on Antithrombotic Therapy[3,7]	-	-	98%	99%
Discharged on Statin Medication[3,7]	-	-	91%	94%
Thrombolytic Therapy Timing[3,7]	-	-	54%	66%
Venous Thromboembolism Prophylaxis[1,3]	-	-	91%	94%
Written Stroke Educational Materials Given[3,7]	-	-	82%	88%
Surgical Care Improvement Project				
Appropriate Beta Blocker Usage[2]	414	99%	98%	98%
Appropriate VTP Within 24 Hours[2]	1,063	100%	98%	98%
Controlled Postoperative Blood Glucose[2,7]	-	-	97%	97%
Perioperative Temperature Management[2]	1,200	100%	100%	100%
Prophylactic Antibiotic Selection[2]	892	100%	99%	99%
Prophylactic Antibiotic Selection (Outpatient)	58	100%	98%	98%
Prophylactic Antibiotic Stopped[2]	878	98%	98%	98%
Prophylactic Antibiotic Timing[2]	892	99%	99%	99%
Prophylactic Antibiotic Timing (Outpatient)	57	100%	98%	98%
Urinary Catheter Removal[2]	1,074	100%	98%	97%
Survey of Patients' Hospital Experiences				
Area Around Room 'Always' Quiet at Night	300+	60%	61%	61%
Doctors 'Always' Communicated Well	300+	86%	83%	82%
Home Recovery Information Given	300+	91%	86%	85%
Hospital Given 9 or 10 on 10 Point Scale	300+	84%	74%	71%
Meds 'Always' Explained Before Given	300+	69%	64%	64%
Nurses 'Always' Communicated Well	300+	83%	81%	79%
Pain 'Always' Well Controlled	300+	77%	73%	71%
Room and Bathroom 'Always' Clean	300+	81%	76%	73%
Timely Help 'Always' Received	300+	70%	71%	68%
Would Definitely Recommend Hospital	300+	86%	73%	71%
Use of Medical Imaging				
Cardiac Imaging Stress Test before Surgery	341	5.0%	5.4%	5.3%
Combination Abdominal CT Scan	706	7.4%	9.3%	10.5%
Combination Brain/Sinus CT Scan	450	1.1%	2.6%	2.7%
Combination Chest CT Scan	346	1.7%	4.6%	2.7%
Follow-up Mammogram/Ultrasound	1,259	6.9%	8.4%	8.8%
Lumbar Spine MRI for Low Back Pain	123	40.7%	38.7%	37.2%

Indiana University Health Ball Memorial Hospital

2401 University Ave
Muncie, IN 47303
Phone: 765-747-3111
Fax: 765-747-3404
URL: www.accesschs.org/baal-memorial-l
Type: Acute Care Hospitals
Emergency Services: Yes
Ownership: Voluntary non-profit - Private
Beds: 350

Key Personnel:

Operating Room. . . . . Shirley Foster
CEO/President. . . . . Michael Haley
Quality Assurance . . . . Mike Hawkins
Cardiac Laboratory. . . . . Marian Kritcer
Infection Control. . . . . Michael Langona
Radiology. . . . . Charles Leiphart, MD
Emergency Room . . . . John Nahre, MD
Intensive Care Unit. . . . . Alexis Neal

Measure	Cases	This Hosp.	State Avg.	U.S. Avg.
Blood Clot Prevention and Treatment				
Anticoagulation Overlap Therapy[2]	133	95%	92%	93%
ICU Venous Thromboembolism Prophylaxis[2]	77	94%	91%	92%
Incidence of Potentially Preventable VTE[2]	28	7%	10%	10%
UFH with Dosages/Platelet Monitoring[2]	96	100%	95%	97%
Venous Thromboembolism Prophylaxis[2]	318	88%	83%	85%
Warfarin Therapy Discharge Instructions[2]	102	75%	71%	75%
Chest Pain/Possible Heart Attack Care				
Aspirin Given Within 24 Hours of Arrival[3,7]	-	-	96%	96%
Fibrinolytic Meds Within 30 Min. of Arrival[5]	-	-	48%	58%
Average Time to ECG (minutes)[3,7]	-	-	6	7
Average Time to Transfer (minutes)[5]	-	-	46	60
Children's Asthma Care				
Received Home Management Plan of Care	-	-	-	88%
Received Reliever Medication	-	-	-	100%
Received Systemic Corticosteroids	-	-	-	100%
Emergency Department				
Admittance Decision Time (minutes)[2]	569	109	80	98
Head CT Results Within 45 Min. of Arrival[1]	-	-	60%	57%
Patients Who Left ER Before Being Seen	61,367	4%	2%	2%
Time from ER Arrival to Admit. (minutes)[2]	573	300	241	274
Time from ER Arrival to Discharge (minutes)	403	174	122	134
Time in ER Before Being Evaluated (minutes)	453	32	22	26
Time to Pain Meds for Fractures (minutes)	170	61	52	57
Heart Attack Care				
Aspirin Given at Discharge	381	98%	99%	99%
Fibrinolytic Meds Within 30 Min. of Arrival[7]	-	-	67%	54%
PCI Within 90 Minutes of Arrival	70	99%	97%	96%
Statin Prescribed at Discharge	373	100%	99%	98%
Heart Failure Care				
ACE Inhibitor or ARB for LVSD[2]	74	91%	97%	97%
Discharge Instructions Given[2]	218	100%	95%	94%
Evaluation of LVS Function[2]	275	100%	99%	99%
Medicare Spending				
Medicare Spending per Patient (ratio)	-	1.01	1.01	0.98
Pneumonia Care				
Appropriate Initial Antibiotic Given[2]	70	99%	95%	95%
Blood Culture Timing[2]	131	96%	98%	98%
Pregnancy and Delivery Care				
Newborn Deliveries Scheduled Early[2]	31	10%	5%	6%
Preventive Care				
Immunization for Influenza[2]	560	95%	91%	90%
Immunization for Pneumonia[2]	670	92%	92%	92%
Stroke Care				
Anticoagulation Therapy for Atrial Fibrillation[2]	13	100%	94%	95%
Antithrombotic Therapy Timing[2]	84	98%	97%	98%
Assessed for Rehabilitation[2]	101	100%	96%	97%
Discharged on Antithrombotic Therapy[2]	89	100%	98%	99%
Discharged on Statin Medication[2]	61	95%	91%	94%
Thrombolytic Therapy Timing[1,2]	-	-	54%	66%
Venous Thromboembolism Prophylaxis[2]	107	98%	91%	94%
Written Stroke Educational Materials Given[2]	56	84%	82%	88%
Surgical Care Improvement Project				
Appropriate Beta Blocker Usage[2]	388	99%	98%	98%
Appropriate VTP Within 24 Hours[2]	755	99%	98%	98%
Controlled Postoperative Blood Glucose[2]	116	99%	97%	97%
Perioperative Temperature Management[2]	838	100%	100%	100%
Prophylactic Antibiotic Selection[2]	790	100%	99%	99%
Prophylactic Antibiotic Selection (Outpatient)	419	99%	98%	98%
Prophylactic Antibiotic Stopped[2]	778	99%	98%	98%
Prophylactic Antibiotic Timing[2]	790	99%	99%	99%
Prophylactic Antibiotic Timing (Outpatient)	420	100%	98%	98%
Urinary Catheter Removal[2]	764	99%	98%	97%
Survey of Patients' Hospital Experiences				
Area Around Room 'Always' Quiet at Night	300+	59%	61%	61%
Doctors 'Always' Communicated Well	300+	78%	83%	82%
Home Recovery Information Given	300+	83%	86%	85%
Hospital Given 9 or 10 on 10 Point Scale	300+	67%	74%	71%
Meds 'Always' Explained Before Given	300+	62%	64%	64%
Nurses 'Always' Communicated Well	300+	79%	81%	79%
Pain 'Always' Well Controlled	300+	72%	73%	71%
Room and Bathroom 'Always' Clean	300+	72%	76%	73%
Timely Help 'Always' Received	300+	63%	71%	68%
Would Definitely Recommend Hospital	300+	61%	73%	71%
Use of Medical Imaging				
Cardiac Imaging Stress Test before Surgery	419	5.7%	5.4%	5.3%
Combination Abdominal CT Scan	1,302	2.2%	9.3%	10.5%
Combination Brain/Sinus CT Scan	1,175	2.5%	2.6%	2.7%
Combination Chest CT Scan	1,034	1.0%	4.6%	2.7%
Follow-up Mammogram/Ultrasound	2,414	8.2%	8.4%	8.8%
Lumbar Spine MRI for Low Back Pain	86	39.5%	38.7%	37.2%

Community Hospital

901 Macarthur Blvd
Munster, IN 46321
Phone: 219-836-1600
Fax: 219-836-6380
URL: www.comhs.org/community
Type: Acute Care Hospitals
Emergency Services: Yes
Ownership: Voluntary non-profit - Private
Beds: 354

Key Personnel:

Quality Assurance . . . . Patricia Baldwin
Emergency Room . . . . Robert L Cavens, MD
President/CEO. . . . . Donald P. Fesko

Measure	Cases	This Hosp.	State Avg.	U.S. Avg.
Blood Clot Prevention and Treatment				
Anticoagulation Overlap Therapy[2]	124	96%	92%	93%
ICU Venous Thromboembolism Prophylaxis[2]	71	93%	91%	92%
Incidence of Potentially Preventable VTE[2]	11	0%	10%	10%
UFH with Dosages/Platelet Monitoring[2]	68	100%	95%	97%
Venous Thromboembolism Prophylaxis[2]	340	87%	83%	85%
Warfarin Therapy Discharge Instructions[2]	83	94%	71%	75%
Chest Pain/Possible Heart Attack Care				
Aspirin Given Within 24 Hours of Arrival[5]	-	-	96%	96%
Fibrinolytic Meds Within 30 Min. of Arrival[5]	-	-	48%	58%
Average Time to ECG (minutes)[5]	-	-	6	7
Average Time to Transfer (minutes)[5]	-	-	46	60
Children's Asthma Care				
Received Home Management Plan of Care	-	-	-	88%
Received Reliever Medication	-	-	-	100%
Received Systemic Corticosteroids	-	-	-	100%
Emergency Department				
Admittance Decision Time (minutes)[2]	649	146	80	98
Head CT Results Within 45 Min. of Arrival[1]	-	-	60%	57%
Patients Who Left ER Before Being Seen	65,403	1%	2%	2%
Time from ER Arrival to Admit. (minutes)[2]	649	274	241	274
Time from ER Arrival to Discharge (minutes)	381	129	122	134
Time in ER Before Being Evaluated (minutes)	425	29	22	26
Time to Pain Meds for Fractures (minutes)	164	45	52	57
Heart Attack Care				
Aspirin Given at Discharge	170	99%	99%	99%
Fibrinolytic Meds Within 30 Min. of Arrival[7]	-	-	67%	54%
PCI Within 90 Minutes of Arrival	32	100%	97%	96%
Statin Prescribed at Discharge	169	98%	99%	98%
Heart Failure Care				
ACE Inhibitor or ARB for LVSD[2]	81	89%	97%	97%
Discharge Instructions Given[2]	266	98%	95%	94%
Evaluation of LVS Function[2]	322	100%	99%	99%
Medicare Spending				
Medicare Spending per Patient (ratio)	-	1.06	1.01	0.98
Pneumonia Care				
Appropriate Initial Antibiotic Given[2]	76	96%	95%	95%
Blood Culture Timing[2]	158	99%	98%	98%

NOTE: Hospital profiles are in alphabetical order by state, then city, then hospital within the city; Rankings exclude hospitals with less than 25 cases except for patient surveys which excludes hospitals with less than 100 cases; (a) 100-299 cases; (1) The number of cases/patients is too few to report; (2) Data submitted were based on a sample of cases/patients; (3) Results are based on a shorter time period than required; (4) Data suppressed by CMS for one or more quarters; (5) Results are not available for this reporting period; (6) Fewer than 100 patients completed the HCAHPS survey; (7) No cases met the criteria for this measure; (8) The lower limit of the confidence interval cannot be calculated if the number of observed infections equals zero; (9) No data are available from the state/territory for this reporting period; (10) The scores shown reflect fewer than 50 completed surveys; (11) There were discrepancies in the data collection process; (12) This measure does not apply to this hospital for this reporting period; (13) Results cannot be calculated for this reporting period; (14) The results for this state are combined with nearby states to protect confidentiality; Please refer to the User's Guide for a full explanation of data.

Measure	Cases	This Hosp.	State Avg.	U.S. Avg.
Pregnancy and Delivery Care				
Newborn Deliveries Scheduled Early[2]	41	10%	5%	6%
Preventive Care				
Immunization for Influenza[2]	565	97%	91%	90%
Immunization for Pneumonia[2]	774	99%	92%	92%
Stroke Care				
Anticoagulation Therapy for Atrial Fibrillation	15	87%	94%	95%
Antithrombotic Therapy Timing	177	99%	97%	98%
Assessed for Rehabilitation	205	82%	96%	97%
Discharged on Antithrombotic Therapy	180	92%	98%	99%
Discharged on Statin Medication	126	78%	91%	94%
Thrombolytic Therapy Timing[1]	-	-	54%	66%
Venous Thromboembolism Prophylaxis	212	84%	91%	94%
Written Stroke Educational Materials Given	114	100%	82%	88%
Surgical Care Improvement Project				
Appropriate Beta Blocker Usage[2]	278	98%	98%	98%
Appropriate VTP Within 24 Hours[2]	446	94%	98%	98%
Controlled Postoperative Blood Glucose[2]	161	98%	97%	97%
Perioperative Temperature Management[2]	556	100%	100%	100%
Prophylactic Antibiotic Selection[2]	527	99%	99%	99%
Prophylactic Antibiotic Selection (Outpatient)	496	99%	98%	98%
Prophylactic Antibiotic Stopped[2]	506	98%	98%	98%
Prophylactic Antibiotic Timing[2]	528	99%	99%	99%
Prophylactic Antibiotic Timing (Outpatient)	497	97%	98%	98%
Urinary Catheter Removal[2]	317	92%	98%	97%
Survey of Patients' Hospital Experiences				
Area Around Room 'Always' Quiet at Night	300+	55%	61%	61%
Doctors 'Always' Communicated Well	300+	80%	83%	82%
Home Recovery Information Given	300+	85%	86%	85%
Hospital Given 9 or 10 on 10 Point Scale	300+	78%	74%	71%
Meds 'Always' Explained Before Given	300+	66%	64%	64%
Nurses 'Always' Communicated Well	300+	84%	81%	79%
Pain 'Always' Well Controlled	300+	75%	73%	71%
Room and Bathroom 'Always' Clean	300+	78%	76%	73%
Timely Help 'Always' Received	300+	73%	71%	68%
Would Definitely Recommend Hospital	300+	80%	73%	71%
Use of Medical Imaging				
Cardiac Imaging Stress Test before Surgery	503	8.9%	5.4%	5.3%
Combination Abdominal CT Scan	2,212	6.0%	9.3%	10.5%
Combination Brain/Sinus CT Scan	1,608	2.4%	2.6%	2.7%
Combination Chest CT Scan	1,243	0.6%	4.6%	2.7%
Follow-up Mammogram/Ultrasound	3,447	8.8%	8.4%	8.8%
Lumbar Spine MRI for Low Back Pain	354	37.3%	38.7%	37.2%

Franciscan Healthcare - Munster

701 Superior Ave
Munster, IN 46321
Phone: 219-922-4200
Type: Acute Care Hospitals
Emergency Services: No
Ownership: Voluntary non-profit - Private
Beds: 63

Measure	Cases	This Hosp.	State Avg.	U.S. Avg.
Blood Clot Prevention and Treatment				
Anticoagulation Overlap Therapy	20	90%	92%	93%
ICU Venous Thromboembolism Prophylaxis	64	92%	91%	92%
Incidence of Potentially Preventable VTE[1]	-	-	10%	10%
UFH with Dosages/Platelet Monitoring	13	100%	95%	97%
Venous Thromboembolism Prophylaxis	382	91%	83%	85%
Warfarin Therapy Discharge Instructions	17	100%	71%	75%
Chest Pain/Possible Heart Attack Care				
Aspirin Given Within 24 Hours of Arrival[5]	-	-	96%	96%
Fibrinolytic Meds Within 30 Min. of Arrival[5]	-	-	48%	58%
Average Time to ECG (minutes)[5]	-	-	6	7
Average Time to Transfer (minutes)[5]	-	-	46	60
Children's Asthma Care				
Received Home Management Plan of Care	-	-	-	88%
Received Reliever Medication	-	-	-	100%
Received Systemic Corticosteroids	-	-	-	100%
Emergency Department				
Admittance Decision Time (minutes)[7]	-	-	80	98
Head CT Results Within 45 Min. of Arrival[5]	-	-	60%	57%
Patients Who Left ER Before Being Seen[5]	-	-	2%	2%
Time from ER Arrival to Admit. (minutes)[7]	-	-	241	274
Time from ER Arrival to Discharge (minutes)[5]	-	-	122	134
Time in ER Before Being Evaluated (minutes)[5]	-	-	22	26
Time to Pain Meds for Fractures (minutes)[5]	-	-	52	57
Heart Attack Care				
Aspirin Given at Discharge[1,3]	-	-	99%	99%
Fibrinolytic Meds Within 30 Min. of Arrival[3,7]	-	-	67%	54%
PCI Within 90 Minutes of Arrival[3,7]	-	-	97%	96%
Statin Prescribed at Discharge[1,3]	-	-	99%	98%
Heart Failure Care				
ACE Inhibitor or ARB for LVSD	17	100%	97%	97%
Discharge Instructions Given	38	89%	95%	94%
Evaluation of LVS Function	42	100%	99%	99%
Medicare Spending				
Medicare Spending per Patient (ratio)	-	0.99	1.01	0.98
Pneumonia Care				
Appropriate Initial Antibiotic Given	18	100%	95%	95%
Blood Culture Timing[7]	-	-	98%	98%
Pregnancy and Delivery Care				
Newborn Deliveries Scheduled Early[7]	-	-	5%	6%
Preventive Care				
Immunization for Influenza	447	99%	91%	90%
Immunization for Pneumonia	625	99%	92%	92%
Stroke Care				
Anticoagulation Therapy for Atrial Fibrillation[1]	-	-	94%	95%
Antithrombotic Therapy Timing[1]	-	-	97%	98%
Assessed for Rehabilitation[1]	-	-	96%	97%
Discharged on Antithrombotic Therapy[1]	-	-	98%	99%
Discharged on Statin Medication[1]	-	-	91%	94%
Thrombolytic Therapy Timing[7]	-	-	54%	66%
Venous Thromboembolism Prophylaxis[1]	-	-	91%	94%
Written Stroke Educational Materials Given[1]	-	-	82%	88%
Surgical Care Improvement Project				
Appropriate Beta Blocker Usage	39	97%	98%	98%
Appropriate VTP Within 24 Hours	96	99%	98%	98%
Controlled Postoperative Blood Glucose	11	91%	97%	97%
Perioperative Temperature Management	102	100%	100%	100%
Prophylactic Antibiotic Selection	79	97%	99%	99%
Prophylactic Antibiotic Selection (Outpatient)	88	99%	98%	98%
Prophylactic Antibiotic Stopped	74	100%	98%	98%
Prophylactic Antibiotic Timing	79	97%	99%	99%
Prophylactic Antibiotic Timing (Outpatient)	89	99%	98%	98%
Urinary Catheter Removal	59	98%	98%	97%
Survey of Patients' Hospital Experiences				
Area Around Room 'Always' Quiet at Night	300+	71%	61%	61%
Doctors 'Always' Communicated Well	300+	83%	83%	82%
Home Recovery Information Given	300+	84%	86%	85%
Hospital Given 9 or 10 on 10 Point Scale	300+	72%	74%	71%
Meds 'Always' Explained Before Given	300+	64%	64%	64%
Nurses 'Always' Communicated Well	300+	84%	81%	79%
Pain 'Always' Well Controlled	300+	71%	73%	71%
Room and Bathroom 'Always' Clean	300+	72%	76%	73%
Timely Help 'Always' Received	300+	74%	71%	68%
Would Definitely Recommend Hospital	300+	75%	73%	71%
Use of Medical Imaging				
Cardiac Imaging Stress Test before Surgery	82	3.7%	5.4%	5.3%
Combination Abdominal CT Scan	451	42.6%	9.3%	10.5%
Combination Brain/Sinus CT Scan[1]	-	-	2.6%	2.7%
Combination Chest CT Scan	602	1.8%	4.6%	2.7%
Follow-up Mammogram/Ultrasound	856	8.8%	8.4%	8.8%
Lumbar Spine MRI for Low Back Pain	134	42.5%	38.7%	37.2%

Floyd Memorial Hospital & Health Services

1850 State St
New Albany, IN 47150
Phone: 812-949-5500
Fax: 812-949-5607
URL: www.floydmedical.org
Type: Acute Care Hospitals
Emergency Services: Yes
Ownership: Government - Local
Beds: 245

Key Personnel:

Radiology. . . . . Damon Andrew Black, MD
Operating Room. . . . . Paul Bennett Brock
Pediatric Ambulatory Care . . . . . . Stuart Eldridge, MD
Pediatric In-Patient Care . . . . Stuart Eldridge, MD
CEO/President. . . . . Bryant R Hanson
Emergency Room . . . . Ruth Heideman
Quality Assurance . . . . Carol Mullen, RN

Measure	Cases	This Hosp.	State Avg.	U.S. Avg.
Blood Clot Prevention and Treatment				
Anticoagulation Overlap Therapy[2]	105	99%	92%	93%
ICU Venous Thromboembolism Prophylaxis[2]	53	98%	91%	92%
Incidence of Potentially Preventable VTE[2]	23	26%	10%	10%
UFH with Dosages/Platelet Monitoring[2]	28	100%	95%	97%
Venous Thromboembolism Prophylaxis[2]	393	72%	83%	85%
Warfarin Therapy Discharge Instructions[2]	73	100%	71%	75%
Chest Pain/Possible Heart Attack Care				
Aspirin Given Within 24 Hours of Arrival[1,3]	-	-	96%	96%
Fibrinolytic Meds Within 30 Min. of Arrival[5]	-	-	48%	58%
Average Time to ECG (minutes)[1,3]	-	-	6	7
Average Time to Transfer (minutes)[5]	-	-	46	60
Children's Asthma Care				
Received Home Management Plan of Care	-	-	-	88%
Received Reliever Medication	-	-	-	100%
Received Systemic Corticosteroids	-	-	-	100%
Emergency Department				
Admittance Decision Time (minutes)[2]	577	83	80	98
Head CT Results Within 45 Min. of Arrival	15	20%	60%	57%
Patients Who Left ER Before Being Seen	45,882	2%	2%	2%
Time from ER Arrival to Admit. (minutes)[2]	791	252	241	274
Time from ER Arrival to Discharge (minutes)	414	141	122	134
Time in ER Before Being Evaluated (minutes)	354	35	22	26
Time to Pain Meds for Fractures (minutes)	173	70	52	57
Heart Attack Care				
Aspirin Given at Discharge	338	100%	99%	99%
Fibrinolytic Meds Within 30 Min. of Arrival[7]	-	-	67%	54%
PCI Within 90 Minutes of Arrival	53	81%	97%	96%
Statin Prescribed at Discharge	314	98%	99%	98%
Heart Failure Care				
ACE Inhibitor or ARB for LVSD	104	97%	97%	97%
Discharge Instructions Given	298	92%	95%	94%
Evaluation of LVS Function	402	99%	99%	99%
Medicare Spending				
Medicare Spending per Patient (ratio)	-	1.01	1.01	0.98
Pneumonia Care				
Appropriate Initial Antibiotic Given	230	97%	95%	95%
Blood Culture Timing	410	96%	98%	98%
Pregnancy and Delivery Care				
Newborn Deliveries Scheduled Early	66	12%	5%	6%
Preventive Care				
Immunization for Influenza[2]	617	83%	91%	90%
Immunization for Pneumonia[2]	864	90%	92%	92%
Stroke Care				
Anticoagulation Therapy for Atrial Fibrillation	14	100%	94%	95%
Antithrombotic Therapy Timing	147	100%	97%	98%
Assessed for Rehabilitation	172	96%	96%	97%
Discharged on Antithrombotic Therapy	158	100%	98%	99%
Discharged on Statin Medication	130	83%	91%	94%
Thrombolytic Therapy Timing[1]	-	-	54%	66%
Venous Thromboembolism Prophylaxis	170	89%	91%	94%
Written Stroke Educational Materials Given	108	53%	82%	88%
Surgical Care Improvement Project				
Appropriate Beta Blocker Usage	398	100%	98%	98%
Appropriate VTP Within 24 Hours	596	99%	98%	98%
Controlled Postoperative Blood Glucose	216	99%	97%	97%
Perioperative Temperature Management	739	100%	100%	100%
Prophylactic Antibiotic Selection	594	99%	99%	99%
Prophylactic Antibiotic Selection (Outpatient)	311	84%	98%	98%
Prophylactic Antibiotic Stopped	582	98%	98%	98%
Prophylactic Antibiotic Timing	594	98%	99%	99%
Prophylactic Antibiotic Timing (Outpatient)	319	97%	98%	98%
Urinary Catheter Removal	569	100%	98%	97%
Survey of Patients' Hospital Experiences				
Area Around Room 'Always' Quiet at Night	(a)	62%	61%	61%
Doctors 'Always' Communicated Well	(a)	85%	83%	82%
Home Recovery Information Given	(a)	85%	86%	85%
Hospital Given 9 or 10 on 10 Point Scale	(a)	81%	74%	71%
Meds 'Always' Explained Before Given	(a)	66%	64%	64%
Nurses 'Always' Communicated Well	(a)	84%	81%	79%
Pain 'Always' Well Controlled	(a)	77%	73%	71%

NOTE: Hospital profiles are in alphabetical order by state, then city, then hospital within the city; Rankings exclude hospitals with less than 25 cases except for patient surveys which excludes hospitals with less than 100 cases; (a) 100-299 cases; (1) The number of cases/patients is too few to report; (2) Data submitted were based on a sample of cases/patients; (3) Results are based on a shorter time period than required; (4) Data suppressed by CMS for one or more quarters; (5) Results are not available for this reporting period; (6) Fewer than 100 patients completed the HCAHPS survey; (7) No cases met the criteria for this measure; (8) The lower limit of the confidence interval cannot be calculated if the number of observed infections equals zero; (9) No data are available from the state/territory for this reporting period; (10) The scores shown reflect fewer than 50 completed surveys; (11) There were discrepancies in the data collection process; (12) This measure does not apply to this hospital for this reporting period; (13) Results cannot be calculated for this reporting period; (14) The results for this state are combined with nearby states to protect confidentiality; Please refer to the User's Guide for a full explanation of data.

Measure	Cases	This Hosp.	State Avg.	U.S. Avg.
Room and Bathroom 'Always' Clean	(a)	76%	76%	73%
Timely Help 'Always' Received	(a)	77%	71%	68%
Would Definitely Recommend Hospital	(a)	80%	73%	71%
Use of Medical Imaging				
Cardiac Imaging Stress Test before Surgery	529	7.9%	5.4%	5.3%
Combination Abdominal CT Scan	1,145	20.7%	9.3%	10.5%
Combination Brain/Sinus CT Scan	837	1.9%	2.6%	2.7%
Combination Chest CT Scan	914	5.8%	4.6%	2.7%
Follow-up Mammogram/Ultrasound	1,849	9.2%	8.4%	8.8%
Lumbar Spine MRI for Low Back Pain	223	37.7%	38.7%	37.2%

Physicians' Medical Center

4023 Reas Ln
New Albany, IN 47150
Phone: 812-206-7660
URL: www.pmcdev.interactivemedialab.com
Type: Acute Care Hospitals
Emergency Services: No
Ownership: Physician

Measure	Cases	This Hosp.	State Avg.	U.S. Avg.
Blood Clot Prevention and Treatment				
Anticoagulation Overlap Therapy[7]	-	-	92%	93%
ICU Venous Thromboembolism Prophylaxis[7]	-	-	91%	92%
Incidence of Potentially Preventable VTE[7]	-	-	10%	10%
UFH with Dosages/Platelet Monitoring[7]	-	-	95%	97%
Venous Thromboembolism Prophylaxis[7]	-	-	83%	85%
Warfarin Therapy Discharge Instructions[7]	-	-	71%	75%
Chest Pain/Possible Heart Attack Care				
Aspirin Given Within 24 Hours of Arrival[5]	-	-	96%	96%
Fibrinolytic Meds Within 30 Min. of Arrival[5]	-	-	48%	58%
Average Time to ECG (minutes)[5]	-	-	6	7
Average Time to Transfer (minutes)[5]	-	-	46	60
Children's Asthma Care				
Received Home Management Plan of Care	-	-	-	88%
Received Reliever Medication	-	-	-	100%
Received Systemic Corticosteroids	-	-	-	100%
Emergency Department				
Admittance Decision Time (minutes)[2,7]	-	-	80	98
Head CT Results Within 45 Min. of Arrival[5]	-	-	60%	57%
Patients Who Left ER Before Being Seen[5]	-	-	2%	2%
Time from ER Arrival to Admit. (minutes)[2,7]	-	-	241	274
Time from ER Arrival to Discharge (minutes)[5]	-	-	122	134
Time in ER Before Being Evaluated (minutes)[5]	-	-	22	26
Time to Pain Meds for Fractures (minutes)[5]	-	-	52	57
Heart Attack Care				
Aspirin Given at Discharge[5]	-	-	99%	99%
Fibrinolytic Meds Within 30 Min. of Arrival[5]	-	-	67%	54%
PCI Within 90 Minutes of Arrival[5]	-	-	97%	96%
Statin Prescribed at Discharge[5]	-	-	99%	98%
Heart Failure Care				
ACE Inhibitor or ARB for LVSD[5]	-	-	97%	97%
Discharge Instructions Given[5]	-	-	95%	94%
Evaluation of LVS Function[5]	-	-	99%	99%
Medicare Spending				
Medicare Spending per Patient (ratio)	-	0.86	1.01	0.98
Pneumonia Care				
Appropriate Initial Antibiotic Given[5]	-	-	95%	95%
Blood Culture Timing[5]	-	-	98%	98%
Pregnancy and Delivery Care				
Newborn Deliveries Scheduled Early[2,7]	-	-	5%	6%
Preventive Care				
Immunization for Influenza[2]	128	85%	91%	90%
Immunization for Pneumonia[2]	60	87%	92%	92%
Stroke Care				
Anticoagulation Therapy for Atrial Fibrillation[5]	-	-	94%	95%
Antithrombotic Therapy Timing[5]	-	-	97%	98%
Assessed for Rehabilitation[5]	-	-	96%	97%
Discharged on Antithrombotic Therapy[5]	-	-	98%	99%
Discharged on Statin Medication[5]	-	-	91%	94%
Thrombolytic Therapy Timing[5]	-	-	54%	66%
Venous Thromboembolism Prophylaxis[5]	-	-	91%	94%
Written Stroke Educational Materials Given[5]	-	-	82%	88%
Surgical Care Improvement Project				
Appropriate Beta Blocker Usage[1,2]	-	-	98%	98%
Appropriate VTP Within 24 Hours[2]	55	98%	98%	98%
Controlled Postoperative Blood Glucose[2,7]	-	-	97%	97%
Perioperative Temperature Management[2]	97	89%	100%	100%
Prophylactic Antibiotic Selection[2]	77	88%	99%	99%
Prophylactic Antibiotic Selection (Outpatient)	182	83%	98%	98%
Prophylactic Antibiotic Stopped[2]	76	91%	98%	98%
Prophylactic Antibiotic Timing[2]	78	88%	99%	99%
Prophylactic Antibiotic Timing (Outpatient)	171	97%	98%	98%
Urinary Catheter Removal[2]	32	100%	98%	97%
Survey of Patients' Hospital Experiences				
Area Around Room 'Always' Quiet at Night	(a)	87%	61%	61%
Doctors 'Always' Communicated Well	(a)	82%	83%	82%
Home Recovery Information Given	(a)	84%	86%	85%
Hospital Given 9 or 10 on 10 Point Scale	(a)	83%	74%	71%
Meds 'Always' Explained Before Given	(a)	72%	64%	64%
Nurses 'Always' Communicated Well	(a)	85%	81%	79%
Pain 'Always' Well Controlled	(a)	77%	73%	71%
Room and Bathroom 'Always' Clean	(a)	79%	76%	73%
Timely Help 'Always' Received	(a)	85%	71%	68%
Would Definitely Recommend Hospital	(a)	79%	73%	71%
Use of Medical Imaging				
Cardiac Imaging Stress Test before Surgery[7]	-	-	5.4%	5.3%
Combination Abdominal CT Scan[7]	-	-	9.3%	10.5%
Combination Brain/Sinus CT Scan[7]	-	-	2.6%	2.7%
Combination Chest CT Scan[7]	-	-	4.6%	2.7%
Follow-up Mammogram/Ultrasound[7]	-	-	8.4%	8.8%
Lumbar Spine MRI for Low Back Pain[7]	-	-	38.7%	37.2%

Henry County Memorial Hospital

1000 N 16th St
New Castle, IN 47362
Phone: 765-521-0890
Fax: 765-521-1555
URL: www.hcmhcares.org
Type: Acute Care Hospitals
Emergency Services: Yes
Ownership: Government - Local
Beds: 107

Key Personnel:
Quality Assurance . . . . Chuck Butler
Operating Room. . . . . Sandy Campbell, RN
Emergency Room . . . . Mark Doyle
Radiology. . . . . Randall Fields
President . . . . Paul Janssen

Measure	Cases	This Hosp.	State Avg.	U.S. Avg.
Blood Clot Prevention and Treatment				
Anticoagulation Overlap Therapy[2]	27	93%	92%	93%
ICU Venous Thromboembolism Prophylaxis[2]	70	99%	91%	92%
Incidence of Potentially Preventable VTE[1,2]	-	-	10%	10%
UFH with Dosages/Platelet Monitoring[1,2]	-	-	95%	97%
Venous Thromboembolism Prophylaxis[2]	140	94%	83%	85%
Warfarin Therapy Discharge Instructions[2]	23	87%	71%	75%
Chest Pain/Possible Heart Attack Care				
Aspirin Given Within 24 Hours of Arrival	124	95%	96%	96%
Fibrinolytic Meds Within 30 Min. of Arrival[7]	-	-	48%	58%
Average Time to ECG (minutes)	132	2	6	7
Average Time to Transfer (minutes)	18	26	46	60
Children's Asthma Care				
Received Home Management Plan of Care	-	-	-	88%
Received Reliever Medication	-	-	-	100%
Received Systemic Corticosteroids	-	-	-	100%
Emergency Department				
Admittance Decision Time (minutes)[2]	374	60	80	98
Head CT Results Within 45 Min. of Arrival	16	62%	60%	57%
Patients Who Left ER Before Being Seen	18,058	2%	2%	2%
Time from ER Arrival to Admit. (minutes)[2]	385	213	241	274
Time from ER Arrival to Discharge (minutes)	274	136	122	134
Time in ER Before Being Evaluated (minutes)	353	22	22	26
Time to Pain Meds for Fractures (minutes)	93	42	52	57
Heart Attack Care				
Aspirin Given at Discharge[1]	-	-	99%	99%
Fibrinolytic Meds Within 30 Min. of Arrival[7]	-	-	67%	54%
PCI Within 90 Minutes of Arrival[7]	-	-	97%	96%
Statin Prescribed at Discharge[1]	-	-	99%	98%
Heart Failure Care				
ACE Inhibitor or ARB for LVSD	13	100%	97%	97%
Discharge Instructions Given	39	95%	95%	94%
Evaluation of LVS Function	55	100%	99%	99%
Medicare Spending				
Medicare Spending per Patient (ratio)	-	1.03	1.01	0.98
Pneumonia Care				
Appropriate Initial Antibiotic Given	97	98%	95%	95%
Blood Culture Timing	123	100%	98%	98%
Pregnancy and Delivery Care				
Newborn Deliveries Scheduled Early	20	10%	5%	6%
Preventive Care				
Immunization for Influenza[2]	289	100%	91%	90%
Immunization for Pneumonia[2]	459	100%	92%	92%
Stroke Care				
Anticoagulation Therapy for Atrial Fibrillation[5]	-	-	94%	95%
Antithrombotic Therapy Timing[5]	-	-	97%	98%
Assessed for Rehabilitation[5]	-	-	96%	97%
Discharged on Antithrombotic Therapy[5]	-	-	98%	99%
Discharged on Statin Medication[5]	-	-	91%	94%
Thrombolytic Therapy Timing[5]	-	-	54%	66%
Venous Thromboembolism Prophylaxis[5]	-	-	91%	94%
Written Stroke Educational Materials Given[5]	-	-	82%	88%
Surgical Care Improvement Project				
Appropriate Beta Blocker Usage	128	98%	98%	98%
Appropriate VTP Within 24 Hours	323	100%	98%	98%
Controlled Postoperative Blood Glucose[7]	-	-	97%	97%
Perioperative Temperature Management	350	100%	100%	100%
Prophylactic Antibiotic Selection	283	100%	99%	99%
Prophylactic Antibiotic Selection (Outpatient)	100	99%	98%	98%
Prophylactic Antibiotic Stopped	279	99%	98%	98%
Prophylactic Antibiotic Timing	283	100%	99%	99%
Prophylactic Antibiotic Timing (Outpatient)	100	100%	98%	98%
Urinary Catheter Removal	91	99%	98%	97%
Survey of Patients' Hospital Experiences				
Area Around Room 'Always' Quiet at Night	300+	59%	61%	61%
Doctors 'Always' Communicated Well	300+	83%	83%	82%
Home Recovery Information Given	300+	89%	86%	85%
Hospital Given 9 or 10 on 10 Point Scale	300+	77%	74%	71%
Meds 'Always' Explained Before Given	300+	71%	64%	64%
Nurses 'Always' Communicated Well	300+	85%	81%	79%
Pain 'Always' Well Controlled	300+	73%	73%	71%
Room and Bathroom 'Always' Clean	300+	80%	76%	73%
Timely Help 'Always' Received	300+	71%	71%	68%
Would Definitely Recommend Hospital	300+	75%	73%	71%
Use of Medical Imaging				
Cardiac Imaging Stress Test before Surgery	308	10.1%	5.4%	5.3%
Combination Abdominal CT Scan	687	9.0%	9.3%	10.5%
Combination Brain/Sinus CT Scan	591	1.7%	2.6%	2.7%
Combination Chest CT Scan	217	9.7%	4.6%	2.7%
Follow-up Mammogram/Ultrasound	916	5.2%	8.4%	8.8%
Lumbar Spine MRI for Low Back Pain	60	43.3%	38.7%	37.2%

The Heart Hospital at Deaconess Gateway

4007 Gateway Blvd
Newburgh, IN 47630
Phone: 812-842-4784
URL: www.deaconess.com
Type: Acute Care Hospitals
Emergency Services: No
Ownership: Proprietary
Beds: 145

Measure	Cases	This Hosp.	State Avg.	U.S. Avg.
Blood Clot Prevention and Treatment				
Anticoagulation Overlap Therapy[1,2]	-	-	92%	93%
ICU Venous Thromboembolism Prophylaxis[2]	70	89%	91%	92%
Incidence of Potentially Preventable VTE[2,7]	-	-	10%	10%
UFH with Dosages/Platelet Monitoring[1,2]	-	-	95%	97%
Venous Thromboembolism Prophylaxis[2]	130	80%	83%	85%
Warfarin Therapy Discharge Instructions[1,2]	-	-	71%	75%
Chest Pain/Possible Heart Attack Care				
Aspirin Given Within 24 Hours of Arrival[5]	-	-	96%	96%
Fibrinolytic Meds Within 30 Min. of Arrival[5]	-	-	48%	58%
Average Time to ECG (minutes)[5]	-	-	6	7
Average Time to Transfer (minutes)[5]	-	-	46	60
Children's Asthma Care				
Received Home Management Plan of Care	-	-	-	88%
Received Reliever Medication	-	-	-	100%

NOTE: Hospital profiles are in alphabetical order by state, then city, then hospital within the city; Rankings exclude hospitals with less than 25 cases except for patient surveys which excludes hospitals with less than 100 cases; (a) 100-299 cases; (1) The number of cases/patients is too few to report; (2) Data submitted were based on a sample of cases/patients; (3) Results are based on a shorter time period than required; (4) Data suppressed by CMS for one or more quarters; (5) Results are not available for this reporting period; (6) Fewer than 100 patients completed the HCAHPS survey; (7) No cases met the criteria for this measure; (8) The lower limit of the confidence interval cannot be calculated if the number of observed infections equals zero; (9) No data are available from the state/territory for this reporting period; (10) The scores shown reflect fewer than 50 completed surveys; (11) There were discrepancies in the data collection process; (12) This measure does not apply to this hospital for this reporting period; (13) Results cannot be calculated for this reporting period; (14) The results for this state are combined with nearby states to protect confidentiality; Please refer to the User's Guide for a full explanation of data.

Received Systemic Corticosteroids	-	-	-	100%
Emergency Department				
Admittance Decision Time (minutes)[2,7]	-	-	80	98
Head CT Results Within 45 Min. of Arrival[5]	-	-	60%	57%
Patients Who Left ER Before Being Seen[5]	-	-	2%	2%
Time from ER Arrival to Admit. (minutes)[2,7]	-	-	241	274
Time from ER Arrival to Discharge (minutes)[5]	-	-	122	134
Time in ER Before Being Evaluated (minutes)[5]	-	-	22	26
Time to Pain Meds for Fractures (minutes)[5]	-	-	52	57
Heart Attack Care				
Aspirin Given at Discharge	294	100%	99%	99%
Fibrinolytic Meds Within 30 Min. of Arrival[7]	-	-	67%	54%
PCI Within 90 Minutes of Arrival[7]	-	-	97%	96%
Statin Prescribed at Discharge	286	99%	99%	98%
Heart Failure Care				
ACE Inhibitor or ARB for LVSD	31	97%	97%	97%
Discharge Instructions Given	54	83%	95%	94%
Evaluation of LVS Function	61	100%	99%	99%
Medicare Spending				
Medicare Spending per Patient (ratio)	-	1.00	1.01	0.98
Pneumonia Care				
Appropriate Initial Antibiotic Given[3,7]	-	-	95%	95%
Blood Culture Timing[3,7]	-	-	98%	98%
Pregnancy and Delivery Care				
Newborn Deliveries Scheduled Early[7]	-	-	5%	6%
Preventive Care				
Immunization for Influenza[2]	308	97%	91%	90%
Immunization for Pneumonia[2]	503	95%	92%	92%
Stroke Care				
Anticoagulation Therapy for Atrial Fibrillation[7]	-	-	94%	95%
Antithrombotic Therapy Timing[7]	-	-	97%	98%
Assessed for Rehabilitation[7]	-	-	96%	97%
Discharged on Antithrombotic Therapy[7]	-	-	98%	99%
Discharged on Statin Medication[7]	-	-	91%	94%
Thrombolytic Therapy Timing[7]	-	-	54%	66%
Venous Thromboembolism Prophylaxis[7]	-	-	91%	94%
Written Stroke Educational Materials Given[7]	-	-	82%	88%
Surgical Care Improvement Project				
Appropriate Beta Blocker Usage[2]	191	100%	98%	98%
Appropriate VTP Within 24 Hours[2]	13	85%	98%	98%
Controlled Postoperative Blood Glucose[2]	280	98%	97%	97%
Perioperative Temperature Management[2]	24	100%	100%	100%
Prophylactic Antibiotic Selection[2]	205	100%	99%	99%
Prophylactic Antibiotic Selection (Outpatient)	420	99%	98%	98%
Prophylactic Antibiotic Stopped[2]	199	97%	98%	98%
Prophylactic Antibiotic Timing[2]	205	100%	99%	99%
Prophylactic Antibiotic Timing (Outpatient)	420	99%	98%	98%
Urinary Catheter Removal[2]	259	100%	98%	97%
Survey of Patients' Hospital Experiences				
Area Around Room 'Always' Quiet at Night	300+	70%	61%	61%
Doctors 'Always' Communicated Well	300+	85%	83%	82%
Home Recovery Information Given	300+	88%	86%	85%
Hospital Given 9 or 10 on 10 Point Scale	300+	88%	74%	71%
Meds 'Always' Explained Before Given	300+	65%	64%	64%
Nurses 'Always' Communicated Well	300+	85%	81%	79%
Pain 'Always' Well Controlled	300+	77%	73%	71%
Room and Bathroom 'Always' Clean	300+	71%	76%	73%
Timely Help 'Always' Received	300+	78%	71%	68%
Would Definitely Recommend Hospital	300+	89%	73%	71%
Use of Medical Imaging				
Cardiac Imaging Stress Test before Surgery	123	5.7%	5.4%	5.3%
Combination Abdominal CT Scan[7]	-	-	9.3%	10.5%
Combination Brain/Sinus CT Scan[1]	-	-	2.6%	2.7%
Combination Chest CT Scan[1]	-	-	4.6%	2.7%
Follow-up Mammogram/Ultrasound[7]	-	-	8.4%	8.8%
Lumbar Spine MRI for Low Back Pain[7]	-	-	38.7%	37.2%

The Women's Hospital

4199 Gateway Blvd
Newburgh, IN 47630
URL: www.deaconess.com
Type: Acute Care Hospitals
Ownership: Proprietary
Phone: 812-842-4200
Emergency Services: No

Key Personnel:
CEO/President. . . . . Linda White

Measure	Cases	This Hosp.	State Avg.	U.S. Avg.
Blood Clot Prevention and Treatment				
Anticoagulation Overlap Therapy[1]	-	-	92%	93%
ICU Venous Thromboembolism Prophylaxis[7]	-	-	91%	92%
Incidence of Potentially Preventable VTE[7]	-	-	10%	10%
UFH with Dosages/Platelet Monitoring[7]	-	-	95%	97%
Venous Thromboembolism Prophylaxis	25	80%	83%	85%
Warfarin Therapy Discharge Instructions[1]	-	-	71%	75%
Chest Pain/Possible Heart Attack Care				
Aspirin Given Within 24 Hours of Arrival[5]	-	-	96%	96%
Fibrinolytic Meds Within 30 Min. of Arrival[5]	-	-	48%	58%
Average Time to ECG (minutes)[5]	-	-	6	7
Average Time to Transfer (minutes)[5]	-	-	46	60
Children's Asthma Care				
Received Home Management Plan of Care	-	-	-	88%
Received Reliever Medication	-	-	-	100%
Received Systemic Corticosteroids	-	-	-	100%
Emergency Department				
Admittance Decision Time (minutes)[2]	120	32	80	98
Head CT Results Within 45 Min. of Arrival[5]	-	-	60%	57%
Patients Who Left ER Before Being Seen	4,117	0%	2%	2%
Time from ER Arrival to Admit. (minutes)[2]	127	97	241	274
Time from ER Arrival to Discharge (minutes)	434	143	122	134
Time in ER Before Being Evaluated (minutes)	452	10	22	26
Time to Pain Meds for Fractures (minutes)[5]	-	-	52	57
Heart Attack Care				
Aspirin Given at Discharge[5]	-	-	99%	99%
Fibrinolytic Meds Within 30 Min. of Arrival[5]	-	-	67%	54%
PCI Within 90 Minutes of Arrival[5]	-	-	97%	96%
Statin Prescribed at Discharge[5]	-	-	99%	98%
Heart Failure Care				
ACE Inhibitor or ARB for LVSD[5]	-	-	97%	97%
Discharge Instructions Given[5]	-	-	95%	94%
Evaluation of LVS Function[5]	-	-	99%	99%
Medicare Spending				
Medicare Spending per Patient (ratio)	-	0.99	1.01	0.98
Pneumonia Care				
Appropriate Initial Antibiotic Given[5]	-	-	95%	95%
Blood Culture Timing[5]	-	-	98%	98%
Pregnancy and Delivery Care				
Newborn Deliveries Scheduled Early[2]	62	24%	5%	6%
Preventive Care				
Immunization for Influenza[2]	390	98%	91%	90%
Immunization for Pneumonia[2]	17	59%	92%	92%
Stroke Care				
Anticoagulation Therapy for Atrial Fibrillation[5]	-	-	94%	95%
Antithrombotic Therapy Timing[5]	-	-	97%	98%
Assessed for Rehabilitation[5]	-	-	96%	97%
Discharged on Antithrombotic Therapy[5]	-	-	98%	99%
Discharged on Statin Medication[5]	-	-	91%	94%
Thrombolytic Therapy Timing[5]	-	-	54%	66%
Venous Thromboembolism Prophylaxis[5]	-	-	91%	94%
Written Stroke Educational Materials Given[5]	-	-	82%	88%
Surgical Care Improvement Project				
Appropriate Beta Blocker Usage	11	91%	98%	98%
Appropriate VTP Within 24 Hours	89	94%	98%	98%
Controlled Postoperative Blood Glucose[7]	-	-	97%	97%
Perioperative Temperature Management	92	100%	100%	100%
Prophylactic Antibiotic Selection	54	100%	99%	99%
Prophylactic Antibiotic Selection (Outpatient)	476	100%	98%	98%
Prophylactic Antibiotic Stopped	52	94%	98%	98%
Prophylactic Antibiotic Timing	54	98%	99%	99%
Prophylactic Antibiotic Timing (Outpatient)	476	98%	98%	98%
Urinary Catheter Removal[1]	-	-	98%	97%
Survey of Patients' Hospital Experiences				
Area Around Room 'Always' Quiet at Night	300+	71%	61%	61%
Doctors 'Always' Communicated Well	300+	81%	83%	82%
Home Recovery Information Given	300+	88%	86%	85%
Hospital Given 9 or 10 on 10 Point Scale	300+	83%	74%	71%
Meds 'Always' Explained Before Given	300+	63%	64%	64%
Nurses 'Always' Communicated Well	300+	83%	81%	79%
Pain 'Always' Well Controlled	300+	71%	73%	71%
Room and Bathroom 'Always' Clean	300+	82%	76%	73%
Timely Help 'Always' Received	300+	67%	71%	68%
Would Definitely Recommend Hospital	300+	83%	73%	71%
Use of Medical Imaging				
Cardiac Imaging Stress Test before Surgery[7]	-	-	5.4%	5.3%
Combination Abdominal CT Scan[1]	-	-	9.3%	10.5%
Combination Brain/Sinus CT Scan[7]	-	-	2.6%	2.7%
Combination Chest CT Scan[7]	-	-	4.6%	2.7%
Follow-up Mammogram/Ultrasound[7]	-	-	8.4%	8.8%
Lumbar Spine MRI for Low Back Pain[7]	-	-	38.7%	37.2%

Riverview Hospital

395 Westfield Rd
Noblesville, IN 46060
URL: www.riverviewhospital.org
Type: Acute Care Hospitals
Ownership: Government - Local
Phone: 317-776-7108
Fax: 317-776-7134
Emergency Services: Yes
Beds: 161

Key Personnel:
Radiology. . . . . Eric Beltz
CEO/President. . . . . Patricia K Fox
Patient Relations . . . . Jared Stark

Measure	Cases	This Hosp.	State Avg.	U.S. Avg.
Blood Clot Prevention and Treatment				
Anticoagulation Overlap Therapy[2]	29	97%	92%	93%
ICU Venous Thromboembolism Prophylaxis[2]	126	100%	91%	92%
Incidence of Potentially Preventable VTE[1,2]	-	-	10%	10%
UFH with Dosages/Platelet Monitoring[1,2]	-	-	95%	97%
Venous Thromboembolism Prophylaxis[2]	242	100%	83%	85%
Warfarin Therapy Discharge Instructions[2]	15	100%	71%	75%
Chest Pain/Possible Heart Attack Care				
Aspirin Given Within 24 Hours of Arrival[1,3]	-	-	96%	96%
Fibrinolytic Meds Within 30 Min. of Arrival[5]	-	-	48%	58%
Average Time to ECG (minutes)[1,3]	-	-	6	7
Average Time to Transfer (minutes)[5]	-	-	46	60
Children's Asthma Care				
Received Home Management Plan of Care	-	-	-	88%
Received Reliever Medication	-	-	-	100%
Received Systemic Corticosteroids	-	-	-	100%
Emergency Department				
Admittance Decision Time (minutes)[2]	742	66	80	98
Head CT Results Within 45 Min. of Arrival[1]	-	-	60%	57%
Patients Who Left ER Before Being Seen	22,679	0%	2%	2%
Time from ER Arrival to Admit. (minutes)[2]	749	197	241	274
Time from ER Arrival to Discharge (minutes)	385	101	122	134
Time in ER Before Being Evaluated (minutes)	398	21	22	26
Time to Pain Meds for Fractures (minutes)	105	54	52	57
Heart Attack Care				
Aspirin Given at Discharge	80	100%	99%	99%
Fibrinolytic Meds Within 30 Min. of Arrival[7]	-	-	67%	54%
PCI Within 90 Minutes of Arrival	24	100%	97%	96%
Statin Prescribed at Discharge	77	100%	99%	98%
Heart Failure Care				
ACE Inhibitor or ARB for LVSD	21	100%	97%	97%
Discharge Instructions Given	73	96%	95%	94%
Evaluation of LVS Function	93	99%	99%	99%
Medicare Spending				
Medicare Spending per Patient (ratio)	-	1.03	1.01	0.98
Pneumonia Care				
Appropriate Initial Antibiotic Given	106	92%	95%	95%
Blood Culture Timing	161	99%	98%	98%
Pregnancy and Delivery Care				
Newborn Deliveries Scheduled Early[2]	24	25%	5%	6%
Preventive Care				
Immunization for Influenza[2]	471	97%	91%	90%
Immunization for Pneumonia[2]	782	98%	92%	92%
Stroke Care				

NOTE: Hospital profiles are in alphabetical order by state, then city, then hospital within the city; Rankings exclude hospitals with less than 25 cases except for patient surveys which excludes hospitals with less than 100 cases; (a) 100-299 cases; (1) The number of cases/patients is too few to report; (2) Data submitted were based on a sample of cases/patients; (3) Results are based on a shorter time period than required; (4) Data suppressed by CMS for one or more quarters; (5) Results are not available for this reporting period; (6) Fewer than 100 patients completed the HCAHPS survey; (7) No cases met the criteria for this measure; (8) The lower limit of the confidence interval cannot be calculated if the number of observed infections equals zero; (9) No data are available from the state/territory for this reporting period; (10) The scores shown reflect fewer than 50 completed surveys; (11) There were discrepancies in the data collection process; (12) This measure does not apply to this hospital for this reporting period; (13) Results cannot be calculated for this reporting period; (14) The results for this state are combined with nearby states to protect confidentiality; Please refer to the User's Guide for a full explanation of data.

Measure	Cases	This Hosp.	State Avg.	U.S. Avg.
Anticoagulation Therapy for Atrial Fibrillation[1]	-	-	94%	95%
Antithrombotic Therapy Timing	41	100%	97%	98%
Assessed for Rehabilitation	40	100%	96%	97%
Discharged on Antithrombotic Therapy	40	100%	98%	99%
Discharged on Statin Medication	36	81%	91%	94%
Thrombolytic Therapy Timing[1]	-	-	54%	66%
Venous Thromboembolism Prophylaxis	45	100%	91%	94%
Written Stroke Educational Materials Given	15	33%	82%	88%
Surgical Care Improvement Project				
Appropriate Beta Blocker Usage	156	93%	98%	98%
Appropriate VTP Within 24 Hours	518	97%	98%	98%
Controlled Postoperative Blood Glucose	21	95%	97%	97%
Perioperative Temperature Management	607	100%	100%	100%
Prophylactic Antibiotic Selection	482	100%	99%	99%
Prophylactic Antibiotic Selection (Outpatient)	101	100%	98%	98%
Prophylactic Antibiotic Stopped	475	98%	98%	98%
Prophylactic Antibiotic Timing	482	99%	99%	99%
Prophylactic Antibiotic Timing (Outpatient)	101	100%	98%	98%
Urinary Catheter Removal	445	100%	98%	97%
Survey of Patients' Hospital Experiences				
Area Around Room 'Always' Quiet at Night	300+	59%	61%	61%
Doctors 'Always' Communicated Well	300+	83%	83%	82%
Home Recovery Information Given	300+	87%	86%	85%
Hospital Given 9 or 10 on 10 Point Scale	300+	73%	74%	71%
Meds 'Always' Explained Before Given	300+	64%	64%	64%
Nurses 'Always' Communicated Well	300+	77%	81%	79%
Pain 'Always' Well Controlled	300+	70%	73%	71%
Room and Bathroom 'Always' Clean	300+	70%	76%	73%
Timely Help 'Always' Received	300+	62%	71%	68%
Would Definitely Recommend Hospital	300+	73%	73%	71%
Use of Medical Imaging				
Cardiac Imaging Stress Test before Surgery	177	6.8%	5.4%	5.3%
Combination Abdominal CT Scan	661	7.0%	9.3%	10.5%
Combination Brain/Sinus CT Scan[1]	-	-	2.6%	2.7%
Combination Chest CT Scan	595	0.5%	4.6%	2.7%
Follow-up Mammogram/Ultrasound	1,076	10.8%	8.4%	8.8%
Lumbar Spine MRI for Low Back Pain	143	41.3%	38.7%	37.2%

Saint Vincent Jennings Hospital

301 Henry St
North Vernon, IN 47265
Phone: 812-352-4200
Fax: 812-352-4201
URL: www.stvincent.org/faccen/jennings
Type: Critical Access Hospitals
Emergency Services: Yes
Ownership: Voluntary non-profit - Church
Beds: 25

Key Personnel:

Chief of Medical Staff . . . . Rashid Alsabeh, MD
Quality Assurance . . . . John D Doyle
Radiology. . . . . Thomas M Ralston, MD
CEO/President. . . . . Anthony R Tersigni, EdD

Measure	Cases	This Hosp.	State Avg.	U.S. Avg.
Blood Clot Prevention and Treatment				
Anticoagulation Overlap Therapy[5]	-	-	92%	93%
ICU Venous Thromboembolism Prophylaxis[5]	-	-	91%	92%
Incidence of Potentially Preventable VTE[5]	-	-	10%	10%
UFH with Dosages/Platelet Monitoring[5]	-	-	95%	97%
Venous Thromboembolism Prophylaxis[5]	-	-	83%	85%
Warfarin Therapy Discharge Instructions[5]	-	-	71%	75%
Chest Pain/Possible Heart Attack Care				
Aspirin Given Within 24 Hours of Arrival[3]	19	84%	96%	96%
Fibrinolytic Meds Within 30 Min. of Arrival[3,7]	-	-	48%	58%
Average Time to ECG (minutes)[3]	22	8	6	7
Average Time to Transfer (minutes)[1,3]	-	-	46	60
Children's Asthma Care				
Received Home Management Plan of Care	-	-	-	88%
Received Reliever Medication	-	-	-	100%
Received Systemic Corticosteroids	-	-	-	100%
Emergency Department				
Admittance Decision Time (minutes)[5]	-	-	80	98
Head CT Results Within 45 Min. of Arrival[5]	-	-	60%	57%
Patients Who Left ER Before Being Seen	9,254	1%	2%	2%
Time from ER Arrival to Admit. (minutes)[5]	-	-	241	274
Time from ER Arrival to Discharge (minutes)[5]	-	-	122	134
Time in ER Before Being Evaluated (minutes)[5]	-	-	22	26
Time to Pain Meds for Fractures (minutes)[5]	-	-	52	57
Heart Attack Care				
Aspirin Given at Discharge[5]	-	-	99%	99%
Fibrinolytic Meds Within 30 Min. of Arrival[5]	-	-	67%	54%
PCI Within 90 Minutes of Arrival[5]	-	-	97%	96%
Statin Prescribed at Discharge[5]	-	-	99%	98%
Heart Failure Care				
ACE Inhibitor or ARB for LVSD	13	85%	97%	97%
Discharge Instructions Given[1]	-	-	95%	94%
Evaluation of LVS Function	13	100%	99%	99%
Medicare Spending				
Medicare Spending per Patient (ratio)			1.01	0.98
Pneumonia Care				
Appropriate Initial Antibiotic Given	35	80%	95%	95%
Blood Culture Timing	43	91%	98%	98%
Pregnancy and Delivery Care				
Newborn Deliveries Scheduled Early[5]	-	-	5%	6%
Preventive Care				
Immunization for Influenza[5]	-	-	91%	90%
Immunization for Pneumonia[5]	-	-	92%	92%
Stroke Care				
Anticoagulation Therapy for Atrial Fibrillation[5]	-	-	94%	95%
Antithrombotic Therapy Timing[5]	-	-	97%	98%
Assessed for Rehabilitation[5]	-	-	96%	97%
Discharged on Antithrombotic Therapy[5]	-	-	98%	99%
Discharged on Statin Medication[5]	-	-	91%	94%
Thrombolytic Therapy Timing[5]	-	-	54%	66%
Venous Thromboembolism Prophylaxis[5]	-	-	91%	94%
Written Stroke Educational Materials Given[5]	-	-	82%	88%
Surgical Care Improvement Project				
Appropriate Beta Blocker Usage[5]	-	-	98%	98%
Appropriate VTP Within 24 Hours[5]	-	-	98%	98%
Controlled Postoperative Blood Glucose[5]	-	-	97%	97%
Perioperative Temperature Management[5]	-	-	100%	100%
Prophylactic Antibiotic Selection[5]	-	-	99%	99%
Prophylactic Antibiotic Selection (Outpatient)[1,3]	-	-	98%	98%
Prophylactic Antibiotic Stopped[5]	-	-	98%	98%
Prophylactic Antibiotic Timing[5]	-	-	99%	99%
Prophylactic Antibiotic Timing (Outpatient)[1,3]	-	-	98%	98%
Urinary Catheter Removal[5]	-	-	98%	97%
Survey of Patients' Hospital Experiences				
Area Around Room 'Always' Quiet at Night[6]	<100	73%	61%	61%
Doctors 'Always' Communicated Well[6]	<100	84%	83%	82%
Home Recovery Information Given[6]	<100	84%	86%	85%
Hospital Given 9 or 10 on 10 Point Scale[6]	<100	73%	74%	71%
Meds 'Always' Explained Before Given[6]	<100	85%	64%	64%
Nurses 'Always' Communicated Well[6]	<100	82%	81%	79%
Pain 'Always' Well Controlled[6]	<100	80%	73%	71%
Room and Bathroom 'Always' Clean[6]	<100	87%	76%	73%
Timely Help 'Always' Received[6]	<100	83%	71%	68%
Would Definitely Recommend Hospital[6]	<100	72%	73%	71%
Use of Medical Imaging				
Cardiac Imaging Stress Test before Surgery	55	3.6%	5.4%	5.3%
Combination Abdominal CT Scan	243	4.5%	9.3%	10.5%
Combination Brain/Sinus CT Scan	259	1.2%	2.6%	2.7%
Combination Chest CT Scan	74	2.7%	4.6%	2.7%
Follow-up Mammogram/Ultrasound	285	15.4%	8.4%	8.8%
Lumbar Spine MRI for Low Back Pain[1]	-	-	38.7%	37.2%

Indiana University Health Paoli Hospital

642 W Hospital Rd
Paoli, IN 47454
Phone: 812-723-2811
Type: Critical Access Hospitals
Emergency Services: Yes
Ownership: Voluntary non-profit - Private

Measure	Cases	This Hosp.	State Avg.	U.S. Avg.
Blood Clot Prevention and Treatment				
Anticoagulation Overlap Therapy[5]	-	-	92%	93%
ICU Venous Thromboembolism Prophylaxis[5]	-	-	91%	92%
Incidence of Potentially Preventable VTE[5]	-	-	10%	10%
UFH with Dosages/Platelet Monitoring[5]	-	-	95%	97%
Venous Thromboembolism Prophylaxis[5]	-	-	83%	85%
Warfarin Therapy Discharge Instructions[5]	-	-	71%	75%
Chest Pain/Possible Heart Attack Care				
Aspirin Given Within 24 Hours of Arrival[5]	-	-	96%	96%
Fibrinolytic Meds Within 30 Min. of Arrival[5]	-	-	48%	58%
Average Time to ECG (minutes)[5]	-	-	6	7
Average Time to Transfer (minutes)[5]	-	-	46	60
Children's Asthma Care				
Received Home Management Plan of Care	-	-	-	88%
Received Reliever Medication	-	-	-	100%
Received Systemic Corticosteroids	-	-	-	100%
Emergency Department				
Admittance Decision Time (minutes)[5]	-	-	80	98
Head CT Results Within 45 Min. of Arrival[5]	-	-	60%	57%
Patients Who Left ER Before Being Seen	10,793	1%	2%	2%
Time from ER Arrival to Admit. (minutes)[5]	-	-	241	274
Time from ER Arrival to Discharge (minutes)[5]	-	-	122	134
Time in ER Before Being Evaluated (minutes)[5]	-	-	22	26
Time to Pain Meds for Fractures (minutes)[5]	-	-	52	57
Heart Attack Care				
Aspirin Given at Discharge[5]	-	-	99%	99%
Fibrinolytic Meds Within 30 Min. of Arrival[5]	-	-	67%	54%
PCI Within 90 Minutes of Arrival[5]	-	-	97%	96%
Statin Prescribed at Discharge[5]	-	-	99%	98%
Heart Failure Care				
ACE Inhibitor or ARB for LVSD[1]	-	-	97%	97%
Discharge Instructions Given[1]	-	-	95%	94%
Evaluation of LVS Function[1]	-	-	99%	99%
Medicare Spending				
Medicare Spending per Patient (ratio)		-	1.01	0.98
Pneumonia Care				
Appropriate Initial Antibiotic Given	19	84%	95%	95%
Blood Culture Timing	36	100%	98%	98%
Pregnancy and Delivery Care				
Newborn Deliveries Scheduled Early[5]	-	-	5%	6%
Preventive Care				
Immunization for Influenza[5]	-	-	91%	90%
Immunization for Pneumonia[5]	-	-	92%	92%
Stroke Care				
Anticoagulation Therapy for Atrial Fibrillation[5]	-	-	94%	95%
Antithrombotic Therapy Timing[5]	-	-	97%	98%
Assessed for Rehabilitation[5]	-	-	96%	97%
Discharged on Antithrombotic Therapy[5]	-	-	98%	99%
Discharged on Statin Medication[5]	-	-	91%	94%
Thrombolytic Therapy Timing[5]	-	-	54%	66%
Venous Thromboembolism Prophylaxis[5]	-	-	91%	94%
Written Stroke Educational Materials Given[5]	-	-	82%	88%
Surgical Care Improvement Project				
Appropriate Beta Blocker Usage[3,7]	-	-	98%	98%
Appropriate VTP Within 24 Hours[1,3]	-	-	98%	98%
Controlled Postoperative Blood Glucose[3,7]	-	-	97%	97%
Perioperative Temperature Management[1,3]	-	-	100%	100%
Prophylactic Antibiotic Selection[1,3]	-	-	99%	99%
Prophylactic Antibiotic Selection (Outpatient)[5]	-	-	98%	98%
Prophylactic Antibiotic Stopped[1,3]	-	-	98%	98%
Prophylactic Antibiotic Timing[1,3]	-	-	99%	99%
Prophylactic Antibiotic Timing (Outpatient)[5]	-	-	98%	98%
Urinary Catheter Removal[3,7]	-	-	98%	97%
Survey of Patients' Hospital Experiences				
Area Around Room 'Always' Quiet at Night[6]	<100	57%	61%	61%
Doctors 'Always' Communicated Well[6]	<100	86%	83%	82%
Home Recovery Information Given[6]	<100	91%	86%	85%
Hospital Given 9 or 10 on 10 Point Scale[6]	<100	73%	74%	71%
Meds 'Always' Explained Before Given[6]	<100	59%	64%	64%
Nurses 'Always' Communicated Well[6]	<100	82%	81%	79%
Pain 'Always' Well Controlled[6]	<100	78%	73%	71%
Room and Bathroom 'Always' Clean[6]	<100	79%	76%	73%
Timely Help 'Always' Received[6]	<100	79%	71%	68%
Would Definitely Recommend Hospital[6]	<100	67%	73%	71%
Use of Medical Imaging				
Cardiac Imaging Stress Test before Surgery[7]	-	-	5.4%	5.3%
Combination Abdominal CT Scan	336	1.5%	9.3%	10.5%
Combination Brain/Sinus CT Scan[1]	-	-	2.6%	2.7%
Combination Chest CT Scan	142	1.4%	4.6%	2.7%

NOTE: Hospital profiles are in alphabetical order by state, then city, then hospital within the city; Rankings exclude hospitals with less than 25 cases except for patient surveys which excludes hospitals with less than 100 cases; (a) 100-299 cases; (1) The number of cases/patients is too few to report; (2) Data submitted were based on a sample of cases/patients; (3) Results are based on a shorter time period than required; (4) Data suppressed by CMS for one or more quarters; (5) Results are not available for this reporting period; (6) Fewer than 100 patients completed the HCAHPS survey; (7) No cases met the criteria for this measure; (8) The lower limit of the confidence interval cannot be calculated if the number of observed infections equals zero; (9) No data are available from the state/territory for this reporting period; (10) The scores shown reflect fewer than 50 completed surveys; (11) There were discrepancies in the data collection process; (12) This measure does not apply to this hospital for this reporting period; (13) Results cannot be calculated for this reporting period; (14) The results for this state are combined with nearby states to protect confidentiality; Please refer to the User's Guide for a full explanation of data.

Follow-up Mammogram/Ultrasound	244	9.8%	8.4%	8.8%
Lumbar Spine MRI for Low Back Pain[1]	-	-	38.7%	37.2%

Dukes Memorial Hospital

275 W 12th St
Peru, IN 46970
URL: www.dukesmemorialhosp.com
Type: Critical Access Hospitals
Ownership: Voluntary non-profit - Private

Phone: 765-472-8000
Fax: 765-473-8244
Emergency Services: Yes
Beds: 158

Key Personnel:
Infection Control. . . . . Gail Berkheiser
CEO/President. . . . . Mike Funk
Emergency Room . . . . Fran Owens
Intensive Care Unit. . . . . Sally Piper
Chief of Medical Staff . . . . Neil J Stalker

Measure	Cases	This Hosp.	State Avg.	U.S. Avg.
Blood Clot Prevention and Treatment				
Anticoagulation Overlap Therapy[1,2]	-	-	92%	93%
ICU Venous Thromboembolism Prophylaxis[2]	45	100%	91%	92%
Incidence of Potentially Preventable VTE[2,7]	-	-	10%	10%
UFH with Dosages/Platelet Monitoring[1,2]	-	-	95%	97%
Venous Thromboembolism Prophylaxis[2]	206	96%	83%	85%
Warfarin Therapy Discharge Instructions[1,2]	-	-	71%	75%
Chest Pain/Possible Heart Attack Care				
Aspirin Given Within 24 Hours of Arrival	63	98%	96%	96%
Fibrinolytic Meds Within 30 Min. of Arrival[7]	-	-	48%	58%
Average Time to ECG (minutes)	65	7	6	7
Average Time to Transfer (minutes)[1]	-	-	46	60
Children's Asthma Care				
Received Home Management Plan of Care	-	-	-	88%
Received Reliever Medication	-	-	-	100%
Received Systemic Corticosteroids	-	-	-	100%
Emergency Department				
Admittance Decision Time (minutes)[2]	317	77	80	98
Head CT Results Within 45 Min. of Arrival	11	91%	60%	57%
Patients Who Left ER Before Being Seen	11,250	3%	2%	2%
Time from ER Arrival to Admit. (minutes)[2]	334	242	241	274
Time from ER Arrival to Discharge (minutes)	363	126	122	134
Time in ER Before Being Evaluated (minutes)	401	21	22	26
Time to Pain Meds for Fractures (minutes)	53	45	52	57
Heart Attack Care				
Aspirin Given at Discharge	22	100%	99%	99%
Fibrinolytic Meds Within 30 Min. of Arrival[7]	-	-	67%	54%
PCI Within 90 Minutes of Arrival[7]	-	-	97%	96%
Statin Prescribed at Discharge	22	100%	99%	98%
Heart Failure Care				
ACE Inhibitor or ARB for LVSD[1]	-	-	97%	97%
Discharge Instructions Given	15	93%	95%	94%
Evaluation of LVS Function	22	100%	99%	99%
Medicare Spending				
Medicare Spending per Patient (ratio)	-	-	1.01	0.98
Pneumonia Care				
Appropriate Initial Antibiotic Given	29	90%	95%	95%
Blood Culture Timing	31	100%	98%	98%
Pregnancy and Delivery Care				
Newborn Deliveries Scheduled Early[2]	23	0%	5%	6%
Preventive Care				
Immunization for Influenza[2]	283	96%	91%	90%
Immunization for Pneumonia[2]	341	99%	92%	92%
Stroke Care				
Anticoagulation Therapy for Atrial Fibrillation[7]	-	-	94%	95%
Antithrombotic Therapy Timing[1]	-	-	97%	98%
Assessed for Rehabilitation[1]	-	-	96%	97%
Discharged on Antithrombotic Therapy[1]	-	-	98%	99%
Discharged on Statin Medication[1]	-	-	91%	94%
Thrombolytic Therapy Timing[7]	-	-	54%	66%
Venous Thromboembolism Prophylaxis[1]	-	-	91%	94%
Written Stroke Educational Materials Given[1]	-	-	82%	88%
Surgical Care Improvement Project				
Appropriate Beta Blocker Usage	13	100%	98%	98%
Appropriate VTP Within 24 Hours	35	100%	98%	98%
Controlled Postoperative Blood Glucose[7]	-	-	97%	97%
Perioperative Temperature Management	39	100%	100%	100%
Prophylactic Antibiotic Selection	23	100%	99%	99%
Prophylactic Antibiotic Selection (Outpatient)	33	100%	98%	98%
Prophylactic Antibiotic Stopped	20	90%	98%	98%
Prophylactic Antibiotic Timing	23	100%	99%	99%
Prophylactic Antibiotic Timing (Outpatient)	33	100%	98%	98%
Urinary Catheter Removal[1]	-	-	98%	97%
Survey of Patients' Hospital Experiences				
Area Around Room 'Always' Quiet at Night	(a)	57%	61%	61%
Doctors 'Always' Communicated Well	(a)	85%	83%	82%
Home Recovery Information Given	(a)	86%	86%	85%
Hospital Given 9 or 10 on 10 Point Scale	(a)	66%	74%	71%
Meds 'Always' Explained Before Given	(a)	63%	64%	64%
Nurses 'Always' Communicated Well	(a)	80%	81%	79%
Pain 'Always' Well Controlled	(a)	71%	73%	71%
Room and Bathroom 'Always' Clean	(a)	73%	76%	73%
Timely Help 'Always' Received	(a)	68%	71%	68%
Would Definitely Recommend Hospital	(a)	65%	73%	71%
Use of Medical Imaging				
Cardiac Imaging Stress Test before Surgery	153	6.5%	5.4%	5.3%
Combination Abdominal CT Scan	225	1.8%	9.3%	10.5%
Combination Brain/Sinus CT Scan[1]	-	-	2.6%	2.7%
Combination Chest CT Scan	167	1.2%	4.6%	2.7%
Follow-up Mammogram/Ultrasound	201	6.5%	8.4%	8.8%
Lumbar Spine MRI for Low Back Pain[1]	-	-	38.7%	37.2%

Saint Joseph Regional Medical Center - Plymouth

1915 Lake Ave
Plymouth, IN 46563
URL: www.sjmed.com
Type: Acute Care Hospitals
Ownership: Voluntary non-profit - Church

Phone: 574-948-4000
Fax: 574-935-2250
Emergency Services: Yes
Beds: 58

Key Personnel:
Chief of Medical Staff. . . . . Stephen Anderson, MD, MMM, FACP
Quality Assurance . . . . Tammy Awland
Emergency Room . . . . Joan Hum
CEO/President. . . . . Loretta Schmidt
Chair/CEO . . . . John Zeglis

Measure	Cases	This Hosp.	State Avg.	U.S. Avg.
Blood Clot Prevention and Treatment				
Anticoagulation Overlap Therapy[1,2]	-	-	92%	93%
ICU Venous Thromboembolism Prophylaxis[2]	61	82%	91%	92%
Incidence of Potentially Preventable VTE[1,2]	-	-	10%	10%
UFH with Dosages/Platelet Monitoring[1,2]	-	-	95%	97%
Venous Thromboembolism Prophylaxis[2]	117	70%	83%	85%
Warfarin Therapy Discharge Instructions[1,2]	-	-	71%	75%
Chest Pain/Possible Heart Attack Care				
Aspirin Given Within 24 Hours of Arrival	41	100%	96%	96%
Fibrinolytic Meds Within 30 Min. of Arrival[1]	-	-	48%	58%
Average Time to ECG (minutes)	41	14	6	7
Average Time to Transfer (minutes)[7]	-	-	46	60
Children's Asthma Care				
Received Home Management Plan of Care	-	-	-	88%
Received Reliever Medication	-	-	-	100%
Received Systemic Corticosteroids	-	-	-	100%
Emergency Department				
Admittance Decision Time (minutes)[2]	328	42	80	98
Head CT Results Within 45 Min. of Arrival[1]	-	-	60%	57%
Patients Who Left ER Before Being Seen	15,767	1%	2%	2%
Time from ER Arrival to Admit. (minutes)[2]	329	197	241	274
Time from ER Arrival to Discharge (minutes)	397	108	122	134
Time in ER Before Being Evaluated (minutes)	430	10	22	26
Time to Pain Meds for Fractures (minutes)	81	48	52	57
Heart Attack Care				
Aspirin Given at Discharge	39	100%	99%	99%
Fibrinolytic Meds Within 30 Min. of Arrival[7]	-	-	67%	54%
PCI Within 90 Minutes of Arrival[7]	-	-	97%	96%
Statin Prescribed at Discharge	39	100%	99%	98%
Heart Failure Care				
ACE Inhibitor or ARB for LVSD	12	100%	97%	97%
Discharge Instructions Given	43	98%	95%	94%
Evaluation of LVS Function	59	100%	99%	99%
Medicare Spending				
Medicare Spending per Patient (ratio)	-	0.98	1.01	0.98
Pneumonia Care				
Appropriate Initial Antibiotic Given	57	100%	95%	95%
Blood Culture Timing	101	100%	98%	98%
Pregnancy and Delivery Care				
Newborn Deliveries Scheduled Early[2]	25	4%	5%	6%
Preventive Care				
Immunization for Influenza[2]	256	96%	91%	90%
Immunization for Pneumonia[2]	329	92%	92%	92%
Stroke Care				
Anticoagulation Therapy for Atrial Fibrillation[1]	-	-	94%	95%
Antithrombotic Therapy Timing	20	100%	97%	98%
Assessed for Rehabilitation	22	95%	96%	97%
Discharged on Antithrombotic Therapy	22	100%	98%	99%
Discharged on Statin Medication	18	94%	91%	94%
Thrombolytic Therapy Timing[7]	-	-	54%	66%
Venous Thromboembolism Prophylaxis	20	95%	91%	94%
Written Stroke Educational Materials Given	14	79%	82%	88%
Surgical Care Improvement Project				
Appropriate Beta Blocker Usage	37	100%	98%	98%
Appropriate VTP Within 24 Hours	78	97%	98%	98%
Controlled Postoperative Blood Glucose[7]	-	-	97%	97%
Perioperative Temperature Management	144	100%	100%	100%
Prophylactic Antibiotic Selection	110	100%	99%	99%
Prophylactic Antibiotic Selection (Outpatient)	26	100%	98%	98%
Prophylactic Antibiotic Stopped	108	100%	98%	98%
Prophylactic Antibiotic Timing	110	99%	99%	99%
Prophylactic Antibiotic Timing (Outpatient)	26	100%	98%	98%
Urinary Catheter Removal	15	93%	98%	97%
Survey of Patients' Hospital Experiences				
Area Around Room 'Always' Quiet at Night	300+	57%	61%	61%
Doctors 'Always' Communicated Well	300+	79%	83%	82%
Home Recovery Information Given	300+	88%	86%	85%
Hospital Given 9 or 10 on 10 Point Scale	300+	74%	74%	71%
Meds 'Always' Explained Before Given	300+	60%	64%	64%
Nurses 'Always' Communicated Well	300+	80%	81%	79%
Pain 'Always' Well Controlled	300+	75%	73%	71%
Room and Bathroom 'Always' Clean	300+	71%	76%	73%
Timely Help 'Always' Received	300+	69%	71%	68%
Would Definitely Recommend Hospital	300+	70%	73%	71%
Use of Medical Imaging				
Cardiac Imaging Stress Test before Surgery	196	2.6%	5.4%	5.3%
Combination Abdominal CT Scan	404	4.7%	9.3%	10.5%
Combination Brain/Sinus CT Scan[1]	-	-	2.6%	2.7%
Combination Chest CT Scan	246	0.0%	4.6%	2.7%
Follow-up Mammogram/Ultrasound	508	7.3%	8.4%	8.8%
Lumbar Spine MRI for Low Back Pain[1]	-	-	38.7%	37.2%

Jay County Hospital

500 W Votaw St
Portland, IN 47371
URL: www.jaycountyhospital.com
Type: Critical Access Hospitals
Ownership: Government - Local

Phone: 260-726-7131
Fax: 260-726-1986
Emergency Services: Yes
Beds: 25

Key Personnel:
Operating Room. . . . . Herman Burgermeister
Infection Control. . . . . Emma Gayle Collins
Cardiology . . . . Frank Conte, MD
Chief of Medical Staff . . . . Ellen Countryman
CEO/President. . . . . Dave Hyatt
Intensive Care Unit. . . . . Jane Jobe
Anesthesiology. . . . . John F Martig
Emergency Room . . . . Robert Robinson, MD

Measure	Cases	This Hosp.	State Avg.	U.S. Avg.
Blood Clot Prevention and Treatment				
Anticoagulation Overlap Therapy[1]	-	-	92%	93%
ICU Venous Thromboembolism Prophylaxis[7]	-	-	91%	92%
Incidence of Potentially Preventable VTE[7]	-	-	10%	10%
UFH with Dosages/Platelet Monitoring[1]	-	-	95%	97%
Venous Thromboembolism Prophylaxis	295	96%	83%	85%
Warfarin Therapy Discharge Instructions[1]	-	-	71%	75%
Chest Pain/Possible Heart Attack Care				
Aspirin Given Within 24 Hours of Arrival	53	94%	96%	96%
Fibrinolytic Meds Within 30 Min. of Arrival[7]	-	-	48%	58%
Average Time to ECG (minutes)	57	2	6	7
Average Time to Transfer (minutes)[7]	-	-	46	60

NOTE: Hospital profiles are in alphabetical order by state, then city, then hospital within the city; Rankings exclude hospitals with less than 25 cases except for patient surveys which excludes hospitals with less than 100 cases; (a) 100-299 cases; (1) The number of cases/patients is too few to report; (2) Data submitted were based on a sample of cases/patients; (3) Results are based on a shorter time period than required; (4) Data suppressed by CMS for one or more quarters; (5) Results are not available for this reporting period; (6) Fewer than 100 patients completed the HCAHPS survey; (7) No cases met the criteria for this measure; (8) The lower limit of the confidence interval cannot be calculated if the number of observed infections equals zero; (9) No data are available from the state/territory for this reporting period; (10) The scores shown reflect fewer than 50 completed surveys; (11) There were discrepancies in the data collection process; (12) This measure does not apply to this hospital for this reporting period; (13) Results cannot be calculated for this reporting period; (14) The results for this state are combined with nearby states to protect confidentiality; Please refer to the User's Guide for a full explanation of data.

Measure	Cases	This Hosp.	State Avg.	U.S. Avg.
Children's Asthma Care				
Received Home Management Plan of Care	-	-	-	88%
Received Reliever Medication	-	-	-	100%
Received Systemic Corticosteroids	-	-	-	100%
Emergency Department				
Admittance Decision Time (minutes)	528	55	80	98
Head CT Results Within 45 Min. of Arrival[1,3]	-	-	60%	57%
Patients Who Left ER Before Being Seen	10,233	1%	2%	2%
Time from ER Arrival to Admit. (minutes)	562	220	241	274
Time from ER Arrival to Discharge (minutes)[3]	642	121	122	134
Time in ER Before Being Evaluated (minutes)[3]	700	16	22	26
Time to Pain Meds for Fractures (minutes)[3]	14	38	52	57
Heart Attack Care				
Aspirin Given at Discharge[5]	-	-	99%	99%
Fibrinolytic Meds Within 30 Min. of Arrival[5]	-	-	67%	54%
PCI Within 90 Minutes of Arrival[5]	-	-	97%	96%
Statin Prescribed at Discharge[5]	-	-	99%	98%
Heart Failure Care				
ACE Inhibitor or ARB for LVSD[1]	-	-	97%	97%
Discharge Instructions Given[1]	-	-	95%	94%
Evaluation of LVS Function	12	92%	99%	99%
Medicare Spending				
Medicare Spending per Patient (ratio)	-	-	1.01	0.98
Pneumonia Care				
Appropriate Initial Antibiotic Given	44	95%	95%	95%
Blood Culture Timing	43	93%	98%	98%
Pregnancy and Delivery Care				
Newborn Deliveries Scheduled Early[5]	-	-	5%	6%
Preventive Care				
Immunization for Influenza	582	95%	91%	90%
Immunization for Pneumonia	752	97%	92%	92%
Stroke Care				
Anticoagulation Therapy for Atrial Fibrillation[5]	-	-	94%	95%
Antithrombotic Therapy Timing[5]	-	-	97%	98%
Assessed for Rehabilitation[5]	-	-	96%	97%
Discharged on Antithrombotic Therapy[5]	-	-	98%	99%
Discharged on Statin Medication[5]	-	-	91%	94%
Thrombolytic Therapy Timing[5]	-	-	54%	66%
Venous Thromboembolism Prophylaxis[5]	-	-	91%	94%
Written Stroke Educational Materials Given[5]	-	-	82%	88%
Surgical Care Improvement Project				
Appropriate Beta Blocker Usage[3,7]	-	-	98%	98%
Appropriate VTP Within 24 Hours	35	69%	98%	98%
Controlled Postoperative Blood Glucose[3,7]	-	-	97%	97%
Perioperative Temperature Management	42	98%	100%	100%
Prophylactic Antibiotic Selection	31	97%	99%	99%
Prophylactic Antibiotic Selection (Outpatient)[1,3]	-	-	98%	98%
Prophylactic Antibiotic Stopped	31	100%	98%	98%
Prophylactic Antibiotic Timing	31	100%	99%	99%
Prophylactic Antibiotic Timing (Outpatient)[1,3]	-	-	98%	98%
Urinary Catheter Removal	17	100%	98%	97%
Survey of Patients' Hospital Experiences				
Area Around Room 'Always' Quiet at Night	300+	72%	61%	61%
Doctors 'Always' Communicated Well	300+	85%	83%	82%
Home Recovery Information Given	300+	85%	86%	85%
Hospital Given 9 or 10 on 10 Point Scale	300+	78%	74%	71%
Meds 'Always' Explained Before Given	300+	67%	64%	64%
Nurses 'Always' Communicated Well	300+	83%	81%	79%
Pain 'Always' Well Controlled	300+	76%	73%	71%
Room and Bathroom 'Always' Clean	300+	74%	76%	73%
Timely Help 'Always' Received	300+	77%	71%	68%
Would Definitely Recommend Hospital	300+	72%	73%	71%
Use of Medical Imaging				
Cardiac Imaging Stress Test before Surgery[1]	-	-	5.4%	5.3%
Combination Abdominal CT Scan	305	1.3%	9.3%	10.5%
Combination Brain/Sinus CT Scan[1]	-	-	2.6%	2.7%
Combination Chest CT Scan	170	0.0%	4.6%	2.7%
Follow-up Mammogram/Ultrasound	343	15.2%	8.4%	8.8%
Lumbar Spine MRI for Low Back Pain	43	44.2%	38.7%	37.2%

Gibson General Hospital

1808 Sherman Dr
Princeton, IN 47670
Type: Critical Access Hospitals
Ownership: Voluntary non-profit - Private
Phone: 812-385-3401
Fax: 812-385-9323
Emergency Services: Yes
Beds: 109

Key Personnel:
Emergency Room . . . . Richard Griffin, Dir
Quality Assurance . . . . Lynette Klostermann
Chief of Medical Staff . . . . Krishna Murthy, MD
President/CEO . . . . Emmett C. Schuster

Measure	Cases	This Hosp.	State Avg.	U.S. Avg.
Blood Clot Prevention and Treatment				
Anticoagulation Overlap Therapy[5]	-	-	92%	93%
ICU Venous Thromboembolism Prophylaxis[5]	-	-	91%	92%
Incidence of Potentially Preventable VTE[5]	-	-	10%	10%
UFH with Dosages/Platelet Monitoring[5]	-	-	95%	97%
Venous Thromboembolism Prophylaxis[5]	-	-	83%	85%
Warfarin Therapy Discharge Instructions[5]	-	-	71%	75%
Chest Pain/Possible Heart Attack Care				
Aspirin Given Within 24 Hours of Arrival[5]	-	-	96%	96%
Fibrinolytic Meds Within 30 Min. of Arrival[5]	-	-	48%	58%
Average Time to ECG (minutes)[5]	-	-	6	7
Average Time to Transfer (minutes)[5]	-	-	46	60
Children's Asthma Care				
Received Home Management Plan of Care	-	-	-	88%
Received Reliever Medication	-	-	-	100%
Received Systemic Corticosteroids	-	-	-	100%
Emergency Department				
Admittance Decision Time (minutes)[5]	-	-	80	98
Head CT Results Within 45 Min. of Arrival[5]	-	-	60%	57%
Patients Who Left ER Before Being Seen	12,643	1%	2%	2%
Time from ER Arrival to Admit. (minutes)[5]	-	-	241	274
Time from ER Arrival to Discharge (minutes)[5]	-	-	122	134
Time in ER Before Being Evaluated (minutes)[5]	-	-	22	26
Time to Pain Meds for Fractures (minutes)[5]	-	-	52	57
Heart Attack Care				
Aspirin Given at Discharge[5]	-	-	99%	99%
Fibrinolytic Meds Within 30 Min. of Arrival[5]	-	-	67%	54%
PCI Within 90 Minutes of Arrival[5]	-	-	97%	96%
Statin Prescribed at Discharge[5]	-	-	99%	98%
Heart Failure Care				
ACE Inhibitor or ARB for LVSD[1]	-	-	97%	97%
Discharge Instructions Given	14	93%	95%	94%
Evaluation of LVS Function	28	93%	99%	99%
Medicare Spending				
Medicare Spending per Patient (ratio)	-	-	1.01	0.98
Pneumonia Care				
Appropriate Initial Antibiotic Given	20	100%	95%	95%
Blood Culture Timing	34	94%	98%	98%
Pregnancy and Delivery Care				
Newborn Deliveries Scheduled Early[5]	-	-	5%	6%
Preventive Care				
Immunization for Influenza[5]	-	-	91%	90%
Immunization for Pneumonia[5]	-	-	92%	92%
Stroke Care				
Anticoagulation Therapy for Atrial Fibrillation[5]	-	-	94%	95%
Antithrombotic Therapy Timing[5]	-	-	97%	98%
Assessed for Rehabilitation[5]	-	-	96%	97%
Discharged on Antithrombotic Therapy[5]	-	-	98%	99%
Discharged on Statin Medication[5]	-	-	91%	94%
Thrombolytic Therapy Timing[5]	-	-	54%	66%
Venous Thromboembolism Prophylaxis[5]	-	-	91%	94%
Written Stroke Educational Materials Given[5]	-	-	82%	88%
Surgical Care Improvement Project				
Appropriate Beta Blocker Usage[5]	-	-	98%	98%
Appropriate VTP Within 24 Hours[5]	-	-	98%	98%
Controlled Postoperative Blood Glucose[5]	-	-	97%	97%
Perioperative Temperature Management[5]	-	-	100%	100%
Prophylactic Antibiotic Selection[5]	-	-	99%	99%
Prophylactic Antibiotic Selection (Outpatient)[5]	-	-	98%	98%
Prophylactic Antibiotic Stopped[5]	-	-	98%	98%
Prophylactic Antibiotic Timing[5]	-	-	99%	99%
Prophylactic Antibiotic Timing (Outpatient)[5]	-	-	98%	98%
Urinary Catheter Removal[5]	-	-	98%	97%
Survey of Patients' Hospital Experiences				
Area Around Room 'Always' Quiet at Night	(a)	72%	61%	61%
Doctors 'Always' Communicated Well	(a)	89%	83%	82%
Home Recovery Information Given	(a)	88%	86%	85%
Hospital Given 9 or 10 on 10 Point Scale	(a)	74%	74%	71%
Meds 'Always' Explained Before Given	(a)	72%	64%	64%
Nurses 'Always' Communicated Well	(a)	89%	81%	79%
Pain 'Always' Well Controlled	(a)	81%	73%	71%
Room and Bathroom 'Always' Clean	(a)	80%	76%	73%
Timely Help 'Always' Received	(a)	82%	71%	68%
Would Definitely Recommend Hospital	(a)	72%	73%	71%
Use of Medical Imaging				
Cardiac Imaging Stress Test before Surgery[1]	-	-	5.4%	5.3%
Combination Abdominal CT Scan	205	8.8%	9.3%	10.5%
Combination Brain/Sinus CT Scan[1]	-	-	2.6%	2.7%
Combination Chest CT Scan	69	17.4%	4.6%	2.7%
Follow-up Mammogram/Ultrasound	227	16.3%	8.4%	8.8%
Lumbar Spine MRI for Low Back Pain[1]	-	-	38.7%	37.2%

Jasper County Hospital

1104 E Grace St
Rensselaer, IN 47978
URL: www.jchh.com
Type: Critical Access Hospitals
Ownership: Government - Local
Phone: 219-866-5141
Fax: 219-866-3234
Emergency Services: Yes
Beds: 86

Key Personnel:
Chief of Medical Staff . . . . Robert Darnady
Emergency Room . . . . Debra Ellis
Quality Assurance . . . . Bill Hollerman
CEO/President. . . . . Tim Schreeg

Measure	Cases	This Hosp.	State Avg.	U.S. Avg.
Blood Clot Prevention and Treatment				
Anticoagulation Overlap Therapy[5]	-	-	92%	93%
ICU Venous Thromboembolism Prophylaxis[5]	-	-	91%	92%
Incidence of Potentially Preventable VTE[5]	-	-	10%	10%
UFH with Dosages/Platelet Monitoring[5]	-	-	95%	97%
Venous Thromboembolism Prophylaxis[5]	-	-	83%	85%
Warfarin Therapy Discharge Instructions[5]	-	-	71%	75%
Chest Pain/Possible Heart Attack Care				
Aspirin Given Within 24 Hours of Arrival	55	96%	96%	96%
Fibrinolytic Meds Within 30 Min. of Arrival[7]	-	-	48%	58%
Average Time to ECG (minutes)	56	6	6	7
Average Time to Transfer (minutes)[1]	-	-	46	60
Children's Asthma Care				
Received Home Management Plan of Care	-	-	-	88%
Received Reliever Medication	-	-	-	100%
Received Systemic Corticosteroids	-	-	-	100%
Emergency Department				
Admittance Decision Time (minutes)[3]	47	75	80	98
Head CT Results Within 45 Min. of Arrival[1,3]	-	-	60%	57%
Patients Who Left ER Before Being Seen	9,903	1%	2%	2%
Time from ER Arrival to Admit. (minutes)[3]	47	184	241	274
Time from ER Arrival to Discharge (minutes)	8,320	101	122	134
Time in ER Before Being Evaluated (minutes)	8,983	21	22	26
Time to Pain Meds for Fractures (minutes)	40	68	52	57
Heart Attack Care				
Aspirin Given at Discharge[1]	-	-	99%	99%
Fibrinolytic Meds Within 30 Min. of Arrival[7]	-	-	67%	54%
PCI Within 90 Minutes of Arrival[3,7]	-	-	97%	96%
Statin Prescribed at Discharge[1]	-	-	99%	98%
Heart Failure Care				
ACE Inhibitor or ARB for LVSD[1]	-	-	97%	97%
Discharge Instructions Given	36	78%	95%	94%
Evaluation of LVS Function	67	97%	99%	99%
Medicare Spending				
Medicare Spending per Patient (ratio)	-	-	1.01	0.98
Pneumonia Care				
Appropriate Initial Antibiotic Given	32	91%	95%	95%
Blood Culture Timing	40	100%	98%	98%
Pregnancy and Delivery Care				
Newborn Deliveries Scheduled Early[3,7]	-	-	5%	6%
Preventive Care				

NOTE: Hospital profiles are in alphabetical order by state, then city, then hospital within the city; Rankings exclude hospitals with less than 25 cases except for patient surveys which excludes hospitals with less than 100 cases; (a) 100-299 cases; (1) The number of cases/patients is too few to report; (2) Data submitted were based on a sample of cases/patients; (3) Results are based on a shorter time period than required; (4) Data suppressed by CMS for one or more quarters; (5) Results are not available for this reporting period; (6) Fewer than 100 patients completed the HCAHPS survey; (7) No cases met the criteria for this measure; (8) The lower limit of the confidence interval cannot be calculated if the number of observed infections equals zero; (9) No data are available from the state/territory for this reporting period; (10) The scores shown reflect fewer than 50 completed surveys; (11) There were discrepancies in the data collection process; (12) This measure does not apply to this hospital for this reporting period; (13) Results cannot be calculated for this reporting period; (14) The results for this state are combined with nearby states to protect confidentiality; Please refer to the User's Guide for a full explanation of data.

Measure	Cases	This Hosp.	State Avg.	U.S. Avg.
Immunization for Influenza[5]	-	-	91%	90%
Immunization for Pneumonia[5]	-	-	92%	92%
Stroke Care				
Anticoagulation Therapy for Atrial Fibrillation[5]	-	-	94%	95%
Antithrombotic Therapy Timing[5]	-	-	97%	98%
Assessed for Rehabilitation[5]	-	-	96%	97%
Discharged on Antithrombotic Therapy[5]	-	-	98%	99%
Discharged on Statin Medication[5]	-	-	91%	94%
Thrombolytic Therapy Timing[5]	-	-	54%	66%
Venous Thromboembolism Prophylaxis[5]	-	-	91%	94%
Written Stroke Educational Materials Given[5]	-	-	82%	88%
Surgical Care Improvement Project				
Appropriate Beta Blocker Usage[5]	-	-	98%	98%
Appropriate VTP Within 24 Hours[3]	19	100%	98%	98%
Controlled Postoperative Blood Glucose[5]	-	-	97%	97%
Perioperative Temperature Management[3]	21	100%	100%	100%
Prophylactic Antibiotic Selection[3]	17	71%	99%	99%
Prophylactic Antibiotic Selection (Outpatient)	22	91%	98%	98%
Prophylactic Antibiotic Stopped[3]	17	94%	98%	98%
Prophylactic Antibiotic Timing[3]	17	94%	99%	99%
Prophylactic Antibiotic Timing (Outpatient)	27	78%	98%	98%
Urinary Catheter Removal[1,3]	-	-	98%	97%
Survey of Patients' Hospital Experiences				
Area Around Room 'Always' Quiet at Night	(a)	45%	61%	61%
Doctors 'Always' Communicated Well	(a)	80%	83%	82%
Home Recovery Information Given	(a)	80%	86%	85%
Hospital Given 9 or 10 on 10 Point Scale	(a)	59%	74%	71%
Meds 'Always' Explained Before Given	(a)	59%	64%	64%
Nurses 'Always' Communicated Well	(a)	75%	81%	79%
Pain 'Always' Well Controlled	(a)	69%	73%	71%
Room and Bathroom 'Always' Clean	(a)	73%	76%	73%
Timely Help 'Always' Received	(a)	58%	71%	68%
Would Definitely Recommend Hospital	(a)	47%	73%	71%
Use of Medical Imaging				
Cardiac Imaging Stress Test before Surgery[1]	-	-	5.4%	5.3%
Combination Abdominal CT Scan	257	5.1%	9.3%	10.5%
Combination Brain/Sinus CT Scan[1]	-	-	2.6%	2.7%
Combination Chest CT Scan	148	0.0%	4.6%	2.7%
Follow-up Mammogram/Ultrasound	252	5.6%	8.4%	8.8%
Lumbar Spine MRI for Low Back Pain	47	53.2%	38.7%	37.2%

Reid Hospital & Health Care Services

1100 Reid Pkwy
Richmond, IN 47374
URL: www.reidhosp.com
Phone: 765-983-3000
Fax: 765-983-3219
Type: Acute Care Hospitals
Ownership: Voluntary non-profit - Private
Emergency Services: Yes
Beds: 233

Key Personnel:
Chief of Medical Staff . . . . Rohit Barva, MD
Operating Room. . . . . Christy Brewer
Quality Assurance . . . . Marilee Crosby
Radiology. . . . . Eugene Ditullio
Coronary Care . . . . Alyson Harrell
CEO/President. . . . . Craig Kinyon
Cardiac Laboratory. . . . . Jeanette Sullivan

Measure	Cases	This Hosp.	State Avg.	U.S. Avg.
Blood Clot Prevention and Treatment				
Anticoagulation Overlap Therapy[2]	67	99%	92%	93%
ICU Venous Thromboembolism Prophylaxis[2]	97	95%	91%	92%
Incidence of Potentially Preventable VTE[1,2]	-	-	10%	10%
UFH with Dosages/Platelet Monitoring[2]	16	100%	95%	97%
Venous Thromboembolism Prophylaxis[2]	329	95%	83%	85%
Warfarin Therapy Discharge Instructions[2]	44	93%	71%	75%
Chest Pain/Possible Heart Attack Care				
Aspirin Given Within 24 Hours of Arrival[5]	-	-	96%	96%
Fibrinolytic Meds Within 30 Min. of Arrival[5]	-	-	48%	58%
Average Time to ECG (minutes)[5]	-	-	6	7
Average Time to Transfer (minutes)[5]	-	-	46	60
Children's Asthma Care				
Received Home Management Plan of Care	-	-	-	88%
Received Reliever Medication	-	-	-	100%
Received Systemic Corticosteroids	-	-	-	100%
Emergency Department				
Admittance Decision Time (minutes)[2]	676	69	80	98
Head CT Results Within 45 Min. of Arrival[1,3]	-	-	60%	57%
Patients Who Left ER Before Being Seen	46,877	0%	2%	2%
Time from ER Arrival to Admit. (minutes)[2]	747	237	241	274
Time from ER Arrival to Discharge (minutes)	367	133	122	134
Time in ER Before Being Evaluated (minutes)	369	37	22	26
Time to Pain Meds for Fractures (minutes)	117	59	52	57
Heart Attack Care				
Aspirin Given at Discharge	386	99%	99%	99%
Fibrinolytic Meds Within 30 Min. of Arrival[7]	-	-	67%	54%
PCI Within 90 Minutes of Arrival	52	98%	97%	96%
Statin Prescribed at Discharge	387	99%	99%	98%
Heart Failure Care				
ACE Inhibitor or ARB for LVSD	75	96%	97%	97%
Discharge Instructions Given	276	94%	95%	94%
Evaluation of LVS Function	387	100%	99%	99%
Medicare Spending				
Medicare Spending per Patient (ratio)	-	1.01	1.01	0.98
Pneumonia Care				
Appropriate Initial Antibiotic Given	239	98%	95%	95%
Blood Culture Timing	435	100%	98%	98%
Pregnancy and Delivery Care				
Newborn Deliveries Scheduled Early	62	13%	5%	6%
Preventive Care				
Immunization for Influenza[2]	569	83%	91%	90%
Immunization for Pneumonia[2]	846	95%	92%	92%
Stroke Care				
Anticoagulation Therapy for Atrial Fibrillation	18	100%	94%	95%
Antithrombotic Therapy Timing	138	97%	97%	98%
Assessed for Rehabilitation	142	99%	96%	97%
Discharged on Antithrombotic Therapy	133	98%	98%	99%
Discharged on Statin Medication	98	89%	91%	94%
Thrombolytic Therapy Timing[1]	-	-	54%	66%
Venous Thromboembolism Prophylaxis	150	98%	91%	94%
Written Stroke Educational Materials Given	63	89%	82%	88%
Surgical Care Improvement Project				
Appropriate Beta Blocker Usage	338	100%	98%	98%
Appropriate VTP Within 24 Hours	662	99%	98%	98%
Controlled Postoperative Blood Glucose	162	98%	97%	97%
Perioperative Temperature Management	775	100%	100%	100%
Prophylactic Antibiotic Selection	693	100%	99%	99%
Prophylactic Antibiotic Selection (Outpatient)	417	100%	98%	98%
Prophylactic Antibiotic Stopped	652	99%	98%	98%
Prophylactic Antibiotic Timing	693	100%	99%	99%
Prophylactic Antibiotic Timing (Outpatient)	418	99%	98%	98%
Urinary Catheter Removal	518	98%	98%	97%
Survey of Patients' Hospital Experiences				
Area Around Room 'Always' Quiet at Night	300+	60%	61%	61%
Doctors 'Always' Communicated Well	300+	81%	83%	82%
Home Recovery Information Given	300+	89%	86%	85%
Hospital Given 9 or 10 on 10 Point Scale	300+	73%	74%	71%
Meds 'Always' Explained Before Given	300+	66%	64%	64%
Nurses 'Always' Communicated Well	300+	79%	81%	79%
Pain 'Always' Well Controlled	300+	69%	73%	71%
Room and Bathroom 'Always' Clean	300+	80%	76%	73%
Timely Help 'Always' Received	300+	66%	71%	68%
Would Definitely Recommend Hospital	300+	70%	73%	71%
Use of Medical Imaging				
Cardiac Imaging Stress Test before Surgery	1,023	4.7%	5.4%	5.3%
Combination Abdominal CT Scan	1,707	6.5%	9.3%	10.5%
Combination Brain/Sinus CT Scan	991	2.3%	2.6%	2.7%
Combination Chest CT Scan	985	0.7%	4.6%	2.7%
Follow-up Mammogram/Ultrasound	2,102	6.1%	8.4%	8.8%
Lumbar Spine MRI for Low Back Pain	311	36.3%	38.7%	37.2%

Woodlawn Hospital

1400 E 9th St
Rochester, IN 46975
Phone: 574-223-3141
Type: Critical Access Hospitals
Emergency Services: Yes
Ownership: Government - Local

Measure	Cases	This Hosp.	State Avg.	U.S. Avg.
Blood Clot Prevention and Treatment				
Anticoagulation Overlap Therapy[5]	-	-	92%	93%
ICU Venous Thromboembolism Prophylaxis[5]	-	-	91%	92%
Incidence of Potentially Preventable VTE[5]	-	-	10%	10%
UFH with Dosages/Platelet Monitoring[5]	-	-	95%	97%
Venous Thromboembolism Prophylaxis[5]	-	-	83%	85%
Warfarin Therapy Discharge Instructions[5]	-	-	71%	75%
Chest Pain/Possible Heart Attack Care				
Aspirin Given Within 24 Hours of Arrival[5]	-	-	96%	96%
Fibrinolytic Meds Within 30 Min. of Arrival[5]	-	-	48%	58%
Average Time to ECG (minutes)[5]	-	-	6	7
Average Time to Transfer (minutes)[5]	-	-	46	60
Children's Asthma Care				
Received Home Management Plan of Care	-	-	-	88%
Received Reliever Medication	-	-	-	100%
Received Systemic Corticosteroids	-	-	-	100%
Emergency Department				
Admittance Decision Time (minutes)[5]	-	-	80	98
Head CT Results Within 45 Min. of Arrival[5]	-	-	60%	57%
Patients Who Left ER Before Being Seen	7,519	0%	2%	2%
Time from ER Arrival to Admit. (minutes)[5]	-	-	241	274
Time from ER Arrival to Discharge (minutes)[5]	-	-	122	134
Time in ER Before Being Evaluated (minutes)[5]	-	-	22	26
Time to Pain Meds for Fractures (minutes)[5]	-	-	52	57
Heart Attack Care				
Aspirin Given at Discharge[5]	-	-	99%	99%
Fibrinolytic Meds Within 30 Min. of Arrival[5]	-	-	67%	54%
PCI Within 90 Minutes of Arrival[5]	-	-	97%	96%
Statin Prescribed at Discharge[5]	-	-	99%	98%
Heart Failure Care				
ACE Inhibitor or ARB for LVSD[1]	-	-	97%	97%
Discharge Instructions Given	30	100%	95%	94%
Evaluation of LVS Function	36	69%	99%	99%
Medicare Spending				
Medicare Spending per Patient (ratio)	-	-	1.01	0.98
Pneumonia Care				
Appropriate Initial Antibiotic Given	48	81%	95%	95%
Blood Culture Timing	45	76%	98%	98%
Pregnancy and Delivery Care				
Newborn Deliveries Scheduled Early[5]	-	-	5%	6%
Preventive Care				
Immunization for Influenza[5]	-	-	91%	90%
Immunization for Pneumonia[5]	-	-	92%	92%
Stroke Care				
Anticoagulation Therapy for Atrial Fibrillation[5]	-	-	94%	95%
Antithrombotic Therapy Timing[5]	-	-	97%	98%
Assessed for Rehabilitation[5]	-	-	96%	97%
Discharged on Antithrombotic Therapy[5]	-	-	98%	99%
Discharged on Statin Medication[5]	-	-	91%	94%
Thrombolytic Therapy Timing[5]	-	-	54%	66%
Venous Thromboembolism Prophylaxis[5]	-	-	91%	94%
Written Stroke Educational Materials Given[5]	-	-	82%	88%
Surgical Care Improvement Project				
Appropriate Beta Blocker Usage[5]	-	-	98%	98%
Appropriate VTP Within 24 Hours[5]	-	-	98%	98%
Controlled Postoperative Blood Glucose[5]	-	-	97%	97%
Perioperative Temperature Management[5]	-	-	100%	100%
Prophylactic Antibiotic Selection[5]	-	-	99%	99%
Prophylactic Antibiotic Selection (Outpatient)[5]	-	-	98%	98%
Prophylactic Antibiotic Stopped[5]	-	-	98%	98%
Prophylactic Antibiotic Timing[5]	-	-	99%	99%
Prophylactic Antibiotic Timing (Outpatient)[5]	-	-	98%	98%
Urinary Catheter Removal[5]	-	-	98%	97%
Survey of Patients' Hospital Experiences				
Area Around Room 'Always' Quiet at Night	(a)	65%	61%	61%
Doctors 'Always' Communicated Well	(a)	87%	83%	82%
Home Recovery Information Given	(a)	93%	86%	85%
Hospital Given 9 or 10 on 10 Point Scale	(a)	75%	74%	71%
Meds 'Always' Explained Before Given	(a)	70%	64%	64%
Nurses 'Always' Communicated Well	(a)	83%	81%	79%
Pain 'Always' Well Controlled	(a)	75%	73%	71%
Room and Bathroom 'Always' Clean	(a)	77%	76%	73%
Timely Help 'Always' Received	(a)	72%	71%	68%
Would Definitely Recommend Hospital	(a)	77%	73%	71%

NOTE: Hospital profiles are in alphabetical order by state, then city, then hospital within the city; Rankings exclude hospitals with less than 25 cases except for patient surveys which excludes hospitals with less than 100 cases; (a) 100-299 cases; (1) The number of cases/patients is too few to report; (2) Data submitted were based on a sample of cases/patients; (3) Results are based on a shorter time period than required; (4) Data suppressed by CMS for one or more quarters; (5) Results are not available for this reporting period; (6) Fewer than 100 patients completed the HCAHPS survey; (7) No cases met the criteria for this measure; (8) The lower limit of the confidence interval cannot be calculated if the number of observed infections equals zero; (9) No data are available from the state/territory for this reporting period; (10) The scores shown reflect fewer than 50 completed surveys; (11) There were discrepancies in the data collection process; (12) This measure does not apply to this hospital for this reporting period; (13) Results cannot be calculated for this reporting period; (14) The results for this state are combined with nearby states to protect confidentiality; Please refer to the User's Guide for a full explanation of data.

Use of Medical Imaging				
Cardiac Imaging Stress Test before Surgery[1]	-	-	5.4%	5.3%
Combination Abdominal CT Scan	196	3.6%	9.3%	10.5%
Combination Brain/Sinus CT Scan	202	1.0%	2.6%	2.7%
Combination Chest CT Scan	146	2.1%	4.6%	2.7%
Follow-up Mammogram/Ultrasound	180	5.6%	8.4%	8.8%
Lumbar Spine MRI for Low Back Pain[1]	-	-	38.7%	37.2%

Rush Memorial Hospital

1300 N Main St
Rushville, IN 46173
E-mail: info@rushmemorial.com
URL: www.rushmemorial.com
Type: Critical Access Hospitals
Ownership: Government - Local

Phone: 765-932-7513
Fax: 765-932-7523
Emergency Services: Yes
Beds: 25

Key Personnel:
Radiology. . . . . Terry Aker
Pediatrics. . . . . Janet Foster
Chief of Medical Staff . . . . Ava Moore
Operating Room. . . . . Kathy Newkirk
Quality Assurance . . . . Linda Noble
CEO/President. . . . . Brad Smith
Emergency Room . . . . Carrie Tressler
Infection Control. . . . . Carol Tulley MT ASCP

Measure	Cases	This Hosp.	State Avg.	U.S. Avg.
Blood Clot Prevention and Treatment				
Anticoagulation Overlap Therapy[1]	-	-	92%	93%
ICU Venous Thromboembolism Prophylaxis[7]	-	-	91%	92%
Incidence of Potentially Preventable VTE[7]	-	-	10%	10%
UFH with Dosages/Platelet Monitoring[7]	-	-	95%	97%
Venous Thromboembolism Prophylaxis	240	12%	83%	85%
Warfarin Therapy Discharge Instructions[1]	-	-	71%	75%
Chest Pain/Possible Heart Attack Care				
Aspirin Given Within 24 Hours of Arrival	50	100%	96%	96%
Fibrinolytic Meds Within 30 Min. of Arrival[7]	-	-	48%	58%
Average Time to ECG (minutes)	51	12	6	7
Average Time to Transfer (minutes)	19	92	46	60
Children's Asthma Care				
Received Home Management Plan of Care	-	-	-	88%
Received Reliever Medication	-	-	-	100%
Received Systemic Corticosteroids	-	-	-	100%
Emergency Department				
Admittance Decision Time (minutes)[2]	220	45	80	98
Head CT Results Within 45 Min. of Arrival[1,3]	-	-	60%	57%
Patients Who Left ER Before Being Seen	9,992	1%	2%	2%
Time from ER Arrival to Admit. (minutes)[2]	242	198	241	274
Time from ER Arrival to Discharge (minutes)[5]	-	-	122	134
Time in ER Before Being Evaluated (minutes)[5]	-	-	22	26
Time to Pain Meds for Fractures (minutes)	31	34	52	57
Heart Attack Care				
Aspirin Given at Discharge[1,3]	-	-	99%	99%
Fibrinolytic Meds Within 30 Min. of Arrival[3,7]	-	-	67%	54%
PCI Within 90 Minutes of Arrival[5]	-	-	97%	96%
Statin Prescribed at Discharge[1,3]	-	-	99%	98%
Heart Failure Care				
ACE Inhibitor or ARB for LVSD[1]	-	-	97%	97%
Discharge Instructions Given	14	86%	95%	94%
Evaluation of LVS Function	22	64%	99%	99%
Medicare Spending				
Medicare Spending per Patient (ratio)	-	-	1.01	0.98
Pneumonia Care				
Appropriate Initial Antibiotic Given[7]	-	-	95%	95%
Blood Culture Timing[7]	-	-	98%	98%
Pregnancy and Delivery Care				
Newborn Deliveries Scheduled Early[3,7]	-	-	5%	6%
Preventive Care				
Immunization for Influenza[2]	207	78%	91%	90%
Immunization for Pneumonia[2]	301	83%	92%	92%
Stroke Care				
Anticoagulation Therapy for Atrial Fibrillation[3,7]	-	-	94%	95%
Antithrombotic Therapy Timing[1,3]	-	-	97%	98%
Assessed for Rehabilitation[1,3]	-	-	96%	97%
Discharged on Antithrombotic Therapy[1,3]	-	-	98%	99%
Discharged on Statin Medication[1,3]	-	-	91%	94%
Thrombolytic Therapy Timing[1,3]	-	-	54%	66%
Venous Thromboembolism Prophylaxis[1,3]	-	-	91%	94%
Written Stroke Educational Materials Given[1,3]	-	-	82%	88%
Surgical Care Improvement Project				
Appropriate Beta Blocker Usage[3,7]	-	-	98%	98%
Appropriate VTP Within 24 Hours[1,3]	-	-	98%	98%
Controlled Postoperative Blood Glucose[3,7]	-	-	97%	97%
Perioperative Temperature Management[1,3]	-	-	100%	100%
Prophylactic Antibiotic Selection[1,3]	-	-	99%	99%
Prophylactic Antibiotic Selection (Outpatient)[3,7]	-	-	98%	98%
Prophylactic Antibiotic Stopped[1,3]	-	-	98%	98%
Prophylactic Antibiotic Timing[1,3]	-	-	99%	99%
Prophylactic Antibiotic Timing (Outpatient)[1,3]	-	-	98%	98%
Urinary Catheter Removal[1,3]	-	-	98%	97%
Survey of Patients' Hospital Experiences				
Area Around Room 'Always' Quiet at Night	(a)	62%	61%	61%
Doctors 'Always' Communicated Well	(a)	86%	83%	82%
Home Recovery Information Given	(a)	80%	86%	85%
Hospital Given 9 or 10 on 10 Point Scale	(a)	66%	74%	71%
Meds 'Always' Explained Before Given	(a)	65%	64%	64%
Nurses 'Always' Communicated Well	(a)	82%	81%	79%
Pain 'Always' Well Controlled	(a)	76%	73%	71%
Room and Bathroom 'Always' Clean	(a)	82%	76%	73%
Timely Help 'Always' Received	(a)	77%	71%	68%
Would Definitely Recommend Hospital	(a)	67%	73%	71%
Use of Medical Imaging				
Cardiac Imaging Stress Test before Surgery	74	6.8%	5.4%	5.3%
Combination Abdominal CT Scan	192	7.3%	9.3%	10.5%
Combination Brain/Sinus CT Scan	180	0.0%	2.6%	2.7%
Combination Chest CT Scan	81	6.2%	4.6%	2.7%
Follow-up Mammogram/Ultrasound	218	2.8%	8.4%	8.8%
Lumbar Spine MRI for Low Back Pain[1]	-	-	38.7%	37.2%

Saint Vincent Salem Hospital

911 N Shelby St
Salem, IN 47167
Type: Critical Access Hospitals
Ownership: Voluntary non-profit - Private

Phone: 812-883-5881
Fax: 812-883-8563
Emergency Services: Yes
Beds: 70

Key Personnel:
Radiology. . . . . Abdelrahman Abdalla
Operating Room. . . . . Doris Biddle
Chief of Medical Staff . . . . Rizwan Khan, MD
CEO/President. . . . . Randy Lindauer
Intensive Care Unit. . . . . Patty Saxton
Quality Assurance . . . . Jim Steggeman
Infection Control. . . . . Lisa Woodward

Measure	Cases	This Hosp.	State Avg.	U.S. Avg.
Blood Clot Prevention and Treatment				
Anticoagulation Overlap Therapy[5]	-	-	92%	93%
ICU Venous Thromboembolism Prophylaxis[5]	-	-	91%	92%
Incidence of Potentially Preventable VTE[5]	-	-	10%	10%
UFH with Dosages/Platelet Monitoring[5]	-	-	95%	97%
Venous Thromboembolism Prophylaxis[5]	-	-	83%	85%
Warfarin Therapy Discharge Instructions[5]	-	-	71%	75%
Chest Pain/Possible Heart Attack Care				
Aspirin Given Within 24 Hours of Arrival[3]	22	68%	96%	96%
Fibrinolytic Meds Within 30 Min. of Arrival[1,3]	-	-	48%	58%
Average Time to ECG (minutes)[3]	24	8	6	7
Average Time to Transfer (minutes)[1,3]	-	-	46	60
Children's Asthma Care				
Received Home Management Plan of Care	-	-	-	88%
Received Reliever Medication	-	-	-	100%
Received Systemic Corticosteroids	-	-	-	100%
Emergency Department				
Admittance Decision Time (minutes)[2,3]	50	15	80	98
Head CT Results Within 45 Min. of Arrival[1,3]	-	-	60%	57%
Patients Who Left ER Before Being Seen	8,285	1%	2%	2%
Time from ER Arrival to Admit. (minutes)[2,3]	50	182	241	274
Time from ER Arrival to Discharge (minutes)[3]	257	117	122	134
Time in ER Before Being Evaluated (minutes)[3]	214	20	22	26
Time to Pain Meds for Fractures (minutes)[3]	39	54	52	57
Heart Attack Care				
Aspirin Given at Discharge[1,3]	-	-	99%	99%
Fibrinolytic Meds Within 30 Min. of Arrival[3,7]	-	-	67%	54%
PCI Within 90 Minutes of Arrival[3,7]	-	-	97%	96%
Statin Prescribed at Discharge[1,3]	-	-	99%	98%
Heart Failure Care				
ACE Inhibitor or ARB for LVSD[1]	-	-	97%	97%
Discharge Instructions Given[1]	-	-	95%	94%
Evaluation of LVS Function[1]	-	-	99%	99%
Medicare Spending				
Medicare Spending per Patient (ratio)	-	-	1.01	0.98
Pneumonia Care				
Appropriate Initial Antibiotic Given	31	94%	95%	95%
Blood Culture Timing	28	100%	98%	98%
Pregnancy and Delivery Care				
Newborn Deliveries Scheduled Early[3,7]	-	-	5%	6%
Preventive Care				
Immunization for Influenza[2,3]	78	86%	91%	90%
Immunization for Pneumonia[2,3]	141	93%	92%	92%
Stroke Care				
Anticoagulation Therapy for Atrial Fibrillation[3,7]	-	-	94%	95%
Antithrombotic Therapy Timing[3,7]	-	-	97%	98%
Assessed for Rehabilitation[1,3]	-	-	96%	97%
Discharged on Antithrombotic Therapy[1,3]	-	-	98%	99%
Discharged on Statin Medication[3,7]	-	-	91%	94%
Thrombolytic Therapy Timing[3,7]	-	-	54%	66%
Venous Thromboembolism Prophylaxis[1,3]	-	-	91%	94%
Written Stroke Educational Materials Given[1,3]	-	-	82%	88%
Surgical Care Improvement Project				
Appropriate Beta Blocker Usage[1,3]	-	-	98%	98%
Appropriate VTP Within 24 Hours[1,3]	-	-	98%	98%
Controlled Postoperative Blood Glucose[3,7]	-	-	97%	97%
Perioperative Temperature Management[1,3]	-	-	100%	100%
Prophylactic Antibiotic Selection[1,3]	-	-	99%	99%
Prophylactic Antibiotic Selection (Outpatient)[3,7]	-	-	98%	98%
Prophylactic Antibiotic Stopped[1,3]	-	-	98%	98%
Prophylactic Antibiotic Timing[1,3]	-	-	99%	99%
Prophylactic Antibiotic Timing (Outpatient)[1,3]	-	-	98%	98%
Urinary Catheter Removal[1,3]	-	-	98%	97%
Survey of Patients' Hospital Experiences				
Area Around Room 'Always' Quiet at Night[6]	<100	65%	61%	61%
Doctors 'Always' Communicated Well[6]	<100	81%	83%	82%
Home Recovery Information Given[6]	<100	87%	86%	85%
Hospital Given 9 or 10 on 10 Point Scale[6]	<100	62%	74%	71%
Meds 'Always' Explained Before Given[6]	<100	75%	64%	64%
Nurses 'Always' Communicated Well[6]	<100	85%	81%	79%
Pain 'Always' Well Controlled[6]	<100	80%	73%	71%
Room and Bathroom 'Always' Clean[6]	<100	71%	76%	73%
Timely Help 'Always' Received[6]	<100	74%	71%	68%
Would Definitely Recommend Hospital[6]	<100	69%	73%	71%
Use of Medical Imaging				
Cardiac Imaging Stress Test before Surgery	105	6.7%	5.4%	5.3%
Combination Abdominal CT Scan	182	4.4%	9.3%	10.5%
Combination Brain/Sinus CT Scan[1]	-	-	2.6%	2.7%
Combination Chest CT Scan	99	4.0%	4.6%	2.7%
Follow-up Mammogram/Ultrasound	180	9.4%	8.4%	8.8%
Lumbar Spine MRI for Low Back Pain	37	54.1%	38.7%	37.2%

Scott Memorial Hospital

1451 N Gardner St
Scottsburg, IN 47170
E-mail: jwells@hsonline.net
URL: www.scottmemorial.com
Type: Critical Access Hospitals
Ownership: Voluntary non-profit - Other

Phone: 812-752-3456
Fax: 812-752-5884
Emergency Services: Yes
Beds: 90

Key Personnel:
Chief of Medical Staff . . . . Shane Avery
Patient Relations . . . . Cindy Bush
CEO/President. . . . . William Cooke, M
Emergency Room . . . . John Croasdell, MD
CEO/President. . . . . Mike Everett
Patient Relations . . . . Dawn Mays
Cardiac Laboratory. . . . . Zaka Rahman
Quality Assurance . . . . Cheryl Stultz, RN

Measure	Cases	This Hosp.	State Avg.	U.S. Avg.
Blood Clot Prevention and Treatment				
Anticoagulation Overlap Therapy[1,2]	-	-	92%	93%

NOTE: Hospital profiles are in alphabetical order by state, then city, then hospital within the city; Rankings exclude hospitals with less than 25 cases except for patient surveys which excludes hospitals with less than 100 cases; (a) 100-299 cases; (1) The number of cases/patients is too few to report; (2) Data submitted were based on a sample of cases/patients; (3) Results are based on a shorter time period than required; (4) Data suppressed by CMS for one or more quarters; (5) Results are not available for this reporting period; (6) Fewer than 100 patients completed the HCAHPS survey; (7) No cases met the criteria for this measure; (8) The lower limit of the confidence interval cannot be calculated if the number of observed infections equals zero; (9) No data are available from the state/territory for this reporting period; (10) The scores shown reflect fewer than 50 completed surveys; (11) There were discrepancies in the data collection process; (12) This measure does not apply to this hospital for this reporting period; (13) Results cannot be calculated for this reporting period; (14) The results for this state are combined with nearby states to protect confidentiality; Please refer to the User's Guide for a full explanation of data.

Measure	Cases	This Hosp.	State Avg.	U.S. Avg.
ICU Venous Thromboembolism Prophylaxis[2]	35	94%	91%	92%
Incidence of Potentially Preventable VTE[1,2]	-	-	10%	10%
UFH with Dosages/Platelet Monitoring[1,2]	-	-	95%	97%
Venous Thromboembolism Prophylaxis[2]	92	87%	83%	85%
Warfarin Therapy Discharge Instructions[1,2]	-	-	71%	75%
Chest Pain/Possible Heart Attack Care				
Aspirin Given Within 24 Hours of Arrival	-	-	96%	96%
Fibrinolytic Meds Within 30 Min. of Arrival	-	-	48%	58%
Average Time to ECG (minutes)	-	-	6	7
Average Time to Transfer (minutes)	-	-	46	60
Children's Asthma Care				
Received Home Management Plan of Care	-	-	-	88%
Received Reliever Medication	-	-	-	100%
Received Systemic Corticosteroids	-	-	-	100%
Emergency Department				
Admittance Decision Time (minutes)[5]	-	-	80	98
Head CT Results Within 45 Min. of Arrival	-	-	60%	57%
Patients Who Left ER Before Being Seen	-	-	2%	2%
Time from ER Arrival to Admit. (minutes)[5]	-	-	241	274
Time from ER Arrival to Discharge (minutes)	-	-	122	134
Time in ER Before Being Evaluated (minutes)	-	-	22	26
Time to Pain Meds for Fractures (minutes)	-	-	52	57
Heart Attack Care				
Aspirin Given at Discharge[5]	-	-	99%	99%
Fibrinolytic Meds Within 30 Min. of Arrival[5]	-	-	67%	54%
PCI Within 90 Minutes of Arrival[5]	-	-	97%	96%
Statin Prescribed at Discharge[5]	-	-	99%	98%
Heart Failure Care				
ACE Inhibitor or ARB for LVSD[1]	-	-	97%	97%
Discharge Instructions Given	25	76%	95%	94%
Evaluation of LVS Function	36	97%	99%	99%
Medicare Spending				
Medicare Spending per Patient (ratio)	-	-	1.01	0.98
Pneumonia Care				
Appropriate Initial Antibiotic Given	74	93%	95%	95%
Blood Culture Timing	83	93%	98%	98%
Pregnancy and Delivery Care				
Newborn Deliveries Scheduled Early[1,3]	-	-	5%	6%
Preventive Care				
Immunization for Influenza[5]	-	-	91%	90%
Immunization for Pneumonia[5]	-	-	92%	92%
Stroke Care				
Anticoagulation Therapy for Atrial Fibrillation[5]	-	-	94%	95%
Antithrombotic Therapy Timing[5]	-	-	97%	98%
Assessed for Rehabilitation[5]	-	-	96%	97%
Discharged on Antithrombotic Therapy[5]	-	-	98%	99%
Discharged on Statin Medication[5]	-	-	91%	94%
Thrombolytic Therapy Timing[5]	-	-	54%	66%
Venous Thromboembolism Prophylaxis[5]	-	-	91%	94%
Written Stroke Educational Materials Given[5]	-	-	82%	88%
Surgical Care Improvement Project				
Appropriate Beta Blocker Usage[5]	-	-	98%	98%
Appropriate VTP Within 24 Hours[5]	-	-	98%	98%
Controlled Postoperative Blood Glucose[5]	-	-	97%	97%
Perioperative Temperature Management[5]	-	-	100%	100%
Prophylactic Antibiotic Selection[5]	-	-	99%	99%
Prophylactic Antibiotic Selection (Outpatient)	-	-	98%	98%
Prophylactic Antibiotic Stopped[5]	-	-	98%	98%
Prophylactic Antibiotic Timing[5]	-	-	99%	99%
Prophylactic Antibiotic Timing (Outpatient)	-	-	98%	98%
Urinary Catheter Removal[5]	-	-	98%	97%
Survey of Patients' Hospital Experiences				
Area Around Room 'Always' Quiet at Night	(a)	60%	61%	61%
Doctors 'Always' Communicated Well	(a)	82%	83%	82%
Home Recovery Information Given	(a)	85%	86%	85%
Hospital Given 9 or 10 on 10 Point Scale	(a)	75%	74%	71%
Meds 'Always' Explained Before Given	(a)	77%	64%	64%
Nurses 'Always' Communicated Well	(a)	84%	81%	79%
Pain 'Always' Well Controlled	(a)	70%	73%	71%
Room and Bathroom 'Always' Clean	(a)	79%	76%	73%
Timely Help 'Always' Received	(a)	79%	71%	68%
Would Definitely Recommend Hospital	(a)	68%	73%	71%
Use of Medical Imaging				
Cardiac Imaging Stress Test before Surgery	-	-	5.4%	5.3%
Combination Abdominal CT Scan	-	-	9.3%	10.5%
Combination Brain/Sinus CT Scan	-	-	2.6%	2.7%
Combination Chest CT Scan	-	-	4.6%	2.7%
Follow-up Mammogram/Ultrasound	-	-	8.4%	8.8%
Lumbar Spine MRI for Low Back Pain	-	-	38.7%	37.2%

Schneck Medical Center

411 W Tipton St
Seymour, IN 47274
E-mail: info@schneckmed.org
URL: www.schneckmed.org
Type: Acute Care Hospitals
Ownership: Government - Local
Phone: 812-522-2349
Fax: 812-522-0544
Emergency Services: Yes
Beds: 166

Key Personnel:
CEO/President. . . . . Gary A Meyer, MHA
Infection Control. . . . . Judy Tape

Measure	Cases	This Hosp.	State Avg.	U.S. Avg.
Blood Clot Prevention and Treatment				
Anticoagulation Overlap Therapy[2]	16	100%	92%	93%
ICU Venous Thromboembolism Prophylaxis[2]	54	100%	91%	92%
Incidence of Potentially Preventable VTE[1,2]	-	-	10%	10%
UFH with Dosages/Platelet Monitoring[1,2]	-	-	95%	97%
Venous Thromboembolism Prophylaxis[2]	219	97%	83%	85%
Warfarin Therapy Discharge Instructions[1,2]	-	-	71%	75%
Chest Pain/Possible Heart Attack Care				
Aspirin Given Within 24 Hours of Arrival	170	97%	96%	96%
Fibrinolytic Meds Within 30 Min. of Arrival[7]	-	-	48%	58%
Average Time to ECG (minutes)	177	5	6	7
Average Time to Transfer (minutes)	20	18	46	60
Children's Asthma Care				
Received Home Management Plan of Care	-	-	-	88%
Received Reliever Medication	-	-	-	100%
Received Systemic Corticosteroids	-	-	-	100%
Emergency Department				
Admittance Decision Time (minutes)[2]	315	44	80	98
Head CT Results Within 45 Min. of Arrival[1]	-	-	60%	57%
Patients Who Left ER Before Being Seen	29,743	2%	2%	2%
Time from ER Arrival to Admit. (minutes)[2]	350	195	241	274
Time from ER Arrival to Discharge (minutes)	351	87	122	134
Time in ER Before Being Evaluated (minutes)	358	20	22	26
Time to Pain Meds for Fractures (minutes)	65	42	52	57
Heart Attack Care				
Aspirin Given at Discharge[1]	-	-	99%	99%
Fibrinolytic Meds Within 30 Min. of Arrival[7]	-	-	67%	54%
PCI Within 90 Minutes of Arrival[7]	-	-	97%	96%
Statin Prescribed at Discharge[1]	-	-	99%	98%
Heart Failure Care				
ACE Inhibitor or ARB for LVSD	17	100%	97%	97%
Discharge Instructions Given	37	100%	95%	94%
Evaluation of LVS Function	62	100%	99%	99%
Medicare Spending				
Medicare Spending per Patient (ratio)	-	0.91	1.01	0.98
Pneumonia Care				
Appropriate Initial Antibiotic Given	81	96%	95%	95%
Blood Culture Timing	94	98%	98%	98%
Pregnancy and Delivery Care				
Newborn Deliveries Scheduled Early[2]	76	12%	5%	6%
Preventive Care				
Immunization for Influenza[2]	361	99%	91%	90%
Immunization for Pneumonia[2]	381	97%	92%	92%
Stroke Care				
Anticoagulation Therapy for Atrial Fibrillation[1]	-	-	94%	95%
Antithrombotic Therapy Timing	39	100%	97%	98%
Assessed for Rehabilitation	40	98%	96%	97%
Discharged on Antithrombotic Therapy	39	95%	98%	99%
Discharged on Statin Medication	33	88%	91%	94%
Thrombolytic Therapy Timing[1]	-	-	54%	66%
Venous Thromboembolism Prophylaxis	40	100%	91%	94%
Written Stroke Educational Materials Given	19	63%	82%	88%
Surgical Care Improvement Project				
Appropriate Beta Blocker Usage	84	96%	98%	98%
Appropriate VTP Within 24 Hours	251	99%	98%	98%
Controlled Postoperative Blood Glucose[7]	-	-	97%	97%
Perioperative Temperature Management	267	100%	100%	100%
Prophylactic Antibiotic Selection	178	99%	99%	99%
Prophylactic Antibiotic Selection (Outpatient)	141	97%	98%	98%
Prophylactic Antibiotic Stopped	167	98%	98%	98%
Prophylactic Antibiotic Timing	179	98%	99%	99%
Prophylactic Antibiotic Timing (Outpatient)	140	99%	98%	98%
Urinary Catheter Removal	46	98%	98%	97%
Survey of Patients' Hospital Experiences				
Area Around Room 'Always' Quiet at Night	300+	68%	61%	61%
Doctors 'Always' Communicated Well	300+	86%	83%	82%
Home Recovery Information Given	300+	85%	86%	85%
Hospital Given 9 or 10 on 10 Point Scale	300+	77%	74%	71%
Meds 'Always' Explained Before Given	300+	68%	64%	64%
Nurses 'Always' Communicated Well	300+	85%	81%	79%
Pain 'Always' Well Controlled	300+	78%	73%	71%
Room and Bathroom 'Always' Clean	300+	81%	76%	73%
Timely Help 'Always' Received	300+	74%	71%	68%
Would Definitely Recommend Hospital	300+	75%	73%	71%
Use of Medical Imaging				
Cardiac Imaging Stress Test before Surgery	220	3.6%	5.4%	5.3%
Combination Abdominal CT Scan	593	3.0%	9.3%	10.5%
Combination Brain/Sinus CT Scan[1]	-	-	2.6%	2.7%
Combination Chest CT Scan	359	0.3%	4.6%	2.7%
Follow-up Mammogram/Ultrasound	657	11.4%	8.4%	8.8%
Lumbar Spine MRI for Low Back Pain	103	47.6%	38.7%	37.2%

Major Hospital

150 W Washington St
Shelbyville, IN 46176
E-mail: info@majorhospital.org
URL: www.majorhospital.org
Type: Acute Care Hospitals
Ownership: Government - Local
Phone: 317-392-3211
Fax: 317-398-5253
Emergency Services: Yes
Beds: 89

Key Personnel:
Cardiology . . . . Sunil Advani
Pediatrics. . . . . Angela Bulm
Anesthesiology. . . . . David D Darding, MD
Pediatrics. . . . . Evan Eckart
CEO/President. . . . . Anthony B Lennen
Radiology. . . . . Scott R Miller, MD
Pulmonology . . . . Robert G Shellman
Chief of Medical Staff. . . . . Ed Stone, MD

Measure	Cases	This Hosp.	State Avg.	U.S. Avg.
Blood Clot Prevention and Treatment				
Anticoagulation Overlap Therapy[2]	24	92%	92%	93%
ICU Venous Thromboembolism Prophylaxis[2]	65	97%	91%	92%
Incidence of Potentially Preventable VTE[1,2]	-	-	10%	10%
UFH with Dosages/Platelet Monitoring[1,2]	-	-	95%	97%
Venous Thromboembolism Prophylaxis[2]	249	93%	83%	85%
Warfarin Therapy Discharge Instructions[2]	13	100%	71%	75%
Chest Pain/Possible Heart Attack Care				
Aspirin Given Within 24 Hours of Arrival	44	93%	96%	96%
Fibrinolytic Meds Within 30 Min. of Arrival[7]	-	-	48%	58%
Average Time to ECG (minutes)	46	4	6	7
Average Time to Transfer (minutes)	17	40	46	60
Children's Asthma Care				
Received Home Management Plan of Care	-	-	-	88%
Received Reliever Medication	-	-	-	100%
Received Systemic Corticosteroids	-	-	-	100%
Emergency Department				
Admittance Decision Time (minutes)[2]	467	37	80	98
Head CT Results Within 45 Min. of Arrival[1]	-	-	60%	57%
Patients Who Left ER Before Being Seen	23,279	2%	2%	2%
Time from ER Arrival to Admit. (minutes)[2]	470	212	241	274
Time from ER Arrival to Discharge (minutes)	460	138	122	134
Time in ER Before Being Evaluated (minutes)	477	5	22	26
Time to Pain Meds for Fractures (minutes)	78	51	52	57
Heart Attack Care				
Aspirin Given at Discharge[1]	-	-	99%	99%
Fibrinolytic Meds Within 30 Min. of Arrival[7]	-	-	67%	54%
PCI Within 90 Minutes of Arrival[7]	-	-	97%	96%
Statin Prescribed at Discharge[1]	-	-	99%	98%

NOTE: Hospital profiles are in alphabetical order by state, then city, then hospital within the city; Rankings exclude hospitals with less than 25 cases except for patient surveys which excludes hospitals with less than 100 cases; (a) 100-299 cases; (1) The number of cases/patients is too few to report; (2) Data submitted were based on a sample of cases/patients; (3) Results are based on a shorter time period than required; (4) Data suppressed by CMS for one or more quarters; (5) Results are not available for this reporting period; (6) Fewer than 100 patients completed the HCAHPS survey; (7) No cases met the criteria for this measure; (8) The lower limit of the confidence interval cannot be calculated if the number of observed infections equals zero; (9) No data are available from the state/territory for this reporting period; (10) The scores shown reflect fewer than 50 completed surveys; (11) There were discrepancies in the data collection process; (12) This measure does not apply to this hospital for this reporting period; (13) Results cannot be calculated for this reporting period; (14) The results for this state are combined with nearby states to protect confidentiality; Please refer to the User's Guide for a full explanation of data.

Measure	Cases	This Hosp.	State Avg.	U.S. Avg.
Heart Failure Care				
ACE Inhibitor or ARB for LVSD	26	100%	97%	97%
Discharge Instructions Given	72	97%	95%	94%
Evaluation of LVS Function	87	100%	99%	99%
Medicare Spending				
Medicare Spending per Patient (ratio)	-	1.02	1.01	0.98
Pneumonia Care				
Appropriate Initial Antibiotic Given	58	95%	95%	95%
Blood Culture Timing	115	99%	98%	98%
Pregnancy and Delivery Care				
Newborn Deliveries Scheduled Early[2]	16	0%	5%	6%
Preventive Care				
Immunization for Influenza[2]	334	98%	91%	90%
Immunization for Pneumonia[2]	405	99%	92%	92%
Stroke Care				
Anticoagulation Therapy for Atrial Fibrillation[1]	-	-	94%	95%
Antithrombotic Therapy Timing	35	100%	97%	98%
Assessed for Rehabilitation	35	91%	96%	97%
Discharged on Antithrombotic Therapy	33	100%	98%	99%
Discharged on Statin Medication	22	95%	91%	94%
Thrombolytic Therapy Timing[1]	-	-	54%	66%
Venous Thromboembolism Prophylaxis	40	100%	91%	94%
Written Stroke Educational Materials Given	18	100%	82%	88%
Surgical Care Improvement Project				
Appropriate Beta Blocker Usage	65	98%	98%	98%
Appropriate VTP Within 24 Hours	167	100%	98%	98%
Controlled Postoperative Blood Glucose[7]	-	-	97%	97%
Perioperative Temperature Management	197	99%	100%	100%
Prophylactic Antibiotic Selection	143	100%	99%	99%
Prophylactic Antibiotic Selection (Outpatient)	13	100%	98%	98%
Prophylactic Antibiotic Stopped	139	99%	98%	98%
Prophylactic Antibiotic Timing	143	100%	99%	99%
Prophylactic Antibiotic Timing (Outpatient)	13	100%	98%	98%
Urinary Catheter Removal	139	100%	98%	97%
Survey of Patients' Hospital Experiences				
Area Around Room 'Always' Quiet at Night	300+	58%	61%	61%
Doctors 'Always' Communicated Well	300+	84%	83%	82%
Home Recovery Information Given	300+	89%	86%	85%
Hospital Given 9 or 10 on 10 Point Scale	300+	75%	74%	71%
Meds 'Always' Explained Before Given	300+	67%	64%	64%
Nurses 'Always' Communicated Well	300+	83%	81%	79%
Pain 'Always' Well Controlled	300+	74%	73%	71%
Room and Bathroom 'Always' Clean	300+	82%	76%	73%
Timely Help 'Always' Received	300+	75%	71%	68%
Would Definitely Recommend Hospital	300+	71%	73%	71%
Use of Medical Imaging				
Cardiac Imaging Stress Test before Surgery	253	5.1%	5.4%	5.3%
Combination Abdominal CT Scan	461	13.7%	9.3%	10.5%
Combination Brain/Sinus CT Scan[1]	-	-	2.6%	2.7%
Combination Chest CT Scan	308	12.7%	4.6%	2.7%
Follow-up Mammogram/Ultrasound	676	3.7%	8.4%	8.8%
Lumbar Spine MRI for Low Back Pain	95	34.7%	38.7%	37.2%

Memorial Hospital of South Bend

615 N Michigan St
South Bend, IN 46601
Phone: 574-647-1000
Fax: 574-647-3670
E-mail: ltatum@memorialsb.org
URL: www.qualityoflife.org
Type: Acute Care Hospitals
Emergency Services: Yes
Ownership: Voluntary non-profit - Private
Beds: 526

Key Personnel:
Chair/CEO . . . . Thomas Burish, PhD
Radiology. . . . . Gerard DuPrat, MD
Pediatric Ambulatory Care . . . . . . Michael Hudson, MD
Pediatric In-Patient Care . . . . Michael Hudson, MD
Infection Control. . . . . Susan Kraska
Chief of Medical Staff . . . . John Mathis, MD
Quality Assurance . . . . Becky Starzynski
Operating Room. . . . . Charlotte Zircher

Measure	Cases	This Hosp.	State Avg.	U.S. Avg.
Blood Clot Prevention and Treatment				
Anticoagulation Overlap Therapy[2]	131	85%	92%	93%
ICU Venous Thromboembolism Prophylaxis[2]	38	95%	91%	92%
Incidence of Potentially Preventable VTE[2]	27	0%	10%	10%
UFH with Dosages/Platelet Monitoring[2]	74	73%	95%	97%
Venous Thromboembolism Prophylaxis[2]	306	89%	83%	85%
Warfarin Therapy Discharge Instructions[2]	109	46%	71%	75%
Chest Pain/Possible Heart Attack Care				
Aspirin Given Within 24 Hours of Arrival[5]	-	-	96%	96%
Fibrinolytic Meds Within 30 Min. of Arrival[5]	-	-	48%	58%
Average Time to ECG (minutes)[5]	-	-	6	7
Average Time to Transfer (minutes)[5]	-	-	46	60
Children's Asthma Care				
Received Home Management Plan of Care	-	-	-	88%
Received Reliever Medication	-	-	-	100%
Received Systemic Corticosteroids	-	-	-	100%
Emergency Department				
Admittance Decision Time (minutes)[2]	373	91	80	98
Head CT Results Within 45 Min. of Arrival[1]	-	-	60%	57%
Patients Who Left ER Before Being Seen	56,583	1%	2%	2%
Time from ER Arrival to Admit. (minutes)[2]	398	252	241	274
Time from ER Arrival to Discharge (minutes)	441	197	122	134
Time in ER Before Being Evaluated (minutes)	467	68	22	26
Time to Pain Meds for Fractures (minutes)	182	86	52	57
Heart Attack Care				
Aspirin Given at Discharge	301	99%	99%	99%
Fibrinolytic Meds Within 30 Min. of Arrival[7]	-	-	67%	54%
PCI Within 90 Minutes of Arrival	68	99%	97%	96%
Statin Prescribed at Discharge	304	98%	99%	98%
Heart Failure Care				
ACE Inhibitor or ARB for LVSD	104	100%	97%	97%
Discharge Instructions Given	314	99%	95%	94%
Evaluation of LVS Function	399	100%	99%	99%
Medicare Spending				
Medicare Spending per Patient (ratio)	-	0.98	1.01	0.98
Pneumonia Care				
Appropriate Initial Antibiotic Given	188	95%	95%	95%
Blood Culture Timing	311	100%	98%	98%
Pregnancy and Delivery Care				
Newborn Deliveries Scheduled Early	184	4%	5%	6%
Preventive Care				
Immunization for Influenza[2]	517	99%	91%	90%
Immunization for Pneumonia[2]	509	96%	92%	92%
Stroke Care				
Anticoagulation Therapy for Atrial Fibrillation	22	100%	94%	95%
Antithrombotic Therapy Timing	146	97%	97%	98%
Assessed for Rehabilitation	194	99%	96%	97%
Discharged on Antithrombotic Therapy	163	97%	98%	99%
Discharged on Statin Medication	133	91%	91%	94%
Thrombolytic Therapy Timing	24	79%	54%	66%
Venous Thromboembolism Prophylaxis	203	97%	91%	94%
Written Stroke Educational Materials Given	89	92%	82%	88%
Surgical Care Improvement Project				
Appropriate Beta Blocker Usage[2]	231	98%	98%	98%
Appropriate VTP Within 24 Hours[2]	405	97%	98%	98%
Controlled Postoperative Blood Glucose[2]	156	99%	97%	97%
Perioperative Temperature Management[2]	600	100%	100%	100%
Prophylactic Antibiotic Selection[2]	573	100%	99%	99%
Prophylactic Antibiotic Selection (Outpatient)	530	98%	98%	98%
Prophylactic Antibiotic Stopped[2]	557	98%	98%	98%
Prophylactic Antibiotic Timing[2]	575	100%	99%	99%
Prophylactic Antibiotic Timing (Outpatient)	531	99%	98%	98%
Urinary Catheter Removal[2]	227	91%	98%	97%
Survey of Patients' Hospital Experiences				
Area Around Room 'Always' Quiet at Night	300+	47%	61%	61%
Doctors 'Always' Communicated Well	300+	80%	83%	82%
Home Recovery Information Given	300+	88%	86%	85%
Hospital Given 9 or 10 on 10 Point Scale	300+	75%	74%	71%
Meds 'Always' Explained Before Given	300+	60%	64%	64%
Nurses 'Always' Communicated Well	300+	80%	81%	79%
Pain 'Always' Well Controlled	300+	70%	73%	71%
Room and Bathroom 'Always' Clean	300+	72%	76%	73%
Timely Help 'Always' Received	300+	72%	71%	68%
Would Definitely Recommend Hospital	300+	80%	73%	71%
Use of Medical Imaging				
Cardiac Imaging Stress Test before Surgery	583	4.8%	5.4%	5.3%
Combination Abdominal CT Scan	863	5.9%	9.3%	10.5%
Combination Brain/Sinus CT Scan	861	1.6%	2.6%	2.7%
Combination Chest CT Scan	505	3.2%	4.6%	2.7%
Follow-up Mammogram/Ultrasound	2,166	6.6%	8.4%	8.8%
Lumbar Spine MRI for Low Back Pain[1]	-	-	38.7%	37.2%

Sullivan County Community Hospital

2200 N Section St
Sullivan, IN 47882
Phone: 812-268-4311
Fax: 812-268-2570
E-mail: denisebrashear@schosp.com
URL: www.schosp.com
Type: Critical Access Hospitals
Emergency Services: Yes
Ownership: Government - Local
Beds: 34

Key Personnel:
Chief of Medical Staff . . . . Gene Bourgasser, MD
Infection Control. . . . . Marti Bradbury, RN
Intensive Care Unit. . . . . Marian Bynum, RN
CEO . . . . Michelle Franklin
Operating Room. . . . . Marilyn Fuson
Radiology. . . . . Stan Hobbs
Quality Assurance . . . . Susan Pershing
Patient Relations . . . . Michelle Smith

Measure	Cases	This Hosp.	State Avg.	U.S. Avg.
Blood Clot Prevention and Treatment				
Anticoagulation Overlap Therapy[5]	-	-	92%	93%
ICU Venous Thromboembolism Prophylaxis[5]	-	-	91%	92%
Incidence of Potentially Preventable VTE[5]	-	-	10%	10%
UFH with Dosages/Platelet Monitoring[5]	-	-	95%	97%
Venous Thromboembolism Prophylaxis[5]	-	-	83%	85%
Warfarin Therapy Discharge Instructions[5]	-	-	71%	75%
Chest Pain/Possible Heart Attack Care				
Aspirin Given Within 24 Hours of Arrival	54	96%	96%	96%
Fibrinolytic Meds Within 30 Min. of Arrival[7]	-	-	48%	58%
Average Time to ECG (minutes)	57	5	6	7
Average Time to Transfer (minutes)[1]	-	-	46	60
Children's Asthma Care				
Received Home Management Plan of Care	-	-	-	88%
Received Reliever Medication	-	-	-	100%
Received Systemic Corticosteroids	-	-	-	100%
Emergency Department				
Admittance Decision Time (minutes)[5]	-	-	80	98
Head CT Results Within 45 Min. of Arrival[1]	-	-	60%	57%
Patients Who Left ER Before Being Seen	8,839	1%	2%	2%
Time from ER Arrival to Admit. (minutes)[5]	-	-	241	274
Time from ER Arrival to Discharge (minutes)[5]	-	-	122	134
Time in ER Before Being Evaluated (minutes)[5]	-	-	22	26
Time to Pain Meds for Fractures (minutes)	42	45	52	57
Heart Attack Care				
Aspirin Given at Discharge[1]	-	-	99%	99%
Fibrinolytic Meds Within 30 Min. of Arrival[7]	-	-	67%	54%
PCI Within 90 Minutes of Arrival[7]	-	-	97%	96%
Statin Prescribed at Discharge[1]	-	-	99%	98%
Heart Failure Care				
ACE Inhibitor or ARB for LVSD	12	58%	97%	97%
Discharge Instructions Given	26	85%	95%	94%
Evaluation of LVS Function	41	95%	99%	99%
Medicare Spending				
Medicare Spending per Patient (ratio)	-	-	1.01	0.98
Pneumonia Care				
Appropriate Initial Antibiotic Given	33	97%	95%	95%
Blood Culture Timing	58	93%	98%	98%
Pregnancy and Delivery Care				
Newborn Deliveries Scheduled Early[5]	-	-	5%	6%
Preventive Care				
Immunization for Influenza[5]	-	-	91%	90%
Immunization for Pneumonia[5]	-	-	92%	92%
Stroke Care				
Anticoagulation Therapy for Atrial Fibrillation[5]	-	-	94%	95%
Antithrombotic Therapy Timing[5]	-	-	97%	98%
Assessed for Rehabilitation[5]	-	-	96%	97%
Discharged on Antithrombotic Therapy[5]	-	-	98%	99%
Discharged on Statin Medication[5]	-	-	91%	94%
Thrombolytic Therapy Timing[5]	-	-	54%	66%
Venous Thromboembolism Prophylaxis[5]	-	-	91%	94%

NOTE: Hospital profiles are in alphabetical order by state, then city, then hospital within the city; Rankings exclude hospitals with less than 25 cases except for patient surveys which excludes hospitals with less than 100 cases; (a) 100-299 cases; (1) The number of cases/patients is too few to report; (2) Data submitted were based on a sample of cases/patients; (3) Results are based on a shorter time period than required; (4) Data suppressed by CMS for one or more quarters; (5) Results are not available for this reporting period; (6) Fewer than 100 patients completed the HCAHPS survey; (7) No cases met the criteria for this measure; (8) The lower limit of the confidence interval cannot be calculated if the number of observed infections equals zero; (9) No data are available from the state/territory for this reporting period; (10) The scores shown reflect fewer than 50 completed surveys; (11) There were discrepancies in the data collection process; (12) This measure does not apply to this hospital for this reporting period; (13) Results cannot be calculated for this reporting period; (14) The results for this state are combined with nearby states to protect confidentiality; Please refer to the User's Guide for a full explanation of data.

Measure	Cases	This Hosp.	State Avg.	U.S. Avg.
Written Stroke Educational Materials Given[5]	-	-	82%	88%
Surgical Care Improvement Project				
Appropriate Beta Blocker Usage[1]	-	-	98%	98%
Appropriate VTP Within 24 Hours	17	94%	98%	98%
Controlled Postoperative Blood Glucose[3,7]	-	-	97%	97%
Perioperative Temperature Management	18	100%	100%	100%
Prophylactic Antibiotic Selection	15	100%	99%	99%
Prophylactic Antibiotic Selection (Outpatient)[3,7]	-	-	98%	98%
Prophylactic Antibiotic Stopped	13	85%	98%	98%
Prophylactic Antibiotic Timing	15	87%	99%	99%
Prophylactic Antibiotic Timing (Outpatient)[3,7]	-	-	98%	98%
Urinary Catheter Removal[1]	-	-	98%	97%
Survey of Patients' Hospital Experiences				
Area Around Room 'Always' Quiet at Night	(a)	59%	61%	61%
Doctors 'Always' Communicated Well	(a)	85%	83%	82%
Home Recovery Information Given	(a)	87%	86%	85%
Hospital Given 9 or 10 on 10 Point Scale	(a)	72%	74%	71%
Meds 'Always' Explained Before Given	(a)	70%	64%	64%
Nurses 'Always' Communicated Well	(a)	81%	81%	79%
Pain 'Always' Well Controlled	(a)	75%	73%	71%
Room and Bathroom 'Always' Clean	(a)	76%	76%	73%
Timely Help 'Always' Received	(a)	76%	71%	68%
Would Definitely Recommend Hospital	(a)	68%	73%	71%
Use of Medical Imaging				
Cardiac Imaging Stress Test before Surgery[1]	-	-	5.4%	5.3%
Combination Abdominal CT Scan	324	18.5%	9.3%	10.5%
Combination Brain/Sinus CT Scan[1]	-	-	2.6%	2.7%
Combination Chest CT Scan	145	3.4%	4.6%	2.7%
Follow-up Mammogram/Ultrasound	232	3.4%	8.4%	8.8%
Lumbar Spine MRI for Low Back Pain[1]	-	-	38.7%	37.2%

Perry County Memorial Hospital

One Hospital Rd
Tell City, IN 47586
URL: www.pchospital.org
Phone: 812-547-7011
Fax: 573-547-3776
Type: Critical Access Hospitals
Ownership: Voluntary non-profit - Other
Emergency Services: Yes
Beds: 38

Key Personnel:
Radiology. . . . . Janice Aaron
Quality Assurance . . . . Sandra Calvert
Coronary Care . . . . Carolyn Hawkns
Infection Control. . . . . Connie Simpson
CEO/President. . . . . Joseph A. Stuber
Operating Room. . . . . Earla Williams

Measure	Cases	This Hosp.	State Avg.	U.S. Avg.
Blood Clot Prevention and Treatment				
Anticoagulation Overlap Therapy[5]	-	-	92%	93%
ICU Venous Thromboembolism Prophylaxis[5]	-	-	91%	92%
Incidence of Potentially Preventable VTE[5]	-	-	10%	10%
UFH with Dosages/Platelet Monitoring[5]	-	-	95%	97%
Venous Thromboembolism Prophylaxis[5]	-	-	83%	85%
Warfarin Therapy Discharge Instructions[5]	-	-	71%	75%
Chest Pain/Possible Heart Attack Care				
Aspirin Given Within 24 Hours of Arrival	50	92%	96%	96%
Fibrinolytic Meds Within 30 Min. of Arrival[1]	-	-	48%	58%
Average Time to ECG (minutes)	56	8	6	7
Average Time to Transfer (minutes)[1]	-	-	46	60
Children's Asthma Care				
Received Home Management Plan of Care	-	-	-	88%
Received Reliever Medication	-	-	-	100%
Received Systemic Corticosteroids	-	-	-	100%
Emergency Department				
Admittance Decision Time (minutes)[5]	-	-	80	98
Head CT Results Within 45 Min. of Arrival[5]	-	-	60%	57%
Patients Who Left ER Before Being Seen	13,120	1%	2%	2%
Time from ER Arrival to Admit. (minutes)[5]	-	-	241	274
Time from ER Arrival to Discharge (minutes)[5]	-	-	122	134
Time in ER Before Being Evaluated (minutes)[5]	-	-	22	26
Time to Pain Meds for Fractures (minutes)[5]	-	-	52	57
Heart Attack Care				
Aspirin Given at Discharge[1]	-	-	99%	99%
Fibrinolytic Meds Within 30 Min. of Arrival[7]	-	-	67%	54%
PCI Within 90 Minutes of Arrival[7]	-	-	97%	96%
Statin Prescribed at Discharge[1]	-	-	99%	98%
Heart Failure Care				
ACE Inhibitor or ARB for LVSD	17	65%	97%	97%
Discharge Instructions Given	37	73%	95%	94%
Evaluation of LVS Function	21	95%	99%	99%
Medicare Spending				
Medicare Spending per Patient (ratio)	-	-	1.01	0.98
Pneumonia Care				
Appropriate Initial Antibiotic Given	43	95%	95%	95%
Blood Culture Timing	66	95%	98%	98%
Pregnancy and Delivery Care				
Newborn Deliveries Scheduled Early[5]	-	-	5%	6%
Preventive Care				
Immunization for Influenza[5]	-	-	91%	90%
Immunization for Pneumonia[5]	-	-	92%	92%
Stroke Care				
Anticoagulation Therapy for Atrial Fibrillation[5]	-	-	94%	95%
Antithrombotic Therapy Timing[5]	-	-	97%	98%
Assessed for Rehabilitation[5]	-	-	96%	97%
Discharged on Antithrombotic Therapy[5]	-	-	98%	99%
Discharged on Statin Medication[5]	-	-	91%	94%
Thrombolytic Therapy Timing[5]	-	-	54%	66%
Venous Thromboembolism Prophylaxis[5]	-	-	91%	94%
Written Stroke Educational Materials Given[5]	-	-	82%	88%
Surgical Care Improvement Project				
Appropriate Beta Blocker Usage[5]	-	-	98%	98%
Appropriate VTP Within 24 Hours[1]	-	-	98%	98%
Controlled Postoperative Blood Glucose[3,7]	-	-	97%	97%
Perioperative Temperature Management[5]	-	-	100%	100%
Prophylactic Antibiotic Selection[1]	-	-	99%	99%
Prophylactic Antibiotic Selection (Outpatient)[1,3]	-	-	98%	98%
Prophylactic Antibiotic Stopped[1]	-	-	98%	98%
Prophylactic Antibiotic Timing[1]	-	-	99%	99%
Prophylactic Antibiotic Timing (Outpatient)[1,3]	-	-	98%	98%
Urinary Catheter Removal[7]	-	-	98%	97%
Survey of Patients' Hospital Experiences				
Area Around Room 'Always' Quiet at Night	(a)	64%	61%	61%
Doctors 'Always' Communicated Well	(a)	84%	83%	82%
Home Recovery Information Given	(a)	86%	86%	85%
Hospital Given 9 or 10 on 10 Point Scale	(a)	72%	74%	71%
Meds 'Always' Explained Before Given	(a)	72%	64%	64%
Nurses 'Always' Communicated Well	(a)	86%	81%	79%
Pain 'Always' Well Controlled	(a)	80%	73%	71%
Room and Bathroom 'Always' Clean	(a)	84%	76%	73%
Timely Help 'Always' Received	(a)	85%	71%	68%
Would Definitely Recommend Hospital	(a)	66%	73%	71%
Use of Medical Imaging				
Cardiac Imaging Stress Test before Surgery	103	7.8%	5.4%	5.3%
Combination Abdominal CT Scan	318	32.4%	9.3%	10.5%
Combination Brain/Sinus CT Scan	308	6.5%	2.6%	2.7%
Combination Chest CT Scan	107	20.6%	4.6%	2.7%
Follow-up Mammogram/Ultrasound	317	6.6%	8.4%	8.8%
Lumbar Spine MRI for Low Back Pain[1]	-	-	38.7%	37.2%

Terre Haute Regional Hospital

3901 S Seventh St
Terre Haute, IN 47802
URL: www.regionalhospital.com
Phone: 812-232-0021
Fax: 812-237-9514
Type: Acute Care Hospitals
Ownership: Proprietary
Emergency Services: Yes
Beds: 278

Key Personnel:
Radiology. . . . . Bruce Adamson
CEO/President. . . . . Mary Ann Conroy
Infection Control. . . . . Diana Bowden
Quality Assurance . . . . Marsha Ciolli
Coronary Care . . . . Deb Girton
Emergency Room . . . . Julie VanOven
Operating Room. . . . . Kim Vester

Measure	Cases	This Hosp.	State Avg.	U.S. Avg.
Blood Clot Prevention and Treatment				
Anticoagulation Overlap Therapy[2]	25	100%	92%	93%
ICU Venous Thromboembolism Prophylaxis[2]	88	100%	91%	92%
Incidence of Potentially Preventable VTE[1,2]	-	-	10%	10%
UFH with Dosages/Platelet Monitoring[1,2]	-	-	95%	97%
Venous Thromboembolism Prophylaxis[2]	302	99%	83%	85%
Warfarin Therapy Discharge Instructions[2]	13	100%	71%	75%
Chest Pain/Possible Heart Attack Care				
Aspirin Given Within 24 Hours of Arrival[1,3]	-	-	96%	96%
Fibrinolytic Meds Within 30 Min. of Arrival[5]	-	-	48%	58%
Average Time to ECG (minutes)[1,3]	-	-	6	7
Average Time to Transfer (minutes)[5]	-	-	46	60
Children's Asthma Care				
Received Home Management Plan of Care	-	-	-	88%
Received Reliever Medication	-	-	-	100%
Received Systemic Corticosteroids	-	-	-	100%
Emergency Department				
Admittance Decision Time (minutes)[2]	458	60	80	98
Head CT Results Within 45 Min. of Arrival[1]	-	-	60%	57%
Patients Who Left ER Before Being Seen	21,385	0%	2%	2%
Time from ER Arrival to Admit. (minutes)[2]	460	210	241	274
Time from ER Arrival to Discharge (minutes)	404	123	122	134
Time in ER Before Being Evaluated (minutes)	460	17	22	26
Time to Pain Meds for Fractures (minutes)	59	33	52	57
Heart Attack Care				
Aspirin Given at Discharge	172	100%	99%	99%
Fibrinolytic Meds Within 30 Min. of Arrival[7]	-	-	67%	54%
PCI Within 90 Minutes of Arrival	14	100%	97%	96%
Statin Prescribed at Discharge	168	100%	99%	98%
Heart Failure Care				
ACE Inhibitor or ARB for LVSD	48	100%	97%	97%
Discharge Instructions Given	146	98%	95%	94%
Evaluation of LVS Function	190	100%	99%	99%
Medicare Spending				
Medicare Spending per Patient (ratio)	-	1.02	1.01	0.98
Pneumonia Care				
Appropriate Initial Antibiotic Given	64	97%	95%	95%
Blood Culture Timing	98	100%	98%	98%
Pregnancy and Delivery Care				
Newborn Deliveries Scheduled Early[2]	49	0%	5%	6%
Preventive Care				
Immunization for Influenza[2]	531	100%	91%	90%
Immunization for Pneumonia[2]	763	100%	92%	92%
Stroke Care				
Anticoagulation Therapy for Atrial Fibrillation[1]	-	-	94%	95%
Antithrombotic Therapy Timing	24	96%	97%	98%
Assessed for Rehabilitation	23	96%	96%	97%
Discharged on Antithrombotic Therapy	21	100%	98%	99%
Discharged on Statin Medication	18	100%	91%	94%
Thrombolytic Therapy Timing[1]	-	-	54%	66%
Venous Thromboembolism Prophylaxis	26	100%	91%	94%
Written Stroke Educational Materials Given	11	82%	82%	88%
Surgical Care Improvement Project				
Appropriate Beta Blocker Usage	118	100%	98%	98%
Appropriate VTP Within 24 Hours	200	100%	98%	98%
Controlled Postoperative Blood Glucose	38	100%	97%	97%
Perioperative Temperature Management	247	100%	100%	100%
Prophylactic Antibiotic Selection	196	99%	99%	99%
Prophylactic Antibiotic Selection (Outpatient)	121	98%	98%	98%
Prophylactic Antibiotic Stopped	153	99%	98%	98%
Prophylactic Antibiotic Timing	196	100%	99%	99%
Prophylactic Antibiotic Timing (Outpatient)	121	99%	98%	98%
Urinary Catheter Removal	128	99%	98%	97%
Survey of Patients' Hospital Experiences				
Area Around Room 'Always' Quiet at Night	300+	55%	61%	61%
Doctors 'Always' Communicated Well	300+	80%	83%	82%
Home Recovery Information Given	300+	87%	86%	85%
Hospital Given 9 or 10 on 10 Point Scale	300+	73%	74%	71%
Meds 'Always' Explained Before Given	300+	61%	64%	64%
Nurses 'Always' Communicated Well	300+	78%	81%	79%
Pain 'Always' Well Controlled	300+	71%	73%	71%
Room and Bathroom 'Always' Clean	300+	78%	76%	73%
Timely Help 'Always' Received	300+	66%	71%	68%
Would Definitely Recommend Hospital	300+	75%	73%	71%
Use of Medical Imaging				
Cardiac Imaging Stress Test before Surgery	142	6.3%	5.4%	5.3%
Combination Abdominal CT Scan	453	4.0%	9.3%	10.5%
Combination Brain/Sinus CT Scan[1]	-	-	2.6%	2.7%

NOTE: Hospital profiles are in alphabetical order by state, then city, then hospital within the city; Rankings exclude hospitals with less than 25 cases except for patient surveys which excludes hospitals with less than 100 cases; (a) 100-299 cases; (1) The number of cases/patients is too few to report; (2) Data submitted were based on a sample of cases/patients; (3) Results are based on a shorter time period than required; (4) Data suppressed by CMS for one or more quarters; (5) Results are not available for this reporting period; (6) Fewer than 100 patients completed the HCAHPS survey; (7) No cases met the criteria for this measure; (8) The lower limit of the confidence interval cannot be calculated if the number of observed infections equals zero; (9) No data are available from the state/territory for this reporting period; (10) The scores shown reflect fewer than 50 completed surveys; (11) There were discrepancies in the data collection process; (12) This measure does not apply to this hospital for this reporting period; (13) Results cannot be calculated for this reporting period; (14) The results for this state are combined with nearby states to protect confidentiality; Please refer to the User's Guide for a full explanation of data.

Combination Chest CT Scan	441	0.7%	4.6%	2.7%
Follow-up Mammogram/Ultrasound	511	10.4%	8.4%	8.8%
Lumbar Spine MRI for Low Back Pain[1]	-	-	38.7%	37.2%

Union Hospital

1606 N Seventh St
Terre Haute, IN 47804
Phone: 812-238-7606
URL: www.uhhg.org
Type: Acute Care Hospitals
Emergency Services: Yes
Ownership: Voluntary non-profit - Other
Key Personnel:
CEO/President. . . . . Steven M. Holman, FACHE
Quality Assurance . . . . Jeanette Spradlin

Measure	Cases	This Hosp.	State Avg.	U.S. Avg.
Blood Clot Prevention and Treatment				
Anticoagulation Overlap Therapy[2]	112	98%	92%	93%
ICU Venous Thromboembolism Prophylaxis[2]	145	100%	91%	92%
Incidence of Potentially Preventable VTE[2]	13	0%	10%	10%
UFH with Dosages/Platelet Monitoring[1,2]	-	-	95%	97%
Venous Thromboembolism Prophylaxis[2]	561	87%	83%	85%
Warfarin Therapy Discharge Instructions[2]	72	97%	71%	75%
Chest Pain/Possible Heart Attack Care				
Aspirin Given Within 24 Hours of Arrival[1,3]	-	-	96%	96%
Fibrinolytic Meds Within 30 Min. of Arrival[3,7]	-	-	48%	58%
Average Time to ECG (minutes)[1,3]	-	-	6	7
Average Time to Transfer (minutes)[3,7]	-	-	46	60
Children's Asthma Care				
Received Home Management Plan of Care	-	-	-	88%
Received Reliever Medication	-	-	-	100%
Received Systemic Corticosteroids	-	-	-	100%
Emergency Department				
Admittance Decision Time (minutes)[2]	686	83	80	98
Head CT Results Within 45 Min. of Arrival	16	81%	60%	57%
Patients Who Left ER Before Being Seen	54,263	0%	2%	2%
Time from ER Arrival to Admit. (minutes)[2]	745	232	241	274
Time from ER Arrival to Discharge (minutes)	526	137	122	134
Time in ER Before Being Evaluated (minutes)	469	11	22	26
Time to Pain Meds for Fractures (minutes)	170	49	52	57
Heart Attack Care				
Aspirin Given at Discharge	535	100%	99%	99%
Fibrinolytic Meds Within 30 Min. of Arrival[7]	-	-	67%	54%
PCI Within 90 Minutes of Arrival	61	95%	97%	96%
Statin Prescribed at Discharge	499	99%	99%	98%
Heart Failure Care				
ACE Inhibitor or ARB for LVSD	159	99%	97%	97%
Discharge Instructions Given	391	92%	95%	94%
Evaluation of LVS Function	511	100%	99%	99%
Medicare Spending				
Medicare Spending per Patient (ratio)	-	1.03	1.01	0.98
Pneumonia Care				
Appropriate Initial Antibiotic Given	320	96%	95%	95%
Blood Culture Timing	358	98%	98%	98%
Pregnancy and Delivery Care				
Newborn Deliveries Scheduled Early	178	8%	5%	6%
Preventive Care				
Immunization for Influenza[2]	695	77%	91%	90%
Immunization for Pneumonia[2]	900	84%	92%	92%
Stroke Care				
Anticoagulation Therapy for Atrial Fibrillation	23	96%	94%	95%
Antithrombotic Therapy Timing	146	100%	97%	98%
Assessed for Rehabilitation	171	99%	96%	97%
Discharged on Antithrombotic Therapy	152	100%	98%	99%
Discharged on Statin Medication	113	93%	91%	94%
Thrombolytic Therapy Timing[1]	-	-	54%	66%
Venous Thromboembolism Prophylaxis	170	97%	91%	94%
Written Stroke Educational Materials Given	83	90%	82%	88%
Surgical Care Improvement Project				
Appropriate Beta Blocker Usage	453	97%	98%	98%
Appropriate VTP Within 24 Hours	765	98%	98%	98%
Controlled Postoperative Blood Glucose	175	98%	97%	97%
Perioperative Temperature Management	886	100%	100%	100%
Prophylactic Antibiotic Selection	718	100%	99%	99%
Prophylactic Antibiotic Selection (Outpatient)	675	97%	98%	98%
Prophylactic Antibiotic Stopped	676	98%	98%	98%
Prophylactic Antibiotic Timing	724	99%	99%	99%
Prophylactic Antibiotic Timing (Outpatient)	673	99%	98%	98%
Urinary Catheter Removal	677	96%	98%	97%
Survey of Patients' Hospital Experiences				
Area Around Room 'Always' Quiet at Night	300+	61%	61%	61%
Doctors 'Always' Communicated Well	300+	75%	83%	82%
Home Recovery Information Given	300+	90%	86%	85%
Hospital Given 9 or 10 on 10 Point Scale	300+	75%	74%	71%
Meds 'Always' Explained Before Given	300+	59%	64%	64%
Nurses 'Always' Communicated Well	300+	77%	81%	79%
Pain 'Always' Well Controlled	300+	67%	73%	71%
Room and Bathroom 'Always' Clean	300+	77%	76%	73%
Timely Help 'Always' Received	300+	66%	71%	68%
Would Definitely Recommend Hospital	300+	78%	73%	71%
Use of Medical Imaging				
Cardiac Imaging Stress Test before Surgery	81	1.2%	5.4%	5.3%
Combination Abdominal CT Scan	1,953	18.8%	9.3%	10.5%
Combination Brain/Sinus CT Scan	1,474	3.3%	2.6%	2.7%
Combination Chest CT Scan	1,322	15.0%	4.6%	2.7%
Follow-up Mammogram/Ultrasound	2,668	8.2%	8.4%	8.8%
Lumbar Spine MRI for Low Back Pain	230	40.4%	38.7%	37.2%

Indiana University Health Tipton Hospital

1000 S Main St
Tipton, IN 46072
Phone: 765-675-8500
Fax: 765-675-8222
URL: www.tiptonhospital.org
Type: Critical Access Hospitals
Emergency Services: Yes
Ownership: Government - Local
Beds: 102
Key Personnel:
Radiology. . . . . Shamim Babchuk
CEO . . . . William R. Cast, MD
Infection Control. . . . . Trina Delph
Quality Assurance . . . . Trina Delph
Chief of Medical Staff. . . . . Vincent Delumpa, MD
Operating Room. . . . . Vincent Delumpa
Intensive Care Unit. . . . . JoEllen Scott
Patient Relations . . . . JoEllen Scott, RN

Measure	Cases	This Hosp.	State Avg.	U.S. Avg.
Blood Clot Prevention and Treatment				
Anticoagulation Overlap Therapy	12	100%	92%	93%
ICU Venous Thromboembolism Prophylaxis	103	89%	91%	92%
Incidence of Potentially Preventable VTE[7]	-	-	10%	10%
UFH with Dosages/Platelet Monitoring[7]	-	-	95%	97%
Venous Thromboembolism Prophylaxis	389	85%	83%	85%
Warfarin Therapy Discharge Instructions[1]	-	-	71%	75%
Chest Pain/Possible Heart Attack Care				
Aspirin Given Within 24 Hours of Arrival	30	100%	96%	96%
Fibrinolytic Meds Within 30 Min. of Arrival[7]	-	-	48%	58%
Average Time to ECG (minutes)	30	6	6	7
Average Time to Transfer (minutes)[1]	-	-	46	60
Children's Asthma Care				
Received Home Management Plan of Care	-	-	-	88%
Received Reliever Medication	-	-	-	100%
Received Systemic Corticosteroids	-	-	-	100%
Emergency Department				
Admittance Decision Time (minutes)	543	75	80	98
Head CT Results Within 45 Min. of Arrival[1]	-	-	60%	57%
Patients Who Left ER Before Being Seen	5,899	0%	2%	2%
Time from ER Arrival to Admit. (minutes)	553	215	241	274
Time from ER Arrival to Discharge (minutes)	430	106	122	134
Time in ER Before Being Evaluated (minutes)	399	15	22	26
Time to Pain Meds for Fractures (minutes)	19	33	52	57
Heart Attack Care				
Aspirin Given at Discharge[1]	-	-	99%	99%
Fibrinolytic Meds Within 30 Min. of Arrival[7]	-	-	67%	54%
PCI Within 90 Minutes of Arrival[7]	-	-	97%	96%
Statin Prescribed at Discharge[1]	-	-	99%	98%
Heart Failure Care				
ACE Inhibitor or ARB for LVSD[1]	-	-	97%	97%
Discharge Instructions Given	16	88%	95%	94%
Evaluation of LVS Function	31	100%	99%	99%
Medicare Spending				
Medicare Spending per Patient (ratio)	-	-	1.01	0.98
Pneumonia Care				
Appropriate Initial Antibiotic Given	53	96%	95%	95%
Blood Culture Timing	65	100%	98%	98%
Pregnancy and Delivery Care				
Newborn Deliveries Scheduled Early[5]	-	-	5%	6%
Preventive Care				
Immunization for Influenza	434	87%	91%	90%
Immunization for Pneumonia	702	91%	92%	92%
Stroke Care				
Anticoagulation Therapy for Atrial Fibrillation[3,7]	-	-	94%	95%
Antithrombotic Therapy Timing[1,3]	-	-	97%	98%
Assessed for Rehabilitation[1,3]	-	-	96%	97%
Discharged on Antithrombotic Therapy[1,3]	-	-	98%	99%
Discharged on Statin Medication[1,3]	-	-	91%	94%
Thrombolytic Therapy Timing[3,7]	-	-	54%	66%
Venous Thromboembolism Prophylaxis[1,3]	-	-	91%	94%
Written Stroke Educational Materials Given[1,3]	-	-	82%	88%
Surgical Care Improvement Project				
Appropriate Beta Blocker Usage	38	97%	98%	98%
Appropriate VTP Within 24 Hours	138	100%	98%	98%
Controlled Postoperative Blood Glucose[3,7]	-	-	97%	97%
Perioperative Temperature Management	145	100%	100%	100%
Prophylactic Antibiotic Selection	111	99%	99%	99%
Prophylactic Antibiotic Selection (Outpatient)	21	76%	98%	98%
Prophylactic Antibiotic Stopped	111	100%	98%	98%
Prophylactic Antibiotic Timing	111	100%	99%	99%
Prophylactic Antibiotic Timing (Outpatient)	21	100%	98%	98%
Urinary Catheter Removal	128	100%	98%	97%
Survey of Patients' Hospital Experiences				
Area Around Room 'Always' Quiet at Night	(a)	63%	61%	61%
Doctors 'Always' Communicated Well	(a)	89%	83%	82%
Home Recovery Information Given	(a)	85%	86%	85%
Hospital Given 9 or 10 on 10 Point Scale	(a)	82%	74%	71%
Meds 'Always' Explained Before Given	(a)	68%	64%	64%
Nurses 'Always' Communicated Well	(a)	82%	81%	79%
Pain 'Always' Well Controlled	(a)	75%	73%	71%
Room and Bathroom 'Always' Clean	(a)	83%	76%	73%
Timely Help 'Always' Received	(a)	68%	71%	68%
Would Definitely Recommend Hospital	(a)	74%	73%	71%
Use of Medical Imaging				
Cardiac Imaging Stress Test before Surgery	122	5.7%	5.4%	5.3%
Combination Abdominal CT Scan	193	7.8%	9.3%	10.5%
Combination Brain/Sinus CT Scan[1]	-	-	2.6%	2.7%
Combination Chest CT Scan	128	3.1%	4.6%	2.7%
Follow-up Mammogram/Ultrasound	341	17.0%	8.4%	8.8%
Lumbar Spine MRI for Low Back Pain[1]	-	-	38.7%	37.2%

Porter Regional Hospital

85 East Us Hwy 6
Valparaiso, IN 46383
Phone: 219-983-8300
Fax: 219-463-4882
URL: www.portermemorial.org
Type: Acute Care Hospitals
Emergency Services: Yes
Ownership: Proprietary
Beds: 402
Key Personnel:
Quality Assurance . . . . Michelle Back, RN
Infection Control. . . . . Julie Downey, RN
Radiology. . . . . Anil Kothari, MD
Chief of Medical Staff . . . . Doug A Mazurek, MD
Pediatric In-Patient Care . . . . Jeffrey Miller, MD
Operating Room. . . . . Rose Mary Mroz
CEO/President. . . . . Johnathan Nalli

Measure	Cases	This Hosp.	State Avg.	U.S. Avg.
Blood Clot Prevention and Treatment				
Anticoagulation Overlap Therapy[2]	84	73%	92%	93%
ICU Venous Thromboembolism Prophylaxis[2]	97	82%	91%	92%
Incidence of Potentially Preventable VTE[2]	29	14%	10%	10%
UFH with Dosages/Platelet Monitoring[2]	65	100%	95%	97%
Venous Thromboembolism Prophylaxis[2]	438	81%	83%	85%
Warfarin Therapy Discharge Instructions[2]	68	26%	71%	75%
Chest Pain/Possible Heart Attack Care				
Aspirin Given Within 24 Hours of Arrival[1,3]	-	-	96%	96%
Fibrinolytic Meds Within 30 Min. of Arrival[5]	-	-	48%	58%
Average Time to ECG (minutes)[1,3]	-	-	6	7
Average Time to Transfer (minutes)[5]	-	-	46	60

NOTE: Hospital profiles are in alphabetical order by state, then city, then hospital within the city; Rankings exclude hospitals with less than 25 cases except for patient surveys which excludes hospitals with less than 100 cases; (a) 100-299 cases; (1) The number of cases/patients is too few to report; (2) Data submitted were based on a sample of cases/patients; (3) Results are based on a shorter time period than required; (4) Data suppressed by CMS for one or more quarters; (5) Results are not available for this reporting period; (6) Fewer than 100 patients completed the HCAHPS survey; (7) No cases met the criteria for this measure; (8) The lower limit of the confidence interval cannot be calculated if the number of observed infections equals zero; (9) No data are available from the state/territory for this reporting period; (10) The scores shown reflect fewer than 50 completed surveys; (11) There were discrepancies in the data collection process; (12) This measure does not apply to this hospital for this reporting period; (13) Results cannot be calculated for this reporting period; (14) The results for this state are combined with nearby states to protect confidentiality; Please refer to the User's Guide for a full explanation of data.

Children's Asthma Care				
Received Home Management Plan of Care	-	-	-	88%
Received Reliever Medication	-	-	-	100%
Received Systemic Corticosteroids	-	-	-	100%
Emergency Department				
Admittance Decision Time (minutes)[2]	829	76	80	98
Head CT Results Within 45 Min. of Arrival[1]	-	-	60%	57%
Patients Who Left ER Before Being Seen	54,995	0%	2%	2%
Time from ER Arrival to Admit. (minutes)[2]	863	239	241	274
Time from ER Arrival to Discharge (minutes)	392	130	122	134
Time in ER Before Being Evaluated (minutes)	403	17	22	26
Time to Pain Meds for Fractures (minutes)	304	54	52	57
Heart Attack Care				
Aspirin Given at Discharge	287	100%	99%	99%
Fibrinolytic Meds Within 30 Min. of Arrival[7]	-	-	67%	54%
PCI Within 90 Minutes of Arrival	49	100%	97%	96%
Statin Prescribed at Discharge	279	100%	99%	98%
Heart Failure Care				
ACE Inhibitor or ARB for LVSD	116	100%	97%	97%
Discharge Instructions Given	294	100%	95%	94%
Evaluation of LVS Function	369	100%	99%	99%
Medicare Spending				
Medicare Spending per Patient (ratio)	-	1.03	1.01	0.98
Pneumonia Care				
Appropriate Initial Antibiotic Given	163	96%	95%	95%
Blood Culture Timing	364	99%	98%	98%
Pregnancy and Delivery Care				
Newborn Deliveries Scheduled Early[2]	24	4%	5%	6%
Preventive Care				
Immunization for Influenza[2]	696	93%	91%	90%
Immunization for Pneumonia[2]	875	95%	92%	92%
Stroke Care				
Anticoagulation Therapy for Atrial Fibrillation	24	96%	94%	95%
Antithrombotic Therapy Timing	121	96%	97%	98%
Assessed for Rehabilitation	127	83%	96%	97%
Discharged on Antithrombotic Therapy	120	98%	98%	99%
Discharged on Statin Medication	99	95%	91%	94%
Thrombolytic Therapy Timing	26	50%	54%	66%
Venous Thromboembolism Prophylaxis	142	88%	91%	94%
Written Stroke Educational Materials Given	73	97%	82%	88%
Surgical Care Improvement Project				
Appropriate Beta Blocker Usage	413	97%	98%	98%
Appropriate VTP Within 24 Hours	353	98%	98%	98%
Controlled Postoperative Blood Glucose	98	99%	97%	97%
Perioperative Temperature Management	1,061	100%	100%	100%
Prophylactic Antibiotic Selection	779	99%	99%	99%
Prophylactic Antibiotic Selection (Outpatient)	407	100%	98%	98%
Prophylactic Antibiotic Stopped	765	99%	98%	98%
Prophylactic Antibiotic Timing	779	99%	99%	99%
Prophylactic Antibiotic Timing (Outpatient)	411	98%	98%	98%
Urinary Catheter Removal	296	98%	98%	97%
Survey of Patients' Hospital Experiences				
Area Around Room 'Always' Quiet at Night	300+	60%	61%	61%
Doctors 'Always' Communicated Well	300+	79%	83%	82%
Home Recovery Information Given	300+	86%	86%	85%
Hospital Given 9 or 10 on 10 Point Scale	300+	72%	74%	71%
Meds 'Always' Explained Before Given	300+	56%	64%	64%
Nurses 'Always' Communicated Well	300+	78%	81%	79%
Pain 'Always' Well Controlled	300+	70%	73%	71%
Room and Bathroom 'Always' Clean	300+	73%	76%	73%
Timely Help 'Always' Received	300+	58%	71%	68%
Would Definitely Recommend Hospital	300+	72%	73%	71%
Use of Medical Imaging				
Cardiac Imaging Stress Test before Surgery	239	4.2%	5.4%	5.3%
Combination Abdominal CT Scan	1,295	17.3%	9.3%	10.5%
Combination Brain/Sinus CT Scan	1,045	3.0%	2.6%	2.7%
Combination Chest CT Scan	883	10.1%	4.6%	2.7%
Follow-up Mammogram/Ultrasound	1,780	6.2%	8.4%	8.8%
Lumbar Spine MRI for Low Back Pain	227	34.8%	38.7%	37.2%

Good Samaritan Hospital

520 S 7th St
Vincennes, IN 47591
Phone: 812-882-5220
URL: www.gshvin.org
Type: Acute Care Hospitals
Emergency Services: Yes
Ownership: Voluntary non-profit - Other

Key Personnel:
Radiology. Gary Chavis
President/CEO. . . . . Robert McLin

Measure	Cases	This Hosp.	State Avg.	U.S. Avg.
Blood Clot Prevention and Treatment				
Anticoagulation Overlap Therapy[2]	44	66%	92%	93%
ICU Venous Thromboembolism Prophylaxis[2]	67	85%	91%	92%
Incidence of Potentially Preventable VTE[1,2]	-	-	10%	10%
UFH with Dosages/Platelet Monitoring[2]	31	100%	95%	97%
Venous Thromboembolism Prophylaxis[2]	348	82%	83%	85%
Warfarin Therapy Discharge Instructions[2]	37	81%	71%	75%
Chest Pain/Possible Heart Attack Care				
Aspirin Given Within 24 Hours of Arrival[1]	-	-	96%	96%
Fibrinolytic Meds Within 30 Min. of Arrival[3,7]	-	-	48%	58%
Average Time to ECG (minutes)[1]	-	-	6	7
Average Time to Transfer (minutes)[3,7]	-	-	46	60
Children's Asthma Care				
Received Home Management Plan of Care	-	-	-	88%
Received Reliever Medication	-	-	-	100%
Received Systemic Corticosteroids	-	-	-	100%
Emergency Department				
Admittance Decision Time (minutes)[2]	685	66	80	98
Head CT Results Within 45 Min. of Arrival	20	70%	60%	57%
Patients Who Left ER Before Being Seen	35,950	0%	2%	2%
Time from ER Arrival to Admit. (minutes)[2]	705	194	241	274
Time from ER Arrival to Discharge (minutes)	373	112	122	134
Time in ER Before Being Evaluated (minutes)	391	24	22	26
Time to Pain Meds for Fractures (minutes)	127	51	52	57
Heart Attack Care				
Aspirin Given at Discharge	115	100%	99%	99%
Fibrinolytic Meds Within 30 Min. of Arrival[7]	-	-	67%	54%
PCI Within 90 Minutes of Arrival	24	96%	97%	96%
Statin Prescribed at Discharge	111	95%	99%	98%
Heart Failure Care				
ACE Inhibitor or ARB for LVSD	80	95%	97%	97%
Discharge Instructions Given	170	83%	95%	94%
Evaluation of LVS Function	231	99%	99%	99%
Medicare Spending				
Medicare Spending per Patient (ratio)	-	0.99	1.01	0.98
Pneumonia Care				
Appropriate Initial Antibiotic Given	137	98%	95%	95%
Blood Culture Timing	248	99%	98%	98%
Pregnancy and Delivery Care				
Newborn Deliveries Scheduled Early	44	9%	5%	6%
Preventive Care				
Immunization for Influenza[2]	561	99%	91%	90%
Immunization for Pneumonia[2]	802	99%	92%	92%
Stroke Care				
Anticoagulation Therapy for Atrial Fibrillation	20	95%	94%	95%
Antithrombotic Therapy Timing	104	100%	97%	98%
Assessed for Rehabilitation	107	97%	96%	97%
Discharged on Antithrombotic Therapy	102	100%	98%	99%
Discharged on Statin Medication	85	93%	91%	94%
Thrombolytic Therapy Timing[1]	-	-	54%	66%
Venous Thromboembolism Prophylaxis	107	99%	91%	94%
Written Stroke Educational Materials Given	53	89%	82%	88%
Surgical Care Improvement Project				
Appropriate Beta Blocker Usage	158	100%	98%	98%
Appropriate VTP Within 24 Hours	389	100%	98%	98%
Controlled Postoperative Blood Glucose[7]	-	-	97%	97%
Perioperative Temperature Management	461	100%	100%	100%
Prophylactic Antibiotic Selection	332	100%	99%	99%
Prophylactic Antibiotic Selection (Outpatient)	152	98%	98%	98%
Prophylactic Antibiotic Stopped	316	99%	98%	98%
Prophylactic Antibiotic Timing	332	100%	99%	99%
Prophylactic Antibiotic Timing (Outpatient)	153	97%	98%	98%
Urinary Catheter Removal	114	96%	98%	97%
Survey of Patients' Hospital Experiences				
Area Around Room 'Always' Quiet at Night	300+	57%	61%	61%
Doctors 'Always' Communicated Well	300+	86%	83%	82%
Home Recovery Information Given	300+	90%	86%	85%
Hospital Given 9 or 10 on 10 Point Scale	300+	78%	74%	71%
Meds 'Always' Explained Before Given	300+	67%	64%	64%
Nurses 'Always' Communicated Well	300+	87%	81%	79%
Pain 'Always' Well Controlled	300+	77%	73%	71%
Room and Bathroom 'Always' Clean	300+	88%	76%	73%
Timely Help 'Always' Received	300+	76%	71%	68%
Would Definitely Recommend Hospital	300+	78%	73%	71%
Use of Medical Imaging				
Cardiac Imaging Stress Test before Surgery	506	5.5%	5.4%	5.3%
Combination Abdominal CT Scan	1,049	31.4%	9.3%	10.5%
Combination Brain/Sinus CT Scan	820	2.3%	2.6%	2.7%
Combination Chest CT Scan	501	34.9%	4.6%	2.7%
Follow-up Mammogram/Ultrasound	1,729	5.4%	8.4%	8.8%
Lumbar Spine MRI for Low Back Pain	176	43.2%	38.7%	37.2%

Wabash County Hospital

710 N East St
Wabash, IN 46992
Phone: 260-563-3131
Fax: 260-569-2410
URL: www.wchospital.com
Type: Critical Access Hospitals
Emergency Services: Yes
Ownership: Government - Local
Beds: 25

Key Personnel:
CEO/President. . . . . Marilyn Custer-Mitchell
Emergency Room . . . . Jonathan Grandstaff-Dunp
Operating Room. . . . . Bill Planck, RN
Chief of Medical Staff . . . . Joseph Rudolph
Quality Assurance . . . . Richard Tucker
Infection Control. . . . . Mike Vogel, RN
Radiology. James Wehrenber, MD
Intensive Care Unit. . . . . Sandy Wright, RN

Measure	Cases	This Hosp.	State Avg.	U.S. Avg.
Blood Clot Prevention and Treatment				
Anticoagulation Overlap Therapy[1,2]	-	-	92%	93%
ICU Venous Thromboembolism Prophylaxis[2]	17	100%	91%	92%
Incidence of Potentially Preventable VTE[1,2]	-	-	10%	10%
UFH with Dosages/Platelet Monitoring[1,2]	-	-	95%	97%
Venous Thromboembolism Prophylaxis[2]	52	96%	83%	85%
Warfarin Therapy Discharge Instructions[1,2]	-	-	71%	75%
Chest Pain/Possible Heart Attack Care				
Aspirin Given Within 24 Hours of Arrival[3]	31	100%	96%	96%
Fibrinolytic Meds Within 30 Min. of Arrival[3,7]	-	-	48%	58%
Average Time to ECG (minutes)[3]	42	7	6	7
Average Time to Transfer (minutes)[1,3]	-	-	46	60
Children's Asthma Care				
Received Home Management Plan of Care	-	-	-	88%
Received Reliever Medication	-	-	-	100%
Received Systemic Corticosteroids	-	-	-	100%
Emergency Department				
Admittance Decision Time (minutes)[5]	-	-	80	98
Head CT Results Within 45 Min. of Arrival[5]	-	-	60%	57%
Patients Who Left ER Before Being Seen	10,724	1%	2%	2%
Time from ER Arrival to Admit. (minutes)[5]	-	-	241	274
Time from ER Arrival to Discharge (minutes)[5]	-	-	122	134
Time in ER Before Being Evaluated (minutes)[5]	-	-	22	26
Time to Pain Meds for Fractures (minutes)[5]	-	-	52	57
Heart Attack Care				
Aspirin Given at Discharge[1,3]	-	-	99%	99%
Fibrinolytic Meds Within 30 Min. of Arrival[3,7]	-	-	67%	54%
PCI Within 90 Minutes of Arrival[3,7]	-	-	97%	96%
Statin Prescribed at Discharge[1,3]	-	-	99%	98%
Heart Failure Care				
ACE Inhibitor or ARB for LVSD[1]	-	-	97%	97%
Discharge Instructions Given	11	82%	95%	94%
Evaluation of LVS Function	26	100%	99%	99%
Medicare Spending				
Medicare Spending per Patient (ratio)	-	-	1.01	0.98
Pneumonia Care				
Appropriate Initial Antibiotic Given	23	87%	95%	95%
Blood Culture Timing	34	97%	98%	98%
Pregnancy and Delivery Care				

NOTE: Hospital profiles are in alphabetical order by state, then city, then hospital within the city; Rankings exclude hospitals with less than 25 cases except for patient surveys which excludes hospitals with less than 100 cases; (a) 100-299 cases; (1) The number of cases/patients is too few to report; (2) Data submitted were based on a sample of cases/patients; (3) Results are based on a shorter time period than required; (4) Data suppressed by CMS for one or more quarters; (5) Results are not available for this reporting period; (6) Fewer than 100 patients completed the HCAHPS survey; (7) No cases met the criteria for this measure; (8) The lower limit of the confidence interval cannot be calculated if the number of observed infections equals zero; (9) No data are available from the state/territory for this reporting period; (10) The scores shown reflect fewer than 50 completed surveys; (11) There were discrepancies in the data collection process; (12) This measure does not apply to this hospital for this reporting period; (13) Results cannot be calculated for this reporting period; (14) The results for this state are combined with nearby states to protect confidentiality; Please refer to the User's Guide for a full explanation of data.

Measure	Cases	This Hosp.	State Avg.	U.S. Avg.
Newborn Deliveries Scheduled Early[5]	-	-	5%	6%
Preventive Care				
Immunization for Influenza[5]	-	-	91%	90%
Immunization for Pneumonia[5]	-	-	92%	92%
Stroke Care				
Anticoagulation Therapy for Atrial Fibrillation[1]	-	-	94%	95%
Antithrombotic Therapy Timing[1]	-	-	97%	98%
Assessed for Rehabilitation[1]	-	-	96%	97%
Discharged on Antithrombotic Therapy[1]	-	-	98%	99%
Discharged on Statin Medication[1]	-	-	91%	94%
Thrombolytic Therapy Timing[7]	-	-	54%	66%
Venous Thromboembolism Prophylaxis[1]	-	-	91%	94%
Written Stroke Educational Materials Given[1]	-	-	82%	88%
Surgical Care Improvement Project				
Appropriate Beta Blocker Usage	20	100%	98%	98%
Appropriate VTP Within 24 Hours	66	97%	98%	98%
Controlled Postoperative Blood Glucose[3,7]	-	-	97%	97%
Perioperative Temperature Management	70	100%	100%	100%
Prophylactic Antibiotic Selection	60	98%	99%	99%
Prophylactic Antibiotic Selection (Outpatient)[3]	24	88%	98%	98%
Prophylactic Antibiotic Stopped	60	100%	98%	98%
Prophylactic Antibiotic Timing	60	95%	99%	99%
Prophylactic Antibiotic Timing (Outpatient)[3]	24	92%	98%	98%
Urinary Catheter Removal	42	98%	98%	97%
Survey of Patients' Hospital Experiences				
Area Around Room 'Always' Quiet at Night	(a)	64%	61%	61%
Doctors 'Always' Communicated Well	(a)	85%	83%	82%
Home Recovery Information Given	(a)	82%	86%	85%
Hospital Given 9 or 10 on 10 Point Scale	(a)	74%	74%	71%
Meds 'Always' Explained Before Given	(a)	69%	64%	64%
Nurses 'Always' Communicated Well	(a)	84%	81%	79%
Pain 'Always' Well Controlled	(a)	71%	73%	71%
Room and Bathroom 'Always' Clean	(a)	84%	76%	73%
Timely Help 'Always' Received	(a)	81%	71%	68%
Would Definitely Recommend Hospital	(a)	64%	73%	71%
Use of Medical Imaging				
Cardiac Imaging Stress Test before Surgery	114	4.4%	5.4%	5.3%
Combination Abdominal CT Scan	260	6.2%	9.3%	10.5%
Combination Brain/Sinus CT Scan[1]	-	-	2.6%	2.7%
Combination Chest CT Scan	129	0.8%	4.6%	2.7%
Follow-up Mammogram/Ultrasound	387	7.0%	8.4%	8.8%
Lumbar Spine MRI for Low Back Pain	59	27.1%	38.7%	37.2%

Kosciusko Community Hospital

2101 E Dubois Dr
Warsaw, IN 46580
Phone: 574-267-3200
Fax: 574-372-7816
URL: www.kch.com
Type: Acute Care Hospitals
Emergency Services: Yes
Ownership: Proprietary
Beds: 72

Key Personnel:

Radiology. . . . . Steph Damon
Chief of Medical Staff. . . . . Gregory Haase, DO
Intensive Care Unit. . . . . Gregory Haase, DO
Anesthesiology. . . . . John Hilgenberg, MD
Infection Control. . . . . Thomas Kocoshis, MD
Emergency Room . . . . Linda Law, MD
CEO/President. . . . . Steve Miller

Measure	Cases	This Hosp.	State Avg.	U.S. Avg.
Blood Clot Prevention and Treatment				
Anticoagulation Overlap Therapy[2]	32	97%	92%	93%
ICU Venous Thromboembolism Prophylaxis[2]	52	100%	91%	92%
Incidence of Potentially Preventable VTE[1,2]	-	-	10%	10%
UFH with Dosages/Platelet Monitoring[2]	20	100%	95%	97%
Venous Thromboembolism Prophylaxis[2]	303	97%	83%	85%
Warfarin Therapy Discharge Instructions[2]	21	100%	71%	75%
Chest Pain/Possible Heart Attack Care				
Aspirin Given Within 24 Hours of Arrival	76	100%	96%	96%
Fibrinolytic Meds Within 30 Min. of Arrival[7]	-	-	48%	58%
Average Time to ECG (minutes)	78	3	6	7
Average Time to Transfer (minutes)	16	39	46	60
Children's Asthma Care				
Received Home Management Plan of Care	-	-	-	88%
Received Reliever Medication	-	-	-	100%
Received Systemic Corticosteroids	-	-	-	100%
Emergency Department				
Admittance Decision Time (minutes)[2]	580	70	80	98
Head CT Results Within 45 Min. of Arrival[1]	-	-	60%	57%
Patients Who Left ER Before Being Seen	24,296	1%	2%	2%
Time from ER Arrival to Admit. (minutes)[2]	580	262	241	274
Time from ER Arrival to Discharge (minutes)	395	142	122	134
Time in ER Before Being Evaluated (minutes)	401	26	22	26
Time to Pain Meds for Fractures (minutes)	90	56	52	57
Heart Attack Care				
Aspirin Given at Discharge	20	100%	99%	99%
Fibrinolytic Meds Within 30 Min. of Arrival[7]	-	-	67%	54%
PCI Within 90 Minutes of Arrival[7]	-	-	97%	96%
Statin Prescribed at Discharge	17	100%	99%	98%
Heart Failure Care				
ACE Inhibitor or ARB for LVSD	22	100%	97%	97%
Discharge Instructions Given	87	93%	95%	94%
Evaluation of LVS Function	118	100%	99%	99%
Medicare Spending				
Medicare Spending per Patient (ratio)	-	0.97	1.01	0.98
Pneumonia Care				
Appropriate Initial Antibiotic Given	79	99%	95%	95%
Blood Culture Timing	135	99%	98%	98%
Pregnancy and Delivery Care				
Newborn Deliveries Scheduled Early[2]	28	11%	5%	6%
Preventive Care				
Immunization for Influenza[2]	442	97%	91%	90%
Immunization for Pneumonia[2]	489	98%	92%	92%
Stroke Care				
Anticoagulation Therapy for Atrial Fibrillation[1]	-	-	94%	95%
Antithrombotic Therapy Timing	34	100%	97%	98%
Assessed for Rehabilitation	40	100%	96%	97%
Discharged on Antithrombotic Therapy	40	100%	98%	99%
Discharged on Statin Medication	29	100%	91%	94%
Thrombolytic Therapy Timing[7]	-	-	54%	66%
Venous Thromboembolism Prophylaxis	35	91%	91%	94%
Written Stroke Educational Materials Given	21	100%	82%	88%
Surgical Care Improvement Project				
Appropriate Beta Blocker Usage	77	100%	98%	98%
Appropriate VTP Within 24 Hours	230	100%	98%	98%
Controlled Postoperative Blood Glucose[7]	-	-	97%	97%
Perioperative Temperature Management	267	100%	100%	100%
Prophylactic Antibiotic Selection	207	100%	99%	99%
Prophylactic Antibiotic Selection (Outpatient)	59	100%	98%	98%
Prophylactic Antibiotic Stopped	207	98%	98%	98%
Prophylactic Antibiotic Timing	207	100%	99%	99%
Prophylactic Antibiotic Timing (Outpatient)	59	100%	98%	98%
Urinary Catheter Removal	38	97%	98%	97%
Survey of Patients' Hospital Experiences				
Area Around Room 'Always' Quiet at Night	300+	64%	61%	61%
Doctors 'Always' Communicated Well	300+	81%	83%	82%
Home Recovery Information Given	300+	87%	86%	85%
Hospital Given 9 or 10 on 10 Point Scale	300+	68%	74%	71%
Meds 'Always' Explained Before Given	300+	65%	64%	64%
Nurses 'Always' Communicated Well	300+	76%	81%	79%
Pain 'Always' Well Controlled	300+	71%	73%	71%
Room and Bathroom 'Always' Clean	300+	72%	76%	73%
Timely Help 'Always' Received	300+	63%	71%	68%
Would Definitely Recommend Hospital	300+	66%	73%	71%
Use of Medical Imaging				
Cardiac Imaging Stress Test before Surgery	113	3.5%	5.4%	5.3%
Combination Abdominal CT Scan	573	3.0%	9.3%	10.5%
Combination Brain/Sinus CT Scan[1]	-	-	2.6%	2.7%
Combination Chest CT Scan	326	0.9%	4.6%	2.7%
Follow-up Mammogram/Ultrasound	669	4.5%	8.4%	8.8%
Lumbar Spine MRI for Low Back Pain	108	35.2%	38.7%	37.2%

Daviess Community Hospital

1314 E Walnut St
Washington, IN 47501
Phone: 812-254-2760
Fax: 812-254-8897
E-mail: msmith@dchosp.org
URL: www.dchosp.org
Type: Acute Care Hospitals
Emergency Services: Yes
Ownership: Voluntary non-profit - Other
Beds: 120

Key Personnel:

CEO . . . . David Bixler
Radiology. . . . . E M Cha, MD
Quality Assurance . . . . Mark Dame
Cardiac Laboratory. . . . . Phillip Dawkins, MD
Chief of Medical Staff. . . . . James Filler
CEO/President. . . . . Gary G Kendrick
Infection Control. . . . . Carol Matteson
Operating Room. . . . . Shirley Yoder

Measure	Cases	This Hosp.	State Avg.	U.S. Avg.
Blood Clot Prevention and Treatment				
Anticoagulation Overlap Therapy[2]	13	62%	92%	93%
ICU Venous Thromboembolism Prophylaxis[2]	70	77%	91%	92%
Incidence of Potentially Preventable VTE[1,2]	-	-	10%	10%
UFH with Dosages/Platelet Monitoring[1,2]	-	-	95%	97%
Venous Thromboembolism Prophylaxis[2]	176	75%	83%	85%
Warfarin Therapy Discharge Instructions[2]	11	18%	71%	75%
Chest Pain/Possible Heart Attack Care				
Aspirin Given Within 24 Hours of Arrival	53	96%	96%	96%
Fibrinolytic Meds Within 30 Min. of Arrival[7]	-	-	48%	58%
Average Time to ECG (minutes)	56	6	6	7
Average Time to Transfer (minutes)	15	40	46	60
Children's Asthma Care				
Received Home Management Plan of Care	-	-	-	88%
Received Reliever Medication	-	-	-	100%
Received Systemic Corticosteroids	-	-	-	100%
Emergency Department				
Admittance Decision Time (minutes)[2]	351	59	80	98
Head CT Results Within 45 Min. of Arrival[1]	-	-	60%	57%
Patients Who Left ER Before Being Seen	13,650	1%	2%	2%
Time from ER Arrival to Admit. (minutes)[2]	363	191	241	274
Time from ER Arrival to Discharge (minutes)	423	100	122	134
Time in ER Before Being Evaluated (minutes)	517	16	22	26
Time to Pain Meds for Fractures (minutes)	46	32	52	57
Heart Attack Care				
Aspirin Given at Discharge[1]	-	-	99%	99%
Fibrinolytic Meds Within 30 Min. of Arrival[7]	-	-	67%	54%
PCI Within 90 Minutes of Arrival[7]	-	-	97%	96%
Statin Prescribed at Discharge[1]	-	-	99%	98%
Heart Failure Care				
ACE Inhibitor or ARB for LVSD[1]	-	-	97%	97%
Discharge Instructions Given	30	80%	95%	94%
Evaluation of LVS Function	40	88%	99%	99%
Medicare Spending				
Medicare Spending per Patient (ratio)	-	1.22	1.01	0.98
Pneumonia Care				
Appropriate Initial Antibiotic Given	53	92%	95%	95%
Blood Culture Timing	79	97%	98%	98%
Pregnancy and Delivery Care				
Newborn Deliveries Scheduled Early	76	32%	5%	6%
Preventive Care				
Immunization for Influenza[2]	432	69%	91%	90%
Immunization for Pneumonia[2]	352	86%	92%	92%
Stroke Care				
Anticoagulation Therapy for Atrial Fibrillation[1]	-	-	94%	95%
Antithrombotic Therapy Timing	22	100%	97%	98%
Assessed for Rehabilitation	23	100%	96%	97%
Discharged on Antithrombotic Therapy	22	86%	98%	99%
Discharged on Statin Medication	19	74%	91%	94%
Thrombolytic Therapy Timing[1]	-	-	54%	66%
Venous Thromboembolism Prophylaxis	23	87%	91%	94%
Written Stroke Educational Materials Given[1]	-	-	82%	88%
Surgical Care Improvement Project				
Appropriate Beta Blocker Usage	16	88%	98%	98%
Appropriate VTP Within 24 Hours	42	88%	98%	98%
Controlled Postoperative Blood Glucose[7]	-	-	97%	97%
Perioperative Temperature Management	56	100%	100%	100%

NOTE: Hospital profiles are in alphabetical order by state, then city, then hospital within the city; Rankings exclude hospitals with less than 25 cases except for patient surveys which excludes hospitals with less than 100 cases; (a) 100-299 cases; (1) The number of cases/patients is too few to report; (2) Data submitted were based on a sample of cases/patients; (3) Results are based on a shorter time period than required; (4) Data suppressed by CMS for one or more quarters; (5) Results are not available for this reporting period; (6) Fewer than 100 patients completed the HCAHPS survey; (7) No cases met the criteria for this measure; (8) The lower limit of the confidence interval cannot be calculated if the number of observed infections equals zero; (9) No data are available from the state/territory for this reporting period; (10) The scores shown reflect fewer than 50 completed surveys; (11) There were discrepancies in the data collection process; (12) This measure does not apply to this hospital for this reporting period; (13) Results cannot be calculated for this reporting period; (14) The results for this state are combined with nearby states to protect confidentiality; Please refer to the User's Guide for a full explanation of data.

Measure	Cases	This Hosp.	State Avg.	U.S. Avg.
Prophylactic Antibiotic Selection	36	97%	99%	99%
Prophylactic Antibiotic Selection (Outpatient)	77	88%	98%	98%
Prophylactic Antibiotic Stopped	31	84%	98%	98%
Prophylactic Antibiotic Timing	36	89%	99%	99%
Prophylactic Antibiotic Timing (Outpatient)	77	95%	98%	98%
Urinary Catheter Removal	37	95%	98%	97%
Survey of Patients' Hospital Experiences				
Area Around Room 'Always' Quiet at Night	300+	57%	61%	61%
Doctors 'Always' Communicated Well	300+	79%	83%	82%
Home Recovery Information Given	300+	88%	86%	85%
Hospital Given 9 or 10 on 10 Point Scale	300+	64%	74%	71%
Meds 'Always' Explained Before Given	300+	64%	64%	64%
Nurses 'Always' Communicated Well	300+	79%	81%	79%
Pain 'Always' Well Controlled	300+	70%	73%	71%
Room and Bathroom 'Always' Clean	300+	67%	76%	73%
Timely Help 'Always' Received	300+	72%	71%	68%
Would Definitely Recommend Hospital	300+	58%	73%	71%
Use of Medical Imaging				
Cardiac Imaging Stress Test before Surgery	129	2.3%	5.4%	5.3%
Combination Abdominal CT Scan	271	4.1%	9.3%	10.5%
Combination Brain/Sinus CT Scan	301	5.3%	2.6%	2.7%
Combination Chest CT Scan	141	3.5%	4.6%	2.7%
Follow-up Mammogram/Ultrasound	455	13.8%	8.4%	8.8%
Lumbar Spine MRI for Low Back Pain	52	44.2%	38.7%	37.2%

Saint Vincent Williamsport Hospital

412 N Monroe St Phone: 765-762-4000
Williamsport, IN 47993 Fax: 765-762-4126
URL: www.stvincent.org
Type: Critical Access Hospitals Emergency Services: Yes
Ownership: Voluntary non-profit - Church Beds: 16

Key Personnel:
Emergency Room . . . . H Brenner, MD
Operating Room. . . . . Chad J Davis
Quality Assurance . . . . John D Doyle
Chief of Medical Staff . . . . Tahir Hafeez, MD
CEO . . . . Jonathan Nalli

Measure	Cases	This Hosp.	State Avg.	U.S. Avg.
Blood Clot Prevention and Treatment				
Anticoagulation Overlap Therapy[1]	-	-	92%	93%
ICU Venous Thromboembolism Prophylaxis[7]	-	-	91%	92%
Incidence of Potentially Preventable VTE[7]	-	-	10%	10%
UFH with Dosages/Platelet Monitoring[7]	-	-	95%	97%
Venous Thromboembolism Prophylaxis	387	91%	83%	85%
Warfarin Therapy Discharge Instructions[1]	-	-	71%	75%
Chest Pain/Possible Heart Attack Care				
Aspirin Given Within 24 Hours of Arrival	43	98%	96%	96%
Fibrinolytic Meds Within 30 Min. of Arrival[7]	-	-	48%	58%
Average Time to ECG (minutes)	46	8	6	7
Average Time to Transfer (minutes)[1]	-	-	46	60
Children's Asthma Care				
Received Home Management Plan of Care	-	-	-	88%
Received Reliever Medication	-	-	-	100%
Received Systemic Corticosteroids	-	-	-	100%
Emergency Department				
Admittance Decision Time (minutes)	395	74	80	98
Head CT Results Within 45 Min. of Arrival[5]	-	-	60%	57%
Patients Who Left ER Before Being Seen	11,563	0%	2%	2%
Time from ER Arrival to Admit. (minutes)	395	196	241	274
Time from ER Arrival to Discharge (minutes)[5]	-	-	122	134
Time in ER Before Being Evaluated (minutes)[5]	-	-	22	26
Time to Pain Meds for Fractures (minutes)[5]	-	-	52	57
Heart Attack Care				
Aspirin Given at Discharge[1,3]	-	-	99%	99%
Fibrinolytic Meds Within 30 Min. of Arrival[3,7]	-	-	67%	54%
PCI Within 90 Minutes of Arrival[3,7]	-	-	97%	96%
Statin Prescribed at Discharge[1,3]	-	-	99%	98%
Heart Failure Care				
ACE Inhibitor or ARB for LVSD[1]	-	-	97%	97%
Discharge Instructions Given	28	100%	95%	94%
Evaluation of LVS Function	45	98%	99%	99%
Medicare Spending				
Medicare Spending per Patient (ratio)	-	-	1.01	0.98
Pneumonia Care				
Appropriate Initial Antibiotic Given	39	85%	95%	95%
Blood Culture Timing	44	100%	98%	98%
Pregnancy and Delivery Care				
Newborn Deliveries Scheduled Early[5]	-	-	5%	6%
Preventive Care				
Immunization for Influenza	333	98%	91%	90%
Immunization for Pneumonia	546	98%	92%	92%
Stroke Care				
Anticoagulation Therapy for Atrial Fibrillation[1]	-	-	94%	95%
Antithrombotic Therapy Timing[1]	-	-	97%	98%
Assessed for Rehabilitation[1]	-	-	96%	97%
Discharged on Antithrombotic Therapy[1]	-	-	98%	99%
Discharged on Statin Medication[1]	-	-	91%	94%
Thrombolytic Therapy Timing[7]	-	-	54%	66%
Venous Thromboembolism Prophylaxis[1]	-	-	91%	94%
Written Stroke Educational Materials Given[1]	-	-	82%	88%
Surgical Care Improvement Project				
Appropriate Beta Blocker Usage[1,3]	-	-	98%	98%
Appropriate VTP Within 24 Hours[3,7]	-	-	98%	98%
Controlled Postoperative Blood Glucose[5]	-	-	97%	97%
Perioperative Temperature Management[1,3]	-	-	100%	100%
Prophylactic Antibiotic Selection[1,3]	-	-	99%	99%
Prophylactic Antibiotic Selection (Outpatient)	17	94%	98%	98%
Prophylactic Antibiotic Stopped[1,3]	-	-	98%	98%
Prophylactic Antibiotic Timing[1,3]	-	-	99%	99%
Prophylactic Antibiotic Timing (Outpatient)	17	100%	98%	98%
Urinary Catheter Removal[3,7]	-	-	98%	97%
Survey of Patients' Hospital Experiences				
Area Around Room 'Always' Quiet at Night	(a)	57%	61%	61%
Doctors 'Always' Communicated Well	(a)	87%	83%	82%
Home Recovery Information Given	(a)	85%	86%	85%
Hospital Given 9 or 10 on 10 Point Scale	(a)	73%	74%	71%
Meds 'Always' Explained Before Given	(a)	59%	64%	64%
Nurses 'Always' Communicated Well	(a)	81%	81%	79%
Pain 'Always' Well Controlled	(a)	69%	73%	71%
Room and Bathroom 'Always' Clean	(a)	75%	76%	73%
Timely Help 'Always' Received	(a)	82%	71%	68%
Would Definitely Recommend Hospital	(a)	64%	73%	71%
Use of Medical Imaging				
Cardiac Imaging Stress Test before Surgery[7]	-	-	5.4%	5.3%
Combination Abdominal CT Scan	236	3.8%	9.3%	10.5%
Combination Brain/Sinus CT Scan	272	1.1%	2.6%	2.7%
Combination Chest CT Scan	88	0.0%	4.6%	2.7%
Follow-up Mammogram/Ultrasound	143	8.4%	8.4%	8.8%
Lumbar Spine MRI for Low Back Pain	49	36.7%	38.7%	37.2%

Pulaski Memorial Hospital

616 E 13th St Phone: 574-946-2100
Winamac, IN 46996
Type: Critical Access Hospitals Emergency Services: Yes
Ownership: Government - Local

Measure	Cases	This Hosp.	State Avg.	U.S. Avg.
Blood Clot Prevention and Treatment				
Anticoagulation Overlap Therapy[1]	-	-	92%	93%
ICU Venous Thromboembolism Prophylaxis[7]	-	-	91%	92%
Incidence of Potentially Preventable VTE[7]	-	-	10%	10%
UFH with Dosages/Platelet Monitoring[1]	-	-	95%	97%
Venous Thromboembolism Prophylaxis	227	93%	83%	85%
Warfarin Therapy Discharge Instructions[1]	-	-	71%	75%
Chest Pain/Possible Heart Attack Care				
Aspirin Given Within 24 Hours of Arrival	51	82%	96%	96%
Fibrinolytic Meds Within 30 Min. of Arrival[7]	-	-	48%	58%
Average Time to ECG (minutes)	55	6	6	7
Average Time to Transfer (minutes)[1]	-	-	46	60
Children's Asthma Care				
Received Home Management Plan of Care	-	-	-	88%
Received Reliever Medication	-	-	-	100%
Received Systemic Corticosteroids	-	-	-	100%
Emergency Department				
Admittance Decision Time (minutes)	333	61	80	98
Head CT Results Within 45 Min. of Arrival[5]	-	-	60%	57%
Patients Who Left ER Before Being Seen	4,986	0%	2%	2%
Time from ER Arrival to Admit. (minutes)	336	224	241	274
Time from ER Arrival to Discharge (minutes)[5]	-	-	122	134
Time in ER Before Being Evaluated (minutes)[5]	-	-	22	26
Time to Pain Meds for Fractures (minutes)[5]	-	-	52	57
Heart Attack Care				
Aspirin Given at Discharge[1,3]	-	-	99%	99%
Fibrinolytic Meds Within 30 Min. of Arrival[5]	-	-	67%	54%
PCI Within 90 Minutes of Arrival[5]	-	-	97%	96%
Statin Prescribed at Discharge[1,3]	-	-	99%	98%
Heart Failure Care				
ACE Inhibitor or ARB for LVSD[1]	-	-	97%	97%
Discharge Instructions Given	15	93%	95%	94%
Evaluation of LVS Function	26	96%	99%	99%
Medicare Spending				
Medicare Spending per Patient (ratio)	-	-	1.01	0.98
Pneumonia Care				
Appropriate Initial Antibiotic Given	26	96%	95%	95%
Blood Culture Timing	34	97%	98%	98%
Pregnancy and Delivery Care				
Newborn Deliveries Scheduled Early[1,3]	-	-	5%	6%
Preventive Care				
Immunization for Influenza	246	96%	91%	90%
Immunization for Pneumonia	311	97%	92%	92%
Stroke Care				
Anticoagulation Therapy for Atrial Fibrillation[1]	-	-	94%	95%
Antithrombotic Therapy Timing[1]	-	-	97%	98%
Assessed for Rehabilitation[1]	-	-	96%	97%
Discharged on Antithrombotic Therapy[1]	-	-	98%	99%
Discharged on Statin Medication[1]	-	-	91%	94%
Thrombolytic Therapy Timing[7]	-	-	54%	66%
Venous Thromboembolism Prophylaxis[1]	-	-	91%	94%
Written Stroke Educational Materials Given[1]	-	-	82%	88%
Surgical Care Improvement Project				
Appropriate Beta Blocker Usage	16	88%	98%	98%
Appropriate VTP Within 24 Hours	25	100%	98%	98%
Controlled Postoperative Blood Glucose[3,7]	-	-	97%	97%
Perioperative Temperature Management	34	100%	100%	100%
Prophylactic Antibiotic Selection	24	100%	99%	99%
Prophylactic Antibiotic Selection (Outpatient)[3,7]	-	-	98%	98%
Prophylactic Antibiotic Stopped	23	91%	98%	98%
Prophylactic Antibiotic Timing	24	100%	99%	99%
Prophylactic Antibiotic Timing (Outpatient)[3,7]	-	-	98%	98%
Urinary Catheter Removal	11	82%	98%	97%
Survey of Patients' Hospital Experiences				
Area Around Room 'Always' Quiet at Night	(a)	65%	61%	61%
Doctors 'Always' Communicated Well	(a)	84%	83%	82%
Home Recovery Information Given	(a)	91%	86%	85%
Hospital Given 9 or 10 on 10 Point Scale	(a)	82%	74%	71%
Meds 'Always' Explained Before Given	(a)	67%	64%	64%
Nurses 'Always' Communicated Well	(a)	84%	81%	79%
Pain 'Always' Well Controlled	(a)	78%	73%	71%
Room and Bathroom 'Always' Clean	(a)	76%	76%	73%
Timely Help 'Always' Received	(a)	82%	71%	68%
Would Definitely Recommend Hospital	(a)	76%	73%	71%
Use of Medical Imaging				
Cardiac Imaging Stress Test before Surgery[1]	-	-	5.4%	5.3%
Combination Abdominal CT Scan	173	32.9%	9.3%	10.5%
Combination Brain/Sinus CT Scan	144	0.0%	2.6%	2.7%
Combination Chest CT Scan	86	29.1%	4.6%	2.7%
Follow-up Mammogram/Ultrasound	203	6.9%	8.4%	8.8%
Lumbar Spine MRI for Low Back Pain[1]	-	-	38.7%	37.2%

Saint Vincent Randolph Hospital

473 E Greenville Ave Phone: 765-584-0004
Winchester, IN 47394 Fax: 765-584-0066
URL: www.stvincent.org
Type: Critical Access Hospitals Emergency Services: No
Ownership: Voluntary non-profit - Private Beds: 25

Key Personnel:
Chief of Medical Staff . . . . Troy A Abbot
Radiology. . . . . Peter D Arfken
Quality Assurance . . . . John D Doyle
Emergency Room . . . . Harry Moynihan, MD
CEO . . . . Jonathan Nalli

NOTE: Hospital profiles are in alphabetical order by state, then city, then hospital within the city; Rankings exclude hospitals with less than 25 cases except for patient surveys which excludes hospitals with less than 100 cases; (a) 100-299 cases; (1) The number of cases/patients is too few to report; (2) Data submitted were based on a sample of cases/patients; (3) Results are based on a shorter time period than required; (4) Data suppressed by CMS for one or more quarters; (5) Results are not available for this reporting period; (6) Fewer than 100 patients completed the HCAHPS survey; (7) No cases met the criteria for this measure; (8) The lower limit of the confidence interval cannot be calculated if the number of observed infections equals zero; (9) No data are available from the state/territory for this reporting period; (10) The scores shown reflect fewer than 50 completed surveys; (11) There were discrepancies in the data collection process; (12) This measure does not apply to this hospital for this reporting period; (13) Results cannot be calculated for this reporting period; (14) The results for this state are combined with nearby states to protect confidentiality; Please refer to the User's Guide for a full explanation of data.

Measure	Cases	This Hosp.	State Avg.	U.S. Avg.
Blood Clot Prevention and Treatment				
Anticoagulation Overlap Therapy[7]	-	-	92%	93%
ICU Venous Thromboembolism Prophylaxis[7]	-	-	91%	92%
Incidence of Potentially Preventable VTE[7]	-	-	10%	10%
UFH with Dosages/Platelet Monitoring[7]	-	-	95%	97%
Venous Thromboembolism Prophylaxis	321	59%	83%	85%
Warfarin Therapy Discharge Instructions[1]	-	-	71%	75%
Chest Pain/Possible Heart Attack Care				
Aspirin Given Within 24 Hours of Arrival	57	91%	96%	96%
Fibrinolytic Meds Within 30 Min. of Arrival[7]	-	-	48%	58%
Average Time to ECG (minutes)	57	7	6	7
Average Time to Transfer (minutes)[1]	-	-	46	60
Children's Asthma Care				
Received Home Management Plan of Care	-	-	-	88%
Received Reliever Medication	-	-	-	100%
Received Systemic Corticosteroids	-	-	-	100%
Emergency Department				
Admittance Decision Time (minutes)[2]	278	100	80	98
Head CT Results Within 45 Min. of Arrival[5]	-	-	60%	57%
Patients Who Left ER Before Being Seen	11,797	0%	2%	2%
Time from ER Arrival to Admit. (minutes)[2]	298	270	241	274
Time from ER Arrival to Discharge (minutes)	343	137	122	134
Time in ER Before Being Evaluated (minutes)	373	35	22	26
Time to Pain Meds for Fractures (minutes)[5]	-	-	52	57
Heart Attack Care				
Aspirin Given at Discharge[1,3]	-	-	99%	99%
Fibrinolytic Meds Within 30 Min. of Arrival[5]	-	-	67%	54%
PCI Within 90 Minutes of Arrival[5]	-	-	97%	96%
Statin Prescribed at Discharge[1,3]	-	-	99%	98%
Heart Failure Care				
ACE Inhibitor or ARB for LVSD[1]	-	-	97%	97%
Discharge Instructions Given	13	100%	95%	94%
Evaluation of LVS Function	28	100%	99%	99%
Medicare Spending				
Medicare Spending per Patient (ratio)	-	-	1.01	0.98
Pneumonia Care				
Appropriate Initial Antibiotic Given	32	97%	95%	95%
Blood Culture Timing	44	91%	98%	98%
Pregnancy and Delivery Care				
Newborn Deliveries Scheduled Early[2,3]	26	0%	5%	6%
Preventive Care				
Immunization for Influenza[2]	336	92%	91%	90%
Immunization for Pneumonia[2]	341	96%	92%	92%
Stroke Care				
Anticoagulation Therapy for Atrial Fibrillation[7]	-	-	94%	95%
Antithrombotic Therapy Timing[1]	-	-	97%	98%
Assessed for Rehabilitation[1]	-	-	96%	97%
Discharged on Antithrombotic Therapy[1]	-	-	98%	99%
Discharged on Statin Medication[1]	-	-	91%	94%
Thrombolytic Therapy Timing[1]	-	-	54%	66%
Venous Thromboembolism Prophylaxis[1]	-	-	91%	94%
Written Stroke Educational Materials Given[7]	-	-	82%	88%
Surgical Care Improvement Project				
Appropriate Beta Blocker Usage[1]	-	-	98%	98%
Appropriate VTP Within 24 Hours	18	94%	98%	98%
Controlled Postoperative Blood Glucose[7]	-	-	97%	97%
Perioperative Temperature Management	23	100%	100%	100%
Prophylactic Antibiotic Selection	17	94%	99%	99%
Prophylactic Antibiotic Selection (Outpatient)[3]	17	100%	98%	98%
Prophylactic Antibiotic Stopped	17	94%	98%	98%
Prophylactic Antibiotic Timing	17	100%	99%	99%
Prophylactic Antibiotic Timing (Outpatient)[3]	18	94%	98%	98%
Urinary Catheter Removal[1]	-	-	98%	97%
Survey of Patients' Hospital Experiences				
Area Around Room 'Always' Quiet at Night	(a)	62%	61%	61%
Doctors 'Always' Communicated Well	(a)	85%	83%	82%
Home Recovery Information Given	(a)	87%	86%	85%
Hospital Given 9 or 10 on 10 Point Scale	(a)	70%	74%	71%
Meds 'Always' Explained Before Given	(a)	66%	64%	64%
Nurses 'Always' Communicated Well	(a)	81%	81%	79%
Pain 'Always' Well Controlled	(a)	71%	73%	71%
Room and Bathroom 'Always' Clean	(a)	70%	76%	73%
Timely Help 'Always' Received	(a)	70%	71%	68%
Would Definitely Recommend Hospital	(a)	68%	73%	71%
Use of Medical Imaging				
Cardiac Imaging Stress Test before Surgery[7]	-	-	5.4%	5.3%
Combination Abdominal CT Scan	268	5.2%	9.3%	10.5%
Combination Brain/Sinus CT Scan[1]	-	-	2.6%	2.7%
Combination Chest CT Scan	178	8.4%	4.6%	2.7%
Follow-up Mammogram/Ultrasound	315	6.0%	8.4%	8.8%
Lumbar Spine MRI for Low Back Pain[1]	-	-	38.7%	37.2%

NOTE: Hospital profiles are in alphabetical order by state, then city, then hospital within the city; Rankings exclude hospitals with less than 25 cases except for patient surveys which excludes hospitals with less than 100 cases; (a) 100-299 cases; (1) The number of cases/patients is too few to report; (2) Data submitted were based on a sample of cases/patients; (3) Results are based on a shorter time period than required; (4) Data suppressed by CMS for one or more quarters; (5) Results are not available for this reporting period; (6) Fewer than 100 patients completed the HCAHPS survey; (7) No cases met the criteria for this measure; (8) The lower limit of the confidence interval cannot be calculated if the number of observed infections equals zero; (9) No data are available from the state/territory for this reporting period; (10) The scores shown reflect fewer than 50 completed surveys; (11) There were discrepancies in the data collection process; (12) This measure does not apply to this hospital for this reporting period; (13) Results cannot be calculated for this reporting period; (14) The results for this state are combined with nearby states to protect confidentiality; Please refer to the User's Guide for a full explanation of data.

Blood Clot Prevention and Treatment

Anticoagulation Overlap Therapy

Hospital Name	City	Rate	Cases
Finley Hospital[2]	Dubuque	100%	44
Mary Greeley Medical Center[2]	Ames	100%	73
Trinity Regional Medical Center[2]	Fort Dodge	100%	43
Mercy Medical Center - North Iowa[2]	Mason City	99%	84
Saint Luke's Regional Medical Center[2]	Sioux City	98%	44
Mercy Medical Center - Des Moines[2]	Des Moines	97%	235
Saint Luke's Hospital[2]	Cedar Rapids	97%	116
Trinity Bettendorf[2]	Bettendorf	97%	31
Alegent Health Mercy Hospital[2]	Council Bluffs	96%	49
University of Iowa Hospital & Clinics[2]	Iowa City	96%	112
Genesis Medical Center - Davenport[2]	Davenport	94%	143
Ottumwa Regional Health Center[2]	Ottumwa	93%	29
Covenant Medical Center[2]	Waterloo	92%	48
Great River Medical Center[2]	West Burlington	91%	53
Iowa Lutheran Hospital[2]	Des Moines	91%	47
Allen Hospital[2]	Waterloo	90%	69
Iowa Methodist Medical Center[2]	Des Moines	90%	154
Mercy Hospital[2]	Iowa City	90%	69
Mercy Medical Center - Cedar Rapids[2]	Cedar Rapids	90%	84
Mercy Medical Center - Clinton[2]	Clinton	90%	40
Mercy Medical Center - Dubuque[2]	Dubuque	88%	60
Mercy Medical Center - Sioux City[2]	Sioux City	87%	71

ICU Venous Thromboembolism Prophylaxis

Hospital Name	City	Rate	Cases
Grinnell Regional Medical Center[2]	Grinnell	100%	32
Mary Greeley Medical Center[2]	Ames	100%	67
Trinity Muscatine[2]	Muscatine	100%	30
Saint Luke's Hospital[2]	Cedar Rapids	99%	98
Alegent Health Mercy Hospital[2]	Council Bluffs	98%	53
Fort Madison Community Hospital[2]	Fort Madison	98%	54
Iowa Methodist Medical Center[2]	Des Moines	98%	84
Mercy Medical Center - Cedar Rapids[2]	Cedar Rapids	98%	62
Genesis Medical Center - Davenport[2]	Davenport	97%	73
Mercy Medical Center - North Iowa[2]	Mason City	95%	81
Methodist Jennie Edmundson[2]	Council Bluffs	95%	108
Keokuk Area Hospital	Keokuk	94%	125
Mercy Hospital[2]	Iowa City	93%	55
Mercy Medical Center - Clinton[2]	Clinton	93%	98
Mercy Medical Center - Dubuque[2]	Dubuque	92%	38
Trinity Bettendorf[2]	Bettendorf	92%	37
Mercy Medical Center - Des Moines[2]	Des Moines	91%	149
Iowa Lutheran Hospital[2]	Des Moines	90%	60
Mercy Medical Center - Sioux City[2]	Sioux City	90%	68
University of Iowa Hospital & Clinics[2]	Iowa City	90%	107
Saint Luke's Regional Medical Center[2]	Sioux City	89%	84
Great River Medical Center[2]	West Burlington	86%	78
Broadlawns Medical Center[2]	Des Moines	85%	123
Trinity Regional Medical Center[2]	Fort Dodge	85%	91
Finley Hospital[2]	Dubuque	84%	90
Allen Hospital[2]	Waterloo	82%	62
Marshalltown Medical & Surgical Center[2]	Marshalltown	82%	120
Covenant Medical Center[2]	Waterloo	81%	52
Ottumwa Regional Health Center[2]	Ottumwa	80%	79

Incidence of Potentially Preventable VTE

Hospital Name	City	Rate	Cases
University of Iowa Hospital & Clinics[2]	Iowa City	12%	48
Mercy Medical Center - Des Moines[2]	Des Moines	15%	39

UFH with Dosages/Platelet Count Monitoring

Hospital Name	City	Rate	Cases
Alegent Health Mercy Hospital[2]	Council Bluffs	100%	40
Allen Hospital[2]	Waterloo	100%	39
Genesis Medical Center - Davenport[2]	Davenport	100%	100
Great River Medical Center[2]	West Burlington	100%	46
Mercy Medical Center - Cedar Rapids[2]	Cedar Rapids	100%	70
Mercy Medical Center - Clinton[2]	Clinton	100%	34
Mercy Medical Center - North Iowa[2]	Mason City	100%	44
Saint Luke's Hospital[2]	Cedar Rapids	100%	101
University of Iowa Hospital & Clinics[2]	Iowa City	100%	123
Iowa Methodist Medical Center[2]	Des Moines	99%	80
Mercy Medical Center - Des Moines[2]	Des Moines	99%	72

Venous Thromboembolism Prophylaxis

Hospital Name	City	Rate	Cases
Grinnell Regional Medical Center[2]	Grinnell	100%	96
Trinity Muscatine[2]	Muscatine	100%	137
Saint Luke's Hospital[2]	Cedar Rapids	99%	253
Fort Madison Community Hospital[2]	Fort Madison	98%	129
Mercy Medical Center - North Iowa[2]	Mason City	97%	287
Keokuk Area Hospital	Keokuk	96%	480
Alegent Health Comm Mem Hosp	Missouri Valley	95%	114
Alegent Health Mercy Hospital[3]	Corning	95%	56
Genesis Medical Center - Davenport[2]	Davenport	95%	310
Waverly Health Center[3]	Waverly	95%	38
Mercy Medical Center - Dubuque[2]	Dubuque	94%	284
Mary Greeley Medical Center[2]	Ames	93%	347
Mercy Medical Center - Clinton[2]	Clinton	93%	337
Trinity Bettendorf[2]	Bettendorf	93%	208
Trinity Regional Medical Center[2]	Fort Dodge	93%	290
Methodist Jennie Edmundson[2]	Council Bluffs	92%	402
Alegent Health Mercy Hospital[2]	Council Bluffs	91%	192
Allen Hospital[2]	Waterloo	89%	307
Finley Hospital[2]	Dubuque	89%	271
Great River Medical Center[2]	West Burlington	89%	285
Floyd County Memorial Hospital[2]	Charles City	88%	120
Lakes Regional Healthcare[2]	Spirit Lake	88%	103
Mercy Hospital[2]	Iowa City	87%	299
Mercy Medical Center - Cedar Rapids[2]	Cedar Rapids	87%	302
Iowa Lutheran Hospital[2]	Des Moines	85%	281
Covenant Medical Center[2]	Waterloo	83%	210
Marshalltown Medical & Surgical Center[2]	Marshalltown	83%	280
Genesis Medical Center - Dewitt	Dewitt	82%	55
Iowa Methodist Medical Center[2]	Des Moines	82%	294
Skiff Medical Center[2]	Newton	81%	236
Mercy Medical Center - Sioux City[2]	Sioux City	80%	320
University of Iowa Hospital & Clinics[2]	Iowa City	80%	282
Saint Luke's Regional Medical Center[2]	Sioux City	79%	263
Mercy Medical Center - Des Moines[2]	Des Moines	78%	456
Spencer Municipal Hospital[2]	Spencer	74%	152
Mahaska Health Partnership[2,3]	Oskaloosa	73%	26
Ottumwa Regional Health Center[2]	Ottumwa	71%	178
Sartori Memorial Hospital[2]	Cedar Falls	70%	80
Broadlawns Medical Center[2]	Des Moines	67%	91
Pella Regional Health Center[2,3]	Pella	59%	32
Dallas County Hospital[2]	Perry	50%	103
St Anthony Reg Hosp & Nursing Home[2]	Carroll	43%	92

Warfarin Therapy Discharge Instructions

Hospital Name	City	Rate	Cases
Great River Medical Center[2]	West Burlington	100%	41
Mercy Medical Center - Cedar Rapids[2]	Cedar Rapids	100%	64
Mercy Hospital[2]	Iowa City	98%	58
Mercy Medical Center - Dubuque[2]	Dubuque	98%	47
Mary Greeley Medical Center[2]	Ames	94%	49
Allen Hospital[2]	Waterloo	93%	54
Iowa Lutheran Hospital[2]	Des Moines	92%	40
University of Iowa Hospital & Clinics[2]	Iowa City	86%	85
Alegent Health Mercy Hospital[2]	Council Bluffs	85%	40
Finley Hospital[2]	Dubuque	85%	33
Mercy Medical Center - Sioux City[2]	Sioux City	83%	52
Genesis Medical Center - Davenport[2]	Davenport	82%	114
Mercy Medical Center - North Iowa[2]	Mason City	81%	59
Trinity Bettendorf[2]	Bettendorf	79%	29
Mercy Medical Center - Clinton[2]	Clinton	77%	26
Iowa Methodist Medical Center[2]	Des Moines	74%	129
Saint Luke's Regional Medical Center[2]	Sioux City	61%	36
Saint Luke's Hospital[2]	Cedar Rapids	60%	99
Mercy Medical Center - Des Moines[2]	Des Moines	57%	184
Trinity Regional Medical Center[2]	Fort Dodge	51%	37
Covenant Medical Center[2]	Waterloo	32%	38

Chest Pain/Possible Heart Attack Care

Aspirin Given Within 24 Hours of Arrival

Hospital Name	City	Rate	Cases
Boone County Hospital	Boone	100%	35
Buchanan County Health Center[3]	Independence	100%	27
Cass County Memorial Hospital	Atlantic	100%	37
Fort Madison Community Hospital	Fort Madison	100%	34
Great River Medical Center	West Burlington	100%	38
Grinnell Regional Medical Center	Grinnell	100%	41
Pella Regional Health Center	Pella	100%	44
Skiff Medical Center	Newton	100%	57
Trinity Muscatine	Muscatine	100%	66
Waverly Health Center[3]	Waverly	100%	35
Broadlawns Medical Center	Des Moines	98%	48
Genesis Medical Center - Dewitt	Dewitt	98%	40
St Anthony Reg Hosp & Nursing Home	Carroll	98%	49
Ottumwa Regional Health Center	Ottumwa	96%	52
Grundy County Memorial Hospital	Grundy Center	95%	38
Spencer Municipal Hospital	Spencer	95%	39
Keokuk Area Hospital	Keokuk	93%	44
Floyd County Memorial Hospital	Charles City	92%	49
Lakes Regional Healthcare	Spirit Lake	91%	65

Average Time to ECG (minutes)

Hospital Name	City	Min.	Cases
Genesis Medical Center - Dewitt	Dewitt	2	41
Lakes Regional Healthcare	Spirit Lake	2	66
Buchanan County Health Center[3]	Independence	3	30
Pella Regional Health Center	Pella	3	47
Floyd County Memorial Hospital	Charles City	4	51
Fort Madison Community Hospital	Fort Madison	4	35
Grundy County Memorial Hospital	Grundy Center	4	38
Mercy Medical Center - Clinton	Clinton	4	28
Trinity Muscatine	Muscatine	4	66
Broadlawns Medical Center	Des Moines	5	49
Cass County Memorial Hospital	Atlantic	5	37
Skiff Medical Center	Newton	5	58
Great River Medical Center	West Burlington	6	38
Keokuk Area Hospital	Keokuk	6	45
St Anthony Reg Hosp & Nursing Home	Carroll	7	49
Ottumwa Regional Health Center	Ottumwa	8	51
Spencer Municipal Hospital	Spencer	8	40
Waverly Health Center[3]	Waverly	8	38
Winneshiek Medical Center	Decorah	8	26
Grinnell Regional Medical Center	Grinnell	9	43
Boone County Hospital	Boone	12	39

Children's Asthma Care

No hospitals met the 25 case threshold.

Emergency Department

Admittance Decision Time (minutes)

Hospital Name	City	Min.	Cases
St Anthony Reg Hosp & Nursing Home[2]	Carroll	23	135
Genesis Medical Center - Dewitt	Dewitt	29	81
Sartori Memorial Hospital[2]	Cedar Falls	29	311
Floyd County Memorial Hospital[2]	Charles City	33	234
Trinity Regional Medical Center[2]	Fort Dodge	36	466
Grundy County Memorial Hospital[2]	Grundy Center	38	66
Spencer Municipal Hospital[2]	Spencer	38	194
Waverly Health Center[2,3]	Waverly	39	179
Dallas County Hospital[2]	Perry	40	85
Avera Holy Family Hospital[2]	Estherville	42	332
Fort Madison Community Hospital[2]	Fort Madison	42	318
Mercy Medical Center - Dubuque[2]	Dubuque	43	406
Methodist Jennie Edmundson[2]	Council Bluffs	43	325
Lakes Regional Healthcare[2]	Spirit Lake	44	255
Pella Regional Health Center[2,3]	Pella	47	120
Mercy Medical Center - Clinton[2]	Clinton	49	527
Mercy Medical Center - North Iowa[2]	Mason City	49	406
Grinnell Regional Medical Center[2]	Grinnell	50	195
Mary Greeley Medical Center[2]	Ames	51	448
Covenant Medical Center[2]	Waterloo	52	368
Alegent Health Mercy Hospital[2]	Council Bluffs	54	430
Keokuk Area Hospital	Keokuk	54	656
Great River Medical Center[2]	West Burlington	55	668
Knoxville Hospital & Clinics[2,3]	Knoxville	55	168
Skiff Medical Center[2]	Newton	55	254
Marshalltown Medical & Surgical Center[2]	Marshalltown	58	416
Trinity Bettendorf[2]	Bettendorf	63	235
Mercy Medical Center - Cedar Rapids[2]	Cedar Rapids	65	591
Saint Luke's Regional Medical Center[2]	Sioux City	65	430
Finley Hospital[2]	Dubuque	66	474
Mercy Medical Center - Des Moines[2]	Des Moines	69	456
Iowa Lutheran Hospital[2]	Des Moines	76	464
Iowa Methodist Medical Center[2]	Des Moines	76	338
Mercy Medical Center - Sioux City[2]	Sioux City	82	619
Genesis Medical Center - Davenport[2]	Davenport	83	375
Mercy Hospital[2]	Iowa City	83	477
Saint Luke's Hospital[2]	Cedar Rapids	84	423
Allen Hospital[2]	Waterloo	90	513
Trinity Muscatine[2]	Muscatine	93	325
Ottumwa Regional Health Center[2]	Ottumwa	94	347
University of Iowa Hospital & Clinics[2]	Iowa City	106	244
Broadlawns Medical Center[2]	Des Moines	156	163

Head CT Results Within 45 Minutes of Arrival

Hospital Name	City	Rate	Cases
Mercy Medical Center - Clinton	Clinton	66%	35

Patients Who Left ER Before Being Seen

Hospital Name	City	Rate	Cases
Alegent Health Mercy Hospital	Council Bluffs	0%	30713
Avera Holy Family Hospital	Estherville	0%	4123
Dallas County Hospital	Perry	0%	4886
Floyd County Memorial Hospital	Charles City	0%	5735
Genesis Medical Center - Dewitt	Dewitt	0%	4651
Grinnell Regional Medical Center	Grinnell	0%	10626
Horn Memorial Hospital	Ida Grove	0%	5846
Iowa Lutheran Hospital	Des Moines	0%	12170
Jackson County Regional Health Center	Maquoketa	0%	5333
Keokuk County Health Center	Sigourney	0%	2009
Lakes Regional Healthcare	Spirit Lake	0%	7069
Mary Greeley Medical Center	Ames	0%	25238
Mercy Medical Center - Dubuque	Dubuque	0%	22311
Methodist Jennie Edmundson	Council Bluffs	0%	19973
St Anthony Reg Hosp & Nursing Home	Carroll	0%	6565

NOTE: Hospital profiles are in alphabetical order by state, then city, then hospital within the city; Rankings exclude hospitals with less than 25 cases except for patient surveys which excludes hospitals with less than 100 cases; (a) 100-299 cases; (1) The number of cases/patients is too few to report; (2) Data submitted were based on a sample of cases/patients; (3) Results are based on a shorter time period than required; (4) Data suppressed by CMS for one or more quarters; (5) Results are not available for this reporting period; (6) Fewer than 100 patients completed the HCAHPS survey; (7) No cases met the criteria for this measure; (8) The lower limit of the confidence interval cannot be calculated if the number of observed infections equals zero; (9) No data are available from the state/territory for this reporting period; (10) The scores shown reflect fewer than 50 completed surveys; (11) There were discrepancies in the data collection process; (12) This measure does not apply to this hospital for this reporting period; (13) Results cannot be calculated for this reporting period; (14) The results for this state are combined with nearby states to protect confidentiality; Please refer to the User's Guide for a full explanation of data.

Saint Luke's Hospital	Cedar Rapids	0%	55467
Spencer Municipal Hospital	Spencer	0%	7888
Trinity Regional Medical Center	Fort Dodge	0%	22531
Van Diest Medical Center	Webster City	0%	6054
Winneshiek Medical Center	Decorah	0%	4784
Allen Hospital	Waterloo	1%	34560
Covenant Medical Center	Waterloo	1%	30822
Genesis Medical Center - Davenport	Davenport	1%	77039
Great River Medical Center	West Burlington	1%	32992
Iowa Methodist Medical Center	Des Moines	1%	30202
Keokuk Area Hospital	Keokuk	1%	12758
Marengo Memorial Hospital	Marengo	1%	3261
Mercy Hospital	Iowa City	1%	21454
Mercy Hosp of Franciscan Sisters	Oelwein	1%	5581
Mercy Medical Center - Cedar Rapids	Cedar Rapids	1%	48009
Mercy Medical Center - Clinton	Clinton	1%	23318
Mercy Medical Center - North Iowa	Mason City	1%	33358
Mercy Medical Center - Sioux City	Sioux City	1%	30860
Ottumwa Regional Health Center	Ottumwa	1%	22953
Palmer Lutheran Health Center	West Union	1%	3594
Sartori Memorial Hospital	Cedar Falls	1%	7287
Skiff Medical Center	Newton	1%	9164
Trinity Bettendorf	Bettendorf	1%	20596
Trinity Muscatine	Muscatine	1%	15565
Finley Hospital	Dubuque	2%	24348
Fort Madison Community Hospital	Fort Madison	2%	13835
Mercy Medical Center - Des Moines	Des Moines	2%	74432
Saint Luke's Regional Medical Center	Sioux City	2%	30038
University of Iowa Hospital & Clinics	Iowa City	2%	64562
Marshalltown Medical & Surgical Center	Marshalltown	3%	19529
Broadlawns Medical Center	Des Moines	4%	35980

Time from ER Arrival to Being Admitted (minutes)

Hospital Name	City	Min.	Cases
Genesis Medical Center - Dewitt	Dewitt	152	81
Dallas County Hospital[2]	Perry	154	110
Grundy County Memorial Hospital[2]	Grundy Center	159	66
Pella Regional Health Center[2,3]	Pella	160	124
St Anthony Reg Hosp & Nursing Home[2]	Carroll	161	140
Knoxville Hospital & Clinics[2,3]	Knoxville	162	168
Lakes Regional Healthcare[2]	Spirit Lake	165	265
Grinnell Regional Medical Center[2]	Grinnell	166	200
Avera Holy Family Hospital[2]	Estherville	167	360
Trinity Regional Medical Center[2]	Fort Dodge	168	475
Methodist Jennie Edmundson[2]	Council Bluffs	169	325
Alegent Health Mercy Hospital[2]	Council Bluffs	172	444
Mary Greeley Medical Center[2]	Ames	173	457
Spencer Municipal Hospital[2]	Spencer	174	201
Fort Madison Community Hospital[2]	Fort Madison	177	334
Floyd County Memorial Hospital[2]	Charles City	178	236
Great River Medical Center[2]	West Burlington	181	721
Trinity Bettendorf[2]	Bettendorf	185	239
Mercy Medical Center - Clinton[2]	Clinton	186	568
Keokuk Area Hospital	Keokuk	187	742
Marshalltown Medical & Surgical Center[2]	Marshalltown	195	426
Mercy Medical Center - Dubuque[2]	Dubuque	196	488
Sartori Memorial Hospital[2]	Cedar Falls	197	315
Mercy Medical Center - Sioux City[2]	Sioux City	198	669
Skiff Medical Center[2]	Newton	199	255
Allen Hospital[2]	Waterloo	206	518
Covenant Medical Center[2]	Waterloo	212	370
Mercy Hospital[2]	Iowa City	214	498
Mercy Medical Center - Cedar Rapids[2]	Cedar Rapids	215	609
Mercy Medical Center - North Iowa[2]	Mason City	215	415
Waverly Health Center[2,3]	Waverly	217	179
Finley Hospital[2]	Dubuque	226	480
Saint Luke's Regional Medical Center[2]	Sioux City	226	444
Trinity Muscatine[2]	Muscatine	232	337
Saint Luke's Hospital[2]	Cedar Rapids	235	427
Iowa Methodist Medical Center[2]	Des Moines	240	350
Iowa Lutheran Hospital[2]	Des Moines	243	472
Mercy Medical Center - Des Moines[2]	Des Moines	244	507
Genesis Medical Center - Davenport[2]	Davenport	250	433
University of Iowa Hospital & Clinics[2]	Iowa City	278	252
Ottumwa Regional Health Center[2]	Ottumwa	280	363
Broadlawns Medical Center[2]	Des Moines	328	200

Time from ER Arrival to Discharge (minutes)

Hospital Name	City	Min.	Cases
Keokuk County Health Center[3]	Sigourney	71	149
Dallas County Hospital[3]	Perry	76	956
Spencer Municipal Hospital	Spencer	78	361
Genesis Medical Center - Dewitt	Dewitt	81	367
Knoxville Hospital & Clinics[3]	Knoxville	84	136
Boone County Hospital	Boone	86	573
St Anthony Reg Hosp & Nursing Home	Carroll	87	432
Mahaska Health Partnership[3]	Oskaloosa	88	248
Floyd County Memorial Hospital	Charles City	90	192
Grinnell Regional Medical Center	Grinnell	90	332
Great River Medical Center	West Burlington	91	379

Stewart Memorial Community Hospital[3]	Lake City	92	852
Fort Madison Community Hospital	Fort Madison	93	357
Keokuk Area Hospital	Keokuk	94	1320
Lakes Regional Healthcare	Spirit Lake	100	370
Mercy Medical Center - Dubuque	Dubuque	101	484
Mary Greeley Medical Center	Ames	102	368
Finley Hospital	Dubuque	103	361
Skiff Medical Center	Newton	103	256
Methodist Jennie Edmundson	Council Bluffs	106	1266
Alegent Health Mercy Hospital	Council Bluffs	110	381
Marshalltown Medical & Surgical Center	Marshalltown	113	310
Sartori Memorial Hospital	Cedar Falls	114	376
Mercy Medical Center - Clinton	Clinton	116	326
Mercy Medical Center - Sioux City	Sioux City	118	406
Trinity Muscatine	Muscatine	118	322
Trinity Regional Medical Center	Fort Dodge	118	352
Trinity Bettendorf	Bettendorf	120	365
Mercy Medical Center - Cedar Rapids	Cedar Rapids	122	367
Genesis Medical Center - Davenport	Davenport	129	387
Mercy Hospital	Iowa City	129	381
Covenant Medical Center	Waterloo	133	382
Mercy Medical Center - North Iowa	Mason City	133	452
Iowa Lutheran Hospital	Des Moines	137	336
Ottumwa Regional Health Center	Ottumwa	138	338
Saint Luke's Hospital	Cedar Rapids	138	353
Broadlawns Medical Center	Des Moines	140	438
Saint Luke's Regional Medical Center	Sioux City	140	362
Iowa Methodist Medical Center	Des Moines	145	369
Mercy Medical Center - Des Moines	Des Moines	149	475
Allen Hospital	Waterloo	160	343
Waverly Health Center[3]	Waverly	164	29
University of Iowa Hospital & Clinics	Iowa City	168	356

Time in ER Before Being Evaluated (minutes)

Hospital Name	City	Min.	Cases
Spencer Municipal Hospital	Spencer	0	417
Mercy Medical Center - Clinton	Clinton	5	430
Mercy Medical Center - Dubuque	Dubuque	5	541
Mercy Medical Center - Sioux City	Sioux City	10	442
Stewart Memorial Community Hospital[3]	Lake City	10	869
Genesis Medical Center - Dewitt	Dewitt	12	417
Keokuk County Health Center[3]	Sigourney	12	182
Skiff Medical Center	Newton	13	383
Floyd County Memorial Hospital	Charles City	14	334
Mary Greeley Medical Center	Ames	15	404
Trinity Bettendorf	Bettendorf	16	379
Mercy Medical Center - North Iowa	Mason City	17	502
Trinity Muscatine	Muscatine	17	442
Knoxville Hospital & Clinics[3]	Knoxville	18	138
Sartori Memorial Hospital	Cedar Falls	18	410
Great River Medical Center	West Burlington	20	387
Mercy Medical Center - Cedar Rapids	Cedar Rapids	20	367
Dallas County Hospital[3]	Perry	21	1026
Lakes Regional Healthcare	Spirit Lake	21	529
Covenant Medical Center	Waterloo	22	413
Greater Regional Medical Center[3]	Creston	22	54
Mahaska Health Partnership[3]	Oskaloosa	23	282
Boone County Hospital	Boone	24	632
Keokuk Area Hospital	Keokuk	24	1186
Ottumwa Regional Health Center	Ottumwa	25	379
Grinnell Regional Medical Center	Grinnell	26	366
Finley Hospital	Dubuque	28	370
Mercy Medical Center - Des Moines	Des Moines	29	503
St Anthony Reg Hosp & Nursing Home	Carroll	29	495
Saint Luke's Regional Medical Center	Sioux City	29	300
Trinity Regional Medical Center	Fort Dodge	29	213
Allen Hospital	Waterloo	30	373
Fort Madison Community Hospital	Fort Madison	30	384
Genesis Medical Center - Davenport	Davenport	30	404
Marshalltown Medical & Surgical Center	Marshalltown	30	377
Mercy Hospital	Iowa City	30	388
Methodist Jennie Edmundson	Council Bluffs	30	1403
Broadlawns Medical Center	Des Moines	36	527
Iowa Lutheran Hospital	Des Moines	36	200
Iowa Methodist Medical Center	Des Moines	36	244
Alegent Health Mercy Hospital	Council Bluffs	37	306
Saint Luke's Hospital	Cedar Rapids	37	371

Time to Pain Meds for Bone Fractures (minutes)

Hospital Name	City	Min.	Cases
Genesis Medical Center - Dewitt	Dewitt	27	27
Fort Madison Community Hospital	Fort Madison	34	43
Trinity Muscatine	Muscatine	36	72
Mary Greeley Medical Center	Ames	37	87
Trinity Bettendorf	Bettendorf	38	90
Iowa Methodist Medical Center	Des Moines	39	198
Saint Luke's Hospital	Cedar Rapids	39	199
Covenant Medical Center	Waterloo	40	52
Finley Hospital	Dubuque	40	84
Great River Medical Center	West Burlington	40	79

Sartori Memorial Hospital	Cedar Falls	40	25
Boone County Hospital	Boone	41	45
Grinnell Regional Medical Center	Grinnell	41	49
St Anthony Reg Hosp & Nursing Home	Carroll	43	35
Alegent Health Mercy Hospital	Council Bluffs	44	80
Keokuk Area Hospital	Keokuk	44	33
Mercy Medical Center - Dubuque	Dubuque	44	77
Spencer Municipal Hospital	Spencer	44	28
Lakes Regional Healthcare	Spirit Lake	45	49
Mercy Medical Center - Des Moines	Des Moines	45	139
Methodist Jennie Edmundson	Council Bluffs	45	65
Ottumwa Regional Health Center	Ottumwa	45	70
Skiff Medical Center	Newton	45	45
Allen Hospital	Waterloo	46	77
Mahaska Health Partnership[3]	Oskaloosa	48	27
Marshalltown Medical & Surgical Center	Marshalltown	48	100
Mercy Medical Center - Clinton	Clinton	48	114
Mercy Medical Center - Cedar Rapids	Cedar Rapids	51	115
Saint Luke's Regional Medical Center	Sioux City	52	133
Trinity Regional Medical Center	Fort Dodge	52	78
Genesis Medical Center - Davenport	Davenport	54	154
Iowa Lutheran Hospital	Des Moines	55	61
Mercy Medical Center - North Iowa	Mason City	55	125
University of Iowa Hospital & Clinics	Iowa City	61	150
Broadlawns Medical Center	Des Moines	68	56
Mercy Hospital	Iowa City	71	107
Mercy Medical Center - Sioux City	Sioux City	73	67

Heart Attack Care

Aspirin Given at Discharge

Hospital Name	City	Rate	Cases
Alegent Health Mercy Hospital	Council Bluffs	100%	98
Allen Hospital	Waterloo	100%	253
Covenant Medical Center	Waterloo	100%	109
Genesis Medical Center - Davenport[2]	Davenport	100%	294
Iowa City VA Medical Center	Iowa City	100%	25
Iowa Lutheran Hospital[2]	Des Moines	100%	90
Marshalltown Medical & Surgical Center	Marshalltown	100%	52
Mary Greeley Medical Center	Ames	100%	153
Mercy Hospital	Iowa City	100%	187
Mercy Medical Center - Cedar Rapids	Cedar Rapids	100%	165
Mercy Medical Center - Clinton[2]	Clinton	100%	111
Mercy Medical Center - Des Moines[2]	Des Moines	100%	313
Mercy Medical Center - Dubuque	Dubuque	100%	208
Mercy Medical Center - Sioux City	Sioux City	100%	319
Methodist Jennie Edmundson	Council Bluffs	100%	97
Saint Luke's Hospital	Cedar Rapids	100%	325
Trinity Regional Medical Center	Fort Dodge	100%	167
University of Iowa Hospital & Clinics	Iowa City	100%	337
Great River Medical Center	West Burlington	99%	150
Iowa Methodist Medical Center[2]	Des Moines	99%	260
Mercy Medical Center - North Iowa	Mason City	99%	240
Ottumwa Regional Health Center	Ottumwa	99%	78
Finley Hospital	Dubuque	98%	81
Saint Luke's Regional Medical Center	Sioux City	98%	104
Trinity Bettendorf	Bettendorf	98%	61

PCI Within 90 Minutes of Arrival

Hospital Name	City	Rate	Cases
Alegent Health Mercy Hospital	Council Bluffs	100%	29
Mercy Hospital	Iowa City	100%	33
Mercy Medical Center - Cedar Rapids	Cedar Rapids	100%	27
Mercy Medical Center - Des Moines[2]	Des Moines	100%	37
Saint Luke's Hospital	Cedar Rapids	100%	46
Genesis Medical Center - Davenport[2]	Davenport	98%	40
Iowa Methodist Medical Center[2]	Des Moines	94%	36
Mercy Medical Center - Sioux City	Sioux City	94%	35
Allen Hospital	Waterloo	92%	37
Mercy Medical Center - Dubuque	Dubuque	88%	33

Statin Prescribed at Discharge

Hospital Name	City	Rate	Cases
Allen Hospital	Waterloo	100%	240
Genesis Medical Center - Davenport[2]	Davenport	100%	272
Marshalltown Medical & Surgical Center	Marshalltown	100%	50
Mary Greeley Medical Center	Ames	100%	147
Mercy Medical Center - Sioux City	Sioux City	100%	316
Methodist Jennie Edmundson	Council Bluffs	100%	95
Alegent Health Mercy Hospital	Council Bluffs	99%	96
Iowa Lutheran Hospital[2]	Des Moines	99%	87
Iowa Methodist Medical Center[2]	Des Moines	99%	247
Mercy Hospital	Iowa City	99%	176
Mercy Medical Center - Cedar Rapids	Cedar Rapids	99%	155
Mercy Medical Center - Clinton[2]	Clinton	99%	103
Mercy Medical Center - Des Moines[2]	Des Moines	99%	304
Mercy Medical Center - Dubuque	Dubuque	99%	189
Saint Luke's Hospital	Cedar Rapids	99%	307
Trinity Regional Medical Center	Fort Dodge	99%	158

NOTE: Hospital profiles are in alphabetical order by state, then city, then hospital within the city; Rankings exclude hospitals with less than 25 cases except for patient surveys which excludes hospitals with less than 100 cases; (a) 100-299 cases; (1) The number of cases/patients is too few to report; (2) Data submitted were based on a sample of cases/patients; (3) Results are based on a shorter time period than required; (4) Data suppressed by CMS for one or more quarters; (5) Results are not available for this reporting period; (6) Fewer than 100 patients completed the HCAHPS survey; (7) No cases met the criteria for this measure; (8) The lower limit of the confidence interval cannot be calculated if the number of observed infections equals zero; (9) No data are available from the state/territory for this reporting period; (10) The scores shown reflect fewer than 50 completed surveys; (11) There were discrepancies in the data collection process; (12) This measure does not apply to this hospital for this reporting period; (13) Results cannot be calculated for this reporting period; (14) The results for this state are combined with nearby states to protect confidentiality; Please refer to the User's Guide for a full explanation of data.

Hospital Name	City	Rate	Cases
University of Iowa Hospital & Clinics	Iowa City	99%	324
Covenant Medical Center	Waterloo	98%	107
Mercy Medical Center - North Iowa	Mason City	98%	239
Saint Luke's Regional Medical Center	Sioux City	98%	100
Great River Medical Center	West Burlington	97%	133
Finley Hospital	Dubuque	96%	80
Ottumwa Regional Health Center	Ottumwa	93%	68
Trinity Bettendorf	Bettendorf	91%	55

Heart Failure Care

ACE Inhibitor or ARB for LVSD

Hospital Name	City	Rate	Cases
Finley Hospital	Dubuque	100%	27
Genesis Medical Center - Davenport[2]	Davenport	100%	82
Great River Medical Center	West Burlington	100%	34
Mary Greeley Medical Center	Ames	100%	33
Mercy Medical Center - Cedar Rapids[2]	Cedar Rapids	100%	44
Mercy Medical Center - Des Moines[2]	Des Moines	100%	71
Mercy Medical Center - Dubuque	Dubuque	100%	27
Saint Luke's Hospital	Cedar Rapids	100%	68
Trinity Regional Medical Center	Fort Dodge	100%	38
Iowa Lutheran Hospital[2]	Des Moines	98%	48
Methodist Jennie Edmundson	Council Bluffs	97%	37
University of Iowa Hospital & Clinics[2]	Iowa City	96%	112
Mercy Hospital	Iowa City	95%	38
Mercy Medical Center - North Iowa	Mason City	95%	95
Saint Luke's Regional Medical Center	Sioux City	95%	37
Allen Hospital	Waterloo	94%	77
Iowa City VA Medical Center	Iowa City	93%	45
Ottumwa Regional Health Center	Ottumwa	93%	30
Iowa Methodist Medical Center[2]	Des Moines	92%	71
Mercy Medical Center - Sioux City	Sioux City	90%	60

Discharge Instructions Given

Hospital Name	City	Rate	Cases
Fort Madison Community Hospital	Fort Madison	100%	39
Mary Greeley Medical Center	Ames	100%	127
Spencer Municipal Hospital	Spencer	100%	30
Trinity Muscatine	Muscatine	100%	25
Alegent Health Mercy Hospital	Council Bluffs	99%	87
Mercy Hospital	Iowa City	99%	138
Mercy Medical Center - Clinton	Clinton	99%	81
Mercy Medical Center - Des Moines[2]	Des Moines	99%	259
Genesis Medical Center - Davenport[2]	Davenport	98%	200
Iowa City VA Medical Center	Iowa City	98%	96
Trinity Regional Medical Center	Fort Dodge	98%	120
Great River Medical Center	West Burlington	97%	95
Mercy Medical Center - Sioux City	Sioux City	97%	155
Saint Luke's Hospital	Cedar Rapids	97%	238
Mercy Medical Center - Cedar Rapids[2]	Cedar Rapids	96%	170
Mercy Medical Center - Dubuque	Dubuque	96%	119
Allen Hospital	Waterloo	95%	293
Trinity Bettendorf[2]	Bettendorf	95%	40
University of Iowa Hospital & Clinics[2]	Iowa City	95%	233
Mercy Medical Center - North Iowa	Mason City	94%	209
Saint Luke's Regional Medical Center	Sioux City	94%	105
Iowa Methodist Medical Center[2]	Des Moines	90%	198
VA Central Iowa Healthcare System	Des Moines	90%	42
Van Diest Medical Center	Webster City	89%	35
Methodist Jennie Edmundson	Council Bluffs	88%	85
Finley Hospital	Dubuque	87%	102
Iowa Lutheran Hospital[2]	Des Moines	87%	127
Keokuk Area Hospital	Keokuk	86%	36
Covenant Medical Center	Waterloo	82%	99
Boone County Hospital	Boone	64%	33
Ottumwa Regional Health Center	Ottumwa	64%	91

Evaluation of LVS Function

Hospital Name	City	Rate	Cases
Alegent Health Mercy Hospital	Council Bluffs	100%	116
Broadlawns Medical Center	Des Moines	100%	30
Fort Madison Community Hospital	Fort Madison	100%	54
Genesis Medical Center - Davenport[2]	Davenport	100%	284
Great River Medical Center	West Burlington	100%	127
Grinnell Regional Medical Center[2]	Grinnell	100%	40
Iowa City VA Medical Center	Iowa City	100%	108
Marshalltown Medical & Surgical Center	Marshalltown	100%	43
Mary Greeley Medical Center	Ames	100%	174
Mercy Medical Center - Cedar Rapids[2]	Cedar Rapids	100%	231
Mercy Medical Center - Clinton	Clinton	100%	120
Mercy Medical Center - Des Moines[2]	Des Moines	100%	337
Mercy Medical Center - North Iowa	Mason City	100%	317
Myrtue Medical Center[2]	Harlan	100%	33
Ottumwa Regional Health Center	Ottumwa	100%	120
Saint Luke's Hospital	Cedar Rapids	100%	299
Spencer Municipal Hospital	Spencer	100%	39
Trinity Muscatine	Muscatine	100%	34
University of Iowa Hospital & Clinics[2]	Iowa City	100%	276
Allen Hospital	Waterloo	99%	384
Covenant Medical Center	Waterloo	99%	147
Iowa Lutheran Hospital[2]	Des Moines	99%	162
Iowa Methodist Medical Center[2]	Des Moines	99%	246
Keokuk Area Hospital	Keokuk	99%	71
Mercy Medical Center - Dubuque	Dubuque	99%	170
Mercy Medical Center - Sioux City	Sioux City	99%	194
Methodist Jennie Edmundson	Council Bluffs	99%	122
Saint Luke's Regional Medical Center	Sioux City	99%	125
Trinity Regional Medical Center	Fort Dodge	99%	150
Trinity Bettendorf[2]	Bettendorf	98%	57
VA Central Iowa Healthcare System	Des Moines	98%	58
Avera Holy Family Hospital[2]	Estherville	97%	37
Jefferson County Health Center	Fairfield	96%	28
Mercy Hospital	Iowa City	96%	176
Finley Hospital	Dubuque	95%	138
St Anthony Reg Hosp & Nursing Home	Carroll	95%	37
Pella Regional Health Center	Pella	94%	35
Boone County Hospital	Boone	92%	51
Montgomery County Memorial Hospital	Red Oak	91%	35
Skiff Medical Center[2]	Newton	90%	41
Van Diest Medical Center	Webster City	87%	55
Washington County Hospital & Clinics	Washington	81%	27
Floyd County Memorial Hospital[2]	Charles City	66%	38
Clarinda Regional Health Center[3]	Clarinda	62%	32

Medicare Spending

Medicare Spending per Patient (ratio)

Hospital Name	City	Ratio	Cases
Broadlawns Medical Center	Des Moines	0.80	-
Fort Madison Community Hospital	Fort Madison	0.82	-
Grinnell Regional Medical Center	Grinnell	0.83	-
Marshalltown Medical & Surgical Center	Marshalltown	0.84	-
Mercy Hospital	Iowa City	0.84	-
Skiff Medical Center	Newton	0.85	-
Spencer Municipal Hospital	Spencer	0.85	-
Great River Medical Center	West Burlington	0.86	-
Lakes Regional Healthcare	Spirit Lake	0.88	-
Keokuk Area Hospital	Keokuk	0.89	-
Allen Hospital	Waterloo	0.90	-
Iowa Lutheran Hospital	Des Moines	0.90	-
Mary Greeley Medical Center	Ames	0.90	-
Mercy Medical Center - Cedar Rapids	Cedar Rapids	0.90	-
Mercy Medical Center - Dubuque	Dubuque	0.90	-
St Anthony Reg Hosp & Nursing Home	Carroll	0.90	-
Mercy Medical Center - North Iowa	Mason City	0.91	-
Methodist Jennie Edmundson	Council Bluffs	0.91	-
Ottumwa Regional Health Center	Ottumwa	0.91	-
Trinity Bettendorf	Bettendorf	0.92	-
Trinity Regional Medical Center	Fort Dodge	0.92	-
Alegent Health Mercy Hospital	Council Bluffs	0.93	-
Mercy Medical Center - Des Moines	Des Moines	0.93	-
Saint Luke's Hospital	Cedar Rapids	0.93	-
Saint Luke's Regional Medical Center	Sioux City	0.93	-
Genesis Medical Center - Davenport	Davenport	0.94	-
Iowa Methodist Medical Center	Des Moines	0.94	-
Mercy Medical Center - Sioux City	Sioux City	0.96	-
Trinity Muscatine	Muscatine	0.96	-
Covenant Medical Center	Waterloo	0.98	-
University of Iowa Hospital & Clinics	Iowa City	0.98	-
Mercy Medical Center - Clinton	Clinton	0.99	-
Finley Hospital	Dubuque	1.00	-
Sartori Memorial Hospital	Cedar Falls	1.01	-

Pneumonia Care

Appropriate Initial Antibiotic Given

Hospital Name	City	Rate	Cases
Broadlawns Medical Center	Des Moines	100%	48
Genesis Medical Center - Davenport[2]	Davenport	100%	101
Lucas County Health Center	Chariton	100%	26
Mary Greeley Medical Center	Ames	100%	106
Myrtue Medical Center	Harlan	100%	31
Ottumwa Regional Health Center	Ottumwa	100%	47
Winneshiek Medical Center	Decorah	100%	39
Alegent Health Mercy Hospital	Council Bluffs	99%	79
Mercy Hospital	Iowa City	99%	97
Mercy Medical Center - Clinton[2]	Clinton	99%	136
Mercy Medical Center - Des Moines[2]	Des Moines	99%	80
Great River Medical Center	West Burlington	98%	106
Mercy Medical Center - Dubuque	Dubuque	98%	85
Mercy Medical Center - Sioux City	Sioux City	98%	97
Saint Luke's Regional Medical Center	Sioux City	98%	139
Trinity Muscatine	Muscatine	98%	47
Buchanan County Health Center	Independence	97%	31
Finley Hospital[2]	Dubuque	97%	67
Iowa Lutheran Hospital[2]	Des Moines	97%	94
Mahaska Health Partnership[3]	Oskaloosa	97%	31
Marshalltown Medical & Surgical Center	Marshalltown	97%	68
Veterans Memorial Hospital	Waukon	97%	29
Allen Hospital[2]	Waterloo	96%	107
Fort Madison Community Hospital	Fort Madison	96%	73
Grinnell Regional Medical Center[2]	Grinnell	96%	46
Jefferson County Health Center	Fairfield	96%	45
Mercy Medical Center - North Iowa	Mason City	96%	123
Sartori Memorial Hospital	Cedar Falls	96%	25
Methodist Jennie Edmundson	Council Bluffs	95%	86
Spencer Municipal Hospital	Spencer	95%	43
Trinity Bettendorf[2]	Bettendorf	95%	79
Boone County Hospital	Boone	94%	33
Lakes Regional Healthcare	Spirit Lake	94%	50
Regional Medical Center	Manchester	94%	31
Trinity Regional Medical Center	Fort Dodge	94%	114
Covenant Medical Center	Waterloo	93%	76
Iowa City VA Medical Center	Iowa City	93%	28
Keokuk Area Hospital	Keokuk	93%	54
Mercy Medical Center - Cedar Rapids[2]	Cedar Rapids	93%	60
Pella Regional Health Center	Pella	93%	29
Stewart Memorial Community Hospital	Lake City	93%	30
VA Central Iowa Healthcare System	Des Moines	91%	43
Clarinda Regional Health Center[3]	Clarinda	88%	34
Saint Luke's Hospital[2]	Cedar Rapids	88%	68
Sanford Sheldon Medical Center	Sheldon	88%	34
Cass County Memorial Hospital	Atlantic	85%	26
Skiff Medical Center[2]	Newton	84%	32
Iowa Methodist Medical Center[2]	Des Moines	82%	57
Washington County Hospital & Clinics	Washington	81%	37
St Anthony Reg Hosp & Nursing Home	Carroll	80%	41
Jones Regional Medical Center	Anamosa	79%	34
Henry County Health Center	Mount Pleasant	78%	27
Van Diest Medical Center	Webster City	76%	29
Palo Alto County Hospital	Emmetsburg	70%	37

Blood Culture Timing

Hospital Name	City	Rate	Cases
Alegent Health Comm Mem Hosp	Missouri Valley	100%	32
Alegent Health Mercy Hospital	Council Bluffs	100%	131
Broadlawns Medical Center	Des Moines	100%	44
Cass County Memorial Hospital	Atlantic	100%	28
Genesis Medical Center - Davenport[2]	Davenport	100%	153
Great River Medical Center	West Burlington	100%	178
Horn Memorial Hospital	Ida Grove	100%	26
Iowa Methodist Medical Center[2]	Des Moines	100%	92
Jefferson County Health Center	Fairfield	100%	32
Lucas County Health Center	Chariton	100%	25
Mahaska Health Partnership[3]	Oskaloosa	100%	41
Marshalltown Medical & Surgical Center	Marshalltown	100%	96
Mary Greeley Medical Center	Ames	100%	165
Mercy Medical Center - Des Moines[2]	Des Moines	100%	193
Mercy Medical Center - North Iowa	Mason City	100%	221
Methodist Jennie Edmundson	Council Bluffs	100%	175
Myrtue Medical Center	Harlan	100%	52
St Anthony Reg Hosp & Nursing Home	Carroll	100%	36
Skiff Medical Center[2]	Newton	100%	50
Trinity Regional Medical Center	Fort Dodge	100%	192
Waverly Health Center[3]	Waverly	100%	26
Allen Hospital[2]	Waterloo	99%	210
Fort Madison Community Hospital	Fort Madison	99%	76
Iowa Lutheran Hospital[2]	Des Moines	99%	134
Mercy Hospital	Iowa City	99%	169
Mercy Medical Center - Cedar Rapids[2]	Cedar Rapids	99%	135
Mercy Medical Center - Clinton[2]	Clinton	99%	207
Mercy Medical Center - Sioux City	Sioux City	99%	141
Trinity Bettendorf[2]	Bettendorf	99%	118
Boone County Hospital	Boone	98%	56
Covenant Medical Center	Waterloo	98%	129
Floyd Valley Hospital[2]	Le Mars	98%	45
Grinnell Regional Medical Center[2]	Grinnell	98%	63
Iowa City VA Medical Center	Iowa City	98%	42
Keokuk Area Hospital	Keokuk	98%	60
Lakes Regional Healthcare	Spirit Lake	98%	54
Saint Luke's Hospital[2]	Cedar Rapids	98%	84
Saint Luke's Regional Medical Center	Sioux City	98%	208
Buchanan County Health Center	Independence	97%	35
Finley Hospital[2]	Dubuque	97%	138
Mercy Medical Center - Dubuque	Dubuque	97%	119
Montgomery County Memorial Hospital	Red Oak	97%	33
Sartori Memorial Hospital	Cedar Falls	97%	32
Spencer Municipal Hospital	Spencer	97%	59
Trinity Muscatine	Muscatine	97%	77
VA Central Iowa Healthcare System	Des Moines	97%	72
Winneshiek Medical Center	Decorah	97%	60
Regional Medical Center	Manchester	96%	52
Ottumwa Regional Health Center	Ottumwa	95%	66
Pella Regional Health Center	Pella	95%	44
Henry County Health Center	Mount Pleasant	94%	33
University of Iowa Hospital & Clinics[2]	Iowa City	93%	86
Washington County Hospital & Clinics	Washington	91%	32
Shenandoah Medical Center	Shenandoah	89%	28
Jones Regional Medical Center	Anamosa	87%	46

NOTE: Hospital profiles are in alphabetical order by state, then city, then hospital within the city; Rankings exclude hospitals with less than 25 cases except for patient surveys which excludes hospitals with less than 100 cases; (a) 100-299 cases; (1) The number of cases/patients is too few to report; (2) Data submitted were based on a sample of cases/patients; (3) Results are based on a shorter time period than required; (4) Data suppressed by CMS for one or more quarters; (5) Results are not available for this reporting period; (6) Fewer than 100 patients completed the HCAHPS survey; (7) No cases met the criteria for this measure; (8) The lower limit of the confidence interval cannot be calculated if the number of observed infections equals zero; (9) No data are available from the state/territory for this reporting period; (10) The scores shown reflect fewer than 50 completed surveys; (11) There were discrepancies in the data collection process; (12) This measure does not apply to this hospital for this reporting period; (13) Results cannot be calculated for this reporting period; (14) The results for this state are combined with nearby states to protect confidentiality; Please refer to the User's Guide for a full explanation of data.

Hospital Name	City	Rate	Cases
Van Diest Medical Center	Webster City	85%	27
Iowa Specialty Hospital - Clarion[2]	Clarion	68%	28

Pregnancy and Delivery Care

Newborns whose Deliveries were Scheduled Early

Hospital Name	City	Rate	Cases
Broadlawns Medical Center	Des Moines	0%	32
Iowa Methodist Medical Center[2]	Des Moines	0%	73
Marshalltown Medical & Surgical Center	Marshalltown	0%	89
Mercy Medical Center - Cedar Rapids[2]	Cedar Rapids	0%	32
Mercy Medical Center - Dubuque	Dubuque	0%	61
Mercy Medical Center - North Iowa[2]	Mason City	0%	40
Methodist Jennie Edmundson	Council Bluffs	0%	26
Ottumwa Regional Health Center	Ottumwa	0%	70
Saint Luke's Hospital[2]	Cedar Rapids	0%	32
Trinity Muscatine	Muscatine	0%	50
Mary Greeley Medical Center	Ames	2%	113
Finley Hospital[2]	Dubuque	3%	30
Iowa Lutheran Hospital[2]	Des Moines	3%	31
Mercy Medical Center - Clinton	Clinton	3%	37
St Anthony Reg Hosp & Nursing Home[2]	Carroll	3%	34
Saint Luke's Regional Medical Center[2]	Sioux City	3%	34
Mercy Medical Center - Des Moines[2]	Des Moines	6%	109
Mercy Medical Center - Sioux City[2]	Sioux City	6%	34
Covenant Medical Center[2]	Waterloo	7%	30
Genesis Medical Center - Davenport[2]	Davenport	7%	30
Mercy Hospital	Iowa City	13%	140
Great River Medical Center[2]	West Burlington	15%	27

Preventive Care

Immunization for Influenza

Hospital Name	City	Rate	Cases
Fort Madison Community Hospital[2]	Fort Madison	99%	373
Grundy County Memorial Hospital[2]	Grundy Center	99%	99
Mercy Medical Center - Clinton[2]	Clinton	99%	539
Mercy Medical Center - Sioux City[2]	Sioux City	99%	669
Grinnell Regional Medical Center[2]	Grinnell	98%	250
Mercy Medical Center - Dubuque[2]	Dubuque	98%	598
Alegent Health Mercy Hospital[2]	Council Bluffs	97%	581
Marshalltown Medical & Surgical Center[2]	Marshalltown	97%	302
Mary Greeley Medical Center[2]	Ames	97%	559
Trinity Muscatine[2]	Muscatine	97%	288
Keokuk Area Hospital	Keokuk	96%	664
Saint Luke's Regional Medical Center[2]	Sioux City	96%	490
Skiff Medical Center[2]	Newton	96%	293
Veterans Memorial Hospital	Waukon	96%	47
Allen Hospital[2]	Waterloo	95%	508
Floyd County Memorial Hospital[2]	Charles City	95%	120
Genesis Medical Center - Davenport[2]	Davenport	95%	542
Mercy Hospital[2]	Iowa City	95%	532
Mercy Medical Center - Des Moines[2]	Des Moines	94%	764
Trinity Regional Medical Center[2]	Fort Dodge	94%	427
Avera Holy Family Hospital[2]	Estherville	93%	287
Hegg Memorial Health Center[2]	Rock Valley	93%	27
Lakes Regional Healthcare[2]	Spirit Lake	93%	289
Sartori Memorial Hospital[2]	Cedar Falls	93%	285
Jackson County Regional Health Center	Maquoketa	92%	72
Mercy Medical Center - Cedar Rapids[2]	Cedar Rapids	92%	564
Mercy Medical Center - North Iowa[2]	Mason City	92%	610
Jefferson County Health Center[2]	Fairfield	91%	82
Finley Hospital[2]	Dubuque	90%	428
Great River Medical Center[2]	West Burlington	90%	553
Iowa Lutheran Hospital[2]	Des Moines	88%	485
University of Iowa Hospital & Clinics[2]	Iowa City	88%	544
Broadlawns Medical Center[2]	Des Moines	87%	320
Covenant Medical Center[2]	Waterloo	87%	502
Genesis Medical Center - Dewitt	Dewitt	87%	39
Knoxville Hospital & Clinics[3]	Knoxville	87%	118
Iowa Methodist Medical Center[2]	Des Moines	85%	494
Saint Luke's Hospital[2]	Cedar Rapids	85%	483
Spencer Municipal Hospital[2]	Spencer	84%	289
Methodist Jennie Edmundson[2]	Council Bluffs	83%	372
Van Diest Medical Center	Webster City	82%	38
Trinity Bettendorf[2]	Bettendorf	76%	339
Waverly Health Center[2,3]	Waverly	76%	78
Dallas County Hospital[2]	Perry	75%	59
Ottumwa Regional Health Center[2]	Ottumwa	75%	291
St Anthony Reg Hosp & Nursing Home[2]	Carroll	33%	276
Pella Regional Health Center[2,3]	Pella	13%	126

Immunization for Pneumonia

Hospital Name	City	Rate	Cases
Hegg Memorial Health Center[2,3]	Rock Valley	100%	26
Fort Madison Community Hospital[2]	Fort Madison	99%	395
Genesis Medical Center - Dewitt	Dewitt	99%	77
Grundy County Memorial Hospital[2]	Grundy Center	99%	146
Mercy Medical Center - Clinton[2]	Clinton	99%	731
Trinity Muscatine[2]	Muscatine	99%	344
Grinnell Regional Medical Center[2]	Grinnell	98%	296
Mercy Medical Center - Sioux City[2]	Sioux City	98%	838
Skiff Medical Center[2]	Newton	98%	379
Washington County Hospital & Clinics[3]	Washington	98%	133
Keokuk Area Hospital	Keokuk	97%	888
Mercy Medical Center - Dubuque[2]	Dubuque	97%	659
Van Diest Medical Center[3]	Webster City	97%	33
Allen Hospital[2]	Waterloo	96%	698
Genesis Medical Center - Davenport[2]	Davenport	95%	722
Jackson County Regional Health Center	Maquoketa	95%	98
Marshalltown Medical & Surgical Center[2]	Marshalltown	95%	456
Mary Greeley Medical Center[2]	Ames	95%	636
Alegent Health Mercy Hospital[2]	Council Bluffs	94%	495
Lakes Regional Healthcare[2]	Spirit Lake	94%	362
Mercy Medical Center - Cedar Rapids[2]	Cedar Rapids	94%	763
Mercy Medical Center - Des Moines[2]	Des Moines	94%	861
Myrtue Medical Center[2,3]	Harlan	94%	69
Avera Holy Family Hospital[2]	Estherville	93%	377
Trinity Regional Medical Center[2]	Fort Dodge	93%	510
Veterans Memorial Hospital	Waukon	93%	81
Great River Medical Center[2]	West Burlington	92%	724
Sartori Memorial Hospital[2]	Cedar Falls	92%	406
Saint Luke's Regional Medical Center[2]	Sioux City	91%	453
Spencer Municipal Hospital[2]	Spencer	91%	286
Floyd County Memorial Hospital[2]	Charles City	90%	238
Waverly Health Center[2,3]	Waverly	90%	125
Mercy Medical Center - North Iowa[2]	Mason City	89%	731
Iowa Lutheran Hospital[2]	Des Moines	88%	660
Mercy Hospital[2]	Iowa City	88%	655
Saint Luke's Hospital[2]	Cedar Rapids	87%	530
Covenant Medical Center[2]	Waterloo	86%	449
Finley Hospital[2]	Dubuque	86%	533
University of Iowa Hospital & Clinics[2]	Iowa City	85%	497
Knoxville Hospital & Clinics[3]	Knoxville	84%	271
Trinity Bettendorf[2]	Bettendorf	82%	369
Iowa Methodist Medical Center[2]	Des Moines	81%	540
Jefferson County Health Center[2]	Fairfield	79%	131
Pella Regional Health Center[2,3]	Pella	79%	210
Methodist Jennie Edmundson[2]	Council Bluffs	74%	510
Broadlawns Medical Center[2]	Des Moines	67%	183
Ottumwa Regional Health Center[2]	Ottumwa	66%	361
Dallas County Hospital[2]	Perry	64%	121
St Anthony Reg Hosp & Nursing Home[2]	Carroll	64%	295

Stroke Care

Anticoagulation Therapy for Atrial Fibrillation

Hospital Name	City	Rate	Cases
Genesis Medical Center - Davenport	Davenport	100%	40
Mercy Hospital	Iowa City	88%	25

Antithrombotic Therapy Timing

Hospital Name	City	Rate	Cases
Alegent Health Mercy Hospital	Council Bluffs	100%	37
Mercy Hospital	Iowa City	100%	95
Mercy Medical Center - Des Moines[2]	Des Moines	100%	78
Mercy Medical Center - Sioux City	Sioux City	100%	74
Methodist Jennie Edmundson	Council Bluffs	100%	34
Saint Luke's Regional Medical Center[2]	Sioux City	100%	41
Trinity Regional Medical Center[2]	Fort Dodge	100%	27
Genesis Medical Center - Davenport	Davenport	99%	174
Mercy Medical Center - Dubuque	Dubuque	99%	80
Great River Medical Center	West Burlington	98%	47
Mary Greeley Medical Center	Ames	98%	63
Mercy Medical Center - Cedar Rapids	Cedar Rapids	98%	59
Saint Luke's Hospital[2]	Cedar Rapids	98%	89
Mercy Medical Center - North Iowa	Mason City	96%	72
University of Iowa Hospital & Clinics[2]	Iowa City	95%	55
Allen Hospital[2]	Waterloo	94%	48
Finley Hospital[2]	Dubuque	94%	51
Iowa Lutheran Hospital[2]	Des Moines	94%	50
Iowa Methodist Medical Center[2]	Des Moines	93%	59
Marshalltown Medical & Surgical Center	Marshalltown	93%	28

Assessed for Rehabilitation

Hospital Name	City	Rate	Cases
Alegent Health Mercy Hospital	Council Bluffs	100%	53
Covenant Medical Center	Waterloo	100%	25
Genesis Medical Center - Davenport	Davenport	100%	213
Great River Medical Center	West Burlington	100%	53
Mercy Medical Center - Cedar Rapids	Cedar Rapids	100%	98
Mercy Medical Center - North Iowa	Mason City	100%	105
Allen Hospital[2]	Waterloo	98%	81
Mercy Hospital	Iowa City	98%	105
Mercy Medical Center - Dubuque	Dubuque	98%	103
Saint Luke's Regional Medical Center[2]	Sioux City	98%	57
Mary Greeley Medical Center	Ames	97%	78
Mercy Medical Center - Des Moines[2]	Des Moines	97%	108
Methodist Jennie Edmundson	Council Bluffs	97%	39
Saint Luke's Hospital[2]	Cedar Rapids	97%	122
Mercy Medical Center - Sioux City	Sioux City	96%	93
Trinity Regional Medical Center[2]	Fort Dodge	96%	28
University of Iowa Hospital & Clinics[2]	Iowa City	96%	114
Iowa Methodist Medical Center[2]	Des Moines	95%	83
Iowa Lutheran Hospital[2]	Des Moines	93%	54
Marshalltown Medical & Surgical Center	Marshalltown	91%	33
Finley Hospital[2]	Dubuque	90%	41

Discharged on Antithrombotic Therapy

Hospital Name	City	Rate	Cases
Alegent Health Mercy Hospital	Council Bluffs	100%	44
Genesis Medical Center - Davenport	Davenport	100%	205
Great River Medical Center	West Burlington	100%	50
Iowa Lutheran Hospital[2]	Des Moines	100%	44
Marshalltown Medical & Surgical Center	Marshalltown	100%	31
Mary Greeley Medical Center	Ames	100%	74
Mercy Hospital	Iowa City	100%	105
Mercy Medical Center - Dubuque	Dubuque	100%	99
Mercy Medical Center - North Iowa	Mason City	100%	86
Mercy Medical Center - Sioux City	Sioux City	100%	78
Methodist Jennie Edmundson	Council Bluffs	100%	35
Saint Luke's Regional Medical Center[2]	Sioux City	100%	51
Trinity Regional Medical Center[2]	Fort Dodge	100%	27
University of Iowa Hospital & Clinics[2]	Iowa City	100%	75
Mercy Medical Center - Des Moines[2]	Des Moines	99%	91
Iowa Methodist Medical Center[2]	Des Moines	98%	66
Mercy Medical Center - Cedar Rapids	Cedar Rapids	98%	92
Saint Luke's Hospital[2]	Cedar Rapids	97%	114
Allen Hospital[2]	Waterloo	96%	74
Finley Hospital[2]	Dubuque	92%	37

Discharged on Statin Medication

Hospital Name	City	Rate	Cases
Alegent Health Mercy Hospital	Council Bluffs	100%	33
Great River Medical Center	West Burlington	100%	39
Mercy Medical Center - North Iowa	Mason City	100%	62
Genesis Medical Center - Davenport	Davenport	98%	161
Saint Luke's Hospital[2]	Cedar Rapids	98%	100
Saint Luke's Regional Medical Center[2]	Sioux City	98%	41
Mercy Hospital	Iowa City	96%	75
Mercy Medical Center - Cedar Rapids	Cedar Rapids	96%	70
Mercy Medical Center - Dubuque	Dubuque	95%	76
Mercy Medical Center - Sioux City	Sioux City	95%	61
Iowa Lutheran Hospital[2]	Des Moines	94%	35
Iowa Methodist Medical Center[2]	Des Moines	94%	50
University of Iowa Hospital & Clinics[2]	Iowa City	94%	47
Mary Greeley Medical Center	Ames	92%	60
Mercy Medical Center - Des Moines[2]	Des Moines	92%	73
Methodist Jennie Edmundson	Council Bluffs	90%	31
Allen Hospital[2]	Waterloo	84%	63
Finley Hospital[2]	Dubuque	77%	30

Thrombolytic Therapy Timing

Hospital Name	City	Rate	Cases
Allen Hospital[2]	Waterloo	63%	30

Venous Thromboembolism (VTE) Prophylaxis

Hospital Name	City	Rate	Cases
Mercy Medical Center - Dubuque	Dubuque	100%	89
University of Iowa Hospital & Clinics[2]	Iowa City	99%	125
Great River Medical Center	West Burlington	98%	52
Mercy Medical Center - North Iowa	Mason City	98%	97
Alegent Health Mercy Hospital	Council Bluffs	96%	50
Genesis Medical Center - Davenport	Davenport	96%	204
Mary Greeley Medical Center	Ames	96%	75
Saint Luke's Hospital[2]	Cedar Rapids	95%	104
Iowa Lutheran Hospital[2]	Des Moines	94%	53
Mercy Medical Center - Cedar Rapids	Cedar Rapids	94%	84
Finley Hospital[2]	Dubuque	93%	56
Mercy Medical Center - Des Moines[2]	Des Moines	93%	107
Mercy Medical Center - Sioux City	Sioux City	93%	102
Methodist Jennie Edmundson	Council Bluffs	93%	43
Saint Luke's Regional Medical Center[2]	Sioux City	93%	60
Trinity Regional Medical Center[2]	Fort Dodge	93%	29
Mercy Hospital	Iowa City	92%	108
Marshalltown Medical & Surgical Center	Marshalltown	90%	29
Allen Hospital[2]	Waterloo	89%	73
Iowa Methodist Medical Center[2]	Des Moines	82%	80

Written Stroke Educational Materials Given

Hospital Name	City	Rate	Cases
Alegent Health Mercy Hospital	Council Bluffs	100%	36
Mercy Medical Center - Cedar Rapids	Cedar Rapids	100%	45
Mercy Medical Center - Sioux City	Sioux City	98%	40
Saint Luke's Regional Medical Center[2]	Sioux City	97%	31
Mercy Medical Center - Dubuque	Dubuque	95%	55
Mercy Hospital	Iowa City	91%	66

NOTE: Hospital profiles are in alphabetical order by state, then city, then hospital within the city; Rankings exclude hospitals with less than 25 cases except for patient surveys which excludes hospitals with less than 100 cases; (a) 100-299 cases; (1) The number of cases/patients is too few to report; (2) Data submitted were based on a sample of cases/patients; (3) Results are based on a shorter time period than required; (4) Data suppressed by CMS for one or more quarters; (5) Results are not available for this reporting period; (6) Fewer than 100 patients completed the HCAHPS survey; (7) No cases met the criteria for this measure; (8) The lower limit of the confidence interval cannot be calculated if the number of observed infections equals zero; (9) No data are available from the state/territory for this reporting period; (10) The scores shown reflect fewer than 50 completed surveys; (11) There were discrepancies in the data collection process; (12) This measure does not apply to this hospital for this reporting period; (13) Results cannot be calculated for this reporting period; (14) The results for this state are combined with nearby states to protect confidentiality; Please refer to the User's Guide for a full explanation of data.

Hospital Name	City	Rate	Cases
Mercy Medical Center - North Iowa	Mason City	91%	47
Mary Greeley Medical Center	Ames	89%	37
University of Iowa Hospital & Clinics[2]	Iowa City	89%	56
Allen Hospital[2]	Waterloo	85%	39
Finley Hospital[2]	Dubuque	85%	27
Genesis Medical Center - Davenport	Davenport	85%	122
Saint Luke's Hospital[2]	Cedar Rapids	85%	72
Iowa Methodist Medical Center[2]	Des Moines	54%	41
Mercy Medical Center - Des Moines[2]	Des Moines	47%	62
Iowa Lutheran Hospital[2]	Des Moines	39%	28

Surgical Care Improvement Project

Appropriate Beta Blocker Usage

Hospital Name	City	Rate	Cases
Finley Hospital[2]	Dubuque	100%	126
Fort Madison Community Hospital	Fort Madison	100%	32
Iowa Lutheran Hospital[2]	Des Moines	100%	49
Iowa Specialty Hospital - Clarion	Clarion	100%	54
Marshalltown Medical & Surgical Center	Marshalltown	100%	35
Mary Greeley Medical Center	Ames	100%	194
Mercy Medical Center - Clinton	Clinton	100%	72
Mercy Medical Center - Dubuque[2]	Dubuque	100%	161
Mercy Medical Center - Sioux City	Sioux City	100%	295
Methodist Jennie Edmundson	Council Bluffs	100%	68
Skiff Medical Center[2]	Newton	100%	36
Spencer Municipal Hospital[2]	Spencer	100%	75
Trinity Bettendorf[2]	Bettendorf	100%	88
Alegent Health Mercy Hospital[2]	Council Bluffs	99%	122
Genesis Medical Center - Davenport[2]	Davenport	99%	222
Great River Medical Center	West Burlington	99%	217
Mercy Medical Center - Des Moines[2]	Des Moines	99%	310
Saint Luke's Hospital[2]	Cedar Rapids	99%	209
Saint Luke's Regional Medical Center[2]	Sioux City	99%	193
Sartori Memorial Hospital	Cedar Falls	99%	69
VA Central Iowa Healthcare System[2]	Des Moines	99%	86
Allen Hospital[2]	Waterloo	98%	249
Covenant Medical Center	Waterloo	98%	134
Iowa Methodist Medical Center[2]	Des Moines	98%	150
Mercy Medical Center - North Iowa	Mason City	98%	361
St Anthony Reg Hosp & Nursing Home[2]	Carroll	98%	91
University of Iowa Hospital & Clinics[2]	Iowa City	98%	235
Mahaska Health Partnership	Oskaloosa	97%	35
Mercy Hospital	Iowa City	97%	397
Mercy Medical Center - Cedar Rapids[2]	Cedar Rapids	97%	105
Trinity Regional Medical Center[2]	Fort Dodge	97%	86
Lakes Regional Healthcare	Spirit Lake	96%	26
Trinity Muscatine	Muscatine	96%	27
Iowa City VA Medical Center[2]	Iowa City	92%	123
Ottumwa Regional Health Center	Ottumwa	89%	64
Broadlawns Medical Center	Des Moines	77%	26

Appropriate VTP Within 24 Hours

Hospital Name	City	Rate	Cases
Finley Hospital[2]	Dubuque	100%	357
Floyd Valley Hospital	Le Mars	100%	70
Fort Madison Community Hospital	Fort Madison	100%	87
Grinnell Regional Medical Center	Grinnell	100%	76
Grundy County Memorial Hospital	Grundy Center	100%	47
Mahaska Health Partnership	Oskaloosa	100%	87
Marshalltown Medical & Surgical Center	Marshalltown	100%	94
Mary Greeley Medical Center	Ames	100%	613
Mercy Medical Center - Cedar Rapids[2]	Cedar Rapids	100%	240
Mercy Medical Center - Clinton	Clinton	100%	148
Saint Luke's Hospital[2]	Cedar Rapids	100%	221
Spencer Municipal Hospital[2]	Spencer	100%	202
Trinity Muscatine	Muscatine	100%	66
Waverly Health Center[3]	Waverly	100%	27
Alegent Health Mercy Hospital[2]	Council Bluffs	99%	371
Allen Hospital[2]	Waterloo	99%	388
Great River Medical Center	West Burlington	99%	518
Iowa City VA Medical Center[2]	Iowa City	99%	239
Iowa Specialty Hospital - Clarion	Clarion	99%	210
Mercy Medical Center - Dubuque[2]	Dubuque	99%	370
Mercy Medical Center - North Iowa	Mason City	99%	816
Mercy Medical Center - Sioux City	Sioux City	99%	506
Methodist Jennie Edmundson	Council Bluffs	99%	261
Saint Luke's Regional Medical Center[2]	Sioux City	99%	602
Sartori Memorial Hospital	Cedar Falls	99%	198
Skiff Medical Center[2]	Newton	99%	118
Trinity Bettendorf[2]	Bettendorf	99%	156
Trinity Regional Medical Center[2]	Fort Dodge	99%	173
University of Iowa Hospital & Clinics[2]	Iowa City	99%	399
Covenant Medical Center	Waterloo	98%	332
Genesis Medical Center - Davenport[2]	Davenport	98%	428
Iowa Methodist Medical Center[2]	Des Moines	98%	389
Mercy Hospital	Iowa City	98%	1103
Mercy Medical Center - Des Moines[2]	Des Moines	97%	536
Ottumwa Regional Health Center	Ottumwa	97%	145
Pella Regional Health Center	Pella	96%	76

Hospital Name	City	Rate	Cases
Broadlawns Medical Center	Des Moines	95%	133
VA Central Iowa Healthcare System[2]	Des Moines	95%	145
Winneshiek Medical Center	Decorah	95%	57
Buena Vista Regional Medical Center	Storm Lake	94%	50
Iowa Lutheran Hospital[2]	Des Moines	94%	255
Mercy Medical Center - Centerville	Centerville	93%	44
Stewart Memorial Community Hospital	Lake City	93%	29
St Anthony Reg Hosp & Nursing Home[2]	Carroll	90%	238
Lakes Regional Healthcare	Spirit Lake	89%	70
Veterans Memorial Hospital	Waukon	89%	28
Boone County Hospital	Boone	87%	53
Greene County Medical Center	Jefferson	84%	31
Jefferson County Health Center	Fairfield	69%	26

Controlled Postoperative Blood Glucose

Hospital Name	City	Rate	Cases
Allen Hospital[2]	Waterloo	98%	126
Mercy Medical Center - Sioux City	Sioux City	98%	61
University of Iowa Hospital & Clinics[2]	Iowa City	97%	109
Iowa Methodist Medical Center[2]	Des Moines	96%	101
Mercy Hospital	Iowa City	96%	99
Mercy Medical Center - Des Moines[2]	Des Moines	96%	158
Mercy Medical Center - Dubuque[2]	Dubuque	96%	52
Mercy Medical Center - North Iowa	Mason City	96%	106
Genesis Medical Center - Davenport[2]	Davenport	95%	110
Saint Luke's Hospital[2]	Cedar Rapids	95%	128

Perioperative Temperature Management

Hospital Name	City	Rate	Cases
Alegent Health Mercy Hospital[2]	Council Bluffs	100%	441
Broadlawns Medical Center	Des Moines	100%	158
Buena Vista Regional Medical Center	Storm Lake	100%	58
Covenant Medical Center	Waterloo	100%	370
Finley Hospital[2]	Dubuque	100%	399
Floyd Valley Hospital	Le Mars	100%	80
Fort Madison Community Hospital	Fort Madison	100%	98
Genesis Medical Center - Davenport[2]	Davenport	100%	552
Great River Medical Center	West Burlington	100%	570
Grundy County Memorial Hospital	Grundy Center	100%	49
Iowa City VA Medical Center[2]	Iowa City	100%	275
Iowa Lutheran Hospital[2]	Des Moines	100%	292
Iowa Methodist Medical Center[2]	Des Moines	100%	500
Iowa Specialty Hospital - Clarion	Clarion	100%	236
Jefferson County Health Center	Fairfield	100%	25
Mahaska Health Partnership	Oskaloosa	100%	96
Marshalltown Medical & Surgical Center	Marshalltown	100%	108
Mary Greeley Medical Center	Ames	100%	659
Mercy Hospital	Iowa City	100%	1204
Mercy Medical Center - Cedar Rapids[2]	Cedar Rapids	100%	300
Mercy Medical Center - Centerville	Centerville	100%	49
Mercy Medical Center - Des Moines[2]	Des Moines	100%	681
Mercy Medical Center - Dubuque[2]	Dubuque	100%	399
Mercy Medical Center - North Iowa	Mason City	100%	903
Mercy Medical Center - Sioux City	Sioux City	100%	659
Methodist Jennie Edmundson	Council Bluffs	100%	322
Pella Regional Health Center	Pella	100%	83
Saint Luke's Regional Medical Center[2]	Sioux City	100%	682
Sartori Memorial Hospital	Cedar Falls	100%	210
Skiff Medical Center[2]	Newton	100%	130
Spencer Municipal Hospital[2]	Spencer	100%	214
Stewart Memorial Community Hospital	Lake City	100%	32
Trinity Bettendorf[2]	Bettendorf	100%	277
Trinity Muscatine	Muscatine	100%	88
Trinity Regional Medical Center[2]	Fort Dodge	100%	246
University of Iowa Hospital & Clinics[2]	Iowa City	100%	530
Veterans Memorial Hospital	Waukon	100%	29
Waverly Health Center[3]	Waverly	100%	29
Winneshiek Medical Center	Decorah	100%	65
Allen Hospital[2]	Waterloo	99%	466
Mercy Medical Center - Clinton	Clinton	99%	175
Ottumwa Regional Health Center	Ottumwa	99%	158
St Anthony Reg Hosp & Nursing Home[2]	Carroll	99%	252
Saint Luke's Hospital[2]	Cedar Rapids	99%	330
VA Central Iowa Healthcare System[2]	Des Moines	99%	166
Boone County Hospital	Boone	98%	53
Grinnell Regional Medical Center	Grinnell	98%	82
Greene County Medical Center	Jefferson	97%	34
Lakes Regional Healthcare	Spirit Lake	94%	82

Prophylactic Antibiotic Selection

Hospital Name	City	Rate	Cases
Alegent Health Mercy Hospital[2]	Council Bluffs	100%	263
Boone County Hospital	Boone	100%	39
Fort Madison Community Hospital	Fort Madison	100%	82
Genesis Medical Center - Davenport[2]	Davenport	100%	456
Grundy County Memorial Hospital	Grundy Center	100%	48
Mahaska Health Partnership	Oskaloosa	100%	76
Marshalltown Medical & Surgical Center	Marshalltown	100%	76
Mary Greeley Medical Center	Ames	100%	458
Mercy Medical Center - Cedar Rapids[2]	Cedar Rapids	100%	192
Mercy Medical Center - Dubuque[2]	Dubuque	100%	333
Methodist Jennie Edmundson	Council Bluffs	100%	224
Orange City Area Health System	Orange City	100%	54
Ottumwa Regional Health Center	Ottumwa	100%	118
Saint Luke's Hospital[2]	Cedar Rapids	100%	318
Skiff Medical Center[2]	Newton	100%	109
Stewart Memorial Community Hospital	Lake City	100%	28
Trinity Muscatine	Muscatine	100%	45
Trinity Regional Medical Center[2]	Fort Dodge	100%	181
University of Iowa Hospital & Clinics[2]	Iowa City	100%	394
Winneshiek Medical Center	Decorah	100%	58
Allen Hospital[2]	Waterloo	99%	385
Broadlawns Medical Center	Des Moines	99%	117
Covenant Medical Center	Waterloo	99%	237
Finley Hospital[2]	Dubuque	99%	325
Great River Medical Center	West Burlington	99%	402
Iowa City VA Medical Center	Iowa City	99%	185
Iowa Methodist Medical Center[2]	Des Moines	99%	399
Mercy Hospital	Iowa City	99%	1049
Mercy Medical Center - Clinton	Clinton	99%	107
Mercy Medical Center - Des Moines[2]	Des Moines	99%	521
Mercy Medical Center - North Iowa	Mason City	99%	713
Mercy Medical Center - Sioux City	Sioux City	99%	332
St Anthony Reg Hosp & Nursing Home[2]	Carroll	99%	188
Saint Luke's Regional Medical Center[2]	Sioux City	99%	499
Sartori Memorial Hospital	Cedar Falls	99%	156
Spencer Municipal Hospital[2]	Spencer	99%	160
Trinity Bettendorf[2]	Bettendorf	99%	195
Buena Vista Regional Medical Center	Storm Lake	98%	53
Floyd Valley Hospital	Le Mars	98%	61
Pella Regional Health Center	Pella	98%	47
VA Central Iowa Healthcare System	Des Moines	98%	123
Lakes Regional Healthcare	Spirit Lake	97%	69
Mercy Medical Center - Centerville	Centerville	97%	34
Iowa Lutheran Hospital[2]	Des Moines	95%	174
Iowa Specialty Hospital - Clarion	Clarion	93%	29
Greene County Medical Center	Jefferson	90%	30
Veterans Memorial Hospital	Waukon	72%	25

Prophylactic Antibiotic Selection (Outpatient)

Hospital Name	City	Rate	Cases
Alegent Health Mercy Hospital	Council Bluffs	100%	102
Finley Hospital	Dubuque	100%	111
Mahaska Health Partnership[3]	Oskaloosa	100%	29
Marshalltown Medical & Surgical Center	Marshalltown	100%	44
Saint Luke's Hospital	Cedar Rapids	100%	560
Trinity Muscatine	Muscatine	100%	36
Waverly Health Center[3]	Waverly	100%	27
Winneshiek Medical Center	Decorah	100%	59
Genesis Medical Center - Davenport	Davenport	99%	540
Iowa Lutheran Hospital	Des Moines	99%	186
Mary Greeley Medical Center	Ames	99%	398
Mercy Medical Center - Cedar Rapids	Cedar Rapids	99%	708
Mercy Medical Center - Des Moines	Des Moines	99%	709
Mercy Medical Center - Dubuque	Dubuque	99%	302
Mercy Medical Center - Sioux City	Sioux City	99%	158
Trinity Regional Medical Center	Fort Dodge	99%	163
University of Iowa Hospital & Clinics	Iowa City	99%	647
Covenant Medical Center	Waterloo	98%	404
Great River Medical Center	West Burlington	98%	233
Mercy Hospital	Iowa City	98%	449
Mercy Medical Center - North Iowa	Mason City	98%	997
Ottumwa Regional Health Center	Ottumwa	98%	149
Allen Hospital	Waterloo	97%	439
Iowa Methodist Medical Center	Des Moines	97%	589
Mercy Medical Center - Clinton	Clinton	97%	79
Pella Regional Health Center	Pella	97%	117
Saint Luke's Regional Medical Center	Sioux City	97%	193
Spencer Municipal Hospital	Spencer	97%	143
Trinity Bettendorf	Bettendorf	97%	118
Fort Madison Community Hospital	Fort Madison	96%	48
Methodist Jennie Edmundson	Council Bluffs	96%	213

Prophylactic Antibiotic Stopped

Hospital Name	City	Rate	Cases
Alegent Health Mercy Hospital[2]	Council Bluffs	100%	249
Boone County Hospital	Boone	100%	39
Floyd Valley Hospital	Le Mars	100%	60
Grundy County Memorial Hospital	Grundy Center	100%	48
Mary Greeley Medical Center	Ames	100%	450
Mercy Medical Center - Clinton	Clinton	100%	103
Pella Regional Health Center	Pella	100%	46
Skiff Medical Center[2]	Newton	100%	108
Stewart Memorial Community Hospital	Lake City	100%	28
Fort Madison Community Hospital	Fort Madison	99%	81
Mercy Medical Center - Des Moines[2]	Des Moines	99%	503
Mercy Medical Center - Dubuque[2]	Dubuque	99%	332
Mercy Medical Center - North Iowa	Mason City	99%	687
Methodist Jennie Edmundson	Council Bluffs	99%	217
Sartori Memorial Hospital	Cedar Falls	99%	156

NOTE: Hospital profiles are in alphabetical order by state, then city, then hospital within the city; Rankings exclude hospitals with less than 25 cases except for patient surveys which excludes hospitals with less than 100 cases; (a) 100-299 cases; (1) The number of cases/patients is too few to report; (2) Data submitted were based on a sample of cases/patients; (3) Results are based on a shorter time period than required; (4) Data suppressed by CMS for one or more quarters; (5) Results are not available for this reporting period; (6) Fewer than 100 patients completed the HCAHPS survey; (7) No cases met the criteria for this measure; (8) The lower limit of the confidence interval cannot be calculated if the number of observed infections equals zero; (9) No data are available from the state/territory for this reporting period; (10) The scores shown reflect fewer than 50 completed surveys; (11) There were discrepancies in the data collection process; (12) This measure does not apply to this hospital for this reporting period; (13) Results cannot be calculated for this reporting period; (14) The results for this state are combined with nearby states to protect confidentiality; Please refer to the User's Guide for a full explanation of data.

Allen Hospital[2]	Waterloo	98%	383
Genesis Medical Center - Davenport[2]	Davenport	98%	428
Great River Medical Center	West Burlington	98%	397
Mercy Hospital	Iowa City	98%	1026
Mercy Medical Center - Cedar Rapids[2]	Cedar Rapids	98%	190
Mercy Medical Center - Sioux City	Sioux City	98%	316
Saint Luke's Regional Medical Center[2]	Sioux City	98%	484
Spencer Municipal Hospital[2]	Spencer	98%	159
University of Iowa Hospital & Clinics[2]	Iowa City	98%	378
VA Central Iowa Healthcare System	Des Moines	98%	120
Winneshiek Medical Center	Decorah	98%	58
Broadlawns Medical Center	Des Moines	97%	115
Covenant Medical Center	Waterloo	97%	228
Finley Hospital[2]	Dubuque	97%	324
Iowa Methodist Medical Center[2]	Des Moines	97%	386
Marshalltown Medical & Surgical Center	Marshalltown	97%	73
Mercy Medical Center - Centerville	Centerville	97%	31
Buena Vista Regional Medical Center	Storm Lake	96%	51
Iowa Lutheran Hospital[2]	Des Moines	96%	171
Mahaska Health Partnership	Oskaloosa	96%	73
Saint Luke's Hospital[2]	Cedar Rapids	95%	306
Trinity Bettendorf[2]	Bettendorf	95%	192
Trinity Regional Medical Center[2]	Fort Dodge	95%	175
Orange City Area Health System	Orange City	94%	53
St Anthony Reg Hosp & Nursing Home[2]	Carroll	94%	187
Greene County Medical Center	Jefferson	93%	30
Iowa Specialty Hospital - Clarion	Clarion	93%	29
Ottumwa Regional Health Center	Ottumwa	93%	113
Iowa City VA Medical Center	Iowa City	92%	184
Lakes Regional Healthcare	Spirit Lake	90%	68
Trinity Muscatine	Muscatine	89%	37

Prophylactic Antibiotic Timing

Hospital Name	City	Rate	Cases
Alegent Health Mercy Hospital[2]	Council Bluffs	100%	263
Covenant Medical Center	Waterloo	100%	237
Finley Hospital[2]	Dubuque	100%	326
Fort Madison Community Hospital	Fort Madison	100%	82
Grundy County Memorial Hospital	Grundy Center	100%	48
Mahaska Health Partnership	Oskaloosa	100%	76
Marshalltown Medical & Surgical Center	Marshalltown	100%	105
Mary Greeley Medical Center	Ames	100%	458
Orange City Area Health System	Orange City	100%	54
Sartori Memorial Hospital	Cedar Falls	100%	156
Trinity Muscatine	Muscatine	100%	45
Genesis Medical Center - Davenport[2]	Davenport	99%	458
Great River Medical Center	West Burlington	99%	402
Iowa Lutheran Hospital[2]	Des Moines	99%	174
Mercy Hospital	Iowa City	99%	1049
Mercy Medical Center - Dubuque[2]	Dubuque	99%	334
Mercy Medical Center - Sioux City	Sioux City	99%	332
Saint Luke's Regional Medical Center[2]	Sioux City	99%	499
Skiff Medical Center[2]	Newton	99%	109
Spencer Municipal Hospital[2]	Spencer	99%	160
Trinity Bettendorf[2]	Bettendorf	99%	195
Allen Hospital[2]	Waterloo	98%	390
Iowa City VA Medical Center	Iowa City	98%	185
Mercy Medical Center - Clinton	Clinton	98%	107
Mercy Medical Center - North Iowa	Mason City	98%	713
Methodist Jennie Edmundson	Council Bluffs	98%	225
Pella Regional Health Center	Pella	98%	47
Saint Luke's Hospital[2]	Cedar Rapids	98%	318
Trinity Regional Medical Center[2]	Fort Dodge	98%	181
University of Iowa Hospital & Clinics[2]	Iowa City	98%	396
Floyd Valley Hospital	Le Mars	97%	62
Iowa Methodist Medical Center[2]	Des Moines	97%	399
Mercy Medical Center - Cedar Rapids[2]	Cedar Rapids	97%	192
Mercy Medical Center - Centerville	Centerville	97%	34
St Anthony Reg Hosp & Nursing Home[2]	Carroll	97%	188
Winneshiek Medical Center	Decorah	97%	58
Lakes Regional Healthcare	Spirit Lake	96%	69
Mercy Medical Center - Des Moines[2]	Des Moines	96%	521
Buena Vista Regional Medical Center	Storm Lake	94%	53
Iowa Specialty Hospital - Clarion	Clarion	93%	29
VA Central Iowa Healthcare System	Des Moines	93%	124
Broadlawns Medical Center	Des Moines	92%	117
Ottumwa Regional Health Center	Ottumwa	91%	118
Greene County Medical Center	Jefferson	87%	30
Stewart Memorial Community Hospital	Lake City	86%	29
Boone County Hospital	Boone	85%	40
Veterans Memorial Hospital	Waukon	80%	25

Prophylactic Antibiotic Timing (Outpatient)

Hospital Name	City	Rate	Cases
Fort Madison Community Hospital	Fort Madison	100%	39
Mahaska Health Partnership[3]	Oskaloosa	100%	29
Marshalltown Medical & Surgical Center	Marshalltown	100%	44
Mary Greeley Medical Center	Ames	100%	390
Mercy Medical Center - Clinton	Clinton	100%	79
Mercy Medical Center - Dubuque	Dubuque	100%	300

Pella Regional Health Center	Pella	100%	117
Alegent Health Mercy Hospital	Council Bluffs	99%	103
Covenant Medical Center	Waterloo	99%	404
Genesis Medical Center - Davenport	Davenport	99%	542
Iowa Methodist Medical Center	Des Moines	99%	589
Mercy Hospital	Iowa City	99%	449
Saint Luke's Hospital	Cedar Rapids	99%	561
Great River Medical Center	West Burlington	98%	233
Iowa Lutheran Hospital	Des Moines	98%	188
Mercy Medical Center - North Iowa	Mason City	98%	1003
Trinity Bettendorf	Bettendorf	98%	119
Mercy Medical Center - Cedar Rapids	Cedar Rapids	97%	721
Mercy Medical Center - Des Moines	Des Moines	97%	708
Trinity Muscatine	Muscatine	97%	35
Trinity Regional Medical Center	Fort Dodge	97%	163
University of Iowa Hospital & Clinics	Iowa City	97%	572
Allen Hospital	Waterloo	96%	445
Spencer Municipal Hospital	Spencer	96%	139
Waverly Health Center[3]	Waverly	96%	28
Finley Hospital	Dubuque	95%	111
Methodist Jennie Edmundson	Council Bluffs	95%	217
Ottumwa Regional Health Center	Ottumwa	95%	151
Saint Luke's Regional Medical Center	Sioux City	95%	196
Winneshiek Medical Center	Decorah	93%	27
Mercy Medical Center - Sioux City	Sioux City	90%	164

Urinary Catheter Removal

Hospital Name	City	Rate	Cases
Buena Vista Regional Medical Center	Storm Lake	100%	40
Fort Madison Community Hospital	Fort Madison	100%	94
Great River Medical Center	West Burlington	100%	448
Lakes Regional Healthcare	Spirit Lake	100%	73
Mercy Medical Center - Clinton	Clinton	100%	123
Mercy Medical Center - Dubuque[2]	Dubuque	100%	363
Sartori Memorial Hospital	Cedar Falls	100%	172
Spencer Municipal Hospital[2]	Spencer	100%	176
Trinity Bettendorf[2]	Bettendorf	100%	63
Trinity Muscatine	Muscatine	100%	41
Alegent Health Mercy Hospital[2]	Council Bluffs	99%	255
Allen Hospital[2]	Waterloo	99%	160
Finley Hospital[2]	Dubuque	99%	329
Genesis Medical Center - Davenport[2]	Davenport	99%	319
Iowa Methodist Medical Center[2]	Des Moines	99%	379
Mahaska Health Partnership	Oskaloosa	99%	79
Mary Greeley Medical Center	Ames	99%	119
Mercy Hospital	Iowa City	99%	1172
Methodist Jennie Edmundson	Council Bluffs	99%	223
University of Iowa Hospital & Clinics[2]	Iowa City	99%	346
Grinnell Regional Medical Center	Grinnell	98%	47
Covenant Medical Center	Waterloo	97%	228
Mercy Medical Center - Cedar Rapids[2]	Cedar Rapids	97%	64
Mercy Medical Center - Sioux City	Sioux City	97%	251
VA Central Iowa Healthcare System[2]	Des Moines	97%	106
Broadlawns Medical Center	Des Moines	96%	81
Iowa Lutheran Hospital[2]	Des Moines	96%	172
Marshalltown Medical & Surgical Center	Marshalltown	96%	28
Mercy Medical Center - Des Moines[2]	Des Moines	96%	249
Ottumwa Regional Health Center	Ottumwa	96%	78
Trinity Regional Medical Center[2]	Fort Dodge	96%	151
Winneshiek Medical Center	Decorah	96%	27
Pella Regional Health Center	Pella	95%	39
Iowa City VA Medical Center[2]	Iowa City	93%	208
St Anthony Reg Hosp & Nursing Home[2]	Carroll	92%	154
Mercy Medical Center - North Iowa	Mason City	90%	209
Saint Luke's Hospital[2]	Cedar Rapids	89%	190
Greene County Medical Center	Jefferson	88%	25
Saint Luke's Regional Medical Center[2]	Sioux City	77%	133

Survey of Patients' Hospital Experiences

Area Around Room 'Always' Quiet at Night

Hospital Name	City	Rate	Cases
Grundy County Memorial Hospital[11]	Grundy Center	83%	(a)
Orange City Area Health System	Orange City	79%	(a)
Jefferson County Health Center	Fairfield	77%	(a)
Waverly Health Center	Waverly	76%	(a)
Sartori Memorial Hospital	Cedar Falls	75%	300+
Clarinda Regional Health Center	Clarinda	73%	(a)
Osceola Community Hospital	Sibley	72%	(a)
Greater Regional Medical Center	Creston	71%	(a)
Pella Regional Health Center	Pella	71%	300+
Floyd County Memorial Hospital	Charles City	70%	(a)
Grinnell Regional Medical Center	Grinnell	70%	300+
St Anthony Reg Hosp & Nursing Home	Carroll	70%	(a)
Iowa Specialty Hospital - Clarion	Clarion	69%	300+
Crawford County Memorial Hospital	Denison	68%	(a)
Floyd Valley Hospital	Le Mars	68%	(a)
Spencer Municipal Hospital	Spencer	68%	300+
Trinity Bettendorf	Bettendorf	68%	300+
Washington County Hospital & Clinics	Washington	68%	(a)

Cass County Memorial Hospital	Atlantic	66%	(a)
Mercy Medical Center - Cedar Rapids	Cedar Rapids	66%	300+
Iowa Methodist Medical Center	Des Moines	65%	300+
Keokuk Area Hospital	Keokuk	65%	(a)
Avera Holy Family Hospital	Estherville	64%	(a)
Winneshiek Medical Center	Decorah	64%	(a)
Alegent Health Mercy Hospital	Council Bluffs	63%	300+
Great River Medical Center	West Burlington	63%	300+
Stewart Memorial Community Hospital	Lake City	63%	(a)
Covenant Medical Center[11]	Waterloo	62%	300+
Myrtue Medical Center	Harlan	62%	(a)
Saint Luke's Hospital	Cedar Rapids	62%	300+
Sioux Ctr Comm Hosp & Health Ctr	Sioux Center	62%	(a)
Burgess Health Center	Onawa	61%	(a)
Mercy Medical Center - Dubuque	Dubuque	61%	300+
Van Diest Medical Center	Webster City	61%	(a)
Finley Hospital	Dubuque	60%	300+
Lakes Regional Healthcare	Spirit Lake	60%	(a)
Montgomery County Memorial Hospital	Red Oak	60%	(a)
Ottumwa Regional Health Center	Ottumwa	60%	300+
Skiff Medical Center	Newton	60%	300+
Boone County Hospital	Boone	59%	(a)
Iowa Lutheran Hospital	Des Moines	59%	300+
Marshalltown Medical & Surgical Center	Marshalltown	59%	300+
Mercy Medical Center - Clinton	Clinton	59%	300+
Broadlawns Medical Center	Des Moines	58%	300+
Fort Madison Community Hospital	Fort Madison	58%	300+
Trinity Regional Medical Center	Fort Dodge	58%	300+
Allen Hospital	Waterloo	57%	300+
Mary Greeley Medical Center	Ames	57%	300+
Mercy Medical Center - Des Moines	Des Moines	57%	300+
Knoxville Hospital & Clinics	Knoxville	56%	(a)
Mercy Hospital	Iowa City	56%	300+
Sanford Sheldon Medical Center	Sheldon	56%	(a)
Shenandoah Medical Center	Shenandoah	56%	(a)
Mercy Medical Center - Sioux City	Sioux City	55%	300+
Methodist Jennie Edmundson	Council Bluffs	55%	300+
Mahaska Health Partnership	Oskaloosa	54%	(a)
Saint Luke's Regional Medical Center	Sioux City	54%	300+
Mercy Medical Center - North Iowa	Mason City	53%	300+
Trinity Muscatine	Muscatine	51%	300+
Genesis Medical Center - Davenport	Davenport	49%	300+
Mercy Medical Center - Centerville	Centerville	48%	(a)
University of Iowa Hospital & Clinics	Iowa City	45%	300+

Doctors 'Always' Communicated Well

Hospital Name	City	Rate	Cases
Greater Regional Medical Center	Creston	92%	(a)
Orange City Area Health System	Orange City	91%	(a)
Pella Regional Health Center	Pella	91%	300+
Floyd County Memorial Hospital	Charles City	90%	(a)
Mahaska Health Partnership	Oskaloosa	90%	(a)
Burgess Health Center	Onawa	89%	(a)
Knoxville Hospital & Clinics	Knoxville	89%	(a)
Montgomery County Memorial Hospital	Red Oak	89%	(a)
Avera Holy Family Hospital	Estherville	88%	(a)
Mercy Hospital	Iowa City	88%	300+
Myrtue Medical Center	Harlan	88%	(a)
Stewart Memorial Community Hospital	Lake City	88%	(a)
Boone County Hospital	Boone	87%	(a)
Floyd Valley Hospital	Le Mars	87%	(a)
Grundy County Memorial Hospital[11]	Grundy Center	87%	(a)
Iowa Specialty Hospital - Clarion	Clarion	87%	300+
Methodist Jennie Edmundson	Council Bluffs	87%	300+
Cass County Memorial Hospital	Atlantic	86%	(a)
Jefferson County Health Center	Fairfield	86%	(a)
St Anthony Reg Hosp & Nursing Home	Carroll	86%	(a)
Crawford County Memorial Hospital	Denison	85%	(a)
Keokuk Area Hospital	Keokuk	85%	(a)
Sioux Ctr Comm Hosp & Health Ctr	Sioux Center	85%	(a)
Skiff Medical Center	Newton	85%	300+
Winneshiek Medical Center	Decorah	85%	(a)
Fort Madison Community Hospital	Fort Madison	84%	300+
Grinnell Regional Medical Center	Grinnell	84%	300+
Lakes Regional Healthcare	Spirit Lake	84%	(a)
Mary Greeley Medical Center	Ames	84%	300+
Waverly Health Center	Waverly	84%	(a)
Clarinda Regional Health Center	Clarinda	83%	(a)
Mercy Medical Center - Centerville	Centerville	83%	(a)
Osceola Community Hospital	Sibley	83%	(a)
Spencer Municipal Hospital	Spencer	83%	300+
Trinity Muscatine	Muscatine	83%	300+
Finley Hospital	Dubuque	82%	300+
Mercy Medical Center - Dubuque	Dubuque	82%	300+
Sartori Memorial Hospital	Cedar Falls	82%	300+
Shenandoah Medical Center	Shenandoah	82%	(a)
Sanford Sheldon Medical Center	Sheldon	81%	(a)
Washington County Hospital & Clinics	Washington	81%	(a)
Great River Medical Center	West Burlington	80%	300+
Iowa Methodist Medical Center	Des Moines	80%	300+
Mercy Medical Center - Cedar Rapids	Cedar Rapids	80%	300+

NOTE: Hospital profiles are in alphabetical order by state, then city, then hospital within the city; Rankings exclude hospitals with less than 25 cases except for patient surveys which excludes hospitals with less than 100 cases; (a) 100-299 cases; (1) The number of cases/patients is too few to report; (2) Data submitted were based on a sample of cases/patients; (3) Results are based on a shorter time period than required; (4) Data suppressed by CMS for one or more quarters; (5) Results are not available for this reporting period; (6) Fewer than 100 patients completed the HCAHPS survey; (7) No cases met the criteria for this measure; (8) The lower limit of the confidence interval cannot be calculated if the number of observed infections equals zero; (9) No data are available from the state/territory for this reporting period; (10) The scores shown reflect fewer than 50 completed surveys; (11) There were discrepancies in the data collection process; (12) This measure does not apply to this hospital for this reporting period; (13) Results cannot be calculated for this reporting period; (14) The results for this state are combined with nearby states to protect confidentiality; Please refer to the User's Guide for a full explanation of data.

Trinity Regional Medical Center	Fort Dodge	80%	300+
Van Diest Medical Center	Webster City	80%	(a)
Alegent Health Mercy Hospital	Council Bluffs	79%	300+
Broadlawns Medical Center	Des Moines	79%	300+
Covenant Medical Center[11]	Waterloo	79%	300+
Mercy Medical Center - Clinton	Clinton	79%	300+
Genesis Medical Center - Davenport	Davenport	78%	300+
Marshalltown Medical & Surgical Center	Marshalltown	78%	300+
Mercy Medical Center - Sioux City	Sioux City	78%	300+
Saint Luke's Hospital	Cedar Rapids	78%	300+
Trinity Bettendorf	Bettendorf	78%	300+
Iowa Lutheran Hospital	Des Moines	77%	300+
Mercy Medical Center - North Iowa	Mason City	77%	300+
Saint Luke's Regional Medical Center	Sioux City	77%	300+
University of Iowa Hospital & Clinics	Iowa City	77%	300+
Mercy Medical Center - Des Moines	Des Moines	76%	300+
Allen Hospital	Waterloo	75%	300+
Ottumwa Regional Health Center	Ottumwa	73%	300+

Home Recovery Information Given

Hospital Name	City	Rate	Cases
Avera Holy Family Hospital	Estherville	94%	(a)
Myrtue Medical Center	Harlan	93%	(a)
Montgomery County Memorial Hospital	Red Oak	92%	(a)
Allen Hospital	Waterloo	91%	300+
Cass County Memorial Hospital	Atlantic	91%	(a)
Finley Hospital	Dubuque	91%	300+
Grundy County Memorial Hospital[11]	Grundy Center	91%	(a)
Mercy Medical Center - Dubuque	Dubuque	91%	300+
Methodist Jennie Edmundson	Council Bluffs	91%	300+
Pella Regional Health Center	Pella	91%	300+
Trinity Regional Medical Center	Fort Dodge	91%	300+
Waverly Health Center	Waverly	91%	(a)
Burgess Health Center	Onawa	90%	(a)
Fort Madison Community Hospital	Fort Madison	90%	300+
Grinnell Regional Medical Center	Grinnell	90%	300+
Lakes Regional Healthcare	Spirit Lake	90%	(a)
Mercy Medical Center - North Iowa	Mason City	90%	300+
Sioux Ctr Comm Hosp & Health Ctr	Sioux Center	90%	(a)
Spencer Municipal Hospital	Spencer	90%	300+
Alegent Health Mercy Hospital	Council Bluffs	89%	300+
Boone County Hospital	Boone	89%	(a)
Floyd Valley Hospital	Le Mars	89%	(a)
Iowa Lutheran Hospital	Des Moines	89%	300+
Mary Greeley Medical Center	Ames	89%	300+
Mercy Hospital	Iowa City	89%	300+
Saint Luke's Hospital	Cedar Rapids	89%	300+
University of Iowa Hospital & Clinics	Iowa City	89%	300+
Floyd County Memorial Hospital	Charles City	88%	(a)
Iowa Specialty Hospital - Clarion	Clarion	88%	300+
Saint Luke's Regional Medical Center	Sioux City	88%	300+
Stewart Memorial Community Hospital	Lake City	88%	(a)
Winneshiek Medical Center	Decorah	88%	(a)
Marshalltown Medical & Surgical Center	Marshalltown	87%	300+
Mercy Medical Center - Clinton	Clinton	87%	300+
Mercy Medical Center - Des Moines	Des Moines	87%	300+
Mercy Medical Center - Sioux City	Sioux City	87%	300+
Orange City Area Health System	Orange City	87%	(a)
St Anthony Reg Hosp & Nursing Home	Carroll	87%	(a)
Skiff Medical Center	Newton	87%	300+
Trinity Bettendorf	Bettendorf	87%	300+
Covenant Medical Center[11]	Waterloo	86%	300+
Great River Medical Center	West Burlington	86%	300+
Iowa Methodist Medical Center	Des Moines	86%	300+
Jefferson County Health Center	Fairfield	86%	(a)
Mercy Medical Center - Cedar Rapids	Cedar Rapids	86%	300+
Washington County Hospital & Clinics	Washington	86%	(a)
Crawford County Memorial Hospital	Denison	85%	(a)
Genesis Medical Center - Davenport	Davenport	85%	300+
Keokuk Area Hospital	Keokuk	85%	(a)
Mahaska Health Partnership	Oskaloosa	85%	(a)
Trinity Muscatine	Muscatine	85%	300+
Clarinda Regional Health Center	Clarinda	84%	(a)
Knoxville Hospital & Clinics	Knoxville	84%	(a)
Osceola Community Hospital	Sibley	84%	(a)
Shenandoah Medical Center	Shenandoah	84%	(a)
Greater Regional Medical Center	Creston	83%	(a)
Sanford Sheldon Medical Center	Sheldon	83%	(a)
Mercy Medical Center - Centerville	Centerville	82%	(a)
Sartori Memorial Hospital	Cedar Falls	81%	300+
Broadlawns Medical Center	Des Moines	80%	300+
Ottumwa Regional Health Center	Ottumwa	78%	300+
Van Diest Medical Center	Webster City	76%	(a)

Hospital Given 9 or 10 on 10 Point Scale

Hospital Name	City	Rate	Cases
Orange City Area Health System	Orange City	92%	(a)
Grundy County Memorial Hospital[11]	Grundy Center	89%	(a)
Pella Regional Health Center	Pella	88%	300+
Jefferson County Health Center	Fairfield	86%	(a)
Burgess Health Center	Onawa	85%	(a)
Iowa Specialty Hospital - Clarion	Clarion	84%	300+
Stewart Memorial Community Hospital	Lake City	84%	(a)
Floyd County Memorial Hospital	Charles City	83%	(a)
Waverly Health Center	Waverly	83%	(a)
Sioux Ctr Comm Hosp & Health Ctr	Sioux Center	81%	(a)
Mary Greeley Medical Center	Ames	80%	300+
Fort Madison Community Hospital	Fort Madison	79%	300+
Cass County Memorial Hospital	Atlantic	78%	(a)
Crawford County Memorial Hospital	Denison	78%	(a)
Mercy Medical Center - Dubuque	Dubuque	78%	300+
Osceola Community Hospital	Sibley	78%	(a)
Saint Luke's Hospital	Cedar Rapids	78%	300+
Floyd Valley Hospital	Le Mars	77%	(a)
Grinnell Regional Medical Center	Grinnell	77%	300+
Mercy Medical Center - Cedar Rapids	Cedar Rapids	77%	300+
St Anthony Reg Hosp & Nursing Home	Carroll	77%	(a)
Spencer Municipal Hospital	Spencer	77%	300+
Trinity Bettendorf	Bettendorf	77%	300+
Iowa Lutheran Hospital	Des Moines	76%	300+
Myrtue Medical Center	Harlan	76%	(a)
Skiff Medical Center	Newton	76%	300+
Finley Hospital	Dubuque	75%	300+
Greater Regional Medical Center	Creston	75%	(a)
Iowa Methodist Medical Center	Des Moines	75%	300+
Keokuk Area Hospital	Keokuk	75%	(a)
Lakes Regional Healthcare	Spirit Lake	75%	(a)
Montgomery County Memorial Hospital	Red Oak	75%	(a)
Avera Holy Family Hospital	Estherville	74%	(a)
Clarinda Regional Health Center	Clarinda	74%	(a)
Alegent Health Mercy Hospital	Council Bluffs	73%	300+
Methodist Jennie Edmundson	Council Bluffs	73%	300+
University of Iowa Hospital & Clinics	Iowa City	73%	300+
Winneshiek Medical Center	Decorah	73%	(a)
Knoxville Hospital & Clinics	Knoxville	72%	(a)
Mercy Hospital	Iowa City	72%	300+
Sanford Sheldon Medical Center	Sheldon	72%	(a)
Washington County Hospital & Clinics	Washington	72%	(a)
Saint Luke's Regional Medical Center	Sioux City	71%	300+
Trinity Regional Medical Center	Fort Dodge	71%	300+
Boone County Hospital	Boone	70%	(a)
Covenant Medical Center[11]	Waterloo	70%	300+
Genesis Medical Center - Davenport	Davenport	70%	300+
Great River Medical Center	West Burlington	70%	300+
Mercy Medical Center - North Iowa	Mason City	70%	300+
Sartori Memorial Hospital	Cedar Falls	70%	300+
Mercy Medical Center - Clinton	Clinton	69%	300+
Mercy Medical Center - Sioux City	Sioux City	69%	300+
Mahaska Health Partnership	Oskaloosa	68%	(a)
Mercy Medical Center - Des Moines	Des Moines	68%	300+
Marshalltown Medical & Surgical Center	Marshalltown	67%	300+
Allen Hospital	Waterloo	66%	300+
Broadlawns Medical Center	Des Moines	66%	300+
Mercy Medical Center - Centerville	Centerville	66%	(a)
Trinity Muscatine	Muscatine	64%	300+
Shenandoah Medical Center	Shenandoah	62%	(a)
Van Diest Medical Center	Webster City	61%	(a)
Ottumwa Regional Health Center	Ottumwa	47%	300+

Meds 'Always' Explained Before Given

Hospital Name	City	Rate	Cases
Stewart Memorial Community Hospital	Lake City	82%	(a)
Grundy County Memorial Hospital[11]	Grundy Center	80%	(a)
Winneshiek Medical Center	Decorah	73%	(a)
Crawford County Memorial Hospital	Denison	71%	(a)
Floyd County Memorial Hospital	Charles City	71%	(a)
Grinnell Regional Medical Center	Grinnell	71%	300+
Iowa Specialty Hospital - Clarion	Clarion	71%	300+
Keokuk Area Hospital	Keokuk	70%	(a)
Pella Regional Health Center	Pella	70%	300+
Spencer Municipal Hospital	Spencer	70%	300+
Waverly Health Center	Waverly	70%	(a)
Cass County Memorial Hospital	Atlantic	69%	(a)
Mary Greeley Medical Center	Ames	69%	300+
Orange City Area Health System	Orange City	69%	(a)
Burgess Health Center	Onawa	67%	(a)
Greater Regional Medical Center	Creston	67%	(a)
Jefferson County Health Center	Fairfield	67%	(a)
Lakes Regional Healthcare	Spirit Lake	67%	(a)
Methodist Jennie Edmundson	Council Bluffs	67%	300+
Myrtue Medical Center	Harlan	67%	(a)
Knoxville Hospital & Clinics	Knoxville	66%	(a)
Mahaska Health Partnership	Oskaloosa	66%	(a)
Mercy Medical Center - Dubuque	Dubuque	66%	300+
St Anthony Reg Hosp & Nursing Home	Carroll	66%	(a)
Skiff Medical Center	Newton	66%	300+
Finley Hospital	Dubuque	65%	300+
Mercy Hospital	Iowa City	65%	300+
Montgomery County Memorial Hospital	Red Oak	65%	(a)
Saint Luke's Hospital	Cedar Rapids	65%	300+
Alegent Health Mercy Hospital	Council Bluffs	64%	300+
Fort Madison Community Hospital	Fort Madison	64%	300+
Genesis Medical Center - Davenport	Davenport	64%	300+
Great River Medical Center	West Burlington	64%	300+
Sioux Ctr Comm Hosp & Health Ctr	Sioux Center	64%	(a)
Trinity Muscatine	Muscatine	64%	300+
Trinity Regional Medical Center	Fort Dodge	64%	300+
Washington County Hospital & Clinics	Washington	64%	(a)
Avera Holy Family Hospital	Estherville	63%	(a)
Iowa Lutheran Hospital	Des Moines	63%	300+
Mercy Medical Center - Cedar Rapids	Cedar Rapids	63%	300+
Mercy Medical Center - Clinton	Clinton	63%	300+
Mercy Medical Center - Des Moines	Des Moines	63%	300+
Boone County Hospital	Boone	62%	(a)
Marshalltown Medical & Surgical Center	Marshalltown	62%	300+
Osceola Community Hospital	Sibley	62%	(a)
Sanford Sheldon Medical Center	Sheldon	62%	(a)
Sartori Memorial Hospital	Cedar Falls	62%	300+
Shenandoah Medical Center	Shenandoah	62%	(a)
Trinity Bettendorf	Bettendorf	62%	300+
Iowa Methodist Medical Center	Des Moines	61%	300+
Mercy Medical Center - North Iowa	Mason City	61%	300+
Mercy Medical Center - Sioux City	Sioux City	61%	300+
Saint Luke's Regional Medical Center	Sioux City	61%	300+
Clarinda Regional Health Center	Clarinda	60%	(a)
Covenant Medical Center[11]	Waterloo	60%	300+
Floyd Valley Hospital	Le Mars	60%	(a)
Broadlawns Medical Center	Des Moines	59%	300+
University of Iowa Hospital & Clinics	Iowa City	59%	300+
Allen Hospital	Waterloo	57%	300+
Mercy Medical Center - Centerville	Centerville	57%	(a)
Van Diest Medical Center	Webster City	51%	(a)
Ottumwa Regional Health Center	Ottumwa	47%	300+

Nurses 'Always' Communicated Well

Hospital Name	City	Rate	Cases
Grundy County Memorial Hospital[11]	Grundy Center	91%	(a)
Floyd County Memorial Hospital	Charles City	88%	(a)
Jefferson County Health Center	Fairfield	88%	(a)
Orange City Area Health System	Orange City	88%	(a)
Stewart Memorial Community Hospital	Lake City	87%	(a)
Fort Madison Community Hospital	Fort Madison	85%	300+
Waverly Health Center	Waverly	85%	(a)
Cass County Memorial Hospital	Atlantic	84%	(a)
Grinnell Regional Medical Center	Grinnell	84%	300+
Iowa Specialty Hospital - Clarion	Clarion	84%	300+
Burgess Health Center	Onawa	83%	(a)
Floyd Valley Hospital	Le Mars	83%	(a)
Knoxville Hospital & Clinics	Knoxville	83%	(a)
Greater Regional Medical Center	Creston	82%	(a)
Montgomery County Memorial Hospital	Red Oak	82%	(a)
Osceola Community Hospital	Sibley	82%	(a)
Pella Regional Health Center	Pella	82%	300+
St Anthony Reg Hosp & Nursing Home	Carroll	82%	(a)
Sioux Ctr Comm Hosp & Health Ctr	Sioux Center	82%	(a)
Trinity Regional Medical Center	Fort Dodge	82%	300+
Avera Holy Family Hospital	Estherville	81%	(a)
Crawford County Memorial Hospital	Denison	81%	(a)
Keokuk Area Hospital	Keokuk	81%	(a)
Mahaska Health Partnership	Oskaloosa	81%	(a)
Mary Greeley Medical Center	Ames	81%	300+
Mercy Medical Center - Dubuque	Dubuque	81%	300+
Methodist Jennie Edmundson	Council Bluffs	81%	300+
Myrtue Medical Center	Harlan	81%	(a)
Skiff Medical Center	Newton	81%	300+
Spencer Municipal Hospital	Spencer	81%	300+
Trinity Muscatine	Muscatine	81%	300+
Boone County Hospital	Boone	80%	(a)
Clarinda Regional Health Center	Clarinda	80%	(a)
Iowa Lutheran Hospital	Des Moines	80%	300+
Mercy Medical Center - Clinton	Clinton	80%	300+
Washington County Hospital & Clinics	Washington	80%	(a)
Alegent Health Mercy Hospital	Council Bluffs	79%	300+
Finley Hospital	Dubuque	79%	300+
Genesis Medical Center - Davenport	Davenport	79%	300+
Lakes Regional Healthcare	Spirit Lake	79%	(a)
Mercy Hospital	Iowa City	79%	300+
Mercy Medical Center - Cedar Rapids	Cedar Rapids	79%	300+
Saint Luke's Hospital	Cedar Rapids	79%	300+
Sartori Memorial Hospital	Cedar Falls	79%	300+
Winneshiek Medical Center	Decorah	79%	(a)
Great River Medical Center	West Burlington	78%	300+
Marshalltown Medical & Surgical Center	Marshalltown	78%	300+
Sanford Sheldon Medical Center	Sheldon	78%	(a)
Trinity Bettendorf	Bettendorf	78%	300+
Mercy Medical Center - North Iowa	Mason City	77%	300+
University of Iowa Hospital & Clinics	Iowa City	77%	300+
Iowa Methodist Medical Center	Des Moines	76%	300+
Mercy Medical Center - Centerville	Centerville	76%	(a)
Mercy Medical Center - Des Moines	Des Moines	76%	300+
Saint Luke's Regional Medical Center	Sioux City	76%	300+
Broadlawns Medical Center	Des Moines	75%	300+

NOTE: Hospital profiles are in alphabetical order by state, then city, then hospital within the city; Rankings exclude hospitals with less than 25 cases except for patient surveys which excludes hospitals with less than 100 cases; (a) 100-299 cases; (1) The number of cases/patients is too few to report; (2) Data submitted were based on a sample of cases/patients; (3) Results are based on a shorter time period than required; (4) Data suppressed by CMS for one or more quarters; (5) Results are not available for this reporting period; (6) Fewer than 100 patients completed the HCAHPS survey; (7) No cases met the criteria for this measure; (8) The lower limit of the confidence interval cannot be calculated if the number of observed infections equals zero; (9) No data are available from the state/territory for this reporting period; (10) The scores shown reflect fewer than 50 completed surveys; (11) There were discrepancies in the data collection process; (12) This measure does not apply to this hospital for this reporting period; (13) Results cannot be calculated for this reporting period; (14) The results for this state are combined with nearby states to protect confidentiality; Please refer to the User's Guide for a full explanation of data.

Shenandoah Medical Center	Shenandoah	75%	(a)
Allen Hospital	Waterloo	74%	300+
Covenant Medical Center[11]	Waterloo	74%	300+
Mercy Medical Center - Sioux City	Sioux City	74%	300+
Van Diest Medical Center	Webster City	71%	(a)
Ottumwa Regional Health Center	Ottumwa	67%	300+

Pain 'Always' Well Controlled

Hospital Name	City	Rate	Cases
Osceola Community Hospital	Sibley	78%	(a)
Sioux Ctr Comm Hosp & Health Ctr	Sioux Center	78%	(a)
Stewart Memorial Community Hospital	Lake City	78%	(a)
Orange City Area Health System	Orange City	77%	(a)
Floyd County Memorial Hospital	Charles City	76%	(a)
Washington County Hospital & Clinics	Washington	76%	(a)
Waverly Health Center	Waverly	76%	(a)
Crawford County Memorial Hospital	Denison	75%	(a)
Grinnell Regional Medical Center	Grinnell	75%	300+
Grundy County Memorial Hospital[11]	Grundy Center	75%	(a)
Iowa Specialty Hospital - Clarion	Clarion	75%	300+
Jefferson County Health Center	Fairfield	75%	(a)
Burgess Health Center	Onawa	74%	(a)
Cass County Memorial Hospital	Atlantic	74%	(a)
Mary Greeley Medical Center	Ames	74%	300+
Pella Regional Health Center	Pella	74%	300+
Trinity Muscatine	Muscatine	74%	300+
Clarinda Regional Health Center	Clarinda	73%	(a)
Floyd Valley Hospital	Le Mars	73%	(a)
Keokuk Area Hospital	Keokuk	72%	(a)
Methodist Jennie Edmundson	Council Bluffs	72%	300+
St Anthony Reg Hosp & Nursing Home	Carroll	72%	(a)
Alegent Health Mercy Hospital	Council Bluffs	71%	300+
Knoxville Hospital & Clinics	Knoxville	71%	(a)
Mercy Medical Center - Dubuque	Dubuque	71%	300+
Saint Luke's Hospital	Cedar Rapids	71%	300+
Spencer Municipal Hospital	Spencer	71%	300+
Finley Hospital	Dubuque	70%	300+
Fort Madison Community Hospital	Fort Madison	70%	300+
Genesis Medical Center - Davenport	Davenport	70%	300+
Greater Regional Medical Center	Creston	70%	(a)
Lakes Regional Healthcare	Spirit Lake	70%	(a)
Montgomery County Memorial Hospital	Red Oak	70%	(a)
Trinity Regional Medical Center	Fort Dodge	70%	300+
Boone County Hospital	Boone	69%	(a)
Great River Medical Center	West Burlington	69%	300+
Mercy Hospital	Iowa City	69%	300+
Mercy Medical Center - Cedar Rapids	Cedar Rapids	69%	300+
Sanford Sheldon Medical Center	Sheldon	69%	(a)
Iowa Lutheran Hospital	Des Moines	68%	300+
Iowa Methodist Medical Center	Des Moines	68%	300+
Mahaska Health Partnership	Oskaloosa	68%	(a)
Marshalltown Medical & Surgical Center	Marshalltown	68%	300+
Mercy Medical Center - Clinton	Clinton	68%	300+
Saint Luke's Regional Medical Center	Sioux City	68%	300+
Skiff Medical Center	Newton	68%	300+
Trinity Bettendorf	Bettendorf	68%	300+
Van Diest Medical Center	Webster City	68%	(a)
Avera Holy Family Hospital	Estherville	67%	(a)
Broadlawns Medical Center	Des Moines	67%	300+
Covenant Medical Center[11]	Waterloo	67%	300+
Mercy Medical Center - Des Moines	Des Moines	67%	300+
Mercy Medical Center - North Iowa	Mason City	67%	300+
University of Iowa Hospital & Clinics	Iowa City	67%	300+
Winneshiek Medical Center	Decorah	67%	(a)
Mercy Medical Center - Sioux City	Sioux City	66%	300+
Sartori Memorial Hospital	Cedar Falls	65%	300+
Allen Hospital	Waterloo	64%	300+
Mercy Medical Center - Centerville	Centerville	63%	(a)
Myrtue Medical Center	Harlan	60%	(a)
Ottumwa Regional Health Center	Ottumwa	60%	300+
Shenandoah Medical Center	Shenandoah	59%	(a)

Room and Bathroom 'Always' Clean

Hospital Name	City	Rate	Cases
Stewart Memorial Community Hospital	Lake City	98%	(a)
Osceola Community Hospital	Sibley	92%	(a)
Grundy County Memorial Hospital[11]	Grundy Center	91%	(a)
Orange City Area Health System	Orange City	89%	(a)
Floyd County Memorial Hospital	Charles City	87%	(a)
Pella Regional Health Center	Pella	87%	300+
Grinnell Regional Medical Center	Grinnell	86%	300+
Jefferson County Health Center	Fairfield	86%	(a)
Iowa Specialty Hospital - Clarion	Clarion	85%	300+
Keokuk Area Hospital	Keokuk	85%	(a)
Waverly Health Center	Waverly	84%	(a)
Winneshiek Medical Center	Decorah	84%	(a)
Burgess Health Center	Onawa	83%	(a)
Floyd Valley Hospital	Le Mars	83%	(a)
Greater Regional Medical Center	Creston	83%	(a)
Van Diest Medical Center	Webster City	83%	(a)
Crawford County Memorial Hospital	Denison	82%	(a)
Fort Madison Community Hospital	Fort Madison	82%	300+
St Anthony Reg Hosp & Nursing Home	Carroll	82%	(a)
Clarinda Regional Health Center	Clarinda	80%	(a)
Mercy Medical Center - Centerville	Centerville	80%	(a)
Spencer Municipal Hospital	Spencer	80%	300+
Cass County Memorial Hospital	Atlantic	79%	(a)
Trinity Regional Medical Center	Fort Dodge	78%	300+
Mary Greeley Medical Center	Ames	77%	300+
Sioux Ctr Comm Hosp & Health Ctr	Sioux Center	77%	(a)
Trinity Bettendorf	Bettendorf	77%	300+
Washington County Hospital & Clinics	Washington	77%	(a)
Avera Holy Family Hospital	Estherville	76%	(a)
Boone County Hospital	Boone	76%	(a)
Lakes Regional Healthcare	Spirit Lake	76%	(a)
Marshalltown Medical & Surgical Center	Marshalltown	76%	300+
Myrtue Medical Center	Harlan	76%	(a)
Trinity Muscatine	Muscatine	76%	300+
Covenant Medical Center[11]	Waterloo	75%	300+
Genesis Medical Center - Davenport	Davenport	75%	300+
Great River Medical Center	West Burlington	75%	300+
Knoxville Hospital & Clinics	Knoxville	75%	(a)
Mercy Medical Center - Cedar Rapids	Cedar Rapids	75%	300+
Montgomery County Memorial Hospital	Red Oak	75%	(a)
Mercy Medical Center - Dubuque	Dubuque	74%	300+
Saint Luke's Hospital	Cedar Rapids	74%	300+
Alegent Health Mercy Hospital	Council Bluffs	73%	300+
Broadlawns Medical Center	Des Moines	73%	300+
Finley Hospital	Dubuque	73%	300+
Iowa Methodist Medical Center	Des Moines	73%	300+
Mahaska Health Partnership	Oskaloosa	73%	(a)
Iowa Lutheran Hospital	Des Moines	72%	300+
Ottumwa Regional Health Center	Ottumwa	72%	300+
Allen Hospital	Waterloo	71%	300+
Mercy Hospital	Iowa City	71%	300+
Mercy Medical Center - North Iowa	Mason City	71%	300+
Methodist Jennie Edmundson	Council Bluffs	71%	300+
Saint Luke's Regional Medical Center	Sioux City	71%	300+
Mercy Medical Center - Sioux City	Sioux City	70%	300+
Sanford Sheldon Medical Center	Sheldon	70%	(a)
Sartori Memorial Hospital	Cedar Falls	70%	300+
Mercy Medical Center - Clinton	Clinton	69%	300+
Skiff Medical Center	Newton	69%	300+
Mercy Medical Center - Des Moines	Des Moines	67%	300+
University of Iowa Hospital & Clinics	Iowa City	67%	300+
Shenandoah Medical Center	Shenandoah	60%	(a)

Timely Help 'Always' Received

Hospital Name	City	Rate	Cases
Grundy County Memorial Hospital[11]	Grundy Center	84%	(a)
Orange City Area Health System	Orange City	80%	(a)
Knoxville Hospital & Clinics	Knoxville	79%	(a)
Greater Regional Medical Center	Creston	78%	(a)
Cass County Memorial Hospital	Atlantic	77%	(a)
Floyd County Memorial Hospital	Charles City	77%	(a)
Montgomery County Memorial Hospital	Red Oak	77%	(a)
Waverly Health Center	Waverly	76%	(a)
Jefferson County Health Center	Fairfield	75%	(a)
Osceola Community Hospital	Sibley	75%	(a)
Pella Regional Health Center	Pella	75%	300+
Iowa Specialty Hospital - Clarion	Clarion	74%	300+
Sanford Sheldon Medical Center	Sheldon	74%	(a)
Trinity Muscatine	Muscatine	74%	300+
Burgess Health Center	Onawa	73%	(a)
Clarinda Regional Health Center	Clarinda	72%	(a)
Grinnell Regional Medical Center	Grinnell	72%	300+
Spencer Municipal Hospital	Spencer	72%	300+
Keokuk Area Hospital	Keokuk	71%	(a)
St Anthony Reg Hosp & Nursing Home	Carroll	71%	(a)
Stewart Memorial Community Hospital	Lake City	71%	(a)
Trinity Regional Medical Center	Fort Dodge	71%	300+
Washington County Hospital & Clinics	Washington	71%	(a)
Boone County Hospital	Boone	70%	(a)
Sioux Ctr Comm Hosp & Health Ctr	Sioux Center	70%	(a)
Skiff Medical Center	Newton	70%	300+
Avera Holy Family Hospital	Estherville	69%	(a)
Crawford County Memorial Hospital	Denison	69%	(a)
Floyd Valley Hospital	Le Mars	69%	(a)
Saint Luke's Hospital	Cedar Rapids	69%	300+
Trinity Bettendorf	Bettendorf	69%	300+
Fort Madison Community Hospital	Fort Madison	68%	300+
Lakes Regional Healthcare	Spirit Lake	68%	(a)
Mercy Medical Center - Dubuque	Dubuque	68%	300+
Marshalltown Medical & Surgical Center	Marshalltown	67%	300+
Finley Hospital	Dubuque	66%	300+
Genesis Medical Center - Davenport	Davenport	66%	300+
Mahaska Health Partnership	Oskaloosa	66%	(a)
Winneshiek Medical Center	Decorah	66%	(a)
Great River Medical Center	West Burlington	65%	300+
Mercy Hospital	Iowa City	65%	300+
Mercy Medical Center - North Iowa	Mason City	65%	300+
Methodist Jennie Edmundson	Council Bluffs	65%	300+
Mercy Medical Center - Clinton	Clinton	64%	300+
Iowa Lutheran Hospital	Des Moines	63%	300+
Mary Greeley Medical Center	Ames	63%	300+
Saint Luke's Regional Medical Center	Sioux City	63%	300+
Covenant Medical Center[11]	Waterloo	62%	300+
Iowa Methodist Medical Center	Des Moines	62%	300+
Alegent Health Mercy Hospital	Council Bluffs	61%	300+
Myrtue Medical Center	Harlan	61%	(a)
Broadlawns Medical Center	Des Moines	60%	300+
Mercy Medical Center - Cedar Rapids	Cedar Rapids	60%	300+
Mercy Medical Center - Sioux City	Sioux City	60%	300+
Shenandoah Medical Center	Shenandoah	60%	(a)
University of Iowa Hospital & Clinics	Iowa City	58%	300+
Allen Hospital	Waterloo	57%	300+
Mercy Medical Center - Centerville	Centerville	57%	(a)
Mercy Medical Center - Des Moines	Des Moines	55%	300+
Ottumwa Regional Health Center	Ottumwa	54%	300+
Sartori Memorial Hospital	Cedar Falls	54%	300+
Van Diest Medical Center	Webster City	53%	(a)

Would Definitely Recommend Hospital

Hospital Name	City	Rate	Cases
Orange City Area Health System	Orange City	92%	(a)
Grundy County Memorial Hospital[11]	Grundy Center	87%	(a)
Stewart Memorial Community Hospital	Lake City	86%	(a)
Pella Regional Health Center	Pella	85%	300+
Jefferson County Health Center	Fairfield	84%	(a)
Sioux Ctr Comm Hosp & Health Ctr	Sioux Center	83%	(a)
Burgess Health Center	Onawa	82%	(a)
Iowa Specialty Hospital - Clarion	Clarion	82%	300+
Mary Greeley Medical Center	Ames	82%	300+
Floyd County Memorial Hospital	Charles City	81%	(a)
Waverly Health Center	Waverly	81%	(a)
Iowa Methodist Medical Center	Des Moines	80%	300+
Mercy Medical Center - Cedar Rapids	Cedar Rapids	80%	300+
Fort Madison Community Hospital	Fort Madison	79%	300+
Mercy Medical Center - Dubuque	Dubuque	79%	300+
St Anthony Reg Hosp & Nursing Home	Carroll	79%	(a)
Saint Luke's Hospital	Cedar Rapids	79%	300+
Trinity Bettendorf	Bettendorf	79%	300+
Finley Hospital	Dubuque	78%	300+
Iowa Lutheran Hospital	Des Moines	78%	300+
Mercy Hospital	Iowa City	78%	300+
Floyd Valley Hospital	Le Mars	77%	(a)
Saint Luke's Regional Medical Center	Sioux City	77%	300+
Spencer Municipal Hospital	Spencer	77%	300+
University of Iowa Hospital & Clinics	Iowa City	77%	300+
Greater Regional Medical Center	Creston	76%	(a)
Methodist Jennie Edmundson	Council Bluffs	76%	300+
Alegent Health Mercy Hospital	Council Bluffs	75%	300+
Osceola Community Hospital	Sibley	75%	(a)
Winneshiek Medical Center	Decorah	75%	(a)
Cass County Memorial Hospital	Atlantic	74%	(a)
Myrtue Medical Center	Harlan	74%	(a)
Skiff Medical Center	Newton	74%	300+
Covenant Medical Center[11]	Waterloo	73%	300+
Grinnell Regional Medical Center	Grinnell	73%	300+
Knoxville Hospital & Clinics	Knoxville	73%	(a)
Montgomery County Memorial Hospital	Red Oak	73%	(a)
Washington County Hospital & Clinics	Washington	73%	(a)
Genesis Medical Center - Davenport	Davenport	72%	300+
Mercy Medical Center - Des Moines	Des Moines	72%	300+
Avera Holy Family Hospital	Estherville	71%	(a)
Boone County Hospital	Boone	71%	(a)
Lakes Regional Healthcare	Spirit Lake	71%	(a)
Mercy Medical Center - Sioux City	Sioux City	71%	300+
Sanford Sheldon Medical Center	Sheldon	71%	(a)
Allen Hospital	Waterloo	70%	300+
Crawford County Memorial Hospital	Denison	69%	(a)
Sartori Memorial Hospital	Cedar Falls	69%	300+
Keokuk Area Hospital	Keokuk	68%	(a)
Mahaska Health Partnership	Oskaloosa	68%	(a)
Great River Medical Center	West Burlington	67%	300+
Mercy Medical Center - North Iowa	Mason City	67%	300+
Trinity Regional Medical Center	Fort Dodge	67%	300+
Clarinda Regional Health Center	Clarinda	66%	(a)
Mercy Medical Center - Clinton	Clinton	64%	300+
Shenandoah Medical Center	Shenandoah	63%	(a)
Broadlawns Medical Center	Des Moines	62%	300+
Trinity Muscatine	Muscatine	61%	300+
Van Diest Medical Center	Webster City	61%	(a)
Marshalltown Medical & Surgical Center	Marshalltown	60%	300+
Mercy Medical Center - Centerville	Centerville	58%	(a)
Ottumwa Regional Health Center	Ottumwa	40%	300+

NOTE: Hospital profiles are in alphabetical order by state, then city, then hospital within the city; Rankings exclude hospitals with less than 25 cases except for patient surveys which excludes hospitals with less than 100 cases; (a) 100-299 cases; (1) The number of cases/patients is too few to report; (2) Data submitted were based on a sample of cases/patients; (3) Results are based on a shorter time period than required; (4) Data suppressed by CMS for one or more quarters; (5) Results are not available for this reporting period; (6) Fewer than 100 patients completed the HCAHPS survey; (7) No cases met the criteria for this measure; (8) The lower limit of the confidence interval cannot be calculated if the number of observed infections equals zero; (9) No data are available from the state/territory for this reporting period; (10) The scores shown reflect fewer than 50 completed surveys; (11) There were discrepancies in the data collection process; (12) This measure does not apply to this hospital for this reporting period; (13) Results cannot be calculated for this reporting period; (14) The results for this state are combined with nearby states to protect confidentiality; Please refer to the User's Guide for a full explanation of data.

Use of Medical Imaging

Cardiac Imaging Stress Test before OP Surgery

Hospital Name	City	Rate	Cases
Iowa Methodist Medical Center	Des Moines	0.0%	49
Skiff Medical Center	Newton	0.9%	116
Knoxville Hospital & Clinics	Knoxville	1.7%	60
Marshalltown Medical & Surgical Center	Marshalltown	1.8%	57
Orange City Area Health System	Orange City	2.6%	76
Greater Regional Medical Center	Creston	2.7%	73
Mitchell County Regional Health	Osage	2.8%	71
Iowa Specialty Hospital - Belmond	Belmond	2.9%	69
Mary Greeley Medical Center	Ames	3.0%	101
Iowa Specialty Hospital - Clarion	Clarion	3.4%	88
Genesis Medical Center - Davenport	Davenport	3.6%	631
Grinnell Regional Medical Center	Grinnell	3.7%	109
Ottumwa Regional Health Center	Ottumwa	3.8%	52
Allen Hospital	Waterloo	4.1%	412
Mercy Hospital	Iowa City	4.2%	96
University of Iowa Hospital & Clinics	Iowa City	4.2%	432
Fort Madison Community Hospital	Fort Madison	4.3%	161
Mercy Medical Center - New Hampton	New Hampton	4.3%	46
Covenant Medical Center	Waterloo	4.4%	472
Alegent Health Mercy Hospital	Council Bluffs	4.6%	346
Mercy Medical Center - Clinton	Clinton	4.7%	106
Mercy Medical Center - Sioux City	Sioux City	4.7%	212
Finley Hospital	Dubuque	4.8%	124
Mercy Medical Center - Cedar Rapids	Cedar Rapids	4.8%	84
Pella Regional Health Center	Pella	4.9%	143
Mercy Medical Center - Des Moines	Des Moines	5.3%	2013
Kossuth Regional Health Center	Algona	5.4%	111
Mercy Medical Center - North Iowa	Mason City	5.4%	928
Boone County Hospital	Boone	6.2%	81
Trinity Muscatine	Muscatine	6.4%	188
Great River Medical Center	West Burlington	7.4%	487
Methodist Jennie Edmundson	Council Bluffs	7.5%	133

Combination Abdominal CT Scan

Hospital Name	City	Rate	Cases
Mercy Hosp of Franciscan Sisters	Oelwein	0.0%	95
Stewart Memorial Community Hospital	Lake City	0.0%	111
Mercy Medical Center - Clinton	Clinton	0.4%	232
Trinity Muscatine	Muscatine	0.7%	278
Trinity Regional Medical Center	Fort Dodge	0.7%	434
Saint Luke's Regional Medical Center	Sioux City	0.8%	240
Dallas County Hospital	Perry	1.2%	85
Genesis Medical Center - Davenport	Davenport	1.2%	1292
Palmer Lutheran Health Center	West Union	1.4%	141
Community Mem Hosp Med Ctr	Sumner	1.5%	66
Genesis Medical Center - Dewitt	Dewitt	1.5%	65
Marshalltown Medical & Surgical Center	Marshalltown	2.2%	224
Mercy Medical Center - Dubuque	Dubuque	2.3%	264
Loring Hospital	Sac City	2.7%	73
St Anthony Reg Hosp & Nursing Home	Carroll	2.7%	293
Allen Hospital	Waterloo	2.9%	977
Grundy County Memorial Hospital	Grundy Center	2.9%	104
Mary Greeley Medical Center	Ames	3.0%	333
Mercy Medical Center - Des Moines	Des Moines	3.0%	1716
Greene County Medical Center	Jefferson	3.2%	62
Covenant Medical Center	Waterloo	3.3%	636
Buchanan County Health Center	Independence	3.4%	146
Skiff Medical Center	Newton	3.5%	226
Sartori Memorial Hospital	Cedar Falls	3.6%	168
Humboldt County Memorial Hospital	Humboldt	3.7%	82
Waverly Health Center	Waverly	3.7%	349
Trinity Bettendorf	Bettendorf	3.8%	293
Van Diest Medical Center	Webster City	3.9%	203
Audubon County Memorial Hospital	Audubon	4.0%	50
Methodist Jennie Edmundson	Council Bluffs	4.1%	540
University of Iowa Hospital & Clinics	Iowa City	4.1%	2163
Jackson County Regional Health Center	Maquoketa	4.3%	92
Marengo Memorial Hospital	Marengo	4.3%	47
Iowa Lutheran Hospital	Des Moines	4.4%	365
Mitchell County Regional Health	Osage	4.6%	130
Montgomery County Memorial Hospital	Red Oak	4.6%	218
Mercy Medical Center - Cedar Rapids	Cedar Rapids	5.0%	1113
Lucas County Health Center	Chariton	5.2%	77
Floyd County Memorial Hospital	Charles City	5.3%	170
Mercy Hospital	Iowa City	5.3%	549
Washington County Hospital & Clinics	Washington	5.3%	131
Keokuk Area Hospital	Keokuk	5.7%	174
Burgess Health Center	Onawa	5.9%	136
Wayne County Hospital	Corydon	6.1%	114
Finley Hospital	Dubuque	6.2%	258
Mercy Medical Center - North Iowa	Mason City	6.2%	1075
Greater Regional Medical Center	Creston	6.4%	281
Jones Regional Medical Center	Anamosa	6.6%	198
Sanford Sheldon Medical Center	Sheldon	6.6%	122
Jefferson County Health Center	Fairfield	6.7%	134
Alegent Health Mercy Hospital	Council Bluffs	7.2%	499
Saint Luke's Hospital	Cedar Rapids	7.2%	725
Regional Medical Center	Manchester	7.3%	287
Mercy Medical Center - New Hampton	New Hampton	7.4%	95
Ringgold County Hospital	Mount Ayr	7.4%	81
Hancock County Health System	Britt	8.0%	88
Crawford County Memorial Hospital	Denison	8.1%	136
Shenandoah Medical Center	Shenandoah	8.2%	255
Guthrie County Hospital	Guthrie Center	9.0%	67
Iowa Methodist Medical Center	Des Moines	9.2%	579
Davis County Hospital	Bloomfield	9.4%	106
Hegg Memorial Health Center	Rock Valley	9.4%	64
Grinnell Regional Medical Center	Grinnell	9.7%	237
Knoxville Hospital & Clinics	Knoxville	10.0%	170
Horn Memorial Hospital	Ida Grove	10.7%	103
Clarinda Regional Health Center	Clarinda	10.9%	175
Kossuth Regional Health Center	Algona	11.2%	125
Avera Holy Family Hospital	Estherville	12.2%	74
Orange City Area Health System	Orange City	14.1%	128
Winneshiek Medical Center	Decorah	14.6%	198
Myrtue Medical Center	Harlan	15.2%	197
Alegent Health Mercy Hospital	Corning	15.3%	131
Lakes Regional Healthcare	Spirit Lake	20.7%	116
Iowa Specialty Hospital - Belmond	Belmond	25.6%	78
Spencer Municipal Hospital	Spencer	26.1%	295
Buena Vista Regional Medical Center	Storm Lake	26.4%	140
Mercy Medical Center - Sioux City	Sioux City	30.1%	491
Pella Regional Health Center	Pella	33.3%	240
Osceola Community Hospital	Sibley	33.9%	59
Van Buren County Hospital	Keosauqua	40.9%	44
Cass County Memorial Hospital	Atlantic	41.3%	184
Ottumwa Regional Health Center	Ottumwa	43.3%	379
Pocahontas Community Hospital	Pocahontas	44.8%	67
Sanford Rock Rapids Medical Center	Rock Rapids	47.9%	48
Great River Medical Center	West Burlington	52.1%	874
Iowa Specialty Hospital - Clarion	Clarion	55.3%	170
Mahaska Health Partnership	Oskaloosa	57.1%	212
Adair County Memorial Hospital	Greenfield	65.2%	66
Fort Madison Community Hospital	Fort Madison	66.7%	249
Boone County Hospital	Boone	68.5%	165
Henry County Health Center	Mount Pleasant	72.4%	192
Monroe County Hospital	Albia	77.3%	88

Combination Brain/Sinus CT Scan

Hospital Name	City	Rate	Cases
Adair County Memorial Hospital	Greenfield	0.0%	77
Baum Harmon Mercy Hospital	Primghar	0.0%	34
Central Community Hospital	Elkader	0.0%	49
Community Mem Hosp Med Ctr	Sumner	0.0%	83
Greene County Medical Center	Jefferson	0.0%	68
Hawarden Community Hospital	Hawarden	0.0%	40
Jones Regional Medical Center	Anamosa	0.0%	174
Keokuk County Health Center	Sigourney	0.0%	42
Manning Regional Healthcare Center	Manning	0.0%	32
Osceola Community Hospital	Sibley	0.0%	44
Sanford Rock Rapids Medical Center	Rock Rapids	0.0%	75
Sioux Ctr Comm Hosp & Health Ctr	Sioux Center	0.0%	52
Van Buren County Hospital	Keosauqua	0.0%	69
Henry County Health Center	Mount Pleasant	0.4%	235
Floyd County Memorial Hospital	Charles City	0.5%	219
Buchanan County Health Center	Independence	0.6%	160
Montgomery County Memorial Hospital	Red Oak	0.6%	175
Spencer Municipal Hospital	Spencer	0.6%	157
Knoxville Hospital & Clinics	Knoxville	0.7%	139
Loring Hospital	Sac City	0.7%	147
Mahaska Health Partnership	Oskaloosa	0.7%	267
Jefferson County Health Center	Fairfield	0.8%	260
Methodist Jennie Edmundson	Council Bluffs	0.8%	380
Skiff Medical Center	Newton	0.8%	236
Mercy Medical Center - Sioux City	Sioux City	0.9%	326
Finley Hospital	Dubuque	1.0%	294
Washington County Hospital & Clinics	Washington	1.0%	194
Clarinda Regional Health Center	Clarinda	1.1%	186
Saint Luke's Hospital	Cedar Rapids	1.1%	750
Genesis Medical Center - Davenport	Davenport	1.2%	1083
Mercy Medical Center - Cedar Rapids	Cedar Rapids	1.6%	878
Trinity Bettendorf	Bettendorf	1.6%	312
Mercy Medical Center - Clinton	Clinton	1.7%	467
University of Iowa Hospital & Clinics	Iowa City	1.7%	653
Mary Greeley Medical Center	Ames	1.8%	450
Covenant Medical Center	Waterloo	1.9%	636
Mercy Medical Center - North Iowa	Mason City	1.9%	680
Mercy Medical Center - Des Moines	Des Moines	2.2%	1291
Iowa Methodist Medical Center	Des Moines	2.3%	782
Great River Medical Center	West Burlington	2.4%	738
Allen Hospital	Waterloo	2.5%	871
Fort Madison Community Hospital	Fort Madison	4.8%	209

Combination Chest CT Scan

Hospital Name	City	Rate	Cases
Alegent Health Mercy Hospital	Council Bluffs	0.0%	229
Allen Hospital	Waterloo	0.0%	604
Buchanan County Health Center	Independence	0.0%	82
Floyd County Memorial Hospital	Charles City	0.0%	56
Guthrie County Hospital	Guthrie Center	0.0%	45
Hancock County Health System	Britt	0.0%	45
Jackson County Regional Health Center	Maquoketa	0.0%	52
Keokuk Area Hospital	Keokuk	0.0%	96
Kossuth Regional Health Center	Algona	0.0%	107
Marshalltown Medical & Surgical Center	Marshalltown	0.0%	117
Mercy Hosp of Franciscan Sisters	Oelwein	0.0%	51
Mitchell County Regional Health	Osage	0.0%	87
Ottumwa Regional Health Center	Ottumwa	0.0%	283
Palmer Lutheran Health Center	West Union	0.0%	91
Pella Regional Health Center	Pella	0.0%	124
Saint Luke's Regional Medical Center	Sioux City	0.0%	71
Sartori Memorial Hospital	Cedar Falls	0.0%	75
Trinity Bettendorf	Bettendorf	0.0%	122
Trinity Muscatine	Muscatine	0.0%	110
Winneshiek Medical Center	Decorah	0.0%	50
Mercy Hospital	Iowa City	0.2%	473
University of Iowa Hospital & Clinics	Iowa City	0.3%	2060
Mercy Medical Center - Dubuque	Dubuque	0.7%	149
Waverly Health Center	Waverly	0.7%	145
Mary Greeley Medical Center	Ames	0.8%	131
Mercy Medical Center - North Iowa	Mason City	0.8%	1138
Skiff Medical Center	Newton	0.8%	130
Covenant Medical Center	Waterloo	0.9%	342
Methodist Jennie Edmundson	Council Bluffs	0.9%	352
Trinity Regional Medical Center	Fort Dodge	1.0%	390
Fort Madison Community Hospital	Fort Madison	1.1%	186
Mercy Medical Center - Sioux City	Sioux City	1.1%	176
Iowa Lutheran Hospital	Des Moines	1.2%	252
Genesis Medical Center - Davenport	Davenport	1.3%	1158
Mercy Medical Center - New Hampton	New Hampton	1.4%	69
Jefferson County Health Center	Fairfield	1.5%	65
St Anthony Reg Hosp & Nursing Home	Carroll	1.5%	197
Mercy Medical Center - Cedar Rapids	Cedar Rapids	1.7%	877
Greater Regional Medical Center	Creston	1.8%	164
Grinnell Regional Medical Center	Grinnell	2.0%	101
Clarinda Regional Health Center	Clarinda	2.3%	88
Saint Luke's Hospital	Cedar Rapids	2.3%	660
Mahaska Health Partnership	Oskaloosa	3.0%	66
Mercy Medical Center - Clinton	Clinton	3.0%	100
Great River Medical Center	West Burlington	3.2%	592
Iowa Methodist Medical Center	Des Moines	4.0%	199
Mercy Medical Center - Des Moines	Des Moines	4.2%	1360
Jones Regional Medical Center	Anamosa	4.5%	112
Regional Medical Center	Manchester	4.5%	156
Montgomery County Memorial Hospital	Red Oak	4.8%	168
Shenandoah Medical Center	Shenandoah	5.2%	211
Boone County Hospital	Boone	5.3%	76
Washington County Hospital & Clinics	Washington	5.3%	57
Van Diest Medical Center	Webster City	5.6%	90
Burgess Health Center	Onawa	6.3%	63
Myrtue Medical Center	Harlan	6.4%	78
Finley Hospital	Dubuque	7.1%	70
Humboldt County Memorial Hospital	Humboldt	7.5%	67
Sanford Sheldon Medical Center	Sheldon	8.7%	69
Henry County Health Center	Mount Pleasant	9.1%	77
Buena Vista Regional Medical Center	Storm Lake	10.1%	69
Knoxville Hospital & Clinics	Knoxville	12.0%	75
Crawford County Memorial Hospital	Denison	15.5%	84
Alegent Health Mercy Hospital	Corning	17.5%	80
Cass County Memorial Hospital	Atlantic	22.4%	147
Spencer Municipal Hospital	Spencer	28.2%	227
Pocahontas Community Hospital	Pocahontas	31.4%	51
Iowa Specialty Hospital - Clarion	Clarion	41.0%	100

Follow-up Mammogram/Ultrasound

A follow-up rate near zero may indicate missed cancer; a rate higher than 14% may mean there is unnecessary follow up.

Hospital Name	City	Rate	Cases
Wayne County Hospital	Corydon	0.5%	203
Avera Holy Family Hospital	Estherville	0.6%	316
Baum Harmon Mercy Hospital	Primghar	1.1%	88
Winneshiek Medical Center	Decorah	1.1%	374
Buena Vista Regional Medical Center	Storm Lake	1.6%	512
Davis County Hospital	Bloomfield	1.6%	192
Mahaska Health Partnership	Oskaloosa	2.1%	525
Monroe County Hospital	Albia	2.4%	211
Van Buren County Hospital	Keosauqua	2.4%	82
Ottumwa Regional Health Center	Ottumwa	2.5%	1021
Ringgold County Hospital	Mount Ayr	2.6%	196
Knoxville Hospital & Clinics	Knoxville	2.9%	278
Alegent Health Mercy Hospital	Corning	3.0%	300
Lucas County Health Center	Chariton	3.1%	229
Keokuk Area Hospital	Keokuk	3.2%	532
Alegent Health Mercy Hospital	Council Bluffs	3.5%	849
Stewart Memorial Community Hospital	Lake City	3.9%	332
Lakes Regional Healthcare	Spirit Lake	4.0%	425
Adair County Memorial Hospital	Greenfield	4.3%	139

NOTE: Hospital profiles are in alphabetical order by state, then city, then hospital within the city; Rankings exclude hospitals with less than 25 cases except for patient surveys which excludes hospitals with less than 100 cases; (a) 100-299 cases; (1) The number of cases/patients is too few to report; (2) Data submitted were based on a sample of cases/patients; (3) Results are based on a shorter time period than required; (4) Data suppressed by CMS for one or more quarters; (5) Results are not available for this reporting period; (6) Fewer than 100 patients completed the HCAHPS survey; (7) No cases met the criteria for this measure; (8) The lower limit of the confidence interval cannot be calculated if the number of observed infections equals zero; (9) No data are available from the state/territory for this reporting period; (10) The scores shown reflect fewer than 50 completed surveys; (11) There were discrepancies in the data collection process; (12) This measure does not apply to this hospital for this reporting period; (13) Results cannot be calculated for this reporting period; (14) The results for this state are combined with nearby states to protect confidentiality; Please refer to the User's Guide for a full explanation of data.

Buchanan County Health Center	Independence	4.4%	251
Burgess Health Center	Onawa	4.5%	312
Hancock County Health System	Britt	4.5%	264
Loring Hospital	Sac City	5.0%	241
Waverly Health Center	Waverly	5.0%	714
St Anthony Reg Hosp & Nursing Home	Carroll	5.1%	448
Clarinda Regional Health Center	Clarinda	5.3%	262
Henry County Health Center	Mount Pleasant	5.4%	425
Manning Regional Healthcare Center	Manning	5.5%	73
Audubon County Memorial Hospital	Audubon	5.6%	142
Regional Medical Center	Manchester	5.6%	534
Mercy Medical Center - New Hampton	New Hampton	5.8%	347
Pella Regional Health Center	Pella	5.8%	844
Trinity Muscatine	Muscatine	5.8%	624
Community Mem Hosp Med Ctr	Sumner	5.9%	101
Jefferson County Health Center	Fairfield	6.0%	348
Dallas County Hospital	Perry	6.1%	181
Myrtue Medical Center	Harlan	6.1%	472
Osceola Community Hospital	Sibley	6.1%	231
Genesis Medical Center - Dewitt	Dewitt	6.2%	259
Mercy Medical Center - Des Moines	Des Moines	6.3%	3436
Skiff Medical Center	Newton	6.3%	685
Jackson County Regional Health Center	Maquoketa	6.6%	425
Finley Hospital	Dubuque	7.0%	215
Mitchell County Regional Health	Osage	7.0%	342
Mercy Medical Center - Sioux City	Sioux City	7.2%	405
Sartori Memorial Hospital	Cedar Falls	7.2%	543
Great River Medical Center	West Burlington	7.3%	1597
Pocahontas Community Hospital	Pocahontas	7.5%	133
Trinity Bettendorf	Bettendorf	7.5%	429
Central Community Hospital	Elkader	7.6%	132
Sanford Sheldon Medical Center	Sheldon	7.6%	353
Spencer Municipal Hospital	Spencer	7.6%	713
Saint Luke's Hospital	Cedar Rapids	7.7%	1769
Floyd County Memorial Hospital	Charles City	7.9%	504
Kossuth Regional Health Center	Algona	7.9%	430
Mercy Hospital	Iowa City	8.1%	1551
Mercy Medical Center - Cedar Rapids	Cedar Rapids	8.1%	2974
Genesis Medical Center - Davenport	Davenport	8.3%	3817
Humboldt County Memorial Hospital	Humboldt	8.3%	242
Mercy Medical Center - North Iowa	Mason City	8.3%	3017
Orange City Area Health System	Orange City	8.4%	431
Washington County Hospital & Clinics	Washington	8.5%	363
Cass County Memorial Hospital	Atlantic	8.8%	434
Grundy County Memorial Hospital	Grundy Center	8.8%	283
George C Grape Community Hospital	Hamburg	8.9%	101
Jones Regional Medical Center	Anamosa	9.1%	274
Montgomery County Memorial Hospital	Red Oak	9.3%	548
Mercy Medical Center - Clinton	Clinton	9.4%	415
Crawford County Memorial Hospital	Denison	9.5%	379
Iowa Lutheran Hospital	Des Moines	10.1%	1095
Sanford Rock Rapids Medical Center	Rock Rapids	10.3%	145
Covenant Medical Center	Waterloo	10.8%	1348
Shenandoah Medical Center	Shenandoah	10.8%	251
Methodist Jennie Edmundson	Council Bluffs	10.9%	1156
Grinnell Regional Medical Center	Grinnell	11.2%	520
Sioux Ctr Comm Hosp & Health Ctr	Sioux Center	11.2%	196
Guthrie County Hospital	Guthrie Center	11.5%	183
Iowa Specialty Hospital - Clarion	Clarion	11.5%	330
Hegg Memorial Health Center	Rock Valley	11.8%	153
University of Iowa Hospital & Clinics	Iowa City	11.9%	1440
Boone County Hospital	Boone	12.0%	450
Greene County Medical Center	Jefferson	12.2%	335
Horn Memorial Hospital	Ida Grove	12.3%	114
Fort Madison Community Hospital	Fort Madison	12.4%	604
Greater Regional Medical Center	Creston	13.5%	527
Allen Hospital	Waterloo	14.1%	2666
Mercy Hosp of Franciscan Sisters	Oelwein	14.4%	201
Mary Greeley Medical Center	Ames	15.4%	272
Hawarden Community Hospital	Hawarden	16.4%	110
Marshalltown Medical & Surgical Center	Marshalltown	17.7%	818
Broadlawns Medical Center	Des Moines	18.3%	164
Iowa Specialty Hospital - Belmond	Belmond	18.6%	113

Lumbar Spine MRI for Low Back Pain

Hospital Name	City	Rate	Cases
St Anthony Reg Hosp & Nursing Home	Carroll	20.5%	73
Lakes Regional Healthcare	Spirit Lake	24.6%	57
Ottumwa Regional Health Center	Ottumwa	25.4%	63
Allen Hospital	Waterloo	27.2%	239
Covenant Medical Center	Waterloo	27.7%	148
Waverly Health Center	Waverly	29.0%	69
Trinity Muscatine	Muscatine	29.1%	55
Mercy Medical Center - Des Moines	Des Moines	29.2%	233
Sartori Memorial Hospital	Cedar Falls	29.2%	89
University of Iowa Hospital & Clinics	Iowa City	30.4%	115
Methodist Jennie Edmundson	Council Bluffs	30.8%	91
Saint Luke's Hospital	Cedar Rapids	31.8%	223
Spencer Municipal Hospital	Spencer	32.1%	53
Finley Hospital	Dubuque	32.9%	146
Mercy Medical Center - Cedar Rapids	Cedar Rapids	33.7%	303
Trinity Regional Medical Center	Fort Dodge	33.7%	101
Genesis Medical Center - Davenport	Davenport	33.9%	274
Skiff Medical Center	Newton	33.9%	56
Fort Madison Community Hospital	Fort Madison	34.7%	72
Great River Medical Center	West Burlington	35.3%	167
Iowa Lutheran Hospital	Des Moines	35.8%	81
Iowa Specialty Hospital - Clarion	Clarion	36.4%	66
Mercy Hospital	Iowa City	38.1%	118
Cass County Memorial Hospital	Atlantic	38.6%	44
Jefferson County Health Center	Fairfield	39.0%	41
Alegent Health Mercy Hospital	Council Bluffs	41.0%	117
Iowa Methodist Medical Center	Des Moines	42.5%	40
Crawford County Memorial Hospital	Denison	44.7%	47
Grinnell Regional Medical Center	Grinnell	46.2%	39
Mercy Medical Center - Sioux City	Sioux City	50.0%	62

NOTE: Hospital profiles are in alphabetical order by state, then city, then hospital within the city; Rankings exclude hospitals with less than 25 cases except for patient surveys which excludes hospitals with less than 100 cases; (a) 100-299 cases; (1) The number of cases/patients is too few to report; (2) Data submitted were based on a sample of cases/patients; (3) Results are based on a shorter time period than required; (4) Data suppressed by CMS for one or more quarters; (5) Results are not available for this reporting period; (6) Fewer than 100 patients completed the HCAHPS survey; (7) No cases met the criteria for this measure; (8) The lower limit of the confidence interval cannot be calculated if the number of observed infections equals zero; (9) No data are available from the state/territory for this reporting period; (10) The scores shown reflect fewer than 50 completed surveys; (11) There were discrepancies in the data collection process; (12) This measure does not apply to this hospital for this reporting period; (13) Results cannot be calculated for this reporting period; (14) The results for this state are combined with nearby states to protect confidentiality; Please refer to the User's Guide for a full explanation of data.

Monroe County Hospital

6580 165th Street
Albia, IA 52531
URL: www.mchalbia.com
Type: Critical Access Hospitals
Ownership: Govt - Hospital Dist/Auth
Phone: 641-932-2134
Fax: 641-932-1671
Emergency Services: Yes
Beds: 46

Key Personnel:
Emergency Room . . . . Jaime Beaumont
Operating Room. . . . . Wanda Campbell, RN
Quality Assurance . . . . Angela Freeman, RN
Chief of Medical Staff . . . . Gerald Itaasll, DO
Radiology. . . . . Jenny Klyn, MD
Infection Control. . . . . Jane Koffman, RN
Ambulatory Care . . . . Brad Leedom
CEO/President. . . . . Greg Paris

Measure	Cases	This Hosp.	State Avg.	U.S. Avg.
Blood Clot Prevention and Treatment				
Anticoagulation Overlap Therapy[5]	-	-	94%	93%
ICU Venous Thromboembolism Prophylaxis[5]	-	-	90%	92%
Incidence of Potentially Preventable VTE[5]	-	-	8%	10%
UFH with Dosages/Platelet Monitoring[5]	-	-	99%	97%
Venous Thromboembolism Prophylaxis[5]	-	-	87%	85%
Warfarin Therapy Discharge Instructions[5]	-	-	77%	75%
Chest Pain/Possible Heart Attack Care				
Aspirin Given Within 24 Hours of Arrival[5]	-	-	97%	96%
Fibrinolytic Meds Within 30 Min. of Arrival[5]	-	-	49%	58%
Average Time to ECG (minutes)[5]	-	-	5	7
Average Time to Transfer (minutes)[5]	-	-	58	60
Children's Asthma Care				
Received Home Management Plan of Care	-	-	-	88%
Received Reliever Medication	-	-	-	100%
Received Systemic Corticosteroids	-	-	-	100%
Emergency Department				
Admittance Decision Time (minutes)[5]	-	-	58	98
Head CT Results Within 45 Min. of Arrival[5]	-	-	55%	57%
Patients Who Left ER Before Being Seen[5]	-	-	1%	2%
Time from ER Arrival to Admit. (minutes)[5]	-	-	202	274
Time from ER Arrival to Discharge (minutes)[5]	-	-	108	134
Time in ER Before Being Evaluated (minutes)[5]	-	-	21	26
Time to Pain Meds for Fractures (minutes)[5]	-	-	46	57
Heart Attack Care				
Aspirin Given at Discharge[5]	-	-	100%	99%
Fibrinolytic Meds Within 30 Min. of Arrival[5]	-	-	-	54%
PCI Within 90 Minutes of Arrival[5]	-	-	94%	96%
Statin Prescribed at Discharge[5]	-	-	98%	98%
Heart Failure Care				
ACE Inhibitor or ARB for LVSD[1,3]	-	-	95%	97%
Discharge Instructions Given[1,3]	-	-	93%	94%
Evaluation of LVS Function[1,3]	-	-	97%	99%
Medicare Spending				
Medicare Spending per Patient (ratio)	-	-	0.91	0.98
Pneumonia Care				
Appropriate Initial Antibiotic Given[1]	-	-	93%	95%
Blood Culture Timing[1]	-	-	98%	98%
Pregnancy and Delivery Care				
Newborn Deliveries Scheduled Early[5]	-	-	4%	6%
Preventive Care				
Immunization for Influenza[5]	-	-	91%	90%
Immunization for Pneumonia[1,3]	-	-	90%	92%
Stroke Care				
Anticoagulation Therapy for Atrial Fibrillation[3,7]	-	-	95%	95%
Antithrombotic Therapy Timing[1,3]	-	-	98%	98%
Assessed for Rehabilitation[1,3]	-	-	97%	97%
Discharged on Antithrombotic Therapy[1,3]	-	-	99%	99%
Discharged on Statin Medication[1,3]	-	-	92%	94%
Thrombolytic Therapy Timing[3,7]	-	-	64%	66%
Venous Thromboembolism Prophylaxis[1,3]	-	-	93%	94%
Written Stroke Educational Materials Given[3,7]	-	-	82%	88%
Surgical Care Improvement Project				
Appropriate Beta Blocker Usage[1]	-	-	98%	98%
Appropriate VTP Within 24 Hours[1]	-	-	98%	98%
Controlled Postoperative Blood Glucose[7]	-	-	96%	97%
Perioperative Temperature Management[1]	-	-	100%	100%
Prophylactic Antibiotic Selection[1]	-	-	99%	99%
Prophylactic Antibiotic Selection (Outpatient)[5]	-	-	98%	98%
Prophylactic Antibiotic Stopped[1]	-	-	98%	98%
Prophylactic Antibiotic Timing[1]	-	-	98%	99%
Prophylactic Antibiotic Timing (Outpatient)[5]	-	-	98%	98%
Urinary Catheter Removal[1]	-	-	97%	97%
Survey of Patients' Hospital Experiences				
Area Around Room 'Always' Quiet at Night[5]	-	-	63%	61%
Doctors 'Always' Communicated Well[5]	-	-	84%	82%
Home Recovery Information Given[5]	-	-	88%	85%
Hospital Given 9 or 10 on 10 Point Scale[5]	-	-	75%	71%
Meds 'Always' Explained Before Given[5]	-	-	66%	64%
Nurses 'Always' Communicated Well[5]	-	-	81%	79%
Pain 'Always' Well Controlled[5]	-	-	71%	71%
Room and Bathroom 'Always' Clean[5]	-	-	79%	73%
Timely Help 'Always' Received[5]	-	-	70%	68%
Would Definitely Recommend Hospital[5]	-	-	74%	71%
Use of Medical Imaging				
Cardiac Imaging Stress Test before Surgery[7]	-	-	4.8%	5.3%
Combination Abdominal CT Scan	88	77.3%	11.5%	10.5%
Combination Brain/Sinus CT Scan[1]	-	-	1.8%	2.7%
Combination Chest CT Scan[1]	-	-	3.5%	2.7%
Follow-up Mammogram/Ultrasound	211	2.4%	7.9%	8.8%
Lumbar Spine MRI for Low Back Pain[1]	-	-	32.2%	37.2%

Kossuth Regional Health Center

1515 South Phillips Street
Algona, IA 50511
URL: www.krhc.com
Type: Critical Access Hospitals
Ownership: Government - Local
Phone: 515-295-2451
Fax: 515-295-7089
Emergency Services: Yes
Beds: 24

Key Personnel:
Chief of Medical Staff . . . . Burt J Bottsen
CEO/President. . . . . Scott Curtis
Infection Control. . . . . Martha Hoffman
Radiology. . . . . Kate Mayer
Anesthesiology. . . . . Joe Miller
Operating Room. . . . . Lori Reding

Measure	Cases	This Hosp.	State Avg.	U.S. Avg.
Blood Clot Prevention and Treatment				
Anticoagulation Overlap Therapy[5]	-	-	94%	93%
ICU Venous Thromboembolism Prophylaxis[5]	-	-	90%	92%
Incidence of Potentially Preventable VTE[5]	-	-	8%	10%
UFH with Dosages/Platelet Monitoring[5]	-	-	99%	97%
Venous Thromboembolism Prophylaxis[5]	-	-	87%	85%
Warfarin Therapy Discharge Instructions[5]	-	-	77%	75%
Chest Pain/Possible Heart Attack Care				
Aspirin Given Within 24 Hours of Arrival[1,3]	-	-	97%	96%
Fibrinolytic Meds Within 30 Min. of Arrival[1,3]	-	-	49%	58%
Average Time to ECG (minutes)[1,3]	-	-	5	7
Average Time to Transfer (minutes)[3,7]	-	-	58	60
Children's Asthma Care				
Received Home Management Plan of Care	-	-	-	88%
Received Reliever Medication	-	-	-	100%
Received Systemic Corticosteroids	-	-	-	100%
Emergency Department				
Admittance Decision Time (minutes)[5]	-	-	58	98
Head CT Results Within 45 Min. of Arrival[5]	-	-	55%	57%
Patients Who Left ER Before Being Seen[5]	-	-	1%	2%
Time from ER Arrival to Admit. (minutes)[5]	-	-	202	274
Time from ER Arrival to Discharge (minutes)[5]	-	-	108	134
Time in ER Before Being Evaluated (minutes)[5]	-	-	21	26
Time to Pain Meds for Fractures (minutes)[5]	-	-	46	57
Heart Attack Care				
Aspirin Given at Discharge[5]	-	-	100%	99%
Fibrinolytic Meds Within 30 Min. of Arrival[5]	-	-	-	54%
PCI Within 90 Minutes of Arrival[5]	-	-	94%	96%
Statin Prescribed at Discharge[5]	-	-	98%	98%
Heart Failure Care				
ACE Inhibitor or ARB for LVSD[1,3]	-	-	95%	97%
Discharge Instructions Given[1,3]	-	-	93%	94%
Evaluation of LVS Function[1,3]	-	-	97%	99%
Medicare Spending				
Medicare Spending per Patient (ratio)	-	-	0.91	0.98
Pneumonia Care				
Appropriate Initial Antibiotic Given[1,3]	-	-	93%	95%
Blood Culture Timing[1,3]	-	-	98%	98%
Pregnancy and Delivery Care				
Newborn Deliveries Scheduled Early[5]	-	-	4%	6%
Preventive Care				
Immunization for Influenza[5]	-	-	91%	90%
Immunization for Pneumonia[5]	-	-	90%	92%
Stroke Care				
Anticoagulation Therapy for Atrial Fibrillation[5]	-	-	95%	95%
Antithrombotic Therapy Timing[5]	-	-	98%	98%
Assessed for Rehabilitation[5]	-	-	97%	97%
Discharged on Antithrombotic Therapy[5]	-	-	99%	99%
Discharged on Statin Medication[5]	-	-	92%	94%
Thrombolytic Therapy Timing[5]	-	-	64%	66%
Venous Thromboembolism Prophylaxis[5]	-	-	93%	94%
Written Stroke Educational Materials Given[5]	-	-	82%	88%
Surgical Care Improvement Project				
Appropriate Beta Blocker Usage[5]	-	-	98%	98%
Appropriate VTP Within 24 Hours[5]	-	-	98%	98%
Controlled Postoperative Blood Glucose[5]	-	-	96%	97%
Perioperative Temperature Management[5]	-	-	100%	100%
Prophylactic Antibiotic Selection[5]	-	-	99%	99%
Prophylactic Antibiotic Selection (Outpatient)[1,3]	-	-	98%	98%
Prophylactic Antibiotic Stopped[5]	-	-	98%	98%
Prophylactic Antibiotic Timing[5]	-	-	98%	99%
Prophylactic Antibiotic Timing (Outpatient)[1,3]	-	-	98%	98%
Urinary Catheter Removal[5]	-	-	97%	97%
Survey of Patients' Hospital Experiences				
Area Around Room 'Always' Quiet at Night[5]	-	-	63%	61%
Doctors 'Always' Communicated Well[5]	-	-	84%	82%
Home Recovery Information Given[5]	-	-	88%	85%
Hospital Given 9 or 10 on 10 Point Scale[5]	-	-	75%	71%
Meds 'Always' Explained Before Given[5]	-	-	66%	64%
Nurses 'Always' Communicated Well[5]	-	-	81%	79%
Pain 'Always' Well Controlled[5]	-	-	71%	71%
Room and Bathroom 'Always' Clean[5]	-	-	79%	73%
Timely Help 'Always' Received[5]	-	-	70%	68%
Would Definitely Recommend Hospital[5]	-	-	74%	71%
Use of Medical Imaging				
Cardiac Imaging Stress Test before Surgery	111	5.4%	4.8%	5.3%
Combination Abdominal CT Scan	125	11.2%	11.5%	10.5%
Combination Brain/Sinus CT Scan[1]	-	-	1.8%	2.7%
Combination Chest CT Scan	107	0.0%	3.5%	2.7%
Follow-up Mammogram/Ultrasound	430	7.9%	7.9%	8.8%
Lumbar Spine MRI for Low Back Pain[1]	-	-	32.2%	37.2%

Mary Greeley Medical Center

1111 Duff Avenue
Ames, IA 50010
E-mail: yourhealth.mgmc@mgmc.com
URL: www.mgmc.org
Type: Acute Care Hospitals
Ownership: Government - Local
Phone: 515-239-2011
Fax: 515-239-2007
Emergency Services: Yes
Beds: 220

Key Personnel:
CEO/President. . . . . Brian Dieter
Infection Control. . . . . Betty Fosse
Quality Assurance . . . . Darla Handsaker
Operating Room. . . . . Christine Holcomb
Emergency Room . . . . Leslie Miller
Chief of Medical Staff . . . . John Paschen, MD
Radiology. . . . . Sue Scoles

Measure	Cases	This Hosp.	State Avg.	U.S. Avg.
Blood Clot Prevention and Treatment				
Anticoagulation Overlap Therapy[2]	73	100%	94%	93%
ICU Venous Thromboembolism Prophylaxis[2]	67	100%	90%	92%
Incidence of Potentially Preventable VTE[2]	14	0%	8%	10%
UFH with Dosages/Platelet Monitoring[1,2]	-	-	99%	97%
Venous Thromboembolism Prophylaxis[2]	347	93%	87%	85%
Warfarin Therapy Discharge Instructions[2]	49	94%	77%	75%
Chest Pain/Possible Heart Attack Care				
Aspirin Given Within 24 Hours of Arrival[1]	-	-	97%	96%
Fibrinolytic Meds Within 30 Min. of Arrival[3,7]	-	-	49%	58%
Average Time to ECG (minutes)[1]	-	-	5	7
Average Time to Transfer (minutes)[1,3]	-	-	58	60

NOTE: Hospital profiles are in alphabetical order by state, then city, then hospital within the city; Rankings exclude hospitals with less than 25 cases except for patient surveys which excludes hospitals with less than 100 cases; (a) 100-299 cases; (1) The number of cases/patients is too few to report; (2) Data submitted were based on a sample of cases/patients; (3) Results are based on a shorter time period than required; (4) Data suppressed by CMS for one or more quarters; (5) Results are not available for this reporting period; (6) Fewer than 100 patients completed the HCAHPS survey; (7) No cases met the criteria for this measure; (8) The lower limit of the confidence interval cannot be calculated if the number of observed infections equals zero; (9) No data are available from the state/territory for this reporting period; (10) The scores shown reflect fewer than 50 completed surveys; (11) There were discrepancies in the data collection process; (12) This measure does not apply to this hospital for this reporting period; (13) Results cannot be calculated for this reporting period; (14) The results for this state are combined with nearby states to protect confidentiality; Please refer to the User's Guide for a full explanation of data.

Measure	Cases	This Hosp.	State Avg.	U.S. Avg.
Children's Asthma Care				
Received Home Management Plan of Care	-	-	-	88%
Received Reliever Medication	-	-	-	100%
Received Systemic Corticosteroids	-	-	-	100%
Emergency Department				
Admittance Decision Time (minutes)[2]	448	51	58	98
Head CT Results Within 45 Min. of Arrival[1]	-	-	55%	57%
Patients Who Left ER Before Being Seen	25,238	0%	1%	2%
Time from ER Arrival to Admit. (minutes)[2]	457	173	202	274
Time from ER Arrival to Discharge (minutes)	368	102	108	134
Time in ER Before Being Evaluated (minutes)	404	15	21	26
Time to Pain Meds for Fractures (minutes)	87	37	46	57
Heart Attack Care				
Aspirin Given at Discharge	153	100%	100%	99%
Fibrinolytic Meds Within 30 Min. of Arrival[7]	-	-	-	54%
PCI Within 90 Minutes of Arrival	23	91%	94%	96%
Statin Prescribed at Discharge	147	100%	98%	98%
Heart Failure Care				
ACE Inhibitor or ARB for LVSD	33	100%	95%	97%
Discharge Instructions Given	127	100%	93%	94%
Evaluation of LVS Function	174	100%	97%	99%
Medicare Spending				
Medicare Spending per Patient (ratio)	-	0.90	0.91	0.98
Pneumonia Care				
Appropriate Initial Antibiotic Given	106	100%	93%	95%
Blood Culture Timing	165	100%	98%	98%
Pregnancy and Delivery Care				
Newborn Deliveries Scheduled Early	113	2%	4%	6%
Preventive Care				
Immunization for Influenza[2]	559	97%	91%	90%
Immunization for Pneumonia[2]	636	95%	90%	92%
Stroke Care				
Anticoagulation Therapy for Atrial Fibrillation	14	100%	95%	95%
Antithrombotic Therapy Timing	63	98%	98%	98%
Assessed for Rehabilitation	78	97%	97%	97%
Discharged on Antithrombotic Therapy	74	100%	99%	99%
Discharged on Statin Medication	60	92%	92%	94%
Thrombolytic Therapy Timing[1]	-	-	64%	66%
Venous Thromboembolism Prophylaxis	75	96%	93%	94%
Written Stroke Educational Materials Given	37	89%	82%	88%
Surgical Care Improvement Project				
Appropriate Beta Blocker Usage	194	100%	98%	98%
Appropriate VTP Within 24 Hours	613	100%	98%	98%
Controlled Postoperative Blood Glucose[7]	-	-	96%	97%
Perioperative Temperature Management	659	100%	100%	100%
Prophylactic Antibiotic Selection	458	100%	99%	99%
Prophylactic Antibiotic Selection (Outpatient)	398	99%	98%	98%
Prophylactic Antibiotic Stopped	450	100%	98%	98%
Prophylactic Antibiotic Timing	458	100%	98%	99%
Prophylactic Antibiotic Timing (Outpatient)	390	100%	98%	98%
Urinary Catheter Removal	119	99%	97%	97%
Survey of Patients' Hospital Experiences				
Area Around Room 'Always' Quiet at Night	300+	57%	63%	61%
Doctors 'Always' Communicated Well	300+	84%	84%	82%
Home Recovery Information Given	300+	89%	88%	85%
Hospital Given 9 or 10 on 10 Point Scale	300+	80%	75%	71%
Meds 'Always' Explained Before Given	300+	69%	66%	64%
Nurses 'Always' Communicated Well	300+	81%	81%	79%
Pain 'Always' Well Controlled	300+	74%	71%	71%
Room and Bathroom 'Always' Clean	300+	77%	79%	73%
Timely Help 'Always' Received	300+	63%	70%	68%
Would Definitely Recommend Hospital	300+	82%	74%	71%
Use of Medical Imaging				
Cardiac Imaging Stress Test before Surgery	101	3.0%	4.8%	5.3%
Combination Abdominal CT Scan	333	3.0%	11.5%	10.5%
Combination Brain/Sinus CT Scan	450	1.8%	1.8%	2.7%
Combination Chest CT Scan	131	0.8%	3.5%	2.7%
Follow-up Mammogram/Ultrasound	272	15.4%	7.9%	8.8%
Lumbar Spine MRI for Low Back Pain[1]	-	-	32.2%	37.2%

Jones Regional Medical Center

1795 Highway 64 East
Anamosa, IA 52205
Phone: 319-462-6131
Fax: 319-462-4689
E-mail: secrisdr@castlukes.com
URL: www.jonesregional.org
Type: Critical Access Hospitals
Emergency Services: Yes
Ownership: Voluntary non-profit - Private
Beds: 25

Key Personnel:
CEO . . . . Eric Briesemeister
Radiology. . . . . Cara Forbes
Quality Assurance . . . . Carla Huber
Emergency Room . . . . M Weston

Measure	Cases	This Hosp.	State Avg.	U.S. Avg.
Blood Clot Prevention and Treatment				
Anticoagulation Overlap Therapy[5]	-	-	94%	93%
ICU Venous Thromboembolism Prophylaxis[5]	-	-	90%	92%
Incidence of Potentially Preventable VTE[5]	-	-	8%	10%
UFH with Dosages/Platelet Monitoring[5]	-	-	99%	97%
Venous Thromboembolism Prophylaxis[5]	-	-	87%	85%
Warfarin Therapy Discharge Instructions[5]	-	-	77%	75%
Chest Pain/Possible Heart Attack Care				
Aspirin Given Within 24 Hours of Arrival[5]	-	-	97%	96%
Fibrinolytic Meds Within 30 Min. of Arrival[5]	-	-	49%	58%
Average Time to ECG (minutes)[5]	-	-	5	7
Average Time to Transfer (minutes)[5]	-	-	58	60
Children's Asthma Care				
Received Home Management Plan of Care	-	-	-	88%
Received Reliever Medication	-	-	-	100%
Received Systemic Corticosteroids	-	-	-	100%
Emergency Department				
Admittance Decision Time (minutes)[5]	-	-	58	98
Head CT Results Within 45 Min. of Arrival[5]	-	-	55%	57%
Patients Who Left ER Before Being Seen[5]	-	-	1%	2%
Time from ER Arrival to Admit. (minutes)[5]	-	-	202	274
Time from ER Arrival to Discharge (minutes)[5]	-	-	108	134
Time in ER Before Being Evaluated (minutes)[5]	-	-	21	26
Time to Pain Meds for Fractures (minutes)[5]	-	-	46	57
Heart Attack Care				
Aspirin Given at Discharge[5]	-	-	100%	99%
Fibrinolytic Meds Within 30 Min. of Arrival[5]	-	-	-	54%
PCI Within 90 Minutes of Arrival[5]	-	-	94%	96%
Statin Prescribed at Discharge[5]	-	-	98%	98%
Heart Failure Care				
ACE Inhibitor or ARB for LVSD[1]	-	-	95%	97%
Discharge Instructions Given	12	100%	93%	94%
Evaluation of LVS Function	21	90%	97%	99%
Medicare Spending				
Medicare Spending per Patient (ratio)	-	-	0.91	0.98
Pneumonia Care				
Appropriate Initial Antibiotic Given	34	79%	93%	95%
Blood Culture Timing	46	87%	98%	98%
Pregnancy and Delivery Care				
Newborn Deliveries Scheduled Early[5]	-	-	4%	6%
Preventive Care				
Immunization for Influenza[5]	-	-	91%	90%
Immunization for Pneumonia[5]	-	-	90%	92%
Stroke Care				
Anticoagulation Therapy for Atrial Fibrillation[5]	-	-	95%	95%
Antithrombotic Therapy Timing[5]	-	-	98%	98%
Assessed for Rehabilitation[5]	-	-	97%	97%
Discharged on Antithrombotic Therapy[5]	-	-	99%	99%
Discharged on Statin Medication[5]	-	-	92%	94%
Thrombolytic Therapy Timing[5]	-	-	64%	66%
Venous Thromboembolism Prophylaxis[5]	-	-	93%	94%
Written Stroke Educational Materials Given[5]	-	-	82%	88%
Surgical Care Improvement Project				
Appropriate Beta Blocker Usage[5]	-	-	98%	98%
Appropriate VTP Within 24 Hours[5]	-	-	98%	98%
Controlled Postoperative Blood Glucose[5]	-	-	96%	97%
Perioperative Temperature Management[5]	-	-	100%	100%
Prophylactic Antibiotic Selection[5]	-	-	99%	99%
Prophylactic Antibiotic Selection (Outpatient)[5]	-	-	98%	98%
Prophylactic Antibiotic Stopped[5]	-	-	98%	98%
Prophylactic Antibiotic Timing[5]	-	-	98%	99%
Prophylactic Antibiotic Timing (Outpatient)[5]	-	-	98%	98%
Urinary Catheter Removal[5]	-	-	97%	97%
Survey of Patients' Hospital Experiences				
Area Around Room 'Always' Quiet at Night[5]	-	-	63%	61%
Doctors 'Always' Communicated Well[5]	-	-	84%	82%
Home Recovery Information Given[5]	-	-	88%	85%
Hospital Given 9 or 10 on 10 Point Scale[5]	-	-	75%	71%
Meds 'Always' Explained Before Given[5]	-	-	66%	64%
Nurses 'Always' Communicated Well[5]	-	-	81%	79%
Pain 'Always' Well Controlled[5]	-	-	71%	71%
Room and Bathroom 'Always' Clean[5]	-	-	79%	73%
Timely Help 'Always' Received[5]	-	-	70%	68%
Would Definitely Recommend Hospital[5]	-	-	74%	71%
Use of Medical Imaging				
Cardiac Imaging Stress Test before Surgery[1]	-	-	4.8%	5.3%
Combination Abdominal CT Scan	198	6.6%	11.5%	10.5%
Combination Brain/Sinus CT Scan	174	0.0%	1.8%	2.7%
Combination Chest CT Scan	112	4.5%	3.5%	2.7%
Follow-up Mammogram/Ultrasound	274	9.1%	7.9%	8.8%
Lumbar Spine MRI for Low Back Pain[1]	-	-	32.2%	37.2%

Cass County Memorial Hospital

1501 East Tenth Street
Atlantic, IA 50022
Phone: 712-243-3250
Type: Critical Access Hospitals
Emergency Services: Yes
Ownership: Government - Local

Key Personnel:
Cardiology . . . . Venkata Alla, M.D.
Radiology. . . . . Jeremy Baum, M.D.
Emergency Room . . . . Patricia Goodemote, M.D.
CEO . . . . Todd Hudspeth
Pulmonology . . . . Jason Mohr, M.D.

Measure	Cases	This Hosp.	State Avg.	U.S. Avg.
Blood Clot Prevention and Treatment				
Anticoagulation Overlap Therapy[5]	-	-	94%	93%
ICU Venous Thromboembolism Prophylaxis[5]	-	-	90%	92%
Incidence of Potentially Preventable VTE[5]	-	-	8%	10%
UFH with Dosages/Platelet Monitoring[5]	-	-	99%	97%
Venous Thromboembolism Prophylaxis[5]	-	-	87%	85%
Warfarin Therapy Discharge Instructions[5]	-	-	77%	75%
Chest Pain/Possible Heart Attack Care				
Aspirin Given Within 24 Hours of Arrival	37	100%	97%	96%
Fibrinolytic Meds Within 30 Min. of Arrival[7]	-	-	49%	58%
Average Time to ECG (minutes)	37	5	5	7
Average Time to Transfer (minutes)[1]	-	-	58	60
Children's Asthma Care				
Received Home Management Plan of Care	-	-	-	88%
Received Reliever Medication	-	-	-	100%
Received Systemic Corticosteroids	-	-	-	100%
Emergency Department				
Admittance Decision Time (minutes)[5]	-	-	58	98
Head CT Results Within 45 Min. of Arrival[1,3]	-	-	55%	57%
Patients Who Left ER Before Being Seen[5]	-	-	1%	2%
Time from ER Arrival to Admit. (minutes)[5]	-	-	202	274
Time from ER Arrival to Discharge (minutes)[5]	-	-	108	134
Time in ER Before Being Evaluated (minutes)[5]	-	-	21	26
Time to Pain Meds for Fractures (minutes)[5]	-	-	46	57
Heart Attack Care				
Aspirin Given at Discharge[3,7]	-	-	100%	99%
Fibrinolytic Meds Within 30 Min. of Arrival[3,7]	-	-	-	54%
PCI Within 90 Minutes of Arrival[3,7]	-	-	94%	96%
Statin Prescribed at Discharge[3,7]	-	-	98%	98%
Heart Failure Care				
ACE Inhibitor or ARB for LVSD[1]	-	-	95%	97%
Discharge Instructions Given[1]	-	-	93%	94%
Evaluation of LVS Function[1]	-	-	97%	99%
Medicare Spending				
Medicare Spending per Patient (ratio)	-	-	0.91	0.98
Pneumonia Care				
Appropriate Initial Antibiotic Given	26	85%	93%	95%
Blood Culture Timing	28	100%	98%	98%
Pregnancy and Delivery Care				

NOTE: Hospital profiles are in alphabetical order by state, then city, then hospital within the city; Rankings exclude hospitals with less than 25 cases except for patient surveys which excludes hospitals with less than 100 cases; (a) 100-299 cases; (1) The number of cases/patients is too few to report; (2) Data submitted were based on a sample of cases/patients; (3) Results are based on a shorter time period than required; (4) Data suppressed by CMS for one or more quarters; (5) Results are not available for this reporting period; (6) Fewer than 100 patients completed the HCAHPS survey; (7) No cases met the criteria for this measure; (8) The lower limit of the confidence interval cannot be calculated if the number of observed infections equals zero; (9) No data are available from the state/territory for this reporting period; (10) The scores shown reflect fewer than 50 completed surveys; (11) There were discrepancies in the data collection process; (12) This measure does not apply to this hospital for this reporting period; (13) Results cannot be calculated for this reporting period; (14) The results for this state are combined with nearby states to protect confidentiality; Please refer to the User's Guide for a full explanation of data.

Measure	Cases	This Hosp.	State Avg.	U.S. Avg.
Newborn Deliveries Scheduled Early[5]	-	-	4%	6%
Preventive Care				
Immunization for Influenza[5]	-	-	91%	90%
Immunization for Pneumonia[5]	-	-	90%	92%
Stroke Care				
Anticoagulation Therapy for Atrial Fibrillation[1,3]	-	-	95%	95%
Antithrombotic Therapy Timing[1,3]	-	-	98%	98%
Assessed for Rehabilitation[1,3]	-	-	97%	97%
Discharged on Antithrombotic Therapy[1,3]	-	-	99%	99%
Discharged on Statin Medication[1,3]	-	-	92%	94%
Thrombolytic Therapy Timing[3,7]	-	-	64%	66%
Venous Thromboembolism Prophylaxis[1,3]	-	-	93%	94%
Written Stroke Educational Materials Given[3,7]	-	-	82%	88%
Surgical Care Improvement Project				
Appropriate Beta Blocker Usage[1]	-	-	98%	98%
Appropriate VTP Within 24 Hours[1]	-	-	98%	98%
Controlled Postoperative Blood Glucose[7]	-	-	96%	97%
Perioperative Temperature Management[1]	-	-	100%	100%
Prophylactic Antibiotic Selection[1]	-	-	99%	99%
Prophylactic Antibiotic Selection (Outpatient)[5]	-	-	98%	98%
Prophylactic Antibiotic Stopped[1]	-	-	98%	98%
Prophylactic Antibiotic Timing[1]	-	-	98%	99%
Prophylactic Antibiotic Timing (Outpatient)[5]	-	-	98%	98%
Urinary Catheter Removal[1]	-	-	97%	97%
Survey of Patients' Hospital Experiences				
Area Around Room 'Always' Quiet at Night	(a)	66%	63%	61%
Doctors 'Always' Communicated Well	(a)	86%	84%	82%
Home Recovery Information Given	(a)	91%	88%	85%
Hospital Given 9 or 10 on 10 Point Scale	(a)	78%	75%	71%
Meds 'Always' Explained Before Given	(a)	69%	66%	64%
Nurses 'Always' Communicated Well	(a)	84%	81%	79%
Pain 'Always' Well Controlled	(a)	74%	71%	71%
Room and Bathroom 'Always' Clean	(a)	79%	79%	73%
Timely Help 'Always' Received	(a)	77%	70%	68%
Would Definitely Recommend Hospital	(a)	74%	74%	71%
Use of Medical Imaging				
Cardiac Imaging Stress Test before Surgery[1]	-	-	4.8%	5.3%
Combination Abdominal CT Scan	184	41.3%	11.5%	10.5%
Combination Brain/Sinus CT Scan[1]	-	-	1.8%	2.7%
Combination Chest CT Scan	147	22.4%	3.5%	2.7%
Follow-up Mammogram/Ultrasound	434	8.8%	7.9%	8.8%
Lumbar Spine MRI for Low Back Pain	44	38.6%	32.2%	37.2%

Audubon County Memorial Hospital

515 Pacific Street
Audubon, IA 50025
Phone: 712-563-2611
Fax: 712-563-5277
E-mail: acmhhosp@netins.net
URL: www.acmhhosp.org
Type: Critical Access Hospitals
Emergency Services: Yes
Ownership: Government - Local
Beds: 25

Key Personnel:

Operating Room. . . . . Ronald Cheney, RN
Quality Assurance . . . . Melissa Christensen
Chief of Medical Staff. . . . . James M Cunningham, DO
Ambulatory Care . . . . Julie Hoffman, RN
Infection Control. . . . . Holly Kjergaard, RN
Anesthesiology. . . . . David Moffitt, CRNA
CEO/President. . . . . Thomas Smith
Emergency Room . . . . Bonnie Tigges, RN

Measure	Cases	This Hosp.	State Avg.	U.S. Avg.
Blood Clot Prevention and Treatment				
Anticoagulation Overlap Therapy[5]	-	-	94%	93%
ICU Venous Thromboembolism Prophylaxis[5]	-	-	90%	92%
Incidence of Potentially Preventable VTE[5]	-	-	8%	10%
UFH with Dosages/Platelet Monitoring[5]	-	-	99%	97%
Venous Thromboembolism Prophylaxis[5]	-	-	87%	85%
Warfarin Therapy Discharge Instructions[5]	-	-	77%	75%
Chest Pain/Possible Heart Attack Care				
Aspirin Given Within 24 Hours of Arrival[3]	11	91%	97%	96%
Fibrinolytic Meds Within 30 Min. of Arrival[1,3]	-	-	49%	58%
Average Time to ECG (minutes)[1,3]	-	-	5	7
Average Time to Transfer (minutes)[1,3]	-	-	58	60
Children's Asthma Care				
Received Home Management Plan of Care	-	-	-	88%
Received Reliever Medication	-	-	-	100%
Received Systemic Corticosteroids	-	-	-	100%
Emergency Department				
Admittance Decision Time (minutes)[5]	-	-	58	98
Head CT Results Within 45 Min. of Arrival[1,3]	-	-	55%	57%
Patients Who Left ER Before Being Seen[5]	-	-	1%	2%
Time from ER Arrival to Admit. (minutes)[5]	-	-	202	274
Time from ER Arrival to Discharge (minutes)[5]	-	-	108	134
Time in ER Before Being Evaluated (minutes)[5]	-	-	21	26
Time to Pain Meds for Fractures (minutes)[5]	-	-	46	57
Heart Attack Care				
Aspirin Given at Discharge[5]	-	-	100%	99%
Fibrinolytic Meds Within 30 Min. of Arrival[5]	-	-	-	54%
PCI Within 90 Minutes of Arrival[5]	-	-	94%	96%
Statin Prescribed at Discharge[5]	-	-	98%	98%
Heart Failure Care				
ACE Inhibitor or ARB for LVSD[3,7]	-	-	95%	97%
Discharge Instructions Given[1,3]	-	-	93%	94%
Evaluation of LVS Function[1,3]	-	-	97%	99%
Medicare Spending				
Medicare Spending per Patient (ratio)	-	-	0.91	0.98
Pneumonia Care				
Appropriate Initial Antibiotic Given[1,3]	-	-	93%	95%
Blood Culture Timing[1,3]	-	-	98%	98%
Pregnancy and Delivery Care				
Newborn Deliveries Scheduled Early[5]	-	-	4%	6%
Preventive Care				
Immunization for Influenza[5]	-	-	91%	90%
Immunization for Pneumonia[5]	-	-	90%	92%
Stroke Care				
Anticoagulation Therapy for Atrial Fibrillation[5]	-	-	95%	95%
Antithrombotic Therapy Timing[5]	-	-	98%	98%
Assessed for Rehabilitation[5]	-	-	97%	97%
Discharged on Antithrombotic Therapy[5]	-	-	99%	99%
Discharged on Statin Medication[5]	-	-	92%	94%
Thrombolytic Therapy Timing[5]	-	-	64%	66%
Venous Thromboembolism Prophylaxis[5]	-	-	93%	94%
Written Stroke Educational Materials Given[5]	-	-	82%	88%
Surgical Care Improvement Project				
Appropriate Beta Blocker Usage[5]	-	-	98%	98%
Appropriate VTP Within 24 Hours[5]	-	-	98%	98%
Controlled Postoperative Blood Glucose[5]	-	-	96%	97%
Perioperative Temperature Management[5]	-	-	100%	100%
Prophylactic Antibiotic Selection[5]	-	-	99%	99%
Prophylactic Antibiotic Selection (Outpatient)[5]	-	-	98%	98%
Prophylactic Antibiotic Stopped[5]	-	-	98%	98%
Prophylactic Antibiotic Timing[5]	-	-	98%	99%
Prophylactic Antibiotic Timing (Outpatient)[5]	-	-	98%	98%
Urinary Catheter Removal[5]	-	-	97%	97%
Survey of Patients' Hospital Experiences				
Area Around Room 'Always' Quiet at Night[10]	<100	47%	63%	61%
Doctors 'Always' Communicated Well[10]	<100	98%	84%	82%
Home Recovery Information Given[10]	<100	94%	88%	85%
Hospital Given 9 or 10 on 10 Point Scale[10]	<100	90%	75%	71%
Meds 'Always' Explained Before Given[10]	<100	89%	66%	64%
Nurses 'Always' Communicated Well[10]	<100	97%	81%	79%
Pain 'Always' Well Controlled[10]	<100	86%	71%	71%
Room and Bathroom 'Always' Clean[10]	<100	99%	79%	73%
Timely Help 'Always' Received[10]	<100	86%	70%	68%
Would Definitely Recommend Hospital[10]	<100	79%	74%	71%
Use of Medical Imaging				
Cardiac Imaging Stress Test before Surgery[1]	-	-	4.8%	5.3%
Combination Abdominal CT Scan	50	4.0%	11.5%	10.5%
Combination Brain/Sinus CT Scan[1]	-	-	1.8%	2.7%
Combination Chest CT Scan[1]	-	-	3.5%	2.7%
Follow-up Mammogram/Ultrasound	142	5.6%	7.9%	8.8%
Lumbar Spine MRI for Low Back Pain[1]	-	-	32.2%	37.2%

Iowa Specialty Hospital - Belmond

403 First Street Se
Belmond, IA 50421
Phone: 641-444-3223
Fax: 641-444-4895
URL: www.belmondmedicalcenter.com
Type: Critical Access Hospitals
Emergency Services: Yes
Ownership: Government - Local
Beds: 22

Key Personnel:

Cardiac Laboratory. . . . . Monica Christensen
Chief of Medical Staff . . . . Lindy C Estwell
CEO/President. . . . . Nancy Gabrielson
Quality Assurance . . . . Denise Hiscocks
Infection Control. . . . . Stacey Ritter
Operating Room. . . . . Stacey Ritter
Ambulatory Care . . . . Janet Rockow

Measure	Cases	This Hosp.	State Avg.	U.S. Avg.
Blood Clot Prevention and Treatment				
Anticoagulation Overlap Therapy[5]	-	-	94%	93%
ICU Venous Thromboembolism Prophylaxis[5]	-	-	90%	92%
Incidence of Potentially Preventable VTE[5]	-	-	8%	10%
UFH with Dosages/Platelet Monitoring[5]	-	-	99%	97%
Venous Thromboembolism Prophylaxis[5]	-	-	87%	85%
Warfarin Therapy Discharge Instructions[5]	-	-	77%	75%
Chest Pain/Possible Heart Attack Care				
Aspirin Given Within 24 Hours of Arrival[1,3]	-	-	97%	96%
Fibrinolytic Meds Within 30 Min. of Arrival[5]	-	-	49%	58%
Average Time to ECG (minutes)[1,3]	-	-	5	7
Average Time to Transfer (minutes)[5]	-	-	58	60
Children's Asthma Care				
Received Home Management Plan of Care	-	-	-	88%
Received Reliever Medication	-	-	-	100%
Received Systemic Corticosteroids	-	-	-	100%
Emergency Department				
Admittance Decision Time (minutes)[5]	-	-	58	98
Head CT Results Within 45 Min. of Arrival[5]	-	-	55%	57%
Patients Who Left ER Before Being Seen[5]	-	-	1%	2%
Time from ER Arrival to Admit. (minutes)[5]	-	-	202	274
Time from ER Arrival to Discharge (minutes)[5]	-	-	108	134
Time in ER Before Being Evaluated (minutes)[5]	-	-	21	26
Time to Pain Meds for Fractures (minutes)[5]	-	-	46	57
Heart Attack Care				
Aspirin Given at Discharge[5]	-	-	100%	99%
Fibrinolytic Meds Within 30 Min. of Arrival[5]	-	-	-	54%
PCI Within 90 Minutes of Arrival[5]	-	-	94%	96%
Statin Prescribed at Discharge[5]	-	-	98%	98%
Heart Failure Care				
ACE Inhibitor or ARB for LVSD[1,3]	-	-	95%	97%
Discharge Instructions Given[1,3]	-	-	93%	94%
Evaluation of LVS Function[1,3]	-	-	97%	99%
Medicare Spending				
Medicare Spending per Patient (ratio)	-	-	0.91	0.98
Pneumonia Care				
Appropriate Initial Antibiotic Given[3,7]	-	-	93%	95%
Blood Culture Timing[1,3]	-	-	98%	98%
Pregnancy and Delivery Care				
Newborn Deliveries Scheduled Early[5]	-	-	4%	6%
Preventive Care				
Immunization for Influenza[5]	-	-	91%	90%
Immunization for Pneumonia[5]	-	-	90%	92%
Stroke Care				
Anticoagulation Therapy for Atrial Fibrillation[5]	-	-	95%	95%
Antithrombotic Therapy Timing[5]	-	-	98%	98%
Assessed for Rehabilitation[5]	-	-	97%	97%
Discharged on Antithrombotic Therapy[5]	-	-	99%	99%
Discharged on Statin Medication[5]	-	-	92%	94%
Thrombolytic Therapy Timing[5]	-	-	64%	66%
Venous Thromboembolism Prophylaxis[5]	-	-	93%	94%
Written Stroke Educational Materials Given[5]	-	-	82%	88%
Surgical Care Improvement Project				
Appropriate Beta Blocker Usage[3,7]	-	-	98%	98%
Appropriate VTP Within 24 Hours[1,3]	-	-	98%	98%
Controlled Postoperative Blood Glucose[3,7]	-	-	96%	97%
Perioperative Temperature Management[1,3]	-	-	100%	100%
Prophylactic Antibiotic Selection[3,7]	-	-	99%	99%
Prophylactic Antibiotic Selection (Outpatient)[5]	-	-	98%	98%

NOTE: Hospital profiles are in alphabetical order by state, then city, then hospital within the city; Rankings exclude hospitals with less than 25 cases except for patient surveys which excludes hospitals with less than 100 cases; (a) 100-299 cases; (1) The number of cases/patients is too few to report; (2) Data submitted were based on a sample of cases/patients; (3) Results are based on a shorter time period than required; (4) Data suppressed by CMS for one or more quarters; (5) Results are not available for this reporting period; (6) Fewer than 100 patients completed the HCAHPS survey; (7) No cases met the criteria for this measure; (8) The lower limit of the confidence interval cannot be calculated if the number of observed infections equals zero; (9) No data are available from the state/territory for this reporting period; (10) The scores shown reflect fewer than 50 completed surveys; (11) There were discrepancies in the data collection process; (12) This measure does not apply to this hospital for this reporting period; (13) Results cannot be calculated for this reporting period; (14) The results for this state are combined with nearby states to protect confidentiality; Please refer to the User's Guide for a full explanation of data.

Measure	Cases	This Hosp.	State Avg.	U.S. Avg.
Prophylactic Antibiotic Stopped[3,7]	-	-	98%	98%
Prophylactic Antibiotic Timing[3,7]	-	-	98%	99%
Prophylactic Antibiotic Timing (Outpatient)[5]	-	-	98%	98%
Urinary Catheter Removal[1,3]	-	-	97%	97%
Survey of Patients' Hospital Experiences				
Area Around Room 'Always' Quiet at Night[6]	<100	85%	63%	61%
Doctors 'Always' Communicated Well[6]	<100	88%	84%	82%
Home Recovery Information Given[6]	<100	81%	88%	85%
Hospital Given 9 or 10 on 10 Point Scale[6]	<100	86%	75%	71%
Meds 'Always' Explained Before Given[6]	<100	68%	66%	64%
Nurses 'Always' Communicated Well[6]	<100	85%	81%	79%
Pain 'Always' Well Controlled[6]	<100	70%	71%	71%
Room and Bathroom 'Always' Clean[6]	<100	91%	79%	73%
Timely Help 'Always' Received[6]	<100	79%	70%	68%
Would Definitely Recommend Hospital[6]	<100	87%	74%	71%
Use of Medical Imaging				
Cardiac Imaging Stress Test before Surgery	69	2.9%	4.8%	5.3%
Combination Abdominal CT Scan	78	25.6%	11.5%	10.5%
Combination Brain/Sinus CT Scan[1]	-	-	1.8%	2.7%
Combination Chest CT Scan[1]	-	-	3.5%	2.7%
Follow-up Mammogram/Ultrasound	113	18.6%	7.9%	8.8%
Lumbar Spine MRI for Low Back Pain[1]	-	-	32.2%	37.2%

Trinity Bettendorf

4500 Utica Ridge Road
Bettendorf, IA 52722
Phone: 563-742-5000
Fax: 563-779-2260
URL: www.trinityqc.com
Type: Acute Care Hospitals
Emergency Services: Yes
Ownership: Voluntary non-profit - Private
Beds: 150

Key Personnel:
Emergency Room .... Julie Anderson-Sudda
Cardiac Laboratory............ Mike Dessert
Patient Relations .... Liza Kline
Radiology............ Kent S Quinn
CEO/President............ Richard A. Seidler
Quality Assurance .... Diana Zogg

Measure	Cases	This Hosp.	State Avg.	U.S. Avg.
Blood Clot Prevention and Treatment				
Anticoagulation Overlap Therapy[2]	31	97%	94%	93%
ICU Venous Thromboembolism Prophylaxis[2]	37	92%	90%	92%
Incidence of Potentially Preventable VTE[2,7]	-	-	8%	10%
UFH with Dosages/Platelet Monitoring[1,2]	-	-	99%	97%
Venous Thromboembolism Prophylaxis[2]	208	93%	87%	85%
Warfarin Therapy Discharge Instructions[2]	29	79%	77%	75%
Chest Pain/Possible Heart Attack Care				
Aspirin Given Within 24 Hours of Arrival[1,3]	-	-	97%	96%
Fibrinolytic Meds Within 30 Min. of Arrival[3,7]	-	-	49%	58%
Average Time to ECG (minutes)[1,3]	-	-	5	7
Average Time to Transfer (minutes)[3,7]	-	-	58	60
Children's Asthma Care				
Received Home Management Plan of Care	-	-	-	88%
Received Reliever Medication	-	-	-	100%
Received Systemic Corticosteroids	-	-	-	100%
Emergency Department				
Admittance Decision Time (minutes)[2]	235	63	58	98
Head CT Results Within 45 Min. of Arrival[1]	-	-	55%	57%
Patients Who Left ER Before Being Seen	20,596	1%	1%	2%
Time from ER Arrival to Admit. (minutes)[2]	239	185	202	274
Time from ER Arrival to Discharge (minutes)	365	120	108	134
Time in ER Before Being Evaluated (minutes)	379	16	21	26
Time to Pain Meds for Fractures (minutes)	90	38	46	57
Heart Attack Care				
Aspirin Given at Discharge	61	98%	100%	99%
Fibrinolytic Meds Within 30 Min. of Arrival[7]	-	-	-	54%
PCI Within 90 Minutes of Arrival	13	100%	94%	96%
Statin Prescribed at Discharge	55	91%	98%	98%
Heart Failure Care				
ACE Inhibitor or ARB for LVSD[2]	15	87%	95%	97%
Discharge Instructions Given[2]	40	95%	93%	94%
Evaluation of LVS Function[2]	57	98%	97%	99%
Medicare Spending				
Medicare Spending per Patient (ratio)	-	0.92	0.91	0.98
Pneumonia Care				
Appropriate Initial Antibiotic Given[2]	79	95%	93%	95%
Blood Culture Timing[2]	118	99%	98%	98%
Pregnancy and Delivery Care				
Newborn Deliveries Scheduled Early[2]	20	0%	4%	6%
Preventive Care				
Immunization for Influenza[2]	339	76%	91%	90%
Immunization for Pneumonia[2]	369	82%	90%	92%
Stroke Care				
Anticoagulation Therapy for Atrial Fibrillation[1,2]	-	-	95%	95%
Antithrombotic Therapy Timing[2]	15	100%	98%	98%
Assessed for Rehabilitation[2]	19	89%	97%	97%
Discharged on Antithrombotic Therapy[2]	18	94%	99%	99%
Discharged on Statin Medication[2]	13	77%	92%	94%
Thrombolytic Therapy Timing[1,2]	-	-	64%	66%
Venous Thromboembolism Prophylaxis[2]	16	88%	93%	94%
Written Stroke Educational Materials Given[2]	14	79%	82%	88%
Surgical Care Improvement Project				
Appropriate Beta Blocker Usage[2]	88	100%	98%	98%
Appropriate VTP Within 24 Hours[2]	156	99%	98%	98%
Controlled Postoperative Blood Glucose[2,7]	-	-	96%	97%
Perioperative Temperature Management[2]	277	100%	100%	100%
Prophylactic Antibiotic Selection[2]	195	99%	99%	99%
Prophylactic Antibiotic Selection (Outpatient)	118	97%	98%	98%
Prophylactic Antibiotic Stopped[2]	192	95%	98%	98%
Prophylactic Antibiotic Timing[2]	195	99%	98%	99%
Prophylactic Antibiotic Timing (Outpatient)	119	98%	98%	98%
Urinary Catheter Removal[2]	63	100%	97%	97%
Survey of Patients' Hospital Experiences				
Area Around Room 'Always' Quiet at Night	300+	68%	63%	61%
Doctors 'Always' Communicated Well	300+	78%	84%	82%
Home Recovery Information Given	300+	87%	88%	85%
Hospital Given 9 or 10 on 10 Point Scale	300+	77%	75%	71%
Meds 'Always' Explained Before Given	300+	62%	66%	64%
Nurses 'Always' Communicated Well	300+	78%	81%	79%
Pain 'Always' Well Controlled	300+	68%	71%	71%
Room and Bathroom 'Always' Clean	300+	77%	79%	73%
Timely Help 'Always' Received	300+	69%	70%	68%
Would Definitely Recommend Hospital	300+	79%	74%	71%
Use of Medical Imaging				
Cardiac Imaging Stress Test before Surgery[1]	-	-	4.8%	5.3%
Combination Abdominal CT Scan	293	3.8%	11.5%	10.5%
Combination Brain/Sinus CT Scan	312	1.6%	1.8%	2.7%
Combination Chest CT Scan	122	0.0%	3.5%	2.7%
Follow-up Mammogram/Ultrasound	429	7.5%	7.9%	8.8%
Lumbar Spine MRI for Low Back Pain[1]	-	-	32.2%	37.2%

Davis County Hospital

509 North Madison Street
Bloomfield, IA 52537
Phone: 641-664-2145
Fax: 641-664-1669
E-mail: webmaster@daviscountyhospital.org
URL: www.daviscountyhospital.org
Type: Critical Access Hospitals
Emergency Services: Yes
Ownership: Govt - Hospital Dist/Auth
Beds: 57

Key Personnel:
Quality Assurance .... Shelly Bassett
CEO/President............ Deborah Herzberg
Infection Control............ Joan Morris
Operating Room............ Jake Settles
Surgery .... Jake Settles, DO
Emergency Room .... Theresa Tuvera
Chief of Medical Staff............ Donald R Wirtanen, DO

Measure	Cases	This Hosp.	State Avg.	U.S. Avg.
Blood Clot Prevention and Treatment				
Anticoagulation Overlap Therapy[5]	-	-	94%	93%
ICU Venous Thromboembolism Prophylaxis[5]	-	-	90%	92%
Incidence of Potentially Preventable VTE[5]	-	-	8%	10%
UFH with Dosages/Platelet Monitoring[5]	-	-	99%	97%
Venous Thromboembolism Prophylaxis[5]	-	-	87%	85%
Warfarin Therapy Discharge Instructions[5]	-	-	77%	75%
Chest Pain/Possible Heart Attack Care				
Aspirin Given Within 24 Hours of Arrival[5]	-	-	97%	96%
Fibrinolytic Meds Within 30 Min. of Arrival[5]	-	-	49%	58%
Average Time to ECG (minutes)[5]	-	-	5	7
Average Time to Transfer (minutes)[5]	-	-	58	60
Children's Asthma Care				
Received Home Management Plan of Care	-	-	-	88%
Received Reliever Medication	-	-	-	100%
Received Systemic Corticosteroids	-	-	-	100%
Emergency Department				
Admittance Decision Time (minutes)[5]	-	-	58	98
Head CT Results Within 45 Min. of Arrival[5]	-	-	55%	57%
Patients Who Left ER Before Being Seen[5]	-	-	1%	2%
Time from ER Arrival to Admit. (minutes)[5]	-	-	202	274
Time from ER Arrival to Discharge (minutes)[5]	-	-	108	134
Time in ER Before Being Evaluated (minutes)[5]	-	-	21	26
Time to Pain Meds for Fractures (minutes)[5]	-	-	46	57
Heart Attack Care				
Aspirin Given at Discharge[5]	-	-	100%	99%
Fibrinolytic Meds Within 30 Min. of Arrival[5]	-	-	-	54%
PCI Within 90 Minutes of Arrival[5]	-	-	94%	96%
Statin Prescribed at Discharge[5]	-	-	98%	98%
Heart Failure Care				
ACE Inhibitor or ARB for LVSD[3,7]	-	-	95%	97%
Discharge Instructions Given[3,7]	-	-	93%	94%
Evaluation of LVS Function[3,7]	-	-	97%	99%
Medicare Spending				
Medicare Spending per Patient (ratio)	-	-	0.91	0.98
Pneumonia Care				
Appropriate Initial Antibiotic Given[1,3]	-	-	93%	95%
Blood Culture Timing[1,3]	-	-	98%	98%
Pregnancy and Delivery Care				
Newborn Deliveries Scheduled Early[5]	-	-	4%	6%
Preventive Care				
Immunization for Influenza[5]	-	-	91%	90%
Immunization for Pneumonia[5]	-	-	90%	92%
Stroke Care				
Anticoagulation Therapy for Atrial Fibrillation[5]	-	-	95%	95%
Antithrombotic Therapy Timing[5]	-	-	98%	98%
Assessed for Rehabilitation[5]	-	-	97%	97%
Discharged on Antithrombotic Therapy[5]	-	-	99%	99%
Discharged on Statin Medication[5]	-	-	92%	94%
Thrombolytic Therapy Timing[5]	-	-	64%	66%
Venous Thromboembolism Prophylaxis[5]	-	-	93%	94%
Written Stroke Educational Materials Given[5]	-	-	82%	88%
Surgical Care Improvement Project				
Appropriate Beta Blocker Usage[5]	-	-	98%	98%
Appropriate VTP Within 24 Hours[5]	-	-	98%	98%
Controlled Postoperative Blood Glucose[5]	-	-	96%	97%
Perioperative Temperature Management[5]	-	-	100%	100%
Prophylactic Antibiotic Selection[5]	-	-	99%	99%
Prophylactic Antibiotic Selection (Outpatient)[5]	-	-	98%	98%
Prophylactic Antibiotic Stopped[5]	-	-	98%	98%
Prophylactic Antibiotic Timing[5]	-	-	98%	99%
Prophylactic Antibiotic Timing (Outpatient)[5]	-	-	98%	98%
Urinary Catheter Removal[5]	-	-	97%	97%
Survey of Patients' Hospital Experiences				
Area Around Room 'Always' Quiet at Night[6]	<100	62%	63%	61%
Doctors 'Always' Communicated Well[6]	<100	80%	84%	82%
Home Recovery Information Given[6]	<100	91%	88%	85%
Hospital Given 9 or 10 on 10 Point Scale[6]	<100	71%	75%	71%
Meds 'Always' Explained Before Given[6]	<100	57%	66%	64%
Nurses 'Always' Communicated Well[6]	<100	74%	81%	79%
Pain 'Always' Well Controlled[6]	<100	61%	71%	71%
Room and Bathroom 'Always' Clean[6]	<100	80%	79%	73%
Timely Help 'Always' Received[6]	<100	75%	70%	68%
Would Definitely Recommend Hospital[6]	<100	69%	74%	71%
Use of Medical Imaging				
Cardiac Imaging Stress Test before Surgery[1]	-	-	4.8%	5.3%
Combination Abdominal CT Scan	106	9.4%	11.5%	10.5%
Combination Brain/Sinus CT Scan[1]	-	-	1.8%	2.7%
Combination Chest CT Scan[1]	-	-	3.5%	2.7%
Follow-up Mammogram/Ultrasound	192	1.6%	7.9%	8.8%
Lumbar Spine MRI for Low Back Pain[1]	-	-	32.2%	37.2%

NOTE: Hospital profiles are in alphabetical order by state, then city, then hospital within the city; Rankings exclude hospitals with less than 25 cases except for patient surveys which excludes hospitals with less than 100 cases; (a) 100-299 cases; (1) The number of cases/patients is too few to report; (2) Data submitted were based on a sample of cases/patients; (3) Results are based on a shorter time period than required; (4) Data suppressed by CMS for one or more quarters; (5) Results are not available for this reporting period; (6) Fewer than 100 patients completed the HCAHPS survey; (7) No cases met the criteria for this measure; (8) The lower limit of the confidence interval cannot be calculated if the number of observed infections equals zero; (9) No data are available from the state/territory for this reporting period; (10) The scores shown reflect fewer than 50 completed surveys; (11) There were discrepancies in the data collection process; (12) This measure does not apply to this hospital for this reporting period; (13) Results cannot be calculated for this reporting period; (14) The results for this state are combined with nearby states to protect confidentiality; Please refer to the User's Guide for a full explanation of data.

Boone County Hospital

1015 Union Street
Boone, IA 50036
Phone: 515-432-3140
Fax: 515-433-8926
E-mail: dibaltimore@boonecountyhospital.com.
URL: www.boonehospital.com

Type: Critical Access Hospitals
Emergency Services: Yes
Ownership: Voluntary non-profit - Other
Beds: 57

Key Personnel:

Chief of Medical Staff.......... Tammy Chance, D.O.
Radiology................... Craig Freeman
Operating Room.............. Laura Krieger
Infection Control............. Karlene Millang
Emergency Room .... Deana Purdy
Patient Relations .... Jackie Reutter
Quality Assurance .... Jackie Reutter
CEO/President............... Joe Smith

Measure	Cases	This Hosp.	State Avg.	U.S. Avg.
Blood Clot Prevention and Treatment				
Anticoagulation Overlap Therapy[5]	-	-	94%	93%
ICU Venous Thromboembolism Prophylaxis[5]	-	-	90%	92%
Incidence of Potentially Preventable VTE[5]	-	-	8%	10%
UFH with Dosages/Platelet Monitoring[5]	-	-	99%	97%
Venous Thromboembolism Prophylaxis[5]	-	-	87%	85%
Warfarin Therapy Discharge Instructions[5]	-	-	77%	75%
Chest Pain/Possible Heart Attack Care				
Aspirin Given Within 24 Hours of Arrival	35	100%	97%	96%
Fibrinolytic Meds Within 30 Min. of Arrival[7]	-	-	49%	58%
Average Time to ECG (minutes)	39	12	5	7
Average Time to Transfer (minutes)[1]	-	-	58	60
Children's Asthma Care				
Received Home Management Plan of Care	-	-	-	88%
Received Reliever Medication	-	-	-	100%
Received Systemic Corticosteroids	-	-	-	100%
Emergency Department				
Admittance Decision Time (minutes)[5]	-	-	58	98
Head CT Results Within 45 Min. of Arrival[1]	-	-	55%	57%
Patients Who Left ER Before Being Seen[5]	-	-	1%	2%
Time from ER Arrival to Admit. (minutes)[5]	-	-	202	274
Time from ER Arrival to Discharge (minutes)	573	86	108	134
Time in ER Before Being Evaluated (minutes)	632	24	21	26
Time to Pain Meds for Fractures (minutes)	45	41	46	57
Heart Attack Care				
Aspirin Given at Discharge[1]	-	-	100%	99%
Fibrinolytic Meds Within 30 Min. of Arrival[7]	-	-	-	54%
PCI Within 90 Minutes of Arrival[7]	-	-	94%	96%
Statin Prescribed at Discharge[1]	-	-	98%	98%
Heart Failure Care				
ACE Inhibitor or ARB for LVSD[1]	-	-	95%	97%
Discharge Instructions Given	33	64%	93%	94%
Evaluation of LVS Function	51	92%	97%	99%
Medicare Spending				
Medicare Spending per Patient (ratio)	-	-	0.91	0.98
Pneumonia Care				
Appropriate Initial Antibiotic Given	33	94%	93%	95%
Blood Culture Timing	56	98%	98%	98%
Pregnancy and Delivery Care				
Newborn Deliveries Scheduled Early[5]	-	-	4%	6%
Preventive Care				
Immunization for Influenza[5]	-	-	91%	90%
Immunization for Pneumonia[5]	-	-	90%	92%
Stroke Care				
Anticoagulation Therapy for Atrial Fibrillation[5]	-	-	95%	95%
Antithrombotic Therapy Timing[5]	-	-	98%	98%
Assessed for Rehabilitation[5]	-	-	97%	97%
Discharged on Antithrombotic Therapy[5]	-	-	99%	99%
Discharged on Statin Medication[5]	-	-	92%	94%
Thrombolytic Therapy Timing[5]	-	-	64%	66%
Venous Thromboembolism Prophylaxis[5]	-	-	93%	94%
Written Stroke Educational Materials Given[5]	-	-	82%	88%
Surgical Care Improvement Project				
Appropriate Beta Blocker Usage	12	92%	98%	98%
Appropriate VTP Within 24 Hours	53	87%	98%	98%
Controlled Postoperative Blood Glucose[7]	-	-	96%	97%
Perioperative Temperature Management	53	98%	100%	100%
Prophylactic Antibiotic Selection	39	100%	99%	99%
Prophylactic Antibiotic Selection (Outpatient)[1,3]	-	-	98%	98%
Prophylactic Antibiotic Stopped	39	100%	98%	98%
Prophylactic Antibiotic Timing	40	85%	98%	99%
Prophylactic Antibiotic Timing (Outpatient)[1,3]	-	-	98%	98%
Urinary Catheter Removal[1]	-	-	97%	97%
Survey of Patients' Hospital Experiences				
Area Around Room 'Always' Quiet at Night	(a)	59%	63%	61%
Doctors 'Always' Communicated Well	(a)	87%	84%	82%
Home Recovery Information Given	(a)	89%	88%	85%
Hospital Given 9 or 10 on 10 Point Scale	(a)	70%	75%	71%
Meds 'Always' Explained Before Given	(a)	62%	66%	64%
Nurses 'Always' Communicated Well	(a)	80%	81%	79%
Pain 'Always' Well Controlled	(a)	69%	71%	71%
Room and Bathroom 'Always' Clean	(a)	76%	79%	73%
Timely Help 'Always' Received	(a)	70%	70%	68%
Would Definitely Recommend Hospital	(a)	71%	74%	71%
Use of Medical Imaging				
Cardiac Imaging Stress Test before Surgery	81	6.2%	4.8%	5.3%
Combination Abdominal CT Scan	165	68.5%	11.5%	10.5%
Combination Brain/Sinus CT Scan[1]	-	-	1.8%	2.7%
Combination Chest CT Scan	76	5.3%	3.5%	2.7%
Follow-up Mammogram/Ultrasound	450	12.0%	7.9%	8.8%
Lumbar Spine MRI for Low Back Pain[1]	-	-	32.2%	37.2%

Hancock County Health System

532 1st Saint Nw
Britt, IA 50423
Phone: 641-843-5000
Fax: 641-843-5100
URL: www.hancockmemhospital.com

Type: Critical Access Hospitals
Emergency Services: Yes
Ownership: Voluntary non-profit - Other
Beds: 25

Key Personnel:

Infection Control.............. Robin Bartlett
Radiology.................... Byron Beasley, MD
Chief of Medical Staff.......... Lyle Fuller, MD
CEO/President............... Vance Jackson
Emergency Room .... Bonnie Wilhite
Operating Room.............. Bonnie Wilhite
Patient Relations .... Andrea Wilson
Quality Assurance .... Laura Zwiefel, DON

Measure	Cases	This Hosp.	State Avg.	U.S. Avg.
Blood Clot Prevention and Treatment				
Anticoagulation Overlap Therapy[5]	-	-	94%	93%
ICU Venous Thromboembolism Prophylaxis[5]	-	-	90%	92%
Incidence of Potentially Preventable VTE[5]	-	-	8%	10%
UFH with Dosages/Platelet Monitoring[5]	-	-	99%	97%
Venous Thromboembolism Prophylaxis[5]	-	-	87%	85%
Warfarin Therapy Discharge Instructions[5]	-	-	77%	75%
Chest Pain/Possible Heart Attack Care				
Aspirin Given Within 24 Hours of Arrival[5]	-	-	97%	96%
Fibrinolytic Meds Within 30 Min. of Arrival[5]	-	-	49%	58%
Average Time to ECG (minutes)[5]	-	-	5	7
Average Time to Transfer (minutes)[5]	-	-	58	60
Children's Asthma Care				
Received Home Management Plan of Care	-	-	-	88%
Received Reliever Medication	-	-	-	100%
Received Systemic Corticosteroids	-	-	-	100%
Emergency Department				
Admittance Decision Time (minutes)[5]	-	-	58	98
Head CT Results Within 45 Min. of Arrival[5]	-	-	55%	57%
Patients Who Left ER Before Being Seen[5]	-	-	1%	2%
Time from ER Arrival to Admit. (minutes)[5]	-	-	202	274
Time from ER Arrival to Discharge (minutes)[5]	-	-	108	134
Time in ER Before Being Evaluated (minutes)[5]	-	-	21	26
Time to Pain Meds for Fractures (minutes)[5]	-	-	46	57
Heart Attack Care				
Aspirin Given at Discharge[5]	-	-	100%	99%
Fibrinolytic Meds Within 30 Min. of Arrival[5]	-	-	-	54%
PCI Within 90 Minutes of Arrival[5]	-	-	94%	96%
Statin Prescribed at Discharge[5]	-	-	98%	98%
Heart Failure Care				
ACE Inhibitor or ARB for LVSD[1]	-	-	95%	97%
Discharge Instructions Given[1]	-	-	93%	94%
Evaluation of LVS Function[1]	-	-	97%	99%
Medicare Spending				
Medicare Spending per Patient (ratio)	-	-	0.91	0.98
Pneumonia Care				
Appropriate Initial Antibiotic Given[1]	-	-	93%	95%
Blood Culture Timing	21	100%	98%	98%
Pregnancy and Delivery Care				
Newborn Deliveries Scheduled Early[5]	-	-	4%	6%
Preventive Care				
Immunization for Influenza[5]	-	-	91%	90%
Immunization for Pneumonia[5]	-	-	90%	92%
Stroke Care				
Anticoagulation Therapy for Atrial Fibrillation[5]	-	-	95%	95%
Antithrombotic Therapy Timing[5]	-	-	98%	98%
Assessed for Rehabilitation[5]	-	-	97%	97%
Discharged on Antithrombotic Therapy[5]	-	-	99%	99%
Discharged on Statin Medication[5]	-	-	92%	94%
Thrombolytic Therapy Timing[5]	-	-	64%	66%
Venous Thromboembolism Prophylaxis[5]	-	-	93%	94%
Written Stroke Educational Materials Given[5]	-	-	82%	88%
Surgical Care Improvement Project				
Appropriate Beta Blocker Usage[5]	-	-	98%	98%
Appropriate VTP Within 24 Hours[5]	-	-	98%	98%
Controlled Postoperative Blood Glucose[5]	-	-	96%	97%
Perioperative Temperature Management[5]	-	-	100%	100%
Prophylactic Antibiotic Selection[5]	-	-	99%	99%
Prophylactic Antibiotic Selection (Outpatient)[5]	-	-	98%	98%
Prophylactic Antibiotic Stopped[5]	-	-	98%	98%
Prophylactic Antibiotic Timing[5]	-	-	98%	99%
Prophylactic Antibiotic Timing (Outpatient)[5]	-	-	98%	98%
Urinary Catheter Removal[5]	-	-	97%	97%
Survey of Patients' Hospital Experiences				
Area Around Room 'Always' Quiet at Night[5]	-	-	63%	61%
Doctors 'Always' Communicated Well[5]	-	-	84%	82%
Home Recovery Information Given[5]	-	-	88%	85%
Hospital Given 9 or 10 on 10 Point Scale[5]	-	-	75%	71%
Meds 'Always' Explained Before Given[5]	-	-	66%	64%
Nurses 'Always' Communicated Well[5]	-	-	81%	79%
Pain 'Always' Well Controlled[5]	-	-	71%	71%
Room and Bathroom 'Always' Clean[5]	-	-	79%	73%
Timely Help 'Always' Received[5]	-	-	70%	68%
Would Definitely Recommend Hospital[5]	-	-	74%	71%
Use of Medical Imaging				
Cardiac Imaging Stress Test before Surgery[1]	-	-	4.8%	5.3%
Combination Abdominal CT Scan	88	8.0%	11.5%	10.5%
Combination Brain/Sinus CT Scan[1]	-	-	1.8%	2.7%
Combination Chest CT Scan	45	0.0%	3.5%	2.7%
Follow-up Mammogram/Ultrasound	264	4.5%	7.9%	8.8%
Lumbar Spine MRI for Low Back Pain[1]	-	-	32.2%	37.2%

Saint Anthony Regional Hospital & Nursing Home

311 South Clark Street
Carroll, IA 51401
Phone: 712-792-3581
Fax: 712-792-2124
URL: www.stanthonyhospital.org

Type: Acute Care Hospitals
Emergency Services: Yes
Ownership: Voluntary non-profit - Church
Beds: 178

Key Personnel:

Pediatrics.................... Karla Cheney, M.D.
Quality Assurance .... Lynda Dorweiler
Operating Room.............. Cindy Erickson
Chief of Medical Staff.......... Lou Ann Lease
Radiology.................... Robert McCleeary
Patient Relations .... Cheri Pheulen
CEO/President............... Gary P Riedmann
Emergency Room .... Sheryll Stolman

Measure	Cases	This Hosp.	State Avg.	U.S. Avg.
Blood Clot Prevention and Treatment				
Anticoagulation Overlap Therapy[2]	11	64%	94%	93%
ICU Venous Thromboembolism Prophylaxis[2]	14	64%	90%	92%
Incidence of Potentially Preventable VTE[2,7]	-	-	8%	10%
UFH with Dosages/Platelet Monitoring[1,2]	-	-	99%	97%
Venous Thromboembolism Prophylaxis[2]	92	43%	87%	85%
Warfarin Therapy Discharge Instructions[2]	11	91%	77%	75%
Chest Pain/Possible Heart Attack Care				
Aspirin Given Within 24 Hours of Arrival	49	98%	97%	96%

NOTE: Hospital profiles are in alphabetical order by state, then city, then hospital within the city; Rankings exclude hospitals with less than 25 cases except for patient surveys which excludes hospitals with less than 100 cases; (a) 100-299 cases; (1) The number of cases/patients is too few to report; (2) Data submitted were based on a sample of cases/patients; (3) Results are based on a shorter time period than required; (4) Data suppressed by CMS for one or more quarters; (5) Results are not available for this reporting period; (6) Fewer than 100 patients completed the HCAHPS survey; (7) No cases met the criteria for this measure; (8) The lower limit of the confidence interval cannot be calculated if the number of observed infections equals zero; (9) No data are available from the state/territory for this reporting period; (10) The scores shown reflect fewer than 50 completed surveys; (11) There were discrepancies in the data collection process; (12) This measure does not apply to this hospital for this reporting period; (13) Results cannot be calculated for this reporting period; (14) The results for this state are combined with nearby states to protect confidentiality; Please refer to the User's Guide for a full explanation of data.

Measure	Cases	This Hosp.	State Avg.	U.S. Avg.
Fibrinolytic Meds Within 30 Min. of Arrival[1]	-	-	49%	58%
Average Time to ECG (minutes)	49	7	5	7
Average Time to Transfer (minutes)[1]	-	-	58	60
Children's Asthma Care				
Received Home Management Plan of Care	-	-	-	88%
Received Reliever Medication	-	-	-	100%
Received Systemic Corticosteroids	-	-	-	100%
Emergency Department				
Admittance Decision Time (minutes)[2]	135	23	58	98
Head CT Results Within 45 Min. of Arrival[1]	-	-	55%	57%
Patients Who Left ER Before Being Seen	6,565	0%	1%	2%
Time from ER Arrival to Admit. (minutes)[2]	140	161	202	274
Time from ER Arrival to Discharge (minutes)	432	87	108	134
Time in ER Before Being Evaluated (minutes)	495	29	21	26
Time to Pain Meds for Fractures (minutes)	35	43	46	57
Heart Attack Care				
Aspirin Given at Discharge[1]	-	-	100%	99%
Fibrinolytic Meds Within 30 Min. of Arrival[7]	-	-	-	54%
PCI Within 90 Minutes of Arrival[7]	-	-	94%	96%
Statin Prescribed at Discharge[1]	-	-	98%	98%
Heart Failure Care				
ACE Inhibitor or ARB for LVSD[1]	-	-	95%	97%
Discharge Instructions Given	23	83%	93%	94%
Evaluation of LVS Function	37	95%	97%	99%
Medicare Spending				
Medicare Spending per Patient (ratio)	-	0.90	0.91	0.98
Pneumonia Care				
Appropriate Initial Antibiotic Given	41	80%	93%	95%
Blood Culture Timing	36	100%	98%	98%
Pregnancy and Delivery Care				
Newborn Deliveries Scheduled Early[2]	34	3%	4%	6%
Preventive Care				
Immunization for Influenza[2]	276	33%	91%	90%
Immunization for Pneumonia[2]	295	64%	90%	92%
Stroke Care				
Anticoagulation Therapy for Atrial Fibrillation[1]	-	-	95%	95%
Antithrombotic Therapy Timing[1]	-	-	98%	98%
Assessed for Rehabilitation	11	100%	97%	97%
Discharged on Antithrombotic Therapy[1]	-	-	99%	99%
Discharged on Statin Medication[1]	-	-	92%	94%
Thrombolytic Therapy Timing[1]	-	-	64%	66%
Venous Thromboembolism Prophylaxis	12	75%	93%	94%
Written Stroke Educational Materials Given[1]	-	-	82%	88%
Surgical Care Improvement Project				
Appropriate Beta Blocker Usage[2]	91	98%	98%	98%
Appropriate VTP Within 24 Hours[2]	238	90%	98%	98%
Controlled Postoperative Blood Glucose[2,7]	-	-	96%	97%
Perioperative Temperature Management[2]	252	99%	100%	100%
Prophylactic Antibiotic Selection[2]	188	99%	99%	99%
Prophylactic Antibiotic Selection (Outpatient)	12	92%	98%	98%
Prophylactic Antibiotic Stopped[2]	187	94%	98%	98%
Prophylactic Antibiotic Timing[2]	188	97%	98%	99%
Prophylactic Antibiotic Timing (Outpatient)	13	92%	98%	98%
Urinary Catheter Removal[2]	154	92%	97%	97%
Survey of Patients' Hospital Experiences				
Area Around Room 'Always' Quiet at Night	(a)	70%	63%	61%
Doctors 'Always' Communicated Well	(a)	86%	84%	82%
Home Recovery Information Given	(a)	87%	88%	85%
Hospital Given 9 or 10 on 10 Point Scale	(a)	77%	75%	71%
Meds 'Always' Explained Before Given	(a)	66%	66%	64%
Nurses 'Always' Communicated Well	(a)	82%	81%	79%
Pain 'Always' Well Controlled	(a)	72%	71%	71%
Room and Bathroom 'Always' Clean	(a)	82%	79%	73%
Timely Help 'Always' Received	(a)	71%	70%	68%
Would Definitely Recommend Hospital	(a)	79%	74%	71%
Use of Medical Imaging				
Cardiac Imaging Stress Test before Surgery[7]	-	-	4.8%	5.3%
Combination Abdominal CT Scan	293	2.7%	11.5%	10.5%
Combination Brain/Sinus CT Scan[1]	-	-	1.8%	2.7%
Combination Chest CT Scan	197	1.5%	3.5%	2.7%
Follow-up Mammogram/Ultrasound	448	5.1%	7.9%	8.8%
Lumbar Spine MRI for Low Back Pain	73	20.5%	32.2%	37.2%

Sartori Memorial Hospital

515 College Street
Cedar Falls, IA 50613
E-mail: schaeferk@covhealth.com
URL: www.covhealth.com/sartori.asp
Type: Acute Care Hospitals
Ownership: Voluntary non-profit - Church

Phone: 319-268-3000
Fax: 319-268-3270
Emergency Services: Yes
Beds: 100

Key Personnel:
Emergency Room . . . . Maureen Beckman, RN
CEO/President. . . . . Sherri Greenwood
Quality Assurance . . . . Kari Kemmer
Infection Control. . . . . Nancy Kiehne, RN
Intensive Care Unit. . . . . Denise Lampman, RN
Operating Room. . . . . Linda Meier, RN
Chief of Medical Staff. . . . . Carl Vanderkooi

Measure	Cases	This Hosp.	State Avg.	U.S. Avg.
Blood Clot Prevention and Treatment				
Anticoagulation Overlap Therapy[2]	15	100%	94%	93%
ICU Venous Thromboembolism Prophylaxis[2]	12	50%	90%	92%
Incidence of Potentially Preventable VTE[1,2]	-	-	8%	10%
UFH with Dosages/Platelet Monitoring[1,2]	-	-	99%	97%
Venous Thromboembolism Prophylaxis[2]	80	70%	87%	85%
Warfarin Therapy Discharge Instructions[1,2]	-	-	77%	75%
Chest Pain/Possible Heart Attack Care				
Aspirin Given Within 24 Hours of Arrival[1,3]	-	-	97%	96%
Fibrinolytic Meds Within 30 Min. of Arrival[3,7]	-	-	49%	58%
Average Time to ECG (minutes)[1,3]	-	-	5	7
Average Time to Transfer (minutes)[1,3]	-	-	58	60
Children's Asthma Care				
Received Home Management Plan of Care	-	-	-	88%
Received Reliever Medication	-	-	-	100%
Received Systemic Corticosteroids	-	-	-	100%
Emergency Department				
Admittance Decision Time (minutes)[2]	311	29	58	98
Head CT Results Within 45 Min. of Arrival[1]	-	-	55%	57%
Patients Who Left ER Before Being Seen	7,287	1%	1%	2%
Time from ER Arrival to Admit. (minutes)[2]	315	197	202	274
Time from ER Arrival to Discharge (minutes)	376	114	108	134
Time in ER Before Being Evaluated (minutes)	410	18	21	26
Time to Pain Meds for Fractures (minutes)	25	40	46	57
Heart Attack Care				
Aspirin Given at Discharge[3,7]	-	-	100%	99%
Fibrinolytic Meds Within 30 Min. of Arrival[3,7]	-	-	-	54%
PCI Within 90 Minutes of Arrival[3,7]	-	-	94%	96%
Statin Prescribed at Discharge[3,7]	-	-	98%	98%
Heart Failure Care				
ACE Inhibitor or ARB for LVSD[1]	-	-	95%	97%
Discharge Instructions Given	16	69%	93%	94%
Evaluation of LVS Function	24	100%	97%	99%
Medicare Spending				
Medicare Spending per Patient (ratio)	-	1.01	0.91	0.98
Pneumonia Care				
Appropriate Initial Antibiotic Given	25	96%	93%	95%
Blood Culture Timing	32	97%	98%	98%
Pregnancy and Delivery Care				
Newborn Deliveries Scheduled Early[7]	-	-	4%	6%
Preventive Care				
Immunization for Influenza[2]	285	93%	91%	90%
Immunization for Pneumonia[2]	406	92%	90%	92%
Stroke Care				
Anticoagulation Therapy for Atrial Fibrillation[1]	-	-	95%	95%
Antithrombotic Therapy Timing[1]	-	-	98%	98%
Assessed for Rehabilitation[1]	-	-	97%	97%
Discharged on Antithrombotic Therapy[1]	-	-	99%	99%
Discharged on Statin Medication[1]	-	-	92%	94%
Thrombolytic Therapy Timing[1]	-	-	64%	66%
Venous Thromboembolism Prophylaxis[1]	-	-	93%	94%
Written Stroke Educational Materials Given[1]	-	-	82%	88%
Surgical Care Improvement Project				
Appropriate Beta Blocker Usage	69	99%	98%	98%
Appropriate VTP Within 24 Hours	198	99%	98%	98%
Controlled Postoperative Blood Glucose[7]	-	-	96%	97%
Perioperative Temperature Management	210	100%	100%	100%
Prophylactic Antibiotic Selection	156	99%	99%	99%
Prophylactic Antibiotic Selection (Outpatient)[1,3]	-	-	98%	98%
Prophylactic Antibiotic Stopped	156	99%	98%	98%
Prophylactic Antibiotic Timing	156	100%	98%	99%
Prophylactic Antibiotic Timing (Outpatient)[1,3]	-	-	98%	98%
Urinary Catheter Removal	172	100%	97%	97%
Survey of Patients' Hospital Experiences				
Area Around Room 'Always' Quiet at Night	300+	75%	63%	61%
Doctors 'Always' Communicated Well	300+	82%	84%	82%
Home Recovery Information Given	300+	81%	88%	85%
Hospital Given 9 or 10 on 10 Point Scale	300+	70%	75%	71%
Meds 'Always' Explained Before Given	300+	62%	66%	64%
Nurses 'Always' Communicated Well	300+	79%	81%	79%
Pain 'Always' Well Controlled	300+	65%	71%	71%
Room and Bathroom 'Always' Clean	300+	70%	79%	73%
Timely Help 'Always' Received	300+	54%	70%	68%
Would Definitely Recommend Hospital	300+	69%	74%	71%
Use of Medical Imaging				
Cardiac Imaging Stress Test before Surgery[1]	-	-	4.8%	5.3%
Combination Abdominal CT Scan	168	3.6%	11.5%	10.5%
Combination Brain/Sinus CT Scan[1]	-	-	1.8%	2.7%
Combination Chest CT Scan	75	0.0%	3.5%	2.7%
Follow-up Mammogram/Ultrasound	543	7.2%	7.9%	8.8%
Lumbar Spine MRI for Low Back Pain	89	29.2%	32.2%	37.2%

Mercy Medical Center - Cedar Rapids

701 10th Street Se
Cedar Rapids, IA 52403
URL: www.mercycare.org
Type: Acute Care Hospitals
Ownership: Voluntary non-profit - Church

Phone: 319-398-6011
Fax: 319-398-6912
Emergency Services: Yes
Beds: 430

Key Personnel:
CEO/President. . . . . Timothy L. Charles
Emergency Room . . . . Sue Courts
Operating Room. . . . . Betty DeBrower
Chief of Medical Staff. . . . . Margie Ebel
Intensive Care Unit. . . . . Rose Hutchcroft, RN
Quality Assurance . . . . Kathy Krusie
Infection Control. . . . . Jolene Utt

Measure	Cases	This Hosp.	State Avg.	U.S. Avg.
Blood Clot Prevention and Treatment				
Anticoagulation Overlap Therapy[2]	84	90%	94%	93%
ICU Venous Thromboembolism Prophylaxis[2]	62	98%	90%	92%
Incidence of Potentially Preventable VTE[1,2]	-	-	8%	10%
UFH with Dosages/Platelet Monitoring[2]	70	100%	99%	97%
Venous Thromboembolism Prophylaxis[2]	302	87%	87%	85%
Warfarin Therapy Discharge Instructions[2]	64	100%	77%	75%
Chest Pain/Possible Heart Attack Care				
Aspirin Given Within 24 Hours of Arrival[1,3]	-	-	97%	96%
Fibrinolytic Meds Within 30 Min. of Arrival[3,7]	-	-	49%	58%
Average Time to ECG (minutes)[1,3]	-	-	5	7
Average Time to Transfer (minutes)[3,7]	-	-	58	60
Children's Asthma Care				
Received Home Management Plan of Care	-	-	-	88%
Received Reliever Medication	-	-	-	100%
Received Systemic Corticosteroids	-	-	-	100%
Emergency Department				
Admittance Decision Time (minutes)[2]	591	65	58	98
Head CT Results Within 45 Min. of Arrival	14	79%	55%	57%
Patients Who Left ER Before Being Seen	48,009	1%	1%	2%
Time from ER Arrival to Admit. (minutes)[2]	609	215	202	274
Time from ER Arrival to Discharge (minutes)	367	122	108	134
Time in ER Before Being Evaluated (minutes)	367	20	21	26
Time to Pain Meds for Fractures (minutes)	115	51	46	57
Heart Attack Care				
Aspirin Given at Discharge	165	100%	100%	99%
Fibrinolytic Meds Within 30 Min. of Arrival[7]	-	-	-	54%
PCI Within 90 Minutes of Arrival	27	100%	94%	96%
Statin Prescribed at Discharge	155	99%	98%	98%
Heart Failure Care				
ACE Inhibitor or ARB for LVSD[2]	44	100%	95%	97%
Discharge Instructions Given[2]	170	96%	93%	94%
Evaluation of LVS Function[2]	231	100%	97%	99%
Medicare Spending				
Medicare Spending per Patient (ratio)	-	0.90	0.91	0.98

NOTE: Hospital profiles are in alphabetical order by state, then city, then hospital within the city; Rankings exclude hospitals with less than 25 cases except for patient surveys which excludes hospitals with less than 100 cases; (a) 100-299 cases; (1) The number of cases/patients is too few to report; (2) Data submitted were based on a sample of cases/patients; (3) Results are based on a shorter time period than required; (4) Data suppressed by CMS for one or more quarters; (5) Results are not available for this reporting period; (6) Fewer than 100 patients completed the HCAHPS survey; (7) No cases met the criteria for this measure; (8) The lower limit of the confidence interval cannot be calculated if the number of observed infections equals zero; (9) No data are available from the state/territory for this reporting period; (10) The scores shown reflect fewer than 50 completed surveys; (11) There were discrepancies in the data collection process; (12) This measure does not apply to this hospital for this reporting period; (13) Results cannot be calculated for this reporting period; (14) The results for this state are combined with nearby states to protect confidentiality; Please refer to the User's Guide for a full explanation of data.

Measure	Cases	This Hosp.	State Avg.	U.S. Avg.
Pneumonia Care				
Appropriate Initial Antibiotic Given[2]	60	93%	93%	95%
Blood Culture Timing[2]	135	99%	98%	98%
Pregnancy and Delivery Care				
Newborn Deliveries Scheduled Early[2]	32	0%	4%	6%
Preventive Care				
Immunization for Influenza[2]	564	92%	91%	90%
Immunization for Pneumonia[2]	763	94%	90%	92%
Stroke Care				
Anticoagulation Therapy for Atrial Fibrillation	19	95%	95%	95%
Antithrombotic Therapy Timing	59	98%	98%	98%
Assessed for Rehabilitation	98	100%	97%	97%
Discharged on Antithrombotic Therapy	92	98%	99%	99%
Discharged on Statin Medication	70	96%	92%	94%
Thrombolytic Therapy Timing	15	100%	64%	66%
Venous Thromboembolism Prophylaxis	84	94%	93%	94%
Written Stroke Educational Materials Given	45	100%	82%	88%
Surgical Care Improvement Project				
Appropriate Beta Blocker Usage[2]	105	97%	98%	98%
Appropriate VTP Within 24 Hours[2]	240	100%	98%	98%
Controlled Postoperative Blood Glucose[2,7]	-	-	96%	97%
Perioperative Temperature Management[2]	300	100%	100%	100%
Prophylactic Antibiotic Selection[2]	192	100%	99%	99%
Prophylactic Antibiotic Selection (Outpatient)	708	99%	98%	98%
Prophylactic Antibiotic Stopped[2]	190	98%	98%	98%
Prophylactic Antibiotic Timing[2]	192	97%	98%	99%
Prophylactic Antibiotic Timing (Outpatient)	721	97%	98%	98%
Urinary Catheter Removal[2]	64	97%	97%	97%
Survey of Patients' Hospital Experiences				
Area Around Room 'Always' Quiet at Night	300+	66%	63%	61%
Doctors 'Always' Communicated Well	300+	80%	84%	82%
Home Recovery Information Given	300+	86%	88%	85%
Hospital Given 9 or 10 on 10 Point Scale	300+	77%	75%	71%
Meds 'Always' Explained Before Given	300+	63%	66%	64%
Nurses 'Always' Communicated Well	300+	79%	81%	79%
Pain 'Always' Well Controlled	300+	69%	71%	71%
Room and Bathroom 'Always' Clean	300+	75%	79%	73%
Timely Help 'Always' Received	300+	60%	70%	68%
Would Definitely Recommend Hospital	300+	80%	74%	71%
Use of Medical Imaging				
Cardiac Imaging Stress Test before Surgery	84	4.8%	4.8%	5.3%
Combination Abdominal CT Scan	1,113	5.0%	11.5%	10.5%
Combination Brain/Sinus CT Scan	878	1.6%	1.8%	2.7%
Combination Chest CT Scan	877	1.7%	3.5%	2.7%
Follow-up Mammogram/Ultrasound	2,974	8.1%	7.9%	8.8%
Lumbar Spine MRI for Low Back Pain	303	33.7%	32.2%	37.2%

Saint Luke's Hospital

1026 A Ave Ne
Cedar Rapids, IA 52402
Phone: 319-369-7211
Fax: 319-369-8036
URL: www.crstlukes.com
Type: Acute Care Hospitals
Emergency Services: Yes
Ownership: Voluntary non-profit - Private
Beds: 560

Key Personnel:

Infection Control. . . . . Brenda Depue
Radiology. . . . . Michael Harleman
Quality Assurance . . . . Sherrie Justice
Chief of Medical Staff. . . . . James R LaMorgese, MD
Operating Room. . . . . Janna Petersen
Pediatric Ambulatory Care . . . . . . Stephen Roth
Pediatric In-Patient Care . . . . Stephen Roth
CEO/President. . . . . Theodore Townsend

Measure	Cases	This Hosp.	State Avg.	U.S. Avg.
Blood Clot Prevention and Treatment				
Anticoagulation Overlap Therapy[2]	116	97%	94%	93%
ICU Venous Thromboembolism Prophylaxis[2]	98	99%	90%	92%
Incidence of Potentially Preventable VTE[2]	11	0%	8%	10%
UFH with Dosages/Platelet Monitoring[2]	101	100%	99%	97%
Venous Thromboembolism Prophylaxis[2]	253	99%	87%	85%
Warfarin Therapy Discharge Instructions[2]	99	60%	77%	75%
Chest Pain/Possible Heart Attack Care				
Aspirin Given Within 24 Hours of Arrival[1,3]	-	-	97%	96%
Fibrinolytic Meds Within 30 Min. of Arrival[5]	-	-	49%	58%
Average Time to ECG (minutes)[1,3]	-	-	5	7
Average Time to Transfer (minutes)[5]	-	-	58	60
Children's Asthma Care				
Received Home Management Plan of Care	-	-	-	88%
Received Reliever Medication	-	-	-	100%
Received Systemic Corticosteroids	-	-	-	100%
Emergency Department				
Admittance Decision Time (minutes)[2]	423	84	58	98
Head CT Results Within 45 Min. of Arrival	15	33%	55%	57%
Patients Who Left ER Before Being Seen	55,467	0%	1%	2%
Time from ER Arrival to Admit. (minutes)[2]	427	235	202	274
Time from ER Arrival to Discharge (minutes)	353	138	108	134
Time in ER Before Being Evaluated (minutes)	371	37	21	26
Time to Pain Meds for Fractures (minutes)	199	39	46	57
Heart Attack Care				
Aspirin Given at Discharge	325	100%	100%	99%
Fibrinolytic Meds Within 30 Min. of Arrival[7]	-	-	-	54%
PCI Within 90 Minutes of Arrival	46	100%	94%	96%
Statin Prescribed at Discharge	307	99%	98%	98%
Heart Failure Care				
ACE Inhibitor or ARB for LVSD	68	100%	95%	97%
Discharge Instructions Given	238	97%	93%	94%
Evaluation of LVS Function	299	100%	97%	99%
Medicare Spending				
Medicare Spending per Patient (ratio)	-	0.93	0.91	0.98
Pneumonia Care				
Appropriate Initial Antibiotic Given[2]	68	88%	93%	95%
Blood Culture Timing[2]	84	98%	98%	98%
Pregnancy and Delivery Care				
Newborn Deliveries Scheduled Early[2]	32	0%	4%	6%
Preventive Care				
Immunization for Influenza[2]	483	85%	91%	90%
Immunization for Pneumonia[2]	530	87%	90%	92%
Stroke Care				
Anticoagulation Therapy for Atrial Fibrillation[2]	18	89%	95%	95%
Antithrombotic Therapy Timing[2]	89	98%	98%	98%
Assessed for Rehabilitation[2]	122	97%	97%	97%
Discharged on Antithrombotic Therapy[2]	114	97%	99%	99%
Discharged on Statin Medication[2]	100	98%	92%	94%
Thrombolytic Therapy Timing[2]	20	70%	64%	66%
Venous Thromboembolism Prophylaxis[2]	104	95%	93%	94%
Written Stroke Educational Materials Given[2]	72	85%	82%	88%
Surgical Care Improvement Project				
Appropriate Beta Blocker Usage[2]	209	99%	98%	98%
Appropriate VTP Within 24 Hours[2]	221	100%	98%	98%
Controlled Postoperative Blood Glucose[2]	128	95%	96%	97%
Perioperative Temperature Management[2]	330	99%	100%	100%
Prophylactic Antibiotic Selection[2]	318	100%	99%	99%
Prophylactic Antibiotic Selection (Outpatient)	560	100%	98%	98%
Prophylactic Antibiotic Stopped[2]	306	95%	98%	98%
Prophylactic Antibiotic Timing[2]	318	98%	98%	99%
Prophylactic Antibiotic Timing (Outpatient)	561	99%	98%	98%
Urinary Catheter Removal[2]	190	89%	97%	97%
Survey of Patients' Hospital Experiences				
Area Around Room 'Always' Quiet at Night	300+	62%	63%	61%
Doctors 'Always' Communicated Well	300+	78%	84%	82%
Home Recovery Information Given	300+	89%	88%	85%
Hospital Given 9 or 10 on 10 Point Scale	300+	78%	75%	71%
Meds 'Always' Explained Before Given	300+	65%	66%	64%
Nurses 'Always' Communicated Well	300+	79%	81%	79%
Pain 'Always' Well Controlled	300+	71%	71%	71%
Room and Bathroom 'Always' Clean	300+	74%	79%	73%
Timely Help 'Always' Received	300+	69%	70%	68%
Would Definitely Recommend Hospital	300+	79%	74%	71%
Use of Medical Imaging				
Cardiac Imaging Stress Test before Surgery[1]	-	-	4.8%	5.3%
Combination Abdominal CT Scan	725	7.2%	11.5%	10.5%
Combination Brain/Sinus CT Scan	750	1.1%	1.8%	2.7%
Combination Chest CT Scan	660	2.3%	3.5%	2.7%
Follow-up Mammogram/Ultrasound	1,769	7.7%	7.9%	8.8%
Lumbar Spine MRI for Low Back Pain	223	31.8%	32.2%	37.2%

Mercy Medical Center - Centerville

One Saint Joseph's Drive
Centerville, IA 52544
Phone: 641-437-4111
Fax: 641-437-3422
URL: www.mercycenterville.org
Type: Critical Access Hospitals
Emergency Services: Yes
Ownership: Voluntary non-profit - Private
Beds: 54

Key Personnel:

Radiology. . . . . Don Breit
Cardiac Laboratory. . . . . Thomas Brown
Quality Assurance . . . . Tonya Clawson
CEO/President. . . . . Scott Grodsky
Chief of Medical Staff . . . . Carl Rouse
Emergency Room . . . . Mary Lou Sales, RN
Operating Room. . . . . Kathy Woolums, RN

Measure	Cases	This Hosp.	State Avg.	U.S. Avg.
Blood Clot Prevention and Treatment				
Anticoagulation Overlap Therapy[5]	-	-	94%	93%
ICU Venous Thromboembolism Prophylaxis[5]	-	-	90%	92%
Incidence of Potentially Preventable VTE[5]	-	-	8%	10%
UFH with Dosages/Platelet Monitoring[5]	-	-	99%	97%
Venous Thromboembolism Prophylaxis[5]	-	-	87%	85%
Warfarin Therapy Discharge Instructions[5]	-	-	77%	75%
Chest Pain/Possible Heart Attack Care				
Aspirin Given Within 24 Hours of Arrival	-	-	97%	96%
Fibrinolytic Meds Within 30 Min. of Arrival	-	-	49%	58%
Average Time to ECG (minutes)	-	-	5	7
Average Time to Transfer (minutes)	-	-	58	60
Children's Asthma Care				
Received Home Management Plan of Care	-	-	-	88%
Received Reliever Medication	-	-	-	100%
Received Systemic Corticosteroids	-	-	-	100%
Emergency Department				
Admittance Decision Time (minutes)[5]	-	-	58	98
Head CT Results Within 45 Min. of Arrival	-	-	55%	57%
Patients Who Left ER Before Being Seen	-	-	1%	2%
Time from ER Arrival to Admit. (minutes)[5]	-	-	202	274
Time from ER Arrival to Discharge (minutes)	-	-	108	134
Time in ER Before Being Evaluated (minutes)	-	-	21	26
Time to Pain Meds for Fractures (minutes)	-	-	46	57
Heart Attack Care				
Aspirin Given at Discharge[1]	-	-	100%	99%
Fibrinolytic Meds Within 30 Min. of Arrival[7]	-	-	-	54%
PCI Within 90 Minutes of Arrival[7]	-	-	94%	96%
Statin Prescribed at Discharge[1]	-	-	98%	98%
Heart Failure Care				
ACE Inhibitor or ARB for LVSD[1]	-	-	95%	97%
Discharge Instructions Given	12	92%	93%	94%
Evaluation of LVS Function	22	100%	97%	99%
Medicare Spending				
Medicare Spending per Patient (ratio)	-	-	0.91	0.98
Pneumonia Care				
Appropriate Initial Antibiotic Given	20	95%	93%	95%
Blood Culture Timing	18	89%	98%	98%
Pregnancy and Delivery Care				
Newborn Deliveries Scheduled Early[5]	-	-	4%	6%
Preventive Care				
Immunization for Influenza[5]	-	-	91%	90%
Immunization for Pneumonia[5]	-	-	90%	92%
Stroke Care				
Anticoagulation Therapy for Atrial Fibrillation[5]	-	-	95%	95%
Antithrombotic Therapy Timing[5]	-	-	98%	98%
Assessed for Rehabilitation[5]	-	-	97%	97%
Discharged on Antithrombotic Therapy[5]	-	-	99%	99%
Discharged on Statin Medication[5]	-	-	92%	94%
Thrombolytic Therapy Timing[5]	-	-	64%	66%
Venous Thromboembolism Prophylaxis[5]	-	-	93%	94%
Written Stroke Educational Materials Given[5]	-	-	82%	88%
Surgical Care Improvement Project				
Appropriate Beta Blocker Usage[1]	-	-	98%	98%
Appropriate VTP Within 24 Hours	44	93%	98%	98%
Controlled Postoperative Blood Glucose[7]	-	-	96%	97%
Perioperative Temperature Management	49	100%	100%	100%
Prophylactic Antibiotic Selection	34	97%	99%	99%
Prophylactic Antibiotic Selection (Outpatient)	-	-	98%	98%

NOTE: Hospital profiles are in alphabetical order by state, then city, then hospital within the city; Rankings exclude hospitals with less than 25 cases except for patient surveys which excludes hospitals with less than 100 cases; (a) 100-299 cases; (1) The number of cases/patients is too few to report; (2) Data submitted were based on a sample of cases/patients; (3) Results are based on a shorter time period than required; (4) Data suppressed by CMS for one or more quarters; (5) Results are not available for this reporting period; (6) Fewer than 100 patients completed the HCAHPS survey; (7) No cases met the criteria for this measure; (8) The lower limit of the confidence interval cannot be calculated if the number of observed infections equals zero; (9) No data are available from the state/territory for this reporting period; (10) The scores shown reflect fewer than 50 completed surveys; (11) There were discrepancies in the data collection process; (12) This measure does not apply to this hospital for this reporting period; (13) Results cannot be calculated for this reporting period; (14) The results for this state are combined with nearby states to protect confidentiality; Please refer to the User's Guide for a full explanation of data.

Measure	Cases	This Hosp.	State Avg.	U.S. Avg.
Prophylactic Antibiotic Stopped	31	97%	98%	98%
Prophylactic Antibiotic Timing	34	97%	98%	99%
Prophylactic Antibiotic Timing (Outpatient)	-	-	98%	98%
Urinary Catheter Removal	15	53%	97%	97%
Survey of Patients' Hospital Experiences				
Area Around Room 'Always' Quiet at Night	(a)	48%	63%	61%
Doctors 'Always' Communicated Well	(a)	83%	84%	82%
Home Recovery Information Given	(a)	82%	88%	85%
Hospital Given 9 or 10 on 10 Point Scale	(a)	66%	75%	71%
Meds 'Always' Explained Before Given	(a)	57%	66%	64%
Nurses 'Always' Communicated Well	(a)	76%	81%	79%
Pain 'Always' Well Controlled	(a)	63%	71%	71%
Room and Bathroom 'Always' Clean	(a)	80%	79%	73%
Timely Help 'Always' Received	(a)	57%	70%	68%
Would Definitely Recommend Hospital	(a)	58%	74%	71%
Use of Medical Imaging				
Cardiac Imaging Stress Test before Surgery	-	-	4.8%	5.3%
Combination Abdominal CT Scan	-	-	11.5%	10.5%
Combination Brain/Sinus CT Scan	-	-	1.8%	2.7%
Combination Chest CT Scan	-	-	3.5%	2.7%
Follow-up Mammogram/Ultrasound	-	-	7.9%	8.8%
Lumbar Spine MRI for Low Back Pain	-	-	32.2%	37.2%

Lucas County Health Center

1200 North 7th Street
Chariton, IA 50049
URL: www.lchcia.com
Type: Critical Access Hospitals
Ownership: Voluntary non-profit - Other
Phone: 641-774-3000
Fax: 641-774-3296
Emergency Services: Yes
Beds: 56

Key Personnel:
Radiology. . . . . Robert V Filippone
CEO/President. . . . . Veronica Fuhs
Quality Assurance . . . . Veronica Fuhs
Emergency Room . . . . Michael Gorski
Chair/CEO. . . . . Betty Hansen
Chief of Medical Staff. . . . . Dr. Christy Manganello, MD
Operating Room. . . . . Becky McCorkle

Measure	Cases	This Hosp.	State Avg.	U.S. Avg.
Blood Clot Prevention and Treatment				
Anticoagulation Overlap Therapy[5]	-	-	94%	93%
ICU Venous Thromboembolism Prophylaxis[5]	-	-	90%	92%
Incidence of Potentially Preventable VTE[5]	-	-	8%	10%
UFH with Dosages/Platelet Monitoring[5]	-	-	99%	97%
Venous Thromboembolism Prophylaxis[5]	-	-	87%	85%
Warfarin Therapy Discharge Instructions[5]	-	-	77%	75%
Chest Pain/Possible Heart Attack Care				
Aspirin Given Within 24 Hours of Arrival[3]	21	100%	97%	96%
Fibrinolytic Meds Within 30 Min. of Arrival[3,7]	-	-	49%	58%
Average Time to ECG (minutes)[3]	22	4	5	7
Average Time to Transfer (minutes)[1,3]	-	-	58	60
Children's Asthma Care				
Received Home Management Plan of Care	-	-	-	88%
Received Reliever Medication	-	-	-	100%
Received Systemic Corticosteroids	-	-	-	100%
Emergency Department				
Admittance Decision Time (minutes)[5]	-	-	58	98
Head CT Results Within 45 Min. of Arrival[1,3]	-	-	55%	57%
Patients Who Left ER Before Being Seen[5]	-	-	1%	2%
Time from ER Arrival to Admit. (minutes)[5]	-	-	202	274
Time from ER Arrival to Discharge (minutes)[5]	-	-	108	134
Time in ER Before Being Evaluated (minutes)[5]	-	-	21	26
Time to Pain Meds for Fractures (minutes)[5]	-	-	46	57
Heart Attack Care				
Aspirin Given at Discharge[5]	-	-	100%	99%
Fibrinolytic Meds Within 30 Min. of Arrival[5]	-	-	-	54%
PCI Within 90 Minutes of Arrival[5]	-	-	94%	96%
Statin Prescribed at Discharge[5]	-	-	98%	98%
Heart Failure Care				
ACE Inhibitor or ARB for LVSD[7]	-	-	95%	97%
Discharge Instructions Given[1]	-	-	93%	94%
Evaluation of LVS Function[1]	-	-	97%	99%
Medicare Spending				
Medicare Spending per Patient (ratio)	-	-	0.91	0.98
Pneumonia Care				
Appropriate Initial Antibiotic Given	26	100%	93%	95%
Blood Culture Timing	25	100%	98%	98%
Pregnancy and Delivery Care				
Newborn Deliveries Scheduled Early[5]	-	-	4%	6%
Preventive Care				
Immunization for Influenza[5]	-	-	91%	90%
Immunization for Pneumonia[5]	-	-	90%	92%
Stroke Care				
Anticoagulation Therapy for Atrial Fibrillation[3,7]	-	-	95%	95%
Antithrombotic Therapy Timing[1,3]	-	-	98%	98%
Assessed for Rehabilitation[1,3]	-	-	97%	97%
Discharged on Antithrombotic Therapy[1,3]	-	-	99%	99%
Discharged on Statin Medication[1,3]	-	-	92%	94%
Thrombolytic Therapy Timing[3,7]	-	-	64%	66%
Venous Thromboembolism Prophylaxis[1,3]	-	-	93%	94%
Written Stroke Educational Materials Given[3,7]	-	-	82%	88%
Surgical Care Improvement Project				
Appropriate Beta Blocker Usage[5]	-	-	98%	98%
Appropriate VTP Within 24 Hours[5]	-	-	98%	98%
Controlled Postoperative Blood Glucose[5]	-	-	96%	97%
Perioperative Temperature Management[5]	-	-	100%	100%
Prophylactic Antibiotic Selection[5]	-	-	99%	99%
Prophylactic Antibiotic Selection (Outpatient)[5]	-	-	98%	98%
Prophylactic Antibiotic Stopped[5]	-	-	98%	98%
Prophylactic Antibiotic Timing[5]	-	-	98%	99%
Prophylactic Antibiotic Timing (Outpatient)[5]	-	-	98%	98%
Urinary Catheter Removal[5]	-	-	97%	97%
Survey of Patients' Hospital Experiences				
Area Around Room 'Always' Quiet at Night[5]	-	-	63%	61%
Doctors 'Always' Communicated Well[5]	-	-	84%	82%
Home Recovery Information Given[5]	-	-	88%	85%
Hospital Given 9 or 10 on 10 Point Scale[5]	-	-	75%	71%
Meds 'Always' Explained Before Given[5]	-	-	66%	64%
Nurses 'Always' Communicated Well[5]	-	-	81%	79%
Pain 'Always' Well Controlled[5]	-	-	71%	71%
Room and Bathroom 'Always' Clean[5]	-	-	79%	73%
Timely Help 'Always' Received[5]	-	-	70%	68%
Would Definitely Recommend Hospital[5]	-	-	74%	71%
Use of Medical Imaging				
Cardiac Imaging Stress Test before Surgery[1]	-	-	4.8%	5.3%
Combination Abdominal CT Scan	77	5.2%	11.5%	10.5%
Combination Brain/Sinus CT Scan[1]	-	-	1.8%	2.7%
Combination Chest CT Scan[1]	-	-	3.5%	2.7%
Follow-up Mammogram/Ultrasound	229	3.1%	7.9%	8.8%
Lumbar Spine MRI for Low Back Pain[1]	-	-	32.2%	37.2%

Floyd County Memorial Hospital

800 11th St
Charles City, IA 50616
URL: www.fcmc.us.com
Type: Critical Access Hospitals
Ownership: Government - Local
Phone: 641-228-6830
Emergency Services: Yes

Measure	Cases	This Hosp.	State Avg.	U.S. Avg.
Blood Clot Prevention and Treatment				
Anticoagulation Overlap Therapy[1,2]	-	-	94%	93%
ICU Venous Thromboembolism Prophylaxis[2,7]	-	-	90%	92%
Incidence of Potentially Preventable VTE[2,7]	-	-	8%	10%
UFH with Dosages/Platelet Monitoring[1,2]	-	-	99%	97%
Venous Thromboembolism Prophylaxis[2]	120	88%	87%	85%
Warfarin Therapy Discharge Instructions[1,2]	-	-	77%	75%
Chest Pain/Possible Heart Attack Care				
Aspirin Given Within 24 Hours of Arrival	49	92%	97%	96%
Fibrinolytic Meds Within 30 Min. of Arrival[1]	-	-	49%	58%
Average Time to ECG (minutes)	51	4	5	7
Average Time to Transfer (minutes)[1]	-	-	58	60
Children's Asthma Care				
Received Home Management Plan of Care	-	-	-	88%
Received Reliever Medication	-	-	-	100%
Received Systemic Corticosteroids	-	-	-	100%
Emergency Department				
Admittance Decision Time (minutes)[2]	234	33	58	98
Head CT Results Within 45 Min. of Arrival[1]	-	-	55%	57%
Patients Who Left ER Before Being Seen	5,735	0%	1%	2%
Time from ER Arrival to Admit. (minutes)[2]	236	178	202	274
Time from ER Arrival to Discharge (minutes)	192	90	108	134
Time in ER Before Being Evaluated (minutes)	334	14	21	26
Time to Pain Meds for Fractures (minutes)	17	52	46	57
Heart Attack Care				
Aspirin Given at Discharge[1,2]	-	-	100%	99%
Fibrinolytic Meds Within 30 Min. of Arrival[2,7]	-	-	-	54%
PCI Within 90 Minutes of Arrival[2,7]	-	-	94%	96%
Statin Prescribed at Discharge[1,2]	-	-	98%	98%
Heart Failure Care				
ACE Inhibitor or ARB for LVSD[1,2]	-	-	95%	97%
Discharge Instructions Given[2]	15	87%	93%	94%
Evaluation of LVS Function[2]	38	66%	97%	99%
Medicare Spending				
Medicare Spending per Patient (ratio)	-	-	0.91	0.98
Pneumonia Care				
Appropriate Initial Antibiotic Given[2]	24	54%	93%	95%
Blood Culture Timing[2]	19	95%	98%	98%
Pregnancy and Delivery Care				
Newborn Deliveries Scheduled Early[5]	-	-	4%	6%
Preventive Care				
Immunization for Influenza[2]	120	95%	91%	90%
Immunization for Pneumonia[2]	238	90%	90%	92%
Stroke Care				
Anticoagulation Therapy for Atrial Fibrillation[1,2]	-	-	95%	95%
Antithrombotic Therapy Timing[1,2]	-	-	98%	98%
Assessed for Rehabilitation[1,2]	-	-	97%	97%
Discharged on Antithrombotic Therapy[1,2]	-	-	99%	99%
Discharged on Statin Medication[1,2]	-	-	92%	94%
Thrombolytic Therapy Timing[2,7]	-	-	64%	66%
Venous Thromboembolism Prophylaxis[2]	11	73%	93%	94%
Written Stroke Educational Materials Given[1,2]	-	-	82%	88%
Surgical Care Improvement Project				
Appropriate Beta Blocker Usage[1,2]	-	-	98%	98%
Appropriate VTP Within 24 Hours[2]	15	93%	98%	98%
Controlled Postoperative Blood Glucose[2,7]	-	-	96%	97%
Perioperative Temperature Management[2]	16	100%	100%	100%
Prophylactic Antibiotic Selection[1,2]	-	-	99%	99%
Prophylactic Antibiotic Selection (Outpatient)[5]	-	-	98%	98%
Prophylactic Antibiotic Stopped[1,2]	-	-	98%	98%
Prophylactic Antibiotic Timing[1,2]	-	-	98%	99%
Prophylactic Antibiotic Timing (Outpatient)[5]	-	-	98%	98%
Urinary Catheter Removal[2]	11	82%	97%	97%
Survey of Patients' Hospital Experiences				
Area Around Room 'Always' Quiet at Night	(a)	70%	63%	61%
Doctors 'Always' Communicated Well	(a)	90%	84%	82%
Home Recovery Information Given	(a)	88%	88%	85%
Hospital Given 9 or 10 on 10 Point Scale	(a)	83%	75%	71%
Meds 'Always' Explained Before Given	(a)	71%	66%	64%
Nurses 'Always' Communicated Well	(a)	88%	81%	79%
Pain 'Always' Well Controlled	(a)	76%	71%	71%
Room and Bathroom 'Always' Clean	(a)	87%	79%	73%
Timely Help 'Always' Received	(a)	77%	70%	68%
Would Definitely Recommend Hospital	(a)	81%	74%	71%
Use of Medical Imaging				
Cardiac Imaging Stress Test before Surgery[1]	-	-	4.8%	5.3%
Combination Abdominal CT Scan	170	5.3%	11.5%	10.5%
Combination Brain/Sinus CT Scan	219	0.5%	1.8%	2.7%
Combination Chest CT Scan	56	0.0%	3.5%	2.7%
Follow-up Mammogram/Ultrasound	504	7.9%	7.9%	8.8%
Lumbar Spine MRI for Low Back Pain[1]	-	-	32.2%	37.2%

Cherokee Regional Medical Center

300 Sioux Valley Drive
Cherokee, IA 51012
E-mail: webmaster@cherokeermc.org
URL: www.cherokeermc.org
Type: Critical Access Hospitals
Ownership: Voluntary non-profit - Private
Phone: 712-225-5101
Fax: 712-225-6870
Emergency Services: Yes
Beds: 25

Key Personnel:
Radiology. . . . . Jeanna Bergendahl
CEO/President. . . . . John M Comstock
Operating Room. . . . . Dondee Halverson
Infection Control. . . . . Susie Haselhoff

NOTE: Hospital profiles are in alphabetical order by state, then city, then hospital within the city; Rankings exclude hospitals with less than 25 cases except for patient surveys which excludes hospitals with less than 100 cases; (a) 100-299 cases; (1) The number of cases/patients is too few to report; (2) Data submitted were based on a sample of cases/patients; (3) Results are based on a shorter time period than required; (4) Data suppressed by CMS for one or more quarters; (5) Results are not available for this reporting period; (6) Fewer than 100 patients completed the HCAHPS survey; (7) No cases met the criteria for this measure; (8) The lower limit of the confidence interval cannot be calculated if the number of observed infections equals zero; (9) No data are available from the state/territory for this reporting period; (10) The scores shown reflect fewer than 50 completed surveys; (11) There were discrepancies in the data collection process; (12) This measure does not apply to this hospital for this reporting period; (13) Results cannot be calculated for this reporting period; (14) The results for this state are combined with nearby states to protect confidentiality; Please refer to the User's Guide for a full explanation of data.

Quality Assurance . . . . Susie Hasolhoff
Coronary Care . . . . Wesley Parker, MD
Chief of Medical Staff . . . . Timothy G Rice

Measure	Cases	This Hosp.	State Avg.	U.S. Avg.
Blood Clot Prevention and Treatment				
Anticoagulation Overlap Therapy[5]	-	-	94%	93%
ICU Venous Thromboembolism Prophylaxis[5]	-	-	90%	92%
Incidence of Potentially Preventable VTE[5]	-	-	8%	10%
UFH with Dosages/Platelet Monitoring[5]	-	-	99%	97%
Venous Thromboembolism Prophylaxis[5]	-	-	87%	85%
Warfarin Therapy Discharge Instructions[5]	-	-	77%	75%
Chest Pain/Possible Heart Attack Care				
Aspirin Given Within 24 Hours of Arrival	-	-	97%	96%
Fibrinolytic Meds Within 30 Min. of Arrival	-	-	49%	58%
Average Time to ECG (minutes)	-	-	5	7
Average Time to Transfer (minutes)	-	-	58	60
Children's Asthma Care				
Received Home Management Plan of Care	-	-	-	88%
Received Reliever Medication	-	-	-	100%
Received Systemic Corticosteroids	-	-	-	100%
Emergency Department				
Admittance Decision Time (minutes)[5]	-	-	58	98
Head CT Results Within 45 Min. of Arrival	-	-	55%	57%
Patients Who Left ER Before Being Seen	-	-	1%	2%
Time from ER Arrival to Admit. (minutes)[5]	-	-	202	274
Time from ER Arrival to Discharge (minutes)	-	-	108	134
Time in ER Before Being Evaluated (minutes)	-	-	21	26
Time to Pain Meds for Fractures (minutes)	-	-	46	57
Heart Attack Care				
Aspirin Given at Discharge[5]	-	-	100%	99%
Fibrinolytic Meds Within 30 Min. of Arrival[5]	-	-	-	54%
PCI Within 90 Minutes of Arrival[5]	-	-	94%	96%
Statin Prescribed at Discharge[5]	-	-	98%	98%
Heart Failure Care				
ACE Inhibitor or ARB for LVSD[1,3]	-	-	95%	97%
Discharge Instructions Given[1,3]	-	-	93%	94%
Evaluation of LVS Function[3]	17	94%	97%	99%
Medicare Spending				
Medicare Spending per Patient (ratio)	-	-	0.91	0.98
Pneumonia Care				
Appropriate Initial Antibiotic Given[2,3]	23	87%	93%	95%
Blood Culture Timing[1,2]	-	-	98%	98%
Pregnancy and Delivery Care				
Newborn Deliveries Scheduled Early[5]	-	-	4%	6%
Preventive Care				
Immunization for Influenza[5]	-	-	91%	90%
Immunization for Pneumonia[5]	-	-	90%	92%
Stroke Care				
Anticoagulation Therapy for Atrial Fibrillation[5]	-	-	95%	95%
Antithrombotic Therapy Timing[5]	-	-	98%	98%
Assessed for Rehabilitation[5]	-	-	97%	97%
Discharged on Antithrombotic Therapy[5]	-	-	99%	99%
Discharged on Statin Medication[5]	-	-	92%	94%
Thrombolytic Therapy Timing[5]	-	-	64%	66%
Venous Thromboembolism Prophylaxis[5]	-	-	93%	94%
Written Stroke Educational Materials Given[5]	-	-	82%	88%
Surgical Care Improvement Project				
Appropriate Beta Blocker Usage[5]	-	-	98%	98%
Appropriate VTP Within 24 Hours[5]	-	-	98%	98%
Controlled Postoperative Blood Glucose[5]	-	-	96%	97%
Perioperative Temperature Management[5]	-	-	100%	100%
Prophylactic Antibiotic Selection[5]	-	-	99%	99%
Prophylactic Antibiotic Selection (Outpatient)	-	-	98%	98%
Prophylactic Antibiotic Stopped[5]	-	-	98%	98%
Prophylactic Antibiotic Timing[5]	-	-	98%	99%
Prophylactic Antibiotic Timing (Outpatient)	-	-	98%	98%
Urinary Catheter Removal[5]	-	-	97%	97%
Survey of Patients' Hospital Experiences				
Area Around Room 'Always' Quiet at Night[5]	-	-	63%	61%
Doctors 'Always' Communicated Well[5]	-	-	84%	82%
Home Recovery Information Given[5]	-	-	88%	85%
Hospital Given 9 or 10 on 10 Point Scale[5]	-	-	75%	71%
Meds 'Always' Explained Before Given[5]	-	-	66%	64%
Nurses 'Always' Communicated Well[5]	-	-	81%	79%
Pain 'Always' Well Controlled[5]	-	-	71%	71%
Room and Bathroom 'Always' Clean[5]	-	-	79%	73%
Timely Help 'Always' Received[5]	-	-	70%	68%
Would Definitely Recommend Hospital[5]	-	-	74%	71%
Use of Medical Imaging				
Cardiac Imaging Stress Test before Surgery	-	-	4.8%	5.3%
Combination Abdominal CT Scan	-	-	11.5%	10.5%
Combination Brain/Sinus CT Scan	-	-	1.8%	2.7%
Combination Chest CT Scan	-	-	3.5%	2.7%
Follow-up Mammogram/Ultrasound	-	-	7.9%	8.8%
Lumbar Spine MRI for Low Back Pain	-	-	32.2%	37.2%

Clarinda Regional Health Center

220 Essie Davison Drive
Clarinda, IA 51632
Phone: 712-542-2176
Fax: 712-542-3380
E-mail: rudys@clarinda.heartland.net
URL: www.clarindahealth.com
Type: Critical Access Hospitals
Emergency Services: Yes
Ownership: Government - Local
Beds: 47

Key Personnel:
Quality Assurance . . . . Janice Brown
Chief of Medical Staff . . . . Robert Clemons
Radiology . . . . Greg Jones
Emergency Room . . . . Cris Meacham
Chair/CEO . . . . Ron Richardson
CEO/President . . . . Chris Stipe
Operating Room . . . . Jan Weakly

Measure	Cases	This Hosp.	State Avg.	U.S. Avg.
Blood Clot Prevention and Treatment				
Anticoagulation Overlap Therapy[5]	-	-	94%	93%
ICU Venous Thromboembolism Prophylaxis[5]	-	-	90%	92%
Incidence of Potentially Preventable VTE[5]	-	-	8%	10%
UFH with Dosages/Platelet Monitoring[5]	-	-	99%	97%
Venous Thromboembolism Prophylaxis[5]	-	-	87%	85%
Warfarin Therapy Discharge Instructions[5]	-	-	77%	75%
Chest Pain/Possible Heart Attack Care				
Aspirin Given Within 24 Hours of Arrival[5]	-	-	97%	96%
Fibrinolytic Meds Within 30 Min. of Arrival[5]	-	-	49%	58%
Average Time to ECG (minutes)[5]	-	-	5	7
Average Time to Transfer (minutes)[5]	-	-	58	60
Children's Asthma Care				
Received Home Management Plan of Care	-	-	-	88%
Received Reliever Medication	-	-	-	100%
Received Systemic Corticosteroids	-	-	-	100%
Emergency Department				
Admittance Decision Time (minutes)[5]	-	-	58	98
Head CT Results Within 45 Min. of Arrival[5]	-	-	55%	57%
Patients Who Left ER Before Being Seen[5]	-	-	1%	2%
Time from ER Arrival to Admit. (minutes)[5]	-	-	202	274
Time from ER Arrival to Discharge (minutes)[5]	-	-	108	134
Time in ER Before Being Evaluated (minutes)[5]	-	-	21	26
Time to Pain Meds for Fractures (minutes)[5]	-	-	46	57
Heart Attack Care				
Aspirin Given at Discharge[5]	-	-	100%	99%
Fibrinolytic Meds Within 30 Min. of Arrival[5]	-	-	-	54%
PCI Within 90 Minutes of Arrival[5]	-	-	94%	96%
Statin Prescribed at Discharge[5]	-	-	98%	98%
Heart Failure Care				
ACE Inhibitor or ARB for LVSD[1,3]	-	-	95%	97%
Discharge Instructions Given[3]	22	95%	93%	94%
Evaluation of LVS Function[3]	32	62%	97%	99%
Medicare Spending				
Medicare Spending per Patient (ratio)	-	-	0.91	0.98
Pneumonia Care				
Appropriate Initial Antibiotic Given[3]	34	88%	93%	95%
Blood Culture Timing[3]	21	95%	98%	98%
Pregnancy and Delivery Care				
Newborn Deliveries Scheduled Early[5]	-	-	4%	6%
Preventive Care				
Immunization for Influenza[5]	-	-	91%	90%
Immunization for Pneumonia[5]	-	-	90%	92%
Stroke Care				
Anticoagulation Therapy for Atrial Fibrillation[5]	-	-	95%	95%
Antithrombotic Therapy Timing[5]	-	-	98%	98%
Assessed for Rehabilitation[5]	-	-	97%	97%
Discharged on Antithrombotic Therapy[5]	-	-	99%	99%
Discharged on Statin Medication[5]	-	-	92%	94%
Thrombolytic Therapy Timing[5]	-	-	64%	66%
Venous Thromboembolism Prophylaxis[5]	-	-	93%	94%
Written Stroke Educational Materials Given[5]	-	-	82%	88%
Surgical Care Improvement Project				
Appropriate Beta Blocker Usage[5]	-	-	98%	98%
Appropriate VTP Within 24 Hours[5]	-	-	98%	98%
Controlled Postoperative Blood Glucose[5]	-	-	96%	97%
Perioperative Temperature Management[5]	-	-	100%	100%
Prophylactic Antibiotic Selection[5]	-	-	99%	99%
Prophylactic Antibiotic Selection (Outpatient)[5]	-	-	98%	98%
Prophylactic Antibiotic Stopped[5]	-	-	98%	98%
Prophylactic Antibiotic Timing[5]	-	-	98%	99%
Prophylactic Antibiotic Timing (Outpatient)[5]	-	-	98%	98%
Urinary Catheter Removal[5]	-	-	97%	97%
Survey of Patients' Hospital Experiences				
Area Around Room 'Always' Quiet at Night	(a)	73%	63%	61%
Doctors 'Always' Communicated Well	(a)	83%	84%	82%
Home Recovery Information Given	(a)	84%	88%	85%
Hospital Given 9 or 10 on 10 Point Scale	(a)	74%	75%	71%
Meds 'Always' Explained Before Given	(a)	60%	66%	64%
Nurses 'Always' Communicated Well	(a)	80%	81%	79%
Pain 'Always' Well Controlled	(a)	73%	71%	71%
Room and Bathroom 'Always' Clean	(a)	80%	79%	73%
Timely Help 'Always' Received	(a)	72%	70%	68%
Would Definitely Recommend Hospital	(a)	66%	74%	71%
Use of Medical Imaging				
Cardiac Imaging Stress Test before Surgery[1]	-	-	4.8%	5.3%
Combination Abdominal CT Scan	175	10.9%	11.5%	10.5%
Combination Brain/Sinus CT Scan	186	1.1%	1.8%	2.7%
Combination Chest CT Scan	88	2.3%	3.5%	2.7%
Follow-up Mammogram/Ultrasound	262	5.3%	7.9%	8.8%
Lumbar Spine MRI for Low Back Pain[1]	-	-	32.2%	37.2%

Iowa Specialty Hospital - Clarion

1316 South Main Street
Clarion, IA 50525
Phone: 515-532-2811
Fax: 515-532-3443
E-mail: wmc@wrightmed.com
URL: www.wrightmed.com
Type: Critical Access Hospitals
Emergency Services: Yes
Ownership: Government - Local
Beds: 25

Key Personnel:
Quality Assurance . . . . Nancy Bakker, RN
Radiology . . . . Abby Kirstein
Operating Room . . . . Robin Meyer, RN
Patient Relations . . . . Annette Odlando
Emergency Room . . . . Vinnette PA-C, PA-C
CEO . . . . Steve Simonin
Chief of Medical Staff . . . . Dustin Smith, MD
Infection Control . . . . Tara Wagner, RN

Measure	Cases	This Hosp.	State Avg.	U.S. Avg.
Blood Clot Prevention and Treatment				
Anticoagulation Overlap Therapy[5]	-	-	94%	93%
ICU Venous Thromboembolism Prophylaxis[5]	-	-	90%	92%
Incidence of Potentially Preventable VTE[5]	-	-	8%	10%
UFH with Dosages/Platelet Monitoring[5]	-	-	99%	97%
Venous Thromboembolism Prophylaxis[5]	-	-	87%	85%
Warfarin Therapy Discharge Instructions[5]	-	-	77%	75%
Chest Pain/Possible Heart Attack Care				
Aspirin Given Within 24 Hours of Arrival[1,3]	-	-	97%	96%
Fibrinolytic Meds Within 30 Min. of Arrival[5]	-	-	49%	58%
Average Time to ECG (minutes)[1,3]	-	-	5	7
Average Time to Transfer (minutes)[5]	-	-	58	60
Children's Asthma Care				
Received Home Management Plan of Care	-	-	-	88%
Received Reliever Medication	-	-	-	100%
Received Systemic Corticosteroids	-	-	-	100%
Emergency Department				
Admittance Decision Time (minutes)[5]	-	-	58	98
Head CT Results Within 45 Min. of Arrival[5]	-	-	55%	57%

NOTE: Hospital profiles are in alphabetical order by state, then city, then hospital within the city; Rankings exclude hospitals with less than 25 cases except for patient surveys which excludes hospitals with less than 100 cases; (a) 100-299 cases; (1) The number of cases/patients is too few to report; (2) Data submitted were based on a sample of cases/patients; (3) Results are based on a shorter time period than required; (4) Data suppressed by CMS for one or more quarters; (5) Results are not available for this reporting period; (6) Fewer than 100 patients completed the HCAHPS survey; (7) No cases met the criteria for this measure; (8) The lower limit of the confidence interval cannot be calculated if the number of observed infections equals zero; (9) No data are available from the state/territory for this reporting period; (10) The scores shown reflect fewer than 50 completed surveys; (11) There were discrepancies in the data collection process; (12) This measure does not apply to this hospital for this reporting period; (13) Results cannot be calculated for this reporting period; (14) The results for this state are combined with nearby states to protect confidentiality; Please refer to the User's Guide for a full explanation of data.

Measure	Cases	This Hosp.	State Avg.	U.S. Avg.
Patients Who Left ER Before Being Seen[5]	-	-	1%	2%
Time from ER Arrival to Admit. (minutes)[5]	-	-	202	274
Time from ER Arrival to Discharge (minutes)[5]	-	-	108	134
Time in ER Before Being Evaluated (minutes)[5]	-	-	21	26
Time to Pain Meds for Fractures (minutes)[5]	-	-	46	57
Heart Attack Care				
Aspirin Given at Discharge[5]	-	-	100%	99%
Fibrinolytic Meds Within 30 Min. of Arrival[5]	-	-	-	54%
PCI Within 90 Minutes of Arrival[5]	-	-	94%	96%
Statin Prescribed at Discharge[5]	-	-	98%	98%
Heart Failure Care				
ACE Inhibitor or ARB for LVSD[5]	-	-	95%	97%
Discharge Instructions Given[5]	-	-	93%	94%
Evaluation of LVS Function[5]	-	-	97%	99%
Medicare Spending				
Medicare Spending per Patient (ratio)	-	-	0.91	0.98
Pneumonia Care				
Appropriate Initial Antibiotic Given[1,2]	-	-	93%	95%
Blood Culture Timing[2]	28	68%	98%	98%
Pregnancy and Delivery Care				
Newborn Deliveries Scheduled Early[5]	-	-	4%	6%
Preventive Care				
Immunization for Influenza[5]	-	-	91%	90%
Immunization for Pneumonia[5]	-	-	90%	92%
Stroke Care				
Anticoagulation Therapy for Atrial Fibrillation[5]	-	-	95%	95%
Antithrombotic Therapy Timing[5]	-	-	98%	98%
Assessed for Rehabilitation[5]	-	-	97%	97%
Discharged on Antithrombotic Therapy[5]	-	-	99%	99%
Discharged on Statin Medication[5]	-	-	92%	94%
Thrombolytic Therapy Timing[5]	-	-	64%	66%
Venous Thromboembolism Prophylaxis[5]	-	-	93%	94%
Written Stroke Educational Materials Given[5]	-	-	82%	88%
Surgical Care Improvement Project				
Appropriate Beta Blocker Usage	54	100%	98%	98%
Appropriate VTP Within 24 Hours	210	99%	98%	98%
Controlled Postoperative Blood Glucose[7]	-	-	96%	97%
Perioperative Temperature Management	236	100%	100%	100%
Prophylactic Antibiotic Selection	29	93%	99%	99%
Prophylactic Antibiotic Selection (Outpatient)[5]	-	-	98%	98%
Prophylactic Antibiotic Stopped	29	93%	98%	98%
Prophylactic Antibiotic Timing	29	93%	98%	99%
Prophylactic Antibiotic Timing (Outpatient)[5]	-	-	98%	98%
Urinary Catheter Removal[1]	-	-	97%	97%
Survey of Patients' Hospital Experiences				
Area Around Room 'Always' Quiet at Night	300+	69%	63%	61%
Doctors 'Always' Communicated Well	300+	87%	84%	82%
Home Recovery Information Given	300+	88%	88%	85%
Hospital Given 9 or 10 on 10 Point Scale	300+	84%	75%	71%
Meds 'Always' Explained Before Given	300+	71%	66%	64%
Nurses 'Always' Communicated Well	300+	84%	81%	79%
Pain 'Always' Well Controlled	300+	75%	71%	71%
Room and Bathroom 'Always' Clean	300+	85%	79%	73%
Timely Help 'Always' Received	300+	74%	70%	68%
Would Definitely Recommend Hospital	300+	82%	74%	71%
Use of Medical Imaging				
Cardiac Imaging Stress Test before Surgery	88	3.4%	4.8%	5.3%
Combination Abdominal CT Scan	170	55.3%	11.5%	10.5%
Combination Brain/Sinus CT Scan[1]	-	-	1.8%	2.7%
Combination Chest CT Scan	100	41.0%	3.5%	2.7%
Follow-up Mammogram/Ultrasound	330	11.5%	7.9%	8.8%
Lumbar Spine MRI for Low Back Pain	66	36.4%	32.2%	37.2%

Mercy Medical Center - Clinton

1410 North 4th Street
Clinton, IA 52732
URL: www.mercyclinton.com
Phone: 563-244-5555
Fax: 563-244-5592
Type: Acute Care Hospitals
Ownership: Voluntary non-profit - Church
Emergency Services: Yes
Beds: 359

Key Personnel:
Operating Room. . . . . Kim Bush
Radiology. . . . . Juergen Holl, MD
Quality Assurance . . . . Lisa Hoppe
CEO/President. . . . . Donna Oliver

Measure	Cases	This Hosp.	State Avg.	U.S. Avg.
Blood Clot Prevention and Treatment				
Anticoagulation Overlap Therapy[2]	40	90%	94%	93%
ICU Venous Thromboembolism Prophylaxis[2]	98	93%	90%	92%
Incidence of Potentially Preventable VTE[1,2]	-	-	8%	10%
UFH with Dosages/Platelet Monitoring[2]	34	100%	99%	97%
Venous Thromboembolism Prophylaxis[2]	337	93%	87%	85%
Warfarin Therapy Discharge Instructions[2]	26	77%	77%	75%
Chest Pain/Possible Heart Attack Care				
Aspirin Given Within 24 Hours of Arrival	24	88%	97%	96%
Fibrinolytic Meds Within 30 Min. of Arrival[3,7]	-	-	49%	58%
Average Time to ECG (minutes)	28	4	5	7
Average Time to Transfer (minutes)[3,7]	-	-	58	60
Children's Asthma Care				
Received Home Management Plan of Care	-	-	-	88%
Received Reliever Medication	-	-	-	100%
Received Systemic Corticosteroids	-	-	-	100%
Emergency Department				
Admittance Decision Time (minutes)[2]	527	49	58	98
Head CT Results Within 45 Min. of Arrival	35	66%	55%	57%
Patients Who Left ER Before Being Seen	23,318	1%	1%	2%
Time from ER Arrival to Admit. (minutes)[2]	568	186	202	274
Time from ER Arrival to Discharge (minutes)	326	116	108	134
Time in ER Before Being Evaluated (minutes)	430	5	21	26
Time to Pain Meds for Fractures (minutes)	114	48	46	57
Heart Attack Care				
Aspirin Given at Discharge[2]	111	100%	100%	99%
Fibrinolytic Meds Within 30 Min. of Arrival[2,7]	-	-	-	54%
PCI Within 90 Minutes of Arrival[2]	22	100%	94%	96%
Statin Prescribed at Discharge[2]	103	99%	98%	98%
Heart Failure Care				
ACE Inhibitor or ARB for LVSD	23	100%	95%	97%
Discharge Instructions Given	81	99%	93%	94%
Evaluation of LVS Function	120	100%	97%	99%
Medicare Spending				
Medicare Spending per Patient (ratio)	-	0.99	0.91	0.98
Pneumonia Care				
Appropriate Initial Antibiotic Given[2]	136	99%	93%	95%
Blood Culture Timing[2]	207	99%	98%	98%
Pregnancy and Delivery Care				
Newborn Deliveries Scheduled Early	37	3%	4%	6%
Preventive Care				
Immunization for Influenza[2]	539	99%	91%	90%
Immunization for Pneumonia[2]	731	99%	90%	92%
Stroke Care				
Anticoagulation Therapy for Atrial Fibrillation[1,2]	-	-	95%	95%
Antithrombotic Therapy Timing[2]	15	100%	98%	98%
Assessed for Rehabilitation[2]	15	100%	97%	97%
Discharged on Antithrombotic Therapy[2]	13	100%	99%	99%
Discharged on Statin Medication[1,2]	-	-	92%	94%
Thrombolytic Therapy Timing[1,2]	-	-	64%	66%
Venous Thromboembolism Prophylaxis[2]	16	100%	93%	94%
Written Stroke Educational Materials Given[1,2]	-	-	82%	88%
Surgical Care Improvement Project				
Appropriate Beta Blocker Usage	72	100%	98%	98%
Appropriate VTP Within 24 Hours	148	100%	98%	98%
Controlled Postoperative Blood Glucose[7]	-	-	96%	97%
Perioperative Temperature Management	175	99%	100%	100%
Prophylactic Antibiotic Selection	107	99%	99%	99%
Prophylactic Antibiotic Selection (Outpatient)	79	97%	98%	98%
Prophylactic Antibiotic Stopped	103	100%	98%	98%
Prophylactic Antibiotic Timing	107	98%	98%	99%
Prophylactic Antibiotic Timing (Outpatient)	79	100%	98%	98%
Urinary Catheter Removal	123	100%	97%	97%
Survey of Patients' Hospital Experiences				
Area Around Room 'Always' Quiet at Night	300+	59%	63%	61%
Doctors 'Always' Communicated Well	300+	79%	84%	82%
Home Recovery Information Given	300+	87%	88%	85%
Hospital Given 9 or 10 on 10 Point Scale	300+	69%	75%	71%
Meds 'Always' Explained Before Given	300+	63%	66%	64%
Nurses 'Always' Communicated Well	300+	80%	81%	79%
Pain 'Always' Well Controlled	300+	68%	71%	71%
Room and Bathroom 'Always' Clean	300+	69%	79%	73%
Timely Help 'Always' Received	300+	64%	70%	68%
Would Definitely Recommend Hospital	300+	64%	74%	71%
Use of Medical Imaging				
Cardiac Imaging Stress Test before Surgery	106	4.7%	4.8%	5.3%
Combination Abdominal CT Scan	232	0.4%	11.5%	10.5%
Combination Brain/Sinus CT Scan	467	1.7%	1.8%	2.7%
Combination Chest CT Scan	100	3.0%	3.5%	2.7%
Follow-up Mammogram/Ultrasound	415	9.4%	7.9%	8.8%
Lumbar Spine MRI for Low Back Pain[1]	-	-	32.2%	37.2%

Alegent Health Mercy Hospital

603 Rosary Drive
Corning, IA 50841
URL: www.alegent.com
Phone: 641-322-3121
Fax: 641-322-3616
Type: Critical Access Hospitals
Ownership: Voluntary non-profit - Private
Emergency Services: Yes
Beds: 22

Key Personnel:
Emergency Room . . . . Richard Alarid
Cardiac Laboratory. . . . . Rosy Bissell
CEO/President. . . . . Richard Rolston, M.D., F.A.A.P.

Measure	Cases	This Hosp.	State Avg.	U.S. Avg.
Blood Clot Prevention and Treatment				
Anticoagulation Overlap Therapy[1,3]	-	-	94%	93%
ICU Venous Thromboembolism Prophylaxis[3,7]	-	-	90%	92%
Incidence of Potentially Preventable VTE[3,7]	-	-	8%	10%
UFH with Dosages/Platelet Monitoring[3,7]	-	-	99%	97%
Venous Thromboembolism Prophylaxis[3]	56	95%	87%	85%
Warfarin Therapy Discharge Instructions[1,3]	-	-	77%	75%
Chest Pain/Possible Heart Attack Care				
Aspirin Given Within 24 Hours of Arrival	14	100%	97%	96%
Fibrinolytic Meds Within 30 Min. of Arrival[7]	-	-	49%	58%
Average Time to ECG (minutes)	13	9	5	7
Average Time to Transfer (minutes)[7]	-	-	58	60
Children's Asthma Care				
Received Home Management Plan of Care	-	-	-	88%
Received Reliever Medication	-	-	-	100%
Received Systemic Corticosteroids	-	-	-	100%
Emergency Department				
Admittance Decision Time (minutes)[5]	-	-	58	98
Head CT Results Within 45 Min. of Arrival[5]	-	-	55%	57%
Patients Who Left ER Before Being Seen[5]	-	-	1%	2%
Time from ER Arrival to Admit. (minutes)[5]	-	-	202	274
Time from ER Arrival to Discharge (minutes)[5]	-	-	108	134
Time in ER Before Being Evaluated (minutes)[5]	-	-	21	26
Time to Pain Meds for Fractures (minutes)[5]	-	-	46	57
Heart Attack Care				
Aspirin Given at Discharge[1,3]	-	-	100%	99%
Fibrinolytic Meds Within 30 Min. of Arrival[3,7]	-	-	-	54%
PCI Within 90 Minutes of Arrival[3,7]	-	-	94%	96%
Statin Prescribed at Discharge[1,3]	-	-	98%	98%
Heart Failure Care				
ACE Inhibitor or ARB for LVSD[1]	-	-	95%	97%
Discharge Instructions Given[1]	-	-	93%	94%
Evaluation of LVS Function[1]	-	-	97%	99%
Medicare Spending				
Medicare Spending per Patient (ratio)	-	-	0.91	0.98
Pneumonia Care				
Appropriate Initial Antibiotic Given	13	100%	93%	95%
Blood Culture Timing[1]	-	-	98%	98%
Pregnancy and Delivery Care				
Newborn Deliveries Scheduled Early[5]	-	-	4%	6%
Preventive Care				
Immunization for Influenza[5]	-	-	91%	90%
Immunization for Pneumonia[5]	-	-	90%	92%
Stroke Care				
Anticoagulation Therapy for Atrial Fibrillation[5]	-	-	95%	95%
Antithrombotic Therapy Timing[5]	-	-	98%	98%
Assessed for Rehabilitation[5]	-	-	97%	97%
Discharged on Antithrombotic Therapy[5]	-	-	99%	99%
Discharged on Statin Medication[5]	-	-	92%	94%
Thrombolytic Therapy Timing[5]	-	-	64%	66%
Venous Thromboembolism Prophylaxis[5]	-	-	93%	94%

NOTE: Hospital profiles are in alphabetical order by state, then city, then hospital within the city; Rankings exclude hospitals with less than 25 cases except for patient surveys which excludes hospitals with less than 100 cases; (a) 100-299 cases; (1) The number of cases/patients is too few to report; (2) Data submitted were based on a sample of cases/patients; (3) Results are based on a shorter time period than required; (4) Data suppressed by CMS for one or more quarters; (5) Results are not available for this reporting period; (6) Fewer than 100 patients completed the HCAHPS survey; (7) No cases met the criteria for this measure; (8) The lower limit of the confidence interval cannot be calculated if the number of observed infections equals zero; (9) No data are available from the state/territory for this reporting period; (10) The scores shown reflect fewer than 50 completed surveys; (11) There were discrepancies in the data collection process; (12) This measure does not apply to this hospital for this reporting period; (13) Results cannot be calculated for this reporting period; (14) The results for this state are combined with nearby states to protect confidentiality; Please refer to the User's Guide for a full explanation of data.

Measure	Cases	This Hosp.	State Avg.	U.S. Avg.
Written Stroke Educational Materials Given[5]	-	-	82%	88%
Surgical Care Improvement Project				
Appropriate Beta Blocker Usage[1]	-	-	98%	98%
Appropriate VTP Within 24 Hours[1]	-	-	98%	98%
Controlled Postoperative Blood Glucose[7]	-	-	96%	97%
Perioperative Temperature Management[1]	-	-	100%	100%
Prophylactic Antibiotic Selection[1]	-	-	99%	99%
Prophylactic Antibiotic Selection (Outpatient)[1,3]	-	-	98%	98%
Prophylactic Antibiotic Stopped[1]	-	-	98%	98%
Prophylactic Antibiotic Timing[1]	-	-	98%	99%
Prophylactic Antibiotic Timing (Outpatient)[1,3]	-	-	98%	98%
Urinary Catheter Removal[1]	-	-	97%	97%
Survey of Patients' Hospital Experiences				
Area Around Room 'Always' Quiet at Night[6]	<100	74%	63%	61%
Doctors 'Always' Communicated Well[6]	<100	87%	84%	82%
Home Recovery Information Given[6]	<100	95%	88%	85%
Hospital Given 9 or 10 on 10 Point Scale[6]	<100	84%	75%	71%
Meds 'Always' Explained Before Given[6]	<100	67%	66%	64%
Nurses 'Always' Communicated Well[6]	<100	86%	81%	79%
Pain 'Always' Well Controlled[6]	<100	79%	71%	71%
Room and Bathroom 'Always' Clean[6]	<100	81%	79%	73%
Timely Help 'Always' Received[6]	<100	87%	70%	68%
Would Definitely Recommend Hospital[6]	<100	82%	74%	71%
Use of Medical Imaging				
Cardiac Imaging Stress Test before Surgery[1]	-	-	4.8%	5.3%
Combination Abdominal CT Scan	131	15.3%	11.5%	10.5%
Combination Brain/Sinus CT Scan[1]	-	-	1.8%	2.7%
Combination Chest CT Scan	80	17.5%	3.5%	2.7%
Follow-up Mammogram/Ultrasound	300	3.0%	7.9%	8.8%
Lumbar Spine MRI for Low Back Pain[1]	-	-	32.2%	37.2%

Wayne County Hospital

417 South East Street
Corydon, IA 50060
Type: Critical Access Hospitals
Ownership: Voluntary non-profit - Other
Phone: 641-872-2260
Fax: 641-872-3116
Emergency Services: Yes
Beds: 28

Key Personnel:
Coronary Care . . . . Martin Aronow
Chief of Medical Staff . . . . Joel Baker
Operating Room . . . . Carol Brown
Radiology . . . . Louis K Madison
Quality Assurance . . . . Kelli McCarty
Emergency Room . . . . Daren PS
CEO . . . . Daren L. Relph, PS-CCP

Measure	Cases	This Hosp.	State Avg.	U.S. Avg.
Blood Clot Prevention and Treatment				
Anticoagulation Overlap Therapy[5]	-	-	94%	93%
ICU Venous Thromboembolism Prophylaxis[5]	-	-	90%	92%
Incidence of Potentially Preventable VTE[5]	-	-	8%	10%
UFH with Dosages/Platelet Monitoring[5]	-	-	99%	97%
Venous Thromboembolism Prophylaxis[5]	-	-	87%	85%
Warfarin Therapy Discharge Instructions[5]	-	-	77%	75%
Chest Pain/Possible Heart Attack Care				
Aspirin Given Within 24 Hours of Arrival[5]	-	-	97%	96%
Fibrinolytic Meds Within 30 Min. of Arrival[5]	-	-	49%	58%
Average Time to ECG (minutes)[5]	-	-	5	7
Average Time to Transfer (minutes)[5]	-	-	58	60
Children's Asthma Care				
Received Home Management Plan of Care	-	-	-	88%
Received Reliever Medication	-	-	-	100%
Received Systemic Corticosteroids	-	-	-	100%
Emergency Department				
Admittance Decision Time (minutes)[5]	-	-	58	98
Head CT Results Within 45 Min. of Arrival[5]	-	-	55%	57%
Patients Who Left ER Before Being Seen[5]	-	-	1%	2%
Time from ER Arrival to Admit. (minutes)[5]	-	-	202	274
Time from ER Arrival to Discharge (minutes)[5]	-	-	108	134
Time in ER Before Being Evaluated (minutes)[5]	-	-	21	26
Time to Pain Meds for Fractures (minutes)[5]	-	-	46	57
Heart Attack Care				
Aspirin Given at Discharge[5]	-	-	100%	99%
Fibrinolytic Meds Within 30 Min. of Arrival[5]	-	-	-	54%
PCI Within 90 Minutes of Arrival[5]	-	-	94%	96%
Statin Prescribed at Discharge[5]	-	-	98%	98%
Heart Failure Care				
ACE Inhibitor or ARB for LVSD[1,3]	-	-	95%	97%
Discharge Instructions Given[1,3]	-	-	93%	94%
Evaluation of LVS Function[1,3]	-	-	97%	99%
Medicare Spending				
Medicare Spending per Patient (ratio)	-	-	0.91	0.98
Pneumonia Care				
Appropriate Initial Antibiotic Given[1,3]	-	-	93%	95%
Blood Culture Timing[1,3]	-	-	98%	98%
Pregnancy and Delivery Care				
Newborn Deliveries Scheduled Early[5]	-	-	4%	6%
Preventive Care				
Immunization for Influenza[5]	-	-	91%	90%
Immunization for Pneumonia[5]	-	-	90%	92%
Stroke Care				
Anticoagulation Therapy for Atrial Fibrillation[5]	-	-	95%	95%
Antithrombotic Therapy Timing[5]	-	-	98%	98%
Assessed for Rehabilitation[5]	-	-	97%	97%
Discharged on Antithrombotic Therapy[5]	-	-	99%	99%
Discharged on Statin Medication[5]	-	-	92%	94%
Thrombolytic Therapy Timing[5]	-	-	64%	66%
Venous Thromboembolism Prophylaxis[5]	-	-	93%	94%
Written Stroke Educational Materials Given[5]	-	-	82%	88%
Surgical Care Improvement Project				
Appropriate Beta Blocker Usage[1,3]	-	-	98%	98%
Appropriate VTP Within 24 Hours[1,3]	-	-	98%	98%
Controlled Postoperative Blood Glucose[3,7]	-	-	96%	97%
Perioperative Temperature Management[1,3]	-	-	100%	100%
Prophylactic Antibiotic Selection[1,3]	-	-	99%	99%
Prophylactic Antibiotic Selection (Outpatient)[5]	-	-	98%	98%
Prophylactic Antibiotic Stopped[1,3]	-	-	98%	98%
Prophylactic Antibiotic Timing[1,3]	-	-	98%	99%
Prophylactic Antibiotic Timing (Outpatient)[5]	-	-	98%	98%
Urinary Catheter Removal[1,3]	-	-	97%	97%
Survey of Patients' Hospital Experiences				
Area Around Room 'Always' Quiet at Night[5]	-	-	63%	61%
Doctors 'Always' Communicated Well[5]	-	-	84%	82%
Home Recovery Information Given[5]	-	-	88%	85%
Hospital Given 9 or 10 on 10 Point Scale[5]	-	-	75%	71%
Meds 'Always' Explained Before Given[5]	-	-	66%	64%
Nurses 'Always' Communicated Well[5]	-	-	81%	79%
Pain 'Always' Well Controlled[5]	-	-	71%	71%
Room and Bathroom 'Always' Clean[5]	-	-	79%	73%
Timely Help 'Always' Received[5]	-	-	70%	68%
Would Definitely Recommend Hospital[5]	-	-	74%	71%
Use of Medical Imaging				
Cardiac Imaging Stress Test before Surgery[1]	-	-	4.8%	5.3%
Combination Abdominal CT Scan	114	6.1%	11.5%	10.5%
Combination Brain/Sinus CT Scan[1]	-	-	1.8%	2.7%
Combination Chest CT Scan[1]	-	-	3.5%	2.7%
Follow-up Mammogram/Ultrasound	203	0.5%	7.9%	8.8%
Lumbar Spine MRI for Low Back Pain[1]	-	-	32.2%	37.2%

Alegent Health Mercy Hospital

800 Mercy Drive
Council Bluffs, IA 51503
URL: www.alegent.com/mercy
Type: Acute Care Hospitals
Ownership: Voluntary non-profit - Private
Phone: 712-328-5000
Fax: 712-328-5088
Emergency Services: Yes
Beds: 324

Key Personnel:
Operating Room . . . . Robin Allen
Quality Assurance . . . . Connie Blietz
Emergency Room . . . . Joe Hoagbin, MD
Radiology . . . . Matthew M Jaksha
CEO/President . . . . Cliff Robertson, MD, MBA
Chief of Medical Staff . . . . Cary Ward, MD

Measure	Cases	This Hosp.	State Avg.	U.S. Avg.
Blood Clot Prevention and Treatment				
Anticoagulation Overlap Therapy[2]	49	96%	94%	93%
ICU Venous Thromboembolism Prophylaxis[2]	53	98%	90%	92%
Incidence of Potentially Preventable VTE[1,2]	-	-	8%	10%
UFH with Dosages/Platelet Monitoring[2]	40	100%	99%	97%
Venous Thromboembolism Prophylaxis[2]	192	91%	87%	85%
Warfarin Therapy Discharge Instructions[2]	40	85%	77%	75%
Chest Pain/Possible Heart Attack Care				
Aspirin Given Within 24 Hours of Arrival[1,3]	-	-	97%	96%
Fibrinolytic Meds Within 30 Min. of Arrival[3,7]	-	-	49%	58%
Average Time to ECG (minutes)[1,3]	-	-	5	7
Average Time to Transfer (minutes)[3,7]	-	-	58	60
Children's Asthma Care				
Received Home Management Plan of Care	-	-	-	88%
Received Reliever Medication	-	-	-	100%
Received Systemic Corticosteroids	-	-	-	100%
Emergency Department				
Admittance Decision Time (minutes)[2]	430	54	58	98
Head CT Results Within 45 Min. of Arrival[1]	-	-	55%	57%
Patients Who Left ER Before Being Seen	30,713	0%	1%	2%
Time from ER Arrival to Admit. (minutes)[2]	444	172	202	274
Time from ER Arrival to Discharge (minutes)	381	110	108	134
Time in ER Before Being Evaluated (minutes)	306	37	21	26
Time to Pain Meds for Fractures (minutes)	80	44	46	57
Heart Attack Care				
Aspirin Given at Discharge	98	100%	100%	99%
Fibrinolytic Meds Within 30 Min. of Arrival[7]	-	-	-	54%
PCI Within 90 Minutes of Arrival	29	100%	94%	96%
Statin Prescribed at Discharge	96	99%	98%	98%
Heart Failure Care				
ACE Inhibitor or ARB for LVSD	22	100%	95%	97%
Discharge Instructions Given	87	99%	93%	94%
Evaluation of LVS Function	116	100%	97%	99%
Medicare Spending				
Medicare Spending per Patient (ratio)	-	0.93	0.91	0.98
Pneumonia Care				
Appropriate Initial Antibiotic Given	79	99%	93%	95%
Blood Culture Timing	131	100%	98%	98%
Pregnancy and Delivery Care				
Newborn Deliveries Scheduled Early[2]	21	0%	4%	6%
Preventive Care				
Immunization for Influenza[2]	581	97%	91%	90%
Immunization for Pneumonia[2]	495	94%	90%	92%
Stroke Care				
Anticoagulation Therapy for Atrial Fibrillation[1]	-	-	95%	95%
Antithrombotic Therapy Timing	37	100%	98%	98%
Assessed for Rehabilitation	53	100%	97%	97%
Discharged on Antithrombotic Therapy	44	100%	99%	99%
Discharged on Statin Medication	33	100%	92%	94%
Thrombolytic Therapy Timing[1]	-	-	64%	66%
Venous Thromboembolism Prophylaxis	50	96%	93%	94%
Written Stroke Educational Materials Given	36	100%	82%	88%
Surgical Care Improvement Project				
Appropriate Beta Blocker Usage[2]	122	99%	98%	98%
Appropriate VTP Within 24 Hours[2]	371	99%	98%	98%
Controlled Postoperative Blood Glucose[2,7]	-	-	96%	97%
Perioperative Temperature Management[2]	441	100%	100%	100%
Prophylactic Antibiotic Selection[2]	263	100%	99%	99%
Prophylactic Antibiotic Selection (Outpatient)	102	100%	98%	98%
Prophylactic Antibiotic Stopped[2]	249	100%	98%	98%
Prophylactic Antibiotic Timing[2]	263	100%	98%	99%
Prophylactic Antibiotic Timing (Outpatient)	103	99%	98%	98%
Urinary Catheter Removal[2]	255	99%	97%	97%
Survey of Patients' Hospital Experiences				
Area Around Room 'Always' Quiet at Night	300+	63%	63%	61%
Doctors 'Always' Communicated Well	300+	79%	84%	82%
Home Recovery Information Given	300+	89%	88%	85%
Hospital Given 9 or 10 on 10 Point Scale	300+	73%	75%	71%
Meds 'Always' Explained Before Given	300+	64%	66%	64%
Nurses 'Always' Communicated Well	300+	79%	81%	79%
Pain 'Always' Well Controlled	300+	71%	71%	71%
Room and Bathroom 'Always' Clean	300+	73%	79%	73%
Timely Help 'Always' Received	300+	61%	70%	68%
Would Definitely Recommend Hospital	300+	75%	74%	71%
Use of Medical Imaging				
Cardiac Imaging Stress Test before Surgery	346	4.6%	4.8%	5.3%
Combination Abdominal CT Scan	499	7.2%	11.5%	10.5%
Combination Brain/Sinus CT Scan[1]	-	-	1.8%	2.7%
Combination Chest CT Scan	229	0.0%	3.5%	2.7%

NOTE: Hospital profiles are in alphabetical order by state, then city, then hospital within the city; Rankings exclude hospitals with less than 25 cases except for patient surveys which excludes hospitals with less than 100 cases; (a) 100-299 cases; (1) The number of cases/patients is too few to report; (2) Data submitted were based on a sample of cases/patients; (3) Results are based on a shorter time period than required; (4) Data suppressed by CMS for one or more quarters; (5) Results are not available for this reporting period; (6) Fewer than 100 patients completed the HCAHPS survey; (7) No cases met the criteria for this measure; (8) The lower limit of the confidence interval cannot be calculated if the number of observed infections equals zero; (9) No data are available from the state/territory for this reporting period; (10) The scores shown reflect fewer than 50 completed surveys; (11) There were discrepancies in the data collection process; (12) This measure does not apply to this hospital for this reporting period; (13) Results cannot be calculated for this reporting period; (14) The results for this state are combined with nearby states to protect confidentiality; Please refer to the User's Guide for a full explanation of data.

Measure	Cases	This Hosp.	State Avg.	U.S. Avg.
Follow-up Mammogram/Ultrasound	849	3.5%	7.9%	8.8%
Lumbar Spine MRI for Low Back Pain	117	41.0%	32.2%	37.2%

Methodist Jennie Edmundson

933 East Pierce Street
Council Bluffs, IA 51503
Phone: 712-396-6000
Fax: 712-396-7617
URL: www.bestcare.org
Type: Acute Care Hospitals
Emergency Services: Yes
Ownership: Voluntary non-profit - Private
Beds: 118

Key Personnel:

Operating Room. . . . . Patrick Ahrens, RN
Radiology. . . . . Jason A Arthur
CEO/President. . . . . John M. Fraser
Quality Assurance . . . . Kathy Mashanic
Chief of Medical Staff. . . . . John A Okerbloom, MD

Measure	Cases	This Hosp.	State Avg.	U.S. Avg.
Blood Clot Prevention and Treatment				
Anticoagulation Overlap Therapy[2]	18	83%	94%	93%
ICU Venous Thromboembolism Prophylaxis[2]	108	95%	90%	92%
Incidence of Potentially Preventable VTE[1,2]	-	-	8%	10%
UFH with Dosages/Platelet Monitoring[1,2]	-	-	99%	97%
Venous Thromboembolism Prophylaxis[2]	402	92%	87%	85%
Warfarin Therapy Discharge Instructions[2]	14	100%	77%	75%
Chest Pain/Possible Heart Attack Care				
Aspirin Given Within 24 Hours of Arrival[1,3]	-	-	97%	96%
Fibrinolytic Meds Within 30 Min. of Arrival[5]	-	-	49%	58%
Average Time to ECG (minutes)[1,3]	-	-	5	7
Average Time to Transfer (minutes)[5]	-	-	58	60
Children's Asthma Care				
Received Home Management Plan of Care	-	-	-	88%
Received Reliever Medication	-	-	-	100%
Received Systemic Corticosteroids	-	-	-	100%
Emergency Department				
Admittance Decision Time (minutes)[2]	325	43	58	98
Head CT Results Within 45 Min. of Arrival[1]	-	-	55%	57%
Patients Who Left ER Before Being Seen	19,973	0%	1%	2%
Time from ER Arrival to Admit. (minutes)[2]	325	169	202	274
Time from ER Arrival to Discharge (minutes)	1,266	106	108	134
Time in ER Before Being Evaluated (minutes)	1,403	30	21	26
Time to Pain Meds for Fractures (minutes)	65	45	46	57
Heart Attack Care				
Aspirin Given at Discharge	97	100%	100%	99%
Fibrinolytic Meds Within 30 Min. of Arrival[7]	-	-	-	54%
PCI Within 90 Minutes of Arrival	16	88%	94%	96%
Statin Prescribed at Discharge	95	100%	98%	98%
Heart Failure Care				
ACE Inhibitor or ARB for LVSD	37	97%	95%	97%
Discharge Instructions Given	85	88%	93%	94%
Evaluation of LVS Function	122	99%	97%	99%
Medicare Spending				
Medicare Spending per Patient (ratio)	-	0.91	0.91	0.98
Pneumonia Care				
Appropriate Initial Antibiotic Given	86	95%	93%	95%
Blood Culture Timing	175	100%	98%	98%
Pregnancy and Delivery Care				
Newborn Deliveries Scheduled Early	26	0%	4%	6%
Preventive Care				
Immunization for Influenza[2]	372	83%	91%	90%
Immunization for Pneumonia[2]	510	74%	90%	92%
Stroke Care				
Anticoagulation Therapy for Atrial Fibrillation[1]	-	-	95%	95%
Antithrombotic Therapy Timing	34	100%	98%	98%
Assessed for Rehabilitation	39	97%	97%	97%
Discharged on Antithrombotic Therapy	35	100%	99%	99%
Discharged on Statin Medication	31	90%	92%	94%
Thrombolytic Therapy Timing[1]	-	-	64%	66%
Venous Thromboembolism Prophylaxis	43	93%	93%	94%
Written Stroke Educational Materials Given	18	100%	82%	88%
Surgical Care Improvement Project				
Appropriate Beta Blocker Usage	68	100%	98%	98%
Appropriate VTP Within 24 Hours	261	99%	98%	98%
Controlled Postoperative Blood Glucose[7]	-	-	96%	97%
Perioperative Temperature Management	322	100%	100%	100%
Prophylactic Antibiotic Selection	224	100%	99%	99%
Prophylactic Antibiotic Selection (Outpatient)	213	96%	98%	98%
Prophylactic Antibiotic Stopped	217	99%	98%	98%
Prophylactic Antibiotic Timing	225	98%	98%	99%
Prophylactic Antibiotic Timing (Outpatient)	217	95%	98%	98%
Urinary Catheter Removal	223	99%	97%	97%
Survey of Patients' Hospital Experiences				
Area Around Room 'Always' Quiet at Night	300+	55%	63%	61%
Doctors 'Always' Communicated Well	300+	87%	84%	82%
Home Recovery Information Given	300+	91%	88%	85%
Hospital Given 9 or 10 on 10 Point Scale	300+	73%	75%	71%
Meds 'Always' Explained Before Given	300+	67%	66%	64%
Nurses 'Always' Communicated Well	300+	81%	81%	79%
Pain 'Always' Well Controlled	300+	72%	71%	71%
Room and Bathroom 'Always' Clean	300+	71%	79%	73%
Timely Help 'Always' Received	300+	65%	70%	68%
Would Definitely Recommend Hospital	300+	76%	74%	71%
Use of Medical Imaging				
Cardiac Imaging Stress Test before Surgery	133	7.5%	4.8%	5.3%
Combination Abdominal CT Scan	540	4.1%	11.5%	10.5%
Combination Brain/Sinus CT Scan	380	0.8%	1.8%	2.7%
Combination Chest CT Scan	352	0.9%	3.5%	2.7%
Follow-up Mammogram/Ultrasound	1,156	10.9%	7.9%	8.8%
Lumbar Spine MRI for Low Back Pain	91	30.8%	32.2%	37.2%

Regional Health Services of Howard County

235 8th Avenue West
Cresco, IA 52136
Phone: 563-547-2101
Fax: 563-547-4223
URL: www.rhshc.com
Type: Critical Access Hospitals
Emergency Services: Yes
Ownership: Voluntary non-profit - Other
Beds: 32

Key Personnel:

Operating Room. . . . . Julie Andera
CEO/President. . . . . David J Hartberg
Quality Assurance . . . . Lois Reinhart
Chief of Medical Staff. . . . . Kathy Strike

Measure	Cases	This Hosp.	State Avg.	U.S. Avg.
Blood Clot Prevention and Treatment				
Anticoagulation Overlap Therapy[5]	-	-	94%	93%
ICU Venous Thromboembolism Prophylaxis[5]	-	-	90%	92%
Incidence of Potentially Preventable VTE[5]	-	-	8%	10%
UFH with Dosages/Platelet Monitoring[5]	-	-	99%	97%
Venous Thromboembolism Prophylaxis[5]	-	-	87%	85%
Warfarin Therapy Discharge Instructions[5]	-	-	77%	75%
Chest Pain/Possible Heart Attack Care				
Aspirin Given Within 24 Hours of Arrival	-	-	97%	96%
Fibrinolytic Meds Within 30 Min. of Arrival	-	-	49%	58%
Average Time to ECG (minutes)	-	-	5	7
Average Time to Transfer (minutes)	-	-	58	60
Children's Asthma Care				
Received Home Management Plan of Care	-	-	-	88%
Received Reliever Medication	-	-	-	100%
Received Systemic Corticosteroids	-	-	-	100%
Emergency Department				
Admittance Decision Time (minutes)[5]	-	-	58	98
Head CT Results Within 45 Min. of Arrival	-	-	55%	57%
Patients Who Left ER Before Being Seen	-	-	1%	2%
Time from ER Arrival to Admit. (minutes)[5]	-	-	202	274
Time from ER Arrival to Discharge (minutes)	-	-	108	134
Time in ER Before Being Evaluated (minutes)	-	-	21	26
Time to Pain Meds for Fractures (minutes)	-	-	46	57
Heart Attack Care				
Aspirin Given at Discharge[5]	-	-	100%	99%
Fibrinolytic Meds Within 30 Min. of Arrival[5]	-	-	-	54%
PCI Within 90 Minutes of Arrival[5]	-	-	94%	96%
Statin Prescribed at Discharge[5]	-	-	98%	98%
Heart Failure Care				
ACE Inhibitor or ARB for LVSD[3,7]	-	-	95%	97%
Discharge Instructions Given[3,7]	-	-	93%	94%
Evaluation of LVS Function[3,7]	-	-	97%	99%
Medicare Spending				
Medicare Spending per Patient (ratio)	-	-	0.91	0.98
Pneumonia Care				
Appropriate Initial Antibiotic Given[1,3]	-	-	93%	95%
Blood Culture Timing[3]	14	86%	98%	98%
Pregnancy and Delivery Care				
Newborn Deliveries Scheduled Early[5]	-	-	4%	6%
Preventive Care				
Immunization for Influenza[5]	-	-	91%	90%
Immunization for Pneumonia[5]	-	-	90%	92%
Stroke Care				
Anticoagulation Therapy for Atrial Fibrillation[5]	-	-	95%	95%
Antithrombotic Therapy Timing[5]	-	-	98%	98%
Assessed for Rehabilitation[5]	-	-	97%	97%
Discharged on Antithrombotic Therapy[5]	-	-	99%	99%
Discharged on Statin Medication[5]	-	-	92%	94%
Thrombolytic Therapy Timing[5]	-	-	64%	66%
Venous Thromboembolism Prophylaxis[5]	-	-	93%	94%
Written Stroke Educational Materials Given[5]	-	-	82%	88%
Surgical Care Improvement Project				
Appropriate Beta Blocker Usage[5]	-	-	98%	98%
Appropriate VTP Within 24 Hours[5]	-	-	98%	98%
Controlled Postoperative Blood Glucose[5]	-	-	96%	97%
Perioperative Temperature Management[5]	-	-	100%	100%
Prophylactic Antibiotic Selection[5]	-	-	99%	99%
Prophylactic Antibiotic Selection (Outpatient)	-	-	98%	98%
Prophylactic Antibiotic Stopped[5]	-	-	98%	98%
Prophylactic Antibiotic Timing[5]	-	-	98%	99%
Prophylactic Antibiotic Timing (Outpatient)	-	-	98%	98%
Urinary Catheter Removal[5]	-	-	97%	97%
Survey of Patients' Hospital Experiences				
Area Around Room 'Always' Quiet at Night[5]	-	-	63%	61%
Doctors 'Always' Communicated Well[5]	-	-	84%	82%
Home Recovery Information Given[5]	-	-	88%	85%
Hospital Given 9 or 10 on 10 Point Scale[5]	-	-	75%	71%
Meds 'Always' Explained Before Given[5]	-	-	66%	64%
Nurses 'Always' Communicated Well[5]	-	-	81%	79%
Pain 'Always' Well Controlled[5]	-	-	71%	71%
Room and Bathroom 'Always' Clean[5]	-	-	79%	73%
Timely Help 'Always' Received[5]	-	-	70%	68%
Would Definitely Recommend Hospital[5]	-	-	74%	71%
Use of Medical Imaging				
Cardiac Imaging Stress Test before Surgery	-	-	4.8%	5.3%
Combination Abdominal CT Scan	-	-	11.5%	10.5%
Combination Brain/Sinus CT Scan	-	-	1.8%	2.7%
Combination Chest CT Scan	-	-	3.5%	2.7%
Follow-up Mammogram/Ultrasound	-	-	7.9%	8.8%
Lumbar Spine MRI for Low Back Pain	-	-	32.2%	37.2%

Greater Regional Medical Center

1700 West Townline Road
Creston, IA 50801
Phone: 641-782-7091
Fax: 641-782-3866
Type: Critical Access Hospitals
Emergency Services: Yes
Ownership: Government - Local
Beds: 25

Key Personnel:

Anesthesiology. . . . . Greg Anderson, MSN, CRNA
Infection Control. . . . . Nancy Anthony
Quality Assurance . . . . Kenya Heffner
Radiology. . . . . Todd Kucera, MD
Surgery . . . . Robert Kuhl, MD
CEO/President. . . . . Monte Neitzel
Chief of Medical Staff. . . . . Steve Reeves, MD

Measure	Cases	This Hosp.	State Avg.	U.S. Avg.
Blood Clot Prevention and Treatment				
Anticoagulation Overlap Therapy[5]	-	-	94%	93%
ICU Venous Thromboembolism Prophylaxis[5]	-	-	90%	92%
Incidence of Potentially Preventable VTE[5]	-	-	8%	10%
UFH with Dosages/Platelet Monitoring[5]	-	-	99%	97%
Venous Thromboembolism Prophylaxis[5]	-	-	87%	85%
Warfarin Therapy Discharge Instructions[5]	-	-	77%	75%
Chest Pain/Possible Heart Attack Care				
Aspirin Given Within 24 Hours of Arrival[1,3]	-	-	97%	96%
Fibrinolytic Meds Within 30 Min. of Arrival[5]	-	-	49%	58%
Average Time to ECG (minutes)[1,3]	-	-	5	7
Average Time to Transfer (minutes)[5]	-	-	58	60
Children's Asthma Care				
Received Home Management Plan of Care	-	-	-	88%
Received Reliever Medication	-	-	-	100%

NOTE: Hospital profiles are in alphabetical order by state, then city, then hospital within the city; Rankings exclude hospitals with less than 25 cases except for patient surveys which excludes hospitals with less than 100 cases; (a) 100-299 cases; (1) The number of cases/patients is too few to report; (2) Data submitted were based on a sample of cases/patients; (3) Results are based on a shorter time period than required; (4) Data suppressed by CMS for one or more quarters; (5) Results are not available for this reporting period; (6) Fewer than 100 patients completed the HCAHPS survey; (7) No cases met the criteria for this measure; (8) The lower limit of the confidence interval cannot be calculated if the number of observed infections equals zero; (9) No data are available from the state/territory for this reporting period; (10) The scores shown reflect fewer than 50 completed surveys; (11) There were discrepancies in the data collection process; (12) This measure does not apply to this hospital for this reporting period; (13) Results cannot be calculated for this reporting period; (14) The results for this state are combined with nearby states to protect confidentiality; Please refer to the User's Guide for a full explanation of data.

Measure	Cases	This Hosp.	State Avg.	U.S. Avg.
Received Systemic Corticosteroids	-	-	-	100%
Emergency Department				
Admittance Decision Time (minutes)[5]	-	-	58	98
Head CT Results Within 45 Min. of Arrival[5]	-	-	55%	57%
Patients Who Left ER Before Being Seen[5]	-	-	1%	2%
Time from ER Arrival to Admit. (minutes)[5]	-	-	202	274
Time from ER Arrival to Discharge (minutes)[1,3]	-	-	108	134
Time in ER Before Being Evaluated (minutes)[3]	54	22	21	26
Time to Pain Meds for Fractures (minutes)[5]	-	-	46	57
Heart Attack Care				
Aspirin Given at Discharge[5]	-	-	100%	99%
Fibrinolytic Meds Within 30 Min. of Arrival[5]	-	-	-	54%
PCI Within 90 Minutes of Arrival[5]	-	-	94%	96%
Statin Prescribed at Discharge[5]	-	-	98%	98%
Heart Failure Care				
ACE Inhibitor or ARB for LVSD[5]	-	-	95%	97%
Discharge Instructions Given[5]	-	-	93%	94%
Evaluation of LVS Function[5]	-	-	97%	99%
Medicare Spending				
Medicare Spending per Patient (ratio)	-	-	0.91	0.98
Pneumonia Care				
Appropriate Initial Antibiotic Given[5]	-	-	93%	95%
Blood Culture Timing[5]	-	-	98%	98%
Pregnancy and Delivery Care				
Newborn Deliveries Scheduled Early[5]	-	-	4%	6%
Preventive Care				
Immunization for Influenza[5]	-	-	91%	90%
Immunization for Pneumonia[5]	-	-	90%	92%
Stroke Care				
Anticoagulation Therapy for Atrial Fibrillation[5]	-	-	95%	95%
Antithrombotic Therapy Timing[5]	-	-	98%	98%
Assessed for Rehabilitation[5]	-	-	97%	97%
Discharged on Antithrombotic Therapy[5]	-	-	99%	99%
Discharged on Statin Medication[5]	-	-	92%	94%
Thrombolytic Therapy Timing[5]	-	-	64%	66%
Venous Thromboembolism Prophylaxis[5]	-	-	93%	94%
Written Stroke Educational Materials Given[5]	-	-	82%	88%
Surgical Care Improvement Project				
Appropriate Beta Blocker Usage[5]	-	-	98%	98%
Appropriate VTP Within 24 Hours[5]	-	-	98%	98%
Controlled Postoperative Blood Glucose[5]	-	-	96%	97%
Perioperative Temperature Management[5]	-	-	100%	100%
Prophylactic Antibiotic Selection[5]	-	-	99%	99%
Prophylactic Antibiotic Selection (Outpatient)[5]	-	-	98%	98%
Prophylactic Antibiotic Stopped[5]	-	-	98%	98%
Prophylactic Antibiotic Timing[5]	-	-	98%	99%
Prophylactic Antibiotic Timing (Outpatient)[5]	-	-	98%	98%
Urinary Catheter Removal[5]	-	-	97%	97%
Survey of Patients' Hospital Experiences				
Area Around Room 'Always' Quiet at Night	(a)	71%	63%	61%
Doctors 'Always' Communicated Well	(a)	92%	84%	82%
Home Recovery Information Given	(a)	83%	88%	85%
Hospital Given 9 or 10 on 10 Point Scale	(a)	75%	75%	71%
Meds 'Always' Explained Before Given	(a)	67%	66%	64%
Nurses 'Always' Communicated Well	(a)	82%	81%	79%
Pain 'Always' Well Controlled	(a)	70%	71%	71%
Room and Bathroom 'Always' Clean	(a)	83%	79%	73%
Timely Help 'Always' Received	(a)	78%	70%	68%
Would Definitely Recommend Hospital	(a)	76%	74%	71%
Use of Medical Imaging				
Cardiac Imaging Stress Test before Surgery	73	2.7%	4.8%	5.3%
Combination Abdominal CT Scan	281	6.4%	11.5%	10.5%
Combination Brain/Sinus CT Scan[1]	-	-	1.8%	2.7%
Combination Chest CT Scan	164	1.8%	3.5%	2.7%
Follow-up Mammogram/Ultrasound	527	13.5%	7.9%	8.8%
Lumbar Spine MRI for Low Back Pain[1]	-	-	32.2%	37.2%

Genesis Medical Center - Davenport

1227 East Rusholme Street
Davenport, IA 52803
Phone: 563-421-1000
Fax: 563-421-6279
URL: www.genesishealth.com
Type: Acute Care Hospitals
Emergency Services: Yes
Ownership: Voluntary non-profit - Other
Beds: 502

Key Personnel:
Infection Control. . . . . Lisa Caffery
Pediatric Ambulatory Care . . . . . . Cindy Chapman
Quality Assurance . . . . Lori Crane
CEO/President. . . . . Doug Cropper
Chief of Medical Staff. . . . . Joseph Lohmuller, MD, MS, FACS
Operating Room. . . . . Rob Nelson, MD
Radiology. . . . . Janet Stensrud

Measure	Cases	This Hosp.	State Avg.	U.S. Avg.
Blood Clot Prevention and Treatment				
Anticoagulation Overlap Therapy[2]	143	94%	94%	93%
ICU Venous Thromboembolism Prophylaxis[2]	73	97%	90%	92%
Incidence of Potentially Preventable VTE[2]	18	11%	8%	10%
UFH with Dosages/Platelet Monitoring[2]	100	100%	99%	97%
Venous Thromboembolism Prophylaxis[2]	310	95%	87%	85%
Warfarin Therapy Discharge Instructions[2]	114	82%	77%	75%
Chest Pain/Possible Heart Attack Care				
Aspirin Given Within 24 Hours of Arrival[1]	-	-	97%	96%
Fibrinolytic Meds Within 30 Min. of Arrival[5]	-	-	49%	58%
Average Time to ECG (minutes)[1]	-	-	5	7
Average Time to Transfer (minutes)[5]	-	-	58	60
Children's Asthma Care				
Received Home Management Plan of Care	-	-	-	88%
Received Reliever Medication	-	-	-	100%
Received Systemic Corticosteroids	-	-	-	100%
Emergency Department				
Admittance Decision Time (minutes)[2]	375	83	58	98
Head CT Results Within 45 Min. of Arrival	11	64%	55%	57%
Patients Who Left ER Before Being Seen	77,039	1%	1%	2%
Time from ER Arrival to Admit. (minutes)[2]	433	250	202	274
Time from ER Arrival to Discharge (minutes)	387	129	108	134
Time in ER Before Being Evaluated (minutes)	404	30	21	26
Time to Pain Meds for Fractures (minutes)	154	54	46	57
Heart Attack Care				
Aspirin Given at Discharge[2]	294	100%	100%	99%
Fibrinolytic Meds Within 30 Min. of Arrival[2,7]	-	-	-	54%
PCI Within 90 Minutes of Arrival[2]	40	98%	94%	96%
Statin Prescribed at Discharge[2]	272	100%	98%	98%
Heart Failure Care				
ACE Inhibitor or ARB for LVSD[2]	82	100%	95%	97%
Discharge Instructions Given[2]	200	98%	93%	94%
Evaluation of LVS Function[2]	284	100%	97%	99%
Medicare Spending				
Medicare Spending per Patient (ratio)	-	0.94	0.91	0.98
Pneumonia Care				
Appropriate Initial Antibiotic Given[2]	101	100%	93%	95%
Blood Culture Timing[2]	153	100%	98%	98%
Pregnancy and Delivery Care				
Newborn Deliveries Scheduled Early[2]	30	7%	4%	6%
Preventive Care				
Immunization for Influenza[2]	542	95%	91%	90%
Immunization for Pneumonia[2]	722	95%	90%	92%
Stroke Care				
Anticoagulation Therapy for Atrial Fibrillation	40	100%	95%	95%
Antithrombotic Therapy Timing	174	99%	98%	98%
Assessed for Rehabilitation	213	100%	97%	97%
Discharged on Antithrombotic Therapy	205	100%	99%	99%
Discharged on Statin Medication	161	98%	92%	94%
Thrombolytic Therapy Timing	20	90%	64%	66%
Venous Thromboembolism Prophylaxis	204	96%	93%	94%
Written Stroke Educational Materials Given	122	85%	82%	88%
Surgical Care Improvement Project				
Appropriate Beta Blocker Usage[2]	222	99%	98%	98%
Appropriate VTP Within 24 Hours[2]	428	98%	98%	98%
Controlled Postoperative Blood Glucose[2]	110	95%	96%	97%
Perioperative Temperature Management[2]	552	100%	100%	100%
Prophylactic Antibiotic Selection[2]	456	100%	99%	99%
Prophylactic Antibiotic Selection (Outpatient)	540	99%	98%	98%
Prophylactic Antibiotic Stopped[2]	428	98%	98%	98%
Prophylactic Antibiotic Timing[2]	458	99%	98%	99%
Prophylactic Antibiotic Timing (Outpatient)	542	99%	98%	98%
Urinary Catheter Removal[2]	319	99%	97%	97%
Survey of Patients' Hospital Experiences				
Area Around Room 'Always' Quiet at Night	300+	49%	63%	61%
Doctors 'Always' Communicated Well	300+	78%	84%	82%
Home Recovery Information Given	300+	85%	88%	85%
Hospital Given 9 or 10 on 10 Point Scale	300+	70%	75%	71%
Meds 'Always' Explained Before Given	300+	64%	66%	64%
Nurses 'Always' Communicated Well	300+	79%	81%	79%
Pain 'Always' Well Controlled	300+	70%	71%	71%
Room and Bathroom 'Always' Clean	300+	75%	79%	73%
Timely Help 'Always' Received	300+	66%	70%	68%
Would Definitely Recommend Hospital	300+	72%	74%	71%
Use of Medical Imaging				
Cardiac Imaging Stress Test before Surgery	631	3.6%	4.8%	5.3%
Combination Abdominal CT Scan	1,292	1.2%	11.5%	10.5%
Combination Brain/Sinus CT Scan	1,083	1.2%	1.8%	2.7%
Combination Chest CT Scan	1,158	1.3%	3.5%	2.7%
Follow-up Mammogram/Ultrasound	3,817	8.3%	7.9%	8.8%
Lumbar Spine MRI for Low Back Pain	274	33.9%	32.2%	37.2%

Winneshiek Medical Center

901 Montgomery Street
Decorah, IA 52101
Phone: 563-382-2911
Fax: 563-387-3102
URL: www.winmedical.org
Type: Critical Access Hospitals
Emergency Services: Yes
Ownership: Government - Local
Beds: 83

Key Personnel:
Emergency Room . . . . Larry Barthel, MD
Emergency Room . . . . Tudy Belay
CEO/President. . . . . Ben Grimstad
Emergency Room . . . . Paul Jakopin
Radiology. . . . . David Jensen
Surgery . . . . Hamid Kakavandi, RN
Quality Assurance . . . . Linda Klimesh

Measure	Cases	This Hosp.	State Avg.	U.S. Avg.
Blood Clot Prevention and Treatment				
Anticoagulation Overlap Therapy[5]	-	-	94%	93%
ICU Venous Thromboembolism Prophylaxis[5]	-	-	90%	92%
Incidence of Potentially Preventable VTE[5]	-	-	8%	10%
UFH with Dosages/Platelet Monitoring[5]	-	-	99%	97%
Venous Thromboembolism Prophylaxis[5]	-	-	87%	85%
Warfarin Therapy Discharge Instructions[5]	-	-	77%	75%
Chest Pain/Possible Heart Attack Care				
Aspirin Given Within 24 Hours of Arrival	24	100%	97%	96%
Fibrinolytic Meds Within 30 Min. of Arrival[1]	-	-	49%	58%
Average Time to ECG (minutes)	26	8	5	7
Average Time to Transfer (minutes)[7]	-	-	58	60
Children's Asthma Care				
Received Home Management Plan of Care	-	-	-	88%
Received Reliever Medication	-	-	-	100%
Received Systemic Corticosteroids	-	-	-	100%
Emergency Department				
Admittance Decision Time (minutes)[5]	-	-	58	98
Head CT Results Within 45 Min. of Arrival[5]	-	-	55%	57%
Patients Who Left ER Before Being Seen	4,784	0%	1%	2%
Time from ER Arrival to Admit. (minutes)[5]	-	-	202	274
Time from ER Arrival to Discharge (minutes)[5]	-	-	108	134
Time in ER Before Being Evaluated (minutes)[5]	-	-	21	26
Time to Pain Meds for Fractures (minutes)[5]	-	-	46	57
Heart Attack Care				
Aspirin Given at Discharge[2]	13	100%	100%	99%
Fibrinolytic Meds Within 30 Min. of Arrival[2,7]	-	-	-	54%
PCI Within 90 Minutes of Arrival[2,7]	-	-	94%	96%
Statin Prescribed at Discharge[2]	11	91%	98%	98%
Heart Failure Care				
ACE Inhibitor or ARB for LVSD[1]	-	-	95%	97%
Discharge Instructions Given	15	100%	93%	94%
Evaluation of LVS Function	23	100%	97%	99%
Medicare Spending				
Medicare Spending per Patient (ratio)	-	-	0.91	0.98
Pneumonia Care				

NOTE: Hospital profiles are in alphabetical order by state, then city, then hospital within the city; Rankings exclude hospitals with less than 25 cases except for patient surveys which excludes hospitals with less than 100 cases; (a) 100-299 cases; (1) The number of cases/patients is too few to report; (2) Data submitted were based on a sample of cases/patients; (3) Results are based on a shorter time period than required; (4) Data suppressed by CMS for one or more quarters; (5) Results are not available for this reporting period; (6) Fewer than 100 patients completed the HCAHPS survey; (7) No cases met the criteria for this measure; (8) The lower limit of the confidence interval cannot be calculated if the number of observed infections equals zero; (9) No data are available from the state/territory for this reporting period; (10) The scores shown reflect fewer than 50 completed surveys; (11) There were discrepancies in the data collection process; (12) This measure does not apply to this hospital for this reporting period; (13) Results cannot be calculated for this reporting period; (14) The results for this state are combined with nearby states to protect confidentiality; Please refer to the User's Guide for a full explanation of data.

Measure	Cases	This Hosp.	State Avg.	U.S. Avg.
Appropriate Initial Antibiotic Given	39	100%	93%	95%
Blood Culture Timing	60	97%	98%	98%
Pregnancy and Delivery Care				
Newborn Deliveries Scheduled Early[5]	-	-	4%	6%
Preventive Care				
Immunization for Influenza[5]	-	-	91%	90%
Immunization for Pneumonia[5]	-	-	90%	92%
Stroke Care				
Anticoagulation Therapy for Atrial Fibrillation[5]	-	-	95%	95%
Antithrombotic Therapy Timing[5]	-	-	98%	98%
Assessed for Rehabilitation[5]	-	-	97%	97%
Discharged on Antithrombotic Therapy[5]	-	-	99%	99%
Discharged on Statin Medication[5]	-	-	92%	94%
Thrombolytic Therapy Timing[5]	-	-	64%	66%
Venous Thromboembolism Prophylaxis[5]	-	-	93%	94%
Written Stroke Educational Materials Given[5]	-	-	82%	88%
Surgical Care Improvement Project				
Appropriate Beta Blocker Usage	13	100%	98%	98%
Appropriate VTP Within 24 Hours	57	95%	98%	98%
Controlled Postoperative Blood Glucose[7]	-	-	96%	97%
Perioperative Temperature Management	65	100%	100%	100%
Prophylactic Antibiotic Selection	58	100%	99%	99%
Prophylactic Antibiotic Selection (Outpatient)	59	100%	98%	98%
Prophylactic Antibiotic Stopped	58	98%	98%	98%
Prophylactic Antibiotic Timing	58	97%	98%	99%
Prophylactic Antibiotic Timing (Outpatient)	27	93%	98%	98%
Urinary Catheter Removal	27	96%	97%	97%
Survey of Patients' Hospital Experiences				
Area Around Room 'Always' Quiet at Night	(a)	64%	63%	61%
Doctors 'Always' Communicated Well	(a)	85%	84%	82%
Home Recovery Information Given	(a)	88%	88%	85%
Hospital Given 9 or 10 on 10 Point Scale	(a)	73%	75%	71%
Meds 'Always' Explained Before Given	(a)	73%	66%	64%
Nurses 'Always' Communicated Well	(a)	79%	81%	79%
Pain 'Always' Well Controlled	(a)	67%	71%	71%
Room and Bathroom 'Always' Clean	(a)	84%	79%	73%
Timely Help 'Always' Received	(a)	66%	70%	68%
Would Definitely Recommend Hospital	(a)	75%	74%	71%
Use of Medical Imaging				
Cardiac Imaging Stress Test before Surgery[1]	-	-	4.8%	5.3%
Combination Abdominal CT Scan	198	14.6%	11.5%	10.5%
Combination Brain/Sinus CT Scan[1]	-	-	1.8%	2.7%
Combination Chest CT Scan	50	0.0%	3.5%	2.7%
Follow-up Mammogram/Ultrasound	374	1.1%	7.9%	8.8%
Lumbar Spine MRI for Low Back Pain[1]	-	-	32.2%	37.2%

Crawford County Memorial Hospital

100 Medical Parkway
Denison, IA 51442
Phone: 712-265-2500
Fax: 712-263-1711
E-mail: edgast@ccmhia.com
URL: www.ccmhia.com
Type: Critical Access Hospitals
Emergency Services: Yes
Ownership: Voluntary non-profit - Other
Beds: 72

Key Personnel:

Quality Assurance . . . . Nancy Bielenberg
Radiology. . . . . Kari Boyens
CEO . . . . Bill Bruce
Operating Room. . . . . Linda Christensen
Cardiology . . . . Venkata M.Alla, MD, BS
Emergency Room . . . . Laurie Powers

Measure	Cases	This Hosp.	State Avg.	U.S. Avg.
Blood Clot Prevention and Treatment				
Anticoagulation Overlap Therapy[5]	-	-	94%	93%
ICU Venous Thromboembolism Prophylaxis[5]	-	-	90%	92%
Incidence of Potentially Preventable VTE[5]	-	-	8%	10%
UFH with Dosages/Platelet Monitoring[5]	-	-	99%	97%
Venous Thromboembolism Prophylaxis[5]	-	-	87%	85%
Warfarin Therapy Discharge Instructions[5]	-	-	77%	75%
Chest Pain/Possible Heart Attack Care				
Aspirin Given Within 24 Hours of Arrival[5]	-	-	97%	96%
Fibrinolytic Meds Within 30 Min. of Arrival[5]	-	-	49%	58%
Average Time to ECG (minutes)[5]	-	-	5	7
Average Time to Transfer (minutes)[5]	-	-	58	60
Children's Asthma Care				
Received Home Management Plan of Care	-	-	-	88%
Received Reliever Medication	-	-	-	100%
Received Systemic Corticosteroids	-	-	-	100%
Emergency Department				
Admittance Decision Time (minutes)[5]	-	-	58	98
Head CT Results Within 45 Min. of Arrival[5]	-	-	55%	57%
Patients Who Left ER Before Being Seen[5]	-	-	1%	2%
Time from ER Arrival to Admit. (minutes)[5]	-	-	202	274
Time from ER Arrival to Discharge (minutes)[5]	-	-	108	134
Time in ER Before Being Evaluated (minutes)[5]	-	-	21	26
Time to Pain Meds for Fractures (minutes)[5]	-	-	46	57
Heart Attack Care				
Aspirin Given at Discharge[5]	-	-	100%	99%
Fibrinolytic Meds Within 30 Min. of Arrival[5]	-	-	-	54%
PCI Within 90 Minutes of Arrival[5]	-	-	94%	96%
Statin Prescribed at Discharge[5]	-	-	98%	98%
Heart Failure Care				
ACE Inhibitor or ARB for LVSD[5]	-	-	95%	97%
Discharge Instructions Given[5]	-	-	93%	94%
Evaluation of LVS Function[5]	-	-	97%	99%
Medicare Spending				
Medicare Spending per Patient (ratio)	-	-	0.91	0.98
Pneumonia Care				
Appropriate Initial Antibiotic Given[5]	-	-	93%	95%
Blood Culture Timing[5]	-	-	98%	98%
Pregnancy and Delivery Care				
Newborn Deliveries Scheduled Early[5]	-	-	4%	6%
Preventive Care				
Immunization for Influenza[5]	-	-	91%	90%
Immunization for Pneumonia[5]	-	-	90%	92%
Stroke Care				
Anticoagulation Therapy for Atrial Fibrillation[5]	-	-	95%	95%
Antithrombotic Therapy Timing[5]	-	-	98%	98%
Assessed for Rehabilitation[5]	-	-	97%	97%
Discharged on Antithrombotic Therapy[5]	-	-	99%	99%
Discharged on Statin Medication[5]	-	-	92%	94%
Thrombolytic Therapy Timing[5]	-	-	64%	66%
Venous Thromboembolism Prophylaxis[5]	-	-	93%	94%
Written Stroke Educational Materials Given[5]	-	-	82%	88%
Surgical Care Improvement Project				
Appropriate Beta Blocker Usage[5]	-	-	98%	98%
Appropriate VTP Within 24 Hours[5]	-	-	98%	98%
Controlled Postoperative Blood Glucose[5]	-	-	96%	97%
Perioperative Temperature Management[5]	-	-	100%	100%
Prophylactic Antibiotic Selection[5]	-	-	99%	99%
Prophylactic Antibiotic Selection (Outpatient)[5]	-	-	98%	98%
Prophylactic Antibiotic Stopped[5]	-	-	98%	98%
Prophylactic Antibiotic Timing[5]	-	-	98%	99%
Prophylactic Antibiotic Timing (Outpatient)[5]	-	-	98%	98%
Urinary Catheter Removal[5]	-	-	97%	97%
Survey of Patients' Hospital Experiences				
Area Around Room 'Always' Quiet at Night	(a)	68%	63%	61%
Doctors 'Always' Communicated Well	(a)	85%	84%	82%
Home Recovery Information Given	(a)	85%	88%	85%
Hospital Given 9 or 10 on 10 Point Scale	(a)	78%	75%	71%
Meds 'Always' Explained Before Given	(a)	71%	66%	64%
Nurses 'Always' Communicated Well	(a)	81%	81%	79%
Pain 'Always' Well Controlled	(a)	75%	71%	71%
Room and Bathroom 'Always' Clean	(a)	82%	79%	73%
Timely Help 'Always' Received	(a)	69%	70%	68%
Would Definitely Recommend Hospital	(a)	69%	74%	71%
Use of Medical Imaging				
Cardiac Imaging Stress Test before Surgery[1]	-	-	4.8%	5.3%
Combination Abdominal CT Scan	136	8.1%	11.5%	10.5%
Combination Brain/Sinus CT Scan[1]	-	-	1.8%	2.7%
Combination Chest CT Scan	84	15.5%	3.5%	2.7%
Follow-up Mammogram/Ultrasound	379	9.5%	7.9%	8.8%
Lumbar Spine MRI for Low Back Pain	47	44.7%	32.2%	37.2%

Broadlawns Medical Center

1801 Hickman Road
Des Moines, IA 50314
Phone: 515-282-2200
Fax: 515-282-5785
E-mail: externalrelations@broadlawns.org
URL: www.broadlawns.org
Type: Acute Care Hospitals
Emergency Services: Yes
Ownership: Voluntary non-profit - Other
Beds: 200

Key Personnel:

Operating Room. . . . . Dapka Baccam
Emergency Room . . . . Ryan Bakke, DO
Pediatric Ambulatory Care . . . . . . Scott Barron, DO
Quality Assurance . . . . Kay Brom
Anesthesiology. . . . . Jason DeWilde, CRNA
President/CEO. . . . . Jody Jenner, RN, FACHE
Chief of Medical Staff . . . . Vincent Mandracchia, DPM, MHA
Radiology. . . . . Dwight Rafferty, MD

Measure	Cases	This Hosp.	State Avg.	U.S. Avg.
Blood Clot Prevention and Treatment				
Anticoagulation Overlap Therapy[2]	22	100%	94%	93%
ICU Venous Thromboembolism Prophylaxis[2]	123	85%	90%	92%
Incidence of Potentially Preventable VTE[1,2]	-	-	8%	10%
UFH with Dosages/Platelet Monitoring[1,2]	-	-	99%	97%
Venous Thromboembolism Prophylaxis[2]	91	67%	87%	85%
Warfarin Therapy Discharge Instructions[2]	19	26%	77%	75%
Chest Pain/Possible Heart Attack Care				
Aspirin Given Within 24 Hours of Arrival	48	98%	97%	96%
Fibrinolytic Meds Within 30 Min. of Arrival[7]	-	-	49%	58%
Average Time to ECG (minutes)	49	5	5	7
Average Time to Transfer (minutes)[1]	-	-	58	60
Children's Asthma Care				
Received Home Management Plan of Care	-	-	-	88%
Received Reliever Medication	-	-	-	100%
Received Systemic Corticosteroids	-	-	-	100%
Emergency Department				
Admittance Decision Time (minutes)[2]	163	156	58	98
Head CT Results Within 45 Min. of Arrival[1]	-	-	55%	57%
Patients Who Left ER Before Being Seen	35,980	4%	1%	2%
Time from ER Arrival to Admit. (minutes)[2]	200	328	202	274
Time from ER Arrival to Discharge (minutes)	438	140	108	134
Time in ER Before Being Evaluated (minutes)	527	36	21	26
Time to Pain Meds for Fractures (minutes)	56	68	46	57
Heart Attack Care				
Aspirin Given at Discharge[1]	-	-	100%	99%
Fibrinolytic Meds Within 30 Min. of Arrival[7]	-	-	-	54%
PCI Within 90 Minutes of Arrival[7]	-	-	94%	96%
Statin Prescribed at Discharge[7]	-	-	98%	98%
Heart Failure Care				
ACE Inhibitor or ARB for LVSD	17	100%	95%	97%
Discharge Instructions Given	24	67%	93%	94%
Evaluation of LVS Function	30	100%	97%	99%
Medicare Spending				
Medicare Spending per Patient (ratio)	-	0.80	0.91	0.98
Pneumonia Care				
Appropriate Initial Antibiotic Given	48	100%	93%	95%
Blood Culture Timing	44	100%	98%	98%
Pregnancy and Delivery Care				
Newborn Deliveries Scheduled Early	32	0%	4%	6%
Preventive Care				
Immunization for Influenza[2]	320	87%	91%	90%
Immunization for Pneumonia[2]	183	67%	90%	92%
Stroke Care				
Anticoagulation Therapy for Atrial Fibrillation[1]	-	-	95%	95%
Antithrombotic Therapy Timing	17	88%	98%	98%
Assessed for Rehabilitation	16	100%	97%	97%
Discharged on Antithrombotic Therapy	16	94%	99%	99%
Discharged on Statin Medication[1]	-	-	92%	94%
Thrombolytic Therapy Timing[7]	-	-	64%	66%
Venous Thromboembolism Prophylaxis	17	88%	93%	94%
Written Stroke Educational Materials Given[1]	-	-	82%	88%
Surgical Care Improvement Project				
Appropriate Beta Blocker Usage	26	77%	98%	98%
Appropriate VTP Within 24 Hours	133	95%	98%	98%
Controlled Postoperative Blood Glucose[7]	-	-	96%	97%
Perioperative Temperature Management	158	100%	100%	100%

NOTE: Hospital profiles are in alphabetical order by state, then city, then hospital within the city; Rankings exclude hospitals with less than 25 cases except for patient surveys which excludes hospitals with less than 100 cases; (a) 100-299 cases; (1) The number of cases/patients is too few to report; (2) Data submitted were based on a sample of cases/patients; (3) Results are based on a shorter time period than required; (4) Data suppressed by CMS for one or more quarters; (5) Results are not available for this reporting period; (6) Fewer than 100 patients completed the HCAHPS survey; (7) No cases met the criteria for this measure; (8) The lower limit of the confidence interval cannot be calculated if the number of observed infections equals zero; (9) No data are available from the state/territory for this reporting period; (10) The scores shown reflect fewer than 50 completed surveys; (11) There were discrepancies in the data collection process; (12) This measure does not apply to this hospital for this reporting period; (13) Results cannot be calculated for this reporting period; (14) The results for this state are combined with nearby states to protect confidentiality; Please refer to the User's Guide for a full explanation of data.

Prophylactic Antibiotic Selection	117	99%	99%	99%
Prophylactic Antibiotic Selection (Outpatient)	23	87%	98%	98%
Prophylactic Antibiotic Stopped	115	97%	98%	98%
Prophylactic Antibiotic Timing	117	92%	98%	99%
Prophylactic Antibiotic Timing (Outpatient)	23	91%	98%	98%
Urinary Catheter Removal	81	96%	97%	97%
Survey of Patients' Hospital Experiences				
Area Around Room 'Always' Quiet at Night	300+	58%	63%	61%
Doctors 'Always' Communicated Well	300+	79%	84%	82%
Home Recovery Information Given	300+	80%	88%	85%
Hospital Given 9 or 10 on 10 Point Scale	300+	66%	75%	71%
Meds 'Always' Explained Before Given	300+	59%	66%	64%
Nurses 'Always' Communicated Well	300+	75%	81%	79%
Pain 'Always' Well Controlled	300+	67%	71%	71%
Room and Bathroom 'Always' Clean	300+	73%	79%	73%
Timely Help 'Always' Received	300+	60%	70%	68%
Would Definitely Recommend Hospital	300+	62%	74%	71%
Use of Medical Imaging				
Cardiac Imaging Stress Test before Surgery[1]	-	-	4.8%	5.3%
Combination Abdominal CT Scan[1]	-	-	11.5%	10.5%
Combination Brain/Sinus CT Scan[1]	-	-	1.8%	2.7%
Combination Chest CT Scan[1]	-	-	3.5%	2.7%
Follow-up Mammogram/Ultrasound	164	18.3%	7.9%	8.8%
Lumbar Spine MRI for Low Back Pain[1]	-	-	32.2%	37.2%

Iowa Lutheran Hospital

700 East University Avenue
Des Moines, IA 50316
URL: www.ihsdesmoines.org
Phone: 515-263-5612
Fax: 515-241-5994
Type: Acute Care Hospitals
Emergency Services: Yes
Ownership: Voluntary non-profit - Private
Beds: 465

Key Personnel:
Chief of Medical Staff.......... Daniel Allen, MD, FACP
Emergency Room .... Pam Ballard
Patient Relations .... Vicki Berberich
CEO/President............... Eric Crowell
Quality Assurance .... Deb Moyer
Operating Room.............. Karen Powell
Radiology.................. Kent S Quinn, MD

Measure	Cases	This Hosp.	State Avg.	U.S. Avg.
Blood Clot Prevention and Treatment				
Anticoagulation Overlap Therapy[2]	47	91%	94%	93%
ICU Venous Thromboembolism Prophylaxis[2]	60	90%	90%	92%
Incidence of Potentially Preventable VTE[1,2]	-	-	8%	10%
UFH with Dosages/Platelet Monitoring[2]	13	100%	99%	97%
Venous Thromboembolism Prophylaxis[2]	281	85%	87%	85%
Warfarin Therapy Discharge Instructions[2]	40	92%	77%	75%
Chest Pain/Possible Heart Attack Care				
Aspirin Given Within 24 Hours of Arrival[1,3]	-	-	97%	96%
Fibrinolytic Meds Within 30 Min. of Arrival[3,7]	-	-	49%	58%
Average Time to ECG (minutes)[1,3]	-	-	5	7
Average Time to Transfer (minutes)[1,3]	-	-	58	60
Children's Asthma Care				
Received Home Management Plan of Care	-	-	-	88%
Received Reliever Medication	-	-	-	100%
Received Systemic Corticosteroids	-	-	-	100%
Emergency Department				
Admittance Decision Time (minutes)[2]	464	76	58	98
Head CT Results Within 45 Min. of Arrival[1]	-	-	55%	57%
Patients Who Left ER Before Being Seen	12,170	0%	1%	2%
Time from ER Arrival to Admit. (minutes)[2]	472	243	202	274
Time from ER Arrival to Discharge (minutes)	336	137	108	134
Time in ER Before Being Evaluated (minutes)	200	36	21	26
Time to Pain Meds for Fractures (minutes)	61	55	46	57
Heart Attack Care				
Aspirin Given at Discharge[2]	90	100%	100%	99%
Fibrinolytic Meds Within 30 Min. of Arrival[2,7]	-	-	-	54%
PCI Within 90 Minutes of Arrival[1,2]	-	-	94%	96%
Statin Prescribed at Discharge[2]	87	99%	98%	98%
Heart Failure Care				
ACE Inhibitor or ARB for LVSD[2]	48	98%	95%	97%
Discharge Instructions Given[2]	127	87%	93%	94%
Evaluation of LVS Function[2]	162	99%	97%	99%
Medicare Spending				
Medicare Spending per Patient (ratio)	-	0.90	0.91	0.98
Pneumonia Care				
Appropriate Initial Antibiotic Given[2]	94	97%	93%	95%
Blood Culture Timing[2]	134	99%	98%	98%
Pregnancy and Delivery Care				
Newborn Deliveries Scheduled Early[2]	31	3%	4%	6%
Preventive Care				
Immunization for Influenza[2]	485	88%	91%	90%
Immunization for Pneumonia[2]	660	88%	90%	92%
Stroke Care				
Anticoagulation Therapy for Atrial Fibrillation[1,2]	-	-	95%	95%
Antithrombotic Therapy Timing[2]	50	94%	98%	98%
Assessed for Rehabilitation[2]	54	93%	97%	97%
Discharged on Antithrombotic Therapy[2]	44	100%	99%	99%
Discharged on Statin Medication[2]	35	94%	92%	94%
Thrombolytic Therapy Timing[1,2]	-	-	64%	66%
Venous Thromboembolism Prophylaxis[2]	53	94%	93%	94%
Written Stroke Educational Materials Given[2]	28	39%	82%	88%
Surgical Care Improvement Project				
Appropriate Beta Blocker Usage[2]	49	100%	98%	98%
Appropriate VTP Within 24 Hours[2]	255	94%	98%	98%
Controlled Postoperative Blood Glucose[2,7]	-	-	96%	97%
Perioperative Temperature Management[2]	292	100%	100%	100%
Prophylactic Antibiotic Selection[2]	174	95%	99%	99%
Prophylactic Antibiotic Selection (Outpatient)	186	99%	98%	98%
Prophylactic Antibiotic Stopped[2]	171	96%	98%	98%
Prophylactic Antibiotic Timing[2]	174	99%	98%	99%
Prophylactic Antibiotic Timing (Outpatient)	188	98%	98%	98%
Urinary Catheter Removal[2]	172	96%	97%	97%
Survey of Patients' Hospital Experiences				
Area Around Room 'Always' Quiet at Night	300+	59%	63%	61%
Doctors 'Always' Communicated Well	300+	77%	84%	82%
Home Recovery Information Given	300+	89%	88%	85%
Hospital Given 9 or 10 on 10 Point Scale	300+	76%	75%	71%
Meds 'Always' Explained Before Given	300+	63%	66%	64%
Nurses 'Always' Communicated Well	300+	80%	81%	79%
Pain 'Always' Well Controlled	300+	68%	71%	71%
Room and Bathroom 'Always' Clean	300+	72%	79%	73%
Timely Help 'Always' Received	300+	63%	70%	68%
Would Definitely Recommend Hospital	300+	78%	74%	71%
Use of Medical Imaging				
Cardiac Imaging Stress Test before Surgery[1]	-	-	4.8%	5.3%
Combination Abdominal CT Scan	365	4.4%	11.5%	10.5%
Combination Brain/Sinus CT Scan[1]	-	-	1.8%	2.7%
Combination Chest CT Scan	252	1.2%	3.5%	2.7%
Follow-up Mammogram/Ultrasound	1,095	10.1%	7.9%	8.8%
Lumbar Spine MRI for Low Back Pain	81	35.8%	32.2%	37.2%

Iowa Methodist Medical Center

1200 Pleasant Street
Des Moines, IA 50309
URL: www.iowahealth.org
Phone: 515-241-6212
Fax: 515-241-8580
Type: Acute Care Hospitals
Emergency Services: Yes
Ownership: Voluntary non-profit - Private
Beds: 373

Key Personnel:
CEO/President............... Eric Crowell
Cardiac Laboratory............ Steve House
Chief of Medical Staff.......... Dr Josephson
Surgery..................... Daniel Kollmorgen, MD
Pediatrics.................. Richard Robus, MD
Emergency Room .... Lynda Schumaker

Measure	Cases	This Hosp.	State Avg.	U.S. Avg.
Blood Clot Prevention and Treatment				
Anticoagulation Overlap Therapy[2]	154	90%	94%	93%
ICU Venous Thromboembolism Prophylaxis[2]	84	98%	90%	92%
Incidence of Potentially Preventable VTE[2]	16	0%	8%	10%
UFH with Dosages/Platelet Monitoring[2]	80	99%	99%	97%
Venous Thromboembolism Prophylaxis[2]	294	82%	87%	85%
Warfarin Therapy Discharge Instructions[2]	129	74%	77%	75%
Chest Pain/Possible Heart Attack Care				
Aspirin Given Within 24 Hours of Arrival[1,3]	-	-	97%	96%
Fibrinolytic Meds Within 30 Min. of Arrival[5]	-	-	49%	58%
Average Time to ECG (minutes)[1,3]	-	-	5	7
Average Time to Transfer (minutes)[5]	-	-	58	60
Children's Asthma Care				
Received Home Management Plan of Care	-	-	-	88%
Received Reliever Medication	-	-	-	100%
Received Systemic Corticosteroids	-	-	-	100%
Emergency Department				
Admittance Decision Time (minutes)[2]	338	76	58	98
Head CT Results Within 45 Min. of Arrival[1]	-	-	55%	57%
Patients Who Left ER Before Being Seen	30,202	1%	1%	2%
Time from ER Arrival to Admit. (minutes)[2]	350	240	202	274
Time from ER Arrival to Discharge (minutes)	369	145	108	134
Time in ER Before Being Evaluated (minutes)	244	36	21	26
Time to Pain Meds for Fractures (minutes)	198	39	46	57
Heart Attack Care				
Aspirin Given at Discharge[2]	260	99%	100%	99%
Fibrinolytic Meds Within 30 Min. of Arrival[2,7]	-	-	-	54%
PCI Within 90 Minutes of Arrival[2]	36	94%	94%	96%
Statin Prescribed at Discharge[2]	247	99%	98%	98%
Heart Failure Care				
ACE Inhibitor or ARB for LVSD[2]	71	92%	95%	97%
Discharge Instructions Given[2]	198	90%	93%	94%
Evaluation of LVS Function[2]	246	99%	97%	99%
Medicare Spending				
Medicare Spending per Patient (ratio)	-	0.94	0.91	0.98
Pneumonia Care				
Appropriate Initial Antibiotic Given[2]	57	82%	93%	95%
Blood Culture Timing[2]	92	100%	98%	98%
Pregnancy and Delivery Care				
Newborn Deliveries Scheduled Early[2]	73	0%	4%	6%
Preventive Care				
Immunization for Influenza[2]	494	85%	91%	90%
Immunization for Pneumonia[2]	540	81%	90%	92%
Stroke Care				
Anticoagulation Therapy for Atrial Fibrillation[2]	13	100%	95%	95%
Antithrombotic Therapy Timing[2]	59	93%	98%	98%
Assessed for Rehabilitation[2]	83	95%	97%	97%
Discharged on Antithrombotic Therapy[2]	66	98%	99%	99%
Discharged on Statin Medication[2]	50	94%	92%	94%
Thrombolytic Therapy Timing[1,2]	-	-	64%	66%
Venous Thromboembolism Prophylaxis[2]	80	82%	93%	94%
Written Stroke Educational Materials Given[2]	41	54%	82%	88%
Surgical Care Improvement Project				
Appropriate Beta Blocker Usage[2]	150	98%	98%	98%
Appropriate VTP Within 24 Hours[2]	389	98%	98%	98%
Controlled Postoperative Blood Glucose[2]	101	96%	96%	97%
Perioperative Temperature Management[2]	500	100%	100%	100%
Prophylactic Antibiotic Selection[2]	399	99%	99%	99%
Prophylactic Antibiotic Selection (Outpatient)	589	97%	98%	98%
Prophylactic Antibiotic Stopped[2]	386	97%	98%	98%
Prophylactic Antibiotic Timing[2]	399	97%	98%	99%
Prophylactic Antibiotic Timing (Outpatient)	589	99%	98%	98%
Urinary Catheter Removal[2]	379	99%	97%	97%
Survey of Patients' Hospital Experiences				
Area Around Room 'Always' Quiet at Night	300+	65%	63%	61%
Doctors 'Always' Communicated Well	300+	80%	84%	82%
Home Recovery Information Given	300+	86%	88%	85%
Hospital Given 9 or 10 on 10 Point Scale	300+	75%	75%	71%
Meds 'Always' Explained Before Given	300+	61%	66%	64%
Nurses 'Always' Communicated Well	300+	76%	81%	79%
Pain 'Always' Well Controlled	300+	68%	71%	71%
Room and Bathroom 'Always' Clean	300+	73%	79%	73%
Timely Help 'Always' Received	300+	62%	70%	68%
Would Definitely Recommend Hospital	300+	80%	74%	71%
Use of Medical Imaging				
Cardiac Imaging Stress Test before Surgery	49	0.0%	4.8%	5.3%
Combination Abdominal CT Scan	579	9.2%	11.5%	10.5%
Combination Brain/Sinus CT Scan	782	2.3%	1.8%	2.7%
Combination Chest CT Scan	199	4.0%	3.5%	2.7%
Follow-up Mammogram/Ultrasound[7]	-	-	7.9%	8.8%
Lumbar Spine MRI for Low Back Pain	40	42.5%	32.2%	37.2%

NOTE: Hospital profiles are in alphabetical order by state, then city, then hospital within the city; Rankings exclude hospitals with less than 25 cases except for patient surveys which excludes hospitals with less than 100 cases; (a) 100-299 cases; (1) The number of cases/patients is too few to report; (2) Data submitted were based on a sample of cases/patients; (3) Results are based on a shorter time period than required; (4) Data suppressed by CMS for one or more quarters; (5) Results are not available for this reporting period; (6) Fewer than 100 patients completed the HCAHPS survey; (7) No cases met the criteria for this measure; (8) The lower limit of the confidence interval cannot be calculated if the number of observed infections equals zero; (9) No data are available from the state/territory for this reporting period; (10) The scores shown reflect fewer than 50 completed surveys; (11) There were discrepancies in the data collection process; (12) This measure does not apply to this hospital for this reporting period; (13) Results cannot be calculated for this reporting period; (14) The results for this state are combined with nearby states to protect confidentiality; Please refer to the User's Guide for a full explanation of data.

Mercy Medical Center - Des Moines

1111 6th Ave
Des Moines, IA 50314
Phone: 515-247-3121
Fax: 515-643-8498
URL: www.mercydesmoines.org
Type: Acute Care Hospitals
Emergency Services: Yes
Ownership: Voluntary non-profit - Private
Beds: 673

Key Personnel:

Infection Control. . . . . Connie Grout
Pediatric Ambulatory Care . . . . . . Sayeed Hussain, MD
Pediatric In-Patient Care . . . . Sayeed Hussain, MD
Radiology. . . . . Ruben Koehler, MD
Operating Room. . . . . Sharon Meadowcroft
Chief of Medical Staff. . . . . RoseMary Mullin
Quality Assurance . . . . Jeff Sutting
CEO/President. . . . . David Vellinga

Measure	Cases	This Hosp.	State Avg.	U.S. Avg.
Blood Clot Prevention and Treatment				
Anticoagulation Overlap Therapy[2]	235	97%	94%	93%
ICU Venous Thromboembolism Prophylaxis[2]	149	91%	90%	92%
Incidence of Potentially Preventable VTE[2]	39	15%	8%	10%
UFH with Dosages/Platelet Monitoring[2]	72	99%	99%	97%
Venous Thromboembolism Prophylaxis[2]	456	78%	87%	85%
Warfarin Therapy Discharge Instructions[2]	184	57%	77%	75%
Chest Pain/Possible Heart Attack Care				
Aspirin Given Within 24 Hours of Arrival[1,3]	-	-	97%	96%
Fibrinolytic Meds Within 30 Min. of Arrival[3,7]	-	-	49%	58%
Average Time to ECG (minutes)[1,3]	-	-	5	7
Average Time to Transfer (minutes)[3,7]	-	-	58	60
Children's Asthma Care				
Received Home Management Plan of Care	-	-	-	88%
Received Reliever Medication	-	-	-	100%
Received Systemic Corticosteroids	-	-	-	100%
Emergency Department				
Admittance Decision Time (minutes)[2]	456	69	58	98
Head CT Results Within 45 Min. of Arrival[1]	-	-	55%	57%
Patients Who Left ER Before Being Seen	74,432	2%	1%	2%
Time from ER Arrival to Admit. (minutes)[2]	507	244	202	274
Time from ER Arrival to Discharge (minutes)	475	149	108	134
Time in ER Before Being Evaluated (minutes)	503	29	21	26
Time to Pain Meds for Fractures (minutes)	139	45	46	57
Heart Attack Care				
Aspirin Given at Discharge[2]	313	100%	100%	99%
Fibrinolytic Meds Within 30 Min. of Arrival[2,7]	-	-	-	54%
PCI Within 90 Minutes of Arrival[2]	37	100%	94%	96%
Statin Prescribed at Discharge[2]	304	99%	98%	98%
Heart Failure Care				
ACE Inhibitor or ARB for LVSD[2]	71	100%	95%	97%
Discharge Instructions Given[2]	259	99%	93%	94%
Evaluation of LVS Function[2]	337	100%	97%	99%
Medicare Spending				
Medicare Spending per Patient (ratio)	-	0.93	0.91	0.98
Pneumonia Care				
Appropriate Initial Antibiotic Given[2]	80	99%	93%	95%
Blood Culture Timing[2]	193	100%	98%	98%
Pregnancy and Delivery Care				
Newborn Deliveries Scheduled Early[2]	109	6%	4%	6%
Preventive Care				
Immunization for Influenza[2]	764	94%	91%	90%
Immunization for Pneumonia[2]	861	94%	90%	92%
Stroke Care				
Anticoagulation Therapy for Atrial Fibrillation[2]	21	95%	95%	95%
Antithrombotic Therapy Timing[2]	78	100%	98%	98%
Assessed for Rehabilitation[2]	108	97%	97%	97%
Discharged on Antithrombotic Therapy[2]	91	99%	99%	99%
Discharged on Statin Medication[2]	73	92%	92%	94%
Thrombolytic Therapy Timing[2]	13	77%	64%	66%
Venous Thromboembolism Prophylaxis[2]	107	93%	93%	94%
Written Stroke Educational Materials Given[2]	62	47%	82%	88%
Surgical Care Improvement Project				
Appropriate Beta Blocker Usage[2]	310	99%	98%	98%
Appropriate VTP Within 24 Hours[2]	536	97%	98%	98%
Controlled Postoperative Blood Glucose[2]	158	96%	96%	97%
Perioperative Temperature Management[2]	681	100%	100%	100%
Prophylactic Antibiotic Selection[2]	521	99%	99%	99%
Prophylactic Antibiotic Selection (Outpatient)	709	99%	98%	98%
Prophylactic Antibiotic Stopped[2]	503	99%	98%	98%
Prophylactic Antibiotic Timing[2]	521	96%	98%	99%
Prophylactic Antibiotic Timing (Outpatient)	708	97%	98%	98%
Urinary Catheter Removal[2]	249	96%	97%	97%
Survey of Patients' Hospital Experiences				
Area Around Room 'Always' Quiet at Night	300+	57%	63%	61%
Doctors 'Always' Communicated Well	300+	76%	84%	82%
Home Recovery Information Given	300+	87%	88%	85%
Hospital Given 9 or 10 on 10 Point Scale	300+	68%	75%	71%
Meds 'Always' Explained Before Given	300+	63%	66%	64%
Nurses 'Always' Communicated Well	300+	76%	81%	79%
Pain 'Always' Well Controlled	300+	67%	71%	71%
Room and Bathroom 'Always' Clean	300+	67%	79%	73%
Timely Help 'Always' Received	300+	55%	70%	68%
Would Definitely Recommend Hospital	300+	72%	74%	71%
Use of Medical Imaging				
Cardiac Imaging Stress Test before Surgery	2,013	5.3%	4.8%	5.3%
Combination Abdominal CT Scan	1,716	3.0%	11.5%	10.5%
Combination Brain/Sinus CT Scan	1,291	2.2%	1.8%	2.7%
Combination Chest CT Scan	1,360	4.2%	3.5%	2.7%
Follow-up Mammogram/Ultrasound	3,436	6.3%	7.9%	8.8%
Lumbar Spine MRI for Low Back Pain	233	29.2%	32.2%	37.2%

VA Central Iowa Healthcare System

3600 30th Street
Des Moines, IA 50310
Phone: 515-699-5999
Fax: 515-699-5862
URL: www.va.gov/sta/guide/home.asp
Type: Acute Care - VA
Emergency Services: No
Ownership: Government Federal
Beds: 327

Key Personnel:

Chief of Medical Staff. . . . . Fredrick Bahls, MD, Ph.D.
CEO/President. . . . . Donald Cooper
Operating Room. . . . . Jeanne Knight
Infection Control. . . . . Barbara Livingston
Quality Assurance . . . . Janelle Runearson
Radiology. . . . . Nita Shirodkar, MD

Measure	Cases	This Hosp.	State Avg.	U.S. Avg.
Blood Clot Prevention and Treatment				
Anticoagulation Overlap Therapy	-	-	94%	93%
ICU Venous Thromboembolism Prophylaxis	-	-	90%	92%
Incidence of Potentially Preventable VTE	-	-	8%	10%
UFH with Dosages/Platelet Monitoring	-	-	99%	97%
Venous Thromboembolism Prophylaxis	-	-	87%	85%
Warfarin Therapy Discharge Instructions	-	-	77%	75%
Chest Pain/Possible Heart Attack Care				
Aspirin Given Within 24 Hours of Arrival	-	-	97%	96%
Fibrinolytic Meds Within 30 Min. of Arrival	-	-	49%	58%
Average Time to ECG (minutes)	-	-	5	7
Average Time to Transfer (minutes)	-	-	58	60
Children's Asthma Care				
Received Home Management Plan of Care	-	-	-	88%
Received Reliever Medication	-	-	-	100%
Received Systemic Corticosteroids	-	-	-	100%
Emergency Department				
Admittance Decision Time (minutes)	-	-	58	98
Head CT Results Within 45 Min. of Arrival	-	-	55%	57%
Patients Who Left ER Before Being Seen	-	-	1%	2%
Time from ER Arrival to Admit. (minutes)	-	-	202	274
Time from ER Arrival to Discharge (minutes)	-	-	108	134
Time in ER Before Being Evaluated (minutes)	-	-	21	26
Time to Pain Meds for Fractures (minutes)	-	-	46	57
Heart Attack Care				
Aspirin Given at Discharge[5]	-	-	100%	99%
Fibrinolytic Meds Within 30 Min. of Arrival[5]	-	-	-	54%
PCI Within 90 Minutes of Arrival[5]	-	-	94%	96%
Statin Prescribed at Discharge[5]	-	-	98%	98%
Heart Failure Care				
ACE Inhibitor or ARB for LVSD[1]	18	100%	95%	97%
Discharge Instructions Given	42	90%	93%	94%
Evaluation of LVS Function	58	98%	97%	99%
Medicare Spending				
Medicare Spending per Patient (ratio)	-	-	0.91	0.98
Pneumonia Care				
Appropriate Initial Antibiotic Given	43	91%	93%	95%
Blood Culture Timing	72	97%	98%	98%
Pregnancy and Delivery Care				
Newborn Deliveries Scheduled Early	-	-	4%	6%
Preventive Care				
Immunization for Influenza[5]	-	-	91%	90%
Immunization for Pneumonia[5]	-	-	90%	92%
Stroke Care				
Anticoagulation Therapy for Atrial Fibrillation	-	-	95%	95%
Antithrombotic Therapy Timing	-	-	98%	98%
Assessed for Rehabilitation	-	-	97%	97%
Discharged on Antithrombotic Therapy	-	-	99%	99%
Discharged on Statin Medication	-	-	92%	94%
Thrombolytic Therapy Timing	-	-	64%	66%
Venous Thromboembolism Prophylaxis	-	-	93%	94%
Written Stroke Educational Materials Given	-	-	82%	88%
Surgical Care Improvement Project				
Appropriate Beta Blocker Usage[2]	86	99%	98%	98%
Appropriate VTP Within 24 Hours[2]	145	95%	98%	98%
Controlled Postoperative Blood Glucose[5]	-	-	96%	97%
Perioperative Temperature Management[2]	166	99%	100%	100%
Prophylactic Antibiotic Selection	123	98%	99%	99%
Prophylactic Antibiotic Selection (Outpatient)	-	-	98%	98%
Prophylactic Antibiotic Stopped	120	98%	98%	98%
Prophylactic Antibiotic Timing	124	93%	98%	99%
Prophylactic Antibiotic Timing (Outpatient)	-	-	98%	98%
Urinary Catheter Removal[2]	106	97%	97%	97%
Survey of Patients' Hospital Experiences				
Area Around Room 'Always' Quiet at Night	-	-	63%	61%
Doctors 'Always' Communicated Well	-	-	84%	82%
Home Recovery Information Given	-	-	88%	85%
Hospital Given 9 or 10 on 10 Point Scale	-	-	75%	71%
Meds 'Always' Explained Before Given	-	-	66%	64%
Nurses 'Always' Communicated Well	-	-	81%	79%
Pain 'Always' Well Controlled	-	-	71%	71%
Room and Bathroom 'Always' Clean	-	-	79%	73%
Timely Help 'Always' Received	-	-	70%	68%
Would Definitely Recommend Hospital	-	-	74%	71%
Use of Medical Imaging				
Cardiac Imaging Stress Test before Surgery	-	-	4.8%	5.3%
Combination Abdominal CT Scan	-	-	11.5%	10.5%
Combination Brain/Sinus CT Scan	-	-	1.8%	2.7%
Combination Chest CT Scan	-	-	3.5%	2.7%
Follow-up Mammogram/Ultrasound	-	-	7.9%	8.8%
Lumbar Spine MRI for Low Back Pain	-	-	32.2%	37.2%

Genesis Medical Center - Dewitt

1118 11th Street
Dewitt, IA 52742
Phone: 563-659-4200
URL: www.genesishealth.com
Type: Critical Access Hospitals
Emergency Services: Yes
Ownership: Voluntary non-profit - Private

Key Personnel:

President/CEO. . . . . Jeffrey M Cooper

Measure	Cases	This Hosp.	State Avg.	U.S. Avg.
Blood Clot Prevention and Treatment				
Anticoagulation Overlap Therapy[1]	-	-	94%	93%
ICU Venous Thromboembolism Prophylaxis[7]	-	-	90%	92%
Incidence of Potentially Preventable VTE[7]	-	-	8%	10%
UFH with Dosages/Platelet Monitoring[1]	-	-	99%	97%
Venous Thromboembolism Prophylaxis	55	82%	87%	85%
Warfarin Therapy Discharge Instructions[1]	-	-	77%	75%
Chest Pain/Possible Heart Attack Care				
Aspirin Given Within 24 Hours of Arrival	40	98%	97%	96%
Fibrinolytic Meds Within 30 Min. of Arrival[7]	-	-	49%	58%
Average Time to ECG (minutes)	41	2	5	7
Average Time to Transfer (minutes)	12	44	58	60
Children's Asthma Care				
Received Home Management Plan of Care	-	-	-	88%
Received Reliever Medication	-	-	-	100%
Received Systemic Corticosteroids	-	-	-	100%
Emergency Department				
Admittance Decision Time (minutes)	81	29	58	98

NOTE: Hospital profiles are in alphabetical order by state, then city, then hospital within the city; Rankings exclude hospitals with less than 25 cases except for patient surveys which excludes hospitals with less than 100 cases; (a) 100-299 cases; (1) The number of cases/patients is too few to report; (2) Data submitted were based on a sample of cases/patients; (3) Results are based on a shorter time period than required; (4) Data suppressed by CMS for one or more quarters; (5) Results are not available for this reporting period; (6) Fewer than 100 patients completed the HCAHPS survey; (7) No cases met the criteria for this measure; (8) The lower limit of the confidence interval cannot be calculated if the number of observed infections equals zero; (9) No data are available from the state/territory for this reporting period; (10) The scores shown reflect fewer than 50 completed surveys; (11) There were discrepancies in the data collection process; (12) This measure does not apply to this hospital for this reporting period; (13) Results cannot be calculated for this reporting period; (14) The results for this state are combined with nearby states to protect confidentiality; Please refer to the User's Guide for a full explanation of data.

Measure	Cases	This Hosp.	State Avg.	U.S. Avg.
Head CT Results Within 45 Min. of Arrival[1]	-	-	55%	57%
Patients Who Left ER Before Being Seen	4,651	0%	1%	2%
Time from ER Arrival to Admit. (minutes)	81	152	202	274
Time from ER Arrival to Discharge (minutes)	367	81	108	134
Time in ER Before Being Evaluated (minutes)	417	12	21	26
Time to Pain Meds for Fractures (minutes)	27	27	46	57
Heart Attack Care				
Aspirin Given at Discharge[3,7]	-	-	100%	99%
Fibrinolytic Meds Within 30 Min. of Arrival[3,7]	-	-	-	54%
PCI Within 90 Minutes of Arrival[3,7]	-	-	94%	96%
Statin Prescribed at Discharge[3,7]	-	-	98%	98%
Heart Failure Care				
ACE Inhibitor or ARB for LVSD[1]	-	-	95%	97%
Discharge Instructions Given[1]	-	-	93%	94%
Evaluation of LVS Function[1]	-	-	97%	99%
Medicare Spending				
Medicare Spending per Patient (ratio)	-	-	0.91	0.98
Pneumonia Care				
Appropriate Initial Antibiotic Given[1]	-	-	93%	95%
Blood Culture Timing[1]	-	-	98%	98%
Pregnancy and Delivery Care				
Newborn Deliveries Scheduled Early[7]	-	-	4%	6%
Preventive Care				
Immunization for Influenza	39	87%	91%	90%
Immunization for Pneumonia	77	99%	90%	92%
Stroke Care				
Anticoagulation Therapy for Atrial Fibrillation[3,7]	-	-	95%	95%
Antithrombotic Therapy Timing[3,7]	-	-	98%	98%
Assessed for Rehabilitation[3,7]	-	-	97%	97%
Discharged on Antithrombotic Therapy[3,7]	-	-	99%	99%
Discharged on Statin Medication[3,7]	-	-	92%	94%
Thrombolytic Therapy Timing[3,7]	-	-	64%	66%
Venous Thromboembolism Prophylaxis[3,7]	-	-	93%	94%
Written Stroke Educational Materials Given[3,7]	-	-	82%	88%
Surgical Care Improvement Project				
Appropriate Beta Blocker Usage[5]	-	-	98%	98%
Appropriate VTP Within 24 Hours[5]	-	-	98%	98%
Controlled Postoperative Blood Glucose[5]	-	-	96%	97%
Perioperative Temperature Management[5]	-	-	100%	100%
Prophylactic Antibiotic Selection[5]	-	-	99%	99%
Prophylactic Antibiotic Selection (Outpatient)[1,3]	-	-	98%	98%
Prophylactic Antibiotic Stopped[5]	-	-	98%	98%
Prophylactic Antibiotic Timing[5]	-	-	98%	99%
Prophylactic Antibiotic Timing (Outpatient)[1,3]	-	-	98%	98%
Urinary Catheter Removal[5]	-	-	97%	97%
Survey of Patients' Hospital Experiences				
Area Around Room 'Always' Quiet at Night[5]	-	-	63%	61%
Doctors 'Always' Communicated Well[5]	-	-	84%	82%
Home Recovery Information Given[5]	-	-	88%	85%
Hospital Given 9 or 10 on 10 Point Scale[5]	-	-	75%	71%
Meds 'Always' Explained Before Given[5]	-	-	66%	64%
Nurses 'Always' Communicated Well[5]	-	-	81%	79%
Pain 'Always' Well Controlled[5]	-	-	71%	71%
Room and Bathroom 'Always' Clean[5]	-	-	79%	73%
Timely Help 'Always' Received[5]	-	-	70%	68%
Would Definitely Recommend Hospital[5]	-	-	74%	71%
Use of Medical Imaging				
Cardiac Imaging Stress Test before Surgery[7]	-	-	4.8%	5.3%
Combination Abdominal CT Scan	65	1.5%	11.5%	10.5%
Combination Brain/Sinus CT Scan[1]	-	-	1.8%	2.7%
Combination Chest CT Scan[1]	-	-	3.5%	2.7%
Follow-up Mammogram/Ultrasound	259	6.2%	7.9%	8.8%
Lumbar Spine MRI for Low Back Pain[1]	-	-	32.2%	37.2%

Finley Hospital

350 North Grandview Avenue — Phone: 563-582-1881
Dubuque, IA 52001 — Fax: 563-589-2620
E-mail: cr@finleyhospital.org
URL: www.finleyhospital.org
Type: Acute Care Hospitals — Emergency Services: Yes
Ownership: Voluntary non-profit - Private — Beds: 158

Key Personnel:
Chief of Medical Staff.......... Thomas J Benda, Jr, MD
Operating Room.............. Lavern Bird
CEO/President............... David Brandon, FACHE
Cardiac Laboratory............ Patty Dissell
Radiology.................. Gregory R Grotz, MD
Quality Assurance .... Ronda Kirkeguard
Pediatric Ambulatory Care ...... R Michael McGill, MD
Pediatric In-Patient Care .... R Michael McGill, MD

Measure	Cases	This Hosp.	State Avg.	U.S. Avg.
Blood Clot Prevention and Treatment				
Anticoagulation Overlap Therapy[2]	44	100%	94%	93%
ICU Venous Thromboembolism Prophylaxis[2]	90	84%	90%	92%
Incidence of Potentially Preventable VTE[1,2]	-	-	8%	10%
UFH with Dosages/Platelet Monitoring[1,2]	-	-	99%	97%
Venous Thromboembolism Prophylaxis[2]	271	89%	87%	85%
Warfarin Therapy Discharge Instructions[2]	33	85%	77%	75%
Chest Pain/Possible Heart Attack Care				
Aspirin Given Within 24 Hours of Arrival[1,3]	-	-	97%	96%
Fibrinolytic Meds Within 30 Min. of Arrival[3,7]	-	-	49%	58%
Average Time to ECG (minutes)[1,3]	-	-	5	7
Average Time to Transfer (minutes)[3,7]	-	-	58	60
Children's Asthma Care				
Received Home Management Plan of Care	-	-	-	88%
Received Reliever Medication	-	-	-	100%
Received Systemic Corticosteroids	-	-	-	100%
Emergency Department				
Admittance Decision Time (minutes)[2]	474	66	58	98
Head CT Results Within 45 Min. of Arrival[1]	-	-	55%	57%
Patients Who Left ER Before Being Seen	24,348	2%	1%	2%
Time from ER Arrival to Admit. (minutes)[2]	480	226	202	274
Time from ER Arrival to Discharge (minutes)	361	103	108	134
Time in ER Before Being Evaluated (minutes)	370	28	21	26
Time to Pain Meds for Fractures (minutes)	84	40	46	57
Heart Attack Care				
Aspirin Given at Discharge	81	98%	100%	99%
Fibrinolytic Meds Within 30 Min. of Arrival[7]	-	-	-	54%
PCI Within 90 Minutes of Arrival	19	100%	94%	96%
Statin Prescribed at Discharge	80	96%	98%	98%
Heart Failure Care				
ACE Inhibitor or ARB for LVSD	27	100%	95%	97%
Discharge Instructions Given	102	87%	93%	94%
Evaluation of LVS Function	138	95%	97%	99%
Medicare Spending				
Medicare Spending per Patient (ratio)	-	1.00	0.91	0.98
Pneumonia Care				
Appropriate Initial Antibiotic Given[2]	67	97%	93%	95%
Blood Culture Timing[2]	138	97%	98%	98%
Pregnancy and Delivery Care				
Newborn Deliveries Scheduled Early[2]	30	3%	4%	6%
Preventive Care				
Immunization for Influenza[2]	428	90%	91%	90%
Immunization for Pneumonia[2]	533	86%	90%	92%
Stroke Care				
Anticoagulation Therapy for Atrial Fibrillation[1,2]	-	-	95%	95%
Antithrombotic Therapy Timing[2]	51	94%	98%	98%
Assessed for Rehabilitation[2]	41	90%	97%	97%
Discharged on Antithrombotic Therapy[2]	37	92%	99%	99%
Discharged on Statin Medication[2]	30	77%	92%	94%
Thrombolytic Therapy Timing[1,2]	-	-	64%	66%
Venous Thromboembolism Prophylaxis[2]	56	93%	93%	94%
Written Stroke Educational Materials Given[2]	27	85%	82%	88%
Surgical Care Improvement Project				
Appropriate Beta Blocker Usage[2]	126	100%	98%	98%
Appropriate VTP Within 24 Hours[2]	357	100%	98%	98%
Controlled Postoperative Blood Glucose[2,7]	-	-	96%	97%
Perioperative Temperature Management[2]	399	100%	100%	100%
Prophylactic Antibiotic Selection[2]	325	99%	99%	99%
Prophylactic Antibiotic Selection (Outpatient)	111	100%	98%	98%
Prophylactic Antibiotic Stopped[2]	324	97%	98%	98%
Prophylactic Antibiotic Timing[2]	326	100%	98%	99%
Prophylactic Antibiotic Timing (Outpatient)	111	95%	98%	98%
Urinary Catheter Removal[2]	329	99%	97%	97%
Survey of Patients' Hospital Experiences				
Area Around Room 'Always' Quiet at Night	300+	60%	63%	61%
Doctors 'Always' Communicated Well	300+	82%	84%	82%
Home Recovery Information Given	300+	91%	88%	85%
Hospital Given 9 or 10 on 10 Point Scale	300+	75%	75%	71%
Meds 'Always' Explained Before Given	300+	65%	66%	64%
Nurses 'Always' Communicated Well	300+	79%	81%	79%
Pain 'Always' Well Controlled	300+	70%	71%	71%
Room and Bathroom 'Always' Clean	300+	73%	79%	73%
Timely Help 'Always' Received	300+	66%	70%	68%
Would Definitely Recommend Hospital	300+	78%	74%	71%
Use of Medical Imaging				
Cardiac Imaging Stress Test before Surgery	124	4.8%	4.8%	5.3%
Combination Abdominal CT Scan	258	6.2%	11.5%	10.5%
Combination Brain/Sinus CT Scan	294	1.0%	1.8%	2.7%
Combination Chest CT Scan	70	7.1%	3.5%	2.7%
Follow-up Mammogram/Ultrasound	215	7.0%	7.9%	8.8%
Lumbar Spine MRI for Low Back Pain	146	32.9%	32.2%	37.2%

Mercy Medical Center - Dubuque

250 Mercy Drive — Phone: 563-589-8000
Dubuque, IA 52001
URL: www.mercydubuque.com
Type: Acute Care Hospitals — Emergency Services: Yes
Ownership: Voluntary non-profit - Church

Measure	Cases	This Hosp.	State Avg.	U.S. Avg.
Blood Clot Prevention and Treatment				
Anticoagulation Overlap Therapy[2]	60	88%	94%	93%
ICU Venous Thromboembolism Prophylaxis[2]	38	92%	90%	92%
Incidence of Potentially Preventable VTE[1,2]	-	-	8%	10%
UFH with Dosages/Platelet Monitoring[2]	19	100%	99%	97%
Venous Thromboembolism Prophylaxis[2]	284	94%	87%	85%
Warfarin Therapy Discharge Instructions[2]	47	98%	77%	75%
Chest Pain/Possible Heart Attack Care				
Aspirin Given Within 24 Hours of Arrival[1]	-	-	97%	96%
Fibrinolytic Meds Within 30 Min. of Arrival[5]	-	-	49%	58%
Average Time to ECG (minutes)[1]	-	-	5	7
Average Time to Transfer (minutes)[5]	-	-	58	60
Children's Asthma Care				
Received Home Management Plan of Care	-	-	-	88%
Received Reliever Medication	-	-	-	100%
Received Systemic Corticosteroids	-	-	-	100%
Emergency Department				
Admittance Decision Time (minutes)[2]	406	43	58	98
Head CT Results Within 45 Min. of Arrival[1]	-	-	55%	57%
Patients Who Left ER Before Being Seen	22,311	0%	1%	2%
Time from ER Arrival to Admit. (minutes)[2]	488	196	202	274
Time from ER Arrival to Discharge (minutes)	484	101	108	134
Time in ER Before Being Evaluated (minutes)	541	5	21	26
Time to Pain Meds for Fractures (minutes)	77	44	46	57
Heart Attack Care				
Aspirin Given at Discharge	208	100%	100%	99%
Fibrinolytic Meds Within 30 Min. of Arrival[7]	-	-	-	54%
PCI Within 90 Minutes of Arrival	33	88%	94%	96%
Statin Prescribed at Discharge	189	99%	98%	98%
Heart Failure Care				
ACE Inhibitor or ARB for LVSD	27	100%	95%	97%
Discharge Instructions Given	119	96%	93%	94%
Evaluation of LVS Function	170	99%	97%	99%
Medicare Spending				
Medicare Spending per Patient (ratio)	-	0.90	0.91	0.98
Pneumonia Care				
Appropriate Initial Antibiotic Given	85	98%	93%	95%
Blood Culture Timing	119	97%	98%	98%
Pregnancy and Delivery Care				
Newborn Deliveries Scheduled Early	61	0%	4%	6%
Preventive Care				
Immunization for Influenza[2]	598	98%	91%	90%
Immunization for Pneumonia[2]	659	97%	90%	92%
Stroke Care				
Anticoagulation Therapy for Atrial Fibrillation	19	95%	95%	95%
Antithrombotic Therapy Timing	80	99%	98%	98%
Assessed for Rehabilitation	103	98%	97%	97%
Discharged on Antithrombotic Therapy	99	100%	99%	99%
Discharged on Statin Medication	76	95%	92%	94%

NOTE: Hospital profiles are in alphabetical order by state, then city, then hospital within the city; Rankings exclude hospitals with less than 25 cases except for patient surveys which excludes hospitals with less than 100 cases; (a) 100-299 cases; (1) The number of cases/patients is too few to report; (2) Data submitted were based on a sample of cases/patients; (3) Results are based on a shorter time period than required; (4) Data suppressed by CMS for one or more quarters; (5) Results are not available for this reporting period; (6) Fewer than 100 patients completed the HCAHPS survey; (7) No cases met the criteria for this measure; (8) The lower limit of the confidence interval cannot be calculated if the number of observed infections equals zero; (9) No data are available from the state/territory for this reporting period; (10) The scores shown reflect fewer than 50 completed surveys; (11) There were discrepancies in the data collection process; (12) This measure does not apply to this hospital for this reporting period; (13) Results cannot be calculated for this reporting period; (14) The results for this state are combined with nearby states to protect confidentiality; Please refer to the User's Guide for a full explanation of data.

Measure	Cases	This Hosp.	State Avg.	U.S. Avg.
Thrombolytic Therapy Timing	12	58%	64%	66%
Venous Thromboembolism Prophylaxis	89	100%	93%	94%
Written Stroke Educational Materials Given	55	95%	82%	88%
Surgical Care Improvement Project				
Appropriate Beta Blocker Usage[2]	161	100%	98%	98%
Appropriate VTP Within 24 Hours[2]	370	99%	98%	98%
Controlled Postoperative Blood Glucose[2]	52	96%	96%	97%
Perioperative Temperature Management[2]	399	100%	100%	100%
Prophylactic Antibiotic Selection[2]	333	100%	99%	99%
Prophylactic Antibiotic Selection (Outpatient)	302	99%	98%	98%
Prophylactic Antibiotic Stopped[2]	332	99%	98%	98%
Prophylactic Antibiotic Timing[2]	334	99%	98%	99%
Prophylactic Antibiotic Timing (Outpatient)	300	100%	98%	98%
Urinary Catheter Removal[2]	363	100%	97%	97%
Survey of Patients' Hospital Experiences				
Area Around Room 'Always' Quiet at Night	300+	61%	63%	61%
Doctors 'Always' Communicated Well	300+	82%	84%	82%
Home Recovery Information Given	300+	91%	88%	85%
Hospital Given 9 or 10 on 10 Point Scale	300+	78%	75%	71%
Meds 'Always' Explained Before Given	300+	66%	66%	64%
Nurses 'Always' Communicated Well	300+	81%	81%	79%
Pain 'Always' Well Controlled	300+	71%	71%	71%
Room and Bathroom 'Always' Clean	300+	74%	79%	73%
Timely Help 'Always' Received	300+	68%	70%	68%
Would Definitely Recommend Hospital	300+	79%	74%	71%
Use of Medical Imaging				
Cardiac Imaging Stress Test before Surgery[1]	-	-	4.8%	5.3%
Combination Abdominal CT Scan	264	2.3%	11.5%	10.5%
Combination Brain/Sinus CT Scan[1]	-	-	1.8%	2.7%
Combination Chest CT Scan	149	0.7%	3.5%	2.7%
Follow-up Mammogram/Ultrasound[1]	-	-	7.9%	8.8%
Lumbar Spine MRI for Low Back Pain[1]	-	-	32.2%	37.2%

Mercy Medical Center - Dyersville

1111 3rd Street Sw
Dyersville, IA 52040
Phone: 563-875-7101
Fax: 563-875-2904
Type: Critical Access Hospitals
Emergency Services: Yes
Ownership: Voluntary non-profit - Private
Beds: 95

Key Personnel:
CEO/President. . . . . Rusty Knight
Operating Room. . . . . Diane Schroeder

Measure	Cases	This Hosp.	State Avg.	U.S. Avg.
Blood Clot Prevention and Treatment				
Anticoagulation Overlap Therapy[5]	-	-	94%	93%
ICU Venous Thromboembolism Prophylaxis[5]	-	-	90%	92%
Incidence of Potentially Preventable VTE[5]	-	-	8%	10%
UFH with Dosages/Platelet Monitoring[5]	-	-	99%	97%
Venous Thromboembolism Prophylaxis[5]	-	-	87%	85%
Warfarin Therapy Discharge Instructions[5]	-	-	77%	75%
Chest Pain/Possible Heart Attack Care				
Aspirin Given Within 24 Hours of Arrival	-	-	97%	96%
Fibrinolytic Meds Within 30 Min. of Arrival	-	-	49%	58%
Average Time to ECG (minutes)	-	-	5	7
Average Time to Transfer (minutes)	-	-	58	60
Children's Asthma Care				
Received Home Management Plan of Care	-	-	-	88%
Received Reliever Medication	-	-	-	100%
Received Systemic Corticosteroids	-	-	-	100%
Emergency Department				
Admittance Decision Time (minutes)[5]	-	-	58	98
Head CT Results Within 45 Min. of Arrival	-	-	55%	57%
Patients Who Left ER Before Being Seen	-	-	1%	2%
Time from ER Arrival to Admit. (minutes)[5]	-	-	202	274
Time from ER Arrival to Discharge (minutes)	-	-	108	134
Time in ER Before Being Evaluated (minutes)	-	-	21	26
Time to Pain Meds for Fractures (minutes)	-	-	46	57
Heart Attack Care				
Aspirin Given at Discharge[5]	-	-	100%	99%
Fibrinolytic Meds Within 30 Min. of Arrival[5]	-	-	-	54%
PCI Within 90 Minutes of Arrival[5]	-	-	94%	96%
Statin Prescribed at Discharge[5]	-	-	98%	98%
Heart Failure Care				
ACE Inhibitor or ARB for LVSD[1,3]	-	-	95%	97%
Discharge Instructions Given[1,3]	-	-	93%	94%
Evaluation of LVS Function[1,3]	-	-	97%	99%
Medicare Spending				
Medicare Spending per Patient (ratio)	-	-	0.91	0.98
Pneumonia Care				
Appropriate Initial Antibiotic Given[1,3]	-	-	93%	95%
Blood Culture Timing[1,3]	-	-	98%	98%
Pregnancy and Delivery Care				
Newborn Deliveries Scheduled Early[5]	-	-	4%	6%
Preventive Care				
Immunization for Influenza[5]	-	-	91%	90%
Immunization for Pneumonia[5]	-	-	90%	92%
Stroke Care				
Anticoagulation Therapy for Atrial Fibrillation[5]	-	-	95%	95%
Antithrombotic Therapy Timing[5]	-	-	98%	98%
Assessed for Rehabilitation[5]	-	-	97%	97%
Discharged on Antithrombotic Therapy[5]	-	-	99%	99%
Discharged on Statin Medication[5]	-	-	92%	94%
Thrombolytic Therapy Timing[5]	-	-	64%	66%
Venous Thromboembolism Prophylaxis[5]	-	-	93%	94%
Written Stroke Educational Materials Given[5]	-	-	82%	88%
Surgical Care Improvement Project				
Appropriate Beta Blocker Usage[5]	-	-	98%	98%
Appropriate VTP Within 24 Hours[5]	-	-	98%	98%
Controlled Postoperative Blood Glucose[5]	-	-	96%	97%
Perioperative Temperature Management[5]	-	-	100%	100%
Prophylactic Antibiotic Selection[5]	-	-	99%	99%
Prophylactic Antibiotic Selection (Outpatient)	-	-	98%	98%
Prophylactic Antibiotic Stopped[5]	-	-	98%	98%
Prophylactic Antibiotic Timing[5]	-	-	98%	99%
Prophylactic Antibiotic Timing (Outpatient)	-	-	98%	98%
Urinary Catheter Removal[5]	-	-	97%	97%
Survey of Patients' Hospital Experiences				
Area Around Room 'Always' Quiet at Night[5]	-	-	63%	61%
Doctors 'Always' Communicated Well[5]	-	-	84%	82%
Home Recovery Information Given[5]	-	-	88%	85%
Hospital Given 9 or 10 on 10 Point Scale[5]	-	-	75%	71%
Meds 'Always' Explained Before Given[5]	-	-	66%	64%
Nurses 'Always' Communicated Well[5]	-	-	81%	79%
Pain 'Always' Well Controlled[5]	-	-	71%	71%
Room and Bathroom 'Always' Clean[5]	-	-	79%	73%
Timely Help 'Always' Received[5]	-	-	70%	68%
Would Definitely Recommend Hospital[5]	-	-	74%	71%
Use of Medical Imaging				
Cardiac Imaging Stress Test before Surgery	-	-	4.8%	5.3%
Combination Abdominal CT Scan	-	-	11.5%	10.5%
Combination Brain/Sinus CT Scan	-	-	1.8%	2.7%
Combination Chest CT Scan	-	-	3.5%	2.7%
Follow-up Mammogram/Ultrasound	-	-	7.9%	8.8%
Lumbar Spine MRI for Low Back Pain	-	-	32.2%	37.2%

Central Community Hospital

901 Davidson Street Nw
Elkader, IA 52043
Phone: 563-245-7000
Fax: 563-245-7080
Type: Critical Access Hospitals
Emergency Services: Yes
Ownership: Voluntary non-profit - Private
Beds: 25

Key Personnel:
Infection Control. . . . . Ann Burds
Radiology. . . . . Ken Dettburn
Quality Assurance . . . . Lisa Marson
Emergency Room . . . . Natalie Shea
Operating Room. . . . . Lori Vlazny, RN
CEO/President. . . . . Fran Zichal
Chief of Medical Staff. . . . . Kenneth Zichal, MD

Measure	Cases	This Hosp.	State Avg.	U.S. Avg.
Blood Clot Prevention and Treatment				
Anticoagulation Overlap Therapy[5]	-	-	94%	93%
ICU Venous Thromboembolism Prophylaxis[5]	-	-	90%	92%
Incidence of Potentially Preventable VTE[5]	-	-	8%	10%
UFH with Dosages/Platelet Monitoring[5]	-	-	99%	97%
Venous Thromboembolism Prophylaxis[5]	-	-	87%	85%
Warfarin Therapy Discharge Instructions[5]	-	-	77%	75%
Chest Pain/Possible Heart Attack Care				
Aspirin Given Within 24 Hours of Arrival[5]	-	-	97%	96%
Fibrinolytic Meds Within 30 Min. of Arrival[5]	-	-	49%	58%
Average Time to ECG (minutes)[5]	-	-	5	7
Average Time to Transfer (minutes)[5]	-	-	58	60
Children's Asthma Care				
Received Home Management Plan of Care	-	-	-	88%
Received Reliever Medication	-	-	-	100%
Received Systemic Corticosteroids	-	-	-	100%
Emergency Department				
Admittance Decision Time (minutes)[5]	-	-	58	98
Head CT Results Within 45 Min. of Arrival[5]	-	-	55%	57%
Patients Who Left ER Before Being Seen[5]	-	-	1%	2%
Time from ER Arrival to Admit. (minutes)[5]	-	-	202	274
Time from ER Arrival to Discharge (minutes)[5]	-	-	108	134
Time in ER Before Being Evaluated (minutes)[5]	-	-	21	26
Time to Pain Meds for Fractures (minutes)[5]	-	-	46	57
Heart Attack Care				
Aspirin Given at Discharge[1,3]	-	-	100%	99%
Fibrinolytic Meds Within 30 Min. of Arrival[5]	-	-	-	54%
PCI Within 90 Minutes of Arrival[5]	-	-	94%	96%
Statin Prescribed at Discharge[1,3]	-	-	98%	98%
Heart Failure Care				
ACE Inhibitor or ARB for LVSD[1,3]	-	-	95%	97%
Discharge Instructions Given[1,3]	-	-	93%	94%
Evaluation of LVS Function[1,3]	-	-	97%	99%
Medicare Spending				
Medicare Spending per Patient (ratio)	-	-	0.91	0.98
Pneumonia Care				
Appropriate Initial Antibiotic Given[1,3]	-	-	93%	95%
Blood Culture Timing[1,3]	-	-	98%	98%
Pregnancy and Delivery Care				
Newborn Deliveries Scheduled Early[5]	-	-	4%	6%
Preventive Care				
Immunization for Influenza[5]	-	-	91%	90%
Immunization for Pneumonia[5]	-	-	90%	92%
Stroke Care				
Anticoagulation Therapy for Atrial Fibrillation[5]	-	-	95%	95%
Antithrombotic Therapy Timing[5]	-	-	98%	98%
Assessed for Rehabilitation[5]	-	-	97%	97%
Discharged on Antithrombotic Therapy[5]	-	-	99%	99%
Discharged on Statin Medication[5]	-	-	92%	94%
Thrombolytic Therapy Timing[5]	-	-	64%	66%
Venous Thromboembolism Prophylaxis[5]	-	-	93%	94%
Written Stroke Educational Materials Given[5]	-	-	82%	88%
Surgical Care Improvement Project				
Appropriate Beta Blocker Usage[5]	-	-	98%	98%
Appropriate VTP Within 24 Hours[5]	-	-	98%	98%
Controlled Postoperative Blood Glucose[5]	-	-	96%	97%
Perioperative Temperature Management[5]	-	-	100%	100%
Prophylactic Antibiotic Selection[5]	-	-	99%	99%
Prophylactic Antibiotic Selection (Outpatient)[5]	-	-	98%	98%
Prophylactic Antibiotic Stopped[5]	-	-	98%	98%
Prophylactic Antibiotic Timing[5]	-	-	98%	99%
Prophylactic Antibiotic Timing (Outpatient)[5]	-	-	98%	98%
Urinary Catheter Removal[5]	-	-	97%	97%
Survey of Patients' Hospital Experiences				
Area Around Room 'Always' Quiet at Night[5]	-	-	63%	61%
Doctors 'Always' Communicated Well[5]	-	-	84%	82%
Home Recovery Information Given[5]	-	-	88%	85%
Hospital Given 9 or 10 on 10 Point Scale[5]	-	-	75%	71%
Meds 'Always' Explained Before Given[5]	-	-	66%	64%
Nurses 'Always' Communicated Well[5]	-	-	81%	79%
Pain 'Always' Well Controlled[5]	-	-	71%	71%
Room and Bathroom 'Always' Clean[5]	-	-	79%	73%
Timely Help 'Always' Received[5]	-	-	70%	68%
Would Definitely Recommend Hospital[5]	-	-	74%	71%
Use of Medical Imaging				
Cardiac Imaging Stress Test before Surgery[1]	-	-	4.8%	5.3%
Combination Abdominal CT Scan[1]	-	-	11.5%	10.5%
Combination Brain/Sinus CT Scan	49	0.0%	1.8%	2.7%
Combination Chest CT Scan[1]	-	-	3.5%	2.7%
Follow-up Mammogram/Ultrasound	132	7.6%	7.9%	8.8%
Lumbar Spine MRI for Low Back Pain[1]	-	-	32.2%	37.2%

NOTE: Hospital profiles are in alphabetical order by state, then city, then hospital within the city; Rankings exclude hospitals with less than 25 cases except for patient surveys which excludes hospitals with less than 100 cases; (a) 100-299 cases; (1) The number of cases/patients is too few to report; (2) Data submitted were based on a sample of cases/patients; (3) Results are based on a shorter time period than required; (4) Data suppressed by CMS for one or more quarters; (5) Results are not available for this reporting period; (6) Fewer than 100 patients completed the HCAHPS survey; (7) No cases met the criteria for this measure; (8) The lower limit of the confidence interval cannot be calculated if the number of observed infections equals zero; (9) No data are available from the state/territory for this reporting period; (10) The scores shown reflect fewer than 50 completed surveys; (11) There were discrepancies in the data collection process; (12) This measure does not apply to this hospital for this reporting period; (13) Results cannot be calculated for this reporting period; (14) The results for this state are combined with nearby states to protect confidentiality; Please refer to the User's Guide for a full explanation of data.

Palo Alto County Hospital

3201 1st Street
Emmetsburg, IA 50536
URL: www.pachs.com
Type: Critical Access Hospitals
Ownership: Voluntary non-profit - Other

Phone: 712-852-5500
Fax: 712-852-5508

Emergency Services: Yes
Beds: 47

Key Personnel:
President . . . . Kris Ausborn
Chief of Medical Staff . . . . Patricia A Banwart
Ambulatory Care . . . . Sheryl Darling, EMS
Operating Room. . . . . Melanie Flynn
Radiology. . . . . Melissa Hospelhorn
Emergency Room . . . . Kim Kerr
CEO/President. . . . . Thomas J Lee
Quality Assurance . . . . Kathey Mehan

Measure	Cases	This Hosp.	State Avg.	U.S. Avg.
Blood Clot Prevention and Treatment				
Anticoagulation Overlap Therapy[5]	-	-	94%	93%
ICU Venous Thromboembolism Prophylaxis[5]	-	-	90%	92%
Incidence of Potentially Preventable VTE[5]	-	-	8%	10%
UFH with Dosages/Platelet Monitoring[5]	-	-	99%	97%
Venous Thromboembolism Prophylaxis[5]	-	-	87%	85%
Warfarin Therapy Discharge Instructions[5]	-	-	77%	75%
Chest Pain/Possible Heart Attack Care				
Aspirin Given Within 24 Hours of Arrival	-	-	97%	96%
Fibrinolytic Meds Within 30 Min. of Arrival	-	-	49%	58%
Average Time to ECG (minutes)	-	-	5	7
Average Time to Transfer (minutes)	-	-	58	60
Children's Asthma Care				
Received Home Management Plan of Care	-	-	-	88%
Received Reliever Medication	-	-	-	100%
Received Systemic Corticosteroids	-	-	-	100%
Emergency Department				
Admittance Decision Time (minutes)[5]	-	-	58	98
Head CT Results Within 45 Min. of Arrival	-	-	55%	57%
Patients Who Left ER Before Being Seen	-	-	1%	2%
Time from ER Arrival to Admit. (minutes)[5]	-	-	202	274
Time from ER Arrival to Discharge (minutes)	-	-	108	134
Time in ER Before Being Evaluated (minutes)	-	-	21	26
Time to Pain Meds for Fractures (minutes)	-	-	46	57
Heart Attack Care				
Aspirin Given at Discharge[5]	-	-	100%	99%
Fibrinolytic Meds Within 30 Min. of Arrival[5]	-	-	-	54%
PCI Within 90 Minutes of Arrival[5]	-	-	94%	96%
Statin Prescribed at Discharge[5]	-	-	98%	98%
Heart Failure Care				
ACE Inhibitor or ARB for LVSD[5]	-	-	95%	97%
Discharge Instructions Given[5]	-	-	93%	94%
Evaluation of LVS Function[5]	-	-	97%	99%
Medicare Spending				
Medicare Spending per Patient (ratio)	-	-	0.91	0.98
Pneumonia Care				
Appropriate Initial Antibiotic Given	37	70%	93%	95%
Blood Culture Timing	16	100%	98%	98%
Pregnancy and Delivery Care				
Newborn Deliveries Scheduled Early[5]	-	-	4%	6%
Preventive Care				
Immunization for Influenza[5]	-	-	91%	90%
Immunization for Pneumonia[5]	-	-	90%	92%
Stroke Care				
Anticoagulation Therapy for Atrial Fibrillation[5]	-	-	95%	95%
Antithrombotic Therapy Timing[5]	-	-	98%	98%
Assessed for Rehabilitation[5]	-	-	97%	97%
Discharged on Antithrombotic Therapy[5]	-	-	99%	99%
Discharged on Statin Medication[5]	-	-	92%	94%
Thrombolytic Therapy Timing[5]	-	-	64%	66%
Venous Thromboembolism Prophylaxis[5]	-	-	93%	94%
Written Stroke Educational Materials Given[5]	-	-	82%	88%
Surgical Care Improvement Project				
Appropriate Beta Blocker Usage[5]	-	-	98%	98%
Appropriate VTP Within 24 Hours[5]	-	-	98%	98%
Controlled Postoperative Blood Glucose[5]	-	-	96%	97%
Perioperative Temperature Management[5]	-	-	100%	100%
Prophylactic Antibiotic Selection[5]	-	-	99%	99%
Prophylactic Antibiotic Selection (Outpatient)	-	-	98%	98%
Prophylactic Antibiotic Stopped[5]	-	-	98%	98%
Prophylactic Antibiotic Timing[5]	-	-	98%	99%
Prophylactic Antibiotic Timing (Outpatient)	-	-	98%	98%
Urinary Catheter Removal[5]	-	-	97%	97%
Survey of Patients' Hospital Experiences				
Area Around Room 'Always' Quiet at Night[5]	-	-	63%	61%
Doctors 'Always' Communicated Well[5]	-	-	84%	82%
Home Recovery Information Given[5]	-	-	88%	85%
Hospital Given 9 or 10 on 10 Point Scale[5]	-	-	75%	71%
Meds 'Always' Explained Before Given[5]	-	-	66%	64%
Nurses 'Always' Communicated Well[5]	-	-	81%	79%
Pain 'Always' Well Controlled[5]	-	-	71%	71%
Room and Bathroom 'Always' Clean[5]	-	-	79%	73%
Timely Help 'Always' Received[5]	-	-	70%	68%
Would Definitely Recommend Hospital[5]	-	-	74%	71%
Use of Medical Imaging				
Cardiac Imaging Stress Test before Surgery	-	-	4.8%	5.3%
Combination Abdominal CT Scan	-	-	11.5%	10.5%
Combination Brain/Sinus CT Scan	-	-	1.8%	2.7%
Combination Chest CT Scan	-	-	3.5%	2.7%
Follow-up Mammogram/Ultrasound	-	-	7.9%	8.8%
Lumbar Spine MRI for Low Back Pain	-	-	32.2%	37.2%

Avera Holy Family Hospital

826 North 8th Street
Estherville, IA 51334
URL: www.averaholyfamily.org
Type: Critical Access Hospitals
Ownership: Voluntary non-profit - Church

Phone: 712-362-2631
Fax: 712-362-2636

Emergency Services: Yes
Beds: 25

Key Personnel:
Chief of Medical Staff . . . . Randy Asman
Patient Relations . . . . John Belk
CEO/President. . . . . Bill Bumgarner
Radiology. . . . . Robert P DeClark
Intensive Care Unit. . . . . Nancy Diekmann
Operating Room. . . . . Joyce Graettinger
Infection Control . . . . Annesley Gunderson
Quality Assurance . . . . Cathi Scharnberg

Measure	Cases	This Hosp.	State Avg.	U.S. Avg.
Blood Clot Prevention and Treatment				
Anticoagulation Overlap Therapy[1,2]	-	-	94%	93%
ICU Venous Thromboembolism Prophylaxis[2,3]	-	-	90%	92%
Incidence of Potentially Preventable VTE[2,3]	-	-	8%	10%
UFH with Dosages/Platelet Monitoring[1,2]	-	-	99%	97%
Venous Thromboembolism Prophylaxis[1,2]	-	-	87%	85%
Warfarin Therapy Discharge Instructions[1,2]	-	-	77%	75%
Chest Pain/Possible Heart Attack Care				
Aspirin Given Within 24 Hours of Arrival[1,3]	-	-	97%	96%
Fibrinolytic Meds Within 30 Min. of Arrival[3,7]	-	-	49%	58%
Average Time to ECG (minutes)[1,3]	-	-	5	7
Average Time to Transfer (minutes)[3,7]	-	-	58	60
Children's Asthma Care				
Received Home Management Plan of Care	-	-	-	88%
Received Reliever Medication	-	-	-	100%
Received Systemic Corticosteroids	-	-	-	100%
Emergency Department				
Admittance Decision Time (minutes)[2]	332	42	58	98
Head CT Results Within 45 Min. of Arrival[1,3]	-	-	55%	57%
Patients Who Left ER Before Being Seen	4,123	0%	1%	2%
Time from ER Arrival to Admit. (minutes)[2]	360	167	202	274
Time from ER Arrival to Discharge (minutes)[5]	-	-	108	134
Time in ER Before Being Evaluated (minutes)[5]	-	-	21	26
Time to Pain Meds for Fractures (minutes)[3]	18	87	46	57
Heart Attack Care				
Aspirin Given at Discharge[1]	-	-	100%	99%
Fibrinolytic Meds Within 30 Min. of Arrival[7]	-	-	-	54%
PCI Within 90 Minutes of Arrival[7]	-	-	94%	96%
Statin Prescribed at Discharge[1]	-	-	98%	98%
Heart Failure Care				
ACE Inhibitor or ARB for LVSD[1,2]	-	-	95%	97%
Discharge Instructions Given[2]	17	100%	93%	94%
Evaluation of LVS Function[2]	37	97%	97%	99%
Medicare Spending				
Medicare Spending per Patient (ratio)	-	-	0.91	0.98
Pneumonia Care				
Appropriate Initial Antibiotic Given[2]	18	94%	93%	95%
Blood Culture Timing[1,2]	-	-	98%	98%
Pregnancy and Delivery Care				
Newborn Deliveries Scheduled Early[1,3]	-	-	4%	6%
Preventive Care				
Immunization for Influenza[2]	287	93%	91%	90%
Immunization for Pneumonia[2]	377	93%	90%	92%
Stroke Care				
Anticoagulation Therapy for Atrial Fibrillation[1,3]	-	-	95%	95%
Antithrombotic Therapy Timing[1,3]	-	-	98%	98%
Assessed for Rehabilitation[1,3]	-	-	97%	97%
Discharged on Antithrombotic Therapy[1,3]	-	-	99%	99%
Discharged on Statin Medication[1,3]	-	-	92%	94%
Thrombolytic Therapy Timing[1,3]	-	-	64%	66%
Venous Thromboembolism Prophylaxis[1,3]	-	-	93%	94%
Written Stroke Educational Materials Given[1,3]	-	-	82%	88%
Surgical Care Improvement Project				
Appropriate Beta Blocker Usage[1]	-	-	98%	98%
Appropriate VTP Within 24 Hours	16	100%	98%	98%
Controlled Postoperative Blood Glucose[7]	-	-	96%	97%
Perioperative Temperature Management	21	100%	100%	100%
Prophylactic Antibiotic Selection	19	100%	99%	99%
Prophylactic Antibiotic Selection (Outpatient)[1,3]	-	-	98%	98%
Prophylactic Antibiotic Stopped	19	100%	98%	98%
Prophylactic Antibiotic Timing	19	89%	98%	99%
Prophylactic Antibiotic Timing (Outpatient)[1,3]	-	-	98%	98%
Urinary Catheter Removal	21	100%	97%	97%
Survey of Patients' Hospital Experiences				
Area Around Room 'Always' Quiet at Night	(a)	64%	63%	61%
Doctors 'Always' Communicated Well	(a)	88%	84%	82%
Home Recovery Information Given	(a)	94%	88%	85%
Hospital Given 9 or 10 on 10 Point Scale	(a)	74%	75%	71%
Meds 'Always' Explained Before Given	(a)	63%	66%	64%
Nurses 'Always' Communicated Well	(a)	81%	81%	79%
Pain 'Always' Well Controlled	(a)	67%	71%	71%
Room and Bathroom 'Always' Clean	(a)	76%	79%	73%
Timely Help 'Always' Received	(a)	69%	70%	68%
Would Definitely Recommend Hospital	(a)	71%	74%	71%
Use of Medical Imaging				
Cardiac Imaging Stress Test before Surgery[1]	-	-	4.8%	5.3%
Combination Abdominal CT Scan	74	12.2%	11.5%	10.5%
Combination Brain/Sinus CT Scan[1]	-	-	1.8%	2.7%
Combination Chest CT Scan[1]	-	-	3.5%	2.7%
Follow-up Mammogram/Ultrasound	316	0.6%	7.9%	8.8%
Lumbar Spine MRI for Low Back Pain[1]	-	-	32.2%	37.2%

Jefferson County Health Center

2000 S Main
Fairfield, IA 52556
URL: www.jchospital.org
Type: Critical Access Hospitals
Ownership: Government - Local

Phone: 641-472-4111
Fax: 641-469-4375

Emergency Services: Yes
Beds: 67

Key Personnel:
CEO/President. . . . . Deb Cardin
Chief of Medical Staff . . . . Deb Cardin
Emergency Room . . . . Michael Eisner
Quality Assurance . . . . Kim Woods, RN

Measure	Cases	This Hosp.	State Avg.	U.S. Avg.
Blood Clot Prevention and Treatment				
Anticoagulation Overlap Therapy[5]	-	-	94%	93%
ICU Venous Thromboembolism Prophylaxis[5]	-	-	90%	92%
Incidence of Potentially Preventable VTE[5]	-	-	8%	10%
UFH with Dosages/Platelet Monitoring[5]	-	-	99%	97%
Venous Thromboembolism Prophylaxis[5]	-	-	87%	85%
Warfarin Therapy Discharge Instructions[5]	-	-	77%	75%
Chest Pain/Possible Heart Attack Care				
Aspirin Given Within 24 Hours of Arrival	12	100%	97%	96%
Fibrinolytic Meds Within 30 Min. of Arrival[7]	-	-	49%	58%
Average Time to ECG (minutes)	12	4	5	7
Average Time to Transfer (minutes)[7]	-	-	58	60
Children's Asthma Care				

NOTE: Hospital profiles are in alphabetical order by state, then city, then hospital within the city; Rankings exclude hospitals with less than 25 cases except for patient surveys which excludes hospitals with less than 100 cases; (a) 100-299 cases; (1) The number of cases/patients is too few to report; (2) Data submitted were based on a sample of cases/patients; (3) Results are based on a shorter time period than required; (4) Data suppressed by CMS for one or more quarters; (5) Results are not available for this reporting period; (6) Fewer than 100 patients completed the HCAHPS survey; (7) No cases met the criteria for this measure; (8) The lower limit of the confidence interval cannot be calculated if the number of observed infections equals zero; (9) No data are available from the state/territory for this reporting period; (10) The scores shown reflect fewer than 50 completed surveys; (11) There were discrepancies in the data collection process; (12) This measure does not apply to this hospital for this reporting period; (13) Results cannot be calculated for this reporting period; (14) The results for this state are combined with nearby states to protect confidentiality; Please refer to the User's Guide for a full explanation of data.

Received Home Management Plan of Care	-	-	-	88%
Received Reliever Medication	-	-	-	100%
Received Systemic Corticosteroids	-	-	-	100%
Emergency Department				
Admittance Decision Time (minutes)[5]	-	-	58	98
Head CT Results Within 45 Min. of Arrival[5]	-	-	55%	57%
Patients Who Left ER Before Being Seen[5]	-	-	1%	2%
Time from ER Arrival to Admit. (minutes)[5]	-	-	202	274
Time from ER Arrival to Discharge (minutes)[5]	-	-	108	134
Time in ER Before Being Evaluated (minutes)[5]	-	-	21	26
Time to Pain Meds for Fractures (minutes)[5]	-	-	46	57
Heart Attack Care				
Aspirin Given at Discharge[5]	-	-	100%	99%
Fibrinolytic Meds Within 30 Min. of Arrival[5]	-	-	-	54%
PCI Within 90 Minutes of Arrival[5]	-	-	94%	96%
Statin Prescribed at Discharge[5]	-	-	98%	98%
Heart Failure Care				
ACE Inhibitor or ARB for LVSD[1]	-	-	95%	97%
Discharge Instructions Given	15	87%	93%	94%
Evaluation of LVS Function	28	96%	97%	99%
Medicare Spending				
Medicare Spending per Patient (ratio)	-	-	0.91	0.98
Pneumonia Care				
Appropriate Initial Antibiotic Given	45	96%	93%	95%
Blood Culture Timing	32	100%	98%	98%
Pregnancy and Delivery Care				
Newborn Deliveries Scheduled Early[5]	-	-	4%	6%
Preventive Care				
Immunization for Influenza[2]	82	91%	91%	90%
Immunization for Pneumonia[2]	131	79%	90%	92%
Stroke Care				
Anticoagulation Therapy for Atrial Fibrillation[5]	-	-	95%	95%
Antithrombotic Therapy Timing[5]	-	-	98%	98%
Assessed for Rehabilitation[5]	-	-	97%	97%
Discharged on Antithrombotic Therapy[5]	-	-	99%	99%
Discharged on Statin Medication[5]	-	-	92%	94%
Thrombolytic Therapy Timing[5]	-	-	64%	66%
Venous Thromboembolism Prophylaxis[5]	-	-	93%	94%
Written Stroke Educational Materials Given[5]	-	-	82%	88%
Surgical Care Improvement Project				
Appropriate Beta Blocker Usage[1]	-	-	98%	98%
Appropriate VTP Within 24 Hours	26	69%	98%	98%
Controlled Postoperative Blood Glucose[7]	-	-	96%	97%
Perioperative Temperature Management	25	100%	100%	100%
Prophylactic Antibiotic Selection	14	93%	99%	99%
Prophylactic Antibiotic Selection (Outpatient)[5]	-	-	98%	98%
Prophylactic Antibiotic Stopped	12	42%	98%	98%
Prophylactic Antibiotic Timing	14	100%	98%	99%
Prophylactic Antibiotic Timing (Outpatient)[5]	-	-	98%	98%
Urinary Catheter Removal	13	100%	97%	97%
Survey of Patients' Hospital Experiences				
Area Around Room 'Always' Quiet at Night	(a)	77%	63%	61%
Doctors 'Always' Communicated Well	(a)	86%	84%	82%
Home Recovery Information Given	(a)	86%	88%	85%
Hospital Given 9 or 10 on 10 Point Scale	(a)	86%	75%	71%
Meds 'Always' Explained Before Given	(a)	67%	66%	64%
Nurses 'Always' Communicated Well	(a)	88%	81%	79%
Pain 'Always' Well Controlled	(a)	75%	71%	71%
Room and Bathroom 'Always' Clean	(a)	86%	79%	73%
Timely Help 'Always' Received	(a)	75%	70%	68%
Would Definitely Recommend Hospital	(a)	84%	74%	71%
Use of Medical Imaging				
Cardiac Imaging Stress Test before Surgery[1]	-	-	4.8%	5.3%
Combination Abdominal CT Scan	134	6.7%	11.5%	10.5%
Combination Brain/Sinus CT Scan	260	0.8%	1.8%	2.7%
Combination Chest CT Scan	65	1.5%	3.5%	2.7%
Follow-up Mammogram/Ultrasound	348	6.0%	7.9%	8.8%
Lumbar Spine MRI for Low Back Pain	41	39.0%	32.2%	37.2%

Trinity Regional Medical Center

802 Kenyon Rd
Fort Dodge, IA 50501
URL: www.trmc.org
Type: Acute Care Hospitals
Ownership: Voluntary non-profit - Private
Phone: 515-573-3101
Fax: 515-573-8710
Emergency Services: Yes
Beds: 200

Key Personnel:
Chief of Medical Staff.......... Kenneth Adams, DO
Quality Assurance .... Steve Gibson
Pediatric Ambulatory Care ...... Joan Hisler
Pediatric In-Patient Care .... Joan Hisler
Radiology.................... Keith Lacey
Infection Control.............. Linda Opheim
Coronary Care .... Sheryl Rogers
CEO/President................ Tom Tibbits

Measure	Cases	This Hosp.	State Avg.	U.S. Avg.
Blood Clot Prevention and Treatment				
Anticoagulation Overlap Therapy[2]	43	100%	94%	93%
ICU Venous Thromboembolism Prophylaxis[2]	91	85%	90%	92%
Incidence of Potentially Preventable VTE[1,2]	-	-	8%	10%
UFH with Dosages/Platelet Monitoring[1,2]	-	-	99%	97%
Venous Thromboembolism Prophylaxis[2]	290	93%	87%	85%
Warfarin Therapy Discharge Instructions[2]	37	51%	77%	75%
Chest Pain/Possible Heart Attack Care				
Aspirin Given Within 24 Hours of Arrival[1,3]	-	-	97%	96%
Fibrinolytic Meds Within 30 Min. of Arrival[5]	-	-	49%	58%
Average Time to ECG (minutes)[1,3]	-	-	5	7
Average Time to Transfer (minutes)[5]	-	-	58	60
Children's Asthma Care				
Received Home Management Plan of Care	-	-	-	88%
Received Reliever Medication	-	-	-	100%
Received Systemic Corticosteroids	-	-	-	100%
Emergency Department				
Admittance Decision Time (minutes)[2]	466	36	58	98
Head CT Results Within 45 Min. of Arrival	13	62%	55%	57%
Patients Who Left ER Before Being Seen	22,531	0%	1%	2%
Time from ER Arrival to Admit. (minutes)[2]	475	168	202	274
Time from ER Arrival to Discharge (minutes)	352	118	108	134
Time in ER Before Being Evaluated (minutes)	213	29	21	26
Time to Pain Meds for Fractures (minutes)	78	52	46	57
Heart Attack Care				
Aspirin Given at Discharge	167	100%	100%	99%
Fibrinolytic Meds Within 30 Min. of Arrival[7]	-	-	-	54%
PCI Within 90 Minutes of Arrival	17	94%	94%	96%
Statin Prescribed at Discharge	158	99%	98%	98%
Heart Failure Care				
ACE Inhibitor or ARB for LVSD	38	100%	95%	97%
Discharge Instructions Given	120	98%	93%	94%
Evaluation of LVS Function	150	99%	97%	99%
Medicare Spending				
Medicare Spending per Patient (ratio)	-	0.92	0.91	0.98
Pneumonia Care				
Appropriate Initial Antibiotic Given	114	94%	93%	95%
Blood Culture Timing	192	100%	98%	98%
Pregnancy and Delivery Care				
Newborn Deliveries Scheduled Early[2]	22	0%	4%	6%
Preventive Care				
Immunization for Influenza[2]	427	94%	91%	90%
Immunization for Pneumonia[2]	510	93%	90%	92%
Stroke Care				
Anticoagulation Therapy for Atrial Fibrillation[1,2]	-	-	95%	95%
Antithrombotic Therapy Timing[2]	27	100%	98%	98%
Assessed for Rehabilitation[2]	28	96%	97%	97%
Discharged on Antithrombotic Therapy[2]	27	100%	99%	99%
Discharged on Statin Medication[2]	19	89%	92%	94%
Thrombolytic Therapy Timing[2,7]	-	-	64%	66%
Venous Thromboembolism Prophylaxis[2]	29	93%	93%	94%
Written Stroke Educational Materials Given[2]	19	84%	82%	88%
Surgical Care Improvement Project				
Appropriate Beta Blocker Usage[2]	86	97%	98%	98%
Appropriate VTP Within 24 Hours[2]	173	99%	98%	98%
Controlled Postoperative Blood Glucose[2]	12	100%	96%	97%
Perioperative Temperature Management[2]	246	100%	100%	100%
Prophylactic Antibiotic Selection[2]	181	100%	99%	99%
Prophylactic Antibiotic Selection (Outpatient)	163	99%	98%	98%
Prophylactic Antibiotic Stopped[2]	175	95%	98%	98%
Prophylactic Antibiotic Timing[2]	181	98%	98%	99%
Prophylactic Antibiotic Timing (Outpatient)	163	97%	98%	98%
Urinary Catheter Removal[2]	151	96%	97%	97%
Survey of Patients' Hospital Experiences				
Area Around Room 'Always' Quiet at Night	300+	58%	63%	61%
Doctors 'Always' Communicated Well	300+	80%	84%	82%
Home Recovery Information Given	300+	91%	88%	85%
Hospital Given 9 or 10 on 10 Point Scale	300+	71%	75%	71%
Meds 'Always' Explained Before Given	300+	64%	66%	64%
Nurses 'Always' Communicated Well	300+	82%	81%	79%
Pain 'Always' Well Controlled	300+	70%	71%	71%
Room and Bathroom 'Always' Clean	300+	78%	79%	73%
Timely Help 'Always' Received	300+	71%	70%	68%
Would Definitely Recommend Hospital	300+	67%	74%	71%
Use of Medical Imaging				
Cardiac Imaging Stress Test before Surgery[1]	-	-	4.8%	5.3%
Combination Abdominal CT Scan	434	0.7%	11.5%	10.5%
Combination Brain/Sinus CT Scan[1]	-	-	1.8%	2.7%
Combination Chest CT Scan	390	1.0%	3.5%	2.7%
Follow-up Mammogram/Ultrasound[7]	-	-	7.9%	8.8%
Lumbar Spine MRI for Low Back Pain	101	33.7%	32.2%	37.2%

Fort Madison Community Hospital

5445 Ave O
Fort Madison, IA 52627
E-mail: jplatt@fmchosp.com
URL: www.fmchosp.com
Type: Acute Care Hospitals
Ownership: Voluntary non-profit - Private
Phone: 319-372-6530
Fax: 319-372-9119
Emergency Services: Yes
Beds: 50

Key Personnel:
President.................... Deanna Barr
Radiology.................... Steven Davis, MD
Emergency Room .... Christina Goebel
Quality Assurance .... Meredith Griffith
Chief of Medical Staff......... David Wenger Keller, MD
CEO/President................ C James Platt
CEO .... C. James Platt

Measure	Cases	This Hosp.	State Avg.	U.S. Avg.
Blood Clot Prevention and Treatment				
Anticoagulation Overlap Therapy[1,2]	-	-	94%	93%
ICU Venous Thromboembolism Prophylaxis[2]	54	98%	90%	92%
Incidence of Potentially Preventable VTE[2,7]	-	-	8%	10%
UFH with Dosages/Platelet Monitoring[1,2]	-	-	99%	97%
Venous Thromboembolism Prophylaxis[2]	129	98%	87%	85%
Warfarin Therapy Discharge Instructions[1,2]	-	-	77%	75%
Chest Pain/Possible Heart Attack Care				
Aspirin Given Within 24 Hours of Arrival	34	100%	97%	96%
Fibrinolytic Meds Within 30 Min. of Arrival[1]	-	-	49%	58%
Average Time to ECG (minutes)	35	4	5	7
Average Time to Transfer (minutes)[1]	-	-	58	60
Children's Asthma Care				
Received Home Management Plan of Care	-	-	-	88%
Received Reliever Medication	-	-	-	100%
Received Systemic Corticosteroids	-	-	-	100%
Emergency Department				
Admittance Decision Time (minutes)[2]	318	42	58	98
Head CT Results Within 45 Min. of Arrival	12	58%	55%	57%
Patients Who Left ER Before Being Seen	13,835	2%	1%	2%
Time from ER Arrival to Admit. (minutes)[2]	334	177	202	274
Time from ER Arrival to Discharge (minutes)	357	93	108	134
Time in ER Before Being Evaluated (minutes)	384	30	21	26
Time to Pain Meds for Fractures (minutes)	43	34	46	57
Heart Attack Care				
Aspirin Given at Discharge	11	100%	100%	99%
Fibrinolytic Meds Within 30 Min. of Arrival[7]	-	-	-	54%
PCI Within 90 Minutes of Arrival[7]	-	-	94%	96%
Statin Prescribed at Discharge[1]	-	-	98%	98%
Heart Failure Care				
ACE Inhibitor or ARB for LVSD	15	100%	95%	97%
Discharge Instructions Given	39	100%	93%	94%
Evaluation of LVS Function	54	100%	97%	99%
Medicare Spending				

NOTE: Hospital profiles are in alphabetical order by state, then city, then hospital within the city; Rankings exclude hospitals with less than 25 cases except for patient surveys which excludes hospitals with less than 100 cases; (a) 100-299 cases; (1) The number of cases/patients is too few to report; (2) Data submitted were based on a sample of cases/patients; (3) Results are based on a shorter time period than required; (4) Data suppressed by CMS for one or more quarters; (5) Results are not available for this reporting period; (6) Fewer than 100 patients completed the HCAHPS survey; (7) No cases met the criteria for this measure; (8) The lower limit of the confidence interval cannot be calculated if the number of observed infections equals zero; (9) No data are available from the state/territory for this reporting period; (10) The scores shown reflect fewer than 50 completed surveys; (11) There were discrepancies in the data collection process; (12) This measure does not apply to this hospital for this reporting period; (13) Results cannot be calculated for this reporting period; (14) The results for this state are combined with nearby states to protect confidentiality; Please refer to the User's Guide for a full explanation of data.

Measure	Cases	This Hosp.	State Avg.	U.S. Avg.
Medicare Spending per Patient (ratio)	-	0.82	0.91	0.98
Pneumonia Care				
Appropriate Initial Antibiotic Given	73	96%	93%	95%
Blood Culture Timing	76	99%	98%	98%
Pregnancy and Delivery Care				
Newborn Deliveries Scheduled Early[2]	23	4%	4%	6%
Preventive Care				
Immunization for Influenza[2]	373	99%	91%	90%
Immunization for Pneumonia[2]	395	99%	90%	92%
Stroke Care				
Anticoagulation Therapy for Atrial Fibrillation[7]	-	-	95%	95%
Antithrombotic Therapy Timing[1]	-	-	98%	98%
Assessed for Rehabilitation[1]	-	-	97%	97%
Discharged on Antithrombotic Therapy[1]	-	-	99%	99%
Discharged on Statin Medication[1]	-	-	92%	94%
Thrombolytic Therapy Timing[7]	-	-	64%	66%
Venous Thromboembolism Prophylaxis[1]	-	-	93%	94%
Written Stroke Educational Materials Given[1]	-	-	82%	88%
Surgical Care Improvement Project				
Appropriate Beta Blocker Usage	32	100%	98%	98%
Appropriate VTP Within 24 Hours	87	100%	98%	98%
Controlled Postoperative Blood Glucose[7]	-	-	96%	97%
Perioperative Temperature Management	98	100%	100%	100%
Prophylactic Antibiotic Selection	82	100%	99%	99%
Prophylactic Antibiotic Selection (Outpatient)	48	96%	98%	98%
Prophylactic Antibiotic Stopped	81	99%	98%	98%
Prophylactic Antibiotic Timing	82	100%	98%	99%
Prophylactic Antibiotic Timing (Outpatient)	39	100%	98%	98%
Urinary Catheter Removal	94	100%	97%	97%
Survey of Patients' Hospital Experiences				
Area Around Room 'Always' Quiet at Night	300+	58%	63%	61%
Doctors 'Always' Communicated Well	300+	84%	84%	82%
Home Recovery Information Given	300+	90%	88%	85%
Hospital Given 9 or 10 on 10 Point Scale	300+	79%	75%	71%
Meds 'Always' Explained Before Given	300+	64%	66%	64%
Nurses 'Always' Communicated Well	300+	85%	81%	79%
Pain 'Always' Well Controlled	300+	70%	71%	71%
Room and Bathroom 'Always' Clean	300+	82%	79%	73%
Timely Help 'Always' Received	300+	68%	70%	68%
Would Definitely Recommend Hospital	300+	79%	74%	71%
Use of Medical Imaging				
Cardiac Imaging Stress Test before Surgery	161	4.3%	4.8%	5.3%
Combination Abdominal CT Scan	249	66.7%	11.5%	10.5%
Combination Brain/Sinus CT Scan	209	4.8%	1.8%	2.7%
Combination Chest CT Scan	186	1.1%	3.5%	2.7%
Follow-up Mammogram/Ultrasound	604	12.4%	7.9%	8.8%
Lumbar Spine MRI for Low Back Pain	72	34.7%	32.2%	37.2%

Adair County Memorial Hospital

609 Se Kent
Greenfield, IA 50849
Phone: 641-743-2123
Fax: 641-743-2610
URL: www.adaircountyhealthsystem.org
Type: Critical Access Hospitals
Emergency Services: Yes
Ownership: Voluntary non-profit - Other
Beds: 31

Key Personnel:
Operating Room. . . . . Marvel Blazer, RN
Quality Assurance . . . . Jan Livingston
CEO . . . . Angela Mortoza
Chief of Medical Staff. . . . . Troy Renaud
Infection Control. . . . . Deb Tindle, RN

Measure	Cases	This Hosp.	State Avg.	U.S. Avg.
Blood Clot Prevention and Treatment				
Anticoagulation Overlap Therapy[5]	-	-	94%	93%
ICU Venous Thromboembolism Prophylaxis[5]	-	-	90%	92%
Incidence of Potentially Preventable VTE[5]	-	-	8%	10%
UFH with Dosages/Platelet Monitoring[5]	-	-	99%	97%
Venous Thromboembolism Prophylaxis[5]	-	-	87%	85%
Warfarin Therapy Discharge Instructions[5]	-	-	77%	75%
Chest Pain/Possible Heart Attack Care				
Aspirin Given Within 24 Hours of Arrival[1]	-	-	97%	96%
Fibrinolytic Meds Within 30 Min. of Arrival[3,7]	-	-	49%	58%
Average Time to ECG (minutes)	11	5	5	7
Average Time to Transfer (minutes)[1,3]	-	-	58	60
Children's Asthma Care				
Received Home Management Plan of Care	-	-	-	88%
Received Reliever Medication	-	-	-	100%
Received Systemic Corticosteroids	-	-	-	100%
Emergency Department				
Admittance Decision Time (minutes)[5]	-	-	58	98
Head CT Results Within 45 Min. of Arrival[1]	-	-	55%	57%
Patients Who Left ER Before Being Seen[5]	-	-	1%	2%
Time from ER Arrival to Admit. (minutes)[5]	-	-	202	274
Time from ER Arrival to Discharge (minutes)[5]	-	-	108	134
Time in ER Before Being Evaluated (minutes)[5]	-	-	21	26
Time to Pain Meds for Fractures (minutes)[5]	-	-	46	57
Heart Attack Care				
Aspirin Given at Discharge[5]	-	-	100%	99%
Fibrinolytic Meds Within 30 Min. of Arrival[5]	-	-	-	54%
PCI Within 90 Minutes of Arrival[5]	-	-	94%	96%
Statin Prescribed at Discharge[5]	-	-	98%	98%
Heart Failure Care				
ACE Inhibitor or ARB for LVSD[1,3]	-	-	95%	97%
Discharge Instructions Given[1,3]	-	-	93%	94%
Evaluation of LVS Function[1,3]	-	-	97%	99%
Medicare Spending				
Medicare Spending per Patient (ratio)	-	-	0.91	0.98
Pneumonia Care				
Appropriate Initial Antibiotic Given[1,2]	-	-	93%	95%
Blood Culture Timing[2]	15	100%	98%	98%
Pregnancy and Delivery Care				
Newborn Deliveries Scheduled Early[5]	-	-	4%	6%
Preventive Care				
Immunization for Influenza[5]	-	-	91%	90%
Immunization for Pneumonia[5]	-	-	90%	92%
Stroke Care				
Anticoagulation Therapy for Atrial Fibrillation[5]	-	-	95%	95%
Antithrombotic Therapy Timing[5]	-	-	98%	98%
Assessed for Rehabilitation[5]	-	-	97%	97%
Discharged on Antithrombotic Therapy[5]	-	-	99%	99%
Discharged on Statin Medication[5]	-	-	92%	94%
Thrombolytic Therapy Timing[5]	-	-	64%	66%
Venous Thromboembolism Prophylaxis[5]	-	-	93%	94%
Written Stroke Educational Materials Given[5]	-	-	82%	88%
Surgical Care Improvement Project				
Appropriate Beta Blocker Usage[5]	-	-	98%	98%
Appropriate VTP Within 24 Hours[5]	-	-	98%	98%
Controlled Postoperative Blood Glucose[5]	-	-	96%	97%
Perioperative Temperature Management[5]	-	-	100%	100%
Prophylactic Antibiotic Selection[5]	-	-	99%	99%
Prophylactic Antibiotic Selection (Outpatient)[5]	-	-	98%	98%
Prophylactic Antibiotic Stopped[5]	-	-	98%	98%
Prophylactic Antibiotic Timing[5]	-	-	98%	99%
Prophylactic Antibiotic Timing (Outpatient)[5]	-	-	98%	98%
Urinary Catheter Removal[5]	-	-	97%	97%
Survey of Patients' Hospital Experiences				
Area Around Room 'Always' Quiet at Night[5]	-	-	63%	61%
Doctors 'Always' Communicated Well[5]	-	-	84%	82%
Home Recovery Information Given[5]	-	-	88%	85%
Hospital Given 9 or 10 on 10 Point Scale[5]	-	-	75%	71%
Meds 'Always' Explained Before Given[5]	-	-	66%	64%
Nurses 'Always' Communicated Well[5]	-	-	81%	79%
Pain 'Always' Well Controlled[5]	-	-	71%	71%
Room and Bathroom 'Always' Clean[5]	-	-	79%	73%
Timely Help 'Always' Received[5]	-	-	70%	68%
Would Definitely Recommend Hospital[5]	-	-	74%	71%
Use of Medical Imaging				
Cardiac Imaging Stress Test before Surgery[1]	-	-	4.8%	5.3%
Combination Abdominal CT Scan	66	65.2%	11.5%	10.5%
Combination Brain/Sinus CT Scan	77	0.0%	1.8%	2.7%
Combination Chest CT Scan[1]	-	-	3.5%	2.7%
Follow-up Mammogram/Ultrasound	139	4.3%	7.9%	8.8%
Lumbar Spine MRI for Low Back Pain[1]	-	-	32.2%	37.2%

Grinnell Regional Medical Center

210 Fourth Avenue
Grinnell, IA 50112
Phone: 641-236-7511
Fax: 641-236-2995
URL: www.grmc.us
Type: Acute Care Hospitals
Emergency Services: Yes
Ownership: Voluntary non-profit - Private
Beds: 81

Key Personnel:
Chief of Medical Staff . . . . Roy Doorebos, MD
Radiology. . . . . William D Heggen
CEO/President. . . . . Todd C Linden
Operating Room. . . . . Deb Reding
Anesthesiology. . . . . James Schuh, MD

Measure	Cases	This Hosp.	State Avg.	U.S. Avg.
Blood Clot Prevention and Treatment				
Anticoagulation Overlap Therapy[1,2]	-	-	94%	93%
ICU Venous Thromboembolism Prophylaxis[2]	32	100%	90%	92%
Incidence of Potentially Preventable VTE[2,7]	-	-	8%	10%
UFH with Dosages/Platelet Monitoring[2,7]	-	-	99%	97%
Venous Thromboembolism Prophylaxis[2]	96	100%	87%	85%
Warfarin Therapy Discharge Instructions[1,2]	-	-	77%	75%
Chest Pain/Possible Heart Attack Care				
Aspirin Given Within 24 Hours of Arrival	41	100%	97%	96%
Fibrinolytic Meds Within 30 Min. of Arrival[1]	-	-	49%	58%
Average Time to ECG (minutes)	43	9	5	7
Average Time to Transfer (minutes)[1]	-	-	58	60
Children's Asthma Care				
Received Home Management Plan of Care	-	-	-	88%
Received Reliever Medication	-	-	-	100%
Received Systemic Corticosteroids	-	-	-	100%
Emergency Department				
Admittance Decision Time (minutes)[2]	195	50	58	98
Head CT Results Within 45 Min. of Arrival[1]	-	-	55%	57%
Patients Who Left ER Before Being Seen	10,626	0%	1%	2%
Time from ER Arrival to Admit. (minutes)[2]	200	166	202	274
Time from ER Arrival to Discharge (minutes)	332	90	108	134
Time in ER Before Being Evaluated (minutes)	366	26	21	26
Time to Pain Meds for Fractures (minutes)	49	41	46	57
Heart Attack Care				
Aspirin Given at Discharge[1]	-	-	100%	99%
Fibrinolytic Meds Within 30 Min. of Arrival[7]	-	-	-	54%
PCI Within 90 Minutes of Arrival[7]	-	-	94%	96%
Statin Prescribed at Discharge[1]	-	-	98%	98%
Heart Failure Care				
ACE Inhibitor or ARB for LVSD[1,2]	-	-	95%	97%
Discharge Instructions Given[2]	19	95%	93%	94%
Evaluation of LVS Function[2]	40	100%	97%	99%
Medicare Spending				
Medicare Spending per Patient (ratio)	-	0.83	0.91	0.98
Pneumonia Care				
Appropriate Initial Antibiotic Given[2]	46	96%	93%	95%
Blood Culture Timing[2]	63	98%	98%	98%
Pregnancy and Delivery Care				
Newborn Deliveries Scheduled Early	14	0%	4%	6%
Preventive Care				
Immunization for Influenza[2]	250	98%	91%	90%
Immunization for Pneumonia[2]	296	98%	90%	92%
Stroke Care				
Anticoagulation Therapy for Atrial Fibrillation[1]	-	-	95%	95%
Antithrombotic Therapy Timing	15	93%	98%	98%
Assessed for Rehabilitation	15	100%	97%	97%
Discharged on Antithrombotic Therapy	15	100%	99%	99%
Discharged on Statin Medication[1]	-	-	92%	94%
Thrombolytic Therapy Timing[1]	-	-	64%	66%
Venous Thromboembolism Prophylaxis	16	100%	93%	94%
Written Stroke Educational Materials Given[1]	-	-	82%	88%
Surgical Care Improvement Project				
Appropriate Beta Blocker Usage	16	94%	98%	98%
Appropriate VTP Within 24 Hours	76	100%	98%	98%
Controlled Postoperative Blood Glucose[7]	-	-	96%	97%
Perioperative Temperature Management	82	98%	100%	100%
Prophylactic Antibiotic Selection	21	95%	99%	99%
Prophylactic Antibiotic Selection (Outpatient)	13	92%	98%	98%
Prophylactic Antibiotic Stopped	17	82%	98%	98%

NOTE: Hospital profiles are in alphabetical order by state, then city, then hospital within the city; Rankings exclude hospitals with less than 25 cases except for patient surveys which excludes hospitals with less than 100 cases; (a) 100-299 cases; (1) The number of cases/patients is too few to report; (2) Data submitted were based on a sample of cases/patients; (3) Results are based on a shorter time period than required; (4) Data suppressed by CMS for one or more quarters; (5) Results are not available for this reporting period; (6) Fewer than 100 patients completed the HCAHPS survey; (7) No cases met the criteria for this measure; (8) The lower limit of the confidence interval cannot be calculated if the number of observed infections equals zero; (9) No data are available from the state/territory for this reporting period; (10) The scores shown reflect fewer than 50 completed surveys; (11) There were discrepancies in the data collection process; (12) This measure does not apply to this hospital for this reporting period; (13) Results cannot be calculated for this reporting period; (14) The results for this state are combined with nearby states to protect confidentiality; Please refer to the User's Guide for a full explanation of data.

Measure	Cases	This Hosp.	State Avg.	U.S. Avg.
Prophylactic Antibiotic Timing	21	90%	98%	99%
Prophylactic Antibiotic Timing (Outpatient)	13	100%	98%	98%
Urinary Catheter Removal	47	98%	97%	97%
Survey of Patients' Hospital Experiences				
Area Around Room 'Always' Quiet at Night	300+	70%	63%	61%
Doctors 'Always' Communicated Well	300+	84%	84%	82%
Home Recovery Information Given	300+	90%	88%	85%
Hospital Given 9 or 10 on 10 Point Scale	300+	77%	75%	71%
Meds 'Always' Explained Before Given	300+	71%	66%	64%
Nurses 'Always' Communicated Well	300+	84%	81%	79%
Pain 'Always' Well Controlled	300+	75%	71%	71%
Room and Bathroom 'Always' Clean	300+	86%	79%	73%
Timely Help 'Always' Received	300+	72%	70%	68%
Would Definitely Recommend Hospital	300+	73%	74%	71%
Use of Medical Imaging				
Cardiac Imaging Stress Test before Surgery	109	3.7%	4.8%	5.3%
Combination Abdominal CT Scan	237	9.7%	11.5%	10.5%
Combination Brain/Sinus CT Scan[1]	-	-	1.8%	2.7%
Combination Chest CT Scan	101	2.0%	3.5%	2.7%
Follow-up Mammogram/Ultrasound	520	11.2%	7.9%	8.8%
Lumbar Spine MRI for Low Back Pain	39	46.2%	32.2%	37.2%

Grundy County Memorial Hospital

201 East J Avenue
Grundy Center, IA 50638
Phone: 319-824-5421
Fax: 319-824-3337
E-mail: janicem@gcmuni.net
URL: www.grundyhospital.com
Type: Critical Access Hospitals
Emergency Services: Yes
Ownership: Voluntary non-profit - Other
Beds: 80

Key Personnel:
Emergency Room . . . . Elizabeth Ash, RN
Operating Room. . . . . Elizabeth Ash
Chief of Medical Staff. . . . . Ryan Bingman, MD
CEO/President. . . . . Pamela K Delagardelle

Measure	Cases	This Hosp.	State Avg.	U.S. Avg.
Blood Clot Prevention and Treatment				
Anticoagulation Overlap Therapy[5]	-	-	94%	93%
ICU Venous Thromboembolism Prophylaxis[5]	-	-	90%	92%
Incidence of Potentially Preventable VTE[5]	-	-	8%	10%
UFH with Dosages/Platelet Monitoring[5]	-	-	99%	97%
Venous Thromboembolism Prophylaxis[5]	-	-	87%	85%
Warfarin Therapy Discharge Instructions[5]	-	-	77%	75%
Chest Pain/Possible Heart Attack Care				
Aspirin Given Within 24 Hours of Arrival	38	95%	97%	96%
Fibrinolytic Meds Within 30 Min. of Arrival[7]	-	-	49%	58%
Average Time to ECG (minutes)	38	4	5	7
Average Time to Transfer (minutes)[7]	-	-	58	60
Children's Asthma Care				
Received Home Management Plan of Care	-	-	-	88%
Received Reliever Medication	-	-	-	100%
Received Systemic Corticosteroids	-	-	-	100%
Emergency Department				
Admittance Decision Time (minutes)[2]	66	38	58	98
Head CT Results Within 45 Min. of Arrival[1,3]	-	-	55%	57%
Patients Who Left ER Before Being Seen[5]	-	-	1%	2%
Time from ER Arrival to Admit. (minutes)[2]	66	159	202	274
Time from ER Arrival to Discharge (minutes)[5]	-	-	108	134
Time in ER Before Being Evaluated (minutes)[5]	-	-	21	26
Time to Pain Meds for Fractures (minutes)[5]	-	-	46	57
Heart Attack Care				
Aspirin Given at Discharge[5]	-	-	100%	99%
Fibrinolytic Meds Within 30 Min. of Arrival[5]	-	-	-	54%
PCI Within 90 Minutes of Arrival[5]	-	-	94%	96%
Statin Prescribed at Discharge[5]	-	-	98%	98%
Heart Failure Care				
ACE Inhibitor or ARB for LVSD[7]	-	-	95%	97%
Discharge Instructions Given[1]	-	-	93%	94%
Evaluation of LVS Function[1]	-	-	97%	99%
Medicare Spending				
Medicare Spending per Patient (ratio)	-	-	0.91	0.98
Pneumonia Care				
Appropriate Initial Antibiotic Given[1]	-	-	93%	95%
Blood Culture Timing[1]	-	-	98%	98%
Pregnancy and Delivery Care				
Newborn Deliveries Scheduled Early[5]	-	-	4%	6%
Preventive Care				
Immunization for Influenza[2]	99	99%	91%	90%
Immunization for Pneumonia[2]	146	99%	90%	92%
Stroke Care				
Anticoagulation Therapy for Atrial Fibrillation[5]	-	-	95%	95%
Antithrombotic Therapy Timing[5]	-	-	98%	98%
Assessed for Rehabilitation[5]	-	-	97%	97%
Discharged on Antithrombotic Therapy[5]	-	-	99%	99%
Discharged on Statin Medication[5]	-	-	92%	94%
Thrombolytic Therapy Timing[5]	-	-	64%	66%
Venous Thromboembolism Prophylaxis[5]	-	-	93%	94%
Written Stroke Educational Materials Given[5]	-	-	82%	88%
Surgical Care Improvement Project				
Appropriate Beta Blocker Usage	14	100%	98%	98%
Appropriate VTP Within 24 Hours	47	100%	98%	98%
Controlled Postoperative Blood Glucose[7]	-	-	96%	97%
Perioperative Temperature Management	49	100%	100%	100%
Prophylactic Antibiotic Selection	48	100%	99%	99%
Prophylactic Antibiotic Selection (Outpatient)[5]	-	-	98%	98%
Prophylactic Antibiotic Stopped	48	100%	98%	98%
Prophylactic Antibiotic Timing	48	100%	98%	99%
Prophylactic Antibiotic Timing (Outpatient)[5]	-	-	98%	98%
Urinary Catheter Removal[1]	-	-	97%	97%
Survey of Patients' Hospital Experiences				
Area Around Room 'Always' Quiet at Night[11]	(a)	83%	63%	61%
Doctors 'Always' Communicated Well[11]	(a)	87%	84%	82%
Home Recovery Information Given[11]	(a)	91%	88%	85%
Hospital Given 9 or 10 on 10 Point Scale[11]	(a)	89%	75%	71%
Meds 'Always' Explained Before Given[11]	(a)	80%	66%	64%
Nurses 'Always' Communicated Well[11]	(a)	91%	81%	79%
Pain 'Always' Well Controlled[11]	(a)	75%	71%	71%
Room and Bathroom 'Always' Clean[11]	(a)	91%	79%	73%
Timely Help 'Always' Received[11]	(a)	84%	70%	68%
Would Definitely Recommend Hospital[11]	(a)	87%	74%	71%
Use of Medical Imaging				
Cardiac Imaging Stress Test before Surgery[7]	-	-	4.8%	5.3%
Combination Abdominal CT Scan	104	2.9%	11.5%	10.5%
Combination Brain/Sinus CT Scan[1]	-	-	1.8%	2.7%
Combination Chest CT Scan[1]	-	-	3.5%	2.7%
Follow-up Mammogram/Ultrasound	283	8.8%	7.9%	8.8%
Lumbar Spine MRI for Low Back Pain[1]	-	-	32.2%	37.2%

Guthrie County Hospital

710 North 12th Street
Guthrie Center, IA 50115
Phone: 641-332-2201
Fax: 641-332-2702
URL: www.gcho.org
Type: Critical Access Hospitals
Emergency Services: Yes
Ownership: Voluntary non-profit - Other
Beds: 25

Key Personnel:
Chief of Medical Staff. . . . . Steven Bascom
Quality Assurance . . . . Kristi Carper
Operating Room. . . . . Nancy Coffman
Infection Control. . . . . Christine Drake
Radiology. . . . . Sarah Madsen
Anesthesiology. . . . . Steve Navarro
CEO . . . . Patrick Petersen

Measure	Cases	This Hosp.	State Avg.	U.S. Avg.
Blood Clot Prevention and Treatment				
Anticoagulation Overlap Therapy	-	-	94%	93%
ICU Venous Thromboembolism Prophylaxis	-	-	90%	92%
Incidence of Potentially Preventable VTE	-	-	8%	10%
UFH with Dosages/Platelet Monitoring	-	-	99%	97%
Venous Thromboembolism Prophylaxis	-	-	87%	85%
Warfarin Therapy Discharge Instructions	-	-	77%	75%
Chest Pain/Possible Heart Attack Care				
Aspirin Given Within 24 Hours of Arrival[5]	-	-	97%	96%
Fibrinolytic Meds Within 30 Min. of Arrival[5]	-	-	49%	58%
Average Time to ECG (minutes)[5]	-	-	5	7
Average Time to Transfer (minutes)[5]	-	-	58	60
Children's Asthma Care				
Received Home Management Plan of Care	-	-	-	88%
Received Reliever Medication	-	-	-	100%
Received Systemic Corticosteroids	-	-	-	100%
Emergency Department				
Admittance Decision Time (minutes)	-	-	58	98
Head CT Results Within 45 Min. of Arrival[5]	-	-	55%	57%
Patients Who Left ER Before Being Seen[5]	-	-	1%	2%
Time from ER Arrival to Admit. (minutes)	-	-	202	274
Time from ER Arrival to Discharge (minutes)[5]	-	-	108	134
Time in ER Before Being Evaluated (minutes)[5]	-	-	21	26
Time to Pain Meds for Fractures (minutes)[5]	-	-	46	57
Heart Attack Care				
Aspirin Given at Discharge	-	-	100%	99%
Fibrinolytic Meds Within 30 Min. of Arrival	-	-	-	54%
PCI Within 90 Minutes of Arrival	-	-	94%	96%
Statin Prescribed at Discharge	-	-	98%	98%
Heart Failure Care				
ACE Inhibitor or ARB for LVSD	-	-	95%	97%
Discharge Instructions Given	-	-	93%	94%
Evaluation of LVS Function	-	-	97%	99%
Medicare Spending				
Medicare Spending per Patient (ratio)	-	-	0.91	0.98
Pneumonia Care				
Appropriate Initial Antibiotic Given	-	-	93%	95%
Blood Culture Timing	-	-	98%	98%
Pregnancy and Delivery Care				
Newborn Deliveries Scheduled Early	-	-	4%	6%
Preventive Care				
Immunization for Influenza	-	-	91%	90%
Immunization for Pneumonia	-	-	90%	92%
Stroke Care				
Anticoagulation Therapy for Atrial Fibrillation	-	-	95%	95%
Antithrombotic Therapy Timing	-	-	98%	98%
Assessed for Rehabilitation	-	-	97%	97%
Discharged on Antithrombotic Therapy	-	-	99%	99%
Discharged on Statin Medication	-	-	92%	94%
Thrombolytic Therapy Timing	-	-	64%	66%
Venous Thromboembolism Prophylaxis	-	-	93%	94%
Written Stroke Educational Materials Given	-	-	82%	88%
Surgical Care Improvement Project				
Appropriate Beta Blocker Usage	-	-	98%	98%
Appropriate VTP Within 24 Hours	-	-	98%	98%
Controlled Postoperative Blood Glucose	-	-	96%	97%
Perioperative Temperature Management	-	-	100%	100%
Prophylactic Antibiotic Selection	-	-	99%	99%
Prophylactic Antibiotic Selection (Outpatient)[5]	-	-	98%	98%
Prophylactic Antibiotic Stopped	-	-	98%	98%
Prophylactic Antibiotic Timing	-	-	98%	99%
Prophylactic Antibiotic Timing (Outpatient)[5]	-	-	98%	98%
Urinary Catheter Removal	-	-	97%	97%
Survey of Patients' Hospital Experiences				
Area Around Room 'Always' Quiet at Night	-	-	63%	61%
Doctors 'Always' Communicated Well	-	-	84%	82%
Home Recovery Information Given	-	-	88%	85%
Hospital Given 9 or 10 on 10 Point Scale	-	-	75%	71%
Meds 'Always' Explained Before Given	-	-	66%	64%
Nurses 'Always' Communicated Well	-	-	81%	79%
Pain 'Always' Well Controlled	-	-	71%	71%
Room and Bathroom 'Always' Clean	-	-	79%	73%
Timely Help 'Always' Received	-	-	70%	68%
Would Definitely Recommend Hospital	-	-	74%	71%
Use of Medical Imaging				
Cardiac Imaging Stress Test before Surgery[1]	-	-	4.8%	5.3%
Combination Abdominal CT Scan	67	9.0%	11.5%	10.5%
Combination Brain/Sinus CT Scan[1]	-	-	1.8%	2.7%
Combination Chest CT Scan	45	0.0%	3.5%	2.7%
Follow-up Mammogram/Ultrasound	183	11.5%	7.9%	8.8%
Lumbar Spine MRI for Low Back Pain[1]	-	-	32.2%	37.2%

Guttenberg Municipal Hospital

200 Main Street
Guttenberg, IA 52052
Phone: 563-252-1121
Fax: 563-252-3120
URL: www.guttenberghospital.org
Type: Critical Access Hospitals
Emergency Services: Yes
Ownership: Government - Local
Beds: 25

Key Personnel:
Emergency Room . . . . Jeff Ashline, PA-C

NOTE: Hospital profiles are in alphabetical order by state, then city, then hospital within the city; Rankings exclude hospitals with less than 25 cases except for patient surveys which excludes hospitals with less than 100 cases; (a) 100-299 cases; (1) The number of cases/patients is too few to report; (2) Data submitted were based on a sample of cases/patients; (3) Results are based on a shorter time period than required; (4) Data suppressed by CMS for one or more quarters; (5) Results are not available for this reporting period; (6) Fewer than 100 patients completed the HCAHPS survey; (7) No cases met the criteria for this measure; (8) The lower limit of the confidence interval cannot be calculated if the number of observed infections equals zero; (9) No data are available from the state/territory for this reporting period; (10) The scores shown reflect fewer than 50 completed surveys; (11) There were discrepancies in the data collection process; (12) This measure does not apply to this hospital for this reporting period; (13) Results cannot be calculated for this reporting period; (14) The results for this state are combined with nearby states to protect confidentiality; Please refer to the User's Guide for a full explanation of data.

Chief of Medical Staff.......... Will Chance, DO
Infection Control.............. Robin Esmann
CEO/President................ Kim Gau
Radiology.................... Lori Kann
Cardiac Laboratory............ Danelle Krapfl
Operating Room.............. Deb Preston

Measure	Cases	This Hosp.	State Avg.	U.S. Avg.
Blood Clot Prevention and Treatment				
Anticoagulation Overlap Therapy[5]	-	-	94%	93%
ICU Venous Thromboembolism Prophylaxis[5]	-	-	90%	92%
Incidence of Potentially Preventable VTE[5]	-	-	8%	10%
UFH with Dosages/Platelet Monitoring[5]	-	-	99%	97%
Venous Thromboembolism Prophylaxis[5]	-	-	87%	85%
Warfarin Therapy Discharge Instructions[5]	-	-	77%	75%
Chest Pain/Possible Heart Attack Care				
Aspirin Given Within 24 Hours of Arrival	-	-	97%	96%
Fibrinolytic Meds Within 30 Min. of Arrival	-	-	49%	58%
Average Time to ECG (minutes)	-	-	5	7
Average Time to Transfer (minutes)	-	-	58	60
Children's Asthma Care				
Received Home Management Plan of Care	-	-	-	88%
Received Reliever Medication	-	-	-	100%
Received Systemic Corticosteroids	-	-	-	100%
Emergency Department				
Admittance Decision Time (minutes)[5]	-	-	58	98
Head CT Results Within 45 Min. of Arrival	-	-	55%	57%
Patients Who Left ER Before Being Seen	-	-	1%	2%
Time from ER Arrival to Admit. (minutes)[5]	-	-	202	274
Time from ER Arrival to Discharge (minutes)	-	-	108	134
Time in ER Before Being Evaluated (minutes)	-	-	21	26
Time to Pain Meds for Fractures (minutes)	-	-	46	57
Heart Attack Care				
Aspirin Given at Discharge[1,3]	-	-	100%	99%
Fibrinolytic Meds Within 30 Min. of Arrival[3,7]	-	-	-	54%
PCI Within 90 Minutes of Arrival[3,7]	-	-	94%	96%
Statin Prescribed at Discharge[1,3]	-	-	98%	98%
Heart Failure Care				
ACE Inhibitor or ARB for LVSD[1]	-	-	95%	97%
Discharge Instructions Given[1]	-	-	93%	94%
Evaluation of LVS Function[1]	-	-	97%	99%
Medicare Spending				
Medicare Spending per Patient (ratio)	-	-	0.91	0.98
Pneumonia Care				
Appropriate Initial Antibiotic Given	19	100%	93%	95%
Blood Culture Timing	22	100%	98%	98%
Pregnancy and Delivery Care				
Newborn Deliveries Scheduled Early[5]	-	-	4%	6%
Preventive Care				
Immunization for Influenza[5]	-	-	91%	90%
Immunization for Pneumonia[5]	-	-	90%	92%
Stroke Care				
Anticoagulation Therapy for Atrial Fibrillation[5]	-	-	95%	95%
Antithrombotic Therapy Timing[5]	-	-	98%	98%
Assessed for Rehabilitation[5]	-	-	97%	97%
Discharged on Antithrombotic Therapy[5]	-	-	99%	99%
Discharged on Statin Medication[5]	-	-	92%	94%
Thrombolytic Therapy Timing[5]	-	-	64%	66%
Venous Thromboembolism Prophylaxis[5]	-	-	93%	94%
Written Stroke Educational Materials Given[5]	-	-	82%	88%
Surgical Care Improvement Project				
Appropriate Beta Blocker Usage[1]	-	-	98%	98%
Appropriate VTP Within 24 Hours[1]	-	-	98%	98%
Controlled Postoperative Blood Glucose[7]	-	-	96%	97%
Perioperative Temperature Management[1]	-	-	100%	100%
Prophylactic Antibiotic Selection[1]	-	-	99%	99%
Prophylactic Antibiotic Selection (Outpatient)	-	-	98%	98%
Prophylactic Antibiotic Stopped[1]	-	-	98%	98%
Prophylactic Antibiotic Timing[1]	-	-	98%	99%
Prophylactic Antibiotic Timing (Outpatient)	-	-	98%	98%
Urinary Catheter Removal[7]	-	-	97%	97%
Survey of Patients' Hospital Experiences				
Area Around Room 'Always' Quiet at Night[6]	<100	74%	63%	61%
Doctors 'Always' Communicated Well[6]	<100	90%	84%	82%
Home Recovery Information Given[6]	<100	90%	88%	85%
Hospital Given 9 or 10 on 10 Point Scale[6]	<100	93%	75%	71%
Meds 'Always' Explained Before Given[6]	<100	79%	66%	64%
Nurses 'Always' Communicated Well[6]	<100	90%	81%	79%
Pain 'Always' Well Controlled[6]	<100	81%	71%	71%
Room and Bathroom 'Always' Clean[6]	<100	92%	79%	73%
Timely Help 'Always' Received[6]	<100	87%	70%	68%
Would Definitely Recommend Hospital[6]	<100	90%	74%	71%
Use of Medical Imaging				
Cardiac Imaging Stress Test before Surgery	-	-	4.8%	5.3%
Combination Abdominal CT Scan	-	-	11.5%	10.5%
Combination Brain/Sinus CT Scan	-	-	1.8%	2.7%
Combination Chest CT Scan	-	-	3.5%	2.7%
Follow-up Mammogram/Ultrasound	-	-	7.9%	8.8%
Lumbar Spine MRI for Low Back Pain	-	-	32.2%	37.2%

George C Grape Community Hospital

2959 Us Highway 275
Hamburg, IA 51640
Phone: 712-382-1515
Type: Critical Access Hospitals
Emergency Services: Yes
Ownership: Voluntary non-profit - Private

Measure	Cases	This Hosp.	State Avg.	U.S. Avg.
Blood Clot Prevention and Treatment				
Anticoagulation Overlap Therapy	-	-	94%	93%
ICU Venous Thromboembolism Prophylaxis	-	-	90%	92%
Incidence of Potentially Preventable VTE	-	-	8%	10%
UFH with Dosages/Platelet Monitoring	-	-	99%	97%
Venous Thromboembolism Prophylaxis	-	-	87%	85%
Warfarin Therapy Discharge Instructions	-	-	77%	75%
Chest Pain/Possible Heart Attack Care				
Aspirin Given Within 24 Hours of Arrival	11	91%	97%	96%
Fibrinolytic Meds Within 30 Min. of Arrival[3,7]	-	-	49%	58%
Average Time to ECG (minutes)[1]	-	-	5	7
Average Time to Transfer (minutes)[3,7]	-	-	58	60
Children's Asthma Care				
Received Home Management Plan of Care	-	-	-	88%
Received Reliever Medication	-	-	-	100%
Received Systemic Corticosteroids	-	-	-	100%
Emergency Department				
Admittance Decision Time (minutes)	-	-	58	98
Head CT Results Within 45 Min. of Arrival[5]	-	-	55%	57%
Patients Who Left ER Before Being Seen[5]	-	-	1%	2%
Time from ER Arrival to Admit. (minutes)	-	-	202	274
Time from ER Arrival to Discharge (minutes)[5]	-	-	108	134
Time in ER Before Being Evaluated (minutes)[5]	-	-	21	26
Time to Pain Meds for Fractures (minutes)[5]	-	-	46	57
Heart Attack Care				
Aspirin Given at Discharge	-	-	100%	99%
Fibrinolytic Meds Within 30 Min. of Arrival	-	-	-	54%
PCI Within 90 Minutes of Arrival	-	-	94%	96%
Statin Prescribed at Discharge	-	-	98%	98%
Heart Failure Care				
ACE Inhibitor or ARB for LVSD	-	-	95%	97%
Discharge Instructions Given	-	-	93%	94%
Evaluation of LVS Function	-	-	97%	99%
Medicare Spending				
Medicare Spending per Patient (ratio)	-	-	0.91	0.98
Pneumonia Care				
Appropriate Initial Antibiotic Given	-	-	93%	95%
Blood Culture Timing	-	-	98%	98%
Pregnancy and Delivery Care				
Newborn Deliveries Scheduled Early	-	-	4%	6%
Preventive Care				
Immunization for Influenza	-	-	91%	90%
Immunization for Pneumonia	-	-	90%	92%
Stroke Care				
Anticoagulation Therapy for Atrial Fibrillation	-	-	95%	95%
Antithrombotic Therapy Timing	-	-	98%	98%
Assessed for Rehabilitation	-	-	97%	97%
Discharged on Antithrombotic Therapy	-	-	99%	99%
Discharged on Statin Medication	-	-	92%	94%
Thrombolytic Therapy Timing	-	-	64%	66%
Venous Thromboembolism Prophylaxis	-	-	93%	94%
Written Stroke Educational Materials Given	-	-	82%	88%
Surgical Care Improvement Project				
Appropriate Beta Blocker Usage	-	-	98%	98%
Appropriate VTP Within 24 Hours	-	-	98%	98%
Controlled Postoperative Blood Glucose	-	-	96%	97%
Perioperative Temperature Management	-	-	100%	100%
Prophylactic Antibiotic Selection	-	-	99%	99%
Prophylactic Antibiotic Selection (Outpatient)[5]	-	-	98%	98%
Prophylactic Antibiotic Stopped	-	-	98%	98%
Prophylactic Antibiotic Timing	-	-	98%	99%
Prophylactic Antibiotic Timing (Outpatient)[5]	-	-	98%	98%
Urinary Catheter Removal	-	-	97%	97%
Survey of Patients' Hospital Experiences				
Area Around Room 'Always' Quiet at Night	-	-	63%	61%
Doctors 'Always' Communicated Well	-	-	84%	82%
Home Recovery Information Given	-	-	88%	85%
Hospital Given 9 or 10 on 10 Point Scale	-	-	75%	71%
Meds 'Always' Explained Before Given	-	-	66%	64%
Nurses 'Always' Communicated Well	-	-	81%	79%
Pain 'Always' Well Controlled	-	-	71%	71%
Room and Bathroom 'Always' Clean	-	-	79%	73%
Timely Help 'Always' Received	-	-	70%	68%
Would Definitely Recommend Hospital	-	-	74%	71%
Use of Medical Imaging				
Cardiac Imaging Stress Test before Surgery[1]	-	-	4.8%	5.3%
Combination Abdominal CT Scan[1]	-	-	11.5%	10.5%
Combination Brain/Sinus CT Scan[1]	-	-	1.8%	2.7%
Combination Chest CT Scan[1]	-	-	3.5%	2.7%
Follow-up Mammogram/Ultrasound	101	8.9%	7.9%	8.8%
Lumbar Spine MRI for Low Back Pain[1]	-	-	32.2%	37.2%

Franklin General Hospital

1720 Central Avenue East
Hampton, IA 50441
Phone: 641-456-5000
Fax: 641-456-5020
URL: www.franklingeneral.com
Type: Critical Access Hospitals
Emergency Services: Yes
Ownership: Government - Local
Beds: 77

Key Personnel:

Cardiology.................. Byron Beasley, DO
Cardiology.................. Samuel Congella, DO
Chief of Medical Staff.......... Brian J Hansen
Surgery.................... Harsha Jaywardena
Cardiology.................. James Reeder, DO
Cardiology.................. Rajinder Verma, DO

Measure	Cases	This Hosp.	State Avg.	U.S. Avg.
Blood Clot Prevention and Treatment				
Anticoagulation Overlap Therapy[5]	-	-	94%	93%
ICU Venous Thromboembolism Prophylaxis[5]	-	-	90%	92%
Incidence of Potentially Preventable VTE[5]	-	-	8%	10%
UFH with Dosages/Platelet Monitoring[5]	-	-	99%	97%
Venous Thromboembolism Prophylaxis[5]	-	-	87%	85%
Warfarin Therapy Discharge Instructions[5]	-	-	77%	75%
Chest Pain/Possible Heart Attack Care				
Aspirin Given Within 24 Hours of Arrival	-	-	97%	96%
Fibrinolytic Meds Within 30 Min. of Arrival	-	-	49%	58%
Average Time to ECG (minutes)	-	-	5	7
Average Time to Transfer (minutes)	-	-	58	60
Children's Asthma Care				
Received Home Management Plan of Care	-	-	-	88%
Received Reliever Medication	-	-	-	100%
Received Systemic Corticosteroids	-	-	-	100%
Emergency Department				
Admittance Decision Time (minutes)[5]	-	-	58	98
Head CT Results Within 45 Min. of Arrival	-	-	55%	57%
Patients Who Left ER Before Being Seen	-	-	1%	2%
Time from ER Arrival to Admit. (minutes)[5]	-	-	202	274
Time from ER Arrival to Discharge (minutes)	-	-	108	134
Time in ER Before Being Evaluated (minutes)	-	-	21	26
Time to Pain Meds for Fractures (minutes)	-	-	46	57
Heart Attack Care				
Aspirin Given at Discharge[5]	-	-	100%	99%
Fibrinolytic Meds Within 30 Min. of Arrival[5]	-	-	-	54%
PCI Within 90 Minutes of Arrival[5]	-	-	94%	96%

NOTE: Hospital profiles are in alphabetical order by state, then city, then hospital within the city; Rankings exclude hospitals with less than 25 cases except for patient surveys which excludes hospitals with less than 100 cases; (a) 100-299 cases; (1) The number of cases/patients is too few to report; (2) Data submitted were based on a sample of cases/patients; (3) Results are based on a shorter time period than required; (4) Data suppressed by CMS for one or more quarters; (5) Results are not available for this reporting period; (6) Fewer than 100 patients completed the HCAHPS survey; (7) No cases met the criteria for this measure; (8) The lower limit of the confidence interval cannot be calculated if the number of observed infections equals zero; (9) No data are available from the state/territory for this reporting period; (10) The scores shown reflect fewer than 50 completed surveys; (11) There were discrepancies in the data collection process; (12) This measure does not apply to this hospital for this reporting period; (13) Results cannot be calculated for this reporting period; (14) The results for this state are combined with nearby states to protect confidentiality; Please refer to the User's Guide for a full explanation of data.

Measure	Cases	This Hosp.	State Avg.	U.S. Avg.
Statin Prescribed at Discharge[5]	-	-	98%	98%
Heart Failure Care				
ACE Inhibitor or ARB for LVSD[5]	-	-	95%	97%
Discharge Instructions Given[5]	-	-	93%	94%
Evaluation of LVS Function[5]	-	-	97%	99%
Medicare Spending				
Medicare Spending per Patient (ratio)	-	-	0.91	0.98
Pneumonia Care				
Appropriate Initial Antibiotic Given	23	65%	93%	95%
Blood Culture Timing[1]	-	-	98%	98%
Pregnancy and Delivery Care				
Newborn Deliveries Scheduled Early[5]	-	-	4%	6%
Preventive Care				
Immunization for Influenza[5]	-	-	91%	90%
Immunization for Pneumonia[5]	-	-	90%	92%
Stroke Care				
Anticoagulation Therapy for Atrial Fibrillation[5]	-	-	95%	95%
Antithrombotic Therapy Timing[5]	-	-	98%	98%
Assessed for Rehabilitation[5]	-	-	97%	97%
Discharged on Antithrombotic Therapy[5]	-	-	99%	99%
Discharged on Statin Medication[5]	-	-	92%	94%
Thrombolytic Therapy Timing[5]	-	-	64%	66%
Venous Thromboembolism Prophylaxis[5]	-	-	93%	94%
Written Stroke Educational Materials Given[5]	-	-	82%	88%
Surgical Care Improvement Project				
Appropriate Beta Blocker Usage[5]	-	-	98%	98%
Appropriate VTP Within 24 Hours[5]	-	-	98%	98%
Controlled Postoperative Blood Glucose[5]	-	-	96%	97%
Perioperative Temperature Management[5]	-	-	100%	100%
Prophylactic Antibiotic Selection[5]	-	-	99%	99%
Prophylactic Antibiotic Selection (Outpatient)	-	-	98%	98%
Prophylactic Antibiotic Stopped[5]	-	-	98%	98%
Prophylactic Antibiotic Timing[5]	-	-	98%	99%
Prophylactic Antibiotic Timing (Outpatient)	-	-	98%	98%
Urinary Catheter Removal[5]	-	-	97%	97%
Survey of Patients' Hospital Experiences				
Area Around Room 'Always' Quiet at Night[5]	-	-	63%	61%
Doctors 'Always' Communicated Well[5]	-	-	84%	82%
Home Recovery Information Given[5]	-	-	88%	85%
Hospital Given 9 or 10 on 10 Point Scale[5]	-	-	75%	71%
Meds 'Always' Explained Before Given[5]	-	-	66%	64%
Nurses 'Always' Communicated Well[5]	-	-	81%	79%
Pain 'Always' Well Controlled[5]	-	-	71%	71%
Room and Bathroom 'Always' Clean[5]	-	-	79%	73%
Timely Help 'Always' Received[5]	-	-	70%	68%
Would Definitely Recommend Hospital[5]	-	-	74%	71%
Use of Medical Imaging				
Cardiac Imaging Stress Test before Surgery	-	-	4.8%	5.3%
Combination Abdominal CT Scan	-	-	11.5%	10.5%
Combination Brain/Sinus CT Scan	-	-	1.8%	2.7%
Combination Chest CT Scan	-	-	3.5%	2.7%
Follow-up Mammogram/Ultrasound	-	-	7.9%	8.8%
Lumbar Spine MRI for Low Back Pain	-	-	32.2%	37.2%

Myrtue Medical Center

1213 Garfield Avenue
Harlan, IA 51537
URL: www.shelbycohealth.com
Phone: 712-755-5161
Fax: 712-755-2640
Type: Critical Access Hospitals
Emergency Services: Yes
Ownership: Voluntary non-profit - Other
Beds: 52

Key Personnel:
Operating Room. . . . . Pat Boettger
Administrator . . . . Kim Burchett
Chairman/CEO . . . . Carmen Hosack
CEO . . . . Barry Jacobsen
Chief of Medical Staff. . . . . Don Klilgaard
Emergency Room . . . . Scott Markham
CEO/President. . . . . Mark Woodring
Quality Assurance . . . . Judy Zea

Measure	Cases	This Hosp.	State Avg.	U.S. Avg.
Blood Clot Prevention and Treatment				
Anticoagulation Overlap Therapy[5]	-	-	94%	93%
ICU Venous Thromboembolism Prophylaxis[5]	-	-	90%	92%
Incidence of Potentially Preventable VTE[5]	-	-	8%	10%
UFH with Dosages/Platelet Monitoring[5]	-	-	99%	97%
Venous Thromboembolism Prophylaxis[5]	-	-	87%	85%
Warfarin Therapy Discharge Instructions[5]	-	-	77%	75%
Chest Pain/Possible Heart Attack Care				
Aspirin Given Within 24 Hours of Arrival[1,3]	-	-	97%	96%
Fibrinolytic Meds Within 30 Min. of Arrival[3,7]	-	-	49%	58%
Average Time to ECG (minutes)[1,3]	-	-	5	7
Average Time to Transfer (minutes)[1,3]	-	-	58	60
Children's Asthma Care				
Received Home Management Plan of Care	-	-	-	88%
Received Reliever Medication	-	-	-	100%
Received Systemic Corticosteroids	-	-	-	100%
Emergency Department				
Admittance Decision Time (minutes)[5]	-	-	58	98
Head CT Results Within 45 Min. of Arrival[5]	-	-	55%	57%
Patients Who Left ER Before Being Seen[5]	-	-	1%	2%
Time from ER Arrival to Admit. (minutes)[5]	-	-	202	274
Time from ER Arrival to Discharge (minutes)[5]	-	-	108	134
Time in ER Before Being Evaluated (minutes)[5]	-	-	21	26
Time to Pain Meds for Fractures (minutes)[5]	-	-	46	57
Heart Attack Care				
Aspirin Given at Discharge[5]	-	-	100%	99%
Fibrinolytic Meds Within 30 Min. of Arrival[5]	-	-	-	54%
PCI Within 90 Minutes of Arrival[5]	-	-	94%	96%
Statin Prescribed at Discharge[5]	-	-	98%	98%
Heart Failure Care				
ACE Inhibitor or ARB for LVSD[1,2]	-	-	95%	97%
Discharge Instructions Given[2]	14	100%	93%	94%
Evaluation of LVS Function[2]	33	100%	97%	99%
Medicare Spending				
Medicare Spending per Patient (ratio)	-	-	0.91	0.98
Pneumonia Care				
Appropriate Initial Antibiotic Given	31	100%	93%	95%
Blood Culture Timing	52	100%	98%	98%
Pregnancy and Delivery Care				
Newborn Deliveries Scheduled Early[5]	-	-	4%	6%
Preventive Care				
Immunization for Influenza[2,3]	23	96%	91%	90%
Immunization for Pneumonia[2,3]	69	94%	90%	92%
Stroke Care				
Anticoagulation Therapy for Atrial Fibrillation[5]	-	-	95%	95%
Antithrombotic Therapy Timing[5]	-	-	98%	98%
Assessed for Rehabilitation[5]	-	-	97%	97%
Discharged on Antithrombotic Therapy[5]	-	-	99%	99%
Discharged on Statin Medication[5]	-	-	92%	94%
Thrombolytic Therapy Timing[5]	-	-	64%	66%
Venous Thromboembolism Prophylaxis[5]	-	-	93%	94%
Written Stroke Educational Materials Given[5]	-	-	82%	88%
Surgical Care Improvement Project				
Appropriate Beta Blocker Usage[1,2]	-	-	98%	98%
Appropriate VTP Within 24 Hours[1,2]	-	-	98%	98%
Controlled Postoperative Blood Glucose[2,3]	-	-	96%	97%
Perioperative Temperature Management[1,2]	-	-	100%	100%
Prophylactic Antibiotic Selection[1,2]	-	-	99%	99%
Prophylactic Antibiotic Selection (Outpatient)[1,3]	-	-	98%	98%
Prophylactic Antibiotic Stopped[1,2]	-	-	98%	98%
Prophylactic Antibiotic Timing[1,2]	-	-	98%	99%
Prophylactic Antibiotic Timing (Outpatient)[1,3]	-	-	98%	98%
Urinary Catheter Removal[1,2]	-	-	97%	97%
Survey of Patients' Hospital Experiences				
Area Around Room 'Always' Quiet at Night	(a)	62%	63%	61%
Doctors 'Always' Communicated Well	(a)	88%	84%	82%
Home Recovery Information Given	(a)	93%	88%	85%
Hospital Given 9 or 10 on 10 Point Scale	(a)	76%	75%	71%
Meds 'Always' Explained Before Given	(a)	67%	66%	64%
Nurses 'Always' Communicated Well	(a)	81%	81%	79%
Pain 'Always' Well Controlled	(a)	60%	71%	71%
Room and Bathroom 'Always' Clean	(a)	76%	79%	73%
Timely Help 'Always' Received	(a)	61%	70%	68%
Would Definitely Recommend Hospital	(a)	74%	74%	71%
Use of Medical Imaging				
Cardiac Imaging Stress Test before Surgery[1]	-	-	4.8%	5.3%
Combination Abdominal CT Scan	197	15.2%	11.5%	10.5%
Combination Brain/Sinus CT Scan[1]	-	-	1.8%	2.7%
Combination Chest CT Scan	78	6.4%	3.5%	2.7%
Follow-up Mammogram/Ultrasound	472	6.1%	7.9%	8.8%
Lumbar Spine MRI for Low Back Pain[1]	-	-	32.2%	37.2%

Hawarden Community Hospital

1111 11th Street
Hawarden, IA 51023
E-mail: commhosp@acsnet.com
URL: www.acsnet.com
Phone: 712-551-3100
Fax: 712-551-3106
Type: Critical Access Hospitals
Emergency Services: Yes
Ownership: Voluntary non-profit - Other
Beds: 18

Key Personnel:
Quality Assurance . . . . Ruth Dickmann
CEO/President. . . . . Chad Markham
Coronary Care . . . . Jeanna Negaard
Chief of Medical Staff. . . . . Dale Nystrom
Emergency Room . . . . Lorna Westra

Measure	Cases	This Hosp.	State Avg.	U.S. Avg.
Blood Clot Prevention and Treatment				
Anticoagulation Overlap Therapy[5]	-	-	94%	93%
ICU Venous Thromboembolism Prophylaxis[5]	-	-	90%	92%
Incidence of Potentially Preventable VTE[5]	-	-	8%	10%
UFH with Dosages/Platelet Monitoring[5]	-	-	99%	97%
Venous Thromboembolism Prophylaxis[5]	-	-	87%	85%
Warfarin Therapy Discharge Instructions[5]	-	-	77%	75%
Chest Pain/Possible Heart Attack Care				
Aspirin Given Within 24 Hours of Arrival[5]	-	-	97%	96%
Fibrinolytic Meds Within 30 Min. of Arrival[5]	-	-	49%	58%
Average Time to ECG (minutes)[5]	-	-	5	7
Average Time to Transfer (minutes)[5]	-	-	58	60
Children's Asthma Care				
Received Home Management Plan of Care	-	-	-	88%
Received Reliever Medication	-	-	-	100%
Received Systemic Corticosteroids	-	-	-	100%
Emergency Department				
Admittance Decision Time (minutes)[5]	-	-	58	98
Head CT Results Within 45 Min. of Arrival[5]	-	-	55%	57%
Patients Who Left ER Before Being Seen[5]	-	-	1%	2%
Time from ER Arrival to Admit. (minutes)[5]	-	-	202	274
Time from ER Arrival to Discharge (minutes)[5]	-	-	108	134
Time in ER Before Being Evaluated (minutes)[5]	-	-	21	26
Time to Pain Meds for Fractures (minutes)[5]	-	-	46	57
Heart Attack Care				
Aspirin Given at Discharge[5]	-	-	100%	99%
Fibrinolytic Meds Within 30 Min. of Arrival[5]	-	-	-	54%
PCI Within 90 Minutes of Arrival[5]	-	-	94%	96%
Statin Prescribed at Discharge[5]	-	-	98%	98%
Heart Failure Care				
ACE Inhibitor or ARB for LVSD[1,3]	-	-	95%	97%
Discharge Instructions Given[3,7]	-	-	93%	94%
Evaluation of LVS Function[1,3]	-	-	97%	99%
Medicare Spending				
Medicare Spending per Patient (ratio)	-	-	0.91	0.98
Pneumonia Care				
Appropriate Initial Antibiotic Given	11	82%	93%	95%
Blood Culture Timing[1]	-	-	98%	98%
Pregnancy and Delivery Care				
Newborn Deliveries Scheduled Early[5]	-	-	4%	6%
Preventive Care				
Immunization for Influenza[5]	-	-	91%	90%
Immunization for Pneumonia[5]	-	-	90%	92%
Stroke Care				
Anticoagulation Therapy for Atrial Fibrillation[5]	-	-	95%	95%
Antithrombotic Therapy Timing[5]	-	-	98%	98%
Assessed for Rehabilitation[5]	-	-	97%	97%
Discharged on Antithrombotic Therapy[5]	-	-	99%	99%
Discharged on Statin Medication[5]	-	-	92%	94%
Thrombolytic Therapy Timing[5]	-	-	64%	66%
Venous Thromboembolism Prophylaxis[5]	-	-	93%	94%
Written Stroke Educational Materials Given[5]	-	-	82%	88%
Surgical Care Improvement Project				
Appropriate Beta Blocker Usage[5]	-	-	98%	98%

NOTE: Hospital profiles are in alphabetical order by state, then city, then hospital within the city; Rankings exclude hospitals with less than 25 cases except for patient surveys which excludes hospitals with less than 100 cases; (a) 100-299 cases; (1) The number of cases/patients is too few to report; (2) Data submitted were based on a sample of cases/patients; (3) Results are based on a shorter time period than required; (4) Data suppressed by CMS for one or more quarters; (5) Results are not available for this reporting period; (6) Fewer than 100 patients completed the HCAHPS survey; (7) No cases met the criteria for this measure; (8) The lower limit of the confidence interval cannot be calculated if the number of observed infections equals zero; (9) No data are available from the state/territory for this reporting period; (10) The scores shown reflect fewer than 50 completed surveys; (11) There were discrepancies in the data collection process; (12) This measure does not apply to this hospital for this reporting period; (13) Results cannot be calculated for this reporting period; (14) The results for this state are combined with nearby states to protect confidentiality; Please refer to the User's Guide for a full explanation of data.

Measure	Cases	This Hosp.	State Avg.	U.S. Avg.
Appropriate VTP Within 24 Hours[5]	-	-	98%	98%
Controlled Postoperative Blood Glucose[5]	-	-	96%	97%
Perioperative Temperature Management[5]	-	-	100%	100%
Prophylactic Antibiotic Selection[5]	-	-	99%	99%
Prophylactic Antibiotic Selection (Outpatient)[5]	-	-	98%	98%
Prophylactic Antibiotic Stopped[5]	-	-	98%	98%
Prophylactic Antibiotic Timing[5]	-	-	98%	99%
Prophylactic Antibiotic Timing (Outpatient)[5]	-	-	98%	98%
Urinary Catheter Removal[5]	-	-	97%	97%
Survey of Patients' Hospital Experiences				
Area Around Room 'Always' Quiet at Night[10]	<100	48%	63%	61%
Doctors 'Always' Communicated Well[10]	<100	85%	84%	82%
Home Recovery Information Given[10]	<100	92%	88%	85%
Hospital Given 9 or 10 on 10 Point Scale[10]	<100	69%	75%	71%
Meds 'Always' Explained Before Given[10]	<100	72%	66%	64%
Nurses 'Always' Communicated Well[10]	<100	86%	81%	79%
Pain 'Always' Well Controlled[10]	<100	91%	71%	71%
Room and Bathroom 'Always' Clean[10]	<100	81%	79%	73%
Timely Help 'Always' Received[10]	<100	90%	70%	68%
Would Definitely Recommend Hospital[10]	<100	78%	74%	71%
Use of Medical Imaging				
Cardiac Imaging Stress Test before Surgery[7]	-	-	4.8%	5.3%
Combination Abdominal CT Scan[1]	-	-	11.5%	10.5%
Combination Brain/Sinus CT Scan	40	0.0%	1.8%	2.7%
Combination Chest CT Scan[1]	-	-	3.5%	2.7%
Follow-up Mammogram/Ultrasound	110	16.4%	7.9%	8.8%
Lumbar Spine MRI for Low Back Pain[1]	-	-	32.2%	37.2%

Humboldt County Memorial Hospital

1000 North 15th Street
Humboldt, IA 50548
Phone: 515-332-4200
Type: Critical Access Hospitals
Emergency Services: Yes
Ownership: Government - Local

Measure	Cases	This Hosp.	State Avg.	U.S. Avg.
Blood Clot Prevention and Treatment				
Anticoagulation Overlap Therapy	-	-	94%	93%
ICU Venous Thromboembolism Prophylaxis	-	-	90%	92%
Incidence of Potentially Preventable VTE	-	-	8%	10%
UFH with Dosages/Platelet Monitoring	-	-	99%	97%
Venous Thromboembolism Prophylaxis	-	-	87%	85%
Warfarin Therapy Discharge Instructions	-	-	77%	75%
Chest Pain/Possible Heart Attack Care				
Aspirin Given Within 24 Hours of Arrival[5]	-	-	97%	96%
Fibrinolytic Meds Within 30 Min. of Arrival[5]	-	-	49%	58%
Average Time to ECG (minutes)[5]	-	-	5	7
Average Time to Transfer (minutes)[5]	-	-	58	60
Children's Asthma Care				
Received Home Management Plan of Care	-	-	-	88%
Received Reliever Medication	-	-	-	100%
Received Systemic Corticosteroids	-	-	-	100%
Emergency Department				
Admittance Decision Time (minutes)	-	-	58	98
Head CT Results Within 45 Min. of Arrival[5]	-	-	55%	57%
Patients Who Left ER Before Being Seen[5]	-	-	1%	2%
Time from ER Arrival to Admit. (minutes)	-	-	202	274
Time from ER Arrival to Discharge (minutes)[5]	-	-	108	134
Time in ER Before Being Evaluated (minutes)[5]	-	-	21	26
Time to Pain Meds for Fractures (minutes)[5]	-	-	46	57
Heart Attack Care				
Aspirin Given at Discharge	-	-	100%	99%
Fibrinolytic Meds Within 30 Min. of Arrival	-	-	-	54%
PCI Within 90 Minutes of Arrival	-	-	94%	96%
Statin Prescribed at Discharge	-	-	98%	98%
Heart Failure Care				
ACE Inhibitor or ARB for LVSD	-	-	95%	97%
Discharge Instructions Given	-	-	93%	94%
Evaluation of LVS Function	-	-	97%	99%
Medicare Spending				
Medicare Spending per Patient (ratio)	-	-	0.91	0.98
Pneumonia Care				
Appropriate Initial Antibiotic Given	-	-	93%	95%
Blood Culture Timing	-	-	98%	98%
Pregnancy and Delivery Care				
Newborn Deliveries Scheduled Early	-	-	4%	6%
Preventive Care				
Immunization for Influenza	-	-	91%	90%
Immunization for Pneumonia	-	-	90%	92%
Stroke Care				
Anticoagulation Therapy for Atrial Fibrillation	-	-	95%	95%
Antithrombotic Therapy Timing	-	-	98%	98%
Assessed for Rehabilitation	-	-	97%	97%
Discharged on Antithrombotic Therapy	-	-	99%	99%
Discharged on Statin Medication	-	-	92%	94%
Thrombolytic Therapy Timing	-	-	64%	66%
Venous Thromboembolism Prophylaxis	-	-	93%	94%
Written Stroke Educational Materials Given	-	-	82%	88%
Surgical Care Improvement Project				
Appropriate Beta Blocker Usage	-	-	98%	98%
Appropriate VTP Within 24 Hours	-	-	98%	98%
Controlled Postoperative Blood Glucose	-	-	96%	97%
Perioperative Temperature Management	-	-	100%	100%
Prophylactic Antibiotic Selection	-	-	99%	99%
Prophylactic Antibiotic Selection (Outpatient)[5]	-	-	98%	98%
Prophylactic Antibiotic Stopped	-	-	98%	98%
Prophylactic Antibiotic Timing	-	-	98%	99%
Prophylactic Antibiotic Timing (Outpatient)[5]	-	-	98%	98%
Urinary Catheter Removal	-	-	97%	97%
Survey of Patients' Hospital Experiences				
Area Around Room 'Always' Quiet at Night	-	-	63%	61%
Doctors 'Always' Communicated Well	-	-	84%	82%
Home Recovery Information Given	-	-	88%	85%
Hospital Given 9 or 10 on 10 Point Scale	-	-	75%	71%
Meds 'Always' Explained Before Given	-	-	66%	64%
Nurses 'Always' Communicated Well	-	-	81%	79%
Pain 'Always' Well Controlled	-	-	71%	71%
Room and Bathroom 'Always' Clean	-	-	79%	73%
Timely Help 'Always' Received	-	-	70%	68%
Would Definitely Recommend Hospital	-	-	74%	71%
Use of Medical Imaging				
Cardiac Imaging Stress Test before Surgery[1]	-	-	4.8%	5.3%
Combination Abdominal CT Scan	82	3.7%	11.5%	10.5%
Combination Brain/Sinus CT Scan[1]	-	-	1.8%	2.7%
Combination Chest CT Scan	67	7.5%	3.5%	2.7%
Follow-up Mammogram/Ultrasound	242	8.3%	7.9%	8.8%
Lumbar Spine MRI for Low Back Pain[1]	-	-	32.2%	37.2%

Horn Memorial Hospital

701 E 2nd St
Ida Grove, IA 51445
Phone: 712-364-3311
Fax: 712-364-3363
E-mail: maugsburger@hornmemorialhospital.org
URL: www.hornmemorialhospital.org
Type: Critical Access Hospitals
Emergency Services: Yes
Ownership: Voluntary non-profit - Private
Beds: 25

Key Personnel:

CEO/President. . . . . Marc Augsburger
Cardiac Laboratory. . . . . Jean Cipperley
Radiology. . . . . Jerri Downs
Quality Assurance . . . . Haether Gann
Infection Control. . . . . Robin Lorenzen
Chief of Medical Staff. . . . . Albert Veltri
Operating Room. . . . . Jill Webb

Measure	Cases	This Hosp.	State Avg.	U.S. Avg.
Blood Clot Prevention and Treatment				
Anticoagulation Overlap Therapy[5]	-	-	94%	93%
ICU Venous Thromboembolism Prophylaxis[5]	-	-	90%	92%
Incidence of Potentially Preventable VTE[5]	-	-	8%	10%
UFH with Dosages/Platelet Monitoring[5]	-	-	99%	97%
Venous Thromboembolism Prophylaxis[5]	-	-	87%	85%
Warfarin Therapy Discharge Instructions[5]	-	-	77%	75%
Chest Pain/Possible Heart Attack Care				
Aspirin Given Within 24 Hours of Arrival[1]	-	-	97%	96%
Fibrinolytic Meds Within 30 Min. of Arrival[1,3]	-	-	49%	58%
Average Time to ECG (minutes)[1]	-	-	5	7
Average Time to Transfer (minutes)[3,7]	-	-	58	60
Children's Asthma Care				
Received Home Management Plan of Care	-	-	-	88%
Received Reliever Medication	-	-	-	100%
Received Systemic Corticosteroids	-	-	-	100%
Emergency Department				
Admittance Decision Time (minutes)[5]	-	-	58	98
Head CT Results Within 45 Min. of Arrival[1,3]	-	-	55%	57%
Patients Who Left ER Before Being Seen	5,846	0%	1%	2%
Time from ER Arrival to Admit. (minutes)[5]	-	-	202	274
Time from ER Arrival to Discharge (minutes)[5]	-	-	108	134
Time in ER Before Being Evaluated (minutes)[5]	-	-	21	26
Time to Pain Meds for Fractures (minutes)[5]	-	-	46	57
Heart Attack Care				
Aspirin Given at Discharge[5]	-	-	100%	99%
Fibrinolytic Meds Within 30 Min. of Arrival[5]	-	-	-	54%
PCI Within 90 Minutes of Arrival[5]	-	-	94%	96%
Statin Prescribed at Discharge[5]	-	-	98%	98%
Heart Failure Care				
ACE Inhibitor or ARB for LVSD[1]	-	-	95%	97%
Discharge Instructions Given[1]	-	-	93%	94%
Evaluation of LVS Function	14	71%	97%	99%
Medicare Spending				
Medicare Spending per Patient (ratio)	-	-	0.91	0.98
Pneumonia Care				
Appropriate Initial Antibiotic Given	20	70%	93%	95%
Blood Culture Timing	26	100%	98%	98%
Pregnancy and Delivery Care				
Newborn Deliveries Scheduled Early[5]	-	-	4%	6%
Preventive Care				
Immunization for Influenza[5]	-	-	91%	90%
Immunization for Pneumonia[5]	-	-	90%	92%
Stroke Care				
Anticoagulation Therapy for Atrial Fibrillation[5]	-	-	95%	95%
Antithrombotic Therapy Timing[5]	-	-	98%	98%
Assessed for Rehabilitation[5]	-	-	97%	97%
Discharged on Antithrombotic Therapy[5]	-	-	99%	99%
Discharged on Statin Medication[5]	-	-	92%	94%
Thrombolytic Therapy Timing[5]	-	-	64%	66%
Venous Thromboembolism Prophylaxis[5]	-	-	93%	94%
Written Stroke Educational Materials Given[5]	-	-	82%	88%
Surgical Care Improvement Project				
Appropriate Beta Blocker Usage[3,7]	-	-	98%	98%
Appropriate VTP Within 24 Hours[1,3]	-	-	98%	98%
Controlled Postoperative Blood Glucose[3,7]	-	-	96%	97%
Perioperative Temperature Management[1,3]	-	-	100%	100%
Prophylactic Antibiotic Selection[1,3]	-	-	99%	99%
Prophylactic Antibiotic Selection (Outpatient)[5]	-	-	98%	98%
Prophylactic Antibiotic Stopped[1,3]	-	-	98%	98%
Prophylactic Antibiotic Timing[1,3]	-	-	98%	99%
Prophylactic Antibiotic Timing (Outpatient)[5]	-	-	98%	98%
Urinary Catheter Removal[1,3]	-	-	97%	97%
Survey of Patients' Hospital Experiences				
Area Around Room 'Always' Quiet at Night[5]	-	-	63%	61%
Doctors 'Always' Communicated Well[5]	-	-	84%	82%
Home Recovery Information Given[5]	-	-	88%	85%
Hospital Given 9 or 10 on 10 Point Scale[5]	-	-	75%	71%
Meds 'Always' Explained Before Given[5]	-	-	66%	64%
Nurses 'Always' Communicated Well[5]	-	-	81%	79%
Pain 'Always' Well Controlled[5]	-	-	71%	71%
Room and Bathroom 'Always' Clean[5]	-	-	79%	73%
Timely Help 'Always' Received[5]	-	-	70%	68%
Would Definitely Recommend Hospital[5]	-	-	74%	71%
Use of Medical Imaging				
Cardiac Imaging Stress Test before Surgery[7]	-	-	4.8%	5.3%
Combination Abdominal CT Scan	103	10.7%	11.5%	10.5%
Combination Brain/Sinus CT Scan[1]	-	-	1.8%	2.7%
Combination Chest CT Scan[1]	-	-	3.5%	2.7%
Follow-up Mammogram/Ultrasound	114	12.3%	7.9%	8.8%
Lumbar Spine MRI for Low Back Pain[1]	-	-	32.2%	37.2%

NOTE: Hospital profiles are in alphabetical order by state, then city, then hospital within the city; Rankings exclude hospitals with less than 25 cases except for patient surveys which excludes hospitals with less than 100 cases; (a) 100-299 cases; (1) The number of cases/patients is too few to report; (2) Data submitted were based on a sample of cases/patients; (3) Results are based on a shorter time period than required; (4) Data suppressed by CMS for one or more quarters; (5) Results are not available for this reporting period; (6) Fewer than 100 patients completed the HCAHPS survey; (7) No cases met the criteria for this measure; (8) The lower limit of the confidence interval cannot be calculated if the number of observed infections equals zero; (9) No data are available from the state/territory for this reporting period; (10) The scores shown reflect fewer than 50 completed surveys; (11) There were discrepancies in the data collection process; (12) This measure does not apply to this hospital for this reporting period; (13) Results cannot be calculated for this reporting period; (14) The results for this state are combined with nearby states to protect confidentiality; Please refer to the User's Guide for a full explanation of data.

Buchanan County Health Center

1600 First Saint East
Independence, IA 50644
URL: www.bchealth.info
Type: Critical Access Hospitals
Ownership: Voluntary non-profit - Other

Phone: 319-332-0999
Fax: 319-334-6149
Emergency Services: Yes
Beds: 84

Key Personnel:
Pulmonology . . . . Kevin Carpenter
Emergency Room . . . . Roslind Gibbs
Cardiology . . . . Keith Kopec
Cardiology . . . . Khalid Mohammad
Quality Assurance . . . . Kathy Post
CEO/President. . . . . Bob Richard
Cardiology . . . . Abbie Schaa

Measure	Cases	This Hosp.	State Avg.	U.S. Avg.
Blood Clot Prevention and Treatment				
Anticoagulation Overlap Therapy[5]	-	-	94%	93%
ICU Venous Thromboembolism Prophylaxis[5]	-	-	90%	92%
Incidence of Potentially Preventable VTE[5]	-	-	8%	10%
UFH with Dosages/Platelet Monitoring[5]	-	-	99%	97%
Venous Thromboembolism Prophylaxis[5]	-	-	87%	85%
Warfarin Therapy Discharge Instructions[5]	-	-	77%	75%
Chest Pain/Possible Heart Attack Care				
Aspirin Given Within 24 Hours of Arrival[3]	27	100%	97%	96%
Fibrinolytic Meds Within 30 Min. of Arrival[5]	-	-	49%	58%
Average Time to ECG (minutes)[3]	30	3	5	7
Average Time to Transfer (minutes)[5]	-	-	58	60
Children's Asthma Care				
Received Home Management Plan of Care	-	-	-	88%
Received Reliever Medication	-	-	-	100%
Received Systemic Corticosteroids	-	-	-	100%
Emergency Department				
Admittance Decision Time (minutes)[5]	-	-	58	98
Head CT Results Within 45 Min. of Arrival[5]	-	-	55%	57%
Patients Who Left ER Before Being Seen[5]	-	-	1%	2%
Time from ER Arrival to Admit. (minutes)[5]	-	-	202	274
Time from ER Arrival to Discharge (minutes)[5]	-	-	108	134
Time in ER Before Being Evaluated (minutes)[5]	-	-	21	26
Time to Pain Meds for Fractures (minutes)[5]	-	-	46	57
Heart Attack Care				
Aspirin Given at Discharge[5]	-	-	100%	99%
Fibrinolytic Meds Within 30 Min. of Arrival[5]	-	-	-	54%
PCI Within 90 Minutes of Arrival[5]	-	-	94%	96%
Statin Prescribed at Discharge[5]	-	-	98%	98%
Heart Failure Care				
ACE Inhibitor or ARB for LVSD[1]	-	-	95%	97%
Discharge Instructions Given	12	83%	93%	94%
Evaluation of LVS Function	14	64%	97%	99%
Medicare Spending				
Medicare Spending per Patient (ratio)	-	-	0.91	0.98
Pneumonia Care				
Appropriate Initial Antibiotic Given	31	97%	93%	95%
Blood Culture Timing	35	97%	98%	98%
Pregnancy and Delivery Care				
Newborn Deliveries Scheduled Early[5]	-	-	4%	6%
Preventive Care				
Immunization for Influenza[5]	-	-	91%	90%
Immunization for Pneumonia[5]	-	-	90%	92%
Stroke Care				
Anticoagulation Therapy for Atrial Fibrillation[5]	-	-	95%	95%
Antithrombotic Therapy Timing[5]	-	-	98%	98%
Assessed for Rehabilitation[5]	-	-	97%	97%
Discharged on Antithrombotic Therapy[5]	-	-	99%	99%
Discharged on Statin Medication[5]	-	-	92%	94%
Thrombolytic Therapy Timing[5]	-	-	64%	66%
Venous Thromboembolism Prophylaxis[5]	-	-	93%	94%
Written Stroke Educational Materials Given[5]	-	-	82%	88%
Surgical Care Improvement Project				
Appropriate Beta Blocker Usage[1]	-	-	98%	98%
Appropriate VTP Within 24 Hours[1]	-	-	98%	98%
Controlled Postoperative Blood Glucose[7]	-	-	96%	97%
Perioperative Temperature Management[1]	-	-	100%	100%
Prophylactic Antibiotic Selection[1]	-	-	99%	99%
Prophylactic Antibiotic Selection (Outpatient)[5]	-	-	98%	98%
Prophylactic Antibiotic Stopped[1]	-	-	98%	98%
Prophylactic Antibiotic Timing[1]	-	-	98%	99%
Prophylactic Antibiotic Timing (Outpatient)[5]	-	-	98%	98%
Urinary Catheter Removal[1]	-	-	97%	97%
Survey of Patients' Hospital Experiences				
Area Around Room 'Always' Quiet at Night[6]	<100	52%	63%	61%
Doctors 'Always' Communicated Well[6]	<100	85%	84%	82%
Home Recovery Information Given[6]	<100	84%	88%	85%
Hospital Given 9 or 10 on 10 Point Scale[6]	<100	52%	75%	71%
Meds 'Always' Explained Before Given[6]	<100	60%	66%	64%
Nurses 'Always' Communicated Well[6]	<100	70%	81%	79%
Pain 'Always' Well Controlled[6]	<100	74%	71%	71%
Room and Bathroom 'Always' Clean[6]	<100	71%	79%	73%
Timely Help 'Always' Received[6]	<100	77%	70%	68%
Would Definitely Recommend Hospital[6]	<100	50%	74%	71%
Use of Medical Imaging				
Cardiac Imaging Stress Test before Surgery[7]	-	-	4.8%	5.3%
Combination Abdominal CT Scan	146	3.4%	11.5%	10.5%
Combination Brain/Sinus CT Scan	160	0.6%	1.8%	2.7%
Combination Chest CT Scan	82	0.0%	3.5%	2.7%
Follow-up Mammogram/Ultrasound	251	4.4%	7.9%	8.8%
Lumbar Spine MRI for Low Back Pain[1]	-	-	32.2%	37.2%

Iowa City VA Medical Center

601 Highway 6 West
Iowa City, IA 52246
URL: www.va.gov/sta/guide/home.asp
Type: Acute Care - VA
Ownership: Government Federal

Phone: 319-338-0581
Fax: 319-339-7171
Emergency Services: No
Beds: 93

Key Personnel:
Operating Room. . . . . Betty Bream, RN
Radiology. . . . . David Bushnell, MD
Chief of Medical Staff. . . . . John Cowdery, MD
Intensive Care Unit. . . . . Kevin Dellsperger, MD
Infection Control. . . . . Mary Fredrickson, RN
Quality Assurance . . . . Natalie Good
CEO/President. . . . . Barry Sharp, RN
Emergency Room . . . . Rodney Zeitler, MD

Measure	Cases	This Hosp.	State Avg.	U.S. Avg.
Blood Clot Prevention and Treatment				
Anticoagulation Overlap Therapy	-	-	94%	93%
ICU Venous Thromboembolism Prophylaxis	-	-	90%	92%
Incidence of Potentially Preventable VTE	-	-	8%	10%
UFH with Dosages/Platelet Monitoring	-	-	99%	97%
Venous Thromboembolism Prophylaxis	-	-	87%	85%
Warfarin Therapy Discharge Instructions	-	-	77%	75%
Chest Pain/Possible Heart Attack Care				
Aspirin Given Within 24 Hours of Arrival	-	-	97%	96%
Fibrinolytic Meds Within 30 Min. of Arrival	-	-	49%	58%
Average Time to ECG (minutes)	-	-	5	7
Average Time to Transfer (minutes)	-	-	58	60
Children's Asthma Care				
Received Home Management Plan of Care	-	-	-	88%
Received Reliever Medication	-	-	-	100%
Received Systemic Corticosteroids	-	-	-	100%
Emergency Department				
Admittance Decision Time (minutes)	-	-	58	98
Head CT Results Within 45 Min. of Arrival	-	-	55%	57%
Patients Who Left ER Before Being Seen	-	-	1%	2%
Time from ER Arrival to Admit. (minutes)	-	-	202	274
Time from ER Arrival to Discharge (minutes)	-	-	108	134
Time in ER Before Being Evaluated (minutes)	-	-	21	26
Time to Pain Meds for Fractures (minutes)	-	-	46	57
Heart Attack Care				
Aspirin Given at Discharge	25	100%	100%	99%
Fibrinolytic Meds Within 30 Min. of Arrival[5]	-	-	-	54%
PCI Within 90 Minutes of Arrival[5]	-	-	94%	96%
Statin Prescribed at Discharge[1]	24	96%	98%	98%
Heart Failure Care				
ACE Inhibitor or ARB for LVSD	45	93%	95%	97%
Discharge Instructions Given	96	98%	93%	94%
Evaluation of LVS Function	108	100%	97%	99%
Medicare Spending				
Medicare Spending per Patient (ratio)	-	-	0.91	0.98
Pneumonia Care				
Appropriate Initial Antibiotic Given	28	93%	93%	95%
Blood Culture Timing	42	98%	98%	98%
Pregnancy and Delivery Care				
Newborn Deliveries Scheduled Early	-	-	4%	6%
Preventive Care				
Immunization for Influenza[5]	-	-	91%	90%
Immunization for Pneumonia[5]	-	-	90%	92%
Stroke Care				
Anticoagulation Therapy for Atrial Fibrillation	-	-	95%	95%
Antithrombotic Therapy Timing	-	-	98%	98%
Assessed for Rehabilitation	-	-	97%	97%
Discharged on Antithrombotic Therapy	-	-	99%	99%
Discharged on Statin Medication	-	-	92%	94%
Thrombolytic Therapy Timing	-	-	64%	66%
Venous Thromboembolism Prophylaxis	-	-	93%	94%
Written Stroke Educational Materials Given	-	-	82%	88%
Surgical Care Improvement Project				
Appropriate Beta Blocker Usage[2]	123	92%	98%	98%
Appropriate VTP Within 24 Hours[2]	239	99%	98%	98%
Controlled Postoperative Blood Glucose[5]	-	-	96%	97%
Perioperative Temperature Management[2]	275	100%	100%	100%
Prophylactic Antibiotic Selection	185	99%	99%	99%
Prophylactic Antibiotic Selection (Outpatient)	-	-	98%	98%
Prophylactic Antibiotic Stopped	184	92%	98%	98%
Prophylactic Antibiotic Timing	185	98%	98%	99%
Prophylactic Antibiotic Timing (Outpatient)	-	-	98%	98%
Urinary Catheter Removal[2]	208	93%	97%	97%
Survey of Patients' Hospital Experiences				
Area Around Room 'Always' Quiet at Night	-	-	63%	61%
Doctors 'Always' Communicated Well	-	-	84%	82%
Home Recovery Information Given	-	-	88%	85%
Hospital Given 9 or 10 on 10 Point Scale	-	-	75%	71%
Meds 'Always' Explained Before Given	-	-	66%	64%
Nurses 'Always' Communicated Well	-	-	81%	79%
Pain 'Always' Well Controlled	-	-	71%	71%
Room and Bathroom 'Always' Clean	-	-	79%	73%
Timely Help 'Always' Received	-	-	70%	68%
Would Definitely Recommend Hospital	-	-	74%	71%
Use of Medical Imaging				
Cardiac Imaging Stress Test before Surgery	-	-	4.8%	5.3%
Combination Abdominal CT Scan	-	-	11.5%	10.5%
Combination Brain/Sinus CT Scan	-	-	1.8%	2.7%
Combination Chest CT Scan	-	-	3.5%	2.7%
Follow-up Mammogram/Ultrasound	-	-	7.9%	8.8%
Lumbar Spine MRI for Low Back Pain	-	-	32.2%	37.2%

Mercy Hospital

500 E Market Street
Iowa City, IA 52245
URL: www.mercyiowacity.org
Type: Acute Care Hospitals
Ownership: Voluntary non-profit - Church

Phone: 319-339-0300
Fax: 319-339-3788
Emergency Services: Yes
Beds: 240

Key Personnel:
Radiology. . . . . Heidi Berns
Quality Assurance . . . . Barb Griswold
Coronary Care . . . . Mike Lebsack
Operating Room. . . . . Sid Mills
CEO/President. . . . . Ronald R Reed
Chief of Medical Staff. . . . . Pete Wallace

Measure	Cases	This Hosp.	State Avg.	U.S. Avg.
Blood Clot Prevention and Treatment				
Anticoagulation Overlap Therapy[2]	69	90%	94%	93%
ICU Venous Thromboembolism Prophylaxis[2]	55	93%	90%	92%
Incidence of Potentially Preventable VTE[1,2]	-	-	8%	10%
UFH with Dosages/Platelet Monitoring[2]	14	50%	99%	97%
Venous Thromboembolism Prophylaxis[2]	299	87%	87%	85%
Warfarin Therapy Discharge Instructions[2]	58	98%	77%	75%
Chest Pain/Possible Heart Attack Care				
Aspirin Given Within 24 Hours of Arrival[3,7]	-	-	97%	96%
Fibrinolytic Meds Within 30 Min. of Arrival[5]	-	-	49%	58%
Average Time to ECG (minutes)[3,7]	-	-	5	7
Average Time to Transfer (minutes)[5]	-	-	58	60
Children's Asthma Care				

NOTE: *Hospital profiles are in alphabetical order by state, then city, then hospital within the city; Rankings exclude hospitals with less than 25 cases except for patient surveys which excludes hospitals with less than 100 cases; (a) 100-299 cases; (1) The number of cases/patients is too few to report; (2) Data submitted were based on a sample of cases/patients; (3) Results are based on a shorter time period than required; (4) Data suppressed by CMS for one or more quarters; (5) Results are not available for this reporting period; (6) Fewer than 100 patients completed the HCAHPS survey; (7) No cases met the criteria for this measure; (8) The lower limit of the confidence interval cannot be calculated if the number of observed infections equals zero; (9) No data are available from the state/territory for this reporting period; (10) The scores shown reflect fewer than 50 completed surveys; (11) There were discrepancies in the data collection process; (12) This measure does not apply to this hospital for this reporting period; (13) Results cannot be calculated for this reporting period; (14) The results for this state are combined with nearby states to protect confidentiality; Please refer to the User's Guide for a full explanation of data.*

Measure	Cases	This Hosp.	State Avg.	U.S. Avg.
Received Home Management Plan of Care	-	-	-	88%
Received Reliever Medication	-	-	-	100%
Received Systemic Corticosteroids	-	-	-	100%
Emergency Department				
Admittance Decision Time (minutes)[2]	477	83	58	98
Head CT Results Within 45 Min. of Arrival[1]	-	-	55%	57%
Patients Who Left ER Before Being Seen	21,454	1%	1%	2%
Time from ER Arrival to Admit. (minutes)[2]	498	214	202	274
Time from ER Arrival to Discharge (minutes)	381	129	108	134
Time in ER Before Being Evaluated (minutes)	388	30	21	26
Time to Pain Meds for Fractures (minutes)	107	71	46	57
Heart Attack Care				
Aspirin Given at Discharge	187	100%	100%	99%
Fibrinolytic Meds Within 30 Min. of Arrival[7]	-	-	-	54%
PCI Within 90 Minutes of Arrival	33	100%	94%	96%
Statin Prescribed at Discharge	176	99%	98%	98%
Heart Failure Care				
ACE Inhibitor or ARB for LVSD	38	95%	95%	97%
Discharge Instructions Given	138	99%	93%	94%
Evaluation of LVS Function	176	96%	97%	99%
Medicare Spending				
Medicare Spending per Patient (ratio)	-	0.84	0.91	0.98
Pneumonia Care				
Appropriate Initial Antibiotic Given	97	99%	93%	95%
Blood Culture Timing	169	99%	98%	98%
Pregnancy and Delivery Care				
Newborn Deliveries Scheduled Early	140	13%	4%	6%
Preventive Care				
Immunization for Influenza[2]	532	95%	91%	90%
Immunization for Pneumonia[2]	655	88%	90%	92%
Stroke Care				
Anticoagulation Therapy for Atrial Fibrillation	25	88%	95%	95%
Antithrombotic Therapy Timing	95	100%	98%	98%
Assessed for Rehabilitation	105	98%	97%	97%
Discharged on Antithrombotic Therapy	105	100%	99%	99%
Discharged on Statin Medication	75	96%	92%	94%
Thrombolytic Therapy Timing	11	91%	64%	66%
Venous Thromboembolism Prophylaxis	108	92%	93%	94%
Written Stroke Educational Materials Given	66	91%	82%	88%
Surgical Care Improvement Project				
Appropriate Beta Blocker Usage	397	97%	98%	98%
Appropriate VTP Within 24 Hours	1,103	98%	98%	98%
Controlled Postoperative Blood Glucose	99	96%	96%	97%
Perioperative Temperature Management	1,204	100%	100%	100%
Prophylactic Antibiotic Selection	1,049	99%	99%	99%
Prophylactic Antibiotic Selection (Outpatient)	449	98%	98%	98%
Prophylactic Antibiotic Stopped	1,026	98%	98%	98%
Prophylactic Antibiotic Timing	1,049	99%	98%	99%
Prophylactic Antibiotic Timing (Outpatient)	449	99%	98%	98%
Urinary Catheter Removal	1,172	99%	97%	97%
Survey of Patients' Hospital Experiences				
Area Around Room 'Always' Quiet at Night	300+	56%	63%	61%
Doctors 'Always' Communicated Well	300+	88%	84%	82%
Home Recovery Information Given	300+	89%	88%	85%
Hospital Given 9 or 10 on 10 Point Scale	300+	72%	75%	71%
Meds 'Always' Explained Before Given	300+	65%	66%	64%
Nurses 'Always' Communicated Well	300+	79%	81%	79%
Pain 'Always' Well Controlled	300+	69%	71%	71%
Room and Bathroom 'Always' Clean	300+	71%	79%	73%
Timely Help 'Always' Received	300+	65%	70%	68%
Would Definitely Recommend Hospital	300+	78%	74%	71%
Use of Medical Imaging				
Cardiac Imaging Stress Test before Surgery	96	4.2%	4.8%	5.3%
Combination Abdominal CT Scan	549	5.3%	11.5%	10.5%
Combination Brain/Sinus CT Scan[1]	-	-	1.8%	2.7%
Combination Chest CT Scan	473	0.2%	3.5%	2.7%
Follow-up Mammogram/Ultrasound	1,551	8.1%	7.9%	8.8%
Lumbar Spine MRI for Low Back Pain	118	38.1%	32.2%	37.2%

University of Iowa Hospital & Clinics

200 Hawkins Drive
Iowa City, IA 52242
URL: www.uihealthcare.com
Phone: 319-356-1616
Fax: 319-356-3862
Type: Acute Care Hospitals
Ownership: Government - State
Emergency Services: Yes
Beds: 705

Key Personnel:

Pediatric Ambulatory Care . . . . . . Michael Artman, MD
Radiology. . . . . Laurie Fajardo, MD
Infection Control. . . . . Loreen Herwaldt, MD
CEO/President. . . . . Ken Kates
Operating Room. . . . . Toni Mueller RN, RN, MSN
Chief of Medical Staff. . . . . Eva Tsalikian, MD

Measure	Cases	This Hosp.	State Avg.	U.S. Avg.
Blood Clot Prevention and Treatment				
Anticoagulation Overlap Therapy[2]	112	96%	94%	93%
ICU Venous Thromboembolism Prophylaxis[2]	107	90%	90%	92%
Incidence of Potentially Preventable VTE[2]	48	12%	8%	10%
UFH with Dosages/Platelet Monitoring[2]	123	100%	99%	97%
Venous Thromboembolism Prophylaxis[2]	282	80%	87%	85%
Warfarin Therapy Discharge Instructions[2]	85	86%	77%	75%
Chest Pain/Possible Heart Attack Care				
Aspirin Given Within 24 Hours of Arrival[5]	-	-	97%	96%
Fibrinolytic Meds Within 30 Min. of Arrival[5]	-	-	49%	58%
Average Time to ECG (minutes)[5]	-	-	5	7
Average Time to Transfer (minutes)[5]	-	-	58	60
Children's Asthma Care				
Received Home Management Plan of Care	-	-	-	88%
Received Reliever Medication	-	-	-	100%
Received Systemic Corticosteroids	-	-	-	100%
Emergency Department				
Admittance Decision Time (minutes)[2]	244	106	58	98
Head CT Results Within 45 Min. of Arrival[1]	-	-	55%	57%
Patients Who Left ER Before Being Seen	64,562	2%	1%	2%
Time from ER Arrival to Admit. (minutes)[2]	252	278	202	274
Time from ER Arrival to Discharge (minutes)	356	168	108	134
Time in ER Before Being Evaluated (minutes)[7]	-	-	21	26
Time to Pain Meds for Fractures (minutes)	150	61	46	57
Heart Attack Care				
Aspirin Given at Discharge	337	100%	100%	99%
Fibrinolytic Meds Within 30 Min. of Arrival[7]	-	-	-	54%
PCI Within 90 Minutes of Arrival	23	78%	94%	96%
Statin Prescribed at Discharge	324	99%	98%	98%
Heart Failure Care				
ACE Inhibitor or ARB for LVSD[2]	112	96%	95%	97%
Discharge Instructions Given[2]	233	95%	93%	94%
Evaluation of LVS Function[2]	276	100%	97%	99%
Medicare Spending				
Medicare Spending per Patient (ratio)	-	0.98	0.91	0.98
Pneumonia Care				
Appropriate Initial Antibiotic Given[2]	21	95%	93%	95%
Blood Culture Timing[2]	86	93%	98%	98%
Pregnancy and Delivery Care				
Newborn Deliveries Scheduled Early[2]	12	8%	4%	6%
Preventive Care				
Immunization for Influenza[2]	544	88%	91%	90%
Immunization for Pneumonia[2]	497	85%	90%	92%
Stroke Care				
Anticoagulation Therapy for Atrial Fibrillation[1,2]	-	-	95%	95%
Antithrombotic Therapy Timing[2]	55	95%	98%	98%
Assessed for Rehabilitation[2]	114	96%	97%	97%
Discharged on Antithrombotic Therapy[2]	75	100%	99%	99%
Discharged on Statin Medication[2]	47	94%	92%	94%
Thrombolytic Therapy Timing[1,2]	-	-	64%	66%
Venous Thromboembolism Prophylaxis[2]	125	99%	93%	94%
Written Stroke Educational Materials Given[2]	56	89%	82%	88%
Surgical Care Improvement Project				
Appropriate Beta Blocker Usage[2]	235	98%	98%	98%
Appropriate VTP Within 24 Hours[2]	399	99%	98%	98%
Controlled Postoperative Blood Glucose[2]	109	97%	96%	97%
Perioperative Temperature Management[2]	530	100%	100%	100%
Prophylactic Antibiotic Selection[2]	394	100%	99%	99%
Prophylactic Antibiotic Selection (Outpatient)	647	99%	98%	98%
Prophylactic Antibiotic Stopped[2]	378	98%	98%	98%
Prophylactic Antibiotic Timing[2]	396	98%	98%	99%
Prophylactic Antibiotic Timing (Outpatient)	572	97%	98%	98%
Urinary Catheter Removal[2]	346	99%	97%	97%
Survey of Patients' Hospital Experiences				
Area Around Room 'Always' Quiet at Night	300+	45%	63%	61%
Doctors 'Always' Communicated Well	300+	77%	84%	82%
Home Recovery Information Given	300+	89%	88%	85%
Hospital Given 9 or 10 on 10 Point Scale	300+	73%	75%	71%
Meds 'Always' Explained Before Given	300+	59%	66%	64%
Nurses 'Always' Communicated Well	300+	77%	81%	79%
Pain 'Always' Well Controlled	300+	67%	71%	71%
Room and Bathroom 'Always' Clean	300+	67%	79%	73%
Timely Help 'Always' Received	300+	58%	70%	68%
Would Definitely Recommend Hospital	300+	77%	74%	71%
Use of Medical Imaging				
Cardiac Imaging Stress Test before Surgery	432	4.2%	4.8%	5.3%
Combination Abdominal CT Scan	2,163	4.1%	11.5%	10.5%
Combination Brain/Sinus CT Scan	653	1.7%	1.8%	2.7%
Combination Chest CT Scan	2,060	0.3%	3.5%	2.7%
Follow-up Mammogram/Ultrasound	1,440	11.9%	7.9%	8.8%
Lumbar Spine MRI for Low Back Pain	115	30.4%	32.2%	37.2%

Hansen Family Hospital

920 South Oak Street
Iowa Falls, IA 50126
URL: www.emhia.com
Phone: 641-648-4631
Fax: 641-648-2850
Type: Critical Access Hospitals
Ownership: Government - Local
Emergency Services: Yes
Beds: 40

Key Personnel:

Chief of Medical Staff. . . . . Joseph Brunkhorst, MD
Intensive Care Unit. . . . . Susan Copp
Infection Control. . . . . Ann Holmguard
CEO/President. . . . . Cherelle Montanya
Quality Assurance . . . . Katie Ricks
Anesthesiology. . . . . Barb Roby

Measure	Cases	This Hosp.	State Avg.	U.S. Avg.
Blood Clot Prevention and Treatment				
Anticoagulation Overlap Therapy[5]	-	-	94%	93%
ICU Venous Thromboembolism Prophylaxis[5]	-	-	90%	92%
Incidence of Potentially Preventable VTE[5]	-	-	8%	10%
UFH with Dosages/Platelet Monitoring[5]	-	-	99%	97%
Venous Thromboembolism Prophylaxis[5]	-	-	87%	85%
Warfarin Therapy Discharge Instructions[5]	-	-	77%	75%
Chest Pain/Possible Heart Attack Care				
Aspirin Given Within 24 Hours of Arrival	-	-	97%	96%
Fibrinolytic Meds Within 30 Min. of Arrival	-	-	49%	58%
Average Time to ECG (minutes)	-	-	5	7
Average Time to Transfer (minutes)	-	-	58	60
Children's Asthma Care				
Received Home Management Plan of Care	-	-	-	88%
Received Reliever Medication	-	-	-	100%
Received Systemic Corticosteroids	-	-	-	100%
Emergency Department				
Admittance Decision Time (minutes)[5]	-	-	58	98
Head CT Results Within 45 Min. of Arrival	-	-	55%	57%
Patients Who Left ER Before Being Seen	-	-	1%	2%
Time from ER Arrival to Admit. (minutes)[5]	-	-	202	274
Time from ER Arrival to Discharge (minutes)	-	-	108	134
Time in ER Before Being Evaluated (minutes)	-	-	21	26
Time to Pain Meds for Fractures (minutes)	-	-	46	57
Heart Attack Care				
Aspirin Given at Discharge[5]	-	-	100%	99%
Fibrinolytic Meds Within 30 Min. of Arrival[5]	-	-	-	54%
PCI Within 90 Minutes of Arrival[5]	-	-	94%	96%
Statin Prescribed at Discharge[5]	-	-	98%	98%
Heart Failure Care				
ACE Inhibitor or ARB for LVSD[3,7]	-	-	95%	97%
Discharge Instructions Given[1,3]	-	-	93%	94%
Evaluation of LVS Function[1,3]	-	-	97%	99%
Medicare Spending				
Medicare Spending per Patient (ratio)	-	-	0.91	0.98
Pneumonia Care				
Appropriate Initial Antibiotic Given[5]	-	-	93%	95%
Blood Culture Timing[5]	-	-	98%	98%

NOTE: Hospital profiles are in alphabetical order by state, then city, then hospital within the city; Rankings exclude hospitals with less than 25 cases except for patient surveys which excludes hospitals with less than 100 cases; (a) 100-299 cases; (1) The number of cases/patients is too few to report; (2) Data submitted were based on a sample of cases/patients; (3) Results are based on a shorter time period than required; (4) Data suppressed by CMS for one or more quarters; (5) Results are not available for this reporting period; (6) Fewer than 100 patients completed the HCAHPS survey; (7) No cases met the criteria for this measure; (8) The lower limit of the confidence interval cannot be calculated if the number of observed infections equals zero; (9) No data are available from the state/territory for this reporting period; (10) The scores shown reflect fewer than 50 completed surveys; (11) There were discrepancies in the data collection process; (12) This measure does not apply to this hospital for this reporting period; (13) Results cannot be calculated for this reporting period; (14) The results for this state are combined with nearby states to protect confidentiality; Please refer to the User's Guide for a full explanation of data.

Measure	Cases	This Hosp.	State Avg.	U.S. Avg.
Pregnancy and Delivery Care				
Newborn Deliveries Scheduled Early[5]	-	-	4%	6%
Preventive Care				
Immunization for Influenza[5]	-	-	91%	90%
Immunization for Pneumonia[5]	-	-	90%	92%
Stroke Care				
Anticoagulation Therapy for Atrial Fibrillation[5]	-	-	95%	95%
Antithrombotic Therapy Timing[5]	-	-	98%	98%
Assessed for Rehabilitation[5]	-	-	97%	97%
Discharged on Antithrombotic Therapy[5]	-	-	99%	99%
Discharged on Statin Medication[5]	-	-	92%	94%
Thrombolytic Therapy Timing[5]	-	-	64%	66%
Venous Thromboembolism Prophylaxis[5]	-	-	93%	94%
Written Stroke Educational Materials Given[5]	-	-	82%	88%
Surgical Care Improvement Project				
Appropriate Beta Blocker Usage[5]	-	-	98%	98%
Appropriate VTP Within 24 Hours[5]	-	-	98%	98%
Controlled Postoperative Blood Glucose[5]	-	-	96%	97%
Perioperative Temperature Management[5]	-	-	100%	100%
Prophylactic Antibiotic Selection[5]	-	-	99%	99%
Prophylactic Antibiotic Selection (Outpatient)	-	-	98%	98%
Prophylactic Antibiotic Stopped[5]	-	-	98%	98%
Prophylactic Antibiotic Timing[5]	-	-	98%	99%
Prophylactic Antibiotic Timing (Outpatient)	-	-	98%	98%
Urinary Catheter Removal[5]	-	-	97%	97%
Survey of Patients' Hospital Experiences				
Area Around Room 'Always' Quiet at Night[5]	-	-	63%	61%
Doctors 'Always' Communicated Well[5]	-	-	84%	82%
Home Recovery Information Given[5]	-	-	88%	85%
Hospital Given 9 or 10 on 10 Point Scale[5]	-	-	75%	71%
Meds 'Always' Explained Before Given[5]	-	-	66%	64%
Nurses 'Always' Communicated Well[5]	-	-	81%	79%
Pain 'Always' Well Controlled[5]	-	-	71%	71%
Room and Bathroom 'Always' Clean[5]	-	-	79%	73%
Timely Help 'Always' Received[5]	-	-	70%	68%
Would Definitely Recommend Hospital[5]	-	-	74%	71%
Use of Medical Imaging				
Cardiac Imaging Stress Test before Surgery	-	-	4.8%	5.3%
Combination Abdominal CT Scan	-	-	11.5%	10.5%
Combination Brain/Sinus CT Scan	-	-	1.8%	2.7%
Combination Chest CT Scan	-	-	3.5%	2.7%
Follow-up Mammogram/Ultrasound	-	-	7.9%	8.8%
Lumbar Spine MRI for Low Back Pain	-	-	32.2%	37.2%

Greene County Medical Center

1000 West Lincolnway
Jefferson, IA 50129
Phone: 515-386-2114
Fax: 515-386-3695
URL: www.gcmchealth.com
Type: Critical Access Hospitals
Emergency Services: Yes
Ownership: Government - Local
Beds: 127

Key Personnel:

Patient Relations . . . . Jacque Andrew
CEO/President. . . . . Karen Bossard
Chief of Medical Staff . . . . Monica L Burgett, MD
Infection Control. . . . . Amy Love
Quality Assurance . . . . Amy Love
Emergency Room . . . . Jeri Reese, RN
Chairman/CEO . . . . Jim Schieisman
Operating Room. . . . . Kraig Tweed

Measure	Cases	This Hosp.	State Avg.	U.S. Avg.
Blood Clot Prevention and Treatment				
Anticoagulation Overlap Therapy[5]	-	-	94%	93%
ICU Venous Thromboembolism Prophylaxis[5]	-	-	90%	92%
Incidence of Potentially Preventable VTE[5]	-	-	8%	10%
UFH with Dosages/Platelet Monitoring[5]	-	-	99%	97%
Venous Thromboembolism Prophylaxis[5]	-	-	87%	85%
Warfarin Therapy Discharge Instructions[5]	-	-	77%	75%
Chest Pain/Possible Heart Attack Care				
Aspirin Given Within 24 Hours of Arrival[5]	-	-	97%	96%
Fibrinolytic Meds Within 30 Min. of Arrival[5]	-	-	49%	58%
Average Time to ECG (minutes)[5]	-	-	5	7
Average Time to Transfer (minutes)[5]	-	-	58	60
Children's Asthma Care				
Received Home Management Plan of Care	-	-	-	88%
Received Reliever Medication	-	-	-	100%
Received Systemic Corticosteroids	-	-	-	100%
Emergency Department				
Admittance Decision Time (minutes)[5]	-	-	58	98
Head CT Results Within 45 Min. of Arrival[5]	-	-	55%	57%
Patients Who Left ER Before Being Seen[5]	-	-	1%	2%
Time from ER Arrival to Admit. (minutes)[5]	-	-	202	274
Time from ER Arrival to Discharge (minutes)[5]	-	-	108	134
Time in ER Before Being Evaluated (minutes)[5]	-	-	21	26
Time to Pain Meds for Fractures (minutes)[5]	-	-	46	57
Heart Attack Care				
Aspirin Given at Discharge[1,3]	-	-	100%	99%
Fibrinolytic Meds Within 30 Min. of Arrival[3,7]	-	-	-	54%
PCI Within 90 Minutes of Arrival[3,7]	-	-	94%	96%
Statin Prescribed at Discharge[1,3]	-	-	98%	98%
Heart Failure Care				
ACE Inhibitor or ARB for LVSD[1,3]	-	-	95%	97%
Discharge Instructions Given[1,3]	-	-	93%	94%
Evaluation of LVS Function[1,3]	-	-	97%	99%
Medicare Spending				
Medicare Spending per Patient (ratio)	-	-	0.91	0.98
Pneumonia Care				
Appropriate Initial Antibiotic Given	12	42%	93%	95%
Blood Culture Timing	11	73%	98%	98%
Pregnancy and Delivery Care				
Newborn Deliveries Scheduled Early[5]	-	-	4%	6%
Preventive Care				
Immunization for Influenza[5]	-	-	91%	90%
Immunization for Pneumonia[5]	-	-	90%	92%
Stroke Care				
Anticoagulation Therapy for Atrial Fibrillation[5]	-	-	95%	95%
Antithrombotic Therapy Timing[5]	-	-	98%	98%
Assessed for Rehabilitation[5]	-	-	97%	97%
Discharged on Antithrombotic Therapy[5]	-	-	99%	99%
Discharged on Statin Medication[5]	-	-	92%	94%
Thrombolytic Therapy Timing[5]	-	-	64%	66%
Venous Thromboembolism Prophylaxis[5]	-	-	93%	94%
Written Stroke Educational Materials Given[5]	-	-	82%	88%
Surgical Care Improvement Project				
Appropriate Beta Blocker Usage[1]	-	-	98%	98%
Appropriate VTP Within 24 Hours	31	84%	98%	98%
Controlled Postoperative Blood Glucose[7]	-	-	96%	97%
Perioperative Temperature Management	34	97%	100%	100%
Prophylactic Antibiotic Selection	30	90%	99%	99%
Prophylactic Antibiotic Selection (Outpatient)[5]	-	-	98%	98%
Prophylactic Antibiotic Stopped	30	93%	98%	98%
Prophylactic Antibiotic Timing	30	87%	98%	99%
Prophylactic Antibiotic Timing (Outpatient)[5]	-	-	98%	98%
Urinary Catheter Removal	25	88%	97%	97%
Survey of Patients' Hospital Experiences				
Area Around Room 'Always' Quiet at Night[5]	-	-	63%	61%
Doctors 'Always' Communicated Well[5]	-	-	84%	82%
Home Recovery Information Given[5]	-	-	88%	85%
Hospital Given 9 or 10 on 10 Point Scale[5]	-	-	75%	71%
Meds 'Always' Explained Before Given[5]	-	-	66%	64%
Nurses 'Always' Communicated Well[5]	-	-	81%	79%
Pain 'Always' Well Controlled[5]	-	-	71%	71%
Room and Bathroom 'Always' Clean[5]	-	-	79%	73%
Timely Help 'Always' Received[5]	-	-	70%	68%
Would Definitely Recommend Hospital[5]	-	-	74%	71%
Use of Medical Imaging				
Cardiac Imaging Stress Test before Surgery[1]	-	-	4.8%	5.3%
Combination Abdominal CT Scan	62	3.2%	11.5%	10.5%
Combination Brain/Sinus CT Scan	68	0.0%	1.8%	2.7%
Combination Chest CT Scan[1]	-	-	3.5%	2.7%
Follow-up Mammogram/Ultrasound	335	12.2%	7.9%	8.8%
Lumbar Spine MRI for Low Back Pain[1]	-	-	32.2%	37.2%

Keokuk Area Hospital

1600 Morgan Street
Keokuk, IA 52632
Phone: 319-524-7150
Fax: 319-524-5317
URL: www.keokukhealthsystems.org
Type: Acute Care Hospitals
Emergency Services: Yes
Ownership: Voluntary non-profit - Private
Beds: 120

Key Personnel:

Pediatric Ambulatory Care . . . . . . Barbara Clark
Pediatric In-Patient Care . . . . Barbara Clark
Chief of Medical Staff . . . . Brigitte Cormier, MD
Radiology. . . . . William Fulcher
Quality Assurance . . . . Susie Lowe, RN
Operating Room. . . . . Dwain Stone
Infection Control. . . . . Ardath Tweedy, RN
CEO/President. . . . . Allan W Zastrow

Measure	Cases	This Hosp.	State Avg.	U.S. Avg.
Blood Clot Prevention and Treatment				
Anticoagulation Overlap Therapy	16	75%	94%	93%
ICU Venous Thromboembolism Prophylaxis	125	94%	90%	92%
Incidence of Potentially Preventable VTE[7]	-	-	8%	10%
UFH with Dosages/Platelet Monitoring[1]	-	-	99%	97%
Venous Thromboembolism Prophylaxis	480	96%	87%	85%
Warfarin Therapy Discharge Instructions	11	100%	77%	75%
Chest Pain/Possible Heart Attack Care				
Aspirin Given Within 24 Hours of Arrival	44	93%	97%	96%
Fibrinolytic Meds Within 30 Min. of Arrival[1]	-	-	49%	58%
Average Time to ECG (minutes)	45	6	5	7
Average Time to Transfer (minutes)[1]	-	-	58	60
Children's Asthma Care				
Received Home Management Plan of Care	-	-	-	88%
Received Reliever Medication	-	-	-	100%
Received Systemic Corticosteroids	-	-	-	100%
Emergency Department				
Admittance Decision Time (minutes)	656	54	58	98
Head CT Results Within 45 Min. of Arrival[1]	-	-	55%	57%
Patients Who Left ER Before Being Seen	12,758	1%	1%	2%
Time from ER Arrival to Admit. (minutes)	742	187	202	274
Time from ER Arrival to Discharge (minutes)	1,320	94	108	134
Time in ER Before Being Evaluated (minutes)	1,186	24	21	26
Time to Pain Meds for Fractures (minutes)	33	44	46	57
Heart Attack Care				
Aspirin Given at Discharge[1]	-	-	100%	99%
Fibrinolytic Meds Within 30 Min. of Arrival[7]	-	-	-	54%
PCI Within 90 Minutes of Arrival[7]	-	-	94%	96%
Statin Prescribed at Discharge[1]	-	-	98%	98%
Heart Failure Care				
ACE Inhibitor or ARB for LVSD	13	92%	95%	97%
Discharge Instructions Given	36	86%	93%	94%
Evaluation of LVS Function	71	99%	97%	99%
Medicare Spending				
Medicare Spending per Patient (ratio)	-	0.89	0.91	0.98
Pneumonia Care				
Appropriate Initial Antibiotic Given	54	93%	93%	95%
Blood Culture Timing	60	98%	98%	98%
Pregnancy and Delivery Care				
Newborn Deliveries Scheduled Early	24	33%	4%	6%
Preventive Care				
Immunization for Influenza	664	96%	91%	90%
Immunization for Pneumonia	888	97%	90%	92%
Stroke Care				
Anticoagulation Therapy for Atrial Fibrillation[1]	-	-	95%	95%
Antithrombotic Therapy Timing[1]	-	-	98%	98%
Assessed for Rehabilitation	11	91%	97%	97%
Discharged on Antithrombotic Therapy	11	100%	99%	99%
Discharged on Statin Medication	11	64%	92%	94%
Thrombolytic Therapy Timing[7]	-	-	64%	66%
Venous Thromboembolism Prophylaxis	11	100%	93%	94%
Written Stroke Educational Materials Given[1]	-	-	82%	88%
Surgical Care Improvement Project				
Appropriate Beta Blocker Usage[1]	-	-	98%	98%
Appropriate VTP Within 24 Hours	19	84%	98%	98%
Controlled Postoperative Blood Glucose[7]	-	-	96%	97%
Perioperative Temperature Management	20	100%	100%	100%
Prophylactic Antibiotic Selection	13	92%	99%	99%

NOTE: Hospital profiles are in alphabetical order by state, then city, then hospital within the city; Rankings exclude hospitals with less than 25 cases except for patient surveys which excludes hospitals with less than 100 cases; (a) 100-299 cases; (1) The number of cases/patients is too few to report; (2) Data submitted were based on a sample of cases/patients; (3) Results are based on a shorter time period than required; (4) Data suppressed by CMS for one or more quarters; (5) Results are not available for this reporting period; (6) Fewer than 100 patients completed the HCAHPS survey; (7) No cases met the criteria for this measure; (8) The lower limit of the confidence interval cannot be calculated if the number of observed infections equals zero; (9) No data are available from the state/territory for this reporting period; (10) The scores shown reflect fewer than 50 completed surveys; (11) There were discrepancies in the data collection process; (12) This measure does not apply to this hospital for this reporting period; (13) Results cannot be calculated for this reporting period; (14) The results for this state are combined with nearby states to protect confidentiality; Please refer to the User's Guide for a full explanation of data.

Measure	Cases	This Hosp.	State Avg.	U.S. Avg.
Prophylactic Antibiotic Selection (Outpatient)[1,3]	-	-	98%	98%
Prophylactic Antibiotic Stopped	13	92%	98%	98%
Prophylactic Antibiotic Timing	13	100%	98%	99%
Prophylactic Antibiotic Timing (Outpatient)[1,3]	-	-	98%	98%
Urinary Catheter Removal	11	73%	97%	97%
Survey of Patients' Hospital Experiences				
Area Around Room 'Always' Quiet at Night	(a)	65%	63%	61%
Doctors 'Always' Communicated Well	(a)	85%	84%	82%
Home Recovery Information Given	(a)	85%	88%	85%
Hospital Given 9 or 10 on 10 Point Scale	(a)	75%	75%	71%
Meds 'Always' Explained Before Given	(a)	70%	66%	64%
Nurses 'Always' Communicated Well	(a)	81%	81%	79%
Pain 'Always' Well Controlled	(a)	72%	71%	71%
Room and Bathroom 'Always' Clean	(a)	85%	79%	73%
Timely Help 'Always' Received	(a)	71%	70%	68%
Would Definitely Recommend Hospital	(a)	68%	74%	71%
Use of Medical Imaging				
Cardiac Imaging Stress Test before Surgery[1]	-	-	4.8%	5.3%
Combination Abdominal CT Scan	174	5.7%	11.5%	10.5%
Combination Brain/Sinus CT Scan[1]	-	-	1.8%	2.7%
Combination Chest CT Scan	96	0.0%	3.5%	2.7%
Follow-up Mammogram/Ultrasound	532	3.2%	7.9%	8.8%
Lumbar Spine MRI for Low Back Pain[1]	-	-	32.2%	37.2%

Van Buren County Hospital

304 Franklin Street
Keosauqua, IA 52565
URL: www.netins.net/showcase/forhealth
Type: Critical Access Hospitals
Ownership: Voluntary non-profit - Other

Phone: 319-293-3171
Fax: 319-293-3142
Emergency Services: Yes
Beds: 25

Key Personnel:
Radiology. . . . . Betsy Caviness
Operating Room. . . . . Barbara Hirschler, RN
Emergency Room . . . . Vicki L Robertson, RN, DON
CEO/President. . . . . Lisa Schnedler

Measure	Cases	This Hosp.	State Avg.	U.S. Avg.
Blood Clot Prevention and Treatment				
Anticoagulation Overlap Therapy[5]	-	-	94%	93%
ICU Venous Thromboembolism Prophylaxis[5]	-	-	90%	92%
Incidence of Potentially Preventable VTE[5]	-	-	8%	10%
UFH with Dosages/Platelet Monitoring[5]	-	-	99%	97%
Venous Thromboembolism Prophylaxis[5]	-	-	87%	85%
Warfarin Therapy Discharge Instructions[5]	-	-	77%	75%
Chest Pain/Possible Heart Attack Care				
Aspirin Given Within 24 Hours of Arrival[5]	-	-	97%	96%
Fibrinolytic Meds Within 30 Min. of Arrival[5]	-	-	49%	58%
Average Time to ECG (minutes)[5]	-	-	5	7
Average Time to Transfer (minutes)[5]	-	-	58	60
Children's Asthma Care				
Received Home Management Plan of Care	-	-	-	88%
Received Reliever Medication	-	-	-	100%
Received Systemic Corticosteroids	-	-	-	100%
Emergency Department				
Admittance Decision Time (minutes)[5]	-	-	58	98
Head CT Results Within 45 Min. of Arrival[5]	-	-	55%	57%
Patients Who Left ER Before Being Seen[5]	-	-	1%	2%
Time from ER Arrival to Admit. (minutes)[5]	-	-	202	274
Time from ER Arrival to Discharge (minutes)[5]	-	-	108	134
Time in ER Before Being Evaluated (minutes)[5]	-	-	21	26
Time to Pain Meds for Fractures (minutes)[5]	-	-	46	57
Heart Attack Care				
Aspirin Given at Discharge[5]	-	-	100%	99%
Fibrinolytic Meds Within 30 Min. of Arrival[5]	-	-	-	54%
PCI Within 90 Minutes of Arrival[5]	-	-	94%	96%
Statin Prescribed at Discharge[5]	-	-	98%	98%
Heart Failure Care				
ACE Inhibitor or ARB for LVSD[1,3]	-	-	95%	97%
Discharge Instructions Given[1,3]	-	-	93%	94%
Evaluation of LVS Function[1,3]	-	-	97%	99%
Medicare Spending				
Medicare Spending per Patient (ratio)	-	-	0.91	0.98
Pneumonia Care				
Appropriate Initial Antibiotic Given[1]	-	-	93%	95%
Blood Culture Timing[1]	-	-	98%	98%
Pregnancy and Delivery Care				
Newborn Deliveries Scheduled Early[5]	-	-	4%	6%
Preventive Care				
Immunization for Influenza[5]	-	-	91%	90%
Immunization for Pneumonia[5]	-	-	90%	92%
Stroke Care				
Anticoagulation Therapy for Atrial Fibrillation[5]	-	-	95%	95%
Antithrombotic Therapy Timing[5]	-	-	98%	98%
Assessed for Rehabilitation[5]	-	-	97%	97%
Discharged on Antithrombotic Therapy[5]	-	-	99%	99%
Discharged on Statin Medication[5]	-	-	92%	94%
Thrombolytic Therapy Timing[5]	-	-	64%	66%
Venous Thromboembolism Prophylaxis[5]	-	-	93%	94%
Written Stroke Educational Materials Given[5]	-	-	82%	88%
Surgical Care Improvement Project				
Appropriate Beta Blocker Usage[5]	-	-	98%	98%
Appropriate VTP Within 24 Hours[5]	-	-	98%	98%
Controlled Postoperative Blood Glucose[5]	-	-	96%	97%
Perioperative Temperature Management[5]	-	-	100%	100%
Prophylactic Antibiotic Selection[5]	-	-	99%	99%
Prophylactic Antibiotic Selection (Outpatient)[5]	-	-	98%	98%
Prophylactic Antibiotic Stopped[5]	-	-	98%	98%
Prophylactic Antibiotic Timing[5]	-	-	98%	99%
Prophylactic Antibiotic Timing (Outpatient)[5]	-	-	98%	98%
Urinary Catheter Removal[5]	-	-	97%	97%
Survey of Patients' Hospital Experiences				
Area Around Room 'Always' Quiet at Night[5]	-	-	63%	61%
Doctors 'Always' Communicated Well[5]	-	-	84%	82%
Home Recovery Information Given[5]	-	-	88%	85%
Hospital Given 9 or 10 on 10 Point Scale[5]	-	-	75%	71%
Meds 'Always' Explained Before Given[5]	-	-	66%	64%
Nurses 'Always' Communicated Well[5]	-	-	81%	79%
Pain 'Always' Well Controlled[5]	-	-	71%	71%
Room and Bathroom 'Always' Clean[5]	-	-	79%	73%
Timely Help 'Always' Received[5]	-	-	70%	68%
Would Definitely Recommend Hospital[5]	-	-	74%	71%
Use of Medical Imaging				
Cardiac Imaging Stress Test before Surgery[1]	-	-	4.8%	5.3%
Combination Abdominal CT Scan	44	40.9%	11.5%	10.5%
Combination Brain/Sinus CT Scan	69	0.0%	1.8%	2.7%
Combination Chest CT Scan[1]	-	-	3.5%	2.7%
Follow-up Mammogram/Ultrasound	82	2.4%	7.9%	8.8%
Lumbar Spine MRI for Low Back Pain[1]	-	-	32.2%	37.2%

Knoxville Hospital & Clinics

1002 South Lincoln Street
Knoxville, IA 50138
URL: www.kach.org
Type: Critical Access Hospitals
Ownership: Voluntary non-profit - Private

Phone: 641-842-2151
Emergency Services: Yes
Beds: 25

Key Personnel:
Emergency Room . . . . Melody Abell
Radiology. . . . . Amy Heimbaugh
CEO . . . . Kevin Kincaid
Administrator . . . . Brain Sims
Operating Room. . . . . Amy Zoutte, RN

Measure	Cases	This Hosp.	State Avg.	U.S. Avg.
Blood Clot Prevention and Treatment				
Anticoagulation Overlap Therapy[5]	-	-	94%	93%
ICU Venous Thromboembolism Prophylaxis[5]	-	-	90%	92%
Incidence of Potentially Preventable VTE[5]	-	-	8%	10%
UFH with Dosages/Platelet Monitoring[5]	-	-	99%	97%
Venous Thromboembolism Prophylaxis[5]	-	-	87%	85%
Warfarin Therapy Discharge Instructions[5]	-	-	77%	75%
Chest Pain/Possible Heart Attack Care				
Aspirin Given Within 24 Hours of Arrival[3]	16	100%	97%	96%
Fibrinolytic Meds Within 30 Min. of Arrival[3,7]	-	-	49%	58%
Average Time to ECG (minutes)[3]	19	4	5	7
Average Time to Transfer (minutes)[1,3]	-	-	58	60
Children's Asthma Care				
Received Home Management Plan of Care	-	-	-	88%
Received Reliever Medication	-	-	-	100%
Received Systemic Corticosteroids	-	-	-	100%
Emergency Department				
Admittance Decision Time (minutes)[2,3]	168	55	58	98
Head CT Results Within 45 Min. of Arrival[1,3]	-	-	55%	57%
Patients Who Left ER Before Being Seen[5]	-	-	1%	2%
Time from ER Arrival to Admit. (minutes)[2,3]	168	162	202	274
Time from ER Arrival to Discharge (minutes)[3]	136	84	108	134
Time in ER Before Being Evaluated (minutes)[3]	138	18	21	26
Time to Pain Meds for Fractures (minutes)[3]	24	14	46	57
Heart Attack Care				
Aspirin Given at Discharge[5]	-	-	100%	99%
Fibrinolytic Meds Within 30 Min. of Arrival[5]	-	-	-	54%
PCI Within 90 Minutes of Arrival[5]	-	-	94%	96%
Statin Prescribed at Discharge[5]	-	-	98%	98%
Heart Failure Care				
ACE Inhibitor or ARB for LVSD[1,3]	-	-	95%	97%
Discharge Instructions Given[1,3]	-	-	93%	94%
Evaluation of LVS Function[1,3]	-	-	97%	99%
Medicare Spending				
Medicare Spending per Patient (ratio)	-	-	0.91	0.98
Pneumonia Care				
Appropriate Initial Antibiotic Given[3]	15	80%	93%	95%
Blood Culture Timing[3]	18	83%	98%	98%
Pregnancy and Delivery Care				
Newborn Deliveries Scheduled Early[5]	-	-	4%	6%
Preventive Care				
Immunization for Influenza[3]	118	87%	91%	90%
Immunization for Pneumonia[3]	271	84%	90%	92%
Stroke Care				
Anticoagulation Therapy for Atrial Fibrillation[5]	-	-	95%	95%
Antithrombotic Therapy Timing[5]	-	-	98%	98%
Assessed for Rehabilitation[5]	-	-	97%	97%
Discharged on Antithrombotic Therapy[5]	-	-	99%	99%
Discharged on Statin Medication[5]	-	-	92%	94%
Thrombolytic Therapy Timing[5]	-	-	64%	66%
Venous Thromboembolism Prophylaxis[5]	-	-	93%	94%
Written Stroke Educational Materials Given[5]	-	-	82%	88%
Surgical Care Improvement Project				
Appropriate Beta Blocker Usage[1,3]	-	-	98%	98%
Appropriate VTP Within 24 Hours[1,3]	-	-	98%	98%
Controlled Postoperative Blood Glucose[3,7]	-	-	96%	97%
Perioperative Temperature Management[1,3]	-	-	100%	100%
Prophylactic Antibiotic Selection[1,3]	-	-	99%	99%
Prophylactic Antibiotic Selection (Outpatient)[1,3]	-	-	98%	98%
Prophylactic Antibiotic Stopped[1,3]	-	-	98%	98%
Prophylactic Antibiotic Timing[1,3]	-	-	98%	99%
Prophylactic Antibiotic Timing (Outpatient)[1,3]	-	-	98%	98%
Urinary Catheter Removal[1,3]	-	-	97%	97%
Survey of Patients' Hospital Experiences				
Area Around Room 'Always' Quiet at Night	(a)	56%	63%	61%
Doctors 'Always' Communicated Well	(a)	89%	84%	82%
Home Recovery Information Given	(a)	84%	88%	85%
Hospital Given 9 or 10 on 10 Point Scale	(a)	72%	75%	71%
Meds 'Always' Explained Before Given	(a)	66%	66%	64%
Nurses 'Always' Communicated Well	(a)	83%	81%	79%
Pain 'Always' Well Controlled	(a)	71%	71%	71%
Room and Bathroom 'Always' Clean	(a)	75%	79%	73%
Timely Help 'Always' Received	(a)	79%	70%	68%
Would Definitely Recommend Hospital	(a)	73%	74%	71%
Use of Medical Imaging				
Cardiac Imaging Stress Test before Surgery	60	1.7%	4.8%	5.3%
Combination Abdominal CT Scan	170	10.0%	11.5%	10.5%
Combination Brain/Sinus CT Scan	139	0.7%	1.8%	2.7%
Combination Chest CT Scan	75	12.0%	3.5%	2.7%
Follow-up Mammogram/Ultrasound	278	2.9%	7.9%	8.8%
Lumbar Spine MRI for Low Back Pain[1]	-	-	32.2%	37.2%

NOTE: Hospital profiles are in alphabetical order by state, then city, then hospital within the city; Rankings exclude hospitals with less than 25 cases except for patient surveys which excludes hospitals with less than 100 cases; (a) 100-299 cases; (1) The number of cases/patients is too few to report; (2) Data submitted were based on a sample of cases/patients; (3) Results are based on a shorter time period than required; (4) Data suppressed by CMS for one or more quarters; (5) Results are not available for this reporting period; (6) Fewer than 100 patients completed the HCAHPS survey; (7) No cases met the criteria for this measure; (8) The lower limit of the confidence interval cannot be calculated if the number of observed infections equals zero; (9) No data are available from the state/territory for this reporting period; (10) The scores shown reflect fewer than 50 completed surveys; (11) There were discrepancies in the data collection process; (12) This measure does not apply to this hospital for this reporting period; (13) Results cannot be calculated for this reporting period; (14) The results for this state are combined with nearby states to protect confidentiality; Please refer to the User's Guide for a full explanation of data.

Stewart Memorial Community Hospital

1301 West Main Street Phone: 712-464-3171
Lake City, IA 51449 Fax: 712-464-3269
URL: www.stewartmemorial.org
Type: Critical Access Hospitals Emergency Services: Yes
Ownership: Voluntary non-profit - Private Beds: 56

Key Personnel:
CEO/President. . . . . Heather Cain
Anesthesiology. . . . . Perry Henley
Operating Room. . . . . Kevin Hibbett
Emergency Room . . . . Obediah Kahn
Surgery . . . . Marc Miller, DO
Radiology. . . . . Mary Reiter
Chair/CEO . . . . Chuck Schmitt
Chief of Medical Staff . . . . Elsie Verbik

Measure	Cases	This Hosp.	State Avg.	U.S. Avg.
Blood Clot Prevention and Treatment				
Anticoagulation Overlap Therapy[1]	-	-	94%	93%
ICU Venous Thromboembolism Prophylaxis[7]	-	-	90%	92%
Incidence of Potentially Preventable VTE[7]	-	-	8%	10%
UFH with Dosages/Platelet Monitoring[1]	-	-	99%	97%
Venous Thromboembolism Prophylaxis[7]	-	-	87%	85%
Warfarin Therapy Discharge Instructions[1]	-	-	77%	75%
Chest Pain/Possible Heart Attack Care				
Aspirin Given Within 24 Hours of Arrival[5]	-	-	97%	96%
Fibrinolytic Meds Within 30 Min. of Arrival[5]	-	-	49%	58%
Average Time to ECG (minutes)[5]	-	-	5	7
Average Time to Transfer (minutes)[5]	-	-	58	60
Children's Asthma Care				
Received Home Management Plan of Care	-	-	-	88%
Received Reliever Medication	-	-	-	100%
Received Systemic Corticosteroids	-	-	-	100%
Emergency Department				
Admittance Decision Time (minutes)[5]	-	-	58	98
Head CT Results Within 45 Min. of Arrival[5]	-	-	55%	57%
Patients Who Left ER Before Being Seen[5]	-	-	1%	2%
Time from ER Arrival to Admit. (minutes)[5]	-	-	202	274
Time from ER Arrival to Discharge (minutes)[3]	852	92	108	134
Time in ER Before Being Evaluated (minutes)[3]	869	10	21	26
Time to Pain Meds for Fractures (minutes)[5]	-	-	46	57
Heart Attack Care				
Aspirin Given at Discharge[1,3]	-	-	100%	99%
Fibrinolytic Meds Within 30 Min. of Arrival[3,7]	-	-	-	54%
PCI Within 90 Minutes of Arrival[3,7]	-	-	94%	96%
Statin Prescribed at Discharge[1,3]	-	-	98%	98%
Heart Failure Care				
ACE Inhibitor or ARB for LVSD[1]	-	-	95%	97%
Discharge Instructions Given[1]	-	-	93%	94%
Evaluation of LVS Function	14	86%	97%	99%
Medicare Spending				
Medicare Spending per Patient (ratio)	-	-	0.91	0.98
Pneumonia Care				
Appropriate Initial Antibiotic Given	30	93%	93%	95%
Blood Culture Timing	23	100%	98%	98%
Pregnancy and Delivery Care				
Newborn Deliveries Scheduled Early[5]	-	-	4%	6%
Preventive Care				
Immunization for Influenza[5]	-	-	91%	90%
Immunization for Pneumonia[5]	-	-	90%	92%
Stroke Care				
Anticoagulation Therapy for Atrial Fibrillation[7]	-	-	95%	95%
Antithrombotic Therapy Timing[1]	-	-	98%	98%
Assessed for Rehabilitation[1]	-	-	97%	97%
Discharged on Antithrombotic Therapy[1]	-	-	99%	99%
Discharged on Statin Medication[1]	-	-	92%	94%
Thrombolytic Therapy Timing[7]	-	-	64%	66%
Venous Thromboembolism Prophylaxis[1]	-	-	93%	94%
Written Stroke Educational Materials Given[7]	-	-	82%	88%
Surgical Care Improvement Project				
Appropriate Beta Blocker Usage[1]	-	-	98%	98%
Appropriate VTP Within 24 Hours	29	93%	98%	98%
Controlled Postoperative Blood Glucose[7]	-	-	96%	97%
Perioperative Temperature Management	32	100%	100%	100%
Prophylactic Antibiotic Selection	28	100%	99%	99%
Prophylactic Antibiotic Selection (Outpatient)[5]	-	-	98%	98%
Prophylactic Antibiotic Stopped	28	100%	98%	98%
Prophylactic Antibiotic Timing	29	86%	98%	99%
Prophylactic Antibiotic Timing (Outpatient)[5]	-	-	98%	98%
Urinary Catheter Removal	16	88%	97%	97%
Survey of Patients' Hospital Experiences				
Area Around Room 'Always' Quiet at Night		(a)	63%	63%	61%
Doctors 'Always' Communicated Well		(a)	88%	84%	82%
Home Recovery Information Given		(a)	88%	88%	85%
Hospital Given 9 or 10 on 10 Point Scale		(a)	84%	75%	71%
Meds 'Always' Explained Before Given		(a)	82%	66%	64%
Nurses 'Always' Communicated Well		(a)	87%	81%	79%
Pain 'Always' Well Controlled		(a)	78%	71%	71%
Room and Bathroom 'Always' Clean		(a)	98%	79%	73%
Timely Help 'Always' Received		(a)	71%	70%	68%
Would Definitely Recommend Hospital		(a)	86%	74%	71%
Use of Medical Imaging				
Cardiac Imaging Stress Test before Surgery[1]	-	-	4.8%	5.3%
Combination Abdominal CT Scan	111	0.0%	11.5%	10.5%
Combination Brain/Sinus CT Scan[1]	-	-	1.8%	2.7%
Combination Chest CT Scan[1]	-	-	3.5%	2.7%
Follow-up Mammogram/Ultrasound	332	3.9%	7.9%	8.8%
Lumbar Spine MRI for Low Back Pain[1]	-	-	32.2%	37.2%

Floyd Valley Hospital

714 Lincoln Saint Ne Phone: 712-546-7871
Le Mars, IA 51031 Fax: 712-546-3352
URL: www.floydvalleyhospital.org
Type: Critical Access Hospitals Emergency Services: Yes
Ownership: Voluntary non-profit - Other Beds: 44

Key Personnel:
Quality Assurance . . . . Renge Detrick
Cardiac Laboratory. . . . . Lavonne Galles
Hemotology Center . . . . Liz Kurth, RN
Infection Control. . . . . Robert Norfolk
Chief of Medical Staff . . . . Paul Parmelee, DO
Anesthesiology. . . . . Gary Tillman
Operating Room. . . . . Gina Vacuna
Patient Relations . . . . Lisa Wiese

Measure	Cases	This Hosp.	State Avg.	U.S. Avg.
Blood Clot Prevention and Treatment				
Anticoagulation Overlap Therapy[5]	-	-	94%	93%
ICU Venous Thromboembolism Prophylaxis[5]	-	-	90%	92%
Incidence of Potentially Preventable VTE[5]	-	-	8%	10%
UFH with Dosages/Platelet Monitoring[5]	-	-	99%	97%
Venous Thromboembolism Prophylaxis[5]	-	-	87%	85%
Warfarin Therapy Discharge Instructions[5]	-	-	77%	75%
Chest Pain/Possible Heart Attack Care				
Aspirin Given Within 24 Hours of Arrival	-	-	97%	96%
Fibrinolytic Meds Within 30 Min. of Arrival	-	-	49%	58%
Average Time to ECG (minutes)	-	-	5	7
Average Time to Transfer (minutes)	-	-	58	60
Children's Asthma Care				
Received Home Management Plan of Care	-	-	-	88%
Received Reliever Medication	-	-	-	100%
Received Systemic Corticosteroids	-	-	-	100%
Emergency Department				
Admittance Decision Time (minutes)[5]	-	-	58	98
Head CT Results Within 45 Min. of Arrival	-	-	55%	57%
Patients Who Left ER Before Being Seen	-	-	1%	2%
Time from ER Arrival to Admit. (minutes)[5]	-	-	202	274
Time from ER Arrival to Discharge (minutes)	-	-	108	134
Time in ER Before Being Evaluated (minutes)	-	-	21	26
Time to Pain Meds for Fractures (minutes)	-	-	46	57
Heart Attack Care				
Aspirin Given at Discharge[5]	-	-	100%	99%
Fibrinolytic Meds Within 30 Min. of Arrival[5]	-	-	-	54%
PCI Within 90 Minutes of Arrival[5]	-	-	94%	96%
Statin Prescribed at Discharge[5]	-	-	98%	98%
Heart Failure Care				
ACE Inhibitor or ARB for LVSD[1,3]	-	-	95%	97%
Discharge Instructions Given[3]	15	93%	93%	94%
Evaluation of LVS Function[3]	23	78%	97%	99%
Medicare Spending				
Medicare Spending per Patient (ratio)	-	-	0.91	0.98
Pneumonia Care				
Appropriate Initial Antibiotic Given[2]	23	91%	93%	95%
Blood Culture Timing[2]	45	98%	98%	98%
Pregnancy and Delivery Care				
Newborn Deliveries Scheduled Early[5]	-	-	4%	6%
Preventive Care				
Immunization for Influenza[5]	-	-	91%	90%
Immunization for Pneumonia[5]	-	-	90%	92%
Stroke Care				
Anticoagulation Therapy for Atrial Fibrillation[5]	-	-	95%	95%
Antithrombotic Therapy Timing[5]	-	-	98%	98%
Assessed for Rehabilitation[5]	-	-	97%	97%
Discharged on Antithrombotic Therapy[5]	-	-	99%	99%
Discharged on Statin Medication[5]	-	-	92%	94%
Thrombolytic Therapy Timing[5]	-	-	64%	66%
Venous Thromboembolism Prophylaxis[5]	-	-	93%	94%
Written Stroke Educational Materials Given[5]	-	-	82%	88%
Surgical Care Improvement Project				
Appropriate Beta Blocker Usage	17	88%	98%	98%
Appropriate VTP Within 24 Hours	70	100%	98%	98%
Controlled Postoperative Blood Glucose[3,7]	-	-	96%	97%
Perioperative Temperature Management	80	100%	100%	100%
Prophylactic Antibiotic Selection	61	98%	99%	99%
Prophylactic Antibiotic Selection (Outpatient)	-	-	98%	98%
Prophylactic Antibiotic Stopped	60	100%	98%	98%
Prophylactic Antibiotic Timing	62	97%	98%	99%
Prophylactic Antibiotic Timing (Outpatient)	-	-	98%	98%
Urinary Catheter Removal[1]	-	-	97%	97%
Survey of Patients' Hospital Experiences				
Area Around Room 'Always' Quiet at Night	(a)	68%	63%	61%
Doctors 'Always' Communicated Well	(a)	87%	84%	82%
Home Recovery Information Given	(a)	89%	88%	85%
Hospital Given 9 or 10 on 10 Point Scale	(a)	77%	75%	71%
Meds 'Always' Explained Before Given	(a)	60%	66%	64%
Nurses 'Always' Communicated Well	(a)	83%	81%	79%
Pain 'Always' Well Controlled	(a)	73%	71%	71%
Room and Bathroom 'Always' Clean	(a)	83%	79%	73%
Timely Help 'Always' Received	(a)	69%	70%	68%
Would Definitely Recommend Hospital	(a)	77%	74%	71%
Use of Medical Imaging				
Cardiac Imaging Stress Test before Surgery	-	-	4.8%	5.3%
Combination Abdominal CT Scan	-	-	11.5%	10.5%
Combination Brain/Sinus CT Scan	-	-	1.8%	2.7%
Combination Chest CT Scan	-	-	3.5%	2.7%
Follow-up Mammogram/Ultrasound	-	-	7.9%	8.8%
Lumbar Spine MRI for Low Back Pain	-	-	32.2%	37.2%

Decatur County Hospital

1405 Nw Church Street Phone: 641-446-4871
Leon, IA 50144 Fax: 641-446-2201
URL: www.decaturcountyhospital.org
Type: Critical Access Hospitals Emergency Services: Yes
Ownership: Govt - Hospital Dist/Auth Beds: 60

Key Personnel:
CEO/President. . . . . Suzanne L. Cooner

Measure	Cases	This Hosp.	State Avg.	U.S. Avg.
Blood Clot Prevention and Treatment				
Anticoagulation Overlap Therapy[5]	-	-	94%	93%
ICU Venous Thromboembolism Prophylaxis[5]	-	-	90%	92%
Incidence of Potentially Preventable VTE[5]	-	-	8%	10%
UFH with Dosages/Platelet Monitoring[5]	-	-	99%	97%
Venous Thromboembolism Prophylaxis[5]	-	-	87%	85%
Warfarin Therapy Discharge Instructions[5]	-	-	77%	75%
Chest Pain/Possible Heart Attack Care				
Aspirin Given Within 24 Hours of Arrival	-	-	97%	96%
Fibrinolytic Meds Within 30 Min. of Arrival	-	-	49%	58%
Average Time to ECG (minutes)	-	-	5	7
Average Time to Transfer (minutes)	-	-	58	60
Children's Asthma Care				
Received Home Management Plan of Care	-	-	-	88%
Received Reliever Medication	-	-	-	100%
Received Systemic Corticosteroids	-	-	-	100%

NOTE: Hospital profiles are in alphabetical order by state, then city, then hospital within the city; Rankings exclude hospitals with less than 25 cases except for patient surveys which excludes hospitals with less than 100 cases; (a) 100-299 cases; (1) The number of cases/patients is too few to report; (2) Data submitted were based on a sample of cases/patients; (3) Results are based on a shorter time period than required; (4) Data suppressed by CMS for one or more quarters; (5) Results are not available for this reporting period; (6) Fewer than 100 patients completed the HCAHPS survey; (7) No cases met the criteria for this measure; (8) The lower limit of the confidence interval cannot be calculated if the number of observed infections equals zero; (9) No data are available from the state/territory for this reporting period; (10) The scores shown reflect fewer than 50 completed surveys; (11) There were discrepancies in the data collection process; (12) This measure does not apply to this hospital for this reporting period; (13) Results cannot be calculated for this reporting period; (14) The results for this state are combined with nearby states to protect confidentiality; Please refer to the User's Guide for a full explanation of data.

Measure	Cases	This Hosp.	State Avg.	U.S. Avg.
Emergency Department				
Admittance Decision Time (minutes)[5]	-	-	58	98
Head CT Results Within 45 Min. of Arrival	-	-	55%	57%
Patients Who Left ER Before Being Seen	-	-	1%	2%
Time from ER Arrival to Admit. (minutes)[5]	-	-	202	274
Time from ER Arrival to Discharge (minutes)	-	-	108	134
Time in ER Before Being Evaluated (minutes)	-	-	21	26
Time to Pain Meds for Fractures (minutes)	-	-	46	57
Heart Attack Care				
Aspirin Given at Discharge[5]	-	-	100%	99%
Fibrinolytic Meds Within 30 Min. of Arrival[5]	-	-	-	54%
PCI Within 90 Minutes of Arrival[5]	-	-	94%	96%
Statin Prescribed at Discharge[5]	-	-	98%	98%
Heart Failure Care				
ACE Inhibitor or ARB for LVSD[5]	-	-	95%	97%
Discharge Instructions Given[5]	-	-	93%	94%
Evaluation of LVS Function[5]	-	-	97%	99%
Medicare Spending				
Medicare Spending per Patient (ratio)	-	-	0.91	0.98
Pneumonia Care				
Appropriate Initial Antibiotic Given[5]	-	-	93%	95%
Blood Culture Timing[5]	-	-	98%	98%
Pregnancy and Delivery Care				
Newborn Deliveries Scheduled Early[5]	-	-	4%	6%
Preventive Care				
Immunization for Influenza[5]	-	-	91%	90%
Immunization for Pneumonia[5]	-	-	90%	92%
Stroke Care				
Anticoagulation Therapy for Atrial Fibrillation[5]	-	-	95%	95%
Antithrombotic Therapy Timing[5]	-	-	98%	98%
Assessed for Rehabilitation[5]	-	-	97%	97%
Discharged on Antithrombotic Therapy[5]	-	-	99%	99%
Discharged on Statin Medication[5]	-	-	92%	94%
Thrombolytic Therapy Timing[5]	-	-	64%	66%
Venous Thromboembolism Prophylaxis[5]	-	-	93%	94%
Written Stroke Educational Materials Given[5]	-	-	82%	88%
Surgical Care Improvement Project				
Appropriate Beta Blocker Usage[5]	-	-	98%	98%
Appropriate VTP Within 24 Hours[5]	-	-	98%	98%
Controlled Postoperative Blood Glucose[5]	-	-	96%	97%
Perioperative Temperature Management[5]	-	-	100%	100%
Prophylactic Antibiotic Selection[5]	-	-	99%	99%
Prophylactic Antibiotic Selection (Outpatient)	-	-	98%	98%
Prophylactic Antibiotic Stopped[5]	-	-	98%	98%
Prophylactic Antibiotic Timing[5]	-	-	98%	99%
Prophylactic Antibiotic Timing (Outpatient)	-	-	98%	98%
Urinary Catheter Removal[5]	-	-	97%	97%
Survey of Patients' Hospital Experiences				
Area Around Room 'Always' Quiet at Night[5]	-	-	63%	61%
Doctors 'Always' Communicated Well[5]	-	-	84%	82%
Home Recovery Information Given[5]	-	-	88%	85%
Hospital Given 9 or 10 on 10 Point Scale[5]	-	-	75%	71%
Meds 'Always' Explained Before Given[5]	-	-	66%	64%
Nurses 'Always' Communicated Well[5]	-	-	81%	79%
Pain 'Always' Well Controlled[5]	-	-	71%	71%
Room and Bathroom 'Always' Clean[5]	-	-	79%	73%
Timely Help 'Always' Received[5]	-	-	70%	68%
Would Definitely Recommend Hospital[5]	-	-	74%	71%
Use of Medical Imaging				
Cardiac Imaging Stress Test before Surgery	-	-	4.8%	5.3%
Combination Abdominal CT Scan	-	-	11.5%	10.5%
Combination Brain/Sinus CT Scan	-	-	1.8%	2.7%
Combination Chest CT Scan	-	-	3.5%	2.7%
Follow-up Mammogram/Ultrasound	-	-	7.9%	8.8%
Lumbar Spine MRI for Low Back Pain	-	-	32.2%	37.2%

Regional Medical Center

709 W Main Street
Manchester, IA 52057
Phone: 563-927-3232
Fax: 563-927-7444
E-mail: information@regmedctr.org
URL: www.regmedctr.org
Type: Critical Access Hospitals
Emergency Services: Yes
Ownership: Government - Local

Key Personnel:
Chief of Medical Staff . . . . R Ried Boom
CEO/President. . . . . Lon Butikofer, RN
Operating Room. . . . . Carol Jebens, RN
Quality Assurance . . . . Joan Wessels, RN

Measure	Cases	This Hosp.	State Avg.	U.S. Avg.
Blood Clot Prevention and Treatment				
Anticoagulation Overlap Therapy[5]	-	-	94%	93%
ICU Venous Thromboembolism Prophylaxis[5]	-	-	90%	92%
Incidence of Potentially Preventable VTE[5]	-	-	8%	10%
UFH with Dosages/Platelet Monitoring[5]	-	-	99%	97%
Venous Thromboembolism Prophylaxis[5]	-	-	87%	85%
Warfarin Therapy Discharge Instructions[5]	-	-	77%	75%
Chest Pain/Possible Heart Attack Care				
Aspirin Given Within 24 Hours of Arrival[5]	-	-	97%	96%
Fibrinolytic Meds Within 30 Min. of Arrival[5]	-	-	49%	58%
Average Time to ECG (minutes)[5]	-	-	5	7
Average Time to Transfer (minutes)[5]	-	-	58	60
Children's Asthma Care				
Received Home Management Plan of Care	-	-	-	88%
Received Reliever Medication	-	-	-	100%
Received Systemic Corticosteroids	-	-	-	100%
Emergency Department				
Admittance Decision Time (minutes)[5]	-	-	58	98
Head CT Results Within 45 Min. of Arrival[5]	-	-	55%	57%
Patients Who Left ER Before Being Seen[5]	-	-	1%	2%
Time from ER Arrival to Admit. (minutes)[5]	-	-	202	274
Time from ER Arrival to Discharge (minutes)[5]	-	-	108	134
Time in ER Before Being Evaluated (minutes)[5]	-	-	21	26
Time to Pain Meds for Fractures (minutes)[5]	-	-	46	57
Heart Attack Care				
Aspirin Given at Discharge[5]	-	-	100%	99%
Fibrinolytic Meds Within 30 Min. of Arrival[5]	-	-	-	54%
PCI Within 90 Minutes of Arrival[5]	-	-	94%	96%
Statin Prescribed at Discharge[5]	-	-	98%	98%
Heart Failure Care				
ACE Inhibitor or ARB for LVSD[1]	-	-	95%	97%
Discharge Instructions Given[1]	-	-	93%	94%
Evaluation of LVS Function	16	100%	97%	99%
Medicare Spending				
Medicare Spending per Patient (ratio)	-	-	0.91	0.98
Pneumonia Care				
Appropriate Initial Antibiotic Given	31	94%	93%	95%
Blood Culture Timing	52	96%	98%	98%
Pregnancy and Delivery Care				
Newborn Deliveries Scheduled Early[5]	-	-	4%	6%
Preventive Care				
Immunization for Influenza[5]	-	-	91%	90%
Immunization for Pneumonia[5]	-	-	90%	92%
Stroke Care				
Anticoagulation Therapy for Atrial Fibrillation[5]	-	-	95%	95%
Antithrombotic Therapy Timing[5]	-	-	98%	98%
Assessed for Rehabilitation[5]	-	-	97%	97%
Discharged on Antithrombotic Therapy[5]	-	-	99%	99%
Discharged on Statin Medication[5]	-	-	92%	94%
Thrombolytic Therapy Timing[5]	-	-	64%	66%
Venous Thromboembolism Prophylaxis[5]	-	-	93%	94%
Written Stroke Educational Materials Given[5]	-	-	82%	88%
Surgical Care Improvement Project				
Appropriate Beta Blocker Usage[5]	-	-	98%	98%
Appropriate VTP Within 24 Hours[5]	-	-	98%	98%
Controlled Postoperative Blood Glucose[5]	-	-	96%	97%
Perioperative Temperature Management[5]	-	-	100%	100%
Prophylactic Antibiotic Selection[5]	-	-	99%	99%
Prophylactic Antibiotic Selection (Outpatient)[5]	-	-	98%	98%
Prophylactic Antibiotic Stopped[5]	-	-	98%	98%
Prophylactic Antibiotic Timing[5]	-	-	98%	99%
Prophylactic Antibiotic Timing (Outpatient)[5]	-	-	98%	98%
Urinary Catheter Removal[5]	-	-	97%	97%
Survey of Patients' Hospital Experiences				
Area Around Room 'Always' Quiet at Night[6]	-	-	63%	61%
Doctors 'Always' Communicated Well[5]	-	-	84%	82%
Home Recovery Information Given[5]	-	-	88%	85%
Hospital Given 9 or 10 on 10 Point Scale[5]	-	-	75%	71%
Meds 'Always' Explained Before Given[5]	-	-	66%	64%
Nurses 'Always' Communicated Well[5]	-	-	81%	79%
Pain 'Always' Well Controlled[5]	-	-	71%	71%
Room and Bathroom 'Always' Clean[5]	-	-	79%	73%
Timely Help 'Always' Received[5]	-	-	70%	68%
Would Definitely Recommend Hospital[5]	-	-	74%	71%
Use of Medical Imaging				
Cardiac Imaging Stress Test before Surgery[7]	-	-	4.8%	5.3%
Combination Abdominal CT Scan	287	7.3%	11.5%	10.5%
Combination Brain/Sinus CT Scan[1]	-	-	1.8%	2.7%
Combination Chest CT Scan	156	4.5%	3.5%	2.7%
Follow-up Mammogram/Ultrasound	534	5.6%	7.9%	8.8%
Lumbar Spine MRI for Low Back Pain[1]	-	-	32.2%	37.2%

Manning Regional Healthcare Center

410 Main Street
Manning, IA 51455
Phone: 712-655-2072
Fax: 712-655-2216
URL: www.mrhcia.com
Type: Critical Access Hospitals
Emergency Services: Yes
Ownership: Voluntary non-profit - Private
Beds: 73

Key Personnel:
Emergency Room . . . . Cynthia Genzen
CEO/President. . . . . Jeanne Goche
Quality Assurance . . . . Kim Jahn
Operating Room. . . . . Josh A Smith
Cardiology . . . . Kyle Ulvelling, MD

Measure	Cases	This Hosp.	State Avg.	U.S. Avg.
Blood Clot Prevention and Treatment				
Anticoagulation Overlap Therapy[5]	-	-	94%	93%
ICU Venous Thromboembolism Prophylaxis[5]	-	-	90%	92%
Incidence of Potentially Preventable VTE[5]	-	-	8%	10%
UFH with Dosages/Platelet Monitoring[5]	-	-	99%	97%
Venous Thromboembolism Prophylaxis[5]	-	-	87%	85%
Warfarin Therapy Discharge Instructions[5]	-	-	77%	75%
Chest Pain/Possible Heart Attack Care				
Aspirin Given Within 24 Hours of Arrival[1,3]	-	-	97%	96%
Fibrinolytic Meds Within 30 Min. of Arrival[3,7]	-	-	49%	58%
Average Time to ECG (minutes)[1,3]	-	-	5	7
Average Time to Transfer (minutes)[1,3]	-	-	58	60
Children's Asthma Care				
Received Home Management Plan of Care	-	-	-	88%
Received Reliever Medication	-	-	-	100%
Received Systemic Corticosteroids	-	-	-	100%
Emergency Department				
Admittance Decision Time (minutes)[5]	-	-	58	98
Head CT Results Within 45 Min. of Arrival[1,3]	-	-	55%	57%
Patients Who Left ER Before Being Seen[5]	-	-	1%	2%
Time from ER Arrival to Admit. (minutes)[5]	-	-	202	274
Time from ER Arrival to Discharge (minutes)[5]	-	-	108	134
Time in ER Before Being Evaluated (minutes)[5]	-	-	21	26
Time to Pain Meds for Fractures (minutes)[1,3]	-	-	46	57
Heart Attack Care				
Aspirin Given at Discharge[3,7]	-	-	100%	99%
Fibrinolytic Meds Within 30 Min. of Arrival[3,7]	-	-	-	54%
PCI Within 90 Minutes of Arrival[3,7]	-	-	94%	96%
Statin Prescribed at Discharge[3,7]	-	-	98%	98%
Heart Failure Care				
ACE Inhibitor or ARB for LVSD[3,7]	-	-	95%	97%
Discharge Instructions Given[1,3]	-	-	93%	94%
Evaluation of LVS Function[1,3]	-	-	97%	99%
Medicare Spending				
Medicare Spending per Patient (ratio)	-	-	0.91	0.98
Pneumonia Care				
Appropriate Initial Antibiotic Given	14	86%	93%	95%
Blood Culture Timing[1]	-	-	98%	98%
Pregnancy and Delivery Care				

NOTE: Hospital profiles are in alphabetical order by state, then city, then hospital within the city; Rankings exclude hospitals with less than 25 cases except for patient surveys which excludes hospitals with less than 100 cases; (a) 100-299 cases; (1) The number of cases/patients is too few to report; (2) Data submitted were based on a sample of cases/patients; (3) Results are based on a shorter time period than required; (4) Data suppressed by CMS for one or more quarters; (5) Results are not available for this reporting period; (6) Fewer than 100 patients completed the HCAHPS survey; (7) No cases met the criteria for this measure; (8) The lower limit of the confidence interval cannot be calculated if the number of observed infections equals zero; (9) No data are available from the state/territory for this reporting period; (10) The scores shown reflect fewer than 50 completed surveys; (11) There were discrepancies in the data collection process; (12) This measure does not apply to this hospital for this reporting period; (13) Results cannot be calculated for this reporting period; (14) The results for this state are combined with nearby states to protect confidentiality; Please refer to the User's Guide for a full explanation of data.

Measure	Cases	This Hosp.	State Avg.	U.S. Avg.
Newborn Deliveries Scheduled Early[5]	-	-	4%	6%
Preventive Care				
Immunization for Influenza[5]	-	-	91%	90%
Immunization for Pneumonia[5]	-	-	90%	92%
Stroke Care				
Anticoagulation Therapy for Atrial Fibrillation[5]	-	-	95%	95%
Antithrombotic Therapy Timing[5]	-	-	98%	98%
Assessed for Rehabilitation[5]	-	-	97%	97%
Discharged on Antithrombotic Therapy[5]	-	-	99%	99%
Discharged on Statin Medication[5]	-	-	92%	94%
Thrombolytic Therapy Timing[5]	-	-	64%	66%
Venous Thromboembolism Prophylaxis[5]	-	-	93%	94%
Written Stroke Educational Materials Given[5]	-	-	82%	88%
Surgical Care Improvement Project				
Appropriate Beta Blocker Usage[3,7]	-	-	98%	98%
Appropriate VTP Within 24 Hours[3,7]	-	-	98%	98%
Controlled Postoperative Blood Glucose[3,7]	-	-	96%	97%
Perioperative Temperature Management[3,7]	-	-	100%	100%
Prophylactic Antibiotic Selection[1,3]	-	-	99%	99%
Prophylactic Antibiotic Selection (Outpatient)[1,3]	-	-	98%	98%
Prophylactic Antibiotic Stopped[1,3]	-	-	98%	98%
Prophylactic Antibiotic Timing[1,3]	-	-	98%	99%
Prophylactic Antibiotic Timing (Outpatient)[1,3]	-	-	98%	98%
Urinary Catheter Removal[3,7]	-	-	97%	97%
Survey of Patients' Hospital Experiences				
Area Around Room 'Always' Quiet at Night[6]	<100	65%	63%	61%
Doctors 'Always' Communicated Well[6]	<100	90%	84%	82%
Home Recovery Information Given[6]	<100	88%	88%	85%
Hospital Given 9 or 10 on 10 Point Scale[6]	<100	77%	75%	71%
Meds 'Always' Explained Before Given[6]	<100	73%	66%	64%
Nurses 'Always' Communicated Well[6]	<100	83%	81%	79%
Pain 'Always' Well Controlled[6]	<100	66%	71%	71%
Room and Bathroom 'Always' Clean[6]	<100	79%	79%	73%
Timely Help 'Always' Received[6]	<100	80%	70%	68%
Would Definitely Recommend Hospital[6]	<100	74%	74%	71%
Use of Medical Imaging				
Cardiac Imaging Stress Test before Surgery[7]	-	-	4.8%	5.3%
Combination Abdominal CT Scan[1]	-	-	11.5%	10.5%
Combination Brain/Sinus CT Scan	32	0.0%	1.8%	2.7%
Combination Chest CT Scan[1]	-	-	3.5%	2.7%
Follow-up Mammogram/Ultrasound	73	5.5%	7.9%	8.8%
Lumbar Spine MRI for Low Back Pain[1]	-	-	32.2%	37.2%

Jackson County Regional Health Center

700 W Grove St
Maquoketa, IA 52060
Phone: 563-652-2474
Fax: 563-652-4018
Type: Critical Access Hospitals
Emergency Services: Yes
Ownership: Government - Local
Beds: 61

Key Personnel:
CEO/President . . . . Curt Coleman, JCRHC
Chief of Medical Staff . . . . Curt Giswein, MD
Radiology . . . . Eric Jahn, MT (ASCP)
Operating Room . . . . Chris Johnson
Infection Control . . . . Sandra Rockwell
Emergency Room . . . . Cheryl Wagner

Measure	Cases	This Hosp.	State Avg.	U.S. Avg.
Blood Clot Prevention and Treatment				
Anticoagulation Overlap Therapy[5]	-	-	94%	93%
ICU Venous Thromboembolism Prophylaxis[5]	-	-	90%	92%
Incidence of Potentially Preventable VTE[5]	-	-	8%	10%
UFH with Dosages/Platelet Monitoring[5]	-	-	99%	97%
Venous Thromboembolism Prophylaxis[5]	-	-	87%	85%
Warfarin Therapy Discharge Instructions[5]	-	-	77%	75%
Chest Pain/Possible Heart Attack Care				
Aspirin Given Within 24 Hours of Arrival[5]	-	-	97%	96%
Fibrinolytic Meds Within 30 Min. of Arrival[5]	-	-	49%	58%
Average Time to ECG (minutes)[5]	-	-	5	7
Average Time to Transfer (minutes)[5]	-	-	58	60
Children's Asthma Care				
Received Home Management Plan of Care	-	-	-	88%
Received Reliever Medication	-	-	-	100%
Received Systemic Corticosteroids	-	-	-	100%
Emergency Department				
Admittance Decision Time (minutes)[5]	-	-	58	98
Head CT Results Within 45 Min. of Arrival[5]	-	-	55%	57%
Patients Who Left ER Before Being Seen	5,333	0%	1%	2%
Time from ER Arrival to Admit. (minutes)[5]	-	-	202	274
Time from ER Arrival to Discharge (minutes)[5]	-	-	108	134
Time in ER Before Being Evaluated (minutes)[5]	-	-	21	26
Time to Pain Meds for Fractures (minutes)[5]	-	-	46	57
Heart Attack Care				
Aspirin Given at Discharge[5]	-	-	100%	99%
Fibrinolytic Meds Within 30 Min. of Arrival[5]	-	-	-	54%
PCI Within 90 Minutes of Arrival[5]	-	-	94%	96%
Statin Prescribed at Discharge[5]	-	-	98%	98%
Heart Failure Care				
ACE Inhibitor or ARB for LVSD[3,7]	-	-	95%	97%
Discharge Instructions Given[1,3]	-	-	93%	94%
Evaluation of LVS Function[1,3]	-	-	97%	99%
Medicare Spending				
Medicare Spending per Patient (ratio)	-	-	0.91	0.98
Pneumonia Care				
Appropriate Initial Antibiotic Given	15	87%	93%	95%
Blood Culture Timing	19	89%	98%	98%
Pregnancy and Delivery Care				
Newborn Deliveries Scheduled Early[5]	-	-	4%	6%
Preventive Care				
Immunization for Influenza	72	92%	91%	90%
Immunization for Pneumonia	98	95%	90%	92%
Stroke Care				
Anticoagulation Therapy for Atrial Fibrillation[5]	-	-	95%	95%
Antithrombotic Therapy Timing[5]	-	-	98%	98%
Assessed for Rehabilitation[5]	-	-	97%	97%
Discharged on Antithrombotic Therapy[5]	-	-	99%	99%
Discharged on Statin Medication[5]	-	-	92%	94%
Thrombolytic Therapy Timing[5]	-	-	64%	66%
Venous Thromboembolism Prophylaxis[5]	-	-	93%	94%
Written Stroke Educational Materials Given[5]	-	-	82%	88%
Surgical Care Improvement Project				
Appropriate Beta Blocker Usage[5]	-	-	98%	98%
Appropriate VTP Within 24 Hours[5]	-	-	98%	98%
Controlled Postoperative Blood Glucose[5]	-	-	96%	97%
Perioperative Temperature Management[5]	-	-	100%	100%
Prophylactic Antibiotic Selection[5]	-	-	99%	99%
Prophylactic Antibiotic Selection (Outpatient)[5]	-	-	98%	98%
Prophylactic Antibiotic Stopped[5]	-	-	98%	98%
Prophylactic Antibiotic Timing[5]	-	-	98%	99%
Prophylactic Antibiotic Timing (Outpatient)[5]	-	-	98%	98%
Urinary Catheter Removal[5]	-	-	97%	97%
Survey of Patients' Hospital Experiences				
Area Around Room 'Always' Quiet at Night[5]	-	-	63%	61%
Doctors 'Always' Communicated Well[5]	-	-	84%	82%
Home Recovery Information Given[5]	-	-	88%	85%
Hospital Given 9 or 10 on 10 Point Scale[5]	-	-	75%	71%
Meds 'Always' Explained Before Given[5]	-	-	66%	64%
Nurses 'Always' Communicated Well[5]	-	-	81%	79%
Pain 'Always' Well Controlled[5]	-	-	71%	71%
Room and Bathroom 'Always' Clean[5]	-	-	79%	73%
Timely Help 'Always' Received[5]	-	-	70%	68%
Would Definitely Recommend Hospital[5]	-	-	74%	71%
Use of Medical Imaging				
Cardiac Imaging Stress Test before Surgery[7]	-	-	4.8%	5.3%
Combination Abdominal CT Scan	92	4.3%	11.5%	10.5%
Combination Brain/Sinus CT Scan[1]	-	-	1.8%	2.7%
Combination Chest CT Scan	52	0.0%	3.5%	2.7%
Follow-up Mammogram/Ultrasound	425	6.6%	7.9%	8.8%
Lumbar Spine MRI for Low Back Pain[1]	-	-	32.2%	37.2%

Marengo Memorial Hospital

300 W May St
Marengo, IA 52301
URL: www.marengohospital.org
Phone: 319-642-5543
Fax: 319-642-8007
Type: Critical Access Hospitals
Emergency Services: Yes
Ownership: Government - Local
Beds: 25

Key Personnel:
Emergency Room . . . . Lisa Eckholm
Chief of Medical Staff . . . . Endriss Estime
CEO . . . . Barry Goettsch, FACHE
Infection Control . . . . Sharon Schulte, RN
Pediatrics . . . . Heidi Wauters

Measure	Cases	This Hosp.	State Avg.	U.S. Avg.
Blood Clot Prevention and Treatment				
Anticoagulation Overlap Therapy[5]	-	-	94%	93%
ICU Venous Thromboembolism Prophylaxis[5]	-	-	90%	92%
Incidence of Potentially Preventable VTE[5]	-	-	8%	10%
UFH with Dosages/Platelet Monitoring[5]	-	-	99%	97%
Venous Thromboembolism Prophylaxis[5]	-	-	87%	85%
Warfarin Therapy Discharge Instructions[5]	-	-	77%	75%
Chest Pain/Possible Heart Attack Care				
Aspirin Given Within 24 Hours of Arrival[1,3]	-	-	97%	96%
Fibrinolytic Meds Within 30 Min. of Arrival[3,7]	-	-	49%	58%
Average Time to ECG (minutes)[1,3]	-	-	5	7
Average Time to Transfer (minutes)[3,7]	-	-	58	60
Children's Asthma Care				
Received Home Management Plan of Care	-	-	-	88%
Received Reliever Medication	-	-	-	100%
Received Systemic Corticosteroids	-	-	-	100%
Emergency Department				
Admittance Decision Time (minutes)[5]	-	-	58	98
Head CT Results Within 45 Min. of Arrival[1,3]	-	-	55%	57%
Patients Who Left ER Before Being Seen	3,261	1%	1%	2%
Time from ER Arrival to Admit. (minutes)[5]	-	-	202	274
Time from ER Arrival to Discharge (minutes)[5]	-	-	108	134
Time in ER Before Being Evaluated (minutes)[5]	-	-	21	26
Time to Pain Meds for Fractures (minutes)[5]	-	-	46	57
Heart Attack Care				
Aspirin Given at Discharge[5]	-	-	100%	99%
Fibrinolytic Meds Within 30 Min. of Arrival[5]	-	-	-	54%
PCI Within 90 Minutes of Arrival[5]	-	-	94%	96%
Statin Prescribed at Discharge[5]	-	-	98%	98%
Heart Failure Care				
ACE Inhibitor or ARB for LVSD[1,3]	-	-	95%	97%
Discharge Instructions Given[1,3]	-	-	93%	94%
Evaluation of LVS Function[1,3]	-	-	97%	99%
Medicare Spending				
Medicare Spending per Patient (ratio)	-	-	0.91	0.98
Pneumonia Care				
Appropriate Initial Antibiotic Given[1,3]	-	-	93%	95%
Blood Culture Timing[1,3]	-	-	98%	98%
Pregnancy and Delivery Care				
Newborn Deliveries Scheduled Early[5]	-	-	4%	6%
Preventive Care				
Immunization for Influenza[5]	-	-	91%	90%
Immunization for Pneumonia[5]	-	-	90%	92%
Stroke Care				
Anticoagulation Therapy for Atrial Fibrillation[5]	-	-	95%	95%
Antithrombotic Therapy Timing[5]	-	-	98%	98%
Assessed for Rehabilitation[5]	-	-	97%	97%
Discharged on Antithrombotic Therapy[5]	-	-	99%	99%
Discharged on Statin Medication[5]	-	-	92%	94%
Thrombolytic Therapy Timing[5]	-	-	64%	66%
Venous Thromboembolism Prophylaxis[5]	-	-	93%	94%
Written Stroke Educational Materials Given[5]	-	-	82%	88%
Surgical Care Improvement Project				
Appropriate Beta Blocker Usage[5]	-	-	98%	98%
Appropriate VTP Within 24 Hours[5]	-	-	98%	98%
Controlled Postoperative Blood Glucose[5]	-	-	96%	97%
Perioperative Temperature Management[5]	-	-	100%	100%
Prophylactic Antibiotic Selection[5]	-	-	99%	99%
Prophylactic Antibiotic Selection (Outpatient)[5]	-	-	98%	98%
Prophylactic Antibiotic Stopped[5]	-	-	98%	98%
Prophylactic Antibiotic Timing[5]	-	-	98%	99%
Prophylactic Antibiotic Timing (Outpatient)[5]	-	-	98%	98%
Urinary Catheter Removal[5]	-	-	97%	97%
Survey of Patients' Hospital Experiences				
Area Around Room 'Always' Quiet at Night[6]	<100	65%	63%	61%
Doctors 'Always' Communicated Well[6]	<100	85%	84%	82%
Home Recovery Information Given[6]	<100	91%	88%	85%
Hospital Given 9 or 10 on 10 Point Scale[6]	<100	79%	75%	71%

NOTE: Hospital profiles are in alphabetical order by state, then city, then hospital within the city; Rankings exclude hospitals with less than 25 cases except for patient surveys which excludes hospitals with less than 100 cases; (a) 100-299 cases; (1) The number of cases/patients is too few to report; (2) Data submitted were based on a sample of cases/patients; (3) Results are based on a shorter time period than required; (4) Data suppressed by CMS for one or more quarters; (5) Results are not available for this reporting period; (6) Fewer than 100 patients completed the HCAHPS survey; (7) No cases met the criteria for this measure; (8) The lower limit of the confidence interval cannot be calculated if the number of observed infections equals zero; (9) No data are available from the state/territory for this reporting period; (10) The scores shown reflect fewer than 50 completed surveys; (11) There were discrepancies in the data collection process; (12) This measure does not apply to this hospital for this reporting period; (13) Results cannot be calculated for this reporting period; (14) The results for this state are combined with nearby states to protect confidentiality; Please refer to the User's Guide for a full explanation of data.

Measure	Cases	This Hosp.	State Avg.	U.S. Avg.
Meds 'Always' Explained Before Given[6]	<100	66%	66%	64%
Nurses 'Always' Communicated Well[6]	<100	84%	81%	79%
Pain 'Always' Well Controlled[6]	<100	73%	71%	71%
Room and Bathroom 'Always' Clean[6]	<100	92%	79%	73%
Timely Help 'Always' Received[6]	<100	78%	70%	68%
Would Definitely Recommend Hospital[6]	<100	89%	74%	71%
Use of Medical Imaging				
Cardiac Imaging Stress Test before Surgery[7]	-	-	4.8%	5.3%
Combination Abdominal CT Scan	47	4.3%	11.5%	10.5%
Combination Brain/Sinus CT Scan[1]	-	-	1.8%	2.7%
Combination Chest CT Scan[1]	-	-	3.5%	2.7%
Follow-up Mammogram/Ultrasound[7]	-	-	7.9%	8.8%
Lumbar Spine MRI for Low Back Pain[1]	-	-	32.2%	37.2%

Marshalltown Medical & Surgical Center

3 South 4th Avenue
Marshalltown, IA 50158
Phone: 641-754-5151
Fax: 641-753-2570
URL: www.everydaychampions.org
Type: Acute Care Hospitals
Emergency Services: Yes
Ownership: Voluntary non-profit - Private
Beds: 176

Key Personnel:
Radiology. . . . . Richard Bedont
Operating Room. . . . . Thomas Foley
CEO/President. . . . . John Hughes, FACHE
Chief of Medical Staff . . . . Gary Peasley
Quality Assurance . . . . Larae Schelling
Pediatric Ambulatory Care . . . . . . Chris Schill
Pediatric In-Patient Care . . . . Chris Schill
Emergency Room . . . . Donna Schuster

Measure	Cases	This Hosp.	State Avg.	U.S. Avg.
Blood Clot Prevention and Treatment				
Anticoagulation Overlap Therapy[2]	22	100%	94%	93%
ICU Venous Thromboembolism Prophylaxis[2]	120	82%	90%	92%
Incidence of Potentially Preventable VTE[1,2]	-	-	8%	10%
UFH with Dosages/Platelet Monitoring[1,2]	-	-	99%	97%
Venous Thromboembolism Prophylaxis[2]	280	83%	87%	85%
Warfarin Therapy Discharge Instructions[2]	21	100%	77%	75%
Chest Pain/Possible Heart Attack Care				
Aspirin Given Within 24 Hours of Arrival[1]	-	-	97%	96%
Fibrinolytic Meds Within 30 Min. of Arrival[3,7]	-	-	49%	58%
Average Time to ECG (minutes)[1]	-	-	5	7
Average Time to Transfer (minutes)[3,7]	-	-	58	60
Children's Asthma Care				
Received Home Management Plan of Care	-	-	-	88%
Received Reliever Medication	-	-	-	100%
Received Systemic Corticosteroids	-	-	-	100%
Emergency Department				
Admittance Decision Time (minutes)[2]	416	58	58	98
Head CT Results Within 45 Min. of Arrival	13	54%	55%	57%
Patients Who Left ER Before Being Seen	19,529	3%	1%	2%
Time from ER Arrival to Admit. (minutes)[2]	426	195	202	274
Time from ER Arrival to Discharge (minutes)	310	113	108	134
Time in ER Before Being Evaluated (minutes)	377	30	21	26
Time to Pain Meds for Fractures (minutes)	100	48	46	57
Heart Attack Care				
Aspirin Given at Discharge	52	100%	100%	99%
Fibrinolytic Meds Within 30 Min. of Arrival[7]	-	-	-	54%
PCI Within 90 Minutes of Arrival	23	87%	94%	96%
Statin Prescribed at Discharge	50	100%	98%	98%
Heart Failure Care				
ACE Inhibitor or ARB for LVSD[1]	-	-	95%	97%
Discharge Instructions Given	24	83%	93%	94%
Evaluation of LVS Function	43	100%	97%	99%
Medicare Spending				
Medicare Spending per Patient (ratio)	-	0.84	0.91	0.98
Pneumonia Care				
Appropriate Initial Antibiotic Given	68	97%	93%	95%
Blood Culture Timing	96	100%	98%	98%
Pregnancy and Delivery Care				
Newborn Deliveries Scheduled Early	89	0%	4%	6%
Preventive Care				
Immunization for Influenza[2]	302	97%	91%	90%
Immunization for Pneumonia[2]	456	95%	90%	92%
Stroke Care				
Anticoagulation Therapy for Atrial Fibrillation[1]	-	-	95%	95%
Antithrombotic Therapy Timing	28	93%	98%	98%
Assessed for Rehabilitation	33	91%	97%	97%
Discharged on Antithrombotic Therapy	31	100%	99%	99%
Discharged on Statin Medication	21	100%	92%	94%
Thrombolytic Therapy Timing[7]	-	-	64%	66%
Venous Thromboembolism Prophylaxis	29	90%	93%	94%
Written Stroke Educational Materials Given	18	72%	82%	88%
Surgical Care Improvement Project				
Appropriate Beta Blocker Usage	35	100%	98%	98%
Appropriate VTP Within 24 Hours	94	100%	98%	98%
Controlled Postoperative Blood Glucose[7]	-	-	96%	97%
Perioperative Temperature Management	108	100%	100%	100%
Prophylactic Antibiotic Selection	76	100%	99%	99%
Prophylactic Antibiotic Selection (Outpatient)	44	100%	98%	98%
Prophylactic Antibiotic Stopped	73	97%	98%	98%
Prophylactic Antibiotic Timing	76	100%	98%	99%
Prophylactic Antibiotic Timing (Outpatient)	44	100%	98%	98%
Urinary Catheter Removal	28	96%	97%	97%
Survey of Patients' Hospital Experiences				
Area Around Room 'Always' Quiet at Night	300+	59%	63%	61%
Doctors 'Always' Communicated Well	300+	78%	84%	82%
Home Recovery Information Given	300+	87%	88%	85%
Hospital Given 9 or 10 on 10 Point Scale	300+	67%	75%	71%
Meds 'Always' Explained Before Given	300+	62%	66%	64%
Nurses 'Always' Communicated Well	300+	78%	81%	79%
Pain 'Always' Well Controlled	300+	68%	71%	71%
Room and Bathroom 'Always' Clean	300+	76%	79%	73%
Timely Help 'Always' Received	300+	67%	70%	68%
Would Definitely Recommend Hospital	300+	60%	74%	71%
Use of Medical Imaging				
Cardiac Imaging Stress Test before Surgery	57	1.8%	4.8%	5.3%
Combination Abdominal CT Scan	224	2.2%	11.5%	10.5%
Combination Brain/Sinus CT Scan[1]	-	-	1.8%	2.7%
Combination Chest CT Scan	117	0.0%	3.5%	2.7%
Follow-up Mammogram/Ultrasound	818	17.7%	7.9%	8.8%
Lumbar Spine MRI for Low Back Pain[1]	-	-	32.2%	37.2%

Mercy Medical Center - North Iowa

1000 Fourth Street Sw
Mason City, IA 50401
Phone: 641-428-7000
Fax: 641-422-7827
URL: www.mercynorthiowa.com
Type: Acute Care Hospitals
Emergency Services: Yes
Ownership: Voluntary non-profit - Church
Beds: 346

Key Personnel:
CEO/President. . . . . James G Fitzpatrick
Emergency Room . . . . Paul Leavens
Chief of Medical Staff . . . . Ron Moeller, MD

Measure	Cases	This Hosp.	State Avg.	U.S. Avg.
Blood Clot Prevention and Treatment				
Anticoagulation Overlap Therapy[2]	84	99%	94%	93%
ICU Venous Thromboembolism Prophylaxis[2]	81	95%	90%	92%
Incidence of Potentially Preventable VTE[2]	13	0%	8%	10%
UFH with Dosages/Platelet Monitoring[2]	44	100%	99%	97%
Venous Thromboembolism Prophylaxis[2]	287	97%	87%	85%
Warfarin Therapy Discharge Instructions[2]	59	81%	77%	75%
Chest Pain/Possible Heart Attack Care				
Aspirin Given Within 24 Hours of Arrival[1,3]	-	-	97%	96%
Fibrinolytic Meds Within 30 Min. of Arrival[3,7]	-	-	49%	58%
Average Time to ECG (minutes)[1,3]	-	-	5	7
Average Time to Transfer (minutes)[3,7]	-	-	58	60
Children's Asthma Care				
Received Home Management Plan of Care	-	-	-	88%
Received Reliever Medication	-	-	-	100%
Received Systemic Corticosteroids	-	-	-	100%
Emergency Department				
Admittance Decision Time (minutes)[2]	406	49	58	98
Head CT Results Within 45 Min. of Arrival[1]	-	-	55%	57%
Patients Who Left ER Before Being Seen	33,358	1%	1%	2%
Time from ER Arrival to Admit. (minutes)[2]	415	215	202	274
Time from ER Arrival to Discharge (minutes)	452	133	108	134
Time in ER Before Being Evaluated (minutes)	502	17	21	26
Time to Pain Meds for Fractures (minutes)	125	55	46	57
Heart Attack Care				
Aspirin Given at Discharge	240	99%	100%	99%
Fibrinolytic Meds Within 30 Min. of Arrival[1]	-	-	-	54%
PCI Within 90 Minutes of Arrival	16	88%	94%	96%
Statin Prescribed at Discharge	239	98%	98%	98%
Heart Failure Care				
ACE Inhibitor or ARB for LVSD	95	95%	95%	97%
Discharge Instructions Given	209	94%	93%	94%
Evaluation of LVS Function	317	100%	97%	99%
Medicare Spending				
Medicare Spending per Patient (ratio)	-	0.91	0.91	0.98
Pneumonia Care				
Appropriate Initial Antibiotic Given	123	96%	93%	95%
Blood Culture Timing	221	100%	98%	98%
Pregnancy and Delivery Care				
Newborn Deliveries Scheduled Early[2]	40	0%	4%	6%
Preventive Care				
Immunization for Influenza[2]	610	92%	91%	90%
Immunization for Pneumonia[2]	731	89%	90%	92%
Stroke Care				
Anticoagulation Therapy for Atrial Fibrillation	18	94%	95%	95%
Antithrombotic Therapy Timing	72	96%	98%	98%
Assessed for Rehabilitation	105	100%	97%	97%
Discharged on Antithrombotic Therapy	86	100%	99%	99%
Discharged on Statin Medication	62	100%	92%	94%
Thrombolytic Therapy Timing[1]	-	-	64%	66%
Venous Thromboembolism Prophylaxis	97	98%	93%	94%
Written Stroke Educational Materials Given	47	91%	82%	88%
Surgical Care Improvement Project				
Appropriate Beta Blocker Usage	361	98%	98%	98%
Appropriate VTP Within 24 Hours	816	99%	98%	98%
Controlled Postoperative Blood Glucose	106	96%	96%	97%
Perioperative Temperature Management	903	100%	100%	100%
Prophylactic Antibiotic Selection	713	99%	99%	99%
Prophylactic Antibiotic Selection (Outpatient)	997	98%	98%	98%
Prophylactic Antibiotic Stopped	687	99%	98%	98%
Prophylactic Antibiotic Timing	713	98%	98%	99%
Prophylactic Antibiotic Timing (Outpatient)	1,003	98%	98%	98%
Urinary Catheter Removal	209	90%	97%	97%
Survey of Patients' Hospital Experiences				
Area Around Room 'Always' Quiet at Night	300+	53%	63%	61%
Doctors 'Always' Communicated Well	300+	77%	84%	82%
Home Recovery Information Given	300+	90%	88%	85%
Hospital Given 9 or 10 on 10 Point Scale	300+	70%	75%	71%
Meds 'Always' Explained Before Given	300+	61%	66%	64%
Nurses 'Always' Communicated Well	300+	77%	81%	79%
Pain 'Always' Well Controlled	300+	67%	71%	71%
Room and Bathroom 'Always' Clean	300+	71%	79%	73%
Timely Help 'Always' Received	300+	65%	70%	68%
Would Definitely Recommend Hospital	300+	67%	74%	71%
Use of Medical Imaging				
Cardiac Imaging Stress Test before Surgery	928	5.4%	4.8%	5.3%
Combination Abdominal CT Scan	1,075	6.2%	11.5%	10.5%
Combination Brain/Sinus CT Scan	680	1.9%	1.8%	2.7%
Combination Chest CT Scan	1,138	0.8%	3.5%	2.7%
Follow-up Mammogram/Ultrasound	3,017	8.3%	7.9%	8.8%
Lumbar Spine MRI for Low Back Pain[1]	-	-	32.2%	37.2%

Alegent Health Community Memorial Hospital

631 N 8th St
Missouri Valley, IA 51555
Phone: 712-642-2784
Fax: 712-642-2760
URL: www.alegent.org
Type: Critical Access Hospitals
Emergency Services: Yes
Ownership: Voluntary non-profit - Private
Beds: 25

Key Personnel:
Radiology. . . . . Kimberly Apker
Patient Relations . . . . Marjorie Clark
Quality Assurance . . . . Anne Hansen, RN
Chief of Medical Staff . . . . Jeffrey Jacobs, MD
President. . . . . Colleen Kannaday
Infection Control. . . . . Sue Peschel, RN
Emergency Room . . . . Joseph T Piccolo, MD
Anesthesiology. . . . . Tom Rice, CRNA

Measure	Cases	This Hosp.	State Avg.	U.S. Avg.

NOTE: Hospital profiles are in alphabetical order by state, then city, then hospital within the city; Rankings exclude hospitals with less than 25 cases except for patient surveys which excludes hospitals with less than 100 cases; (a) 100-299 cases; (1) The number of cases/patients is too few to report; (2) Data submitted were based on a sample of cases/patients; (3) Results are based on a shorter time period than required; (4) Data suppressed by CMS for one or more quarters; (5) Results are not available for this reporting period; (6) Fewer than 100 patients completed the HCAHPS survey; (7) No cases met the criteria for this measure; (8) The lower limit of the confidence interval cannot be calculated if the number of observed infections equals zero; (9) No data are available from the state/territory for this reporting period; (10) The scores shown reflect fewer than 50 completed surveys; (11) There were discrepancies in the data collection process; (12) This measure does not apply to this hospital for this reporting period; (13) Results cannot be calculated for this reporting period; (14) The results for this state are combined with nearby states to protect confidentiality; Please refer to the User's Guide for a full explanation of data.

Measure	Cases	This Hosp.	State Avg.	U.S. Avg.
Blood Clot Prevention and Treatment				
Anticoagulation Overlap Therapy[1]	-	-	94%	93%
ICU Venous Thromboembolism Prophylaxis[7]	-	-	90%	92%
Incidence of Potentially Preventable VTE[7]	-	-	8%	10%
UFH with Dosages/Platelet Monitoring[7]	-	-	99%	97%
Venous Thromboembolism Prophylaxis	114	95%	87%	85%
Warfarin Therapy Discharge Instructions[1]	-	-	77%	75%
Chest Pain/Possible Heart Attack Care				
Aspirin Given Within 24 Hours of Arrival	-	-	97%	96%
Fibrinolytic Meds Within 30 Min. of Arrival	-	-	49%	58%
Average Time to ECG (minutes)	-	-	5	7
Average Time to Transfer (minutes)	-	-	58	60
Children's Asthma Care				
Received Home Management Plan of Care	-	-	-	88%
Received Reliever Medication	-	-	-	100%
Received Systemic Corticosteroids	-	-	-	100%
Emergency Department				
Admittance Decision Time (minutes)[5]	-	-	58	98
Head CT Results Within 45 Min. of Arrival	-	-	55%	57%
Patients Who Left ER Before Being Seen	-	-	1%	2%
Time from ER Arrival to Admit. (minutes)[5]	-	-	202	274
Time from ER Arrival to Discharge (minutes)	-	-	108	134
Time in ER Before Being Evaluated (minutes)	-	-	21	26
Time to Pain Meds for Fractures (minutes)	-	-	46	57
Heart Attack Care				
Aspirin Given at Discharge[1,3]	-	-	100%	99%
Fibrinolytic Meds Within 30 Min. of Arrival[3,7]	-	-	-	54%
PCI Within 90 Minutes of Arrival[3,7]	-	-	94%	96%
Statin Prescribed at Discharge[1,3]	-	-	98%	98%
Heart Failure Care				
ACE Inhibitor or ARB for LVSD[1]	-	-	95%	97%
Discharge Instructions Given[1]	-	-	93%	94%
Evaluation of LVS Function	16	100%	97%	99%
Medicare Spending				
Medicare Spending per Patient (ratio)	-	-	0.91	0.98
Pneumonia Care				
Appropriate Initial Antibiotic Given	22	100%	93%	95%
Blood Culture Timing	32	100%	98%	98%
Pregnancy and Delivery Care				
Newborn Deliveries Scheduled Early[5]	-	-	4%	6%
Preventive Care				
Immunization for Influenza[5]	-	-	91%	90%
Immunization for Pneumonia[5]	-	-	90%	92%
Stroke Care				
Anticoagulation Therapy for Atrial Fibrillation[5]	-	-	95%	95%
Antithrombotic Therapy Timing[5]	-	-	98%	98%
Assessed for Rehabilitation[5]	-	-	97%	97%
Discharged on Antithrombotic Therapy[5]	-	-	99%	99%
Discharged on Statin Medication[5]	-	-	92%	94%
Thrombolytic Therapy Timing[5]	-	-	64%	66%
Venous Thromboembolism Prophylaxis[5]	-	-	93%	94%
Written Stroke Educational Materials Given[5]	-	-	82%	88%
Surgical Care Improvement Project				
Appropriate Beta Blocker Usage[5]	-	-	98%	98%
Appropriate VTP Within 24 Hours[5]	-	-	98%	98%
Controlled Postoperative Blood Glucose[5]	-	-	96%	97%
Perioperative Temperature Management[5]	-	-	100%	100%
Prophylactic Antibiotic Selection[5]	-	-	99%	99%
Prophylactic Antibiotic Selection (Outpatient)	-	-	98%	98%
Prophylactic Antibiotic Stopped[5]	-	-	98%	98%
Prophylactic Antibiotic Timing[5]	-	-	98%	99%
Prophylactic Antibiotic Timing (Outpatient)	-	-	98%	98%
Urinary Catheter Removal[5]	-	-	97%	97%
Survey of Patients' Hospital Experiences				
Area Around Room 'Always' Quiet at Night[6]	<100	60%	63%	61%
Doctors 'Always' Communicated Well[6]	<100	85%	84%	82%
Home Recovery Information Given[6]	<100	93%	88%	85%
Hospital Given 9 or 10 on 10 Point Scale[6]	<100	83%	75%	71%
Meds 'Always' Explained Before Given[6]	<100	60%	66%	64%
Nurses 'Always' Communicated Well[6]	<100	82%	81%	79%
Pain 'Always' Well Controlled[6]	<100	67%	71%	71%
Room and Bathroom 'Always' Clean[6]	<100	78%	79%	73%
Timely Help 'Always' Received[6]	<100	75%	70%	68%
Would Definitely Recommend Hospital[6]	<100	75%	74%	71%
Use of Medical Imaging				
Cardiac Imaging Stress Test before Surgery	-	-	4.8%	5.3%
Combination Abdominal CT Scan	-	-	11.5%	10.5%
Combination Brain/Sinus CT Scan	-	-	1.8%	2.7%
Combination Chest CT Scan	-	-	3.5%	2.7%
Follow-up Mammogram/Ultrasound	-	-	7.9%	8.8%
Lumbar Spine MRI for Low Back Pain	-	-	32.2%	37.2%

Ringgold County Hospital

504 North Cleveland Street
Mount Ayr, IA 50854
Type: Critical Access Hospitals
Ownership: Government - Local
Phone: 641-464-3226
Fax: 641-464-4420
Emergency Services: Yes
Beds: 46

Key Personnel:
Chairman/CEO . . . . Kathi Braby
Ambulatory Care . . . . Joe Dukes
Chief of Medical Staff . . . . Dane Johnson, DO
Operating Room. . . . . Dane Johnson, RN
CEO/President . . . . Gordon W Winkler
Administrator . . . . Gordon W. Winkler

Measure	Cases	This Hosp.	State Avg.	U.S. Avg.
Blood Clot Prevention and Treatment				
Anticoagulation Overlap Therapy[5]	-	-	94%	93%
ICU Venous Thromboembolism Prophylaxis[5]	-	-	90%	92%
Incidence of Potentially Preventable VTE[5]	-	-	8%	10%
UFH with Dosages/Platelet Monitoring[5]	-	-	99%	97%
Venous Thromboembolism Prophylaxis[5]	-	-	87%	85%
Warfarin Therapy Discharge Instructions[5]	-	-	77%	75%
Chest Pain/Possible Heart Attack Care				
Aspirin Given Within 24 Hours of Arrival[5]	-	-	97%	96%
Fibrinolytic Meds Within 30 Min. of Arrival[5]	-	-	49%	58%
Average Time to ECG (minutes)[5]	-	-	5	7
Average Time to Transfer (minutes)[5]	-	-	58	60
Children's Asthma Care				
Received Home Management Plan of Care	-	-	-	88%
Received Reliever Medication	-	-	-	100%
Received Systemic Corticosteroids	-	-	-	100%
Emergency Department				
Admittance Decision Time (minutes)[5]	-	-	58	98
Head CT Results Within 45 Min. of Arrival[5]	-	-	55%	57%
Patients Who Left ER Before Being Seen[5]	-	-	1%	2%
Time from ER Arrival to Admit. (minutes)[5]	-	-	202	274
Time from ER Arrival to Discharge (minutes)[5]	-	-	108	134
Time in ER Before Being Evaluated (minutes)[5]	-	-	21	26
Time to Pain Meds for Fractures (minutes)[5]	-	-	46	57
Heart Attack Care				
Aspirin Given at Discharge[5]	-	-	100%	99%
Fibrinolytic Meds Within 30 Min. of Arrival[5]	-	-	-	54%
PCI Within 90 Minutes of Arrival[5]	-	-	94%	96%
Statin Prescribed at Discharge[5]	-	-	98%	98%
Heart Failure Care				
ACE Inhibitor or ARB for LVSD[1,3]	-	-	95%	97%
Discharge Instructions Given[1,3]	-	-	93%	94%
Evaluation of LVS Function[1,3]	-	-	97%	99%
Medicare Spending				
Medicare Spending per Patient (ratio)	-	-	0.91	0.98
Pneumonia Care				
Appropriate Initial Antibiotic Given[1,3]	-	-	93%	95%
Blood Culture Timing[1,3]	-	-	98%	98%
Pregnancy and Delivery Care				
Newborn Deliveries Scheduled Early[5]	-	-	4%	6%
Preventive Care				
Immunization for Influenza[5]	-	-	91%	90%
Immunization for Pneumonia[5]	-	-	90%	92%
Stroke Care				
Anticoagulation Therapy for Atrial Fibrillation[5]	-	-	95%	95%
Antithrombotic Therapy Timing[5]	-	-	98%	98%
Assessed for Rehabilitation[5]	-	-	97%	97%
Discharged on Antithrombotic Therapy[5]	-	-	99%	99%
Discharged on Statin Medication[5]	-	-	92%	94%
Thrombolytic Therapy Timing[5]	-	-	64%	66%
Venous Thromboembolism Prophylaxis[5]	-	-	93%	94%
Written Stroke Educational Materials Given[5]	-	-	82%	88%
Surgical Care Improvement Project				
Appropriate Beta Blocker Usage[5]	-	-	98%	98%
Appropriate VTP Within 24 Hours[5]	-	-	98%	98%
Controlled Postoperative Blood Glucose[5]	-	-	96%	97%
Perioperative Temperature Management[5]	-	-	100%	100%
Prophylactic Antibiotic Selection[5]	-	-	99%	99%
Prophylactic Antibiotic Selection (Outpatient)[5]	-	-	98%	98%
Prophylactic Antibiotic Stopped[5]	-	-	98%	98%
Prophylactic Antibiotic Timing[5]	-	-	98%	99%
Prophylactic Antibiotic Timing (Outpatient)[5]	-	-	98%	98%
Urinary Catheter Removal[5]	-	-	97%	97%
Survey of Patients' Hospital Experiences				
Area Around Room 'Always' Quiet at Night[6]	<100	67%	63%	61%
Doctors 'Always' Communicated Well[6]	<100	81%	84%	82%
Home Recovery Information Given[6]	<100	87%	88%	85%
Hospital Given 9 or 10 on 10 Point Scale[6]	<100	75%	75%	71%
Meds 'Always' Explained Before Given[6]	<100	68%	66%	64%
Nurses 'Always' Communicated Well[6]	<100	83%	81%	79%
Pain 'Always' Well Controlled[6]	<100	61%	71%	71%
Room and Bathroom 'Always' Clean[6]	<100	77%	79%	73%
Timely Help 'Always' Received[6]	<100	78%	70%	68%
Would Definitely Recommend Hospital[6]	<100	80%	74%	71%
Use of Medical Imaging				
Cardiac Imaging Stress Test before Surgery[1]	-	-	4.8%	5.3%
Combination Abdominal CT Scan	81	7.4%	11.5%	10.5%
Combination Brain/Sinus CT Scan[1]	-	-	1.8%	2.7%
Combination Chest CT Scan[1]	-	-	3.5%	2.7%
Follow-up Mammogram/Ultrasound	196	2.6%	7.9%	8.8%
Lumbar Spine MRI for Low Back Pain[1]	-	-	32.2%	37.2%

Henry County Health Center

407 S White St
Mount Pleasant, IA 52641
E-mail: miller@hchc.org
URL: www.hchc.org
Type: Critical Access Hospitals
Ownership: Government - Local
Phone: 319-385-3141
Fax: 319-385-6731
Emergency Services: Yes
Beds: 99

Key Personnel:
Chief of Medical Staff . . . . Cheryl Christensen
CEO/President. . . . . Rob Gardner
Operating Room. . . . . Becky Johnson, RN
Emergency Room . . . . Vicky Oge, RN
Quality Assurance . . . . Lois Roth, RN

Measure	Cases	This Hosp.	State Avg.	U.S. Avg.
Blood Clot Prevention and Treatment				
Anticoagulation Overlap Therapy[5]	-	-	94%	93%
ICU Venous Thromboembolism Prophylaxis[5]	-	-	90%	92%
Incidence of Potentially Preventable VTE[5]	-	-	8%	10%
UFH with Dosages/Platelet Monitoring[5]	-	-	99%	97%
Venous Thromboembolism Prophylaxis[5]	-	-	87%	85%
Warfarin Therapy Discharge Instructions[5]	-	-	77%	75%
Chest Pain/Possible Heart Attack Care				
Aspirin Given Within 24 Hours of Arrival[5]	-	-	97%	96%
Fibrinolytic Meds Within 30 Min. of Arrival[5]	-	-	49%	58%
Average Time to ECG (minutes)[5]	-	-	5	7
Average Time to Transfer (minutes)[5]	-	-	58	60
Children's Asthma Care				
Received Home Management Plan of Care	-	-	-	88%
Received Reliever Medication	-	-	-	100%
Received Systemic Corticosteroids	-	-	-	100%
Emergency Department				
Admittance Decision Time (minutes)[5]	-	-	58	98
Head CT Results Within 45 Min. of Arrival[5]	-	-	55%	57%
Patients Who Left ER Before Being Seen[5]	-	-	1%	2%
Time from ER Arrival to Admit. (minutes)[5]	-	-	202	274
Time from ER Arrival to Discharge (minutes)[5]	-	-	108	134
Time in ER Before Being Evaluated (minutes)[5]	-	-	21	26
Time to Pain Meds for Fractures (minutes)[5]	-	-	46	57
Heart Attack Care				
Aspirin Given at Discharge[1,3]	-	-	100%	99%
Fibrinolytic Meds Within 30 Min. of Arrival[3,7]	-	-	-	54%
PCI Within 90 Minutes of Arrival[3,7]	-	-	94%	96%
Statin Prescribed at Discharge[1,3]	-	-	98%	98%

NOTE: Hospital profiles are in alphabetical order by state, then city, then hospital within the city; Rankings exclude hospitals with less than 25 cases except for patient surveys which excludes hospitals with less than 100 cases; (a) 100-299 cases; (1) The number of cases/patients is too few to report; (2) Data submitted were based on a sample of cases/patients; (3) Results are based on a shorter time period than required; (4) Data suppressed by CMS for one or more quarters; (5) Results are not available for this reporting period; (6) Fewer than 100 patients completed the HCAHPS survey; (7) No cases met the criteria for this measure; (8) The lower limit of the confidence interval cannot be calculated if the number of observed infections equals zero; (9) No data are available from the state/territory for this reporting period; (10) The scores shown reflect fewer than 50 completed surveys; (11) There were discrepancies in the data collection process; (12) This measure does not apply to this hospital for this reporting period; (13) Results cannot be calculated for this reporting period; (14) The results for this state are combined with nearby states to protect confidentiality; Please refer to the User's Guide for a full explanation of data.

Measure	Cases	This Hosp.	State Avg.	U.S. Avg.
Heart Failure Care				
ACE Inhibitor or ARB for LVSD[1]	-	-	95%	97%
Discharge Instructions Given[1]	-	-	93%	94%
Evaluation of LVS Function	11	82%	97%	99%
Medicare Spending				
Medicare Spending per Patient (ratio)	-	-	0.91	0.98
Pneumonia Care				
Appropriate Initial Antibiotic Given	27	78%	93%	95%
Blood Culture Timing	33	94%	98%	98%
Pregnancy and Delivery Care				
Newborn Deliveries Scheduled Early[5]	-	-	4%	6%
Preventive Care				
Immunization for Influenza[5]	-	-	91%	90%
Immunization for Pneumonia[5]	-	-	90%	92%
Stroke Care				
Anticoagulation Therapy for Atrial Fibrillation[5]	-	-	95%	95%
Antithrombotic Therapy Timing[5]	-	-	98%	98%
Assessed for Rehabilitation[5]	-	-	97%	97%
Discharged on Antithrombotic Therapy[5]	-	-	99%	99%
Discharged on Statin Medication[5]	-	-	92%	94%
Thrombolytic Therapy Timing[5]	-	-	64%	66%
Venous Thromboembolism Prophylaxis[5]	-	-	93%	94%
Written Stroke Educational Materials Given[5]	-	-	82%	88%
Surgical Care Improvement Project				
Appropriate Beta Blocker Usage[5]	-	-	98%	98%
Appropriate VTP Within 24 Hours[5]	-	-	98%	98%
Controlled Postoperative Blood Glucose[5]	-	-	96%	97%
Perioperative Temperature Management[5]	-	-	100%	100%
Prophylactic Antibiotic Selection[5]	-	-	99%	99%
Prophylactic Antibiotic Selection (Outpatient)[5]	-	-	98%	98%
Prophylactic Antibiotic Stopped[5]	-	-	98%	98%
Prophylactic Antibiotic Timing[5]	-	-	98%	99%
Prophylactic Antibiotic Timing (Outpatient)[5]	-	-	98%	98%
Urinary Catheter Removal[5]	-	-	97%	97%
Survey of Patients' Hospital Experiences				
Area Around Room 'Always' Quiet at Night[6]	<100	72%	63%	61%
Doctors 'Always' Communicated Well[6]	<100	78%	84%	82%
Home Recovery Information Given[6]	<100	84%	88%	85%
Hospital Given 9 or 10 on 10 Point Scale[6]	<100	69%	75%	71%
Meds 'Always' Explained Before Given[6]	<100	64%	66%	64%
Nurses 'Always' Communicated Well[6]	<100	76%	81%	79%
Pain 'Always' Well Controlled[6]	<100	65%	71%	71%
Room and Bathroom 'Always' Clean[6]	<100	74%	79%	73%
Timely Help 'Always' Received[6]	<100	64%	70%	68%
Would Definitely Recommend Hospital[6]	<100	61%	74%	71%
Use of Medical Imaging				
Cardiac Imaging Stress Test before Surgery[1]	-	-	4.8%	5.3%
Combination Abdominal CT Scan	192	72.4%	11.5%	10.5%
Combination Brain/Sinus CT Scan	235	0.4%	1.8%	2.7%
Combination Chest CT Scan	77	9.1%	3.5%	2.7%
Follow-up Mammogram/Ultrasound	425	5.4%	7.9%	8.8%
Lumbar Spine MRI for Low Back Pain[1]	-	-	32.2%	37.2%

Trinity Muscatine

1518 Mulberry Avenue
Muscatine, IA 52761
Phone: 563-264-9100
Fax: 563-264-9463
E-mail: tvanwey@unityiowa.org
URL: www.unityiowa.com
Type: Acute Care Hospitals
Emergency Services: Yes
Ownership: Voluntary non-profit - Private
Beds: 80

Key Personnel:
Intensive Care Unit. . . . . Pam Askew, RN
Cardiology . . . . Mark G Berry
Patient Relations . . . . Zerita Hadden-Hudson
Cardiology . . . . David Hall, RN
Anesthesiology. . . . . M Sami Iqbal, DO
CEO/President. . . . . Vincent A Keane
Anesthesiology. . . . . Mark D Kline, RN
Hemotology Center . . . . Rajani Rangray

Measure	Cases	This Hosp.	State Avg.	U.S. Avg.
Blood Clot Prevention and Treatment				
Anticoagulation Overlap Therapy[2]	11	91%	94%	93%
ICU Venous Thromboembolism Prophylaxis[2]	30	100%	90%	92%
Incidence of Potentially Preventable VTE[1,2]	-	-	8%	10%
UFH with Dosages/Platelet Monitoring[2,7]	-	-	99%	97%
Venous Thromboembolism Prophylaxis[2]	137	100%	87%	85%
Warfarin Therapy Discharge Instructions[1,2]	-	-	77%	75%
Chest Pain/Possible Heart Attack Care				
Aspirin Given Within 24 Hours of Arrival	66	100%	97%	96%
Fibrinolytic Meds Within 30 Min. of Arrival[7]	-	-	49%	58%
Average Time to ECG (minutes)	66	4	5	7
Average Time to Transfer (minutes)	15	34	58	60
Children's Asthma Care				
Received Home Management Plan of Care	-	-	-	88%
Received Reliever Medication	-	-	-	100%
Received Systemic Corticosteroids	-	-	-	100%
Emergency Department				
Admittance Decision Time (minutes)[2]	325	93	58	98
Head CT Results Within 45 Min. of Arrival	13	23%	55%	57%
Patients Who Left ER Before Being Seen	15,565	1%	1%	2%
Time from ER Arrival to Admit. (minutes)[2]	337	232	202	274
Time from ER Arrival to Discharge (minutes)	322	118	108	134
Time in ER Before Being Evaluated (minutes)	442	17	21	26
Time to Pain Meds for Fractures (minutes)	72	36	46	57
Heart Attack Care				
Aspirin Given at Discharge[1]	-	-	100%	99%
Fibrinolytic Meds Within 30 Min. of Arrival[7]	-	-	-	54%
PCI Within 90 Minutes of Arrival[7]	-	-	94%	96%
Statin Prescribed at Discharge[1]	-	-	98%	98%
Heart Failure Care				
ACE Inhibitor or ARB for LVSD	12	100%	95%	97%
Discharge Instructions Given	25	100%	93%	94%
Evaluation of LVS Function	34	100%	97%	99%
Medicare Spending				
Medicare Spending per Patient (ratio)	-	0.96	0.91	0.98
Pneumonia Care				
Appropriate Initial Antibiotic Given	47	98%	93%	95%
Blood Culture Timing	77	97%	98%	98%
Pregnancy and Delivery Care				
Newborn Deliveries Scheduled Early	50	0%	4%	6%
Preventive Care				
Immunization for Influenza[2]	288	97%	91%	90%
Immunization for Pneumonia[2]	344	99%	90%	92%
Stroke Care				
Anticoagulation Therapy for Atrial Fibrillation[1]	-	-	95%	95%
Antithrombotic Therapy Timing[1]	-	-	98%	98%
Assessed for Rehabilitation[1]	-	-	97%	97%
Discharged on Antithrombotic Therapy[1]	-	-	99%	99%
Discharged on Statin Medication[1]	-	-	92%	94%
Thrombolytic Therapy Timing[7]	-	-	64%	66%
Venous Thromboembolism Prophylaxis[1]	-	-	93%	94%
Written Stroke Educational Materials Given[1]	-	-	82%	88%
Surgical Care Improvement Project				
Appropriate Beta Blocker Usage	27	96%	98%	98%
Appropriate VTP Within 24 Hours	66	100%	98%	98%
Controlled Postoperative Blood Glucose[7]	-	-	96%	97%
Perioperative Temperature Management	88	100%	100%	100%
Prophylactic Antibiotic Selection	45	100%	99%	99%
Prophylactic Antibiotic Selection (Outpatient)	36	100%	98%	98%
Prophylactic Antibiotic Stopped	37	89%	98%	98%
Prophylactic Antibiotic Timing	45	100%	98%	99%
Prophylactic Antibiotic Timing (Outpatient)	35	97%	98%	98%
Urinary Catheter Removal	41	100%	97%	97%
Survey of Patients' Hospital Experiences				
Area Around Room 'Always' Quiet at Night	300+	51%	63%	61%
Doctors 'Always' Communicated Well	300+	83%	84%	82%
Home Recovery Information Given	300+	85%	88%	85%
Hospital Given 9 or 10 on 10 Point Scale	300+	64%	75%	71%
Meds 'Always' Explained Before Given	300+	64%	66%	64%
Nurses 'Always' Communicated Well	300+	81%	81%	79%
Pain 'Always' Well Controlled	300+	74%	71%	71%
Room and Bathroom 'Always' Clean	300+	76%	79%	73%
Timely Help 'Always' Received	300+	74%	70%	68%
Would Definitely Recommend Hospital	300+	61%	74%	71%
Use of Medical Imaging				
Cardiac Imaging Stress Test before Surgery	188	6.4%	4.8%	5.3%
Combination Abdominal CT Scan	278	0.7%	11.5%	10.5%
Combination Brain/Sinus CT Scan[1]	-	-	1.8%	2.7%
Combination Chest CT Scan	110	0.0%	3.5%	2.7%
Follow-up Mammogram/Ultrasound	624	5.8%	7.9%	8.8%
Lumbar Spine MRI for Low Back Pain	55	29.1%	32.2%	37.2%

Story County Hospital

640 South 19th Street
Nevada, IA 50201
Phone: 515-382-2111
Fax: 515-382-6617
URL: www.scmcnevada.org
Type: Critical Access Hospitals
Emergency Services: Yes
Ownership: Government - Local
Beds: 122

Key Personnel:
Chairman/CEO . . . . Dave Anderson
Chief of Medical Staff. . . . . Alison Carleton
Operating Room. . . . . Marcia Engler
Quality Assurance . . . . Julie Schreitmueller
Emergency Room . . . . Lisa Whitaker
Radiology. . . . . Cindy White
CEO/President. . . . . Todd M Willert

Measure	Cases	This Hosp.	State Avg.	U.S. Avg.
Blood Clot Prevention and Treatment				
Anticoagulation Overlap Therapy[5]	-	-	94%	93%
ICU Venous Thromboembolism Prophylaxis[5]	-	-	90%	92%
Incidence of Potentially Preventable VTE[5]	-	-	8%	10%
UFH with Dosages/Platelet Monitoring[5]	-	-	99%	97%
Venous Thromboembolism Prophylaxis[5]	-	-	87%	85%
Warfarin Therapy Discharge Instructions[5]	-	-	77%	75%
Chest Pain/Possible Heart Attack Care				
Aspirin Given Within 24 Hours of Arrival	-	-	97%	96%
Fibrinolytic Meds Within 30 Min. of Arrival	-	-	49%	58%
Average Time to ECG (minutes)	-	-	5	7
Average Time to Transfer (minutes)	-	-	58	60
Children's Asthma Care				
Received Home Management Plan of Care	-	-	-	88%
Received Reliever Medication	-	-	-	100%
Received Systemic Corticosteroids	-	-	-	100%
Emergency Department				
Admittance Decision Time (minutes)[5]	-	-	58	98
Head CT Results Within 45 Min. of Arrival	-	-	55%	57%
Patients Who Left ER Before Being Seen	-	-	1%	2%
Time from ER Arrival to Admit. (minutes)[5]	-	-	202	274
Time from ER Arrival to Discharge (minutes)	-	-	108	134
Time in ER Before Being Evaluated (minutes)	-	-	21	26
Time to Pain Meds for Fractures (minutes)	-	-	46	57
Heart Attack Care				
Aspirin Given at Discharge[5]	-	-	100%	99%
Fibrinolytic Meds Within 30 Min. of Arrival[5]	-	-	-	54%
PCI Within 90 Minutes of Arrival[5]	-	-	94%	96%
Statin Prescribed at Discharge[5]	-	-	98%	98%
Heart Failure Care				
ACE Inhibitor or ARB for LVSD[1,3]	-	-	95%	97%
Discharge Instructions Given[1,3]	-	-	93%	94%
Evaluation of LVS Function[1,3]	-	-	97%	99%
Medicare Spending				
Medicare Spending per Patient (ratio)	-	-	0.91	0.98
Pneumonia Care				
Appropriate Initial Antibiotic Given[1,3]	-	-	93%	95%
Blood Culture Timing[1,3]	-	-	98%	98%
Pregnancy and Delivery Care				
Newborn Deliveries Scheduled Early[5]	-	-	4%	6%
Preventive Care				
Immunization for Influenza[5]	-	-	91%	90%
Immunization for Pneumonia[5]	-	-	90%	92%
Stroke Care				
Anticoagulation Therapy for Atrial Fibrillation[5]	-	-	95%	95%
Antithrombotic Therapy Timing[5]	-	-	98%	98%
Assessed for Rehabilitation[5]	-	-	97%	97%
Discharged on Antithrombotic Therapy[5]	-	-	99%	99%
Discharged on Statin Medication[5]	-	-	92%	94%
Thrombolytic Therapy Timing[5]	-	-	64%	66%
Venous Thromboembolism Prophylaxis[5]	-	-	93%	94%
Written Stroke Educational Materials Given[5]	-	-	82%	88%
Surgical Care Improvement Project				

NOTE: Hospital profiles are in alphabetical order by state, then city, then hospital within the city; Rankings exclude hospitals with less than 25 cases except for patient surveys which excludes hospitals with less than 100 cases; (a) 100-299 cases; (1) The number of cases/patients is too few to report; (2) Data submitted were based on a sample of cases/patients; (3) Results are based on a shorter time period than required; (4) Data suppressed by CMS for one or more quarters; (5) Results are not available for this reporting period; (6) Fewer than 100 patients completed the HCAHPS survey; (7) No cases met the criteria for this measure; (8) The lower limit of the confidence interval cannot be calculated if the number of observed infections equals zero; (9) No data are available from the state/territory for this reporting period; (10) The scores shown reflect fewer than 50 completed surveys; (11) There were discrepancies in the data collection process; (12) This measure does not apply to this hospital for this reporting period; (13) Results cannot be calculated for this reporting period; (14) The results for this state are combined with nearby states to protect confidentiality; Please refer to the User's Guide for a full explanation of data.

Measure	Cases	This Hosp.	State Avg.	U.S. Avg.
Appropriate Beta Blocker Usage[1,3]	-	-	98%	98%
Appropriate VTP Within 24 Hours[1,3]	-	-	98%	98%
Controlled Postoperative Blood Glucose[3,7]	-	-	96%	97%
Perioperative Temperature Management[3]	13	100%	100%	100%
Prophylactic Antibiotic Selection[3]	12	100%	99%	99%
Prophylactic Antibiotic Selection (Outpatient)	-	-	98%	98%
Prophylactic Antibiotic Stopped[3]	12	92%	98%	98%
Prophylactic Antibiotic Timing[3]	12	92%	98%	99%
Prophylactic Antibiotic Timing (Outpatient)	-	-	98%	98%
Urinary Catheter Removal[3,7]	-	-	97%	97%
Survey of Patients' Hospital Experiences				
Area Around Room 'Always' Quiet at Night[10]	<100	65%	63%	61%
Doctors 'Always' Communicated Well[10]	<100	89%	84%	82%
Home Recovery Information Given[10]	<100	89%	88%	85%
Hospital Given 9 or 10 on 10 Point Scale[10]	<100	78%	75%	71%
Meds 'Always' Explained Before Given[10]	<100	68%	66%	64%
Nurses 'Always' Communicated Well[10]	<100	80%	81%	79%
Pain 'Always' Well Controlled[10]	<100	64%	71%	71%
Room and Bathroom 'Always' Clean[10]	<100	78%	79%	73%
Timely Help 'Always' Received[10]	<100	63%	70%	68%
Would Definitely Recommend Hospital[10]	<100	84%	74%	71%
Use of Medical Imaging				
Cardiac Imaging Stress Test before Surgery	-	-	4.8%	5.3%
Combination Abdominal CT Scan	-	-	11.5%	10.5%
Combination Brain/Sinus CT Scan	-	-	1.8%	2.7%
Combination Chest CT Scan	-	-	3.5%	2.7%
Follow-up Mammogram/Ultrasound	-	-	7.9%	8.8%
Lumbar Spine MRI for Low Back Pain	-	-	32.2%	37.2%

Mercy Medical Center - New Hampton

308 North Maple Avenue
New Hampton, IA 50659
Phone: 641-394-4121
Fax: 641-394-2328
URL: www.mercynewhampton.com
Type: Critical Access Hospitals
Emergency Services: Yes
Ownership: Voluntary non-profit - Church
Beds: 18

Key Personnel:

Chief of Medical Staff . . . . Luke Brinkman, DO
Emergency Room . . . . Jessie Duman
Infection Control. . . . . Sharon Heiring, RN
Pulmonology . . . . Gary Levinson
CEO/President. . . . . Bruce Roesler

Measure	Cases	This Hosp.	State Avg.	U.S. Avg.
Blood Clot Prevention and Treatment				
Anticoagulation Overlap Therapy[5]	-	-	94%	93%
ICU Venous Thromboembolism Prophylaxis[5]	-	-	90%	92%
Incidence of Potentially Preventable VTE[5]	-	-	8%	10%
UFH with Dosages/Platelet Monitoring[5]	-	-	99%	97%
Venous Thromboembolism Prophylaxis[5]	-	-	87%	85%
Warfarin Therapy Discharge Instructions[5]	-	-	77%	75%
Chest Pain/Possible Heart Attack Care				
Aspirin Given Within 24 Hours of Arrival[5]	-	-	97%	96%
Fibrinolytic Meds Within 30 Min. of Arrival[5]	-	-	49%	58%
Average Time to ECG (minutes)[5]	-	-	5	7
Average Time to Transfer (minutes)[5]	-	-	58	60
Children's Asthma Care				
Received Home Management Plan of Care	-	-	-	88%
Received Reliever Medication	-	-	-	100%
Received Systemic Corticosteroids	-	-	-	100%
Emergency Department				
Admittance Decision Time (minutes)[5]	-	-	58	98
Head CT Results Within 45 Min. of Arrival[5]	-	-	55%	57%
Patients Who Left ER Before Being Seen[5]	-	-	1%	2%
Time from ER Arrival to Admit. (minutes)[5]	-	-	202	274
Time from ER Arrival to Discharge (minutes)[5]	-	-	108	134
Time in ER Before Being Evaluated (minutes)[5]	-	-	21	26
Time to Pain Meds for Fractures (minutes)[5]	-	-	46	57
Heart Attack Care				
Aspirin Given at Discharge[1,3]	-	-	100%	99%
Fibrinolytic Meds Within 30 Min. of Arrival[3,7]	-	-	-	54%
PCI Within 90 Minutes of Arrival[3,7]	-	-	94%	96%
Statin Prescribed at Discharge[1,3]	-	-	98%	98%
Heart Failure Care				
ACE Inhibitor or ARB for LVSD[1]	-	-	95%	97%
Discharge Instructions Given[1]	-	-	93%	94%
Evaluation of LVS Function[1]	-	-	97%	99%
Medicare Spending				
Medicare Spending per Patient (ratio)	-	-	0.91	0.98
Pneumonia Care				
Appropriate Initial Antibiotic Given[1]	-	-	93%	95%
Blood Culture Timing	14	100%	98%	98%
Pregnancy and Delivery Care				
Newborn Deliveries Scheduled Early[5]	-	-	4%	6%
Preventive Care				
Immunization for Influenza[5]	-	-	91%	90%
Immunization for Pneumonia[5]	-	-	90%	92%
Stroke Care				
Anticoagulation Therapy for Atrial Fibrillation[5]	-	-	95%	95%
Antithrombotic Therapy Timing[5]	-	-	98%	98%
Assessed for Rehabilitation[5]	-	-	97%	97%
Discharged on Antithrombotic Therapy[5]	-	-	99%	99%
Discharged on Statin Medication[5]	-	-	92%	94%
Thrombolytic Therapy Timing[5]	-	-	64%	66%
Venous Thromboembolism Prophylaxis[5]	-	-	93%	94%
Written Stroke Educational Materials Given[5]	-	-	82%	88%
Surgical Care Improvement Project				
Appropriate Beta Blocker Usage[5]	-	-	98%	98%
Appropriate VTP Within 24 Hours[5]	-	-	98%	98%
Controlled Postoperative Blood Glucose[5]	-	-	96%	97%
Perioperative Temperature Management[5]	-	-	100%	100%
Prophylactic Antibiotic Selection[5]	-	-	99%	99%
Prophylactic Antibiotic Selection (Outpatient)[5]	-	-	98%	98%
Prophylactic Antibiotic Stopped[5]	-	-	98%	98%
Prophylactic Antibiotic Timing[5]	-	-	98%	99%
Prophylactic Antibiotic Timing (Outpatient)[5]	-	-	98%	98%
Urinary Catheter Removal[5]	-	-	97%	97%
Survey of Patients' Hospital Experiences				
Area Around Room 'Always' Quiet at Night[5]	-	-	63%	61%
Doctors 'Always' Communicated Well[5]	-	-	84%	82%
Home Recovery Information Given[5]	-	-	88%	85%
Hospital Given 9 or 10 on 10 Point Scale[5]	-	-	75%	71%
Meds 'Always' Explained Before Given[5]	-	-	66%	64%
Nurses 'Always' Communicated Well[5]	-	-	81%	79%
Pain 'Always' Well Controlled[5]	-	-	71%	71%
Room and Bathroom 'Always' Clean[5]	-	-	79%	73%
Timely Help 'Always' Received[5]	-	-	70%	68%
Would Definitely Recommend Hospital[5]	-	-	74%	71%
Use of Medical Imaging				
Cardiac Imaging Stress Test before Surgery	46	4.3%	4.8%	5.3%
Combination Abdominal CT Scan	95	7.4%	11.5%	10.5%
Combination Brain/Sinus CT Scan[1]	-	-	1.8%	2.7%
Combination Chest CT Scan	69	1.4%	3.5%	2.7%
Follow-up Mammogram/Ultrasound	347	5.8%	7.9%	8.8%
Lumbar Spine MRI for Low Back Pain[1]	-	-	32.2%	37.2%

Skiff Medical Center

204 North 4th Avenue East
Newton, IA 50208
Phone: 641-792-1273
Fax: 641-792-4603
E-mail: info@skiffmed.com
URL: www.skiffmed.com
Type: Acute Care Hospitals
Emergency Services: Yes
Ownership: Government - Local
Beds: 68

Key Personnel:

CEO/President. . . . . Brett Altman
Quality Assurance . . . . Robert Campbell
Emergency Room . . . . Susan Carzoli, RN
Chief of Medical Staff . . . . Tammy Chance, DO
Infection Control. . . . . Lisa Guldberg, RN BSN
Radiology. . . . . Jane Hettinger
Operating Room. . . . . Ann Polking, RN
Patient Relations . . . . Steve Wilbur

Measure	Cases	This Hosp.	State Avg.	U.S. Avg.
Blood Clot Prevention and Treatment				
Anticoagulation Overlap Therapy[2]	13	92%	94%	93%
ICU Venous Thromboembolism Prophylaxis[2]	19	74%	90%	92%
Incidence of Potentially Preventable VTE[1,2]	-	-	8%	10%
UFH with Dosages/Platelet Monitoring[1,2]	-	-	99%	97%
Venous Thromboembolism Prophylaxis[2]	236	81%	87%	85%
Warfarin Therapy Discharge Instructions[2]	11	91%	77%	75%
Chest Pain/Possible Heart Attack Care				
Aspirin Given Within 24 Hours of Arrival	57	100%	97%	96%
Fibrinolytic Meds Within 30 Min. of Arrival[7]	-	-	49%	58%
Average Time to ECG (minutes)	58	5	5	7
Average Time to Transfer (minutes)[1]	-	-	58	60
Children's Asthma Care				
Received Home Management Plan of Care	-	-	-	88%
Received Reliever Medication	-	-	-	100%
Received Systemic Corticosteroids	-	-	-	100%
Emergency Department				
Admittance Decision Time (minutes)[2]	254	55	58	98
Head CT Results Within 45 Min. of Arrival[1]	-	-	55%	57%
Patients Who Left ER Before Being Seen	9,164	1%	1%	2%
Time from ER Arrival to Admit. (minutes)[2]	255	199	202	274
Time from ER Arrival to Discharge (minutes)	256	103	108	134
Time in ER Before Being Evaluated (minutes)	383	13	21	26
Time to Pain Meds for Fractures (minutes)	45	45	46	57
Heart Attack Care				
Aspirin Given at Discharge[1,3]	-	-	100%	99%
Fibrinolytic Meds Within 30 Min. of Arrival[3,7]	-	-	-	54%
PCI Within 90 Minutes of Arrival[3,7]	-	-	94%	96%
Statin Prescribed at Discharge[1,3]	-	-	98%	98%
Heart Failure Care				
ACE Inhibitor or ARB for LVSD[1,2]	-	-	95%	97%
Discharge Instructions Given[2]	24	79%	93%	94%
Evaluation of LVS Function[2]	41	90%	97%	99%
Medicare Spending				
Medicare Spending per Patient (ratio)	-	0.85	0.91	0.98
Pneumonia Care				
Appropriate Initial Antibiotic Given[2]	32	84%	93%	95%
Blood Culture Timing[2]	50	100%	98%	98%
Pregnancy and Delivery Care				
Newborn Deliveries Scheduled Early[1,2]	-	-	4%	6%
Preventive Care				
Immunization for Influenza[2]	293	96%	91%	90%
Immunization for Pneumonia[2]	379	98%	90%	92%
Stroke Care				
Anticoagulation Therapy for Atrial Fibrillation[1]	-	-	95%	95%
Antithrombotic Therapy Timing	14	93%	98%	98%
Assessed for Rehabilitation	17	100%	97%	97%
Discharged on Antithrombotic Therapy	16	94%	99%	99%
Discharged on Statin Medication	17	59%	92%	94%
Thrombolytic Therapy Timing[1]	-	-	64%	66%
Venous Thromboembolism Prophylaxis	16	81%	93%	94%
Written Stroke Educational Materials Given[1]	-	-	82%	88%
Surgical Care Improvement Project				
Appropriate Beta Blocker Usage[2]	36	100%	98%	98%
Appropriate VTP Within 24 Hours[2]	118	99%	98%	98%
Controlled Postoperative Blood Glucose[2,7]	-	-	96%	97%
Perioperative Temperature Management[2]	130	100%	100%	100%
Prophylactic Antibiotic Selection[2]	109	100%	99%	99%
Prophylactic Antibiotic Selection (Outpatient)	22	100%	98%	98%
Prophylactic Antibiotic Stopped[2]	108	100%	98%	98%
Prophylactic Antibiotic Timing[2]	109	99%	98%	99%
Prophylactic Antibiotic Timing (Outpatient)	22	100%	98%	98%
Urinary Catheter Removal[2]	23	87%	97%	97%
Survey of Patients' Hospital Experiences				
Area Around Room 'Always' Quiet at Night	300+	60%	63%	61%
Doctors 'Always' Communicated Well	300+	85%	84%	82%
Home Recovery Information Given	300+	87%	88%	85%
Hospital Given 9 or 10 on 10 Point Scale	300+	76%	75%	71%
Meds 'Always' Explained Before Given	300+	66%	66%	64%
Nurses 'Always' Communicated Well	300+	81%	81%	79%
Pain 'Always' Well Controlled	300+	68%	71%	71%
Room and Bathroom 'Always' Clean	300+	69%	79%	73%
Timely Help 'Always' Received	300+	70%	70%	68%
Would Definitely Recommend Hospital	300+	74%	74%	71%
Use of Medical Imaging				
Cardiac Imaging Stress Test before Surgery	116	0.9%	4.8%	5.3%
Combination Abdominal CT Scan	226	3.5%	11.5%	10.5%
Combination Brain/Sinus CT Scan	236	0.8%	1.8%	2.7%

NOTE: Hospital profiles are in alphabetical order by state, then city, then hospital within the city; Rankings exclude hospitals with less than 25 cases except for patient surveys which excludes hospitals with less than 100 cases; (a) 100-299 cases; (1) The number of cases/patients is too few to report; (2) Data submitted were based on a sample of cases/patients; (3) Results are based on a shorter time period than required; (4) Data suppressed by CMS for one or more quarters; (5) Results are not available for this reporting period; (6) Fewer than 100 patients completed the HCAHPS survey; (7) No cases met the criteria for this measure; (8) The lower limit of the confidence interval cannot be calculated if the number of observed infections equals zero; (9) No data are available from the state/territory for this reporting period; (10) The scores shown reflect fewer than 50 completed surveys; (11) There were discrepancies in the data collection process; (12) This measure does not apply to this hospital for this reporting period; (13) Results cannot be calculated for this reporting period; (14) The results for this state are combined with nearby states to protect confidentiality; Please refer to the User's Guide for a full explanation of data.

Measure	Cases	This Hosp.	State Avg.	U.S. Avg.
Combination Chest CT Scan	130	0.8%	3.5%	2.7%
Follow-up Mammogram/Ultrasound	685	6.3%	7.9%	8.8%
Lumbar Spine MRI for Low Back Pain	56	33.9%	32.2%	37.2%

Mercy Hospital of Franciscan Sisters - Oelwein

201 Eighth Avenue Se
Oelwein, IA 50662
Phone: 319-283-6000
Fax: 319-283-6004
URL: www.covhealth.com
Type: Critical Access Hospitals
Emergency Services: Yes
Ownership: Voluntary non-profit - Other
Beds: 64

Key Personnel:
Chief of Medical Staff. . . . . Michael Atherley
Quality Assurance . . . . DeAnne Fox, RN
CEO/President. . . . . Katherine Hintz
Operating Room. . . . . Anthony Leo, RN
Emergency Room . . . . Judy Malget, RN

Measure	Cases	This Hosp.	State Avg.	U.S. Avg.
Blood Clot Prevention and Treatment				
Anticoagulation Overlap Therapy[5]	-	-	94%	93%
ICU Venous Thromboembolism Prophylaxis[5]	-	-	90%	92%
Incidence of Potentially Preventable VTE[5]	-	-	8%	10%
UFH with Dosages/Platelet Monitoring[5]	-	-	99%	97%
Venous Thromboembolism Prophylaxis[5]	-	-	87%	85%
Warfarin Therapy Discharge Instructions[5]	-	-	77%	75%
Chest Pain/Possible Heart Attack Care				
Aspirin Given Within 24 Hours of Arrival[3]	14	93%	97%	96%
Fibrinolytic Meds Within 30 Min. of Arrival[3,7]	-	-	49%	58%
Average Time to ECG (minutes)[3]	16	5	5	7
Average Time to Transfer (minutes)[3,7]	-	-	58	60
Children's Asthma Care				
Received Home Management Plan of Care	-	-	-	88%
Received Reliever Medication	-	-	-	100%
Received Systemic Corticosteroids	-	-	-	100%
Emergency Department				
Admittance Decision Time (minutes)[5]	-	-	58	98
Head CT Results Within 45 Min. of Arrival[5]	-	-	55%	57%
Patients Who Left ER Before Being Seen	5,581	1%	1%	2%
Time from ER Arrival to Admit. (minutes)[5]	-	-	202	274
Time from ER Arrival to Discharge (minutes)[5]	-	-	108	134
Time in ER Before Being Evaluated (minutes)[5]	-	-	21	26
Time to Pain Meds for Fractures (minutes)[5]	-	-	46	57
Heart Attack Care				
Aspirin Given at Discharge[5]	-	-	100%	99%
Fibrinolytic Meds Within 30 Min. of Arrival[5]	-	-	-	54%
PCI Within 90 Minutes of Arrival[5]	-	-	94%	96%
Statin Prescribed at Discharge[5]	-	-	98%	98%
Heart Failure Care				
ACE Inhibitor or ARB for LVSD[7]	-	-	95%	97%
Discharge Instructions Given[1]	-	-	93%	94%
Evaluation of LVS Function[1]	-	-	97%	99%
Medicare Spending				
Medicare Spending per Patient (ratio)	-	-	0.91	0.98
Pneumonia Care				
Appropriate Initial Antibiotic Given[1]	-	-	93%	95%
Blood Culture Timing[1]	-	-	98%	98%
Pregnancy and Delivery Care				
Newborn Deliveries Scheduled Early[3,7]	-	-	4%	6%
Preventive Care				
Immunization for Influenza[5]	-	-	91%	90%
Immunization for Pneumonia[5]	-	-	90%	92%
Stroke Care				
Anticoagulation Therapy for Atrial Fibrillation[5]	-	-	95%	95%
Antithrombotic Therapy Timing[5]	-	-	98%	98%
Assessed for Rehabilitation[5]	-	-	97%	97%
Discharged on Antithrombotic Therapy[5]	-	-	99%	99%
Discharged on Statin Medication[5]	-	-	92%	94%
Thrombolytic Therapy Timing[5]	-	-	64%	66%
Venous Thromboembolism Prophylaxis[5]	-	-	93%	94%
Written Stroke Educational Materials Given[5]	-	-	82%	88%
Surgical Care Improvement Project				
Appropriate Beta Blocker Usage[5]	-	-	98%	98%
Appropriate VTP Within 24 Hours[5]	-	-	98%	98%
Controlled Postoperative Blood Glucose[5]	-	-	96%	97%
Perioperative Temperature Management[5]	-	-	100%	100%
Prophylactic Antibiotic Selection[5]	-	-	99%	99%
Prophylactic Antibiotic Selection (Outpatient)[5]	-	-	98%	98%
Prophylactic Antibiotic Stopped[5]	-	-	98%	98%
Prophylactic Antibiotic Timing[5]	-	-	98%	99%
Prophylactic Antibiotic Timing (Outpatient)[5]	-	-	98%	98%
Urinary Catheter Removal[5]	-	-	97%	97%
Survey of Patients' Hospital Experiences				
Area Around Room 'Always' Quiet at Night[10]	<100	61%	63%	61%
Doctors 'Always' Communicated Well[10]	<100	64%	84%	82%
Home Recovery Information Given[10]	<100	83%	88%	85%
Hospital Given 9 or 10 on 10 Point Scale[10]	<100	64%	75%	71%
Meds 'Always' Explained Before Given[10]	<100	72%	66%	64%
Nurses 'Always' Communicated Well[10]	<100	76%	81%	79%
Pain 'Always' Well Controlled[10]	<100	74%	71%	71%
Room and Bathroom 'Always' Clean[10]	<100	79%	79%	73%
Timely Help 'Always' Received[10]	<100	67%	70%	68%
Would Definitely Recommend Hospital[10]	<100	60%	74%	71%
Use of Medical Imaging				
Cardiac Imaging Stress Test before Surgery[7]	-	-	4.8%	5.3%
Combination Abdominal CT Scan	95	0.0%	11.5%	10.5%
Combination Brain/Sinus CT Scan[1]	-	-	1.8%	2.7%
Combination Chest CT Scan	51	0.0%	3.5%	2.7%
Follow-up Mammogram/Ultrasound	201	14.4%	7.9%	8.8%
Lumbar Spine MRI for Low Back Pain[1]	-	-	32.2%	37.2%

Burgess Health Center

1600 Diamond Street
Onawa, IA 51040
Phone: 712-423-2311
Fax: 712-423-3500
URL: www.burgesshc.org
Type: Critical Access Hospitals
Emergency Services: Yes
Ownership: Voluntary non-profit - Private
Beds: 48

Key Personnel:
Infection Control. . . . . Rose Bunstead, RN
Cardiology . . . . Alegent Creighton
Radiology. . . . . Robert Faulk
Emergency Room . . . . John L Garred, Jr, MD
Chief of Medical Staff. . . . . John L Garred Sr, Sr, MD
Pediatric In-Patient Care . . . . Anne Hansen
Quality Assurance . . . . Kim Leif

Measure	Cases	This Hosp.	State Avg.	U.S. Avg.
Blood Clot Prevention and Treatment				
Anticoagulation Overlap Therapy[5]	-	-	94%	93%
ICU Venous Thromboembolism Prophylaxis[5]	-	-	90%	92%
Incidence of Potentially Preventable VTE[5]	-	-	8%	10%
UFH with Dosages/Platelet Monitoring[5]	-	-	99%	97%
Venous Thromboembolism Prophylaxis[5]	-	-	87%	85%
Warfarin Therapy Discharge Instructions[5]	-	-	77%	75%
Chest Pain/Possible Heart Attack Care				
Aspirin Given Within 24 Hours of Arrival[5]	-	-	97%	96%
Fibrinolytic Meds Within 30 Min. of Arrival[5]	-	-	49%	58%
Average Time to ECG (minutes)[5]	-	-	5	7
Average Time to Transfer (minutes)[5]	-	-	58	60
Children's Asthma Care				
Received Home Management Plan of Care	-	-	-	88%
Received Reliever Medication	-	-	-	100%
Received Systemic Corticosteroids	-	-	-	100%
Emergency Department				
Admittance Decision Time (minutes)[5]	-	-	58	98
Head CT Results Within 45 Min. of Arrival[5]	-	-	55%	57%
Patients Who Left ER Before Being Seen[5]	-	-	1%	2%
Time from ER Arrival to Admit. (minutes)[5]	-	-	202	274
Time from ER Arrival to Discharge (minutes)[5]	-	-	108	134
Time in ER Before Being Evaluated (minutes)[5]	-	-	21	26
Time to Pain Meds for Fractures (minutes)[5]	-	-	46	57
Heart Attack Care				
Aspirin Given at Discharge[5]	-	-	100%	99%
Fibrinolytic Meds Within 30 Min. of Arrival[5]	-	-	-	54%
PCI Within 90 Minutes of Arrival[5]	-	-	94%	96%
Statin Prescribed at Discharge[5]	-	-	98%	98%
Heart Failure Care				
ACE Inhibitor or ARB for LVSD[5]	-	-	95%	97%
Discharge Instructions Given[5]	-	-	93%	94%
Evaluation of LVS Function[5]	-	-	97%	99%
Medicare Spending				
Medicare Spending per Patient (ratio)	-	-	0.91	0.98
Pneumonia Care				
Appropriate Initial Antibiotic Given[5]	-	-	93%	95%
Blood Culture Timing[5]	-	-	98%	98%
Pregnancy and Delivery Care				
Newborn Deliveries Scheduled Early[5]	-	-	4%	6%
Preventive Care				
Immunization for Influenza[5]	-	-	91%	90%
Immunization for Pneumonia[5]	-	-	90%	92%
Stroke Care				
Anticoagulation Therapy for Atrial Fibrillation[5]	-	-	95%	95%
Antithrombotic Therapy Timing[5]	-	-	98%	98%
Assessed for Rehabilitation[5]	-	-	97%	97%
Discharged on Antithrombotic Therapy[5]	-	-	99%	99%
Discharged on Statin Medication[5]	-	-	92%	94%
Thrombolytic Therapy Timing[5]	-	-	64%	66%
Venous Thromboembolism Prophylaxis[5]	-	-	93%	94%
Written Stroke Educational Materials Given[5]	-	-	82%	88%
Surgical Care Improvement Project				
Appropriate Beta Blocker Usage[5]	-	-	98%	98%
Appropriate VTP Within 24 Hours[5]	-	-	98%	98%
Controlled Postoperative Blood Glucose[5]	-	-	96%	97%
Perioperative Temperature Management[5]	-	-	100%	100%
Prophylactic Antibiotic Selection[5]	-	-	99%	99%
Prophylactic Antibiotic Selection (Outpatient)[5]	-	-	98%	98%
Prophylactic Antibiotic Stopped[5]	-	-	98%	98%
Prophylactic Antibiotic Timing[5]	-	-	98%	99%
Prophylactic Antibiotic Timing (Outpatient)[5]	-	-	98%	98%
Urinary Catheter Removal[5]	-	-	97%	97%
Survey of Patients' Hospital Experiences				
Area Around Room 'Always' Quiet at Night	(a)	61%	63%	61%
Doctors 'Always' Communicated Well	(a)	89%	84%	82%
Home Recovery Information Given	(a)	90%	88%	85%
Hospital Given 9 or 10 on 10 Point Scale	(a)	85%	75%	71%
Meds 'Always' Explained Before Given	(a)	67%	66%	64%
Nurses 'Always' Communicated Well	(a)	83%	81%	79%
Pain 'Always' Well Controlled	(a)	74%	71%	71%
Room and Bathroom 'Always' Clean	(a)	83%	79%	73%
Timely Help 'Always' Received	(a)	73%	70%	68%
Would Definitely Recommend Hospital	(a)	82%	74%	71%
Use of Medical Imaging				
Cardiac Imaging Stress Test before Surgery[7]	-	-	4.8%	5.3%
Combination Abdominal CT Scan	136	5.9%	11.5%	10.5%
Combination Brain/Sinus CT Scan[1]	-	-	1.8%	2.7%
Combination Chest CT Scan	63	6.3%	3.5%	2.7%
Follow-up Mammogram/Ultrasound	312	4.5%	7.9%	8.8%
Lumbar Spine MRI for Low Back Pain[1]	-	-	32.2%	37.2%

Orange City Area Health System

1000 Lincoln Circle Se
Orange City, IA 51041
Phone: 712-737-4984
Fax: 712-737-5252
URL: www.ochealthsystem.org
Type: Critical Access Hospitals
Emergency Services: Yes
Ownership: Voluntary non-profit - Other
Beds: 68

Key Personnel:
Infection Control. . . . . Val Droog
Quality Assurance . . . . Val Droog
CEO/President. . . . . Martin W Guthmiller
Patient Relations . . . . Melinda Kentfield
Operating Room. . . . . Steven C Locker
Emergency Room . . . . Amy Van Beck
Radiology. . . . . Nicholas de Vries
Chief of Medical Staff. . . . . John Weber, MD

Measure	Cases	This Hosp.	State Avg.	U.S. Avg.
Blood Clot Prevention and Treatment				
Anticoagulation Overlap Therapy[5]	-	-	94%	93%
ICU Venous Thromboembolism Prophylaxis[5]	-	-	90%	92%
Incidence of Potentially Preventable VTE[5]	-	-	8%	10%
UFH with Dosages/Platelet Monitoring[5]	-	-	99%	97%
Venous Thromboembolism Prophylaxis[5]	-	-	87%	85%
Warfarin Therapy Discharge Instructions[5]	-	-	77%	75%
Chest Pain/Possible Heart Attack Care				
Aspirin Given Within 24 Hours of Arrival[1,3]	-	-	97%	96%
Fibrinolytic Meds Within 30 Min. of Arrival[5]	-	-	49%	58%

NOTE: Hospital profiles are in alphabetical order by state, then city, then hospital within the city; Rankings exclude hospitals with less than 25 cases except for patient surveys which excludes hospitals with less than 100 cases; (a) 100-299 cases; (1) The number of cases/patients is too few to report; (2) Data submitted were based on a sample of cases/patients; (3) Results are based on a shorter time period than required; (4) Data suppressed by CMS for one or more quarters; (5) Results are not available for this reporting period; (6) Fewer than 100 patients completed the HCAHPS survey; (7) No cases met the criteria for this measure; (8) The lower limit of the confidence interval cannot be calculated if the number of observed infections equals zero; (9) No data are available from the state/territory for this reporting period; (10) The scores shown reflect fewer than 50 completed surveys; (11) There were discrepancies in the data collection process; (12) This measure does not apply to this hospital for this reporting period; (13) Results cannot be calculated for this reporting period; (14) The results for this state are combined with nearby states to protect confidentiality; Please refer to the User's Guide for a full explanation of data.

Measure	Cases	This Hosp.	State Avg.	U.S. Avg.
Average Time to ECG (minutes)[1,3]	-	-	5	7
Average Time to Transfer (minutes)[5]	-	-	58	60
Children's Asthma Care				
Received Home Management Plan of Care	-	-	-	88%
Received Reliever Medication	-	-	-	100%
Received Systemic Corticosteroids	-	-	-	100%
Emergency Department				
Admittance Decision Time (minutes)[3,7]	-	-	58	98
Head CT Results Within 45 Min. of Arrival[5]	-	-	55%	57%
Patients Who Left ER Before Being Seen[5]	-	-	1%	2%
Time from ER Arrival to Admit. (minutes)[3,7]	-	-	202	274
Time from ER Arrival to Discharge (minutes)[5]	-	-	108	134
Time in ER Before Being Evaluated (minutes)[5]	-	-	21	26
Time to Pain Meds for Fractures (minutes)[5]	-	-	46	57
Heart Attack Care				
Aspirin Given at Discharge[1,3]	-	-	100%	99%
Fibrinolytic Meds Within 30 Min. of Arrival[5]	-	-	-	54%
PCI Within 90 Minutes of Arrival[5]	-	-	94%	96%
Statin Prescribed at Discharge[1,3]	-	-	98%	98%
Heart Failure Care				
ACE Inhibitor or ARB for LVSD[1]	-	-	95%	97%
Discharge Instructions Given	12	100%	93%	94%
Evaluation of LVS Function	13	100%	97%	99%
Medicare Spending				
Medicare Spending per Patient (ratio)	-	-	0.91	0.98
Pneumonia Care				
Appropriate Initial Antibiotic Given[1]	-	-	93%	95%
Blood Culture Timing[1]	-	-	98%	98%
Pregnancy and Delivery Care				
Newborn Deliveries Scheduled Early[5]	-	-	4%	6%
Preventive Care				
Immunization for Influenza[5]	-	-	91%	90%
Immunization for Pneumonia[5]	-	-	90%	92%
Stroke Care				
Anticoagulation Therapy for Atrial Fibrillation[5]	-	-	95%	95%
Antithrombotic Therapy Timing[5]	-	-	98%	98%
Assessed for Rehabilitation[5]	-	-	97%	97%
Discharged on Antithrombotic Therapy[5]	-	-	99%	99%
Discharged on Statin Medication[5]	-	-	92%	94%
Thrombolytic Therapy Timing[5]	-	-	64%	66%
Venous Thromboembolism Prophylaxis[5]	-	-	93%	94%
Written Stroke Educational Materials Given[5]	-	-	82%	88%
Surgical Care Improvement Project				
Appropriate Beta Blocker Usage	13	100%	98%	98%
Appropriate VTP Within 24 Hours[3]	16	100%	98%	98%
Controlled Postoperative Blood Glucose[3,7]	-	-	96%	97%
Perioperative Temperature Management[3,7]	-	-	100%	100%
Prophylactic Antibiotic Selection	54	100%	99%	99%
Prophylactic Antibiotic Selection (Outpatient)[1,3]	-	-	98%	98%
Prophylactic Antibiotic Stopped	53	94%	98%	98%
Prophylactic Antibiotic Timing	54	100%	98%	99%
Prophylactic Antibiotic Timing (Outpatient)[1,3]	-	-	98%	98%
Urinary Catheter Removal[1,3]	-	-	97%	97%
Survey of Patients' Hospital Experiences				
Area Around Room 'Always' Quiet at Night	(a)	79%	63%	61%
Doctors 'Always' Communicated Well	(a)	91%	84%	82%
Home Recovery Information Given	(a)	87%	88%	85%
Hospital Given 9 or 10 on 10 Point Scale	(a)	92%	75%	71%
Meds 'Always' Explained Before Given	(a)	69%	66%	64%
Nurses 'Always' Communicated Well	(a)	88%	81%	79%
Pain 'Always' Well Controlled	(a)	77%	71%	71%
Room and Bathroom 'Always' Clean	(a)	89%	79%	73%
Timely Help 'Always' Received	(a)	80%	70%	68%
Would Definitely Recommend Hospital	(a)	92%	74%	71%
Use of Medical Imaging				
Cardiac Imaging Stress Test before Surgery	76	2.6%	4.8%	5.3%
Combination Abdominal CT Scan	128	14.1%	11.5%	10.5%
Combination Brain/Sinus CT Scan[1]	-	-	1.8%	2.7%
Combination Chest CT Scan[1]	-	-	3.5%	2.7%
Follow-up Mammogram/Ultrasound	431	8.4%	7.9%	8.8%
Lumbar Spine MRI for Low Back Pain[1]	-	-	32.2%	37.2%

Mitchell County Regional Health

616 North Eighth Street
Osage, IA 50461
Type: Critical Access Hospitals
Ownership: Voluntary non-profit - Other
Phone: 641-732-6000
Emergency Services: Yes

Measure	Cases	This Hosp.	State Avg.	U.S. Avg.
Blood Clot Prevention and Treatment				
Anticoagulation Overlap Therapy	-	-	94%	93%
ICU Venous Thromboembolism Prophylaxis	-	-	90%	92%
Incidence of Potentially Preventable VTE	-	-	8%	10%
UFH with Dosages/Platelet Monitoring	-	-	99%	97%
Venous Thromboembolism Prophylaxis	-	-	87%	85%
Warfarin Therapy Discharge Instructions	-	-	77%	75%
Chest Pain/Possible Heart Attack Care				
Aspirin Given Within 24 Hours of Arrival	11	100%	97%	96%
Fibrinolytic Meds Within 30 Min. of Arrival[1]	-	-	49%	58%
Average Time to ECG (minutes)	11	8	5	7
Average Time to Transfer (minutes)[1]	-	-	58	60
Children's Asthma Care				
Received Home Management Plan of Care	-	-	-	88%
Received Reliever Medication	-	-	-	100%
Received Systemic Corticosteroids	-	-	-	100%
Emergency Department				
Admittance Decision Time (minutes)	-	-	58	98
Head CT Results Within 45 Min. of Arrival[5]	-	-	55%	57%
Patients Who Left ER Before Being Seen[5]	-	-	1%	2%
Time from ER Arrival to Admit. (minutes)	-	-	202	274
Time from ER Arrival to Discharge (minutes)[5]	-	-	108	134
Time in ER Before Being Evaluated (minutes)[5]	-	-	21	26
Time to Pain Meds for Fractures (minutes)[5]	-	-	46	57
Heart Attack Care				
Aspirin Given at Discharge	-	-	100%	99%
Fibrinolytic Meds Within 30 Min. of Arrival	-	-	-	54%
PCI Within 90 Minutes of Arrival	-	-	94%	96%
Statin Prescribed at Discharge	-	-	98%	98%
Heart Failure Care				
ACE Inhibitor or ARB for LVSD	-	-	95%	97%
Discharge Instructions Given	-	-	93%	94%
Evaluation of LVS Function	-	-	97%	99%
Medicare Spending				
Medicare Spending per Patient (ratio)	-	-	0.91	0.98
Pneumonia Care				
Appropriate Initial Antibiotic Given	-	-	93%	95%
Blood Culture Timing	-	-	98%	98%
Pregnancy and Delivery Care				
Newborn Deliveries Scheduled Early	-	-	4%	6%
Preventive Care				
Immunization for Influenza	-	-	91%	90%
Immunization for Pneumonia	-	-	90%	92%
Stroke Care				
Anticoagulation Therapy for Atrial Fibrillation	-	-	95%	95%
Antithrombotic Therapy Timing	-	-	98%	98%
Assessed for Rehabilitation	-	-	97%	97%
Discharged on Antithrombotic Therapy	-	-	99%	99%
Discharged on Statin Medication	-	-	92%	94%
Thrombolytic Therapy Timing	-	-	64%	66%
Venous Thromboembolism Prophylaxis	-	-	93%	94%
Written Stroke Educational Materials Given	-	-	82%	88%
Surgical Care Improvement Project				
Appropriate Beta Blocker Usage	-	-	98%	98%
Appropriate VTP Within 24 Hours	-	-	98%	98%
Controlled Postoperative Blood Glucose	-	-	96%	97%
Perioperative Temperature Management	-	-	100%	100%
Prophylactic Antibiotic Selection	-	-	99%	99%
Prophylactic Antibiotic Selection (Outpatient)[5]	-	-	98%	98%
Prophylactic Antibiotic Stopped	-	-	98%	98%
Prophylactic Antibiotic Timing	-	-	98%	99%
Prophylactic Antibiotic Timing (Outpatient)[5]	-	-	98%	98%
Urinary Catheter Removal	-	-	97%	97%
Survey of Patients' Hospital Experiences				
Area Around Room 'Always' Quiet at Night	-	-	63%	61%
Doctors 'Always' Communicated Well	-	-	84%	82%
Home Recovery Information Given	-	-	88%	85%
Hospital Given 9 or 10 on 10 Point Scale	-	-	75%	71%
Meds 'Always' Explained Before Given	-	-	66%	64%
Nurses 'Always' Communicated Well	-	-	81%	79%
Pain 'Always' Well Controlled	-	-	71%	71%
Room and Bathroom 'Always' Clean	-	-	79%	73%
Timely Help 'Always' Received	-	-	70%	68%
Would Definitely Recommend Hospital	-	-	74%	71%
Use of Medical Imaging				
Cardiac Imaging Stress Test before Surgery	71	2.8%	4.8%	5.3%
Combination Abdominal CT Scan	130	4.6%	11.5%	10.5%
Combination Brain/Sinus CT Scan[1]	-	-	1.8%	2.7%
Combination Chest CT Scan	87	0.0%	3.5%	2.7%
Follow-up Mammogram/Ultrasound	342	7.0%	7.9%	8.8%
Lumbar Spine MRI for Low Back Pain[1]	-	-	32.2%	37.2%

Clarke County Hospital

800 S Fillmore St
Osceola, IA 50213
URL: www.clarkehosp.org
Type: Critical Access Hospitals
Ownership: Government - Local
Phone: 641-342-2184
Fax: 641-342-5378
Emergency Services: Yes
Beds: 55

Key Personnel:

Cardiac Laboratory. . . . . Peggie Dumber
CEO/President. . . . . Brian Evans
Radiology. . . . . Robert Filippone
Emergency Room . . . . Neline Halls
Chief of Medical Staff . . . . Vicki Irvin
Infection Control. . . . . Cindy Johnson
Quality Assurance . . . . Deb Lundquist

Measure	Cases	This Hosp.	State Avg.	U.S. Avg.
Blood Clot Prevention and Treatment				
Anticoagulation Overlap Therapy[5]	-	-	94%	93%
ICU Venous Thromboembolism Prophylaxis[5]	-	-	90%	92%
Incidence of Potentially Preventable VTE[5]	-	-	8%	10%
UFH with Dosages/Platelet Monitoring[5]	-	-	99%	97%
Venous Thromboembolism Prophylaxis[5]	-	-	87%	85%
Warfarin Therapy Discharge Instructions[5]	-	-	77%	75%
Chest Pain/Possible Heart Attack Care				
Aspirin Given Within 24 Hours of Arrival	-	-	97%	96%
Fibrinolytic Meds Within 30 Min. of Arrival	-	-	49%	58%
Average Time to ECG (minutes)	-	-	5	7
Average Time to Transfer (minutes)	-	-	58	60
Children's Asthma Care				
Received Home Management Plan of Care	-	-	-	88%
Received Reliever Medication	-	-	-	100%
Received Systemic Corticosteroids	-	-	-	100%
Emergency Department				
Admittance Decision Time (minutes)[5]	-	-	58	98
Head CT Results Within 45 Min. of Arrival	-	-	55%	57%
Patients Who Left ER Before Being Seen	-	-	1%	2%
Time from ER Arrival to Admit. (minutes)[5]	-	-	202	274
Time from ER Arrival to Discharge (minutes)	-	-	108	134
Time in ER Before Being Evaluated (minutes)	-	-	21	26
Time to Pain Meds for Fractures (minutes)	-	-	46	57
Heart Attack Care				
Aspirin Given at Discharge[5]	-	-	100%	99%
Fibrinolytic Meds Within 30 Min. of Arrival[5]	-	-	-	54%
PCI Within 90 Minutes of Arrival[5]	-	-	94%	96%
Statin Prescribed at Discharge[5]	-	-	98%	98%
Heart Failure Care				
ACE Inhibitor or ARB for LVSD[1]	-	-	95%	97%
Discharge Instructions Given[1]	-	-	93%	94%
Evaluation of LVS Function[1]	-	-	97%	99%
Medicare Spending				
Medicare Spending per Patient (ratio)	-	-	0.91	0.98
Pneumonia Care				
Appropriate Initial Antibiotic Given[1]	-	-	93%	95%
Blood Culture Timing	15	100%	98%	98%
Pregnancy and Delivery Care				
Newborn Deliveries Scheduled Early[5]	-	-	4%	6%
Preventive Care				
Immunization for Influenza[5]	-	-	91%	90%
Immunization for Pneumonia[5]	-	-	90%	92%

NOTE: Hospital profiles are in alphabetical order by state, then city, then hospital within the city; Rankings exclude hospitals with less than 25 cases except for patient surveys which excludes hospitals with less than 100 cases; (a) 100-299 cases; (1) The number of cases/patients is too few to report; (2) Data submitted were based on a sample of cases/patients; (3) Results are based on a shorter time period than required; (4) Data suppressed by CMS for one or more quarters; (5) Results are not available for this reporting period; (6) Fewer than 100 patients completed the HCAHPS survey; (7) No cases met the criteria for this measure; (8) The lower limit of the confidence interval cannot be calculated if the number of observed infections equals zero; (9) No data are available from the state/territory for this reporting period; (10) The scores shown reflect fewer than 50 completed surveys; (11) There were discrepancies in the data collection process; (12) This measure does not apply to this hospital for this reporting period; (13) Results cannot be calculated for this reporting period; (14) The results for this state are combined with nearby states to protect confidentiality; Please refer to the User's Guide for a full explanation of data.

Measure	Cases	This Hosp.	State Avg.	U.S. Avg.
Stroke Care				
Anticoagulation Therapy for Atrial Fibrillation[5]	-	-	95%	95%
Antithrombotic Therapy Timing[5]	-	-	98%	98%
Assessed for Rehabilitation[5]	-	-	97%	97%
Discharged on Antithrombotic Therapy[5]	-	-	99%	99%
Discharged on Statin Medication[5]	-	-	92%	94%
Thrombolytic Therapy Timing[5]	-	-	64%	66%
Venous Thromboembolism Prophylaxis[5]	-	-	93%	94%
Written Stroke Educational Materials Given[5]	-	-	82%	88%
Surgical Care Improvement Project				
Appropriate Beta Blocker Usage[5]	-	-	98%	98%
Appropriate VTP Within 24 Hours[5]	-	-	98%	98%
Controlled Postoperative Blood Glucose[5]	-	-	96%	97%
Perioperative Temperature Management[5]	-	-	100%	100%
Prophylactic Antibiotic Selection[5]	-	-	99%	99%
Prophylactic Antibiotic Selection (Outpatient)	-	-	98%	98%
Prophylactic Antibiotic Stopped[5]	-	-	98%	98%
Prophylactic Antibiotic Timing[5]	-	-	98%	99%
Prophylactic Antibiotic Timing (Outpatient)	-	-	98%	98%
Urinary Catheter Removal[5]	-	-	97%	97%
Survey of Patients' Hospital Experiences				
Area Around Room 'Always' Quiet at Night[6]	<100	86%	63%	61%
Doctors 'Always' Communicated Well[6]	<100	96%	84%	82%
Home Recovery Information Given[6]	<100	98%	88%	85%
Hospital Given 9 or 10 on 10 Point Scale[6]	<100	85%	75%	71%
Meds 'Always' Explained Before Given[6]	<100	85%	66%	64%
Nurses 'Always' Communicated Well[6]	<100	93%	81%	79%
Pain 'Always' Well Controlled[6]	<100	84%	71%	71%
Room and Bathroom 'Always' Clean[6]	<100	93%	79%	73%
Timely Help 'Always' Received[6]	<100	85%	70%	68%
Would Definitely Recommend Hospital[6]	<100	86%	74%	71%
Use of Medical Imaging				
Cardiac Imaging Stress Test before Surgery	-	-	4.8%	5.3%
Combination Abdominal CT Scan	-	-	11.5%	10.5%
Combination Brain/Sinus CT Scan	-	-	1.8%	2.7%
Combination Chest CT Scan	-	-	3.5%	2.7%
Follow-up Mammogram/Ultrasound	-	-	7.9%	8.8%
Lumbar Spine MRI for Low Back Pain	-	-	32.2%	37.2%

Mahaska Health Partnership

1229 C Avenue East
Oskaloosa, IA 52577
Phone: 641-672-3100
Fax: 641-672-3153
URL: www.mahaskahospital.com
Type: Critical Access Hospitals
Emergency Services: Yes
Ownership: Voluntary non-profit - Other
Beds: 69

Key Personnel:
Radiology. . . . . Akhtar Ashraf
Operating Room. . . . . Timothy Breon
Quality Assurance . . . . Steve Conner
Chief of Medical Staff. . . . . Shawn Dawson
Cardiac Laboratory. . . . . Faye Drosg
Infection Control. . . . . Julie Gibbons
Emergency Room . . . . Matt Whitis

Measure	Cases	This Hosp.	State Avg.	U.S. Avg.
Blood Clot Prevention and Treatment				
Anticoagulation Overlap Therapy[1,2]	-	-	94%	93%
ICU Venous Thromboembolism Prophylaxis[1,2]	-	-	90%	92%
Incidence of Potentially Preventable VTE[2,3]	-	-	8%	10%
UFH with Dosages/Platelet Monitoring[2,3]	-	-	99%	97%
Venous Thromboembolism Prophylaxis[2,3]	26	73%	87%	85%
Warfarin Therapy Discharge Instructions[1,2]	-	-	77%	75%
Chest Pain/Possible Heart Attack Care				
Aspirin Given Within 24 Hours of Arrival[3]	16	100%	97%	96%
Fibrinolytic Meds Within 30 Min. of Arrival[1,3]	-	-	49%	58%
Average Time to ECG (minutes)[3]	17	4	5	7
Average Time to Transfer (minutes)[1,3]	-	-	58	60
Children's Asthma Care				
Received Home Management Plan of Care	-	-	-	88%
Received Reliever Medication	-	-	-	100%
Received Systemic Corticosteroids	-	-	-	100%
Emergency Department				
Admittance Decision Time (minutes)[5]	-	-	58	98
Head CT Results Within 45 Min. of Arrival[1,3]	-	-	55%	57%
Patients Who Left ER Before Being Seen[5]	-	-	1%	2%
Time from ER Arrival to Admit. (minutes)[5]	-	-	202	274
Time from ER Arrival to Discharge (minutes)[3]	248	88	108	134
Time in ER Before Being Evaluated (minutes)[3]	282	23	21	26
Time to Pain Meds for Fractures (minutes)[3]	27	48	46	57
Heart Attack Care				
Aspirin Given at Discharge[5]	-	-	100%	99%
Fibrinolytic Meds Within 30 Min. of Arrival[5]	-	-	-	54%
PCI Within 90 Minutes of Arrival[5]	-	-	94%	96%
Statin Prescribed at Discharge[5]	-	-	98%	98%
Heart Failure Care				
ACE Inhibitor or ARB for LVSD[1,3]	-	-	95%	97%
Discharge Instructions Given[3]	12	100%	93%	94%
Evaluation of LVS Function[3]	17	100%	97%	99%
Medicare Spending				
Medicare Spending per Patient (ratio)	-	-	0.91	0.98
Pneumonia Care				
Appropriate Initial Antibiotic Given[3]	31	97%	93%	95%
Blood Culture Timing[3]	41	100%	98%	98%
Pregnancy and Delivery Care				
Newborn Deliveries Scheduled Early[5]	-	-	4%	6%
Preventive Care				
Immunization for Influenza[5]	-	-	91%	90%
Immunization for Pneumonia[5]	-	-	90%	92%
Stroke Care				
Anticoagulation Therapy for Atrial Fibrillation[5]	-	-	95%	95%
Antithrombotic Therapy Timing[5]	-	-	98%	98%
Assessed for Rehabilitation[5]	-	-	97%	97%
Discharged on Antithrombotic Therapy[5]	-	-	99%	99%
Discharged on Statin Medication[5]	-	-	92%	94%
Thrombolytic Therapy Timing[5]	-	-	64%	66%
Venous Thromboembolism Prophylaxis[5]	-	-	93%	94%
Written Stroke Educational Materials Given[5]	-	-	82%	88%
Surgical Care Improvement Project				
Appropriate Beta Blocker Usage	35	97%	98%	98%
Appropriate VTP Within 24 Hours	87	100%	98%	98%
Controlled Postoperative Blood Glucose[7]	-	-	96%	97%
Perioperative Temperature Management	96	100%	100%	100%
Prophylactic Antibiotic Selection	76	100%	99%	99%
Prophylactic Antibiotic Selection (Outpatient)[3]	29	100%	98%	98%
Prophylactic Antibiotic Stopped	73	96%	98%	98%
Prophylactic Antibiotic Timing	76	100%	98%	99%
Prophylactic Antibiotic Timing (Outpatient)[3]	29	100%	98%	98%
Urinary Catheter Removal	79	99%	97%	97%
Survey of Patients' Hospital Experiences				
Area Around Room 'Always' Quiet at Night	(a)	54%	63%	61%
Doctors 'Always' Communicated Well	(a)	90%	84%	82%
Home Recovery Information Given	(a)	85%	88%	85%
Hospital Given 9 or 10 on 10 Point Scale	(a)	68%	75%	71%
Meds 'Always' Explained Before Given	(a)	66%	66%	64%
Nurses 'Always' Communicated Well	(a)	81%	81%	79%
Pain 'Always' Well Controlled	(a)	68%	71%	71%
Room and Bathroom 'Always' Clean	(a)	73%	79%	73%
Timely Help 'Always' Received	(a)	66%	70%	68%
Would Definitely Recommend Hospital	(a)	68%	74%	71%
Use of Medical Imaging				
Cardiac Imaging Stress Test before Surgery[1]	-	-	4.8%	5.3%
Combination Abdominal CT Scan	212	57.1%	11.5%	10.5%
Combination Brain/Sinus CT Scan	267	0.7%	1.8%	2.7%
Combination Chest CT Scan	66	3.0%	3.5%	2.7%
Follow-up Mammogram/Ultrasound	525	2.1%	7.9%	8.8%
Lumbar Spine MRI for Low Back Pain[1]	-	-	32.2%	37.2%

Ottumwa Regional Health Center

1001 E Pennsylvania
Ottumwa, IA 52501
Phone: 641-682-7511
Fax: 641-684-3154
E-mail: webmaster@orhc.com
URL: www.orhc.com
Type: Acute Care Hospitals
Emergency Services: Yes
Ownership: Proprietary
Beds: 250

Key Personnel:
Operating Room. . . . . Brenda Jeffers
Radiology. . . . . Lynn Manning
Quality Assurance . . . . Curt Mecks
CEO/President. . . . . Tom Siemers
Infection Control. . . . . Paula Simplot
Chief of Medical Staff. . . . . Kenneth Wayne

Measure	Cases	This Hosp.	State Avg.	U.S. Avg.
Blood Clot Prevention and Treatment				
Anticoagulation Overlap Therapy[2]	29	93%	94%	93%
ICU Venous Thromboembolism Prophylaxis[2]	79	80%	90%	92%
Incidence of Potentially Preventable VTE[1,2]	-	-	8%	10%
UFH with Dosages/Platelet Monitoring[2]	16	100%	99%	97%
Venous Thromboembolism Prophylaxis[2]	178	71%	87%	85%
Warfarin Therapy Discharge Instructions[2]	18	72%	77%	75%
Chest Pain/Possible Heart Attack Care				
Aspirin Given Within 24 Hours of Arrival	52	96%	97%	96%
Fibrinolytic Meds Within 30 Min. of Arrival[1]	-	-	49%	58%
Average Time to ECG (minutes)	51	8	5	7
Average Time to Transfer (minutes)[1]	-	-	58	60
Children's Asthma Care				
Received Home Management Plan of Care	-	-	-	88%
Received Reliever Medication	-	-	-	100%
Received Systemic Corticosteroids	-	-	-	100%
Emergency Department				
Admittance Decision Time (minutes)[2]	347	94	58	98
Head CT Results Within 45 Min. of Arrival	15	80%	55%	57%
Patients Who Left ER Before Being Seen	22,953	1%	1%	2%
Time from ER Arrival to Admit. (minutes)[2]	363	280	202	274
Time from ER Arrival to Discharge (minutes)	338	138	108	134
Time in ER Before Being Evaluated (minutes)	379	25	21	26
Time to Pain Meds for Fractures (minutes)	70	45	46	57
Heart Attack Care				
Aspirin Given at Discharge	78	99%	100%	99%
Fibrinolytic Meds Within 30 Min. of Arrival[1]	-	-	-	54%
PCI Within 90 Minutes of Arrival[1]	-	-	94%	96%
Statin Prescribed at Discharge	68	93%	98%	98%
Heart Failure Care				
ACE Inhibitor or ARB for LVSD	30	93%	95%	97%
Discharge Instructions Given	91	64%	93%	94%
Evaluation of LVS Function	120	100%	97%	99%
Medicare Spending				
Medicare Spending per Patient (ratio)	-	0.91	0.91	0.98
Pneumonia Care				
Appropriate Initial Antibiotic Given	47	100%	93%	95%
Blood Culture Timing	66	95%	98%	98%
Pregnancy and Delivery Care				
Newborn Deliveries Scheduled Early	70	0%	4%	6%
Preventive Care				
Immunization for Influenza[2]	291	75%	91%	90%
Immunization for Pneumonia[2]	361	66%	90%	92%
Stroke Care				
Anticoagulation Therapy for Atrial Fibrillation[7]	-	-	95%	95%
Antithrombotic Therapy Timing[1]	-	-	98%	98%
Assessed for Rehabilitation[1]	-	-	97%	97%
Discharged on Antithrombotic Therapy[1]	-	-	99%	99%
Discharged on Statin Medication[1]	-	-	92%	94%
Thrombolytic Therapy Timing[7]	-	-	64%	66%
Venous Thromboembolism Prophylaxis[1]	-	-	93%	94%
Written Stroke Educational Materials Given[1]	-	-	82%	88%
Surgical Care Improvement Project				
Appropriate Beta Blocker Usage	64	89%	98%	98%
Appropriate VTP Within 24 Hours	145	97%	98%	98%
Controlled Postoperative Blood Glucose[7]	-	-	96%	97%
Perioperative Temperature Management	158	99%	100%	100%
Prophylactic Antibiotic Selection	118	100%	99%	99%
Prophylactic Antibiotic Selection (Outpatient)	149	98%	98%	98%
Prophylactic Antibiotic Stopped	113	93%	98%	98%
Prophylactic Antibiotic Timing	118	91%	98%	99%
Prophylactic Antibiotic Timing (Outpatient)	151	95%	98%	98%
Urinary Catheter Removal	78	96%	97%	97%
Survey of Patients' Hospital Experiences				
Area Around Room 'Always' Quiet at Night	300+	60%	63%	61%
Doctors 'Always' Communicated Well	300+	73%	84%	82%
Home Recovery Information Given	300+	78%	88%	85%
Hospital Given 9 or 10 on 10 Point Scale	300+	47%	75%	71%
Meds 'Always' Explained Before Given	300+	47%	66%	64%

NOTE: Hospital profiles are in alphabetical order by state, then city, then hospital within the city; Rankings exclude hospitals with less than 25 cases except for patient surveys which excludes hospitals with less than 100 cases; (a) 100-299 cases; (1) The number of cases/patients is too few to report; (2) Data submitted were based on a sample of cases/patients; (3) Results are based on a shorter time period than required; (4) Data suppressed by CMS for one or more quarters; (5) Results are not available for this reporting period; (6) Fewer than 100 patients completed the HCAHPS survey; (7) No cases met the criteria for this measure; (8) The lower limit of the confidence interval cannot be calculated if the number of observed infections equals zero; (9) No data are available from the state/territory for this reporting period; (10) The scores shown reflect fewer than 50 completed surveys; (11) There were discrepancies in the data collection process; (12) This measure does not apply to this hospital for this reporting period; (13) Results cannot be calculated for this reporting period; (14) The results for this state are combined with nearby states to protect confidentiality; Please refer to the User's Guide for a full explanation of data.

Nurses 'Always' Communicated Well	300+	67%	81%	79%
Pain 'Always' Well Controlled	300+	60%	71%	71%
Room and Bathroom 'Always' Clean	300+	72%	79%	73%
Timely Help 'Always' Received	300+	54%	70%	68%
Would Definitely Recommend Hospital	300+	40%	74%	71%
Use of Medical Imaging				
Cardiac Imaging Stress Test before Surgery	52	3.8%	4.8%	5.3%
Combination Abdominal CT Scan	379	43.3%	11.5%	10.5%
Combination Brain/Sinus CT Scan[1]	-	-	1.8%	2.7%
Combination Chest CT Scan	283	0.0%	3.5%	2.7%
Follow-up Mammogram/Ultrasound	1,021	2.5%	7.9%	8.8%
Lumbar Spine MRI for Low Back Pain	63	25.4%	32.2%	37.2%

Pella Regional Health Center

404 Jefferson Street
Pella, IA 50219
E-mail: info@pellahealth.org
URL: www.pellahealth.org
Phone: 641-628-3150
Fax: 641-628-8901
Type: Critical Access Hospitals
Ownership: Voluntary non-profit - Other
Emergency Services: Yes
Beds: 47

Key Personnel:
Quality Assurance . . . . Barb Braafhart
Chief of Medical Staff . . . . Jeffrey Hartung, MD
Radiology . . . . Lee Henry, DO
CEO/President . . . . Bob Kroese
Operating Room . . . . Matt Morgan, RN
Cardiac Laboratory . . . . Sherilyn Nickel
Infection Control . . . . Cheryl Thomson, RN

Measure	Cases	This Hosp.	State Avg.	U.S. Avg.
Blood Clot Prevention and Treatment				
Anticoagulation Overlap Therapy[1,2]	-	-	94%	93%
ICU Venous Thromboembolism Prophylaxis[1,2]	-	-	90%	92%
Incidence of Potentially Preventable VTE[1,2]	-	-	8%	10%
UFH with Dosages/Platelet Monitoring[1,2]	-	-	99%	97%
Venous Thromboembolism Prophylaxis[2,3]	32	59%	87%	85%
Warfarin Therapy Discharge Instructions[1,2]	-	-	77%	75%
Chest Pain/Possible Heart Attack Care				
Aspirin Given Within 24 Hours of Arrival	44	100%	97%	96%
Fibrinolytic Meds Within 30 Min. of Arrival[7]	-	-	49%	58%
Average Time to ECG (minutes)	47	3	5	7
Average Time to Transfer (minutes)[1]	-	-	58	60
Children's Asthma Care				
Received Home Management Plan of Care	-	-	-	88%
Received Reliever Medication	-	-	-	100%
Received Systemic Corticosteroids	-	-	-	100%
Emergency Department				
Admittance Decision Time (minutes)[2,3]	120	47	58	98
Head CT Results Within 45 Min. of Arrival[5]	-	-	55%	57%
Patients Who Left ER Before Being Seen[5]	-	-	1%	2%
Time from ER Arrival to Admit. (minutes)[2,3]	124	160	202	274
Time from ER Arrival to Discharge (minutes)[5]	-	-	108	134
Time in ER Before Being Evaluated (minutes)[5]	-	-	21	26
Time to Pain Meds for Fractures (minutes)[5]	-	-	46	57
Heart Attack Care				
Aspirin Given at Discharge[5]	-	-	100%	99%
Fibrinolytic Meds Within 30 Min. of Arrival[5]	-	-	-	54%
PCI Within 90 Minutes of Arrival[5]	-	-	94%	96%
Statin Prescribed at Discharge[5]	-	-	98%	98%
Heart Failure Care				
ACE Inhibitor or ARB for LVSD[1]	-	-	95%	97%
Discharge Instructions Given	20	95%	93%	94%
Evaluation of LVS Function	35	94%	97%	99%
Medicare Spending				
Medicare Spending per Patient (ratio)	-	-	0.91	0.98
Pneumonia Care				
Appropriate Initial Antibiotic Given	29	93%	93%	95%
Blood Culture Timing	44	95%	98%	98%
Pregnancy and Delivery Care				
Newborn Deliveries Scheduled Early[5]	-	-	4%	6%
Preventive Care				
Immunization for Influenza[2,3]	126	13%	91%	90%
Immunization for Pneumonia[2,3]	210	79%	90%	92%
Stroke Care				
Anticoagulation Therapy for Atrial Fibrillation[3,7]	-	-	95%	95%
Antithrombotic Therapy Timing[3,7]	-	-	98%	98%
Assessed for Rehabilitation[1,3]	-	-	97%	97%
Discharged on Antithrombotic Therapy[1,3]	-	-	99%	99%
Discharged on Statin Medication[3,7]	-	-	92%	94%
Thrombolytic Therapy Timing[3,7]	-	-	64%	66%
Venous Thromboembolism Prophylaxis[3,7]	-	-	93%	94%
Written Stroke Educational Materials Given[1,3]	-	-	82%	88%
Surgical Care Improvement Project				
Appropriate Beta Blocker Usage	23	87%	98%	98%
Appropriate VTP Within 24 Hours	76	96%	98%	98%
Controlled Postoperative Blood Glucose[3,7]	-	-	96%	97%
Perioperative Temperature Management	83	100%	100%	100%
Prophylactic Antibiotic Selection	47	98%	99%	99%
Prophylactic Antibiotic Selection (Outpatient)	117	97%	98%	98%
Prophylactic Antibiotic Stopped	46	100%	98%	98%
Prophylactic Antibiotic Timing	47	98%	98%	99%
Prophylactic Antibiotic Timing (Outpatient)	117	100%	98%	98%
Urinary Catheter Removal	39	95%	97%	97%
Survey of Patients' Hospital Experiences				
Area Around Room 'Always' Quiet at Night	300+	71%	63%	61%
Doctors 'Always' Communicated Well	300+	91%	84%	82%
Home Recovery Information Given	300+	91%	88%	85%
Hospital Given 9 or 10 on 10 Point Scale	300+	88%	75%	71%
Meds 'Always' Explained Before Given	300+	70%	66%	64%
Nurses 'Always' Communicated Well	300+	82%	81%	79%
Pain 'Always' Well Controlled	300+	74%	71%	71%
Room and Bathroom 'Always' Clean	300+	87%	79%	73%
Timely Help 'Always' Received	300+	75%	70%	68%
Would Definitely Recommend Hospital	300+	85%	74%	71%
Use of Medical Imaging				
Cardiac Imaging Stress Test before Surgery	143	4.9%	4.8%	5.3%
Combination Abdominal CT Scan	240	33.3%	11.5%	10.5%
Combination Brain/Sinus CT Scan[1]	-	-	1.8%	2.7%
Combination Chest CT Scan	124	0.0%	3.5%	2.7%
Follow-up Mammogram/Ultrasound	844	5.8%	7.9%	8.8%
Lumbar Spine MRI for Low Back Pain[1]	-	-	32.2%	37.2%

Dallas County Hospital

610 Tenth Street
Perry, IA 50220
URL: www.dallascohospital.org
Phone: 515-465-3547
Fax: 515-465-2922
Type: Critical Access Hospitals
Ownership: Voluntary non-profit - Other
Emergency Services: Yes
Beds: 25

Key Personnel:
Emergency Room . . . . Katie Heldt, RN
Operating Room . . . . Katie Heldt, RN
Infection Control . . . . Candace Jackson
Quality Assurance . . . . Candace Jackson
Chief of Medical Staff . . . . Steven C Johnson, MD
CEO . . . . Matt Wille

Measure	Cases	This Hosp.	State Avg.	U.S. Avg.
Blood Clot Prevention and Treatment				
Anticoagulation Overlap Therapy[1,2]	-	-	94%	93%
ICU Venous Thromboembolism Prophylaxis[2,7]	-	-	90%	92%
Incidence of Potentially Preventable VTE[2,7]	-	-	8%	10%
UFH with Dosages/Platelet Monitoring[1,2]	-	-	99%	97%
Venous Thromboembolism Prophylaxis[2]	103	50%	87%	85%
Warfarin Therapy Discharge Instructions[1,2]	-	-	77%	75%
Chest Pain/Possible Heart Attack Care				
Aspirin Given Within 24 Hours of Arrival[3]	14	100%	97%	96%
Fibrinolytic Meds Within 30 Min. of Arrival[3,7]	-	-	49%	58%
Average Time to ECG (minutes)[3]	14	4	5	7
Average Time to Transfer (minutes)[1,3]	-	-	58	60
Children's Asthma Care				
Received Home Management Plan of Care	-	-	-	88%
Received Reliever Medication	-	-	-	100%
Received Systemic Corticosteroids	-	-	-	100%
Emergency Department				
Admittance Decision Time (minutes)[2]	85	40	58	98
Head CT Results Within 45 Min. of Arrival[1,3]	-	-	55%	57%
Patients Who Left ER Before Being Seen	4,886	0%	1%	2%
Time from ER Arrival to Admit. (minutes)[2]	110	154	202	274
Time from ER Arrival to Discharge (minutes)[3]	956	76	108	134
Time in ER Before Being Evaluated (minutes)[3]	1,026	21	21	26
Time to Pain Meds for Fractures (minutes)[3]	19	28	46	57
Heart Attack Care				
Aspirin Given at Discharge[1,3]	-	-	100%	99%
Fibrinolytic Meds Within 30 Min. of Arrival[3,7]	-	-	-	54%
PCI Within 90 Minutes of Arrival[3,7]	-	-	94%	96%
Statin Prescribed at Discharge[1,3]	-	-	98%	98%
Heart Failure Care				
ACE Inhibitor or ARB for LVSD[1]	-	-	95%	97%
Discharge Instructions Given[1]	-	-	93%	94%
Evaluation of LVS Function[1]	-	-	97%	99%
Medicare Spending				
Medicare Spending per Patient (ratio)	-	-	0.91	0.98
Pneumonia Care				
Appropriate Initial Antibiotic Given	12	92%	93%	95%
Blood Culture Timing	22	100%	98%	98%
Pregnancy and Delivery Care				
Newborn Deliveries Scheduled Early[3,7]	-	-	4%	6%
Preventive Care				
Immunization for Influenza[2]	59	75%	91%	90%
Immunization for Pneumonia[2]	121	64%	90%	92%
Stroke Care				
Anticoagulation Therapy for Atrial Fibrillation[3,7]	-	-	95%	95%
Antithrombotic Therapy Timing[1,3]	-	-	98%	98%
Assessed for Rehabilitation[1,3]	-	-	97%	97%
Discharged on Antithrombotic Therapy[1,3]	-	-	99%	99%
Discharged on Statin Medication[1,3]	-	-	92%	94%
Thrombolytic Therapy Timing[1,3]	-	-	64%	66%
Venous Thromboembolism Prophylaxis[1,3]	-	-	93%	94%
Written Stroke Educational Materials Given[1,3]	-	-	82%	88%
Surgical Care Improvement Project				
Appropriate Beta Blocker Usage[5]	-	-	98%	98%
Appropriate VTP Within 24 Hours[5]	-	-	98%	98%
Controlled Postoperative Blood Glucose[5]	-	-	96%	97%
Perioperative Temperature Management[5]	-	-	100%	100%
Prophylactic Antibiotic Selection[5]	-	-	99%	99%
Prophylactic Antibiotic Selection (Outpatient)[5]	-	-	98%	98%
Prophylactic Antibiotic Stopped[5]	-	-	98%	98%
Prophylactic Antibiotic Timing[5]	-	-	98%	99%
Prophylactic Antibiotic Timing (Outpatient)[5]	-	-	98%	98%
Urinary Catheter Removal[5]	-	-	97%	97%
Survey of Patients' Hospital Experiences				
Area Around Room 'Always' Quiet at Night[6]	<100	68%	63%	61%
Doctors 'Always' Communicated Well[6]	<100	84%	84%	82%
Home Recovery Information Given[6]	<100	87%	88%	85%
Hospital Given 9 or 10 on 10 Point Scale[6]	<100	84%	75%	71%
Meds 'Always' Explained Before Given[6]	<100	67%	66%	64%
Nurses 'Always' Communicated Well[6]	<100	89%	81%	79%
Pain 'Always' Well Controlled[6]	<100	74%	71%	71%
Room and Bathroom 'Always' Clean[6]	<100	88%	79%	73%
Timely Help 'Always' Received[6]	<100	80%	70%	68%
Would Definitely Recommend Hospital[6]	<100	72%	74%	71%
Use of Medical Imaging				
Cardiac Imaging Stress Test before Surgery[7]	-	-	4.8%	5.3%
Combination Abdominal CT Scan	85	1.2%	11.5%	10.5%
Combination Brain/Sinus CT Scan[1]	-	-	1.8%	2.7%
Combination Chest CT Scan[1]	-	-	3.5%	2.7%
Follow-up Mammogram/Ultrasound	181	6.1%	7.9%	8.8%
Lumbar Spine MRI for Low Back Pain[1]	-	-	32.2%	37.2%

Pocahontas Community Hospital

606 N W 7th Street
Pocahontas, IA 50574
Phone: 712-335-3501
Type: Critical Access Hospitals
Ownership: Government - Local
Emergency Services: Yes

Measure	Cases	This Hosp.	State Avg.	U.S. Avg.
Blood Clot Prevention and Treatment				
Anticoagulation Overlap Therapy	-	-	94%	93%
ICU Venous Thromboembolism Prophylaxis	-	-	90%	92%
Incidence of Potentially Preventable VTE	-	-	8%	10%
UFH with Dosages/Platelet Monitoring	-	-	99%	97%
Venous Thromboembolism Prophylaxis	-	-	87%	85%
Warfarin Therapy Discharge Instructions	-	-	77%	75%

NOTE: Hospital profiles are in alphabetical order by state, then city, then hospital within the city; Rankings exclude hospitals with less than 25 cases except for patient surveys which excludes hospitals with less than 100 cases; (a) 100-299 cases; (1) The number of cases/patients is too few to report; (2) Data submitted were based on a sample of cases/patients; (3) Results are based on a shorter time period than required; (4) Data suppressed by CMS for one or more quarters; (5) Results are not available for this reporting period; (6) Fewer than 100 patients completed the HCAHPS survey; (7) No cases met the criteria for this measure; (8) The lower limit of the confidence interval cannot be calculated if the number of observed infections equals zero; (9) No data are available from the state/territory for this reporting period; (10) The scores shown reflect fewer than 50 completed surveys; (11) There were discrepancies in the data collection process; (12) This measure does not apply to this hospital for this reporting period; (13) Results cannot be calculated for this reporting period; (14) The results for this state are combined with nearby states to protect confidentiality; Please refer to the User's Guide for a full explanation of data.

Chest Pain/Possible Heart Attack Care				
Aspirin Given Within 24 Hours of Arrival[5]	-	-	97%	96%
Fibrinolytic Meds Within 30 Min. of Arrival[5]	-	-	49%	58%
Average Time to ECG (minutes)[5]	-	-	5	7
Average Time to Transfer (minutes)[5]	-	-	58	60
Children's Asthma Care				
Received Home Management Plan of Care	-	-	-	88%
Received Reliever Medication	-	-	-	100%
Received Systemic Corticosteroids	-	-	-	100%
Emergency Department				
Admittance Decision Time (minutes)	-	-	58	98
Head CT Results Within 45 Min. of Arrival[5]	-	-	55%	57%
Patients Who Left ER Before Being Seen[5]	-	-	1%	2%
Time from ER Arrival to Admit. (minutes)	-	-	202	274
Time from ER Arrival to Discharge (minutes)[5]	-	-	108	134
Time in ER Before Being Evaluated (minutes)[5]	-	-	21	26
Time to Pain Meds for Fractures (minutes)[5]	-	-	46	57
Heart Attack Care				
Aspirin Given at Discharge	-	-	100%	99%
Fibrinolytic Meds Within 30 Min. of Arrival	-	-	-	54%
PCI Within 90 Minutes of Arrival	-	-	94%	96%
Statin Prescribed at Discharge	-	-	98%	98%
Heart Failure Care				
ACE Inhibitor or ARB for LVSD	-	-	95%	97%
Discharge Instructions Given	-	-	93%	94%
Evaluation of LVS Function	-	-	97%	99%
Medicare Spending				
Medicare Spending per Patient (ratio)	-	-	0.91	0.98
Pneumonia Care				
Appropriate Initial Antibiotic Given	-	-	93%	95%
Blood Culture Timing	-	-	98%	98%
Pregnancy and Delivery Care				
Newborn Deliveries Scheduled Early	-	-	4%	6%
Preventive Care				
Immunization for Influenza	-	-	91%	90%
Immunization for Pneumonia	-	-	90%	92%
Stroke Care				
Anticoagulation Therapy for Atrial Fibrillation	-	-	95%	95%
Antithrombotic Therapy Timing	-	-	98%	98%
Assessed for Rehabilitation	-	-	97%	97%
Discharged on Antithrombotic Therapy	-	-	99%	99%
Discharged on Statin Medication	-	-	92%	94%
Thrombolytic Therapy Timing	-	-	64%	66%
Venous Thromboembolism Prophylaxis	-	-	93%	94%
Written Stroke Educational Materials Given	-	-	82%	88%
Surgical Care Improvement Project				
Appropriate Beta Blocker Usage	-	-	98%	98%
Appropriate VTP Within 24 Hours	-	-	98%	98%
Controlled Postoperative Blood Glucose	-	-	96%	97%
Perioperative Temperature Management	-	-	100%	100%
Prophylactic Antibiotic Selection	-	-	99%	99%
Prophylactic Antibiotic Selection (Outpatient)[5]	-	-	98%	98%
Prophylactic Antibiotic Stopped	-	-	98%	98%
Prophylactic Antibiotic Timing	-	-	98%	99%
Prophylactic Antibiotic Timing (Outpatient)[5]	-	-	98%	98%
Urinary Catheter Removal	-	-	97%	97%
Survey of Patients' Hospital Experiences				
Area Around Room 'Always' Quiet at Night	-	-	63%	61%
Doctors 'Always' Communicated Well	-	-	84%	82%
Home Recovery Information Given	-	-	88%	85%
Hospital Given 9 or 10 on 10 Point Scale	-	-	75%	71%
Meds 'Always' Explained Before Given	-	-	66%	64%
Nurses 'Always' Communicated Well	-	-	81%	79%
Pain 'Always' Well Controlled	-	-	71%	71%
Room and Bathroom 'Always' Clean	-	-	79%	73%
Timely Help 'Always' Received	-	-	70%	68%
Would Definitely Recommend Hospital	-	-	74%	71%
Use of Medical Imaging				
Cardiac Imaging Stress Test before Surgery[7]	-	-	4.8%	5.3%
Combination Abdominal CT Scan	67	44.8%	11.5%	10.5%
Combination Brain/Sinus CT Scan[1]	-	-	1.8%	2.7%
Combination Chest CT Scan	51	31.4%	3.5%	2.7%
Follow-up Mammogram/Ultrasound	133	7.5%	7.9%	8.8%
Lumbar Spine MRI for Low Back Pain[1]	-	-	32.2%	37.2%

Baum Harmon Mercy Hospital

255 N Welch Avenue
Primghar, IA 51245
URL: www.baumharmon.org
Type: Critical Access Hospitals
Ownership: Voluntary non-profit - Church
Phone: 712-957-2300
Fax: 712-757-0300
Emergency Services: Yes
Beds: 14

Key Personnel:
Emergency Room . . . . Linda Bindner
Operating Room. . . . . Linda Bindner
Chief of Medical Staff . . . . Shailosh Desai, MD
Radiology. . . . . Amy Halverson
Ambulatory Care . . . . Shirley Lenhart
Infection Control. . . . . Tracy Lenz
Quality Assurance . . . . Allyson Thomas
President . . . . Marty Webe

Measure	Cases	This Hosp.	State Avg.	U.S. Avg.
Blood Clot Prevention and Treatment				
Anticoagulation Overlap Therapy[5]	-	-	94%	93%
ICU Venous Thromboembolism Prophylaxis[5]	-	-	90%	92%
Incidence of Potentially Preventable VTE[5]	-	-	8%	10%
UFH with Dosages/Platelet Monitoring[5]	-	-	99%	97%
Venous Thromboembolism Prophylaxis[5]	-	-	87%	85%
Warfarin Therapy Discharge Instructions[5]	-	-	77%	75%
Chest Pain/Possible Heart Attack Care				
Aspirin Given Within 24 Hours of Arrival[5]	-	-	97%	96%
Fibrinolytic Meds Within 30 Min. of Arrival[5]	-	-	49%	58%
Average Time to ECG (minutes)[5]	-	-	5	7
Average Time to Transfer (minutes)[5]	-	-	58	60
Children's Asthma Care				
Received Home Management Plan of Care	-	-	-	88%
Received Reliever Medication	-	-	-	100%
Received Systemic Corticosteroids	-	-	-	100%
Emergency Department				
Admittance Decision Time (minutes)[5]	-	-	58	98
Head CT Results Within 45 Min. of Arrival[5]	-	-	55%	57%
Patients Who Left ER Before Being Seen[5]	-	-	1%	2%
Time from ER Arrival to Admit. (minutes)[5]	-	-	202	274
Time from ER Arrival to Discharge (minutes)[5]	-	-	108	134
Time in ER Before Being Evaluated (minutes)[5]	-	-	21	26
Time to Pain Meds for Fractures (minutes)[5]	-	-	46	57
Heart Attack Care				
Aspirin Given at Discharge[5]	-	-	100%	99%
Fibrinolytic Meds Within 30 Min. of Arrival[5]	-	-	-	54%
PCI Within 90 Minutes of Arrival[5]	-	-	94%	96%
Statin Prescribed at Discharge[5]	-	-	98%	98%
Heart Failure Care				
ACE Inhibitor or ARB for LVSD[5]	-	-	95%	97%
Discharge Instructions Given[5]	-	-	93%	94%
Evaluation of LVS Function[5]	-	-	97%	99%
Medicare Spending				
Medicare Spending per Patient (ratio)	-	-	0.91	0.98
Pneumonia Care				
Appropriate Initial Antibiotic Given[5]	-	-	93%	95%
Blood Culture Timing[5]	-	-	98%	98%
Pregnancy and Delivery Care				
Newborn Deliveries Scheduled Early[5]	-	-	4%	6%
Preventive Care				
Immunization for Influenza[5]	-	-	91%	90%
Immunization for Pneumonia[5]	-	-	90%	92%
Stroke Care				
Anticoagulation Therapy for Atrial Fibrillation[5]	-	-	95%	95%
Antithrombotic Therapy Timing[5]	-	-	98%	98%
Assessed for Rehabilitation[5]	-	-	97%	97%
Discharged on Antithrombotic Therapy[5]	-	-	99%	99%
Discharged on Statin Medication[5]	-	-	92%	94%
Thrombolytic Therapy Timing[5]	-	-	64%	66%
Venous Thromboembolism Prophylaxis[5]	-	-	93%	94%
Written Stroke Educational Materials Given[5]	-	-	82%	88%
Surgical Care Improvement Project				
Appropriate Beta Blocker Usage[5]	-	-	98%	98%
Appropriate VTP Within 24 Hours[5]	-	-	98%	98%
Controlled Postoperative Blood Glucose[5]	-	-	96%	97%
Perioperative Temperature Management[5]	-	-	100%	100%
Prophylactic Antibiotic Selection[5]	-	-	99%	99%
Prophylactic Antibiotic Selection (Outpatient)[5]	-	-	98%	98%
Prophylactic Antibiotic Stopped[5]	-	-	98%	98%
Prophylactic Antibiotic Timing[5]	-	-	98%	99%
Prophylactic Antibiotic Timing (Outpatient)[5]	-	-	98%	98%
Urinary Catheter Removal[5]	-	-	97%	97%
Survey of Patients' Hospital Experiences				
Area Around Room 'Always' Quiet at Night[5]	-	-	63%	61%
Doctors 'Always' Communicated Well[5]	-	-	84%	82%
Home Recovery Information Given[5]	-	-	88%	85%
Hospital Given 9 or 10 on 10 Point Scale[5]	-	-	75%	71%
Meds 'Always' Explained Before Given[5]	-	-	66%	64%
Nurses 'Always' Communicated Well[5]	-	-	81%	79%
Pain 'Always' Well Controlled[5]	-	-	71%	71%
Room and Bathroom 'Always' Clean[5]	-	-	79%	73%
Timely Help 'Always' Received[5]	-	-	70%	68%
Would Definitely Recommend Hospital[5]	-	-	74%	71%
Use of Medical Imaging				
Cardiac Imaging Stress Test before Surgery[7]	-	-	4.8%	5.3%
Combination Abdominal CT Scan[1]	-	-	11.5%	10.5%
Combination Brain/Sinus CT Scan	34	0.0%	1.8%	2.7%
Combination Chest CT Scan[1]	-	-	3.5%	2.7%
Follow-up Mammogram/Ultrasound	88	1.1%	7.9%	8.8%
Lumbar Spine MRI for Low Back Pain[1]	-	-	32.2%	37.2%

Montgomery County Memorial Hospital

2301 Eastern Avenue
Red Oak, IA 51566
URL: www.mcmh.org
Type: Critical Access Hospitals
Ownership: Government - Local
Phone: 712-623-7000
Fax: 712-623-7180
Emergency Services: Yes
Beds: 40

Key Personnel:
Chief of Medical Staff . . . . Edward Grass
Operating Room. . . . . Jane King
Quality Assurance . . . . Ron Kloewer
CEO . . . . Allen E Pohren
Radiology. . . . . Peggy Reed

Measure	Cases	This Hosp.	State Avg.	U.S. Avg.
Blood Clot Prevention and Treatment				
Anticoagulation Overlap Therapy[5]	-	-	94%	93%
ICU Venous Thromboembolism Prophylaxis[5]	-	-	90%	92%
Incidence of Potentially Preventable VTE[5]	-	-	8%	10%
UFH with Dosages/Platelet Monitoring[5]	-	-	99%	97%
Venous Thromboembolism Prophylaxis[5]	-	-	87%	85%
Warfarin Therapy Discharge Instructions[5]	-	-	77%	75%
Chest Pain/Possible Heart Attack Care				
Aspirin Given Within 24 Hours of Arrival[1,3]	-	-	97%	96%
Fibrinolytic Meds Within 30 Min. of Arrival[1,3]	-	-	49%	58%
Average Time to ECG (minutes)[3]	12	12	5	7
Average Time to Transfer (minutes)[1,3]	-	-	58	60
Children's Asthma Care				
Received Home Management Plan of Care	-	-	-	88%
Received Reliever Medication	-	-	-	100%
Received Systemic Corticosteroids	-	-	-	100%
Emergency Department				
Admittance Decision Time (minutes)[5]	-	-	58	98
Head CT Results Within 45 Min. of Arrival[1,3]	-	-	55%	57%
Patients Who Left ER Before Being Seen[5]	-	-	1%	2%
Time from ER Arrival to Admit. (minutes)[5]	-	-	202	274
Time from ER Arrival to Discharge (minutes)[5]	-	-	108	134
Time in ER Before Being Evaluated (minutes)[5]	-	-	21	26
Time to Pain Meds for Fractures (minutes)[5]	-	-	46	57
Heart Attack Care				
Aspirin Given at Discharge[1]	-	-	100%	99%
Fibrinolytic Meds Within 30 Min. of Arrival[7]	-	-	-	54%
PCI Within 90 Minutes of Arrival[7]	-	-	94%	96%
Statin Prescribed at Discharge[1]	-	-	98%	98%
Heart Failure Care				
ACE Inhibitor or ARB for LVSD[1]	-	-	95%	97%
Discharge Instructions Given	20	95%	93%	94%
Evaluation of LVS Function	35	91%	97%	99%

NOTE: Hospital profiles are in alphabetical order by state, then city, then hospital within the city; Rankings exclude hospitals with less than 25 cases except for patient surveys which excludes hospitals with less than 100 cases; (a) 100-299 cases; (1) The number of cases/patients is too few to report; (2) Data submitted were based on a sample of cases/patients; (3) Results are based on a shorter time period than required; (4) Data suppressed by CMS for one or more quarters; (5) Results are not available for this reporting period; (6) Fewer than 100 patients completed the HCAHPS survey; (7) No cases met the criteria for this measure; (8) The lower limit of the confidence interval cannot be calculated if the number of observed infections equals zero; (9) No data are available from the state/territory for this reporting period; (10) The scores shown reflect fewer than 50 completed surveys; (11) There were discrepancies in the data collection process; (12) This measure does not apply to this hospital for this reporting period; (13) Results cannot be calculated for this reporting period; (14) The results for this state are combined with nearby states to protect confidentiality; Please refer to the User's Guide for a full explanation of data.

Measure	Cases	This Hosp.	State Avg.	U.S. Avg.
Medicare Spending				
Medicare Spending per Patient (ratio)	-	-	0.91	0.98
Pneumonia Care				
Appropriate Initial Antibiotic Given	20	85%	93%	95%
Blood Culture Timing	33	97%	98%	98%
Pregnancy and Delivery Care				
Newborn Deliveries Scheduled Early[5]	-	-	4%	6%
Preventive Care				
Immunization for Influenza[5]	-	-	91%	90%
Immunization for Pneumonia[5]	-	-	90%	92%
Stroke Care				
Anticoagulation Therapy for Atrial Fibrillation[1,3]	-	-	95%	95%
Antithrombotic Therapy Timing[1,3]	-	-	98%	98%
Assessed for Rehabilitation[1,3]	-	-	97%	97%
Discharged on Antithrombotic Therapy[1,3]	-	-	99%	99%
Discharged on Statin Medication[1,3]	-	-	92%	94%
Thrombolytic Therapy Timing[1,3]	-	-	64%	66%
Venous Thromboembolism Prophylaxis[1,3]	-	-	93%	94%
Written Stroke Educational Materials Given[1,3]	-	-	82%	88%
Surgical Care Improvement Project				
Appropriate Beta Blocker Usage[1]	-	-	98%	98%
Appropriate VTP Within 24 Hours	16	69%	98%	98%
Controlled Postoperative Blood Glucose[7]	-	-	96%	97%
Perioperative Temperature Management	19	100%	100%	100%
Prophylactic Antibiotic Selection	11	91%	99%	99%
Prophylactic Antibiotic Selection (Outpatient)[5]	-	-	98%	98%
Prophylactic Antibiotic Stopped	11	100%	98%	98%
Prophylactic Antibiotic Timing	11	100%	98%	99%
Prophylactic Antibiotic Timing (Outpatient)[5]	-	-	98%	98%
Urinary Catheter Removal[1]	-	-	97%	97%
Survey of Patients' Hospital Experiences				
Area Around Room 'Always' Quiet at Night	(a)	60%	63%	61%
Doctors 'Always' Communicated Well	(a)	89%	84%	82%
Home Recovery Information Given	(a)	92%	88%	85%
Hospital Given 9 or 10 on 10 Point Scale	(a)	75%	75%	71%
Meds 'Always' Explained Before Given	(a)	65%	66%	64%
Nurses 'Always' Communicated Well	(a)	82%	81%	79%
Pain 'Always' Well Controlled	(a)	70%	71%	71%
Room and Bathroom 'Always' Clean	(a)	75%	79%	73%
Timely Help 'Always' Received	(a)	77%	70%	68%
Would Definitely Recommend Hospital	(a)	73%	74%	71%
Use of Medical Imaging				
Cardiac Imaging Stress Test before Surgery[1]	-	-	4.8%	5.3%
Combination Abdominal CT Scan	218	4.6%	11.5%	10.5%
Combination Brain/Sinus CT Scan	175	0.6%	1.8%	2.7%
Combination Chest CT Scan	168	4.8%	3.5%	2.7%
Follow-up Mammogram/Ultrasound	548	9.3%	7.9%	8.8%
Lumbar Spine MRI for Low Back Pain[1]	-	-	32.2%	37.2%

Sanford Rock Rapids Medical Center

801 South Greene Street
Rock Rapids, IA 51246
Phone: 712-472-2591
Fax: 712-472-2552
URL: www.merrillpioneer.org
Type: Critical Access Hospitals
Emergency Services: Yes
Ownership: Voluntary non-profit - Private
Beds: 25

Key Personnel:

Infection Control. . . . . Linda Brinkhous
Emergency Room . . . . Cathy Huff
Operating Room. . . . . William Jongewaard
CEO/President. . . . . Kelby K. Krabbenhoft
Chief of Medical Staff. . . . . David Springer, MD
Radiology. . . . . Robert Thorbrogger

Measure	Cases	This Hosp.	State Avg.	U.S. Avg.
Blood Clot Prevention and Treatment				
Anticoagulation Overlap Therapy[5]	-	-	94%	93%
ICU Venous Thromboembolism Prophylaxis[5]	-	-	90%	92%
Incidence of Potentially Preventable VTE[5]	-	-	8%	10%
UFH with Dosages/Platelet Monitoring[5]	-	-	99%	97%
Venous Thromboembolism Prophylaxis[5]	-	-	87%	85%
Warfarin Therapy Discharge Instructions[5]	-	-	77%	75%
Chest Pain/Possible Heart Attack Care				
Aspirin Given Within 24 Hours of Arrival[5]	-	-	97%	96%
Fibrinolytic Meds Within 30 Min. of Arrival[5]	-	-	49%	58%
Average Time to ECG (minutes)[5]	-	-	5	7
Average Time to Transfer (minutes)[5]	-	-	58	60
Children's Asthma Care				
Received Home Management Plan of Care	-	-	-	88%
Received Reliever Medication	-	-	-	100%
Received Systemic Corticosteroids	-	-	-	100%
Emergency Department				
Admittance Decision Time (minutes)[5]	-	-	58	98
Head CT Results Within 45 Min. of Arrival[5]	-	-	55%	57%
Patients Who Left ER Before Being Seen[5]	-	-	1%	2%
Time from ER Arrival to Admit. (minutes)[5]	-	-	202	274
Time from ER Arrival to Discharge (minutes)[5]	-	-	108	134
Time in ER Before Being Evaluated (minutes)[5]	-	-	21	26
Time to Pain Meds for Fractures (minutes)[5]	-	-	46	57
Heart Attack Care				
Aspirin Given at Discharge[1,3]	-	-	100%	99%
Fibrinolytic Meds Within 30 Min. of Arrival[3,7]	-	-	-	54%
PCI Within 90 Minutes of Arrival[3,7]	-	-	94%	96%
Statin Prescribed at Discharge[1,3]	-	-	98%	98%
Heart Failure Care				
ACE Inhibitor or ARB for LVSD[1,3]	-	-	95%	97%
Discharge Instructions Given[1,3]	-	-	93%	94%
Evaluation of LVS Function[1,3]	-	-	97%	99%
Medicare Spending				
Medicare Spending per Patient (ratio)	-	-	0.91	0.98
Pneumonia Care				
Appropriate Initial Antibiotic Given[1]	-	-	93%	95%
Blood Culture Timing[1]	-	-	98%	98%
Pregnancy and Delivery Care				
Newborn Deliveries Scheduled Early[5]	-	-	4%	6%
Preventive Care				
Immunization for Influenza[5]	-	-	91%	90%
Immunization for Pneumonia[5]	-	-	90%	92%
Stroke Care				
Anticoagulation Therapy for Atrial Fibrillation[5]	-	-	95%	95%
Antithrombotic Therapy Timing[5]	-	-	98%	98%
Assessed for Rehabilitation[5]	-	-	97%	97%
Discharged on Antithrombotic Therapy[5]	-	-	99%	99%
Discharged on Statin Medication[5]	-	-	92%	94%
Thrombolytic Therapy Timing[5]	-	-	64%	66%
Venous Thromboembolism Prophylaxis[5]	-	-	93%	94%
Written Stroke Educational Materials Given[5]	-	-	82%	88%
Surgical Care Improvement Project				
Appropriate Beta Blocker Usage[1]	-	-	98%	98%
Appropriate VTP Within 24 Hours[1]	-	-	98%	98%
Controlled Postoperative Blood Glucose[7]	-	-	96%	97%
Perioperative Temperature Management[1]	-	-	100%	100%
Prophylactic Antibiotic Selection[1]	-	-	99%	99%
Prophylactic Antibiotic Selection (Outpatient)[5]	-	-	98%	98%
Prophylactic Antibiotic Stopped[1]	-	-	98%	98%
Prophylactic Antibiotic Timing[1]	-	-	98%	99%
Prophylactic Antibiotic Timing (Outpatient)[5]	-	-	98%	98%
Urinary Catheter Removal[1]	-	-	97%	97%
Survey of Patients' Hospital Experiences				
Area Around Room 'Always' Quiet at Night[6]	<100	61%	63%	61%
Doctors 'Always' Communicated Well[6]	<100	89%	84%	82%
Home Recovery Information Given[6]	<100	82%	88%	85%
Hospital Given 9 or 10 on 10 Point Scale[6]	<100	83%	75%	71%
Meds 'Always' Explained Before Given[6]	<100	63%	66%	64%
Nurses 'Always' Communicated Well[6]	<100	89%	81%	79%
Pain 'Always' Well Controlled[6]	<100	79%	71%	71%
Room and Bathroom 'Always' Clean[6]	<100	84%	79%	73%
Timely Help 'Always' Received[6]	<100	83%	70%	68%
Would Definitely Recommend Hospital[6]	<100	80%	74%	71%
Use of Medical Imaging				
Cardiac Imaging Stress Test before Surgery[1]	-	-	4.8%	5.3%
Combination Abdominal CT Scan	48	47.9%	11.5%	10.5%
Combination Brain/Sinus CT Scan	75	0.0%	1.8%	2.7%
Combination Chest CT Scan[1]	-	-	3.5%	2.7%
Follow-up Mammogram/Ultrasound	145	10.3%	7.9%	8.8%
Lumbar Spine MRI for Low Back Pain[1]	-	-	32.2%	37.2%

Hegg Memorial Health Center

1202 21st Avenue
Rock Valley, IA 51247
Phone: 712-476-8000
Fax: 712-476-8090
URL: www.heggmemorialhealthcenter.org
Type: Critical Access Hospitals
Emergency Services: Yes
Ownership: Voluntary non-profit - Private
Beds: 123

Key Personnel:

Radiology. . . . . Tami Berkenpas
Quality Assurance . . . . Stacey Jumbeck
Chief of Medical Staff . . . . Brad Kamstra
Operating Room. . . . . Alma Post
CEO/President. . . . . Glenn Zevenbergen

Measure	Cases	This Hosp.	State Avg.	U.S. Avg.
Blood Clot Prevention and Treatment				
Anticoagulation Overlap Therapy[5]	-	-	94%	93%
ICU Venous Thromboembolism Prophylaxis[5]	-	-	90%	92%
Incidence of Potentially Preventable VTE[5]	-	-	8%	10%
UFH with Dosages/Platelet Monitoring[5]	-	-	99%	97%
Venous Thromboembolism Prophylaxis[5]	-	-	87%	85%
Warfarin Therapy Discharge Instructions[5]	-	-	77%	75%
Chest Pain/Possible Heart Attack Care				
Aspirin Given Within 24 Hours of Arrival[1,3]	-	-	97%	96%
Fibrinolytic Meds Within 30 Min. of Arrival[5]	-	-	49%	58%
Average Time to ECG (minutes)[1,3]	-	-	5	7
Average Time to Transfer (minutes)[5]	-	-	58	60
Children's Asthma Care				
Received Home Management Plan of Care	-	-	-	88%
Received Reliever Medication	-	-	-	100%
Received Systemic Corticosteroids	-	-	-	100%
Emergency Department				
Admittance Decision Time (minutes)[5]	-	-	58	98
Head CT Results Within 45 Min. of Arrival[5]	-	-	55%	57%
Patients Who Left ER Before Being Seen[5]	-	-	1%	2%
Time from ER Arrival to Admit. (minutes)[5]	-	-	202	274
Time from ER Arrival to Discharge (minutes)[5]	-	-	108	134
Time in ER Before Being Evaluated (minutes)[5]	-	-	21	26
Time to Pain Meds for Fractures (minutes)[5]	-	-	46	57
Heart Attack Care				
Aspirin Given at Discharge[5]	-	-	100%	99%
Fibrinolytic Meds Within 30 Min. of Arrival[5]	-	-	-	54%
PCI Within 90 Minutes of Arrival[5]	-	-	94%	96%
Statin Prescribed at Discharge[5]	-	-	98%	98%
Heart Failure Care				
ACE Inhibitor or ARB for LVSD[3,7]	-	-	95%	97%
Discharge Instructions Given[3,7]	-	-	93%	94%
Evaluation of LVS Function[1,3]	-	-	97%	99%
Medicare Spending				
Medicare Spending per Patient (ratio)	-	-	0.91	0.98
Pneumonia Care				
Appropriate Initial Antibiotic Given[3]	11	100%	93%	95%
Blood Culture Timing[1,3]	-	-	98%	98%
Pregnancy and Delivery Care				
Newborn Deliveries Scheduled Early[5]	-	-	4%	6%
Preventive Care				
Immunization for Influenza[2]	27	93%	91%	90%
Immunization for Pneumonia[2,3]	26	100%	90%	92%
Stroke Care				
Anticoagulation Therapy for Atrial Fibrillation[5]	-	-	95%	95%
Antithrombotic Therapy Timing[5]	-	-	98%	98%
Assessed for Rehabilitation[5]	-	-	97%	97%
Discharged on Antithrombotic Therapy[5]	-	-	99%	99%
Discharged on Statin Medication[5]	-	-	92%	94%
Thrombolytic Therapy Timing[5]	-	-	64%	66%
Venous Thromboembolism Prophylaxis[5]	-	-	93%	94%
Written Stroke Educational Materials Given[5]	-	-	82%	88%
Surgical Care Improvement Project				
Appropriate Beta Blocker Usage[3,7]	-	-	98%	98%
Appropriate VTP Within 24 Hours[1,3]	-	-	98%	98%
Controlled Postoperative Blood Glucose[3,7]	-	-	96%	97%
Perioperative Temperature Management[1,3]	-	-	100%	100%
Prophylactic Antibiotic Selection[1,3]	-	-	99%	99%
Prophylactic Antibiotic Selection (Outpatient)[5]	-	-	98%	98%
Prophylactic Antibiotic Stopped[1,3]	-	-	98%	98%

NOTE: Hospital profiles are in alphabetical order by state, then city, then hospital within the city; Rankings exclude hospitals with less than 25 cases except for patient surveys which excludes hospitals with less than 100 cases; (a) 100-299 cases; (1) The number of cases/patients is too few to report; (2) Data submitted were based on a sample of cases/patients; (3) Results are based on a shorter time period than required; (4) Data suppressed by CMS for one or more quarters; (5) Results are not available for this reporting period; (6) Fewer than 100 patients completed the HCAHPS survey; (7) No cases met the criteria for this measure; (8) The lower limit of the confidence interval cannot be calculated if the number of observed infections equals zero; (9) No data are available from the state/territory for this reporting period; (10) The scores shown reflect fewer than 50 completed surveys; (11) There were discrepancies in the data collection process; (12) This measure does not apply to this hospital for this reporting period; (13) Results cannot be calculated for this reporting period; (14) The results for this state are combined with nearby states to protect confidentiality; Please refer to the User's Guide for a full explanation of data.

Measure	Cases	This Hosp.	State Avg.	U.S. Avg.
Prophylactic Antibiotic Timing[1,3]	-	-	98%	99%
Prophylactic Antibiotic Timing (Outpatient)[5]	-	-	98%	98%
Urinary Catheter Removal[1,3]	-	-	97%	97%
Survey of Patients' Hospital Experiences				
Area Around Room 'Always' Quiet at Night[6]	<100	63%	63%	61%
Doctors 'Always' Communicated Well[6]	<100	89%	84%	82%
Home Recovery Information Given[6]	<100	92%	88%	85%
Hospital Given 9 or 10 on 10 Point Scale[6]	<100	82%	75%	71%
Meds 'Always' Explained Before Given[6]	<100	68%	66%	64%
Nurses 'Always' Communicated Well[6]	<100	79%	81%	79%
Pain 'Always' Well Controlled[6]	<100	69%	71%	71%
Room and Bathroom 'Always' Clean[6]	<100	77%	79%	73%
Timely Help 'Always' Received[6]	<100	72%	70%	68%
Would Definitely Recommend Hospital[6]	<100	81%	74%	71%
Use of Medical Imaging				
Cardiac Imaging Stress Test before Surgery[1]	-	-	4.8%	5.3%
Combination Abdominal CT Scan	64	9.4%	11.5%	10.5%
Combination Brain/Sinus CT Scan[1]	-	-	1.8%	2.7%
Combination Chest CT Scan[1]	-	-	3.5%	2.7%
Follow-up Mammogram/Ultrasound	153	11.8%	7.9%	8.8%
Lumbar Spine MRI for Low Back Pain[1]	-	-	32.2%	37.2%

Loring Hospital

211 Highland Avenue PO Box 217
Sac City, IA 50583
Phone: 712-662-7105
Type: Critical Access Hospitals
Emergency Services: Yes
Ownership: Voluntary non-profit - Private

Measure	Cases	This Hosp.	State Avg.	U.S. Avg.
Blood Clot Prevention and Treatment				
Anticoagulation Overlap Therapy[5]	-	-	94%	93%
ICU Venous Thromboembolism Prophylaxis[5]	-	-	90%	92%
Incidence of Potentially Preventable VTE[5]	-	-	8%	10%
UFH with Dosages/Platelet Monitoring[5]	-	-	99%	97%
Venous Thromboembolism Prophylaxis[5]	-	-	87%	85%
Warfarin Therapy Discharge Instructions[5]	-	-	77%	75%
Chest Pain/Possible Heart Attack Care				
Aspirin Given Within 24 Hours of Arrival[5]	-	-	97%	96%
Fibrinolytic Meds Within 30 Min. of Arrival[5]	-	-	49%	58%
Average Time to ECG (minutes)[5]	-	-	5	7
Average Time to Transfer (minutes)[5]	-	-	58	60
Children's Asthma Care				
Received Home Management Plan of Care	-	-	-	88%
Received Reliever Medication	-	-	-	100%
Received Systemic Corticosteroids	-	-	-	100%
Emergency Department				
Admittance Decision Time (minutes)[5]	-	-	58	98
Head CT Results Within 45 Min. of Arrival[5]	-	-	55%	57%
Patients Who Left ER Before Being Seen[5]	-	-	1%	2%
Time from ER Arrival to Admit. (minutes)[5]	-	-	202	274
Time from ER Arrival to Discharge (minutes)[5]	-	-	108	134
Time in ER Before Being Evaluated (minutes)[5]	-	-	21	26
Time to Pain Meds for Fractures (minutes)[5]	-	-	46	57
Heart Attack Care				
Aspirin Given at Discharge[1,3]	-	-	100%	99%
Fibrinolytic Meds Within 30 Min. of Arrival[3,7]	-	-	-	54%
PCI Within 90 Minutes of Arrival[5]	-	-	94%	96%
Statin Prescribed at Discharge[1,3]	-	-	98%	98%
Heart Failure Care				
ACE Inhibitor or ARB for LVSD[1]	-	-	95%	97%
Discharge Instructions Given[1]	-	-	93%	94%
Evaluation of LVS Function	18	83%	97%	99%
Medicare Spending				
Medicare Spending per Patient (ratio)	-	-	0.91	0.98
Pneumonia Care				
Appropriate Initial Antibiotic Given	16	69%	93%	95%
Blood Culture Timing[1]	-	-	98%	98%
Pregnancy and Delivery Care				
Newborn Deliveries Scheduled Early[5]	-	-	4%	6%
Preventive Care				
Immunization for Influenza[5]	-	-	91%	90%
Immunization for Pneumonia[5]	-	-	90%	92%
Stroke Care				
Anticoagulation Therapy for Atrial Fibrillation[5]	-	-	95%	95%
Antithrombotic Therapy Timing[5]	-	-	98%	98%
Assessed for Rehabilitation[5]	-	-	97%	97%
Discharged on Antithrombotic Therapy[5]	-	-	99%	99%
Discharged on Statin Medication[5]	-	-	92%	94%
Thrombolytic Therapy Timing[5]	-	-	64%	66%
Venous Thromboembolism Prophylaxis[5]	-	-	93%	94%
Written Stroke Educational Materials Given[5]	-	-	82%	88%
Surgical Care Improvement Project				
Appropriate Beta Blocker Usage[5]	-	-	98%	98%
Appropriate VTP Within 24 Hours[5]	-	-	98%	98%
Controlled Postoperative Blood Glucose[5]	-	-	96%	97%
Perioperative Temperature Management[5]	-	-	100%	100%
Prophylactic Antibiotic Selection[5]	-	-	99%	99%
Prophylactic Antibiotic Selection (Outpatient)[5]	-	-	98%	98%
Prophylactic Antibiotic Stopped[5]	-	-	98%	98%
Prophylactic Antibiotic Timing[5]	-	-	98%	99%
Prophylactic Antibiotic Timing (Outpatient)[5]	-	-	98%	98%
Urinary Catheter Removal[5]	-	-	97%	97%
Survey of Patients' Hospital Experiences				
Area Around Room 'Always' Quiet at Night[5]	-	-	63%	61%
Doctors 'Always' Communicated Well[5]	-	-	84%	82%
Home Recovery Information Given[5]	-	-	88%	85%
Hospital Given 9 or 10 on 10 Point Scale[5]	-	-	75%	71%
Meds 'Always' Explained Before Given[5]	-	-	66%	64%
Nurses 'Always' Communicated Well[5]	-	-	81%	79%
Pain 'Always' Well Controlled[5]	-	-	71%	71%
Room and Bathroom 'Always' Clean[5]	-	-	79%	73%
Timely Help 'Always' Received[5]	-	-	70%	68%
Would Definitely Recommend Hospital[5]	-	-	74%	71%
Use of Medical Imaging				
Cardiac Imaging Stress Test before Surgery[7]	-	-	4.8%	5.3%
Combination Abdominal CT Scan	73	2.7%	11.5%	10.5%
Combination Brain/Sinus CT Scan	147	0.7%	1.8%	2.7%
Combination Chest CT Scan[1]	-	-	3.5%	2.7%
Follow-up Mammogram/Ultrasound	241	5.0%	7.9%	8.8%
Lumbar Spine MRI for Low Back Pain[1]	-	-	32.2%	37.2%

Sanford Sheldon Medical Center

118 North 7th Avenue
Sheldon, IA 51201
Phone: 712-324-5041
Fax: 712-324-6015
URL: www.nwiowahealthcenter.org
Type: Critical Access Hospitals
Emergency Services: Yes
Ownership: Voluntary non-profit - Private
Beds: 28

Key Personnel:
Emergency Room . . . . Kathy Altena, RN
Chief of Medical Staff . . . . Amy M Badberg
Operating Room. . . . . William Jongewaard
CEO/President. . . . . Charles R Miller
Quality Assurance . . . . Beverly Scholten

Measure	Cases	This Hosp.	State Avg.	U.S. Avg.
Blood Clot Prevention and Treatment				
Anticoagulation Overlap Therapy[5]	-	-	94%	93%
ICU Venous Thromboembolism Prophylaxis[5]	-	-	90%	92%
Incidence of Potentially Preventable VTE[5]	-	-	8%	10%
UFH with Dosages/Platelet Monitoring[5]	-	-	99%	97%
Venous Thromboembolism Prophylaxis[5]	-	-	87%	85%
Warfarin Therapy Discharge Instructions[5]	-	-	77%	75%
Chest Pain/Possible Heart Attack Care				
Aspirin Given Within 24 Hours of Arrival[5]	-	-	97%	96%
Fibrinolytic Meds Within 30 Min. of Arrival[5]	-	-	49%	58%
Average Time to ECG (minutes)[5]	-	-	5	7
Average Time to Transfer (minutes)[5]	-	-	58	60
Children's Asthma Care				
Received Home Management Plan of Care	-	-	-	88%
Received Reliever Medication	-	-	-	100%
Received Systemic Corticosteroids	-	-	-	100%
Emergency Department				
Admittance Decision Time (minutes)[5]	-	-	58	98
Head CT Results Within 45 Min. of Arrival[5]	-	-	55%	57%
Patients Who Left ER Before Being Seen[5]	-	-	1%	2%
Time from ER Arrival to Admit. (minutes)[5]	-	-	202	274
Time from ER Arrival to Discharge (minutes)[5]	-	-	108	134
Time in ER Before Being Evaluated (minutes)[5]	-	-	21	26
Time to Pain Meds for Fractures (minutes)[5]	-	-	46	57
Heart Attack Care				
Aspirin Given at Discharge[5]	-	-	100%	99%
Fibrinolytic Meds Within 30 Min. of Arrival[5]	-	-	-	54%
PCI Within 90 Minutes of Arrival[5]	-	-	94%	96%
Statin Prescribed at Discharge[5]	-	-	98%	98%
Heart Failure Care				
ACE Inhibitor or ARB for LVSD[1]	-	-	95%	97%
Discharge Instructions Given[1]	-	-	93%	94%
Evaluation of LVS Function	15	80%	97%	99%
Medicare Spending				
Medicare Spending per Patient (ratio)	-	-	0.91	0.98
Pneumonia Care				
Appropriate Initial Antibiotic Given	34	88%	93%	95%
Blood Culture Timing	18	89%	98%	98%
Pregnancy and Delivery Care				
Newborn Deliveries Scheduled Early[5]	-	-	4%	6%
Preventive Care				
Immunization for Influenza[5]	-	-	91%	90%
Immunization for Pneumonia[5]	-	-	90%	92%
Stroke Care				
Anticoagulation Therapy for Atrial Fibrillation[5]	-	-	95%	95%
Antithrombotic Therapy Timing[5]	-	-	98%	98%
Assessed for Rehabilitation[5]	-	-	97%	97%
Discharged on Antithrombotic Therapy[5]	-	-	99%	99%
Discharged on Statin Medication[5]	-	-	92%	94%
Thrombolytic Therapy Timing[5]	-	-	64%	66%
Venous Thromboembolism Prophylaxis[5]	-	-	93%	94%
Written Stroke Educational Materials Given[5]	-	-	82%	88%
Surgical Care Improvement Project				
Appropriate Beta Blocker Usage[5]	-	-	98%	98%
Appropriate VTP Within 24 Hours[5]	-	-	98%	98%
Controlled Postoperative Blood Glucose[5]	-	-	96%	97%
Perioperative Temperature Management[5]	-	-	100%	100%
Prophylactic Antibiotic Selection[5]	-	-	99%	99%
Prophylactic Antibiotic Selection (Outpatient)[5]	-	-	98%	98%
Prophylactic Antibiotic Stopped[5]	-	-	98%	98%
Prophylactic Antibiotic Timing[5]	-	-	98%	99%
Prophylactic Antibiotic Timing (Outpatient)[5]	-	-	98%	98%
Urinary Catheter Removal[5]	-	-	97%	97%
Survey of Patients' Hospital Experiences				
Area Around Room 'Always' Quiet at Night	(a)	56%	63%	61%
Doctors 'Always' Communicated Well	(a)	81%	84%	82%
Home Recovery Information Given	(a)	83%	88%	85%
Hospital Given 9 or 10 on 10 Point Scale	(a)	72%	75%	71%
Meds 'Always' Explained Before Given	(a)	62%	66%	64%
Nurses 'Always' Communicated Well	(a)	78%	81%	79%
Pain 'Always' Well Controlled	(a)	69%	71%	71%
Room and Bathroom 'Always' Clean	(a)	70%	79%	73%
Timely Help 'Always' Received	(a)	74%	70%	68%
Would Definitely Recommend Hospital	(a)	71%	74%	71%
Use of Medical Imaging				
Cardiac Imaging Stress Test before Surgery[1]	-	-	4.8%	5.3%
Combination Abdominal CT Scan	122	6.6%	11.5%	10.5%
Combination Brain/Sinus CT Scan[1]	-	-	1.8%	2.7%
Combination Chest CT Scan	69	8.7%	3.5%	2.7%
Follow-up Mammogram/Ultrasound	353	7.6%	7.9%	8.8%
Lumbar Spine MRI for Low Back Pain[1]	-	-	32.2%	37.2%

Shenandoah Medical Center

300 Pershing Avenue
Shenandoah, IA 51601
Phone: 712-246-1230
Fax: 712-246-4737
URL: www.shenandoahmedcenter.com
Type: Critical Access Hospitals
Emergency Services: Yes
Ownership: Voluntary non-profit - Private
Beds: 88

Key Personnel:
Chief of Medical Staff . . . . John Bowery
Emergency Room . . . . Tammy Franks
Intensive Care Unit. . . . . Dana Grady
Radiology. . . . . Linda Head
Operating Room. . . . . Hamid Kakavandi
CEO/President. . . . . Susan McGough
Quality Assurance . . . . Jo McKeown

NOTE: Hospital profiles are in alphabetical order by state, then city, then hospital within the city; Rankings exclude hospitals with less than 25 cases except for patient surveys which excludes hospitals with less than 100 cases; (a) 100-299 cases; (1) The number of cases/patients is too few to report; (2) Data submitted were based on a sample of cases/patients; (3) Results are based on a shorter time period than required; (4) Data suppressed by CMS for one or more quarters; (5) Results are not available for this reporting period; (6) Fewer than 100 patients completed the HCAHPS survey; (7) No cases met the criteria for this measure; (8) The lower limit of the confidence interval cannot be calculated if the number of observed infections equals zero; (9) No data are available from the state/territory for this reporting period; (10) The scores shown reflect fewer than 50 completed surveys; (11) There were discrepancies in the data collection process; (12) This measure does not apply to this hospital for this reporting period; (13) Results cannot be calculated for this reporting period; (14) The results for this state are combined with nearby states to protect confidentiality; Please refer to the User's Guide for a full explanation of data.

Measure	Cases	This Hosp.	State Avg.	U.S. Avg.
Blood Clot Prevention and Treatment				
Anticoagulation Overlap Therapy[5]	-	-	94%	93%
ICU Venous Thromboembolism Prophylaxis[5]	-	-	90%	92%
Incidence of Potentially Preventable VTE[5]	-	-	8%	10%
UFH with Dosages/Platelet Monitoring[5]	-	-	99%	97%
Venous Thromboembolism Prophylaxis[5]	-	-	87%	85%
Warfarin Therapy Discharge Instructions[5]	-	-	77%	75%
Chest Pain/Possible Heart Attack Care				
Aspirin Given Within 24 Hours of Arrival	20	95%	97%	96%
Fibrinolytic Meds Within 30 Min. of Arrival[3,7]	-	-	49%	58%
Average Time to ECG (minutes)	20	7	5	7
Average Time to Transfer (minutes)[1,3]	-	-	58	60
Children's Asthma Care				
Received Home Management Plan of Care	-	-	-	88%
Received Reliever Medication	-	-	-	100%
Received Systemic Corticosteroids	-	-	-	100%
Emergency Department				
Admittance Decision Time (minutes)[5]	-	-	58	98
Head CT Results Within 45 Min. of Arrival[5]	-	-	55%	57%
Patients Who Left ER Before Being Seen[5]	-	-	1%	2%
Time from ER Arrival to Admit. (minutes)[5]	-	-	202	274
Time from ER Arrival to Discharge (minutes)[5]	-	-	108	134
Time in ER Before Being Evaluated (minutes)[5]	-	-	21	26
Time to Pain Meds for Fractures (minutes)[5]	-	-	46	57
Heart Attack Care				
Aspirin Given at Discharge[5]	-	-	100%	99%
Fibrinolytic Meds Within 30 Min. of Arrival[5]	-	-	-	54%
PCI Within 90 Minutes of Arrival[5]	-	-	94%	96%
Statin Prescribed at Discharge[5]	-	-	98%	98%
Heart Failure Care				
ACE Inhibitor or ARB for LVSD[1]	-	-	95%	97%
Discharge Instructions Given[1]	-	-	93%	94%
Evaluation of LVS Function[1]	-	-	97%	99%
Medicare Spending				
Medicare Spending per Patient (ratio)	-	-	0.91	0.98
Pneumonia Care				
Appropriate Initial Antibiotic Given	24	96%	93%	95%
Blood Culture Timing	28	89%	98%	98%
Pregnancy and Delivery Care				
Newborn Deliveries Scheduled Early[5]	-	-	4%	6%
Preventive Care				
Immunization for Influenza[5]	-	-	91%	90%
Immunization for Pneumonia[5]	-	-	90%	92%
Stroke Care				
Anticoagulation Therapy for Atrial Fibrillation[5]	-	-	95%	95%
Antithrombotic Therapy Timing[5]	-	-	98%	98%
Assessed for Rehabilitation[5]	-	-	97%	97%
Discharged on Antithrombotic Therapy[5]	-	-	99%	99%
Discharged on Statin Medication[5]	-	-	92%	94%
Thrombolytic Therapy Timing[5]	-	-	64%	66%
Venous Thromboembolism Prophylaxis[5]	-	-	93%	94%
Written Stroke Educational Materials Given[5]	-	-	82%	88%
Surgical Care Improvement Project				
Appropriate Beta Blocker Usage[1]	-	-	98%	98%
Appropriate VTP Within 24 Hours[1]	-	-	98%	98%
Controlled Postoperative Blood Glucose[7]	-	-	96%	97%
Perioperative Temperature Management	13	92%	100%	100%
Prophylactic Antibiotic Selection	11	91%	99%	99%
Prophylactic Antibiotic Selection (Outpatient)[5]	-	-	98%	98%
Prophylactic Antibiotic Stopped	11	100%	98%	98%
Prophylactic Antibiotic Timing	11	100%	98%	99%
Prophylactic Antibiotic Timing (Outpatient)[5]	-	-	98%	98%
Urinary Catheter Removal[1]	-	-	97%	97%
Survey of Patients' Hospital Experiences				
Area Around Room 'Always' Quiet at Night	(a)	56%	63%	61%
Doctors 'Always' Communicated Well	(a)	82%	84%	82%
Home Recovery Information Given	(a)	84%	88%	85%
Hospital Given 9 or 10 on 10 Point Scale	(a)	62%	75%	71%
Meds 'Always' Explained Before Given	(a)	62%	66%	64%
Nurses 'Always' Communicated Well	(a)	75%	81%	79%
Pain 'Always' Well Controlled	(a)	59%	71%	71%
Room and Bathroom 'Always' Clean	(a)	60%	79%	73%
Timely Help 'Always' Received	(a)	60%	70%	68%
Would Definitely Recommend Hospital	(a)	63%	74%	71%
Use of Medical Imaging				
Cardiac Imaging Stress Test before Surgery[1]	-	-	4.8%	5.3%
Combination Abdominal CT Scan	255	8.2%	11.5%	10.5%
Combination Brain/Sinus CT Scan[1]	-	-	1.8%	2.7%
Combination Chest CT Scan	211	5.2%	3.5%	2.7%
Follow-up Mammogram/Ultrasound	251	10.8%	7.9%	8.8%
Lumbar Spine MRI for Low Back Pain[1]	-	-	32.2%	37.2%

Osceola Community Hospital

600 9th Avenue North
Sibley, IA 51249
URL: www.osceolacommunityhospital.org
Type: Critical Access Hospitals
Ownership: Voluntary non-profit - Private
Phone: 712-754-2574
Fax: 712-754-3782
Emergency Services: Yes
Beds: 32

Key Personnel:
CEO/President. . . . . Janet Dykstra
Operating Room. . . . . Pauline Van Engen
Chief of Medical Staff . . . . William Hicks
Quality Assurance . . . . Sherry McElroy
Radiology. . . . . R W Thorbrogger

Measure	Cases	This Hosp.	State Avg.	U.S. Avg.
Blood Clot Prevention and Treatment				
Anticoagulation Overlap Therapy[5]	-	-	94%	93%
ICU Venous Thromboembolism Prophylaxis[5]	-	-	90%	92%
Incidence of Potentially Preventable VTE[5]	-	-	8%	10%
UFH with Dosages/Platelet Monitoring[5]	-	-	99%	97%
Venous Thromboembolism Prophylaxis[5]	-	-	87%	85%
Warfarin Therapy Discharge Instructions[5]	-	-	77%	75%
Chest Pain/Possible Heart Attack Care				
Aspirin Given Within 24 Hours of Arrival[5]	-	-	97%	96%
Fibrinolytic Meds Within 30 Min. of Arrival[5]	-	-	49%	58%
Average Time to ECG (minutes)[5]	-	-	5	7
Average Time to Transfer (minutes)[5]	-	-	58	60
Children's Asthma Care				
Received Home Management Plan of Care	-	-	-	88%
Received Reliever Medication	-	-	-	100%
Received Systemic Corticosteroids	-	-	-	100%
Emergency Department				
Admittance Decision Time (minutes)[5]	-	-	58	98
Head CT Results Within 45 Min. of Arrival[5]	-	-	55%	57%
Patients Who Left ER Before Being Seen[5]	-	-	1%	2%
Time from ER Arrival to Admit. (minutes)[5]	-	-	202	274
Time from ER Arrival to Discharge (minutes)[5]	-	-	108	134
Time in ER Before Being Evaluated (minutes)[5]	-	-	21	26
Time to Pain Meds for Fractures (minutes)[5]	-	-	46	57
Heart Attack Care				
Aspirin Given at Discharge[5]	-	-	100%	99%
Fibrinolytic Meds Within 30 Min. of Arrival[5]	-	-	-	54%
PCI Within 90 Minutes of Arrival[5]	-	-	94%	96%
Statin Prescribed at Discharge[5]	-	-	98%	98%
Heart Failure Care				
ACE Inhibitor or ARB for LVSD[1]	-	-	95%	97%
Discharge Instructions Given	14	64%	93%	94%
Evaluation of LVS Function	18	78%	97%	99%
Medicare Spending				
Medicare Spending per Patient (ratio)	-	-	0.91	0.98
Pneumonia Care				
Appropriate Initial Antibiotic Given	16	94%	93%	95%
Blood Culture Timing[1]	-	-	98%	98%
Pregnancy and Delivery Care				
Newborn Deliveries Scheduled Early[5]	-	-	4%	6%
Preventive Care				
Immunization for Influenza[5]	-	-	91%	90%
Immunization for Pneumonia[5]	-	-	90%	92%
Stroke Care				
Anticoagulation Therapy for Atrial Fibrillation[5]	-	-	95%	95%
Antithrombotic Therapy Timing[5]	-	-	98%	98%
Assessed for Rehabilitation[5]	-	-	97%	97%
Discharged on Antithrombotic Therapy[5]	-	-	99%	99%
Discharged on Statin Medication[5]	-	-	92%	94%
Thrombolytic Therapy Timing[5]	-	-	64%	66%
Venous Thromboembolism Prophylaxis[5]	-	-	93%	94%
Written Stroke Educational Materials Given[5]	-	-	82%	88%
Surgical Care Improvement Project				
Appropriate Beta Blocker Usage[3,7]	-	-	98%	98%
Appropriate VTP Within 24 Hours[1,3]	-	-	98%	98%
Controlled Postoperative Blood Glucose[3,7]	-	-	96%	97%
Perioperative Temperature Management[1,3]	-	-	100%	100%
Prophylactic Antibiotic Selection[1,3]	-	-	99%	99%
Prophylactic Antibiotic Selection (Outpatient)[5]	-	-	98%	98%
Prophylactic Antibiotic Stopped[1,3]	-	-	98%	98%
Prophylactic Antibiotic Timing[1,3]	-	-	98%	99%
Prophylactic Antibiotic Timing (Outpatient)[5]	-	-	98%	98%
Urinary Catheter Removal[1,3]	-	-	97%	97%
Survey of Patients' Hospital Experiences				
Area Around Room 'Always' Quiet at Night	(a)	72%	63%	61%
Doctors 'Always' Communicated Well	(a)	83%	84%	82%
Home Recovery Information Given	(a)	84%	88%	85%
Hospital Given 9 or 10 on 10 Point Scale	(a)	78%	75%	71%
Meds 'Always' Explained Before Given	(a)	62%	66%	64%
Nurses 'Always' Communicated Well	(a)	82%	81%	79%
Pain 'Always' Well Controlled	(a)	78%	71%	71%
Room and Bathroom 'Always' Clean	(a)	92%	79%	73%
Timely Help 'Always' Received	(a)	75%	70%	68%
Would Definitely Recommend Hospital	(a)	75%	74%	71%
Use of Medical Imaging				
Cardiac Imaging Stress Test before Surgery[1]	-	-	4.8%	5.3%
Combination Abdominal CT Scan	59	33.9%	11.5%	10.5%
Combination Brain/Sinus CT Scan	44	0.0%	1.8%	2.7%
Combination Chest CT Scan[1]	-	-	3.5%	2.7%
Follow-up Mammogram/Ultrasound	231	6.1%	7.9%	8.8%
Lumbar Spine MRI for Low Back Pain[1]	-	-	32.2%	37.2%

Keokuk County Health Center

23019 Highway 149
Sigourney, IA 52591
Type: Critical Access Hospitals
Ownership: Voluntary non-profit - Other
Phone: 641-622-2720
Emergency Services: Yes

Measure	Cases	This Hosp.	State Avg.	U.S. Avg.
Blood Clot Prevention and Treatment				
Anticoagulation Overlap Therapy	-	-	94%	93%
ICU Venous Thromboembolism Prophylaxis	-	-	90%	92%
Incidence of Potentially Preventable VTE	-	-	8%	10%
UFH with Dosages/Platelet Monitoring	-	-	99%	97%
Venous Thromboembolism Prophylaxis	-	-	87%	85%
Warfarin Therapy Discharge Instructions	-	-	77%	75%
Chest Pain/Possible Heart Attack Care				
Aspirin Given Within 24 Hours of Arrival[1,3]	-	-	97%	96%
Fibrinolytic Meds Within 30 Min. of Arrival[3,7]	-	-	49%	58%
Average Time to ECG (minutes)[1,3]	-	-	5	7
Average Time to Transfer (minutes)[1,3]	-	-	58	60
Children's Asthma Care				
Received Home Management Plan of Care	-	-	-	88%
Received Reliever Medication	-	-	-	100%
Received Systemic Corticosteroids	-	-	-	100%
Emergency Department				
Admittance Decision Time (minutes)	-	-	58	98
Head CT Results Within 45 Min. of Arrival[5]	-	-	55%	57%
Patients Who Left ER Before Being Seen	2,009	0%	1%	2%
Time from ER Arrival to Admit. (minutes)	-	-	202	274
Time from ER Arrival to Discharge (minutes)[3]	149	71	108	134
Time in ER Before Being Evaluated (minutes)[3]	182	12	21	26
Time to Pain Meds for Fractures (minutes)[1,3]	-	-	46	57
Heart Attack Care				
Aspirin Given at Discharge	-	-	100%	99%
Fibrinolytic Meds Within 30 Min. of Arrival	-	-	-	54%
PCI Within 90 Minutes of Arrival	-	-	94%	96%
Statin Prescribed at Discharge	-	-	98%	98%
Heart Failure Care				
ACE Inhibitor or ARB for LVSD	-	-	95%	97%
Discharge Instructions Given	-	-	93%	94%
Evaluation of LVS Function	-	-	97%	99%
Medicare Spending				

NOTE: Hospital profiles are in alphabetical order by state, then city, then hospital within the city; Rankings exclude hospitals with less than 25 cases except for patient surveys which excludes hospitals with less than 100 cases; (a) 100-299 cases; (1) The number of cases/patients is too few to report; (2) Data submitted were based on a sample of cases/patients; (3) Results are based on a shorter time period than required; (4) Data suppressed by CMS for one or more quarters; (5) Results are not available for this reporting period; (6) Fewer than 100 patients completed the HCAHPS survey; (7) No cases met the criteria for this measure; (8) The lower limit of the confidence interval cannot be calculated if the number of observed infections equals zero; (9) No data are available from the state/territory for this reporting period; (10) The scores shown reflect fewer than 50 completed surveys; (11) There were discrepancies in the data collection process; (12) This measure does not apply to this hospital for this reporting period; (13) Results cannot be calculated for this reporting period; (14) The results for this state are combined with nearby states to protect confidentiality; Please refer to the User's Guide for a full explanation of data.

Measure	Cases	This Hosp.	State Avg.	U.S. Avg.
Medicare Spending per Patient (ratio)	-	-	0.91	0.98
Pneumonia Care				
Appropriate Initial Antibiotic Given	-	-	93%	95%
Blood Culture Timing	-	-	98%	98%
Pregnancy and Delivery Care				
Newborn Deliveries Scheduled Early	-	-	4%	6%
Preventive Care				
Immunization for Influenza	-	-	91%	90%
Immunization for Pneumonia	-	-	90%	92%
Stroke Care				
Anticoagulation Therapy for Atrial Fibrillation	-	-	95%	95%
Antithrombotic Therapy Timing	-	-	98%	98%
Assessed for Rehabilitation	-	-	97%	97%
Discharged on Antithrombotic Therapy	-	-	99%	99%
Discharged on Statin Medication	-	-	92%	94%
Thrombolytic Therapy Timing	-	-	64%	66%
Venous Thromboembolism Prophylaxis	-	-	93%	94%
Written Stroke Educational Materials Given	-	-	82%	88%
Surgical Care Improvement Project				
Appropriate Beta Blocker Usage	-	-	98%	98%
Appropriate VTP Within 24 Hours	-	-	98%	98%
Controlled Postoperative Blood Glucose	-	-	96%	97%
Perioperative Temperature Management	-	-	100%	100%
Prophylactic Antibiotic Selection	-	-	99%	99%
Prophylactic Antibiotic Selection (Outpatient)[5]	-	-	98%	98%
Prophylactic Antibiotic Stopped	-	-	98%	98%
Prophylactic Antibiotic Timing	-	-	98%	99%
Prophylactic Antibiotic Timing (Outpatient)[5]	-	-	98%	98%
Urinary Catheter Removal	-	-	97%	97%
Survey of Patients' Hospital Experiences				
Area Around Room 'Always' Quiet at Night	-	-	63%	61%
Doctors 'Always' Communicated Well	-	-	84%	82%
Home Recovery Information Given	-	-	88%	85%
Hospital Given 9 or 10 on 10 Point Scale	-	-	75%	71%
Meds 'Always' Explained Before Given	-	-	66%	64%
Nurses 'Always' Communicated Well	-	-	81%	79%
Pain 'Always' Well Controlled	-	-	71%	71%
Room and Bathroom 'Always' Clean	-	-	79%	73%
Timely Help 'Always' Received	-	-	70%	68%
Would Definitely Recommend Hospital	-	-	74%	71%
Use of Medical Imaging				
Cardiac Imaging Stress Test before Surgery[7]	-	-	4.8%	5.3%
Combination Abdominal CT Scan[1]	-	-	11.5%	10.5%
Combination Brain/Sinus CT Scan	42	0.0%	1.8%	2.7%
Combination Chest CT Scan[1]	-	-	3.5%	2.7%
Follow-up Mammogram/Ultrasound[7]	-	-	7.9%	8.8%
Lumbar Spine MRI for Low Back Pain[7]	-	-	32.2%	37.2%

Sioux Center Community Hospital & Health Center

605 South Main Avenue
Sioux Center, IA 51250
URL: www.schospital.org
Type: Critical Access Hospitals
Ownership: Voluntary non-profit - Private
Phone: 712-722-1271
Fax: 712-722-0787
Emergency Services: No
Beds: 90

Key Personnel:
Radiology. . . . . Robert P DeClark
Quality Assurance . . . . Sheryl Hulstein
CEO/President. . . . . Kayleen Lee
Chief of Medical Staff . . . . Mary McClung

Measure	Cases	This Hosp.	State Avg.	U.S. Avg.
Blood Clot Prevention and Treatment				
Anticoagulation Overlap Therapy[5]	-	-	94%	93%
ICU Venous Thromboembolism Prophylaxis[5]	-	-	90%	92%
Incidence of Potentially Preventable VTE[5]	-	-	8%	10%
UFH with Dosages/Platelet Monitoring[5]	-	-	99%	97%
Venous Thromboembolism Prophylaxis[5]	-	-	87%	85%
Warfarin Therapy Discharge Instructions[5]	-	-	77%	75%
Chest Pain/Possible Heart Attack Care				
Aspirin Given Within 24 Hours of Arrival[5]	-	-	97%	96%
Fibrinolytic Meds Within 30 Min. of Arrival[5]	-	-	49%	58%
Average Time to ECG (minutes)[5]	-	-	5	7
Average Time to Transfer (minutes)[5]	-	-	58	60
Children's Asthma Care				
Received Home Management Plan of Care	-	-	-	88%
Received Reliever Medication	-	-	-	100%
Received Systemic Corticosteroids	-	-	-	100%
Emergency Department				
Admittance Decision Time (minutes)[5]	-	-	58	98
Head CT Results Within 45 Min. of Arrival[5]	-	-	55%	57%
Patients Who Left ER Before Being Seen[5]	-	-	1%	2%
Time from ER Arrival to Admit. (minutes)[5]	-	-	202	274
Time from ER Arrival to Discharge (minutes)[5]	-	-	108	134
Time in ER Before Being Evaluated (minutes)[5]	-	-	21	26
Time to Pain Meds for Fractures (minutes)[5]	-	-	46	57
Heart Attack Care				
Aspirin Given at Discharge[5]	-	-	100%	99%
Fibrinolytic Meds Within 30 Min. of Arrival[5]	-	-	-	54%
PCI Within 90 Minutes of Arrival[5]	-	-	94%	96%
Statin Prescribed at Discharge[5]	-	-	98%	98%
Heart Failure Care				
ACE Inhibitor or ARB for LVSD[3,7]	-	-	95%	97%
Discharge Instructions Given[1,3]	-	-	93%	94%
Evaluation of LVS Function[1,3]	-	-	97%	99%
Medicare Spending				
Medicare Spending per Patient (ratio)	-	-	0.91	0.98
Pneumonia Care				
Appropriate Initial Antibiotic Given[1]	-	-	93%	95%
Blood Culture Timing[1]	-	-	98%	98%
Pregnancy and Delivery Care				
Newborn Deliveries Scheduled Early[5]	-	-	4%	6%
Preventive Care				
Immunization for Influenza[5]	-	-	91%	90%
Immunization for Pneumonia[5]	-	-	90%	92%
Stroke Care				
Anticoagulation Therapy for Atrial Fibrillation[5]	-	-	95%	95%
Antithrombotic Therapy Timing[5]	-	-	98%	98%
Assessed for Rehabilitation[5]	-	-	97%	97%
Discharged on Antithrombotic Therapy[5]	-	-	99%	99%
Discharged on Statin Medication[5]	-	-	92%	94%
Thrombolytic Therapy Timing[5]	-	-	64%	66%
Venous Thromboembolism Prophylaxis[5]	-	-	93%	94%
Written Stroke Educational Materials Given[5]	-	-	82%	88%
Surgical Care Improvement Project				
Appropriate Beta Blocker Usage[1,3]	-	-	98%	98%
Appropriate VTP Within 24 Hours[1,3]	-	-	98%	98%
Controlled Postoperative Blood Glucose[3,7]	-	-	96%	97%
Perioperative Temperature Management[1,3]	-	-	100%	100%
Prophylactic Antibiotic Selection[1,3]	-	-	99%	99%
Prophylactic Antibiotic Selection (Outpatient)[5]	-	-	98%	98%
Prophylactic Antibiotic Stopped[1,3]	-	-	98%	98%
Prophylactic Antibiotic Timing[1,3]	-	-	98%	99%
Prophylactic Antibiotic Timing (Outpatient)[5]	-	-	98%	98%
Urinary Catheter Removal[1,3]	-	-	97%	97%
Survey of Patients' Hospital Experiences				
Area Around Room 'Always' Quiet at Night	(a)	62%	63%	61%
Doctors 'Always' Communicated Well	(a)	85%	84%	82%
Home Recovery Information Given	(a)	90%	88%	85%
Hospital Given 9 or 10 on 10 Point Scale	(a)	81%	75%	71%
Meds 'Always' Explained Before Given	(a)	64%	66%	64%
Nurses 'Always' Communicated Well	(a)	82%	81%	79%
Pain 'Always' Well Controlled	(a)	78%	71%	71%
Room and Bathroom 'Always' Clean	(a)	77%	79%	73%
Timely Help 'Always' Received	(a)	70%	70%	68%
Would Definitely Recommend Hospital	(a)	83%	74%	71%
Use of Medical Imaging				
Cardiac Imaging Stress Test before Surgery[1]	-	-	4.8%	5.3%
Combination Abdominal CT Scan[1]	-	-	11.5%	10.5%
Combination Brain/Sinus CT Scan	52	0.0%	1.8%	2.7%
Combination Chest CT Scan[1]	-	-	3.5%	2.7%
Follow-up Mammogram/Ultrasound	196	11.2%	7.9%	8.8%
Lumbar Spine MRI for Low Back Pain[1]	-	-	32.2%	37.2%

Mercy Medical Center - Sioux City

801 5th St
Sioux City, IA 51101
URL: www.mercysiouxcity.com
Type: Acute Care Hospitals
Ownership: Voluntary non-profit - Private
Phone: 712-279-2010
Fax: 712-279-5624
Emergency Services: Yes
Beds: 483

Key Personnel:
Radiology. . . . . Jonathan C Beeler, MD
Pediatric Ambulatory Care . . . . . . Vijay Chawala, MD
Pediatric In-Patient Care . . . . Vijay Chawala, MD
CEO/President. . . . . James Fitzpatrick
Coronary Care . . . . Mitchell Horowitz, MD
Quality Assurance . . . . Chris Kelly
Chief of Medical Staff . . . . Jerome Pierson, MD
Infection Control. . . . . Diane Priekfat

Measure	Cases	This Hosp.	State Avg.	U.S. Avg.
Blood Clot Prevention and Treatment				
Anticoagulation Overlap Therapy[2]	71	87%	94%	93%
ICU Venous Thromboembolism Prophylaxis[2]	68	90%	90%	92%
Incidence of Potentially Preventable VTE[1,2]	-	-	8%	10%
UFH with Dosages/Platelet Monitoring[2]	20	100%	99%	97%
Venous Thromboembolism Prophylaxis[2]	320	80%	87%	85%
Warfarin Therapy Discharge Instructions[2]	52	83%	77%	75%
Chest Pain/Possible Heart Attack Care				
Aspirin Given Within 24 Hours of Arrival[5]	-	-	97%	96%
Fibrinolytic Meds Within 30 Min. of Arrival[5]	-	-	49%	58%
Average Time to ECG (minutes)[5]	-	-	5	7
Average Time to Transfer (minutes)[5]	-	-	58	60
Children's Asthma Care				
Received Home Management Plan of Care	-	-	-	88%
Received Reliever Medication	-	-	-	100%
Received Systemic Corticosteroids	-	-	-	100%
Emergency Department				
Admittance Decision Time (minutes)[2]	619	82	58	98
Head CT Results Within 45 Min. of Arrival[3,7]	-	-	55%	57%
Patients Who Left ER Before Being Seen	30,860	1%	1%	2%
Time from ER Arrival to Admit. (minutes)[2]	669	198	202	274
Time from ER Arrival to Discharge (minutes)	406	118	108	134
Time in ER Before Being Evaluated (minutes)	442	10	21	26
Time to Pain Meds for Fractures (minutes)	67	73	46	57
Heart Attack Care				
Aspirin Given at Discharge	319	100%	100%	99%
Fibrinolytic Meds Within 30 Min. of Arrival[7]	-	-	-	54%
PCI Within 90 Minutes of Arrival	35	94%	94%	96%
Statin Prescribed at Discharge	316	100%	98%	98%
Heart Failure Care				
ACE Inhibitor or ARB for LVSD	60	90%	95%	97%
Discharge Instructions Given	155	97%	93%	94%
Evaluation of LVS Function	194	99%	97%	99%
Medicare Spending				
Medicare Spending per Patient (ratio)	-	0.96	0.91	0.98
Pneumonia Care				
Appropriate Initial Antibiotic Given	97	98%	93%	95%
Blood Culture Timing	141	99%	98%	98%
Pregnancy and Delivery Care				
Newborn Deliveries Scheduled Early[2]	34	6%	4%	6%
Preventive Care				
Immunization for Influenza[2]	669	99%	91%	90%
Immunization for Pneumonia[2]	838	98%	90%	92%
Stroke Care				
Anticoagulation Therapy for Atrial Fibrillation	11	91%	95%	95%
Antithrombotic Therapy Timing	74	100%	98%	98%
Assessed for Rehabilitation	93	96%	97%	97%
Discharged on Antithrombotic Therapy	78	100%	99%	99%
Discharged on Statin Medication	61	95%	92%	94%
Thrombolytic Therapy Timing[1]	-	-	64%	66%
Venous Thromboembolism Prophylaxis	102	93%	93%	94%
Written Stroke Educational Materials Given	40	98%	82%	88%
Surgical Care Improvement Project				
Appropriate Beta Blocker Usage	295	100%	98%	98%
Appropriate VTP Within 24 Hours	506	99%	98%	98%
Controlled Postoperative Blood Glucose	61	98%	96%	97%
Perioperative Temperature Management	659	100%	100%	100%
Prophylactic Antibiotic Selection	332	99%	99%	99%

NOTE: Hospital profiles are in alphabetical order by state, then city, then hospital within the city; Rankings exclude hospitals with less than 25 cases except for patient surveys which excludes hospitals with less than 100 cases; (a) 100-299 cases; (1) The number of cases/patients is too few to report; (2) Data submitted were based on a sample of cases/patients; (3) Results are based on a shorter time period than required; (4) Data suppressed by CMS for one or more quarters; (5) Results are not available for this reporting period; (6) Fewer than 100 patients completed the HCAHPS survey; (7) No cases met the criteria for this measure; (8) The lower limit of the confidence interval cannot be calculated if the number of observed infections equals zero; (9) No data are available from the state/territory for this reporting period; (10) The scores shown reflect fewer than 50 completed surveys; (11) There were discrepancies in the data collection process; (12) This measure does not apply to this hospital for this reporting period; (13) Results cannot be calculated for this reporting period; (14) The results for this state are combined with nearby states to protect confidentiality; Please refer to the User's Guide for a full explanation of data.

Measure	Cases	This Hosp.	State Avg.	U.S. Avg.
Prophylactic Antibiotic Selection (Outpatient)	158	99%	98%	98%
Prophylactic Antibiotic Stopped	316	98%	98%	98%
Prophylactic Antibiotic Timing	332	99%	98%	99%
Prophylactic Antibiotic Timing (Outpatient)	164	90%	98%	98%
Urinary Catheter Removal	251	97%	97%	97%
Survey of Patients' Hospital Experiences				
Area Around Room 'Always' Quiet at Night	300+	55%	63%	61%
Doctors 'Always' Communicated Well	300+	78%	84%	82%
Home Recovery Information Given	300+	87%	88%	85%
Hospital Given 9 or 10 on 10 Point Scale	300+	69%	75%	71%
Meds 'Always' Explained Before Given	300+	61%	66%	64%
Nurses 'Always' Communicated Well	300+	74%	81%	79%
Pain 'Always' Well Controlled	300+	66%	71%	71%
Room and Bathroom 'Always' Clean	300+	70%	79%	73%
Timely Help 'Always' Received	300+	60%	70%	68%
Would Definitely Recommend Hospital	300+	71%	74%	71%
Use of Medical Imaging				
Cardiac Imaging Stress Test before Surgery	212	4.7%	4.8%	5.3%
Combination Abdominal CT Scan	491	30.1%	11.5%	10.5%
Combination Brain/Sinus CT Scan	326	0.9%	1.8%	2.7%
Combination Chest CT Scan	176	1.1%	3.5%	2.7%
Follow-up Mammogram/Ultrasound	405	7.2%	7.9%	8.8%
Lumbar Spine MRI for Low Back Pain	62	50.0%	32.2%	37.2%

Saint Luke's Regional Medical Center

2720 Stone Park Boulevard
Sioux City, IA 51104
URL: www.stlukes.org
Type: Acute Care Hospitals
Ownership: Voluntary non-profit - Private
Phone: 712-279-3500
Fax: 712-279-7958
Emergency Services: Yes
Beds: 353

Key Personnel:

Operating Room. . . . . Becky Arnburg, RN
Emergency Room . . . . Paul Berger, MD
Anesthesiology. . . . . Paul Burke, DO
Chief of Medical Staff. . . . . Richard Hildebrand, DO
Quality Assurance . . . . Raeann Isaacson
Pediatric Ambulatory Care . . . . . . Colleen Johnson, RN
Pediatric In-Patient Care . . . . Colleen Johnson, RN
Infection Control. . . . . Dee Pedersen, RN

Measure	Cases	This Hosp.	State Avg.	U.S. Avg.
Blood Clot Prevention and Treatment				
Anticoagulation Overlap Therapy[2]	44	98%	94%	93%
ICU Venous Thromboembolism Prophylaxis[2]	84	89%	90%	92%
Incidence of Potentially Preventable VTE[1,2]	-	-	8%	10%
UFH with Dosages/Platelet Monitoring[1,2]	-	-	99%	97%
Venous Thromboembolism Prophylaxis[2]	263	79%	87%	85%
Warfarin Therapy Discharge Instructions[2]	36	61%	77%	75%
Chest Pain/Possible Heart Attack Care				
Aspirin Given Within 24 Hours of Arrival[5]	-	-	97%	96%
Fibrinolytic Meds Within 30 Min. of Arrival[5]	-	-	49%	58%
Average Time to ECG (minutes)[5]	-	-	5	7
Average Time to Transfer (minutes)[5]	-	-	58	60
Children's Asthma Care				
Received Home Management Plan of Care	-	-	-	88%
Received Reliever Medication	-	-	-	100%
Received Systemic Corticosteroids	-	-	-	100%
Emergency Department				
Admittance Decision Time (minutes)[2]	430	65	58	98
Head CT Results Within 45 Min. of Arrival[3,7]	-	-	55%	57%
Patients Who Left ER Before Being Seen	30,038	2%	1%	2%
Time from ER Arrival to Admit. (minutes)[2]	444	226	202	274
Time from ER Arrival to Discharge (minutes)	362	140	108	134
Time in ER Before Being Evaluated (minutes)	300	29	21	26
Time to Pain Meds for Fractures (minutes)	133	52	46	57
Heart Attack Care				
Aspirin Given at Discharge	104	98%	100%	99%
Fibrinolytic Meds Within 30 Min. of Arrival[7]	-	-	-	54%
PCI Within 90 Minutes of Arrival[1]	-	-	94%	96%
Statin Prescribed at Discharge	100	98%	98%	98%
Heart Failure Care				
ACE Inhibitor or ARB for LVSD	37	95%	95%	97%
Discharge Instructions Given	105	94%	93%	94%
Evaluation of LVS Function	125	99%	97%	99%
Medicare Spending				
Medicare Spending per Patient (ratio)	-	0.93	0.91	0.98
Pneumonia Care				
Appropriate Initial Antibiotic Given	139	98%	93%	95%
Blood Culture Timing	208	98%	98%	98%
Pregnancy and Delivery Care				
Newborn Deliveries Scheduled Early[2]	34	3%	4%	6%
Preventive Care				
Immunization for Influenza[2]	490	96%	91%	90%
Immunization for Pneumonia[2]	453	91%	90%	92%
Stroke Care				
Anticoagulation Therapy for Atrial Fibrillation[1,2]	-	-	95%	95%
Antithrombotic Therapy Timing[2]	41	100%	98%	98%
Assessed for Rehabilitation[2]	57	98%	97%	97%
Discharged on Antithrombotic Therapy[2]	51	100%	99%	99%
Discharged on Statin Medication[2]	41	98%	92%	94%
Thrombolytic Therapy Timing[1,2]	-	-	64%	66%
Venous Thromboembolism Prophylaxis[2]	60	93%	93%	94%
Written Stroke Educational Materials Given[2]	31	97%	82%	88%
Surgical Care Improvement Project				
Appropriate Beta Blocker Usage[2]	193	99%	98%	98%
Appropriate VTP Within 24 Hours[2]	602	99%	98%	98%
Controlled Postoperative Blood Glucose[2,7]	-	-	96%	97%
Perioperative Temperature Management[2]	682	100%	100%	100%
Prophylactic Antibiotic Selection[2]	499	99%	99%	99%
Prophylactic Antibiotic Selection (Outpatient)	193	97%	98%	98%
Prophylactic Antibiotic Stopped[2]	484	98%	98%	98%
Prophylactic Antibiotic Timing[2]	499	99%	98%	99%
Prophylactic Antibiotic Timing (Outpatient)	196	95%	98%	98%
Urinary Catheter Removal[2]	133	77%	97%	97%
Survey of Patients' Hospital Experiences				
Area Around Room 'Always' Quiet at Night	300+	54%	63%	61%
Doctors 'Always' Communicated Well	300+	77%	84%	82%
Home Recovery Information Given	300+	88%	88%	85%
Hospital Given 9 or 10 on 10 Point Scale	300+	71%	75%	71%
Meds 'Always' Explained Before Given	300+	61%	66%	64%
Nurses 'Always' Communicated Well	300+	76%	81%	79%
Pain 'Always' Well Controlled	300+	68%	71%	71%
Room and Bathroom 'Always' Clean	300+	71%	79%	73%
Timely Help 'Always' Received	300+	63%	70%	68%
Would Definitely Recommend Hospital	300+	77%	74%	71%
Use of Medical Imaging				
Cardiac Imaging Stress Test before Surgery[1]	-	-	4.8%	5.3%
Combination Abdominal CT Scan	240	0.8%	11.5%	10.5%
Combination Brain/Sinus CT Scan[1]	-	-	1.8%	2.7%
Combination Chest CT Scan	71	0.0%	3.5%	2.7%
Follow-up Mammogram/Ultrasound[7]	-	-	7.9%	8.8%
Lumbar Spine MRI for Low Back Pain[1]	-	-	32.2%	37.2%

Spencer Municipal Hospital

1200 1st Avenue East
Spencer, IA 51301
E-mail: ddoorn@spencerhospital.org
URL: www.spencerhospital.org
Type: Acute Care Hospitals
Ownership: Government - Local
Phone: 712-264-8300
Fax: 712-264-6404
Emergency Services: Yes
Beds: 99

Key Personnel:

Emergency Room . . . . Deb Brodersen
Radiology. . . . . Charles Crouch
CEO/President. . . . . Jason Harrington
Operating Room. . . . . Jeffre Helmink
Chief of Medical Staff . . . . John Hill

Measure	Cases	This Hosp.	State Avg.	U.S. Avg.
Blood Clot Prevention and Treatment				
Anticoagulation Overlap Therapy[1,2]	-	-	94%	93%
ICU Venous Thromboembolism Prophylaxis[2]	24	75%	90%	92%
Incidence of Potentially Preventable VTE[2,7]	-	-	8%	10%
UFH with Dosages/Platelet Monitoring[1,2]	-	-	99%	97%
Venous Thromboembolism Prophylaxis[2]	152	74%	87%	85%
Warfarin Therapy Discharge Instructions[1,2]	-	-	77%	75%
Chest Pain/Possible Heart Attack Care				
Aspirin Given Within 24 Hours of Arrival	39	95%	97%	96%
Fibrinolytic Meds Within 30 Min. of Arrival[1]	-	-	49%	58%
Average Time to ECG (minutes)	40	8	5	7
Average Time to Transfer (minutes)[1]	-	-	58	60
Children's Asthma Care				
Received Home Management Plan of Care	-	-	-	88%
Received Reliever Medication	-	-	-	100%
Received Systemic Corticosteroids	-	-	-	100%
Emergency Department				
Admittance Decision Time (minutes)[2]	194	38	58	98
Head CT Results Within 45 Min. of Arrival[1,3]	-	-	55%	57%
Patients Who Left ER Before Being Seen	7,888	0%	1%	2%
Time from ER Arrival to Admit. (minutes)[2]	201	174	202	274
Time from ER Arrival to Discharge (minutes)	361	78	108	134
Time in ER Before Being Evaluated (minutes)	417	0	21	26
Time to Pain Meds for Fractures (minutes)	28	44	46	57
Heart Attack Care				
Aspirin Given at Discharge[5]	-	-	100%	99%
Fibrinolytic Meds Within 30 Min. of Arrival[5]	-	-	-	54%
PCI Within 90 Minutes of Arrival[5]	-	-	94%	96%
Statin Prescribed at Discharge[5]	-	-	98%	98%
Heart Failure Care				
ACE Inhibitor or ARB for LVSD[1]	-	-	95%	97%
Discharge Instructions Given	30	100%	93%	94%
Evaluation of LVS Function	39	100%	97%	99%
Medicare Spending				
Medicare Spending per Patient (ratio)	-	0.85	0.91	0.98
Pneumonia Care				
Appropriate Initial Antibiotic Given	43	95%	93%	95%
Blood Culture Timing	59	97%	98%	98%
Pregnancy and Delivery Care				
Newborn Deliveries Scheduled Early	18	17%	4%	6%
Preventive Care				
Immunization for Influenza[2]	289	84%	91%	90%
Immunization for Pneumonia[2]	286	91%	90%	92%
Stroke Care				
Anticoagulation Therapy for Atrial Fibrillation[3,7]	-	-	95%	95%
Antithrombotic Therapy Timing[1,3]	-	-	98%	98%
Assessed for Rehabilitation[1,3]	-	-	97%	97%
Discharged on Antithrombotic Therapy[1,3]	-	-	99%	99%
Discharged on Statin Medication[1,3]	-	-	92%	94%
Thrombolytic Therapy Timing[3,7]	-	-	64%	66%
Venous Thromboembolism Prophylaxis[1,3]	-	-	93%	94%
Written Stroke Educational Materials Given[1,3]	-	-	82%	88%
Surgical Care Improvement Project				
Appropriate Beta Blocker Usage[2]	75	100%	98%	98%
Appropriate VTP Within 24 Hours[2]	202	100%	98%	98%
Controlled Postoperative Blood Glucose[2,7]	-	-	96%	97%
Perioperative Temperature Management[2]	214	100%	100%	100%
Prophylactic Antibiotic Selection[2]	160	99%	99%	99%
Prophylactic Antibiotic Selection (Outpatient)	143	97%	98%	98%
Prophylactic Antibiotic Stopped[2]	159	98%	98%	98%
Prophylactic Antibiotic Timing[2]	160	99%	98%	99%
Prophylactic Antibiotic Timing (Outpatient)	139	96%	98%	98%
Urinary Catheter Removal[2]	176	100%	97%	97%
Survey of Patients' Hospital Experiences				
Area Around Room 'Always' Quiet at Night	300+	68%	63%	61%
Doctors 'Always' Communicated Well	300+	83%	84%	82%
Home Recovery Information Given	300+	90%	88%	85%
Hospital Given 9 or 10 on 10 Point Scale	300+	77%	75%	71%
Meds 'Always' Explained Before Given	300+	70%	66%	64%
Nurses 'Always' Communicated Well	300+	81%	81%	79%
Pain 'Always' Well Controlled	300+	71%	71%	71%
Room and Bathroom 'Always' Clean	300+	80%	79%	73%
Timely Help 'Always' Received	300+	72%	70%	68%
Would Definitely Recommend Hospital	300+	77%	74%	71%
Use of Medical Imaging				
Cardiac Imaging Stress Test before Surgery[1]	-	-	4.8%	5.3%
Combination Abdominal CT Scan	295	26.1%	11.5%	10.5%
Combination Brain/Sinus CT Scan	157	0.6%	1.8%	2.7%
Combination Chest CT Scan	227	28.2%	3.5%	2.7%
Follow-up Mammogram/Ultrasound	713	7.6%	7.9%	8.8%
Lumbar Spine MRI for Low Back Pain	53	32.1%	32.2%	37.2%

NOTE: Hospital profiles are in alphabetical order by state, then city, then hospital within the city; Rankings exclude hospitals with less than 25 cases except for patient surveys which excludes hospitals with less than 100 cases; (a) 100-299 cases; (1) The number of cases/patients is too few to report; (2) Data submitted were based on a sample of cases/patients; (3) Results are based on a shorter time period than required; (4) Data suppressed by CMS for one or more quarters; (5) Results are not available for this reporting period; (6) Fewer than 100 patients completed the HCAHPS survey; (7) No cases met the criteria for this measure; (8) The lower limit of the confidence interval cannot be calculated if the number of observed infections equals zero; (9) No data are available from the state/territory for this reporting period; (10) The scores shown reflect fewer than 50 completed surveys; (11) There were discrepancies in the data collection process; (12) This measure does not apply to this hospital for this reporting period; (13) Results cannot be calculated for this reporting period; (14) The results for this state are combined with nearby states to protect confidentiality; Please refer to the User's Guide for a full explanation of data.

Lakes Regional Healthcare

2301 Highway 71
Spirit Lake, IA 51360
URL: www.lakeshealth.org
Type: Acute Care Hospitals
Ownership: Government - Local

Phone: 712-336-1230
Fax: 712-336-8626

Emergency Services: Yes
Beds: 49

Key Personnel:
Chief of Medical Staff.......... Andrew Brevik
CEO/President............... Jason Harrington
Operating Room.............. Jeffre Helmink
Emergency Room .... Geoff Messerole
Radiology.................. Jim Myerly
Chairman/CEO .... Denny Perry
President.................. Brian Sohn

Measure	Cases	This Hosp.	State Avg.	U.S. Avg.
Blood Clot Prevention and Treatment				
Anticoagulation Overlap Therapy[1,2]	-	-	94%	93%
ICU Venous Thromboembolism Prophylaxis[2]	19	100%	90%	92%
Incidence of Potentially Preventable VTE[1,2]	-	-	8%	10%
UFH with Dosages/Platelet Monitoring[2,7]	-	-	99%	97%
Venous Thromboembolism Prophylaxis[2]	103	88%	87%	85%
Warfarin Therapy Discharge Instructions[1,2]	-	-	77%	75%
Chest Pain/Possible Heart Attack Care				
Aspirin Given Within 24 Hours of Arrival	65	91%	97%	96%
Fibrinolytic Meds Within 30 Min. of Arrival[1]	-	-	49%	58%
Average Time to ECG (minutes)	66	2	5	7
Average Time to Transfer (minutes)[7]	-	-	58	60
Children's Asthma Care				
Received Home Management Plan of Care	-	-	-	88%
Received Reliever Medication	-	-	-	100%
Received Systemic Corticosteroids	-	-	-	100%
Emergency Department				
Admittance Decision Time (minutes)[2]	255	44	58	98
Head CT Results Within 45 Min. of Arrival	15	47%	55%	57%
Patients Who Left ER Before Being Seen	7,069	0%	1%	2%
Time from ER Arrival to Admit. (minutes)[2]	265	165	202	274
Time from ER Arrival to Discharge (minutes)	370	100	108	134
Time in ER Before Being Evaluated (minutes)	529	21	21	26
Time to Pain Meds for Fractures (minutes)	49	45	46	57
Heart Attack Care				
Aspirin Given at Discharge[1]	-	-	100%	99%
Fibrinolytic Meds Within 30 Min. of Arrival[7]	-	-	-	54%
PCI Within 90 Minutes of Arrival[7]	-	-	94%	96%
Statin Prescribed at Discharge[1]	-	-	98%	98%
Heart Failure Care				
ACE Inhibitor or ARB for LVSD[1]	-	-	95%	97%
Discharge Instructions Given	13	92%	93%	94%
Evaluation of LVS Function	19	89%	97%	99%
Medicare Spending				
Medicare Spending per Patient (ratio)	-	0.88	0.91	0.98
Pneumonia Care				
Appropriate Initial Antibiotic Given	50	94%	93%	95%
Blood Culture Timing	54	98%	98%	98%
Pregnancy and Delivery Care				
Newborn Deliveries Scheduled Early	15	20%	4%	6%
Preventive Care				
Immunization for Influenza[2]	289	93%	91%	90%
Immunization for Pneumonia[2]	362	94%	90%	92%
Stroke Care				
Anticoagulation Therapy for Atrial Fibrillation[1]	-	-	95%	95%
Antithrombotic Therapy Timing[1]	-	-	98%	98%
Assessed for Rehabilitation[1]	-	-	97%	97%
Discharged on Antithrombotic Therapy[1]	-	-	99%	99%
Discharged on Statin Medication[1]	-	-	92%	94%
Thrombolytic Therapy Timing[1]	-	-	64%	66%
Venous Thromboembolism Prophylaxis	11	45%	93%	94%
Written Stroke Educational Materials Given[1]	-	-	82%	88%
Surgical Care Improvement Project				
Appropriate Beta Blocker Usage	26	96%	98%	98%
Appropriate VTP Within 24 Hours	70	89%	98%	98%
Controlled Postoperative Blood Glucose[7]	-	-	96%	97%
Perioperative Temperature Management	82	94%	100%	100%
Prophylactic Antibiotic Selection	69	97%	99%	99%
Prophylactic Antibiotic Selection (Outpatient)	17	94%	98%	98%
Prophylactic Antibiotic Stopped	68	90%	98%	98%
Prophylactic Antibiotic Timing	69	96%	98%	99%
Prophylactic Antibiotic Timing (Outpatient)	17	100%	98%	98%
Urinary Catheter Removal	73	100%	97%	97%
Survey of Patients' Hospital Experiences				
Area Around Room 'Always' Quiet at Night	(a)	60%	63%	61%
Doctors 'Always' Communicated Well	(a)	84%	84%	82%
Home Recovery Information Given	(a)	90%	88%	85%
Hospital Given 9 or 10 on 10 Point Scale	(a)	75%	75%	71%
Meds 'Always' Explained Before Given	(a)	67%	66%	64%
Nurses 'Always' Communicated Well	(a)	79%	81%	79%
Pain 'Always' Well Controlled	(a)	70%	71%	71%
Room and Bathroom 'Always' Clean	(a)	76%	79%	73%
Timely Help 'Always' Received	(a)	68%	70%	68%
Would Definitely Recommend Hospital	(a)	71%	74%	71%
Use of Medical Imaging				
Cardiac Imaging Stress Test before Surgery[1]	-	-	4.8%	5.3%
Combination Abdominal CT Scan	116	20.7%	11.5%	10.5%
Combination Brain/Sinus CT Scan[1]	-	-	1.8%	2.7%
Combination Chest CT Scan[1]	-	-	3.5%	2.7%
Follow-up Mammogram/Ultrasound	425	4.0%	7.9%	8.8%
Lumbar Spine MRI for Low Back Pain	57	24.6%	32.2%	37.2%

Buena Vista Regional Medical Center

1525 West 5th Street
Storm Lake, IA 50588
E-mail: marketing-info@bvrmc.org
URL: www.bvrmc.org
Type: Critical Access Hospitals
Ownership: Government - Local

Phone: 712-732-4030
Fax: 712-213-1233

Emergency Services: Yes
Beds: 54

Key Personnel:
Chief of Medical Staff.......... David Archer
CEO/President............... Steven Colerick
Quality Assurance .... Kathy Collins
Operating Room.............. Jason Dierking
Radiology.................. Ingrid Franze
Emergency Room .... Denise Haisch
Infection Control............ Judy Kropf

Measure	Cases	This Hosp.	State Avg.	U.S. Avg.
Blood Clot Prevention and Treatment				
Anticoagulation Overlap Therapy[5]	-	-	94%	93%
ICU Venous Thromboembolism Prophylaxis[5]	-	-	90%	92%
Incidence of Potentially Preventable VTE[5]	-	-	8%	10%
UFH with Dosages/Platelet Monitoring[5]	-	-	99%	97%
Venous Thromboembolism Prophylaxis[5]	-	-	87%	85%
Warfarin Therapy Discharge Instructions[5]	-	-	77%	75%
Chest Pain/Possible Heart Attack Care				
Aspirin Given Within 24 Hours of Arrival[5]	-	-	97%	96%
Fibrinolytic Meds Within 30 Min. of Arrival[5]	-	-	49%	58%
Average Time to ECG (minutes)[5]	-	-	5	7
Average Time to Transfer (minutes)[5]	-	-	58	60
Children's Asthma Care				
Received Home Management Plan of Care	-	-	-	88%
Received Reliever Medication	-	-	-	100%
Received Systemic Corticosteroids	-	-	-	100%
Emergency Department				
Admittance Decision Time (minutes)[5]	-	-	58	98
Head CT Results Within 45 Min. of Arrival[5]	-	-	55%	57%
Patients Who Left ER Before Being Seen[5]	-	-	1%	2%
Time from ER Arrival to Admit. (minutes)[5]	-	-	202	274
Time from ER Arrival to Discharge (minutes)[5]	-	-	108	134
Time in ER Before Being Evaluated (minutes)[5]	-	-	21	26
Time to Pain Meds for Fractures (minutes)[5]	-	-	46	57
Heart Attack Care				
Aspirin Given at Discharge[1,3]	-	-	100%	99%
Fibrinolytic Meds Within 30 Min. of Arrival[3,7]	-	-	-	54%
PCI Within 90 Minutes of Arrival[3,7]	-	-	94%	96%
Statin Prescribed at Discharge[1,3]	-	-	98%	98%
Heart Failure Care				
ACE Inhibitor or ARB for LVSD[1]	-	-	95%	97%
Discharge Instructions Given[1]	-	-	93%	94%
Evaluation of LVS Function	12	75%	97%	99%
Medicare Spending				
Medicare Spending per Patient (ratio)	-	-	0.91	0.98
Pneumonia Care				
Appropriate Initial Antibiotic Given	11	91%	93%	95%
Blood Culture Timing	11	100%	98%	98%
Pregnancy and Delivery Care				
Newborn Deliveries Scheduled Early[5]	-	-	4%	6%
Preventive Care				
Immunization for Influenza[5]	-	-	91%	90%
Immunization for Pneumonia[5]	-	-	90%	92%
Stroke Care				
Anticoagulation Therapy for Atrial Fibrillation[5]	-	-	95%	95%
Antithrombotic Therapy Timing[5]	-	-	98%	98%
Assessed for Rehabilitation[5]	-	-	97%	97%
Discharged on Antithrombotic Therapy[5]	-	-	99%	99%
Discharged on Statin Medication[5]	-	-	92%	94%
Thrombolytic Therapy Timing[5]	-	-	64%	66%
Venous Thromboembolism Prophylaxis[5]	-	-	93%	94%
Written Stroke Educational Materials Given[5]	-	-	82%	88%
Surgical Care Improvement Project				
Appropriate Beta Blocker Usage	11	100%	98%	98%
Appropriate VTP Within 24 Hours	50	94%	98%	98%
Controlled Postoperative Blood Glucose[7]	-	-	96%	97%
Perioperative Temperature Management	58	100%	100%	100%
Prophylactic Antibiotic Selection	53	98%	99%	99%
Prophylactic Antibiotic Selection (Outpatient)[5]	-	-	98%	98%
Prophylactic Antibiotic Stopped	51	96%	98%	98%
Prophylactic Antibiotic Timing	53	94%	98%	99%
Prophylactic Antibiotic Timing (Outpatient)[5]	-	-	98%	98%
Urinary Catheter Removal	40	100%	97%	97%
Survey of Patients' Hospital Experiences				
Area Around Room 'Always' Quiet at Night[5]	-	-	63%	61%
Doctors 'Always' Communicated Well[5]	-	-	84%	82%
Home Recovery Information Given[5]	-	-	88%	85%
Hospital Given 9 or 10 on 10 Point Scale[5]	-	-	75%	71%
Meds 'Always' Explained Before Given[5]	-	-	66%	64%
Nurses 'Always' Communicated Well[5]	-	-	81%	79%
Pain 'Always' Well Controlled[5]	-	-	71%	71%
Room and Bathroom 'Always' Clean[5]	-	-	79%	73%
Timely Help 'Always' Received[5]	-	-	70%	68%
Would Definitely Recommend Hospital[5]	-	-	74%	71%
Use of Medical Imaging				
Cardiac Imaging Stress Test before Surgery[1]	-	-	4.8%	5.3%
Combination Abdominal CT Scan	140	26.4%	11.5%	10.5%
Combination Brain/Sinus CT Scan[1]	-	-	1.8%	2.7%
Combination Chest CT Scan	69	10.1%	3.5%	2.7%
Follow-up Mammogram/Ultrasound	512	1.6%	7.9%	8.8%
Lumbar Spine MRI for Low Back Pain[1]	-	-	32.2%	37.2%

Community Memorial Hospital Medical Center

909 West First Street
Sumner, IA 50674
Type: Critical Access Hospitals
Ownership: Voluntary non-profit - Private

Phone: 563-578-3275

Emergency Services: Yes

Measure	Cases	This Hosp.	State Avg.	U.S. Avg.
Blood Clot Prevention and Treatment				
Anticoagulation Overlap Therapy[5]	-	-	94%	93%
ICU Venous Thromboembolism Prophylaxis[5]	-	-	90%	92%
Incidence of Potentially Preventable VTE[5]	-	-	8%	10%
UFH with Dosages/Platelet Monitoring[5]	-	-	99%	97%
Venous Thromboembolism Prophylaxis[5]	-	-	87%	85%
Warfarin Therapy Discharge Instructions[5]	-	-	77%	75%
Chest Pain/Possible Heart Attack Care				
Aspirin Given Within 24 Hours of Arrival	12	100%	97%	96%
Fibrinolytic Meds Within 30 Min. of Arrival[3,7]	-	-	49%	58%
Average Time to ECG (minutes)	11	7	5	7
Average Time to Transfer (minutes)[1,3]	-	-	58	60
Children's Asthma Care				
Received Home Management Plan of Care	-	-	-	88%
Received Reliever Medication	-	-	-	100%
Received Systemic Corticosteroids	-	-	-	100%
Emergency Department				
Admittance Decision Time (minutes)[5]	-	-	58	98
Head CT Results Within 45 Min. of Arrival[5]	-	-	55%	57%

NOTE: Hospital profiles are in alphabetical order by state, then city, then hospital within the city; Rankings exclude hospitals with less than 25 cases except for patient surveys which excludes hospitals with less than 100 cases; (a) 100-299 cases; (1) The number of cases/patients is too few to report; (2) Data submitted were based on a sample of cases/patients; (3) Results are based on a shorter time period than required; (4) Data suppressed by CMS for one or more quarters; (5) Results are not available for this reporting period; (6) Fewer than 100 patients completed the HCAHPS survey; (7) No cases met the criteria for this measure; (8) The lower limit of the confidence interval cannot be calculated if the number of observed infections equals zero; (9) No data are available from the state/territory for this reporting period; (10) The scores shown reflect fewer than 50 completed surveys; (11) There were discrepancies in the data collection process; (12) This measure does not apply to this hospital for this reporting period; (13) Results cannot be calculated for this reporting period; (14) The results for this state are combined with nearby states to protect confidentiality; Please refer to the User's Guide for a full explanation of data.

Measure	Cases	This Hosp.	State Avg.	U.S. Avg.
Patients Who Left ER Before Being Seen[5]	-	-	1%	2%
Time from ER Arrival to Admit. (minutes)[5]	-	-	202	274
Time from ER Arrival to Discharge (minutes)[5]	-	-	108	134
Time in ER Before Being Evaluated (minutes)[5]	-	-	21	26
Time to Pain Meds for Fractures (minutes)[5]	-	-	46	57
Heart Attack Care				
Aspirin Given at Discharge[5]	-	-	100%	99%
Fibrinolytic Meds Within 30 Min. of Arrival[5]	-	-	-	54%
PCI Within 90 Minutes of Arrival[5]	-	-	94%	96%
Statin Prescribed at Discharge[5]	-	-	98%	98%
Heart Failure Care				
ACE Inhibitor or ARB for LVSD[3,7]	-	-	95%	97%
Discharge Instructions Given[1,3]	-	-	93%	94%
Evaluation of LVS Function[1,3]	-	-	97%	99%
Medicare Spending				
Medicare Spending per Patient (ratio)	-	-	0.91	0.98
Pneumonia Care				
Appropriate Initial Antibiotic Given	13	92%	93%	95%
Blood Culture Timing[1]	-	-	98%	98%
Pregnancy and Delivery Care				
Newborn Deliveries Scheduled Early[5]	-	-	4%	6%
Preventive Care				
Immunization for Influenza[5]	-	-	91%	90%
Immunization for Pneumonia[5]	-	-	90%	92%
Stroke Care				
Anticoagulation Therapy for Atrial Fibrillation[5]	-	-	95%	95%
Antithrombotic Therapy Timing[5]	-	-	98%	98%
Assessed for Rehabilitation[5]	-	-	97%	97%
Discharged on Antithrombotic Therapy[5]	-	-	99%	99%
Discharged on Statin Medication[5]	-	-	92%	94%
Thrombolytic Therapy Timing[5]	-	-	64%	66%
Venous Thromboembolism Prophylaxis[5]	-	-	93%	94%
Written Stroke Educational Materials Given[5]	-	-	82%	88%
Surgical Care Improvement Project				
Appropriate Beta Blocker Usage[5]	-	-	98%	98%
Appropriate VTP Within 24 Hours[5]	-	-	98%	98%
Controlled Postoperative Blood Glucose[5]	-	-	96%	97%
Perioperative Temperature Management[5]	-	-	100%	100%
Prophylactic Antibiotic Selection[5]	-	-	99%	99%
Prophylactic Antibiotic Selection (Outpatient)[5]	-	-	98%	98%
Prophylactic Antibiotic Stopped[5]	-	-	98%	98%
Prophylactic Antibiotic Timing[5]	-	-	98%	99%
Prophylactic Antibiotic Timing (Outpatient)[5]	-	-	98%	98%
Urinary Catheter Removal[5]	-	-	97%	97%
Survey of Patients' Hospital Experiences				
Area Around Room 'Always' Quiet at Night[5]	-	-	63%	61%
Doctors 'Always' Communicated Well[5]	-	-	84%	82%
Home Recovery Information Given[5]	-	-	88%	85%
Hospital Given 9 or 10 on 10 Point Scale[5]	-	-	75%	71%
Meds 'Always' Explained Before Given[5]	-	-	66%	64%
Nurses 'Always' Communicated Well[5]	-	-	81%	79%
Pain 'Always' Well Controlled[5]	-	-	71%	71%
Room and Bathroom 'Always' Clean[5]	-	-	79%	73%
Timely Help 'Always' Received[5]	-	-	70%	68%
Would Definitely Recommend Hospital[5]	-	-	74%	71%
Use of Medical Imaging				
Cardiac Imaging Stress Test before Surgery[7]	-	-	4.8%	5.3%
Combination Abdominal CT Scan	66	1.5%	11.5%	10.5%
Combination Brain/Sinus CT Scan	83	0.0%	1.8%	2.7%
Combination Chest CT Scan[1]	-	-	3.5%	2.7%
Follow-up Mammogram/Ultrasound	101	5.9%	7.9%	8.8%
Lumbar Spine MRI for Low Back Pain[1]	-	-	32.2%	37.2%

Virginia Gay Hospital

502 North 9th Avenue Phone: 319-472-6200
Vinton, IA 52349
Type: Critical Access Hospitals Emergency Services: Yes
Ownership: Voluntary non-profit - Private

Measure	Cases	This Hosp.	State Avg.	U.S. Avg.
Blood Clot Prevention and Treatment				
Anticoagulation Overlap Therapy[3,7]	-	-	94%	93%
ICU Venous Thromboembolism Prophylaxis[3,7]	-	-	90%	92%
Incidence of Potentially Preventable VTE[3,7]	-	-	8%	10%
UFH with Dosages/Platelet Monitoring[3,7]	-	-	99%	97%
Venous Thromboembolism Prophylaxis[1,3]	-	-	87%	85%
Warfarin Therapy Discharge Instructions[3,7]	-	-	77%	75%
Chest Pain/Possible Heart Attack Care				
Aspirin Given Within 24 Hours of Arrival	-	-	97%	96%
Fibrinolytic Meds Within 30 Min. of Arrival	-	-	49%	58%
Average Time to ECG (minutes)	-	-	5	7
Average Time to Transfer (minutes)	-	-	58	60
Children's Asthma Care				
Received Home Management Plan of Care	-	-	-	88%
Received Reliever Medication	-	-	-	100%
Received Systemic Corticosteroids	-	-	-	100%
Emergency Department				
Admittance Decision Time (minutes)[1,3]	-	-	58	98
Head CT Results Within 45 Min. of Arrival	-	-	55%	57%
Patients Who Left ER Before Being Seen	-	-	1%	2%
Time from ER Arrival to Admit. (minutes)[1,3]	-	-	202	274
Time from ER Arrival to Discharge (minutes)	-	-	108	134
Time in ER Before Being Evaluated (minutes)	-	-	21	26
Time to Pain Meds for Fractures (minutes)	-	-	46	57
Heart Attack Care				
Aspirin Given at Discharge[3,7]	-	-	100%	99%
Fibrinolytic Meds Within 30 Min. of Arrival[3,7]	-	-	-	54%
PCI Within 90 Minutes of Arrival[3,7]	-	-	94%	96%
Statin Prescribed at Discharge[3,7]	-	-	98%	98%
Heart Failure Care				
ACE Inhibitor or ARB for LVSD[3,7]	-	-	95%	97%
Discharge Instructions Given[1,3]	-	-	93%	94%
Evaluation of LVS Function[1,3]	-	-	97%	99%
Medicare Spending				
Medicare Spending per Patient (ratio)	-	-	0.91	0.98
Pneumonia Care				
Appropriate Initial Antibiotic Given[1,3]	-	-	93%	95%
Blood Culture Timing[1,3]	-	-	98%	98%
Pregnancy and Delivery Care				
Newborn Deliveries Scheduled Early[5]	-	-	4%	6%
Preventive Care				
Immunization for Influenza[5]	-	-	91%	90%
Immunization for Pneumonia[5]	-	-	90%	92%
Stroke Care				
Anticoagulation Therapy for Atrial Fibrillation[5]	-	-	95%	95%
Antithrombotic Therapy Timing[5]	-	-	98%	98%
Assessed for Rehabilitation[5]	-	-	97%	97%
Discharged on Antithrombotic Therapy[5]	-	-	99%	99%
Discharged on Statin Medication[5]	-	-	92%	94%
Thrombolytic Therapy Timing[5]	-	-	64%	66%
Venous Thromboembolism Prophylaxis[5]	-	-	93%	94%
Written Stroke Educational Materials Given[5]	-	-	82%	88%
Surgical Care Improvement Project				
Appropriate Beta Blocker Usage[1,3]	-	-	98%	98%
Appropriate VTP Within 24 Hours[3,7]	-	-	98%	98%
Controlled Postoperative Blood Glucose[3,7]	-	-	96%	97%
Perioperative Temperature Management[1,3]	-	-	100%	100%
Prophylactic Antibiotic Selection[3,7]	-	-	99%	99%
Prophylactic Antibiotic Selection (Outpatient)	-	-	98%	98%
Prophylactic Antibiotic Stopped[3,7]	-	-	98%	98%
Prophylactic Antibiotic Timing[3,7]	-	-	98%	99%
Prophylactic Antibiotic Timing (Outpatient)	-	-	98%	98%
Urinary Catheter Removal[1,3]	-	-	97%	97%
Survey of Patients' Hospital Experiences				
Area Around Room 'Always' Quiet at Night[5]	-	-	63%	61%
Doctors 'Always' Communicated Well[5]	-	-	84%	82%
Home Recovery Information Given[5]	-	-	88%	85%
Hospital Given 9 or 10 on 10 Point Scale[5]	-	-	75%	71%
Meds 'Always' Explained Before Given[5]	-	-	66%	64%
Nurses 'Always' Communicated Well[5]	-	-	81%	79%
Pain 'Always' Well Controlled[5]	-	-	71%	71%
Room and Bathroom 'Always' Clean[5]	-	-	79%	73%
Timely Help 'Always' Received[5]	-	-	70%	68%
Would Definitely Recommend Hospital[5]	-	-	74%	71%
Use of Medical Imaging				
Cardiac Imaging Stress Test before Surgery	-	-	4.8%	5.3%
Combination Abdominal CT Scan	-	-	11.5%	10.5%
Combination Brain/Sinus CT Scan	-	-	1.8%	2.7%
Combination Chest CT Scan	-	-	3.5%	2.7%
Follow-up Mammogram/Ultrasound	-	-	7.9%	8.8%
Lumbar Spine MRI for Low Back Pain	-	-	32.2%	37.2%

Washington County Hospital & Clinics

400 East Polk Street Phone: 319-653-5481
Washington, IA 52353 Fax: 319-653-3401
URL: www.wchc.org
Type: Critical Access Hospitals Emergency Services: Yes
Ownership: Government - State Beds: 91

Key Personnel:
Radiology. . . . . Douglas Boatman
Emergency Room . . . . Cathy Buffington
CEO/President. . . . . Don Patterson
Chief of Medical Staff . . . . Robin Plattenberger-
Quality Assurance . . . . Kathy Richardson
Operating Room. . . . . Frank Sanfiel

Measure	Cases	This Hosp.	State Avg.	U.S. Avg.
Blood Clot Prevention and Treatment				
Anticoagulation Overlap Therapy[5]	-	-	94%	93%
ICU Venous Thromboembolism Prophylaxis[5]	-	-	90%	92%
Incidence of Potentially Preventable VTE[5]	-	-	8%	10%
UFH with Dosages/Platelet Monitoring[5]	-	-	99%	97%
Venous Thromboembolism Prophylaxis[5]	-	-	87%	85%
Warfarin Therapy Discharge Instructions[5]	-	-	77%	75%
Chest Pain/Possible Heart Attack Care				
Aspirin Given Within 24 Hours of Arrival[5]	-	-	97%	96%
Fibrinolytic Meds Within 30 Min. of Arrival[5]	-	-	49%	58%
Average Time to ECG (minutes)[5]	-	-	5	7
Average Time to Transfer (minutes)[5]	-	-	58	60
Children's Asthma Care				
Received Home Management Plan of Care	-	-	-	88%
Received Reliever Medication	-	-	-	100%
Received Systemic Corticosteroids	-	-	-	100%
Emergency Department				
Admittance Decision Time (minutes)[5]	-	-	58	98
Head CT Results Within 45 Min. of Arrival[5]	-	-	55%	57%
Patients Who Left ER Before Being Seen[5]	-	-	1%	2%
Time from ER Arrival to Admit. (minutes)[5]	-	-	202	274
Time from ER Arrival to Discharge (minutes)[5]	-	-	108	134
Time in ER Before Being Evaluated (minutes)[5]	-	-	21	26
Time to Pain Meds for Fractures (minutes)[5]	-	-	46	57
Heart Attack Care				
Aspirin Given at Discharge[1,3]	-	-	100%	99%
Fibrinolytic Meds Within 30 Min. of Arrival[1,3]	-	-	-	54%
PCI Within 90 Minutes of Arrival[3,7]	-	-	94%	96%
Statin Prescribed at Discharge[1,3]	-	-	98%	98%
Heart Failure Care				
ACE Inhibitor or ARB for LVSD	11	91%	95%	97%
Discharge Instructions Given[1]	-	-	93%	94%
Evaluation of LVS Function	27	81%	97%	99%
Medicare Spending				
Medicare Spending per Patient (ratio)	-	-	0.91	0.98
Pneumonia Care				
Appropriate Initial Antibiotic Given	37	81%	93%	95%
Blood Culture Timing	32	91%	98%	98%
Pregnancy and Delivery Care				
Newborn Deliveries Scheduled Early[5]	-	-	4%	6%
Preventive Care				
Immunization for Influenza[5]	-	-	91%	90%
Immunization for Pneumonia[3]	133	98%	90%	92%
Stroke Care				
Anticoagulation Therapy for Atrial Fibrillation[5]	-	-	95%	95%
Antithrombotic Therapy Timing[5]	-	-	98%	98%
Assessed for Rehabilitation[5]	-	-	97%	97%
Discharged on Antithrombotic Therapy[5]	-	-	99%	99%
Discharged on Statin Medication[5]	-	-	92%	94%
Thrombolytic Therapy Timing[5]	-	-	64%	66%
Venous Thromboembolism Prophylaxis[5]	-	-	93%	94%
Written Stroke Educational Materials Given[5]	-	-	82%	88%
Surgical Care Improvement Project				

NOTE: Hospital profiles are in alphabetical order by state, then city, then hospital within the city; Rankings exclude hospitals with less than 25 cases except for patient surveys which excludes hospitals with less than 100 cases; (a) 100-299 cases; (1) The number of cases/patients is too few to report; (2) Data submitted were based on a sample of cases/patients; (3) Results are based on a shorter time period than required; (4) Data suppressed by CMS for one or more quarters; (5) Results are not available for this reporting period; (6) Fewer than 100 patients completed the HCAHPS survey; (7) No cases met the criteria for this measure; (8) The lower limit of the confidence interval cannot be calculated if the number of observed infections equals zero; (9) No data are available from the state/territory for this reporting period; (10) The scores shown reflect fewer than 50 completed surveys; (11) There were discrepancies in the data collection process; (12) This measure does not apply to this hospital for this reporting period; (13) Results cannot be calculated for this reporting period; (14) The results for this state are combined with nearby states to protect confidentiality; Please refer to the User's Guide for a full explanation of data.

Measure	Cases	This Hosp.	State Avg.	U.S. Avg.
Appropriate Beta Blocker Usage[7]	-	-	98%	98%
Appropriate VTP Within 24 Hours[1]	-	-	98%	98%
Controlled Postoperative Blood Glucose[7]	-	-	96%	97%
Perioperative Temperature Management[1]	-	-	100%	100%
Prophylactic Antibiotic Selection[1]	-	-	99%	99%
Prophylactic Antibiotic Selection (Outpatient)[5]	-	-	98%	98%
Prophylactic Antibiotic Stopped[1]	-	-	98%	98%
Prophylactic Antibiotic Timing[1]	-	-	98%	99%
Prophylactic Antibiotic Timing (Outpatient)[5]	-	-	98%	98%
Urinary Catheter Removal[1]	-	-	97%	97%
Survey of Patients' Hospital Experiences				
Area Around Room 'Always' Quiet at Night	(a)	68%	63%	61%
Doctors 'Always' Communicated Well	(a)	81%	84%	82%
Home Recovery Information Given	(a)	86%	88%	85%
Hospital Given 9 or 10 on 10 Point Scale	(a)	72%	75%	71%
Meds 'Always' Explained Before Given	(a)	64%	66%	64%
Nurses 'Always' Communicated Well	(a)	80%	81%	79%
Pain 'Always' Well Controlled	(a)	76%	71%	71%
Room and Bathroom 'Always' Clean	(a)	77%	79%	73%
Timely Help 'Always' Received	(a)	71%	70%	68%
Would Definitely Recommend Hospital	(a)	73%	74%	71%
Use of Medical Imaging				
Cardiac Imaging Stress Test before Surgery[1]		-	4.8%	5.3%
Combination Abdominal CT Scan	131	5.3%	11.5%	10.5%
Combination Brain/Sinus CT Scan	194	1.0%	1.8%	2.7%
Combination Chest CT Scan	57	5.3%	3.5%	2.7%
Follow-up Mammogram/Ultrasound	363	8.5%	7.9%	8.8%
Lumbar Spine MRI for Low Back Pain[1]	-	-	32.2%	37.2%

Allen Hospital

1825 Logan Avenue
Waterloo, IA 50703
URL: www.allenhospital.org
Type: Acute Care Hospitals
Ownership: Voluntary non-profit - Private
Phone: 319-235-3941
Fax: 319-235-3461
Emergency Services: Yes
Beds: 234

Key Personnel:
Pediatric In-Patient Care .... Dee Van Beiser
Infection Control.............. Bill Farmer
Quality Assurance .... Bill Farmer
Coronary Care................ Deb Gingrich
Chief of Medical Staff.......... Thomas S Gorsche, MD
Pediatric Ambulatory Care ...... Vonice Hoffman
Radiology................... Kent S Quinn
CEO/President............... Richard A Seidler

Measure	Cases	This Hosp.	State Avg.	U.S. Avg.
Blood Clot Prevention and Treatment				
Anticoagulation Overlap Therapy[2]	69	90%	94%	93%
ICU Venous Thromboembolism Prophylaxis[2]	62	82%	90%	92%
Incidence of Potentially Preventable VTE[2]	14	0%	8%	10%
UFH with Dosages/Platelet Monitoring[2]	39	100%	99%	97%
Venous Thromboembolism Prophylaxis[2]	307	89%	87%	85%
Warfarin Therapy Discharge Instructions[2]	54	93%	77%	75%
Chest Pain/Possible Heart Attack Care				
Aspirin Given Within 24 Hours of Arrival[1,3]	-	-	97%	96%
Fibrinolytic Meds Within 30 Min. of Arrival[5]	-	-	49%	58%
Average Time to ECG (minutes)[1,3]	-	-	5	7
Average Time to Transfer (minutes)[5]	-	-	58	60
Children's Asthma Care				
Received Home Management Plan of Care	-	-	-	88%
Received Reliever Medication	-	-	-	100%
Received Systemic Corticosteroids	-	-	-	100%
Emergency Department				
Admittance Decision Time (minutes)[2]	513	90	58	98
Head CT Results Within 45 Min. of Arrival	15	80%	55%	57%
Patients Who Left ER Before Being Seen	34,560	1%	1%	2%
Time from ER Arrival to Admit. (minutes)[2]	518	206	202	274
Time from ER Arrival to Discharge (minutes)	343	160	108	134
Time in ER Before Being Evaluated (minutes)	373	30	21	26
Time to Pain Meds for Fractures (minutes)	77	46	46	57
Heart Attack Care				
Aspirin Given at Discharge	253	100%	100%	99%
Fibrinolytic Meds Within 30 Min. of Arrival[7]	-	-	-	54%
PCI Within 90 Minutes of Arrival	37	92%	94%	96%
Statin Prescribed at Discharge	240	100%	98%	98%
Heart Failure Care				
ACE Inhibitor or ARB for LVSD	77	94%	95%	97%
Discharge Instructions Given	293	95%	93%	94%
Evaluation of LVS Function	384	99%	97%	99%
Medicare Spending				
Medicare Spending per Patient (ratio)	-	0.90	0.91	0.98
Pneumonia Care				
Appropriate Initial Antibiotic Given[2]	107	96%	93%	95%
Blood Culture Timing[2]	210	99%	98%	98%
Pregnancy and Delivery Care				
Newborn Deliveries Scheduled Early[2]	17	0%	4%	6%
Preventive Care				
Immunization for Influenza[2]	508	95%	91%	90%
Immunization for Pneumonia[2]	698	96%	90%	92%
Stroke Care				
Anticoagulation Therapy for Atrial Fibrillation[2]	11	91%	95%	95%
Antithrombotic Therapy Timing[2]	48	94%	98%	98%
Assessed for Rehabilitation[2]	81	98%	97%	97%
Discharged on Antithrombotic Therapy[2]	74	96%	99%	99%
Discharged on Statin Medication[2]	63	84%	92%	94%
Thrombolytic Therapy Timing[2]	30	63%	64%	66%
Venous Thromboembolism Prophylaxis[2]	73	89%	93%	94%
Written Stroke Educational Materials Given[2]	39	85%	82%	88%
Surgical Care Improvement Project				
Appropriate Beta Blocker Usage[2]	249	98%	98%	98%
Appropriate VTP Within 24 Hours[2]	388	99%	98%	98%
Controlled Postoperative Blood Glucose[2]	126	98%	96%	97%
Perioperative Temperature Management[2]	466	99%	100%	100%
Prophylactic Antibiotic Selection[2]	385	99%	99%	99%
Prophylactic Antibiotic Selection (Outpatient)	439	97%	98%	98%
Prophylactic Antibiotic Stopped[2]	383	98%	98%	98%
Prophylactic Antibiotic Timing[2]	390	98%	98%	99%
Prophylactic Antibiotic Timing (Outpatient)	445	96%	98%	98%
Urinary Catheter Removal[2]	160	99%	97%	97%
Survey of Patients' Hospital Experiences				
Area Around Room 'Always' Quiet at Night	300+	57%	63%	61%
Doctors 'Always' Communicated Well	300+	75%	84%	82%
Home Recovery Information Given	300+	91%	88%	85%
Hospital Given 9 or 10 on 10 Point Scale	300+	66%	75%	71%
Meds 'Always' Explained Before Given	300+	57%	66%	64%
Nurses 'Always' Communicated Well	300+	74%	81%	79%
Pain 'Always' Well Controlled	300+	64%	71%	71%
Room and Bathroom 'Always' Clean	300+	71%	79%	73%
Timely Help 'Always' Received	300+	57%	70%	68%
Would Definitely Recommend Hospital	300+	70%	74%	71%
Use of Medical Imaging				
Cardiac Imaging Stress Test before Surgery	412	4.1%	4.8%	5.3%
Combination Abdominal CT Scan	977	2.9%	11.5%	10.5%
Combination Brain/Sinus CT Scan	871	2.5%	1.8%	2.7%
Combination Chest CT Scan	604	0.0%	3.5%	2.7%
Follow-up Mammogram/Ultrasound	2,666	14.1%	7.9%	8.8%
Lumbar Spine MRI for Low Back Pain	239	27.2%	32.2%	37.2%

Covenant Medical Center

3421 West Ninth Street
Waterloo, IA 50702
URL: www.covhealth.com
Type: Acute Care Hospitals
Ownership: Voluntary non-profit - Church
Phone: 319-272-8000
Fax: 319-272-7313
Emergency Services: Yes
Beds: 366

Key Personnel:
Pediatric In-Patient Care .... Siddiq Arab, MD
Chief of Medical Staff.......... Cassandra Foensr, MD
Radiology................... Lawrence Furlong, MD
Intensive Care Unit............ Denise Lampman, RN
Operating Room.............. Niki Maas
Pediatric Ambulatory Care ...... Stephen Riggs, MD
Infection Control.............. Nancy Schuler
Quality Assurance .... Nancy Schuler, RN

Measure	Cases	This Hosp.	State Avg.	U.S. Avg.
Blood Clot Prevention and Treatment				
Anticoagulation Overlap Therapy[2]	48	92%	94%	93%
ICU Venous Thromboembolism Prophylaxis[2]	52	81%	90%	92%
Incidence of Potentially Preventable VTE[1,2]	-	-	8%	10%
UFH with Dosages/Platelet Monitoring[1,2]	-	-	99%	97%
Venous Thromboembolism Prophylaxis[2]	210	83%	87%	85%
Warfarin Therapy Discharge Instructions[2]	38	32%	77%	75%
Chest Pain/Possible Heart Attack Care				
Aspirin Given Within 24 Hours of Arrival[1,3]	-	-	97%	96%
Fibrinolytic Meds Within 30 Min. of Arrival[3,7]	-	-	49%	58%
Average Time to ECG (minutes)[1,3]	-	-	5	7
Average Time to Transfer (minutes)[3,7]	-	-	58	60
Children's Asthma Care				
Received Home Management Plan of Care	-	-	-	88%
Received Reliever Medication	-	-	-	100%
Received Systemic Corticosteroids	-	-	-	100%
Emergency Department				
Admittance Decision Time (minutes)[2]	368	52	58	98
Head CT Results Within 45 Min. of Arrival	14	71%	55%	57%
Patients Who Left ER Before Being Seen	30,822	1%	1%	2%
Time from ER Arrival to Admit. (minutes)[2]	370	212	202	274
Time from ER Arrival to Discharge (minutes)	382	133	108	134
Time in ER Before Being Evaluated (minutes)	413	22	21	26
Time to Pain Meds for Fractures (minutes)	52	40	46	57
Heart Attack Care				
Aspirin Given at Discharge	109	100%	100%	99%
Fibrinolytic Meds Within 30 Min. of Arrival[7]	-	-	-	54%
PCI Within 90 Minutes of Arrival	19	89%	94%	96%
Statin Prescribed at Discharge	107	98%	98%	98%
Heart Failure Care				
ACE Inhibitor or ARB for LVSD	16	100%	95%	97%
Discharge Instructions Given	99	82%	93%	94%
Evaluation of LVS Function	147	99%	97%	99%
Medicare Spending				
Medicare Spending per Patient (ratio)	-	0.98	0.91	0.98
Pneumonia Care				
Appropriate Initial Antibiotic Given	76	93%	93%	95%
Blood Culture Timing	129	98%	98%	98%
Pregnancy and Delivery Care				
Newborn Deliveries Scheduled Early[2]	30	7%	4%	6%
Preventive Care				
Immunization for Influenza[2]	502	87%	91%	90%
Immunization for Pneumonia[2]	449	86%	90%	92%
Stroke Care				
Anticoagulation Therapy for Atrial Fibrillation[1]	-	-	95%	95%
Antithrombotic Therapy Timing	15	100%	98%	98%
Assessed for Rehabilitation	25	100%	97%	97%
Discharged on Antithrombotic Therapy	23	100%	99%	99%
Discharged on Statin Medication	21	86%	92%	94%
Thrombolytic Therapy Timing[1]	-	-	64%	66%
Venous Thromboembolism Prophylaxis	16	69%	93%	94%
Written Stroke Educational Materials Given	17	47%	82%	88%
Surgical Care Improvement Project				
Appropriate Beta Blocker Usage	134	98%	98%	98%
Appropriate VTP Within 24 Hours	332	98%	98%	98%
Controlled Postoperative Blood Glucose[7]	-	-	96%	97%
Perioperative Temperature Management	370	100%	100%	100%
Prophylactic Antibiotic Selection	237	99%	99%	99%
Prophylactic Antibiotic Selection (Outpatient)	404	98%	98%	98%
Prophylactic Antibiotic Stopped	228	97%	98%	98%
Prophylactic Antibiotic Timing	237	100%	98%	99%
Prophylactic Antibiotic Timing (Outpatient)	404	99%	98%	98%
Urinary Catheter Removal	228	97%	97%	97%
Survey of Patients' Hospital Experiences				
Area Around Room 'Always' Quiet at Night[11]	300+	62%	63%	61%
Doctors 'Always' Communicated Well[11]	300+	79%	84%	82%
Home Recovery Information Given[11]	300+	86%	88%	85%
Hospital Given 9 or 10 on 10 Point Scale[11]	300+	70%	75%	71%
Meds 'Always' Explained Before Given[11]	300+	60%	66%	64%
Nurses 'Always' Communicated Well[11]	300+	74%	81%	79%
Pain 'Always' Well Controlled[11]	300+	67%	71%	71%
Room and Bathroom 'Always' Clean[11]	300+	75%	79%	73%
Timely Help 'Always' Received[11]	300+	62%	70%	68%
Would Definitely Recommend Hospital[11]	300+	73%	74%	71%
Use of Medical Imaging				
Cardiac Imaging Stress Test before Surgery	472	4.4%	4.8%	5.3%
Combination Abdominal CT Scan	636	3.3%	11.5%	10.5%

NOTE: Hospital profiles are in alphabetical order by state, then city, then hospital within the city; Rankings exclude hospitals with less than 25 cases except for patient surveys which excludes hospitals with less than 100 cases; (a) 100-299 cases; (1) The number of cases/patients is too few to report; (2) Data submitted were based on a sample of cases/patients; (3) Results are based on a shorter time period than required; (4) Data suppressed by CMS for one or more quarters; (5) Results are not available for this reporting period; (6) Fewer than 100 patients completed the HCAHPS survey; (7) No cases met the criteria for this measure; (8) The lower limit of the confidence interval cannot be calculated if the number of observed infections equals zero; (9) No data are available from the state/territory for this reporting period; (10) The scores shown reflect fewer than 50 completed surveys; (11) There were discrepancies in the data collection process; (12) This measure does not apply to this hospital for this reporting period; (13) Results cannot be calculated for this reporting period; (14) The results for this state are combined with nearby states to protect confidentiality; Please refer to the User's Guide for a full explanation of data.

Measure	Cases	This Hosp.	State Avg.	U.S. Avg.
Combination Brain/Sinus CT Scan	636	1.9%	1.8%	2.7%
Combination Chest CT Scan	342	0.9%	3.5%	2.7%
Follow-up Mammogram/Ultrasound	1,348	10.8%	7.9%	8.8%
Lumbar Spine MRI for Low Back Pain	148	27.7%	32.2%	37.2%

Veterans Memorial Hospital

40 1st Street Se
Waukon, IA 52172
Phone: 563-568-3411
Fax: 563-568-5550
URL: www.vmhospital.com
Type: Critical Access Hospitals
Emergency Services: Yes
Ownership: Government - Local
Beds: 25

Key Personnel:

Chief of Medical Staff.......... Larry Bartel
Emergency Room .... Diane Butikofer
Quality Assurance .... Fred Mathews
CEO .... Michael D Myers
Cardiac Laboratory............ Lynn Ohara
Operating Room............... Barb Wilkes, RN

Measure	Cases	This Hosp.	State Avg.	U.S. Avg.
Blood Clot Prevention and Treatment				
Anticoagulation Overlap Therapy[5]	-	-	94%	93%
ICU Venous Thromboembolism Prophylaxis[5]	-	-	90%	92%
Incidence of Potentially Preventable VTE[5]	-	-	8%	10%
UFH with Dosages/Platelet Monitoring[5]	-	-	99%	97%
Venous Thromboembolism Prophylaxis[5]	-	-	87%	85%
Warfarin Therapy Discharge Instructions[5]	-	-	77%	75%
Chest Pain/Possible Heart Attack Care				
Aspirin Given Within 24 Hours of Arrival	-	-	97%	96%
Fibrinolytic Meds Within 30 Min. of Arrival	-	-	49%	58%
Average Time to ECG (minutes)	-	-	5	7
Average Time to Transfer (minutes)	-	-	58	60
Children's Asthma Care				
Received Home Management Plan of Care	-	-	-	88%
Received Reliever Medication	-	-	-	100%
Received Systemic Corticosteroids	-	-	-	100%
Emergency Department				
Admittance Decision Time (minutes)[5]	-	-	58	98
Head CT Results Within 45 Min. of Arrival	-	-	55%	57%
Patients Who Left ER Before Being Seen	-	-	1%	2%
Time from ER Arrival to Admit. (minutes)[5]	-	-	202	274
Time from ER Arrival to Discharge (minutes)	-	-	108	134
Time in ER Before Being Evaluated (minutes)	-	-	21	26
Time to Pain Meds for Fractures (minutes)	-	-	46	57
Heart Attack Care				
Aspirin Given at Discharge[1]	-	-	100%	99%
Fibrinolytic Meds Within 30 Min. of Arrival[7]	-	-	-	54%
PCI Within 90 Minutes of Arrival[7]	-	-	94%	96%
Statin Prescribed at Discharge[1]	-	-	98%	98%
Heart Failure Care				
ACE Inhibitor or ARB for LVSD[1]	-	-	95%	97%
Discharge Instructions Given[1]	-	-	93%	94%
Evaluation of LVS Function	12	83%	97%	99%
Medicare Spending				
Medicare Spending per Patient (ratio)	-	-	0.91	0.98
Pneumonia Care				
Appropriate Initial Antibiotic Given	29	97%	93%	95%
Blood Culture Timing	24	100%	98%	98%
Pregnancy and Delivery Care				
Newborn Deliveries Scheduled Early[5]	-	-	4%	6%
Preventive Care				
Immunization for Influenza	47	96%	91%	90%
Immunization for Pneumonia	81	93%	90%	92%
Stroke Care				
Anticoagulation Therapy for Atrial Fibrillation[5]	-	-	95%	95%
Antithrombotic Therapy Timing[5]	-	-	98%	98%
Assessed for Rehabilitation[5]	-	-	97%	97%
Discharged on Antithrombotic Therapy[5]	-	-	99%	99%
Discharged on Statin Medication[5]	-	-	92%	94%
Thrombolytic Therapy Timing[5]	-	-	64%	66%
Venous Thromboembolism Prophylaxis[5]	-	-	93%	94%
Written Stroke Educational Materials Given[5]	-	-	82%	88%
Surgical Care Improvement Project				
Appropriate Beta Blocker Usage[1]	-	-	98%	98%
Appropriate VTP Within 24 Hours	28	89%	98%	98%
Controlled Postoperative Blood Glucose[7]	-	-	96%	97%
Perioperative Temperature Management	29	100%	100%	100%
Prophylactic Antibiotic Selection	25	72%	99%	99%
Prophylactic Antibiotic Selection (Outpatient)	-	-	98%	98%
Prophylactic Antibiotic Stopped	24	92%	98%	98%
Prophylactic Antibiotic Timing	25	80%	98%	99%
Prophylactic Antibiotic Timing (Outpatient)	-	-	98%	98%
Urinary Catheter Removal[1]	-	-	97%	97%
Survey of Patients' Hospital Experiences				
Area Around Room 'Always' Quiet at Night[5]	-	-	63%	61%
Doctors 'Always' Communicated Well[5]	-	-	84%	82%
Home Recovery Information Given[5]	-	-	88%	85%
Hospital Given 9 or 10 on 10 Point Scale[5]	-	-	75%	71%
Meds 'Always' Explained Before Given[5]	-	-	66%	64%
Nurses 'Always' Communicated Well[5]	-	-	81%	79%
Pain 'Always' Well Controlled[5]	-	-	71%	71%
Room and Bathroom 'Always' Clean[5]	-	-	79%	73%
Timely Help 'Always' Received[5]	-	-	70%	68%
Would Definitely Recommend Hospital[5]	-	-	74%	71%
Use of Medical Imaging				
Cardiac Imaging Stress Test before Surgery	-	-	4.8%	5.3%
Combination Abdominal CT Scan	-	-	11.5%	10.5%
Combination Brain/Sinus CT Scan	-	-	1.8%	2.7%
Combination Chest CT Scan	-	-	3.5%	2.7%
Follow-up Mammogram/Ultrasound	-	-	7.9%	8.8%
Lumbar Spine MRI for Low Back Pain	-	-	32.2%	37.2%

Waverly Health Center

312 9th Street Sw
Waverly, IA 50677
Phone: 319-352-4120
Fax: 319-352-3992
E-mail: aflessner@wavhosp.org
URL: www.waverlyhealthcenter.org
Type: Critical Access Hospitals
Emergency Services: Yes
Ownership: Government - Local
Beds: 45

Key Personnel:

Radiology..................... Rajeev Anugu
Infection Control............. Dixie Kramer
Pediatric Ambulatory Care .... David Rathe, DO
Pediatric In-Patient Care .... David Rathe, DO
Quality Assurance .... Carol Stone
Chief of Medical Staff.......... Terrie Thurm
CEO/President............... Michael Trachta
Operating Room.............. Lisa Warne

Measure	Cases	This Hosp.	State Avg.	U.S. Avg.
Blood Clot Prevention and Treatment				
Anticoagulation Overlap Therapy[1,3]	-	-	94%	93%
ICU Venous Thromboembolism Prophylaxis[3,7]	-	-	90%	92%
Incidence of Potentially Preventable VTE[3,7]	-	-	8%	10%
UFH with Dosages/Platelet Monitoring[1,3]	-	-	99%	97%
Venous Thromboembolism Prophylaxis[3]	38	95%	87%	85%
Warfarin Therapy Discharge Instructions[1,3]	-	-	77%	75%
Chest Pain/Possible Heart Attack Care				
Aspirin Given Within 24 Hours of Arrival[3]	35	100%	97%	96%
Fibrinolytic Meds Within 30 Min. of Arrival[3,7]	-	-	49%	58%
Average Time to ECG (minutes)[3]	38	8	5	7
Average Time to Transfer (minutes)[1,3]	-	-	58	60
Children's Asthma Care				
Received Home Management Plan of Care	-	-	-	88%
Received Reliever Medication	-	-	-	100%
Received Systemic Corticosteroids	-	-	-	100%
Emergency Department				
Admittance Decision Time (minutes)[2,3]	179	39	58	98
Head CT Results Within 45 Min. of Arrival[5]	-	-	55%	57%
Patients Who Left ER Before Being Seen[5]	-	-	1%	2%
Time from ER Arrival to Admit. (minutes)[2,3]	179	217	202	274
Time from ER Arrival to Discharge (minutes)[3]	29	164	108	134
Time in ER Before Being Evaluated (minutes)[3]	19	28	21	26
Time to Pain Meds for Fractures (minutes)[5]	-	-	46	57
Heart Attack Care				
Aspirin Given at Discharge[1,3]	-	-	100%	99%
Fibrinolytic Meds Within 30 Min. of Arrival[3,7]	-	-	-	54%
PCI Within 90 Minutes of Arrival[3,7]	-	-	94%	96%
Statin Prescribed at Discharge[1,3]	-	-	98%	98%
Heart Failure Care				
ACE Inhibitor or ARB for LVSD[1,3]	-	-	95%	97%
Discharge Instructions Given[1,3]	-	-	93%	94%
Evaluation of LVS Function[1,3]	-	-	97%	99%
Medicare Spending				
Medicare Spending per Patient (ratio)	-	-	0.91	0.98
Pneumonia Care				
Appropriate Initial Antibiotic Given[1,3]	-	-	93%	95%
Blood Culture Timing[3]	26	100%	98%	98%
Pregnancy and Delivery Care				
Newborn Deliveries Scheduled Early[5]	-	-	4%	6%
Preventive Care				
Immunization for Influenza[2,3]	78	76%	91%	90%
Immunization for Pneumonia[2,3]	125	90%	90%	92%
Stroke Care				
Anticoagulation Therapy for Atrial Fibrillation[5]	-	-	95%	95%
Antithrombotic Therapy Timing[5]	-	-	98%	98%
Assessed for Rehabilitation[5]	-	-	97%	97%
Discharged on Antithrombotic Therapy[5]	-	-	99%	99%
Discharged on Statin Medication[5]	-	-	92%	94%
Thrombolytic Therapy Timing[5]	-	-	64%	66%
Venous Thromboembolism Prophylaxis[5]	-	-	93%	94%
Written Stroke Educational Materials Given[5]	-	-	82%	88%
Surgical Care Improvement Project				
Appropriate Beta Blocker Usage[1,3]	-	-	98%	98%
Appropriate VTP Within 24 Hours[3]	27	100%	98%	98%
Controlled Postoperative Blood Glucose[3,7]	-	-	96%	97%
Perioperative Temperature Management[3]	29	100%	100%	100%
Prophylactic Antibiotic Selection[3]	24	100%	99%	99%
Prophylactic Antibiotic Selection (Outpatient)[3]	27	100%	98%	98%
Prophylactic Antibiotic Stopped[3]	23	100%	98%	98%
Prophylactic Antibiotic Timing[3]	24	100%	98%	99%
Prophylactic Antibiotic Timing (Outpatient)[3]	28	96%	98%	98%
Urinary Catheter Removal[1,3]	-	-	97%	97%
Survey of Patients' Hospital Experiences				
Area Around Room 'Always' Quiet at Night	(a)	76%	63%	61%
Doctors 'Always' Communicated Well	(a)	84%	84%	82%
Home Recovery Information Given	(a)	91%	88%	85%
Hospital Given 9 or 10 on 10 Point Scale	(a)	83%	75%	71%
Meds 'Always' Explained Before Given	(a)	70%	66%	64%
Nurses 'Always' Communicated Well	(a)	85%	81%	79%
Pain 'Always' Well Controlled	(a)	76%	71%	71%
Room and Bathroom 'Always' Clean	(a)	84%	79%	73%
Timely Help 'Always' Received	(a)	76%	70%	68%
Would Definitely Recommend Hospital	(a)	81%	74%	71%
Use of Medical Imaging				
Cardiac Imaging Stress Test before Surgery[1]	-	-	4.8%	5.3%
Combination Abdominal CT Scan	349	3.7%	11.5%	10.5%
Combination Brain/Sinus CT Scan[1]	-	-	1.8%	2.7%
Combination Chest CT Scan	145	0.7%	3.5%	2.7%
Follow-up Mammogram/Ultrasound	714	5.0%	7.9%	8.8%
Lumbar Spine MRI for Low Back Pain	69	29.0%	32.2%	37.2%

Van Diest Medical Center

2350 Hospital Drive
Webster City, IA 50595
Phone: 515-832-9400
URL: www.hamiltonhospital.com
Type: Critical Access Hospitals
Emergency Services: Yes
Ownership: Government - Local
Beds: 25

Measure	Cases	This Hosp.	State Avg.	U.S. Avg.
Blood Clot Prevention and Treatment				
Anticoagulation Overlap Therapy[5]	-	-	94%	93%
ICU Venous Thromboembolism Prophylaxis[5]	-	-	90%	92%
Incidence of Potentially Preventable VTE[5]	-	-	8%	10%
UFH with Dosages/Platelet Monitoring[5]	-	-	99%	97%
Venous Thromboembolism Prophylaxis[5]	-	-	87%	85%
Warfarin Therapy Discharge Instructions[5]	-	-	77%	75%
Chest Pain/Possible Heart Attack Care				
Aspirin Given Within 24 Hours of Arrival[5]	-	-	97%	96%
Fibrinolytic Meds Within 30 Min. of Arrival[5]	-	-	49%	58%
Average Time to ECG (minutes)[5]	-	-	5	7
Average Time to Transfer (minutes)[5]	-	-	58	60
Children's Asthma Care				

NOTE: Hospital profiles are in alphabetical order by state, then city, then hospital within the city; Rankings exclude hospitals with less than 25 cases except for patient surveys which excludes hospitals with less than 100 cases; (a) 100-299 cases; (1) The number of cases/patients is too few to report; (2) Data submitted were based on a sample of cases/patients; (3) Results are based on a shorter time period than required; (4) Data suppressed by CMS for one or more quarters; (5) Results are not available for this reporting period; (6) Fewer than 100 patients completed the HCAHPS survey; (7) No cases met the criteria for this measure; (8) The lower limit of the confidence interval cannot be calculated if the number of observed infections equals zero; (9) No data are available from the state/territory for this reporting period; (10) The scores shown reflect fewer than 50 completed surveys; (11) There were discrepancies in the data collection process; (12) This measure does not apply to this hospital for this reporting period; (13) Results cannot be calculated for this reporting period; (14) The results for this state are combined with nearby states to protect confidentiality; Please refer to the User's Guide for a full explanation of data.

Received Home Management Plan of Care	-	-	-	88%
Received Reliever Medication	-	-	-	100%
Received Systemic Corticosteroids	-	-	-	100%
Emergency Department				
Admittance Decision Time (minutes)[5]	-	-	58	98
Head CT Results Within 45 Min. of Arrival[5]	-	-	55%	57%
Patients Who Left ER Before Being Seen	6,054	0%	1%	2%
Time from ER Arrival to Admit. (minutes)[5]	-	-	202	274
Time from ER Arrival to Discharge (minutes)[5]	-	-	108	134
Time in ER Before Being Evaluated (minutes)[5]	-	-	21	26
Time to Pain Meds for Fractures (minutes)[5]	-	-	46	57
Heart Attack Care				
Aspirin Given at Discharge[3,7]	-	-	100%	99%
Fibrinolytic Meds Within 30 Min. of Arrival[3,7]	-	-	-	54%
PCI Within 90 Minutes of Arrival[3,7]	-	-	94%	96%
Statin Prescribed at Discharge[3,7]	-	-	98%	98%
Heart Failure Care				
ACE Inhibitor or ARB for LVSD[1]	-	-	95%	97%
Discharge Instructions Given	35	89%	93%	94%
Evaluation of LVS Function	55	87%	97%	99%
Medicare Spending				
Medicare Spending per Patient (ratio)	-	-	0.91	0.98
Pneumonia Care				
Appropriate Initial Antibiotic Given	29	76%	93%	95%
Blood Culture Timing	27	85%	98%	98%
Pregnancy and Delivery Care				
Newborn Deliveries Scheduled Early[5]	-	-	4%	6%
Preventive Care				
Immunization for Influenza	38	82%	91%	90%
Immunization for Pneumonia[3]	33	97%	90%	92%
Stroke Care				
Anticoagulation Therapy for Atrial Fibrillation[5]	-	-	95%	95%
Antithrombotic Therapy Timing[5]	-	-	98%	98%
Assessed for Rehabilitation[5]	-	-	97%	97%
Discharged on Antithrombotic Therapy[5]	-	-	99%	99%
Discharged on Statin Medication[5]	-	-	92%	94%
Thrombolytic Therapy Timing[5]	-	-	64%	66%
Venous Thromboembolism Prophylaxis[5]	-	-	93%	94%
Written Stroke Educational Materials Given[5]	-	-	82%	88%
Surgical Care Improvement Project				
Appropriate Beta Blocker Usage[1,3]	-	-	98%	98%
Appropriate VTP Within 24 Hours[1,3]	-	-	98%	98%
Controlled Postoperative Blood Glucose[3,7]	-	-	96%	97%
Perioperative Temperature Management[1,3]	-	-	100%	100%
Prophylactic Antibiotic Selection[1,3]	-	-	99%	99%
Prophylactic Antibiotic Selection (Outpatient)[5]	-	-	98%	98%
Prophylactic Antibiotic Stopped[1,3]	-	-	98%	98%
Prophylactic Antibiotic Timing[1,3]	-	-	98%	99%
Prophylactic Antibiotic Timing (Outpatient)[5]	-	-	98%	98%
Urinary Catheter Removal[3,7]	-	-	97%	97%
Survey of Patients' Hospital Experiences				
Area Around Room 'Always' Quiet at Night	(a)	61%	63%	61%
Doctors 'Always' Communicated Well	(a)	80%	84%	82%
Home Recovery Information Given	(a)	76%	88%	85%
Hospital Given 9 or 10 on 10 Point Scale	(a)	61%	75%	71%
Meds 'Always' Explained Before Given	(a)	51%	66%	64%
Nurses 'Always' Communicated Well	(a)	71%	81%	79%
Pain 'Always' Well Controlled	(a)	68%	71%	71%
Room and Bathroom 'Always' Clean	(a)	83%	79%	73%
Timely Help 'Always' Received	(a)	53%	70%	68%
Would Definitely Recommend Hospital	(a)	61%	74%	71%
Use of Medical Imaging				
Cardiac Imaging Stress Test before Surgery[1]	-	-	4.8%	5.3%
Combination Abdominal CT Scan	203	3.9%	11.5%	10.5%
Combination Brain/Sinus CT Scan[1]	-	-	1.8%	2.7%
Combination Chest CT Scan	90	5.6%	3.5%	2.7%
Follow-up Mammogram/Ultrasound[1]	-	-	7.9%	8.8%
Lumbar Spine MRI for Low Back Pain[1]	-	-	32.2%	37.2%

Great River Medical Center

1221 South Gear Avenue
West Burlington, IA 52655
URL: www.greatrivermedical.org
Phone: 319-768-1000
Fax: 319-768-3306
Type: Acute Care Hospitals
Emergency Services: Yes
Ownership: Voluntary non-profit - Private
Beds: 378

Key Personnel:

Radiology. Donald Gale, MD
Operating Room. . . . . Ann Hannum, RN
Chief of Medical Staff. . . . . Doug Peters, MD
CEO/President. . . . . Mark Richardson
Intensive Care Unit. . . . . Edna Smull, MD
Emergency Room . . . . James Vandenberg, MD
Quality Assurance . . . . Tom Zimmerman

Measure	Cases	This Hosp.	State Avg.	U.S. Avg.
Blood Clot Prevention and Treatment				
Anticoagulation Overlap Therapy[2]	53	91%	94%	93%
ICU Venous Thromboembolism Prophylaxis[2]	78	86%	90%	92%
Incidence of Potentially Preventable VTE[1,2]	-	-	8%	10%
UFH with Dosages/Platelet Monitoring[2]	46	100%	99%	97%
Venous Thromboembolism Prophylaxis[2]	285	89%	87%	85%
Warfarin Therapy Discharge Instructions[2]	41	100%	77%	75%
Chest Pain/Possible Heart Attack Care				
Aspirin Given Within 24 Hours of Arrival	38	100%	97%	96%
Fibrinolytic Meds Within 30 Min. of Arrival[1]	-	-	49%	58%
Average Time to ECG (minutes)	38	6	5	7
Average Time to Transfer (minutes)[1]	-	-	58	60
Children's Asthma Care				
Received Home Management Plan of Care	-	-	-	88%
Received Reliever Medication	-	-	-	100%
Received Systemic Corticosteroids	-	-	-	100%
Emergency Department				
Admittance Decision Time (minutes)[2]	668	55	58	98
Head CT Results Within 45 Min. of Arrival	21	71%	55%	57%
Patients Who Left ER Before Being Seen	32,992	1%	1%	2%
Time from ER Arrival to Admit. (minutes)[2]	721	181	202	274
Time from ER Arrival to Discharge (minutes)	379	91	108	134
Time in ER Before Being Evaluated (minutes)	387	20	21	26
Time to Pain Meds for Fractures (minutes)	79	40	46	57
Heart Attack Care				
Aspirin Given at Discharge	150	99%	100%	99%
Fibrinolytic Meds Within 30 Min. of Arrival[7]	-	-	-	54%
PCI Within 90 Minutes of Arrival	17	88%	94%	96%
Statin Prescribed at Discharge	133	97%	98%	98%
Heart Failure Care				
ACE Inhibitor or ARB for LVSD	34	100%	95%	97%
Discharge Instructions Given	95	97%	93%	94%
Evaluation of LVS Function	127	100%	97%	99%
Medicare Spending				
Medicare Spending per Patient (ratio)	-	0.86	0.91	0.98
Pneumonia Care				
Appropriate Initial Antibiotic Given	106	98%	93%	95%
Blood Culture Timing	178	100%	98%	98%
Pregnancy and Delivery Care				
Newborn Deliveries Scheduled Early[2]	27	15%	4%	6%
Preventive Care				
Immunization for Influenza[2]	553	90%	91%	90%
Immunization for Pneumonia[2]	724	92%	90%	92%
Stroke Care				
Anticoagulation Therapy for Atrial Fibrillation[1]	-	-	95%	95%
Antithrombotic Therapy Timing	47	98%	98%	98%
Assessed for Rehabilitation	53	100%	97%	97%
Discharged on Antithrombotic Therapy	50	100%	99%	99%
Discharged on Statin Medication	39	100%	92%	94%
Thrombolytic Therapy Timing[7]	-	-	64%	66%
Venous Thromboembolism Prophylaxis	52	98%	93%	94%
Written Stroke Educational Materials Given	23	100%	82%	88%
Surgical Care Improvement Project				
Appropriate Beta Blocker Usage	217	99%	98%	98%
Appropriate VTP Within 24 Hours	518	99%	98%	98%
Controlled Postoperative Blood Glucose[7]	-	-	96%	97%
Perioperative Temperature Management	570	100%	100%	100%
Prophylactic Antibiotic Selection	402	99%	99%	99%
Prophylactic Antibiotic Selection (Outpatient)	233	98%	98%	98%
Prophylactic Antibiotic Stopped	397	98%	98%	98%
Prophylactic Antibiotic Timing	402	99%	98%	99%
Prophylactic Antibiotic Timing (Outpatient)	233	98%	98%	98%
Urinary Catheter Removal	448	100%	97%	97%
Survey of Patients' Hospital Experiences				
Area Around Room 'Always' Quiet at Night	300+	63%	63%	61%
Doctors 'Always' Communicated Well	300+	80%	84%	82%
Home Recovery Information Given	300+	86%	88%	85%
Hospital Given 9 or 10 on 10 Point Scale	300+	70%	75%	71%
Meds 'Always' Explained Before Given	300+	64%	66%	64%
Nurses 'Always' Communicated Well	300+	78%	81%	79%
Pain 'Always' Well Controlled	300+	69%	71%	71%
Room and Bathroom 'Always' Clean	300+	75%	79%	73%
Timely Help 'Always' Received	300+	65%	70%	68%
Would Definitely Recommend Hospital	300+	67%	74%	71%
Use of Medical Imaging				
Cardiac Imaging Stress Test before Surgery	487	7.4%	4.8%	5.3%
Combination Abdominal CT Scan	874	52.1%	11.5%	10.5%
Combination Brain/Sinus CT Scan	738	2.4%	1.8%	2.7%
Combination Chest CT Scan	592	3.2%	3.5%	2.7%
Follow-up Mammogram/Ultrasound	1,597	7.3%	7.9%	8.8%
Lumbar Spine MRI for Low Back Pain	167	35.3%	32.2%	37.2%

Palmer Lutheran Health Center

112 Jefferson Street
West Union, IA 52175
Phone: 563-422-3811
Fax: 563-422-3664
Type: Critical Access Hospitals
Emergency Services: Yes
Ownership: Voluntary non-profit - Private
Beds: 25

Key Personnel:

Quality Assurance . . . . Julie Ball
Chief of Medical Staff. . . . . Chaudri Rasool
Operating Room. . . . . Sue Schneider, RN
CEO . . . . Steve Stark
Emergency Room . . . . Jon Suddarth, RN

Measure	Cases	This Hosp.	State Avg.	U.S. Avg.
Blood Clot Prevention and Treatment				
Anticoagulation Overlap Therapy[5]	-	-	94%	93%
ICU Venous Thromboembolism Prophylaxis[5]	-	-	90%	92%
Incidence of Potentially Preventable VTE[5]	-	-	8%	10%
UFH with Dosages/Platelet Monitoring[5]	-	-	99%	97%
Venous Thromboembolism Prophylaxis[5]	-	-	87%	85%
Warfarin Therapy Discharge Instructions[5]	-	-	77%	75%
Chest Pain/Possible Heart Attack Care				
Aspirin Given Within 24 Hours of Arrival[5]	-	-	97%	96%
Fibrinolytic Meds Within 30 Min. of Arrival[5]	-	-	49%	58%
Average Time to ECG (minutes)[5]	-	-	5	7
Average Time to Transfer (minutes)[5]	-	-	58	60
Children's Asthma Care				
Received Home Management Plan of Care	-	-	-	88%
Received Reliever Medication	-	-	-	100%
Received Systemic Corticosteroids	-	-	-	100%
Emergency Department				
Admittance Decision Time (minutes)[5]	-	-	58	98
Head CT Results Within 45 Min. of Arrival[5]	-	-	55%	57%
Patients Who Left ER Before Being Seen	3,594	1%	1%	2%
Time from ER Arrival to Admit. (minutes)[5]	-	-	202	274
Time from ER Arrival to Discharge (minutes)[5]	-	-	108	134
Time in ER Before Being Evaluated (minutes)[5]	-	-	21	26
Time to Pain Meds for Fractures (minutes)[5]	-	-	46	57
Heart Attack Care				
Aspirin Given at Discharge[5]	-	-	100%	99%
Fibrinolytic Meds Within 30 Min. of Arrival[5]	-	-	-	54%
PCI Within 90 Minutes of Arrival[5]	-	-	94%	96%
Statin Prescribed at Discharge[5]	-	-	98%	98%
Heart Failure Care				
ACE Inhibitor or ARB for LVSD[1]	-	-	95%	97%
Discharge Instructions Given[1]	-	-	93%	94%
Evaluation of LVS Function[1]	-	-	97%	99%
Medicare Spending				
Medicare Spending per Patient (ratio)	-	-	0.91	0.98
Pneumonia Care				
Appropriate Initial Antibiotic Given	17	88%	93%	95%
Blood Culture Timing	21	100%	98%	98%

NOTE: Hospital profiles are in alphabetical order by state, then city, then hospital within the city; Rankings exclude hospitals with less than 25 cases except for patient surveys which excludes hospitals with less than 100 cases; (a) 100-299 cases; (1) The number of cases/patients is too few to report; (2) Data submitted were based on a sample of cases/patients; (3) Results are based on a shorter time period than required; (4) Data suppressed by CMS for one or more quarters; (5) Results are not available for this reporting period; (6) Fewer than 100 patients completed the HCAHPS survey; (7) No cases met the criteria for this measure; (8) The lower limit of the confidence interval cannot be calculated if the number of observed infections equals zero; (9) No data are available from the state/territory for this reporting period; (10) The scores shown reflect fewer than 50 completed surveys; (11) There were discrepancies in the data collection process; (12) This measure does not apply to this hospital for this reporting period; (13) Results cannot be calculated for this reporting period; (14) The results for this state are combined with nearby states to protect confidentiality; Please refer to the User's Guide for a full explanation of data.

Pregnancy and Delivery Care				
Newborn Deliveries Scheduled Early[5]	-	-	4%	6%
Preventive Care				
Immunization for Influenza[5]	-	-	91%	90%
Immunization for Pneumonia[5]	-	-	90%	92%
Stroke Care				
Anticoagulation Therapy for Atrial Fibrillation[5]	-	-	95%	95%
Antithrombotic Therapy Timing[5]	-	-	98%	98%
Assessed for Rehabilitation[5]	-	-	97%	97%
Discharged on Antithrombotic Therapy[5]	-	-	99%	99%
Discharged on Statin Medication[5]	-	-	92%	94%
Thrombolytic Therapy Timing[5]	-	-	64%	66%
Venous Thromboembolism Prophylaxis[5]	-	-	93%	94%
Written Stroke Educational Materials Given[5]	-	-	82%	88%
Surgical Care Improvement Project				
Appropriate Beta Blocker Usage[5]	-	-	98%	98%
Appropriate VTP Within 24 Hours[5]	-	-	98%	98%
Controlled Postoperative Blood Glucose[5]	-	-	96%	97%
Perioperative Temperature Management[5]	-	-	100%	100%
Prophylactic Antibiotic Selection[5]	-	-	99%	99%
Prophylactic Antibiotic Selection (Outpatient)[5]	-	-	98%	98%
Prophylactic Antibiotic Stopped[5]	-	-	98%	98%
Prophylactic Antibiotic Timing[5]	-	-	98%	99%
Prophylactic Antibiotic Timing (Outpatient)[5]	-	-	98%	98%
Urinary Catheter Removal[5]	-	-	97%	97%
Survey of Patients' Hospital Experiences				
Area Around Room 'Always' Quiet at Night[5]	-	-	63%	61%
Doctors 'Always' Communicated Well[5]	-	-	84%	82%
Home Recovery Information Given[5]	-	-	88%	85%
Hospital Given 9 or 10 on 10 Point Scale[5]	-	-	75%	71%
Meds 'Always' Explained Before Given[5]	-	-	66%	64%
Nurses 'Always' Communicated Well[5]	-	-	81%	79%
Pain 'Always' Well Controlled[5]	-	-	71%	71%
Room and Bathroom 'Always' Clean[5]	-	-	79%	73%
Timely Help 'Always' Received[5]	-	-	70%	68%
Would Definitely Recommend Hospital[5]	-	-	74%	71%
Use of Medical Imaging				
Cardiac Imaging Stress Test before Surgery[1]	-	-	4.8%	5.3%
Combination Abdominal CT Scan	141	1.4%	11.5%	10.5%
Combination Brain/Sinus CT Scan[1]	-	-	1.8%	2.7%
Combination Chest CT Scan	91	0.0%	3.5%	2.7%
Follow-up Mammogram/Ultrasound[7]	-	-	7.9%	8.8%
Lumbar Spine MRI for Low Back Pain[1]	-	-	32.2%	37.2%

Madison County Memorial Hospital

300 West Hutchings Street
Winterset, IA 50273
Phone: 515-462-2373
Fax: 515-462-5008
URL: www.madisonhealth.com
Type: Critical Access Hospitals
Ownership: Government - Local
Emergency Services: Yes
Beds: 31

Key Personnel:
Chief of Medical Staff.......... Sherrie Broadbent
Emergency Room .... Cindy Frank
CEO .... Marcia Hendricks, RN, MHA, FACHE
Operating Room.............. Janet Loomis
Quality Assurance .... Terri Simmons

Measure	Cases	This Hosp.	State Avg.	U.S. Avg.
Blood Clot Prevention and Treatment				
Anticoagulation Overlap Therapy[5]	-	-	94%	93%
ICU Venous Thromboembolism Prophylaxis[5]	-	-	90%	92%
Incidence of Potentially Preventable VTE[5]	-	-	8%	10%
UFH with Dosages/Platelet Monitoring[5]	-	-	99%	97%
Venous Thromboembolism Prophylaxis[5]	-	-	87%	85%
Warfarin Therapy Discharge Instructions[5]	-	-	77%	75%
Chest Pain/Possible Heart Attack Care				
Aspirin Given Within 24 Hours of Arrival	-	-	97%	96%
Fibrinolytic Meds Within 30 Min. of Arrival	-	-	49%	58%
Average Time to ECG (minutes)	-	-	5	7
Average Time to Transfer (minutes)	-	-	58	60
Children's Asthma Care				
Received Home Management Plan of Care	-	-	-	88%
Received Reliever Medication	-	-	-	100%
Received Systemic Corticosteroids	-	-	-	100%
Emergency Department				
Admittance Decision Time (minutes)[5]	-	-	58	98
Head CT Results Within 45 Min. of Arrival	-	-	55%	57%
Patients Who Left ER Before Being Seen	-	-	1%	2%
Time from ER Arrival to Admit. (minutes)[5]	-	-	202	274
Time from ER Arrival to Discharge (minutes)	-	-	108	134
Time in ER Before Being Evaluated (minutes)	-	-	21	26
Time to Pain Meds for Fractures (minutes)	-	-	46	57
Heart Attack Care				
Aspirin Given at Discharge[1,3]	-	-	100%	99%
Fibrinolytic Meds Within 30 Min. of Arrival[3,7]	-	-	-	54%
PCI Within 90 Minutes of Arrival[3,7]	-	-	94%	96%
Statin Prescribed at Discharge[1,3]	-	-	98%	98%
Heart Failure Care				
ACE Inhibitor or ARB for LVSD[1]	-	-	95%	97%
Discharge Instructions Given	13	77%	93%	94%
Evaluation of LVS Function	15	67%	97%	99%
Medicare Spending				
Medicare Spending per Patient (ratio)	-	-	0.91	0.98
Pneumonia Care				
Appropriate Initial Antibiotic Given	16	38%	93%	95%
Blood Culture Timing	17	82%	98%	98%
Pregnancy and Delivery Care				
Newborn Deliveries Scheduled Early[5]	-	-	4%	6%
Preventive Care				
Immunization for Influenza[5]	-	-	91%	90%
Immunization for Pneumonia[5]	-	-	90%	92%
Stroke Care				
Anticoagulation Therapy for Atrial Fibrillation[5]	-	-	95%	95%
Antithrombotic Therapy Timing[5]	-	-	98%	98%
Assessed for Rehabilitation[5]	-	-	97%	97%
Discharged on Antithrombotic Therapy[5]	-	-	99%	99%
Discharged on Statin Medication[5]	-	-	92%	94%
Thrombolytic Therapy Timing[5]	-	-	64%	66%
Venous Thromboembolism Prophylaxis[5]	-	-	93%	94%
Written Stroke Educational Materials Given[5]	-	-	82%	88%
Surgical Care Improvement Project				
Appropriate Beta Blocker Usage[5]	-	-	98%	98%
Appropriate VTP Within 24 Hours[5]	-	-	98%	98%
Controlled Postoperative Blood Glucose[5]	-	-	96%	97%
Perioperative Temperature Management[5]	-	-	100%	100%
Prophylactic Antibiotic Selection[5]	-	-	99%	99%
Prophylactic Antibiotic Selection (Outpatient)	-	-	98%	98%
Prophylactic Antibiotic Stopped[5]	-	-	98%	98%
Prophylactic Antibiotic Timing[5]	-	-	98%	99%
Prophylactic Antibiotic Timing (Outpatient)	-	-	98%	98%
Urinary Catheter Removal[5]	-	-	97%	97%
Survey of Patients' Hospital Experiences				
Area Around Room 'Always' Quiet at Night[6]	<100	81%	63%	61%
Doctors 'Always' Communicated Well[6]	<100	88%	84%	82%
Home Recovery Information Given[6]	<100	95%	88%	85%
Hospital Given 9 or 10 on 10 Point Scale[6]	<100	85%	75%	71%
Meds 'Always' Explained Before Given[6]	<100	82%	66%	64%
Nurses 'Always' Communicated Well[6]	<100	84%	81%	79%
Pain 'Always' Well Controlled[6]	<100	74%	71%	71%
Room and Bathroom 'Always' Clean[6]	<100	76%	79%	73%
Timely Help 'Always' Received[6]	<100	75%	70%	68%
Would Definitely Recommend Hospital[6]	<100	90%	74%	71%
Use of Medical Imaging				
Cardiac Imaging Stress Test before Surgery	-	-	4.8%	5.3%
Combination Abdominal CT Scan	-	-	11.5%	10.5%
Combination Brain/Sinus CT Scan	-	-	1.8%	2.7%
Combination Chest CT Scan	-	-	3.5%	2.7%
Follow-up Mammogram/Ultrasound	-	-	7.9%	8.8%
Lumbar Spine MRI for Low Back Pain	-	-	32.2%	37.2%

NOTE: Hospital profiles are in alphabetical order by state, then city, then hospital within the city; Rankings exclude hospitals with less than 25 cases except for patient surveys which excludes hospitals with less than 100 cases; (a) 100-299 cases; (1) The number of cases/patients is too few to report; (2) Data submitted were based on a sample of cases/patients; (3) Results are based on a shorter time period than required; (4) Data suppressed by CMS for one or more quarters; (5) Results are not available for this reporting period; (6) Fewer than 100 patients completed the HCAHPS survey; (7) No cases met the criteria for this measure; (8) The lower limit of the confidence interval cannot be calculated if the number of observed infections equals zero; (9) No data are available from the state/territory for this reporting period; (10) The scores shown reflect fewer than 50 completed surveys; (11) There were discrepancies in the data collection process; (12) This measure does not apply to this hospital for this reporting period; (13) Results cannot be calculated for this reporting period; (14) The results for this state are combined with nearby states to protect confidentiality; Please refer to the User's Guide for a full explanation of data.

Blood Clot Prevention and Treatment

Anticoagulation Overlap Therapy

Hospital Name	City	Rate	Cases
Lawrence Memorial Hospital[2]	Lawrence	100%	31
Overland Park Regional Medical Center[2]	Overland Park	100%	63
Wesley Medical Center[2]	Wichita	100%	132
Shawnee Mission Medical Center[2]	Shawnee Miss.	99%	145
University of Kansas Hospital[2]	Kansas City	98%	173
Menorah Medical Center[2]	Overland Park	97%	35
Mercy Regional Health Center[2]	Manhattan	97%	31
Hays Medical Center[2]	Hays	96%	47
Providence Medical Center[2]	Kansas City	95%	61
Olathe Medical Center[2]	Olathe	94%	63
Newton Medical Center[2]	Newton	93%	42
Saint Francis Health Center[2]	Topeka	92%	76
Salina Regional Health Center[2]	Salina	92%	64
Via Christi Hospitals Wichita[2]	Wichita	92%	170
Saint Luke's South Hospital[2]	Overland Park	91%	33
Stormont - Vail Healthcare[2]	Topeka	90%	116
Hutchinson Regional Medical Center[2]	Hutchinson	78%	55

ICU Venous Thromboembolism Prophylaxis

Hospital Name	City	Rate	Cases
Kansas Medical Center[2]	Andover	100%	70
Labette Health[2]	Parsons	100%	34
Menorah Medical Center[2]	Overland Park	100%	80
Overland Park Regional Medical Center[2]	Overland Park	100%	133
Stormont - Vail Healthcare[2]	Topeka	100%	94
Via Christi Hospital Pittsburg[2]	Pittsburg	100%	67
Wesley Medical Center[2]	Wichita	100%	195
Saint Catherine Hospital[2]	Garden City	99%	109
Shawnee Mission Medical Center[2]	Shawnee Miss.	98%	50
Southwest Medical Center[2]	Liberal	98%	45
Via Christi Hospitals Wichita[2]	Wichita	98%	151
Western Plains Medical Complex[2]	Dodge City	98%	107
University of Kansas Hospital[2]	Kansas City	97%	100
Via Christi Hospital Wichita Saint Teresa[2]	Wichita	97%	31
Ransom Memorial Hospital[2]	Ottawa	96%	25
Saint John Hospital[2]	Leavenworth	96%	50
Mercy Hospital - Fort Scott[2]	Fort Scott	95%	39
Saint Francis Health Center[2]	Topeka	95%	88
Newman Regional Health[2]	Emporia	94%	35
Lawrence Memorial Hospital[2]	Lawrence	93%	30
Saint Luke's Cushing Hospital[2]	Leavenworth	93%	29
Kansas Heart Hospital[2]	Wichita	92%	195
McPherson Hospital[2]	Mcpherson	92%	75
Providence Medical Center[2]	Kansas City	92%	80
Salina Regional Health Center[2]	Salina	90%	78
Mercy Hospital Independence[2]	Independence	88%	33
Newton Medical Center[2]	Newton	87%	46
Hays Medical Center[2]	Hays	86%	73
Coffeyville Regional Medical Center[2]	Coffeyville	85%	54
Olathe Medical Center[2]	Olathe	85%	74
Geary Community Hospital[2]	Junction City	82%	65
William Newton Hospital	Winfield	76%	34
Pratt Regional Medical Center[2]	Pratt	72%	25
Mercy Regional Health Center[2]	Manhattan	67%	60
Morton County Hospital[2]	Elkhart	66%	29
Saint Luke's South Hospital[2]	Overland Park	65%	48
Hutchinson Regional Medical Center[2]	Hutchinson	50%	134

Incidence of Potentially Preventable VTE

Hospital Name	City	Rate	Cases
Via Christi Hospitals Wichita[2]	Wichita	3%	30
University of Kansas Hospital[2]	Kansas City	4%	84

UFH with Dosages/Platelet Count Monitoring

Hospital Name	City	Rate	Cases
Overland Park Regional Medical Center[2]	Overland Park	100%	60
Providence Medical Center[2]	Kansas City	100%	42
Saint Francis Health Center[2]	Topeka	100%	54
Stormont - Vail Healthcare[2]	Topeka	100%	97
Via Christi Hospitals Wichita[2]	Wichita	100%	94
Wesley Medical Center[2]	Wichita	100%	56
Hays Medical Center[2]	Hays	97%	29
Via Christi Hospital Pittsburg[2]	Pittsburg	96%	26
University of Kansas Hospital[2]	Kansas City	92%	144

Venous Thromboembolism Prophylaxis

Hospital Name	City	Rate	Cases
Allen County Regional Hospital[2,3]	Iola	100%	74
Kansas Spine & Specialty Hospital[2]	Wichita	100%	243
Overland Park Regional Medical Center[2]	Overland Park	100%	278
Wesley Medical Center[2]	Wichita	100%	279
Menorah Medical Center[2]	Overland Park	99%	302
Miami County Medical Center	Paola	98%	165
Stormont - Vail Healthcare[2]	Topeka	98%	330
Via Christi Hospitals Wichita[2]	Wichita	98%	215
Ransom Memorial Hospital[2]	Ottawa	97%	117
Saint Luke's Cushing Hospital[2]	Leavenworth	97%	76
Via Christi Hospital Wichita Saint Teresa[2]	Wichita	97%	123
Southwest Medical Center[2]	Liberal	95%	78
Via Christi Hospital Pittsburg[2]	Pittsburg	95%	237
University of Kansas Hospital[2]	Kansas City	93%	318
Providence Medical Center[2]	Kansas City	92%	356
Saint Catherine Hospital[2]	Garden City	92%	228
Lawrence Memorial Hospital[2]	Lawrence	91%	320
Western Plains Medical Complex[2]	Dodge City	91%	87
Saint Francis Health Center[2]	Topeka	90%	345
Mercy Hospital - Fort Scott[2]	Fort Scott	89%	106
Labette Health[2]	Parsons	88%	181
Nemaha Valley Community Hospital	Seneca	88%	32
Olathe Medical Center[2]	Olathe	86%	298
Saint John Hospital[2]	Leavenworth	86%	66
Shawnee Mission Medical Center[2]	Shawnee Miss.	86%	333
Newton Medical Center[2]	Newton	85%	172
McPherson Hospital[2]	Mcpherson	83%	236
Susan B Allen Memorial Hospital[2]	El Dorado	83%	122
Salina Regional Health Center[2]	Salina	81%	320
Anderson County Hospital	Garnett	80%	41
Coffeyville Regional Medical Center[2]	Coffeyville	79%	136
Saint Luke's South Hospital[2]	Overland Park	78%	278
Hays Medical Center[2]	Hays	77%	329
Newman Regional Health[2]	Emporia	77%	143
Kansas Heart Hospital[2]	Wichita	76%	143
Hospital District #6 of Harper County	Anthony	75%	106
Community Hosp-Onaga/St Marys Campus[2]	Onaga	74%	186
Saint Luke Hospital & Living Center	Marion	73%	62
Geary Community Hospital[2]	Junction City	72%	105
Doctors Hospital	Leawood	71%	28
Mercy Hospital Independence[2]	Independence	66%	73
South Central Kansas Medical Center[2]	Arkansas City	66%	76
Mercy Regional Health Center[2]	Manhattan	63%	308
Pratt Regional Medical Center[2]	Pratt	54%	52
William Newton Hospital	Winfield	53%	283
Great Bend Regional Hospital[2]	Great Bend	48%	95
Hutchinson Regional Medical Center[2]	Hutchinson	41%	365
Morton County Hospital[2]	Elkhart	28%	190
Mercy Hospital[2]	Moundridge	24%	109
Sumner Regional Medical Center[2]	Wellington	23%	169
Coffey County Hospital[2]	Burlington	21%	116
Harper Hospital District No 5	Harper	6%	49
Bob Wilson Memorial Grant County Hospital[2]	Ulysses	0%	113

Warfarin Therapy Discharge Instructions

Hospital Name	City	Rate	Cases
Overland Park Regional Medical Center[2]	Overland Park	100%	34
Saint Francis Health Center[2]	Topeka	100%	54
Wesley Medical Center[2]	Wichita	100%	99
Providence Medical Center[2]	Kansas City	97%	38
Shawnee Mission Medical Center[2]	Shawnee Miss.	97%	113
Via Christi Hospitals Wichita[2]	Wichita	92%	124
Hutchinson Regional Medical Center[2]	Hutchinson	84%	38
Olathe Medical Center[2]	Olathe	80%	54
University of Kansas Hospital[2]	Kansas City	79%	126
Lawrence Memorial Hospital[2]	Lawrence	77%	26
Stormont - Vail Healthcare[2]	Topeka	67%	82
Salina Regional Health Center[2]	Salina	62%	50
Newton Medical Center[2]	Newton	57%	28
Saint Luke's South Hospital[2]	Overland Park	52%	27
Hays Medical Center[2]	Hays	42%	36

Chest Pain/Possible Heart Attack Care

Aspirin Given Within 24 Hours of Arrival

Hospital Name	City	Rate	Cases
Labette Health	Parsons	100%	39
Newton Medical Center	Newton	100%	46
Ransom Memorial Hospital	Ottawa	100%	28
Susan B Allen Memorial Hospital	El Dorado	100%	80
William Newton Hospital	Winfield	99%	73
Great Bend Regional Hospital	Great Bend	98%	45
Newman Regional Health	Emporia	98%	84
Mercy Hospital - Fort Scott	Fort Scott	97%	31
Miami County Medical Center	Paola	96%	26
Saint Luke's Cushing Hospital	Leavenworth	96%	27
South Central Kansas Medical Center	Arkansas City	96%	27
McPherson Hospital	Mcpherson	95%	64
Mercy Hospital Independence	Independence	95%	64
Geary Community Hospital	Junction City	94%	34
Neosho Memorial Regional Medical Center	Chanute	93%	44
Southwest Medical Center	Liberal	90%	48
Via Christi Hospital Wichita Saint Teresa	Wichita	89%	37
Clay County Medical Center	Clay Center	84%	25

Average Time to ECG (minutes)

Hospital Name	City	Min.	Cases
Mercy Hospital Independence	Independence	1	60
Newman Regional Health	Emporia	4	86
Susan B Allen Memorial Hospital	El Dorado	4	84
William Newton Hospital	Winfield	4	76
South Central Kansas Medical Center	Arkansas City	5	30
Labette Health	Parsons	6	40
Neosho Memorial Regional Medical Center	Chanute	7	46
Ransom Memorial Hospital	Ottawa	7	31
Newton Medical Center	Newton	8	48
Coffeyville Regional Medical Center	Coffeyville	9	25
Geary Community Hospital	Junction City	9	35
Miami County Medical Center	Paola	9	26
Mercy Hospital - Fort Scott	Fort Scott	10	29
Saint Luke's Cushing Hospital	Leavenworth	10	28
Via Christi Hospital Wichita Saint Teresa	Wichita	10	36
McPherson Hospital	Mcpherson	14	63
Great Bend Regional Hospital	Great Bend	15	46
Southwest Medical Center	Liberal	17	49

Children's Asthma Care

Received Home Management Plan of Care

Hospital Name	City	Rate	Cases
Wesley Medical Center	Wichita	98%	133
Children's Mercy South[2]	Overland Park	90%	231

Received Reliever Medication

Hospital Name	City	Rate	Cases
Children's Mercy South[2]	Overland Park	100%	236
Wesley Medical Center	Wichita	100%	134

Received Systemic Corticosteroids

Hospital Name	City	Rate	Cases
Children's Mercy South[2]	Overland Park	100%	232
Wesley Medical Center	Wichita	100%	134

Emergency Department

Admittance Decision Time (minutes)

Hospital Name	City	Min.	Cases
Community Hosp-Onaga/St Marys Campus[2]	Onaga	0	113
Ellsworth County Medical Center[2]	Ellsworth	0	126
Harper Hospital District No 5[3]	Harper	0	67
Herington Municipal Hospital[2]	Herington	0	126
Mercy Hospital[2]	Moundridge	0	82
Nemaha Valley Community Hospital	Seneca	0	64
Comanche County Hospital	Coldwater	10	32
Holton Community Hospital	Holton	10	59
Rawlins County Health Center[3]	Atwood	10	28
Hospital District #6 of Harper County	Anthony	15	84
Saint Luke Hospital & Living Center	Marion	15	43
Pawnee Valley Community Hospital[3]	Larned	18	27
Graham County Hospital	Hill City	19	111
Citizens Medical Center[3]	Colby	20	91
Ness County Hospital District #2	Ness City	20	53
Pratt Regional Medical Center[2]	Pratt	25	214
Sumner Regional Medical Center	Wellington	27	54
Girard Medical Center[2]	Girard	30	309
Mercy Maude Norton Hospital[2,3]	Columbus	30	31
Morton County Hospital[2]	Elkhart	30	133
Stormont - Vail Healthcare[2]	Topeka	34	575
Coffey County Hospital[2]	Burlington	35	110
Allen County Regional Hospital[2,3]	Iola	38	205
Fredonia Regional Hospital	Fredonia	40	100
Mitchell County Hospital Health Systems[3]	Beloit	40	27
Clara Barton Hospital[2]	Hoisington	42	145
Miami County Medical Center	Paola	43	254
Great Bend Regional Hospital[2]	Great Bend	44	60
Mercy Hospital Independence[2]	Independence	45	212
Ransom Memorial Hospital[2]	Ottawa	45	238
William Newton Hospital[2]	Winfield	48	288
Kansas Medical Center[2]	Andover	49	163
Newton Medical Center	Newton	50	877
South Central Kansas Medical Center[2]	Arkansas City	50	158
Lawrence Memorial Hospital[2]	Lawrence	51	650
Bob Wilson Memorial Grant County Hospital[2]	Ulysses	52	84
Saint Luke's Cushing Hospital[2]	Leavenworth	54	136
Menorah Medical Center[2]	Overland Park	55	345
Newman Regional Health[2]	Emporia	55	250
Saint Catherine Hospital[2]	Garden City	55	243
Via Christi Hospital Pittsburg[2]	Pittsburg	56	356
Neosho Memorial Regional Medical Center[2]	Chanute	60	261
Wesley Medical Center[2]	Wichita	60	580
Olathe Medical Center[2]	Olathe	62	604
Hays Medical Center[2]	Hays	63	227
McPherson Hospital[2]	Mcpherson	63	291

NOTE: Hospital profiles are in alphabetical order by state, then city, then hospital within the city; Rankings exclude hospitals with less than 25 cases except for patient surveys which excludes hospitals with less than 100 cases; (a) 100-299 cases; (1) The number of cases/patients is too few to report; (2) Data submitted were based on a sample of cases/patients; (3) Results are based on a shorter time period than required; (4) Data suppressed by CMS for one or more quarters; (5) Results are not available for this reporting period; (6) Fewer than 100 patients completed the HCAHPS survey; (7) No cases met the criteria for this measure; (8) The lower limit of the confidence interval cannot be calculated if the number of observed infections equals zero; (9) No data are available from the state/territory for this reporting period; (10) The scores shown reflect fewer than 50 completed surveys; (11) There were discrepancies in the data collection process; (12) This measure does not apply to this hospital for this reporting period; (13) Results cannot be calculated for this reporting period; (14) The results for this state are combined with nearby states to protect confidentiality; Please refer to the User's Guide for a full explanation of data.

Via Christi Hospital Wichita Saint Teresa[2]	Wichita	64	250
Overland Park Regional Medical Center[2]	Overland Park	65	603
Salina Regional Health Center[2]	Salina	66	312
Saint John Hospital[2]	Leavenworth	67	365
Labette Health[2]	Parsons	68	268
Geary Community Hospital[2]	Junction City	70	147
Hutchinson Regional Medical Center[2]	Hutchinson	70	456
Susan B Allen Memorial Hospital[2]	El Dorado	70	200
Southwest Medical Center[2]	Liberal	72	112
Via Christi Hospitals Wichita[2]	Wichita	73	409
Mercy Hospital - Fort Scott[2]	Fort Scott	74	232
Saint Luke's South Hospital[2]	Overland Park	74	452
Mercy Regional Health Center[2]	Manhattan	78	336
Providence Medical Center[2]	Kansas City	81	807
Western Plains Medical Complex[2]	Dodge City	83	195
Saint Francis Health Center[2]	Topeka	84	561
Shawnee Mission Medical Center[2]	Shawnee Miss.	87	372
Coffeyville Regional Medical Center[2]	Coffeyville	126	206
University of Kansas Hospital[2]	Kansas City	148	427

Patients Who Left ER Before Being Seen

Hospital Name	City	Rate	Cases
Bob Wilson Memorial Grant County Hospital	Ulysses	0%	2849
Coffey County Hospital	Burlington	0%	3910
Mercy Hospital	Moundridge	0%	927
Mercy Hospital Independence	Independence	0%	8846
Morton County Hospital	Elkhart	0%	2391
Neosho Memorial Regional Medical Center	Chanute	0%	9118
Newman Regional Health	Emporia	0%	10742
Pratt Regional Medical Center	Pratt	0%	6210
Saint John Hospital	Leavenworth	0%	10544
Shawnee Mission Medical Center	Shawnee Miss.	0%	68942
South Central Kansas Medical Center	Arkansas City	0%	7269
Via Christi Hospital Wichita Saint Teresa	Wichita	0%	13468
Coffeyville Regional Medical Center	Coffeyville	1%	8074
Edwards County Hospital	Kinsley	1%	896
Fredonia Regional Hospital	Fredonia	1%	2340
Great Bend Regional Hospital	Great Bend	1%	8008
Hays Medical Center	Hays	1%	14408
Hutchinson Regional Medical Center	Hutchinson	1%	24777
Kansas Medical Center	Andover	1%	6831
Labette Health	Parsons	1%	11817
Lawrence Memorial Hospital	Lawrence	1%	37271
McPherson Hospital	Mcpherson	1%	4011
Meade District Hospital	Meade	1%	1224
Menorah Medical Center	Overland Park	1%	14527
Mercy Regional Health Center	Manhattan	1%	21276
Miami County Medical Center	Paola	1%	10098
Newton Medical Center	Newton	1%	13307
Olathe Medical Center	Olathe	1%	42363
Saint Catherine Hospital	Garden City	1%	15498
Stormont - Vail Healthcare	Topeka	1%	63191
Sumner Regional Medical Center	Wellington	1%	3982
Susan B Allen Memorial Hospital	El Dorado	1%	13479
Western Plains Medical Complex	Dodge City	1%	9667
William Newton Hospital	Winfield	1%	9130
Overland Park Regional Medical Center	Overland Park	2%	22696
Ransom Memorial Hospital	Ottawa	2%	10772
Saint Francis Health Center	Topeka	2%	33958
Saint Luke's South Hospital	Overland Park	2%	15999
Salina Regional Health Center	Salina	2%	30407
Via Christi Hospital Pittsburg	Pittsburg	2%	15151
Wesley Medical Center	Wichita	2%	92131
Mercy Hospital - Fort Scott	Fort Scott	3%	6900
Providence Medical Center	Kansas City	3%	36616
Saint Luke's Cushing Hospital	Leavenworth	3%	11499
Southwest Medical Center	Liberal	3%	9534
Via Christi Hospitals Wichita	Wichita	3%	123061
University of Kansas Hospital	Kansas City	4%	49301
Ellsworth County Medical Center	Ellsworth	8%	2762
Geary Community Hospital	Junction City	9%	14078

Time from ER Arrival to Being Admitted (minutes)

Hospital Name	City	Min.	Cases
Harper Hospital District No 5[3]	Harper	15	67
Comanche County Hospital	Coldwater	61	32
Ness County Hospital District #2	Ness City	72	54
Graham County Hospital	Hill City	74	111
Saint Luke Hospital & Living Center	Marion	75	43
Nemaha Valley Community Hospital	Seneca	92	64
Morton County Hospital[2]	Elkhart	94	132
Rawlins County Health Center[3]	Atwood	94	28
Fredonia Regional Hospital	Fredonia	95	124
Community Hosp-Onaga/St Marys Campus[2]	Onaga	100	138
Mercy Hospital[2]	Moundridge	100	84
Coffey County Hospital[2]	Burlington	102	200
Osborne County Memorial Hospital[3]	Osborne	104	29
Hospital District #6 of Harper County	Anthony	105	101
Citizens Medical Center[3]	Colby	115	118
Herington Municipal Hospital[2]	Herington	116	126
Bob Wilson Memorial Grant County Hospital[2]	Ulysses	117	93
Ellsworth County Medical Center[2]	Ellsworth	129	135
Mercy Maude Norton Hospital[2,3]	Columbus	131	31
Pratt Regional Medical Center[2]	Pratt	132	224
South Central Kansas Medical Center[2]	Arkansas City	140	174
Kansas Medical Center[2]	Andover	143	165
Mitchell County Hospital Health Systems[3]	Beloit	145	27
Sumner Regional Medical Center	Wellington	145	66
Clay County Medical Center	Clay Center	150	47
Holton Community Hospital	Holton	150	71
Great Bend Regional Hospital[2]	Great Bend	155	120
Pawnee Valley Community Hospital[3]	Larned	155	27
Allen County Regional Hospital[2,3]	Iola	156	230
Via Christi Hospital Wichita Saint Teresa[2]	Wichita	158	252
Saint Catherine Hospital[2]	Garden City	163	257
Girard Medical Center[2]	Girard	166	330
Coffeyville Regional Medical Center[2]	Coffeyville	172	230
Mercy Hospital - Fort Scott[2]	Fort Scott	172	245
Overland Park Regional Medical Center[2]	Overland Park	172	604
Mercy Hospital Independence[2]	Independence	174	237
Via Christi Hospital Pittsburg[2]	Pittsburg	174	358
Neosho Memorial Regional Medical Center[2]	Chanute	175	284
Newton Medical Center	Newton	176	893
Hays Medical Center[2]	Hays	177	346
Salina Regional Health Center[2]	Salina	178	334
Via Christi Hospitals Wichita[2]	Wichita	180	421
Wesley Medical Center[2]	Wichita	180	580
Saint Luke's Cushing Hospital[2]	Leavenworth	181	153
Ransom Memorial Hospital[2]	Ottawa	184	249
Susan B Allen Memorial Hospital[2]	El Dorado	184	200
Clara Barton Hospital[2]	Hoisington	188	160
Southwest Medical Center[2]	Liberal	189	115
Lawrence Memorial Hospital[2]	Lawrence	194	654
Miami County Medical Center	Paola	194	260
Olathe Medical Center[2]	Olathe	196	608
Menorah Medical Center[2]	Overland Park	198	345
Newman Regional Health[2]	Emporia	200	254
Saint John Hospital[2]	Leavenworth	200	372
Hutchinson Regional Medical Center[2]	Hutchinson	203	499
William Newton Hospital[2]	Winfield	205	289
Mercy Regional Health Center[2]	Manhattan	206	373
Western Plains Medical Complex[2]	Dodge City	222	196
Saint Luke's South Hospital[2]	Overland Park	226	455
McPherson Hospital[2]	Mcpherson	227	306
Labette Health[2]	Parsons	230	274
Stormont - Vail Healthcare[2]	Topeka	234	583
Shawnee Mission Medical Center[2]	Shawnee Miss.	241	385
Providence Medical Center[2]	Kansas City	247	807
Saint Francis Health Center[2]	Topeka	248	563
Geary Community Hospital[2]	Junction City	265	150
University of Kansas Hospital[2]	Kansas City	367	428

Time from ER Arrival to Discharge (minutes)

Hospital Name	City	Min.	Cases
Coffey County Hospital	Burlington	59	275
Pratt Regional Medical Center	Pratt	61	1243
Allen County Regional Hospital[3]	Iola	62	252
Great Bend Regional Hospital	Great Bend	65	379
Kansas Medical Center	Andover	67	376
Bob Wilson Memorial Grant County Hospital	Ulysses	72	311
Hiawatha Community Hospital[3]	Hiawatha	73	86
South Central Kansas Medical Center	Arkansas City	74	300
Clay County Medical Center[3]	Clay Center	76	127
Ellsworth County Medical Center	Ellsworth	78	203
Mercy Hospital	Moundridge	80	207
Sumner Regional Medical Center	Wellington	80	384
Morton County Hospital	Elkhart	82	185
Community Hosp-Onaga/St Marys Campus	Onaga	85	353
Mercy Maude Norton Hospital[3]	Columbus	87	70
Via Christi Hospital Wichita Saint Teresa	Wichita	90	380
Saint John Hospital	Leavenworth	93	348
Miami County Medical Center	Paola	95	373
Saint Catherine Hospital	Garden City	96	598
William Newton Hospital	Winfield	97	253
Mercy Hospital - Fort Scott	Fort Scott	98	349
Norton County Hospital[3]	Norton	98	25
Susan B Allen Memorial Hospital	El Dorado	98	425
McPherson Hospital	Mcpherson	99	297
Saint Luke's Cushing Hospital	Leavenworth	99	360
Mercy Hospital Independence	Independence	102	362
Edwards County Hospital[3]	Kinsley	104	26
Ransom Memorial Hospital	Ottawa	104	420
Coffeyville Regional Medical Center	Coffeyville	106	341
Western Plains Medical Complex	Dodge City	106	383
Providence Medical Center	Kansas City	109	398
Hutchinson Regional Medical Center	Hutchinson	110	556
Mercy Regional Health Center	Manhattan	112	360
Clara Barton Hospital	Hoisington	113	229
Wesley Medical Center	Wichita	114	474
Salina Regional Health Center	Salina	116	346
Via Christi Hospital Pittsburg	Pittsburg	117	328
Hays Medical Center	Hays	118	374
Newman Regional Health	Emporia	118	407
Labette Health	Parsons	119	937
Via Christi Hospitals Wichita	Wichita	119	351
Newton Medical Center	Newton	123	10344
Olathe Medical Center	Olathe	124	387
Southwest Medical Center	Liberal	128	356
Overland Park Regional Medical Center	Overland Park	136	480
Shawnee Mission Medical Center	Shawnee Miss.	137	365
Saint Luke's South Hospital	Overland Park	140	369
Geary Community Hospital	Junction City	141	375
Menorah Medical Center	Overland Park	142	416
Lawrence Memorial Hospital	Lawrence	144	426
Saint Francis Health Center	Topeka	148	362
Stormont - Vail Healthcare	Topeka	162	445
University of Kansas Hospital	Kansas City	190	342

Time in ER Before Being Evaluated (minutes)

Hospital Name	City	Min.	Cases
Allen County Regional Hospital[3]	Iola	7	293
Salina Regional Health Center	Salina	7	379
Pratt Regional Medical Center	Pratt	8	1288
Coffeyville Regional Medical Center	Coffeyville	9	380
Saint John Hospital	Leavenworth	9	374
Overland Park Regional Medical Center	Overland Park	11	507
Community Hosp-Onaga/St Marys Campus	Onaga	13	416
Great Bend Regional Hospital	Great Bend	13	306
South Central Kansas Medical Center	Arkansas City	13	384
Coffey County Hospital	Burlington	15	265
Graham County Hospital	Hill City	15	92
Mercy Hospital - Fort Scott	Fort Scott	15	381
Via Christi Hospital Wichita Saint Teresa	Wichita	15	415
Mercy Regional Health Center	Manhattan	16	324
Anderson County Hospital	Garnett	17	37
Lawrence Memorial Hospital	Lawrence	17	449
Menorah Medical Center	Overland Park	17	478
Miami County Medical Center	Paola	17	404
Mercy Maude Norton Hospital[3]	Columbus	18	83
Newton Medical Center	Newton	18	11566
Providence Medical Center	Kansas City	18	418
William Newton Hospital	Winfield	18	385
Mercy Hospital Independence	Independence	19	390
Newman Regional Health	Emporia	19	472
Stormont - Vail Healthcare	Topeka	19	431
Western Plains Medical Complex	Dodge City	19	422
Edwards County Hospital[3]	Kinsley	20	29
Olathe Medical Center	Olathe	20	411
Ransom Memorial Hospital	Ottawa	21	453
Clara Barton Hospital	Hoisington	22	256
Hays Medical Center	Hays	22	362
Kansas Medical Center	Andover	22	362
McPherson Hospital	Mcpherson	22	289
Norton County Hospital[3]	Norton	22	42
Susan B Allen Memorial Hospital	El Dorado	22	478
Wesley Medical Center	Wichita	22	515
Mercy Hospital	Moundridge	23	258
Via Christi Hospitals Wichita	Wichita	23	376
Ellsworth County Medical Center	Ellsworth	24	216
Saint Catherine Hospital	Garden City	24	595
Clay County Medical Center[3]	Clay Center	25	133
Via Christi Hospital Pittsburg	Pittsburg	26	293
Hiawatha Community Hospital[3]	Hiawatha	28	83
Saint Luke's Cushing Hospital	Leavenworth	28	301
Saint Luke's South Hospital	Overland Park	28	130
Bob Wilson Memorial Grant County Hospital	Ulysses	30	294
Saint Francis Health Center	Topeka	31	382
Morton County Hospital	Elkhart	33	197
Labette Health	Parsons	34	983
Southwest Medical Center	Liberal	35	400
University of Kansas Hospital	Kansas City	35	353
Shawnee Mission Medical Center	Shawnee Miss.	37	200
Hutchinson Regional Medical Center	Hutchinson	41	372
Geary Community Hospital	Junction City	44	364
Sumner Regional Medical Center	Wellington	44	435

Time to Pain Meds for Bone Fractures (minutes)

Hospital Name	City	Min.	Cases
South Central Kansas Medical Center	Arkansas City	31	45
Great Bend Regional Hospital	Great Bend	32	44
Menorah Medical Center	Overland Park	32	46
Via Christi Hospital Wichita Saint Teresa	Wichita	34	63
Lawrence Memorial Hospital	Lawrence	35	176
Kansas Medical Center	Andover	38	70
Overland Park Regional Medical Center	Overland Park	38	109
Susan B Allen Memorial Hospital	El Dorado	39	53
Providence Medical Center	Kansas City	42	118
Saint Luke's Cushing Hospital	Leavenworth	42	49
Shawnee Mission Medical Center	Shawnee Miss.	42	239
Saint John Hospital	Leavenworth	43	51
Olathe Medical Center	Olathe	44	180

NOTE: Hospital profiles are in alphabetical order by state, then city, then hospital within the city; Rankings exclude hospitals with less than 25 cases except for patient surveys which excludes hospitals with less than 100 cases; (a) 100-299 cases; (1) The number of cases/patients is too few to report; (2) Data submitted were based on a sample of cases/patients; (3) Results are based on a shorter time period than required; (4) Data suppressed by CMS for one or more quarters; (5) Results are not available for this reporting period; (6) Fewer than 100 patients completed the HCAHPS survey; (7) No cases met the criteria for this measure; (8) The lower limit of the confidence interval cannot be calculated if the number of observed infections equals zero; (9) No data are available from the state/territory for this reporting period; (10) The scores shown reflect fewer than 50 completed surveys; (11) There were discrepancies in the data collection process; (12) This measure does not apply to this hospital for this reporting period; (13) Results cannot be calculated for this reporting period; (14) The results for this state are combined with nearby states to protect confidentiality; Please refer to the User's Guide for a full explanation of data.

Salina Regional Health Center	Salina	45	114
Stormont - Vail Healthcare	Topeka	45	187
Coffeyville Regional Medical Center	Coffeyville	46	37
Geary Community Hospital	Junction City	46	50
William Newton Hospital	Winfield	46	28
Saint Catherine Hospital	Garden City	47	71
Hays Medical Center	Hays	48	60
Miami County Medical Center	Paola	48	48
Ransom Memorial Hospital	Ottawa	49	39
Wesley Medical Center	Wichita	49	312
Mercy Regional Health Center	Manhattan	52	84
Newman Regional Health	Emporia	52	50
Via Christi Hospitals Wichita	Wichita	53	163
Western Plains Medical Complex	Dodge City	53	36
McPherson Hospital	Mcpherson	57	28
Saint Francis Health Center	Topeka	57	91
Via Christi Hospital Pittsburg	Pittsburg	57	41
Hutchinson Regional Medical Center	Hutchinson	59	108
Labette Health	Parsons	59	49
Saint Luke's South Hospital	Overland Park	60	50
Newton Medical Center	Newton	62	102
Southwest Medical Center	Liberal	78	36
University of Kansas Hospital	Kansas City	78	136

Heart Attack Care

Aspirin Given at Discharge

Hospital Name	City	Rate	Cases
Hutchinson Regional Medical Center	Hutchinson	100%	152
Kansas Heart Hospital[2]	Wichita	100%	224
Kansas Medical Center[2]	Andover	100%	191
Lawrence Memorial Hospital	Lawrence	100%	106
Mercy Regional Health Center	Manhattan	100%	115
Newton Medical Center	Newton	100%	25
Olathe Medical Center	Olathe	100%	238
Overland Park Regional Medical Center	Overland Park	100%	111
Saint Catherine Hospital	Garden City	100%	38
Saint Francis Health Center	Topeka	100%	162
Saint Luke's South Hospital	Overland Park	100%	74
Stormont - Vail Healthcare	Topeka	100%	313
University of Kansas Hospital	Kansas City	100%	254
Wesley Medical Center[2]	Wichita	100%	287
Western Plains Medical Complex	Dodge City	100%	33
Wichita VA Medical Center	Wichita	100%	35
Hays Medical Center[2]	Hays	99%	198
Providence Medical Center	Kansas City	99%	158
Salina Regional Health Center	Salina	99%	153
Shawnee Mission Medical Center[2]	Shawnee Miss.	99%	205
Via Christi Hospital Pittsburg	Pittsburg	99%	73
Via Christi Hospitals Wichita[2]	Wichita	99%	301
Menorah Medical Center[2]	Overland Park	98%	55

PCI Within 90 Minutes of Arrival

Hospital Name	City	Rate	Cases
Lawrence Memorial Hospital	Lawrence	100%	25
Olathe Medical Center	Olathe	100%	37
Overland Park Regional Medical Center	Overland Park	100%	28
University of Kansas Hospital	Kansas City	100%	26
Wesley Medical Center[2]	Wichita	100%	40
Via Christi Hospitals Wichita[2]	Wichita	99%	68
Shawnee Mission Medical Center[2]	Shawnee Miss.	98%	58
Stormont - Vail Healthcare	Topeka	98%	45
Providence Medical Center	Kansas City	97%	30
Hutchinson Regional Medical Center	Hutchinson	96%	27

Statin Prescribed at Discharge

Hospital Name	City	Rate	Cases
Hutchinson Regional Medical Center	Hutchinson	100%	138
Kansas Heart Hospital[2]	Wichita	100%	208
Kansas Medical Center[2]	Andover	100%	190
Lawrence Memorial Hospital	Lawrence	100%	103
Menorah Medical Center[2]	Overland Park	100%	51
Newton Medical Center	Newton	100%	26
Olathe Medical Center	Olathe	100%	236
Overland Park Regional Medical Center	Overland Park	100%	112
Providence Medical Center	Kansas City	100%	146
Saint Catherine Hospital	Garden City	100%	37
Saint Francis Health Center	Topeka	100%	151
Shawnee Mission Medical Center[2]	Shawnee Miss.	100%	204
Stormont - Vail Healthcare	Topeka	100%	299
University of Kansas Hospital	Kansas City	100%	241
Wesley Medical Center[2]	Wichita	100%	259
Western Plains Medical Complex	Dodge City	100%	32
Wichita VA Medical Center	Wichita	100%	25
Saint Luke's South Hospital	Overland Park	99%	71
Salina Regional Health Center	Salina	99%	148
Via Christi Hospitals Wichita[2]	Wichita	99%	278
Hays Medical Center[2]	Hays	98%	200
Mercy Regional Health Center	Manhattan	98%	109

Via Christi Hospital Pittsburg	Pittsburg	98%	61

Heart Failure Care

ACE Inhibitor or ARB for LVSD

Hospital Name	City	Rate	Cases
Hutchinson Regional Medical Center	Hutchinson	100%	62
Kansas Medical Center	Andover	100%	37
Lawrence Memorial Hospital	Lawrence	100%	28
Overland Park Regional Medical Center	Overland Park	100%	48
Providence Medical Center	Kansas City	100%	143
Saint Francis Health Center	Topeka	100%	65
Saint Luke's South Hospital	Overland Park	100%	26
Salina Regional Health Center	Salina	100%	32
Shawnee Mission Medical Center[2]	Shawnee Miss.	100%	100
Stormont - Vail Healthcare	Topeka	100%	120
Wesley Medical Center[2]	Wichita	100%	69
Wichita VA Medical Center	Wichita	100%	32
Olathe Medical Center	Olathe	99%	84
University of Kansas Hospital	Kansas City	99%	126
Kansas Heart Hospital[2]	Wichita	98%	56
Mercy Regional Health Center	Manhattan	98%	48
Via Christi Hospitals Wichita[2]	Wichita	97%	66
VA Eastern Kansas Healthcare System	Leavenworth	96%	25
Hays Medical Center	Hays	88%	56
Newman Regional Health	Emporia	88%	26

Discharge Instructions Given

Hospital Name	City	Rate	Cases
Kansas Medical Center	Andover	100%	77
Lawrence Memorial Hospital	Lawrence	100%	117
Neosho Memorial Regional Medical Center[2]	Chanute	100%	26
Newman Regional Health	Emporia	100%	31
Saint Catherine Hospital	Garden City	100%	32
Saint John Hospital	Leavenworth	100%	26
Stormont - Vail Healthcare	Topeka	100%	331
Via Christi Hospital Wichita Saint Teresa[2]	Wichita	100%	26
Wesley Medical Center[2]	Wichita	100%	226
Western Plains Medical Complex	Dodge City	100%	26
Wichita VA Medical Center	Wichita	100%	77
Menorah Medical Center[2]	Overland Park	99%	85
Shawnee Mission Medical Center[2]	Shawnee Miss.	99%	221
Providence Medical Center	Kansas City	98%	262
Hutchinson Regional Medical Center	Hutchinson	97%	113
Overland Park Regional Medical Center	Overland Park	97%	131
Saint Francis Health Center	Topeka	97%	157
University of Kansas Hospital	Kansas City	97%	344
Via Christi Hospitals Wichita[2]	Wichita	97%	217
Susan B Allen Memorial Hospital	El Dorado	96%	26
VA Eastern Kansas Healthcare System	Leavenworth	96%	75
Coffeyville Regional Medical Center	Coffeyville	95%	37
Olathe Medical Center	Olathe	95%	199
Coffey County Hospital	Burlington	94%	32
Kansas Heart Hospital[2]	Wichita	93%	139
Saint Luke's South Hospital	Overland Park	93%	105
Labette Health	Parsons	90%	30
Mercy Regional Health Center	Manhattan	90%	67
Salina Regional Health Center	Salina	86%	73
Mercy Hospital - Fort Scott	Fort Scott	83%	30
Via Christi Hospital Pittsburg	Pittsburg	81%	62
Hays Medical Center	Hays	78%	141
Newton Medical Center	Newton	76%	42

Evaluation of LVS Function

Hospital Name	City	Rate	Cases
Hutchinson Regional Medical Center	Hutchinson	100%	146
Kansas Heart Hospital[2]	Wichita	100%	160
Kansas Medical Center	Andover	100%	108
Labette Health	Parsons	100%	45
Lawrence Memorial Hospital	Lawrence	100%	148
Menorah Medical Center[2]	Overland Park	100%	137
Mercy Hospital - Fort Scott	Fort Scott	100%	41
Mercy Regional Health Center	Manhattan	100%	92
Neosho Memorial Regional Medical Center[2]	Chanute	100%	45
Newman Regional Health	Emporia	100%	52
Olathe Medical Center	Olathe	100%	255
Overland Park Regional Medical Center	Overland Park	100%	187
Providence Medical Center	Kansas City	100%	332
Saint Catherine Hospital	Garden City	100%	46
Saint Francis Health Center	Topeka	100%	204
Saint John Hospital	Leavenworth	100%	35
Saint Luke's South Hospital	Overland Park	100%	147
Salina Regional Health Center	Salina	100%	97
Shawnee Mission Medical Center[2]	Shawnee Miss.	100%	275
Stormont - Vail Healthcare	Topeka	100%	425
Susan B Allen Memorial Hospital	El Dorado	100%	44
University of Kansas Hospital	Kansas City	100%	403
Via Christi Hospital Pittsburg	Pittsburg	100%	86
Via Christi Hospital Wichita Saint Teresa[2]	Wichita	100%	42

Via Christi Hospitals Wichita[2]	Wichita	100%	311
Wesley Medical Center[2]	Wichita	100%	291
Western Plains Medical Complex	Dodge City	100%	44
Wichita VA Medical Center	Wichita	100%	84
Hays Medical Center	Hays	99%	180
VA Eastern Kansas Healthcare System	Leavenworth	99%	90
Coffeyville Regional Medical Center	Coffeyville	98%	65
Newton Medical Center	Newton	97%	74
Ransom Memorial Hospital	Ottawa	97%	29
Girard Medical Center	Girard	96%	25
Coffey County Hospital	Burlington	93%	46
Mercy Hospital Independence	Independence	92%	25
Southwest Medical Center	Liberal	92%	26
Atchison Hospital	Atchison	89%	28
McPherson Hospital[2]	Mcpherson	79%	28
Cloud County Health Center	Concordia	50%	26

Medicare Spending

Medicare Spending per Patient (ratio)

Hospital Name	City	Ratio	Cases
Morton County Hospital	Elkhart	0.71	-
Bob Wilson Memorial Grant County Hospital	Ulysses	0.74	-
Mercy Hospital	Moundridge	0.77	-
Summit Surgical	Hutchinson	0.81	-
Salina Surgical Hospital	Salina	0.84	-
Kansas Surgery & Recovery Center	Wichita	0.85	-
Manhattan Surgical Hospital	Manhattan	0.85	-
Coffey County Hospital	Burlington	0.86	-
Doctors Hospital	Leawood	0.88	-
Kansas Heart Hospital	Wichita	0.88	-
Southwest Medical Center	Liberal	0.88	-
Labette Health	Parsons	0.89	-
Newton Medical Center	Newton	0.89	-
Coffeyville Regional Medical Center	Coffeyville	0.90	-
Kansas City Orthopaedic Institute	Leawood	0.90	-
Lawrence Memorial Hospital	Lawrence	0.90	-
Western Plains Medical Complex	Dodge City	0.90	-
Kansas Spine & Specialty Hospital	Wichita	0.91	-
Ransom Memorial Hospital	Ottawa	0.91	-
Saint Luke's Cushing Hospital	Leavenworth	0.91	-
Sumner Regional Medical Center	Wellington	0.91	-
Geary Community Hospital	Junction City	0.92	-
McPherson Hospital	Mcpherson	0.93	-
Mercy Hospital Independence	Independence	0.93	-
Via Christi Hospital Pittsburg	Pittsburg	0.93	-
Kansas Medical Center	Andover	0.94	-
Miami County Medical Center	Paola	0.94	-
Newman Regional Health	Emporia	0.94	-
Pratt Regional Medical Center	Pratt	0.94	-
South Central Kansas Medical Center	Arkansas City	0.94	-
Mercy Hospital - Fort Scott	Fort Scott	0.95	-
Saint Catherine Hospital	Garden City	0.95	-
Susan B Allen Memorial Hospital	El Dorado	0.96	-
Great Bend Regional Hospital	Great Bend	0.97	-
Hutchinson Regional Medical Center	Hutchinson	0.97	-
Hays Medical Center	Hays	0.98	-
University of Kansas Hospital	Kansas City	0.98	-
Via Christi Hospitals Wichita	Wichita	0.98	-
Mercy Regional Health Center	Manhattan	0.99	-
Olathe Medical Center	Olathe	0.99	-
Saint John Hospital	Leavenworth	0.99	-
Saint Luke's South Hospital	Overland Park	0.99	-
Via Christi Hospital Wichita Saint Teresa	Wichita	0.99	-
Stormont - Vail Healthcare	Topeka	1.00	-
Wesley Medical Center	Wichita	1.00	-
Salina Regional Health Center	Salina	1.01	-
Providence Medical Center	Kansas City	1.02	-
Saint Francis Health Center	Topeka	1.03	-
Shawnee Mission Medical Center	Shawnee Miss.	1.03	-
Menorah Medical Center	Overland Park	1.04	-
Overland Park Regional Medical Center	Overland Park	1.04	-
Minimally Invasive Surgery Hospital	Lenexa	1.66	-

Pneumonia Care

Appropriate Initial Antibiotic Given

Hospital Name	City	Rate	Cases
Geary Community Hospital	Junction City	100%	37
Hutchinson Regional Medical Center	Hutchinson	100%	112
Lawrence Memorial Hospital	Lawrence	100%	111
Menorah Medical Center[2]	Overland Park	100%	67
Mercy Hospital - Fort Scott	Fort Scott	100%	42
Mercy Regional Health Center	Manhattan	100%	57
Olathe Medical Center	Olathe	100%	116
Ransom Memorial Hospital	Ottawa	100%	46
Wesley Medical Center[2]	Wichita	100%	54
Wichita VA Medical Center	Wichita	100%	28
Providence Medical Center	Kansas City	99%	108
Via Christi Hospital Wichita Saint Teresa[2]	Wichita	99%	89

NOTE: Hospital profiles are in alphabetical order by state, then city, then hospital within the city; Rankings exclude hospitals with less than 25 cases except for patient surveys which excludes hospitals with less than 100 cases; (a) 100-299 cases; (1) The number of cases/patients is too few to report; (2) Data submitted were based on a sample of cases/patients; (3) Results are based on a shorter time period than required; (4) Data suppressed by CMS for one or more quarters; (5) Results are not available for this reporting period; (6) Fewer than 100 patients completed the HCAHPS survey; (7) No cases met the criteria for this measure; (8) The lower limit of the confidence interval cannot be calculated if the number of observed infections equals zero; (9) No data are available from the state/territory for this reporting period; (10) The scores shown reflect fewer than 50 completed surveys; (11) There were discrepancies in the data collection process; (12) This measure does not apply to this hospital for this reporting period; (13) Results cannot be calculated for this reporting period; (14) The results for this state are combined with nearby states to protect confidentiality; Please refer to the User's Guide for a full explanation of data.

Hospital Name	City	Rate	Cases
McPherson Hospital[2]	Mcpherson	98%	44
Overland Park Regional Medical Center	Overland Park	98%	85
Saint Catherine Hospital	Garden City	98%	48
Shawnee Mission Medical Center[2]	Shawnee Miss.	98%	104
University of Kansas Hospital	Kansas City	98%	125
Via Christi Hospital Pittsburg	Pittsburg	98%	85
William Newton Hospital[2]	Winfield	98%	40
Newton Medical Center	Newton	97%	67
Saint Francis Health Center	Topeka	97%	117
Stormont - Vail Healthcare	Topeka	97%	228
Newman Regional Health	Emporia	96%	50
Salina Regional Health Center	Salina	96%	124
Coffey County Hospital	Burlington	95%	37
Saint Luke's South Hospital	Overland Park	95%	93
Susan B Allen Memorial Hospital	El Dorado	95%	85
VA Eastern Kansas Healthcare System	Leavenworth	95%	57
Via Christi Hospitals Wichita[2]	Wichita	95%	107
Western Plains Medical Complex	Dodge City	95%	38
Hays Medical Center[2]	Hays	94%	36
Neosho Memorial Regional Medical Center[2]	Chanute	94%	78
South Central Kansas Medical Center[2]	Arkansas City	94%	33
Labette Health	Parsons	93%	30
Atchison Hospital	Atchison	92%	59
Southwest Medical Center	Liberal	92%	36
Cloud County Health Center	Concordia	88%	43
Kingman Community Hospital	Kingman	88%	26
Saint Luke's Cushing Hospital	Leavenworth	86%	28
Coffeyville Regional Medical Center	Coffeyville	84%	44
Great Bend Regional Hospital[2]	Great Bend	84%	38
Girard Medical Center	Girard	76%	25
Pratt Regional Medical Center[2]	Pratt	75%	57
Republic County Hospital[2,3]	Belleville	72%	25

Blood Culture Timing

Hospital Name	City	Rate	Cases
Girard Medical Center	Girard	100%	38
Kansas Medical Center	Andover	100%	34
Menorah Medical Center[2]	Overland Park	100%	109
Mercy Hospital - Fort Scott	Fort Scott	100%	42
Mercy Hospital Independence	Independence	100%	33
Mercy Regional Health Center	Manhattan	100%	111
Neosho Memorial Regional Medical Center[2]	Chanute	100%	115
Newton Medical Center	Newton	100%	92
Saint John Hospital	Leavenworth	100%	26
Saint Luke's Cushing Hospital	Leavenworth	100%	38
Salina Regional Health Center	Salina	100%	185
Shawnee Mission Medical Center[2]	Shawnee Miss.	100%	143
Stormont - Vail Healthcare	Topeka	100%	425
Susan B Allen Memorial Hospital	El Dorado	100%	81
Trego County Lemke Memorial Hospital	Wa Keeney	100%	30
University of Kansas Hospital	Kansas City	100%	328
VA Eastern Kansas Healthcare System	Leavenworth	100%	91
Wesley Medical Center[2]	Wichita	100%	69
Western Plains Medical Complex	Dodge City	100%	56
Wichita VA Medical Center	Wichita	100%	72
William Newton Hospital[2]	Winfield	100%	29
Hutchinson Regional Medical Center	Hutchinson	99%	140
Lawrence Memorial Hospital	Lawrence	99%	247
Olathe Medical Center	Olathe	99%	198
Overland Park Regional Medical Center	Overland Park	99%	136
Saint Francis Health Center	Topeka	99%	147
Saint Luke's South Hospital	Overland Park	99%	109
Via Christi Hospital Pittsburg	Pittsburg	99%	142
Via Christi Hospitals Wichita[2]	Wichita	99%	134
Atchison Hospital	Atchison	98%	65
Pratt Regional Medical Center[2]	Pratt	98%	54
Providence Medical Center	Kansas City	98%	219
Via Christi Hospital Wichita Saint Teresa[2]	Wichita	98%	91
Saint Catherine Hospital	Garden City	97%	61
Coffeyville Regional Medical Center	Coffeyville	96%	56
Memorial Hospital	Abilene	96%	25
Newman Regional Health	Emporia	96%	49
Southwest Medical Center	Liberal	96%	25
Hays Medical Center[2]	Hays	95%	60
Labette Health	Parsons	94%	51
Geary Community Hospital	Junction City	93%	29
Ransom Memorial Hospital	Ottawa	90%	69
South Central Kansas Medical Center[2]	Arkansas City	90%	29
McPherson Hospital[2]	Mcpherson	86%	51

Pregnancy and Delivery Care

Newborns whose Deliveries were Scheduled Early

Hospital Name	City	Rate	Cases
McPherson Hospital[2]	Mcpherson	0%	36
Menorah Medical Center[2]	Overland Park	0%	26
Mercy Regional Health Center	Manhattan	0%	84
Overland Park Regional Medical Center[2]	Overland Park	0%	42
Providence Medical Center[2]	Kansas City	0%	29
Via Christi Hospital Pittsburg	Pittsburg	0%	51
Via Christi Hospitals Wichita[2]	Wichita	0%	45
Western Plains Medical Complex[2]	Dodge City	0%	27
William Newton Hospital	Winfield	0%	43
Wesley Medical Center[2]	Wichita	1%	98
Hutchinson Regional Medical Center	Hutchinson	2%	60
Olathe Medical Center[2]	Olathe	2%	49
Saint Francis Health Center[2]	Topeka	2%	42
Great Bend Regional Hospital	Great Bend	3%	60
Labette Health	Parsons	4%	25
Stormont - Vail Healthcare	Topeka	4%	156
Salina Regional Health Center	Salina	5%	99
Lawrence Memorial Hospital	Lawrence	6%	72
Saint Luke's South Hospital[2]	Overland Park	6%	31
Newton Medical Center	Newton	9%	32
Mercy Hospital - Fort Scott[2]	Fort Scott	10%	29
Southwest Medical Center[2]	Liberal	11%	55
Susan B Allen Memorial Hospital[2]	El Dorado	12%	43
Saint Catherine Hospital	Garden City	38%	56
Hays Medical Center	Hays	46%	100
Shawnee Mission Medical Center[2]	Shawnee Miss.	60%	123

Preventive Care

Immunization for Influenza

Hospital Name	City	Rate	Cases
Allen County Regional Hospital[2]	Iola	100%	239
Kansas Medical Center[2]	Andover	100%	303
Menorah Medical Center[2]	Overland Park	100%	544
Overland Park Regional Medical Center[2]	Overland Park	100%	478
Stormont - Vail Healthcare[2]	Topeka	100%	616
Summit Surgical	Hutchinson	100%	109
Kansas Heart Hospital[2]	Wichita	99%	308
Ransom Memorial Hospital[2]	Ottawa	99%	297
Salina Surgical Hospital	Salina	99%	296
South Central Kansas Medical Center[2]	Arkansas City	99%	228
Wesley Medical Center[2]	Wichita	99%	653
Kansas City Orthopaedic Institute	Leawood	98%	372
Mercy Hospital - Fort Scott[2]	Fort Scott	98%	253
Miami County Medical Center	Paola	98%	201
Via Christi Hospital Pittsburg[2]	Pittsburg	98%	341
Western Plains Medical Complex[2]	Dodge City	98%	272
William Newton Hospital	Winfield	98%	292
Holton Community Hospital	Holton	97%	75
Lawrence Memorial Hospital[2]	Lawrence	97%	524
Manhattan Surgical Hospital	Manhattan	97%	212
Mercy Regional Health Center[2]	Manhattan	96%	463
Saint Luke's Cushing Hospital[2]	Leavenworth	96%	366
Shawnee Mission Medical Center[2]	Shawnee Miss.	96%	508
University of Kansas Hospital[2]	Kansas City	96%	548
Clay County Medical Center	Clay Center	95%	43
Mercy Hospital Independence[2]	Independence	95%	236
Susan B Allen Memorial Hospital[2]	El Dorado	95%	244
Kansas Spine & Specialty Hospital[2]	Wichita	94%	302
Mitchell County Hospital Health Systems[3]	Beloit	94%	34
Olathe Medical Center[2]	Olathe	94%	539
Providence Medical Center[2]	Kansas City	94%	594
Saint John Hospital[2]	Leavenworth	94%	267
Via Christi Hospital Wichita Saint Teresa[2]	Wichita	93%	288
Via Christi Hospitals Wichita[2]	Wichita	93%	512
Minimally Invasive Surgery Hospital[2]	Lenexa	92%	59
Southwest Medical Center[2]	Liberal	91%	220
Coffeyville Regional Medical Center[2]	Coffeyville	90%	271
Girard Medical Center[2]	Girard	90%	235
Salina Regional Health Center[2]	Salina	90%	489
Coffey County Hospital[2]	Burlington	89%	296
Hays Medical Center[2]	Hays	89%	531
Cloud County Health Center	Concordia	88%	49
Ellsworth County Medical Center[2]	Ellsworth	88%	74
Pawnee Valley Community Hospital	Larned	88%	34
Fredonia Regional Hospital	Fredonia	87%	188
Labette Health[2]	Parsons	87%	297
Pratt Regional Medical Center[2]	Pratt	87%	295
Saint Luke's South Hospital[2]	Overland Park	87%	497
Neosho Memorial Regional Medical Center[2]	Chanute	86%	292
Hutchinson Regional Medical Center[2]	Hutchinson	85%	580
Saint Catherine Hospital[2]	Garden City	85%	371
Saint Luke Hospital & Living Center	Marion	83%	41
Community Hosp-Onaga/St Marys Campus	Onaga	82%	217
Ottawa County Health Center[2]	Minneapolis	82%	71
Morton County Hospital[2]	Elkhart	81%	151
Nemaha Valley Community Hospital	Seneca	81%	77
Newton Medical Center	Newton	80%	1273
Republic County Hospital[2]	Belleville	79%	283
Geary Community Hospital[2]	Junction City	77%	219
McPherson Hospital[2]	Mcpherson	75%	341
Saint Francis Health Center[2]	Topeka	74%	518
Citizens Medical Center[3]	Colby	72%	54
Mercy Hospital	Moundridge	72%	118
Graham County Hospital	Hill City	70%	145
Clara Barton Hospital	Hoisington	68%	69
Newman Regional Health[2]	Emporia	68%	269
Great Bend Regional Hospital[2]	Great Bend	65%	279
Doctors Hospital	Leawood	56%	64
Hospital District #6 of Harper County	Anthony	51%	93
Sumner Regional Medical Center	Wellington	50%	197
Bob Wilson Memorial Grant County Hospital[2]	Ulysses	48%	171
Kansas Surgery & Recovery Center[2]	Wichita	46%	308
Ness County Hospital District #2	Ness City	45%	31
Harper Hospital District No 5[3]	Harper	43%	30
Herington Municipal Hospital	Herington	32%	68
Osborne County Memorial Hospital[3]	Osborne	25%	56

Immunization for Pneumonia

Hospital Name	City	Rate	Cases
Kansas Medical Center[2]	Andover	100%	497
Menorah Medical Center[2]	Overland Park	100%	690
Stormont - Vail Healthcare[2]	Topeka	100%	747
Western Plains Medical Complex[2]	Dodge City	100%	244
Kansas Heart Hospital[2]	Wichita	99%	527
Mercy Hospital - Fort Scott[2]	Fort Scott	99%	309
Mercy Hospital Independence[2]	Independence	99%	264
Miami County Medical Center	Paola	99%	279
Overland Park Regional Medical Center[2]	Overland Park	99%	472
Salina Surgical Hospital	Salina	99%	398
Shawnee Mission Medical Center[2]	Shawnee Miss.	99%	527
Summit Surgical	Hutchinson	99%	125
Allen County Regional Hospital[2,3]	Iola	98%	214
South Central Kansas Medical Center[2]	Arkansas City	98%	211
Wesley Medical Center[2]	Wichita	98%	570
Ransom Memorial Hospital[2]	Ottawa	97%	384
Saint John Hospital[2]	Leavenworth	97%	416
Saint Luke's Cushing Hospital[2]	Leavenworth	97%	287
Via Christi Hospital Pittsburg[2]	Pittsburg	97%	380
William Newton Hospital	Winfield	97%	414
Kansas City Orthopaedic Institute	Leawood	96%	392
Salina Regional Health Center[2]	Salina	96%	630
University of Kansas Hospital[2]	Kansas City	95%	625
Clay County Medical Center[2]	Clay Center	94%	71
Olathe Medical Center[2]	Olathe	94%	707
Saint Luke's South Hospital[2]	Overland Park	94%	563
Coffey County Hospital[2]	Burlington	93%	334
Lawrence Memorial Hospital[2]	Lawrence	93%	572
Ottawa County Health Center[2]	Minneapolis	93%	94
Providence Medical Center[2]	Kansas City	93%	852
Susan B Allen Memorial Hospital[2]	El Dorado	93%	284
Via Christi Hospital Wichita Saint Teresa[2]	Wichita	93%	366
Fredonia Regional Hospital	Fredonia	92%	270
Mercy Regional Health Center[2]	Manhattan	92%	504
Neosho Memorial Regional Medical Center[2]	Chanute	92%	339
Via Christi Hospitals Wichita[2]	Wichita	92%	601
Holton Community Hospital	Holton	91%	120
Manhattan Surgical Hospital	Manhattan	91%	141
Southwest Medical Center[2]	Liberal	91%	129
Community Hosp-Onaga/St Marys Campus	Onaga	90%	289
Mitchell County Hospital Health Systems[3]	Beloit	90%	30
Cloud County Health Center[2]	Concordia	89%	101
Girard Medical Center[2]	Girard	89%	386
Hays Medical Center[2]	Hays	89%	686
Kansas Spine & Specialty Hospital[2]	Wichita	88%	324
Labette Health[2]	Parsons	88%	357
Pratt Regional Medical Center[2]	Pratt	88%	361
Hutchinson Regional Medical Center[2]	Hutchinson	87%	820
Saint Catherine Hospital[2]	Garden City	87%	344
Coffeyville Regional Medical Center[2]	Coffeyville	86%	395
Nemaha Valley Community Hospital	Seneca	86%	107
Newton Medical Center	Newton	86%	1490
Ellsworth County Medical Center[2]	Ellsworth	85%	144
Mercy Hospital	Moundridge	85%	129
Newman Regional Health[2]	Emporia	85%	329
Republic County Hospital[2,3]	Belleville	84%	294
Morton County Hospital[2]	Elkhart	83%	228
Saint Luke Hospital & Living Center	Marion	82%	67
Clara Barton Hospital[2]	Hoisington	81%	100
Kansas Surgery & Recovery Center[2]	Wichita	81%	409
Geary Community Hospital[2]	Junction City	79%	242
McPherson Hospital[2]	Mcpherson	79%	439
Graham County Hospital	Hill City	78%	222
Saint Francis Health Center[2]	Topeka	77%	716
Norton County Hospital[2,3]	Norton	70%	33
Great Bend Regional Hospital[2]	Great Bend	69%	307
Medicine Lodge Memorial Hospital[2,3]	Medicine Lodge	68%	38
Sumner Regional Medical Center[2]	Wellington	67%	206
Bob Wilson Memorial Grant County Hospital[2]	Ulysses	65%	139
Pawnee Valley Community Hospital[3]	Larned	65%	34
Citizens Medical Center[3]	Colby	63%	131
Doctors Hospital	Leawood	62%	93
Hospital District #6 of Harper County	Anthony	59%	129
Decatur County Hospital[3]	Oberlin	58%	33
Ashland Health Center[3]	Ashland	55%	33
Herington Municipal Hospital	Herington	42%	98
Harper Hospital District No 5[3]	Harper	41%	86

NOTE: Hospital profiles are in alphabetical order by state, then city, then hospital within the city; Rankings exclude hospitals with less than 25 cases except for patient surveys which excludes hospitals with less than 100 cases; (a) 100-299 cases; (1) The number of cases/patients is too few to report; (2) Data submitted were based on a sample of cases/patients; (3) Results are based on a shorter time period than required; (4) Data suppressed by CMS for one or more quarters; (5) Results are not available for this reporting period; (6) Fewer than 100 patients completed the HCAHPS survey; (7) No cases met the criteria for this measure; (8) The lower limit of the confidence interval cannot be calculated if the number of observed infections equals zero; (9) No data are available from the state/territory for this reporting period; (10) The scores shown reflect fewer than 50 completed surveys; (11) There were discrepancies in the data collection process; (12) This measure does not apply to this hospital for this reporting period; (13) Results cannot be calculated for this reporting period; (14) The results for this state are combined with nearby states to protect confidentiality; Please refer to the User's Guide for a full explanation of data.

Hospital Name	City	Rate	Cases
Ness County Hospital District #2	Ness City	36%	50
Osborne County Memorial Hospital[3]	Osborne	35%	65
Rush County Memorial Hospital[3]	La Crosse	9%	35
Hospital District #1 of Rice County[3]	Lyons	7%	28

Stroke Care

Anticoagulation Therapy for Atrial Fibrillation

Hospital Name	City	Rate	Cases
Stormont - Vail Healthcare	Topeka	89%	37

Antithrombotic Therapy Timing

Hospital Name	City	Rate	Cases
Lawrence Memorial Hospital	Lawrence	100%	38
Menorah Medical Center[2]	Overland Park	100%	37
Mercy Regional Health Center	Manhattan	100%	33
Olathe Medical Center	Olathe	100%	87
Overland Park Regional Medical Center	Overland Park	100%	55
Saint Francis Health Center	Topeka	100%	93
Saint Luke's South Hospital	Overland Park	100%	27
Stormont - Vail Healthcare	Topeka	100%	165
University of Kansas Hospital[2]	Kansas City	100%	61
Wesley Medical Center[2]	Wichita	100%	93
Coffeyville Regional Medical Center	Coffeyville	97%	31
Hays Medical Center	Hays	97%	30
Providence Medical Center	Kansas City	97%	92
Shawnee Mission Medical Center	Shawnee Miss.	97%	117
Newman Regional Health	Emporia	96%	28
Salina Regional Health Center	Salina	96%	73
Via Christi Hospitals Wichita[2]	Wichita	95%	94
Hutchinson Regional Medical Center	Hutchinson	91%	47

Assessed for Rehabilitation

Hospital Name	City	Rate	Cases
Lawrence Memorial Hospital	Lawrence	100%	59
Menorah Medical Center[2]	Overland Park	100%	53
Newman Regional Health	Emporia	100%	26
Overland Park Regional Medical Center	Overland Park	100%	66
Saint Francis Health Center	Topeka	100%	106
Stormont - Vail Healthcare	Topeka	100%	219
University of Kansas Hospital[2]	Kansas City	100%	104
Wesley Medical Center[2]	Wichita	100%	105
Providence Medical Center	Kansas City	99%	113
Olathe Medical Center	Olathe	98%	104
Mercy Regional Health Center	Manhattan	97%	38
Shawnee Mission Medical Center	Shawnee Miss.	97%	152
Via Christi Hospitals Wichita[2]	Wichita	97%	132
Salina Regional Health Center	Salina	95%	85
Coffeyville Regional Medical Center	Coffeyville	94%	34
Hays Medical Center	Hays	94%	36
Hutchinson Regional Medical Center	Hutchinson	94%	50
Saint Luke's South Hospital	Overland Park	92%	39

Discharged on Antithrombotic Therapy

Hospital Name	City	Rate	Cases
Hays Medical Center	Hays	100%	36
Lawrence Memorial Hospital	Lawrence	100%	57
Menorah Medical Center[2]	Overland Park	100%	45
Mercy Regional Health Center	Manhattan	100%	37
Olathe Medical Center	Olathe	100%	92
Overland Park Regional Medical Center	Overland Park	100%	58
Providence Medical Center	Kansas City	100%	102
Saint Francis Health Center	Topeka	100%	97
Stormont - Vail Healthcare	Topeka	100%	199
University of Kansas Hospital[2]	Kansas City	100%	73
Wesley Medical Center[2]	Wichita	100%	89
Shawnee Mission Medical Center	Shawnee Miss.	98%	136
Via Christi Hospitals Wichita[2]	Wichita	98%	99
Coffeyville Regional Medical Center	Coffeyville	97%	32
Saint Luke's South Hospital	Overland Park	97%	39
Hutchinson Regional Medical Center	Hutchinson	96%	49
Newman Regional Health	Emporia	96%	25
Salina Regional Health Center	Salina	96%	77

Discharged on Statin Medication

Hospital Name	City	Rate	Cases
Lawrence Memorial Hospital	Lawrence	100%	42
Menorah Medical Center[2]	Overland Park	100%	34
Olathe Medical Center	Olathe	100%	64
Overland Park Regional Medical Center	Overland Park	100%	42
Saint Francis Health Center	Topeka	100%	78
Wesley Medical Center[2]	Wichita	100%	62
Stormont - Vail Healthcare	Topeka	99%	152
Providence Medical Center	Kansas City	98%	84
Shawnee Mission Medical Center	Shawnee Miss.	98%	97
University of Kansas Hospital[2]	Kansas City	97%	58
Via Christi Hospitals Wichita[2]	Wichita	95%	85
Hays Medical Center	Hays	90%	31

Hospital Name	City	Rate	Cases
Saint Luke's South Hospital	Overland Park	83%	29
Salina Regional Health Center	Salina	76%	67
Hutchinson Regional Medical Center	Hutchinson	69%	39
Coffeyville Regional Medical Center	Coffeyville	55%	33
Newman Regional Health	Emporia	48%	25

Thrombolytic Therapy Timing

Hospital Name	City	Rate	Cases
Stormont - Vail Healthcare	Topeka	92%	26

Venous Thromboembolism (VTE) Prophylaxis

Hospital Name	City	Rate	Cases
Lawrence Memorial Hospital	Lawrence	100%	46
Menorah Medical Center[2]	Overland Park	100%	48
Overland Park Regional Medical Center	Overland Park	100%	73
Saint Francis Health Center	Topeka	100%	117
Stormont - Vail Healthcare	Topeka	100%	227
University of Kansas Hospital[2]	Kansas City	100%	103
Wesley Medical Center[2]	Wichita	100%	114
Via Christi Hospitals Wichita[2]	Wichita	99%	145
Olathe Medical Center	Olathe	98%	102
Saint Luke's South Hospital	Overland Park	96%	28
Coffeyville Regional Medical Center	Coffeyville	95%	37
Providence Medical Center	Kansas City	95%	114
Salina Regional Health Center	Salina	92%	85
Shawnee Mission Medical Center	Shawnee Miss.	92%	147
Mercy Regional Health Center	Manhattan	89%	38
Hays Medical Center	Hays	83%	35
Newman Regional Health	Emporia	83%	29
Hutchinson Regional Medical Center	Hutchinson	56%	50

Written Stroke Educational Materials Given

Hospital Name	City	Rate	Cases
Stormont - Vail Healthcare	Topeka	100%	90
Providence Medical Center	Kansas City	98%	59
Wesley Medical Center[2]	Wichita	98%	56
Overland Park Regional Medical Center	Overland Park	97%	32
Saint Francis Health Center	Topeka	96%	47
Shawnee Mission Medical Center	Shawnee Miss.	95%	78
Via Christi Hospitals Wichita[2]	Wichita	95%	60
Lawrence Memorial Hospital	Lawrence	94%	36
University of Kansas Hospital[2]	Kansas City	90%	60
Olathe Medical Center	Olathe	89%	65
Salina Regional Health Center	Salina	53%	43

Surgical Care Improvement Project

Appropriate Beta Blocker Usage

Hospital Name	City	Rate	Cases
Kansas Heart Hospital[2]	Wichita	100%	212
Kansas Medical Center[2]	Andover	100%	124
Kansas Spine & Specialty Hospital[2]	Wichita	100%	30
Kansas Surgery & Recovery Center[2]	Wichita	100%	50
Overland Park Regional Medical Center[2]	Overland Park	100%	147
Saint Catherine Hospital	Garden City	100%	71
Saint Francis Health Center[2]	Topeka	100%	264
Saint Luke's South Hospital	Overland Park	100%	199
Summit Surgical	Hutchinson	100%	41
University of Kansas Hospital[2]	Kansas City	100%	202
Via Christi Hospital Wichita Saint Teresa[2]	Wichita	100%	49
Wesley Medical Center[2]	Wichita	100%	245
Hutchinson Regional Medical Center	Hutchinson	99%	212
Mercy Regional Health Center	Manhattan	99%	134
Newton Medical Center	Newton	99%	95
Salina Regional Health Center[2]	Salina	99%	269
Stormont - Vail Healthcare[2]	Topeka	99%	422
Via Christi Hospital Pittsburg	Pittsburg	99%	77
Via Christi Hospitals Wichita[2]	Wichita	99%	197
Hays Medical Center[2]	Hays	98%	159
Lawrence Memorial Hospital	Lawrence	98%	156
Olathe Medical Center[2]	Olathe	98%	203
Pratt Regional Medical Center[2]	Pratt	98%	58
Salina Surgical Hospital	Salina	98%	157
Shawnee Mission Medical Center[2]	Shawnee Miss.	98%	217
Great Bend Regional Hospital[2]	Great Bend	97%	72
Labette Health	Parsons	97%	143
Coffeyville Regional Medical Center	Coffeyville	96%	49
Manhattan Surgical Hospital	Manhattan	95%	39
Menorah Medical Center[2]	Overland Park	95%	161
Newman Regional Health	Emporia	95%	42
Providence Medical Center[2]	Kansas City	95%	176
Western Plains Medical Complex	Dodge City	91%	32
Wichita VA Medical Center[2]	Wichita	91%	56

Appropriate VTP Within 24 Hours

Hospital Name	City	Rate	Cases
Hutchinson Regional Medical Center	Hutchinson	100%	445
Kansas City Orthopaedic Institute[2]	Leawood	100%	188

Hospital Name	City	Rate	Cases
Kansas Medical Center[2]	Andover	100%	187
Kansas Surgery & Recovery Center[2]	Wichita	100%	219
Manhattan Surgical Hospital	Manhattan	100%	118
Meade District Hospital	Meade	100%	38
Mercy Hospital - Fort Scott	Fort Scott	100%	67
Miami County Medical Center	Paola	100%	50
Olathe Medical Center[2]	Olathe	100%	468
Pratt Regional Medical Center[2]	Pratt	100%	186
Providence Medical Center[2]	Kansas City	100%	459
Saint Francis Health Center[2]	Topeka	100%	633
Saint Luke's South Hospital	Overland Park	100%	729
William Newton Hospital	Winfield	100%	42
Coffeyville Regional Medical Center	Coffeyville	99%	136
Lawrence Memorial Hospital	Lawrence	99%	556
Menorah Medical Center[2]	Overland Park	99%	405
Mercy Regional Health Center	Manhattan	99%	347
Newman Regional Health	Emporia	99%	125
Overland Park Regional Medical Center[2]	Overland Park	99%	380
Salina Regional Health Center[2]	Salina	99%	416
Salina Surgical Hospital	Salina	99%	512
Stormont - Vail Healthcare[2]	Topeka	99%	937
Summit Surgical	Hutchinson	99%	172
Via Christi Hospital Wichita Saint Teresa[2]	Wichita	99%	165
Wesley Medical Center[2]	Wichita	99%	500
Great Bend Regional Hospital[2]	Great Bend	98%	253
Kansas Spine & Specialty Hospital[2]	Wichita	98%	102
Labette Health	Parsons	98%	478
Saint Catherine Hospital	Garden City	98%	277
Shawnee Mission Medical Center[2]	Shawnee Miss.	98%	449
Western Plains Medical Complex	Dodge City	98%	97
Coffey County Hospital	Burlington	97%	31
Neosho Memorial Regional Medical Center[2]	Chanute	97%	33
University of Kansas Hospital[2]	Kansas City	97%	397
Via Christi Hospitals Wichita[2]	Wichita	97%	382
Wichita VA Medical Center[2]	Wichita	97%	147
Geary Community Hospital	Junction City	96%	106
Hays Medical Center[2]	Hays	96%	313
Newton Medical Center	Newton	96%	282
South Central Kansas Medical Center[2]	Arkansas City	96%	55
Southwest Medical Center	Liberal	96%	73
Via Christi Hospital Pittsburg	Pittsburg	96%	203
Mercy Hospital Independence	Independence	95%	38
Ransom Memorial Hospital	Ottawa	95%	87
Saint Luke's Cushing Hospital	Leavenworth	94%	36
Susan B Allen Memorial Hospital	El Dorado	94%	51
Girard Medical Center	Girard	92%	26
Atchison Hospital	Atchison	91%	69
Clara Barton Hospital	Hoisington	91%	32

Controlled Postoperative Blood Glucose

Hospital Name	City	Rate	Cases
Kansas Medical Center[2]	Andover	100%	131
Menorah Medical Center[2]	Overland Park	100%	53
University of Kansas Hospital[2]	Kansas City	99%	129
Via Christi Hospitals Wichita[2]	Wichita	99%	144
Hutchinson Regional Medical Center	Hutchinson	98%	124
Providence Medical Center[2]	Kansas City	98%	52
Saint Francis Health Center[2]	Topeka	98%	104
Stormont - Vail Healthcare[2]	Topeka	98%	187
Wesley Medical Center[2]	Wichita	98%	173
Kansas Heart Hospital[2]	Wichita	97%	321
Salina Regional Health Center[2]	Salina	97%	73
Shawnee Mission Medical Center[2]	Shawnee Miss.	97%	137
Overland Park Regional Medical Center[2]	Overland Park	96%	45
Hays Medical Center[2]	Hays	95%	61
Olathe Medical Center[2]	Olathe	91%	103

Perioperative Temperature Management

Hospital Name	City	Rate	Cases
Atchison Hospital	Atchison	100%	73
Clara Barton Hospital	Hoisington	100%	35
Coffeyville Regional Medical Center	Coffeyville	100%	152
Girard Medical Center	Girard	100%	31
Great Bend Regional Hospital[2]	Great Bend	100%	280
Hays Medical Center[2]	Hays	100%	404
Hutchinson Regional Medical Center	Hutchinson	100%	551
Kansas City Orthopaedic Institute[2]	Leawood	100%	197
Kansas Heart Hospital[2]	Wichita	100%	81
Kansas Medical Center[2]	Andover	100%	324
Kansas Surgery & Recovery Center[2]	Wichita	100%	220
Labette Health	Parsons	100%	518
Lawrence Memorial Hospital	Lawrence	100%	649
Manhattan Surgical Hospital	Manhattan	100%	325
Meade District Hospital	Meade	100%	40
Menorah Medical Center[2]	Overland Park	100%	486
Mercy Hospital - Fort Scott	Fort Scott	100%	71
Mercy Hospital Independence	Independence	100%	39
Mercy Regional Health Center	Manhattan	100%	393
Miami County Medical Center	Paola	100%	51
Neosho Memorial Regional Medical Center[2]	Chanute	100%	37

NOTE: Hospital profiles are in alphabetical order by state, then city, then hospital within the city; Rankings exclude hospitals with less than 25 cases except for patient surveys which excludes hospitals with less than 100 cases; (a) 100-299 cases; (1) The number of cases/patients is too few to report; (2) Data submitted were based on a sample of cases/patients; (3) Results are based on a shorter time period than required; (4) Data suppressed by CMS for one or more quarters; (5) Results are not available for this reporting period; (6) Fewer than 100 patients completed the HCAHPS survey; (7) No cases met the criteria for this measure; (8) The lower limit of the confidence interval cannot be calculated if the number of observed infections equals zero; (9) No data are available from the state/territory for this reporting period; (10) The scores shown reflect fewer than 50 completed surveys; (11) There were discrepancies in the data collection process; (12) This measure does not apply to this hospital for this reporting period; (13) Results cannot be calculated for this reporting period; (14) The results for this state are combined with nearby states to protect confidentiality; Please refer to the User's Guide for a full explanation of data.

Hospital Name	City	Rate	Cases
Newman Regional Health	Emporia	100%	137
Newton Medical Center	Newton	100%	301
Olathe Medical Center[2]	Olathe	100%	542
Overland Park Regional Medical Center[2]	Overland Park	100%	453
Pratt Regional Medical Center[2]	Pratt	100%	202
Providence Medical Center[2]	Kansas City	100%	514
Ransom Memorial Hospital	Ottawa	100%	103
Saint Francis Health Center[2]	Topeka	100%	704
Saint Luke's Cushing Hospital	Leavenworth	100%	66
Saint Luke's South Hospital	Overland Park	100%	789
Salina Regional Health Center[2]	Salina	100%	611
Salina Surgical Hospital	Salina	100%	549
Shawnee Mission Medical Center[2]	Shawnee Miss.	100%	543
South Central Kansas Medical Center[2]	Arkansas City	100%	57
Southwest Medical Center	Liberal	100%	77
Stormont - Vail Healthcare[2]	Topeka	100%	1030
Summit Surgical	Hutchinson	100%	211
Susan B Allen Memorial Hospital	El Dorado	100%	77
University of Kansas Hospital[2]	Kansas City	100%	493
Via Christi Hospital Pittsburg	Pittsburg	100%	241
Via Christi Hospital Wichita Saint Teresa[2]	Wichita	100%	186
Via Christi Hospitals Wichita[2]	Wichita	100%	493
Wesley Medical Center[2]	Wichita	100%	646
Western Plains Medical Complex	Dodge City	100%	112
Wichita VA Medical Center[2]	Wichita	100%	162
Geary Community Hospital	Junction City	99%	120
Saint Catherine Hospital	Garden City	99%	314
Kansas Spine & Specialty Hospital[2]	Wichita	98%	110
William Newton Hospital	Winfield	98%	45
Coffey County Hospital	Burlington	97%	32

Prophylactic Antibiotic Selection

Hospital Name	City	Rate	Cases
Coffey County Hospital	Burlington	100%	26
Girard Medical Center	Girard	100%	27
Kansas City Orthopaedic Institute[2]	Leawood	100%	148
Kansas Heart Hospital[2]	Wichita	100%	323
Kansas Medical Center[2]	Andover	100%	286
Kansas Spine & Specialty Hospital[2]	Wichita	100%	99
Kansas Surgery & Recovery Center[2]	Wichita	100%	155
Labette Health	Parsons	100%	439
Manhattan Surgical Hospital	Manhattan	100%	314
Menorah Medical Center[2]	Overland Park	100%	364
Mercy Hospital - Fort Scott	Fort Scott	100%	52
Miami County Medical Center	Paola	100%	43
Newman Regional Health	Emporia	100%	79
Overland Park Regional Medical Center[2]	Overland Park	100%	355
Saint Luke's South Hospital	Overland Park	100%	620
Stormont - Vail Healthcare[2]	Topeka	100%	963
Via Christi Hospitals Wichita[2]	Wichita	100%	427
Coffeyville Regional Medical Center	Coffeyville	99%	96
Geary Community Hospital	Junction City	99%	100
Hays Medical Center[2]	Hays	99%	315
Hutchinson Regional Medical Center	Hutchinson	99%	459
Lawrence Memorial Hospital	Lawrence	99%	506
Mercy Regional Health Center	Manhattan	99%	252
Olathe Medical Center[2]	Olathe	99%	432
Saint Francis Health Center[2]	Topeka	99%	614
Salina Regional Health Center[2]	Salina	99%	302
Salina Surgical Hospital	Salina	99%	506
Shawnee Mission Medical Center[2]	Shawnee Miss.	99%	441
Summit Surgical	Hutchinson	99%	209
University of Kansas Hospital[2]	Kansas City	99%	418
Via Christi Hospital Wichita Saint Teresa[2]	Wichita	99%	145
Wesley Medical Center[2]	Wichita	99%	528
Wichita VA Medical Center	Wichita	99%	119
Newton Medical Center	Newton	98%	212
Pratt Regional Medical Center[2]	Pratt	98%	162
Providence Medical Center[2]	Kansas City	98%	423
Saint Catherine Hospital	Garden City	98%	223
Saint Luke's Cushing Hospital	Leavenworth	98%	52
Atchison Hospital	Atchison	97%	61
Clara Barton Hospital	Hoisington	97%	32
Great Bend Regional Hospital[2]	Great Bend	97%	244
Western Plains Medical Complex	Dodge City	97%	73
Ransom Memorial Hospital	Ottawa	96%	75
Via Christi Hospital Pittsburg	Pittsburg	96%	160
Susan B Allen Memorial Hospital	El Dorado	93%	61
William Newton Hospital	Winfield	92%	37
Southwest Medical Center	Liberal	88%	51
Meade District Hospital	Meade	87%	38
South Central Kansas Medical Center[2]	Arkansas City	86%	37

Prophylactic Antibiotic Selection (Outpatient)

Hospital Name	City	Rate	Cases
Kansas Heart Hospital	Wichita	100%	278
Kansas Medical Center	Andover	100%	335
Kansas Spine & Specialty Hospital	Wichita	100%	426
Kansas Surgery & Recovery Center	Wichita	100%	55
Manhattan Surgical Hospital	Manhattan	100%	95

Hospital Name	City	Rate	Cases
Mercy Hospital - Fort Scott	Fort Scott	100%	48
Mercy Regional Health Center	Manhattan	100%	66
Overland Park Regional Medical Center	Overland Park	100%	550
Coffeyville Regional Medical Center	Coffeyville	99%	119
Hutchinson Regional Medical Center	Hutchinson	99%	246
Labette Health	Parsons	99%	79
Menorah Medical Center	Overland Park	99%	465
Providence Medical Center	Kansas City	99%	255
Saint Francis Health Center	Topeka	99%	557
Saint Luke's South Hospital	Overland Park	99%	153
Salina Surgical Hospital	Salina	99%	231
Stormont - Vail Healthcare	Topeka	99%	841
Susan B Allen Memorial Hospital	El Dorado	99%	68
University of Kansas Hospital	Kansas City	99%	621
Via Christi Hospitals Wichita	Wichita	99%	628
Wesley Medical Center	Wichita	99%	785
Lawrence Memorial Hospital	Lawrence	98%	188
Newman Regional Health	Emporia	98%	62
Saint Catherine Hospital	Garden City	98%	64
Shawnee Mission Medical Center	Shawnee Miss.	98%	566
Via Christi Hospital Pittsburg	Pittsburg	98%	124
Newton Medical Center	Newton	97%	179
Neosho Memorial Regional Medical Center	Chanute	96%	67
Western Plains Medical Complex	Dodge City	96%	73
Hays Medical Center	Hays	95%	306
Southwest Medical Center	Liberal	95%	185
Olathe Medical Center	Olathe	94%	415
Salina Regional Health Center	Salina	93%	302
South Central Kansas Medical Center	Arkansas City	90%	48
Ransom Memorial Hospital	Ottawa	88%	60

Prophylactic Antibiotic Stopped

Hospital Name	City	Rate	Cases
Clara Barton Hospital	Hoisington	100%	32
Kansas Medical Center[2]	Andover	100%	280
Kansas Surgery & Recovery Center[2]	Wichita	100%	155
Lawrence Memorial Hospital	Lawrence	100%	504
Meade District Hospital	Meade	100%	38
Mercy Hospital - Fort Scott	Fort Scott	100%	50
Miami County Medical Center	Paola	100%	40
Newman Regional Health	Emporia	100%	74
Saint Francis Health Center[2]	Topeka	100%	607
Saint Luke's South Hospital	Overland Park	100%	612
Salina Surgical Hospital	Salina	100%	505
Shawnee Mission Medical Center[2]	Shawnee Miss.	100%	405
Summit Surgical	Hutchinson	100%	209
Wesley Medical Center[2]	Wichita	100%	511
William Newton Hospital	Winfield	100%	37
Kansas City Orthopaedic Institute[2]	Leawood	99%	148
Kansas Heart Hospital[2]	Wichita	99%	316
Labette Health	Parsons	99%	431
Manhattan Surgical Hospital	Manhattan	99%	314
Menorah Medical Center[2]	Overland Park	99%	354
Mercy Regional Health Center	Manhattan	99%	245
Overland Park Regional Medical Center[2]	Overland Park	99%	348
Providence Medical Center[2]	Kansas City	99%	420
Ransom Memorial Hospital	Ottawa	99%	74
Salina Regional Health Center[2]	Salina	99%	281
Stormont - Vail Healthcare[2]	Topeka	99%	947
University of Kansas Hospital[2]	Kansas City	99%	415
Via Christi Hospitals Wichita[2]	Wichita	99%	418
Wichita VA Medical Center	Wichita	99%	116
Coffeyville Regional Medical Center	Coffeyville	98%	83
Hutchinson Regional Medical Center	Hutchinson	98%	430
Pratt Regional Medical Center[2]	Pratt	98%	159
Saint Luke's Cushing Hospital	Leavenworth	98%	52
Via Christi Hospital Pittsburg	Pittsburg	98%	152
Hays Medical Center[2]	Hays	97%	302
Newton Medical Center	Newton	97%	202
South Central Kansas Medical Center[2]	Arkansas City	97%	36
Susan B Allen Memorial Hospital	El Dorado	97%	59
Olathe Medical Center[2]	Olathe	96%	418
Atchison Hospital	Atchison	95%	58
Kansas Spine & Specialty Hospital[2]	Wichita	94%	99
Via Christi Hospital Wichita Saint Teresa[2]	Wichita	94%	139
Western Plains Medical Complex	Dodge City	94%	67
Geary Community Hospital	Junction City	93%	97
Girard Medical Center	Girard	93%	27
Coffey County Hospital	Burlington	92%	25
Great Bend Regional Hospital[2]	Great Bend	87%	241
Southwest Medical Center	Liberal	81%	43
Saint Catherine Hospital	Garden City	74%	219

Prophylactic Antibiotic Timing

Hospital Name	City	Rate	Cases
Coffeyville Regional Medical Center	Coffeyville	100%	96
Girard Medical Center	Girard	100%	27
Hutchinson Regional Medical Center	Hutchinson	100%	461
Kansas Medical Center[2]	Andover	100%	286
Kansas Surgery & Recovery Center[2]	Wichita	100%	155

Hospital Name	City	Rate	Cases
Labette Health	Parsons	100%	439
Lawrence Memorial Hospital	Lawrence	100%	506
Menorah Medical Center[2]	Overland Park	100%	363
Miami County Medical Center	Paola	100%	43
Newman Regional Health	Emporia	100%	79
Overland Park Regional Medical Center[2]	Overland Park	100%	355
Providence Medical Center[2]	Kansas City	100%	425
Saint Francis Health Center[2]	Topeka	100%	614
Saint Luke's South Hospital	Overland Park	100%	620
South Central Kansas Medical Center[2]	Arkansas City	100%	37
Stormont - Vail Healthcare[2]	Topeka	100%	966
Susan B Allen Memorial Hospital	El Dorado	100%	61
Via Christi Hospital Pittsburg	Pittsburg	100%	160
Via Christi Hospitals Wichita[2]	Wichita	100%	428
Wesley Medical Center[2]	Wichita	100%	531
Western Plains Medical Complex	Dodge City	100%	73
Wichita VA Medical Center	Wichita	100%	119
Hays Medical Center[2]	Hays	99%	318
Kansas City Orthopaedic Institute[2]	Leawood	99%	148
Kansas Heart Hospital[2]	Wichita	99%	324
Kansas Spine & Specialty Hospital[2]	Wichita	99%	99
Manhattan Surgical Hospital	Manhattan	99%	314
Olathe Medical Center[2]	Olathe	99%	432
Pratt Regional Medical Center[2]	Pratt	99%	162
Salina Regional Health Center[2]	Salina	99%	302
Salina Surgical Hospital	Salina	99%	506
Shawnee Mission Medical Center[2]	Shawnee Miss.	99%	443
Summit Surgical	Hutchinson	99%	209
University of Kansas Hospital[2]	Kansas City	99%	420
Via Christi Hospital Wichita Saint Teresa[2]	Wichita	99%	145
Geary Community Hospital	Junction City	98%	100
Mercy Hospital - Fort Scott	Fort Scott	98%	52
Mercy Regional Health Center	Manhattan	98%	252
Saint Luke's Cushing Hospital	Leavenworth	98%	53
Clara Barton Hospital	Hoisington	97%	32
Ransom Memorial Hospital	Ottawa	97%	75
Great Bend Regional Hospital[2]	Great Bend	96%	244
Saint Catherine Hospital	Garden City	96%	224
Meade District Hospital	Meade	95%	38
Newton Medical Center	Newton	93%	214
Coffey County Hospital	Burlington	92%	26
William Newton Hospital	Winfield	92%	37
Southwest Medical Center	Liberal	88%	52
Atchison Hospital	Atchison	82%	62

Prophylactic Antibiotic Timing (Outpatient)

Hospital Name	City	Rate	Cases
Coffeyville Regional Medical Center	Coffeyville	100%	107
Kansas Medical Center	Andover	100%	335
Kansas Surgery & Recovery Center	Wichita	100%	55
Salina Surgical Hospital	Salina	100%	226
South Central Kansas Medical Center	Arkansas City	100%	48
Wesley Medical Center	Wichita	100%	787
Kansas Heart Hospital	Wichita	99%	278
Kansas Spine & Specialty Hospital	Wichita	99%	426
Labette Health	Parsons	99%	80
Menorah Medical Center	Overland Park	99%	466
Overland Park Regional Medical Center	Overland Park	99%	553
Providence Medical Center	Kansas City	99%	253
Saint Luke's South Hospital	Overland Park	99%	153
Stormont - Vail Healthcare	Topeka	99%	843
Susan B Allen Memorial Hospital	El Dorado	99%	68
Via Christi Hospitals Wichita	Wichita	99%	635
Western Plains Medical Complex	Dodge City	99%	74
Hutchinson Regional Medical Center	Hutchinson	98%	249
Lawrence Memorial Hospital	Lawrence	98%	134
Manhattan Surgical Hospital	Manhattan	98%	97
Mercy Hospital - Fort Scott	Fort Scott	98%	48
Newman Regional Health	Emporia	98%	62
Olathe Medical Center	Olathe	98%	418
Shawnee Mission Medical Center	Shawnee Miss.	98%	570
Via Christi Hospital Pittsburg	Pittsburg	98%	126
Mercy Regional Health Center	Manhattan	97%	67
Saint Catherine Hospital	Garden City	97%	66
University of Kansas Hospital	Kansas City	97%	623
Saint Francis Health Center	Topeka	96%	567
Neosho Memorial Regional Medical Center	Chanute	95%	63
Salina Regional Health Center	Salina	95%	300
Southwest Medical Center	Liberal	95%	185
Newton Medical Center	Newton	94%	181
Ransom Memorial Hospital	Ottawa	91%	44
Hays Medical Center	Hays	81%	277

Urinary Catheter Removal

Hospital Name	City	Rate	Cases
Coffey County Hospital	Burlington	100%	31
Hutchinson Regional Medical Center	Hutchinson	100%	398
Kansas Medical Center[2]	Andover	100%	257
Lawrence Memorial Hospital	Lawrence	100%	514
Manhattan Surgical Hospital	Manhattan	100%	53

NOTE: Hospital profiles are in alphabetical order by state, then city, then hospital within the city; Rankings exclude hospitals with less than 25 cases except for patient surveys which excludes hospitals with less than 100 cases; (a) 100-299 cases; (1) The number of cases/patients is too few to report; (2) Data submitted were based on a sample of cases/patients; (3) Results are based on a shorter time period than required; (4) Data suppressed by CMS for one or more quarters; (5) Results are not available for this reporting period; (6) Fewer than 100 patients completed the HCAHPS survey; (7) No cases met the criteria for this measure; (8) The lower limit of the confidence interval cannot be calculated if the number of observed infections equals zero; (9) No data are available from the state/territory for this reporting period; (10) The scores shown reflect fewer than 50 completed surveys; (11) There were discrepancies in the data collection process; (12) This measure does not apply to this hospital for this reporting period; (13) Results cannot be calculated for this reporting period; (14) The results for this state are combined with nearby states to protect confidentiality; Please refer to the User's Guide for a full explanation of data.

Menorah Medical Center[2]	Overland Park	100%	181
Mercy Regional Health Center	Manhattan	100%	200
Miami County Medical Center	Paola	100%	29
Saint Francis Health Center[2]	Topeka	100%	587
Saint Luke's Cushing Hospital	Leavenworth	100%	27
Saint Luke's South Hospital	Overland Park	100%	70
Salina Surgical Hospital	Salina	100%	35
Southwest Medical Center	Liberal	100%	42
Summit Surgical	Hutchinson	100%	166
Susan B Allen Memorial Hospital	El Dorado	100%	31
Wesley Medical Center[2]	Wichita	100%	303
Wichita VA Medical Center[2]	Wichita	100%	27
Kansas Heart Hospital[2]	Wichita	99%	268
Pratt Regional Medical Center[2]	Pratt	99%	177
Shawnee Mission Medical Center[2]	Shawnee Miss.	99%	239
Via Christi Hospital Wichita Saint Teresa[2]	Wichita	99%	170
Geary Community Hospital	Junction City	98%	94
Meade District Hospital	Meade	98%	41
Salina Regional Health Center[2]	Salina	98%	210
South Central Kansas Medical Center[2]	Arkansas City	98%	46
Via Christi Hospitals Wichita[2]	Wichita	98%	266
Mercy Hospital - Fort Scott	Fort Scott	97%	30
Ransom Memorial Hospital	Ottawa	97%	62
Stormont - Vail Healthcare[2]	Topeka	97%	382
Coffeyville Regional Medical Center	Coffeyville	96%	83
Newman Regional Health	Emporia	96%	90
Olathe Medical Center[2]	Olathe	96%	396
Overland Park Regional Medical Center[2]	Overland Park	96%	155
University of Kansas Hospital[2]	Kansas City	96%	337
Via Christi Hospital Pittsburg	Pittsburg	96%	98
Hays Medical Center[2]	Hays	95%	235
Western Plains Medical Complex	Dodge City	95%	55
Labette Health	Parsons	94%	132
Providence Medical Center[2]	Kansas City	93%	182
Atchison Hospital	Atchison	92%	61
Newton Medical Center	Newton	92%	257
Great Bend Regional Hospital[2]	Great Bend	85%	156
Saint Catherine Hospital	Garden City	66%	162

Survey of Patients' Hospital Experiences

Area Around Room 'Always' Quiet at Night

Hospital Name	City	Rate	Cases
Manhattan Surgical Hospital	Manhattan	94%	(a)
Miami County Medical Center	Paola	82%	(a)
Salina Surgical Hospital	Salina	81%	300+
Via Christi Hospital Wichita Saint Teresa	Wichita	80%	300+
Kansas Surgery & Recovery Center	Wichita	76%	300+
Atchison Hospital	Atchison	73%	(a)
Mercy Hospital - Fort Scott[11]	Fort Scott	73%	300+
Kansas Spine & Specialty Hospital	Wichita	72%	300+
Coffey County Hospital	Burlington	71%	(a)
Kansas City Orthopaedic Institute	Leawood	70%	300+
Saint John Hospital	Leavenworth	69%	(a)
Kansas Medical Center	Andover	68%	300+
Memorial Hospital	Abilene	68%	(a)
Saint Catherine Hospital	Garden City	68%	300+
Saint Luke's Cushing Hospital	Leavenworth	68%	(a)
Hays Medical Center	Hays	67%	300+
Shawnee Mission Medical Center[11]	Shawnee Miss.	67%	300+
Geary Community Hospital	Junction City	66%	300+
Kansas Heart Hospital	Wichita	66%	300+
McPherson Hospital	Mcpherson	66%	(a)
Great Bend Regional Hospital	Great Bend	65%	300+
Mercy Hospital Independence[11]	Independence	65%	(a)
Mercy Regional Health Center	Manhattan	65%	300+
Ransom Memorial Hospital	Ottawa	65%	300+
University of Kansas Hospital	Kansas City	65%	300+
Neosho Memorial Regional Medical Center	Chanute	64%	300+
Providence Medical Center	Kansas City	64%	300+
Stormont - Vail Healthcare	Topeka	64%	300+
Coffeyville Regional Medical Center	Coffeyville	62%	300+
Pratt Regional Medical Center	Pratt	62%	300+
Susan B Allen Memorial Hospital	El Dorado	62%	300+
William Newton Hospital	Winfield	62%	(a)
South Central Kansas Medical Center	Arkansas City	61%	(a)
Via Christi Hospital Pittsburg	Pittsburg	61%	300+
Kingman Community Hospital	Kingman	60%	(a)
Labette Health	Parsons	60%	300+
Olathe Medical Center	Olathe	60%	300+
Saint Luke's South Hospital	Overland Park	60%	300+
Lawrence Memorial Hospital	Lawrence	59%	300+
Newman Regional Health	Emporia	59%	300+
Salina Regional Health Center[11]	Salina	59%	300+
Menorah Medical Center	Overland Park	58%	300+
Wesley Medical Center	Wichita	58%	300+
Southwest Medical Center	Liberal	57%	300+
Newton Medical Center	Newton	56%	300+
Saint Francis Health Center	Topeka	56%	300+
Citizens Medical Center	Colby	54%	(a)
Republic County Hospital	Belleville	54%	(a)
Western Plains Medical Complex	Dodge City	53%	300+
Overland Park Regional Medical Center	Overland Park	52%	300+
Via Christi Hospitals Wichita	Wichita	50%	300+
Hutchinson Regional Medical Center	Hutchinson	43%	300+

Doctors 'Always' Communicated Well

Hospital Name	City	Rate	Cases
Manhattan Surgical Hospital	Manhattan	92%	(a)
Coffey County Hospital	Burlington	90%	(a)
Kansas City Orthopaedic Institute	Leawood	89%	300+
Neosho Memorial Regional Medical Center	Chanute	89%	300+
Republic County Hospital	Belleville	88%	(a)
Salina Surgical Hospital	Salina	87%	300+
Via Christi Hospital Wichita Saint Teresa	Wichita	87%	300+
Atchison Hospital	Atchison	86%	(a)
Kansas Surgery & Recovery Center	Wichita	86%	300+
Kingman Community Hospital	Kingman	86%	(a)
Labette Health	Parsons	86%	300+
McPherson Hospital	Mcpherson	86%	(a)
Mercy Hospital - Fort Scott[11]	Fort Scott	86%	300+
Pratt Regional Medical Center	Pratt	86%	300+
Ransom Memorial Hospital	Ottawa	86%	300+
South Central Kansas Medical Center	Arkansas City	86%	(a)
Susan B Allen Memorial Hospital	El Dorado	86%	300+
Geary Community Hospital	Junction City	85%	300+
Memorial Hospital	Abilene	85%	(a)
Miami County Medical Center	Paola	85%	(a)
Newman Regional Health	Emporia	85%	300+
Citizens Medical Center	Colby	84%	(a)
Mercy Hospital Independence[11]	Independence	84%	(a)
Mercy Regional Health Center	Manhattan	84%	300+
Saint Luke's Cushing Hospital	Leavenworth	84%	(a)
Hays Medical Center	Hays	83%	300+
Kansas Heart Hospital	Wichita	83%	300+
Newton Medical Center	Newton	83%	300+
Kansas Medical Center	Andover	82%	300+
Kansas Spine & Specialty Hospital	Wichita	82%	300+
Lawrence Memorial Hospital	Lawrence	82%	300+
Olathe Medical Center	Olathe	82%	300+
Salina Regional Health Center[11]	Salina	82%	300+
Southwest Medical Center	Liberal	82%	300+
Via Christi Hospital Pittsburg	Pittsburg	82%	300+
Coffeyville Regional Medical Center	Coffeyville	81%	300+
Great Bend Regional Hospital	Great Bend	81%	300+
Saint Catherine Hospital	Garden City	81%	300+
Shawnee Mission Medical Center[11]	Shawnee Miss.	81%	300+
William Newton Hospital	Winfield	81%	(a)
Stormont - Vail Healthcare	Topeka	80%	300+
University of Kansas Hospital	Kansas City	80%	300+
Wesley Medical Center	Wichita	80%	300+
Menorah Medical Center	Overland Park	79%	300+
Overland Park Regional Medical Center	Overland Park	79%	300+
Saint Francis Health Center	Topeka	79%	300+
Saint John Hospital	Leavenworth	79%	(a)
Providence Medical Center	Kansas City	78%	300+
Saint Luke's South Hospital	Overland Park	78%	300+
Via Christi Hospitals Wichita	Wichita	76%	300+
Western Plains Medical Complex	Dodge City	76%	300+
Hutchinson Regional Medical Center	Hutchinson	72%	300+

Home Recovery Information Given

Hospital Name	City	Rate	Cases
Kansas City Orthopaedic Institute	Leawood	94%	300+
Manhattan Surgical Hospital	Manhattan	93%	(a)
Miami County Medical Center	Paola	92%	(a)
Neosho Memorial Regional Medical Center	Chanute	92%	300+
Kansas Medical Center	Andover	91%	300+
University of Kansas Hospital	Kansas City	91%	300+
Geary Community Hospital	Junction City	90%	300+
Olathe Medical Center	Olathe	90%	300+
Salina Surgical Hospital	Salina	90%	300+
South Central Kansas Medical Center	Arkansas City	90%	(a)
Stormont - Vail Healthcare	Topeka	90%	300+
Hays Medical Center	Hays	89%	300+
Labette Health	Parsons	89%	300+
Lawrence Memorial Hospital	Lawrence	89%	300+
Newton Medical Center	Newton	89%	300+
Pratt Regional Medical Center	Pratt	89%	300+
Saint Luke's Cushing Hospital	Leavenworth	89%	(a)
Salina Regional Health Center[11]	Salina	89%	300+
Shawnee Mission Medical Center[11]	Shawnee Miss.	89%	300+
Southwest Medical Center	Liberal	89%	300+
Atchison Hospital	Atchison	88%	(a)
Kansas Surgery & Recovery Center	Wichita	88%	300+
Menorah Medical Center	Overland Park	88%	300+
Mercy Hospital - Fort Scott[11]	Fort Scott	88%	300+
Saint Luke's South Hospital	Overland Park	88%	300+
Memorial Hospital	Abilene	87%	(a)
Overland Park Regional Medical Center	Overland Park	87%	300+
Coffey County Hospital	Burlington	86%	(a)
Kansas Spine & Specialty Hospital	Wichita	86%	300+
Mercy Hospital Independence[11]	Independence	86%	(a)
Newman Regional Health	Emporia	86%	300+
Ransom Memorial Hospital	Ottawa	86%	300+
Republic County Hospital	Belleville	86%	(a)
Saint Francis Health Center	Topeka	86%	300+
Susan B Allen Memorial Hospital	El Dorado	86%	300+
Via Christi Hospital Pittsburg	Pittsburg	86%	300+
Via Christi Hospital Wichita Saint Teresa	Wichita	85%	300+
Wesley Medical Center	Wichita	85%	300+
Coffeyville Regional Medical Center	Coffeyville	84%	300+
Great Bend Regional Hospital	Great Bend	84%	300+
Kansas Heart Hospital	Wichita	84%	300+
Kingman Community Hospital	Kingman	84%	(a)
Mercy Regional Health Center	Manhattan	84%	300+
Citizens Medical Center	Colby	83%	(a)
Providence Medical Center	Kansas City	83%	300+
William Newton Hospital	Winfield	83%	(a)
Saint Catherine Hospital	Garden City	82%	300+
Saint John Hospital	Leavenworth	82%	(a)
Via Christi Hospitals Wichita	Wichita	82%	300+
Hutchinson Regional Medical Center	Hutchinson	81%	300+
McPherson Hospital	Mcpherson	79%	(a)
Western Plains Medical Complex	Dodge City	78%	300+

Hospital Given 9 or 10 on 10 Point Scale

Hospital Name	City	Rate	Cases
Manhattan Surgical Hospital	Manhattan	92%	(a)
Salina Surgical Hospital	Salina	92%	300+
Via Christi Hospital Wichita Saint Teresa	Wichita	89%	300+
Kansas Heart Hospital	Wichita	88%	300+
Kansas City Orthopaedic Institute	Leawood	87%	300+
Kansas Surgery & Recovery Center	Wichita	84%	300+
Kingman Community Hospital	Kingman	83%	(a)
Neosho Memorial Regional Medical Center	Chanute	82%	300+
Shawnee Mission Medical Center[11]	Shawnee Miss.	82%	300+
University of Kansas Hospital	Kansas City	82%	300+
Coffey County Hospital	Burlington	81%	(a)
Kansas Medical Center	Andover	80%	300+
Kansas Spine & Specialty Hospital	Wichita	79%	300+
Miami County Medical Center	Paola	78%	(a)
Memorial Hospital	Abilene	77%	(a)
Mercy Hospital - Fort Scott[11]	Fort Scott	77%	300+
Citizens Medical Center	Colby	76%	(a)
Hays Medical Center	Hays	76%	300+
Stormont - Vail Healthcare	Topeka	76%	300+
Susan B Allen Memorial Hospital	El Dorado	76%	300+
William Newton Hospital	Winfield	76%	(a)
Lawrence Memorial Hospital	Lawrence	75%	300+
Mercy Regional Health Center	Manhattan	75%	300+
Olathe Medical Center	Olathe	75%	300+
Republic County Hospital	Belleville	75%	(a)
Salina Regional Health Center[11]	Salina	75%	300+
Newton Medical Center	Newton	74%	300+
Saint Luke's South Hospital	Overland Park	74%	300+
South Central Kansas Medical Center	Arkansas City	74%	(a)
Geary Community Hospital	Junction City	73%	300+
Great Bend Regional Hospital	Great Bend	73%	300+
Mercy Hospital Independence[11]	Independence	73%	(a)
Saint Luke's Cushing Hospital	Leavenworth	73%	(a)
Labette Health	Parsons	72%	300+
Pratt Regional Medical Center	Pratt	72%	300+
Ransom Memorial Hospital	Ottawa	72%	300+
Saint Francis Health Center	Topeka	72%	300+
Saint John Hospital	Leavenworth	71%	(a)
Southwest Medical Center	Liberal	71%	300+
Atchison Hospital	Atchison	70%	(a)
Coffeyville Regional Medical Center	Coffeyville	70%	300+
McPherson Hospital	Mcpherson	69%	(a)
Menorah Medical Center	Overland Park	69%	300+
Saint Catherine Hospital	Garden City	69%	300+
Providence Medical Center	Kansas City	68%	300+
Via Christi Hospital Pittsburg	Pittsburg	68%	300+
Via Christi Hospitals Wichita	Wichita	68%	300+
Wesley Medical Center	Wichita	68%	300+
Newman Regional Health	Emporia	67%	300+
Overland Park Regional Medical Center	Overland Park	67%	300+
Hutchinson Regional Medical Center	Hutchinson	58%	300+
Western Plains Medical Complex	Dodge City	57%	300+

Meds 'Always' Explained Before Given

Hospital Name	City	Rate	Cases
Miami County Medical Center	Paola	83%	(a)
Manhattan Surgical Hospital	Manhattan	79%	(a)
Kansas City Orthopaedic Institute	Leawood	78%	300+
Neosho Memorial Regional Medical Center	Chanute	75%	300+
Saint Luke's Cushing Hospital	Leavenworth	74%	(a)
Salina Surgical Hospital	Salina	73%	300+
Citizens Medical Center	Colby	72%	(a)

NOTE: Hospital profiles are in alphabetical order by state, then city, then hospital within the city; Rankings exclude hospitals with less than 25 cases except for patient surveys which excludes hospitals with less than 100 cases; (a) 100-299 cases; (1) The number of cases/patients is too few to report; (2) Data submitted were based on a sample of cases/patients; (3) Results are based on a shorter time period than required; (4) Data suppressed by CMS for one or more quarters; (5) Results are not available for this reporting period; (6) Fewer than 100 patients completed the HCAHPS survey; (7) No cases met the criteria for this measure; (8) The lower limit of the confidence interval cannot be calculated if the number of observed infections equals zero; (9) No data are available from the state/territory for this reporting period; (10) The scores shown reflect fewer than 50 completed surveys; (11) There were discrepancies in the data collection process; (12) This measure does not apply to this hospital for this reporting period; (13) Results cannot be calculated for this reporting period; (14) The results for this state are combined with nearby states to protect confidentiality; Please refer to the User's Guide for a full explanation of data.

Hospital Name	City	Rate	Cases
Coffey County Hospital	Burlington	71%	(a)
Mercy Hospital - Fort Scott[11]	Fort Scott	71%	300+
William Newton Hospital	Winfield	71%	(a)
Memorial Hospital	Abilene	70%	(a)
Kansas Surgery & Recovery Center	Wichita	69%	300+
Kansas Medical Center	Andover	68%	300+
Kingman Community Hospital	Kingman	68%	(a)
Via Christi Hospital Wichita Saint Teresa	Wichita	68%	300+
Kansas Spine & Specialty Hospital	Wichita	67%	300+
Newman Regional Health	Emporia	67%	300+
Ransom Memorial Hospital	Ottawa	67%	300+
Shawnee Mission Medical Center[11]	Shawnee Miss.	67%	300+
South Central Kansas Medical Center	Arkansas City	67%	(a)
Geary Community Hospital	Junction City	66%	300+
Hays Medical Center	Hays	66%	300+
Mercy Hospital Independence[11]	Independence	66%	(a)
Coffeyville Regional Medical Center	Coffeyville	65%	300+
Kansas Heart Hospital	Wichita	65%	300+
Lawrence Memorial Hospital	Lawrence	65%	300+
Republic County Hospital	Belleville	65%	(a)
Salina Regional Health Center[11]	Salina	65%	300+
Atchison Hospital	Atchison	64%	(a)
Pratt Regional Medical Center	Pratt	64%	300+
Southwest Medical Center	Liberal	64%	300+
Stormont - Vail Healthcare	Topeka	64%	300+
Via Christi Hospital Pittsburg	Pittsburg	64%	300+
University of Kansas Hospital	Kansas City	63%	300+
Labette Health	Parsons	62%	300+
McPherson Hospital	Mcpherson	62%	(a)
Mercy Regional Health Center	Manhattan	62%	300+
Saint Catherine Hospital	Garden City	62%	300+
Saint Francis Health Center	Topeka	62%	300+
Susan B Allen Memorial Hospital	El Dorado	62%	300+
Great Bend Regional Hospital	Great Bend	61%	300+
Olathe Medical Center	Olathe	61%	300+
Saint Luke's South Hospital	Overland Park	60%	300+
Newton Medical Center	Newton	59%	300+
Overland Park Regional Medical Center	Overland Park	59%	300+
Providence Medical Center	Kansas City	59%	300+
Menorah Medical Center	Overland Park	58%	300+
Via Christi Hospitals Wichita	Wichita	58%	300+
Saint John Hospital	Leavenworth	57%	(a)
Wesley Medical Center	Wichita	57%	300+
Western Plains Medical Complex	Dodge City	53%	300+
Hutchinson Regional Medical Center	Hutchinson	52%	300+

Nurses 'Always' Communicated Well

Hospital Name	City	Rate	Cases
Manhattan Surgical Hospital	Manhattan	91%	(a)
Salina Surgical Hospital	Salina	90%	300+
Kansas City Orthopaedic Institute	Leawood	88%	300+
Miami County Medical Center	Paola	86%	(a)
Neosho Memorial Regional Medical Center	Chanute	86%	300+
Coffey County Hospital	Burlington	85%	(a)
McPherson Hospital	Mcpherson	85%	(a)
Memorial Hospital	Abilene	85%	(a)
Via Christi Hospital Wichita Saint Teresa	Wichita	85%	300+
Citizens Medical Center	Colby	84%	(a)
Kansas Heart Hospital	Wichita	84%	300+
Kansas Surgery & Recovery Center	Wichita	84%	300+
William Newton Hospital	Winfield	84%	(a)
Kingman Community Hospital	Kingman	83%	(a)
Mercy Hospital - Fort Scott[11]	Fort Scott	82%	300+
Pratt Regional Medical Center	Pratt	82%	300+
Saint Luke's Cushing Hospital	Leavenworth	82%	(a)
Shawnee Mission Medical Center[11]	Shawnee Miss.	82%	300+
University of Kansas Hospital	Kansas City	82%	300+
Mercy Regional Health Center	Manhattan	81%	300+
Newman Regional Health	Emporia	81%	300+
Mercy Hospital Independence[11]	Independence	80%	(a)
South Central Kansas Medical Center	Arkansas City	80%	(a)
Susan B Allen Memorial Hospital	El Dorado	80%	300+
Via Christi Hospital Pittsburg	Pittsburg	80%	300+
Hays Medical Center	Hays	79%	300+
Labette Health	Parsons	79%	300+
Lawrence Memorial Hospital	Lawrence	79%	300+
Ransom Memorial Hospital	Ottawa	79%	300+
Salina Regional Health Center[11]	Salina	79%	300+
Atchison Hospital	Atchison	78%	(a)
Coffeyville Regional Medical Center	Coffeyville	78%	300+
Great Bend Regional Hospital	Great Bend	78%	300+
Kansas Medical Center	Andover	78%	300+
Kansas Spine & Specialty Hospital	Wichita	78%	300+
Olathe Medical Center	Olathe	78%	300+
Saint Francis Health Center	Topeka	78%	300+
Saint John Hospital	Leavenworth	78%	(a)
Southwest Medical Center	Liberal	78%	300+
Stormont - Vail Healthcare	Topeka	78%	300+
Geary Community Hospital	Junction City	77%	300+
Newton Medical Center	Newton	77%	300+
Overland Park Regional Medical Center	Overland Park	76%	300+
Providence Medical Center	Kansas City	76%	300+
Saint Catherine Hospital	Garden City	76%	300+
Via Christi Hospitals Wichita	Wichita	75%	300+
Republic County Hospital	Belleville	74%	(a)
Saint Luke's South Hospital	Overland Park	74%	300+
Menorah Medical Center	Overland Park	73%	300+
Wesley Medical Center	Wichita	73%	300+
Western Plains Medical Complex	Dodge City	70%	300+
Hutchinson Regional Medical Center	Hutchinson	69%	300+

Pain 'Always' Well Controlled

Hospital Name	City	Rate	Cases
Manhattan Surgical Hospital	Manhattan	86%	(a)
Miami County Medical Center	Paola	80%	(a)
Kansas City Orthopaedic Institute	Leawood	79%	300+
McPherson Hospital	Mcpherson	79%	(a)
Kingman Community Hospital	Kingman	78%	(a)
Memorial Hospital	Abilene	78%	(a)
Salina Surgical Hospital	Salina	78%	300+
Via Christi Hospital Wichita Saint Teresa	Wichita	78%	300+
Kansas Heart Hospital	Wichita	77%	300+
Neosho Memorial Regional Medical Center	Chanute	77%	300+
Mercy Hospital - Fort Scott[11]	Fort Scott	75%	300+
Coffey County Hospital	Burlington	74%	(a)
Coffeyville Regional Medical Center	Coffeyville	74%	300+
Atchison Hospital	Atchison	73%	(a)
Citizens Medical Center	Colby	73%	(a)
Mercy Regional Health Center	Manhattan	73%	300+
Newman Regional Health	Emporia	73%	300+
Shawnee Mission Medical Center[11]	Shawnee Miss.	73%	300+
University of Kansas Hospital	Kansas City	73%	300+
Hays Medical Center	Hays	72%	300+
Kansas Spine & Specialty Hospital	Wichita	72%	300+
Kansas Surgery & Recovery Center	Wichita	72%	300+
Pratt Regional Medical Center	Pratt	72%	300+
Geary Community Hospital	Junction City	71%	300+
Via Christi Hospital Pittsburg	Pittsburg	71%	300+
William Newton Hospital	Winfield	71%	(a)
Mercy Hospital Independence[11]	Independence	70%	(a)
Olathe Medical Center	Olathe	70%	300+
Overland Park Regional Medical Center	Overland Park	70%	300+
Salina Regional Health Center[11]	Salina	70%	300+
South Central Kansas Medical Center	Arkansas City	70%	(a)
Southwest Medical Center	Liberal	70%	300+
Great Bend Regional Hospital	Great Bend	69%	300+
Providence Medical Center	Kansas City	69%	300+
Saint Francis Health Center	Topeka	69%	300+
Saint Luke's Cushing Hospital	Leavenworth	69%	(a)
Kansas Medical Center	Andover	68%	300+
Labette Health	Parsons	68%	300+
Lawrence Memorial Hospital	Lawrence	68%	300+
Menorah Medical Center	Overland Park	68%	300+
Newton Medical Center	Newton	68%	300+
Ransom Memorial Hospital	Ottawa	68%	300+
Stormont - Vail Healthcare	Topeka	68%	300+
Susan B Allen Memorial Hospital	El Dorado	68%	300+
Saint Catherine Hospital	Garden City	67%	300+
Saint John Hospital	Leavenworth	67%	(a)
Wesley Medical Center	Wichita	67%	300+
Via Christi Hospitals Wichita	Wichita	66%	300+
Saint Luke's South Hospital	Overland Park	63%	300+
Hutchinson Regional Medical Center	Hutchinson	62%	300+
Western Plains Medical Complex	Dodge City	61%	300+
Republic County Hospital	Belleville	60%	(a)

Room and Bathroom 'Always' Clean

Hospital Name	City	Rate	Cases
Kansas Heart Hospital	Wichita	89%	300+
Manhattan Surgical Hospital	Manhattan	86%	(a)
Neosho Memorial Regional Medical Center	Chanute	86%	300+
Republic County Hospital	Belleville	84%	(a)
Salina Surgical Hospital	Salina	84%	300+
Kansas Surgery & Recovery Center	Wichita	83%	300+
Coffey County Hospital	Burlington	82%	(a)
Miami County Medical Center	Paola	82%	(a)
Shawnee Mission Medical Center[11]	Shawnee Miss.	82%	300+
Kansas City Orthopaedic Institute	Leawood	81%	300+
Kingman Community Hospital	Kingman	81%	(a)
South Central Kansas Medical Center	Arkansas City	79%	(a)
Memorial Hospital	Abilene	78%	(a)
Newman Regional Health	Emporia	77%	300+
Saint Catherine Hospital	Garden City	77%	300+
Kansas Medical Center	Andover	76%	300+
Pratt Regional Medical Center	Pratt	76%	300+
William Newton Hospital	Winfield	76%	(a)
Coffeyville Regional Medical Center	Coffeyville	75%	300+
Labette Health	Parsons	75%	300+
Mercy Hospital - Fort Scott[11]	Fort Scott	75%	300+
Ransom Memorial Hospital	Ottawa	75%	300+
Saint Luke's Cushing Hospital	Leavenworth	75%	(a)
Susan B Allen Memorial Hospital	El Dorado	75%	300+
Via Christi Hospital Wichita Saint Teresa	Wichita	75%	300+
Great Bend Regional Hospital	Great Bend	74%	300+
McPherson Hospital	Mcpherson	74%	(a)
Salina Regional Health Center[11]	Salina	74%	300+
Southwest Medical Center	Liberal	74%	300+
Hays Medical Center	Hays	73%	300+
Newton Medical Center	Newton	73%	300+
Mercy Regional Health Center	Manhattan	72%	300+
Providence Medical Center	Kansas City	72%	300+
Citizens Medical Center	Colby	71%	(a)
Geary Community Hospital	Junction City	71%	300+
Lawrence Memorial Hospital	Lawrence	71%	300+
Saint John Hospital	Leavenworth	71%	(a)
Stormont - Vail Healthcare	Topeka	71%	300+
Atchison Hospital	Atchison	69%	(a)
Saint Francis Health Center	Topeka	69%	300+
University of Kansas Hospital	Kansas City	69%	300+
Via Christi Hospital Pittsburg	Pittsburg	69%	300+
Kansas Spine & Specialty Hospital	Wichita	68%	300+
Mercy Hospital Independence[11]	Independence	68%	(a)
Via Christi Hospitals Wichita	Wichita	68%	300+
Olathe Medical Center	Olathe	67%	300+
Saint Luke's South Hospital	Overland Park	65%	300+
Western Plains Medical Complex	Dodge City	65%	300+
Wesley Medical Center	Wichita	64%	300+
Hutchinson Regional Medical Center	Hutchinson	63%	300+
Menorah Medical Center	Overland Park	63%	300+
Overland Park Regional Medical Center	Overland Park	58%	300+

Timely Help 'Always' Received

Hospital Name	City	Rate	Cases
Manhattan Surgical Hospital	Manhattan	91%	(a)
Salina Surgical Hospital	Salina	88%	300+
Kansas City Orthopaedic Institute	Leawood	87%	300+
Miami County Medical Center	Paola	85%	(a)
Saint John Hospital	Leavenworth	78%	(a)
Kansas Heart Hospital	Wichita	77%	300+
Mercy Hospital - Fort Scott[11]	Fort Scott	77%	300+
Kingman Community Hospital	Kingman	75%	(a)
Citizens Medical Center	Colby	74%	(a)
Coffey County Hospital	Burlington	74%	(a)
Kansas Surgery & Recovery Center	Wichita	74%	300+
Pratt Regional Medical Center	Pratt	74%	300+
William Newton Hospital	Winfield	74%	(a)
Great Bend Regional Hospital	Great Bend	73%	300+
Saint Luke's Cushing Hospital	Leavenworth	73%	(a)
Via Christi Hospital Wichita Saint Teresa	Wichita	73%	300+
University of Kansas Hospital	Kansas City	72%	300+
Atchison Hospital	Atchison	71%	(a)
Neosho Memorial Regional Medical Center	Chanute	71%	300+
Susan B Allen Memorial Hospital	El Dorado	71%	300+
Labette Health	Parsons	70%	300+
McPherson Hospital	Mcpherson	70%	(a)
Mercy Regional Health Center	Manhattan	70%	300+
Ransom Memorial Hospital	Ottawa	70%	300+
South Central Kansas Medical Center	Arkansas City	70%	(a)
Mercy Hospital Independence[11]	Independence	69%	(a)
Kansas Medical Center	Andover	68%	300+
Memorial Hospital	Abilene	68%	(a)
Newman Regional Health	Emporia	68%	300+
Shawnee Mission Medical Center[11]	Shawnee Miss.	68%	300+
Stormont - Vail Healthcare	Topeka	68%	300+
Geary Community Hospital	Junction City	67%	300+
Kansas Spine & Specialty Hospital	Wichita	67%	300+
Lawrence Memorial Hospital	Lawrence	67%	300+
Olathe Medical Center	Olathe	67%	300+
Hays Medical Center	Hays	66%	300+
Newton Medical Center	Newton	66%	300+
Providence Medical Center	Kansas City	65%	300+
Republic County Hospital	Belleville	65%	(a)
Southwest Medical Center	Liberal	65%	300+
Coffeyville Regional Medical Center	Coffeyville	64%	300+
Saint Luke's South Hospital	Overland Park	64%	300+
Salina Regional Health Center[11]	Salina	64%	300+
Via Christi Hospital Pittsburg	Pittsburg	64%	300+
Saint Francis Health Center	Topeka	63%	300+
Saint Catherine Hospital	Garden City	61%	300+
Hutchinson Regional Medical Center	Hutchinson	60%	300+
Menorah Medical Center	Overland Park	59%	300+
Overland Park Regional Medical Center	Overland Park	58%	300+
Via Christi Hospitals Wichita	Wichita	57%	300+
Western Plains Medical Complex	Dodge City	56%	300+
Wesley Medical Center	Wichita	55%	300+

Would Definitely Recommend Hospital

Hospital Name	City	Rate	Cases
Manhattan Surgical Hospital	Manhattan	93%	(a)
Salina Surgical Hospital	Salina	92%	300+
Kansas Heart Hospital	Wichita	90%	300+

NOTE: Hospital profiles are in alphabetical order by state, then city, then hospital within the city; Rankings exclude hospitals with less than 25 cases except for patient surveys which excludes hospitals with less than 100 cases; (a) 100-299 cases; (1) The number of cases/patients is too few to report; (2) Data submitted were based on a sample of cases/patients; (3) Results are based on a shorter time period than required; (4) Data suppressed by CMS for one or more quarters; (5) Results are not available for this reporting period; (6) Fewer than 100 patients completed the HCAHPS survey; (7) No cases met the criteria for this measure; (8) The lower limit of the confidence interval cannot be calculated if the number of observed infections equals zero; (9) No data are available from the state/territory for this reporting period; (10) The scores shown reflect fewer than 50 completed surveys; (11) There were discrepancies in the data collection process; (12) This measure does not apply to this hospital for this reporting period; (13) Results cannot be calculated for this reporting period; (14) The results for this state are combined with nearby states to protect confidentiality; Please refer to the User's Guide for a full explanation of data.

Kansas City Orthopaedic Institute	Leawood	89%	300+
Via Christi Hospital Wichita Saint Teresa	Wichita	88%	300+
Kansas Surgery & Recovery Center	Wichita	87%	300+
University of Kansas Hospital	Kansas City	85%	300+
Coffey County Hospital	Burlington	84%	(a)
Shawnee Mission Medical Center[11]	Shawnee Miss.	84%	300+
Republic County Hospital	Belleville	83%	(a)
Kansas Medical Center	Andover	81%	300+
Neosho Memorial Regional Medical Center	Chanute	81%	300+
Kingman Community Hospital	Kingman	80%	(a)
Kansas Spine & Specialty Hospital	Wichita	79%	300+
Saint Luke's South Hospital	Overland Park	79%	300+
Stormont - Vail Healthcare	Topeka	79%	300+
Olathe Medical Center	Olathe	78%	300+
Newton Medical Center	Newton	77%	300+
William Newton Hospital	Winfield	77%	(a)
Citizens Medical Center	Colby	76%	(a)
Mercy Regional Health Center	Manhattan	75%	300+
Pratt Regional Medical Center	Pratt	75%	300+
Saint Francis Health Center	Topeka	75%	300+
Salina Regional Health Center[11]	Salina	75%	300+
Great Bend Regional Hospital	Great Bend	74%	300+
Hays Medical Center	Hays	74%	300+
Lawrence Memorial Hospital	Lawrence	74%	300+
Susan B Allen Memorial Hospital	El Dorado	74%	300+
Memorial Hospital	Abilene	73%	(a)
Miami County Medical Center	Paola	73%	(a)
Ransom Memorial Hospital	Ottawa	73%	300+
Saint Luke's Cushing Hospital	Leavenworth	73%	(a)
Saint John Hospital	Leavenworth	71%	(a)
South Central Kansas Medical Center	Arkansas City	71%	(a)
Geary Community Hospital	Junction City	70%	300+
Labette Health	Parsons	70%	300+
Via Christi Hospitals Wichita	Wichita	70%	300+
Wesley Medical Center	Wichita	70%	300+
Menorah Medical Center	Overland Park	69%	300+
Overland Park Regional Medical Center	Overland Park	69%	300+
Southwest Medical Center	Liberal	69%	300+
Mercy Hospital - Fort Scott[11]	Fort Scott	68%	300+
Atchison Hospital	Atchison	67%	(a)
Via Christi Hospital Pittsburg	Pittsburg	67%	300+
Providence Medical Center	Kansas City	66%	300+
Coffeyville Regional Medical Center	Coffeyville	65%	300+
Mercy Hospital Independence[11]	Independence	65%	(a)
Saint Catherine Hospital	Garden City	64%	300+
Newman Regional Health	Emporia	63%	300+
McPherson Hospital	Mcpherson	61%	(a)
Hutchinson Regional Medical Center	Hutchinson	58%	300+
Western Plains Medical Complex	Dodge City	52%	300+

Use of Medical Imaging

Cardiac Imaging Stress Test before OP Surgery

Hospital Name	City	Rate	Cases
Smith County Memorial Hospital	Smith Center	0.0%	51
Susan B Allen Memorial Hospital	El Dorado	0.8%	130
Southwest Medical Center	Liberal	1.8%	169
Fredonia Regional Hospital	Fredonia	1.9%	52
Kansas Heart Hospital	Wichita	1.9%	155
Miami County Medical Center	Paola	2.2%	93
Saint Luke's Cushing Hospital	Leavenworth	2.2%	45
Geary Community Hospital	Junction City	2.5%	121
Newton Medical Center	Newton	3.1%	129
Shawnee Mission Medical Center	Shawnee Miss.	3.1%	392
Coffeyville Regional Medical Center	Coffeyville	3.4%	147
Coffey County Hospital	Burlington	3.5%	113
Via Christi Hospitals Wichita	Wichita	3.7%	435
Via Christi Hospital Pittsburg	Pittsburg	3.9%	458
Hays Medical Center	Hays	4.3%	510
Saint Luke's South Hospital	Overland Park	4.3%	392
Clay County Medical Center	Clay Center	4.4%	91
Newman Regional Health	Emporia	4.5%	89
Labette Health	Parsons	4.7%	358
Neosho Memorial Regional Medical Center	Chanute	4.7%	169
Overland Park Regional Medical Center	Overland Park	4.8%	273
Pratt Regional Medical Center	Pratt	4.8%	188
Wesley Medical Center	Wichita	4.8%	124
Menorah Medical Center	Overland Park	4.9%	448
Via Christi Hospital Wichita Saint Teresa	Wichita	4.9%	82
Salina Regional Health Center	Salina	5.1%	78
Stormont - Vail Healthcare	Topeka	5.2%	1619
Community Hosp-Onaga/St Marys Campus	Onaga	5.3%	57
Mercy Hospital Independence	Independence	5.3%	75
Providence Medical Center	Kansas City	5.3%	303
Saint Catherine Hospital	Garden City	5.5%	274
Mercy Hospital - Fort Scott	Fort Scott	5.6%	125
Olathe Medical Center	Olathe	5.6%	444
Ransom Memorial Hospital	Ottawa	5.6%	124
Saint Francis Health Center	Topeka	5.7%	719
Kansas Medical Center	Andover	6.0%	183
Hutchinson Regional Medical Center	Hutchinson	6.2%	97
Lawrence Memorial Hospital	Lawrence	6.2%	450
Holton Community Hospital	Holton	6.4%	110
Hiawatha Community Hospital	Hiawatha	6.6%	91
University of Kansas Hospital	Kansas City	7.1%	2166
William Newton Hospital	Winfield	7.2%	97
Mercy Regional Health Center	Manhattan	7.4%	215

Combination Abdominal CT Scan

Hospital Name	City	Rate	Cases
Hutchinson Regional Medical Center	Hutchinson	0.6%	344
Girard Medical Center	Girard	1.0%	105
Susan B Allen Memorial Hospital	El Dorado	1.1%	465
Providence Medical Center	Kansas City	1.7%	404
Olathe Medical Center	Olathe	2.6%	661
Miami County Medical Center	Paola	2.7%	182
Lawrence Memorial Hospital	Lawrence	3.0%	1089
Wesley Medical Center	Wichita	3.0%	1128
Ransom Memorial Hospital	Ottawa	3.2%	253
Geary Community Hospital	Junction City	3.5%	258
Sabetha Community Hospital	Sabetha	3.7%	82
Saint John Hospital	Leavenworth	3.8%	185
Mercy Regional Health Center	Manhattan	3.9%	431
Western Plains Medical Complex	Dodge City	4.0%	126
Overland Park Regional Medical Center	Overland Park	4.2%	330
Community Hosp-Onaga/St Marys Campus	Onaga	4.6%	131
Ellsworth County Medical Center	Ellsworth	5.1%	137
Decatur County Hospital	Oberlin	5.2%	58
Neosho Memorial Regional Medical Center	Chanute	5.5%	399
Stormont - Vail Healthcare	Topeka	6.1%	2206
Saint Francis Health Center	Topeka	6.8%	1105
Saint Luke's South Hospital	Overland Park	8.9%	518
Newman Regional Health	Emporia	10.7%	485
Mercy Hospital Independence	Independence	11.3%	204
Holton Community Hospital	Holton	11.6%	95
Great Bend Regional Hospital	Great Bend	12.7%	488
Norton County Hospital	Norton	12.9%	70
Salina Regional Health Center	Salina	13.1%	733
Coffeyville Regional Medical Center	Coffeyville	13.4%	336
Menorah Medical Center	Overland Park	13.5%	620
Shawnee Mission Medical Center	Shawnee Miss.	14.0%	1006
Meade District Hospital	Meade	14.1%	71
Coffey County Hospital	Burlington	14.3%	84
University of Kansas Hospital	Kansas City	15.7%	3475
Southwest Medical Center	Liberal	16.2%	222
Mercy Hospital - Fort Scott	Fort Scott	16.7%	282
Saint Catherine Hospital	Garden City	20.7%	425
Via Christi Hospital Pittsburg	Pittsburg	22.6%	478
Saint Luke's Cushing Hospital	Leavenworth	23.0%	209
Allen County Regional Hospital	Iola	27.3%	187
Smith County Memorial Hospital	Smith Center	28.3%	60
Graham County Hospital	Hill City	30.2%	63
Kansas Medical Center	Andover	30.5%	128
Clay County Medical Center	Clay Center	32.9%	164
Anderson County Hospital	Garnett	35.2%	108
Clara Barton Hospital	Hoisington	37.6%	141
Newton Medical Center	Newton	40.3%	330
South Central Kansas Medical Center	Arkansas City	41.4%	145
Hays Medical Center	Hays	45.2%	598
Morton County Hospital	Elkhart	48.8%	41
Via Christi Hospitals Wichita	Wichita	50.3%	1550
McPherson Hospital	Mcpherson	53.8%	266
Via Christi Hospital Wichita Saint Teresa	Wichita	58.6%	256
William Newton Hospital	Winfield	65.0%	277
Pratt Regional Medical Center	Pratt	68.6%	159
Sumner Regional Medical Center	Wellington	69.6%	135
Hiawatha Community Hospital	Hiawatha	75.8%	128
Labette Health	Parsons	75.8%	400
Fredonia Regional Hospital	Fredonia	76.3%	131

Combination Brain/Sinus CT Scan

Hospital Name	City	Rate	Cases
Clara Barton Hospital	Hoisington	0.0%	102
Hillsboro Community Hospital	Hillsboro	0.0%	34
Kansas Spine & Specialty Hospital	Wichita	0.0%	67
Meade District Hospital	Meade	0.0%	40
Sabetha Community Hospital	Sabetha	0.0%	44
Mercy Hospital Independence	Independence	0.5%	199
Mercy Hospital - Fort Scott	Fort Scott	0.7%	272
Saint Catherine Hospital	Garden City	1.0%	200
Susan B Allen Memorial Hospital	El Dorado	1.5%	330
Stormont - Vail Healthcare	Topeka	1.9%	1540
Wesley Medical Center	Wichita	2.2%	975
Shawnee Mission Medical Center	Shawnee Miss.	2.3%	1150
Lawrence Memorial Hospital	Lawrence	2.6%	821
Via Christi Hospitals Wichita	Wichita	3.1%	1539
University of Kansas Hospital	Kansas City	3.8%	755
Olathe Medical Center	Olathe	4.3%	605
Overland Park Regional Medical Center	Overland Park	4.3%	391
Saint Francis Health Center	Topeka	4.6%	745
Geary Community Hospital	Junction City	5.2%	192
Menorah Medical Center	Overland Park	5.4%	463
Via Christi Hospital Pittsburg	Pittsburg	5.9%	358
Decatur County Hospital	Oberlin	14.6%	41

Combination Chest CT Scan

Hospital Name	City	Rate	Cases
Coffeyville Regional Medical Center	Coffeyville	0.0%	197
Decatur County Hospital	Oberlin	0.0%	58
Ellsworth County Medical Center	Ellsworth	0.0%	74
Geary Community Hospital	Junction City	0.0%	216
Hutchinson Regional Medical Center	Hutchinson	0.0%	78
Labette Health	Parsons	0.0%	308
Lawrence Memorial Hospital	Lawrence	0.0%	744
Mercy Regional Health Center	Manhattan	0.0%	389
Newman Regional Health	Emporia	0.0%	339
Ransom Memorial Hospital	Ottawa	0.0%	180
Sabetha Community Hospital	Sabetha	0.0%	46
Saint Catherine Hospital	Garden City	0.0%	277
Susan B Allen Memorial Hospital	El Dorado	0.0%	312
Olathe Medical Center	Olathe	0.2%	653
Salina Regional Health Center	Salina	0.2%	513
Providence Medical Center	Kansas City	0.3%	310
University of Kansas Hospital	Kansas City	0.3%	4371
Newton Medical Center	Newton	0.5%	205
William Newton Hospital	Winfield	0.6%	173
Overland Park Regional Medical Center	Overland Park	0.8%	266
Saint Francis Health Center	Topeka	0.8%	647
Saint Luke's South Hospital	Overland Park	0.8%	238
Menorah Medical Center	Overland Park	0.9%	569
Stormont - Vail Healthcare	Topeka	0.9%	1369
Wesley Medical Center	Wichita	0.9%	585
Saint Luke's Cushing Hospital	Leavenworth	1.1%	91
South Central Kansas Medical Center	Arkansas City	1.1%	94
Hays Medical Center	Hays	1.2%	812
Fredonia Regional Hospital	Fredonia	1.3%	78
Holton Community Hospital	Holton	1.6%	64
Clay County Medical Center	Clay Center	1.7%	173
Saint John Hospital	Leavenworth	1.8%	113
Western Plains Medical Complex	Dodge City	2.0%	51
Allen County Regional Hospital	Iola	2.1%	97
Anderson County Hospital	Garnett	2.1%	47
Miami County Medical Center	Paola	2.5%	80
Hiawatha Community Hospital	Hiawatha	2.6%	78
Mercy Hospital Independence	Independence	3.3%	121
Wamego Health Center	Wamego	3.4%	58
McPherson Hospital	Mcpherson	4.2%	213
Community Hosp-Onaga/St Marys Campus	Onaga	5.0%	80
Neosho Memorial Regional Medical Center	Chanute	5.7%	261
Norton County Hospital	Norton	5.9%	68
Shawnee Mission Medical Center	Shawnee Miss.	6.5%	368
Great Bend Regional Hospital	Great Bend	9.0%	401
Clara Barton Hospital	Hoisington	12.1%	91
Graham County Hospital	Hill City	12.2%	74
Via Christi Hospitals Wichita	Wichita	12.4%	677
Southwest Medical Center	Liberal	14.4%	118
Mercy Hospital - Fort Scott	Fort Scott	16.1%	186
Via Christi Hospital Pittsburg	Pittsburg	16.6%	259
Sumner Regional Medical Center	Wellington	19.7%	66
Kansas Medical Center	Andover	20.4%	93
Pratt Regional Medical Center	Pratt	27.3%	150
Via Christi Hospital Wichita Saint Teresa	Wichita	27.5%	91

Follow-up Mammogram/Ultrasound

A follow-up rate near zero may indicate missed cancer; a rate higher than 14% may mean there is unnecessary follow up.

Hospital Name	City	Rate	Cases
Sumner Regional Medical Center	Wellington	1.1%	273
Clara Barton Hospital	Hoisington	1.4%	138
Saint Catherine Hospital	Garden City	1.6%	437
Bob Wilson Memorial Grant County Hospital	Ulysses	2.8%	106
Neosho Memorial Regional Medical Center	Chanute	2.9%	552
Southwest Medical Center	Liberal	3.1%	324
Saint Francis Health Center	Topeka	3.4%	2493
Allen County Regional Hospital	Iola	4.3%	232
Anderson County Hospital	Garnett	4.5%	247
Girard Medical Center	Girard	4.5%	176
Edwards County Hospital	Kinsley	4.7%	86
Saint Luke's Cushing Hospital	Leavenworth	4.7%	425
Labette Health	Parsons	4.9%	535
South Central Kansas Medical Center	Arkansas City	5.0%	259
Norton County Hospital	Norton	5.1%	256
Coffey County Hospital	Burlington	5.3%	378
Geary Community Hospital	Junction City	5.5%	669
Holton Community Hospital	Holton	5.6%	267
Shawnee Mission Medical Center	Shawnee Miss.	5.9%	2198
Saint Luke's South Hospital	Overland Park	6.5%	874
Ransom Memorial Hospital	Ottawa	6.6%	529
Western Plains Medical Complex	Dodge City	6.6%	228
Lawrence Memorial Hospital	Lawrence	6.8%	2576

NOTE: Hospital profiles are in alphabetical order by state, then city, then hospital within the city; Rankings exclude hospitals with less than 25 cases except for patient surveys which excludes hospitals with less than 100 cases; (a) 100-299 cases; (1) The number of cases/patients is too few to report; (2) Data submitted were based on a sample of cases/patients; (3) Results are based on a shorter time period than required; (4) Data suppressed by CMS for one or more quarters; (5) Results are not available for this reporting period; (6) Fewer than 100 patients completed the HCAHPS survey; (7) No cases met the criteria for this measure; (8) The lower limit of the confidence interval cannot be calculated if the number of observed infections equals zero; (9) No data are available from the state/territory for this reporting period; (10) The scores shown reflect fewer than 50 completed surveys; (11) There were discrepancies in the data collection process; (12) This measure does not apply to this hospital for this reporting period; (13) Results cannot be calculated for this reporting period; (14) The results for this state are combined with nearby states to protect confidentiality; Please refer to the User's Guide for a full explanation of data.

Newton Medical Center	Newton	6.9%	1000
Hiawatha Community Hospital	Hiawatha	7.6%	276
William Newton Hospital	Winfield	8.0%	572
Clay County Medical Center	Clay Center	8.1%	321
University of Kansas Hospital	Kansas City	8.1%	2091
Wamego Health Center	Wamego	8.2%	182
Menorah Medical Center	Overland Park	8.4%	1169
Ellsworth County Medical Center	Ellsworth	8.6%	139
Mercy Regional Health Center	Manhattan	8.6%	1489
Wesley Medical Center	Wichita	8.6%	232
Hays Medical Center	Hays	8.7%	1086
Saint John Hospital	Leavenworth	8.8%	296
Via Christi Hospitals Wichita	Wichita	8.8%	900
Meade District Hospital	Meade	9.0%	89
Olathe Medical Center	Olathe	9.3%	1656
Mercy Maude Norton Hospital	Columbus	9.4%	224
McPherson Hospital	Mcpherson	9.5%	410
Mercy Hospital Independence	Independence	9.7%	403
Graham County Hospital	Hill City	10.1%	99
Fredonia Regional Hospital	Fredonia	10.2%	127
Smith County Memorial Hospital	Smith Center	10.6%	170
Mercy Hospital - Fort Scott	Fort Scott	10.7%	391
Providence Medical Center	Kansas City	11.0%	445
Community Hosp-Onaga/St Marys Campus	Onaga	11.6%	164
Salina Regional Health Center	Salina	11.6%	318
Coffeyville Regional Medical Center	Coffeyville	11.8%	465
Miami County Medical Center	Paola	11.8%	501
Overland Park Regional Medical Center	Overland Park	11.8%	439
Sabetha Community Hospital	Sabetha	11.8%	170
Via Christi Hospital Pittsburg	Pittsburg	14.4%	773
Newman Regional Health	Emporia	14.5%	303
Pratt Regional Medical Center	Pratt	18.7%	476
Susan B Allen Memorial Hospital	El Dorado	24.0%	501

Lumbar Spine MRI for Low Back Pain

Hospital Name	City	Rate	Cases
Ransom Memorial Hospital	Ottawa	29.8%	57
University of Kansas Hospital	Kansas City	31.5%	200
Salina Regional Health Center	Salina	31.7%	164
Newton Medical Center	Newton	33.0%	94
Menorah Medical Center	Overland Park	34.8%	132
Kansas City Orthopaedic Institute	Leawood	35.1%	151
Kansas Surgery & Recovery Center	Wichita	35.5%	121
Doctors Hospital	Leawood	35.7%	56
Great Bend Regional Hospital	Great Bend	36.0%	89
Coffeyville Regional Medical Center	Coffeyville	36.5%	104
Newman Regional Health	Emporia	37.1%	140
Saint Francis Health Center	Topeka	37.4%	382
Kansas Spine & Specialty Hospital	Wichita	37.9%	87
Via Christi Hospital Pittsburg	Pittsburg	38.0%	71
Stormont - Vail Healthcare	Topeka	38.4%	609
Coffey County Hospital	Burlington	38.6%	44
Saint Luke's South Hospital	Overland Park	38.9%	90
South Central Kansas Medical Center	Arkansas City	39.4%	66
Wesley Medical Center	Wichita	40.5%	74
Mercy Hospital - Fort Scott	Fort Scott	41.0%	61
Pratt Regional Medical Center	Pratt	41.1%	95
Mercy Regional Health Center	Manhattan	41.7%	48
Shawnee Mission Medical Center	Shawnee Miss.	41.8%	194
Neosho Memorial Regional Medical Center	Chanute	42.0%	81
Olathe Medical Center	Olathe	42.3%	246
Providence Medical Center	Kansas City	42.3%	52
Lawrence Memorial Hospital	Lawrence	42.9%	191
Saint Catherine Hospital	Garden City	43.2%	74
Mercy Hospital Independence	Independence	43.5%	46
Hays Medical Center	Hays	43.7%	119
Susan B Allen Memorial Hospital	El Dorado	44.2%	129
Geary Community Hospital	Junction City	45.5%	44
Southwest Medical Center	Liberal	45.7%	46
William Newton Hospital	Winfield	45.8%	59
Miami County Medical Center	Paola	46.0%	50
Clay County Medical Center	Clay Center	46.2%	52
Overland Park Regional Medical Center	Overland Park	48.0%	50
Labette Health	Parsons	49.4%	83

NOTE: Hospital profiles are in alphabetical order by state, then city, then hospital within the city; Rankings exclude hospitals with less than 25 cases except for patient surveys which excludes hospitals with less than 100 cases; (a) 100-299 cases; (1) The number of cases/patients is too few to report; (2) Data submitted were based on a sample of cases/patients; (3) Results are based on a shorter time period than required; (4) Data suppressed by CMS for one or more quarters; (5) Results are not available for this reporting period; (6) Fewer than 100 patients completed the HCAHPS survey; (7) No cases met the criteria for this measure; (8) The lower limit of the confidence interval cannot be calculated if the number of observed infections equals zero; (9) No data are available from the state/territory for this reporting period; (10) The scores shown reflect fewer than 50 completed surveys; (11) There were discrepancies in the data collection process; (12) This measure does not apply to this hospital for this reporting period; (13) Results cannot be calculated for this reporting period; (14) The results for this state are combined with nearby states to protect confidentiality; Please refer to the User's Guide for a full explanation of data.

Memorial Hospital

511 Ne 10th St
Abilene, KS 67410
Phone: 785-263-6610
Fax: 785-263-6622
URL: www.mhsks.org
Type: Critical Access Hospitals
Emergency Services: Yes
Ownership: Govt - Hospital Dist/Auth
Beds: 25

Key Personnel:
Radiology. . . . . Jim Bartin
Operating Room. . . . . Marcus Gann, MD
Infection Control. . . . . Carol Landis, RN
Chief of Medical Staff. . . . . Chantel Long, MD
CEO/President. . . . . Mark A Miller
Quality Assurance . . . . Sara Rosebrook
Emergency Room . . . . Carol Ross

Measure	Cases	This Hosp.	State Avg.	U.S. Avg.
Blood Clot Prevention and Treatment				
Anticoagulation Overlap Therapy[5]	-	-	94%	93%
ICU Venous Thromboembolism Prophylaxis[5]	-	-	91%	92%
Incidence of Potentially Preventable VTE[5]	-	-	8%	10%
UFH with Dosages/Platelet Monitoring[5]	-	-	98%	97%
Venous Thromboembolism Prophylaxis[5]	-	-	79%	85%
Warfarin Therapy Discharge Instructions[5]	-	-	84%	75%
Chest Pain/Possible Heart Attack Care				
Aspirin Given Within 24 Hours of Arrival	-	-	94%	96%
Fibrinolytic Meds Within 30 Min. of Arrival	-	-	41%	58%
Average Time to ECG (minutes)	-	-	8	7
Average Time to Transfer (minutes)	-	-	57	60
Children's Asthma Care				
Received Home Management Plan of Care	-	-	-	88%
Received Reliever Medication	-	-	-	100%
Received Systemic Corticosteroids	-	-	-	100%
Emergency Department				
Admittance Decision Time (minutes)[5]	-	-	57	98
Head CT Results Within 45 Min. of Arrival	-	-	53%	57%
Patients Who Left ER Before Being Seen	-	-	2%	2%
Time from ER Arrival to Admit. (minutes)[5]	-	-	185	274
Time from ER Arrival to Discharge (minutes)	-	-	104	134
Time in ER Before Being Evaluated (minutes)	-	-	18	26
Time to Pain Meds for Fractures (minutes)	-	-	47	57
Heart Attack Care				
Aspirin Given at Discharge[3,7]	-	-	99%	99%
Fibrinolytic Meds Within 30 Min. of Arrival[3,7]	-	-	-	54%
PCI Within 90 Minutes of Arrival[3,7]	-	-	97%	96%
Statin Prescribed at Discharge[3,7]	-	-	99%	98%
Heart Failure Care				
ACE Inhibitor or ARB for LVSD[1]	-	-	95%	97%
Discharge Instructions Given[1]	-	-	91%	94%
Evaluation of LVS Function	22	50%	94%	99%
Medicare Spending				
Medicare Spending per Patient (ratio)	-	-	0.94	0.98
Pneumonia Care				
Appropriate Initial Antibiotic Given	20	80%	92%	95%
Blood Culture Timing	25	96%	98%	98%
Pregnancy and Delivery Care				
Newborn Deliveries Scheduled Early[5]	-	-	12%	6%
Preventive Care				
Immunization for Influenza[5]	-	-	88%	90%
Immunization for Pneumonia[5]	-	-	90%	92%
Stroke Care				
Anticoagulation Therapy for Atrial Fibrillation[5]	-	-	88%	95%
Antithrombotic Therapy Timing[5]	-	-	97%	98%
Assessed for Rehabilitation[5]	-	-	97%	97%
Discharged on Antithrombotic Therapy[5]	-	-	98%	99%
Discharged on Statin Medication[5]	-	-	88%	94%
Thrombolytic Therapy Timing[5]	-	-	68%	66%
Venous Thromboembolism Prophylaxis[5]	-	-	93%	94%
Written Stroke Educational Materials Given[5]	-	-	84%	88%
Surgical Care Improvement Project				
Appropriate Beta Blocker Usage[5]	-	-	98%	98%
Appropriate VTP Within 24 Hours[5]	-	-	98%	98%
Controlled Postoperative Blood Glucose[5]	-	-	98%	97%
Perioperative Temperature Management[5]	-	-	100%	100%
Prophylactic Antibiotic Selection[5]	-	-	99%	99%
Prophylactic Antibiotic Selection (Outpatient)	-	-	98%	98%
Prophylactic Antibiotic Stopped[5]	-	-	98%	98%
Prophylactic Antibiotic Timing[5]	-	-	99%	99%
Prophylactic Antibiotic Timing (Outpatient)	-	-	98%	98%
Urinary Catheter Removal[5]	-	-	97%	97%
Survey of Patients' Hospital Experiences				
Area Around Room 'Always' Quiet at Night	(a)	68%	65%	61%
Doctors 'Always' Communicated Well	(a)	85%	85%	82%
Home Recovery Information Given	(a)	87%	86%	85%
Hospital Given 9 or 10 on 10 Point Scale	(a)	77%	76%	71%
Meds 'Always' Explained Before Given	(a)	70%	66%	64%
Nurses 'Always' Communicated Well	(a)	85%	81%	79%
Pain 'Always' Well Controlled	(a)	78%	72%	71%
Room and Bathroom 'Always' Clean	(a)	78%	76%	73%
Timely Help 'Always' Received	(a)	68%	72%	68%
Would Definitely Recommend Hospital	(a)	73%	75%	71%
Use of Medical Imaging				
Cardiac Imaging Stress Test before Surgery	-	-	5%	5.3%
Combination Abdominal CT Scan	-	-	19%	10.5%
Combination Brain/Sinus CT Scan	-	-	2.9%	2.7%
Combination Chest CT Scan	-	-	3.9%	2.7%
Follow-up Mammogram/Ultrasound	-	-	7.8%	8.8%
Lumbar Spine MRI for Low Back Pain	-	-	40.2%	37.2%

Kansas Medical Center

1124 West 21st Street
Andover, KS 67002
Phone: 316-300-4000
URL: www.ksmedcenter.com
Type: Acute Care Hospitals
Emergency Services: Yes
Ownership: Proprietary
Beds: 60

Measure	Cases	This Hosp.	State Avg.	U.S. Avg.
Blood Clot Prevention and Treatment				
Anticoagulation Overlap Therapy[2]	21	100%	94%	93%
ICU Venous Thromboembolism Prophylaxis[2]	70	100%	91%	92%
Incidence of Potentially Preventable VTE[1,2]	-	-	8%	10%
UFH with Dosages/Platelet Monitoring[2]	20	100%	98%	97%
Venous Thromboembolism Prophylaxis[2]	18	100%	79%	85%
Warfarin Therapy Discharge Instructions[2]	17	100%	84%	75%
Chest Pain/Possible Heart Attack Care				
Aspirin Given Within 24 Hours of Arrival[1,3]	-	-	94%	96%
Fibrinolytic Meds Within 30 Min. of Arrival[3,7]	-	-	41%	58%
Average Time to ECG (minutes)[1,3]	-	-	8	7
Average Time to Transfer (minutes)[3,7]	-	-	57	60
Children's Asthma Care				
Received Home Management Plan of Care	-	-	-	88%
Received Reliever Medication	-	-	-	100%
Received Systemic Corticosteroids	-	-	-	100%
Emergency Department				
Admittance Decision Time (minutes)[2]	163	49	57	98
Head CT Results Within 45 Min. of Arrival[1]	-	-	53%	57%
Patients Who Left ER Before Being Seen	6,831	1%	2%	2%
Time from ER Arrival to Admit. (minutes)[2]	165	143	185	274
Time from ER Arrival to Discharge (minutes)	376	67	104	134
Time in ER Before Being Evaluated (minutes)	362	22	18	26
Time to Pain Meds for Fractures (minutes)	70	38	47	57
Heart Attack Care				
Aspirin Given at Discharge[2]	191	100%	99%	99%
Fibrinolytic Meds Within 30 Min. of Arrival[2,7]	-	-	-	54%
PCI Within 90 Minutes of Arrival[1,2]	-	-	97%	96%
Statin Prescribed at Discharge[2]	190	100%	99%	98%
Heart Failure Care				
ACE Inhibitor or ARB for LVSD	37	100%	95%	97%
Discharge Instructions Given	77	100%	91%	94%
Evaluation of LVS Function	108	100%	94%	99%
Medicare Spending				
Medicare Spending per Patient (ratio)	-	0.94	0.94	0.98
Pneumonia Care				
Appropriate Initial Antibiotic Given	22	100%	92%	95%
Blood Culture Timing	34	100%	98%	98%
Pregnancy and Delivery Care				
Newborn Deliveries Scheduled Early[2,7]	-	-	12%	6%
Preventive Care				
Immunization for Influenza[2]	303	100%	88%	90%
Immunization for Pneumonia[2]	497	100%	90%	92%
Stroke Care				
Anticoagulation Therapy for Atrial Fibrillation[1]	-	-	88%	95%
Antithrombotic Therapy Timing[1]	-	-	97%	98%
Assessed for Rehabilitation[1]	-	-	97%	97%
Discharged on Antithrombotic Therapy[1]	-	-	98%	99%
Discharged on Statin Medication[1]	-	-	88%	94%
Thrombolytic Therapy Timing[7]	-	-	68%	66%
Venous Thromboembolism Prophylaxis[1]	-	-	93%	94%
Written Stroke Educational Materials Given[1]	-	-	84%	88%
Surgical Care Improvement Project				
Appropriate Beta Blocker Usage[2]	124	100%	98%	98%
Appropriate VTP Within 24 Hours[2]	187	100%	98%	98%
Controlled Postoperative Blood Glucose[2]	131	100%	98%	97%
Perioperative Temperature Management[2]	324	100%	100%	100%
Prophylactic Antibiotic Selection[2]	286	100%	99%	99%
Prophylactic Antibiotic Selection (Outpatient)	335	100%	98%	98%
Prophylactic Antibiotic Stopped[2]	280	100%	98%	98%
Prophylactic Antibiotic Timing[2]	286	100%	99%	99%
Prophylactic Antibiotic Timing (Outpatient)	335	100%	98%	98%
Urinary Catheter Removal[2]	257	100%	97%	97%
Survey of Patients' Hospital Experiences				
Area Around Room 'Always' Quiet at Night	300+	68%	65%	61%
Doctors 'Always' Communicated Well	300+	82%	85%	82%
Home Recovery Information Given	300+	91%	86%	85%
Hospital Given 9 or 10 on 10 Point Scale	300+	80%	76%	71%
Meds 'Always' Explained Before Given	300+	68%	66%	64%
Nurses 'Always' Communicated Well	300+	78%	81%	79%
Pain 'Always' Well Controlled	300+	68%	72%	71%
Room and Bathroom 'Always' Clean	300+	76%	76%	73%
Timely Help 'Always' Received	300+	68%	72%	68%
Would Definitely Recommend Hospital	300+	81%	75%	71%
Use of Medical Imaging				
Cardiac Imaging Stress Test before Surgery	183	6.0%	5%	5.3%
Combination Abdominal CT Scan	128	30.5%	19%	10.5%
Combination Brain/Sinus CT Scan[1]	-	-	2.9%	2.7%
Combination Chest CT Scan	93	20.4%	3.9%	2.7%
Follow-up Mammogram/Ultrasound[7]	-	-	7.8%	8.8%
Lumbar Spine MRI for Low Back Pain[7]	-	-	40.2%	37.2%

Hospital District #6 of Harper County

1101 E Spring Street
Anthony, KS 67003
Phone: 620-842-5111
Type: Critical Access Hospitals
Emergency Services: Yes
Ownership: Govt - Hospital Dist/Auth

Measure	Cases	This Hosp.	State Avg.	U.S. Avg.
Blood Clot Prevention and Treatment				
Anticoagulation Overlap Therapy[7]	-	-	94%	93%
ICU Venous Thromboembolism Prophylaxis[7]	-	-	91%	92%
Incidence of Potentially Preventable VTE[7]	-	-	8%	10%
UFH with Dosages/Platelet Monitoring[7]	-	-	98%	97%
Venous Thromboembolism Prophylaxis	106	75%	79%	85%
Warfarin Therapy Discharge Instructions[7]	-	-	84%	75%
Chest Pain/Possible Heart Attack Care				
Aspirin Given Within 24 Hours of Arrival	-	-	94%	96%
Fibrinolytic Meds Within 30 Min. of Arrival	-	-	41%	58%
Average Time to ECG (minutes)	-	-	8	7
Average Time to Transfer (minutes)	-	-	57	60
Children's Asthma Care				
Received Home Management Plan of Care	-	-	-	88%
Received Reliever Medication	-	-	-	100%
Received Systemic Corticosteroids	-	-	-	100%
Emergency Department				
Admittance Decision Time (minutes)	84	15	57	98
Head CT Results Within 45 Min. of Arrival	-	-	53%	57%
Patients Who Left ER Before Being Seen	-	-	2%	2%
Time from ER Arrival to Admit. (minutes)	101	105	185	274
Time from ER Arrival to Discharge (minutes)	-	-	104	134
Time in ER Before Being Evaluated (minutes)	-	-	18	26
Time to Pain Meds for Fractures (minutes)	-	-	47	57
Heart Attack Care				
Aspirin Given at Discharge[1,3]	-	-	99%	99%

NOTE: Hospital profiles are in alphabetical order by state, then city, then hospital within the city; Rankings exclude hospitals with less than 25 cases except for patient surveys which excludes hospitals with less than 100 cases; (a) 100-299 cases; (1) The number of cases/patients is too few to report; (2) Data submitted were based on a sample of cases/patients; (3) Results are based on a shorter time period than required; (4) Data suppressed by CMS for one or more quarters; (5) Results are not available for this reporting period; (6) Fewer than 100 patients completed the HCAHPS survey; (7) No cases met the criteria for this measure; (8) The lower limit of the confidence interval cannot be calculated if the number of observed infections equals zero; (9) No data are available from the state/territory for this reporting period; (10) The scores shown reflect fewer than 50 completed surveys; (11) There were discrepancies in the data collection process; (12) This measure does not apply to this hospital for this reporting period; (13) Results cannot be calculated for this reporting period; (14) The results for this state are combined with nearby states to protect confidentiality; Please refer to the User's Guide for a full explanation of data.

Measure	Cases	This Hosp.	State Avg.	U.S. Avg.
Fibrinolytic Meds Within 30 Min. of Arrival[3,7]	-	-	-	54%
PCI Within 90 Minutes of Arrival[3,7]	-	-	97%	96%
Statin Prescribed at Discharge[1,3]	-	-	99%	98%
Heart Failure Care				
ACE Inhibitor or ARB for LVSD[7]	-	-	95%	97%
Discharge Instructions Given[1]	-	-	91%	94%
Evaluation of LVS Function	13	46%	94%	99%
Medicare Spending				
Medicare Spending per Patient (ratio)	-	-	0.94	0.98
Pneumonia Care				
Appropriate Initial Antibiotic Given[1,3]	-	-	92%	95%
Blood Culture Timing[3,7]	-	-	98%	98%
Pregnancy and Delivery Care				
Newborn Deliveries Scheduled Early[3,7]	-	-	12%	6%
Preventive Care				
Immunization for Influenza	93	51%	88%	90%
Immunization for Pneumonia	129	59%	90%	92%
Stroke Care				
Anticoagulation Therapy for Atrial Fibrillation[3,7]	-	-	88%	95%
Antithrombotic Therapy Timing[1,3]	-	-	97%	98%
Assessed for Rehabilitation[1,3]	-	-	97%	97%
Discharged on Antithrombotic Therapy[1,3]	-	-	98%	99%
Discharged on Statin Medication[1,3]	-	-	88%	94%
Thrombolytic Therapy Timing[1,3]	-	-	68%	66%
Venous Thromboembolism Prophylaxis[1,3]	-	-	93%	94%
Written Stroke Educational Materials Given[3,7]	-	-	84%	88%
Surgical Care Improvement Project				
Appropriate Beta Blocker Usage[5]	-	-	98%	98%
Appropriate VTP Within 24 Hours[5]	-	-	98%	98%
Controlled Postoperative Blood Glucose[5]	-	-	98%	97%
Perioperative Temperature Management[5]	-	-	100%	100%
Prophylactic Antibiotic Selection[5]	-	-	99%	99%
Prophylactic Antibiotic Selection (Outpatient)	-	-	98%	98%
Prophylactic Antibiotic Stopped[5]	-	-	98%	98%
Prophylactic Antibiotic Timing[5]	-	-	99%	99%
Prophylactic Antibiotic Timing (Outpatient)	-	-	98%	98%
Urinary Catheter Removal[5]	-	-	97%	97%
Survey of Patients' Hospital Experiences				
Area Around Room 'Always' Quiet at Night[5]	-	-	65%	61%
Doctors 'Always' Communicated Well[5]	-	-	85%	82%
Home Recovery Information Given[5]	-	-	86%	85%
Hospital Given 9 or 10 on 10 Point Scale[5]	-	-	76%	71%
Meds 'Always' Explained Before Given[5]	-	-	66%	64%
Nurses 'Always' Communicated Well[5]	-	-	81%	79%
Pain 'Always' Well Controlled[5]	-	-	72%	71%
Room and Bathroom 'Always' Clean[5]	-	-	76%	73%
Timely Help 'Always' Received[5]	-	-	72%	68%
Would Definitely Recommend Hospital[5]	-	-	75%	71%
Use of Medical Imaging				
Cardiac Imaging Stress Test before Surgery	-	-	5%	5.3%
Combination Abdominal CT Scan	-	-	19%	10.5%
Combination Brain/Sinus CT Scan	-	-	2.9%	2.7%
Combination Chest CT Scan	-	-	3.9%	2.7%
Follow-up Mammogram/Ultrasound	-	-	7.8%	8.8%
Lumbar Spine MRI for Low Back Pain	-	-	40.2%	37.2%

South Central Kansas Medical Center

6401 Patterson Parkway
Arkansas City, KS 67005
E-mail: ceo@sckrmc.com
URL: www.sckrmc.com
Phone: 620-442-2500
Fax: 620-441-5966
Type: Acute Care Hospitals
Ownership: Government - Local
Emergency Services: Yes
Beds: 85

Key Personnel:
Surgery .... Tyson Blatchford
Cardiology .... Gregory R Boxberger
CEO/President.............. Phyllis Macy-Mills
Cardiology .... Whitney Reader
Surgery .... Chandy Samuel
Chief of Medical Staff.......... Kamran Shahzada, MD

Measure	Cases	This Hosp.	State Avg.	U.S. Avg.
Blood Clot Prevention and Treatment				
Anticoagulation Overlap Therapy[1,2]	-	-	94%	93%
ICU Venous Thromboembolism Prophylaxis[2]	13	69%	91%	92%
Incidence of Potentially Preventable VTE[1,2]	-	-	8%	10%
UFH with Dosages/Platelet Monitoring[2,7]	-	-	98%	97%
Venous Thromboembolism Prophylaxis[2]	76	66%	79%	85%
Warfarin Therapy Discharge Instructions[1,2]	-	-	84%	75%
Chest Pain/Possible Heart Attack Care				
Aspirin Given Within 24 Hours of Arrival	27	96%	94%	96%
Fibrinolytic Meds Within 30 Min. of Arrival[1]	-	-	41%	58%
Average Time to ECG (minutes)	30	5	8	7
Average Time to Transfer (minutes)[1]	-	-	57	60
Children's Asthma Care				
Received Home Management Plan of Care	-	-	-	88%
Received Reliever Medication	-	-	-	100%
Received Systemic Corticosteroids	-	-	-	100%
Emergency Department				
Admittance Decision Time (minutes)[2]	158	50	57	98
Head CT Results Within 45 Min. of Arrival[1,3]	-	-	53%	57%
Patients Who Left ER Before Being Seen	7,269	0%	2%	2%
Time from ER Arrival to Admit. (minutes)[2]	174	140	185	274
Time from ER Arrival to Discharge (minutes)	300	74	104	134
Time in ER Before Being Evaluated (minutes)	384	13	18	26
Time to Pain Meds for Fractures (minutes)	45	31	47	57
Heart Attack Care				
Aspirin Given at Discharge[5]	-	-	99%	99%
Fibrinolytic Meds Within 30 Min. of Arrival[5]	-	-	-	54%
PCI Within 90 Minutes of Arrival[5]	-	-	97%	96%
Statin Prescribed at Discharge[5]	-	-	99%	98%
Heart Failure Care				
ACE Inhibitor or ARB for LVSD[1,3]	-	-	95%	97%
Discharge Instructions Given[1,3]	-	-	91%	94%
Evaluation of LVS Function[1,3]	-	-	94%	99%
Medicare Spending				
Medicare Spending per Patient (ratio)	-	0.94	0.94	0.98
Pneumonia Care				
Appropriate Initial Antibiotic Given[2]	33	94%	92%	95%
Blood Culture Timing[2]	29	90%	98%	98%
Pregnancy and Delivery Care				
Newborn Deliveries Scheduled Early	17	0%	12%	6%
Preventive Care				
Immunization for Influenza[2]	228	99%	88%	90%
Immunization for Pneumonia[2]	211	98%	90%	92%
Stroke Care				
Anticoagulation Therapy for Atrial Fibrillation[1,3]	-	-	88%	95%
Antithrombotic Therapy Timing[1,3]	-	-	97%	98%
Assessed for Rehabilitation[1,3]	-	-	97%	97%
Discharged on Antithrombotic Therapy[1,3]	-	-	98%	99%
Discharged on Statin Medication[1,3]	-	-	88%	94%
Thrombolytic Therapy Timing[1,3]	-	-	68%	66%
Venous Thromboembolism Prophylaxis[1,3]	-	-	93%	94%
Written Stroke Educational Materials Given[3,7]	-	-	84%	88%
Surgical Care Improvement Project				
Appropriate Beta Blocker Usage[2]	13	77%	98%	98%
Appropriate VTP Within 24 Hours[2]	55	96%	98%	98%
Controlled Postoperative Blood Glucose[2,7]	-	-	98%	97%
Perioperative Temperature Management[2]	57	100%	100%	100%
Prophylactic Antibiotic Selection[2]	37	86%	99%	99%
Prophylactic Antibiotic Selection (Outpatient)	48	90%	98%	98%
Prophylactic Antibiotic Stopped[2]	36	97%	98%	98%
Prophylactic Antibiotic Timing[2]	37	100%	99%	99%
Prophylactic Antibiotic Timing (Outpatient)	48	100%	98%	98%
Urinary Catheter Removal[2]	46	98%	97%	97%
Survey of Patients' Hospital Experiences				
Area Around Room 'Always' Quiet at Night	(a)	61%	65%	61%
Doctors 'Always' Communicated Well	(a)	86%	85%	82%
Home Recovery Information Given	(a)	90%	86%	85%
Hospital Given 9 or 10 on 10 Point Scale	(a)	74%	76%	71%
Meds 'Always' Explained Before Given	(a)	67%	66%	64%
Nurses 'Always' Communicated Well	(a)	80%	81%	79%
Pain 'Always' Well Controlled	(a)	70%	72%	71%
Room and Bathroom 'Always' Clean	(a)	79%	76%	73%
Timely Help 'Always' Received	(a)	70%	72%	68%
Would Definitely Recommend Hospital	(a)	71%	75%	71%
Use of Medical Imaging				
Cardiac Imaging Stress Test before Surgery[1]	-	-	5%	5.3%
Combination Abdominal CT Scan	145	41.4%	19%	10.5%
Combination Brain/Sinus CT Scan[1]	-	-	2.9%	2.7%
Combination Chest CT Scan	94	1.1%	3.9%	2.7%
Follow-up Mammogram/Ultrasound	259	5.0%	7.8%	8.8%
Lumbar Spine MRI for Low Back Pain	66	39.4%	40.2%	37.2%

Ashland Health Center

709 Oak Street
Ashland, KS 67831
URL: www.phn.org
Phone: 620-635-2241
Fax: 620-635-2229
Type: Critical Access Hospitals
Ownership: Govt - Hospital Dist/Auth
Emergency Services: No
Beds: 47

Key Personnel:
CEO .... Benjamin Anderson
CEO/President.................. Daryl Marshall
Emergency Room .... Michelle Moore
Quality Assurance .... Michelle Moore
Cardiac Laboratory............ Samuel Todd Stephens, MD
Chief of Medical Staff.......... Samuel Todd Stephens

Measure	Cases	This Hosp.	State Avg.	U.S. Avg.
Blood Clot Prevention and Treatment				
Anticoagulation Overlap Therapy[5]	-	-	94%	93%
ICU Venous Thromboembolism Prophylaxis[5]	-	-	91%	92%
Incidence of Potentially Preventable VTE[5]	-	-	8%	10%
UFH with Dosages/Platelet Monitoring[5]	-	-	98%	97%
Venous Thromboembolism Prophylaxis[5]	-	-	79%	85%
Warfarin Therapy Discharge Instructions[5]	-	-	84%	75%
Chest Pain/Possible Heart Attack Care				
Aspirin Given Within 24 Hours of Arrival	-	-	94%	96%
Fibrinolytic Meds Within 30 Min. of Arrival	-	-	41%	58%
Average Time to ECG (minutes)	-	-	8	7
Average Time to Transfer (minutes)	-	-	57	60
Children's Asthma Care				
Received Home Management Plan of Care	-	-	-	88%
Received Reliever Medication	-	-	-	100%
Received Systemic Corticosteroids	-	-	-	100%
Emergency Department				
Admittance Decision Time (minutes)[3]	18	8	57	98
Head CT Results Within 45 Min. of Arrival	-	-	53%	57%
Patients Who Left ER Before Being Seen	-	-	2%	2%
Time from ER Arrival to Admit. (minutes)[3]	21	105	185	274
Time from ER Arrival to Discharge (minutes)	-	-	104	134
Time in ER Before Being Evaluated (minutes)	-	-	18	26
Time to Pain Meds for Fractures (minutes)	-	-	47	57
Heart Attack Care				
Aspirin Given at Discharge[5]	-	-	99%	99%
Fibrinolytic Meds Within 30 Min. of Arrival[5]	-	-	-	54%
PCI Within 90 Minutes of Arrival[5]	-	-	97%	96%
Statin Prescribed at Discharge[5]	-	-	99%	98%
Heart Failure Care				
ACE Inhibitor or ARB for LVSD[1,3]	-	-	95%	97%
Discharge Instructions Given[1,3]	-	-	91%	94%
Evaluation of LVS Function[1,3]	-	-	94%	99%
Medicare Spending				
Medicare Spending per Patient (ratio)	-	-	0.94	0.98
Pneumonia Care				
Appropriate Initial Antibiotic Given[1,3]	-	-	92%	95%
Blood Culture Timing[1,3]	-	-	98%	98%
Pregnancy and Delivery Care				
Newborn Deliveries Scheduled Early[5]	-	-	12%	6%
Preventive Care				
Immunization for Influenza[3]	13	92%	88%	90%
Immunization for Pneumonia[3]	33	55%	90%	92%
Stroke Care				
Anticoagulation Therapy for Atrial Fibrillation[5]	-	-	88%	95%
Antithrombotic Therapy Timing[5]	-	-	97%	98%
Assessed for Rehabilitation[5]	-	-	97%	97%
Discharged on Antithrombotic Therapy[5]	-	-	98%	99%
Discharged on Statin Medication[5]	-	-	88%	94%
Thrombolytic Therapy Timing[5]	-	-	68%	66%
Venous Thromboembolism Prophylaxis[5]	-	-	93%	94%
Written Stroke Educational Materials Given[5]	-	-	84%	88%
Surgical Care Improvement Project				

NOTE: Hospital profiles are in alphabetical order by state, then city, then hospital within the city; Rankings exclude hospitals with less than 25 cases except for patient surveys which excludes hospitals with less than 100 cases; (a) 100-299 cases; (1) The number of cases/patients is too few to report; (2) Data submitted were based on a sample of cases/patients; (3) Results are based on a shorter time period than required; (4) Data suppressed by CMS for one or more quarters; (5) Results are not available for this reporting period; (6) Fewer than 100 patients completed the HCAHPS survey; (7) No cases met the criteria for this measure; (8) The lower limit of the confidence interval cannot be calculated if the number of observed infections equals zero; (9) No data are available from the state/territory for this reporting period; (10) The scores shown reflect fewer than 50 completed surveys; (11) There were discrepancies in the data collection process; (12) This measure does not apply to this hospital for this reporting period; (13) Results cannot be calculated for this reporting period; (14) The results for this state are combined with nearby states to protect confidentiality; Please refer to the User's Guide for a full explanation of data.

Measure	Cases	This Hosp.	State Avg.	U.S. Avg.
Appropriate Beta Blocker Usage[5]	-	-	98%	98%
Appropriate VTP Within 24 Hours[5]	-	-	98%	98%
Controlled Postoperative Blood Glucose[5]	-	-	98%	97%
Perioperative Temperature Management[5]	-	-	100%	100%
Prophylactic Antibiotic Selection[5]	-	-	99%	99%
Prophylactic Antibiotic Selection (Outpatient)	-	-	98%	98%
Prophylactic Antibiotic Stopped[5]	-	-	98%	98%
Prophylactic Antibiotic Timing[5]	-	-	99%	99%
Prophylactic Antibiotic Timing (Outpatient)	-	-	98%	98%
Urinary Catheter Removal[5]	-	-	97%	97%
Survey of Patients' Hospital Experiences				
Area Around Room 'Always' Quiet at Night[5]	-	-	65%	61%
Doctors 'Always' Communicated Well[5]	-	-	85%	82%
Home Recovery Information Given[5]	-	-	86%	85%
Hospital Given 9 or 10 on 10 Point Scale[5]	-	-	76%	71%
Meds 'Always' Explained Before Given[5]	-	-	66%	64%
Nurses 'Always' Communicated Well[5]	-	-	81%	79%
Pain 'Always' Well Controlled[5]	-	-	72%	71%
Room and Bathroom 'Always' Clean[5]	-	-	76%	73%
Timely Help 'Always' Received[5]	-	-	72%	68%
Would Definitely Recommend Hospital[5]	-	-	75%	71%
Use of Medical Imaging				
Cardiac Imaging Stress Test before Surgery	-	-	5%	5.3%
Combination Abdominal CT Scan	-	-	19%	10.5%
Combination Brain/Sinus CT Scan	-	-	2.9%	2.7%
Combination Chest CT Scan	-	-	3.9%	2.7%
Follow-up Mammogram/Ultrasound	-	-	7.8%	8.8%
Lumbar Spine MRI for Low Back Pain	-	-	40.2%	37.2%

Atchison Hospital

800 Ravin Hill Drive
Atchison, KS 66002
Phone: 913-360-5581
Fax: 913-367-2913
Type: Critical Access Hospitals
Emergency Services: Yes
Ownership: Voluntary non-profit - Private
Beds: 115

Key Personnel:

Infection Control. . . . . Jim Brown
Quality Assurance . . . . Kathy Butler
Patient Relations . . . . Susan Gilkison
CEO . . . . John Jacobson
Operating Room. . . . . Jean Ober
Chief of Medical Staff. . . . . Scott Rossow, DO
Radiology. . . . . Maryann Scholz
Intensive Care Unit. . . . . Lora Willming

Measure	Cases	This Hosp.	State Avg.	U.S. Avg.
Blood Clot Prevention and Treatment				
Anticoagulation Overlap Therapy[5]	-	-	94%	93%
ICU Venous Thromboembolism Prophylaxis[5]	-	-	91%	92%
Incidence of Potentially Preventable VTE[5]	-	-	8%	10%
UFH with Dosages/Platelet Monitoring[5]	-	-	98%	97%
Venous Thromboembolism Prophylaxis[5]	-	-	79%	85%
Warfarin Therapy Discharge Instructions[5]	-	-	84%	75%
Chest Pain/Possible Heart Attack Care				
Aspirin Given Within 24 Hours of Arrival	-	-	94%	96%
Fibrinolytic Meds Within 30 Min. of Arrival	-	-	41%	58%
Average Time to ECG (minutes)	-	-	8	7
Average Time to Transfer (minutes)	-	-	57	60
Children's Asthma Care				
Received Home Management Plan of Care	-	-	-	88%
Received Reliever Medication	-	-	-	100%
Received Systemic Corticosteroids	-	-	-	100%
Emergency Department				
Admittance Decision Time (minutes)[5]	-	-	57	98
Head CT Results Within 45 Min. of Arrival	-	-	53%	57%
Patients Who Left ER Before Being Seen	-	-	2%	2%
Time from ER Arrival to Admit. (minutes)[5]	-	-	185	274
Time from ER Arrival to Discharge (minutes)	-	-	104	134
Time in ER Before Being Evaluated (minutes)	-	-	18	26
Time to Pain Meds for Fractures (minutes)	-	-	47	57
Heart Attack Care				
Aspirin Given at Discharge[5]	-	-	99%	99%
Fibrinolytic Meds Within 30 Min. of Arrival[5]	-	-	-	54%
PCI Within 90 Minutes of Arrival[5]	-	-	97%	96%
Statin Prescribed at Discharge[5]	-	-	99%	98%
Heart Failure Care				
ACE Inhibitor or ARB for LVSD[1]	-	-	95%	97%
Discharge Instructions Given	16	88%	91%	94%
Evaluation of LVS Function	28	89%	94%	99%
Medicare Spending				
Medicare Spending per Patient (ratio)	-	-	0.94	0.98
Pneumonia Care				
Appropriate Initial Antibiotic Given	59	92%	92%	95%
Blood Culture Timing	65	98%	98%	98%
Pregnancy and Delivery Care				
Newborn Deliveries Scheduled Early[5]	-	-	12%	6%
Preventive Care				
Immunization for Influenza[5]	-	-	88%	90%
Immunization for Pneumonia[5]	-	-	90%	92%
Stroke Care				
Anticoagulation Therapy for Atrial Fibrillation[5]	-	-	88%	95%
Antithrombotic Therapy Timing[5]	-	-	97%	98%
Assessed for Rehabilitation[5]	-	-	97%	97%
Discharged on Antithrombotic Therapy[5]	-	-	98%	99%
Discharged on Statin Medication[5]	-	-	88%	94%
Thrombolytic Therapy Timing[5]	-	-	68%	66%
Venous Thromboembolism Prophylaxis[5]	-	-	93%	94%
Written Stroke Educational Materials Given[5]	-	-	84%	88%
Surgical Care Improvement Project				
Appropriate Beta Blocker Usage	17	94%	98%	98%
Appropriate VTP Within 24 Hours	69	91%	98%	98%
Controlled Postoperative Blood Glucose[7]	-	-	98%	97%
Perioperative Temperature Management	73	100%	100%	100%
Prophylactic Antibiotic Selection	61	97%	99%	99%
Prophylactic Antibiotic Selection (Outpatient)	-	-	98%	98%
Prophylactic Antibiotic Stopped	58	95%	98%	98%
Prophylactic Antibiotic Timing	62	82%	99%	99%
Prophylactic Antibiotic Timing (Outpatient)	-	-	98%	98%
Urinary Catheter Removal	61	92%	97%	97%
Survey of Patients' Hospital Experiences				
Area Around Room 'Always' Quiet at Night	(a)	73%	65%	61%
Doctors 'Always' Communicated Well	(a)	86%	85%	82%
Home Recovery Information Given	(a)	88%	86%	85%
Hospital Given 9 or 10 on 10 Point Scale	(a)	70%	76%	71%
Meds 'Always' Explained Before Given	(a)	64%	66%	64%
Nurses 'Always' Communicated Well	(a)	78%	81%	79%
Pain 'Always' Well Controlled	(a)	73%	72%	71%
Room and Bathroom 'Always' Clean	(a)	69%	76%	73%
Timely Help 'Always' Received	(a)	71%	72%	68%
Would Definitely Recommend Hospital	(a)	67%	75%	71%
Use of Medical Imaging				
Cardiac Imaging Stress Test before Surgery	-	-	5%	5.3%
Combination Abdominal CT Scan	-	-	19%	10.5%
Combination Brain/Sinus CT Scan	-	-	2.9%	2.7%
Combination Chest CT Scan	-	-	3.9%	2.7%
Follow-up Mammogram/Ultrasound	-	-	7.8%	8.8%
Lumbar Spine MRI for Low Back Pain	-	-	40.2%	37.2%

Rawlins County Health Center

707 Grant St
Atwood, KS 67730
Phone: 785-626-3211
Type: Critical Access Hospitals
Emergency Services: Yes
Ownership: Voluntary non-profit - Other

Measure	Cases	This Hosp.	State Avg.	U.S. Avg.
Blood Clot Prevention and Treatment				
Anticoagulation Overlap Therapy[5]	-	-	94%	93%
ICU Venous Thromboembolism Prophylaxis[5]	-	-	91%	92%
Incidence of Potentially Preventable VTE[5]	-	-	8%	10%
UFH with Dosages/Platelet Monitoring[5]	-	-	98%	97%
Venous Thromboembolism Prophylaxis[5]	-	-	79%	85%
Warfarin Therapy Discharge Instructions[5]	-	-	84%	75%
Chest Pain/Possible Heart Attack Care				
Aspirin Given Within 24 Hours of Arrival	-	-	94%	96%
Fibrinolytic Meds Within 30 Min. of Arrival	-	-	41%	58%
Average Time to ECG (minutes)	-	-	8	7
Average Time to Transfer (minutes)	-	-	57	60
Children's Asthma Care				
Received Home Management Plan of Care	-	-	-	88%
Received Reliever Medication	-	-	-	100%
Received Systemic Corticosteroids	-	-	-	100%
Emergency Department				
Admittance Decision Time (minutes)[3]	28	10	57	98
Head CT Results Within 45 Min. of Arrival	-	-	53%	57%
Patients Who Left ER Before Being Seen	-	-	2%	2%
Time from ER Arrival to Admit. (minutes)[3]	28	94	185	274
Time from ER Arrival to Discharge (minutes)	-	-	104	134
Time in ER Before Being Evaluated (minutes)	-	-	18	26
Time to Pain Meds for Fractures (minutes)	-	-	47	57
Heart Attack Care				
Aspirin Given at Discharge[3,7]	-	-	99%	99%
Fibrinolytic Meds Within 30 Min. of Arrival[3,7]	-	-	-	54%
PCI Within 90 Minutes of Arrival[3,7]	-	-	97%	96%
Statin Prescribed at Discharge[3,7]	-	-	99%	98%
Heart Failure Care				
ACE Inhibitor or ARB for LVSD[3,7]	-	-	95%	97%
Discharge Instructions Given[1,3]	-	-	91%	94%
Evaluation of LVS Function[1,3]	-	-	94%	99%
Medicare Spending				
Medicare Spending per Patient (ratio)	-	-	0.94	0.98
Pneumonia Care				
Appropriate Initial Antibiotic Given[1]	-	-	92%	95%
Blood Culture Timing[1]	-	-	98%	98%
Pregnancy and Delivery Care				
Newborn Deliveries Scheduled Early[5]	-	-	12%	6%
Preventive Care				
Immunization for Influenza[5]	-	-	88%	90%
Immunization for Pneumonia[3]	24	46%	90%	92%
Stroke Care				
Anticoagulation Therapy for Atrial Fibrillation[5]	-	-	88%	95%
Antithrombotic Therapy Timing[5]	-	-	97%	98%
Assessed for Rehabilitation[5]	-	-	97%	97%
Discharged on Antithrombotic Therapy[5]	-	-	98%	99%
Discharged on Statin Medication[5]	-	-	88%	94%
Thrombolytic Therapy Timing[5]	-	-	68%	66%
Venous Thromboembolism Prophylaxis[5]	-	-	93%	94%
Written Stroke Educational Materials Given[5]	-	-	84%	88%
Surgical Care Improvement Project				
Appropriate Beta Blocker Usage[5]	-	-	98%	98%
Appropriate VTP Within 24 Hours[5]	-	-	98%	98%
Controlled Postoperative Blood Glucose[5]	-	-	98%	97%
Perioperative Temperature Management[5]	-	-	100%	100%
Prophylactic Antibiotic Selection[5]	-	-	99%	99%
Prophylactic Antibiotic Selection (Outpatient)	-	-	98%	98%
Prophylactic Antibiotic Stopped[5]	-	-	98%	98%
Prophylactic Antibiotic Timing[5]	-	-	99%	99%
Prophylactic Antibiotic Timing (Outpatient)	-	-	98%	98%
Urinary Catheter Removal[5]	-	-	97%	97%
Survey of Patients' Hospital Experiences				
Area Around Room 'Always' Quiet at Night[5]	-	-	65%	61%
Doctors 'Always' Communicated Well[5]	-	-	85%	82%
Home Recovery Information Given[5]	-	-	86%	85%
Hospital Given 9 or 10 on 10 Point Scale[5]	-	-	76%	71%
Meds 'Always' Explained Before Given[5]	-	-	66%	64%
Nurses 'Always' Communicated Well[5]	-	-	81%	79%
Pain 'Always' Well Controlled[5]	-	-	72%	71%
Room and Bathroom 'Always' Clean[5]	-	-	76%	73%
Timely Help 'Always' Received[5]	-	-	72%	68%
Would Definitely Recommend Hospital[5]	-	-	75%	71%
Use of Medical Imaging				
Cardiac Imaging Stress Test before Surgery	-	-	5%	5.3%
Combination Abdominal CT Scan	-	-	19%	10.5%
Combination Brain/Sinus CT Scan	-	-	2.9%	2.7%
Combination Chest CT Scan	-	-	3.9%	2.7%
Follow-up Mammogram/Ultrasound	-	-	7.8%	8.8%
Lumbar Spine MRI for Low Back Pain	-	-	40.2%	37.2%

NOTE: Hospital profiles are in alphabetical order by state, then city, then hospital within the city; Rankings exclude hospitals with less than 25 cases except for patient surveys which excludes hospitals with less than 100 cases; (a) 100-299 cases; (1) The number of cases/patients is too few to report; (2) Data submitted were based on a sample of cases/patients; (3) Results are based on a shorter time period than required; (4) Data suppressed by CMS for one or more quarters; (5) Results are not available for this reporting period; (6) Fewer than 100 patients completed the HCAHPS survey; (7) No cases met the criteria for this measure; (8) The lower limit of the confidence interval cannot be calculated if the number of observed infections equals zero; (9) No data are available from the state/territory for this reporting period; (10) The scores shown reflect fewer than 50 completed surveys; (11) There were discrepancies in the data collection process; (12) This measure does not apply to this hospital for this reporting period; (13) Results cannot be calculated for this reporting period; (14) The results for this state are combined with nearby states to protect confidentiality; Please refer to the User's Guide for a full explanation of data.

Republic County Hospital

2420 G Street Phone: 785-527-2254
Belleville, KS 66935 Fax: 785-527-2324
E-mail: rchospital1@nckcn.com
URL: www.republiccountyhospital.org
Type: Critical Access Hospitals Emergency Services: Yes
Ownership: Voluntary non-profit - Private Beds: 63
Key Personnel:
Radiology. Linda Elliott
Anesthesiology. . . . . Dr. Robert Holt
CEO/President. . . . . Blaine Miller

Measure	Cases	This Hosp.	State Avg.	U.S. Avg.
Blood Clot Prevention and Treatment				
Anticoagulation Overlap Therapy[5]	-	-	94%	93%
ICU Venous Thromboembolism Prophylaxis[5]	-	-	91%	92%
Incidence of Potentially Preventable VTE[5]	-	-	8%	10%
UFH with Dosages/Platelet Monitoring[5]	-	-	98%	97%
Venous Thromboembolism Prophylaxis[5]	-	-	79%	85%
Warfarin Therapy Discharge Instructions[5]	-	-	84%	75%
Chest Pain/Possible Heart Attack Care				
Aspirin Given Within 24 Hours of Arrival	-	-	94%	96%
Fibrinolytic Meds Within 30 Min. of Arrival	-	-	41%	58%
Average Time to ECG (minutes)	-	-	8	7
Average Time to Transfer (minutes)	-	-	57	60
Children's Asthma Care				
Received Home Management Plan of Care	-	-	-	88%
Received Reliever Medication	-	-	-	100%
Received Systemic Corticosteroids	-	-	-	100%
Emergency Department				
Admittance Decision Time (minutes)[5]	-	-	57	98
Head CT Results Within 45 Min. of Arrival	-	-	53%	57%
Patients Who Left ER Before Being Seen	-	-	2%	2%
Time from ER Arrival to Admit. (minutes)[5]	-	-	185	274
Time from ER Arrival to Discharge (minutes)	-	-	104	134
Time in ER Before Being Evaluated (minutes)	-	-	18	26
Time to Pain Meds for Fractures (minutes)	-	-	47	57
Heart Attack Care				
Aspirin Given at Discharge[1,2]	-	-	99%	99%
Fibrinolytic Meds Within 30 Min. of Arrival[2,3]	-	-	-	54%
PCI Within 90 Minutes of Arrival[2,3]	-	-	97%	96%
Statin Prescribed at Discharge[1,2]	-	-	99%	98%
Heart Failure Care				
ACE Inhibitor or ARB for LVSD[1,2]	-	-	95%	97%
Discharge Instructions Given[1,2]	-	-	91%	94%
Evaluation of LVS Function[1,2]	-	-	94%	99%
Medicare Spending				
Medicare Spending per Patient (ratio)	-	-	0.94	0.98
Pneumonia Care				
Appropriate Initial Antibiotic Given[2,3]	25	72%	92%	95%
Blood Culture Timing[1,2]	-	-	98%	98%
Pregnancy and Delivery Care				
Newborn Deliveries Scheduled Early[5]	-	-	12%	6%
Preventive Care				
Immunization for Influenza[2]	283	79%	88%	90%
Immunization for Pneumonia[2,3]	294	84%	90%	92%
Stroke Care				
Anticoagulation Therapy for Atrial Fibrillation[5]	-	-	88%	95%
Antithrombotic Therapy Timing[5]	-	-	97%	98%
Assessed for Rehabilitation[5]	-	-	97%	97%
Discharged on Antithrombotic Therapy[5]	-	-	98%	99%
Discharged on Statin Medication[5]	-	-	88%	94%
Thrombolytic Therapy Timing[5]	-	-	68%	66%
Venous Thromboembolism Prophylaxis[5]	-	-	93%	94%
Written Stroke Educational Materials Given[5]	-	-	84%	88%
Surgical Care Improvement Project				
Appropriate Beta Blocker Usage[1,3]	-	-	98%	98%
Appropriate VTP Within 24 Hours[1,3]	-	-	98%	98%
Controlled Postoperative Blood Glucose[3,7]	-	-	98%	97%
Perioperative Temperature Management[1,3]	-	-	100%	100%
Prophylactic Antibiotic Selection[1,3]	-	-	99%	99%
Prophylactic Antibiotic Selection (Outpatient)	-	-	98%	98%
Prophylactic Antibiotic Stopped[1,3]	-	-	98%	98%
Prophylactic Antibiotic Timing[1,3]	-	-	99%	99%
Prophylactic Antibiotic Timing (Outpatient)	-	-	98%	98%
Urinary Catheter Removal[1,3]	-	-	97%	97%
Survey of Patients' Hospital Experiences				
Area Around Room 'Always' Quiet at Night	(a)	54%	65%	61%
Doctors 'Always' Communicated Well	(a)	88%	85%	82%
Home Recovery Information Given	(a)	86%	86%	85%
Hospital Given 9 or 10 on 10 Point Scale	(a)	75%	76%	71%
Meds 'Always' Explained Before Given	(a)	65%	66%	64%
Nurses 'Always' Communicated Well	(a)	74%	81%	79%
Pain 'Always' Well Controlled	(a)	60%	72%	71%
Room and Bathroom 'Always' Clean	(a)	84%	76%	73%
Timely Help 'Always' Received	(a)	65%	72%	68%
Would Definitely Recommend Hospital	(a)	83%	75%	71%
Use of Medical Imaging				
Cardiac Imaging Stress Test before Surgery	-	-	5%	5.3%
Combination Abdominal CT Scan	-	-	19%	10.5%
Combination Brain/Sinus CT Scan	-	-	2.9%	2.7%
Combination Chest CT Scan	-	-	3.9%	2.7%
Follow-up Mammogram/Ultrasound	-	-	7.8%	8.8%
Lumbar Spine MRI for Low Back Pain	-	-	40.2%	37.2%

Mitchell County Hospital Health Systems

400 W 8th Street PO Box 399 Phone: 785-738-2266
Beloit, KS 67420 Fax: 785-738-9503
URL: www.gpha.com
Type: Critical Access Hospitals Emergency Services: Yes
Ownership: Government - Local Beds: 99
Key Personnel:
CEO/President. . . . . Dave Dellasega
Chair/CEO . . . . Thomas E. Keller
Emergency Room . . . . Mary Grey
Radiology. . . . . Richard J Kueker

Measure	Cases	This Hosp.	State Avg.	U.S. Avg.
Blood Clot Prevention and Treatment				
Anticoagulation Overlap Therapy[5]	-	-	94%	93%
ICU Venous Thromboembolism Prophylaxis[5]	-	-	91%	92%
Incidence of Potentially Preventable VTE[5]	-	-	8%	10%
UFH with Dosages/Platelet Monitoring[5]	-	-	98%	97%
Venous Thromboembolism Prophylaxis[5]	-	-	79%	85%
Warfarin Therapy Discharge Instructions[5]	-	-	84%	75%
Chest Pain/Possible Heart Attack Care				
Aspirin Given Within 24 Hours of Arrival	-	-	94%	96%
Fibrinolytic Meds Within 30 Min. of Arrival	-	-	41%	58%
Average Time to ECG (minutes)	-	-	8	7
Average Time to Transfer (minutes)	-	-	57	60
Children's Asthma Care				
Received Home Management Plan of Care	-	-	-	88%
Received Reliever Medication	-	-	-	100%
Received Systemic Corticosteroids	-	-	-	100%
Emergency Department				
Admittance Decision Time (minutes)[3]	27	40	57	98
Head CT Results Within 45 Min. of Arrival	-	-	53%	57%
Patients Who Left ER Before Being Seen	-	-	2%	2%
Time from ER Arrival to Admit. (minutes)[3]	27	145	185	274
Time from ER Arrival to Discharge (minutes)	-	-	104	134
Time in ER Before Being Evaluated (minutes)	-	-	18	26
Time to Pain Meds for Fractures (minutes)	-	-	47	57
Heart Attack Care				
Aspirin Given at Discharge[1,3]	-	-	99%	99%
Fibrinolytic Meds Within 30 Min. of Arrival[3,7]	-	-	-	54%
PCI Within 90 Minutes of Arrival[3,7]	-	-	97%	96%
Statin Prescribed at Discharge[1,3]	-	-	99%	98%
Heart Failure Care				
ACE Inhibitor or ARB for LVSD[1,3]	-	-	95%	97%
Discharge Instructions Given[1,3]	-	-	91%	94%
Evaluation of LVS Function[1,3]	-	-	94%	99%
Medicare Spending				
Medicare Spending per Patient (ratio)	-	-	0.94	0.98
Pneumonia Care				
Appropriate Initial Antibiotic Given[3]	19	79%	92%	95%
Blood Culture Timing[3]	16	100%	98%	98%
Pregnancy and Delivery Care				
Newborn Deliveries Scheduled Early[5]	-	-	12%	6%
Preventive Care				
Immunization for Influenza[3]	34	94%	88%	90%
Immunization for Pneumonia[3]	30	90%	90%	92%
Stroke Care				
Anticoagulation Therapy for Atrial Fibrillation[5]	-	-	88%	95%
Antithrombotic Therapy Timing[5]	-	-	97%	98%
Assessed for Rehabilitation[5]	-	-	97%	97%
Discharged on Antithrombotic Therapy[5]	-	-	98%	99%
Discharged on Statin Medication[5]	-	-	88%	94%
Thrombolytic Therapy Timing[5]	-	-	68%	66%
Venous Thromboembolism Prophylaxis[5]	-	-	93%	94%
Written Stroke Educational Materials Given[5]	-	-	84%	88%
Surgical Care Improvement Project				
Appropriate Beta Blocker Usage[5]	-	-	98%	98%
Appropriate VTP Within 24 Hours[5]	-	-	98%	98%
Controlled Postoperative Blood Glucose[5]	-	-	98%	97%
Perioperative Temperature Management[5]	-	-	100%	100%
Prophylactic Antibiotic Selection[5]	-	-	99%	99%
Prophylactic Antibiotic Selection (Outpatient)	-	-	98%	98%
Prophylactic Antibiotic Stopped[5]	-	-	98%	98%
Prophylactic Antibiotic Timing[5]	-	-	99%	99%
Prophylactic Antibiotic Timing (Outpatient)	-	-	98%	98%
Urinary Catheter Removal[5]	-	-	97%	97%
Survey of Patients' Hospital Experiences				
Area Around Room 'Always' Quiet at Night[5]	-	-	65%	61%
Doctors 'Always' Communicated Well[5]	-	-	85%	82%
Home Recovery Information Given[5]	-	-	86%	85%
Hospital Given 9 or 10 on 10 Point Scale[5]	-	-	76%	71%
Meds 'Always' Explained Before Given[5]	-	-	66%	64%
Nurses 'Always' Communicated Well[5]	-	-	81%	79%
Pain 'Always' Well Controlled[5]	-	-	72%	71%
Room and Bathroom 'Always' Clean[5]	-	-	76%	73%
Timely Help 'Always' Received[5]	-	-	72%	68%
Would Definitely Recommend Hospital[5]	-	-	75%	71%
Use of Medical Imaging				
Cardiac Imaging Stress Test before Surgery	-	-	5%	5.3%
Combination Abdominal CT Scan	-	-	19%	10.5%
Combination Brain/Sinus CT Scan	-	-	2.9%	2.7%
Combination Chest CT Scan	-	-	3.9%	2.7%
Follow-up Mammogram/Ultrasound	-	-	7.8%	8.8%
Lumbar Spine MRI for Low Back Pain	-	-	40.2%	37.2%

Coffey County Hospital

801 North 4th Street Phone: 620-364-2121
Burlington, KS 66839 Fax: 620-364-2605
URL: www.coffeyhealth.org
Type: Acute Care Hospitals Emergency Services: Yes
Ownership: Government - Local Beds: 78
Key Personnel:
CEO/President. . . . . Dennis George
Radiology. . . . . Kevin Hughes
Patient Relations . . . . Krystal Nicholson
Chief of Medical Staff . . . . John Shell, MD
Emergency Room . . . . John Shell
Quality Assurance . . . . Rebecca Thurman
Infection Control. . . . . Elaine Weston, RN
Operating Room. . . . . Sherry Young

Measure	Cases	This Hosp.	State Avg.	U.S. Avg.
Blood Clot Prevention and Treatment				
Anticoagulation Overlap Therapy[1,2]	-	-	94%	93%
ICU Venous Thromboembolism Prophylaxis[1,2]	-	-	91%	92%
Incidence of Potentially Preventable VTE[1,2]	-	-	8%	10%
UFH with Dosages/Platelet Monitoring[2,7]	-	-	98%	97%
Venous Thromboembolism Prophylaxis[2]	116	21%	79%	85%
Warfarin Therapy Discharge Instructions[1,2]	-	-	84%	75%
Chest Pain/Possible Heart Attack Care				
Aspirin Given Within 24 Hours of Arrival[1,3]	-	-	94%	96%
Fibrinolytic Meds Within 30 Min. of Arrival[3,7]	-	-	41%	58%
Average Time to ECG (minutes)[1,3]	-	-	8	7
Average Time to Transfer (minutes)[3,7]	-	-	57	60
Children's Asthma Care				
Received Home Management Plan of Care	-	-	-	88%
Received Reliever Medication	-	-	-	100%
Received Systemic Corticosteroids	-	-	-	100%

NOTE: Hospital profiles are in alphabetical order by state, then city, then hospital within the city; Rankings exclude hospitals with less than 25 cases except for patient surveys which excludes hospitals with less than 100 cases; (a) 100-299 cases; (1) The number of cases/patients is too few to report; (2) Data submitted were based on a sample of cases/patients; (3) Results are based on a shorter time period than required; (4) Data suppressed by CMS for one or more quarters; (5) Results are not available for this reporting period; (6) Fewer than 100 patients completed the HCAHPS survey; (7) No cases met the criteria for this measure; (8) The lower limit of the confidence interval cannot be calculated if the number of observed infections equals zero; (9) No data are available from the state/territory for this reporting period; (10) The scores shown reflect fewer than 50 completed surveys; (11) There were discrepancies in the data collection process; (12) This measure does not apply to this hospital for this reporting period; (13) Results cannot be calculated for this reporting period; (14) The results for this state are combined with nearby states to protect confidentiality; Please refer to the User's Guide for a full explanation of data.

Measure	Cases	This Hosp.	State Avg.	U.S. Avg.
Emergency Department				
Admittance Decision Time (minutes)[2]	110	35	57	98
Head CT Results Within 45 Min. of Arrival[5]	-	-	53%	57%
Patients Who Left ER Before Being Seen	3,910	0%	2%	2%
Time from ER Arrival to Admit. (minutes)[2]	200	102	185	274
Time from ER Arrival to Discharge (minutes)	275	59	104	134
Time in ER Before Being Evaluated (minutes)	265	15	18	26
Time to Pain Meds for Fractures (minutes)[3]	16	32	47	57
Heart Attack Care				
Aspirin Given at Discharge[5]	-	-	99%	99%
Fibrinolytic Meds Within 30 Min. of Arrival[5]	-	-	-	54%
PCI Within 90 Minutes of Arrival[5]	-	-	97%	96%
Statin Prescribed at Discharge[5]	-	-	99%	98%
Heart Failure Care				
ACE Inhibitor or ARB for LVSD[1]	-	-	95%	97%
Discharge Instructions Given	32	94%	91%	94%
Evaluation of LVS Function	46	93%	94%	99%
Medicare Spending				
Medicare Spending per Patient (ratio)	-	0.86	0.94	0.98
Pneumonia Care				
Appropriate Initial Antibiotic Given	37	95%	92%	95%
Blood Culture Timing	11	91%	98%	98%
Pregnancy and Delivery Care				
Newborn Deliveries Scheduled Early[2]	15	0%	12%	6%
Preventive Care				
Immunization for Influenza[2]	296	89%	88%	90%
Immunization for Pneumonia[2]	334	93%	90%	92%
Stroke Care				
Anticoagulation Therapy for Atrial Fibrillation[5]	-	-	88%	95%
Antithrombotic Therapy Timing[5]	-	-	97%	98%
Assessed for Rehabilitation[5]	-	-	97%	97%
Discharged on Antithrombotic Therapy[5]	-	-	98%	99%
Discharged on Statin Medication[5]	-	-	88%	94%
Thrombolytic Therapy Timing[5]	-	-	68%	66%
Venous Thromboembolism Prophylaxis[5]	-	-	93%	94%
Written Stroke Educational Materials Given[5]	-	-	84%	88%
Surgical Care Improvement Project				
Appropriate Beta Blocker Usage[1]	-	-	98%	98%
Appropriate VTP Within 24 Hours	31	97%	98%	98%
Controlled Postoperative Blood Glucose[7]	-	-	98%	97%
Perioperative Temperature Management	32	97%	100%	100%
Prophylactic Antibiotic Selection	26	100%	99%	99%
Prophylactic Antibiotic Selection (Outpatient)[5]	-	-	98%	98%
Prophylactic Antibiotic Stopped	25	92%	98%	98%
Prophylactic Antibiotic Timing	26	92%	99%	99%
Prophylactic Antibiotic Timing (Outpatient)[5]	-	-	98%	98%
Urinary Catheter Removal	31	100%	97%	97%
Survey of Patients' Hospital Experiences				
Area Around Room 'Always' Quiet at Night	(a)	71%	65%	61%
Doctors 'Always' Communicated Well	(a)	90%	85%	82%
Home Recovery Information Given	(a)	86%	86%	85%
Hospital Given 9 or 10 on 10 Point Scale	(a)	81%	76%	71%
Meds 'Always' Explained Before Given	(a)	71%	66%	64%
Nurses 'Always' Communicated Well	(a)	85%	81%	79%
Pain 'Always' Well Controlled	(a)	74%	72%	71%
Room and Bathroom 'Always' Clean	(a)	82%	76%	73%
Timely Help 'Always' Received	(a)	74%	72%	68%
Would Definitely Recommend Hospital	(a)	84%	75%	71%
Use of Medical Imaging				
Cardiac Imaging Stress Test before Surgery	113	3.5%	5%	5.3%
Combination Abdominal CT Scan	84	14.3%	19%	10.5%
Combination Brain/Sinus CT Scan[1]	-	-	2.9%	2.7%
Combination Chest CT Scan[1]	-	-	3.9%	2.7%
Follow-up Mammogram/Ultrasound	378	5.3%	7.8%	8.8%
Lumbar Spine MRI for Low Back Pain	44	38.6%	40.2%	37.2%

Neosho Memorial Regional Medical Center

629 South Plummer Phone: 620-431-4000
Chanute, KS 66720 Fax: 620-431-7556
URL: www.nmrmc.com
Type: Critical Access Hospitals Emergency Services: Yes
Ownership: Government - Local Beds: 97

Key Personnel:
CEO/President. . . . . Murray L Brown
Operating Room. . . . . Billy Browne, RN
Intensive Care Unit. . . . . Sandy Froemming, RN
Quality Assurance . . . . Sandy Froemming, RN
Emergency Room . . . . Pat Lucke, RN
Chief of Medical Staff. . . . . DeAnna Vaugh, MD
Infection Control. . . . . Kathy Wicker, RN
Radiology. . . . . Mark Witaczack

Measure	Cases	This Hosp.	State Avg.	U.S. Avg.
Blood Clot Prevention and Treatment				
Anticoagulation Overlap Therapy[1,3]	-	-	94%	93%
ICU Venous Thromboembolism Prophylaxis[3,7]	-	-	91%	92%
Incidence of Potentially Preventable VTE[3,7]	-	-	8%	10%
UFH with Dosages/Platelet Monitoring[3,7]	-	-	98%	97%
Venous Thromboembolism Prophylaxis[3,7]	-	-	79%	85%
Warfarin Therapy Discharge Instructions[1,3]	-	-	84%	75%
Chest Pain/Possible Heart Attack Care				
Aspirin Given Within 24 Hours of Arrival	44	93%	94%	96%
Fibrinolytic Meds Within 30 Min. of Arrival[1]	-	-	41%	58%
Average Time to ECG (minutes)	46	7	8	7
Average Time to Transfer (minutes)[7]	-	-	57	60
Children's Asthma Care				
Received Home Management Plan of Care	-	-	-	88%
Received Reliever Medication	-	-	-	100%
Received Systemic Corticosteroids	-	-	-	100%
Emergency Department				
Admittance Decision Time (minutes)[2]	261	60	57	98
Head CT Results Within 45 Min. of Arrival[5]	-	-	53%	57%
Patients Who Left ER Before Being Seen	9,118	0%	2%	2%
Time from ER Arrival to Admit. (minutes)[2]	284	175	185	274
Time from ER Arrival to Discharge (minutes)[5]	-	-	104	134
Time in ER Before Being Evaluated (minutes)[5]	-	-	18	26
Time to Pain Meds for Fractures (minutes)[5]	-	-	47	57
Heart Attack Care				
Aspirin Given at Discharge[1,2]	-	-	99%	99%
Fibrinolytic Meds Within 30 Min. of Arrival[2,3]	-	-	-	54%
PCI Within 90 Minutes of Arrival[2,3]	-	-	97%	96%
Statin Prescribed at Discharge[1,2]	-	-	99%	98%
Heart Failure Care				
ACE Inhibitor or ARB for LVSD[2]	16	88%	95%	97%
Discharge Instructions Given[2]	26	100%	91%	94%
Evaluation of LVS Function[2]	45	100%	94%	99%
Medicare Spending				
Medicare Spending per Patient (ratio)	-	-	0.94	0.98
Pneumonia Care				
Appropriate Initial Antibiotic Given[2]	78	94%	92%	95%
Blood Culture Timing[2]	115	100%	98%	98%
Pregnancy and Delivery Care				
Newborn Deliveries Scheduled Early[5]	-	-	12%	6%
Preventive Care				
Immunization for Influenza[2]	292	86%	88%	90%
Immunization for Pneumonia[2]	339	92%	90%	92%
Stroke Care				
Anticoagulation Therapy for Atrial Fibrillation[1,2]	-	-	88%	95%
Antithrombotic Therapy Timing[2,3]	12	92%	97%	98%
Assessed for Rehabilitation[2,3]	11	91%	97%	97%
Discharged on Antithrombotic Therapy[2,3]	11	91%	98%	99%
Discharged on Statin Medication[2,3]	11	55%	88%	94%
Thrombolytic Therapy Timing[1,2]	-	-	68%	66%
Venous Thromboembolism Prophylaxis[2,3]	13	46%	93%	94%
Written Stroke Educational Materials Given[1,2]	-	-	84%	88%
Surgical Care Improvement Project				
Appropriate Beta Blocker Usage[1,2]	-	-	98%	98%
Appropriate VTP Within 24 Hours[2]	33	97%	98%	98%
Controlled Postoperative Blood Glucose[2,3]	-	-	98%	97%
Perioperative Temperature Management[2]	37	100%	100%	100%
Prophylactic Antibiotic Selection[2]	15	93%	99%	99%
Prophylactic Antibiotic Selection (Outpatient)	67	96%	98%	98%
Prophylactic Antibiotic Stopped[2]	13	100%	98%	98%
Prophylactic Antibiotic Timing[2]	15	100%	99%	99%
Prophylactic Antibiotic Timing (Outpatient)	63	95%	98%	98%
Urinary Catheter Removal[1,2]	-	-	97%	97%
Survey of Patients' Hospital Experiences				
Area Around Room 'Always' Quiet at Night	300+	64%	65%	61%
Doctors 'Always' Communicated Well	300+	89%	85%	82%
Home Recovery Information Given	300+	92%	86%	85%
Hospital Given 9 or 10 on 10 Point Scale	300+	82%	76%	71%
Meds 'Always' Explained Before Given	300+	75%	66%	64%
Nurses 'Always' Communicated Well	300+	86%	81%	79%
Pain 'Always' Well Controlled	300+	77%	72%	71%
Room and Bathroom 'Always' Clean	300+	86%	76%	73%
Timely Help 'Always' Received	300+	71%	72%	68%
Would Definitely Recommend Hospital	300+	81%	75%	71%
Use of Medical Imaging				
Cardiac Imaging Stress Test before Surgery	169	4.7%	5%	5.3%
Combination Abdominal CT Scan	399	5.5%	19%	10.5%
Combination Brain/Sinus CT Scan[1]	-	-	2.9%	2.7%
Combination Chest CT Scan	261	5.7%	3.9%	2.7%
Follow-up Mammogram/Ultrasound	552	2.9%	7.8%	8.8%
Lumbar Spine MRI for Low Back Pain	81	42.0%	40.2%	37.2%

Clay County Medical Center

617 Liberty Phone: 785-632-2144
Clay Center, KS 67432
Type: Critical Access Hospitals Emergency Services: Yes
Ownership: Government - Local

Key Personnel:
CEO/President. . . . . Ron Bender
Anesthesiology. . . . . Scott Husted
Radiology. . . . . James Peterson

Measure	Cases	This Hosp.	State Avg.	U.S. Avg.
Blood Clot Prevention and Treatment				
Anticoagulation Overlap Therapy[5]	-	-	94%	93%
ICU Venous Thromboembolism Prophylaxis[5]	-	-	91%	92%
Incidence of Potentially Preventable VTE[5]	-	-	8%	10%
UFH with Dosages/Platelet Monitoring[5]	-	-	98%	97%
Venous Thromboembolism Prophylaxis[5]	-	-	79%	85%
Warfarin Therapy Discharge Instructions[5]	-	-	84%	75%
Chest Pain/Possible Heart Attack Care				
Aspirin Given Within 24 Hours of Arrival	25	84%	94%	96%
Fibrinolytic Meds Within 30 Min. of Arrival[1,3]	-	-	41%	58%
Average Time to ECG (minutes)	24	14	8	7
Average Time to Transfer (minutes)[1,3]	-	-	57	60
Children's Asthma Care				
Received Home Management Plan of Care	-	-	-	88%
Received Reliever Medication	-	-	-	100%
Received Systemic Corticosteroids	-	-	-	100%
Emergency Department				
Admittance Decision Time (minutes)	14	38	57	98
Head CT Results Within 45 Min. of Arrival[5]	-	-	53%	57%
Patients Who Left ER Before Being Seen[5]	-	-	2%	2%
Time from ER Arrival to Admit. (minutes)	47	150	185	274
Time from ER Arrival to Discharge (minutes)[3]	127	76	104	134
Time in ER Before Being Evaluated (minutes)[3]	133	25	18	26
Time to Pain Meds for Fractures (minutes)[5]	-	-	47	57
Heart Attack Care				
Aspirin Given at Discharge[1,3]	-	-	99%	99%
Fibrinolytic Meds Within 30 Min. of Arrival[1,3]	-	-	-	54%
PCI Within 90 Minutes of Arrival[3,7]	-	-	97%	96%
Statin Prescribed at Discharge[1,3]	-	-	99%	98%
Heart Failure Care				
ACE Inhibitor or ARB for LVSD[1]	-	-	95%	97%
Discharge Instructions Given[1]	-	-	91%	94%
Evaluation of LVS Function	15	33%	94%	99%
Medicare Spending				
Medicare Spending per Patient (ratio)	-	-	0.94	0.98
Pneumonia Care				
Appropriate Initial Antibiotic Given[1]	-	-	92%	95%
Blood Culture Timing[1]	-	-	98%	98%
Pregnancy and Delivery Care				
Newborn Deliveries Scheduled Early[5]	-	-	12%	6%
Preventive Care				
Immunization for Influenza	43	95%	88%	90%
Immunization for Pneumonia[2]	71	94%	90%	92%
Stroke Care				
Anticoagulation Therapy for Atrial Fibrillation[5]	-	-	88%	95%
Antithrombotic Therapy Timing[5]	-	-	97%	98%

NOTE: Hospital profiles are in alphabetical order by state, then city, then hospital within the city; Rankings exclude hospitals with less than 25 cases except for patient surveys which excludes hospitals with less than 100 cases; (a) 100-299 cases; (1) The number of cases/patients is too few to report; (2) Data submitted were based on a sample of cases/patients; (3) Results are based on a shorter time period than required; (4) Data suppressed by CMS for one or more quarters; (5) Results are not available for this reporting period; (6) Fewer than 100 patients completed the HCAHPS survey; (7) No cases met the criteria for this measure; (8) The lower limit of the confidence interval cannot be calculated if the number of observed infections equals zero; (9) No data are available from the state/territory for this reporting period; (10) The scores shown reflect fewer than 50 completed surveys; (11) There were discrepancies in the data collection process; (12) This measure does not apply to this hospital for this reporting period; (13) Results cannot be calculated for this reporting period; (14) The results for this state are combined with nearby states to protect confidentiality; Please refer to the User's Guide for a full explanation of data.

Measure	Cases	This Hosp.	State Avg.	U.S. Avg.
Assessed for Rehabilitation[5]	-	-	97%	97%
Discharged on Antithrombotic Therapy[5]	-	-	98%	99%
Discharged on Statin Medication[5]	-	-	88%	94%
Thrombolytic Therapy Timing[5]	-	-	68%	66%
Venous Thromboembolism Prophylaxis[5]	-	-	93%	94%
Written Stroke Educational Materials Given[5]	-	-	84%	88%
Surgical Care Improvement Project				
Appropriate Beta Blocker Usage[5]	-	-	98%	98%
Appropriate VTP Within 24 Hours[5]	-	-	98%	98%
Controlled Postoperative Blood Glucose[5]	-	-	98%	97%
Perioperative Temperature Management[5]	-	-	100%	100%
Prophylactic Antibiotic Selection[5]	-	-	99%	99%
Prophylactic Antibiotic Selection (Outpatient)[5]	-	-	98%	98%
Prophylactic Antibiotic Stopped[5]	-	-	98%	98%
Prophylactic Antibiotic Timing[5]	-	-	99%	99%
Prophylactic Antibiotic Timing (Outpatient)[5]	-	-	98%	98%
Urinary Catheter Removal[5]	-	-	97%	97%
Survey of Patients' Hospital Experiences				
Area Around Room 'Always' Quiet at Night[5]	-	-	65%	61%
Doctors 'Always' Communicated Well[5]	-	-	85%	82%
Home Recovery Information Given[5]	-	-	86%	85%
Hospital Given 9 or 10 on 10 Point Scale[5]	-	-	76%	71%
Meds 'Always' Explained Before Given[5]	-	-	66%	64%
Nurses 'Always' Communicated Well[5]	-	-	81%	79%
Pain 'Always' Well Controlled[5]	-	-	72%	71%
Room and Bathroom 'Always' Clean[5]	-	-	76%	73%
Timely Help 'Always' Received[5]	-	-	72%	68%
Would Definitely Recommend Hospital[5]	-	-	75%	71%
Use of Medical Imaging				
Cardiac Imaging Stress Test before Surgery	91	4.4%	5%	5.3%
Combination Abdominal CT Scan	164	32.9%	19%	10.5%
Combination Brain/Sinus CT Scan[1]	-	-	2.9%	2.7%
Combination Chest CT Scan	173	1.7%	3.9%	2.7%
Follow-up Mammogram/Ultrasound	321	8.1%	7.8%	8.8%
Lumbar Spine MRI for Low Back Pain	52	46.2%	40.2%	37.2%

Coffeyville Regional Medical Center

1400 W 4th St
Coffeyville, KS 67337
Phone: 620-251-1200
Fax: 620-252-1562
E-mail: humanresources@crmcinc.com
URL: www.crmcinc.com
Type: Acute Care Hospitals
Emergency Services: Yes
Ownership: Government - Local
Beds: 148

Key Personnel:

CEO . . . . Jim Chromik
Chairman/CEO . . . . Dr. Raymond Hawley
CEO/President. . . . . Jerry Marquette
Quality Assurance . . . . Laura Robson
Chief of Medical Staff. . . . . Tiru M Venkat
Radiology. . . . . Donald White

Measure	Cases	This Hosp.	State Avg.	U.S. Avg.
Blood Clot Prevention and Treatment				
Anticoagulation Overlap Therapy[2]	13	85%	94%	93%
ICU Venous Thromboembolism Prophylaxis[2]	54	85%	91%	92%
Incidence of Potentially Preventable VTE[1,2]	-	-	8%	10%
UFH with Dosages/Platelet Monitoring[1,2]	-	-	98%	97%
Venous Thromboembolism Prophylaxis[2]	136	79%	79%	85%
Warfarin Therapy Discharge Instructions[1,2]	-	-	84%	75%
Chest Pain/Possible Heart Attack Care				
Aspirin Given Within 24 Hours of Arrival	24	83%	94%	96%
Fibrinolytic Meds Within 30 Min. of Arrival[3,7]	-	-	41%	58%
Average Time to ECG (minutes)	25	9	8	7
Average Time to Transfer (minutes)[1,3]	-	-	57	60
Children's Asthma Care				
Received Home Management Plan of Care	-	-	-	88%
Received Reliever Medication	-	-	-	100%
Received Systemic Corticosteroids	-	-	-	100%
Emergency Department				
Admittance Decision Time (minutes)[2]	206	126	57	98
Head CT Results Within 45 Min. of Arrival	13	15%	53%	57%
Patients Who Left ER Before Being Seen	8,074	1%	2%	2%
Time from ER Arrival to Admit. (minutes)[2]	230	172	185	274
Time from ER Arrival to Discharge (minutes)	341	106	104	134
Time in ER Before Being Evaluated (minutes)	380	9	18	26
Time to Pain Meds for Fractures (minutes)	37	46	47	57
Heart Attack Care				
Aspirin Given at Discharge[1]	-	-	99%	99%
Fibrinolytic Meds Within 30 Min. of Arrival[7]	-	-	-	54%
PCI Within 90 Minutes of Arrival[7]	-	-	97%	96%
Statin Prescribed at Discharge[1]	-	-	99%	98%
Heart Failure Care				
ACE Inhibitor or ARB for LVSD	19	79%	95%	97%
Discharge Instructions Given	37	95%	91%	94%
Evaluation of LVS Function	65	98%	94%	99%
Medicare Spending				
Medicare Spending per Patient (ratio)	-	0.90	0.94	0.98
Pneumonia Care				
Appropriate Initial Antibiotic Given	44	84%	92%	95%
Blood Culture Timing	56	96%	98%	98%
Pregnancy and Delivery Care				
Newborn Deliveries Scheduled Early[2]	14	14%	12%	6%
Preventive Care				
Immunization for Influenza[2]	271	90%	88%	90%
Immunization for Pneumonia[2]	395	86%	90%	92%
Stroke Care				
Anticoagulation Therapy for Atrial Fibrillation[1]	-	-	88%	95%
Antithrombotic Therapy Timing	31	97%	97%	98%
Assessed for Rehabilitation	34	94%	97%	97%
Discharged on Antithrombotic Therapy	32	97%	98%	99%
Discharged on Statin Medication	33	55%	88%	94%
Thrombolytic Therapy Timing[1]	-	-	68%	66%
Venous Thromboembolism Prophylaxis	37	95%	93%	94%
Written Stroke Educational Materials Given	17	6%	84%	88%
Surgical Care Improvement Project				
Appropriate Beta Blocker Usage	49	96%	98%	98%
Appropriate VTP Within 24 Hours	136	99%	98%	98%
Controlled Postoperative Blood Glucose[7]	-	-	98%	97%
Perioperative Temperature Management	152	100%	100%	100%
Prophylactic Antibiotic Selection	96	99%	99%	99%
Prophylactic Antibiotic Selection (Outpatient)	119	99%	98%	98%
Prophylactic Antibiotic Stopped	83	98%	98%	98%
Prophylactic Antibiotic Timing	96	100%	99%	99%
Prophylactic Antibiotic Timing (Outpatient)	107	100%	98%	98%
Urinary Catheter Removal	83	96%	97%	97%
Survey of Patients' Hospital Experiences				
Area Around Room 'Always' Quiet at Night	300+	62%	65%	61%
Doctors 'Always' Communicated Well	300+	81%	85%	82%
Home Recovery Information Given	300+	84%	86%	85%
Hospital Given 9 or 10 on 10 Point Scale	300+	70%	76%	71%
Meds 'Always' Explained Before Given	300+	65%	66%	64%
Nurses 'Always' Communicated Well	300+	78%	81%	79%
Pain 'Always' Well Controlled	300+	74%	72%	71%
Room and Bathroom 'Always' Clean	300+	75%	76%	73%
Timely Help 'Always' Received	300+	64%	72%	68%
Would Definitely Recommend Hospital	300+	65%	75%	71%
Use of Medical Imaging				
Cardiac Imaging Stress Test before Surgery	147	3.4%	5%	5.3%
Combination Abdominal CT Scan	336	13.4%	19%	10.5%
Combination Brain/Sinus CT Scan[1]	-	-	2.9%	2.7%
Combination Chest CT Scan	197	0.0%	3.9%	2.7%
Follow-up Mammogram/Ultrasound	465	11.8%	7.8%	8.8%
Lumbar Spine MRI for Low Back Pain	104	36.5%	40.2%	37.2%

Citizens Medical Center

100 E College Drive
Colby, KS 67701
Phone: 785-462-7511
Type: Critical Access Hospitals
Emergency Services: Yes
Ownership: Voluntary non-profit - Private

Measure	Cases	This Hosp.	State Avg.	U.S. Avg.
Blood Clot Prevention and Treatment				
Anticoagulation Overlap Therapy[1,3]	-	-	94%	93%
ICU Venous Thromboembolism Prophylaxis[3,7]	-	-	91%	92%
Incidence of Potentially Preventable VTE[3,7]	-	-	8%	10%
UFH with Dosages/Platelet Monitoring[3,7]	-	-	98%	97%
Venous Thromboembolism Prophylaxis[1,3]	-	-	79%	85%
Warfarin Therapy Discharge Instructions[1,3]	-	-	84%	75%
Chest Pain/Possible Heart Attack Care				
Aspirin Given Within 24 Hours of Arrival	-	-	94%	96%
Fibrinolytic Meds Within 30 Min. of Arrival	-	-	41%	58%
Average Time to ECG (minutes)	-	-	8	7
Average Time to Transfer (minutes)	-	-	57	60
Children's Asthma Care				
Received Home Management Plan of Care	-	-	-	88%
Received Reliever Medication	-	-	-	100%
Received Systemic Corticosteroids	-	-	-	100%
Emergency Department				
Admittance Decision Time (minutes)[3]	91	20	57	98
Head CT Results Within 45 Min. of Arrival	-	-	53%	57%
Patients Who Left ER Before Being Seen	-	-	2%	2%
Time from ER Arrival to Admit. (minutes)[3]	118	115	185	274
Time from ER Arrival to Discharge (minutes)	-	-	104	134
Time in ER Before Being Evaluated (minutes)	-	-	18	26
Time to Pain Meds for Fractures (minutes)	-	-	47	57
Heart Attack Care				
Aspirin Given at Discharge[1,3]	-	-	99%	99%
Fibrinolytic Meds Within 30 Min. of Arrival[3,7]	-	-	-	54%
PCI Within 90 Minutes of Arrival[3,7]	-	-	97%	96%
Statin Prescribed at Discharge[1,3]	-	-	99%	98%
Heart Failure Care				
ACE Inhibitor or ARB for LVSD[1,3]	-	-	95%	97%
Discharge Instructions Given[1,3]	-	-	91%	94%
Evaluation of LVS Function[3]	12	50%	94%	99%
Medicare Spending				
Medicare Spending per Patient (ratio)	-	-	0.94	0.98
Pneumonia Care				
Appropriate Initial Antibiotic Given[1]	-	-	92%	95%
Blood Culture Timing[1]	-	-	98%	98%
Pregnancy and Delivery Care				
Newborn Deliveries Scheduled Early[5]	-	-	12%	6%
Preventive Care				
Immunization for Influenza[3]	54	72%	88%	90%
Immunization for Pneumonia[3]	131	63%	90%	92%
Stroke Care				
Anticoagulation Therapy for Atrial Fibrillation[1,3]	-	-	88%	95%
Antithrombotic Therapy Timing[1,3]	-	-	97%	98%
Assessed for Rehabilitation[1,3]	-	-	97%	97%
Discharged on Antithrombotic Therapy[1,3]	-	-	98%	99%
Discharged on Statin Medication[1,3]	-	-	88%	94%
Thrombolytic Therapy Timing[3,7]	-	-	68%	66%
Venous Thromboembolism Prophylaxis[1,3]	-	-	93%	94%
Written Stroke Educational Materials Given[1,3]	-	-	84%	88%
Surgical Care Improvement Project				
Appropriate Beta Blocker Usage[5]	-	-	98%	98%
Appropriate VTP Within 24 Hours[5]	-	-	98%	98%
Controlled Postoperative Blood Glucose[5]	-	-	98%	97%
Perioperative Temperature Management[5]	-	-	100%	100%
Prophylactic Antibiotic Selection[5]	-	-	99%	99%
Prophylactic Antibiotic Selection (Outpatient)	-	-	98%	98%
Prophylactic Antibiotic Stopped[5]	-	-	98%	98%
Prophylactic Antibiotic Timing[5]	-	-	99%	99%
Prophylactic Antibiotic Timing (Outpatient)	-	-	98%	98%
Urinary Catheter Removal[5]	-	-	97%	97%
Survey of Patients' Hospital Experiences				
Area Around Room 'Always' Quiet at Night	(a)	54%	65%	61%
Doctors 'Always' Communicated Well	(a)	84%	85%	82%
Home Recovery Information Given	(a)	83%	86%	85%
Hospital Given 9 or 10 on 10 Point Scale	(a)	76%	76%	71%
Meds 'Always' Explained Before Given	(a)	72%	66%	64%
Nurses 'Always' Communicated Well	(a)	84%	81%	79%
Pain 'Always' Well Controlled	(a)	73%	72%	71%
Room and Bathroom 'Always' Clean	(a)	71%	76%	73%
Timely Help 'Always' Received	(a)	74%	72%	68%
Would Definitely Recommend Hospital	(a)	76%	75%	71%
Use of Medical Imaging				
Cardiac Imaging Stress Test before Surgery	-	-	5%	5.3%
Combination Abdominal CT Scan	-	-	19%	10.5%
Combination Brain/Sinus CT Scan	-	-	2.9%	2.7%
Combination Chest CT Scan	-	-	3.9%	2.7%

NOTE: Hospital profiles are in alphabetical order by state, then city, then hospital within the city; Rankings exclude hospitals with less than 25 cases except for patient surveys which excludes hospitals with less than 100 cases; (a) 100-299 cases; (1) The number of cases/patients is too few to report; (2) Data submitted were based on a sample of cases/patients; (3) Results are based on a shorter time period than required; (4) Data suppressed by CMS for one or more quarters; (5) Results are not available for this reporting period; (6) Fewer than 100 patients completed the HCAHPS survey; (7) No cases met the criteria for this measure; (8) The lower limit of the confidence interval cannot be calculated if the number of observed infections equals zero; (9) No data are available from the state/territory for this reporting period; (10) The scores shown reflect fewer than 50 completed surveys; (11) There were discrepancies in the data collection process; (12) This measure does not apply to this hospital for this reporting period; (13) Results cannot be calculated for this reporting period; (14) The results for this state are combined with nearby states to protect confidentiality; Please refer to the User's Guide for a full explanation of data.

Follow-up Mammogram/Ultrasound	-	-	7.8%	8.8%
Lumbar Spine MRI for Low Back Pain	-	-	40.2%	37.2%

Comanche County Hospital

2nd & Frisco Street
Coldwater, KS 67029
URL: www.gpha.com
Type: Critical Access Hospitals
Ownership: Government - Local
Phone: 620-582-2144
Fax: 620-582-2572
Emergency Services: Yes
Beds: 14

Measure	Cases	This Hosp.	State Avg.	U.S. Avg.
Blood Clot Prevention and Treatment				
Anticoagulation Overlap Therapy[5]	-	-	94%	93%
ICU Venous Thromboembolism Prophylaxis[5]	-	-	91%	92%
Incidence of Potentially Preventable VTE[5]	-	-	8%	10%
UFH with Dosages/Platelet Monitoring[5]	-	-	98%	97%
Venous Thromboembolism Prophylaxis[5]	-	-	79%	85%
Warfarin Therapy Discharge Instructions[5]	-	-	84%	75%
Chest Pain/Possible Heart Attack Care				
Aspirin Given Within 24 Hours of Arrival	-	-	94%	96%
Fibrinolytic Meds Within 30 Min. of Arrival	-	-	41%	58%
Average Time to ECG (minutes)	-	-	8	7
Average Time to Transfer (minutes)	-	-	57	60
Children's Asthma Care				
Received Home Management Plan of Care	-	-	-	88%
Received Reliever Medication	-	-	-	100%
Received Systemic Corticosteroids	-	-	-	100%
Emergency Department				
Admittance Decision Time (minutes)	32	10	57	98
Head CT Results Within 45 Min. of Arrival	-	-	53%	57%
Patients Who Left ER Before Being Seen	-	-	2%	2%
Time from ER Arrival to Admit. (minutes)	32	61	185	274
Time from ER Arrival to Discharge (minutes)	-	-	104	134
Time in ER Before Being Evaluated (minutes)	-	-	18	26
Time to Pain Meds for Fractures (minutes)	-	-	47	57
Heart Attack Care				
Aspirin Given at Discharge[5]	-	-	99%	99%
Fibrinolytic Meds Within 30 Min. of Arrival[5]	-	-	-	54%
PCI Within 90 Minutes of Arrival[5]	-	-	97%	96%
Statin Prescribed at Discharge[5]	-	-	99%	98%
Heart Failure Care				
ACE Inhibitor or ARB for LVSD[5]	-	-	95%	97%
Discharge Instructions Given[5]	-	-	91%	94%
Evaluation of LVS Function[5]	-	-	94%	99%
Medicare Spending				
Medicare Spending per Patient (ratio)	-	-	0.94	0.98
Pneumonia Care				
Appropriate Initial Antibiotic Given[1]	-	-	92%	95%
Blood Culture Timing[1]	-	-	98%	98%
Pregnancy and Delivery Care				
Newborn Deliveries Scheduled Early[5]	-	-	12%	6%
Preventive Care				
Immunization for Influenza	18	78%	88%	90%
Immunization for Pneumonia	21	43%	90%	92%
Stroke Care				
Anticoagulation Therapy for Atrial Fibrillation[5]	-	-	88%	95%
Antithrombotic Therapy Timing[5]	-	-	97%	98%
Assessed for Rehabilitation[5]	-	-	97%	97%
Discharged on Antithrombotic Therapy[5]	-	-	98%	99%
Discharged on Statin Medication[5]	-	-	88%	94%
Thrombolytic Therapy Timing[5]	-	-	68%	66%
Venous Thromboembolism Prophylaxis[5]	-	-	93%	94%
Written Stroke Educational Materials Given[5]	-	-	84%	88%
Surgical Care Improvement Project				
Appropriate Beta Blocker Usage[5]	-	-	98%	98%
Appropriate VTP Within 24 Hours[5]	-	-	98%	98%
Controlled Postoperative Blood Glucose[5]	-	-	98%	97%
Perioperative Temperature Management[5]	-	-	100%	100%
Prophylactic Antibiotic Selection[5]	-	-	99%	99%
Prophylactic Antibiotic Selection (Outpatient)	-	-	98%	98%
Prophylactic Antibiotic Stopped[5]	-	-	98%	98%
Prophylactic Antibiotic Timing[5]	-	-	99%	99%
Prophylactic Antibiotic Timing (Outpatient)	-	-	98%	98%
Urinary Catheter Removal[5]	-	-	97%	97%
Survey of Patients' Hospital Experiences				
Area Around Room 'Always' Quiet at Night[5]	-	-	65%	61%
Doctors 'Always' Communicated Well[5]	-	-	85%	82%
Home Recovery Information Given[5]	-	-	86%	85%
Hospital Given 9 or 10 on 10 Point Scale[5]	-	-	76%	71%
Meds 'Always' Explained Before Given[5]	-	-	66%	64%
Nurses 'Always' Communicated Well[5]	-	-	81%	79%
Pain 'Always' Well Controlled[5]	-	-	72%	71%
Room and Bathroom 'Always' Clean[5]	-	-	76%	73%
Timely Help 'Always' Received[5]	-	-	72%	68%
Would Definitely Recommend Hospital[5]	-	-	75%	71%
Use of Medical Imaging				
Cardiac Imaging Stress Test before Surgery	-	-	5%	5.3%
Combination Abdominal CT Scan	-	-	19%	10.5%
Combination Brain/Sinus CT Scan	-	-	2.9%	2.7%
Combination Chest CT Scan	-	-	3.9%	2.7%
Follow-up Mammogram/Ultrasound	-	-	7.8%	8.8%
Lumbar Spine MRI for Low Back Pain	-	-	40.2%	37.2%

Mercy Maude Norton Hospital

220 N Pennsylvania Avenue
Columbus, KS 66725
Type: Critical Access Hospitals
Ownership: Voluntary non-profit - Church
Phone: 620-429-2545
Emergency Services: Yes

Measure	Cases	This Hosp.	State Avg.	U.S. Avg.
Blood Clot Prevention and Treatment				
Anticoagulation Overlap Therapy[7]	-	-	94%	93%
ICU Venous Thromboembolism Prophylaxis[7]	-	-	91%	92%
Incidence of Potentially Preventable VTE[7]	-	-	8%	10%
UFH with Dosages/Platelet Monitoring[7]	-	-	98%	97%
Venous Thromboembolism Prophylaxis	16	69%	79%	85%
Warfarin Therapy Discharge Instructions[7]	-	-	84%	75%
Chest Pain/Possible Heart Attack Care				
Aspirin Given Within 24 Hours of Arrival[1,3]	-	-	94%	96%
Fibrinolytic Meds Within 30 Min. of Arrival[3,7]	-	-	41%	58%
Average Time to ECG (minutes)[1,3]	-	-	8	7
Average Time to Transfer (minutes)[3,7]	-	-	57	60
Children's Asthma Care				
Received Home Management Plan of Care	-	-	-	88%
Received Reliever Medication	-	-	-	100%
Received Systemic Corticosteroids	-	-	-	100%
Emergency Department				
Admittance Decision Time (minutes)[2,3]	31	30	57	98
Head CT Results Within 45 Min. of Arrival[5]	-	-	53%	57%
Patients Who Left ER Before Being Seen[5]	-	-	2%	2%
Time from ER Arrival to Admit. (minutes)[2,3]	31	131	185	274
Time from ER Arrival to Discharge (minutes)[3]	70	87	104	134
Time in ER Before Being Evaluated (minutes)[3]	83	18	18	26
Time to Pain Meds for Fractures (minutes)[1,3]	-	-	47	57
Heart Attack Care				
Aspirin Given at Discharge[5]	-	-	99%	99%
Fibrinolytic Meds Within 30 Min. of Arrival[5]	-	-	-	54%
PCI Within 90 Minutes of Arrival[5]	-	-	97%	96%
Statin Prescribed at Discharge[5]	-	-	99%	98%
Heart Failure Care				
ACE Inhibitor or ARB for LVSD[1,3]	-	-	95%	97%
Discharge Instructions Given[1,3]	-	-	91%	94%
Evaluation of LVS Function[1,3]	-	-	94%	99%
Medicare Spending				
Medicare Spending per Patient (ratio)	-	-	0.94	0.98
Pneumonia Care				
Appropriate Initial Antibiotic Given[1,2]	-	-	92%	95%
Blood Culture Timing[1,2]	-	-	98%	98%
Pregnancy and Delivery Care				
Newborn Deliveries Scheduled Early[5]	-	-	12%	6%
Preventive Care				
Immunization for Influenza[3]	15	47%	88%	90%
Immunization for Pneumonia[3]	22	73%	90%	92%
Stroke Care				
Anticoagulation Therapy for Atrial Fibrillation[3,7]	-	-	88%	95%
Antithrombotic Therapy Timing[3,7]	-	-	97%	98%
Assessed for Rehabilitation[3,7]	-	-	97%	97%
Discharged on Antithrombotic Therapy[3,7]	-	-	98%	99%
Discharged on Statin Medication[3,7]	-	-	88%	94%
Thrombolytic Therapy Timing[3,7]	-	-	68%	66%
Venous Thromboembolism Prophylaxis[3,7]	-	-	93%	94%
Written Stroke Educational Materials Given[3,7]	-	-	84%	88%
Surgical Care Improvement Project				
Appropriate Beta Blocker Usage[5]	-	-	98%	98%
Appropriate VTP Within 24 Hours[5]	-	-	98%	98%
Controlled Postoperative Blood Glucose[5]	-	-	98%	97%
Perioperative Temperature Management[5]	-	-	100%	100%
Prophylactic Antibiotic Selection[5]	-	-	99%	99%
Prophylactic Antibiotic Selection (Outpatient)[5]	-	-	98%	98%
Prophylactic Antibiotic Stopped[5]	-	-	98%	98%
Prophylactic Antibiotic Timing[5]	-	-	99%	99%
Prophylactic Antibiotic Timing (Outpatient)[5]	-	-	98%	98%
Urinary Catheter Removal[5]	-	-	97%	97%
Survey of Patients' Hospital Experiences				
Area Around Room 'Always' Quiet at Night[5]	-	-	65%	61%
Doctors 'Always' Communicated Well[5]	-	-	85%	82%
Home Recovery Information Given[5]	-	-	86%	85%
Hospital Given 9 or 10 on 10 Point Scale[5]	-	-	76%	71%
Meds 'Always' Explained Before Given[5]	-	-	66%	64%
Nurses 'Always' Communicated Well[5]	-	-	81%	79%
Pain 'Always' Well Controlled[5]	-	-	72%	71%
Room and Bathroom 'Always' Clean[5]	-	-	76%	73%
Timely Help 'Always' Received[5]	-	-	72%	68%
Would Definitely Recommend Hospital[5]	-	-	75%	71%
Use of Medical Imaging				
Cardiac Imaging Stress Test before Surgery[7]	-	-	5%	5.3%
Combination Abdominal CT Scan[7]	-	-	19%	10.5%
Combination Brain/Sinus CT Scan[7]	-	-	2.9%	2.7%
Combination Chest CT Scan[7]	-	-	3.9%	2.7%
Follow-up Mammogram/Ultrasound	224	9.4%	7.8%	8.8%
Lumbar Spine MRI for Low Back Pain[7]	-	-	40.2%	37.2%

Cloud County Health Center

1100 Highland Drive
Concordia, KS 66901
URL: www.cchc.com
Type: Critical Access Hospitals
Ownership: Voluntary non-profit - Private
Phone: 785-243-1234
Fax: 785-243-8411
Emergency Services: Yes
Beds: 25

Key Personnel:

President/CEO. . . . . Don Bates
Operating Room. . . . . Muhammad Butt, MD
Quality Assurance . . . . Lisa Hasenbank
Emergency Room . . . . Dana Jordan
Chief of Medical Staff . . . . Travis Jordan, DO
Radiology. . . . . Richard J Kueker
Intensive Care Unit. . . . . Laura Otte

Measure	Cases	This Hosp.	State Avg.	U.S. Avg.
Blood Clot Prevention and Treatment				
Anticoagulation Overlap Therapy[5]	-	-	94%	93%
ICU Venous Thromboembolism Prophylaxis[5]	-	-	91%	92%
Incidence of Potentially Preventable VTE[5]	-	-	8%	10%
UFH with Dosages/Platelet Monitoring[5]	-	-	98%	97%
Venous Thromboembolism Prophylaxis[5]	-	-	79%	85%
Warfarin Therapy Discharge Instructions[5]	-	-	84%	75%
Chest Pain/Possible Heart Attack Care				
Aspirin Given Within 24 Hours of Arrival	-	-	94%	96%
Fibrinolytic Meds Within 30 Min. of Arrival	-	-	41%	58%
Average Time to ECG (minutes)	-	-	8	7
Average Time to Transfer (minutes)	-	-	57	60
Children's Asthma Care				
Received Home Management Plan of Care	-	-	-	88%
Received Reliever Medication	-	-	-	100%
Received Systemic Corticosteroids	-	-	-	100%
Emergency Department				
Admittance Decision Time (minutes)[5]	-	-	57	98
Head CT Results Within 45 Min. of Arrival	-	-	53%	57%
Patients Who Left ER Before Being Seen	-	-	2%	2%
Time from ER Arrival to Admit. (minutes)[5]	-	-	185	274
Time from ER Arrival to Discharge (minutes)	-	-	104	134
Time in ER Before Being Evaluated (minutes)	-	-	18	26

NOTE: Hospital profiles are in alphabetical order by state, then city, then hospital within the city; Rankings exclude hospitals with less than 25 cases except for patient surveys which excludes hospitals with less than 100 cases; (a) 100-299 cases; (1) The number of cases/patients is too few to report; (2) Data submitted were based on a sample of cases/patients; (3) Results are based on a shorter time period than required; (4) Data suppressed by CMS for one or more quarters; (5) Results are not available for this reporting period; (6) Fewer than 100 patients completed the HCAHPS survey; (7) No cases met the criteria for this measure; (8) The lower limit of the confidence interval cannot be calculated if the number of observed infections equals zero; (9) No data are available from the state/territory for this reporting period; (10) The scores shown reflect fewer than 50 completed surveys; (11) There were discrepancies in the data collection process; (12) This measure does not apply to this hospital for this reporting period; (13) Results cannot be calculated for this reporting period; (14) The results for this state are combined with nearby states to protect confidentiality; Please refer to the User's Guide for a full explanation of data.

Measure	Cases	This Hosp.	State Avg.	U.S. Avg.
Time to Pain Meds for Fractures (minutes)	-	-	47	57
Heart Attack Care				
Aspirin Given at Discharge[5]	-	-	99%	99%
Fibrinolytic Meds Within 30 Min. of Arrival[5]	-	-	-	54%
PCI Within 90 Minutes of Arrival[5]	-	-	97%	96%
Statin Prescribed at Discharge[5]	-	-	99%	98%
Heart Failure Care				
ACE Inhibitor or ARB for LVSD[1]	-	-	95%	97%
Discharge Instructions Given	16	88%	91%	94%
Evaluation of LVS Function	26	50%	94%	99%
Medicare Spending				
Medicare Spending per Patient (ratio)	-	-	0.94	0.98
Pneumonia Care				
Appropriate Initial Antibiotic Given	43	88%	92%	95%
Blood Culture Timing	16	75%	98%	98%
Pregnancy and Delivery Care				
Newborn Deliveries Scheduled Early[5]	-	-	12%	6%
Preventive Care				
Immunization for Influenza	49	88%	88%	90%
Immunization for Pneumonia[2]	101	89%	90%	92%
Stroke Care				
Anticoagulation Therapy for Atrial Fibrillation[1]	-	-	88%	95%
Antithrombotic Therapy Timing[1]	-	-	97%	98%
Assessed for Rehabilitation[1]	-	-	97%	97%
Discharged on Antithrombotic Therapy[1]	-	-	98%	99%
Discharged on Statin Medication[1]	-	-	88%	94%
Thrombolytic Therapy Timing[1]	-	-	68%	66%
Venous Thromboembolism Prophylaxis[1]	-	-	93%	94%
Written Stroke Educational Materials Given[1]	-	-	84%	88%
Surgical Care Improvement Project				
Appropriate Beta Blocker Usage[5]	-	-	98%	98%
Appropriate VTP Within 24 Hours[5]	-	-	98%	98%
Controlled Postoperative Blood Glucose[5]	-	-	98%	97%
Perioperative Temperature Management[5]	-	-	100%	100%
Prophylactic Antibiotic Selection[5]	-	-	99%	99%
Prophylactic Antibiotic Selection (Outpatient)	-	-	98%	98%
Prophylactic Antibiotic Stopped[5]	-	-	98%	98%
Prophylactic Antibiotic Timing[5]	-	-	99%	99%
Prophylactic Antibiotic Timing (Outpatient)	-	-	98%	98%
Urinary Catheter Removal[5]	-	-	97%	97%
Survey of Patients' Hospital Experiences				
Area Around Room 'Always' Quiet at Night[5]	-	-	65%	61%
Doctors 'Always' Communicated Well[5]	-	-	85%	82%
Home Recovery Information Given[5]	-	-	86%	85%
Hospital Given 9 or 10 on 10 Point Scale[5]	-	-	76%	71%
Meds 'Always' Explained Before Given[5]	-	-	66%	64%
Nurses 'Always' Communicated Well[5]	-	-	81%	79%
Pain 'Always' Well Controlled[5]	-	-	72%	71%
Room and Bathroom 'Always' Clean[5]	-	-	76%	73%
Timely Help 'Always' Received[5]	-	-	72%	68%
Would Definitely Recommend Hospital[5]	-	-	75%	71%
Use of Medical Imaging				
Cardiac Imaging Stress Test before Surgery	-	-	5%	5.3%
Combination Abdominal CT Scan	-	-	19%	10.5%
Combination Brain/Sinus CT Scan	-	-	2.9%	2.7%
Combination Chest CT Scan	-	-	3.9%	2.7%
Follow-up Mammogram/Ultrasound	-	-	7.8%	8.8%
Lumbar Spine MRI for Low Back Pain	-	-	40.2%	37.2%

Morris County Hospital

600 N Washington St
Council Grove, KS 66846
Phone: 620-767-6811
Fax: 620-767-5611
URL: www.mrchosp.com
Type: Critical Access Hospitals
Emergency Services: Yes
Ownership: Government - Local
Beds: 28
Key Personnel:
Chief of Medical Staff.......... Daniel R Frese
Emergency Room .... Joel Hornung
Radiology.................. Stephen M Knecht
CEO/President............... James H Reagan Jr, MD

Measure	Cases	This Hosp.	State Avg.	U.S. Avg.
Blood Clot Prevention and Treatment				
Anticoagulation Overlap Therapy[5]	-	-	94%	93%
ICU Venous Thromboembolism Prophylaxis[5]	-	-	91%	92%
Incidence of Potentially Preventable VTE[5]	-	-	8%	10%
UFH with Dosages/Platelet Monitoring[5]	-	-	98%	97%
Venous Thromboembolism Prophylaxis[5]	-	-	79%	85%
Warfarin Therapy Discharge Instructions[5]	-	-	84%	75%
Chest Pain/Possible Heart Attack Care				
Aspirin Given Within 24 Hours of Arrival	-	-	94%	96%
Fibrinolytic Meds Within 30 Min. of Arrival	-	-	41%	58%
Average Time to ECG (minutes)	-	-	8	7
Average Time to Transfer (minutes)	-	-	57	60
Children's Asthma Care				
Received Home Management Plan of Care	-	-	-	88%
Received Reliever Medication	-	-	-	100%
Received Systemic Corticosteroids	-	-	-	100%
Emergency Department				
Admittance Decision Time (minutes)[5]	-	-	57	98
Head CT Results Within 45 Min. of Arrival	-	-	53%	57%
Patients Who Left ER Before Being Seen	-	-	2%	2%
Time from ER Arrival to Admit. (minutes)[5]	-	-	185	274
Time from ER Arrival to Discharge (minutes)	-	-	104	134
Time in ER Before Being Evaluated (minutes)	-	-	18	26
Time to Pain Meds for Fractures (minutes)	-	-	47	57
Heart Attack Care				
Aspirin Given at Discharge[1,3]	-	-	99%	99%
Fibrinolytic Meds Within 30 Min. of Arrival[3,7]	-	-	-	54%
PCI Within 90 Minutes of Arrival[3,7]	-	-	97%	96%
Statin Prescribed at Discharge[1,3]	-	-	99%	98%
Heart Failure Care				
ACE Inhibitor or ARB for LVSD[1]	-	-	95%	97%
Discharge Instructions Given	16	44%	91%	94%
Evaluation of LVS Function	21	81%	94%	99%
Medicare Spending				
Medicare Spending per Patient (ratio)	-	-	0.94	0.98
Pneumonia Care				
Appropriate Initial Antibiotic Given	11	100%	92%	95%
Blood Culture Timing[7]	-	-	98%	98%
Pregnancy and Delivery Care				
Newborn Deliveries Scheduled Early[5]	-	-	12%	6%
Preventive Care				
Immunization for Influenza[5]	-	-	88%	90%
Immunization for Pneumonia[5]	-	-	90%	92%
Stroke Care				
Anticoagulation Therapy for Atrial Fibrillation[5]	-	-	88%	95%
Antithrombotic Therapy Timing[5]	-	-	97%	98%
Assessed for Rehabilitation[5]	-	-	97%	97%
Discharged on Antithrombotic Therapy[5]	-	-	98%	99%
Discharged on Statin Medication[5]	-	-	88%	94%
Thrombolytic Therapy Timing[5]	-	-	68%	66%
Venous Thromboembolism Prophylaxis[5]	-	-	93%	94%
Written Stroke Educational Materials Given[5]	-	-	84%	88%
Surgical Care Improvement Project				
Appropriate Beta Blocker Usage[5]	-	-	98%	98%
Appropriate VTP Within 24 Hours[5]	-	-	98%	98%
Controlled Postoperative Blood Glucose[5]	-	-	98%	97%
Perioperative Temperature Management[5]	-	-	100%	100%
Prophylactic Antibiotic Selection[5]	-	-	99%	99%
Prophylactic Antibiotic Selection (Outpatient)	-	-	98%	98%
Prophylactic Antibiotic Stopped[5]	-	-	98%	98%
Prophylactic Antibiotic Timing[5]	-	-	99%	99%
Prophylactic Antibiotic Timing (Outpatient)	-	-	98%	98%
Urinary Catheter Removal[5]	-	-	97%	97%
Survey of Patients' Hospital Experiences				
Area Around Room 'Always' Quiet at Night[6]	<100	72%	65%	61%
Doctors 'Always' Communicated Well[6]	<100	86%	85%	82%
Home Recovery Information Given[6]	<100	78%	86%	85%
Hospital Given 9 or 10 on 10 Point Scale[6]	<100	87%	76%	71%
Meds 'Always' Explained Before Given[6]	<100	67%	66%	64%
Nurses 'Always' Communicated Well[6]	<100	84%	81%	79%
Pain 'Always' Well Controlled[6]	<100	68%	72%	71%
Room and Bathroom 'Always' Clean[6]	<100	75%	76%	73%
Timely Help 'Always' Received[6]	<100	82%	72%	68%
Would Definitely Recommend Hospital[6]	<100	77%	75%	71%
Use of Medical Imaging				
Cardiac Imaging Stress Test before Surgery	-	-	5%	5.3%
Combination Abdominal CT Scan	-	-	19%	10.5%
Combination Brain/Sinus CT Scan	-	-	2.9%	2.7%
Combination Chest CT Scan	-	-	3.9%	2.7%
Follow-up Mammogram/Ultrasound	-	-	7.8%	8.8%
Lumbar Spine MRI for Low Back Pain	-	-	40.2%	37.2%

Western Plains Medical Complex

3001 Avenue A
Dodge City, KS 67801
Phone: 620-225-8400
Fax: 620-225-8403
URL: www.westernplainsmc.com
Type: Acute Care Hospitals
Emergency Services: Yes
Ownership: Proprietary
Beds: 110
Key Personnel:
Radiology.................. Carl Fieser
Chief of Medical Staff.......... R C Trotter, MD
CEO/President............... John E Walker
Emergency Room .... Phillis Williams

Measure	Cases	This Hosp.	State Avg.	U.S. Avg.
Blood Clot Prevention and Treatment				
Anticoagulation Overlap Therapy[2]	16	100%	94%	93%
ICU Venous Thromboembolism Prophylaxis[2]	107	98%	91%	92%
Incidence of Potentially Preventable VTE[2,7]	-	-	8%	10%
UFH with Dosages/Platelet Monitoring[1,2]	-	-	98%	97%
Venous Thromboembolism Prophylaxis[2]	87	91%	79%	85%
Warfarin Therapy Discharge Instructions[2]	11	100%	84%	75%
Chest Pain/Possible Heart Attack Care				
Aspirin Given Within 24 Hours of Arrival[1,3]	-	-	94%	96%
Fibrinolytic Meds Within 30 Min. of Arrival[3,7]	-	-	41%	58%
Average Time to ECG (minutes)[1,3]	-	-	8	7
Average Time to Transfer (minutes)[3,7]	-	-	57	60
Children's Asthma Care				
Received Home Management Plan of Care	-	-	-	88%
Received Reliever Medication	-	-	-	100%
Received Systemic Corticosteroids	-	-	-	100%
Emergency Department				
Admittance Decision Time (minutes)[2]	195	83	57	98
Head CT Results Within 45 Min. of Arrival[1,3]	-	-	53%	57%
Patients Who Left ER Before Being Seen	9,667	1%	2%	2%
Time from ER Arrival to Admit. (minutes)[2]	196	222	185	274
Time from ER Arrival to Discharge (minutes)	383	106	104	134
Time in ER Before Being Evaluated (minutes)	422	19	18	26
Time to Pain Meds for Fractures (minutes)	36	53	47	57
Heart Attack Care				
Aspirin Given at Discharge	33	100%	99%	99%
Fibrinolytic Meds Within 30 Min. of Arrival[7]	-	-	-	54%
PCI Within 90 Minutes of Arrival[1]	-	-	97%	96%
Statin Prescribed at Discharge	32	100%	99%	98%
Heart Failure Care				
ACE Inhibitor or ARB for LVSD	13	100%	95%	97%
Discharge Instructions Given	26	100%	91%	94%
Evaluation of LVS Function	44	100%	94%	99%
Medicare Spending				
Medicare Spending per Patient (ratio)	-	0.90	0.94	0.98
Pneumonia Care				
Appropriate Initial Antibiotic Given	38	95%	92%	95%
Blood Culture Timing	56	100%	98%	98%
Pregnancy and Delivery Care				
Newborn Deliveries Scheduled Early[2]	27	0%	12%	6%
Preventive Care				
Immunization for Influenza[2]	272	98%	88%	90%
Immunization for Pneumonia[2]	244	100%	90%	92%
Stroke Care				
Anticoagulation Therapy for Atrial Fibrillation[7]	-	-	88%	95%
Antithrombotic Therapy Timing[1]	-	-	97%	98%
Assessed for Rehabilitation[1]	-	-	97%	97%
Discharged on Antithrombotic Therapy[1]	-	-	98%	99%
Discharged on Statin Medication[1]	-	-	88%	94%
Thrombolytic Therapy Timing[7]	-	-	68%	66%
Venous Thromboembolism Prophylaxis	11	100%	93%	94%
Written Stroke Educational Materials Given[1]	-	-	84%	88%
Surgical Care Improvement Project				

NOTE: Hospital profiles are in alphabetical order by state, then city, then hospital within the city; Rankings exclude hospitals with less than 25 cases except for patient surveys which excludes hospitals with less than 100 cases; (a) 100-299 cases; (1) The number of cases/patients is too few to report; (2) Data submitted were based on a sample of cases/patients; (3) Results are based on a shorter time period than required; (4) Data suppressed by CMS for one or more quarters; (5) Results are not available for this reporting period; (6) Fewer than 100 patients completed the HCAHPS survey; (7) No cases met the criteria for this measure; (8) The lower limit of the confidence interval cannot be calculated if the number of observed infections equals zero; (9) No data are available from the state/territory for this reporting period; (10) The scores shown reflect fewer than 50 completed surveys; (11) There were discrepancies in the data collection process; (12) This measure does not apply to this hospital for this reporting period; (13) Results cannot be calculated for this reporting period; (14) The results for this state are combined with nearby states to protect confidentiality; Please refer to the User's Guide for a full explanation of data.

Measure	Cases	This Hosp.	State Avg.	U.S. Avg.
Appropriate Beta Blocker Usage	32	91%	98%	98%
Appropriate VTP Within 24 Hours	97	98%	98%	98%
Controlled Postoperative Blood Glucose[7]	-	-	98%	97%
Perioperative Temperature Management	112	100%	100%	100%
Prophylactic Antibiotic Selection	73	97%	99%	99%
Prophylactic Antibiotic Selection (Outpatient)	73	96%	98%	98%
Prophylactic Antibiotic Stopped	67	94%	98%	98%
Prophylactic Antibiotic Timing	73	100%	99%	99%
Prophylactic Antibiotic Timing (Outpatient)	74	99%	98%	98%
Urinary Catheter Removal	55	95%	97%	97%
Survey of Patients' Hospital Experiences				
Area Around Room 'Always' Quiet at Night	300+	53%	65%	61%
Doctors 'Always' Communicated Well	300+	76%	85%	82%
Home Recovery Information Given	300+	78%	86%	85%
Hospital Given 9 or 10 on 10 Point Scale	300+	57%	76%	71%
Meds 'Always' Explained Before Given	300+	53%	66%	64%
Nurses 'Always' Communicated Well	300+	70%	81%	79%
Pain 'Always' Well Controlled	300+	61%	72%	71%
Room and Bathroom 'Always' Clean	300+	65%	76%	73%
Timely Help 'Always' Received	300+	56%	72%	68%
Would Definitely Recommend Hospital	300+	52%	75%	71%
Use of Medical Imaging				
Cardiac Imaging Stress Test before Surgery[1]	-	-	5%	5.3%
Combination Abdominal CT Scan	126	4.0%	19%	10.5%
Combination Brain/Sinus CT Scan[1]	-	-	2.9%	2.7%
Combination Chest CT Scan	51	2.0%	3.9%	2.7%
Follow-up Mammogram/Ultrasound	228	6.6%	7.8%	8.8%
Lumbar Spine MRI for Low Back Pain[1]	-	-	40.2%	37.2%

Susan B Allen Memorial Hospital

720 W Central St
El Dorado, KS 67042
URL: www.sbamh.com
Phone: 316-322-4557
Fax: 316-321-2916
Type: Acute Care Hospitals
Ownership: Voluntary non-profit - Private
Emergency Services: Yes
Beds: 103

Key Personnel:

President/CEO. . . . . Gayle Arnett
Chief of Medical Staff. . . . . Cathy N Cooper
Radiology. . . . . Hilary Zarnow, MD/FACR

Measure	Cases	This Hosp.	State Avg.	U.S. Avg.
Blood Clot Prevention and Treatment				
Anticoagulation Overlap Therapy[1,2]	-	-	94%	93%
ICU Venous Thromboembolism Prophylaxis[2]	23	96%	91%	92%
Incidence of Potentially Preventable VTE[1,2]	-	-	8%	10%
UFH with Dosages/Platelet Monitoring[1,2]	-	-	98%	97%
Venous Thromboembolism Prophylaxis[2]	122	83%	79%	85%
Warfarin Therapy Discharge Instructions[1,2]	-	-	84%	75%
Chest Pain/Possible Heart Attack Care				
Aspirin Given Within 24 Hours of Arrival	80	100%	94%	96%
Fibrinolytic Meds Within 30 Min. of Arrival[7]	-	-	41%	58%
Average Time to ECG (minutes)	84	4	8	7
Average Time to Transfer (minutes)	12	26	57	60
Children's Asthma Care				
Received Home Management Plan of Care	-	-	-	88%
Received Reliever Medication	-	-	-	100%
Received Systemic Corticosteroids	-	-	-	100%
Emergency Department				
Admittance Decision Time (minutes)[2]	200	70	57	98
Head CT Results Within 45 Min. of Arrival	16	50%	53%	57%
Patients Who Left ER Before Being Seen	13,479	1%	2%	2%
Time from ER Arrival to Admit. (minutes)[2]	200	184	185	274
Time from ER Arrival to Discharge (minutes)	425	98	104	134
Time in ER Before Being Evaluated (minutes)	478	22	18	26
Time to Pain Meds for Fractures (minutes)	53	39	47	57
Heart Attack Care				
Aspirin Given at Discharge[1,3]	-	-	99%	99%
Fibrinolytic Meds Within 30 Min. of Arrival[3,7]	-	-	-	54%
PCI Within 90 Minutes of Arrival[3,7]	-	-	97%	96%
Statin Prescribed at Discharge[1,3]	-	-	99%	98%
Heart Failure Care				
ACE Inhibitor or ARB for LVSD[1]	-	-	95%	97%
Discharge Instructions Given	26	96%	91%	94%
Evaluation of LVS Function	44	100%	94%	99%
Medicare Spending				
Medicare Spending per Patient (ratio)	-	0.96	0.94	0.98
Pneumonia Care				
Appropriate Initial Antibiotic Given	85	95%	92%	95%
Blood Culture Timing	81	100%	98%	98%
Pregnancy and Delivery Care				
Newborn Deliveries Scheduled Early[2]	43	12%	12%	6%
Preventive Care				
Immunization for Influenza[2]	244	95%	88%	90%
Immunization for Pneumonia[2]	284	93%	90%	92%
Stroke Care				
Anticoagulation Therapy for Atrial Fibrillation[1]	-	-	88%	95%
Antithrombotic Therapy Timing	18	94%	97%	98%
Assessed for Rehabilitation	19	100%	97%	97%
Discharged on Antithrombotic Therapy	18	100%	98%	99%
Discharged on Statin Medication	13	54%	88%	94%
Thrombolytic Therapy Timing[1]	-	-	68%	66%
Venous Thromboembolism Prophylaxis	17	76%	93%	94%
Written Stroke Educational Materials Given[1]	-	-	84%	88%
Surgical Care Improvement Project				
Appropriate Beta Blocker Usage	13	100%	98%	98%
Appropriate VTP Within 24 Hours	51	94%	98%	98%
Controlled Postoperative Blood Glucose[7]	-	-	98%	97%
Perioperative Temperature Management	77	100%	100%	100%
Prophylactic Antibiotic Selection	61	93%	99%	99%
Prophylactic Antibiotic Selection (Outpatient)	68	99%	98%	98%
Prophylactic Antibiotic Stopped	59	97%	98%	98%
Prophylactic Antibiotic Timing	61	100%	99%	99%
Prophylactic Antibiotic Timing (Outpatient)	68	99%	98%	98%
Urinary Catheter Removal	31	100%	97%	97%
Survey of Patients' Hospital Experiences				
Area Around Room 'Always' Quiet at Night	300+	62%	65%	61%
Doctors 'Always' Communicated Well	300+	86%	85%	82%
Home Recovery Information Given	300+	86%	86%	85%
Hospital Given 9 or 10 on 10 Point Scale	300+	76%	76%	71%
Meds 'Always' Explained Before Given	300+	62%	66%	64%
Nurses 'Always' Communicated Well	300+	80%	81%	79%
Pain 'Always' Well Controlled	300+	68%	72%	71%
Room and Bathroom 'Always' Clean	300+	75%	76%	73%
Timely Help 'Always' Received	300+	71%	72%	68%
Would Definitely Recommend Hospital	300+	74%	75%	71%
Use of Medical Imaging				
Cardiac Imaging Stress Test before Surgery	130	0.8%	5%	5.3%
Combination Abdominal CT Scan	465	1.1%	19%	10.5%
Combination Brain/Sinus CT Scan	330	1.5%	2.9%	2.7%
Combination Chest CT Scan	312	0.0%	3.9%	2.7%
Follow-up Mammogram/Ultrasound	501	24.0%	7.8%	8.8%
Lumbar Spine MRI for Low Back Pain	129	44.2%	40.2%	37.2%

Morton County Hospital

445 N Hilltop
Elkhart, KS 67950
URL: www.mchswecare.com
Phone: 620-697-2141
Fax: 620-697-4766
Type: Acute Care Hospitals
Ownership: Voluntary non-profit - Other
Emergency Services: Yes
Beds: 120

Key Personnel:

Radiology. . . . . Mindano Beltran
CEO/President. . . . . Leonard Hernandez
Chief of Medical Staff. . . . . Dominador Perido, MD
Surgery . . . . Dominador T. Perido, MD

Measure	Cases	This Hosp.	State Avg.	U.S. Avg.
Blood Clot Prevention and Treatment				
Anticoagulation Overlap Therapy[1,2]	-	-	94%	93%
ICU Venous Thromboembolism Prophylaxis[2]	29	66%	91%	92%
Incidence of Potentially Preventable VTE[2,7]	-	-	8%	10%
UFH with Dosages/Platelet Monitoring[2,7]	-	-	98%	97%
Venous Thromboembolism Prophylaxis[2]	190	28%	79%	85%
Warfarin Therapy Discharge Instructions[1,2]	-	-	84%	75%
Chest Pain/Possible Heart Attack Care				
Aspirin Given Within 24 Hours of Arrival[1,3]	-	-	94%	96%
Fibrinolytic Meds Within 30 Min. of Arrival[5]	-	-	41%	58%
Average Time to ECG (minutes)[1,3]	-	-	8	7
Average Time to Transfer (minutes)[5]	-	-	57	60
Children's Asthma Care				
Received Home Management Plan of Care	-	-	-	88%
Received Reliever Medication	-	-	-	100%
Received Systemic Corticosteroids	-	-	-	100%
Emergency Department				
Admittance Decision Time (minutes)[2]	133	30	57	98
Head CT Results Within 45 Min. of Arrival[5]	-	-	53%	57%
Patients Who Left ER Before Being Seen	2,391	0%	2%	2%
Time from ER Arrival to Admit. (minutes)[2]	132	94	185	274
Time from ER Arrival to Discharge (minutes)	185	82	104	134
Time in ER Before Being Evaluated (minutes)	197	33	18	26
Time to Pain Meds for Fractures (minutes)[1]	-	-	47	57
Heart Attack Care				
Aspirin Given at Discharge[1,2]	-	-	99%	99%
Fibrinolytic Meds Within 30 Min. of Arrival[2,3]	-	-	-	54%
PCI Within 90 Minutes of Arrival[2,3]	-	-	97%	96%
Statin Prescribed at Discharge[1,2]	-	-	99%	98%
Heart Failure Care				
ACE Inhibitor or ARB for LVSD[1,2]	-	-	95%	97%
Discharge Instructions Given[2]	12	25%	91%	94%
Evaluation of LVS Function[2]	21	57%	94%	99%
Medicare Spending				
Medicare Spending per Patient (ratio)	-	0.71	0.94	0.98
Pneumonia Care				
Appropriate Initial Antibiotic Given[2]	12	25%	92%	95%
Blood Culture Timing[1,2]	-	-	98%	98%
Pregnancy and Delivery Care				
Newborn Deliveries Scheduled Early[7]	-	-	12%	6%
Preventive Care				
Immunization for Influenza[2]	151	81%	88%	90%
Immunization for Pneumonia[2]	228	83%	90%	92%
Stroke Care				
Anticoagulation Therapy for Atrial Fibrillation[2,3]	-	-	88%	95%
Antithrombotic Therapy Timing[1,2]	-	-	97%	98%
Assessed for Rehabilitation[1,2]	-	-	97%	97%
Discharged on Antithrombotic Therapy[1,2]	-	-	98%	99%
Discharged on Statin Medication[1,2]	-	-	88%	94%
Thrombolytic Therapy Timing[2,3]	-	-	68%	66%
Venous Thromboembolism Prophylaxis[1,2]	-	-	93%	94%
Written Stroke Educational Materials Given[2,3]	-	-	84%	88%
Surgical Care Improvement Project				
Appropriate Beta Blocker Usage[2,3]	-	-	98%	98%
Appropriate VTP Within 24 Hours[2,3]	-	-	98%	98%
Controlled Postoperative Blood Glucose[2,3]	-	-	98%	97%
Perioperative Temperature Management[1,2]	-	-	100%	100%
Prophylactic Antibiotic Selection[2,3]	-	-	99%	99%
Prophylactic Antibiotic Selection (Outpatient)[1,3]	-	-	98%	98%
Prophylactic Antibiotic Stopped[2,3]	-	-	98%	98%
Prophylactic Antibiotic Timing[2,3]	-	-	99%	99%
Prophylactic Antibiotic Timing (Outpatient)[1,3]	-	-	98%	98%
Urinary Catheter Removal[2,3]	-	-	97%	97%
Survey of Patients' Hospital Experiences				
Area Around Room 'Always' Quiet at Night[6]	<100	43%	65%	61%
Doctors 'Always' Communicated Well[6]	<100	76%	85%	82%
Home Recovery Information Given[6]	<100	89%	86%	85%
Hospital Given 9 or 10 on 10 Point Scale[6]	<100	59%	76%	71%
Meds 'Always' Explained Before Given[6]	<100	53%	66%	64%
Nurses 'Always' Communicated Well[6]	<100	71%	81%	79%
Pain 'Always' Well Controlled[6]	<100	73%	72%	71%
Room and Bathroom 'Always' Clean[6]	<100	67%	76%	73%
Timely Help 'Always' Received[6]	<100	71%	72%	68%
Would Definitely Recommend Hospital[6]	<100	61%	75%	71%
Use of Medical Imaging				
Cardiac Imaging Stress Test before Surgery[1]	-	-	5%	5.3%
Combination Abdominal CT Scan	41	48.8%	19%	10.5%
Combination Brain/Sinus CT Scan[1]	-	-	2.9%	2.7%
Combination Chest CT Scan[1]	-	-	3.9%	2.7%
Follow-up Mammogram/Ultrasound[1]	-	-	7.8%	8.8%
Lumbar Spine MRI for Low Back Pain[1]	-	-	40.2%	37.2%

NOTE: Hospital profiles are in alphabetical order by state, then city, then hospital within the city; Rankings exclude hospitals with less than 25 cases except for patient surveys which excludes hospitals with less than 100 cases; (a) 100-299 cases; (1) The number of cases/patients is too few to report; (2) Data submitted were based on a sample of cases/patients; (3) Results are based on a shorter time period than required; (4) Data suppressed by CMS for one or more quarters; (5) Results are not available for this reporting period; (6) Fewer than 100 patients completed the HCAHPS survey; (7) No cases met the criteria for this measure; (8) The lower limit of the confidence interval cannot be calculated if the number of observed infections equals zero; (9) No data are available from the state/territory for this reporting period; (10) The scores shown reflect fewer than 50 completed surveys; (11) There were discrepancies in the data collection process; (12) This measure does not apply to this hospital for this reporting period; (13) Results cannot be calculated for this reporting period; (14) The results for this state are combined with nearby states to protect confidentiality; Please refer to the User's Guide for a full explanation of data.

Ellinwood District Hospital

605 N Main Street
Ellinwood, KS 67526
Phone: 620-564-2548
Type: Critical Access Hospitals
Emergency Services: Yes
Ownership: Govt - Hospital Dist/Auth

Measure	Cases	This Hosp.	State Avg.	U.S. Avg.
Blood Clot Prevention and Treatment				
Anticoagulation Overlap Therapy[5]	-	-	94%	93%
ICU Venous Thromboembolism Prophylaxis[5]	-	-	91%	92%
Incidence of Potentially Preventable VTE[5]	-	-	8%	10%
UFH with Dosages/Platelet Monitoring[5]	-	-	98%	97%
Venous Thromboembolism Prophylaxis[5]	-	-	79%	85%
Warfarin Therapy Discharge Instructions[5]	-	-	84%	75%
Chest Pain/Possible Heart Attack Care				
Aspirin Given Within 24 Hours of Arrival	-	-	94%	96%
Fibrinolytic Meds Within 30 Min. of Arrival	-	-	41%	58%
Average Time to ECG (minutes)	-	-	8	7
Average Time to Transfer (minutes)	-	-	57	60
Children's Asthma Care				
Received Home Management Plan of Care	-	-	-	88%
Received Reliever Medication	-	-	-	100%
Received Systemic Corticosteroids	-	-	-	100%
Emergency Department				
Admittance Decision Time (minutes)[5]	-	-	57	98
Head CT Results Within 45 Min. of Arrival	-	-	53%	57%
Patients Who Left ER Before Being Seen	-	-	2%	2%
Time from ER Arrival to Admit. (minutes)[5]	-	-	185	274
Time from ER Arrival to Discharge (minutes)	-	-	104	134
Time in ER Before Being Evaluated (minutes)	-	-	18	26
Time to Pain Meds for Fractures (minutes)	-	-	47	57
Heart Attack Care				
Aspirin Given at Discharge[5]	-	-	99%	99%
Fibrinolytic Meds Within 30 Min. of Arrival[5]	-	-	-	54%
PCI Within 90 Minutes of Arrival[5]	-	-	97%	96%
Statin Prescribed at Discharge[5]	-	-	99%	98%
Heart Failure Care				
ACE Inhibitor or ARB for LVSD[1,3]	-	-	95%	97%
Discharge Instructions Given[1,3]	-	-	91%	94%
Evaluation of LVS Function[1,3]	-	-	94%	99%
Medicare Spending				
Medicare Spending per Patient (ratio)	-	-	0.94	0.98
Pneumonia Care				
Appropriate Initial Antibiotic Given[7]	-	-	92%	95%
Blood Culture Timing[7]	-	-	98%	98%
Pregnancy and Delivery Care				
Newborn Deliveries Scheduled Early[5]	-	-	12%	6%
Preventive Care				
Immunization for Influenza[1,3]	-	-	88%	90%
Immunization for Pneumonia[1,3]	-	-	90%	92%
Stroke Care				
Anticoagulation Therapy for Atrial Fibrillation[5]	-	-	88%	95%
Antithrombotic Therapy Timing[5]	-	-	97%	98%
Assessed for Rehabilitation[5]	-	-	97%	97%
Discharged on Antithrombotic Therapy[5]	-	-	98%	99%
Discharged on Statin Medication[5]	-	-	88%	94%
Thrombolytic Therapy Timing[5]	-	-	68%	66%
Venous Thromboembolism Prophylaxis[5]	-	-	93%	94%
Written Stroke Educational Materials Given[5]	-	-	84%	88%
Surgical Care Improvement Project				
Appropriate Beta Blocker Usage[5]	-	-	98%	98%
Appropriate VTP Within 24 Hours[5]	-	-	98%	98%
Controlled Postoperative Blood Glucose[5]	-	-	98%	97%
Perioperative Temperature Management[5]	-	-	100%	100%
Prophylactic Antibiotic Selection[5]	-	-	99%	99%
Prophylactic Antibiotic Selection (Outpatient)	-	-	98%	98%
Prophylactic Antibiotic Stopped[5]	-	-	98%	98%
Prophylactic Antibiotic Timing[5]	-	-	99%	99%
Prophylactic Antibiotic Timing (Outpatient)	-	-	98%	98%
Urinary Catheter Removal[5]	-	-	97%	97%
Survey of Patients' Hospital Experiences				
Area Around Room 'Always' Quiet at Night[5]	-	-	65%	61%
Doctors 'Always' Communicated Well[5]	-	-	85%	82%
Home Recovery Information Given[5]	-	-	86%	85%
Hospital Given 9 or 10 on 10 Point Scale[5]	-	-	76%	71%
Meds 'Always' Explained Before Given[5]	-	-	66%	64%
Nurses 'Always' Communicated Well[5]	-	-	81%	79%
Pain 'Always' Well Controlled[5]	-	-	72%	71%
Room and Bathroom 'Always' Clean[5]	-	-	76%	73%
Timely Help 'Always' Received[5]	-	-	72%	68%
Would Definitely Recommend Hospital[5]	-	-	75%	71%
Use of Medical Imaging				
Cardiac Imaging Stress Test before Surgery	-	-	5%	5.3%
Combination Abdominal CT Scan	-	-	19%	10.5%
Combination Brain/Sinus CT Scan	-	-	2.9%	2.7%
Combination Chest CT Scan	-	-	3.9%	2.7%
Follow-up Mammogram/Ultrasound	-	-	7.8%	8.8%
Lumbar Spine MRI for Low Back Pain	-	-	40.2%	37.2%

Ellsworth County Medical Center

1604 Aylward Avenue
Ellsworth, KS 67439
Phone: 785-472-3111
Fax: 785-472-5760
URL: www.ewmed.com
Type: Critical Access Hospitals
Emergency Services: Yes
Ownership: Government - Local
Beds: 20

Key Personnel:
Cardiology . . . . Michael Hagely, MD
CEO/President. . . . . Roger Masse
Radiology. . . . . Randy Packard
Quality Assurance . . . . Teresa Pearson
Emergency Room . . . . Tammy Stefek
Chief of Medical Staff . . . . Ronald Whitmer, DO
Infection Control. . . . . Sue Wolf

Measure	Cases	This Hosp.	State Avg.	U.S. Avg.
Blood Clot Prevention and Treatment				
Anticoagulation Overlap Therapy[1,3]	-	-	94%	93%
ICU Venous Thromboembolism Prophylaxis[3,7]	-	-	91%	92%
Incidence of Potentially Preventable VTE[3,7]	-	-	8%	10%
UFH with Dosages/Platelet Monitoring[1,3]	-	-	98%	97%
Venous Thromboembolism Prophylaxis[3,7]	-	-	79%	85%
Warfarin Therapy Discharge Instructions[1,3]	-	-	84%	75%
Chest Pain/Possible Heart Attack Care				
Aspirin Given Within 24 Hours of Arrival[1,3]	-	-	94%	96%
Fibrinolytic Meds Within 30 Min. of Arrival[1,3]	-	-	41%	58%
Average Time to ECG (minutes)[1,3]	-	-	8	7
Average Time to Transfer (minutes)[1,3]	-	-	57	60
Children's Asthma Care				
Received Home Management Plan of Care	-	-	-	88%
Received Reliever Medication	-	-	-	100%
Received Systemic Corticosteroids	-	-	-	100%
Emergency Department				
Admittance Decision Time (minutes)[2]	126	0	57	98
Head CT Results Within 45 Min. of Arrival[1,3]	-	-	53%	57%
Patients Who Left ER Before Being Seen	2,762	8%	2%	2%
Time from ER Arrival to Admit. (minutes)[2]	135	129	185	274
Time from ER Arrival to Discharge (minutes)	203	78	104	134
Time in ER Before Being Evaluated (minutes)	216	24	18	26
Time to Pain Meds for Fractures (minutes)[1,3]	-	-	47	57
Heart Attack Care				
Aspirin Given at Discharge[1,3]	-	-	99%	99%
Fibrinolytic Meds Within 30 Min. of Arrival[3,7]	-	-	-	54%
PCI Within 90 Minutes of Arrival[3,7]	-	-	97%	96%
Statin Prescribed at Discharge[1,3]	-	-	99%	98%
Heart Failure Care				
ACE Inhibitor or ARB for LVSD[1,2]	-	-	95%	97%
Discharge Instructions Given[2]	16	50%	91%	94%
Evaluation of LVS Function[2]	18	56%	94%	99%
Medicare Spending				
Medicare Spending per Patient (ratio)	-	-	0.94	0.98
Pneumonia Care				
Appropriate Initial Antibiotic Given	16	81%	92%	95%
Blood Culture Timing	11	100%	98%	98%
Pregnancy and Delivery Care				
Newborn Deliveries Scheduled Early[5]	-	-	12%	6%
Preventive Care				
Immunization for Influenza[2]	74	88%	88%	90%
Immunization for Pneumonia[2]	144	85%	90%	92%
Stroke Care				
Anticoagulation Therapy for Atrial Fibrillation[1,3]	-	-	88%	95%
Antithrombotic Therapy Timing[1,3]	-	-	97%	98%
Assessed for Rehabilitation[1,3]	-	-	97%	97%
Discharged on Antithrombotic Therapy[1,3]	-	-	98%	99%
Discharged on Statin Medication[1,3]	-	-	88%	94%
Thrombolytic Therapy Timing[1,3]	-	-	68%	66%
Venous Thromboembolism Prophylaxis[1,3]	-	-	93%	94%
Written Stroke Educational Materials Given[1,3]	-	-	84%	88%
Surgical Care Improvement Project				
Appropriate Beta Blocker Usage[5]	-	-	98%	98%
Appropriate VTP Within 24 Hours[5]	-	-	98%	98%
Controlled Postoperative Blood Glucose[5]	-	-	98%	97%
Perioperative Temperature Management[5]	-	-	100%	100%
Prophylactic Antibiotic Selection[5]	-	-	99%	99%
Prophylactic Antibiotic Selection (Outpatient)[5]	-	-	98%	98%
Prophylactic Antibiotic Stopped[5]	-	-	98%	98%
Prophylactic Antibiotic Timing[5]	-	-	99%	99%
Prophylactic Antibiotic Timing (Outpatient)[5]	-	-	98%	98%
Urinary Catheter Removal[5]	-	-	97%	97%
Survey of Patients' Hospital Experiences				
Area Around Room 'Always' Quiet at Night[6]	<100	56%	65%	61%
Doctors 'Always' Communicated Well[6]	<100	91%	85%	82%
Home Recovery Information Given[6]	<100	76%	86%	85%
Hospital Given 9 or 10 on 10 Point Scale[6]	<100	79%	76%	71%
Meds 'Always' Explained Before Given[6]	<100	59%	66%	64%
Nurses 'Always' Communicated Well[6]	<100	81%	81%	79%
Pain 'Always' Well Controlled[6]	<100	64%	72%	71%
Room and Bathroom 'Always' Clean[6]	<100	93%	76%	73%
Timely Help 'Always' Received[6]	<100	84%	72%	68%
Would Definitely Recommend Hospital[6]	<100	82%	75%	71%
Use of Medical Imaging				
Cardiac Imaging Stress Test before Surgery[7]	-	-	5%	5.3%
Combination Abdominal CT Scan	137	5.1%	19%	10.5%
Combination Brain/Sinus CT Scan[1]	-	-	2.9%	2.7%
Combination Chest CT Scan	74	0.0%	3.9%	2.7%
Follow-up Mammogram/Ultrasound	139	8.6%	7.8%	8.8%
Lumbar Spine MRI for Low Back Pain[1]	-	-	40.2%	37.2%

Newman Regional Health

1201 West 12th Avenue
Emporia, KS 66801
Phone: 620-343-6800
Fax: 620-341-7801
URL: www.newmanrh.org
Type: Acute Care Hospitals
Emergency Services: Yes
Ownership: Government - Local
Beds: 178

Key Personnel:
Chief of Medical Staff . . . . Cy K Anderson, MD
Quality Assurance . . . . Kathie Butcher
Operating Room. . . . . Robert Dorsey
Pediatric In-Patient Care . . . . Amy Jarvis
Radiology. . . . . Stephen M Knecht
Cardiac Laboratory. . . . . Jim Pelch
Infection Control. . . . . Jami White
CEO . . . . Robert Wright

Measure	Cases	This Hosp.	State Avg.	U.S. Avg.
Blood Clot Prevention and Treatment				
Anticoagulation Overlap Therapy[2]	19	100%	94%	93%
ICU Venous Thromboembolism Prophylaxis[2]	35	94%	91%	92%
Incidence of Potentially Preventable VTE[1,2]	-	-	8%	10%
UFH with Dosages/Platelet Monitoring[2]	13	100%	98%	97%
Venous Thromboembolism Prophylaxis[2]	143	77%	79%	85%
Warfarin Therapy Discharge Instructions[2]	15	73%	84%	75%
Chest Pain/Possible Heart Attack Care				
Aspirin Given Within 24 Hours of Arrival	84	98%	94%	96%
Fibrinolytic Meds Within 30 Min. of Arrival[1,3]	-	-	41%	58%
Average Time to ECG (minutes)	86	4	8	7
Average Time to Transfer (minutes)[3]	16	40	57	60
Children's Asthma Care				
Received Home Management Plan of Care	-	-	-	88%
Received Reliever Medication	-	-	-	100%
Received Systemic Corticosteroids	-	-	-	100%
Emergency Department				
Admittance Decision Time (minutes)[2]	250	55	57	98
Head CT Results Within 45 Min. of Arrival	12	50%	53%	57%

NOTE: Hospital profiles are in alphabetical order by state, then city, then hospital within the city; Rankings exclude hospitals with less than 25 cases except for patient surveys which excludes hospitals with less than 100 cases; (a) 100-299 cases; (1) The number of cases/patients is too few to report; (2) Data submitted were based on a sample of cases/patients; (3) Results are based on a shorter time period than required; (4) Data suppressed by CMS for one or more quarters; (5) Results are not available for this reporting period; (6) Fewer than 100 patients completed the HCAHPS survey; (7) No cases met the criteria for this measure; (8) The lower limit of the confidence interval cannot be calculated if the number of observed infections equals zero; (9) No data are available from the state/territory for this reporting period; (10) The scores shown reflect fewer than 50 completed surveys; (11) There were discrepancies in the data collection process; (12) This measure does not apply to this hospital for this reporting period; (13) Results cannot be calculated for this reporting period; (14) The results for this state are combined with nearby states to protect confidentiality; Please refer to the User's Guide for a full explanation of data.

Patients Who Left ER Before Being Seen	10,742	0%	2%	2%
Time from ER Arrival to Admit. (minutes)[2]	254	200	185	274
Time from ER Arrival to Discharge (minutes)	407	118	104	134
Time in ER Before Being Evaluated (minutes)	472	19	18	26
Time to Pain Meds for Fractures (minutes)	50	52	47	57
Heart Attack Care				
Aspirin Given at Discharge	23	100%	99%	99%
Fibrinolytic Meds Within 30 Min. of Arrival[7]	-	-	-	54%
PCI Within 90 Minutes of Arrival[1]	-	-	97%	96%
Statin Prescribed at Discharge	21	95%	99%	98%
Heart Failure Care				
ACE Inhibitor or ARB for LVSD	26	88%	95%	97%
Discharge Instructions Given	31	100%	91%	94%
Evaluation of LVS Function	52	100%	94%	99%
Medicare Spending				
Medicare Spending per Patient (ratio)	-	0.94	0.94	0.98
Pneumonia Care				
Appropriate Initial Antibiotic Given	50	96%	92%	95%
Blood Culture Timing	49	96%	98%	98%
Pregnancy and Delivery Care				
Newborn Deliveries Scheduled Early[2]	20	0%	12%	6%
Preventive Care				
Immunization for Influenza[2]	269	68%	88%	90%
Immunization for Pneumonia[2]	329	85%	90%	92%
Stroke Care				
Anticoagulation Therapy for Atrial Fibrillation[1]	-	-	88%	95%
Antithrombotic Therapy Timing	28	96%	97%	98%
Assessed for Rehabilitation	26	100%	97%	97%
Discharged on Antithrombotic Therapy	25	96%	98%	99%
Discharged on Statin Medication	25	48%	88%	94%
Thrombolytic Therapy Timing[1]	-	-	68%	66%
Venous Thromboembolism Prophylaxis	29	83%	93%	94%
Written Stroke Educational Materials Given[1]	-	-	84%	88%
Surgical Care Improvement Project				
Appropriate Beta Blocker Usage	42	95%	98%	98%
Appropriate VTP Within 24 Hours	125	99%	98%	98%
Controlled Postoperative Blood Glucose[7]	-	-	98%	97%
Perioperative Temperature Management	137	100%	100%	100%
Prophylactic Antibiotic Selection	79	100%	99%	99%
Prophylactic Antibiotic Selection (Outpatient)	62	98%	98%	98%
Prophylactic Antibiotic Stopped	74	100%	98%	98%
Prophylactic Antibiotic Timing	79	100%	99%	99%
Prophylactic Antibiotic Timing (Outpatient)	62	98%	98%	98%
Urinary Catheter Removal	90	96%	97%	97%
Survey of Patients' Hospital Experiences				
Area Around Room 'Always' Quiet at Night	300+	59%	65%	61%
Doctors 'Always' Communicated Well	300+	85%	85%	82%
Home Recovery Information Given	300+	86%	86%	85%
Hospital Given 9 or 10 on 10 Point Scale	300+	67%	76%	71%
Meds 'Always' Explained Before Given	300+	67%	66%	64%
Nurses 'Always' Communicated Well	300+	81%	81%	79%
Pain 'Always' Well Controlled	300+	73%	72%	71%
Room and Bathroom 'Always' Clean	300+	77%	76%	73%
Timely Help 'Always' Received	300+	68%	72%	68%
Would Definitely Recommend Hospital	300+	63%	75%	71%
Use of Medical Imaging				
Cardiac Imaging Stress Test before Surgery	89	4.5%	5%	5.3%
Combination Abdominal CT Scan	485	10.7%	19%	10.5%
Combination Brain/Sinus CT Scan[1]	-	-	2.9%	2.7%
Combination Chest CT Scan	339	0.0%	3.9%	2.7%
Follow-up Mammogram/Ultrasound	303	14.5%	7.8%	8.8%
Lumbar Spine MRI for Low Back Pain	140	37.1%	40.2%	37.2%

Greenwood County Hospital

100 W 16th Street
Eureka, KS 67045
Phone: 620-583-7451
Fax: 620-583-6884
Type: Critical Access Hospitals
Emergency Services: Yes
Ownership: Government - Local
Beds: 25
Key Personnel:
CEO .... Thomas Henton, Administrattor

Measure	Cases	This Hosp.	State Avg.	U.S. Avg.
Blood Clot Prevention and Treatment				
Anticoagulation Overlap Therapy[5]	-	-	94%	93%
ICU Venous Thromboembolism Prophylaxis[5]	-	-	91%	92%
Incidence of Potentially Preventable VTE[5]	-	-	8%	10%
UFH with Dosages/Platelet Monitoring[5]	-	-	98%	97%
Venous Thromboembolism Prophylaxis[5]	-	-	79%	85%
Warfarin Therapy Discharge Instructions[5]	-	-	84%	75%
Chest Pain/Possible Heart Attack Care				
Aspirin Given Within 24 Hours of Arrival	-	-	94%	96%
Fibrinolytic Meds Within 30 Min. of Arrival	-	-	41%	58%
Average Time to ECG (minutes)	-	-	8	7
Average Time to Transfer (minutes)	-	-	57	60
Children's Asthma Care				
Received Home Management Plan of Care	-	-	-	88%
Received Reliever Medication	-	-	-	100%
Received Systemic Corticosteroids	-	-	-	100%
Emergency Department				
Admittance Decision Time (minutes)[5]	-	-	57	98
Head CT Results Within 45 Min. of Arrival	-	-	53%	57%
Patients Who Left ER Before Being Seen	-	-	2%	2%
Time from ER Arrival to Admit. (minutes)[5]	-	-	185	274
Time from ER Arrival to Discharge (minutes)	-	-	104	134
Time in ER Before Being Evaluated (minutes)	-	-	18	26
Time to Pain Meds for Fractures (minutes)	-	-	47	57
Heart Attack Care				
Aspirin Given at Discharge[1,3]	-	-	99%	99%
Fibrinolytic Meds Within 30 Min. of Arrival[3,7]	-	-	-	54%
PCI Within 90 Minutes of Arrival[3,7]	-	-	97%	96%
Statin Prescribed at Discharge[1,3]	-	-	99%	98%
Heart Failure Care				
ACE Inhibitor or ARB for LVSD[3,7]	-	-	95%	97%
Discharge Instructions Given[1,3]	-	-	91%	94%
Evaluation of LVS Function[3]	16	19%	94%	99%
Medicare Spending				
Medicare Spending per Patient (ratio)	-	-	0.94	0.98
Pneumonia Care				
Appropriate Initial Antibiotic Given[1,3]	-	-	92%	95%
Blood Culture Timing[1,3]	-	-	98%	98%
Pregnancy and Delivery Care				
Newborn Deliveries Scheduled Early[5]	-	-	12%	6%
Preventive Care				
Immunization for Influenza[5]	-	-	88%	90%
Immunization for Pneumonia[5]	-	-	90%	92%
Stroke Care				
Anticoagulation Therapy for Atrial Fibrillation[5]	-	-	88%	95%
Antithrombotic Therapy Timing[5]	-	-	97%	98%
Assessed for Rehabilitation[5]	-	-	97%	97%
Discharged on Antithrombotic Therapy[5]	-	-	98%	99%
Discharged on Statin Medication[5]	-	-	88%	94%
Thrombolytic Therapy Timing[5]	-	-	68%	66%
Venous Thromboembolism Prophylaxis[5]	-	-	93%	94%
Written Stroke Educational Materials Given[5]	-	-	84%	88%
Surgical Care Improvement Project				
Appropriate Beta Blocker Usage[5]	-	-	98%	98%
Appropriate VTP Within 24 Hours[5]	-	-	98%	98%
Controlled Postoperative Blood Glucose[5]	-	-	98%	97%
Perioperative Temperature Management[5]	-	-	100%	100%
Prophylactic Antibiotic Selection[5]	-	-	99%	99%
Prophylactic Antibiotic Selection (Outpatient)	-	-	98%	98%
Prophylactic Antibiotic Stopped[5]	-	-	98%	98%
Prophylactic Antibiotic Timing[5]	-	-	99%	99%
Prophylactic Antibiotic Timing (Outpatient)	-	-	98%	98%
Urinary Catheter Removal[5]	-	-	97%	97%
Survey of Patients' Hospital Experiences				
Area Around Room 'Always' Quiet at Night[5]	-	-	65%	61%
Doctors 'Always' Communicated Well[5]	-	-	85%	82%
Home Recovery Information Given[5]	-	-	86%	85%
Hospital Given 9 or 10 on 10 Point Scale[5]	-	-	76%	71%
Meds 'Always' Explained Before Given[5]	-	-	66%	64%
Nurses 'Always' Communicated Well[5]	-	-	81%	79%
Pain 'Always' Well Controlled[5]	-	-	72%	71%
Room and Bathroom 'Always' Clean[5]	-	-	76%	73%
Timely Help 'Always' Received[5]	-	-	72%	68%
Would Definitely Recommend Hospital[5]	-	-	75%	71%
Use of Medical Imaging				
Cardiac Imaging Stress Test before Surgery	-	-	5%	5.3%
Combination Abdominal CT Scan	-	-	19%	10.5%
Combination Brain/Sinus CT Scan	-	-	2.9%	2.7%
Combination Chest CT Scan	-	-	3.9%	2.7%
Follow-up Mammogram/Ultrasound	-	-	7.8%	8.8%
Lumbar Spine MRI for Low Back Pain	-	-	40.2%	37.2%

Mercy Hospital - Fort Scott

401 Woodland Hills Blvd
Phone: 620-223-7057
Fort Scott, KS 66701
URL: www.mercy.net
Type: Acute Care Hospitals
Emergency Services: Yes
Ownership: Voluntary non-profit - Church
Key Personnel:
Operating Room. . . . . Ralph Hall
Radiology. . . . . Becky Williams

Measure	Cases	This Hosp.	State Avg.	U.S. Avg.
Blood Clot Prevention and Treatment				
Anticoagulation Overlap Therapy[2]	11	82%	94%	93%
ICU Venous Thromboembolism Prophylaxis[2]	39	95%	91%	92%
Incidence of Potentially Preventable VTE[1,2]	-	-	8%	10%
UFH with Dosages/Platelet Monitoring[1,2]	-	-	98%	97%
Venous Thromboembolism Prophylaxis[2]	106	89%	79%	85%
Warfarin Therapy Discharge Instructions[1,2]	-	-	84%	75%
Chest Pain/Possible Heart Attack Care				
Aspirin Given Within 24 Hours of Arrival	31	97%	94%	96%
Fibrinolytic Meds Within 30 Min. of Arrival[1]	-	-	41%	58%
Average Time to ECG (minutes)	29	10	8	7
Average Time to Transfer (minutes)[1]	-	-	57	60
Children's Asthma Care				
Received Home Management Plan of Care	-	-	-	88%
Received Reliever Medication	-	-	-	100%
Received Systemic Corticosteroids	-	-	-	100%
Emergency Department				
Admittance Decision Time (minutes)[2]	232	74	57	98
Head CT Results Within 45 Min. of Arrival[1]	-	-	53%	57%
Patients Who Left ER Before Being Seen	6,900	3%	2%	2%
Time from ER Arrival to Admit. (minutes)[2]	245	172	185	274
Time from ER Arrival to Discharge (minutes)	349	98	104	134
Time in ER Before Being Evaluated (minutes)	381	15	18	26
Time to Pain Meds for Fractures (minutes)	23	30	47	57
Heart Attack Care				
Aspirin Given at Discharge[1]	-	-	99%	99%
Fibrinolytic Meds Within 30 Min. of Arrival[7]	-	-	-	54%
PCI Within 90 Minutes of Arrival[7]	-	-	97%	96%
Statin Prescribed at Discharge[1]	-	-	99%	98%
Heart Failure Care				
ACE Inhibitor or ARB for LVSD	14	86%	95%	97%
Discharge Instructions Given	30	83%	91%	94%
Evaluation of LVS Function	41	100%	94%	99%
Medicare Spending				
Medicare Spending per Patient (ratio)	-	0.95	0.94	0.98
Pneumonia Care				
Appropriate Initial Antibiotic Given	42	100%	92%	95%
Blood Culture Timing	42	100%	98%	98%
Pregnancy and Delivery Care				
Newborn Deliveries Scheduled Early[2]	29	10%	12%	6%
Preventive Care				
Immunization for Influenza[2]	253	98%	88%	90%
Immunization for Pneumonia[2]	309	99%	90%	92%
Stroke Care				
Anticoagulation Therapy for Atrial Fibrillation[1]	-	-	88%	95%
Antithrombotic Therapy Timing[1]	-	-	97%	98%
Assessed for Rehabilitation[1]	-	-	97%	97%
Discharged on Antithrombotic Therapy[1]	-	-	98%	99%
Discharged on Statin Medication[1]	-	-	88%	94%
Thrombolytic Therapy Timing[1]	-	-	68%	66%
Venous Thromboembolism Prophylaxis[1]	-	-	93%	94%
Written Stroke Educational Materials Given[1]	-	-	84%	88%
Surgical Care Improvement Project				
Appropriate Beta Blocker Usage	17	82%	98%	98%

NOTE: Hospital profiles are in alphabetical order by state, then city, then hospital within the city; Rankings exclude hospitals with less than 25 cases except for patient surveys which excludes hospitals with less than 100 cases; (a) 100-299 cases; (1) The number of cases/patients is too few to report; (2) Data submitted were based on a sample of cases/patients; (3) Results are based on a shorter time period than required; (4) Data suppressed by CMS for one or more quarters; (5) Results are not available for this reporting period; (6) Fewer than 100 patients completed the HCAHPS survey; (7) No cases met the criteria for this measure; (8) The lower limit of the confidence interval cannot be calculated if the number of observed infections equals zero; (9) No data are available from the state/territory for this reporting period; (10) The scores shown reflect fewer than 50 completed surveys; (11) There were discrepancies in the data collection process; (12) This measure does not apply to this hospital for this reporting period; (13) Results cannot be calculated for this reporting period; (14) The results for this state are combined with nearby states to protect confidentiality; Please refer to the User's Guide for a full explanation of data.

Measure	Cases	This Hosp.	State Avg.	U.S. Avg.
Appropriate VTP Within 24 Hours	67	100%	98%	98%
Controlled Postoperative Blood Glucose[7]	-	-	98%	97%
Perioperative Temperature Management	71	100%	100%	100%
Prophylactic Antibiotic Selection	52	100%	99%	99%
Prophylactic Antibiotic Selection (Outpatient)	48	100%	98%	98%
Prophylactic Antibiotic Stopped	50	100%	98%	98%
Prophylactic Antibiotic Timing	52	98%	99%	99%
Prophylactic Antibiotic Timing (Outpatient)	48	98%	98%	98%
Urinary Catheter Removal	30	97%	97%	97%
Survey of Patients' Hospital Experiences				
Area Around Room 'Always' Quiet at Night[11]	300+	73%	65%	61%
Doctors 'Always' Communicated Well[11]	300+	86%	85%	82%
Home Recovery Information Given[11]	300+	88%	86%	85%
Hospital Given 9 or 10 on 10 Point Scale[11]	300+	77%	76%	71%
Meds 'Always' Explained Before Given[11]	300+	71%	66%	64%
Nurses 'Always' Communicated Well[11]	300+	82%	81%	79%
Pain 'Always' Well Controlled[11]	300+	75%	72%	71%
Room and Bathroom 'Always' Clean[11]	300+	75%	76%	73%
Timely Help 'Always' Received[11]	300+	77%	72%	68%
Would Definitely Recommend Hospital[11]	300+	68%	75%	71%
Use of Medical Imaging				
Cardiac Imaging Stress Test before Surgery	125	5.6%	5%	5.3%
Combination Abdominal CT Scan	282	16.7%	19%	10.5%
Combination Brain/Sinus CT Scan	272	0.7%	2.9%	2.7%
Combination Chest CT Scan	186	16.1%	3.9%	2.7%
Follow-up Mammogram/Ultrasound	391	10.7%	7.8%	8.8%
Lumbar Spine MRI for Low Back Pain	61	41.0%	40.2%	37.2%

Fredonia Regional Hospital

1527 Madison
Fredonia, KS 66736
Phone: 620-378-2121
Fax: 620-378-3169
URL: www.gpha.com
Type: Critical Access Hospitals
Emergency Services: Yes
Ownership: Government - Local
Beds: 25

Key Personnel:
Chief of Medical Staff.......... Oswaldo Bacami
Emergency Room............. Kim Buttler
CEO/President............... Terry Deschaine
Infection Control.............. Darrell Odell

Measure	Cases	This Hosp.	State Avg.	U.S. Avg.
Blood Clot Prevention and Treatment				
Anticoagulation Overlap Therapy[5]	-	-	94%	93%
ICU Venous Thromboembolism Prophylaxis[5]	-	-	91%	92%
Incidence of Potentially Preventable VTE[5]	-	-	8%	10%
UFH with Dosages/Platelet Monitoring[5]	-	-	98%	97%
Venous Thromboembolism Prophylaxis[5]	-	-	79%	85%
Warfarin Therapy Discharge Instructions[5]	-	-	84%	75%
Chest Pain/Possible Heart Attack Care				
Aspirin Given Within 24 Hours of Arrival[1,3]	-	-	94%	96%
Fibrinolytic Meds Within 30 Min. of Arrival[3,7]	-	-	41%	58%
Average Time to ECG (minutes)[1,3]	-	-	8	7
Average Time to Transfer (minutes)[1,3]	-	-	57	60
Children's Asthma Care				
Received Home Management Plan of Care	-	-	-	88%
Received Reliever Medication	-	-	-	100%
Received Systemic Corticosteroids	-	-	-	100%
Emergency Department				
Admittance Decision Time (minutes)	100	40	57	98
Head CT Results Within 45 Min. of Arrival[5]	-	-	53%	57%
Patients Who Left ER Before Being Seen	2,340	1%	2%	2%
Time from ER Arrival to Admit. (minutes)	124	95	185	274
Time from ER Arrival to Discharge (minutes)[5]	-	-	104	134
Time in ER Before Being Evaluated (minutes)[5]	-	-	18	26
Time to Pain Meds for Fractures (minutes)[5]	-	-	47	57
Heart Attack Care				
Aspirin Given at Discharge[1,3]	-	-	99%	99%
Fibrinolytic Meds Within 30 Min. of Arrival[3,7]	-	-	-	54%
PCI Within 90 Minutes of Arrival[3,7]	-	-	97%	96%
Statin Prescribed at Discharge[1,3]	-	-	99%	98%
Heart Failure Care				
ACE Inhibitor or ARB for LVSD[1,3]	-	-	95%	97%
Discharge Instructions Given[1,3]	-	-	91%	94%
Evaluation of LVS Function[1,3]	-	-	94%	99%
Medicare Spending				
Medicare Spending per Patient (ratio)	-	-	0.94	0.98
Pneumonia Care				
Appropriate Initial Antibiotic Given	18	89%	92%	95%
Blood Culture Timing[1]	-	-	98%	98%
Pregnancy and Delivery Care				
Newborn Deliveries Scheduled Early[5]	-	-	12%	6%
Preventive Care				
Immunization for Influenza	188	87%	88%	90%
Immunization for Pneumonia	270	92%	90%	92%
Stroke Care				
Anticoagulation Therapy for Atrial Fibrillation[5]	-	-	88%	95%
Antithrombotic Therapy Timing[5]	-	-	97%	98%
Assessed for Rehabilitation[5]	-	-	97%	97%
Discharged on Antithrombotic Therapy[5]	-	-	98%	99%
Discharged on Statin Medication[5]	-	-	88%	94%
Thrombolytic Therapy Timing[5]	-	-	68%	66%
Venous Thromboembolism Prophylaxis[5]	-	-	93%	94%
Written Stroke Educational Materials Given[5]	-	-	84%	88%
Surgical Care Improvement Project				
Appropriate Beta Blocker Usage[5]	-	-	98%	98%
Appropriate VTP Within 24 Hours[5]	-	-	98%	98%
Controlled Postoperative Blood Glucose[5]	-	-	98%	97%
Perioperative Temperature Management[5]	-	-	100%	100%
Prophylactic Antibiotic Selection[5]	-	-	99%	99%
Prophylactic Antibiotic Selection (Outpatient)[5]	-	-	98%	98%
Prophylactic Antibiotic Stopped[5]	-	-	98%	98%
Prophylactic Antibiotic Timing[5]	-	-	99%	99%
Prophylactic Antibiotic Timing (Outpatient)[5]	-	-	98%	98%
Urinary Catheter Removal[5]	-	-	97%	97%
Survey of Patients' Hospital Experiences				
Area Around Room 'Always' Quiet at Night[5]	-	-	65%	61%
Doctors 'Always' Communicated Well[5]	-	-	85%	82%
Home Recovery Information Given[5]	-	-	86%	85%
Hospital Given 9 or 10 on 10 Point Scale[5]	-	-	76%	71%
Meds 'Always' Explained Before Given[5]	-	-	66%	64%
Nurses 'Always' Communicated Well[5]	-	-	81%	79%
Pain 'Always' Well Controlled[5]	-	-	72%	71%
Room and Bathroom 'Always' Clean[5]	-	-	76%	73%
Timely Help 'Always' Received[5]	-	-	72%	68%
Would Definitely Recommend Hospital[5]	-	-	75%	71%
Use of Medical Imaging				
Cardiac Imaging Stress Test before Surgery	52	1.9%	5%	5.3%
Combination Abdominal CT Scan	131	76.3%	19%	10.5%
Combination Brain/Sinus CT Scan[1]	-	-	2.9%	2.7%
Combination Chest CT Scan	78	1.3%	3.9%	2.7%
Follow-up Mammogram/Ultrasound	127	10.2%	7.8%	8.8%
Lumbar Spine MRI for Low Back Pain[1]	-	-	40.2%	37.2%

Premier Surgical Institute

1619 K Highway 66, PO Box 127
Galena, KS 66739
Phone: 620-783-1732
Type: Acute Care Hospitals
Emergency Services: No
Ownership: Government - Local

Measure	Cases	This Hosp.	State Avg.	U.S. Avg.
Blood Clot Prevention and Treatment				
Anticoagulation Overlap Therapy[5]	-	-	94%	93%
ICU Venous Thromboembolism Prophylaxis[5]	-	-	91%	92%
Incidence of Potentially Preventable VTE[5]	-	-	8%	10%
UFH with Dosages/Platelet Monitoring[5]	-	-	98%	97%
Venous Thromboembolism Prophylaxis[5]	-	-	79%	85%
Warfarin Therapy Discharge Instructions[5]	-	-	84%	75%
Chest Pain/Possible Heart Attack Care				
Aspirin Given Within 24 Hours of Arrival[5]	-	-	94%	96%
Fibrinolytic Meds Within 30 Min. of Arrival[5]	-	-	41%	58%
Average Time to ECG (minutes)[5]	-	-	8	7
Average Time to Transfer (minutes)[5]	-	-	57	60
Children's Asthma Care				
Received Home Management Plan of Care	-	-	-	88%
Received Reliever Medication	-	-	-	100%
Received Systemic Corticosteroids	-	-	-	100%
Emergency Department				
Admittance Decision Time (minutes)[5]	-	-	57	98
Head CT Results Within 45 Min. of Arrival[5]	-	-	53%	57%
Patients Who Left ER Before Being Seen[5]	-	-	2%	2%
Time from ER Arrival to Admit. (minutes)[5]	-	-	185	274
Time from ER Arrival to Discharge (minutes)[5]	-	-	104	134
Time in ER Before Being Evaluated (minutes)[5]	-	-	18	26
Time to Pain Meds for Fractures (minutes)[5]	-	-	47	57
Heart Attack Care				
Aspirin Given at Discharge[5]	-	-	99%	99%
Fibrinolytic Meds Within 30 Min. of Arrival[5]	-	-	-	54%
PCI Within 90 Minutes of Arrival[5]	-	-	97%	96%
Statin Prescribed at Discharge[5]	-	-	99%	98%
Heart Failure Care				
ACE Inhibitor or ARB for LVSD[5]	-	-	95%	97%
Discharge Instructions Given[5]	-	-	91%	94%
Evaluation of LVS Function[5]	-	-	94%	99%
Medicare Spending				
Medicare Spending per Patient (ratio)	-	-	0.94	0.98
Pneumonia Care				
Appropriate Initial Antibiotic Given[5]	-	-	92%	95%
Blood Culture Timing[5]	-	-	98%	98%
Pregnancy and Delivery Care				
Newborn Deliveries Scheduled Early[5]	-	-	12%	6%
Preventive Care				
Immunization for Influenza[5]	-	-	88%	90%
Immunization for Pneumonia[5]	-	-	90%	92%
Stroke Care				
Anticoagulation Therapy for Atrial Fibrillation[5]	-	-	88%	95%
Antithrombotic Therapy Timing[5]	-	-	97%	98%
Assessed for Rehabilitation[5]	-	-	97%	97%
Discharged on Antithrombotic Therapy[5]	-	-	98%	99%
Discharged on Statin Medication[5]	-	-	88%	94%
Thrombolytic Therapy Timing[5]	-	-	68%	66%
Venous Thromboembolism Prophylaxis[5]	-	-	93%	94%
Written Stroke Educational Materials Given[5]	-	-	84%	88%
Surgical Care Improvement Project				
Appropriate Beta Blocker Usage[5]	-	-	98%	98%
Appropriate VTP Within 24 Hours[5]	-	-	98%	98%
Controlled Postoperative Blood Glucose[5]	-	-	98%	97%
Perioperative Temperature Management[5]	-	-	100%	100%
Prophylactic Antibiotic Selection[5]	-	-	99%	99%
Prophylactic Antibiotic Selection (Outpatient)[5]	-	-	98%	98%
Prophylactic Antibiotic Stopped[5]	-	-	98%	98%
Prophylactic Antibiotic Timing[5]	-	-	99%	99%
Prophylactic Antibiotic Timing (Outpatient)[5]	-	-	98%	98%
Urinary Catheter Removal[5]	-	-	97%	97%
Survey of Patients' Hospital Experiences				
Area Around Room 'Always' Quiet at Night[5]	-	-	65%	61%
Doctors 'Always' Communicated Well[5]	-	-	85%	82%
Home Recovery Information Given[5]	-	-	86%	85%
Hospital Given 9 or 10 on 10 Point Scale[5]	-	-	76%	71%
Meds 'Always' Explained Before Given[5]	-	-	66%	64%
Nurses 'Always' Communicated Well[5]	-	-	81%	79%
Pain 'Always' Well Controlled[5]	-	-	72%	71%
Room and Bathroom 'Always' Clean[5]	-	-	76%	73%
Timely Help 'Always' Received[5]	-	-	72%	68%
Would Definitely Recommend Hospital[5]	-	-	75%	71%
Use of Medical Imaging				
Cardiac Imaging Stress Test before Surgery[7]	-	-	5%	5.3%
Combination Abdominal CT Scan[7]	-	-	19%	10.5%
Combination Brain/Sinus CT Scan[7]	-	-	2.9%	2.7%
Combination Chest CT Scan[7]	-	-	3.9%	2.7%
Follow-up Mammogram/Ultrasound[7]	-	-	7.8%	8.8%
Lumbar Spine MRI for Low Back Pain[7]	-	-	40.2%	37.2%

Saint Catherine Hospital

401 East Spruce
Garden City, KS 67846
Phone: 620-272-2561
Fax: 620-272-2528
URL: www.stcath-hosp.org
Type: Acute Care Hospitals
Emergency Services: Yes
Ownership: Voluntary non-profit - Church

Key Personnel:
Chief of Medical Staff.......... James Bruno
Quality Assurance............ Nancy Killion

NOTE: Hospital profiles are in alphabetical order by state, then city, then hospital within the city; Rankings exclude hospitals with less than 25 cases except for patient surveys which excludes hospitals with less than 100 cases; (a) 100-299 cases; (1) The number of cases/patients is too few to report; (2) Data submitted were based on a sample of cases/patients; (3) Results are based on a shorter time period than required; (4) Data suppressed by CMS for one or more quarters; (5) Results are not available for this reporting period; (6) Fewer than 100 patients completed the HCAHPS survey; (7) No cases met the criteria for this measure; (8) The lower limit of the confidence interval cannot be calculated if the number of observed infections equals zero; (9) No data are available from the state/territory for this reporting period; (10) The scores shown reflect fewer than 50 completed surveys; (11) There were discrepancies in the data collection process; (12) This measure does not apply to this hospital for this reporting period; (13) Results cannot be calculated for this reporting period; (14) The results for this state are combined with nearby states to protect confidentiality; Please refer to the User's Guide for a full explanation of data.

Radiology. Soen Liong
CEO/President. . . . . Scott Taylor

Measure	Cases	This Hosp.	State Avg.	U.S. Avg.
Blood Clot Prevention and Treatment				
Anticoagulation Overlap Therapy[2]	22	100%	94%	93%
ICU Venous Thromboembolism Prophylaxis[2]	109	99%	91%	92%
Incidence of Potentially Preventable VTE[2,7]	-	-	8%	10%
UFH with Dosages/Platelet Monitoring[2]	12	100%	98%	97%
Venous Thromboembolism Prophylaxis[2]	228	92%	79%	85%
Warfarin Therapy Discharge Instructions[2]	19	100%	84%	75%
Chest Pain/Possible Heart Attack Care				
Aspirin Given Within 24 Hours of Arrival	15	93%	94%	96%
Fibrinolytic Meds Within 30 Min. of Arrival[7]	-	-	41%	58%
Average Time to ECG (minutes)	15	27	8	7
Average Time to Transfer (minutes)[1]	-	-	57	60
Children's Asthma Care				
Received Home Management Plan of Care	-	-	-	88%
Received Reliever Medication	-	-	-	100%
Received Systemic Corticosteroids	-	-	-	100%
Emergency Department				
Admittance Decision Time (minutes)[2]	243	55	57	98
Head CT Results Within 45 Min. of Arrival[1]	-	-	53%	57%
Patients Who Left ER Before Being Seen	15,498	1%	2%	2%
Time from ER Arrival to Admit. (minutes)[2]	257	163	185	274
Time from ER Arrival to Discharge (minutes)	598	96	104	134
Time in ER Before Being Evaluated (minutes)	595	24	18	26
Time to Pain Meds for Fractures (minutes)	71	47	47	57
Heart Attack Care				
Aspirin Given at Discharge	38	100%	99%	99%
Fibrinolytic Meds Within 30 Min. of Arrival[7]	-	-	-	54%
PCI Within 90 Minutes of Arrival[1]	-	-	97%	96%
Statin Prescribed at Discharge	37	100%	99%	98%
Heart Failure Care				
ACE Inhibitor or ARB for LVSD	13	100%	95%	97%
Discharge Instructions Given	32	100%	91%	94%
Evaluation of LVS Function	46	100%	94%	99%
Medicare Spending				
Medicare Spending per Patient (ratio)	-	0.95	0.94	0.98
Pneumonia Care				
Appropriate Initial Antibiotic Given	48	98%	92%	95%
Blood Culture Timing	61	97%	98%	98%
Pregnancy and Delivery Care				
Newborn Deliveries Scheduled Early	56	38%	12%	6%
Preventive Care				
Immunization for Influenza[2]	371	85%	88%	90%
Immunization for Pneumonia[2]	344	87%	90%	92%
Stroke Care				
Anticoagulation Therapy for Atrial Fibrillation[1]	-	-	88%	95%
Antithrombotic Therapy Timing[1]	-	-	97%	98%
Assessed for Rehabilitation[1]	-	-	97%	97%
Discharged on Antithrombotic Therapy[1]	-	-	98%	99%
Discharged on Statin Medication[1]	-	-	88%	94%
Thrombolytic Therapy Timing[7]	-	-	68%	66%
Venous Thromboembolism Prophylaxis[1]	-	-	93%	94%
Written Stroke Educational Materials Given[1]	-	-	84%	88%
Surgical Care Improvement Project				
Appropriate Beta Blocker Usage	71	100%	98%	98%
Appropriate VTP Within 24 Hours	277	98%	98%	98%
Controlled Postoperative Blood Glucose[7]	-	-	98%	97%
Perioperative Temperature Management	314	99%	100%	100%
Prophylactic Antibiotic Selection	223	98%	99%	99%
Prophylactic Antibiotic Selection (Outpatient)	64	98%	98%	98%
Prophylactic Antibiotic Stopped	219	74%	98%	98%
Prophylactic Antibiotic Timing	224	96%	99%	99%
Prophylactic Antibiotic Timing (Outpatient)	66	97%	98%	98%
Urinary Catheter Removal	162	66%	97%	97%
Survey of Patients' Hospital Experiences				
Area Around Room 'Always' Quiet at Night	300+	68%	65%	61%
Doctors 'Always' Communicated Well	300+	81%	85%	82%
Home Recovery Information Given	300+	82%	86%	85%
Hospital Given 9 or 10 on 10 Point Scale	300+	69%	76%	71%
Meds 'Always' Explained Before Given	300+	62%	66%	64%
Nurses 'Always' Communicated Well	300+	76%	81%	79%
Pain 'Always' Well Controlled	300+	67%	72%	71%
Room and Bathroom 'Always' Clean	300+	77%	76%	73%
Timely Help 'Always' Received	300+	61%	72%	68%
Would Definitely Recommend Hospital	300+	64%	75%	71%
Use of Medical Imaging				
Cardiac Imaging Stress Test before Surgery	274	5.5%	5%	5.3%
Combination Abdominal CT Scan	425	20.7%	19%	10.5%
Combination Brain/Sinus CT Scan	200	1.0%	2.9%	2.7%
Combination Chest CT Scan	277	0.0%	3.9%	2.7%
Follow-up Mammogram/Ultrasound	437	1.6%	7.8%	8.8%
Lumbar Spine MRI for Low Back Pain	74	43.2%	40.2%	37.2%

Anderson County Hospital

421 S Maple
Garnett, KS 66032
URL: www.saintlukeshealthsystem.org
Type: Critical Access Hospitals
Ownership: Government - Local
Phone: 785-204-4000
Fax: 785-448-3118
Emergency Services: Yes
Beds: 25

Key Personnel:
Pediatric In-Patient Care . . . . Beth Anderson
CEO/President. . . . . Dennis A Hachenberg, FACHE

Measure	Cases	This Hosp.	State Avg.	U.S. Avg.
Blood Clot Prevention and Treatment				
Anticoagulation Overlap Therapy[7]	-	-	94%	93%
ICU Venous Thromboembolism Prophylaxis[3,7]	-	-	91%	92%
Incidence of Potentially Preventable VTE[7]	-	-	8%	10%
UFH with Dosages/Platelet Monitoring[7]	-	-	98%	97%
Venous Thromboembolism Prophylaxis	41	80%	79%	85%
Warfarin Therapy Discharge Instructions[7]	-	-	84%	75%
Chest Pain/Possible Heart Attack Care				
Aspirin Given Within 24 Hours of Arrival[3]	24	96%	94%	96%
Fibrinolytic Meds Within 30 Min. of Arrival[3,7]	-	-	41%	58%
Average Time to ECG (minutes)[3]	24	9	8	7
Average Time to Transfer (minutes)[3,7]	-	-	57	60
Children's Asthma Care				
Received Home Management Plan of Care	-	-	-	88%
Received Reliever Medication	-	-	-	100%
Received Systemic Corticosteroids	-	-	-	100%
Emergency Department				
Admittance Decision Time (minutes)[5]	-	-	57	98
Head CT Results Within 45 Min. of Arrival[5]	-	-	53%	57%
Patients Who Left ER Before Being Seen[5]	-	-	2%	2%
Time from ER Arrival to Admit. (minutes)[5]	-	-	185	274
Time from ER Arrival to Discharge (minutes)[1]	-	-	104	134
Time in ER Before Being Evaluated (minutes)	37	17	18	26
Time to Pain Meds for Fractures (minutes)[5]	-	-	47	57
Heart Attack Care				
Aspirin Given at Discharge[5]	-	-	99%	99%
Fibrinolytic Meds Within 30 Min. of Arrival[5]	-	-	-	54%
PCI Within 90 Minutes of Arrival[5]	-	-	97%	96%
Statin Prescribed at Discharge[5]	-	-	99%	98%
Heart Failure Care				
ACE Inhibitor or ARB for LVSD[1,3]	-	-	95%	97%
Discharge Instructions Given[1,3]	-	-	91%	94%
Evaluation of LVS Function[1,3]	-	-	94%	99%
Medicare Spending				
Medicare Spending per Patient (ratio)	-	-	0.94	0.98
Pneumonia Care				
Appropriate Initial Antibiotic Given[1]	-	-	92%	95%
Blood Culture Timing[1]	-	-	98%	98%
Pregnancy and Delivery Care				
Newborn Deliveries Scheduled Early[5]	-	-	12%	6%
Preventive Care				
Immunization for Influenza[5]	-	-	88%	90%
Immunization for Pneumonia[5]	-	-	90%	92%
Stroke Care				
Anticoagulation Therapy for Atrial Fibrillation[5]	-	-	88%	95%
Antithrombotic Therapy Timing[5]	-	-	97%	98%
Assessed for Rehabilitation[5]	-	-	97%	97%
Discharged on Antithrombotic Therapy[5]	-	-	98%	99%
Discharged on Statin Medication[5]	-	-	88%	94%
Thrombolytic Therapy Timing[5]	-	-	68%	66%
Venous Thromboembolism Prophylaxis[5]	-	-	93%	94%
Written Stroke Educational Materials Given[5]	-	-	84%	88%
Surgical Care Improvement Project				
Appropriate Beta Blocker Usage[5]	-	-	98%	98%
Appropriate VTP Within 24 Hours[5]	-	-	98%	98%
Controlled Postoperative Blood Glucose[5]	-	-	98%	97%
Perioperative Temperature Management[5]	-	-	100%	100%
Prophylactic Antibiotic Selection[5]	-	-	99%	99%
Prophylactic Antibiotic Selection (Outpatient)[5]	-	-	98%	98%
Prophylactic Antibiotic Stopped[5]	-	-	98%	98%
Prophylactic Antibiotic Timing[5]	-	-	99%	99%
Prophylactic Antibiotic Timing (Outpatient)[5]	-	-	98%	98%
Urinary Catheter Removal[5]	-	-	97%	97%
Survey of Patients' Hospital Experiences				
Area Around Room 'Always' Quiet at Night[10]	<100	77%	65%	61%
Doctors 'Always' Communicated Well[10]	<100	93%	85%	82%
Home Recovery Information Given[10]	<100	91%	86%	85%
Hospital Given 9 or 10 on 10 Point Scale[10]	<100	84%	76%	71%
Meds 'Always' Explained Before Given[10]	<100	81%	66%	64%
Nurses 'Always' Communicated Well[10]	<100	90%	81%	79%
Pain 'Always' Well Controlled[10]	<100	80%	72%	71%
Room and Bathroom 'Always' Clean[10]	<100	93%	76%	73%
Timely Help 'Always' Received[10]	<100	92%	72%	68%
Would Definitely Recommend Hospital[10]	<100	85%	75%	71%
Use of Medical Imaging				
Cardiac Imaging Stress Test before Surgery[1]	-	-	5%	5.3%
Combination Abdominal CT Scan	108	35.2%	19%	10.5%
Combination Brain/Sinus CT Scan[1]	-	-	2.9%	2.7%
Combination Chest CT Scan	47	2.1%	3.9%	2.7%
Follow-up Mammogram/Ultrasound	247	4.5%	7.8%	8.8%
Lumbar Spine MRI for Low Back Pain[1]	-	-	40.2%	37.2%

Girard Medical Center

302 North Hospital Drive
Girard, KS 66743
Type: Critical Access Hospitals
Ownership: Government - Local
Phone: 620-724-8291
Fax: 620-724-6332
Emergency Services: Yes
Beds: 38

Key Personnel:
Infection Control. . . . . Karen Brooks
Operating Room. . . . . Carol Diskin, RN
Chief of Medical Staff. . . . . Mindi Garner, DO
Patient Relations . . . . Joyce Geier
Quality Assurance . . . . Joyce Geier
CEO/President. . . . . Michael Payne
Coronary Care . . . . Don Shull
Intensive Care Unit. . . . . Donald Shull

Measure	Cases	This Hosp.	State Avg.	U.S. Avg.
Blood Clot Prevention and Treatment				
Anticoagulation Overlap Therapy[5]	-	-	94%	93%
ICU Venous Thromboembolism Prophylaxis[5]	-	-	91%	92%
Incidence of Potentially Preventable VTE[5]	-	-	8%	10%
UFH with Dosages/Platelet Monitoring[5]	-	-	98%	97%
Venous Thromboembolism Prophylaxis[5]	-	-	79%	85%
Warfarin Therapy Discharge Instructions[5]	-	-	84%	75%
Chest Pain/Possible Heart Attack Care				
Aspirin Given Within 24 Hours of Arrival[5]	-	-	94%	96%
Fibrinolytic Meds Within 30 Min. of Arrival[5]	-	-	41%	58%
Average Time to ECG (minutes)[5]	-	-	8	7
Average Time to Transfer (minutes)[5]	-	-	57	60
Children's Asthma Care				
Received Home Management Plan of Care	-	-	-	88%
Received Reliever Medication	-	-	-	100%
Received Systemic Corticosteroids	-	-	-	100%
Emergency Department				
Admittance Decision Time (minutes)[2]	309	30	57	98
Head CT Results Within 45 Min. of Arrival[5]	-	-	53%	57%
Patients Who Left ER Before Being Seen[5]	-	-	2%	2%
Time from ER Arrival to Admit. (minutes)[2]	330	166	185	274
Time from ER Arrival to Discharge (minutes)[5]	-	-	104	134
Time in ER Before Being Evaluated (minutes)[5]	-	-	18	26
Time to Pain Meds for Fractures (minutes)[5]	-	-	47	57
Heart Attack Care				
Aspirin Given at Discharge[1,3]	-	-	99%	99%
Fibrinolytic Meds Within 30 Min. of Arrival[5]	-	-	-	54%

NOTE: Hospital profiles are in alphabetical order by state, then city, then hospital within the city; Rankings exclude hospitals with less than 25 cases except for patient surveys which excludes hospitals with less than 100 cases; (a) 100-299 cases; (1) The number of cases/patients is too few to report; (2) Data submitted were based on a sample of cases/patients; (3) Results are based on a shorter time period than required; (4) Data suppressed by CMS for one or more quarters; (5) Results are not available for this reporting period; (6) Fewer than 100 patients completed the HCAHPS survey; (7) No cases met the criteria for this measure; (8) The lower limit of the confidence interval cannot be calculated if the number of observed infections equals zero; (9) No data are available from the state/territory for this reporting period; (10) The scores shown reflect fewer than 50 completed surveys; (11) There were discrepancies in the data collection process; (12) This measure does not apply to this hospital for this reporting period; (13) Results cannot be calculated for this reporting period; (14) The results for this state are combined with nearby states to protect confidentiality; Please refer to the User's Guide for a full explanation of data.

PCI Within 90 Minutes of Arrival[5]	-	-	97%	96%
Statin Prescribed at Discharge[1,3]	-	-	99%	98%
Heart Failure Care				
ACE Inhibitor or ARB for LVSD[1]	-	-	95%	97%
Discharge Instructions Given	13	100%	91%	94%
Evaluation of LVS Function	25	96%	94%	99%
Medicare Spending				
Medicare Spending per Patient (ratio)	-	-	0.94	0.98
Pneumonia Care				
Appropriate Initial Antibiotic Given	25	76%	92%	95%
Blood Culture Timing	38	100%	98%	98%
Pregnancy and Delivery Care				
Newborn Deliveries Scheduled Early[5]	-	-	12%	6%
Preventive Care				
Immunization for Influenza[2]	235	90%	88%	90%
Immunization for Pneumonia[2]	386	89%	90%	92%
Stroke Care				
Anticoagulation Therapy for Atrial Fibrillation[5]	-	-	88%	95%
Antithrombotic Therapy Timing[5]	-	-	97%	98%
Assessed for Rehabilitation[5]	-	-	97%	97%
Discharged on Antithrombotic Therapy[5]	-	-	98%	99%
Discharged on Statin Medication[5]	-	-	88%	94%
Thrombolytic Therapy Timing[5]	-	-	68%	66%
Venous Thromboembolism Prophylaxis[5]	-	-	93%	94%
Written Stroke Educational Materials Given[5]	-	-	84%	88%
Surgical Care Improvement Project				
Appropriate Beta Blocker Usage[1]	-	-	98%	98%
Appropriate VTP Within 24 Hours	26	92%	98%	98%
Controlled Postoperative Blood Glucose[3,7]	-	-	98%	97%
Perioperative Temperature Management	31	100%	100%	100%
Prophylactic Antibiotic Selection	27	100%	99%	99%
Prophylactic Antibiotic Selection (Outpatient)[5]	-	-	98%	98%
Prophylactic Antibiotic Stopped	27	93%	98%	98%
Prophylactic Antibiotic Timing	27	100%	99%	99%
Prophylactic Antibiotic Timing (Outpatient)[5]	-	-	98%	98%
Urinary Catheter Removal	19	89%	97%	97%
Survey of Patients' Hospital Experiences				
Area Around Room 'Always' Quiet at Night[6]	<100	67%	65%	61%
Doctors 'Always' Communicated Well[6]	<100	91%	85%	82%
Home Recovery Information Given[6]	<100	82%	86%	85%
Hospital Given 9 or 10 on 10 Point Scale[6]	<100	85%	76%	71%
Meds 'Always' Explained Before Given[6]	<100	74%	66%	64%
Nurses 'Always' Communicated Well[6]	<100	84%	81%	79%
Pain 'Always' Well Controlled[6]	<100	75%	72%	71%
Room and Bathroom 'Always' Clean[6]	<100	87%	76%	73%
Timely Help 'Always' Received[6]	<100	80%	72%	68%
Would Definitely Recommend Hospital[6]	<100	82%	75%	71%
Use of Medical Imaging				
Cardiac Imaging Stress Test before Surgery[7]	-	-	5%	5.3%
Combination Abdominal CT Scan	105	1.0%	19%	10.5%
Combination Brain/Sinus CT Scan[1]	-	-	2.9%	2.7%
Combination Chest CT Scan[1]	-	-	3.9%	2.7%
Follow-up Mammogram/Ultrasound	176	4.5%	7.8%	8.8%
Lumbar Spine MRI for Low Back Pain[1]	-	-	40.2%	37.2%

Goodland Regional Medical Center

220 West Second Street
Goodland, KS 67735
Phone: 785-890-3625
Fax: 785-890-7209
Type: Critical Access Hospitals
Emergency Services: Yes
Ownership: Government - Local
Beds: 25

Key Personnel:

Operating Room. . . . . Florida Cruz, RN
Chief of Medical Staff. . . . . Travis Daise, MD
Quality Assurance . . . . Mary Ann Elliott, RN
Emergency Room . . . . Kathy Erickson, RN
Radiology. . . . . Carl W Fieser, ARRT
Infection Control. . . . . Karen Hooker, RRT
Patient Relations . . . . Brenda McCants
CEO . . . . Marion A. Tony Thompson, FACHE

Measure	Cases	This Hosp.	State Avg.	U.S. Avg.
Blood Clot Prevention and Treatment				
Anticoagulation Overlap Therapy[5]	-	-	94%	93%
ICU Venous Thromboembolism Prophylaxis[5]	-	-	91%	92%
Incidence of Potentially Preventable VTE[5]	-	-	8%	10%
UFH with Dosages/Platelet Monitoring[5]	-	-	98%	97%
Venous Thromboembolism Prophylaxis[5]	-	-	79%	85%
Warfarin Therapy Discharge Instructions[5]	-	-	84%	75%
Chest Pain/Possible Heart Attack Care				
Aspirin Given Within 24 Hours of Arrival	-	-	94%	96%
Fibrinolytic Meds Within 30 Min. of Arrival	-	-	41%	58%
Average Time to ECG (minutes)	-	-	8	7
Average Time to Transfer (minutes)	-	-	57	60
Children's Asthma Care				
Received Home Management Plan of Care	-	-	-	88%
Received Reliever Medication	-	-	-	100%
Received Systemic Corticosteroids	-	-	-	100%
Emergency Department				
Admittance Decision Time (minutes)[5]	-	-	57	98
Head CT Results Within 45 Min. of Arrival	-	-	53%	57%
Patients Who Left ER Before Being Seen	-	-	2%	2%
Time from ER Arrival to Admit. (minutes)[5]	-	-	185	274
Time from ER Arrival to Discharge (minutes)	-	-	104	134
Time in ER Before Being Evaluated (minutes)	-	-	18	26
Time to Pain Meds for Fractures (minutes)	-	-	47	57
Heart Attack Care				
Aspirin Given at Discharge[5]	-	-	99%	99%
Fibrinolytic Meds Within 30 Min. of Arrival[5]	-	-	-	54%
PCI Within 90 Minutes of Arrival[5]	-	-	97%	96%
Statin Prescribed at Discharge[5]	-	-	99%	98%
Heart Failure Care				
ACE Inhibitor or ARB for LVSD[1]	-	-	95%	97%
Discharge Instructions Given[1]	-	-	91%	94%
Evaluation of LVS Function	12	58%	94%	99%
Medicare Spending				
Medicare Spending per Patient (ratio)	-	-	0.94	0.98
Pneumonia Care				
Appropriate Initial Antibiotic Given	13	77%	92%	95%
Blood Culture Timing[7]	-	-	98%	98%
Pregnancy and Delivery Care				
Newborn Deliveries Scheduled Early[5]	-	-	12%	6%
Preventive Care				
Immunization for Influenza[5]	-	-	88%	90%
Immunization for Pneumonia[5]	-	-	90%	92%
Stroke Care				
Anticoagulation Therapy for Atrial Fibrillation[5]	-	-	88%	95%
Antithrombotic Therapy Timing[5]	-	-	97%	98%
Assessed for Rehabilitation[5]	-	-	97%	97%
Discharged on Antithrombotic Therapy[5]	-	-	98%	99%
Discharged on Statin Medication[5]	-	-	88%	94%
Thrombolytic Therapy Timing[5]	-	-	68%	66%
Venous Thromboembolism Prophylaxis[5]	-	-	93%	94%
Written Stroke Educational Materials Given[5]	-	-	84%	88%
Surgical Care Improvement Project				
Appropriate Beta Blocker Usage[5]	-	-	98%	98%
Appropriate VTP Within 24 Hours[5]	-	-	98%	98%
Controlled Postoperative Blood Glucose[5]	-	-	98%	97%
Perioperative Temperature Management[5]	-	-	100%	100%
Prophylactic Antibiotic Selection[5]	-	-	99%	99%
Prophylactic Antibiotic Selection (Outpatient)	-	-	98%	98%
Prophylactic Antibiotic Stopped[5]	-	-	98%	98%
Prophylactic Antibiotic Timing[5]	-	-	99%	99%
Prophylactic Antibiotic Timing (Outpatient)	-	-	98%	98%
Urinary Catheter Removal[5]	-	-	97%	97%
Survey of Patients' Hospital Experiences				
Area Around Room 'Always' Quiet at Night[5]	-	-	65%	61%
Doctors 'Always' Communicated Well[5]	-	-	85%	82%
Home Recovery Information Given[5]	-	-	86%	85%
Hospital Given 9 or 10 on 10 Point Scale[5]	-	-	76%	71%
Meds 'Always' Explained Before Given[5]	-	-	66%	64%
Nurses 'Always' Communicated Well[5]	-	-	81%	79%
Pain 'Always' Well Controlled[5]	-	-	72%	71%
Room and Bathroom 'Always' Clean[5]	-	-	76%	73%
Timely Help 'Always' Received[5]	-	-	72%	68%
Would Definitely Recommend Hospital[5]	-	-	75%	71%
Use of Medical Imaging				
Cardiac Imaging Stress Test before Surgery	-	-	5%	5.3%
Combination Abdominal CT Scan	-	-	19%	10.5%
Combination Brain/Sinus CT Scan	-	-	2.9%	2.7%
Combination Chest CT Scan	-	-	3.9%	2.7%
Follow-up Mammogram/Ultrasound	-	-	7.8%	8.8%
Lumbar Spine MRI for Low Back Pain	-	-	40.2%	37.2%

Great Bend Regional Hospital

514 Cleveland Street
Great Bend, KS 67530
Phone: 620-792-8833
Fax: 6207921448
URL: www.greatbendsurgical.com
Type: Acute Care Hospitals
Emergency Services: Yes
Ownership: Proprietary
Beds: 9

Key Personnel:

Administrator . . . . Pam Chambers
CEO . . . . Brent Hanson
Radiology. . . . . Gary McKee, MD
Anesthesiology. . . . . Garret Rebel, CRNA
Pediatrics. . . . . Gerasimos Stavens, MD

Measure	Cases	This Hosp.	State Avg.	U.S. Avg.
Blood Clot Prevention and Treatment				
Anticoagulation Overlap Therapy[1,2]	-	-	94%	93%
ICU Venous Thromboembolism Prophylaxis[1,2]	-	-	91%	92%
Incidence of Potentially Preventable VTE[1,2]	-	-	8%	10%
UFH with Dosages/Platelet Monitoring[2,7]	-	-	98%	97%
Venous Thromboembolism Prophylaxis[2]	95	48%	79%	85%
Warfarin Therapy Discharge Instructions[1,2]	-	-	84%	75%
Chest Pain/Possible Heart Attack Care				
Aspirin Given Within 24 Hours of Arrival	45	98%	94%	96%
Fibrinolytic Meds Within 30 Min. of Arrival[1]	-	-	41%	58%
Average Time to ECG (minutes)	46	15	8	7
Average Time to Transfer (minutes)[1]	-	-	57	60
Children's Asthma Care				
Received Home Management Plan of Care	-	-	-	88%
Received Reliever Medication	-	-	-	100%
Received Systemic Corticosteroids	-	-	-	100%
Emergency Department				
Admittance Decision Time (minutes)[2]	60	44	57	98
Head CT Results Within 45 Min. of Arrival[1]	-	-	53%	57%
Patients Who Left ER Before Being Seen	8,008	1%	2%	2%
Time from ER Arrival to Admit. (minutes)[2]	120	155	185	274
Time from ER Arrival to Discharge (minutes)	379	65	104	134
Time in ER Before Being Evaluated (minutes)	306	13	18	26
Time to Pain Meds for Fractures (minutes)	44	32	47	57
Heart Attack Care				
Aspirin Given at Discharge[1,3]	-	-	99%	99%
Fibrinolytic Meds Within 30 Min. of Arrival[3,7]	-	-	-	54%
PCI Within 90 Minutes of Arrival[3,7]	-	-	97%	96%
Statin Prescribed at Discharge[1,3]	-	-	99%	98%
Heart Failure Care				
ACE Inhibitor or ARB for LVSD[7]	-	-	95%	97%
Discharge Instructions Given[1]	-	-	91%	94%
Evaluation of LVS Function[1]	-	-	94%	99%
Medicare Spending				
Medicare Spending per Patient (ratio)	-	0.97	0.94	0.98
Pneumonia Care				
Appropriate Initial Antibiotic Given[2]	38	84%	92%	95%
Blood Culture Timing[2]	22	95%	98%	98%
Pregnancy and Delivery Care				
Newborn Deliveries Scheduled Early	60	3%	12%	6%
Preventive Care				
Immunization for Influenza[2]	279	65%	88%	90%
Immunization for Pneumonia[2]	307	69%	90%	92%
Stroke Care				
Anticoagulation Therapy for Atrial Fibrillation[1]	-	-	88%	95%
Antithrombotic Therapy Timing[1]	-	-	97%	98%
Assessed for Rehabilitation[1]	-	-	97%	97%
Discharged on Antithrombotic Therapy[1]	-	-	98%	99%
Discharged on Statin Medication[1]	-	-	88%	94%
Thrombolytic Therapy Timing[7]	-	-	68%	66%
Venous Thromboembolism Prophylaxis[1]	-	-	93%	94%
Written Stroke Educational Materials Given[1]	-	-	84%	88%
Surgical Care Improvement Project				
Appropriate Beta Blocker Usage[2]	72	97%	98%	98%
Appropriate VTP Within 24 Hours[2]	253	98%	98%	98%

NOTE: Hospital profiles are in alphabetical order by state, then city, then hospital within the city; Rankings exclude hospitals with less than 25 cases except for patient surveys which excludes hospitals with less than 100 cases; (a) 100-299 cases; (1) The number of cases/patients is too few to report; (2) Data submitted were based on a sample of cases/patients; (3) Results are based on a shorter time period than required; (4) Data suppressed by CMS for one or more quarters; (5) Results are not available for this reporting period; (6) Fewer than 100 patients completed the HCAHPS survey; (7) No cases met the criteria for this measure; (8) The lower limit of the confidence interval cannot be calculated if the number of observed infections equals zero; (9) No data are available from the state/territory for this reporting period; (10) The scores shown reflect fewer than 50 completed surveys; (11) There were discrepancies in the data collection process; (12) This measure does not apply to this hospital for this reporting period; (13) Results cannot be calculated for this reporting period; (14) The results for this state are combined with nearby states to protect confidentiality; Please refer to the User's Guide for a full explanation of data.

Measure	Cases	This Hosp.	State Avg.	U.S. Avg.
Controlled Postoperative Blood Glucose[2,7]	-	-	98%	97%
Perioperative Temperature Management[2]	280	100%	100%	100%
Prophylactic Antibiotic Selection[2]	244	97%	99%	99%
Prophylactic Antibiotic Selection (Outpatient)[1,3]	-	-	98%	98%
Prophylactic Antibiotic Stopped[2]	241	87%	98%	98%
Prophylactic Antibiotic Timing[2]	244	96%	99%	99%
Prophylactic Antibiotic Timing (Outpatient)[1,3]	-	-	98%	98%
Urinary Catheter Removal[2]	156	85%	97%	97%
Survey of Patients' Hospital Experiences				
Area Around Room 'Always' Quiet at Night	300+	65%	65%	61%
Doctors 'Always' Communicated Well	300+	81%	85%	82%
Home Recovery Information Given	300+	84%	86%	85%
Hospital Given 9 or 10 on 10 Point Scale	300+	73%	76%	71%
Meds 'Always' Explained Before Given	300+	61%	66%	64%
Nurses 'Always' Communicated Well	300+	78%	81%	79%
Pain 'Always' Well Controlled	300+	69%	72%	71%
Room and Bathroom 'Always' Clean	300+	74%	76%	73%
Timely Help 'Always' Received	300+	73%	72%	68%
Would Definitely Recommend Hospital	300+	74%	75%	71%
Use of Medical Imaging				
Cardiac Imaging Stress Test before Surgery[1]	-	-	5%	5.3%
Combination Abdominal CT Scan	488	12.7%	19%	10.5%
Combination Brain/Sinus CT Scan[1]	-	-	2.9%	2.7%
Combination Chest CT Scan	401	9.0%	3.9%	2.7%
Follow-up Mammogram/Ultrasound[7]	-	-	7.8%	8.8%
Lumbar Spine MRI for Low Back Pain	89	36.0%	40.2%	37.2%

Hanover Hospital

205 S Hanover Street
Hanover, KS 66945
Phone: 785-337-2214
Type: Critical Access Hospitals
Emergency Services: Yes
Ownership: Govt - Hospital Dist/Auth

Measure	Cases	This Hosp.	State Avg.	U.S. Avg.
Blood Clot Prevention and Treatment				
Anticoagulation Overlap Therapy[5]	-	-	94%	93%
ICU Venous Thromboembolism Prophylaxis[5]	-	-	91%	92%
Incidence of Potentially Preventable VTE[5]	-	-	8%	10%
UFH with Dosages/Platelet Monitoring[5]	-	-	98%	97%
Venous Thromboembolism Prophylaxis[5]	-	-	79%	85%
Warfarin Therapy Discharge Instructions[5]	-	-	84%	75%
Chest Pain/Possible Heart Attack Care				
Aspirin Given Within 24 Hours of Arrival	-	-	94%	96%
Fibrinolytic Meds Within 30 Min. of Arrival	-	-	41%	58%
Average Time to ECG (minutes)	-	-	8	7
Average Time to Transfer (minutes)	-	-	57	60
Children's Asthma Care				
Received Home Management Plan of Care	-	-	-	88%
Received Reliever Medication	-	-	-	100%
Received Systemic Corticosteroids	-	-	-	100%
Emergency Department				
Admittance Decision Time (minutes)[3,7]	-	-	57	98
Head CT Results Within 45 Min. of Arrival	-	-	53%	57%
Patients Who Left ER Before Being Seen	-	-	2%	2%
Time from ER Arrival to Admit. (minutes)[3,7]	-	-	185	274
Time from ER Arrival to Discharge (minutes)	-	-	104	134
Time in ER Before Being Evaluated (minutes)	-	-	18	26
Time to Pain Meds for Fractures (minutes)	-	-	47	57
Heart Attack Care				
Aspirin Given at Discharge[5]	-	-	99%	99%
Fibrinolytic Meds Within 30 Min. of Arrival[5]	-	-	-	54%
PCI Within 90 Minutes of Arrival[5]	-	-	97%	96%
Statin Prescribed at Discharge[5]	-	-	99%	98%
Heart Failure Care				
ACE Inhibitor or ARB for LVSD[3,7]	-	-	95%	97%
Discharge Instructions Given[3,7]	-	-	91%	94%
Evaluation of LVS Function[1,3]	-	-	94%	99%
Medicare Spending				
Medicare Spending per Patient (ratio)	-	-	0.94	0.98
Pneumonia Care				
Appropriate Initial Antibiotic Given[1,2]	-	-	92%	95%
Blood Culture Timing[1,2]	-	-	98%	98%
Pregnancy and Delivery Care				
Newborn Deliveries Scheduled Early[5]	-	-	12%	6%
Preventive Care				
Immunization for Influenza	13	92%	88%	90%
Immunization for Pneumonia[2]	18	89%	90%	92%
Stroke Care				
Anticoagulation Therapy for Atrial Fibrillation[5]	-	-	88%	95%
Antithrombotic Therapy Timing[5]	-	-	97%	98%
Assessed for Rehabilitation[5]	-	-	97%	97%
Discharged on Antithrombotic Therapy[5]	-	-	98%	99%
Discharged on Statin Medication[5]	-	-	88%	94%
Thrombolytic Therapy Timing[5]	-	-	68%	66%
Venous Thromboembolism Prophylaxis[5]	-	-	93%	94%
Written Stroke Educational Materials Given[5]	-	-	84%	88%
Surgical Care Improvement Project				
Appropriate Beta Blocker Usage[5]	-	-	98%	98%
Appropriate VTP Within 24 Hours[5]	-	-	98%	98%
Controlled Postoperative Blood Glucose[5]	-	-	98%	97%
Perioperative Temperature Management[5]	-	-	100%	100%
Prophylactic Antibiotic Selection[5]	-	-	99%	99%
Prophylactic Antibiotic Selection (Outpatient)	-	-	98%	98%
Prophylactic Antibiotic Stopped[5]	-	-	98%	98%
Prophylactic Antibiotic Timing[5]	-	-	99%	99%
Prophylactic Antibiotic Timing (Outpatient)	-	-	98%	98%
Urinary Catheter Removal[5]	-	-	97%	97%
Survey of Patients' Hospital Experiences				
Area Around Room 'Always' Quiet at Night[5]	-	-	65%	61%
Doctors 'Always' Communicated Well[5]	-	-	85%	82%
Home Recovery Information Given[5]	-	-	86%	85%
Hospital Given 9 or 10 on 10 Point Scale[5]	-	-	76%	71%
Meds 'Always' Explained Before Given[5]	-	-	66%	64%
Nurses 'Always' Communicated Well[5]	-	-	81%	79%
Pain 'Always' Well Controlled[5]	-	-	72%	71%
Room and Bathroom 'Always' Clean[5]	-	-	76%	73%
Timely Help 'Always' Received[5]	-	-	72%	68%
Would Definitely Recommend Hospital[5]	-	-	75%	71%
Use of Medical Imaging				
Cardiac Imaging Stress Test before Surgery	-	-	5%	5.3%
Combination Abdominal CT Scan	-	-	19%	10.5%
Combination Brain/Sinus CT Scan	-	-	2.9%	2.7%
Combination Chest CT Scan	-	-	3.9%	2.7%
Follow-up Mammogram/Ultrasound	-	-	7.8%	8.8%
Lumbar Spine MRI for Low Back Pain	-	-	40.2%	37.2%

Harper Hospital District No 5

700 West 13th
Harper, KS 67058
Phone: 620-896-7324
Fax: 620-896-7127
URL: www.harperhosp.com
Type: Critical Access Hospitals
Emergency Services: Yes
Ownership: Govt - Hospital Dist/Auth
Beds: 38

Key Personnel:
Chief of Medical Staff . . . . Ralph Bellar
Cardiology . . . . Roger Bond, MD
CEO/President. . . . . Kim Cinelli
Emergency Room . . . . Martha Ediger
Chairman/CEO . . . . Bob Hightree
Operating Room. . . . . Donald Ransom, DO
Surgery . . . . Donald Ransom, DO
Infection Control. . . . . Nearaj Vasishtha

Measure	Cases	This Hosp.	State Avg.	U.S. Avg.
Blood Clot Prevention and Treatment				
Anticoagulation Overlap Therapy[1]	-	-	94%	93%
ICU Venous Thromboembolism Prophylaxis[7]	-	-	91%	92%
Incidence of Potentially Preventable VTE[7]	-	-	8%	10%
UFH with Dosages/Platelet Monitoring[7]	-	-	98%	97%
Venous Thromboembolism Prophylaxis	49	6%	79%	85%
Warfarin Therapy Discharge Instructions[1]	-	-	84%	75%
Chest Pain/Possible Heart Attack Care				
Aspirin Given Within 24 Hours of Arrival	-	-	94%	96%
Fibrinolytic Meds Within 30 Min. of Arrival	-	-	41%	58%
Average Time to ECG (minutes)	-	-	8	7
Average Time to Transfer (minutes)	-	-	57	60
Children's Asthma Care				
Received Home Management Plan of Care	-	-	-	88%
Received Reliever Medication	-	-	-	100%
Received Systemic Corticosteroids	-	-	-	100%
Emergency Department				
Admittance Decision Time (minutes)[3]	67	0	57	98
Head CT Results Within 45 Min. of Arrival	-	-	53%	57%
Patients Who Left ER Before Being Seen	-	-	2%	2%
Time from ER Arrival to Admit. (minutes)[3]	67	15	185	274
Time from ER Arrival to Discharge (minutes)	-	-	104	134
Time in ER Before Being Evaluated (minutes)	-	-	18	26
Time to Pain Meds for Fractures (minutes)	-	-	47	57
Heart Attack Care				
Aspirin Given at Discharge[5]	-	-	99%	99%
Fibrinolytic Meds Within 30 Min. of Arrival[5]	-	-	-	54%
PCI Within 90 Minutes of Arrival[5]	-	-	97%	96%
Statin Prescribed at Discharge[5]	-	-	99%	98%
Heart Failure Care				
ACE Inhibitor or ARB for LVSD[1,3]	-	-	95%	97%
Discharge Instructions Given[1,3]	-	-	91%	94%
Evaluation of LVS Function[1,3]	-	-	94%	99%
Medicare Spending				
Medicare Spending per Patient (ratio)	-	-	0.94	0.98
Pneumonia Care				
Appropriate Initial Antibiotic Given[3]	11	91%	92%	95%
Blood Culture Timing[1,3]	-	-	98%	98%
Pregnancy and Delivery Care				
Newborn Deliveries Scheduled Early[5]	-	-	12%	6%
Preventive Care				
Immunization for Influenza[3]	30	43%	88%	90%
Immunization for Pneumonia[3]	86	41%	90%	92%
Stroke Care				
Anticoagulation Therapy for Atrial Fibrillation[5]	-	-	88%	95%
Antithrombotic Therapy Timing[5]	-	-	97%	98%
Assessed for Rehabilitation[5]	-	-	97%	97%
Discharged on Antithrombotic Therapy[5]	-	-	98%	99%
Discharged on Statin Medication[5]	-	-	88%	94%
Thrombolytic Therapy Timing[5]	-	-	68%	66%
Venous Thromboembolism Prophylaxis[5]	-	-	93%	94%
Written Stroke Educational Materials Given[5]	-	-	84%	88%
Surgical Care Improvement Project				
Appropriate Beta Blocker Usage[3,7]	-	-	98%	98%
Appropriate VTP Within 24 Hours[1,3]	-	-	98%	98%
Controlled Postoperative Blood Glucose[3,7]	-	-	98%	97%
Perioperative Temperature Management[1,3]	-	-	100%	100%
Prophylactic Antibiotic Selection[3,7]	-	-	99%	99%
Prophylactic Antibiotic Selection (Outpatient)	-	-	98%	98%
Prophylactic Antibiotic Stopped[3,7]	-	-	98%	98%
Prophylactic Antibiotic Timing[3,7]	-	-	99%	99%
Prophylactic Antibiotic Timing (Outpatient)	-	-	98%	98%
Urinary Catheter Removal[1,3]	-	-	97%	97%
Survey of Patients' Hospital Experiences				
Area Around Room 'Always' Quiet at Night[5]	-	-	65%	61%
Doctors 'Always' Communicated Well[5]	-	-	85%	82%
Home Recovery Information Given[5]	-	-	86%	85%
Hospital Given 9 or 10 on 10 Point Scale[5]	-	-	76%	71%
Meds 'Always' Explained Before Given[5]	-	-	66%	64%
Nurses 'Always' Communicated Well[5]	-	-	81%	79%
Pain 'Always' Well Controlled[5]	-	-	72%	71%
Room and Bathroom 'Always' Clean[5]	-	-	76%	73%
Timely Help 'Always' Received[5]	-	-	72%	68%
Would Definitely Recommend Hospital[5]	-	-	75%	71%
Use of Medical Imaging				
Cardiac Imaging Stress Test before Surgery	-	-	5%	5.3%
Combination Abdominal CT Scan	-	-	19%	10.5%
Combination Brain/Sinus CT Scan	-	-	2.9%	2.7%
Combination Chest CT Scan	-	-	3.9%	2.7%
Follow-up Mammogram/Ultrasound	-	-	7.8%	8.8%
Lumbar Spine MRI for Low Back Pain	-	-	40.2%	37.2%

NOTE: Hospital profiles are in alphabetical order by state, then city, then hospital within the city; Rankings exclude hospitals with less than 25 cases except for patient surveys which excludes hospitals with less than 100 cases; (a) 100-299 cases; (1) The number of cases/patients is too few to report; (2) Data submitted were based on a sample of cases/patients; (3) Results are based on a shorter time period than required; (4) Data suppressed by CMS for one or more quarters; (5) Results are not available for this reporting period; (6) Fewer than 100 patients completed the HCAHPS survey; (7) No cases met the criteria for this measure; (8) The lower limit of the confidence interval cannot be calculated if the number of observed infections equals zero; (9) No data are available from the state/territory for this reporting period; (10) The scores shown reflect fewer than 50 completed surveys; (11) There were discrepancies in the data collection process; (12) This measure does not apply to this hospital for this reporting period; (13) Results cannot be calculated for this reporting period; (14) The results for this state are combined with nearby states to protect confidentiality; Please refer to the User's Guide for a full explanation of data.

Hays Medical Center

2220 Canterbury Drive Phone: 785-623-5000
Hays, KS 67601 Fax: 785-623-5627
URL: www.haysmed.com
Type: Acute Care Hospitals Emergency Services: Yes
Ownership: Voluntary non-profit - Other Beds: 158

Key Personnel:
CEO/President. . . . . John H Jeter
Chief of Medical Staff. . . . . Larry Watts, MD
Radiology. . . . . Michael Wright

Measure	Cases	This Hosp.	State Avg.	U.S. Avg.
Blood Clot Prevention and Treatment				
Anticoagulation Overlap Therapy[2]	47	96%	94%	93%
ICU Venous Thromboembolism Prophylaxis[2]	73	86%	91%	92%
Incidence of Potentially Preventable VTE[1,2]	-	-	8%	10%
UFH with Dosages/Platelet Monitoring[2]	29	97%	98%	97%
Venous Thromboembolism Prophylaxis[2]	329	77%	79%	85%
Warfarin Therapy Discharge Instructions[2]	36	42%	84%	75%
Chest Pain/Possible Heart Attack Care				
Aspirin Given Within 24 Hours of Arrival[5]	-	-	94%	96%
Fibrinolytic Meds Within 30 Min. of Arrival[5]	-	-	41%	58%
Average Time to ECG (minutes)[5]	-	-	8	7
Average Time to Transfer (minutes)[5]	-	-	57	60
Children's Asthma Care				
Received Home Management Plan of Care	-	-	-	88%
Received Reliever Medication	-	-	-	100%
Received Systemic Corticosteroids	-	-	-	100%
Emergency Department				
Admittance Decision Time (minutes)[2]	227	63	57	98
Head CT Results Within 45 Min. of Arrival[1]	-	-	53%	57%
Patients Who Left ER Before Being Seen	14,408	1%	2%	2%
Time from ER Arrival to Admit. (minutes)[2]	346	177	185	274
Time from ER Arrival to Discharge (minutes)	374	118	104	134
Time in ER Before Being Evaluated (minutes)	362	22	18	26
Time to Pain Meds for Fractures (minutes)	60	48	47	57
Heart Attack Care				
Aspirin Given at Discharge[2]	198	99%	99%	99%
Fibrinolytic Meds Within 30 Min. of Arrival[1,2]	-	-	-	54%
PCI Within 90 Minutes of Arrival[1,2]	-	-	97%	96%
Statin Prescribed at Discharge[2]	200	98%	99%	98%
Heart Failure Care				
ACE Inhibitor or ARB for LVSD	56	88%	95%	97%
Discharge Instructions Given	141	78%	91%	94%
Evaluation of LVS Function	180	99%	94%	99%
Medicare Spending				
Medicare Spending per Patient (ratio)	-	0.98	0.94	0.98
Pneumonia Care				
Appropriate Initial Antibiotic Given[2]	36	94%	92%	95%
Blood Culture Timing[2]	60	95%	98%	98%
Pregnancy and Delivery Care				
Newborn Deliveries Scheduled Early	100	46%	12%	6%
Preventive Care				
Immunization for Influenza[2]	531	89%	88%	90%
Immunization for Pneumonia[2]	686	89%	90%	92%
Stroke Care				
Anticoagulation Therapy for Atrial Fibrillation[1]	-	-	88%	95%
Antithrombotic Therapy Timing	30	97%	97%	98%
Assessed for Rehabilitation	36	94%	97%	97%
Discharged on Antithrombotic Therapy	36	100%	98%	99%
Discharged on Statin Medication	31	90%	88%	94%
Thrombolytic Therapy Timing[1]	-	-	68%	66%
Venous Thromboembolism Prophylaxis	35	83%	93%	94%
Written Stroke Educational Materials Given	21	71%	84%	88%
Surgical Care Improvement Project				
Appropriate Beta Blocker Usage[2]	159	98%	98%	98%
Appropriate VTP Within 24 Hours[2]	313	96%	98%	98%
Controlled Postoperative Blood Glucose[2]	61	95%	98%	97%
Perioperative Temperature Management[2]	404	100%	100%	100%
Prophylactic Antibiotic Selection[2]	315	99%	99%	99%
Prophylactic Antibiotic Selection (Outpatient)	306	95%	98%	98%
Prophylactic Antibiotic Stopped[2]	302	97%	98%	98%
Prophylactic Antibiotic Timing[2]	318	99%	99%	99%
Prophylactic Antibiotic Timing (Outpatient)	277	81%	98%	98%
Urinary Catheter Removal[2]	235	95%	97%	97%
Survey of Patients' Hospital Experiences				
Area Around Room 'Always' Quiet at Night	300+	67%	65%	61%
Doctors 'Always' Communicated Well	300+	83%	85%	82%
Home Recovery Information Given	300+	89%	86%	85%
Hospital Given 9 or 10 on 10 Point Scale	300+	76%	76%	71%
Meds 'Always' Explained Before Given	300+	66%	66%	64%
Nurses 'Always' Communicated Well	300+	79%	81%	79%
Pain 'Always' Well Controlled	300+	72%	72%	71%
Room and Bathroom 'Always' Clean	300+	73%	76%	73%
Timely Help 'Always' Received	300+	66%	72%	68%
Would Definitely Recommend Hospital	300+	74%	75%	71%
Use of Medical Imaging				
Cardiac Imaging Stress Test before Surgery	510	4.3%	5%	5.3%
Combination Abdominal CT Scan	598	45.2%	19%	10.5%
Combination Brain/Sinus CT Scan[1]	-	-	2.9%	2.7%
Combination Chest CT Scan	812	1.2%	3.9%	2.7%
Follow-up Mammogram/Ultrasound	1,086	8.7%	7.8%	8.8%
Lumbar Spine MRI for Low Back Pain	119	43.7%	40.2%	37.2%

Herington Municipal Hospital

100 E Helen Street Phone: 785-258-2207
Herington, KS 67449 Fax: 785-258-5127
Type: Critical Access Hospitals Emergency Services: Yes
Ownership: Voluntary non-profit - Other Beds: 25

Key Personnel:
Infection Control. . . . . Marge Bergstrom, RN
CEO . . . . Michael J., Ryan
Chief of Medical Staff. . . . . John Mosier
Radiology. . . . . Mary Schroeder
Quality Assurance . . . . Mary Steiner, RN
Emergency Room . . . . Rose Stimac, RN
Operating Room. . . . . Rose Stimac, RN

Measure	Cases	This Hosp.	State Avg.	U.S. Avg.
Blood Clot Prevention and Treatment				
Anticoagulation Overlap Therapy[3,7]	-	-	94%	93%
ICU Venous Thromboembolism Prophylaxis[3,7]	-	-	91%	92%
Incidence of Potentially Preventable VTE[3,7]	-	-	8%	10%
UFH with Dosages/Platelet Monitoring[1,3]	-	-	98%	97%
Venous Thromboembolism Prophylaxis[3,7]	-	-	79%	85%
Warfarin Therapy Discharge Instructions[1,3]	-	-	84%	75%
Chest Pain/Possible Heart Attack Care				
Aspirin Given Within 24 Hours of Arrival	-	-	94%	96%
Fibrinolytic Meds Within 30 Min. of Arrival	-	-	41%	58%
Average Time to ECG (minutes)	-	-	8	7
Average Time to Transfer (minutes)	-	-	57	60
Children's Asthma Care				
Received Home Management Plan of Care	-	-	-	88%
Received Reliever Medication	-	-	-	100%
Received Systemic Corticosteroids	-	-	-	100%
Emergency Department				
Admittance Decision Time (minutes)[2]	126	0	57	98
Head CT Results Within 45 Min. of Arrival	-	-	53%	57%
Patients Who Left ER Before Being Seen	-	-	2%	2%
Time from ER Arrival to Admit. (minutes)[2]	126	116	185	274
Time from ER Arrival to Discharge (minutes)	-	-	104	134
Time in ER Before Being Evaluated (minutes)	-	-	18	26
Time to Pain Meds for Fractures (minutes)	-	-	47	57
Heart Attack Care				
Aspirin Given at Discharge[1,3]	-	-	99%	99%
Fibrinolytic Meds Within 30 Min. of Arrival[3,7]	-	-	-	54%
PCI Within 90 Minutes of Arrival[3,7]	-	-	97%	96%
Statin Prescribed at Discharge[1,3]	-	-	99%	98%
Heart Failure Care				
ACE Inhibitor or ARB for LVSD[1]	-	-	95%	97%
Discharge Instructions Given[1]	-	-	91%	94%
Evaluation of LVS Function[1]	-	-	94%	99%
Medicare Spending				
Medicare Spending per Patient (ratio)	-	-	0.94	0.98
Pneumonia Care				
Appropriate Initial Antibiotic Given[1]	-	-	92%	95%
Blood Culture Timing[1]	-	-	98%	98%
Pregnancy and Delivery Care				
Newborn Deliveries Scheduled Early[5]	-	-	12%	6%
Preventive Care				
Immunization for Influenza	68	32%	88%	90%
Immunization for Pneumonia	98	42%	90%	92%
Stroke Care				
Anticoagulation Therapy for Atrial Fibrillation[5]	-	-	88%	95%
Antithrombotic Therapy Timing[5]	-	-	97%	98%
Assessed for Rehabilitation[5]	-	-	97%	97%
Discharged on Antithrombotic Therapy[5]	-	-	98%	99%
Discharged on Statin Medication[5]	-	-	88%	94%
Thrombolytic Therapy Timing[5]	-	-	68%	66%
Venous Thromboembolism Prophylaxis[5]	-	-	93%	94%
Written Stroke Educational Materials Given[5]	-	-	84%	88%
Surgical Care Improvement Project				
Appropriate Beta Blocker Usage[5]	-	-	98%	98%
Appropriate VTP Within 24 Hours[5]	-	-	98%	98%
Controlled Postoperative Blood Glucose[5]	-	-	98%	97%
Perioperative Temperature Management[5]	-	-	100%	100%
Prophylactic Antibiotic Selection[5]	-	-	99%	99%
Prophylactic Antibiotic Selection (Outpatient)	-	-	98%	98%
Prophylactic Antibiotic Stopped[5]	-	-	98%	98%
Prophylactic Antibiotic Timing[5]	-	-	99%	99%
Prophylactic Antibiotic Timing (Outpatient)	-	-	98%	98%
Urinary Catheter Removal[5]	-	-	97%	97%
Survey of Patients' Hospital Experiences				
Area Around Room 'Always' Quiet at Night[5]	-	-	65%	61%
Doctors 'Always' Communicated Well[5]	-	-	85%	82%
Home Recovery Information Given[5]	-	-	86%	85%
Hospital Given 9 or 10 on 10 Point Scale[5]	-	-	76%	71%
Meds 'Always' Explained Before Given[5]	-	-	66%	64%
Nurses 'Always' Communicated Well[5]	-	-	81%	79%
Pain 'Always' Well Controlled[5]	-	-	72%	71%
Room and Bathroom 'Always' Clean[5]	-	-	76%	73%
Timely Help 'Always' Received[5]	-	-	72%	68%
Would Definitely Recommend Hospital[5]	-	-	75%	71%
Use of Medical Imaging				
Cardiac Imaging Stress Test before Surgery	-	-	5%	5.3%
Combination Abdominal CT Scan	-	-	19%	10.5%
Combination Brain/Sinus CT Scan	-	-	2.9%	2.7%
Combination Chest CT Scan	-	-	3.9%	2.7%
Follow-up Mammogram/Ultrasound	-	-	7.8%	8.8%
Lumbar Spine MRI for Low Back Pain	-	-	40.2%	37.2%

Hiawatha Community Hospital

300 Utah Street Phone: 785-742-6283
Hiawatha, KS 66434
Type: Critical Access Hospitals Emergency Services: Yes
Ownership: Voluntary non-profit - Private

Measure	Cases	This Hosp.	State Avg.	U.S. Avg.
Blood Clot Prevention and Treatment				
Anticoagulation Overlap Therapy[5]	-	-	94%	93%
ICU Venous Thromboembolism Prophylaxis[5]	-	-	91%	92%
Incidence of Potentially Preventable VTE[5]	-	-	8%	10%
UFH with Dosages/Platelet Monitoring[5]	-	-	98%	97%
Venous Thromboembolism Prophylaxis[5]	-	-	79%	85%
Warfarin Therapy Discharge Instructions[5]	-	-	84%	75%
Chest Pain/Possible Heart Attack Care				
Aspirin Given Within 24 Hours of Arrival[1,3]	-	-	94%	96%
Fibrinolytic Meds Within 30 Min. of Arrival[1,3]	-	-	41%	58%
Average Time to ECG (minutes)[1,3]	-	-	8	7
Average Time to Transfer (minutes)[1,3]	-	-	57	60
Children's Asthma Care				
Received Home Management Plan of Care	-	-	-	88%
Received Reliever Medication	-	-	-	100%
Received Systemic Corticosteroids	-	-	-	100%
Emergency Department				
Admittance Decision Time (minutes)[5]	-	-	57	98
Head CT Results Within 45 Min. of Arrival[1,3]	-	-	53%	57%
Patients Who Left ER Before Being Seen[5]	-	-	2%	2%
Time from ER Arrival to Admit. (minutes)[5]	-	-	185	274
Time from ER Arrival to Discharge (minutes)[3]	86	73	104	134
Time in ER Before Being Evaluated (minutes)[3]	83	28	18	26
Time to Pain Meds for Fractures (minutes)[1,3]	-	-	47	57

NOTE: Hospital profiles are in alphabetical order by state, then city, then hospital within the city; Rankings exclude hospitals with less than 25 cases except for patient surveys which excludes hospitals with less than 100 cases; (a) 100-299 cases; (1) The number of cases/patients is too few to report; (2) Data submitted were based on a sample of cases/patients; (3) Results are based on a shorter time period than required; (4) Data suppressed by CMS for one or more quarters; (5) Results are not available for this reporting period; (6) Fewer than 100 patients completed the HCAHPS survey; (7) No cases met the criteria for this measure; (8) The lower limit of the confidence interval cannot be calculated if the number of observed infections equals zero; (9) No data are available from the state/territory for this reporting period; (10) The scores shown reflect fewer than 50 completed surveys; (11) There were discrepancies in the data collection process; (12) This measure does not apply to this hospital for this reporting period; (13) Results cannot be calculated for this reporting period; (14) The results for this state are combined with nearby states to protect confidentiality; Please refer to the User's Guide for a full explanation of data.

Measure	Cases	This Hosp.	State Avg.	U.S. Avg.
Heart Attack Care				
Aspirin Given at Discharge[3,7]	-	-	99%	99%
Fibrinolytic Meds Within 30 Min. of Arrival[3,7]	-	-	-	54%
PCI Within 90 Minutes of Arrival[3,7]	-	-	97%	96%
Statin Prescribed at Discharge[3,7]	-	-	99%	98%
Heart Failure Care				
ACE Inhibitor or ARB for LVSD[1,3]	-	-	95%	97%
Discharge Instructions Given[3]	13	77%	91%	94%
Evaluation of LVS Function[3]	22	68%	94%	99%
Medicare Spending				
Medicare Spending per Patient (ratio)	-	-	0.94	0.98
Pneumonia Care				
Appropriate Initial Antibiotic Given[3]	20	85%	92%	95%
Blood Culture Timing[3]	12	92%	98%	98%
Pregnancy and Delivery Care				
Newborn Deliveries Scheduled Early[5]	-	-	12%	6%
Preventive Care				
Immunization for Influenza[5]	-	-	88%	90%
Immunization for Pneumonia[5]	-	-	90%	92%
Stroke Care				
Anticoagulation Therapy for Atrial Fibrillation[5]	-	-	88%	95%
Antithrombotic Therapy Timing[5]	-	-	97%	98%
Assessed for Rehabilitation[5]	-	-	97%	97%
Discharged on Antithrombotic Therapy[5]	-	-	98%	99%
Discharged on Statin Medication[5]	-	-	88%	94%
Thrombolytic Therapy Timing[5]	-	-	68%	66%
Venous Thromboembolism Prophylaxis[5]	-	-	93%	94%
Written Stroke Educational Materials Given[5]	-	-	84%	88%
Surgical Care Improvement Project				
Appropriate Beta Blocker Usage[1,3]	-	-	98%	98%
Appropriate VTP Within 24 Hours[1,3]	-	-	98%	98%
Controlled Postoperative Blood Glucose[3,7]	-	-	98%	97%
Perioperative Temperature Management[3]	11	100%	100%	100%
Prophylactic Antibiotic Selection[1,3]	-	-	99%	99%
Prophylactic Antibiotic Selection (Outpatient)[5]	-	-	98%	98%
Prophylactic Antibiotic Stopped[1,3]	-	-	98%	98%
Prophylactic Antibiotic Timing[1,3]	-	-	99%	99%
Prophylactic Antibiotic Timing (Outpatient)[5]	-	-	98%	98%
Urinary Catheter Removal[1,3]	-	-	97%	97%
Survey of Patients' Hospital Experiences				
Area Around Room 'Always' Quiet at Night[5]	-	-	65%	61%
Doctors 'Always' Communicated Well[5]	-	-	85%	82%
Home Recovery Information Given[5]	-	-	86%	85%
Hospital Given 9 or 10 on 10 Point Scale[5]	-	-	76%	71%
Meds 'Always' Explained Before Given[5]	-	-	66%	64%
Nurses 'Always' Communicated Well[5]	-	-	81%	79%
Pain 'Always' Well Controlled[5]	-	-	72%	71%
Room and Bathroom 'Always' Clean[5]	-	-	76%	73%
Timely Help 'Always' Received[5]	-	-	72%	68%
Would Definitely Recommend Hospital[5]	-	-	75%	71%
Use of Medical Imaging				
Cardiac Imaging Stress Test before Surgery	91	6.6%	5%	5.3%
Combination Abdominal CT Scan	128	75.8%	19%	10.5%
Combination Brain/Sinus CT Scan[1]	-	-	2.9%	2.7%
Combination Chest CT Scan	78	2.6%	3.9%	2.7%
Follow-up Mammogram/Ultrasound	276	7.6%	7.8%	8.8%
Lumbar Spine MRI for Low Back Pain[1]	-	-	40.2%	37.2%

Graham County Hospital

304 West Prout Street
Hill City, KS 67642
Phone: 785-421-2121
Fax: 785-421-2034
Type: Critical Access Hospitals
Ownership: Government - Local
Emergency Services: Yes
Beds: 25

Key Personnel:
CEO/President. . . . . Doug Newman
Quality Assurance . . . . Kathy Richmeier

Measure	Cases	This Hosp.	State Avg.	U.S. Avg.
Blood Clot Prevention and Treatment				
Anticoagulation Overlap Therapy[1,3]	-	-	94%	93%
ICU Venous Thromboembolism Prophylaxis[3,7]	-	-	91%	92%
Incidence of Potentially Preventable VTE[3,7]	-	-	8%	10%
UFH with Dosages/Platelet Monitoring[3,7]	-	-	98%	97%
Venous Thromboembolism Prophylaxis[3,7]	-	-	79%	85%
Warfarin Therapy Discharge Instructions[1,3]	-	-	84%	75%
Chest Pain/Possible Heart Attack Care				
Aspirin Given Within 24 Hours of Arrival	15	87%	94%	96%
Fibrinolytic Meds Within 30 Min. of Arrival[1,3]	-	-	41%	58%
Average Time to ECG (minutes)	15	10	8	7
Average Time to Transfer (minutes)[3,7]	-	-	57	60
Children's Asthma Care				
Received Home Management Plan of Care	-	-	-	88%
Received Reliever Medication	-	-	-	100%
Received Systemic Corticosteroids	-	-	-	100%
Emergency Department				
Admittance Decision Time (minutes)	111	19	57	98
Head CT Results Within 45 Min. of Arrival[5]	-	-	53%	57%
Patients Who Left ER Before Being Seen[5]	-	-	2%	2%
Time from ER Arrival to Admit. (minutes)	111	74	185	274
Time from ER Arrival to Discharge (minutes)[1]	-	-	104	134
Time in ER Before Being Evaluated (minutes)	92	15	18	26
Time to Pain Meds for Fractures (minutes)[1,3]	-	-	47	57
Heart Attack Care				
Aspirin Given at Discharge[3,7]	-	-	99%	99%
Fibrinolytic Meds Within 30 Min. of Arrival[3,7]	-	-	-	54%
PCI Within 90 Minutes of Arrival[3,7]	-	-	97%	96%
Statin Prescribed at Discharge[3,7]	-	-	99%	98%
Heart Failure Care				
ACE Inhibitor or ARB for LVSD[1]	-	-	95%	97%
Discharge Instructions Given[1]	-	-	91%	94%
Evaluation of LVS Function	18	61%	94%	99%
Medicare Spending				
Medicare Spending per Patient (ratio)	-	-	0.94	0.98
Pneumonia Care				
Appropriate Initial Antibiotic Given[1]	-	-	92%	95%
Blood Culture Timing[1]	-	-	98%	98%
Pregnancy and Delivery Care				
Newborn Deliveries Scheduled Early[5]	-	-	12%	6%
Preventive Care				
Immunization for Influenza	145	70%	88%	90%
Immunization for Pneumonia	222	78%	90%	92%
Stroke Care				
Anticoagulation Therapy for Atrial Fibrillation[3,7]	-	-	88%	95%
Antithrombotic Therapy Timing[1,3]	-	-	97%	98%
Assessed for Rehabilitation[1,3]	-	-	97%	97%
Discharged on Antithrombotic Therapy[1,3]	-	-	98%	99%
Discharged on Statin Medication[1,3]	-	-	88%	94%
Thrombolytic Therapy Timing[3,7]	-	-	68%	66%
Venous Thromboembolism Prophylaxis[1,3]	-	-	93%	94%
Written Stroke Educational Materials Given[1,3]	-	-	84%	88%
Surgical Care Improvement Project				
Appropriate Beta Blocker Usage[5]	-	-	98%	98%
Appropriate VTP Within 24 Hours[5]	-	-	98%	98%
Controlled Postoperative Blood Glucose[5]	-	-	98%	97%
Perioperative Temperature Management[5]	-	-	100%	100%
Prophylactic Antibiotic Selection[5]	-	-	99%	99%
Prophylactic Antibiotic Selection (Outpatient)[5]	-	-	98%	98%
Prophylactic Antibiotic Stopped[5]	-	-	98%	98%
Prophylactic Antibiotic Timing[5]	-	-	99%	99%
Prophylactic Antibiotic Timing (Outpatient)[5]	-	-	98%	98%
Urinary Catheter Removal[5]	-	-	97%	97%
Survey of Patients' Hospital Experiences				
Area Around Room 'Always' Quiet at Night[5]	-	-	65%	61%
Doctors 'Always' Communicated Well[5]	-	-	85%	82%
Home Recovery Information Given[5]	-	-	86%	85%
Hospital Given 9 or 10 on 10 Point Scale[5]	-	-	76%	71%
Meds 'Always' Explained Before Given[5]	-	-	66%	64%
Nurses 'Always' Communicated Well[5]	-	-	81%	79%
Pain 'Always' Well Controlled[5]	-	-	72%	71%
Room and Bathroom 'Always' Clean[5]	-	-	76%	73%
Timely Help 'Always' Received[5]	-	-	72%	68%
Would Definitely Recommend Hospital[5]	-	-	75%	71%
Use of Medical Imaging				
Cardiac Imaging Stress Test before Surgery[1]	-	-	5%	5.3%
Combination Abdominal CT Scan	63	30.2%	19%	10.5%
Combination Brain/Sinus CT Scan[1]	-	-	2.9%	2.7%
Combination Chest CT Scan	74	12.2%	3.9%	2.7%
Follow-up Mammogram/Ultrasound	99	10.1%	7.8%	8.8%
Lumbar Spine MRI for Low Back Pain[1]	-	-	40.2%	37.2%

Hillsboro Community Hospital

701 S Main Street
Hillsboro, KS 67063
Phone: 620-947-3114
Fax: 620-947-5690
E-mail: comf@southwind.net
URL: www.hillsboromedicalcenter.org
Type: Critical Access Hospitals
Ownership: Proprietary
Emergency Services: Yes
Beds: 79

Key Personnel:
Chief of Medical Staff. . . . . A Randal Claassen
Emergency Room . . . . Jan Fenske, RN
Infection Control. . . . . Cayle Goertzen, MT
Quality Assurance . . . . Ken Johnson, RT
Radiology. . . . . Billie Kueser
Anesthesiology. . . . . Bob Reese, CRNA
CEO/President. . . . . Michael Ryan

Measure	Cases	This Hosp.	State Avg.	U.S. Avg.
Blood Clot Prevention and Treatment				
Anticoagulation Overlap Therapy[5]	-	-	94%	93%
ICU Venous Thromboembolism Prophylaxis[5]	-	-	91%	92%
Incidence of Potentially Preventable VTE[5]	-	-	8%	10%
UFH with Dosages/Platelet Monitoring[5]	-	-	98%	97%
Venous Thromboembolism Prophylaxis[5]	-	-	79%	85%
Warfarin Therapy Discharge Instructions[5]	-	-	84%	75%
Chest Pain/Possible Heart Attack Care				
Aspirin Given Within 24 Hours of Arrival[5]	-	-	94%	96%
Fibrinolytic Meds Within 30 Min. of Arrival[5]	-	-	41%	58%
Average Time to ECG (minutes)[5]	-	-	8	7
Average Time to Transfer (minutes)[5]	-	-	57	60
Children's Asthma Care				
Received Home Management Plan of Care	-	-	-	88%
Received Reliever Medication	-	-	-	100%
Received Systemic Corticosteroids	-	-	-	100%
Emergency Department				
Admittance Decision Time (minutes)[5]	-	-	57	98
Head CT Results Within 45 Min. of Arrival[5]	-	-	53%	57%
Patients Who Left ER Before Being Seen[5]	-	-	2%	2%
Time from ER Arrival to Admit. (minutes)[5]	-	-	185	274
Time from ER Arrival to Discharge (minutes)[5]	-	-	104	134
Time in ER Before Being Evaluated (minutes)[5]	-	-	18	26
Time to Pain Meds for Fractures (minutes)[5]	-	-	47	57
Heart Attack Care				
Aspirin Given at Discharge[5]	-	-	99%	99%
Fibrinolytic Meds Within 30 Min. of Arrival[5]	-	-	-	54%
PCI Within 90 Minutes of Arrival[5]	-	-	97%	96%
Statin Prescribed at Discharge[5]	-	-	99%	98%
Heart Failure Care				
ACE Inhibitor or ARB for LVSD[5]	-	-	95%	97%
Discharge Instructions Given[5]	-	-	91%	94%
Evaluation of LVS Function[5]	-	-	94%	99%
Medicare Spending				
Medicare Spending per Patient (ratio)	-	-	0.94	0.98
Pneumonia Care				
Appropriate Initial Antibiotic Given[5]	-	-	92%	95%
Blood Culture Timing[5]	-	-	98%	98%
Pregnancy and Delivery Care				
Newborn Deliveries Scheduled Early[5]	-	-	12%	6%
Preventive Care				
Immunization for Influenza[5]	-	-	88%	90%
Immunization for Pneumonia[5]	-	-	90%	92%
Stroke Care				
Anticoagulation Therapy for Atrial Fibrillation[5]	-	-	88%	95%
Antithrombotic Therapy Timing[5]	-	-	97%	98%
Assessed for Rehabilitation[5]	-	-	97%	97%
Discharged on Antithrombotic Therapy[5]	-	-	98%	99%
Discharged on Statin Medication[5]	-	-	88%	94%
Thrombolytic Therapy Timing[5]	-	-	68%	66%
Venous Thromboembolism Prophylaxis[5]	-	-	93%	94%
Written Stroke Educational Materials Given[5]	-	-	84%	88%
Surgical Care Improvement Project				
Appropriate Beta Blocker Usage[5]	-	-	98%	98%

NOTE: Hospital profiles are in alphabetical order by state, then city, then hospital within the city; Rankings exclude hospitals with less than 25 cases except for patient surveys which excludes hospitals with less than 100 cases; (a) 100-299 cases; (1) The number of cases/patients is too few to report; (2) Data submitted were based on a sample of cases/patients; (3) Results are based on a shorter time period than required; (4) Data suppressed by CMS for one or more quarters; (5) Results are not available for this reporting period; (6) Fewer than 100 patients completed the HCAHPS survey; (7) No cases met the criteria for this measure; (8) The lower limit of the confidence interval cannot be calculated if the number of observed infections equals zero; (9) No data are available from the state/territory for this reporting period; (10) The scores shown reflect fewer than 50 completed surveys; (11) There were discrepancies in the data collection process; (12) This measure does not apply to this hospital for this reporting period; (13) Results cannot be calculated for this reporting period; (14) The results for this state are combined with nearby states to protect confidentiality; Please refer to the User's Guide for a full explanation of data.

Appropriate VTP Within 24 Hours[5]	-	-	98%	98%
Controlled Postoperative Blood Glucose[5]	-	-	98%	97%
Perioperative Temperature Management[5]	-	-	100%	100%
Prophylactic Antibiotic Selection[5]	-	-	99%	99%
Prophylactic Antibiotic Selection (Outpatient)[5]	-	-	98%	98%
Prophylactic Antibiotic Stopped[5]	-	-	98%	98%
Prophylactic Antibiotic Timing[5]	-	-	99%	99%
Prophylactic Antibiotic Timing (Outpatient)[5]	-	-	98%	98%
Urinary Catheter Removal[5]	-	-	97%	97%
Survey of Patients' Hospital Experiences				
Area Around Room 'Always' Quiet at Night[5]	-	-	65%	61%
Doctors 'Always' Communicated Well[5]	-	-	85%	82%
Home Recovery Information Given[5]	-	-	86%	85%
Hospital Given 9 or 10 on 10 Point Scale[5]	-	-	76%	71%
Meds 'Always' Explained Before Given[5]	-	-	66%	64%
Nurses 'Always' Communicated Well[5]	-	-	81%	79%
Pain 'Always' Well Controlled[5]	-	-	72%	71%
Room and Bathroom 'Always' Clean[5]	-	-	76%	73%
Timely Help 'Always' Received[5]	-	-	72%	68%
Would Definitely Recommend Hospital[5]	-	-	75%	71%
Use of Medical Imaging				
Cardiac Imaging Stress Test before Surgery[7]	-	-	5%	5.3%
Combination Abdominal CT Scan[1]	-	-	19%	10.5%
Combination Brain/Sinus CT Scan	34	0.0%	2.9%	2.7%
Combination Chest CT Scan[1]	-	-	3.9%	2.7%
Follow-up Mammogram/Ultrasound[7]	-	-	7.8%	8.8%
Lumbar Spine MRI for Low Back Pain[1]	-	-	40.2%	37.2%

Clara Barton Hospital

250 W 9th Street
Hoisington, KS 67544
Phone: 620-653-2114
Fax: 620-653-2350
URL: www.clarabartonhospital.org
Type: Critical Access Hospitals
Emergency Services: Yes
Ownership: Voluntary non-profit - Private
Beds: 48

Key Personnel:
Operating Room. . . . . Robert Arnold, RN
Chair/CEO . . . . Troy Bailey
Radiology. Robert Bowerman
CEO/President. . . . . Curt Colson, CHE
Quality Assurance . . . . Colletta Debes, RN
Infection Control. . . . . Stacey Dolechek
Chief of Medical Staff . . . . Dr. Nathan Knackstedt, DO

Measure	Cases	This Hosp.	State Avg.	U.S. Avg.
Blood Clot Prevention and Treatment				
Anticoagulation Overlap Therapy[5]	-	-	94%	93%
ICU Venous Thromboembolism Prophylaxis[5]	-	-	91%	92%
Incidence of Potentially Preventable VTE[5]	-	-	8%	10%
UFH with Dosages/Platelet Monitoring[5]	-	-	98%	97%
Venous Thromboembolism Prophylaxis[5]	-	-	79%	85%
Warfarin Therapy Discharge Instructions[5]	-	-	84%	75%
Chest Pain/Possible Heart Attack Care				
Aspirin Given Within 24 Hours of Arrival[1]	-	-	94%	96%
Fibrinolytic Meds Within 30 Min. of Arrival[5]	-	-	41%	58%
Average Time to ECG (minutes)[1]	-	-	8	7
Average Time to Transfer (minutes)[5]	-	-	57	60
Children's Asthma Care				
Received Home Management Plan of Care	-	-	-	88%
Received Reliever Medication	-	-	-	100%
Received Systemic Corticosteroids	-	-	-	100%
Emergency Department				
Admittance Decision Time (minutes)[2]	145	42	57	98
Head CT Results Within 45 Min. of Arrival[1,3]	-	-	53%	57%
Patients Who Left ER Before Being Seen[5]	-	-	2%	2%
Time from ER Arrival to Admit. (minutes)[2]	160	188	185	274
Time from ER Arrival to Discharge (minutes)	229	113	104	134
Time in ER Before Being Evaluated (minutes)	256	22	18	26
Time to Pain Meds for Fractures (minutes)[5]	-	-	47	57
Heart Attack Care				
Aspirin Given at Discharge[5]	-	-	99%	99%
Fibrinolytic Meds Within 30 Min. of Arrival[5]	-	-	-	54%
PCI Within 90 Minutes of Arrival[5]	-	-	97%	96%
Statin Prescribed at Discharge[5]	-	-	99%	98%
Heart Failure Care				
ACE Inhibitor or ARB for LVSD[1,3]	-	-	95%	97%
Discharge Instructions Given[1,3]	-	-	91%	94%
Evaluation of LVS Function[1,3]	-	-	94%	99%
Medicare Spending				
Medicare Spending per Patient (ratio)	-	-	0.94	0.98
Pneumonia Care				
Appropriate Initial Antibiotic Given	16	75%	92%	95%
Blood Culture Timing[1]	-	-	98%	98%
Pregnancy and Delivery Care				
Newborn Deliveries Scheduled Early[5]	-	-	12%	6%
Preventive Care				
Immunization for Influenza	69	68%	88%	90%
Immunization for Pneumonia[2]	100	81%	90%	92%
Stroke Care				
Anticoagulation Therapy for Atrial Fibrillation[5]	-	-	88%	95%
Antithrombotic Therapy Timing[5]	-	-	97%	98%
Assessed for Rehabilitation[5]	-	-	97%	97%
Discharged on Antithrombotic Therapy[5]	-	-	98%	99%
Discharged on Statin Medication[5]	-	-	88%	94%
Thrombolytic Therapy Timing[5]	-	-	68%	66%
Venous Thromboembolism Prophylaxis[5]	-	-	93%	94%
Written Stroke Educational Materials Given[5]	-	-	84%	88%
Surgical Care Improvement Project				
Appropriate Beta Blocker Usage[1]	-	-	98%	98%
Appropriate VTP Within 24 Hours	32	91%	98%	98%
Controlled Postoperative Blood Glucose[7]	-	-	98%	97%
Perioperative Temperature Management	35	100%	100%	100%
Prophylactic Antibiotic Selection	32	97%	99%	99%
Prophylactic Antibiotic Selection (Outpatient)[5]	-	-	98%	98%
Prophylactic Antibiotic Stopped	32	100%	98%	98%
Prophylactic Antibiotic Timing	32	97%	99%	99%
Prophylactic Antibiotic Timing (Outpatient)[5]	-	-	98%	98%
Urinary Catheter Removal[1]	-	-	97%	97%
Survey of Patients' Hospital Experiences				
Area Around Room 'Always' Quiet at Night[5]	-	-	65%	61%
Doctors 'Always' Communicated Well[5]	-	-	85%	82%
Home Recovery Information Given[5]	-	-	86%	85%
Hospital Given 9 or 10 on 10 Point Scale[5]	-	-	76%	71%
Meds 'Always' Explained Before Given[5]	-	-	66%	64%
Nurses 'Always' Communicated Well[5]	-	-	81%	79%
Pain 'Always' Well Controlled[5]	-	-	72%	71%
Room and Bathroom 'Always' Clean[5]	-	-	76%	73%
Timely Help 'Always' Received[5]	-	-	72%	68%
Would Definitely Recommend Hospital[5]	-	-	75%	71%
Use of Medical Imaging				
Cardiac Imaging Stress Test before Surgery[1]	-	-	5%	5.3%
Combination Abdominal CT Scan	141	37.6%	19%	10.5%
Combination Brain/Sinus CT Scan	102	0.0%	2.9%	2.7%
Combination Chest CT Scan	91	12.1%	3.9%	2.7%
Follow-up Mammogram/Ultrasound	138	1.4%	7.8%	8.8%
Lumbar Spine MRI for Low Back Pain[1]	-	-	40.2%	37.2%

Holton Community Hospital

1110 Columbine Dr
Holton, KS 66436
Phone: 785-364-2116
Type: Critical Access Hospitals
Emergency Services: Yes
Ownership: Voluntary non-profit - Private

Key Personnel:
Radiology. . . . . Deb Davies
Cardiac Laboratory. . . . . Beth Nelson
CEO . . . . Carrie Saia
Operating Room. . . . . April Zeller

Measure	Cases	This Hosp.	State Avg.	U.S. Avg.
Blood Clot Prevention and Treatment				
Anticoagulation Overlap Therapy[5]	-	-	94%	93%
ICU Venous Thromboembolism Prophylaxis[5]	-	-	91%	92%
Incidence of Potentially Preventable VTE[5]	-	-	8%	10%
UFH with Dosages/Platelet Monitoring[5]	-	-	98%	97%
Venous Thromboembolism Prophylaxis[5]	-	-	79%	85%
Warfarin Therapy Discharge Instructions[5]	-	-	84%	75%
Chest Pain/Possible Heart Attack Care				
Aspirin Given Within 24 Hours of Arrival	19	95%	94%	96%
Fibrinolytic Meds Within 30 Min. of Arrival[3,7]	-	-	41%	58%
Average Time to ECG (minutes)	22	8	8	7
Average Time to Transfer (minutes)[1,3]	-	-	57	60
Children's Asthma Care				
Received Home Management Plan of Care	-	-	-	88%
Received Reliever Medication	-	-	-	100%
Received Systemic Corticosteroids	-	-	-	100%
Emergency Department				
Admittance Decision Time (minutes)	59	10	57	98
Head CT Results Within 45 Min. of Arrival[5]	-	-	53%	57%
Patients Who Left ER Before Being Seen[5]	-	-	2%	2%
Time from ER Arrival to Admit. (minutes)	71	150	185	274
Time from ER Arrival to Discharge (minutes)[5]	-	-	104	134
Time in ER Before Being Evaluated (minutes)[5]	-	-	18	26
Time to Pain Meds for Fractures (minutes)[5]	-	-	47	57
Heart Attack Care				
Aspirin Given at Discharge[5]	-	-	99%	99%
Fibrinolytic Meds Within 30 Min. of Arrival[5]	-	-	-	54%
PCI Within 90 Minutes of Arrival[5]	-	-	97%	96%
Statin Prescribed at Discharge[5]	-	-	99%	98%
Heart Failure Care				
ACE Inhibitor or ARB for LVSD[1,3]	-	-	95%	97%
Discharge Instructions Given[1,3]	-	-	91%	94%
Evaluation of LVS Function[3]	12	92%	94%	99%
Medicare Spending				
Medicare Spending per Patient (ratio)	-	-	0.94	0.98
Pneumonia Care				
Appropriate Initial Antibiotic Given	16	81%	92%	95%
Blood Culture Timing[1]	-	-	98%	98%
Pregnancy and Delivery Care				
Newborn Deliveries Scheduled Early[5]	-	-	12%	6%
Preventive Care				
Immunization for Influenza	75	97%	88%	90%
Immunization for Pneumonia	120	91%	90%	92%
Stroke Care				
Anticoagulation Therapy for Atrial Fibrillation[5]	-	-	88%	95%
Antithrombotic Therapy Timing[5]	-	-	97%	98%
Assessed for Rehabilitation[5]	-	-	97%	97%
Discharged on Antithrombotic Therapy[5]	-	-	98%	99%
Discharged on Statin Medication[5]	-	-	88%	94%
Thrombolytic Therapy Timing[5]	-	-	68%	66%
Venous Thromboembolism Prophylaxis[5]	-	-	93%	94%
Written Stroke Educational Materials Given[5]	-	-	84%	88%
Surgical Care Improvement Project				
Appropriate Beta Blocker Usage[5]	-	-	98%	98%
Appropriate VTP Within 24 Hours[5]	-	-	98%	98%
Controlled Postoperative Blood Glucose[5]	-	-	98%	97%
Perioperative Temperature Management[5]	-	-	100%	100%
Prophylactic Antibiotic Selection[5]	-	-	99%	99%
Prophylactic Antibiotic Selection (Outpatient)[1,3]	-	-	98%	98%
Prophylactic Antibiotic Stopped[5]	-	-	98%	98%
Prophylactic Antibiotic Timing[5]	-	-	99%	99%
Prophylactic Antibiotic Timing (Outpatient)[1,3]	-	-	98%	98%
Urinary Catheter Removal[5]	-	-	97%	97%
Survey of Patients' Hospital Experiences				
Area Around Room 'Always' Quiet at Night[10]	<100	72%	65%	61%
Doctors 'Always' Communicated Well[10]	<100	96%	85%	82%
Home Recovery Information Given[10]	<100	90%	86%	85%
Hospital Given 9 or 10 on 10 Point Scale[10]	<100	74%	76%	71%
Meds 'Always' Explained Before Given[10]	<100	67%	66%	64%
Nurses 'Always' Communicated Well[10]	<100	90%	81%	79%
Pain 'Always' Well Controlled[10]	<100	81%	72%	71%
Room and Bathroom 'Always' Clean[10]	<100	71%	76%	73%
Timely Help 'Always' Received[10]	<100	72%	72%	68%
Would Definitely Recommend Hospital[10]	<100	66%	75%	71%
Use of Medical Imaging				
Cardiac Imaging Stress Test before Surgery	110	6.4%	5%	5.3%
Combination Abdominal CT Scan	95	11.6%	19%	10.5%
Combination Brain/Sinus CT Scan[1]	-	-	2.9%	2.7%
Combination Chest CT Scan	64	1.6%	3.9%	2.7%
Follow-up Mammogram/Ultrasound	267	5.6%	7.8%	8.8%
Lumbar Spine MRI for Low Back Pain[1]	-	-	40.2%	37.2%

NOTE: Hospital profiles are in alphabetical order by state, then city, then hospital within the city; Rankings exclude hospitals with less than 25 cases except for patient surveys which excludes hospitals with less than 100 cases; (a) 100-299 cases; (1) The number of cases/patients is too few to report; (2) Data submitted were based on a sample of cases/patients; (3) Results are based on a shorter time period than required; (4) Data suppressed by CMS for one or more quarters; (5) Results are not available for this reporting period; (6) Fewer than 100 patients completed the HCAHPS survey; (7) No cases met the criteria for this measure; (8) The lower limit of the confidence interval cannot be calculated if the number of observed infections equals zero; (9) No data are available from the state/territory for this reporting period; (10) The scores shown reflect fewer than 50 completed surveys; (11) There were discrepancies in the data collection process; (12) This measure does not apply to this hospital for this reporting period; (13) Results cannot be calculated for this reporting period; (14) The results for this state are combined with nearby states to protect confidentiality; Please refer to the User's Guide for a full explanation of data.

Horton Community Hospital

240 West 18th Street
Horton, KS 66439
Phone: 785-486-2642
Type: Critical Access Hospitals
Emergency Services: Yes
Ownership: Proprietary

Measure	Cases	This Hosp.	State Avg.	U.S. Avg.
Blood Clot Prevention and Treatment				
Anticoagulation Overlap Therapy	-	-	94%	93%
ICU Venous Thromboembolism Prophylaxis	-	-	91%	92%
Incidence of Potentially Preventable VTE	-	-	8%	10%
UFH with Dosages/Platelet Monitoring	-	-	98%	97%
Venous Thromboembolism Prophylaxis	-	-	79%	85%
Warfarin Therapy Discharge Instructions	-	-	84%	75%
Chest Pain/Possible Heart Attack Care				
Aspirin Given Within 24 Hours of Arrival[5]	-	-	94%	96%
Fibrinolytic Meds Within 30 Min. of Arrival[5]	-	-	41%	58%
Average Time to ECG (minutes)[5]	-	-	8	7
Average Time to Transfer (minutes)[5]	-	-	57	60
Children's Asthma Care				
Received Home Management Plan of Care	-	-	-	88%
Received Reliever Medication	-	-	-	100%
Received Systemic Corticosteroids	-	-	-	100%
Emergency Department				
Admittance Decision Time (minutes)	-	-	57	98
Head CT Results Within 45 Min. of Arrival[5]	-	-	53%	57%
Patients Who Left ER Before Being Seen[5]	-	-	2%	2%
Time from ER Arrival to Admit. (minutes)	-	-	185	274
Time from ER Arrival to Discharge (minutes)[5]	-	-	104	134
Time in ER Before Being Evaluated (minutes)[5]	-	-	18	26
Time to Pain Meds for Fractures (minutes)[5]	-	-	47	57
Heart Attack Care				
Aspirin Given at Discharge	-	-	99%	99%
Fibrinolytic Meds Within 30 Min. of Arrival	-	-	-	54%
PCI Within 90 Minutes of Arrival	-	-	97%	96%
Statin Prescribed at Discharge	-	-	99%	98%
Heart Failure Care				
ACE Inhibitor or ARB for LVSD	-	-	95%	97%
Discharge Instructions Given	-	-	91%	94%
Evaluation of LVS Function	-	-	94%	99%
Medicare Spending				
Medicare Spending per Patient (ratio)	-	-	0.94	0.98
Pneumonia Care				
Appropriate Initial Antibiotic Given	-	-	92%	95%
Blood Culture Timing	-	-	98%	98%
Pregnancy and Delivery Care				
Newborn Deliveries Scheduled Early	-	-	12%	6%
Preventive Care				
Immunization for Influenza	-	-	88%	90%
Immunization for Pneumonia	-	-	90%	92%
Stroke Care				
Anticoagulation Therapy for Atrial Fibrillation	-	-	88%	95%
Antithrombotic Therapy Timing	-	-	97%	98%
Assessed for Rehabilitation	-	-	97%	97%
Discharged on Antithrombotic Therapy	-	-	98%	99%
Discharged on Statin Medication	-	-	88%	94%
Thrombolytic Therapy Timing	-	-	68%	66%
Venous Thromboembolism Prophylaxis	-	-	93%	94%
Written Stroke Educational Materials Given	-	-	84%	88%
Surgical Care Improvement Project				
Appropriate Beta Blocker Usage	-	-	98%	98%
Appropriate VTP Within 24 Hours	-	-	98%	98%
Controlled Postoperative Blood Glucose	-	-	98%	97%
Perioperative Temperature Management	-	-	100%	100%
Prophylactic Antibiotic Selection	-	-	99%	99%
Prophylactic Antibiotic Selection (Outpatient)[5]	-	-	98%	98%
Prophylactic Antibiotic Stopped	-	-	98%	98%
Prophylactic Antibiotic Timing	-	-	99%	99%
Prophylactic Antibiotic Timing (Outpatient)[5]	-	-	98%	98%
Urinary Catheter Removal	-	-	97%	97%
Survey of Patients' Hospital Experiences				
Area Around Room 'Always' Quiet at Night	-	-	65%	61%
Doctors 'Always' Communicated Well	-	-	85%	82%
Home Recovery Information Given	-	-	86%	85%
Hospital Given 9 or 10 on 10 Point Scale	-	-	76%	71%
Meds 'Always' Explained Before Given	-	-	66%	64%
Nurses 'Always' Communicated Well	-	-	81%	79%
Pain 'Always' Well Controlled	-	-	72%	71%
Room and Bathroom 'Always' Clean	-	-	76%	73%
Timely Help 'Always' Received	-	-	72%	68%
Would Definitely Recommend Hospital	-	-	75%	71%
Use of Medical Imaging				
Cardiac Imaging Stress Test before Surgery[1]	-	-	5%	5.3%
Combination Abdominal CT Scan[1]	-	-	19%	10.5%
Combination Brain/Sinus CT Scan[1]	-	-	2.9%	2.7%
Combination Chest CT Scan[1]	-	-	3.9%	2.7%
Follow-up Mammogram/Ultrasound[1]	-	-	7.8%	8.8%
Lumbar Spine MRI for Low Back Pain[1]	-	-	40.2%	37.2%

Sheridan County Hospital

826 18th Street
Hoxie, KS 67740
Phone: 785-675-3281
URL: www.sheridanhospital.org
Type: Critical Access Hospitals
Emergency Services: Yes
Ownership: Government - Local

Key Personnel:

Radiology. . . . . Daniel R. Alzheimer, M.D.
Pediatrics. . . . . Mary I. Bowers, M.D.
Cardiology . . . . Michael W. Brennan, M.D.
Anesthesiology. . . . . Bradley G. Hanebrink, D.O.
CEO . . . . Mike McCafferty

Measure	Cases	This Hosp.	State Avg.	U.S. Avg.
Blood Clot Prevention and Treatment				
Anticoagulation Overlap Therapy[5]	-	-	94%	93%
ICU Venous Thromboembolism Prophylaxis[5]	-	-	91%	92%
Incidence of Potentially Preventable VTE[5]	-	-	8%	10%
UFH with Dosages/Platelet Monitoring[5]	-	-	98%	97%
Venous Thromboembolism Prophylaxis[5]	-	-	79%	85%
Warfarin Therapy Discharge Instructions[5]	-	-	84%	75%
Chest Pain/Possible Heart Attack Care				
Aspirin Given Within 24 Hours of Arrival	-	-	94%	96%
Fibrinolytic Meds Within 30 Min. of Arrival	-	-	41%	58%
Average Time to ECG (minutes)	-	-	8	7
Average Time to Transfer (minutes)	-	-	57	60
Children's Asthma Care				
Received Home Management Plan of Care	-	-	-	88%
Received Reliever Medication	-	-	-	100%
Received Systemic Corticosteroids	-	-	-	100%
Emergency Department				
Admittance Decision Time (minutes)[5]	-	-	57	98
Head CT Results Within 45 Min. of Arrival	-	-	53%	57%
Patients Who Left ER Before Being Seen	-	-	2%	2%
Time from ER Arrival to Admit. (minutes)[5]	-	-	185	274
Time from ER Arrival to Discharge (minutes)	-	-	104	134
Time in ER Before Being Evaluated (minutes)	-	-	18	26
Time to Pain Meds for Fractures (minutes)	-	-	47	57
Heart Attack Care				
Aspirin Given at Discharge[3,7]	-	-	99%	99%
Fibrinolytic Meds Within 30 Min. of Arrival[3,7]	-	-	-	54%
PCI Within 90 Minutes of Arrival[3,7]	-	-	97%	96%
Statin Prescribed at Discharge[3,7]	-	-	99%	98%
Heart Failure Care				
ACE Inhibitor or ARB for LVSD[3,7]	-	-	95%	97%
Discharge Instructions Given[1,3]	-	-	91%	94%
Evaluation of LVS Function[1,3]	-	-	94%	99%
Medicare Spending				
Medicare Spending per Patient (ratio)	-	-	0.94	0.98
Pneumonia Care				
Appropriate Initial Antibiotic Given[1]	-	-	92%	95%
Blood Culture Timing[7]	-	-	98%	98%
Pregnancy and Delivery Care				
Newborn Deliveries Scheduled Early[5]	-	-	12%	6%
Preventive Care				
Immunization for Influenza[1,3]	-	-	88%	90%
Immunization for Pneumonia[1,3]	-	-	90%	92%
Stroke Care				
Anticoagulation Therapy for Atrial Fibrillation[5]	-	-	88%	95%
Antithrombotic Therapy Timing[5]	-	-	97%	98%
Assessed for Rehabilitation[5]	-	-	97%	97%
Discharged on Antithrombotic Therapy[5]	-	-	98%	99%
Discharged on Statin Medication[5]	-	-	88%	94%
Thrombolytic Therapy Timing[5]	-	-	68%	66%
Venous Thromboembolism Prophylaxis[5]	-	-	93%	94%
Written Stroke Educational Materials Given[5]	-	-	84%	88%
Surgical Care Improvement Project				
Appropriate Beta Blocker Usage[5]	-	-	98%	98%
Appropriate VTP Within 24 Hours[5]	-	-	98%	98%
Controlled Postoperative Blood Glucose[5]	-	-	98%	97%
Perioperative Temperature Management[5]	-	-	100%	100%
Prophylactic Antibiotic Selection[5]	-	-	99%	99%
Prophylactic Antibiotic Selection (Outpatient)	-	-	98%	98%
Prophylactic Antibiotic Stopped[5]	-	-	98%	98%
Prophylactic Antibiotic Timing[5]	-	-	99%	99%
Prophylactic Antibiotic Timing (Outpatient)	-	-	98%	98%
Urinary Catheter Removal[5]	-	-	97%	97%
Survey of Patients' Hospital Experiences				
Area Around Room 'Always' Quiet at Night[5]	-	-	65%	61%
Doctors 'Always' Communicated Well[5]	-	-	85%	82%
Home Recovery Information Given[5]	-	-	86%	85%
Hospital Given 9 or 10 on 10 Point Scale[5]	-	-	76%	71%
Meds 'Always' Explained Before Given[5]	-	-	66%	64%
Nurses 'Always' Communicated Well[5]	-	-	81%	79%
Pain 'Always' Well Controlled[5]	-	-	72%	71%
Room and Bathroom 'Always' Clean[5]	-	-	76%	73%
Timely Help 'Always' Received[5]	-	-	72%	68%
Would Definitely Recommend Hospital[5]	-	-	75%	71%
Use of Medical Imaging				
Cardiac Imaging Stress Test before Surgery	-	-	5%	5.3%
Combination Abdominal CT Scan	-	-	19%	10.5%
Combination Brain/Sinus CT Scan	-	-	2.9%	2.7%
Combination Chest CT Scan	-	-	3.9%	2.7%
Follow-up Mammogram/Ultrasound	-	-	7.8%	8.8%
Lumbar Spine MRI for Low Back Pain	-	-	40.2%	37.2%

Stevens County Hospital

1006 S Jackson
Hugoton, KS 67951
Phone: 620-544-6178
Type: Critical Access Hospitals
Emergency Services: Yes
Ownership: Government - Local

Measure	Cases	This Hosp.	State Avg.	U.S. Avg.
Blood Clot Prevention and Treatment				
Anticoagulation Overlap Therapy[5]	-	-	94%	93%
ICU Venous Thromboembolism Prophylaxis[5]	-	-	91%	92%
Incidence of Potentially Preventable VTE[5]	-	-	8%	10%
UFH with Dosages/Platelet Monitoring[5]	-	-	98%	97%
Venous Thromboembolism Prophylaxis[5]	-	-	79%	85%
Warfarin Therapy Discharge Instructions[5]	-	-	84%	75%
Chest Pain/Possible Heart Attack Care				
Aspirin Given Within 24 Hours of Arrival	-	-	94%	96%
Fibrinolytic Meds Within 30 Min. of Arrival	-	-	41%	58%
Average Time to ECG (minutes)	-	-	8	7
Average Time to Transfer (minutes)	-	-	57	60
Children's Asthma Care				
Received Home Management Plan of Care	-	-	-	88%
Received Reliever Medication	-	-	-	100%
Received Systemic Corticosteroids	-	-	-	100%
Emergency Department				
Admittance Decision Time (minutes)[1,3]	-	-	57	98
Head CT Results Within 45 Min. of Arrival	-	-	53%	57%
Patients Who Left ER Before Being Seen	-	-	2%	2%
Time from ER Arrival to Admit. (minutes)[1,3]	-	-	185	274
Time from ER Arrival to Discharge (minutes)	-	-	104	134
Time in ER Before Being Evaluated (minutes)	-	-	18	26
Time to Pain Meds for Fractures (minutes)	-	-	47	57
Heart Attack Care				
Aspirin Given at Discharge[5]	-	-	99%	99%
Fibrinolytic Meds Within 30 Min. of Arrival[5]	-	-	-	54%
PCI Within 90 Minutes of Arrival[5]	-	-	97%	96%
Statin Prescribed at Discharge[5]	-	-	99%	98%

NOTE: Hospital profiles are in alphabetical order by state, then city, then hospital within the city; Rankings exclude hospitals with less than 25 cases except for patient surveys which excludes hospitals with less than 100 cases; (a) 100-299 cases; (1) The number of cases/patients is too few to report; (2) Data submitted were based on a sample of cases/patients; (3) Results are based on a shorter time period than required; (4) Data suppressed by CMS for one or more quarters; (5) Results are not available for this reporting period; (6) Fewer than 100 patients completed the HCAHPS survey; (7) No cases met the criteria for this measure; (8) The lower limit of the confidence interval cannot be calculated if the number of observed infections equals zero; (9) No data are available from the state/territory for this reporting period; (10) The scores shown reflect fewer than 50 completed surveys; (11) There were discrepancies in the data collection process; (12) This measure does not apply to this hospital for this reporting period; (13) Results cannot be calculated for this reporting period; (14) The results for this state are combined with nearby states to protect confidentiality; Please refer to the User's Guide for a full explanation of data.

Measure	Cases	This Hosp.	State Avg.	U.S. Avg.
Heart Failure Care				
ACE Inhibitor or ARB for LVSD[1,3]	-	-	95%	97%
Discharge Instructions Given[1,3]	-	-	91%	94%
Evaluation of LVS Function[1,3]	-	-	94%	99%
Medicare Spending				
Medicare Spending per Patient (ratio)	-	-	0.94	0.98
Pneumonia Care				
Appropriate Initial Antibiotic Given[3]	13	31%	92%	95%
Blood Culture Timing[1,3]	-	-	98%	98%
Pregnancy and Delivery Care				
Newborn Deliveries Scheduled Early[5]	-	-	12%	6%
Preventive Care				
Immunization for Influenza[1,3]	-	-	88%	90%
Immunization for Pneumonia[3]	23	61%	90%	92%
Stroke Care				
Anticoagulation Therapy for Atrial Fibrillation[5]	-	-	88%	95%
Antithrombotic Therapy Timing[5]	-	-	97%	98%
Assessed for Rehabilitation[5]	-	-	97%	97%
Discharged on Antithrombotic Therapy[5]	-	-	98%	99%
Discharged on Statin Medication[5]	-	-	88%	94%
Thrombolytic Therapy Timing[5]	-	-	68%	66%
Venous Thromboembolism Prophylaxis[5]	-	-	93%	94%
Written Stroke Educational Materials Given[5]	-	-	84%	88%
Surgical Care Improvement Project				
Appropriate Beta Blocker Usage[5]	-	-	98%	98%
Appropriate VTP Within 24 Hours[5]	-	-	98%	98%
Controlled Postoperative Blood Glucose[5]	-	-	98%	97%
Perioperative Temperature Management[5]	-	-	100%	100%
Prophylactic Antibiotic Selection[5]	-	-	99%	99%
Prophylactic Antibiotic Selection (Outpatient)	-	-	98%	98%
Prophylactic Antibiotic Stopped[5]	-	-	98%	98%
Prophylactic Antibiotic Timing[5]	-	-	99%	99%
Prophylactic Antibiotic Timing (Outpatient)	-	-	98%	98%
Urinary Catheter Removal[5]	-	-	97%	97%
Survey of Patients' Hospital Experiences				
Area Around Room 'Always' Quiet at Night[5]	-	-	65%	61%
Doctors 'Always' Communicated Well[5]	-	-	85%	82%
Home Recovery Information Given[5]	-	-	86%	85%
Hospital Given 9 or 10 on 10 Point Scale[5]	-	-	76%	71%
Meds 'Always' Explained Before Given[5]	-	-	66%	64%
Nurses 'Always' Communicated Well[5]	-	-	81%	79%
Pain 'Always' Well Controlled[5]	-	-	72%	71%
Room and Bathroom 'Always' Clean[5]	-	-	76%	73%
Timely Help 'Always' Received[5]	-	-	72%	68%
Would Definitely Recommend Hospital[5]	-	-	75%	71%
Use of Medical Imaging				
Cardiac Imaging Stress Test before Surgery	-	-	5%	5.3%
Combination Abdominal CT Scan	-	-	19%	10.5%
Combination Brain/Sinus CT Scan	-	-	2.9%	2.7%
Combination Chest CT Scan	-	-	3.9%	2.7%
Follow-up Mammogram/Ultrasound	-	-	7.8%	8.8%
Lumbar Spine MRI for Low Back Pain	-	-	40.2%	37.2%

Hutchinson Regional Medical Center

1701 E 23rd Avenue
Hutchinson, KS 67502
Phone: 620-665-2001
Fax: 620-513-3811
E-mail: info@hhosp.com
URL: www.hutchinsonhospital.com
Type: Acute Care Hospitals
Ownership: Proprietary
Emergency Services: Yes
Beds: 200
Key Personnel:
CEO/President. . . . . Mark Norrell

Measure	Cases	This Hosp.	State Avg.	U.S. Avg.
Blood Clot Prevention and Treatment				
Anticoagulation Overlap Therapy[2]	55	78%	94%	93%
ICU Venous Thromboembolism Prophylaxis[2]	134	50%	91%	92%
Incidence of Potentially Preventable VTE[2]	16	69%	8%	10%
UFH with Dosages/Platelet Monitoring[1,2]	-	-	98%	97%
Venous Thromboembolism Prophylaxis[2]	365	41%	79%	85%
Warfarin Therapy Discharge Instructions[2]	38	84%	84%	75%
Chest Pain/Possible Heart Attack Care				
Aspirin Given Within 24 Hours of Arrival[1]	-	-	94%	96%
Fibrinolytic Meds Within 30 Min. of Arrival[5]	-	-	41%	58%
Average Time to ECG (minutes)[1]	-	-	8	7
Average Time to Transfer (minutes)[5]	-	-	57	60
Children's Asthma Care				
Received Home Management Plan of Care	-	-	-	88%
Received Reliever Medication	-	-	-	100%
Received Systemic Corticosteroids	-	-	-	100%
Emergency Department				
Admittance Decision Time (minutes)[2]	456	70	57	98
Head CT Results Within 45 Min. of Arrival	12	67%	53%	57%
Patients Who Left ER Before Being Seen	24,777	1%	2%	2%
Time from ER Arrival to Admit. (minutes)[2]	499	203	185	274
Time from ER Arrival to Discharge (minutes)	556	110	104	134
Time in ER Before Being Evaluated (minutes)	372	41	18	26
Time to Pain Meds for Fractures (minutes)	108	59	47	57
Heart Attack Care				
Aspirin Given at Discharge	152	100%	99%	99%
Fibrinolytic Meds Within 30 Min. of Arrival[7]	-	-	-	54%
PCI Within 90 Minutes of Arrival	27	96%	97%	96%
Statin Prescribed at Discharge	138	100%	99%	98%
Heart Failure Care				
ACE Inhibitor or ARB for LVSD	62	100%	95%	97%
Discharge Instructions Given	113	97%	91%	94%
Evaluation of LVS Function	146	100%	94%	99%
Medicare Spending				
Medicare Spending per Patient (ratio)	-	0.97	0.94	0.98
Pneumonia Care				
Appropriate Initial Antibiotic Given	112	100%	92%	95%
Blood Culture Timing	140	99%	98%	98%
Pregnancy and Delivery Care				
Newborn Deliveries Scheduled Early	60	2%	12%	6%
Preventive Care				
Immunization for Influenza[2]	580	85%	88%	90%
Immunization for Pneumonia[2]	820	87%	90%	92%
Stroke Care				
Anticoagulation Therapy for Atrial Fibrillation[1]	-	-	88%	95%
Antithrombotic Therapy Timing	47	91%	97%	98%
Assessed for Rehabilitation	50	94%	97%	97%
Discharged on Antithrombotic Therapy	49	96%	98%	99%
Discharged on Statin Medication	39	69%	88%	94%
Thrombolytic Therapy Timing[1]	-	-	68%	66%
Venous Thromboembolism Prophylaxis	50	56%	93%	94%
Written Stroke Educational Materials Given	24	50%	84%	88%
Surgical Care Improvement Project				
Appropriate Beta Blocker Usage	212	99%	98%	98%
Appropriate VTP Within 24 Hours	445	100%	98%	98%
Controlled Postoperative Blood Glucose	124	98%	98%	97%
Perioperative Temperature Management	551	100%	100%	100%
Prophylactic Antibiotic Selection	459	99%	99%	99%
Prophylactic Antibiotic Selection (Outpatient)	246	99%	98%	98%
Prophylactic Antibiotic Stopped	430	98%	98%	98%
Prophylactic Antibiotic Timing	461	100%	99%	99%
Prophylactic Antibiotic Timing (Outpatient)	249	98%	98%	98%
Urinary Catheter Removal	398	100%	97%	97%
Survey of Patients' Hospital Experiences				
Area Around Room 'Always' Quiet at Night	300+	43%	65%	61%
Doctors 'Always' Communicated Well	300+	72%	85%	82%
Home Recovery Information Given	300+	81%	86%	85%
Hospital Given 9 or 10 on 10 Point Scale	300+	58%	76%	71%
Meds 'Always' Explained Before Given	300+	52%	66%	64%
Nurses 'Always' Communicated Well	300+	69%	81%	79%
Pain 'Always' Well Controlled	300+	62%	72%	71%
Room and Bathroom 'Always' Clean	300+	63%	76%	73%
Timely Help 'Always' Received	300+	60%	72%	68%
Would Definitely Recommend Hospital	300+	58%	75%	71%
Use of Medical Imaging				
Cardiac Imaging Stress Test before Surgery	97	6.2%	5%	5.3%
Combination Abdominal CT Scan	344	0.6%	19%	10.5%
Combination Brain/Sinus CT Scan[1]	-	-	2.9%	2.7%
Combination Chest CT Scan	78	0.0%	3.9%	2.7%
Follow-up Mammogram/Ultrasound[7]	-	-	7.8%	8.8%
Lumbar Spine MRI for Low Back Pain[1]	-	-	40.2%	37.2%

Summit Surgical

1818 East 23rd Avenue
Hutchinson, KS 67502
Phone: 620-662-6000
URL: www.summitks.com
Type: Acute Care Hospitals
Ownership: Physician
Emergency Services: No
Beds: 6

Measure	Cases	This Hosp.	State Avg.	U.S. Avg.
Blood Clot Prevention and Treatment				
Anticoagulation Overlap Therapy[7]	-	-	94%	93%
ICU Venous Thromboembolism Prophylaxis[7]	-	-	91%	92%
Incidence of Potentially Preventable VTE[7]	-	-	8%	10%
UFH with Dosages/Platelet Monitoring[7]	-	-	98%	97%
Venous Thromboembolism Prophylaxis[1]	-	-	79%	85%
Warfarin Therapy Discharge Instructions[7]	-	-	84%	75%
Chest Pain/Possible Heart Attack Care				
Aspirin Given Within 24 Hours of Arrival[5]	-	-	94%	96%
Fibrinolytic Meds Within 30 Min. of Arrival[5]	-	-	41%	58%
Average Time to ECG (minutes)[5]	-	-	8	7
Average Time to Transfer (minutes)[5]	-	-	57	60
Children's Asthma Care				
Received Home Management Plan of Care	-	-	-	88%
Received Reliever Medication	-	-	-	100%
Received Systemic Corticosteroids	-	-	-	100%
Emergency Department				
Admittance Decision Time (minutes)[7]	-	-	57	98
Head CT Results Within 45 Min. of Arrival[5]	-	-	53%	57%
Patients Who Left ER Before Being Seen[5]	-	-	2%	2%
Time from ER Arrival to Admit. (minutes)[7]	-	-	185	274
Time from ER Arrival to Discharge (minutes)[5]	-	-	104	134
Time in ER Before Being Evaluated (minutes)[5]	-	-	18	26
Time to Pain Meds for Fractures (minutes)[5]	-	-	47	57
Heart Attack Care				
Aspirin Given at Discharge[5]	-	-	99%	99%
Fibrinolytic Meds Within 30 Min. of Arrival[5]	-	-	-	54%
PCI Within 90 Minutes of Arrival[5]	-	-	97%	96%
Statin Prescribed at Discharge[5]	-	-	99%	98%
Heart Failure Care				
ACE Inhibitor or ARB for LVSD[5]	-	-	95%	97%
Discharge Instructions Given[5]	-	-	91%	94%
Evaluation of LVS Function[5]	-	-	94%	99%
Medicare Spending				
Medicare Spending per Patient (ratio)	-	0.81	0.94	0.98
Pneumonia Care				
Appropriate Initial Antibiotic Given[5]	-	-	92%	95%
Blood Culture Timing[5]	-	-	98%	98%
Pregnancy and Delivery Care				
Newborn Deliveries Scheduled Early[7]	-	-	12%	6%
Preventive Care				
Immunization for Influenza	109	100%	88%	90%
Immunization for Pneumonia	125	99%	90%	92%
Stroke Care				
Anticoagulation Therapy for Atrial Fibrillation[5]	-	-	88%	95%
Antithrombotic Therapy Timing[5]	-	-	97%	98%
Assessed for Rehabilitation[5]	-	-	97%	97%
Discharged on Antithrombotic Therapy[5]	-	-	98%	99%
Discharged on Statin Medication[5]	-	-	88%	94%
Thrombolytic Therapy Timing[5]	-	-	68%	66%
Venous Thromboembolism Prophylaxis[5]	-	-	93%	94%
Written Stroke Educational Materials Given[5]	-	-	84%	88%
Surgical Care Improvement Project				
Appropriate Beta Blocker Usage	41	100%	98%	98%
Appropriate VTP Within 24 Hours	172	99%	98%	98%
Controlled Postoperative Blood Glucose[7]	-	-	98%	97%
Perioperative Temperature Management	211	100%	100%	100%
Prophylactic Antibiotic Selection	209	99%	99%	99%
Prophylactic Antibiotic Selection (Outpatient)[1,3]	-	-	98%	98%
Prophylactic Antibiotic Stopped	209	100%	98%	98%
Prophylactic Antibiotic Timing	209	99%	99%	99%
Prophylactic Antibiotic Timing (Outpatient)[1,3]	-	-	98%	98%
Urinary Catheter Removal	166	100%	97%	97%
Survey of Patients' Hospital Experiences				
Area Around Room 'Always' Quiet at Night[6]	<100	86%	65%	61%

NOTE: Hospital profiles are in alphabetical order by state, then city, then hospital within the city; Rankings exclude hospitals with less than 25 cases except for patient surveys which excludes hospitals with less than 100 cases; (a) 100-299 cases; (1) The number of cases/patients is too few to report; (2) Data submitted were based on a sample of cases/patients; (3) Results are based on a shorter time period than required; (4) Data suppressed by CMS for one or more quarters; (5) Results are not available for this reporting period; (6) Fewer than 100 patients completed the HCAHPS survey; (7) No cases met the criteria for this measure; (8) The lower limit of the confidence interval cannot be calculated if the number of observed infections equals zero; (9) No data are available from the state/territory for this reporting period; (10) The scores shown reflect fewer than 50 completed surveys; (11) There were discrepancies in the data collection process; (12) This measure does not apply to this hospital for this reporting period; (13) Results cannot be calculated for this reporting period; (14) The results for this state are combined with nearby states to protect confidentiality; Please refer to the User's Guide for a full explanation of data.

Doctors 'Always' Communicated Well[6]	<100	86%	85%	82%
Home Recovery Information Given[6]	<100	93%	86%	85%
Hospital Given 9 or 10 on 10 Point Scale[6]	<100	90%	76%	71%
Meds 'Always' Explained Before Given[6]	<100	72%	66%	64%
Nurses 'Always' Communicated Well[6]	<100	87%	81%	79%
Pain 'Always' Well Controlled[6]	<100	76%	72%	71%
Room and Bathroom 'Always' Clean[6]	<100	85%	76%	73%
Timely Help 'Always' Received[6]	<100	85%	72%	68%
Would Definitely Recommend Hospital[6]	<100	87%	75%	71%
Use of Medical Imaging				
Cardiac Imaging Stress Test before Surgery[7]	-	-	5%	5.3%
Combination Abdominal CT Scan[7]	-	-	19%	10.5%
Combination Brain/Sinus CT Scan[7]	-	-	2.9%	2.7%
Combination Chest CT Scan[7]	-	-	3.9%	2.7%
Follow-up Mammogram/Ultrasound[7]	-	-	7.8%	8.8%
Lumbar Spine MRI for Low Back Pain[7]	-	-	40.2%	37.2%

Mercy Hospital Independence

800 West Myrtle Street
Independence, KS 67301
Phone: 620-331-2200
Fax: 620-332-3270
Type: Acute Care Hospitals
Emergency Services: Yes
Ownership: Voluntary non-profit - Church
Beds: 93

Key Personnel:
Quality Assurance . . . . Eric Asmussen
Emergency Room . . . . Charles Empson, MD
Infection Control. . . . . Michelle Foreman
Intensive Care Unit. . . . . Michelle Foreman
Operating Room. . . . . Ralph Hall
Radiology. . . . . Kevin Hamm, MD
Chief of Medical Staff. . . . . Cathey Henisey
CEO/President. . . . . John Woodrich

Measure	Cases	This Hosp.	State Avg.	U.S. Avg.
Blood Clot Prevention and Treatment				
Anticoagulation Overlap Therapy[1,2]	-	-	94%	93%
ICU Venous Thromboembolism Prophylaxis[2]	33	88%	91%	92%
Incidence of Potentially Preventable VTE[1,2]	-	-	8%	10%
UFH with Dosages/Platelet Monitoring[2,7]	-	-	98%	97%
Venous Thromboembolism Prophylaxis[2]	73	66%	79%	85%
Warfarin Therapy Discharge Instructions[1,2]	-	-	84%	75%
Chest Pain/Possible Heart Attack Care				
Aspirin Given Within 24 Hours of Arrival	64	95%	94%	96%
Fibrinolytic Meds Within 30 Min. of Arrival[7]	-	-	41%	58%
Average Time to ECG (minutes)	60	1	8	7
Average Time to Transfer (minutes)[1]	-	-	57	60
Children's Asthma Care				
Received Home Management Plan of Care	-	-	-	88%
Received Reliever Medication	-	-	-	100%
Received Systemic Corticosteroids	-	-	-	100%
Emergency Department				
Admittance Decision Time (minutes)[2]	212	45	57	98
Head CT Results Within 45 Min. of Arrival[1]	-	-	53%	57%
Patients Who Left ER Before Being Seen	8,846	0%	2%	2%
Time from ER Arrival to Admit. (minutes)[2]	237	174	185	274
Time from ER Arrival to Discharge (minutes)	362	102	104	134
Time in ER Before Being Evaluated (minutes)	390	19	18	26
Time to Pain Meds for Fractures (minutes)	19	31	47	57
Heart Attack Care				
Aspirin Given at Discharge[1,3]	-	-	99%	99%
Fibrinolytic Meds Within 30 Min. of Arrival[3,7]	-	-	-	54%
PCI Within 90 Minutes of Arrival[3,7]	-	-	97%	96%
Statin Prescribed at Discharge[1,3]	-	-	99%	98%
Heart Failure Care				
ACE Inhibitor or ARB for LVSD[1]	-	-	95%	97%
Discharge Instructions Given	15	87%	91%	94%
Evaluation of LVS Function	25	92%	94%	99%
Medicare Spending				
Medicare Spending per Patient (ratio)	-	0.93	0.94	0.98
Pneumonia Care				
Appropriate Initial Antibiotic Given	16	94%	92%	95%
Blood Culture Timing	33	100%	98%	98%
Pregnancy and Delivery Care				
Newborn Deliveries Scheduled Early[2]	14	14%	12%	6%
Preventive Care				
Immunization for Influenza[2]	236	95%	88%	90%
Immunization for Pneumonia[2]	264	99%	90%	92%
Stroke Care				
Anticoagulation Therapy for Atrial Fibrillation[7]	-	-	88%	95%
Antithrombotic Therapy Timing[1]	-	-	97%	98%
Assessed for Rehabilitation[1]	-	-	97%	97%
Discharged on Antithrombotic Therapy[1]	-	-	98%	99%
Discharged on Statin Medication[1]	-	-	88%	94%
Thrombolytic Therapy Timing[1]	-	-	68%	66%
Venous Thromboembolism Prophylaxis[1]	-	-	93%	94%
Written Stroke Educational Materials Given[1]	-	-	84%	88%
Surgical Care Improvement Project				
Appropriate Beta Blocker Usage[1]	-	-	98%	98%
Appropriate VTP Within 24 Hours	38	95%	98%	98%
Controlled Postoperative Blood Glucose[7]	-	-	98%	97%
Perioperative Temperature Management	39	100%	100%	100%
Prophylactic Antibiotic Selection	19	95%	99%	99%
Prophylactic Antibiotic Selection (Outpatient)[1,3]	-	-	98%	98%
Prophylactic Antibiotic Stopped	19	100%	98%	98%
Prophylactic Antibiotic Timing	19	100%	99%	99%
Prophylactic Antibiotic Timing (Outpatient)[1,3]	-	-	98%	98%
Urinary Catheter Removal	15	80%	97%	97%
Survey of Patients' Hospital Experiences				
Area Around Room 'Always' Quiet at Night[11]	(a)	65%	65%	61%
Doctors 'Always' Communicated Well[11]	(a)	84%	85%	82%
Home Recovery Information Given[11]	(a)	86%	86%	85%
Hospital Given 9 or 10 on 10 Point Scale[11]	(a)	73%	76%	71%
Meds 'Always' Explained Before Given[11]	(a)	66%	66%	64%
Nurses 'Always' Communicated Well[11]	(a)	80%	81%	79%
Pain 'Always' Well Controlled[11]	(a)	70%	72%	71%
Room and Bathroom 'Always' Clean[11]	(a)	68%	76%	73%
Timely Help 'Always' Received[11]	(a)	69%	72%	68%
Would Definitely Recommend Hospital[11]	(a)	65%	75%	71%
Use of Medical Imaging				
Cardiac Imaging Stress Test before Surgery	75	5.3%	5%	5.3%
Combination Abdominal CT Scan	204	11.3%	19%	10.5%
Combination Brain/Sinus CT Scan	199	0.5%	2.9%	2.7%
Combination Chest CT Scan	121	3.3%	3.9%	2.7%
Follow-up Mammogram/Ultrasound	403	9.7%	7.8%	8.8%
Lumbar Spine MRI for Low Back Pain	46	43.5%	40.2%	37.2%

Allen County Regional Hospital

101 South 1st Street
Iola, KS 66749
Phone: 620-365-1021
Fax: 620-365-1140
URL: www.allencountyhospital.com
Type: Critical Access Hospitals
Emergency Services: Yes
Ownership: Proprietary
Beds: 25

Key Personnel:
CEO/President. . . . . Jennifer Jackman

Measure	Cases	This Hosp.	State Avg.	U.S. Avg.
Blood Clot Prevention and Treatment				
Anticoagulation Overlap Therapy[1,2]	-	-	94%	93%
ICU Venous Thromboembolism Prophylaxis[1,2]	-	-	91%	92%
Incidence of Potentially Preventable VTE[2,3]	-	-	8%	10%
UFH with Dosages/Platelet Monitoring[2,3]	-	-	98%	97%
Venous Thromboembolism Prophylaxis[2,3]	74	100%	79%	85%
Warfarin Therapy Discharge Instructions[1,2]	-	-	84%	75%
Chest Pain/Possible Heart Attack Care				
Aspirin Given Within 24 Hours of Arrival[3]	22	100%	94%	96%
Fibrinolytic Meds Within 30 Min. of Arrival[1,3]	-	-	41%	58%
Average Time to ECG (minutes)[3]	23	5	8	7
Average Time to Transfer (minutes)[3,7]	-	-	57	60
Children's Asthma Care				
Received Home Management Plan of Care	-	-	-	88%
Received Reliever Medication	-	-	-	100%
Received Systemic Corticosteroids	-	-	-	100%
Emergency Department				
Admittance Decision Time (minutes)[2,3]	205	38	57	98
Head CT Results Within 45 Min. of Arrival[3,7]	-	-	53%	57%
Patients Who Left ER Before Being Seen[5]	-	-	2%	2%
Time from ER Arrival to Admit. (minutes)[2,3]	230	156	185	274
Time from ER Arrival to Discharge (minutes)[3]	252	62	104	134
Time in ER Before Being Evaluated (minutes)[3]	293	7	18	26
Time to Pain Meds for Fractures (minutes)[3]	15	28	47	57
Heart Attack Care				
Aspirin Given at Discharge[5]	-	-	99%	99%
Fibrinolytic Meds Within 30 Min. of Arrival[5]	-	-	-	54%
PCI Within 90 Minutes of Arrival[5]	-	-	97%	96%
Statin Prescribed at Discharge[5]	-	-	99%	98%
Heart Failure Care				
ACE Inhibitor or ARB for LVSD[1,3]	-	-	95%	97%
Discharge Instructions Given[1,3]	-	-	91%	94%
Evaluation of LVS Function[1,3]	-	-	94%	99%
Medicare Spending				
Medicare Spending per Patient (ratio)	-	-	0.94	0.98
Pneumonia Care				
Appropriate Initial Antibiotic Given[3]	13	92%	92%	95%
Blood Culture Timing[3]	19	100%	98%	98%
Pregnancy and Delivery Care				
Newborn Deliveries Scheduled Early[1,2]	-	-	12%	6%
Preventive Care				
Immunization for Influenza[2]	239	100%	88%	90%
Immunization for Pneumonia[2,3]	214	98%	90%	92%
Stroke Care				
Anticoagulation Therapy for Atrial Fibrillation[1,2]	-	-	88%	95%
Antithrombotic Therapy Timing[1,2]	-	-	97%	98%
Assessed for Rehabilitation[1,2]	-	-	97%	97%
Discharged on Antithrombotic Therapy[1,2]	-	-	98%	99%
Discharged on Statin Medication[1,2]	-	-	88%	94%
Thrombolytic Therapy Timing[2,3]	-	-	68%	66%
Venous Thromboembolism Prophylaxis[1,2]	-	-	93%	94%
Written Stroke Educational Materials Given[1,2]	-	-	84%	88%
Surgical Care Improvement Project				
Appropriate Beta Blocker Usage[3,7]	-	-	98%	98%
Appropriate VTP Within 24 Hours[1,3]	-	-	98%	98%
Controlled Postoperative Blood Glucose[3,7]	-	-	98%	97%
Perioperative Temperature Management[1,3]	-	-	100%	100%
Prophylactic Antibiotic Selection[3,7]	-	-	99%	99%
Prophylactic Antibiotic Selection (Outpatient)[3,7]	-	-	98%	98%
Prophylactic Antibiotic Stopped[3,7]	-	-	98%	98%
Prophylactic Antibiotic Timing[3,7]	-	-	99%	99%
Prophylactic Antibiotic Timing (Outpatient)[3,7]	-	-	98%	98%
Urinary Catheter Removal[1,3]	-	-	97%	97%
Survey of Patients' Hospital Experiences				
Area Around Room 'Always' Quiet at Night[6]	<100	61%	65%	61%
Doctors 'Always' Communicated Well[6]	<100	83%	85%	82%
Home Recovery Information Given[6]	<100	83%	86%	85%
Hospital Given 9 or 10 on 10 Point Scale[6]	<100	62%	76%	71%
Meds 'Always' Explained Before Given[6]	<100	64%	66%	64%
Nurses 'Always' Communicated Well[6]	<100	77%	81%	79%
Pain 'Always' Well Controlled[6]	<100	68%	72%	71%
Room and Bathroom 'Always' Clean[6]	<100	72%	76%	73%
Timely Help 'Always' Received[6]	<100	70%	72%	68%
Would Definitely Recommend Hospital[6]	<100	56%	75%	71%
Use of Medical Imaging				
Cardiac Imaging Stress Test before Surgery[7]	-	-	5%	5.3%
Combination Abdominal CT Scan	187	27.3%	19%	10.5%
Combination Brain/Sinus CT Scan[1]	-	-	2.9%	2.7%
Combination Chest CT Scan	97	2.1%	3.9%	2.7%
Follow-up Mammogram/Ultrasound	232	4.3%	7.8%	8.8%
Lumbar Spine MRI for Low Back Pain[1]	-	-	40.2%	37.2%

Hodgeman County Health Center

809 Bramley
Jetmore, KS 67854
Phone: 620-357-8361
Fax: 620-357-6120
E-mail: vbamberger@hchconline.org
URL: www.hchconline.org
Type: Critical Access Hospitals
Emergency Services: Yes
Ownership: Government - Local
Beds: 52

Key Personnel:
Infection Control. . . . . Nancy Ferguson, RN
Quality Assurance . . . . Nancy Ferguson, RN
Operating Room. . . . . Julie Schraeder
Chief of Medical Staff. . . . . Richard Alan Snodgrass
Emergency Room . . . . Gail Tucker
Intensive Care Unit. . . . . Gail Tucker

Measure	Cases	This Hosp.	State Avg.	U.S. Avg.
Blood Clot Prevention and Treatment				

NOTE: Hospital profiles are in alphabetical order by state, then city, then hospital within the city; Rankings exclude hospitals with less than 25 cases except for patient surveys which excludes hospitals with less than 100 cases; (a) 100-299 cases; (1) The number of cases/patients is too few to report; (2) Data submitted were based on a sample of cases/patients; (3) Results are based on a shorter time period than required; (4) Data suppressed by CMS for one or more quarters; (5) Results are not available for this reporting period; (6) Fewer than 100 patients completed the HCAHPS survey; (7) No cases met the criteria for this measure; (8) The lower limit of the confidence interval cannot be calculated if the number of observed infections equals zero; (9) No data are available from the state/territory for this reporting period; (10) The scores shown reflect fewer than 50 completed surveys; (11) There were discrepancies in the data collection process; (12) This measure does not apply to this hospital for this reporting period; (13) Results cannot be calculated for this reporting period; (14) The results for this state are combined with nearby states to protect confidentiality; Please refer to the User's Guide for a full explanation of data.

Measure	Cases	This Hosp.	State Avg.	U.S. Avg.
Anticoagulation Overlap Therapy[5]	-	-	94%	93%
ICU Venous Thromboembolism Prophylaxis[5]	-	-	91%	92%
Incidence of Potentially Preventable VTE[5]	-	-	8%	10%
UFH with Dosages/Platelet Monitoring[5]	-	-	98%	97%
Venous Thromboembolism Prophylaxis[5]	-	-	79%	85%
Warfarin Therapy Discharge Instructions[5]	-	-	84%	75%
Chest Pain/Possible Heart Attack Care				
Aspirin Given Within 24 Hours of Arrival	-	-	94%	96%
Fibrinolytic Meds Within 30 Min. of Arrival	-	-	41%	58%
Average Time to ECG (minutes)	-	-	8	7
Average Time to Transfer (minutes)	-	-	57	60
Children's Asthma Care				
Received Home Management Plan of Care	-	-	-	88%
Received Reliever Medication	-	-	-	100%
Received Systemic Corticosteroids	-	-	-	100%
Emergency Department				
Admittance Decision Time (minutes)[5]	-	-	57	98
Head CT Results Within 45 Min. of Arrival	-	-	53%	57%
Patients Who Left ER Before Being Seen	-	-	2%	2%
Time from ER Arrival to Admit. (minutes)[5]	-	-	185	274
Time from ER Arrival to Discharge (minutes)	-	-	104	134
Time in ER Before Being Evaluated (minutes)	-	-	18	26
Time to Pain Meds for Fractures (minutes)	-	-	47	57
Heart Attack Care				
Aspirin Given at Discharge[5]	-	-	99%	99%
Fibrinolytic Meds Within 30 Min. of Arrival[5]	-	-	-	54%
PCI Within 90 Minutes of Arrival[5]	-	-	97%	96%
Statin Prescribed at Discharge[5]	-	-	99%	98%
Heart Failure Care				
ACE Inhibitor or ARB for LVSD[5]	-	-	95%	97%
Discharge Instructions Given[5]	-	-	91%	94%
Evaluation of LVS Function[5]	-	-	94%	99%
Medicare Spending				
Medicare Spending per Patient (ratio)	-	-	0.94	0.98
Pneumonia Care				
Appropriate Initial Antibiotic Given[1,3]	-	-	92%	95%
Blood Culture Timing[3,7]	-	-	98%	98%
Pregnancy and Delivery Care				
Newborn Deliveries Scheduled Early[5]	-	-	12%	6%
Preventive Care				
Immunization for Influenza[5]	-	-	88%	90%
Immunization for Pneumonia[5]	-	-	90%	92%
Stroke Care				
Anticoagulation Therapy for Atrial Fibrillation[5]	-	-	88%	95%
Antithrombotic Therapy Timing[5]	-	-	97%	98%
Assessed for Rehabilitation[5]	-	-	97%	97%
Discharged on Antithrombotic Therapy[5]	-	-	98%	99%
Discharged on Statin Medication[5]	-	-	88%	94%
Thrombolytic Therapy Timing[5]	-	-	68%	66%
Venous Thromboembolism Prophylaxis[5]	-	-	93%	94%
Written Stroke Educational Materials Given[5]	-	-	84%	88%
Surgical Care Improvement Project				
Appropriate Beta Blocker Usage[5]	-	-	98%	98%
Appropriate VTP Within 24 Hours[5]	-	-	98%	98%
Controlled Postoperative Blood Glucose[5]	-	-	98%	97%
Perioperative Temperature Management[5]	-	-	100%	100%
Prophylactic Antibiotic Selection[5]	-	-	99%	99%
Prophylactic Antibiotic Selection (Outpatient)	-	-	98%	98%
Prophylactic Antibiotic Stopped[5]	-	-	98%	98%
Prophylactic Antibiotic Timing[5]	-	-	99%	99%
Prophylactic Antibiotic Timing (Outpatient)	-	-	98%	98%
Urinary Catheter Removal[5]	-	-	97%	97%
Survey of Patients' Hospital Experiences				
Area Around Room 'Always' Quiet at Night[5]	-	-	65%	61%
Doctors 'Always' Communicated Well[5]	-	-	85%	82%
Home Recovery Information Given[5]	-	-	86%	85%
Hospital Given 9 or 10 on 10 Point Scale[5]	-	-	76%	71%
Meds 'Always' Explained Before Given[5]	-	-	66%	64%
Nurses 'Always' Communicated Well[5]	-	-	81%	79%
Pain 'Always' Well Controlled[5]	-	-	72%	71%
Room and Bathroom 'Always' Clean[5]	-	-	76%	73%
Timely Help 'Always' Received[5]	-	-	72%	68%
Would Definitely Recommend Hospital[5]	-	-	75%	71%
Use of Medical Imaging				
Cardiac Imaging Stress Test before Surgery	-	-	5%	5.3%
Combination Abdominal CT Scan	-	-	19%	10.5%
Combination Brain/Sinus CT Scan	-	-	2.9%	2.7%
Combination Chest CT Scan	-	-	3.9%	2.7%
Follow-up Mammogram/Ultrasound	-	-	7.8%	8.8%
Lumbar Spine MRI for Low Back Pain	-	-	40.2%	37.2%

Stanton County Hospital

404 N Chestnut
Johnson, KS 67855
Phone: 620-492-6250
Type: Critical Access Hospitals
Emergency Services: Yes
Ownership: Government - Local

Measure	Cases	This Hosp.	State Avg.	U.S. Avg.
Blood Clot Prevention and Treatment				
Anticoagulation Overlap Therapy[5]	-	-	94%	93%
ICU Venous Thromboembolism Prophylaxis[5]	-	-	91%	92%
Incidence of Potentially Preventable VTE[5]	-	-	8%	10%
UFH with Dosages/Platelet Monitoring[5]	-	-	98%	97%
Venous Thromboembolism Prophylaxis[5]	-	-	79%	85%
Warfarin Therapy Discharge Instructions[5]	-	-	84%	75%
Chest Pain/Possible Heart Attack Care				
Aspirin Given Within 24 Hours of Arrival	-	-	94%	96%
Fibrinolytic Meds Within 30 Min. of Arrival	-	-	41%	58%
Average Time to ECG (minutes)	-	-	8	7
Average Time to Transfer (minutes)	-	-	57	60
Children's Asthma Care				
Received Home Management Plan of Care	-	-	-	88%
Received Reliever Medication	-	-	-	100%
Received Systemic Corticosteroids	-	-	-	100%
Emergency Department				
Admittance Decision Time (minutes)[3,7]	-	-	57	98
Head CT Results Within 45 Min. of Arrival	-	-	53%	57%
Patients Who Left ER Before Being Seen	-	-	2%	2%
Time from ER Arrival to Admit. (minutes)[3,7]	-	-	185	274
Time from ER Arrival to Discharge (minutes)	-	-	104	134
Time in ER Before Being Evaluated (minutes)	-	-	18	26
Time to Pain Meds for Fractures (minutes)	-	-	47	57
Heart Attack Care				
Aspirin Given at Discharge[5]	-	-	99%	99%
Fibrinolytic Meds Within 30 Min. of Arrival[5]	-	-	-	54%
PCI Within 90 Minutes of Arrival[5]	-	-	97%	96%
Statin Prescribed at Discharge[5]	-	-	99%	98%
Heart Failure Care				
ACE Inhibitor or ARB for LVSD[3,7]	-	-	95%	97%
Discharge Instructions Given[1,3]	-	-	91%	94%
Evaluation of LVS Function[1,3]	-	-	94%	99%
Medicare Spending				
Medicare Spending per Patient (ratio)	-	-	0.94	0.98
Pneumonia Care				
Appropriate Initial Antibiotic Given[1,3]	-	-	92%	95%
Blood Culture Timing[3,7]	-	-	98%	98%
Pregnancy and Delivery Care				
Newborn Deliveries Scheduled Early[5]	-	-	12%	6%
Preventive Care				
Immunization for Influenza[1]	-	-	88%	90%
Immunization for Pneumonia[1]	-	-	90%	92%
Stroke Care				
Anticoagulation Therapy for Atrial Fibrillation[5]	-	-	88%	95%
Antithrombotic Therapy Timing[5]	-	-	97%	98%
Assessed for Rehabilitation[5]	-	-	97%	97%
Discharged on Antithrombotic Therapy[5]	-	-	98%	99%
Discharged on Statin Medication[5]	-	-	88%	94%
Thrombolytic Therapy Timing[5]	-	-	68%	66%
Venous Thromboembolism Prophylaxis[5]	-	-	93%	94%
Written Stroke Educational Materials Given[5]	-	-	84%	88%
Surgical Care Improvement Project				
Appropriate Beta Blocker Usage[5]	-	-	98%	98%
Appropriate VTP Within 24 Hours[5]	-	-	98%	98%
Controlled Postoperative Blood Glucose[5]	-	-	98%	97%
Perioperative Temperature Management[5]	-	-	100%	100%
Prophylactic Antibiotic Selection[5]	-	-	99%	99%
Prophylactic Antibiotic Selection (Outpatient)	-	-	98%	98%
Prophylactic Antibiotic Stopped[5]	-	-	98%	98%
Prophylactic Antibiotic Timing[5]	-	-	99%	99%
Prophylactic Antibiotic Timing (Outpatient)	-	-	98%	98%
Urinary Catheter Removal[5]	-	-	97%	97%
Survey of Patients' Hospital Experiences				
Area Around Room 'Always' Quiet at Night[5]	-	-	65%	61%
Doctors 'Always' Communicated Well[5]	-	-	85%	82%
Home Recovery Information Given[5]	-	-	86%	85%
Hospital Given 9 or 10 on 10 Point Scale[5]	-	-	76%	71%
Meds 'Always' Explained Before Given[5]	-	-	66%	64%
Nurses 'Always' Communicated Well[5]	-	-	81%	79%
Pain 'Always' Well Controlled[5]	-	-	72%	71%
Room and Bathroom 'Always' Clean[5]	-	-	76%	73%
Timely Help 'Always' Received[5]	-	-	72%	68%
Would Definitely Recommend Hospital[5]	-	-	75%	71%
Use of Medical Imaging				
Cardiac Imaging Stress Test before Surgery	-	-	5%	5.3%
Combination Abdominal CT Scan	-	-	19%	10.5%
Combination Brain/Sinus CT Scan	-	-	2.9%	2.7%
Combination Chest CT Scan	-	-	3.9%	2.7%
Follow-up Mammogram/Ultrasound	-	-	7.8%	8.8%
Lumbar Spine MRI for Low Back Pain	-	-	40.2%	37.2%

Geary Community Hospital

1102 Saint Mary's Road
Junction City, KS 66441
Phone: 785-210-3301
Fax: 785-238-5278
E-mail: ceo@gchks.org
URL: www.gchks.org
Type: Acute Care Hospitals
Emergency Services: Yes
Ownership: Government - Local
Beds: 92

Key Personnel:
Quality Assurance . . . . Elaine Becker, RN
Chief of Medical Staff . . . . Charles Bollman, MD
CEO/President. . . . . David K Bradley, CHE
Infection Control. . . . . Sandy Grant, RN
Operating Room. . . . . Karen Roles, RN
Radiology. . . . . Pat Small
Pediatric Ambulatory Care . . . . . . Monika Strauhal, MD

Measure	Cases	This Hosp.	State Avg.	U.S. Avg.
Blood Clot Prevention and Treatment				
Anticoagulation Overlap Therapy[1,2]	-	-	94%	93%
ICU Venous Thromboembolism Prophylaxis[2]	65	82%	91%	92%
Incidence of Potentially Preventable VTE[2,7]	-	-	8%	10%
UFH with Dosages/Platelet Monitoring[1,2]	-	-	98%	97%
Venous Thromboembolism Prophylaxis[2]	105	72%	79%	85%
Warfarin Therapy Discharge Instructions[1,2]	-	-	84%	75%
Chest Pain/Possible Heart Attack Care				
Aspirin Given Within 24 Hours of Arrival	34	94%	94%	96%
Fibrinolytic Meds Within 30 Min. of Arrival[7]	-	-	41%	58%
Average Time to ECG (minutes)	35	9	8	7
Average Time to Transfer (minutes)[1]	-	-	57	60
Children's Asthma Care				
Received Home Management Plan of Care	-	-	-	88%
Received Reliever Medication	-	-	-	100%
Received Systemic Corticosteroids	-	-	-	100%
Emergency Department				
Admittance Decision Time (minutes)[2]	147	70	57	98
Head CT Results Within 45 Min. of Arrival[1]	-	-	53%	57%
Patients Who Left ER Before Being Seen	14,078	9%	2%	2%
Time from ER Arrival to Admit. (minutes)[2]	150	265	185	274
Time from ER Arrival to Discharge (minutes)	375	141	104	134
Time in ER Before Being Evaluated (minutes)	364	44	18	26
Time to Pain Meds for Fractures (minutes)	50	46	47	57
Heart Attack Care				
Aspirin Given at Discharge[1,3]	-	-	99%	99%
Fibrinolytic Meds Within 30 Min. of Arrival[3,7]	-	-	-	54%
PCI Within 90 Minutes of Arrival[3,7]	-	-	97%	96%
Statin Prescribed at Discharge[1,3]	-	-	99%	98%
Heart Failure Care				
ACE Inhibitor or ARB for LVSD[1]	-	-	95%	97%
Discharge Instructions Given	20	70%	91%	94%
Evaluation of LVS Function	23	74%	94%	99%

NOTE: Hospital profiles are in alphabetical order by state, then city, then hospital within the city; Rankings exclude hospitals with less than 25 cases except for patient surveys which excludes hospitals with less than 100 cases; (a) 100-299 cases; (1) The number of cases/patients is too few to report; (2) Data submitted were based on a sample of cases/patients; (3) Results are based on a shorter time period than required; (4) Data suppressed by CMS for one or more quarters; (5) Results are not available for this reporting period; (6) Fewer than 100 patients completed the HCAHPS survey; (7) No cases met the criteria for this measure; (8) The lower limit of the confidence interval cannot be calculated if the number of observed infections equals zero; (9) No data are available from the state/territory for this reporting period; (10) The scores shown reflect fewer than 50 completed surveys; (11) There were discrepancies in the data collection process; (12) This measure does not apply to this hospital for this reporting period; (13) Results cannot be calculated for this reporting period; (14) The results for this state are combined with nearby states to protect confidentiality; Please refer to the User's Guide for a full explanation of data.

Measure	Cases	This Hosp.	State Avg.	U.S. Avg.
Medicare Spending				
Medicare Spending per Patient (ratio)	-	0.92	0.94	0.98
Pneumonia Care				
Appropriate Initial Antibiotic Given	37	100%	92%	95%
Blood Culture Timing	29	93%	98%	98%
Pregnancy and Delivery Care				
Newborn Deliveries Scheduled Early	24	0%	12%	6%
Preventive Care				
Immunization for Influenza[2]	219	77%	88%	90%
Immunization for Pneumonia[2]	242	79%	90%	92%
Stroke Care				
Anticoagulation Therapy for Atrial Fibrillation[1]	-	-	88%	95%
Antithrombotic Therapy Timing	15	87%	97%	98%
Assessed for Rehabilitation	14	93%	97%	97%
Discharged on Antithrombotic Therapy	14	86%	98%	99%
Discharged on Statin Medication	14	57%	88%	94%
Thrombolytic Therapy Timing[1]	-	-	68%	66%
Venous Thromboembolism Prophylaxis	18	83%	93%	94%
Written Stroke Educational Materials Given[1]	-	-	84%	88%
Surgical Care Improvement Project				
Appropriate Beta Blocker Usage	21	95%	98%	98%
Appropriate VTP Within 24 Hours	106	96%	98%	98%
Controlled Postoperative Blood Glucose[7]	-	-	98%	97%
Perioperative Temperature Management	120	99%	100%	100%
Prophylactic Antibiotic Selection	100	99%	99%	99%
Prophylactic Antibiotic Selection (Outpatient)	13	100%	98%	98%
Prophylactic Antibiotic Stopped	97	93%	98%	98%
Prophylactic Antibiotic Timing	100	98%	99%	99%
Prophylactic Antibiotic Timing (Outpatient)	13	85%	98%	98%
Urinary Catheter Removal	94	98%	97%	97%
Survey of Patients' Hospital Experiences				
Area Around Room 'Always' Quiet at Night	300+	66%	65%	61%
Doctors 'Always' Communicated Well	300+	85%	85%	82%
Home Recovery Information Given	300+	90%	86%	85%
Hospital Given 9 or 10 on 10 Point Scale	300+	73%	76%	71%
Meds 'Always' Explained Before Given	300+	66%	66%	64%
Nurses 'Always' Communicated Well	300+	77%	81%	79%
Pain 'Always' Well Controlled	300+	71%	72%	71%
Room and Bathroom 'Always' Clean	300+	71%	76%	73%
Timely Help 'Always' Received	300+	67%	72%	68%
Would Definitely Recommend Hospital	300+	70%	75%	71%
Use of Medical Imaging				
Cardiac Imaging Stress Test before Surgery	121	2.5%	5%	5.3%
Combination Abdominal CT Scan	258	3.5%	19%	10.5%
Combination Brain/Sinus CT Scan	192	5.2%	2.9%	2.7%
Combination Chest CT Scan	216	0.0%	3.9%	2.7%
Follow-up Mammogram/Ultrasound	669	5.5%	7.8%	8.8%
Lumbar Spine MRI for Low Back Pain	44	45.5%	40.2%	37.2%

Providence Medical Center

8929 Parallel Parkway
Kansas City, KS 66112
Phone: 913-596-3930
Fax: 913-596-4324
URL: www.providence-health.org
Type: Acute Care Hospitals
Emergency Services: Yes
Ownership: Voluntary non-profit - Church
Beds: 400

Key Personnel:

Emergency Room . . . . Victoria C Allison, MD
Quality Assurance . . . . Julie Bogart
Radiology. . . . . William H Brooks
Operating Room. . . . . Scott D Ellison
Intensive Care Unit. . . . . Patty Geiger
CEO/President. . . . . Randall Nyp
Chairman/CEO . . . . Dr. Prem Reddy, MD, FACC, FCCP
Patient Relations . . . . Vicki Short

Measure	Cases	This Hosp.	State Avg.	U.S. Avg.
Blood Clot Prevention and Treatment				
Anticoagulation Overlap Therapy[2]	61	95%	94%	93%
ICU Venous Thromboembolism Prophylaxis[2]	80	92%	91%	92%
Incidence of Potentially Preventable VTE[2]	14	7%	8%	10%
UFH with Dosages/Platelet Monitoring[2]	42	100%	98%	97%
Venous Thromboembolism Prophylaxis[2]	356	92%	79%	85%
Warfarin Therapy Discharge Instructions[2]	38	97%	84%	75%
Chest Pain/Possible Heart Attack Care				
Aspirin Given Within 24 Hours of Arrival[5]	-	-	94%	96%
Fibrinolytic Meds Within 30 Min. of Arrival[5]	-	-	41%	58%
Average Time to ECG (minutes)[5]	-	-	8	7
Average Time to Transfer (minutes)[5]	-	-	57	60
Children's Asthma Care				
Received Home Management Plan of Care	-	-	-	88%
Received Reliever Medication	-	-	-	100%
Received Systemic Corticosteroids	-	-	-	100%
Emergency Department				
Admittance Decision Time (minutes)[2]	807	81	57	98
Head CT Results Within 45 Min. of Arrival[1,3]	-	-	53%	57%
Patients Who Left ER Before Being Seen	36,616	3%	2%	2%
Time from ER Arrival to Admit. (minutes)[2]	807	247	185	274
Time from ER Arrival to Discharge (minutes)	398	109	104	134
Time in ER Before Being Evaluated (minutes)	418	18	18	26
Time to Pain Meds for Fractures (minutes)	118	42	47	57
Heart Attack Care				
Aspirin Given at Discharge	158	99%	99%	99%
Fibrinolytic Meds Within 30 Min. of Arrival[7]	-	-	-	54%
PCI Within 90 Minutes of Arrival	30	97%	97%	96%
Statin Prescribed at Discharge	146	100%	99%	98%
Heart Failure Care				
ACE Inhibitor or ARB for LVSD	143	100%	95%	97%
Discharge Instructions Given	262	98%	91%	94%
Evaluation of LVS Function	332	100%	94%	99%
Medicare Spending				
Medicare Spending per Patient (ratio)	-	1.02	0.94	0.98
Pneumonia Care				
Appropriate Initial Antibiotic Given	108	99%	92%	95%
Blood Culture Timing	219	98%	98%	98%
Pregnancy and Delivery Care				
Newborn Deliveries Scheduled Early[2]	29	0%	12%	6%
Preventive Care				
Immunization for Influenza[2]	594	94%	88%	90%
Immunization for Pneumonia[2]	852	93%	90%	92%
Stroke Care				
Anticoagulation Therapy for Atrial Fibrillation	12	92%	88%	95%
Antithrombotic Therapy Timing	92	97%	97%	98%
Assessed for Rehabilitation	113	99%	97%	97%
Discharged on Antithrombotic Therapy	102	100%	98%	99%
Discharged on Statin Medication	84	98%	88%	94%
Thrombolytic Therapy Timing[1]	-	-	68%	66%
Venous Thromboembolism Prophylaxis	114	95%	93%	94%
Written Stroke Educational Materials Given	59	98%	84%	88%
Surgical Care Improvement Project				
Appropriate Beta Blocker Usage[2]	176	95%	98%	98%
Appropriate VTP Within 24 Hours[2]	459	100%	98%	98%
Controlled Postoperative Blood Glucose[2]	52	98%	98%	97%
Perioperative Temperature Management[2]	514	100%	100%	100%
Prophylactic Antibiotic Selection[2]	423	98%	99%	99%
Prophylactic Antibiotic Selection (Outpatient)	255	99%	98%	98%
Prophylactic Antibiotic Stopped[2]	420	99%	98%	98%
Prophylactic Antibiotic Timing[2]	425	100%	99%	99%
Prophylactic Antibiotic Timing (Outpatient)	253	99%	98%	98%
Urinary Catheter Removal[2]	182	93%	97%	97%
Survey of Patients' Hospital Experiences				
Area Around Room 'Always' Quiet at Night	300+	64%	65%	61%
Doctors 'Always' Communicated Well	300+	78%	85%	82%
Home Recovery Information Given	300+	83%	86%	85%
Hospital Given 9 or 10 on 10 Point Scale	300+	68%	76%	71%
Meds 'Always' Explained Before Given	300+	59%	66%	64%
Nurses 'Always' Communicated Well	300+	76%	81%	79%
Pain 'Always' Well Controlled	300+	69%	72%	71%
Room and Bathroom 'Always' Clean	300+	72%	76%	73%
Timely Help 'Always' Received	300+	65%	72%	68%
Would Definitely Recommend Hospital	300+	66%	75%	71%
Use of Medical Imaging				
Cardiac Imaging Stress Test before Surgery	303	5.3%	5%	5.3%
Combination Abdominal CT Scan	404	1.7%	19%	10.5%
Combination Brain/Sinus CT Scan[1]	-	-	2.9%	2.7%
Combination Chest CT Scan	310	0.3%	3.9%	2.7%
Follow-up Mammogram/Ultrasound	445	11.0%	7.8%	8.8%
Lumbar Spine MRI for Low Back Pain	52	42.3%	40.2%	37.2%

University of Kansas Hospital

3901 Rainbow Blvd
Kansas City, KS 66103
Phone: 913-588-7332
Fax: 913-588-5863
URL: www.kumc.edu
Type: Acute Care Hospitals
Emergency Services: Yes
Ownership: Govt - Hospital Dist/Auth
Beds: 620

Key Personnel:

CEO/President. . . . . Irene Cumming
Quality Assurance . . . . Robin Heckelbeck
Radiology. . . . . Mary Monroe
Pediatric Ambulatory Care . . . . . . Cynthia Sparks
Pediatric In-Patient Care . . . . Cynthia Sparks
Operating Room. . . . . Laurie Wood
Infection Control. . . . . Daivd Woods

Measure	Cases	This Hosp.	State Avg.	U.S. Avg.
Blood Clot Prevention and Treatment				
Anticoagulation Overlap Therapy[2]	173	98%	94%	93%
ICU Venous Thromboembolism Prophylaxis[2]	100	97%	91%	92%
Incidence of Potentially Preventable VTE[2]	84	4%	8%	10%
UFH with Dosages/Platelet Monitoring[2]	144	92%	98%	97%
Venous Thromboembolism Prophylaxis[2]	318	93%	79%	85%
Warfarin Therapy Discharge Instructions[2]	126	79%	84%	75%
Chest Pain/Possible Heart Attack Care				
Aspirin Given Within 24 Hours of Arrival[5]	-	-	94%	96%
Fibrinolytic Meds Within 30 Min. of Arrival[5]	-	-	41%	58%
Average Time to ECG (minutes)[5]	-	-	8	7
Average Time to Transfer (minutes)[5]	-	-	57	60
Children's Asthma Care				
Received Home Management Plan of Care	-	-	-	88%
Received Reliever Medication	-	-	-	100%
Received Systemic Corticosteroids	-	-	-	100%
Emergency Department				
Admittance Decision Time (minutes)[2]	427	148	57	98
Head CT Results Within 45 Min. of Arrival[1,3]	-	-	53%	57%
Patients Who Left ER Before Being Seen	49,301	4%	2%	2%
Time from ER Arrival to Admit. (minutes)[2]	428	367	185	274
Time from ER Arrival to Discharge (minutes)	342	190	104	134
Time in ER Before Being Evaluated (minutes)	353	35	18	26
Time to Pain Meds for Fractures (minutes)	136	78	47	57
Heart Attack Care				
Aspirin Given at Discharge	254	100%	99%	99%
Fibrinolytic Meds Within 30 Min. of Arrival[7]	-	-	-	54%
PCI Within 90 Minutes of Arrival	26	100%	97%	96%
Statin Prescribed at Discharge	241	100%	99%	98%
Heart Failure Care				
ACE Inhibitor or ARB for LVSD	126	99%	95%	97%
Discharge Instructions Given	344	97%	91%	94%
Evaluation of LVS Function	403	100%	94%	99%
Medicare Spending				
Medicare Spending per Patient (ratio)	-	0.98	0.94	0.98
Pneumonia Care				
Appropriate Initial Antibiotic Given	125	98%	92%	95%
Blood Culture Timing	328	100%	98%	98%
Pregnancy and Delivery Care				
Newborn Deliveries Scheduled Early[2]	20	0%	12%	6%
Preventive Care				
Immunization for Influenza[2]	548	96%	88%	90%
Immunization for Pneumonia[2]	625	95%	90%	92%
Stroke Care				
Anticoagulation Therapy for Atrial Fibrillation[1,2]	-	-	88%	95%
Antithrombotic Therapy Timing[2]	61	100%	97%	98%
Assessed for Rehabilitation[2]	104	100%	97%	97%
Discharged on Antithrombotic Therapy[2]	73	100%	98%	99%
Discharged on Statin Medication[2]	58	97%	88%	94%
Thrombolytic Therapy Timing[1,2]	-	-	68%	66%
Venous Thromboembolism Prophylaxis[2]	103	100%	93%	94%
Written Stroke Educational Materials Given[2]	60	90%	84%	88%
Surgical Care Improvement Project				
Appropriate Beta Blocker Usage[2]	202	100%	98%	98%
Appropriate VTP Within 24 Hours[2]	397	97%	98%	98%
Controlled Postoperative Blood Glucose[2]	129	99%	98%	97%
Perioperative Temperature Management[2]	493	100%	100%	100%

NOTE: Hospital profiles are in alphabetical order by state, then city, then hospital within the city; Rankings exclude hospitals with less than 25 cases except for patient surveys which excludes hospitals with less than 100 cases; (a) 100-299 cases; (1) The number of cases/patients is too few to report; (2) Data submitted were based on a sample of cases/patients; (3) Results are based on a shorter time period than required; (4) Data suppressed by CMS for one or more quarters; (5) Results are not available for this reporting period; (6) Fewer than 100 patients completed the HCAHPS survey; (7) No cases met the criteria for this measure; (8) The lower limit of the confidence interval cannot be calculated if the number of observed infections equals zero; (9) No data are available from the state/territory for this reporting period; (10) The scores shown reflect fewer than 50 completed surveys; (11) There were discrepancies in the data collection process; (12) This measure does not apply to this hospital for this reporting period; (13) Results cannot be calculated for this reporting period; (14) The results for this state are combined with nearby states to protect confidentiality; Please refer to the User's Guide for a full explanation of data.

Prophylactic Antibiotic Selection[2]	418	99%	99%	99%
Prophylactic Antibiotic Selection (Outpatient)	621	99%	98%	98%
Prophylactic Antibiotic Stopped[2]	415	99%	98%	98%
Prophylactic Antibiotic Timing[2]	420	99%	99%	99%
Prophylactic Antibiotic Timing (Outpatient)	623	97%	98%	98%
Urinary Catheter Removal[2]	337	96%	97%	97%
Survey of Patients' Hospital Experiences				
Area Around Room 'Always' Quiet at Night	300+	65%	65%	61%
Doctors 'Always' Communicated Well	300+	80%	85%	82%
Home Recovery Information Given	300+	91%	86%	85%
Hospital Given 9 or 10 on 10 Point Scale	300+	82%	76%	71%
Meds 'Always' Explained Before Given	300+	63%	66%	64%
Nurses 'Always' Communicated Well	300+	82%	81%	79%
Pain 'Always' Well Controlled	300+	73%	72%	71%
Room and Bathroom 'Always' Clean	300+	69%	76%	73%
Timely Help 'Always' Received	300+	72%	72%	68%
Would Definitely Recommend Hospital	300+	85%	75%	71%
Use of Medical Imaging				
Cardiac Imaging Stress Test before Surgery	2,166	7.1%	5%	5.3%
Combination Abdominal CT Scan	3,475	15.7%	19%	10.5%
Combination Brain/Sinus CT Scan	755	3.8%	2.9%	2.7%
Combination Chest CT Scan	4,371	0.3%	3.9%	2.7%
Follow-up Mammogram/Ultrasound	2,091	8.1%	7.8%	8.8%
Lumbar Spine MRI for Low Back Pain	200	31.5%	40.2%	37.2%

Kingman Community Hospital

750 W Ave D
Kingman, KS 67068
Phone: 620-532-3147
Fax: 620-532-5221
E-mail: nvhs@ink.org
URL: www.nvhsinc.com
Type: Critical Access Hospitals
Emergency Services: Yes
Ownership: Voluntary non-profit - Private
Beds: 50

Key Personnel:

Quality Assurance . . . . Gayle Easley, BSN
Radiology. . . . . Connie Johnson
Emergency Room . . . . Nita McFarland
Chief of Medical Staff . . . . Victoria Moots, DO
CEO/President. . . . . Gary Tiller
Infection Control. . . . . Nancy Wilson, RN

Measure	Cases	This Hosp.	State Avg.	U.S. Avg.
Blood Clot Prevention and Treatment				
Anticoagulation Overlap Therapy[5]	-	-	94%	93%
ICU Venous Thromboembolism Prophylaxis[5]	-	-	91%	92%
Incidence of Potentially Preventable VTE[5]	-	-	8%	10%
UFH with Dosages/Platelet Monitoring[5]	-	-	98%	97%
Venous Thromboembolism Prophylaxis[5]	-	-	79%	85%
Warfarin Therapy Discharge Instructions[5]	-	-	84%	75%
Chest Pain/Possible Heart Attack Care				
Aspirin Given Within 24 Hours of Arrival	-	-	94%	96%
Fibrinolytic Meds Within 30 Min. of Arrival	-	-	41%	58%
Average Time to ECG (minutes)	-	-	8	7
Average Time to Transfer (minutes)	-	-	57	60
Children's Asthma Care				
Received Home Management Plan of Care	-	-	-	88%
Received Reliever Medication	-	-	-	100%
Received Systemic Corticosteroids	-	-	-	100%
Emergency Department				
Admittance Decision Time (minutes)[5]	-	-	57	98
Head CT Results Within 45 Min. of Arrival	-	-	53%	57%
Patients Who Left ER Before Being Seen	-	-	2%	2%
Time from ER Arrival to Admit. (minutes)[5]	-	-	185	274
Time from ER Arrival to Discharge (minutes)	-	-	104	134
Time in ER Before Being Evaluated (minutes)	-	-	18	26
Time to Pain Meds for Fractures (minutes)	-	-	47	57
Heart Attack Care				
Aspirin Given at Discharge[5]	-	-	99%	99%
Fibrinolytic Meds Within 30 Min. of Arrival[5]	-	-	-	54%
PCI Within 90 Minutes of Arrival[5]	-	-	97%	96%
Statin Prescribed at Discharge[5]	-	-	99%	98%
Heart Failure Care				
ACE Inhibitor or ARB for LVSD[1,3]	-	-	95%	97%
Discharge Instructions Given[1,3]	-	-	91%	94%
Evaluation of LVS Function[1,3]	-	-	94%	99%
Medicare Spending				
Medicare Spending per Patient (ratio)	-	-	0.94	0.98
Pneumonia Care				
Appropriate Initial Antibiotic Given	26	88%	92%	95%
Blood Culture Timing	13	85%	98%	98%
Pregnancy and Delivery Care				
Newborn Deliveries Scheduled Early[5]	-	-	12%	6%
Preventive Care				
Immunization for Influenza[5]	-	-	88%	90%
Immunization for Pneumonia[5]	-	-	90%	92%
Stroke Care				
Anticoagulation Therapy for Atrial Fibrillation[5]	-	-	88%	95%
Antithrombotic Therapy Timing[5]	-	-	97%	98%
Assessed for Rehabilitation[5]	-	-	97%	97%
Discharged on Antithrombotic Therapy[5]	-	-	98%	99%
Discharged on Statin Medication[5]	-	-	88%	94%
Thrombolytic Therapy Timing[5]	-	-	68%	66%
Venous Thromboembolism Prophylaxis[5]	-	-	93%	94%
Written Stroke Educational Materials Given[5]	-	-	84%	88%
Surgical Care Improvement Project				
Appropriate Beta Blocker Usage[3,7]	-	-	98%	98%
Appropriate VTP Within 24 Hours[1,3]	-	-	98%	98%
Controlled Postoperative Blood Glucose[5]	-	-	98%	97%
Perioperative Temperature Management[1,3]	-	-	100%	100%
Prophylactic Antibiotic Selection[1,3]	-	-	99%	99%
Prophylactic Antibiotic Selection (Outpatient)	-	-	98%	98%
Prophylactic Antibiotic Stopped[1,3]	-	-	98%	98%
Prophylactic Antibiotic Timing[1,3]	-	-	99%	99%
Prophylactic Antibiotic Timing (Outpatient)	-	-	98%	98%
Urinary Catheter Removal[3,7]	-	-	97%	97%
Survey of Patients' Hospital Experiences				
Area Around Room 'Always' Quiet at Night	(a)	60%	65%	61%
Doctors 'Always' Communicated Well	(a)	86%	85%	82%
Home Recovery Information Given	(a)	84%	86%	85%
Hospital Given 9 or 10 on 10 Point Scale	(a)	83%	76%	71%
Meds 'Always' Explained Before Given	(a)	68%	66%	64%
Nurses 'Always' Communicated Well	(a)	83%	81%	79%
Pain 'Always' Well Controlled	(a)	78%	72%	71%
Room and Bathroom 'Always' Clean	(a)	81%	76%	73%
Timely Help 'Always' Received	(a)	75%	72%	68%
Would Definitely Recommend Hospital	(a)	80%	75%	71%
Use of Medical Imaging				
Cardiac Imaging Stress Test before Surgery	-	-	5%	5.3%
Combination Abdominal CT Scan	-	-	19%	10.5%
Combination Brain/Sinus CT Scan	-	-	2.9%	2.7%
Combination Chest CT Scan	-	-	3.9%	2.7%
Follow-up Mammogram/Ultrasound	-	-	7.8%	8.8%
Lumbar Spine MRI for Low Back Pain	-	-	40.2%	37.2%

Edwards County Hospital

620 West Eighth Street
Kinsley, KS 67547
Phone: 620-659-3621
URL: www.edwardscohospital.com
Type: Critical Access Hospitals
Emergency Services: Yes
Ownership: Government - Local

Key Personnel:

CEO . . . . Bob Krickbaum
Radiology. . . . . Janna Simmons

Measure	Cases	This Hosp.	State Avg.	U.S. Avg.
Blood Clot Prevention and Treatment				
Anticoagulation Overlap Therapy[5]	-	-	94%	93%
ICU Venous Thromboembolism Prophylaxis[5]	-	-	91%	92%
Incidence of Potentially Preventable VTE[5]	-	-	8%	10%
UFH with Dosages/Platelet Monitoring[5]	-	-	98%	97%
Venous Thromboembolism Prophylaxis[5]	-	-	79%	85%
Warfarin Therapy Discharge Instructions[5]	-	-	84%	75%
Chest Pain/Possible Heart Attack Care				
Aspirin Given Within 24 Hours of Arrival[1,3]	-	-	94%	96%
Fibrinolytic Meds Within 30 Min. of Arrival[5]	-	-	41%	58%
Average Time to ECG (minutes)[1,3]	-	-	8	7
Average Time to Transfer (minutes)[5]	-	-	57	60
Children's Asthma Care				
Received Home Management Plan of Care	-	-	-	88%
Received Reliever Medication	-	-	-	100%
Received Systemic Corticosteroids	-	-	-	100%
Emergency Department				
Admittance Decision Time (minutes)[5]	-	-	57	98
Head CT Results Within 45 Min. of Arrival[5]	-	-	53%	57%
Patients Who Left ER Before Being Seen	896	1%	2%	2%
Time from ER Arrival to Admit. (minutes)[5]	-	-	185	274
Time from ER Arrival to Discharge (minutes)[3]	26	104	104	134
Time in ER Before Being Evaluated (minutes)[3]	29	20	18	26
Time to Pain Meds for Fractures (minutes)[5]	-	-	47	57
Heart Attack Care				
Aspirin Given at Discharge[5]	-	-	99%	99%
Fibrinolytic Meds Within 30 Min. of Arrival[5]	-	-	-	54%
PCI Within 90 Minutes of Arrival[5]	-	-	97%	96%
Statin Prescribed at Discharge[5]	-	-	99%	98%
Heart Failure Care				
ACE Inhibitor or ARB for LVSD[3,7]	-	-	95%	97%
Discharge Instructions Given[1,3]	-	-	91%	94%
Evaluation of LVS Function[1,3]	-	-	94%	99%
Medicare Spending				
Medicare Spending per Patient (ratio)	-	-	0.94	0.98
Pneumonia Care				
Appropriate Initial Antibiotic Given[1]	-	-	92%	95%
Blood Culture Timing[7]	-	-	98%	98%
Pregnancy and Delivery Care				
Newborn Deliveries Scheduled Early[5]	-	-	12%	6%
Preventive Care				
Immunization for Influenza[5]	-	-	88%	90%
Immunization for Pneumonia[5]	-	-	90%	92%
Stroke Care				
Anticoagulation Therapy for Atrial Fibrillation[5]	-	-	88%	95%
Antithrombotic Therapy Timing[5]	-	-	97%	98%
Assessed for Rehabilitation[5]	-	-	97%	97%
Discharged on Antithrombotic Therapy[5]	-	-	98%	99%
Discharged on Statin Medication[5]	-	-	88%	94%
Thrombolytic Therapy Timing[5]	-	-	68%	66%
Venous Thromboembolism Prophylaxis[5]	-	-	93%	94%
Written Stroke Educational Materials Given[5]	-	-	84%	88%
Surgical Care Improvement Project				
Appropriate Beta Blocker Usage[5]	-	-	98%	98%
Appropriate VTP Within 24 Hours[5]	-	-	98%	98%
Controlled Postoperative Blood Glucose[5]	-	-	98%	97%
Perioperative Temperature Management[5]	-	-	100%	100%
Prophylactic Antibiotic Selection[5]	-	-	99%	99%
Prophylactic Antibiotic Selection (Outpatient)[5]	-	-	98%	98%
Prophylactic Antibiotic Stopped[5]	-	-	98%	98%
Prophylactic Antibiotic Timing[5]	-	-	99%	99%
Prophylactic Antibiotic Timing (Outpatient)[5]	-	-	98%	98%
Urinary Catheter Removal[5]	-	-	97%	97%
Survey of Patients' Hospital Experiences				
Area Around Room 'Always' Quiet at Night[5]	-	-	65%	61%
Doctors 'Always' Communicated Well[5]	-	-	85%	82%
Home Recovery Information Given[5]	-	-	86%	85%
Hospital Given 9 or 10 on 10 Point Scale[5]	-	-	76%	71%
Meds 'Always' Explained Before Given[5]	-	-	66%	64%
Nurses 'Always' Communicated Well[5]	-	-	81%	79%
Pain 'Always' Well Controlled[5]	-	-	72%	71%
Room and Bathroom 'Always' Clean[5]	-	-	76%	73%
Timely Help 'Always' Received[5]	-	-	72%	68%
Would Definitely Recommend Hospital[5]	-	-	75%	71%
Use of Medical Imaging				
Cardiac Imaging Stress Test before Surgery[1]	-	-	5%	5.3%
Combination Abdominal CT Scan[1]	-	-	19%	10.5%
Combination Brain/Sinus CT Scan[1]	-	-	2.9%	2.7%
Combination Chest CT Scan[1]	-	-	3.9%	2.7%
Follow-up Mammogram/Ultrasound	86	4.7%	7.8%	8.8%
Lumbar Spine MRI for Low Back Pain[1]	-	-	40.2%	37.2%

Kiowa District Hospital

1002 4th Street
Kiowa, KS 67070
Phone: 620-825-4131
Fax: 620-825-4667
Type: Critical Access Hospitals
Emergency Services: Yes
Ownership: Govt - Hospital Dist/Auth
Beds: 24

Key Personnel:

Anesthesiology. . . . . Jerry Darger

NOTE: Hospital profiles are in alphabetical order by state, then city, then hospital within the city; Rankings exclude hospitals with less than 25 cases except for patient surveys which excludes hospitals with less than 100 cases; (a) 100-299 cases; (1) The number of cases/patients is too few to report; (2) Data submitted were based on a sample of cases/patients; (3) Results are based on a shorter time period than required; (4) Data suppressed by CMS for one or more quarters; (5) Results are not available for this reporting period; (6) Fewer than 100 patients completed the HCAHPS survey; (7) No cases met the criteria for this measure; (8) The lower limit of the confidence interval cannot be calculated if the number of observed infections equals zero; (9) No data are available from the state/territory for this reporting period; (10) The scores shown reflect fewer than 50 completed surveys; (11) There were discrepancies in the data collection process; (12) This measure does not apply to this hospital for this reporting period; (13) Results cannot be calculated for this reporting period; (14) The results for this state are combined with nearby states to protect confidentiality; Please refer to the User's Guide for a full explanation of data.

Emergency Room . . . . Patty McNamar
Infection Control . . . . Patty McNamar
CEO/President . . . . Brian Stacey
Chief of Medical Staff . . . . Paul Wilhelm, MD
Quality Assurance . . . . Kathy Winters

Measure	Cases	This Hosp.	State Avg.	U.S. Avg.
Blood Clot Prevention and Treatment				
Anticoagulation Overlap Therapy[5]	-	-	94%	93%
ICU Venous Thromboembolism Prophylaxis[5]	-	-	91%	92%
Incidence of Potentially Preventable VTE[5]	-	-	8%	10%
UFH with Dosages/Platelet Monitoring[5]	-	-	98%	97%
Venous Thromboembolism Prophylaxis[5]	-	-	79%	85%
Warfarin Therapy Discharge Instructions[5]	-	-	84%	75%
Chest Pain/Possible Heart Attack Care				
Aspirin Given Within 24 Hours of Arrival[1,3]	-	-	94%	96%
Fibrinolytic Meds Within 30 Min. of Arrival[1,3]	-	-	41%	58%
Average Time to ECG (minutes)[1,3]	-	-	8	7
Average Time to Transfer (minutes)[3,7]	-	-	57	60
Children's Asthma Care				
Received Home Management Plan of Care	-	-	-	88%
Received Reliever Medication	-	-	-	100%
Received Systemic Corticosteroids	-	-	-	100%
Emergency Department				
Admittance Decision Time (minutes)[5]	-	-	57	98
Head CT Results Within 45 Min. of Arrival[5]	-	-	53%	57%
Patients Who Left ER Before Being Seen[5]	-	-	2%	2%
Time from ER Arrival to Admit. (minutes)[5]	-	-	185	274
Time from ER Arrival to Discharge (minutes)[5]	-	-	104	134
Time in ER Before Being Evaluated (minutes)[5]	-	-	18	26
Time to Pain Meds for Fractures (minutes)[5]	-	-	47	57
Heart Attack Care				
Aspirin Given at Discharge[5]	-	-	99%	99%
Fibrinolytic Meds Within 30 Min. of Arrival[5]	-	-	-	54%
PCI Within 90 Minutes of Arrival[5]	-	-	97%	96%
Statin Prescribed at Discharge[5]	-	-	99%	98%
Heart Failure Care				
ACE Inhibitor or ARB for LVSD[5]	-	-	95%	97%
Discharge Instructions Given[5]	-	-	91%	94%
Evaluation of LVS Function[5]	-	-	94%	99%
Medicare Spending				
Medicare Spending per Patient (ratio)	-	-	0.94	0.98
Pneumonia Care				
Appropriate Initial Antibiotic Given[1,2]	-	-	92%	95%
Blood Culture Timing[2,7]	-	-	98%	98%
Pregnancy and Delivery Care				
Newborn Deliveries Scheduled Early[5]	-	-	12%	6%
Preventive Care				
Immunization for Influenza[5]	-	-	88%	90%
Immunization for Pneumonia[5]	-	-	90%	92%
Stroke Care				
Anticoagulation Therapy for Atrial Fibrillation[5]	-	-	88%	95%
Antithrombotic Therapy Timing[5]	-	-	97%	98%
Assessed for Rehabilitation[5]	-	-	97%	97%
Discharged on Antithrombotic Therapy[5]	-	-	98%	99%
Discharged on Statin Medication[5]	-	-	88%	94%
Thrombolytic Therapy Timing[5]	-	-	68%	66%
Venous Thromboembolism Prophylaxis[5]	-	-	93%	94%
Written Stroke Educational Materials Given[5]	-	-	84%	88%
Surgical Care Improvement Project				
Appropriate Beta Blocker Usage[5]	-	-	98%	98%
Appropriate VTP Within 24 Hours[5]	-	-	98%	98%
Controlled Postoperative Blood Glucose[5]	-	-	98%	97%
Perioperative Temperature Management[5]	-	-	100%	100%
Prophylactic Antibiotic Selection[5]	-	-	99%	99%
Prophylactic Antibiotic Selection (Outpatient)[5]	-	-	98%	98%
Prophylactic Antibiotic Stopped[5]	-	-	98%	98%
Prophylactic Antibiotic Timing[5]	-	-	99%	99%
Prophylactic Antibiotic Timing (Outpatient)[5]	-	-	98%	98%
Urinary Catheter Removal[5]	-	-	97%	97%
Survey of Patients' Hospital Experiences				
Area Around Room 'Always' Quiet at Night[5]	-	-	65%	61%
Doctors 'Always' Communicated Well[5]	-	-	85%	82%
Home Recovery Information Given[5]	-	-	86%	85%
Hospital Given 9 or 10 on 10 Point Scale[5]	-	-	76%	71%
Meds 'Always' Explained Before Given[5]	-	-	66%	64%
Nurses 'Always' Communicated Well[5]	-	-	81%	79%
Pain 'Always' Well Controlled[5]	-	-	72%	71%
Room and Bathroom 'Always' Clean[5]	-	-	76%	73%
Timely Help 'Always' Received[5]	-	-	72%	68%
Would Definitely Recommend Hospital[5]	-	-	75%	71%
Use of Medical Imaging				
Cardiac Imaging Stress Test before Surgery[7]	-	-	5%	5.3%
Combination Abdominal CT Scan[1]	-	-	19%	10.5%
Combination Brain/Sinus CT Scan[1]	-	-	2.9%	2.7%
Combination Chest CT Scan[1]	-	-	3.9%	2.7%
Follow-up Mammogram/Ultrasound[7]	-	-	7.8%	8.8%
Lumbar Spine MRI for Low Back Pain[1]	-	-	40.2%	37.2%

Rush County Memorial Hospital

801 Locust St
La Crosse, KS 67548
Phone: 785-222-2545
Type: Critical Access Hospitals
Emergency Services: Yes
Ownership: Government - Local

Measure	Cases	This Hosp.	State Avg.	U.S. Avg.
Blood Clot Prevention and Treatment				
Anticoagulation Overlap Therapy[2,3]	-	-	94%	93%
ICU Venous Thromboembolism Prophylaxis[2,3]	-	-	91%	92%
Incidence of Potentially Preventable VTE[2,3]	-	-	8%	10%
UFH with Dosages/Platelet Monitoring[2,3]	-	-	98%	97%
Venous Thromboembolism Prophylaxis[1,2]	-	-	79%	85%
Warfarin Therapy Discharge Instructions[2,3]	-	-	84%	75%
Chest Pain/Possible Heart Attack Care				
Aspirin Given Within 24 Hours of Arrival	-	-	94%	96%
Fibrinolytic Meds Within 30 Min. of Arrival	-	-	41%	58%
Average Time to ECG (minutes)	-	-	8	7
Average Time to Transfer (minutes)	-	-	57	60
Children's Asthma Care				
Received Home Management Plan of Care	-	-	-	88%
Received Reliever Medication	-	-	-	100%
Received Systemic Corticosteroids	-	-	-	100%
Emergency Department				
Admittance Decision Time (minutes)[3,7]	-	-	57	98
Head CT Results Within 45 Min. of Arrival	-	-	53%	57%
Patients Who Left ER Before Being Seen	-	-	2%	2%
Time from ER Arrival to Admit. (minutes)[3,7]	-	-	185	274
Time from ER Arrival to Discharge (minutes)	-	-	104	134
Time in ER Before Being Evaluated (minutes)	-	-	18	26
Time to Pain Meds for Fractures (minutes)	-	-	47	57
Heart Attack Care				
Aspirin Given at Discharge[5]	-	-	99%	99%
Fibrinolytic Meds Within 30 Min. of Arrival[5]	-	-	-	54%
PCI Within 90 Minutes of Arrival[5]	-	-	97%	96%
Statin Prescribed at Discharge[5]	-	-	99%	98%
Heart Failure Care				
ACE Inhibitor or ARB for LVSD[3,7]	-	-	95%	97%
Discharge Instructions Given[3,7]	-	-	91%	94%
Evaluation of LVS Function[1,3]	-	-	94%	99%
Medicare Spending				
Medicare Spending per Patient (ratio)	-	-	0.94	0.98
Pneumonia Care				
Appropriate Initial Antibiotic Given[1,2]	-	-	92%	95%
Blood Culture Timing[2,3]	-	-	98%	98%
Pregnancy and Delivery Care				
Newborn Deliveries Scheduled Early[5]	-	-	12%	6%
Preventive Care				
Immunization for Influenza[1,3]	-	-	88%	90%
Immunization for Pneumonia[3]	35	9%	90%	92%
Stroke Care				
Anticoagulation Therapy for Atrial Fibrillation[5]	-	-	88%	95%
Antithrombotic Therapy Timing[5]	-	-	97%	98%
Assessed for Rehabilitation[5]	-	-	97%	97%
Discharged on Antithrombotic Therapy[5]	-	-	98%	99%
Discharged on Statin Medication[5]	-	-	88%	94%
Thrombolytic Therapy Timing[5]	-	-	68%	66%
Venous Thromboembolism Prophylaxis[5]	-	-	93%	94%
Written Stroke Educational Materials Given[5]	-	-	84%	88%
Surgical Care Improvement Project				
Appropriate Beta Blocker Usage[5]	-	-	98%	98%
Appropriate VTP Within 24 Hours[5]	-	-	98%	98%
Controlled Postoperative Blood Glucose[5]	-	-	98%	97%
Perioperative Temperature Management[5]	-	-	100%	100%
Prophylactic Antibiotic Selection[5]	-	-	99%	99%
Prophylactic Antibiotic Selection (Outpatient)	-	-	98%	98%
Prophylactic Antibiotic Stopped[5]	-	-	98%	98%
Prophylactic Antibiotic Timing[5]	-	-	99%	99%
Prophylactic Antibiotic Timing (Outpatient)	-	-	98%	98%
Urinary Catheter Removal[5]	-	-	97%	97%
Survey of Patients' Hospital Experiences				
Area Around Room 'Always' Quiet at Night[5]	-	-	65%	61%
Doctors 'Always' Communicated Well[5]	-	-	85%	82%
Home Recovery Information Given[5]	-	-	86%	85%
Hospital Given 9 or 10 on 10 Point Scale[5]	-	-	76%	71%
Meds 'Always' Explained Before Given[5]	-	-	66%	64%
Nurses 'Always' Communicated Well[5]	-	-	81%	79%
Pain 'Always' Well Controlled[5]	-	-	72%	71%
Room and Bathroom 'Always' Clean[5]	-	-	76%	73%
Timely Help 'Always' Received[5]	-	-	72%	68%
Would Definitely Recommend Hospital[5]	-	-	75%	71%
Use of Medical Imaging				
Cardiac Imaging Stress Test before Surgery	-	-	5%	5.3%
Combination Abdominal CT Scan	-	-	19%	10.5%
Combination Brain/Sinus CT Scan	-	-	2.9%	2.7%
Combination Chest CT Scan	-	-	3.9%	2.7%
Follow-up Mammogram/Ultrasound	-	-	7.8%	8.8%
Lumbar Spine MRI for Low Back Pain	-	-	40.2%	37.2%

Kearny County Hospital

500 Thorpe Street
Lakin, KS 67860
Phone: 620-355-7111
Fax: 620-355-1527
URL: www.kearnycountyhospital.com
Type: Critical Access Hospitals
Emergency Services: No
Ownership: Government - Local
Beds: 90

Key Personnel:

Infection Control . . . . Ken Barnett, RN

Measure	Cases	This Hosp.	State Avg.	U.S. Avg.
Blood Clot Prevention and Treatment				
Anticoagulation Overlap Therapy[5]	-	-	94%	93%
ICU Venous Thromboembolism Prophylaxis[5]	-	-	91%	92%
Incidence of Potentially Preventable VTE[5]	-	-	8%	10%
UFH with Dosages/Platelet Monitoring[5]	-	-	98%	97%
Venous Thromboembolism Prophylaxis[5]	-	-	79%	85%
Warfarin Therapy Discharge Instructions[5]	-	-	84%	75%
Chest Pain/Possible Heart Attack Care				
Aspirin Given Within 24 Hours of Arrival	-	-	94%	96%
Fibrinolytic Meds Within 30 Min. of Arrival	-	-	41%	58%
Average Time to ECG (minutes)	-	-	8	7
Average Time to Transfer (minutes)	-	-	57	60
Children's Asthma Care				
Received Home Management Plan of Care	-	-	-	88%
Received Reliever Medication	-	-	-	100%
Received Systemic Corticosteroids	-	-	-	100%
Emergency Department				
Admittance Decision Time (minutes)[5]	-	-	57	98
Head CT Results Within 45 Min. of Arrival	-	-	53%	57%
Patients Who Left ER Before Being Seen	-	-	2%	2%
Time from ER Arrival to Admit. (minutes)[5]	-	-	185	274
Time from ER Arrival to Discharge (minutes)	-	-	104	134
Time in ER Before Being Evaluated (minutes)	-	-	18	26
Time to Pain Meds for Fractures (minutes)	-	-	47	57
Heart Attack Care				
Aspirin Given at Discharge[3,7]	-	-	99%	99%
Fibrinolytic Meds Within 30 Min. of Arrival[3,7]	-	-	-	54%
PCI Within 90 Minutes of Arrival[3,7]	-	-	97%	96%
Statin Prescribed at Discharge[3,7]	-	-	99%	98%
Heart Failure Care				
ACE Inhibitor or ARB for LVSD[3,7]	-	-	95%	97%
Discharge Instructions Given[1,3]	-	-	91%	94%

NOTE: Hospital profiles are in alphabetical order by state, then city, then hospital within the city; Rankings exclude hospitals with less than 25 cases except for patient surveys which excludes hospitals with less than 100 cases; (a) 100-299 cases; (1) The number of cases/patients is too few to report; (2) Data submitted were based on a sample of cases/patients; (3) Results are based on a shorter time period than required; (4) Data suppressed by CMS for one or more quarters; (5) Results are not available for this reporting period; (6) Fewer than 100 patients completed the HCAHPS survey; (7) No cases met the criteria for this measure; (8) The lower limit of the confidence interval cannot be calculated if the number of observed infections equals zero; (9) No data are available from the state/territory for this reporting period; (10) The scores shown reflect fewer than 50 completed surveys; (11) There were discrepancies in the data collection process; (12) This measure does not apply to this hospital for this reporting period; (13) Results cannot be calculated for this reporting period; (14) The results for this state are combined with nearby states to protect confidentiality; Please refer to the User's Guide for a full explanation of data.

Measure	Cases	This Hosp.	State Avg.	U.S. Avg.
Evaluation of LVS Function[1,3]	-	-	94%	99%
Medicare Spending				
Medicare Spending per Patient (ratio)	-	-	0.94	0.98
Pneumonia Care				
Appropriate Initial Antibiotic Given[1,3]	-	-	92%	95%
Blood Culture Timing[1,3]	-	-	98%	98%
Pregnancy and Delivery Care				
Newborn Deliveries Scheduled Early[5]	-	-	12%	6%
Preventive Care				
Immunization for Influenza[5]	-	-	88%	90%
Immunization for Pneumonia[5]	-	-	90%	92%
Stroke Care				
Anticoagulation Therapy for Atrial Fibrillation[5]	-	-	88%	95%
Antithrombotic Therapy Timing[5]	-	-	97%	98%
Assessed for Rehabilitation[5]	-	-	97%	97%
Discharged on Antithrombotic Therapy[5]	-	-	98%	99%
Discharged on Statin Medication[5]	-	-	88%	94%
Thrombolytic Therapy Timing[5]	-	-	68%	66%
Venous Thromboembolism Prophylaxis[5]	-	-	93%	94%
Written Stroke Educational Materials Given[5]	-	-	84%	88%
Surgical Care Improvement Project				
Appropriate Beta Blocker Usage[5]	-	-	98%	98%
Appropriate VTP Within 24 Hours[5]	-	-	98%	98%
Controlled Postoperative Blood Glucose[5]	-	-	98%	97%
Perioperative Temperature Management[5]	-	-	100%	100%
Prophylactic Antibiotic Selection[5]	-	-	99%	99%
Prophylactic Antibiotic Selection (Outpatient)	-	-	98%	98%
Prophylactic Antibiotic Stopped[5]	-	-	98%	98%
Prophylactic Antibiotic Timing[5]	-	-	99%	99%
Prophylactic Antibiotic Timing (Outpatient)	-	-	98%	98%
Urinary Catheter Removal[5]	-	-	97%	97%
Survey of Patients' Hospital Experiences				
Area Around Room 'Always' Quiet at Night[5]	-	-	65%	61%
Doctors 'Always' Communicated Well[5]	-	-	85%	82%
Home Recovery Information Given[5]	-	-	86%	85%
Hospital Given 9 or 10 on 10 Point Scale[5]	-	-	76%	71%
Meds 'Always' Explained Before Given[5]	-	-	66%	64%
Nurses 'Always' Communicated Well[5]	-	-	81%	79%
Pain 'Always' Well Controlled[5]	-	-	72%	71%
Room and Bathroom 'Always' Clean[5]	-	-	76%	73%
Timely Help 'Always' Received[5]	-	-	72%	68%
Would Definitely Recommend Hospital[5]	-	-	75%	71%
Use of Medical Imaging				
Cardiac Imaging Stress Test before Surgery	-	-	5%	5.3%
Combination Abdominal CT Scan	-	-	19%	10.5%
Combination Brain/Sinus CT Scan	-	-	2.9%	2.7%
Combination Chest CT Scan	-	-	3.9%	2.7%
Follow-up Mammogram/Ultrasound	-	-	7.8%	8.8%
Lumbar Spine MRI for Low Back Pain	-	-	40.2%	37.2%

Pawnee Valley Community Hospital

923 Carroll Avenue
Larned, KS 67550
Phone: 620-285-3162
Type: Critical Access Hospitals
Emergency Services: Yes
Ownership: Government - Local

Measure	Cases	This Hosp.	State Avg.	U.S. Avg.
Blood Clot Prevention and Treatment				
Anticoagulation Overlap Therapy[5]	-	-	94%	93%
ICU Venous Thromboembolism Prophylaxis[5]	-	-	91%	92%
Incidence of Potentially Preventable VTE[5]	-	-	8%	10%
UFH with Dosages/Platelet Monitoring[5]	-	-	98%	97%
Venous Thromboembolism Prophylaxis[5]	-	-	79%	85%
Warfarin Therapy Discharge Instructions[5]	-	-	84%	75%
Chest Pain/Possible Heart Attack Care				
Aspirin Given Within 24 Hours of Arrival[5]	-	-	94%	96%
Fibrinolytic Meds Within 30 Min. of Arrival[5]	-	-	41%	58%
Average Time to ECG (minutes)[5]	-	-	8	7
Average Time to Transfer (minutes)[5]	-	-	57	60
Children's Asthma Care				
Received Home Management Plan of Care	-	-	-	88%
Received Reliever Medication	-	-	-	100%
Received Systemic Corticosteroids	-	-	-	100%
Emergency Department				
Admittance Decision Time (minutes)[3]	27	18	57	98
Head CT Results Within 45 Min. of Arrival[5]	-	-	53%	57%
Patients Who Left ER Before Being Seen[5]	-	-	2%	2%
Time from ER Arrival to Admit. (minutes)[3]	27	155	185	274
Time from ER Arrival to Discharge (minutes)[5]	-	-	104	134
Time in ER Before Being Evaluated (minutes)[5]	-	-	18	26
Time to Pain Meds for Fractures (minutes)[5]	-	-	47	57
Heart Attack Care				
Aspirin Given at Discharge[1,3]	-	-	99%	99%
Fibrinolytic Meds Within 30 Min. of Arrival[3,7]	-	-	-	54%
PCI Within 90 Minutes of Arrival[3,7]	-	-	97%	96%
Statin Prescribed at Discharge[1,3]	-	-	99%	98%
Heart Failure Care				
ACE Inhibitor or ARB for LVSD[7]	-	-	95%	97%
Discharge Instructions Given[1]	-	-	91%	94%
Evaluation of LVS Function	14	7%	94%	99%
Medicare Spending				
Medicare Spending per Patient (ratio)		-	0.94	0.98
Pneumonia Care				
Appropriate Initial Antibiotic Given[1]	-	-	92%	95%
Blood Culture Timing	11	100%	98%	98%
Pregnancy and Delivery Care				
Newborn Deliveries Scheduled Early[5]	-	-	12%	6%
Preventive Care				
Immunization for Influenza	34	88%	88%	90%
Immunization for Pneumonia[3]	34	65%	90%	92%
Stroke Care				
Anticoagulation Therapy for Atrial Fibrillation[5]	-	-	88%	95%
Antithrombotic Therapy Timing[5]	-	-	97%	98%
Assessed for Rehabilitation[5]	-	-	97%	97%
Discharged on Antithrombotic Therapy[5]	-	-	98%	99%
Discharged on Statin Medication[5]	-	-	88%	94%
Thrombolytic Therapy Timing[5]	-	-	68%	66%
Venous Thromboembolism Prophylaxis[5]	-	-	93%	94%
Written Stroke Educational Materials Given[5]	-	-	84%	88%
Surgical Care Improvement Project				
Appropriate Beta Blocker Usage[5]	-	-	98%	98%
Appropriate VTP Within 24 Hours[5]	-	-	98%	98%
Controlled Postoperative Blood Glucose[5]	-	-	98%	97%
Perioperative Temperature Management[5]	-	-	100%	100%
Prophylactic Antibiotic Selection[5]	-	-	99%	99%
Prophylactic Antibiotic Selection (Outpatient)[5]	-	-	98%	98%
Prophylactic Antibiotic Stopped[5]	-	-	98%	98%
Prophylactic Antibiotic Timing[5]	-	-	99%	99%
Prophylactic Antibiotic Timing (Outpatient)[5]	-	-	98%	98%
Urinary Catheter Removal[5]	-	-	97%	97%
Survey of Patients' Hospital Experiences				
Area Around Room 'Always' Quiet at Night[5]	-	-	65%	61%
Doctors 'Always' Communicated Well[5]	-	-	85%	82%
Home Recovery Information Given[5]	-	-	86%	85%
Hospital Given 9 or 10 on 10 Point Scale[5]	-	-	76%	71%
Meds 'Always' Explained Before Given[5]	-	-	66%	64%
Nurses 'Always' Communicated Well[5]	-	-	81%	79%
Pain 'Always' Well Controlled[5]	-	-	72%	71%
Room and Bathroom 'Always' Clean[5]	-	-	76%	73%
Timely Help 'Always' Received[5]	-	-	72%	68%
Would Definitely Recommend Hospital[5]	-	-	75%	71%
Use of Medical Imaging				
Cardiac Imaging Stress Test before Surgery[5]	-	-	5%	5.3%
Combination Abdominal CT Scan[5]	-	-	19%	10.5%
Combination Brain/Sinus CT Scan[5]	-	-	2.9%	2.7%
Combination Chest CT Scan[5]	-	-	3.9%	2.7%
Follow-up Mammogram/Ultrasound[5]	-	-	7.8%	8.8%
Lumbar Spine MRI for Low Back Pain[5]	-	-	40.2%	37.2%

Lawrence Memorial Hospital

325 Maine Street
Lawrence, KS 66044
URL: www.lmh.org
Phone: 785-505-6100
Fax: 785-749-6126
Type: Acute Care Hospitals
Emergency Services: Yes
Ownership: Government - Local
Beds: 173

Key Personnel:

Intensive Care Unit. . . . . Carol Cockrett
Operating Room. . . . . Dale Denning
Emergency Room . . . . Darin Elo, RN, BSN
Chief of Medical Staff . . . . Eric Huerter, MD
Anesthesiology. . . . . Christopher Malikfs, MD
CEO/President. . . . . Gene Meyer
Infection Control. . . . . Janet Wehrle

Measure	Cases	This Hosp.	State Avg.	U.S. Avg.
Blood Clot Prevention and Treatment				
Anticoagulation Overlap Therapy[2]	31	100%	94%	93%
ICU Venous Thromboembolism Prophylaxis[2]	30	93%	91%	92%
Incidence of Potentially Preventable VTE[1,2]	-	-	8%	10%
UFH with Dosages/Platelet Monitoring[1,2]	-	-	98%	97%
Venous Thromboembolism Prophylaxis[2]	320	91%	79%	85%
Warfarin Therapy Discharge Instructions[2]	26	77%	84%	75%
Chest Pain/Possible Heart Attack Care				
Aspirin Given Within 24 Hours of Arrival	17	100%	94%	96%
Fibrinolytic Meds Within 30 Min. of Arrival[3,7]	-	-	41%	58%
Average Time to ECG (minutes)	17	0	8	7
Average Time to Transfer (minutes)[1,3]	-	-	57	60
Children's Asthma Care				
Received Home Management Plan of Care	-	-	-	88%
Received Reliever Medication	-	-	-	100%
Received Systemic Corticosteroids	-	-	-	100%
Emergency Department				
Admittance Decision Time (minutes)[2]	650	51	57	98
Head CT Results Within 45 Min. of Arrival	14	79%	53%	57%
Patients Who Left ER Before Being Seen	37,271	1%	2%	2%
Time from ER Arrival to Admit. (minutes)[2]	654	194	185	274
Time from ER Arrival to Discharge (minutes)	426	144	104	134
Time in ER Before Being Evaluated (minutes)	449	17	18	26
Time to Pain Meds for Fractures (minutes)	176	35	47	57
Heart Attack Care				
Aspirin Given at Discharge	106	100%	99%	99%
Fibrinolytic Meds Within 30 Min. of Arrival[7]	-	-	-	54%
PCI Within 90 Minutes of Arrival	25	100%	97%	96%
Statin Prescribed at Discharge	103	100%	99%	98%
Heart Failure Care				
ACE Inhibitor or ARB for LVSD	28	100%	95%	97%
Discharge Instructions Given	117	100%	91%	94%
Evaluation of LVS Function	148	100%	94%	99%
Medicare Spending				
Medicare Spending per Patient (ratio)	-	0.90	0.94	0.98
Pneumonia Care				
Appropriate Initial Antibiotic Given	111	100%	92%	95%
Blood Culture Timing	247	99%	98%	98%
Pregnancy and Delivery Care				
Newborn Deliveries Scheduled Early	72	6%	12%	6%
Preventive Care				
Immunization for Influenza[2]	524	97%	88%	90%
Immunization for Pneumonia[2]	572	93%	90%	92%
Stroke Care				
Anticoagulation Therapy for Atrial Fibrillation[1]	-	-	88%	95%
Antithrombotic Therapy Timing	38	100%	97%	98%
Assessed for Rehabilitation	59	100%	97%	97%
Discharged on Antithrombotic Therapy	57	100%	98%	99%
Discharged on Statin Medication	42	100%	88%	94%
Thrombolytic Therapy Timing	12	100%	68%	66%
Venous Thromboembolism Prophylaxis	46	100%	93%	94%
Written Stroke Educational Materials Given	36	94%	84%	88%
Surgical Care Improvement Project				
Appropriate Beta Blocker Usage	156	98%	98%	98%
Appropriate VTP Within 24 Hours	556	99%	98%	98%
Controlled Postoperative Blood Glucose[7]	-	-	98%	97%
Perioperative Temperature Management	649	100%	100%	100%
Prophylactic Antibiotic Selection	506	99%	99%	99%
Prophylactic Antibiotic Selection (Outpatient)	188	98%	98%	98%
Prophylactic Antibiotic Stopped	504	100%	98%	98%
Prophylactic Antibiotic Timing	506	100%	99%	99%
Prophylactic Antibiotic Timing (Outpatient)	134	98%	98%	98%
Urinary Catheter Removal	514	100%	97%	97%
Survey of Patients' Hospital Experiences				
Area Around Room 'Always' Quiet at Night	300+	59%	65%	61%
Doctors 'Always' Communicated Well	300+	82%	85%	82%

NOTE: Hospital profiles are in alphabetical order by state, then city, then hospital within the city; Rankings exclude hospitals with less than 25 cases except for patient surveys which excludes hospitals with less than 100 cases; (a) 100-299 cases; (1) The number of cases/patients is too few to report; (2) Data submitted were based on a sample of cases/patients; (3) Results are based on a shorter time period than required; (4) Data suppressed by CMS for one or more quarters; (5) Results are not available for this reporting period; (6) Fewer than 100 patients completed the HCAHPS survey; (7) No cases met the criteria for this measure; (8) The lower limit of the confidence interval cannot be calculated if the number of observed infections equals zero; (9) No data are available from the state/territory for this reporting period; (10) The scores shown reflect fewer than 50 completed surveys; (11) There were discrepancies in the data collection process; (12) This measure does not apply to this hospital for this reporting period; (13) Results cannot be calculated for this reporting period; (14) The results for this state are combined with nearby states to protect confidentiality; Please refer to the User's Guide for a full explanation of data.

Measure	Cases	This Hosp.	State Avg.	U.S. Avg.
Home Recovery Information Given	300+	89%	86%	85%
Hospital Given 9 or 10 on 10 Point Scale	300+	75%	76%	71%
Meds 'Always' Explained Before Given	300+	65%	66%	64%
Nurses 'Always' Communicated Well	300+	79%	81%	79%
Pain 'Always' Well Controlled	300+	68%	72%	71%
Room and Bathroom 'Always' Clean	300+	71%	76%	73%
Timely Help 'Always' Received	300+	67%	72%	68%
Would Definitely Recommend Hospital	300+	74%	75%	71%
Use of Medical Imaging				
Cardiac Imaging Stress Test before Surgery	450	6.2%	5%	5.3%
Combination Abdominal CT Scan	1,089	3.0%	19%	10.5%
Combination Brain/Sinus CT Scan	821	2.6%	2.9%	2.7%
Combination Chest CT Scan	744	0.0%	3.9%	2.7%
Follow-up Mammogram/Ultrasound	2,576	6.8%	7.8%	8.8%
Lumbar Spine MRI for Low Back Pain	191	42.9%	40.2%	37.2%

Saint John Hospital

3500 South 4th Street
Leavenworth, KS 66048
URL: www.providence-health.org
Phone: 913-596-3930
Fax: 913-680-6013
Type: Acute Care Hospitals
Ownership: Voluntary non-profit - Other
Emergency Services: Yes
Beds: 76

Key Personnel:
Chairman/CEO . . . . Prem Dorsey
Quality Assurance . . . . Lynda Grimm
Operating Room. . . . . Brenda Johnson
Pediatric Ambulatory Care . . . . . . Jeffrey Lawhead, MD
Pediatric In-Patient Care . . . . Jeffrey Lawhead, MD
Chief of Medical Staff. . . . . Greg Madsen
Infection Control. . . . . Barbara McNett, RN
Intensive Care Unit. . . . . Donna Steward, MD

Measure	Cases	This Hosp.	State Avg.	U.S. Avg.
Blood Clot Prevention and Treatment				
Anticoagulation Overlap Therapy[1,2]	-	-	94%	93%
ICU Venous Thromboembolism Prophylaxis[2]	50	96%	91%	92%
Incidence of Potentially Preventable VTE[1,2]	-	-	8%	10%
UFH with Dosages/Platelet Monitoring[1,2]	-	-	98%	97%
Venous Thromboembolism Prophylaxis[2]	66	86%	79%	85%
Warfarin Therapy Discharge Instructions[1,2]	-	-	84%	75%
Chest Pain/Possible Heart Attack Care				
Aspirin Given Within 24 Hours of Arrival	19	100%	94%	96%
Fibrinolytic Meds Within 30 Min. of Arrival[3,7]	-	-	41%	58%
Average Time to ECG (minutes)	20	12	8	7
Average Time to Transfer (minutes)[1,3]	-	-	57	60
Children's Asthma Care				
Received Home Management Plan of Care	-	-	-	88%
Received Reliever Medication	-	-	-	100%
Received Systemic Corticosteroids	-	-	-	100%
Emergency Department				
Admittance Decision Time (minutes)[2]	365	67	57	98
Head CT Results Within 45 Min. of Arrival[3,7]	-	-	53%	57%
Patients Who Left ER Before Being Seen	10,544	0%	2%	2%
Time from ER Arrival to Admit. (minutes)[2]	372	200	185	274
Time from ER Arrival to Discharge (minutes)	348	93	104	134
Time in ER Before Being Evaluated (minutes)	374	9	18	26
Time to Pain Meds for Fractures (minutes)	51	43	47	57
Heart Attack Care				
Aspirin Given at Discharge[1]	-	-	99%	99%
Fibrinolytic Meds Within 30 Min. of Arrival[7]	-	-	-	54%
PCI Within 90 Minutes of Arrival[7]	-	-	97%	96%
Statin Prescribed at Discharge[1]	-	-	99%	98%
Heart Failure Care				
ACE Inhibitor or ARB for LVSD[1]	-	-	95%	97%
Discharge Instructions Given	26	100%	91%	94%
Evaluation of LVS Function	35	100%	94%	99%
Medicare Spending				
Medicare Spending per Patient (ratio)	-	0.99	0.94	0.98
Pneumonia Care				
Appropriate Initial Antibiotic Given	16	100%	92%	95%
Blood Culture Timing	26	100%	98%	98%
Pregnancy and Delivery Care				
Newborn Deliveries Scheduled Early[1,2]	-	-	12%	6%
Preventive Care				
Immunization for Influenza[2]	267	94%	88%	90%
Immunization for Pneumonia[2]	416	97%	90%	92%
Stroke Care				
Anticoagulation Therapy for Atrial Fibrillation[1]	-	-	88%	95%
Antithrombotic Therapy Timing[1]	-	-	97%	98%
Assessed for Rehabilitation[1]	-	-	97%	97%
Discharged on Antithrombotic Therapy[1]	-	-	98%	99%
Discharged on Statin Medication[1]	-	-	88%	94%
Thrombolytic Therapy Timing[1]	-	-	68%	66%
Venous Thromboembolism Prophylaxis[1]	-	-	93%	94%
Written Stroke Educational Materials Given[1]	-	-	84%	88%
Surgical Care Improvement Project				
Appropriate Beta Blocker Usage[1]	-	-	98%	98%
Appropriate VTP Within 24 Hours[1]	-	-	98%	98%
Controlled Postoperative Blood Glucose[7]	-	-	98%	97%
Perioperative Temperature Management[1]	-	-	100%	100%
Prophylactic Antibiotic Selection[1]	-	-	99%	99%
Prophylactic Antibiotic Selection (Outpatient)	11	91%	98%	98%
Prophylactic Antibiotic Stopped[1]	-	-	98%	98%
Prophylactic Antibiotic Timing[1]	-	-	99%	99%
Prophylactic Antibiotic Timing (Outpatient)	12	92%	98%	98%
Urinary Catheter Removal[1]	-	-	97%	97%
Survey of Patients' Hospital Experiences				
Area Around Room 'Always' Quiet at Night	(a)	69%	65%	61%
Doctors 'Always' Communicated Well	(a)	79%	85%	82%
Home Recovery Information Given	(a)	82%	86%	85%
Hospital Given 9 or 10 on 10 Point Scale	(a)	71%	76%	71%
Meds 'Always' Explained Before Given	(a)	57%	66%	64%
Nurses 'Always' Communicated Well	(a)	78%	81%	79%
Pain 'Always' Well Controlled	(a)	67%	72%	71%
Room and Bathroom 'Always' Clean	(a)	71%	76%	73%
Timely Help 'Always' Received	(a)	78%	72%	68%
Would Definitely Recommend Hospital	(a)	71%	75%	71%
Use of Medical Imaging				
Cardiac Imaging Stress Test before Surgery[1]	-	-	5%	5.3%
Combination Abdominal CT Scan	185	3.8%	19%	10.5%
Combination Brain/Sinus CT Scan[1]	-	-	2.9%	2.7%
Combination Chest CT Scan	113	1.8%	3.9%	2.7%
Follow-up Mammogram/Ultrasound	296	8.8%	7.8%	8.8%
Lumbar Spine MRI for Low Back Pain[1]	-	-	40.2%	37.2%

Saint Luke's Cushing Hospital

711 Marshall Street
Leavenworth, KS 66048
URL: www.saintlukeshealthsystem.org
Phone: 913-684-1102
Fax: 913-684-1390
Type: Acute Care Hospitals
Ownership: Voluntary non-profit - Private
Emergency Services: Yes
Beds: 74

Key Personnel:
CEO/President. . . . . Ron Baker
Emergency Room . . . . Jonathan Finks
Chief of Medical Staff . . . . Dr Habib
Radiology. . . . . John H MacMillan

Measure	Cases	This Hosp.	State Avg.	U.S. Avg.
Blood Clot Prevention and Treatment				
Anticoagulation Overlap Therapy[1,2]	-	-	94%	93%
ICU Venous Thromboembolism Prophylaxis[2]	29	93%	91%	92%
Incidence of Potentially Preventable VTE[1,2]	-	-	8%	10%
UFH with Dosages/Platelet Monitoring[1,2]	-	-	98%	97%
Venous Thromboembolism Prophylaxis[2]	76	97%	79%	85%
Warfarin Therapy Discharge Instructions[1,2]	-	-	84%	75%
Chest Pain/Possible Heart Attack Care				
Aspirin Given Within 24 Hours of Arrival	27	96%	94%	96%
Fibrinolytic Meds Within 30 Min. of Arrival[7]	-	-	41%	58%
Average Time to ECG (minutes)	28	10	8	7
Average Time to Transfer (minutes)[1]	-	-	57	60
Children's Asthma Care				
Received Home Management Plan of Care	-	-	-	88%
Received Reliever Medication	-	-	-	100%
Received Systemic Corticosteroids	-	-	-	100%
Emergency Department				
Admittance Decision Time (minutes)[2]	136	54	57	98
Head CT Results Within 45 Min. of Arrival[1]	-	-	53%	57%
Patients Who Left ER Before Being Seen	11,499	3%	2%	2%
Time from ER Arrival to Admit. (minutes)[2]	153	181	185	274
Time from ER Arrival to Discharge (minutes)	360	99	104	134
Time in ER Before Being Evaluated (minutes)	301	28	18	26
Time to Pain Meds for Fractures (minutes)	49	42	47	57
Heart Attack Care				
Aspirin Given at Discharge[1,3]	-	-	99%	99%
Fibrinolytic Meds Within 30 Min. of Arrival[3,7]	-	-	-	54%
PCI Within 90 Minutes of Arrival[3,7]	-	-	97%	96%
Statin Prescribed at Discharge[1,3]	-	-	99%	98%
Heart Failure Care				
ACE Inhibitor or ARB for LVSD[1]	-	-	95%	97%
Discharge Instructions Given	16	94%	91%	94%
Evaluation of LVS Function	22	100%	94%	99%
Medicare Spending				
Medicare Spending per Patient (ratio)	-	0.91	0.94	0.98
Pneumonia Care				
Appropriate Initial Antibiotic Given	28	86%	92%	95%
Blood Culture Timing	38	100%	98%	98%
Pregnancy and Delivery Care				
Newborn Deliveries Scheduled Early	17	0%	12%	6%
Preventive Care				
Immunization for Influenza[2]	366	96%	88%	90%
Immunization for Pneumonia[2]	287	97%	90%	92%
Stroke Care				
Anticoagulation Therapy for Atrial Fibrillation[3,7]	-	-	88%	95%
Antithrombotic Therapy Timing[1,3]	-	-	97%	98%
Assessed for Rehabilitation[1,3]	-	-	97%	97%
Discharged on Antithrombotic Therapy[1,3]	-	-	98%	99%
Discharged on Statin Medication[1,3]	-	-	88%	94%
Thrombolytic Therapy Timing[3,7]	-	-	68%	66%
Venous Thromboembolism Prophylaxis[1,3]	-	-	93%	94%
Written Stroke Educational Materials Given[1,3]	-	-	84%	88%
Surgical Care Improvement Project				
Appropriate Beta Blocker Usage	11	91%	98%	98%
Appropriate VTP Within 24 Hours	36	94%	98%	98%
Controlled Postoperative Blood Glucose[7]	-	-	98%	97%
Perioperative Temperature Management	66	100%	100%	100%
Prophylactic Antibiotic Selection	52	98%	99%	99%
Prophylactic Antibiotic Selection (Outpatient)	11	100%	98%	98%
Prophylactic Antibiotic Stopped	52	98%	98%	98%
Prophylactic Antibiotic Timing	53	98%	99%	99%
Prophylactic Antibiotic Timing (Outpatient)	11	100%	98%	98%
Urinary Catheter Removal	27	100%	97%	97%
Survey of Patients' Hospital Experiences				
Area Around Room 'Always' Quiet at Night	(a)	68%	65%	61%
Doctors 'Always' Communicated Well	(a)	84%	85%	82%
Home Recovery Information Given	(a)	89%	86%	85%
Hospital Given 9 or 10 on 10 Point Scale	(a)	73%	76%	71%
Meds 'Always' Explained Before Given	(a)	74%	66%	64%
Nurses 'Always' Communicated Well	(a)	82%	81%	79%
Pain 'Always' Well Controlled	(a)	69%	72%	71%
Room and Bathroom 'Always' Clean	(a)	75%	76%	73%
Timely Help 'Always' Received	(a)	73%	72%	68%
Would Definitely Recommend Hospital	(a)	73%	75%	71%
Use of Medical Imaging				
Cardiac Imaging Stress Test before Surgery	45	2.2%	5%	5.3%
Combination Abdominal CT Scan	209	23.0%	19%	10.5%
Combination Brain/Sinus CT Scan[1]	-	-	2.9%	2.7%
Combination Chest CT Scan	91	1.1%	3.9%	2.7%
Follow-up Mammogram/Ultrasound	425	4.7%	7.8%	8.8%
Lumbar Spine MRI for Low Back Pain[1]	-	-	40.2%	37.2%

VA Eastern Kansas Healthcare System

4101 S. 4th Street
Leavenworth, KS 66048
URL: www.leavenworth.va.gov
Phone: 913-682-2000
Fax: 785-350-4474
Type: Acute Care - VA
Ownership: Government Federal
Emergency Services: No
Beds: 197

Key Personnel:
Patient Relations . . . . Rebecca M Garcia, RN, MSN
Operating Room. . . . . Chris Haller, MD
CEO/President. . . . . Judy K McKee, FACHE
Radiology. . . . . M G Rao, MD
Chief of Medical Staff . . . . Rajeev Trehan, MD/MBBS

NOTE: Hospital profiles are in alphabetical order by state, then city, then hospital within the city; Rankings exclude hospitals with less than 25 cases except for patient surveys which excludes hospitals with less than 100 cases; (a) 100-299 cases; (1) The number of cases/patients is too few to report; (2) Data submitted were based on a sample of cases/patients; (3) Results are based on a shorter time period than required; (4) Data suppressed by CMS for one or more quarters; (5) Results are not available for this reporting period; (6) Fewer than 100 patients completed the HCAHPS survey; (7) No cases met the criteria for this measure; (8) The lower limit of the confidence interval cannot be calculated if the number of observed infections equals zero; (9) No data are available from the state/territory for this reporting period; (10) The scores shown reflect fewer than 50 completed surveys; (11) There were discrepancies in the data collection process; (12) This measure does not apply to this hospital for this reporting period; (13) Results cannot be calculated for this reporting period; (14) The results for this state are combined with nearby states to protect confidentiality; Please refer to the User's Guide for a full explanation of data.

Measure	Cases	This Hosp.	State Avg.	U.S. Avg.
Blood Clot Prevention and Treatment				
Anticoagulation Overlap Therapy	-	-	94%	93%
ICU Venous Thromboembolism Prophylaxis	-	-	91%	92%
Incidence of Potentially Preventable VTE	-	-	8%	10%
UFH with Dosages/Platelet Monitoring	-	-	98%	97%
Venous Thromboembolism Prophylaxis	-	-	79%	85%
Warfarin Therapy Discharge Instructions	-	-	84%	75%
Chest Pain/Possible Heart Attack Care				
Aspirin Given Within 24 Hours of Arrival	-	-	94%	96%
Fibrinolytic Meds Within 30 Min. of Arrival	-	-	41%	58%
Average Time to ECG (minutes)	-	-	8	7
Average Time to Transfer (minutes)	-	-	57	60
Children's Asthma Care				
Received Home Management Plan of Care	-	-	-	88%
Received Reliever Medication	-	-	-	100%
Received Systemic Corticosteroids	-	-	-	100%
Emergency Department				
Admittance Decision Time (minutes)	-	-	57	98
Head CT Results Within 45 Min. of Arrival	-	-	53%	57%
Patients Who Left ER Before Being Seen	-	-	2%	2%
Time from ER Arrival to Admit. (minutes)	-	-	185	274
Time from ER Arrival to Discharge (minutes)	-	-	104	134
Time in ER Before Being Evaluated (minutes)	-	-	18	26
Time to Pain Meds for Fractures (minutes)	-	-	47	57
Heart Attack Care				
Aspirin Given at Discharge[1]	-	-	99%	99%
Fibrinolytic Meds Within 30 Min. of Arrival[5]	-	-	-	54%
PCI Within 90 Minutes of Arrival[5]	-	-	97%	96%
Statin Prescribed at Discharge[1]	-	-	99%	98%
Heart Failure Care				
ACE Inhibitor or ARB for LVSD	25	96%	95%	97%
Discharge Instructions Given	75	96%	91%	94%
Evaluation of LVS Function	90	99%	94%	99%
Medicare Spending				
Medicare Spending per Patient (ratio)	-	-	0.94	0.98
Pneumonia Care				
Appropriate Initial Antibiotic Given	57	95%	92%	95%
Blood Culture Timing	91	100%	98%	98%
Pregnancy and Delivery Care				
Newborn Deliveries Scheduled Early	-	-	12%	6%
Preventive Care				
Immunization for Influenza[5]	-	-	88%	90%
Immunization for Pneumonia[5]	-	-	90%	92%
Stroke Care				
Anticoagulation Therapy for Atrial Fibrillation	-	-	88%	95%
Antithrombotic Therapy Timing	-	-	97%	98%
Assessed for Rehabilitation	-	-	97%	97%
Discharged on Antithrombotic Therapy	-	-	98%	99%
Discharged on Statin Medication	-	-	88%	94%
Thrombolytic Therapy Timing	-	-	68%	66%
Venous Thromboembolism Prophylaxis	-	-	93%	94%
Written Stroke Educational Materials Given	-	-	84%	88%
Surgical Care Improvement Project				
Appropriate Beta Blocker Usage[1,2]	-	-	98%	98%
Appropriate VTP Within 24 Hours[1,2]	-	-	98%	98%
Controlled Postoperative Blood Glucose[5]	-	-	98%	97%
Perioperative Temperature Management[1,2]	-	-	100%	100%
Prophylactic Antibiotic Selection[1]	-	-	99%	99%
Prophylactic Antibiotic Selection (Outpatient)	-	-	98%	98%
Prophylactic Antibiotic Stopped[1]	-	-	98%	98%
Prophylactic Antibiotic Timing[1]	-	-	99%	99%
Prophylactic Antibiotic Timing (Outpatient)	-	-	98%	98%
Urinary Catheter Removal[1,2]	-	-	97%	97%
Survey of Patients' Hospital Experiences				
Area Around Room 'Always' Quiet at Night	-	-	65%	61%
Doctors 'Always' Communicated Well	-	-	85%	82%
Home Recovery Information Given	-	-	86%	85%
Hospital Given 9 or 10 on 10 Point Scale	-	-	76%	71%
Meds 'Always' Explained Before Given	-	-	66%	64%
Nurses 'Always' Communicated Well	-	-	81%	79%
Pain 'Always' Well Controlled	-	-	72%	71%
Room and Bathroom 'Always' Clean	-	-	76%	73%
Timely Help 'Always' Received	-	-	72%	68%
Would Definitely Recommend Hospital	-	-	75%	71%
Use of Medical Imaging				
Cardiac Imaging Stress Test before Surgery	-	-	5%	5.3%
Combination Abdominal CT Scan	-	-	19%	10.5%
Combination Brain/Sinus CT Scan	-	-	2.9%	2.7%
Combination Chest CT Scan	-	-	3.9%	2.7%
Follow-up Mammogram/Ultrasound	-	-	7.8%	8.8%
Lumbar Spine MRI for Low Back Pain	-	-	40.2%	37.2%

Doctors Hospital

4901 College Blvd
Leawood, KS 66211
Type: Acute Care Hospitals
Ownership: Proprietary
Phone: 913-529-1801
Emergency Services: Yes

Measure	Cases	This Hosp.	State Avg.	U.S. Avg.
Blood Clot Prevention and Treatment				
Anticoagulation Overlap Therapy[7]	-	-	94%	93%
ICU Venous Thromboembolism Prophylaxis[7]	-	-	91%	92%
Incidence of Potentially Preventable VTE[7]	-	-	8%	10%
UFH with Dosages/Platelet Monitoring[7]	-	-	98%	97%
Venous Thromboembolism Prophylaxis	28	71%	79%	85%
Warfarin Therapy Discharge Instructions[7]	-	-	84%	75%
Chest Pain/Possible Heart Attack Care				
Aspirin Given Within 24 Hours of Arrival[5]	-	-	94%	96%
Fibrinolytic Meds Within 30 Min. of Arrival[5]	-	-	41%	58%
Average Time to ECG (minutes)[5]	-	-	8	7
Average Time to Transfer (minutes)[5]	-	-	57	60
Children's Asthma Care				
Received Home Management Plan of Care	-	-	-	88%
Received Reliever Medication	-	-	-	100%
Received Systemic Corticosteroids	-	-	-	100%
Emergency Department				
Admittance Decision Time (minutes)[7]	-	-	57	98
Head CT Results Within 45 Min. of Arrival[5]	-	-	53%	57%
Patients Who Left ER Before Being Seen[5]	-	-	2%	2%
Time from ER Arrival to Admit. (minutes)[7]	-	-	185	274
Time from ER Arrival to Discharge (minutes)[5]	-	-	104	134
Time in ER Before Being Evaluated (minutes)[5]	-	-	18	26
Time to Pain Meds for Fractures (minutes)[5]	-	-	47	57
Heart Attack Care				
Aspirin Given at Discharge[5]	-	-	99%	99%
Fibrinolytic Meds Within 30 Min. of Arrival[5]	-	-	-	54%
PCI Within 90 Minutes of Arrival[5]	-	-	97%	96%
Statin Prescribed at Discharge[5]	-	-	99%	98%
Heart Failure Care				
ACE Inhibitor or ARB for LVSD[5]	-	-	95%	97%
Discharge Instructions Given[5]	-	-	91%	94%
Evaluation of LVS Function[5]	-	-	94%	99%
Medicare Spending				
Medicare Spending per Patient (ratio)	-	0.88	0.94	0.98
Pneumonia Care				
Appropriate Initial Antibiotic Given[5]	-	-	92%	95%
Blood Culture Timing[5]	-	-	98%	98%
Pregnancy and Delivery Care				
Newborn Deliveries Scheduled Early[7]	-	-	12%	6%
Preventive Care				
Immunization for Influenza	64	56%	88%	90%
Immunization for Pneumonia	93	62%	90%	92%
Stroke Care				
Anticoagulation Therapy for Atrial Fibrillation[5]	-	-	88%	95%
Antithrombotic Therapy Timing[5]	-	-	97%	98%
Assessed for Rehabilitation[5]	-	-	97%	97%
Discharged on Antithrombotic Therapy[5]	-	-	98%	99%
Discharged on Statin Medication[5]	-	-	88%	94%
Thrombolytic Therapy Timing[5]	-	-	68%	66%
Venous Thromboembolism Prophylaxis[5]	-	-	93%	94%
Written Stroke Educational Materials Given[5]	-	-	84%	88%
Surgical Care Improvement Project				
Appropriate Beta Blocker Usage[1,3]	-	-	98%	98%
Appropriate VTP Within 24 Hours[1,3]	-	-	98%	98%
Controlled Postoperative Blood Glucose[3,7]	-	-	98%	97%
Perioperative Temperature Management[1,3]	-	-	100%	100%
Prophylactic Antibiotic Selection[1,3]	-	-	99%	99%
Prophylactic Antibiotic Selection (Outpatient)	14	100%	98%	98%
Prophylactic Antibiotic Stopped[1,3]	-	-	98%	98%
Prophylactic Antibiotic Timing[1,3]	-	-	99%	99%
Prophylactic Antibiotic Timing (Outpatient)	14	93%	98%	98%
Urinary Catheter Removal[1,3]	-	-	97%	97%
Survey of Patients' Hospital Experiences				
Area Around Room 'Always' Quiet at Night[10]	<100	80%	65%	61%
Doctors 'Always' Communicated Well[10]	<100	81%	85%	82%
Home Recovery Information Given[10]	<100	90%	86%	85%
Hospital Given 9 or 10 on 10 Point Scale[10]	<100	92%	76%	71%
Meds 'Always' Explained Before Given[10]	<100	69%	66%	64%
Nurses 'Always' Communicated Well[10]	<100	85%	81%	79%
Pain 'Always' Well Controlled[10]	<100	78%	72%	71%
Room and Bathroom 'Always' Clean[10]	<100	81%	76%	73%
Timely Help 'Always' Received[10]	<100	80%	72%	68%
Would Definitely Recommend Hospital[10]	<100	79%	75%	71%
Use of Medical Imaging				
Cardiac Imaging Stress Test before Surgery[7]	-	-	5%	5.3%
Combination Abdominal CT Scan[7]	-	-	19%	10.5%
Combination Brain/Sinus CT Scan[7]	-	-	2.9%	2.7%
Combination Chest CT Scan[7]	-	-	3.9%	2.7%
Follow-up Mammogram/Ultrasound[7]	-	-	7.8%	8.8%
Lumbar Spine MRI for Low Back Pain	56	35.7%	40.2%	37.2%

Kansas City Orthopaedic Institute

3651 College Blvd
Leawood, KS 66211
URL: www.kcoi.com
Type: Acute Care Hospitals
Ownership: Physician
Phone: 913-319-7633
Fax: 816-531-5313
Emergency Services: No
Beds: 9

Measure	Cases	This Hosp.	State Avg.	U.S. Avg.
Blood Clot Prevention and Treatment				
Anticoagulation Overlap Therapy[7]	-	-	94%	93%
ICU Venous Thromboembolism Prophylaxis[7]	-	-	91%	92%
Incidence of Potentially Preventable VTE[7]	-	-	8%	10%
UFH with Dosages/Platelet Monitoring[7]	-	-	98%	97%
Venous Thromboembolism Prophylaxis	12	92%	79%	85%
Warfarin Therapy Discharge Instructions[7]	-	-	84%	75%
Chest Pain/Possible Heart Attack Care				
Aspirin Given Within 24 Hours of Arrival[5]	-	-	94%	96%
Fibrinolytic Meds Within 30 Min. of Arrival[5]	-	-	41%	58%
Average Time to ECG (minutes)[5]	-	-	8	7
Average Time to Transfer (minutes)[5]	-	-	57	60
Children's Asthma Care				
Received Home Management Plan of Care	-	-	-	88%
Received Reliever Medication	-	-	-	100%
Received Systemic Corticosteroids	-	-	-	100%
Emergency Department				
Admittance Decision Time (minutes)[7]	-	-	57	98
Head CT Results Within 45 Min. of Arrival[5]	-	-	53%	57%
Patients Who Left ER Before Being Seen[5]	-	-	2%	2%
Time from ER Arrival to Admit. (minutes)[7]	-	-	185	274
Time from ER Arrival to Discharge (minutes)[5]	-	-	104	134
Time in ER Before Being Evaluated (minutes)[5]	-	-	18	26
Time to Pain Meds for Fractures (minutes)[5]	-	-	47	57
Heart Attack Care				
Aspirin Given at Discharge[5]	-	-	99%	99%
Fibrinolytic Meds Within 30 Min. of Arrival[5]	-	-	-	54%
PCI Within 90 Minutes of Arrival[5]	-	-	97%	96%
Statin Prescribed at Discharge[5]	-	-	99%	98%
Heart Failure Care				
ACE Inhibitor or ARB for LVSD[5]	-	-	95%	97%
Discharge Instructions Given[5]	-	-	91%	94%
Evaluation of LVS Function[5]	-	-	94%	99%
Medicare Spending				
Medicare Spending per Patient (ratio)	-	0.90	0.94	0.98
Pneumonia Care				
Appropriate Initial Antibiotic Given[5]	-	-	92%	95%
Blood Culture Timing[5]	-	-	98%	98%

NOTE: Hospital profiles are in alphabetical order by state, then city, then hospital within the city; Rankings exclude hospitals with less than 25 cases except for patient surveys which excludes hospitals with less than 100 cases; (a) 100-299 cases; (1) The number of cases/patients is too few to report; (2) Data submitted were based on a sample of cases/patients; (3) Results are based on a shorter time period than required; (4) Data suppressed by CMS for one or more quarters; (5) Results are not available for this reporting period; (6) Fewer than 100 patients completed the HCAHPS survey; (7) No cases met the criteria for this measure; (8) The lower limit of the confidence interval cannot be calculated if the number of observed infections equals zero; (9) No data are available from the state/territory for this reporting period; (10) The scores shown reflect fewer than 50 completed surveys; (11) There were discrepancies in the data collection process; (12) This measure does not apply to this hospital for this reporting period; (13) Results cannot be calculated for this reporting period; (14) The results for this state are combined with nearby states to protect confidentiality; Please refer to the User's Guide for a full explanation of data.

Measure	Cases	This Hosp.	State Avg.	U.S. Avg.
Pregnancy and Delivery Care				
Newborn Deliveries Scheduled Early[7]	-	-	12%	6%
Preventive Care				
Immunization for Influenza	372	98%	88%	90%
Immunization for Pneumonia	392	96%	90%	92%
Stroke Care				
Anticoagulation Therapy for Atrial Fibrillation[5]	-	-	88%	95%
Antithrombotic Therapy Timing[5]	-	-	97%	98%
Assessed for Rehabilitation[5]	-	-	97%	97%
Discharged on Antithrombotic Therapy[5]	-	-	98%	99%
Discharged on Statin Medication[5]	-	-	88%	94%
Thrombolytic Therapy Timing[5]	-	-	68%	66%
Venous Thromboembolism Prophylaxis[5]	-	-	93%	94%
Written Stroke Educational Materials Given[5]	-	-	84%	88%
Surgical Care Improvement Project				
Appropriate Beta Blocker Usage[2]	23	100%	98%	98%
Appropriate VTP Within 24 Hours[2]	188	100%	98%	98%
Controlled Postoperative Blood Glucose[2,7]	-	-	98%	97%
Perioperative Temperature Management[2]	197	100%	100%	100%
Prophylactic Antibiotic Selection[2]	148	100%	99%	99%
Prophylactic Antibiotic Selection (Outpatient)[5]	-	-	98%	98%
Prophylactic Antibiotic Stopped[2]	148	99%	98%	98%
Prophylactic Antibiotic Timing[2]	148	99%	99%	99%
Prophylactic Antibiotic Timing (Outpatient)[5]	-	-	98%	98%
Urinary Catheter Removal[1,2]	-	-	97%	97%
Survey of Patients' Hospital Experiences				
Area Around Room 'Always' Quiet at Night	300+	70%	65%	61%
Doctors 'Always' Communicated Well	300+	89%	85%	82%
Home Recovery Information Given	300+	94%	86%	85%
Hospital Given 9 or 10 on 10 Point Scale	300+	87%	76%	71%
Meds 'Always' Explained Before Given	300+	78%	66%	64%
Nurses 'Always' Communicated Well	300+	88%	81%	79%
Pain 'Always' Well Controlled	300+	79%	72%	71%
Room and Bathroom 'Always' Clean	300+	81%	76%	73%
Timely Help 'Always' Received	300+	87%	72%	68%
Would Definitely Recommend Hospital	300+	89%	75%	71%
Use of Medical Imaging				
Cardiac Imaging Stress Test before Surgery[7]	-	-	5%	5.3%
Combination Abdominal CT Scan[7]	-	-	19%	10.5%
Combination Brain/Sinus CT Scan[7]	-	-	2.9%	2.7%
Combination Chest CT Scan[7]	-	-	3.9%	2.7%
Follow-up Mammogram/Ultrasound[7]	-	-	7.8%	8.8%
Lumbar Spine MRI for Low Back Pain	151	35.1%	40.2%	37.2%

Minimally Invasive Surgery Hospital

11217 Lakeview Avenue
Lenexa, KS 66219
Phone: 913-322-7401
Type: Acute Care Hospitals
Emergency Services: No
Ownership: Proprietary

Measure	Cases	This Hosp.	State Avg.	U.S. Avg.
Blood Clot Prevention and Treatment				
Anticoagulation Overlap Therapy[2,7]	-	-	94%	93%
ICU Venous Thromboembolism Prophylaxis[2,7]	-	-	91%	92%
Incidence of Potentially Preventable VTE[2,7]	-	-	8%	10%
UFH with Dosages/Platelet Monitoring[2,7]	-	-	98%	97%
Venous Thromboembolism Prophylaxis[1,2]	-	-	79%	85%
Warfarin Therapy Discharge Instructions[2,7]	-	-	84%	75%
Chest Pain/Possible Heart Attack Care				
Aspirin Given Within 24 Hours of Arrival[5]	-	-	94%	96%
Fibrinolytic Meds Within 30 Min. of Arrival[5]	-	-	41%	58%
Average Time to ECG (minutes)[5]	-	-	8	7
Average Time to Transfer (minutes)[5]	-	-	57	60
Children's Asthma Care				
Received Home Management Plan of Care	-	-	-	88%
Received Reliever Medication	-	-	-	100%
Received Systemic Corticosteroids	-	-	-	100%
Emergency Department				
Admittance Decision Time (minutes)[2,7]	-	-	57	98
Head CT Results Within 45 Min. of Arrival[5]	-	-	53%	57%
Patients Who Left ER Before Being Seen[5]	-	-	2%	2%
Time from ER Arrival to Admit. (minutes)[2,7]	-	-	185	274
Time from ER Arrival to Discharge (minutes)[5]	-	-	104	134
Time in ER Before Being Evaluated (minutes)[5]	-	-	18	26
Time to Pain Meds for Fractures (minutes)[5]	-	-	47	57
Heart Attack Care				
Aspirin Given at Discharge[5]	-	-	99%	99%
Fibrinolytic Meds Within 30 Min. of Arrival[5]	-	-	-	54%
PCI Within 90 Minutes of Arrival[5]	-	-	97%	96%
Statin Prescribed at Discharge[5]	-	-	99%	98%
Heart Failure Care				
ACE Inhibitor or ARB for LVSD[5]	-	-	95%	97%
Discharge Instructions Given[5]	-	-	91%	94%
Evaluation of LVS Function[5]	-	-	94%	99%
Medicare Spending				
Medicare Spending per Patient (ratio)	-	1.66	0.94	0.98
Pneumonia Care				
Appropriate Initial Antibiotic Given[5]	-	-	92%	95%
Blood Culture Timing[5]	-	-	98%	98%
Pregnancy and Delivery Care				
Newborn Deliveries Scheduled Early[2,7]	-	-	12%	6%
Preventive Care				
Immunization for Influenza[2]	59	92%	88%	90%
Immunization for Pneumonia[2]	22	91%	90%	92%
Stroke Care				
Anticoagulation Therapy for Atrial Fibrillation[5]	-	-	88%	95%
Antithrombotic Therapy Timing[5]	-	-	97%	98%
Assessed for Rehabilitation[5]	-	-	97%	97%
Discharged on Antithrombotic Therapy[5]	-	-	98%	99%
Discharged on Statin Medication[5]	-	-	88%	94%
Thrombolytic Therapy Timing[5]	-	-	68%	66%
Venous Thromboembolism Prophylaxis[5]	-	-	93%	94%
Written Stroke Educational Materials Given[5]	-	-	84%	88%
Surgical Care Improvement Project				
Appropriate Beta Blocker Usage[2,3]	-	-	98%	98%
Appropriate VTP Within 24 Hours[2,3]	-	-	98%	98%
Controlled Postoperative Blood Glucose[2,3]	-	-	98%	97%
Perioperative Temperature Management[1,2]	-	-	100%	100%
Prophylactic Antibiotic Selection[2,3]	-	-	99%	99%
Prophylactic Antibiotic Selection (Outpatient)[5]	-	-	98%	98%
Prophylactic Antibiotic Stopped[2,3]	-	-	98%	98%
Prophylactic Antibiotic Timing[2,3]	-	-	99%	99%
Prophylactic Antibiotic Timing (Outpatient)[5]	-	-	98%	98%
Urinary Catheter Removal[2,3]	-	-	97%	97%
Survey of Patients' Hospital Experiences				
Area Around Room 'Always' Quiet at Night[6]	<100	81%	65%	61%
Doctors 'Always' Communicated Well[6]	<100	90%	85%	82%
Home Recovery Information Given[6]	<100	94%	86%	85%
Hospital Given 9 or 10 on 10 Point Scale[6]	<100	85%	76%	71%
Meds 'Always' Explained Before Given[6]	<100	90%	66%	64%
Nurses 'Always' Communicated Well[6]	<100	91%	81%	79%
Pain 'Always' Well Controlled[6]	<100	74%	72%	71%
Room and Bathroom 'Always' Clean[6]	<100	82%	76%	73%
Timely Help 'Always' Received[6]	<100	92%	72%	68%
Would Definitely Recommend Hospital[6]	<100	84%	75%	71%
Use of Medical Imaging				
Cardiac Imaging Stress Test before Surgery[7]	-	-	5%	5.3%
Combination Abdominal CT Scan[1]	-	-	19%	10.5%
Combination Brain/Sinus CT Scan[1]	-	-	2.9%	2.7%
Combination Chest CT Scan[1]	-	-	3.9%	2.7%
Follow-up Mammogram/Ultrasound[7]	-	-	7.8%	8.8%
Lumbar Spine MRI for Low Back Pain[7]	-	-	40.2%	37.2%

Wichita County Health Center

211 E Earl Street
Leoti, KS 67861
Phone: 620-375-2233
Fax: 620-375-2248
Type: Critical Access Hospitals
Emergency Services: No
Ownership: Government - Local
Beds: 39

Key Personnel:
Chair/CEO.................. Russell Berning
CEO/President.............. Tyson Sterling
Radiology.................. Martha Vallejo
Infection Control.......... Beverly White, RN
Quality Assurance.......... Beverly White, RN

Measure	Cases	This Hosp.	State Avg.	U.S. Avg.
Blood Clot Prevention and Treatment				
Anticoagulation Overlap Therapy[5]	-	-	94%	93%
ICU Venous Thromboembolism Prophylaxis[5]	-	-	91%	92%
Incidence of Potentially Preventable VTE[5]	-	-	8%	10%
UFH with Dosages/Platelet Monitoring[5]	-	-	98%	97%
Venous Thromboembolism Prophylaxis[5]	-	-	79%	85%
Warfarin Therapy Discharge Instructions[5]	-	-	84%	75%
Chest Pain/Possible Heart Attack Care				
Aspirin Given Within 24 Hours of Arrival	-	-	94%	96%
Fibrinolytic Meds Within 30 Min. of Arrival	-	-	41%	58%
Average Time to ECG (minutes)	-	-	8	7
Average Time to Transfer (minutes)	-	-	57	60
Children's Asthma Care				
Received Home Management Plan of Care	-	-	-	88%
Received Reliever Medication	-	-	-	100%
Received Systemic Corticosteroids	-	-	-	100%
Emergency Department				
Admittance Decision Time (minutes)[1,3]	-	-	57	98
Head CT Results Within 45 Min. of Arrival	-	-	53%	57%
Patients Who Left ER Before Being Seen	-	-	2%	2%
Time from ER Arrival to Admit. (minutes)[1,3]	-	-	185	274
Time from ER Arrival to Discharge (minutes)	-	-	104	134
Time in ER Before Being Evaluated (minutes)	-	-	18	26
Time to Pain Meds for Fractures (minutes)	-	-	47	57
Heart Attack Care				
Aspirin Given at Discharge[5]	-	-	99%	99%
Fibrinolytic Meds Within 30 Min. of Arrival[5]	-	-	-	54%
PCI Within 90 Minutes of Arrival[5]	-	-	97%	96%
Statin Prescribed at Discharge[5]	-	-	99%	98%
Heart Failure Care				
ACE Inhibitor or ARB for LVSD[5]	-	-	95%	97%
Discharge Instructions Given[5]	-	-	91%	94%
Evaluation of LVS Function[5]	-	-	94%	99%
Medicare Spending				
Medicare Spending per Patient (ratio)	-	-	0.94	0.98
Pneumonia Care				
Appropriate Initial Antibiotic Given[1,3]	-	-	92%	95%
Blood Culture Timing[1,3]	-	-	98%	98%
Pregnancy and Delivery Care				
Newborn Deliveries Scheduled Early[5]	-	-	12%	6%
Preventive Care				
Immunization for Influenza[1,3]	-	-	88%	90%
Immunization for Pneumonia[1,3]	-	-	90%	92%
Stroke Care				
Anticoagulation Therapy for Atrial Fibrillation[5]	-	-	88%	95%
Antithrombotic Therapy Timing[5]	-	-	97%	98%
Assessed for Rehabilitation[5]	-	-	97%	97%
Discharged on Antithrombotic Therapy[5]	-	-	98%	99%
Discharged on Statin Medication[5]	-	-	88%	94%
Thrombolytic Therapy Timing[5]	-	-	68%	66%
Venous Thromboembolism Prophylaxis[5]	-	-	93%	94%
Written Stroke Educational Materials Given[5]	-	-	84%	88%
Surgical Care Improvement Project				
Appropriate Beta Blocker Usage[5]	-	-	98%	98%
Appropriate VTP Within 24 Hours[5]	-	-	98%	98%
Controlled Postoperative Blood Glucose[5]	-	-	98%	97%
Perioperative Temperature Management[5]	-	-	100%	100%
Prophylactic Antibiotic Selection[5]	-	-	99%	99%
Prophylactic Antibiotic Selection (Outpatient)	-	-	98%	98%
Prophylactic Antibiotic Stopped[5]	-	-	98%	98%
Prophylactic Antibiotic Timing[5]	-	-	99%	99%
Prophylactic Antibiotic Timing (Outpatient)	-	-	98%	98%
Urinary Catheter Removal[5]	-	-	97%	97%
Survey of Patients' Hospital Experiences				
Area Around Room 'Always' Quiet at Night[5]	-	-	65%	61%
Doctors 'Always' Communicated Well[5]	-	-	85%	82%
Home Recovery Information Given[5]	-	-	86%	85%
Hospital Given 9 or 10 on 10 Point Scale[5]	-	-	76%	71%
Meds 'Always' Explained Before Given[5]	-	-	66%	64%
Nurses 'Always' Communicated Well[5]	-	-	81%	79%
Pain 'Always' Well Controlled[5]	-	-	72%	71%
Room and Bathroom 'Always' Clean[5]	-	-	76%	73%
Timely Help 'Always' Received[5]	-	-	72%	68%

NOTE: Hospital profiles are in alphabetical order by state, then city, then hospital within the city; Rankings exclude hospitals with less than 25 cases except for patient surveys which excludes hospitals with less than 100 cases; (a) 100-299 cases; (1) The number of cases/patients is too few to report; (2) Data submitted were based on a sample of cases/patients; (3) Results are based on a shorter time period than required; (4) Data suppressed by CMS for one or more quarters; (5) Results are not available for this reporting period; (6) Fewer than 100 patients completed the HCAHPS survey; (7) No cases met the criteria for this measure; (8) The lower limit of the confidence interval cannot be calculated if the number of observed infections equals zero; (9) No data are available from the state/territory for this reporting period; (10) The scores shown reflect fewer than 50 completed surveys; (11) There were discrepancies in the data collection process; (12) This measure does not apply to this hospital for this reporting period; (13) Results cannot be calculated for this reporting period; (14) The results for this state are combined with nearby states to protect confidentiality; Please refer to the User's Guide for a full explanation of data.

Would Definitely Recommend Hospital[5]	-	-	75%	71%
Use of Medical Imaging				
Cardiac Imaging Stress Test before Surgery	-	-	5%	5.3%
Combination Abdominal CT Scan	-	-	19%	10.5%
Combination Brain/Sinus CT Scan	-	-	2.9%	2.7%
Combination Chest CT Scan	-	-	3.9%	2.7%
Follow-up Mammogram/Ultrasound	-	-	7.8%	8.8%
Lumbar Spine MRI for Low Back Pain	-	-	40.2%	37.2%

Southwest Medical Center

315 West 15th Street
Liberal, KS 67901
Phone: 620-629-6291
URL: www.swmedcenter.com
Type: Acute Care Hospitals
Emergency Services: Yes
Ownership: Government - Local
Beds: 80

Key Personnel:
President/CEO. . . . . Norman T Lambert

Measure	Cases	This Hosp.	State Avg.	U.S. Avg.
Blood Clot Prevention and Treatment				
Anticoagulation Overlap Therapy[2]	13	54%	94%	93%
ICU Venous Thromboembolism Prophylaxis[2]	45	98%	91%	92%
Incidence of Potentially Preventable VTE[1,2]	-	-	8%	10%
UFH with Dosages/Platelet Monitoring[2,7]	-	-	98%	97%
Venous Thromboembolism Prophylaxis[2]	78	95%	79%	85%
Warfarin Therapy Discharge Instructions[2]	11	100%	84%	75%
Chest Pain/Possible Heart Attack Care				
Aspirin Given Within 24 Hours of Arrival	48	90%	94%	96%
Fibrinolytic Meds Within 30 Min. of Arrival[1,3]	-	-	41%	58%
Average Time to ECG (minutes)	49	17	8	7
Average Time to Transfer (minutes)[1,3]	-	-	57	60
Children's Asthma Care				
Received Home Management Plan of Care	-	-	-	88%
Received Reliever Medication	-	-	-	100%
Received Systemic Corticosteroids	-	-	-	100%
Emergency Department				
Admittance Decision Time (minutes)[2]	112	72	57	98
Head CT Results Within 45 Min. of Arrival[1]	-	-	53%	57%
Patients Who Left ER Before Being Seen	9,534	3%	2%	2%
Time from ER Arrival to Admit. (minutes)[2]	115	189	185	274
Time from ER Arrival to Discharge (minutes)	356	128	104	134
Time in ER Before Being Evaluated (minutes)	400	35	18	26
Time to Pain Meds for Fractures (minutes)	36	78	47	57
Heart Attack Care				
Aspirin Given at Discharge[1]	-	-	99%	99%
Fibrinolytic Meds Within 30 Min. of Arrival[7]	-	-	-	54%
PCI Within 90 Minutes of Arrival[7]	-	-	97%	96%
Statin Prescribed at Discharge[1]	-	-	99%	98%
Heart Failure Care				
ACE Inhibitor or ARB for LVSD[1]	-	-	95%	97%
Discharge Instructions Given	21	90%	91%	94%
Evaluation of LVS Function	26	92%	94%	99%
Medicare Spending				
Medicare Spending per Patient (ratio)	-	0.88	0.94	0.98
Pneumonia Care				
Appropriate Initial Antibiotic Given	36	92%	92%	95%
Blood Culture Timing	25	96%	98%	98%
Pregnancy and Delivery Care				
Newborn Deliveries Scheduled Early[2]	55	11%	12%	6%
Preventive Care				
Immunization for Influenza[2]	220	91%	88%	90%
Immunization for Pneumonia[2]	129	91%	90%	92%
Stroke Care				
Anticoagulation Therapy for Atrial Fibrillation[1]	-	-	88%	95%
Antithrombotic Therapy Timing[1]	-	-	97%	98%
Assessed for Rehabilitation[1]	-	-	97%	97%
Discharged on Antithrombotic Therapy[1]	-	-	98%	99%
Discharged on Statin Medication[1]	-	-	88%	94%
Thrombolytic Therapy Timing[1]	-	-	68%	66%
Venous Thromboembolism Prophylaxis[1]	-	-	93%	94%
Written Stroke Educational Materials Given[1]	-	-	84%	88%
Surgical Care Improvement Project				
Appropriate Beta Blocker Usage	22	91%	98%	98%
Appropriate VTP Within 24 Hours	73	96%	98%	98%
Controlled Postoperative Blood Glucose[7]	-	-	98%	97%
Perioperative Temperature Management	77	100%	100%	100%
Prophylactic Antibiotic Selection	51	88%	99%	99%
Prophylactic Antibiotic Selection (Outpatient)	185	95%	98%	98%
Prophylactic Antibiotic Stopped	43	81%	98%	98%
Prophylactic Antibiotic Timing	52	88%	99%	99%
Prophylactic Antibiotic Timing (Outpatient)	185	95%	98%	98%
Urinary Catheter Removal	42	100%	97%	97%
Survey of Patients' Hospital Experiences				
Area Around Room 'Always' Quiet at Night	300+	57%	65%	61%
Doctors 'Always' Communicated Well	300+	82%	85%	82%
Home Recovery Information Given	300+	89%	86%	85%
Hospital Given 9 or 10 on 10 Point Scale	300+	71%	76%	71%
Meds 'Always' Explained Before Given	300+	64%	66%	64%
Nurses 'Always' Communicated Well	300+	78%	81%	79%
Pain 'Always' Well Controlled	300+	70%	72%	71%
Room and Bathroom 'Always' Clean	300+	74%	76%	73%
Timely Help 'Always' Received	300+	65%	72%	68%
Would Definitely Recommend Hospital	300+	69%	75%	71%
Use of Medical Imaging				
Cardiac Imaging Stress Test before Surgery	169	1.8%	5%	5.3%
Combination Abdominal CT Scan	222	16.2%	19%	10.5%
Combination Brain/Sinus CT Scan[1]	-	-	2.9%	2.7%
Combination Chest CT Scan	118	14.4%	3.9%	2.7%
Follow-up Mammogram/Ultrasound	324	3.1%	7.8%	8.8%
Lumbar Spine MRI for Low Back Pain	46	45.7%	40.2%	37.2%

Lindsborg Community Hospital

605 W Lincoln Street
Lindsborg, KS 67456
Phone: 785-227-3308
Fax: 785-227-4130
E-mail: lch@lindsborghospital.org
URL: www.lindsborghospital.org
Type: Critical Access Hospitals
Emergency Services: Yes
Ownership: Voluntary non-profit - Private
Beds: 25

Key Personnel:
Radiology. Anna Anderson
Chief of Medical Staff. . . . . Susan Chrislip
Emergency Room . . . . Beth Hedberg, RN
Infection Control. . . . . Beth Hedberg, RN
Surgery . . . . Tracy Littrell
Administrator . . . . Larry VanDerWege
Operating Room. . . . . Joanie Worthen, RN, B
Quality Assurance . . . . Joanie Worthen, RN, B

Measure	Cases	This Hosp.	State Avg.	U.S. Avg.
Blood Clot Prevention and Treatment				
Anticoagulation Overlap Therapy[5]	-	-	94%	93%
ICU Venous Thromboembolism Prophylaxis[5]	-	-	91%	92%
Incidence of Potentially Preventable VTE[5]	-	-	8%	10%
UFH with Dosages/Platelet Monitoring[5]	-	-	98%	97%
Venous Thromboembolism Prophylaxis[5]	-	-	79%	85%
Warfarin Therapy Discharge Instructions[5]	-	-	84%	75%
Chest Pain/Possible Heart Attack Care				
Aspirin Given Within 24 Hours of Arrival	-	-	94%	96%
Fibrinolytic Meds Within 30 Min. of Arrival	-	-	41%	58%
Average Time to ECG (minutes)	-	-	8	7
Average Time to Transfer (minutes)	-	-	57	60
Children's Asthma Care				
Received Home Management Plan of Care	-	-	-	88%
Received Reliever Medication	-	-	-	100%
Received Systemic Corticosteroids	-	-	-	100%
Emergency Department				
Admittance Decision Time (minutes)[5]	-	-	57	98
Head CT Results Within 45 Min. of Arrival	-	-	53%	57%
Patients Who Left ER Before Being Seen	-	-	2%	2%
Time from ER Arrival to Admit. (minutes)[5]	-	-	185	274
Time from ER Arrival to Discharge (minutes)	-	-	104	134
Time in ER Before Being Evaluated (minutes)	-	-	18	26
Time to Pain Meds for Fractures (minutes)	-	-	47	57
Heart Attack Care				
Aspirin Given at Discharge[5]	-	-	99%	99%
Fibrinolytic Meds Within 30 Min. of Arrival[5]	-	-	-	54%
PCI Within 90 Minutes of Arrival[5]	-	-	97%	96%
Statin Prescribed at Discharge[5]	-	-	99%	98%
Heart Failure Care				
ACE Inhibitor or ARB for LVSD[3,7]	-	-	95%	97%
Discharge Instructions Given[1,3]	-	-	91%	94%
Evaluation of LVS Function[1,3]	-	-	94%	99%
Medicare Spending				
Medicare Spending per Patient (ratio)	-	-	0.94	0.98
Pneumonia Care				
Appropriate Initial Antibiotic Given[1]	-	-	92%	95%
Blood Culture Timing[1]	-	-	98%	98%
Pregnancy and Delivery Care				
Newborn Deliveries Scheduled Early[5]	-	-	12%	6%
Preventive Care				
Immunization for Influenza[5]	-	-	88%	90%
Immunization for Pneumonia[5]	-	-	90%	92%
Stroke Care				
Anticoagulation Therapy for Atrial Fibrillation[5]	-	-	88%	95%
Antithrombotic Therapy Timing[5]	-	-	97%	98%
Assessed for Rehabilitation[5]	-	-	97%	97%
Discharged on Antithrombotic Therapy[5]	-	-	98%	99%
Discharged on Statin Medication[5]	-	-	88%	94%
Thrombolytic Therapy Timing[5]	-	-	68%	66%
Venous Thromboembolism Prophylaxis[5]	-	-	93%	94%
Written Stroke Educational Materials Given[5]	-	-	84%	88%
Surgical Care Improvement Project				
Appropriate Beta Blocker Usage[5]	-	-	98%	98%
Appropriate VTP Within 24 Hours[5]	-	-	98%	98%
Controlled Postoperative Blood Glucose[5]	-	-	98%	97%
Perioperative Temperature Management[5]	-	-	100%	100%
Prophylactic Antibiotic Selection[5]	-	-	99%	99%
Prophylactic Antibiotic Selection (Outpatient)	-	-	98%	98%
Prophylactic Antibiotic Stopped[5]	-	-	98%	98%
Prophylactic Antibiotic Timing[5]	-	-	99%	99%
Prophylactic Antibiotic Timing (Outpatient)	-	-	98%	98%
Urinary Catheter Removal[5]	-	-	97%	97%
Survey of Patients' Hospital Experiences				
Area Around Room 'Always' Quiet at Night[5]	-	-	65%	61%
Doctors 'Always' Communicated Well[5]	-	-	85%	82%
Home Recovery Information Given[5]	-	-	86%	85%
Hospital Given 9 or 10 on 10 Point Scale[5]	-	-	76%	71%
Meds 'Always' Explained Before Given[5]	-	-	66%	64%
Nurses 'Always' Communicated Well[5]	-	-	81%	79%
Pain 'Always' Well Controlled[5]	-	-	72%	71%
Room and Bathroom 'Always' Clean[5]	-	-	76%	73%
Timely Help 'Always' Received[5]	-	-	72%	68%
Would Definitely Recommend Hospital[5]	-	-	75%	71%
Use of Medical Imaging				
Cardiac Imaging Stress Test before Surgery	-	-	5%	5.3%
Combination Abdominal CT Scan	-	-	19%	10.5%
Combination Brain/Sinus CT Scan	-	-	2.9%	2.7%
Combination Chest CT Scan	-	-	3.9%	2.7%
Follow-up Mammogram/Ultrasound	-	-	7.8%	8.8%
Lumbar Spine MRI for Low Back Pain	-	-	40.2%	37.2%

Hospital District #1 of Rice County

619 South Clark Avenue
Lyons, KS 67554
Phone: 620-257-5173
Type: Critical Access Hospitals
Emergency Services: No
Ownership: Govt - Hospital Dist/Auth

Measure	Cases	This Hosp.	State Avg.	U.S. Avg.
Blood Clot Prevention and Treatment				
Anticoagulation Overlap Therapy[5]	-	-	94%	93%
ICU Venous Thromboembolism Prophylaxis[5]	-	-	91%	92%
Incidence of Potentially Preventable VTE[5]	-	-	8%	10%
UFH with Dosages/Platelet Monitoring[5]	-	-	98%	97%
Venous Thromboembolism Prophylaxis[5]	-	-	79%	85%
Warfarin Therapy Discharge Instructions[5]	-	-	84%	75%
Chest Pain/Possible Heart Attack Care				
Aspirin Given Within 24 Hours of Arrival	-	-	94%	96%
Fibrinolytic Meds Within 30 Min. of Arrival	-	-	41%	58%
Average Time to ECG (minutes)	-	-	8	7
Average Time to Transfer (minutes)	-	-	57	60
Children's Asthma Care				
Received Home Management Plan of Care	-	-	-	88%

NOTE: Hospital profiles are in alphabetical order by state, then city, then hospital within the city; Rankings exclude hospitals with less than 25 cases except for patient surveys which excludes hospitals with less than 100 cases; (a) 100-299 cases; (1) The number of cases/patients is too few to report; (2) Data submitted were based on a sample of cases/patients; (3) Results are based on a shorter time period than required; (4) Data suppressed by CMS for one or more quarters; (5) Results are not available for this reporting period; (6) Fewer than 100 patients completed the HCAHPS survey; (7) No cases met the criteria for this measure; (8) The lower limit of the confidence interval cannot be calculated if the number of observed infections equals zero; (9) No data are available from the state/territory for this reporting period; (10) The scores shown reflect fewer than 50 completed surveys; (11) There were discrepancies in the data collection process; (12) This measure does not apply to this hospital for this reporting period; (13) Results cannot be calculated for this reporting period; (14) The results for this state are combined with nearby states to protect confidentiality; Please refer to the User's Guide for a full explanation of data.

Measure	Cases	This Hosp.	State Avg.	U.S. Avg.
Received Reliever Medication	-	-	-	100%
Received Systemic Corticosteroids	-	-	-	100%
Emergency Department				
Admittance Decision Time (minutes)[1,3]	-	-	57	98
Head CT Results Within 45 Min. of Arrival	-	-	53%	57%
Patients Who Left ER Before Being Seen	-	-	2%	2%
Time from ER Arrival to Admit. (minutes)[3]	22	106	185	274
Time from ER Arrival to Discharge (minutes)	-	-	104	134
Time in ER Before Being Evaluated (minutes)	-	-	18	26
Time to Pain Meds for Fractures (minutes)	-	-	47	57
Heart Attack Care				
Aspirin Given at Discharge[5]	-	-	99%	99%
Fibrinolytic Meds Within 30 Min. of Arrival[5]	-	-	-	54%
PCI Within 90 Minutes of Arrival[5]	-	-	97%	96%
Statin Prescribed at Discharge[5]	-	-	99%	98%
Heart Failure Care				
ACE Inhibitor or ARB for LVSD[5]	-	-	95%	97%
Discharge Instructions Given[5]	-	-	91%	94%
Evaluation of LVS Function[5]	-	-	94%	99%
Medicare Spending				
Medicare Spending per Patient (ratio)	-	-	0.94	0.98
Pneumonia Care				
Appropriate Initial Antibiotic Given	11	82%	92%	95%
Blood Culture Timing[1]	-	-	98%	98%
Pregnancy and Delivery Care				
Newborn Deliveries Scheduled Early[5]	-	-	12%	6%
Preventive Care				
Immunization for Influenza[5]	-	-	88%	90%
Immunization for Pneumonia[3]	28	7%	90%	92%
Stroke Care				
Anticoagulation Therapy for Atrial Fibrillation[5]	-	-	88%	95%
Antithrombotic Therapy Timing[5]	-	-	97%	98%
Assessed for Rehabilitation[5]	-	-	97%	97%
Discharged on Antithrombotic Therapy[5]	-	-	98%	99%
Discharged on Statin Medication[5]	-	-	88%	94%
Thrombolytic Therapy Timing[5]	-	-	68%	66%
Venous Thromboembolism Prophylaxis[5]	-	-	93%	94%
Written Stroke Educational Materials Given[5]	-	-	84%	88%
Surgical Care Improvement Project				
Appropriate Beta Blocker Usage[5]	-	-	98%	98%
Appropriate VTP Within 24 Hours[5]	-	-	98%	98%
Controlled Postoperative Blood Glucose[5]	-	-	98%	97%
Perioperative Temperature Management[5]	-	-	100%	100%
Prophylactic Antibiotic Selection[5]	-	-	99%	99%
Prophylactic Antibiotic Selection (Outpatient)	-	-	98%	98%
Prophylactic Antibiotic Stopped[5]	-	-	98%	98%
Prophylactic Antibiotic Timing[5]	-	-	99%	99%
Prophylactic Antibiotic Timing (Outpatient)	-	-	98%	98%
Urinary Catheter Removal[5]	-	-	97%	97%
Survey of Patients' Hospital Experiences				
Area Around Room 'Always' Quiet at Night[5]	-	-	65%	61%
Doctors 'Always' Communicated Well[5]	-	-	85%	82%
Home Recovery Information Given[5]	-	-	86%	85%
Hospital Given 9 or 10 on 10 Point Scale[5]	-	-	76%	71%
Meds 'Always' Explained Before Given[5]	-	-	66%	64%
Nurses 'Always' Communicated Well[5]	-	-	81%	79%
Pain 'Always' Well Controlled[5]	-	-	72%	71%
Room and Bathroom 'Always' Clean[5]	-	-	76%	73%
Timely Help 'Always' Received[5]	-	-	72%	68%
Would Definitely Recommend Hospital[5]	-	-	75%	71%
Use of Medical Imaging				
Cardiac Imaging Stress Test before Surgery	-	-	5%	5.3%
Combination Abdominal CT Scan	-	-	19%	10.5%
Combination Brain/Sinus CT Scan	-	-	2.9%	2.7%
Combination Chest CT Scan	-	-	3.9%	2.7%
Follow-up Mammogram/Ultrasound	-	-	7.8%	8.8%
Lumbar Spine MRI for Low Back Pain	-	-	40.2%	37.2%

Manhattan Surgical Hospital

1829 College Avenue
Manhattan, KS 66502
Phone: 785-776-5100
URL: www.manhattansurgical.com
Type: Acute Care Hospitals
Emergency Services: No
Ownership: Physician

Measure	Cases	This Hosp.	State Avg.	U.S. Avg.
Blood Clot Prevention and Treatment				
Anticoagulation Overlap Therapy[7]	-	-	94%	93%
ICU Venous Thromboembolism Prophylaxis[7]	-	-	91%	92%
Incidence of Potentially Preventable VTE[7]	-	-	8%	10%
UFH with Dosages/Platelet Monitoring[7]	-	-	98%	97%
Venous Thromboembolism Prophylaxis	12	100%	79%	85%
Warfarin Therapy Discharge Instructions[7]	-	-	84%	75%
Chest Pain/Possible Heart Attack Care				
Aspirin Given Within 24 Hours of Arrival[5]	-	-	94%	96%
Fibrinolytic Meds Within 30 Min. of Arrival[5]	-	-	41%	58%
Average Time to ECG (minutes)[5]	-	-	8	7
Average Time to Transfer (minutes)[5]	-	-	57	60
Children's Asthma Care				
Received Home Management Plan of Care	-	-	-	88%
Received Reliever Medication	-	-	-	100%
Received Systemic Corticosteroids	-	-	-	100%
Emergency Department				
Admittance Decision Time (minutes)[7]	-	-	57	98
Head CT Results Within 45 Min. of Arrival[5]	-	-	53%	57%
Patients Who Left ER Before Being Seen[5]	-	-	2%	2%
Time from ER Arrival to Admit. (minutes)[7]	-	-	185	274
Time from ER Arrival to Discharge (minutes)[5]	-	-	104	134
Time in ER Before Being Evaluated (minutes)[5]	-	-	18	26
Time to Pain Meds for Fractures (minutes)[5]	-	-	47	57
Heart Attack Care				
Aspirin Given at Discharge[5]	-	-	99%	99%
Fibrinolytic Meds Within 30 Min. of Arrival[5]	-	-	-	54%
PCI Within 90 Minutes of Arrival[5]	-	-	97%	96%
Statin Prescribed at Discharge[5]	-	-	99%	98%
Heart Failure Care				
ACE Inhibitor or ARB for LVSD[5]	-	-	95%	97%
Discharge Instructions Given[5]	-	-	91%	94%
Evaluation of LVS Function[5]	-	-	94%	99%
Medicare Spending				
Medicare Spending per Patient (ratio)	-	0.85	0.94	0.98
Pneumonia Care				
Appropriate Initial Antibiotic Given[5]	-	-	92%	95%
Blood Culture Timing[5]	-	-	98%	98%
Pregnancy and Delivery Care				
Newborn Deliveries Scheduled Early[7]	-	-	12%	6%
Preventive Care				
Immunization for Influenza	212	97%	88%	90%
Immunization for Pneumonia	141	91%	90%	92%
Stroke Care				
Anticoagulation Therapy for Atrial Fibrillation[5]	-	-	88%	95%
Antithrombotic Therapy Timing[5]	-	-	97%	98%
Assessed for Rehabilitation[5]	-	-	97%	97%
Discharged on Antithrombotic Therapy[5]	-	-	98%	99%
Discharged on Statin Medication[5]	-	-	88%	94%
Thrombolytic Therapy Timing[5]	-	-	68%	66%
Venous Thromboembolism Prophylaxis[5]	-	-	93%	94%
Written Stroke Educational Materials Given[5]	-	-	84%	88%
Surgical Care Improvement Project				
Appropriate Beta Blocker Usage	39	95%	98%	98%
Appropriate VTP Within 24 Hours	118	100%	98%	98%
Controlled Postoperative Blood Glucose[7]	-	-	98%	97%
Perioperative Temperature Management	325	100%	100%	100%
Prophylactic Antibiotic Selection	314	100%	99%	99%
Prophylactic Antibiotic Selection (Outpatient)	95	100%	98%	98%
Prophylactic Antibiotic Stopped	314	99%	98%	98%
Prophylactic Antibiotic Timing	314	99%	99%	99%
Prophylactic Antibiotic Timing (Outpatient)	97	98%	98%	98%
Urinary Catheter Removal	53	100%	97%	97%
Survey of Patients' Hospital Experiences				
Area Around Room 'Always' Quiet at Night	(a)	94%	65%	61%
Doctors 'Always' Communicated Well	(a)	92%	85%	82%
Home Recovery Information Given	(a)	93%	86%	85%
Hospital Given 9 or 10 on 10 Point Scale	(a)	92%	76%	71%
Meds 'Always' Explained Before Given	(a)	79%	66%	64%
Nurses 'Always' Communicated Well	(a)	91%	81%	79%
Pain 'Always' Well Controlled	(a)	86%	72%	71%
Room and Bathroom 'Always' Clean	(a)	86%	76%	73%
Timely Help 'Always' Received	(a)	91%	72%	68%
Would Definitely Recommend Hospital	(a)	93%	75%	71%
Use of Medical Imaging				
Cardiac Imaging Stress Test before Surgery[7]	-	-	5%	5.3%
Combination Abdominal CT Scan[7]	-	-	19%	10.5%
Combination Brain/Sinus CT Scan[7]	-	-	2.9%	2.7%
Combination Chest CT Scan[7]	-	-	3.9%	2.7%
Follow-up Mammogram/Ultrasound[7]	-	-	7.8%	8.8%
Lumbar Spine MRI for Low Back Pain[7]	-	-	40.2%	37.2%

Mercy Regional Health Center

1823 College Ave
Manhattan, KS 66502
Phone: 785-776-2831
Fax: 785-776-2804
URL: www.mercyregional.org
Type: Acute Care Hospitals
Emergency Services: Yes
Ownership: Voluntary non-profit - Church
Beds: 150

Key Personnel:
CEO/President. . . . . John Broberg
Cardiac Laboratory. . . . . Don Hedden
Pediatric In-Patient Care . . . . Dawn Julian
Quality Assurance . . . . Denise Klimek
Infection Control. . . . . Vivian Nutsch
Chief of Medical Staff . . . . Joe Philipp
Operating Room. . . . . Dante Wheat
Radiology. . . . . Gary Whitlock

Measure	Cases	This Hosp.	State Avg.	U.S. Avg.
Blood Clot Prevention and Treatment				
Anticoagulation Overlap Therapy[2]	31	97%	94%	93%
ICU Venous Thromboembolism Prophylaxis[2]	60	67%	91%	92%
Incidence of Potentially Preventable VTE[1,2]	-	-	8%	10%
UFH with Dosages/Platelet Monitoring[2]	12	100%	98%	97%
Venous Thromboembolism Prophylaxis[2]	308	63%	79%	85%
Warfarin Therapy Discharge Instructions[2]	20	95%	84%	75%
Chest Pain/Possible Heart Attack Care				
Aspirin Given Within 24 Hours of Arrival[1,3]	-	-	94%	96%
Fibrinolytic Meds Within 30 Min. of Arrival[3,7]	-	-	41%	58%
Average Time to ECG (minutes)[1,3]	-	-	8	7
Average Time to Transfer (minutes)[3,7]	-	-	57	60
Children's Asthma Care				
Received Home Management Plan of Care	-	-	-	88%
Received Reliever Medication	-	-	-	100%
Received Systemic Corticosteroids	-	-	-	100%
Emergency Department				
Admittance Decision Time (minutes)[2]	336	78	57	98
Head CT Results Within 45 Min. of Arrival[1]	-	-	53%	57%
Patients Who Left ER Before Being Seen	21,276	1%	2%	2%
Time from ER Arrival to Admit. (minutes)[2]	373	206	185	274
Time from ER Arrival to Discharge (minutes)	360	112	104	134
Time in ER Before Being Evaluated (minutes)	324	16	18	26
Time to Pain Meds for Fractures (minutes)	84	52	47	57
Heart Attack Care				
Aspirin Given at Discharge	115	100%	99%	99%
Fibrinolytic Meds Within 30 Min. of Arrival[7]	-	-	-	54%
PCI Within 90 Minutes of Arrival	13	92%	97%	96%
Statin Prescribed at Discharge	109	98%	99%	98%
Heart Failure Care				
ACE Inhibitor or ARB for LVSD	48	98%	95%	97%
Discharge Instructions Given	67	90%	91%	94%
Evaluation of LVS Function	92	100%	94%	99%
Medicare Spending				
Medicare Spending per Patient (ratio)	-	0.99	0.94	0.98
Pneumonia Care				
Appropriate Initial Antibiotic Given	57	100%	92%	95%
Blood Culture Timing	111	100%	98%	98%
Pregnancy and Delivery Care				
Newborn Deliveries Scheduled Early	84	0%	12%	6%
Preventive Care				

NOTE: Hospital profiles are in alphabetical order by state, then city, then hospital within the city; Rankings exclude hospitals with less than 25 cases except for patient surveys which excludes hospitals with less than 100 cases; (a) 100-299 cases; (1) The number of cases/patients is too few to report; (2) Data submitted were based on a sample of cases/patients; (3) Results are based on a shorter time period than required; (4) Data suppressed by CMS for one or more quarters; (5) Results are not available for this reporting period; (6) Fewer than 100 patients completed the HCAHPS survey; (7) No cases met the criteria for this measure; (8) The lower limit of the confidence interval cannot be calculated if the number of observed infections equals zero; (9) No data are available from the state/territory for this reporting period; (10) The scores shown reflect fewer than 50 completed surveys; (11) There were discrepancies in the data collection process; (12) This measure does not apply to this hospital for this reporting period; (13) Results cannot be calculated for this reporting period; (14) The results for this state are combined with nearby states to protect confidentiality; Please refer to the User's Guide for a full explanation of data.

Measure	Cases	This Hosp.	State Avg.	U.S. Avg.
Immunization for Influenza[2]	463	96%	88%	90%
Immunization for Pneumonia[2]	504	92%	90%	92%
Stroke Care				
Anticoagulation Therapy for Atrial Fibrillation[1]	-	-	88%	95%
Antithrombotic Therapy Timing	33	100%	97%	98%
Assessed for Rehabilitation	38	97%	97%	97%
Discharged on Antithrombotic Therapy	37	100%	98%	99%
Discharged on Statin Medication	22	86%	88%	94%
Thrombolytic Therapy Timing[1]	-	-	68%	66%
Venous Thromboembolism Prophylaxis	38	89%	93%	94%
Written Stroke Educational Materials Given	11	73%	84%	88%
Surgical Care Improvement Project				
Appropriate Beta Blocker Usage	134	99%	98%	98%
Appropriate VTP Within 24 Hours	347	99%	98%	98%
Controlled Postoperative Blood Glucose[7]	-	-	98%	97%
Perioperative Temperature Management	393	100%	100%	100%
Prophylactic Antibiotic Selection	252	99%	99%	99%
Prophylactic Antibiotic Selection (Outpatient)	66	100%	98%	98%
Prophylactic Antibiotic Stopped	245	99%	98%	98%
Prophylactic Antibiotic Timing	252	98%	99%	99%
Prophylactic Antibiotic Timing (Outpatient)	67	97%	98%	98%
Urinary Catheter Removal	200	100%	97%	97%
Survey of Patients' Hospital Experiences				
Area Around Room 'Always' Quiet at Night	300+	65%	65%	61%
Doctors 'Always' Communicated Well	300+	84%	85%	82%
Home Recovery Information Given	300+	84%	86%	85%
Hospital Given 9 or 10 on 10 Point Scale	300+	75%	76%	71%
Meds 'Always' Explained Before Given	300+	62%	66%	64%
Nurses 'Always' Communicated Well	300+	81%	81%	79%
Pain 'Always' Well Controlled	300+	73%	72%	71%
Room and Bathroom 'Always' Clean	300+	72%	76%	73%
Timely Help 'Always' Received	300+	70%	72%	68%
Would Definitely Recommend Hospital	300+	75%	75%	71%
Use of Medical Imaging				
Cardiac Imaging Stress Test before Surgery	215	7.4%	5%	5.3%
Combination Abdominal CT Scan	431	3.9%	19%	10.5%
Combination Brain/Sinus CT Scan[1]	-	-	2.9%	2.7%
Combination Chest CT Scan	389	0.0%	3.9%	2.7%
Follow-up Mammogram/Ultrasound	1,489	8.6%	7.8%	8.8%
Lumbar Spine MRI for Low Back Pain	48	41.7%	40.2%	37.2%

Saint Luke Hospital & Living Center

535 South Freebron
Marion, KS 66861
URL: www.slhmarion.org
Type: Critical Access Hospitals
Ownership: Govt - Hospital Dist/Auth
Phone: 620-382-2177
Fax: 620-382-9104
Emergency Services: Yes
Beds: 54

Key Personnel:
CEO/President............Jeremy Armstrong
Chairman/CEO ....Mike Connell
CEO ....Jeremy Ensey
Operating Room............Clayton Fetsch
Quality Assurance ....Vickie Guetersloh
Chief of Medical Staff............Don Hudson
Emergency Room ....Linda Kennedy
Anesthesiology............Bruce Skiles CRNA

Measure	Cases	This Hosp.	State Avg.	U.S. Avg.
Blood Clot Prevention and Treatment				
Anticoagulation Overlap Therapy[7]	-	-	94%	93%
ICU Venous Thromboembolism Prophylaxis[7]	-	-	91%	92%
Incidence of Potentially Preventable VTE[7]	-	-	8%	10%
UFH with Dosages/Platelet Monitoring[7]	-	-	98%	97%
Venous Thromboembolism Prophylaxis	62	73%	79%	85%
Warfarin Therapy Discharge Instructions[7]	-	-	84%	75%
Chest Pain/Possible Heart Attack Care				
Aspirin Given Within 24 Hours of Arrival	-	-	94%	96%
Fibrinolytic Meds Within 30 Min. of Arrival	-	-	41%	58%
Average Time to ECG (minutes)	-	-	8	7
Average Time to Transfer (minutes)	-	-	57	60
Children's Asthma Care				
Received Home Management Plan of Care	-	-	-	88%
Received Reliever Medication	-	-	-	100%
Received Systemic Corticosteroids	-	-	-	100%
Emergency Department				
Admittance Decision Time (minutes)	43	15	57	98
Head CT Results Within 45 Min. of Arrival	-	-	53%	57%
Patients Who Left ER Before Being Seen	-	-	2%	2%
Time from ER Arrival to Admit. (minutes)	43	75	185	274
Time from ER Arrival to Discharge (minutes)	-	-	104	134
Time in ER Before Being Evaluated (minutes)	-	-	18	26
Time to Pain Meds for Fractures (minutes)	-	-	47	57
Heart Attack Care				
Aspirin Given at Discharge[5]	-	-	99%	99%
Fibrinolytic Meds Within 30 Min. of Arrival[5]	-	-	-	54%
PCI Within 90 Minutes of Arrival[5]	-	-	97%	96%
Statin Prescribed at Discharge[5]	-	-	99%	98%
Heart Failure Care				
ACE Inhibitor or ARB for LVSD[1,3]	-	-	95%	97%
Discharge Instructions Given[1,3]	-	-	91%	94%
Evaluation of LVS Function[1,3]	-	-	94%	99%
Medicare Spending				
Medicare Spending per Patient (ratio)	-	-	0.94	0.98
Pneumonia Care				
Appropriate Initial Antibiotic Given	13	92%	92%	95%
Blood Culture Timing[1]	-	-	98%	98%
Pregnancy and Delivery Care				
Newborn Deliveries Scheduled Early[2,3]	-	-	12%	6%
Preventive Care				
Immunization for Influenza	41	83%	88%	90%
Immunization for Pneumonia	67	82%	90%	92%
Stroke Care				
Anticoagulation Therapy for Atrial Fibrillation[3,7]	-	-	88%	95%
Antithrombotic Therapy Timing[1,3]	-	-	97%	98%
Assessed for Rehabilitation[1,3]	-	-	97%	97%
Discharged on Antithrombotic Therapy[1,3]	-	-	98%	99%
Discharged on Statin Medication[1,3]	-	-	88%	94%
Thrombolytic Therapy Timing[1,3]	-	-	68%	66%
Venous Thromboembolism Prophylaxis[1,3]	-	-	93%	94%
Written Stroke Educational Materials Given[1,3]	-	-	84%	88%
Surgical Care Improvement Project				
Appropriate Beta Blocker Usage[5]	-	-	98%	98%
Appropriate VTP Within 24 Hours[5]	-	-	98%	98%
Controlled Postoperative Blood Glucose[5]	-	-	98%	97%
Perioperative Temperature Management[5]	-	-	100%	100%
Prophylactic Antibiotic Selection[5]	-	-	99%	99%
Prophylactic Antibiotic Selection (Outpatient)	-	-	98%	98%
Prophylactic Antibiotic Stopped[5]	-	-	98%	98%
Prophylactic Antibiotic Timing[5]	-	-	99%	99%
Prophylactic Antibiotic Timing (Outpatient)	-	-	98%	98%
Urinary Catheter Removal[5]	-	-	97%	97%
Survey of Patients' Hospital Experiences				
Area Around Room 'Always' Quiet at Night[5]	-	-	65%	61%
Doctors 'Always' Communicated Well[5]	-	-	85%	82%
Home Recovery Information Given[5]	-	-	86%	85%
Hospital Given 9 or 10 on 10 Point Scale[5]	-	-	76%	71%
Meds 'Always' Explained Before Given[5]	-	-	66%	64%
Nurses 'Always' Communicated Well[5]	-	-	81%	79%
Pain 'Always' Well Controlled[5]	-	-	72%	71%
Room and Bathroom 'Always' Clean[5]	-	-	76%	73%
Timely Help 'Always' Received[5]	-	-	72%	68%
Would Definitely Recommend Hospital[5]	-	-	75%	71%
Use of Medical Imaging				
Cardiac Imaging Stress Test before Surgery	-	-	5%	5.3%
Combination Abdominal CT Scan	-	-	19%	10.5%
Combination Brain/Sinus CT Scan	-	-	2.9%	2.7%
Combination Chest CT Scan	-	-	3.9%	2.7%
Follow-up Mammogram/Ultrasound	-	-	7.8%	8.8%
Lumbar Spine MRI for Low Back Pain	-	-	40.2%	37.2%

Community Memorial Healthcare

708 N 18th Street
Marysville, KS 66508
Type: Critical Access Hospitals
Ownership: Voluntary non-profit - Private
Phone: 785-562-2311
Emergency Services: Yes

Measure	Cases	This Hosp.	State Avg.	U.S. Avg.
Blood Clot Prevention and Treatment				
Anticoagulation Overlap Therapy[5]	-	-	94%	93%
ICU Venous Thromboembolism Prophylaxis[5]	-	-	91%	92%
Incidence of Potentially Preventable VTE[5]	-	-	8%	10%
UFH with Dosages/Platelet Monitoring[5]	-	-	98%	97%
Venous Thromboembolism Prophylaxis[5]	-	-	79%	85%
Warfarin Therapy Discharge Instructions[5]	-	-	84%	75%
Chest Pain/Possible Heart Attack Care				
Aspirin Given Within 24 Hours of Arrival	-	-	94%	96%
Fibrinolytic Meds Within 30 Min. of Arrival	-	-	41%	58%
Average Time to ECG (minutes)	-	-	8	7
Average Time to Transfer (minutes)	-	-	57	60
Children's Asthma Care				
Received Home Management Plan of Care	-	-	-	88%
Received Reliever Medication	-	-	-	100%
Received Systemic Corticosteroids	-	-	-	100%
Emergency Department				
Admittance Decision Time (minutes)[5]	-	-	57	98
Head CT Results Within 45 Min. of Arrival	-	-	53%	57%
Patients Who Left ER Before Being Seen	-	-	2%	2%
Time from ER Arrival to Admit. (minutes)[5]	-	-	185	274
Time from ER Arrival to Discharge (minutes)	-	-	104	134
Time in ER Before Being Evaluated (minutes)	-	-	18	26
Time to Pain Meds for Fractures (minutes)	-	-	47	57
Heart Attack Care				
Aspirin Given at Discharge[5]	-	-	99%	99%
Fibrinolytic Meds Within 30 Min. of Arrival[5]	-	-	-	54%
PCI Within 90 Minutes of Arrival[5]	-	-	97%	96%
Statin Prescribed at Discharge[5]	-	-	99%	98%
Heart Failure Care				
ACE Inhibitor or ARB for LVSD[1]	-	-	95%	97%
Discharge Instructions Given	13	0%	91%	94%
Evaluation of LVS Function	22	68%	94%	99%
Medicare Spending				
Medicare Spending per Patient (ratio)	-	-	0.94	0.98
Pneumonia Care				
Appropriate Initial Antibiotic Given	20	85%	92%	95%
Blood Culture Timing[1]	-	-	98%	98%
Pregnancy and Delivery Care				
Newborn Deliveries Scheduled Early[5]	-	-	12%	6%
Preventive Care				
Immunization for Influenza[5]	-	-	88%	90%
Immunization for Pneumonia[5]	-	-	90%	92%
Stroke Care				
Anticoagulation Therapy for Atrial Fibrillation[5]	-	-	88%	95%
Antithrombotic Therapy Timing[5]	-	-	97%	98%
Assessed for Rehabilitation[5]	-	-	97%	97%
Discharged on Antithrombotic Therapy[5]	-	-	98%	99%
Discharged on Statin Medication[5]	-	-	88%	94%
Thrombolytic Therapy Timing[5]	-	-	68%	66%
Venous Thromboembolism Prophylaxis[5]	-	-	93%	94%
Written Stroke Educational Materials Given[5]	-	-	84%	88%
Surgical Care Improvement Project				
Appropriate Beta Blocker Usage[5]	-	-	98%	98%
Appropriate VTP Within 24 Hours[5]	-	-	98%	98%
Controlled Postoperative Blood Glucose[5]	-	-	98%	97%
Perioperative Temperature Management[5]	-	-	100%	100%
Prophylactic Antibiotic Selection[5]	-	-	99%	99%
Prophylactic Antibiotic Selection (Outpatient)	-	-	98%	98%
Prophylactic Antibiotic Stopped[5]	-	-	98%	98%
Prophylactic Antibiotic Timing[5]	-	-	99%	99%
Prophylactic Antibiotic Timing (Outpatient)	-	-	98%	98%
Urinary Catheter Removal[5]	-	-	97%	97%
Survey of Patients' Hospital Experiences				
Area Around Room 'Always' Quiet at Night[5]	-	-	65%	61%
Doctors 'Always' Communicated Well[5]	-	-	85%	82%
Home Recovery Information Given[5]	-	-	86%	85%
Hospital Given 9 or 10 on 10 Point Scale[5]	-	-	76%	71%
Meds 'Always' Explained Before Given[5]	-	-	66%	64%
Nurses 'Always' Communicated Well[5]	-	-	81%	79%
Pain 'Always' Well Controlled[5]	-	-	72%	71%
Room and Bathroom 'Always' Clean[5]	-	-	76%	73%
Timely Help 'Always' Received[5]	-	-	72%	68%

NOTE: Hospital profiles are in alphabetical order by state, then city, then hospital within the city; Rankings exclude hospitals with less than 25 cases except for patient surveys which excludes hospitals with less than 100 cases; (a) 100-299 cases; (1) The number of cases/patients is too few to report; (2) Data submitted were based on a sample of cases/patients; (3) Results are based on a shorter time period than required; (4) Data suppressed by CMS for one or more quarters; (5) Results are not available for this reporting period; (6) Fewer than 100 patients completed the HCAHPS survey; (7) No cases met the criteria for this measure; (8) The lower limit of the confidence interval cannot be calculated if the number of observed infections equals zero; (9) No data are available from the state/territory for this reporting period; (10) The scores shown reflect fewer than 50 completed surveys; (11) There were discrepancies in the data collection process; (12) This measure does not apply to this hospital for this reporting period; (13) Results cannot be calculated for this reporting period; (14) The results for this state are combined with nearby states to protect confidentiality; Please refer to the User's Guide for a full explanation of data.

Measure	Cases	This Hosp.	State Avg.	U.S. Avg.
Would Definitely Recommend Hospital[5]	-	-	75%	71%
Use of Medical Imaging				
Cardiac Imaging Stress Test before Surgery	-	-	5%	5.3%
Combination Abdominal CT Scan	-	-	19%	10.5%
Combination Brain/Sinus CT Scan	-	-	2.9%	2.7%
Combination Chest CT Scan	-	-	3.9%	2.7%
Follow-up Mammogram/Ultrasound	-	-	7.8%	8.8%
Lumbar Spine MRI for Low Back Pain	-	-	40.2%	37.2%

McPherson Hospital

1000 Hospital Drive
Mcpherson, KS 67460
Phone: 620-241-2250
Fax: 620-245-9153
Type: Acute Care Hospitals
Emergency Services: Yes
Ownership: Voluntary non-profit - Private
Beds: 70

Key Personnel:
Quality Assurance . . . . Terri Gehring
Chief of Medical Staff . . . . Trish Goad
Infection Control . . . . Kathy Rishel
Intensive Care Unit . . . . Cheryl Vincent, RN
CEO/President . . . . Rex Walk
Emergency Room . . . . Richard L Watson

Measure	Cases	This Hosp.	State Avg.	U.S. Avg.
Blood Clot Prevention and Treatment				
Anticoagulation Overlap Therapy[1,2]	-	-	94%	93%
ICU Venous Thromboembolism Prophylaxis[2]	75	92%	91%	92%
Incidence of Potentially Preventable VTE[1,2]	-	-	8%	10%
UFH with Dosages/Platelet Monitoring[1,2]	-	-	98%	97%
Venous Thromboembolism Prophylaxis[2]	236	83%	79%	85%
Warfarin Therapy Discharge Instructions[1,2]	-	-	84%	75%
Chest Pain/Possible Heart Attack Care				
Aspirin Given Within 24 Hours of Arrival	64	95%	94%	96%
Fibrinolytic Meds Within 30 Min. of Arrival[7]	-	-	41%	58%
Average Time to ECG (minutes)	63	14	8	7
Average Time to Transfer (minutes)	18	84	57	60
Children's Asthma Care				
Received Home Management Plan of Care	-	-	-	88%
Received Reliever Medication	-	-	-	100%
Received Systemic Corticosteroids	-	-	-	100%
Emergency Department				
Admittance Decision Time (minutes)[2]	291	63	57	98
Head CT Results Within 45 Min. of Arrival[1]	-	-	53%	57%
Patients Who Left ER Before Being Seen	4,011	1%	2%	2%
Time from ER Arrival to Admit. (minutes)[2]	306	227	185	274
Time from ER Arrival to Discharge (minutes)	297	99	104	134
Time in ER Before Being Evaluated (minutes)	289	22	18	26
Time to Pain Meds for Fractures (minutes)	28	57	47	57
Heart Attack Care				
Aspirin Given at Discharge[1,2]	-	-	99%	99%
Fibrinolytic Meds Within 30 Min. of Arrival[2,7]	-	-	-	54%
PCI Within 90 Minutes of Arrival[2,7]	-	-	97%	96%
Statin Prescribed at Discharge[1,2]	-	-	99%	98%
Heart Failure Care				
ACE Inhibitor or ARB for LVSD[1,2]	-	-	95%	97%
Discharge Instructions Given[2]	14	79%	91%	94%
Evaluation of LVS Function[2]	28	79%	94%	99%
Medicare Spending				
Medicare Spending per Patient (ratio)	-	0.93	0.94	0.98
Pneumonia Care				
Appropriate Initial Antibiotic Given[2]	44	98%	92%	95%
Blood Culture Timing[2]	51	86%	98%	98%
Pregnancy and Delivery Care				
Newborn Deliveries Scheduled Early[2]	36	0%	12%	6%
Preventive Care				
Immunization for Influenza[2]	341	75%	88%	90%
Immunization for Pneumonia[2]	439	79%	90%	92%
Stroke Care				
Anticoagulation Therapy for Atrial Fibrillation[1,2]	-	-	88%	95%
Antithrombotic Therapy Timing[1,2]	-	-	97%	98%
Assessed for Rehabilitation[1,2]	-	-	97%	97%
Discharged on Antithrombotic Therapy[1,2]	-	-	98%	99%
Discharged on Statin Medication[1,2]	-	-	88%	94%
Thrombolytic Therapy Timing[1,2]	-	-	68%	66%
Venous Thromboembolism Prophylaxis[1,2]	-	-	93%	94%
Written Stroke Educational Materials Given[1,2]	-	-	84%	88%
Surgical Care Improvement Project				
Appropriate Beta Blocker Usage[1,2]	-	-	98%	98%
Appropriate VTP Within 24 Hours[2]	20	75%	98%	98%
Controlled Postoperative Blood Glucose[2,7]	-	-	98%	97%
Perioperative Temperature Management[2]	22	77%	100%	100%
Prophylactic Antibiotic Selection[2,7]	-	-	99%	99%
Prophylactic Antibiotic Selection (Outpatient)[1,3]	-	-	98%	98%
Prophylactic Antibiotic Stopped[2,7]	-	-	98%	98%
Prophylactic Antibiotic Timing[2,7]	-	-	99%	99%
Prophylactic Antibiotic Timing (Outpatient)[1,3]	-	-	98%	98%
Urinary Catheter Removal[2]	13	100%	97%	97%
Survey of Patients' Hospital Experiences				
Area Around Room 'Always' Quiet at Night	(a)	66%	65%	61%
Doctors 'Always' Communicated Well	(a)	86%	85%	82%
Home Recovery Information Given	(a)	79%	86%	85%
Hospital Given 9 or 10 on 10 Point Scale	(a)	69%	76%	71%
Meds 'Always' Explained Before Given	(a)	62%	66%	64%
Nurses 'Always' Communicated Well	(a)	85%	81%	79%
Pain 'Always' Well Controlled	(a)	79%	72%	71%
Room and Bathroom 'Always' Clean	(a)	74%	76%	73%
Timely Help 'Always' Received	(a)	70%	72%	68%
Would Definitely Recommend Hospital	(a)	61%	75%	71%
Use of Medical Imaging				
Cardiac Imaging Stress Test before Surgery[1]	-	-	5%	5.3%
Combination Abdominal CT Scan	266	53.8%	19%	10.5%
Combination Brain/Sinus CT Scan[1]	-	-	2.9%	2.7%
Combination Chest CT Scan	213	4.2%	3.9%	2.7%
Follow-up Mammogram/Ultrasound	410	9.5%	7.8%	8.8%
Lumbar Spine MRI for Low Back Pain[1]	-	-	40.2%	37.2%

Meade District Hospital

510 E Carthage
Meade, KS 67864
Phone: 620-873-2141
Fax: 620-873-2576
URL: www.meadehospital.com
Type: Critical Access Hospitals
Emergency Services: Yes
Ownership: Govt - Hospital Dist/Auth

Key Personnel:
Radiology . . . . Brad Bird ARRT
Operating Room . . . . Jane Chance, RN
CEO/President . . . . Mickey Thomas

Measure	Cases	This Hosp.	State Avg.	U.S. Avg.
Blood Clot Prevention and Treatment				
Anticoagulation Overlap Therapy[5]	-	-	94%	93%
ICU Venous Thromboembolism Prophylaxis[5]	-	-	91%	92%
Incidence of Potentially Preventable VTE[5]	-	-	8%	10%
UFH with Dosages/Platelet Monitoring[5]	-	-	98%	97%
Venous Thromboembolism Prophylaxis[5]	-	-	79%	85%
Warfarin Therapy Discharge Instructions[5]	-	-	84%	75%
Chest Pain/Possible Heart Attack Care				
Aspirin Given Within 24 Hours of Arrival[5]	-	-	94%	96%
Fibrinolytic Meds Within 30 Min. of Arrival[5]	-	-	41%	58%
Average Time to ECG (minutes)[5]	-	-	8	7
Average Time to Transfer (minutes)[5]	-	-	57	60
Children's Asthma Care				
Received Home Management Plan of Care	-	-	-	88%
Received Reliever Medication	-	-	-	100%
Received Systemic Corticosteroids	-	-	-	100%
Emergency Department				
Admittance Decision Time (minutes)[5]	-	-	57	98
Head CT Results Within 45 Min. of Arrival[5]	-	-	53%	57%
Patients Who Left ER Before Being Seen	1,224	1%	2%	2%
Time from ER Arrival to Admit. (minutes)[5]	-	-	185	274
Time from ER Arrival to Discharge (minutes)[5]	-	-	104	134
Time in ER Before Being Evaluated (minutes)[5]	-	-	18	26
Time to Pain Meds for Fractures (minutes)[5]	-	-	47	57
Heart Attack Care				
Aspirin Given at Discharge[3,7]	-	-	99%	99%
Fibrinolytic Meds Within 30 Min. of Arrival[3,7]	-	-	-	54%
PCI Within 90 Minutes of Arrival[3,7]	-	-	97%	96%
Statin Prescribed at Discharge[3,7]	-	-	99%	98%
Heart Failure Care				
ACE Inhibitor or ARB for LVSD[1]	-	-	95%	97%
Discharge Instructions Given[1]	-	-	91%	94%
Evaluation of LVS Function	20	90%	94%	99%
Medicare Spending				
Medicare Spending per Patient (ratio)	-	-	0.94	0.98
Pneumonia Care				
Appropriate Initial Antibiotic Given	22	68%	92%	95%
Blood Culture Timing[1]	-	-	98%	98%
Pregnancy and Delivery Care				
Newborn Deliveries Scheduled Early[5]	-	-	12%	6%
Preventive Care				
Immunization for Influenza[5]	-	-	88%	90%
Immunization for Pneumonia[5]	-	-	90%	92%
Stroke Care				
Anticoagulation Therapy for Atrial Fibrillation[5]	-	-	88%	95%
Antithrombotic Therapy Timing[5]	-	-	97%	98%
Assessed for Rehabilitation[5]	-	-	97%	97%
Discharged on Antithrombotic Therapy[5]	-	-	98%	99%
Discharged on Statin Medication[5]	-	-	88%	94%
Thrombolytic Therapy Timing[5]	-	-	68%	66%
Venous Thromboembolism Prophylaxis[5]	-	-	93%	94%
Written Stroke Educational Materials Given[5]	-	-	84%	88%
Surgical Care Improvement Project				
Appropriate Beta Blocker Usage[1]	-	-	98%	98%
Appropriate VTP Within 24 Hours	38	100%	98%	98%
Controlled Postoperative Blood Glucose[7]	-	-	98%	97%
Perioperative Temperature Management	40	100%	100%	100%
Prophylactic Antibiotic Selection	38	87%	99%	99%
Prophylactic Antibiotic Selection (Outpatient)[5]	-	-	98%	98%
Prophylactic Antibiotic Stopped	38	100%	98%	98%
Prophylactic Antibiotic Timing	38	95%	99%	99%
Prophylactic Antibiotic Timing (Outpatient)[5]	-	-	98%	98%
Urinary Catheter Removal	41	98%	97%	97%
Survey of Patients' Hospital Experiences				
Area Around Room 'Always' Quiet at Night[6]	<100	67%	65%	61%
Doctors 'Always' Communicated Well[6]	<100	92%	85%	82%
Home Recovery Information Given[6]	<100	92%	86%	85%
Hospital Given 9 or 10 on 10 Point Scale[6]	<100	86%	76%	71%
Meds 'Always' Explained Before Given[6]	<100	80%	66%	64%
Nurses 'Always' Communicated Well[6]	<100	89%	81%	79%
Pain 'Always' Well Controlled[6]	<100	78%	72%	71%
Room and Bathroom 'Always' Clean[6]	<100	84%	76%	73%
Timely Help 'Always' Received[6]	<100	83%	72%	68%
Would Definitely Recommend Hospital[6]	<100	83%	75%	71%
Use of Medical Imaging				
Cardiac Imaging Stress Test before Surgery[1]	-	-	5%	5.3%
Combination Abdominal CT Scan	71	14.1%	19%	10.5%
Combination Brain/Sinus CT Scan	40	0.0%	2.9%	2.7%
Combination Chest CT Scan[1]	-	-	3.9%	2.7%
Follow-up Mammogram/Ultrasound	89	9.0%	7.8%	8.8%
Lumbar Spine MRI for Low Back Pain[1]	-	-	40.2%	37.2%

Medicine Lodge Memorial Hospital

710 N Walnut Street
Medicine Lodge, KS 67104
Phone: 620-886-3771
Type: Critical Access Hospitals
Emergency Services: Yes
Ownership: Govt - Hospital Dist/Auth

Measure	Cases	This Hosp.	State Avg.	U.S. Avg.
Blood Clot Prevention and Treatment				
Anticoagulation Overlap Therapy[5]	-	-	94%	93%
ICU Venous Thromboembolism Prophylaxis[5]	-	-	91%	92%
Incidence of Potentially Preventable VTE[5]	-	-	8%	10%
UFH with Dosages/Platelet Monitoring[5]	-	-	98%	97%
Venous Thromboembolism Prophylaxis[5]	-	-	79%	85%
Warfarin Therapy Discharge Instructions[5]	-	-	84%	75%
Chest Pain/Possible Heart Attack Care				
Aspirin Given Within 24 Hours of Arrival	-	-	94%	96%
Fibrinolytic Meds Within 30 Min. of Arrival	-	-	41%	58%
Average Time to ECG (minutes)	-	-	8	7
Average Time to Transfer (minutes)	-	-	57	60
Children's Asthma Care				
Received Home Management Plan of Care	-	-	-	88%
Received Reliever Medication	-	-	-	100%
Received Systemic Corticosteroids	-	-	-	100%

NOTE: Hospital profiles are in alphabetical order by state, then city, then hospital within the city; Rankings exclude hospitals with less than 25 cases except for patient surveys which excludes hospitals with less than 100 cases; (a) 100-299 cases; (1) The number of cases/patients is too few to report; (2) Data submitted were based on a sample of cases/patients; (3) Results are based on a shorter time period than required; (4) Data suppressed by CMS for one or more quarters; (5) Results are not available for this reporting period; (6) Fewer than 100 patients completed the HCAHPS survey; (7) No cases met the criteria for this measure; (8) The lower limit of the confidence interval cannot be calculated if the number of observed infections equals zero; (9) No data are available from the state/territory for this reporting period; (10) The scores shown reflect fewer than 50 completed surveys; (11) There were discrepancies in the data collection process; (12) This measure does not apply to this hospital for this reporting period; (13) Results cannot be calculated for this reporting period; (14) The results for this state are combined with nearby states to protect confidentiality; Please refer to the User's Guide for a full explanation of data.

Emergency Department				
Admittance Decision Time (minutes)[1,3]	-	-	57	98
Head CT Results Within 45 Min. of Arrival	-	-	53%	57%
Patients Who Left ER Before Being Seen	-	-	2%	2%
Time from ER Arrival to Admit. (minutes)[1,3]	-	-	185	274
Time from ER Arrival to Discharge (minutes)	-	-	104	134
Time in ER Before Being Evaluated (minutes)	-	-	18	26
Time to Pain Meds for Fractures (minutes)	-	-	47	57
Heart Attack Care				
Aspirin Given at Discharge[5]	-	-	99%	99%
Fibrinolytic Meds Within 30 Min. of Arrival[5]	-	-	-	54%
PCI Within 90 Minutes of Arrival[5]	-	-	97%	96%
Statin Prescribed at Discharge[5]	-	-	99%	98%
Heart Failure Care				
ACE Inhibitor or ARB for LVSD[1,3]	-	-	95%	97%
Discharge Instructions Given[1,3]	-	-	91%	94%
Evaluation of LVS Function[1,3]	-	-	94%	99%
Medicare Spending				
Medicare Spending per Patient (ratio)	-	-	0.94	0.98
Pneumonia Care				
Appropriate Initial Antibiotic Given[1,3]	-	-	92%	95%
Blood Culture Timing[1,3]	-	-	98%	98%
Pregnancy and Delivery Care				
Newborn Deliveries Scheduled Early[5]	-	-	12%	6%
Preventive Care				
Immunization for Influenza[3]	18	72%	88%	90%
Immunization for Pneumonia[2,3]	38	68%	90%	92%
Stroke Care				
Anticoagulation Therapy for Atrial Fibrillation[5]	-	-	88%	95%
Antithrombotic Therapy Timing[5]	-	-	97%	98%
Assessed for Rehabilitation[5]	-	-	97%	97%
Discharged on Antithrombotic Therapy[5]	-	-	98%	99%
Discharged on Statin Medication[5]	-	-	88%	94%
Thrombolytic Therapy Timing[5]	-	-	68%	66%
Venous Thromboembolism Prophylaxis[5]	-	-	93%	94%
Written Stroke Educational Materials Given[5]	-	-	84%	88%
Surgical Care Improvement Project				
Appropriate Beta Blocker Usage[5]	-	-	98%	98%
Appropriate VTP Within 24 Hours[5]	-	-	98%	98%
Controlled Postoperative Blood Glucose[5]	-	-	98%	97%
Perioperative Temperature Management[5]	-	-	100%	100%
Prophylactic Antibiotic Selection[5]	-	-	99%	99%
Prophylactic Antibiotic Selection (Outpatient)	-	-	98%	98%
Prophylactic Antibiotic Stopped[5]	-	-	98%	98%
Prophylactic Antibiotic Timing[5]	-	-	99%	99%
Prophylactic Antibiotic Timing (Outpatient)	-	-	98%	98%
Urinary Catheter Removal[5]	-	-	97%	97%
Survey of Patients' Hospital Experiences				
Area Around Room 'Always' Quiet at Night[5]	-	-	65%	61%
Doctors 'Always' Communicated Well[5]	-	-	85%	82%
Home Recovery Information Given[5]	-	-	86%	85%
Hospital Given 9 or 10 on 10 Point Scale[5]	-	-	76%	71%
Meds 'Always' Explained Before Given[5]	-	-	66%	64%
Nurses 'Always' Communicated Well[5]	-	-	81%	79%
Pain 'Always' Well Controlled[5]	-	-	72%	71%
Room and Bathroom 'Always' Clean[5]	-	-	76%	73%
Timely Help 'Always' Received[5]	-	-	72%	68%
Would Definitely Recommend Hospital[5]	-	-	75%	71%
Use of Medical Imaging				
Cardiac Imaging Stress Test before Surgery	-	-	5%	5.3%
Combination Abdominal CT Scan	-	-	19%	10.5%
Combination Brain/Sinus CT Scan	-	-	2.9%	2.7%
Combination Chest CT Scan	-	-	3.9%	2.7%
Follow-up Mammogram/Ultrasound	-	-	7.8%	8.8%
Lumbar Spine MRI for Low Back Pain	-	-	40.2%	37.2%

Ottawa County Health Center

215 E 8th Street
Minneapolis, KS 67467
Type: Critical Access Hospitals
Ownership: Government - Local

Phone: 785-392-2122
Fax: 785-392-2852
Emergency Services: Yes
Beds: 25

Key Personnel:
Quality Assurance . . . . Debbie Comfort
CEO/President. . . . . Joy Reed

Measure	Cases	This Hosp.	State Avg.	U.S. Avg.
Blood Clot Prevention and Treatment				
Anticoagulation Overlap Therapy[5]	-	-	94%	93%
ICU Venous Thromboembolism Prophylaxis[5]	-	-	91%	92%
Incidence of Potentially Preventable VTE[5]	-	-	8%	10%
UFH with Dosages/Platelet Monitoring[5]	-	-	98%	97%
Venous Thromboembolism Prophylaxis[5]	-	-	79%	85%
Warfarin Therapy Discharge Instructions[5]	-	-	84%	75%
Chest Pain/Possible Heart Attack Care				
Aspirin Given Within 24 Hours of Arrival[5]	-	-	94%	96%
Fibrinolytic Meds Within 30 Min. of Arrival[1,3]	-	-	41%	58%
Average Time to ECG (minutes)[1,3]	-	-	8	7
Average Time to Transfer (minutes)[1,3]	-	-	57	60
Children's Asthma Care				
Received Home Management Plan of Care	-	-	-	88%
Received Reliever Medication	-	-	-	100%
Received Systemic Corticosteroids	-	-	-	100%
Emergency Department				
Admittance Decision Time (minutes)[5]	-	-	57	98
Head CT Results Within 45 Min. of Arrival[5]	-	-	53%	57%
Patients Who Left ER Before Being Seen[5]	-	-	2%	2%
Time from ER Arrival to Admit. (minutes)[5]	-	-	185	274
Time from ER Arrival to Discharge (minutes)[5]	-	-	104	134
Time in ER Before Being Evaluated (minutes)[5]	-	-	18	26
Time to Pain Meds for Fractures (minutes)[5]	-	-	47	57
Heart Attack Care				
Aspirin Given at Discharge[5]	-	-	99%	99%
Fibrinolytic Meds Within 30 Min. of Arrival[5]	-	-	-	54%
PCI Within 90 Minutes of Arrival[5]	-	-	97%	96%
Statin Prescribed at Discharge[5]	-	-	99%	98%
Heart Failure Care				
ACE Inhibitor or ARB for LVSD[2,3]	-	-	95%	97%
Discharge Instructions Given[1,2]	-	-	91%	94%
Evaluation of LVS Function[1,2]	-	-	94%	99%
Medicare Spending				
Medicare Spending per Patient (ratio)	-	-	0.94	0.98
Pneumonia Care				
Appropriate Initial Antibiotic Given[2]	11	82%	92%	95%
Blood Culture Timing[1,2]	-	-	98%	98%
Pregnancy and Delivery Care				
Newborn Deliveries Scheduled Early[5]	-	-	12%	6%
Preventive Care				
Immunization for Influenza[2]	71	82%	88%	90%
Immunization for Pneumonia[2]	94	93%	90%	92%
Stroke Care				
Anticoagulation Therapy for Atrial Fibrillation[5]	-	-	88%	95%
Antithrombotic Therapy Timing[5]	-	-	97%	98%
Assessed for Rehabilitation[5]	-	-	97%	97%
Discharged on Antithrombotic Therapy[5]	-	-	98%	99%
Discharged on Statin Medication[5]	-	-	88%	94%
Thrombolytic Therapy Timing[5]	-	-	68%	66%
Venous Thromboembolism Prophylaxis[5]	-	-	93%	94%
Written Stroke Educational Materials Given[5]	-	-	84%	88%
Surgical Care Improvement Project				
Appropriate Beta Blocker Usage[5]	-	-	98%	98%
Appropriate VTP Within 24 Hours[5]	-	-	98%	98%
Controlled Postoperative Blood Glucose[5]	-	-	98%	97%
Perioperative Temperature Management[5]	-	-	100%	100%
Prophylactic Antibiotic Selection[5]	-	-	99%	99%
Prophylactic Antibiotic Selection (Outpatient)[5]	-	-	98%	98%
Prophylactic Antibiotic Stopped[5]	-	-	98%	98%
Prophylactic Antibiotic Timing[5]	-	-	99%	99%
Prophylactic Antibiotic Timing (Outpatient)[5]	-	-	98%	98%
Urinary Catheter Removal[5]	-	-	97%	97%
Survey of Patients' Hospital Experiences				
Area Around Room 'Always' Quiet at Night[5]	-	-	65%	61%
Doctors 'Always' Communicated Well[5]	-	-	85%	82%
Home Recovery Information Given[5]	-	-	86%	85%
Hospital Given 9 or 10 on 10 Point Scale[5]	-	-	76%	71%
Meds 'Always' Explained Before Given[5]	-	-	66%	64%
Nurses 'Always' Communicated Well[5]	-	-	81%	79%
Pain 'Always' Well Controlled[5]	-	-	72%	71%
Room and Bathroom 'Always' Clean[5]	-	-	76%	73%
Timely Help 'Always' Received[5]	-	-	72%	68%
Would Definitely Recommend Hospital[5]	-	-	75%	71%
Use of Medical Imaging				
Cardiac Imaging Stress Test before Surgery[7]	-	-	5%	5.3%
Combination Abdominal CT Scan[7]	-	-	19%	10.5%
Combination Brain/Sinus CT Scan[7]	-	-	2.9%	2.7%
Combination Chest CT Scan[7]	-	-	3.9%	2.7%
Follow-up Mammogram/Ultrasound[7]	-	-	7.8%	8.8%
Lumbar Spine MRI for Low Back Pain[7]	-	-	40.2%	37.2%

Minneola District Hospital #2

212 Main
Minneola, KS 67865
Type: Critical Access Hospitals
Ownership: Govt - Hospital Dist/Auth

Phone: 620-885-4264
Emergency Services: Yes

Measure	Cases	This Hosp.	State Avg.	U.S. Avg.
Blood Clot Prevention and Treatment				
Anticoagulation Overlap Therapy[5]	-	-	94%	93%
ICU Venous Thromboembolism Prophylaxis[5]	-	-	91%	92%
Incidence of Potentially Preventable VTE[5]	-	-	8%	10%
UFH with Dosages/Platelet Monitoring[5]	-	-	98%	97%
Venous Thromboembolism Prophylaxis[5]	-	-	79%	85%
Warfarin Therapy Discharge Instructions[5]	-	-	84%	75%
Chest Pain/Possible Heart Attack Care				
Aspirin Given Within 24 Hours of Arrival	-	-	94%	96%
Fibrinolytic Meds Within 30 Min. of Arrival	-	-	41%	58%
Average Time to ECG (minutes)	-	-	8	7
Average Time to Transfer (minutes)	-	-	57	60
Children's Asthma Care				
Received Home Management Plan of Care	-	-	-	88%
Received Reliever Medication	-	-	-	100%
Received Systemic Corticosteroids	-	-	-	100%
Emergency Department				
Admittance Decision Time (minutes)[5]	-	-	57	98
Head CT Results Within 45 Min. of Arrival	-	-	53%	57%
Patients Who Left ER Before Being Seen	-	-	2%	2%
Time from ER Arrival to Admit. (minutes)[5]	-	-	185	274
Time from ER Arrival to Discharge (minutes)	-	-	104	134
Time in ER Before Being Evaluated (minutes)	-	-	18	26
Time to Pain Meds for Fractures (minutes)	-	-	47	57
Heart Attack Care				
Aspirin Given at Discharge[5]	-	-	99%	99%
Fibrinolytic Meds Within 30 Min. of Arrival[5]	-	-	-	54%
PCI Within 90 Minutes of Arrival[5]	-	-	97%	96%
Statin Prescribed at Discharge[5]	-	-	99%	98%
Heart Failure Care				
ACE Inhibitor or ARB for LVSD[1,3]	-	-	95%	97%
Discharge Instructions Given[1,3]	-	-	91%	94%
Evaluation of LVS Function[1,3]	-	-	94%	99%
Medicare Spending				
Medicare Spending per Patient (ratio)	-	-	0.94	0.98
Pneumonia Care				
Appropriate Initial Antibiotic Given[1]	-	-	92%	95%
Blood Culture Timing[1]	-	-	98%	98%
Pregnancy and Delivery Care				
Newborn Deliveries Scheduled Early[5]	-	-	12%	6%
Preventive Care				
Immunization for Influenza[5]	-	-	88%	90%
Immunization for Pneumonia[5]	-	-	90%	92%
Stroke Care				
Anticoagulation Therapy for Atrial Fibrillation[5]	-	-	88%	95%
Antithrombotic Therapy Timing[5]	-	-	97%	98%
Assessed for Rehabilitation[5]	-	-	97%	97%
Discharged on Antithrombotic Therapy[5]	-	-	98%	99%
Discharged on Statin Medication[5]	-	-	88%	94%
Thrombolytic Therapy Timing[5]	-	-	68%	66%
Venous Thromboembolism Prophylaxis[5]	-	-	93%	94%
Written Stroke Educational Materials Given[5]	-	-	84%	88%
Surgical Care Improvement Project				
Appropriate Beta Blocker Usage[5]	-	-	98%	98%
Appropriate VTP Within 24 Hours[5]	-	-	98%	98%

NOTE: Hospital profiles are in alphabetical order by state, then city, then hospital within the city; Rankings exclude hospitals with less than 25 cases except for patient surveys which excludes hospitals with less than 100 cases; (a) 100-299 cases; (1) The number of cases/patients is too few to report; (2) Data submitted were based on a sample of cases/patients; (3) Results are based on a shorter time period than required; (4) Data suppressed by CMS for one or more quarters; (5) Results are not available for this reporting period; (6) Fewer than 100 patients completed the HCAHPS survey; (7) No cases met the criteria for this measure; (8) The lower limit of the confidence interval cannot be calculated if the number of observed infections equals zero; (9) No data are available from the state/territory for this reporting period; (10) The scores shown reflect fewer than 50 completed surveys; (11) There were discrepancies in the data collection process; (12) This measure does not apply to this hospital for this reporting period; (13) Results cannot be calculated for this reporting period; (14) The results for this state are combined with nearby states to protect confidentiality; Please refer to the User's Guide for a full explanation of data.

Measure	Cases	This Hosp.	State Avg.	U.S. Avg.
Controlled Postoperative Blood Glucose[5]	-	-	98%	97%
Perioperative Temperature Management[5]	-	-	100%	100%
Prophylactic Antibiotic Selection[5]	-	-	99%	99%
Prophylactic Antibiotic Selection (Outpatient)	-	-	98%	98%
Prophylactic Antibiotic Stopped[5]	-	-	98%	98%
Prophylactic Antibiotic Timing[5]	-	-	99%	99%
Prophylactic Antibiotic Timing (Outpatient)	-	-	98%	98%
Urinary Catheter Removal[5]	-	-	97%	97%
Survey of Patients' Hospital Experiences				
Area Around Room 'Always' Quiet at Night[5]	-	-	65%	61%
Doctors 'Always' Communicated Well[5]	-	-	85%	82%
Home Recovery Information Given[5]	-	-	86%	85%
Hospital Given 9 or 10 on 10 Point Scale[5]	-	-	76%	71%
Meds 'Always' Explained Before Given[5]	-	-	66%	64%
Nurses 'Always' Communicated Well[5]	-	-	81%	79%
Pain 'Always' Well Controlled[5]	-	-	72%	71%
Room and Bathroom 'Always' Clean[5]	-	-	76%	73%
Timely Help 'Always' Received[5]	-	-	72%	68%
Would Definitely Recommend Hospital[5]	-	-	75%	71%
Use of Medical Imaging				
Cardiac Imaging Stress Test before Surgery	-	-	5%	5.3%
Combination Abdominal CT Scan	-	-	19%	10.5%
Combination Brain/Sinus CT Scan	-	-	2.9%	2.7%
Combination Chest CT Scan	-	-	3.9%	2.7%
Follow-up Mammogram/Ultrasound	-	-	7.8%	8.8%
Lumbar Spine MRI for Low Back Pain	-	-	40.2%	37.2%

Mercy Hospital

218 E Pack St
Moundridge, KS 67107
Phone: 620-345-6391
Fax: 620-345-6344
Type: Acute Care Hospitals
Emergency Services: Yes
Ownership: Voluntary non-profit - Church
Beds: 21

Key Personnel:
Quality Assurance .... Verla Friesen, RN, RM
Coronary Care .... Karen Ratzlaff
Emergency Room .... Donnella Unruh, RN

Measure	Cases	This Hosp.	State Avg.	U.S. Avg.
Blood Clot Prevention and Treatment				
Anticoagulation Overlap Therapy[2,7]	-	-	94%	93%
ICU Venous Thromboembolism Prophylaxis[2,7]	-	-	91%	92%
Incidence of Potentially Preventable VTE[2,7]	-	-	8%	10%
UFH with Dosages/Platelet Monitoring[2,7]	-	-	98%	97%
Venous Thromboembolism Prophylaxis[2]	109	24%	79%	85%
Warfarin Therapy Discharge Instructions[2,7]	-	-	84%	75%
Chest Pain/Possible Heart Attack Care				
Aspirin Given Within 24 Hours of Arrival[5]	-	-	94%	96%
Fibrinolytic Meds Within 30 Min. of Arrival[5]	-	-	41%	58%
Average Time to ECG (minutes)[5]	-	-	8	7
Average Time to Transfer (minutes)[5]	-	-	57	60
Children's Asthma Care				
Received Home Management Plan of Care	-	-	-	88%
Received Reliever Medication	-	-	-	100%
Received Systemic Corticosteroids	-	-	-	100%
Emergency Department				
Admittance Decision Time (minutes)[2]	82	0	57	98
Head CT Results Within 45 Min. of Arrival[5]	-	-	53%	57%
Patients Who Left ER Before Being Seen	927	0%	2%	2%
Time from ER Arrival to Admit. (minutes)[2]	84	100	185	274
Time from ER Arrival to Discharge (minutes)	207	80	104	134
Time in ER Before Being Evaluated (minutes)	258	23	18	26
Time to Pain Meds for Fractures (minutes)[5]	-	-	47	57
Heart Attack Care				
Aspirin Given at Discharge[3,7]	-	-	99%	99%
Fibrinolytic Meds Within 30 Min. of Arrival[3,7]	-	-	-	54%
PCI Within 90 Minutes of Arrival[3,7]	-	-	97%	96%
Statin Prescribed at Discharge[3,7]	-	-	99%	98%
Heart Failure Care				
ACE Inhibitor or ARB for LVSD[1]	-	-	95%	97%
Discharge Instructions Given[1]	-	-	91%	94%
Evaluation of LVS Function	14	100%	94%	99%
Medicare Spending				
Medicare Spending per Patient (ratio)	-	0.77	0.94	0.98
Pneumonia Care				
Appropriate Initial Antibiotic Given[1]	-	-	92%	95%
Blood Culture Timing[1]	-	-	98%	98%
Pregnancy and Delivery Care				
Newborn Deliveries Scheduled Early[1]	-	-	12%	6%
Preventive Care				
Immunization for Influenza	118	72%	88%	90%
Immunization for Pneumonia	129	85%	90%	92%
Stroke Care				
Anticoagulation Therapy for Atrial Fibrillation[5]	-	-	88%	95%
Antithrombotic Therapy Timing[5]	-	-	97%	98%
Assessed for Rehabilitation[5]	-	-	97%	97%
Discharged on Antithrombotic Therapy[5]	-	-	98%	99%
Discharged on Statin Medication[5]	-	-	88%	94%
Thrombolytic Therapy Timing[5]	-	-	68%	66%
Venous Thromboembolism Prophylaxis[5]	-	-	93%	94%
Written Stroke Educational Materials Given[5]	-	-	84%	88%
Surgical Care Improvement Project				
Appropriate Beta Blocker Usage[5]	-	-	98%	98%
Appropriate VTP Within 24 Hours[5]	-	-	98%	98%
Controlled Postoperative Blood Glucose[5]	-	-	98%	97%
Perioperative Temperature Management[5]	-	-	100%	100%
Prophylactic Antibiotic Selection[5]	-	-	99%	99%
Prophylactic Antibiotic Selection (Outpatient)[5]	-	-	98%	98%
Prophylactic Antibiotic Stopped[5]	-	-	98%	98%
Prophylactic Antibiotic Timing[5]	-	-	99%	99%
Prophylactic Antibiotic Timing (Outpatient)[5]	-	-	98%	98%
Urinary Catheter Removal[5]	-	-	97%	97%
Survey of Patients' Hospital Experiences				
Area Around Room 'Always' Quiet at Night[6]	<100	77%	65%	61%
Doctors 'Always' Communicated Well[6]	<100	98%	85%	82%
Home Recovery Information Given[6]	<100	86%	86%	85%
Hospital Given 9 or 10 on 10 Point Scale[6]	<100	92%	76%	71%
Meds 'Always' Explained Before Given[6]	<100	66%	66%	64%
Nurses 'Always' Communicated Well[6]	<100	88%	81%	79%
Pain 'Always' Well Controlled[6]	<100	68%	72%	71%
Room and Bathroom 'Always' Clean[6]	<100	91%	76%	73%
Timely Help 'Always' Received[6]	<100	83%	72%	68%
Would Definitely Recommend Hospital[6]	<100	91%	75%	71%
Use of Medical Imaging				
Cardiac Imaging Stress Test before Surgery[7]	-	-	5%	5.3%
Combination Abdominal CT Scan[7]	-	-	19%	10.5%
Combination Brain/Sinus CT Scan[7]	-	-	2.9%	2.7%
Combination Chest CT Scan[7]	-	-	3.9%	2.7%
Follow-up Mammogram/Ultrasound[7]	-	-	7.8%	8.8%
Lumbar Spine MRI for Low Back Pain[7]	-	-	40.2%	37.2%

Wilson Medical Center

Reece Campus 2600 Ottawa Road
Neodesha, KS 66757
Phone: 620-325-8369
Fax: 620-325-2907
URL: www.wilsoncountyhospital.org
Type: Critical Access Hospitals
Emergency Services: Yes
Ownership: Voluntary non-profit - Other
Beds: 38

Key Personnel:
Chief of Medical Staff .... Amy Cunningham
CEO/President .... John Gutschenritter

Measure	Cases	This Hosp.	State Avg.	U.S. Avg.
Blood Clot Prevention and Treatment				
Anticoagulation Overlap Therapy[5]	-	-	94%	93%
ICU Venous Thromboembolism Prophylaxis[5]	-	-	91%	92%
Incidence of Potentially Preventable VTE[5]	-	-	8%	10%
UFH with Dosages/Platelet Monitoring[5]	-	-	98%	97%
Venous Thromboembolism Prophylaxis[5]	-	-	79%	85%
Warfarin Therapy Discharge Instructions[5]	-	-	84%	75%
Chest Pain/Possible Heart Attack Care				
Aspirin Given Within 24 Hours of Arrival	-	-	94%	96%
Fibrinolytic Meds Within 30 Min. of Arrival	-	-	41%	58%
Average Time to ECG (minutes)	-	-	8	7
Average Time to Transfer (minutes)	-	-	57	60
Children's Asthma Care				
Received Home Management Plan of Care	-	-	-	88%
Received Reliever Medication	-	-	-	100%
Received Systemic Corticosteroids	-	-	-	100%
Emergency Department				
Admittance Decision Time (minutes)[5]	-	-	57	98
Head CT Results Within 45 Min. of Arrival	-	-	53%	57%
Patients Who Left ER Before Being Seen	-	-	2%	2%
Time from ER Arrival to Admit. (minutes)[5]	-	-	185	274
Time from ER Arrival to Discharge (minutes)	-	-	104	134
Time in ER Before Being Evaluated (minutes)	-	-	18	26
Time to Pain Meds for Fractures (minutes)	-	-	47	57
Heart Attack Care				
Aspirin Given at Discharge[5]	-	-	99%	99%
Fibrinolytic Meds Within 30 Min. of Arrival[5]	-	-	-	54%
PCI Within 90 Minutes of Arrival[5]	-	-	97%	96%
Statin Prescribed at Discharge[5]	-	-	99%	98%
Heart Failure Care				
ACE Inhibitor or ARB for LVSD[3,7]	-	-	95%	97%
Discharge Instructions Given[1,3]	-	-	91%	94%
Evaluation of LVS Function[1,3]	-	-	94%	99%
Medicare Spending				
Medicare Spending per Patient (ratio)	-	-	0.94	0.98
Pneumonia Care				
Appropriate Initial Antibiotic Given	14	50%	92%	95%
Blood Culture Timing	11	73%	98%	98%
Pregnancy and Delivery Care				
Newborn Deliveries Scheduled Early[5]	-	-	12%	6%
Preventive Care				
Immunization for Influenza[5]	-	-	88%	90%
Immunization for Pneumonia[5]	-	-	90%	92%
Stroke Care				
Anticoagulation Therapy for Atrial Fibrillation[5]	-	-	88%	95%
Antithrombotic Therapy Timing[5]	-	-	97%	98%
Assessed for Rehabilitation[5]	-	-	97%	97%
Discharged on Antithrombotic Therapy[5]	-	-	98%	99%
Discharged on Statin Medication[5]	-	-	88%	94%
Thrombolytic Therapy Timing[5]	-	-	68%	66%
Venous Thromboembolism Prophylaxis[5]	-	-	93%	94%
Written Stroke Educational Materials Given[5]	-	-	84%	88%
Surgical Care Improvement Project				
Appropriate Beta Blocker Usage[5]	-	-	98%	98%
Appropriate VTP Within 24 Hours[5]	-	-	98%	98%
Controlled Postoperative Blood Glucose[5]	-	-	98%	97%
Perioperative Temperature Management[5]	-	-	100%	100%
Prophylactic Antibiotic Selection[5]	-	-	99%	99%
Prophylactic Antibiotic Selection (Outpatient)	-	-	98%	98%
Prophylactic Antibiotic Stopped[5]	-	-	98%	98%
Prophylactic Antibiotic Timing[5]	-	-	99%	99%
Prophylactic Antibiotic Timing (Outpatient)	-	-	98%	98%
Urinary Catheter Removal[5]	-	-	97%	97%
Survey of Patients' Hospital Experiences				
Area Around Room 'Always' Quiet at Night[6]	<100	82%	65%	61%
Doctors 'Always' Communicated Well[6]	<100	94%	85%	82%
Home Recovery Information Given[6]	<100	90%	86%	85%
Hospital Given 9 or 10 on 10 Point Scale[6]	<100	83%	76%	71%
Meds 'Always' Explained Before Given[6]	<100	70%	66%	64%
Nurses 'Always' Communicated Well[6]	<100	87%	81%	79%
Pain 'Always' Well Controlled[6]	<100	83%	72%	71%
Room and Bathroom 'Always' Clean[6]	<100	88%	76%	73%
Timely Help 'Always' Received[6]	<100	82%	72%	68%
Would Definitely Recommend Hospital[6]	<100	83%	75%	71%
Use of Medical Imaging				
Cardiac Imaging Stress Test before Surgery	-	-	5%	5.3%
Combination Abdominal CT Scan	-	-	19%	10.5%
Combination Brain/Sinus CT Scan	-	-	2.9%	2.7%
Combination Chest CT Scan	-	-	3.9%	2.7%
Follow-up Mammogram/Ultrasound	-	-	7.8%	8.8%
Lumbar Spine MRI for Low Back Pain	-	-	40.2%	37.2%

Ness County Hospital District #2

312 Custer Street
Ness City, KS 67560
Phone: 785-798-2291
Fax: 785-798-3435
E-mail: nesshosp@gbta.net
Type: Critical Access Hospitals
Emergency Services: Yes
Ownership: Government - Local
Beds: 20

Key Personnel:
Quality Assurance .... Susan Kuehn
Infection Control.............. Brenda Sutton, RN

NOTE: Hospital profiles are in alphabetical order by state, then city, then hospital within the city; Rankings exclude hospitals with less than 25 cases except for patient surveys which excludes hospitals with less than 100 cases; (a) 100-299 cases; (1) The number of cases/patients is too few to report; (2) Data submitted were based on a sample of cases/patients; (3) Results are based on a shorter time period than required; (4) Data suppressed by CMS for one or more quarters; (5) Results are not available for this reporting period; (6) Fewer than 100 patients completed the HCAHPS survey; (7) No cases met the criteria for this measure; (8) The lower limit of the confidence interval cannot be calculated if the number of observed infections equals zero; (9) No data are available from the state/territory for this reporting period; (10) The scores shown reflect fewer than 50 completed surveys; (11) There were discrepancies in the data collection process; (12) This measure does not apply to this hospital for this reporting period; (13) Results cannot be calculated for this reporting period; (14) The results for this state are combined with nearby states to protect confidentiality; Please refer to the User's Guide for a full explanation of data.

Emergency Room . . . . Brenda Wassinger

Measure	Cases	This Hosp.	State Avg.	U.S. Avg.
Blood Clot Prevention and Treatment				
Anticoagulation Overlap Therapy[5]	-	-	94%	93%
ICU Venous Thromboembolism Prophylaxis[5]	-	-	91%	92%
Incidence of Potentially Preventable VTE[5]	-	-	8%	10%
UFH with Dosages/Platelet Monitoring[5]	-	-	98%	97%
Venous Thromboembolism Prophylaxis[5]	-	-	79%	85%
Warfarin Therapy Discharge Instructions[5]	-	-	84%	75%
Chest Pain/Possible Heart Attack Care				
Aspirin Given Within 24 Hours of Arrival	-	-	94%	96%
Fibrinolytic Meds Within 30 Min. of Arrival	-	-	41%	58%
Average Time to ECG (minutes)	-	-	8	7
Average Time to Transfer (minutes)	-	-	57	60
Children's Asthma Care				
Received Home Management Plan of Care	-	-	-	88%
Received Reliever Medication	-	-	-	100%
Received Systemic Corticosteroids	-	-	-	100%
Emergency Department				
Admittance Decision Time (minutes)	53	20	57	98
Head CT Results Within 45 Min. of Arrival	-	-	53%	57%
Patients Who Left ER Before Being Seen	-	-	2%	2%
Time from ER Arrival to Admit. (minutes)	54	72	185	274
Time from ER Arrival to Discharge (minutes)	-	-	104	134
Time in ER Before Being Evaluated (minutes)	-	-	18	26
Time to Pain Meds for Fractures (minutes)	-	-	47	57
Heart Attack Care				
Aspirin Given at Discharge[5]	-	-	99%	99%
Fibrinolytic Meds Within 30 Min. of Arrival[5]	-	-	-	54%
PCI Within 90 Minutes of Arrival[5]	-	-	97%	96%
Statin Prescribed at Discharge[5]	-	-	99%	98%
Heart Failure Care				
ACE Inhibitor or ARB for LVSD[3,7]	-	-	95%	97%
Discharge Instructions Given[1,3]	-	-	91%	94%
Evaluation of LVS Function[1,3]	-	-	94%	99%
Medicare Spending				
Medicare Spending per Patient (ratio)	-	-	0.94	0.98
Pneumonia Care				
Appropriate Initial Antibiotic Given[1]	-	-	92%	95%
Blood Culture Timing[1]	-	-	98%	98%
Pregnancy and Delivery Care				
Newborn Deliveries Scheduled Early[5]	-	-	12%	6%
Preventive Care				
Immunization for Influenza	31	45%	88%	90%
Immunization for Pneumonia	50	36%	90%	92%
Stroke Care				
Anticoagulation Therapy for Atrial Fibrillation[5]	-	-	88%	95%
Antithrombotic Therapy Timing[5]	-	-	97%	98%
Assessed for Rehabilitation[5]	-	-	97%	97%
Discharged on Antithrombotic Therapy[5]	-	-	98%	99%
Discharged on Statin Medication[5]	-	-	88%	94%
Thrombolytic Therapy Timing[5]	-	-	68%	66%
Venous Thromboembolism Prophylaxis[5]	-	-	93%	94%
Written Stroke Educational Materials Given[5]	-	-	84%	88%
Surgical Care Improvement Project				
Appropriate Beta Blocker Usage[5]	-	-	98%	98%
Appropriate VTP Within 24 Hours[5]	-	-	98%	98%
Controlled Postoperative Blood Glucose[5]	-	-	98%	97%
Perioperative Temperature Management[5]	-	-	100%	100%
Prophylactic Antibiotic Selection[5]	-	-	99%	99%
Prophylactic Antibiotic Selection (Outpatient)	-	-	98%	98%
Prophylactic Antibiotic Stopped[5]	-	-	98%	98%
Prophylactic Antibiotic Timing[5]	-	-	99%	99%
Prophylactic Antibiotic Timing (Outpatient)	-	-	98%	98%
Urinary Catheter Removal[5]	-	-	97%	97%
Survey of Patients' Hospital Experiences				
Area Around Room 'Always' Quiet at Night[5]	-	-	65%	61%
Doctors 'Always' Communicated Well[5]	-	-	85%	82%
Home Recovery Information Given[5]	-	-	86%	85%
Hospital Given 9 or 10 on 10 Point Scale[5]	-	-	76%	71%
Meds 'Always' Explained Before Given[5]	-	-	66%	64%
Nurses 'Always' Communicated Well[5]	-	-	81%	79%
Pain 'Always' Well Controlled[5]	-	-	72%	71%
Room and Bathroom 'Always' Clean[5]	-	-	76%	73%
Timely Help 'Always' Received[5]	-	-	72%	68%
Would Definitely Recommend Hospital[5]	-	-	75%	71%
Use of Medical Imaging				
Cardiac Imaging Stress Test before Surgery	-	-	5%	5.3%
Combination Abdominal CT Scan	-	-	19%	10.5%
Combination Brain/Sinus CT Scan	-	-	2.9%	2.7%
Combination Chest CT Scan	-	-	3.9%	2.7%
Follow-up Mammogram/Ultrasound	-	-	7.8%	8.8%
Lumbar Spine MRI for Low Back Pain	-	-	40.2%	37.2%

Newton Medical Center

600 Medical Center Drive
Newton, KS 67114
Phone: 316-804-6001
Fax: 316-804-6260
E-mail: nmcinfor@newmedctr.org
URL: www.newtonmedicalcenter.com
Type: Acute Care Hospitals
Emergency Services: Yes
Ownership: Voluntary non-profit - Private
Beds: 103

Key Personnel:
Chief of Medical Staff. . . . . Joseph Aiyenowo
Radiology. . . . . Maj-Beth Biernacki
CEO/President. . . . . Steven G Kelly, FACHE

Measure	Cases	This Hosp.	State Avg.	U.S. Avg.
Blood Clot Prevention and Treatment				
Anticoagulation Overlap Therapy[2]	42	93%	94%	93%
ICU Venous Thromboembolism Prophylaxis[2]	46	87%	91%	92%
Incidence of Potentially Preventable VTE[1,2]	-	-	8%	10%
UFH with Dosages/Platelet Monitoring[2]	12	100%	98%	97%
Venous Thromboembolism Prophylaxis[2]	172	85%	79%	85%
Warfarin Therapy Discharge Instructions[2]	28	57%	84%	75%
Chest Pain/Possible Heart Attack Care				
Aspirin Given Within 24 Hours of Arrival	46	100%	94%	96%
Fibrinolytic Meds Within 30 Min. of Arrival[1]	-	-	41%	58%
Average Time to ECG (minutes)	48	8	8	7
Average Time to Transfer (minutes)[1]	-	-	57	60
Children's Asthma Care				
Received Home Management Plan of Care	-	-	-	88%
Received Reliever Medication	-	-	-	100%
Received Systemic Corticosteroids	-	-	-	100%
Emergency Department				
Admittance Decision Time (minutes)	877	50	57	98
Head CT Results Within 45 Min. of Arrival[1]	-	-	53%	57%
Patients Who Left ER Before Being Seen	13,307	1%	2%	2%
Time from ER Arrival to Admit. (minutes)	893	176	185	274
Time from ER Arrival to Discharge (minutes)	10,344	123	104	134
Time in ER Before Being Evaluated (minutes)	11,566	18	18	26
Time to Pain Meds for Fractures (minutes)	102	62	47	57
Heart Attack Care				
Aspirin Given at Discharge	25	100%	99%	99%
Fibrinolytic Meds Within 30 Min. of Arrival[7]	-	-	-	54%
PCI Within 90 Minutes of Arrival[1]	-	-	97%	96%
Statin Prescribed at Discharge	26	100%	99%	98%
Heart Failure Care				
ACE Inhibitor or ARB for LVSD	11	100%	95%	97%
Discharge Instructions Given	42	76%	91%	94%
Evaluation of LVS Function	74	97%	94%	99%
Medicare Spending				
Medicare Spending per Patient (ratio)	-	0.89	0.94	0.98
Pneumonia Care				
Appropriate Initial Antibiotic Given	67	97%	92%	95%
Blood Culture Timing	92	100%	98%	98%
Pregnancy and Delivery Care				
Newborn Deliveries Scheduled Early	32	9%	12%	6%
Preventive Care				
Immunization for Influenza	1,273	80%	88%	90%
Immunization for Pneumonia	1,490	86%	90%	92%
Stroke Care				
Anticoagulation Therapy for Atrial Fibrillation[1]	-	-	88%	95%
Antithrombotic Therapy Timing	13	100%	97%	98%
Assessed for Rehabilitation	19	100%	97%	97%
Discharged on Antithrombotic Therapy	17	59%	98%	99%
Discharged on Statin Medication	16	56%	88%	94%
Thrombolytic Therapy Timing[7]	-	-	68%	66%
Venous Thromboembolism Prophylaxis	16	56%	93%	94%
Written Stroke Educational Materials Given[1]	-	-	84%	88%
Surgical Care Improvement Project				
Appropriate Beta Blocker Usage	95	99%	98%	98%
Appropriate VTP Within 24 Hours	282	96%	98%	98%
Controlled Postoperative Blood Glucose[7]	-	-	98%	97%
Perioperative Temperature Management	301	100%	100%	100%
Prophylactic Antibiotic Selection	212	98%	99%	99%
Prophylactic Antibiotic Selection (Outpatient)	179	97%	98%	98%
Prophylactic Antibiotic Stopped	202	97%	98%	98%
Prophylactic Antibiotic Timing	214	93%	99%	99%
Prophylactic Antibiotic Timing (Outpatient)	181	94%	98%	98%
Urinary Catheter Removal	257	92%	97%	97%
Survey of Patients' Hospital Experiences				
Area Around Room 'Always' Quiet at Night	300+	56%	65%	61%
Doctors 'Always' Communicated Well	300+	83%	85%	82%
Home Recovery Information Given	300+	89%	86%	85%
Hospital Given 9 or 10 on 10 Point Scale	300+	74%	76%	71%
Meds 'Always' Explained Before Given	300+	59%	66%	64%
Nurses 'Always' Communicated Well	300+	77%	81%	79%
Pain 'Always' Well Controlled	300+	68%	72%	71%
Room and Bathroom 'Always' Clean	300+	73%	76%	73%
Timely Help 'Always' Received	300+	66%	72%	68%
Would Definitely Recommend Hospital	300+	77%	75%	71%
Use of Medical Imaging				
Cardiac Imaging Stress Test before Surgery	129	3.1%	5%	5.3%
Combination Abdominal CT Scan	330	40.3%	19%	10.5%
Combination Brain/Sinus CT Scan[1]	-	-	2.9%	2.7%
Combination Chest CT Scan	205	0.5%	3.9%	2.7%
Follow-up Mammogram/Ultrasound	1,000	6.9%	7.8%	8.8%
Lumbar Spine MRI for Low Back Pain	94	33.0%	40.2%	37.2%

Norton County Hospital

102 E Holme Street
Norton, KS 67654
Phone: 785-877-3351
Fax: 785-877-2841
E-mail: ntcohoso@ruraltel.net
Type: Critical Access Hospitals
Emergency Services: Yes
Ownership: Government - Local
Beds: 43

Key Personnel:
Emergency Room . . . . Georgia Brier
Chief of Medical Staff . . . . Glenda Maurer, MD
CEO/President. . . . . Richard Miller
Quality Assurance . . . . Lyn Thiele

Measure	Cases	This Hosp.	State Avg.	U.S. Avg.
Blood Clot Prevention and Treatment				
Anticoagulation Overlap Therapy[1,3]	-	-	94%	93%
ICU Venous Thromboembolism Prophylaxis[3,7]	-	-	91%	92%
Incidence of Potentially Preventable VTE[3,7]	-	-	8%	10%
UFH with Dosages/Platelet Monitoring[1,3]	-	-	98%	97%
Venous Thromboembolism Prophylaxis[3,7]	-	-	79%	85%
Warfarin Therapy Discharge Instructions[1,3]	-	-	84%	75%
Chest Pain/Possible Heart Attack Care				
Aspirin Given Within 24 Hours of Arrival[1,3]	-	-	94%	96%
Fibrinolytic Meds Within 30 Min. of Arrival[3,7]	-	-	41%	58%
Average Time to ECG (minutes)[1,3]	-	-	8	7
Average Time to Transfer (minutes)[3,7]	-	-	57	60
Children's Asthma Care				
Received Home Management Plan of Care	-	-	-	88%
Received Reliever Medication	-	-	-	100%
Received Systemic Corticosteroids	-	-	-	100%
Emergency Department				
Admittance Decision Time (minutes)[2,3]	-	-	57	98
Head CT Results Within 45 Min. of Arrival[3,7]	-	-	53%	57%
Patients Who Left ER Before Being Seen[5]	-	-	2%	2%
Time from ER Arrival to Admit. (minutes)[2,3]	19	109	185	274
Time from ER Arrival to Discharge (minutes)[3]	25	98	104	134
Time in ER Before Being Evaluated (minutes)[3]	42	22	18	26
Time to Pain Meds for Fractures (minutes)[1,3]	-	-	47	57
Heart Attack Care				
Aspirin Given at Discharge[5]	-	-	99%	99%
Fibrinolytic Meds Within 30 Min. of Arrival[5]	-	-	-	54%

NOTE: Hospital profiles are in alphabetical order by state, then city, then hospital within the city; Rankings exclude hospitals with less than 25 cases except for patient surveys which excludes hospitals with less than 100 cases; (a) 100-299 cases; (1) The number of cases/patients is too few to report; (2) Data submitted were based on a sample of cases/patients; (3) Results are based on a shorter time period than required; (4) Data suppressed by CMS for one or more quarters; (5) Results are not available for this reporting period; (6) Fewer than 100 patients completed the HCAHPS survey; (7) No cases met the criteria for this measure; (8) The lower limit of the confidence interval cannot be calculated if the number of observed infections equals zero; (9) No data are available from the state/territory for this reporting period; (10) The scores shown reflect fewer than 50 completed surveys; (11) There were discrepancies in the data collection process; (12) This measure does not apply to this hospital for this reporting period; (13) Results cannot be calculated for this reporting period; (14) The results for this state are combined with nearby states to protect confidentiality; Please refer to the User's Guide for a full explanation of data.

Measure	Cases	This Hosp.	State Avg.	U.S. Avg.
PCI Within 90 Minutes of Arrival[5]	-	-	97%	96%
Statin Prescribed at Discharge[5]	-	-	99%	98%
Heart Failure Care				
ACE Inhibitor or ARB for LVSD[2,3]	-	-	95%	97%
Discharge Instructions Given[1,2]	-	-	91%	94%
Evaluation of LVS Function[1,2]	-	-	94%	99%
Medicare Spending				
Medicare Spending per Patient (ratio)	-	-	0.94	0.98
Pneumonia Care				
Appropriate Initial Antibiotic Given[1,3]	-	-	92%	95%
Blood Culture Timing[1,3]	-	-	98%	98%
Pregnancy and Delivery Care				
Newborn Deliveries Scheduled Early[5]	-	-	12%	6%
Preventive Care				
Immunization for Influenza[5]	-	-	88%	90%
Immunization for Pneumonia[2,3]	33	70%	90%	92%
Stroke Care				
Anticoagulation Therapy for Atrial Fibrillation[5]	-	-	88%	95%
Antithrombotic Therapy Timing[5]	-	-	97%	98%
Assessed for Rehabilitation[5]	-	-	97%	97%
Discharged on Antithrombotic Therapy[5]	-	-	98%	99%
Discharged on Statin Medication[5]	-	-	88%	94%
Thrombolytic Therapy Timing[5]	-	-	68%	66%
Venous Thromboembolism Prophylaxis[5]	-	-	93%	94%
Written Stroke Educational Materials Given[5]	-	-	84%	88%
Surgical Care Improvement Project				
Appropriate Beta Blocker Usage[5]	-	-	98%	98%
Appropriate VTP Within 24 Hours[5]	-	-	98%	98%
Controlled Postoperative Blood Glucose[5]	-	-	98%	97%
Perioperative Temperature Management[5]	-	-	100%	100%
Prophylactic Antibiotic Selection[5]	-	-	99%	99%
Prophylactic Antibiotic Selection (Outpatient)[5]	-	-	98%	98%
Prophylactic Antibiotic Stopped[5]	-	-	98%	98%
Prophylactic Antibiotic Timing[5]	-	-	99%	99%
Prophylactic Antibiotic Timing (Outpatient)[5]	-	-	98%	98%
Urinary Catheter Removal[5]	-	-	97%	97%
Survey of Patients' Hospital Experiences				
Area Around Room 'Always' Quiet at Night[5]	-	-	65%	61%
Doctors 'Always' Communicated Well[5]	-	-	85%	82%
Home Recovery Information Given[5]	-	-	86%	85%
Hospital Given 9 or 10 on 10 Point Scale[5]	-	-	76%	71%
Meds 'Always' Explained Before Given[5]	-	-	66%	64%
Nurses 'Always' Communicated Well[5]	-	-	81%	79%
Pain 'Always' Well Controlled[5]	-	-	72%	71%
Room and Bathroom 'Always' Clean[5]	-	-	76%	73%
Timely Help 'Always' Received[5]	-	-	72%	68%
Would Definitely Recommend Hospital[5]	-	-	75%	71%
Use of Medical Imaging				
Cardiac Imaging Stress Test before Surgery[1]	-	-	5%	5.3%
Combination Abdominal CT Scan	70	12.9%	19%	10.5%
Combination Brain/Sinus CT Scan[1]	-	-	2.9%	2.7%
Combination Chest CT Scan	68	5.9%	3.9%	2.7%
Follow-up Mammogram/Ultrasound	256	5.1%	7.8%	8.8%
Lumbar Spine MRI for Low Back Pain[1]	-	-	40.2%	37.2%

Decatur County Hospital

810 W Columbia Street
Oberlin, KS 67749
Phone: 785-475-2208
Type: Critical Access Hospitals
Emergency Services: Yes
Ownership: Government - Local

Measure	Cases	This Hosp.	State Avg.	U.S. Avg.
Blood Clot Prevention and Treatment				
Anticoagulation Overlap Therapy[5]	-	-	94%	93%
ICU Venous Thromboembolism Prophylaxis[5]	-	-	91%	92%
Incidence of Potentially Preventable VTE[5]	-	-	8%	10%
UFH with Dosages/Platelet Monitoring[5]	-	-	98%	97%
Venous Thromboembolism Prophylaxis[5]	-	-	79%	85%
Warfarin Therapy Discharge Instructions[5]	-	-	84%	75%
Chest Pain/Possible Heart Attack Care				
Aspirin Given Within 24 Hours of Arrival[5]	-	-	94%	96%
Fibrinolytic Meds Within 30 Min. of Arrival[5]	-	-	41%	58%
Average Time to ECG (minutes)[5]	-	-	8	7
Average Time to Transfer (minutes)[5]	-	-	57	60
Children's Asthma Care				
Received Home Management Plan of Care	-	-	-	88%
Received Reliever Medication	-	-	-	100%
Received Systemic Corticosteroids	-	-	-	100%
Emergency Department				
Admittance Decision Time (minutes)[3]	16	16	57	98
Head CT Results Within 45 Min. of Arrival[5]	-	-	53%	57%
Patients Who Left ER Before Being Seen[5]	-	-	2%	2%
Time from ER Arrival to Admit. (minutes)[3]	16	104	185	274
Time from ER Arrival to Discharge (minutes)[5]	-	-	104	134
Time in ER Before Being Evaluated (minutes)[5]	-	-	18	26
Time to Pain Meds for Fractures (minutes)[5]	-	-	47	57
Heart Attack Care				
Aspirin Given at Discharge[5]	-	-	99%	99%
Fibrinolytic Meds Within 30 Min. of Arrival[5]	-	-	-	54%
PCI Within 90 Minutes of Arrival[5]	-	-	97%	96%
Statin Prescribed at Discharge[5]	-	-	99%	98%
Heart Failure Care				
ACE Inhibitor or ARB for LVSD[1,3]	-	-	95%	97%
Discharge Instructions Given[1,3]	-	-	91%	94%
Evaluation of LVS Function[1,3]	-	-	94%	99%
Medicare Spending				
Medicare Spending per Patient (ratio)	-	-	0.94	0.98
Pneumonia Care				
Appropriate Initial Antibiotic Given[1,3]	-	-	92%	95%
Blood Culture Timing[3,7]	-	-	98%	98%
Pregnancy and Delivery Care				
Newborn Deliveries Scheduled Early[5]	-	-	12%	6%
Preventive Care				
Immunization for Influenza[5]	-	-	88%	90%
Immunization for Pneumonia[3]	33	58%	90%	92%
Stroke Care				
Anticoagulation Therapy for Atrial Fibrillation[5]	-	-	88%	95%
Antithrombotic Therapy Timing[5]	-	-	97%	98%
Assessed for Rehabilitation[5]	-	-	97%	97%
Discharged on Antithrombotic Therapy[5]	-	-	98%	99%
Discharged on Statin Medication[5]	-	-	88%	94%
Thrombolytic Therapy Timing[5]	-	-	68%	66%
Venous Thromboembolism Prophylaxis[5]	-	-	93%	94%
Written Stroke Educational Materials Given[5]	-	-	84%	88%
Surgical Care Improvement Project				
Appropriate Beta Blocker Usage[5]	-	-	98%	98%
Appropriate VTP Within 24 Hours[5]	-	-	98%	98%
Controlled Postoperative Blood Glucose[5]	-	-	98%	97%
Perioperative Temperature Management[5]	-	-	100%	100%
Prophylactic Antibiotic Selection[5]	-	-	99%	99%
Prophylactic Antibiotic Selection (Outpatient)[5]	-	-	98%	98%
Prophylactic Antibiotic Stopped[5]	-	-	98%	98%
Prophylactic Antibiotic Timing[5]	-	-	99%	99%
Prophylactic Antibiotic Timing (Outpatient)[5]	-	-	98%	98%
Urinary Catheter Removal[5]	-	-	97%	97%
Survey of Patients' Hospital Experiences				
Area Around Room 'Always' Quiet at Night[5]	-	-	65%	61%
Doctors 'Always' Communicated Well[5]	-	-	85%	82%
Home Recovery Information Given[5]	-	-	86%	85%
Hospital Given 9 or 10 on 10 Point Scale[5]	-	-	76%	71%
Meds 'Always' Explained Before Given[5]	-	-	66%	64%
Nurses 'Always' Communicated Well[5]	-	-	81%	79%
Pain 'Always' Well Controlled[5]	-	-	72%	71%
Room and Bathroom 'Always' Clean[5]	-	-	76%	73%
Timely Help 'Always' Received[5]	-	-	72%	68%
Would Definitely Recommend Hospital[5]	-	-	75%	71%
Use of Medical Imaging				
Cardiac Imaging Stress Test before Surgery[1]	-	-	5%	5.3%
Combination Abdominal CT Scan	58	5.2%	19%	10.5%
Combination Brain/Sinus CT Scan	41	14.6%	2.9%	2.7%
Combination Chest CT Scan	58	0.0%	3.9%	2.7%
Follow-up Mammogram/Ultrasound[1]	-	-	7.8%	8.8%
Lumbar Spine MRI for Low Back Pain[1]	-	-	40.2%	37.2%

Olathe Medical Center

20333 West 151st Street
Olathe, KS 66061
Phone: 913-791-4200
Fax: 913-791-4393
URL: www.ohsi.com
Type: Acute Care Hospitals
Emergency Services: Yes
Ownership: Voluntary non-profit - Private
Beds: 200

Key Personnel:

Radiology . . . . Donald J Boss
Intensive Care Unit . . . . Carol Cleek
Infection Control . . . . Elaine Fitzmaurice
Emergency Room . . . . Cindy Kolich
Cardiac Laboratory . . . . Kit Power
Quality Assurance . . . . Nancy Schnegelberger
Chief of Medical Staff . . . . Bruce Snider, MD
Operating Room . . . . Dave Wayatt

Measure	Cases	This Hosp.	State Avg.	U.S. Avg.
Blood Clot Prevention and Treatment				
Anticoagulation Overlap Therapy[2]	63	94%	94%	93%
ICU Venous Thromboembolism Prophylaxis[2]	74	85%	91%	92%
Incidence of Potentially Preventable VTE[1,2]	-	-	8%	10%
UFH with Dosages/Platelet Monitoring[2]	18	100%	98%	97%
Venous Thromboembolism Prophylaxis[2]	298	86%	79%	85%
Warfarin Therapy Discharge Instructions[2]	54	80%	84%	75%
Chest Pain/Possible Heart Attack Care				
Aspirin Given Within 24 Hours of Arrival[1,3]	-	-	94%	96%
Fibrinolytic Meds Within 30 Min. of Arrival[5]	-	-	41%	58%
Average Time to ECG (minutes)[1,3]	-	-	8	7
Average Time to Transfer (minutes)[5]	-	-	57	60
Children's Asthma Care				
Received Home Management Plan of Care	-	-	-	88%
Received Reliever Medication	-	-	-	100%
Received Systemic Corticosteroids	-	-	-	100%
Emergency Department				
Admittance Decision Time (minutes)[2]	604	62	57	98
Head CT Results Within 45 Min. of Arrival[1]	-	-	53%	57%
Patients Who Left ER Before Being Seen	42,363	1%	2%	2%
Time from ER Arrival to Admit. (minutes)[2]	608	196	185	274
Time from ER Arrival to Discharge (minutes)	387	124	104	134
Time in ER Before Being Evaluated (minutes)	411	20	18	26
Time to Pain Meds for Fractures (minutes)	180	44	47	57
Heart Attack Care				
Aspirin Given at Discharge	238	100%	99%	99%
Fibrinolytic Meds Within 30 Min. of Arrival[7]	-	-	-	54%
PCI Within 90 Minutes of Arrival	37	100%	97%	96%
Statin Prescribed at Discharge	236	100%	99%	98%
Heart Failure Care				
ACE Inhibitor or ARB for LVSD	84	99%	95%	97%
Discharge Instructions Given	199	95%	91%	94%
Evaluation of LVS Function	255	100%	94%	99%
Medicare Spending				
Medicare Spending per Patient (ratio)	-	0.99	0.94	0.98
Pneumonia Care				
Appropriate Initial Antibiotic Given	116	100%	92%	95%
Blood Culture Timing	198	99%	98%	98%
Pregnancy and Delivery Care				
Newborn Deliveries Scheduled Early[2]	49	2%	12%	6%
Preventive Care				
Immunization for Influenza[2]	539	94%	88%	90%
Immunization for Pneumonia[2]	707	94%	90%	92%
Stroke Care				
Anticoagulation Therapy for Atrial Fibrillation	14	93%	88%	95%
Antithrombotic Therapy Timing	87	100%	97%	98%
Assessed for Rehabilitation	104	98%	97%	97%
Discharged on Antithrombotic Therapy	92	100%	98%	99%
Discharged on Statin Medication	64	100%	88%	94%
Thrombolytic Therapy Timing[1]	-	-	68%	66%
Venous Thromboembolism Prophylaxis	102	98%	93%	94%
Written Stroke Educational Materials Given	65	89%	84%	88%
Surgical Care Improvement Project				
Appropriate Beta Blocker Usage[2]	203	98%	98%	98%
Appropriate VTP Within 24 Hours[2]	468	100%	98%	98%
Controlled Postoperative Blood Glucose[2]	103	91%	98%	97%
Perioperative Temperature Management[2]	542	100%	100%	100%
Prophylactic Antibiotic Selection[2]	432	99%	99%	99%

NOTE: Hospital profiles are in alphabetical order by state, then city, then hospital within the city; Rankings exclude hospitals with less than 25 cases except for patient surveys which excludes hospitals with less than 100 cases; (a) 100-299 cases; (1) The number of cases/patients is too few to report; (2) Data submitted were based on a sample of cases/patients; (3) Results are based on a shorter time period than required; (4) Data suppressed by CMS for one or more quarters; (5) Results are not available for this reporting period; (6) Fewer than 100 patients completed the HCAHPS survey; (7) No cases met the criteria for this measure; (8) The lower limit of the confidence interval cannot be calculated if the number of observed infections equals zero; (9) No data are available from the state/territory for this reporting period; (10) The scores shown reflect fewer than 50 completed surveys; (11) There were discrepancies in the data collection process; (12) This measure does not apply to this hospital for this reporting period; (13) Results cannot be calculated for this reporting period; (14) The results for this state are combined with nearby states to protect confidentiality; Please refer to the User's Guide for a full explanation of data.

Measure	Cases	This Hosp.	State Avg.	U.S. Avg.
Prophylactic Antibiotic Selection (Outpatient)	415	94%	98%	98%
Prophylactic Antibiotic Stopped[2]	418	96%	98%	98%
Prophylactic Antibiotic Timing[2]	432	99%	99%	99%
Prophylactic Antibiotic Timing (Outpatient)	418	98%	98%	98%
Urinary Catheter Removal[2]	396	96%	97%	97%
Survey of Patients' Hospital Experiences				
Area Around Room 'Always' Quiet at Night	300+	60%	65%	61%
Doctors 'Always' Communicated Well	300+	82%	85%	82%
Home Recovery Information Given	300+	90%	86%	85%
Hospital Given 9 or 10 on 10 Point Scale	300+	75%	76%	71%
Meds 'Always' Explained Before Given	300+	61%	66%	64%
Nurses 'Always' Communicated Well	300+	78%	81%	79%
Pain 'Always' Well Controlled	300+	70%	72%	71%
Room and Bathroom 'Always' Clean	300+	67%	76%	73%
Timely Help 'Always' Received	300+	67%	72%	68%
Would Definitely Recommend Hospital	300+	78%	75%	71%
Use of Medical Imaging				
Cardiac Imaging Stress Test before Surgery	444	5.6%	5%	5.3%
Combination Abdominal CT Scan	661	2.6%	19%	10.5%
Combination Brain/Sinus CT Scan	605	4.3%	2.9%	2.7%
Combination Chest CT Scan	653	0.2%	3.9%	2.7%
Follow-up Mammogram/Ultrasound	1,656	9.3%	7.8%	8.8%
Lumbar Spine MRI for Low Back Pain	246	42.3%	40.2%	37.2%

Community Hospital - Onaga & Saint Marys Campus

120 West 8th Street
Onaga, KS 66521
URL: www.chcs-ks.org
Type: Critical Access Hospitals
Ownership: Voluntary non-profit - Private

Phone: 785-889-4272
Fax: 785-889-7163
Emergency Services: Yes
Beds: 30

Key Personnel:
Pediatric Ambulatory Care . . . . . . Elaine Becker
Pediatric In-Patient Care . . . . Elaine Becker
Emergency Room . . . . Mary Matzke
Patient Relations . . . . Melinda May, RN
CEO/President. . . . . Greg Unruh
Infection Control. . . . . Cathy VanDonge
Quality Assurance . . . . Pam Wilkie
Chief of Medical Staff. . . . . Nancy J Zidek

Measure	Cases	This Hosp.	State Avg.	U.S. Avg.
Blood Clot Prevention and Treatment				
Anticoagulation Overlap Therapy[1,2]	-	-	94%	93%
ICU Venous Thromboembolism Prophylaxis[2,7]	-	-	91%	92%
Incidence of Potentially Preventable VTE[1,2]	-	-	8%	10%
UFH with Dosages/Platelet Monitoring[2,7]	-	-	98%	97%
Venous Thromboembolism Prophylaxis[2]	186	74%	79%	85%
Warfarin Therapy Discharge Instructions[2,7]	-	-	84%	75%
Chest Pain/Possible Heart Attack Care				
Aspirin Given Within 24 Hours of Arrival[1,3]	-	-	94%	96%
Fibrinolytic Meds Within 30 Min. of Arrival[3,7]	-	-	41%	58%
Average Time to ECG (minutes)[1,3]	-	-	8	7
Average Time to Transfer (minutes)[1,3]	-	-	57	60
Children's Asthma Care				
Received Home Management Plan of Care	-	-	-	88%
Received Reliever Medication	-	-	-	100%
Received Systemic Corticosteroids	-	-	-	100%
Emergency Department				
Admittance Decision Time (minutes)[2]	113	0	57	98
Head CT Results Within 45 Min. of Arrival[1,3]	-	-	53%	57%
Patients Who Left ER Before Being Seen[5]	-	-	2%	2%
Time from ER Arrival to Admit. (minutes)[2]	138	100	185	274
Time from ER Arrival to Discharge (minutes)	353	85	104	134
Time in ER Before Being Evaluated (minutes)	416	13	18	26
Time to Pain Meds for Fractures (minutes)[5]	-	-	47	57
Heart Attack Care				
Aspirin Given at Discharge[5]	-	-	99%	99%
Fibrinolytic Meds Within 30 Min. of Arrival[5]	-	-	-	54%
PCI Within 90 Minutes of Arrival[5]	-	-	97%	96%
Statin Prescribed at Discharge[5]	-	-	99%	98%
Heart Failure Care				
ACE Inhibitor or ARB for LVSD[1]	-	-	95%	97%
Discharge Instructions Given[1]	-	-	91%	94%
Evaluation of LVS Function	20	100%	94%	99%
Medicare Spending				
Medicare Spending per Patient (ratio)	-	-	0.94	0.98
Pneumonia Care				
Appropriate Initial Antibiotic Given	20	70%	92%	95%
Blood Culture Timing[1]	-	-	98%	98%
Pregnancy and Delivery Care				
Newborn Deliveries Scheduled Early[5]	-	-	12%	6%
Preventive Care				
Immunization for Influenza	217	82%	88%	90%
Immunization for Pneumonia	289	90%	90%	92%
Stroke Care				
Anticoagulation Therapy for Atrial Fibrillation[1,3]	-	-	88%	95%
Antithrombotic Therapy Timing[1,3]	-	-	97%	98%
Assessed for Rehabilitation[1,3]	-	-	97%	97%
Discharged on Antithrombotic Therapy[1,3]	-	-	98%	99%
Discharged on Statin Medication[1,3]	-	-	88%	94%
Thrombolytic Therapy Timing[1,3]	-	-	68%	66%
Venous Thromboembolism Prophylaxis[1,3]	-	-	93%	94%
Written Stroke Educational Materials Given[1,3]	-	-	84%	88%
Surgical Care Improvement Project				
Appropriate Beta Blocker Usage[5]	-	-	98%	98%
Appropriate VTP Within 24 Hours[5]	-	-	98%	98%
Controlled Postoperative Blood Glucose[5]	-	-	98%	97%
Perioperative Temperature Management[5]	-	-	100%	100%
Prophylactic Antibiotic Selection[5]	-	-	99%	99%
Prophylactic Antibiotic Selection (Outpatient)[5]	-	-	98%	98%
Prophylactic Antibiotic Stopped[5]	-	-	98%	98%
Prophylactic Antibiotic Timing[5]	-	-	99%	99%
Prophylactic Antibiotic Timing (Outpatient)[5]	-	-	98%	98%
Urinary Catheter Removal[5]	-	-	97%	97%
Survey of Patients' Hospital Experiences				
Area Around Room 'Always' Quiet at Night[6]	<100	59%	65%	61%
Doctors 'Always' Communicated Well[6]	<100	90%	85%	82%
Home Recovery Information Given[6]	<100	85%	86%	85%
Hospital Given 9 or 10 on 10 Point Scale[6]	<100	72%	76%	71%
Meds 'Always' Explained Before Given[6]	<100	65%	66%	64%
Nurses 'Always' Communicated Well[6]	<100	85%	81%	79%
Pain 'Always' Well Controlled[6]	<100	77%	72%	71%
Room and Bathroom 'Always' Clean[6]	<100	79%	76%	73%
Timely Help 'Always' Received[6]	<100	73%	72%	68%
Would Definitely Recommend Hospital[6]	<100	77%	75%	71%
Use of Medical Imaging				
Cardiac Imaging Stress Test before Surgery	57	5.3%	5%	5.3%
Combination Abdominal CT Scan	131	4.6%	19%	10.5%
Combination Brain/Sinus CT Scan[1]	-	-	2.9%	2.7%
Combination Chest CT Scan	80	5.0%	3.9%	2.7%
Follow-up Mammogram/Ultrasound	164	11.6%	7.8%	8.8%
Lumbar Spine MRI for Low Back Pain[1]	-	-	40.2%	37.2%

Osborne County Memorial Hospital

424 W New Hampshire Street
Osborne, KS 67473
URL: www.ocmh.org
Type: Critical Access Hospitals
Ownership: Government - Local

Phone: 785-346-2121
Fax: 785-346-5498
Emergency Services: Yes
Beds: 25

Key Personnel:
Chief of Medical Staff . . . . Barbara Brown
CEO/President. . . . . Roger John

Measure	Cases	This Hosp.	State Avg.	U.S. Avg.
Blood Clot Prevention and Treatment				
Anticoagulation Overlap Therapy[5]	-	-	94%	93%
ICU Venous Thromboembolism Prophylaxis[5]	-	-	91%	92%
Incidence of Potentially Preventable VTE[5]	-	-	8%	10%
UFH with Dosages/Platelet Monitoring[5]	-	-	98%	97%
Venous Thromboembolism Prophylaxis[5]	-	-	79%	85%
Warfarin Therapy Discharge Instructions[5]	-	-	84%	75%
Chest Pain/Possible Heart Attack Care				
Aspirin Given Within 24 Hours of Arrival	-	-	94%	96%
Fibrinolytic Meds Within 30 Min. of Arrival	-	-	41%	58%
Average Time to ECG (minutes)	-	-	8	7
Average Time to Transfer (minutes)	-	-	57	60
Children's Asthma Care				
Received Home Management Plan of Care	-	-	-	88%
Received Reliever Medication	-	-	-	100%
Received Systemic Corticosteroids	-	-	-	100%
Emergency Department				
Admittance Decision Time (minutes)[3]	20	5	57	98
Head CT Results Within 45 Min. of Arrival	-	-	53%	57%
Patients Who Left ER Before Being Seen	-	-	2%	2%
Time from ER Arrival to Admit. (minutes)[3]	29	104	185	274
Time from ER Arrival to Discharge (minutes)	-	-	104	134
Time in ER Before Being Evaluated (minutes)	-	-	18	26
Time to Pain Meds for Fractures (minutes)	-	-	47	57
Heart Attack Care				
Aspirin Given at Discharge[5]	-	-	99%	99%
Fibrinolytic Meds Within 30 Min. of Arrival[5]	-	-	-	54%
PCI Within 90 Minutes of Arrival[5]	-	-	97%	96%
Statin Prescribed at Discharge[5]	-	-	99%	98%
Heart Failure Care				
ACE Inhibitor or ARB for LVSD[3,7]	-	-	95%	97%
Discharge Instructions Given[1,3]	-	-	91%	94%
Evaluation of LVS Function[1,3]	-	-	94%	99%
Medicare Spending				
Medicare Spending per Patient (ratio)	-	-	0.94	0.98
Pneumonia Care				
Appropriate Initial Antibiotic Given[1,3]	-	-	92%	95%
Blood Culture Timing[3,7]	-	-	98%	98%
Pregnancy and Delivery Care				
Newborn Deliveries Scheduled Early[5]	-	-	12%	6%
Preventive Care				
Immunization for Influenza[3]	56	25%	88%	90%
Immunization for Pneumonia[3]	65	35%	90%	92%
Stroke Care				
Anticoagulation Therapy for Atrial Fibrillation[3,7]	-	-	88%	95%
Antithrombotic Therapy Timing[1,3]	-	-	97%	98%
Assessed for Rehabilitation[3,7]	-	-	97%	97%
Discharged on Antithrombotic Therapy[3,7]	-	-	98%	99%
Discharged on Statin Medication[3,7]	-	-	88%	94%
Thrombolytic Therapy Timing[3,7]	-	-	68%	66%
Venous Thromboembolism Prophylaxis[1,3]	-	-	93%	94%
Written Stroke Educational Materials Given[3,7]	-	-	84%	88%
Surgical Care Improvement Project				
Appropriate Beta Blocker Usage[5]	-	-	98%	98%
Appropriate VTP Within 24 Hours[5]	-	-	98%	98%
Controlled Postoperative Blood Glucose[5]	-	-	98%	97%
Perioperative Temperature Management[5]	-	-	100%	100%
Prophylactic Antibiotic Selection[5]	-	-	99%	99%
Prophylactic Antibiotic Selection (Outpatient)	-	-	98%	98%
Prophylactic Antibiotic Stopped[5]	-	-	98%	98%
Prophylactic Antibiotic Timing[5]	-	-	99%	99%
Prophylactic Antibiotic Timing (Outpatient)	-	-	98%	98%
Urinary Catheter Removal[5]	-	-	97%	97%
Survey of Patients' Hospital Experiences				
Area Around Room 'Always' Quiet at Night[5]	-	-	65%	61%
Doctors 'Always' Communicated Well[5]	-	-	85%	82%
Home Recovery Information Given[5]	-	-	86%	85%
Hospital Given 9 or 10 on 10 Point Scale[5]	-	-	76%	71%
Meds 'Always' Explained Before Given[5]	-	-	66%	64%
Nurses 'Always' Communicated Well[5]	-	-	81%	79%
Pain 'Always' Well Controlled[5]	-	-	72%	71%
Room and Bathroom 'Always' Clean[5]	-	-	76%	73%
Timely Help 'Always' Received[5]	-	-	72%	68%
Would Definitely Recommend Hospital[5]	-	-	75%	71%
Use of Medical Imaging				
Cardiac Imaging Stress Test before Surgery	-	-	5%	5.3%
Combination Abdominal CT Scan	-	-	19%	10.5%
Combination Brain/Sinus CT Scan	-	-	2.9%	2.7%
Combination Chest CT Scan	-	-	3.9%	2.7%
Follow-up Mammogram/Ultrasound	-	-	7.8%	8.8%
Lumbar Spine MRI for Low Back Pain	-	-	40.2%	37.2%

Oswego Community Hospital

800 Barker Drive
Oswego, KS 67356
Type: Critical Access Hospitals
Ownership: Proprietary

Phone: 620-795-2921
Fax: 620-795-3094
Emergency Services: Yes
Beds: 12

Key Personnel:
Chief of Medical Staff . . . . Stanley Haag, MD

NOTE: Hospital profiles are in alphabetical order by state, then city, then hospital within the city; Rankings exclude hospitals with less than 25 cases except for patient surveys which excludes hospitals with less than 100 cases; (a) 100-299 cases; (1) The number of cases/patients is too few to report; (2) Data submitted were based on a sample of cases/patients; (3) Results are based on a shorter time period than required; (4) Data suppressed by CMS for one or more quarters; (5) Results are not available for this reporting period; (6) Fewer than 100 patients completed the HCAHPS survey; (7) No cases met the criteria for this measure; (8) The lower limit of the confidence interval cannot be calculated if the number of observed infections equals zero; (9) No data are available from the state/territory for this reporting period; (10) The scores shown reflect fewer than 50 completed surveys; (11) There were discrepancies in the data collection process; (12) This measure does not apply to this hospital for this reporting period; (13) Results cannot be calculated for this reporting period; (14) The results for this state are combined with nearby states to protect confidentiality; Please refer to the User's Guide for a full explanation of data.

Measure	Cases	This Hosp.	State Avg.	U.S. Avg.
Blood Clot Prevention and Treatment				
Anticoagulation Overlap Therapy[5]	-	-	94%	93%
ICU Venous Thromboembolism Prophylaxis[5]	-	-	91%	92%
Incidence of Potentially Preventable VTE[5]	-	-	8%	10%
UFH with Dosages/Platelet Monitoring[5]	-	-	98%	97%
Venous Thromboembolism Prophylaxis[5]	-	-	79%	85%
Warfarin Therapy Discharge Instructions[5]	-	-	84%	75%
Chest Pain/Possible Heart Attack Care				
Aspirin Given Within 24 Hours of Arrival	-	-	94%	96%
Fibrinolytic Meds Within 30 Min. of Arrival	-	-	41%	58%
Average Time to ECG (minutes)	-	-	8	7
Average Time to Transfer (minutes)	-	-	57	60
Children's Asthma Care				
Received Home Management Plan of Care	-	-	-	88%
Received Reliever Medication	-	-	-	100%
Received Systemic Corticosteroids	-	-	-	100%
Emergency Department				
Admittance Decision Time (minutes)[1,3]	-	-	57	98
Head CT Results Within 45 Min. of Arrival	-	-	53%	57%
Patients Who Left ER Before Being Seen	-	-	2%	2%
Time from ER Arrival to Admit. (minutes)[1,3]	-	-	185	274
Time from ER Arrival to Discharge (minutes)	-	-	104	134
Time in ER Before Being Evaluated (minutes)	-	-	18	26
Time to Pain Meds for Fractures (minutes)	-	-	47	57
Heart Attack Care				
Aspirin Given at Discharge[5]	-	-	99%	99%
Fibrinolytic Meds Within 30 Min. of Arrival[5]	-	-	-	54%
PCI Within 90 Minutes of Arrival[5]	-	-	97%	96%
Statin Prescribed at Discharge[5]	-	-	99%	98%
Heart Failure Care				
ACE Inhibitor or ARB for LVSD[3,7]	-	-	95%	97%
Discharge Instructions Given[3,7]	-	-	91%	94%
Evaluation of LVS Function[1,3]	-	-	94%	99%
Medicare Spending				
Medicare Spending per Patient (ratio)	-	-	0.94	0.98
Pneumonia Care				
Appropriate Initial Antibiotic Given[1,3]	-	-	92%	95%
Blood Culture Timing[3,7]	-	-	98%	98%
Pregnancy and Delivery Care				
Newborn Deliveries Scheduled Early[5]	-	-	12%	6%
Preventive Care				
Immunization for Influenza[5]	-	-	88%	90%
Immunization for Pneumonia[1,3]	-	-	90%	92%
Stroke Care				
Anticoagulation Therapy for Atrial Fibrillation[5]	-	-	88%	95%
Antithrombotic Therapy Timing[5]	-	-	97%	98%
Assessed for Rehabilitation[5]	-	-	97%	97%
Discharged on Antithrombotic Therapy[5]	-	-	98%	99%
Discharged on Statin Medication[5]	-	-	88%	94%
Thrombolytic Therapy Timing[5]	-	-	68%	66%
Venous Thromboembolism Prophylaxis[5]	-	-	93%	94%
Written Stroke Educational Materials Given[5]	-	-	84%	88%
Surgical Care Improvement Project				
Appropriate Beta Blocker Usage[5]	-	-	98%	98%
Appropriate VTP Within 24 Hours[5]	-	-	98%	98%
Controlled Postoperative Blood Glucose[5]	-	-	98%	97%
Perioperative Temperature Management[5]	-	-	100%	100%
Prophylactic Antibiotic Selection[5]	-	-	99%	99%
Prophylactic Antibiotic Selection (Outpatient)	-	-	98%	98%
Prophylactic Antibiotic Stopped[5]	-	-	98%	98%
Prophylactic Antibiotic Timing[5]	-	-	99%	99%
Prophylactic Antibiotic Timing (Outpatient)	-	-	98%	98%
Urinary Catheter Removal[5]	-	-	97%	97%
Survey of Patients' Hospital Experiences				
Area Around Room 'Always' Quiet at Night[5]	-	-	65%	61%
Doctors 'Always' Communicated Well[5]	-	-	85%	82%
Home Recovery Information Given[5]	-	-	86%	85%
Hospital Given 9 or 10 on 10 Point Scale[5]	-	-	76%	71%
Meds 'Always' Explained Before Given[5]	-	-	66%	64%
Nurses 'Always' Communicated Well[5]	-	-	81%	79%
Pain 'Always' Well Controlled[5]	-	-	72%	71%
Room and Bathroom 'Always' Clean[5]	-	-	76%	73%
Timely Help 'Always' Received[5]	-	-	72%	68%
Would Definitely Recommend Hospital[5]	-	-	75%	71%
Use of Medical Imaging				
Cardiac Imaging Stress Test before Surgery	-	-	5%	5.3%
Combination Abdominal CT Scan	-	-	19%	10.5%
Combination Brain/Sinus CT Scan	-	-	2.9%	2.7%
Combination Chest CT Scan	-	-	3.9%	2.7%
Follow-up Mammogram/Ultrasound	-	-	7.8%	8.8%
Lumbar Spine MRI for Low Back Pain	-	-	40.2%	37.2%

Ransom Memorial Hospital

1301 S Main Street
Ottawa, KS 66067
URL: www.ransom.org
Type: Acute Care Hospitals
Ownership: Government - Local
Phone: 785-229-8308
Fax: 785-242-8339
Emergency Services: Yes
Beds: 55

Key Personnel:
Operating Room. . . . . Rick Coffman
CEO/President. . . . . Larry Felix
Radiology. . . . . Kelly Z. Hart, MD
Surgery . . . . Rodney T. McCalla, MD
Emergency Room . . . . Thomas S. Mitchell, MD
Infection Control. . . . . Linda Reed
Patient Relations . . . . Susan Ward
Quality Assurance . . . . Susan Ward

Measure	Cases	This Hosp.	State Avg.	U.S. Avg.
Blood Clot Prevention and Treatment				
Anticoagulation Overlap Therapy[1,2]	-	-	94%	93%
ICU Venous Thromboembolism Prophylaxis[2]	25	96%	91%	92%
Incidence of Potentially Preventable VTE[1,2]	-	-	8%	10%
UFH with Dosages/Platelet Monitoring[2,7]	-	-	98%	97%
Venous Thromboembolism Prophylaxis[2]	117	97%	79%	85%
Warfarin Therapy Discharge Instructions[1,2]	-	-	84%	75%
Chest Pain/Possible Heart Attack Care				
Aspirin Given Within 24 Hours of Arrival	28	100%	94%	96%
Fibrinolytic Meds Within 30 Min. of Arrival[7]	-	-	41%	58%
Average Time to ECG (minutes)	31	7	8	7
Average Time to Transfer (minutes)[1]	-	-	57	60
Children's Asthma Care				
Received Home Management Plan of Care	-	-	-	88%
Received Reliever Medication	-	-	-	100%
Received Systemic Corticosteroids	-	-	-	100%
Emergency Department				
Admittance Decision Time (minutes)[2]	238	45	57	98
Head CT Results Within 45 Min. of Arrival[1]	-	-	53%	57%
Patients Who Left ER Before Being Seen	10,772	2%	2%	2%
Time from ER Arrival to Admit. (minutes)[2]	249	184	185	274
Time from ER Arrival to Discharge (minutes)	420	104	104	134
Time in ER Before Being Evaluated (minutes)	453	21	18	26
Time to Pain Meds for Fractures (minutes)	39	49	47	57
Heart Attack Care				
Aspirin Given at Discharge[3,7]	-	-	99%	99%
Fibrinolytic Meds Within 30 Min. of Arrival[3,7]	-	-	-	54%
PCI Within 90 Minutes of Arrival[3,7]	-	-	97%	96%
Statin Prescribed at Discharge[3,7]	-	-	99%	98%
Heart Failure Care				
ACE Inhibitor or ARB for LVSD[1]	-	-	95%	97%
Discharge Instructions Given	16	75%	91%	94%
Evaluation of LVS Function	29	97%	94%	99%
Medicare Spending				
Medicare Spending per Patient (ratio)	-	0.91	0.94	0.98
Pneumonia Care				
Appropriate Initial Antibiotic Given	46	100%	92%	95%
Blood Culture Timing	69	90%	98%	98%
Pregnancy and Delivery Care				
Newborn Deliveries Scheduled Early[2]	15	7%	12%	6%
Preventive Care				
Immunization for Influenza[2]	297	99%	88%	90%
Immunization for Pneumonia[2]	384	97%	90%	92%
Stroke Care				
Anticoagulation Therapy for Atrial Fibrillation[3,7]	-	-	88%	95%
Antithrombotic Therapy Timing[1,3]	-	-	97%	98%
Assessed for Rehabilitation[1,3]	-	-	97%	97%
Discharged on Antithrombotic Therapy[1,3]	-	-	98%	99%
Discharged on Statin Medication[1,3]	-	-	88%	94%
Thrombolytic Therapy Timing[3,7]	-	-	68%	66%
Venous Thromboembolism Prophylaxis[1,3]	-	-	93%	94%
Written Stroke Educational Materials Given[1,3]	-	-	84%	88%
Surgical Care Improvement Project				
Appropriate Beta Blocker Usage	23	96%	98%	98%
Appropriate VTP Within 24 Hours	87	95%	98%	98%
Controlled Postoperative Blood Glucose[7]	-	-	98%	97%
Perioperative Temperature Management	103	100%	100%	100%
Prophylactic Antibiotic Selection	75	96%	99%	99%
Prophylactic Antibiotic Selection (Outpatient)	60	88%	98%	98%
Prophylactic Antibiotic Stopped	74	99%	98%	98%
Prophylactic Antibiotic Timing	75	97%	99%	99%
Prophylactic Antibiotic Timing (Outpatient)	44	91%	98%	98%
Urinary Catheter Removal	62	97%	97%	97%
Survey of Patients' Hospital Experiences				
Area Around Room 'Always' Quiet at Night	300+	65%	65%	61%
Doctors 'Always' Communicated Well	300+	86%	85%	82%
Home Recovery Information Given	300+	86%	86%	85%
Hospital Given 9 or 10 on 10 Point Scale	300+	72%	76%	71%
Meds 'Always' Explained Before Given	300+	67%	66%	64%
Nurses 'Always' Communicated Well	300+	79%	81%	79%
Pain 'Always' Well Controlled	300+	68%	72%	71%
Room and Bathroom 'Always' Clean	300+	75%	76%	73%
Timely Help 'Always' Received	300+	70%	72%	68%
Would Definitely Recommend Hospital	300+	73%	75%	71%
Use of Medical Imaging				
Cardiac Imaging Stress Test before Surgery	124	5.6%	5%	5.3%
Combination Abdominal CT Scan	253	3.2%	19%	10.5%
Combination Brain/Sinus CT Scan[1]	-	-	2.9%	2.7%
Combination Chest CT Scan	180	0.0%	3.9%	2.7%
Follow-up Mammogram/Ultrasound	529	6.6%	7.8%	8.8%
Lumbar Spine MRI for Low Back Pain	57	29.8%	40.2%	37.2%

Children's Mercy South

5808 W 110th Street
Overland Park, KS 66211
Type: Childrens
Ownership: Voluntary non-profit - Private
Phone: 913-234-3000
Emergency Services: No

Measure	Cases	This Hosp.	State Avg.	U.S. Avg.
Blood Clot Prevention and Treatment				
Anticoagulation Overlap Therapy[5]	-	-	94%	93%
ICU Venous Thromboembolism Prophylaxis[5]	-	-	91%	92%
Incidence of Potentially Preventable VTE[5]	-	-	8%	10%
UFH with Dosages/Platelet Monitoring[5]	-	-	98%	97%
Venous Thromboembolism Prophylaxis[5]	-	-	79%	85%
Warfarin Therapy Discharge Instructions[5]	-	-	84%	75%
Chest Pain/Possible Heart Attack Care				
Aspirin Given Within 24 Hours of Arrival	-	-	94%	96%
Fibrinolytic Meds Within 30 Min. of Arrival	-	-	41%	58%
Average Time to ECG (minutes)	-	-	8	7
Average Time to Transfer (minutes)	-	-	57	60
Children's Asthma Care				
Received Home Management Plan of Care[2]	231	90%	-	88%
Received Reliever Medication[2]	236	100%	-	100%
Received Systemic Corticosteroids[2]	232	100%	-	100%
Emergency Department				
Admittance Decision Time (minutes)[5]	-	-	57	98
Head CT Results Within 45 Min. of Arrival	-	-	53%	57%
Patients Who Left ER Before Being Seen	-	-	2%	2%
Time from ER Arrival to Admit. (minutes)[5]	-	-	185	274
Time from ER Arrival to Discharge (minutes)	-	-	104	134
Time in ER Before Being Evaluated (minutes)	-	-	18	26
Time to Pain Meds for Fractures (minutes)	-	-	47	57
Heart Attack Care				
Aspirin Given at Discharge[5]	-	-	99%	99%
Fibrinolytic Meds Within 30 Min. of Arrival[5]	-	-	-	54%
PCI Within 90 Minutes of Arrival[5]	-	-	97%	96%
Statin Prescribed at Discharge[5]	-	-	99%	98%
Heart Failure Care				
ACE Inhibitor or ARB for LVSD[5]	-	-	95%	97%

NOTE: Hospital profiles are in alphabetical order by state, then city, then hospital within the city; Rankings exclude hospitals with less than 25 cases except for patient surveys which excludes hospitals with less than 100 cases; (a) 100-299 cases; (1) The number of cases/patients is too few to report; (2) Data submitted were based on a sample of cases/patients; (3) Results are based on a shorter time period than required; (4) Data suppressed by CMS for one or more quarters; (5) Results are not available for this reporting period; (6) Fewer than 100 patients completed the HCAHPS survey; (7) No cases met the criteria for this measure; (8) The lower limit of the confidence interval cannot be calculated if the number of observed infections equals zero; (9) No data are available from the state/territory for this reporting period; (10) The scores shown reflect fewer than 50 completed surveys; (11) There were discrepancies in the data collection process; (12) This measure does not apply to this hospital for this reporting period; (13) Results cannot be calculated for this reporting period; (14) The results for this state are combined with nearby states to protect confidentiality; Please refer to the User's Guide for a full explanation of data.

Measure	Cases	This Hosp.	State Avg.	U.S. Avg.
Discharge Instructions Given[5]	-	-	91%	94%
Evaluation of LVS Function[5]	-	-	94%	99%
Medicare Spending				
Medicare Spending per Patient (ratio)	-	-	0.94	0.98
Pneumonia Care				
Appropriate Initial Antibiotic Given[5]	-	-	92%	95%
Blood Culture Timing[5]	-	-	98%	98%
Pregnancy and Delivery Care				
Newborn Deliveries Scheduled Early[5]	-	-	12%	6%
Preventive Care				
Immunization for Influenza[5]	-	-	88%	90%
Immunization for Pneumonia[5]	-	-	90%	92%
Stroke Care				
Anticoagulation Therapy for Atrial Fibrillation[5]	-	-	88%	95%
Antithrombotic Therapy Timing[5]	-	-	97%	98%
Assessed for Rehabilitation[5]	-	-	97%	97%
Discharged on Antithrombotic Therapy[5]	-	-	98%	99%
Discharged on Statin Medication[5]	-	-	88%	94%
Thrombolytic Therapy Timing[5]	-	-	68%	66%
Venous Thromboembolism Prophylaxis[5]	-	-	93%	94%
Written Stroke Educational Materials Given[5]	-	-	84%	88%
Surgical Care Improvement Project				
Appropriate Beta Blocker Usage[5]	-	-	98%	98%
Appropriate VTP Within 24 Hours[5]	-	-	98%	98%
Controlled Postoperative Blood Glucose[5]	-	-	98%	97%
Perioperative Temperature Management[5]	-	-	100%	100%
Prophylactic Antibiotic Selection[5]	-	-	99%	99%
Prophylactic Antibiotic Selection (Outpatient)	-	-	98%	98%
Prophylactic Antibiotic Stopped[5]	-	-	98%	98%
Prophylactic Antibiotic Timing[5]	-	-	99%	99%
Prophylactic Antibiotic Timing (Outpatient)	-	-	98%	98%
Urinary Catheter Removal[5]	-	-	97%	97%
Survey of Patients' Hospital Experiences				
Area Around Room 'Always' Quiet at Night[5]	-	-	65%	61%
Doctors 'Always' Communicated Well[5]	-	-	85%	82%
Home Recovery Information Given[5]	-	-	86%	85%
Hospital Given 9 or 10 on 10 Point Scale[5]	-	-	76%	71%
Meds 'Always' Explained Before Given[5]	-	-	66%	64%
Nurses 'Always' Communicated Well[5]	-	-	81%	79%
Pain 'Always' Well Controlled[5]	-	-	72%	71%
Room and Bathroom 'Always' Clean[5]	-	-	76%	73%
Timely Help 'Always' Received[5]	-	-	72%	68%
Would Definitely Recommend Hospital[5]	-	-	75%	71%
Use of Medical Imaging				
Cardiac Imaging Stress Test before Surgery	-	-	5%	5.3%
Combination Abdominal CT Scan	-	-	19%	10.5%
Combination Brain/Sinus CT Scan	-	-	2.9%	2.7%
Combination Chest CT Scan	-	-	3.9%	2.7%
Follow-up Mammogram/Ultrasound	-	-	7.8%	8.8%
Lumbar Spine MRI for Low Back Pain	-	-	40.2%	37.2%

Menorah Medical Center

5721 West 119th Street
Overland Park, KS 66209
Phone: 913-498-6773
Fax: 913-498-7106
URL: www.menorahmedicalcenter.com
Type: Acute Care Hospitals
Emergency Services: Yes
Ownership: Voluntary non-profit - Other
Beds: 158
Key Personnel:
CEO/President. . . . . Steven Wilkinson

Measure	Cases	This Hosp.	State Avg.	U.S. Avg.
Blood Clot Prevention and Treatment				
Anticoagulation Overlap Therapy[2]	35	97%	94%	93%
ICU Venous Thromboembolism Prophylaxis[2]	80	100%	91%	92%
Incidence of Potentially Preventable VTE[2]	21	0%	8%	10%
UFH with Dosages/Platelet Monitoring[2]	23	100%	98%	97%
Venous Thromboembolism Prophylaxis[2]	302	99%	79%	85%
Warfarin Therapy Discharge Instructions[2]	16	100%	84%	75%
Chest Pain/Possible Heart Attack Care				
Aspirin Given Within 24 Hours of Arrival[5]	-	-	94%	96%
Fibrinolytic Meds Within 30 Min. of Arrival[5]	-	-	41%	58%
Average Time to ECG (minutes)[5]	-	-	8	7
Average Time to Transfer (minutes)[5]	-	-	57	60
Children's Asthma Care				
Received Home Management Plan of Care	-	-	-	88%
Received Reliever Medication	-	-	-	100%
Received Systemic Corticosteroids	-	-	-	100%
Emergency Department				
Admittance Decision Time (minutes)[2]	345	55	57	98
Head CT Results Within 45 Min. of Arrival[1]	-	-	53%	57%
Patients Who Left ER Before Being Seen	14,527	1%	2%	2%
Time from ER Arrival to Admit. (minutes)[2]	345	198	185	274
Time from ER Arrival to Discharge (minutes)	416	142	104	134
Time in ER Before Being Evaluated (minutes)	478	17	18	26
Time to Pain Meds for Fractures (minutes)	46	32	47	57
Heart Attack Care				
Aspirin Given at Discharge[2]	55	98%	99%	99%
Fibrinolytic Meds Within 30 Min. of Arrival[2,7]	-	-	-	54%
PCI Within 90 Minutes of Arrival[2]	11	100%	97%	96%
Statin Prescribed at Discharge[2]	51	100%	99%	98%
Heart Failure Care				
ACE Inhibitor or ARB for LVSD[2]	21	100%	95%	97%
Discharge Instructions Given[2]	85	99%	91%	94%
Evaluation of LVS Function[2]	137	100%	94%	99%
Medicare Spending				
Medicare Spending per Patient (ratio)	-	1.04	0.94	0.98
Pneumonia Care				
Appropriate Initial Antibiotic Given[2]	67	100%	92%	95%
Blood Culture Timing[2]	109	100%	98%	98%
Pregnancy and Delivery Care				
Newborn Deliveries Scheduled Early[2]	26	0%	12%	6%
Preventive Care				
Immunization for Influenza[2]	544	100%	88%	90%
Immunization for Pneumonia[2]	690	100%	90%	92%
Stroke Care				
Anticoagulation Therapy for Atrial Fibrillation[1,2]	-	-	88%	95%
Antithrombotic Therapy Timing[2]	37	100%	97%	98%
Assessed for Rehabilitation[2]	53	100%	97%	97%
Discharged on Antithrombotic Therapy[2]	45	100%	98%	99%
Discharged on Statin Medication[2]	34	100%	88%	94%
Thrombolytic Therapy Timing[1,2]	-	-	68%	66%
Venous Thromboembolism Prophylaxis[2]	48	100%	93%	94%
Written Stroke Educational Materials Given[2]	21	100%	84%	88%
Surgical Care Improvement Project				
Appropriate Beta Blocker Usage[2]	161	95%	98%	98%
Appropriate VTP Within 24 Hours[2]	405	99%	98%	98%
Controlled Postoperative Blood Glucose[2]	53	100%	98%	97%
Perioperative Temperature Management[2]	486	100%	100%	100%
Prophylactic Antibiotic Selection[2]	364	100%	99%	99%
Prophylactic Antibiotic Selection (Outpatient)	465	99%	98%	98%
Prophylactic Antibiotic Stopped[2]	354	99%	98%	98%
Prophylactic Antibiotic Timing[2]	363	100%	99%	99%
Prophylactic Antibiotic Timing (Outpatient)	466	99%	98%	98%
Urinary Catheter Removal[2]	181	100%	97%	97%
Survey of Patients' Hospital Experiences				
Area Around Room 'Always' Quiet at Night	300+	58%	65%	61%
Doctors 'Always' Communicated Well	300+	79%	85%	82%
Home Recovery Information Given	300+	88%	86%	85%
Hospital Given 9 or 10 on 10 Point Scale	300+	69%	76%	71%
Meds 'Always' Explained Before Given	300+	58%	66%	64%
Nurses 'Always' Communicated Well	300+	73%	81%	79%
Pain 'Always' Well Controlled	300+	68%	72%	71%
Room and Bathroom 'Always' Clean	300+	63%	76%	73%
Timely Help 'Always' Received	300+	59%	72%	68%
Would Definitely Recommend Hospital	300+	69%	75%	71%
Use of Medical Imaging				
Cardiac Imaging Stress Test before Surgery	448	4.9%	5%	5.3%
Combination Abdominal CT Scan	620	13.5%	19%	10.5%
Combination Brain/Sinus CT Scan	463	5.4%	2.9%	2.7%
Combination Chest CT Scan	569	0.9%	3.9%	2.7%
Follow-up Mammogram/Ultrasound	1,169	8.4%	7.8%	8.8%
Lumbar Spine MRI for Low Back Pain	132	34.8%	40.2%	37.2%

Overland Park Regional Medical Center

10500 Quivira Road
Overland Park, KS 66215
Phone: 913-541-5301
Fax: 913-541-5790
URL: www.oprmc.com
Type: Acute Care Hospitals
Emergency Services: Yes
Ownership: Proprietary
Beds: 236
Key Personnel:
Radiology. . . . . James R Bergh
CEO/President. . . . . Kevin J Hicks

Measure	Cases	This Hosp.	State Avg.	U.S. Avg.
Blood Clot Prevention and Treatment				
Anticoagulation Overlap Therapy[2]	63	100%	94%	93%
ICU Venous Thromboembolism Prophylaxis[2]	133	100%	91%	92%
Incidence of Potentially Preventable VTE[2]	17	0%	8%	10%
UFH with Dosages/Platelet Monitoring[2]	60	100%	98%	97%
Venous Thromboembolism Prophylaxis[2]	278	100%	79%	85%
Warfarin Therapy Discharge Instructions[2]	34	100%	84%	75%
Chest Pain/Possible Heart Attack Care				
Aspirin Given Within 24 Hours of Arrival[1,3]	-	-	94%	96%
Fibrinolytic Meds Within 30 Min. of Arrival[5]	-	-	41%	58%
Average Time to ECG (minutes)[1,3]	-	-	8	7
Average Time to Transfer (minutes)[5]	-	-	57	60
Children's Asthma Care				
Received Home Management Plan of Care	-	-	-	88%
Received Reliever Medication	-	-	-	100%
Received Systemic Corticosteroids	-	-	-	100%
Emergency Department				
Admittance Decision Time (minutes)[2]	603	65	57	98
Head CT Results Within 45 Min. of Arrival[1]	-	-	53%	57%
Patients Who Left ER Before Being Seen	22,696	2%	2%	2%
Time from ER Arrival to Admit. (minutes)[2]	604	172	185	274
Time from ER Arrival to Discharge (minutes)	480	136	104	134
Time in ER Before Being Evaluated (minutes)	507	11	18	26
Time to Pain Meds for Fractures (minutes)	109	38	47	57
Heart Attack Care				
Aspirin Given at Discharge	111	100%	99%	99%
Fibrinolytic Meds Within 30 Min. of Arrival[7]	-	-	-	54%
PCI Within 90 Minutes of Arrival	28	100%	97%	96%
Statin Prescribed at Discharge	112	100%	99%	98%
Heart Failure Care				
ACE Inhibitor or ARB for LVSD	48	100%	95%	97%
Discharge Instructions Given	131	97%	91%	94%
Evaluation of LVS Function	187	100%	94%	99%
Medicare Spending				
Medicare Spending per Patient (ratio)	-	1.04	0.94	0.98
Pneumonia Care				
Appropriate Initial Antibiotic Given	85	98%	92%	95%
Blood Culture Timing	136	99%	98%	98%
Pregnancy and Delivery Care				
Newborn Deliveries Scheduled Early[2]	42	0%	12%	6%
Preventive Care				
Immunization for Influenza[2]	478	100%	88%	90%
Immunization for Pneumonia[2]	472	99%	90%	92%
Stroke Care				
Anticoagulation Therapy for Atrial Fibrillation[1]	-	-	88%	95%
Antithrombotic Therapy Timing	55	100%	97%	98%
Assessed for Rehabilitation	66	100%	97%	97%
Discharged on Antithrombotic Therapy	58	100%	98%	99%
Discharged on Statin Medication	42	100%	88%	94%
Thrombolytic Therapy Timing[1]	-	-	68%	66%
Venous Thromboembolism Prophylaxis	73	100%	93%	94%
Written Stroke Educational Materials Given	32	97%	84%	88%
Surgical Care Improvement Project				
Appropriate Beta Blocker Usage[2]	147	100%	98%	98%
Appropriate VTP Within 24 Hours[2]	380	99%	98%	98%
Controlled Postoperative Blood Glucose[2]	45	96%	98%	97%
Perioperative Temperature Management[2]	453	100%	100%	100%
Prophylactic Antibiotic Selection[2]	355	100%	99%	99%
Prophylactic Antibiotic Selection (Outpatient)	550	100%	98%	98%
Prophylactic Antibiotic Stopped[2]	348	99%	98%	98%
Prophylactic Antibiotic Timing[2]	355	100%	99%	99%
Prophylactic Antibiotic Timing (Outpatient)	553	99%	98%	98%
Urinary Catheter Removal[2]	155	96%	97%	97%

NOTE: Hospital profiles are in alphabetical order by state, then city, then hospital within the city; Rankings exclude hospitals with less than 25 cases except for patient surveys which excludes hospitals with less than 100 cases; (a) 100-299 cases; (1) The number of cases/patients is too few to report; (2) Data submitted were based on a sample of cases/patients; (3) Results are based on a shorter time period than required; (4) Data suppressed by CMS for one or more quarters; (5) Results are not available for this reporting period; (6) Fewer than 100 patients completed the HCAHPS survey; (7) No cases met the criteria for this measure; (8) The lower limit of the confidence interval cannot be calculated if the number of observed infections equals zero; (9) No data are available from the state/territory for this reporting period; (10) The scores shown reflect fewer than 50 completed surveys; (11) There were discrepancies in the data collection process; (12) This measure does not apply to this hospital for this reporting period; (13) Results cannot be calculated for this reporting period; (14) The results for this state are combined with nearby states to protect confidentiality; Please refer to the User's Guide for a full explanation of data.

Measure	Cases	This Hosp.	State Avg.	U.S. Avg.
Survey of Patients' Hospital Experiences				
Area Around Room 'Always' Quiet at Night	300+	52%	65%	61%
Doctors 'Always' Communicated Well	300+	79%	85%	82%
Home Recovery Information Given	300+	87%	86%	85%
Hospital Given 9 or 10 on 10 Point Scale	300+	67%	76%	71%
Meds 'Always' Explained Before Given	300+	59%	66%	64%
Nurses 'Always' Communicated Well	300+	76%	81%	79%
Pain 'Always' Well Controlled	300+	70%	72%	71%
Room and Bathroom 'Always' Clean	300+	58%	76%	73%
Timely Help 'Always' Received	300+	58%	72%	68%
Would Definitely Recommend Hospital	300+	69%	75%	71%
Use of Medical Imaging				
Cardiac Imaging Stress Test before Surgery	273	4.8%	5%	5.3%
Combination Abdominal CT Scan	330	4.2%	19%	10.5%
Combination Brain/Sinus CT Scan	391	4.3%	2.9%	2.7%
Combination Chest CT Scan	266	0.8%	3.9%	2.7%
Follow-up Mammogram/Ultrasound	439	11.8%	7.8%	8.8%
Lumbar Spine MRI for Low Back Pain	50	48.0%	40.2%	37.2%

Saint Luke's South Hospital

12300 Metcalf Avenue
Overland Park, KS 66213
Phone: 913-317-7904
Fax: 913-317-7672
URL: www.saintlukeshealthsystem.org
Type: Acute Care Hospitals
Emergency Services: Yes
Ownership: Voluntary non-profit - Other
Beds: 89

Key Personnel:
Radiology. . . . . David Marcus
CEO/President. . . . . Julie Quirin

Measure	Cases	This Hosp.	State Avg.	U.S. Avg.
Blood Clot Prevention and Treatment				
Anticoagulation Overlap Therapy[2]	33	91%	94%	93%
ICU Venous Thromboembolism Prophylaxis[2]	48	65%	91%	92%
Incidence of Potentially Preventable VTE[1,2]	-	-	8%	10%
UFH with Dosages/Platelet Monitoring[2]	23	100%	98%	97%
Venous Thromboembolism Prophylaxis[2]	278	78%	79%	85%
Warfarin Therapy Discharge Instructions[2]	27	52%	84%	75%
Chest Pain/Possible Heart Attack Care				
Aspirin Given Within 24 Hours of Arrival[1,3]	-	-	94%	96%
Fibrinolytic Meds Within 30 Min. of Arrival[3,7]	-	-	41%	58%
Average Time to ECG (minutes)[1,3]	-	-	8	7
Average Time to Transfer (minutes)[3,7]	-	-	57	60
Children's Asthma Care				
Received Home Management Plan of Care	-	-	-	88%
Received Reliever Medication	-	-	-	100%
Received Systemic Corticosteroids	-	-	-	100%
Emergency Department				
Admittance Decision Time (minutes)[2]	452	74	57	98
Head CT Results Within 45 Min. of Arrival	21	71%	53%	57%
Patients Who Left ER Before Being Seen	15,999	2%	2%	2%
Time from ER Arrival to Admit. (minutes)[2]	455	226	185	274
Time from ER Arrival to Discharge (minutes)	369	140	104	134
Time in ER Before Being Evaluated (minutes)	130	28	18	26
Time to Pain Meds for Fractures (minutes)	50	60	47	57
Heart Attack Care				
Aspirin Given at Discharge	74	100%	99%	99%
Fibrinolytic Meds Within 30 Min. of Arrival[7]	-	-	-	54%
PCI Within 90 Minutes of Arrival	15	100%	97%	96%
Statin Prescribed at Discharge	71	99%	99%	98%
Heart Failure Care				
ACE Inhibitor or ARB for LVSD	26	100%	95%	97%
Discharge Instructions Given	105	93%	91%	94%
Evaluation of LVS Function	147	100%	94%	99%
Medicare Spending				
Medicare Spending per Patient (ratio)	-	0.99	0.94	0.98
Pneumonia Care				
Appropriate Initial Antibiotic Given	93	95%	92%	95%
Blood Culture Timing	109	99%	98%	98%
Pregnancy and Delivery Care				
Newborn Deliveries Scheduled Early[2]	31	6%	12%	6%
Preventive Care				
Immunization for Influenza[2]	497	87%	88%	90%
Immunization for Pneumonia[2]	563	94%	90%	92%
Stroke Care				
Anticoagulation Therapy for Atrial Fibrillation[1]	-	-	88%	95%
Antithrombotic Therapy Timing	27	100%	97%	98%
Assessed for Rehabilitation	39	92%	97%	97%
Discharged on Antithrombotic Therapy	39	97%	98%	99%
Discharged on Statin Medication	29	83%	88%	94%
Thrombolytic Therapy Timing[1]	-	-	68%	66%
Venous Thromboembolism Prophylaxis	28	96%	93%	94%
Written Stroke Educational Materials Given	22	77%	84%	88%
Surgical Care Improvement Project				
Appropriate Beta Blocker Usage	199	100%	98%	98%
Appropriate VTP Within 24 Hours	729	100%	98%	98%
Controlled Postoperative Blood Glucose[7]	-	-	98%	97%
Perioperative Temperature Management	789	100%	100%	100%
Prophylactic Antibiotic Selection	620	100%	99%	99%
Prophylactic Antibiotic Selection (Outpatient)	153	99%	98%	98%
Prophylactic Antibiotic Stopped	612	100%	98%	98%
Prophylactic Antibiotic Timing	620	100%	99%	99%
Prophylactic Antibiotic Timing (Outpatient)	153	99%	98%	98%
Urinary Catheter Removal	70	100%	97%	97%
Survey of Patients' Hospital Experiences				
Area Around Room 'Always' Quiet at Night	300+	60%	65%	61%
Doctors 'Always' Communicated Well	300+	78%	85%	82%
Home Recovery Information Given	300+	88%	86%	85%
Hospital Given 9 or 10 on 10 Point Scale	300+	74%	76%	71%
Meds 'Always' Explained Before Given	300+	60%	66%	64%
Nurses 'Always' Communicated Well	300+	74%	81%	79%
Pain 'Always' Well Controlled	300+	63%	72%	71%
Room and Bathroom 'Always' Clean	300+	65%	76%	73%
Timely Help 'Always' Received	300+	64%	72%	68%
Would Definitely Recommend Hospital	300+	79%	75%	71%
Use of Medical Imaging				
Cardiac Imaging Stress Test before Surgery	392	4.3%	5%	5.3%
Combination Abdominal CT Scan	518	8.9%	19%	10.5%
Combination Brain/Sinus CT Scan[1]	-	-	2.9%	2.7%
Combination Chest CT Scan	238	0.8%	3.9%	2.7%
Follow-up Mammogram/Ultrasound	874	6.5%	7.8%	8.8%
Lumbar Spine MRI for Low Back Pain	90	38.9%	40.2%	37.2%

Miami County Medical Center

2100 Baptiste Drive
Paola, KS 66071
Phone: 913-557-4385
Fax: 913-294-5919
URL: www.olathehealth.org
Type: Acute Care Hospitals
Emergency Services: Yes
Ownership: Govt - Hospital Dist/Auth
Beds: 39

Key Personnel:
Infection Control. . . . . Kathy Auten
Operating Room. . . . . Sharon Bell
Chief of Medical Staff . . . . Jack Campbell
CEO/President. . . . . Frank H Devocelle
Cardiology . . . . Basem Kayali, MD
Surgery . . . . Daniel R. Perry, MD
Emergency Room . . . . Daniel Ross, MD
Quality Assurance . . . . Jerry Wiesner

Measure	Cases	This Hosp.	State Avg.	U.S. Avg.
Blood Clot Prevention and Treatment				
Anticoagulation Overlap Therapy[1]	-	-	94%	93%
ICU Venous Thromboembolism Prophylaxis[7]	-	-	91%	92%
Incidence of Potentially Preventable VTE[7]	-	-	8%	10%
UFH with Dosages/Platelet Monitoring[7]	-	-	98%	97%
Venous Thromboembolism Prophylaxis	165	98%	79%	85%
Warfarin Therapy Discharge Instructions[1]	-	-	84%	75%
Chest Pain/Possible Heart Attack Care				
Aspirin Given Within 24 Hours of Arrival	26	96%	94%	96%
Fibrinolytic Meds Within 30 Min. of Arrival[7]	-	-	41%	58%
Average Time to ECG (minutes)	26	9	8	7
Average Time to Transfer (minutes)[1]	-	-	57	60
Children's Asthma Care				
Received Home Management Plan of Care	-	-	-	88%
Received Reliever Medication	-	-	-	100%
Received Systemic Corticosteroids	-	-	-	100%
Emergency Department				
Admittance Decision Time (minutes)	254	43	57	98
Head CT Results Within 45 Min. of Arrival[1]	-	-	53%	57%
Patients Who Left ER Before Being Seen	10,098	1%	2%	2%
Time from ER Arrival to Admit. (minutes)	260	194	185	274
Time from ER Arrival to Discharge (minutes)	373	95	104	134
Time in ER Before Being Evaluated (minutes)	404	17	18	26
Time to Pain Meds for Fractures (minutes)	48	48	47	57
Heart Attack Care				
Aspirin Given at Discharge[5]	-	-	99%	99%
Fibrinolytic Meds Within 30 Min. of Arrival[5]	-	-	-	54%
PCI Within 90 Minutes of Arrival[5]	-	-	97%	96%
Statin Prescribed at Discharge[5]	-	-	99%	98%
Heart Failure Care				
ACE Inhibitor or ARB for LVSD[1]	-	-	95%	97%
Discharge Instructions Given[1]	-	-	91%	94%
Evaluation of LVS Function	14	100%	94%	99%
Medicare Spending				
Medicare Spending per Patient (ratio)	-	0.94	0.94	0.98
Pneumonia Care				
Appropriate Initial Antibiotic Given	13	100%	92%	95%
Blood Culture Timing	20	95%	98%	98%
Pregnancy and Delivery Care				
Newborn Deliveries Scheduled Early[7]	-	-	12%	6%
Preventive Care				
Immunization for Influenza	201	98%	88%	90%
Immunization for Pneumonia	279	99%	90%	92%
Stroke Care				
Anticoagulation Therapy for Atrial Fibrillation[3,7]	-	-	88%	95%
Antithrombotic Therapy Timing[1,3]	-	-	97%	98%
Assessed for Rehabilitation[1,3]	-	-	97%	97%
Discharged on Antithrombotic Therapy[1,3]	-	-	98%	99%
Discharged on Statin Medication[1,3]	-	-	88%	94%
Thrombolytic Therapy Timing[3,7]	-	-	68%	66%
Venous Thromboembolism Prophylaxis[1,3]	-	-	93%	94%
Written Stroke Educational Materials Given[1,3]	-	-	84%	88%
Surgical Care Improvement Project				
Appropriate Beta Blocker Usage	15	100%	98%	98%
Appropriate VTP Within 24 Hours	50	100%	98%	98%
Controlled Postoperative Blood Glucose[7]	-	-	98%	97%
Perioperative Temperature Management	51	100%	100%	100%
Prophylactic Antibiotic Selection	43	100%	99%	99%
Prophylactic Antibiotic Selection (Outpatient)[1,3]	-	-	98%	98%
Prophylactic Antibiotic Stopped	40	100%	98%	98%
Prophylactic Antibiotic Timing	43	100%	99%	99%
Prophylactic Antibiotic Timing (Outpatient)[1,3]	-	-	98%	98%
Urinary Catheter Removal	29	100%	97%	97%
Survey of Patients' Hospital Experiences				
Area Around Room 'Always' Quiet at Night	(a)	82%	65%	61%
Doctors 'Always' Communicated Well	(a)	85%	85%	82%
Home Recovery Information Given	(a)	92%	86%	85%
Hospital Given 9 or 10 on 10 Point Scale	(a)	78%	76%	71%
Meds 'Always' Explained Before Given	(a)	83%	66%	64%
Nurses 'Always' Communicated Well	(a)	86%	81%	79%
Pain 'Always' Well Controlled	(a)	80%	72%	71%
Room and Bathroom 'Always' Clean	(a)	82%	76%	73%
Timely Help 'Always' Received	(a)	85%	72%	68%
Would Definitely Recommend Hospital	(a)	73%	75%	71%
Use of Medical Imaging				
Cardiac Imaging Stress Test before Surgery	93	2.2%	5%	5.3%
Combination Abdominal CT Scan	182	2.7%	19%	10.5%
Combination Brain/Sinus CT Scan[1]	-	-	2.9%	2.7%
Combination Chest CT Scan	80	2.5%	3.9%	2.7%
Follow-up Mammogram/Ultrasound	501	11.8%	7.8%	8.8%
Lumbar Spine MRI for Low Back Pain	50	46.0%	40.2%	37.2%

Labette Health

1902 South Us Hwy 59
Parsons, KS 67357
Phone: 620-421-4880
Fax: 620-421-5042
URL: www.lcmc.com
Type: Acute Care Hospitals
Emergency Services: Yes
Ownership: Government - Local
Beds: 109

Key Personnel:
Patient Relations . . . . Janet Ball
Radiology. . . . . Robert Gibbs
Infection Control. . . . . Carol Hale
Quality Assurance . . . . Debra Herrman
Intensive Care Unit. . . . . Kathy McKinney
Chief of Medical Staff . . . . Dr Rothstein

NOTE: Hospital profiles are in alphabetical order by state, then city, then hospital within the city; Rankings exclude hospitals with less than 25 cases except for patient surveys which excludes hospitals with less than 100 cases; (a) 100-299 cases; (1) The number of cases/patients is too few to report; (2) Data submitted were based on a sample of cases/patients; (3) Results are based on a shorter time period than required; (4) Data suppressed by CMS for one or more quarters; (5) Results are not available for this reporting period; (6) Fewer than 100 patients completed the HCAHPS survey; (7) No cases met the criteria for this measure; (8) The lower limit of the confidence interval cannot be calculated if the number of observed infections equals zero; (9) No data are available from the state/territory for this reporting period; (10) The scores shown reflect fewer than 50 completed surveys; (11) There were discrepancies in the data collection process; (12) This measure does not apply to this hospital for this reporting period; (13) Results cannot be calculated for this reporting period; (14) The results for this state are combined with nearby states to protect confidentiality; Please refer to the User's Guide for a full explanation of data.

President . . . . Vincent Schibi
Operating Room. . . . . JoDee Witty

Measure	Cases	This Hosp.	State Avg.	U.S. Avg.
Blood Clot Prevention and Treatment				
Anticoagulation Overlap Therapy[2]	11	100%	94%	93%
ICU Venous Thromboembolism Prophylaxis[2]	34	100%	91%	92%
Incidence of Potentially Preventable VTE[1,2]	-	-	8%	10%
UFH with Dosages/Platelet Monitoring[1,2]	-	-	98%	97%
Venous Thromboembolism Prophylaxis[2]	181	88%	79%	85%
Warfarin Therapy Discharge Instructions[2]	11	100%	84%	75%
Chest Pain/Possible Heart Attack Care				
Aspirin Given Within 24 Hours of Arrival	39	100%	94%	96%
Fibrinolytic Meds Within 30 Min. of Arrival[1]	-	-	41%	58%
Average Time to ECG (minutes)	40	6	8	7
Average Time to Transfer (minutes)[1]	-	-	57	60
Children's Asthma Care				
Received Home Management Plan of Care	-	-	-	88%
Received Reliever Medication	-	-	-	100%
Received Systemic Corticosteroids	-	-	-	100%
Emergency Department				
Admittance Decision Time (minutes)[2]	268	68	57	98
Head CT Results Within 45 Min. of Arrival[1]	-	-	53%	57%
Patients Who Left ER Before Being Seen	11,817	1%	2%	2%
Time from ER Arrival to Admit. (minutes)[2]	274	230	185	274
Time from ER Arrival to Discharge (minutes)	937	119	104	134
Time in ER Before Being Evaluated (minutes)	983	34	18	26
Time to Pain Meds for Fractures (minutes)	49	59	47	57
Heart Attack Care				
Aspirin Given at Discharge[1,3]	-	-	99%	99%
Fibrinolytic Meds Within 30 Min. of Arrival[3,7]	-	-	-	54%
PCI Within 90 Minutes of Arrival[3,7]	-	-	97%	96%
Statin Prescribed at Discharge[1,3]	-	-	99%	98%
Heart Failure Care				
ACE Inhibitor or ARB for LVSD	15	27%	95%	97%
Discharge Instructions Given	30	90%	91%	94%
Evaluation of LVS Function	45	100%	94%	99%
Medicare Spending				
Medicare Spending per Patient (ratio)	-	0.89	0.94	0.98
Pneumonia Care				
Appropriate Initial Antibiotic Given	30	93%	92%	95%
Blood Culture Timing	51	94%	98%	98%
Pregnancy and Delivery Care				
Newborn Deliveries Scheduled Early	25	4%	12%	6%
Preventive Care				
Immunization for Influenza[2]	297	87%	88%	90%
Immunization for Pneumonia[2]	357	88%	90%	92%
Stroke Care				
Anticoagulation Therapy for Atrial Fibrillation[1]	-	-	88%	95%
Antithrombotic Therapy Timing	24	92%	97%	98%
Assessed for Rehabilitation	21	90%	97%	97%
Discharged on Antithrombotic Therapy	21	90%	98%	99%
Discharged on Statin Medication	18	94%	88%	94%
Thrombolytic Therapy Timing[7]	-	-	68%	66%
Venous Thromboembolism Prophylaxis	22	77%	93%	94%
Written Stroke Educational Materials Given[1]	-	-	84%	88%
Surgical Care Improvement Project				
Appropriate Beta Blocker Usage	143	97%	98%	98%
Appropriate VTP Within 24 Hours	478	98%	98%	98%
Controlled Postoperative Blood Glucose[7]	-	-	98%	97%
Perioperative Temperature Management	518	100%	100%	100%
Prophylactic Antibiotic Selection	439	100%	99%	99%
Prophylactic Antibiotic Selection (Outpatient)	79	99%	98%	98%
Prophylactic Antibiotic Stopped	431	99%	98%	98%
Prophylactic Antibiotic Timing	439	100%	99%	99%
Prophylactic Antibiotic Timing (Outpatient)	80	99%	98%	98%
Urinary Catheter Removal	132	94%	97%	97%
Survey of Patients' Hospital Experiences				
Area Around Room 'Always' Quiet at Night	300+	60%	65%	61%
Doctors 'Always' Communicated Well	300+	86%	85%	82%
Home Recovery Information Given	300+	89%	86%	85%
Hospital Given 9 or 10 on 10 Point Scale	300+	72%	76%	71%
Meds 'Always' Explained Before Given	300+	62%	66%	64%
Nurses 'Always' Communicated Well	300+	79%	81%	79%
Pain 'Always' Well Controlled	300+	68%	72%	71%
Room and Bathroom 'Always' Clean	300+	75%	76%	73%
Timely Help 'Always' Received	300+	70%	72%	68%
Would Definitely Recommend Hospital	300+	70%	75%	71%
Use of Medical Imaging				
Cardiac Imaging Stress Test before Surgery	358	4.7%	5%	5.3%
Combination Abdominal CT Scan	400	75.8%	19%	10.5%
Combination Brain/Sinus CT Scan[1]	-	-	2.9%	2.7%
Combination Chest CT Scan	308	0.0%	3.9%	2.7%
Follow-up Mammogram/Ultrasound	535	4.9%	7.8%	8.8%
Lumbar Spine MRI for Low Back Pain	83	49.4%	40.2%	37.2%

Phillips County Hospital

1150 State Street
Phillipsburg, KS 67661
Type: Critical Access Hospitals
Ownership: Government - Local
Phone: 785-543-5226
Fax: 785-543-6272
Emergency Services: Yes
Beds: 62

Key Personnel:

Operating Room. . . . . Hazel Ames
Quality Assurance . . . . Hazel Ames
CEO/President. . . . . Heather Harper
Chairman/CEO . . . . Art Henrickson

Measure	Cases	This Hosp.	State Avg.	U.S. Avg.
Blood Clot Prevention and Treatment				
Anticoagulation Overlap Therapy[5]	-	-	94%	93%
ICU Venous Thromboembolism Prophylaxis[5]	-	-	91%	92%
Incidence of Potentially Preventable VTE[5]	-	-	8%	10%
UFH with Dosages/Platelet Monitoring[5]	-	-	98%	97%
Venous Thromboembolism Prophylaxis[5]	-	-	79%	85%
Warfarin Therapy Discharge Instructions[5]	-	-	84%	75%
Chest Pain/Possible Heart Attack Care				
Aspirin Given Within 24 Hours of Arrival	-	-	94%	96%
Fibrinolytic Meds Within 30 Min. of Arrival	-	-	41%	58%
Average Time to ECG (minutes)	-	-	8	7
Average Time to Transfer (minutes)	-	-	57	60
Children's Asthma Care				
Received Home Management Plan of Care	-	-	-	88%
Received Reliever Medication	-	-	-	100%
Received Systemic Corticosteroids	-	-	-	100%
Emergency Department				
Admittance Decision Time (minutes)[3]	12	30	57	98
Head CT Results Within 45 Min. of Arrival	-	-	53%	57%
Patients Who Left ER Before Being Seen	-	-	2%	2%
Time from ER Arrival to Admit. (minutes)[3]	12	188	185	274
Time from ER Arrival to Discharge (minutes)	-	-	104	134
Time in ER Before Being Evaluated (minutes)	-	-	18	26
Time to Pain Meds for Fractures (minutes)	-	-	47	57
Heart Attack Care				
Aspirin Given at Discharge[5]	-	-	99%	99%
Fibrinolytic Meds Within 30 Min. of Arrival[5]	-	-	-	54%
PCI Within 90 Minutes of Arrival[5]	-	-	97%	96%
Statin Prescribed at Discharge[5]	-	-	99%	98%
Heart Failure Care				
ACE Inhibitor or ARB for LVSD[3,7]	-	-	95%	97%
Discharge Instructions Given[3,7]	-	-	91%	94%
Evaluation of LVS Function[1,3]	-	-	94%	99%
Medicare Spending				
Medicare Spending per Patient (ratio)	-	-	0.94	0.98
Pneumonia Care				
Appropriate Initial Antibiotic Given[1]	-	-	92%	95%
Blood Culture Timing[1]	-	-	98%	98%
Pregnancy and Delivery Care				
Newborn Deliveries Scheduled Early[5]	-	-	12%	6%
Preventive Care				
Immunization for Influenza[5]	-	-	88%	90%
Immunization for Pneumonia[3]	18	50%	90%	92%
Stroke Care				
Anticoagulation Therapy for Atrial Fibrillation[5]	-	-	88%	95%
Antithrombotic Therapy Timing[5]	-	-	97%	98%
Assessed for Rehabilitation[5]	-	-	97%	97%
Discharged on Antithrombotic Therapy[5]	-	-	98%	99%
Discharged on Statin Medication[5]	-	-	88%	94%
Thrombolytic Therapy Timing[5]	-	-	68%	66%
Venous Thromboembolism Prophylaxis[5]	-	-	93%	94%
Written Stroke Educational Materials Given[5]	-	-	84%	88%
Surgical Care Improvement Project				
Appropriate Beta Blocker Usage[5]	-	-	98%	98%
Appropriate VTP Within 24 Hours[5]	-	-	98%	98%
Controlled Postoperative Blood Glucose[5]	-	-	98%	97%
Perioperative Temperature Management[5]	-	-	100%	100%
Prophylactic Antibiotic Selection[5]	-	-	99%	99%
Prophylactic Antibiotic Selection (Outpatient)	-	-	98%	98%
Prophylactic Antibiotic Stopped[5]	-	-	98%	98%
Prophylactic Antibiotic Timing[5]	-	-	99%	99%
Prophylactic Antibiotic Timing (Outpatient)	-	-	98%	98%
Urinary Catheter Removal[5]	-	-	97%	97%
Survey of Patients' Hospital Experiences				
Area Around Room 'Always' Quiet at Night[5]	-	-	65%	61%
Doctors 'Always' Communicated Well[5]	-	-	85%	82%
Home Recovery Information Given[5]	-	-	86%	85%
Hospital Given 9 or 10 on 10 Point Scale[5]	-	-	76%	71%
Meds 'Always' Explained Before Given[5]	-	-	66%	64%
Nurses 'Always' Communicated Well[5]	-	-	81%	79%
Pain 'Always' Well Controlled[5]	-	-	72%	71%
Room and Bathroom 'Always' Clean[5]	-	-	76%	73%
Timely Help 'Always' Received[5]	-	-	72%	68%
Would Definitely Recommend Hospital[5]	-	-	75%	71%
Use of Medical Imaging				
Cardiac Imaging Stress Test before Surgery	-	-	5%	5.3%
Combination Abdominal CT Scan	-	-	19%	10.5%
Combination Brain/Sinus CT Scan	-	-	2.9%	2.7%
Combination Chest CT Scan	-	-	3.9%	2.7%
Follow-up Mammogram/Ultrasound	-	-	7.8%	8.8%
Lumbar Spine MRI for Low Back Pain	-	-	40.2%	37.2%

Via Christi Hospital Pittsburg

1 Mt Carmel Way
Pittsburg, KS 66762
URL: www.via-christi.org
Type: Acute Care Hospitals
Ownership: Voluntary non-profit - Private
Phone: 620-231-6100
Emergency Services: Yes
Beds: 188

Measure	Cases	This Hosp.	State Avg.	U.S. Avg.
Blood Clot Prevention and Treatment				
Anticoagulation Overlap Therapy[2]	18	100%	94%	93%
ICU Venous Thromboembolism Prophylaxis[2]	67	100%	91%	92%
Incidence of Potentially Preventable VTE[1,2]	-	-	8%	10%
UFH with Dosages/Platelet Monitoring[2]	26	96%	98%	97%
Venous Thromboembolism Prophylaxis[2]	237	95%	79%	85%
Warfarin Therapy Discharge Instructions[2]	15	100%	84%	75%
Chest Pain/Possible Heart Attack Care				
Aspirin Given Within 24 Hours of Arrival	15	100%	94%	96%
Fibrinolytic Meds Within 30 Min. of Arrival[7]	-	-	41%	58%
Average Time to ECG (minutes)	17	7	8	7
Average Time to Transfer (minutes)[1]	-	-	57	60
Children's Asthma Care				
Received Home Management Plan of Care	-	-	-	88%
Received Reliever Medication	-	-	-	100%
Received Systemic Corticosteroids	-	-	-	100%
Emergency Department				
Admittance Decision Time (minutes)[2]	356	56	57	98
Head CT Results Within 45 Min. of Arrival[1]	-	-	53%	57%
Patients Who Left ER Before Being Seen	15,151	2%	2%	2%
Time from ER Arrival to Admit. (minutes)[2]	358	174	185	274
Time from ER Arrival to Discharge (minutes)	328	117	104	134
Time in ER Before Being Evaluated (minutes)	293	26	18	26
Time to Pain Meds for Fractures (minutes)	41	57	47	57
Heart Attack Care				
Aspirin Given at Discharge	73	99%	99%	99%
Fibrinolytic Meds Within 30 Min. of Arrival[7]	-	-	-	54%
PCI Within 90 Minutes of Arrival	14	100%	97%	96%
Statin Prescribed at Discharge	61	98%	99%	98%
Heart Failure Care				
ACE Inhibitor or ARB for LVSD	21	95%	95%	97%
Discharge Instructions Given	62	81%	91%	94%

NOTE: Hospital profiles are in alphabetical order by state, then city, then hospital within the city; Rankings exclude hospitals with less than 25 cases except for patient surveys which excludes hospitals with less than 100 cases; (a) 100-299 cases; (1) The number of cases/patients is too few to report; (2) Data submitted were based on a sample of cases/patients; (3) Results are based on a shorter time period than required; (4) Data suppressed by CMS for one or more quarters; (5) Results are not available for this reporting period; (6) Fewer than 100 patients completed the HCAHPS survey; (7) No cases met the criteria for this measure; (8) The lower limit of the confidence interval cannot be calculated if the number of observed infections equals zero; (9) No data are available from the state/territory for this reporting period; (10) The scores shown reflect fewer than 50 completed surveys; (11) There were discrepancies in the data collection process; (12) This measure does not apply to this hospital for this reporting period; (13) Results cannot be calculated for this reporting period; (14) The results for this state are combined with nearby states to protect confidentiality; Please refer to the User's Guide for a full explanation of data.

Measure	Cases	This Hosp.	State Avg.	U.S. Avg.
Evaluation of LVS Function	86	100%	94%	99%
Medicare Spending				
Medicare Spending per Patient (ratio)	-	0.93	0.94	0.98
Pneumonia Care				
Appropriate Initial Antibiotic Given	85	98%	92%	95%
Blood Culture Timing	142	99%	98%	98%
Pregnancy and Delivery Care				
Newborn Deliveries Scheduled Early	51	0%	12%	6%
Preventive Care				
Immunization for Influenza[2]	341	98%	88%	90%
Immunization for Pneumonia[2]	380	97%	90%	92%
Stroke Care				
Anticoagulation Therapy for Atrial Fibrillation[1]	-	-	88%	95%
Antithrombotic Therapy Timing	21	100%	97%	98%
Assessed for Rehabilitation	22	86%	97%	97%
Discharged on Antithrombotic Therapy	20	100%	98%	99%
Discharged on Statin Medication	16	94%	88%	94%
Thrombolytic Therapy Timing[1]	-	-	68%	66%
Venous Thromboembolism Prophylaxis	22	100%	93%	94%
Written Stroke Educational Materials Given[1]	-	-	84%	88%
Surgical Care Improvement Project				
Appropriate Beta Blocker Usage	77	99%	98%	98%
Appropriate VTP Within 24 Hours	203	96%	98%	98%
Controlled Postoperative Blood Glucose[7]	-	-	98%	97%
Perioperative Temperature Management	241	100%	100%	100%
Prophylactic Antibiotic Selection	160	96%	99%	99%
Prophylactic Antibiotic Selection (Outpatient)	124	98%	98%	98%
Prophylactic Antibiotic Stopped	152	98%	98%	98%
Prophylactic Antibiotic Timing	160	100%	99%	99%
Prophylactic Antibiotic Timing (Outpatient)	126	98%	98%	98%
Urinary Catheter Removal	98	96%	97%	97%
Survey of Patients' Hospital Experiences				
Area Around Room 'Always' Quiet at Night	300+	61%	65%	61%
Doctors 'Always' Communicated Well	300+	82%	85%	82%
Home Recovery Information Given	300+	86%	86%	85%
Hospital Given 9 or 10 on 10 Point Scale	300+	68%	76%	71%
Meds 'Always' Explained Before Given	300+	64%	66%	64%
Nurses 'Always' Communicated Well	300+	80%	81%	79%
Pain 'Always' Well Controlled	300+	71%	72%	71%
Room and Bathroom 'Always' Clean	300+	69%	76%	73%
Timely Help 'Always' Received	300+	64%	72%	68%
Would Definitely Recommend Hospital	300+	67%	75%	71%
Use of Medical Imaging				
Cardiac Imaging Stress Test before Surgery	458	3.9%	5%	5.3%
Combination Abdominal CT Scan	478	22.6%	19%	10.5%
Combination Brain/Sinus CT Scan	358	5.9%	2.9%	2.7%
Combination Chest CT Scan	259	16.6%	3.9%	2.7%
Follow-up Mammogram/Ultrasound	773	14.4%	7.8%	8.8%
Lumbar Spine MRI for Low Back Pain	71	38.0%	40.2%	37.2%

Pratt Regional Medical Center

200 Commodore St
Pratt, KS 67124
E-mail: spage@prmc.org
URL: www.prmc.org
Type: Acute Care Hospitals
Ownership: Voluntary non-profit - Private
Phone: 620-450-1160
Fax: 620-672-2113
Emergency Services: Yes
Beds: 84

Key Personnel:
Radiology. . . . . Connie Adelhardt
Chair/CEO . . . . J Wakon Fowler
Intensive Care Unit. . . . . Brandi Graf
Operating Room. . . . . Brandi Graf
Infection Control. . . . . Cecile Pearce, RN
Quality Assurance . . . . Marla Rose
Chairman/CEO . . . . Rich Sanders
Surgery . . . . Jason Wiltshire, MD

Measure	Cases	This Hosp.	State Avg.	U.S. Avg.
Blood Clot Prevention and Treatment				
Anticoagulation Overlap Therapy[2]	16	69%	94%	93%
ICU Venous Thromboembolism Prophylaxis[2]	25	72%	91%	92%
Incidence of Potentially Preventable VTE[1,2]	-	-	8%	10%
UFH with Dosages/Platelet Monitoring[1,2]	-	-	98%	97%
Venous Thromboembolism Prophylaxis[2]	52	54%	79%	85%
Warfarin Therapy Discharge Instructions[1,2]	-	-	84%	75%
Chest Pain/Possible Heart Attack Care				
Aspirin Given Within 24 Hours of Arrival[3]	18	94%	94%	96%
Fibrinolytic Meds Within 30 Min. of Arrival[3,7]	-	-	41%	58%
Average Time to ECG (minutes)[3]	18	9	8	7
Average Time to Transfer (minutes)[3,7]	-	-	57	60
Children's Asthma Care				
Received Home Management Plan of Care	-	-	-	88%
Received Reliever Medication	-	-	-	100%
Received Systemic Corticosteroids	-	-	-	100%
Emergency Department				
Admittance Decision Time (minutes)[2]	214	25	57	98
Head CT Results Within 45 Min. of Arrival[1,3]	-	-	53%	57%
Patients Who Left ER Before Being Seen	6,210	0%	2%	2%
Time from ER Arrival to Admit. (minutes)[2]	224	132	185	274
Time from ER Arrival to Discharge (minutes)	1,243	61	104	134
Time in ER Before Being Evaluated (minutes)	1,288	8	18	26
Time to Pain Meds for Fractures (minutes)	19	40	47	57
Heart Attack Care				
Aspirin Given at Discharge[5]	-	-	99%	99%
Fibrinolytic Meds Within 30 Min. of Arrival[5]	-	-	-	54%
PCI Within 90 Minutes of Arrival[5]	-	-	97%	96%
Statin Prescribed at Discharge[5]	-	-	99%	98%
Heart Failure Care				
ACE Inhibitor or ARB for LVSD[1,2]	-	-	95%	97%
Discharge Instructions Given[2,3]	14	79%	91%	94%
Evaluation of LVS Function[2,3]	20	70%	94%	99%
Medicare Spending				
Medicare Spending per Patient (ratio)	-	0.94	0.94	0.98
Pneumonia Care				
Appropriate Initial Antibiotic Given[2]	57	75%	92%	95%
Blood Culture Timing[2]	54	98%	98%	98%
Pregnancy and Delivery Care				
Newborn Deliveries Scheduled Early	23	39%	12%	6%
Preventive Care				
Immunization for Influenza[2]	295	87%	88%	90%
Immunization for Pneumonia[2]	361	88%	90%	92%
Stroke Care				
Anticoagulation Therapy for Atrial Fibrillation[1,3]	-	-	88%	95%
Antithrombotic Therapy Timing[1,3]	-	-	97%	98%
Assessed for Rehabilitation[1,3]	-	-	97%	97%
Discharged on Antithrombotic Therapy[1,3]	-	-	98%	99%
Discharged on Statin Medication[1,3]	-	-	88%	94%
Thrombolytic Therapy Timing[1,3]	-	-	68%	66%
Venous Thromboembolism Prophylaxis[1,3]	-	-	93%	94%
Written Stroke Educational Materials Given[1,3]	-	-	84%	88%
Surgical Care Improvement Project				
Appropriate Beta Blocker Usage[2]	58	98%	98%	98%
Appropriate VTP Within 24 Hours[2]	186	100%	98%	98%
Controlled Postoperative Blood Glucose[2,7]	-	-	98%	97%
Perioperative Temperature Management[2]	202	100%	100%	100%
Prophylactic Antibiotic Selection[2]	162	98%	99%	99%
Prophylactic Antibiotic Selection (Outpatient)	16	94%	98%	98%
Prophylactic Antibiotic Stopped[2]	159	98%	98%	98%
Prophylactic Antibiotic Timing[2]	162	99%	99%	99%
Prophylactic Antibiotic Timing (Outpatient)	16	94%	98%	98%
Urinary Catheter Removal[2]	177	99%	97%	97%
Survey of Patients' Hospital Experiences				
Area Around Room 'Always' Quiet at Night	300+	62%	65%	61%
Doctors 'Always' Communicated Well	300+	86%	85%	82%
Home Recovery Information Given	300+	89%	86%	85%
Hospital Given 9 or 10 on 10 Point Scale	300+	72%	76%	71%
Meds 'Always' Explained Before Given	300+	64%	66%	64%
Nurses 'Always' Communicated Well	300+	82%	81%	79%
Pain 'Always' Well Controlled	300+	72%	72%	71%
Room and Bathroom 'Always' Clean	300+	76%	76%	73%
Timely Help 'Always' Received	300+	74%	72%	68%
Would Definitely Recommend Hospital	300+	75%	75%	71%
Use of Medical Imaging				
Cardiac Imaging Stress Test before Surgery	188	4.8%	5%	5.3%
Combination Abdominal CT Scan	159	68.6%	19%	10.5%
Combination Brain/Sinus CT Scan[1]	-	-	2.9%	2.7%
Combination Chest CT Scan	150	27.3%	3.9%	2.7%
Follow-up Mammogram/Ultrasound	476	18.7%	7.8%	8.8%
Lumbar Spine MRI for Low Back Pain	95	41.1%	40.2%	37.2%

Gove County Medical Center

520 West 5th Street
Quinter, KS 67752
Type: Critical Access Hospitals
Ownership: Voluntary non-profit - Other
Phone: 785-754-3341
Fax: 785-754-3329
Emergency Services: No
Beds: 21

Key Personnel:
CEO/President. . . . . Paul Davis

Measure	Cases	This Hosp.	State Avg.	U.S. Avg.
Blood Clot Prevention and Treatment				
Anticoagulation Overlap Therapy[5]	-	-	94%	93%
ICU Venous Thromboembolism Prophylaxis[5]	-	-	91%	92%
Incidence of Potentially Preventable VTE[5]	-	-	8%	10%
UFH with Dosages/Platelet Monitoring[5]	-	-	98%	97%
Venous Thromboembolism Prophylaxis[5]	-	-	79%	85%
Warfarin Therapy Discharge Instructions[5]	-	-	84%	75%
Chest Pain/Possible Heart Attack Care				
Aspirin Given Within 24 Hours of Arrival	-	-	94%	96%
Fibrinolytic Meds Within 30 Min. of Arrival	-	-	41%	58%
Average Time to ECG (minutes)	-	-	8	7
Average Time to Transfer (minutes)	-	-	57	60
Children's Asthma Care				
Received Home Management Plan of Care	-	-	-	88%
Received Reliever Medication	-	-	-	100%
Received Systemic Corticosteroids	-	-	-	100%
Emergency Department				
Admittance Decision Time (minutes)[5]	-	-	57	98
Head CT Results Within 45 Min. of Arrival	-	-	53%	57%
Patients Who Left ER Before Being Seen	-	-	2%	2%
Time from ER Arrival to Admit. (minutes)[5]	-	-	185	274
Time from ER Arrival to Discharge (minutes)	-	-	104	134
Time in ER Before Being Evaluated (minutes)	-	-	18	26
Time to Pain Meds for Fractures (minutes)	-	-	47	57
Heart Attack Care				
Aspirin Given at Discharge[5]	-	-	99%	99%
Fibrinolytic Meds Within 30 Min. of Arrival[5]	-	-	-	54%
PCI Within 90 Minutes of Arrival[5]	-	-	97%	96%
Statin Prescribed at Discharge[5]	-	-	99%	98%
Heart Failure Care				
ACE Inhibitor or ARB for LVSD[3,7]	-	-	95%	97%
Discharge Instructions Given[1,3]	-	-	91%	94%
Evaluation of LVS Function[1,3]	-	-	94%	99%
Medicare Spending				
Medicare Spending per Patient (ratio)	-	-	0.94	0.98
Pneumonia Care				
Appropriate Initial Antibiotic Given[1,3]	-	-	92%	95%
Blood Culture Timing[1,3]	-	-	98%	98%
Pregnancy and Delivery Care				
Newborn Deliveries Scheduled Early[5]	-	-	12%	6%
Preventive Care				
Immunization for Influenza[5]	-	-	88%	90%
Immunization for Pneumonia[5]	-	-	90%	92%
Stroke Care				
Anticoagulation Therapy for Atrial Fibrillation[5]	-	-	88%	95%
Antithrombotic Therapy Timing[5]	-	-	97%	98%
Assessed for Rehabilitation[5]	-	-	97%	97%
Discharged on Antithrombotic Therapy[5]	-	-	98%	99%
Discharged on Statin Medication[5]	-	-	88%	94%
Thrombolytic Therapy Timing[5]	-	-	68%	66%
Venous Thromboembolism Prophylaxis[5]	-	-	93%	94%
Written Stroke Educational Materials Given[5]	-	-	84%	88%
Surgical Care Improvement Project				
Appropriate Beta Blocker Usage[5]	-	-	98%	98%
Appropriate VTP Within 24 Hours[5]	-	-	98%	98%
Controlled Postoperative Blood Glucose[5]	-	-	98%	97%
Perioperative Temperature Management[5]	-	-	100%	100%
Prophylactic Antibiotic Selection[5]	-	-	99%	99%
Prophylactic Antibiotic Selection (Outpatient)	-	-	98%	98%
Prophylactic Antibiotic Stopped[5]	-	-	98%	98%
Prophylactic Antibiotic Timing[5]	-	-	99%	99%
Prophylactic Antibiotic Timing (Outpatient)	-	-	98%	98%

NOTE: Hospital profiles are in alphabetical order by state, then city, then hospital within the city; Rankings exclude hospitals with less than 25 cases except for patient surveys which excludes hospitals with less than 100 cases; (a) 100-299 cases; (1) The number of cases/patients is too few to report; (2) Data submitted were based on a sample of cases/patients; (3) Results are based on a shorter time period than required; (4) Data suppressed by CMS for one or more quarters; (5) Results are not available for this reporting period; (6) Fewer than 100 patients completed the HCAHPS survey; (7) No cases met the criteria for this measure; (8) The lower limit of the confidence interval cannot be calculated if the number of observed infections equals zero; (9) No data are available from the state/territory for this reporting period; (10) The scores shown reflect fewer than 50 completed surveys; (11) There were discrepancies in the data collection process; (12) This measure does not apply to this hospital for this reporting period; (13) Results cannot be calculated for this reporting period; (14) The results for this state are combined with nearby states to protect confidentiality; Please refer to the User's Guide for a full explanation of data.

Measure	Cases	This Hosp.	State Avg.	U.S. Avg.
Urinary Catheter Removal[5]	-	-	97%	97%
Survey of Patients' Hospital Experiences				
Area Around Room 'Always' Quiet at Night[5]	-	-	65%	61%
Doctors 'Always' Communicated Well[5]	-	-	85%	82%
Home Recovery Information Given[5]	-	-	86%	85%
Hospital Given 9 or 10 on 10 Point Scale[5]	-	-	76%	71%
Meds 'Always' Explained Before Given[5]	-	-	66%	64%
Nurses 'Always' Communicated Well[5]	-	-	81%	79%
Pain 'Always' Well Controlled[5]	-	-	72%	71%
Room and Bathroom 'Always' Clean[5]	-	-	76%	73%
Timely Help 'Always' Received[5]	-	-	72%	68%
Would Definitely Recommend Hospital[5]	-	-	75%	71%
Use of Medical Imaging				
Cardiac Imaging Stress Test before Surgery	-	-	5%	5.3%
Combination Abdominal CT Scan	-	-	19%	10.5%
Combination Brain/Sinus CT Scan	-	-	2.9%	2.7%
Combination Chest CT Scan	-	-	3.9%	2.7%
Follow-up Mammogram/Ultrasound	-	-	7.8%	8.8%
Lumbar Spine MRI for Low Back Pain	-	-	40.2%	37.2%

Grisell Memorial Hospital

210 South Vermont Avenue
Ransom, KS 67572
Type: Critical Access Hospitals
Ownership: Govt - Hospital Dist/Auth
Phone: 785-731-2231
Fax: 785-731-2895
Emergency Services: Yes
Beds: 46

Key Personnel:
Chief of Medical Staff.......... Allen McLean, MD
Emergency Room .... Allen McLean, MD
Administrator .... Kris Ochs
CEO/President................ Kris Ochs
Quality Assurance .... Carol Ryan

Measure	Cases	This Hosp.	State Avg.	U.S. Avg.
Blood Clot Prevention and Treatment				
Anticoagulation Overlap Therapy[5]	-	-	94%	93%
ICU Venous Thromboembolism Prophylaxis[5]	-	-	91%	92%
Incidence of Potentially Preventable VTE[5]	-	-	8%	10%
UFH with Dosages/Platelet Monitoring[5]	-	-	98%	97%
Venous Thromboembolism Prophylaxis[5]	-	-	79%	85%
Warfarin Therapy Discharge Instructions[5]	-	-	84%	75%
Chest Pain/Possible Heart Attack Care				
Aspirin Given Within 24 Hours of Arrival[1,3]	-	-	94%	96%
Fibrinolytic Meds Within 30 Min. of Arrival[5]	-	-	41%	58%
Average Time to ECG (minutes)[1,3]	-	-	8	7
Average Time to Transfer (minutes)[5]	-	-	57	60
Children's Asthma Care				
Received Home Management Plan of Care	-	-	-	88%
Received Reliever Medication	-	-	-	100%
Received Systemic Corticosteroids	-	-	-	100%
Emergency Department				
Admittance Decision Time (minutes)[5]	-	-	57	98
Head CT Results Within 45 Min. of Arrival[5]	-	-	53%	57%
Patients Who Left ER Before Being Seen[5]	-	-	2%	2%
Time from ER Arrival to Admit. (minutes)[5]	-	-	185	274
Time from ER Arrival to Discharge (minutes)[5]	-	-	104	134
Time in ER Before Being Evaluated (minutes)[5]	-	-	18	26
Time to Pain Meds for Fractures (minutes)[5]	-	-	47	57
Heart Attack Care				
Aspirin Given at Discharge[5]	-	-	99%	99%
Fibrinolytic Meds Within 30 Min. of Arrival[5]	-	-	-	54%
PCI Within 90 Minutes of Arrival[5]	-	-	97%	96%
Statin Prescribed at Discharge[5]	-	-	99%	98%
Heart Failure Care				
ACE Inhibitor or ARB for LVSD[3,7]	-	-	95%	97%
Discharge Instructions Given[3,7]	-	-	91%	94%
Evaluation of LVS Function[1,3]	-	-	94%	99%
Medicare Spending				
Medicare Spending per Patient (ratio)	-	-	0.94	0.98
Pneumonia Care				
Appropriate Initial Antibiotic Given[1]	-	-	92%	95%
Blood Culture Timing[1]	-	-	98%	98%
Pregnancy and Delivery Care				
Newborn Deliveries Scheduled Early[5]	-	-	12%	6%
Preventive Care				
Immunization for Influenza[5]	-	-	88%	90%
Immunization for Pneumonia[5]	-	-	90%	92%
Stroke Care				
Anticoagulation Therapy for Atrial Fibrillation[5]	-	-	88%	95%
Antithrombotic Therapy Timing[5]	-	-	97%	98%
Assessed for Rehabilitation[5]	-	-	97%	97%
Discharged on Antithrombotic Therapy[5]	-	-	98%	99%
Discharged on Statin Medication[5]	-	-	88%	94%
Thrombolytic Therapy Timing[5]	-	-	68%	66%
Venous Thromboembolism Prophylaxis[5]	-	-	93%	94%
Written Stroke Educational Materials Given[5]	-	-	84%	88%
Surgical Care Improvement Project				
Appropriate Beta Blocker Usage[5]	-	-	98%	98%
Appropriate VTP Within 24 Hours[5]	-	-	98%	98%
Controlled Postoperative Blood Glucose[5]	-	-	98%	97%
Perioperative Temperature Management[5]	-	-	100%	100%
Prophylactic Antibiotic Selection[5]	-	-	99%	99%
Prophylactic Antibiotic Selection (Outpatient)[5]	-	-	98%	98%
Prophylactic Antibiotic Stopped[5]	-	-	98%	98%
Prophylactic Antibiotic Timing[5]	-	-	99%	99%
Prophylactic Antibiotic Timing (Outpatient)[5]	-	-	98%	98%
Urinary Catheter Removal[5]	-	-	97%	97%
Survey of Patients' Hospital Experiences				
Area Around Room 'Always' Quiet at Night[5]	-	-	65%	61%
Doctors 'Always' Communicated Well[5]	-	-	85%	82%
Home Recovery Information Given[5]	-	-	86%	85%
Hospital Given 9 or 10 on 10 Point Scale[5]	-	-	76%	71%
Meds 'Always' Explained Before Given[5]	-	-	66%	64%
Nurses 'Always' Communicated Well[5]	-	-	81%	79%
Pain 'Always' Well Controlled[5]	-	-	72%	71%
Room and Bathroom 'Always' Clean[5]	-	-	76%	73%
Timely Help 'Always' Received[5]	-	-	72%	68%
Would Definitely Recommend Hospital[5]	-	-	75%	71%
Use of Medical Imaging				
Cardiac Imaging Stress Test before Surgery[7]	-	-	5%	5.3%
Combination Abdominal CT Scan[7]	-	-	19%	10.5%
Combination Brain/Sinus CT Scan[7]	-	-	2.9%	2.7%
Combination Chest CT Scan[7]	-	-	3.9%	2.7%
Follow-up Mammogram/Ultrasound[1]	-	-	7.8%	8.8%
Lumbar Spine MRI for Low Back Pain[1]	-	-	40.2%	37.2%

Russell Regional Hospital

200 S Main Street
Russell, KS 67665
URL: www.russellhospital.org
Type: Critical Access Hospitals
Ownership: Voluntary non-profit - Private
Phone: 785-483-3131
Fax: 785-483-2037
Emergency Services: Yes
Beds: 25

Key Personnel:
Operating Room.............. Janet Cable, RN
Infection Control............. Kay Haywood, RN
Quality Assurance .... Kay Haywood, RN
Chief of Medical Staff.......... Earl Merkel, MD
Anesthesiology................ Darrell Millon
Emergency Room .... Kay Steinert, RN

Measure	Cases	This Hosp.	State Avg.	U.S. Avg.
Blood Clot Prevention and Treatment				
Anticoagulation Overlap Therapy[5]	-	-	94%	93%
ICU Venous Thromboembolism Prophylaxis[5]	-	-	91%	92%
Incidence of Potentially Preventable VTE[5]	-	-	8%	10%
UFH with Dosages/Platelet Monitoring[5]	-	-	98%	97%
Venous Thromboembolism Prophylaxis[5]	-	-	79%	85%
Warfarin Therapy Discharge Instructions[5]	-	-	84%	75%
Chest Pain/Possible Heart Attack Care				
Aspirin Given Within 24 Hours of Arrival	-	-	94%	96%
Fibrinolytic Meds Within 30 Min. of Arrival	-	-	41%	58%
Average Time to ECG (minutes)	-	-	8	7
Average Time to Transfer (minutes)	-	-	57	60
Children's Asthma Care				
Received Home Management Plan of Care	-	-	-	88%
Received Reliever Medication	-	-	-	100%
Received Systemic Corticosteroids	-	-	-	100%
Emergency Department				
Admittance Decision Time (minutes)[5]	-	-	57	98
Head CT Results Within 45 Min. of Arrival	-	-	53%	57%
Patients Who Left ER Before Being Seen	-	-	2%	2%
Time from ER Arrival to Admit. (minutes)[5]	-	-	185	274
Time from ER Arrival to Discharge (minutes)	-	-	104	134
Time in ER Before Being Evaluated (minutes)	-	-	18	26
Time to Pain Meds for Fractures (minutes)	-	-	47	57
Heart Attack Care				
Aspirin Given at Discharge[5]	-	-	99%	99%
Fibrinolytic Meds Within 30 Min. of Arrival[5]	-	-	-	54%
PCI Within 90 Minutes of Arrival[5]	-	-	97%	96%
Statin Prescribed at Discharge[5]	-	-	99%	98%
Heart Failure Care				
ACE Inhibitor or ARB for LVSD[3,7]	-	-	95%	97%
Discharge Instructions Given[1,3]	-	-	91%	94%
Evaluation of LVS Function[1,3]	-	-	94%	99%
Medicare Spending				
Medicare Spending per Patient (ratio)	-	-	0.94	0.98
Pneumonia Care				
Appropriate Initial Antibiotic Given[1]	-	-	92%	95%
Blood Culture Timing[1]	-	-	98%	98%
Pregnancy and Delivery Care				
Newborn Deliveries Scheduled Early[5]	-	-	12%	6%
Preventive Care				
Immunization for Influenza[5]	-	-	88%	90%
Immunization for Pneumonia[5]	-	-	90%	92%
Stroke Care				
Anticoagulation Therapy for Atrial Fibrillation[5]	-	-	88%	95%
Antithrombotic Therapy Timing[5]	-	-	97%	98%
Assessed for Rehabilitation[5]	-	-	97%	97%
Discharged on Antithrombotic Therapy[5]	-	-	98%	99%
Discharged on Statin Medication[5]	-	-	88%	94%
Thrombolytic Therapy Timing[5]	-	-	68%	66%
Venous Thromboembolism Prophylaxis[5]	-	-	93%	94%
Written Stroke Educational Materials Given[5]	-	-	84%	88%
Surgical Care Improvement Project				
Appropriate Beta Blocker Usage[5]	-	-	98%	98%
Appropriate VTP Within 24 Hours[5]	-	-	98%	98%
Controlled Postoperative Blood Glucose[5]	-	-	98%	97%
Perioperative Temperature Management[5]	-	-	100%	100%
Prophylactic Antibiotic Selection[5]	-	-	99%	99%
Prophylactic Antibiotic Selection (Outpatient)	-	-	98%	98%
Prophylactic Antibiotic Stopped[5]	-	-	98%	98%
Prophylactic Antibiotic Timing[5]	-	-	99%	99%
Prophylactic Antibiotic Timing (Outpatient)	-	-	98%	98%
Urinary Catheter Removal[5]	-	-	97%	97%
Survey of Patients' Hospital Experiences				
Area Around Room 'Always' Quiet at Night[5]	-	-	65%	61%
Doctors 'Always' Communicated Well[5]	-	-	85%	82%
Home Recovery Information Given[5]	-	-	86%	85%
Hospital Given 9 or 10 on 10 Point Scale[5]	-	-	76%	71%
Meds 'Always' Explained Before Given[5]	-	-	66%	64%
Nurses 'Always' Communicated Well[5]	-	-	81%	79%
Pain 'Always' Well Controlled[5]	-	-	72%	71%
Room and Bathroom 'Always' Clean[5]	-	-	76%	73%
Timely Help 'Always' Received[5]	-	-	72%	68%
Would Definitely Recommend Hospital[5]	-	-	75%	71%
Use of Medical Imaging				
Cardiac Imaging Stress Test before Surgery	-	-	5%	5.3%
Combination Abdominal CT Scan	-	-	19%	10.5%
Combination Brain/Sinus CT Scan	-	-	2.9%	2.7%
Combination Chest CT Scan	-	-	3.9%	2.7%
Follow-up Mammogram/Ultrasound	-	-	7.8%	8.8%
Lumbar Spine MRI for Low Back Pain	-	-	40.2%	37.2%

Sabetha Community Hospital

14th & Oregon
Sabetha, KS 66534
Type: Critical Access Hospitals
Ownership: Voluntary non-profit - Private
Phone: 785-284-2121
Fax: 785-284-2516
Emergency Services: Yes
Beds: 27

Key Personnel:
CEO/President................ Rita Buurman
Patient Relations .... Linnae Coker

Measure	Cases	This Hosp.	State Avg.	U.S. Avg.
Blood Clot Prevention and Treatment				

NOTE: Hospital profiles are in alphabetical order by state, then city, then hospital within the city; Rankings exclude hospitals with less than 25 cases except for patient surveys which excludes hospitals with less than 100 cases; (a) 100-299 cases; (1) The number of cases/patients is too few to report; (2) Data submitted were based on a sample of cases/patients; (3) Results are based on a shorter time period than required; (4) Data suppressed by CMS for one or more quarters; (5) Results are not available for this reporting period; (6) Fewer than 100 patients completed the HCAHPS survey; (7) No cases met the criteria for this measure; (8) The lower limit of the confidence interval cannot be calculated if the number of observed infections equals zero; (9) No data are available from the state/territory for this reporting period; (10) The scores shown reflect fewer than 50 completed surveys; (11) There were discrepancies in the data collection process; (12) This measure does not apply to this hospital for this reporting period; (13) Results cannot be calculated for this reporting period; (14) The results for this state are combined with nearby states to protect confidentiality; Please refer to the User's Guide for a full explanation of data.

Measure	Cases	This Hosp.	State Avg.	U.S. Avg.
Anticoagulation Overlap Therapy[5]	-	-	94%	93%
ICU Venous Thromboembolism Prophylaxis[5]	-	-	91%	92%
Incidence of Potentially Preventable VTE[5]	-	-	8%	10%
UFH with Dosages/Platelet Monitoring[5]	-	-	98%	97%
Venous Thromboembolism Prophylaxis[5]	-	-	79%	85%
Warfarin Therapy Discharge Instructions[5]	-	-	84%	75%
Chest Pain/Possible Heart Attack Care				
Aspirin Given Within 24 Hours of Arrival[5]	-	-	94%	96%
Fibrinolytic Meds Within 30 Min. of Arrival[5]	-	-	41%	58%
Average Time to ECG (minutes)[5]	-	-	8	7
Average Time to Transfer (minutes)[5]	-	-	57	60
Children's Asthma Care				
Received Home Management Plan of Care	-	-	-	88%
Received Reliever Medication	-	-	-	100%
Received Systemic Corticosteroids	-	-	-	100%
Emergency Department				
Admittance Decision Time (minutes)[5]	-	-	57	98
Head CT Results Within 45 Min. of Arrival[5]	-	-	53%	57%
Patients Who Left ER Before Being Seen[5]	-	-	2%	2%
Time from ER Arrival to Admit. (minutes)[5]	-	-	185	274
Time from ER Arrival to Discharge (minutes)[5]	-	-	104	134
Time in ER Before Being Evaluated (minutes)[5]	-	-	18	26
Time to Pain Meds for Fractures (minutes)[5]	-	-	47	57
Heart Attack Care				
Aspirin Given at Discharge[5]	-	-	99%	99%
Fibrinolytic Meds Within 30 Min. of Arrival[5]	-	-	-	54%
PCI Within 90 Minutes of Arrival[5]	-	-	97%	96%
Statin Prescribed at Discharge[5]	-	-	99%	98%
Heart Failure Care				
ACE Inhibitor or ARB for LVSD[1]	-	-	95%	97%
Discharge Instructions Given[1]	-	-	91%	94%
Evaluation of LVS Function[1]	-	-	94%	99%
Medicare Spending				
Medicare Spending per Patient (ratio)	-	-	0.94	0.98
Pneumonia Care				
Appropriate Initial Antibiotic Given[1,3]	-	-	92%	95%
Blood Culture Timing[1,3]	-	-	98%	98%
Pregnancy and Delivery Care				
Newborn Deliveries Scheduled Early[5]	-	-	12%	6%
Preventive Care				
Immunization for Influenza[5]	-	-	88%	90%
Immunization for Pneumonia[5]	-	-	90%	92%
Stroke Care				
Anticoagulation Therapy for Atrial Fibrillation[5]	-	-	88%	95%
Antithrombotic Therapy Timing[5]	-	-	97%	98%
Assessed for Rehabilitation[5]	-	-	97%	97%
Discharged on Antithrombotic Therapy[5]	-	-	98%	99%
Discharged on Statin Medication[5]	-	-	88%	94%
Thrombolytic Therapy Timing[5]	-	-	68%	66%
Venous Thromboembolism Prophylaxis[5]	-	-	93%	94%
Written Stroke Educational Materials Given[5]	-	-	84%	88%
Surgical Care Improvement Project				
Appropriate Beta Blocker Usage[1,3]	-	-	98%	98%
Appropriate VTP Within 24 Hours[1,3]	-	-	98%	98%
Controlled Postoperative Blood Glucose[3,7]	-	-	98%	97%
Perioperative Temperature Management[1,3]	-	-	100%	100%
Prophylactic Antibiotic Selection[1,3]	-	-	99%	99%
Prophylactic Antibiotic Selection (Outpatient)[5]	-	-	98%	98%
Prophylactic Antibiotic Stopped[1,3]	-	-	98%	98%
Prophylactic Antibiotic Timing[1,3]	-	-	99%	99%
Prophylactic Antibiotic Timing (Outpatient)[5]	-	-	98%	98%
Urinary Catheter Removal[1,3]	-	-	97%	97%
Survey of Patients' Hospital Experiences				
Area Around Room 'Always' Quiet at Night[6]	<100	62%	65%	61%
Doctors 'Always' Communicated Well[6]	<100	90%	85%	82%
Home Recovery Information Given[6]	<100	90%	86%	85%
Hospital Given 9 or 10 on 10 Point Scale[6]	<100	79%	76%	71%
Meds 'Always' Explained Before Given[6]	<100	68%	66%	64%
Nurses 'Always' Communicated Well[6]	<100	83%	81%	79%
Pain 'Always' Well Controlled[6]	<100	66%	72%	71%
Room and Bathroom 'Always' Clean[6]	<100	74%	76%	73%
Timely Help 'Always' Received[6]	<100	73%	72%	68%
Would Definitely Recommend Hospital[6]	<100	83%	75%	71%
Use of Medical Imaging				
Cardiac Imaging Stress Test before Surgery[1]	-	-	5%	5.3%
Combination Abdominal CT Scan	82	3.7%	19%	10.5%
Combination Brain/Sinus CT Scan	44	0.0%	2.9%	2.7%
Combination Chest CT Scan	46	0.0%	3.9%	2.7%
Follow-up Mammogram/Ultrasound	170	11.8%	7.8%	8.8%
Lumbar Spine MRI for Low Back Pain[1]	-	-	40.2%	37.2%

Cheyenne County Hospital

210 West 1st Street
Saint Francis, KS 67756
Phone: 785-332-2104
Fax: 785-332-3255
E-mail: llacy@cheyennecountyhospital.com
URL: www.cheyennecountyhospital.com
Type: Critical Access Hospitals
Emergency Services: Yes
Ownership: Government - Local
Beds: 16

Key Personnel:

Quality Assurance . . . . JoAnn Klre
CEO/President. . . . . Leslie Lacey
Emergency Room . . . . Tenille Lee, RN
Operating Room. . . . . Amelia Zuege
Anesthesiology. . . . . Kim Zweygardt, CRNA

Measure	Cases	This Hosp.	State Avg.	U.S. Avg.
Blood Clot Prevention and Treatment				
Anticoagulation Overlap Therapy[5]	-	-	94%	93%
ICU Venous Thromboembolism Prophylaxis[5]	-	-	91%	92%
Incidence of Potentially Preventable VTE[5]	-	-	8%	10%
UFH with Dosages/Platelet Monitoring[5]	-	-	98%	97%
Venous Thromboembolism Prophylaxis[5]	-	-	79%	85%
Warfarin Therapy Discharge Instructions[5]	-	-	84%	75%
Chest Pain/Possible Heart Attack Care				
Aspirin Given Within 24 Hours of Arrival	-	-	94%	96%
Fibrinolytic Meds Within 30 Min. of Arrival	-	-	41%	58%
Average Time to ECG (minutes)	-	-	8	7
Average Time to Transfer (minutes)	-	-	57	60
Children's Asthma Care				
Received Home Management Plan of Care	-	-	-	88%
Received Reliever Medication	-	-	-	100%
Received Systemic Corticosteroids	-	-	-	100%
Emergency Department				
Admittance Decision Time (minutes)[1,3]	-	-	57	98
Head CT Results Within 45 Min. of Arrival	-	-	53%	57%
Patients Who Left ER Before Being Seen	-	-	2%	2%
Time from ER Arrival to Admit. (minutes)[1,3]	-	-	185	274
Time from ER Arrival to Discharge (minutes)	-	-	104	134
Time in ER Before Being Evaluated (minutes)	-	-	18	26
Time to Pain Meds for Fractures (minutes)	-	-	47	57
Heart Attack Care				
Aspirin Given at Discharge[1,3]	-	-	99%	99%
Fibrinolytic Meds Within 30 Min. of Arrival[3,7]	-	-	-	54%
PCI Within 90 Minutes of Arrival[3,7]	-	-	97%	96%
Statin Prescribed at Discharge[1,3]	-	-	99%	98%
Heart Failure Care				
ACE Inhibitor or ARB for LVSD[1,3]	-	-	95%	97%
Discharge Instructions Given[3,7]	-	-	91%	94%
Evaluation of LVS Function[1,3]	-	-	94%	99%
Medicare Spending				
Medicare Spending per Patient (ratio)	-	-	0.94	0.98
Pneumonia Care				
Appropriate Initial Antibiotic Given[1]	-	-	92%	95%
Blood Culture Timing[1]	-	-	98%	98%
Pregnancy and Delivery Care				
Newborn Deliveries Scheduled Early[5]	-	-	12%	6%
Preventive Care				
Immunization for Influenza[5]	-	-	88%	90%
Immunization for Pneumonia[1,3]	-	-	90%	92%
Stroke Care				
Anticoagulation Therapy for Atrial Fibrillation[5]	-	-	88%	95%
Antithrombotic Therapy Timing[5]	-	-	97%	98%
Assessed for Rehabilitation[5]	-	-	97%	97%
Discharged on Antithrombotic Therapy[5]	-	-	98%	99%
Discharged on Statin Medication[5]	-	-	88%	94%
Thrombolytic Therapy Timing[5]	-	-	68%	66%
Venous Thromboembolism Prophylaxis[5]	-	-	93%	94%
Written Stroke Educational Materials Given[5]	-	-	84%	88%
Surgical Care Improvement Project				
Appropriate Beta Blocker Usage[5]	-	-	98%	98%
Appropriate VTP Within 24 Hours[5]	-	-	98%	98%
Controlled Postoperative Blood Glucose[5]	-	-	98%	97%
Perioperative Temperature Management[5]	-	-	100%	100%
Prophylactic Antibiotic Selection[5]	-	-	99%	99%
Prophylactic Antibiotic Selection (Outpatient)	-	-	98%	98%
Prophylactic Antibiotic Stopped[5]	-	-	98%	98%
Prophylactic Antibiotic Timing[5]	-	-	99%	99%
Prophylactic Antibiotic Timing (Outpatient)	-	-	98%	98%
Urinary Catheter Removal[5]	-	-	97%	97%
Survey of Patients' Hospital Experiences				
Area Around Room 'Always' Quiet at Night[5]	-	-	65%	61%
Doctors 'Always' Communicated Well[5]	-	-	85%	82%
Home Recovery Information Given[5]	-	-	86%	85%
Hospital Given 9 or 10 on 10 Point Scale[5]	-	-	76%	71%
Meds 'Always' Explained Before Given[5]	-	-	66%	64%
Nurses 'Always' Communicated Well[5]	-	-	81%	79%
Pain 'Always' Well Controlled[5]	-	-	72%	71%
Room and Bathroom 'Always' Clean[5]	-	-	76%	73%
Timely Help 'Always' Received[5]	-	-	72%	68%
Would Definitely Recommend Hospital[5]	-	-	75%	71%
Use of Medical Imaging				
Cardiac Imaging Stress Test before Surgery	-	-	5%	5.3%
Combination Abdominal CT Scan	-	-	19%	10.5%
Combination Brain/Sinus CT Scan	-	-	2.9%	2.7%
Combination Chest CT Scan	-	-	3.9%	2.7%
Follow-up Mammogram/Ultrasound	-	-	7.8%	8.8%
Lumbar Spine MRI for Low Back Pain	-	-	40.2%	37.2%

Salina Regional Health Center

400 South Santa Fe Avenue
Salina, KS 67401
Phone: 785-452-7000
Fax: 785-452-6963
E-mail: srhc@midusa.net
URL: www.srhc.com
Type: Acute Care Hospitals
Emergency Services: Yes
Ownership: Voluntary non-profit - Private
Beds: 385

Key Personnel:

Quality Assurance . . . . Melda Allen
Radiology. . . . . Andrew M Brittan
Pediatric Ambulatory Care . . . . . . Deb Hyman
Pediatric In-Patient Care . . . . Deb Hyman
Chief of Medical Staff . . . . Mark Mikinski, MD
Infection Control. . . . . Kelli Olson
CEO/President. . . . . Randy Peterson
Operating Room. . . . . David E Smith

Measure	Cases	This Hosp.	State Avg.	U.S. Avg.
Blood Clot Prevention and Treatment				
Anticoagulation Overlap Therapy[2]	64	92%	94%	93%
ICU Venous Thromboembolism Prophylaxis[2]	78	90%	91%	92%
Incidence of Potentially Preventable VTE[1,2]	-	-	8%	10%
UFH with Dosages/Platelet Monitoring[2]	18	89%	98%	97%
Venous Thromboembolism Prophylaxis[2]	320	81%	79%	85%
Warfarin Therapy Discharge Instructions[2]	50	62%	84%	75%
Chest Pain/Possible Heart Attack Care				
Aspirin Given Within 24 Hours of Arrival[1,3]	-	-	94%	96%
Fibrinolytic Meds Within 30 Min. of Arrival[5]	-	-	41%	58%
Average Time to ECG (minutes)[1,3]	-	-	8	7
Average Time to Transfer (minutes)[5]	-	-	57	60
Children's Asthma Care				
Received Home Management Plan of Care	-	-	-	88%
Received Reliever Medication	-	-	-	100%
Received Systemic Corticosteroids	-	-	-	100%
Emergency Department				
Admittance Decision Time (minutes)[2]	312	66	57	98
Head CT Results Within 45 Min. of Arrival[1]	-	-	53%	57%
Patients Who Left ER Before Being Seen	30,407	2%	2%	2%
Time from ER Arrival to Admit. (minutes)[2]	334	178	185	274
Time from ER Arrival to Discharge (minutes)	346	116	104	134
Time in ER Before Being Evaluated (minutes)	379	7	18	26
Time to Pain Meds for Fractures (minutes)	114	45	47	57
Heart Attack Care				
Aspirin Given at Discharge	153	99%	99%	99%

NOTE: Hospital profiles are in alphabetical order by state, then city, then hospital within the city; Rankings exclude hospitals with less than 25 cases except for patient surveys which excludes hospitals with less than 100 cases; (a) 100-299 cases; (1) The number of cases/patients is too few to report; (2) Data submitted were based on a sample of cases/patients; (3) Results are based on a shorter time period than required; (4) Data suppressed by CMS for one or more quarters; (5) Results are not available for this reporting period; (6) Fewer than 100 patients completed the HCAHPS survey; (7) No cases met the criteria for this measure; (8) The lower limit of the confidence interval cannot be calculated if the number of observed infections equals zero; (9) No data are available from the state/territory for this reporting period; (10) The scores shown reflect fewer than 50 completed surveys; (11) There were discrepancies in the data collection process; (12) This measure does not apply to this hospital for this reporting period; (13) Results cannot be calculated for this reporting period; (14) The results for this state are combined with nearby states to protect confidentiality; Please refer to the User's Guide for a full explanation of data.

Measure	Cases	This Hosp.	State Avg.	U.S. Avg.
Fibrinolytic Meds Within 30 Min. of Arrival[7]	-	-	-	54%
PCI Within 90 Minutes of Arrival	21	95%	97%	96%
Statin Prescribed at Discharge	148	99%	99%	98%
Heart Failure Care				
ACE Inhibitor or ARB for LVSD	32	100%	95%	97%
Discharge Instructions Given	73	86%	91%	94%
Evaluation of LVS Function	97	100%	94%	99%
Medicare Spending				
Medicare Spending per Patient (ratio)	-	1.01	0.94	0.98
Pneumonia Care				
Appropriate Initial Antibiotic Given	124	96%	92%	95%
Blood Culture Timing	185	100%	98%	98%
Pregnancy and Delivery Care				
Newborn Deliveries Scheduled Early	99	5%	12%	6%
Preventive Care				
Immunization for Influenza[2]	489	90%	88%	90%
Immunization for Pneumonia[2]	630	96%	90%	92%
Stroke Care				
Anticoagulation Therapy for Atrial Fibrillation	15	93%	88%	95%
Antithrombotic Therapy Timing	73	96%	97%	98%
Assessed for Rehabilitation	85	95%	97%	97%
Discharged on Antithrombotic Therapy	77	96%	98%	99%
Discharged on Statin Medication	67	76%	88%	94%
Thrombolytic Therapy Timing[1]	-	-	68%	66%
Venous Thromboembolism Prophylaxis	85	92%	93%	94%
Written Stroke Educational Materials Given	43	53%	84%	88%
Surgical Care Improvement Project				
Appropriate Beta Blocker Usage[2]	269	99%	98%	98%
Appropriate VTP Within 24 Hours[2]	416	99%	98%	98%
Controlled Postoperative Blood Glucose[2]	73	97%	98%	97%
Perioperative Temperature Management[2]	611	100%	100%	100%
Prophylactic Antibiotic Selection[2]	302	99%	99%	99%
Prophylactic Antibiotic Selection (Outpatient)	302	93%	98%	98%
Prophylactic Antibiotic Stopped[2]	281	99%	98%	98%
Prophylactic Antibiotic Timing[2]	302	99%	99%	99%
Prophylactic Antibiotic Timing (Outpatient)	300	95%	98%	98%
Urinary Catheter Removal[2]	210	98%	97%	97%
Survey of Patients' Hospital Experiences				
Area Around Room 'Always' Quiet at Night[11]	300+	59%	65%	61%
Doctors 'Always' Communicated Well[11]	300+	82%	85%	82%
Home Recovery Information Given[11]	300+	89%	86%	85%
Hospital Given 9 or 10 on 10 Point Scale[11]	300+	75%	76%	71%
Meds 'Always' Explained Before Given[11]	300+	65%	66%	64%
Nurses 'Always' Communicated Well[11]	300+	79%	81%	79%
Pain 'Always' Well Controlled[11]	300+	70%	72%	71%
Room and Bathroom 'Always' Clean[11]	300+	74%	76%	73%
Timely Help 'Always' Received[11]	300+	64%	72%	68%
Would Definitely Recommend Hospital[11]	300+	75%	75%	71%
Use of Medical Imaging				
Cardiac Imaging Stress Test before Surgery	78	5.1%	5%	5.3%
Combination Abdominal CT Scan	733	13.1%	19%	10.5%
Combination Brain/Sinus CT Scan[1]	-	-	2.9%	2.7%
Combination Chest CT Scan	513	0.2%	3.9%	2.7%
Follow-up Mammogram/Ultrasound	318	11.6%	7.8%	8.8%
Lumbar Spine MRI for Low Back Pain	164	31.7%	40.2%	37.2%

Salina Surgical Hospital

401 South Santa Fe Avenue Phone: 785-827-0610
Salina, KS 67401
URL: www.salinasurgical.com
Type: Acute Care Hospitals Emergency Services: No
Ownership: Proprietary Beds: 16
Key Personnel:
CEO/President. . . . . James Sergeant

Measure	Cases	This Hosp.	State Avg.	U.S. Avg.
Blood Clot Prevention and Treatment				
Anticoagulation Overlap Therapy[7]	-	-	94%	93%
ICU Venous Thromboembolism Prophylaxis[7]	-	-	91%	92%
Incidence of Potentially Preventable VTE[7]	-	-	8%	10%
UFH with Dosages/Platelet Monitoring[7]	-	-	98%	97%
Venous Thromboembolism Prophylaxis	22	73%	79%	85%
Warfarin Therapy Discharge Instructions[7]	-	-	84%	75%
Chest Pain/Possible Heart Attack Care				
Aspirin Given Within 24 Hours of Arrival[5]	-	-	94%	96%
Fibrinolytic Meds Within 30 Min. of Arrival[5]	-	-	41%	58%
Average Time to ECG (minutes)[5]	-	-	8	7
Average Time to Transfer (minutes)[5]	-	-	57	60
Children's Asthma Care				
Received Home Management Plan of Care	-	-	-	88%
Received Reliever Medication	-	-	-	100%
Received Systemic Corticosteroids	-	-	-	100%
Emergency Department				
Admittance Decision Time (minutes)[7]	-	-	57	98
Head CT Results Within 45 Min. of Arrival[5]	-	-	53%	57%
Patients Who Left ER Before Being Seen[1]	-	-	2%	2%
Time from ER Arrival to Admit. (minutes)[7]	-	-	185	274
Time from ER Arrival to Discharge (minutes)[5]	-	-	104	134
Time in ER Before Being Evaluated (minutes)[5]	-	-	18	26
Time to Pain Meds for Fractures (minutes)[5]	-	-	47	57
Heart Attack Care				
Aspirin Given at Discharge[5]	-	-	99%	99%
Fibrinolytic Meds Within 30 Min. of Arrival[5]	-	-	-	54%
PCI Within 90 Minutes of Arrival[5]	-	-	97%	96%
Statin Prescribed at Discharge[5]	-	-	99%	98%
Heart Failure Care				
ACE Inhibitor or ARB for LVSD[5]	-	-	95%	97%
Discharge Instructions Given[5]	-	-	91%	94%
Evaluation of LVS Function[5]	-	-	94%	99%
Medicare Spending				
Medicare Spending per Patient (ratio)	-	0.84	0.94	0.98
Pneumonia Care				
Appropriate Initial Antibiotic Given[5]	-	-	92%	95%
Blood Culture Timing[5]	-	-	98%	98%
Pregnancy and Delivery Care				
Newborn Deliveries Scheduled Early[7]	-	-	12%	6%
Preventive Care				
Immunization for Influenza	296	99%	88%	90%
Immunization for Pneumonia	398	99%	90%	92%
Stroke Care				
Anticoagulation Therapy for Atrial Fibrillation[7]	-	-	88%	95%
Antithrombotic Therapy Timing[7]	-	-	97%	98%
Assessed for Rehabilitation[7]	-	-	97%	97%
Discharged on Antithrombotic Therapy[7]	-	-	98%	99%
Discharged on Statin Medication[7]	-	-	88%	94%
Thrombolytic Therapy Timing[7]	-	-	68%	66%
Venous Thromboembolism Prophylaxis[7]	-	-	93%	94%
Written Stroke Educational Materials Given[7]	-	-	84%	88%
Surgical Care Improvement Project				
Appropriate Beta Blocker Usage	157	98%	98%	98%
Appropriate VTP Within 24 Hours	512	99%	98%	98%
Controlled Postoperative Blood Glucose[7]	-	-	98%	97%
Perioperative Temperature Management	549	100%	100%	100%
Prophylactic Antibiotic Selection	506	99%	99%	99%
Prophylactic Antibiotic Selection (Outpatient)	231	99%	98%	98%
Prophylactic Antibiotic Stopped	505	100%	98%	98%
Prophylactic Antibiotic Timing	506	99%	99%	99%
Prophylactic Antibiotic Timing (Outpatient)	226	100%	98%	98%
Urinary Catheter Removal	35	100%	97%	97%
Survey of Patients' Hospital Experiences				
Area Around Room 'Always' Quiet at Night	300+	81%	65%	61%
Doctors 'Always' Communicated Well	300+	87%	85%	82%
Home Recovery Information Given	300+	90%	86%	85%
Hospital Given 9 or 10 on 10 Point Scale	300+	92%	76%	71%
Meds 'Always' Explained Before Given	300+	73%	66%	64%
Nurses 'Always' Communicated Well	300+	90%	81%	79%
Pain 'Always' Well Controlled	300+	78%	72%	71%
Room and Bathroom 'Always' Clean	300+	84%	76%	73%
Timely Help 'Always' Received	300+	88%	72%	68%
Would Definitely Recommend Hospital	300+	92%	75%	71%
Use of Medical Imaging				
Cardiac Imaging Stress Test before Surgery[7]	-	-	5%	5.3%
Combination Abdominal CT Scan[7]	-	-	19%	10.5%
Combination Brain/Sinus CT Scan[7]	-	-	2.9%	2.7%
Combination Chest CT Scan[7]	-	-	3.9%	2.7%
Follow-up Mammogram/Ultrasound[7]	-	-	7.8%	8.8%
Lumbar Spine MRI for Low Back Pain[7]	-	-	40.2%	37.2%

Satanta District Hospital

Cheyenne & Apache Phone: 620-649-2761
Satanta, KS 67870
Type: Critical Access Hospitals Emergency Services: Yes
Ownership: Govt - Hospital Dist/Auth

Measure	Cases	This Hosp.	State Avg.	U.S. Avg.
Blood Clot Prevention and Treatment				
Anticoagulation Overlap Therapy[5]	-	-	94%	93%
ICU Venous Thromboembolism Prophylaxis[5]	-	-	91%	92%
Incidence of Potentially Preventable VTE[5]	-	-	8%	10%
UFH with Dosages/Platelet Monitoring[5]	-	-	98%	97%
Venous Thromboembolism Prophylaxis[5]	-	-	79%	85%
Warfarin Therapy Discharge Instructions[5]	-	-	84%	75%
Chest Pain/Possible Heart Attack Care				
Aspirin Given Within 24 Hours of Arrival	-	-	94%	96%
Fibrinolytic Meds Within 30 Min. of Arrival	-	-	41%	58%
Average Time to ECG (minutes)	-	-	8	7
Average Time to Transfer (minutes)	-	-	57	60
Children's Asthma Care				
Received Home Management Plan of Care	-	-	-	88%
Received Reliever Medication	-	-	-	100%
Received Systemic Corticosteroids	-	-	-	100%
Emergency Department				
Admittance Decision Time (minutes)[5]	-	-	57	98
Head CT Results Within 45 Min. of Arrival	-	-	53%	57%
Patients Who Left ER Before Being Seen	-	-	2%	2%
Time from ER Arrival to Admit. (minutes)[5]	-	-	185	274
Time from ER Arrival to Discharge (minutes)	-	-	104	134
Time in ER Before Being Evaluated (minutes)	-	-	18	26
Time to Pain Meds for Fractures (minutes)	-	-	47	57
Heart Attack Care				
Aspirin Given at Discharge[3,7]	-	-	99%	99%
Fibrinolytic Meds Within 30 Min. of Arrival[3,7]	-	-	-	54%
PCI Within 90 Minutes of Arrival[3,7]	-	-	97%	96%
Statin Prescribed at Discharge[3,7]	-	-	99%	98%
Heart Failure Care				
ACE Inhibitor or ARB for LVSD[3,7]	-	-	95%	97%
Discharge Instructions Given[1,3]	-	-	91%	94%
Evaluation of LVS Function[1,3]	-	-	94%	99%
Medicare Spending				
Medicare Spending per Patient (ratio)	-	-	0.94	0.98
Pneumonia Care				
Appropriate Initial Antibiotic Given[1]	-	-	92%	95%
Blood Culture Timing[1]	-	-	98%	98%
Pregnancy and Delivery Care				
Newborn Deliveries Scheduled Early[5]	-	-	12%	6%
Preventive Care				
Immunization for Influenza[5]	-	-	88%	90%
Immunization for Pneumonia[5]	-	-	90%	92%
Stroke Care				
Anticoagulation Therapy for Atrial Fibrillation[5]	-	-	88%	95%
Antithrombotic Therapy Timing[5]	-	-	97%	98%
Assessed for Rehabilitation[5]	-	-	97%	97%
Discharged on Antithrombotic Therapy[5]	-	-	98%	99%
Discharged on Statin Medication[5]	-	-	88%	94%
Thrombolytic Therapy Timing[5]	-	-	68%	66%
Venous Thromboembolism Prophylaxis[5]	-	-	93%	94%
Written Stroke Educational Materials Given[5]	-	-	84%	88%
Surgical Care Improvement Project				
Appropriate Beta Blocker Usage[5]	-	-	98%	98%
Appropriate VTP Within 24 Hours[5]	-	-	98%	98%
Controlled Postoperative Blood Glucose[5]	-	-	98%	97%
Perioperative Temperature Management[5]	-	-	100%	100%
Prophylactic Antibiotic Selection[5]	-	-	99%	99%
Prophylactic Antibiotic Selection (Outpatient)	-	-	98%	98%
Prophylactic Antibiotic Stopped[5]	-	-	98%	98%
Prophylactic Antibiotic Timing[5]	-	-	99%	99%
Prophylactic Antibiotic Timing (Outpatient)	-	-	98%	98%
Urinary Catheter Removal[5]	-	-	97%	97%
Survey of Patients' Hospital Experiences				

NOTE: Hospital profiles are in alphabetical order by state, then city, then hospital within the city; Rankings exclude hospitals with less than 25 cases except for patient surveys which excludes hospitals with less than 100 cases; (a) 100-299 cases; (1) The number of cases/patients is too few to report; (2) Data submitted were based on a sample of cases/patients; (3) Results are based on a shorter time period than required; (4) Data suppressed by CMS for one or more quarters; (5) Results are not available for this reporting period; (6) Fewer than 100 patients completed the HCAHPS survey; (7) No cases met the criteria for this measure; (8) The lower limit of the confidence interval cannot be calculated if the number of observed infections equals zero; (9) No data are available from the state/territory for this reporting period; (10) The scores shown reflect fewer than 50 completed surveys; (11) There were discrepancies in the data collection process; (12) This measure does not apply to this hospital for this reporting period; (13) Results cannot be calculated for this reporting period; (14) The results for this state are combined with nearby states to protect confidentiality; Please refer to the User's Guide for a full explanation of data.

Measure	Cases	This Hosp.	State Avg.	U.S. Avg.
Area Around Room 'Always' Quiet at Night[5]	-	-	65%	61%
Doctors 'Always' Communicated Well[5]	-	-	85%	82%
Home Recovery Information Given[5]	-	-	86%	85%
Hospital Given 9 or 10 on 10 Point Scale[5]	-	-	76%	71%
Meds 'Always' Explained Before Given[5]	-	-	66%	64%
Nurses 'Always' Communicated Well[5]	-	-	81%	79%
Pain 'Always' Well Controlled[5]	-	-	72%	71%
Room and Bathroom 'Always' Clean[5]	-	-	76%	73%
Timely Help 'Always' Received[5]	-	-	72%	68%
Would Definitely Recommend Hospital[5]	-	-	75%	71%
Use of Medical Imaging				
Cardiac Imaging Stress Test before Surgery	-	-	5%	5.3%
Combination Abdominal CT Scan	-	-	19%	10.5%
Combination Brain/Sinus CT Scan	-	-	2.9%	2.7%
Combination Chest CT Scan	-	-	3.9%	2.7%
Follow-up Mammogram/Ultrasound	-	-	7.8%	8.8%
Lumbar Spine MRI for Low Back Pain	-	-	40.2%	37.2%

Scott County Hospital

201 Albert Avenue
Scott City, KS 67871
Phone: 620-872-5811
Fax: 620-872-7193
URL: www.scotthospital.net
Type: Critical Access Hospitals
Emergency Services: Yes
Ownership: Voluntary non-profit - Private
Beds: 27
Key Personnel:
Infection Control. . . . . Thea Beckman
President/CEO. . . . . Mark Burnett
Chief of Medical Staff. . . . . Christian Cupp
Intensive Care Unit. . . . . Jenie Griswold
Operating Room. . . . . Deanna Kennedy

Measure	Cases	This Hosp.	State Avg.	U.S. Avg.
Blood Clot Prevention and Treatment				
Anticoagulation Overlap Therapy[5]	-	-	94%	93%
ICU Venous Thromboembolism Prophylaxis[5]	-	-	91%	92%
Incidence of Potentially Preventable VTE[5]	-	-	8%	10%
UFH with Dosages/Platelet Monitoring[5]	-	-	98%	97%
Venous Thromboembolism Prophylaxis[5]	-	-	79%	85%
Warfarin Therapy Discharge Instructions[5]	-	-	84%	75%
Chest Pain/Possible Heart Attack Care				
Aspirin Given Within 24 Hours of Arrival	-	-	94%	96%
Fibrinolytic Meds Within 30 Min. of Arrival	-	-	41%	58%
Average Time to ECG (minutes)	-	-	8	7
Average Time to Transfer (minutes)	-	-	57	60
Children's Asthma Care				
Received Home Management Plan of Care	-	-	-	88%
Received Reliever Medication	-	-	-	100%
Received Systemic Corticosteroids	-	-	-	100%
Emergency Department				
Admittance Decision Time (minutes)[5]	-	-	57	98
Head CT Results Within 45 Min. of Arrival	-	-	53%	57%
Patients Who Left ER Before Being Seen	-	-	2%	2%
Time from ER Arrival to Admit. (minutes)[5]	-	-	185	274
Time from ER Arrival to Discharge (minutes)	-	-	104	134
Time in ER Before Being Evaluated (minutes)	-	-	18	26
Time to Pain Meds for Fractures (minutes)	-	-	47	57
Heart Attack Care				
Aspirin Given at Discharge[5]	-	-	99%	99%
Fibrinolytic Meds Within 30 Min. of Arrival[5]	-	-	-	54%
PCI Within 90 Minutes of Arrival[5]	-	-	97%	96%
Statin Prescribed at Discharge[5]	-	-	99%	98%
Heart Failure Care				
ACE Inhibitor or ARB for LVSD[1,2]	-	-	95%	97%
Discharge Instructions Given[1,2]	-	-	91%	94%
Evaluation of LVS Function[2,3]	17	24%	94%	99%
Medicare Spending				
Medicare Spending per Patient (ratio)	-	-	0.94	0.98
Pneumonia Care				
Appropriate Initial Antibiotic Given[1,3]	-	-	92%	95%
Blood Culture Timing[1,3]	-	-	98%	98%
Pregnancy and Delivery Care				
Newborn Deliveries Scheduled Early[5]	-	-	12%	6%
Preventive Care				
Immunization for Influenza[5]	-	-	88%	90%
Immunization for Pneumonia[5]	-	-	90%	92%
Stroke Care				
Anticoagulation Therapy for Atrial Fibrillation[5]	-	-	88%	95%
Antithrombotic Therapy Timing[5]	-	-	97%	98%
Assessed for Rehabilitation[5]	-	-	97%	97%
Discharged on Antithrombotic Therapy[5]	-	-	98%	99%
Discharged on Statin Medication[5]	-	-	88%	94%
Thrombolytic Therapy Timing[5]	-	-	68%	66%
Venous Thromboembolism Prophylaxis[5]	-	-	93%	94%
Written Stroke Educational Materials Given[5]	-	-	84%	88%
Surgical Care Improvement Project				
Appropriate Beta Blocker Usage[5]	-	-	98%	98%
Appropriate VTP Within 24 Hours[5]	-	-	98%	98%
Controlled Postoperative Blood Glucose[5]	-	-	98%	97%
Perioperative Temperature Management[5]	-	-	100%	100%
Prophylactic Antibiotic Selection[5]	-	-	99%	99%
Prophylactic Antibiotic Selection (Outpatient)	-	-	98%	98%
Prophylactic Antibiotic Stopped[5]	-	-	98%	98%
Prophylactic Antibiotic Timing[5]	-	-	99%	99%
Prophylactic Antibiotic Timing (Outpatient)	-	-	98%	98%
Urinary Catheter Removal[5]	-	-	97%	97%
Survey of Patients' Hospital Experiences				
Area Around Room 'Always' Quiet at Night[5]	-	-	65%	61%
Doctors 'Always' Communicated Well[5]	-	-	85%	82%
Home Recovery Information Given[5]	-	-	86%	85%
Hospital Given 9 or 10 on 10 Point Scale[5]	-	-	76%	71%
Meds 'Always' Explained Before Given[5]	-	-	66%	64%
Nurses 'Always' Communicated Well[5]	-	-	81%	79%
Pain 'Always' Well Controlled[5]	-	-	72%	71%
Room and Bathroom 'Always' Clean[5]	-	-	76%	73%
Timely Help 'Always' Received[5]	-	-	72%	68%
Would Definitely Recommend Hospital[5]	-	-	75%	71%
Use of Medical Imaging				
Cardiac Imaging Stress Test before Surgery	-	-	5%	5.3%
Combination Abdominal CT Scan	-	-	19%	10.5%
Combination Brain/Sinus CT Scan	-	-	2.9%	2.7%
Combination Chest CT Scan	-	-	3.9%	2.7%
Follow-up Mammogram/Ultrasound	-	-	7.8%	8.8%
Lumbar Spine MRI for Low Back Pain	-	-	40.2%	37.2%

Sedan City Hospital

300 North Street
Sedan, KS 67361
Phone: 620-725-3115
Fax: 620-725-3297
Type: Critical Access Hospitals
Emergency Services: Yes
Ownership: Government - Local
Beds: 25
Key Personnel:
Quality Assurance . . . . Candy Kairchmer
Chief of Medical Staff. . . . . James McDermott, DO
Emergency Room . . . . James Mcdermott, DO

Measure	Cases	This Hosp.	State Avg.	U.S. Avg.
Blood Clot Prevention and Treatment				
Anticoagulation Overlap Therapy[5]	-	-	94%	93%
ICU Venous Thromboembolism Prophylaxis[5]	-	-	91%	92%
Incidence of Potentially Preventable VTE[5]	-	-	8%	10%
UFH with Dosages/Platelet Monitoring[5]	-	-	98%	97%
Venous Thromboembolism Prophylaxis[5]	-	-	79%	85%
Warfarin Therapy Discharge Instructions[5]	-	-	84%	75%
Chest Pain/Possible Heart Attack Care				
Aspirin Given Within 24 Hours of Arrival	-	-	94%	96%
Fibrinolytic Meds Within 30 Min. of Arrival	-	-	41%	58%
Average Time to ECG (minutes)	-	-	8	7
Average Time to Transfer (minutes)	-	-	57	60
Children's Asthma Care				
Received Home Management Plan of Care	-	-	-	88%
Received Reliever Medication	-	-	-	100%
Received Systemic Corticosteroids	-	-	-	100%
Emergency Department				
Admittance Decision Time (minutes)[5]	-	-	57	98
Head CT Results Within 45 Min. of Arrival	-	-	53%	57%
Patients Who Left ER Before Being Seen	-	-	2%	2%
Time from ER Arrival to Admit. (minutes)[5]	-	-	185	274
Time from ER Arrival to Discharge (minutes)	-	-	104	134
Time in ER Before Being Evaluated (minutes)	-	-	18	26
Time to Pain Meds for Fractures (minutes)	-	-	47	57
Heart Attack Care				
Aspirin Given at Discharge[5]	-	-	99%	99%
Fibrinolytic Meds Within 30 Min. of Arrival[5]	-	-	-	54%
PCI Within 90 Minutes of Arrival[5]	-	-	97%	96%
Statin Prescribed at Discharge[5]	-	-	99%	98%
Heart Failure Care				
ACE Inhibitor or ARB for LVSD[3,7]	-	-	95%	97%
Discharge Instructions Given[1,3]	-	-	91%	94%
Evaluation of LVS Function[1,3]	-	-	94%	99%
Medicare Spending				
Medicare Spending per Patient (ratio)	-	-	0.94	0.98
Pneumonia Care				
Appropriate Initial Antibiotic Given[1,3]	-	-	92%	95%
Blood Culture Timing[3,7]	-	-	98%	98%
Pregnancy and Delivery Care				
Newborn Deliveries Scheduled Early[5]	-	-	12%	6%
Preventive Care				
Immunization for Influenza[5]	-	-	88%	90%
Immunization for Pneumonia[5]	-	-	90%	92%
Stroke Care				
Anticoagulation Therapy for Atrial Fibrillation[5]	-	-	88%	95%
Antithrombotic Therapy Timing[5]	-	-	97%	98%
Assessed for Rehabilitation[5]	-	-	97%	97%
Discharged on Antithrombotic Therapy[5]	-	-	98%	99%
Discharged on Statin Medication[5]	-	-	88%	94%
Thrombolytic Therapy Timing[5]	-	-	68%	66%
Venous Thromboembolism Prophylaxis[5]	-	-	93%	94%
Written Stroke Educational Materials Given[5]	-	-	84%	88%
Surgical Care Improvement Project				
Appropriate Beta Blocker Usage[5]	-	-	98%	98%
Appropriate VTP Within 24 Hours[5]	-	-	98%	98%
Controlled Postoperative Blood Glucose[5]	-	-	98%	97%
Perioperative Temperature Management[5]	-	-	100%	100%
Prophylactic Antibiotic Selection[5]	-	-	99%	99%
Prophylactic Antibiotic Selection (Outpatient)	-	-	98%	98%
Prophylactic Antibiotic Stopped[5]	-	-	98%	98%
Prophylactic Antibiotic Timing[5]	-	-	99%	99%
Prophylactic Antibiotic Timing (Outpatient)	-	-	98%	98%
Urinary Catheter Removal[5]	-	-	97%	97%
Survey of Patients' Hospital Experiences				
Area Around Room 'Always' Quiet at Night[5]	-	-	65%	61%
Doctors 'Always' Communicated Well[5]	-	-	85%	82%
Home Recovery Information Given[5]	-	-	86%	85%
Hospital Given 9 or 10 on 10 Point Scale[5]	-	-	76%	71%
Meds 'Always' Explained Before Given[5]	-	-	66%	64%
Nurses 'Always' Communicated Well[5]	-	-	81%	79%
Pain 'Always' Well Controlled[5]	-	-	72%	71%
Room and Bathroom 'Always' Clean[5]	-	-	76%	73%
Timely Help 'Always' Received[5]	-	-	72%	68%
Would Definitely Recommend Hospital[5]	-	-	75%	71%
Use of Medical Imaging				
Cardiac Imaging Stress Test before Surgery	-	-	5%	5.3%
Combination Abdominal CT Scan	-	-	19%	10.5%
Combination Brain/Sinus CT Scan	-	-	2.9%	2.7%
Combination Chest CT Scan	-	-	3.9%	2.7%
Follow-up Mammogram/Ultrasound	-	-	7.8%	8.8%
Lumbar Spine MRI for Low Back Pain	-	-	40.2%	37.2%

Nemaha Valley Community Hospital

1600 Community Dr
Seneca, KS 66538
Phone: 785-336-6181
Fax: 785-336-3052
Type: Critical Access Hospitals
Emergency Services: Yes
Ownership: Voluntary non-profit - Private
Beds: 24
Key Personnel:
CEO/President. . . . . Stan Regehr
Infection Control. . . . . Donna Stallbaum

Measure	Cases	This Hosp.	State Avg.	U.S. Avg.
Blood Clot Prevention and Treatment				
Anticoagulation Overlap Therapy[7]	-	-	94%	93%
ICU Venous Thromboembolism Prophylaxis[7]	-	-	91%	92%
Incidence of Potentially Preventable VTE[7]	-	-	8%	10%
UFH with Dosages/Platelet Monitoring[7]	-	-	98%	97%
Venous Thromboembolism Prophylaxis	32	88%	79%	85%

NOTE: Hospital profiles are in alphabetical order by state, then city, then hospital within the city; Rankings exclude hospitals with less than 25 cases except for patient surveys which excludes hospitals with less than 100 cases; (a) 100-299 cases; (1) The number of cases/patients is too few to report; (2) Data submitted were based on a sample of cases/patients; (3) Results are based on a shorter time period than required; (4) Data suppressed by CMS for one or more quarters; (5) Results are not available for this reporting period; (6) Fewer than 100 patients completed the HCAHPS survey; (7) No cases met the criteria for this measure; (8) The lower limit of the confidence interval cannot be calculated if the number of observed infections equals zero; (9) No data are available from the state/territory for this reporting period; (10) The scores shown reflect fewer than 50 completed surveys; (11) There were discrepancies in the data collection process; (12) This measure does not apply to this hospital for this reporting period; (13) Results cannot be calculated for this reporting period; (14) The results for this state are combined with nearby states to protect confidentiality; Please refer to the User's Guide for a full explanation of data.

Measure	Cases	This Hosp.	State Avg.	U.S. Avg.
Warfarin Therapy Discharge Instructions[7]	-	-	84%	75%
Chest Pain/Possible Heart Attack Care				
Aspirin Given Within 24 Hours of Arrival	-	-	94%	96%
Fibrinolytic Meds Within 30 Min. of Arrival	-	-	41%	58%
Average Time to ECG (minutes)	-	-	8	7
Average Time to Transfer (minutes)	-	-	57	60
Children's Asthma Care				
Received Home Management Plan of Care	-	-	-	88%
Received Reliever Medication	-	-	-	100%
Received Systemic Corticosteroids	-	-	-	100%
Emergency Department				
Admittance Decision Time (minutes)	64	0	57	98
Head CT Results Within 45 Min. of Arrival	-	-	53%	57%
Patients Who Left ER Before Being Seen	-	-	2%	2%
Time from ER Arrival to Admit. (minutes)	64	92	185	274
Time from ER Arrival to Discharge (minutes)	-	-	104	134
Time in ER Before Being Evaluated (minutes)	-	-	18	26
Time to Pain Meds for Fractures (minutes)	-	-	47	57
Heart Attack Care				
Aspirin Given at Discharge[3,7]	-	-	99%	99%
Fibrinolytic Meds Within 30 Min. of Arrival[3,7]	-	-	-	54%
PCI Within 90 Minutes of Arrival[3,7]	-	-	97%	96%
Statin Prescribed at Discharge[1,3]	-	-	99%	98%
Heart Failure Care				
ACE Inhibitor or ARB for LVSD[1,3]	-	-	95%	97%
Discharge Instructions Given[1,3]	-	-	91%	94%
Evaluation of LVS Function[1,3]	-	-	94%	99%
Medicare Spending				
Medicare Spending per Patient (ratio)	-	-	0.94	0.98
Pneumonia Care				
Appropriate Initial Antibiotic Given	15	87%	92%	95%
Blood Culture Timing[1]	-	-	98%	98%
Pregnancy and Delivery Care				
Newborn Deliveries Scheduled Early[5]	-	-	12%	6%
Preventive Care				
Immunization for Influenza	77	81%	88%	90%
Immunization for Pneumonia	107	86%	90%	92%
Stroke Care				
Anticoagulation Therapy for Atrial Fibrillation[5]	-	-	88%	95%
Antithrombotic Therapy Timing[5]	-	-	97%	98%
Assessed for Rehabilitation[5]	-	-	97%	97%
Discharged on Antithrombotic Therapy[5]	-	-	98%	99%
Discharged on Statin Medication[5]	-	-	88%	94%
Thrombolytic Therapy Timing[5]	-	-	68%	66%
Venous Thromboembolism Prophylaxis[5]	-	-	93%	94%
Written Stroke Educational Materials Given[5]	-	-	84%	88%
Surgical Care Improvement Project				
Appropriate Beta Blocker Usage[3,7]	-	-	98%	98%
Appropriate VTP Within 24 Hours[1,3]	-	-	98%	98%
Controlled Postoperative Blood Glucose[3,7]	-	-	98%	97%
Perioperative Temperature Management[1,3]	-	-	100%	100%
Prophylactic Antibiotic Selection[3,7]	-	-	99%	99%
Prophylactic Antibiotic Selection (Outpatient)	-	-	98%	98%
Prophylactic Antibiotic Stopped[3,7]	-	-	98%	98%
Prophylactic Antibiotic Timing[3,7]	-	-	99%	99%
Prophylactic Antibiotic Timing (Outpatient)	-	-	98%	98%
Urinary Catheter Removal[1,3]	-	-	97%	97%
Survey of Patients' Hospital Experiences				
Area Around Room 'Always' Quiet at Night[5]	-	-	65%	61%
Doctors 'Always' Communicated Well[5]	-	-	85%	82%
Home Recovery Information Given[5]	-	-	86%	85%
Hospital Given 9 or 10 on 10 Point Scale[5]	-	-	76%	71%
Meds 'Always' Explained Before Given[5]	-	-	66%	64%
Nurses 'Always' Communicated Well[5]	-	-	81%	79%
Pain 'Always' Well Controlled[5]	-	-	72%	71%
Room and Bathroom 'Always' Clean[5]	-	-	76%	73%
Timely Help 'Always' Received[5]	-	-	72%	68%
Would Definitely Recommend Hospital[5]	-	-	75%	71%
Use of Medical Imaging				
Cardiac Imaging Stress Test before Surgery	-	-	5%	5.3%
Combination Abdominal CT Scan	-	-	19%	10.5%
Combination Brain/Sinus CT Scan	-	-	2.9%	2.7%
Combination Chest CT Scan	-	-	3.9%	2.7%
Follow-up Mammogram/Ultrasound	-	-	7.8%	8.8%
Lumbar Spine MRI for Low Back Pain	-	-	40.2%	37.2%

Shawnee Mission Medical Center

9100 W 74th Street
Shawnee Mission, KS 66204
E-mail: webmaster@shawneemission.org
URL: www.shawneemission.org
Type: Acute Care Hospitals
Ownership: Voluntary non-profit - Church
Phone: 913-676-2151
Fax: 913-676-7724
Emergency Services: Yes
Beds: 383

Key Personnel:
Chief of Medical Staff . . . . Robin Harrold
Coronary Care . . . . Louise Rada
CEO/President . . . . Samuel H Turner, Sr

Measure	Cases	This Hosp.	State Avg.	U.S. Avg.
Blood Clot Prevention and Treatment				
Anticoagulation Overlap Therapy[2]	145	99%	94%	93%
ICU Venous Thromboembolism Prophylaxis[2]	50	98%	91%	92%
Incidence of Potentially Preventable VTE[2]	24	21%	8%	10%
UFH with Dosages/Platelet Monitoring[2]	14	100%	98%	97%
Venous Thromboembolism Prophylaxis[2]	333	86%	79%	85%
Warfarin Therapy Discharge Instructions[2]	113	97%	84%	75%
Chest Pain/Possible Heart Attack Care				
Aspirin Given Within 24 Hours of Arrival[3,7]	-	-	94%	96%
Fibrinolytic Meds Within 30 Min. of Arrival[5]	-	-	41%	58%
Average Time to ECG (minutes)[3,7]	-	-	8	7
Average Time to Transfer (minutes)[5]	-	-	57	60
Children's Asthma Care				
Received Home Management Plan of Care	-	-	-	88%
Received Reliever Medication	-	-	-	100%
Received Systemic Corticosteroids	-	-	-	100%
Emergency Department				
Admittance Decision Time (minutes)[2]	372	87	57	98
Head CT Results Within 45 Min. of Arrival[1]	-	-	53%	57%
Patients Who Left ER Before Being Seen	68,942	0%	2%	2%
Time from ER Arrival to Admit. (minutes)[2]	385	241	185	274
Time from ER Arrival to Discharge (minutes)	365	137	104	134
Time in ER Before Being Evaluated (minutes)	200	37	18	26
Time to Pain Meds for Fractures (minutes)	239	42	47	57
Heart Attack Care				
Aspirin Given at Discharge[2]	205	99%	99%	99%
Fibrinolytic Meds Within 30 Min. of Arrival[2,7]	-	-	-	54%
PCI Within 90 Minutes of Arrival[2]	58	98%	97%	96%
Statin Prescribed at Discharge[2]	204	100%	99%	98%
Heart Failure Care				
ACE Inhibitor or ARB for LVSD[2]	100	100%	95%	97%
Discharge Instructions Given[2]	221	99%	91%	94%
Evaluation of LVS Function[2]	275	100%	94%	99%
Medicare Spending				
Medicare Spending per Patient (ratio)	-	1.03	0.94	0.98
Pneumonia Care				
Appropriate Initial Antibiotic Given[2]	104	98%	92%	95%
Blood Culture Timing[2]	143	100%	98%	98%
Pregnancy and Delivery Care				
Newborn Deliveries Scheduled Early[2]	123	60%	12%	6%
Preventive Care				
Immunization for Influenza[2]	508	96%	88%	90%
Immunization for Pneumonia[2]	527	99%	90%	92%
Stroke Care				
Anticoagulation Therapy for Atrial Fibrillation	19	89%	88%	95%
Antithrombotic Therapy Timing	117	97%	97%	98%
Assessed for Rehabilitation	152	97%	97%	97%
Discharged on Antithrombotic Therapy	136	98%	98%	99%
Discharged on Statin Medication	97	98%	88%	94%
Thrombolytic Therapy Timing	21	81%	68%	66%
Venous Thromboembolism Prophylaxis	147	92%	93%	94%
Written Stroke Educational Materials Given	78	95%	84%	88%
Surgical Care Improvement Project				
Appropriate Beta Blocker Usage[2]	217	98%	98%	98%
Appropriate VTP Within 24 Hours[2]	449	98%	98%	98%
Controlled Postoperative Blood Glucose[2]	137	97%	98%	97%
Perioperative Temperature Management[2]	543	100%	100%	100%
Prophylactic Antibiotic Selection[2]	441	99%	99%	99%
Prophylactic Antibiotic Selection (Outpatient)	566	98%	98%	98%
Prophylactic Antibiotic Stopped[2]	405	100%	98%	98%
Prophylactic Antibiotic Timing[2]	443	99%	99%	99%
Prophylactic Antibiotic Timing (Outpatient)	570	98%	98%	98%
Urinary Catheter Removal[2]	239	99%	97%	97%
Survey of Patients' Hospital Experiences				
Area Around Room 'Always' Quiet at Night[11]	300+	67%	65%	61%
Doctors 'Always' Communicated Well[11]	300+	81%	85%	82%
Home Recovery Information Given[11]	300+	89%	86%	85%
Hospital Given 9 or 10 on 10 Point Scale[11]	300+	82%	76%	71%
Meds 'Always' Explained Before Given[11]	300+	67%	66%	64%
Nurses 'Always' Communicated Well[11]	300+	82%	81%	79%
Pain 'Always' Well Controlled[11]	300+	73%	72%	71%
Room and Bathroom 'Always' Clean[11]	300+	82%	76%	73%
Timely Help 'Always' Received[11]	300+	68%	72%	68%
Would Definitely Recommend Hospital[11]	300+	84%	75%	71%
Use of Medical Imaging				
Cardiac Imaging Stress Test before Surgery	392	3.1%	5%	5.3%
Combination Abdominal CT Scan	1,006	14.0%	19%	10.5%
Combination Brain/Sinus CT Scan	1,150	2.3%	2.9%	2.7%
Combination Chest CT Scan	368	6.5%	3.9%	2.7%
Follow-up Mammogram/Ultrasound	2,198	5.9%	7.8%	8.8%
Lumbar Spine MRI for Low Back Pain	194	41.8%	40.2%	37.2%

Smith County Memorial Hospital

614 South Main Street
Smith Center, KS 66967
URL: www.smithcohosp.org
Type: Critical Access Hospitals
Ownership: Government - Local
Phone: 785-282-6845
Fax: 785-282-6331
Emergency Services: No
Beds: 25

Key Personnel:
Chief of Medical Staff . . . . Joe Barnes
Quality Assurance . . . . Julie Haresnape
Cardiac Laboratory. . . . . Paula Hayes, RN
Infection Control. . . . . Karen Herndon
CEO/President. . . . . Carolyn Hess, RN
Operating Room. . . . . Chris Horn, RN
Emergency Room . . . . Laura Kingsbury, RN
Radiology. . . . . Kayla Wolf

Measure	Cases	This Hosp.	State Avg.	U.S. Avg.
Blood Clot Prevention and Treatment				
Anticoagulation Overlap Therapy[5]	-	-	94%	93%
ICU Venous Thromboembolism Prophylaxis[5]	-	-	91%	92%
Incidence of Potentially Preventable VTE[5]	-	-	8%	10%
UFH with Dosages/Platelet Monitoring[5]	-	-	98%	97%
Venous Thromboembolism Prophylaxis[5]	-	-	79%	85%
Warfarin Therapy Discharge Instructions[5]	-	-	84%	75%
Chest Pain/Possible Heart Attack Care				
Aspirin Given Within 24 Hours of Arrival[1,3]	-	-	94%	96%
Fibrinolytic Meds Within 30 Min. of Arrival[3,7]	-	-	41%	58%
Average Time to ECG (minutes)[1,3]	-	-	8	7
Average Time to Transfer (minutes)[3,7]	-	-	57	60
Children's Asthma Care				
Received Home Management Plan of Care	-	-	-	88%
Received Reliever Medication	-	-	-	100%
Received Systemic Corticosteroids	-	-	-	100%
Emergency Department				
Admittance Decision Time (minutes)[5]	-	-	57	98
Head CT Results Within 45 Min. of Arrival[1,3]	-	-	53%	57%
Patients Who Left ER Before Being Seen[5]	-	-	2%	2%
Time from ER Arrival to Admit. (minutes)[5]	-	-	185	274
Time from ER Arrival to Discharge (minutes)[5]	-	-	104	134
Time in ER Before Being Evaluated (minutes)[5]	-	-	18	26
Time to Pain Meds for Fractures (minutes)[1,3]	-	-	47	57
Heart Attack Care				
Aspirin Given at Discharge[1,3]	-	-	99%	99%
Fibrinolytic Meds Within 30 Min. of Arrival[3,7]	-	-	-	54%
PCI Within 90 Minutes of Arrival[3,7]	-	-	97%	96%
Statin Prescribed at Discharge[1,3]	-	-	99%	98%
Heart Failure Care				
ACE Inhibitor or ARB for LVSD[7]	-	-	95%	97%
Discharge Instructions Given[1]	-	-	91%	94%
Evaluation of LVS Function	14	50%	94%	99%

NOTE: Hospital profiles are in alphabetical order by state, then city, then hospital within the city; Rankings exclude hospitals with less than 25 cases except for patient surveys which excludes hospitals with less than 100 cases; (a) 100-299 cases; (1) The number of cases/patients is too few to report; (2) Data submitted were based on a sample of cases/patients; (3) Results are based on a shorter time period than required; (4) Data suppressed by CMS for one or more quarters; (5) Results are not available for this reporting period; (6) Fewer than 100 patients completed the HCAHPS survey; (7) No cases met the criteria for this measure; (8) The lower limit of the confidence interval cannot be calculated if the number of observed infections equals zero; (9) No data are available from the state/territory for this reporting period; (10) The scores shown reflect fewer than 50 completed surveys; (11) There were discrepancies in the data collection process; (12) This measure does not apply to this hospital for this reporting period; (13) Results cannot be calculated for this reporting period; (14) The results for this state are combined with nearby states to protect confidentiality; Please refer to the User's Guide for a full explanation of data.

Measure	Cases	This Hosp.	State Avg.	U.S. Avg.
Medicare Spending				
Medicare Spending per Patient (ratio)	-	-	0.94	0.98
Pneumonia Care				
Appropriate Initial Antibiotic Given	21	86%	92%	95%
Blood Culture Timing[1]	-	-	98%	98%
Pregnancy and Delivery Care				
Newborn Deliveries Scheduled Early[5]	-	-	12%	6%
Preventive Care				
Immunization for Influenza[5]	-	-	88%	90%
Immunization for Pneumonia[5]	-	-	90%	92%
Stroke Care				
Anticoagulation Therapy for Atrial Fibrillation[5]	-	-	88%	95%
Antithrombotic Therapy Timing[5]	-	-	97%	98%
Assessed for Rehabilitation[5]	-	-	97%	97%
Discharged on Antithrombotic Therapy[5]	-	-	98%	99%
Discharged on Statin Medication[5]	-	-	88%	94%
Thrombolytic Therapy Timing[5]	-	-	68%	66%
Venous Thromboembolism Prophylaxis[5]	-	-	93%	94%
Written Stroke Educational Materials Given[5]	-	-	84%	88%
Surgical Care Improvement Project				
Appropriate Beta Blocker Usage[5]	-	-	98%	98%
Appropriate VTP Within 24 Hours[5]	-	-	98%	98%
Controlled Postoperative Blood Glucose[5]	-	-	98%	97%
Perioperative Temperature Management[5]	-	-	100%	100%
Prophylactic Antibiotic Selection[5]	-	-	99%	99%
Prophylactic Antibiotic Selection (Outpatient)[1,3]	-	-	98%	98%
Prophylactic Antibiotic Stopped[5]	-	-	98%	98%
Prophylactic Antibiotic Timing[5]	-	-	99%	99%
Prophylactic Antibiotic Timing (Outpatient)[1,3]	-	-	98%	98%
Urinary Catheter Removal[5]	-	-	97%	97%
Survey of Patients' Hospital Experiences				
Area Around Room 'Always' Quiet at Night[5]	-	-	65%	61%
Doctors 'Always' Communicated Well[5]	-	-	85%	82%
Home Recovery Information Given[5]	-	-	86%	85%
Hospital Given 9 or 10 on 10 Point Scale[5]	-	-	76%	71%
Meds 'Always' Explained Before Given[5]	-	-	66%	64%
Nurses 'Always' Communicated Well[5]	-	-	81%	79%
Pain 'Always' Well Controlled[5]	-	-	72%	71%
Room and Bathroom 'Always' Clean[5]	-	-	76%	73%
Timely Help 'Always' Received[5]	-	-	72%	68%
Would Definitely Recommend Hospital[5]	-	-	75%	71%
Use of Medical Imaging				
Cardiac Imaging Stress Test before Surgery	51	0.0%	5%	5.3%
Combination Abdominal CT Scan	60	28.3%	19%	10.5%
Combination Brain/Sinus CT Scan[1]	-	-	2.9%	2.7%
Combination Chest CT Scan[1]	-	-	3.9%	2.7%
Follow-up Mammogram/Ultrasound	170	10.6%	7.8%	8.8%
Lumbar Spine MRI for Low Back Pain[1]	-	-	40.2%	37.2%

Stafford County Hospital

502 S Buckeye
Stafford, KS 67578
Phone: 620-234-5221
Type: Critical Access Hospitals
Emergency Services: Yes
Ownership: Government - Local

Measure	Cases	This Hosp.	State Avg.	U.S. Avg.
Blood Clot Prevention and Treatment				
Anticoagulation Overlap Therapy[5]	-	-	94%	93%
ICU Venous Thromboembolism Prophylaxis[5]	-	-	91%	92%
Incidence of Potentially Preventable VTE[5]	-	-	8%	10%
UFH with Dosages/Platelet Monitoring[5]	-	-	98%	97%
Venous Thromboembolism Prophylaxis[5]	-	-	79%	85%
Warfarin Therapy Discharge Instructions[5]	-	-	84%	75%
Chest Pain/Possible Heart Attack Care				
Aspirin Given Within 24 Hours of Arrival	-	-	94%	96%
Fibrinolytic Meds Within 30 Min. of Arrival	-	-	41%	58%
Average Time to ECG (minutes)	-	-	8	7
Average Time to Transfer (minutes)	-	-	57	60
Children's Asthma Care				
Received Home Management Plan of Care	-	-	-	88%
Received Reliever Medication	-	-	-	100%
Received Systemic Corticosteroids	-	-	-	100%
Emergency Department				
Admittance Decision Time (minutes)[5]	-	-	57	98
Head CT Results Within 45 Min. of Arrival	-	-	53%	57%
Patients Who Left ER Before Being Seen	-	-	2%	2%
Time from ER Arrival to Admit. (minutes)[5]	-	-	185	274
Time from ER Arrival to Discharge (minutes)	-	-	104	134
Time in ER Before Being Evaluated (minutes)	-	-	18	26
Time to Pain Meds for Fractures (minutes)	-	-	47	57
Heart Attack Care				
Aspirin Given at Discharge[5]	-	-	99%	99%
Fibrinolytic Meds Within 30 Min. of Arrival[5]	-	-	-	54%
PCI Within 90 Minutes of Arrival[5]	-	-	97%	96%
Statin Prescribed at Discharge[5]	-	-	99%	98%
Heart Failure Care				
ACE Inhibitor or ARB for LVSD[5]	-	-	95%	97%
Discharge Instructions Given[5]	-	-	91%	94%
Evaluation of LVS Function[5]	-	-	94%	99%
Medicare Spending				
Medicare Spending per Patient (ratio)	-	-	0.94	0.98
Pneumonia Care				
Appropriate Initial Antibiotic Given[3,7]	-	-	92%	95%
Blood Culture Timing[3,7]	-	-	98%	98%
Pregnancy and Delivery Care				
Newborn Deliveries Scheduled Early[5]	-	-	12%	6%
Preventive Care				
Immunization for Influenza[5]	-	-	88%	90%
Immunization for Pneumonia[5]	-	-	90%	92%
Stroke Care				
Anticoagulation Therapy for Atrial Fibrillation[5]	-	-	88%	95%
Antithrombotic Therapy Timing[5]	-	-	97%	98%
Assessed for Rehabilitation[5]	-	-	97%	97%
Discharged on Antithrombotic Therapy[5]	-	-	98%	99%
Discharged on Statin Medication[5]	-	-	88%	94%
Thrombolytic Therapy Timing[5]	-	-	68%	66%
Venous Thromboembolism Prophylaxis[5]	-	-	93%	94%
Written Stroke Educational Materials Given[5]	-	-	84%	88%
Surgical Care Improvement Project				
Appropriate Beta Blocker Usage[5]	-	-	98%	98%
Appropriate VTP Within 24 Hours[5]	-	-	98%	98%
Controlled Postoperative Blood Glucose[5]	-	-	98%	97%
Perioperative Temperature Management[5]	-	-	100%	100%
Prophylactic Antibiotic Selection[5]	-	-	99%	99%
Prophylactic Antibiotic Selection (Outpatient)	-	-	98%	98%
Prophylactic Antibiotic Stopped[5]	-	-	98%	98%
Prophylactic Antibiotic Timing[5]	-	-	99%	99%
Prophylactic Antibiotic Timing (Outpatient)	-	-	98%	98%
Urinary Catheter Removal[5]	-	-	97%	97%
Survey of Patients' Hospital Experiences				
Area Around Room 'Always' Quiet at Night[5]	-	-	65%	61%
Doctors 'Always' Communicated Well[5]	-	-	85%	82%
Home Recovery Information Given[5]	-	-	86%	85%
Hospital Given 9 or 10 on 10 Point Scale[5]	-	-	76%	71%
Meds 'Always' Explained Before Given[5]	-	-	66%	64%
Nurses 'Always' Communicated Well[5]	-	-	81%	79%
Pain 'Always' Well Controlled[5]	-	-	72%	71%
Room and Bathroom 'Always' Clean[5]	-	-	76%	73%
Timely Help 'Always' Received[5]	-	-	72%	68%
Would Definitely Recommend Hospital[5]	-	-	75%	71%
Use of Medical Imaging				
Cardiac Imaging Stress Test before Surgery	-	-	5%	5.3%
Combination Abdominal CT Scan	-	-	19%	10.5%
Combination Brain/Sinus CT Scan	-	-	2.9%	2.7%
Combination Chest CT Scan	-	-	3.9%	2.7%
Follow-up Mammogram/Ultrasound	-	-	7.8%	8.8%
Lumbar Spine MRI for Low Back Pain	-	-	40.2%	37.2%

Hamilton County Hospital

700 North Huser
Syracuse, KS 67878
Phone: 620-384-7461
Fax: 620-384-5500
URL: www.hamiltoncountyhospital.net
Type: Critical Access Hospitals
Emergency Services: Yes
Ownership: Government - Local
Beds: 25

Key Personnel:

CEO . . . . Bryan Coffey
Operating Room. . . . . Loraine Durler, RN
Quality Assurance . . . . Loraine Durler, RN
Radiology. . . . . Fred Nichols
Emergency Room . . . . Joseph Rehal, MD

Measure	Cases	This Hosp.	State Avg.	U.S. Avg.
Blood Clot Prevention and Treatment				
Anticoagulation Overlap Therapy[5]	-	-	94%	93%
ICU Venous Thromboembolism Prophylaxis[5]	-	-	91%	92%
Incidence of Potentially Preventable VTE[5]	-	-	8%	10%
UFH with Dosages/Platelet Monitoring[5]	-	-	98%	97%
Venous Thromboembolism Prophylaxis[5]	-	-	79%	85%
Warfarin Therapy Discharge Instructions[5]	-	-	84%	75%
Chest Pain/Possible Heart Attack Care				
Aspirin Given Within 24 Hours of Arrival	-	-	94%	96%
Fibrinolytic Meds Within 30 Min. of Arrival	-	-	41%	58%
Average Time to ECG (minutes)	-	-	8	7
Average Time to Transfer (minutes)	-	-	57	60
Children's Asthma Care				
Received Home Management Plan of Care	-	-	-	88%
Received Reliever Medication	-	-	-	100%
Received Systemic Corticosteroids	-	-	-	100%
Emergency Department				
Admittance Decision Time (minutes)[5]	-	-	57	98
Head CT Results Within 45 Min. of Arrival	-	-	53%	57%
Patients Who Left ER Before Being Seen	-	-	2%	2%
Time from ER Arrival to Admit. (minutes)[5]	-	-	185	274
Time from ER Arrival to Discharge (minutes)	-	-	104	134
Time in ER Before Being Evaluated (minutes)	-	-	18	26
Time to Pain Meds for Fractures (minutes)	-	-	47	57
Heart Attack Care				
Aspirin Given at Discharge[1,3]	-	-	99%	99%
Fibrinolytic Meds Within 30 Min. of Arrival[3,7]	-	-	-	54%
PCI Within 90 Minutes of Arrival[3,7]	-	-	97%	96%
Statin Prescribed at Discharge[1,3]	-	-	99%	98%
Heart Failure Care				
ACE Inhibitor or ARB for LVSD[7]	-	-	95%	97%
Discharge Instructions Given[1]	-	-	91%	94%
Evaluation of LVS Function[1]	-	-	94%	99%
Medicare Spending				
Medicare Spending per Patient (ratio)	-	-	0.94	0.98
Pneumonia Care				
Appropriate Initial Antibiotic Given[2]	14	79%	92%	95%
Blood Culture Timing[1,2]	-	-	98%	98%
Pregnancy and Delivery Care				
Newborn Deliveries Scheduled Early[5]	-	-	12%	6%
Preventive Care				
Immunization for Influenza[5]	-	-	88%	90%
Immunization for Pneumonia[5]	-	-	90%	92%
Stroke Care				
Anticoagulation Therapy for Atrial Fibrillation[5]	-	-	88%	95%
Antithrombotic Therapy Timing[5]	-	-	97%	98%
Assessed for Rehabilitation[5]	-	-	97%	97%
Discharged on Antithrombotic Therapy[5]	-	-	98%	99%
Discharged on Statin Medication[5]	-	-	88%	94%
Thrombolytic Therapy Timing[5]	-	-	68%	66%
Venous Thromboembolism Prophylaxis[5]	-	-	93%	94%
Written Stroke Educational Materials Given[5]	-	-	84%	88%
Surgical Care Improvement Project				
Appropriate Beta Blocker Usage[5]	-	-	98%	98%
Appropriate VTP Within 24 Hours[5]	-	-	98%	98%
Controlled Postoperative Blood Glucose[5]	-	-	98%	97%
Perioperative Temperature Management[5]	-	-	100%	100%
Prophylactic Antibiotic Selection[5]	-	-	99%	99%
Prophylactic Antibiotic Selection (Outpatient)	-	-	98%	98%
Prophylactic Antibiotic Stopped[5]	-	-	98%	98%
Prophylactic Antibiotic Timing[5]	-	-	99%	99%
Prophylactic Antibiotic Timing (Outpatient)	-	-	98%	98%
Urinary Catheter Removal[5]	-	-	97%	97%
Survey of Patients' Hospital Experiences				
Area Around Room 'Always' Quiet at Night[5]	-	-	65%	61%
Doctors 'Always' Communicated Well[5]	-	-	85%	82%
Home Recovery Information Given[5]	-	-	86%	85%
Hospital Given 9 or 10 on 10 Point Scale[5]	-	-	76%	71%

NOTE: Hospital profiles are in alphabetical order by state, then city, then hospital within the city; Rankings exclude hospitals with less than 25 cases except for patient surveys which excludes hospitals with less than 100 cases; (a) 100-299 cases; (1) The number of cases/patients is too few to report; (2) Data submitted were based on a sample of cases/patients; (3) Results are based on a shorter time period than required; (4) Data suppressed by CMS for one or more quarters; (5) Results are not available for this reporting period; (6) Fewer than 100 patients completed the HCAHPS survey; (7) No cases met the criteria for this measure; (8) The lower limit of the confidence interval cannot be calculated if the number of observed infections equals zero; (9) No data are available from the state/territory for this reporting period; (10) The scores shown reflect fewer than 50 completed surveys; (11) There were discrepancies in the data collection process; (12) This measure does not apply to this hospital for this reporting period; (13) Results cannot be calculated for this reporting period; (14) The results for this state are combined with nearby states to protect confidentiality; Please refer to the User's Guide for a full explanation of data.

Measure	Cases	This Hosp.	State Avg.	U.S. Avg.
Meds 'Always' Explained Before Given[5]	-	-	66%	64%
Nurses 'Always' Communicated Well[5]	-	-	81%	79%
Pain 'Always' Well Controlled[5]	-	-	72%	71%
Room and Bathroom 'Always' Clean[5]	-	-	76%	73%
Timely Help 'Always' Received[5]	-	-	72%	68%
Would Definitely Recommend Hospital[5]	-	-	75%	71%
Use of Medical Imaging				
Cardiac Imaging Stress Test before Surgery	-	-	5%	5.3%
Combination Abdominal CT Scan	-	-	19%	10.5%
Combination Brain/Sinus CT Scan	-	-	2.9%	2.7%
Combination Chest CT Scan	-	-	3.9%	2.7%
Follow-up Mammogram/Ultrasound	-	-	7.8%	8.8%
Lumbar Spine MRI for Low Back Pain	-	-	40.2%	37.2%

Saint Francis Health Center

1700 Sw 7th Street
Topeka, KS 66606
Phone: 785-295-8000
Fax: 785-295-7854
E-mail: cr@stfrancistopeka.org
URL: www.stfrancistopeka.org
Type: Acute Care Hospitals
Emergency Services: Yes
Ownership: Voluntary non-profit - Church
Beds: 378

Key Personnel:
Operating Room. . . . . Bernita Berntsen, RN
Coronary Care . . . . Moussa Elbayoumy
CEO/President. . . . . Robert Erickson
Chief of Medical Staff . . . . Tom Hamilton, DO
Infection Control. . . . . Nancy Krohe
Chair/CEO . . . . Greg Schwerdt

Measure	Cases	This Hosp.	State Avg.	U.S. Avg.
Blood Clot Prevention and Treatment				
Anticoagulation Overlap Therapy[2]	76	92%	94%	93%
ICU Venous Thromboembolism Prophylaxis[2]	88	95%	91%	92%
Incidence of Potentially Preventable VTE[1,2]	-	-	8%	10%
UFH with Dosages/Platelet Monitoring[2]	54	100%	98%	97%
Venous Thromboembolism Prophylaxis[2]	345	90%	79%	85%
Warfarin Therapy Discharge Instructions[2]	54	100%	84%	75%
Chest Pain/Possible Heart Attack Care				
Aspirin Given Within 24 Hours of Arrival[5]	-	-	94%	96%
Fibrinolytic Meds Within 30 Min. of Arrival[5]	-	-	41%	58%
Average Time to ECG (minutes)[5]	-	-	8	7
Average Time to Transfer (minutes)[5]	-	-	57	60
Children's Asthma Care				
Received Home Management Plan of Care	-	-	-	88%
Received Reliever Medication	-	-	-	100%
Received Systemic Corticosteroids	-	-	-	100%
Emergency Department				
Admittance Decision Time (minutes)[2]	561	84	57	98
Head CT Results Within 45 Min. of Arrival[1,3]	-	-	53%	57%
Patients Who Left ER Before Being Seen	33,958	2%	2%	2%
Time from ER Arrival to Admit. (minutes)[2]	563	248	185	274
Time from ER Arrival to Discharge (minutes)	362	148	104	134
Time in ER Before Being Evaluated (minutes)	382	31	18	26
Time to Pain Meds for Fractures (minutes)	91	57	47	57
Heart Attack Care				
Aspirin Given at Discharge	162	100%	99%	99%
Fibrinolytic Meds Within 30 Min. of Arrival[7]	-	-	-	54%
PCI Within 90 Minutes of Arrival	21	100%	97%	96%
Statin Prescribed at Discharge	151	100%	99%	98%
Heart Failure Care				
ACE Inhibitor or ARB for LVSD	65	100%	95%	97%
Discharge Instructions Given	157	97%	91%	94%
Evaluation of LVS Function	204	100%	94%	99%
Medicare Spending				
Medicare Spending per Patient (ratio)	-	1.03	0.94	0.98
Pneumonia Care				
Appropriate Initial Antibiotic Given	117	97%	92%	95%
Blood Culture Timing	147	99%	98%	98%
Pregnancy and Delivery Care				
Newborn Deliveries Scheduled Early[2]	42	2%	12%	6%
Preventive Care				
Immunization for Influenza[2]	518	74%	88%	90%
Immunization for Pneumonia[2]	716	77%	90%	92%
Stroke Care				
Anticoagulation Therapy for Atrial Fibrillation	11	100%	88%	95%
Antithrombotic Therapy Timing	93	100%	97%	98%
Assessed for Rehabilitation	106	100%	97%	97%
Discharged on Antithrombotic Therapy	97	100%	98%	99%
Discharged on Statin Medication	78	100%	88%	94%
Thrombolytic Therapy Timing[1]	-	-	68%	66%
Venous Thromboembolism Prophylaxis	117	100%	93%	94%
Written Stroke Educational Materials Given	47	96%	84%	88%
Surgical Care Improvement Project				
Appropriate Beta Blocker Usage[2]	264	100%	98%	98%
Appropriate VTP Within 24 Hours[2]	633	100%	98%	98%
Controlled Postoperative Blood Glucose[2]	104	98%	98%	97%
Perioperative Temperature Management[2]	704	100%	100%	100%
Prophylactic Antibiotic Selection[2]	614	99%	99%	99%
Prophylactic Antibiotic Selection (Outpatient)	557	99%	98%	98%
Prophylactic Antibiotic Stopped[2]	607	100%	98%	98%
Prophylactic Antibiotic Timing[2]	614	100%	99%	99%
Prophylactic Antibiotic Timing (Outpatient)	567	96%	98%	98%
Urinary Catheter Removal[2]	587	100%	97%	97%
Survey of Patients' Hospital Experiences				
Area Around Room 'Always' Quiet at Night	300+	56%	65%	61%
Doctors 'Always' Communicated Well	300+	79%	85%	82%
Home Recovery Information Given	300+	86%	86%	85%
Hospital Given 9 or 10 on 10 Point Scale	300+	72%	76%	71%
Meds 'Always' Explained Before Given	300+	62%	66%	64%
Nurses 'Always' Communicated Well	300+	78%	81%	79%
Pain 'Always' Well Controlled	300+	69%	72%	71%
Room and Bathroom 'Always' Clean	300+	69%	76%	73%
Timely Help 'Always' Received	300+	63%	72%	68%
Would Definitely Recommend Hospital	300+	75%	75%	71%
Use of Medical Imaging				
Cardiac Imaging Stress Test before Surgery	719	5.7%	5%	5.3%
Combination Abdominal CT Scan	1,105	6.8%	19%	10.5%
Combination Brain/Sinus CT Scan	745	4.6%	2.9%	2.7%
Combination Chest CT Scan	647	0.8%	3.9%	2.7%
Follow-up Mammogram/Ultrasound	2,493	3.4%	7.8%	8.8%
Lumbar Spine MRI for Low Back Pain	382	37.4%	40.2%	37.2%

Stormont - Vail Healthcare

1500 Sw 10th St
Topeka, KS 66604
Phone: 785-354-6121
Fax: 785-354-5123
URL: www.stormontvail.org
Type: Acute Care Hospitals
Emergency Services: Yes
Ownership: Voluntary non-profit - Private
Beds: 586

Key Personnel:
Operating Room. . . . . Jane Asher, RN
Radiology. . . . . James Kilmartin, MD
Quality Assurance . . . . Mike Lummis
Chief of Medical Staff . . . . Kent Palmberg, MD
Patient Relations . . . . Carol Perry, RN
CEO/President. . . . . Randy Peterson
Emergency Room . . . . Dorothy Rice, RN

Measure	Cases	This Hosp.	State Avg.	U.S. Avg.
Blood Clot Prevention and Treatment				
Anticoagulation Overlap Therapy[2]	116	90%	94%	93%
ICU Venous Thromboembolism Prophylaxis[2]	94	100%	91%	92%
Incidence of Potentially Preventable VTE[1,2]	-	-	8%	10%
UFH with Dosages/Platelet Monitoring[2]	97	100%	98%	97%
Venous Thromboembolism Prophylaxis[2]	330	98%	79%	85%
Warfarin Therapy Discharge Instructions[2]	82	67%	84%	75%
Chest Pain/Possible Heart Attack Care				
Aspirin Given Within 24 Hours of Arrival[3,7]	-	-	94%	96%
Fibrinolytic Meds Within 30 Min. of Arrival[5]	-	-	41%	58%
Average Time to ECG (minutes)[3,7]	-	-	8	7
Average Time to Transfer (minutes)[5]	-	-	57	60
Children's Asthma Care				
Received Home Management Plan of Care	-	-	-	88%
Received Reliever Medication	-	-	-	100%
Received Systemic Corticosteroids	-	-	-	100%
Emergency Department				
Admittance Decision Time (minutes)[2]	575	34	57	98
Head CT Results Within 45 Min. of Arrival[1]	-	-	53%	57%
Patients Who Left ER Before Being Seen	63,191	1%	2%	2%
Time from ER Arrival to Admit. (minutes)[2]	583	234	185	274
Time from ER Arrival to Discharge (minutes)	445	162	104	134
Time in ER Before Being Evaluated (minutes)	431	19	18	26
Time to Pain Meds for Fractures (minutes)	187	45	47	57
Heart Attack Care				
Aspirin Given at Discharge	313	100%	99%	99%
Fibrinolytic Meds Within 30 Min. of Arrival[7]	-	-	-	54%
PCI Within 90 Minutes of Arrival	45	98%	97%	96%
Statin Prescribed at Discharge	299	100%	99%	98%
Heart Failure Care				
ACE Inhibitor or ARB for LVSD	120	100%	95%	97%
Discharge Instructions Given	331	100%	91%	94%
Evaluation of LVS Function	425	100%	94%	99%
Medicare Spending				
Medicare Spending per Patient (ratio)	-	1.00	0.94	0.98
Pneumonia Care				
Appropriate Initial Antibiotic Given	228	97%	92%	95%
Blood Culture Timing	425	100%	98%	98%
Pregnancy and Delivery Care				
Newborn Deliveries Scheduled Early	156	4%	12%	6%
Preventive Care				
Immunization for Influenza[2]	616	100%	88%	90%
Immunization for Pneumonia[2]	747	100%	90%	92%
Stroke Care				
Anticoagulation Therapy for Atrial Fibrillation	37	89%	88%	95%
Antithrombotic Therapy Timing	165	100%	97%	98%
Assessed for Rehabilitation	219	100%	97%	97%
Discharged on Antithrombotic Therapy	199	100%	98%	99%
Discharged on Statin Medication	152	99%	88%	94%
Thrombolytic Therapy Timing	26	92%	68%	66%
Venous Thromboembolism Prophylaxis	227	100%	93%	94%
Written Stroke Educational Materials Given	90	100%	84%	88%
Surgical Care Improvement Project				
Appropriate Beta Blocker Usage[2]	422	99%	98%	98%
Appropriate VTP Within 24 Hours[2]	937	99%	98%	98%
Controlled Postoperative Blood Glucose[2]	187	98%	98%	97%
Perioperative Temperature Management[2]	1,030	100%	100%	100%
Prophylactic Antibiotic Selection[2]	963	100%	99%	99%
Prophylactic Antibiotic Selection (Outpatient)	841	99%	98%	98%
Prophylactic Antibiotic Stopped[2]	947	99%	98%	98%
Prophylactic Antibiotic Timing[2]	966	100%	99%	99%
Prophylactic Antibiotic Timing (Outpatient)	843	99%	98%	98%
Urinary Catheter Removal[2]	382	97%	97%	97%
Survey of Patients' Hospital Experiences				
Area Around Room 'Always' Quiet at Night	300+	64%	65%	61%
Doctors 'Always' Communicated Well	300+	80%	85%	82%
Home Recovery Information Given	300+	90%	86%	85%
Hospital Given 9 or 10 on 10 Point Scale	300+	76%	76%	71%
Meds 'Always' Explained Before Given	300+	64%	66%	64%
Nurses 'Always' Communicated Well	300+	78%	81%	79%
Pain 'Always' Well Controlled	300+	68%	72%	71%
Room and Bathroom 'Always' Clean	300+	71%	76%	73%
Timely Help 'Always' Received	300+	68%	72%	68%
Would Definitely Recommend Hospital	300+	79%	75%	71%
Use of Medical Imaging				
Cardiac Imaging Stress Test before Surgery	1,619	5.2%	5%	5.3%
Combination Abdominal CT Scan	2,206	6.1%	19%	10.5%
Combination Brain/Sinus CT Scan	1,540	1.9%	2.9%	2.7%
Combination Chest CT Scan	1,369	0.9%	3.9%	2.7%
Follow-up Mammogram/Ultrasound[7]	-	-	7.8%	8.8%
Lumbar Spine MRI for Low Back Pain	609	38.4%	40.2%	37.2%

Greeley County Health Services

506 3rd Street
Tribune, KS 67879
Phone: 620-376-4221
Fax: 620-376-2406
Type: Critical Access Hospitals
Emergency Services: Yes
Ownership: Government - Local
Beds: 18

Key Personnel:
CEO/President. . . . . Todd Burch
Quality Assurance . . . . Lisa Larkin, RN
Chief of Medical Staff . . . . Robert P Moser, MD
Emergency Room . . . . Robert P Moser, MD
Infection Control. . . . . Linda Peterson, RN

Measure	Cases	This Hosp.	State Avg.	U.S. Avg.
Blood Clot Prevention and Treatment				

NOTE: Hospital profiles are in alphabetical order by state, then city, then hospital within the city; Rankings exclude hospitals with less than 25 cases except for patient surveys which excludes hospitals with less than 100 cases; (a) 100-299 cases; (1) The number of cases/patients is too few to report; (2) Data submitted were based on a sample of cases/patients; (3) Results are based on a shorter time period than required; (4) Data suppressed by CMS for one or more quarters; (5) Results are not available for this reporting period; (6) Fewer than 100 patients completed the HCAHPS survey; (7) No cases met the criteria for this measure; (8) The lower limit of the confidence interval cannot be calculated if the number of observed infections equals zero; (9) No data are available from the state/territory for this reporting period; (10) The scores shown reflect fewer than 50 completed surveys; (11) There were discrepancies in the data collection process; (12) This measure does not apply to this hospital for this reporting period; (13) Results cannot be calculated for this reporting period; (14) The results for this state are combined with nearby states to protect confidentiality; Please refer to the User's Guide for a full explanation of data.

Measure	Cases	This Hosp.	State Avg.	U.S. Avg.
Anticoagulation Overlap Therapy[5]	-	-	94%	93%
ICU Venous Thromboembolism Prophylaxis[5]	-	-	91%	92%
Incidence of Potentially Preventable VTE[5]	-	-	8%	10%
UFH with Dosages/Platelet Monitoring[5]	-	-	98%	97%
Venous Thromboembolism Prophylaxis[5]	-	-	79%	85%
Warfarin Therapy Discharge Instructions[5]	-	-	84%	75%
Chest Pain/Possible Heart Attack Care				
Aspirin Given Within 24 Hours of Arrival	-	-	94%	96%
Fibrinolytic Meds Within 30 Min. of Arrival	-	-	41%	58%
Average Time to ECG (minutes)	-	-	8	7
Average Time to Transfer (minutes)	-	-	57	60
Children's Asthma Care				
Received Home Management Plan of Care	-	-	-	88%
Received Reliever Medication	-	-	-	100%
Received Systemic Corticosteroids	-	-	-	100%
Emergency Department				
Admittance Decision Time (minutes)[5]	-	-	57	98
Head CT Results Within 45 Min. of Arrival	-	-	53%	57%
Patients Who Left ER Before Being Seen	-	-	2%	2%
Time from ER Arrival to Admit. (minutes)[5]	-	-	185	274
Time from ER Arrival to Discharge (minutes)	-	-	104	134
Time in ER Before Being Evaluated (minutes)	-	-	18	26
Time to Pain Meds for Fractures (minutes)	-	-	47	57
Heart Attack Care				
Aspirin Given at Discharge[1,3]	-	-	99%	99%
Fibrinolytic Meds Within 30 Min. of Arrival[3,7]	-	-	-	54%
PCI Within 90 Minutes of Arrival[3,7]	-	-	97%	96%
Statin Prescribed at Discharge[1,3]	-	-	99%	98%
Heart Failure Care				
ACE Inhibitor or ARB for LVSD[1]	-	-	95%	97%
Discharge Instructions Given[1]	-	-	91%	94%
Evaluation of LVS Function[1]	-	-	94%	99%
Medicare Spending				
Medicare Spending per Patient (ratio)	-	-	0.94	0.98
Pneumonia Care				
Appropriate Initial Antibiotic Given[1]	-	-	92%	95%
Blood Culture Timing[1]	-	-	98%	98%
Pregnancy and Delivery Care				
Newborn Deliveries Scheduled Early[5]	-	-	12%	6%
Preventive Care				
Immunization for Influenza[5]	-	-	88%	90%
Immunization for Pneumonia[5]	-	-	90%	92%
Stroke Care				
Anticoagulation Therapy for Atrial Fibrillation[5]	-	-	88%	95%
Antithrombotic Therapy Timing[5]	-	-	97%	98%
Assessed for Rehabilitation[5]	-	-	97%	97%
Discharged on Antithrombotic Therapy[5]	-	-	98%	99%
Discharged on Statin Medication[5]	-	-	88%	94%
Thrombolytic Therapy Timing[5]	-	-	68%	66%
Venous Thromboembolism Prophylaxis[5]	-	-	93%	94%
Written Stroke Educational Materials Given[5]	-	-	84%	88%
Surgical Care Improvement Project				
Appropriate Beta Blocker Usage[5]	-	-	98%	98%
Appropriate VTP Within 24 Hours[5]	-	-	98%	98%
Controlled Postoperative Blood Glucose[5]	-	-	98%	97%
Perioperative Temperature Management[5]	-	-	100%	100%
Prophylactic Antibiotic Selection[5]	-	-	99%	99%
Prophylactic Antibiotic Selection (Outpatient)	-	-	98%	98%
Prophylactic Antibiotic Stopped[5]	-	-	98%	98%
Prophylactic Antibiotic Timing[5]	-	-	99%	99%
Prophylactic Antibiotic Timing (Outpatient)	-	-	98%	98%
Urinary Catheter Removal[5]	-	-	97%	97%
Survey of Patients' Hospital Experiences				
Area Around Room 'Always' Quiet at Night[6]	<100	61%	65%	61%
Doctors 'Always' Communicated Well[6]	<100	88%	85%	82%
Home Recovery Information Given[6]	<100	71%	86%	85%
Hospital Given 9 or 10 on 10 Point Scale[6]	<100	80%	76%	71%
Meds 'Always' Explained Before Given[6]	<100	71%	66%	64%
Nurses 'Always' Communicated Well[6]	<100	80%	81%	79%
Pain 'Always' Well Controlled[6]	<100	73%	72%	71%
Room and Bathroom 'Always' Clean[6]	<100	87%	76%	73%
Timely Help 'Always' Received[6]	<100	80%	72%	68%
Would Definitely Recommend Hospital[6]	<100	85%	75%	71%
Use of Medical Imaging				
Cardiac Imaging Stress Test before Surgery	-	-	5%	5.3%
Combination Abdominal CT Scan	-	-	19%	10.5%
Combination Brain/Sinus CT Scan	-	-	2.9%	2.7%
Combination Chest CT Scan	-	-	3.9%	2.7%
Follow-up Mammogram/Ultrasound	-	-	7.8%	8.8%
Lumbar Spine MRI for Low Back Pain	-	-	40.2%	37.2%

Bob Wilson Memorial Grant County Hospital

415 N Main Street
Ulysses, KS 67880
URL: www.bwmgch.com
Type: Acute Care Hospitals
Ownership: Government - Local
Phone: 620-356-1266
Fax: 620-356-2302
Emergency Services: Yes
Beds: 46

Key Personnel:
CEO/President. . . . . Steve Daniel
CEO . . . . Art Frable
Quality Assurance . . . . Karoala Nicholas

Measure	Cases	This Hosp.	State Avg.	U.S. Avg.
Blood Clot Prevention and Treatment				
Anticoagulation Overlap Therapy[1,2]	-	-	94%	93%
ICU Venous Thromboembolism Prophylaxis[2,7]	-	-	91%	92%
Incidence of Potentially Preventable VTE[2,7]	-	-	8%	10%
UFH with Dosages/Platelet Monitoring[2,7]	-	-	98%	97%
Venous Thromboembolism Prophylaxis[2]	113	0%	79%	85%
Warfarin Therapy Discharge Instructions[1,2]	-	-	84%	75%
Chest Pain/Possible Heart Attack Care				
Aspirin Given Within 24 Hours of Arrival	14	100%	94%	96%
Fibrinolytic Meds Within 30 Min. of Arrival[1]	-	-	41%	58%
Average Time to ECG (minutes)	13	11	8	7
Average Time to Transfer (minutes)[7]	-	-	57	60
Children's Asthma Care				
Received Home Management Plan of Care	-	-	-	88%
Received Reliever Medication	-	-	-	100%
Received Systemic Corticosteroids	-	-	-	100%
Emergency Department				
Admittance Decision Time (minutes)[2]	84	52	57	98
Head CT Results Within 45 Min. of Arrival[1,3]	-	-	53%	57%
Patients Who Left ER Before Being Seen	2,849	0%	2%	2%
Time from ER Arrival to Admit. (minutes)[2]	93	117	185	274
Time from ER Arrival to Discharge (minutes)	311	72	104	134
Time in ER Before Being Evaluated (minutes)	294	30	18	26
Time to Pain Meds for Fractures (minutes)	21	60	47	57
Heart Attack Care				
Aspirin Given at Discharge[5]	-	-	99%	99%
Fibrinolytic Meds Within 30 Min. of Arrival[5]	-	-	-	54%
PCI Within 90 Minutes of Arrival[5]	-	-	97%	96%
Statin Prescribed at Discharge[5]	-	-	99%	98%
Heart Failure Care				
ACE Inhibitor or ARB for LVSD[1,2]	-	-	95%	97%
Discharge Instructions Given[1,2]	-	-	91%	94%
Evaluation of LVS Function[1,2]	-	-	94%	99%
Medicare Spending				
Medicare Spending per Patient (ratio)	-	0.74	0.94	0.98
Pneumonia Care				
Appropriate Initial Antibiotic Given[1,2]	-	-	92%	95%
Blood Culture Timing[1,2]	-	-	98%	98%
Pregnancy and Delivery Care				
Newborn Deliveries Scheduled Early[2]	15	27%	12%	6%
Preventive Care				
Immunization for Influenza[2]	171	48%	88%	90%
Immunization for Pneumonia[2]	139	65%	90%	92%
Stroke Care				
Anticoagulation Therapy for Atrial Fibrillation[3,7]	-	-	88%	95%
Antithrombotic Therapy Timing[1,3]	-	-	97%	98%
Assessed for Rehabilitation[1,3]	-	-	97%	97%
Discharged on Antithrombotic Therapy[1,3]	-	-	98%	99%
Discharged on Statin Medication[1,3]	-	-	88%	94%
Thrombolytic Therapy Timing[1,3]	-	-	68%	66%
Venous Thromboembolism Prophylaxis[1,3]	-	-	93%	94%
Written Stroke Educational Materials Given[1,3]	-	-	84%	88%
Surgical Care Improvement Project				
Appropriate Beta Blocker Usage[1,2]	-	-	98%	98%
Appropriate VTP Within 24 Hours[1,2]	-	-	98%	98%
Controlled Postoperative Blood Glucose[2,3]	-	-	98%	97%
Perioperative Temperature Management[1,2]	-	-	100%	100%
Prophylactic Antibiotic Selection[1,2]	-	-	99%	99%
Prophylactic Antibiotic Selection (Outpatient)[5]	-	-	98%	98%
Prophylactic Antibiotic Stopped[1,2]	-	-	98%	98%
Prophylactic Antibiotic Timing[1,2]	-	-	99%	99%
Prophylactic Antibiotic Timing (Outpatient)[5]	-	-	98%	98%
Urinary Catheter Removal[1,2]	-	-	97%	97%
Survey of Patients' Hospital Experiences				
Area Around Room 'Always' Quiet at Night[6]	<100	65%	65%	61%
Doctors 'Always' Communicated Well[6]	<100	78%	85%	82%
Home Recovery Information Given[6]	<100	72%	86%	85%
Hospital Given 9 or 10 on 10 Point Scale[6]	<100	53%	76%	71%
Meds 'Always' Explained Before Given[6]	<100	65%	66%	64%
Nurses 'Always' Communicated Well[6]	<100	77%	81%	79%
Pain 'Always' Well Controlled[6]	<100	64%	72%	71%
Room and Bathroom 'Always' Clean[6]	<100	75%	76%	73%
Timely Help 'Always' Received[6]	<100	76%	72%	68%
Would Definitely Recommend Hospital[6]	<100	58%	75%	71%
Use of Medical Imaging				
Cardiac Imaging Stress Test before Surgery[7]	-	-	5%	5.3%
Combination Abdominal CT Scan[1]	-	-	19%	10.5%
Combination Brain/Sinus CT Scan[1]	-	-	2.9%	2.7%
Combination Chest CT Scan[1]	-	-	3.9%	2.7%
Follow-up Mammogram/Ultrasound	106	2.8%	7.8%	8.8%
Lumbar Spine MRI for Low Back Pain[1]	-	-	40.2%	37.2%

Trego County Lemke Memorial Hospital

320 Thirteenth St
Wa Keeney, KS 67672
Type: Critical Access Hospitals
Ownership: Government - Local
Phone: 785-743-2182
Fax: 785-743-6317
Emergency Services: Yes
Beds: 25

Key Personnel:
Pulmonology . . . . Kent B. Berquist, MD
Quality Assurance . . . . Lavonne Finck
Emergency Room . . . . Judy Hearting
Operating Room. . . . . Judy Hearting
Cardiology . . . . Mohammed Janif
CEO/President. . . . . Stacey Malson
Infection Control. . . . . Mary Jo McClannahan
Radiology. . . . . Brian Shaw

Measure	Cases	This Hosp.	State Avg.	U.S. Avg.
Blood Clot Prevention and Treatment				
Anticoagulation Overlap Therapy[5]	-	-	94%	93%
ICU Venous Thromboembolism Prophylaxis[5]	-	-	91%	92%
Incidence of Potentially Preventable VTE[5]	-	-	8%	10%
UFH with Dosages/Platelet Monitoring[5]	-	-	98%	97%
Venous Thromboembolism Prophylaxis[5]	-	-	79%	85%
Warfarin Therapy Discharge Instructions[5]	-	-	84%	75%
Chest Pain/Possible Heart Attack Care				
Aspirin Given Within 24 Hours of Arrival	-	-	94%	96%
Fibrinolytic Meds Within 30 Min. of Arrival	-	-	41%	58%
Average Time to ECG (minutes)	-	-	8	7
Average Time to Transfer (minutes)	-	-	57	60
Children's Asthma Care				
Received Home Management Plan of Care	-	-	-	88%
Received Reliever Medication	-	-	-	100%
Received Systemic Corticosteroids	-	-	-	100%
Emergency Department				
Admittance Decision Time (minutes)[5]	-	-	57	98
Head CT Results Within 45 Min. of Arrival	-	-	53%	57%
Patients Who Left ER Before Being Seen	-	-	2%	2%
Time from ER Arrival to Admit. (minutes)[5]	-	-	185	274
Time from ER Arrival to Discharge (minutes)	-	-	104	134
Time in ER Before Being Evaluated (minutes)	-	-	18	26
Time to Pain Meds for Fractures (minutes)	-	-	47	57
Heart Attack Care				
Aspirin Given at Discharge[5]	-	-	99%	99%
Fibrinolytic Meds Within 30 Min. of Arrival[5]	-	-	-	54%
PCI Within 90 Minutes of Arrival[5]	-	-	97%	96%
Statin Prescribed at Discharge[5]	-	-	99%	98%
Heart Failure Care				

NOTE: Hospital profiles are in alphabetical order by state, then city, then hospital within the city; Rankings exclude hospitals with less than 25 cases except for patient surveys which excludes hospitals with less than 100 cases; (a) 100-299 cases; (1) The number of cases/patients is too few to report; (2) Data submitted were based on a sample of cases/patients; (3) Results are based on a shorter time period than required; (4) Data suppressed by CMS for one or more quarters; (5) Results are not available for this reporting period; (6) Fewer than 100 patients completed the HCAHPS survey; (7) No cases met the criteria for this measure; (8) The lower limit of the confidence interval cannot be calculated if the number of observed infections equals zero; (9) No data are available from the state/territory for this reporting period; (10) The scores shown reflect fewer than 50 completed surveys; (11) There were discrepancies in the data collection process; (12) This measure does not apply to this hospital for this reporting period; (13) Results cannot be calculated for this reporting period; (14) The results for this state are combined with nearby states to protect confidentiality; Please refer to the User's Guide for a full explanation of data.

Measure	Cases	This Hosp.	State Avg.	U.S. Avg.
ACE Inhibitor or ARB for LVSD[7]	-	-	95%	97%
Discharge Instructions Given[1]	-	-	91%	94%
Evaluation of LVS Function	16	81%	94%	99%
Medicare Spending				
Medicare Spending per Patient (ratio)	-	-	0.94	0.98
Pneumonia Care				
Appropriate Initial Antibiotic Given	23	70%	92%	95%
Blood Culture Timing	30	100%	98%	98%
Pregnancy and Delivery Care				
Newborn Deliveries Scheduled Early[5]	-	-	12%	6%
Preventive Care				
Immunization for Influenza[5]	-	-	88%	90%
Immunization for Pneumonia[5]	-	-	90%	92%
Stroke Care				
Anticoagulation Therapy for Atrial Fibrillation[5]	-	-	88%	95%
Antithrombotic Therapy Timing[5]	-	-	97%	98%
Assessed for Rehabilitation[5]	-	-	97%	97%
Discharged on Antithrombotic Therapy[5]	-	-	98%	99%
Discharged on Statin Medication[5]	-	-	88%	94%
Thrombolytic Therapy Timing[5]	-	-	68%	66%
Venous Thromboembolism Prophylaxis[5]	-	-	93%	94%
Written Stroke Educational Materials Given[5]	-	-	84%	88%
Surgical Care Improvement Project				
Appropriate Beta Blocker Usage[5]	-	-	98%	98%
Appropriate VTP Within 24 Hours[5]	-	-	98%	98%
Controlled Postoperative Blood Glucose[5]	-	-	98%	97%
Perioperative Temperature Management[5]	-	-	100%	100%
Prophylactic Antibiotic Selection[5]	-	-	99%	99%
Prophylactic Antibiotic Selection (Outpatient)	-	-	98%	98%
Prophylactic Antibiotic Stopped[5]	-	-	98%	98%
Prophylactic Antibiotic Timing[5]	-	-	99%	99%
Prophylactic Antibiotic Timing (Outpatient)	-	-	98%	98%
Urinary Catheter Removal[5]	-	-	97%	97%
Survey of Patients' Hospital Experiences				
Area Around Room 'Always' Quiet at Night[6]	<100	54%	65%	61%
Doctors 'Always' Communicated Well[6]	<100	89%	85%	82%
Home Recovery Information Given[6]	<100	88%	86%	85%
Hospital Given 9 or 10 on 10 Point Scale[6]	<100	77%	76%	71%
Meds 'Always' Explained Before Given[6]	<100	61%	66%	64%
Nurses 'Always' Communicated Well[6]	<100	82%	81%	79%
Pain 'Always' Well Controlled[6]	<100	71%	72%	71%
Room and Bathroom 'Always' Clean[6]	<100	76%	76%	73%
Timely Help 'Always' Received[6]	<100	72%	72%	68%
Would Definitely Recommend Hospital[6]	<100	85%	75%	71%
Use of Medical Imaging				
Cardiac Imaging Stress Test before Surgery	-	-	5%	5.3%
Combination Abdominal CT Scan	-	-	19%	10.5%
Combination Brain/Sinus CT Scan	-	-	2.9%	2.7%
Combination Chest CT Scan	-	-	3.9%	2.7%
Follow-up Mammogram/Ultrasound	-	-	7.8%	8.8%
Lumbar Spine MRI for Low Back Pain	-	-	40.2%	37.2%

Wamego Health Center

711 Genn Drive
Wamego, KS 66547
URL: www.wamegocityhospital.com
Type: Critical Access Hospitals
Ownership: Voluntary non-profit - Private

Phone: 785-458-7201
Fax: 785-456-6916
Emergency Services: Yes
Beds: 26

Measure	Cases	This Hosp.	State Avg.	U.S. Avg.
Blood Clot Prevention and Treatment				
Anticoagulation Overlap Therapy[5]	-	-	94%	93%
ICU Venous Thromboembolism Prophylaxis[5]	-	-	91%	92%
Incidence of Potentially Preventable VTE[5]	-	-	8%	10%
UFH with Dosages/Platelet Monitoring[5]	-	-	98%	97%
Venous Thromboembolism Prophylaxis[5]	-	-	79%	85%
Warfarin Therapy Discharge Instructions[5]	-	-	84%	75%
Chest Pain/Possible Heart Attack Care				
Aspirin Given Within 24 Hours of Arrival[5]	-	-	94%	96%
Fibrinolytic Meds Within 30 Min. of Arrival[5]	-	-	41%	58%
Average Time to ECG (minutes)[5]	-	-	8	7
Average Time to Transfer (minutes)[5]	-	-	57	60
Children's Asthma Care				
Received Home Management Plan of Care	-	-	-	88%
Received Reliever Medication	-	-	-	100%
Received Systemic Corticosteroids	-	-	-	100%
Emergency Department				
Admittance Decision Time (minutes)[5]	-	-	57	98
Head CT Results Within 45 Min. of Arrival[5]	-	-	53%	57%
Patients Who Left ER Before Being Seen[5]	-	-	2%	2%
Time from ER Arrival to Admit. (minutes)[5]	-	-	185	274
Time from ER Arrival to Discharge (minutes)[5]	-	-	104	134
Time in ER Before Being Evaluated (minutes)[5]	-	-	18	26
Time to Pain Meds for Fractures (minutes)[5]	-	-	47	57
Heart Attack Care				
Aspirin Given at Discharge[5]	-	-	99%	99%
Fibrinolytic Meds Within 30 Min. of Arrival[5]	-	-	-	54%
PCI Within 90 Minutes of Arrival[5]	-	-	97%	96%
Statin Prescribed at Discharge[5]	-	-	99%	98%
Heart Failure Care				
ACE Inhibitor or ARB for LVSD[3,7]	-	-	95%	97%
Discharge Instructions Given[1,3]	-	-	91%	94%
Evaluation of LVS Function[1,3]	-	-	94%	99%
Medicare Spending				
Medicare Spending per Patient (ratio)	-	-	0.94	0.98
Pneumonia Care				
Appropriate Initial Antibiotic Given[1]	-	-	92%	95%
Blood Culture Timing[1]	-	-	98%	98%
Pregnancy and Delivery Care				
Newborn Deliveries Scheduled Early[5]	-	-	12%	6%
Preventive Care				
Immunization for Influenza[5]	-	-	88%	90%
Immunization for Pneumonia[5]	-	-	90%	92%
Stroke Care				
Anticoagulation Therapy for Atrial Fibrillation[5]	-	-	88%	95%
Antithrombotic Therapy Timing[5]	-	-	97%	98%
Assessed for Rehabilitation[5]	-	-	97%	97%
Discharged on Antithrombotic Therapy[5]	-	-	98%	99%
Discharged on Statin Medication[5]	-	-	88%	94%
Thrombolytic Therapy Timing[5]	-	-	68%	66%
Venous Thromboembolism Prophylaxis[5]	-	-	93%	94%
Written Stroke Educational Materials Given[5]	-	-	84%	88%
Surgical Care Improvement Project				
Appropriate Beta Blocker Usage[5]	-	-	98%	98%
Appropriate VTP Within 24 Hours[5]	-	-	98%	98%
Controlled Postoperative Blood Glucose[5]	-	-	98%	97%
Perioperative Temperature Management[5]	-	-	100%	100%
Prophylactic Antibiotic Selection[5]	-	-	99%	99%
Prophylactic Antibiotic Selection (Outpatient)[5]	-	-	98%	98%
Prophylactic Antibiotic Stopped[5]	-	-	98%	98%
Prophylactic Antibiotic Timing[5]	-	-	99%	99%
Prophylactic Antibiotic Timing (Outpatient)[5]	-	-	98%	98%
Urinary Catheter Removal[5]	-	-	97%	97%
Survey of Patients' Hospital Experiences				
Area Around Room 'Always' Quiet at Night[10]	<100	70%	65%	61%
Doctors 'Always' Communicated Well[10]	<100	91%	85%	82%
Home Recovery Information Given[10]	<100	91%	86%	85%
Hospital Given 9 or 10 on 10 Point Scale[10]	<100	87%	76%	71%
Meds 'Always' Explained Before Given[10]	<100	80%	66%	64%
Nurses 'Always' Communicated Well[10]	<100	88%	81%	79%
Pain 'Always' Well Controlled[10]	<100	64%	72%	71%
Room and Bathroom 'Always' Clean[10]	<100	88%	76%	73%
Timely Help 'Always' Received[10]	<100	80%	72%	68%
Would Definitely Recommend Hospital[10]	<100	84%	75%	71%
Use of Medical Imaging				
Cardiac Imaging Stress Test before Surgery[7]	-	-	5%	5.3%
Combination Abdominal CT Scan[1]	-	-	19%	10.5%
Combination Brain/Sinus CT Scan[1]	-	-	2.9%	2.7%
Combination Chest CT Scan	58	3.4%	3.9%	2.7%
Follow-up Mammogram/Ultrasound	182	8.2%	7.8%	8.8%
Lumbar Spine MRI for Low Back Pain[1]	-	-	40.2%	37.2%

Washington County Hospital

304 E 3rd Street
Washington, KS 66968
Type: Critical Access Hospitals
Ownership: Government - Local

Phone: 785-325-2211
Fax: 785-325-3224
Emergency Services: Yes
Beds: 27

Key Personnel:
Chief of Medical Staff . . . . David Hodgson
CEO/President . . . . Everett Lutjemeier
Quality Assurance . . . . Clifford Steward
Emergency Room . . . . Marry Walter

Measure	Cases	This Hosp.	State Avg.	U.S. Avg.
Blood Clot Prevention and Treatment				
Anticoagulation Overlap Therapy[5]	-	-	94%	93%
ICU Venous Thromboembolism Prophylaxis[5]	-	-	91%	92%
Incidence of Potentially Preventable VTE[5]	-	-	8%	10%
UFH with Dosages/Platelet Monitoring[5]	-	-	98%	97%
Venous Thromboembolism Prophylaxis[5]	-	-	79%	85%
Warfarin Therapy Discharge Instructions[5]	-	-	84%	75%
Chest Pain/Possible Heart Attack Care				
Aspirin Given Within 24 Hours of Arrival	-	-	94%	96%
Fibrinolytic Meds Within 30 Min. of Arrival	-	-	41%	58%
Average Time to ECG (minutes)	-	-	8	7
Average Time to Transfer (minutes)	-	-	57	60
Children's Asthma Care				
Received Home Management Plan of Care	-	-	-	88%
Received Reliever Medication	-	-	-	100%
Received Systemic Corticosteroids	-	-	-	100%
Emergency Department				
Admittance Decision Time (minutes)[5]	-	-	57	98
Head CT Results Within 45 Min. of Arrival	-	-	53%	57%
Patients Who Left ER Before Being Seen	-	-	2%	2%
Time from ER Arrival to Admit. (minutes)[5]	-	-	185	274
Time from ER Arrival to Discharge (minutes)	-	-	104	134
Time in ER Before Being Evaluated (minutes)	-	-	18	26
Time to Pain Meds for Fractures (minutes)	-	-	47	57
Heart Attack Care				
Aspirin Given at Discharge[5]	-	-	99%	99%
Fibrinolytic Meds Within 30 Min. of Arrival[5]	-	-	-	54%
PCI Within 90 Minutes of Arrival[5]	-	-	97%	96%
Statin Prescribed at Discharge[5]	-	-	99%	98%
Heart Failure Care				
ACE Inhibitor or ARB for LVSD[5]	-	-	95%	97%
Discharge Instructions Given[5]	-	-	91%	94%
Evaluation of LVS Function[5]	-	-	94%	99%
Medicare Spending				
Medicare Spending per Patient (ratio)	-	-	0.94	0.98
Pneumonia Care				
Appropriate Initial Antibiotic Given	14	86%	92%	95%
Blood Culture Timing[7]	-	-	98%	98%
Pregnancy and Delivery Care				
Newborn Deliveries Scheduled Early[5]	-	-	12%	6%
Preventive Care				
Immunization for Influenza[5]	-	-	88%	90%
Immunization for Pneumonia[5]	-	-	90%	92%
Stroke Care				
Anticoagulation Therapy for Atrial Fibrillation[5]	-	-	88%	95%
Antithrombotic Therapy Timing[5]	-	-	97%	98%
Assessed for Rehabilitation[5]	-	-	97%	97%
Discharged on Antithrombotic Therapy[5]	-	-	98%	99%
Discharged on Statin Medication[5]	-	-	88%	94%
Thrombolytic Therapy Timing[5]	-	-	68%	66%
Venous Thromboembolism Prophylaxis[5]	-	-	93%	94%
Written Stroke Educational Materials Given[5]	-	-	84%	88%
Surgical Care Improvement Project				
Appropriate Beta Blocker Usage[5]	-	-	98%	98%
Appropriate VTP Within 24 Hours[5]	-	-	98%	98%
Controlled Postoperative Blood Glucose[5]	-	-	98%	97%
Perioperative Temperature Management[5]	-	-	100%	100%
Prophylactic Antibiotic Selection[5]	-	-	99%	99%
Prophylactic Antibiotic Selection (Outpatient)	-	-	98%	98%
Prophylactic Antibiotic Stopped[5]	-	-	98%	98%
Prophylactic Antibiotic Timing[5]	-	-	99%	99%
Prophylactic Antibiotic Timing (Outpatient)	-	-	98%	98%

NOTE: Hospital profiles are in alphabetical order by state, then city, then hospital within the city; Rankings exclude hospitals with less than 25 cases except for patient surveys which excludes hospitals with less than 100 cases; (a) 100-299 cases; (1) The number of cases/patients is too few to report; (2) Data submitted were based on a sample of cases/patients; (3) Results are based on a shorter time period than required; (4) Data suppressed by CMS for one or more quarters; (5) Results are not available for this reporting period; (6) Fewer than 100 patients completed the HCAHPS survey; (7) No cases met the criteria for this measure; (8) The lower limit of the confidence interval cannot be calculated if the number of observed infections equals zero; (9) No data are available from the state/territory for this reporting period; (10) The scores shown reflect fewer than 50 completed surveys; (11) There were discrepancies in the data collection process; (12) This measure does not apply to this hospital for this reporting period; (13) Results cannot be calculated for this reporting period; (14) The results for this state are combined with nearby states to protect confidentiality; Please refer to the User's Guide for a full explanation of data.

Measure	Cases	This Hosp.	State Avg.	U.S. Avg.
Urinary Catheter Removal[5]	-	-	97%	97%
Survey of Patients' Hospital Experiences				
Area Around Room 'Always' Quiet at Night[5]	-	-	65%	61%
Doctors 'Always' Communicated Well[5]	-	-	85%	82%
Home Recovery Information Given[5]	-	-	86%	85%
Hospital Given 9 or 10 on 10 Point Scale[5]	-	-	76%	71%
Meds 'Always' Explained Before Given[5]	-	-	66%	64%
Nurses 'Always' Communicated Well[5]	-	-	81%	79%
Pain 'Always' Well Controlled[5]	-	-	72%	71%
Room and Bathroom 'Always' Clean[5]	-	-	76%	73%
Timely Help 'Always' Received[5]	-	-	72%	68%
Would Definitely Recommend Hospital[5]	-	-	75%	71%
Use of Medical Imaging				
Cardiac Imaging Stress Test before Surgery	-	-	5%	5.3%
Combination Abdominal CT Scan	-	-	19%	10.5%
Combination Brain/Sinus CT Scan	-	-	2.9%	2.7%
Combination Chest CT Scan	-	-	3.9%	2.7%
Follow-up Mammogram/Ultrasound	-	-	7.8%	8.8%
Lumbar Spine MRI for Low Back Pain	-	-	40.2%	37.2%

Sumner Regional Medical Center

1323 North A St
Wellington, KS 67152
Phone: 620-399-1299
Fax: 620-326-2225
URL: www.srmcks.org
Type: Acute Care Hospitals
Emergency Services: Yes
Ownership: Government - Local
Beds: 80

Key Personnel:
Chief of Medical Staff.......... Larry Anderson
Chairman/CEO .... Fred Hinman, PhD
Radiology.................. Neil Rosenquist
Quality Assurance .... Susan Runyan

Measure	Cases	This Hosp.	State Avg.	U.S. Avg.
Blood Clot Prevention and Treatment				
Anticoagulation Overlap Therapy[1,2]	-	-	94%	93%
ICU Venous Thromboembolism Prophylaxis[1,2]	-	-	91%	92%
Incidence of Potentially Preventable VTE[2,7]	-	-	8%	10%
UFH with Dosages/Platelet Monitoring[2,7]	-	-	98%	97%
Venous Thromboembolism Prophylaxis[2]	169	23%	79%	85%
Warfarin Therapy Discharge Instructions[1,2]	-	-	84%	75%
Chest Pain/Possible Heart Attack Care				
Aspirin Given Within 24 Hours of Arrival	24	79%	94%	96%
Fibrinolytic Meds Within 30 Min. of Arrival[1,3]	-	-	41%	58%
Average Time to ECG (minutes)	23	13	8	7
Average Time to Transfer (minutes)[3,7]	-	-	57	60
Children's Asthma Care				
Received Home Management Plan of Care	-	-	-	88%
Received Reliever Medication	-	-	-	100%
Received Systemic Corticosteroids	-	-	-	100%
Emergency Department				
Admittance Decision Time (minutes)	54	27	57	98
Head CT Results Within 45 Min. of Arrival[1,3]	-	-	53%	57%
Patients Who Left ER Before Being Seen	3,982	1%	2%	2%
Time from ER Arrival to Admit. (minutes)	66	145	185	274
Time from ER Arrival to Discharge (minutes)	384	80	104	134
Time in ER Before Being Evaluated (minutes)	435	44	18	26
Time to Pain Meds for Fractures (minutes)	20	56	47	57
Heart Attack Care				
Aspirin Given at Discharge[3,7]	-	-	99%	99%
Fibrinolytic Meds Within 30 Min. of Arrival[3,7]	-	-	-	54%
PCI Within 90 Minutes of Arrival[3,7]	-	-	97%	96%
Statin Prescribed at Discharge[3,7]	-	-	99%	98%
Heart Failure Care				
ACE Inhibitor or ARB for LVSD[3,7]	-	-	95%	97%
Discharge Instructions Given[1,3]	-	-	91%	94%
Evaluation of LVS Function[1,3]	-	-	94%	99%
Medicare Spending				
Medicare Spending per Patient (ratio)	-	0.91	0.94	0.98
Pneumonia Care				
Appropriate Initial Antibiotic Given	23	70%	92%	95%
Blood Culture Timing[1]	-	-	98%	98%
Pregnancy and Delivery Care				
Newborn Deliveries Scheduled Early	19	16%	12%	6%
Preventive Care				
Immunization for Influenza	197	50%	88%	90%
Immunization for Pneumonia[2]	206	67%	90%	92%
Stroke Care				
Anticoagulation Therapy for Atrial Fibrillation[3,7]	-	-	88%	95%
Antithrombotic Therapy Timing[1,3]	-	-	97%	98%
Assessed for Rehabilitation[1,3]	-	-	97%	97%
Discharged on Antithrombotic Therapy[1,3]	-	-	98%	99%
Discharged on Statin Medication[1,3]	-	-	88%	94%
Thrombolytic Therapy Timing[1,3]	-	-	68%	66%
Venous Thromboembolism Prophylaxis[1,3]	-	-	93%	94%
Written Stroke Educational Materials Given[3,7]	-	-	84%	88%
Surgical Care Improvement Project				
Appropriate Beta Blocker Usage[5]	-	-	98%	98%
Appropriate VTP Within 24 Hours[5]	-	-	98%	98%
Controlled Postoperative Blood Glucose[5]	-	-	98%	97%
Perioperative Temperature Management[5]	-	-	100%	100%
Prophylactic Antibiotic Selection[5]	-	-	99%	99%
Prophylactic Antibiotic Selection (Outpatient)[5]	-	-	98%	98%
Prophylactic Antibiotic Stopped[5]	-	-	98%	98%
Prophylactic Antibiotic Timing[5]	-	-	99%	99%
Prophylactic Antibiotic Timing (Outpatient)[5]	-	-	98%	98%
Urinary Catheter Removal[5]	-	-	97%	97%
Survey of Patients' Hospital Experiences				
Area Around Room 'Always' Quiet at Night[6]	<100	54%	65%	61%
Doctors 'Always' Communicated Well[6]	<100	86%	85%	82%
Home Recovery Information Given[6]	<100	81%	86%	85%
Hospital Given 9 or 10 on 10 Point Scale[6]	<100	54%	76%	71%
Meds 'Always' Explained Before Given[6]	<100	56%	66%	64%
Nurses 'Always' Communicated Well[6]	<100	74%	81%	79%
Pain 'Always' Well Controlled[6]	<100	67%	72%	71%
Room and Bathroom 'Always' Clean[6]	<100	65%	76%	73%
Timely Help 'Always' Received[6]	<100	67%	72%	68%
Would Definitely Recommend Hospital[6]	<100	64%	75%	71%
Use of Medical Imaging				
Cardiac Imaging Stress Test before Surgery[7]	-	-	5%	5.3%
Combination Abdominal CT Scan	135	69.6%	19%	10.5%
Combination Brain/Sinus CT Scan[1]	-	-	2.9%	2.7%
Combination Chest CT Scan	66	19.7%	3.9%	2.7%
Follow-up Mammogram/Ultrasound	273	1.1%	7.8%	8.8%
Lumbar Spine MRI for Low Back Pain[1]	-	-	40.2%	37.2%

Kansas Heart Hospital

3601 North Webb Road
Wichita, KS 67226
Phone: 316-630-5000
Fax: 316-630-5050
URL: www.kansasheart.com
Type: Acute Care Hospitals
Emergency Services: No
Ownership: Proprietary
Beds: 54

Key Personnel:
CEO/President.............. Thomas L Aschom, MD
Chairman/CEO .... Gregory F. Duck, MD
Intensive Care Unit........... Sandy McClune, RN
Quality Assurance .... Nancy Miller, RN BSN, MA
Surgery .... Carla Nelson, RN
Radiology.................. Deb Sikes, RDCS, RVT

Measure	Cases	This Hosp.	State Avg.	U.S. Avg.
Blood Clot Prevention and Treatment				
Anticoagulation Overlap Therapy[2]	18	100%	94%	93%
ICU Venous Thromboembolism Prophylaxis[2]	195	92%	91%	92%
Incidence of Potentially Preventable VTE[1,2]	-	-	8%	10%
UFH with Dosages/Platelet Monitoring[2]	18	100%	98%	97%
Venous Thromboembolism Prophylaxis[2]	143	76%	79%	85%
Warfarin Therapy Discharge Instructions[2]	14	100%	84%	75%
Chest Pain/Possible Heart Attack Care				
Aspirin Given Within 24 Hours of Arrival[5]	-	-	94%	96%
Fibrinolytic Meds Within 30 Min. of Arrival[5]	-	-	41%	58%
Average Time to ECG (minutes)[5]	-	-	8	7
Average Time to Transfer (minutes)[5]	-	-	57	60
Children's Asthma Care				
Received Home Management Plan of Care	-	-	-	88%
Received Reliever Medication	-	-	-	100%
Received Systemic Corticosteroids	-	-	-	100%
Emergency Department				
Admittance Decision Time (minutes)[2,7]	-	-	57	98
Head CT Results Within 45 Min. of Arrival[5]	-	-	53%	57%
Patients Who Left ER Before Being Seen[5]	-	-	2%	2%
Time from ER Arrival to Admit. (minutes)[2,7]	-	-	185	274
Time from ER Arrival to Discharge (minutes)[5]	-	-	104	134
Time in ER Before Being Evaluated (minutes)[5]	-	-	18	26
Time to Pain Meds for Fractures (minutes)[5]	-	-	47	57
Heart Attack Care				
Aspirin Given at Discharge[2]	224	100%	99%	99%
Fibrinolytic Meds Within 30 Min. of Arrival[2,7]	-	-	-	54%
PCI Within 90 Minutes of Arrival[1,2]	-	-	97%	96%
Statin Prescribed at Discharge[2]	208	100%	99%	98%
Heart Failure Care				
ACE Inhibitor or ARB for LVSD[2]	56	98%	95%	97%
Discharge Instructions Given[2]	139	93%	91%	94%
Evaluation of LVS Function[2]	160	100%	94%	99%
Medicare Spending				
Medicare Spending per Patient (ratio)	-	0.88	0.94	0.98
Pneumonia Care				
Appropriate Initial Antibiotic Given[7]	-	-	92%	95%
Blood Culture Timing[7]	-	-	98%	98%
Pregnancy and Delivery Care				
Newborn Deliveries Scheduled Early[7]	-	-	12%	6%
Preventive Care				
Immunization for Influenza[2]	308	99%	88%	90%
Immunization for Pneumonia[2]	527	99%	90%	92%
Stroke Care				
Anticoagulation Therapy for Atrial Fibrillation[1,2]	-	-	88%	95%
Antithrombotic Therapy Timing[1,2]	-	-	97%	98%
Assessed for Rehabilitation[1,2]	-	-	97%	97%
Discharged on Antithrombotic Therapy[1,2]	-	-	98%	99%
Discharged on Statin Medication[1,2]	-	-	88%	94%
Thrombolytic Therapy Timing[2,7]	-	-	68%	66%
Venous Thromboembolism Prophylaxis[1,2]	-	-	93%	94%
Written Stroke Educational Materials Given[1,2]	-	-	84%	88%
Surgical Care Improvement Project				
Appropriate Beta Blocker Usage[2]	212	100%	98%	98%
Appropriate VTP Within 24 Hours[2]	19	100%	98%	98%
Controlled Postoperative Blood Glucose[2]	321	97%	98%	97%
Perioperative Temperature Management[2]	81	100%	100%	100%
Prophylactic Antibiotic Selection[2]	323	100%	99%	99%
Prophylactic Antibiotic Selection (Outpatient)	278	100%	98%	98%
Prophylactic Antibiotic Stopped[2]	316	99%	98%	98%
Prophylactic Antibiotic Timing[2]	324	99%	99%	99%
Prophylactic Antibiotic Timing (Outpatient)	278	99%	98%	98%
Urinary Catheter Removal[2]	268	99%	97%	97%
Survey of Patients' Hospital Experiences				
Area Around Room 'Always' Quiet at Night	300+	66%	65%	61%
Doctors 'Always' Communicated Well	300+	83%	85%	82%
Home Recovery Information Given	300+	84%	86%	85%
Hospital Given 9 or 10 on 10 Point Scale	300+	88%	76%	71%
Meds 'Always' Explained Before Given	300+	65%	66%	64%
Nurses 'Always' Communicated Well	300+	84%	81%	79%
Pain 'Always' Well Controlled	300+	77%	72%	71%
Room and Bathroom 'Always' Clean	300+	89%	76%	73%
Timely Help 'Always' Received	300+	77%	72%	68%
Would Definitely Recommend Hospital	300+	90%	75%	71%
Use of Medical Imaging				
Cardiac Imaging Stress Test before Surgery	155	1.9%	5%	5.3%
Combination Abdominal CT Scan[1]	-	-	19%	10.5%
Combination Brain/Sinus CT Scan[1]	-	-	2.9%	2.7%
Combination Chest CT Scan[1]	-	-	3.9%	2.7%
Follow-up Mammogram/Ultrasound[7]	-	-	7.8%	8.8%
Lumbar Spine MRI for Low Back Pain[7]	-	-	40.2%	37.2%

Kansas Spine & Specialty Hospital

3333 North Webb Road
Wichita, KS 67226
Phone: 316-462-5326
Type: Acute Care Hospitals
Emergency Services: No
Ownership: Physician
Beds: 22

Key Personnel:
Radiology.................... Thomas D. Cox, M.D.
Anesthesiology................ Gregory Meister, MD
CEO/President................ Thomas M Schmitt

Measure	Cases	This Hosp.	State Avg.	U.S. Avg.

NOTE: Hospital profiles are in alphabetical order by state, then city, then hospital within the city; Rankings exclude hospitals with less than 25 cases except for patient surveys which excludes hospitals with less than 100 cases; (a) 100-299 cases; (1) The number of cases/patients is too few to report; (2) Data submitted were based on a sample of cases/patients; (3) Results are based on a shorter time period than required; (4) Data suppressed by CMS for one or more quarters; (5) Results are not available for this reporting period; (6) Fewer than 100 patients completed the HCAHPS survey; (7) No cases met the criteria for this measure; (8) The lower limit of the confidence interval cannot be calculated if the number of observed infections equals zero; (9) No data are available from the state/territory for this reporting period; (10) The scores shown reflect fewer than 50 completed surveys; (11) There were discrepancies in the data collection process; (12) This measure does not apply to this hospital for this reporting period; (13) Results cannot be calculated for this reporting period; (14) The results for this state are combined with nearby states to protect confidentiality; Please refer to the User's Guide for a full explanation of data.

Measure	Cases	This Hosp.	State Avg.	U.S. Avg.
Blood Clot Prevention and Treatment				
Anticoagulation Overlap Therapy[2,7]	-	-	94%	93%
ICU Venous Thromboembolism Prophylaxis[2,7]	-	-	91%	92%
Incidence of Potentially Preventable VTE[2,7]	-	-	8%	10%
UFH with Dosages/Platelet Monitoring[2,7]	-	-	98%	97%
Venous Thromboembolism Prophylaxis[2]	243	100%	79%	85%
Warfarin Therapy Discharge Instructions[2,7]	-	-	84%	75%
Chest Pain/Possible Heart Attack Care				
Aspirin Given Within 24 Hours of Arrival[5]	-	-	94%	96%
Fibrinolytic Meds Within 30 Min. of Arrival[5]	-	-	41%	58%
Average Time to ECG (minutes)[5]	-	-	8	7
Average Time to Transfer (minutes)[5]	-	-	57	60
Children's Asthma Care				
Received Home Management Plan of Care	-	-	-	88%
Received Reliever Medication	-	-	-	100%
Received Systemic Corticosteroids	-	-	-	100%
Emergency Department				
Admittance Decision Time (minutes)[2,7]	-	-	57	98
Head CT Results Within 45 Min. of Arrival[5]	-	-	53%	57%
Patients Who Left ER Before Being Seen[5]	-	-	2%	2%
Time from ER Arrival to Admit. (minutes)[2,7]	-	-	185	274
Time from ER Arrival to Discharge (minutes)[5]	-	-	104	134
Time in ER Before Being Evaluated (minutes)[5]	-	-	18	26
Time to Pain Meds for Fractures (minutes)[5]	-	-	47	57
Heart Attack Care				
Aspirin Given at Discharge[5]	-	-	99%	99%
Fibrinolytic Meds Within 30 Min. of Arrival[5]	-	-	-	54%
PCI Within 90 Minutes of Arrival[5]	-	-	97%	96%
Statin Prescribed at Discharge[5]	-	-	99%	98%
Heart Failure Care				
ACE Inhibitor or ARB for LVSD[5]	-	-	95%	97%
Discharge Instructions Given[5]	-	-	91%	94%
Evaluation of LVS Function[5]	-	-	94%	99%
Medicare Spending				
Medicare Spending per Patient (ratio)	-	0.91	0.94	0.98
Pneumonia Care				
Appropriate Initial Antibiotic Given[5]	-	-	92%	95%
Blood Culture Timing[5]	-	-	98%	98%
Pregnancy and Delivery Care				
Newborn Deliveries Scheduled Early[7]	-	-	12%	6%
Preventive Care				
Immunization for Influenza[2]	302	94%	88%	90%
Immunization for Pneumonia[2]	324	88%	90%	92%
Stroke Care				
Anticoagulation Therapy for Atrial Fibrillation[5]	-	-	88%	95%
Antithrombotic Therapy Timing[5]	-	-	97%	98%
Assessed for Rehabilitation[5]	-	-	97%	97%
Discharged on Antithrombotic Therapy[5]	-	-	98%	99%
Discharged on Statin Medication[5]	-	-	88%	94%
Thrombolytic Therapy Timing[5]	-	-	68%	66%
Venous Thromboembolism Prophylaxis[5]	-	-	93%	94%
Written Stroke Educational Materials Given[5]	-	-	84%	88%
Surgical Care Improvement Project				
Appropriate Beta Blocker Usage[2]	30	100%	98%	98%
Appropriate VTP Within 24 Hours[2]	102	98%	98%	98%
Controlled Postoperative Blood Glucose[2,7]	-	-	98%	97%
Perioperative Temperature Management[2]	110	98%	100%	100%
Prophylactic Antibiotic Selection[2]	99	100%	99%	99%
Prophylactic Antibiotic Selection (Outpatient)	426	100%	98%	98%
Prophylactic Antibiotic Stopped[2]	99	94%	98%	98%
Prophylactic Antibiotic Timing[2]	99	99%	99%	99%
Prophylactic Antibiotic Timing (Outpatient)	426	99%	98%	98%
Urinary Catheter Removal[1,2]	-	-	97%	97%
Survey of Patients' Hospital Experiences				
Area Around Room 'Always' Quiet at Night	300+	72%	65%	61%
Doctors 'Always' Communicated Well	300+	82%	85%	82%
Home Recovery Information Given	300+	86%	86%	85%
Hospital Given 9 or 10 on 10 Point Scale	300+	79%	76%	71%
Meds 'Always' Explained Before Given	300+	67%	66%	64%
Nurses 'Always' Communicated Well	300+	78%	81%	79%
Pain 'Always' Well Controlled	300+	72%	72%	71%
Room and Bathroom 'Always' Clean	300+	68%	76%	73%
Timely Help 'Always' Received	300+	67%	72%	68%
Would Definitely Recommend Hospital	300+	79%	75%	71%
Use of Medical Imaging				
Cardiac Imaging Stress Test before Surgery[7]	-	-	5%	5.3%
Combination Abdominal CT Scan[1]	-	-	19%	10.5%
Combination Brain/Sinus CT Scan	67	0.0%	2.9%	2.7%
Combination Chest CT Scan[1]	-	-	3.9%	2.7%
Follow-up Mammogram/Ultrasound[7]	-	-	7.8%	8.8%
Lumbar Spine MRI for Low Back Pain	87	37.9%	40.2%	37.2%

Kansas Surgery & Recovery Center

2770 North Webb Road
Wichita, KS 67226
Phone: 316-634-0090
Fax: 316-634-0005
URL: www.ksrc.org
Type: Acute Care Hospitals
Ownership: Proprietary
Emergency Services: No
Beds: 24

Key Personnel:
Radiology. . . . . Timithy C Benning
Anesthesiology. . . . . Michael Caughlin
Radiology. . . . . Amanda Zernickow

Measure	Cases	This Hosp.	State Avg.	U.S. Avg.
Blood Clot Prevention and Treatment				
Anticoagulation Overlap Therapy[2,7]	-	-	94%	93%
ICU Venous Thromboembolism Prophylaxis[2,7]	-	-	91%	92%
Incidence of Potentially Preventable VTE[2,7]	-	-	8%	10%
UFH with Dosages/Platelet Monitoring[2,7]	-	-	98%	97%
Venous Thromboembolism Prophylaxis[2]	22	100%	79%	85%
Warfarin Therapy Discharge Instructions[2,7]	-	-	84%	75%
Chest Pain/Possible Heart Attack Care				
Aspirin Given Within 24 Hours of Arrival[5]	-	-	94%	96%
Fibrinolytic Meds Within 30 Min. of Arrival[5]	-	-	41%	58%
Average Time to ECG (minutes)[5]	-	-	8	7
Average Time to Transfer (minutes)[5]	-	-	57	60
Children's Asthma Care				
Received Home Management Plan of Care	-	-	-	88%
Received Reliever Medication	-	-	-	100%
Received Systemic Corticosteroids	-	-	-	100%
Emergency Department				
Admittance Decision Time (minutes)[2,7]	-	-	57	98
Head CT Results Within 45 Min. of Arrival[5]	-	-	53%	57%
Patients Who Left ER Before Being Seen[5]	-	-	2%	2%
Time from ER Arrival to Admit. (minutes)[2,7]	-	-	185	274
Time from ER Arrival to Discharge (minutes)[5]	-	-	104	134
Time in ER Before Being Evaluated (minutes)[5]	-	-	18	26
Time to Pain Meds for Fractures (minutes)[5]	-	-	47	57
Heart Attack Care				
Aspirin Given at Discharge[5]	-	-	99%	99%
Fibrinolytic Meds Within 30 Min. of Arrival[5]	-	-	-	54%
PCI Within 90 Minutes of Arrival[5]	-	-	97%	96%
Statin Prescribed at Discharge[5]	-	-	99%	98%
Heart Failure Care				
ACE Inhibitor or ARB for LVSD[5]	-	-	95%	97%
Discharge Instructions Given[5]	-	-	91%	94%
Evaluation of LVS Function[5]	-	-	94%	99%
Medicare Spending				
Medicare Spending per Patient (ratio)	-	0.85	0.94	0.98
Pneumonia Care				
Appropriate Initial Antibiotic Given[5]	-	-	92%	95%
Blood Culture Timing[5]	-	-	98%	98%
Pregnancy and Delivery Care				
Newborn Deliveries Scheduled Early[7]	-	-	12%	6%
Preventive Care				
Immunization for Influenza[2]	308	46%	88%	90%
Immunization for Pneumonia[2]	409	81%	90%	92%
Stroke Care				
Anticoagulation Therapy for Atrial Fibrillation[5]	-	-	88%	95%
Antithrombotic Therapy Timing[5]	-	-	97%	98%
Assessed for Rehabilitation[5]	-	-	97%	97%
Discharged on Antithrombotic Therapy[5]	-	-	98%	99%
Discharged on Statin Medication[5]	-	-	88%	94%
Thrombolytic Therapy Timing[5]	-	-	68%	66%
Venous Thromboembolism Prophylaxis[5]	-	-	93%	94%
Written Stroke Educational Materials Given[5]	-	-	84%	88%
Surgical Care Improvement Project				
Appropriate Beta Blocker Usage[2]	50	100%	98%	98%
Appropriate VTP Within 24 Hours[2]	219	100%	98%	98%
Controlled Postoperative Blood Glucose[2,7]	-	-	98%	97%
Perioperative Temperature Management[2]	220	100%	100%	100%
Prophylactic Antibiotic Selection[2]	155	100%	99%	99%
Prophylactic Antibiotic Selection (Outpatient)	55	100%	98%	98%
Prophylactic Antibiotic Stopped[2]	155	100%	98%	98%
Prophylactic Antibiotic Timing[2]	155	100%	99%	99%
Prophylactic Antibiotic Timing (Outpatient)	55	100%	98%	98%
Urinary Catheter Removal[2,7]	-	-	97%	97%
Survey of Patients' Hospital Experiences				
Area Around Room 'Always' Quiet at Night	300+	76%	65%	61%
Doctors 'Always' Communicated Well	300+	86%	85%	82%
Home Recovery Information Given	300+	88%	86%	85%
Hospital Given 9 or 10 on 10 Point Scale	300+	84%	76%	71%
Meds 'Always' Explained Before Given	300+	69%	66%	64%
Nurses 'Always' Communicated Well	300+	84%	81%	79%
Pain 'Always' Well Controlled	300+	72%	72%	71%
Room and Bathroom 'Always' Clean	300+	83%	76%	73%
Timely Help 'Always' Received	300+	74%	72%	68%
Would Definitely Recommend Hospital	300+	87%	75%	71%
Use of Medical Imaging				
Cardiac Imaging Stress Test before Surgery[7]	-	-	5%	5.3%
Combination Abdominal CT Scan[1]	-	-	19%	10.5%
Combination Brain/Sinus CT Scan[7]	-	-	2.9%	2.7%
Combination Chest CT Scan[1]	-	-	3.9%	2.7%
Follow-up Mammogram/Ultrasound[7]	-	-	7.8%	8.8%
Lumbar Spine MRI for Low Back Pain	121	35.5%	40.2%	37.2%

Via Christi Hospital Wichita Saint Teresa

14800 West Saint Teresa
Wichita, KS 67235
Phone: 316-796-7800
URL: www.via-christi.org
Type: Acute Care Hospitals
Ownership: Voluntary non-profit - Church
Emergency Services: Yes
Beds: 68

Measure	Cases	This Hosp.	State Avg.	U.S. Avg.
Blood Clot Prevention and Treatment				
Anticoagulation Overlap Therapy[2]	16	94%	94%	93%
ICU Venous Thromboembolism Prophylaxis[2]	31	97%	91%	92%
Incidence of Potentially Preventable VTE[1,2]	-	-	8%	10%
UFH with Dosages/Platelet Monitoring[1,2]	-	-	98%	97%
Venous Thromboembolism Prophylaxis[2]	123	97%	79%	85%
Warfarin Therapy Discharge Instructions[1,2]	-	-	84%	75%
Chest Pain/Possible Heart Attack Care				
Aspirin Given Within 24 Hours of Arrival	37	89%	94%	96%
Fibrinolytic Meds Within 30 Min. of Arrival[7]	-	-	41%	58%
Average Time to ECG (minutes)	36	10	8	7
Average Time to Transfer (minutes)[7]	-	-	57	60
Children's Asthma Care				
Received Home Management Plan of Care	-	-	-	88%
Received Reliever Medication	-	-	-	100%
Received Systemic Corticosteroids	-	-	-	100%
Emergency Department				
Admittance Decision Time (minutes)[2]	250	64	57	98
Head CT Results Within 45 Min. of Arrival[1]	-	-	53%	57%
Patients Who Left ER Before Being Seen	13,468	0%	2%	2%
Time from ER Arrival to Admit. (minutes)[2]	252	158	185	274
Time from ER Arrival to Discharge (minutes)	380	90	104	134
Time in ER Before Being Evaluated (minutes)	415	15	18	26
Time to Pain Meds for Fractures (minutes)	63	34	47	57
Heart Attack Care				
Aspirin Given at Discharge[1,2]	-	-	99%	99%
Fibrinolytic Meds Within 30 Min. of Arrival[2,7]	-	-	-	54%
PCI Within 90 Minutes of Arrival[2,7]	-	-	97%	96%
Statin Prescribed at Discharge[1,2]	-	-	99%	98%
Heart Failure Care				
ACE Inhibitor or ARB for LVSD[2]	16	94%	95%	97%
Discharge Instructions Given[2]	26	100%	91%	94%
Evaluation of LVS Function[2]	42	100%	94%	99%
Medicare Spending				
Medicare Spending per Patient (ratio)	-	0.99	0.94	0.98

NOTE: Hospital profiles are in alphabetical order by state, then city, then hospital within the city; Rankings exclude hospitals with less than 25 cases except for patient surveys which excludes hospitals with less than 100 cases; (a) 100-299 cases; (1) The number of cases/patients is too few to report; (2) Data submitted were based on a sample of cases/patients; (3) Results are based on a shorter time period than required; (4) Data suppressed by CMS for one or more quarters; (5) Results are not available for this reporting period; (6) Fewer than 100 patients completed the HCAHPS survey; (7) No cases met the criteria for this measure; (8) The lower limit of the confidence interval cannot be calculated if the number of observed infections equals zero; (9) No data are available from the state/territory for this reporting period; (10) The scores shown reflect fewer than 50 completed surveys; (11) There were discrepancies in the data collection process; (12) This measure does not apply to this hospital for this reporting period; (13) Results cannot be calculated for this reporting period; (14) The results for this state are combined with nearby states to protect confidentiality; Please refer to the User's Guide for a full explanation of data.

Measure	Cases	This Hosp.	State Avg.	U.S. Avg.
Pneumonia Care				
Appropriate Initial Antibiotic Given[2]	89	99%	92%	95%
Blood Culture Timing[2]	91	98%	98%	98%
Pregnancy and Delivery Care				
Newborn Deliveries Scheduled Early[2]	13	0%	12%	6%
Preventive Care				
Immunization for Influenza[2]	288	93%	88%	90%
Immunization for Pneumonia[2]	366	93%	90%	92%
Stroke Care				
Anticoagulation Therapy for Atrial Fibrillation[1,2]	-	-	88%	95%
Antithrombotic Therapy Timing[2]	15	100%	97%	98%
Assessed for Rehabilitation[2]	22	100%	97%	97%
Discharged on Antithrombotic Therapy[2]	21	100%	98%	99%
Discharged on Statin Medication[2]	18	61%	88%	94%
Thrombolytic Therapy Timing[1,2]	-	-	68%	66%
Venous Thromboembolism Prophylaxis[2]	14	93%	93%	94%
Written Stroke Educational Materials Given[2]	16	75%	84%	88%
Surgical Care Improvement Project				
Appropriate Beta Blocker Usage[2]	49	100%	98%	98%
Appropriate VTP Within 24 Hours[2]	165	99%	98%	98%
Controlled Postoperative Blood Glucose[2,7]	-	-	98%	97%
Perioperative Temperature Management[2]	186	100%	100%	100%
Prophylactic Antibiotic Selection[2]	145	99%	99%	99%
Prophylactic Antibiotic Selection (Outpatient)[3]	15	100%	98%	98%
Prophylactic Antibiotic Stopped[2]	139	94%	98%	98%
Prophylactic Antibiotic Timing[2]	145	99%	99%	99%
Prophylactic Antibiotic Timing (Outpatient)[3]	15	100%	98%	98%
Urinary Catheter Removal[2]	170	99%	97%	97%
Survey of Patients' Hospital Experiences				
Area Around Room 'Always' Quiet at Night	300+	80%	65%	61%
Doctors 'Always' Communicated Well	300+	87%	85%	82%
Home Recovery Information Given	300+	85%	86%	85%
Hospital Given 9 or 10 on 10 Point Scale	300+	89%	76%	71%
Meds 'Always' Explained Before Given	300+	68%	66%	64%
Nurses 'Always' Communicated Well	300+	85%	81%	79%
Pain 'Always' Well Controlled	300+	78%	72%	71%
Room and Bathroom 'Always' Clean	300+	75%	76%	73%
Timely Help 'Always' Received	300+	73%	72%	68%
Would Definitely Recommend Hospital	300+	88%	75%	71%
Use of Medical Imaging				
Cardiac Imaging Stress Test before Surgery	82	4.9%	5%	5.3%
Combination Abdominal CT Scan	256	58.6%	19%	10.5%
Combination Brain/Sinus CT Scan[1]	-	-	2.9%	2.7%
Combination Chest CT Scan	91	27.5%	3.9%	2.7%
Follow-up Mammogram/Ultrasound[7]	-	-	7.8%	8.8%
Lumbar Spine MRI for Low Back Pain[1]	-	-	40.2%	37.2%

Via Christi Hospitals Wichita

929 North Saint Francis Street
Wichita, KS 67214
Phone: 316-268-5000
Fax: 316-291-4570
URL: www.via-christi.org
Type: Acute Care Hospitals
Emergency Services: Yes
Ownership: Voluntary non-profit - Church
Beds: 840

Key Personnel:
Radiology. . . . . Jon Anders, MD
Anesthesiology. . . . . Bryan Black, MD
Hemotology Center . . . . Shaker R Dakhil, MD, FACP
Infection Control. . . . . Susan Hendrickson
Patient Relations . . . . Susan Hendriskson
CEO/President. . . . . Michalene Maringer
Emergency Room . . . . Cindy Prine
Pediatric In-Patient Care . . . . Dimitrios E Stephanopoulos, MD, FAAP

Measure	Cases	This Hosp.	State Avg.	U.S. Avg.
Blood Clot Prevention and Treatment				
Anticoagulation Overlap Therapy[2]	170	92%	94%	93%
ICU Venous Thromboembolism Prophylaxis[2]	151	98%	91%	92%
Incidence of Potentially Preventable VTE[2]	30	3%	8%	10%
UFH with Dosages/Platelet Monitoring[2]	94	100%	98%	97%
Venous Thromboembolism Prophylaxis[2]	215	98%	79%	85%
Warfarin Therapy Discharge Instructions[2]	124	92%	84%	75%
Chest Pain/Possible Heart Attack Care				
Aspirin Given Within 24 Hours of Arrival[5]	-	-	94%	96%
Fibrinolytic Meds Within 30 Min. of Arrival[5]	-	-	41%	58%
Average Time to ECG (minutes)[5]	-	-	8	7
Average Time to Transfer (minutes)[5]	-	-	57	60
Children's Asthma Care				
Received Home Management Plan of Care	-	-	-	88%
Received Reliever Medication	-	-	-	100%
Received Systemic Corticosteroids	-	-	-	100%
Emergency Department				
Admittance Decision Time (minutes)[2]	409	73	57	98
Head CT Results Within 45 Min. of Arrival[1]	-	-	53%	57%
Patients Who Left ER Before Being Seen	>100k	3%	2%	2%
Time from ER Arrival to Admit. (minutes)[2]	421	180	185	274
Time from ER Arrival to Discharge (minutes)	351	119	104	134
Time in ER Before Being Evaluated (minutes)	376	23	18	26
Time to Pain Meds for Fractures (minutes)	163	53	47	57
Heart Attack Care				
Aspirin Given at Discharge[2]	301	99%	99%	99%
Fibrinolytic Meds Within 30 Min. of Arrival[2,7]	-	-	-	54%
PCI Within 90 Minutes of Arrival[2]	68	99%	97%	96%
Statin Prescribed at Discharge[2]	278	99%	99%	98%
Heart Failure Care				
ACE Inhibitor or ARB for LVSD[2]	66	97%	95%	97%
Discharge Instructions Given[2]	217	97%	91%	94%
Evaluation of LVS Function[2]	311	100%	94%	99%
Medicare Spending				
Medicare Spending per Patient (ratio)	-	0.98	0.94	0.98
Pneumonia Care				
Appropriate Initial Antibiotic Given[2]	107	95%	92%	95%
Blood Culture Timing[2]	134	99%	98%	98%
Pregnancy and Delivery Care				
Newborn Deliveries Scheduled Early[2]	45	0%	12%	6%
Preventive Care				
Immunization for Influenza[2]	512	93%	88%	90%
Immunization for Pneumonia[2]	601	92%	90%	92%
Stroke Care				
Anticoagulation Therapy for Atrial Fibrillation[2]	17	59%	88%	95%
Antithrombotic Therapy Timing[2]	94	95%	97%	98%
Assessed for Rehabilitation[2]	132	97%	97%	97%
Discharged on Antithrombotic Therapy[2]	99	98%	98%	99%
Discharged on Statin Medication[2]	85	95%	88%	94%
Thrombolytic Therapy Timing[1,2]	-	-	68%	66%
Venous Thromboembolism Prophylaxis[2]	145	99%	93%	94%
Written Stroke Educational Materials Given[2]	60	95%	84%	88%
Surgical Care Improvement Project				
Appropriate Beta Blocker Usage[2]	197	99%	98%	98%
Appropriate VTP Within 24 Hours[2]	382	97%	98%	98%
Controlled Postoperative Blood Glucose[2]	144	99%	98%	97%
Perioperative Temperature Management[2]	493	100%	100%	100%
Prophylactic Antibiotic Selection[2]	427	100%	99%	99%
Prophylactic Antibiotic Selection (Outpatient)	628	99%	98%	98%
Prophylactic Antibiotic Stopped[2]	418	99%	98%	98%
Prophylactic Antibiotic Timing[2]	428	100%	99%	99%
Prophylactic Antibiotic Timing (Outpatient)	635	99%	98%	98%
Urinary Catheter Removal[2]	266	98%	97%	97%
Survey of Patients' Hospital Experiences				
Area Around Room 'Always' Quiet at Night	300+	50%	65%	61%
Doctors 'Always' Communicated Well	300+	76%	85%	82%
Home Recovery Information Given	300+	82%	86%	85%
Hospital Given 9 or 10 on 10 Point Scale	300+	68%	76%	71%
Meds 'Always' Explained Before Given	300+	58%	66%	64%
Nurses 'Always' Communicated Well	300+	75%	81%	79%
Pain 'Always' Well Controlled	300+	66%	72%	71%
Room and Bathroom 'Always' Clean	300+	68%	76%	73%
Timely Help 'Always' Received	300+	57%	72%	68%
Would Definitely Recommend Hospital	300+	70%	75%	71%
Use of Medical Imaging				
Cardiac Imaging Stress Test before Surgery	435	3.7%	5%	5.3%
Combination Abdominal CT Scan	1,550	50.3%	19%	10.5%
Combination Brain/Sinus CT Scan	1,539	3.1%	2.9%	2.7%
Combination Chest CT Scan	677	12.4%	3.9%	2.7%
Follow-up Mammogram/Ultrasound	900	8.8%	7.8%	8.8%
Lumbar Spine MRI for Low Back Pain[1]	-	-	40.2%	37.2%

Wesley Medical Center

550 N Hillside Street
Wichita, KS 67214
Phone: 316-962-2000
Fax: 316-962-7076
URL: www.wesleymc.com
Type: Acute Care Hospitals
Emergency Services: Yes
Ownership: Proprietary
Beds: 760

Key Personnel:
Radiology. . . . . Richard Ahlstrand, MD
Operating Room. . . . . Sue Ebertowski, RN
Chief of Medical Staff . . . . Dr. Francie Ekengren
Emergency Room . . . . Diane Lippolt
Anesthesiology. . . . . Robert McKay, MD
Pediatric In-Patient Care . . . . Curt Pickert, MD
CEO/President. . . . . Hugh Tappan

Measure	Cases	This Hosp.	State Avg.	U.S. Avg.
Blood Clot Prevention and Treatment				
Anticoagulation Overlap Therapy[2]	132	100%	94%	93%
ICU Venous Thromboembolism Prophylaxis[2]	195	100%	91%	92%
Incidence of Potentially Preventable VTE[2]	24	0%	8%	10%
UFH with Dosages/Platelet Monitoring[2]	56	100%	98%	97%
Venous Thromboembolism Prophylaxis[2]	279	100%	79%	85%
Warfarin Therapy Discharge Instructions[2]	99	100%	84%	75%
Chest Pain/Possible Heart Attack Care				
Aspirin Given Within 24 Hours of Arrival[3]	17	100%	94%	96%
Fibrinolytic Meds Within 30 Min. of Arrival[3,7]	-	-	41%	58%
Average Time to ECG (minutes)[3]	17	10	8	7
Average Time to Transfer (minutes)[3,7]	-	-	57	60
Children's Asthma Care				
Received Home Management Plan of Care	133	98%	-	88%
Received Reliever Medication	134	100%	-	100%
Received Systemic Corticosteroids	134	100%	-	100%
Emergency Department				
Admittance Decision Time (minutes)[2]	580	60	57	98
Head CT Results Within 45 Min. of Arrival[1]	-	-	53%	57%
Patients Who Left ER Before Being Seen	92,131	2%	2%	2%
Time from ER Arrival to Admit. (minutes)[2]	580	180	185	274
Time from ER Arrival to Discharge (minutes)	474	114	104	134
Time in ER Before Being Evaluated (minutes)	515	22	18	26
Time to Pain Meds for Fractures (minutes)	312	49	47	57
Heart Attack Care				
Aspirin Given at Discharge[2]	287	100%	99%	99%
Fibrinolytic Meds Within 30 Min. of Arrival[2,7]	-	-	-	54%
PCI Within 90 Minutes of Arrival[2]	40	100%	97%	96%
Statin Prescribed at Discharge[2]	259	100%	99%	98%
Heart Failure Care				
ACE Inhibitor or ARB for LVSD[2]	69	100%	95%	97%
Discharge Instructions Given[2]	226	100%	91%	94%
Evaluation of LVS Function[2]	291	100%	94%	99%
Medicare Spending				
Medicare Spending per Patient (ratio)	-	1.00	0.94	0.98
Pneumonia Care				
Appropriate Initial Antibiotic Given[2]	54	100%	92%	95%
Blood Culture Timing[2]	69	100%	98%	98%
Pregnancy and Delivery Care				
Newborn Deliveries Scheduled Early[2]	98	1%	12%	6%
Preventive Care				
Immunization for Influenza[2]	653	99%	88%	90%
Immunization for Pneumonia[2]	570	98%	90%	92%
Stroke Care				
Anticoagulation Therapy for Atrial Fibrillation[2]	11	100%	88%	95%
Antithrombotic Therapy Timing[2]	93	100%	97%	98%
Assessed for Rehabilitation[2]	105	100%	97%	97%
Discharged on Antithrombotic Therapy[2]	89	100%	98%	99%
Discharged on Statin Medication[2]	62	100%	88%	94%
Thrombolytic Therapy Timing[1,2]	-	-	68%	66%
Venous Thromboembolism Prophylaxis[2]	114	100%	93%	94%
Written Stroke Educational Materials Given[2]	56	98%	84%	88%
Surgical Care Improvement Project				
Appropriate Beta Blocker Usage[2]	245	100%	98%	98%
Appropriate VTP Within 24 Hours[2]	500	99%	98%	98%
Controlled Postoperative Blood Glucose[2]	173	98%	98%	97%
Perioperative Temperature Management[2]	646	100%	100%	100%
Prophylactic Antibiotic Selection[2]	528	99%	99%	99%
Prophylactic Antibiotic Selection (Outpatient)	785	99%	98%	98%

NOTE: Hospital profiles are in alphabetical order by state, then city, then hospital within the city; Rankings exclude hospitals with less than 25 cases except for patient surveys which excludes hospitals with less than 100 cases; (a) 100-299 cases; (1) The number of cases/patients is too few to report; (2) Data submitted were based on a sample of cases/patients; (3) Results are based on a shorter time period than required; (4) Data suppressed by CMS for one or more quarters; (5) Results are not available for this reporting period; (6) Fewer than 100 patients completed the HCAHPS survey; (7) No cases met the criteria for this measure; (8) The lower limit of the confidence interval cannot be calculated if the number of observed infections equals zero; (9) No data are available from the state/territory for this reporting period; (10) The scores shown reflect fewer than 50 completed surveys; (11) There were discrepancies in the data collection process; (12) This measure does not apply to this hospital for this reporting period; (13) Results cannot be calculated for this reporting period; (14) The results for this state are combined with nearby states to protect confidentiality; Please refer to the User's Guide for a full explanation of data.

Prophylactic Antibiotic Stopped[2]	511	100%	98%	98%
Prophylactic Antibiotic Timing[2]	531	100%	99%	99%
Prophylactic Antibiotic Timing (Outpatient)	787	100%	98%	98%
Urinary Catheter Removal[2]	303	100%	97%	97%
Survey of Patients' Hospital Experiences				
Area Around Room 'Always' Quiet at Night	300+	58%	65%	61%
Doctors 'Always' Communicated Well	300+	80%	85%	82%
Home Recovery Information Given	300+	85%	86%	85%
Hospital Given 9 or 10 on 10 Point Scale	300+	68%	76%	71%
Meds 'Always' Explained Before Given	300+	57%	66%	64%
Nurses 'Always' Communicated Well	300+	73%	81%	79%
Pain 'Always' Well Controlled	300+	67%	72%	71%
Room and Bathroom 'Always' Clean	300+	64%	76%	73%
Timely Help 'Always' Received	300+	55%	72%	68%
Would Definitely Recommend Hospital	300+	70%	75%	71%
Use of Medical Imaging				
Cardiac Imaging Stress Test before Surgery	124	4.8%	5%	5.3%
Combination Abdominal CT Scan	1,128	3.0%	19%	10.5%
Combination Brain/Sinus CT Scan	975	2.2%	2.9%	2.7%
Combination Chest CT Scan	585	0.9%	3.9%	2.7%
Follow-up Mammogram/Ultrasound	232	8.6%	7.8%	8.8%
Lumbar Spine MRI for Low Back Pain	74	40.5%	40.2%	37.2%

Wichita VA Medical Center

5500 E. Kellog
Wichita, KS 67218
Phone: 316-685-2221
Fax: 316-651-3666
URL: www.wichita.va.gov
Type: Acute Care - VA
Emergency Services: No
Ownership: Government Federal
Beds: 72

Key Personnel:
Patient Relations . . . . Linda Guhr
Intensive Care Unit. . . . . Zubair Hassan, MD
Chief of Medical Staff. . . . . Kent Murray, MD
CEO/President. . . . . Thomas Sanders, FACHE

Measure	Cases	This Hosp.	State Avg.	U.S. Avg.
Blood Clot Prevention and Treatment				
Anticoagulation Overlap Therapy	-	-	94%	93%
ICU Venous Thromboembolism Prophylaxis	-	-	91%	92%
Incidence of Potentially Preventable VTE	-	-	8%	10%
UFH with Dosages/Platelet Monitoring	-	-	98%	97%
Venous Thromboembolism Prophylaxis	-	-	79%	85%
Warfarin Therapy Discharge Instructions	-	-	84%	75%
Chest Pain/Possible Heart Attack Care				
Aspirin Given Within 24 Hours of Arrival	-	-	94%	96%
Fibrinolytic Meds Within 30 Min. of Arrival	-	-	41%	58%
Average Time to ECG (minutes)	-	-	8	7
Average Time to Transfer (minutes)	-	-	57	60
Children's Asthma Care				
Received Home Management Plan of Care	-	-	-	88%
Received Reliever Medication	-	-	-	100%
Received Systemic Corticosteroids	-	-	-	100%
Emergency Department				
Admittance Decision Time (minutes)	-	-	57	98
Head CT Results Within 45 Min. of Arrival	-	-	53%	57%
Patients Who Left ER Before Being Seen	-	-	2%	2%
Time from ER Arrival to Admit. (minutes)	-	-	185	274
Time from ER Arrival to Discharge (minutes)	-	-	104	134
Time in ER Before Being Evaluated (minutes)	-	-	18	26
Time to Pain Meds for Fractures (minutes)	-	-	47	57
Heart Attack Care				
Aspirin Given at Discharge	35	100%	99%	99%
Fibrinolytic Meds Within 30 Min. of Arrival[5]	-	-	-	54%
PCI Within 90 Minutes of Arrival[1]	-	-	97%	96%
Statin Prescribed at Discharge	25	100%	99%	98%
Heart Failure Care				
ACE Inhibitor or ARB for LVSD	32	100%	95%	97%
Discharge Instructions Given	77	100%	91%	94%
Evaluation of LVS Function	84	100%	94%	99%
Medicare Spending				
Medicare Spending per Patient (ratio)	-	-	0.94	0.98
Pneumonia Care				
Appropriate Initial Antibiotic Given	28	100%	92%	95%
Blood Culture Timing	72	100%	98%	98%
Pregnancy and Delivery Care				
Newborn Deliveries Scheduled Early	-	-	12%	6%
Preventive Care				
Immunization for Influenza[5]	-	-	88%	90%
Immunization for Pneumonia[5]	-	-	90%	92%
Stroke Care				
Anticoagulation Therapy for Atrial Fibrillation	-	-	88%	95%
Antithrombotic Therapy Timing	-	-	97%	98%
Assessed for Rehabilitation	-	-	97%	97%
Discharged on Antithrombotic Therapy	-	-	98%	99%
Discharged on Statin Medication	-	-	88%	94%
Thrombolytic Therapy Timing	-	-	68%	66%
Venous Thromboembolism Prophylaxis	-	-	93%	94%
Written Stroke Educational Materials Given	-	-	84%	88%
Surgical Care Improvement Project				
Appropriate Beta Blocker Usage[2]	56	91%	98%	98%
Appropriate VTP Within 24 Hours[2]	147	97%	98%	98%
Controlled Postoperative Blood Glucose[5]	-	-	98%	97%
Perioperative Temperature Management[2]	162	100%	100%	100%
Prophylactic Antibiotic Selection	119	99%	99%	99%
Prophylactic Antibiotic Selection (Outpatient)	-	-	98%	98%
Prophylactic Antibiotic Stopped	116	99%	98%	98%
Prophylactic Antibiotic Timing	119	100%	99%	99%
Prophylactic Antibiotic Timing (Outpatient)	-	-	98%	98%
Urinary Catheter Removal[2]	27	100%	97%	97%
Survey of Patients' Hospital Experiences				
Area Around Room 'Always' Quiet at Night	-	-	65%	61%
Doctors 'Always' Communicated Well	-	-	85%	82%
Home Recovery Information Given	-	-	86%	85%
Hospital Given 9 or 10 on 10 Point Scale	-	-	76%	71%
Meds 'Always' Explained Before Given	-	-	66%	64%
Nurses 'Always' Communicated Well	-	-	81%	79%
Pain 'Always' Well Controlled	-	-	72%	71%
Room and Bathroom 'Always' Clean	-	-	76%	73%
Timely Help 'Always' Received	-	-	72%	68%
Would Definitely Recommend Hospital	-	-	75%	71%
Use of Medical Imaging				
Cardiac Imaging Stress Test before Surgery	-	-	5%	5.3%
Combination Abdominal CT Scan	-	-	19%	10.5%
Combination Brain/Sinus CT Scan	-	-	2.9%	2.7%
Combination Chest CT Scan	-	-	3.9%	2.7%
Follow-up Mammogram/Ultrasound	-	-	7.8%	8.8%
Lumbar Spine MRI for Low Back Pain	-	-	40.2%	37.2%

Jefferson County Memorial Hospital

408 Delaware St
Winchester, KS 66097
Phone: 913-774-4340
Fax: 913-774-8605
URL: www.jcmhospital.org
Type: Critical Access Hospitals
Emergency Services: Yes
Ownership: Voluntary non-profit - Private
Beds: 25

Key Personnel:
Chief of Medical Staff. . . . . Larry Campbell
CEO/President. . . . . Joye H Huston, RN, M

Measure	Cases	This Hosp.	State Avg.	U.S. Avg.
Blood Clot Prevention and Treatment				
Anticoagulation Overlap Therapy[5]	-	-	94%	93%
ICU Venous Thromboembolism Prophylaxis[5]	-	-	91%	92%
Incidence of Potentially Preventable VTE[5]	-	-	8%	10%
UFH with Dosages/Platelet Monitoring[5]	-	-	98%	97%
Venous Thromboembolism Prophylaxis[5]	-	-	79%	85%
Warfarin Therapy Discharge Instructions[5]	-	-	84%	75%
Chest Pain/Possible Heart Attack Care				
Aspirin Given Within 24 Hours of Arrival	-	-	94%	96%
Fibrinolytic Meds Within 30 Min. of Arrival	-	-	41%	58%
Average Time to ECG (minutes)	-	-	8	7
Average Time to Transfer (minutes)	-	-	57	60
Children's Asthma Care				
Received Home Management Plan of Care	-	-	-	88%
Received Reliever Medication	-	-	-	100%
Received Systemic Corticosteroids	-	-	-	100%
Emergency Department				
Admittance Decision Time (minutes)[5]	-	-	57	98
Head CT Results Within 45 Min. of Arrival	-	-	53%	57%
Patients Who Left ER Before Being Seen	-	-	2%	2%
Time from ER Arrival to Admit. (minutes)[5]	-	-	185	274
Time from ER Arrival to Discharge (minutes)	-	-	104	134
Time in ER Before Being Evaluated (minutes)	-	-	18	26
Time to Pain Meds for Fractures (minutes)	-	-	47	57
Heart Attack Care				
Aspirin Given at Discharge[5]	-	-	99%	99%
Fibrinolytic Meds Within 30 Min. of Arrival[5]	-	-	-	54%
PCI Within 90 Minutes of Arrival[5]	-	-	97%	96%
Statin Prescribed at Discharge[5]	-	-	99%	98%
Heart Failure Care				
ACE Inhibitor or ARB for LVSD[5]	-	-	95%	97%
Discharge Instructions Given[5]	-	-	91%	94%
Evaluation of LVS Function[5]	-	-	94%	99%
Medicare Spending				
Medicare Spending per Patient (ratio)	-	-	0.94	0.98
Pneumonia Care				
Appropriate Initial Antibiotic Given[5]	-	-	92%	95%
Blood Culture Timing[5]	-	-	98%	98%
Pregnancy and Delivery Care				
Newborn Deliveries Scheduled Early[5]	-	-	12%	6%
Preventive Care				
Immunization for Influenza[5]	-	-	88%	90%
Immunization for Pneumonia[5]	-	-	90%	92%
Stroke Care				
Anticoagulation Therapy for Atrial Fibrillation[5]	-	-	88%	95%
Antithrombotic Therapy Timing[5]	-	-	97%	98%
Assessed for Rehabilitation[5]	-	-	97%	97%
Discharged on Antithrombotic Therapy[5]	-	-	98%	99%
Discharged on Statin Medication[5]	-	-	88%	94%
Thrombolytic Therapy Timing[5]	-	-	68%	66%
Venous Thromboembolism Prophylaxis[5]	-	-	93%	94%
Written Stroke Educational Materials Given[5]	-	-	84%	88%
Surgical Care Improvement Project				
Appropriate Beta Blocker Usage[5]	-	-	98%	98%
Appropriate VTP Within 24 Hours[5]	-	-	98%	98%
Controlled Postoperative Blood Glucose[5]	-	-	98%	97%
Perioperative Temperature Management[5]	-	-	100%	100%
Prophylactic Antibiotic Selection[5]	-	-	99%	99%
Prophylactic Antibiotic Selection (Outpatient)	-	-	98%	98%
Prophylactic Antibiotic Stopped[5]	-	-	98%	98%
Prophylactic Antibiotic Timing[5]	-	-	99%	99%
Prophylactic Antibiotic Timing (Outpatient)	-	-	98%	98%
Urinary Catheter Removal[5]	-	-	97%	97%
Survey of Patients' Hospital Experiences				
Area Around Room 'Always' Quiet at Night[5]	-	-	65%	61%
Doctors 'Always' Communicated Well[5]	-	-	85%	82%
Home Recovery Information Given[5]	-	-	86%	85%
Hospital Given 9 or 10 on 10 Point Scale[5]	-	-	76%	71%
Meds 'Always' Explained Before Given[5]	-	-	66%	64%
Nurses 'Always' Communicated Well[5]	-	-	81%	79%
Pain 'Always' Well Controlled[5]	-	-	72%	71%
Room and Bathroom 'Always' Clean[5]	-	-	76%	73%
Timely Help 'Always' Received[5]	-	-	72%	68%
Would Definitely Recommend Hospital[5]	-	-	75%	71%
Use of Medical Imaging				
Cardiac Imaging Stress Test before Surgery	-	-	5%	5.3%
Combination Abdominal CT Scan	-	-	19%	10.5%
Combination Brain/Sinus CT Scan	-	-	2.9%	2.7%
Combination Chest CT Scan	-	-	3.9%	2.7%
Follow-up Mammogram/Ultrasound	-	-	7.8%	8.8%
Lumbar Spine MRI for Low Back Pain	-	-	40.2%	37.2%

William Newton Hospital

1300 East Fifth Avenue
Winfield, KS 67156
Phone: 620-221-2300
Fax: 620-221-3594
URL: www.wnmh.org
Type: Critical Access Hospitals
Emergency Services: Yes
Ownership: Government - Local
Beds: 25

Key Personnel:
Chief of Medical Staff . . . . Tom Embers
Emergency Room . . . . Greg Faimon, MD
Intensive Care Unit. . . . . Barbara Humpert, RN
Quality Assurance . . . . Jamie Kaiser, RN
Infection Control. . . . . Linda King, RN

NOTE: Hospital profiles are in alphabetical order by state, then city, then hospital within the city; Rankings exclude hospitals with less than 25 cases except for patient surveys which excludes hospitals with less than 100 cases; (a) 100-299 cases; (1) The number of cases/patients is too few to report; (2) Data submitted were based on a sample of cases/patients; (3) Results are based on a shorter time period than required; (4) Data suppressed by CMS for one or more quarters; (5) Results are not available for this reporting period; (6) Fewer than 100 patients completed the HCAHPS survey; (7) No cases met the criteria for this measure; (8) The lower limit of the confidence interval cannot be calculated if the number of observed infections equals zero; (9) No data are available from the state/territory for this reporting period; (10) The scores shown reflect fewer than 50 completed surveys; (11) There were discrepancies in the data collection process; (12) This measure does not apply to this hospital for this reporting period; (13) Results cannot be calculated for this reporting period; (14) The results for this state are combined with nearby states to protect confidentiality; Please refer to the User's Guide for a full explanation of data.

CEO .... J. Ben Quinton
Operating Room............... Amy Soto, RN

Measure	Cases	This Hosp.	State Avg.	U.S. Avg.
Blood Clot Prevention and Treatment				
Anticoagulation Overlap Therapy[1]	-	-	94%	93%
ICU Venous Thromboembolism Prophylaxis	34	76%	91%	92%
Incidence of Potentially Preventable VTE[7]	-	-	8%	10%
UFH with Dosages/Platelet Monitoring[7]	-	-	98%	97%
Venous Thromboembolism Prophylaxis	283	53%	79%	85%
Warfarin Therapy Discharge Instructions[1]	-	-	84%	75%
Chest Pain/Possible Heart Attack Care				
Aspirin Given Within 24 Hours of Arrival	73	99%	94%	96%
Fibrinolytic Meds Within 30 Min. of Arrival[1]	-	-	41%	58%
Average Time to ECG (minutes)	76	4	8	7
Average Time to Transfer (minutes)[1]	-	-	57	60
Children's Asthma Care				
Received Home Management Plan of Care	-	-	-	88%
Received Reliever Medication	-	-	-	100%
Received Systemic Corticosteroids	-	-	-	100%
Emergency Department				
Admittance Decision Time (minutes)[2]	288	48	57	98
Head CT Results Within 45 Min. of Arrival[1]	-	-	53%	57%
Patients Who Left ER Before Being Seen	9,130	1%	2%	2%
Time from ER Arrival to Admit. (minutes)[2]	289	205	185	274
Time from ER Arrival to Discharge (minutes)	253	97	104	134
Time in ER Before Being Evaluated (minutes)	385	18	18	26
Time to Pain Meds for Fractures (minutes)	28	46	47	57
Heart Attack Care				
Aspirin Given at Discharge[1,3]	-	-	99%	99%
Fibrinolytic Meds Within 30 Min. of Arrival[3,7]	-	-	-	54%
PCI Within 90 Minutes of Arrival[3,7]	-	-	97%	96%
Statin Prescribed at Discharge[1,3]	-	-	99%	98%
Heart Failure Care				
ACE Inhibitor or ARB for LVSD[1]	-	-	95%	97%
Discharge Instructions Given[1]	-	-	91%	94%
Evaluation of LVS Function[1]	-	-	94%	99%
Medicare Spending				
Medicare Spending per Patient (ratio)	-	-	0.94	0.98
Pneumonia Care				
Appropriate Initial Antibiotic Given[2]	40	98%	92%	95%
Blood Culture Timing[2]	29	100%	98%	98%
Pregnancy and Delivery Care				
Newborn Deliveries Scheduled Early	43	0%	12%	6%
Preventive Care				
Immunization for Influenza	292	98%	88%	90%
Immunization for Pneumonia	414	97%	90%	92%
Stroke Care				
Anticoagulation Therapy for Atrial Fibrillation[1]	-	-	88%	95%
Antithrombotic Therapy Timing[1]	-	-	97%	98%
Assessed for Rehabilitation[1]	-	-	97%	97%
Discharged on Antithrombotic Therapy[1]	-	-	98%	99%
Discharged on Statin Medication[1]	-	-	88%	94%
Thrombolytic Therapy Timing[1]	-	-	68%	66%
Venous Thromboembolism Prophylaxis[1]	-	-	93%	94%
Written Stroke Educational Materials Given[1]	-	-	84%	88%
Surgical Care Improvement Project				
Appropriate Beta Blocker Usage[1]	-	-	98%	98%
Appropriate VTP Within 24 Hours	42	100%	98%	98%
Controlled Postoperative Blood Glucose[7]	-	-	98%	97%
Perioperative Temperature Management	45	98%	100%	100%
Prophylactic Antibiotic Selection	37	92%	99%	99%
Prophylactic Antibiotic Selection (Outpatient)	20	100%	98%	98%
Prophylactic Antibiotic Stopped	37	100%	98%	98%
Prophylactic Antibiotic Timing	37	92%	99%	99%
Prophylactic Antibiotic Timing (Outpatient)	20	95%	98%	98%
Urinary Catheter Removal	16	75%	97%	97%
Survey of Patients' Hospital Experiences				
Area Around Room 'Always' Quiet at Night	(a)	62%	65%	61%
Doctors 'Always' Communicated Well	(a)	81%	85%	82%
Home Recovery Information Given	(a)	83%	86%	85%
Hospital Given 9 or 10 on 10 Point Scale	(a)	76%	76%	71%
Meds 'Always' Explained Before Given	(a)	71%	66%	64%
Nurses 'Always' Communicated Well	(a)	84%	81%	79%
Pain 'Always' Well Controlled	(a)	71%	72%	71%
Room and Bathroom 'Always' Clean	(a)	76%	76%	73%
Timely Help 'Always' Received	(a)	74%	72%	68%
Would Definitely Recommend Hospital	(a)	77%	75%	71%
Use of Medical Imaging				
Cardiac Imaging Stress Test before Surgery	97	7.2%	5%	5.3%
Combination Abdominal CT Scan	277	65.0%	19%	10.5%
Combination Brain/Sinus CT Scan[1]	-	-	2.9%	2.7%
Combination Chest CT Scan	173	0.6%	3.9%	2.7%
Follow-up Mammogram/Ultrasound	572	8.0%	7.8%	8.8%
Lumbar Spine MRI for Low Back Pain	59	45.8%	40.2%	37.2%

NOTE: Hospital profiles are in alphabetical order by state, then city, then hospital within the city; Rankings exclude hospitals with less than 25 cases except for patient surveys which excludes hospitals with less than 100 cases; (a) 100-299 cases; (1) The number of cases/patients is too few to report; (2) Data submitted were based on a sample of cases/patients; (3) Results are based on a shorter time period than required; (4) Data suppressed by CMS for one or more quarters; (5) Results are not available for this reporting period; (6) Fewer than 100 patients completed the HCAHPS survey; (7) No cases met the criteria for this measure; (8) The lower limit of the confidence interval cannot be calculated if the number of observed infections equals zero; (9) No data are available from the state/territory for this reporting period; (10) The scores shown reflect fewer than 50 completed surveys; (11) There were discrepancies in the data collection process; (12) This measure does not apply to this hospital for this reporting period; (13) Results cannot be calculated for this reporting period; (14) The results for this state are combined with nearby states to protect confidentiality; Please refer to the User's Guide for a full explanation of data.

Blood Clot Prevention and Treatment

Anticoagulation Overlap Therapy

Hospital Name	City	Rate	Cases
Beaumont Health System[2]	Royal Oak	100%	336
Holland Community Hospital[2]	Holland	100%	48
Mclaren Bay Region[2]	Bay City	100%	92
Mclaren Lapeer Region[2]	Lapeer	100%	66
Mercy Health Partners - Mercy Campus[2]	Muskegon	100%	107
Mercy Hospital - Cadillac[2]	Cadillac	100%	35
Mercy Hospital - Grayling[2]	Grayling	100%	28
Spectrum Health Zeeland Comm Hosp[2]	Zeeland	100%	31
William Beaumont Hospital - Troy[2]	Troy	100%	227
Borgess Medical Center[2]	Kalamazoo	99%	137
Detroit Receiving Hosp & U Health Ctr[2]	Detroit	99%	105
Edward W Sparrow Hospital[2]	Lansing	99%	161
Henry Ford Hospital[2]	Detroit	99%	255
Huron Valley - Sinai Hospital[2]	Commerce Twp	99%	67
Mercy Memorial Hospital System[2]	Monroe	99%	69
Harper University Hospital[2]	Detroit	98%	82
Saint Mary's Health Care[2]	Grand Rapids	98%	114
University of Michigan Health System[2]	Ann Arbor	98%	233
Beaumont Health System[2]	Grosse Pointe	97%	104
Mclaren - Greater Lansing[2]	Lansing	97%	103
Mclaren Oakland[2]	Pontiac	97%	31
Oaklawn Hospital[2]	Marshall	97%	35
Allegiance Health[2]	Jackson	96%	127
Emma L Bixby Medical Center[2]	Adrian	96%	26
Mclaren Flint[2]	Flint	96%	192
Mercy Health Hackley Campus[2]	Muskegon	96%	52
Midmichigan Medical Center - Midland[2]	Midland	95%	104
Saint Joseph Mercy Hospital[2]	Ann Arbor	95%	261
Saint Joseph Mercy Livingston Hospital[2]	Howell	95%	39
Henry Ford Macomb Hospital[2]	Clinton Twp	94%	146
Marquette General Hospital[2]	Marquette	94%	49
Munson Medical Center[2]	Traverse City	94%	112
Providence Hospital & Medical Centers[2]	Southfield	94%	304
Saint John Hospital & Medical Center[2]	Detroit	94%	178
Sinai - Grace Hospital[2]	Detroit	94%	141
Spectrum Health United Memorial[2]	Greenville	94%	32
Covenant Medical Center[2]	Saginaw	93%	192
Henry Ford Wyandotte Hospital[2]	Wyandotte	93%	183
Mclaren - Northern Michigan[2]	Petoskey	93%	46
Henry Ford West Bloomfield Hospital[2]	W Bloomfield	92%	119
Mclaren Macomb[2]	Mount Clemens	92%	95
Saint Joseph Mercy Oakland[2]	Pontiac	92%	113
Botsford Hospital[2]	Farmington Hills	91%	149
Crittenton Hospital Medical Center[2]	Rochester	91%	87
Bronson Methodist Hospital[2]	Kalamazoo	89%	176
Port Huron Hospital[2]	Port Huron	89%	93
Saint Mary Mercy Hospital[2]	Livonia	89%	163
Bronson Battle Creek Hospital[2]	Battle Creek	88%	77
Oakwood Hospital - Taylor[2]	Taylor	87%	54
St John Macomb-Oakland Hosp[2]	Warren	87%	213
Alpena Regional Medical Center[2]	Alpena	86%	28
Hurley Medical Center[2]	Flint	86%	66
Metro Health Hospital[2]	Wyoming	86%	64
Spectrum Health - Butterworth Campus[2]	Grand Rapids	86%	310
Memorial Healthcare[2]	Owosso	85%	33
Oakwood Hospital - Southshore[2]	Trenton	81%	98
Garden City Hospital[2]	Garden City	80%	54
Lakeland Hospital - Saint Joseph[2]	Saint Joseph	70%	118
Saint Mary's of Michigan Medical Center[2]	Saginaw	66%	104
Genesys Reg Med Ctr-Health Park[2]	Grand Blanc	61%	227
West Branch Regional Medical Center[2]	West Branch	54%	26
Oakwood Hospital - Dearborn[2]	Dearborn	53%	186
Community Health Center of Branch County[2]	Coldwater	52%	25
Mclaren Central Michigan[2]	Mount Pleasant	48%	44
Oakwood Hospital - Wayne[2]	Wayne	38%	69

ICU Venous Thromboembolism Prophylaxis

Hospital Name	City	Rate	Cases
Botsford Hospital[2]	Farmington Hills	100%	28
Chelsea Community Hospital[2]	Chelsea	100%	38
Dickinson County Memorial Hospital[2]	Iron Mountain	100%	34
Garden City Hospital[2]	Garden City	100%	65
Henry Ford Macomb Hospital[2]	Clinton Twp	100%	51
Mclaren - Greater Lansing[2]	Lansing	100%	31
Mclaren Bay Region[2]	Bay City	100%	91
Mclaren Lapeer Region[2]	Lapeer	100%	79
Mclaren Macomb[2]	Mount Clemens	100%	69
Mercy Hospital - Grayling[2]	Grayling	100%	49
Mercy Memorial Hospital System[2]	Monroe	100%	47
North Ottawa Community Health Center[2]	Grand Haven	100%	49
Saint John Hospital & Medical Center[2]	Detroit	100%	77
St John Macomb-Oakland Hosp[2]	Warren	100%	49
Sinai - Grace Hospital[2]	Detroit	100%	45
Spectrum Health - Reed City Campus[2]	Reed City	100%	26
William Beaumont Hospital - Troy[2]	Troy	100%	46
Crittenton Hospital Medical Center[2]	Rochester	99%	79

Hospital Name	City	Rate	Cases
Henry Ford Hospital[2]	Detroit	99%	133
Mclaren - Northern Michigan[2]	Petoskey	99%	89
Mclaren Flint[2]	Flint	99%	74
University of Michigan Health System[2]	Ann Arbor	99%	85
Alpena Regional Medical Center[2]	Alpena	98%	48
Beaumont Health System[2]	Grosse Pointe	98%	47
Borgess Medical Center[2]	Kalamazoo	98%	62
Mclaren Oakland[2]	Pontiac	98%	62
Providence Hospital & Medical Centers[2]	Southfield	98%	102
Saint Mary's Health Care[2]	Grand Rapids	98%	45
Spectrum Health United Memorial[2]	Greenville	98%	50
Harper University Hospital[2]	Detroit	97%	94
Huron Valley - Sinai Hospital[2]	Commerce Twp	97%	35
Mclaren Central Michigan[2]	Mount Pleasant	97%	63
Midmichigan Medical Center - Clare[2]	Clare	97%	30
Saint Joseph Mercy Oakland[2]	Pontiac	97%	90
Saint Mary Mercy Hospital[2]	Livonia	97%	36
Spectrum Health Big Rapids Hospital[2]	Big Rapids	97%	37
Henry Ford West Bloomfield Hospital[2]	W Bloomfield	96%	97
Memorial Healthcare[2]	Owosso	96%	56
Mercy Hospital - Cadillac[2]	Cadillac	96%	51
Metro Health Hospital[2]	Wyoming	96%	52
Munson Medical Center[2]	Traverse City	96%	26
Saint Joseph Mercy Hospital[2]	Ann Arbor	96%	51
Covenant Medical Center[2]	Saginaw	95%	115
Detroit Receiving Hosp & U Health Ctr[2]	Detroit	95%	115
Oaklawn Hospital[2]	Marshall	95%	38
Otsego Memorial Hospital[2]	Gaylord	95%	97
Allegiance Health[2]	Jackson	94%	35
Beaumont Health System[2]	Royal Oak	94%	47
Edward W Sparrow Hospital[2]	Lansing	94%	82
Memorial Medical Center of West Michigan[2]	Ludington	94%	48
Saint Mary's of Michigan Medical Center[2]	Saginaw	94%	136
Spectrum Health Gerber Memorial[2]	Fremont	94%	62
Bronson Battle Creek Hospital[2]	Battle Creek	93%	82
Emma L Bixby Medical Center[2]	Adrian	93%	82
Mercy Health Partners - Mercy Campus[2]	Muskegon	93%	116
Spectrum Health - Butterworth Campus[2]	Grand Rapids	93%	59
Henry Ford Wyandotte Hospital[2]	Wyandotte	92%	64
Hurley Medical Center[2]	Flint	92%	84
Midmichigan Medical Center - Midland[2]	Midland	92%	90
Portage Health[2]	Hancock	92%	26
Oakwood Hospital - Southshore[2]	Trenton	91%	54
Port Huron Hospital[2]	Port Huron	91%	54
Mercy Health Hackley Campus[2]	Muskegon	90%	90
Karmanos Cancer Center[2]	Detroit	89%	35
Oakwood Hospital - Taylor[2]	Taylor	89%	64
Pennock Hospital[2]	Hastings	88%	25
Genesys Reg Med Ctr-Health Park[2]	Grand Blanc	87%	119
Oakwood Hospital - Dearborn[2]	Dearborn	86%	74
Three Rivers Health[2]	Three Rivers	86%	92
Hillsdale Community Health Center[2]	Hillsdale	85%	26
Oakwood Hospital - Wayne[2]	Wayne	85%	98
Midmichigan Medical Center - Gratiot[2]	Alma	84%	64
Promedica Herrick Hospital[2]	Tecumseh	84%	25
Lakeland Hospital - Saint Joseph[2]	Saint Joseph	83%	36
Marquette General Hospital[2]	Marquette	83%	103
Saint Joseph Mercy Port Huron[2]	Port Huron	80%	79
Chippewa County War Memorial Hospital[2]	Sault Ste Marie	77%	64
Bronson Methodist Hospital[2]	Kalamazoo	71%	65
West Branch Regional Medical Center[2]	West Branch	62%	76
Community Health Center of Branch County[2]	Coldwater	59%	34

Incidence of Potentially Preventable VTE

Hospital Name	City	Rate	Cases
Saint John Hospital & Medical Center[2]	Detroit	0%	48
St John Macomb-Oakland Hosp[2]	Warren	0%	41
William Beaumont Hospital - Troy[2]	Troy	0%	31
Spectrum Health - Butterworth Campus[2]	Grand Rapids	1%	67
Providence Hospital & Medical Centers[2]	Southfield	2%	62
Covenant Medical Center[2]	Saginaw	3%	32
Henry Ford Hospital[2]	Detroit	3%	111
University of Michigan Health System[2]	Ann Arbor	4%	84
Beaumont Health System[2]	Royal Oak	5%	127
Detroit Receiving Hosp & U Health Ctr[2]	Detroit	6%	31
Henry Ford West Bloomfield Hospital[2]	W Bloomfield	6%	35
Henry Ford Wyandotte Hospital[2]	Wyandotte	6%	35
Saint Joseph Mercy Hospital[2]	Ann Arbor	7%	42
Henry Ford Macomb Hospital[2]	Clinton Twp	10%	30
Sinai - Grace Hospital[2]	Detroit	11%	45
Saint Mary Mercy Hospital[2]	Livonia	15%	33
Bronson Methodist Hospital[2]	Kalamazoo	18%	38
Genesys Reg Med Ctr-Health Park[2]	Grand Blanc	23%	64

UFH with Dosages/Platelet Count Monitoring

Hospital Name	City	Rate	Cases
Alpena Regional Medical Center[2]	Alpena	100%	26
Beaumont Health System[2]	Grosse Pointe	100%	90
Beaumont Health System[2]	Royal Oak	100%	407
Borgess Medical Center[2]	Kalamazoo	100%	140
Botsford Hospital[2]	Farmington Hills	100%	180
Crittenton Hospital Medical Center[2]	Rochester	100%	88
Detroit Receiving Hosp & U Health Ctr[2]	Detroit	100%	69
Harper University Hospital[2]	Detroit	100%	72
Henry Ford Hospital[2]	Detroit	100%	320
Henry Ford Macomb Hospital[2]	Clinton Twp	100%	155
Henry Ford Wyandotte Hospital[2]	Wyandotte	100%	168
Holland Community Hospital[2]	Holland	100%	39
Huron Valley - Sinai Hospital[2]	Commerce Twp	100%	69
Mclaren - Northern Michigan[2]	Petoskey	100%	44
Mclaren Bay Region[2]	Bay City	100%	95
Mclaren Central Michigan[2]	Mount Pleasant	100%	45
Mclaren Lapeer Region[2]	Lapeer	100%	67
Mclaren Macomb[2]	Mount Clemens	100%	58
Mercy Health Hackley Campus[2]	Muskegon	100%	32
Mercy Health Partners - Mercy Campus[2]	Muskegon	100%	97
Mercy Hospital - Cadillac[2]	Cadillac	100%	28
Mercy Memorial Hospital System[2]	Monroe	100%	33
Metro Health Hospital[2]	Wyoming	100%	59
Midmichigan Medical Center - Midland[2]	Midland	100%	83
Munson Medical Center[2]	Traverse City	100%	84
Oaklawn Hospital[2]	Marshall	100%	27
Oakwood Hospital - Dearborn[2]	Dearborn	100%	202
Oakwood Hospital - Southshore[2]	Trenton	100%	107
Oakwood Hospital - Taylor[2]	Taylor	100%	55
Oakwood Hospital - Wayne[2]	Wayne	100%	81
Saint John Hospital & Medical Center[2]	Detroit	100%	189
St John Macomb-Oakland Hosp[2]	Warren	100%	229
Saint Joseph Mercy Hospital[2]	Ann Arbor	100%	290
Saint Joseph Mercy Livingston Hospital[2]	Howell	100%	36
Saint Joseph Mercy Oakland[2]	Pontiac	100%	135
Saint Mary Mercy Hospital[2]	Livonia	100%	134
Saint Mary's Health Care[2]	Grand Rapids	100%	85
Sinai - Grace Hospital[2]	Detroit	100%	91
Spectrum Health - Butterworth Campus[2]	Grand Rapids	100%	328
William Beaumont Hospital - Troy[2]	Troy	100%	256
Mclaren - Greater Lansing[2]	Lansing	99%	88
Providence Hospital & Medical Centers[2]	Southfield	99%	363
Saint Mary's of Michigan Medical Center[2]	Saginaw	99%	103
Allegiance Health[2]	Jackson	98%	164
Bronson Battle Creek Hospital[2]	Battle Creek	98%	60
Edward W Sparrow Hospital[2]	Lansing	98%	172
Genesys Reg Med Ctr-Health Park[2]	Grand Blanc	98%	245
Hurley Medical Center[2]	Flint	98%	60
Port Huron Hospital[2]	Port Huron	98%	94
Henry Ford West Bloomfield Hospital[2]	W Bloomfield	97%	139
Mclaren Oakland[2]	Pontiac	97%	37
University of Michigan Health System[2]	Ann Arbor	97%	287
Lakeland Hospital - Saint Joseph[2]	Saint Joseph	95%	104
Mclaren Flint[2]	Flint	91%	219
Community Health Center of Branch County[2]	Coldwater	74%	27
Bronson Methodist Hospital[2]	Kalamazoo	69%	184
Garden City Hospital[2]	Garden City	43%	72
Covenant Medical Center[2]	Saginaw	38%	174

Venous Thromboembolism Prophylaxis

Hospital Name	City	Rate	Cases
Holland Community Hospital[2]	Holland	99%	341
Mclaren Lapeer Region[2]	Lapeer	99%	330
Mercy Memorial Hospital System[2]	Monroe	99%	371
Straith Hospital For Special Surgery	Southfield	99%	447
Chelsea Community Hospital[2]	Chelsea	98%	242
Mclaren - Greater Lansing[2]	Lansing	98%	330
Mclaren Bay Region[2]	Bay City	98%	306
Mercy Hospital - Cadillac[2]	Cadillac	98%	318
Mercy Hospital - Grayling[2]	Grayling	98%	223
Botsford Hospital[2]	Farmington Hills	97%	352
Mclaren - Northern Michigan[2]	Petoskey	97%	305
Memorial Medical Center of West Michigan[2]	Ludington	97%	141
North Ottawa Community Health Center[2]	Grand Haven	97%	105
Southeast Michigan Surgical Hospital	Warren	97%	31
Spectrum Health United Memorial[2]	Greenville	97%	182
University of Michigan Health System[2]	Ann Arbor	97%	359
Mclaren Oakland[2]	Pontiac	96%	335
Portage Health[2]	Hancock	96%	81
Saint John Hospital & Medical Center[2]	Detroit	96%	372
Saint Mary's Health Care[2]	Grand Rapids	96%	308
Spectrum Health Big Rapids Hospital[2]	Big Rapids	96%	124
Spectrum Health United Mem-Kelsey Camp[2]	Lakeview	96%	124
Covenant Medical Center[2]	Saginaw	95%	330
Dickinson County Memorial Hospital[2]	Iron Mountain	95%	242
Providence Hospital & Medical Centers[2]	Southfield	95%	720
Spectrum Health Zeeland Comm Hosp[2]	Zeeland	95%	160
Alpena Regional Medical Center[2]	Alpena	94%	334
Garden City Hospital[2]	Garden City	94%	361
Spectrum Health Gerber Memorial[2]	Fremont	94%	212
Detroit Receiving Hosp & U Health Ctr[2]	Detroit	93%	288
Huron Medical Center[2]	Bad Axe	93%	94
Mercy Health Hackley Campus[2]	Muskegon	93%	258
Midmichigan Medical Center - Clare[2]	Clare	93%	137
St John Macomb-Oakland Hosp[2]	Warren	93%	401

NOTE: Hospital profiles are in alphabetical order by state, then city, then hospital within the city; Rankings exclude hospitals with less than 25 cases except for patient surveys which excludes hospitals with less than 100 cases; (a) 100-299 cases; (1) The number of cases/patients is too few to report; (2) Data submitted were based on a sample of cases/patients; (3) Results are based on a shorter time period than required; (4) Data suppressed by CMS for one or more quarters; (5) Results are not available for this reporting period; (6) Fewer than 100 patients completed the HCAHPS survey; (7) No cases met the criteria for this measure; (8) The lower limit of the confidence interval cannot be calculated if the number of observed infections equals zero; (9) No data are available from the state/territory for this reporting period; (10) The scores shown reflect fewer than 50 completed surveys; (11) There were discrepancies in the data collection process; (12) This measure does not apply to this hospital for this reporting period; (13) Results cannot be calculated for this reporting period; (14) The results for this state are combined with nearby states to protect confidentiality; Please refer to the User's Guide for a full explanation of data.

Hospital Name	City	Rate	Cases
South Haven Community Hospital[2]	South Haven	93%	120
Tawas Saint Joseph Hospital[2]	Tawas City	93%	95
Beaumont Health System[2]	Grosse Pointe	92%	374
Crittenton Hospital Medical Center[2]	Rochester	92%	309
Henry Ford Hospital[2]	Detroit	92%	318
Hillsdale Community Health Center[2]	Hillsdale	92%	105
Mclaren Macomb[2]	Mount Clemens	92%	369
Metro Health Hospital[2]	Wyoming	92%	328
Midmichigan Medical Center - Midland[2]	Midland	92%	311
Oakland Regional Hospital	Southfield	92%	251
Oaklawn Hospital[2]	Marshall	92%	169
Saint Joseph Mercy Livingston Hospital[2]	Howell	92%	326
Chippewa County War Memorial Hospital[2]	Sault Ste Marie	91%	218
Harper University Hospital[2]	Detroit	91%	358
Huron Valley - Sinai Hospital[2]	Commerce Twp	91%	345
Marquette General Hospital[2]	Marquette	91%	222
Mercy Health Partners - Mercy Campus[2]	Muskegon	91%	301
Saint Joseph Mercy Hospital[2]	Ann Arbor	91%	403
Bronson Battle Creek Hospital[2]	Battle Creek	90%	362
Emma L Bixby Medical Center[2]	Adrian	90%	229
Munson Medical Center[2]	Traverse City	90%	430
Three Rivers Health[2]	Three Rivers	90%	582
William Beaumont Hospital - Troy[2]	Troy	90%	355
Beaumont Health System[2]	Royal Oak	89%	383
Memorial Healthcare[2]	Owosso	89%	203
Sinai - Grace Hospital[2]	Detroit	89%	387
Allegiance Health[2]	Jackson	88%	365
Otsego Memorial Hospital[2]	Gaylord	88%	160
Saint Joseph Mercy Oakland[2]	Pontiac	88%	344
Spectrum Health - Reed City Campus[2]	Reed City	88%	90
Hurley Medical Center[2]	Flint	87%	328
Mclaren Flint[2]	Flint	87%	312
Edward W Sparrow Hospital[2]	Lansing	86%	442
Henry Ford West Bloomfield Hospital[2]	W Bloomfield	86%	306
Promedica Herrick Hospital[2]	Tecumseh	85%	71
Lakeland Hospital - Saint Joseph[2]	Saint Joseph	84%	343
Saint Mary Mercy Hospital[2]	Livonia	84%	402
Spectrum Health - Butterworth Campus[2]	Grand Rapids	84%	322
Henry Ford Macomb Hospital[2]	Clinton Twp	83%	372
Oakwood Hospital - Taylor[2]	Taylor	83%	320
Pennock Hospital[2]	Hastings	83%	187
Sparrow Ionia Hospital[2]	Ionia	83%	161
Mclaren Central Michigan[2]	Mount Pleasant	82%	271
Saint John River District Hospital[2]	East China	82%	148
Bronson Methodist Hospital[2]	Kalamazoo	80%	362
Midmichigan Medical Center - Gratiot[2]	Alma	80%	346
Sturgis Hospital[2]	Sturgis	80%	109
Saint Mary's of Michigan Medical Center[2]	Saginaw	79%	315
Carson City Hospital[2]	Carson City	78%	110
Henry Ford Wyandotte Hospital[2]	Wyandotte	78%	365
Borgess Medical Center[2]	Kalamazoo	77%	331
Sparrow Clinton Hospital[2]	Saint Johns	75%	306
Doctors' Hospital of Michigan[2,3]	Pontiac	73%	96
Oakwood Hospital - Dearborn[2]	Dearborn	71%	345
Marlette Regional Hospital[2]	Marlette	69%	108
Genesys Reg Med Ctr-Health Park[2]	Grand Blanc	67%	366
Saint Joseph Mercy Port Huron[2]	Port Huron	66%	316
Karmanos Cancer Center[2]	Detroit	64%	365
Oakwood Hospital - Southshore[2]	Trenton	64%	363
Lakeland Community Hospital - Watervliet[2]	Watervliet	62%	64
Port Huron Hospital[2]	Port Huron	62%	351
Oakwood Hospital - Wayne[2]	Wayne	53%	339
Mercy Health Lakeshore Campus[2]	Shelby	42%	69
Community Health Center of Branch County[2]	Coldwater	41%	270
West Branch Regional Medical Center[2]	West Branch	38%	130
Saint Mary's Standish Community Hospital[2]	Standish	32%	82

Warfarin Therapy Discharge Instructions

Hospital Name	City	Rate	Cases
Holland Community Hospital[2]	Holland	100%	35
Mclaren - Greater Lansing[2]	Lansing	100%	94
Memorial Healthcare[2]	Owosso	100%	27
West Branch Regional Medical Center[2]	West Branch	100%	26
William Beaumont Hospital - Troy[2]	Troy	99%	152
Providence Hospital & Medical Centers[2]	Southfield	98%	226
Mercy Hospital - Cadillac[2]	Cadillac	97%	32
Mercy Memorial Hospital System[2]	Monroe	97%	39
Edward W Sparrow Hospital[2]	Lansing	96%	124
Mclaren Lapeer Region[2]	Lapeer	96%	57
Beaumont Health System[2]	Royal Oak	95%	219
Henry Ford Wyandotte Hospital[2]	Wyandotte	94%	143
Mclaren Bay Region[2]	Bay City	94%	65
Huron Valley - Sinai Hospital[2]	Commerce Twp	93%	54
Oaklawn Hospital[2]	Marshall	93%	30
Mclaren Central Michigan[2]	Mount Pleasant	91%	32
Beaumont Health System[2]	Grosse Pointe	90%	80
Bronson Methodist Hospital[2]	Kalamazoo	90%	133
Henry Ford Macomb Hospital[2]	Clinton Twp	90%	105
Mercy Health Partners - Mercy Campus[2]	Muskegon	90%	73
Midmichigan Medical Center - Midland[2]	Midland	89%	89
Port Huron Hospital[2]	Port Huron	86%	64
Botsford Hospital[2]	Farmington Hills	83%	117
University of Michigan Health System[2]	Ann Arbor	82%	180
Mercy Health Hackley Campus[2]	Muskegon	81%	37
St John Macomb-Oakland Hosp[2]	Warren	81%	151
Spectrum Health United Memorial[2]	Greenville	81%	26
Crittenton Hospital Medical Center[2]	Rochester	80%	60
Detroit Receiving Hosp & U Health Ctr[2]	Detroit	79%	68
Mclaren Flint[2]	Flint	78%	139
Henry Ford West Bloomfield Hospital[2]	W Bloomfield	77%	83
Saint Joseph Mercy Oakland[2]	Pontiac	76%	86
Saint Mary Mercy Hospital[2]	Livonia	75%	113
Borgess Medical Center[2]	Kalamazoo	74%	101
Henry Ford Hospital[2]	Detroit	74%	199
Saint John Hospital & Medical Center[2]	Detroit	74%	123
Mclaren - Northern Michigan[2]	Petoskey	72%	32
Allegiance Health[2]	Jackson	71%	102
Oakwood Hospital - Dearborn[2]	Dearborn	70%	106
Harper University Hospital[2]	Detroit	69%	51
Oakwood Hospital - Wayne[2]	Wayne	65%	34
Saint Mary's Health Care[2]	Grand Rapids	63%	91
Hurley Medical Center[2]	Flint	60%	50
Spectrum Health - Butterworth Campus[2]	Grand Rapids	59%	239
Covenant Medical Center[2]	Saginaw	57%	141
Bronson Battle Creek Hospital[2]	Battle Creek	54%	59
Mclaren Macomb[2]	Mount Clemens	49%	69
Sinai - Grace Hospital[2]	Detroit	47%	98
Saint Joseph Mercy Livingston Hospital[2]	Howell	36%	36
Munson Medical Center[2]	Traverse City	33%	88
Saint Mary's of Michigan Medical Center[2]	Saginaw	32%	75
Metro Health Hospital[2]	Wyoming	29%	55
Saint Joseph Mercy Hospital[2]	Ann Arbor	25%	208
Lakeland Hospital - Saint Joseph[2]	Saint Joseph	22%	97
Marquette General Hospital[2]	Marquette	20%	40
Genesys Reg Med Ctr-Health Park[2]	Grand Blanc	19%	162
Oakwood Hospital - Southshore[2]	Trenton	3%	76
Oakwood Hospital - Taylor[2]	Taylor	0%	33

Chest Pain/Possible Heart Attack Care

Aspirin Given Within 24 Hours of Arrival

Hospital Name	City	Rate	Cases
Alpena Regional Medical Center	Alpena	100%	95
Aspirus Grand View Hospital	Ironwood	100%	50
Baraga County Memorial Hospital	L' Anse	100%	35
Detroit Receiving Hosp & U Health Ctr	Detroit	100%	166
Garden City Hospital	Garden City	100%	29
Hayes Green Beach Memorial Hospital	Charlotte	100%	39
Hills & Dales General Hospital	Cass City	100%	39
Holland Community Hospital	Holland	100%	37
Huron Medical Center	Bad Axe	100%	27
Kalkaska Memorial Health Center	Kalkaska	100%	68
Mclaren Lapeer Region	Lapeer	100%	83
Mercy Memorial Hospital System	Monroe	100%	68
Midmichigan Medical Center - Gladwin	Gladwin	100%	144
Oaklawn Hospital	Marshall	100%	271
Oakwood Hospital - Southshore	Trenton	100%	56
Saint John Hospital & Medical Center	Detroit	100%	40
Saint Joseph Mercy Port Huron	Port Huron	100%	30
Sparrow Clinton Hospital	Saint Johns	100%	29
Spectrum Health United Mem-Kelsey Camp	Lakeview	100%	35
Spectrum Health Zeeland Comm Hosp	Zeeland	100%	78
West Shore Medical Center	Manistee	100%	59
Carson City Hospital	Carson City	99%	72
Dickinson County Memorial Hospital	Iron Mountain	99%	72
Mclaren Oakland	Pontiac	99%	86
Spectrum Health Big Rapids Hospital	Big Rapids	99%	138
Eaton Rapids Medical Center	Eaton Rapids	98%	60
Marlette Regional Hospital	Marlette	98%	53
Mclaren Central Michigan	Mount Pleasant	98%	63
Midmichigan Medical Center - Clare	Clare	98%	130
Midmichigan Medical Center - Gratiot	Alma	98%	110
Northstar Health System	Iron River	98%	42
Oakwood Hospital - Taylor	Taylor	98%	59
Oakwood Hospital - Wayne	Wayne	98%	48
Portage Health	Hancock	98%	51
Saint Francis Hospital	Escanaba	98%	66
St John Macomb-Oakland Hosp	Warren	98%	65
Saint John River District Hospital	East China	98%	55
Scheurer Hospital	Pigeon	98%	52
Spectrum Health United Memorial	Greenville	98%	127
Chelsea Community Hospital	Chelsea	97%	91
Mercy Hospital - Grayling	Grayling	97%	169
Promedica Herrick Hospital	Tecumseh	97%	70
South Haven Community Hospital	South Haven	97%	78
Spectrum Health Gerber Memorial	Fremont	97%	115
Tawas Saint Joseph Hospital	Tawas City	97%	180
West Branch Regional Medical Center	West Branch	97%	79
Bell Hospital	Ishpeming	96%	27
Chippewa County War Memorial Hospital	Sault Ste Marie	96%	84
Emma L Bixby Medical Center	Adrian	96%	188
Lakeland Community Hospital - Watervliet	Watervliet	96%	25
Memorial Healthcare	Owosso	96%	93
Memorial Medical Center of West Michigan	Ludington	96%	77
Otsego Memorial Hospital	Gaylord	96%	105
Paul Oliver Memorial Hospital	Frankfort	96%	55
Pennock Hospital	Hastings	96%	49
Saint Mary Mercy Hospital	Livonia	96%	49
Henry Ford Hospital	Detroit	95%	38
Henry Ford Wyandotte Hospital	Wyandotte	95%	105
Saint Mary's Standish Community Hospital	Standish	95%	132
Bronson Battle Creek Hospital	Battle Creek	94%	140
Community Health Center of Branch County	Coldwater	94%	187
North Ottawa Community Health Center	Grand Haven	94%	77
Schoolcraft Memorial Hospital	Manistique	94%	35
Spectrum Health - Reed City Campus	Reed City	94%	106
Allegan General Hospital	Allegan	93%	58
Allegiance Health	Jackson	93%	29
Caro Community Hospital	Caro	92%	51
Hillsdale Community Health Center	Hillsdale	92%	89
Mercy Health Hackley Campus	Muskegon	92%	53
Mercy Hospital - Cadillac	Cadillac	92%	78
Saint Joseph Mercy Livingston Hospital	Howell	92%	155
Sturgis Hospital	Sturgis	91%	65
Mercy Health Lakeshore Campus	Shelby	77%	30
Three Rivers Health	Three Rivers	73%	237

Fibrinolytic Meds Within 30 Minutes of Arrival

Hospital Name	City	Rate	Cases
Tawas Saint Joseph Hospital	Tawas City	59%	27

Average Time to ECG (minutes)

Hospital Name	City	Min.	Cases
Sturgis Hospital	Sturgis	0	72
Marlette Regional Hospital	Marlette	2	50
Kalkaska Memorial Health Center	Kalkaska	3	72
Oakwood Hospital - Southshore	Trenton	3	55
Saint John River District Hospital	East China	3	55
Helen Newberry Joy Hospital	Newberry	4	25
Mclaren Lapeer Region	Lapeer	4	83
Oaklawn Hospital	Marshall	4	283
Saint Joseph Mercy Port Huron	Port Huron	4	30
Tawas Saint Joseph Hospital	Tawas City	4	182
Eaton Rapids Medical Center	Eaton Rapids	5	65
Hillsdale Community Health Center	Hillsdale	5	93
Mercy Hospital - Grayling	Grayling	5	173
Mercy Memorial Hospital System	Monroe	5	68
Oakwood Hospital - Taylor	Taylor	5	60
Saint John Hospital & Medical Center	Detroit	5	41
Spectrum Health - Reed City Campus	Reed City	5	110
Spectrum Health United Memorial	Greenville	5	131
Chelsea Community Hospital	Chelsea	6	92
Emma L Bixby Medical Center	Adrian	6	191
Garden City Hospital	Garden City	6	30
Mclaren Central Michigan	Mount Pleasant	6	66
North Ottawa Community Health Center	Grand Haven	6	82
Oakwood Hospital - Wayne	Wayne	6	53
Saint Joseph Mercy Livingston Hospital	Howell	6	158
Scheurer Hospital	Pigeon	6	54
Schoolcraft Memorial Hospital	Manistique	6	36
Sparrow Clinton Hospital	Saint Johns	6	30
West Shore Medical Center	Manistee	6	61
Aspirus Grand View Hospital	Ironwood	7	50
Carson City Hospital	Carson City	7	77
Henry Ford Wyandotte Hospital	Wyandotte	7	107
Hills & Dales General Hospital	Cass City	7	39
Holland Community Hospital	Holland	7	39
Lakeland Community Hospital - Watervliet	Watervliet	7	25
Mclaren Oakland	Pontiac	7	86
Midmichigan Medical Center - Clare	Clare	7	136
Otsego Memorial Hospital	Gaylord	7	106
Paul Oliver Memorial Hospital	Frankfort	7	56
Pennock Hospital	Hastings	7	50
Promedica Herrick Hospital	Tecumseh	7	74
St John Macomb-Oakland Hosp	Warren	7	67
Spectrum Health United Mem-Kelsey Camp	Lakeview	7	36
Alpena Regional Medical Center	Alpena	8	95
Hayes Green Beach Memorial Hospital	Charlotte	8	39
Huron Medical Center	Bad Axe	8	27
Mercy Hospital - Cadillac	Cadillac	8	81
Midmichigan Medical Center - Gratiot	Alma	8	116
Northstar Health System	Iron River	8	42
Portage Health	Hancock	8	52
Spectrum Health Big Rapids Hospital	Big Rapids	8	144
Allegiance Health	Jackson	9	29
Caro Community Hospital	Caro	9	53
Memorial Healthcare	Owosso	9	96
Memorial Medical Center of West Michigan	Ludington	9	79
Spectrum Health Gerber Memorial	Fremont	9	123
Spectrum Health Zeeland Comm Hosp	Zeeland	9	80
Baraga County Memorial Hospital	L' Anse	10	35

NOTE: Hospital profiles are in alphabetical order by state, then city, then hospital within the city; Rankings exclude hospitals with less than 25 cases except for patient surveys which excludes hospitals with less than 100 cases; (a) 100-299 cases; (1) The number of cases/patients is too few to report; (2) Data submitted were based on a sample of cases/patients; (3) Results are based on a shorter time period than required; (4) Data suppressed by CMS for one or more quarters; (5) Results are not available for this reporting period; (6) Fewer than 100 patients completed the HCAHPS survey; (7) No cases met the criteria for this measure; (8) The lower limit of the confidence interval cannot be calculated if the number of observed infections equals zero; (9) No data are available from the state/territory for this reporting period; (10) The scores shown reflect fewer than 50 completed surveys; (11) There were discrepancies in the data collection process; (12) This measure does not apply to this hospital for this reporting period; (13) Results cannot be calculated for this reporting period; (14) The results for this state are combined with nearby states to protect confidentiality; Please refer to the User's Guide for a full explanation of data.

Bronson Battle Creek Hospital	Battle Creek	10	145
Dickinson County Memorial Hospital	Iron Mountain	10	73
Henry Ford Hospital	Detroit	10	38
Midmichigan Medical Center - Gladwin	Gladwin	10	154
Saint Francis Hospital	Escanaba	10	68
Saint Mary Mercy Hospital	Livonia	10	50
South Haven Community Hospital	South Haven	10	82
Three Rivers Health	Three Rivers	10	250
West Branch Regional Medical Center	West Branch	10	81
Allegan General Hospital	Allegan	11	60
Bell Hospital	Ishpeming	12	27
Community Health Center of Branch County	Coldwater	12	196
Mercy Health Hackley Campus	Muskegon	12	54
Chippewa County War Memorial Hospital	Sault Ste Marie	13	85
Detroit Receiving Hosp & U Health Ctr	Detroit	14	167
Mercy Health Lakeshore Campus	Shelby	14	34
Saint Mary's Standish Community Hospital	Standish	20	133

Average Time to Transfer (minutes)

Hospital Name	City	Min.	Cases
Mclaren Lapeer Region	Lapeer	29	27
Bronson Battle Creek Hospital	Battle Creek	63	25

Children's Asthma Care

Received Home Management Plan of Care

Hospital Name	City	Rate	Cases
Bronson Methodist Hospital	Kalamazoo	96%	74
Children's Hospital of Michigan[2]	Detroit	95%	371
Spectrum Health - Butterworth Campus	Grand Rapids	95%	164

Received Reliever Medication

Hospital Name	City	Rate	Cases
Bronson Methodist Hospital	Kalamazoo	100%	75
Children's Hospital of Michigan[2]	Detroit	100%	372
Spectrum Health - Butterworth Campus	Grand Rapids	99%	164

Received Systemic Corticosteroids

Hospital Name	City	Rate	Cases
Bronson Methodist Hospital	Kalamazoo	100%	75
Children's Hospital of Michigan[2]	Detroit	100%	372
Spectrum Health - Butterworth Campus	Grand Rapids	99%	164

Emergency Department

Admittance Decision Time (minutes)

Hospital Name	City	Min.	Cases
Lakeland Community Hospital - Watervliet[2]	Watervliet	37	282
Sparrow Clinton Hospital[2]	Saint Johns	45	542
Carson City Hospital[2]	Carson City	46	184
Portage Health[2]	Hancock	48	249
Saint Francis Hospital[2]	Escanaba	49	426
Pennock Hospital[2]	Hastings	50	242
Sturgis Hospital[2]	Sturgis	50	173
Metro Health Hospital[2]	Wyoming	52	585
Spectrum Health United Mem-Kelsey Camp	Lakeview	52	145
Tawas Saint Joseph Hospital[2]	Tawas City	52	286
Marlette Regional Hospital[2]	Marlette	54	335
Bell Hospital[2]	Ishpeming	55	105
Memorial Healthcare[2]	Owosso	57	368
Sparrow Ionia Hospital[2]	Ionia	57	481
Memorial Medical Center of West Michigan[2]	Ludington	60	351
Three Rivers Health[2]	Three Rivers	60	349
Chippewa County War Memorial Hospital[2]	Sault Ste Marie	62	405
Holland Community Hospital[2]	Holland	62	531
Mclaren Bay Region[2]	Bay City	64	482
Saint John River District Hospital[2]	East China	65	150
West Branch Regional Medical Center[2]	West Branch	65	174
Chelsea Community Hospital[2]	Chelsea	66	253
Hills & Dales General Hospital	Cass City	67	419
Bronson Battle Creek Hospital[2]	Battle Creek	68	603
Dickinson County Memorial Hospital[2]	Iron Mountain	68	332
Midmichigan Medical Center - Gratiot[2]	Alma	70	428
Midmichigan Medical Center - Clare[2]	Clare	71	482
Oaklawn Hospital[2]	Marshall	71	283
Mclaren Central Michigan[2]	Mount Pleasant	73	417
Spectrum Health Big Rapids Hospital[2]	Big Rapids	73	301
Huron Valley - Sinai Hospital[2]	Commerce Twp	74	564
Huron Medical Center[2]	Bad Axe	75	172
Detroit Receiving Hosp & U Health Ctr[2]	Detroit	77	759
Promedica Herrick Hospital[2]	Tecumseh	77	419
Harper University Hospital[2]	Detroit	78	252
Beaumont Health System[2]	Royal Oak	80	576
Hillsdale Community Health Center[2]	Hillsdale	80	395
Spectrum Health United Memorial[2]	Greenville	80	336
Saint Joseph Mercy Port Huron[2]	Port Huron	84	478
Edward W Sparrow Hospital[2]	Lansing	85	941
Sinai - Grace Hospital[2]	Detroit	86	520
Port Huron Hospital[2]	Port Huron	88	572
Saint John Hospital & Medical Center[2]	Detroit	88	579
Lakeland Hospital - Saint Joseph[2]	Saint Joseph	90	618
Midmichigan Medical Center - Midland[2]	Midland	92	519
Saint Joseph Mercy Livingston Hospital[2]	Howell	92	570
South Haven Community Hospital[2]	South Haven	94	277
Saint Mary Mercy Hospital[2]	Livonia	95	721
Saint Mary's Health Care[2]	Grand Rapids	96	404
Mercy Health Hackley Campus[2]	Muskegon	98	312
Oakwood Hospital - Southshore[2]	Trenton	99	797
Spectrum Health - Butterworth Campus[2]	Grand Rapids	101	449
Emma L Bixby Medical Center[2]	Adrian	102	414
Spectrum Health Zeeland Comm Hosp[2]	Zeeland	102	224
Allegiance Health[2]	Jackson	105	781
Beaumont Health System[2]	Grosse Pointe	105	755
Botsford Hospital[2]	Farmington Hills	106	865
Mercy Memorial Hospital System[2]	Monroe	108	726
Oakwood Hospital - Wayne[2]	Wayne	108	800
Crittenton Hospital Medical Center[2]	Rochester	110	632
North Ottawa Community Health Center[2]	Grand Haven	112	301
Saint Joseph Mercy Hospital[2]	Ann Arbor	112	583
Alpena Regional Medical Center[2]	Alpena	114	589
Otsego Memorial Hospital[2]	Gaylord	117	221
Covenant Medical Center[2]	Saginaw	118	766
Oakwood Hospital - Taylor[2]	Taylor	119	593
Bronson Methodist Hospital[2]	Kalamazoo	120	482
Mercy Hospital - Cadillac[2]	Cadillac	124	524
Saint Mary's of Michigan Medical Center[2]	Saginaw	124	523
Doctors' Hospital of Michigan[2,3]	Pontiac	125	119
Providence Hospital & Medical Centers[2]	Southfield	127	1281
Henry Ford Macomb Hospital[2]	Clinton Twp	129	649
Mercy Health Partners - Mercy Campus[2]	Muskegon	130	508
St John Macomb-Oakland Hosp[2]	Warren	130	840
Saint Joseph Mercy Oakland[2]	Pontiac	132	567
Spectrum Health Gerber Memorial[2]	Fremont	132	412
Mclaren - Northern Michigan[2]	Petoskey	133	481
William Beaumont Hospital - Troy[2]	Troy	138	661
Community Health Center of Branch County[2]	Coldwater	139	165
Mclaren Macomb[2]	Mount Clemens	139	525
Marquette General Hospital[2]	Marquette	142	200
Borgess Medical Center[2]	Kalamazoo	144	506
Mercy Hospital - Grayling[2]	Grayling	147	507
Mclaren Lapeer Region[2]	Lapeer	150	858
Hurley Medical Center[2]	Flint	158	542
Mclaren Oakland[2]	Pontiac	164	519
Mclaren Flint[2]	Flint	165	723
Mclaren - Greater Lansing[2]	Lansing	167	339
Genesys Reg Med Ctr-Health Park[2]	Grand Blanc	168	735
Oakwood Hospital - Dearborn[2]	Dearborn	168	636
Henry Ford Hospital[2]	Detroit	172	628
Munson Medical Center[2]	Traverse City	177	523
Garden City Hospital[2]	Garden City	204	867
University of Michigan Health System[2]	Ann Arbor	213	529
Henry Ford Wyandotte Hospital[2]	Wyandotte	218	738
Henry Ford West Bloomfield Hospital[2]	W Bloomfield	236	566

Head CT Results Within 45 Minutes of Arrival

Hospital Name	City	Rate	Cases
Saint Joseph Mercy Livingston Hospital	Howell	88%	33
Henry Ford Wyandotte Hospital	Wyandotte	67%	33
St John Macomb-Oakland Hosp	Warren	40%	50
Genesys Reg Med Ctr-Health Park	Grand Blanc	13%	39

Patients Who Left ER Before Being Seen

Hospital Name	City	Rate	Cases
Borgess - Lee Memorial Hospital	Dowagiac	0%	5058
Carson City Hospital	Carson City	0%	13544
Covenant Medical Center	Saginaw	0%	88793
Henry Ford Macomb Hospital	Clinton Twp	0%	71171
Henry Ford Wyandotte Hospital	Wyandotte	0%	93821
Holland Community Hospital	Holland	0%	44109
Huron Medical Center	Bad Axe	0%	7162
Huron Valley - Sinai Hospital	Commerce Twp	0%	33716
Mackinac Straits Hospital & Health Center	Saint Ignace	0%	5631
Marquette General Hospital	Marquette	0%	25338
Mclaren Lapeer Region	Lapeer	0%	30425
Mclaren Macomb	Mount Clemens	0%	64826
North Ottawa Community Health Center	Grand Haven	0%	17113
Portage Health	Hancock	0%	13424
Saint John River District Hospital	East China	0%	12409
Saint Joseph Mercy Livingston Hospital	Howell	0%	47535
Saint Mary's Health Care	Grand Rapids	0%	62942
Spectrum Health Zeeland Comm Hosp	Zeeland	0%	22256
Allegiance Health	Jackson	1%	81072
Alpena Regional Medical Center	Alpena	1%	22540
Beaumont Health System	Royal Oak	1%	119950
Bronson Methodist Hospital	Kalamazoo	1%	94713
Chelsea Community Hospital	Chelsea	1%	17222
Community Health Center of Branch County	Coldwater	1%	24850
Crittenton Hospital Medical Center	Rochester	1%	29773
Detroit Receiving Hosp & U Health Ctr	Detroit	1%	104694
Dickinson County Memorial Hospital	Iron Mountain	1%	18847
Emma L Bixby Medical Center	Adrian	1%	34185
Genesys Reg Med Ctr-Health Park	Grand Blanc	1%	64075
Harper University Hospital	Detroit	1%	40222
Henry Ford West Bloomfield Hospital	W Bloomfield	1%	39507
Hillsdale Community Health Center	Hillsdale	1%	25643
Mclaren - Northern Michigan	Petoskey	1%	28832
Mclaren Bay Region	Bay City	1%	44062
Mclaren Central Michigan	Mount Pleasant	1%	31677
Mclaren Oakland	Pontiac	1%	53668
Memorial Medical Center of West Michigan	Ludington	1%	25440
Mercy Health Hackley Campus	Muskegon	1%	61613
Mercy Hospital - Grayling	Grayling	1%	20702
Mercy Memorial Hospital System	Monroe	1%	47169
Midmichigan Medical Center - Gratiot	Alma	1%	21483
Midmichigan Medical Center - Midland	Midland	1%	36764
Munson Medical Center	Traverse City	1%	25657
Oaklawn Hospital	Marshall	1%	22966
Oakwood Hospital - Southshore	Trenton	1%	30111
Providence Hospital & Medical Centers	Southfield	1%	112364
Saint John Hospital & Medical Center	Detroit	1%	120928
Sinai - Grace Hospital	Detroit	1%	102706
South Haven Community Hospital	South Haven	1%	14363
Spectrum Health - Butterworth Campus	Grand Rapids	1%	190840
Spectrum Health Big Rapids Hospital	Big Rapids	1%	23791
Spectrum Health Gerber Memorial	Fremont	1%	24676
Spectrum Health United Memorial	Greenville	1%	27296
Sturgis Hospital	Sturgis	1%	15568
Tawas Saint Joseph Hospital	Tawas City	1%	16843
Three Rivers Health	Three Rivers	1%	20605
William Beaumont Hospital - Troy	Troy	1%	79773
Beaumont Health System	Grosse Pointe	2%	35153
Borgess Medical Center	Kalamazoo	2%	55230
Botsford Hospital	Farmington Hills	2%	44118
Chippewa County War Memorial Hospital	Sault Ste Marie	2%	17121
Edward W Sparrow Hospital	Lansing	2%	130599
Garden City Hospital	Garden City	2%	51303
Henry Ford Hospital	Detroit	2%	192401
Mclaren Flint	Flint	2%	67081
Memorial Healthcare	Owosso	2%	28610
Mercy Health Partners - Mercy Campus	Muskegon	2%	47072
Mercy Hospital - Cadillac	Cadillac	2%	22329
Otsego Memorial Hospital	Gaylord	2%	13910
Pennock Hospital	Hastings	2%	18102
St John Macomb-Oakland Hosp	Warren	2%	104623
Saint Joseph Mercy Hospital	Ann Arbor	2%	97263
Saint Joseph Mercy Oakland	Pontiac	2%	53567
Saint Joseph Mercy Port Huron	Port Huron	2%	11101
Saint Mary Mercy Hospital	Livonia	2%	42745
Saint Mary's of Michigan Medical Center	Saginaw	2%	53811
University of Michigan Health System	Ann Arbor	2%	97196
Lakeland Community Hospital - Watervliet	Watervliet	3%	11542
Lakeland Hospital - Saint Joseph	Saint Joseph	3%	69855
Metro Health Hospital	Wyoming	3%	32356
Midmichigan Medical Center - Clare	Clare	3%	15575
Bronson Battle Creek Hospital	Battle Creek	4%	51249
Hurley Medical Center	Flint	4%	99803
Mclaren - Greater Lansing	Lansing	4%	44750
Oakwood Hospital - Dearborn	Dearborn	4%	76743
Oakwood Hospital - Taylor	Taylor	4%	31654
Port Huron Hospital	Port Huron	4%	40108
West Branch Regional Medical Center	West Branch	4%	16318
Oakwood Hospital - Wayne	Wayne	7%	41400

Time from ER Arrival to Being Admitted (minutes)

Hospital Name	City	Min.	Cases
Detroit Receiving Hosp & U Health Ctr[2]	Detroit	173	763
Carson City Hospital[2]	Carson City	180	209
Metro Health Hospital[2]	Wyoming	195	637
Marlette Regional Hospital[2]	Marlette	200	440
Portage Health[2]	Hancock	201	275
Sturgis Hospital[2]	Sturgis	208	186
Lakeland Community Hospital - Watervliet[2]	Watervliet	210	282
Saint John River District Hospital[2]	East China	210	321
Huron Valley - Sinai Hospital[2]	Commerce Twp	212	587
Tawas Saint Joseph Hospital[2]	Tawas City	213	297
Holland Community Hospital[2]	Holland	215	534
Sparrow Ionia Hospital[2]	Ionia	216	495
Promedica Herrick Hospital[2]	Tecumseh	217	419
Hills & Dales General Hospital	Cass City	219	419
Huron Medical Center[2]	Bad Axe	220	178
Mclaren Central Michigan[2]	Mount Pleasant	228	425
Dickinson County Memorial Hospital[2]	Iron Mountain	230	346
Sparrow Clinton Hospital[2]	Saint Johns	230	544
Spectrum Health United Mem-Kelsey Camp	Lakeview	232	155
Three Rivers Health[2]	Three Rivers	232	367
Hillsdale Community Health Center[2]	Hillsdale	234	422
Saint Francis Hospital[2]	Escanaba	234	465
Harper University Hospital[2]	Detroit	237	290
Covenant Medical Center[2]	Saginaw	238	767

NOTE: Hospital profiles are in alphabetical order by state, then city, then hospital within the city; Rankings exclude hospitals with less than 25 cases except for patient surveys which excludes hospitals with less than 100 cases; (a) 100-299 cases; (1) The number of cases/patients is too few to report; (2) Data submitted were based on a sample of cases/patients; (3) Results are based on a shorter time period than required; (4) Data suppressed by CMS for one or more quarters; (5) Results are not available for this reporting period; (6) Fewer than 100 patients completed the HCAHPS survey; (7) No cases met the criteria for this measure; (8) The lower limit of the confidence interval cannot be calculated if the number of observed infections equals zero; (9) No data are available from the state/territory for this reporting period; (10) The scores shown reflect fewer than 50 completed surveys; (11) There were discrepancies in the data collection process; (12) This measure does not apply to this hospital for this reporting period; (13) Results cannot be calculated for this reporting period; (14) The results for this state are combined with nearby states to protect confidentiality; Please refer to the User's Guide for a full explanation of data.

Chippewa County War Memorial Hospital[2]	Sault Ste Marie	240	408
Spectrum Health United Memorial[2]	Greenville	240	337
Saint Joseph Mercy Port Huron[2]	Port Huron	243	479
Midmichigan Medical Center - Midland[2]	Midland	245	545
Bell Hospital[2]	Ishpeming	246	114
Pennock Hospital[2]	Hastings	246	248
Midmichigan Medical Center - Clare[2]	Clare	248	546
Oaklawn Hospital[2]	Marshall	251	291
Mclaren Bay Region[2]	Bay City	253	498
Saint Mary's Health Care[2]	Grand Rapids	253	404
Spectrum Health - Butterworth Campus[2]	Grand Rapids	254	454
Mclaren - Northern Michigan[2]	Petoskey	256	488
Midmichigan Medical Center - Gratiot[2]	Alma	257	477
Memorial Healthcare[2]	Owosso	261	376
Emma L Bixby Medical Center[2]	Adrian	262	414
Spectrum Health Zeeland Comm Hosp[2]	Zeeland	263	229
Community Health Center of Branch County[2]	Coldwater	265	385
Mclaren Oakland[2]	Pontiac	265	537
Spectrum Health Big Rapids Hospital[2]	Big Rapids	267	302
Memorial Medical Center of West Michigan[2]	Ludington	271	357
North Ottawa Community Health Center[2]	Grand Haven	271	306
Alpena Regional Medical Center[2]	Alpena	272	601
Bronson Battle Creek Hospital[2]	Battle Creek	274	617
Saint Joseph Mercy Livingston Hospital[2]	Howell	275	578
Lakeland Hospital - Saint Joseph[2]	Saint Joseph	279	623
Botsford Hospital[2]	Farmington Hills	280	865
Otsego Memorial Hospital[2]	Gaylord	283	241
Marquette General Hospital[2]	Marquette	284	216
Crittenton Hospital Medical Center[2]	Rochester	285	633
Mercy Health Hackley Campus[2]	Muskegon	286	315
Beaumont Health System[2]	Grosse Pointe	288	757
Doctors' Hospital of Michigan[2,3]	Pontiac	288	128
Mercy Memorial Hospital System[2]	Monroe	288	741
Port Huron Hospital[2]	Port Huron	288	585
Spectrum Health Gerber Memorial[2]	Fremont	290	420
West Branch Regional Medical Center[2]	West Branch	296	195
Mercy Hospital - Cadillac[2]	Cadillac	297	539
Mercy Health Partners - Mercy Campus[2]	Muskegon	298	518
Saint John Hospital & Medical Center[2]	Detroit	298	604
Allegiance Health[2]	Jackson	302	784
Borgess Medical Center[2]	Kalamazoo	302	510
Sinai - Grace Hospital[2]	Detroit	302	603
Chelsea Community Hospital[2]	Chelsea	304	263
Saint Mary's of Michigan Medical Center[2]	Saginaw	305	563
Mercy Hospital - Grayling[2]	Grayling	307	508
Saint Mary Mercy Hospital[2]	Livonia	309	748
Mclaren Macomb[2]	Mount Clemens	311	593
Bronson Methodist Hospital[2]	Kalamazoo	314	504
Beaumont Health System[2]	Royal Oak	318	577
Edward W Sparrow Hospital[2]	Lansing	319	955
Providence Hospital & Medical Centers[2]	Southfield	321	1300
Saint Joseph Mercy Oakland[2]	Pontiac	322	618
South Haven Community Hospital[2]	South Haven	325	278
Henry Ford West Bloomfield Hospital[2]	W Bloomfield	326	568
Munson Medical Center[2]	Traverse City	326	532
Mclaren Lapeer Region[2]	Lapeer	327	858
Saint Joseph Mercy Hospital[2]	Ann Arbor	337	594
St John Macomb-Oakland Hosp[2]	Warren	338	848
Henry Ford Macomb Hospital[2]	Clinton Twp	340	700
Oakwood Hospital - Southshore[2]	Trenton	347	797
Oakwood Hospital - Taylor[2]	Taylor	351	593
Oakwood Hospital - Wayne[2]	Wayne	352	800
William Beaumont Hospital - Troy[2]	Troy	352	664
Genesys Reg Med Ctr-Health Park[2]	Grand Blanc	364	791
Hurley Medical Center[2]	Flint	407	551
Henry Ford Wyandotte Hospital[2]	Wyandotte	408	764
Mclaren - Greater Lansing[2]	Lansing	416	578
University of Michigan Health System[2]	Ann Arbor	416	534
Henry Ford Hospital[2]	Detroit	417	629
Mclaren Flint[2]	Flint	426	747
Oakwood Hospital - Dearborn[2]	Dearborn	434	642
Garden City Hospital[2]	Garden City	452	867

Time from ER Arrival to Discharge (minutes)

Hospital Name	City	Min.	Cases
Caro Community Hospital	Caro	69	345
Aspirus Keweenaw Hospital	Laurium	70	354
McKenzie Health System	Sandusky	74	359
Marlette Regional Hospital	Marlette	77	307
Mclaren Oakland	Pontiac	79	334
Paul Oliver Memorial Hospital	Frankfort	79	348
Portage Health	Hancock	79	398
Baraga County Memorial Hospital	L' Anse	80	257
Saint Mary's Standish Community Hospital	Standish	80	371
Mercy Health Hackley Campus	Muskegon	84	366
Mercy Health Lakeshore Campus	Shelby	85	355
Northstar Health System	Iron River	85	412
Aspirus Ontonagon Hospital	Ontonagon	88	238
Memorial Medical Center of West Michigan	Ludington	90	566
Scheurer Hospital	Pigeon	90	376
Emma L Bixby Medical Center	Adrian	91	326
Promedica Herrick Hospital	Tecumseh	91	321
Carson City Hospital	Carson City	92	428
Spectrum Health - Reed City Campus	Reed City	93	396
West Shore Medical Center	Manistee	94	360
Huron Medical Center	Bad Axe	95	352
Schoolcraft Memorial Hospital	Manistique	95	1275
Kalkaska Memorial Health Center	Kalkaska	96	465
Saint John River District Hospital	East China	96	350
Sparrow Ionia Hospital	Ionia	96	435
Sturgis Hospital	Sturgis	96	332
Eaton Rapids Medical Center	Eaton Rapids	99	421
Mercy Memorial Hospital System	Monroe	99	493
Mackinac Straits Hospital & Health Center	Saint Ignace	100	1222
Tawas Saint Joseph Hospital	Tawas City	100	377
Three Rivers Health	Three Rivers	101	602
Lakeland Community Hospital - Watervliet	Watervliet	102	363
Bell Hospital	Ishpeming	103	986
Community Health Center of Branch County	Coldwater	103	325
North Ottawa Community Health Center	Grand Haven	104	424
Detroit Receiving Hosp & U Health Ctr	Detroit	106	272
Mclaren Central Michigan	Mount Pleasant	106	404
Spectrum Health Zeeland Comm Hosp	Zeeland	106	354
Marquette General Hospital	Marquette	107	341
Munising Memorial Hospital	Munising	108	291
Mclaren - Northern Michigan	Petoskey	109	366
Borgess - Lee Memorial Hospital	Dowagiac	110	484
Doctors' Hospital of Michigan[3]	Pontiac	110	149
Hills & Dales General Hospital	Cass City	110	282
Saint Joseph Mercy Port Huron	Port Huron	110	363
Hillsdale Community Health Center	Hillsdale	111	251
Metro Health Hospital	Wyoming	111	465
Spectrum Health United Mem-Kelsey Camp	Lakeview	112	382
Botsford Hospital	Farmington Hills	114	364
Sparrow Clinton Hospital	Saint Johns	114	445
Bronson Lakeview Hospital	Paw Paw	115	399
Spectrum Health United Memorial	Greenville	115	463
Henry Ford Wyandotte Hospital	Wyandotte	118	376
Saint Joseph Mercy Livingston Hospital	Howell	119	415
Oaklawn Hospital	Marshall	121	333
Holland Community Hospital	Holland	122	376
Spectrum Health Big Rapids Hospital	Big Rapids	122	444
Charlevoix Area Hospital	Charlevoix	124	328
Dickinson County Memorial Hospital	Iron Mountain	124	381
Otsego Memorial Hospital	Gaylord	124	330
Spectrum Health - Butterworth Campus	Grand Rapids	124	1364
Spectrum Health Gerber Memorial	Fremont	126	430
Memorial Healthcare	Owosso	127	402
Saint John Hospital & Medical Center	Detroit	127	341
Allegan General Hospital	Allegan	128	361
Lakeland Hospital - Saint Joseph	Saint Joseph	128	359
Saint Mary's of Michigan Medical Center	Saginaw	128	369
Huron Valley - Sinai Hospital	Commerce Twp	130	344
Mclaren Macomb	Mount Clemens	130	382
Mercy Health Partners - Mercy Campus	Muskegon	130	361
Saint Mary's Health Care	Grand Rapids	131	338
Port Huron Hospital	Port Huron	133	414
Deckerville Community Hospital	Deckerville	135	171
Chippewa County War Memorial Hospital	Sault Ste Marie	136	310
Harbor Beach Community Hospital	Harbor Beach	138	266
Sheridan Community Hospital	Sheridan	138	1178
Alpena Regional Medical Center	Alpena	139	388
Midmichigan Medical Center - Gladwin	Gladwin	139	404
Mclaren Bay Region	Bay City	140	436
Bronson Methodist Hospital	Kalamazoo	141	450
Oakwood Hospital - Wayne	Wayne	142	334
Harper University Hospital	Detroit	144	424
Pennock Hospital	Hastings	144	400
South Haven Community Hospital	South Haven	147	439
Mclaren Lapeer Region	Lapeer	151	345
Borgess Medical Center	Kalamazoo	153	517
Henry Ford Hospital	Detroit	153	377
Saint Joseph Mercy Oakland	Pontiac	154	354
Saint Francis Hospital	Escanaba	155	399
Providence Hospital & Medical Centers	Southfield	156	720
Garden City Hospital	Garden City	157	1053
Hayes Green Beach Memorial Hospital	Charlotte	157	412
Helen Newberry Joy Hospital	Newberry	157	341
Sinai - Grace Hospital	Detroit	158	328
Mercy Hospital - Cadillac	Cadillac	159	401
Munson Medical Center	Traverse City	159	393
Henry Ford West Bloomfield Hospital	W Bloomfield	160	382
Mercy Hospital - Grayling	Grayling	161	351
Midmichigan Medical Center - Gratiot	Alma	161	427
Bronson Battle Creek Hospital	Battle Creek	162	364
Crittenton Hospital Medical Center	Rochester	162	332
Saint Joseph Mercy Hospital	Ann Arbor	163	403
Hurley Medical Center	Flint	164	324
Allegiance Health	Jackson	165	394
Midmichigan Medical Center - Midland	Midland	166	420
Covenant Medical Center	Saginaw	168	419
Midmichigan Medical Center - Clare	Clare	168	406
West Branch Regional Medical Center	West Branch	168	377
Oakwood Hospital - Taylor	Taylor	173	332
St John Macomb-Oakland Hosp	Warren	174	357
William Beaumont Hospital - Troy	Troy	174	325
Beaumont Health System	Grosse Pointe	175	357
Chelsea Community Hospital	Chelsea	179	383
Genesys Reg Med Ctr-Health Park	Grand Blanc	181	373
Beaumont Health System	Royal Oak	182	325
Henry Ford Macomb Hospital	Clinton Twp	185	329
Mclaren Flint	Flint	187	348
Edward W Sparrow Hospital	Lansing	192	2819
Mclaren - Greater Lansing	Lansing	197	321
Oakwood Hospital - Southshore	Trenton	198	338
Saint Mary Mercy Hospital	Livonia	205	352
Oakwood Hospital - Dearborn	Dearborn	251	331
University of Michigan Health System	Ann Arbor	259	421

Time in ER Before Being Evaluated (minutes)

Hospital Name	City	Min.	Cases
Detroit Receiving Hosp & U Health Ctr	Detroit	0	261
Sinai - Grace Hospital	Detroit	0	249
Promedica Herrick Hospital	Tecumseh	2	384
Emma L Bixby Medical Center	Adrian	6	382
Metro Health Hospital	Wyoming	6	365
Harper University Hospital	Detroit	7	91
Henry Ford Macomb Hospital	Clinton Twp	7	371
Mercy Health Lakeshore Campus	Shelby	8	382
Harbor Beach Community Hospital	Harbor Beach	10	356
Helen Newberry Joy Hospital	Newberry	10	310
Saint Mary's Health Care	Grand Rapids	10	382
Mercy Health Hackley Campus	Muskegon	11	378
Spectrum Health - Reed City Campus	Reed City	11	328
Aspirus Ontonagon Hospital	Ontonagon	12	272
Marlette Regional Hospital	Marlette	12	426
McKenzie Health System	Sandusky	12	385
Mercy Memorial Hospital System	Monroe	12	573
Paul Oliver Memorial Hospital	Frankfort	12	368
Saint Joseph Mercy Livingston Hospital	Howell	12	484
Borgess - Lee Memorial Hospital	Dowagiac	14	589
Botsford Hospital	Farmington Hills	14	384
Chelsea Community Hospital	Chelsea	14	415
Huron Medical Center	Bad Axe	14	381
Portage Health	Hancock	14	442
Aspirus Keweenaw Hospital	Laurium	15	339
Baraga County Memorial Hospital	L' Anse	15	317
Covenant Medical Center	Saginaw	15	443
Deckerville Community Hospital	Deckerville	15	214
Holland Community Hospital	Holland	15	403
Caro Community Hospital	Caro	16	379
Carson City Hospital	Carson City	16	489
Mackinac Straits Hospital & Health Center	Saint Ignace	16	1354
Mclaren Macomb	Mount Clemens	16	407
Mercy Health Partners - Mercy Campus	Muskegon	16	364
Saint Joseph Mercy Port Huron	Port Huron	16	399
Schoolcraft Memorial Hospital	Manistique	16	1360
Spectrum Health United Mem-Kelsey Camp	Lakeview	16	297
Mclaren - Northern Michigan	Petoskey	17	405
Mclaren Oakland	Pontiac	17	324
Scheurer Hospital	Pigeon	17	412
Sparrow Ionia Hospital	Ionia	17	483
Beaumont Health System	Grosse Pointe	18	397
Huron Valley - Sinai Hospital	Commerce Twp	18	78
Kalkaska Memorial Health Center	Kalkaska	18	534
Lakeland Hospital - Saint Joseph	Saint Joseph	18	378
North Ottawa Community Health Center	Grand Haven	18	430
Otsego Memorial Hospital	Gaylord	18	374
Saint John River District Hospital	East China	18	345
Spectrum Health Gerber Memorial	Fremont	18	356
Spectrum Health Zeeland Comm Hosp	Zeeland	18	246
Munson Medical Center	Traverse City	19	454
Saint Mary Mercy Hospital	Livonia	19	472
Spectrum Health United Memorial	Greenville	19	370
Borgess Medical Center	Kalamazoo	20	597
Northstar Health System	Iron River	20	390
Providence Hospital & Medical Centers	Southfield	20	822
Saint Joseph Mercy Hospital	Ann Arbor	20	482
Saint Joseph Mercy Oakland	Pontiac	20	405
Lakeland Community Hospital - Watervliet	Watervliet	21	386
Spectrum Health - Butterworth Campus	Grand Rapids	21	846
Bronson Lakeview Hospital	Paw Paw	22	411
Crittenton Hospital Medical Center	Rochester	22	406
Saint John Hospital & Medical Center	Detroit	22	411
Hillsdale Community Health Center	Hillsdale	23	340
Mclaren Lapeer Region	Lapeer	23	372
Munising Memorial Hospital	Munising	23	251
Saint Mary's Standish Community Hospital	Standish	23	425
Sturgis Hospital	Sturgis	23	355
Marquette General Hospital	Marquette	24	327
Oaklawn Hospital	Marshall	24	383
Port Huron Hospital	Port Huron	24	451
West Shore Medical Center	Manistee	24	131

NOTE: Hospital profiles are in alphabetical order by state, then city, then hospital within the city; Rankings exclude hospitals with less than 25 cases except for patient surveys which excludes hospitals with less than 100 cases; (a) 100-299 cases; (1) The number of cases/patients is too few to report; (2) Data submitted were based on a sample of cases/patients; (3) Results are based on a shorter time period than required; (4) Data suppressed by CMS for one or more quarters; (5) Results are not available for this reporting period; (6) Fewer than 100 patients completed the HCAHPS survey; (7) No cases met the criteria for this measure; (8) The lower limit of the confidence interval cannot be calculated if the number of observed infections equals zero; (9) No data are available from the state/territory for this reporting period; (10) The scores shown reflect fewer than 50 completed surveys; (11) There were discrepancies in the data collection process; (12) This measure does not apply to this hospital for this reporting period; (13) Results cannot be calculated for this reporting period; (14) The results for this state are combined with nearby states to protect confidentiality; Please refer to the User's Guide for a full explanation of data.

Memorial Medical Center of West Michigan	Ludington	25	582
Doctors' Hospital of Michigan[3]	Pontiac	26	161
Hills & Dales General Hospital	Cass City	26	395
Oakwood Hospital - Southshore	Trenton	26	383
St John Macomb-Oakland Hosp	Warren	26	411
Tawas Saint Joseph Hospital	Tawas City	26	411
Charlevoix Area Hospital	Charlevoix	27	377
Dickinson County Memorial Hospital	Iron Mountain	27	417
Garden City Hospital	Garden City	27	1191
Henry Ford West Bloomfield Hospital	W Bloomfield	27	395
Mercy Hospital - Cadillac	Cadillac	27	439
Saint Francis Hospital	Escanaba	27	426
Allegan General Hospital	Allegan	28	444
Beaumont Health System	Royal Oak	28	308
Bell Hospital	Ishpeming	28	579
Bronson Methodist Hospital	Kalamazoo	28	375
Eaton Rapids Medical Center	Eaton Rapids	28	459
Mclaren Central Michigan	Mount Pleasant	28	420
Mercy Hospital - Grayling	Grayling	28	376
Three Rivers Health	Three Rivers	28	682
University of Michigan Health System	Ann Arbor	28	533
Bronson Battle Creek Hospital	Battle Creek	30	404
South Haven Community Hospital	South Haven	30	522
Spectrum Health Big Rapids Hospital	Big Rapids	30	440
West Branch Regional Medical Center	West Branch	30	447
Midmichigan Medical Center - Gratiot	Alma	31	320
Oakwood Hospital - Wayne	Wayne	31	381
Community Health Center of Branch County	Coldwater	32	265
Oakwood Hospital - Taylor	Taylor	32	362
Midmichigan Medical Center - Gladwin	Gladwin	33	369
Sheridan Community Hospital	Sheridan	33	1283
Allegiance Health	Jackson	36	414
Mclaren Bay Region	Bay City	36	419
Memorial Healthcare	Owosso	36	425
Midmichigan Medical Center - Clare	Clare	36	320
Henry Ford Hospital	Detroit	37	356
Mclaren Flint	Flint	37	383
Saint Mary's of Michigan Medical Center	Saginaw	38	371
William Beaumont Hospital - Troy	Troy	38	310
Edward W Sparrow Hospital	Lansing	39	3030
Hayes Green Beach Memorial Hospital	Charlotte	39	430
Sparrow Clinton Hospital	Saint Johns	39	472
Pennock Hospital	Hastings	41	417
Henry Ford Wyandotte Hospital	Wyandotte	42	371
Chippewa County War Memorial Hospital	Sault Ste Marie	44	280
Alpena Regional Medical Center	Alpena	46	336
Oakwood Hospital - Dearborn	Dearborn	46	365
Genesys Reg Med Ctr-Health Park	Grand Blanc	47	362
Mclaren - Greater Lansing	Lansing	53	369
Hurley Medical Center	Flint	54	183
Midmichigan Medical Center - Midland	Midland	56	436

Time to Pain Meds for Bone Fractures (minutes)

Hospital Name	City	Min.	Cases
Spectrum Health - Butterworth Campus	Grand Rapids	22	485
Sparrow Ionia Hospital[3]	Ionia	32	49
Portage Health	Hancock	34	41
Saint John River District Hospital	East China	35	51
Carson City Hospital	Carson City	36	53
North Ottawa Community Health Center	Grand Haven	36	112
Huron Medical Center	Bad Axe	37	45
Huron Valley - Sinai Hospital	Commerce Twp	37	138
Beaumont Health System	Grosse Pointe	38	57
Holland Community Hospital	Holland	38	230
Mercy Memorial Hospital System	Monroe	38	143
Spectrum Health Gerber Memorial	Fremont	39	99
Promedica Herrick Hospital	Tecumseh	40	60
Spectrum Health Zeeland Comm Hosp	Zeeland	40	88
Three Rivers Health	Three Rivers	40	83
Mercy Health Hackley Campus	Muskegon	42	144
Saint Joseph Mercy Oakland	Pontiac	42	106
Metro Health Hospital	Wyoming	43	253
Spectrum Health United Mem-Kelsey Camp	Lakeview	43	50
Spectrum Health United Memorial	Greenville	43	165
Sturgis Hospital	Sturgis	43	77
Dickinson County Memorial Hospital	Iron Mountain	44	70
Henry Ford Wyandotte Hospital	Wyandotte	44	250
Memorial Medical Center of West Michigan	Ludington	44	108
Saint Joseph Mercy Livingston Hospital	Howell	44	174
Providence Hospital & Medical Centers	Southfield	45	332
Saint Mary's of Michigan Medical Center	Saginaw	47	122
South Haven Community Hospital	South Haven	47	61
Tawas Saint Joseph Hospital	Tawas City	47	72
Bronson Lakeview Hospital[3]	Paw Paw	48	32
Mclaren Central Michigan	Mount Pleasant	48	111
Mclaren Macomb	Mount Clemens	48	153
Pennock Hospital	Hastings	48	72
Saint Francis Hospital	Escanaba	48	98
Mclaren - Northern Michigan	Petoskey	49	191
Lakeland Community Hospital - Watervliet	Watervliet	50	55
Marquette General Hospital	Marquette	50	66
Mclaren Oakland	Pontiac	50	161
Otsego Memorial Hospital	Gaylord	50	96
Saint Joseph Mercy Port Huron	Port Huron	50	81
Detroit Receiving Hosp & U Health Ctr	Detroit	51	161
Mclaren Lapeer Region	Lapeer	51	147
Spectrum Health - Reed City Campus[3]	Reed City	51	41
Chelsea Community Hospital	Chelsea	52	86
Mercy Hospital - Cadillac	Cadillac	52	146
Spectrum Health Big Rapids Hospital	Big Rapids	52	49
Emma L Bixby Medical Center	Adrian	53	172
Munson Medical Center	Traverse City	53	146
Mercy Health Partners - Mercy Campus	Muskegon	54	105
Botsford Hospital	Farmington Hills	55	179
Covenant Medical Center	Saginaw	56	220
Oakwood Hospital - Southshore	Trenton	56	98
Saint Joseph Mercy Hospital	Ann Arbor	56	242
Allegiance Health	Jackson	57	217
Harper University Hospital	Detroit	57	65
Henry Ford Macomb Hospital	Clinton Twp	57	160
Oakwood Hospital - Wayne	Wayne	57	142
West Shore Medical Center[3]	Manistee	57	43
William Beaumont Hospital - Troy	Troy	57	185
Bell Hospital	Ishpeming	59	28
Hayes Green Beach Memorial Hospital[3]	Charlotte	59	52
Lakeland Hospital - Saint Joseph	Saint Joseph	60	249
Memorial Healthcare	Owosso	60	88
Mercy Hospital - Grayling	Grayling	60	76
Oakwood Hospital - Taylor	Taylor	60	83
Saint John Hospital & Medical Center	Detroit	61	229
Community Health Center of Branch County	Coldwater	62	97
Midmichigan Medical Center - Clare	Clare	62	99
Oaklawn Hospital	Marshall	62	92
Sinai - Grace Hospital	Detroit	62	146
West Branch Regional Medical Center	West Branch	62	76
Chippewa County War Memorial Hospital	Sault Ste Marie	63	66
Borgess Medical Center	Kalamazoo	64	130
Hillsdale Community Health Center	Hillsdale	64	86
Port Huron Hospital	Port Huron	64	199
Crittenton Hospital Medical Center	Rochester	65	210
Mclaren Bay Region	Bay City	65	93
Saint Mary Mercy Hospital	Livonia	65	184
Bronson Methodist Hospital	Kalamazoo	66	410
Genesys Reg Med Ctr-Health Park	Grand Blanc	66	415
Midmichigan Medical Center - Gladwin	Gladwin	66	73
University of Michigan Health System	Ann Arbor	66	164
Beaumont Health System	Royal Oak	67	182
Midmichigan Medical Center - Midland	Midland	67	147
Mclaren Flint	Flint	68	217
Midmichigan Medical Center - Gratiot	Alma	68	81
St John Macomb-Oakland Hosp	Warren	68	330
Bronson Battle Creek Hospital	Battle Creek	70	156
Saint Mary's Health Care	Grand Rapids	71	262
Henry Ford Hospital	Detroit	72	232
Alpena Regional Medical Center	Alpena	73	111
Edward W Sparrow Hospital	Lansing	74	318
Henry Ford West Bloomfield Hospital	W Bloomfield	74	116
Hurley Medical Center	Flint	74	261
Garden City Hospital	Garden City	76	130
Mclaren - Greater Lansing	Lansing	82	132
Oakwood Hospital - Dearborn	Dearborn	82	209

Heart Attack Care

Aspirin Given at Discharge

Hospital Name	City	Rate	Cases
Alpena Regional Medical Center	Alpena	100%	26
Beaumont Health System	Grosse Pointe	100%	85
Beaumont Health System	Royal Oak	100%	850
Botsford Hospital	Farmington Hills	100%	102
Bronson Battle Creek Hospital	Battle Creek	100%	42
Covenant Medical Center	Saginaw	100%	509
Crittenton Hospital Medical Center	Rochester	100%	123
Detroit Receiving Hosp & U Health Ctr	Detroit	100%	205
Edward W Sparrow Hospital	Lansing	100%	540
Genesys Reg Med Ctr-Health Park	Grand Blanc	100%	465
Harper University Hospital	Detroit	100%	458
Henry Ford Macomb Hospital	Clinton Twp	100%	439
Holland Community Hospital	Holland	100%	89
Marquette General Hospital	Marquette	100%	420
Mclaren - Northern Michigan	Petoskey	100%	358
Mclaren Bay Region	Bay City	100%	402
Mclaren Flint	Flint	100%	576
Mclaren Lapeer Region[2]	Lapeer	100%	51
Mercy Health Partners - Mercy Campus[2]	Muskegon	100%	289
Mercy Memorial Hospital System	Monroe	100%	80
Metro Health Hospital	Wyoming	100%	135
Munson Medical Center[2]	Traverse City	100%	347
Oakwood Hospital - Wayne	Wayne	100%	90
Providence Hospital & Medical Centers	Southfield	100%	469
Saint John Hospital & Medical Center	Detroit	100%	403
St John Macomb-Oakland Hosp	Warren	100%	359
Saint Joseph Mercy Hospital	Ann Arbor	100%	690
Saint Joseph Mercy Oakland[2]	Pontiac	100%	327
Saint Joseph Mercy Port Huron	Port Huron	100%	27
Saint Mary's Health Care	Grand Rapids	100%	112
Sinai - Grace Hospital	Detroit	100%	336
Spectrum Health - Butterworth Campus	Grand Rapids	100%	939
University of Michigan Health System	Ann Arbor	100%	340
William Beaumont Hospital - Troy	Troy	100%	475
Allegiance Health[2]	Jackson	99%	314
Bronson Methodist Hospital	Kalamazoo	99%	391
Garden City Hospital	Garden City	99%	141
Henry Ford Hospital	Detroit	99%	715
Henry Ford West Bloomfield Hospital	W Bloomfield	99%	135
Lakeland Hospital - Saint Joseph	Saint Joseph	99%	301
Mclaren - Greater Lansing	Lansing	99%	204
Midmichigan Medical Center - Midland	Midland	99%	514
Saint Mary Mercy Hospital	Livonia	99%	162
Saint Mary's of Michigan Medical Center[2]	Saginaw	99%	290
Borgess Medical Center	Kalamazoo	98%	649
Hurley Medical Center	Flint	98%	115
Huron Valley - Sinai Hospital	Commerce Twp	98%	137
Mclaren Macomb	Mount Clemens	98%	368
Port Huron Hospital	Port Huron	98%	354
VA Ann Arbor Healthcare System	Ann Arbor	98%	61
Oakwood Hospital - Dearborn[2]	Dearborn	97%	269
Oakwood Hospital - Southshore	Trenton	97%	70
Chippewa County War Memorial Hospital	Sault Ste Marie	96%	25
Midmichigan Medical Center - Gratiot	Alma	93%	30
Henry Ford Wyandotte Hospital[2]	Wyandotte	92%	192

PCI Within 90 Minutes of Arrival

Hospital Name	City	Rate	Cases
Crittenton Hospital Medical Center	Rochester	100%	27
Henry Ford Macomb Hospital	Clinton Twp	100%	72
Huron Valley - Sinai Hospital	Commerce Twp	100%	44
Oakwood Hospital - Southshore	Trenton	100%	30
Oakwood Hospital - Wayne	Wayne	100%	32
Port Huron Hospital	Port Huron	100%	50
St John Macomb-Oakland Hosp	Warren	100%	72
Sinai - Grace Hospital	Detroit	100%	25
Beaumont Health System	Royal Oak	99%	85
Genesys Reg Med Ctr-Health Park	Grand Blanc	99%	79
Mclaren Flint	Flint	99%	90
Saint John Hospital & Medical Center	Detroit	99%	75
William Beaumont Hospital - Troy	Troy	99%	79
Henry Ford Hospital	Detroit	98%	47
Holland Community Hospital	Holland	97%	30
Metro Health Hospital	Wyoming	97%	39
Munson Medical Center[2]	Traverse City	97%	29
Saint Joseph Mercy Oakland[2]	Pontiac	97%	68
Borgess Medical Center	Kalamazoo	96%	68
Marquette General Hospital	Marquette	96%	28
Spectrum Health - Butterworth Campus	Grand Rapids	96%	114
Allegiance Health[2]	Jackson	95%	63
Covenant Medical Center	Saginaw	95%	57
Saint Joseph Mercy Hospital	Ann Arbor	95%	94
University of Michigan Health System	Ann Arbor	95%	60
Bronson Methodist Hospital	Kalamazoo	94%	71
Edward W Sparrow Hospital	Lansing	94%	70
Mclaren Bay Region	Bay City	94%	54
Mclaren Macomb	Mount Clemens	94%	80
Henry Ford Wyandotte Hospital[2]	Wyandotte	93%	29
Lakeland Hospital - Saint Joseph	Saint Joseph	93%	41
Mercy Health Partners - Mercy Campus[2]	Muskegon	93%	41
Oakwood Hospital - Dearborn[2]	Dearborn	93%	27
Mclaren - Greater Lansing	Lansing	92%	26
Saint Mary's Health Care	Grand Rapids	92%	36
Midmichigan Medical Center - Midland	Midland	91%	44
Saint Mary Mercy Hospital	Livonia	90%	49
Providence Hospital & Medical Centers	Southfield	89%	71
Hurley Medical Center	Flint	88%	33
Garden City Hospital	Garden City	84%	49
Saint Mary's of Michigan Medical Center[2]	Saginaw	72%	25

Statin Prescribed at Discharge

Hospital Name	City	Rate	Cases
Beaumont Health System	Grosse Pointe	100%	81
Beaumont Health System	Royal Oak	100%	806
Detroit Receiving Hosp & U Health Ctr	Detroit	100%	209
Edward W Sparrow Hospital	Lansing	100%	541
Henry Ford Macomb Hospital	Clinton Twp	100%	412
Holland Community Hospital	Holland	100%	83
Marquette General Hospital	Marquette	100%	412
Mclaren - Northern Michigan	Petoskey	100%	353
Metro Health Hospital	Wyoming	100%	130
Munson Medical Center[2]	Traverse City	100%	312
Saint Joseph Mercy Hospital	Ann Arbor	100%	681
Saint Joseph Mercy Oakland[2]	Pontiac	100%	310
University of Michigan Health System	Ann Arbor	100%	330

NOTE: Hospital profiles are in alphabetical order by state, then city, then hospital within the city; Rankings exclude hospitals with less than 25 cases except for patient surveys which excludes hospitals with less than 100 cases; (a) 100-299 cases; (1) The number of cases/patients is too few to report; (2) Data submitted were based on a sample of cases/patients; (3) Results are based on a shorter time period than required; (4) Data suppressed by CMS for one or more quarters; (5) Results are not available for this reporting period; (6) Fewer than 100 patients completed the HCAHPS survey; (7) No cases met the criteria for this measure; (8) The lower limit of the confidence interval cannot be calculated if the number of observed infections equals zero; (9) No data are available from the state/territory for this reporting period; (10) The scores shown reflect fewer than 50 completed surveys; (11) There were discrepancies in the data collection process; (12) This measure does not apply to this hospital for this reporting period; (13) Results cannot be calculated for this reporting period; (14) The results for this state are combined with nearby states to protect confidentiality; Please refer to the User's Guide for a full explanation of data.

VA Ann Arbor Healthcare System	Ann Arbor	100%	61
William Beaumont Hospital - Troy	Troy	100%	464
Borgess Medical Center	Kalamazoo	99%	626
Botsford Hospital	Farmington Hills	99%	110
Covenant Medical Center	Saginaw	99%	493
Crittenton Hospital Medical Center	Rochester	99%	114
Genesys Reg Med Ctr-Health Park	Grand Blanc	99%	460
Harper University Hospital	Detroit	99%	461
Lakeland Hospital - Saint Joseph	Saint Joseph	99%	282
Mclaren Flint	Flint	99%	557
Mercy Health Partners - Mercy Campus[2]	Muskegon	99%	280
Mercy Memorial Hospital System	Monroe	99%	71
Oakwood Hospital - Southshore	Trenton	99%	68
Providence Hospital & Medical Centers	Southfield	99%	459
Saint John Hospital & Medical Center	Detroit	99%	400
St John Macomb-Oakland Hosp	Warren	99%	351
Sinai - Grace Hospital	Detroit	99%	336
Spectrum Health - Butterworth Campus	Grand Rapids	99%	915
Allegiance Health[2]	Jackson	98%	287
Bronson Methodist Hospital	Kalamazoo	98%	368
Henry Ford Hospital	Detroit	98%	701
Henry Ford West Bloomfield Hospital	W Bloomfield	98%	132
Mclaren - Greater Lansing	Lansing	98%	200
Mclaren Bay Region	Bay City	98%	403
Midmichigan Medical Center - Midland	Midland	98%	506
Port Huron Hospital	Port Huron	98%	349
Saint Mary's Health Care	Grand Rapids	98%	115
Bronson Battle Creek Hospital	Battle Creek	97%	36
Garden City Hospital	Garden City	97%	144
Hurley Medical Center	Flint	97%	115
Huron Valley - Sinai Hospital	Commerce Twp	97%	131
Oakwood Hospital - Wayne	Wayne	97%	94
Saint Mary Mercy Hospital	Livonia	97%	159
Saint Mary's of Michigan Medical Center[2]	Saginaw	97%	287
Mclaren Lapeer Region[2]	Lapeer	96%	48
Mclaren Macomb	Mount Clemens	94%	361
Oakwood Hospital - Dearborn[2]	Dearborn	91%	270
Henry Ford Wyandotte Hospital[2]	Wyandotte	90%	174
Midmichigan Medical Center - Gratiot	Alma	61%	33

Heart Failure Care

ACE Inhibitor or ARB for LVSD

Hospital Name	City	Rate	Cases
Beaumont Health System	Grosse Pointe	100%	128
Beaumont Health System	Royal Oak	100%	418
Crittenton Hospital Medical Center	Rochester	100%	92
Henry Ford Macomb Hospital[2]	Clinton Twp	100%	67
Holland Community Hospital	Holland	100%	57
Marquette General Hospital	Marquette	100%	53
Mclaren Central Michigan	Mount Pleasant	100%	35
Mercy Hospital - Grayling	Grayling	100%	28
Mercy Memorial Hospital System	Monroe	100%	61
Metro Health Hospital	Wyoming	100%	52
Oakwood Hospital - Southshore[2]	Trenton	100%	58
Oakwood Hospital - Taylor	Taylor	100%	51
St John Macomb-Oakland Hosp	Warren	100%	272
Saint Joseph Mercy Livingston Hospital	Howell	100%	27
Saint Joseph Mercy Oakland[2]	Pontiac	100%	100
Saint Joseph Mercy Port Huron	Port Huron	100%	30
William Beaumont Hospital - Troy	Troy	100%	191
Borgess Medical Center	Kalamazoo	99%	150
Detroit Receiving Hosp & U Health Ctr	Detroit	99%	192
Harper University Hospital	Detroit	99%	274
Mclaren - Northern Michigan	Petoskey	99%	73
Oakwood Hospital - Dearborn[2]	Dearborn	99%	93
Port Huron Hospital	Port Huron	99%	81
Saint John Hospital & Medical Center	Detroit	99%	334
Saint Joseph Mercy Hospital	Ann Arbor	99%	181
Spectrum Health - Butterworth Campus	Grand Rapids	99%	302
University of Michigan Health System	Ann Arbor	99%	261
Covenant Medical Center	Saginaw	98%	154
Genesys Reg Med Ctr-Health Park	Grand Blanc	98%	146
Huron Valley - Sinai Hospital	Commerce Twp	98%	64
Bronson Battle Creek Hospital	Battle Creek	97%	60
Detroit (John D. Dingell) VA Med Ctr	Detroit	97%	66
Mclaren Flint	Flint	97%	246
Midmichigan Medical Center - Gratiot	Alma	97%	31
Providence Hospital & Medical Centers	Southfield	97%	338
Saint Mary Mercy Hospital	Livonia	97%	137
Sinai - Grace Hospital	Detroit	97%	283
Mclaren Oakland	Pontiac	96%	55
Mercy Health Hackley Campus	Muskegon	96%	27
Botsford Hospital	Farmington Hills	95%	119
Chippewa County War Memorial Hospital	Sault Ste Marie	94%	33
Edward W Sparrow Hospital	Lansing	94%	210
Henry Ford Hospital[2]	Detroit	94%	116
Henry Ford West Bloomfield Hospital	W Bloomfield	94%	64
Lakeland Hospital - Saint Joseph[2]	Saint Joseph	94%	100
Midmichigan Medical Center - Clare	Clare	94%	31
Allegiance Health[2]	Jackson	93%	86
Mclaren Lapeer Region[2]	Lapeer	93%	44
Munson Medical Center[2]	Traverse City	93%	90
Oakwood Hospital - Wayne	Wayne	93%	67
VA Ann Arbor Healthcare System	Ann Arbor	93%	54
Alpena Regional Medical Center	Alpena	92%	26
Mercy Hospital - Cadillac	Cadillac	92%	49
Saint Mary's of Michigan Medical Center[2]	Saginaw	91%	92
Garden City Hospital	Garden City	90%	67
Mclaren Macomb	Mount Clemens	90%	122
Mercy Health Partners - Mercy Campus[2]	Muskegon	90%	73
Bronson Methodist Hospital	Kalamazoo	89%	130
Henry Ford Wyandotte Hospital[2]	Wyandotte	89%	56
Mclaren - Greater Lansing	Lansing	89%	117
Mclaren Bay Region	Bay City	89%	148
Saint Mary's Health Care[2]	Grand Rapids	89%	64
Hurley Medical Center[2]	Flint	87%	109
West Branch Regional Medical Center	West Branch	85%	34
Midmichigan Medical Center - Midland	Midland	80%	74

Discharge Instructions Given

Hospital Name	City	Rate	Cases
Beaumont Health System	Grosse Pointe	100%	361
Beaumont Health System	Royal Oak	100%	1160
Borgess Medical Center	Kalamazoo	100%	433
Carson City Hospital	Carson City	100%	28
Chelsea Community Hospital	Chelsea	100%	67
Crittenton Hospital Medical Center	Rochester	100%	214
Hayes Green Beach Memorial Hospital	Charlotte	100%	29
Henry Ford Hospital[2]	Detroit	100%	273
Henry Ford Wyandotte Hospital[2]	Wyandotte	100%	248
Holland Community Hospital	Holland	100%	127
Huron Medical Center	Bad Axe	100%	27
Pennock Hospital	Hastings	100%	57
Providence Hospital & Medical Centers	Southfield	100%	893
Saint Francis Hospital	Escanaba	100%	31
Saint John Hospital & Medical Center	Detroit	100%	861
St John Macomb-Oakland Hosp	Warren	100%	719
Saint Joseph Mercy Oakland[2]	Pontiac	100%	262
Sparrow Clinton Hospital	Saint Johns	100%	34
VA Ann Arbor Healthcare System	Ann Arbor	100%	153
William Beaumont Hospital - Troy	Troy	100%	579
Botsford Hospital	Farmington Hills	99%	335
Detroit Receiving Hosp & U Health Ctr	Detroit	99%	383
Garden City Hospital	Garden City	99%	288
Harper University Hospital	Detroit	99%	637
Henry Ford West Bloomfield Hospital	W Bloomfield	99%	239
Mercy Hospital - Grayling	Grayling	99%	95
Saint Joseph Mercy Port Huron	Port Huron	99%	112
University of Michigan Health System	Ann Arbor	99%	718
Community Health Center of Branch County	Coldwater	98%	82
Mclaren - Northern Michigan	Petoskey	98%	223
Mercy Hospital - Cadillac	Cadillac	98%	120
Saint Joseph Mercy Hospital	Ann Arbor	98%	613
Sinai - Grace Hospital	Detroit	98%	583
Spectrum Health - Butterworth Campus	Grand Rapids	98%	971
Spectrum Health Gerber Memorial	Fremont	98%	49
Tawas Saint Joseph Hospital	Tawas City	98%	42
Allegan General Hospital	Allegan	97%	31
Henry Ford Macomb Hospital[2]	Clinton Twp	97%	229
Mclaren Central Michigan	Mount Pleasant	97%	122
Mclaren Oakland	Pontiac	97%	106
Metro Health Hospital	Wyoming	97%	175
Munson Medical Center[2]	Traverse City	97%	286
Oakwood Hospital - Southshore[2]	Trenton	97%	177
Saint Mary's Health Care[2]	Grand Rapids	97%	240
Spectrum Health Big Rapids Hospital	Big Rapids	97%	63
Spectrum Health United Memorial	Greenville	97%	77
Sturgis Hospital	Sturgis	97%	37
Three Rivers Health	Three Rivers	97%	61
Bronson Battle Creek Hospital	Battle Creek	96%	208
Huron Valley - Sinai Hospital	Commerce Twp	96%	244
Mercy Memorial Hospital System	Monroe	96%	142
Midmichigan Medical Center - Clare	Clare	96%	95
Midmichigan Medical Center - Gladwin	Gladwin	96%	57
Oaklawn Hospital	Marshall	96%	56
Saint Mary Mercy Hospital	Livonia	96%	320
Mclaren Lapeer Region[2]	Lapeer	95%	169
Mclaren Flint	Flint	94%	771
Oakwood Hospital - Taylor	Taylor	94%	88
Otsego Memorial Hospital	Gaylord	94%	33
Saint John River District Hospital	East China	94%	48
Lakeland Hospital - Saint Joseph[2]	Saint Joseph	93%	263
Saint Joseph Mercy Livingston Hospital	Howell	93%	105
Spectrum Health Zeeland Comm Hosp	Zeeland	93%	56
Aspirus Keweenaw Hospital	Laurium	92%	25
Edward W Sparrow Hospital	Lansing	92%	533
Mclaren Bay Region	Bay City	92%	393
Alpena Regional Medical Center	Alpena	91%	137
Memorial Healthcare	Owosso	90%	41
Midmichigan Medical Center - Gratiot	Alma	90%	132
Detroit (John D. Dingell) VA Med Ctr	Detroit	89%	131
Port Huron Hospital	Port Huron	89%	233
Covenant Medical Center	Saginaw	88%	512
Iron Mountain MI VA Medical Center	Iron Mountain	87%	30
Marquette General Hospital	Marquette	87%	164
Oakwood Hospital - Wayne	Wayne	87%	156
Allegiance Health[2]	Jackson	86%	287
Genesys Reg Med Ctr-Health Park	Grand Blanc	86%	500
Mercy Health Hackley Campus	Muskegon	86%	57
West Branch Regional Medical Center	West Branch	86%	83
Bronson Methodist Hospital	Kalamazoo	85%	398
Mercy Health Partners - Mercy Campus[2]	Muskegon	85%	214
Promedica Herrick Hospital	Tecumseh	85%	39
Hillsdale Community Health Center	Hillsdale	84%	56
Memorial Medical Center of West Michigan	Ludington	84%	58
Oakwood Hospital - Dearborn[2]	Dearborn	83%	205
Dickinson County Memorial Hospital	Iron Mountain	82%	72
Saint Mary's of Michigan Medical Center[2]	Saginaw	81%	242
West Shore Medical Center	Manistee	81%	36
Hurley Medical Center[2]	Flint	80%	251
Mclaren Macomb	Mount Clemens	80%	340
Midmichigan Medical Center - Midland	Midland	80%	338
Chippewa County War Memorial Hospital	Sault Ste Marie	78%	81
Emma L Bixby Medical Center	Adrian	77%	69
Northstar Health System	Iron River	73%	26
Mclaren - Greater Lansing	Lansing	72%	298
Marlette Regional Hospital	Marlette	63%	27

Evaluation of LVS Function

Hospital Name	City	Rate	Cases
Allegan General Hospital	Allegan	100%	36
Allegiance Health[2]	Jackson	100%	353
Alpena Regional Medical Center	Alpena	100%	162
Aspirus Grand View Hospital	Ironwood	100%	36
Aspirus Keweenaw Hospital	Laurium	100%	30
Beaumont Health System	Grosse Pointe	100%	410
Beaumont Health System	Royal Oak	100%	1402
Borgess - Lee Memorial Hospital	Dowagiac	100%	27
Botsford Hospital	Farmington Hills	100%	427
Bronson Battle Creek Hospital	Battle Creek	100%	273
Bronson Lakeview Hospital	Paw Paw	100%	28
Bronson Methodist Hospital	Kalamazoo	100%	464
Carson City Hospital	Carson City	100%	36
Chelsea Community Hospital	Chelsea	100%	79
Covenant Medical Center	Saginaw	100%	625
Crittenton Hospital Medical Center	Rochester	100%	283
Detroit Receiving Hosp & U Health Ctr	Detroit	100%	443
Emma L Bixby Medical Center	Adrian	100%	104
Genesys Reg Med Ctr-Health Park	Grand Blanc	100%	616
Harper University Hospital	Detroit	100%	721
Hayes Green Beach Memorial Hospital	Charlotte	100%	37
Henry Ford Hospital[2]	Detroit	100%	311
Henry Ford Macomb Hospital[2]	Clinton Twp	100%	294
Hillsdale Community Health Center	Hillsdale	100%	69
Holland Community Hospital	Holland	100%	164
Huron Valley - Sinai Hospital	Commerce Twp	100%	315
Iron Mountain MI VA Medical Center	Iron Mountain	100%	36
Lakeland Hospital - Saint Joseph[2]	Saint Joseph	100%	318
Mclaren - Northern Michigan	Petoskey	100%	247
Mclaren Macomb	Mount Clemens	100%	409
Memorial Medical Center of West Michigan	Ludington	100%	72
Mercy Health Hackley Campus	Muskegon	100%	74
Mercy Health Partners - Mercy Campus[2]	Muskegon	100%	249
Mercy Hospital - Grayling	Grayling	100%	113
Mercy Memorial Hospital System	Monroe	100%	211
Metro Health Hospital	Wyoming	100%	209
Midmichigan Medical Center - Gladwin	Gladwin	100%	75
Midmichigan Medical Center - Midland	Midland	100%	399
Munson Medical Center[2]	Traverse City	100%	330
North Ottawa Community Health Center	Grand Haven	100%	33
Oaklawn Hospital	Marshall	100%	65
Oakwood Hospital - Southshore[2]	Trenton	100%	217
Oakwood Hospital - Taylor	Taylor	100%	141
Pennock Hospital	Hastings	100%	80
Port Huron Hospital	Port Huron	100%	303
Promedica Herrick Hospital	Tecumseh	100%	50
Providence Hospital & Medical Centers	Southfield	100%	1067
Saint Francis Hospital	Escanaba	100%	44
Saint John Hospital & Medical Center	Detroit	100%	1021
St John Macomb-Oakland Hosp	Warren	100%	878
Saint John River District Hospital	East China	100%	58
Saint Joseph Mercy Hospital	Ann Arbor	100%	758
Saint Joseph Mercy Livingston Hospital	Howell	100%	138
Saint Joseph Mercy Oakland[2]	Pontiac	100%	323
Saint Joseph Mercy Port Huron	Port Huron	100%	151
Saint Mary Mercy Hospital	Livonia	100%	482
Saint Mary's of Michigan Medical Center[2]	Saginaw	100%	292
Sinai - Grace Hospital	Detroit	100%	678
Spectrum Health - Butterworth Campus	Grand Rapids	100%	1180
Spectrum Health Big Rapids Hospital	Big Rapids	100%	72
Spectrum Health Gerber Memorial	Fremont	100%	60

NOTE: Hospital profiles are in alphabetical order by state, then city, then hospital within the city; Rankings exclude hospitals with less than 25 cases except for patient surveys which excludes hospitals with less than 100 cases; (a) 100-299 cases; (1) The number of cases/patients is too few to report; (2) Data submitted were based on a sample of cases/patients; (3) Results are based on a shorter time period than required; (4) Data suppressed by CMS for one or more quarters; (5) Results are not available for this reporting period; (6) Fewer than 100 patients completed the HCAHPS survey; (7) No cases met the criteria for this measure; (8) The lower limit of the confidence interval cannot be calculated if the number of observed infections equals zero; (9) No data are available from the state/territory for this reporting period; (10) The scores shown reflect fewer than 50 completed surveys; (11) There were discrepancies in the data collection process; (12) This measure does not apply to this hospital for this reporting period; (13) Results cannot be calculated for this reporting period; (14) The results for this state are combined with nearby states to protect confidentiality; Please refer to the User's Guide for a full explanation of data.

Hospital Name	City	Rate	Cases
Spectrum Health United Memorial	Greenville	100%	102
Spectrum Health Zeeland Comm Hosp	Zeeland	100%	70
University of Michigan Health System	Ann Arbor	100%	826
VA Ann Arbor Healthcare System	Ann Arbor	100%	164
William Beaumont Hospital - Troy	Troy	100%	720
Borgess Medical Center	Kalamazoo	99%	533
Community Health Center of Branch County	Coldwater	99%	102
Detroit (John D. Dingell) VA Med Ctr	Detroit	99%	137
Dickinson County Memorial Hospital	Iron Mountain	99%	99
Garden City Hospital	Garden City	99%	366
Henry Ford Wyandotte Hospital[2]	Wyandotte	99%	297
Marquette General Hospital	Marquette	99%	197
Mclaren - Greater Lansing	Lansing	99%	345
Mclaren Central Michigan	Mount Pleasant	99%	157
Mclaren Flint	Flint	99%	929
Mclaren Lapeer Region[2]	Lapeer	99%	216
Midmichigan Medical Center - Clare	Clare	99%	110
Midmichigan Medical Center - Gratiot	Alma	99%	174
Saint Mary's Health Care[2]	Grand Rapids	99%	306
Chippewa County War Memorial Hospital	Sault Ste Marie	98%	97
Edward W Sparrow Hospital	Lansing	98%	675
Henry Ford West Bloomfield Hospital	W Bloomfield	98%	324
Mclaren Oakland	Pontiac	98%	130
Memorial Healthcare	Owosso	98%	56
Mercy Hospital - Cadillac	Cadillac	98%	131
Otsego Memorial Hospital	Gaylord	98%	42
Sparrow Clinton Hospital	Saint Johns	98%	49
Tawas Saint Joseph Hospital	Tawas City	98%	52
West Shore Medical Center	Manistee	98%	41
Mclaren Bay Region	Bay City	97%	477
Oakwood Hospital - Dearborn[2]	Dearborn	97%	272
Oakwood Hospital - Wayne	Wayne	97%	190
Three Rivers Health	Three Rivers	97%	72
South Haven Community Hospital	South Haven	96%	28
Sturgis Hospital	Sturgis	96%	51
Hurley Medical Center[2]	Flint	95%	285
Huron Medical Center	Bad Axe	95%	37
West Branch Regional Medical Center	West Branch	94%	96
Northstar Health System	Iron River	93%	55
Marlette Regional Hospital	Marlette	74%	31

Medicare Spending

Medicare Spending per Patient (ratio)

Hospital Name	City	Ratio	Cases
Brighton Hospital	Brighton	0.73	-
Portage Health	Hancock	0.87	-
Huron Medical Center	Bad Axe	0.88	-
Mercy Hospital - Cadillac	Cadillac	0.88	-
Midmichigan Medical Center - Clare	Clare	0.88	-
Spectrum Health Gerber Memorial	Fremont	0.88	-
Spectrum Health Big Rapids Hospital	Big Rapids	0.89	-
Chippewa County War Memorial Hospital	Sault Ste Marie	0.90	-
Mclaren Lapeer Region	Lapeer	0.90	-
Memorial Medical Center of West Michigan	Ludington	0.90	-
Mercy Hospital - Grayling	Grayling	0.90	-
Midmichigan Medical Center - Midland	Midland	0.90	-
Munson Medical Center	Traverse City	0.90	-
Pennock Hospital	Hastings	0.90	-
Healthsource Saginaw	Saginaw	0.91	-
Otsego Memorial Hospital	Gaylord	0.91	-
South Haven Community Hospital	South Haven	0.91	-
Spectrum Health United Memorial	Greenville	0.91	-
Spectrum Health Zeeland Comm Hosp	Zeeland	0.91	-
Tawas Saint Joseph Hospital	Tawas City	0.91	-
Holland Community Hospital	Holland	0.92	-
Oaklawn Hospital	Marshall	0.92	-
Borgess Medical Center	Kalamazoo	0.93	-
Bronson Methodist Hospital	Kalamazoo	0.93	-
Dickinson County Memorial Hospital	Iron Mountain	0.93	-
Mclaren Central Michigan	Mount Pleasant	0.93	-
Metro Health Hospital	Wyoming	0.93	-
North Ottawa Community Health Center	Grand Haven	0.93	-
Carson City Hospital	Carson City	0.94	-
Chelsea Community Hospital	Chelsea	0.94	-
Mclaren - Greater Lansing	Lansing	0.94	-
Mclaren - Northern Michigan	Petoskey	0.94	-
Oakland Regional Hospital	Southfield	0.94	-
Port Huron Hospital	Port Huron	0.94	-
Saint Joseph Mercy Livingston Hospital	Howell	0.94	-
Saint Mary's Health Care	Grand Rapids	0.94	-
Emma L Bixby Medical Center	Adrian	0.95	-
Genesys Reg Med Ctr-Health Park	Grand Blanc	0.95	-
Lakeland Hospital - Saint Joseph	Saint Joseph	0.95	-
Marquette General Hospital	Marquette	0.95	-
Memorial Healthcare	Owosso	0.95	-
Saint Joseph Mercy Port Huron	Port Huron	0.95	-
Sturgis Hospital	Sturgis	0.95	-
Three Rivers Health	Three Rivers	0.95	-
Community Health Center of Branch County	Coldwater	0.96	-
Doctors' Hospital of Michigan	Pontiac	0.96	-
Lakeland Community Hospital - Watervliet	Watervliet	0.96	-
Mclaren Flint	Flint	0.96	-
Allegiance Health	Jackson	0.97	-
Mclaren Macomb	Mount Clemens	0.97	-
Midmichigan Medical Center - Gratiot	Alma	0.97	-
Saint Joseph Mercy Hospital	Ann Arbor	0.97	-
Spectrum Health - Butterworth Campus	Grand Rapids	0.97	-
Covenant Medical Center	Saginaw	0.98	-
Edward W Sparrow Hospital	Lansing	0.98	-
Henry Ford Hospital	Detroit	0.98	-
Hurley Medical Center	Flint	0.98	-
Mercy Health Partners - Mercy Campus	Muskegon	0.98	-
Providence Hospital & Medical Centers	Southfield	0.98	-
West Branch Regional Medical Center	West Branch	0.98	-
Beaumont Health System	Grosse Pointe	0.99	-
Bronson Battle Creek Hospital	Battle Creek	0.99	-
Harper University Hospital	Detroit	0.99	-
Henry Ford Wyandotte Hospital	Wyandotte	0.99	-
Hillsdale Community Health Center	Hillsdale	0.99	-
Mercy Health Hackley Campus	Muskegon	0.99	-
Saint John River District Hospital	East China	0.99	-
Mclaren Bay Region	Bay City	1.00	-
Saint Mary's of Michigan Medical Center	Saginaw	1.00	-
University of Michigan Health System	Ann Arbor	1.00	-
Detroit Receiving Hosp & U Health Ctr	Detroit	1.01	-
Henry Ford West Bloomfield Hospital	W Bloomfield	1.01	-
Huron Valley - Sinai Hospital	Commerce Twp	1.01	-
Karmanos Cancer Center	Detroit	1.01	-
Mclaren Oakland	Pontiac	1.01	-
William Beaumont Hospital - Troy	Troy	1.01	-
Alpena Regional Medical Center	Alpena	1.02	-
Beaumont Health System	Royal Oak	1.02	-
Oakwood Hospital - Dearborn	Dearborn	1.02	-
Oakwood Hospital - Southshore	Trenton	1.02	-
Saint John Hospital & Medical Center	Detroit	1.02	-
Saint Joseph Mercy Oakland	Pontiac	1.02	-
Mercy Memorial Hospital System	Monroe	1.03	-
Crittenton Hospital Medical Center	Rochester	1.04	-
Henry Ford Macomb Hospital	Clinton Twp	1.04	-
St John Macomb-Oakland Hosp	Warren	1.04	-
Sinai - Grace Hospital	Detroit	1.04	-
Botsford Hospital	Farmington Hills	1.05	-
Saint Mary Mercy Hospital	Livonia	1.06	-
Garden City Hospital	Garden City	1.07	-
Oakwood Hospital - Wayne	Wayne	1.07	-
Oakwood Hospital - Taylor	Taylor	1.10	-
Straith Hospital For Special Surgery	Southfield	1.11	-

Pneumonia Care

Appropriate Initial Antibiotic Given

Hospital Name	City	Rate	Cases
Allegan General Hospital	Allegan	100%	56
Beaumont Health System	Grosse Pointe	100%	155
Bronson Lakeview Hospital	Paw Paw	100%	65
Detroit (John D. Dingell) VA Med Ctr	Detroit	100%	31
Detroit Receiving Hosp & U Health Ctr	Detroit	100%	86
Marquette General Hospital	Marquette	100%	61
Mclaren Lapeer Region[2]	Lapeer	100%	94
Mercy Hospital - Grayling	Grayling	100%	75
Oaklawn Hospital	Marshall	100%	68
Otsego Memorial Hospital	Gaylord	100%	59
Promedica Herrick Hospital	Tecumseh	100%	32
Saint Francis Hospital	Escanaba	100%	35
Saint Joseph Mercy Port Huron[2]	Port Huron	100%	79
Saint Mary's of Michigan Medical Center[2]	Saginaw	100%	45
Scheurer Hospital	Pigeon	100%	35
Spectrum Health United Mem-Kelsey Camp	Lakeview	100%	34
VA Ann Arbor Healthcare System	Ann Arbor	100%	29
West Shore Medical Center	Manistee	100%	54
William Beaumont Hospital - Troy[2]	Troy	100%	124
Beaumont Health System[2]	Royal Oak	99%	88
Chelsea Community Hospital	Chelsea	99%	71
Crittenton Hospital Medical Center	Rochester	99%	115
Emma L Bixby Medical Center[2]	Adrian	99%	75
Holland Community Hospital	Holland	99%	163
Huron Valley - Sinai Hospital	Commerce Twp	99%	105
Metro Health Hospital[2]	Wyoming	99%	101
Munson Medical Center[2]	Traverse City	99%	114
Saint John Hospital & Medical Center	Detroit	99%	235
Saint Joseph Mercy Oakland[2]	Pontiac	99%	98
Saint Mary's Health Care[2]	Grand Rapids	99%	113
Spectrum Health Big Rapids Hospital	Big Rapids	99%	68
Spectrum Health Zeeland Comm Hosp	Zeeland	99%	74
Allegiance Health[2]	Jackson	98%	105
Borgess Medical Center[2]	Kalamazoo	98%	132
Botsford Hospital	Farmington Hills	98%	180
Carson City Hospital	Carson City	98%	41
Dickinson County Memorial Hospital	Iron Mountain	98%	65
Genesys Reg Med Ctr-Health Park	Grand Blanc	98%	390
Mclaren - Northern Michigan	Petoskey	98%	89
Mclaren Flint[2]	Flint	98%	178
Mercy Memorial Hospital System	Monroe	98%	191
Midmichigan Medical Center - Gratiot	Alma	98%	64
Providence Hospital & Medical Centers	Southfield	98%	394
Spectrum Health - Reed City Campus	Reed City	98%	53
Tawas Saint Joseph Hospital	Tawas City	98%	49
University of Michigan Health System	Ann Arbor	98%	143
Bronson Methodist Hospital	Kalamazoo	97%	227
Edward W Sparrow Hospital[2]	Lansing	97%	287
Garden City Hospital	Garden City	97%	147
Hillsdale Community Health Center	Hillsdale	97%	91
Huron Medical Center[2]	Bad Axe	97%	37
Mercy Health Partners - Mercy Campus[2]	Muskegon	97%	73
Mercy Hospital - Cadillac	Cadillac	97%	114
Oakwood Hospital - Southshore[2]	Trenton	97%	102
Port Huron Hospital	Port Huron	97%	147
St John Macomb-Oakland Hosp	Warren	97%	417
Saint Joseph Mercy Livingston Hospital	Howell	97%	95
Sinai - Grace Hospital	Detroit	97%	183
South Haven Community Hospital	South Haven	97%	39
Sparrow Ionia Hospital	Ionia	97%	34
Spectrum Health - Butterworth Campus[2]	Grand Rapids	97%	138
Covenant Medical Center	Saginaw	96%	253
Harper University Hospital	Detroit	96%	74
Henry Ford Hospital[2]	Detroit	96%	47
Henry Ford Macomb Hospital[2]	Clinton Twp	96%	127
Marlette Regional Hospital	Marlette	96%	27
Saint Mary's Standish Community Hospital	Standish	96%	28
Spectrum Health Gerber Memorial	Fremont	96%	98
Bronson Battle Creek Hospital[2]	Battle Creek	95%	151
Lakeland Community Hospital - Watervliet	Watervliet	95%	42
Mclaren Bay Region	Bay City	95%	133
Mclaren Oakland	Pontiac	95%	74
Memorial Medical Center of West Michigan	Ludington	95%	96
Midmichigan Medical Center - Midland	Midland	95%	169
Oakwood Hospital - Taylor[2]	Taylor	95%	81
Saint Joseph Mercy Hospital	Ann Arbor	95%	287
Saint Mary Mercy Hospital	Livonia	95%	222
McKenzie Health System	Sandusky	94%	33
Midmichigan Medical Center - Clare	Clare	94%	62
Oakwood Hospital - Dearborn[2]	Dearborn	94%	96
Pennock Hospital	Hastings	94%	87
Saint John River District Hospital	East China	94%	63
Alpena Regional Medical Center	Alpena	93%	140
Lakeland Hospital - Saint Joseph[2]	Saint Joseph	93%	75
Mclaren Macomb	Mount Clemens	93%	238
Memorial Healthcare	Owosso	93%	89
Mercy Health Hackley Campus[2]	Muskegon	93%	92
Spectrum Health United Memorial	Greenville	93%	92
Hurley Medical Center[2]	Flint	92%	75
Mclaren Central Michigan	Mount Pleasant	92%	106
Oakwood Hospital - Wayne[2]	Wayne	92%	93
Bell Hospital	Ishpeming	91%	34
Three Rivers Health	Three Rivers	91%	58
Chippewa County War Memorial Hospital	Sault Ste Marie	90%	100
Community Health Center of Branch County	Coldwater	90%	119
Henry Ford Wyandotte Hospital[2]	Wyandotte	90%	73
Borgess - Lee Memorial Hospital	Dowagiac	89%	36
Hills & Dales General Hospital	Cass City	87%	39
Aspirus Grand View Hospital	Ironwood	85%	61
Mclaren - Greater Lansing	Lansing	85%	176
North Ottawa Community Health Center	Grand Haven	85%	40
Schoolcraft Memorial Hospital	Manistique	85%	39
Henry Ford West Bloomfield Hospital[2]	W Bloomfield	83%	71
Sturgis Hospital	Sturgis	79%	42
West Branch Regional Medical Center[2]	West Branch	73%	64

Blood Culture Timing

Hospital Name	City	Rate	Cases
Aspirus Keweenaw Hospital	Laurium	100%	44
Beaumont Health System	Grosse Pointe	100%	233
Botsford Hospital	Farmington Hills	100%	364
Carson City Hospital	Carson City	100%	64
Charlevoix Area Hospital	Charlevoix	100%	28
Crittenton Hospital Medical Center	Rochester	100%	243
Detroit (John D. Dingell) VA Med Ctr	Detroit	100%	65
Emma L Bixby Medical Center[2]	Adrian	100%	162
Garden City Hospital	Garden City	100%	270
Hayes Green Beach Memorial Hospital	Charlotte	100%	66
Hillsdale Community Health Center	Hillsdale	100%	145
Holland Community Hospital	Holland	100%	303
Huron Valley - Sinai Hospital	Commerce Twp	100%	220
Iron Mountain MI VA Medical Center	Iron Mountain	100%	26
McKenzie Health System	Sandusky	100%	44
Mclaren Oakland	Pontiac	100%	111
Mercy Health Hackley Campus[2]	Muskegon	100%	152
Oaklawn Hospital	Marshall	100%	104
Pennock Hospital	Hastings	100%	122
Promedica Herrick Hospital	Tecumseh	100%	47

NOTE: Hospital profiles are in alphabetical order by state, then city, then hospital within the city; Rankings exclude hospitals with less than 25 cases except for patient surveys which excludes hospitals with less than 100 cases; (a) 100-299 cases; (1) The number of cases/patients is too few to report; (2) Data submitted were based on a sample of cases/patients; (3) Results are based on a shorter time period than required; (4) Data suppressed by CMS for one or more quarters; (5) Results are not available for this reporting period; (6) Fewer than 100 patients completed the HCAHPS survey; (7) No cases met the criteria for this measure; (8) The lower limit of the confidence interval cannot be calculated if the number of observed infections equals zero; (9) No data are available from the state/territory for this reporting period; (10) The scores shown reflect fewer than 50 completed surveys; (11) There were discrepancies in the data collection process; (12) This measure does not apply to this hospital for this reporting period; (13) Results cannot be calculated for this reporting period; (14) The results for this state are combined with nearby states to protect confidentiality; Please refer to the User's Guide for a full explanation of data.

Providence Hospital & Medical Centers	Southfield	100%	450
Saint Francis Hospital	Escanaba	100%	79
Saint John Hospital & Medical Center	Detroit	100%	231
St John Macomb-Oakland Hosp	Warren	100%	468
Saint Joseph Mercy Port Huron[2]	Port Huron	100%	138
Spectrum Health - Butterworth Campus[2]	Grand Rapids	100%	271
William Beaumont Hospital - Troy[2]	Troy	100%	184
Allegiance Health[2]	Jackson	99%	139
Aspirus Grand View Hospital	Ironwood	99%	98
Community Health Center of Branch County	Coldwater	99%	166
Detroit Receiving Hosp & U Health Ctr	Detroit	99%	450
Henry Ford Hospital[2]	Detroit	99%	140
Henry Ford Wyandotte Hospital[2]	Wyandotte	99%	113
Lakeland Hospital - Saint Joseph[2]	Saint Joseph	99%	137
Marquette General Hospital	Marquette	99%	112
Memorial Medical Center of West Michigan	Ludington	99%	174
Mercy Hospital - Grayling	Grayling	99%	121
Midmichigan Medical Center - Clare	Clare	99%	94
Midmichigan Medical Center - Midland	Midland	99%	284
Munson Medical Center[2]	Traverse City	99%	201
Oakwood Hospital - Dearborn[2]	Dearborn	99%	111
Oakwood Hospital - Taylor[2]	Taylor	99%	171
Port Huron Hospital	Port Huron	99%	271
Saint John River District Hospital	East China	99%	77
Saint Joseph Mercy Oakland[2]	Pontiac	99%	101
Saint Mary Mercy Hospital	Livonia	99%	356
Saint Mary's Health Care[2]	Grand Rapids	99%	145
Spectrum Health Big Rapids Hospital	Big Rapids	99%	109
Spectrum Health United Memorial	Greenville	99%	205
Beaumont Health System[2]	Royal Oak	98%	122
Bell Hospital	Ishpeming	98%	56
Borgess - Lee Memorial Hospital	Dowagiac	98%	40
Bronson Battle Creek Hospital[2]	Battle Creek	98%	245
Bronson Lakeview Hospital	Paw Paw	98%	87
Bronson Methodist Hospital	Kalamazoo	98%	404
Covenant Medical Center	Saginaw	98%	571
Dickinson County Memorial Hospital	Iron Mountain	98%	107
Genesys Reg Med Ctr-Health Park	Grand Blanc	98%	562
Harper University Hospital	Detroit	98%	218
Henry Ford Macomb Hospital[2]	Clinton Twp	98%	222
Memorial Healthcare	Owosso	98%	124
Mercy Health Partners - Mercy Campus[2]	Muskegon	98%	157
Mercy Memorial Hospital System	Monroe	98%	262
Oakwood Hospital - Wayne[2]	Wayne	98%	180
Saint Joseph Mercy Hospital	Ann Arbor	98%	378
Tawas Saint Joseph Hospital	Tawas City	98%	86
University of Michigan Health System	Ann Arbor	98%	350
VA Ann Arbor Healthcare System	Ann Arbor	98%	66
Allegan General Hospital	Allegan	97%	68
Alpena Regional Medical Center	Alpena	97%	222
Borgess Medical Center[2]	Kalamazoo	97%	269
Chelsea Community Hospital	Chelsea	97%	102
Edward W Sparrow Hospital[2]	Lansing	97%	549
Huron Medical Center[2]	Bad Axe	97%	67
Mclaren Lapeer Region[2]	Lapeer	97%	146
Metro Health Hospital[2]	Wyoming	97%	223
Midmichigan Medical Center - Gladwin	Gladwin	97%	38
North Ottawa Community Health Center	Grand Haven	97%	67
Oakwood Hospital - Southshore[2]	Trenton	97%	124
Portage Health	Hancock	97%	37
Saint Joseph Mercy Livingston Hospital	Howell	97%	187
Sparrow Clinton Hospital	Saint Johns	97%	34
Spectrum Health - Reed City Campus	Reed City	97%	90
Spectrum Health United Mem-Kelsey Camp	Lakeview	97%	34
Sturgis Hospital	Sturgis	97%	70
West Shore Medical Center	Manistee	97%	75
Chippewa County War Memorial Hospital	Sault Ste Marie	96%	155
Helen Newberry Joy Hospital	Newberry	96%	27
Henry Ford West Bloomfield Hospital[2]	W Bloomfield	96%	192
Lakeland Community Hospital - Watervliet	Watervliet	96%	48
Mclaren - Northern Michigan	Petoskey	96%	181
Mclaren Flint[2]	Flint	96%	47
Mercy Hospital - Cadillac	Cadillac	96%	180
Midmichigan Medical Center - Gratiot	Alma	96%	104
Otsego Memorial Hospital	Gaylord	96%	102
Schoolcraft Memorial Hospital	Manistique	96%	49
Sinai - Grace Hospital	Detroit	96%	399
South Haven Community Hospital	South Haven	96%	55
Spectrum Health Gerber Memorial	Fremont	96%	148
Mclaren Bay Region	Bay City	95%	171
Northstar Health System	Iron River	95%	43
Spectrum Health Zeeland Comm Hosp	Zeeland	95%	133
Mclaren Central Michigan	Mount Pleasant	94%	117
Mclaren Macomb	Mount Clemens	94%	377
Saint Mary's of Michigan Medical Center[2]	Saginaw	94%	141
Sparrow Ionia Hospital	Ionia	93%	42
Three Rivers Health	Three Rivers	93%	87
Hurley Medical Center[2]	Flint	92%	88
Hills & Dales General Hospital	Cass City	90%	29
Saint Mary's Standish Community Hospital	Standish	90%	39
West Branch Regional Medical Center[2]	West Branch	89%	76
Mclaren - Greater Lansing	Lansing	87%	194
Eaton Rapids Medical Center	Eaton Rapids	82%	28
Marlette Regional Hospital	Marlette	80%	46

Pregnancy and Delivery Care

Newborns whose Deliveries were Scheduled Early

Hospital Name	City	Rate	Cases
Bronson Methodist Hospital	Kalamazoo	0%	208
Dickinson County Memorial Hospital[2]	Iron Mountain	0%	31
Edward W Sparrow Hospital[2]	Lansing	0%	239
Garden City Hospital	Garden City	0%	49
Mclaren Bay Region[2]	Bay City	0%	66
Mclaren Central Michigan[2]	Mount Pleasant	0%	30
Memorial Healthcare[2]	Owosso	0%	26
Mercy Health Hackley Campus[2]	Muskegon	0%	27
Mercy Memorial Hospital System	Monroe	0%	68
Munson Medical Center[2]	Traverse City	0%	28
Oakwood Hospital - Dearborn[2]	Dearborn	0%	658
Oakwood Hospital - Wayne[2]	Wayne	0%	168
Saint Joseph Mercy Oakland	Pontiac	0%	342
Saint Mary's Health Care[2]	Grand Rapids	0%	184
Henry Ford West Bloomfield Hospital	W Bloomfield	1%	109
Holland Community Hospital	Holland	1%	126
Oakwood Hospital - Southshore[2]	Trenton	1%	134
Spectrum Health - Butterworth Campus[2]	Grand Rapids	1%	77
University of Michigan Health System	Ann Arbor	1%	203
Genesys Reg Med Ctr-Health Park[2]	Grand Blanc	2%	339
Henry Ford Hospital	Detroit	2%	214
Henry Ford Macomb Hospital	Clinton Twp	2%	180
Henry Ford Wyandotte Hospital	Wyandotte	2%	146
Midmichigan Medical Center - Midland[2]	Midland	2%	114
Port Huron Hospital[2]	Port Huron	2%	123
Providence Hospital & Medical Centers	Southfield	2%	394
Saint Joseph Mercy Hospital[2]	Ann Arbor	2%	56
Allegiance Health[2]	Jackson	3%	37
Botsford Hospital[2]	Farmington Hills	3%	32
Bronson Battle Creek Hospital[2]	Battle Creek	3%	32
Crittenton Hospital Medical Center	Rochester	3%	70
Memorial Medical Center of West Michigan[2]	Ludington	3%	32
Saint John River District Hospital	East China	3%	33
Spectrum Health Zeeland Comm Hosp[2]	Zeeland	3%	35
Sturgis Hospital[2]	Sturgis	3%	38
Beaumont Health System[2]	Royal Oak	4%	51
Covenant Medical Center	Saginaw	4%	367
Emma L Bixby Medical Center[2]	Adrian	4%	26
Mclaren Lapeer Region[2]	Lapeer	4%	26
Metro Health Hospital	Wyoming	4%	122
Saint John Hospital & Medical Center	Detroit	4%	280
Saint Mary Mercy Hospital[2]	Livonia	4%	27
Mercy Hospital - Grayling	Grayling	5%	37
William Beaumont Hospital - Troy[2]	Troy	5%	66
Huron Valley - Sinai Hospital[2]	Commerce Twp	7%	42
Mclaren - Northern Michigan	Petoskey	7%	75
Mclaren Flint	Flint	7%	55
Mclaren Macomb	Mount Clemens	7%	100
St John Macomb-Oakland Hosp	Warren	8%	103
South Haven Community Hospital[2]	South Haven	8%	25
Harper University Hospital[2]	Detroit	9%	43
Carson City Hospital[2]	Carson City	10%	31
Midmichigan Medical Center - Gratiot[2]	Alma	10%	68
Beaumont Health System[2]	Grosse Pointe	12%	26
Hurley Medical Center[2]	Flint	15%	48
Mclaren - Greater Lansing[2]	Lansing	15%	81
Spectrum Health United Memorial[2]	Greenville	17%	58
Hillsdale Community Health Center[2]	Hillsdale	44%	149

Preventive Care

Immunization for Influenza

Hospital Name	City	Rate	Cases
North Ottawa Community Health Center[2]	Grand Haven	100%	240
Hillsdale Community Health Center[2]	Hillsdale	99%	307
Holland Community Hospital[2]	Holland	99%	515
Mclaren Central Michigan[2]	Mount Pleasant	99%	361
Mercy Memorial Hospital System[2]	Monroe	99%	539
Saint Francis Hospital[2]	Escanaba	99%	347
Saint Joseph Mercy Oakland[2]	Pontiac	99%	570
Alpena Regional Medical Center[2]	Alpena	98%	415
Huron Valley - Sinai Hospital[2]	Commerce Twp	98%	546
Oaklawn Hospital[2]	Marshall	98%	366
Otsego Memorial Hospital[2]	Gaylord	98%	255
Saint Joseph Mercy Livingston Hospital[2]	Howell	98%	403
Straith Hospital For Special Surgery[2]	Southfield	98%	285
Tawas Saint Joseph Hospital[2]	Tawas City	98%	258
Covenant Medical Center[2]	Saginaw	97%	524
Harper University Hospital[2]	Detroit	97%	487
Marlette Regional Hospital[2,3]	Marlette	97%	135
Midmichigan Medical Center - Clare[2]	Clare	97%	322
Munson Medical Center[2]	Traverse City	97%	605
Oakwood Hospital - Southshore[2]	Trenton	97%	539
Saint John Hospital & Medical Center[2]	Detroit	97%	555
South Haven Community Hospital[2]	South Haven	97%	266
Spectrum Health Gerber Memorial[2]	Fremont	97%	407
Beaumont Health System[2]	Grosse Pointe	96%	594
Carson City Hospital[2]	Carson City	96%	258
Crittenton Hospital Medical Center[2]	Rochester	96%	570
Lakeland Community Hospital - Watervliet[2]	Watervliet	96%	254
Port Huron Hospital[2]	Port Huron	96%	559
Portage Health[2]	Hancock	96%	244
Saint Mary's Health Care[2]	Grand Rapids	96%	527
Sinai - Grace Hospital[2]	Detroit	96%	554
Spectrum Health United Mem-Kelsey Camp	Lakeview	96%	107
Spectrum Health Zeeland Comm Hosp[2]	Zeeland	96%	224
Sturgis Hospital[2]	Sturgis	96%	234
William Beaumont Hospital - Troy[2]	Troy	96%	570
Beaumont Health System[2]	Royal Oak	95%	578
Bronson Battle Creek Hospital[2]	Battle Creek	95%	574
Chelsea Community Hospital[2]	Chelsea	95%	354
Community Health Center of Branch County[2]	Coldwater	95%	351
Dickinson County Memorial Hospital[2]	Iron Mountain	95%	289
Mclaren Bay Region[2]	Bay City	95%	566
Mclaren Oakland[2]	Pontiac	95%	438
Promedica Herrick Hospital[2]	Tecumseh	95%	287
Providence Hospital & Medical Centers[2]	Southfield	95%	1113
Saint John River District Hospital[2]	East China	95%	261
Spectrum Health United Memorial[2]	Greenville	95%	269
Detroit Receiving Hosp & U Health Ctr[2]	Detroit	94%	598
Huron Medical Center[2]	Bad Axe	94%	271
Mclaren Lapeer Region[2]	Lapeer	94%	555
Mclaren Macomb[2]	Mount Clemens	94%	602
Memorial Medical Center of West Michigan[2]	Ludington	94%	265
Mercy Hospital - Grayling[2]	Grayling	94%	294
Metro Health Hospital[2]	Wyoming	94%	536
St John Macomb-Oakland Hosp[2]	Warren	93%	584
Saint Mary's of Michigan Medical Center[2]	Saginaw	93%	614
Spectrum Health Big Rapids Hospital[2]	Big Rapids	93%	310
Allegan General Hospital	Allegan	92%	165
Borgess Medical Center[2]	Kalamazoo	92%	553
Garden City Hospital[2]	Garden City	92%	550
Lakeland Hospital - Saint Joseph[2]	Saint Joseph	92%	532
Mercy Hospital - Cadillac[2]	Cadillac	92%	323
Pennock Hospital[2]	Hastings	92%	266
Spectrum Health - Butterworth Campus[2]	Grand Rapids	92%	531
Allegiance Health[2]	Jackson	91%	558
Emma L Bixby Medical Center[2]	Adrian	91%	369
Mclaren - Northern Michigan[2]	Petoskey	91%	578
Oakwood Hospital - Taylor[2]	Taylor	91%	581
Saint Joseph Mercy Hospital[2]	Ann Arbor	91%	623
Mclaren Flint[2]	Flint	90%	571
Mercy Health Partners - Mercy Campus[2]	Muskegon	90%	588
Mercy Health Hackley Campus[2]	Muskegon	89%	473
Saint Mary Mercy Hospital[2]	Livonia	88%	667
Saginaw VA Medical Center[2,3]	Saginaw	87%	133
Botsford Hospital[2]	Farmington Hills	86%	546
Bronson Methodist Hospital[2]	Kalamazoo	86%	650
Henry Ford Wyandotte Hospital[2]	Wyandotte	86%	563
Marquette General Hospital[2]	Marquette	86%	534
Mclaren - Greater Lansing[2]	Lansing	86%	566
University of Michigan Health System[2]	Ann Arbor	86%	576
Edward W Sparrow Hospital[2]	Lansing	85%	743
Henry Ford West Bloomfield Hospital[2]	W Bloomfield	84%	525
Three Rivers Health[2]	Three Rivers	84%	261
Bronson Lakeview Hospital[3]	Paw Paw	83%	248
Healthsource Saginaw[2]	Saginaw	82%	191
Henry Ford Macomb Hospital[2]	Clinton Twp	81%	573
Hills & Dales General Hospital	Cass City	81%	235
Oakland Regional Hospital	Southfield	78%	196
Doctors' Hospital of Michigan[2]	Pontiac	76%	105
Chippewa County War Memorial Hospital[2]	Sault Ste Marie	73%	293
Memorial Healthcare[2]	Owosso	73%	331
Henry Ford Hospital[2]	Detroit	72%	539
Saint Joseph Mercy Port Huron[2]	Port Huron	72%	425
Hurley Medical Center[2]	Flint	70%	509
West Branch Regional Medical Center[2]	West Branch	66%	288
Oakwood Hospital - Wayne[2]	Wayne	65%	532
Southeast Michigan Surgical Hospital	Warren	61%	84
Midmichigan Medical Center - Gratiot[2]	Alma	60%	448
Genesys Reg Med Ctr-Health Park[2]	Grand Blanc	58%	625
Midmichigan Medical Center - Midland[2]	Midland	56%	553
Oakwood Hospital - Dearborn[2]	Dearborn	56%	523
Karmanos Cancer Center[2]	Detroit	52%	367
Brighton Hospital[2]	Brighton	33%	281

Immunization for Pneumonia

Hospital Name	City	Rate	Cases
Holland Community Hospital[2]	Holland	100%	561
Hillsdale Community Health Center[2]	Hillsdale	99%	490
Huron Medical Center[2]	Bad Axe	99%	289
Mercy Memorial Hospital System[2]	Monroe	99%	671
Midmichigan Medical Center - Clare[2]	Clare	99%	522

NOTE: Hospital profiles are in alphabetical order by state, then city, then hospital within the city; Rankings exclude hospitals with less than 25 cases except for patient surveys which excludes hospitals with less than 100 cases; (a) 100-299 cases; (1) The number of cases/patients is too few to report; (2) Data submitted were based on a sample of cases/patients; (3) Results are based on a shorter time period than required; (4) Data suppressed by CMS for one or more quarters; (5) Results are not available for this reporting period; (6) Fewer than 100 patients completed the HCAHPS survey; (7) No cases met the criteria for this measure; (8) The lower limit of the confidence interval cannot be calculated if the number of observed infections equals zero; (9) No data are available from the state/territory for this reporting period; (10) The scores shown reflect fewer than 50 completed surveys; (11) There were discrepancies in the data collection process; (12) This measure does not apply to this hospital for this reporting period; (13) Results cannot be calculated for this reporting period; (14) The results for this state are combined with nearby states to protect confidentiality; Please refer to the User's Guide for a full explanation of data.

Saint Joseph Mercy Oakland[2]	Pontiac	99%	746
Sturgis Hospital[2]	Sturgis	99%	274
Community Health Center of Branch County[2]	Coldwater	98%	444
Dickinson County Memorial Hospital[2]	Iron Mountain	98%	368
Lakeland Community Hospital - Watervliet[2]	Watervliet	98%	392
Mclaren Central Michigan[2]	Mount Pleasant	98%	463
Memorial Medical Center of West Michigan[2]	Ludington	98%	314
North Ottawa Community Health Center[2]	Grand Haven	98%	262
Port Huron Hospital[2]	Port Huron	98%	705
Saginaw VA Medical Center[2,3]	Saginaw	98%	281
Spectrum Health Gerber Memorial[2]	Fremont	98%	494
Spectrum Health United Mem-Kelsey Camp	Lakeview	98%	172
Spectrum Health United Memorial[2]	Greenville	98%	360
Carson City Hospital[2]	Carson City	97%	267
Covenant Medical Center[2]	Saginaw	97%	689
Harper University Hospital[2]	Detroit	97%	538
Huron Valley - Sinai Hospital[2]	Commerce Twp	97%	644
Oaklawn Hospital[2]	Marshall	97%	375
Otsego Memorial Hospital[2]	Gaylord	97%	307
Saint Francis Hospital[2]	Escanaba	97%	465
Saint John River District Hospital[2]	East China	97%	338
Saint Joseph Mercy Livingston Hospital[2]	Howell	97%	577
South Haven Community Hospital[2]	South Haven	97%	266
Spectrum Health Zeeland Comm Hosp[2]	Zeeland	97%	265
Straith Hospital For Special Surgery[2]	Southfield	97%	562
Alpena Regional Medical Center[2]	Alpena	96%	603
Chelsea Community Hospital[2]	Chelsea	96%	426
Mercy Hospital - Grayling[2]	Grayling	96%	434
Portage Health[2]	Hancock	96%	251
Beaumont Health System[2]	Grosse Pointe	95%	864
Mclaren Bay Region[2]	Bay City	95%	777
Oakwood Hospital - Taylor[2]	Taylor	95%	798
Pennock Hospital[2]	Hastings	95%	362
Sinai - Grace Hospital[2]	Detroit	95%	734
Spectrum Health - Butterworth Campus[2]	Grand Rapids	95%	534
William Beaumont Hospital - Troy[2]	Troy	95%	759
Crittenton Hospital Medical Center[2]	Rochester	94%	708
Marlette Regional Hospital[2,3]	Marlette	94%	324
Oakwood Hospital - Southshore[2]	Trenton	94%	762
Providence Hospital & Medical Centers[2]	Southfield	94%	1429
Saint Joseph Mercy Hospital[2]	Ann Arbor	94%	769
Beaumont Health System[2]	Royal Oak	93%	794
Mclaren Macomb[2]	Mount Clemens	93%	796
Mercy Hospital - Cadillac[2]	Cadillac	93%	461
Metro Health Hospital[2]	Wyoming	93%	552
Munson Medical Center[2]	Traverse City	93%	801
Promedica Herrick Hospital[2]	Tecumseh	93%	466
Tawas Saint Joseph Hospital[2]	Tawas City	93%	305
Allegan General Hospital	Allegan	92%	263
Allegiance Health[2]	Jackson	92%	708
Detroit Receiving Hosp & U Health Ctr[2]	Detroit	92%	713
Garden City Hospital[2]	Garden City	92%	709
Mclaren Flint[2]	Flint	92%	846
Mclaren Lapeer Region[2]	Lapeer	92%	750
Saint John Hospital & Medical Center[2]	Detroit	92%	656
St John Macomb-Oakland Hosp[2]	Warren	92%	862
Saint Mary's Health Care[2]	Grand Rapids	92%	611
Aspirus Ontonagon Hospital[3]	Ontonagon	91%	85
Borgess Medical Center[2]	Kalamazoo	91%	777
Emma L Bixby Medical Center[2]	Adrian	91%	430
Mclaren Oakland[2]	Pontiac	91%	576
Spectrum Health Big Rapids Hospital[2]	Big Rapids	91%	339
Bronson Battle Creek Hospital[2]	Battle Creek	90%	802
Mclaren - Northern Michigan[2]	Petoskey	90%	803
Oakwood Hospital - Wayne[2]	Wayne	89%	701
University of Michigan Health System[2]	Ann Arbor	89%	534
Bronson Methodist Hospital[2]	Kalamazoo	88%	673
Lakeland Hospital - Saint Joseph[2]	Saint Joseph	88%	722
Mercy Health Partners - Mercy Campus[2]	Muskegon	88%	972
Chippewa County War Memorial Hospital[2]	Sault Ste Marie	87%	373
Botsford Hospital[2]	Farmington Hills	86%	723
Mercy Health Hackley Campus[2]	Muskegon	86%	411
Saint Mary Mercy Hospital[2]	Livonia	86%	903
Marquette General Hospital[2]	Marquette	85%	639
Memorial Healthcare[2]	Owosso	85%	388
Saint Mary's of Michigan Medical Center[2]	Saginaw	85%	881
Scheurer Hospital[2,3]	Pigeon	85%	253
Oakland Regional Hospital	Southfield	84%	325
Edward W Sparrow Hospital[2]	Lansing	83%	956
Hayes Green Beach Memorial Hospital[2,3]	Charlotte	83%	213
Hills & Dales General Hospital	Cass City	83%	343
Henry Ford Macomb Hospital[2]	Clinton Twp	82%	751
Henry Ford West Bloomfield Hospital[2]	W Bloomfield	82%	655
Henry Ford Wyandotte Hospital[2]	Wyandotte	82%	737
Bronson Lakeview Hospital[2,3]	Paw Paw	81%	462
Three Rivers Health[2]	Three Rivers	80%	389
Mclaren - Greater Lansing[2]	Lansing	78%	759
Doctors' Hospital of Michigan[2,3]	Pontiac	77%	179
Midmichigan Medical Center - Gratiot[2]	Alma	76%	568
Oakwood Hospital - Dearborn[2]	Dearborn	76%	635
Saint Joseph Mercy Port Huron[2]	Port Huron	75%	631
Southeast Michigan Surgical Hospital	Warren	75%	44
Hurley Medical Center[2]	Flint	73%	458
Midmichigan Medical Center - Midland[2]	Midland	73%	758
West Branch Regional Medical Center[2]	West Branch	72%	475
Henry Ford Hospital[2]	Detroit	71%	687
Karmanos Cancer Center[2]	Detroit	65%	391
Genesys Reg Med Ctr-Health Park[2]	Grand Blanc	62%	808

Stroke Care

Anticoagulation Therapy for Atrial Fibrillation

Hospital Name	City	Rate	Cases
Beaumont Health System[2]	Royal Oak	100%	42
Bronson Methodist Hospital	Kalamazoo	100%	34
Covenant Medical Center	Saginaw	100%	25
Edward W Sparrow Hospital	Lansing	100%	33
Henry Ford Hospital	Detroit	100%	38
Henry Ford Macomb Hospital	Clinton Twp	100%	33
Mclaren - Northern Michigan	Petoskey	100%	25
Saint Joseph Mercy Oakland	Pontiac	100%	39
William Beaumont Hospital - Troy	Troy	100%	36
Mclaren Bay Region	Bay City	97%	33
St John Macomb-Oakland Hosp	Warren	97%	31
Lakeland Hospital - Saint Joseph	Saint Joseph	96%	27
Saint John Hospital & Medical Center	Detroit	96%	52
Spectrum Health - Butterworth Campus	Grand Rapids	92%	100
University of Michigan Health System	Ann Arbor	92%	37
Providence Hospital & Medical Centers	Southfield	89%	36
Henry Ford West Bloomfield Hospital	W Bloomfield	88%	26
Mclaren Macomb[2]	Mount Clemens	76%	37
Mclaren Flint[2]	Flint	73%	33

Antithrombotic Therapy Timing

Hospital Name	City	Rate	Cases
Beaumont Health System	Grosse Pointe	100%	70
Covenant Medical Center	Saginaw	100%	218
Dickinson County Memorial Hospital	Iron Mountain	100%	25
Edward W Sparrow Hospital	Lansing	100%	241
Garden City Hospital[2]	Garden City	100%	110
Holland Community Hospital	Holland	100%	80
Marquette General Hospital[2]	Marquette	100%	60
Mclaren Lapeer Region[2]	Lapeer	100%	56
Mclaren Oakland	Pontiac	100%	44
Mercy Health Partners - Mercy Campus[2]	Muskegon	100%	69
Mercy Hospital - Grayling[2]	Grayling	100%	43
Metro Health Hospital	Wyoming	100%	84
Munson Medical Center[2]	Traverse City	100%	99
North Ottawa Community Health Center	Grand Haven	100%	25
Saint Joseph Mercy Livingston Hospital[2]	Howell	100%	41
Spectrum Health United Memorial	Greenville	100%	25
William Beaumont Hospital - Troy	Troy	100%	220
Botsford Hospital	Farmington Hills	99%	141
Lakeland Hospital - Saint Joseph	Saint Joseph	99%	169
Mercy Memorial Hospital System	Monroe	99%	74
St John Macomb-Oakland Hosp	Warren	99%	222
Saint Joseph Mercy Hospital[2]	Ann Arbor	99%	75
Beaumont Health System[2]	Royal Oak	98%	292
Detroit Receiving Hosp & U Health Ctr	Detroit	98%	130
Genesys Reg Med Ctr-Health Park[2]	Grand Blanc	98%	107
Harper University Hospital	Detroit	98%	60
Hurley Medical Center[2]	Flint	98%	105
Mclaren - Northern Michigan	Petoskey	98%	131
Mclaren Macomb[2]	Mount Clemens	98%	129
Mercy Health Hackley Campus[2]	Muskegon	98%	90
Providence Hospital & Medical Centers	Southfield	98%	303
Saint Joseph Mercy Oakland	Pontiac	98%	207
Saint Joseph Mercy Port Huron	Port Huron	98%	60
Saint Mary Mercy Hospital[2]	Livonia	98%	97
Sinai - Grace Hospital	Detroit	98%	225
Spectrum Health - Butterworth Campus	Grand Rapids	98%	460
Allegiance Health[2]	Jackson	97%	97
Borgess Medical Center[2]	Kalamazoo	97%	58
Chelsea Community Hospital	Chelsea	97%	33
Emma L Bixby Medical Center	Adrian	97%	36
Henry Ford Wyandotte Hospital[2]	Wyandotte	97%	102
Mclaren - Greater Lansing	Lansing	97%	118
Mclaren Bay Region	Bay City	97%	129
Mclaren Central Michigan	Mount Pleasant	97%	35
Midmichigan Medical Center - Gratiot	Alma	97%	34
Saint John Hospital & Medical Center	Detroit	97%	335
Bronson Methodist Hospital	Kalamazoo	96%	214
Henry Ford Macomb Hospital	Clinton Twp	96%	199
Midmichigan Medical Center - Midland	Midland	96%	89
Saint Mary's of Michigan Medical Center[2]	Saginaw	96%	69
University of Michigan Health System	Ann Arbor	96%	167
Alpena Regional Medical Center	Alpena	95%	61
Crittenton Hospital Medical Center	Rochester	95%	79
Henry Ford Hospital	Detroit	95%	378
Oakwood Hospital - Southshore[2]	Trenton	95%	74
Henry Ford West Bloomfield Hospital	W Bloomfield	94%	129
Oakwood Hospital - Taylor	Taylor	94%	50
Saint Mary's Health Care	Grand Rapids	94%	72
Huron Valley - Sinai Hospital	Commerce Twp	93%	56
Mclaren Flint[2]	Flint	93%	152
Port Huron Hospital	Port Huron	93%	107
Hillsdale Community Health Center	Hillsdale	92%	38
Oakwood Hospital - Dearborn[2]	Dearborn	92%	79
Oakwood Hospital - Wayne[2]	Wayne	92%	62
Otsego Memorial Hospital	Gaylord	92%	25
Bronson Battle Creek Hospital	Battle Creek	90%	79
Chippewa County War Memorial Hospital	Sault Ste Marie	90%	30
Community Health Center of Branch County	Coldwater	83%	35

Assessed for Rehabilitation

Hospital Name	City	Rate	Cases
Beaumont Health System	Grosse Pointe	100%	75
Beaumont Health System[2]	Royal Oak	100%	370
Botsford Hospital	Farmington Hills	100%	143
Chelsea Community Hospital	Chelsea	100%	36
Emma L Bixby Medical Center	Adrian	100%	39
Holland Community Hospital	Holland	100%	92
Lakeland Hospital - Saint Joseph	Saint Joseph	100%	195
Mclaren Lapeer Region[2]	Lapeer	100%	66
Memorial Healthcare	Owosso	100%	27
Mercy Health Partners - Mercy Campus[2]	Muskegon	100%	73
Mercy Hospital - Cadillac	Cadillac	100%	29
Mercy Hospital - Grayling[2]	Grayling	100%	50
North Ottawa Community Health Center	Grand Haven	100%	31
St John Macomb-Oakland Hosp	Warren	100%	209
Saint Mary Mercy Hospital[2]	Livonia	100%	104
Saint Mary's Health Care	Grand Rapids	100%	110
Spectrum Health Big Rapids Hospital	Big Rapids	100%	28
Spectrum Health United Memorial	Greenville	100%	28
William Beaumont Hospital - Troy	Troy	100%	265
Covenant Medical Center	Saginaw	99%	270
Detroit Receiving Hosp & U Health Ctr	Detroit	99%	194
Edward W Sparrow Hospital	Lansing	99%	363
Harper University Hospital	Detroit	99%	83
Mclaren - Northern Michigan	Petoskey	99%	144
Mclaren Bay Region	Bay City	99%	165
Mercy Health Hackley Campus[2]	Muskegon	99%	111
Metro Health Hospital	Wyoming	99%	120
Oakwood Hospital - Dearborn[2]	Dearborn	99%	96
Saint John Hospital & Medical Center	Detroit	99%	430
Saint Joseph Mercy Oakland	Pontiac	99%	280
Sinai - Grace Hospital	Detroit	99%	285
Allegiance Health[2]	Jackson	98%	114
Henry Ford Macomb Hospital	Clinton Twp	98%	221
Marquette General Hospital[2]	Marquette	98%	104
Munson Medical Center[2]	Traverse City	98%	126
Providence Hospital & Medical Centers	Southfield	98%	422
Spectrum Health - Butterworth Campus	Grand Rapids	98%	642
Bronson Methodist Hospital	Kalamazoo	97%	311
Dickinson County Memorial Hospital	Iron Mountain	97%	33
Garden City Hospital[2]	Garden City	97%	140
Henry Ford West Bloomfield Hospital	W Bloomfield	97%	159
Mclaren - Greater Lansing	Lansing	97%	119
Mercy Memorial Hospital System	Monroe	97%	76
Saint Joseph Mercy Hospital[2]	Ann Arbor	97%	106
Saint Joseph Mercy Port Huron	Port Huron	97%	60
Spectrum Health Gerber Memorial	Fremont	97%	33
Midmichigan Medical Center - Midland	Midland	96%	113
Saint Joseph Mercy Livingston Hospital[2]	Howell	96%	49
Saint Mary's of Michigan Medical Center[2]	Saginaw	96%	103
University of Michigan Health System	Ann Arbor	96%	326
Bronson Battle Creek Hospital	Battle Creek	95%	86
Crittenton Hospital Medical Center	Rochester	95%	115
Henry Ford Hospital	Detroit	95%	530
Mclaren Oakland	Pontiac	94%	48
Oakwood Hospital - Wayne[2]	Wayne	94%	68
Alpena Regional Medical Center	Alpena	93%	69
Genesys Reg Med Ctr-Health Park[2]	Grand Blanc	93%	115
Hurley Medical Center[2]	Flint	93%	133
Huron Valley - Sinai Hospital	Commerce Twp	92%	74
Mclaren Flint[2]	Flint	92%	178
Oakwood Hospital - Southshore[2]	Trenton	92%	85
Port Huron Hospital	Port Huron	92%	107
Borgess Medical Center[2]	Kalamazoo	91%	80
Mclaren Central Michigan	Mount Pleasant	91%	43
Midmichigan Medical Center - Gratiot	Alma	91%	33
Henry Ford Wyandotte Hospital[2]	Wyandotte	90%	116
Hillsdale Community Health Center	Hillsdale	90%	41
Oakwood Hospital - Taylor	Taylor	90%	50
Chippewa County War Memorial Hospital	Sault Ste Marie	81%	32
Mclaren Macomb[2]	Mount Clemens	81%	163
Community Health Center of Branch County	Coldwater	59%	41

Discharged on Antithrombotic Therapy

Hospital Name	City	Rate	Cases
Allegiance Health[2]	Jackson	100%	99

NOTE: Hospital profiles are in alphabetical order by state, then city, then hospital within the city; Rankings exclude hospitals with less than 25 cases except for patient surveys which excludes hospitals with less than 100 cases; (a) 100-299 cases; (1) The number of cases/patients is too few to report; (2) Data submitted were based on a sample of cases/patients; (3) Results are based on a shorter time period than required; (4) Data suppressed by CMS for one or more quarters; (5) Results are not available for this reporting period; (6) Fewer than 100 patients completed the HCAHPS survey; (7) No cases met the criteria for this measure; (8) The lower limit of the confidence interval cannot be calculated if the number of observed infections equals zero; (9) No data are available from the state/territory for this reporting period; (10) The scores shown reflect fewer than 50 completed surveys; (11) There were discrepancies in the data collection process; (12) This measure does not apply to this hospital for this reporting period; (13) Results cannot be calculated for this reporting period; (14) The results for this state are combined with nearby states to protect confidentiality; Please refer to the User's Guide for a full explanation of data.

Beaumont Health System	Grosse Pointe	100%	72
Beaumont Health System[2]	Royal Oak	100%	303
Borgess Medical Center[2]	Kalamazoo	100%	69
Chelsea Community Hospital	Chelsea	100%	34
Chippewa County War Memorial Hospital	Sault Ste Marie	100%	32
Covenant Medical Center	Saginaw	100%	226
Dickinson County Memorial Hospital	Iron Mountain	100%	29
Emma L Bixby Medical Center	Adrian	100%	39
Garden City Hospital[2]	Garden City	100%	128
Henry Ford Hospital	Detroit	100%	441
Holland Community Hospital	Holland	100%	87
Marquette General Hospital[2]	Marquette	100%	88
Mclaren - Northern Michigan	Petoskey	100%	136
Mclaren Central Michigan	Mount Pleasant	100%	39
Mclaren Lapeer Region[2]	Lapeer	100%	60
Memorial Healthcare	Owosso	100%	25
Mercy Health Partners - Mercy Campus[2]	Muskegon	100%	71
Mercy Hospital - Cadillac	Cadillac	100%	28
Mercy Hospital - Grayling[2]	Grayling	100%	48
Mercy Memorial Hospital System	Monroe	100%	74
Metro Health Hospital	Wyoming	100%	103
Midmichigan Medical Center - Gratiot	Alma	100%	33
Midmichigan Medical Center - Midland	Midland	100%	98
North Ottawa Community Health Center	Grand Haven	100%	30
Saint John Hospital & Medical Center	Detroit	100%	368
St John Macomb-Oakland Hosp	Warren	100%	204
Saint Joseph Mercy Hospital[2]	Ann Arbor	100%	96
Saint Joseph Mercy Oakland	Pontiac	100%	248
Saint Joseph Mercy Port Huron	Port Huron	100%	59
Saint Mary Mercy Hospital[2]	Livonia	100%	95
Sinai - Grace Hospital	Detroit	100%	237
Spectrum Health Gerber Memorial	Fremont	100%	32
Spectrum Health United Memorial	Greenville	100%	27
University of Michigan Health System	Ann Arbor	100%	216
William Beaumont Hospital - Troy	Troy	100%	246
Bronson Battle Creek Hospital	Battle Creek	99%	84
Crittenton Hospital Medical Center	Rochester	99%	105
Detroit Receiving Hosp & U Health Ctr	Detroit	99%	154
Edward W Sparrow Hospital	Lansing	99%	298
Harper University Hospital	Detroit	99%	68
Henry Ford Macomb Hospital	Clinton Twp	99%	206
Henry Ford West Bloomfield Hospital	W Bloomfield	99%	147
Huron Valley - Sinai Hospital	Commerce Twp	99%	69
Lakeland Hospital - Saint Joseph	Saint Joseph	99%	179
Mclaren Bay Region	Bay City	99%	142
Munson Medical Center[2]	Traverse City	99%	116
Providence Hospital & Medical Centers	Southfield	99%	336
Saint Mary's of Michigan Medical Center[2]	Saginaw	99%	79
Spectrum Health - Butterworth Campus	Grand Rapids	99%	524
Bronson Methodist Hospital	Kalamazoo	98%	256
Mclaren - Greater Lansing	Lansing	98%	119
Mclaren Macomb[2]	Mount Clemens	98%	146
Mclaren Oakland	Pontiac	98%	46
Mercy Health Hackley Campus[2]	Muskegon	98%	90
Saint Joseph Mercy Livingston Hospital[2]	Howell	98%	49
Botsford Hospital	Farmington Hills	97%	125
Genesys Reg Med Ctr-Health Park[2]	Grand Blanc	97%	108
Hillsdale Community Health Center	Hillsdale	97%	39
Oakwood Hospital - Southshore[2]	Trenton	97%	78
Alpena Regional Medical Center	Alpena	96%	67
Mclaren Flint[2]	Flint	96%	157
Saint Mary's Health Care	Grand Rapids	96%	98
Spectrum Health Big Rapids Hospital	Big Rapids	96%	26
Oakwood Hospital - Wayne[2]	Wayne	95%	66
Port Huron Hospital	Port Huron	95%	100
Oakwood Hospital - Dearborn[2]	Dearborn	94%	85
Henry Ford Wyandotte Hospital[2]	Wyandotte	92%	109
Hurley Medical Center[2]	Flint	92%	117
Oakwood Hospital - Taylor	Taylor	86%	49
Community Health Center of Branch County	Coldwater	82%	40

Discharged on Statin Medication

Hospital Name	City	Rate	Cases
Beaumont Health System	Grosse Pointe	100%	57
Beaumont Health System[2]	Royal Oak	100%	237
Borgess Medical Center[2]	Kalamazoo	100%	57
Holland Community Hospital	Holland	100%	61
Marquette General Hospital[2]	Marquette	100%	73
Mclaren - Northern Michigan	Petoskey	100%	98
Mercy Health Partners - Mercy Campus[2]	Muskegon	100%	58
Mercy Hospital - Cadillac	Cadillac	100%	28
Mercy Hospital - Grayling[2]	Grayling	100%	41
Munson Medical Center[2]	Traverse City	100%	84
Saint Joseph Mercy Hospital[2]	Ann Arbor	100%	82
Saint Joseph Mercy Oakland	Pontiac	100%	197
William Beaumont Hospital - Troy	Troy	100%	184
Detroit Receiving Hosp & U Health Ctr	Detroit	99%	112
Henry Ford Hospital	Detroit	99%	340
Mclaren - Greater Lansing	Lansing	99%	81
Providence Hospital & Medical Centers	Southfield	99%	247
Saint John Hospital & Medical Center	Detroit	99%	313
University of Michigan Health System	Ann Arbor	99%	159
Bronson Methodist Hospital	Kalamazoo	98%	204
Lakeland Hospital - Saint Joseph	Saint Joseph	98%	128
Midmichigan Medical Center - Midland	Midland	98%	80
St John Macomb-Oakland Hosp	Warren	98%	159
Spectrum Health - Butterworth Campus	Grand Rapids	98%	406
Chelsea Community Hospital	Chelsea	96%	25
Garden City Hospital[2]	Garden City	96%	94
Harper University Hospital	Detroit	96%	50
Mercy Memorial Hospital System	Monroe	96%	46
Spectrum Health Gerber Memorial	Fremont	96%	27
Crittenton Hospital Medical Center	Rochester	95%	80
Edward W Sparrow Hospital	Lansing	95%	229
Henry Ford Macomb Hospital	Clinton Twp	95%	163
Henry Ford West Bloomfield Hospital	W Bloomfield	95%	122
Mclaren Flint[2]	Flint	95%	138
Saint Joseph Mercy Livingston Hospital[2]	Howell	95%	40
Sinai - Grace Hospital	Detroit	95%	166
Alpena Regional Medical Center	Alpena	94%	54
Covenant Medical Center	Saginaw	94%	171
Mclaren Lapeer Region[2]	Lapeer	94%	48
Mercy Health Hackley Campus[2]	Muskegon	94%	78
Metro Health Hospital	Wyoming	94%	81
Saint Mary Mercy Hospital[2]	Livonia	94%	85
Saint Mary's Health Care	Grand Rapids	94%	63
Allegiance Health[2]	Jackson	93%	76
Bronson Battle Creek Hospital	Battle Creek	92%	72
Mclaren Bay Region	Bay City	91%	116
Mclaren Oakland	Pontiac	91%	34
Huron Valley - Sinai Hospital	Commerce Twp	90%	59
Oakwood Hospital - Dearborn[2]	Dearborn	90%	71
Saint Mary's of Michigan Medical Center[2]	Saginaw	90%	67
Genesys Reg Med Ctr-Health Park[2]	Grand Blanc	89%	89
Mclaren Macomb[2]	Mount Clemens	88%	125
Botsford Hospital	Farmington Hills	87%	106
Mclaren Central Michigan	Mount Pleasant	86%	36
Henry Ford Wyandotte Hospital[2]	Wyandotte	85%	91
Port Huron Hospital	Port Huron	85%	79
Emma L Bixby Medical Center	Adrian	84%	32
Hillsdale Community Health Center	Hillsdale	83%	30
Hurley Medical Center[2]	Flint	82%	83
Midmichigan Medical Center - Gratiot	Alma	81%	26
Oakwood Hospital - Wayne[2]	Wayne	81%	53
Chippewa County War Memorial Hospital	Sault Ste Marie	73%	26
Oakwood Hospital - Southshore[2]	Trenton	73%	67
Saint Joseph Mercy Port Huron	Port Huron	73%	49
Oakwood Hospital - Taylor	Taylor	68%	41
Community Health Center of Branch County	Coldwater	47%	34

Thrombolytic Therapy Timing

Hospital Name	City	Rate	Cases
Bronson Methodist Hospital	Kalamazoo	88%	32
Edward W Sparrow Hospital	Lansing	88%	42
Saint John Hospital & Medical Center	Detroit	88%	26
Sinai - Grace Hospital	Detroit	72%	25
Detroit Receiving Hosp & U Health Ctr	Detroit	70%	27
Spectrum Health - Butterworth Campus	Grand Rapids	70%	37
Mclaren Macomb[2]	Mount Clemens	48%	25
Metro Health Hospital	Wyoming	48%	25

Venous Thromboembolism (VTE) Prophylaxis

Hospital Name	City	Rate	Cases
Holland Community Hospital	Holland	100%	96
Mclaren - Northern Michigan	Petoskey	100%	161
Mclaren Lapeer Region[2]	Lapeer	100%	73
Mercy Hospital - Cadillac	Cadillac	100%	28
Mercy Memorial Hospital System	Monroe	100%	81
North Ottawa Community Health Center	Grand Haven	100%	27
Saint Joseph Mercy Oakland	Pontiac	100%	319
Spectrum Health Big Rapids Hospital	Big Rapids	100%	25
University of Michigan Health System	Ann Arbor	100%	325
Beaumont Health System	Grosse Pointe	99%	75
Beaumont Health System[2]	Royal Oak	99%	391
Bronson Battle Creek Hospital	Battle Creek	99%	80
Metro Health Hospital	Wyoming	99%	105
Providence Hospital & Medical Centers	Southfield	99%	436
Detroit Receiving Hosp & U Health Ctr	Detroit	98%	208
Harper University Hospital	Detroit	98%	82
Henry Ford Hospital	Detroit	98%	536
Mercy Hospital - Grayling[2]	Grayling	98%	48
Saint John Hospital & Medical Center	Detroit	98%	460
St John Macomb-Oakland Hosp	Warren	98%	229
Spectrum Health - Butterworth Campus	Grand Rapids	98%	654
Chelsea Community Hospital	Chelsea	97%	34
Chippewa County War Memorial Hospital	Sault Ste Marie	97%	29
Covenant Medical Center	Saginaw	97%	281
Huron Valley - Sinai Hospital	Commerce Twp	97%	66
Lakeland Hospital - Saint Joseph	Saint Joseph	97%	203
Midmichigan Medical Center - Midland	Midland	97%	115
Saint Joseph Mercy Hospital[2]	Ann Arbor	97%	98
Saint Mary's Health Care	Grand Rapids	97%	109
Sinai - Grace Hospital	Detroit	97%	297
Alpena Regional Medical Center	Alpena	96%	69
Botsford Hospital	Farmington Hills	96%	169
Crittenton Hospital Medical Center	Rochester	96%	106
Edward W Sparrow Hospital	Lansing	96%	361
Henry Ford West Bloomfield Hospital	W Bloomfield	96%	156
Mclaren Oakland	Pontiac	96%	56
Saint Mary Mercy Hospital[2]	Livonia	96%	117
William Beaumont Hospital - Troy	Troy	96%	252
Bronson Methodist Hospital	Kalamazoo	95%	319
Emma L Bixby Medical Center	Adrian	95%	43
Garden City Hospital[2]	Garden City	95%	148
Mclaren - Greater Lansing	Lansing	95%	116
Mercy Health Partners - Mercy Campus[2]	Muskegon	95%	74
Saint Joseph Mercy Livingston Hospital[2]	Howell	95%	39
Saint Mary's of Michigan Medical Center[2]	Saginaw	95%	112
Allegiance Health[2]	Jackson	94%	119
Oakwood Hospital - Dearborn[2]	Dearborn	94%	102
Dickinson County Memorial Hospital	Iron Mountain	93%	28
Mercy Health Hackley Campus[2]	Muskegon	93%	117
Munson Medical Center[2]	Traverse City	93%	135
Mclaren Bay Region	Bay City	92%	178
Borgess Medical Center[2]	Kalamazoo	91%	80
Hurley Medical Center[2]	Flint	91%	142
Henry Ford Macomb Hospital	Clinton Twp	90%	237
Midmichigan Medical Center - Gratiot	Alma	90%	31
Genesys Reg Med Ctr-Health Park[2]	Grand Blanc	89%	119
Mclaren Macomb[2]	Mount Clemens	88%	172
Oakwood Hospital - Taylor	Taylor	86%	49
Hillsdale Community Health Center	Hillsdale	85%	41
Marquette General Hospital[2]	Marquette	85%	98
Henry Ford Wyandotte Hospital[2]	Wyandotte	81%	109
Oakwood Hospital - Wayne[2]	Wayne	78%	68
Mclaren Flint[2]	Flint	77%	180
Mclaren Central Michigan	Mount Pleasant	73%	37
Oakwood Hospital - Southshore[2]	Trenton	69%	89
Port Huron Hospital	Port Huron	69%	120
Saint Joseph Mercy Port Huron	Port Huron	67%	64
Community Health Center of Branch County	Coldwater	46%	37

Written Stroke Educational Materials Given

Hospital Name	City	Rate	Cases
Covenant Medical Center	Saginaw	100%	121
Holland Community Hospital	Holland	100%	43
Lakeland Hospital - Saint Joseph	Saint Joseph	100%	107
Mclaren - Northern Michigan	Petoskey	100%	77
Saint Mary Mercy Hospital[2]	Livonia	100%	54
Saint Joseph Mercy Oakland	Pontiac	99%	124
Bronson Methodist Hospital	Kalamazoo	97%	172
Saint John Hospital & Medical Center	Detroit	97%	221
Beaumont Health System	Grosse Pointe	96%	54
Detroit Receiving Hosp & U Health Ctr	Detroit	96%	107
Metro Health Hospital	Wyoming	96%	82
Hurley Medical Center[2]	Flint	95%	77
Providence Hospital & Medical Centers	Southfield	95%	236
St John Macomb-Oakland Hosp	Warren	95%	121
Spectrum Health - Butterworth Campus	Grand Rapids	95%	324
Crittenton Hospital Medical Center	Rochester	94%	63
Garden City Hospital[2]	Garden City	94%	70
Mclaren - Greater Lansing	Lansing	94%	84
Beaumont Health System[2]	Royal Oak	93%	207
Henry Ford Macomb Hospital	Clinton Twp	93%	110
Munson Medical Center[2]	Traverse City	93%	68
Saint Mary's Health Care	Grand Rapids	93%	59
William Beaumont Hospital - Troy	Troy	93%	147
Harper University Hospital	Detroit	92%	49
Henry Ford Wyandotte Hospital[2]	Wyandotte	92%	77
Saint Joseph Mercy Port Huron	Port Huron	92%	26
Saint Mary's of Michigan Medical Center[2]	Saginaw	91%	58
Borgess Medical Center[2]	Kalamazoo	90%	49
Henry Ford Hospital	Detroit	90%	282
University of Michigan Health System	Ann Arbor	90%	177
Saint Joseph Mercy Hospital[2]	Ann Arbor	89%	53
Allegiance Health[2]	Jackson	88%	58
Edward W Sparrow Hospital	Lansing	88%	204
Mclaren Bay Region	Bay City	88%	82
Oakwood Hospital - Dearborn[2]	Dearborn	88%	57
Sinai - Grace Hospital	Detroit	88%	144
Saint Joseph Mercy Livingston Hospital[2]	Howell	86%	35
Genesys Reg Med Ctr-Health Park[2]	Grand Blanc	84%	70
Henry Ford West Bloomfield Hospital	W Bloomfield	84%	80
Botsford Hospital	Farmington Hills	83%	58
Huron Valley - Sinai Hospital	Commerce Twp	83%	47
Mercy Memorial Hospital System	Monroe	82%	34
Mclaren Oakland	Pontiac	80%	30
Midmichigan Medical Center - Midland	Midland	80%	76
Bronson Battle Creek Hospital	Battle Creek	78%	50
Mercy Hospital - Grayling[2]	Grayling	75%	36
Mclaren Lapeer Region[2]	Lapeer	73%	37
Port Huron Hospital	Port Huron	72%	61

NOTE: Hospital profiles are in alphabetical order by state, then city, then hospital within the city; Rankings exclude hospitals with less than 25 cases except for patient surveys which excludes hospitals with less than 100 cases; (a) 100-299 cases; (1) The number of cases/patients is too few to report; (2) Data submitted were based on a sample of cases/patients; (3) Results are based on a shorter time period than required; (4) Data suppressed by CMS for one or more quarters; (5) Results are not available for this reporting period; (6) Fewer than 100 patients completed the HCAHPS survey; (7) No cases met the criteria for this measure; (8) The lower limit of the confidence interval cannot be calculated if the number of observed infections equals zero; (9) No data are available from the state/territory for this reporting period; (10) The scores shown reflect fewer than 50 completed surveys; (11) There were discrepancies in the data collection process; (12) This measure does not apply to this hospital for this reporting period; (13) Results cannot be calculated for this reporting period; (14) The results for this state are combined with nearby states to protect confidentiality; Please refer to the User's Guide for a full explanation of data.

Mclaren Flint[2]	Flint	66%	114
Oakwood Hospital - Wayne[2]	Wayne	56%	36
Marquette General Hospital[2]	Marquette	52%	56
Mercy Health Hackley Campus[2]	Muskegon	50%	44
Mclaren Macomb[2]	Mount Clemens	37%	94
Oakwood Hospital - Southshore[2]	Trenton	36%	47
Mercy Health Partners - Mercy Campus[2]	Muskegon	35%	40
Oakwood Hospital - Taylor	Taylor	32%	25
Alpena Regional Medical Center	Alpena	19%	32
Community Health Center of Branch County	Coldwater	11%	27

Surgical Care Improvement Project

Appropriate Beta Blocker Usage

Hospital Name	City	Rate	Cases
Bell Hospital[2]	Ishpeming	100%	40
Chelsea Community Hospital[2]	Chelsea	100%	134
Hillsdale Community Health Center	Hillsdale	100%	65
Holland Community Hospital[2]	Holland	100%	222
Huron Medical Center[2]	Bad Axe	100%	38
Lakeland Hospital - Saint Joseph[2]	Saint Joseph	100%	210
Midmichigan Medical Center - Clare	Clare	100%	29
Munson Medical Center[2]	Traverse City	100%	333
Oaklawn Hospital[2]	Marshall	100%	139
Portage Health	Hancock	100%	52
Promedica Herrick Hospital[2]	Tecumseh	100%	35
Providence Hospital & Medical Centers[2]	Southfield	100%	866
St John Macomb-Oakland Hosp[2]	Warren	100%	431
Saint Joseph Mercy Oakland[2]	Pontiac	100%	228
Scheurer Hospital	Pigeon	100%	33
Sparrow Clinton Hospital	Saint Johns	100%	27
Spectrum Health Big Rapids Hospital	Big Rapids	100%	33
West Branch Regional Medical Center[2]	West Branch	100%	61
William Beaumont Hospital - Troy[2]	Troy	100%	210
Allegiance Health[2]	Jackson	99%	249
Beaumont Health System[2]	Royal Oak	99%	303
Borgess Medical Center[2]	Kalamazoo	99%	277
Bronson Battle Creek Hospital[2]	Battle Creek	99%	291
Bronson Methodist Hospital[2]	Kalamazoo	99%	481
Detroit Receiving Hosp & U Health Ctr[2]	Detroit	99%	153
Edward W Sparrow Hospital[2]	Lansing	99%	653
Harper University Hospital[2]	Detroit	99%	188
Henry Ford Macomb Hospital[2]	Clinton Twp	99%	343
Henry Ford West Bloomfield Hospital[2]	W Bloomfield	99%	120
Henry Ford Wyandotte Hospital[2]	Wyandotte	99%	138
Mclaren Flint[2]	Flint	99%	430
Mclaren Oakland[2]	Pontiac	99%	79
Memorial Healthcare[2]	Owosso	99%	92
Mercy Health Partners - Mercy Campus[2]	Muskegon	99%	208
North Ottawa Community Health Center	Grand Haven	99%	68
Oakwood Hospital - Dearborn[2]	Dearborn	99%	224
Oakwood Hospital - Taylor[2]	Taylor	99%	102
Saint John Hospital & Medical Center[2]	Detroit	99%	504
Saint Joseph Mercy Hospital[2]	Ann Arbor	99%	692
Saint Joseph Mercy Port Huron[2]	Port Huron	99%	115
Saint Mary Mercy Hospital	Livonia	99%	259
Saint Mary's Health Care[2]	Grand Rapids	99%	162
Saint Mary's of Michigan Medical Center[2]	Saginaw	99%	216
Spectrum Health - Butterworth Campus[2]	Grand Rapids	99%	298
Alpena Regional Medical Center[2]	Alpena	98%	123
Botsford Hospital[2]	Farmington Hills	98%	173
Carson City Hospital	Carson City	98%	50
Covenant Medical Center[2]	Saginaw	98%	640
Dickinson County Memorial Hospital	Iron Mountain	98%	66
Garden City Hospital	Garden City	98%	140
Mclaren - Greater Lansing[2]	Lansing	98%	165
Mclaren - Northern Michigan[2]	Petoskey	98%	237
Mclaren Central Michigan	Mount Pleasant	98%	66
Mclaren Macomb[2]	Mount Clemens	98%	353
Mercy Hospital - Grayling	Grayling	98%	56
Metro Health Hospital[2]	Wyoming	98%	100
Midmichigan Medical Center - Gratiot	Alma	98%	92
Oakwood Hospital - Wayne[2]	Wayne	98%	65
Sinai - Grace Hospital[2]	Detroit	98%	171
University of Michigan Health System[2]	Ann Arbor	98%	799
Beaumont Health System[2]	Grosse Pointe	97%	166
Chippewa County War Memorial Hospital	Sault Ste Marie	97%	76
Crittenton Hospital Medical Center[2]	Rochester	97%	264
Marquette General Hospital[2]	Marquette	97%	234
Mclaren Bay Region	Bay City	97%	611
Mercy Memorial Hospital System	Monroe	97%	133
Port Huron Hospital	Port Huron	97%	306
Saint John River District Hospital	East China	97%	33
Genesys Reg Med Ctr-Health Park[2]	Grand Blanc	96%	650
Henry Ford Hospital[2]	Detroit	96%	269
Hurley Medical Center[2]	Flint	96%	107
Mercy Health Hackley Campus[2]	Muskegon	96%	106
Mercy Hospital - Cadillac	Cadillac	96%	108
Midmichigan Medical Center - Midland	Midland	96%	472
Otsego Memorial Hospital[2]	Gaylord	96%	53
Saint Joseph Mercy Livingston Hospital	Howell	96%	45
Spectrum Health Zeeland Comm Hosp	Zeeland	96%	69
Tawas Saint Joseph Hospital	Tawas City	96%	56
VA Ann Arbor Healthcare System[2]	Ann Arbor	96%	262
West Shore Medical Center	Manistee	96%	27
Community Health Center of Branch County	Coldwater	95%	55
Detroit (John D. Dingell) VA Med Ctr[2]	Detroit	95%	97
Emma L Bixby Medical Center[2]	Adrian	95%	85
Huron Valley - Sinai Hospital[2]	Commerce Twp	95%	169
Lakeland Community Hospital - Watervliet	Watervliet	95%	42
Memorial Medical Center of West Michigan	Ludington	95%	74
Allegan General Hospital	Allegan	94%	35
Oakwood Hospital - Southshore[2]	Trenton	94%	118
Spectrum Health Gerber Memorial	Fremont	94%	50
Pennock Hospital	Hastings	93%	70
Spectrum Health United Memorial	Greenville	93%	46
Karmanos Cancer Center[2]	Detroit	90%	111
Mclaren Lapeer Region[2]	Lapeer	90%	83
Sturgis Hospital	Sturgis	84%	25

Appropriate VTP Within 24 Hours

Hospital Name	City	Rate	Cases
Allegiance Health[2]	Jackson	100%	428
Aspirus Keweenaw Hospital	Laurium	100%	42
Beaumont Health System[2]	Grosse Pointe	100%	448
Botsford Hospital[2]	Farmington Hills	100%	488
Harper University Hospital[2]	Detroit	100%	310
Hayes Green Beach Memorial Hospital	Charlotte	100%	47
Henry Ford Wyandotte Hospital[2]	Wyandotte	100%	413
Hillsdale Community Health Center	Hillsdale	100%	203
Holland Community Hospital[2]	Holland	100%	527
Lakeland Community Hospital - Watervliet	Watervliet	100%	156
Marlette Regional Hospital	Marlette	100%	26
Mercy Hospital - Grayling	Grayling	100%	200
Mercy Memorial Hospital System	Monroe	100%	304
Munson Medical Center[2]	Traverse City	100%	438
Oakwood Hospital - Taylor[2]	Taylor	100%	269
Port Huron Hospital	Port Huron	100%	641
Portage Health	Hancock	100%	166
Promedica Herrick Hospital[2]	Tecumseh	100%	89
Providence Hospital & Medical Centers[2]	Southfield	100%	2140
Saint Francis Hospital	Escanaba	100%	63
Saint John Hospital & Medical Center[2]	Detroit	100%	976
Saint Joseph Mercy Oakland[2]	Pontiac	100%	479
Saint Joseph Mercy Port Huron[2]	Port Huron	100%	386
Saint Mary Mercy Hospital	Livonia	100%	749
Saint Mary's Health Care[2]	Grand Rapids	100%	413
Sparrow Clinton Hospital	Saint Johns	100%	46
Spectrum Health Zeeland Comm Hosp	Zeeland	100%	166
Sturgis Hospital	Sturgis	100%	89
Tawas Saint Joseph Hospital	Tawas City	100%	140
University of Michigan Health System[2]	Ann Arbor	100%	1266
VA Ann Arbor Healthcare System[2]	Ann Arbor	100%	215
William Beaumont Hospital - Troy[2]	Troy	100%	282
Allegan General Hospital	Allegan	99%	146
Beaumont Health System[2]	Royal Oak	99%	554
Chelsea Community Hospital[2]	Chelsea	99%	782
Covenant Medical Center[2]	Saginaw	99%	1483
Crittenton Hospital Medical Center[2]	Rochester	99%	608
Detroit (John D. Dingell) VA Med Ctr[2]	Detroit	99%	203
Detroit Receiving Hosp & U Health Ctr[2]	Detroit	99%	467
Dickinson County Memorial Hospital	Iron Mountain	99%	244
Henry Ford Hospital[2]	Detroit	99%	449
Henry Ford Macomb Hospital[2]	Clinton Twp	99%	595
Huron Valley - Sinai Hospital[2]	Commerce Twp	99%	549
Lakeland Hospital - Saint Joseph[2]	Saint Joseph	99%	352
Mclaren - Northern Michigan[2]	Petoskey	99%	333
Mclaren Macomb[2]	Mount Clemens	99%	592
Metro Health Hospital[2]	Wyoming	99%	326
North Ottawa Community Health Center	Grand Haven	99%	195
Oaklawn Hospital[2]	Marshall	99%	348
Oakwood Hospital - Dearborn[2]	Dearborn	99%	318
Oakwood Hospital - Southshore[2]	Trenton	99%	285
Oakwood Hospital - Wayne[2]	Wayne	99%	236
Otsego Memorial Hospital[2]	Gaylord	99%	192
St John Macomb-Oakland Hosp[2]	Warren	99%	808
Saint Joseph Mercy Livingston Hospital	Howell	99%	129
Spectrum Health Big Rapids Hospital	Big Rapids	99%	148
Alpena Regional Medical Center[2]	Alpena	98%	293
Bronson Battle Creek Hospital[2]	Battle Creek	98%	752
Carson City Hospital	Carson City	98%	147
Garden City Hospital	Garden City	98%	388
Henry Ford West Bloomfield Hospital[2]	W Bloomfield	98%	359
Huron Medical Center[2]	Bad Axe	98%	116
Karmanos Cancer Center[2]	Detroit	98%	346
Mclaren Bay Region	Bay City	98%	792
Mclaren Flint[2]	Flint	98%	506
Mclaren Oakland[2]	Pontiac	98%	249
Mercy Health Hackley Campus[2]	Muskegon	98%	293
Mercy Health Partners - Mercy Campus[2]	Muskegon	98%	223
Mercy Hospital - Cadillac	Cadillac	98%	326
Midmichigan Medical Center - Midland	Midland	98%	1032
Pennock Hospital	Hastings	98%	248
Saint John River District Hospital	East China	98%	90
Saint Joseph Mercy Hospital[2]	Ann Arbor	98%	1625
Sinai - Grace Hospital[2]	Detroit	98%	391
Spectrum Health - Butterworth Campus[2]	Grand Rapids	98%	579
Spectrum Health Gerber Memorial	Fremont	98%	164
Spectrum Health United Memorial	Greenville	98%	138
Chippewa County War Memorial Hospital	Sault Ste Marie	97%	198
Genesys Reg Med Ctr-Health Park[2]	Grand Blanc	97%	1346
Mclaren Lapeer Region[2]	Lapeer	97%	275
Midmichigan Medical Center - Clare	Clare	97%	63
Midmichigan Medical Center - Gratiot	Alma	97%	204
Saint Mary's of Michigan Medical Center[2]	Saginaw	97%	374
South Haven Community Hospital	South Haven	97%	63
Bell Hospital[2]	Ishpeming	96%	133
Edward W Sparrow Hospital[2]	Lansing	96%	1746
Emma L Bixby Medical Center[2]	Adrian	96%	275
Hurley Medical Center[2]	Flint	96%	334
Mclaren - Greater Lansing[2]	Lansing	96%	279
Bronson Methodist Hospital[2]	Kalamazoo	95%	968
Community Health Center of Branch County	Coldwater	95%	165
Marquette General Hospital[2]	Marquette	95%	353
Memorial Medical Center of West Michigan	Ludington	95%	219
West Branch Regional Medical Center[2]	West Branch	95%	175
Borgess Medical Center[2]	Kalamazoo	93%	255
Mclaren Central Michigan	Mount Pleasant	93%	233
Memorial Healthcare[2]	Owosso	93%	247
West Shore Medical Center	Manistee	92%	96
Scheurer Hospital	Pigeon	89%	94
Hills & Dales General Hospital	Cass City	88%	25
Oakland Regional Hospital	Southfield	63%	52

Controlled Postoperative Blood Glucose

Hospital Name	City	Rate	Cases
Crittenton Hospital Medical Center[2]	Rochester	100%	68
Harper University Hospital[2]	Detroit	100%	71
Port Huron Hospital	Port Huron	100%	103
Sinai - Grace Hospital[2]	Detroit	100%	58
William Beaumont Hospital - Troy[2]	Troy	100%	119
Allegiance Health[2]	Jackson	99%	105
Bronson Methodist Hospital[2]	Kalamazoo	99%	210
Genesys Reg Med Ctr-Health Park[2]	Grand Blanc	99%	180
Henry Ford Macomb Hospital[2]	Clinton Twp	99%	131
Mclaren - Northern Michigan[2]	Petoskey	99%	134
Mclaren Macomb[2]	Mount Clemens	99%	91
Saint John Hospital & Medical Center[2]	Detroit	99%	192
Saint Joseph Mercy Hospital[2]	Ann Arbor	99%	170
Spectrum Health - Butterworth Campus[2]	Grand Rapids	99%	170
University of Michigan Health System[2]	Ann Arbor	99%	668
Beaumont Health System[2]	Royal Oak	98%	133
Borgess Medical Center[2]	Kalamazoo	98%	247
Lakeland Hospital - Saint Joseph[2]	Saint Joseph	98%	96
Mclaren Flint[2]	Flint	98%	263
Providence Hospital & Medical Centers[2]	Southfield	98%	175
Covenant Medical Center[2]	Saginaw	97%	153
Mercy Health Partners - Mercy Campus[2]	Muskegon	97%	118
St John Macomb-Oakland Hosp[2]	Warren	97%	129
Saint Joseph Mercy Oakland[2]	Pontiac	97%	154
Edward W Sparrow Hospital[2]	Lansing	96%	234
Munson Medical Center[2]	Traverse City	96%	179
Oakwood Hospital - Dearborn[2]	Dearborn	96%	127
Henry Ford Hospital[2]	Detroit	95%	136
Marquette General Hospital[2]	Marquette	95%	131
VA Ann Arbor Healthcare System[2]	Ann Arbor	95%	160
Saint Mary's of Michigan Medical Center[2]	Saginaw	94%	130
Mclaren Bay Region	Bay City	93%	408
Mclaren - Greater Lansing[2]	Lansing	91%	110
Midmichigan Medical Center - Midland	Midland	88%	224

Perioperative Temperature Management

Hospital Name	City	Rate	Cases
Allegan General Hospital	Allegan	100%	162
Allegiance Health[2]	Jackson	100%	519
Alpena Regional Medical Center[2]	Alpena	100%	341
Aspirus Grand View Hospital	Ironwood	100%	82
Aspirus Keweenaw Hospital	Laurium	100%	26
Beaumont Health System[2]	Grosse Pointe	100%	564
Beaumont Health System[2]	Royal Oak	100%	703
Bell Hospital[2]	Ishpeming	100%	201
Borgess Medical Center[2]	Kalamazoo	100%	418
Botsford Hospital[2]	Farmington Hills	100%	561
Bronson Battle Creek Hospital[2]	Battle Creek	100%	905
Bronson Methodist Hospital[2]	Kalamazoo	100%	1150
Carson City Hospital	Carson City	100%	158
Chelsea Community Hospital[2]	Chelsea	100%	935
Chippewa County War Memorial Hospital	Sault Ste Marie	100%	222
Community Health Center of Branch County	Coldwater	100%	183
Crittenton Hospital Medical Center[2]	Rochester	100%	764
Detroit Receiving Hosp & U Health Ctr[2]	Detroit	100%	529

NOTE: Hospital profiles are in alphabetical order by state, then city, then hospital within the city; Rankings exclude hospitals with less than 25 cases except for patient surveys which excludes hospitals with less than 100 cases; (a) 100-299 cases; (1) The number of cases/patients is too few to report; (2) Data submitted were based on a sample of cases/patients; (3) Results are based on a shorter time period than required; (4) Data suppressed by CMS for one or more quarters; (5) Results are not available for this reporting period; (6) Fewer than 100 patients completed the HCAHPS survey; (7) No cases met the criteria for this measure; (8) The lower limit of the confidence interval cannot be calculated if the number of observed infections equals zero; (9) No data are available from the state/territory for this reporting period; (10) The scores shown reflect fewer than 50 completed surveys; (11) There were discrepancies in the data collection process; (12) This measure does not apply to this hospital for this reporting period; (13) Results cannot be calculated for this reporting period; (14) The results for this state are combined with nearby states to protect confidentiality; Please refer to the User's Guide for a full explanation of data.

Dickinson County Memorial Hospital	Iron Mountain	100%	280
Edward W Sparrow Hospital[2]	Lansing	100%	2330
Garden City Hospital	Garden City	100%	452
Genesys Reg Med Ctr-Health Park[2]	Grand Blanc	100%	1515
Harper University Hospital[2]	Detroit	100%	432
Hayes Green Beach Memorial Hospital	Charlotte	100%	49
Henry Ford Macomb Hospital[2]	Clinton Twp	100%	768
Henry Ford West Bloomfield Hospital[2]	W Bloomfield	100%	441
Henry Ford Wyandotte Hospital[2]	Wyandotte	100%	481
Hills & Dales General Hospital	Cass City	100%	32
Hillsdale Community Health Center	Hillsdale	100%	220
Holland Community Hospital[2]	Holland	100%	830
Huron Medical Center[2]	Bad Axe	100%	127
Huron Valley - Sinai Hospital[2]	Commerce Twp	100%	693
Karmanos Cancer Center[2]	Detroit	100%	378
Lakeland Community Hospital - Watervliet	Watervliet	100%	161
Lakeland Hospital - Saint Joseph[2]	Saint Joseph	100%	485
Marquette General Hospital[2]	Marquette	100%	475
Mclaren - Northern Michigan[2]	Petoskey	100%	445
Mclaren Bay Region	Bay City	100%	942
Mclaren Central Michigan	Mount Pleasant	100%	271
Mclaren Flint[2]	Flint	100%	697
Mclaren Lapeer Region[2]	Lapeer	100%	299
Mclaren Macomb[2]	Mount Clemens	100%	865
Mclaren Oakland[2]	Pontiac	100%	297
Memorial Healthcare[2]	Owosso	100%	262
Memorial Medical Center of West Michigan	Ludington	100%	248
Mercy Health Hackley Campus[2]	Muskegon	100%	336
Mercy Health Partners - Mercy Campus[2]	Muskegon	100%	364
Mercy Hospital - Cadillac	Cadillac	100%	368
Mercy Hospital - Grayling	Grayling	100%	243
Mercy Memorial Hospital System	Monroe	100%	413
Metro Health Hospital[2]	Wyoming	100%	398
Munson Medical Center[2]	Traverse City	100%	751
North Ottawa Community Health Center	Grand Haven	100%	247
Oaklawn Hospital[2]	Marshall	100%	488
Oakwood Hospital - Dearborn[2]	Dearborn	100%	424
Oakwood Hospital - Southshore[2]	Trenton	100%	354
Oakwood Hospital - Taylor[2]	Taylor	100%	278
Oakwood Hospital - Wayne[2]	Wayne	100%	261
Pennock Hospital	Hastings	100%	286
Portage Health	Hancock	100%	195
Promedica Herrick Hospital[2]	Tecumseh	100%	101
Providence Hospital & Medical Centers[2]	Southfield	100%	2402
Saint Francis Hospital	Escanaba	100%	85
Saint John Hospital & Medical Center[2]	Detroit	100%	1255
St John Macomb-Oakland Hosp[2]	Warren	100%	964
Saint John River District Hospital	East China	100%	105
Saint Joseph Mercy Hospital[2]	Ann Arbor	100%	1878
Saint Joseph Mercy Livingston Hospital	Howell	100%	195
Saint Joseph Mercy Oakland[2]	Pontiac	100%	713
Saint Joseph Mercy Port Huron[2]	Port Huron	100%	407
Saint Mary Mercy Hospital	Livonia	100%	870
Saint Mary's Health Care[2]	Grand Rapids	100%	562
Sinai - Grace Hospital[2]	Detroit	100%	474
South Haven Community Hospital	South Haven	100%	69
Sparrow Clinton Hospital	Saint Johns	100%	55
Spectrum Health - Butterworth Campus[2]	Grand Rapids	100%	755
Spectrum Health Big Rapids Hospital	Big Rapids	100%	157
Spectrum Health Gerber Memorial	Fremont	100%	204
Spectrum Health Zeeland Comm Hosp	Zeeland	100%	222
Sturgis Hospital	Sturgis	100%	105
Tawas Saint Joseph Hospital	Tawas City	100%	161
Three Rivers Health	Three Rivers	100%	26
University of Michigan Health System[2]	Ann Arbor	100%	1567
William Beaumont Hospital - Troy[2]	Troy	100%	399
Covenant Medical Center[2]	Saginaw	99%	1677
Emma L Bixby Medical Center[2]	Adrian	99%	308
Henry Ford Hospital[2]	Detroit	99%	581
Mclaren - Greater Lansing[2]	Lansing	99%	425
Midmichigan Medical Center - Clare	Clare	99%	69
Otsego Memorial Hospital[2]	Gaylord	99%	198
Port Huron Hospital	Port Huron	99%	750
Spectrum Health United Memorial	Greenville	99%	161
VA Ann Arbor Healthcare System[2]	Ann Arbor	99%	312
West Branch Regional Medical Center[2]	West Branch	99%	189
West Shore Medical Center	Manistee	99%	139
Midmichigan Medical Center - Gratiot	Alma	98%	261
Midmichigan Medical Center - Midland	Midland	98%	1218
Saint Mary's of Michigan Medical Center[2]	Saginaw	98%	500
Scheurer Hospital	Pigeon	98%	94
Marlette Regional Hospital	Marlette	97%	29
Oakland Regional Hospital	Southfield	97%	62
Hurley Medical Center[2]	Flint	96%	401
Detroit (John D. Dingell) VA Med Ctr[2]	Detroit	95%	309

Prophylactic Antibiotic Selection

Hospital Name	City	Rate	Cases
Allegiance Health[2]	Jackson	100%	442
Aspirus Grand View Hospital	Ironwood	100%	56
Aspirus Keweenaw Hospital	Laurium	100%	32
Beaumont Health System[2]	Grosse Pointe	100%	402
Borgess Medical Center[2]	Kalamazoo	100%	521
Chelsea Community Hospital[2]	Chelsea	100%	787
Covenant Medical Center[2]	Saginaw	100%	1190
Detroit Receiving Hosp & U Health Ctr[2]	Detroit	100%	398
Henry Ford Macomb Hospital[2]	Clinton Twp	100%	701
Henry Ford West Bloomfield Hospital[2]	W Bloomfield	100%	287
Henry Ford Wyandotte Hospital[2]	Wyandotte	100%	321
Hillsdale Community Health Center	Hillsdale	100%	150
Holland Community Hospital[2]	Holland	100%	693
Huron Valley - Sinai Hospital[2]	Commerce Twp	100%	535
Lakeland Community Hospital - Watervliet	Watervliet	100%	132
Memorial Medical Center of West Michigan	Ludington	100%	163
Mercy Hospital - Grayling	Grayling	100%	203
Mercy Memorial Hospital System	Monroe	100%	266
Midmichigan Medical Center - Midland	Midland	100%	1057
Oakland Regional Hospital	Southfield	100%	41
Oaklawn Hospital[2]	Marshall	100%	338
Oakwood Hospital - Taylor[2]	Taylor	100%	199
Pennock Hospital	Hastings	100%	216
Promedica Herrick Hospital[2]	Tecumseh	100%	72
Providence Hospital & Medical Centers[2]	Southfield	100%	1856
Saint Francis Hospital	Escanaba	100%	51
Saint John Hospital & Medical Center[2]	Detroit	100%	1170
Saint John River District Hospital	East China	100%	76
Saint Joseph Mercy Oakland[2]	Pontiac	100%	490
Saint Joseph Mercy Port Huron[2]	Port Huron	100%	255
Spectrum Health Big Rapids Hospital	Big Rapids	100%	136
Spectrum Health Gerber Memorial	Fremont	100%	149
Spectrum Health United Memorial	Greenville	100%	98
Spectrum Health Zeeland Comm Hosp	Zeeland	100%	151
Sturgis Hospital	Sturgis	100%	73
Tawas Saint Joseph Hospital	Tawas City	100%	130
Beaumont Health System[2]	Royal Oak	99%	554
Bell Hospital[2]	Ishpeming	99%	167
Botsford Hospital[2]	Farmington Hills	99%	420
Bronson Battle Creek Hospital[2]	Battle Creek	99%	693
Bronson Methodist Hospital[2]	Kalamazoo	99%	1060
Carson City Hospital	Carson City	99%	116
Chippewa County War Memorial Hospital	Sault Ste Marie	99%	178
Community Health Center of Branch County	Coldwater	99%	108
Crittenton Hospital Medical Center[2]	Rochester	99%	635
Dickinson County Memorial Hospital	Iron Mountain	99%	217
Edward W Sparrow Hospital[2]	Lansing	99%	1462
Garden City Hospital	Garden City	99%	285
Henry Ford Hospital[2]	Detroit	99%	475
Lakeland Hospital - Saint Joseph[2]	Saint Joseph	99%	424
Marquette General Hospital[2]	Marquette	99%	448
Mclaren - Northern Michigan[2]	Petoskey	99%	405
Mclaren Bay Region	Bay City	99%	935
Mclaren Central Michigan	Mount Pleasant	99%	192
Mclaren Flint[2]	Flint	99%	700
Mclaren Lapeer Region[2]	Lapeer	99%	199
Mclaren Macomb[2]	Mount Clemens	99%	766
Mercy Health Hackley Campus[2]	Muskegon	99%	212
Mercy Health Partners - Mercy Campus[2]	Muskegon	99%	298
Mercy Hospital - Cadillac	Cadillac	99%	287
Metro Health Hospital[2]	Wyoming	99%	239
Munson Medical Center[2]	Traverse City	99%	592
North Ottawa Community Health Center	Grand Haven	99%	180
Oakwood Hospital - Southshore[2]	Trenton	99%	240
Oakwood Hospital - Wayne[2]	Wayne	99%	160
Otsego Memorial Hospital[2]	Gaylord	99%	158
Portage Health	Hancock	99%	148
St John Macomb-Oakland Hosp[2]	Warren	99%	810
Saint Joseph Mercy Hospital[2]	Ann Arbor	99%	1741
Saint Joseph Mercy Livingston Hospital	Howell	99%	144
Saint Mary Mercy Hospital	Livonia	99%	546
Saint Mary's of Michigan Medical Center[2]	Saginaw	99%	387
Scheurer Hospital	Pigeon	99%	78
Sinai - Grace Hospital[2]	Detroit	99%	377
University of Michigan Health System[2]	Ann Arbor	99%	1620
VA Ann Arbor Healthcare System	Ann Arbor	99%	333
West Shore Medical Center	Manistee	99%	74
William Beaumont Hospital - Troy[2]	Troy	99%	360
Allegan General Hospital	Allegan	98%	129
Alpena Regional Medical Center[2]	Alpena	98%	244
Detroit (John D. Dingell) VA Med Ctr	Detroit	98%	183
Emma L Bixby Medical Center[2]	Adrian	98%	210
Genesys Reg Med Ctr-Health Park[2]	Grand Blanc	98%	1378
Hurley Medical Center[2]	Flint	98%	267
Huron Medical Center[2]	Bad Axe	98%	113
Mclaren Oakland[2]	Pontiac	98%	199
Memorial Healthcare[2]	Owosso	98%	187
Oakwood Hospital - Dearborn[2]	Dearborn	98%	370
Port Huron Hospital	Port Huron	98%	637
Saint Mary's Health Care[2]	Grand Rapids	98%	392
Spectrum Health - Butterworth Campus[2]	Grand Rapids	98%	597
Harper University Hospital[2]	Detroit	97%	327
Hayes Green Beach Memorial Hospital	Charlotte	97%	36
Mclaren - Greater Lansing[2]	Lansing	97%	399
Sparrow Clinton Hospital	Saint Johns	97%	39
Hills & Dales General Hospital	Cass City	96%	25
Karmanos Cancer Center[2]	Detroit	96%	135
Midmichigan Medical Center - Clare	Clare	96%	45
South Haven Community Hospital	South Haven	94%	53
Midmichigan Medical Center - Gratiot	Alma	85%	183
West Branch Regional Medical Center[2]	West Branch	50%	168

Prophylactic Antibiotic Selection (Outpatient)

Hospital Name	City	Rate	Cases
Dickinson County Memorial Hospital	Iron Mountain	100%	76
Eaton Rapids Medical Center	Eaton Rapids	100%	46
Holland Community Hospital	Holland	100%	453
Mclaren Bay Region	Bay City	100%	447
Memorial Medical Center of West Michigan	Ludington	100%	59
North Ottawa Community Health Center	Grand Haven	100%	119
Otsego Memorial Hospital	Gaylord	100%	72
Providence Hospital & Medical Centers	Southfield	100%	927
Saint Joseph Mercy Oakland	Pontiac	100%	409
Spectrum Health Big Rapids Hospital	Big Rapids	100%	42
Allegiance Health	Jackson	99%	483
Beaumont Health System	Grosse Pointe	99%	156
Borgess Medical Center	Kalamazoo	99%	897
Bronson Battle Creek Hospital	Battle Creek	99%	238
Carson City Hospital	Carson City	99%	178
Crittenton Hospital Medical Center	Rochester	99%	223
Henry Ford Macomb Hospital	Clinton Twp	99%	409
Huron Valley - Sinai Hospital	Commerce Twp	99%	143
Lakeland Hospital - Saint Joseph	Saint Joseph	99%	288
Mclaren - Northern Michigan	Petoskey	99%	622
Mclaren Flint	Flint	99%	539
Mclaren Macomb	Mount Clemens	99%	279
Mercy Health Hackley Campus	Muskegon	99%	503
Mercy Health Partners - Mercy Campus	Muskegon	99%	477
Mercy Memorial Hospital System	Monroe	99%	200
Metro Health Hospital	Wyoming	99%	724
Oakwood Hospital - Wayne	Wayne	99%	199
Pennock Hospital	Hastings	99%	72
Saint Mary's of Michigan Medical Center	Saginaw	99%	369
Spectrum Health United Memorial	Greenville	99%	67
University of Michigan Health System	Ann Arbor	99%	992
William Beaumont Hospital - Troy	Troy	99%	452
Beaumont Health System	Royal Oak	98%	671
Bronson Methodist Hospital	Kalamazoo	98%	732
Chelsea Community Hospital	Chelsea	98%	87
Henry Ford Wyandotte Hospital	Wyandotte	98%	333
Hurley Medical Center	Flint	98%	222
Marquette General Hospital	Marquette	98%	644
Memorial Healthcare	Owosso	98%	192
Munson Medical Center	Traverse City	98%	522
Oakwood Hospital - Southshore	Trenton	98%	105
Saint John Hospital & Medical Center	Detroit	98%	514
Saint John River District Hospital	East China	98%	53
Saint Joseph Mercy Hospital	Ann Arbor	98%	1193
Saint Joseph Mercy Livingston Hospital	Howell	98%	44
Saint Mary Mercy Hospital	Livonia	98%	253
Saint Mary's Health Care	Grand Rapids	98%	464
Sinai - Grace Hospital	Detroit	98%	387
Covenant Medical Center	Saginaw	97%	781
Harper University Hospital	Detroit	97%	579
Mercy Hospital - Cadillac	Cadillac	97%	36
Midmichigan Medical Center - Gratiot	Alma	97%	71
Oaklawn Hospital	Marshall	97%	63
Oakwood Hospital - Dearborn	Dearborn	97%	366
Port Huron Hospital	Port Huron	97%	217
St John Macomb-Oakland Hosp	Warren	97%	548
West Branch Regional Medical Center	West Branch	97%	58
Community Health Center of Branch County	Coldwater	96%	50
Emma L Bixby Medical Center	Adrian	96%	127
Henry Ford Hospital	Detroit	96%	506
Sturgis Hospital	Sturgis	96%	56
Edward W Sparrow Hospital	Lansing	95%	388
Genesys Reg Med Ctr-Health Park	Grand Blanc	95%	601
Karmanos Cancer Center	Detroit	95%	157
Mercy Hospital - Grayling	Grayling	95%	73
Midmichigan Medical Center - Midland	Midland	95%	620
Portage Health	Hancock	95%	65
Spectrum Health - Butterworth Campus	Grand Rapids	95%	979
Detroit Receiving Hosp & U Health Ctr	Detroit	94%	53
Garden City Hospital	Garden City	94%	140
Huron Medical Center	Bad Axe	94%	64
Spectrum Health Gerber Memorial	Fremont	94%	33
Tawas Saint Joseph Hospital	Tawas City	94%	36
Alpena Regional Medical Center	Alpena	93%	137
Botsford Hospital	Farmington Hills	92%	322
Mclaren Central Michigan	Mount Pleasant	92%	118
Bell Hospital	Ishpeming	91%	70
Henry Ford West Bloomfield Hospital	W Bloomfield	90%	271
Mclaren Oakland	Pontiac	90%	134
Saint Francis Hospital	Escanaba	90%	40
Mclaren Lapeer Region	Lapeer	89%	66

NOTE: Hospital profiles are in alphabetical order by state, then city, then hospital within the city; Rankings exclude hospitals with less than 25 cases except for patient surveys which excludes hospitals with less than 100 cases; (a) 100-299 cases; (1) The number of cases/patients is too few to report; (2) Data submitted were based on a sample of cases/patients; (3) Results are based on a shorter time period than required; (4) Data suppressed by CMS for one or more quarters; (5) Results are not available for this reporting period; (6) Fewer than 100 patients completed the HCAHPS survey; (7) No cases met the criteria for this measure; (8) The lower limit of the confidence interval cannot be calculated if the number of observed infections equals zero; (9) No data are available from the state/territory for this reporting period; (10) The scores shown reflect fewer than 50 completed surveys; (11) There were discrepancies in the data collection process; (12) This measure does not apply to this hospital for this reporting period; (13) Results cannot be calculated for this reporting period; (14) The results for this state are combined with nearby states to protect confidentiality; Please refer to the User's Guide for a full explanation of data.

Hospital Name	City	Rate	Cases
Mclaren - Greater Lansing	Lansing	84%	562
Marlette Regional Hospital	Marlette	58%	26

Prophylactic Antibiotic Stopped

Hospital Name	City	Rate	Cases
Aspirus Grand View Hospital	Ironwood	100%	54
Beaumont Health System[2]	Royal Oak	100%	539
Bronson Battle Creek Hospital[2]	Battle Creek	100%	662
Chelsea Community Hospital[2]	Chelsea	100%	781
Holland Community Hospital[2]	Holland	100%	688
Huron Medical Center[2]	Bad Axe	100%	112
Lakeland Community Hospital - Watervliet	Watervliet	100%	132
Mclaren Central Michigan	Mount Pleasant	100%	191
Midmichigan Medical Center - Clare	Clare	100%	43
Oakland Regional Hospital	Southfield	100%	41
Oaklawn Hospital[2]	Marshall	100%	335
Saint John River District Hospital	East China	100%	74
Saint Joseph Mercy Port Huron[2]	Port Huron	100%	233
South Haven Community Hospital	South Haven	100%	53
William Beaumont Hospital - Troy[2]	Troy	100%	344
Allegiance Health[2]	Jackson	99%	434
Beaumont Health System[2]	Grosse Pointe	99%	391
Borgess Medical Center[2]	Kalamazoo	99%	505
Botsford Hospital[2]	Farmington Hills	99%	416
Community Health Center of Branch County	Coldwater	99%	104
Detroit (John D. Dingell) VA Med Ctr	Detroit	99%	183
Detroit Receiving Hosp & U Health Ctr[2]	Detroit	99%	395
Henry Ford Macomb Hospital[2]	Clinton Twp	99%	684
Henry Ford West Bloomfield Hospital[2]	W Bloomfield	99%	279
Hillsdale Community Health Center	Hillsdale	99%	147
Huron Valley - Sinai Hospital[2]	Commerce Twp	99%	528
Mclaren - Northern Michigan[2]	Petoskey	99%	395
Mclaren Bay Region	Bay City	99%	924
Mercy Health Hackley Campus[2]	Muskegon	99%	203
Mercy Health Partners - Mercy Campus[2]	Muskegon	99%	294
Munson Medical Center[2]	Traverse City	99%	563
Oakwood Hospital - Taylor[2]	Taylor	99%	186
Promedica Herrick Hospital[2]	Tecumseh	99%	68
Providence Hospital & Medical Centers[2]	Southfield	99%	1745
Saint John Hospital & Medical Center[2]	Detroit	99%	1143
St John Macomb-Oakland Hosp[2]	Warren	99%	783
Saint Joseph Mercy Hospital[2]	Ann Arbor	99%	1702
Saint Joseph Mercy Livingston Hospital	Howell	99%	139
Saint Joseph Mercy Oakland[2]	Pontiac	99%	478
Saint Mary Mercy Hospital	Livonia	99%	529
Spectrum Health - Butterworth Campus[2]	Grand Rapids	99%	594
Spectrum Health Gerber Memorial	Fremont	99%	147
Spectrum Health United Memorial	Greenville	99%	98
Spectrum Health Zeeland Comm Hosp	Zeeland	99%	150
West Shore Medical Center	Manistee	99%	73
Alpena Regional Medical Center[2]	Alpena	98%	225
Bell Hospital[2]	Ishpeming	98%	167
Bronson Methodist Hospital[2]	Kalamazoo	98%	1038
Covenant Medical Center[2]	Saginaw	98%	878
Crittenton Hospital Medical Center[2]	Rochester	98%	611
Henry Ford Hospital[2]	Detroit	98%	460
Henry Ford Wyandotte Hospital[2]	Wyandotte	98%	314
Lakeland Hospital - Saint Joseph[2]	Saint Joseph	98%	418
Mclaren - Greater Lansing[2]	Lansing	98%	387
Mclaren Macomb[2]	Mount Clemens	98%	747
Memorial Healthcare[2]	Owosso	98%	184
Memorial Medical Center of West Michigan	Ludington	98%	161
Mercy Hospital - Cadillac	Cadillac	98%	285
Mercy Hospital - Grayling	Grayling	98%	197
Mercy Memorial Hospital System	Monroe	98%	254
North Ottawa Community Health Center	Grand Haven	98%	174
Port Huron Hospital	Port Huron	98%	605
Saint Francis Hospital	Escanaba	98%	49
Saint Mary's Health Care[2]	Grand Rapids	98%	385
Sinai - Grace Hospital[2]	Detroit	98%	353
Spectrum Health Big Rapids Hospital	Big Rapids	98%	134
Tawas Saint Joseph Hospital	Tawas City	98%	130
University of Michigan Health System[2]	Ann Arbor	98%	1558
Aspirus Keweenaw Hospital	Laurium	97%	32
Garden City Hospital	Garden City	97%	279
Genesys Reg Med Ctr-Health Park[2]	Grand Blanc	97%	1347
Marquette General Hospital[2]	Marquette	97%	439
Mclaren Flint[2]	Flint	97%	662
Mclaren Lapeer Region[2]	Lapeer	97%	190
Metro Health Hospital[2]	Wyoming	97%	235
Oakwood Hospital - Southshore[2]	Trenton	97%	237
Oakwood Hospital - Wayne[2]	Wayne	97%	156
Otsego Memorial Hospital[2]	Gaylord	97%	157
Pennock Hospital	Hastings	97%	215
Portage Health	Hancock	97%	141
Chippewa County War Memorial Hospital	Sault Ste Marie	96%	170
Edward W Sparrow Hospital[2]	Lansing	96%	1448
Karmanos Cancer Center[2]	Detroit	96%	122
Mclaren Oakland[2]	Pontiac	96%	188
Midmichigan Medical Center - Midland	Midland	96%	1033
Allegan General Hospital	Allegan	95%	126
Dickinson County Memorial Hospital	Iron Mountain	95%	214
Emma L Bixby Medical Center[2]	Adrian	95%	205
Harper University Hospital[2]	Detroit	95%	309
Hurley Medical Center[2]	Flint	95%	259
Midmichigan Medical Center - Gratiot	Alma	95%	175
Saint Mary's of Michigan Medical Center[2]	Saginaw	95%	365
Hayes Green Beach Memorial Hospital	Charlotte	94%	36
Sturgis Hospital	Sturgis	94%	69
West Branch Regional Medical Center[2]	West Branch	94%	160
Carson City Hospital	Carson City	93%	113
VA Ann Arbor Healthcare System	Ann Arbor	93%	322
Scheurer Hospital	Pigeon	92%	74
Sparrow Clinton Hospital	Saint Johns	92%	39
Oakwood Hospital - Dearborn[2]	Dearborn	90%	360

Prophylactic Antibiotic Timing

Hospital Name	City	Rate	Cases
Aspirus Grand View Hospital	Ironwood	100%	56
Botsford Hospital[2]	Farmington Hills	100%	420
Bronson Methodist Hospital[2]	Kalamazoo	100%	1062
Chelsea Community Hospital[2]	Chelsea	100%	787
Chippewa County War Memorial Hospital	Sault Ste Marie	100%	178
Community Health Center of Branch County	Coldwater	100%	108
Emma L Bixby Medical Center[2]	Adrian	100%	210
Harper University Hospital[2]	Detroit	100%	327
Henry Ford Macomb Hospital[2]	Clinton Twp	100%	702
Hills & Dales General Hospital	Cass City	100%	25
Hillsdale Community Health Center	Hillsdale	100%	150
Holland Community Hospital[2]	Holland	100%	693
Huron Medical Center[2]	Bad Axe	100%	113
Karmanos Cancer Center[2]	Detroit	100%	135
Lakeland Community Hospital - Watervliet	Watervliet	100%	132
Mclaren Oakland[2]	Pontiac	100%	200
Mercy Health Hackley Campus[2]	Muskegon	100%	212
Mercy Health Partners - Mercy Campus[2]	Muskegon	100%	298
Munson Medical Center[2]	Traverse City	100%	592
North Ottawa Community Health Center	Grand Haven	100%	180
Oakwood Hospital - Taylor[2]	Taylor	100%	199
Pennock Hospital	Hastings	100%	216
Providence Hospital & Medical Centers[2]	Southfield	100%	1856
Saint John Hospital & Medical Center[2]	Detroit	100%	1170
Saint Joseph Mercy Oakland[2]	Pontiac	100%	491
Saint Joseph Mercy Port Huron[2]	Port Huron	100%	255
South Haven Community Hospital	South Haven	100%	53
Sparrow Clinton Hospital	Saint Johns	100%	39
Tawas Saint Joseph Hospital	Tawas City	100%	130
University of Michigan Health System[2]	Ann Arbor	100%	1618
West Shore Medical Center	Manistee	100%	74
Allegiance Health[2]	Jackson	99%	442
Beaumont Health System[2]	Grosse Pointe	99%	402
Beaumont Health System[2]	Royal Oak	99%	554
Borgess Medical Center[2]	Kalamazoo	99%	526
Bronson Battle Creek Hospital[2]	Battle Creek	99%	693
Detroit (John D. Dingell) VA Med Ctr	Detroit	99%	183
Detroit Receiving Hosp & U Health Ctr[2]	Detroit	99%	399
Dickinson County Memorial Hospital	Iron Mountain	99%	217
Garden City Hospital	Garden City	99%	285
Genesys Reg Med Ctr-Health Park[2]	Grand Blanc	99%	1379
Henry Ford Hospital[2]	Detroit	99%	476
Hurley Medical Center[2]	Flint	99%	267
Huron Valley - Sinai Hospital[2]	Commerce Twp	99%	535
Lakeland Hospital - Saint Joseph[2]	Saint Joseph	99%	425
Marquette General Hospital[2]	Marquette	99%	449
Mclaren Central Michigan	Mount Pleasant	99%	192
Mclaren Flint[2]	Flint	99%	703
Mclaren Lapeer Region[2]	Lapeer	99%	199
Mercy Hospital - Cadillac	Cadillac	99%	287
Mercy Hospital - Grayling	Grayling	99%	203
Mercy Memorial Hospital System	Monroe	99%	269
Oaklawn Hospital[2]	Marshall	99%	339
Oakwood Hospital - Southshore[2]	Trenton	99%	241
Port Huron Hospital	Port Huron	99%	638
Promedica Herrick Hospital[2]	Tecumseh	99%	72
Saint Joseph Mercy Hospital[2]	Ann Arbor	99%	1743
Saint Joseph Mercy Livingston Hospital	Howell	99%	144
Saint Mary Mercy Hospital	Livonia	99%	546
Saint Mary's of Michigan Medical Center[2]	Saginaw	99%	388
Spectrum Health Zeeland Comm Hosp	Zeeland	99%	151
Sturgis Hospital	Sturgis	99%	73
William Beaumont Hospital - Troy[2]	Troy	99%	362
Alpena Regional Medical Center[2]	Alpena	98%	244
Bell Hospital[2]	Ishpeming	98%	167
Covenant Medical Center[2]	Saginaw	98%	1193
Crittenton Hospital Medical Center[2]	Rochester	98%	635
Henry Ford Wyandotte Hospital[2]	Wyandotte	98%	322
Mclaren - Northern Michigan[2]	Petoskey	98%	405
Mclaren Macomb[2]	Mount Clemens	98%	767
Metro Health Hospital[2]	Wyoming	98%	239
Midmichigan Medical Center - Clare	Clare	98%	45
Midmichigan Medical Center - Midland	Midland	98%	1057
Oakwood Hospital - Wayne[2]	Wayne	98%	161
Saint Francis Hospital	Escanaba	98%	51
Saint Mary's Health Care[2]	Grand Rapids	98%	392
Sinai - Grace Hospital[2]	Detroit	98%	378
Spectrum Health Gerber Memorial	Fremont	98%	149
Allegan General Hospital	Allegan	97%	129
Aspirus Keweenaw Hospital	Laurium	97%	32
Carson City Hospital	Carson City	97%	116
Mclaren - Greater Lansing[2]	Lansing	97%	400
Mclaren Bay Region	Bay City	97%	939
Memorial Healthcare[2]	Owosso	97%	187
Portage Health	Hancock	97%	148
St John Macomb-Oakland Hosp[2]	Warren	97%	811
Scheurer Hospital	Pigeon	97%	78
Spectrum Health United Memorial	Greenville	97%	98
Memorial Medical Center of West Michigan	Ludington	96%	163
Oakwood Hospital - Dearborn[2]	Dearborn	96%	375
Saint John River District Hospital	East China	96%	76
Spectrum Health Big Rapids Hospital	Big Rapids	96%	136
VA Ann Arbor Healthcare System	Ann Arbor	96%	333
Edward W Sparrow Hospital[2]	Lansing	95%	1470
Henry Ford West Bloomfield Hospital[2]	W Bloomfield	95%	287
Oakland Regional Hospital	Southfield	95%	41
Hayes Green Beach Memorial Hospital	Charlotte	94%	36
Otsego Memorial Hospital[2]	Gaylord	94%	159
Midmichigan Medical Center - Gratiot	Alma	92%	185
Spectrum Health - Butterworth Campus[2]	Grand Rapids	92%	616
West Branch Regional Medical Center[2]	West Branch	75%	169

Prophylactic Antibiotic Timing (Outpatient)

Hospital Name	City	Rate	Cases
Allegiance Health	Jackson	100%	474
Botsford Hospital	Farmington Hills	100%	321
Bronson Battle Creek Hospital	Battle Creek	100%	238
Detroit Receiving Hosp & U Health Ctr	Detroit	100%	53
Harper University Hospital	Detroit	100%	525
Holland Community Hospital	Holland	100%	453
Huron Medical Center	Bad Axe	100%	64
Mercy Hospital - Cadillac	Cadillac	100%	36
Mercy Hospital - Grayling	Grayling	100%	64
Oaklawn Hospital	Marshall	100%	63
Pennock Hospital	Hastings	100%	34
Saint Joseph Mercy Oakland	Pontiac	100%	409
Saint Mary's Health Care	Grand Rapids	100%	462
Saint Mary's of Michigan Medical Center	Saginaw	100%	369
Spectrum Health Big Rapids Hospital	Big Rapids	100%	32
Borgess Medical Center	Kalamazoo	99%	899
Carson City Hospital	Carson City	99%	180
Chelsea Community Hospital	Chelsea	99%	84
Crittenton Hospital Medical Center	Rochester	99%	223
Henry Ford Macomb Hospital	Clinton Twp	99%	410
Mclaren Flint	Flint	99%	542
Mercy Health Hackley Campus	Muskegon	99%	485
Mercy Health Partners - Mercy Campus	Muskegon	99%	425
Metro Health Hospital	Wyoming	99%	726
North Ottawa Community Health Center	Grand Haven	99%	78
Saint John Hospital & Medical Center	Detroit	99%	518
William Beaumont Hospital - Troy	Troy	99%	442
Beaumont Health System	Grosse Pointe	98%	151
Beaumont Health System	Royal Oak	98%	634
Bell Hospital	Ishpeming	98%	42
Bronson Methodist Hospital	Kalamazoo	98%	737
Community Health Center of Branch County	Coldwater	98%	51
Henry Ford Wyandotte Hospital	Wyandotte	98%	332
Huron Valley - Sinai Hospital	Commerce Twp	98%	133
Lakeland Hospital - Saint Joseph	Saint Joseph	98%	284
Mclaren Lapeer Region	Lapeer	98%	66
Memorial Medical Center of West Michigan	Ludington	98%	59
Mercy Memorial Hospital System	Monroe	98%	184
Port Huron Hospital	Port Huron	98%	218
Providence Hospital & Medical Centers	Southfield	98%	931
St John Macomb-Oakland Hosp	Warren	98%	550
Saint John River District Hospital	East China	98%	53
Saint Joseph Mercy Hospital	Ann Arbor	98%	1173
Dickinson County Memorial Hospital	Iron Mountain	97%	64
Edward W Sparrow Hospital	Lansing	97%	391
Garden City Hospital	Garden City	97%	143
Mclaren Bay Region	Bay City	97%	449
Memorial Healthcare	Owosso	97%	194
Munson Medical Center	Traverse City	97%	496
Sinai - Grace Hospital	Detroit	97%	385
University of Michigan Health System	Ann Arbor	97%	753
Covenant Medical Center	Saginaw	96%	756
Emma L Bixby Medical Center	Adrian	96%	128
Mclaren - Northern Michigan	Petoskey	96%	628
Mclaren Central Michigan	Mount Pleasant	96%	93
Mclaren Macomb	Mount Clemens	96%	287
Oakwood Hospital - Wayne	Wayne	96%	170
Otsego Memorial Hospital	Gaylord	96%	73
Spectrum Health United Memorial	Greenville	96%	67
Marquette General Hospital	Marquette	95%	533
Saint Francis Hospital	Escanaba	95%	41

NOTE: Hospital profiles are in alphabetical order by state, then city, then hospital within the city; Rankings exclude hospitals with less than 25 cases except for patient surveys which excludes hospitals with less than 100 cases; (a) 100-299 cases; (1) The number of cases/patients is too few to report; (2) Data submitted were based on a sample of cases/patients; (3) Results are based on a shorter time period than required; (4) Data suppressed by CMS for one or more quarters; (5) Results are not available for this reporting period; (6) Fewer than 100 patients completed the HCAHPS survey; (7) No cases met the criteria for this measure; (8) The lower limit of the confidence interval cannot be calculated if the number of observed infections equals zero; (9) No data are available from the state/territory for this reporting period; (10) The scores shown reflect fewer than 50 completed surveys; (11) There were discrepancies in the data collection process; (12) This measure does not apply to this hospital for this reporting period; (13) Results cannot be calculated for this reporting period; (14) The results for this state are combined with nearby states to protect confidentiality; Please refer to the User's Guide for a full explanation of data.

Saint Mary Mercy Hospital	Livonia	95%	257
Spectrum Health - Butterworth Campus	Grand Rapids	95%	986
Tawas Saint Joseph Hospital	Tawas City	95%	37
Hurley Medical Center	Flint	94%	228
Oakwood Hospital - Southshore	Trenton	94%	103
Sturgis Hospital	Sturgis	94%	53
Midmichigan Medical Center - Midland	Midland	93%	629
Alpena Regional Medical Center	Alpena	92%	139
Henry Ford West Bloomfield Hospital	W Bloomfield	92%	119
Mclaren Oakland	Pontiac	92%	136
Oakwood Hospital - Dearborn	Dearborn	92%	364
Spectrum Health Gerber Memorial	Fremont	92%	36
Mclaren - Greater Lansing	Lansing	90%	584
West Branch Regional Medical Center	West Branch	90%	62
Eaton Rapids Medical Center	Eaton Rapids	89%	47
Genesys Reg Med Ctr-Health Park	Grand Blanc	89%	597
Saint Joseph Mercy Livingston Hospital	Howell	87%	30
Henry Ford Hospital	Detroit	82%	234
Marlette Regional Hospital	Marlette	77%	30
Midmichigan Medical Center - Gratiot	Alma	75%	88
Karmanos Cancer Center	Detroit	61%	115

Urinary Catheter Removal

Hospital Name	City	Rate	Cases
Allegiance Health[2]	Jackson	100%	210
Aspirus Keweenaw Hospital	Laurium	100%	30
Beaumont Health System[2]	Royal Oak	100%	475
Bell Hospital[2]	Ishpeming	100%	41
Chelsea Community Hospital[2]	Chelsea	100%	687
Crittenton Hospital Medical Center[2]	Rochester	100%	206
Detroit Receiving Hosp & U Health Ctr[2]	Detroit	100%	481
Dickinson County Memorial Hospital	Iron Mountain	100%	206
Henry Ford Macomb Hospital[2]	Clinton Twp	100%	578
Holland Community Hospital[2]	Holland	100%	92
Huron Valley - Sinai Hospital[2]	Commerce Twp	100%	436
Mercy Hospital - Grayling	Grayling	100%	133
Midmichigan Medical Center - Clare	Clare	100%	61
Oakland Regional Hospital	Southfield	100%	39
Portage Health	Hancock	100%	53
Saint Francis Hospital	Escanaba	100%	40
Saint Joseph Mercy Oakland[2]	Pontiac	100%	395
Saint Joseph Mercy Port Huron[2]	Port Huron	100%	340
South Haven Community Hospital	South Haven	100%	50
Spectrum Health United Memorial	Greenville	100%	108
Spectrum Health Zeeland Comm Hosp	Zeeland	100%	40
West Shore Medical Center	Manistee	100%	87
Beaumont Health System[2]	Grosse Pointe	99%	337
Carson City Hospital	Carson City	99%	97
Covenant Medical Center[2]	Saginaw	99%	529
Lakeland Community Hospital - Watervliet	Watervliet	99%	153
Mclaren Central Michigan	Mount Pleasant	99%	130
Memorial Healthcare[2]	Owosso	99%	224
Mercy Memorial Hospital System	Monroe	99%	122
North Ottawa Community Health Center	Grand Haven	99%	174
Otsego Memorial Hospital[2]	Gaylord	99%	154
Providence Hospital & Medical Centers[2]	Southfield	99%	1656
Saint John Hospital & Medical Center[2]	Detroit	99%	660
St John Macomb-Oakland Hosp[2]	Warren	99%	713
Saint Mary Mercy Hospital	Livonia	99%	559
Spectrum Health Big Rapids Hospital	Big Rapids	99%	121
Tawas Saint Joseph Hospital	Tawas City	99%	121
William Beaumont Hospital - Troy[2]	Troy	99%	313
Allegan General Hospital	Allegan	98%	45
Aspirus Grand View Hospital	Ironwood	98%	46
Borgess Medical Center[2]	Kalamazoo	98%	336
Bronson Battle Creek Hospital[2]	Battle Creek	98%	721
Genesys Reg Med Ctr-Health Park[2]	Grand Blanc	98%	1265
Harper University Hospital[2]	Detroit	98%	232
Mclaren Oakland[2]	Pontiac	98%	220
Mercy Health Partners - Mercy Campus[2]	Muskegon	98%	288
Metro Health Hospital[2]	Wyoming	98%	253
Saint Joseph Mercy Hospital[2]	Ann Arbor	98%	1715
Saint Joseph Mercy Livingston Hospital	Howell	98%	122
Saint Mary's Health Care[2]	Grand Rapids	98%	326
Sinai - Grace Hospital[2]	Detroit	98%	270
Sparrow Clinton Hospital	Saint Johns	98%	42
Spectrum Health - Butterworth Campus[2]	Grand Rapids	98%	607
University of Michigan Health System[2]	Ann Arbor	98%	1479
Botsford Hospital[2]	Farmington Hills	97%	414
Hills & Dales General Hospital	Cass City	97%	29
Huron Medical Center[2]	Bad Axe	97%	110
Lakeland Hospital - Saint Joseph[2]	Saint Joseph	97%	361
Mclaren Flint[2]	Flint	97%	363
Mclaren Macomb[2]	Mount Clemens	97%	592
Oaklawn Hospital[2]	Marshall	97%	175
Oakwood Hospital - Taylor[2]	Taylor	97%	66
Saint John River District Hospital	East China	97%	76
Sturgis Hospital	Sturgis	97%	64
Community Health Center of Branch County	Coldwater	96%	116
Detroit (John D. Dingell) VA Med Ctr[2]	Detroit	96%	92
Garden City Hospital	Garden City	96%	256
Henry Ford West Bloomfield Hospital[2]	W Bloomfield	96%	235
Hillsdale Community Health Center	Hillsdale	96%	161
Mercy Hospital - Cadillac	Cadillac	96%	54
Munson Medical Center[2]	Traverse City	96%	308
Pennock Hospital	Hastings	96%	57
VA Ann Arbor Healthcare System[2]	Ann Arbor	96%	310
Bronson Methodist Hospital[2]	Kalamazoo	95%	655
Henry Ford Hospital[2]	Detroit	95%	407
Mclaren - Northern Michigan[2]	Petoskey	95%	250
Mclaren Lapeer Region[2]	Lapeer	95%	195
Midmichigan Medical Center - Gratiot	Alma	95%	178
Midmichigan Medical Center - Midland	Midland	95%	861
Port Huron Hospital	Port Huron	95%	635
Promedica Herrick Hospital[2]	Tecumseh	95%	81
Alpena Regional Medical Center[2]	Alpena	94%	197
Marquette General Hospital[2]	Marquette	94%	232
Oakwood Hospital - Wayne[2]	Wayne	94%	50
Scheurer Hospital	Pigeon	94%	89
Emma L Bixby Medical Center[2]	Adrian	93%	188
Mercy Health Hackley Campus[2]	Muskegon	93%	89
West Branch Regional Medical Center[2]	West Branch	93%	173
Karmanos Cancer Center[2]	Detroit	92%	87
Chippewa County War Memorial Hospital	Sault Ste Marie	91%	53
Mclaren Bay Region	Bay City	90%	532
Memorial Medical Center of West Michigan	Ludington	89%	57
Oakwood Hospital - Southshore[2]	Trenton	89%	76
Saint Mary's of Michigan Medical Center[2]	Saginaw	87%	287
Edward W Sparrow Hospital[2]	Lansing	86%	740
Henry Ford Wyandotte Hospital[2]	Wyandotte	85%	139
Oakwood Hospital - Dearborn[2]	Dearborn	84%	242
Mclaren - Greater Lansing[2]	Lansing	82%	171
Hurley Medical Center[2]	Flint	78%	107
Marlette Regional Hospital	Marlette	52%	25

Survey of Patients' Hospital Experiences

Area Around Room 'Always' Quiet at Night

Hospital Name	City	Rate	Cases
Chelsea Community Hospital	Chelsea	76%	300+
Borgess - Lee Memorial Hospital	Dowagiac	73%	(a)
Hills & Dales General Hospital	Cass City	73%	(a)
Allegan General Hospital	Allegan	72%	(a)
Carson City Hospital	Carson City	71%	300+
Charlevoix Area Hospital	Charlevoix	71%	300+
Henry Ford West Bloomfield Hospital	W Bloomfield	71%	300+
Mackinac Straits Hospital & Health Center	Saint Ignace	70%	(a)
North Ottawa Community Health Center	Grand Haven	70%	300+
Spectrum Health Zeeland Comm Hosp	Zeeland	70%	300+
Schoolcraft Memorial Hospital	Manistique	69%	(a)
Midmichigan Medical Center - Gladwin	Gladwin	68%	(a)
Baraga County Memorial Hospital	L' Anse	67%	(a)
Hayes Green Beach Memorial Hospital	Charlotte	67%	(a)
Saint John River District Hospital	East China	67%	300+
Lakeland Community Hospital - Watervliet	Watervliet	66%	(a)
Oaklawn Hospital	Marshall	66%	300+
Bronson Lakeview Hospital	Paw Paw	65%	(a)
Promedica Herrick Hospital	Tecumseh	65%	(a)
Saint Mary's Standish Community Hospital	Standish	65%	(a)
Sparrow Ionia Hospital	Ionia	65%	(a)
Tawas Saint Joseph Hospital	Tawas City	65%	300+
West Shore Medical Center	Manistee	65%	(a)
Doctors' Hospital of Michigan	Pontiac	64%	(a)
Marlette Regional Hospital	Marlette	64%	(a)
Metro Health Hospital	Wyoming	64%	300+
Midmichigan Medical Center - Gratiot	Alma	64%	300+
Spectrum Health Big Rapids Hospital	Big Rapids	64%	300+
Aspirus Grand View Hospital	Ironwood	63%	(a)
Dickinson County Memorial Hospital	Iron Mountain	63%	300+
Midmichigan Medical Center - Midland	Midland	63%	300+
Pennock Hospital	Hastings	63%	300+
Saint Joseph Mercy Port Huron	Port Huron	63%	300+
Scheurer Hospital	Pigeon	63%	(a)
South Haven Community Hospital	South Haven	63%	300+
Spectrum Health - Reed City Campus	Reed City	63%	(a)
Harper University Hospital[11]	Detroit	62%	300+
Memorial Healthcare	Owosso	62%	300+
Three Rivers Health	Three Rivers	62%	(a)
Emma L Bixby Medical Center	Adrian	61%	300+
Mercy Hospital - Cadillac	Cadillac	61%	300+
Oakwood Hospital - Southshore	Trenton	61%	300+
Saint Joseph Mercy Livingston Hospital	Howell	61%	300+
Sparrow Clinton Hospital	Saint Johns	61%	(a)
West Branch Regional Medical Center	West Branch	61%	300+
Community Health Center of Branch County	Coldwater	60%	300+
Lakeland Hospital - Saint Joseph	Saint Joseph	60%	300+
Saint Mary's Health Care	Grand Rapids	60%	300+
Sinai - Grace Hospital[11]	Detroit	60%	300+
Sturgis Hospital	Sturgis	60%	300+
Hillsdale Community Health Center	Hillsdale	59%	(a)
Mercy Hospital - Grayling	Grayling	59%	300+
Portage Health	Hancock	59%	300+
Saint Francis Hospital	Escanaba	59%	300+
Spectrum Health United Memorial	Greenville	59%	300+
Aspirus Keweenaw Hospital	Laurium	58%	(a)
Bronson Methodist Hospital	Kalamazoo	58%	300+
Detroit Receiving Hosp & U Health Ctr[11]	Detroit	58%	300+
Huron Valley - Sinai Hospital[11]	Commerce Twp	58%	300+
Karmanos Cancer Center	Detroit	58%	300+
Munson Medical Center	Traverse City	58%	300+
Oakwood Hospital - Taylor	Taylor	58%	300+
Beaumont Health System	Grosse Pointe	57%	300+
Crittenton Hospital Medical Center[11]	Rochester	57%	300+
Mclaren - Greater Lansing	Lansing	57%	300+
Mclaren Central Michigan	Mount Pleasant	57%	300+
Memorial Medical Center of West Michigan	Ludington	57%	300+
Midmichigan Medical Center - Clare	Clare	57%	300+
Saint Joseph Mercy Hospital	Ann Arbor	57%	300+
Spectrum Health Gerber Memorial	Fremont	57%	300+
Borgess Medical Center	Kalamazoo	56%	300+
Chippewa County War Memorial Hospital	Sault Ste Marie	56%	300+
Henry Ford Hospital	Detroit	56%	300+
Mclaren Oakland	Pontiac	56%	300+
Providence Hospital & Medical Centers	Southfield	56%	300+
Spectrum Health - Butterworth Campus[11]	Grand Rapids	56%	300+
Hurley Medical Center	Flint	55%	300+
Huron Medical Center	Bad Axe	55%	300+
Oakwood Hospital - Wayne	Wayne	55%	300+
Port Huron Hospital	Port Huron	55%	300+
Holland Community Hospital	Holland	54%	300+
Mercy Health Partners - Mercy Campus	Muskegon	54%	300+
Saint John Hospital & Medical Center	Detroit	54%	300+
Garden City Hospital	Garden City	53%	300+
Saint Joseph Mercy Oakland	Pontiac	53%	300+
Saint Mary Mercy Hospital	Livonia	53%	300+
Bronson Battle Creek Hospital	Battle Creek	52%	300+
Edward W Sparrow Hospital	Lansing	52%	300+
Mclaren Flint	Flint	52%	300+
Otsego Memorial Hospital	Gaylord	52%	(a)
Allegiance Health	Jackson	51%	300+
Marquette General Hospital	Marquette	51%	300+
Beaumont Health System	Royal Oak	50%	300+
Helen Newberry Joy Hospital	Newberry	50%	(a)
Mclaren Bay Region	Bay City	50%	300+
Mclaren - Northern Michigan	Petoskey	49%	300+
Mclaren Lapeer Region	Lapeer	49%	300+
Oakwood Hospital - Dearborn	Dearborn	49%	300+
University of Michigan Health System	Ann Arbor	49%	300+
Covenant Medical Center	Saginaw	48%	300+
Henry Ford Macomb Hospital	Clinton Twp	48%	300+
Mercy Health Hackley Campus	Muskegon	48%	300+
Mercy Memorial Hospital System	Monroe	48%	300+
Mclaren Macomb	Mount Clemens	47%	300+
Saint Mary's of Michigan Medical Center	Saginaw	47%	300+
Genesys Reg Med Ctr-Health Park	Grand Blanc	46%	300+
St John Macomb-Oakland Hosp	Warren	46%	300+
William Beaumont Hospital - Troy	Troy	46%	300+
Alpena Regional Medical Center	Alpena	45%	300+
Botsford Hospital	Farmington Hills	44%	300+
Henry Ford Wyandotte Hospital	Wyandotte	42%	300+

Doctors 'Always' Communicated Well

Hospital Name	City	Rate	Cases
Aspirus Keweenaw Hospital	Laurium	89%	(a)
Helen Newberry Joy Hospital	Newberry	89%	(a)
Bronson Lakeview Hospital	Paw Paw	88%	(a)
Carson City Hospital	Carson City	87%	300+
Baraga County Memorial Hospital	L' Anse	86%	(a)
Lakeland Community Hospital - Watervliet	Watervliet	86%	(a)
Marlette Regional Hospital	Marlette	86%	(a)
Otsego Memorial Hospital	Gaylord	86%	(a)
Portage Health	Hancock	86%	300+
Sparrow Clinton Hospital	Saint Johns	86%	(a)
Spectrum Health Zeeland Comm Hosp	Zeeland	86%	300+
Allegan General Hospital	Allegan	85%	(a)
Charlevoix Area Hospital	Charlevoix	85%	300+
Saint Mary's Standish Community Hospital	Standish	85%	(a)
Schoolcraft Memorial Hospital	Manistique	85%	(a)
Spectrum Health Big Rapids Hospital	Big Rapids	85%	300+
Chelsea Community Hospital	Chelsea	84%	300+
Emma L Bixby Medical Center	Adrian	84%	300+
Hills & Dales General Hospital	Cass City	84%	(a)
Huron Medical Center	Bad Axe	84%	300+
Mercy Hospital - Cadillac	Cadillac	84%	300+
Saint Francis Hospital	Escanaba	84%	300+
Aspirus Grand View Hospital	Ironwood	83%	(a)
Mackinac Straits Hospital & Health Center	Saint Ignace	83%	(a)
Midmichigan Medical Center - Midland	Midland	83%	300+
Munson Medical Center	Traverse City	83%	300+
Pennock Hospital	Hastings	83%	300+
South Haven Community Hospital	South Haven	83%	300+
West Shore Medical Center	Manistee	83%	(a)

NOTE: Hospital profiles are in alphabetical order by state, then city, then hospital within the city; Rankings exclude hospitals with less than 25 cases except for patient surveys which excludes hospitals with less than 100 cases; (a) 100-299 cases; (1) The number of cases/patients is too few to report; (2) Data submitted were based on a sample of cases/patients; (3) Results are based on a shorter time period than required; (4) Data suppressed by CMS for one or more quarters; (5) Results are not available for this reporting period; (6) Fewer than 100 patients completed the HCAHPS survey; (7) No cases met the criteria for this measure; (8) The lower limit of the confidence interval cannot be calculated if the number of observed infections equals zero; (9) No data are available from the state/territory for this reporting period; (10) The scores shown reflect fewer than 50 completed surveys; (11) There were discrepancies in the data collection process; (12) This measure does not apply to this hospital for this reporting period; (13) Results cannot be calculated for this reporting period; (14) The results for this state are combined with nearby states to protect confidentiality; Please refer to the User's Guide for a full explanation of data.

Hospital Name	City	Rate	Cases
Borgess - Lee Memorial Hospital	Dowagiac	82%	(a)
Bronson Methodist Hospital	Kalamazoo	82%	300+
Dickinson County Memorial Hospital	Iron Mountain	82%	300+
Holland Community Hospital	Holland	82%	300+
Mercy Hospital - Grayling	Grayling	82%	300+
Metro Health Hospital	Wyoming	82%	300+
Midmichigan Medical Center - Gratiot	Alma	82%	300+
Oaklawn Hospital	Marshall	82%	300+
Promedica Herrick Hospital	Tecumseh	82%	(a)
Saint John River District Hospital	East China	82%	300+
Saint Joseph Mercy Livingston Hospital	Howell	82%	300+
Scheurer Hospital	Pigeon	82%	(a)
Spectrum Health United Memorial	Greenville	82%	300+
Sturgis Hospital	Sturgis	82%	300+
Chippewa County War Memorial Hospital	Sault Ste Marie	81%	300+
Lakeland Hospital - Saint Joseph	Saint Joseph	81%	300+
Oakwood Hospital - Southshore	Trenton	81%	300+
Spectrum Health Gerber Memorial	Fremont	81%	300+
Tawas Saint Joseph Hospital	Tawas City	81%	300+
Mclaren - Northern Michigan	Petoskey	80%	300+
Memorial Medical Center of West Michigan	Ludington	80%	300+
North Ottawa Community Health Center	Grand Haven	80%	300+
Oakwood Hospital - Taylor	Taylor	80%	300+
Saint Mary's Health Care	Grand Rapids	80%	300+
Sparrow Ionia Hospital	Ionia	80%	(a)
Beaumont Health System	Grosse Pointe	79%	300+
Community Health Center of Branch County	Coldwater	79%	300+
Covenant Medical Center	Saginaw	79%	300+
Detroit Receiving Hosp & U Health Ctr[11]	Detroit	79%	300+
Harper University Hospital[11]	Detroit	79%	300+
Henry Ford Hospital	Detroit	79%	300+
Henry Ford West Bloomfield Hospital	W Bloomfield	79%	300+
Mclaren Central Michigan	Mount Pleasant	79%	300+
Memorial Healthcare	Owosso	79%	300+
Mercy Health Partners - Mercy Campus	Muskegon	79%	300+
Midmichigan Medical Center - Gladwin	Gladwin	79%	(a)
Providence Hospital & Medical Centers	Southfield	79%	300+
Alpena Regional Medical Center	Alpena	78%	300+
Beaumont Health System	Royal Oak	78%	300+
Borgess Medical Center	Kalamazoo	78%	300+
Botsford Hospital	Farmington Hills	78%	300+
Crittenton Hospital Medical Center[11]	Rochester	78%	300+
Doctors' Hospital of Michigan	Pontiac	78%	(a)
Huron Valley - Sinai Hospital[11]	Commerce Twp	78%	300+
Karmanos Cancer Center	Detroit	78%	300+
Mclaren Bay Region	Bay City	78%	300+
Oakwood Hospital - Dearborn	Dearborn	78%	300+
Saint John Hospital & Medical Center	Detroit	78%	300+
Spectrum Health - Butterworth Campus[11]	Grand Rapids	78%	300+
Spectrum Health - Reed City Campus	Reed City	78%	(a)
University of Michigan Health System	Ann Arbor	78%	300+
Garden City Hospital	Garden City	77%	300+
Hurley Medical Center	Flint	77%	300+
Mercy Health Hackley Campus	Muskegon	77%	300+
Mercy Memorial Hospital System	Monroe	77%	300+
Midmichigan Medical Center - Clare	Clare	77%	300+
Port Huron Hospital	Port Huron	77%	300+
Saint Joseph Mercy Hospital	Ann Arbor	77%	300+
Saint Mary's of Michigan Medical Center	Saginaw	77%	300+
Bronson Battle Creek Hospital	Battle Creek	76%	300+
Edward W Sparrow Hospital	Lansing	76%	300+
Genesys Reg Med Ctr-Health Park	Grand Blanc	76%	300+
Hillsdale Community Health Center	Hillsdale	76%	(a)
Marquette General Hospital	Marquette	76%	300+
Mclaren Lapeer Region	Lapeer	76%	300+
Saint Joseph Mercy Port Huron	Port Huron	76%	300+
Sinai - Grace Hospital[11]	Detroit	76%	300+
West Branch Regional Medical Center	West Branch	76%	300+
William Beaumont Hospital - Troy	Troy	76%	300+
Allegiance Health	Jackson	75%	300+
Hayes Green Beach Memorial Hospital	Charlotte	75%	(a)
Henry Ford Wyandotte Hospital	Wyandotte	75%	300+
Mclaren Macomb	Mount Clemens	75%	300+
Mclaren Oakland	Pontiac	75%	300+
Oakwood Hospital - Wayne	Wayne	75%	300+
Saint Mary Mercy Hospital	Livonia	75%	300+
Henry Ford Macomb Hospital	Clinton Twp	74%	300+
Mclaren Flint	Flint	74%	300+
St John Macomb-Oakland Hosp	Warren	74%	300+
Saint Joseph Mercy Oakland	Pontiac	74%	300+
Mclaren - Greater Lansing	Lansing	73%	300+
Three Rivers Health	Three Rivers	73%	(a)

Home Recovery Information Given

Hospital Name	City	Rate	Cases
Mercy Hospital - Grayling	Grayling	93%	300+
Mackinac Straits Hospital & Health Center	Saint Ignace	92%	(a)
Mercy Hospital - Cadillac	Cadillac	92%	300+
Metro Health Hospital	Wyoming	92%	300+
Pennock Hospital	Hastings	92%	300+
Spectrum Health - Reed City Campus	Reed City	92%	(a)
Spectrum Health Gerber Memorial	Fremont	92%	300+
Spectrum Health United Memorial	Greenville	92%	300+
Chelsea Community Hospital	Chelsea	91%	300+
Oaklawn Hospital	Marshall	91%	300+
Promedica Herrick Hospital	Tecumseh	91%	(a)
Sparrow Clinton Hospital	Saint Johns	91%	(a)
Sparrow Ionia Hospital	Ionia	91%	(a)
Spectrum Health Zeeland Comm Hosp	Zeeland	91%	300+
Allegan General Hospital	Allegan	90%	(a)
Holland Community Hospital	Holland	90%	300+
Karmanos Cancer Center	Detroit	90%	300+
Midmichigan Medical Center - Clare	Clare	90%	300+
Midmichigan Medical Center - Gratiot	Alma	90%	300+
Saint Mary's Health Care	Grand Rapids	90%	300+
Schoolcraft Memorial Hospital	Manistique	90%	(a)
Spectrum Health Big Rapids Hospital	Big Rapids	90%	300+
University of Michigan Health System	Ann Arbor	90%	300+
Bronson Methodist Hospital	Kalamazoo	89%	300+
Hayes Green Beach Memorial Hospital	Charlotte	89%	(a)
Helen Newberry Joy Hospital	Newberry	89%	(a)
Huron Medical Center	Bad Axe	89%	300+
Lakeland Community Hospital - Watervliet	Watervliet	89%	(a)
Marlette Regional Hospital	Marlette	89%	(a)
Mclaren - Northern Michigan	Petoskey	89%	300+
Memorial Healthcare	Owosso	89%	300+
Mercy Health Partners - Mercy Campus	Muskegon	89%	300+
Midmichigan Medical Center - Gladwin	Gladwin	89%	(a)
Midmichigan Medical Center - Midland	Midland	89%	300+
North Ottawa Community Health Center	Grand Haven	89%	300+
Saint Joseph Mercy Livingston Hospital	Howell	89%	300+
Saint Joseph Mercy Port Huron	Port Huron	89%	300+
Saint Mary's Standish Community Hospital	Standish	89%	(a)
Spectrum Health - Butterworth Campus[11]	Grand Rapids	89%	300+
Carson City Hospital	Carson City	88%	300+
Charlevoix Area Hospital	Charlevoix	88%	300+
Chippewa County War Memorial Hospital	Sault Ste Marie	88%	300+
Emma L Bixby Medical Center	Adrian	88%	300+
Hills & Dales General Hospital	Cass City	88%	(a)
Hillsdale Community Health Center	Hillsdale	88%	(a)
Huron Valley - Sinai Hospital[11]	Commerce Twp	88%	300+
Marquette General Hospital	Marquette	88%	300+
Memorial Medical Center of West Michigan	Ludington	88%	300+
Otsego Memorial Hospital	Gaylord	88%	(a)
Saint Francis Hospital	Escanaba	88%	300+
Sturgis Hospital	Sturgis	88%	300+
West Branch Regional Medical Center	West Branch	88%	300+
Alpena Regional Medical Center	Alpena	87%	300+
Aspirus Grand View Hospital	Ironwood	87%	(a)
Aspirus Keweenaw Hospital	Laurium	87%	(a)
Edward W Sparrow Hospital	Lansing	87%	300+
Mclaren Bay Region	Bay City	87%	300+
Mclaren Central Michigan	Mount Pleasant	87%	300+
Mercy Health Hackley Campus	Muskegon	87%	300+
Munson Medical Center	Traverse City	87%	300+
Oakwood Hospital - Taylor	Taylor	87%	300+
Saint Joseph Mercy Hospital	Ann Arbor	87%	300+
Saint Joseph Mercy Oakland	Pontiac	87%	300+
Tawas Saint Joseph Hospital	Tawas City	87%	300+
Beaumont Health System	Royal Oak	86%	300+
Borgess Medical Center	Kalamazoo	86%	300+
Covenant Medical Center	Saginaw	86%	300+
Dickinson County Memorial Hospital	Iron Mountain	86%	300+
Lakeland Hospital - Saint Joseph	Saint Joseph	86%	300+
Saint Mary Mercy Hospital	Livonia	86%	300+
Saint Mary's of Michigan Medical Center	Saginaw	86%	300+
Scheurer Hospital	Pigeon	86%	(a)
South Haven Community Hospital	South Haven	86%	300+
Three Rivers Health	Three Rivers	86%	(a)
West Shore Medical Center	Manistee	86%	(a)
Allegiance Health	Jackson	85%	300+
Beaumont Health System	Grosse Pointe	85%	300+
Bronson Battle Creek Hospital	Battle Creek	85%	300+
Bronson Lakeview Hospital	Paw Paw	85%	(a)
Community Health Center of Branch County	Coldwater	85%	300+
Crittenton Hospital Medical Center[11]	Rochester	85%	300+
Harper University Hospital[11]	Detroit	85%	300+
Mclaren - Greater Lansing	Lansing	85%	300+
Mclaren Flint	Flint	85%	300+
Mclaren Lapeer Region	Lapeer	85%	300+
Mclaren Oakland	Pontiac	85%	300+
Mercy Memorial Hospital System	Monroe	85%	300+
Port Huron Hospital	Port Huron	85%	300+
Portage Health	Hancock	85%	300+
Providence Hospital & Medical Centers	Southfield	85%	300+
Saint John River District Hospital	East China	85%	300+
Baraga County Memorial Hospital	L' Anse	84%	(a)
Botsford Hospital	Farmington Hills	84%	300+
Detroit Receiving Hosp & U Health Ctr[11]	Detroit	84%	300+
Garden City Hospital	Garden City	84%	300+
Genesys Reg Med Ctr-Health Park	Grand Blanc	84%	300+
Henry Ford West Bloomfield Hospital	W Bloomfield	84%	300+
Henry Ford Wyandotte Hospital	Wyandotte	84%	300+
Hurley Medical Center	Flint	84%	300+
Mclaren Macomb	Mount Clemens	84%	300+
William Beaumont Hospital - Troy	Troy	84%	300+
Borgess - Lee Memorial Hospital	Dowagiac	83%	(a)
Henry Ford Hospital	Detroit	83%	300+
Henry Ford Macomb Hospital	Clinton Twp	83%	300+
Oakwood Hospital - Southshore	Trenton	83%	300+
Saint John Hospital & Medical Center	Detroit	83%	300+
Oakwood Hospital - Dearborn	Dearborn	82%	300+
St John Macomb-Oakland Hosp	Warren	82%	300+
Sinai - Grace Hospital[11]	Detroit	81%	300+
Oakwood Hospital - Wayne	Wayne	80%	300+
Doctors' Hospital of Michigan	Pontiac	78%	(a)

Hospital Given 9 or 10 on 10 Point Scale

Hospital Name	City	Rate	Cases
Chelsea Community Hospital	Chelsea	85%	300+
Allegan General Hospital	Allegan	83%	(a)
Metro Health Hospital	Wyoming	83%	300+
Spectrum Health Zeeland Comm Hosp	Zeeland	83%	300+
Bronson Lakeview Hospital	Paw Paw	82%	(a)
Bronson Methodist Hospital	Kalamazoo	82%	300+
Marlette Regional Hospital	Marlette	81%	(a)
Munson Medical Center	Traverse City	81%	300+
Sparrow Clinton Hospital	Saint Johns	81%	(a)
Charlevoix Area Hospital	Charlevoix	80%	300+
Henry Ford West Bloomfield Hospital	W Bloomfield	80%	300+
Lakeland Community Hospital - Watervliet	Watervliet	79%	(a)
Midmichigan Medical Center - Midland	Midland	79%	300+
Portage Health	Hancock	79%	300+
Saint Joseph Mercy Hospital	Ann Arbor	79%	300+
Carson City Hospital	Carson City	78%	300+
Mackinac Straits Hospital & Health Center	Saint Ignace	78%	(a)
Mercy Hospital - Cadillac	Cadillac	78%	300+
North Ottawa Community Health Center	Grand Haven	78%	300+
Schoolcraft Memorial Hospital	Manistique	78%	(a)
Holland Community Hospital	Holland	77%	300+
Oaklawn Hospital	Marshall	77%	300+
Saint Mary's Health Care	Grand Rapids	77%	300+
Spectrum Health Big Rapids Hospital	Big Rapids	77%	300+
Beaumont Health System	Grosse Pointe	76%	300+
Mercy Hospital - Grayling	Grayling	76%	300+
Saint Mary's Standish Community Hospital	Standish	76%	(a)
Scheurer Hospital	Pigeon	76%	(a)
Spectrum Health - Butterworth Campus[11]	Grand Rapids	76%	300+
Spectrum Health United Memorial	Greenville	76%	300+
University of Michigan Health System	Ann Arbor	76%	300+
Otsego Memorial Hospital	Gaylord	75%	(a)
Sparrow Ionia Hospital	Ionia	75%	(a)
Midmichigan Medical Center - Gratiot	Alma	74%	300+
Oakwood Hospital - Southshore	Trenton	74%	300+
Oakwood Hospital - Taylor	Taylor	74%	300+
Pennock Hospital	Hastings	74%	300+
Promedica Herrick Hospital	Tecumseh	74%	(a)
Saint John River District Hospital	East China	74%	300+
West Shore Medical Center	Manistee	74%	(a)
Beaumont Health System	Royal Oak	73%	300+
Borgess Medical Center	Kalamazoo	73%	300+
Chippewa County War Memorial Hospital	Sault Ste Marie	73%	300+
Hills & Dales General Hospital	Cass City	73%	(a)
Lakeland Hospital - Saint Joseph	Saint Joseph	73%	300+
Saint Francis Hospital	Escanaba	73%	300+
Community Health Center of Branch County	Coldwater	72%	300+
Helen Newberry Joy Hospital	Newberry	72%	(a)
Huron Valley - Sinai Hospital[11]	Commerce Twp	72%	300+
Karmanos Cancer Center	Detroit	72%	300+
Spectrum Health Gerber Memorial	Fremont	72%	300+
Sturgis Hospital	Sturgis	72%	300+
Aspirus Keweenaw Hospital	Laurium	71%	(a)
Mclaren - Northern Michigan	Petoskey	71%	300+
South Haven Community Hospital	South Haven	71%	300+
William Beaumont Hospital - Troy	Troy	71%	300+
Borgess - Lee Memorial Hospital	Dowagiac	70%	(a)
Edward W Sparrow Hospital	Lansing	70%	300+
Huron Medical Center	Bad Axe	70%	300+
Memorial Medical Center of West Michigan	Ludington	70%	300+
Providence Hospital & Medical Centers	Southfield	70%	300+
Covenant Medical Center	Saginaw	69%	300+
Crittenton Hospital Medical Center[11]	Rochester	69%	300+
Emma L Bixby Medical Center	Adrian	69%	300+
Mclaren Flint	Flint	69%	300+
Memorial Healthcare	Owosso	69%	300+
Mercy Health Partners - Mercy Campus	Muskegon	69%	300+
Saint Joseph Mercy Livingston Hospital	Howell	69%	300+
Saint Joseph Mercy Oakland	Pontiac	69%	300+
Saint Mary Mercy Hospital	Livonia	69%	300+
Tawas Saint Joseph Hospital	Tawas City	69%	300+
Harper University Hospital[11]	Detroit	68%	300+
Henry Ford Hospital	Detroit	68%	300+
Midmichigan Medical Center - Gladwin	Gladwin	68%	(a)

NOTE: Hospital profiles are in alphabetical order by state, then city, then hospital within the city; Rankings exclude hospitals with less than 25 cases except for patient surveys which excludes hospitals with less than 100 cases; (a) 100-299 cases; (1) The number of cases/patients is too few to report; (2) Data submitted were based on a sample of cases/patients; (3) Results are based on a shorter time period than required; (4) Data suppressed by CMS for one or more quarters; (5) Results are not available for this reporting period; (6) Fewer than 100 patients completed the HCAHPS survey; (7) No cases met the criteria for this measure; (8) The lower limit of the confidence interval cannot be calculated if the number of observed infections equals zero; (9) No data are available from the state/territory for this reporting period; (10) The scores shown reflect fewer than 50 completed surveys; (11) There were discrepancies in the data collection process; (12) This measure does not apply to this hospital for this reporting period; (13) Results cannot be calculated for this reporting period; (14) The results for this state are combined with nearby states to protect confidentiality; Please refer to the User's Guide for a full explanation of data.

Hospital Name	City	Rate	Cases
Port Huron Hospital	Port Huron	68%	300+
Saint Joseph Mercy Port Huron	Port Huron	68%	300+
Genesys Reg Med Ctr-Health Park	Grand Blanc	67%	300+
Hayes Green Beach Memorial Hospital	Charlotte	67%	(a)
Mclaren Central Michigan	Mount Pleasant	67%	300+
Midmichigan Medical Center - Clare	Clare	67%	300+
Oakwood Hospital - Wayne	Wayne	67%	300+
Spectrum Health - Reed City Campus	Reed City	67%	(a)
Baraga County Memorial Hospital	L' Anse	66%	(a)
Dickinson County Memorial Hospital	Iron Mountain	66%	300+
Garden City Hospital	Garden City	66%	300+
Henry Ford Wyandotte Hospital	Wyandotte	66%	300+
Hillsdale Community Health Center	Hillsdale	66%	(a)
Oakwood Hospital - Dearborn	Dearborn	66%	300+
Saint John Hospital & Medical Center	Detroit	66%	300+
Botsford Hospital	Farmington Hills	65%	300+
Hurley Medical Center	Flint	65%	300+
Allegiance Health	Jackson	64%	300+
Detroit Receiving Hosp & U Health Ctr[11]	Detroit	64%	300+
Henry Ford Macomb Hospital	Clinton Twp	64%	300+
Mclaren Bay Region	Bay City	64%	300+
Mclaren Oakland	Pontiac	64%	300+
Three Rivers Health	Three Rivers	64%	(a)
West Branch Regional Medical Center	West Branch	64%	300+
Mercy Health Hackley Campus	Muskegon	63%	300+
Saint Mary's of Michigan Medical Center	Saginaw	63%	300+
Alpena Regional Medical Center	Alpena	62%	300+
Bronson Battle Creek Hospital	Battle Creek	62%	300+
Mclaren Lapeer Region	Lapeer	62%	300+
Mclaren - Greater Lansing	Lansing	61%	300+
Mclaren Macomb	Mount Clemens	61%	300+
Aspirus Grand View Hospital	Ironwood	60%	(a)
St John Macomb-Oakland Hosp	Warren	60%	300+
Marquette General Hospital	Marquette	59%	300+
Mercy Memorial Hospital System	Monroe	58%	300+
Sinai - Grace Hospital[11]	Detroit	54%	300+
Doctors' Hospital of Michigan	Pontiac	53%	(a)

Meds 'Always' Explained Before Given

Hospital Name	City	Rate	Cases
Mackinac Straits Hospital & Health Center	Saint Ignace	80%	(a)
Bronson Lakeview Hospital	Paw Paw	75%	(a)
Saint Francis Hospital	Escanaba	73%	300+
Helen Newberry Joy Hospital	Newberry	72%	(a)
Marlette Regional Hospital	Marlette	72%	(a)
Carson City Hospital	Carson City	71%	300+
Otsego Memorial Hospital	Gaylord	71%	(a)
Scheurer Hospital	Pigeon	71%	(a)
Spectrum Health United Memorial	Greenville	71%	300+
West Shore Medical Center	Manistee	70%	(a)
Allegan General Hospital	Allegan	69%	(a)
Charlevoix Area Hospital	Charlevoix	69%	300+
Lakeland Community Hospital - Watervliet	Watervliet	69%	(a)
Mercy Hospital - Cadillac	Cadillac	69%	300+
Mercy Hospital - Grayling	Grayling	69%	300+
Oaklawn Hospital	Marshall	69%	300+
Aspirus Keweenaw Hospital	Laurium	68%	(a)
Baraga County Memorial Hospital	L' Anse	68%	(a)
Chelsea Community Hospital	Chelsea	68%	300+
Hills & Dales General Hospital	Cass City	68%	(a)
Midmichigan Medical Center - Midland	Midland	68%	300+
Oakwood Hospital - Taylor	Taylor	68%	300+
Saint Mary's Standish Community Hospital	Standish	68%	(a)
Schoolcraft Memorial Hospital	Manistique	68%	(a)
Sparrow Clinton Hospital	Saint Johns	68%	(a)
Spectrum Health Big Rapids Hospital	Big Rapids	68%	300+
Spectrum Health Gerber Memorial	Fremont	68%	300+
Spectrum Health Zeeland Comm Hosp	Zeeland	68%	300+
Community Health Center of Branch County	Coldwater	67%	300+
Midmichigan Medical Center - Gladwin	Gladwin	67%	(a)
Portage Health	Hancock	67%	300+
Chippewa County War Memorial Hospital	Sault Ste Marie	66%	300+
Metro Health Hospital	Wyoming	66%	300+
Midmichigan Medical Center - Clare	Clare	66%	300+
Munson Medical Center	Traverse City	66%	300+
Bronson Methodist Hospital	Kalamazoo	65%	300+
Karmanos Cancer Center	Detroit	65%	300+
Oakwood Hospital - Southshore	Trenton	65%	300+
Promedica Herrick Hospital	Tecumseh	65%	(a)
Saint John River District Hospital	East China	65%	300+
Sparrow Ionia Hospital	Ionia	65%	(a)
Sturgis Hospital	Sturgis	65%	300+
Emma L Bixby Medical Center	Adrian	64%	300+
Lakeland Hospital - Saint Joseph	Saint Joseph	64%	300+
Midmichigan Medical Center - Gratiot	Alma	64%	300+
Saint Joseph Mercy Livingston Hospital	Howell	64%	300+
South Haven Community Hospital	South Haven	64%	300+
Tawas Saint Joseph Hospital	Tawas City	64%	300+
Dickinson County Memorial Hospital	Iron Mountain	63%	300+
Huron Medical Center	Bad Axe	63%	300+
Memorial Healthcare	Owosso	63%	300+
North Ottawa Community Health Center	Grand Haven	63%	300+
Pennock Hospital	Hastings	63%	300+
Saint Mary's Health Care	Grand Rapids	63%	300+
Allegiance Health	Jackson	62%	300+
Edward W Sparrow Hospital	Lansing	62%	300+
Hayes Green Beach Memorial Hospital	Charlotte	62%	(a)
Henry Ford West Bloomfield Hospital	W Bloomfield	62%	300+
Hillsdale Community Health Center	Hillsdale	62%	(a)
Holland Community Hospital	Holland	62%	300+
Mclaren - Northern Michigan	Petoskey	62%	300+
Memorial Medical Center of West Michigan	Ludington	62%	300+
Oakwood Hospital - Dearborn	Dearborn	62%	300+
Spectrum Health - Butterworth Campus[11]	Grand Rapids	62%	300+
Three Rivers Health	Three Rivers	62%	(a)
University of Michigan Health System	Ann Arbor	62%	300+
Garden City Hospital	Garden City	61%	300+
Hurley Medical Center	Flint	61%	300+
Oakwood Hospital - Wayne	Wayne	61%	300+
Port Huron Hospital	Port Huron	61%	300+
Beaumont Health System	Grosse Pointe	60%	300+
Covenant Medical Center	Saginaw	60%	300+
Detroit Receiving Hosp & U Health Ctr[11]	Detroit	60%	300+
Henry Ford Hospital	Detroit	60%	300+
Henry Ford Macomb Hospital	Clinton Twp	60%	300+
Saint Joseph Mercy Hospital	Ann Arbor	60%	300+
West Branch Regional Medical Center	West Branch	60%	300+
Aspirus Grand View Hospital	Ironwood	59%	(a)
Beaumont Health System	Royal Oak	59%	300+
Botsford Hospital	Farmington Hills	59%	300+
Bronson Battle Creek Hospital	Battle Creek	59%	300+
Mclaren Bay Region	Bay City	59%	300+
Mclaren Oakland	Pontiac	59%	300+
Mercy Memorial Hospital System	Monroe	59%	300+
Providence Hospital & Medical Centers	Southfield	59%	300+
Crittenton Hospital Medical Center[11]	Rochester	58%	300+
Harper University Hospital[11]	Detroit	58%	300+
Henry Ford Wyandotte Hospital	Wyandotte	58%	300+
Marquette General Hospital	Marquette	58%	300+
Mclaren Lapeer Region	Lapeer	58%	300+
Mercy Health Partners - Mercy Campus	Muskegon	58%	300+
Saint John Hospital & Medical Center	Detroit	58%	300+
William Beaumont Hospital - Troy	Troy	58%	300+
Alpena Regional Medical Center	Alpena	57%	300+
Genesys Reg Med Ctr-Health Park	Grand Blanc	57%	300+
Mclaren Flint	Flint	57%	300+
Saint Mary Mercy Hospital	Livonia	57%	300+
Borgess Medical Center	Kalamazoo	56%	300+
Huron Valley - Sinai Hospital[11]	Commerce Twp	56%	300+
Mclaren - Greater Lansing	Lansing	56%	300+
Mclaren Central Michigan	Mount Pleasant	56%	300+
St John Macomb-Oakland Hosp	Warren	56%	300+
Saint Joseph Mercy Oakland	Pontiac	56%	300+
Saint Joseph Mercy Port Huron	Port Huron	56%	300+
Spectrum Health - Reed City Campus	Reed City	56%	(a)
Mercy Health Hackley Campus	Muskegon	55%	300+
Borgess - Lee Memorial Hospital	Dowagiac	54%	(a)
Doctors' Hospital of Michigan	Pontiac	54%	(a)
Saint Mary's of Michigan Medical Center	Saginaw	54%	300+
Mclaren Macomb	Mount Clemens	53%	300+
Sinai - Grace Hospital[11]	Detroit	53%	300+

Nurses 'Always' Communicated Well

Hospital Name	City	Rate	Cases
Spectrum Health Zeeland Comm Hosp	Zeeland	86%	300+
Allegan General Hospital	Allegan	85%	(a)
Aspirus Keweenaw Hospital	Laurium	85%	(a)
Bronson Lakeview Hospital	Paw Paw	85%	(a)
Chelsea Community Hospital	Chelsea	85%	300+
Mackinac Straits Hospital & Health Center	Saint Ignace	85%	(a)
Marlette Regional Hospital	Marlette	85%	(a)
Munson Medical Center	Traverse City	85%	300+
Portage Health	Hancock	85%	300+
Scheurer Hospital	Pigeon	85%	(a)
Schoolcraft Memorial Hospital	Manistique	85%	(a)
Hills & Dales General Hospital	Cass City	84%	(a)
Lakeland Community Hospital - Watervliet	Watervliet	84%	(a)
Mercy Hospital - Cadillac	Cadillac	84%	300+
Oakwood Hospital - Taylor	Taylor	84%	300+
Saint Francis Hospital	Escanaba	84%	300+
Sparrow Clinton Hospital	Saint Johns	84%	(a)
Charlevoix Area Hospital	Charlevoix	83%	300+
Chippewa County War Memorial Hospital	Sault Ste Marie	83%	300+
Mercy Hospital - Grayling	Grayling	83%	300+
Midmichigan Medical Center - Midland	Midland	83%	300+
Otsego Memorial Hospital	Gaylord	83%	(a)
Sparrow Ionia Hospital	Ionia	83%	(a)
Borgess - Lee Memorial Hospital	Dowagiac	82%	(a)
Carson City Hospital	Carson City	82%	300+
Community Health Center of Branch County	Coldwater	82%	300+
Karmanos Cancer Center	Detroit	82%	300+
Promedica Herrick Hospital	Tecumseh	82%	(a)
Spectrum Health Big Rapids Hospital	Big Rapids	82%	300+
Spectrum Health United Memorial	Greenville	82%	300+
Sturgis Hospital	Sturgis	82%	300+
West Shore Medical Center	Manistee	82%	(a)
Baraga County Memorial Hospital	L' Anse	81%	(a)
Bronson Methodist Hospital	Kalamazoo	81%	300+
Covenant Medical Center	Saginaw	81%	300+
Helen Newberry Joy Hospital	Newberry	81%	(a)
Memorial Healthcare	Owosso	81%	300+
Midmichigan Medical Center - Gladwin	Gladwin	81%	(a)
Oakwood Hospital - Southshore	Trenton	81%	300+
Pennock Hospital	Hastings	81%	300+
South Haven Community Hospital	South Haven	81%	300+
Spectrum Health - Butterworth Campus[11]	Grand Rapids	81%	300+
Spectrum Health Gerber Memorial	Fremont	81%	300+
Beaumont Health System	Grosse Pointe	80%	300+
Borgess Medical Center	Kalamazoo	80%	300+
Huron Medical Center	Bad Axe	80%	300+
Memorial Medical Center of West Michigan	Ludington	80%	300+
Metro Health Hospital	Wyoming	80%	300+
Midmichigan Medical Center - Gratiot	Alma	80%	300+
Oakwood Hospital - Dearborn	Dearborn	80%	300+
Oakwood Hospital - Wayne	Wayne	80%	300+
Port Huron Hospital	Port Huron	80%	300+
Saint Mary's Health Care	Grand Rapids	80%	300+
Saint Mary's Standish Community Hospital	Standish	80%	(a)
Tawas Saint Joseph Hospital	Tawas City	80%	300+
Dickinson County Memorial Hospital	Iron Mountain	79%	300+
Emma L Bixby Medical Center	Adrian	79%	300+
Lakeland Hospital - Saint Joseph	Saint Joseph	79%	300+
Mclaren - Northern Michigan	Petoskey	79%	300+
Midmichigan Medical Center - Clare	Clare	79%	300+
North Ottawa Community Health Center	Grand Haven	79%	300+
Oaklawn Hospital	Marshall	79%	300+
Saint John River District Hospital	East China	79%	300+
Saint Joseph Mercy Hospital	Ann Arbor	79%	300+
Saint Joseph Mercy Livingston Hospital	Howell	79%	300+
Spectrum Health - Reed City Campus	Reed City	79%	(a)
Edward W Sparrow Hospital	Lansing	78%	300+
Harper University Hospital[11]	Detroit	78%	300+
Henry Ford Macomb Hospital	Clinton Twp	78%	300+
Hillsdale Community Health Center	Hillsdale	78%	(a)
Mercy Memorial Hospital System	Monroe	78%	300+
University of Michigan Health System	Ann Arbor	78%	300+
Allegiance Health	Jackson	77%	300+
Alpena Regional Medical Center	Alpena	77%	300+
Botsford Hospital	Farmington Hills	77%	300+
Crittenton Hospital Medical Center[11]	Rochester	77%	300+
Garden City Hospital	Garden City	77%	300+
Henry Ford West Bloomfield Hospital	W Bloomfield	77%	300+
Holland Community Hospital	Holland	77%	300+
Mclaren Central Michigan	Mount Pleasant	77%	300+
Three Rivers Health	Three Rivers	77%	(a)
William Beaumont Hospital - Troy	Troy	77%	300+
Beaumont Health System	Royal Oak	76%	300+
Mercy Health Partners - Mercy Campus	Muskegon	76%	300+
Providence Hospital & Medical Centers	Southfield	76%	300+
Saint Joseph Mercy Oakland	Pontiac	76%	300+
Saint Mary Mercy Hospital	Livonia	76%	300+
Aspirus Grand View Hospital	Ironwood	75%	(a)
Genesys Reg Med Ctr-Health Park	Grand Blanc	75%	300+
Hayes Green Beach Memorial Hospital	Charlotte	75%	(a)
Henry Ford Hospital	Detroit	75%	300+
Henry Ford Wyandotte Hospital	Wyandotte	75%	300+
Huron Valley - Sinai Hospital[11]	Commerce Twp	75%	300+
Mclaren Bay Region	Bay City	75%	300+
Mclaren Lapeer Region	Lapeer	75%	300+
Saint Joseph Mercy Port Huron	Port Huron	75%	300+
West Branch Regional Medical Center	West Branch	75%	300+
Bronson Battle Creek Hospital	Battle Creek	74%	300+
Detroit Receiving Hosp & U Health Ctr[11]	Detroit	74%	300+
Hurley Medical Center	Flint	74%	300+
Mclaren Flint	Flint	74%	300+
Mclaren Oakland	Pontiac	74%	300+
Saint John Hospital & Medical Center	Detroit	74%	300+
Saint Mary's of Michigan Medical Center	Saginaw	74%	300+
Mclaren - Greater Lansing	Lansing	73%	300+
Mclaren Macomb	Mount Clemens	73%	300+
Sinai - Grace Hospital[11]	Detroit	73%	300+
Mercy Health Hackley Campus	Muskegon	72%	300+
St John Macomb-Oakland Hosp	Warren	72%	300+
Marquette General Hospital	Marquette	71%	300+
Doctors' Hospital of Michigan	Pontiac	68%	(a)

Pain 'Always' Well Controlled

Hospital Name	City	Rate	Cases
Bronson Lakeview Hospital	Paw Paw	83%	(a)
Saint Francis Hospital	Escanaba	80%	300+
Allegan General Hospital	Allegan	79%	(a)
Schoolcraft Memorial Hospital	Manistique	79%	(a)
Scheurer Hospital	Pigeon	78%	(a)

NOTE: Hospital profiles are in alphabetical order by state, then city, then hospital within the city; Rankings exclude hospitals with less than 25 cases except for patient surveys which excludes hospitals with less than 100 cases; (a) 100-299 cases; (1) The number of cases/patients is too few to report; (2) Data submitted were based on a sample of cases/patients; (3) Results are based on a shorter time period than required; (4) Data suppressed by CMS for one or more quarters; (5) Results are not available for this reporting period; (6) Fewer than 100 patients completed the HCAHPS survey; (7) No cases met the criteria for this measure; (8) The lower limit of the confidence interval cannot be calculated if the number of observed infections equals zero; (9) No data are available from the state/territory for this reporting period; (10) The scores shown reflect fewer than 50 completed surveys; (11) There were discrepancies in the data collection process; (12) This measure does not apply to this hospital for this reporting period; (13) Results cannot be calculated for this reporting period; (14) The results for this state are combined with nearby states to protect confidentiality; Please refer to the User's Guide for a full explanation of data.

Hospital Name	City	Rate	Cases
Charlevoix Area Hospital	Charlevoix	77%	300+
Portage Health	Hancock	77%	300+
Carson City Hospital	Carson City	76%	300+
Lakeland Community Hospital - Watervliet	Watervliet	76%	(a)
Mackinac Straits Hospital & Health Center	Saint Ignace	76%	(a)
Munson Medical Center	Traverse City	76%	300+
Oakwood Hospital - Taylor	Taylor	76%	300+
Saint Mary's Standish Community Hospital	Standish	76%	(a)
Sturgis Hospital	Sturgis	76%	300+
Huron Medical Center	Bad Axe	75%	300+
Midmichigan Medical Center - Midland	Midland	75%	300+
Spectrum Health Big Rapids Hospital	Big Rapids	75%	300+
Chippewa County War Memorial Hospital	Sault Ste Marie	74%	300+
Chelsea Community Hospital	Chelsea	73%	300+
Dickinson County Memorial Hospital	Iron Mountain	73%	300+
Hills & Dales General Hospital	Cass City	73%	(a)
Mercy Hospital - Cadillac	Cadillac	73%	300+
Mercy Hospital - Grayling	Grayling	73%	300+
Oakwood Hospital - Southshore	Trenton	73%	300+
Otsego Memorial Hospital	Gaylord	73%	(a)
Spectrum Health - Reed City Campus	Reed City	73%	(a)
Spectrum Health Zeeland Comm Hosp	Zeeland	73%	300+
Aspirus Grand View Hospital	Ironwood	72%	(a)
Aspirus Keweenaw Hospital	Laurium	72%	(a)
Bronson Methodist Hospital	Kalamazoo	72%	300+
Mclaren - Northern Michigan	Petoskey	72%	300+
Metro Health Hospital	Wyoming	72%	300+
Promedica Herrick Hospital	Tecumseh	72%	(a)
Tawas Saint Joseph Hospital	Tawas City	72%	300+
Three Rivers Health	Three Rivers	72%	(a)
Beaumont Health System	Grosse Pointe	71%	300+
Borgess Medical Center	Kalamazoo	71%	300+
Covenant Medical Center	Saginaw	71%	300+
Emma L Bixby Medical Center	Adrian	71%	300+
Garden City Hospital	Garden City	71%	300+
Hayes Green Beach Memorial Hospital	Charlotte	71%	(a)
Holland Community Hospital	Holland	71%	300+
Karmanos Cancer Center	Detroit	71%	300+
Lakeland Hospital - Saint Joseph	Saint Joseph	71%	300+
Mclaren Central Michigan	Mount Pleasant	71%	300+
Memorial Healthcare	Owosso	71%	300+
Midmichigan Medical Center - Clare	Clare	71%	300+
Midmichigan Medical Center - Gladwin	Gladwin	71%	(a)
Oakwood Hospital - Dearborn	Dearborn	71%	300+
Oakwood Hospital - Wayne	Wayne	71%	300+
Pennock Hospital	Hastings	71%	300+
Port Huron Hospital	Port Huron	71%	300+
Saint John River District Hospital	East China	71%	300+
Saint Joseph Mercy Livingston Hospital	Howell	71%	300+
Saint Mary's Health Care	Grand Rapids	71%	300+
South Haven Community Hospital	South Haven	71%	300+
Sparrow Clinton Hospital	Saint Johns	71%	(a)
Spectrum Health United Memorial	Greenville	71%	300+
West Shore Medical Center	Manistee	71%	(a)
Community Health Center of Branch County	Coldwater	70%	300+
Edward W Sparrow Hospital	Lansing	70%	300+
Marlette Regional Hospital	Marlette	70%	(a)
Midmichigan Medical Center - Gratiot	Alma	70%	300+
Oaklawn Hospital	Marshall	70%	300+
Saint Joseph Mercy Hospital	Ann Arbor	70%	300+
Sparrow Ionia Hospital	Ionia	70%	(a)
Spectrum Health - Butterworth Campus[11]	Grand Rapids	70%	300+
Spectrum Health Gerber Memorial	Fremont	70%	300+
William Beaumont Hospital - Troy	Troy	70%	300+
Borgess - Lee Memorial Hospital	Dowagiac	69%	(a)
Botsford Hospital	Farmington Hills	69%	300+
Crittenton Hospital Medical Center[11]	Rochester	69%	300+
Harper University Hospital[11]	Detroit	69%	300+
Henry Ford West Bloomfield Hospital	W Bloomfield	69%	300+
Memorial Medical Center of West Michigan	Ludington	69%	300+
North Ottawa Community Health Center	Grand Haven	69%	300+
Saint Joseph Mercy Port Huron	Port Huron	69%	300+
University of Michigan Health System	Ann Arbor	69%	300+
Bronson Battle Creek Hospital	Battle Creek	68%	300+
Genesys Reg Med Ctr-Health Park	Grand Blanc	68%	300+
Henry Ford Hospital	Detroit	68%	300+
Hillsdale Community Health Center	Hillsdale	68%	(a)
Mclaren Flint	Flint	68%	300+
Saint Mary Mercy Hospital	Livonia	68%	300+
Alpena Regional Medical Center	Alpena	67%	300+
Beaumont Health System	Royal Oak	67%	300+
Detroit Receiving Hosp & U Health Ctr[11]	Detroit	67%	300+
Henry Ford Macomb Hospital	Clinton Twp	67%	300+
Henry Ford Wyandotte Hospital	Wyandotte	67%	300+
Huron Valley - Sinai Hospital[11]	Commerce Twp	67%	300+
Mclaren Bay Region	Bay City	67%	300+
Mercy Health Partners - Mercy Campus	Muskegon	67%	300+
Mercy Memorial Hospital System	Monroe	67%	300+
Providence Hospital & Medical Centers	Southfield	67%	300+
Saint Joseph Mercy Oakland	Pontiac	67%	300+
West Branch Regional Medical Center	West Branch	67%	300+
Allegiance Health	Jackson	66%	300+
Baraga County Memorial Hospital	L'Anse	66%	(a)
Hurley Medical Center	Flint	66%	300+
Mclaren - Greater Lansing	Lansing	66%	300+
Mclaren Lapeer Region	Lapeer	66%	300+
Saint John Hospital & Medical Center	Detroit	66%	300+
Mclaren Oakland	Pontiac	65%	300+
Sinai - Grace Hospital[11]	Detroit	65%	300+
Helen Newberry Joy Hospital	Newberry	64%	(a)
Mclaren Macomb	Mount Clemens	64%	300+
Marquette General Hospital	Marquette	63%	300+
Mercy Health Hackley Campus	Muskegon	63%	300+
St John Macomb-Oakland Hosp	Warren	63%	300+
Saint Mary's of Michigan Medical Center	Saginaw	61%	300+
Doctors' Hospital of Michigan	Pontiac	56%	(a)

Room and Bathroom 'Always' Clean

Hospital Name	City	Rate	Cases
Baraga County Memorial Hospital	L'Anse	88%	(a)
Scheurer Hospital	Pigeon	88%	(a)
Mackinac Straits Hospital & Health Center	Saint Ignace	85%	(a)
Spectrum Health Zeeland Comm Hosp	Zeeland	85%	300+
Dickinson County Memorial Hospital	Iron Mountain	84%	300+
Helen Newberry Joy Hospital	Newberry	84%	(a)
Memorial Healthcare	Owosso	84%	300+
Bronson Lakeview Hospital	Paw Paw	83%	(a)
Portage Health	Hancock	83%	300+
Schoolcraft Memorial Hospital	Manistique	83%	(a)
West Shore Medical Center	Manistee	83%	(a)
Aspirus Keweenaw Hospital	Laurium	82%	(a)
Carson City Hospital	Carson City	82%	300+
Charlevoix Area Hospital	Charlevoix	82%	300+
Marlette Regional Hospital	Marlette	82%	(a)
Spectrum Health United Memorial	Greenville	82%	300+
Allegan General Hospital	Allegan	81%	(a)
Lakeland Community Hospital - Watervliet	Watervliet	80%	(a)
Spectrum Health - Reed City Campus	Reed City	80%	(a)
Chelsea Community Hospital	Chelsea	79%	300+
Hills & Dales General Hospital	Cass City	79%	(a)
Sturgis Hospital	Sturgis	79%	300+
Huron Medical Center	Bad Axe	78%	300+
Saint Francis Hospital	Escanaba	78%	300+
Hayes Green Beach Memorial Hospital	Charlotte	77%	(a)
Otsego Memorial Hospital	Gaylord	77%	(a)
Sparrow Clinton Hospital	Saint Johns	77%	(a)
Sparrow Ionia Hospital	Ionia	77%	(a)
Spectrum Health Gerber Memorial	Fremont	77%	300+
Three Rivers Health	Three Rivers	77%	(a)
Beaumont Health System	Grosse Pointe	76%	300+
North Ottawa Community Health Center	Grand Haven	76%	300+
Oakwood Hospital - Southshore	Trenton	76%	300+
Promedica Herrick Hospital	Tecumseh	76%	(a)
Spectrum Health - Butterworth Campus[11]	Grand Rapids	76%	300+
Holland Community Hospital	Holland	75%	300+
Memorial Medical Center of West Michigan	Ludington	75%	300+
Mercy Hospital - Grayling	Grayling	75%	300+
Metro Health Hospital	Wyoming	75%	300+
Munson Medical Center	Traverse City	75%	300+
Port Huron Hospital	Port Huron	75%	300+
Saint John River District Hospital	East China	75%	300+
Spectrum Health Big Rapids Hospital	Big Rapids	75%	300+
Alpena Regional Medical Center	Alpena	74%	300+
Bronson Methodist Hospital	Kalamazoo	74%	300+
Garden City Hospital	Garden City	74%	300+
Marquette General Hospital	Marquette	74%	300+
Midmichigan Medical Center - Midland	Midland	74%	300+
Oaklawn Hospital	Marshall	74%	300+
Tawas Saint Joseph Hospital	Tawas City	74%	300+
Borgess - Lee Memorial Hospital	Dowagiac	73%	(a)
Hillsdale Community Health Center	Hillsdale	73%	(a)
Lakeland Hospital - Saint Joseph	Saint Joseph	73%	300+
Mclaren Central Michigan	Mount Pleasant	73%	300+
Midmichigan Medical Center - Gratiot	Alma	73%	300+
Saint Joseph Mercy Port Huron	Port Huron	72%	300+
South Haven Community Hospital	South Haven	72%	300+
West Branch Regional Medical Center	West Branch	72%	300+
Community Health Center of Branch County	Coldwater	71%	300+
Emma L Bixby Medical Center	Adrian	71%	300+
Henry Ford West Bloomfield Hospital	W Bloomfield	71%	300+
Mclaren - Northern Michigan	Petoskey	71%	300+
Mercy Hospital - Cadillac	Cadillac	71%	300+
Midmichigan Medical Center - Clare	Clare	71%	300+
Oakwood Hospital - Taylor	Taylor	71%	300+
Oakwood Hospital - Wayne	Wayne	71%	300+
Chippewa County War Memorial Hospital	Sault Ste Marie	70%	300+
Mclaren Oakland	Pontiac	70%	300+
Saint Joseph Mercy Livingston Hospital	Howell	69%	300+
Saint Mary's Health Care	Grand Rapids	69%	300+
Saint Mary's Standish Community Hospital	Standish	69%	(a)
William Beaumont Hospital - Troy	Troy	69%	300+
Bronson Battle Creek Hospital	Battle Creek	68%	300+
Crittenton Hospital Medical Center[11]	Rochester	68%	300+
Karmanos Cancer Center	Detroit	68%	300+
Mclaren Lapeer Region	Lapeer	68%	300+
Midmichigan Medical Center - Gladwin	Gladwin	68%	(a)
Saint Joseph Mercy Hospital	Ann Arbor	68%	300+
Beaumont Health System	Royal Oak	67%	300+
Huron Valley - Sinai Hospital[11]	Commerce Twp	67%	300+
Mercy Memorial Hospital System	Monroe	67%	300+
Oakwood Hospital - Dearborn	Dearborn	67%	300+
Pennock Hospital	Hastings	67%	300+
Saint Mary Mercy Hospital	Livonia	67%	300+
Allegiance Health	Jackson	66%	300+
Borgess Medical Center	Kalamazoo	66%	300+
Covenant Medical Center	Saginaw	66%	300+
Edward W Sparrow Hospital	Lansing	66%	300+
Harper University Hospital[11]	Detroit	66%	300+
Mclaren Flint	Flint	66%	300+
Mercy Health Partners - Mercy Campus	Muskegon	66%	300+
Aspirus Grand View Hospital	Ironwood	65%	(a)
Henry Ford Hospital	Detroit	65%	300+
University of Michigan Health System	Ann Arbor	65%	300+
Genesys Reg Med Ctr-Health Park	Grand Blanc	64%	300+
Henry Ford Wyandotte Hospital	Wyandotte	64%	300+
Mclaren - Greater Lansing	Lansing	64%	300+
Botsford Hospital	Farmington Hills	63%	300+
Mercy Health Hackley Campus	Muskegon	63%	300+
St John Macomb-Oakland Hosp	Warren	63%	300+
Mclaren Bay Region	Bay City	62%	300+
Sinai - Grace Hospital[11]	Detroit	62%	300+
Hurley Medical Center	Flint	61%	300+
Henry Ford Macomb Hospital	Clinton Twp	60%	300+
Saint Mary's of Michigan Medical Center	Saginaw	60%	300+
Providence Hospital & Medical Centers	Southfield	59%	300+
Detroit Receiving Hosp & U Health Ctr[11]	Detroit	58%	300+
Doctors' Hospital of Michigan	Pontiac	58%	(a)
Mclaren Macomb	Mount Clemens	58%	300+
Saint John Hospital & Medical Center	Detroit	58%	300+
Saint Joseph Mercy Oakland	Pontiac	56%	300+

Timely Help 'Always' Received

Hospital Name	City	Rate	Cases
Hills & Dales General Hospital	Cass City	86%	(a)
Carson City Hospital	Carson City	84%	300+
Lakeland Community Hospital - Watervliet	Watervliet	84%	(a)
Schoolcraft Memorial Hospital	Manistique	84%	(a)
Aspirus Keweenaw Hospital	Laurium	82%	(a)
Charlevoix Area Hospital	Charlevoix	82%	300+
Helen Newberry Joy Hospital	Newberry	81%	(a)
Bronson Lakeview Hospital	Paw Paw	80%	(a)
Saint Francis Hospital	Escanaba	80%	300+
Sparrow Ionia Hospital	Ionia	80%	(a)
Saint Mary's Standish Community Hospital	Standish	79%	(a)
Scheurer Hospital	Pigeon	79%	(a)
Portage Health	Hancock	78%	300+
Allegan General Hospital	Allegan	77%	(a)
Mercy Hospital - Cadillac	Cadillac	77%	300+
South Haven Community Hospital	South Haven	77%	300+
Chelsea Community Hospital	Chelsea	76%	300+
Munson Medical Center	Traverse City	76%	300+
Otsego Memorial Hospital	Gaylord	76%	(a)
Sparrow Clinton Hospital	Saint Johns	76%	(a)
Tawas Saint Joseph Hospital	Tawas City	76%	300+
Alpena Regional Medical Center	Alpena	75%	300+
Chippewa County War Memorial Hospital	Sault Ste Marie	75%	300+
Mackinac Straits Hospital & Health Center	Saint Ignace	75%	(a)
Midmichigan Medical Center - Midland	Midland	75%	300+
Oakwood Hospital - Taylor	Taylor	75%	300+
Memorial Medical Center of West Michigan	Ludington	74%	300+
Spectrum Health - Reed City Campus	Reed City	74%	(a)
Spectrum Health Gerber Memorial	Fremont	74%	300+
Baraga County Memorial Hospital	L'Anse	73%	(a)
Mercy Hospital - Grayling	Grayling	73%	300+
Midmichigan Medical Center - Clare	Clare	73%	300+
Midmichigan Medical Center - Gladwin	Gladwin	73%	(a)
North Ottawa Community Health Center	Grand Haven	73%	300+
Spectrum Health Zeeland Comm Hosp	Zeeland	73%	300+
West Shore Medical Center	Manistee	73%	(a)
Huron Medical Center	Bad Axe	72%	300+
Memorial Healthcare	Owosso	72%	300+
Spectrum Health Big Rapids Hospital	Big Rapids	72%	300+
Aspirus Grand View Hospital	Ironwood	71%	(a)
Oakwood Hospital - Southshore	Trenton	71%	300+
Promedica Herrick Hospital	Tecumseh	71%	(a)
Genesys Reg Med Ctr-Health Park	Grand Blanc	70%	300+
Marlette Regional Hospital	Marlette	70%	(a)
Mclaren - Northern Michigan	Petoskey	70%	300+
Saint John River District Hospital	East China	70%	300+
Sturgis Hospital	Sturgis	70%	300+
Bronson Methodist Hospital	Kalamazoo	69%	300+
Dickinson County Memorial Hospital	Iron Mountain	69%	300+
Mclaren Central Michigan	Mount Pleasant	69%	300+

NOTE: Hospital profiles are in alphabetical order by state, then city, then hospital within the city; Rankings exclude hospitals with less than 25 cases except for patient surveys which excludes hospitals with less than 100 cases; (a) 100-299 cases; (1) The number of cases/patients is too few to report; (2) Data submitted were based on a sample of cases/patients; (3) Results are based on a shorter time period than required; (4) Data suppressed by CMS for one or more quarters; (5) Results are not available for this reporting period; (6) Fewer than 100 patients completed the HCAHPS survey; (7) No cases met the criteria for this measure; (8) The lower limit of the confidence interval cannot be calculated if the number of observed infections equals zero; (9) No data are available from the state/territory for this reporting period; (10) The scores shown reflect fewer than 50 completed surveys; (11) There were discrepancies in the data collection process; (12) This measure does not apply to this hospital for this reporting period; (13) Results cannot be calculated for this reporting period; (14) The results for this state are combined with nearby states to protect confidentiality; Please refer to the User's Guide for a full explanation of data.

Hospital Name	City	Rate	Cases
Oaklawn Hospital	Marshall	69%	300+
Saint Joseph Mercy Livingston Hospital	Howell	69%	300+
Three Rivers Health	Three Rivers	69%	(a)
Beaumont Health System	Grosse Pointe	68%	300+
Borgess - Lee Memorial Hospital	Dowagiac	68%	(a)
Garden City Hospital	Garden City	68%	300+
Hillsdale Community Health Center	Hillsdale	68%	(a)
Holland Community Hospital	Holland	68%	300+
Metro Health Hospital	Wyoming	68%	300+
Oakwood Hospital - Wayne	Wayne	68%	300+
Huron Valley - Sinai Hospital[11]	Commerce Twp	67%	300+
Pennock Hospital	Hastings	67%	300+
West Branch Regional Medical Center	West Branch	67%	300+
William Beaumont Hospital - Troy	Troy	67%	300+
Allegiance Health	Jackson	66%	300+
Community Health Center of Branch County	Coldwater	66%	300+
Emma L Bixby Medical Center	Adrian	66%	300+
Hayes Green Beach Memorial Hospital	Charlotte	66%	(a)
Midmichigan Medical Center - Gratiot	Alma	66%	300+
Oakwood Hospital - Dearborn	Dearborn	66%	300+
Port Huron Hospital	Port Huron	66%	300+
Spectrum Health United Memorial	Greenville	66%	300+
Covenant Medical Center	Saginaw	65%	300+
Lakeland Hospital - Saint Joseph	Saint Joseph	65%	300+
Crittenton Hospital Medical Center[11]	Rochester	64%	300+
Edward W Sparrow Hospital	Lansing	64%	300+
Karmanos Cancer Center	Detroit	64%	300+
Saint Joseph Mercy Hospital	Ann Arbor	64%	300+
Saint Mary's Health Care	Grand Rapids	64%	300+
Spectrum Health - Butterworth Campus[11]	Grand Rapids	64%	300+
University of Michigan Health System	Ann Arbor	64%	300+
Botsford Hospital	Farmington Hills	63%	300+
Bronson Battle Creek Hospital	Battle Creek	63%	300+
Henry Ford Macomb Hospital	Clinton Twp	63%	300+
Henry Ford West Bloomfield Hospital	W Bloomfield	63%	300+
Mclaren Lapeer Region	Lapeer	63%	300+
Detroit Receiving Hosp & U Health Ctr[11]	Detroit	62%	300+
Henry Ford Hospital	Detroit	62%	300+
Henry Ford Wyandotte Hospital	Wyandotte	62%	300+
Mclaren Bay Region	Bay City	62%	300+
Mclaren Oakland	Pontiac	62%	300+
Mercy Health Partners - Mercy Campus	Muskegon	62%	300+
Saint Mary Mercy Hospital	Livonia	62%	300+
Beaumont Health System	Royal Oak	61%	300+
Harper University Hospital[11]	Detroit	61%	300+
Marquette General Hospital	Marquette	61%	300+
Mercy Memorial Hospital System	Monroe	61%	300+
Providence Hospital & Medical Centers	Southfield	61%	300+
Saint Joseph Mercy Port Huron	Port Huron	61%	300+
Saint Mary's of Michigan Medical Center	Saginaw	61%	300+
Borgess Medical Center	Kalamazoo	60%	300+
Mclaren Macomb	Mount Clemens	60%	300+
Saint Joseph Mercy Oakland	Pontiac	60%	300+
Hurley Medical Center	Flint	59%	300+
Mclaren - Greater Lansing	Lansing	59%	300+
Mclaren Flint	Flint	59%	300+
Mercy Health Hackley Campus	Muskegon	58%	300+
Saint John Hospital & Medical Center	Detroit	57%	300+
St John Macomb-Oakland Hosp	Warren	56%	300+
Sinai - Grace Hospital[11]	Detroit	56%	300+
Doctors' Hospital of Michigan	Pontiac	48%	(a)

Would Definitely Recommend Hospital

Hospital Name	City	Rate	Cases
Chelsea Community Hospital	Chelsea	87%	300+
Munson Medical Center	Traverse City	87%	300+
Bronson Methodist Hospital	Kalamazoo	85%	300+
Mackinac Straits Hospital & Health Center	Saint Ignace	85%	(a)
Spectrum Health Zeeland Comm Hosp	Zeeland	84%	300+
Charlevoix Area Hospital	Charlevoix	83%	300+
Henry Ford West Bloomfield Hospital	W Bloomfield	82%	300+
Metro Health Hospital	Wyoming	82%	300+
University of Michigan Health System	Ann Arbor	82%	300+
Marlette Regional Hospital	Marlette	81%	(a)
Oaklawn Hospital	Marshall	81%	300+
Saint Joseph Mercy Hospital	Ann Arbor	81%	300+
Midmichigan Medical Center - Midland	Midland	80%	300+
Portage Health	Hancock	80%	300+
Sparrow Clinton Hospital	Saint Johns	80%	(a)
Spectrum Health - Butterworth Campus[11]	Grand Rapids	80%	300+
Carson City Hospital	Carson City	78%	300+
Holland Community Hospital	Holland	78%	300+
Karmanos Cancer Center	Detroit	78%	300+
Saint Mary's Health Care	Grand Rapids	78%	300+
Beaumont Health System	Royal Oak	77%	300+
Mclaren - Northern Michigan	Petoskey	77%	300+
Spectrum Health United Memorial	Greenville	77%	300+
Beaumont Health System	Grosse Pointe	76%	300+
Covenant Medical Center	Saginaw	76%	300+
Hills & Dales General Hospital	Cass City	76%	(a)
Lakeland Community Hospital - Watervliet	Watervliet	76%	(a)
Mercy Hospital - Grayling	Grayling	76%	300+
Scheurer Hospital	Pigeon	76%	(a)
Spectrum Health Big Rapids Hospital	Big Rapids	76%	300+
Allegan General Hospital	Allegan	75%	(a)
Borgess Medical Center	Kalamazoo	75%	300+
Huron Valley - Sinai Hospital[11]	Commerce Twp	75%	300+
Oakwood Hospital - Southshore	Trenton	75%	300+
William Beaumont Hospital - Troy	Troy	75%	300+
Edward W Sparrow Hospital	Lansing	74%	300+
Mercy Hospital - Cadillac	Cadillac	74%	300+
Schoolcraft Memorial Hospital	Manistique	74%	(a)
Bronson Lakeview Hospital	Paw Paw	73%	(a)
Midmichigan Medical Center - Gratiot	Alma	73%	300+
North Ottawa Community Health Center	Grand Haven	73%	300+
Oakwood Hospital - Taylor	Taylor	73%	300+
Promedica Herrick Hospital	Tecumseh	73%	(a)
Aspirus Keweenaw Hospital	Laurium	72%	(a)
Pennock Hospital	Hastings	72%	300+
Providence Hospital & Medical Centers	Southfield	72%	300+
Saint Joseph Mercy Oakland	Pontiac	72%	300+
Chippewa County War Memorial Hospital	Sault Ste Marie	71%	300+
Genesys Reg Med Ctr-Health Park	Grand Blanc	71%	300+
Henry Ford Hospital	Detroit	71%	300+
Huron Medical Center	Bad Axe	71%	300+
Mercy Health Partners - Mercy Campus	Muskegon	71%	300+
Otsego Memorial Hospital	Gaylord	71%	(a)
Lakeland Hospital - Saint Joseph	Saint Joseph	70%	300+
West Shore Medical Center	Manistee	70%	(a)
Community Health Center of Branch County	Coldwater	69%	300+
Hurley Medical Center	Flint	69%	300+
Mclaren Flint	Flint	69%	300+
Saint Joseph Mercy Livingston Hospital	Howell	69%	300+
Saint Joseph Mercy Port Huron	Port Huron	69%	300+
Saint Mary Mercy Hospital	Livonia	69%	300+
Spectrum Health Gerber Memorial	Fremont	69%	300+
Crittenton Hospital Medical Center[11]	Rochester	68%	300+
Harper University Hospital[11]	Detroit	68%	300+
Saint Mary's of Michigan Medical Center	Saginaw	68%	300+
Port Huron Hospital	Port Huron	67%	300+
Saint Francis Hospital	Escanaba	67%	300+
Saint John Hospital & Medical Center	Detroit	67%	300+
Saint Mary's Standish Community Hospital	Standish	67%	(a)
Sturgis Hospital	Sturgis	67%	300+
Tawas Saint Joseph Hospital	Tawas City	67%	300+
Garden City Hospital	Garden City	66%	300+
Henry Ford Macomb Hospital	Clinton Twp	66%	300+
Mclaren - Greater Lansing	Lansing	66%	300+
Oakwood Hospital - Dearborn	Dearborn	66%	300+
Saint John River District Hospital	East China	66%	300+
Spectrum Health - Reed City Campus	Reed City	66%	(a)
Botsford Hospital	Farmington Hills	65%	300+
Detroit Receiving Hosp & U Health Ctr[11]	Detroit	65%	300+
Emma L Bixby Medical Center	Adrian	65%	300+
Henry Ford Wyandotte Hospital	Wyandotte	65%	300+
Mclaren Oakland	Pontiac	65%	300+
Memorial Healthcare	Owosso	65%	300+
Oakwood Hospital - Wayne	Wayne	65%	300+
Baraga County Memorial Hospital	L'Anse	64%	(a)
Borgess - Lee Memorial Hospital	Dowagiac	64%	(a)
Hayes Green Beach Memorial Hospital	Charlotte	64%	(a)
Helen Newberry Joy Hospital	Newberry	64%	(a)
Memorial Medical Center of West Michigan	Ludington	64%	300+
Mercy Health Hackley Campus	Muskegon	64%	300+
Midmichigan Medical Center - Clare	Clare	64%	(a)
West Branch Regional Medical Center	West Branch	64%	300+
Allegiance Health	Jackson	63%	300+
Dickinson County Memorial Hospital	Iron Mountain	63%	300+
Mclaren Bay Region	Bay City	63%	300+
Mclaren Central Michigan	Mount Pleasant	63%	300+
Midmichigan Medical Center - Gladwin	Gladwin	63%	(a)
South Haven Community Hospital	South Haven	63%	300+
Sparrow Ionia Hospital	Ionia	63%	(a)
Mclaren Macomb	Mount Clemens	62%	300+
St John Macomb-Oakland Hosp	Warren	61%	300+
Marquette General Hospital	Marquette	60%	300+
Three Rivers Health	Three Rivers	60%	(a)
Aspirus Grand View Hospital	Ironwood	59%	(a)
Hillsdale Community Health Center	Hillsdale	59%	(a)
Alpena Regional Medical Center	Alpena	58%	300+
Bronson Battle Creek Hospital	Battle Creek	57%	300+
Mclaren Lapeer Region	Lapeer	56%	300+
Doctors' Hospital of Michigan	Pontiac	54%	(a)
Mercy Memorial Hospital System	Monroe	50%	300+
Sinai - Grace Hospital[11]	Detroit	48%	300+

Use of Medical Imaging

Cardiac Imaging Stress Test before OP Surgery

Hospital Name	City	Rate	Cases
Northstar Health System	Iron River	1.3%	75
Borgess - Lee Memorial Hospital	Dowagiac	2.0%	50
Lakeland Hospital - Saint Joseph	Saint Joseph	2.0%	49
Saint Joseph Mercy Port Huron	Port Huron	2.0%	101
Community Health Center of Branch County	Coldwater	2.7%	258
Hayes Green Beach Memorial Hospital	Charlotte	2.8%	144
Chippewa County War Memorial Hospital	Sault Ste Marie	3.0%	302
Mclaren Central Michigan	Mount Pleasant	3.0%	462
Helen Newberry Joy Hospital	Newberry	3.1%	65
Port Huron Hospital	Port Huron	3.1%	228
Three Rivers Health	Three Rivers	3.1%	191
Borgess Medical Center	Kalamazoo	3.4%	1587
Emma L Bixby Medical Center	Adrian	3.4%	267
Saint Joseph Mercy Livingston Hospital	Howell	3.4%	647
North Ottawa Community Health Center	Grand Haven	3.5%	113
South Haven Community Hospital	South Haven	3.5%	114
Bronson Lakeview Hospital	Paw Paw	3.6%	165
Mercy Hospital - Cadillac	Cadillac	3.6%	448
Scheurer Hospital	Pigeon	3.6%	250
Saint Joseph Mercy Hospital	Ann Arbor	3.7%	2341
Allegiance Health	Jackson	3.8%	1069
Marlette Regional Hospital	Marlette	3.8%	260
Mclaren Bay Region	Bay City	3.9%	695
Spectrum Health - Reed City Campus	Reed City	3.9%	129
Mclaren Lapeer Region	Lapeer	4.0%	251
Otsego Memorial Hospital	Gaylord	4.0%	224
Alpena Regional Medical Center	Alpena	4.1%	343
Hills & Dales General Hospital	Cass City	4.1%	97
Midmichigan Medical Center - Gratiot	Alma	4.3%	92
Tawas Saint Joseph Hospital	Tawas City	4.3%	444
Mclaren - Northern Michigan	Petoskey	4.4%	1611
Midmichigan Medical Center - Clare	Clare	4.4%	204
Spectrum Health United Memorial	Greenville	4.4%	321
Charlevoix Area Hospital	Charlevoix	4.5%	111
Edward W Sparrow Hospital	Lansing	4.5%	1865
Oaklawn Hospital	Marshall	4.5%	313
Promedica Herrick Hospital	Tecumseh	4.5%	177
Mercy Hospital - Grayling	Grayling	4.6%	458
Providence Hospital & Medical Centers	Southfield	4.6%	2660
Bell Hospital	Ishpeming	4.7%	85
Bronson Methodist Hospital	Kalamazoo	4.7%	1194
Carson City Hospital	Carson City	4.7%	128
Huron Medical Center	Bad Axe	4.7%	214
Munson Medical Center	Traverse City	4.7%	2620
Henry Ford Hospital	Detroit	4.8%	1094
Memorial Medical Center of West Michigan	Ludington	4.8%	290
Mercy Memorial Hospital System	Monroe	4.8%	126
Mercy Health Partners - Mercy Campus	Muskegon	4.9%	1225
Saint John Hospital & Medical Center	Detroit	4.9%	1028
Saint Mary's of Michigan Medical Center	Saginaw	4.9%	1665
Saint Mary's Standish Community Hospital	Standish	4.9%	162
University of Michigan Health System	Ann Arbor	4.9%	1402
Midmichigan Medical Center - Gladwin	Gladwin	5.0%	222
Beaumont Health System	Royal Oak	5.1%	4313
Holland Community Hospital	Holland	5.1%	235
Spectrum Health - Butterworth Campus	Grand Rapids	5.1%	2108
Mclaren - Greater Lansing	Lansing	5.2%	805
Oakwood Hospital - Taylor	Taylor	5.2%	248
West Shore Medical Center	Manistee	5.2%	173
Covenant Medical Center	Saginaw	5.3%	722
Portage Health	Hancock	5.3%	152
Schoolcraft Memorial Hospital	Manistique	5.3%	94
Henry Ford Macomb Hospital	Clinton Twp	5.4%	661
Saint Joseph Mercy Oakland	Pontiac	5.4%	503
Spectrum Health Zeeland Comm Hosp	Zeeland	5.4%	56
Saint Mary's Health Care	Grand Rapids	5.5%	474
Henry Ford West Bloomfield Hospital	W Bloomfield	5.6%	396
McKenzie Health System	Sandusky	5.6%	71
Metro Health Hospital	Wyoming	5.6%	698
Oakwood Hospital - Southshore	Trenton	5.6%	461
Beaumont Health System	Grosse Pointe	5.7%	457
Bronson Battle Creek Hospital	Battle Creek	5.7%	508
Midmichigan Medical Center - Midland	Midland	5.8%	969
Spectrum Health Gerber Memorial	Fremont	6.0%	250
William Beaumont Hospital - Troy	Troy	6.0%	1206
Mclaren Oakland	Pontiac	6.1%	163
Genesys Reg Med Ctr-Health Park	Grand Blanc	6.2%	726
Harper University Hospital	Detroit	6.2%	485
Henry Ford Wyandotte Hospital	Wyandotte	6.2%	630
St John Macomb-Oakland Hosp	Warren	6.3%	1168
Dickinson County Memorial Hospital	Iron Mountain	6.4%	234
Aspirus Grand View Hospital	Ironwood	6.5%	108
Chelsea Community Hospital	Chelsea	6.5%	276
Hillsdale Community Health Center	Hillsdale	6.5%	168
West Branch Regional Medical Center	West Branch	6.5%	643
Botsford Hospital	Farmington Hills	6.8%	366
Crittenton Hospital Medical Center	Rochester	6.9%	245
Sinai - Grace Hospital	Detroit	6.9%	348
Spectrum Health Big Rapids Hospital	Big Rapids	6.9%	231
Allegan General Hospital	Allegan	7.1%	113
Pennock Hospital	Hastings	7.1%	226
Marquette General Hospital	Marquette	7.2%	759

NOTE: Hospital profiles are in alphabetical order by state, then city, then hospital within the city; Rankings exclude hospitals with less than 25 cases except for patient surveys which excludes hospitals with less than 100 cases; (a) 100-299 cases; (1) The number of cases/patients is too few to report; (2) Data submitted were based on a sample of cases/patients; (3) Results are based on a shorter time period than required; (4) Data suppressed by CMS for one or more quarters; (5) Results are not available for this reporting period; (6) Fewer than 100 patients completed the HCAHPS survey; (7) No cases met the criteria for this measure; (8) The lower limit of the confidence interval cannot be calculated if the number of observed infections equals zero; (9) No data are available from the state/territory for this reporting period; (10) The scores shown reflect fewer than 50 completed surveys; (11) There were discrepancies in the data collection process; (12) This measure does not apply to this hospital for this reporting period; (13) Results cannot be calculated for this reporting period; (14) The results for this state are combined with nearby states to protect confidentiality; Please refer to the User's Guide for a full explanation of data.

Hospital Name	City	Rate	Cases
Oakwood Hospital - Dearborn	Dearborn	7.2%	709
Sparrow Ionia Hospital	Ionia	7.2%	139
Saint Francis Hospital	Escanaba	7.4%	216
Sturgis Hospital	Sturgis	7.5%	307
Huron Valley - Sinai Hospital	Commerce Twp	7.7%	403
Sparrow Clinton Hospital	Saint Johns	7.7%	195
Garden City Hospital	Garden City	8.2%	268
Saint Mary Mercy Hospital	Livonia	8.2%	490
Mclaren Macomb	Mount Clemens	8.6%	384
Saint John River District Hospital	East China	9.0%	111
Oakwood Hospital - Wayne	Wayne	9.6%	427
Memorial Healthcare	Owosso	10.3%	107
Aspirus Keweenaw Hospital	Laurium	12.3%	122

Combination Abdominal CT Scan

Hospital Name	City	Rate	Cases
Marlette Regional Hospital	Marlette	0.4%	282
Oaklawn Hospital	Marshall	1.5%	608
Saint John River District Hospital	East China	1.5%	325
Hurley Medical Center	Flint	1.8%	399
Genesys Reg Med Ctr-Health Park	Grand Blanc	2.0%	1076
Spectrum Health Gerber Memorial	Fremont	2.0%	512
Aspirus Grand View Hospital	Ironwood	2.2%	275
Borgess - Lee Memorial Hospital	Dowagiac	2.2%	276
Sparrow Ionia Hospital	Ionia	2.2%	363
Bronson Battle Creek Hospital	Battle Creek	2.3%	1309
Bronson Lakeview Hospital	Paw Paw	2.3%	391
Hillsdale Community Health Center	Hillsdale	2.4%	509
Spectrum Health - Reed City Campus	Reed City	2.4%	575
Mercy Hospital - Cadillac	Cadillac	2.6%	646
Lakeland Community Hospital - Watervliet	Watervliet	2.7%	256
Pennock Hospital	Hastings	2.7%	376
Spectrum Health United Memorial	Greenville	3.0%	660
Sturgis Hospital	Sturgis	3.0%	368
Kalkaska Memorial Health Center	Kalkaska	3.1%	195
Memorial Healthcare	Owosso	3.1%	685
Mclaren Lapeer Region	Lapeer	3.2%	603
McKenzie Health System	Sandusky	3.4%	204
Midmichigan Medical Center - Clare	Clare	3.4%	531
West Shore Medical Center	Manistee	3.4%	615
Henry Ford Wyandotte Hospital	Wyandotte	3.6%	1316
Port Huron Hospital	Port Huron	3.6%	828
Spectrum Health - Butterworth Campus	Grand Rapids	3.6%	2756
Henry Ford Hospital	Detroit	3.7%	2635
Bronson Methodist Hospital	Kalamazoo	3.9%	1126
Eaton Rapids Medical Center	Eaton Rapids	3.9%	179
Mercy Memorial Hospital System	Monroe	3.9%	851
Midmichigan Medical Center - Gladwin	Gladwin	4.0%	428
Saint Joseph Mercy Livingston Hospital	Howell	4.0%	1054
Spectrum Health Zeeland Comm Hosp	Zeeland	4.1%	195
Mercy Hospital - Grayling	Grayling	4.2%	778
Promedica Herrick Hospital	Tecumseh	4.2%	265
Munson Medical Center	Traverse City	4.4%	1462
Henry Ford West Bloomfield Hospital	W Bloomfield	4.5%	1037
Sparrow Clinton Hospital	Saint Johns	4.5%	404
Edward W Sparrow Hospital	Lansing	4.6%	2268
Mercy Health Lakeshore Campus	Shelby	4.6%	153
Saint Joseph Mercy Port Huron	Port Huron	4.6%	370
Saint Mary Mercy Hospital	Livonia	4.6%	865
Emma L Bixby Medical Center	Adrian	4.8%	587
Beaumont Health System	Royal Oak	4.9%	3712
Providence Hospital & Medical Centers	Southfield	4.9%	2119
Midmichigan Medical Center - Midland	Midland	5.0%	1310
Saint Mary's Health Care	Grand Rapids	5.0%	1356
University of Michigan Health System	Ann Arbor	5.0%	3659
Allegiance Health	Jackson	5.1%	1806
Lakeland Hospital - Saint Joseph	Saint Joseph	5.1%	1530
Mackinac Straits Hospital & Health Center	Saint Ignace	5.2%	193
Allegan General Hospital	Allegan	5.3%	282
Oakwood Hospital - Taylor	Taylor	5.3%	449
Mclaren Central Michigan	Mount Pleasant	5.4%	462
Memorial Medical Center of West Michigan	Ludington	5.4%	610
Mclaren - Northern Michigan	Petoskey	5.5%	1443
Mercy Health Partners - Mercy Campus	Muskegon	5.5%	1199
Holland Community Hospital	Holland	5.9%	573
Botsford Hospital	Farmington Hills	6.0%	1025
Helen Newberry Joy Hospital	Newberry	6.0%	201
Otsego Memorial Hospital	Gaylord	6.2%	518
Sinai - Grace Hospital	Detroit	6.3%	749
Spectrum Health United Mem-Kelsey Camp	Lakeview	6.3%	128
Beaumont Health System	Grosse Pointe	6.5%	855
Oakwood Hospital - Dearborn	Dearborn	6.6%	1755
Borgess Medical Center	Kalamazoo	6.7%	1220
South Haven Community Hospital	South Haven	6.7%	224
William Beaumont Hospital - Troy	Troy	6.7%	2747
Sheridan Community Hospital	Sheridan	7.2%	97
Paul Oliver Memorial Hospital	Frankfort	7.3%	151
Saint Joseph Mercy Hospital	Ann Arbor	7.3%	2275
Three Rivers Health	Three Rivers	7.4%	338
Metro Health Hospital	Wyoming	7.5%	882
Northstar Health System	Iron River	7.8%	217
Carson City Hospital	Carson City	7.9%	239
Mercy Health Hackley Campus	Muskegon	7.9%	693
North Ottawa Community Health Center	Grand Haven	8.1%	210
Saint Mary's Standish Community Hospital	Standish	8.3%	445
Aspirus Ontonagon Hospital	Ontonagon	8.6%	93
Dickinson County Memorial Hospital	Iron Mountain	8.9%	549
Saint John Hospital & Medical Center	Detroit	9.0%	1819
Portage Health	Hancock	9.1%	275
Oakwood Hospital - Wayne	Wayne	9.6%	783
Midmichigan Medical Center - Gratiot	Alma	9.9%	564
Harbor Beach Community Hospital	Harbor Beach	10.1%	69
Chippewa County War Memorial Hospital	Sault Ste Marie	10.3%	465
Community Health Center of Branch County	Coldwater	10.4%	469
Chelsea Community Hospital	Chelsea	10.5%	392
Mclaren - Greater Lansing	Lansing	10.7%	971
Mclaren Bay Region	Bay City	11.2%	1136
Charlevoix Area Hospital	Charlevoix	11.7%	162
Oakwood Hospital - Southshore	Trenton	12.1%	768
Detroit Receiving Hosp & U Health Ctr	Detroit	12.2%	263
Aspirus Keweenaw Hospital	Laurium	12.4%	137
Caro Community Hospital	Caro	12.4%	185
Saint Francis Hospital	Escanaba	12.5%	472
Garden City Hospital	Garden City	13.1%	766
Saint Joseph Mercy Oakland	Pontiac	14.0%	881
Covenant Medical Center	Saginaw	14.2%	1524
Crittenton Hospital Medical Center	Rochester	14.6%	726
Henry Ford Macomb Hospital	Clinton Twp	15.3%	1271
Saint Mary's of Michigan Medical Center	Saginaw	15.4%	1038
Huron Valley - Sinai Hospital	Commerce Twp	15.5%	586
St John Macomb-Oakland Hosp	Warren	15.7%	1650
Munising Memorial Hospital	Munising	15.9%	88
Tawas Saint Joseph Hospital	Tawas City	17.5%	743
Alpena Regional Medical Center	Alpena	17.8%	1023
Harper University Hospital	Detroit	17.8%	805
Mclaren Oakland	Pontiac	20.3%	572
Hills & Dales General Hospital	Cass City	22.3%	211
Scheurer Hospital	Pigeon	23.0%	265
Huron Medical Center	Bad Axe	23.4%	290
West Branch Regional Medical Center	West Branch	23.8%	793
Karmanos Cancer Center	Detroit	25.6%	1891
Mclaren Flint	Flint	26.1%	1863
Spectrum Health Big Rapids Hospital	Big Rapids	26.4%	345
Doctors' Hospital of Michigan	Pontiac	27.5%	142
Mclaren Macomb	Mount Clemens	29.0%	1346
Hayes Green Beach Memorial Hospital	Charlotte	30.1%	405
Marquette General Hospital	Marquette	37.0%	511
Bell Hospital	Ishpeming	41.8%	184
Schoolcraft Memorial Hospital	Manistique	48.2%	139
Baraga County Memorial Hospital	L'Anse	74.2%	89

Combination Brain/Sinus CT Scan

Hospital Name	City	Rate	Cases
Harbor Beach Community Hospital	Harbor Beach	0.0%	107
Kalkaska Memorial Health Center	Kalkaska	0.0%	167
Henry Ford Hospital	Detroit	0.1%	1549
Henry Ford West Bloomfield Hospital	W Bloomfield	0.1%	774
Saint Mary's Standish Community Hospital	Standish	0.4%	280
Chelsea Community Hospital	Chelsea	0.7%	405
Midmichigan Medical Center - Gladwin	Gladwin	0.7%	437
Munising Memorial Hospital	Munising	0.7%	144
Sheridan Community Hospital	Sheridan	0.7%	149
Mercy Health Hackley Campus	Muskegon	0.8%	732
Midmichigan Medical Center - Clare	Clare	0.8%	488
Carson City Hospital	Carson City	0.9%	233
Dickinson County Memorial Hospital	Iron Mountain	0.9%	331
Caro Community Hospital	Caro	1.0%	194
Holland Community Hospital	Holland	1.0%	677
Charlevoix Area Hospital	Charlevoix	1.1%	188
Spectrum Health - Reed City Campus	Reed City	1.1%	438
Allegiance Health	Jackson	1.2%	1348
Mackinac Straits Hospital & Health Center	Saint Ignace	1.2%	163
Saint Joseph Mercy Livingston Hospital	Howell	1.2%	514
William Beaumont Hospital - Troy	Troy	1.2%	1623
Beaumont Health System	Royal Oak	1.3%	1806
University of Michigan Health System	Ann Arbor	1.3%	1260
Alpena Regional Medical Center	Alpena	1.4%	692
Saint Joseph Mercy Hospital	Ann Arbor	1.4%	1116
Saint Joseph Mercy Port Huron	Port Huron	1.4%	367
Detroit Receiving Hosp & U Health Ctr	Detroit	1.5%	585
Providence Hospital & Medical Centers	Southfield	1.5%	1574
Mercy Hospital - Grayling	Grayling	1.6%	689
Covenant Medical Center	Saginaw	1.7%	1126
Crittenton Hospital Medical Center	Rochester	1.7%	484
Genesys Reg Med Ctr-Health Park	Grand Blanc	1.7%	1120
Saint Joseph Mercy Oakland	Pontiac	1.7%	833
West Branch Regional Medical Center	West Branch	1.7%	586
Beaumont Health System	Grosse Pointe	1.8%	673
Marquette General Hospital	Marquette	1.8%	436
Mclaren - Northern Michigan	Petoskey	1.8%	793
Garden City Hospital	Garden City	1.9%	739
Memorial Medical Center of West Michigan	Ludington	1.9%	568
Spectrum Health United Memorial	Greenville	1.9%	565
Bronson Battle Creek Hospital	Battle Creek	2.0%	980
Henry Ford Macomb Hospital	Clinton Twp	2.0%	1326
Metro Health Hospital	Wyoming	2.0%	704
Munson Medical Center	Traverse City	2.0%	1326
Lakeland Hospital - Saint Joseph	Saint Joseph	2.1%	1163
Midmichigan Medical Center - Midland	Midland	2.1%	945
Spectrum Health - Butterworth Campus	Grand Rapids	2.1%	1898
Bronson Methodist Hospital	Kalamazoo	2.2%	1191
Hillsdale Community Health Center	Hillsdale	2.2%	403
Emma L Bixby Medical Center	Adrian	2.3%	574
Henry Ford Wyandotte Hospital	Wyandotte	2.3%	997
Mclaren Central Michigan	Mount Pleasant	2.3%	566
Saint John Hospital & Medical Center	Detroit	2.3%	1469
Saint Mary Mercy Hospital	Livonia	2.3%	968
Borgess Medical Center	Kalamazoo	2.4%	757
Memorial Healthcare	Owosso	2.4%	582
Saint Francis Hospital	Escanaba	2.4%	574
Mclaren Macomb	Mount Clemens	2.5%	957
Midmichigan Medical Center - Gratiot	Alma	2.5%	517
Mclaren Bay Region	Bay City	2.6%	893
Mclaren Flint	Flint	2.6%	1409
Mercy Health Partners - Mercy Campus	Muskegon	2.6%	1122
Port Huron Hospital	Port Huron	2.6%	740
Tawas Saint Joseph Hospital	Tawas City	2.6%	621
St John Macomb-Oakland Hosp	Warren	2.9%	1824
Oakwood Hospital - Dearborn	Dearborn	3.3%	1567
Saint Mary's Health Care	Grand Rapids	3.4%	951
Edward W Sparrow Hospital	Lansing	3.5%	2136
Botsford Hospital	Farmington Hills	3.7%	909
Saint Mary's of Michigan Medical Center	Saginaw	3.8%	1026
Mclaren Lapeer Region	Lapeer	3.9%	671
Oakwood Hospital - Wayne	Wayne	3.9%	983
Chippewa County War Memorial Hospital	Sault Ste Marie	4.2%	429
Hurley Medical Center	Flint	4.2%	595
Mclaren - Greater Lansing	Lansing	4.2%	1009
Sinai - Grace Hospital	Detroit	5.2%	815

Combination Chest CT Scan

Hospital Name	City	Rate	Cases
Allegiance Health	Jackson	0.0%	1463
Bronson Lakeview Hospital	Paw Paw	0.0%	169
Bronson Methodist Hospital	Kalamazoo	0.0%	508
Charlevoix Area Hospital	Charlevoix	0.0%	90
Eaton Rapids Medical Center	Eaton Rapids	0.0%	51
Hurley Medical Center	Flint	0.0%	213
Kalkaska Memorial Health Center	Kalkaska	0.0%	173
Marlette Regional Hospital	Marlette	0.0%	154
Memorial Healthcare	Owosso	0.0%	535
Mercy Hospital - Cadillac	Cadillac	0.0%	465
Mercy Memorial Hospital System	Monroe	0.0%	532
Paul Oliver Memorial Hospital	Frankfort	0.0%	89
Promedica Herrick Hospital	Tecumseh	0.0%	125
Sheridan Community Hospital	Sheridan	0.0%	57
Sparrow Ionia Hospital	Ionia	0.0%	154
Spectrum Health United Mem-Kelsey Camp	Lakeview	0.0%	66
Spectrum Health United Memorial	Greenville	0.0%	474
Bronson Battle Creek Hospital	Battle Creek	0.1%	812
Henry Ford Wyandotte Hospital	Wyandotte	0.1%	1007
Munson Medical Center	Traverse City	0.1%	1043
Beaumont Health System	Grosse Pointe	0.2%	664
Edward W Sparrow Hospital	Lansing	0.2%	1112
Oaklawn Hospital	Marshall	0.2%	410
Mercy Hospital - Grayling	Grayling	0.3%	314
University of Michigan Health System	Ann Arbor	0.3%	4942
Chelsea Community Hospital	Chelsea	0.4%	266
Garden City Hospital	Garden City	0.4%	458
Mclaren Flint	Flint	0.4%	1187
Saint John River District Hospital	East China	0.4%	226
Saint Mary's Health Care	Grand Rapids	0.4%	1142
Mclaren - Greater Lansing	Lansing	0.5%	620
Saint Joseph Mercy Port Huron	Port Huron	0.5%	217
Pennock Hospital	Hastings	0.6%	180
Sparrow Clinton Hospital	Saint Johns	0.6%	157
Spectrum Health Gerber Memorial	Fremont	0.6%	321
Holland Community Hospital	Holland	0.7%	294
Mclaren Lapeer Region	Lapeer	0.8%	355
Port Huron Hospital	Port Huron	0.8%	714
Crittenton Hospital Medical Center	Rochester	0.9%	569
McKenzie Health System	Sandusky	1.0%	97
Mclaren - Northern Michigan	Petoskey	1.0%	1006
Hillsdale Community Health Center	Hillsdale	1.1%	377
Oakwood Hospital - Taylor	Taylor	1.1%	267
Otsego Memorial Hospital	Gaylord	1.1%	368
Providence Hospital & Medical Centers	Southfield	1.1%	1819
South Haven Community Hospital	South Haven	1.1%	92
Borgess - Lee Memorial Hospital	Dowagiac	1.2%	161
Lakeland Hospital - Saint Joseph	Saint Joseph	1.2%	905
Spectrum Health - Butterworth Campus	Grand Rapids	1.2%	1742
Spectrum Health Big Rapids Hospital	Big Rapids	1.2%	338
Oakwood Hospital - Southshore	Trenton	1.3%	546

NOTE: Hospital profiles are in alphabetical order by state, then city, then hospital within the city; Rankings exclude hospitals with less than 25 cases except for patient surveys which excludes hospitals with less than 100 cases; (a) 100-299 cases; (1) The number of cases/patients is too few to report; (2) Data submitted were based on a sample of cases/patients; (3) Results are based on a shorter time period than required; (4) Data suppressed by CMS for one or more quarters; (5) Results are not available for this reporting period; (6) Fewer than 100 patients completed the HCAHPS survey; (7) No cases met the criteria for this measure; (8) The lower limit of the confidence interval cannot be calculated if the number of observed infections equals zero; (9) No data are available from the state/territory for this reporting period; (10) The scores shown reflect fewer than 50 completed surveys; (11) There were discrepancies in the data collection process; (12) This measure does not apply to this hospital for this reporting period; (13) Results cannot be calculated for this reporting period; (14) The results for this state are combined with nearby states to protect confidentiality; Please refer to the User's Guide for a full explanation of data.

Hospital Name	City	Rate	Cases
Aspirus Grand View Hospital	Ironwood	1.4%	147
Midmichigan Medical Center - Midland	Midland	1.4%	916
Dickinson County Memorial Hospital	Iron Mountain	1.5%	409
Baraga County Memorial Hospital	L'Anse	1.7%	58
Botsford Hospital	Farmington Hills	1.7%	898
Sinai - Grace Hospital	Detroit	1.7%	518
Spectrum Health - Reed City Campus	Reed City	1.7%	359
Memorial Medical Center of West Michigan	Ludington	1.8%	542
Sturgis Hospital	Sturgis	1.9%	214
Aspirus Keweenaw Hospital	Laurium	2.1%	96
Helen Newberry Joy Hospital	Newberry	2.1%	145
Mackinac Straits Hospital & Health Center	Saint Ignace	2.1%	143
Portage Health	Hancock	2.1%	188
Beaumont Health System	Royal Oak	2.2%	3884
Three Rivers Health	Three Rivers	2.2%	185
William Beaumont Hospital - Troy	Troy	2.2%	2523
Emma L Bixby Medical Center	Adrian	2.3%	347
Midmichigan Medical Center - Gladwin	Gladwin	2.3%	345
Midmichigan Medical Center - Clare	Clare	2.6%	385
Saint John Hospital & Medical Center	Detroit	2.7%	1130
Mercy Health Lakeshore Campus	Shelby	2.8%	71
Henry Ford Hospital	Detroit	2.9%	2480
Midmichigan Medical Center - Gratiot	Alma	2.9%	419
West Shore Medical Center	Manistee	2.9%	347
Saint Joseph Mercy Livingston Hospital	Howell	3.0%	832
Huron Valley - Sinai Hospital	Commerce Twp	3.1%	513
Munising Memorial Hospital	Munising	3.1%	96
Caro Community Hospital	Caro	3.4%	146
Henry Ford West Bloomfield Hospital	W Bloomfield	3.4%	907
Carson City Hospital	Carson City	3.5%	142
Chippewa County War Memorial Hospital	Sault Ste Marie	3.5%	282
Lakeland Community Hospital - Watervliet	Watervliet	3.7%	81
Borgess Medical Center	Kalamazoo	3.8%	841
Mclaren Bay Region	Bay City	3.8%	841
Saint Joseph Mercy Hospital	Ann Arbor	3.9%	1929
Spectrum Health Zeeland Comm Hosp	Zeeland	3.9%	77
Harbor Beach Community Hospital	Harbor Beach	4.2%	71
Hayes Green Beach Memorial Hospital	Charlotte	4.4%	159
Saint Mary Mercy Hospital	Livonia	4.7%	616
Mclaren Central Michigan	Mount Pleasant	4.9%	306
Metro Health Hospital	Wyoming	5.0%	516
Saint Francis Hospital	Escanaba	5.0%	281
Genesys Reg Med Ctr-Health Park	Grand Blanc	5.1%	454
Karmanos Cancer Center	Detroit	5.1%	2887
Mercy Health Hackley Campus	Muskegon	5.1%	369
Mercy Health Partners - Mercy Campus	Muskegon	5.3%	658
Allegan General Hospital	Allegan	5.5%	128
Bell Hospital	Ishpeming	5.6%	72
Oakwood Hospital - Dearborn	Dearborn	6.0%	1273
Alpena Regional Medical Center	Alpena	6.3%	819
Northstar Health System	Iron River	7.1%	127
Henry Ford Macomb Hospital	Clinton Twp	7.5%	867
St John Macomb-Oakland Hosp	Warren	7.7%	923
Mclaren Oakland	Pontiac	8.5%	388
Scheurer Hospital	Pigeon	8.6%	174
Saint Mary's Standish Community Hospital	Standish	8.7%	208
Oakwood Hospital - Wayne	Wayne	9.0%	499
Covenant Medical Center	Saginaw	9.7%	876
Community Health Center of Branch County	Coldwater	10.2%	266
Harper University Hospital	Detroit	10.9%	524
North Ottawa Community Health Center	Grand Haven	10.9%	192
Detroit Receiving Hosp & U Health Ctr	Detroit	12.6%	175
Saint Joseph Mercy Oakland	Pontiac	12.8%	635
Marquette General Hospital	Marquette	16.3%	386
Tawas Saint Joseph Hospital	Tawas City	18.8%	388
Mclaren Macomb	Mount Clemens	19.5%	922
Saint Mary's of Michigan Medical Center	Saginaw	23.8%	759
West Branch Regional Medical Center	West Branch	26.9%	726
Huron Medical Center	Bad Axe	29.2%	96
Hills & Dales General Hospital	Cass City	31.3%	128
Schoolcraft Memorial Hospital	Manistique	37.3%	102

Follow-up Mammogram/Ultrasound

A follow-up rate near zero may indicate missed cancer; a rate higher than 14% may mean there is unnecessary follow up.

Hospital Name	City	Rate	Cases
Baraga County Memorial Hospital	L'Anse	1.0%	201
Northstar Health System	Iron River	1.0%	289
West Branch Regional Medical Center	West Branch	2.4%	874
Spectrum Health Zeeland Comm Hosp	Zeeland	2.9%	350
Eaton Rapids Medical Center	Eaton Rapids	3.0%	266
Bell Hospital	Ishpeming	3.2%	603
Munising Memorial Hospital	Munising	3.3%	181
Bronson Battle Creek Hospital	Battle Creek	3.7%	2906
Bronson Lakeview Hospital	Paw Paw	3.7%	566
Mclaren - Greater Lansing	Lansing	3.7%	1925
Mclaren Bay Region	Bay City	3.7%	2499
Scheurer Hospital	Pigeon	3.7%	459
Allegiance Health	Jackson	3.8%	3420
Sparrow Clinton Hospital	Saint Johns	3.9%	334
Tawas Saint Joseph Hospital	Tawas City	4.0%	1216
Huron Medical Center	Bad Axe	4.1%	437
West Shore Medical Center	Manistee	4.2%	613
Doctors' Hospital of Michigan	Pontiac	4.3%	328
Mclaren Macomb	Mount Clemens	4.3%	1688
North Ottawa Community Health Center	Grand Haven	4.7%	705
Mercy Health Lakeshore Campus	Shelby	4.8%	435
Saint Mary's Health Care	Grand Rapids	4.9%	1998
Chippewa County War Memorial Hospital	Sault Ste Marie	5.0%	738
Lakeland Hospital - Saint Joseph	Saint Joseph	5.0%	3115
Saint John Hospital & Medical Center	Detroit	5.0%	4116
Marlette Regional Hospital	Marlette	5.1%	395
Three Rivers Health	Three Rivers	5.2%	324
Bronson Methodist Hospital	Kalamazoo	5.3%	1768
Midmichigan Medical Center - Gratiot	Alma	5.4%	1231
Sturgis Hospital	Sturgis	5.4%	537
Botsford Hospital	Farmington Hills	5.6%	1274
Mercy Health Hackley Campus	Muskegon	5.7%	1661
St John Macomb-Oakland Hosp	Warren	5.8%	2132
Dickinson County Memorial Hospital	Iron Mountain	5.9%	846
Mercy Health Partners - Mercy Campus	Muskegon	6.0%	2093
South Haven Community Hospital	South Haven	6.0%	420
Oaklawn Hospital	Marshall	6.2%	1150
Covenant Medical Center	Saginaw	6.3%	3726
Providence Hospital & Medical Centers	Southfield	6.3%	5415
Schoolcraft Memorial Hospital	Manistique	6.3%	382
Midmichigan Medical Center - Clare	Clare	6.7%	1071
Saint Mary's Standish Community Hospital	Standish	6.8%	337
Mclaren Oakland	Pontiac	6.9%	547
Alpena Regional Medical Center	Alpena	7.1%	2027
Mclaren Flint	Flint	7.1%	2478
Saint Francis Hospital	Escanaba	7.1%	828
Mclaren Central Michigan	Mount Pleasant	7.2%	572
Memorial Medical Center of West Michigan	Ludington	7.2%	1123
Emma L Bixby Medical Center	Adrian	7.3%	779
Mclaren - Northern Michigan	Petoskey	7.3%	2547
Hayes Green Beach Memorial Hospital	Charlotte	7.4%	448
Paul Oliver Memorial Hospital	Frankfort	7.4%	530
Saint Joseph Mercy Livingston Hospital	Howell	7.4%	1651
Edward W Sparrow Hospital	Lansing	7.5%	1954
Helen Newberry Joy Hospital	Newberry	7.5%	345
Henry Ford West Bloomfield Hospital	W Bloomfield	7.5%	1204
Saint Mary's of Michigan Medical Center	Saginaw	7.6%	1544
Borgess Medical Center	Kalamazoo	7.7%	2364
Deckerville Community Hospital	Deckerville	7.7%	91
Henry Ford Hospital	Detroit	7.7%	5424
Huron Valley - Sinai Hospital	Commerce Twp	7.7%	1156
Saint Joseph Mercy Hospital	Ann Arbor	7.7%	4728
Garden City Hospital	Garden City	7.8%	632
Kalkaska Memorial Health Center	Kalkaska	7.9%	522
Midmichigan Medical Center - Gladwin	Gladwin	7.9%	818
Pennock Hospital	Hastings	8.0%	841
Community Health Center of Branch County	Coldwater	8.1%	777
Oakwood Hospital - Dearborn	Dearborn	8.1%	2547
Spectrum Health United Mem-Kelsey Camp	Lakeview	8.2%	146
Midmichigan Medical Center - Midland	Midland	8.3%	2797
Sparrow Ionia Hospital	Ionia	8.3%	314
Mercy Hospital - Grayling	Grayling	8.4%	1064
Saint Joseph Mercy Oakland	Pontiac	8.4%	2344
Memorial Healthcare	Owosso	8.6%	1397
Spectrum Health United Memorial	Greenville	8.6%	814
University of Michigan Health System	Ann Arbor	8.8%	3808
Oakwood Hospital - Southshore	Trenton	8.9%	674
Charlevoix Area Hospital	Charlevoix	9.1%	308
Crittenton Hospital Medical Center	Rochester	9.1%	1764
Lakeland Community Hospital - Watervliet	Watervliet	9.1%	395
Mercy Memorial Hospital System	Monroe	9.2%	1365
Spectrum Health - Butterworth Campus	Grand Rapids	9.2%	4684
Hillsdale Community Health Center	Hillsdale	9.3%	767
Oakwood Hospital - Taylor	Taylor	9.3%	745
Munson Medical Center	Traverse City	9.5%	3778
Karmanos Cancer Center	Detroit	9.7%	4019
Mercy Hospital - Cadillac	Cadillac	9.7%	1020
Saint Mary Mercy Hospital	Livonia	9.8%	1535
Aspirus Ontonagon Hospital	Ontonagon	9.9%	162
Promedica Herrick Hospital	Tecumseh	9.9%	1082
Henry Ford Macomb Hospital	Clinton Twp	10.1%	2466
William Beaumont Hospital - Troy	Troy	10.2%	5505
Henry Ford Wyandotte Hospital	Wyandotte	10.4%	1608
Spectrum Health Gerber Memorial	Fremont	10.5%	770
Port Huron Hospital	Port Huron	10.7%	1680
Holland Community Hospital	Holland	10.8%	1367
Chelsea Community Hospital	Chelsea	10.9%	1161
Marquette General Hospital	Marquette	10.9%	1802
Allegan General Hospital	Allegan	11.1%	452
Mackinac Straits Hospital & Health Center	Saint Ignace	11.1%	316
Aspirus Keweenaw Hospital	Laurium	11.4%	237
Portage Health	Hancock	11.5%	530
Borgess - Lee Memorial Hospital	Dowagiac	12.0%	242
Spectrum Health - Reed City Campus	Reed City	12.1%	528
Sheridan Community Hospital	Sheridan	12.4%	186
McKenzie Health System	Sandusky	12.5%	208
Caro Community Hospital	Caro	12.6%	206
Sinai - Grace Hospital	Detroit	12.8%	1363
Oakwood Hospital - Wayne	Wayne	13.0%	1403
Metro Health Hospital	Wyoming	13.2%	1167
Spectrum Health Big Rapids Hospital	Big Rapids	13.2%	612
Otsego Memorial Hospital	Gaylord	13.3%	701
Carson City Hospital	Carson City	13.5%	490
Saint Joseph Mercy Port Huron	Port Huron	14.2%	824
Hurley Medical Center	Flint	14.5%	159
Mclaren Lapeer Region	Lapeer	14.9%	404
Harbor Beach Community Hospital	Harbor Beach	15.1%	106
Beaumont Health System	Grosse Pointe	15.3%	766
Beaumont Health System	Royal Oak	15.7%	8670
Genesys Reg Med Ctr-Health Park	Grand Blanc	17.5%	171
Aspirus Grand View Hospital	Ironwood	20.5%	303
Saint John River District Hospital	East China	20.5%	518
Hills & Dales General Hospital	Cass City	23.5%	166

Lumbar Spine MRI for Low Back Pain

Hospital Name	City	Rate	Cases
Beaumont Health System	Grosse Pointe	24.1%	145
Garden City Hospital	Garden City	25.3%	75
Hillsdale Community Health Center	Hillsdale	28.3%	99
Huron Valley - Sinai Hospital	Commerce Twp	28.4%	109
Hurley Medical Center	Flint	28.6%	63
Oakwood Hospital - Southshore	Trenton	28.6%	98
Harper University Hospital	Detroit	29.0%	193
Oaklawn Hospital	Marshall	29.1%	55
St John Macomb-Oakland Hosp	Warren	29.4%	197
Emma L Bixby Medical Center	Adrian	31.1%	190
Sinai - Grace Hospital	Detroit	31.4%	102
Saint Joseph Mercy Oakland	Pontiac	31.7%	186
William Beaumont Hospital - Troy	Troy	32.0%	535
Mclaren Flint	Flint	32.1%	405
Beaumont Health System	Royal Oak	32.2%	456
University of Michigan Health System	Ann Arbor	32.2%	273
Henry Ford Wyandotte Hospital	Wyandotte	32.5%	249
Midmichigan Medical Center - Midland	Midland	32.6%	427
Sturgis Hospital	Sturgis	32.7%	49
Munson Medical Center	Traverse City	32.8%	357
Chelsea Community Hospital	Chelsea	33.0%	176
Botsford Hospital	Farmington Hills	33.3%	54
Oakwood Hospital - Dearborn	Dearborn	33.3%	204
Bronson Methodist Hospital	Kalamazoo	33.5%	164
Port Huron Hospital	Port Huron	33.5%	188
Henry Ford Macomb Hospital	Clinton Twp	34.0%	194
Saint John Hospital & Medical Center	Detroit	34.0%	203
Mclaren Lapeer Region	Lapeer	34.4%	180
Saint Mary's Health Care	Grand Rapids	34.5%	200
Mercy Memorial Hospital System	Monroe	34.6%	107
Oakwood Hospital - Wayne	Wayne	34.6%	188
Mclaren - Northern Michigan	Petoskey	34.8%	221
Allegiance Health	Jackson	35.3%	380
Saint Mary's of Michigan Medical Center	Saginaw	35.3%	419
Memorial Healthcare	Owosso	35.4%	127
Genesys Reg Med Ctr-Health Park	Grand Blanc	35.7%	258
Saint Joseph Mercy Hospital	Ann Arbor	35.8%	534
Saint Joseph Mercy Livingston Hospital	Howell	36.0%	175
Community Health Center of Branch County	Coldwater	36.1%	61
Bronson Battle Creek Hospital	Battle Creek	36.2%	130
Borgess Medical Center	Kalamazoo	36.3%	620
Mclaren - Greater Lansing	Lansing	36.4%	173
Midmichigan Medical Center - Clare	Clare	36.4%	110
Midmichigan Medical Center - Gratiot	Alma	36.4%	77
Saint Mary Mercy Hospital	Livonia	36.7%	139
Mercy Hospital - Cadillac	Cadillac	36.9%	160
Lakeland Hospital - Saint Joseph	Saint Joseph	37.1%	248
Pennock Hospital	Hastings	37.2%	78
Charlevoix Area Hospital	Charlevoix	37.5%	48
Marquette General Hospital	Marquette	37.6%	213
Providence Hospital & Medical Centers	Southfield	37.6%	396
Sparrow Clinton Hospital	Saint Johns	37.7%	53
Three Rivers Health	Three Rivers	37.7%	53
Mclaren Bay Region	Bay City	37.9%	314
Mercy Health Partners - Mercy Campus	Muskegon	38.2%	424
Alpena Regional Medical Center	Alpena	38.9%	221
Hayes Green Beach Memorial Hospital	Charlotte	38.9%	54
Spectrum Health - Butterworth Campus	Grand Rapids	39.1%	524
Henry Ford Hospital	Detroit	39.5%	286
Covenant Medical Center	Saginaw	40.8%	377
Metro Health Hospital	Wyoming	40.8%	147
West Shore Medical Center	Manistee	41.0%	78
Memorial Medical Center of West Michigan	Ludington	41.1%	124
Oakwood Hospital - Taylor	Taylor	41.2%	51
Mercy Health Hackley Campus	Muskegon	41.5%	142
Mclaren Central Michigan	Mount Pleasant	41.8%	98
Henry Ford West Bloomfield Hospital	W Bloomfield	42.1%	121
Dickinson County Memorial Hospital	Iron Mountain	42.2%	161
Holland Community Hospital	Holland	42.3%	142
Chippewa County War Memorial Hospital	Sault Ste Marie	42.4%	118
Spectrum Health United Memorial	Greenville	42.9%	175

NOTE: Hospital profiles are in alphabetical order by state, then city, then hospital within the city; Rankings exclude hospitals with less than 25 cases except for patient surveys which excludes hospitals with less than 100 cases; (a) 100-299 cases; (1) The number of cases/patients is too few to report; (2) Data submitted were based on a sample of cases/patients; (3) Results are based on a shorter time period than required; (4) Data suppressed by CMS for one or more quarters; (5) Results are not available for this reporting period; (6) Fewer than 100 patients completed the HCAHPS survey; (7) No cases met the criteria for this measure; (8) The lower limit of the confidence interval cannot be calculated if the number of observed infections equals zero; (9) No data are available from the state/territory for this reporting period; (10) The scores shown reflect fewer than 50 completed surveys; (11) There were discrepancies in the data collection process; (12) This measure does not apply to this hospital for this reporting period; (13) Results cannot be calculated for this reporting period; (14) The results for this state are combined with nearby states to protect confidentiality; Please refer to the User's Guide for a full explanation of data.

Saint Francis Hospital	Escanaba	43.4%	106
Midmichigan Medical Center - Gladwin	Gladwin	43.8%	89
Bell Hospital	Ishpeming	44.4%	36
Spectrum Health Big Rapids Hospital	Big Rapids	44.4%	99
Saint Mary's Standish Community Hospital	Standish	44.8%	67
Carson City Hospital	Carson City	45.3%	106
Aspirus Grand View Hospital	Ironwood	45.7%	35
Tawas Saint Joseph Hospital	Tawas City	47.3%	131
Otsego Memorial Hospital	Gaylord	48.4%	161
Mercy Hospital - Grayling	Grayling	49.2%	126
Helen Newberry Joy Hospital	Newberry	50.0%	34
Kalkaska Memorial Health Center	Kalkaska	51.8%	56
West Branch Regional Medical Center	West Branch	53.1%	160
Portage Health	Hancock	53.2%	62
Allegan General Hospital	Allegan	58.5%	41
Spectrum Health - Reed City Campus	Reed City	59.0%	100
Spectrum Health Gerber Memorial	Fremont	59.3%	108
Bronson Lakeview Hospital	Paw Paw	62.1%	58

NOTE: Hospital profiles are in alphabetical order by state, then city, then hospital within the city; Rankings exclude hospitals with less than 25 cases except for patient surveys which excludes hospitals with less than 100 cases; (a) 100-299 cases; (1) The number of cases/patients is too few to report; (2) Data submitted were based on a sample of cases/patients; (3) Results are based on a shorter time period than required; (4) Data suppressed by CMS for one or more quarters; (5) Results are not available for this reporting period; (6) Fewer than 100 patients completed the HCAHPS survey; (7) No cases met the criteria for this measure; (8) The lower limit of the confidence interval cannot be calculated if the number of observed infections equals zero; (9) No data are available from the state/territory for this reporting period; (10) The scores shown reflect fewer than 50 completed surveys; (11) There were discrepancies in the data collection process; (12) This measure does not apply to this hospital for this reporting period; (13) Results cannot be calculated for this reporting period; (14) The results for this state are combined with nearby states to protect confidentiality; Please refer to the User's Guide for a full explanation of data.

Emma L Bixby Medical Center

818 Riverside Avenue
Adrian, MI 49221
URL: www.promedica.org
Type: Acute Care Hospitals
Ownership: Voluntary non-profit - Private
Phone: 517-265-0900
Fax: 517-265-0918
Emergency Services: Yes
Beds: 88

Key Personnel:
Operating Room. . . . . Abdul Arshad
CEO/President. . . . . Randy Oostra
Patient Relations . . . . Sheila Schwartz
Quality Assurance . . . . Linda Yielding

Measure	Cases	This Hosp.	State Avg.	U.S. Avg.
Blood Clot Prevention and Treatment				
Anticoagulation Overlap Therapy[2]	26	96%	90%	93%
ICU Venous Thromboembolism Prophylaxis[2]	82	93%	93%	92%
Incidence of Potentially Preventable VTE[1,2]	-	-	8%	10%
UFH with Dosages/Platelet Monitoring[2]	21	100%	96%	97%
Venous Thromboembolism Prophylaxis[2]	229	90%	87%	85%
Warfarin Therapy Discharge Instructions[2]	16	12%	72%	75%
Chest Pain/Possible Heart Attack Care				
Aspirin Given Within 24 Hours of Arrival	188	96%	96%	96%
Fibrinolytic Meds Within 30 Min. of Arrival[1]	-	-	63%	58%
Average Time to ECG (minutes)	191	6	8	7
Average Time to Transfer (minutes)[1]	-	-	53	60
Children's Asthma Care				
Received Home Management Plan of Care	-	-	-	88%
Received Reliever Medication	-	-	-	100%
Received Systemic Corticosteroids	-	-	-	100%
Emergency Department				
Admittance Decision Time (minutes)[2]	414	102	102	98
Head CT Results Within 45 Min. of Arrival	18	22%	54%	57%
Patients Who Left ER Before Being Seen	34,185	1%	2%	2%
Time from ER Arrival to Admit. (minutes)[2]	414	262	288	274
Time from ER Arrival to Discharge (minutes)	326	91	128	134
Time in ER Before Being Evaluated (minutes)	382	6	22	26
Time to Pain Meds for Fractures (minutes)	172	53	55	57
Heart Attack Care				
Aspirin Given at Discharge	17	94%	99%	99%
Fibrinolytic Meds Within 30 Min. of Arrival[7]	-	-	20%	54%
PCI Within 90 Minutes of Arrival[7]	-	-	95%	96%
Statin Prescribed at Discharge	16	75%	98%	98%
Heart Failure Care				
ACE Inhibitor or ARB for LVSD	21	95%	96%	97%
Discharge Instructions Given	69	77%	94%	94%
Evaluation of LVS Function	104	100%	99%	99%
Medicare Spending				
Medicare Spending per Patient (ratio)	-	0.95	0.96	0.98
Pneumonia Care				
Appropriate Initial Antibiotic Given[2]	75	99%	96%	95%
Blood Culture Timing[2]	162	100%	98%	98%
Pregnancy and Delivery Care				
Newborn Deliveries Scheduled Early[2]	26	4%	3%	6%
Preventive Care				
Immunization for Influenza[2]	369	91%	89%	90%
Immunization for Pneumonia[2]	430	91%	90%	92%
Stroke Care				
Anticoagulation Therapy for Atrial Fibrillation[1]	-	-	92%	95%
Antithrombotic Therapy Timing	36	97%	97%	98%
Assessed for Rehabilitation	39	100%	97%	97%
Discharged on Antithrombotic Therapy	39	100%	99%	99%
Discharged on Statin Medication	32	84%	94%	94%
Thrombolytic Therapy Timing[1]	-	-	69%	66%
Venous Thromboembolism Prophylaxis	43	95%	94%	94%
Written Stroke Educational Materials Given	20	80%	87%	88%
Surgical Care Improvement Project				
Appropriate Beta Blocker Usage[2]	85	95%	98%	98%
Appropriate VTP Within 24 Hours[2]	275	96%	98%	98%
Controlled Postoperative Blood Glucose[2,7]	-	-	97%	97%
Perioperative Temperature Management[2]	308	99%	100%	100%
Prophylactic Antibiotic Selection[2]	210	98%	99%	99%
Prophylactic Antibiotic Selection (Outpatient)	127	96%	97%	98%
Prophylactic Antibiotic Stopped[2]	205	95%	98%	98%
Prophylactic Antibiotic Timing[2]	210	100%	98%	99%
Prophylactic Antibiotic Timing (Outpatient)	128	96%	97%	98%
Urinary Catheter Removal[2]	188	93%	97%	97%
Survey of Patients' Hospital Experiences				
Area Around Room 'Always' Quiet at Night	300+	61%	60%	61%
Doctors 'Always' Communicated Well	300+	84%	81%	82%
Home Recovery Information Given	300+	88%	87%	85%
Hospital Given 9 or 10 on 10 Point Scale	300+	69%	71%	71%
Meds 'Always' Explained Before Given	300+	64%	64%	64%
Nurses 'Always' Communicated Well	300+	79%	80%	79%
Pain 'Always' Well Controlled	300+	71%	71%	71%
Room and Bathroom 'Always' Clean	300+	71%	73%	73%
Timely Help 'Always' Received	300+	66%	70%	68%
Would Definitely Recommend Hospital	300+	65%	71%	71%
Use of Medical Imaging				
Cardiac Imaging Stress Test before Surgery	267	3.4%	5.1%	5.3%
Combination Abdominal CT Scan	587	4.8%	8.7%	10.5%
Combination Brain/Sinus CT Scan	574	2.3%	2.2%	2.7%
Combination Chest CT Scan	347	2.3%	3.6%	2.7%
Follow-up Mammogram/Ultrasound	779	7.3%	8.2%	8.8%
Lumbar Spine MRI for Low Back Pain	190	31.1%	36.9%	37.2%

Allegan General Hospital

555 Linn Street
Allegan, MI 49010
Type: Critical Access Hospitals
Ownership: Voluntary non-profit - Other
Phone: 269-686-4101
Fax: 269-673-4344
Emergency Services: Yes
Beds: 63

Key Personnel:
CEO/President. . . . . Gerald Barbins
Infection Control. . . . . Sandra Brenner
Quality Assurance . . . . Linda Curry
Patient Relations . . . . Grace Gant
Emergency Room . . . . Timothy Hall
Intensive Care Unit. . . . . Timothy Hall
Anesthesiology. . . . . Kenneth Whitcomb
Operating Room. . . . . Phyllis Wilson

Measure	Cases	This Hosp.	State Avg.	U.S. Avg.
Blood Clot Prevention and Treatment				
Anticoagulation Overlap Therapy[5]	-	-	90%	93%
ICU Venous Thromboembolism Prophylaxis[5]	-	-	93%	92%
Incidence of Potentially Preventable VTE[5]	-	-	8%	10%
UFH with Dosages/Platelet Monitoring[5]	-	-	96%	97%
Venous Thromboembolism Prophylaxis[5]	-	-	87%	85%
Warfarin Therapy Discharge Instructions[5]	-	-	72%	75%
Chest Pain/Possible Heart Attack Care				
Aspirin Given Within 24 Hours of Arrival	58	93%	96%	96%
Fibrinolytic Meds Within 30 Min. of Arrival[7]	-	-	63%	58%
Average Time to ECG (minutes)	60	11	8	7
Average Time to Transfer (minutes)[1]	-	-	53	60
Children's Asthma Care				
Received Home Management Plan of Care	-	-	-	88%
Received Reliever Medication	-	-	-	100%
Received Systemic Corticosteroids	-	-	-	100%
Emergency Department				
Admittance Decision Time (minutes)[5]	-	-	102	98
Head CT Results Within 45 Min. of Arrival[5]	-	-	54%	57%
Patients Who Left ER Before Being Seen[5]	-	-	2%	2%
Time from ER Arrival to Admit. (minutes)[5]	-	-	288	274
Time from ER Arrival to Discharge (minutes)	361	128	128	134
Time in ER Before Being Evaluated (minutes)	444	28	22	26
Time to Pain Meds for Fractures (minutes)[5]	-	-	55	57
Heart Attack Care				
Aspirin Given at Discharge[1]	-	-	99%	99%
Fibrinolytic Meds Within 30 Min. of Arrival[7]	-	-	20%	54%
PCI Within 90 Minutes of Arrival[7]	-	-	95%	96%
Statin Prescribed at Discharge[1]	-	-	98%	98%
Heart Failure Care				
ACE Inhibitor or ARB for LVSD[1]	-	-	96%	97%
Discharge Instructions Given	31	97%	94%	94%
Evaluation of LVS Function	36	100%	99%	99%
Medicare Spending				
Medicare Spending per Patient (ratio)	-	-	0.96	0.98
Pneumonia Care				
Appropriate Initial Antibiotic Given	56	100%	96%	95%
Blood Culture Timing	68	97%	98%	98%
Pregnancy and Delivery Care				
Newborn Deliveries Scheduled Early[5]	-	-	3%	6%
Preventive Care				
Immunization for Influenza	165	92%	89%	90%
Immunization for Pneumonia	263	92%	90%	92%
Stroke Care				
Anticoagulation Therapy for Atrial Fibrillation[5]	-	-	92%	95%
Antithrombotic Therapy Timing[5]	-	-	97%	98%
Assessed for Rehabilitation[5]	-	-	97%	97%
Discharged on Antithrombotic Therapy[5]	-	-	99%	99%
Discharged on Statin Medication[5]	-	-	94%	94%
Thrombolytic Therapy Timing[5]	-	-	69%	66%
Venous Thromboembolism Prophylaxis[5]	-	-	94%	94%
Written Stroke Educational Materials Given[5]	-	-	87%	88%
Surgical Care Improvement Project				
Appropriate Beta Blocker Usage	35	94%	98%	98%
Appropriate VTP Within 24 Hours	146	99%	98%	98%
Controlled Postoperative Blood Glucose[7]	-	-	97%	97%
Perioperative Temperature Management	162	100%	100%	100%
Prophylactic Antibiotic Selection	129	98%	99%	99%
Prophylactic Antibiotic Selection (Outpatient)[5]	-	-	97%	98%
Prophylactic Antibiotic Stopped	126	95%	98%	98%
Prophylactic Antibiotic Timing	129	97%	98%	99%
Prophylactic Antibiotic Timing (Outpatient)[5]	-	-	97%	98%
Urinary Catheter Removal	45	98%	97%	97%
Survey of Patients' Hospital Experiences				
Area Around Room 'Always' Quiet at Night	(a)	72%	60%	61%
Doctors 'Always' Communicated Well	(a)	85%	81%	82%
Home Recovery Information Given	(a)	90%	87%	85%
Hospital Given 9 or 10 on 10 Point Scale	(a)	83%	71%	71%
Meds 'Always' Explained Before Given	(a)	69%	64%	64%
Nurses 'Always' Communicated Well	(a)	85%	80%	79%
Pain 'Always' Well Controlled	(a)	79%	71%	71%
Room and Bathroom 'Always' Clean	(a)	81%	73%	73%
Timely Help 'Always' Received	(a)	77%	70%	68%
Would Definitely Recommend Hospital	(a)	75%	71%	71%
Use of Medical Imaging				
Cardiac Imaging Stress Test before Surgery	113	7.1%	5.1%	5.3%
Combination Abdominal CT Scan	282	5.3%	8.7%	10.5%
Combination Brain/Sinus CT Scan[1]	-	-	2.2%	2.7%
Combination Chest CT Scan	128	5.5%	3.6%	2.7%
Follow-up Mammogram/Ultrasound	452	11.1%	8.2%	8.8%
Lumbar Spine MRI for Low Back Pain	41	58.5%	36.9%	37.2%

Midmichigan Medical Center - Gratiot

300 E Warwick Dr
Alma, MI 48801
URL: www.midmichigan.org
Type: Acute Care Hospitals
Ownership: Voluntary non-profit - Private
Phone: 989-463-1101
Fax: 989-463-6948
Emergency Services: Yes
Beds: 142

Key Personnel:
Radiology. . . . . Johannes Buiteweg
Patient Relations . . . . Penny Daniels
Infection Control. . . . . Janet Davis, RN
CEO/President. . . . . Tom Desauw
Quality Assurance . . . . Jill Goodell
Intensive Care Unit. . . . . Glenn King, RN
Emergency Room . . . . Kim Noreen, RN
Operating Room. . . . . Tammy Terrell, RN

Measure	Cases	This Hosp.	State Avg.	U.S. Avg.
Blood Clot Prevention and Treatment				
Anticoagulation Overlap Therapy[2]	18	56%	90%	93%
ICU Venous Thromboembolism Prophylaxis[2]	64	84%	93%	92%
Incidence of Potentially Preventable VTE[1,2]	-	-	8%	10%
UFH with Dosages/Platelet Monitoring[2]	11	100%	96%	97%
Venous Thromboembolism Prophylaxis[2]	346	80%	87%	85%
Warfarin Therapy Discharge Instructions[2]	14	86%	72%	75%
Chest Pain/Possible Heart Attack Care				
Aspirin Given Within 24 Hours of Arrival	110	98%	96%	96%
Fibrinolytic Meds Within 30 Min. of Arrival[1]	-	-	63%	58%
Average Time to ECG (minutes)	116	8	8	7
Average Time to Transfer (minutes)[1]	-	-	53	60
Children's Asthma Care				
Received Home Management Plan of Care	-	-	-	88%

NOTE: Hospital profiles are in alphabetical order by state, then city, then hospital within the city; Rankings exclude hospitals with less than 25 cases except for patient surveys which excludes hospitals with less than 100 cases; (a) 100-299 cases; (1) The number of cases/patients is too few to report; (2) Data submitted were based on a sample of cases/patients; (3) Results are based on a shorter time period than required; (4) Data suppressed by CMS for one or more quarters; (5) Results are not available for this reporting period; (6) Fewer than 100 patients completed the HCAHPS survey; (7) No cases met the criteria for this measure; (8) The lower limit of the confidence interval cannot be calculated if the number of observed infections equals zero; (9) No data are available from the state/territory for this reporting period; (10) The scores shown reflect fewer than 50 completed surveys; (11) There were discrepancies in the data collection process; (12) This measure does not apply to this hospital for this reporting period; (13) Results cannot be calculated for this reporting period; (14) The results for this state are combined with nearby states to protect confidentiality; Please refer to the User's Guide for a full explanation of data.

Measure	Cases	This Hosp.	State Avg.	U.S. Avg.
Received Reliever Medication	-	-	-	100%
Received Systemic Corticosteroids	-	-	-	100%
Emergency Department				
Admittance Decision Time (minutes)[2]	428	70	102	98
Head CT Results Within 45 Min. of Arrival	18	44%	54%	57%
Patients Who Left ER Before Being Seen	21,483	1%	2%	2%
Time from ER Arrival to Admit. (minutes)[2]	477	257	288	274
Time from ER Arrival to Discharge (minutes)	427	161	128	134
Time in ER Before Being Evaluated (minutes)	320	31	22	26
Time to Pain Meds for Fractures (minutes)	81	68	55	57
Heart Attack Care				
Aspirin Given at Discharge	30	93%	99%	99%
Fibrinolytic Meds Within 30 Min. of Arrival[7]	-	-	20%	54%
PCI Within 90 Minutes of Arrival[7]	-	-	95%	96%
Statin Prescribed at Discharge	33	61%	98%	98%
Heart Failure Care				
ACE Inhibitor or ARB for LVSD	31	97%	96%	97%
Discharge Instructions Given	132	90%	94%	94%
Evaluation of LVS Function	174	99%	99%	99%
Medicare Spending				
Medicare Spending per Patient (ratio)	-	0.97	0.96	0.98
Pneumonia Care				
Appropriate Initial Antibiotic Given	64	98%	96%	95%
Blood Culture Timing	104	96%	98%	98%
Pregnancy and Delivery Care				
Newborn Deliveries Scheduled Early[2]	68	10%	3%	6%
Preventive Care				
Immunization for Influenza[2]	448	60%	89%	90%
Immunization for Pneumonia[2]	568	76%	90%	92%
Stroke Care				
Anticoagulation Therapy for Atrial Fibrillation[1]	-	-	92%	95%
Antithrombotic Therapy Timing	34	97%	97%	98%
Assessed for Rehabilitation	33	91%	97%	97%
Discharged on Antithrombotic Therapy	33	100%	99%	99%
Discharged on Statin Medication	26	81%	94%	94%
Thrombolytic Therapy Timing[1]	-	-	69%	66%
Venous Thromboembolism Prophylaxis	31	90%	94%	94%
Written Stroke Educational Materials Given	16	75%	87%	88%
Surgical Care Improvement Project				
Appropriate Beta Blocker Usage	92	98%	98%	98%
Appropriate VTP Within 24 Hours	204	97%	98%	98%
Controlled Postoperative Blood Glucose[7]	-	-	97%	97%
Perioperative Temperature Management	261	98%	100%	100%
Prophylactic Antibiotic Selection	183	85%	99%	99%
Prophylactic Antibiotic Selection (Outpatient)	71	97%	97%	98%
Prophylactic Antibiotic Stopped	175	95%	98%	98%
Prophylactic Antibiotic Timing	185	92%	98%	99%
Prophylactic Antibiotic Timing (Outpatient)	88	75%	97%	98%
Urinary Catheter Removal	178	95%	97%	97%
Survey of Patients' Hospital Experiences				
Area Around Room 'Always' Quiet at Night	300+	64%	60%	61%
Doctors 'Always' Communicated Well	300+	82%	81%	82%
Home Recovery Information Given	300+	90%	87%	85%
Hospital Given 9 or 10 on 10 Point Scale	300+	74%	71%	71%
Meds 'Always' Explained Before Given	300+	64%	64%	64%
Nurses 'Always' Communicated Well	300+	80%	80%	79%
Pain 'Always' Well Controlled	300+	70%	71%	71%
Room and Bathroom 'Always' Clean	300+	73%	73%	73%
Timely Help 'Always' Received	300+	66%	70%	68%
Would Definitely Recommend Hospital	300+	73%	71%	71%
Use of Medical Imaging				
Cardiac Imaging Stress Test before Surgery	92	4.3%	5.1%	5.3%
Combination Abdominal CT Scan	564	9.9%	8.7%	10.5%
Combination Brain/Sinus CT Scan	517	2.5%	2.2%	2.7%
Combination Chest CT Scan	419	2.9%	3.6%	2.7%
Follow-up Mammogram/Ultrasound	1,231	5.4%	8.2%	8.8%
Lumbar Spine MRI for Low Back Pain	77	36.4%	36.9%	37.2%

Alpena Regional Medical Center

1501 W Chisholm St
Alpena, MI 49707
Phone: 989-356-7390
Fax: 989-356-7773
E-mail: info@agh.org
URL: www.agh.org
Type: Acute Care Hospitals
Emergency Services: Yes
Ownership: Proprietary
Beds: 146

Key Personnel:
Anesthesiology. . . . . John Banish, MD
CEO/President. . . . . John McVeety
Chair/CEO . . . . Eric Smith
Pediatric Ambulatory Care . . . . . . Richard F Willis, MD

Measure	Cases	This Hosp.	State Avg.	U.S. Avg.
Blood Clot Prevention and Treatment				
Anticoagulation Overlap Therapy[2]	28	86%	90%	93%
ICU Venous Thromboembolism Prophylaxis[2]	48	98%	93%	92%
Incidence of Potentially Preventable VTE[1,2]	-	-	8%	10%
UFH with Dosages/Platelet Monitoring[2]	26	100%	96%	97%
Venous Thromboembolism Prophylaxis[2]	334	94%	87%	85%
Warfarin Therapy Discharge Instructions[2]	23	87%	72%	75%
Chest Pain/Possible Heart Attack Care				
Aspirin Given Within 24 Hours of Arrival	95	100%	96%	96%
Fibrinolytic Meds Within 30 Min. of Arrival	16	75%	63%	58%
Average Time to ECG (minutes)	95	8	8	7
Average Time to Transfer (minutes)[1]	-	-	53	60
Children's Asthma Care				
Received Home Management Plan of Care	-	-	-	88%
Received Reliever Medication	-	-	-	100%
Received Systemic Corticosteroids	-	-	-	100%
Emergency Department				
Admittance Decision Time (minutes)[2]	589	114	102	98
Head CT Results Within 45 Min. of Arrival[1]	-	-	54%	57%
Patients Who Left ER Before Being Seen	22,540	1%	2%	2%
Time from ER Arrival to Admit. (minutes)[2]	601	272	288	274
Time from ER Arrival to Discharge (minutes)	388	139	128	134
Time in ER Before Being Evaluated (minutes)	336	46	22	26
Time to Pain Meds for Fractures (minutes)	111	73	55	57
Heart Attack Care				
Aspirin Given at Discharge	26	100%	99%	99%
Fibrinolytic Meds Within 30 Min. of Arrival[1]	-	-	20%	54%
PCI Within 90 Minutes of Arrival[7]	-	-	95%	96%
Statin Prescribed at Discharge	23	96%	98%	98%
Heart Failure Care				
ACE Inhibitor or ARB for LVSD	26	92%	96%	97%
Discharge Instructions Given	137	91%	94%	94%
Evaluation of LVS Function	162	100%	99%	99%
Medicare Spending				
Medicare Spending per Patient (ratio)	-	1.02	0.96	0.98
Pneumonia Care				
Appropriate Initial Antibiotic Given	140	93%	96%	95%
Blood Culture Timing	222	97%	98%	98%
Pregnancy and Delivery Care				
Newborn Deliveries Scheduled Early[2]	24	12%	3%	6%
Preventive Care				
Immunization for Influenza[2]	415	98%	89%	90%
Immunization for Pneumonia[2]	603	96%	90%	92%
Stroke Care				
Anticoagulation Therapy for Atrial Fibrillation	18	100%	92%	95%
Antithrombotic Therapy Timing	61	95%	97%	98%
Assessed for Rehabilitation	69	93%	97%	97%
Discharged on Antithrombotic Therapy	67	96%	99%	99%
Discharged on Statin Medication	54	94%	94%	94%
Thrombolytic Therapy Timing	12	75%	69%	66%
Venous Thromboembolism Prophylaxis	69	96%	94%	94%
Written Stroke Educational Materials Given	32	19%	87%	88%
Surgical Care Improvement Project				
Appropriate Beta Blocker Usage[2]	123	98%	98%	98%
Appropriate VTP Within 24 Hours[2]	293	98%	98%	98%
Controlled Postoperative Blood Glucose[2,7]	-	-	97%	97%
Perioperative Temperature Management[2]	341	100%	100%	100%
Prophylactic Antibiotic Selection[2]	244	98%	99%	99%
Prophylactic Antibiotic Selection (Outpatient)	137	93%	97%	98%
Prophylactic Antibiotic Stopped[2]	225	98%	98%	98%
Prophylactic Antibiotic Timing[2]	244	98%	98%	99%
Prophylactic Antibiotic Timing (Outpatient)	139	92%	97%	98%
Urinary Catheter Removal[2]	197	94%	97%	97%
Survey of Patients' Hospital Experiences				
Area Around Room 'Always' Quiet at Night	300+	45%	60%	61%
Doctors 'Always' Communicated Well	300+	78%	81%	82%
Home Recovery Information Given	300+	87%	87%	85%
Hospital Given 9 or 10 on 10 Point Scale	300+	62%	71%	71%
Meds 'Always' Explained Before Given	300+	57%	64%	64%
Nurses 'Always' Communicated Well	300+	77%	80%	79%
Pain 'Always' Well Controlled	300+	67%	71%	71%
Room and Bathroom 'Always' Clean	300+	74%	73%	73%
Timely Help 'Always' Received	300+	75%	70%	68%
Would Definitely Recommend Hospital	300+	58%	71%	71%
Use of Medical Imaging				
Cardiac Imaging Stress Test before Surgery	343	4.1%	5.1%	5.3%
Combination Abdominal CT Scan	1,023	17.8%	8.7%	10.5%
Combination Brain/Sinus CT Scan	692	1.4%	2.2%	2.7%
Combination Chest CT Scan	819	6.3%	3.6%	2.7%
Follow-up Mammogram/Ultrasound	2,027	7.1%	8.2%	8.8%
Lumbar Spine MRI for Low Back Pain	221	38.9%	36.9%	37.2%

Saint Joseph Mercy Hospital

5301 E Huron River Dr
Ann Arbor, MI 48106
Phone: 734-712-3791
Fax: 734-712-7133
URL: www.stjoesannarbor.or
Type: Acute Care Hospitals
Emergency Services: No
Ownership: Voluntary non-profit - Church
Beds: 581

Key Personnel:
Quality Assurance . . . . Dolores Adroiune
Chief of Medical Staff. . . . . Rossana DGrood
Operating Room. . . . . Harriet Hnis
Emergency Room . . . . John McCabe, MD
Cardiac Laboratory. . . . . Mary Poskie

Measure	Cases	This Hosp.	State Avg.	U.S. Avg.
Blood Clot Prevention and Treatment				
Anticoagulation Overlap Therapy[2]	261	95%	90%	93%
ICU Venous Thromboembolism Prophylaxis[2]	51	96%	93%	92%
Incidence of Potentially Preventable VTE[2]	42	7%	8%	10%
UFH with Dosages/Platelet Monitoring[2]	290	100%	96%	97%
Venous Thromboembolism Prophylaxis[2]	403	91%	87%	85%
Warfarin Therapy Discharge Instructions[2]	208	25%	72%	75%
Chest Pain/Possible Heart Attack Care				
Aspirin Given Within 24 Hours of Arrival	22	77%	96%	96%
Fibrinolytic Meds Within 30 Min. of Arrival[3,7]	-	-	63%	58%
Average Time to ECG (minutes)	24	12	8	7
Average Time to Transfer (minutes)[3,7]	-	-	53	60
Children's Asthma Care				
Received Home Management Plan of Care	-	-	-	88%
Received Reliever Medication	-	-	-	100%
Received Systemic Corticosteroids	-	-	-	100%
Emergency Department				
Admittance Decision Time (minutes)[2]	583	112	102	98
Head CT Results Within 45 Min. of Arrival	12	58%	54%	57%
Patients Who Left ER Before Being Seen	97,263	2%	2%	2%
Time from ER Arrival to Admit. (minutes)[2]	594	337	288	274
Time from ER Arrival to Discharge (minutes)	403	163	128	134
Time in ER Before Being Evaluated (minutes)	482	20	22	26
Time to Pain Meds for Fractures (minutes)	242	56	55	57
Heart Attack Care				
Aspirin Given at Discharge	690	100%	99%	99%
Fibrinolytic Meds Within 30 Min. of Arrival[7]	-	-	20%	54%
PCI Within 90 Minutes of Arrival	94	95%	95%	96%
Statin Prescribed at Discharge	681	100%	98%	98%
Heart Failure Care				
ACE Inhibitor or ARB for LVSD	181	99%	96%	97%
Discharge Instructions Given	613	98%	94%	94%
Evaluation of LVS Function	758	100%	99%	99%
Medicare Spending				
Medicare Spending per Patient (ratio)	-	0.97	0.96	0.98
Pneumonia Care				
Appropriate Initial Antibiotic Given	287	95%	96%	95%
Blood Culture Timing	378	98%	98%	98%
Pregnancy and Delivery Care				

NOTE: Hospital profiles are in alphabetical order by state, then city, then hospital within the city; Rankings exclude hospitals with less than 25 cases except for patient surveys which excludes hospitals with less than 100 cases; (a) 100-299 cases; (1) The number of cases/patients is too few to report; (2) Data submitted were based on a sample of cases/patients; (3) Results are based on a shorter time period than required; (4) Data suppressed by CMS for one or more quarters; (5) Results are not available for this reporting period; (6) Fewer than 100 patients completed the HCAHPS survey; (7) No cases met the criteria for this measure; (8) The lower limit of the confidence interval cannot be calculated if the number of observed infections equals zero; (9) No data are available from the state/territory for this reporting period; (10) The scores shown reflect fewer than 50 completed surveys; (11) There were discrepancies in the data collection process; (12) This measure does not apply to this hospital for this reporting period; (13) Results cannot be calculated for this reporting period; (14) The results for this state are combined with nearby states to protect confidentiality; Please refer to the User's Guide for a full explanation of data.

Measure	Cases	This Hosp.	State Avg.	U.S. Avg.
Newborn Deliveries Scheduled Early[2]	56	2%	3%	6%
Preventive Care				
Immunization for Influenza[2]	623	91%	89%	90%
Immunization for Pneumonia[2]	769	94%	90%	92%
Stroke Care				
Anticoagulation Therapy for Atrial Fibrillation[1,2]	-	-	92%	95%
Antithrombotic Therapy Timing[2]	75	99%	97%	98%
Assessed for Rehabilitation[2]	106	97%	97%	97%
Discharged on Antithrombotic Therapy[2]	96	100%	99%	99%
Discharged on Statin Medication[2]	82	100%	94%	94%
Thrombolytic Therapy Timing[2]	17	76%	69%	66%
Venous Thromboembolism Prophylaxis[2]	98	97%	94%	94%
Written Stroke Educational Materials Given[2]	53	89%	87%	88%
Surgical Care Improvement Project				
Appropriate Beta Blocker Usage[2]	692	99%	98%	98%
Appropriate VTP Within 24 Hours[2]	1,625	98%	98%	98%
Controlled Postoperative Blood Glucose[2]	170	99%	97%	97%
Perioperative Temperature Management[2]	1,878	100%	100%	100%
Prophylactic Antibiotic Selection[2]	1,741	99%	99%	99%
Prophylactic Antibiotic Selection (Outpatient)	1,193	98%	97%	98%
Prophylactic Antibiotic Stopped[2]	1,702	99%	98%	98%
Prophylactic Antibiotic Timing[2]	1,743	99%	98%	99%
Prophylactic Antibiotic Timing (Outpatient)	1,173	98%	97%	98%
Urinary Catheter Removal[2]	1,715	98%	97%	97%
Survey of Patients' Hospital Experiences				
Area Around Room 'Always' Quiet at Night	300+	57%	60%	61%
Doctors 'Always' Communicated Well	300+	77%	81%	82%
Home Recovery Information Given	300+	87%	87%	85%
Hospital Given 9 or 10 on 10 Point Scale	300+	79%	71%	71%
Meds 'Always' Explained Before Given	300+	60%	64%	64%
Nurses 'Always' Communicated Well	300+	79%	80%	79%
Pain 'Always' Well Controlled	300+	70%	71%	71%
Room and Bathroom 'Always' Clean	300+	68%	73%	73%
Timely Help 'Always' Received	300+	64%	70%	68%
Would Definitely Recommend Hospital	300+	81%	71%	71%
Use of Medical Imaging				
Cardiac Imaging Stress Test before Surgery	2,341	3.7%	5.1%	5.3%
Combination Abdominal CT Scan	2,275	7.3%	8.7%	10.5%
Combination Brain/Sinus CT Scan	1,116	1.4%	2.2%	2.7%
Combination Chest CT Scan	1,929	3.9%	3.6%	2.7%
Follow-up Mammogram/Ultrasound	4,728	7.7%	8.2%	8.8%
Lumbar Spine MRI for Low Back Pain	534	35.8%	36.9%	37.2%

University of Michigan Health System

1500 E Medical Center Drive, Spc 5474 Phone: 734-764-1505
Ann Arbor, MI 48109
URL: www.med.umich.edu
Type: Acute Care Hospitals Emergency Services: Yes
Ownership: Voluntary non-profit - Private Beds: 930

Key Personnel:

Quality Assurance . . . . S Anderson
Chief of Medical Staff. . . . . D Campbell, MD
Pediatric Ambulatory Care . . . . . . Valerie Castle, MD
Operating Room. . . . . Sheri Dufek
Radiology. . . . . N Reed Dunnick, MD
Infection Control. . . . . Candace Friedman, MPH
CEO/President. . . . . Ora Hirsch Pescovitz, MD

Measure	Cases	This Hosp.	State Avg.	U.S. Avg.
Blood Clot Prevention and Treatment				
Anticoagulation Overlap Therapy[2]	233	98%	90%	93%
ICU Venous Thromboembolism Prophylaxis[2]	85	99%	93%	92%
Incidence of Potentially Preventable VTE[2]	84	4%	8%	10%
UFH with Dosages/Platelet Monitoring[2]	287	97%	96%	97%
Venous Thromboembolism Prophylaxis[2]	359	97%	87%	85%
Warfarin Therapy Discharge Instructions[2]	180	82%	72%	75%
Chest Pain/Possible Heart Attack Care				
Aspirin Given Within 24 Hours of Arrival[5]	-	-	96%	96%
Fibrinolytic Meds Within 30 Min. of Arrival[5]	-	-	63%	58%
Average Time to ECG (minutes)[5]	-	-	8	7
Average Time to Transfer (minutes)[5]	-	-	53	60
Children's Asthma Care				
Received Home Management Plan of Care	-	-	-	88%
Received Reliever Medication	-	-	-	100%
Received Systemic Corticosteroids	-	-	-	100%
Emergency Department				
Admittance Decision Time (minutes)[2]	529	213	102	98
Head CT Results Within 45 Min. of Arrival[1,3]	-	-	54%	57%
Patients Who Left ER Before Being Seen	97,196	2%	2%	2%
Time from ER Arrival to Admit. (minutes)[2]	534	416	288	274
Time from ER Arrival to Discharge (minutes)	421	259	128	134
Time in ER Before Being Evaluated (minutes)	533	28	22	26
Time to Pain Meds for Fractures (minutes)	164	66	55	57
Heart Attack Care				
Aspirin Given at Discharge	340	100%	99%	99%
Fibrinolytic Meds Within 30 Min. of Arrival[7]	-	-	20%	54%
PCI Within 90 Minutes of Arrival	60	95%	95%	96%
Statin Prescribed at Discharge	330	100%	98%	98%
Heart Failure Care				
ACE Inhibitor or ARB for LVSD	261	99%	96%	97%
Discharge Instructions Given	718	99%	94%	94%
Evaluation of LVS Function	826	100%	99%	99%
Medicare Spending				
Medicare Spending per Patient (ratio)	-	1.00	0.96	0.98
Pneumonia Care				
Appropriate Initial Antibiotic Given	143	98%	96%	95%
Blood Culture Timing	350	98%	98%	98%
Pregnancy and Delivery Care				
Newborn Deliveries Scheduled Early	203	1%	3%	6%
Preventive Care				
Immunization for Influenza[2]	576	86%	89%	90%
Immunization for Pneumonia[2]	534	89%	90%	92%
Stroke Care				
Anticoagulation Therapy for Atrial Fibrillation	37	92%	92%	95%
Antithrombotic Therapy Timing	167	96%	97%	98%
Assessed for Rehabilitation	326	96%	97%	97%
Discharged on Antithrombotic Therapy	216	100%	99%	99%
Discharged on Statin Medication	159	99%	94%	94%
Thrombolytic Therapy Timing	13	85%	69%	66%
Venous Thromboembolism Prophylaxis	325	100%	94%	94%
Written Stroke Educational Materials Given	177	90%	87%	88%
Surgical Care Improvement Project				
Appropriate Beta Blocker Usage[2]	799	98%	98%	98%
Appropriate VTP Within 24 Hours[2]	1,266	100%	98%	98%
Controlled Postoperative Blood Glucose[2]	668	99%	97%	97%
Perioperative Temperature Management[2]	1,567	100%	100%	100%
Prophylactic Antibiotic Selection[2]	1,620	99%	99%	99%
Prophylactic Antibiotic Selection (Outpatient)	992	99%	97%	98%
Prophylactic Antibiotic Stopped[2]	1,558	98%	98%	98%
Prophylactic Antibiotic Timing[2]	1,618	100%	98%	99%
Prophylactic Antibiotic Timing (Outpatient)	753	97%	97%	98%
Urinary Catheter Removal[2]	1,479	98%	97%	97%
Survey of Patients' Hospital Experiences				
Area Around Room 'Always' Quiet at Night	300+	49%	60%	61%
Doctors 'Always' Communicated Well	300+	78%	81%	82%
Home Recovery Information Given	300+	90%	87%	85%
Hospital Given 9 or 10 on 10 Point Scale	300+	76%	71%	71%
Meds 'Always' Explained Before Given	300+	62%	64%	64%
Nurses 'Always' Communicated Well	300+	78%	80%	79%
Pain 'Always' Well Controlled	300+	69%	71%	71%
Room and Bathroom 'Always' Clean	300+	65%	73%	73%
Timely Help 'Always' Received	300+	64%	70%	68%
Would Definitely Recommend Hospital	300+	82%	71%	71%
Use of Medical Imaging				
Cardiac Imaging Stress Test before Surgery	1,402	4.9%	5.1%	5.3%
Combination Abdominal CT Scan	3,659	5.0%	8.7%	10.5%
Combination Brain/Sinus CT Scan	1,260	1.3%	2.2%	2.7%
Combination Chest CT Scan	4,942	0.3%	3.6%	2.7%
Follow-up Mammogram/Ultrasound	3,808	8.8%	8.2%	8.8%
Lumbar Spine MRI for Low Back Pain	273	32.2%	36.9%	37.2%

VA Ann Arbor Healthcare System

2215 Fuller Road Phone: 734-769-7100
Ann Arbor, MI 48105 Fax: 734-761-7870
Type: Acute Care - VA Emergency Services: No
Ownership: Government Federal Beds: 132

Key Personnel:

CEO/President. . . . . Lou Ann Atkins
Chief of Medical Staff. . . . . Eric W Young, MD

Measure	Cases	This Hosp.	State Avg.	U.S. Avg.
Blood Clot Prevention and Treatment				
Anticoagulation Overlap Therapy	-	-	90%	93%
ICU Venous Thromboembolism Prophylaxis	-	-	93%	92%
Incidence of Potentially Preventable VTE	-	-	8%	10%
UFH with Dosages/Platelet Monitoring	-	-	96%	97%
Venous Thromboembolism Prophylaxis	-	-	87%	85%
Warfarin Therapy Discharge Instructions	-	-	72%	75%
Chest Pain/Possible Heart Attack Care				
Aspirin Given Within 24 Hours of Arrival	-	-	96%	96%
Fibrinolytic Meds Within 30 Min. of Arrival	-	-	63%	58%
Average Time to ECG (minutes)	-	-	8	7
Average Time to Transfer (minutes)	-	-	53	60
Children's Asthma Care				
Received Home Management Plan of Care	-	-	-	88%
Received Reliever Medication	-	-	-	100%
Received Systemic Corticosteroids	-	-	-	100%
Emergency Department				
Admittance Decision Time (minutes)	-	-	102	98
Head CT Results Within 45 Min. of Arrival	-	-	54%	57%
Patients Who Left ER Before Being Seen	-	-	2%	2%
Time from ER Arrival to Admit. (minutes)	-	-	288	274
Time from ER Arrival to Discharge (minutes)	-	-	128	134
Time in ER Before Being Evaluated (minutes)	-	-	22	26
Time to Pain Meds for Fractures (minutes)	-	-	55	57
Heart Attack Care				
Aspirin Given at Discharge	61	98%	99%	99%
Fibrinolytic Meds Within 30 Min. of Arrival[5]	-	-	20%	54%
PCI Within 90 Minutes of Arrival[1]	-	-	95%	96%
Statin Prescribed at Discharge	61	100%	98%	98%
Heart Failure Care				
ACE Inhibitor or ARB for LVSD	54	93%	96%	97%
Discharge Instructions Given	153	100%	94%	94%
Evaluation of LVS Function	164	100%	99%	99%
Medicare Spending				
Medicare Spending per Patient (ratio)	-	-	0.96	0.98
Pneumonia Care				
Appropriate Initial Antibiotic Given	29	100%	96%	95%
Blood Culture Timing	66	98%	98%	98%
Pregnancy and Delivery Care				
Newborn Deliveries Scheduled Early	-	-	3%	6%
Preventive Care				
Immunization for Influenza[5]	-	-	89%	90%
Immunization for Pneumonia[5]	-	-	90%	92%
Stroke Care				
Anticoagulation Therapy for Atrial Fibrillation	-	-	92%	95%
Antithrombotic Therapy Timing	-	-	97%	98%
Assessed for Rehabilitation	-	-	97%	97%
Discharged on Antithrombotic Therapy	-	-	99%	99%
Discharged on Statin Medication	-	-	94%	94%
Thrombolytic Therapy Timing	-	-	69%	66%
Venous Thromboembolism Prophylaxis	-	-	94%	94%
Written Stroke Educational Materials Given	-	-	87%	88%
Surgical Care Improvement Project				
Appropriate Beta Blocker Usage[2]	262	96%	98%	98%
Appropriate VTP Within 24 Hours[2]	215	100%	98%	98%
Controlled Postoperative Blood Glucose[2]	160	95%	97%	97%
Perioperative Temperature Management[2]	312	99%	100%	100%
Prophylactic Antibiotic Selection	333	99%	99%	99%
Prophylactic Antibiotic Selection (Outpatient)	-	-	97%	98%
Prophylactic Antibiotic Stopped	322	93%	98%	98%
Prophylactic Antibiotic Timing	333	96%	98%	99%
Prophylactic Antibiotic Timing (Outpatient)	-	-	97%	98%
Urinary Catheter Removal[2]	310	96%	97%	97%
Survey of Patients' Hospital Experiences				
Area Around Room 'Always' Quiet at Night	-	-	60%	61%
Doctors 'Always' Communicated Well	-	-	81%	82%
Home Recovery Information Given	-	-	87%	85%
Hospital Given 9 or 10 on 10 Point Scale	-	-	71%	71%
Meds 'Always' Explained Before Given	-	-	64%	64%
Nurses 'Always' Communicated Well	-	-	80%	79%
Pain 'Always' Well Controlled	-	-	71%	71%

NOTE: Hospital profiles are in alphabetical order by state, then city, then hospital within the city; Rankings exclude hospitals with less than 25 cases except for patient surveys which excludes hospitals with less than 100 cases; (a) 100-299 cases; (1) The number of cases/patients is too few to report; (2) Data submitted were based on a sample of cases/patients; (3) Results are based on a shorter time period than required; (4) Data suppressed by CMS for one or more quarters; (5) Results are not available for this reporting period; (6) Fewer than 100 patients completed the HCAHPS survey; (7) No cases met the criteria for this measure; (8) The lower limit of the confidence interval cannot be calculated if the number of observed infections equals zero; (9) No data are available from the state/territory for this reporting period; (10) The scores shown reflect fewer than 50 completed surveys; (11) There were discrepancies in the data collection process; (12) This measure does not apply to this hospital for this reporting period; (13) Results cannot be calculated for this reporting period; (14) The results for this state are combined with nearby states to protect confidentiality; Please refer to the User's Guide for a full explanation of data.

Measure	Cases	This Hosp.	State Avg.	U.S. Avg.
Room and Bathroom 'Always' Clean	-	-	73%	73%
Timely Help 'Always' Received	-	-	70%	68%
Would Definitely Recommend Hospital	-	-	71%	71%
Use of Medical Imaging				
Cardiac Imaging Stress Test before Surgery	-	-	5.1%	5.3%
Combination Abdominal CT Scan	-	-	8.7%	10.5%
Combination Brain/Sinus CT Scan	-	-	2.2%	2.7%
Combination Chest CT Scan	-	-	3.6%	2.7%
Follow-up Mammogram/Ultrasound	-	-	8.2%	8.8%
Lumbar Spine MRI for Low Back Pain	-	-	36.9%	37.2%

Huron Medical Center

1100 South Van Dyke Road
Bad Axe, MI 48413
URL: www.huronmedicalcenter.org
Type: Acute Care Hospitals
Ownership: Voluntary non-profit - Private
Phone: 989-269-9521
Fax: 989-269-7948
Emergency Services: Yes
Beds: 64

Key Personnel:
Quality Assurance . . . . Laura Abraham-Acker
Emergency Room . . . . Bryon Beck
Radiology. . . . . David Carter
Operating Room. . . . . Linda Dumaw
CEO/President. . . . . Jeffery Longbrake
Patient Relations . . . . Len Matestic
Chief of Medical Staff. . . . . Jerome Yaklic

Measure	Cases	This Hosp.	State Avg.	U.S. Avg.
Blood Clot Prevention and Treatment				
Anticoagulation Overlap Therapy[1,2]	-	-	90%	93%
ICU Venous Thromboembolism Prophylaxis[2]	19	100%	93%	92%
Incidence of Potentially Preventable VTE[2,7]	-	-	8%	10%
UFH with Dosages/Platelet Monitoring[2,7]	-	-	96%	97%
Venous Thromboembolism Prophylaxis[2]	94	93%	87%	85%
Warfarin Therapy Discharge Instructions[1,2]	-	-	72%	75%
Chest Pain/Possible Heart Attack Care				
Aspirin Given Within 24 Hours of Arrival	27	100%	96%	96%
Fibrinolytic Meds Within 30 Min. of Arrival[1]	-	-	63%	58%
Average Time to ECG (minutes)	27	8	8	7
Average Time to Transfer (minutes)[7]	-	-	53	60
Children's Asthma Care				
Received Home Management Plan of Care	-	-	-	88%
Received Reliever Medication	-	-	-	100%
Received Systemic Corticosteroids	-	-	-	100%
Emergency Department				
Admittance Decision Time (minutes)[2]	172	75	102	98
Head CT Results Within 45 Min. of Arrival[1]	-	-	54%	57%
Patients Who Left ER Before Being Seen	7,162	0%	2%	2%
Time from ER Arrival to Admit. (minutes)[2]	178	220	288	274
Time from ER Arrival to Discharge (minutes)	352	95	128	134
Time in ER Before Being Evaluated (minutes)	381	14	22	26
Time to Pain Meds for Fractures (minutes)	45	37	55	57
Heart Attack Care				
Aspirin Given at Discharge	13	100%	99%	99%
Fibrinolytic Meds Within 30 Min. of Arrival[7]	-	-	20%	54%
PCI Within 90 Minutes of Arrival[7]	-	-	95%	96%
Statin Prescribed at Discharge	13	100%	98%	98%
Heart Failure Care				
ACE Inhibitor or ARB for LVSD[1]	-	-	96%	97%
Discharge Instructions Given	27	100%	94%	94%
Evaluation of LVS Function	37	95%	99%	99%
Medicare Spending				
Medicare Spending per Patient (ratio)	-	0.88	0.96	0.98
Pneumonia Care				
Appropriate Initial Antibiotic Given[2]	37	97%	96%	95%
Blood Culture Timing[2]	67	97%	98%	98%
Pregnancy and Delivery Care				
Newborn Deliveries Scheduled Early[2]	21	0%	3%	6%
Preventive Care				
Immunization for Influenza[2]	271	94%	89%	90%
Immunization for Pneumonia[2]	289	99%	90%	92%
Stroke Care				
Anticoagulation Therapy for Atrial Fibrillation[1]	-	-	92%	95%
Antithrombotic Therapy Timing	14	100%	97%	98%
Assessed for Rehabilitation	13	85%	97%	97%
Discharged on Antithrombotic Therapy	13	100%	99%	99%
Discharged on Statin Medication	13	92%	94%	94%
Thrombolytic Therapy Timing[7]	-	-	69%	66%
Venous Thromboembolism Prophylaxis	13	92%	94%	94%
Written Stroke Educational Materials Given[1]	-	-	87%	88%
Surgical Care Improvement Project				
Appropriate Beta Blocker Usage[2]	38	100%	98%	98%
Appropriate VTP Within 24 Hours[2]	116	98%	98%	98%
Controlled Postoperative Blood Glucose[2,7]	-	-	97%	97%
Perioperative Temperature Management[2]	127	100%	100%	100%
Prophylactic Antibiotic Selection[2]	113	98%	99%	99%
Prophylactic Antibiotic Selection (Outpatient)	64	94%	97%	98%
Prophylactic Antibiotic Stopped[2]	112	100%	98%	98%
Prophylactic Antibiotic Timing[2]	113	100%	98%	99%
Prophylactic Antibiotic Timing (Outpatient)	64	100%	97%	98%
Urinary Catheter Removal[2]	110	97%	97%	97%
Survey of Patients' Hospital Experiences				
Area Around Room 'Always' Quiet at Night	300+	55%	60%	61%
Doctors 'Always' Communicated Well	300+	84%	81%	82%
Home Recovery Information Given	300+	89%	87%	85%
Hospital Given 9 or 10 on 10 Point Scale	300+	70%	71%	71%
Meds 'Always' Explained Before Given	300+	63%	64%	64%
Nurses 'Always' Communicated Well	300+	80%	80%	79%
Pain 'Always' Well Controlled	300+	75%	71%	71%
Room and Bathroom 'Always' Clean	300+	78%	73%	73%
Timely Help 'Always' Received	300+	72%	70%	68%
Would Definitely Recommend Hospital	300+	71%	71%	71%
Use of Medical Imaging				
Cardiac Imaging Stress Test before Surgery	214	4.7%	5.1%	5.3%
Combination Abdominal CT Scan	290	23.4%	8.7%	10.5%
Combination Brain/Sinus CT Scan[1]	-	-	2.2%	2.7%
Combination Chest CT Scan	96	29.2%	3.6%	2.7%
Follow-up Mammogram/Ultrasound	437	4.1%	8.2%	8.8%
Lumbar Spine MRI for Low Back Pain[7]	-	-	36.9%	37.2%

Battle Creek VA Medical Center

5500 Armstrong Rd.
Battle Creek, MI 49015
URL: www.battlecreek.va.gov
Type: Acute Care - VA
Ownership: Government Federal
Phone: 269-966-5600
Emergency Services: No

Key Personnel:
Infection Control. . . . . Daniel Allen
Radiology. . . . . Jeff Brewster
CEO/President. . . . . Suzanne Klinker
Quality Assurance . . . . Gail M O'Dwyer
Coronary Care . . . . Helen Parkis, RN
Intensive Care Unit. . . . . Nina Santos, RN
Chief of Medical Staff. . . . . Ketan Shah, MD
Emergency Room . . . . Donna Sumrall, RN

Measure	Cases	This Hosp.	State Avg.	U.S. Avg.
Blood Clot Prevention and Treatment				
Anticoagulation Overlap Therapy	-	-	90%	93%
ICU Venous Thromboembolism Prophylaxis	-	-	93%	92%
Incidence of Potentially Preventable VTE	-	-	8%	10%
UFH with Dosages/Platelet Monitoring	-	-	96%	97%
Venous Thromboembolism Prophylaxis	-	-	87%	85%
Warfarin Therapy Discharge Instructions	-	-	72%	75%
Chest Pain/Possible Heart Attack Care				
Aspirin Given Within 24 Hours of Arrival	-	-	96%	96%
Fibrinolytic Meds Within 30 Min. of Arrival	-	-	63%	58%
Average Time to ECG (minutes)	-	-	8	7
Average Time to Transfer (minutes)	-	-	53	60
Children's Asthma Care				
Received Home Management Plan of Care	-	-	-	88%
Received Reliever Medication	-	-	-	100%
Received Systemic Corticosteroids	-	-	-	100%
Emergency Department				
Admittance Decision Time (minutes)	-	-	102	98
Head CT Results Within 45 Min. of Arrival	-	-	54%	57%
Patients Who Left ER Before Being Seen	-	-	2%	2%
Time from ER Arrival to Admit. (minutes)	-	-	288	274
Time from ER Arrival to Discharge (minutes)	-	-	128	134
Time in ER Before Being Evaluated (minutes)	-	-	22	26
Time to Pain Meds for Fractures (minutes)	-	-	55	57
Heart Attack Care				
Aspirin Given at Discharge[5]	-	-	99%	99%
Fibrinolytic Meds Within 30 Min. of Arrival[5]	-	-	20%	54%
PCI Within 90 Minutes of Arrival[5]	-	-	95%	96%
Statin Prescribed at Discharge[5]	-	-	98%	98%
Heart Failure Care				
ACE Inhibitor or ARB for LVSD[1]	-	-	96%	97%
Discharge Instructions Given[1]	21	90%	94%	94%
Evaluation of LVS Function[1]	22	100%	99%	99%
Medicare Spending				
Medicare Spending per Patient (ratio)	-	-	0.96	0.98
Pneumonia Care				
Appropriate Initial Antibiotic Given[1]	18	100%	96%	95%
Blood Culture Timing[5]	-	-	98%	98%
Pregnancy and Delivery Care				
Newborn Deliveries Scheduled Early	-	-	3%	6%
Preventive Care				
Immunization for Influenza[5]	-	-	89%	90%
Immunization for Pneumonia[5]	-	-	90%	92%
Stroke Care				
Anticoagulation Therapy for Atrial Fibrillation	-	-	92%	95%
Antithrombotic Therapy Timing	-	-	97%	98%
Assessed for Rehabilitation	-	-	97%	97%
Discharged on Antithrombotic Therapy	-	-	99%	99%
Discharged on Statin Medication	-	-	94%	94%
Thrombolytic Therapy Timing	-	-	69%	66%
Venous Thromboembolism Prophylaxis	-	-	94%	94%
Written Stroke Educational Materials Given	-	-	87%	88%
Surgical Care Improvement Project				
Appropriate Beta Blocker Usage[5]	-	-	98%	98%
Appropriate VTP Within 24 Hours[5]	-	-	98%	98%
Controlled Postoperative Blood Glucose[5]	-	-	97%	97%
Perioperative Temperature Management[5]	-	-	100%	100%
Prophylactic Antibiotic Selection[5]	-	-	99%	99%
Prophylactic Antibiotic Selection (Outpatient)	-	-	97%	98%
Prophylactic Antibiotic Stopped[5]	-	-	98%	98%
Prophylactic Antibiotic Timing[5]	-	-	98%	99%
Prophylactic Antibiotic Timing (Outpatient)	-	-	97%	98%
Urinary Catheter Removal[5]	-	-	97%	97%
Survey of Patients' Hospital Experiences				
Area Around Room 'Always' Quiet at Night	-	-	60%	61%
Doctors 'Always' Communicated Well	-	-	81%	82%
Home Recovery Information Given	-	-	87%	85%
Hospital Given 9 or 10 on 10 Point Scale	-	-	71%	71%
Meds 'Always' Explained Before Given	-	-	64%	64%
Nurses 'Always' Communicated Well	-	-	80%	79%
Pain 'Always' Well Controlled	-	-	71%	71%
Room and Bathroom 'Always' Clean	-	-	73%	73%
Timely Help 'Always' Received	-	-	70%	68%
Would Definitely Recommend Hospital	-	-	71%	71%
Use of Medical Imaging				
Cardiac Imaging Stress Test before Surgery	-	-	5.1%	5.3%
Combination Abdominal CT Scan	-	-	8.7%	10.5%
Combination Brain/Sinus CT Scan	-	-	2.2%	2.7%
Combination Chest CT Scan	-	-	3.6%	2.7%
Follow-up Mammogram/Ultrasound	-	-	8.2%	8.8%
Lumbar Spine MRI for Low Back Pain	-	-	36.9%	37.2%

Bronson Battle Creek Hospital

300 North Avenue
Battle Creek, MI 49017
URL: www.bchealth.com
Type: Acute Care Hospitals
Ownership: Proprietary
Phone: 269-966-8000
Fax: 269-966-8366
Emergency Services: Yes
Beds: 315

Key Personnel:
Intensive Care Unit. . . . . Annette Beming
CEO/President. . . . . Pat Garrett
Pediatric Ambulatory Care . . . . . . Samuel Grossman, DO
Radiology. . . . . Steven Miltz-Miller, MD
Pediatric In-Patient Care . . . . Shohreh Moazami, MD

Measure	Cases	This Hosp.	State Avg.	U.S. Avg.
Blood Clot Prevention and Treatment				
Anticoagulation Overlap Therapy[2]	77	88%	90%	93%
ICU Venous Thromboembolism Prophylaxis[2]	82	93%	93%	92%

NOTE: Hospital profiles are in alphabetical order by state, then city, then hospital within the city; Rankings exclude hospitals with less than 25 cases except for patient surveys which excludes hospitals with less than 100 cases; (a) 100-299 cases; (1) The number of cases/patients is too few to report; (2) Data submitted were based on a sample of cases/patients; (3) Results are based on a shorter time period than required; (4) Data suppressed by CMS for one or more quarters; (5) Results are not available for this reporting period; (6) Fewer than 100 patients completed the HCAHPS survey; (7) No cases met the criteria for this measure; (8) The lower limit of the confidence interval cannot be calculated if the number of observed infections equals zero; (9) No data are available from the state/territory for this reporting period; (10) The scores shown reflect fewer than 50 completed surveys; (11) There were discrepancies in the data collection process; (12) This measure does not apply to this hospital for this reporting period; (13) Results cannot be calculated for this reporting period; (14) The results for this state are combined with nearby states to protect confidentiality; Please refer to the User's Guide for a full explanation of data.

Measure	Cases	This Hosp.	State Avg.	U.S. Avg.
Incidence of Potentially Preventable VTE[1,2]	-	-	8%	10%
UFH with Dosages/Platelet Monitoring[2]	60	98%	96%	97%
Venous Thromboembolism Prophylaxis[2]	362	90%	87%	85%
Warfarin Therapy Discharge Instructions[2]	59	54%	72%	75%
Chest Pain/Possible Heart Attack Care				
Aspirin Given Within 24 Hours of Arrival	140	94%	96%	96%
Fibrinolytic Meds Within 30 Min. of Arrival[7]	-	-	63%	58%
Average Time to ECG (minutes)	145	10	8	7
Average Time to Transfer (minutes)	25	63	53	60
Children's Asthma Care				
Received Home Management Plan of Care	-	-	-	88%
Received Reliever Medication	-	-	-	100%
Received Systemic Corticosteroids	-	-	-	100%
Emergency Department				
Admittance Decision Time (minutes)[2]	603	68	102	98
Head CT Results Within 45 Min. of Arrival	18	39%	54%	57%
Patients Who Left ER Before Being Seen	51,249	4%	2%	2%
Time from ER Arrival to Admit. (minutes)[2]	617	274	288	274
Time from ER Arrival to Discharge (minutes)	364	162	128	134
Time in ER Before Being Evaluated (minutes)	404	30	22	26
Time to Pain Meds for Fractures (minutes)	156	70	55	57
Heart Attack Care				
Aspirin Given at Discharge	42	100%	99%	99%
Fibrinolytic Meds Within 30 Min. of Arrival[7]	-	-	20%	54%
PCI Within 90 Minutes of Arrival[7]	-	-	95%	96%
Statin Prescribed at Discharge	36	97%	98%	98%
Heart Failure Care				
ACE Inhibitor or ARB for LVSD	60	97%	96%	97%
Discharge Instructions Given	208	96%	94%	94%
Evaluation of LVS Function	273	100%	99%	99%
Medicare Spending				
Medicare Spending per Patient (ratio)	-	0.99	0.96	0.98
Pneumonia Care				
Appropriate Initial Antibiotic Given[2]	151	95%	96%	95%
Blood Culture Timing[2]	245	98%	98%	98%
Pregnancy and Delivery Care				
Newborn Deliveries Scheduled Early[2]	32	3%	3%	6%
Preventive Care				
Immunization for Influenza[2]	574	95%	89%	90%
Immunization for Pneumonia[2]	802	90%	90%	92%
Stroke Care				
Anticoagulation Therapy for Atrial Fibrillation	14	71%	92%	95%
Antithrombotic Therapy Timing	79	90%	97%	98%
Assessed for Rehabilitation	86	95%	97%	97%
Discharged on Antithrombotic Therapy	84	99%	99%	99%
Discharged on Statin Medication	72	92%	94%	94%
Thrombolytic Therapy Timing[1]	-	-	69%	66%
Venous Thromboembolism Prophylaxis	80	99%	94%	94%
Written Stroke Educational Materials Given	50	78%	87%	88%
Surgical Care Improvement Project				
Appropriate Beta Blocker Usage[2]	291	99%	98%	98%
Appropriate VTP Within 24 Hours[2]	752	98%	98%	98%
Controlled Postoperative Blood Glucose[2,7]	-	-	97%	97%
Perioperative Temperature Management[2]	905	100%	100%	100%
Prophylactic Antibiotic Selection[2]	693	99%	99%	99%
Prophylactic Antibiotic Selection (Outpatient)	238	99%	97%	98%
Prophylactic Antibiotic Stopped[2]	662	100%	98%	98%
Prophylactic Antibiotic Timing[2]	693	99%	98%	99%
Prophylactic Antibiotic Timing (Outpatient)	238	100%	97%	98%
Urinary Catheter Removal[2]	721	98%	97%	97%
Survey of Patients' Hospital Experiences				
Area Around Room 'Always' Quiet at Night	300+	52%	60%	61%
Doctors 'Always' Communicated Well	300+	76%	81%	82%
Home Recovery Information Given	300+	85%	87%	85%
Hospital Given 9 or 10 on 10 Point Scale	300+	62%	71%	71%
Meds 'Always' Explained Before Given	300+	59%	64%	64%
Nurses 'Always' Communicated Well	300+	74%	80%	79%
Pain 'Always' Well Controlled	300+	68%	71%	71%
Room and Bathroom 'Always' Clean	300+	68%	73%	73%
Timely Help 'Always' Received	300+	63%	70%	68%
Would Definitely Recommend Hospital	300+	57%	71%	71%
Use of Medical Imaging				
Cardiac Imaging Stress Test before Surgery	508	5.7%	5.1%	5.3%
Combination Abdominal CT Scan	1,309	2.3%	8.7%	10.5%
Combination Brain/Sinus CT Scan	980	2.0%	2.2%	2.7%
Combination Chest CT Scan	812	0.1%	3.6%	2.7%
Follow-up Mammogram/Ultrasound	2,906	3.7%	8.2%	8.8%
Lumbar Spine MRI for Low Back Pain	130	36.2%	36.9%	37.2%

Mclaren Bay Region

1900 Columbus Ave
Bay City, MI 48708
URL: www.baymed.org
Type: Acute Care Hospitals
Ownership: Voluntary non-profit - Other
Phone: 989-894-3000
Fax: 989-894-4464
Emergency Services: Yes
Beds: 415

Key Personnel:
Pediatric Ambulatory Care . . . . . . RE Bickham, MD
Chief of Medical Staff . . . . Christopher Brueck, MD
Infection Control . . . . Karen Frahm, RN
Pediatric In-Patient Care . . . . Carol Jones
Quality Assurance . . . . Jack Miller
Radiology . . . . Dave Nall
Coronary Care . . . . Willa Rousseau
CEO/President . . . . Robert Wright

Measure	Cases	This Hosp.	State Avg.	U.S. Avg.
Blood Clot Prevention and Treatment				
Anticoagulation Overlap Therapy[2]	92	100%	90%	93%
ICU Venous Thromboembolism Prophylaxis[2]	91	100%	93%	92%
Incidence of Potentially Preventable VTE[2]	23	22%	8%	10%
UFH with Dosages/Platelet Monitoring[2]	95	100%	96%	97%
Venous Thromboembolism Prophylaxis[2]	306	98%	87%	85%
Warfarin Therapy Discharge Instructions[2]	65	94%	72%	75%
Chest Pain/Possible Heart Attack Care				
Aspirin Given Within 24 Hours of Arrival[1,3]	-	-	96%	96%
Fibrinolytic Meds Within 30 Min. of Arrival[5]	-	-	63%	58%
Average Time to ECG (minutes)[1,3]	-	-	8	7
Average Time to Transfer (minutes)[5]	-	-	53	60
Children's Asthma Care				
Received Home Management Plan of Care	-	-	-	88%
Received Reliever Medication	-	-	-	100%
Received Systemic Corticosteroids	-	-	-	100%
Emergency Department				
Admittance Decision Time (minutes)[2]	482	64	102	98
Head CT Results Within 45 Min. of Arrival[1]	-	-	54%	57%
Patients Who Left ER Before Being Seen	44,062	1%	2%	2%
Time from ER Arrival to Admit. (minutes)[2]	498	253	288	274
Time from ER Arrival to Discharge (minutes)	436	140	128	134
Time in ER Before Being Evaluated (minutes)	419	36	22	26
Time to Pain Meds for Fractures (minutes)	93	65	55	57
Heart Attack Care				
Aspirin Given at Discharge	402	100%	99%	99%
Fibrinolytic Meds Within 30 Min. of Arrival[7]	-	-	20%	54%
PCI Within 90 Minutes of Arrival	54	94%	95%	96%
Statin Prescribed at Discharge	403	98%	98%	98%
Heart Failure Care				
ACE Inhibitor or ARB for LVSD	148	89%	96%	97%
Discharge Instructions Given	393	92%	94%	94%
Evaluation of LVS Function	477	97%	99%	99%
Medicare Spending				
Medicare Spending per Patient (ratio)	-	1.00	0.96	0.98
Pneumonia Care				
Appropriate Initial Antibiotic Given	133	95%	96%	95%
Blood Culture Timing	171	95%	98%	98%
Pregnancy and Delivery Care				
Newborn Deliveries Scheduled Early[2]	66	0%	3%	6%
Preventive Care				
Immunization for Influenza[2]	566	95%	89%	90%
Immunization for Pneumonia[2]	777	95%	90%	92%
Stroke Care				
Anticoagulation Therapy for Atrial Fibrillation	33	97%	92%	95%
Antithrombotic Therapy Timing	129	97%	97%	98%
Assessed for Rehabilitation	165	99%	97%	97%
Discharged on Antithrombotic Therapy	142	99%	99%	99%
Discharged on Statin Medication	116	91%	94%	94%
Thrombolytic Therapy Timing	11	100%	69%	66%
Venous Thromboembolism Prophylaxis	178	92%	94%	94%
Written Stroke Educational Materials Given	82	88%	87%	88%
Surgical Care Improvement Project				
Appropriate Beta Blocker Usage	611	97%	98%	98%
Appropriate VTP Within 24 Hours	792	98%	98%	98%
Controlled Postoperative Blood Glucose	408	93%	97%	97%
Perioperative Temperature Management	942	100%	100%	100%
Prophylactic Antibiotic Selection	935	99%	99%	99%
Prophylactic Antibiotic Selection (Outpatient)	447	100%	97%	98%
Prophylactic Antibiotic Stopped	924	99%	98%	98%
Prophylactic Antibiotic Timing	939	97%	98%	99%
Prophylactic Antibiotic Timing (Outpatient)	449	97%	97%	98%
Urinary Catheter Removal	532	90%	97%	97%
Survey of Patients' Hospital Experiences				
Area Around Room 'Always' Quiet at Night	300+	50%	60%	61%
Doctors 'Always' Communicated Well	300+	78%	81%	82%
Home Recovery Information Given	300+	87%	87%	85%
Hospital Given 9 or 10 on 10 Point Scale	300+	64%	71%	71%
Meds 'Always' Explained Before Given	300+	59%	64%	64%
Nurses 'Always' Communicated Well	300+	75%	80%	79%
Pain 'Always' Well Controlled	300+	67%	71%	71%
Room and Bathroom 'Always' Clean	300+	62%	73%	73%
Timely Help 'Always' Received	300+	62%	70%	68%
Would Definitely Recommend Hospital	300+	63%	71%	71%
Use of Medical Imaging				
Cardiac Imaging Stress Test before Surgery	695	3.9%	5.1%	5.3%
Combination Abdominal CT Scan	1,136	11.2%	8.7%	10.5%
Combination Brain/Sinus CT Scan	893	2.6%	2.2%	2.7%
Combination Chest CT Scan	841	3.8%	3.6%	2.7%
Follow-up Mammogram/Ultrasound	2,499	3.7%	8.2%	8.8%
Lumbar Spine MRI for Low Back Pain	314	37.9%	36.9%	37.2%

Spectrum Health Big Rapids Hospital

605 Oak Street
Big Rapids, MI 49307
URL: www.mcmc.br.com
Type: Acute Care Hospitals
Ownership: Government - Local
Phone: 231-796-8691
Fax: 231-592-4462
Emergency Services: Yes
Beds: 74

Key Personnel:
Chief of Medical Staff . . . . Charles Brummeler
CEO/President . . . . Sam Daugherty
Quality Assurance . . . . Amanda Jensen
Emergency Room . . . . Virginia Keusch, RN
Radiology . . . . Blase Vitello

Measure	Cases	This Hosp.	State Avg.	U.S. Avg.
Blood Clot Prevention and Treatment				
Anticoagulation Overlap Therapy[2]	22	82%	90%	93%
ICU Venous Thromboembolism Prophylaxis[2]	37	97%	93%	92%
Incidence of Potentially Preventable VTE[1,2]	-	-	8%	10%
UFH with Dosages/Platelet Monitoring[1,2]	-	-	96%	97%
Venous Thromboembolism Prophylaxis[2]	124	96%	87%	85%
Warfarin Therapy Discharge Instructions[2]	19	100%	72%	75%
Chest Pain/Possible Heart Attack Care				
Aspirin Given Within 24 Hours of Arrival	138	99%	96%	96%
Fibrinolytic Meds Within 30 Min. of Arrival[1]	-	-	63%	58%
Average Time to ECG (minutes)	144	8	8	7
Average Time to Transfer (minutes)	19	77	53	60
Children's Asthma Care				
Received Home Management Plan of Care	-	-	-	88%
Received Reliever Medication	-	-	-	100%
Received Systemic Corticosteroids	-	-	-	100%
Emergency Department				
Admittance Decision Time (minutes)[2]	301	73	102	98
Head CT Results Within 45 Min. of Arrival	16	50%	54%	57%
Patients Who Left ER Before Being Seen	23,791	1%	2%	2%
Time from ER Arrival to Admit. (minutes)[2]	302	267	288	274
Time from ER Arrival to Discharge (minutes)	444	122	128	134
Time in ER Before Being Evaluated (minutes)	440	30	22	26
Time to Pain Meds for Fractures (minutes)	49	52	55	57
Heart Attack Care				
Aspirin Given at Discharge[1]	-	-	99%	99%
Fibrinolytic Meds Within 30 Min. of Arrival[7]	-	-	20%	54%
PCI Within 90 Minutes of Arrival[7]	-	-	95%	96%
Statin Prescribed at Discharge[1]	-	-	98%	98%

NOTE: Hospital profiles are in alphabetical order by state, then city, then hospital within the city; Rankings exclude hospitals with less than 25 cases except for patient surveys which excludes hospitals with less than 100 cases; (a) 100-299 cases; (1) The number of cases/patients is too few to report; (2) Data submitted were based on a sample of cases/patients; (3) Results are based on a shorter time period than required; (4) Data suppressed by CMS for one or more quarters; (5) Results are not available for this reporting period; (6) Fewer than 100 patients completed the HCAHPS survey; (7) No cases met the criteria for this measure; (8) The lower limit of the confidence interval cannot be calculated if the number of observed infections equals zero; (9) No data are available from the state/territory for this reporting period; (10) The scores shown reflect fewer than 50 completed surveys; (11) There were discrepancies in the data collection process; (12) This measure does not apply to this hospital for this reporting period; (13) Results cannot be calculated for this reporting period; (14) The results for this state are combined with nearby states to protect confidentiality; Please refer to the User's Guide for a full explanation of data.

Measure	Cases	This Hosp.	State Avg.	U.S. Avg.
Heart Failure Care				
ACE Inhibitor or ARB for LVSD	17	88%	96%	97%
Discharge Instructions Given	63	97%	94%	94%
Evaluation of LVS Function	72	100%	99%	99%
Medicare Spending				
Medicare Spending per Patient (ratio)	-	0.89	0.96	0.98
Pneumonia Care				
Appropriate Initial Antibiotic Given	68	99%	96%	95%
Blood Culture Timing	109	99%	98%	98%
Pregnancy and Delivery Care				
Newborn Deliveries Scheduled Early[2]	21	0%	3%	6%
Preventive Care				
Immunization for Influenza[2]	310	93%	89%	90%
Immunization for Pneumonia[2]	339	91%	90%	92%
Stroke Care				
Anticoagulation Therapy for Atrial Fibrillation[1]	-	-	92%	95%
Antithrombotic Therapy Timing	22	95%	97%	98%
Assessed for Rehabilitation	28	100%	97%	97%
Discharged on Antithrombotic Therapy	26	96%	99%	99%
Discharged on Statin Medication	18	78%	94%	94%
Thrombolytic Therapy Timing[1]	-	-	69%	66%
Venous Thromboembolism Prophylaxis	25	100%	94%	94%
Written Stroke Educational Materials Given	15	93%	87%	88%
Surgical Care Improvement Project				
Appropriate Beta Blocker Usage	33	100%	98%	98%
Appropriate VTP Within 24 Hours	148	99%	98%	98%
Controlled Postoperative Blood Glucose[7]	-	-	97%	97%
Perioperative Temperature Management	157	100%	100%	100%
Prophylactic Antibiotic Selection	136	100%	99%	99%
Prophylactic Antibiotic Selection (Outpatient)	42	100%	97%	98%
Prophylactic Antibiotic Stopped	134	98%	98%	98%
Prophylactic Antibiotic Timing	136	96%	98%	99%
Prophylactic Antibiotic Timing (Outpatient)	32	100%	97%	98%
Urinary Catheter Removal	121	99%	97%	97%
Survey of Patients' Hospital Experiences				
Area Around Room 'Always' Quiet at Night	300+	64%	60%	61%
Doctors 'Always' Communicated Well	300+	85%	81%	82%
Home Recovery Information Given	300+	90%	87%	85%
Hospital Given 9 or 10 on 10 Point Scale	300+	77%	71%	71%
Meds 'Always' Explained Before Given	300+	68%	64%	64%
Nurses 'Always' Communicated Well	300+	82%	80%	79%
Pain 'Always' Well Controlled	300+	75%	71%	71%
Room and Bathroom 'Always' Clean	300+	75%	73%	73%
Timely Help 'Always' Received	300+	72%	70%	68%
Would Definitely Recommend Hospital	300+	76%	71%	71%
Use of Medical Imaging				
Cardiac Imaging Stress Test before Surgery	231	6.9%	5.1%	5.3%
Combination Abdominal CT Scan	345	26.4%	8.7%	10.5%
Combination Brain/Sinus CT Scan[1]	-	-	2.2%	2.7%
Combination Chest CT Scan	338	1.2%	3.6%	2.7%
Follow-up Mammogram/Ultrasound	612	13.2%	8.2%	8.8%
Lumbar Spine MRI for Low Back Pain	99	44.4%	36.9%	37.2%

Brighton Hospital

12851 Grand River Rd
Brighton, MI 48116
Phone: 810-227-1211
Fax: 810-227-1869
E-mail: info@brightonhospital.org
URL: www.stjohn.org/brighton
Type: Acute Care Hospitals
Emergency Services: No
Ownership: Voluntary non-profit - Private
Beds: 63
Key Personnel:
CEO/President. . . . . Denise Bertin-Epp
Chief of Medical Staff. . . . . Michael Brooks, MD

Measure	Cases	This Hosp.	State Avg.	U.S. Avg.
Blood Clot Prevention and Treatment				
Anticoagulation Overlap Therapy[2,7]	-	-	90%	93%
ICU Venous Thromboembolism Prophylaxis[2,7]	-	-	93%	92%
Incidence of Potentially Preventable VTE[2,7]	-	-	8%	10%
UFH with Dosages/Platelet Monitoring[2,7]	-	-	96%	97%
Venous Thromboembolism Prophylaxis[2,7]	-	-	87%	85%
Warfarin Therapy Discharge Instructions[2,7]	-	-	72%	75%
Chest Pain/Possible Heart Attack Care				
Aspirin Given Within 24 Hours of Arrival[5]	-	-	96%	96%
Fibrinolytic Meds Within 30 Min. of Arrival[5]	-	-	63%	58%
Average Time to ECG (minutes)[5]	-	-	8	7
Average Time to Transfer (minutes)[5]	-	-	53	60
Children's Asthma Care				
Received Home Management Plan of Care	-	-	-	88%
Received Reliever Medication	-	-	-	100%
Received Systemic Corticosteroids	-	-	-	100%
Emergency Department				
Admittance Decision Time (minutes)[2,7]	-	-	102	98
Head CT Results Within 45 Min. of Arrival[5]	-	-	54%	57%
Patients Who Left ER Before Being Seen[5]	-	-	2%	2%
Time from ER Arrival to Admit. (minutes)[2,7]	-	-	288	274
Time from ER Arrival to Discharge (minutes)[5]	-	-	128	134
Time in ER Before Being Evaluated (minutes)[5]	-	-	22	26
Time to Pain Meds for Fractures (minutes)[5]	-	-	55	57
Heart Attack Care				
Aspirin Given at Discharge[5]	-	-	99%	99%
Fibrinolytic Meds Within 30 Min. of Arrival[5]	-	-	20%	54%
PCI Within 90 Minutes of Arrival[5]	-	-	95%	96%
Statin Prescribed at Discharge[5]	-	-	98%	98%
Heart Failure Care				
ACE Inhibitor or ARB for LVSD[5]	-	-	96%	97%
Discharge Instructions Given[5]	-	-	94%	94%
Evaluation of LVS Function[5]	-	-	99%	99%
Medicare Spending				
Medicare Spending per Patient (ratio)	-	0.73	0.96	0.98
Pneumonia Care				
Appropriate Initial Antibiotic Given[5]	-	-	96%	95%
Blood Culture Timing[5]	-	-	98%	98%
Pregnancy and Delivery Care				
Newborn Deliveries Scheduled Early[7]	-	-	3%	6%
Preventive Care				
Immunization for Influenza[2]	281	33%	89%	90%
Immunization for Pneumonia[1,2]	-	-	90%	92%
Stroke Care				
Anticoagulation Therapy for Atrial Fibrillation[5]	-	-	92%	95%
Antithrombotic Therapy Timing[5]	-	-	97%	98%
Assessed for Rehabilitation[5]	-	-	97%	97%
Discharged on Antithrombotic Therapy[5]	-	-	99%	99%
Discharged on Statin Medication[5]	-	-	94%	94%
Thrombolytic Therapy Timing[5]	-	-	69%	66%
Venous Thromboembolism Prophylaxis[5]	-	-	94%	94%
Written Stroke Educational Materials Given[5]	-	-	87%	88%
Surgical Care Improvement Project				
Appropriate Beta Blocker Usage[5]	-	-	98%	98%
Appropriate VTP Within 24 Hours[5]	-	-	98%	98%
Controlled Postoperative Blood Glucose[5]	-	-	97%	97%
Perioperative Temperature Management[5]	-	-	100%	100%
Prophylactic Antibiotic Selection[5]	-	-	99%	99%
Prophylactic Antibiotic Selection (Outpatient)[5]	-	-	97%	98%
Prophylactic Antibiotic Stopped[5]	-	-	98%	98%
Prophylactic Antibiotic Timing[5]	-	-	98%	99%
Prophylactic Antibiotic Timing (Outpatient)[5]	-	-	97%	98%
Urinary Catheter Removal[5]	-	-	97%	97%
Survey of Patients' Hospital Experiences				
Area Around Room 'Always' Quiet at Night[1]	-	-	60%	61%
Doctors 'Always' Communicated Well[1]	-	-	81%	82%
Home Recovery Information Given[1]	-	-	87%	85%
Hospital Given 9 or 10 on 10 Point Scale[1]	-	-	71%	71%
Meds 'Always' Explained Before Given[1]	-	-	64%	64%
Nurses 'Always' Communicated Well[1]	-	-	80%	79%
Pain 'Always' Well Controlled[1]	-	-	71%	71%
Room and Bathroom 'Always' Clean[1]	-	-	73%	73%
Timely Help 'Always' Received[1]	-	-	70%	68%
Would Definitely Recommend Hospital[1]	-	-	71%	71%
Use of Medical Imaging				
Cardiac Imaging Stress Test before Surgery[7]	-	-	5.1%	5.3%
Combination Abdominal CT Scan[7]	-	-	8.7%	10.5%
Combination Brain/Sinus CT Scan[7]	-	-	2.2%	2.7%
Combination Chest CT Scan[7]	-	-	3.6%	2.7%
Follow-up Mammogram/Ultrasound[7]	-	-	8.2%	8.8%
Lumbar Spine MRI for Low Back Pain[7]	-	-	36.9%	37.2%

Mercy Hospital - Cadillac

400 Hobart St
Cadillac, MI 49601
Phone: 231-876-7200
Fax: 231-876-7439
E-mail: mercycadillac@trinity-health.org
URL: www.mercycadillac.munsonhealthcare.org
Type: Acute Care Hospitals
Emergency Services: Yes
Ownership: Voluntary non-profit - Church
Beds: 174
Key Personnel:
Emergency Room . . . . Janet Eng
CEO/President. . . . . John H Macleod

Measure	Cases	This Hosp.	State Avg.	U.S. Avg.
Blood Clot Prevention and Treatment				
Anticoagulation Overlap Therapy[2]	35	100%	90%	93%
ICU Venous Thromboembolism Prophylaxis[2]	51	96%	93%	92%
Incidence of Potentially Preventable VTE[1,2]	-	-	8%	10%
UFH with Dosages/Platelet Monitoring[2]	28	100%	96%	97%
Venous Thromboembolism Prophylaxis[2]	318	98%	87%	85%
Warfarin Therapy Discharge Instructions[2]	32	97%	72%	75%
Chest Pain/Possible Heart Attack Care				
Aspirin Given Within 24 Hours of Arrival	78	92%	96%	96%
Fibrinolytic Meds Within 30 Min. of Arrival[1]	-	-	63%	58%
Average Time to ECG (minutes)	81	8	8	7
Average Time to Transfer (minutes)	13	77	53	60
Children's Asthma Care				
Received Home Management Plan of Care	-	-	-	88%
Received Reliever Medication	-	-	-	100%
Received Systemic Corticosteroids	-	-	-	100%
Emergency Department				
Admittance Decision Time (minutes)[2]	524	124	102	98
Head CT Results Within 45 Min. of Arrival	20	35%	54%	57%
Patients Who Left ER Before Being Seen	22,329	2%	2%	2%
Time from ER Arrival to Admit. (minutes)[2]	539	297	288	274
Time from ER Arrival to Discharge (minutes)	401	159	128	134
Time in ER Before Being Evaluated (minutes)	439	27	22	26
Time to Pain Meds for Fractures (minutes)	146	52	55	57
Heart Attack Care				
Aspirin Given at Discharge[1]	-	-	99%	99%
Fibrinolytic Meds Within 30 Min. of Arrival[7]	-	-	20%	54%
PCI Within 90 Minutes of Arrival[7]	-	-	95%	96%
Statin Prescribed at Discharge[1]	-	-	98%	98%
Heart Failure Care				
ACE Inhibitor or ARB for LVSD	49	92%	96%	97%
Discharge Instructions Given	120	98%	94%	94%
Evaluation of LVS Function	131	98%	99%	99%
Medicare Spending				
Medicare Spending per Patient (ratio)	-	0.88	0.96	0.98
Pneumonia Care				
Appropriate Initial Antibiotic Given	114	97%	96%	95%
Blood Culture Timing	180	96%	98%	98%
Pregnancy and Delivery Care				
Newborn Deliveries Scheduled Early[2]	22	0%	3%	6%
Preventive Care				
Immunization for Influenza[2]	323	92%	89%	90%
Immunization for Pneumonia[2]	461	93%	90%	92%
Stroke Care				
Anticoagulation Therapy for Atrial Fibrillation[1]	-	-	92%	95%
Antithrombotic Therapy Timing	23	100%	97%	98%
Assessed for Rehabilitation	29	100%	97%	97%
Discharged on Antithrombotic Therapy	28	100%	99%	99%
Discharged on Statin Medication	28	100%	94%	94%
Thrombolytic Therapy Timing[7]	-	-	69%	66%
Venous Thromboembolism Prophylaxis	28	100%	94%	94%
Written Stroke Educational Materials Given	17	82%	87%	88%
Surgical Care Improvement Project				
Appropriate Beta Blocker Usage	108	96%	98%	98%
Appropriate VTP Within 24 Hours	326	98%	98%	98%
Controlled Postoperative Blood Glucose[7]	-	-	97%	97%
Perioperative Temperature Management	368	100%	100%	100%
Prophylactic Antibiotic Selection	287	99%	99%	99%
Prophylactic Antibiotic Selection (Outpatient)	36	97%	97%	98%
Prophylactic Antibiotic Stopped	285	98%	98%	98%
Prophylactic Antibiotic Timing	287	99%	98%	99%
Prophylactic Antibiotic Timing (Outpatient)	36	100%	97%	98%

NOTE: Hospital profiles are in alphabetical order by state, then city, then hospital within the city; Rankings exclude hospitals with less than 25 cases except for patient surveys which excludes hospitals with less than 100 cases; (a) 100-299 cases; (1) The number of cases/patients is too few to report; (2) Data submitted were based on a sample of cases/patients; (3) Results are based on a shorter time period than required; (4) Data suppressed by CMS for one or more quarters; (5) Results are not available for this reporting period; (6) Fewer than 100 patients completed the HCAHPS survey; (7) No cases met the criteria for this measure; (8) The lower limit of the confidence interval cannot be calculated if the number of observed infections equals zero; (9) No data are available from the state/territory for this reporting period; (10) The scores shown reflect fewer than 50 completed surveys; (11) There were discrepancies in the data collection process; (12) This measure does not apply to this hospital for this reporting period; (13) Results cannot be calculated for this reporting period; (14) The results for this state are combined with nearby states to protect confidentiality; Please refer to the User's Guide for a full explanation of data.

Measure	Cases	This Hosp.	State Avg.	U.S. Avg.
Urinary Catheter Removal	54	96%	97%	97%
Survey of Patients' Hospital Experiences				
Area Around Room 'Always' Quiet at Night	300+	61%	60%	61%
Doctors 'Always' Communicated Well	300+	84%	81%	82%
Home Recovery Information Given	300+	92%	87%	85%
Hospital Given 9 or 10 on 10 Point Scale	300+	78%	71%	71%
Meds 'Always' Explained Before Given	300+	69%	64%	64%
Nurses 'Always' Communicated Well	300+	84%	80%	79%
Pain 'Always' Well Controlled	300+	73%	71%	71%
Room and Bathroom 'Always' Clean	300+	71%	73%	73%
Timely Help 'Always' Received	300+	77%	70%	68%
Would Definitely Recommend Hospital	300+	74%	71%	71%
Use of Medical Imaging				
Cardiac Imaging Stress Test before Surgery	448	3.6%	5.1%	5.3%
Combination Abdominal CT Scan	646	2.6%	8.7%	10.5%
Combination Brain/Sinus CT Scan[1]	-	-	2.2%	2.7%
Combination Chest CT Scan	465	0.0%	3.6%	2.7%
Follow-up Mammogram/Ultrasound	1,020	9.7%	8.2%	8.8%
Lumbar Spine MRI for Low Back Pain	160	36.9%	36.9%	37.2%

Caro Community Hospital

401 N Hooper Street
Caro, MI 48723
Phone: 989-673-3141
Fax: 989-673-8471
Type: Critical Access Hospitals
Emergency Services: Yes
Ownership: Voluntary non-profit - Private
Beds: 25

Key Personnel:
Chief of Medical Staff . . . . A Ferreira, MD
Infection Control . . . . Tammy Gugel
CEO/President . . . . William P Miller
Quality Assurance . . . . Sue Morris, RN

Measure	Cases	This Hosp.	State Avg.	U.S. Avg.
Blood Clot Prevention and Treatment				
Anticoagulation Overlap Therapy[5]	-	-	90%	93%
ICU Venous Thromboembolism Prophylaxis[5]	-	-	93%	92%
Incidence of Potentially Preventable VTE[5]	-	-	8%	10%
UFH with Dosages/Platelet Monitoring[5]	-	-	96%	97%
Venous Thromboembolism Prophylaxis[5]	-	-	87%	85%
Warfarin Therapy Discharge Instructions[5]	-	-	72%	75%
Chest Pain/Possible Heart Attack Care				
Aspirin Given Within 24 Hours of Arrival	51	92%	96%	96%
Fibrinolytic Meds Within 30 Min. of Arrival[1]	-	-	63%	58%
Average Time to ECG (minutes)	53	9	8	7
Average Time to Transfer (minutes)[7]	-	-	53	60
Children's Asthma Care				
Received Home Management Plan of Care	-	-	-	88%
Received Reliever Medication	-	-	-	100%
Received Systemic Corticosteroids	-	-	-	100%
Emergency Department				
Admittance Decision Time (minutes)[5]	-	-	102	98
Head CT Results Within 45 Min. of Arrival[5]	-	-	54%	57%
Patients Who Left ER Before Being Seen[5]	-	-	2%	2%
Time from ER Arrival to Admit. (minutes)[5]	-	-	288	274
Time from ER Arrival to Discharge (minutes)	345	69	128	134
Time in ER Before Being Evaluated (minutes)	379	16	22	26
Time to Pain Meds for Fractures (minutes)[5]	-	-	55	57
Heart Attack Care				
Aspirin Given at Discharge[5]	-	-	99%	99%
Fibrinolytic Meds Within 30 Min. of Arrival[5]	-	-	20%	54%
PCI Within 90 Minutes of Arrival[5]	-	-	95%	96%
Statin Prescribed at Discharge[5]	-	-	98%	98%
Heart Failure Care				
ACE Inhibitor or ARB for LVSD[1,3]	-	-	96%	97%
Discharge Instructions Given[1,3]	-	-	94%	94%
Evaluation of LVS Function[1,3]	-	-	99%	99%
Medicare Spending				
Medicare Spending per Patient (ratio)	-	-	0.96	0.98
Pneumonia Care				
Appropriate Initial Antibiotic Given	11	73%	96%	95%
Blood Culture Timing	21	95%	98%	98%
Pregnancy and Delivery Care				
Newborn Deliveries Scheduled Early[5]	-	-	3%	6%
Preventive Care				
Immunization for Influenza[5]	-	-	89%	90%
Immunization for Pneumonia[5]	-	-	90%	92%
Stroke Care				
Anticoagulation Therapy for Atrial Fibrillation[5]	-	-	92%	95%
Antithrombotic Therapy Timing[5]	-	-	97%	98%
Assessed for Rehabilitation[5]	-	-	97%	97%
Discharged on Antithrombotic Therapy[5]	-	-	99%	99%
Discharged on Statin Medication[5]	-	-	94%	94%
Thrombolytic Therapy Timing[5]	-	-	69%	66%
Venous Thromboembolism Prophylaxis[5]	-	-	94%	94%
Written Stroke Educational Materials Given[5]	-	-	87%	88%
Surgical Care Improvement Project				
Appropriate Beta Blocker Usage[5]	-	-	98%	98%
Appropriate VTP Within 24 Hours[5]	-	-	98%	98%
Controlled Postoperative Blood Glucose[5]	-	-	97%	97%
Perioperative Temperature Management[5]	-	-	100%	100%
Prophylactic Antibiotic Selection[5]	-	-	99%	99%
Prophylactic Antibiotic Selection (Outpatient)[5]	-	-	97%	98%
Prophylactic Antibiotic Stopped[5]	-	-	98%	98%
Prophylactic Antibiotic Timing[5]	-	-	98%	99%
Prophylactic Antibiotic Timing (Outpatient)[5]	-	-	97%	98%
Urinary Catheter Removal[5]	-	-	97%	97%
Survey of Patients' Hospital Experiences				
Area Around Room 'Always' Quiet at Night[10]	<100	69%	60%	61%
Doctors 'Always' Communicated Well[10]	<100	88%	81%	82%
Home Recovery Information Given[10]	<100	88%	87%	85%
Hospital Given 9 or 10 on 10 Point Scale[10]	<100	75%	71%	71%
Meds 'Always' Explained Before Given[10]	<100	65%	64%	64%
Nurses 'Always' Communicated Well[10]	<100	84%	80%	79%
Pain 'Always' Well Controlled[10]	<100	89%	71%	71%
Room and Bathroom 'Always' Clean[10]	<100	78%	73%	73%
Timely Help 'Always' Received[10]	<100	83%	70%	68%
Would Definitely Recommend Hospital[10]	<100	74%	71%	71%
Use of Medical Imaging				
Cardiac Imaging Stress Test before Surgery[1]	-	-	5.1%	5.3%
Combination Abdominal CT Scan	185	12.4%	8.7%	10.5%
Combination Brain/Sinus CT Scan	194	1.0%	2.2%	2.7%
Combination Chest CT Scan	146	3.4%	3.6%	2.7%
Follow-up Mammogram/Ultrasound	206	12.6%	8.2%	8.8%
Lumbar Spine MRI for Low Back Pain[7]	-	-	36.9%	37.2%

Carson City Hospital

406 East Elm St
Carson City, MI 48811
Phone: 989-584-3131
Fax: 989-584-6165
E-mail: bruce@carsoncityhospital.com
URL: www.carsoncityhospital.com
Type: Acute Care Hospitals
Emergency Services: Yes
Ownership: Voluntary non-profit - Other
Beds: 77

Key Personnel:
Pediatric In-Patient Care . . . . Alberto Betancourt, MD
Hemotology Center . . . . Usha S Chamarthy, MD
Anesthesiology. . . . . Michael Mullins, DO
Anesthesiology. . . . . Sally Range, RN
Quality Assurance . . . . Shawn Smith
Cardiology . . . . Joni R Summitt, MD
CEO/President. . . . . Bruce L Traverse

Measure	Cases	This Hosp.	State Avg.	U.S. Avg.
Blood Clot Prevention and Treatment				
Anticoagulation Overlap Therapy[2]	11	100%	90%	93%
ICU Venous Thromboembolism Prophylaxis[1,2]	-	-	93%	92%
Incidence of Potentially Preventable VTE[1,2]	-	-	8%	10%
UFH with Dosages/Platelet Monitoring[1,2]	-	-	96%	97%
Venous Thromboembolism Prophylaxis[2]	110	78%	87%	85%
Warfarin Therapy Discharge Instructions[1,2]	-	-	72%	75%
Chest Pain/Possible Heart Attack Care				
Aspirin Given Within 24 Hours of Arrival	72	99%	96%	96%
Fibrinolytic Meds Within 30 Min. of Arrival[1]	-	-	63%	58%
Average Time to ECG (minutes)	77	7	8	7
Average Time to Transfer (minutes)[1]	-	-	53	60
Children's Asthma Care				
Received Home Management Plan of Care	-	-	-	88%
Received Reliever Medication	-	-	-	100%
Received Systemic Corticosteroids	-	-	-	100%
Emergency Department				
Admittance Decision Time (minutes)[2]	184	46	102	98
Head CT Results Within 45 Min. of Arrival	14	79%	54%	57%
Patients Who Left ER Before Being Seen	13,544	0%	2%	2%
Time from ER Arrival to Admit. (minutes)[2]	209	180	288	274
Time from ER Arrival to Discharge (minutes)	428	92	128	134
Time in ER Before Being Evaluated (minutes)	489	16	22	26
Time to Pain Meds for Fractures (minutes)	53	36	55	57
Heart Attack Care				
Aspirin Given at Discharge[1,3]	-	-	99%	99%
Fibrinolytic Meds Within 30 Min. of Arrival[3,7]	-	-	20%	54%
PCI Within 90 Minutes of Arrival[3,7]	-	-	95%	96%
Statin Prescribed at Discharge[1,3]	-	-	98%	98%
Heart Failure Care				
ACE Inhibitor or ARB for LVSD[1]	-	-	96%	97%
Discharge Instructions Given	28	100%	94%	94%
Evaluation of LVS Function	36	100%	99%	99%
Medicare Spending				
Medicare Spending per Patient (ratio)	-	0.94	0.96	0.98
Pneumonia Care				
Appropriate Initial Antibiotic Given	41	98%	96%	95%
Blood Culture Timing	64	100%	98%	98%
Pregnancy and Delivery Care				
Newborn Deliveries Scheduled Early[2]	31	10%	3%	6%
Preventive Care				
Immunization for Influenza[2]	258	96%	89%	90%
Immunization for Pneumonia[2]	267	97%	90%	92%
Stroke Care				
Anticoagulation Therapy for Atrial Fibrillation[1]	-	-	92%	95%
Antithrombotic Therapy Timing	14	50%	97%	98%
Assessed for Rehabilitation	21	95%	97%	97%
Discharged on Antithrombotic Therapy	21	100%	99%	99%
Discharged on Statin Medication	20	50%	94%	94%
Thrombolytic Therapy Timing[1]	-	-	69%	66%
Venous Thromboembolism Prophylaxis	17	71%	94%	94%
Written Stroke Educational Materials Given[1]	-	-	87%	88%
Surgical Care Improvement Project				
Appropriate Beta Blocker Usage	50	98%	98%	98%
Appropriate VTP Within 24 Hours	147	98%	98%	98%
Controlled Postoperative Blood Glucose[7]	-	-	97%	97%
Perioperative Temperature Management	158	100%	100%	100%
Prophylactic Antibiotic Selection	116	99%	99%	99%
Prophylactic Antibiotic Selection (Outpatient)	178	99%	97%	98%
Prophylactic Antibiotic Stopped	113	93%	98%	98%
Prophylactic Antibiotic Timing	116	97%	98%	99%
Prophylactic Antibiotic Timing (Outpatient)	180	99%	97%	98%
Urinary Catheter Removal	97	99%	97%	97%
Survey of Patients' Hospital Experiences				
Area Around Room 'Always' Quiet at Night	300+	71%	60%	61%
Doctors 'Always' Communicated Well	300+	87%	81%	82%
Home Recovery Information Given	300+	88%	87%	85%
Hospital Given 9 or 10 on 10 Point Scale	300+	78%	71%	71%
Meds 'Always' Explained Before Given	300+	71%	64%	64%
Nurses 'Always' Communicated Well	300+	82%	80%	79%
Pain 'Always' Well Controlled	300+	76%	71%	71%
Room and Bathroom 'Always' Clean	300+	82%	73%	73%
Timely Help 'Always' Received	300+	84%	70%	68%
Would Definitely Recommend Hospital	300+	78%	71%	71%
Use of Medical Imaging				
Cardiac Imaging Stress Test before Surgery	128	4.7%	5.1%	5.3%
Combination Abdominal CT Scan	239	7.9%	8.7%	10.5%
Combination Brain/Sinus CT Scan	233	0.9%	2.2%	2.7%
Combination Chest CT Scan	142	3.5%	3.6%	2.7%
Follow-up Mammogram/Ultrasound	490	13.5%	8.2%	8.8%
Lumbar Spine MRI for Low Back Pain	106	45.3%	36.9%	37.2%

Hills & Dales General Hospital

4675 Hill Street
Cass City, MI 48726
Phone: 989-872-2121
Fax: 989-872-5376
E-mail: publicinfo@hillsanddales.com
URL: www.hillsanddales.com
Type: Critical Access Hospitals
Emergency Services: Yes
Ownership: Voluntary non-profit - Private
Beds: 65

Key Personnel:
Hemotology Center . . . . John Bartnik, MD
Chairman/CEO . . . . Orvil Beecher

NOTE: Hospital profiles are in alphabetical order by state, then city, then hospital within the city; Rankings exclude hospitals with less than 25 cases except for patient surveys which excludes hospitals with less than 100 cases; (a) 100-299 cases; (1) The number of cases/patients is too few to report; (2) Data submitted were based on a sample of cases/patients; (3) Results are based on a shorter time period than required; (4) Data suppressed by CMS for one or more quarters; (5) Results are not available for this reporting period; (6) Fewer than 100 patients completed the HCAHPS survey; (7) No cases met the criteria for this measure; (8) The lower limit of the confidence interval cannot be calculated if the number of observed infections equals zero; (9) No data are available from the state/territory for this reporting period; (10) The scores shown reflect fewer than 50 completed surveys; (11) There were discrepancies in the data collection process; (12) This measure does not apply to this hospital for this reporting period; (13) Results cannot be calculated for this reporting period; (14) The results for this state are combined with nearby states to protect confidentiality; Please refer to the User's Guide for a full explanation of data.

Cardiac Laboratory. . . . . Jeffrey Carney, MD
CEO/President. . . . . Dee McKrow
Surgery . . . . Francis Ozim, MD
Radiology. . . . . Vikram Rao

Measure	Cases	This Hosp.	State Avg.	U.S. Avg.
Blood Clot Prevention and Treatment				
Anticoagulation Overlap Therapy[5]	-	-	90%	93%
ICU Venous Thromboembolism Prophylaxis[5]	-	-	93%	92%
Incidence of Potentially Preventable VTE[5]	-	-	8%	10%
UFH with Dosages/Platelet Monitoring[5]	-	-	96%	97%
Venous Thromboembolism Prophylaxis[5]	-	-	87%	85%
Warfarin Therapy Discharge Instructions[5]	-	-	72%	75%
Chest Pain/Possible Heart Attack Care				
Aspirin Given Within 24 Hours of Arrival	39	100%	96%	96%
Fibrinolytic Meds Within 30 Min. of Arrival[1]	-	-	63%	58%
Average Time to ECG (minutes)	39	7	8	7
Average Time to Transfer (minutes)[1]	-	-	53	60
Children's Asthma Care				
Received Home Management Plan of Care	-	-	-	88%
Received Reliever Medication	-	-	-	100%
Received Systemic Corticosteroids	-	-	-	100%
Emergency Department				
Admittance Decision Time (minutes)	419	67	102	98
Head CT Results Within 45 Min. of Arrival[5]	-	-	54%	57%
Patients Who Left ER Before Being Seen[5]	-	-	2%	2%
Time from ER Arrival to Admit. (minutes)	419	219	288	274
Time from ER Arrival to Discharge (minutes)	282	110	128	134
Time in ER Before Being Evaluated (minutes)	395	26	22	26
Time to Pain Meds for Fractures (minutes)[5]	-	-	55	57
Heart Attack Care				
Aspirin Given at Discharge[1,3]	-	-	99%	99%
Fibrinolytic Meds Within 30 Min. of Arrival[3,7]	-	-	20%	54%
PCI Within 90 Minutes of Arrival[3,7]	-	-	95%	96%
Statin Prescribed at Discharge[1,3]	-	-	98%	98%
Heart Failure Care				
ACE Inhibitor or ARB for LVSD[1]	-	-	96%	97%
Discharge Instructions Given	13	85%	94%	94%
Evaluation of LVS Function	16	75%	99%	99%
Medicare Spending				
Medicare Spending per Patient (ratio)	-	-	0.96	0.98
Pneumonia Care				
Appropriate Initial Antibiotic Given	39	87%	96%	95%
Blood Culture Timing	29	90%	98%	98%
Pregnancy and Delivery Care				
Newborn Deliveries Scheduled Early[5]	-	-	3%	6%
Preventive Care				
Immunization for Influenza	235	81%	89%	90%
Immunization for Pneumonia	343	83%	90%	92%
Stroke Care				
Anticoagulation Therapy for Atrial Fibrillation[5]	-	-	92%	95%
Antithrombotic Therapy Timing[5]	-	-	97%	98%
Assessed for Rehabilitation[5]	-	-	97%	97%
Discharged on Antithrombotic Therapy[5]	-	-	99%	99%
Discharged on Statin Medication[5]	-	-	94%	94%
Thrombolytic Therapy Timing[5]	-	-	69%	66%
Venous Thromboembolism Prophylaxis[5]	-	-	94%	94%
Written Stroke Educational Materials Given[5]	-	-	87%	88%
Surgical Care Improvement Project				
Appropriate Beta Blocker Usage[1]	-	-	98%	98%
Appropriate VTP Within 24 Hours	25	88%	98%	98%
Controlled Postoperative Blood Glucose[7]	-	-	97%	97%
Perioperative Temperature Management	32	100%	100%	100%
Prophylactic Antibiotic Selection	25	96%	99%	99%
Prophylactic Antibiotic Selection (Outpatient)[1,3]	-	-	97%	98%
Prophylactic Antibiotic Stopped	24	100%	98%	98%
Prophylactic Antibiotic Timing	25	100%	98%	99%
Prophylactic Antibiotic Timing (Outpatient)[1,3]	-	-	97%	98%
Urinary Catheter Removal	29	97%	97%	97%
Survey of Patients' Hospital Experiences				
Area Around Room 'Always' Quiet at Night	(a)	73%	60%	61%
Doctors 'Always' Communicated Well	(a)	84%	81%	82%
Home Recovery Information Given	(a)	88%	87%	85%
Hospital Given 9 or 10 on 10 Point Scale	(a)	73%	71%	71%
Meds 'Always' Explained Before Given	(a)	68%	64%	64%
Nurses 'Always' Communicated Well	(a)	84%	80%	79%
Pain 'Always' Well Controlled	(a)	73%	71%	71%
Room and Bathroom 'Always' Clean	(a)	79%	73%	73%
Timely Help 'Always' Received	(a)	86%	70%	68%
Would Definitely Recommend Hospital	(a)	76%	71%	71%
Use of Medical Imaging				
Cardiac Imaging Stress Test before Surgery	97	4.1%	5.1%	5.3%
Combination Abdominal CT Scan	211	22.3%	8.7%	10.5%
Combination Brain/Sinus CT Scan[1]	-	-	2.2%	2.7%
Combination Chest CT Scan	128	31.3%	3.6%	2.7%
Follow-up Mammogram/Ultrasound	166	23.5%	8.2%	8.8%
Lumbar Spine MRI for Low Back Pain[7]	-	-	36.9%	37.2%

Charlevoix Area Hospital

14700 Lakeshore Drive
Charlevoix, MI 49720
Phone: 231-547-4024
Fax: 231-547-8080
Type: Critical Access Hospitals
Emergency Services: Yes
Ownership: Voluntary non-profit - Other
Beds: 50

Key Personnel:
Radiology. . . . . Ralph J Duman
Intensive Care Unit. . . . . James Gels, MD
Operating Room. . . . . Chris Good, RN
CEO/President. . . . . William Jackson
Emergency Room . . . . Dennis Joy
Chief of Medical Staff. . . . . Dennis M Joy, MD
Quality Assurance . . . . Chris Wilhelm
Infection Control. . . . . Karen Withers

Measure	Cases	This Hosp.	State Avg.	U.S. Avg.
Blood Clot Prevention and Treatment				
Anticoagulation Overlap Therapy[5]	-	-	90%	93%
ICU Venous Thromboembolism Prophylaxis[5]	-	-	93%	92%
Incidence of Potentially Preventable VTE[5]	-	-	8%	10%
UFH with Dosages/Platelet Monitoring[5]	-	-	96%	97%
Venous Thromboembolism Prophylaxis[5]	-	-	87%	85%
Warfarin Therapy Discharge Instructions[5]	-	-	72%	75%
Chest Pain/Possible Heart Attack Care				
Aspirin Given Within 24 Hours of Arrival[1,3]	-	-	96%	96%
Fibrinolytic Meds Within 30 Min. of Arrival[3,7]	-	-	63%	58%
Average Time to ECG (minutes)[1,3]	-	-	8	7
Average Time to Transfer (minutes)[3,7]	-	-	53	60
Children's Asthma Care				
Received Home Management Plan of Care	-	-	-	88%
Received Reliever Medication	-	-	-	100%
Received Systemic Corticosteroids	-	-	-	100%
Emergency Department				
Admittance Decision Time (minutes)[5]	-	-	102	98
Head CT Results Within 45 Min. of Arrival[5]	-	-	54%	57%
Patients Who Left ER Before Being Seen[5]	-	-	2%	2%
Time from ER Arrival to Admit. (minutes)[5]	-	-	288	274
Time from ER Arrival to Discharge (minutes)	328	124	128	134
Time in ER Before Being Evaluated (minutes)	377	27	22	26
Time to Pain Meds for Fractures (minutes)[5]	-	-	55	57
Heart Attack Care				
Aspirin Given at Discharge[1,3]	-	-	99%	99%
Fibrinolytic Meds Within 30 Min. of Arrival[3,7]	-	-	20%	54%
PCI Within 90 Minutes of Arrival[3,7]	-	-	95%	96%
Statin Prescribed at Discharge[3,7]	-	-	98%	98%
Heart Failure Care				
ACE Inhibitor or ARB for LVSD[1]	-	-	96%	97%
Discharge Instructions Given[1]	-	-	94%	94%
Evaluation of LVS Function	13	100%	99%	99%
Medicare Spending				
Medicare Spending per Patient (ratio)	-	-	0.96	0.98
Pneumonia Care				
Appropriate Initial Antibiotic Given	19	100%	96%	95%
Blood Culture Timing	28	100%	98%	98%
Pregnancy and Delivery Care				
Newborn Deliveries Scheduled Early[5]	-	-	3%	6%
Preventive Care				
Immunization for Influenza[5]	-	-	89%	90%
Immunization for Pneumonia[5]	-	-	90%	92%
Stroke Care				
Anticoagulation Therapy for Atrial Fibrillation[5]	-	-	92%	95%
Antithrombotic Therapy Timing[5]	-	-	97%	98%
Assessed for Rehabilitation[5]	-	-	97%	97%
Discharged on Antithrombotic Therapy[5]	-	-	99%	99%
Discharged on Statin Medication[5]	-	-	94%	94%
Thrombolytic Therapy Timing[5]	-	-	69%	66%
Venous Thromboembolism Prophylaxis[5]	-	-	94%	94%
Written Stroke Educational Materials Given[5]	-	-	87%	88%
Surgical Care Improvement Project				
Appropriate Beta Blocker Usage[5]	-	-	98%	98%
Appropriate VTP Within 24 Hours[5]	-	-	98%	98%
Controlled Postoperative Blood Glucose[5]	-	-	97%	97%
Perioperative Temperature Management[5]	-	-	100%	100%
Prophylactic Antibiotic Selection[5]	-	-	99%	99%
Prophylactic Antibiotic Selection (Outpatient)[1,3]	-	-	97%	98%
Prophylactic Antibiotic Stopped[5]	-	-	98%	98%
Prophylactic Antibiotic Timing[5]	-	-	98%	99%
Prophylactic Antibiotic Timing (Outpatient)[1,3]	-	-	97%	98%
Urinary Catheter Removal[5]	-	-	97%	97%
Survey of Patients' Hospital Experiences				
Area Around Room 'Always' Quiet at Night	300+	71%	60%	61%
Doctors 'Always' Communicated Well	300+	85%	81%	82%
Home Recovery Information Given	300+	88%	87%	85%
Hospital Given 9 or 10 on 10 Point Scale	300+	80%	71%	71%
Meds 'Always' Explained Before Given	300+	69%	64%	64%
Nurses 'Always' Communicated Well	300+	83%	80%	79%
Pain 'Always' Well Controlled	300+	77%	71%	71%
Room and Bathroom 'Always' Clean	300+	82%	73%	73%
Timely Help 'Always' Received	300+	82%	70%	68%
Would Definitely Recommend Hospital	300+	83%	71%	71%
Use of Medical Imaging				
Cardiac Imaging Stress Test before Surgery	111	4.5%	5.1%	5.3%
Combination Abdominal CT Scan	162	11.7%	8.7%	10.5%
Combination Brain/Sinus CT Scan	188	1.1%	2.2%	2.7%
Combination Chest CT Scan	90	0.0%	3.6%	2.7%
Follow-up Mammogram/Ultrasound	308	9.1%	8.2%	8.8%
Lumbar Spine MRI for Low Back Pain	48	37.5%	36.9%	37.2%

Hayes Green Beach Memorial Hospital

321 E Harris Street
Charlotte, MI 48813
Phone: 517-543-1050
Fax: 517-543-0875
E-mail: mrush@hgbhealth.com
URL: www.hgbhealth.com
Type: Critical Access Hospitals
Emergency Services: Yes
Ownership: Voluntary non-profit - Other
Beds: 45

Key Personnel:
Surgery . . . . Stephanie Almy
Chairman/CEO . . . . Fred Darin, OD
Emergency Room . . . . Sherman Horn
Chief of Medical Staff. . . . . Hugh Lindsey, DO
CEO/President. . . . . Matthew W Rush, CHE
Radiology. . . . . Bing Tai
Anesthesiology. . . . . Douglas Wolford

Measure	Cases	This Hosp.	State Avg.	U.S. Avg.
Blood Clot Prevention and Treatment				
Anticoagulation Overlap Therapy[5]	-	-	90%	93%
ICU Venous Thromboembolism Prophylaxis[5]	-	-	93%	92%
Incidence of Potentially Preventable VTE[5]	-	-	8%	10%
UFH with Dosages/Platelet Monitoring[5]	-	-	96%	97%
Venous Thromboembolism Prophylaxis[5]	-	-	87%	85%
Warfarin Therapy Discharge Instructions[5]	-	-	72%	75%
Chest Pain/Possible Heart Attack Care				
Aspirin Given Within 24 Hours of Arrival	39	100%	96%	96%
Fibrinolytic Meds Within 30 Min. of Arrival[1]	-	-	63%	58%
Average Time to ECG (minutes)	39	8	8	7
Average Time to Transfer (minutes)[1]	-	-	53	60
Children's Asthma Care				
Received Home Management Plan of Care	-	-	-	88%
Received Reliever Medication	-	-	-	100%
Received Systemic Corticosteroids	-	-	-	100%
Emergency Department				
Admittance Decision Time (minutes)[5]	-	-	102	98
Head CT Results Within 45 Min. of Arrival[5]	-	-	54%	57%
Patients Who Left ER Before Being Seen[5]	-	-	2%	2%

NOTE: Hospital profiles are in alphabetical order by state, then city, then hospital within the city; Rankings exclude hospitals with less than 25 cases except for patient surveys which excludes hospitals with less than 100 cases; (a) 100-299 cases; (1) The number of cases/patients is too few to report; (2) Data submitted were based on a sample of cases/patients; (3) Results are based on a shorter time period than required; (4) Data suppressed by CMS for one or more quarters; (5) Results are not available for this reporting period; (6) Fewer than 100 patients completed the HCAHPS survey; (7) No cases met the criteria for this measure; (8) The lower limit of the confidence interval cannot be calculated if the number of observed infections equals zero; (9) No data are available from the state/territory for this reporting period; (10) The scores shown reflect fewer than 50 completed surveys; (11) There were discrepancies in the data collection process; (12) This measure does not apply to this hospital for this reporting period; (13) Results cannot be calculated for this reporting period; (14) The results for this state are combined with nearby states to protect confidentiality; Please refer to the User's Guide for a full explanation of data.

Measure	Cases	This Hosp.	State Avg.	U.S. Avg.
Time from ER Arrival to Admit. (minutes)[5]	-	-	288	274
Time from ER Arrival to Discharge (minutes)	412	157	128	134
Time in ER Before Being Evaluated (minutes)	430	39	22	26
Time to Pain Meds for Fractures (minutes)[3]	52	59	55	57
Heart Attack Care				
Aspirin Given at Discharge[1,3]	-	-	99%	99%
Fibrinolytic Meds Within 30 Min. of Arrival[3,7]	-	-	20%	54%
PCI Within 90 Minutes of Arrival[3,7]	-	-	95%	96%
Statin Prescribed at Discharge[1,3]	-	-	98%	98%
Heart Failure Care				
ACE Inhibitor or ARB for LVSD[1]	-	-	96%	97%
Discharge Instructions Given	29	100%	94%	94%
Evaluation of LVS Function	37	100%	99%	99%
Medicare Spending				
Medicare Spending per Patient (ratio)	-	-	0.96	0.98
Pneumonia Care				
Appropriate Initial Antibiotic Given	23	100%	96%	95%
Blood Culture Timing	66	100%	98%	98%
Pregnancy and Delivery Care				
Newborn Deliveries Scheduled Early[5]	-	-	3%	6%
Preventive Care				
Immunization for Influenza[5]	-	-	89%	90%
Immunization for Pneumonia[2,3]	213	83%	90%	92%
Stroke Care				
Anticoagulation Therapy for Atrial Fibrillation[5]	-	-	92%	95%
Antithrombotic Therapy Timing[5]	-	-	97%	98%
Assessed for Rehabilitation[5]	-	-	97%	97%
Discharged on Antithrombotic Therapy[5]	-	-	99%	99%
Discharged on Statin Medication[5]	-	-	94%	94%
Thrombolytic Therapy Timing[5]	-	-	69%	66%
Venous Thromboembolism Prophylaxis[5]	-	-	94%	94%
Written Stroke Educational Materials Given[5]	-	-	87%	88%
Surgical Care Improvement Project				
Appropriate Beta Blocker Usage[1]	-	-	98%	98%
Appropriate VTP Within 24 Hours	47	100%	98%	98%
Controlled Postoperative Blood Glucose[7]	-	-	97%	97%
Perioperative Temperature Management	49	100%	100%	100%
Prophylactic Antibiotic Selection	36	97%	99%	99%
Prophylactic Antibiotic Selection (Outpatient)	19	100%	97%	98%
Prophylactic Antibiotic Stopped	36	94%	98%	98%
Prophylactic Antibiotic Timing	36	94%	98%	99%
Prophylactic Antibiotic Timing (Outpatient)	19	100%	97%	98%
Urinary Catheter Removal	13	92%	97%	97%
Survey of Patients' Hospital Experiences				
Area Around Room 'Always' Quiet at Night	(a)	67%	60%	61%
Doctors 'Always' Communicated Well	(a)	75%	81%	82%
Home Recovery Information Given	(a)	89%	87%	85%
Hospital Given 9 or 10 on 10 Point Scale	(a)	67%	71%	71%
Meds 'Always' Explained Before Given	(a)	62%	64%	64%
Nurses 'Always' Communicated Well	(a)	75%	80%	79%
Pain 'Always' Well Controlled	(a)	71%	71%	71%
Room and Bathroom 'Always' Clean	(a)	77%	73%	73%
Timely Help 'Always' Received	(a)	66%	70%	68%
Would Definitely Recommend Hospital	(a)	64%	71%	71%
Use of Medical Imaging				
Cardiac Imaging Stress Test before Surgery	144	2.8%	5.1%	5.3%
Combination Abdominal CT Scan	405	30.1%	8.7%	10.5%
Combination Brain/Sinus CT Scan[1]	-	-	2.2%	2.7%
Combination Chest CT Scan	159	4.4%	3.6%	2.7%
Follow-up Mammogram/Ultrasound	448	7.4%	8.2%	8.8%
Lumbar Spine MRI for Low Back Pain	54	38.9%	36.9%	37.2%

Chelsea Community Hospital

775 S Main St
Chelsea, MI 48118
URL: www.cch.org
Phone: 734-475-3911
Fax: 734-475-4066
Type: Acute Care Hospitals
Ownership: Voluntary non-profit - Private
Emergency Services: Yes
Beds: 113

Key Personnel:
Emergency Room . . . . Nancy Fields
CEO/President. . . . . Kathleen Griffiths
Chief of Medical Staff . . . . Lawrence Handelsman

Measure	Cases	This Hosp.	State Avg.	U.S. Avg.
Blood Clot Prevention and Treatment				
Anticoagulation Overlap Therapy[2]	18	100%	90%	93%
ICU Venous Thromboembolism Prophylaxis[2]	38	100%	93%	92%
Incidence of Potentially Preventable VTE[1,2]	-	-	8%	10%
UFH with Dosages/Platelet Monitoring[2]	13	100%	96%	97%
Venous Thromboembolism Prophylaxis[2]	242	98%	87%	85%
Warfarin Therapy Discharge Instructions[2]	20	90%	72%	75%
Chest Pain/Possible Heart Attack Care				
Aspirin Given Within 24 Hours of Arrival	91	97%	96%	96%
Fibrinolytic Meds Within 30 Min. of Arrival[7]	-	-	63%	58%
Average Time to ECG (minutes)	92	6	8	7
Average Time to Transfer (minutes)[1]	-	-	53	60
Children's Asthma Care				
Received Home Management Plan of Care	-	-	-	88%
Received Reliever Medication	-	-	-	100%
Received Systemic Corticosteroids	-	-	-	100%
Emergency Department				
Admittance Decision Time (minutes)[2]	253	66	102	98
Head CT Results Within 45 Min. of Arrival[1]	-	-	54%	57%
Patients Who Left ER Before Being Seen	17,222	1%	2%	2%
Time from ER Arrival to Admit. (minutes)[2]	263	304	288	274
Time from ER Arrival to Discharge (minutes)	383	179	128	134
Time in ER Before Being Evaluated (minutes)	415	14	22	26
Time to Pain Meds for Fractures (minutes)	86	52	55	57
Heart Attack Care				
Aspirin Given at Discharge[1]	-	-	99%	99%
Fibrinolytic Meds Within 30 Min. of Arrival[7]	-	-	20%	54%
PCI Within 90 Minutes of Arrival[7]	-	-	95%	96%
Statin Prescribed at Discharge[1]	-	-	98%	98%
Heart Failure Care				
ACE Inhibitor or ARB for LVSD	18	100%	96%	97%
Discharge Instructions Given	67	100%	94%	94%
Evaluation of LVS Function	79	100%	99%	99%
Medicare Spending				
Medicare Spending per Patient (ratio)	-	0.94	0.96	0.98
Pneumonia Care				
Appropriate Initial Antibiotic Given	71	99%	96%	95%
Blood Culture Timing	102	97%	98%	98%
Pregnancy and Delivery Care				
Newborn Deliveries Scheduled Early[7]	-	-	3%	6%
Preventive Care				
Immunization for Influenza[2]	354	95%	89%	90%
Immunization for Pneumonia[2]	426	96%	90%	92%
Stroke Care				
Anticoagulation Therapy for Atrial Fibrillation[1]	-	-	92%	95%
Antithrombotic Therapy Timing	33	97%	97%	98%
Assessed for Rehabilitation	36	100%	97%	97%
Discharged on Antithrombotic Therapy	34	100%	99%	99%
Discharged on Statin Medication	25	96%	94%	94%
Thrombolytic Therapy Timing[7]	-	-	69%	66%
Venous Thromboembolism Prophylaxis	34	97%	94%	94%
Written Stroke Educational Materials Given	16	75%	87%	88%
Surgical Care Improvement Project				
Appropriate Beta Blocker Usage[2]	134	100%	98%	98%
Appropriate VTP Within 24 Hours[2]	782	99%	98%	98%
Controlled Postoperative Blood Glucose[2,7]	-	-	97%	97%
Perioperative Temperature Management[2]	935	100%	100%	100%
Prophylactic Antibiotic Selection[2]	787	100%	99%	99%
Prophylactic Antibiotic Selection (Outpatient)	87	98%	97%	98%
Prophylactic Antibiotic Stopped[2]	781	100%	98%	98%
Prophylactic Antibiotic Timing[2]	787	100%	98%	99%
Prophylactic Antibiotic Timing (Outpatient)	84	99%	97%	98%
Urinary Catheter Removal[2]	687	100%	97%	97%
Survey of Patients' Hospital Experiences				
Area Around Room 'Always' Quiet at Night	300+	76%	60%	61%
Doctors 'Always' Communicated Well	300+	84%	81%	82%
Home Recovery Information Given	300+	91%	87%	85%
Hospital Given 9 or 10 on 10 Point Scale	300+	85%	71%	71%
Meds 'Always' Explained Before Given	300+	68%	64%	64%
Nurses 'Always' Communicated Well	300+	85%	80%	79%
Pain 'Always' Well Controlled	300+	73%	71%	71%
Room and Bathroom 'Always' Clean	300+	79%	73%	73%
Timely Help 'Always' Received	300+	76%	70%	68%
Would Definitely Recommend Hospital	300+	87%	71%	71%
Use of Medical Imaging				
Cardiac Imaging Stress Test before Surgery	276	6.5%	5.1%	5.3%
Combination Abdominal CT Scan	392	10.5%	8.7%	10.5%
Combination Brain/Sinus CT Scan	405	0.7%	2.2%	2.7%
Combination Chest CT Scan	266	0.4%	3.6%	2.7%
Follow-up Mammogram/Ultrasound	1,161	10.9%	8.2%	8.8%
Lumbar Spine MRI for Low Back Pain	176	33.0%	36.9%	37.2%

Midmichigan Medical Center - Clare

703 N Mcewan St
Clare, MI 48617
URL: www.midmichigan.org
Phone: 989-802-5000
Fax: 989-802-8895
Type: Acute Care Hospitals
Ownership: Voluntary non-profit - Other
Emergency Services: Yes
Beds: 49

Key Personnel:
Coronary Care . . . . Robert Briggs, RN
Operating Room. . . . . Mary Eppert, RN
Surgery . . . . Vivian Ko, DO
Emergency Room . . . . Jose C. Magno, MD
Chief of Medical Staff . . . . Rajani Mallick
Quality Assurance . . . . Penny Parsons
Pediatric In-Patient Care . . . . Bette Shepard, MD
Infection Control. . . . . Bea Van Buskirk, RN

Measure	Cases	This Hosp.	State Avg.	U.S. Avg.
Blood Clot Prevention and Treatment				
Anticoagulation Overlap Therapy[1,2]	-	-	90%	93%
ICU Venous Thromboembolism Prophylaxis[2]	30	97%	93%	92%
Incidence of Potentially Preventable VTE[1,2]	-	-	8%	10%
UFH with Dosages/Platelet Monitoring[1,2]	-	-	96%	97%
Venous Thromboembolism Prophylaxis[2]	137	93%	87%	85%
Warfarin Therapy Discharge Instructions[1,2]	-	-	72%	75%
Chest Pain/Possible Heart Attack Care				
Aspirin Given Within 24 Hours of Arrival	130	98%	96%	96%
Fibrinolytic Meds Within 30 Min. of Arrival[1]	-	-	63%	58%
Average Time to ECG (minutes)	136	7	8	7
Average Time to Transfer (minutes)[1]	-	-	53	60
Children's Asthma Care				
Received Home Management Plan of Care	-	-	-	88%
Received Reliever Medication	-	-	-	100%
Received Systemic Corticosteroids	-	-	-	100%
Emergency Department				
Admittance Decision Time (minutes)[2]	482	71	102	98
Head CT Results Within 45 Min. of Arrival	11	82%	54%	57%
Patients Who Left ER Before Being Seen	15,575	3%	2%	2%
Time from ER Arrival to Admit. (minutes)[2]	546	248	288	274
Time from ER Arrival to Discharge (minutes)	406	168	128	134
Time in ER Before Being Evaluated (minutes)	320	36	22	26
Time to Pain Meds for Fractures (minutes)	99	62	55	57
Heart Attack Care				
Aspirin Given at Discharge	16	100%	99%	99%
Fibrinolytic Meds Within 30 Min. of Arrival[7]	-	-	20%	54%
PCI Within 90 Minutes of Arrival[7]	-	-	95%	96%
Statin Prescribed at Discharge	14	93%	98%	98%
Heart Failure Care				
ACE Inhibitor or ARB for LVSD	31	94%	96%	97%
Discharge Instructions Given	95	96%	94%	94%
Evaluation of LVS Function	110	99%	99%	99%
Medicare Spending				
Medicare Spending per Patient (ratio)	-	0.88	0.96	0.98
Pneumonia Care				
Appropriate Initial Antibiotic Given	62	94%	96%	95%
Blood Culture Timing	94	99%	98%	98%
Pregnancy and Delivery Care				
Newborn Deliveries Scheduled Early[7]	-	-	3%	6%
Preventive Care				
Immunization for Influenza[2]	322	97%	89%	90%
Immunization for Pneumonia[2]	522	99%	90%	92%
Stroke Care				
Anticoagulation Therapy for Atrial Fibrillation[1]	-	-	92%	95%
Antithrombotic Therapy Timing	13	100%	97%	98%
Assessed for Rehabilitation	13	100%	97%	97%
Discharged on Antithrombotic Therapy	13	100%	99%	99%

NOTE: Hospital profiles are in alphabetical order by state, then city, then hospital within the city; Rankings exclude hospitals with less than 25 cases except for patient surveys which excludes hospitals with less than 100 cases; (a) 100-299 cases; (1) The number of cases/patients is too few to report; (2) Data submitted were based on a sample of cases/patients; (3) Results are based on a shorter time period than required; (4) Data suppressed by CMS for one or more quarters; (5) Results are not available for this reporting period; (6) Fewer than 100 patients completed the HCAHPS survey; (7) No cases met the criteria for this measure; (8) The lower limit of the confidence interval cannot be calculated if the number of observed infections equals zero; (9) No data are available from the state/territory for this reporting period; (10) The scores shown reflect fewer than 50 completed surveys; (11) There were discrepancies in the data collection process; (12) This measure does not apply to this hospital for this reporting period; (13) Results cannot be calculated for this reporting period; (14) The results for this state are combined with nearby states to protect confidentiality; Please refer to the User's Guide for a full explanation of data.

Measure	Cases	This Hosp.	State Avg.	U.S. Avg.
Discharged on Statin Medication	12	100%	94%	94%
Thrombolytic Therapy Timing[1]	-	-	69%	66%
Venous Thromboembolism Prophylaxis	14	86%	94%	94%
Written Stroke Educational Materials Given[1]	-	-	87%	88%
Surgical Care Improvement Project				
Appropriate Beta Blocker Usage	29	100%	98%	98%
Appropriate VTP Within 24 Hours	63	97%	98%	98%
Controlled Postoperative Blood Glucose[7]	-	-	97%	97%
Perioperative Temperature Management	69	99%	100%	100%
Prophylactic Antibiotic Selection	45	96%	99%	99%
Prophylactic Antibiotic Selection (Outpatient)[1]	-	-	97%	98%
Prophylactic Antibiotic Stopped	43	100%	98%	98%
Prophylactic Antibiotic Timing	45	98%	98%	99%
Prophylactic Antibiotic Timing (Outpatient)[1]	-	-	97%	98%
Urinary Catheter Removal	61	100%	97%	97%
Survey of Patients' Hospital Experiences				
Area Around Room 'Always' Quiet at Night	300+	57%	60%	61%
Doctors 'Always' Communicated Well	300+	77%	81%	82%
Home Recovery Information Given	300+	90%	87%	85%
Hospital Given 9 or 10 on 10 Point Scale	300+	67%	71%	71%
Meds 'Always' Explained Before Given	300+	66%	64%	64%
Nurses 'Always' Communicated Well	300+	79%	80%	79%
Pain 'Always' Well Controlled	300+	71%	71%	71%
Room and Bathroom 'Always' Clean	300+	71%	73%	73%
Timely Help 'Always' Received	300+	73%	70%	68%
Would Definitely Recommend Hospital	300+	64%	71%	71%
Use of Medical Imaging				
Cardiac Imaging Stress Test before Surgery	204	4.4%	5.1%	5.3%
Combination Abdominal CT Scan	531	3.4%	8.7%	10.5%
Combination Brain/Sinus CT Scan	488	0.8%	2.2%	2.7%
Combination Chest CT Scan	385	2.6%	3.6%	2.7%
Follow-up Mammogram/Ultrasound	1,071	6.7%	8.2%	8.8%
Lumbar Spine MRI for Low Back Pain	110	36.4%	36.9%	37.2%

Henry Ford Macomb Hospital

15855 Nineteen Mile Rd
Clinton Township, MI 48038
Phone: 586-263-2300
Fax: 586-263-2859
URL: www.stjoe-macomb.com
Type: Acute Care Hospitals
Emergency Services: Yes
Ownership: Proprietary
Beds: 435

Key Personnel:
Operating Room. . . . . Susan Assaf
Pediatric In-Patient Care . . . . Allen Balinski, MD
Quality Assurance . . . . Jane Goldfarb
Radiology. . . . . Donna Moir
Infection Control. . . . . Sharon Ritter
CEO/President. . . . . Barbara Rossmann
Chief of Medical Staff . . . . Richard Stone, MD

Measure	Cases	This Hosp.	State Avg.	U.S. Avg.
Blood Clot Prevention and Treatment				
Anticoagulation Overlap Therapy[2]	146	94%	90%	93%
ICU Venous Thromboembolism Prophylaxis[2]	51	100%	93%	92%
Incidence of Potentially Preventable VTE[2]	30	10%	8%	10%
UFH with Dosages/Platelet Monitoring[2]	155	100%	96%	97%
Venous Thromboembolism Prophylaxis[2]	372	83%	87%	85%
Warfarin Therapy Discharge Instructions[2]	105	90%	72%	75%
Chest Pain/Possible Heart Attack Care				
Aspirin Given Within 24 Hours of Arrival[1]	-	-	96%	96%
Fibrinolytic Meds Within 30 Min. of Arrival[3,7]	-	-	63%	58%
Average Time to ECG (minutes)[1]	-	-	8	7
Average Time to Transfer (minutes)[3,7]	-	-	53	60
Children's Asthma Care				
Received Home Management Plan of Care	-	-	-	88%
Received Reliever Medication	-	-	-	100%
Received Systemic Corticosteroids	-	-	-	100%
Emergency Department				
Admittance Decision Time (minutes)[2]	649	129	102	98
Head CT Results Within 45 Min. of Arrival	12	67%	54%	57%
Patients Who Left ER Before Being Seen	71,171	0%	2%	2%
Time from ER Arrival to Admit. (minutes)[2]	700	340	288	274
Time from ER Arrival to Discharge (minutes)	329	185	128	134
Time in ER Before Being Evaluated (minutes)	371	7	22	26
Time to Pain Meds for Fractures (minutes)	160	57	55	57
Heart Attack Care				
Aspirin Given at Discharge	439	100%	99%	99%
Fibrinolytic Meds Within 30 Min. of Arrival[7]	-	-	20%	54%
PCI Within 90 Minutes of Arrival	72	100%	95%	96%
Statin Prescribed at Discharge	412	100%	98%	98%
Heart Failure Care				
ACE Inhibitor or ARB for LVSD[2]	67	100%	96%	97%
Discharge Instructions Given[2]	229	97%	94%	94%
Evaluation of LVS Function[2]	294	100%	99%	99%
Medicare Spending				
Medicare Spending per Patient (ratio)	-	1.04	0.96	0.98
Pneumonia Care				
Appropriate Initial Antibiotic Given[2]	127	96%	96%	95%
Blood Culture Timing[2]	222	98%	98%	98%
Pregnancy and Delivery Care				
Newborn Deliveries Scheduled Early	180	2%	3%	6%
Preventive Care				
Immunization for Influenza[2]	573	81%	89%	90%
Immunization for Pneumonia[2]	751	82%	90%	92%
Stroke Care				
Anticoagulation Therapy for Atrial Fibrillation	33	100%	92%	95%
Antithrombotic Therapy Timing	199	96%	97%	98%
Assessed for Rehabilitation	221	98%	97%	97%
Discharged on Antithrombotic Therapy	206	99%	99%	99%
Discharged on Statin Medication	163	95%	94%	94%
Thrombolytic Therapy Timing	20	90%	69%	66%
Venous Thromboembolism Prophylaxis	237	90%	94%	94%
Written Stroke Educational Materials Given	110	93%	87%	88%
Surgical Care Improvement Project				
Appropriate Beta Blocker Usage[2]	343	99%	98%	98%
Appropriate VTP Within 24 Hours[2]	595	99%	98%	98%
Controlled Postoperative Blood Glucose[2]	131	99%	97%	97%
Perioperative Temperature Management[2]	768	100%	100%	100%
Prophylactic Antibiotic Selection[2]	701	100%	99%	99%
Prophylactic Antibiotic Selection (Outpatient)	409	99%	97%	98%
Prophylactic Antibiotic Stopped[2]	684	99%	98%	98%
Prophylactic Antibiotic Timing[2]	702	100%	98%	99%
Prophylactic Antibiotic Timing (Outpatient)	410	99%	97%	98%
Urinary Catheter Removal[2]	578	100%	97%	97%
Survey of Patients' Hospital Experiences				
Area Around Room 'Always' Quiet at Night	300+	48%	60%	61%
Doctors 'Always' Communicated Well	300+	74%	81%	82%
Home Recovery Information Given	300+	83%	87%	85%
Hospital Given 9 or 10 on 10 Point Scale	300+	64%	71%	71%
Meds 'Always' Explained Before Given	300+	60%	64%	64%
Nurses 'Always' Communicated Well	300+	78%	80%	79%
Pain 'Always' Well Controlled	300+	67%	71%	71%
Room and Bathroom 'Always' Clean	300+	60%	73%	73%
Timely Help 'Always' Received	300+	63%	70%	68%
Would Definitely Recommend Hospital	300+	66%	71%	71%
Use of Medical Imaging				
Cardiac Imaging Stress Test before Surgery	661	5.4%	5.1%	5.3%
Combination Abdominal CT Scan	1,271	15.3%	8.7%	10.5%
Combination Brain/Sinus CT Scan	1,326	2.0%	2.2%	2.7%
Combination Chest CT Scan	867	7.5%	3.6%	2.7%
Follow-up Mammogram/Ultrasound	2,466	10.1%	8.2%	8.8%
Lumbar Spine MRI for Low Back Pain	194	34.0%	36.9%	37.2%

Community Health Center of Branch County

274 E Chicago St
Coldwater, MI 49036
Phone: 517-279-5400
Fax: 517-279-5499
URL: www.chcbc.com
Type: Acute Care Hospitals
Emergency Services: Yes
Ownership: Government - Local
Beds: 96

Key Personnel:
CEO/President. . . . . Randy DeGroot
Pediatric Ambulatory Care . . . . . . Edelwina Dy, MD
Radiology. . . . . John Kirkpatrick, MD
Quality Assurance . . . . Connie Mayers
Infection Control. . . . . Connie Meyer
Pediatric In-Patient Care . . . . Connie Meyer, MD
Coronary Care . . . . Jane Obrochta
Chief of Medical Staff . . . . John Sennish

Measure	Cases	This Hosp.	State Avg.	U.S. Avg.
Blood Clot Prevention and Treatment				
Anticoagulation Overlap Therapy[2]	25	52%	90%	93%
ICU Venous Thromboembolism Prophylaxis[2]	34	59%	93%	92%
Incidence of Potentially Preventable VTE[1,2]	-	-	8%	10%
UFH with Dosages/Platelet Monitoring[2]	27	74%	96%	97%
Venous Thromboembolism Prophylaxis[2]	270	41%	87%	85%
Warfarin Therapy Discharge Instructions[2]	19	79%	72%	75%
Chest Pain/Possible Heart Attack Care				
Aspirin Given Within 24 Hours of Arrival	187	94%	96%	96%
Fibrinolytic Meds Within 30 Min. of Arrival[1]	-	-	63%	58%
Average Time to ECG (minutes)	196	12	8	7
Average Time to Transfer (minutes)[1]	-	-	53	60
Children's Asthma Care				
Received Home Management Plan of Care	-	-	-	88%
Received Reliever Medication	-	-	-	100%
Received Systemic Corticosteroids	-	-	-	100%
Emergency Department				
Admittance Decision Time (minutes)[2]	165	139	102	98
Head CT Results Within 45 Min. of Arrival[1]	-	-	54%	57%
Patients Who Left ER Before Being Seen	24,850	1%	2%	2%
Time from ER Arrival to Admit. (minutes)[2]	385	265	288	274
Time from ER Arrival to Discharge (minutes)	325	103	128	134
Time in ER Before Being Evaluated (minutes)	265	32	22	26
Time to Pain Meds for Fractures (minutes)	97	62	55	57
Heart Attack Care				
Aspirin Given at Discharge	12	100%	99%	99%
Fibrinolytic Meds Within 30 Min. of Arrival[7]	-	-	20%	54%
PCI Within 90 Minutes of Arrival[7]	-	-	95%	96%
Statin Prescribed at Discharge[1]	-	-	98%	98%
Heart Failure Care				
ACE Inhibitor or ARB for LVSD	22	95%	96%	97%
Discharge Instructions Given	82	98%	94%	94%
Evaluation of LVS Function	102	99%	99%	99%
Medicare Spending				
Medicare Spending per Patient (ratio)	-	0.96	0.96	0.98
Pneumonia Care				
Appropriate Initial Antibiotic Given	119	90%	96%	95%
Blood Culture Timing	166	99%	98%	98%
Pregnancy and Delivery Care				
Newborn Deliveries Scheduled Early[2]	20	0%	3%	6%
Preventive Care				
Immunization for Influenza[2]	351	95%	89%	90%
Immunization for Pneumonia[2]	444	98%	90%	92%
Stroke Care				
Anticoagulation Therapy for Atrial Fibrillation	12	25%	92%	95%
Antithrombotic Therapy Timing	35	83%	97%	98%
Assessed for Rehabilitation	41	59%	97%	97%
Discharged on Antithrombotic Therapy	40	82%	99%	99%
Discharged on Statin Medication	34	47%	94%	94%
Thrombolytic Therapy Timing[1]	-	-	69%	66%
Venous Thromboembolism Prophylaxis	37	46%	94%	94%
Written Stroke Educational Materials Given	27	11%	87%	88%
Surgical Care Improvement Project				
Appropriate Beta Blocker Usage	55	95%	98%	98%
Appropriate VTP Within 24 Hours	165	95%	98%	98%
Controlled Postoperative Blood Glucose[7]	-	-	97%	97%
Perioperative Temperature Management	183	100%	100%	100%
Prophylactic Antibiotic Selection	108	99%	99%	99%
Prophylactic Antibiotic Selection (Outpatient)	50	96%	97%	98%
Prophylactic Antibiotic Stopped	104	99%	98%	98%
Prophylactic Antibiotic Timing	108	100%	98%	99%
Prophylactic Antibiotic Timing (Outpatient)	51	98%	97%	98%
Urinary Catheter Removal	116	96%	97%	97%
Survey of Patients' Hospital Experiences				
Area Around Room 'Always' Quiet at Night	300+	60%	60%	61%
Doctors 'Always' Communicated Well	300+	79%	81%	82%
Home Recovery Information Given	300+	85%	87%	85%
Hospital Given 9 or 10 on 10 Point Scale	300+	72%	71%	71%
Meds 'Always' Explained Before Given	300+	67%	64%	64%
Nurses 'Always' Communicated Well	300+	82%	80%	79%
Pain 'Always' Well Controlled	300+	70%	71%	71%
Room and Bathroom 'Always' Clean	300+	71%	73%	73%
Timely Help 'Always' Received	300+	66%	70%	68%

NOTE: Hospital profiles are in alphabetical order by state, then city, then hospital within the city; Rankings exclude hospitals with less than 25 cases except for patient surveys which excludes hospitals with less than 100 cases; (a) 100-299 cases; (1) The number of cases/patients is too few to report; (2) Data submitted were based on a sample of cases/patients; (3) Results are based on a shorter time period than required; (4) Data suppressed by CMS for one or more quarters; (5) Results are not available for this reporting period; (6) Fewer than 100 patients completed the HCAHPS survey; (7) No cases met the criteria for this measure; (8) The lower limit of the confidence interval cannot be calculated if the number of observed infections equals zero; (9) No data are available from the state/territory for this reporting period; (10) The scores shown reflect fewer than 50 completed surveys; (11) There were discrepancies in the data collection process; (12) This measure does not apply to this hospital for this reporting period; (13) Results cannot be calculated for this reporting period; (14) The results for this state are combined with nearby states to protect confidentiality; Please refer to the User's Guide for a full explanation of data.

Would Definitely Recommend Hospital	300+	69%	71%	71%
Use of Medical Imaging				
Cardiac Imaging Stress Test before Surgery	258	2.7%	5.1%	5.3%
Combination Abdominal CT Scan	469	10.4%	8.7%	10.5%
Combination Brain/Sinus CT Scan[1]	-	-	2.2%	2.7%
Combination Chest CT Scan	266	10.2%	3.6%	2.7%
Follow-up Mammogram/Ultrasound	777	8.1%	8.2%	8.8%
Lumbar Spine MRI for Low Back Pain	61	36.1%	36.9%	37.2%

Huron Valley - Sinai Hospital

One William Carls Drive
Commerce Township, MI 48382
URL: www.hvsh.org
Type: Acute Care Hospitals
Ownership: Proprietary
Phone: 248-937-3370
Fax: 248-937-5074
Emergency Services: Yes
Beds: 153

Key Personnel:
Chief of Medical Staff.......... Marc P Bocknek
Radiology.................. John Kelly, DO
CEO/President............... Robert J Yellan

Measure	Cases	This Hosp.	State Avg.	U.S. Avg.
Blood Clot Prevention and Treatment				
Anticoagulation Overlap Therapy[2]	67	99%	90%	93%
ICU Venous Thromboembolism Prophylaxis[2]	35	97%	93%	92%
Incidence of Potentially Preventable VTE[2]	13	0%	8%	10%
UFH with Dosages/Platelet Monitoring[2]	69	100%	96%	97%
Venous Thromboembolism Prophylaxis[2]	345	91%	87%	85%
Warfarin Therapy Discharge Instructions[2]	54	93%	72%	75%
Chest Pain/Possible Heart Attack Care				
Aspirin Given Within 24 Hours of Arrival	21	100%	96%	96%
Fibrinolytic Meds Within 30 Min. of Arrival[3,7]	-	-	63%	58%
Average Time to ECG (minutes)	20	1	8	7
Average Time to Transfer (minutes)[3,7]	-	-	53	60
Children's Asthma Care				
Received Home Management Plan of Care	-	-	-	88%
Received Reliever Medication	-	-	-	100%
Received Systemic Corticosteroids	-	-	-	100%
Emergency Department				
Admittance Decision Time (minutes)[2]	564	74	102	98
Head CT Results Within 45 Min. of Arrival[1]	-	-	54%	57%
Patients Who Left ER Before Being Seen	33,716	0%	2%	2%
Time from ER Arrival to Admit. (minutes)[2]	587	212	288	274
Time from ER Arrival to Discharge (minutes)	344	130	128	134
Time in ER Before Being Evaluated (minutes)	78	18	22	26
Time to Pain Meds for Fractures (minutes)	138	37	55	57
Heart Attack Care				
Aspirin Given at Discharge	137	98%	99%	99%
Fibrinolytic Meds Within 30 Min. of Arrival[7]	-	-	20%	54%
PCI Within 90 Minutes of Arrival	44	100%	95%	96%
Statin Prescribed at Discharge	131	97%	98%	98%
Heart Failure Care				
ACE Inhibitor or ARB for LVSD	64	98%	96%	97%
Discharge Instructions Given	244	96%	94%	94%
Evaluation of LVS Function	315	100%	99%	99%
Medicare Spending				
Medicare Spending per Patient (ratio)	-	1.01	0.96	0.98
Pneumonia Care				
Appropriate Initial Antibiotic Given	105	99%	96%	95%
Blood Culture Timing	220	100%	98%	98%
Pregnancy and Delivery Care				
Newborn Deliveries Scheduled Early[2]	42	7%	3%	6%
Preventive Care				
Immunization for Influenza[2]	546	98%	89%	90%
Immunization for Pneumonia[2]	644	97%	90%	92%
Stroke Care				
Anticoagulation Therapy for Atrial Fibrillation[1]	-	-	92%	95%
Antithrombotic Therapy Timing	56	93%	97%	98%
Assessed for Rehabilitation	74	92%	97%	97%
Discharged on Antithrombotic Therapy	69	99%	99%	99%
Discharged on Statin Medication	59	90%	94%	94%
Thrombolytic Therapy Timing[1]	-	-	69%	66%
Venous Thromboembolism Prophylaxis	66	97%	94%	94%
Written Stroke Educational Materials Given	47	83%	87%	88%
Surgical Care Improvement Project				
Appropriate Beta Blocker Usage[2]	169	95%	98%	98%
Appropriate VTP Within 24 Hours[2]	549	99%	98%	98%
Controlled Postoperative Blood Glucose[2,7]	-	-	97%	97%
Perioperative Temperature Management[2]	693	100%	100%	100%
Prophylactic Antibiotic Selection[2]	535	100%	99%	99%
Prophylactic Antibiotic Selection (Outpatient)	143	99%	97%	98%
Prophylactic Antibiotic Stopped[2]	528	99%	98%	98%
Prophylactic Antibiotic Timing[2]	535	99%	98%	99%
Prophylactic Antibiotic Timing (Outpatient)	133	98%	97%	98%
Urinary Catheter Removal[2]	436	100%	97%	97%
Survey of Patients' Hospital Experiences				
Area Around Room 'Always' Quiet at Night[11]	300+	58%	60%	61%
Doctors 'Always' Communicated Well[11]	300+	78%	81%	82%
Home Recovery Information Given[11]	300+	88%	87%	85%
Hospital Given 9 or 10 on 10 Point Scale[11]	300+	72%	71%	71%
Meds 'Always' Explained Before Given[11]	300+	56%	64%	64%
Nurses 'Always' Communicated Well[11]	300+	75%	80%	79%
Pain 'Always' Well Controlled[11]	300+	67%	71%	71%
Room and Bathroom 'Always' Clean[11]	300+	67%	73%	73%
Timely Help 'Always' Received[11]	300+	67%	70%	68%
Would Definitely Recommend Hospital[11]	300+	75%	71%	71%
Use of Medical Imaging				
Cardiac Imaging Stress Test before Surgery	403	7.7%	5.1%	5.3%
Combination Abdominal CT Scan	586	15.5%	8.7%	10.5%
Combination Brain/Sinus CT Scan[1]	-	-	2.2%	2.7%
Combination Chest CT Scan	513	3.1%	3.6%	2.7%
Follow-up Mammogram/Ultrasound	1,156	7.7%	8.2%	8.8%
Lumbar Spine MRI for Low Back Pain	109	28.4%	36.9%	37.2%

Oakwood Hospital - Dearborn

18101 Oakwood Blvd
Dearborn, MI 48124
E-mail: guestrel@oakwood.org
URL: www.oakwood.org
Type: Acute Care Hospitals
Ownership: Proprietary
Phone: 313-593-7125
Fax: 313-436-2038
Emergency Services: Yes
Beds: 632

Key Personnel:
CEO/President................ Brian Connolly
Chief of Medical Staff.......... Malcolm Henoch, MD

Measure	Cases	This Hosp.	State Avg.	U.S. Avg.
Blood Clot Prevention and Treatment				
Anticoagulation Overlap Therapy[2]	186	53%	90%	93%
ICU Venous Thromboembolism Prophylaxis[2]	74	86%	93%	92%
Incidence of Potentially Preventable VTE[2]	20	0%	8%	10%
UFH with Dosages/Platelet Monitoring[2]	202	100%	96%	97%
Venous Thromboembolism Prophylaxis[2]	345	71%	87%	85%
Warfarin Therapy Discharge Instructions[2]	106	70%	72%	75%
Chest Pain/Possible Heart Attack Care				
Aspirin Given Within 24 Hours of Arrival	14	93%	96%	96%
Fibrinolytic Meds Within 30 Min. of Arrival[3,7]	-	-	63%	58%
Average Time to ECG (minutes)	14	0	8	7
Average Time to Transfer (minutes)[3,7]	-	-	53	60
Children's Asthma Care				
Received Home Management Plan of Care	-	-	-	88%
Received Reliever Medication	-	-	-	100%
Received Systemic Corticosteroids	-	-	-	100%
Emergency Department				
Admittance Decision Time (minutes)[2]	636	168	102	98
Head CT Results Within 45 Min. of Arrival[1]	-	-	54%	57%
Patients Who Left ER Before Being Seen	76,743	4%	2%	2%
Time from ER Arrival to Admit. (minutes)[2]	642	434	288	274
Time from ER Arrival to Discharge (minutes)	331	251	128	134
Time in ER Before Being Evaluated (minutes)	365	46	22	26
Time to Pain Meds for Fractures (minutes)	209	82	55	57
Heart Attack Care				
Aspirin Given at Discharge[2]	269	97%	99%	99%
Fibrinolytic Meds Within 30 Min. of Arrival[2,7]	-	-	20%	54%
PCI Within 90 Minutes of Arrival[2]	27	93%	95%	96%
Statin Prescribed at Discharge[2]	270	91%	98%	98%
Heart Failure Care				
ACE Inhibitor or ARB for LVSD[2]	93	99%	96%	97%
Discharge Instructions Given[2]	205	83%	94%	94%
Evaluation of LVS Function[2]	272	97%	99%	99%
Medicare Spending				
Medicare Spending per Patient (ratio)	-	1.02	0.96	0.98
Pneumonia Care				
Appropriate Initial Antibiotic Given[2]	96	94%	96%	95%
Blood Culture Timing[2]	111	99%	98%	98%
Pregnancy and Delivery Care				
Newborn Deliveries Scheduled Early[2]	658	0%	3%	6%
Preventive Care				
Immunization for Influenza[2]	523	56%	89%	90%
Immunization for Pneumonia[2]	635	76%	90%	92%
Stroke Care				
Anticoagulation Therapy for Atrial Fibrillation[1,2]	-	-	92%	95%
Antithrombotic Therapy Timing[2]	79	92%	97%	98%
Assessed for Rehabilitation[2]	96	99%	97%	97%
Discharged on Antithrombotic Therapy[2]	85	94%	99%	99%
Discharged on Statin Medication[2]	71	90%	94%	94%
Thrombolytic Therapy Timing[1,2]	-	-	69%	66%
Venous Thromboembolism Prophylaxis[2]	102	94%	94%	94%
Written Stroke Educational Materials Given[2]	57	88%	87%	88%
Surgical Care Improvement Project				
Appropriate Beta Blocker Usage[2]	224	99%	98%	98%
Appropriate VTP Within 24 Hours[2]	318	99%	98%	98%
Controlled Postoperative Blood Glucose[2]	127	96%	97%	97%
Perioperative Temperature Management[2]	424	100%	100%	100%
Prophylactic Antibiotic Selection[2]	370	98%	99%	99%
Prophylactic Antibiotic Selection (Outpatient)	366	97%	97%	98%
Prophylactic Antibiotic Stopped[2]	360	90%	98%	98%
Prophylactic Antibiotic Timing[2]	375	96%	98%	99%
Prophylactic Antibiotic Timing (Outpatient)	364	92%	97%	98%
Urinary Catheter Removal[2]	242	84%	97%	97%
Survey of Patients' Hospital Experiences				
Area Around Room 'Always' Quiet at Night	300+	49%	60%	61%
Doctors 'Always' Communicated Well	300+	78%	81%	82%
Home Recovery Information Given	300+	82%	87%	85%
Hospital Given 9 or 10 on 10 Point Scale	300+	66%	71%	71%
Meds 'Always' Explained Before Given	300+	62%	64%	64%
Nurses 'Always' Communicated Well	300+	80%	80%	79%
Pain 'Always' Well Controlled	300+	71%	71%	71%
Room and Bathroom 'Always' Clean	300+	67%	73%	73%
Timely Help 'Always' Received	300+	66%	70%	68%
Would Definitely Recommend Hospital	300+	66%	71%	71%
Use of Medical Imaging				
Cardiac Imaging Stress Test before Surgery	709	7.2%	5.1%	5.3%
Combination Abdominal CT Scan	1,755	6.6%	8.7%	10.5%
Combination Brain/Sinus CT Scan	1,567	3.3%	2.2%	2.7%
Combination Chest CT Scan	1,273	6.0%	3.6%	2.7%
Follow-up Mammogram/Ultrasound	2,547	8.1%	8.2%	8.8%
Lumbar Spine MRI for Low Back Pain	204	33.3%	36.9%	37.2%

Deckerville Community Hospital

3559 Pine St
Deckerville, MI 48427
URL: www.deckervillehosp.org
Type: Critical Access Hospitals
Ownership: Voluntary non-profit - Other
Phone: 810-376-2835
Emergency Services: Yes

Key Personnel:
Emergency Room............ Angie M Connachie
CEO...................... Edward Gamache
Radiology.................. App Arao Mukkamala
Cardiology................. Suresh Tumma

Measure	Cases	This Hosp.	State Avg.	U.S. Avg.
Blood Clot Prevention and Treatment				
Anticoagulation Overlap Therapy[5]	-	-	90%	93%
ICU Venous Thromboembolism Prophylaxis[5]	-	-	93%	92%
Incidence of Potentially Preventable VTE[5]	-	-	8%	10%
UFH with Dosages/Platelet Monitoring[5]	-	-	96%	97%
Venous Thromboembolism Prophylaxis[5]	-	-	87%	85%
Warfarin Therapy Discharge Instructions[5]	-	-	72%	75%
Chest Pain/Possible Heart Attack Care				
Aspirin Given Within 24 Hours of Arrival	22	100%	96%	96%
Fibrinolytic Meds Within 30 Min. of Arrival[1]	-	-	63%	58%
Average Time to ECG (minutes)	20	14	8	7
Average Time to Transfer (minutes)[1]	-	-	53	60

NOTE: Hospital profiles are in alphabetical order by state, then city, then hospital within the city; Rankings exclude hospitals with less than 25 cases except for patient surveys which excludes hospitals with less than 100 cases; (a) 100-299 cases; (1) The number of cases/patients is too few to report; (2) Data submitted were based on a sample of cases/patients; (3) Results are based on a shorter time period than required; (4) Data suppressed by CMS for one or more quarters; (5) Results are not available for this reporting period; (6) Fewer than 100 patients completed the HCAHPS survey; (7) No cases met the criteria for this measure; (8) The lower limit of the confidence interval cannot be calculated if the number of observed infections equals zero; (9) No data are available from the state/territory for this reporting period; (10) The scores shown reflect fewer than 50 completed surveys; (11) There were discrepancies in the data collection process; (12) This measure does not apply to this hospital for this reporting period; (13) Results cannot be calculated for this reporting period; (14) The results for this state are combined with nearby states to protect confidentiality; Please refer to the User's Guide for a full explanation of data.

Measure	Cases	This Hosp.	State Avg.	U.S. Avg.
Children's Asthma Care				
Received Home Management Plan of Care	-	-	-	88%
Received Reliever Medication	-	-	-	100%
Received Systemic Corticosteroids	-	-	-	100%
Emergency Department				
Admittance Decision Time (minutes)[5]	-	-	102	98
Head CT Results Within 45 Min. of Arrival[5]	-	-	54%	57%
Patients Who Left ER Before Being Seen[5]	-	-	2%	2%
Time from ER Arrival to Admit. (minutes)[5]	-	-	288	274
Time from ER Arrival to Discharge (minutes)	171	135	128	134
Time in ER Before Being Evaluated (minutes)	214	15	22	26
Time to Pain Meds for Fractures (minutes)[5]	-	-	55	57
Heart Attack Care				
Aspirin Given at Discharge[5]	-	-	99%	99%
Fibrinolytic Meds Within 30 Min. of Arrival[5]	-	-	20%	54%
PCI Within 90 Minutes of Arrival[5]	-	-	95%	96%
Statin Prescribed at Discharge[5]	-	-	98%	98%
Heart Failure Care				
ACE Inhibitor or ARB for LVSD[3,7]	-	-	96%	97%
Discharge Instructions Given[1,3]	-	-	94%	94%
Evaluation of LVS Function[1,3]	-	-	99%	99%
Medicare Spending				
Medicare Spending per Patient (ratio)	-	-	0.96	0.98
Pneumonia Care				
Appropriate Initial Antibiotic Given[1]	-	-	96%	95%
Blood Culture Timing[1]	-	-	98%	98%
Pregnancy and Delivery Care				
Newborn Deliveries Scheduled Early[5]	-	-	3%	6%
Preventive Care				
Immunization for Influenza[5]	-	-	89%	90%
Immunization for Pneumonia[5]	-	-	90%	92%
Stroke Care				
Anticoagulation Therapy for Atrial Fibrillation[5]	-	-	92%	95%
Antithrombotic Therapy Timing[5]	-	-	97%	98%
Assessed for Rehabilitation[5]	-	-	97%	97%
Discharged on Antithrombotic Therapy[5]	-	-	99%	99%
Discharged on Statin Medication[5]	-	-	94%	94%
Thrombolytic Therapy Timing[5]	-	-	69%	66%
Venous Thromboembolism Prophylaxis[5]	-	-	94%	94%
Written Stroke Educational Materials Given[5]	-	-	87%	88%
Surgical Care Improvement Project				
Appropriate Beta Blocker Usage[5]	-	-	98%	98%
Appropriate VTP Within 24 Hours[5]	-	-	98%	98%
Controlled Postoperative Blood Glucose[5]	-	-	97%	97%
Perioperative Temperature Management[5]	-	-	100%	100%
Prophylactic Antibiotic Selection[5]	-	-	99%	99%
Prophylactic Antibiotic Selection (Outpatient)[5]	-	-	97%	98%
Prophylactic Antibiotic Stopped[5]	-	-	98%	98%
Prophylactic Antibiotic Timing[5]	-	-	98%	99%
Prophylactic Antibiotic Timing (Outpatient)[5]	-	-	97%	98%
Urinary Catheter Removal[5]	-	-	97%	97%
Survey of Patients' Hospital Experiences				
Area Around Room 'Always' Quiet at Night[5]	-	-	60%	61%
Doctors 'Always' Communicated Well[5]	-	-	81%	82%
Home Recovery Information Given[5]	-	-	87%	85%
Hospital Given 9 or 10 on 10 Point Scale[5]	-	-	71%	71%
Meds 'Always' Explained Before Given[5]	-	-	64%	64%
Nurses 'Always' Communicated Well[5]	-	-	80%	79%
Pain 'Always' Well Controlled[5]	-	-	71%	71%
Room and Bathroom 'Always' Clean[5]	-	-	73%	73%
Timely Help 'Always' Received[5]	-	-	70%	68%
Would Definitely Recommend Hospital[5]	-	-	71%	71%
Use of Medical Imaging				
Cardiac Imaging Stress Test before Surgery[7]	-	-	5.1%	5.3%
Combination Abdominal CT Scan[1]	-	-	8.7%	10.5%
Combination Brain/Sinus CT Scan[1]	-	-	2.2%	2.7%
Combination Chest CT Scan[1]	-	-	3.6%	2.7%
Follow-up Mammogram/Ultrasound	91	7.7%	8.2%	8.8%
Lumbar Spine MRI for Low Back Pain[7]	-	-	36.9%	37.2%

Children's Hospital of Michigan

3901 Beaubien
Detroit, MI 48201
Phone: 313-745-5437
Fax: 313-887-5211
URL: www.childrensdmc.org
Type: Childrens
Ownership: Proprietary
Emergency Services: Yes
Beds: 240

Key Personnel:

Infection Control. . . . . Basim Asmar, MD
Chief of Medical Staff . . . . M Safwan Badr
Radiology. . . . . Steven Batipps
CEO/President. . . . . Michael E Duggan, MD
Quality Assurance . . . . Marlene Ercolani

Measure	Cases	This Hosp.	State Avg.	U.S. Avg.
Blood Clot Prevention and Treatment				
Anticoagulation Overlap Therapy[5]	-	-	90%	93%
ICU Venous Thromboembolism Prophylaxis[5]	-	-	93%	92%
Incidence of Potentially Preventable VTE[5]	-	-	8%	10%
UFH with Dosages/Platelet Monitoring[5]	-	-	96%	97%
Venous Thromboembolism Prophylaxis[5]	-	-	87%	85%
Warfarin Therapy Discharge Instructions[5]	-	-	72%	75%
Chest Pain/Possible Heart Attack Care				
Aspirin Given Within 24 Hours of Arrival	-	-	96%	96%
Fibrinolytic Meds Within 30 Min. of Arrival	-	-	63%	58%
Average Time to ECG (minutes)	-	-	8	7
Average Time to Transfer (minutes)	-	-	53	60
Children's Asthma Care				
Received Home Management Plan of Care[2]	371	95%	-	88%
Received Reliever Medication[2]	372	100%	-	100%
Received Systemic Corticosteroids[2]	372	100%	-	100%
Emergency Department				
Admittance Decision Time (minutes)[5]	-	-	102	98
Head CT Results Within 45 Min. of Arrival	-	-	54%	57%
Patients Who Left ER Before Being Seen	-	-	2%	2%
Time from ER Arrival to Admit. (minutes)[5]	-	-	288	274
Time from ER Arrival to Discharge (minutes)	-	-	128	134
Time in ER Before Being Evaluated (minutes)	-	-	22	26
Time to Pain Meds for Fractures (minutes)	-	-	55	57
Heart Attack Care				
Aspirin Given at Discharge[5]	-	-	99%	99%
Fibrinolytic Meds Within 30 Min. of Arrival[5]	-	-	20%	54%
PCI Within 90 Minutes of Arrival[5]	-	-	95%	96%
Statin Prescribed at Discharge[5]	-	-	98%	98%
Heart Failure Care				
ACE Inhibitor or ARB for LVSD[5]	-	-	96%	97%
Discharge Instructions Given[5]	-	-	94%	94%
Evaluation of LVS Function[5]	-	-	99%	99%
Medicare Spending				
Medicare Spending per Patient (ratio)	-	-	0.96	0.98
Pneumonia Care				
Appropriate Initial Antibiotic Given[5]	-	-	96%	95%
Blood Culture Timing[5]	-	-	98%	98%
Pregnancy and Delivery Care				
Newborn Deliveries Scheduled Early[5]	-	-	3%	6%
Preventive Care				
Immunization for Influenza[5]	-	-	89%	90%
Immunization for Pneumonia[5]	-	-	90%	92%
Stroke Care				
Anticoagulation Therapy for Atrial Fibrillation[5]	-	-	92%	95%
Antithrombotic Therapy Timing[5]	-	-	97%	98%
Assessed for Rehabilitation[5]	-	-	97%	97%
Discharged on Antithrombotic Therapy[5]	-	-	99%	99%
Discharged on Statin Medication[5]	-	-	94%	94%
Thrombolytic Therapy Timing[5]	-	-	69%	66%
Venous Thromboembolism Prophylaxis[5]	-	-	94%	94%
Written Stroke Educational Materials Given[5]	-	-	87%	88%
Surgical Care Improvement Project				
Appropriate Beta Blocker Usage[5]	-	-	98%	98%
Appropriate VTP Within 24 Hours[5]	-	-	98%	98%
Controlled Postoperative Blood Glucose[5]	-	-	97%	97%
Perioperative Temperature Management[5]	-	-	100%	100%
Prophylactic Antibiotic Selection[5]	-	-	99%	99%
Prophylactic Antibiotic Selection (Outpatient)	-	-	97%	98%
Prophylactic Antibiotic Stopped[5]	-	-	98%	98%
Prophylactic Antibiotic Timing[5]	-	-	98%	99%
Prophylactic Antibiotic Timing (Outpatient)	-	-	97%	98%
Urinary Catheter Removal[5]	-	-	97%	97%
Survey of Patients' Hospital Experiences				
Area Around Room 'Always' Quiet at Night[5]	-	-	60%	61%
Doctors 'Always' Communicated Well[5]	-	-	81%	82%
Home Recovery Information Given[5]	-	-	87%	85%
Hospital Given 9 or 10 on 10 Point Scale[5]	-	-	71%	71%
Meds 'Always' Explained Before Given[5]	-	-	64%	64%
Nurses 'Always' Communicated Well[5]	-	-	80%	79%
Pain 'Always' Well Controlled[5]	-	-	71%	71%
Room and Bathroom 'Always' Clean[5]	-	-	73%	73%
Timely Help 'Always' Received[5]	-	-	70%	68%
Would Definitely Recommend Hospital[5]	-	-	71%	71%
Use of Medical Imaging				
Cardiac Imaging Stress Test before Surgery	-	-	5.1%	5.3%
Combination Abdominal CT Scan	-	-	8.7%	10.5%
Combination Brain/Sinus CT Scan	-	-	2.2%	2.7%
Combination Chest CT Scan	-	-	3.6%	2.7%
Follow-up Mammogram/Ultrasound	-	-	8.2%	8.8%
Lumbar Spine MRI for Low Back Pain	-	-	36.9%	37.2%

Detroit (John D. Dingell) VA Medical Center

4646 John R.
Detroit, MI 48201
Phone: 313-576-1000
Fax: 313-576-1991
URL: www.detroit.va.gov
Type: Acute Care - VA
Ownership: Government Federal
Emergency Services: No
Beds: 372

Key Personnel:

Intensive Care Unit. . . . . Basim Bubaybo, MD
Quality Assurance . . . . Marvin Dick
Chief of Medical Staff . . . . Scott Gruber, MD
Radiology. . . . . Sue Han, MD
Anesthesiology. . . . . Robert Kozol, MD
Emergency Room . . . . Boaz I Milner, MD
Infection Control. . . . . Ronaldo Supena, MD

Measure	Cases	This Hosp.	State Avg.	U.S. Avg.
Blood Clot Prevention and Treatment				
Anticoagulation Overlap Therapy	-	-	90%	93%
ICU Venous Thromboembolism Prophylaxis	-	-	93%	92%
Incidence of Potentially Preventable VTE	-	-	8%	10%
UFH with Dosages/Platelet Monitoring	-	-	96%	97%
Venous Thromboembolism Prophylaxis	-	-	87%	85%
Warfarin Therapy Discharge Instructions	-	-	72%	75%
Chest Pain/Possible Heart Attack Care				
Aspirin Given Within 24 Hours of Arrival	-	-	96%	96%
Fibrinolytic Meds Within 30 Min. of Arrival	-	-	63%	58%
Average Time to ECG (minutes)	-	-	8	7
Average Time to Transfer (minutes)	-	-	53	60
Children's Asthma Care				
Received Home Management Plan of Care	-	-	-	88%
Received Reliever Medication	-	-	-	100%
Received Systemic Corticosteroids	-	-	-	100%
Emergency Department				
Admittance Decision Time (minutes)	-	-	102	98
Head CT Results Within 45 Min. of Arrival	-	-	54%	57%
Patients Who Left ER Before Being Seen	-	-	2%	2%
Time from ER Arrival to Admit. (minutes)	-	-	288	274
Time from ER Arrival to Discharge (minutes)	-	-	128	134
Time in ER Before Being Evaluated (minutes)	-	-	22	26
Time to Pain Meds for Fractures (minutes)	-	-	55	57
Heart Attack Care				
Aspirin Given at Discharge[1]	-	-	99%	99%
Fibrinolytic Meds Within 30 Min. of Arrival[5]	-	-	20%	54%
PCI Within 90 Minutes of Arrival[5]	-	-	95%	96%
Statin Prescribed at Discharge[1]	-	-	98%	98%
Heart Failure Care				
ACE Inhibitor or ARB for LVSD	66	97%	96%	97%
Discharge Instructions Given	131	89%	94%	94%
Evaluation of LVS Function	137	99%	99%	99%
Medicare Spending				
Medicare Spending per Patient (ratio)	-	-	0.96	0.98
Pneumonia Care				
Appropriate Initial Antibiotic Given	31	100%	96%	95%

NOTE: Hospital profiles are in alphabetical order by state, then city, then hospital within the city; Rankings exclude hospitals with less than 25 cases except for patient surveys which excludes hospitals with less than 100 cases; (a) 100-299 cases; (1) The number of cases/patients is too few to report; (2) Data submitted were based on a sample of cases/patients; (3) Results are based on a shorter time period than required; (4) Data suppressed by CMS for one or more quarters; (5) Results are not available for this reporting period; (6) Fewer than 100 patients completed the HCAHPS survey; (7) No cases met the criteria for this measure; (8) The lower limit of the confidence interval cannot be calculated if the number of observed infections equals zero; (9) No data are available from the state/territory for this reporting period; (10) The scores shown reflect fewer than 50 completed surveys; (11) There were discrepancies in the data collection process; (12) This measure does not apply to this hospital for this reporting period; (13) Results cannot be calculated for this reporting period; (14) The results for this state are combined with nearby states to protect confidentiality; Please refer to the User's Guide for a full explanation of data.

Measure	Cases	This Hosp.	State Avg.	U.S. Avg.
Blood Culture Timing	65	100%	98%	98%
Pregnancy and Delivery Care				
Newborn Deliveries Scheduled Early	-	-	3%	6%
Preventive Care				
Immunization for Influenza[5]	-	-	89%	90%
Immunization for Pneumonia[5]	-	-	90%	92%
Stroke Care				
Anticoagulation Therapy for Atrial Fibrillation	-	-	92%	95%
Antithrombotic Therapy Timing	-	-	97%	98%
Assessed for Rehabilitation	-	-	97%	97%
Discharged on Antithrombotic Therapy	-	-	99%	99%
Discharged on Statin Medication	-	-	94%	94%
Thrombolytic Therapy Timing	-	-	69%	66%
Venous Thromboembolism Prophylaxis	-	-	94%	94%
Written Stroke Educational Materials Given	-	-	87%	88%
Surgical Care Improvement Project				
Appropriate Beta Blocker Usage[2]	97	95%	98%	98%
Appropriate VTP Within 24 Hours[2]	203	99%	98%	98%
Controlled Postoperative Blood Glucose[5]	-	-	97%	97%
Perioperative Temperature Management[2]	309	95%	100%	100%
Prophylactic Antibiotic Selection	183	98%	99%	99%
Prophylactic Antibiotic Selection (Outpatient)	-	-	97%	98%
Prophylactic Antibiotic Stopped	183	99%	98%	98%
Prophylactic Antibiotic Timing	183	99%	98%	99%
Prophylactic Antibiotic Timing (Outpatient)	-	-	97%	98%
Urinary Catheter Removal[2]	92	96%	97%	97%
Survey of Patients' Hospital Experiences				
Area Around Room 'Always' Quiet at Night	-	-	60%	61%
Doctors 'Always' Communicated Well	-	-	81%	82%
Home Recovery Information Given	-	-	87%	85%
Hospital Given 9 or 10 on 10 Point Scale	-	-	71%	71%
Meds 'Always' Explained Before Given	-	-	64%	64%
Nurses 'Always' Communicated Well	-	-	80%	79%
Pain 'Always' Well Controlled	-	-	71%	71%
Room and Bathroom 'Always' Clean	-	-	73%	73%
Timely Help 'Always' Received	-	-	70%	68%
Would Definitely Recommend Hospital	-	-	71%	71%
Use of Medical Imaging				
Cardiac Imaging Stress Test before Surgery	-	-	5.1%	5.3%
Combination Abdominal CT Scan	-	-	8.7%	10.5%
Combination Brain/Sinus CT Scan	-	-	2.2%	2.7%
Combination Chest CT Scan	-	-	3.6%	2.7%
Follow-up Mammogram/Ultrasound	-	-	8.2%	8.8%
Lumbar Spine MRI for Low Back Pain	-	-	36.9%	37.2%

Detroit Receiving Hospital & University Health Center

4201 Saint Antoine Saint - 3m
Detroit, MI 48201
E-mail: lbowman@dmc.org
URL: www.drhuhc.org
Phone: 313-745-3104
Fax: 313-966-7206
Type: Acute Care Hospitals
Ownership: Proprietary
Emergency Services: Yes
Beds: 258

Key Personnel:
Radiology.................. Gail Alexander
Intensive Care Unit............ Sue Ellen Bennett, RN
Infection Control............. Beth Dziekan
Patient Relations .... Patricia E Natale
Quality Assurance .... Margaret Rand
Emergency Room .... Padraic J Sweeny, MD
CEO/President............... Iris A Taylor, PhD RN
Chief of Medical Staff.......... Robert Wilson, MD

Measure	Cases	This Hosp.	State Avg.	U.S. Avg.
Blood Clot Prevention and Treatment				
Anticoagulation Overlap Therapy[2]	105	99%	90%	93%
ICU Venous Thromboembolism Prophylaxis[2]	115	95%	93%	92%
Incidence of Potentially Preventable VTE[2]	31	6%	8%	10%
UFH with Dosages/Platelet Monitoring[2]	69	100%	96%	97%
Venous Thromboembolism Prophylaxis[2]	288	93%	87%	85%
Warfarin Therapy Discharge Instructions[2]	68	79%	72%	75%
Chest Pain/Possible Heart Attack Care				
Aspirin Given Within 24 Hours of Arrival	166	100%	96%	96%
Fibrinolytic Meds Within 30 Min. of Arrival[7]	-	-	63%	58%
Average Time to ECG (minutes)	167	14	8	7
Average Time to Transfer (minutes)	22	30	53	60
Children's Asthma Care				
Received Home Management Plan of Care	-	-	-	88%
Received Reliever Medication	-	-	-	100%
Received Systemic Corticosteroids	-	-	-	100%
Emergency Department				
Admittance Decision Time (minutes)[2]	759	77	102	98
Head CT Results Within 45 Min. of Arrival[1]	-	-	54%	57%
Patients Who Left ER Before Being Seen	>100k	1%	2%	2%
Time from ER Arrival to Admit. (minutes)[2]	763	173	288	274
Time from ER Arrival to Discharge (minutes)	272	106	128	134
Time in ER Before Being Evaluated (minutes)	261	0	22	26
Time to Pain Meds for Fractures (minutes)	161	51	55	57
Heart Attack Care				
Aspirin Given at Discharge	205	100%	99%	99%
Fibrinolytic Meds Within 30 Min. of Arrival[7]	-	-	20%	54%
PCI Within 90 Minutes of Arrival[7]	-	-	95%	96%
Statin Prescribed at Discharge	209	100%	98%	98%
Heart Failure Care				
ACE Inhibitor or ARB for LVSD	192	99%	96%	97%
Discharge Instructions Given	383	99%	94%	94%
Evaluation of LVS Function	443	100%	99%	99%
Medicare Spending				
Medicare Spending per Patient (ratio)	-	1.01	0.96	0.98
Pneumonia Care				
Appropriate Initial Antibiotic Given	86	100%	96%	95%
Blood Culture Timing	450	99%	98%	98%
Pregnancy and Delivery Care				
Newborn Deliveries Scheduled Early[2,7]	-	-	3%	6%
Preventive Care				
Immunization for Influenza[2]	598	94%	89%	90%
Immunization for Pneumonia[2]	713	92%	90%	92%
Stroke Care				
Anticoagulation Therapy for Atrial Fibrillation[1]	-	-	92%	95%
Antithrombotic Therapy Timing	130	98%	97%	98%
Assessed for Rehabilitation	194	99%	97%	97%
Discharged on Antithrombotic Therapy	154	99%	99%	99%
Discharged on Statin Medication	112	99%	94%	94%
Thrombolytic Therapy Timing	27	70%	69%	66%
Venous Thromboembolism Prophylaxis	208	98%	94%	94%
Written Stroke Educational Materials Given	107	96%	87%	88%
Surgical Care Improvement Project				
Appropriate Beta Blocker Usage[2]	153	99%	98%	98%
Appropriate VTP Within 24 Hours[2]	467	99%	98%	98%
Controlled Postoperative Blood Glucose[2,7]	-	-	97%	97%
Perioperative Temperature Management[2]	529	100%	100%	100%
Prophylactic Antibiotic Selection[2]	398	100%	99%	99%
Prophylactic Antibiotic Selection (Outpatient)	53	94%	97%	98%
Prophylactic Antibiotic Stopped[2]	395	99%	98%	98%
Prophylactic Antibiotic Timing[2]	399	99%	98%	99%
Prophylactic Antibiotic Timing (Outpatient)	53	100%	97%	98%
Urinary Catheter Removal[2]	481	100%	97%	97%
Survey of Patients' Hospital Experiences				
Area Around Room 'Always' Quiet at Night[11]	300+	58%	60%	61%
Doctors 'Always' Communicated Well[11]	300+	79%	81%	82%
Home Recovery Information Given[11]	300+	84%	87%	85%
Hospital Given 9 or 10 on 10 Point Scale[11]	300+	64%	71%	71%
Meds 'Always' Explained Before Given[11]	300+	60%	64%	64%
Nurses 'Always' Communicated Well[11]	300+	74%	80%	79%
Pain 'Always' Well Controlled[11]	300+	67%	71%	71%
Room and Bathroom 'Always' Clean[11]	300+	58%	73%	73%
Timely Help 'Always' Received[11]	300+	62%	70%	68%
Would Definitely Recommend Hospital[11]	300+	65%	71%	71%
Use of Medical Imaging				
Cardiac Imaging Stress Test before Surgery[7]	-	-	5.1%	5.3%
Combination Abdominal CT Scan	263	12.2%	8.7%	10.5%
Combination Brain/Sinus CT Scan	585	1.5%	2.2%	2.7%
Combination Chest CT Scan	175	12.6%	3.6%	2.7%
Follow-up Mammogram/Ultrasound[7]	-	-	8.2%	8.8%
Lumbar Spine MRI for Low Back Pain[1]	-	-	36.9%	37.2%

Harper University Hospital

3990 John R Street
Detroit, MI 48201
URL: www.harperhospital.org
Phone: 313-745-6211
Fax: 313-745-1520
Type: Acute Care Hospitals
Ownership: Proprietary
Emergency Services: Yes
Beds: 658

Key Personnel:
Chief of Medical Staff.......... M Safwan Badr, MD
CEO/President............... Micheal Duggan
Radiology.................. Mehendra Shah
Emergency Room .... Patrick Sweeney

Measure	Cases	This Hosp.	State Avg.	U.S. Avg.
Blood Clot Prevention and Treatment				
Anticoagulation Overlap Therapy[2]	82	98%	90%	93%
ICU Venous Thromboembolism Prophylaxis[2]	94	97%	93%	92%
Incidence of Potentially Preventable VTE[2]	23	22%	8%	10%
UFH with Dosages/Platelet Monitoring[2]	72	100%	96%	97%
Venous Thromboembolism Prophylaxis[2]	358	91%	87%	85%
Warfarin Therapy Discharge Instructions[2]	51	69%	72%	75%
Chest Pain/Possible Heart Attack Care				
Aspirin Given Within 24 Hours of Arrival	13	100%	96%	96%
Fibrinolytic Meds Within 30 Min. of Arrival[3,7]	-	-	63%	58%
Average Time to ECG (minutes)	12	0	8	7
Average Time to Transfer (minutes)[3,7]	-	-	53	60
Children's Asthma Care				
Received Home Management Plan of Care	-	-	-	88%
Received Reliever Medication	-	-	-	100%
Received Systemic Corticosteroids	-	-	-	100%
Emergency Department				
Admittance Decision Time (minutes)[2]	252	78	102	98
Head CT Results Within 45 Min. of Arrival[1]	-	-	54%	57%
Patients Who Left ER Before Being Seen	40,222	1%	2%	2%
Time from ER Arrival to Admit. (minutes)[2]	290	237	288	274
Time from ER Arrival to Discharge (minutes)	424	144	128	134
Time in ER Before Being Evaluated (minutes)	91	7	22	26
Time to Pain Meds for Fractures (minutes)	65	57	55	57
Heart Attack Care				
Aspirin Given at Discharge	458	100%	99%	99%
Fibrinolytic Meds Within 30 Min. of Arrival[7]	-	-	20%	54%
PCI Within 90 Minutes of Arrival	21	86%	95%	96%
Statin Prescribed at Discharge	461	99%	98%	98%
Heart Failure Care				
ACE Inhibitor or ARB for LVSD	274	99%	96%	97%
Discharge Instructions Given	637	99%	94%	94%
Evaluation of LVS Function	721	100%	99%	99%
Medicare Spending				
Medicare Spending per Patient (ratio)	-	0.99	0.96	0.98
Pneumonia Care				
Appropriate Initial Antibiotic Given	74	96%	96%	95%
Blood Culture Timing	218	98%	98%	98%
Pregnancy and Delivery Care				
Newborn Deliveries Scheduled Early[2]	43	9%	3%	6%
Preventive Care				
Immunization for Influenza[2]	487	97%	89%	90%
Immunization for Pneumonia[2]	538	97%	90%	92%
Stroke Care				
Anticoagulation Therapy for Atrial Fibrillation[1]	-	-	92%	95%
Antithrombotic Therapy Timing	60	98%	97%	98%
Assessed for Rehabilitation	83	99%	97%	97%
Discharged on Antithrombotic Therapy	68	99%	99%	99%
Discharged on Statin Medication	50	96%	94%	94%
Thrombolytic Therapy Timing[1]	-	-	69%	66%
Venous Thromboembolism Prophylaxis	82	98%	94%	94%
Written Stroke Educational Materials Given	49	92%	87%	88%
Surgical Care Improvement Project				
Appropriate Beta Blocker Usage[2]	188	99%	98%	98%
Appropriate VTP Within 24 Hours[2]	310	100%	98%	98%
Controlled Postoperative Blood Glucose[2]	71	100%	97%	97%
Perioperative Temperature Management[2]	432	100%	100%	100%
Prophylactic Antibiotic Selection[2]	327	97%	99%	99%
Prophylactic Antibiotic Selection (Outpatient)	579	97%	97%	98%
Prophylactic Antibiotic Stopped[2]	309	95%	98%	98%
Prophylactic Antibiotic Timing[2]	327	100%	98%	99%

NOTE: Hospital profiles are in alphabetical order by state, then city, then hospital within the city; Rankings exclude hospitals with less than 25 cases except for patient surveys which excludes hospitals with less than 100 cases; (a) 100-299 cases; (1) The number of cases/patients is too few to report; (2) Data submitted were based on a sample of cases/patients; (3) Results are based on a shorter time period than required; (4) Data suppressed by CMS for one or more quarters; (5) Results are not available for this reporting period; (6) Fewer than 100 patients completed the HCAHPS survey; (7) No cases met the criteria for this measure; (8) The lower limit of the confidence interval cannot be calculated if the number of observed infections equals zero; (9) No data are available from the state/territory for this reporting period; (10) The scores shown reflect fewer than 50 completed surveys; (11) There were discrepancies in the data collection process; (12) This measure does not apply to this hospital for this reporting period; (13) Results cannot be calculated for this reporting period; (14) The results for this state are combined with nearby states to protect confidentiality; Please refer to the User's Guide for a full explanation of data.

Prophylactic Antibiotic Timing (Outpatient)	525	100%	97%	98%
Urinary Catheter Removal[2]	232	98%	97%	97%
Survey of Patients' Hospital Experiences				
Area Around Room 'Always' Quiet at Night[11]	300+	62%	60%	61%
Doctors 'Always' Communicated Well[11]	300+	79%	81%	82%
Home Recovery Information Given[11]	300+	85%	87%	85%
Hospital Given 9 or 10 on 10 Point Scale[11]	300+	68%	71%	71%
Meds 'Always' Explained Before Given[11]	300+	58%	64%	64%
Nurses 'Always' Communicated Well[11]	300+	78%	80%	79%
Pain 'Always' Well Controlled[11]	300+	69%	71%	71%
Room and Bathroom 'Always' Clean[11]	300+	66%	73%	73%
Timely Help 'Always' Received[11]	300+	61%	70%	68%
Would Definitely Recommend Hospital[11]	300+	68%	71%	71%
Use of Medical Imaging				
Cardiac Imaging Stress Test before Surgery	485	6.2%	5.1%	5.3%
Combination Abdominal CT Scan	805	17.8%	8.7%	10.5%
Combination Brain/Sinus CT Scan[1]	-	-	2.2%	2.7%
Combination Chest CT Scan	524	10.9%	3.6%	2.7%
Follow-up Mammogram/Ultrasound[7]	-	-	8.2%	8.8%
Lumbar Spine MRI for Low Back Pain	193	29.0%	36.9%	37.2%

Henry Ford Hospital

2799 W Grand Blvd
Detroit, MI 48202
Phone: 313-916-2600
Fax: 313-916-7236
URL: www.henryfordhospital.com
Type: Acute Care Hospitals
Emergency Services: Yes
Ownership: Voluntary non-profit - Private
Beds: 903

Key Personnel:

Operating Room. . . . . Gaylord D Alexander, MD
Chief of Medical Staff . . . . William Conway, MD
Coronary Care . . . . Michael P Hudson, MD
President . . . . Robert G. Riney
Cardiac Laboratory. . . . . Hani N Sabbah, PhD
Radiology. . . . . Michael Sandler, MD
CEO/President. . . . . Nancy M. Schlichting
Quality Assurance . . . . Irene Turkewycz

Measure	Cases	This Hosp.	State Avg.	U.S. Avg.
Blood Clot Prevention and Treatment				
Anticoagulation Overlap Therapy[2]	255	99%	90%	93%
ICU Venous Thromboembolism Prophylaxis[2]	133	99%	93%	92%
Incidence of Potentially Preventable VTE[2]	111	3%	8%	10%
UFH with Dosages/Platelet Monitoring[2]	320	100%	96%	97%
Venous Thromboembolism Prophylaxis[2]	318	92%	87%	85%
Warfarin Therapy Discharge Instructions[2]	199	74%	72%	75%
Chest Pain/Possible Heart Attack Care				
Aspirin Given Within 24 Hours of Arrival	38	95%	96%	96%
Fibrinolytic Meds Within 30 Min. of Arrival[7]	-	-	63%	58%
Average Time to ECG (minutes)	38	10	8	7
Average Time to Transfer (minutes)[1]	-	-	53	60
Children's Asthma Care				
Received Home Management Plan of Care	-	-	-	88%
Received Reliever Medication	-	-	-	100%
Received Systemic Corticosteroids	-	-	-	100%
Emergency Department				
Admittance Decision Time (minutes)[2]	628	172	102	98
Head CT Results Within 45 Min. of Arrival[1]	-	-	54%	57%
Patients Who Left ER Before Being Seen	>100k	2%	2%	2%
Time from ER Arrival to Admit. (minutes)[2]	629	417	288	274
Time from ER Arrival to Discharge (minutes)	377	153	128	134
Time in ER Before Being Evaluated (minutes)	356	37	22	26
Time to Pain Meds for Fractures (minutes)	232	72	55	57
Heart Attack Care				
Aspirin Given at Discharge	715	99%	99%	99%
Fibrinolytic Meds Within 30 Min. of Arrival[7]	-	-	20%	54%
PCI Within 90 Minutes of Arrival	47	98%	95%	96%
Statin Prescribed at Discharge	701	98%	98%	98%
Heart Failure Care				
ACE Inhibitor or ARB for LVSD[2]	116	94%	96%	97%
Discharge Instructions Given[2]	273	100%	94%	94%
Evaluation of LVS Function[2]	311	100%	99%	99%
Medicare Spending				
Medicare Spending per Patient (ratio)	-	0.98	0.96	0.98
Pneumonia Care				
Appropriate Initial Antibiotic Given[2]	47	96%	96%	95%
Blood Culture Timing[2]	140	99%	98%	98%
Pregnancy and Delivery Care				
Newborn Deliveries Scheduled Early	214	2%	3%	6%
Preventive Care				
Immunization for Influenza[2]	539	72%	89%	90%
Immunization for Pneumonia[2]	687	71%	90%	92%
Stroke Care				
Anticoagulation Therapy for Atrial Fibrillation	38	100%	92%	95%
Antithrombotic Therapy Timing	378	95%	97%	98%
Assessed for Rehabilitation	530	95%	97%	97%
Discharged on Antithrombotic Therapy	441	100%	99%	99%
Discharged on Statin Medication	340	99%	94%	94%
Thrombolytic Therapy Timing	23	91%	69%	66%
Venous Thromboembolism Prophylaxis	536	98%	94%	94%
Written Stroke Educational Materials Given	282	90%	87%	88%
Surgical Care Improvement Project				
Appropriate Beta Blocker Usage[2]	269	96%	98%	98%
Appropriate VTP Within 24 Hours[2]	449	99%	98%	98%
Controlled Postoperative Blood Glucose[2]	136	95%	97%	97%
Perioperative Temperature Management[2]	581	99%	100%	100%
Prophylactic Antibiotic Selection[2]	475	99%	99%	99%
Prophylactic Antibiotic Selection (Outpatient)	506	96%	97%	98%
Prophylactic Antibiotic Stopped[2]	460	98%	98%	98%
Prophylactic Antibiotic Timing[2]	476	99%	98%	99%
Prophylactic Antibiotic Timing (Outpatient)	234	82%	97%	98%
Urinary Catheter Removal[2]	407	95%	97%	97%
Survey of Patients' Hospital Experiences				
Area Around Room 'Always' Quiet at Night	300+	56%	60%	61%
Doctors 'Always' Communicated Well	300+	79%	81%	82%
Home Recovery Information Given	300+	83%	87%	85%
Hospital Given 9 or 10 on 10 Point Scale	300+	68%	71%	71%
Meds 'Always' Explained Before Given	300+	60%	64%	64%
Nurses 'Always' Communicated Well	300+	75%	80%	79%
Pain 'Always' Well Controlled	300+	68%	71%	71%
Room and Bathroom 'Always' Clean	300+	65%	73%	73%
Timely Help 'Always' Received	300+	62%	70%	68%
Would Definitely Recommend Hospital	300+	71%	71%	71%
Use of Medical Imaging				
Cardiac Imaging Stress Test before Surgery	1,094	4.8%	5.1%	5.3%
Combination Abdominal CT Scan	2,635	3.7%	8.7%	10.5%
Combination Brain/Sinus CT Scan	1,549	0.1%	2.2%	2.7%
Combination Chest CT Scan	2,480	2.9%	3.6%	2.7%
Follow-up Mammogram/Ultrasound	5,424	7.7%	8.2%	8.8%
Lumbar Spine MRI for Low Back Pain	286	39.5%	36.9%	37.2%

Karmanos Cancer Center

4100 John R
Detroit, MI 48201
Phone: 800-576-6266
E-mail: info@karmanos.org
URL: www.karmanos.org
Type: Acute Care Hospitals
Emergency Services: No
Ownership: Proprietary
Beds: 123

Key Personnel:

CEO/President. . . . . John C Ruckdeschel

Measure	Cases	This Hosp.	State Avg.	U.S. Avg.
Blood Clot Prevention and Treatment				
Anticoagulation Overlap Therapy[1,2]	-	-	90%	93%
ICU Venous Thromboembolism Prophylaxis[2]	35	89%	93%	92%
Incidence of Potentially Preventable VTE[1,2]	-	-	8%	10%
UFH with Dosages/Platelet Monitoring[1,2]	-	-	96%	97%
Venous Thromboembolism Prophylaxis[2]	365	64%	87%	85%
Warfarin Therapy Discharge Instructions[1,2]	-	-	72%	75%
Chest Pain/Possible Heart Attack Care				
Aspirin Given Within 24 Hours of Arrival[5]	-	-	96%	96%
Fibrinolytic Meds Within 30 Min. of Arrival[5]	-	-	63%	58%
Average Time to ECG (minutes)[5]	-	-	8	7
Average Time to Transfer (minutes)[5]	-	-	53	60
Children's Asthma Care				
Received Home Management Plan of Care	-	-	-	88%
Received Reliever Medication	-	-	-	100%
Received Systemic Corticosteroids	-	-	-	100%
Emergency Department				
Admittance Decision Time (minutes)[2,7]	-	-	102	98
Head CT Results Within 45 Min. of Arrival[5]	-	-	54%	57%
Patients Who Left ER Before Being Seen[5]	-	-	2%	2%
Time from ER Arrival to Admit. (minutes)[2,7]	-	-	288	274
Time from ER Arrival to Discharge (minutes)[5]	-	-	128	134
Time in ER Before Being Evaluated (minutes)[5]	-	-	22	26
Time to Pain Meds for Fractures (minutes)[5]	-	-	55	57
Heart Attack Care				
Aspirin Given at Discharge[1,3]	-	-	99%	99%
Fibrinolytic Meds Within 30 Min. of Arrival[3,7]	-	-	20%	54%
PCI Within 90 Minutes of Arrival[3,7]	-	-	95%	96%
Statin Prescribed at Discharge[1,3]	-	-	98%	98%
Heart Failure Care				
ACE Inhibitor or ARB for LVSD[1]	-	-	96%	97%
Discharge Instructions Given	16	12%	94%	94%
Evaluation of LVS Function	17	100%	99%	99%
Medicare Spending				
Medicare Spending per Patient (ratio)	-	1.01	0.96	0.98
Pneumonia Care				
Appropriate Initial Antibiotic Given[7]	-	-	96%	95%
Blood Culture Timing[7]	-	-	98%	98%
Pregnancy and Delivery Care				
Newborn Deliveries Scheduled Early[7]	-	-	3%	6%
Preventive Care				
Immunization for Influenza[2]	367	52%	89%	90%
Immunization for Pneumonia[2]	391	65%	90%	92%
Stroke Care				
Anticoagulation Therapy for Atrial Fibrillation[1]	-	-	92%	95%
Antithrombotic Therapy Timing[1]	-	-	97%	98%
Assessed for Rehabilitation[1]	-	-	97%	97%
Discharged on Antithrombotic Therapy[1]	-	-	99%	99%
Discharged on Statin Medication[1]	-	-	94%	94%
Thrombolytic Therapy Timing[7]	-	-	69%	66%
Venous Thromboembolism Prophylaxis[1]	-	-	94%	94%
Written Stroke Educational Materials Given[1]	-	-	87%	88%
Surgical Care Improvement Project				
Appropriate Beta Blocker Usage[2]	111	90%	98%	98%
Appropriate VTP Within 24 Hours[2]	346	98%	98%	98%
Controlled Postoperative Blood Glucose[2,7]	-	-	97%	97%
Perioperative Temperature Management[2]	378	100%	100%	100%
Prophylactic Antibiotic Selection[2]	135	96%	99%	99%
Prophylactic Antibiotic Selection (Outpatient)	157	95%	97%	98%
Prophylactic Antibiotic Stopped[2]	122	96%	98%	98%
Prophylactic Antibiotic Timing[2]	135	100%	98%	99%
Prophylactic Antibiotic Timing (Outpatient)	115	61%	97%	98%
Urinary Catheter Removal[2]	87	92%	97%	97%
Survey of Patients' Hospital Experiences				
Area Around Room 'Always' Quiet at Night	300+	58%	60%	61%
Doctors 'Always' Communicated Well	300+	78%	81%	82%
Home Recovery Information Given	300+	90%	87%	85%
Hospital Given 9 or 10 on 10 Point Scale	300+	72%	71%	71%
Meds 'Always' Explained Before Given	300+	65%	64%	64%
Nurses 'Always' Communicated Well	300+	82%	80%	79%
Pain 'Always' Well Controlled	300+	71%	71%	71%
Room and Bathroom 'Always' Clean	300+	68%	73%	73%
Timely Help 'Always' Received	300+	64%	70%	68%
Would Definitely Recommend Hospital	300+	78%	71%	71%
Use of Medical Imaging				
Cardiac Imaging Stress Test before Surgery[7]	-	-	5.1%	5.3%
Combination Abdominal CT Scan	1,891	25.6%	8.7%	10.5%
Combination Brain/Sinus CT Scan[1]	-	-	2.2%	2.7%
Combination Chest CT Scan	2,887	5.1%	3.6%	2.7%
Follow-up Mammogram/Ultrasound	4,019	9.7%	8.2%	8.8%
Lumbar Spine MRI for Low Back Pain[1]	-	-	36.9%	37.2%

Saint John Hospital & Medical Center

22101 Moross Rd
Detroit, MI 48236
Phone: 313-343-4000
URL: www.stjohnprovidence.org
Type: Acute Care Hospitals
Emergency Services: Yes
Ownership: Voluntary non-profit - Church
Beds: 772

Key Personnel:

President . . . . Diane Radloff

Measure	Cases	This Hosp.	State Avg.	U.S. Avg.

NOTE: Hospital profiles are in alphabetical order by state, then city, then hospital within the city; Rankings exclude hospitals with less than 25 cases except for patient surveys which excludes hospitals with less than 100 cases; (a) 100-299 cases; (1) The number of cases/patients is too few to report; (2) Data submitted were based on a sample of cases/patients; (3) Results are based on a shorter time period than required; (4) Data suppressed by CMS for one or more quarters; (5) Results are not available for this reporting period; (6) Fewer than 100 patients completed the HCAHPS survey; (7) No cases met the criteria for this measure; (8) The lower limit of the confidence interval cannot be calculated if the number of observed infections equals zero; (9) No data are available from the state/territory for this reporting period; (10) The scores shown reflect fewer than 50 completed surveys; (11) There were discrepancies in the data collection process; (12) This measure does not apply to this hospital for this reporting period; (13) Results cannot be calculated for this reporting period; (14) The results for this state are combined with nearby states to protect confidentiality; Please refer to the User's Guide for a full explanation of data.

Blood Clot Prevention and Treatment				
Anticoagulation Overlap Therapy[2]	178	94%	90%	93%
ICU Venous Thromboembolism Prophylaxis[2]	77	100%	93%	92%
Incidence of Potentially Preventable VTE[2]	48	0%	8%	10%
UFH with Dosages/Platelet Monitoring[2]	189	100%	96%	97%
Venous Thromboembolism Prophylaxis[2]	372	96%	87%	85%
Warfarin Therapy Discharge Instructions[2]	123	74%	72%	75%
Chest Pain/Possible Heart Attack Care				
Aspirin Given Within 24 Hours of Arrival	40	100%	96%	96%
Fibrinolytic Meds Within 30 Min. of Arrival[7]	-	-	63%	58%
Average Time to ECG (minutes)	41	5	8	7
Average Time to Transfer (minutes)[1]	-	-	53	60
Children's Asthma Care				
Received Home Management Plan of Care	-	-	-	88%
Received Reliever Medication	-	-	-	100%
Received Systemic Corticosteroids	-	-	-	100%
Emergency Department				
Admittance Decision Time (minutes)[2]	579	88	102	98
Head CT Results Within 45 Min. of Arrival[1]	-	-	54%	57%
Patients Who Left ER Before Being Seen	>100k	1%	2%	2%
Time from ER Arrival to Admit. (minutes)[2]	604	298	288	274
Time from ER Arrival to Discharge (minutes)	341	127	128	134
Time in ER Before Being Evaluated (minutes)	411	22	22	26
Time to Pain Meds for Fractures (minutes)	229	61	55	57
Heart Attack Care				
Aspirin Given at Discharge	403	100%	99%	99%
Fibrinolytic Meds Within 30 Min. of Arrival[7]	-	-	20%	54%
PCI Within 90 Minutes of Arrival	75	99%	95%	96%
Statin Prescribed at Discharge	400	99%	98%	98%
Heart Failure Care				
ACE Inhibitor or ARB for LVSD	334	99%	96%	97%
Discharge Instructions Given	861	100%	94%	94%
Evaluation of LVS Function	1,021	100%	99%	99%
Medicare Spending				
Medicare Spending per Patient (ratio)	-	1.02	0.96	0.98
Pneumonia Care				
Appropriate Initial Antibiotic Given	235	99%	96%	95%
Blood Culture Timing	231	100%	98%	98%
Pregnancy and Delivery Care				
Newborn Deliveries Scheduled Early	280	4%	3%	6%
Preventive Care				
Immunization for Influenza[2]	555	97%	89%	90%
Immunization for Pneumonia[2]	656	92%	90%	92%
Stroke Care				
Anticoagulation Therapy for Atrial Fibrillation	52	96%	92%	95%
Antithrombotic Therapy Timing	335	97%	97%	98%
Assessed for Rehabilitation	430	99%	97%	97%
Discharged on Antithrombotic Therapy	368	100%	99%	99%
Discharged on Statin Medication	313	99%	94%	94%
Thrombolytic Therapy Timing	26	88%	69%	66%
Venous Thromboembolism Prophylaxis	460	98%	94%	94%
Written Stroke Educational Materials Given	221	97%	87%	88%
Surgical Care Improvement Project				
Appropriate Beta Blocker Usage[2]	504	99%	98%	98%
Appropriate VTP Within 24 Hours[2]	976	100%	98%	98%
Controlled Postoperative Blood Glucose[2]	192	99%	97%	97%
Perioperative Temperature Management[2]	1,255	100%	100%	100%
Prophylactic Antibiotic Selection[2]	1,170	100%	99%	99%
Prophylactic Antibiotic Selection (Outpatient)	514	98%	97%	98%
Prophylactic Antibiotic Stopped[2]	1,143	99%	98%	98%
Prophylactic Antibiotic Timing[2]	1,170	100%	98%	99%
Prophylactic Antibiotic Timing (Outpatient)	518	99%	97%	98%
Urinary Catheter Removal[2]	660	99%	97%	97%
Survey of Patients' Hospital Experiences				
Area Around Room 'Always' Quiet at Night	300+	54%	60%	61%
Doctors 'Always' Communicated Well	300+	78%	81%	82%
Home Recovery Information Given	300+	83%	87%	85%
Hospital Given 9 or 10 on 10 Point Scale	300+	66%	71%	71%
Meds 'Always' Explained Before Given	300+	58%	64%	64%
Nurses 'Always' Communicated Well	300+	74%	80%	79%
Pain 'Always' Well Controlled	300+	66%	71%	71%
Room and Bathroom 'Always' Clean	300+	58%	73%	73%
Timely Help 'Always' Received	300+	57%	70%	68%
Would Definitely Recommend Hospital	300+	67%	71%	71%
Use of Medical Imaging				
Cardiac Imaging Stress Test before Surgery	1,028	4.9%	5.1%	5.3%
Combination Abdominal CT Scan	1,819	9.0%	8.7%	10.5%
Combination Brain/Sinus CT Scan	1,469	2.3%	2.2%	2.7%
Combination Chest CT Scan	1,130	2.7%	3.6%	2.7%
Follow-up Mammogram/Ultrasound	4,116	5.0%	8.2%	8.8%
Lumbar Spine MRI for Low Back Pain	203	34.0%	36.9%	37.2%

Sinai - Grace Hospital

6071 W Outer Drive
Detroit, MI 48235
URL: www.sinaigrace.org
Type: Acute Care Hospitals
Ownership: Proprietary
Phone: 313-966-3300
Fax: 313-966-3546
Emergency Services: Yes
Beds: 404

Key Personnel:
Quality Assurance . . . . Michelle Bellmore
Operating Room. . . . . Deidra Brown-Cobb
Infection Control. . . . . Sheila Finch
Chief of Medical Staff. . . . . John Haapaniemi, DO
Pediatric Ambulatory Care . . . . . . Anne-Mare Ice, MD
CEO/President. . . . . Conrad Mallett, Jr
Radiology. . . . . Terry Posa
Cardiac Laboratory. . . . . Diane Wehby

Measure	Cases	This Hosp.	State Avg.	U.S. Avg.
Blood Clot Prevention and Treatment				
Anticoagulation Overlap Therapy[2]	141	94%	90%	93%
ICU Venous Thromboembolism Prophylaxis[2]	45	100%	93%	92%
Incidence of Potentially Preventable VTE[2]	45	11%	8%	10%
UFH with Dosages/Platelet Monitoring[2]	91	100%	96%	97%
Venous Thromboembolism Prophylaxis[2]	387	89%	87%	85%
Warfarin Therapy Discharge Instructions[2]	98	47%	72%	75%
Chest Pain/Possible Heart Attack Care				
Aspirin Given Within 24 Hours of Arrival[1]	-	-	96%	96%
Fibrinolytic Meds Within 30 Min. of Arrival[3,7]	-	-	63%	58%
Average Time to ECG (minutes)	11	0	8	7
Average Time to Transfer (minutes)[3,7]	-	-	53	60
Children's Asthma Care				
Received Home Management Plan of Care	-	-	-	88%
Received Reliever Medication	-	-	-	100%
Received Systemic Corticosteroids	-	-	-	100%
Emergency Department				
Admittance Decision Time (minutes)[2]	520	86	102	98
Head CT Results Within 45 Min. of Arrival[1]	-	-	54%	57%
Patients Who Left ER Before Being Seen	>100k	1%	2%	2%
Time from ER Arrival to Admit. (minutes)[2]	603	302	288	274
Time from ER Arrival to Discharge (minutes)	328	158	128	134
Time in ER Before Being Evaluated (minutes)	249	0	22	26
Time to Pain Meds for Fractures (minutes)	146	62	55	57
Heart Attack Care				
Aspirin Given at Discharge	336	100%	99%	99%
Fibrinolytic Meds Within 30 Min. of Arrival[7]	-	-	20%	54%
PCI Within 90 Minutes of Arrival	25	100%	95%	96%
Statin Prescribed at Discharge	336	99%	98%	98%
Heart Failure Care				
ACE Inhibitor or ARB for LVSD	283	97%	96%	97%
Discharge Instructions Given	583	98%	94%	94%
Evaluation of LVS Function	678	100%	99%	99%
Medicare Spending				
Medicare Spending per Patient (ratio)	-	1.04	0.96	0.98
Pneumonia Care				
Appropriate Initial Antibiotic Given	183	97%	96%	95%
Blood Culture Timing	399	96%	98%	98%
Pregnancy and Delivery Care				
Newborn Deliveries Scheduled Early[2]	24	0%	3%	6%
Preventive Care				
Immunization for Influenza[2]	554	96%	89%	90%
Immunization for Pneumonia[2]	734	95%	90%	92%
Stroke Care				
Anticoagulation Therapy for Atrial Fibrillation	11	91%	92%	95%
Antithrombotic Therapy Timing	225	98%	97%	98%
Assessed for Rehabilitation	285	99%	97%	97%
Discharged on Antithrombotic Therapy	237	100%	99%	99%
Discharged on Statin Medication	166	95%	94%	94%
Thrombolytic Therapy Timing	25	72%	69%	66%
Venous Thromboembolism Prophylaxis	297	97%	94%	94%
Written Stroke Educational Materials Given	144	88%	87%	88%
Surgical Care Improvement Project				
Appropriate Beta Blocker Usage[2]	171	98%	98%	98%
Appropriate VTP Within 24 Hours[2]	391	98%	98%	98%
Controlled Postoperative Blood Glucose[2]	58	100%	97%	97%
Perioperative Temperature Management[2]	474	100%	100%	100%
Prophylactic Antibiotic Selection[2]	377	99%	99%	99%
Prophylactic Antibiotic Selection (Outpatient)	387	98%	97%	98%
Prophylactic Antibiotic Stopped[2]	353	98%	98%	98%
Prophylactic Antibiotic Timing[2]	378	98%	98%	99%
Prophylactic Antibiotic Timing (Outpatient)	385	97%	97%	98%
Urinary Catheter Removal[2]	270	98%	97%	97%
Survey of Patients' Hospital Experiences				
Area Around Room 'Always' Quiet at Night[11]	300+	60%	60%	61%
Doctors 'Always' Communicated Well[11]	300+	76%	81%	82%
Home Recovery Information Given[11]	300+	81%	87%	85%
Hospital Given 9 or 10 on 10 Point Scale[11]	300+	54%	71%	71%
Meds 'Always' Explained Before Given[11]	300+	53%	64%	64%
Nurses 'Always' Communicated Well[11]	300+	73%	80%	79%
Pain 'Always' Well Controlled[11]	300+	65%	71%	71%
Room and Bathroom 'Always' Clean[11]	300+	62%	73%	73%
Timely Help 'Always' Received[11]	300+	56%	70%	68%
Would Definitely Recommend Hospital[11]	300+	48%	71%	71%
Use of Medical Imaging				
Cardiac Imaging Stress Test before Surgery	348	6.9%	5.1%	5.3%
Combination Abdominal CT Scan	749	6.3%	8.7%	10.5%
Combination Brain/Sinus CT Scan	815	5.2%	2.2%	2.7%
Combination Chest CT Scan	518	1.7%	3.6%	2.7%
Follow-up Mammogram/Ultrasound	1,363	12.8%	8.2%	8.8%
Lumbar Spine MRI for Low Back Pain	102	31.4%	36.9%	37.2%

Borgess - Lee Memorial Hospital

420 W High Street
Dowagiac, MI 49047
Type: Critical Access Hospitals
Ownership: Voluntary non-profit - Private
Phone: 269-782-8681
Fax: 269-783-3044
Emergency Services: Yes
Beds: 74

Key Personnel:
Intensive Care Unit. . . . . Boonchoo Chang, MD
Infection Control. . . . . Sandy Claborn
Operating Room. . . . . Sandy Claborn
Radiology. . . . . Marcio S Curvelo, MD
Emergency Room . . . . Paul Rehkepf, MD
Pediatric Ambulatory Care . . . . . . Jaime Rodriguez, MD
Chief of Medical Staff. . . . . Mohammad Taqi
Quality Assurance . . . . Marilyn White, RN

Measure	Cases	This Hosp.	State Avg.	U.S. Avg.
Blood Clot Prevention and Treatment				
Anticoagulation Overlap Therapy[5]	-	-	90%	93%
ICU Venous Thromboembolism Prophylaxis[5]	-	-	93%	92%
Incidence of Potentially Preventable VTE[5]	-	-	8%	10%
UFH with Dosages/Platelet Monitoring[5]	-	-	96%	97%
Venous Thromboembolism Prophylaxis[5]	-	-	87%	85%
Warfarin Therapy Discharge Instructions[5]	-	-	72%	75%
Chest Pain/Possible Heart Attack Care				
Aspirin Given Within 24 Hours of Arrival[3]	14	100%	96%	96%
Fibrinolytic Meds Within 30 Min. of Arrival[3,7]	-	-	63%	58%
Average Time to ECG (minutes)[3]	14	6	8	7
Average Time to Transfer (minutes)[1,3]	-	-	53	60
Children's Asthma Care				
Received Home Management Plan of Care	-	-	-	88%
Received Reliever Medication	-	-	-	100%
Received Systemic Corticosteroids	-	-	-	100%
Emergency Department				
Admittance Decision Time (minutes)[5]	-	-	102	98
Head CT Results Within 45 Min. of Arrival[5]	-	-	54%	57%
Patients Who Left ER Before Being Seen	5,058	0%	2%	2%
Time from ER Arrival to Admit. (minutes)[5]	-	-	288	274
Time from ER Arrival to Discharge (minutes)	484	110	128	134
Time in ER Before Being Evaluated (minutes)	589	14	22	26
Time to Pain Meds for Fractures (minutes)[5]	-	-	55	57
Heart Attack Care				

NOTE: *Hospital profiles are in alphabetical order by state, then city, then hospital within the city; Rankings exclude hospitals with less than 25 cases except for patient surveys which excludes hospitals with less than 100 cases; (a) 100-299 cases; (1) The number of cases/patients is too few to report; (2) Data submitted were based on a sample of cases/patients; (3) Results are based on a shorter time period than required; (4) Data suppressed by CMS for one or more quarters; (5) Results are not available for this reporting period; (6) Fewer than 100 patients completed the HCAHPS survey; (7) No cases met the criteria for this measure; (8) The lower limit of the confidence interval cannot be calculated if the number of observed infections equals zero; (9) No data are available from the state/territory for this reporting period; (10) The scores shown reflect fewer than 50 completed surveys; (11) There were discrepancies in the data collection process; (12) This measure does not apply to this hospital for this reporting period; (13) Results cannot be calculated for this reporting period; (14) The results for this state are combined with nearby states to protect confidentiality; Please refer to the User's Guide for a full explanation of data.*

Measure	Cases	This Hosp.	State Avg.	U.S. Avg.
Aspirin Given at Discharge[1,3]	-	-	99%	99%
Fibrinolytic Meds Within 30 Min. of Arrival[3,7]	-	-	20%	54%
PCI Within 90 Minutes of Arrival[3,7]	-	-	95%	96%
Statin Prescribed at Discharge[1,3]	-	-	98%	98%
Heart Failure Care				
ACE Inhibitor or ARB for LVSD[1]	-	-	96%	97%
Discharge Instructions Given	19	74%	94%	94%
Evaluation of LVS Function	27	100%	99%	99%
Medicare Spending				
Medicare Spending per Patient (ratio)	-	-	0.96	0.98
Pneumonia Care				
Appropriate Initial Antibiotic Given	36	89%	96%	95%
Blood Culture Timing	40	98%	98%	98%
Pregnancy and Delivery Care				
Newborn Deliveries Scheduled Early[3,7]	-	-	3%	6%
Preventive Care				
Immunization for Influenza[5]	-	-	89%	90%
Immunization for Pneumonia[5]	-	-	90%	92%
Stroke Care				
Anticoagulation Therapy for Atrial Fibrillation[5]	-	-	92%	95%
Antithrombotic Therapy Timing[5]	-	-	97%	98%
Assessed for Rehabilitation[5]	-	-	97%	97%
Discharged on Antithrombotic Therapy[5]	-	-	99%	99%
Discharged on Statin Medication[5]	-	-	94%	94%
Thrombolytic Therapy Timing[5]	-	-	69%	66%
Venous Thromboembolism Prophylaxis[5]	-	-	94%	94%
Written Stroke Educational Materials Given[5]	-	-	87%	88%
Surgical Care Improvement Project				
Appropriate Beta Blocker Usage[1,3]	-	-	98%	98%
Appropriate VTP Within 24 Hours[1,3]	-	-	98%	98%
Controlled Postoperative Blood Glucose[3,7]	-	-	97%	97%
Perioperative Temperature Management[1,3]	-	-	100%	100%
Prophylactic Antibiotic Selection[1,3]	-	-	99%	99%
Prophylactic Antibiotic Selection (Outpatient)[5]	-	-	97%	98%
Prophylactic Antibiotic Stopped[1,3]	-	-	98%	98%
Prophylactic Antibiotic Timing[1,3]	-	-	98%	99%
Prophylactic Antibiotic Timing (Outpatient)[5]	-	-	97%	98%
Urinary Catheter Removal[1,3]	-	-	97%	97%
Survey of Patients' Hospital Experiences				
Area Around Room 'Always' Quiet at Night	(a)	73%	60%	61%
Doctors 'Always' Communicated Well	(a)	82%	81%	82%
Home Recovery Information Given	(a)	83%	87%	85%
Hospital Given 9 or 10 on 10 Point Scale	(a)	70%	71%	71%
Meds 'Always' Explained Before Given	(a)	54%	64%	64%
Nurses 'Always' Communicated Well	(a)	82%	80%	79%
Pain 'Always' Well Controlled	(a)	69%	71%	71%
Room and Bathroom 'Always' Clean	(a)	73%	73%	73%
Timely Help 'Always' Received	(a)	68%	70%	68%
Would Definitely Recommend Hospital	(a)	64%	71%	71%
Use of Medical Imaging				
Cardiac Imaging Stress Test before Surgery	50	2.0%	5.1%	5.3%
Combination Abdominal CT Scan	276	2.2%	8.7%	10.5%
Combination Brain/Sinus CT Scan[1]	-	-	2.2%	2.7%
Combination Chest CT Scan	161	1.2%	3.6%	2.7%
Follow-up Mammogram/Ultrasound	242	12.0%	8.2%	8.8%
Lumbar Spine MRI for Low Back Pain[1]	-	-	36.9%	37.2%

Saint John River District Hospital

4100 River Rd — Phone: 810-329-7111
East China, MI 48054 — Fax: 810-329-8920
URL: www.stjohn.org
Type: Acute Care Hospitals — Emergency Services: Yes
Ownership: Govt - Hospital Dist/Auth — Beds: 68

Key Personnel:

Infection Control. . . . . Heidi Boadway, RN
Radiology. . . . . Herminio C Calderon, MD
Quality Assurance . . . . John D Doyle
Operating Room. . . . . Andrew K Gavagan, RN
CEO/President. . . . . Patricia Maryland, EdD
Chief of Medical Staff . . . . Michael C Wiemann, DO
Pediatric Ambulatory Care . . . . . . John Zmielko, MD

Measure	Cases	This Hosp.	State Avg.	U.S. Avg.
Blood Clot Prevention and Treatment				
Anticoagulation Overlap Therapy[2]	13	100%	90%	93%
ICU Venous Thromboembolism Prophylaxis[2]	24	100%	93%	92%
Incidence of Potentially Preventable VTE[1,2]	-	-	8%	10%
UFH with Dosages/Platelet Monitoring[2]	14	100%	96%	97%
Venous Thromboembolism Prophylaxis[2]	148	82%	87%	85%
Warfarin Therapy Discharge Instructions[1,2]	-	-	72%	75%
Chest Pain/Possible Heart Attack Care				
Aspirin Given Within 24 Hours of Arrival	55	98%	96%	96%
Fibrinolytic Meds Within 30 Min. of Arrival[7]	-	-	63%	58%
Average Time to ECG (minutes)	55	3	8	7
Average Time to Transfer (minutes)[1]	-	-	53	60
Children's Asthma Care				
Received Home Management Plan of Care	-	-	-	88%
Received Reliever Medication	-	-	-	100%
Received Systemic Corticosteroids	-	-	-	100%
Emergency Department				
Admittance Decision Time (minutes)[2]	150	65	102	98
Head CT Results Within 45 Min. of Arrival	11	64%	54%	57%
Patients Who Left ER Before Being Seen	12,409	0%	2%	2%
Time from ER Arrival to Admit. (minutes)[2]	321	210	288	274
Time from ER Arrival to Discharge (minutes)	350	96	128	134
Time in ER Before Being Evaluated (minutes)	345	18	22	26
Time to Pain Meds for Fractures (minutes)	51	35	55	57
Heart Attack Care				
Aspirin Given at Discharge[1]	-	-	99%	99%
Fibrinolytic Meds Within 30 Min. of Arrival[7]	-	-	20%	54%
PCI Within 90 Minutes of Arrival[7]	-	-	95%	96%
Statin Prescribed at Discharge[1]	-	-	98%	98%
Heart Failure Care				
ACE Inhibitor or ARB for LVSD	16	88%	96%	97%
Discharge Instructions Given	48	94%	94%	94%
Evaluation of LVS Function	58	100%	99%	99%
Medicare Spending				
Medicare Spending per Patient (ratio)	-	0.99	0.96	0.98
Pneumonia Care				
Appropriate Initial Antibiotic Given	63	94%	96%	95%
Blood Culture Timing	77	99%	98%	98%
Pregnancy and Delivery Care				
Newborn Deliveries Scheduled Early	33	3%	3%	6%
Preventive Care				
Immunization for Influenza[2]	261	95%	89%	90%
Immunization for Pneumonia[2]	338	97%	90%	92%
Stroke Care				
Anticoagulation Therapy for Atrial Fibrillation[1]	-	-	92%	95%
Antithrombotic Therapy Timing	21	100%	97%	98%
Assessed for Rehabilitation	19	100%	97%	97%
Discharged on Antithrombotic Therapy	18	100%	99%	99%
Discharged on Statin Medication	15	80%	94%	94%
Thrombolytic Therapy Timing[1]	-	-	69%	66%
Venous Thromboembolism Prophylaxis	22	86%	94%	94%
Written Stroke Educational Materials Given	11	91%	87%	88%
Surgical Care Improvement Project				
Appropriate Beta Blocker Usage	33	97%	98%	98%
Appropriate VTP Within 24 Hours	90	98%	98%	98%
Controlled Postoperative Blood Glucose[7]	-	-	97%	97%
Perioperative Temperature Management	105	100%	100%	100%
Prophylactic Antibiotic Selection	76	100%	99%	99%
Prophylactic Antibiotic Selection (Outpatient)	53	98%	97%	98%
Prophylactic Antibiotic Stopped	74	100%	98%	98%
Prophylactic Antibiotic Timing	76	96%	98%	99%
Prophylactic Antibiotic Timing (Outpatient)	53	98%	97%	98%
Urinary Catheter Removal	76	97%	97%	97%
Survey of Patients' Hospital Experiences				
Area Around Room 'Always' Quiet at Night	300+	67%	60%	61%
Doctors 'Always' Communicated Well	300+	82%	81%	82%
Home Recovery Information Given	300+	85%	87%	85%
Hospital Given 9 or 10 on 10 Point Scale	300+	74%	71%	71%
Meds 'Always' Explained Before Given	300+	65%	64%	64%
Nurses 'Always' Communicated Well	300+	79%	80%	79%
Pain 'Always' Well Controlled	300+	71%	71%	71%
Room and Bathroom 'Always' Clean	300+	75%	73%	73%
Timely Help 'Always' Received	300+	70%	70%	68%
Would Definitely Recommend Hospital	300+	66%	71%	71%
Use of Medical Imaging				
Cardiac Imaging Stress Test before Surgery	111	9.0%	5.1%	5.3%
Combination Abdominal CT Scan	325	1.5%	8.7%	10.5%
Combination Brain/Sinus CT Scan[1]	-	-	2.2%	2.7%
Combination Chest CT Scan	226	0.4%	3.6%	2.7%
Follow-up Mammogram/Ultrasound	518	20.5%	8.2%	8.8%
Lumbar Spine MRI for Low Back Pain[1]	-	-	36.9%	37.2%

Eaton Rapids Medical Center

1500 S Main Street — Phone: 517-663-2671
Eaton Rapids, MI 48827 — Fax: 517-663-4920
URL: www.eatonrapidsmedicalcenter.org
Type: Critical Access Hospitals — Emergency Services: Yes
Ownership: Voluntary non-profit - Private — Beds: 20

Key Personnel:

Radiology. . . . . Pauline Chee
Operating Room. . . . . Jeffrey Deppen
Chief of Medical Staff. . . . . Ashok Gupta
CEO/President. . . . . Timothy J. Johnson

Measure	Cases	This Hosp.	State Avg.	U.S. Avg.
Blood Clot Prevention and Treatment				
Anticoagulation Overlap Therapy[5]	-	-	90%	93%
ICU Venous Thromboembolism Prophylaxis[5]	-	-	93%	92%
Incidence of Potentially Preventable VTE[5]	-	-	8%	10%
UFH with Dosages/Platelet Monitoring[5]	-	-	96%	97%
Venous Thromboembolism Prophylaxis[5]	-	-	87%	85%
Warfarin Therapy Discharge Instructions[5]	-	-	72%	75%
Chest Pain/Possible Heart Attack Care				
Aspirin Given Within 24 Hours of Arrival	60	98%	96%	96%
Fibrinolytic Meds Within 30 Min. of Arrival[1]	-	-	63%	58%
Average Time to ECG (minutes)	65	5	8	7
Average Time to Transfer (minutes)[1]	-	-	53	60
Children's Asthma Care				
Received Home Management Plan of Care	-	-	-	88%
Received Reliever Medication	-	-	-	100%
Received Systemic Corticosteroids	-	-	-	100%
Emergency Department				
Admittance Decision Time (minutes)[5]	-	-	102	98
Head CT Results Within 45 Min. of Arrival[5]	-	-	54%	57%
Patients Who Left ER Before Being Seen[5]	-	-	2%	2%
Time from ER Arrival to Admit. (minutes)[5]	-	-	288	274
Time from ER Arrival to Discharge (minutes)	421	99	128	134
Time in ER Before Being Evaluated (minutes)	459	28	22	26
Time to Pain Meds for Fractures (minutes)[5]	-	-	55	57
Heart Attack Care				
Aspirin Given at Discharge[1]	-	-	99%	99%
Fibrinolytic Meds Within 30 Min. of Arrival[7]	-	-	20%	54%
PCI Within 90 Minutes of Arrival[7]	-	-	95%	96%
Statin Prescribed at Discharge[1]	-	-	98%	98%
Heart Failure Care				
ACE Inhibitor or ARB for LVSD[1]	-	-	96%	97%
Discharge Instructions Given	19	100%	94%	94%
Evaluation of LVS Function	20	95%	99%	99%
Medicare Spending				
Medicare Spending per Patient (ratio)	-	-	0.96	0.98
Pneumonia Care				
Appropriate Initial Antibiotic Given	23	78%	96%	95%
Blood Culture Timing	28	82%	98%	98%
Pregnancy and Delivery Care				
Newborn Deliveries Scheduled Early[5]	-	-	3%	6%
Preventive Care				
Immunization for Influenza[5]	-	-	89%	90%
Immunization for Pneumonia[5]	-	-	90%	92%
Stroke Care				
Anticoagulation Therapy for Atrial Fibrillation[5]	-	-	92%	95%
Antithrombotic Therapy Timing[5]	-	-	97%	98%
Assessed for Rehabilitation[5]	-	-	97%	97%
Discharged on Antithrombotic Therapy[5]	-	-	99%	99%
Discharged on Statin Medication[5]	-	-	94%	94%
Thrombolytic Therapy Timing[5]	-	-	69%	66%
Venous Thromboembolism Prophylaxis[5]	-	-	94%	94%
Written Stroke Educational Materials Given[5]	-	-	87%	88%
Surgical Care Improvement Project				

NOTE: Hospital profiles are in alphabetical order by state, then city, then hospital within the city; Rankings exclude hospitals with less than 25 cases except for patient surveys which excludes hospitals with less than 100 cases; (a) 100-299 cases; (1) The number of cases/patients is too few to report; (2) Data submitted were based on a sample of cases/patients; (3) Results are based on a shorter time period than required; (4) Data suppressed by CMS for one or more quarters; (5) Results are not available for this reporting period; (6) Fewer than 100 patients completed the HCAHPS survey; (7) No cases met the criteria for this measure; (8) The lower limit of the confidence interval cannot be calculated if the number of observed infections equals zero; (9) No data are available from the state/territory for this reporting period; (10) The scores shown reflect fewer than 50 completed surveys; (11) There were discrepancies in the data collection process; (12) This measure does not apply to this hospital for this reporting period; (13) Results cannot be calculated for this reporting period; (14) The results for this state are combined with nearby states to protect confidentiality; Please refer to the User's Guide for a full explanation of data.

Measure	Cases	This Hosp.	State Avg.	U.S. Avg.
Appropriate Beta Blocker Usage[5]	-	-	98%	98%
Appropriate VTP Within 24 Hours[5]	-	-	98%	98%
Controlled Postoperative Blood Glucose[5]	-	-	97%	97%
Perioperative Temperature Management[5]	-	-	100%	100%
Prophylactic Antibiotic Selection[5]	-	-	99%	99%
Prophylactic Antibiotic Selection (Outpatient)	46	100%	97%	98%
Prophylactic Antibiotic Stopped[5]	-	-	98%	98%
Prophylactic Antibiotic Timing[5]	-	-	98%	99%
Prophylactic Antibiotic Timing (Outpatient)	47	89%	97%	98%
Urinary Catheter Removal[5]	-	-	97%	97%
Survey of Patients' Hospital Experiences				
Area Around Room 'Always' Quiet at Night[10]	<100	74%	60%	61%
Doctors 'Always' Communicated Well[10]	<100	83%	81%	82%
Home Recovery Information Given[10]	<100	92%	87%	85%
Hospital Given 9 or 10 on 10 Point Scale[10]	<100	91%	71%	71%
Meds 'Always' Explained Before Given[10]	<100	83%	64%	64%
Nurses 'Always' Communicated Well[10]	<100	93%	80%	79%
Pain 'Always' Well Controlled[10]	<100	81%	71%	71%
Room and Bathroom 'Always' Clean[10]	<100	89%	73%	73%
Timely Help 'Always' Received[10]	<100	86%	70%	68%
Would Definitely Recommend Hospital[10]	<100	92%	71%	71%
Use of Medical Imaging				
Cardiac Imaging Stress Test before Surgery[1]	-	-	5.1%	5.3%
Combination Abdominal CT Scan	179	3.9%	8.7%	10.5%
Combination Brain/Sinus CT Scan[1]	-	-	2.2%	2.7%
Combination Chest CT Scan	51	0.0%	3.6%	2.7%
Follow-up Mammogram/Ultrasound	266	3.0%	8.2%	8.8%
Lumbar Spine MRI for Low Back Pain[1]	-	-	36.9%	37.2%

Saint Francis Hospital

3401 Ludington St
Escanaba, MI 49829
URL: www.osfstfrancis.or
Type: Critical Access Hospitals
Ownership: Voluntary non-profit - Church

Phone: 906-786-3311
Emergency Services: Yes

Measure	Cases	This Hosp.	State Avg.	U.S. Avg.
Blood Clot Prevention and Treatment				
Anticoagulation Overlap Therapy[5]	-	-	90%	93%
ICU Venous Thromboembolism Prophylaxis[5]	-	-	93%	92%
Incidence of Potentially Preventable VTE[5]	-	-	8%	10%
UFH with Dosages/Platelet Monitoring[5]	-	-	96%	97%
Venous Thromboembolism Prophylaxis[5]	-	-	87%	85%
Warfarin Therapy Discharge Instructions[5]	-	-	72%	75%
Chest Pain/Possible Heart Attack Care				
Aspirin Given Within 24 Hours of Arrival	66	98%	96%	96%
Fibrinolytic Meds Within 30 Min. of Arrival[1]	-	-	63%	58%
Average Time to ECG (minutes)	68	10	8	7
Average Time to Transfer (minutes)[1]	-	-	53	60
Children's Asthma Care				
Received Home Management Plan of Care	-	-	-	88%
Received Reliever Medication	-	-	-	100%
Received Systemic Corticosteroids	-	-	-	100%
Emergency Department				
Admittance Decision Time (minutes)[2]	426	49	102	98
Head CT Results Within 45 Min. of Arrival	13	54%	54%	57%
Patients Who Left ER Before Being Seen[5]	-	-	2%	2%
Time from ER Arrival to Admit. (minutes)[2]	465	234	288	274
Time from ER Arrival to Discharge (minutes)	399	155	128	134
Time in ER Before Being Evaluated (minutes)	426	27	22	26
Time to Pain Meds for Fractures (minutes)	98	48	55	57
Heart Attack Care				
Aspirin Given at Discharge[1]	-	-	99%	99%
Fibrinolytic Meds Within 30 Min. of Arrival[7]	-	-	20%	54%
PCI Within 90 Minutes of Arrival[7]	-	-	95%	96%
Statin Prescribed at Discharge[1]	-	-	98%	98%
Heart Failure Care				
ACE Inhibitor or ARB for LVSD	13	100%	96%	97%
Discharge Instructions Given	31	100%	94%	94%
Evaluation of LVS Function	44	100%	99%	99%
Medicare Spending				
Medicare Spending per Patient (ratio)	-	-	0.96	0.98
Pneumonia Care				
Appropriate Initial Antibiotic Given	35	100%	96%	95%
Blood Culture Timing	79	100%	98%	98%
Pregnancy and Delivery Care				
Newborn Deliveries Scheduled Early[5]	-	-	3%	6%
Preventive Care				
Immunization for Influenza[2]	347	99%	89%	90%
Immunization for Pneumonia[2]	465	97%	90%	92%
Stroke Care				
Anticoagulation Therapy for Atrial Fibrillation[5]	-	-	92%	95%
Antithrombotic Therapy Timing[5]	-	-	97%	98%
Assessed for Rehabilitation[5]	-	-	97%	97%
Discharged on Antithrombotic Therapy[5]	-	-	99%	99%
Discharged on Statin Medication[5]	-	-	94%	94%
Thrombolytic Therapy Timing[5]	-	-	69%	66%
Venous Thromboembolism Prophylaxis[5]	-	-	94%	94%
Written Stroke Educational Materials Given[5]	-	-	87%	88%
Surgical Care Improvement Project				
Appropriate Beta Blocker Usage	19	100%	98%	98%
Appropriate VTP Within 24 Hours	63	100%	98%	98%
Controlled Postoperative Blood Glucose[7]	-	-	97%	97%
Perioperative Temperature Management	85	100%	100%	100%
Prophylactic Antibiotic Selection	51	100%	99%	99%
Prophylactic Antibiotic Selection (Outpatient)	40	90%	97%	98%
Prophylactic Antibiotic Stopped	49	98%	98%	98%
Prophylactic Antibiotic Timing	51	98%	98%	99%
Prophylactic Antibiotic Timing (Outpatient)	41	95%	97%	98%
Urinary Catheter Removal	40	100%	97%	97%
Survey of Patients' Hospital Experiences				
Area Around Room 'Always' Quiet at Night	300+	59%	60%	61%
Doctors 'Always' Communicated Well	300+	84%	81%	82%
Home Recovery Information Given	300+	88%	87%	85%
Hospital Given 9 or 10 on 10 Point Scale	300+	73%	71%	71%
Meds 'Always' Explained Before Given	300+	73%	64%	64%
Nurses 'Always' Communicated Well	300+	84%	80%	79%
Pain 'Always' Well Controlled	300+	80%	71%	71%
Room and Bathroom 'Always' Clean	300+	78%	73%	73%
Timely Help 'Always' Received	300+	80%	70%	68%
Would Definitely Recommend Hospital	300+	67%	71%	71%
Use of Medical Imaging				
Cardiac Imaging Stress Test before Surgery	216	7.4%	5.1%	5.3%
Combination Abdominal CT Scan	472	12.5%	8.7%	10.5%
Combination Brain/Sinus CT Scan	574	2.4%	2.2%	2.7%
Combination Chest CT Scan	281	5.0%	3.6%	2.7%
Follow-up Mammogram/Ultrasound	828	7.1%	8.2%	8.8%
Lumbar Spine MRI for Low Back Pain	106	43.4%	36.9%	37.2%

Botsford Hospital

28050 Grand River Avenue
Farmington Hills, MI 48336
URL: www.botsfordsystem.org
Type: Acute Care Hospitals
Ownership: Voluntary non-profit - Private

Phone: 248-471-8000
Fax: 248-615-1125
Emergency Services: Yes
Beds: 330

Key Personnel:
Operating Room. . . . . Rita Julius, RN
CEO/President. . . . . Dr Paul LaCasse
Pediatric In-Patient Care . . . . Harold Margolis, DO
Radiology. . . . . Stephan Morse, DO
Quality Assurance . . . . Judy O'Connor
Chief of Medical Staff . . . . David Susser, DO

Measure	Cases	This Hosp.	State Avg.	U.S. Avg.
Blood Clot Prevention and Treatment				
Anticoagulation Overlap Therapy[2]	149	91%	90%	93%
ICU Venous Thromboembolism Prophylaxis[2]	28	100%	93%	92%
Incidence of Potentially Preventable VTE[2]	21	10%	8%	10%
UFH with Dosages/Platelet Monitoring[2]	180	100%	96%	97%
Venous Thromboembolism Prophylaxis[2]	352	97%	87%	85%
Warfarin Therapy Discharge Instructions[2]	117	83%	72%	75%
Chest Pain/Possible Heart Attack Care				
Aspirin Given Within 24 Hours of Arrival	21	90%	96%	96%
Fibrinolytic Meds Within 30 Min. of Arrival[7]	-	-	63%	58%
Average Time to ECG (minutes)	22	11	8	7
Average Time to Transfer (minutes)[1]	-	-	53	60
Children's Asthma Care				
Received Home Management Plan of Care	-	-	-	88%
Received Reliever Medication	-	-	-	100%
Received Systemic Corticosteroids	-	-	-	100%
Emergency Department				
Admittance Decision Time (minutes)[2]	865	106	102	98
Head CT Results Within 45 Min. of Arrival[1]	-	-	54%	57%
Patients Who Left ER Before Being Seen	44,118	2%	2%	2%
Time from ER Arrival to Admit. (minutes)[2]	865	280	288	274
Time from ER Arrival to Discharge (minutes)	364	114	128	134
Time in ER Before Being Evaluated (minutes)	384	14	22	26
Time to Pain Meds for Fractures (minutes)	179	55	55	57
Heart Attack Care				
Aspirin Given at Discharge	102	100%	99%	99%
Fibrinolytic Meds Within 30 Min. of Arrival[7]	-	-	20%	54%
PCI Within 90 Minutes of Arrival	24	67%	95%	96%
Statin Prescribed at Discharge	110	99%	98%	98%
Heart Failure Care				
ACE Inhibitor or ARB for LVSD	119	95%	96%	97%
Discharge Instructions Given	335	99%	94%	94%
Evaluation of LVS Function	427	100%	99%	99%
Medicare Spending				
Medicare Spending per Patient (ratio)	-	1.05	0.96	0.98
Pneumonia Care				
Appropriate Initial Antibiotic Given	180	98%	96%	95%
Blood Culture Timing	364	100%	98%	98%
Pregnancy and Delivery Care				
Newborn Deliveries Scheduled Early[2]	32	3%	3%	6%
Preventive Care				
Immunization for Influenza[2]	546	86%	89%	90%
Immunization for Pneumonia[2]	723	86%	90%	92%
Stroke Care				
Anticoagulation Therapy for Atrial Fibrillation	13	100%	92%	95%
Antithrombotic Therapy Timing	141	99%	97%	98%
Assessed for Rehabilitation	143	100%	97%	97%
Discharged on Antithrombotic Therapy	125	97%	99%	99%
Discharged on Statin Medication	106	87%	94%	94%
Thrombolytic Therapy Timing[1]	-	-	69%	66%
Venous Thromboembolism Prophylaxis	169	96%	94%	94%
Written Stroke Educational Materials Given	58	83%	87%	88%
Surgical Care Improvement Project				
Appropriate Beta Blocker Usage[2]	173	98%	98%	98%
Appropriate VTP Within 24 Hours[2]	488	100%	98%	98%
Controlled Postoperative Blood Glucose[2,7]	-	-	97%	97%
Perioperative Temperature Management[2]	561	100%	100%	100%
Prophylactic Antibiotic Selection[2]	420	99%	99%	99%
Prophylactic Antibiotic Selection (Outpatient)	322	92%	97%	98%
Prophylactic Antibiotic Stopped[2]	416	99%	98%	98%
Prophylactic Antibiotic Timing[2]	420	100%	98%	99%
Prophylactic Antibiotic Timing (Outpatient)	321	100%	97%	98%
Urinary Catheter Removal[2]	414	97%	97%	97%
Survey of Patients' Hospital Experiences				
Area Around Room 'Always' Quiet at Night	300+	44%	60%	61%
Doctors 'Always' Communicated Well	300+	78%	81%	82%
Home Recovery Information Given	300+	84%	87%	85%
Hospital Given 9 or 10 on 10 Point Scale	300+	65%	71%	71%
Meds 'Always' Explained Before Given	300+	59%	64%	64%
Nurses 'Always' Communicated Well	300+	77%	80%	79%
Pain 'Always' Well Controlled	300+	69%	71%	71%
Room and Bathroom 'Always' Clean	300+	63%	73%	73%
Timely Help 'Always' Received	300+	63%	70%	68%
Would Definitely Recommend Hospital	300+	65%	71%	71%
Use of Medical Imaging				
Cardiac Imaging Stress Test before Surgery	366	6.8%	5.1%	5.3%
Combination Abdominal CT Scan	1,025	6.0%	8.7%	10.5%
Combination Brain/Sinus CT Scan	909	3.7%	2.2%	2.7%
Combination Chest CT Scan	898	1.7%	3.6%	2.7%
Follow-up Mammogram/Ultrasound	1,274	5.6%	8.2%	8.8%
Lumbar Spine MRI for Low Back Pain	54	33.3%	36.9%	37.2%

NOTE: Hospital profiles are in alphabetical order by state, then city, then hospital within the city; Rankings exclude hospitals with less than 25 cases except for patient surveys which excludes hospitals with less than 100 cases; (a) 100-299 cases; (1) The number of cases/patients is too few to report; (2) Data submitted were based on a sample of cases/patients; (3) Results are based on a shorter time period than required; (4) Data suppressed by CMS for one or more quarters; (5) Results are not available for this reporting period; (6) Fewer than 100 patients completed the HCAHPS survey; (7) No cases met the criteria for this measure; (8) The lower limit of the confidence interval cannot be calculated if the number of observed infections equals zero; (9) No data are available from the state/territory for this reporting period; (10) The scores shown reflect fewer than 50 completed surveys; (11) There were discrepancies in the data collection process; (12) This measure does not apply to this hospital for this reporting period; (13) Results cannot be calculated for this reporting period; (14) The results for this state are combined with nearby states to protect confidentiality; Please refer to the User's Guide for a full explanation of data.

Hurley Medical Center

One Hurley Plaza
Flint, MI 48503
Phone: 810-257-9000
Fax: 810-257-9111
URL: www.hurleymc.com
Type: Acute Care Hospitals
Emergency Services: Yes
Ownership: Voluntary non-profit - Other
Beds: 443
Key Personnel:
Quality Assurance . . . . William Smith
CEO/President. . . . . Patrick Wardell

Measure	Cases	This Hosp.	State Avg.	U.S. Avg.
Blood Clot Prevention and Treatment				
Anticoagulation Overlap Therapy[2]	66	86%	90%	93%
ICU Venous Thromboembolism Prophylaxis[2]	84	92%	93%	92%
Incidence of Potentially Preventable VTE[1,2]	-	-	8%	10%
UFH with Dosages/Platelet Monitoring[2]	60	98%	96%	97%
Venous Thromboembolism Prophylaxis[2]	328	87%	87%	85%
Warfarin Therapy Discharge Instructions[2]	50	60%	72%	75%
Chest Pain/Possible Heart Attack Care				
Aspirin Given Within 24 Hours of Arrival[1,3]	-	-	96%	96%
Fibrinolytic Meds Within 30 Min. of Arrival[3,7]	-	-	63%	58%
Average Time to ECG (minutes)[1,3]	-	-	8	7
Average Time to Transfer (minutes)[1,3]	-	-	53	60
Children's Asthma Care				
Received Home Management Plan of Care	-	-	-	88%
Received Reliever Medication	-	-	-	100%
Received Systemic Corticosteroids	-	-	-	100%
Emergency Department				
Admittance Decision Time (minutes)[2]	542	158	102	98
Head CT Results Within 45 Min. of Arrival[1,3]	-	-	54%	57%
Patients Who Left ER Before Being Seen	99,803	4%	2%	2%
Time from ER Arrival to Admit. (minutes)[2]	551	407	288	274
Time from ER Arrival to Discharge (minutes)	324	164	128	134
Time in ER Before Being Evaluated (minutes)	183	54	22	26
Time to Pain Meds for Fractures (minutes)	261	74	55	57
Heart Attack Care				
Aspirin Given at Discharge	115	98%	99%	99%
Fibrinolytic Meds Within 30 Min. of Arrival[7]	-	-	20%	54%
PCI Within 90 Minutes of Arrival	33	88%	95%	96%
Statin Prescribed at Discharge	115	97%	98%	98%
Heart Failure Care				
ACE Inhibitor or ARB for LVSD[2]	109	87%	96%	97%
Discharge Instructions Given[2]	251	80%	94%	94%
Evaluation of LVS Function[2]	285	95%	99%	99%
Medicare Spending				
Medicare Spending per Patient (ratio)	-	0.98	0.96	0.98
Pneumonia Care				
Appropriate Initial Antibiotic Given[2]	75	92%	96%	95%
Blood Culture Timing[2]	88	92%	98%	98%
Pregnancy and Delivery Care				
Newborn Deliveries Scheduled Early[2]	48	15%	3%	6%
Preventive Care				
Immunization for Influenza[2]	509	70%	89%	90%
Immunization for Pneumonia[2]	458	73%	90%	92%
Stroke Care				
Anticoagulation Therapy for Atrial Fibrillation[2]	12	92%	92%	95%
Antithrombotic Therapy Timing[2]	105	98%	97%	98%
Assessed for Rehabilitation[2]	133	93%	97%	97%
Discharged on Antithrombotic Therapy[2]	117	92%	99%	99%
Discharged on Statin Medication[2]	83	82%	94%	94%
Thrombolytic Therapy Timing[2]	12	67%	69%	66%
Venous Thromboembolism Prophylaxis[2]	142	91%	94%	94%
Written Stroke Educational Materials Given[2]	77	95%	87%	88%
Surgical Care Improvement Project				
Appropriate Beta Blocker Usage[2]	107	96%	98%	98%
Appropriate VTP Within 24 Hours[2]	334	96%	98%	98%
Controlled Postoperative Blood Glucose[2,7]	-	-	97%	97%
Perioperative Temperature Management[2]	401	96%	100%	100%
Prophylactic Antibiotic Selection[2]	267	98%	99%	99%
Prophylactic Antibiotic Selection (Outpatient)	222	98%	97%	98%
Prophylactic Antibiotic Stopped[2]	259	95%	98%	98%
Prophylactic Antibiotic Timing[2]	267	99%	98%	99%
Prophylactic Antibiotic Timing (Outpatient)	228	94%	97%	98%
Urinary Catheter Removal[2]	107	78%	97%	97%
Survey of Patients' Hospital Experiences				
Area Around Room 'Always' Quiet at Night	300+	55%	60%	61%
Doctors 'Always' Communicated Well	300+	77%	81%	82%
Home Recovery Information Given	300+	84%	87%	85%
Hospital Given 9 or 10 on 10 Point Scale	300+	65%	71%	71%
Meds 'Always' Explained Before Given	300+	61%	64%	64%
Nurses 'Always' Communicated Well	300+	74%	80%	79%
Pain 'Always' Well Controlled	300+	66%	71%	71%
Room and Bathroom 'Always' Clean	300+	61%	73%	73%
Timely Help 'Always' Received	300+	59%	70%	68%
Would Definitely Recommend Hospital	300+	69%	71%	71%
Use of Medical Imaging				
Cardiac Imaging Stress Test before Surgery[1]	-	-	5.1%	5.3%
Combination Abdominal CT Scan	399	1.8%	8.7%	10.5%
Combination Brain/Sinus CT Scan	595	4.2%	2.2%	2.7%
Combination Chest CT Scan	213	0.0%	3.6%	2.7%
Follow-up Mammogram/Ultrasound	159	14.5%	8.2%	8.8%
Lumbar Spine MRI for Low Back Pain	63	28.6%	36.9%	37.2%

Mclaren Flint

401 S Ballenger Highway
Flint, MI 48532
Phone: 810-342-2000
Fax: 810-342-2428
URL: www.mclaren.org
Type: Acute Care Hospitals
Emergency Services: Yes
Ownership: Voluntary non-profit - Private
Beds: 452
Key Personnel:
Chief of Medical Staff. . . . . Jagdish Bhagat, MD
Radiology. . . . . ML Kahn, MD
CEO/President. . . . . Donald C Kooy
Infection Control. . . . . Janee Macklin
Quality Assurance . . . . Richard Sardelli
Operating Room. . . . . Debra Stephenson
Pediatric Ambulatory Care . . . . . . KE Vobach, MD
Patient Relations . . . . Annetta Wilbon

Measure	Cases	This Hosp.	State Avg.	U.S. Avg.
Blood Clot Prevention and Treatment				
Anticoagulation Overlap Therapy[2]	192	96%	90%	93%
ICU Venous Thromboembolism Prophylaxis[2]	74	99%	93%	92%
Incidence of Potentially Preventable VTE[2]	23	0%	8%	10%
UFH with Dosages/Platelet Monitoring[2]	219	91%	96%	97%
Venous Thromboembolism Prophylaxis[2]	312	87%	87%	85%
Warfarin Therapy Discharge Instructions[2]	139	78%	72%	75%
Chest Pain/Possible Heart Attack Care				
Aspirin Given Within 24 Hours of Arrival[3,7]	-	-	96%	96%
Fibrinolytic Meds Within 30 Min. of Arrival[5]	-	-	63%	58%
Average Time to ECG (minutes)[1,3]	-	-	8	7
Average Time to Transfer (minutes)[5]	-	-	53	60
Children's Asthma Care				
Received Home Management Plan of Care	-	-	-	88%
Received Reliever Medication	-	-	-	100%
Received Systemic Corticosteroids	-	-	-	100%
Emergency Department				
Admittance Decision Time (minutes)[2]	723	165	102	98
Head CT Results Within 45 Min. of Arrival[1]	-	-	54%	57%
Patients Who Left ER Before Being Seen	67,081	2%	2%	2%
Time from ER Arrival to Admit. (minutes)[2]	747	426	288	274
Time from ER Arrival to Discharge (minutes)	348	187	128	134
Time in ER Before Being Evaluated (minutes)	383	37	22	26
Time to Pain Meds for Fractures (minutes)	217	68	55	57
Heart Attack Care				
Aspirin Given at Discharge	576	100%	99%	99%
Fibrinolytic Meds Within 30 Min. of Arrival[7]	-	-	20%	54%
PCI Within 90 Minutes of Arrival	90	99%	95%	96%
Statin Prescribed at Discharge	557	99%	98%	98%
Heart Failure Care				
ACE Inhibitor or ARB for LVSD	246	97%	96%	97%
Discharge Instructions Given	771	94%	94%	94%
Evaluation of LVS Function	929	99%	99%	99%
Medicare Spending				
Medicare Spending per Patient (ratio)	-	0.96	0.96	0.98
Pneumonia Care				
Appropriate Initial Antibiotic Given[2]	178	98%	96%	95%
Blood Culture Timing[2]	47	96%	98%	98%
Pregnancy and Delivery Care				
Newborn Deliveries Scheduled Early	55	7%	3%	6%
Preventive Care				
Immunization for Influenza[2]	571	90%	89%	90%
Immunization for Pneumonia[2]	846	92%	90%	92%
Stroke Care				
Anticoagulation Therapy for Atrial Fibrillation[2]	33	73%	92%	95%
Antithrombotic Therapy Timing[2]	152	93%	97%	98%
Assessed for Rehabilitation[2]	178	92%	97%	97%
Discharged on Antithrombotic Therapy[2]	157	96%	99%	99%
Discharged on Statin Medication[2]	138	95%	94%	94%
Thrombolytic Therapy Timing[2]	22	50%	69%	66%
Venous Thromboembolism Prophylaxis[2]	180	77%	94%	94%
Written Stroke Educational Materials Given[2]	114	66%	87%	88%
Surgical Care Improvement Project				
Appropriate Beta Blocker Usage[2]	430	99%	98%	98%
Appropriate VTP Within 24 Hours[2]	506	98%	98%	98%
Controlled Postoperative Blood Glucose[2]	263	98%	97%	97%
Perioperative Temperature Management[2]	697	100%	100%	100%
Prophylactic Antibiotic Selection[2]	700	99%	99%	99%
Prophylactic Antibiotic Selection (Outpatient)	539	99%	97%	98%
Prophylactic Antibiotic Stopped[2]	662	97%	98%	98%
Prophylactic Antibiotic Timing[2]	703	99%	98%	99%
Prophylactic Antibiotic Timing (Outpatient)	542	99%	97%	98%
Urinary Catheter Removal[2]	363	97%	97%	97%
Survey of Patients' Hospital Experiences				
Area Around Room 'Always' Quiet at Night	300+	52%	60%	61%
Doctors 'Always' Communicated Well	300+	74%	81%	82%
Home Recovery Information Given	300+	85%	87%	85%
Hospital Given 9 or 10 on 10 Point Scale	300+	69%	71%	71%
Meds 'Always' Explained Before Given	300+	57%	64%	64%
Nurses 'Always' Communicated Well	300+	74%	80%	79%
Pain 'Always' Well Controlled	300+	68%	71%	71%
Room and Bathroom 'Always' Clean	300+	66%	73%	73%
Timely Help 'Always' Received	300+	59%	70%	68%
Would Definitely Recommend Hospital	300+	69%	71%	71%
Use of Medical Imaging				
Cardiac Imaging Stress Test before Surgery[1]	-	-	5.1%	5.3%
Combination Abdominal CT Scan	1,863	26.1%	8.7%	10.5%
Combination Brain/Sinus CT Scan	1,409	2.6%	2.2%	2.7%
Combination Chest CT Scan	1,187	0.4%	3.6%	2.7%
Follow-up Mammogram/Ultrasound	2,478	7.1%	8.2%	8.8%
Lumbar Spine MRI for Low Back Pain	405	32.1%	36.9%	37.2%

Paul Oliver Memorial Hospital

224 Park Avenue
Frankfort, MI 49635
Phone: 231-352-2200
Fax: 231-352-9621
E-mail: pomh@mhc.net
URL: www.munsonhealthcare.org
Type: Critical Access Hospitals
Emergency Services: Yes
Ownership: Government - Local
Beds: 48
Key Personnel:
Operating Room. . . . . Angela Anderson, RN
Emergency Room . . . . Donna Clarke, RN
Chair/CEO. . . . . Paul Clulo
Infection Control. . . . . Sandra Honigfort
Patient Relations . . . . Debbie Link
Quality Assurance . . . . Debra Link
Chief of Medical Staff. . . . . Gerard Mahoney
President. . . . . Peter Marinoff

Measure	Cases	This Hosp.	State Avg.	U.S. Avg.
Blood Clot Prevention and Treatment				
Anticoagulation Overlap Therapy[5]	-	-	90%	93%
ICU Venous Thromboembolism Prophylaxis[5]	-	-	93%	92%
Incidence of Potentially Preventable VTE[5]	-	-	8%	10%
UFH with Dosages/Platelet Monitoring[5]	-	-	96%	97%
Venous Thromboembolism Prophylaxis[5]	-	-	87%	85%
Warfarin Therapy Discharge Instructions[5]	-	-	72%	75%
Chest Pain/Possible Heart Attack Care				
Aspirin Given Within 24 Hours of Arrival	55	96%	96%	96%
Fibrinolytic Meds Within 30 Min. of Arrival[7]	-	-	63%	58%
Average Time to ECG (minutes)	56	7	8	7
Average Time to Transfer (minutes)[1]	-	-	53	60
Children's Asthma Care				
Received Home Management Plan of Care	-	-	-	88%

NOTE: Hospital profiles are in alphabetical order by state, then city, then hospital within the city; Rankings exclude hospitals with less than 25 cases except for patient surveys which excludes hospitals with less than 100 cases; (a) 100-299 cases; (1) The number of cases/patients is too few to report; (2) Data submitted were based on a sample of cases/patients; (3) Results are based on a shorter time period than required; (4) Data suppressed by CMS for one or more quarters; (5) Results are not available for this reporting period; (6) Fewer than 100 patients completed the HCAHPS survey; (7) No cases met the criteria for this measure; (8) The lower limit of the confidence interval cannot be calculated if the number of observed infections equals zero; (9) No data are available from the state/territory for this reporting period; (10) The scores shown reflect fewer than 50 completed surveys; (11) There were discrepancies in the data collection process; (12) This measure does not apply to this hospital for this reporting period; (13) Results cannot be calculated for this reporting period; (14) The results for this state are combined with nearby states to protect confidentiality; Please refer to the User's Guide for a full explanation of data.

Measure	Cases	This Hosp.	State Avg.	U.S. Avg.
Received Reliever Medication				100%
Received Systemic Corticosteroids	-		-	100%
Emergency Department				
Admittance Decision Time (minutes)[5]	-	-	102	98
Head CT Results Within 45 Min. of Arrival[5]	-	-	54%	57%
Patients Who Left ER Before Being Seen[5]	-	-	2%	2%
Time from ER Arrival to Admit. (minutes)[5]	-	-	288	274
Time from ER Arrival to Discharge (minutes)	348	79	128	134
Time in ER Before Being Evaluated (minutes)	368	12	22	26
Time to Pain Meds for Fractures (minutes)[5]	-	-	55	57
Heart Attack Care				
Aspirin Given at Discharge[5]	-	-	99%	99%
Fibrinolytic Meds Within 30 Min. of Arrival[5]	-	-	20%	54%
PCI Within 90 Minutes of Arrival[5]	-	-	95%	96%
Statin Prescribed at Discharge[5]	-	-	98%	98%
Heart Failure Care				
ACE Inhibitor or ARB for LVSD[5]	-	-	96%	97%
Discharge Instructions Given[5]	-	-	94%	94%
Evaluation of LVS Function[5]	-	-	99%	99%
Medicare Spending				
Medicare Spending per Patient (ratio)	-	-	0.96	0.98
Pneumonia Care				
Appropriate Initial Antibiotic Given[5]	-	-	96%	95%
Blood Culture Timing[5]	-	-	98%	98%
Pregnancy and Delivery Care				
Newborn Deliveries Scheduled Early[5]	-	-	3%	6%
Preventive Care				
Immunization for Influenza[5]	-	-	89%	90%
Immunization for Pneumonia[5]	-	-	90%	92%
Stroke Care				
Anticoagulation Therapy for Atrial Fibrillation[5]	-	-	92%	95%
Antithrombotic Therapy Timing[5]	-	-	97%	98%
Assessed for Rehabilitation[5]	-	-	97%	97%
Discharged on Antithrombotic Therapy[5]	-	-	99%	99%
Discharged on Statin Medication[5]	-	-	94%	94%
Thrombolytic Therapy Timing[5]	-	-	69%	66%
Venous Thromboembolism Prophylaxis[5]	-	-	94%	94%
Written Stroke Educational Materials Given[5]	-	-	87%	88%
Surgical Care Improvement Project				
Appropriate Beta Blocker Usage[5]	-	-	98%	98%
Appropriate VTP Within 24 Hours[5]	-	-	98%	98%
Controlled Postoperative Blood Glucose[5]	-	-	97%	97%
Perioperative Temperature Management[5]	-	-	100%	100%
Prophylactic Antibiotic Selection[5]	-	-	99%	99%
Prophylactic Antibiotic Selection (Outpatient)[5]	-	-	97%	98%
Prophylactic Antibiotic Stopped[5]	-	-	98%	98%
Prophylactic Antibiotic Timing[5]	-	-	98%	99%
Prophylactic Antibiotic Timing (Outpatient)[5]	-	-	97%	98%
Urinary Catheter Removal[5]	-	-	97%	97%
Survey of Patients' Hospital Experiences				
Area Around Room 'Always' Quiet at Night[5]	-	-	60%	61%
Doctors 'Always' Communicated Well[5]	-	-	81%	82%
Home Recovery Information Given[5]	-	-	87%	85%
Hospital Given 9 or 10 on 10 Point Scale[5]	-	-	71%	71%
Meds 'Always' Explained Before Given[5]	-	-	64%	64%
Nurses 'Always' Communicated Well[5]	-	-	80%	79%
Pain 'Always' Well Controlled[5]	-	-	71%	71%
Room and Bathroom 'Always' Clean[5]	-	-	73%	73%
Timely Help 'Always' Received[5]	-	-	70%	68%
Would Definitely Recommend Hospital[5]	-	-	71%	71%
Use of Medical Imaging				
Cardiac Imaging Stress Test before Surgery[7]	-	-	5.1%	5.3%
Combination Abdominal CT Scan	151	7.3%	8.7%	10.5%
Combination Brain/Sinus CT Scan[1]	-	-	2.2%	2.7%
Combination Chest CT Scan	89	0.0%	3.6%	2.7%
Follow-up Mammogram/Ultrasound	530	7.4%	8.2%	8.8%
Lumbar Spine MRI for Low Back Pain[1]	-	-	36.9%	37.2%

Spectrum Health Gerber Memorial

212 S Sullivan St — Phone: 231-924-3300
Fremont, MI 49412 — Fax: 231-924-1320
E-mail: hr@gmhs.org
URL: www.gmhs.org
Type: Acute Care Hospitals — Emergency Services: Yes
Ownership: Voluntary non-profit - Private — Beds: 77

Key Personnel:
Patient Relations . . . . Sharon Boczkaja
Hemotology Center . . . . Kathy Evans
Infection Control. . . . . Gretchen Farinosi
Chief of Medical Staff. . . . . Douglas Johnson
Radiology. . . . . Joseph Marous
Operating Room. . . . . Marianne Patton
CEO/President. . . . . Randal Stasik
Intensive Care Unit. . . . . Patti Wethington

Measure	Cases	This Hosp.	State Avg.	U.S. Avg.
Blood Clot Prevention and Treatment				
Anticoagulation Overlap Therapy[2]	21	90%	90%	93%
ICU Venous Thromboembolism Prophylaxis[2]	62	94%	93%	92%
Incidence of Potentially Preventable VTE[1,2]	-	-	8%	10%
UFH with Dosages/Platelet Monitoring[2]	13	100%	96%	97%
Venous Thromboembolism Prophylaxis[2]	212	94%	87%	85%
Warfarin Therapy Discharge Instructions[2]	17	94%	72%	75%
Chest Pain/Possible Heart Attack Care				
Aspirin Given Within 24 Hours of Arrival	115	97%	96%	96%
Fibrinolytic Meds Within 30 Min. of Arrival[1]	-	-	63%	58%
Average Time to ECG (minutes)	123	9	8	7
Average Time to Transfer (minutes)[1]	-	-	53	60
Children's Asthma Care				
Received Home Management Plan of Care	-	-	-	88%
Received Reliever Medication	-	-	-	100%
Received Systemic Corticosteroids	-	-	-	100%
Emergency Department				
Admittance Decision Time (minutes)[2]	412	132	102	98
Head CT Results Within 45 Min. of Arrival[1]	-	-	54%	57%
Patients Who Left ER Before Being Seen	24,676	1%	2%	2%
Time from ER Arrival to Admit. (minutes)[2]	420	290	288	274
Time from ER Arrival to Discharge (minutes)	430	126	128	134
Time in ER Before Being Evaluated (minutes)	356	18	22	26
Time to Pain Meds for Fractures (minutes)	99	39	55	57
Heart Attack Care				
Aspirin Given at Discharge[1,3]	-	-	99%	99%
Fibrinolytic Meds Within 30 Min. of Arrival[3,7]	-	-	20%	54%
PCI Within 90 Minutes of Arrival[3,7]	-	-	95%	96%
Statin Prescribed at Discharge[1,3]	-	-	98%	98%
Heart Failure Care				
ACE Inhibitor or ARB for LVSD	11	100%	96%	97%
Discharge Instructions Given	49	98%	94%	94%
Evaluation of LVS Function	60	100%	99%	99%
Medicare Spending				
Medicare Spending per Patient (ratio)	-	0.88	0.96	0.98
Pneumonia Care				
Appropriate Initial Antibiotic Given	98	96%	96%	95%
Blood Culture Timing	148	96%	98%	98%
Pregnancy and Delivery Care				
Newborn Deliveries Scheduled Early[2]	16	0%	3%	6%
Preventive Care				
Immunization for Influenza[2]	407	97%	89%	90%
Immunization for Pneumonia[2]	494	98%	90%	92%
Stroke Care				
Anticoagulation Therapy for Atrial Fibrillation[1]	-	-	92%	95%
Antithrombotic Therapy Timing	23	100%	97%	98%
Assessed for Rehabilitation	33	97%	97%	97%
Discharged on Antithrombotic Therapy	32	100%	99%	99%
Discharged on Statin Medication	27	96%	94%	94%
Thrombolytic Therapy Timing[7]	-	-	69%	66%
Venous Thromboembolism Prophylaxis	23	96%	94%	94%
Written Stroke Educational Materials Given	22	91%	87%	88%
Surgical Care Improvement Project				
Appropriate Beta Blocker Usage	50	94%	98%	98%
Appropriate VTP Within 24 Hours	164	98%	98%	98%
Controlled Postoperative Blood Glucose[7]	-	-	97%	97%
Perioperative Temperature Management	204	100%	100%	100%
Prophylactic Antibiotic Selection	149	100%	99%	99%
Prophylactic Antibiotic Selection (Outpatient)	33	94%	97%	98%
Prophylactic Antibiotic Stopped	147	99%	98%	98%
Prophylactic Antibiotic Timing	149	98%	98%	99%
Prophylactic Antibiotic Timing (Outpatient)	36	92%	97%	98%
Urinary Catheter Removal	18	100%	97%	97%
Survey of Patients' Hospital Experiences				
Area Around Room 'Always' Quiet at Night	300+	57%	60%	61%
Doctors 'Always' Communicated Well	300+	81%	81%	82%
Home Recovery Information Given	300+	92%	87%	85%
Hospital Given 9 or 10 on 10 Point Scale	300+	72%	71%	71%
Meds 'Always' Explained Before Given	300+	68%	64%	64%
Nurses 'Always' Communicated Well	300+	81%	80%	79%
Pain 'Always' Well Controlled	300+	70%	71%	71%
Room and Bathroom 'Always' Clean	300+	77%	73%	73%
Timely Help 'Always' Received	300+	74%	70%	68%
Would Definitely Recommend Hospital	300+	69%	71%	71%
Use of Medical Imaging				
Cardiac Imaging Stress Test before Surgery	250	6.0%	5.1%	5.3%
Combination Abdominal CT Scan	512	2.0%	8.7%	10.5%
Combination Brain/Sinus CT Scan[1]	-	-	2.2%	2.7%
Combination Chest CT Scan	321	0.6%	3.6%	2.7%
Follow-up Mammogram/Ultrasound	770	10.5%	8.2%	8.8%
Lumbar Spine MRI for Low Back Pain	108	59.3%	36.9%	37.2%

Garden City Hospital

6245 Inkster Rd — Phone: 734-421-3300
Garden City, MI 48135 — Fax: 734-421-0593
URL: www.gchosp.org
Type: Acute Care Hospitals — Emergency Services: Yes
Ownership: Voluntary non-profit - Private — Beds: 323

Key Personnel:
Cardiac Laboratory. . . . . Debbie DeMatteis
Operating Room. . . . . Annette Krupa
CEO/President. . . . . Gary R Ley
Quality Assurance . . . . Lisa Sielski
Patient Relations . . . . Malissa Stringer
Radiology. . . . . Jim Williamson

Measure	Cases	This Hosp.	State Avg.	U.S. Avg.
Blood Clot Prevention and Treatment				
Anticoagulation Overlap Therapy[2]	54	80%	90%	93%
ICU Venous Thromboembolism Prophylaxis[2]	65	100%	93%	92%
Incidence of Potentially Preventable VTE[1,2]	-	-	8%	10%
UFH with Dosages/Platelet Monitoring[2]	72	43%	96%	97%
Venous Thromboembolism Prophylaxis[2]	361	94%	87%	85%
Warfarin Therapy Discharge Instructions[2]	24	75%	72%	75%
Chest Pain/Possible Heart Attack Care				
Aspirin Given Within 24 Hours of Arrival	29	100%	96%	96%
Fibrinolytic Meds Within 30 Min. of Arrival[7]	-	-	63%	58%
Average Time to ECG (minutes)	30	6	8	7
Average Time to Transfer (minutes)[7]	-	-	53	60
Children's Asthma Care				
Received Home Management Plan of Care	-	-	-	88%
Received Reliever Medication	-	-	-	100%
Received Systemic Corticosteroids	-	-	-	100%
Emergency Department				
Admittance Decision Time (minutes)[2]	867	204	102	98
Head CT Results Within 45 Min. of Arrival	14	93%	54%	57%
Patients Who Left ER Before Being Seen	51,303	2%	2%	2%
Time from ER Arrival to Admit. (minutes)[2]	867	452	288	274
Time from ER Arrival to Discharge (minutes)	1,053	157	128	134
Time in ER Before Being Evaluated (minutes)	1,191	27	22	26
Time to Pain Meds for Fractures (minutes)	130	76	55	57
Heart Attack Care				
Aspirin Given at Discharge	141	99%	99%	99%
Fibrinolytic Meds Within 30 Min. of Arrival[7]	-	-	20%	54%
PCI Within 90 Minutes of Arrival	49	84%	95%	96%
Statin Prescribed at Discharge	144	97%	98%	98%
Heart Failure Care				
ACE Inhibitor or ARB for LVSD	67	90%	96%	97%
Discharge Instructions Given	288	99%	94%	94%
Evaluation of LVS Function	366	99%	99%	99%
Medicare Spending				
Medicare Spending per Patient (ratio)	-	1.07	0.96	0.98

NOTE: Hospital profiles are in alphabetical order by state, then city, then hospital within the city; Rankings exclude hospitals with less than 25 cases except for patient surveys which excludes hospitals with less than 100 cases; (a) 100-299 cases; (1) The number of cases/patients is too few to report; (2) Data submitted were based on a sample of cases/patients; (3) Results are based on a shorter time period than required; (4) Data suppressed by CMS for one or more quarters; (5) Results are not available for this reporting period; (6) Fewer than 100 patients completed the HCAHPS survey; (7) No cases met the criteria for this measure; (8) The lower limit of the confidence interval cannot be calculated if the number of observed infections equals zero; (9) No data are available from the state/territory for this reporting period; (10) The scores shown reflect fewer than 50 completed surveys; (11) There were discrepancies in the data collection process; (12) This measure does not apply to this hospital for this reporting period; (13) Results cannot be calculated for this reporting period; (14) The results for this state are combined with nearby states to protect confidentiality; Please refer to the User's Guide for a full explanation of data.

Measure	Cases	This Hosp.	State Avg.	U.S. Avg.
Pneumonia Care				
Appropriate Initial Antibiotic Given	147	97%	96%	95%
Blood Culture Timing	270	100%	98%	98%
Pregnancy and Delivery Care				
Newborn Deliveries Scheduled Early	49	0%	3%	6%
Preventive Care				
Immunization for Influenza[2]	550	92%	89%	90%
Immunization for Pneumonia[2]	709	92%	90%	92%
Stroke Care				
Anticoagulation Therapy for Atrial Fibrillation[2]	18	89%	92%	95%
Antithrombotic Therapy Timing[2]	110	100%	97%	98%
Assessed for Rehabilitation[2]	140	97%	97%	97%
Discharged on Antithrombotic Therapy[2]	128	100%	99%	99%
Discharged on Statin Medication[2]	94	96%	94%	94%
Thrombolytic Therapy Timing[2]	14	93%	69%	66%
Venous Thromboembolism Prophylaxis[2]	148	95%	94%	94%
Written Stroke Educational Materials Given[2]	70	94%	87%	88%
Surgical Care Improvement Project				
Appropriate Beta Blocker Usage	140	98%	98%	98%
Appropriate VTP Within 24 Hours	388	98%	98%	98%
Controlled Postoperative Blood Glucose[7]	-	-	97%	97%
Perioperative Temperature Management	452	100%	100%	100%
Prophylactic Antibiotic Selection	285	99%	99%	99%
Prophylactic Antibiotic Selection (Outpatient)	140	94%	97%	98%
Prophylactic Antibiotic Stopped	279	97%	98%	98%
Prophylactic Antibiotic Timing	285	99%	98%	99%
Prophylactic Antibiotic Timing (Outpatient)	143	97%	97%	98%
Urinary Catheter Removal	256	96%	97%	97%
Survey of Patients' Hospital Experiences				
Area Around Room 'Always' Quiet at Night	300+	53%	60%	61%
Doctors 'Always' Communicated Well	300+	77%	81%	82%
Home Recovery Information Given	300+	84%	87%	85%
Hospital Given 9 or 10 on 10 Point Scale	300+	66%	71%	71%
Meds 'Always' Explained Before Given	300+	61%	64%	64%
Nurses 'Always' Communicated Well	300+	77%	80%	79%
Pain 'Always' Well Controlled	300+	71%	71%	71%
Room and Bathroom 'Always' Clean	300+	74%	73%	73%
Timely Help 'Always' Received	300+	68%	70%	68%
Would Definitely Recommend Hospital	300+	66%	71%	71%
Use of Medical Imaging				
Cardiac Imaging Stress Test before Surgery	268	8.2%	5.1%	5.3%
Combination Abdominal CT Scan	766	13.1%	8.7%	10.5%
Combination Brain/Sinus CT Scan	739	1.9%	2.2%	2.7%
Combination Chest CT Scan	458	0.4%	3.6%	2.7%
Follow-up Mammogram/Ultrasound	632	7.8%	8.2%	8.8%
Lumbar Spine MRI for Low Back Pain	75	25.3%	36.9%	37.2%

Otsego Memorial Hospital

825 N Center Ave
Gaylord, MI 49735
Phone: 989-731-2100
Fax: 989-731-7792
E-mail: omh@otsegomemorialhospital.org
URL: www.otsegomemorialhospital.org
Type: Acute Care Hospitals
Emergency Services: Yes
Ownership: Voluntary non-profit - Private
Beds: 53

Key Personnel:

Radiology. . . . . Michael Angileri
Pediatric Ambulatory Care . . . . . . Alida Asencio, MD
Pediatric In-Patient Care . . . . Alida Asencio, MD
Operating Room. . . . . Wendy Frye
Quality Assurance . . . . Maryann Hoffmann
Chief of Medical Staff . . . . David Miner, MD
CEO/President. . . . . David Schuster
Infection Control. . . . . Lisa Stier, RN

Measure	Cases	This Hosp.	State Avg.	U.S. Avg.
Blood Clot Prevention and Treatment				
Anticoagulation Overlap Therapy[1,2]	-	-	90%	93%
ICU Venous Thromboembolism Prophylaxis[2]	97	95%	93%	92%
Incidence of Potentially Preventable VTE[1,2]	-	-	8%	10%
UFH with Dosages/Platelet Monitoring[1,2]	-	-	96%	97%
Venous Thromboembolism Prophylaxis[2]	160	88%	87%	85%
Warfarin Therapy Discharge Instructions[1,2]	-	-	72%	75%
Chest Pain/Possible Heart Attack Care				
Aspirin Given Within 24 Hours of Arrival	105	96%	96%	96%
Fibrinolytic Meds Within 30 Min. of Arrival[1]	-	-	63%	58%
Average Time to ECG (minutes)	106	7	8	7
Average Time to Transfer (minutes)[1]	-	-	53	60
Children's Asthma Care				
Received Home Management Plan of Care	-	-	-	88%
Received Reliever Medication	-	-	-	100%
Received Systemic Corticosteroids	-	-	-	100%
Emergency Department				
Admittance Decision Time (minutes)[2]	221	117	102	98
Head CT Results Within 45 Min. of Arrival[1]	-	-	54%	57%
Patients Who Left ER Before Being Seen	13,910	2%	2%	2%
Time from ER Arrival to Admit. (minutes)[2]	241	283	288	274
Time from ER Arrival to Discharge (minutes)	330	124	128	134
Time in ER Before Being Evaluated (minutes)	374	18	22	26
Time to Pain Meds for Fractures (minutes)	96	50	55	57
Heart Attack Care				
Aspirin Given at Discharge[1,3]	-	-	99%	99%
Fibrinolytic Meds Within 30 Min. of Arrival[3,7]	-	-	20%	54%
PCI Within 90 Minutes of Arrival[3,7]	-	-	95%	96%
Statin Prescribed at Discharge[1,3]	-	-	98%	98%
Heart Failure Care				
ACE Inhibitor or ARB for LVSD	15	87%	96%	97%
Discharge Instructions Given	33	94%	94%	94%
Evaluation of LVS Function	42	98%	99%	99%
Medicare Spending				
Medicare Spending per Patient (ratio)	-	0.91	0.96	0.98
Pneumonia Care				
Appropriate Initial Antibiotic Given	59	100%	96%	95%
Blood Culture Timing	102	96%	98%	98%
Pregnancy and Delivery Care				
Newborn Deliveries Scheduled Early[2]	18	11%	3%	6%
Preventive Care				
Immunization for Influenza[2]	255	98%	89%	90%
Immunization for Pneumonia[2]	307	97%	90%	92%
Stroke Care				
Anticoagulation Therapy for Atrial Fibrillation[1]	-	-	92%	95%
Antithrombotic Therapy Timing	25	92%	97%	98%
Assessed for Rehabilitation	22	100%	97%	97%
Discharged on Antithrombotic Therapy	22	95%	99%	99%
Discharged on Statin Medication	18	94%	94%	94%
Thrombolytic Therapy Timing[1]	-	-	69%	66%
Venous Thromboembolism Prophylaxis	23	83%	94%	94%
Written Stroke Educational Materials Given	11	91%	87%	88%
Surgical Care Improvement Project				
Appropriate Beta Blocker Usage[2]	53	96%	98%	98%
Appropriate VTP Within 24 Hours[2]	192	99%	98%	98%
Controlled Postoperative Blood Glucose[2,7]	-	-	97%	97%
Perioperative Temperature Management[2]	198	99%	100%	100%
Prophylactic Antibiotic Selection[2]	158	99%	99%	99%
Prophylactic Antibiotic Selection (Outpatient)	72	100%	97%	98%
Prophylactic Antibiotic Stopped[2]	157	97%	98%	98%
Prophylactic Antibiotic Timing[2]	159	94%	98%	99%
Prophylactic Antibiotic Timing (Outpatient)	73	96%	97%	98%
Urinary Catheter Removal[2]	154	99%	97%	97%
Survey of Patients' Hospital Experiences				
Area Around Room 'Always' Quiet at Night	(a)	52%	60%	61%
Doctors 'Always' Communicated Well	(a)	86%	81%	82%
Home Recovery Information Given	(a)	88%	87%	85%
Hospital Given 9 or 10 on 10 Point Scale	(a)	75%	71%	71%
Meds 'Always' Explained Before Given	(a)	71%	64%	64%
Nurses 'Always' Communicated Well	(a)	83%	80%	79%
Pain 'Always' Well Controlled	(a)	73%	71%	71%
Room and Bathroom 'Always' Clean	(a)	77%	73%	73%
Timely Help 'Always' Received	(a)	76%	70%	68%
Would Definitely Recommend Hospital	(a)	71%	71%	71%
Use of Medical Imaging				
Cardiac Imaging Stress Test before Surgery	224	4.0%	5.1%	5.3%
Combination Abdominal CT Scan	518	6.2%	8.7%	10.5%
Combination Brain/Sinus CT Scan[1]	-	-	2.2%	2.7%
Combination Chest CT Scan	368	1.1%	3.6%	2.7%
Follow-up Mammogram/Ultrasound	701	13.3%	8.2%	8.8%
Lumbar Spine MRI for Low Back Pain	161	48.4%	36.9%	37.2%

Midmichigan Medical Center - Gladwin

515 Quarter Street
Gladwin, MI 48624
Phone: 989-426-9286
Fax: 989-246-6400
URL: www.midmichigan.org
Type: Critical Access Hospitals
Emergency Services: Yes
Ownership: Voluntary non-profit - Private
Beds: 25

Key Personnel:

Infection Control. . . . . Dana Garafalo
Operating Room. . . . . Christy Gary
CEO/President. . . . . Raymond H Stover
Emergency Room . . . . Donald Willman

Measure	Cases	This Hosp.	State Avg.	U.S. Avg.
Blood Clot Prevention and Treatment				
Anticoagulation Overlap Therapy[5]	-	-	90%	93%
ICU Venous Thromboembolism Prophylaxis[5]	-	-	93%	92%
Incidence of Potentially Preventable VTE[5]	-	-	8%	10%
UFH with Dosages/Platelet Monitoring[5]	-	-	96%	97%
Venous Thromboembolism Prophylaxis[5]	-	-	87%	85%
Warfarin Therapy Discharge Instructions[5]	-	-	72%	75%
Chest Pain/Possible Heart Attack Care				
Aspirin Given Within 24 Hours of Arrival	144	100%	96%	96%
Fibrinolytic Meds Within 30 Min. of Arrival[1]	-	-	63%	58%
Average Time to ECG (minutes)	154	10	8	7
Average Time to Transfer (minutes)[1]	-	-	53	60
Children's Asthma Care				
Received Home Management Plan of Care	-	-	-	88%
Received Reliever Medication	-	-	-	100%
Received Systemic Corticosteroids	-	-	-	100%
Emergency Department				
Admittance Decision Time (minutes)[5]	-	-	102	98
Head CT Results Within 45 Min. of Arrival[1]	-	-	54%	57%
Patients Who Left ER Before Being Seen[5]	-	-	2%	2%
Time from ER Arrival to Admit. (minutes)[5]	-	-	288	274
Time from ER Arrival to Discharge (minutes)	404	139	128	134
Time in ER Before Being Evaluated (minutes)	369	33	22	26
Time to Pain Meds for Fractures (minutes)	73	66	55	57
Heart Attack Care				
Aspirin Given at Discharge[5]	-	-	99%	99%
Fibrinolytic Meds Within 30 Min. of Arrival[5]	-	-	20%	54%
PCI Within 90 Minutes of Arrival[5]	-	-	95%	96%
Statin Prescribed at Discharge[5]	-	-	98%	98%
Heart Failure Care				
ACE Inhibitor or ARB for LVSD	12	100%	96%	97%
Discharge Instructions Given	57	96%	94%	94%
Evaluation of LVS Function	75	100%	99%	99%
Medicare Spending				
Medicare Spending per Patient (ratio)	-	-	0.96	0.98
Pneumonia Care				
Appropriate Initial Antibiotic Given	23	100%	96%	95%
Blood Culture Timing	38	97%	98%	98%
Pregnancy and Delivery Care				
Newborn Deliveries Scheduled Early[3,7]	-	-	3%	6%
Preventive Care				
Immunization for Influenza[5]	-	-	89%	90%
Immunization for Pneumonia[5]	-	-	90%	92%
Stroke Care				
Anticoagulation Therapy for Atrial Fibrillation[5]	-	-	92%	95%
Antithrombotic Therapy Timing[5]	-	-	97%	98%
Assessed for Rehabilitation[5]	-	-	97%	97%
Discharged on Antithrombotic Therapy[5]	-	-	99%	99%
Discharged on Statin Medication[5]	-	-	94%	94%
Thrombolytic Therapy Timing[5]	-	-	69%	66%
Venous Thromboembolism Prophylaxis[5]	-	-	94%	94%
Written Stroke Educational Materials Given[5]	-	-	87%	88%
Surgical Care Improvement Project				
Appropriate Beta Blocker Usage[5]	-	-	98%	98%
Appropriate VTP Within 24 Hours[5]	-	-	98%	98%
Controlled Postoperative Blood Glucose[5]	-	-	97%	97%
Perioperative Temperature Management[5]	-	-	100%	100%
Prophylactic Antibiotic Selection[5]	-	-	99%	99%
Prophylactic Antibiotic Selection (Outpatient)[5]	-	-	97%	98%
Prophylactic Antibiotic Stopped[5]	-	-	98%	98%
Prophylactic Antibiotic Timing[5]	-	-	98%	99%

NOTE: Hospital profiles are in alphabetical order by state, then city, then hospital within the city; Rankings exclude hospitals with less than 25 cases except for patient surveys which excludes hospitals with less than 100 cases; (a) 100-299 cases; (1) The number of cases/patients is too few to report; (2) Data submitted were based on a sample of cases/patients; (3) Results are based on a shorter time period than required; (4) Data suppressed by CMS for one or more quarters; (5) Results are not available for this reporting period; (6) Fewer than 100 patients completed the HCAHPS survey; (7) No cases met the criteria for this measure; (8) The lower limit of the confidence interval cannot be calculated if the number of observed infections equals zero; (9) No data are available from the state/territory for this reporting period; (10) The scores shown reflect fewer than 50 completed surveys; (11) There were discrepancies in the data collection process; (12) This measure does not apply to this hospital for this reporting period; (13) Results cannot be calculated for this reporting period; (14) The results for this state are combined with nearby states to protect confidentiality; Please refer to the User's Guide for a full explanation of data.

Measure	Cases	This Hosp.	State Avg.	U.S. Avg.
Prophylactic Antibiotic Timing (Outpatient)[5]	-	-	97%	98%
Urinary Catheter Removal[5]	-	-	97%	97%
Survey of Patients' Hospital Experiences				
Area Around Room 'Always' Quiet at Night	(a)	68%	60%	61%
Doctors 'Always' Communicated Well	(a)	79%	81%	82%
Home Recovery Information Given	(a)	89%	87%	85%
Hospital Given 9 or 10 on 10 Point Scale	(a)	68%	71%	71%
Meds 'Always' Explained Before Given	(a)	67%	64%	64%
Nurses 'Always' Communicated Well	(a)	81%	80%	79%
Pain 'Always' Well Controlled	(a)	71%	71%	71%
Room and Bathroom 'Always' Clean	(a)	68%	73%	73%
Timely Help 'Always' Received	(a)	73%	70%	68%
Would Definitely Recommend Hospital	(a)	63%	71%	71%
Use of Medical Imaging				
Cardiac Imaging Stress Test before Surgery	222	5.0%	5.1%	5.3%
Combination Abdominal CT Scan	428	4.0%	8.7%	10.5%
Combination Brain/Sinus CT Scan	437	0.7%	2.2%	2.7%
Combination Chest CT Scan	345	2.3%	3.6%	2.7%
Follow-up Mammogram/Ultrasound	818	7.9%	8.2%	8.8%
Lumbar Spine MRI for Low Back Pain	89	43.8%	36.9%	37.2%

Genesys Regional Medical Center - Health Park

One Genesys Parkway
Grand Blanc, MI 48439
Phone: 810-606-5000
Fax: 810-606-6279
URL: www.genesys.org
Type: Acute Care Hospitals
Emergency Services: Yes
Ownership: Voluntary non-profit - Church
Beds: 410

Key Personnel:

CEO/President. . . . . Elizabeth Aderholdt
Cardiac Laboratory. . . . . Paul Brown
Operating Room. . . . . Karen Ferrara
Radiology. . . . . Michael Gedwill
Infection Control. . . . . Pamela Goran
Pediatric Ambulatory Care . . . . . . Kamale Hasan, MD
Quality Assurance . . . . Greg Knuth
Chief of Medical Staff. . . . . Kenneth Steibel, MD

Measure	Cases	This Hosp.	State Avg.	U.S. Avg.
Blood Clot Prevention and Treatment				
Anticoagulation Overlap Therapy[2]	227	61%	90%	93%
ICU Venous Thromboembolism Prophylaxis[2]	119	87%	93%	92%
Incidence of Potentially Preventable VTE[2]	64	23%	8%	10%
UFH with Dosages/Platelet Monitoring[2]	245	98%	96%	97%
Venous Thromboembolism Prophylaxis[2]	366	67%	87%	85%
Warfarin Therapy Discharge Instructions[2]	162	19%	72%	75%
Chest Pain/Possible Heart Attack Care				
Aspirin Given Within 24 Hours of Arrival[5]	-	-	96%	96%
Fibrinolytic Meds Within 30 Min. of Arrival[5]	-	-	63%	58%
Average Time to ECG (minutes)[5]	-	-	8	7
Average Time to Transfer (minutes)[5]	-	-	53	60
Children's Asthma Care				
Received Home Management Plan of Care	-	-	-	88%
Received Reliever Medication	-	-	-	100%
Received Systemic Corticosteroids	-	-	-	100%
Emergency Department				
Admittance Decision Time (minutes)[2]	735	168	102	98
Head CT Results Within 45 Min. of Arrival	39	13%	54%	57%
Patients Who Left ER Before Being Seen	64,075	1%	2%	2%
Time from ER Arrival to Admit. (minutes)[2]	791	364	288	274
Time from ER Arrival to Discharge (minutes)	373	181	128	134
Time in ER Before Being Evaluated (minutes)	362	47	22	26
Time to Pain Meds for Fractures (minutes)	415	66	55	57
Heart Attack Care				
Aspirin Given at Discharge	465	100%	99%	99%
Fibrinolytic Meds Within 30 Min. of Arrival[7]	-	-	20%	54%
PCI Within 90 Minutes of Arrival	79	99%	95%	96%
Statin Prescribed at Discharge	460	99%	98%	98%
Heart Failure Care				
ACE Inhibitor or ARB for LVSD	146	98%	96%	97%
Discharge Instructions Given	500	86%	94%	94%
Evaluation of LVS Function	616	100%	99%	99%
Medicare Spending				
Medicare Spending per Patient (ratio)	-	0.95	0.96	0.98
Pneumonia Care				
Appropriate Initial Antibiotic Given	390	98%	96%	95%
Blood Culture Timing	562	98%	98%	98%
Pregnancy and Delivery Care				
Newborn Deliveries Scheduled Early[2]	339	2%	3%	6%
Preventive Care				
Immunization for Influenza[2]	625	58%	89%	90%
Immunization for Pneumonia[2]	808	62%	90%	92%
Stroke Care				
Anticoagulation Therapy for Atrial Fibrillation[2]	14	86%	92%	95%
Antithrombotic Therapy Timing[2]	107	98%	97%	98%
Assessed for Rehabilitation[2]	115	93%	97%	97%
Discharged on Antithrombotic Therapy[2]	108	97%	99%	99%
Discharged on Statin Medication[2]	89	89%	94%	94%
Thrombolytic Therapy Timing[1,2]	-	-	69%	66%
Venous Thromboembolism Prophylaxis[2]	119	89%	94%	94%
Written Stroke Educational Materials Given[2]	70	84%	87%	88%
Surgical Care Improvement Project				
Appropriate Beta Blocker Usage[2]	650	96%	98%	98%
Appropriate VTP Within 24 Hours[2]	1,346	97%	98%	98%
Controlled Postoperative Blood Glucose[2]	180	99%	97%	97%
Perioperative Temperature Management[2]	1,515	100%	100%	100%
Prophylactic Antibiotic Selection[2]	1,378	98%	99%	99%
Prophylactic Antibiotic Selection (Outpatient)	601	95%	97%	98%
Prophylactic Antibiotic Stopped[2]	1,347	97%	98%	98%
Prophylactic Antibiotic Timing[2]	1,379	99%	98%	99%
Prophylactic Antibiotic Timing (Outpatient)	597	89%	97%	98%
Urinary Catheter Removal[2]	1,265	98%	97%	97%
Survey of Patients' Hospital Experiences				
Area Around Room 'Always' Quiet at Night	300+	46%	60%	61%
Doctors 'Always' Communicated Well	300+	76%	81%	82%
Home Recovery Information Given	300+	84%	87%	85%
Hospital Given 9 or 10 on 10 Point Scale	300+	67%	71%	71%
Meds 'Always' Explained Before Given	300+	57%	64%	64%
Nurses 'Always' Communicated Well	300+	75%	80%	79%
Pain 'Always' Well Controlled	300+	68%	71%	71%
Room and Bathroom 'Always' Clean	300+	64%	73%	73%
Timely Help 'Always' Received	300+	70%	70%	68%
Would Definitely Recommend Hospital	300+	71%	71%	71%
Use of Medical Imaging				
Cardiac Imaging Stress Test before Surgery	726	6.2%	5.1%	5.3%
Combination Abdominal CT Scan	1,076	2.0%	8.7%	10.5%
Combination Brain/Sinus CT Scan	1,120	1.7%	2.2%	2.7%
Combination Chest CT Scan	454	5.1%	3.6%	2.7%
Follow-up Mammogram/Ultrasound	171	17.5%	8.2%	8.8%
Lumbar Spine MRI for Low Back Pain	258	35.7%	36.9%	37.2%

North Ottawa Community Health Center

1309 Sheldon Rd
Grand Haven, MI 49417
Phone: 616-842-3600
Fax: 616-847-5621
URL: www.noch.org
Type: Acute Care Hospitals
Emergency Services: Yes
Ownership: Govt - Hospital Dist/Auth
Beds: 81

Key Personnel:

Pediatric In-Patient Care . . . . Linda Bouman
Radiology. . . . . Lynn S McCurdy
CEO/President. . . . . Michael Payne
Chief of Medical Staff. . . . . M Gary Robertson, MD

Measure	Cases	This Hosp.	State Avg.	U.S. Avg.
Blood Clot Prevention and Treatment				
Anticoagulation Overlap Therapy[2]	22	100%	90%	93%
ICU Venous Thromboembolism Prophylaxis[2]	49	100%	93%	92%
Incidence of Potentially Preventable VTE[2,7]	-	-	8%	10%
UFH with Dosages/Platelet Monitoring[1,2]	-	-	96%	97%
Venous Thromboembolism Prophylaxis[2]	105	97%	87%	85%
Warfarin Therapy Discharge Instructions[2]	19	84%	72%	75%
Chest Pain/Possible Heart Attack Care				
Aspirin Given Within 24 Hours of Arrival	77	94%	96%	96%
Fibrinolytic Meds Within 30 Min. of Arrival[7]	-	-	63%	58%
Average Time to ECG (minutes)	82	6	8	7
Average Time to Transfer (minutes)[1]	-	-	53	60
Children's Asthma Care				
Received Home Management Plan of Care	-	-	-	88%
Received Reliever Medication	-	-	-	100%
Received Systemic Corticosteroids	-	-	-	100%
Emergency Department				
Admittance Decision Time (minutes)[2]	301	112	102	98
Head CT Results Within 45 Min. of Arrival[1]	-	-	54%	57%
Patients Who Left ER Before Being Seen	17,113	0%	2%	2%
Time from ER Arrival to Admit. (minutes)[2]	306	271	288	274
Time from ER Arrival to Discharge (minutes)	424	104	128	134
Time in ER Before Being Evaluated (minutes)	430	18	22	26
Time to Pain Meds for Fractures (minutes)	112	36	55	57
Heart Attack Care				
Aspirin Given at Discharge[1]	-	-	99%	99%
Fibrinolytic Meds Within 30 Min. of Arrival[7]	-	-	20%	54%
PCI Within 90 Minutes of Arrival[7]	-	-	95%	96%
Statin Prescribed at Discharge[1]	-	-	98%	98%
Heart Failure Care				
ACE Inhibitor or ARB for LVSD[1]	-	-	96%	97%
Discharge Instructions Given	22	100%	94%	94%
Evaluation of LVS Function	33	100%	99%	99%
Medicare Spending				
Medicare Spending per Patient (ratio)	-	0.93	0.96	0.98
Pneumonia Care				
Appropriate Initial Antibiotic Given	40	85%	96%	95%
Blood Culture Timing	67	97%	98%	98%
Pregnancy and Delivery Care				
Newborn Deliveries Scheduled Early[2]	24	0%	3%	6%
Preventive Care				
Immunization for Influenza[2]	240	100%	89%	90%
Immunization for Pneumonia[2]	262	98%	90%	92%
Stroke Care				
Anticoagulation Therapy for Atrial Fibrillation[1]	-	-	92%	95%
Antithrombotic Therapy Timing	25	100%	97%	98%
Assessed for Rehabilitation	31	100%	97%	97%
Discharged on Antithrombotic Therapy	30	100%	99%	99%
Discharged on Statin Medication	22	95%	94%	94%
Thrombolytic Therapy Timing[7]	-	-	69%	66%
Venous Thromboembolism Prophylaxis	27	100%	94%	94%
Written Stroke Educational Materials Given	15	93%	87%	88%
Surgical Care Improvement Project				
Appropriate Beta Blocker Usage	68	99%	98%	98%
Appropriate VTP Within 24 Hours	195	99%	98%	98%
Controlled Postoperative Blood Glucose[7]	-	-	97%	97%
Perioperative Temperature Management	247	100%	100%	100%
Prophylactic Antibiotic Selection	180	99%	99%	99%
Prophylactic Antibiotic Selection (Outpatient)	119	100%	97%	98%
Prophylactic Antibiotic Stopped	174	98%	98%	98%
Prophylactic Antibiotic Timing	180	100%	98%	99%
Prophylactic Antibiotic Timing (Outpatient)	78	99%	97%	98%
Urinary Catheter Removal	174	99%	97%	97%
Survey of Patients' Hospital Experiences				
Area Around Room 'Always' Quiet at Night	300+	70%	60%	61%
Doctors 'Always' Communicated Well	300+	80%	81%	82%
Home Recovery Information Given	300+	89%	87%	85%
Hospital Given 9 or 10 on 10 Point Scale	300+	78%	71%	71%
Meds 'Always' Explained Before Given	300+	63%	64%	64%
Nurses 'Always' Communicated Well	300+	79%	80%	79%
Pain 'Always' Well Controlled	300+	69%	71%	71%
Room and Bathroom 'Always' Clean	300+	76%	73%	73%
Timely Help 'Always' Received	300+	73%	70%	68%
Would Definitely Recommend Hospital	300+	73%	71%	71%
Use of Medical Imaging				
Cardiac Imaging Stress Test before Surgery	113	3.5%	5.1%	5.3%
Combination Abdominal CT Scan	210	8.1%	8.7%	10.5%
Combination Brain/Sinus CT Scan[1]	-	-	2.2%	2.7%
Combination Chest CT Scan	192	10.9%	3.6%	2.7%
Follow-up Mammogram/Ultrasound	705	4.7%	8.2%	8.8%
Lumbar Spine MRI for Low Back Pain[1]	-	-	36.9%	37.2%

Saint Mary's Health Care

200 Jefferson Avenue Se
Grand Rapids, MI 49503
Phone: 616-685-5000
Fax: 616-732-3035
URL: www.smhealthcare.org
Type: Acute Care Hospitals
Emergency Services: Yes
Ownership: Voluntary non-profit - Church
Beds: 324

Key Personnel:

CEO/President. . . . . David Blair, MD

NOTE: Hospital profiles are in alphabetical order by state, then city, then hospital within the city; Rankings exclude hospitals with less than 25 cases except for patient surveys which excludes hospitals with less than 100 cases; (a) 100-299 cases; (1) The number of cases/patients is too few to report; (2) Data submitted were based on a sample of cases/patients; (3) Results are based on a shorter time period than required; (4) Data suppressed by CMS for one or more quarters; (5) Results are not available for this reporting period; (6) Fewer than 100 patients completed the HCAHPS survey; (7) No cases met the criteria for this measure; (8) The lower limit of the confidence interval cannot be calculated if the number of observed infections equals zero; (9) No data are available from the state/territory for this reporting period; (10) The scores shown reflect fewer than 50 completed surveys; (11) There were discrepancies in the data collection process; (12) This measure does not apply to this hospital for this reporting period; (13) Results cannot be calculated for this reporting period; (14) The results for this state are combined with nearby states to protect confidentiality; Please refer to the User's Guide for a full explanation of data.

Patient Relations .... Vicki Garrett, RN
Chair/CEO .... Martha Gonzalez-Cortes
Radiology .... Earl Monks
Infection Control .... Mary Neuman, RN
Emergency Room .... Michael Olgren, MD
Quality Assurance .... Barb Vanpattan
Chief of Medical Staff .... Terrance Wright, MD

Measure	Cases	This Hosp.	State Avg.	U.S. Avg.
Blood Clot Prevention and Treatment				
Anticoagulation Overlap Therapy[2]	114	98%	90%	93%
ICU Venous Thromboembolism Prophylaxis[2]	45	98%	93%	92%
Incidence of Potentially Preventable VTE[2]	18	6%	8%	10%
UFH with Dosages/Platelet Monitoring[2]	85	100%	96%	97%
Venous Thromboembolism Prophylaxis[2]	308	96%	87%	85%
Warfarin Therapy Discharge Instructions[2]	91	63%	72%	75%
Chest Pain/Possible Heart Attack Care				
Aspirin Given Within 24 Hours of Arrival[1]	-	-	96%	96%
Fibrinolytic Meds Within 30 Min. of Arrival[3,7]	-	-	63%	58%
Average Time to ECG (minutes)[1]	-	-	8	7
Average Time to Transfer (minutes)[3,7]	-	-	53	60
Children's Asthma Care				
Received Home Management Plan of Care	-	-	-	88%
Received Reliever Medication	-	-	-	100%
Received Systemic Corticosteroids	-	-	-	100%
Emergency Department				
Admittance Decision Time (minutes)[2]	404	96	102	98
Head CT Results Within 45 Min. of Arrival[3,7]	-	-	54%	57%
Patients Who Left ER Before Being Seen	62,942	0%	2%	2%
Time from ER Arrival to Admit. (minutes)[2]	404	253	288	274
Time from ER Arrival to Discharge (minutes)	338	131	128	134
Time in ER Before Being Evaluated (minutes)	382	10	22	26
Time to Pain Meds for Fractures (minutes)	262	71	55	57
Heart Attack Care				
Aspirin Given at Discharge	112	100%	99%	99%
Fibrinolytic Meds Within 30 Min. of Arrival[1]	-	-	20%	54%
PCI Within 90 Minutes of Arrival	36	92%	95%	96%
Statin Prescribed at Discharge	115	98%	98%	98%
Heart Failure Care				
ACE Inhibitor or ARB for LVSD[2]	64	89%	96%	97%
Discharge Instructions Given[2]	240	97%	94%	94%
Evaluation of LVS Function[2]	306	99%	99%	99%
Medicare Spending				
Medicare Spending per Patient (ratio)	-	0.94	0.96	0.98
Pneumonia Care				
Appropriate Initial Antibiotic Given[2]	113	99%	96%	95%
Blood Culture Timing[2]	145	99%	98%	98%
Pregnancy and Delivery Care				
Newborn Deliveries Scheduled Early[2]	184	0%	3%	6%
Preventive Care				
Immunization for Influenza[2]	527	96%	89%	90%
Immunization for Pneumonia[2]	611	92%	90%	92%
Stroke Care				
Anticoagulation Therapy for Atrial Fibrillation	19	100%	92%	95%
Antithrombotic Therapy Timing	72	94%	97%	98%
Assessed for Rehabilitation	110	100%	97%	97%
Discharged on Antithrombotic Therapy	98	96%	99%	99%
Discharged on Statin Medication	63	94%	94%	94%
Thrombolytic Therapy Timing	19	89%	69%	66%
Venous Thromboembolism Prophylaxis	109	97%	94%	94%
Written Stroke Educational Materials Given	59	93%	87%	88%
Surgical Care Improvement Project				
Appropriate Beta Blocker Usage[2]	162	99%	98%	98%
Appropriate VTP Within 24 Hours[2]	413	100%	98%	98%
Controlled Postoperative Blood Glucose[1,2]	-	-	97%	97%
Perioperative Temperature Management[2]	562	100%	100%	100%
Prophylactic Antibiotic Selection[2]	392	98%	99%	99%
Prophylactic Antibiotic Selection (Outpatient)	464	98%	97%	98%
Prophylactic Antibiotic Stopped[2]	385	98%	98%	98%
Prophylactic Antibiotic Timing[2]	392	98%	98%	99%
Prophylactic Antibiotic Timing (Outpatient)	462	100%	97%	98%
Urinary Catheter Removal[2]	326	98%	97%	97%
Survey of Patients' Hospital Experiences				
Area Around Room 'Always' Quiet at Night	300+	60%	60%	61%
Doctors 'Always' Communicated Well	300+	80%	81%	82%
Home Recovery Information Given	300+	90%	87%	85%
Hospital Given 9 or 10 on 10 Point Scale	300+	77%	71%	71%
Meds 'Always' Explained Before Given	300+	63%	64%	64%
Nurses 'Always' Communicated Well	300+	80%	80%	79%
Pain 'Always' Well Controlled	300+	71%	71%	71%
Room and Bathroom 'Always' Clean	300+	69%	73%	73%
Timely Help 'Always' Received	300+	64%	70%	68%
Would Definitely Recommend Hospital	300+	78%	71%	71%
Use of Medical Imaging				
Cardiac Imaging Stress Test before Surgery	474	5.5%	5.1%	5.3%
Combination Abdominal CT Scan	1,356	5.0%	8.7%	10.5%
Combination Brain/Sinus CT Scan	951	3.4%	2.2%	2.7%
Combination Chest CT Scan	1,142	0.4%	3.6%	2.7%
Follow-up Mammogram/Ultrasound	1,998	4.9%	8.2%	8.8%
Lumbar Spine MRI for Low Back Pain	200	34.5%	36.9%	37.2%

Spectrum Health - Butterworth Campus

100 Michigan Saint Ne
Grand Rapids, MI 49503
Phone: 616-391-1774
Fax: 616-391-2780
URL: www.spectrum-health.org
Type: Acute Care Hospitals
Emergency Services: Yes
Ownership: Voluntary non-profit - Private
Beds: 986

Key Personnel:

CEO/President .... Richard C Breon
Quality Assurance .... Nancy Hansen
Pediatric In-Patient Care .... Ronald Hofmann
Radiology .... Charles Luhenton
Cardiac Laboratory .... Marla Niedzwiecki
Infection Control .... Deb Paul
Chief of Medical Staff .... Brian Roelof
Operating Room .... Kathy Shaneberger

Measure	Cases	This Hosp.	State Avg.	U.S. Avg.
Blood Clot Prevention and Treatment				
Anticoagulation Overlap Therapy[2]	310	86%	90%	93%
ICU Venous Thromboembolism Prophylaxis[2]	59	93%	93%	92%
Incidence of Potentially Preventable VTE[2]	67	1%	8%	10%
UFH with Dosages/Platelet Monitoring[2]	328	100%	96%	97%
Venous Thromboembolism Prophylaxis[2]	322	84%	87%	85%
Warfarin Therapy Discharge Instructions[2]	239	59%	72%	75%
Chest Pain/Possible Heart Attack Care				
Aspirin Given Within 24 Hours of Arrival[5]	-	-	96%	96%
Fibrinolytic Meds Within 30 Min. of Arrival[5]	-	-	63%	58%
Average Time to ECG (minutes)[5]	-	-	8	7
Average Time to Transfer (minutes)[5]	-	-	53	60
Children's Asthma Care				
Received Home Management Plan of Care	164	95%	-	88%
Received Reliever Medication	164	99%	-	100%
Received Systemic Corticosteroids	164	99%	-	100%
Emergency Department				
Admittance Decision Time (minutes)[2]	449	101	102	98
Head CT Results Within 45 Min. of Arrival[1]	-	-	54%	57%
Patients Who Left ER Before Being Seen	>100k	1%	2%	2%
Time from ER Arrival to Admit. (minutes)[2]	454	254	288	274
Time from ER Arrival to Discharge (minutes)	1,364	124	128	134
Time in ER Before Being Evaluated (minutes)	846	21	22	26
Time to Pain Meds for Fractures (minutes)	485	22	55	57
Heart Attack Care				
Aspirin Given at Discharge	939	100%	99%	99%
Fibrinolytic Meds Within 30 Min. of Arrival[7]	-	-	20%	54%
PCI Within 90 Minutes of Arrival	114	96%	95%	96%
Statin Prescribed at Discharge	915	99%	98%	98%
Heart Failure Care				
ACE Inhibitor or ARB for LVSD	302	99%	96%	97%
Discharge Instructions Given	971	98%	94%	94%
Evaluation of LVS Function	1,180	100%	99%	99%
Medicare Spending				
Medicare Spending per Patient (ratio)	-	0.97	0.96	0.98
Pneumonia Care				
Appropriate Initial Antibiotic Given[2]	138	97%	96%	95%
Blood Culture Timing[2]	271	100%	98%	98%
Pregnancy and Delivery Care				
Newborn Deliveries Scheduled Early[2]	77	1%	3%	6%
Preventive Care				
Immunization for Influenza[2]	531	92%	89%	90%
Immunization for Pneumonia[2]	534	95%	90%	92%
Stroke Care				
Anticoagulation Therapy for Atrial Fibrillation	100	92%	92%	95%
Antithrombotic Therapy Timing	460	98%	97%	98%
Assessed for Rehabilitation	642	98%	97%	97%
Discharged on Antithrombotic Therapy	524	99%	99%	99%
Discharged on Statin Medication	406	98%	94%	94%
Thrombolytic Therapy Timing	37	70%	69%	66%
Venous Thromboembolism Prophylaxis	654	98%	94%	94%
Written Stroke Educational Materials Given	324	95%	87%	88%
Surgical Care Improvement Project				
Appropriate Beta Blocker Usage[2]	298	99%	98%	98%
Appropriate VTP Within 24 Hours[2]	579	98%	98%	98%
Controlled Postoperative Blood Glucose[2]	170	99%	97%	97%
Perioperative Temperature Management[2]	755	100%	100%	100%
Prophylactic Antibiotic Selection[2]	597	98%	99%	99%
Prophylactic Antibiotic Selection (Outpatient)	979	95%	97%	98%
Prophylactic Antibiotic Stopped[2]	594	99%	98%	98%
Prophylactic Antibiotic Timing[2]	616	92%	98%	99%
Prophylactic Antibiotic Timing (Outpatient)	986	95%	97%	98%
Urinary Catheter Removal[2]	607	98%	97%	97%
Survey of Patients' Hospital Experiences				
Area Around Room 'Always' Quiet at Night[11]	300+	56%	60%	61%
Doctors 'Always' Communicated Well[11]	300+	78%	81%	82%
Home Recovery Information Given[11]	300+	89%	87%	85%
Hospital Given 9 or 10 on 10 Point Scale[11]	300+	76%	71%	71%
Meds 'Always' Explained Before Given[11]	300+	62%	64%	64%
Nurses 'Always' Communicated Well[11]	300+	81%	80%	79%
Pain 'Always' Well Controlled[11]	300+	70%	71%	71%
Room and Bathroom 'Always' Clean[11]	300+	76%	73%	73%
Timely Help 'Always' Received[11]	300+	64%	70%	68%
Would Definitely Recommend Hospital[11]	300+	80%	71%	71%
Use of Medical Imaging				
Cardiac Imaging Stress Test before Surgery	2,108	5.1%	5.1%	5.3%
Combination Abdominal CT Scan	2,756	3.6%	8.7%	10.5%
Combination Brain/Sinus CT Scan	1,898	2.1%	2.2%	2.7%
Combination Chest CT Scan	1,742	1.2%	3.6%	2.7%
Follow-up Mammogram/Ultrasound	4,684	9.2%	8.2%	8.8%
Lumbar Spine MRI for Low Back Pain	524	39.1%	36.9%	37.2%

Mercy Hospital - Grayling

1100 E Michigan Ave
Grayling, MI 49738
Phone: 989-348-5461
Fax: 989-348-0485
URL: www.mercygrayling.munsonhealthcare.org
Type: Acute Care Hospitals
Emergency Services: Yes
Ownership: Voluntary non-profit - Church
Beds: 130

Key Personnel:

Cardiac Laboratory .... Sue Boardman
Emergency Room .... D Gulow, MD
Chief of Medical Staff .... David Hunter
CEO .... Stephen Reimer-Matuzsak

Measure	Cases	This Hosp.	State Avg.	U.S. Avg.
Blood Clot Prevention and Treatment				
Anticoagulation Overlap Therapy[2]	28	100%	90%	93%
ICU Venous Thromboembolism Prophylaxis[2]	49	100%	93%	92%
Incidence of Potentially Preventable VTE[2,7]	-	-	8%	10%
UFH with Dosages/Platelet Monitoring[2]	16	100%	96%	97%
Venous Thromboembolism Prophylaxis[2]	223	98%	87%	85%
Warfarin Therapy Discharge Instructions[2]	24	88%	72%	75%
Chest Pain/Possible Heart Attack Care				
Aspirin Given Within 24 Hours of Arrival	169	97%	96%	96%
Fibrinolytic Meds Within 30 Min. of Arrival[1]	-	-	63%	58%
Average Time to ECG (minutes)	173	5	8	7
Average Time to Transfer (minutes)[1]	-	-	53	60
Children's Asthma Care				
Received Home Management Plan of Care	-	-	-	88%
Received Reliever Medication	-	-	-	100%
Received Systemic Corticosteroids	-	-	-	100%
Emergency Department				
Admittance Decision Time (minutes)[2]	507	147	102	98
Head CT Results Within 45 Min. of Arrival	14	50%	54%	57%
Patients Who Left ER Before Being Seen	20,702	1%	2%	2%

NOTE: Hospital profiles are in alphabetical order by state, then city, then hospital within the city; Rankings exclude hospitals with less than 25 cases except for patient surveys which excludes hospitals with less than 100 cases; (a) 100-299 cases; (1) The number of cases/patients is too few to report; (2) Data submitted were based on a sample of cases/patients; (3) Results are based on a shorter time period than required; (4) Data suppressed by CMS for one or more quarters; (5) Results are not available for this reporting period; (6) Fewer than 100 patients completed the HCAHPS survey; (7) No cases met the criteria for this measure; (8) The lower limit of the confidence interval cannot be calculated if the number of observed infections equals zero; (9) No data are available from the state/territory for this reporting period; (10) The scores shown reflect fewer than 50 completed surveys; (11) There were discrepancies in the data collection process; (12) This measure does not apply to this hospital for this reporting period; (13) Results cannot be calculated for this reporting period; (14) The results for this state are combined with nearby states to protect confidentiality; Please refer to the User's Guide for a full explanation of data.

Measure	Cases	This Hosp.	State Avg.	U.S. Avg.
Time from ER Arrival to Admit. (minutes)[2]	508	307	288	274
Time from ER Arrival to Discharge (minutes)	351	161	128	134
Time in ER Before Being Evaluated (minutes)	376	28	22	26
Time to Pain Meds for Fractures (minutes)	76	60	55	57
Heart Attack Care				
Aspirin Given at Discharge	12	100%	99%	99%
Fibrinolytic Meds Within 30 Min. of Arrival[7]	-	-	20%	54%
PCI Within 90 Minutes of Arrival[7]	-	-	95%	96%
Statin Prescribed at Discharge	11	100%	98%	98%
Heart Failure Care				
ACE Inhibitor or ARB for LVSD	28	100%	96%	97%
Discharge Instructions Given	95	99%	94%	94%
Evaluation of LVS Function	113	100%	99%	99%
Medicare Spending				
Medicare Spending per Patient (ratio)	-	0.90	0.96	0.98
Pneumonia Care				
Appropriate Initial Antibiotic Given	75	100%	96%	95%
Blood Culture Timing	121	99%	98%	98%
Pregnancy and Delivery Care				
Newborn Deliveries Scheduled Early	37	5%	3%	6%
Preventive Care				
Immunization for Influenza[2]	294	94%	89%	90%
Immunization for Pneumonia[2]	434	96%	90%	92%
Stroke Care				
Anticoagulation Therapy for Atrial Fibrillation[1,2]	-	-	92%	95%
Antithrombotic Therapy Timing[2]	43	100%	97%	98%
Assessed for Rehabilitation[2]	50	100%	97%	97%
Discharged on Antithrombotic Therapy[2]	48	100%	99%	99%
Discharged on Statin Medication[2]	41	100%	94%	94%
Thrombolytic Therapy Timing[1,2]	-	-	69%	66%
Venous Thromboembolism Prophylaxis[2]	48	98%	94%	94%
Written Stroke Educational Materials Given[2]	36	75%	87%	88%
Surgical Care Improvement Project				
Appropriate Beta Blocker Usage	56	98%	98%	98%
Appropriate VTP Within 24 Hours	200	100%	98%	98%
Controlled Postoperative Blood Glucose[7]	-	-	97%	97%
Perioperative Temperature Management	243	100%	100%	100%
Prophylactic Antibiotic Selection	203	100%	99%	99%
Prophylactic Antibiotic Selection (Outpatient)	73	95%	97%	98%
Prophylactic Antibiotic Stopped	197	98%	98%	98%
Prophylactic Antibiotic Timing	203	99%	98%	99%
Prophylactic Antibiotic Timing (Outpatient)	64	100%	97%	98%
Urinary Catheter Removal	133	100%	97%	97%
Survey of Patients' Hospital Experiences				
Area Around Room 'Always' Quiet at Night	300+	59%	60%	61%
Doctors 'Always' Communicated Well	300+	82%	81%	82%
Home Recovery Information Given	300+	93%	87%	85%
Hospital Given 9 or 10 on 10 Point Scale	300+	76%	71%	71%
Meds 'Always' Explained Before Given	300+	69%	64%	64%
Nurses 'Always' Communicated Well	300+	83%	80%	79%
Pain 'Always' Well Controlled	300+	73%	71%	71%
Room and Bathroom 'Always' Clean	300+	75%	73%	73%
Timely Help 'Always' Received	300+	73%	70%	68%
Would Definitely Recommend Hospital	300+	76%	71%	71%
Use of Medical Imaging				
Cardiac Imaging Stress Test before Surgery	458	4.6%	5.1%	5.3%
Combination Abdominal CT Scan	778	4.2%	8.7%	10.5%
Combination Brain/Sinus CT Scan	689	1.6%	2.2%	2.7%
Combination Chest CT Scan	314	0.3%	3.6%	2.7%
Follow-up Mammogram/Ultrasound	1,064	8.4%	8.2%	8.8%
Lumbar Spine MRI for Low Back Pain	126	49.2%	36.9%	37.2%

Spectrum Health United Memorial - United Campus

615 S Bower Street
Greenville, MI 48838
E-mail: contactus@umha.org
URL: www.umha.org
Type: Acute Care Hospitals
Ownership: Voluntary non-profit - Other
Phone: 616-754-4691
Fax: 616-754-5054
Emergency Services: Yes
Beds: 105

Key Personnel:
Quality Assurance . . . . Etta Barrera
CEO/President. . . . . Paul Donir
Ambulatory Care . . . . Stephen Romanella

Measure	Cases	This Hosp.	State Avg.	U.S. Avg.
Blood Clot Prevention and Treatment				
Anticoagulation Overlap Therapy[2]	32	94%	90%	93%
ICU Venous Thromboembolism Prophylaxis[2]	50	98%	93%	92%
Incidence of Potentially Preventable VTE[1,2]	-	-	8%	10%
UFH with Dosages/Platelet Monitoring[1,2]	-	-	96%	97%
Venous Thromboembolism Prophylaxis[2]	182	97%	87%	85%
Warfarin Therapy Discharge Instructions[2]	26	81%	72%	75%
Chest Pain/Possible Heart Attack Care				
Aspirin Given Within 24 Hours of Arrival	127	98%	96%	96%
Fibrinolytic Meds Within 30 Min. of Arrival[7]	-	-	63%	58%
Average Time to ECG (minutes)	131	5	8	7
Average Time to Transfer (minutes)	22	41	53	60
Children's Asthma Care				
Received Home Management Plan of Care	-	-	-	88%
Received Reliever Medication	-	-	-	100%
Received Systemic Corticosteroids	-	-	-	100%
Emergency Department				
Admittance Decision Time (minutes)[2]	336	80	102	98
Head CT Results Within 45 Min. of Arrival[1]	-	-	54%	57%
Patients Who Left ER Before Being Seen	27,296	1%	2%	2%
Time from ER Arrival to Admit. (minutes)[2]	337	240	288	274
Time from ER Arrival to Discharge (minutes)	463	115	128	134
Time in ER Before Being Evaluated (minutes)	370	19	22	26
Time to Pain Meds for Fractures (minutes)	165	43	55	57
Heart Attack Care				
Aspirin Given at Discharge[1,3]	-	-	99%	99%
Fibrinolytic Meds Within 30 Min. of Arrival[3,7]	-	-	20%	54%
PCI Within 90 Minutes of Arrival[3,7]	-	-	95%	96%
Statin Prescribed at Discharge[1,3]	-	-	98%	98%
Heart Failure Care				
ACE Inhibitor or ARB for LVSD	18	94%	96%	97%
Discharge Instructions Given	77	97%	94%	94%
Evaluation of LVS Function	102	100%	99%	99%
Medicare Spending				
Medicare Spending per Patient (ratio)	-	0.91	0.96	0.98
Pneumonia Care				
Appropriate Initial Antibiotic Given	92	93%	96%	95%
Blood Culture Timing	205	99%	98%	98%
Pregnancy and Delivery Care				
Newborn Deliveries Scheduled Early[2]	58	17%	3%	6%
Preventive Care				
Immunization for Influenza[2]	269	95%	89%	90%
Immunization for Pneumonia[2]	360	98%	90%	92%
Stroke Care				
Anticoagulation Therapy for Atrial Fibrillation[1]	-	-	92%	95%
Antithrombotic Therapy Timing	25	100%	97%	98%
Assessed for Rehabilitation	28	100%	97%	97%
Discharged on Antithrombotic Therapy	27	100%	99%	99%
Discharged on Statin Medication	23	96%	94%	94%
Thrombolytic Therapy Timing[7]	-	-	69%	66%
Venous Thromboembolism Prophylaxis	24	96%	94%	94%
Written Stroke Educational Materials Given	16	94%	87%	88%
Surgical Care Improvement Project				
Appropriate Beta Blocker Usage	46	93%	98%	98%
Appropriate VTP Within 24 Hours	138	98%	98%	98%
Controlled Postoperative Blood Glucose[7]	-	-	97%	97%
Perioperative Temperature Management	161	99%	100%	100%
Prophylactic Antibiotic Selection	98	100%	99%	99%
Prophylactic Antibiotic Selection (Outpatient)	67	99%	97%	98%
Prophylactic Antibiotic Stopped	98	99%	98%	98%
Prophylactic Antibiotic Timing	98	97%	98%	99%
Prophylactic Antibiotic Timing (Outpatient)	67	96%	97%	98%
Urinary Catheter Removal	108	100%	97%	97%
Survey of Patients' Hospital Experiences				
Area Around Room 'Always' Quiet at Night	300+	59%	60%	61%
Doctors 'Always' Communicated Well	300+	82%	81%	82%
Home Recovery Information Given	300+	92%	87%	85%
Hospital Given 9 or 10 on 10 Point Scale	300+	76%	71%	71%
Meds 'Always' Explained Before Given	300+	71%	64%	64%
Nurses 'Always' Communicated Well	300+	82%	80%	79%
Pain 'Always' Well Controlled	300+	71%	71%	71%
Room and Bathroom 'Always' Clean	300+	82%	73%	73%
Timely Help 'Always' Received	300+	66%	70%	68%
Would Definitely Recommend Hospital	300+	77%	71%	71%
Use of Medical Imaging				
Cardiac Imaging Stress Test before Surgery	321	4.4%	5.1%	5.3%
Combination Abdominal CT Scan	660	3.0%	8.7%	10.5%
Combination Brain/Sinus CT Scan	565	1.9%	2.2%	2.7%
Combination Chest CT Scan	474	0.0%	3.6%	2.7%
Follow-up Mammogram/Ultrasound	814	8.6%	8.2%	8.8%
Lumbar Spine MRI for Low Back Pain	175	42.9%	36.9%	37.2%

Beaumont Health System

468 Cadieux Rd
Grosse Pointe, MI 48230
URL: www.beaumonthospitals.com
Type: Acute Care Hospitals
Ownership: Voluntary non-profit - Private
Phone: 313-343-1000
Fax: 313-343-1327
Emergency Services: Yes
Beds: 289

Key Personnel:
Chief of Medical Staff . . . . Ananias C. Diokno, MD
Hemotology Center . . . . Jackie Fisher
Infection Control. . . . . Suzanne Gardner
Chair/CEO . . . . Stephen R. Howard
CEO/President. . . . . Gene Michalski
Operating Room. . . . . Gail Pietrzyk
Quality Assurance . . . . Barb Stemmer

Measure	Cases	This Hosp.	State Avg.	U.S. Avg.
Blood Clot Prevention and Treatment				
Anticoagulation Overlap Therapy[2]	104	97%	90%	93%
ICU Venous Thromboembolism Prophylaxis[2]	47	98%	93%	92%
Incidence of Potentially Preventable VTE[2]	23	4%	8%	10%
UFH with Dosages/Platelet Monitoring[2]	90	100%	96%	97%
Venous Thromboembolism Prophylaxis[2]	374	92%	87%	85%
Warfarin Therapy Discharge Instructions[2]	80	90%	72%	75%
Chest Pain/Possible Heart Attack Care				
Aspirin Given Within 24 Hours of Arrival[1]	-	-	96%	96%
Fibrinolytic Meds Within 30 Min. of Arrival[3,7]	-	-	63%	58%
Average Time to ECG (minutes)[1]	-	-	8	7
Average Time to Transfer (minutes)[3,7]	-	-	53	60
Children's Asthma Care				
Received Home Management Plan of Care	-	-	-	88%
Received Reliever Medication	-	-	-	100%
Received Systemic Corticosteroids	-	-	-	100%
Emergency Department				
Admittance Decision Time (minutes)[2]	755	105	102	98
Head CT Results Within 45 Min. of Arrival[1,3]	-	-	54%	57%
Patients Who Left ER Before Being Seen	35,153	2%	2%	2%
Time from ER Arrival to Admit. (minutes)[2]	757	288	288	274
Time from ER Arrival to Discharge (minutes)	357	175	128	134
Time in ER Before Being Evaluated (minutes)	397	18	22	26
Time to Pain Meds for Fractures (minutes)	57	38	55	57
Heart Attack Care				
Aspirin Given at Discharge	85	100%	99%	99%
Fibrinolytic Meds Within 30 Min. of Arrival[7]	-	-	20%	54%
PCI Within 90 Minutes of Arrival	14	100%	95%	96%
Statin Prescribed at Discharge	81	100%	98%	98%
Heart Failure Care				
ACE Inhibitor or ARB for LVSD	128	100%	96%	97%
Discharge Instructions Given	361	100%	94%	94%
Evaluation of LVS Function	410	100%	99%	99%
Medicare Spending				
Medicare Spending per Patient (ratio)	-	0.99	0.96	0.98
Pneumonia Care				
Appropriate Initial Antibiotic Given	155	100%	96%	95%
Blood Culture Timing	233	100%	98%	98%
Pregnancy and Delivery Care				
Newborn Deliveries Scheduled Early[2]	26	12%	3%	6%
Preventive Care				
Immunization for Influenza[2]	594	96%	89%	90%
Immunization for Pneumonia[2]	864	95%	90%	92%
Stroke Care				
Anticoagulation Therapy for Atrial Fibrillation[1]	-	-	92%	95%
Antithrombotic Therapy Timing	70	100%	97%	98%
Assessed for Rehabilitation	75	100%	97%	97%
Discharged on Antithrombotic Therapy	72	100%	99%	99%

NOTE: Hospital profiles are in alphabetical order by state, then city, then hospital within the city; Rankings exclude hospitals with less than 25 cases except for patient surveys which excludes hospitals with less than 100 cases; (a) 100-299 cases; (1) The number of cases/patients is too few to report; (2) Data submitted were based on a sample of cases/patients; (3) Results are based on a shorter time period than required; (4) Data suppressed by CMS for one or more quarters; (5) Results are not available for this reporting period; (6) Fewer than 100 patients completed the HCAHPS survey; (7) No cases met the criteria for this measure; (8) The lower limit of the confidence interval cannot be calculated if the number of observed infections equals zero; (9) No data are available from the state/territory for this reporting period; (10) The scores shown reflect fewer than 50 completed surveys; (11) There were discrepancies in the data collection process; (12) This measure does not apply to this hospital for this reporting period; (13) Results cannot be calculated for this reporting period; (14) The results for this state are combined with nearby states to protect confidentiality; Please refer to the User's Guide for a full explanation of data.

Discharged on Statin Medication	57	100%	94%	94%
Thrombolytic Therapy Timing[7]	-	-	69%	66%
Venous Thromboembolism Prophylaxis	75	99%	94%	94%
Written Stroke Educational Materials Given	54	96%	87%	88%
Surgical Care Improvement Project				
Appropriate Beta Blocker Usage[2]	166	97%	98%	98%
Appropriate VTP Within 24 Hours[2]	448	100%	98%	98%
Controlled Postoperative Blood Glucose[2,7]	-	-	97%	97%
Perioperative Temperature Management[2]	564	100%	100%	100%
Prophylactic Antibiotic Selection[2]	402	100%	99%	99%
Prophylactic Antibiotic Selection (Outpatient)	156	99%	97%	98%
Prophylactic Antibiotic Stopped[2]	391	99%	98%	98%
Prophylactic Antibiotic Timing[2]	402	99%	98%	99%
Prophylactic Antibiotic Timing (Outpatient)	151	98%	97%	98%
Urinary Catheter Removal[2]	337	99%	97%	97%
Survey of Patients' Hospital Experiences				
Area Around Room 'Always' Quiet at Night	300+	57%	60%	61%
Doctors 'Always' Communicated Well	300+	79%	81%	82%
Home Recovery Information Given	300+	85%	87%	85%
Hospital Given 9 or 10 on 10 Point Scale	300+	76%	71%	71%
Meds 'Always' Explained Before Given	300+	60%	64%	64%
Nurses 'Always' Communicated Well	300+	80%	80%	79%
Pain 'Always' Well Controlled	300+	71%	71%	71%
Room and Bathroom 'Always' Clean	300+	76%	73%	73%
Timely Help 'Always' Received	300+	68%	70%	68%
Would Definitely Recommend Hospital	300+	76%	71%	71%
Use of Medical Imaging				
Cardiac Imaging Stress Test before Surgery	457	5.7%	5.1%	5.3%
Combination Abdominal CT Scan	855	6.5%	8.7%	10.5%
Combination Brain/Sinus CT Scan	673	1.8%	2.2%	2.7%
Combination Chest CT Scan	664	0.2%	3.6%	2.7%
Follow-up Mammogram/Ultrasound	766	15.3%	8.2%	8.8%
Lumbar Spine MRI for Low Back Pain	145	24.1%	36.9%	37.2%

Portage Health

500 Campus Drive
Hancock, MI 49930
Phone: 906-483-1000
Fax: 906-483-1521
E-mail: jsbigan@phsys.org
URL: www.portagehealth.org
Type: Acute Care Hospitals
Emergency Services: Yes
Ownership: Voluntary non-profit - Other
Beds: 74

Key Personnel:
CEO/President . . . . James Bogan
Pediatric In-Patient Care . . . . Sarah Campbell, MD
Emergency Room . . . . Mary Beth Hines
Chief of Medical Staff . . . . David Kass, MD
Anesthesiology . . . . Kirk R Klemme, MD
Radiology . . . . Ethelbert Lara, MD
Hemotology Center . . . . Savitri Padmanabhan, MD

Measure	Cases	This Hosp.	State Avg.	U.S. Avg.
Blood Clot Prevention and Treatment				
Anticoagulation Overlap Therapy[1,2]	-	-	90%	93%
ICU Venous Thromboembolism Prophylaxis[2]	26	92%	93%	92%
Incidence of Potentially Preventable VTE[2,7]	-	-	8%	10%
UFH with Dosages/Platelet Monitoring[2,7]	-	-	96%	97%
Venous Thromboembolism Prophylaxis[2]	81	96%	87%	85%
Warfarin Therapy Discharge Instructions[1,2]	-	-	72%	75%
Chest Pain/Possible Heart Attack Care				
Aspirin Given Within 24 Hours of Arrival	51	98%	96%	96%
Fibrinolytic Meds Within 30 Min. of Arrival[1]	-	-	63%	58%
Average Time to ECG (minutes)	52	8	8	7
Average Time to Transfer (minutes)[7]	-	-	53	60
Children's Asthma Care				
Received Home Management Plan of Care	-	-	-	88%
Received Reliever Medication	-	-	-	100%
Received Systemic Corticosteroids	-	-	-	100%
Emergency Department				
Admittance Decision Time (minutes)[2]	249	48	102	98
Head CT Results Within 45 Min. of Arrival[1]	-	-	54%	57%
Patients Who Left ER Before Being Seen	13,424	0%	2%	2%
Time from ER Arrival to Admit. (minutes)[2]	275	201	288	274
Time from ER Arrival to Discharge (minutes)	398	79	128	134
Time in ER Before Being Evaluated (minutes)	442	14	22	26
Time to Pain Meds for Fractures (minutes)	41	34	55	57
Heart Attack Care				
Aspirin Given at Discharge[1]	-	-	99%	99%
Fibrinolytic Meds Within 30 Min. of Arrival[7]	-	-	20%	54%
PCI Within 90 Minutes of Arrival[7]	-	-	95%	96%
Statin Prescribed at Discharge[1]	-	-	98%	98%
Heart Failure Care				
ACE Inhibitor or ARB for LVSD[1]	-	-	96%	97%
Discharge Instructions Given	15	100%	94%	94%
Evaluation of LVS Function	19	100%	99%	99%
Medicare Spending				
Medicare Spending per Patient (ratio)	-	0.87	0.96	0.98
Pneumonia Care				
Appropriate Initial Antibiotic Given	19	100%	96%	95%
Blood Culture Timing	37	97%	98%	98%
Pregnancy and Delivery Care				
Newborn Deliveries Scheduled Early[2]	20	0%	3%	6%
Preventive Care				
Immunization for Influenza[2]	244	96%	89%	90%
Immunization for Pneumonia[2]	251	96%	90%	92%
Stroke Care				
Anticoagulation Therapy for Atrial Fibrillation[7]	-	-	92%	95%
Antithrombotic Therapy Timing	15	100%	97%	98%
Assessed for Rehabilitation	19	100%	97%	97%
Discharged on Antithrombotic Therapy	18	100%	99%	99%
Discharged on Statin Medication	13	92%	94%	94%
Thrombolytic Therapy Timing[7]	-	-	69%	66%
Venous Thromboembolism Prophylaxis	17	100%	94%	94%
Written Stroke Educational Materials Given	13	54%	87%	88%
Surgical Care Improvement Project				
Appropriate Beta Blocker Usage	52	100%	98%	98%
Appropriate VTP Within 24 Hours	166	100%	98%	98%
Controlled Postoperative Blood Glucose[7]	-	-	97%	97%
Perioperative Temperature Management	195	100%	100%	100%
Prophylactic Antibiotic Selection	148	99%	99%	99%
Prophylactic Antibiotic Selection (Outpatient)	65	95%	97%	98%
Prophylactic Antibiotic Stopped	141	97%	98%	98%
Prophylactic Antibiotic Timing	148	97%	98%	99%
Prophylactic Antibiotic Timing (Outpatient)	14	93%	97%	98%
Urinary Catheter Removal	53	100%	97%	97%
Survey of Patients' Hospital Experiences				
Area Around Room 'Always' Quiet at Night	300+	59%	60%	61%
Doctors 'Always' Communicated Well	300+	86%	81%	82%
Home Recovery Information Given	300+	85%	87%	85%
Hospital Given 9 or 10 on 10 Point Scale	300+	79%	71%	71%
Meds 'Always' Explained Before Given	300+	67%	64%	64%
Nurses 'Always' Communicated Well	300+	85%	80%	79%
Pain 'Always' Well Controlled	300+	77%	71%	71%
Room and Bathroom 'Always' Clean	300+	83%	73%	73%
Timely Help 'Always' Received	300+	78%	70%	68%
Would Definitely Recommend Hospital	300+	80%	71%	71%
Use of Medical Imaging				
Cardiac Imaging Stress Test before Surgery	152	5.3%	5.1%	5.3%
Combination Abdominal CT Scan	275	9.1%	8.7%	10.5%
Combination Brain/Sinus CT Scan[1]	-	-	2.2%	2.7%
Combination Chest CT Scan	188	2.1%	3.6%	2.7%
Follow-up Mammogram/Ultrasound	530	11.5%	8.2%	8.8%
Lumbar Spine MRI for Low Back Pain	62	53.2%	36.9%	37.2%

Harbor Beach Community Hospital

210 S First St
Harbor Beach, MI 48441
Phone: 989-479-3201
Fax: 989-479-5000
E-mail: admin@hbch.org
URL: www.hbch.org
Type: Critical Access Hospitals
Emergency Services: Yes
Ownership: Voluntary non-profit - Private
Beds: 61

Key Personnel:
CEO/President . . . . Edward Gamache
Chief of Medical Staff . . . . Jaime Tan, MD

Measure	Cases	This Hosp.	State Avg.	U.S. Avg.
Blood Clot Prevention and Treatment				
Anticoagulation Overlap Therapy[5]	-	-	90%	93%
ICU Venous Thromboembolism Prophylaxis[5]	-	-	93%	92%
Incidence of Potentially Preventable VTE[5]	-	-	8%	10%
UFH with Dosages/Platelet Monitoring[5]	-	-	96%	97%
Venous Thromboembolism Prophylaxis[5]	-	-	87%	85%
Warfarin Therapy Discharge Instructions[5]	-	-	72%	75%
Chest Pain/Possible Heart Attack Care				
Aspirin Given Within 24 Hours of Arrival	21	100%	96%	96%
Fibrinolytic Meds Within 30 Min. of Arrival[7]	-	-	63%	58%
Average Time to ECG (minutes)	22	4	8	7
Average Time to Transfer (minutes)[7]	-	-	53	60
Children's Asthma Care				
Received Home Management Plan of Care	-	-	-	88%
Received Reliever Medication	-	-	-	100%
Received Systemic Corticosteroids	-	-	-	100%
Emergency Department				
Admittance Decision Time (minutes)[5]	-	-	102	98
Head CT Results Within 45 Min. of Arrival[5]	-	-	54%	57%
Patients Who Left ER Before Being Seen[5]	-	-	2%	2%
Time from ER Arrival to Admit. (minutes)[5]	-	-	288	274
Time from ER Arrival to Discharge (minutes)	266	138	128	134
Time in ER Before Being Evaluated (minutes)	356	10	22	26
Time to Pain Meds for Fractures (minutes)[5]	-	-	55	57
Heart Attack Care				
Aspirin Given at Discharge[5]	-	-	99%	99%
Fibrinolytic Meds Within 30 Min. of Arrival[5]	-	-	20%	54%
PCI Within 90 Minutes of Arrival[5]	-	-	95%	96%
Statin Prescribed at Discharge[5]	-	-	98%	98%
Heart Failure Care				
ACE Inhibitor or ARB for LVSD[3,7]	-	-	96%	97%
Discharge Instructions Given[1,3]	-	-	94%	94%
Evaluation of LVS Function[1,3]	-	-	99%	99%
Medicare Spending				
Medicare Spending per Patient (ratio)	-	-	0.96	0.98
Pneumonia Care				
Appropriate Initial Antibiotic Given[1]	-	-	96%	95%
Blood Culture Timing[1]	-	-	98%	98%
Pregnancy and Delivery Care				
Newborn Deliveries Scheduled Early[5]	-	-	3%	6%
Preventive Care				
Immunization for Influenza[5]	-	-	89%	90%
Immunization for Pneumonia[5]	-	-	90%	92%
Stroke Care				
Anticoagulation Therapy for Atrial Fibrillation[5]	-	-	92%	95%
Antithrombotic Therapy Timing[5]	-	-	97%	98%
Assessed for Rehabilitation[5]	-	-	97%	97%
Discharged on Antithrombotic Therapy[5]	-	-	99%	99%
Discharged on Statin Medication[5]	-	-	94%	94%
Thrombolytic Therapy Timing[5]	-	-	69%	66%
Venous Thromboembolism Prophylaxis[5]	-	-	94%	94%
Written Stroke Educational Materials Given[5]	-	-	87%	88%
Surgical Care Improvement Project				
Appropriate Beta Blocker Usage[5]	-	-	98%	98%
Appropriate VTP Within 24 Hours[5]	-	-	98%	98%
Controlled Postoperative Blood Glucose[5]	-	-	97%	97%
Perioperative Temperature Management[5]	-	-	100%	100%
Prophylactic Antibiotic Selection[5]	-	-	99%	99%
Prophylactic Antibiotic Selection (Outpatient)[5]	-	-	97%	98%
Prophylactic Antibiotic Stopped[5]	-	-	98%	98%
Prophylactic Antibiotic Timing[5]	-	-	98%	99%
Prophylactic Antibiotic Timing (Outpatient)[5]	-	-	97%	98%
Urinary Catheter Removal[5]	-	-	97%	97%
Survey of Patients' Hospital Experiences				
Area Around Room 'Always' Quiet at Night[3,10]	<100	56%	60%	61%
Doctors 'Always' Communicated Well[3,10]	<100	94%	81%	82%
Home Recovery Information Given[3,10]	<100	96%	87%	85%
Hospital Given 9 or 10 on 10 Point Scale[3,10]	<100	72%	71%	71%
Meds 'Always' Explained Before Given[3,10]	<100	74%	64%	64%
Nurses 'Always' Communicated Well[3,10]	<100	89%	80%	79%
Pain 'Always' Well Controlled[3,10]	<100	94%	71%	71%
Room and Bathroom 'Always' Clean[3,10]	<100	82%	73%	73%
Timely Help 'Always' Received[3,10]	<100	100%	70%	68%
Would Definitely Recommend Hospital[3,10]	<100	69%	71%	71%
Use of Medical Imaging				
Cardiac Imaging Stress Test before Surgery[1]	-	-	5.1%	5.3%

NOTE: Hospital profiles are in alphabetical order by state, then city, then hospital within the city; Rankings exclude hospitals with less than 25 cases except for patient surveys which excludes hospitals with less than 100 cases; (a) 100-299 cases; (1) The number of cases/patients is too few to report; (2) Data submitted were based on a sample of cases/patients; (3) Results are based on a shorter time period than required; (4) Data suppressed by CMS for one or more quarters; (5) Results are not available for this reporting period; (6) Fewer than 100 patients completed the HCAHPS survey; (7) No cases met the criteria for this measure; (8) The lower limit of the confidence interval cannot be calculated if the number of observed infections equals zero; (9) No data are available from the state/territory for this reporting period; (10) The scores shown reflect fewer than 50 completed surveys; (11) There were discrepancies in the data collection process; (12) This measure does not apply to this hospital for this reporting period; (13) Results cannot be calculated for this reporting period; (14) The results for this state are combined with nearby states to protect confidentiality; Please refer to the User's Guide for a full explanation of data.

Measure	Cases	This Hosp.	State Avg.	U.S. Avg.
Combination Abdominal CT Scan	69	10.1%	8.7%	10.5%
Combination Brain/Sinus CT Scan	107	0.0%	2.2%	2.7%
Combination Chest CT Scan	71	4.2%	3.6%	2.7%
Follow-up Mammogram/Ultrasound	106	15.1%	8.2%	8.8%
Lumbar Spine MRI for Low Back Pain[7]	-	-	36.9%	37.2%

Pennock Hospital

1009 W Green St
Hastings, MI 49058
Phone: 269-945-3451
E-mail: info@pennockhealth.com
URL: www.pennockhealth.com
Type: Acute Care Hospitals
Emergency Services: Yes
Ownership: Voluntary non-profit - Other
Beds: 88

Key Personnel:
CEO/President. . . . . Sheryl Lewis Blake
Radiology. . . . . Dennis Bruce
Chief of Medical Staff . . . . Matt Garber, MD
Emergency Room . . . . Natalie Goran
Quality Assurance . . . . Carla Neil
Intensive Care Unit. . . . . Diana Overmire
Operating Room. . . . . Diana Overmire
Infection Control. . . . . Jeanne Pugh

Measure	Cases	This Hosp.	State Avg.	U.S. Avg.
Blood Clot Prevention and Treatment				
Anticoagulation Overlap Therapy[2]	19	68%	90%	93%
ICU Venous Thromboembolism Prophylaxis[2]	25	88%	93%	92%
Incidence of Potentially Preventable VTE[1,2]	-	-	8%	10%
UFH with Dosages/Platelet Monitoring[1,2]	-	-	96%	97%
Venous Thromboembolism Prophylaxis[2]	187	83%	87%	85%
Warfarin Therapy Discharge Instructions[2]	15	73%	72%	75%
Chest Pain/Possible Heart Attack Care				
Aspirin Given Within 24 Hours of Arrival	49	96%	96%	96%
Fibrinolytic Meds Within 30 Min. of Arrival[7]	-	-	63%	58%
Average Time to ECG (minutes)	50	7	8	7
Average Time to Transfer (minutes)[1]	-	-	53	60
Children's Asthma Care				
Received Home Management Plan of Care	-	-	-	88%
Received Reliever Medication	-	-	-	100%
Received Systemic Corticosteroids	-	-	-	100%
Emergency Department				
Admittance Decision Time (minutes)[2]	242	50	102	98
Head CT Results Within 45 Min. of Arrival[1,3]	-	-	54%	57%
Patients Who Left ER Before Being Seen	18,102	2%	2%	2%
Time from ER Arrival to Admit. (minutes)[2]	248	246	288	274
Time from ER Arrival to Discharge (minutes)	400	144	128	134
Time in ER Before Being Evaluated (minutes)	417	41	22	26
Time to Pain Meds for Fractures (minutes)	72	48	55	57
Heart Attack Care				
Aspirin Given at Discharge[1]	-	-	99%	99%
Fibrinolytic Meds Within 30 Min. of Arrival[7]	-	-	20%	54%
PCI Within 90 Minutes of Arrival[7]	-	-	95%	96%
Statin Prescribed at Discharge[1]	-	-	98%	98%
Heart Failure Care				
ACE Inhibitor or ARB for LVSD	19	100%	96%	97%
Discharge Instructions Given	57	100%	94%	94%
Evaluation of LVS Function	80	100%	99%	99%
Medicare Spending				
Medicare Spending per Patient (ratio)	-	0.90	0.96	0.98
Pneumonia Care				
Appropriate Initial Antibiotic Given	87	94%	96%	95%
Blood Culture Timing	122	100%	98%	98%
Pregnancy and Delivery Care				
Newborn Deliveries Scheduled Early[2]	13	8%	3%	6%
Preventive Care				
Immunization for Influenza[2]	266	92%	89%	90%
Immunization for Pneumonia[2]	362	95%	90%	92%
Stroke Care				
Anticoagulation Therapy for Atrial Fibrillation[1]	-	-	92%	95%
Antithrombotic Therapy Timing	21	100%	97%	98%
Assessed for Rehabilitation	21	100%	97%	97%
Discharged on Antithrombotic Therapy	21	100%	99%	99%
Discharged on Statin Medication	18	94%	94%	94%
Thrombolytic Therapy Timing[1]	-	-	69%	66%
Venous Thromboembolism Prophylaxis	21	86%	94%	94%
Written Stroke Educational Materials Given[1]	-	-	87%	88%
Surgical Care Improvement Project				
Appropriate Beta Blocker Usage	70	93%	98%	98%
Appropriate VTP Within 24 Hours	248	98%	98%	98%
Controlled Postoperative Blood Glucose[7]	-	-	97%	97%
Perioperative Temperature Management	286	100%	100%	100%
Prophylactic Antibiotic Selection	216	100%	99%	99%
Prophylactic Antibiotic Selection (Outpatient)	72	99%	97%	98%
Prophylactic Antibiotic Stopped	215	97%	98%	98%
Prophylactic Antibiotic Timing	216	100%	98%	99%
Prophylactic Antibiotic Timing (Outpatient)	34	100%	97%	98%
Urinary Catheter Removal	57	96%	97%	97%
Survey of Patients' Hospital Experiences				
Area Around Room 'Always' Quiet at Night	300+	63%	60%	61%
Doctors 'Always' Communicated Well	300+	83%	81%	82%
Home Recovery Information Given	300+	92%	87%	85%
Hospital Given 9 or 10 on 10 Point Scale	300+	74%	71%	71%
Meds 'Always' Explained Before Given	300+	63%	64%	64%
Nurses 'Always' Communicated Well	300+	81%	80%	79%
Pain 'Always' Well Controlled	300+	71%	71%	71%
Room and Bathroom 'Always' Clean	300+	67%	73%	73%
Timely Help 'Always' Received	300+	67%	70%	68%
Would Definitely Recommend Hospital	300+	72%	71%	71%
Use of Medical Imaging				
Cardiac Imaging Stress Test before Surgery	226	7.1%	5.1%	5.3%
Combination Abdominal CT Scan	376	2.7%	8.7%	10.5%
Combination Brain/Sinus CT Scan[1]	-	-	2.2%	2.7%
Combination Chest CT Scan	180	0.6%	3.6%	2.7%
Follow-up Mammogram/Ultrasound	841	8.0%	8.2%	8.8%
Lumbar Spine MRI for Low Back Pain	78	37.2%	36.9%	37.2%

Hillsdale Community Health Center

168 S Howell Street
Hillsdale, MI 49242
Phone: 517-437-4451
URL: www.hchc.com
Type: Acute Care Hospitals
Emergency Services: Yes
Ownership: Government - Federal
Beds: 65

Key Personnel:
Operating Room. . . . . Denise Baker
Emergency Room . . . . Keith Baron, MD
Intensive Care Unit. . . . . Janice Gutowski
Radiology. . . . . Rocky Saenz
Infection Control. . . . . Debra Shatelrow, RN
Chief of Medical Staff . . . . Pat Sudds
Coronary Care . . . . Doris Whorley
Quality Assurance . . . . Doris Whorley, RN

Measure	Cases	This Hosp.	State Avg.	U.S. Avg.
Blood Clot Prevention and Treatment				
Anticoagulation Overlap Therapy[2]	16	38%	90%	93%
ICU Venous Thromboembolism Prophylaxis[2]	26	85%	93%	92%
Incidence of Potentially Preventable VTE[1,2]	-	-	8%	10%
UFH with Dosages/Platelet Monitoring[1,2]	-	-	96%	97%
Venous Thromboembolism Prophylaxis[2]	105	92%	87%	85%
Warfarin Therapy Discharge Instructions[1,2]	-	-	72%	75%
Chest Pain/Possible Heart Attack Care				
Aspirin Given Within 24 Hours of Arrival	89	92%	96%	96%
Fibrinolytic Meds Within 30 Min. of Arrival[1]	-	-	63%	58%
Average Time to ECG (minutes)	93	5	8	7
Average Time to Transfer (minutes)[1]	-	-	53	60
Children's Asthma Care				
Received Home Management Plan of Care	-	-	-	88%
Received Reliever Medication	-	-	-	100%
Received Systemic Corticosteroids	-	-	-	100%
Emergency Department				
Admittance Decision Time (minutes)[2]	395	80	102	98
Head CT Results Within 45 Min. of Arrival[1]	-	-	54%	57%
Patients Who Left ER Before Being Seen	25,643	1%	2%	2%
Time from ER Arrival to Admit. (minutes)[2]	422	234	288	274
Time from ER Arrival to Discharge (minutes)	251	111	128	134
Time in ER Before Being Evaluated (minutes)	340	23	22	26
Time to Pain Meds for Fractures (minutes)	86	64	55	57
Heart Attack Care				
Aspirin Given at Discharge	20	100%	99%	99%
Fibrinolytic Meds Within 30 Min. of Arrival[7]	-	-	20%	54%
PCI Within 90 Minutes of Arrival[7]	-	-	95%	96%
Statin Prescribed at Discharge	16	94%	98%	98%
Heart Failure Care				
ACE Inhibitor or ARB for LVSD	23	91%	96%	97%
Discharge Instructions Given	56	84%	94%	94%
Evaluation of LVS Function	69	100%	99%	99%
Medicare Spending				
Medicare Spending per Patient (ratio)	-	0.99	0.96	0.98
Pneumonia Care				
Appropriate Initial Antibiotic Given	91	97%	96%	95%
Blood Culture Timing	145	100%	98%	98%
Pregnancy and Delivery Care				
Newborn Deliveries Scheduled Early[2]	149	44%	3%	6%
Preventive Care				
Immunization for Influenza[2]	307	99%	89%	90%
Immunization for Pneumonia[2]	490	99%	90%	92%
Stroke Care				
Anticoagulation Therapy for Atrial Fibrillation[1]	-	-	92%	95%
Antithrombotic Therapy Timing	38	92%	97%	98%
Assessed for Rehabilitation	41	90%	97%	97%
Discharged on Antithrombotic Therapy	39	97%	99%	99%
Discharged on Statin Medication	30	83%	94%	94%
Thrombolytic Therapy Timing[1]	-	-	69%	66%
Venous Thromboembolism Prophylaxis	41	85%	94%	94%
Written Stroke Educational Materials Given	18	61%	87%	88%
Surgical Care Improvement Project				
Appropriate Beta Blocker Usage	65	100%	98%	98%
Appropriate VTP Within 24 Hours	203	100%	98%	98%
Controlled Postoperative Blood Glucose[7]	-	-	97%	97%
Perioperative Temperature Management	220	100%	100%	100%
Prophylactic Antibiotic Selection	150	100%	99%	99%
Prophylactic Antibiotic Selection (Outpatient)[3]	12	92%	97%	98%
Prophylactic Antibiotic Stopped	147	99%	98%	98%
Prophylactic Antibiotic Timing	150	100%	98%	99%
Prophylactic Antibiotic Timing (Outpatient)[3]	12	100%	97%	98%
Urinary Catheter Removal	161	96%	97%	97%
Survey of Patients' Hospital Experiences				
Area Around Room 'Always' Quiet at Night	(a)	59%	60%	61%
Doctors 'Always' Communicated Well	(a)	76%	81%	82%
Home Recovery Information Given	(a)	88%	87%	85%
Hospital Given 9 or 10 on 10 Point Scale	(a)	66%	71%	71%
Meds 'Always' Explained Before Given	(a)	62%	64%	64%
Nurses 'Always' Communicated Well	(a)	78%	80%	79%
Pain 'Always' Well Controlled	(a)	68%	71%	71%
Room and Bathroom 'Always' Clean	(a)	73%	73%	73%
Timely Help 'Always' Received	(a)	68%	70%	68%
Would Definitely Recommend Hospital	(a)	59%	71%	71%
Use of Medical Imaging				
Cardiac Imaging Stress Test before Surgery	168	6.5%	5.1%	5.3%
Combination Abdominal CT Scan	509	2.4%	8.7%	10.5%
Combination Brain/Sinus CT Scan	403	2.2%	2.2%	2.7%
Combination Chest CT Scan	377	1.1%	3.6%	2.7%
Follow-up Mammogram/Ultrasound	767	9.3%	8.2%	8.8%
Lumbar Spine MRI for Low Back Pain	99	28.3%	36.9%	37.2%

Holland Community Hospital

602 Michigan Ave
Holland, MI 49423
Phone: 616-392-5141
Fax: 616-394-3572
E-mail: info@hollandhospital.org
URL: www.hoho.org
Type: Acute Care Hospitals
Emergency Services: Yes
Ownership: Voluntary non-profit - Private
Beds: 205

Key Personnel:
Pediatric Ambulatory Care . . . . . . Kathy Austin
Radiology. . . . . Anthony D Barclay
Quality Assurance . . . . Laurel Barens
Operating Room. . . . . James S Ceton, RN
Infection Control. . . . . Theresa Ellis, RN
Patient Relations . . . . Kathy Henry
CEO/President. . . . . Dale Sowders
Chief of Medical Staff . . . . Anthony Yasick, MD

Measure	Cases	This Hosp.	State Avg.	U.S. Avg.
Blood Clot Prevention and Treatment				
Anticoagulation Overlap Therapy[2]	48	100%	90%	93%

NOTE: Hospital profiles are in alphabetical order by state, then city, then hospital within the city; Rankings exclude hospitals with less than 25 cases except for patient surveys which excludes hospitals with less than 100 cases; (a) 100-299 cases; (1) The number of cases/patients is too few to report; (2) Data submitted were based on a sample of cases/patients; (3) Results are based on a shorter time period than required; (4) Data suppressed by CMS for one or more quarters; (5) Results are not available for this reporting period; (6) Fewer than 100 patients completed the HCAHPS survey; (7) No cases met the criteria for this measure; (8) The lower limit of the confidence interval cannot be calculated if the number of observed infections equals zero; (9) No data are available from the state/territory for this reporting period; (10) The scores shown reflect fewer than 50 completed surveys; (11) There were discrepancies in the data collection process; (12) This measure does not apply to this hospital for this reporting period; (13) Results cannot be calculated for this reporting period; (14) The results for this state are combined with nearby states to protect confidentiality; Please refer to the User's Guide for a full explanation of data.

Measure	Cases	This Hosp.	State Avg.	U.S. Avg.
ICU Venous Thromboembolism Prophylaxis[2]	20	100%	93%	92%
Incidence of Potentially Preventable VTE[1,2]	-	-	8%	10%
UFH with Dosages/Platelet Monitoring[2]	39	100%	96%	97%
Venous Thromboembolism Prophylaxis[2]	341	99%	87%	85%
Warfarin Therapy Discharge Instructions[2]	35	100%	72%	75%
Chest Pain/Possible Heart Attack Care				
Aspirin Given Within 24 Hours of Arrival	37	100%	96%	96%
Fibrinolytic Meds Within 30 Min. of Arrival[7]	-	-	63%	58%
Average Time to ECG (minutes)	39	7	8	7
Average Time to Transfer (minutes)[1]	-	-	53	60
Children's Asthma Care				
Received Home Management Plan of Care	-	-	-	88%
Received Reliever Medication	-	-	-	100%
Received Systemic Corticosteroids	-	-	-	100%
Emergency Department				
Admittance Decision Time (minutes)[2]	531	62	102	98
Head CT Results Within 45 Min. of Arrival[1]	-	-	54%	57%
Patients Who Left ER Before Being Seen	44,109	0%	2%	2%
Time from ER Arrival to Admit. (minutes)[2]	534	215	288	274
Time from ER Arrival to Discharge (minutes)	376	122	128	134
Time in ER Before Being Evaluated (minutes)	403	15	22	26
Time to Pain Meds for Fractures (minutes)	230	38	55	57
Heart Attack Care				
Aspirin Given at Discharge	89	100%	99%	99%
Fibrinolytic Meds Within 30 Min. of Arrival[7]	-	-	20%	54%
PCI Within 90 Minutes of Arrival	30	97%	95%	96%
Statin Prescribed at Discharge	83	100%	98%	98%
Heart Failure Care				
ACE Inhibitor or ARB for LVSD	57	100%	96%	97%
Discharge Instructions Given	127	100%	94%	94%
Evaluation of LVS Function	164	100%	99%	99%
Medicare Spending				
Medicare Spending per Patient (ratio)	-	0.92	0.96	0.98
Pneumonia Care				
Appropriate Initial Antibiotic Given	163	99%	96%	95%
Blood Culture Timing	303	100%	98%	98%
Pregnancy and Delivery Care				
Newborn Deliveries Scheduled Early	126	1%	3%	6%
Preventive Care				
Immunization for Influenza[2]	515	99%	89%	90%
Immunization for Pneumonia[2]	561	100%	90%	92%
Stroke Care				
Anticoagulation Therapy for Atrial Fibrillation	17	100%	92%	95%
Antithrombotic Therapy Timing	80	100%	97%	98%
Assessed for Rehabilitation	92	100%	97%	97%
Discharged on Antithrombotic Therapy	87	100%	99%	99%
Discharged on Statin Medication	61	100%	94%	94%
Thrombolytic Therapy Timing[1]	-	-	69%	66%
Venous Thromboembolism Prophylaxis	96	100%	94%	94%
Written Stroke Educational Materials Given	43	100%	87%	88%
Surgical Care Improvement Project				
Appropriate Beta Blocker Usage[2]	222	100%	98%	98%
Appropriate VTP Within 24 Hours[2]	527	100%	98%	98%
Controlled Postoperative Blood Glucose[2,7]	-	-	97%	97%
Perioperative Temperature Management[2]	830	100%	100%	100%
Prophylactic Antibiotic Selection[2]	693	100%	99%	99%
Prophylactic Antibiotic Selection (Outpatient)	453	100%	97%	98%
Prophylactic Antibiotic Stopped[2]	688	100%	98%	98%
Prophylactic Antibiotic Timing[2]	693	100%	98%	99%
Prophylactic Antibiotic Timing (Outpatient)	453	100%	97%	98%
Urinary Catheter Removal[2]	92	100%	97%	97%
Survey of Patients' Hospital Experiences				
Area Around Room 'Always' Quiet at Night	300+	54%	60%	61%
Doctors 'Always' Communicated Well	300+	82%	81%	82%
Home Recovery Information Given	300+	90%	87%	85%
Hospital Given 9 or 10 on 10 Point Scale	300+	77%	71%	71%
Meds 'Always' Explained Before Given	300+	62%	64%	64%
Nurses 'Always' Communicated Well	300+	77%	80%	79%
Pain 'Always' Well Controlled	300+	71%	71%	71%
Room and Bathroom 'Always' Clean	300+	75%	73%	73%
Timely Help 'Always' Received	300+	68%	70%	68%
Would Definitely Recommend Hospital	300+	78%	71%	71%
Use of Medical Imaging				
Cardiac Imaging Stress Test before Surgery	235	5.1%	5.1%	5.3%
Combination Abdominal CT Scan	573	5.9%	8.7%	10.5%
Combination Brain/Sinus CT Scan	677	1.0%	2.2%	2.7%
Combination Chest CT Scan	294	0.7%	3.6%	2.7%
Follow-up Mammogram/Ultrasound	1,367	10.8%	8.2%	8.8%
Lumbar Spine MRI for Low Back Pain	142	42.3%	36.9%	37.2%

Saint Joseph Mercy Livingston Hospital

620 Byron Rd
Howell, MI 48843
Phone: 517-545-6000
Fax: 517-545-6192
URL: www.sjmh.com
Type: Acute Care Hospitals
Emergency Services: Yes
Ownership: Voluntary non-profit - Other
Beds: 136

Key Personnel:
Quality Assurance .... Peggy Casper
Emergency Room .... Pat Claffey, RN
Infection Control............. Charles Craig, MD
CEO/President............. Garry C. Faja
Chief of Medical Staff.......... Charles Kelly, DO
Operating Room............. Joyce Kessler
Intensive Care Unit............ Fran Rocheleau, RN
Radiology.................. Cheryl Rusk, DO

Measure	Cases	This Hosp.	State Avg.	U.S. Avg.
Blood Clot Prevention and Treatment				
Anticoagulation Overlap Therapy[2]	39	95%	90%	93%
ICU Venous Thromboembolism Prophylaxis[2]	22	82%	93%	92%
Incidence of Potentially Preventable VTE[1,2]	-	-	8%	10%
UFH with Dosages/Platelet Monitoring[2]	36	100%	96%	97%
Venous Thromboembolism Prophylaxis[2]	326	92%	87%	85%
Warfarin Therapy Discharge Instructions[2]	36	36%	72%	75%
Chest Pain/Possible Heart Attack Care				
Aspirin Given Within 24 Hours of Arrival	155	92%	96%	96%
Fibrinolytic Meds Within 30 Min. of Arrival[7]	-	-	63%	58%
Average Time to ECG (minutes)	158	6	8	7
Average Time to Transfer (minutes)	23	39	53	60
Children's Asthma Care				
Received Home Management Plan of Care	-	-	-	88%
Received Reliever Medication	-	-	-	100%
Received Systemic Corticosteroids	-	-	-	100%
Emergency Department				
Admittance Decision Time (minutes)[2]	570	92	102	98
Head CT Results Within 45 Min. of Arrival	33	88%	54%	57%
Patients Who Left ER Before Being Seen	47,535	0%	2%	2%
Time from ER Arrival to Admit. (minutes)[2]	578	275	288	274
Time from ER Arrival to Discharge (minutes)	415	119	128	134
Time in ER Before Being Evaluated (minutes)	484	12	22	26
Time to Pain Meds for Fractures (minutes)	174	44	55	57
Heart Attack Care				
Aspirin Given at Discharge[1]	-	-	99%	99%
Fibrinolytic Meds Within 30 Min. of Arrival[7]	-	-	20%	54%
PCI Within 90 Minutes of Arrival[7]	-	-	95%	96%
Statin Prescribed at Discharge[1]	-	-	98%	98%
Heart Failure Care				
ACE Inhibitor or ARB for LVSD	27	100%	96%	97%
Discharge Instructions Given	105	93%	94%	94%
Evaluation of LVS Function	138	100%	99%	99%
Medicare Spending				
Medicare Spending per Patient (ratio)	-	0.94	0.96	0.98
Pneumonia Care				
Appropriate Initial Antibiotic Given	95	97%	96%	95%
Blood Culture Timing	187	97%	98%	98%
Pregnancy and Delivery Care				
Newborn Deliveries Scheduled Early[7]	-	-	3%	6%
Preventive Care				
Immunization for Influenza[2]	403	98%	89%	90%
Immunization for Pneumonia[2]	577	97%	90%	92%
Stroke Care				
Anticoagulation Therapy for Atrial Fibrillation[1,2]	-	-	92%	95%
Antithrombotic Therapy Timing[2]	41	100%	97%	98%
Assessed for Rehabilitation[2]	49	96%	97%	97%
Discharged on Antithrombotic Therapy[2]	49	98%	99%	99%
Discharged on Statin Medication[2]	40	95%	94%	94%
Thrombolytic Therapy Timing[1,2]	-	-	69%	66%
Venous Thromboembolism Prophylaxis[2]	39	95%	94%	94%
Written Stroke Educational Materials Given[2]	35	86%	87%	88%
Surgical Care Improvement Project				
Appropriate Beta Blocker Usage	45	96%	98%	98%
Appropriate VTP Within 24 Hours	129	99%	98%	98%
Controlled Postoperative Blood Glucose[7]	-	-	97%	97%
Perioperative Temperature Management	195	100%	100%	100%
Prophylactic Antibiotic Selection	144	99%	99%	99%
Prophylactic Antibiotic Selection (Outpatient)	44	98%	97%	98%
Prophylactic Antibiotic Stopped	139	99%	98%	98%
Prophylactic Antibiotic Timing	144	99%	98%	99%
Prophylactic Antibiotic Timing (Outpatient)	30	87%	97%	98%
Urinary Catheter Removal	122	98%	97%	97%
Survey of Patients' Hospital Experiences				
Area Around Room 'Always' Quiet at Night	300+	61%	60%	61%
Doctors 'Always' Communicated Well	300+	82%	81%	82%
Home Recovery Information Given	300+	89%	87%	85%
Hospital Given 9 or 10 on 10 Point Scale	300+	69%	71%	71%
Meds 'Always' Explained Before Given	300+	64%	64%	64%
Nurses 'Always' Communicated Well	300+	79%	80%	79%
Pain 'Always' Well Controlled	300+	71%	71%	71%
Room and Bathroom 'Always' Clean	300+	69%	73%	73%
Timely Help 'Always' Received	300+	69%	70%	68%
Would Definitely Recommend Hospital	300+	69%	71%	71%
Use of Medical Imaging				
Cardiac Imaging Stress Test before Surgery	647	3.4%	5.1%	5.3%
Combination Abdominal CT Scan	1,054	4.0%	8.7%	10.5%
Combination Brain/Sinus CT Scan	514	1.2%	2.2%	2.7%
Combination Chest CT Scan	832	3.0%	3.6%	2.7%
Follow-up Mammogram/Ultrasound	1,651	7.4%	8.2%	8.8%
Lumbar Spine MRI for Low Back Pain	175	36.0%	36.9%	37.2%

Sparrow Ionia Hospital

520 E Washington Street
Ionia, MI 48846
Phone: 616-527-4200
Fax: 616-527-5731
E-mail: ltjalsma@ioniahoapitl.org
URL: www.ioniahospital.org
Type: Critical Access Hospitals
Emergency Services: Yes
Ownership: Voluntary non-profit - Private
Beds: 25

Key Personnel:
Patient Relations .... Ricki Burk, BS, RN
Emergency Room .... Doyle Calley, MD
Quality Assurance .... Barb Dora
Radiology.................. Robert Hills
Chief of Medical Staff.......... Amy B Jentz
Infection Control.............. Cheryl Koon, RN
CEO/President................ Bill Roeser

Measure	Cases	This Hosp.	State Avg.	U.S. Avg.
Blood Clot Prevention and Treatment				
Anticoagulation Overlap Therapy[1,2]	-	-	90%	93%
ICU Venous Thromboembolism Prophylaxis[2,7]	-	-	93%	92%
Incidence of Potentially Preventable VTE[2,7]	-	-	8%	10%
UFH with Dosages/Platelet Monitoring[1,2]	-	-	96%	97%
Venous Thromboembolism Prophylaxis[2]	161	83%	87%	85%
Warfarin Therapy Discharge Instructions[1,2]	-	-	72%	75%
Chest Pain/Possible Heart Attack Care				
Aspirin Given Within 24 Hours of Arrival	23	100%	96%	96%
Fibrinolytic Meds Within 30 Min. of Arrival[7]	-	-	63%	58%
Average Time to ECG (minutes)	24	6	8	7
Average Time to Transfer (minutes)[1]	-	-	53	60
Children's Asthma Care				
Received Home Management Plan of Care	-	-	-	88%
Received Reliever Medication	-	-	-	100%
Received Systemic Corticosteroids	-	-	-	100%
Emergency Department				
Admittance Decision Time (minutes)[2]	481	57	102	98
Head CT Results Within 45 Min. of Arrival[5]	-	-	54%	57%
Patients Who Left ER Before Being Seen[5]	-	-	2%	2%
Time from ER Arrival to Admit. (minutes)[2]	495	216	288	274
Time from ER Arrival to Discharge (minutes)	435	96	128	134
Time in ER Before Being Evaluated (minutes)	483	17	22	26
Time to Pain Meds for Fractures (minutes)[3]	49	32	55	57
Heart Attack Care				
Aspirin Given at Discharge[5]	-	-	99%	99%

NOTE: Hospital profiles are in alphabetical order by state, then city, then hospital within the city; Rankings exclude hospitals with less than 25 cases except for patient surveys which excludes hospitals with less than 100 cases; (a) 100-299 cases; (1) The number of cases/patients is too few to report; (2) Data submitted were based on a sample of cases/patients; (3) Results are based on a shorter time period than required; (4) Data suppressed by CMS for one or more quarters; (5) Results are not available for this reporting period; (6) Fewer than 100 patients completed the HCAHPS survey; (7) No cases met the criteria for this measure; (8) The lower limit of the confidence interval cannot be calculated if the number of observed infections equals zero; (9) No data are available from the state/territory for this reporting period; (10) The scores shown reflect fewer than 50 completed surveys; (11) There were discrepancies in the data collection process; (12) This measure does not apply to this hospital for this reporting period; (13) Results cannot be calculated for this reporting period; (14) The results for this state are combined with nearby states to protect confidentiality; Please refer to the User's Guide for a full explanation of data.

Measure	Cases	This Hosp.	State Avg.	U.S. Avg.
Fibrinolytic Meds Within 30 Min. of Arrival[5]	-	-	20%	54%
PCI Within 90 Minutes of Arrival[5]	-	-	95%	96%
Statin Prescribed at Discharge[5]	-	-	98%	98%
Heart Failure Care				
ACE Inhibitor or ARB for LVSD	12	100%	96%	97%
Discharge Instructions Given	17	100%	94%	94%
Evaluation of LVS Function	21	100%	99%	99%
Medicare Spending				
Medicare Spending per Patient (ratio)	-	-	0.96	0.98
Pneumonia Care				
Appropriate Initial Antibiotic Given	34	97%	96%	95%
Blood Culture Timing	42	93%	98%	98%
Pregnancy and Delivery Care				
Newborn Deliveries Scheduled Early[5]	-	-	3%	6%
Preventive Care				
Immunization for Influenza[5]	-	-	89%	90%
Immunization for Pneumonia[5]	-	-	90%	92%
Stroke Care				
Anticoagulation Therapy for Atrial Fibrillation[5]	-	-	92%	95%
Antithrombotic Therapy Timing[5]	-	-	97%	98%
Assessed for Rehabilitation[5]	-	-	97%	97%
Discharged on Antithrombotic Therapy[5]	-	-	99%	99%
Discharged on Statin Medication[5]	-	-	94%	94%
Thrombolytic Therapy Timing[5]	-	-	69%	66%
Venous Thromboembolism Prophylaxis[5]	-	-	94%	94%
Written Stroke Educational Materials Given[5]	-	-	87%	88%
Surgical Care Improvement Project				
Appropriate Beta Blocker Usage[1]	-	-	98%	98%
Appropriate VTP Within 24 Hours	14	93%	98%	98%
Controlled Postoperative Blood Glucose[7]	-	-	97%	97%
Perioperative Temperature Management	16	100%	100%	100%
Prophylactic Antibiotic Selection[1]	-	-	99%	99%
Prophylactic Antibiotic Selection (Outpatient)[3,7]	-	-	97%	98%
Prophylactic Antibiotic Stopped[1]	-	-	98%	98%
Prophylactic Antibiotic Timing[1]	-	-	98%	99%
Prophylactic Antibiotic Timing (Outpatient)[3,7]	-	-	97%	98%
Urinary Catheter Removal[1]	-	-	97%	97%
Survey of Patients' Hospital Experiences				
Area Around Room 'Always' Quiet at Night	(a)	65%	60%	61%
Doctors 'Always' Communicated Well	(a)	80%	81%	82%
Home Recovery Information Given	(a)	91%	87%	85%
Hospital Given 9 or 10 on 10 Point Scale	(a)	75%	71%	71%
Meds 'Always' Explained Before Given	(a)	65%	64%	64%
Nurses 'Always' Communicated Well	(a)	83%	80%	79%
Pain 'Always' Well Controlled	(a)	70%	71%	71%
Room and Bathroom 'Always' Clean	(a)	77%	73%	73%
Timely Help 'Always' Received	(a)	80%	70%	68%
Would Definitely Recommend Hospital	(a)	63%	71%	71%
Use of Medical Imaging				
Cardiac Imaging Stress Test before Surgery	139	7.2%	5.1%	5.3%
Combination Abdominal CT Scan	363	2.2%	8.7%	10.5%
Combination Brain/Sinus CT Scan[1]	-	-	2.2%	2.7%
Combination Chest CT Scan	154	0.0%	3.6%	2.7%
Follow-up Mammogram/Ultrasound	314	8.3%	8.2%	8.8%
Lumbar Spine MRI for Low Back Pain[1]	-	-	36.9%	37.2%

Dickinson County Memorial Hospital

1721 S Stephenson Ave
Iron Mountain, MI 49801
URL: www.dchs.org
Type: Acute Care Hospitals
Ownership: Government - Local

Phone: 906-774-1313
Fax: 906-776-5791
Emergency Services: Yes
Beds: 96

Key Personnel:
Chief of Medical Staff.......... Daniel Benishek
Radiology.................. Kevin Diehl, DO
Cardiology.................. V. Mahadev, MD
Radiology.................. Bayani Manzano, MD
Radiology.................. Louis Mautone, DO
Quality Assurance .... Mark Rossato
Cardiology.................. Clayton Shaker, MD
Cardiology.................. Barbara Washington, MD

Measure	Cases	This Hosp.	State Avg.	U.S. Avg.
Blood Clot Prevention and Treatment				
Anticoagulation Overlap Therapy[2]	19	95%	90%	93%
ICU Venous Thromboembolism Prophylaxis[2]	34	100%	93%	92%
Incidence of Potentially Preventable VTE[1,2]	-	-	8%	10%
UFH with Dosages/Platelet Monitoring[1,2]	-	-	96%	97%
Venous Thromboembolism Prophylaxis[2]	242	95%	87%	85%
Warfarin Therapy Discharge Instructions[2]	18	94%	72%	75%
Chest Pain/Possible Heart Attack Care				
Aspirin Given Within 24 Hours of Arrival	72	99%	96%	96%
Fibrinolytic Meds Within 30 Min. of Arrival[1]	-	-	63%	58%
Average Time to ECG (minutes)	73	10	8	7
Average Time to Transfer (minutes)[1]	-	-	53	60
Children's Asthma Care				
Received Home Management Plan of Care	-	-	-	88%
Received Reliever Medication	-	-	-	100%
Received Systemic Corticosteroids	-	-	-	100%
Emergency Department				
Admittance Decision Time (minutes)[2]	332	68	102	98
Head CT Results Within 45 Min. of Arrival[1]	-	-	54%	57%
Patients Who Left ER Before Being Seen	18,847	1%	2%	2%
Time from ER Arrival to Admit. (minutes)[2]	346	230	288	274
Time from ER Arrival to Discharge (minutes)	381	124	128	134
Time in ER Before Being Evaluated (minutes)	417	27	22	26
Time to Pain Meds for Fractures (minutes)	70	44	55	57
Heart Attack Care				
Aspirin Given at Discharge	19	100%	99%	99%
Fibrinolytic Meds Within 30 Min. of Arrival[7]	-	-	20%	54%
PCI Within 90 Minutes of Arrival[7]	-	-	95%	96%
Statin Prescribed at Discharge	15	93%	98%	98%
Heart Failure Care				
ACE Inhibitor or ARB for LVSD	15	100%	96%	97%
Discharge Instructions Given	72	82%	94%	94%
Evaluation of LVS Function	99	99%	99%	99%
Medicare Spending				
Medicare Spending per Patient (ratio)	-	0.93	0.96	0.98
Pneumonia Care				
Appropriate Initial Antibiotic Given	65	98%	96%	95%
Blood Culture Timing	107	98%	98%	98%
Pregnancy and Delivery Care				
Newborn Deliveries Scheduled Early[2]	31	0%	3%	6%
Preventive Care				
Immunization for Influenza[2]	289	95%	89%	90%
Immunization for Pneumonia[2]	368	98%	90%	92%
Stroke Care				
Anticoagulation Therapy for Atrial Fibrillation[1]	-	-	92%	95%
Antithrombotic Therapy Timing	25	100%	97%	98%
Assessed for Rehabilitation	33	97%	97%	97%
Discharged on Antithrombotic Therapy	29	100%	99%	99%
Discharged on Statin Medication	23	87%	94%	94%
Thrombolytic Therapy Timing[1]	-	-	69%	66%
Venous Thromboembolism Prophylaxis	28	93%	94%	94%
Written Stroke Educational Materials Given	20	80%	87%	88%
Surgical Care Improvement Project				
Appropriate Beta Blocker Usage	66	98%	98%	98%
Appropriate VTP Within 24 Hours	244	99%	98%	98%
Controlled Postoperative Blood Glucose[7]	-	-	97%	97%
Perioperative Temperature Management	280	100%	100%	100%
Prophylactic Antibiotic Selection	217	99%	99%	99%
Prophylactic Antibiotic Selection (Outpatient)	76	100%	97%	98%
Prophylactic Antibiotic Stopped	214	95%	98%	98%
Prophylactic Antibiotic Timing	217	99%	98%	99%
Prophylactic Antibiotic Timing (Outpatient)	64	97%	97%	98%
Urinary Catheter Removal	206	100%	97%	97%
Survey of Patients' Hospital Experiences				
Area Around Room 'Always' Quiet at Night	300+	63%	60%	61%
Doctors 'Always' Communicated Well	300+	82%	81%	82%
Home Recovery Information Given	300+	86%	87%	85%
Hospital Given 9 or 10 on 10 Point Scale	300+	66%	71%	71%
Meds 'Always' Explained Before Given	300+	63%	64%	64%
Nurses 'Always' Communicated Well	300+	79%	80%	79%
Pain 'Always' Well Controlled	300+	73%	71%	71%
Room and Bathroom 'Always' Clean	300+	84%	73%	73%
Timely Help 'Always' Received	300+	69%	70%	68%
Would Definitely Recommend Hospital	300+	63%	71%	71%
Use of Medical Imaging				
Cardiac Imaging Stress Test before Surgery	234	6.4%	5.1%	5.3%
Combination Abdominal CT Scan	549	8.9%	8.7%	10.5%
Combination Brain/Sinus CT Scan	331	0.9%	2.2%	2.7%
Combination Chest CT Scan	409	1.5%	3.6%	2.7%
Follow-up Mammogram/Ultrasound	846	5.9%	8.2%	8.8%
Lumbar Spine MRI for Low Back Pain	161	42.2%	36.9%	37.2%

Iron Mountain MI VA Medical Center

325 East H Street
Iron Mountain, MI 49801
Type: Acute Care - VA
Ownership: Government Federal

Phone: 906-774-3300
Fax: 906-779-3114
Emergency Services: No
Beds: 61

Key Personnel:
Quality Assurance .... Mary Gagala, RN
Operating Room............. Mary L Limback, MD
Chief of Medical Staff .... Gail M. McNutt, MD

Measure	Cases	This Hosp.	State Avg.	U.S. Avg.
Blood Clot Prevention and Treatment				
Anticoagulation Overlap Therapy	-	-	90%	93%
ICU Venous Thromboembolism Prophylaxis	-	-	93%	92%
Incidence of Potentially Preventable VTE	-	-	8%	10%
UFH with Dosages/Platelet Monitoring	-	-	96%	97%
Venous Thromboembolism Prophylaxis	-	-	87%	85%
Warfarin Therapy Discharge Instructions	-	-	72%	75%
Chest Pain/Possible Heart Attack Care				
Aspirin Given Within 24 Hours of Arrival	-	-	96%	96%
Fibrinolytic Meds Within 30 Min. of Arrival	-	-	63%	58%
Average Time to ECG (minutes)	-	-	8	7
Average Time to Transfer (minutes)	-	-	53	60
Children's Asthma Care				
Received Home Management Plan of Care	-	-	-	88%
Received Reliever Medication	-	-	-	100%
Received Systemic Corticosteroids	-	-	-	100%
Emergency Department				
Admittance Decision Time (minutes)	-	-	102	98
Head CT Results Within 45 Min. of Arrival	-	-	54%	57%
Patients Who Left ER Before Being Seen	-	-	2%	2%
Time from ER Arrival to Admit. (minutes)	-	-	288	274
Time from ER Arrival to Discharge (minutes)	-	-	128	134
Time in ER Before Being Evaluated (minutes)	-	-	22	26
Time to Pain Meds for Fractures (minutes)	-	-	55	57
Heart Attack Care				
Aspirin Given at Discharge[1]	-	-	99%	99%
Fibrinolytic Meds Within 30 Min. of Arrival[5]	-	-	20%	54%
PCI Within 90 Minutes of Arrival[5]	-	-	95%	96%
Statin Prescribed at Discharge[1]	-	-	98%	98%
Heart Failure Care				
ACE Inhibitor or ARB for LVSD[1]	11	91%	96%	97%
Discharge Instructions Given	30	87%	94%	94%
Evaluation of LVS Function	36	100%	99%	99%
Medicare Spending				
Medicare Spending per Patient (ratio)	-	-	0.96	0.98
Pneumonia Care				
Appropriate Initial Antibiotic Given[1]	13	92%	96%	95%
Blood Culture Timing	26	100%	98%	98%
Pregnancy and Delivery Care				
Newborn Deliveries Scheduled Early	-	-	3%	6%
Preventive Care				
Immunization for Influenza[5]	-	-	89%	90%
Immunization for Pneumonia[5]	-	-	90%	92%
Stroke Care				
Anticoagulation Therapy for Atrial Fibrillation	-	-	92%	95%
Antithrombotic Therapy Timing	-	-	97%	98%
Assessed for Rehabilitation	-	-	97%	97%
Discharged on Antithrombotic Therapy	-	-	99%	99%
Discharged on Statin Medication	-	-	94%	94%
Thrombolytic Therapy Timing	-	-	69%	66%
Venous Thromboembolism Prophylaxis	-	-	94%	94%
Written Stroke Educational Materials Given	-	-	87%	88%
Surgical Care Improvement Project				
Appropriate Beta Blocker Usage[5]	-	-	98%	98%
Appropriate VTP Within 24 Hours[5]	-	-	98%	98%

NOTE: Hospital profiles are in alphabetical order by state, then city, then hospital within the city; Rankings exclude hospitals with less than 25 cases except for patient surveys which excludes hospitals with less than 100 cases; (a) 100-299 cases; (1) The number of cases/patients is too few to report; (2) Data submitted were based on a sample of cases/patients; (3) Results are based on a shorter time period than required; (4) Data suppressed by CMS for one or more quarters; (5) Results are not available for this reporting period; (6) Fewer than 100 patients completed the HCAHPS survey; (7) No cases met the criteria for this measure; (8) The lower limit of the confidence interval cannot be calculated if the number of observed infections equals zero; (9) No data are available from the state/territory for this reporting period; (10) The scores shown reflect fewer than 50 completed surveys; (11) There were discrepancies in the data collection process; (12) This measure does not apply to this hospital for this reporting period; (13) Results cannot be calculated for this reporting period; (14) The results for this state are combined with nearby states to protect confidentiality; Please refer to the User's Guide for a full explanation of data.

Measure	Cases	This Hosp.	State Avg.	U.S. Avg.
Controlled Postoperative Blood Glucose[5]	-	-	97%	97%
Perioperative Temperature Management[5]	-	-	100%	100%
Prophylactic Antibiotic Selection[5]	-	-	99%	99%
Prophylactic Antibiotic Selection (Outpatient)	-	-	97%	98%
Prophylactic Antibiotic Stopped[5]	-	-	98%	98%
Prophylactic Antibiotic Timing[5]	-	-	98%	99%
Prophylactic Antibiotic Timing (Outpatient)	-	-	97%	98%
Urinary Catheter Removal[5]	-	-	97%	97%
Survey of Patients' Hospital Experiences				
Area Around Room 'Always' Quiet at Night	-	-	60%	61%
Doctors 'Always' Communicated Well	-	-	81%	82%
Home Recovery Information Given	-	-	87%	85%
Hospital Given 9 or 10 on 10 Point Scale	-	-	71%	71%
Meds 'Always' Explained Before Given	-	-	64%	64%
Nurses 'Always' Communicated Well	-	-	80%	79%
Pain 'Always' Well Controlled	-	-	71%	71%
Room and Bathroom 'Always' Clean	-	-	73%	73%
Timely Help 'Always' Received	-	-	70%	68%
Would Definitely Recommend Hospital	-	-	71%	71%
Use of Medical Imaging				
Cardiac Imaging Stress Test before Surgery	-	-	5.1%	5.3%
Combination Abdominal CT Scan	-	-	8.7%	10.5%
Combination Brain/Sinus CT Scan	-	-	2.2%	2.7%
Combination Chest CT Scan	-	-	3.6%	2.7%
Follow-up Mammogram/Ultrasound	-	-	8.2%	8.8%
Lumbar Spine MRI for Low Back Pain	-	-	36.9%	37.2%

Northstar Health System

1400 W Ice Lake Road
Iron River, MI 49935
Phone: 906-265-6121
Fax: 906-265-9793
URL: www.icch.org
Type: Critical Access Hospitals
Emergency Services: Yes
Ownership: Voluntary non-profit - Other
Beds: 67

Key Personnel:
Radiology. Jane Cook
Infection Control. . . . . Carolyn Dunlap
Quality Assurance . . . . Carolyn Dunlap
Emergency Room . . . . James Grebner, MD
CEO/President. . . . . Connie Kououzos
Intensive Care Unit. . . . . Mary Larson
Chief of Medical Staff. . . . . Nasseem Rizkalla
Operating Room. . . . . Jean Stroud

Measure	Cases	This Hosp.	State Avg.	U.S. Avg.
Blood Clot Prevention and Treatment				
Anticoagulation Overlap Therapy[5]	-	-	90%	93%
ICU Venous Thromboembolism Prophylaxis[5]	-	-	93%	92%
Incidence of Potentially Preventable VTE[5]	-	-	8%	10%
UFH with Dosages/Platelet Monitoring[5]	-	-	96%	97%
Venous Thromboembolism Prophylaxis[5]	-	-	87%	85%
Warfarin Therapy Discharge Instructions[5]	-	-	72%	75%
Chest Pain/Possible Heart Attack Care				
Aspirin Given Within 24 Hours of Arrival	42	98%	96%	96%
Fibrinolytic Meds Within 30 Min. of Arrival[1]	-	-	63%	58%
Average Time to ECG (minutes)	42	8	8	7
Average Time to Transfer (minutes)[7]	-	-	53	60
Children's Asthma Care				
Received Home Management Plan of Care	-	-	-	88%
Received Reliever Medication	-	-	-	100%
Received Systemic Corticosteroids	-	-	-	100%
Emergency Department				
Admittance Decision Time (minutes)[5]	-	-	102	98
Head CT Results Within 45 Min. of Arrival[5]	-	-	54%	57%
Patients Who Left ER Before Being Seen[5]	-	-	2%	2%
Time from ER Arrival to Admit. (minutes)[5]	-	-	288	274
Time from ER Arrival to Discharge (minutes)	412	85	128	134
Time in ER Before Being Evaluated (minutes)	390	20	22	26
Time to Pain Meds for Fractures (minutes)[5]	-	-	55	57
Heart Attack Care				
Aspirin Given at Discharge[1]	-	-	99%	99%
Fibrinolytic Meds Within 30 Min. of Arrival[7]	-	-	20%	54%
PCI Within 90 Minutes of Arrival[7]	-	-	95%	96%
Statin Prescribed at Discharge[1]	-	-	98%	98%
Heart Failure Care				
ACE Inhibitor or ARB for LVSD	16	81%	96%	97%
Discharge Instructions Given	26	73%	94%	94%
Evaluation of LVS Function	55	93%	99%	99%
Medicare Spending				
Medicare Spending per Patient (ratio)	-	-	0.96	0.98
Pneumonia Care				
Appropriate Initial Antibiotic Given	15	53%	96%	95%
Blood Culture Timing	43	95%	98%	98%
Pregnancy and Delivery Care				
Newborn Deliveries Scheduled Early[5]	-	-	3%	6%
Preventive Care				
Immunization for Influenza[5]	-	-	89%	90%
Immunization for Pneumonia[5]	-	-	90%	92%
Stroke Care				
Anticoagulation Therapy for Atrial Fibrillation[5]	-	-	92%	95%
Antithrombotic Therapy Timing[5]	-	-	97%	98%
Assessed for Rehabilitation[5]	-	-	97%	97%
Discharged on Antithrombotic Therapy[5]	-	-	99%	99%
Discharged on Statin Medication[5]	-	-	94%	94%
Thrombolytic Therapy Timing[5]	-	-	69%	66%
Venous Thromboembolism Prophylaxis[5]	-	-	94%	94%
Written Stroke Educational Materials Given[5]	-	-	87%	88%
Surgical Care Improvement Project				
Appropriate Beta Blocker Usage[5]	-	-	98%	98%
Appropriate VTP Within 24 Hours[5]	-	-	98%	98%
Controlled Postoperative Blood Glucose[5]	-	-	97%	97%
Perioperative Temperature Management[5]	-	-	100%	100%
Prophylactic Antibiotic Selection[5]	-	-	99%	99%
Prophylactic Antibiotic Selection (Outpatient)[1,3]	-	-	97%	98%
Prophylactic Antibiotic Stopped[5]	-	-	98%	98%
Prophylactic Antibiotic Timing[5]	-	-	98%	99%
Prophylactic Antibiotic Timing (Outpatient)[1,3]	-	-	97%	98%
Urinary Catheter Removal[5]	-	-	97%	97%
Survey of Patients' Hospital Experiences				
Area Around Room 'Always' Quiet at Night[5]	-	-	60%	61%
Doctors 'Always' Communicated Well[5]	-	-	81%	82%
Home Recovery Information Given[5]	-	-	87%	85%
Hospital Given 9 or 10 on 10 Point Scale[5]	-	-	71%	71%
Meds 'Always' Explained Before Given[5]	-	-	64%	64%
Nurses 'Always' Communicated Well[5]	-	-	80%	79%
Pain 'Always' Well Controlled[5]	-	-	71%	71%
Room and Bathroom 'Always' Clean[5]	-	-	73%	73%
Timely Help 'Always' Received[5]	-	-	70%	68%
Would Definitely Recommend Hospital[5]	-	-	71%	71%
Use of Medical Imaging				
Cardiac Imaging Stress Test before Surgery	75	1.3%	5.1%	5.3%
Combination Abdominal CT Scan	217	7.8%	8.7%	10.5%
Combination Brain/Sinus CT Scan[1]	-	-	2.2%	2.7%
Combination Chest CT Scan	127	7.1%	3.6%	2.7%
Follow-up Mammogram/Ultrasound	289	1.0%	8.2%	8.8%
Lumbar Spine MRI for Low Back Pain[1]	-	-	36.9%	37.2%

Aspirus Grand View Hospital

N10561 Grand View Lane
Ironwood, MI 49938
Phone: 906-932-2525
Fax: 906-932-1921
E-mail: rkimmes@gvhs.org
URL: www.gvhs.org
Type: Critical Access Hospitals
Emergency Services: Yes
Ownership: Voluntary non-profit - Private
Beds: 25

Key Personnel:
Emergency Room . . . . Curtis Buchheit, RN
Operating Room. . . . . Sandra Case, RN
Radiology. Jorge E Arsuaga
Chief of Medical Staff. . . . . Jeffrey Edwards, MD
CEO/President. . . . . David Hartberg
Quality Assurance . . . . Judith Holst
Intensive Care Unit. . . . . Julie Monville, RN
Infection Control. . . . . Jean Peterson, RN

Measure	Cases	This Hosp.	State Avg.	U.S. Avg.
Blood Clot Prevention and Treatment				
Anticoagulation Overlap Therapy[5]	-	-	90%	93%
ICU Venous Thromboembolism Prophylaxis[5]	-	-	93%	92%
Incidence of Potentially Preventable VTE[5]	-	-	8%	10%
UFH with Dosages/Platelet Monitoring[5]	-	-	96%	97%
Venous Thromboembolism Prophylaxis[5]	-	-	87%	85%
Warfarin Therapy Discharge Instructions[5]	-	-	72%	75%
Chest Pain/Possible Heart Attack Care				
Aspirin Given Within 24 Hours of Arrival	50	100%	96%	96%
Fibrinolytic Meds Within 30 Min. of Arrival[1]	-	-	63%	58%
Average Time to ECG (minutes)	50	7	8	7
Average Time to Transfer (minutes)[1]	-	-	53	60
Children's Asthma Care				
Received Home Management Plan of Care	-	-	-	88%
Received Reliever Medication	-	-	-	100%
Received Systemic Corticosteroids	-	-	-	100%
Emergency Department				
Admittance Decision Time (minutes)[5]	-	-	102	98
Head CT Results Within 45 Min. of Arrival[5]	-	-	54%	57%
Patients Who Left ER Before Being Seen[5]	-	-	2%	2%
Time from ER Arrival to Admit. (minutes)[5]	-	-	288	274
Time from ER Arrival to Discharge (minutes)[5]	-	-	128	134
Time in ER Before Being Evaluated (minutes)[5]	-	-	22	26
Time to Pain Meds for Fractures (minutes)[5]	-	-	55	57
Heart Attack Care				
Aspirin Given at Discharge[1]	-	-	99%	99%
Fibrinolytic Meds Within 30 Min. of Arrival[7]	-	-	20%	54%
PCI Within 90 Minutes of Arrival[7]	-	-	95%	96%
Statin Prescribed at Discharge[1]	-	-	98%	98%
Heart Failure Care				
ACE Inhibitor or ARB for LVSD[1]	-	-	96%	97%
Discharge Instructions Given	24	100%	94%	94%
Evaluation of LVS Function	36	100%	99%	99%
Medicare Spending				
Medicare Spending per Patient (ratio)	-	-	0.96	0.98
Pneumonia Care				
Appropriate Initial Antibiotic Given	61	85%	96%	95%
Blood Culture Timing	98	99%	98%	98%
Pregnancy and Delivery Care				
Newborn Deliveries Scheduled Early[5]	-	-	3%	6%
Preventive Care				
Immunization for Influenza[5]	-	-	89%	90%
Immunization for Pneumonia[5]	-	-	90%	92%
Stroke Care				
Anticoagulation Therapy for Atrial Fibrillation[5]	-	-	92%	95%
Antithrombotic Therapy Timing[5]	-	-	97%	98%
Assessed for Rehabilitation[5]	-	-	97%	97%
Discharged on Antithrombotic Therapy[5]	-	-	99%	99%
Discharged on Statin Medication[5]	-	-	94%	94%
Thrombolytic Therapy Timing[5]	-	-	69%	66%
Venous Thromboembolism Prophylaxis[5]	-	-	94%	94%
Written Stroke Educational Materials Given[5]	-	-	87%	88%
Surgical Care Improvement Project				
Appropriate Beta Blocker Usage	21	95%	98%	98%
Appropriate VTP Within 24 Hours[3]	23	100%	98%	98%
Controlled Postoperative Blood Glucose[7]	-	-	97%	97%
Perioperative Temperature Management	82	100%	100%	100%
Prophylactic Antibiotic Selection	56	100%	99%	99%
Prophylactic Antibiotic Selection (Outpatient)[1,3]	-	-	97%	98%
Prophylactic Antibiotic Stopped	54	100%	98%	98%
Prophylactic Antibiotic Timing	56	100%	98%	99%
Prophylactic Antibiotic Timing (Outpatient)[1,3]	-	-	97%	98%
Urinary Catheter Removal	46	98%	97%	97%
Survey of Patients' Hospital Experiences				
Area Around Room 'Always' Quiet at Night	(a)	63%	60%	61%
Doctors 'Always' Communicated Well	(a)	83%	81%	82%
Home Recovery Information Given	(a)	87%	87%	85%
Hospital Given 9 or 10 on 10 Point Scale	(a)	60%	71%	71%
Meds 'Always' Explained Before Given	(a)	59%	64%	64%
Nurses 'Always' Communicated Well	(a)	75%	80%	79%
Pain 'Always' Well Controlled	(a)	72%	71%	71%
Room and Bathroom 'Always' Clean	(a)	65%	73%	73%
Timely Help 'Always' Received	(a)	71%	70%	68%
Would Definitely Recommend Hospital	(a)	59%	71%	71%
Use of Medical Imaging				
Cardiac Imaging Stress Test before Surgery	108	6.5%	5.1%	5.3%
Combination Abdominal CT Scan	275	2.2%	8.7%	10.5%
Combination Brain/Sinus CT Scan[1]	-	-	2.2%	2.7%

NOTE: Hospital profiles are in alphabetical order by state, then city, then hospital within the city; Rankings exclude hospitals with less than 25 cases except for patient surveys which excludes hospitals with less than 100 cases; (a) 100-299 cases; (1) The number of cases/patients is too few to report; (2) Data submitted were based on a sample of cases/patients; (3) Results are based on a shorter time period than required; (4) Data suppressed by CMS for one or more quarters; (5) Results are not available for this reporting period; (6) Fewer than 100 patients completed the HCAHPS survey; (7) No cases met the criteria for this measure; (8) The lower limit of the confidence interval cannot be calculated if the number of observed infections equals zero; (9) No data are available from the state/territory for this reporting period; (10) The scores shown reflect fewer than 50 completed surveys; (11) There were discrepancies in the data collection process; (12) This measure does not apply to this hospital for this reporting period; (13) Results cannot be calculated for this reporting period; (14) The results for this state are combined with nearby states to protect confidentiality; Please refer to the User's Guide for a full explanation of data.

Combination Chest CT Scan	147	1.4%	3.6%	2.7%
Follow-up Mammogram/Ultrasound	303	20.5%	8.2%	8.8%
Lumbar Spine MRI for Low Back Pain	35	45.7%	36.9%	37.2%

Bell Hospital

901 Lakeshore Drive
Ishpeming, MI 49849
E-mail: dedwards@bellmi.org
URL: www.bellhospital.org
Type: Critical Access Hospitals
Ownership: Voluntary non-profit - Private
Phone: 906-486-4431
Fax: 906-485-2136
Emergency Services: Yes
Beds: 69

Key Personnel:
Radiology . . . . Todd Bostwick, MD
Hemotology Center . . . . Cathleen Chen, MD
Quality Assurance . . . . Teresa Howell, RN
Pediatric In-Patient Care . . . . Dr Kurt Lehmann
Radiology . . . . Paul Lyle
Cardiology . . . . David A Pesola, MD, FACC
Anesthesiology. . . . . Joel Slade, MD
Patient Relations . . . . Peg Strickle

Measure	Cases	This Hosp.	State Avg.	U.S. Avg.
Blood Clot Prevention and Treatment				
Anticoagulation Overlap Therapy[5]	-	-	90%	93%
ICU Venous Thromboembolism Prophylaxis[5]	-	-	93%	92%
Incidence of Potentially Preventable VTE[5]	-	-	8%	10%
UFH with Dosages/Platelet Monitoring[5]	-	-	96%	97%
Venous Thromboembolism Prophylaxis[5]	-	-	87%	85%
Warfarin Therapy Discharge Instructions[5]	-	-	72%	75%
Chest Pain/Possible Heart Attack Care				
Aspirin Given Within 24 Hours of Arrival	27	96%	96%	96%
Fibrinolytic Meds Within 30 Min. of Arrival[1]	-	-	63%	58%
Average Time to ECG (minutes)	27	12	8	7
Average Time to Transfer (minutes)[1]	-	-	53	60
Children's Asthma Care				
Received Home Management Plan of Care	-	-	-	88%
Received Reliever Medication	-	-	-	100%
Received Systemic Corticosteroids	-	-	-	100%
Emergency Department				
Admittance Decision Time (minutes)[2]	105	55	102	98
Head CT Results Within 45 Min. of Arrival[1]	-	-	54%	57%
Patients Who Left ER Before Being Seen[5]	-	-	2%	2%
Time from ER Arrival to Admit. (minutes)[2]	114	246	288	274
Time from ER Arrival to Discharge (minutes)	986	103	128	134
Time in ER Before Being Evaluated (minutes)	579	28	22	26
Time to Pain Meds for Fractures (minutes)	28	59	55	57
Heart Attack Care				
Aspirin Given at Discharge[1]	-	-	99%	99%
Fibrinolytic Meds Within 30 Min. of Arrival[7]	-	-	20%	54%
PCI Within 90 Minutes of Arrival[7]	-	-	95%	96%
Statin Prescribed at Discharge[1]	-	-	98%	98%
Heart Failure Care				
ACE Inhibitor or ARB for LVSD[1]	-	-	96%	97%
Discharge Instructions Given[1]	-	-	94%	94%
Evaluation of LVS Function[1]	-	-	99%	99%
Medicare Spending				
Medicare Spending per Patient (ratio)	-	-	0.96	0.98
Pneumonia Care				
Appropriate Initial Antibiotic Given	34	91%	96%	95%
Blood Culture Timing	56	98%	98%	98%
Pregnancy and Delivery Care				
Newborn Deliveries Scheduled Early[5]	-	-	3%	6%
Preventive Care				
Immunization for Influenza[5]	-	-	89%	90%
Immunization for Pneumonia[5]	-	-	90%	92%
Stroke Care				
Anticoagulation Therapy for Atrial Fibrillation[5]	-	-	92%	95%
Antithrombotic Therapy Timing[5]	-	-	97%	98%
Assessed for Rehabilitation[5]	-	-	97%	97%
Discharged on Antithrombotic Therapy[5]	-	-	99%	99%
Discharged on Statin Medication[5]	-	-	94%	94%
Thrombolytic Therapy Timing[5]	-	-	69%	66%
Venous Thromboembolism Prophylaxis[5]	-	-	94%	94%
Written Stroke Educational Materials Given[5]	-	-	87%	88%
Surgical Care Improvement Project				
Appropriate Beta Blocker Usage[2]	40	100%	98%	98%
Appropriate VTP Within 24 Hours[2]	133	96%	98%	98%
Controlled Postoperative Blood Glucose[2,7]	-	-	97%	97%
Perioperative Temperature Management[2]	201	100%	100%	100%
Prophylactic Antibiotic Selection[2]	167	99%	99%	99%
Prophylactic Antibiotic Selection (Outpatient)	70	91%	97%	98%
Prophylactic Antibiotic Stopped[2]	167	98%	98%	98%
Prophylactic Antibiotic Timing[2]	167	98%	98%	99%
Prophylactic Antibiotic Timing (Outpatient)	42	98%	97%	98%
Urinary Catheter Removal[2]	41	100%	97%	97%
Survey of Patients' Hospital Experiences				
Area Around Room 'Always' Quiet at Night[5]	-	-	60%	61%
Doctors 'Always' Communicated Well[5]	-	-	81%	82%
Home Recovery Information Given[5]	-	-	87%	85%
Hospital Given 9 or 10 on 10 Point Scale[5]	-	-	71%	71%
Meds 'Always' Explained Before Given[5]	-	-	64%	64%
Nurses 'Always' Communicated Well[5]	-	-	80%	79%
Pain 'Always' Well Controlled[5]	-	-	71%	71%
Room and Bathroom 'Always' Clean[5]	-	-	73%	73%
Timely Help 'Always' Received[5]	-	-	70%	68%
Would Definitely Recommend Hospital[5]	-	-	71%	71%
Use of Medical Imaging				
Cardiac Imaging Stress Test before Surgery	85	4.7%	5.1%	5.3%
Combination Abdominal CT Scan	184	41.8%	8.7%	10.5%
Combination Brain/Sinus CT Scan[1]	-	-	2.2%	2.7%
Combination Chest CT Scan	72	5.6%	3.6%	2.7%
Follow-up Mammogram/Ultrasound	603	3.2%	8.2%	8.8%
Lumbar Spine MRI for Low Back Pain	36	44.4%	36.9%	37.2%

Allegiance Health

205 N East Ave
Jackson, MI 49201
URL: www.footehealth.org
Type: Acute Care Hospitals
Ownership: Voluntary non-profit - Other
Phone: 517-788-4800
Fax: 517-788-4829
Emergency Services: Yes
Beds: 411

Key Personnel:
President . . . . Georgia Fojtasek, RN, EdD
Patient Relations . . . . Jacalyn Liebowitz, RN
Chief of Medical Staff . . . . John Mogerman, MD
Chairman/CEO . . . . Larry Schultz

Measure	Cases	This Hosp.	State Avg.	U.S. Avg.
Blood Clot Prevention and Treatment				
Anticoagulation Overlap Therapy[2]	127	96%	90%	93%
ICU Venous Thromboembolism Prophylaxis[2]	35	94%	93%	92%
Incidence of Potentially Preventable VTE[2]	13	8%	8%	10%
UFH with Dosages/Platelet Monitoring[2]	164	98%	96%	97%
Venous Thromboembolism Prophylaxis[2]	365	88%	87%	85%
Warfarin Therapy Discharge Instructions[2]	102	71%	72%	75%
Chest Pain/Possible Heart Attack Care				
Aspirin Given Within 24 Hours of Arrival	29	93%	96%	96%
Fibrinolytic Meds Within 30 Min. of Arrival[3,7]	-	-	63%	58%
Average Time to ECG (minutes)	29	9	8	7
Average Time to Transfer (minutes)[3,7]	-	-	53	60
Children's Asthma Care				
Received Home Management Plan of Care	-	-	-	88%
Received Reliever Medication	-	-	-	100%
Received Systemic Corticosteroids	-	-	-	100%
Emergency Department				
Admittance Decision Time (minutes)[2]	781	105	102	98
Head CT Results Within 45 Min. of Arrival	18	56%	54%	57%
Patients Who Left ER Before Being Seen	81,072	1%	2%	2%
Time from ER Arrival to Admit. (minutes)[2]	784	302	288	274
Time from ER Arrival to Discharge (minutes)	394	165	128	134
Time in ER Before Being Evaluated (minutes)	414	36	22	26
Time to Pain Meds for Fractures (minutes)	217	57	55	57
Heart Attack Care				
Aspirin Given at Discharge[2]	314	99%	99%	99%
Fibrinolytic Meds Within 30 Min. of Arrival[2,7]	-	-	20%	54%
PCI Within 90 Minutes of Arrival[2]	63	95%	95%	96%
Statin Prescribed at Discharge[2]	287	98%	98%	98%
Heart Failure Care				
ACE Inhibitor or ARB for LVSD[2]	86	93%	96%	97%
Discharge Instructions Given[2]	287	86%	94%	94%
Evaluation of LVS Function[2]	353	100%	99%	99%
Medicare Spending				
Medicare Spending per Patient (ratio)	-	0.97	0.96	0.98
Pneumonia Care				
Appropriate Initial Antibiotic Given[2]	105	98%	96%	95%
Blood Culture Timing[2]	139	99%	98%	98%
Pregnancy and Delivery Care				
Newborn Deliveries Scheduled Early[2]	37	3%	3%	6%
Preventive Care				
Immunization for Influenza[2]	558	91%	89%	90%
Immunization for Pneumonia[2]	708	92%	90%	92%
Stroke Care				
Anticoagulation Therapy for Atrial Fibrillation[2]	15	93%	92%	95%
Antithrombotic Therapy Timing[2]	97	97%	97%	98%
Assessed for Rehabilitation[2]	114	98%	97%	97%
Discharged on Antithrombotic Therapy[2]	99	100%	99%	99%
Discharged on Statin Medication[2]	76	93%	94%	94%
Thrombolytic Therapy Timing[1,2]	-	-	69%	66%
Venous Thromboembolism Prophylaxis[2]	119	94%	94%	94%
Written Stroke Educational Materials Given[2]	58	88%	87%	88%
Surgical Care Improvement Project				
Appropriate Beta Blocker Usage[2]	249	99%	98%	98%
Appropriate VTP Within 24 Hours[2]	428	100%	98%	98%
Controlled Postoperative Blood Glucose[2]	105	99%	97%	97%
Perioperative Temperature Management[2]	519	100%	100%	100%
Prophylactic Antibiotic Selection[2]	442	100%	99%	99%
Prophylactic Antibiotic Selection (Outpatient)	483	99%	97%	98%
Prophylactic Antibiotic Stopped[2]	434	99%	98%	98%
Prophylactic Antibiotic Timing[2]	442	99%	98%	99%
Prophylactic Antibiotic Timing (Outpatient)	474	100%	97%	98%
Urinary Catheter Removal[2]	210	100%	97%	97%
Survey of Patients' Hospital Experiences				
Area Around Room 'Always' Quiet at Night	300+	51%	60%	61%
Doctors 'Always' Communicated Well	300+	75%	81%	82%
Home Recovery Information Given	300+	85%	87%	85%
Hospital Given 9 or 10 on 10 Point Scale	300+	64%	71%	71%
Meds 'Always' Explained Before Given	300+	62%	64%	64%
Nurses 'Always' Communicated Well	300+	77%	80%	79%
Pain 'Always' Well Controlled	300+	66%	71%	71%
Room and Bathroom 'Always' Clean	300+	66%	73%	73%
Timely Help 'Always' Received	300+	66%	70%	68%
Would Definitely Recommend Hospital	300+	63%	71%	71%
Use of Medical Imaging				
Cardiac Imaging Stress Test before Surgery	1,069	3.8%	5.1%	5.3%
Combination Abdominal CT Scan	1,806	5.1%	8.7%	10.5%
Combination Brain/Sinus CT Scan	1,348	1.2%	2.2%	2.7%
Combination Chest CT Scan	1,463	0.0%	3.6%	2.7%
Follow-up Mammogram/Ultrasound	3,420	3.8%	8.2%	8.8%
Lumbar Spine MRI for Low Back Pain	380	35.3%	36.9%	37.2%

Borgess Medical Center

1521 Gull Road
Kalamazoo, MI 49048
URL: www.borgess.com
Type: Acute Care Hospitals
Ownership: Voluntary non-profit - Other
Phone: 269-226-7000
Fax: 269-226-5966
Emergency Services: Yes
Beds: 424

Key Personnel:
Quality Assurance . . . . Jan Anderson
Cardiac Laboratory. . . . . Sharon Bedecsll, MD
Pediatric In-Patient Care . . . . Kathy Hornbeck, RN
Coronary Care . . . . Steve Marzloff
Infection Control. . . . . Karen Miller
Operating Room. . . . . Rand O'Leary
Chief of Medical Staff . . . . Dale Rowe, MD
CEO/President. . . . . Paul Spaude

Measure	Cases	This Hosp.	State Avg.	U.S. Avg.
Blood Clot Prevention and Treatment				
Anticoagulation Overlap Therapy[2]	137	99%	90%	93%
ICU Venous Thromboembolism Prophylaxis[2]	62	98%	93%	92%
Incidence of Potentially Preventable VTE[2]	18	0%	8%	10%
UFH with Dosages/Platelet Monitoring[2]	140	100%	96%	97%
Venous Thromboembolism Prophylaxis[2]	331	77%	87%	85%
Warfarin Therapy Discharge Instructions[2]	101	74%	72%	75%
Chest Pain/Possible Heart Attack Care				

NOTE: Hospital profiles are in alphabetical order by state, then city, then hospital within the city; Rankings exclude hospitals with less than 25 cases except for patient surveys which excludes hospitals with less than 100 cases; (a) 100-299 cases; (1) The number of cases/patients is too few to report; (2) Data submitted were based on a sample of cases/patients; (3) Results are based on a shorter time period than required; (4) Data suppressed by CMS for one or more quarters; (5) Results are not available for this reporting period; (6) Fewer than 100 patients completed the HCAHPS survey; (7) No cases met the criteria for this measure; (8) The lower limit of the confidence interval cannot be calculated if the number of observed infections equals zero; (9) No data are available from the state/territory for this reporting period; (10) The scores shown reflect fewer than 50 completed surveys; (11) There were discrepancies in the data collection process; (12) This measure does not apply to this hospital for this reporting period; (13) Results cannot be calculated for this reporting period; (14) The results for this state are combined with nearby states to protect confidentiality; Please refer to the User's Guide for a full explanation of data.

Measure	Cases	This Hosp.	State Avg.	U.S. Avg.
Aspirin Given Within 24 Hours of Arrival[1,3]	-	-	96%	96%
Fibrinolytic Meds Within 30 Min. of Arrival[5]	-	-	63%	58%
Average Time to ECG (minutes)[1,3]	-	-	8	7
Average Time to Transfer (minutes)[5]	-	-	53	60
Children's Asthma Care				
Received Home Management Plan of Care	-	-	-	88%
Received Reliever Medication	-	-	-	100%
Received Systemic Corticosteroids	-	-	-	100%
Emergency Department				
Admittance Decision Time (minutes)[2]	506	144	102	98
Head CT Results Within 45 Min. of Arrival[1]	-	-	54%	57%
Patients Who Left ER Before Being Seen	55,230	2%	2%	2%
Time from ER Arrival to Admit. (minutes)[2]	510	302	288	274
Time from ER Arrival to Discharge (minutes)	517	153	128	134
Time in ER Before Being Evaluated (minutes)	597	20	22	26
Time to Pain Meds for Fractures (minutes)	130	64	55	57
Heart Attack Care				
Aspirin Given at Discharge	649	98%	99%	99%
Fibrinolytic Meds Within 30 Min. of Arrival[7]	-	-	20%	54%
PCI Within 90 Minutes of Arrival	68	96%	95%	96%
Statin Prescribed at Discharge	626	99%	98%	98%
Heart Failure Care				
ACE Inhibitor or ARB for LVSD	150	99%	96%	97%
Discharge Instructions Given	433	100%	94%	94%
Evaluation of LVS Function	533	99%	99%	99%
Medicare Spending				
Medicare Spending per Patient (ratio)	-	0.93	0.96	0.98
Pneumonia Care				
Appropriate Initial Antibiotic Given[2]	132	98%	96%	95%
Blood Culture Timing[2]	269	97%	98%	98%
Pregnancy and Delivery Care				
Newborn Deliveries Scheduled Early[1,2]	-	-	3%	6%
Preventive Care				
Immunization for Influenza[2]	553	92%	89%	90%
Immunization for Pneumonia[2]	777	91%	90%	92%
Stroke Care				
Anticoagulation Therapy for Atrial Fibrillation[1,2]	-	-	92%	95%
Antithrombotic Therapy Timing[2]	58	97%	97%	98%
Assessed for Rehabilitation[2]	80	91%	97%	97%
Discharged on Antithrombotic Therapy[2]	69	100%	99%	99%
Discharged on Statin Medication[2]	57	100%	94%	94%
Thrombolytic Therapy Timing[1,2]	-	-	69%	66%
Venous Thromboembolism Prophylaxis[2]	80	91%	94%	94%
Written Stroke Educational Materials Given[2]	49	90%	87%	88%
Surgical Care Improvement Project				
Appropriate Beta Blocker Usage[2]	277	99%	98%	98%
Appropriate VTP Within 24 Hours[2]	255	93%	98%	98%
Controlled Postoperative Blood Glucose[2]	247	98%	97%	97%
Perioperative Temperature Management[2]	418	100%	100%	100%
Prophylactic Antibiotic Selection[2]	521	100%	99%	99%
Prophylactic Antibiotic Selection (Outpatient)	897	99%	97%	98%
Prophylactic Antibiotic Stopped[2]	505	99%	98%	98%
Prophylactic Antibiotic Timing[2]	526	99%	98%	99%
Prophylactic Antibiotic Timing (Outpatient)	899	99%	97%	98%
Urinary Catheter Removal[2]	336	98%	97%	97%
Survey of Patients' Hospital Experiences				
Area Around Room 'Always' Quiet at Night	300+	56%	60%	61%
Doctors 'Always' Communicated Well	300+	78%	81%	82%
Home Recovery Information Given	300+	86%	87%	85%
Hospital Given 9 or 10 on 10 Point Scale	300+	73%	71%	71%
Meds 'Always' Explained Before Given	300+	56%	64%	64%
Nurses 'Always' Communicated Well	300+	80%	80%	79%
Pain 'Always' Well Controlled	300+	71%	71%	71%
Room and Bathroom 'Always' Clean	300+	66%	73%	73%
Timely Help 'Always' Received	300+	60%	70%	68%
Would Definitely Recommend Hospital	300+	75%	71%	71%
Use of Medical Imaging				
Cardiac Imaging Stress Test before Surgery	1,587	3.4%	5.1%	5.3%
Combination Abdominal CT Scan	1,220	6.7%	8.7%	10.5%
Combination Brain/Sinus CT Scan	757	2.4%	2.2%	2.7%
Combination Chest CT Scan	841	3.8%	3.6%	2.7%
Follow-up Mammogram/Ultrasound	2,364	7.7%	8.2%	8.8%
Lumbar Spine MRI for Low Back Pain	620	36.3%	36.9%	37.2%

Bronson Methodist Hospital

601 John Street 42
Kalamazoo, MI 49007
Phone: 269-341-6000
Fax: 269-341-8696
E-mail: bennettk@bronsonhg.org
URL: www.bronsonhealth.com
Type: Acute Care Hospitals
Emergency Services: Yes
Ownership: Voluntary non-profit - Private
Beds: 343

Key Personnel:
Patient Relations . . . . Katie Harrelson, RN MSA
Quality Assurance . . . . Cheryl L Knapp
Chief of Medical Staff . . . . Scott D. Larson, MD
CEO/President . . . . Frank J Sardone
Ambulatory Care . . . . Brook Ward

Measure	Cases	This Hosp.	State Avg.	U.S. Avg.
Blood Clot Prevention and Treatment				
Anticoagulation Overlap Therapy[2]	176	89%	90%	93%
ICU Venous Thromboembolism Prophylaxis[2]	65	71%	93%	92%
Incidence of Potentially Preventable VTE[2]	38	18%	8%	10%
UFH with Dosages/Platelet Monitoring[2]	184	69%	96%	97%
Venous Thromboembolism Prophylaxis[2]	362	80%	87%	85%
Warfarin Therapy Discharge Instructions[2]	133	90%	72%	75%
Chest Pain/Possible Heart Attack Care				
Aspirin Given Within 24 Hours of Arrival[5]	-	-	96%	96%
Fibrinolytic Meds Within 30 Min. of Arrival[5]	-	-	63%	58%
Average Time to ECG (minutes)[5]	-	-	8	7
Average Time to Transfer (minutes)[5]	-	-	53	60
Children's Asthma Care				
Received Home Management Plan of Care	74	96%	-	88%
Received Reliever Medication	75	100%	-	100%
Received Systemic Corticosteroids	75	100%	-	100%
Emergency Department				
Admittance Decision Time (minutes)[2]	482	120	102	98
Head CT Results Within 45 Min. of Arrival	13	0%	54%	57%
Patients Who Left ER Before Being Seen	94,713	1%	2%	2%
Time from ER Arrival to Admit. (minutes)[2]	504	314	288	274
Time from ER Arrival to Discharge (minutes)	450	141	128	134
Time in ER Before Being Evaluated (minutes)	375	28	22	26
Time to Pain Meds for Fractures (minutes)	410	66	55	57
Heart Attack Care				
Aspirin Given at Discharge	391	99%	99%	99%
Fibrinolytic Meds Within 30 Min. of Arrival[7]	-	-	20%	54%
PCI Within 90 Minutes of Arrival	71	94%	95%	96%
Statin Prescribed at Discharge	368	98%	98%	98%
Heart Failure Care				
ACE Inhibitor or ARB for LVSD	130	89%	96%	97%
Discharge Instructions Given	398	85%	94%	94%
Evaluation of LVS Function	464	100%	99%	99%
Medicare Spending				
Medicare Spending per Patient (ratio)	-	0.93	0.96	0.98
Pneumonia Care				
Appropriate Initial Antibiotic Given	227	97%	96%	95%
Blood Culture Timing	404	98%	98%	98%
Pregnancy and Delivery Care				
Newborn Deliveries Scheduled Early	208	0%	3%	6%
Preventive Care				
Immunization for Influenza[2]	650	86%	89%	90%
Immunization for Pneumonia[2]	673	88%	90%	92%
Stroke Care				
Anticoagulation Therapy for Atrial Fibrillation	34	100%	92%	95%
Antithrombotic Therapy Timing	214	96%	97%	98%
Assessed for Rehabilitation	311	97%	97%	97%
Discharged on Antithrombotic Therapy	256	98%	99%	99%
Discharged on Statin Medication	204	98%	94%	94%
Thrombolytic Therapy Timing	32	88%	69%	66%
Venous Thromboembolism Prophylaxis	319	95%	94%	94%
Written Stroke Educational Materials Given	172	97%	87%	88%
Surgical Care Improvement Project				
Appropriate Beta Blocker Usage[2]	481	99%	98%	98%
Appropriate VTP Within 24 Hours[2]	968	95%	98%	98%
Controlled Postoperative Blood Glucose[2]	210	99%	97%	97%
Perioperative Temperature Management[2]	1,150	100%	100%	100%
Prophylactic Antibiotic Selection[2]	1,060	99%	99%	99%
Prophylactic Antibiotic Selection (Outpatient)	732	98%	97%	98%
Prophylactic Antibiotic Stopped[2]	1,038	98%	98%	98%
Prophylactic Antibiotic Timing[2]	1,062	100%	98%	99%
Prophylactic Antibiotic Timing (Outpatient)	737	98%	97%	98%
Urinary Catheter Removal[2]	655	95%	97%	97%
Survey of Patients' Hospital Experiences				
Area Around Room 'Always' Quiet at Night	300+	58%	60%	61%
Doctors 'Always' Communicated Well	300+	82%	81%	82%
Home Recovery Information Given	300+	89%	87%	85%
Hospital Given 9 or 10 on 10 Point Scale	300+	82%	71%	71%
Meds 'Always' Explained Before Given	300+	65%	64%	64%
Nurses 'Always' Communicated Well	300+	81%	80%	79%
Pain 'Always' Well Controlled	300+	72%	71%	71%
Room and Bathroom 'Always' Clean	300+	74%	73%	73%
Timely Help 'Always' Received	300+	69%	70%	68%
Would Definitely Recommend Hospital	300+	85%	71%	71%
Use of Medical Imaging				
Cardiac Imaging Stress Test before Surgery	1,194	4.7%	5.1%	5.3%
Combination Abdominal CT Scan	1,126	3.9%	8.7%	10.5%
Combination Brain/Sinus CT Scan	1,191	2.2%	2.2%	2.7%
Combination Chest CT Scan	508	0.0%	3.6%	2.7%
Follow-up Mammogram/Ultrasound	1,768	5.3%	8.2%	8.8%
Lumbar Spine MRI for Low Back Pain	164	33.5%	36.9%	37.2%

Kalkaska Memorial Health Center

419 S Coral
Kalkaska, MI 49646
Phone: 231-258-7500
Type: Critical Access Hospitals
Emergency Services: Yes
Ownership: Govt - Hospital Dist/Auth

Measure	Cases	This Hosp.	State Avg.	U.S. Avg.
Blood Clot Prevention and Treatment				
Anticoagulation Overlap Therapy[5]	-	-	90%	93%
ICU Venous Thromboembolism Prophylaxis[5]	-	-	93%	92%
Incidence of Potentially Preventable VTE[5]	-	-	8%	10%
UFH with Dosages/Platelet Monitoring[5]	-	-	96%	97%
Venous Thromboembolism Prophylaxis[5]	-	-	87%	85%
Warfarin Therapy Discharge Instructions[5]	-	-	72%	75%
Chest Pain/Possible Heart Attack Care				
Aspirin Given Within 24 Hours of Arrival	68	100%	96%	96%
Fibrinolytic Meds Within 30 Min. of Arrival[1]	-	-	63%	58%
Average Time to ECG (minutes)	72	3	8	7
Average Time to Transfer (minutes)[7]	-	-	53	60
Children's Asthma Care				
Received Home Management Plan of Care	-	-	-	88%
Received Reliever Medication	-	-	-	100%
Received Systemic Corticosteroids	-	-	-	100%
Emergency Department				
Admittance Decision Time (minutes)[5]	-	-	102	98
Head CT Results Within 45 Min. of Arrival[5]	-	-	54%	57%
Patients Who Left ER Before Being Seen[5]	-	-	2%	2%
Time from ER Arrival to Admit. (minutes)[5]	-	-	288	274
Time from ER Arrival to Discharge (minutes)	465	96	128	134
Time in ER Before Being Evaluated (minutes)	534	18	22	26
Time to Pain Meds for Fractures (minutes)[5]	-	-	55	57
Heart Attack Care				
Aspirin Given at Discharge[5]	-	-	99%	99%
Fibrinolytic Meds Within 30 Min. of Arrival[5]	-	-	20%	54%
PCI Within 90 Minutes of Arrival[5]	-	-	95%	96%
Statin Prescribed at Discharge[5]	-	-	98%	98%
Heart Failure Care				
ACE Inhibitor or ARB for LVSD[3,7]	-	-	96%	97%
Discharge Instructions Given[3,7]	-	-	94%	94%
Evaluation of LVS Function[3,7]	-	-	99%	99%
Medicare Spending				
Medicare Spending per Patient (ratio)	-	-	0.96	0.98
Pneumonia Care				
Appropriate Initial Antibiotic Given[1,3]	-	-	96%	95%
Blood Culture Timing[1,3]	-	-	98%	98%
Pregnancy and Delivery Care				
Newborn Deliveries Scheduled Early[5]	-	-	3%	6%
Preventive Care				
Immunization for Influenza[5]	-	-	89%	90%

NOTE: Hospital profiles are in alphabetical order by state, then city, then hospital within the city; Rankings exclude hospitals with less than 25 cases except for patient surveys which excludes hospitals with less than 100 cases; (a) 100-299 cases; (1) The number of cases/patients is too few to report; (2) Data submitted were based on a sample of cases/patients; (3) Results are based on a shorter time period than required; (4) Data suppressed by CMS for one or more quarters; (5) Results are not available for this reporting period; (6) Fewer than 100 patients completed the HCAHPS survey; (7) No cases met the criteria for this measure; (8) The lower limit of the confidence interval cannot be calculated if the number of observed infections equals zero; (9) No data are available from the state/territory for this reporting period; (10) The scores shown reflect fewer than 50 completed surveys; (11) There were discrepancies in the data collection process; (12) This measure does not apply to this hospital for this reporting period; (13) Results cannot be calculated for this reporting period; (14) The results for this state are combined with nearby states to protect confidentiality; Please refer to the User's Guide for a full explanation of data.

Immunization for Pneumonia[5]	-	-	90%	92%
Stroke Care				
Anticoagulation Therapy for Atrial Fibrillation[5]	-	-	92%	95%
Antithrombotic Therapy Timing[5]	-	-	97%	98%
Assessed for Rehabilitation[5]	-	-	97%	97%
Discharged on Antithrombotic Therapy[5]	-	-	99%	99%
Discharged on Statin Medication[5]	-	-	94%	94%
Thrombolytic Therapy Timing[5]	-	-	69%	66%
Venous Thromboembolism Prophylaxis[5]	-	-	94%	94%
Written Stroke Educational Materials Given[5]	-	-	87%	88%
Surgical Care Improvement Project				
Appropriate Beta Blocker Usage[5]	-	-	98%	98%
Appropriate VTP Within 24 Hours[5]	-	-	98%	98%
Controlled Postoperative Blood Glucose[5]	-	-	97%	97%
Perioperative Temperature Management[5]	-	-	100%	100%
Prophylactic Antibiotic Selection[5]	-	-	99%	99%
Prophylactic Antibiotic Selection (Outpatient)[5]	-	-	97%	98%
Prophylactic Antibiotic Stopped[5]	-	-	98%	98%
Prophylactic Antibiotic Timing[5]	-	-	98%	99%
Prophylactic Antibiotic Timing (Outpatient)[5]	-	-	97%	98%
Urinary Catheter Removal[5]	-	-	97%	97%
Survey of Patients' Hospital Experiences				
Area Around Room 'Always' Quiet at Night[5]	-	-	60%	61%
Doctors 'Always' Communicated Well[5]	-	-	81%	82%
Home Recovery Information Given[5]	-	-	87%	85%
Hospital Given 9 or 10 on 10 Point Scale[5]	-	-	71%	71%
Meds 'Always' Explained Before Given[5]	-	-	64%	64%
Nurses 'Always' Communicated Well[5]	-	-	80%	79%
Pain 'Always' Well Controlled[5]	-	-	71%	71%
Room and Bathroom 'Always' Clean[5]	-	-	73%	73%
Timely Help 'Always' Received[5]	-	-	70%	68%
Would Definitely Recommend Hospital[5]	-	-	71%	71%
Use of Medical Imaging				
Cardiac Imaging Stress Test before Surgery[7]	-	-	5.1%	5.3%
Combination Abdominal CT Scan	195	3.1%	8.7%	10.5%
Combination Brain/Sinus CT Scan	167	0.0%	2.2%	2.7%
Combination Chest CT Scan	173	0.0%	3.6%	2.7%
Follow-up Mammogram/Ultrasound	522	7.9%	8.2%	8.8%
Lumbar Spine MRI for Low Back Pain	56	51.8%	36.9%	37.2%

Baraga County Memorial Hospital

18341 Us Highway 41 | Phone: 906-524-3300
L' Anse, MI 49946 | Fax: 906-524-5466
E-mail: flozier@bcmh.org
URL: www.bcmh.org
Type: Critical Access Hospitals | Emergency Services: Yes
Ownership: Government - Local | Beds: 44

Key Personnel:
Ambulatory Care . . . . Mary Grondin, RN
Operating Room. . . . . Mary Grondin, RN
Anesthesiology. . . . . Jerry Hill, CRNA
Radiology. . . . . Dean Jackson, RT
CEO/President. . . . . John Tembreull
Infection Control. . . . . Andrea Uren, RN
Chief of Medical Staff . . . . Craig Vickstrom, MD

Measure	Cases	This Hosp.	State Avg.	U.S. Avg.
Blood Clot Prevention and Treatment				
Anticoagulation Overlap Therapy[5]	-	-	90%	93%
ICU Venous Thromboembolism Prophylaxis[5]	-	-	93%	92%
Incidence of Potentially Preventable VTE[5]	-	-	8%	10%
UFH with Dosages/Platelet Monitoring[5]	-	-	96%	97%
Venous Thromboembolism Prophylaxis[5]	-	-	87%	85%
Warfarin Therapy Discharge Instructions[5]	-	-	72%	75%
Chest Pain/Possible Heart Attack Care				
Aspirin Given Within 24 Hours of Arrival	35	100%	96%	96%
Fibrinolytic Meds Within 30 Min. of Arrival[1]	-	-	63%	58%
Average Time to ECG (minutes)	35	10	8	7
Average Time to Transfer (minutes)[7]	-	-	53	60
Children's Asthma Care				
Received Home Management Plan of Care	-	-	-	88%
Received Reliever Medication	-	-	-	100%
Received Systemic Corticosteroids	-	-	-	100%
Emergency Department				
Admittance Decision Time (minutes)[5]	-	-	102	98
Head CT Results Within 45 Min. of Arrival[5]	-	-	54%	57%
Patients Who Left ER Before Being Seen[5]	-	-	2%	2%
Time from ER Arrival to Admit. (minutes)[5]	-	-	288	274
Time from ER Arrival to Discharge (minutes)	257	80	128	134
Time in ER Before Being Evaluated (minutes)	317	15	22	26
Time to Pain Meds for Fractures (minutes)[5]	-	-	55	57
Heart Attack Care				
Aspirin Given at Discharge[5]	-	-	99%	99%
Fibrinolytic Meds Within 30 Min. of Arrival[5]	-	-	20%	54%
PCI Within 90 Minutes of Arrival[5]	-	-	95%	96%
Statin Prescribed at Discharge[5]	-	-	98%	98%
Heart Failure Care				
ACE Inhibitor or ARB for LVSD[1]	-	-	96%	97%
Discharge Instructions Given	13	77%	94%	94%
Evaluation of LVS Function	14	100%	99%	99%
Medicare Spending				
Medicare Spending per Patient (ratio)	-	-	0.96	0.98
Pneumonia Care				
Appropriate Initial Antibiotic Given	20	70%	96%	95%
Blood Culture Timing	16	100%	98%	98%
Pregnancy and Delivery Care				
Newborn Deliveries Scheduled Early[5]	-	-	3%	6%
Preventive Care				
Immunization for Influenza[5]	-	-	89%	90%
Immunization for Pneumonia[5]	-	-	90%	92%
Stroke Care				
Anticoagulation Therapy for Atrial Fibrillation[5]	-	-	92%	95%
Antithrombotic Therapy Timing[5]	-	-	97%	98%
Assessed for Rehabilitation[5]	-	-	97%	97%
Discharged on Antithrombotic Therapy[5]	-	-	99%	99%
Discharged on Statin Medication[5]	-	-	94%	94%
Thrombolytic Therapy Timing[5]	-	-	69%	66%
Venous Thromboembolism Prophylaxis[5]	-	-	94%	94%
Written Stroke Educational Materials Given[5]	-	-	87%	88%
Surgical Care Improvement Project				
Appropriate Beta Blocker Usage[5]	-	-	98%	98%
Appropriate VTP Within 24 Hours[5]	-	-	98%	98%
Controlled Postoperative Blood Glucose[5]	-	-	97%	97%
Perioperative Temperature Management[5]	-	-	100%	100%
Prophylactic Antibiotic Selection[5]	-	-	99%	99%
Prophylactic Antibiotic Selection (Outpatient)[5]	-	-	97%	98%
Prophylactic Antibiotic Stopped[5]	-	-	98%	98%
Prophylactic Antibiotic Timing[5]	-	-	98%	99%
Prophylactic Antibiotic Timing (Outpatient)[5]	-	-	97%	98%
Urinary Catheter Removal[5]	-	-	97%	97%
Survey of Patients' Hospital Experiences				
Area Around Room 'Always' Quiet at Night	(a)	67%	60%	61%
Doctors 'Always' Communicated Well	(a)	86%	81%	82%
Home Recovery Information Given	(a)	84%	87%	85%
Hospital Given 9 or 10 on 10 Point Scale	(a)	66%	71%	71%
Meds 'Always' Explained Before Given	(a)	68%	64%	64%
Nurses 'Always' Communicated Well	(a)	81%	80%	79%
Pain 'Always' Well Controlled	(a)	66%	71%	71%
Room and Bathroom 'Always' Clean	(a)	88%	73%	73%
Timely Help 'Always' Received	(a)	73%	70%	68%
Would Definitely Recommend Hospital	(a)	64%	71%	71%
Use of Medical Imaging				
Cardiac Imaging Stress Test before Surgery[1]	-	-	5.1%	5.3%
Combination Abdominal CT Scan	89	74.2%	8.7%	10.5%
Combination Brain/Sinus CT Scan[1]	-	-	2.2%	2.7%
Combination Chest CT Scan	58	1.7%	3.6%	2.7%
Follow-up Mammogram/Ultrasound	201	1.0%	8.2%	8.8%
Lumbar Spine MRI for Low Back Pain[1]	-	-	36.9%	37.2%

Spectrum Health United Memorial - Kelsey Campus

418 Washington | Phone: 989-352-7211
Lakeview, MI 48850 | Fax: 616-754-5054
Type: Critical Access Hospitals | Emergency Services: Yes
Ownership: Voluntary non-profit - Other | Beds: 94

Key Personnel:
Quality Assurance . . . . Etta Barrera
CEO/President. . . . . Ken Cegner
Chief of Medical Staff. . . . . M Dewys

Measure	Cases	This Hosp.	State Avg.	U.S. Avg.
Blood Clot Prevention and Treatment				
Anticoagulation Overlap Therapy[1,2]	-	-	90%	93%
ICU Venous Thromboembolism Prophylaxis[2,7]	-	-	93%	92%
Incidence of Potentially Preventable VTE[1,2]	-	-	8%	10%
UFH with Dosages/Platelet Monitoring[1,2]	-	-	96%	97%
Venous Thromboembolism Prophylaxis[2]	124	96%	87%	85%
Warfarin Therapy Discharge Instructions[1,2]	-	-	72%	75%
Chest Pain/Possible Heart Attack Care				
Aspirin Given Within 24 Hours of Arrival	35	100%	96%	96%
Fibrinolytic Meds Within 30 Min. of Arrival[7]	-	-	63%	58%
Average Time to ECG (minutes)	36	7	8	7
Average Time to Transfer (minutes)[7]	-	-	53	60
Children's Asthma Care				
Received Home Management Plan of Care	-	-	-	88%
Received Reliever Medication	-	-	-	100%
Received Systemic Corticosteroids	-	-	-	100%
Emergency Department				
Admittance Decision Time (minutes)	145	52	102	98
Head CT Results Within 45 Min. of Arrival[1,3]	-	-	54%	57%
Patients Who Left ER Before Being Seen[5]	-	-	2%	2%
Time from ER Arrival to Admit. (minutes)	155	232	288	274
Time from ER Arrival to Discharge (minutes)	382	112	128	134
Time in ER Before Being Evaluated (minutes)	297	16	22	26
Time to Pain Meds for Fractures (minutes)	50	43	55	57
Heart Attack Care				
Aspirin Given at Discharge[5]	-	-	99%	99%
Fibrinolytic Meds Within 30 Min. of Arrival[5]	-	-	20%	54%
PCI Within 90 Minutes of Arrival[5]	-	-	95%	96%
Statin Prescribed at Discharge[5]	-	-	98%	98%
Heart Failure Care				
ACE Inhibitor or ARB for LVSD[1]	-	-	96%	97%
Discharge Instructions Given	13	92%	94%	94%
Evaluation of LVS Function	15	100%	99%	99%
Medicare Spending				
Medicare Spending per Patient (ratio)	-	-	0.96	0.98
Pneumonia Care				
Appropriate Initial Antibiotic Given	34	100%	96%	95%
Blood Culture Timing	34	97%	98%	98%
Pregnancy and Delivery Care				
Newborn Deliveries Scheduled Early[5]	-	-	3%	6%
Preventive Care				
Immunization for Influenza	107	96%	89%	90%
Immunization for Pneumonia	172	98%	90%	92%
Stroke Care				
Anticoagulation Therapy for Atrial Fibrillation[3,7]	-	-	92%	95%
Antithrombotic Therapy Timing[1,3]	-	-	97%	98%
Assessed for Rehabilitation[1,3]	-	-	97%	97%
Discharged on Antithrombotic Therapy[1,3]	-	-	99%	99%
Discharged on Statin Medication[3,7]	-	-	94%	94%
Thrombolytic Therapy Timing[3,7]	-	-	69%	66%
Venous Thromboembolism Prophylaxis[1,3]	-	-	94%	94%
Written Stroke Educational Materials Given[3,7]	-	-	87%	88%
Surgical Care Improvement Project				
Appropriate Beta Blocker Usage[5]	-	-	98%	98%
Appropriate VTP Within 24 Hours[5]	-	-	98%	98%
Controlled Postoperative Blood Glucose[5]	-	-	97%	97%
Perioperative Temperature Management[5]	-	-	100%	100%
Prophylactic Antibiotic Selection[5]	-	-	99%	99%
Prophylactic Antibiotic Selection (Outpatient)[5]	-	-	97%	98%
Prophylactic Antibiotic Stopped[5]	-	-	98%	98%
Prophylactic Antibiotic Timing[5]	-	-	98%	99%
Prophylactic Antibiotic Timing (Outpatient)[5]	-	-	97%	98%
Urinary Catheter Removal[5]	-	-	97%	97%
Survey of Patients' Hospital Experiences				
Area Around Room 'Always' Quiet at Night[6]	<100	77%	60%	61%
Doctors 'Always' Communicated Well[6]	<100	83%	81%	82%
Home Recovery Information Given[6]	<100	92%	87%	85%
Hospital Given 9 or 10 on 10 Point Scale[6]	<100	79%	71%	71%
Meds 'Always' Explained Before Given[6]	<100	82%	64%	64%
Nurses 'Always' Communicated Well[6]	<100	88%	80%	79%
Pain 'Always' Well Controlled[6]	<100	88%	71%	71%

NOTE: Hospital profiles are in alphabetical order by state, then city, then hospital within the city; Rankings exclude hospitals with less than 25 cases except for patient surveys which excludes hospitals with less than 100 cases; (a) 100-299 cases; (1) The number of cases/patients is too few to report; (2) Data submitted were based on a sample of cases/patients; (3) Results are based on a shorter time period than required; (4) Data suppressed by CMS for one or more quarters; (5) Results are not available for this reporting period; (6) Fewer than 100 patients completed the HCAHPS survey; (7) No cases met the criteria for this measure; (8) The lower limit of the confidence interval cannot be calculated if the number of observed infections equals zero; (9) No data are available from the state/territory for this reporting period; (10) The scores shown reflect fewer than 50 completed surveys; (11) There were discrepancies in the data collection process; (12) This measure does not apply to this hospital for this reporting period; (13) Results cannot be calculated for this reporting period; (14) The results for this state are combined with nearby states to protect confidentiality; Please refer to the User's Guide for a full explanation of data.

Measure	Cases	This Hosp.	State Avg.	U.S. Avg.
Room and Bathroom 'Always' Clean[6]	<100	90%	73%	73%
Timely Help 'Always' Received[6]	<100	95%	70%	68%
Would Definitely Recommend Hospital[6]	<100	74%	71%	71%
Use of Medical Imaging				
Cardiac Imaging Stress Test before Surgery[1]	-	-	5.1%	5.3%
Combination Abdominal CT Scan	128	6.3%	8.7%	10.5%
Combination Brain/Sinus CT Scan[1]	-	-	2.2%	2.7%
Combination Chest CT Scan	66	0.0%	3.6%	2.7%
Follow-up Mammogram/Ultrasound	146	8.2%	8.2%	8.8%
Lumbar Spine MRI for Low Back Pain[7]	-	-	36.9%	37.2%

Edward W Sparrow Hospital

1215 E Michigan Avenue
Lansing, MI 48912
Phone: 517-364-1000
Fax: 517-364-5050
URL: www.sparrow.org
Type: Acute Care Hospitals
Emergency Services: Yes
Ownership: Voluntary non-profit - Other
Beds: 535

Key Personnel:
Chair/CEO . . . . Greg Brogan
CEO/President. . . . . Joe Damore
Infection Control. . . . . John Dyke, MD
Quality Assurance . . . . John Dyke
Operating Room. . . . . Phyllis Kik, RN

Measure	Cases	This Hosp.	State Avg.	U.S. Avg.
Blood Clot Prevention and Treatment				
Anticoagulation Overlap Therapy[2]	161	99%	90%	93%
ICU Venous Thromboembolism Prophylaxis[2]	82	94%	93%	92%
Incidence of Potentially Preventable VTE[2]	22	14%	8%	10%
UFH with Dosages/Platelet Monitoring[2]	172	98%	96%	97%
Venous Thromboembolism Prophylaxis[2]	442	86%	87%	85%
Warfarin Therapy Discharge Instructions[2]	124	96%	72%	75%
Chest Pain/Possible Heart Attack Care				
Aspirin Given Within 24 Hours of Arrival[1,3]	-	-	96%	96%
Fibrinolytic Meds Within 30 Min. of Arrival[5]	-	-	63%	58%
Average Time to ECG (minutes)[1,3]	-	-	8	7
Average Time to Transfer (minutes)[5]	-	-	53	60
Children's Asthma Care				
Received Home Management Plan of Care	-	-	-	88%
Received Reliever Medication	-	-	-	100%
Received Systemic Corticosteroids	-	-	-	100%
Emergency Department				
Admittance Decision Time (minutes)[2]	941	85	102	98
Head CT Results Within 45 Min. of Arrival[7]	-	-	54%	57%
Patients Who Left ER Before Being Seen	>100k	2%	2%	2%
Time from ER Arrival to Admit. (minutes)[2]	955	319	288	274
Time from ER Arrival to Discharge (minutes)	2,819	192	128	134
Time in ER Before Being Evaluated (minutes)	3,030	39	22	26
Time to Pain Meds for Fractures (minutes)	318	74	55	57
Heart Attack Care				
Aspirin Given at Discharge	540	100%	99%	99%
Fibrinolytic Meds Within 30 Min. of Arrival[7]	-	-	20%	54%
PCI Within 90 Minutes of Arrival	70	94%	95%	96%
Statin Prescribed at Discharge	541	100%	98%	98%
Heart Failure Care				
ACE Inhibitor or ARB for LVSD	210	94%	96%	97%
Discharge Instructions Given	533	92%	94%	94%
Evaluation of LVS Function	675	98%	99%	99%
Medicare Spending				
Medicare Spending per Patient (ratio)	-	0.98	0.96	0.98
Pneumonia Care				
Appropriate Initial Antibiotic Given[2]	287	97%	96%	95%
Blood Culture Timing[2]	549	97%	98%	98%
Pregnancy and Delivery Care				
Newborn Deliveries Scheduled Early[2]	239	0%	3%	6%
Preventive Care				
Immunization for Influenza[2]	743	85%	89%	90%
Immunization for Pneumonia[2]	956	83%	90%	92%
Stroke Care				
Anticoagulation Therapy for Atrial Fibrillation	33	100%	92%	95%
Antithrombotic Therapy Timing	241	100%	97%	98%
Assessed for Rehabilitation	363	99%	97%	97%
Discharged on Antithrombotic Therapy	298	99%	99%	99%
Discharged on Statin Medication	229	95%	94%	94%
Thrombolytic Therapy Timing	42	88%	69%	66%
Venous Thromboembolism Prophylaxis	361	96%	94%	94%
Written Stroke Educational Materials Given	204	88%	87%	88%
Surgical Care Improvement Project				
Appropriate Beta Blocker Usage[2]	653	99%	98%	98%
Appropriate VTP Within 24 Hours[2]	1,746	96%	98%	98%
Controlled Postoperative Blood Glucose[2]	234	96%	97%	97%
Perioperative Temperature Management[2]	2,330	100%	100%	100%
Prophylactic Antibiotic Selection[2]	1,462	99%	99%	99%
Prophylactic Antibiotic Selection (Outpatient)	388	95%	97%	98%
Prophylactic Antibiotic Stopped[2]	1,448	96%	98%	98%
Prophylactic Antibiotic Timing[2]	1,470	95%	98%	99%
Prophylactic Antibiotic Timing (Outpatient)	391	97%	97%	98%
Urinary Catheter Removal[2]	740	86%	97%	97%
Survey of Patients' Hospital Experiences				
Area Around Room 'Always' Quiet at Night	300+	52%	60%	61%
Doctors 'Always' Communicated Well	300+	76%	81%	82%
Home Recovery Information Given	300+	87%	87%	85%
Hospital Given 9 or 10 on 10 Point Scale	300+	70%	71%	71%
Meds 'Always' Explained Before Given	300+	62%	64%	64%
Nurses 'Always' Communicated Well	300+	78%	80%	79%
Pain 'Always' Well Controlled	300+	70%	71%	71%
Room and Bathroom 'Always' Clean	300+	66%	73%	73%
Timely Help 'Always' Received	300+	64%	70%	68%
Would Definitely Recommend Hospital	300+	74%	71%	71%
Use of Medical Imaging				
Cardiac Imaging Stress Test before Surgery	1,865	4.5%	5.1%	5.3%
Combination Abdominal CT Scan	2,268	4.6%	8.7%	10.5%
Combination Brain/Sinus CT Scan	2,136	3.5%	2.2%	2.7%
Combination Chest CT Scan	1,112	0.2%	3.6%	2.7%
Follow-up Mammogram/Ultrasound	1,954	7.5%	8.2%	8.8%
Lumbar Spine MRI for Low Back Pain[1]	-	-	36.9%	37.2%

Mclaren - Greater Lansing

401 W Greenlawn Ave
Lansing, MI 48910
Phone: 517-975-6000
URL: www.mclaren.org
Type: Acute Care Hospitals
Emergency Services: Yes
Ownership: Voluntary non-profit - Private

Key Personnel:
Infection Control. . . . . Theresa Larsen
Quality Assurance . . . . Theresa Larsen

Measure	Cases	This Hosp.	State Avg.	U.S. Avg.
Blood Clot Prevention and Treatment				
Anticoagulation Overlap Therapy[2]	103	97%	90%	93%
ICU Venous Thromboembolism Prophylaxis[2]	31	100%	93%	92%
Incidence of Potentially Preventable VTE[2]	15	13%	8%	10%
UFH with Dosages/Platelet Monitoring[2]	88	99%	96%	97%
Venous Thromboembolism Prophylaxis[2]	330	98%	87%	85%
Warfarin Therapy Discharge Instructions[2]	94	100%	72%	75%
Chest Pain/Possible Heart Attack Care				
Aspirin Given Within 24 Hours of Arrival[1,3]	-	-	96%	96%
Fibrinolytic Meds Within 30 Min. of Arrival[3,7]	-	-	63%	58%
Average Time to ECG (minutes)[1,3]	-	-	8	7
Average Time to Transfer (minutes)[3,7]	-	-	53	60
Children's Asthma Care				
Received Home Management Plan of Care	-	-	-	88%
Received Reliever Medication	-	-	-	100%
Received Systemic Corticosteroids	-	-	-	100%
Emergency Department				
Admittance Decision Time (minutes)[2]	339	167	102	98
Head CT Results Within 45 Min. of Arrival[1]	-	-	54%	57%
Patients Who Left ER Before Being Seen	44,750	4%	2%	2%
Time from ER Arrival to Admit. (minutes)[2]	578	416	288	274
Time from ER Arrival to Discharge (minutes)	321	197	128	134
Time in ER Before Being Evaluated (minutes)	369	53	22	26
Time to Pain Meds for Fractures (minutes)	132	82	55	57
Heart Attack Care				
Aspirin Given at Discharge	204	99%	99%	99%
Fibrinolytic Meds Within 30 Min. of Arrival[7]	-	-	20%	54%
PCI Within 90 Minutes of Arrival	26	92%	95%	96%
Statin Prescribed at Discharge	200	98%	98%	98%
Heart Failure Care				
ACE Inhibitor or ARB for LVSD	117	89%	96%	97%
Discharge Instructions Given	298	72%	94%	94%
Evaluation of LVS Function	345	99%	99%	99%
Medicare Spending				
Medicare Spending per Patient (ratio)	-	0.94	0.96	0.98
Pneumonia Care				
Appropriate Initial Antibiotic Given	176	85%	96%	95%
Blood Culture Timing	194	87%	98%	98%
Pregnancy and Delivery Care				
Newborn Deliveries Scheduled Early[2]	81	15%	3%	6%
Preventive Care				
Immunization for Influenza[2]	566	86%	89%	90%
Immunization for Pneumonia[2]	759	78%	90%	92%
Stroke Care				
Anticoagulation Therapy for Atrial Fibrillation	12	92%	92%	95%
Antithrombotic Therapy Timing	118	97%	97%	98%
Assessed for Rehabilitation	119	97%	97%	97%
Discharged on Antithrombotic Therapy	119	98%	99%	99%
Discharged on Statin Medication	81	99%	94%	94%
Thrombolytic Therapy Timing	14	14%	69%	66%
Venous Thromboembolism Prophylaxis	116	95%	94%	94%
Written Stroke Educational Materials Given	84	94%	87%	88%
Surgical Care Improvement Project				
Appropriate Beta Blocker Usage[2]	165	98%	98%	98%
Appropriate VTP Within 24 Hours[2]	279	96%	98%	98%
Controlled Postoperative Blood Glucose[2]	110	91%	97%	97%
Perioperative Temperature Management[2]	425	99%	100%	100%
Prophylactic Antibiotic Selection[2]	399	97%	99%	99%
Prophylactic Antibiotic Selection (Outpatient)	562	84%	97%	98%
Prophylactic Antibiotic Stopped[2]	387	98%	98%	98%
Prophylactic Antibiotic Timing[2]	400	97%	98%	99%
Prophylactic Antibiotic Timing (Outpatient)	584	90%	97%	98%
Urinary Catheter Removal[2]	171	82%	97%	97%
Survey of Patients' Hospital Experiences				
Area Around Room 'Always' Quiet at Night	300+	57%	60%	61%
Doctors 'Always' Communicated Well	300+	73%	81%	82%
Home Recovery Information Given	300+	85%	87%	85%
Hospital Given 9 or 10 on 10 Point Scale	300+	61%	71%	71%
Meds 'Always' Explained Before Given	300+	56%	64%	64%
Nurses 'Always' Communicated Well	300+	73%	80%	79%
Pain 'Always' Well Controlled	300+	66%	71%	71%
Room and Bathroom 'Always' Clean	300+	64%	73%	73%
Timely Help 'Always' Received	300+	59%	70%	68%
Would Definitely Recommend Hospital	300+	66%	71%	71%
Use of Medical Imaging				
Cardiac Imaging Stress Test before Surgery	805	5.2%	5.1%	5.3%
Combination Abdominal CT Scan	971	10.7%	8.7%	10.5%
Combination Brain/Sinus CT Scan	1,009	4.2%	2.2%	2.7%
Combination Chest CT Scan	620	0.5%	3.6%	2.7%
Follow-up Mammogram/Ultrasound	1,925	3.7%	8.2%	8.8%
Lumbar Spine MRI for Low Back Pain	173	36.4%	36.9%	37.2%

Mclaren Lapeer Region

1375 N Main St
Lapeer, MI 48446
Phone: 810-667-5500
Fax: 810-667-5582
URL: www.lapeerregional.org
Type: Acute Care Hospitals
Emergency Services: Yes
Ownership: Voluntary non-profit - Private
Beds: 185

Key Personnel:
Pediatric Ambulatory Care . . . . . . Mark Braniecki, DO
Pediatric In-Patient Care . . . . Mark Braniecki, DO
CEO/President. . . . . Barton Buxton, EdD
Quality Assurance . . . . Terri Capdeville
Chief of Medical Staff. . . . . Darlin David, MD
Infection Control. . . . . Florence Elston, RN
Radiology. . . . . Richard F Grzybowski, DO
Operating Room. . . . . Robert M Stenz, RN

Measure	Cases	This Hosp.	State Avg.	U.S. Avg.
Blood Clot Prevention and Treatment				
Anticoagulation Overlap Therapy[2]	66	100%	90%	93%
ICU Venous Thromboembolism Prophylaxis[2]	79	100%	93%	92%
Incidence of Potentially Preventable VTE[1,2]	-	-	8%	10%
UFH with Dosages/Platelet Monitoring[2]	67	100%	96%	97%
Venous Thromboembolism Prophylaxis[2]	330	99%	87%	85%
Warfarin Therapy Discharge Instructions[2]	57	96%	72%	75%

NOTE: Hospital profiles are in alphabetical order by state, then city, then hospital within the city; Rankings exclude hospitals with less than 25 cases except for patient surveys which excludes hospitals with less than 100 cases; (a) 100-299 cases; (1) The number of cases/patients is too few to report; (2) Data submitted were based on a sample of cases/patients; (3) Results are based on a shorter time period than required; (4) Data suppressed by CMS for one or more quarters; (5) Results are not available for this reporting period; (6) Fewer than 100 patients completed the HCAHPS survey; (7) No cases met the criteria for this measure; (8) The lower limit of the confidence interval cannot be calculated if the number of observed infections equals zero; (9) No data are available from the state/territory for this reporting period; (10) The scores shown reflect fewer than 50 completed surveys; (11) There were discrepancies in the data collection process; (12) This measure does not apply to this hospital for this reporting period; (13) Results cannot be calculated for this reporting period; (14) The results for this state are combined with nearby states to protect confidentiality; Please refer to the User's Guide for a full explanation of data.

Measure	Cases	This Hosp.	State Avg.	U.S. Avg.
Chest Pain/Possible Heart Attack Care				
Aspirin Given Within 24 Hours of Arrival	83	100%	96%	96%
Fibrinolytic Meds Within 30 Min. of Arrival[7]	-	-	63%	58%
Average Time to ECG (minutes)	83	4	8	7
Average Time to Transfer (minutes)	27	29	53	60
Children's Asthma Care				
Received Home Management Plan of Care	-	-	-	88%
Received Reliever Medication	-	-	-	100%
Received Systemic Corticosteroids	-	-	-	100%
Emergency Department				
Admittance Decision Time (minutes)[2]	858	150	102	98
Head CT Results Within 45 Min. of Arrival[1]	-	-	54%	57%
Patients Who Left ER Before Being Seen	30,425	0%	2%	2%
Time from ER Arrival to Admit. (minutes)[2]	858	327	288	274
Time from ER Arrival to Discharge (minutes)	345	151	128	134
Time in ER Before Being Evaluated (minutes)	372	23	22	26
Time to Pain Meds for Fractures (minutes)	147	51	55	57
Heart Attack Care				
Aspirin Given at Discharge[2]	51	100%	99%	99%
Fibrinolytic Meds Within 30 Min. of Arrival[2,7]	-	-	20%	54%
PCI Within 90 Minutes of Arrival[2,7]	-	-	95%	96%
Statin Prescribed at Discharge[2]	48	96%	98%	98%
Heart Failure Care				
ACE Inhibitor or ARB for LVSD[2]	44	93%	96%	97%
Discharge Instructions Given[2]	169	95%	94%	94%
Evaluation of LVS Function[2]	216	99%	99%	99%
Medicare Spending				
Medicare Spending per Patient (ratio)	-	0.90	0.96	0.98
Pneumonia Care				
Appropriate Initial Antibiotic Given[2]	94	100%	96%	95%
Blood Culture Timing[2]	146	97%	98%	98%
Pregnancy and Delivery Care				
Newborn Deliveries Scheduled Early[2]	26	4%	3%	6%
Preventive Care				
Immunization for Influenza[2]	555	94%	89%	90%
Immunization for Pneumonia[2]	750	92%	90%	92%
Stroke Care				
Anticoagulation Therapy for Atrial Fibrillation[1,2]	-	-	92%	95%
Antithrombotic Therapy Timing[2]	56	100%	97%	98%
Assessed for Rehabilitation[2]	66	100%	97%	97%
Discharged on Antithrombotic Therapy[2]	60	100%	99%	99%
Discharged on Statin Medication[2]	48	94%	94%	94%
Thrombolytic Therapy Timing[1,2]	-	-	69%	66%
Venous Thromboembolism Prophylaxis[2]	73	100%	94%	94%
Written Stroke Educational Materials Given[2]	37	73%	87%	88%
Surgical Care Improvement Project				
Appropriate Beta Blocker Usage[2]	83	90%	98%	98%
Appropriate VTP Within 24 Hours[2]	275	97%	98%	98%
Controlled Postoperative Blood Glucose[2,7]	-	-	97%	97%
Perioperative Temperature Management[2]	299	100%	100%	100%
Prophylactic Antibiotic Selection[2]	199	99%	99%	99%
Prophylactic Antibiotic Selection (Outpatient)	66	89%	97%	98%
Prophylactic Antibiotic Stopped[2]	190	97%	98%	98%
Prophylactic Antibiotic Timing[2]	199	99%	98%	99%
Prophylactic Antibiotic Timing (Outpatient)	66	98%	97%	98%
Urinary Catheter Removal[2]	195	95%	97%	97%
Survey of Patients' Hospital Experiences				
Area Around Room 'Always' Quiet at Night	300+	49%	60%	61%
Doctors 'Always' Communicated Well	300+	76%	81%	82%
Home Recovery Information Given	300+	85%	87%	85%
Hospital Given 9 or 10 on 10 Point Scale	300+	62%	71%	71%
Meds 'Always' Explained Before Given	300+	58%	64%	64%
Nurses 'Always' Communicated Well	300+	75%	80%	79%
Pain 'Always' Well Controlled	300+	66%	71%	71%
Room and Bathroom 'Always' Clean	300+	68%	73%	73%
Timely Help 'Always' Received	300+	63%	70%	68%
Would Definitely Recommend Hospital	300+	56%	71%	71%
Use of Medical Imaging				
Cardiac Imaging Stress Test before Surgery	251	4.0%	5.1%	5.3%
Combination Abdominal CT Scan	603	3.2%	8.7%	10.5%
Combination Brain/Sinus CT Scan	671	3.9%	2.2%	2.7%
Combination Chest CT Scan	355	0.8%	3.6%	2.7%
Follow-up Mammogram/Ultrasound	404	14.9%	8.2%	8.8%
Lumbar Spine MRI for Low Back Pain	180	34.4%	36.9%	37.2%

Aspirus Keweenaw Hospital

205 Osceola
Laurium, MI 49913
Phone: 906-337-6500
Type: Critical Access Hospitals
Emergency Services: Yes
Ownership: Voluntary non-profit - Private

Measure	Cases	This Hosp.	State Avg.	U.S. Avg.
Blood Clot Prevention and Treatment				
Anticoagulation Overlap Therapy[5]	-	-	90%	93%
ICU Venous Thromboembolism Prophylaxis[5]	-	-	93%	92%
Incidence of Potentially Preventable VTE[5]	-	-	8%	10%
UFH with Dosages/Platelet Monitoring[5]	-	-	96%	97%
Venous Thromboembolism Prophylaxis[5]	-	-	87%	85%
Warfarin Therapy Discharge Instructions[5]	-	-	72%	75%
Chest Pain/Possible Heart Attack Care				
Aspirin Given Within 24 Hours of Arrival[1]	-	-	96%	96%
Fibrinolytic Meds Within 30 Min. of Arrival[3,7]	-	-	63%	58%
Average Time to ECG (minutes)[1]	-	-	8	7
Average Time to Transfer (minutes)[3,7]	-	-	53	60
Children's Asthma Care				
Received Home Management Plan of Care	-	-	-	88%
Received Reliever Medication	-	-	-	100%
Received Systemic Corticosteroids	-	-	-	100%
Emergency Department				
Admittance Decision Time (minutes)[5]	-	-	102	98
Head CT Results Within 45 Min. of Arrival[5]	-	-	54%	57%
Patients Who Left ER Before Being Seen[5]	-	-	2%	2%
Time from ER Arrival to Admit. (minutes)[5]	-	-	288	274
Time from ER Arrival to Discharge (minutes)	354	70	128	134
Time in ER Before Being Evaluated (minutes)	339	15	22	26
Time to Pain Meds for Fractures (minutes)[1,3]	-	-	55	57
Heart Attack Care				
Aspirin Given at Discharge[1]	-	-	99%	99%
Fibrinolytic Meds Within 30 Min. of Arrival[7]	-	-	20%	54%
PCI Within 90 Minutes of Arrival[7]	-	-	95%	96%
Statin Prescribed at Discharge[1]	-	-	98%	98%
Heart Failure Care				
ACE Inhibitor or ARB for LVSD[1]	-	-	96%	97%
Discharge Instructions Given	25	92%	94%	94%
Evaluation of LVS Function	30	100%	99%	99%
Medicare Spending				
Medicare Spending per Patient (ratio)	-	-	0.96	0.98
Pneumonia Care				
Appropriate Initial Antibiotic Given	21	90%	96%	95%
Blood Culture Timing	44	100%	98%	98%
Pregnancy and Delivery Care				
Newborn Deliveries Scheduled Early[5]	-	-	3%	6%
Preventive Care				
Immunization for Influenza[5]	-	-	89%	90%
Immunization for Pneumonia[5]	-	-	90%	92%
Stroke Care				
Anticoagulation Therapy for Atrial Fibrillation[5]	-	-	92%	95%
Antithrombotic Therapy Timing[5]	-	-	97%	98%
Assessed for Rehabilitation[5]	-	-	97%	97%
Discharged on Antithrombotic Therapy[5]	-	-	99%	99%
Discharged on Statin Medication[5]	-	-	94%	94%
Thrombolytic Therapy Timing[5]	-	-	69%	66%
Venous Thromboembolism Prophylaxis[5]	-	-	94%	94%
Written Stroke Educational Materials Given[5]	-	-	87%	88%
Surgical Care Improvement Project				
Appropriate Beta Blocker Usage	18	94%	98%	98%
Appropriate VTP Within 24 Hours	42	100%	98%	98%
Controlled Postoperative Blood Glucose[7]	-	-	97%	97%
Perioperative Temperature Management	26	100%	100%	100%
Prophylactic Antibiotic Selection	32	100%	99%	99%
Prophylactic Antibiotic Selection (Outpatient)[5]	-	-	97%	98%
Prophylactic Antibiotic Stopped	32	97%	98%	98%
Prophylactic Antibiotic Timing	32	97%	98%	99%
Prophylactic Antibiotic Timing (Outpatient)[5]	-	-	97%	98%
Urinary Catheter Removal	30	100%	97%	97%
Survey of Patients' Hospital Experiences				
Area Around Room 'Always' Quiet at Night	(a)	58%	60%	61%
Doctors 'Always' Communicated Well	(a)	89%	81%	82%
Home Recovery Information Given	(a)	87%	87%	85%
Hospital Given 9 or 10 on 10 Point Scale	(a)	71%	71%	71%
Meds 'Always' Explained Before Given	(a)	68%	64%	64%
Nurses 'Always' Communicated Well	(a)	85%	80%	79%
Pain 'Always' Well Controlled	(a)	72%	71%	71%
Room and Bathroom 'Always' Clean	(a)	82%	73%	73%
Timely Help 'Always' Received	(a)	82%	70%	68%
Would Definitely Recommend Hospital	(a)	72%	71%	71%
Use of Medical Imaging				
Cardiac Imaging Stress Test before Surgery	122	12.3%	5.1%	5.3%
Combination Abdominal CT Scan	137	12.4%	8.7%	10.5%
Combination Brain/Sinus CT Scan[1]	-	-	2.2%	2.7%
Combination Chest CT Scan	96	2.1%	3.6%	2.7%
Follow-up Mammogram/Ultrasound	237	11.4%	8.2%	8.8%
Lumbar Spine MRI for Low Back Pain[1]	-	-	36.9%	37.2%

Saint Mary Mercy Hospital

36475 Five Mile Road
Livonia, MI 48154
Phone: 734-655-4800
Fax: 734-591-3854
URL: www.stmarymercy.org
Type: Acute Care Hospitals
Emergency Services: Yes
Ownership: Voluntary non-profit - Private
Beds: 304

Key Personnel:
Anesthesiology. . . . . Timothy Cahill, MD
Quality Assurance . . . . Lucy Caramanna
Chief of Medical Staff. . . . . Peter Dews, MD
Radiology. . . . . Christopher Esshaki, MD
Infection Control. . . . . Jennifer L Furman
Surgery . . . . John Iljas, MD
Coronary Care . . . . Butchi B Paidipaty
CEO/President. . . . . David A. Spivey

Measure	Cases	This Hosp.	State Avg.	U.S. Avg.
Blood Clot Prevention and Treatment				
Anticoagulation Overlap Therapy[2]	163	89%	90%	93%
ICU Venous Thromboembolism Prophylaxis[2]	36	97%	93%	92%
Incidence of Potentially Preventable VTE[2]	33	15%	8%	10%
UFH with Dosages/Platelet Monitoring[2]	134	100%	96%	97%
Venous Thromboembolism Prophylaxis[2]	402	84%	87%	85%
Warfarin Therapy Discharge Instructions[2]	113	75%	72%	75%
Chest Pain/Possible Heart Attack Care				
Aspirin Given Within 24 Hours of Arrival	49	96%	96%	96%
Fibrinolytic Meds Within 30 Min. of Arrival[7]	-	-	63%	58%
Average Time to ECG (minutes)	50	10	8	7
Average Time to Transfer (minutes)[1]	-	-	53	60
Children's Asthma Care				
Received Home Management Plan of Care	-	-	-	88%
Received Reliever Medication	-	-	-	100%
Received Systemic Corticosteroids	-	-	-	100%
Emergency Department				
Admittance Decision Time (minutes)[2]	721	95	102	98
Head CT Results Within 45 Min. of Arrival	18	83%	54%	57%
Patients Who Left ER Before Being Seen	42,745	2%	2%	2%
Time from ER Arrival to Admit. (minutes)[2]	748	309	288	274
Time from ER Arrival to Discharge (minutes)	352	205	128	134
Time in ER Before Being Evaluated (minutes)	472	19	22	26
Time to Pain Meds for Fractures (minutes)	184	65	55	57
Heart Attack Care				
Aspirin Given at Discharge	162	99%	99%	99%
Fibrinolytic Meds Within 30 Min. of Arrival[7]	-	-	20%	54%
PCI Within 90 Minutes of Arrival	49	90%	95%	96%
Statin Prescribed at Discharge	159	97%	98%	98%
Heart Failure Care				
ACE Inhibitor or ARB for LVSD	137	97%	96%	97%
Discharge Instructions Given	320	96%	94%	94%
Evaluation of LVS Function	482	100%	99%	99%
Medicare Spending				
Medicare Spending per Patient (ratio)	-	1.06	0.96	0.98
Pneumonia Care				
Appropriate Initial Antibiotic Given	222	95%	96%	95%
Blood Culture Timing	356	99%	98%	98%
Pregnancy and Delivery Care				

NOTE: Hospital profiles are in alphabetical order by state, then city, then hospital within the city; Rankings exclude hospitals with less than 25 cases except for patient surveys which excludes hospitals with less than 100 cases; (a) 100-299 cases; (1) The number of cases/patients is too few to report; (2) Data submitted were based on a sample of cases/patients; (3) Results are based on a shorter time period than required; (4) Data suppressed by CMS for one or more quarters; (5) Results are not available for this reporting period; (6) Fewer than 100 patients completed the HCAHPS survey; (7) No cases met the criteria for this measure; (8) The lower limit of the confidence interval cannot be calculated if the number of observed infections equals zero; (9) No data are available from the state/territory for this reporting period; (10) The scores shown reflect fewer than 50 completed surveys; (11) There were discrepancies in the data collection process; (12) This measure does not apply to this hospital for this reporting period; (13) Results cannot be calculated for this reporting period; (14) The results for this state are combined with nearby states to protect confidentiality; Please refer to the User's Guide for a full explanation of data.

Newborn Deliveries Scheduled Early[2]	27	4%	3%	6%
Preventive Care				
Immunization for Influenza[2]	667	88%	89%	90%
Immunization for Pneumonia[2]	903	86%	90%	92%
Stroke Care				
Anticoagulation Therapy for Atrial Fibrillation[2]	15	93%	92%	95%
Antithrombotic Therapy Timing[2]	97	98%	97%	98%
Assessed for Rehabilitation[2]	104	100%	97%	97%
Discharged on Antithrombotic Therapy[2]	95	100%	99%	99%
Discharged on Statin Medication[2]	85	94%	94%	94%
Thrombolytic Therapy Timing[2]	16	81%	69%	66%
Venous Thromboembolism Prophylaxis[2]	117	96%	94%	94%
Written Stroke Educational Materials Given[2]	54	100%	87%	88%
Surgical Care Improvement Project				
Appropriate Beta Blocker Usage	259	99%	98%	98%
Appropriate VTP Within 24 Hours	749	100%	98%	98%
Controlled Postoperative Blood Glucose[7]	-	-	97%	97%
Perioperative Temperature Management	870	100%	100%	100%
Prophylactic Antibiotic Selection	546	99%	99%	99%
Prophylactic Antibiotic Selection (Outpatient)	253	98%	97%	98%
Prophylactic Antibiotic Stopped	529	99%	98%	98%
Prophylactic Antibiotic Timing	546	99%	98%	99%
Prophylactic Antibiotic Timing (Outpatient)	257	95%	97%	98%
Urinary Catheter Removal	559	99%	97%	97%
Survey of Patients' Hospital Experiences				
Area Around Room 'Always' Quiet at Night	300+	53%	60%	61%
Doctors 'Always' Communicated Well	300+	75%	81%	82%
Home Recovery Information Given	300+	86%	87%	85%
Hospital Given 9 or 10 on 10 Point Scale	300+	69%	71%	71%
Meds 'Always' Explained Before Given	300+	57%	64%	64%
Nurses 'Always' Communicated Well	300+	76%	80%	79%
Pain 'Always' Well Controlled	300+	68%	71%	71%
Room and Bathroom 'Always' Clean	300+	67%	73%	73%
Timely Help 'Always' Received	300+	62%	70%	68%
Would Definitely Recommend Hospital	300+	69%	71%	71%
Use of Medical Imaging				
Cardiac Imaging Stress Test before Surgery	490	8.2%	5.1%	5.3%
Combination Abdominal CT Scan	865	4.6%	8.7%	10.5%
Combination Brain/Sinus CT Scan	968	2.3%	2.2%	2.7%
Combination Chest CT Scan	616	4.7%	3.6%	2.7%
Follow-up Mammogram/Ultrasound	1,535	9.8%	8.2%	8.8%
Lumbar Spine MRI for Low Back Pain	139	36.7%	36.9%	37.2%

Memorial Medical Center of West Michigan

1 N Atkinson Drive
Ludington, MI 49431
Phone: 231-843-2591
Fax: 231-845-1732
E-mail: bobm@mmcwm.com
URL: www.mmcwm.com
Type: Acute Care Hospitals
Emergency Services: Yes
Ownership: Voluntary non-profit - Other

Key Personnel:

Patient Relations . . . . Helen Johnson, RN MSN
Chief of Medical Staff . . . . Allan Nelson, MD
Emergency Room . . . . Steven Strbick, DO
CEO/President . . . . Mark Vipperman, FACHE

Measure	Cases	This Hosp.	State Avg.	U.S. Avg.
Blood Clot Prevention and Treatment				
Anticoagulation Overlap Therapy[2]	23	96%	90%	93%
ICU Venous Thromboembolism Prophylaxis[2]	48	94%	93%	92%
Incidence of Potentially Preventable VTE[2,7]	-	-	8%	10%
UFH with Dosages/Platelet Monitoring[2]	20	100%	96%	97%
Venous Thromboembolism Prophylaxis[2]	141	97%	87%	85%
Warfarin Therapy Discharge Instructions[2]	15	100%	72%	75%
Chest Pain/Possible Heart Attack Care				
Aspirin Given Within 24 Hours of Arrival	77	96%	96%	96%
Fibrinolytic Meds Within 30 Min. of Arrival[1]	-	-	63%	58%
Average Time to ECG (minutes)	79	9	8	7
Average Time to Transfer (minutes)[1]	-	-	53	60
Children's Asthma Care				
Received Home Management Plan of Care	-	-	-	88%
Received Reliever Medication	-	-	-	100%
Received Systemic Corticosteroids	-	-	-	100%
Emergency Department				
Admittance Decision Time (minutes)[2]	351	60	102	98
Head CT Results Within 45 Min. of Arrival	13	100%	54%	57%
Patients Who Left ER Before Being Seen	25,440	1%	2%	2%
Time from ER Arrival to Admit. (minutes)[2]	357	271	288	274
Time from ER Arrival to Discharge (minutes)	566	90	128	134
Time in ER Before Being Evaluated (minutes)	582	25	22	26
Time to Pain Meds for Fractures (minutes)	108	44	55	57
Heart Attack Care				
Aspirin Given at Discharge[1,3]	-	-	99%	99%
Fibrinolytic Meds Within 30 Min. of Arrival[3,7]	-	-	20%	54%
PCI Within 90 Minutes of Arrival[3,7]	-	-	95%	96%
Statin Prescribed at Discharge[1,3]	-	-	98%	98%
Heart Failure Care				
ACE Inhibitor or ARB for LVSD	11	82%	96%	97%
Discharge Instructions Given	58	84%	94%	94%
Evaluation of LVS Function	72	100%	99%	99%
Medicare Spending				
Medicare Spending per Patient (ratio)	-	0.90	0.96	0.98
Pneumonia Care				
Appropriate Initial Antibiotic Given	96	95%	96%	95%
Blood Culture Timing	174	99%	98%	98%
Pregnancy and Delivery Care				
Newborn Deliveries Scheduled Early[2]	32	3%	3%	6%
Preventive Care				
Immunization for Influenza[2]	265	94%	89%	90%
Immunization for Pneumonia[2]	314	98%	90%	92%
Stroke Care				
Anticoagulation Therapy for Atrial Fibrillation[1]	-	-	92%	95%
Antithrombotic Therapy Timing	21	100%	97%	98%
Assessed for Rehabilitation	24	100%	97%	97%
Discharged on Antithrombotic Therapy	22	95%	99%	99%
Discharged on Statin Medication	16	94%	94%	94%
Thrombolytic Therapy Timing[7]	-	-	69%	66%
Venous Thromboembolism Prophylaxis	23	96%	94%	94%
Written Stroke Educational Materials Given	16	88%	87%	88%
Surgical Care Improvement Project				
Appropriate Beta Blocker Usage	74	95%	98%	98%
Appropriate VTP Within 24 Hours	219	95%	98%	98%
Controlled Postoperative Blood Glucose[7]	-	-	97%	97%
Perioperative Temperature Management	248	100%	100%	100%
Prophylactic Antibiotic Selection	163	100%	99%	99%
Prophylactic Antibiotic Selection (Outpatient)	59	100%	97%	98%
Prophylactic Antibiotic Stopped	161	98%	98%	98%
Prophylactic Antibiotic Timing	163	96%	98%	99%
Prophylactic Antibiotic Timing (Outpatient)	59	98%	97%	98%
Urinary Catheter Removal	57	89%	97%	97%
Survey of Patients' Hospital Experiences				
Area Around Room 'Always' Quiet at Night	300+	57%	60%	61%
Doctors 'Always' Communicated Well	300+	80%	81%	82%
Home Recovery Information Given	300+	88%	87%	85%
Hospital Given 9 or 10 on 10 Point Scale	300+	70%	71%	71%
Meds 'Always' Explained Before Given	300+	62%	64%	64%
Nurses 'Always' Communicated Well	300+	80%	80%	79%
Pain 'Always' Well Controlled	300+	69%	71%	71%
Room and Bathroom 'Always' Clean	300+	75%	73%	73%
Timely Help 'Always' Received	300+	74%	70%	68%
Would Definitely Recommend Hospital	300+	64%	71%	71%
Use of Medical Imaging				
Cardiac Imaging Stress Test before Surgery	290	4.8%	5.1%	5.3%
Combination Abdominal CT Scan	610	5.4%	8.7%	10.5%
Combination Brain/Sinus CT Scan	568	1.9%	2.2%	2.7%
Combination Chest CT Scan	542	1.8%	3.6%	2.7%
Follow-up Mammogram/Ultrasound	1,123	7.2%	8.2%	8.8%
Lumbar Spine MRI for Low Back Pain	124	41.1%	36.9%	37.2%

West Shore Medical Center

1465 E Parkdale Avenue
Manistee, MI 49660
Phone: 231-398-1000
Fax: 231-398-1098
URL: www.westshoremedcenter.org
Type: Critical Access Hospitals
Emergency Services: Yes
Ownership: Voluntary non-profit - Other

Key Personnel:

Emergency Room . . . . Donald Albrecht
Quality Assurance . . . . Sandy Arnold
President . . . . James Baker
Operating Room. . . . . Eduardo Barlan
Chief of Medical Staff . . . . Glenn Griffiths
Intensive Care Unit. . . . . Joyce Miler
Radiology. . . . . John Raymond

Measure	Cases	This Hosp.	State Avg.	U.S. Avg.
Blood Clot Prevention and Treatment				
Anticoagulation Overlap Therapy[5]	-	-	90%	93%
ICU Venous Thromboembolism Prophylaxis[5]	-	-	93%	92%
Incidence of Potentially Preventable VTE[5]	-	-	8%	10%
UFH with Dosages/Platelet Monitoring[5]	-	-	96%	97%
Venous Thromboembolism Prophylaxis[5]	-	-	87%	85%
Warfarin Therapy Discharge Instructions[5]	-	-	72%	75%
Chest Pain/Possible Heart Attack Care				
Aspirin Given Within 24 Hours of Arrival	59	100%	96%	96%
Fibrinolytic Meds Within 30 Min. of Arrival[1]	-	-	63%	58%
Average Time to ECG (minutes)	61	6	8	7
Average Time to Transfer (minutes)[1]	-	-	53	60
Children's Asthma Care				
Received Home Management Plan of Care	-	-	-	88%
Received Reliever Medication	-	-	-	100%
Received Systemic Corticosteroids	-	-	-	100%
Emergency Department				
Admittance Decision Time (minutes)[5]	-	-	102	98
Head CT Results Within 45 Min. of Arrival[5]	-	-	54%	57%
Patients Who Left ER Before Being Seen[5]	-	-	2%	2%
Time from ER Arrival to Admit. (minutes)[5]	-	-	288	274
Time from ER Arrival to Discharge (minutes)	360	94	128	134
Time in ER Before Being Evaluated (minutes)	131	24	22	26
Time to Pain Meds for Fractures (minutes)[3]	43	57	55	57
Heart Attack Care				
Aspirin Given at Discharge[1]	-	-	99%	99%
Fibrinolytic Meds Within 30 Min. of Arrival[7]	-	-	20%	54%
PCI Within 90 Minutes of Arrival[7]	-	-	95%	96%
Statin Prescribed at Discharge[1]	-	-	98%	98%
Heart Failure Care				
ACE Inhibitor or ARB for LVSD[1]	-	-	96%	97%
Discharge Instructions Given	36	81%	94%	94%
Evaluation of LVS Function	41	98%	99%	99%
Medicare Spending				
Medicare Spending per Patient (ratio)	-	-	0.96	0.98
Pneumonia Care				
Appropriate Initial Antibiotic Given	54	100%	96%	95%
Blood Culture Timing	75	97%	98%	98%
Pregnancy and Delivery Care				
Newborn Deliveries Scheduled Early[5]	-	-	3%	6%
Preventive Care				
Immunization for Influenza[5]	-	-	89%	90%
Immunization for Pneumonia[5]	-	-	90%	92%
Stroke Care				
Anticoagulation Therapy for Atrial Fibrillation[5]	-	-	92%	95%
Antithrombotic Therapy Timing[5]	-	-	97%	98%
Assessed for Rehabilitation[5]	-	-	97%	97%
Discharged on Antithrombotic Therapy[5]	-	-	99%	99%
Discharged on Statin Medication[5]	-	-	94%	94%
Thrombolytic Therapy Timing[5]	-	-	69%	66%
Venous Thromboembolism Prophylaxis[5]	-	-	94%	94%
Written Stroke Educational Materials Given[5]	-	-	87%	88%
Surgical Care Improvement Project				
Appropriate Beta Blocker Usage	27	96%	98%	98%
Appropriate VTP Within 24 Hours	96	92%	98%	98%
Controlled Postoperative Blood Glucose[7]	-	-	97%	97%
Perioperative Temperature Management	139	99%	100%	100%
Prophylactic Antibiotic Selection	74	99%	99%	99%
Prophylactic Antibiotic Selection (Outpatient)	16	100%	97%	98%
Prophylactic Antibiotic Stopped	73	99%	98%	98%
Prophylactic Antibiotic Timing	74	100%	98%	99%
Prophylactic Antibiotic Timing (Outpatient)	16	100%	97%	98%
Urinary Catheter Removal	87	100%	97%	97%
Survey of Patients' Hospital Experiences				
Area Around Room 'Always' Quiet at Night	(a)	65%	60%	61%
Doctors 'Always' Communicated Well	(a)	83%	81%	82%

NOTE: Hospital profiles are in alphabetical order by state, then city, then hospital within the city; Rankings exclude hospitals with less than 25 cases except for patient surveys which excludes hospitals with less than 100 cases; (a) 100-299 cases; (1) The number of cases/patients is too few to report; (2) Data submitted were based on a sample of cases/patients; (3) Results are based on a shorter time period than required; (4) Data suppressed by CMS for one or more quarters; (5) Results are not available for this reporting period; (6) Fewer than 100 patients completed the HCAHPS survey; (7) No cases met the criteria for this measure; (8) The lower limit of the confidence interval cannot be calculated if the number of observed infections equals zero; (9) No data are available from the state/territory for this reporting period; (10) The scores shown reflect fewer than 50 completed surveys; (11) There were discrepancies in the data collection process; (12) This measure does not apply to this hospital for this reporting period; (13) Results cannot be calculated for this reporting period; (14) The results for this state are combined with nearby states to protect confidentiality; Please refer to the User's Guide for a full explanation of data.

Measure	Cases	This Hosp.	State Avg.	U.S. Avg.
Home Recovery Information Given	(a)	86%	87%	85%
Hospital Given 9 or 10 on 10 Point Scale	(a)	74%	71%	71%
Meds 'Always' Explained Before Given	(a)	70%	64%	64%
Nurses 'Always' Communicated Well	(a)	82%	80%	79%
Pain 'Always' Well Controlled	(a)	71%	71%	71%
Room and Bathroom 'Always' Clean	(a)	83%	73%	73%
Timely Help 'Always' Received	(a)	73%	70%	68%
Would Definitely Recommend Hospital	(a)	70%	71%	71%
Use of Medical Imaging				
Cardiac Imaging Stress Test before Surgery	173	5.2%	5.1%	5.3%
Combination Abdominal CT Scan	615	3.4%	8.7%	10.5%
Combination Brain/Sinus CT Scan[1]	-	-	2.2%	2.7%
Combination Chest CT Scan	347	2.9%	3.6%	2.7%
Follow-up Mammogram/Ultrasound	613	4.2%	8.2%	8.8%
Lumbar Spine MRI for Low Back Pain	78	41.0%	36.9%	37.2%

Schoolcraft Memorial Hospital

7870w Us Highway 2
Manistique, MI 49854
Phone: 906-341-3200
Fax: 906-341-3297
E-mail: ajones@scmh.org
URL: www.scmh.org

Type: Critical Access Hospitals
Emergency Services: Yes
Ownership: Government - Local
Beds: 25

Key Personnel:
CEO/President. . . . . David B Jahn

Measure	Cases	This Hosp.	State Avg.	U.S. Avg.
Blood Clot Prevention and Treatment				
Anticoagulation Overlap Therapy[5]	-	-	90%	93%
ICU Venous Thromboembolism Prophylaxis[5]	-	-	93%	92%
Incidence of Potentially Preventable VTE[5]	-	-	8%	10%
UFH with Dosages/Platelet Monitoring[5]	-	-	96%	97%
Venous Thromboembolism Prophylaxis[5]	-	-	87%	85%
Warfarin Therapy Discharge Instructions[5]	-	-	72%	75%
Chest Pain/Possible Heart Attack Care				
Aspirin Given Within 24 Hours of Arrival	35	94%	96%	96%
Fibrinolytic Meds Within 30 Min. of Arrival[1,3]	-	-	63%	58%
Average Time to ECG (minutes)	36	6	8	7
Average Time to Transfer (minutes)[3,7]	-	-	53	60
Children's Asthma Care				
Received Home Management Plan of Care	-	-	-	88%
Received Reliever Medication	-	-	-	100%
Received Systemic Corticosteroids	-	-	-	100%
Emergency Department				
Admittance Decision Time (minutes)[5]	-	-	102	98
Head CT Results Within 45 Min. of Arrival[5]	-	-	54%	57%
Patients Who Left ER Before Being Seen[5]	-	-	2%	2%
Time from ER Arrival to Admit. (minutes)[5]	-	-	288	274
Time from ER Arrival to Discharge (minutes)	1,275	95	128	134
Time in ER Before Being Evaluated (minutes)	1,360	16	22	26
Time to Pain Meds for Fractures (minutes)[5]	-	-	55	57
Heart Attack Care				
Aspirin Given at Discharge[5]	-	-	99%	99%
Fibrinolytic Meds Within 30 Min. of Arrival[5]	-	-	20%	54%
PCI Within 90 Minutes of Arrival[5]	-	-	95%	96%
Statin Prescribed at Discharge[5]	-	-	98%	98%
Heart Failure Care				
ACE Inhibitor or ARB for LVSD[1]	-	-	96%	97%
Discharge Instructions Given[1]	-	-	94%	94%
Evaluation of LVS Function[1]	-	-	99%	99%
Medicare Spending				
Medicare Spending per Patient (ratio)	-	-	0.96	0.98
Pneumonia Care				
Appropriate Initial Antibiotic Given	39	85%	96%	95%
Blood Culture Timing	49	96%	98%	98%
Pregnancy and Delivery Care				
Newborn Deliveries Scheduled Early[5]	-	-	3%	6%
Preventive Care				
Immunization for Influenza[5]	-	-	89%	90%
Immunization for Pneumonia[5]	-	-	90%	92%
Stroke Care				
Anticoagulation Therapy for Atrial Fibrillation[5]	-	-	92%	95%
Antithrombotic Therapy Timing[5]	-	-	97%	98%
Assessed for Rehabilitation[5]	-	-	97%	97%
Discharged on Antithrombotic Therapy[5]	-	-	99%	99%
Discharged on Statin Medication[5]	-	-	94%	94%
Thrombolytic Therapy Timing[5]	-	-	69%	66%
Venous Thromboembolism Prophylaxis[5]	-	-	94%	94%
Written Stroke Educational Materials Given[5]	-	-	87%	88%
Surgical Care Improvement Project				
Appropriate Beta Blocker Usage[5]	-	-	98%	98%
Appropriate VTP Within 24 Hours[5]	-	-	98%	98%
Controlled Postoperative Blood Glucose[5]	-	-	97%	97%
Perioperative Temperature Management[5]	-	-	100%	100%
Prophylactic Antibiotic Selection[5]	-	-	99%	99%
Prophylactic Antibiotic Selection (Outpatient)[5]	-	-	97%	98%
Prophylactic Antibiotic Stopped[5]	-	-	98%	98%
Prophylactic Antibiotic Timing[5]	-	-	98%	99%
Prophylactic Antibiotic Timing (Outpatient)[5]	-	-	97%	98%
Urinary Catheter Removal[5]	-	-	97%	97%
Survey of Patients' Hospital Experiences				
Area Around Room 'Always' Quiet at Night	(a)	69%	60%	61%
Doctors 'Always' Communicated Well	(a)	85%	81%	82%
Home Recovery Information Given	(a)	90%	87%	85%
Hospital Given 9 or 10 on 10 Point Scale	(a)	78%	71%	71%
Meds 'Always' Explained Before Given	(a)	68%	64%	64%
Nurses 'Always' Communicated Well	(a)	85%	80%	79%
Pain 'Always' Well Controlled	(a)	79%	71%	71%
Room and Bathroom 'Always' Clean	(a)	83%	73%	73%
Timely Help 'Always' Received	(a)	84%	70%	68%
Would Definitely Recommend Hospital	(a)	74%	71%	71%
Use of Medical Imaging				
Cardiac Imaging Stress Test before Surgery	94	5.3%	5.1%	5.3%
Combination Abdominal CT Scan	139	48.2%	8.7%	10.5%
Combination Brain/Sinus CT Scan[1]	-	-	2.2%	2.7%
Combination Chest CT Scan	102	37.3%	3.6%	2.7%
Follow-up Mammogram/Ultrasound	382	6.3%	8.2%	8.8%
Lumbar Spine MRI for Low Back Pain[1]	-	-	36.9%	37.2%

Marlette Regional Hospital

2770 Main Street
Marlette, MI 48453
Phone: 989-635-4000
Fax: 989-635-4027
URL: www.marlettecommunityhospital.com

Type: Critical Access Hospitals
Emergency Services: Yes
Ownership: Voluntary non-profit - Private
Beds: 97

Key Personnel:
Anesthesiology. . . . . Jody Bovenschen
Emergency Room . . . . Susan Brzezinski
Patient Relations . . . . Molly Disteirath
Quality Assurance . . . . Bobbi Jones
Infection Control. . . . . Sharon Kasprzyk, RN
Operating Room. . . . . Mohan Dass Macha
CEO/President. . . . . David S McEwen
Chief of Medical Staff. . . . . William Starbird, MD

Measure	Cases	This Hosp.	State Avg.	U.S. Avg.
Blood Clot Prevention and Treatment				
Anticoagulation Overlap Therapy[1,2]	-	-	90%	93%
ICU Venous Thromboembolism Prophylaxis[1,2]	-	-	93%	92%
Incidence of Potentially Preventable VTE[1,2]	-	-	8%	10%
UFH with Dosages/Platelet Monitoring[1,2]	-	-	96%	97%
Venous Thromboembolism Prophylaxis[2]	108	69%	87%	85%
Warfarin Therapy Discharge Instructions[1,2]	-	-	72%	75%
Chest Pain/Possible Heart Attack Care				
Aspirin Given Within 24 Hours of Arrival	53	98%	96%	96%
Fibrinolytic Meds Within 30 Min. of Arrival[1]	-	-	63%	58%
Average Time to ECG (minutes)	50	2	8	7
Average Time to Transfer (minutes)[1]	-	-	53	60
Children's Asthma Care				
Received Home Management Plan of Care	-	-	-	88%
Received Reliever Medication	-	-	-	100%
Received Systemic Corticosteroids	-	-	-	100%
Emergency Department				
Admittance Decision Time (minutes)[2]	335	54	102	98
Head CT Results Within 45 Min. of Arrival[5]	-	-	54%	57%
Patients Who Left ER Before Being Seen[5]	-	-	2%	2%
Time from ER Arrival to Admit. (minutes)[2]	440	200	288	274
Time from ER Arrival to Discharge (minutes)	307	77	128	134
Time in ER Before Being Evaluated (minutes)	426	12	22	26
Time to Pain Meds for Fractures (minutes)[5]	-	-	55	57
Heart Attack Care				
Aspirin Given at Discharge[1]	-	-	99%	99%
Fibrinolytic Meds Within 30 Min. of Arrival[7]	-	-	20%	54%
PCI Within 90 Minutes of Arrival[7]	-	-	95%	96%
Statin Prescribed at Discharge[1]	-	-	98%	98%
Heart Failure Care				
ACE Inhibitor or ARB for LVSD	13	69%	96%	97%
Discharge Instructions Given	27	63%	94%	94%
Evaluation of LVS Function	31	74%	99%	99%
Medicare Spending				
Medicare Spending per Patient (ratio)	-	-	0.96	0.98
Pneumonia Care				
Appropriate Initial Antibiotic Given	27	96%	96%	95%
Blood Culture Timing	46	80%	98%	98%
Pregnancy and Delivery Care				
Newborn Deliveries Scheduled Early[5]	-	-	3%	6%
Preventive Care				
Immunization for Influenza[2,3]	135	97%	89%	90%
Immunization for Pneumonia[2,3]	324	94%	90%	92%
Stroke Care				
Anticoagulation Therapy for Atrial Fibrillation[1]	-	-	92%	95%
Antithrombotic Therapy Timing[1]	-	-	97%	98%
Assessed for Rehabilitation[1]	-	-	97%	97%
Discharged on Antithrombotic Therapy[1]	-	-	99%	99%
Discharged on Statin Medication[1]	-	-	94%	94%
Thrombolytic Therapy Timing[7]	-	-	69%	66%
Venous Thromboembolism Prophylaxis[1]	-	-	94%	94%
Written Stroke Educational Materials Given[1]	-	-	87%	88%
Surgical Care Improvement Project				
Appropriate Beta Blocker Usage[1]	-	-	98%	98%
Appropriate VTP Within 24 Hours	26	100%	98%	98%
Controlled Postoperative Blood Glucose[7]	-	-	97%	97%
Perioperative Temperature Management	29	97%	100%	100%
Prophylactic Antibiotic Selection	23	96%	99%	99%
Prophylactic Antibiotic Selection (Outpatient)	26	58%	97%	98%
Prophylactic Antibiotic Stopped	22	82%	98%	98%
Prophylactic Antibiotic Timing	23	96%	98%	99%
Prophylactic Antibiotic Timing (Outpatient)	30	77%	97%	98%
Urinary Catheter Removal	25	52%	97%	97%
Survey of Patients' Hospital Experiences				
Area Around Room 'Always' Quiet at Night	(a)	64%	60%	61%
Doctors 'Always' Communicated Well	(a)	86%	81%	82%
Home Recovery Information Given	(a)	89%	87%	85%
Hospital Given 9 or 10 on 10 Point Scale	(a)	81%	71%	71%
Meds 'Always' Explained Before Given	(a)	72%	64%	64%
Nurses 'Always' Communicated Well	(a)	85%	80%	79%
Pain 'Always' Well Controlled	(a)	70%	71%	71%
Room and Bathroom 'Always' Clean	(a)	82%	73%	73%
Timely Help 'Always' Received	(a)	70%	70%	68%
Would Definitely Recommend Hospital	(a)	81%	71%	71%
Use of Medical Imaging				
Cardiac Imaging Stress Test before Surgery	260	3.8%	5.1%	5.3%
Combination Abdominal CT Scan	282	0.4%	8.7%	10.5%
Combination Brain/Sinus CT Scan[1]	-	-	2.2%	2.7%
Combination Chest CT Scan	154	0.0%	3.6%	2.7%
Follow-up Mammogram/Ultrasound	395	5.1%	8.2%	8.8%
Lumbar Spine MRI for Low Back Pain[7]	-	-	36.9%	37.2%

Marquette General Hospital

420 W Magnetic
Marquette, MI 49855
Phone: 906-228-9440
Fax: 906-225-3098
URL: www.mgh.org

Type: Acute Care Hospitals
Emergency Services: Yes
Ownership: Government - Local
Beds: 352

Key Personnel:
Chief of Medical Staff. . . . . Daniel Hardie, MD
CEO/President. . . . . Bill Nemacheck
Chair/CEO . . . . Watson Olson

Measure	Cases	This Hosp.	State Avg.	U.S. Avg.
Blood Clot Prevention and Treatment				
Anticoagulation Overlap Therapy[2]	49	94%	90%	93%
ICU Venous Thromboembolism Prophylaxis[2]	103	83%	93%	92%

NOTE: Hospital profiles are in alphabetical order by state, then city, then hospital within the city; Rankings exclude hospitals with less than 25 cases except for patient surveys which excludes hospitals with less than 100 cases; (a) 100-299 cases; (1) The number of cases/patients is too few to report; (2) Data submitted were based on a sample of cases/patients; (3) Results are based on a shorter time period than required; (4) Data suppressed by CMS for one or more quarters; (5) Results are not available for this reporting period; (6) Fewer than 100 patients completed the HCAHPS survey; (7) No cases met the criteria for this measure; (8) The lower limit of the confidence interval cannot be calculated if the number of observed infections equals zero; (9) No data are available from the state/territory for this reporting period; (10) The scores shown reflect fewer than 50 completed surveys; (11) There were discrepancies in the data collection process; (12) This measure does not apply to this hospital for this reporting period; (13) Results cannot be calculated for this reporting period; (14) The results for this state are combined with nearby states to protect confidentiality; Please refer to the User's Guide for a full explanation of data.

Measure	Cases	This Hosp.	State Avg.	U.S. Avg.
Incidence of Potentially Preventable VTE[1,2]	-	-	8%	10%
UFH with Dosages/Platelet Monitoring[2]	12	33%	96%	97%
Venous Thromboembolism Prophylaxis[2]	222	91%	87%	85%
Warfarin Therapy Discharge Instructions[2]	40	20%	72%	75%
Chest Pain/Possible Heart Attack Care				
Aspirin Given Within 24 Hours of Arrival[1,3]	-	-	96%	96%
Fibrinolytic Meds Within 30 Min. of Arrival[5]	-	-	63%	58%
Average Time to ECG (minutes)[1,3]	-	-	8	7
Average Time to Transfer (minutes)[5]	-	-	53	60
Children's Asthma Care				
Received Home Management Plan of Care	-	-	-	88%
Received Reliever Medication	-	-	-	100%
Received Systemic Corticosteroids	-	-	-	100%
Emergency Department				
Admittance Decision Time (minutes)[2]	200	142	102	98
Head CT Results Within 45 Min. of Arrival[1]	-	-	54%	57%
Patients Who Left ER Before Being Seen	25,338	0%	2%	2%
Time from ER Arrival to Admit. (minutes)[2]	216	284	288	274
Time from ER Arrival to Discharge (minutes)	341	107	128	134
Time in ER Before Being Evaluated (minutes)	327	24	22	26
Time to Pain Meds for Fractures (minutes)	66	50	55	57
Heart Attack Care				
Aspirin Given at Discharge	420	100%	99%	99%
Fibrinolytic Meds Within 30 Min. of Arrival[7]	-	-	20%	54%
PCI Within 90 Minutes of Arrival	28	96%	95%	96%
Statin Prescribed at Discharge	412	100%	98%	98%
Heart Failure Care				
ACE Inhibitor or ARB for LVSD	53	100%	96%	97%
Discharge Instructions Given	164	87%	94%	94%
Evaluation of LVS Function	197	99%	99%	99%
Medicare Spending				
Medicare Spending per Patient (ratio)		0.95	0.96	0.98
Pneumonia Care				
Appropriate Initial Antibiotic Given	61	100%	96%	95%
Blood Culture Timing	112	99%	98%	98%
Pregnancy and Delivery Care				
Newborn Deliveries Scheduled Early[2]	18	6%	3%	6%
Preventive Care				
Immunization for Influenza[2]	534	86%	89%	90%
Immunization for Pneumonia[2]	639	85%	90%	92%
Stroke Care				
Anticoagulation Therapy for Atrial Fibrillation[2]	21	86%	92%	95%
Antithrombotic Therapy Timing[2]	60	100%	97%	98%
Assessed for Rehabilitation[2]	104	98%	97%	97%
Discharged on Antithrombotic Therapy[2]	88	100%	99%	99%
Discharged on Statin Medication[2]	73	100%	94%	94%
Thrombolytic Therapy Timing[1,2]	-	-	69%	66%
Venous Thromboembolism Prophylaxis[2]	98	85%	94%	94%
Written Stroke Educational Materials Given[2]	56	52%	87%	88%
Surgical Care Improvement Project				
Appropriate Beta Blocker Usage[2]	234	97%	98%	98%
Appropriate VTP Within 24 Hours[2]	353	95%	98%	98%
Controlled Postoperative Blood Glucose[2]	131	95%	97%	97%
Perioperative Temperature Management[2]	475	100%	100%	100%
Prophylactic Antibiotic Selection[2]	448	99%	99%	99%
Prophylactic Antibiotic Selection (Outpatient)	644	98%	97%	98%
Prophylactic Antibiotic Stopped[2]	439	97%	98%	98%
Prophylactic Antibiotic Timing[2]	449	99%	98%	99%
Prophylactic Antibiotic Timing (Outpatient)	533	95%	97%	98%
Urinary Catheter Removal[2]	232	94%	97%	97%
Survey of Patients' Hospital Experiences				
Area Around Room 'Always' Quiet at Night	300+	51%	60%	61%
Doctors 'Always' Communicated Well	300+	76%	81%	82%
Home Recovery Information Given	300+	88%	87%	85%
Hospital Given 9 or 10 on 10 Point Scale	300+	59%	71%	71%
Meds 'Always' Explained Before Given	300+	58%	64%	64%
Nurses 'Always' Communicated Well	300+	71%	80%	79%
Pain 'Always' Well Controlled	300+	63%	71%	71%
Room and Bathroom 'Always' Clean	300+	74%	73%	73%
Timely Help 'Always' Received	300+	61%	70%	68%
Would Definitely Recommend Hospital	300+	60%	71%	71%
Use of Medical Imaging				
Cardiac Imaging Stress Test before Surgery	759	7.2%	5.1%	5.3%
Combination Abdominal CT Scan	511	37.0%	8.7%	10.5%
Combination Brain/Sinus CT Scan	436	1.8%	2.2%	2.7%
Combination Chest CT Scan	386	16.3%	3.6%	2.7%
Follow-up Mammogram/Ultrasound	1,802	10.9%	8.2%	8.8%
Lumbar Spine MRI for Low Back Pain	213	37.6%	36.9%	37.2%

Oaklawn Hospital

200 N Madison
Marshall, MI 49068
Phone: 269-781-4271
Fax: 269-781-7117
URL: www.oaklawnhospital.org
Type: Acute Care Hospitals
Emergency Services: Yes
Ownership: Voluntary non-profit - Other
Beds: 94

Key Personnel:

Radiology. . . . . Indraneel Baner, RRT
Operating Room. . . . . Thomas Casale, RN
Intensive Care Unit. . . . . Dr Alcides Gil-Acosta
Anesthesiology. . . . . Rick Gorham
Infection Control. . . . . Pat Jendryka, RN
Emergency Room . . . . Dr David Komasara
Chief of Medical Staff. . . . . George Seifert, MD

Measure	Cases	This Hosp.	State Avg.	U.S. Avg.
Blood Clot Prevention and Treatment				
Anticoagulation Overlap Therapy[2]	35	97%	90%	93%
ICU Venous Thromboembolism Prophylaxis[2]	38	95%	93%	92%
Incidence of Potentially Preventable VTE[1,2]	-	-	8%	10%
UFH with Dosages/Platelet Monitoring[2]	27	100%	96%	97%
Venous Thromboembolism Prophylaxis[2]	169	92%	87%	85%
Warfarin Therapy Discharge Instructions[2]	30	93%	72%	75%
Chest Pain/Possible Heart Attack Care				
Aspirin Given Within 24 Hours of Arrival	271	100%	96%	96%
Fibrinolytic Meds Within 30 Min. of Arrival[7]	-	-	63%	58%
Average Time to ECG (minutes)	283	4	8	7
Average Time to Transfer (minutes)	22	24	53	60
Children's Asthma Care				
Received Home Management Plan of Care	-	-	-	88%
Received Reliever Medication	-	-	-	100%
Received Systemic Corticosteroids	-	-	-	100%
Emergency Department				
Admittance Decision Time (minutes)[2]	283	71	102	98
Head CT Results Within 45 Min. of Arrival	11	64%	54%	57%
Patients Who Left ER Before Being Seen	22,966	1%	2%	2%
Time from ER Arrival to Admit. (minutes)[2]	291	251	288	274
Time from ER Arrival to Discharge (minutes)	333	121	128	134
Time in ER Before Being Evaluated (minutes)	383	24	22	26
Time to Pain Meds for Fractures (minutes)	92	62	55	57
Heart Attack Care				
Aspirin Given at Discharge[1]	-	-	99%	99%
Fibrinolytic Meds Within 30 Min. of Arrival[7]	-	-	20%	54%
PCI Within 90 Minutes of Arrival[7]	-	-	95%	96%
Statin Prescribed at Discharge[1]	-	-	98%	98%
Heart Failure Care				
ACE Inhibitor or ARB for LVSD	17	94%	96%	97%
Discharge Instructions Given	56	96%	94%	94%
Evaluation of LVS Function	65	100%	99%	99%
Medicare Spending				
Medicare Spending per Patient (ratio)	-	0.92	0.96	0.98
Pneumonia Care				
Appropriate Initial Antibiotic Given	68	100%	96%	95%
Blood Culture Timing	104	100%	98%	98%
Pregnancy and Delivery Care				
Newborn Deliveries Scheduled Early[2]	17	0%	3%	6%
Preventive Care				
Immunization for Influenza[2]	366	98%	89%	90%
Immunization for Pneumonia[2]	375	97%	90%	92%
Stroke Care				
Anticoagulation Therapy for Atrial Fibrillation[1]	-	-	92%	95%
Antithrombotic Therapy Timing	12	100%	97%	98%
Assessed for Rehabilitation	20	100%	97%	97%
Discharged on Antithrombotic Therapy	20	95%	99%	99%
Discharged on Statin Medication	15	93%	94%	94%
Thrombolytic Therapy Timing[7]	-	-	69%	66%
Venous Thromboembolism Prophylaxis	14	86%	94%	94%
Written Stroke Educational Materials Given	15	100%	87%	88%
Surgical Care Improvement Project				
Appropriate Beta Blocker Usage[2]	139	100%	98%	98%
Appropriate VTP Within 24 Hours[2]	348	99%	98%	98%
Controlled Postoperative Blood Glucose[2,7]	-	-	97%	97%
Perioperative Temperature Management[2]	488	100%	100%	100%
Prophylactic Antibiotic Selection[2]	338	100%	99%	99%
Prophylactic Antibiotic Selection (Outpatient)	63	97%	97%	98%
Prophylactic Antibiotic Stopped[2]	335	100%	98%	98%
Prophylactic Antibiotic Timing[2]	339	99%	98%	99%
Prophylactic Antibiotic Timing (Outpatient)	63	100%	97%	98%
Urinary Catheter Removal[2]	175	97%	97%	97%
Survey of Patients' Hospital Experiences				
Area Around Room 'Always' Quiet at Night	300+	66%	60%	61%
Doctors 'Always' Communicated Well	300+	82%	81%	82%
Home Recovery Information Given	300+	91%	87%	85%
Hospital Given 9 or 10 on 10 Point Scale	300+	77%	71%	71%
Meds 'Always' Explained Before Given	300+	69%	64%	64%
Nurses 'Always' Communicated Well	300+	79%	80%	79%
Pain 'Always' Well Controlled	300+	70%	71%	71%
Room and Bathroom 'Always' Clean	300+	74%	73%	73%
Timely Help 'Always' Received	300+	69%	70%	68%
Would Definitely Recommend Hospital	300+	81%	71%	71%
Use of Medical Imaging				
Cardiac Imaging Stress Test before Surgery	313	4.5%	5.1%	5.3%
Combination Abdominal CT Scan	608	1.5%	8.7%	10.5%
Combination Brain/Sinus CT Scan[1]	-	-	2.2%	2.7%
Combination Chest CT Scan	410	0.2%	3.6%	2.7%
Follow-up Mammogram/Ultrasound	1,150	6.2%	8.2%	8.8%
Lumbar Spine MRI for Low Back Pain	55	29.1%	36.9%	37.2%

Midmichigan Medical Center - Midland

4000 Wellness Drive
Midland, MI 48670
Phone: 989-839-3000
Fax: 989-839-3307
URL: www.midmichigan.org
Type: Acute Care Hospitals
Emergency Services: Yes
Ownership: Voluntary non-profit - Other
Beds: 250

Key Personnel:

Cardiac Laboratory. . . . . Karen Colkins
Infection Control. . . . . Brenda Dauer, RN
Operating Room. . . . . Cindy Ferdrich
Chief of Medical Staff. . . . . Mark Goethe, MD
Radiology. . . . . Rajnikant Mehta, MD
Quality Assurance . . . . Chandra Morse
CEO/President. . . . . Rick Reynolds
Pediatric In-Patient Care . . . . Denise Schaffert, MD

Measure	Cases	This Hosp.	State Avg.	U.S. Avg.
Blood Clot Prevention and Treatment				
Anticoagulation Overlap Therapy[2]	104	95%	90%	93%
ICU Venous Thromboembolism Prophylaxis[2]	90	92%	93%	92%
Incidence of Potentially Preventable VTE[1,2]	-	-	8%	10%
UFH with Dosages/Platelet Monitoring[2]	83	100%	96%	97%
Venous Thromboembolism Prophylaxis[2]	311	92%	87%	85%
Warfarin Therapy Discharge Instructions[2]	89	89%	72%	75%
Chest Pain/Possible Heart Attack Care				
Aspirin Given Within 24 Hours of Arrival[1,3]	-	-	96%	96%
Fibrinolytic Meds Within 30 Min. of Arrival[5]	-	-	63%	58%
Average Time to ECG (minutes)[1,3]	-	-	8	7
Average Time to Transfer (minutes)[5]	-	-	53	60
Children's Asthma Care				
Received Home Management Plan of Care	-	-	-	88%
Received Reliever Medication	-	-	-	100%
Received Systemic Corticosteroids	-	-	-	100%
Emergency Department				
Admittance Decision Time (minutes)[2]	519	92	102	98
Head CT Results Within 45 Min. of Arrival[1]	-	-	54%	57%
Patients Who Left ER Before Being Seen	36,764	1%	2%	2%
Time from ER Arrival to Admit. (minutes)[2]	545	245	288	274
Time from ER Arrival to Discharge (minutes)	420	166	128	134
Time in ER Before Being Evaluated (minutes)	436	56	22	26
Time to Pain Meds for Fractures (minutes)	147	67	55	57
Heart Attack Care				
Aspirin Given at Discharge	514	99%	99%	99%
Fibrinolytic Meds Within 30 Min. of Arrival[7]	-	-	20%	54%
PCI Within 90 Minutes of Arrival	44	91%	95%	96%

NOTE: Hospital profiles are in alphabetical order by state, then city, then hospital within the city; Rankings exclude hospitals with less than 25 cases except for patient surveys which excludes hospitals with less than 100 cases; (a) 100-299 cases; (1) The number of cases/patients is too few to report; (2) Data submitted were based on a sample of cases/patients; (3) Results are based on a shorter time period than required; (4) Data suppressed by CMS for one or more quarters; (5) Results are not available for this reporting period; (6) Fewer than 100 patients completed the HCAHPS survey; (7) No cases met the criteria for this measure; (8) The lower limit of the confidence interval cannot be calculated if the number of observed infections equals zero; (9) No data are available from the state/territory for this reporting period; (10) The scores shown reflect fewer than 50 completed surveys; (11) There were discrepancies in the data collection process; (12) This measure does not apply to this hospital for this reporting period; (13) Results cannot be calculated for this reporting period; (14) The results for this state are combined with nearby states to protect confidentiality; Please refer to the User's Guide for a full explanation of data.

Measure	Cases	This Hosp.	State Avg.	U.S. Avg.
Statin Prescribed at Discharge	506	98%	98%	98%
Heart Failure Care				
ACE Inhibitor or ARB for LVSD	74	80%	96%	97%
Discharge Instructions Given	338	80%	94%	94%
Evaluation of LVS Function	399	100%	99%	99%
Medicare Spending				
Medicare Spending per Patient (ratio)	-	0.90	0.96	0.98
Pneumonia Care				
Appropriate Initial Antibiotic Given	169	95%	96%	95%
Blood Culture Timing	284	99%	98%	98%
Pregnancy and Delivery Care				
Newborn Deliveries Scheduled Early[2]	114	2%	3%	6%
Preventive Care				
Immunization for Influenza[2]	553	56%	89%	90%
Immunization for Pneumonia[2]	758	73%	90%	92%
Stroke Care				
Anticoagulation Therapy for Atrial Fibrillation	22	77%	92%	95%
Antithrombotic Therapy Timing	89	96%	97%	98%
Assessed for Rehabilitation	113	96%	97%	97%
Discharged on Antithrombotic Therapy	98	100%	99%	99%
Discharged on Statin Medication	80	98%	94%	94%
Thrombolytic Therapy Timing[1]	-	-	69%	66%
Venous Thromboembolism Prophylaxis	115	97%	94%	94%
Written Stroke Educational Materials Given	76	80%	87%	88%
Surgical Care Improvement Project				
Appropriate Beta Blocker Usage	472	96%	98%	98%
Appropriate VTP Within 24 Hours	1,032	98%	98%	98%
Controlled Postoperative Blood Glucose	224	88%	97%	97%
Perioperative Temperature Management	1,218	98%	100%	100%
Prophylactic Antibiotic Selection	1,057	100%	99%	99%
Prophylactic Antibiotic Selection (Outpatient)	620	95%	97%	98%
Prophylactic Antibiotic Stopped	1,033	96%	98%	98%
Prophylactic Antibiotic Timing	1,057	98%	98%	99%
Prophylactic Antibiotic Timing (Outpatient)	629	93%	97%	98%
Urinary Catheter Removal	861	95%	97%	97%
Survey of Patients' Hospital Experiences				
Area Around Room 'Always' Quiet at Night	300+	63%	60%	61%
Doctors 'Always' Communicated Well	300+	83%	81%	82%
Home Recovery Information Given	300+	89%	87%	85%
Hospital Given 9 or 10 on 10 Point Scale	300+	79%	71%	71%
Meds 'Always' Explained Before Given	300+	68%	64%	64%
Nurses 'Always' Communicated Well	300+	83%	80%	79%
Pain 'Always' Well Controlled	300+	75%	71%	71%
Room and Bathroom 'Always' Clean	300+	74%	73%	73%
Timely Help 'Always' Received	300+	75%	70%	68%
Would Definitely Recommend Hospital	300+	80%	71%	71%
Use of Medical Imaging				
Cardiac Imaging Stress Test before Surgery	969	5.8%	5.1%	5.3%
Combination Abdominal CT Scan	1,310	5.0%	8.7%	10.5%
Combination Brain/Sinus CT Scan	945	2.1%	2.2%	2.7%
Combination Chest CT Scan	916	1.4%	3.6%	2.7%
Follow-up Mammogram/Ultrasound	2,797	8.3%	8.2%	8.8%
Lumbar Spine MRI for Low Back Pain	427	32.6%	36.9%	37.2%

Mercy Memorial Hospital System

718 N Macomb St
Monroe, MI 48162
URL: www.mercymemorial.org
Type: Acute Care Hospitals
Ownership: Voluntary non-profit - Other
Phone: 734-240-8400
Fax: 734-241-0032
Emergency Services: Yes
Beds: 238

Key Personnel:
Chief of Medical Staff.......... Danilo Dona
Operating Room.............. Pam Haddix
Emergency Room .... Lynn Lohner
CEO/President............... Annette Phillips
Cardiac Laboratory............ David Rhodes

Measure	Cases	This Hosp.	State Avg.	U.S. Avg.
Blood Clot Prevention and Treatment				
Anticoagulation Overlap Therapy[2]	69	99%	90%	93%
ICU Venous Thromboembolism Prophylaxis[2]	47	100%	93%	92%
Incidence of Potentially Preventable VTE[1,2]	-	-	8%	10%
UFH with Dosages/Platelet Monitoring[2]	33	100%	96%	97%
Venous Thromboembolism Prophylaxis[2]	371	99%	87%	85%
Warfarin Therapy Discharge Instructions[2]	39	97%	72%	75%
Chest Pain/Possible Heart Attack Care				
Aspirin Given Within 24 Hours of Arrival	68	100%	96%	96%
Fibrinolytic Meds Within 30 Min. of Arrival[1]	-	-	63%	58%
Average Time to ECG (minutes)	68	5	8	7
Average Time to Transfer (minutes)[1]	-	-	53	60
Children's Asthma Care				
Received Home Management Plan of Care	-	-	-	88%
Received Reliever Medication	-	-	-	100%
Received Systemic Corticosteroids	-	-	-	100%
Emergency Department				
Admittance Decision Time (minutes)[2]	726	108	102	98
Head CT Results Within 45 Min. of Arrival[1]	-	-	54%	57%
Patients Who Left ER Before Being Seen	47,169	1%	2%	2%
Time from ER Arrival to Admit. (minutes)[2]	741	288	288	274
Time from ER Arrival to Discharge (minutes)	493	99	128	134
Time in ER Before Being Evaluated (minutes)	573	12	22	26
Time to Pain Meds for Fractures (minutes)	143	38	55	57
Heart Attack Care				
Aspirin Given at Discharge	80	100%	99%	99%
Fibrinolytic Meds Within 30 Min. of Arrival[1]	-	-	20%	54%
PCI Within 90 Minutes of Arrival[7]	-	-	95%	96%
Statin Prescribed at Discharge	71	99%	98%	98%
Heart Failure Care				
ACE Inhibitor or ARB for LVSD	61	100%	96%	97%
Discharge Instructions Given	142	96%	94%	94%
Evaluation of LVS Function	211	100%	99%	99%
Medicare Spending				
Medicare Spending per Patient (ratio)	-	1.03	0.96	0.98
Pneumonia Care				
Appropriate Initial Antibiotic Given	191	98%	96%	95%
Blood Culture Timing	262	98%	98%	98%
Pregnancy and Delivery Care				
Newborn Deliveries Scheduled Early	68	0%	3%	6%
Preventive Care				
Immunization for Influenza[2]	539	99%	89%	90%
Immunization for Pneumonia[2]	671	99%	90%	92%
Stroke Care				
Anticoagulation Therapy for Atrial Fibrillation[1]	-	-	92%	95%
Antithrombotic Therapy Timing	74	99%	97%	98%
Assessed for Rehabilitation	76	97%	97%	97%
Discharged on Antithrombotic Therapy	74	100%	99%	99%
Discharged on Statin Medication	46	96%	94%	94%
Thrombolytic Therapy Timing[1]	-	-	69%	66%
Venous Thromboembolism Prophylaxis	81	100%	94%	94%
Written Stroke Educational Materials Given	34	82%	87%	88%
Surgical Care Improvement Project				
Appropriate Beta Blocker Usage	133	97%	98%	98%
Appropriate VTP Within 24 Hours	304	100%	98%	98%
Controlled Postoperative Blood Glucose[7]	-	-	97%	97%
Perioperative Temperature Management	413	100%	100%	100%
Prophylactic Antibiotic Selection	266	100%	99%	99%
Prophylactic Antibiotic Selection (Outpatient)	200	99%	97%	98%
Prophylactic Antibiotic Stopped	254	98%	98%	98%
Prophylactic Antibiotic Timing	269	99%	98%	99%
Prophylactic Antibiotic Timing (Outpatient)	184	98%	97%	98%
Urinary Catheter Removal	122	99%	97%	97%
Survey of Patients' Hospital Experiences				
Area Around Room 'Always' Quiet at Night	300+	48%	60%	61%
Doctors 'Always' Communicated Well	300+	77%	81%	82%
Home Recovery Information Given	300+	85%	87%	85%
Hospital Given 9 or 10 on 10 Point Scale	300+	58%	71%	71%
Meds 'Always' Explained Before Given	300+	59%	64%	64%
Nurses 'Always' Communicated Well	300+	78%	80%	79%
Pain 'Always' Well Controlled	300+	67%	71%	71%
Room and Bathroom 'Always' Clean	300+	67%	73%	73%
Timely Help 'Always' Received	300+	61%	70%	68%
Would Definitely Recommend Hospital	300+	50%	71%	71%
Use of Medical Imaging				
Cardiac Imaging Stress Test before Surgery	126	4.8%	5.1%	5.3%
Combination Abdominal CT Scan	851	3.9%	8.7%	10.5%
Combination Brain/Sinus CT Scan[1]	-	-	2.2%	2.7%
Combination Chest CT Scan	532	0.0%	3.6%	2.7%
Follow-up Mammogram/Ultrasound	1,365	9.2%	8.2%	8.8%
Lumbar Spine MRI for Low Back Pain	107	34.6%	36.9%	37.2%

Mclaren Macomb

1000 Harrington Blvd
Mount Clemens, MI 48043
URL: www.mcrmc.org
Type: Acute Care Hospitals
Ownership: Proprietary
Phone: 586-493-8000
Fax: 586-741-4179
Emergency Services: Yes
Beds: 288

Key Personnel:
Radiology.................. Michele Blair, DO
Emergency Room .... Sue Durst, RN
CEO/President.............. Phil Incarnati
Pediatric Ambulatory Care ...... Bahman Mehdizadeh, MD
Pediatric In-Patient Care .... Bahman Mehdizadeh, MD
Chief of Medical Staff.......... Michael Tawney, DO
Quality Assurance .... Heather Tweed
Chair/CEO.................. Ted B. Wahby

Measure	Cases	This Hosp.	State Avg.	U.S. Avg.
Blood Clot Prevention and Treatment				
Anticoagulation Overlap Therapy[2]	95	92%	90%	93%
ICU Venous Thromboembolism Prophylaxis[2]	69	100%	93%	92%
Incidence of Potentially Preventable VTE[2]	18	0%	8%	10%
UFH with Dosages/Platelet Monitoring[2]	58	100%	96%	97%
Venous Thromboembolism Prophylaxis[2]	369	92%	87%	85%
Warfarin Therapy Discharge Instructions[2]	69	49%	72%	75%
Chest Pain/Possible Heart Attack Care				
Aspirin Given Within 24 Hours of Arrival[1,3]	-	-	96%	96%
Fibrinolytic Meds Within 30 Min. of Arrival[3,7]	-	-	63%	58%
Average Time to ECG (minutes)[1,3]	-	-	8	7
Average Time to Transfer (minutes)[3,7]	-	-	53	60
Children's Asthma Care				
Received Home Management Plan of Care	-	-	-	88%
Received Reliever Medication	-	-	-	100%
Received Systemic Corticosteroids	-	-	-	100%
Emergency Department				
Admittance Decision Time (minutes)[2]	525	139	102	98
Head CT Results Within 45 Min. of Arrival[1]	-	-	54%	57%
Patients Who Left ER Before Being Seen	64,826	0%	2%	2%
Time from ER Arrival to Admit. (minutes)[2]	593	311	288	274
Time from ER Arrival to Discharge (minutes)	382	130	128	134
Time in ER Before Being Evaluated (minutes)	407	16	22	26
Time to Pain Meds for Fractures (minutes)	153	48	55	57
Heart Attack Care				
Aspirin Given at Discharge	368	98%	99%	99%
Fibrinolytic Meds Within 30 Min. of Arrival[7]	-	-	20%	54%
PCI Within 90 Minutes of Arrival	80	94%	95%	96%
Statin Prescribed at Discharge	361	94%	98%	98%
Heart Failure Care				
ACE Inhibitor or ARB for LVSD	122	90%	96%	97%
Discharge Instructions Given	340	80%	94%	94%
Evaluation of LVS Function	409	100%	99%	99%
Medicare Spending				
Medicare Spending per Patient (ratio)	-	0.97	0.96	0.98
Pneumonia Care				
Appropriate Initial Antibiotic Given	238	93%	96%	95%
Blood Culture Timing	377	94%	98%	98%
Pregnancy and Delivery Care				
Newborn Deliveries Scheduled Early	100	7%	3%	6%
Preventive Care				
Immunization for Influenza[2]	602	94%	89%	90%
Immunization for Pneumonia[2]	796	93%	90%	92%
Stroke Care				
Anticoagulation Therapy for Atrial Fibrillation[2]	37	76%	92%	95%
Antithrombotic Therapy Timing[2]	129	98%	97%	98%
Assessed for Rehabilitation[2]	163	81%	97%	97%
Discharged on Antithrombotic Therapy[2]	146	98%	99%	99%
Discharged on Statin Medication[2]	125	88%	94%	94%
Thrombolytic Therapy Timing[2]	25	48%	69%	66%
Venous Thromboembolism Prophylaxis[2]	172	88%	94%	94%
Written Stroke Educational Materials Given[2]	94	37%	87%	88%
Surgical Care Improvement Project				
Appropriate Beta Blocker Usage[2]	353	98%	98%	98%

NOTE: Hospital profiles are in alphabetical order by state, then city, then hospital within the city; Rankings exclude hospitals with less than 25 cases except for patient surveys which excludes hospitals with less than 100 cases; (a) 100-299 cases; (1) The number of cases/patients is too few to report; (2) Data submitted were based on a sample of cases/patients; (3) Results are based on a shorter time period than required; (4) Data suppressed by CMS for one or more quarters; (5) Results are not available for this reporting period; (6) Fewer than 100 patients completed the HCAHPS survey; (7) No cases met the criteria for this measure; (8) The lower limit of the confidence interval cannot be calculated if the number of observed infections equals zero; (9) No data are available from the state/territory for this reporting period; (10) The scores shown reflect fewer than 50 completed surveys; (11) There were discrepancies in the data collection process; (12) This measure does not apply to this hospital for this reporting period; (13) Results cannot be calculated for this reporting period; (14) The results for this state are combined with nearby states to protect confidentiality; Please refer to the User's Guide for a full explanation of data.

Measure	Cases	This Hosp.	State Avg.	U.S. Avg.
Appropriate VTP Within 24 Hours[2]	592	99%	98%	98%
Controlled Postoperative Blood Glucose[2]	91	99%	97%	97%
Perioperative Temperature Management[2]	865	100%	100%	100%
Prophylactic Antibiotic Selection[2]	766	99%	99%	99%
Prophylactic Antibiotic Selection (Outpatient)	279	99%	97%	98%
Prophylactic Antibiotic Stopped[2]	747	98%	98%	98%
Prophylactic Antibiotic Timing[2]	767	98%	98%	99%
Prophylactic Antibiotic Timing (Outpatient)	287	96%	97%	98%
Urinary Catheter Removal[2]	592	97%	97%	97%
Survey of Patients' Hospital Experiences				
Area Around Room 'Always' Quiet at Night	300+	47%	60%	61%
Doctors 'Always' Communicated Well	300+	75%	81%	82%
Home Recovery Information Given	300+	84%	87%	85%
Hospital Given 9 or 10 on 10 Point Scale	300+	61%	71%	71%
Meds 'Always' Explained Before Given	300+	53%	64%	64%
Nurses 'Always' Communicated Well	300+	73%	80%	79%
Pain 'Always' Well Controlled	300+	64%	71%	71%
Room and Bathroom 'Always' Clean	300+	58%	73%	73%
Timely Help 'Always' Received	300+	60%	70%	68%
Would Definitely Recommend Hospital	300+	62%	71%	71%
Use of Medical Imaging				
Cardiac Imaging Stress Test before Surgery	384	8.6%	5.1%	5.3%
Combination Abdominal CT Scan	1,346	29.0%	8.7%	10.5%
Combination Brain/Sinus CT Scan	957	2.5%	2.2%	2.7%
Combination Chest CT Scan	922	19.5%	3.6%	2.7%
Follow-up Mammogram/Ultrasound	1,688	4.3%	8.2%	8.8%
Lumbar Spine MRI for Low Back Pain[7]	-	-	36.9%	37.2%

Mclaren Central Michigan

1221 South Drive
Mount Pleasant, MI 48858
Phone: 989-772-6700
Fax: 989-772-1150
E-mail: mbousley@voyager.net
URL: www.cmch.org
Type: Acute Care Hospitals
Emergency Services: Yes
Ownership: Voluntary non-profit - Private
Beds: 137

Key Personnel:

Radiology. . . . . David Dubriwny
CEO/President. . . . . Bill Lawrence
Chief of Medical Staff. . . . . Ashok Vashishta, MD

Measure	Cases	This Hosp.	State Avg.	U.S. Avg.
Blood Clot Prevention and Treatment				
Anticoagulation Overlap Therapy[2]	44	48%	90%	93%
ICU Venous Thromboembolism Prophylaxis[2]	63	97%	93%	92%
Incidence of Potentially Preventable VTE[1,2]	-	-	8%	10%
UFH with Dosages/Platelet Monitoring[2]	45	100%	96%	97%
Venous Thromboembolism Prophylaxis[2]	271	82%	87%	85%
Warfarin Therapy Discharge Instructions[2]	32	91%	72%	75%
Chest Pain/Possible Heart Attack Care				
Aspirin Given Within 24 Hours of Arrival	63	98%	96%	96%
Fibrinolytic Meds Within 30 Min. of Arrival[1]	-	-	63%	58%
Average Time to ECG (minutes)	66	6	8	7
Average Time to Transfer (minutes)[1]	-	-	53	60
Children's Asthma Care				
Received Home Management Plan of Care	-	-	-	88%
Received Reliever Medication	-	-	-	100%
Received Systemic Corticosteroids	-	-	-	100%
Emergency Department				
Admittance Decision Time (minutes)[2]	417	73	102	98
Head CT Results Within 45 Min. of Arrival[1]	-	-	54%	57%
Patients Who Left ER Before Being Seen	31,677	1%	2%	2%
Time from ER Arrival to Admit. (minutes)[2]	425	228	288	274
Time from ER Arrival to Discharge (minutes)	404	106	128	134
Time in ER Before Being Evaluated (minutes)	420	28	22	26
Time to Pain Meds for Fractures (minutes)	111	48	55	57
Heart Attack Care				
Aspirin Given at Discharge	19	95%	99%	99%
Fibrinolytic Meds Within 30 Min. of Arrival[7]	-	-	20%	54%
PCI Within 90 Minutes of Arrival[7]	-	-	95%	96%
Statin Prescribed at Discharge	20	85%	98%	98%
Heart Failure Care				
ACE Inhibitor or ARB for LVSD	35	100%	96%	97%
Discharge Instructions Given	122	97%	94%	94%
Evaluation of LVS Function	157	99%	99%	99%
Medicare Spending				
Medicare Spending per Patient (ratio)	-	0.93	0.96	0.98
Pneumonia Care				
Appropriate Initial Antibiotic Given	106	92%	96%	95%
Blood Culture Timing	117	94%	98%	98%
Pregnancy and Delivery Care				
Newborn Deliveries Scheduled Early[2]	30	0%	3%	6%
Preventive Care				
Immunization for Influenza[2]	361	99%	89%	90%
Immunization for Pneumonia[2]	463	98%	90%	92%
Stroke Care				
Anticoagulation Therapy for Atrial Fibrillation[1]	-	-	92%	95%
Antithrombotic Therapy Timing	35	97%	97%	98%
Assessed for Rehabilitation	43	91%	97%	97%
Discharged on Antithrombotic Therapy	39	100%	99%	99%
Discharged on Statin Medication	36	86%	94%	94%
Thrombolytic Therapy Timing[1]	-	-	69%	66%
Venous Thromboembolism Prophylaxis	37	73%	94%	94%
Written Stroke Educational Materials Given	22	77%	87%	88%
Surgical Care Improvement Project				
Appropriate Beta Blocker Usage	66	98%	98%	98%
Appropriate VTP Within 24 Hours	233	93%	98%	98%
Controlled Postoperative Blood Glucose[7]	-	-	97%	97%
Perioperative Temperature Management	271	100%	100%	100%
Prophylactic Antibiotic Selection	192	99%	99%	99%
Prophylactic Antibiotic Selection (Outpatient)	118	92%	97%	98%
Prophylactic Antibiotic Stopped	191	100%	98%	98%
Prophylactic Antibiotic Timing	192	99%	98%	99%
Prophylactic Antibiotic Timing (Outpatient)	93	96%	97%	98%
Urinary Catheter Removal	130	99%	97%	97%
Survey of Patients' Hospital Experiences				
Area Around Room 'Always' Quiet at Night	300+	57%	60%	61%
Doctors 'Always' Communicated Well	300+	79%	81%	82%
Home Recovery Information Given	300+	87%	87%	85%
Hospital Given 9 or 10 on 10 Point Scale	300+	67%	71%	71%
Meds 'Always' Explained Before Given	300+	56%	64%	64%
Nurses 'Always' Communicated Well	300+	77%	80%	79%
Pain 'Always' Well Controlled	300+	71%	71%	71%
Room and Bathroom 'Always' Clean	300+	73%	73%	73%
Timely Help 'Always' Received	300+	69%	70%	68%
Would Definitely Recommend Hospital	300+	63%	71%	71%
Use of Medical Imaging				
Cardiac Imaging Stress Test before Surgery	462	3.0%	5.1%	5.3%
Combination Abdominal CT Scan	462	5.4%	8.7%	10.5%
Combination Brain/Sinus CT Scan	566	2.3%	2.2%	2.7%
Combination Chest CT Scan	306	4.9%	3.6%	2.7%
Follow-up Mammogram/Ultrasound	572	7.2%	8.2%	8.8%
Lumbar Spine MRI for Low Back Pain	98	41.8%	36.9%	37.2%

Munising Memorial Hospital

1500 Sand Point Rd
Munising, MI 49862
Phone: 906-387-4110
Type: Critical Access Hospitals
Emergency Services: Yes
Ownership: Voluntary non-profit - Private

Measure	Cases	This Hosp.	State Avg.	U.S. Avg.
Blood Clot Prevention and Treatment				
Anticoagulation Overlap Therapy[5]	-	-	90%	93%
ICU Venous Thromboembolism Prophylaxis[5]	-	-	93%	92%
Incidence of Potentially Preventable VTE[5]	-	-	8%	10%
UFH with Dosages/Platelet Monitoring[5]	-	-	96%	97%
Venous Thromboembolism Prophylaxis[5]	-	-	87%	85%
Warfarin Therapy Discharge Instructions[5]	-	-	72%	75%
Chest Pain/Possible Heart Attack Care				
Aspirin Given Within 24 Hours of Arrival[1,3]	-	-	96%	96%
Fibrinolytic Meds Within 30 Min. of Arrival[3,7]	-	-	63%	58%
Average Time to ECG (minutes)[1,3]	-	-	8	7
Average Time to Transfer (minutes)[1,3]	-	-	53	60
Children's Asthma Care				
Received Home Management Plan of Care	-	-	-	88%
Received Reliever Medication	-	-	-	100%
Received Systemic Corticosteroids	-	-	-	100%
Emergency Department				
Admittance Decision Time (minutes)[5]	-	-	102	98
Head CT Results Within 45 Min. of Arrival[5]	-	-	54%	57%
Patients Who Left ER Before Being Seen[5]	-	-	2%	2%
Time from ER Arrival to Admit. (minutes)[5]	-	-	288	274
Time from ER Arrival to Discharge (minutes)	291	108	128	134
Time in ER Before Being Evaluated (minutes)	251	23	22	26
Time to Pain Meds for Fractures (minutes)[5]	-	-	55	57
Heart Attack Care				
Aspirin Given at Discharge[5]	-	-	99%	99%
Fibrinolytic Meds Within 30 Min. of Arrival[5]	-	-	20%	54%
PCI Within 90 Minutes of Arrival[5]	-	-	95%	96%
Statin Prescribed at Discharge[5]	-	-	98%	98%
Heart Failure Care				
ACE Inhibitor or ARB for LVSD[3,7]	-	-	96%	97%
Discharge Instructions Given[1,3]	-	-	94%	94%
Evaluation of LVS Function[1,3]	-	-	99%	99%
Medicare Spending				
Medicare Spending per Patient (ratio)	-	-	0.96	0.98
Pneumonia Care				
Appropriate Initial Antibiotic Given	14	64%	96%	95%
Blood Culture Timing[1]	-	-	98%	98%
Pregnancy and Delivery Care				
Newborn Deliveries Scheduled Early[5]	-	-	3%	6%
Preventive Care				
Immunization for Influenza[5]	-	-	89%	90%
Immunization for Pneumonia[5]	-	-	90%	92%
Stroke Care				
Anticoagulation Therapy for Atrial Fibrillation[5]	-	-	92%	95%
Antithrombotic Therapy Timing[5]	-	-	97%	98%
Assessed for Rehabilitation[5]	-	-	97%	97%
Discharged on Antithrombotic Therapy[5]	-	-	99%	99%
Discharged on Statin Medication[5]	-	-	94%	94%
Thrombolytic Therapy Timing[5]	-	-	69%	66%
Venous Thromboembolism Prophylaxis[5]	-	-	94%	94%
Written Stroke Educational Materials Given[5]	-	-	87%	88%
Surgical Care Improvement Project				
Appropriate Beta Blocker Usage[5]	-	-	98%	98%
Appropriate VTP Within 24 Hours[5]	-	-	98%	98%
Controlled Postoperative Blood Glucose[5]	-	-	97%	97%
Perioperative Temperature Management[5]	-	-	100%	100%
Prophylactic Antibiotic Selection[5]	-	-	99%	99%
Prophylactic Antibiotic Selection (Outpatient)[5]	-	-	97%	98%
Prophylactic Antibiotic Stopped[5]	-	-	98%	98%
Prophylactic Antibiotic Timing[5]	-	-	98%	99%
Prophylactic Antibiotic Timing (Outpatient)[5]	-	-	97%	98%
Urinary Catheter Removal[5]	-	-	97%	97%
Survey of Patients' Hospital Experiences				
Area Around Room 'Always' Quiet at Night[3,10]	<100	77%	60%	61%
Doctors 'Always' Communicated Well[3,10]	<100	92%	81%	82%
Home Recovery Information Given[3,10]	<100	85%	87%	85%
Hospital Given 9 or 10 on 10 Point Scale[3,10]	<100	67%	71%	71%
Meds 'Always' Explained Before Given[3,10]	<100	94%	64%	64%
Nurses 'Always' Communicated Well[3,10]	<100	90%	80%	79%
Pain 'Always' Well Controlled[3,10]	<100	100%	71%	71%
Room and Bathroom 'Always' Clean[3,10]	<100	98%	73%	73%
Timely Help 'Always' Received[3,10]	<100	80%	70%	68%
Would Definitely Recommend Hospital[3,10]	<100	79%	71%	71%
Use of Medical Imaging				
Cardiac Imaging Stress Test before Surgery[7]	-	-	5.1%	5.3%
Combination Abdominal CT Scan	88	15.9%	8.7%	10.5%
Combination Brain/Sinus CT Scan	144	0.7%	2.2%	2.7%
Combination Chest CT Scan	96	3.1%	3.6%	2.7%
Follow-up Mammogram/Ultrasound	181	3.3%	8.2%	8.8%
Lumbar Spine MRI for Low Back Pain[7]	-	-	36.9%	37.2%

Mercy Health Hackley Campus

1700 Clinton Street
Muskegon, MI 49442
Phone: 231-726-3511
Fax: 231-726-2232
URL: www.hackley.org
Type: Acute Care Hospitals
Emergency Services: Yes
Ownership: Voluntary non-profit - Private
Beds: 181

Key Personnel:

Operating Room. . . . . Brian Gluck
Quality Assurance . . . . Eileen Howe

NOTE: Hospital profiles are in alphabetical order by state, then city, then hospital within the city; Rankings exclude hospitals with less than 25 cases except for patient surveys which excludes hospitals with less than 100 cases; (a) 100-299 cases; (1) The number of cases/patients is too few to report; (2) Data submitted were based on a sample of cases/patients; (3) Results are based on a shorter time period than required; (4) Data suppressed by CMS for one or more quarters; (5) Results are not available for this reporting period; (6) Fewer than 100 patients completed the HCAHPS survey; (7) No cases met the criteria for this measure; (8) The lower limit of the confidence interval cannot be calculated if the number of observed infections equals zero; (9) No data are available from the state/territory for this reporting period; (10) The scores shown reflect fewer than 50 completed surveys; (11) There were discrepancies in the data collection process; (12) This measure does not apply to this hospital for this reporting period; (13) Results cannot be calculated for this reporting period; (14) The results for this state are combined with nearby states to protect confidentiality; Please refer to the User's Guide for a full explanation of data.

Chief of Medical Staff.......... Herbert Miller, MD
CEO/President............... Gordon A Mudler

Measure	Cases	This Hosp.	State Avg.	U.S. Avg.
Blood Clot Prevention and Treatment				
Anticoagulation Overlap Therapy[2]	52	96%	90%	93%
ICU Venous Thromboembolism Prophylaxis[2]	90	90%	93%	92%
Incidence of Potentially Preventable VTE[1,2]	-	-	8%	10%
UFH with Dosages/Platelet Monitoring[2]	32	100%	96%	97%
Venous Thromboembolism Prophylaxis[2]	258	93%	87%	85%
Warfarin Therapy Discharge Instructions[2]	37	81%	72%	75%
Chest Pain/Possible Heart Attack Care				
Aspirin Given Within 24 Hours of Arrival	53	92%	96%	96%
Fibrinolytic Meds Within 30 Min. of Arrival[1]	-	-	63%	58%
Average Time to ECG (minutes)	54	12	8	7
Average Time to Transfer (minutes)	13	54	53	60
Children's Asthma Care				
Received Home Management Plan of Care	-	-	-	88%
Received Reliever Medication	-	-	-	100%
Received Systemic Corticosteroids	-	-	-	100%
Emergency Department				
Admittance Decision Time (minutes)[2]	312	98	102	98
Head CT Results Within 45 Min. of Arrival[1]	-	-	54%	57%
Patients Who Left ER Before Being Seen	61,613	1%	2%	2%
Time from ER Arrival to Admit. (minutes)[2]	315	286	288	274
Time from ER Arrival to Discharge (minutes)	366	84	128	134
Time in ER Before Being Evaluated (minutes)	378	11	22	26
Time to Pain Meds for Fractures (minutes)	144	42	55	57
Heart Attack Care				
Aspirin Given at Discharge[1]	-	-	99%	99%
Fibrinolytic Meds Within 30 Min. of Arrival[7]	-	-	20%	54%
PCI Within 90 Minutes of Arrival[7]	-	-	95%	96%
Statin Prescribed at Discharge[1]	-	-	98%	98%
Heart Failure Care				
ACE Inhibitor or ARB for LVSD	27	96%	96%	97%
Discharge Instructions Given	57	86%	94%	94%
Evaluation of LVS Function	74	100%	99%	99%
Medicare Spending				
Medicare Spending per Patient (ratio)	-	0.99	0.96	0.98
Pneumonia Care				
Appropriate Initial Antibiotic Given[2]	92	93%	96%	95%
Blood Culture Timing[2]	152	100%	98%	98%
Pregnancy and Delivery Care				
Newborn Deliveries Scheduled Early[2]	27	0%	3%	6%
Preventive Care				
Immunization for Influenza[2]	473	89%	89%	90%
Immunization for Pneumonia[2]	411	86%	90%	92%
Stroke Care				
Anticoagulation Therapy for Atrial Fibrillation[2]	20	95%	92%	95%
Antithrombotic Therapy Timing[2]	90	98%	97%	98%
Assessed for Rehabilitation[2]	111	99%	97%	97%
Discharged on Antithrombotic Therapy[2]	90	98%	99%	99%
Discharged on Statin Medication[2]	78	94%	94%	94%
Thrombolytic Therapy Timing[1,2]	-	-	69%	66%
Venous Thromboembolism Prophylaxis[2]	117	93%	94%	94%
Written Stroke Educational Materials Given[2]	44	50%	87%	88%
Surgical Care Improvement Project				
Appropriate Beta Blocker Usage[2]	106	96%	98%	98%
Appropriate VTP Within 24 Hours[2]	293	98%	98%	98%
Controlled Postoperative Blood Glucose[2,7]	-	-	97%	97%
Perioperative Temperature Management[2]	336	100%	100%	100%
Prophylactic Antibiotic Selection[2]	212	99%	99%	99%
Prophylactic Antibiotic Selection (Outpatient)	503	99%	97%	98%
Prophylactic Antibiotic Stopped[2]	203	99%	98%	98%
Prophylactic Antibiotic Timing[2]	212	100%	98%	99%
Prophylactic Antibiotic Timing (Outpatient)	485	99%	97%	98%
Urinary Catheter Removal[2]	89	93%	97%	97%
Survey of Patients' Hospital Experiences				
Area Around Room 'Always' Quiet at Night	300+	48%	60%	61%
Doctors 'Always' Communicated Well	300+	77%	81%	82%
Home Recovery Information Given	300+	87%	87%	85%
Hospital Given 9 or 10 on 10 Point Scale	300+	63%	71%	71%
Meds 'Always' Explained Before Given	300+	55%	64%	64%
Nurses 'Always' Communicated Well	300+	72%	80%	79%
Pain 'Always' Well Controlled	300+	63%	71%	71%
Room and Bathroom 'Always' Clean	300+	63%	73%	73%
Timely Help 'Always' Received	300+	58%	70%	68%
Would Definitely Recommend Hospital	300+	64%	71%	71%
Use of Medical Imaging				
Cardiac Imaging Stress Test before Surgery[1]	-	-	5.1%	5.3%
Combination Abdominal CT Scan	693	7.9%	8.7%	10.5%
Combination Brain/Sinus CT Scan	732	0.8%	2.2%	2.7%
Combination Chest CT Scan	369	5.1%	3.6%	2.7%
Follow-up Mammogram/Ultrasound	1,661	5.7%	8.2%	8.8%
Lumbar Spine MRI for Low Back Pain	142	41.5%	36.9%	37.2%

Mercy Health Partners - Mercy Campus

1500 E Sherman Boulevard
Muskegon, MI 49444
Phone: 231-672-3901
Fax: 231-672-3854
URL: www.mghp.com
Type: Acute Care Hospitals
Emergency Services: Yes
Ownership: Voluntary non-profit - Church
Beds: 282

Key Personnel:
Infection Control................ Kurt Atton
Coronary Care................ Rick Denaie
Quality Assurance............ Julie Erickson
Pediatric Ambulatory Care...... Kathy Halfpap
CEO/President............... Gregory A. Loomis
Operating Room.............. Kathy Shoneberger
Chief of Medical Staff.......... F Remington Sprague, MD
Radiology.................. Richard A. Wilcox, MD

Measure	Cases	This Hosp.	State Avg.	U.S. Avg.
Blood Clot Prevention and Treatment				
Anticoagulation Overlap Therapy[2]	107	100%	90%	93%
ICU Venous Thromboembolism Prophylaxis[2]	116	93%	93%	92%
Incidence of Potentially Preventable VTE[1,2]	-	-	8%	10%
UFH with Dosages/Platelet Monitoring[2]	97	100%	96%	97%
Venous Thromboembolism Prophylaxis[2]	301	91%	87%	85%
Warfarin Therapy Discharge Instructions[2]	73	90%	72%	75%
Chest Pain/Possible Heart Attack Care				
Aspirin Given Within 24 Hours of Arrival[1]	-	-	96%	96%
Fibrinolytic Meds Within 30 Min. of Arrival[3,7]	-	-	63%	58%
Average Time to ECG (minutes)	12	9	8	7
Average Time to Transfer (minutes)[3,7]	-	-	53	60
Children's Asthma Care				
Received Home Management Plan of Care	-	-	-	88%
Received Reliever Medication	-	-	-	100%
Received Systemic Corticosteroids	-	-	-	100%
Emergency Department				
Admittance Decision Time (minutes)[2]	508	130	102	98
Head CT Results Within 45 Min. of Arrival[1]	-	-	54%	57%
Patients Who Left ER Before Being Seen	47,072	2%	2%	2%
Time from ER Arrival to Admit. (minutes)[2]	518	298	288	274
Time from ER Arrival to Discharge (minutes)	361	130	128	134
Time in ER Before Being Evaluated (minutes)	364	16	22	26
Time to Pain Meds for Fractures (minutes)	105	54	55	57
Heart Attack Care				
Aspirin Given at Discharge[2]	289	100%	99%	99%
Fibrinolytic Meds Within 30 Min. of Arrival[2,7]	-	-	20%	54%
PCI Within 90 Minutes of Arrival[2]	41	93%	95%	96%
Statin Prescribed at Discharge[2]	280	99%	98%	98%
Heart Failure Care				
ACE Inhibitor or ARB for LVSD[2]	73	90%	96%	97%
Discharge Instructions Given[2]	214	85%	94%	94%
Evaluation of LVS Function[2]	249	100%	99%	99%
Medicare Spending				
Medicare Spending per Patient (ratio)	-	0.98	0.96	0.98
Pneumonia Care				
Appropriate Initial Antibiotic Given[2]	73	97%	96%	95%
Blood Culture Timing[2]	157	98%	98%	98%
Pregnancy and Delivery Care				
Newborn Deliveries Scheduled Early[7]	-	-	3%	6%
Preventive Care				
Immunization for Influenza[2]	588	90%	89%	90%
Immunization for Pneumonia[2]	972	88%	90%	92%
Stroke Care				
Anticoagulation Therapy for Atrial Fibrillation[2]	11	100%	92%	95%
Antithrombotic Therapy Timing[2]	69	100%	97%	98%
Assessed for Rehabilitation[2]	73	100%	97%	97%
Discharged on Antithrombotic Therapy[2]	71	100%	99%	99%
Discharged on Statin Medication[2]	58	100%	94%	94%
Thrombolytic Therapy Timing[1,2]	-	-	69%	66%
Venous Thromboembolism Prophylaxis[2]	74	95%	94%	94%
Written Stroke Educational Materials Given[2]	40	35%	87%	88%
Surgical Care Improvement Project				
Appropriate Beta Blocker Usage[2]	208	99%	98%	98%
Appropriate VTP Within 24 Hours[2]	223	98%	98%	98%
Controlled Postoperative Blood Glucose[2]	118	97%	97%	97%
Perioperative Temperature Management[2]	364	100%	100%	100%
Prophylactic Antibiotic Selection[2]	298	99%	99%	99%
Prophylactic Antibiotic Selection (Outpatient)	477	99%	97%	98%
Prophylactic Antibiotic Stopped[2]	294	99%	98%	98%
Prophylactic Antibiotic Timing[2]	298	100%	98%	99%
Prophylactic Antibiotic Timing (Outpatient)	425	99%	97%	98%
Urinary Catheter Removal[2]	288	98%	97%	97%
Survey of Patients' Hospital Experiences				
Area Around Room 'Always' Quiet at Night	300+	54%	60%	61%
Doctors 'Always' Communicated Well	300+	79%	81%	82%
Home Recovery Information Given	300+	89%	87%	85%
Hospital Given 9 or 10 on 10 Point Scale	300+	69%	71%	71%
Meds 'Always' Explained Before Given	300+	58%	64%	64%
Nurses 'Always' Communicated Well	300+	76%	80%	79%
Pain 'Always' Well Controlled	300+	67%	71%	71%
Room and Bathroom 'Always' Clean	300+	66%	73%	73%
Timely Help 'Always' Received	300+	62%	70%	68%
Would Definitely Recommend Hospital	300+	71%	71%	71%
Use of Medical Imaging				
Cardiac Imaging Stress Test before Surgery	1,225	4.9%	5.1%	5.3%
Combination Abdominal CT Scan	1,199	5.5%	8.7%	10.5%
Combination Brain/Sinus CT Scan	1,122	2.6%	2.2%	2.7%
Combination Chest CT Scan	658	5.3%	3.6%	2.7%
Follow-up Mammogram/Ultrasound	2,093	6.0%	8.2%	8.8%
Lumbar Spine MRI for Low Back Pain	424	38.2%	36.9%	37.2%

Helen Newberry Joy Hospital

502 W Harrie St
Newberry, MI 49868
Phone: 906-293-9200
Type: Critical Access Hospitals
Emergency Services: Yes
Ownership: Government - Local

Measure	Cases	This Hosp.	State Avg.	U.S. Avg.
Blood Clot Prevention and Treatment				
Anticoagulation Overlap Therapy[5]	-	-	90%	93%
ICU Venous Thromboembolism Prophylaxis[5]	-	-	93%	92%
Incidence of Potentially Preventable VTE[5]	-	-	8%	10%
UFH with Dosages/Platelet Monitoring[5]	-	-	96%	97%
Venous Thromboembolism Prophylaxis[5]	-	-	87%	85%
Warfarin Therapy Discharge Instructions[5]	-	-	72%	75%
Chest Pain/Possible Heart Attack Care				
Aspirin Given Within 24 Hours of Arrival	24	96%	96%	96%
Fibrinolytic Meds Within 30 Min. of Arrival[1]	-	-	63%	58%
Average Time to ECG (minutes)	25	4	8	7
Average Time to Transfer (minutes)[7]	-	-	53	60
Children's Asthma Care				
Received Home Management Plan of Care	-	-	-	88%
Received Reliever Medication	-	-	-	100%
Received Systemic Corticosteroids	-	-	-	100%
Emergency Department				
Admittance Decision Time (minutes)[5]	-	-	102	98
Head CT Results Within 45 Min. of Arrival[5]	-	-	54%	57%
Patients Who Left ER Before Being Seen[5]	-	-	2%	2%
Time from ER Arrival to Admit. (minutes)[5]	-	-	288	274
Time from ER Arrival to Discharge (minutes)	341	157	128	134
Time in ER Before Being Evaluated (minutes)	310	10	22	26
Time to Pain Meds for Fractures (minutes)[5]	-	-	55	57
Heart Attack Care				
Aspirin Given at Discharge[5]	-	-	99%	99%
Fibrinolytic Meds Within 30 Min. of Arrival[5]	-	-	20%	54%
PCI Within 90 Minutes of Arrival[5]	-	-	95%	96%
Statin Prescribed at Discharge[5]	-	-	98%	98%

NOTE: Hospital profiles are in alphabetical order by state, then city, then hospital within the city; Rankings exclude hospitals with less than 25 cases except for patient surveys which excludes hospitals with less than 100 cases; (a) 100-299 cases; (1) The number of cases/patients is too few to report; (2) Data submitted were based on a sample of cases/patients; (3) Results are based on a shorter time period than required; (4) Data suppressed by CMS for one or more quarters; (5) Results are not available for this reporting period; (6) Fewer than 100 patients completed the HCAHPS survey; (7) No cases met the criteria for this measure; (8) The lower limit of the confidence interval cannot be calculated if the number of observed infections equals zero; (9) No data are available from the state/territory for this reporting period; (10) The scores shown reflect fewer than 50 completed surveys; (11) There were discrepancies in the data collection process; (12) This measure does not apply to this hospital for this reporting period; (13) Results cannot be calculated for this reporting period; (14) The results for this state are combined with nearby states to protect confidentiality; Please refer to the User's Guide for a full explanation of data.

Measure	Cases	This Hosp.	State Avg.	U.S. Avg.
Heart Failure Care				
ACE Inhibitor or ARB for LVSD[1]	-	-	96%	97%
Discharge Instructions Given[1]	-	-	94%	94%
Evaluation of LVS Function	17	76%	99%	99%
Medicare Spending				
Medicare Spending per Patient (ratio)	-	-	0.96	0.98
Pneumonia Care				
Appropriate Initial Antibiotic Given	21	95%	96%	95%
Blood Culture Timing	27	96%	98%	98%
Pregnancy and Delivery Care				
Newborn Deliveries Scheduled Early[5]	-	-	3%	6%
Preventive Care				
Immunization for Influenza[5]	-	-	89%	90%
Immunization for Pneumonia[5]	-	-	90%	92%
Stroke Care				
Anticoagulation Therapy for Atrial Fibrillation[5]	-	-	92%	95%
Antithrombotic Therapy Timing[5]	-	-	97%	98%
Assessed for Rehabilitation[5]	-	-	97%	97%
Discharged on Antithrombotic Therapy[5]	-	-	99%	99%
Discharged on Statin Medication[5]	-	-	94%	94%
Thrombolytic Therapy Timing[5]	-	-	69%	66%
Venous Thromboembolism Prophylaxis[5]	-	-	94%	94%
Written Stroke Educational Materials Given[5]	-	-	87%	88%
Surgical Care Improvement Project				
Appropriate Beta Blocker Usage[5]	-	-	98%	98%
Appropriate VTP Within 24 Hours[5]	-	-	98%	98%
Controlled Postoperative Blood Glucose[5]	-	-	97%	97%
Perioperative Temperature Management[5]	-	-	100%	100%
Prophylactic Antibiotic Selection[5]	-	-	99%	99%
Prophylactic Antibiotic Selection (Outpatient)[5]	-	-	97%	98%
Prophylactic Antibiotic Stopped[5]	-	-	98%	98%
Prophylactic Antibiotic Timing[5]	-	-	98%	99%
Prophylactic Antibiotic Timing (Outpatient)[5]	-	-	97%	98%
Urinary Catheter Removal[5]	-	-	97%	97%
Survey of Patients' Hospital Experiences				
Area Around Room 'Always' Quiet at Night	(a)	50%	60%	61%
Doctors 'Always' Communicated Well	(a)	89%	81%	82%
Home Recovery Information Given	(a)	89%	87%	85%
Hospital Given 9 or 10 on 10 Point Scale	(a)	72%	71%	71%
Meds 'Always' Explained Before Given	(a)	72%	64%	64%
Nurses 'Always' Communicated Well	(a)	81%	80%	79%
Pain 'Always' Well Controlled	(a)	64%	71%	71%
Room and Bathroom 'Always' Clean	(a)	84%	73%	73%
Timely Help 'Always' Received	(a)	81%	70%	68%
Would Definitely Recommend Hospital	(a)	64%	71%	71%
Use of Medical Imaging				
Cardiac Imaging Stress Test before Surgery	65	3.1%	5.1%	5.3%
Combination Abdominal CT Scan	201	6.0%	8.7%	10.5%
Combination Brain/Sinus CT Scan[1]	-	-	2.2%	2.7%
Combination Chest CT Scan	145	2.1%	3.6%	2.7%
Follow-up Mammogram/Ultrasound	345	7.5%	8.2%	8.8%
Lumbar Spine MRI for Low Back Pain	34	50.0%	36.9%	37.2%

Aspirus Ontonagon Hospital

601 S Seventh St
Ontonagon, MI 49953
Phone: 906-884-8000
Type: Critical Access Hospitals
Emergency Services: Yes
Ownership: Government - Local

Measure	Cases	This Hosp.	State Avg.	U.S. Avg.
Blood Clot Prevention and Treatment				
Anticoagulation Overlap Therapy[5]	-	-	90%	93%
ICU Venous Thromboembolism Prophylaxis[5]	-	-	93%	92%
Incidence of Potentially Preventable VTE[5]	-	-	8%	10%
UFH with Dosages/Platelet Monitoring[5]	-	-	96%	97%
Venous Thromboembolism Prophylaxis[5]	-	-	87%	85%
Warfarin Therapy Discharge Instructions[5]	-	-	72%	75%
Chest Pain/Possible Heart Attack Care				
Aspirin Given Within 24 Hours of Arrival	14	100%	96%	96%
Fibrinolytic Meds Within 30 Min. of Arrival[1,3]	-	-	63%	58%
Average Time to ECG (minutes)	14	8	8	7
Average Time to Transfer (minutes)[3,7]	-	-	53	60
Children's Asthma Care				
Received Home Management Plan of Care	-	-	-	88%
Received Reliever Medication	-	-	-	100%
Received Systemic Corticosteroids	-	-	-	100%
Emergency Department				
Admittance Decision Time (minutes)[5]	-	-	102	98
Head CT Results Within 45 Min. of Arrival[5]	-	-	54%	57%
Patients Who Left ER Before Being Seen[5]	-	-	2%	2%
Time from ER Arrival to Admit. (minutes)[5]	-	-	288	274
Time from ER Arrival to Discharge (minutes)	238	88	128	134
Time in ER Before Being Evaluated (minutes)	272	12	22	26
Time to Pain Meds for Fractures (minutes)[1,3]	-	-	55	57
Heart Attack Care				
Aspirin Given at Discharge[5]	-	-	99%	99%
Fibrinolytic Meds Within 30 Min. of Arrival[5]	-	-	20%	54%
PCI Within 90 Minutes of Arrival[5]	-	-	95%	96%
Statin Prescribed at Discharge[5]	-	-	98%	98%
Heart Failure Care				
ACE Inhibitor or ARB for LVSD[1]	-	-	96%	97%
Discharge Instructions Given[1]	-	-	94%	94%
Evaluation of LVS Function[1]	-	-	99%	99%
Medicare Spending				
Medicare Spending per Patient (ratio)	-	-	0.96	0.98
Pneumonia Care				
Appropriate Initial Antibiotic Given[1]	-	-	96%	95%
Blood Culture Timing	12	92%	98%	98%
Pregnancy and Delivery Care				
Newborn Deliveries Scheduled Early[5]	-	-	3%	6%
Preventive Care				
Immunization for Influenza[5]	-	-	89%	90%
Immunization for Pneumonia[3]	85	91%	90%	92%
Stroke Care				
Anticoagulation Therapy for Atrial Fibrillation[5]	-	-	92%	95%
Antithrombotic Therapy Timing[5]	-	-	97%	98%
Assessed for Rehabilitation[5]	-	-	97%	97%
Discharged on Antithrombotic Therapy[5]	-	-	99%	99%
Discharged on Statin Medication[5]	-	-	94%	94%
Thrombolytic Therapy Timing[5]	-	-	69%	66%
Venous Thromboembolism Prophylaxis[5]	-	-	94%	94%
Written Stroke Educational Materials Given[5]	-	-	87%	88%
Surgical Care Improvement Project				
Appropriate Beta Blocker Usage	11	100%	98%	98%
Appropriate VTP Within 24 Hours[1]	-	-	98%	98%
Controlled Postoperative Blood Glucose[7]	-	-	97%	97%
Perioperative Temperature Management	19	100%	100%	100%
Prophylactic Antibiotic Selection	18	100%	99%	99%
Prophylactic Antibiotic Selection (Outpatient)[5]	-	-	97%	98%
Prophylactic Antibiotic Stopped	18	100%	98%	98%
Prophylactic Antibiotic Timing	18	100%	98%	99%
Prophylactic Antibiotic Timing (Outpatient)[5]	-	-	97%	98%
Urinary Catheter Removal[7]	-	-	97%	97%
Survey of Patients' Hospital Experiences				
Area Around Room 'Always' Quiet at Night[6]	<100	64%	60%	61%
Doctors 'Always' Communicated Well[6]	<100	85%	81%	82%
Home Recovery Information Given[6]	<100	84%	87%	85%
Hospital Given 9 or 10 on 10 Point Scale[6]	<100	71%	71%	71%
Meds 'Always' Explained Before Given[6]	<100	74%	64%	64%
Nurses 'Always' Communicated Well[6]	<100	90%	80%	79%
Pain 'Always' Well Controlled[6]	<100	77%	71%	71%
Room and Bathroom 'Always' Clean[6]	<100	92%	73%	73%
Timely Help 'Always' Received[6]	<100	83%	70%	68%
Would Definitely Recommend Hospital[6]	<100	70%	71%	71%
Use of Medical Imaging				
Cardiac Imaging Stress Test before Surgery[1]	-	-	5.1%	5.3%
Combination Abdominal CT Scan	93	8.6%	8.7%	10.5%
Combination Brain/Sinus CT Scan[1]	-	-	2.2%	2.7%
Combination Chest CT Scan[1]	-	-	3.6%	2.7%
Follow-up Mammogram/Ultrasound	162	9.9%	8.2%	8.8%
Lumbar Spine MRI for Low Back Pain[7]	-	-	36.9%	37.2%

Memorial Healthcare

826 West King Street
Owosso, MI 48867
URL: www.memorialhealthcare.org
Phone: 989-723-5211
Fax: 989-725-8937
Type: Acute Care Hospitals
Ownership: Voluntary non-profit - Other
Emergency Services: Yes
Beds: 143

Key Personnel:
Infection Control. . . . . Lynn Howes
CEO/President. . . . . Brian L. Long, FACHE
Radiology. . . . . Keith Morrow
Pediatric In-Patient Care . . . . Kathy Roberts
Chief of Medical Staff . . . . Michael Schmidt, DO
Quality Assurance . . . . Sue Spragg
Operating Room. . . . . Vicki Watkins
Cardiac Laboratory. . . . . Kathy Whal

Measure	Cases	This Hosp.	State Avg.	U.S. Avg.
Blood Clot Prevention and Treatment				
Anticoagulation Overlap Therapy[2]	33	85%	90%	93%
ICU Venous Thromboembolism Prophylaxis[2]	56	96%	93%	92%
Incidence of Potentially Preventable VTE[1,2]	-	-	8%	10%
UFH with Dosages/Platelet Monitoring[2]	14	100%	96%	97%
Venous Thromboembolism Prophylaxis[2]	203	89%	87%	85%
Warfarin Therapy Discharge Instructions[2]	27	100%	72%	75%
Chest Pain/Possible Heart Attack Care				
Aspirin Given Within 24 Hours of Arrival	93	96%	96%	96%
Fibrinolytic Meds Within 30 Min. of Arrival[1]	-	-	63%	58%
Average Time to ECG (minutes)	96	9	8	7
Average Time to Transfer (minutes)[1]	-	-	53	60
Children's Asthma Care				
Received Home Management Plan of Care	-	-	-	88%
Received Reliever Medication	-	-	-	100%
Received Systemic Corticosteroids	-	-	-	100%
Emergency Department				
Admittance Decision Time (minutes)[2]	368	57	102	98
Head CT Results Within 45 Min. of Arrival[1]	-	-	54%	57%
Patients Who Left ER Before Being Seen	28,610	2%	2%	2%
Time from ER Arrival to Admit. (minutes)[2]	376	261	288	274
Time from ER Arrival to Discharge (minutes)	402	127	128	134
Time in ER Before Being Evaluated (minutes)	425	36	22	26
Time to Pain Meds for Fractures (minutes)	88	60	55	57
Heart Attack Care				
Aspirin Given at Discharge[1]	-	-	99%	99%
Fibrinolytic Meds Within 30 Min. of Arrival[7]	-	-	20%	54%
PCI Within 90 Minutes of Arrival[7]	-	-	95%	96%
Statin Prescribed at Discharge[1]	-	-	98%	98%
Heart Failure Care				
ACE Inhibitor or ARB for LVSD	14	86%	96%	97%
Discharge Instructions Given	41	90%	94%	94%
Evaluation of LVS Function	56	98%	99%	99%
Medicare Spending				
Medicare Spending per Patient (ratio)	-	0.95	0.96	0.98
Pneumonia Care				
Appropriate Initial Antibiotic Given	89	93%	96%	95%
Blood Culture Timing	124	98%	98%	98%
Pregnancy and Delivery Care				
Newborn Deliveries Scheduled Early[2]	26	0%	3%	6%
Preventive Care				
Immunization for Influenza[2]	331	73%	89%	90%
Immunization for Pneumonia[2]	388	85%	90%	92%
Stroke Care				
Anticoagulation Therapy for Atrial Fibrillation[1]	-	-	92%	95%
Antithrombotic Therapy Timing	21	100%	97%	98%
Assessed for Rehabilitation	27	100%	97%	97%
Discharged on Antithrombotic Therapy	25	100%	99%	99%
Discharged on Statin Medication	23	96%	94%	94%
Thrombolytic Therapy Timing[1]	-	-	69%	66%
Venous Thromboembolism Prophylaxis	22	82%	94%	94%
Written Stroke Educational Materials Given	17	76%	87%	88%
Surgical Care Improvement Project				
Appropriate Beta Blocker Usage[2]	92	99%	98%	98%
Appropriate VTP Within 24 Hours[2]	247	93%	98%	98%
Controlled Postoperative Blood Glucose[2,7]	-	-	97%	97%
Perioperative Temperature Management[2]	262	100%	100%	100%
Prophylactic Antibiotic Selection[2]	187	98%	99%	99%

NOTE: Hospital profiles are in alphabetical order by state, then city, then hospital within the city; Rankings exclude hospitals with less than 25 cases except for patient surveys which excludes hospitals with less than 100 cases; (a) 100-299 cases; (1) The number of cases/patients is too few to report; (2) Data submitted were based on a sample of cases/patients; (3) Results are based on a shorter time period than required; (4) Data suppressed by CMS for one or more quarters; (5) Results are not available for this reporting period; (6) Fewer than 100 patients completed the HCAHPS survey; (7) No cases met the criteria for this measure; (8) The lower limit of the confidence interval cannot be calculated if the number of observed infections equals zero; (9) No data are available from the state/territory for this reporting period; (10) The scores shown reflect fewer than 50 completed surveys; (11) There were discrepancies in the data collection process; (12) This measure does not apply to this hospital for this reporting period; (13) Results cannot be calculated for this reporting period; (14) The results for this state are combined with nearby states to protect confidentiality; Please refer to the User's Guide for a full explanation of data.

Prophylactic Antibiotic Selection (Outpatient)	192	98%	97%	98%
Prophylactic Antibiotic Stopped[2]	184	98%	98%	98%
Prophylactic Antibiotic Timing[2]	187	97%	98%	99%
Prophylactic Antibiotic Timing (Outpatient)	194	97%	97%	98%
Urinary Catheter Removal[2]	224	99%	97%	97%
Survey of Patients' Hospital Experiences				
Area Around Room 'Always' Quiet at Night	300+	62%	60%	61%
Doctors 'Always' Communicated Well	300+	79%	81%	82%
Home Recovery Information Given	300+	89%	87%	85%
Hospital Given 9 or 10 on 10 Point Scale	300+	69%	71%	71%
Meds 'Always' Explained Before Given	300+	63%	64%	64%
Nurses 'Always' Communicated Well	300+	81%	80%	79%
Pain 'Always' Well Controlled	300+	71%	71%	71%
Room and Bathroom 'Always' Clean	300+	84%	73%	73%
Timely Help 'Always' Received	300+	72%	70%	68%
Would Definitely Recommend Hospital	300+	65%	71%	71%
Use of Medical Imaging				
Cardiac Imaging Stress Test before Surgery	107	10.3%	5.1%	5.3%
Combination Abdominal CT Scan	685	3.1%	8.7%	10.5%
Combination Brain/Sinus CT Scan	582	2.4%	2.2%	2.7%
Combination Chest CT Scan	535	0.0%	3.6%	2.7%
Follow-up Mammogram/Ultrasound	1,397	8.6%	8.2%	8.8%
Lumbar Spine MRI for Low Back Pain	127	35.4%	36.9%	37.2%

Bronson Lakeview Hospital

408 Hazen Street
Paw Paw, MI 49079
Type: Critical Access Hospitals
Ownership: Govt - Hospital Dist/Auth
Phone: 269-657-1400
Fax: 269-657-1339
Emergency Services: Yes
Beds: 174

Key Personnel:
Pediatric Ambulatory Care . . . . . . Jay J Bathani, MD
Pediatric In-Patient Care . . . . Jay J Bathani, MD
Infection Control. . . . . Sandra Oszaniec
Chief of Medical Staff. . . . . David B Peirce, MD
CEO/President. . . . . Frank J. Sardone
Quality Assurance . . . . Marijo Snyder, MD, FACOG
Operating Room. . . . . Mary Starkweather
Radiology. . . . . Sue Szakal, MD

Measure	Cases	This Hosp.	State Avg.	U.S. Avg.
Blood Clot Prevention and Treatment				
Anticoagulation Overlap Therapy[5]	-	-	90%	93%
ICU Venous Thromboembolism Prophylaxis[5]	-	-	93%	92%
Incidence of Potentially Preventable VTE[5]	-	-	8%	10%
UFH with Dosages/Platelet Monitoring[5]	-	-	96%	97%
Venous Thromboembolism Prophylaxis[5]	-	-	87%	85%
Warfarin Therapy Discharge Instructions[5]	-	-	72%	75%
Chest Pain/Possible Heart Attack Care				
Aspirin Given Within 24 Hours of Arrival	12	92%	96%	96%
Fibrinolytic Meds Within 30 Min. of Arrival[7]	-	-	63%	58%
Average Time to ECG (minutes)	12	9	8	7
Average Time to Transfer (minutes)[7]	-	-	53	60
Children's Asthma Care				
Received Home Management Plan of Care	-	-	-	88%
Received Reliever Medication	-	-	-	100%
Received Systemic Corticosteroids	-	-	-	100%
Emergency Department				
Admittance Decision Time (minutes)[5]	-	-	102	98
Head CT Results Within 45 Min. of Arrival[5]	-	-	54%	57%
Patients Who Left ER Before Being Seen[5]	-	-	2%	2%
Time from ER Arrival to Admit. (minutes)[5]	-	-	288	274
Time from ER Arrival to Discharge (minutes)	399	115	128	134
Time in ER Before Being Evaluated (minutes)	411	22	22	26
Time to Pain Meds for Fractures (minutes)[3]	32	48	55	57
Heart Attack Care				
Aspirin Given at Discharge[1,3]	-	-	99%	99%
Fibrinolytic Meds Within 30 Min. of Arrival[3,7]	-	-	20%	54%
PCI Within 90 Minutes of Arrival[3,7]	-	-	95%	96%
Statin Prescribed at Discharge[1,3]	-	-	98%	98%
Heart Failure Care				
ACE Inhibitor or ARB for LVSD[1]	-	-	96%	97%
Discharge Instructions Given	24	96%	94%	94%
Evaluation of LVS Function	28	100%	99%	99%
Medicare Spending				
Medicare Spending per Patient (ratio)	-	-	0.96	0.98
Pneumonia Care				
Appropriate Initial Antibiotic Given	65	100%	96%	95%
Blood Culture Timing	87	98%	98%	98%
Pregnancy and Delivery Care				
Newborn Deliveries Scheduled Early[5]	-	-	3%	6%
Preventive Care				
Immunization for Influenza[3]	248	83%	89%	90%
Immunization for Pneumonia[2,3]	462	81%	90%	92%
Stroke Care				
Anticoagulation Therapy for Atrial Fibrillation[5]	-	-	92%	95%
Antithrombotic Therapy Timing[5]	-	-	97%	98%
Assessed for Rehabilitation[5]	-	-	97%	97%
Discharged on Antithrombotic Therapy[5]	-	-	99%	99%
Discharged on Statin Medication[5]	-	-	94%	94%
Thrombolytic Therapy Timing[5]	-	-	69%	66%
Venous Thromboembolism Prophylaxis[5]	-	-	94%	94%
Written Stroke Educational Materials Given[5]	-	-	87%	88%
Surgical Care Improvement Project				
Appropriate Beta Blocker Usage[5]	-	-	98%	98%
Appropriate VTP Within 24 Hours[5]	-	-	98%	98%
Controlled Postoperative Blood Glucose[5]	-	-	97%	97%
Perioperative Temperature Management[5]	-	-	100%	100%
Prophylactic Antibiotic Selection[5]	-	-	99%	99%
Prophylactic Antibiotic Selection (Outpatient)[5]	-	-	97%	98%
Prophylactic Antibiotic Stopped[5]	-	-	98%	98%
Prophylactic Antibiotic Timing[5]	-	-	98%	99%
Prophylactic Antibiotic Timing (Outpatient)[5]	-	-	97%	98%
Urinary Catheter Removal[5]	-	-	97%	97%
Survey of Patients' Hospital Experiences				
Area Around Room 'Always' Quiet at Night	(a)	65%	60%	61%
Doctors 'Always' Communicated Well	(a)	88%	81%	82%
Home Recovery Information Given	(a)	85%	87%	85%
Hospital Given 9 or 10 on 10 Point Scale	(a)	82%	71%	71%
Meds 'Always' Explained Before Given	(a)	75%	64%	64%
Nurses 'Always' Communicated Well	(a)	85%	80%	79%
Pain 'Always' Well Controlled	(a)	83%	71%	71%
Room and Bathroom 'Always' Clean	(a)	83%	73%	73%
Timely Help 'Always' Received	(a)	80%	70%	68%
Would Definitely Recommend Hospital	(a)	73%	71%	71%
Use of Medical Imaging				
Cardiac Imaging Stress Test before Surgery	165	3.6%	5.1%	5.3%
Combination Abdominal CT Scan	391	2.3%	8.7%	10.5%
Combination Brain/Sinus CT Scan[1]	-	-	2.2%	2.7%
Combination Chest CT Scan	169	0.0%	3.6%	2.7%
Follow-up Mammogram/Ultrasound	566	3.7%	8.2%	8.8%
Lumbar Spine MRI for Low Back Pain	58	62.1%	36.9%	37.2%

Mclaren - Northern Michigan

416 Connable Ave
Petoskey, MI 49770
URL: www.northernhealth.org
Type: Acute Care Hospitals
Ownership: Voluntary non-profit - Other
Phone: 231-487-4000
Fax: 231-487-7798
Emergency Services: Yes
Beds: 243

Key Personnel:
Chief of Medical Staff. . . . . John Bednar, MD
Quality Assurance . . . . Ingrid Flemming
Radiology. . . . . William E Henry
CEO/President. . . . . Thomas Mroczkowski

Measure	Cases	This Hosp.	State Avg.	U.S. Avg.
Blood Clot Prevention and Treatment				
Anticoagulation Overlap Therapy[2]	46	93%	90%	93%
ICU Venous Thromboembolism Prophylaxis[2]	89	99%	93%	92%
Incidence of Potentially Preventable VTE[1,2]	-	-	8%	10%
UFH with Dosages/Platelet Monitoring[2]	44	100%	96%	97%
Venous Thromboembolism Prophylaxis[2]	305	97%	87%	85%
Warfarin Therapy Discharge Instructions[2]	32	72%	72%	75%
Chest Pain/Possible Heart Attack Care				
Aspirin Given Within 24 Hours of Arrival[5]	-	-	96%	96%
Fibrinolytic Meds Within 30 Min. of Arrival[5]	-	-	63%	58%
Average Time to ECG (minutes)[5]	-	-	8	7
Average Time to Transfer (minutes)[5]	-	-	53	60
Children's Asthma Care				
Received Home Management Plan of Care	-	-	-	88%
Received Reliever Medication	-	-	-	100%
Received Systemic Corticosteroids	-	-	-	100%
Emergency Department				
Admittance Decision Time (minutes)[2]	481	133	102	98
Head CT Results Within 45 Min. of Arrival[1,3]	-	-	54%	57%
Patients Who Left ER Before Being Seen	28,832	1%	2%	2%
Time from ER Arrival to Admit. (minutes)[2]	488	256	288	274
Time from ER Arrival to Discharge (minutes)	366	109	128	134
Time in ER Before Being Evaluated (minutes)	405	17	22	26
Time to Pain Meds for Fractures (minutes)	191	49	55	57
Heart Attack Care				
Aspirin Given at Discharge	358	100%	99%	99%
Fibrinolytic Meds Within 30 Min. of Arrival[7]	-	-	20%	54%
PCI Within 90 Minutes of Arrival	23	96%	95%	96%
Statin Prescribed at Discharge	353	100%	98%	98%
Heart Failure Care				
ACE Inhibitor or ARB for LVSD	73	99%	96%	97%
Discharge Instructions Given	223	98%	94%	94%
Evaluation of LVS Function	247	100%	99%	99%
Medicare Spending				
Medicare Spending per Patient (ratio)	-	0.94	0.96	0.98
Pneumonia Care				
Appropriate Initial Antibiotic Given	89	98%	96%	95%
Blood Culture Timing	181	96%	98%	98%
Pregnancy and Delivery Care				
Newborn Deliveries Scheduled Early	75	7%	3%	6%
Preventive Care				
Immunization for Influenza[2]	578	91%	89%	90%
Immunization for Pneumonia[2]	803	90%	90%	92%
Stroke Care				
Anticoagulation Therapy for Atrial Fibrillation	25	100%	92%	95%
Antithrombotic Therapy Timing	131	98%	97%	98%
Assessed for Rehabilitation	144	99%	97%	97%
Discharged on Antithrombotic Therapy	136	100%	99%	99%
Discharged on Statin Medication	98	100%	94%	94%
Thrombolytic Therapy Timing	11	91%	69%	66%
Venous Thromboembolism Prophylaxis	161	100%	94%	94%
Written Stroke Educational Materials Given	77	100%	87%	88%
Surgical Care Improvement Project				
Appropriate Beta Blocker Usage[2]	237	98%	98%	98%
Appropriate VTP Within 24 Hours[2]	333	99%	98%	98%
Controlled Postoperative Blood Glucose[2]	134	99%	97%	97%
Perioperative Temperature Management[2]	445	100%	100%	100%
Prophylactic Antibiotic Selection[2]	405	99%	99%	99%
Prophylactic Antibiotic Selection (Outpatient)	622	99%	97%	98%
Prophylactic Antibiotic Stopped[2]	395	99%	98%	98%
Prophylactic Antibiotic Timing[2]	405	98%	98%	99%
Prophylactic Antibiotic Timing (Outpatient)	628	96%	97%	98%
Urinary Catheter Removal[2]	250	95%	97%	97%
Survey of Patients' Hospital Experiences				
Area Around Room 'Always' Quiet at Night	300+	49%	60%	61%
Doctors 'Always' Communicated Well	300+	80%	81%	82%
Home Recovery Information Given	300+	89%	87%	85%
Hospital Given 9 or 10 on 10 Point Scale	300+	71%	71%	71%
Meds 'Always' Explained Before Given	300+	62%	64%	64%
Nurses 'Always' Communicated Well	300+	79%	80%	79%
Pain 'Always' Well Controlled	300+	72%	71%	71%
Room and Bathroom 'Always' Clean	300+	71%	73%	73%
Timely Help 'Always' Received	300+	70%	70%	68%
Would Definitely Recommend Hospital	300+	77%	71%	71%
Use of Medical Imaging				
Cardiac Imaging Stress Test before Surgery	1,611	4.4%	5.1%	5.3%
Combination Abdominal CT Scan	1,443	5.5%	8.7%	10.5%
Combination Brain/Sinus CT Scan	793	1.8%	2.2%	2.7%
Combination Chest CT Scan	1,006	1.0%	3.6%	2.7%
Follow-up Mammogram/Ultrasound	2,547	7.3%	8.2%	8.8%
Lumbar Spine MRI for Low Back Pain	221	34.8%	36.9%	37.2%

NOTE: Hospital profiles are in alphabetical order by state, then city, then hospital within the city; Rankings exclude hospitals with less than 25 cases except for patient surveys which excludes hospitals with less than 100 cases; (a) 100-299 cases; (1) The number of cases/patients is too few to report; (2) Data submitted were based on a sample of cases/patients; (3) Results are based on a shorter time period than required; (4) Data suppressed by CMS for one or more quarters; (5) Results are not available for this reporting period; (6) Fewer than 100 patients completed the HCAHPS survey; (7) No cases met the criteria for this measure; (8) The lower limit of the confidence interval cannot be calculated if the number of observed infections equals zero; (9) No data are available from the state/territory for this reporting period; (10) The scores shown reflect fewer than 50 completed surveys; (11) There were discrepancies in the data collection process; (12) This measure does not apply to this hospital for this reporting period; (13) Results cannot be calculated for this reporting period; (14) The results for this state are combined with nearby states to protect confidentiality; Please refer to the User's Guide for a full explanation of data.

Scheurer Hospital

170 N Caseville Rd
Pigeon, MI 48755
Phone: 989-453-3223
Type: Critical Access Hospitals
Emergency Services: Yes
Ownership: Voluntary non-profit - Other

Measure	Cases	This Hosp.	State Avg.	U.S. Avg.
Blood Clot Prevention and Treatment				
Anticoagulation Overlap Therapy[5]	-	-	90%	93%
ICU Venous Thromboembolism Prophylaxis[5]	-	-	93%	92%
Incidence of Potentially Preventable VTE[5]	-	-	8%	10%
UFH with Dosages/Platelet Monitoring[5]	-	-	96%	97%
Venous Thromboembolism Prophylaxis[5]	-	-	87%	85%
Warfarin Therapy Discharge Instructions[5]	-	-	72%	75%
Chest Pain/Possible Heart Attack Care				
Aspirin Given Within 24 Hours of Arrival	52	98%	96%	96%
Fibrinolytic Meds Within 30 Min. of Arrival[1]	-	-	63%	58%
Average Time to ECG (minutes)	54	6	8	7
Average Time to Transfer (minutes)[1]	-	-	53	60
Children's Asthma Care				
Received Home Management Plan of Care	-	-	-	88%
Received Reliever Medication	-	-	-	100%
Received Systemic Corticosteroids	-	-	-	100%
Emergency Department				
Admittance Decision Time (minutes)[5]	-	-	102	98
Head CT Results Within 45 Min. of Arrival[5]	-	-	54%	57%
Patients Who Left ER Before Being Seen[5]	-	-	2%	2%
Time from ER Arrival to Admit. (minutes)[5]	-	-	288	274
Time from ER Arrival to Discharge (minutes)	376	90	128	134
Time in ER Before Being Evaluated (minutes)	412	17	22	26
Time to Pain Meds for Fractures (minutes)[5]	-	-	55	57
Heart Attack Care				
Aspirin Given at Discharge[5]	-	-	99%	99%
Fibrinolytic Meds Within 30 Min. of Arrival[5]	-	-	20%	54%
PCI Within 90 Minutes of Arrival[5]	-	-	95%	96%
Statin Prescribed at Discharge[5]	-	-	98%	98%
Heart Failure Care				
ACE Inhibitor or ARB for LVSD[1]	-	-	96%	97%
Discharge Instructions Given	12	83%	94%	94%
Evaluation of LVS Function	12	92%	99%	99%
Medicare Spending				
Medicare Spending per Patient (ratio)	-	-	0.96	0.98
Pneumonia Care				
Appropriate Initial Antibiotic Given	35	100%	96%	95%
Blood Culture Timing	21	100%	98%	98%
Pregnancy and Delivery Care				
Newborn Deliveries Scheduled Early[5]	-	-	3%	6%
Preventive Care				
Immunization for Influenza[5]	-	-	89%	90%
Immunization for Pneumonia[2,3]	253	85%	90%	92%
Stroke Care				
Anticoagulation Therapy for Atrial Fibrillation[5]	-	-	92%	95%
Antithrombotic Therapy Timing[5]	-	-	97%	98%
Assessed for Rehabilitation[5]	-	-	97%	97%
Discharged on Antithrombotic Therapy[5]	-	-	99%	99%
Discharged on Statin Medication[5]	-	-	94%	94%
Thrombolytic Therapy Timing[5]	-	-	69%	66%
Venous Thromboembolism Prophylaxis[5]	-	-	94%	94%
Written Stroke Educational Materials Given[5]	-	-	87%	88%
Surgical Care Improvement Project				
Appropriate Beta Blocker Usage	33	100%	98%	98%
Appropriate VTP Within 24 Hours	94	89%	98%	98%
Controlled Postoperative Blood Glucose[7]	-	-	97%	97%
Perioperative Temperature Management	94	98%	100%	100%
Prophylactic Antibiotic Selection	78	99%	99%	99%
Prophylactic Antibiotic Selection (Outpatient)[1,3]	-	-	97%	98%
Prophylactic Antibiotic Stopped	74	92%	98%	98%
Prophylactic Antibiotic Timing	78	97%	98%	99%
Prophylactic Antibiotic Timing (Outpatient)[1,3]	-	-	97%	98%
Urinary Catheter Removal	89	94%	97%	97%
Survey of Patients' Hospital Experiences				
Area Around Room 'Always' Quiet at Night	(a)	63%	60%	61%
Doctors 'Always' Communicated Well	(a)	82%	81%	82%
Home Recovery Information Given	(a)	86%	87%	85%
Hospital Given 9 or 10 on 10 Point Scale	(a)	76%	71%	71%
Meds 'Always' Explained Before Given	(a)	71%	64%	64%
Nurses 'Always' Communicated Well	(a)	85%	80%	79%
Pain 'Always' Well Controlled	(a)	78%	71%	71%
Room and Bathroom 'Always' Clean	(a)	88%	73%	73%
Timely Help 'Always' Received	(a)	79%	70%	68%
Would Definitely Recommend Hospital	(a)	76%	71%	71%
Use of Medical Imaging				
Cardiac Imaging Stress Test before Surgery	250	3.6%	5.1%	5.3%
Combination Abdominal CT Scan	265	23.0%	8.7%	10.5%
Combination Brain/Sinus CT Scan[1]	-	-	2.2%	2.7%
Combination Chest CT Scan	174	8.6%	3.6%	2.7%
Follow-up Mammogram/Ultrasound	459	3.7%	8.2%	8.8%
Lumbar Spine MRI for Low Back Pain[7]	-	-	36.9%	37.2%

Doctors' Hospital of Michigan

461 W Huron St
Pontiac, MI 48341
Phone: 248-857-7200
Fax: 248-857-6801
URL: www.nomc.org
Type: Acute Care Hospitals
Emergency Services: Yes
Ownership: Physician
Beds: 380

Key Personnel:

Quality Assurance . . . . Rodger Chrysler
Anesthesiology. . . . . Y Falick, MD
Radiology. . . . . M Khalid, MD
Chief of Medical Staff. . . . . Bruce Lessien
Emergency Room . . . . Derrek McCallmont, MD
Infection Control. . . . . Luretta Pandya, RN
CEO/President. . . . . John Ponczocha

Measure	Cases	This Hosp.	State Avg.	U.S. Avg.
Blood Clot Prevention and Treatment				
Anticoagulation Overlap Therapy[1,2]	-	-	90%	93%
ICU Venous Thromboembolism Prophylaxis[1,2]	-	-	93%	92%
Incidence of Potentially Preventable VTE[2,3]	-	-	8%	10%
UFH with Dosages/Platelet Monitoring[1,2]	-	-	96%	97%
Venous Thromboembolism Prophylaxis[2,3]	96	73%	87%	85%
Warfarin Therapy Discharge Instructions[1,2]	-	-	72%	75%
Chest Pain/Possible Heart Attack Care				
Aspirin Given Within 24 Hours of Arrival[1,3]	-	-	96%	96%
Fibrinolytic Meds Within 30 Min. of Arrival[3,7]	-	-	63%	58%
Average Time to ECG (minutes)[1,3]	-	-	8	7
Average Time to Transfer (minutes)[1,3]	-	-	53	60
Children's Asthma Care				
Received Home Management Plan of Care	-	-	-	88%
Received Reliever Medication	-	-	-	100%
Received Systemic Corticosteroids	-	-	-	100%
Emergency Department				
Admittance Decision Time (minutes)[2,3]	119	125	102	98
Head CT Results Within 45 Min. of Arrival[5]	-	-	54%	57%
Patients Who Left ER Before Being Seen[5]	-	-	2%	2%
Time from ER Arrival to Admit. (minutes)[2,3]	128	288	288	274
Time from ER Arrival to Discharge (minutes)[3]	149	110	128	134
Time in ER Before Being Evaluated (minutes)[3]	161	26	22	26
Time to Pain Meds for Fractures (minutes)[1,3]	-	-	55	57
Heart Attack Care				
Aspirin Given at Discharge[3,7]	-	-	99%	99%
Fibrinolytic Meds Within 30 Min. of Arrival[3,7]	-	-	20%	54%
PCI Within 90 Minutes of Arrival[3,7]	-	-	95%	96%
Statin Prescribed at Discharge[3,7]	-	-	98%	98%
Heart Failure Care				
ACE Inhibitor or ARB for LVSD[1,2]	-	-	96%	97%
Discharge Instructions Given[1,2]	-	-	94%	94%
Evaluation of LVS Function[1,2]	-	-	99%	99%
Medicare Spending				
Medicare Spending per Patient (ratio)	-	0.96	0.96	0.98
Pneumonia Care				
Appropriate Initial Antibiotic Given[1,2]	-	-	96%	95%
Blood Culture Timing[1,2]	-	-	98%	98%
Pregnancy and Delivery Care				
Newborn Deliveries Scheduled Early[3,7]	-	-	3%	6%
Preventive Care				
Immunization for Influenza[2]	105	76%	89%	90%
Immunization for Pneumonia[2,3]	179	77%	90%	92%
Stroke Care				
Anticoagulation Therapy for Atrial Fibrillation[5]	-	-	92%	95%
Antithrombotic Therapy Timing[5]	-	-	97%	98%
Assessed for Rehabilitation[5]	-	-	97%	97%
Discharged on Antithrombotic Therapy[5]	-	-	99%	99%
Discharged on Statin Medication[5]	-	-	94%	94%
Thrombolytic Therapy Timing[5]	-	-	69%	66%
Venous Thromboembolism Prophylaxis[5]	-	-	94%	94%
Written Stroke Educational Materials Given[5]	-	-	87%	88%
Surgical Care Improvement Project				
Appropriate Beta Blocker Usage[1,3]	-	-	98%	98%
Appropriate VTP Within 24 Hours[1,3]	-	-	98%	98%
Controlled Postoperative Blood Glucose[3,7]	-	-	97%	97%
Perioperative Temperature Management[3]	13	100%	100%	100%
Prophylactic Antibiotic Selection[1,3]	-	-	99%	99%
Prophylactic Antibiotic Selection (Outpatient)[5]	-	-	97%	98%
Prophylactic Antibiotic Stopped[1,3]	-	-	98%	98%
Prophylactic Antibiotic Timing[1,3]	-	-	98%	99%
Prophylactic Antibiotic Timing (Outpatient)[5]	-	-	97%	98%
Urinary Catheter Removal[3]	11	45%	97%	97%
Survey of Patients' Hospital Experiences				
Area Around Room 'Always' Quiet at Night	(a)	64%	60%	61%
Doctors 'Always' Communicated Well	(a)	78%	81%	82%
Home Recovery Information Given	(a)	78%	87%	85%
Hospital Given 9 or 10 on 10 Point Scale	(a)	53%	71%	71%
Meds 'Always' Explained Before Given	(a)	54%	64%	64%
Nurses 'Always' Communicated Well	(a)	68%	80%	79%
Pain 'Always' Well Controlled	(a)	56%	71%	71%
Room and Bathroom 'Always' Clean	(a)	58%	73%	73%
Timely Help 'Always' Received	(a)	48%	70%	68%
Would Definitely Recommend Hospital	(a)	54%	71%	71%
Use of Medical Imaging				
Cardiac Imaging Stress Test before Surgery[1]	-	-	5.1%	5.3%
Combination Abdominal CT Scan	142	27.5%	8.7%	10.5%
Combination Brain/Sinus CT Scan[1]	-	-	2.2%	2.7%
Combination Chest CT Scan[1]	-	-	3.6%	2.7%
Follow-up Mammogram/Ultrasound	328	4.3%	8.2%	8.8%
Lumbar Spine MRI for Low Back Pain[1]	-	-	36.9%	37.2%

Mclaren Oakland

50 North Perry
Pontiac, MI 48342
Phone: 248-338-5000
Fax: 248-338-5667
URL: www.pohmedical.org
Type: Acute Care Hospitals
Emergency Services: Yes
Ownership: Voluntary non-profit - Private
Beds: 308

Key Personnel:

Operating Room. . . . . Jackie Adams, RN
Chief of Medical Staff. . . . . Steve Calkin
Infection Control. . . . . MO Doyle, DO
Radiology. . . . . DA Kellam, DO
Pediatric Ambulatory Care . . . . . . ID Kernis, DO
Pediatric In-Patient Care . . . . ID Kernis, DO
Quality Assurance . . . . Lynn Kirby
CEO/President. . . . . Patrick Lamberti

Measure	Cases	This Hosp.	State Avg.	U.S. Avg.
Blood Clot Prevention and Treatment				
Anticoagulation Overlap Therapy[2]	31	97%	90%	93%
ICU Venous Thromboembolism Prophylaxis[2]	62	98%	93%	92%
Incidence of Potentially Preventable VTE[2]	16	12%	8%	10%
UFH with Dosages/Platelet Monitoring[2]	37	97%	96%	97%
Venous Thromboembolism Prophylaxis[2]	335	96%	87%	85%
Warfarin Therapy Discharge Instructions[2]	12	42%	72%	75%
Chest Pain/Possible Heart Attack Care				
Aspirin Given Within 24 Hours of Arrival	86	99%	96%	96%
Fibrinolytic Meds Within 30 Min. of Arrival[7]	-	-	63%	58%
Average Time to ECG (minutes)	86	7	8	7
Average Time to Transfer (minutes)	13	56	53	60
Children's Asthma Care				
Received Home Management Plan of Care	-	-	-	88%
Received Reliever Medication	-	-	-	100%
Received Systemic Corticosteroids	-	-	-	100%
Emergency Department				
Admittance Decision Time (minutes)[2]	519	164	102	98
Head CT Results Within 45 Min. of Arrival[1]	-	-	54%	57%

NOTE: Hospital profiles are in alphabetical order by state, then city, then hospital within the city; Rankings exclude hospitals with less than 25 cases except for patient surveys which excludes hospitals with less than 100 cases; (a) 100-299 cases; (1) The number of cases/patients is too few to report; (2) Data submitted were based on a sample of cases/patients; (3) Results are based on a shorter time period than required; (4) Data suppressed by CMS for one or more quarters; (5) Results are not available for this reporting period; (6) Fewer than 100 patients completed the HCAHPS survey; (7) No cases met the criteria for this measure; (8) The lower limit of the confidence interval cannot be calculated if the number of observed infections equals zero; (9) No data are available from the state/territory for this reporting period; (10) The scores shown reflect fewer than 50 completed surveys; (11) There were discrepancies in the data collection process; (12) This measure does not apply to this hospital for this reporting period; (13) Results cannot be calculated for this reporting period; (14) The results for this state are combined with nearby states to protect confidentiality; Please refer to the User's Guide for a full explanation of data.

Measure	Cases	This Hosp.	State Avg.	U.S. Avg.
Patients Who Left ER Before Being Seen	53,668	1%	2%	2%
Time from ER Arrival to Admit. (minutes)[2]	537	265	288	274
Time from ER Arrival to Discharge (minutes)	334	79	128	134
Time in ER Before Being Evaluated (minutes)	324	17	22	26
Time to Pain Meds for Fractures (minutes)	161	50	55	57
Heart Attack Care				
Aspirin Given at Discharge	20	90%	99%	99%
Fibrinolytic Meds Within 30 Min. of Arrival[7]	-	-	20%	54%
PCI Within 90 Minutes of Arrival[7]	-	-	95%	96%
Statin Prescribed at Discharge	19	95%	98%	98%
Heart Failure Care				
ACE Inhibitor or ARB for LVSD	55	96%	96%	97%
Discharge Instructions Given	106	97%	94%	94%
Evaluation of LVS Function	130	98%	99%	99%
Medicare Spending				
Medicare Spending per Patient (ratio)	-	1.01	0.96	0.98
Pneumonia Care				
Appropriate Initial Antibiotic Given	74	95%	96%	95%
Blood Culture Timing	111	100%	98%	98%
Pregnancy and Delivery Care				
Newborn Deliveries Scheduled Early[7]	-	-	3%	6%
Preventive Care				
Immunization for Influenza[2]	438	95%	89%	90%
Immunization for Pneumonia[2]	576	91%	90%	92%
Stroke Care				
Anticoagulation Therapy for Atrial Fibrillation[1]	-	-	92%	95%
Antithrombotic Therapy Timing	44	100%	97%	98%
Assessed for Rehabilitation	48	94%	97%	97%
Discharged on Antithrombotic Therapy	46	98%	99%	99%
Discharged on Statin Medication	34	91%	94%	94%
Thrombolytic Therapy Timing[1]	-	-	69%	66%
Venous Thromboembolism Prophylaxis	56	96%	94%	94%
Written Stroke Educational Materials Given	30	80%	87%	88%
Surgical Care Improvement Project				
Appropriate Beta Blocker Usage[2]	79	99%	98%	98%
Appropriate VTP Within 24 Hours[2]	249	98%	98%	98%
Controlled Postoperative Blood Glucose[2,7]	-	-	97%	97%
Perioperative Temperature Management[2]	297	100%	100%	100%
Prophylactic Antibiotic Selection[2]	199	98%	99%	99%
Prophylactic Antibiotic Selection (Outpatient)	134	90%	97%	98%
Prophylactic Antibiotic Stopped[2]	188	96%	98%	98%
Prophylactic Antibiotic Timing[2]	200	100%	98%	99%
Prophylactic Antibiotic Timing (Outpatient)	136	92%	97%	98%
Urinary Catheter Removal[2]	220	98%	97%	97%
Survey of Patients' Hospital Experiences				
Area Around Room 'Always' Quiet at Night	300+	56%	60%	61%
Doctors 'Always' Communicated Well	300+	75%	81%	82%
Home Recovery Information Given	300+	85%	87%	85%
Hospital Given 9 or 10 on 10 Point Scale	300+	64%	71%	71%
Meds 'Always' Explained Before Given	300+	59%	64%	64%
Nurses 'Always' Communicated Well	300+	74%	80%	79%
Pain 'Always' Well Controlled	300+	65%	71%	71%
Room and Bathroom 'Always' Clean	300+	70%	73%	73%
Timely Help 'Always' Received	300+	62%	70%	68%
Would Definitely Recommend Hospital	300+	65%	71%	71%
Use of Medical Imaging				
Cardiac Imaging Stress Test before Surgery	163	6.1%	5.1%	5.3%
Combination Abdominal CT Scan	572	20.3%	8.7%	10.5%
Combination Brain/Sinus CT Scan[1]	-	-	2.2%	2.7%
Combination Chest CT Scan	388	8.5%	3.6%	2.7%
Follow-up Mammogram/Ultrasound	547	6.9%	8.2%	8.8%
Lumbar Spine MRI for Low Back Pain[7]	-	-	36.9%	37.2%

Saint Joseph Mercy Oakland

44405 Woodward Ave
Pontiac, MI 48341
Phone: 248-858-3000
Fax: 248-858-3155
URL: www.stjoesoakland.org
Type: Acute Care Hospitals
Emergency Services: Yes
Ownership: Voluntary non-profit - Private
Beds: 443

Key Personnel:
Pediatric Ambulatory Care . . . . . . Rajendra Desai, MD
Operating Room. . . . . Trudy Lentini
Emergency Room . . . . Mary Jo Malafa
Chief of Medical Staff. . . . . Michael K. Smith, DO, FACOS
Radiology. . . . . Babu Vemuri, MD
CEO/President. . . . . Jack Weiner, FACHE

Measure	Cases	This Hosp.	State Avg.	U.S. Avg.
Blood Clot Prevention and Treatment				
Anticoagulation Overlap Therapy[2]	113	92%	90%	93%
ICU Venous Thromboembolism Prophylaxis[2]	90	97%	93%	92%
Incidence of Potentially Preventable VTE[2]	13	0%	8%	10%
UFH with Dosages/Platelet Monitoring[2]	135	100%	96%	97%
Venous Thromboembolism Prophylaxis[2]	344	88%	87%	85%
Warfarin Therapy Discharge Instructions[2]	86	76%	72%	75%
Chest Pain/Possible Heart Attack Care				
Aspirin Given Within 24 Hours of Arrival[5]	-	-	96%	96%
Fibrinolytic Meds Within 30 Min. of Arrival[5]	-	-	63%	58%
Average Time to ECG (minutes)[5]	-	-	8	7
Average Time to Transfer (minutes)[5]	-	-	53	60
Children's Asthma Care				
Received Home Management Plan of Care	-	-	-	88%
Received Reliever Medication	-	-	-	100%
Received Systemic Corticosteroids	-	-	-	100%
Emergency Department				
Admittance Decision Time (minutes)[2]	567	132	102	98
Head CT Results Within 45 Min. of Arrival[1,3]	-	-	54%	57%
Patients Who Left ER Before Being Seen	53,567	2%	2%	2%
Time from ER Arrival to Admit. (minutes)[2]	618	322	288	274
Time from ER Arrival to Discharge (minutes)	354	154	128	134
Time in ER Before Being Evaluated (minutes)	405	20	22	26
Time to Pain Meds for Fractures (minutes)	106	42	55	57
Heart Attack Care				
Aspirin Given at Discharge[2]	327	100%	99%	99%
Fibrinolytic Meds Within 30 Min. of Arrival[2,7]	-	-	20%	54%
PCI Within 90 Minutes of Arrival[2]	68	97%	95%	96%
Statin Prescribed at Discharge[2]	310	100%	98%	98%
Heart Failure Care				
ACE Inhibitor or ARB for LVSD[2]	100	100%	96%	97%
Discharge Instructions Given[2]	262	100%	94%	94%
Evaluation of LVS Function[2]	323	100%	99%	99%
Medicare Spending				
Medicare Spending per Patient (ratio)	-	1.02	0.96	0.98
Pneumonia Care				
Appropriate Initial Antibiotic Given[2]	98	99%	96%	95%
Blood Culture Timing[2]	101	99%	98%	98%
Pregnancy and Delivery Care				
Newborn Deliveries Scheduled Early	342	0%	3%	6%
Preventive Care				
Immunization for Influenza[2]	570	99%	89%	90%
Immunization for Pneumonia[2]	746	99%	90%	92%
Stroke Care				
Anticoagulation Therapy for Atrial Fibrillation	39	100%	92%	95%
Antithrombotic Therapy Timing	207	98%	97%	98%
Assessed for Rehabilitation	280	99%	97%	97%
Discharged on Antithrombotic Therapy	248	100%	99%	99%
Discharged on Statin Medication	197	100%	94%	94%
Thrombolytic Therapy Timing	21	100%	69%	66%
Venous Thromboembolism Prophylaxis	319	100%	94%	94%
Written Stroke Educational Materials Given	124	99%	87%	88%
Surgical Care Improvement Project				
Appropriate Beta Blocker Usage[2]	228	100%	98%	98%
Appropriate VTP Within 24 Hours[2]	479	100%	98%	98%
Controlled Postoperative Blood Glucose[2]	154	97%	97%	97%
Perioperative Temperature Management[2]	713	100%	100%	100%
Prophylactic Antibiotic Selection[2]	490	100%	99%	99%
Prophylactic Antibiotic Selection (Outpatient)	409	100%	97%	98%
Prophylactic Antibiotic Stopped[2]	478	99%	98%	98%
Prophylactic Antibiotic Timing[2]	491	100%	98%	99%
Prophylactic Antibiotic Timing (Outpatient)	409	100%	97%	98%
Urinary Catheter Removal[2]	395	100%	97%	97%
Survey of Patients' Hospital Experiences				
Area Around Room 'Always' Quiet at Night	300+	53%	60%	61%
Doctors 'Always' Communicated Well	300+	74%	81%	82%
Home Recovery Information Given	300+	87%	87%	85%
Hospital Given 9 or 10 on 10 Point Scale	300+	69%	71%	71%
Meds 'Always' Explained Before Given	300+	56%	64%	64%
Nurses 'Always' Communicated Well	300+	76%	80%	79%
Pain 'Always' Well Controlled	300+	67%	71%	71%
Room and Bathroom 'Always' Clean	300+	56%	73%	73%
Timely Help 'Always' Received	300+	60%	70%	68%
Would Definitely Recommend Hospital	300+	72%	71%	71%
Use of Medical Imaging				
Cardiac Imaging Stress Test before Surgery	503	5.4%	5.1%	5.3%
Combination Abdominal CT Scan	881	14.0%	8.7%	10.5%
Combination Brain/Sinus CT Scan	833	1.7%	2.2%	2.7%
Combination Chest CT Scan	635	12.8%	3.6%	2.7%
Follow-up Mammogram/Ultrasound	2,344	8.4%	8.2%	8.8%
Lumbar Spine MRI for Low Back Pain	186	31.7%	36.9%	37.2%

Port Huron Hospital

1221 Pine Grove Ave
Port Huron, MI 48060
Phone: 810-987-5000
Fax: 810-985-2675
E-mail: phhwebmaster@porthuronhosp.org
URL: www.porthuronhospital.org
Type: Acute Care Hospitals
Emergency Services: Yes
Ownership: Voluntary non-profit - Other
Beds: 186

Key Personnel:
Cardiac Laboratory. . . . . Maryann Barnes
Operating Room. . . . . Frank Brettschneider, DO
Radiology. . . . . F William Coop
CEO/President. . . . . Tom DeFauw
Quality Assurance . . . . Mary Pool
Pediatric Ambulatory Care . . . . . . Kathy Richards
Chief of Medical Staff. . . . . Michael Tawney, DO

Measure	Cases	This Hosp.	State Avg.	U.S. Avg.
Blood Clot Prevention and Treatment				
Anticoagulation Overlap Therapy[2]	93	89%	90%	93%
ICU Venous Thromboembolism Prophylaxis[2]	54	91%	93%	92%
Incidence of Potentially Preventable VTE[2]	13	54%	8%	10%
UFH with Dosages/Platelet Monitoring[2]	94	98%	96%	97%
Venous Thromboembolism Prophylaxis[2]	351	62%	87%	85%
Warfarin Therapy Discharge Instructions[2]	64	86%	72%	75%
Chest Pain/Possible Heart Attack Care				
Aspirin Given Within 24 Hours of Arrival[1,3]	-	-	96%	96%
Fibrinolytic Meds Within 30 Min. of Arrival[3,7]	-	-	63%	58%
Average Time to ECG (minutes)[1,3]	-	-	8	7
Average Time to Transfer (minutes)[3,7]	-	-	53	60
Children's Asthma Care				
Received Home Management Plan of Care	-	-	-	88%
Received Reliever Medication	-	-	-	100%
Received Systemic Corticosteroids	-	-	-	100%
Emergency Department				
Admittance Decision Time (minutes)[2]	572	88	102	98
Head CT Results Within 45 Min. of Arrival	18	67%	54%	57%
Patients Who Left ER Before Being Seen	40,108	4%	2%	2%
Time from ER Arrival to Admit. (minutes)[2]	585	288	288	274
Time from ER Arrival to Discharge (minutes)	414	133	128	134
Time in ER Before Being Evaluated (minutes)	451	24	22	26
Time to Pain Meds for Fractures (minutes)	199	64	55	57
Heart Attack Care				
Aspirin Given at Discharge	354	98%	99%	99%
Fibrinolytic Meds Within 30 Min. of Arrival[7]	-	-	20%	54%
PCI Within 90 Minutes of Arrival	50	100%	95%	96%
Statin Prescribed at Discharge	349	98%	98%	98%
Heart Failure Care				
ACE Inhibitor or ARB for LVSD	81	99%	96%	97%
Discharge Instructions Given	233	89%	94%	94%
Evaluation of LVS Function	303	100%	99%	99%
Medicare Spending				
Medicare Spending per Patient (ratio)	-	0.94	0.96	0.98
Pneumonia Care				
Appropriate Initial Antibiotic Given	147	97%	96%	95%
Blood Culture Timing	271	99%	98%	98%
Pregnancy and Delivery Care				
Newborn Deliveries Scheduled Early[2]	123	2%	3%	6%
Preventive Care				
Immunization for Influenza[2]	559	96%	89%	90%
Immunization for Pneumonia[2]	705	98%	90%	92%
Stroke Care				
Anticoagulation Therapy for Atrial Fibrillation	15	73%	92%	95%

NOTE: Hospital profiles are in alphabetical order by state, then city, then hospital within the city; Rankings exclude hospitals with less than 25 cases except for patient surveys which excludes hospitals with less than 100 cases; (a) 100-299 cases; (1) The number of cases/patients is too few to report; (2) Data submitted were based on a sample of cases/patients; (3) Results are based on a shorter time period than required; (4) Data suppressed by CMS for one or more quarters; (5) Results are not available for this reporting period; (6) Fewer than 100 patients completed the HCAHPS survey; (7) No cases met the criteria for this measure; (8) The lower limit of the confidence interval cannot be calculated if the number of observed infections equals zero; (9) No data are available from the state/territory for this reporting period; (10) The scores shown reflect fewer than 50 completed surveys; (11) There were discrepancies in the data collection process; (12) This measure does not apply to this hospital for this reporting period; (13) Results cannot be calculated for this reporting period; (14) The results for this state are combined with nearby states to protect confidentiality; Please refer to the User's Guide for a full explanation of data.

Measure	Cases	This Hosp.	State Avg.	U.S. Avg.
Antithrombotic Therapy Timing	107	93%	97%	98%
Assessed for Rehabilitation	107	92%	97%	97%
Discharged on Antithrombotic Therapy	100	95%	99%	99%
Discharged on Statin Medication	79	85%	94%	94%
Thrombolytic Therapy Timing[1]	-	-	69%	66%
Venous Thromboembolism Prophylaxis	120	69%	94%	94%
Written Stroke Educational Materials Given	61	72%	87%	88%
Surgical Care Improvement Project				
Appropriate Beta Blocker Usage	306	97%	98%	98%
Appropriate VTP Within 24 Hours	641	100%	98%	98%
Controlled Postoperative Blood Glucose	103	100%	97%	97%
Perioperative Temperature Management	750	99%	100%	100%
Prophylactic Antibiotic Selection	637	98%	99%	99%
Prophylactic Antibiotic Selection (Outpatient)	217	97%	97%	98%
Prophylactic Antibiotic Stopped	605	98%	98%	98%
Prophylactic Antibiotic Timing	638	99%	98%	99%
Prophylactic Antibiotic Timing (Outpatient)	218	98%	97%	98%
Urinary Catheter Removal	635	95%	97%	97%
Survey of Patients' Hospital Experiences				
Area Around Room 'Always' Quiet at Night	300+	55%	60%	61%
Doctors 'Always' Communicated Well	300+	77%	81%	82%
Home Recovery Information Given	300+	85%	87%	85%
Hospital Given 9 or 10 on 10 Point Scale	300+	68%	71%	71%
Meds 'Always' Explained Before Given	300+	61%	64%	64%
Nurses 'Always' Communicated Well	300+	80%	80%	79%
Pain 'Always' Well Controlled	300+	71%	71%	71%
Room and Bathroom 'Always' Clean	300+	75%	73%	73%
Timely Help 'Always' Received	300+	66%	70%	68%
Would Definitely Recommend Hospital	300+	67%	71%	71%
Use of Medical Imaging				
Cardiac Imaging Stress Test before Surgery	228	3.1%	5.1%	5.3%
Combination Abdominal CT Scan	828	3.6%	8.7%	10.5%
Combination Brain/Sinus CT Scan	740	2.6%	2.2%	2.7%
Combination Chest CT Scan	714	0.8%	3.6%	2.7%
Follow-up Mammogram/Ultrasound	1,680	10.7%	8.2%	8.8%
Lumbar Spine MRI for Low Back Pain	188	33.5%	36.9%	37.2%

Saint Joseph Mercy Port Huron

2601 Electric Avenue
Port Huron, MI 48060
Phone: 810-985-1510
Fax: 810-985-1508
URL: www.mercyporthuron.com
Type: Acute Care Hospitals
Ownership: Voluntary non-profit - Church
Emergency Services: Yes
Beds: 119

Key Personnel:
Emergency Room . . . . Jere Baldwin, MD
Chief of Medical Staff. . . . . Robert Camara, DO
Infection Control. . . . . D Heide
Operating Room. . . . . Brenda Miller
Quality Assurance . . . . Julie Schieman
Radiology. . . . . Daniel Shogren
CEO/President. . . . . Rebekah Smith, RN
Intensive Care Unit. . . . . Brian Thick

Measure	Cases	This Hosp.	State Avg.	U.S. Avg.
Blood Clot Prevention and Treatment				
Anticoagulation Overlap Therapy[2]	20	90%	90%	93%
ICU Venous Thromboembolism Prophylaxis[2]	79	80%	93%	92%
Incidence of Potentially Preventable VTE[1,2]	-	-	8%	10%
UFH with Dosages/Platelet Monitoring[2]	17	100%	96%	97%
Venous Thromboembolism Prophylaxis[2]	316	66%	87%	85%
Warfarin Therapy Discharge Instructions[2]	11	100%	72%	75%
Chest Pain/Possible Heart Attack Care				
Aspirin Given Within 24 Hours of Arrival	30	100%	96%	96%
Fibrinolytic Meds Within 30 Min. of Arrival[7]	-	-	63%	58%
Average Time to ECG (minutes)	30	4	8	7
Average Time to Transfer (minutes)	11	67	53	60
Children's Asthma Care				
Received Home Management Plan of Care	-	-	-	88%
Received Reliever Medication	-	-	-	100%
Received Systemic Corticosteroids	-	-	-	100%
Emergency Department				
Admittance Decision Time (minutes)[2]	478	84	102	98
Head CT Results Within 45 Min. of Arrival	13	69%	54%	57%
Patients Who Left ER Before Being Seen	11,101	2%	2%	2%
Time from ER Arrival to Admit. (minutes)[2]	479	243	288	274
Time from ER Arrival to Discharge (minutes)	363	110	128	134
Time in ER Before Being Evaluated (minutes)	399	16	22	26
Time to Pain Meds for Fractures (minutes)	81	50	55	57
Heart Attack Care				
Aspirin Given at Discharge	27	100%	99%	99%
Fibrinolytic Meds Within 30 Min. of Arrival[7]	-	-	20%	54%
PCI Within 90 Minutes of Arrival[7]	-	-	95%	96%
Statin Prescribed at Discharge	23	96%	98%	98%
Heart Failure Care				
ACE Inhibitor or ARB for LVSD	30	100%	96%	97%
Discharge Instructions Given	112	99%	94%	94%
Evaluation of LVS Function	151	100%	99%	99%
Medicare Spending				
Medicare Spending per Patient (ratio)	-	0.95	0.96	0.98
Pneumonia Care				
Appropriate Initial Antibiotic Given[2]	79	100%	96%	95%
Blood Culture Timing[2]	138	100%	98%	98%
Pregnancy and Delivery Care				
Newborn Deliveries Scheduled Early[7]	-	-	3%	6%
Preventive Care				
Immunization for Influenza[2]	425	72%	89%	90%
Immunization for Pneumonia[2]	631	75%	90%	92%
Stroke Care				
Anticoagulation Therapy for Atrial Fibrillation[1]	-	-	92%	95%
Antithrombotic Therapy Timing	60	98%	97%	98%
Assessed for Rehabilitation	60	97%	97%	97%
Discharged on Antithrombotic Therapy	59	100%	99%	99%
Discharged on Statin Medication	49	73%	94%	94%
Thrombolytic Therapy Timing	11	9%	69%	66%
Venous Thromboembolism Prophylaxis	64	67%	94%	94%
Written Stroke Educational Materials Given	26	92%	87%	88%
Surgical Care Improvement Project				
Appropriate Beta Blocker Usage[2]	115	99%	98%	98%
Appropriate VTP Within 24 Hours[2]	386	100%	98%	98%
Controlled Postoperative Blood Glucose[2,7]	-	-	97%	97%
Perioperative Temperature Management[2]	407	100%	100%	100%
Prophylactic Antibiotic Selection[2]	255	100%	99%	99%
Prophylactic Antibiotic Selection (Outpatient)	22	91%	97%	98%
Prophylactic Antibiotic Stopped[2]	233	100%	98%	98%
Prophylactic Antibiotic Timing[2]	255	100%	98%	99%
Prophylactic Antibiotic Timing (Outpatient)	22	100%	97%	98%
Urinary Catheter Removal[2]	340	100%	97%	97%
Survey of Patients' Hospital Experiences				
Area Around Room 'Always' Quiet at Night	300+	63%	60%	61%
Doctors 'Always' Communicated Well	300+	76%	81%	82%
Home Recovery Information Given	300+	89%	87%	85%
Hospital Given 9 or 10 on 10 Point Scale	300+	68%	71%	71%
Meds 'Always' Explained Before Given	300+	56%	64%	64%
Nurses 'Always' Communicated Well	300+	75%	80%	79%
Pain 'Always' Well Controlled	300+	69%	71%	71%
Room and Bathroom 'Always' Clean	300+	72%	73%	73%
Timely Help 'Always' Received	300+	61%	70%	68%
Would Definitely Recommend Hospital	300+	69%	71%	71%
Use of Medical Imaging				
Cardiac Imaging Stress Test before Surgery	101	2.0%	5.1%	5.3%
Combination Abdominal CT Scan	370	4.6%	8.7%	10.5%
Combination Brain/Sinus CT Scan	367	1.4%	2.2%	2.7%
Combination Chest CT Scan	217	0.5%	3.6%	2.7%
Follow-up Mammogram/Ultrasound	824	14.2%	8.2%	8.8%
Lumbar Spine MRI for Low Back Pain[1]	-	-	36.9%	37.2%

Spectrum Health - Reed City Campus

PO Box 75, 300 N Patterson
Reed City, MI 49677
Phone: 231-832-3271
Fax: 231-832-1817
URL: www.spectrum-health.org
Type: Critical Access Hospitals
Ownership: Voluntary non-profit - Private
Emergency Services: Yes
Beds: 106

Key Personnel:
CEO/President. . . . . Tom Kauffman

Measure	Cases	This Hosp.	State Avg.	U.S. Avg.
Blood Clot Prevention and Treatment				
Anticoagulation Overlap Therapy[1,2]	-	-	90%	93%
ICU Venous Thromboembolism Prophylaxis[2]	26	100%	93%	92%
Incidence of Potentially Preventable VTE[2,7]	-	-	8%	10%
UFH with Dosages/Platelet Monitoring[1,2]	-	-	96%	97%
Venous Thromboembolism Prophylaxis[2]	90	88%	87%	85%
Warfarin Therapy Discharge Instructions[1,2]	-	-	72%	75%
Chest Pain/Possible Heart Attack Care				
Aspirin Given Within 24 Hours of Arrival	106	94%	96%	96%
Fibrinolytic Meds Within 30 Min. of Arrival[7]	-	-	63%	58%
Average Time to ECG (minutes)	110	5	8	7
Average Time to Transfer (minutes)	14	42	53	60
Children's Asthma Care				
Received Home Management Plan of Care	-	-	-	88%
Received Reliever Medication	-	-	-	100%
Received Systemic Corticosteroids	-	-	-	100%
Emergency Department				
Admittance Decision Time (minutes)[5]	-	-	102	98
Head CT Results Within 45 Min. of Arrival[1,3]	-	-	54%	57%
Patients Who Left ER Before Being Seen[5]	-	-	2%	2%
Time from ER Arrival to Admit. (minutes)[5]	-	-	288	274
Time from ER Arrival to Discharge (minutes)	396	93	128	134
Time in ER Before Being Evaluated (minutes)	328	11	22	26
Time to Pain Meds for Fractures (minutes)[3]	41	51	55	57
Heart Attack Care				
Aspirin Given at Discharge[1,3]	-	-	99%	99%
Fibrinolytic Meds Within 30 Min. of Arrival[3,7]	-	-	20%	54%
PCI Within 90 Minutes of Arrival[3,7]	-	-	95%	96%
Statin Prescribed at Discharge[1,3]	-	-	98%	98%
Heart Failure Care				
ACE Inhibitor or ARB for LVSD[1]	-	-	96%	97%
Discharge Instructions Given	11	82%	94%	94%
Evaluation of LVS Function	16	100%	99%	99%
Medicare Spending				
Medicare Spending per Patient (ratio)	-	-	0.96	0.98
Pneumonia Care				
Appropriate Initial Antibiotic Given	53	98%	96%	95%
Blood Culture Timing	90	97%	98%	98%
Pregnancy and Delivery Care				
Newborn Deliveries Scheduled Early[5]	-	-	3%	6%
Preventive Care				
Immunization for Influenza[5]	-	-	89%	90%
Immunization for Pneumonia[5]	-	-	90%	92%
Stroke Care				
Anticoagulation Therapy for Atrial Fibrillation[1]	-	-	92%	95%
Antithrombotic Therapy Timing	12	100%	97%	98%
Assessed for Rehabilitation[1]	-	-	97%	97%
Discharged on Antithrombotic Therapy[1]	-	-	99%	99%
Discharged on Statin Medication[1]	-	-	94%	94%
Thrombolytic Therapy Timing[7]	-	-	69%	66%
Venous Thromboembolism Prophylaxis	11	100%	94%	94%
Written Stroke Educational Materials Given[1]	-	-	87%	88%
Surgical Care Improvement Project				
Appropriate Beta Blocker Usage[5]	-	-	98%	98%
Appropriate VTP Within 24 Hours[5]	-	-	98%	98%
Controlled Postoperative Blood Glucose[5]	-	-	97%	97%
Perioperative Temperature Management[5]	-	-	100%	100%
Prophylactic Antibiotic Selection[5]	-	-	99%	99%
Prophylactic Antibiotic Selection (Outpatient)[1,3]	-	-	97%	98%
Prophylactic Antibiotic Stopped[5]	-	-	98%	98%
Prophylactic Antibiotic Timing[5]	-	-	98%	99%
Prophylactic Antibiotic Timing (Outpatient)[1,3]	-	-	97%	98%
Urinary Catheter Removal[5]	-	-	97%	97%
Survey of Patients' Hospital Experiences				
Area Around Room 'Always' Quiet at Night	(a)	63%	60%	61%
Doctors 'Always' Communicated Well	(a)	78%	81%	82%
Home Recovery Information Given	(a)	92%	87%	85%
Hospital Given 9 or 10 on 10 Point Scale	(a)	67%	71%	71%
Meds 'Always' Explained Before Given	(a)	56%	64%	64%
Nurses 'Always' Communicated Well	(a)	79%	80%	79%
Pain 'Always' Well Controlled	(a)	73%	71%	71%
Room and Bathroom 'Always' Clean	(a)	80%	73%	73%
Timely Help 'Always' Received	(a)	74%	70%	68%
Would Definitely Recommend Hospital	(a)	66%	71%	71%
Use of Medical Imaging				

NOTE: Hospital profiles are in alphabetical order by state, then city, then hospital within the city; Rankings exclude hospitals with less than 25 cases except for patient surveys which excludes hospitals with less than 100 cases; (a) 100-299 cases; (1) The number of cases/patients is too few to report; (2) Data submitted were based on a sample of cases/patients; (3) Results are based on a shorter time period than required; (4) Data suppressed by CMS for one or more quarters; (5) Results are not available for this reporting period; (6) Fewer than 100 patients completed the HCAHPS survey; (7) No cases met the criteria for this measure; (8) The lower limit of the confidence interval cannot be calculated if the number of observed infections equals zero; (9) No data are available from the state/territory for this reporting period; (10) The scores shown reflect fewer than 50 completed surveys; (11) There were discrepancies in the data collection process; (12) This measure does not apply to this hospital for this reporting period; (13) Results cannot be calculated for this reporting period; (14) The results for this state are combined with nearby states to protect confidentiality; Please refer to the User's Guide for a full explanation of data.

Cardiac Imaging Stress Test before Surgery	129	3.9%	5.1%	5.3%
Combination Abdominal CT Scan	575	2.4%	8.7%	10.5%
Combination Brain/Sinus CT Scan	438	1.1%	2.2%	2.7%
Combination Chest CT Scan	359	1.7%	3.6%	2.7%
Follow-up Mammogram/Ultrasound	528	12.1%	8.2%	8.8%
Lumbar Spine MRI for Low Back Pain	100	59.0%	36.9%	37.2%

Crittenton Hospital Medical Center

1101 W University Drive
Rochester, MI 48307
URL: www.crittenton.com
Type: Acute Care Hospitals
Ownership: Voluntary non-profit - Private
Phone: 248-652-5000
Fax: 248-650-0353
Emergency Services: Yes
Beds: 290

Key Personnel:
Chairman/CEO .... Robert J. Lenihan, II
CEO/President............... Roy Powell
Chief of Medical Staff.......... Sheryl Wissman, MD

Measure	Cases	This Hosp.	State Avg.	U.S. Avg.
Blood Clot Prevention and Treatment				
Anticoagulation Overlap Therapy[2]	87	91%	90%	93%
ICU Venous Thromboembolism Prophylaxis[2]	79	99%	93%	92%
Incidence of Potentially Preventable VTE[2]	12	0%	8%	10%
UFH with Dosages/Platelet Monitoring[2]	88	100%	96%	97%
Venous Thromboembolism Prophylaxis[2]	309	92%	87%	85%
Warfarin Therapy Discharge Instructions[2]	60	80%	72%	75%
Chest Pain/Possible Heart Attack Care				
Aspirin Given Within 24 Hours of Arrival[1,3]	-	-	96%	96%
Fibrinolytic Meds Within 30 Min. of Arrival[5]	-	-	63%	58%
Average Time to ECG (minutes)[1,3]	-	-	8	7
Average Time to Transfer (minutes)[5]	-	-	53	60
Children's Asthma Care				
Received Home Management Plan of Care	-	-	-	88%
Received Reliever Medication	-	-	-	100%
Received Systemic Corticosteroids	-	-	-	100%
Emergency Department				
Admittance Decision Time (minutes)[2]	632	110	102	98
Head CT Results Within 45 Min. of Arrival[1]	-	-	54%	57%
Patients Who Left ER Before Being Seen	29,773	1%	2%	2%
Time from ER Arrival to Admit. (minutes)[2]	633	285	288	274
Time from ER Arrival to Discharge (minutes)	332	162	128	134
Time in ER Before Being Evaluated (minutes)	406	22	22	26
Time to Pain Meds for Fractures (minutes)	210	65	55	57
Heart Attack Care				
Aspirin Given at Discharge	123	100%	99%	99%
Fibrinolytic Meds Within 30 Min. of Arrival[7]	-	-	20%	54%
PCI Within 90 Minutes of Arrival	27	100%	95%	96%
Statin Prescribed at Discharge	114	99%	98%	98%
Heart Failure Care				
ACE Inhibitor or ARB for LVSD	92	100%	96%	97%
Discharge Instructions Given	214	100%	94%	94%
Evaluation of LVS Function	283	100%	99%	99%
Medicare Spending				
Medicare Spending per Patient (ratio)	-	1.04	0.96	0.98
Pneumonia Care				
Appropriate Initial Antibiotic Given	115	99%	96%	95%
Blood Culture Timing	243	100%	98%	98%
Pregnancy and Delivery Care				
Newborn Deliveries Scheduled Early	70	3%	3%	6%
Preventive Care				
Immunization for Influenza[2]	570	96%	89%	90%
Immunization for Pneumonia[2]	708	94%	90%	92%
Stroke Care				
Anticoagulation Therapy for Atrial Fibrillation	19	100%	92%	95%
Antithrombotic Therapy Timing	79	95%	97%	98%
Assessed for Rehabilitation	115	95%	97%	97%
Discharged on Antithrombotic Therapy	105	99%	99%	99%
Discharged on Statin Medication	80	95%	94%	94%
Thrombolytic Therapy Timing	15	100%	69%	66%
Venous Thromboembolism Prophylaxis	106	96%	94%	94%
Written Stroke Educational Materials Given	63	94%	87%	88%
Surgical Care Improvement Project				
Appropriate Beta Blocker Usage[2]	264	97%	98%	98%
Appropriate VTP Within 24 Hours[2]	608	99%	98%	98%
Controlled Postoperative Blood Glucose[2]	68	100%	97%	97%
Perioperative Temperature Management[2]	764	100%	100%	100%
Prophylactic Antibiotic Selection[2]	635	99%	99%	99%
Prophylactic Antibiotic Selection (Outpatient)	223	99%	97%	98%
Prophylactic Antibiotic Stopped[2]	611	98%	98%	98%
Prophylactic Antibiotic Timing[2]	635	98%	98%	99%
Prophylactic Antibiotic Timing (Outpatient)	223	99%	97%	98%
Urinary Catheter Removal[2]	206	100%	97%	97%
Survey of Patients' Hospital Experiences				
Area Around Room 'Always' Quiet at Night[11]	300+	57%	60%	61%
Doctors 'Always' Communicated Well[11]	300+	78%	81%	82%
Home Recovery Information Given[11]	300+	85%	87%	85%
Hospital Given 9 or 10 on 10 Point Scale[11]	300+	69%	71%	71%
Meds 'Always' Explained Before Given[11]	300+	58%	64%	64%
Nurses 'Always' Communicated Well[11]	300+	77%	80%	79%
Pain 'Always' Well Controlled[11]	300+	69%	71%	71%
Room and Bathroom 'Always' Clean[11]	300+	68%	73%	73%
Timely Help 'Always' Received[11]	300+	64%	70%	68%
Would Definitely Recommend Hospital[11]	300+	68%	71%	71%
Use of Medical Imaging				
Cardiac Imaging Stress Test before Surgery	245	6.9%	5.1%	5.3%
Combination Abdominal CT Scan	726	14.6%	8.7%	10.5%
Combination Brain/Sinus CT Scan	484	1.7%	2.2%	2.7%
Combination Chest CT Scan	569	0.9%	3.6%	2.7%
Follow-up Mammogram/Ultrasound	1,764	9.1%	8.2%	8.8%
Lumbar Spine MRI for Low Back Pain[1]	-	-	36.9%	37.2%

Beaumont Health System

3601 W Thirteen Mile Rd
Royal Oak, MI 48073
URL: www.beaumonthospitals.com
Type: Acute Care Hospitals
Ownership: Proprietary
Phone: 248-898-5000
Fax: 248-551-0854
Emergency Services: Yes
Beds: 1,061

Key Personnel:
Infection Control.............. Jeffrey Bond, MD
Quality Assurance .... Edward R Grima
Chair/CEO...................... Stephen R. Howard
Chief of Medical Staff.......... Ronald B Irwin, MD
Anesthesiology................ N Sean O'Hanian, MD
CEO/President................ Ted Wasson
Emergency Room .... Andrew Wilson, MD

Measure	Cases	This Hosp.	State Avg.	U.S. Avg.
Blood Clot Prevention and Treatment				
Anticoagulation Overlap Therapy[2]	336	100%	90%	93%
ICU Venous Thromboembolism Prophylaxis[2]	47	94%	93%	92%
Incidence of Potentially Preventable VTE[2]	127	5%	8%	10%
UFH with Dosages/Platelet Monitoring[2]	407	100%	96%	97%
Venous Thromboembolism Prophylaxis[2]	383	89%	87%	85%
Warfarin Therapy Discharge Instructions[2]	219	95%	72%	75%
Chest Pain/Possible Heart Attack Care				
Aspirin Given Within 24 Hours of Arrival[1,3]	-	-	96%	96%
Fibrinolytic Meds Within 30 Min. of Arrival[5]	-	-	63%	58%
Average Time to ECG (minutes)[1,3]	-	-	8	7
Average Time to Transfer (minutes)[5]	-	-	53	60
Children's Asthma Care				
Received Home Management Plan of Care	-	-	-	88%
Received Reliever Medication	-	-	-	100%
Received Systemic Corticosteroids	-	-	-	100%
Emergency Department				
Admittance Decision Time (minutes)[2]	576	80	102	98
Head CT Results Within 45 Min. of Arrival[1]	-	-	54%	57%
Patients Who Left ER Before Being Seen	>100k	1%	2%	2%
Time from ER Arrival to Admit. (minutes)[2]	577	318	288	274
Time from ER Arrival to Discharge (minutes)	325	182	128	134
Time in ER Before Being Evaluated (minutes)	308	28	22	26
Time to Pain Meds for Fractures (minutes)	182	67	55	57
Heart Attack Care				
Aspirin Given at Discharge	850	100%	99%	99%
Fibrinolytic Meds Within 30 Min. of Arrival[7]	-	-	20%	54%
PCI Within 90 Minutes of Arrival	85	99%	95%	96%
Statin Prescribed at Discharge	806	100%	98%	98%
Heart Failure Care				
ACE Inhibitor or ARB for LVSD	418	100%	96%	97%
Discharge Instructions Given	1,160	100%	94%	94%
Evaluation of LVS Function	1,402	100%	99%	99%
Medicare Spending				
Medicare Spending per Patient (ratio)	-	1.02	0.96	0.98
Pneumonia Care				
Appropriate Initial Antibiotic Given[2]	88	99%	96%	95%
Blood Culture Timing[2]	122	98%	98%	98%
Pregnancy and Delivery Care				
Newborn Deliveries Scheduled Early[2]	51	4%	3%	6%
Preventive Care				
Immunization for Influenza[2]	578	95%	89%	90%
Immunization for Pneumonia[2]	794	93%	90%	92%
Stroke Care				
Anticoagulation Therapy for Atrial Fibrillation[2]	42	100%	92%	95%
Antithrombotic Therapy Timing[2]	292	98%	97%	98%
Assessed for Rehabilitation[2]	370	100%	97%	97%
Discharged on Antithrombotic Therapy[2]	303	100%	99%	99%
Discharged on Statin Medication[2]	237	100%	94%	94%
Thrombolytic Therapy Timing[1,2]	-	-	69%	66%
Venous Thromboembolism Prophylaxis[2]	391	99%	94%	94%
Written Stroke Educational Materials Given[2]	207	93%	87%	88%
Surgical Care Improvement Project				
Appropriate Beta Blocker Usage[2]	303	99%	98%	98%
Appropriate VTP Within 24 Hours[2]	554	99%	98%	98%
Controlled Postoperative Blood Glucose[2]	133	98%	97%	97%
Perioperative Temperature Management[2]	703	100%	100%	100%
Prophylactic Antibiotic Selection[2]	554	99%	99%	99%
Prophylactic Antibiotic Selection (Outpatient)	671	98%	97%	98%
Prophylactic Antibiotic Stopped[2]	539	100%	98%	98%
Prophylactic Antibiotic Timing[2]	554	99%	98%	99%
Prophylactic Antibiotic Timing (Outpatient)	634	98%	97%	98%
Urinary Catheter Removal[2]	475	100%	97%	97%
Survey of Patients' Hospital Experiences				
Area Around Room 'Always' Quiet at Night	300+	50%	60%	61%
Doctors 'Always' Communicated Well	300+	78%	81%	82%
Home Recovery Information Given	300+	86%	87%	85%
Hospital Given 9 or 10 on 10 Point Scale	300+	73%	71%	71%
Meds 'Always' Explained Before Given	300+	59%	64%	64%
Nurses 'Always' Communicated Well	300+	76%	80%	79%
Pain 'Always' Well Controlled	300+	67%	71%	71%
Room and Bathroom 'Always' Clean	300+	67%	73%	73%
Timely Help 'Always' Received	300+	61%	70%	68%
Would Definitely Recommend Hospital	300+	77%	71%	71%
Use of Medical Imaging				
Cardiac Imaging Stress Test before Surgery	4,313	5.1%	5.1%	5.3%
Combination Abdominal CT Scan	3,712	4.9%	8.7%	10.5%
Combination Brain/Sinus CT Scan	1,806	1.3%	2.2%	2.7%
Combination Chest CT Scan	3,884	2.2%	3.6%	2.7%
Follow-up Mammogram/Ultrasound	8,670	15.7%	8.2%	8.8%
Lumbar Spine MRI for Low Back Pain	456	32.2%	36.9%	37.2%

Covenant Medical Center

1447 N Harrison
Saginaw, MI 48602
URL: www.covenanthealthcare.com
Type: Acute Care Hospitals
Ownership: Voluntary non-profit - Other
Phone: 989-583-4000
Fax: 989-583-6457
Emergency Services: Yes
Beds: 601

Key Personnel:
Operating Room.............. John Germain
Chief of Medical Staff.......... John Kasanovich, MD
Radiology.................... Ginny Latty
CEO/President................ Spencer T Maidlow
Quality Assurance .... Sue Paterson
Intensive Care Unit............ Jan Penney, RN
Emergency Room .... Joesph C Spadafore, MD
Patient Relations .... Alison Van Norman

Measure	Cases	This Hosp.	State Avg.	U.S. Avg.
Blood Clot Prevention and Treatment				
Anticoagulation Overlap Therapy[2]	192	93%	90%	93%
ICU Venous Thromboembolism Prophylaxis[2]	115	95%	93%	92%
Incidence of Potentially Preventable VTE[2]	32	3%	8%	10%
UFH with Dosages/Platelet Monitoring[2]	174	38%	96%	97%
Venous Thromboembolism Prophylaxis[2]	330	95%	87%	85%
Warfarin Therapy Discharge Instructions[2]	141	57%	72%	75%
Chest Pain/Possible Heart Attack Care				

NOTE: Hospital profiles are in alphabetical order by state, then city, then hospital within the city; Rankings exclude hospitals with less than 25 cases except for patient surveys which excludes hospitals with less than 100 cases; (a) 100-299 cases; (1) The number of cases/patients is too few to report; (2) Data submitted were based on a sample of cases/patients; (3) Results are based on a shorter time period than required; (4) Data suppressed by CMS for one or more quarters; (5) Results are not available for this reporting period; (6) Fewer than 100 patients completed the HCAHPS survey; (7) No cases met the criteria for this measure; (8) The lower limit of the confidence interval cannot be calculated if the number of observed infections equals zero; (9) No data are available from the state/territory for this reporting period; (10) The scores shown reflect fewer than 50 completed surveys; (11) There were discrepancies in the data collection process; (12) This measure does not apply to this hospital for this reporting period; (13) Results cannot be calculated for this reporting period; (14) The results for this state are combined with nearby states to protect confidentiality; Please refer to the User's Guide for a full explanation of data.

Aspirin Given Within 24 Hours of Arrival	11	100%	96%	96%
Fibrinolytic Meds Within 30 Min. of Arrival[5]	-	-	63%	58%
Average Time to ECG (minutes)	11	30	8	7
Average Time to Transfer (minutes)[5]	-	-	53	60
Children's Asthma Care				
Received Home Management Plan of Care	-	-	-	88%
Received Reliever Medication	-	-	-	100%
Received Systemic Corticosteroids	-	-	-	100%
Emergency Department				
Admittance Decision Time (minutes)[2]	766	118	102	98
Head CT Results Within 45 Min. of Arrival[1]	-	-	54%	57%
Patients Who Left ER Before Being Seen	88,793	0%	2%	2%
Time from ER Arrival to Admit. (minutes)[2]	767	238	288	274
Time from ER Arrival to Discharge (minutes)	419	168	128	134
Time in ER Before Being Evaluated (minutes)	443	15	22	26
Time to Pain Meds for Fractures (minutes)	220	56	55	57
Heart Attack Care				
Aspirin Given at Discharge	509	100%	99%	99%
Fibrinolytic Meds Within 30 Min. of Arrival[7]	-	-	20%	54%
PCI Within 90 Minutes of Arrival	57	95%	95%	96%
Statin Prescribed at Discharge	493	99%	98%	98%
Heart Failure Care				
ACE Inhibitor or ARB for LVSD	154	98%	96%	97%
Discharge Instructions Given	512	88%	94%	94%
Evaluation of LVS Function	625	100%	99%	99%
Medicare Spending				
Medicare Spending per Patient (ratio)	-	0.98	0.96	0.98
Pneumonia Care				
Appropriate Initial Antibiotic Given	253	96%	96%	95%
Blood Culture Timing	571	98%	98%	98%
Pregnancy and Delivery Care				
Newborn Deliveries Scheduled Early	367	4%	3%	6%
Preventive Care				
Immunization for Influenza[2]	524	97%	89%	90%
Immunization for Pneumonia[2]	689	97%	90%	92%
Stroke Care				
Anticoagulation Therapy for Atrial Fibrillation	25	100%	92%	95%
Antithrombotic Therapy Timing	218	100%	97%	98%
Assessed for Rehabilitation	270	99%	97%	97%
Discharged on Antithrombotic Therapy	226	100%	99%	99%
Discharged on Statin Medication	171	94%	94%	94%
Thrombolytic Therapy Timing	17	76%	69%	66%
Venous Thromboembolism Prophylaxis	281	97%	94%	94%
Written Stroke Educational Materials Given	121	100%	87%	88%
Surgical Care Improvement Project				
Appropriate Beta Blocker Usage[2]	640	98%	98%	98%
Appropriate VTP Within 24 Hours[2]	1,483	99%	98%	98%
Controlled Postoperative Blood Glucose[2]	153	97%	97%	97%
Perioperative Temperature Management[2]	1,677	99%	100%	100%
Prophylactic Antibiotic Selection[2]	1,190	100%	99%	99%
Prophylactic Antibiotic Selection (Outpatient)	781	97%	97%	98%
Prophylactic Antibiotic Stopped[2]	878	98%	98%	98%
Prophylactic Antibiotic Timing[2]	1,193	98%	98%	99%
Prophylactic Antibiotic Timing (Outpatient)	756	96%	97%	98%
Urinary Catheter Removal[2]	529	99%	97%	97%
Survey of Patients' Hospital Experiences				
Area Around Room 'Always' Quiet at Night	300+	48%	60%	61%
Doctors 'Always' Communicated Well	300+	79%	81%	82%
Home Recovery Information Given	300+	86%	87%	85%
Hospital Given 9 or 10 on 10 Point Scale	300+	69%	71%	71%
Meds 'Always' Explained Before Given	300+	60%	64%	64%
Nurses 'Always' Communicated Well	300+	81%	80%	79%
Pain 'Always' Well Controlled	300+	71%	71%	71%
Room and Bathroom 'Always' Clean	300+	66%	73%	73%
Timely Help 'Always' Received	300+	65%	70%	68%
Would Definitely Recommend Hospital	300+	76%	71%	71%
Use of Medical Imaging				
Cardiac Imaging Stress Test before Surgery	722	5.3%	5.1%	5.3%
Combination Abdominal CT Scan	1,524	14.2%	8.7%	10.5%
Combination Brain/Sinus CT Scan	1,126	1.7%	2.2%	2.7%
Combination Chest CT Scan	876	9.7%	3.6%	2.7%
Follow-up Mammogram/Ultrasound	3,726	6.3%	8.2%	8.8%
Lumbar Spine MRI for Low Back Pain	377	40.8%	36.9%	37.2%

Healthsource Saginaw

3340 Hospital Road
Saginaw, MI 48608
Type: Acute Care Hospitals
Ownership: Voluntary non-profit - Other
Phone: 989-790-7888
Fax: 989-790-9297
Emergency Services: Yes
Beds: 317

Key Personnel:
Infection Control. . . . . Sherry Baker
Quality Assurance . . . . Rich Firebaugh
CEO/President. . . . . Lester Heybor Jr
Chief of Medical Staff . . . . D Kuligowsky, MD

Measure	Cases	This Hosp.	State Avg.	U.S. Avg.
Blood Clot Prevention and Treatment				
Anticoagulation Overlap Therapy[2,7]	-	-	90%	93%
ICU Venous Thromboembolism Prophylaxis[2,7]	-	-	93%	92%
Incidence of Potentially Preventable VTE[2,7]	-	-	8%	10%
UFH with Dosages/Platelet Monitoring[2,7]	-	-	96%	97%
Venous Thromboembolism Prophylaxis[2,7]	-	-	87%	85%
Warfarin Therapy Discharge Instructions[2,7]	-	-	72%	75%
Chest Pain/Possible Heart Attack Care				
Aspirin Given Within 24 Hours of Arrival[5]	-	-	96%	96%
Fibrinolytic Meds Within 30 Min. of Arrival[5]	-	-	63%	58%
Average Time to ECG (minutes)[5]	-	-	8	7
Average Time to Transfer (minutes)[5]	-	-	53	60
Children's Asthma Care				
Received Home Management Plan of Care	-	-	-	88%
Received Reliever Medication	-	-	-	100%
Received Systemic Corticosteroids	-	-	-	100%
Emergency Department				
Admittance Decision Time (minutes)[2,7]	-	-	102	98
Head CT Results Within 45 Min. of Arrival[5]	-	-	54%	57%
Patients Who Left ER Before Being Seen[5]	-	-	2%	2%
Time from ER Arrival to Admit. (minutes)[2,7]	-	-	288	274
Time from ER Arrival to Discharge (minutes)[5]	-	-	128	134
Time in ER Before Being Evaluated (minutes)[5]	-	-	22	26
Time to Pain Meds for Fractures (minutes)[5]	-	-	55	57
Heart Attack Care				
Aspirin Given at Discharge[5]	-	-	99%	99%
Fibrinolytic Meds Within 30 Min. of Arrival[5]	-	-	20%	54%
PCI Within 90 Minutes of Arrival[5]	-	-	95%	96%
Statin Prescribed at Discharge[5]	-	-	98%	98%
Heart Failure Care				
ACE Inhibitor or ARB for LVSD[5]	-	-	96%	97%
Discharge Instructions Given[5]	-	-	94%	94%
Evaluation of LVS Function[5]	-	-	99%	99%
Medicare Spending				
Medicare Spending per Patient (ratio)	-	0.91	0.96	0.98
Pneumonia Care				
Appropriate Initial Antibiotic Given[5]	-	-	96%	95%
Blood Culture Timing[5]	-	-	98%	98%
Pregnancy and Delivery Care				
Newborn Deliveries Scheduled Early[7]	-	-	3%	6%
Preventive Care				
Immunization for Influenza[2]	191	82%	89%	90%
Immunization for Pneumonia[2]	15	27%	90%	92%
Stroke Care				
Anticoagulation Therapy for Atrial Fibrillation[5]	-	-	92%	95%
Antithrombotic Therapy Timing[5]	-	-	97%	98%
Assessed for Rehabilitation[5]	-	-	97%	97%
Discharged on Antithrombotic Therapy[5]	-	-	99%	99%
Discharged on Statin Medication[5]	-	-	94%	94%
Thrombolytic Therapy Timing[5]	-	-	69%	66%
Venous Thromboembolism Prophylaxis[5]	-	-	94%	94%
Written Stroke Educational Materials Given[5]	-	-	87%	88%
Surgical Care Improvement Project				
Appropriate Beta Blocker Usage[5]	-	-	98%	98%
Appropriate VTP Within 24 Hours[5]	-	-	98%	98%
Controlled Postoperative Blood Glucose[5]	-	-	97%	97%
Perioperative Temperature Management[5]	-	-	100%	100%
Prophylactic Antibiotic Selection[5]	-	-	99%	99%
Prophylactic Antibiotic Selection (Outpatient)[5]	-	-	97%	98%
Prophylactic Antibiotic Stopped[5]	-	-	98%	98%
Prophylactic Antibiotic Timing[5]	-	-	98%	99%
Prophylactic Antibiotic Timing (Outpatient)[5]	-	-	97%	98%
Urinary Catheter Removal[5]	-	-	97%	97%
Survey of Patients' Hospital Experiences				
Area Around Room 'Always' Quiet at Night[1]	-	-	60%	61%
Doctors 'Always' Communicated Well[1]	-	-	81%	82%
Home Recovery Information Given[1]	-	-	87%	85%
Hospital Given 9 or 10 on 10 Point Scale[1]	-	-	71%	71%
Meds 'Always' Explained Before Given[1]	-	-	64%	64%
Nurses 'Always' Communicated Well[1]	-	-	80%	79%
Pain 'Always' Well Controlled[1]	-	-	71%	71%
Room and Bathroom 'Always' Clean[1]	-	-	73%	73%
Timely Help 'Always' Received[1]	-	-	70%	68%
Would Definitely Recommend Hospital[1]	-	-	71%	71%
Use of Medical Imaging				
Cardiac Imaging Stress Test before Surgery[7]	-	-	5.1%	5.3%
Combination Abdominal CT Scan[7]	-	-	8.7%	10.5%
Combination Brain/Sinus CT Scan[7]	-	-	2.2%	2.7%
Combination Chest CT Scan[7]	-	-	3.6%	2.7%
Follow-up Mammogram/Ultrasound[7]	-	-	8.2%	8.8%
Lumbar Spine MRI for Low Back Pain[7]	-	-	36.9%	37.2%

Saginaw VA Medical Center

1500 Weiss Street
Saginaw, MI 48602
Type: Acute Care - VA
Ownership: Government Federal
Phone: 989-497-2500
Fax: 989-791-2217
Emergency Services: No
Beds: 238

Key Personnel:
Chief of Medical Staff . . . . Menham Lender, MD

Measure	Cases	This Hosp.	State Avg.	U.S. Avg.
Blood Clot Prevention and Treatment				
Anticoagulation Overlap Therapy	-	-	90%	93%
ICU Venous Thromboembolism Prophylaxis	-	-	93%	92%
Incidence of Potentially Preventable VTE	-	-	8%	10%
UFH with Dosages/Platelet Monitoring	-	-	96%	97%
Venous Thromboembolism Prophylaxis	-	-	87%	85%
Warfarin Therapy Discharge Instructions	-	-	72%	75%
Chest Pain/Possible Heart Attack Care				
Aspirin Given Within 24 Hours of Arrival	-	-	96%	96%
Fibrinolytic Meds Within 30 Min. of Arrival	-	-	63%	58%
Average Time to ECG (minutes)	-	-	8	7
Average Time to Transfer (minutes)	-	-	53	60
Children's Asthma Care				
Received Home Management Plan of Care	-	-	-	88%
Received Reliever Medication	-	-	-	100%
Received Systemic Corticosteroids	-	-	-	100%
Emergency Department				
Admittance Decision Time (minutes)	-	-	102	98
Head CT Results Within 45 Min. of Arrival	-	-	54%	57%
Patients Who Left ER Before Being Seen	-	-	2%	2%
Time from ER Arrival to Admit. (minutes)	-	-	288	274
Time from ER Arrival to Discharge (minutes)	-	-	128	134
Time in ER Before Being Evaluated (minutes)	-	-	22	26
Time to Pain Meds for Fractures (minutes)	-	-	55	57
Heart Attack Care				
Aspirin Given at Discharge[5]	-	-	99%	99%
Fibrinolytic Meds Within 30 Min. of Arrival[5]	-	-	20%	54%
PCI Within 90 Minutes of Arrival[5]	-	-	95%	96%
Statin Prescribed at Discharge[5]	-	-	98%	98%
Heart Failure Care				
ACE Inhibitor or ARB for LVSD[1]	-	-	96%	97%
Discharge Instructions Given[1]	15	100%	94%	94%
Evaluation of LVS Function[1]	23	100%	99%	99%
Medicare Spending				
Medicare Spending per Patient (ratio)	-	-	0.96	0.98
Pneumonia Care				
Appropriate Initial Antibiotic Given[1]	17	100%	96%	95%
Blood Culture Timing[5]	-	-	98%	98%
Pregnancy and Delivery Care				
Newborn Deliveries Scheduled Early	-	-	3%	6%
Preventive Care				
Immunization for Influenza[2,3]	133	87%	89%	90%
Immunization for Pneumonia[2,3]	281	98%	90%	92%

NOTE: Hospital profiles are in alphabetical order by state, then city, then hospital within the city; Rankings exclude hospitals with less than 25 cases except for patient surveys which excludes hospitals with less than 100 cases; (a) 100-299 cases; (1) The number of cases/patients is too few to report; (2) Data submitted were based on a sample of cases/patients; (3) Results are based on a shorter time period than required; (4) Data suppressed by CMS for one or more quarters; (5) Results are not available for this reporting period; (6) Fewer than 100 patients completed the HCAHPS survey; (7) No cases met the criteria for this measure; (8) The lower limit of the confidence interval cannot be calculated if the number of observed infections equals zero; (9) No data are available from the state/territory for this reporting period; (10) The scores shown reflect fewer than 50 completed surveys; (11) There were discrepancies in the data collection process; (12) This measure does not apply to this hospital for this reporting period; (13) Results cannot be calculated for this reporting period; (14) The results for this state are combined with nearby states to protect confidentiality; Please refer to the User's Guide for a full explanation of data.

Measure	Cases	This Hosp.	State Avg.	U.S. Avg.
Stroke Care				
Anticoagulation Therapy for Atrial Fibrillation	-	-	92%	95%
Antithrombotic Therapy Timing	-	-	97%	98%
Assessed for Rehabilitation	-	-	97%	97%
Discharged on Antithrombotic Therapy	-	-	99%	99%
Discharged on Statin Medication	-	-	94%	94%
Thrombolytic Therapy Timing	-	-	69%	66%
Venous Thromboembolism Prophylaxis	-	-	94%	94%
Written Stroke Educational Materials Given	-	-	87%	88%
Surgical Care Improvement Project				
Appropriate Beta Blocker Usage[5]	-	-	98%	98%
Appropriate VTP Within 24 Hours[5]	-	-	98%	98%
Controlled Postoperative Blood Glucose[5]	-	-	97%	97%
Perioperative Temperature Management[5]	-	-	100%	100%
Prophylactic Antibiotic Selection[5]	-	-	99%	99%
Prophylactic Antibiotic Selection (Outpatient)	-	-	97%	98%
Prophylactic Antibiotic Stopped[5]	-	-	98%	98%
Prophylactic Antibiotic Timing[5]	-	-	98%	99%
Prophylactic Antibiotic Timing (Outpatient)	-	-	97%	98%
Urinary Catheter Removal[5]	-	-	97%	97%
Survey of Patients' Hospital Experiences				
Area Around Room 'Always' Quiet at Night	-	-	60%	61%
Doctors 'Always' Communicated Well	-	-	81%	82%
Home Recovery Information Given	-	-	87%	85%
Hospital Given 9 or 10 on 10 Point Scale	-	-	71%	71%
Meds 'Always' Explained Before Given	-	-	64%	64%
Nurses 'Always' Communicated Well	-	-	80%	79%
Pain 'Always' Well Controlled	-	-	71%	71%
Room and Bathroom 'Always' Clean	-	-	73%	73%
Timely Help 'Always' Received	-	-	70%	68%
Would Definitely Recommend Hospital	-	-	71%	71%
Use of Medical Imaging				
Cardiac Imaging Stress Test before Surgery	-	-	5.1%	5.3%
Combination Abdominal CT Scan	-	-	8.7%	10.5%
Combination Brain/Sinus CT Scan	-	-	2.2%	2.7%
Combination Chest CT Scan	-	-	3.6%	2.7%
Follow-up Mammogram/Ultrasound	-	-	8.2%	8.8%
Lumbar Spine MRI for Low Back Pain	-	-	36.9%	37.2%

Saint Mary's of Michigan Medical Center

800 S Washington Avenue
Saginaw, MI 48601
URL: www.stmarysofmichigan.org
Type: Acute Care Hospitals
Ownership: Voluntary non-profit - Church
Phone: 989-776-8000
Fax: 989-907-8141
Emergency Services: Yes
Beds: 268

Key Personnel:
Emergency Room . . . . Louise Beyerlein
CEO/President. . . . . John Graham
Chief of Medical Staff . . . . Baghuram Sarvepalli, MD
Radiology. . . . . Gary Stefanko
Quality Assurance . . . . Mary Storm

Measure	Cases	This Hosp.	State Avg.	U.S. Avg.
Blood Clot Prevention and Treatment				
Anticoagulation Overlap Therapy[2]	104	66%	90%	93%
ICU Venous Thromboembolism Prophylaxis[2]	136	94%	93%	92%
Incidence of Potentially Preventable VTE[2]	24	8%	8%	10%
UFH with Dosages/Platelet Monitoring[2]	103	99%	96%	97%
Venous Thromboembolism Prophylaxis[2]	315	79%	87%	85%
Warfarin Therapy Discharge Instructions[2]	75	32%	72%	75%
Chest Pain/Possible Heart Attack Care				
Aspirin Given Within 24 Hours of Arrival[1]	-	-	96%	96%
Fibrinolytic Meds Within 30 Min. of Arrival[5]	-	-	63%	58%
Average Time to ECG (minutes)	11	23	8	7
Average Time to Transfer (minutes)[5]	-	-	53	60
Children's Asthma Care				
Received Home Management Plan of Care	-	-	-	88%
Received Reliever Medication	-	-	-	100%
Received Systemic Corticosteroids	-	-	-	100%
Emergency Department				
Admittance Decision Time (minutes)[2]	523	124	102	98
Head CT Results Within 45 Min. of Arrival[1,3]	-	-	54%	57%
Patients Who Left ER Before Being Seen	53,811	2%	2%	2%
Time from ER Arrival to Admit. (minutes)[2]	563	305	288	274
Time from ER Arrival to Discharge (minutes)	369	128	128	134
Time in ER Before Being Evaluated (minutes)	371	38	22	26
Time to Pain Meds for Fractures (minutes)	122	47	55	57
Heart Attack Care				
Aspirin Given at Discharge[2]	290	99%	99%	99%
Fibrinolytic Meds Within 30 Min. of Arrival[2,7]	-	-	20%	54%
PCI Within 90 Minutes of Arrival[2]	25	72%	95%	96%
Statin Prescribed at Discharge[2]	287	97%	98%	98%
Heart Failure Care				
ACE Inhibitor or ARB for LVSD[2]	92	91%	96%	97%
Discharge Instructions Given[2]	242	81%	94%	94%
Evaluation of LVS Function[2]	292	100%	99%	99%
Medicare Spending				
Medicare Spending per Patient (ratio)	-	1.00	0.96	0.98
Pneumonia Care				
Appropriate Initial Antibiotic Given[2]	45	100%	96%	95%
Blood Culture Timing[2]	141	94%	98%	98%
Pregnancy and Delivery Care				
Newborn Deliveries Scheduled Early[7]	-	-	3%	6%
Preventive Care				
Immunization for Influenza[2]	614	93%	89%	90%
Immunization for Pneumonia[2]	881	85%	90%	92%
Stroke Care				
Anticoagulation Therapy for Atrial Fibrillation[2]	15	93%	92%	95%
Antithrombotic Therapy Timing[2]	69	96%	97%	98%
Assessed for Rehabilitation[2]	103	96%	97%	97%
Discharged on Antithrombotic Therapy[2]	79	99%	99%	99%
Discharged on Statin Medication[2]	67	90%	94%	94%
Thrombolytic Therapy Timing[1,2]	-	-	69%	66%
Venous Thromboembolism Prophylaxis[2]	112	95%	94%	94%
Written Stroke Educational Materials Given[2]	58	91%	87%	88%
Surgical Care Improvement Project				
Appropriate Beta Blocker Usage[2]	216	99%	98%	98%
Appropriate VTP Within 24 Hours[2]	374	97%	98%	98%
Controlled Postoperative Blood Glucose[2]	130	94%	97%	97%
Perioperative Temperature Management[2]	500	98%	100%	100%
Prophylactic Antibiotic Selection[2]	387	99%	99%	99%
Prophylactic Antibiotic Selection (Outpatient)	369	99%	97%	98%
Prophylactic Antibiotic Stopped[2]	365	95%	98%	98%
Prophylactic Antibiotic Timing[2]	388	99%	98%	99%
Prophylactic Antibiotic Timing (Outpatient)	369	100%	97%	98%
Urinary Catheter Removal[2]	287	87%	97%	97%
Survey of Patients' Hospital Experiences				
Area Around Room 'Always' Quiet at Night	300+	47%	60%	61%
Doctors 'Always' Communicated Well	300+	77%	81%	82%
Home Recovery Information Given	300+	86%	87%	85%
Hospital Given 9 or 10 on 10 Point Scale	300+	63%	71%	71%
Meds 'Always' Explained Before Given	300+	54%	64%	64%
Nurses 'Always' Communicated Well	300+	74%	80%	79%
Pain 'Always' Well Controlled	300+	61%	71%	71%
Room and Bathroom 'Always' Clean	300+	60%	73%	73%
Timely Help 'Always' Received	300+	61%	70%	68%
Would Definitely Recommend Hospital	300+	68%	71%	71%
Use of Medical Imaging				
Cardiac Imaging Stress Test before Surgery	1,665	4.9%	5.1%	5.3%
Combination Abdominal CT Scan	1,038	15.4%	8.7%	10.5%
Combination Brain/Sinus CT Scan	1,026	3.8%	2.2%	2.7%
Combination Chest CT Scan	759	23.8%	3.6%	2.7%
Follow-up Mammogram/Ultrasound	1,544	7.6%	8.2%	8.8%
Lumbar Spine MRI for Low Back Pain	419	35.3%	36.9%	37.2%

Mackinac Straits Hospital & Health Center

1140 N State Street
Saint Ignace, MI 49781
URL: www.mackinacstraitshealth.org
Type: Critical Access Hospitals
Ownership: Voluntary non-profit - Private
Phone: 906-643-8585
Emergency Services: Yes

Measure	Cases	This Hosp.	State Avg.	U.S. Avg.
Blood Clot Prevention and Treatment				
Anticoagulation Overlap Therapy[5]	-	-	90%	93%
ICU Venous Thromboembolism Prophylaxis[5]	-	-	93%	92%
Incidence of Potentially Preventable VTE[5]	-	-	8%	10%
UFH with Dosages/Platelet Monitoring[5]	-	-	96%	97%
Venous Thromboembolism Prophylaxis[5]	-	-	87%	85%
Warfarin Therapy Discharge Instructions[5]	-	-	72%	75%
Chest Pain/Possible Heart Attack Care				
Aspirin Given Within 24 Hours of Arrival[3]	12	92%	96%	96%
Fibrinolytic Meds Within 30 Min. of Arrival[3,7]	-	-	63%	58%
Average Time to ECG (minutes)[3]	13	7	8	7
Average Time to Transfer (minutes)[1,3]	-	-	53	60
Children's Asthma Care				
Received Home Management Plan of Care	-	-	-	88%
Received Reliever Medication	-	-	-	100%
Received Systemic Corticosteroids	-	-	-	100%
Emergency Department				
Admittance Decision Time (minutes)[5]	-	-	102	98
Head CT Results Within 45 Min. of Arrival[5]	-	-	54%	57%
Patients Who Left ER Before Being Seen	5,631	0%	2%	2%
Time from ER Arrival to Admit. (minutes)[5]	-	-	288	274
Time from ER Arrival to Discharge (minutes)	1,222	100	128	134
Time in ER Before Being Evaluated (minutes)	1,354	16	22	26
Time to Pain Meds for Fractures (minutes)[5]	-	-	55	57
Heart Attack Care				
Aspirin Given at Discharge[5]	-	-	99%	99%
Fibrinolytic Meds Within 30 Min. of Arrival[5]	-	-	20%	54%
PCI Within 90 Minutes of Arrival[5]	-	-	95%	96%
Statin Prescribed at Discharge[5]	-	-	98%	98%
Heart Failure Care				
ACE Inhibitor or ARB for LVSD[1,3]	-	-	96%	97%
Discharge Instructions Given[1,3]	-	-	94%	94%
Evaluation of LVS Function[1,3]	-	-	99%	99%
Medicare Spending				
Medicare Spending per Patient (ratio)	-	-	0.96	0.98
Pneumonia Care				
Appropriate Initial Antibiotic Given[1]	-	-	96%	95%
Blood Culture Timing	16	100%	98%	98%
Pregnancy and Delivery Care				
Newborn Deliveries Scheduled Early[5]	-	-	3%	6%
Preventive Care				
Immunization for Influenza[5]	-	-	89%	90%
Immunization for Pneumonia[5]	-	-	90%	92%
Stroke Care				
Anticoagulation Therapy for Atrial Fibrillation[5]	-	-	92%	95%
Antithrombotic Therapy Timing[5]	-	-	97%	98%
Assessed for Rehabilitation[5]	-	-	97%	97%
Discharged on Antithrombotic Therapy[5]	-	-	99%	99%
Discharged on Statin Medication[5]	-	-	94%	94%
Thrombolytic Therapy Timing[5]	-	-	69%	66%
Venous Thromboembolism Prophylaxis[5]	-	-	94%	94%
Written Stroke Educational Materials Given[5]	-	-	87%	88%
Surgical Care Improvement Project				
Appropriate Beta Blocker Usage[5]	-	-	98%	98%
Appropriate VTP Within 24 Hours[5]	-	-	98%	98%
Controlled Postoperative Blood Glucose[5]	-	-	97%	97%
Perioperative Temperature Management[5]	-	-	100%	100%
Prophylactic Antibiotic Selection[5]	-	-	99%	99%
Prophylactic Antibiotic Selection (Outpatient)[5]	-	-	97%	98%
Prophylactic Antibiotic Stopped[5]	-	-	98%	98%
Prophylactic Antibiotic Timing[5]	-	-	98%	99%
Prophylactic Antibiotic Timing (Outpatient)[5]	-	-	97%	98%
Urinary Catheter Removal[5]	-	-	97%	97%
Survey of Patients' Hospital Experiences				
Area Around Room 'Always' Quiet at Night	(a)	70%	60%	61%
Doctors 'Always' Communicated Well	(a)	83%	81%	82%
Home Recovery Information Given	(a)	92%	87%	85%
Hospital Given 9 or 10 on 10 Point Scale	(a)	78%	71%	71%
Meds 'Always' Explained Before Given	(a)	80%	64%	64%
Nurses 'Always' Communicated Well	(a)	85%	80%	79%
Pain 'Always' Well Controlled	(a)	76%	71%	71%
Room and Bathroom 'Always' Clean	(a)	85%	73%	73%
Timely Help 'Always' Received	(a)	75%	70%	68%
Would Definitely Recommend Hospital	(a)	85%	71%	71%
Use of Medical Imaging				
Cardiac Imaging Stress Test before Surgery[1]	-	-	5.1%	5.3%

NOTE: Hospital profiles are in alphabetical order by state, then city, then hospital within the city; Rankings exclude hospitals with less than 25 cases except for patient surveys which excludes hospitals with less than 100 cases; (a) 100-299 cases; (1) The number of cases/patients is too few to report; (2) Data submitted were based on a sample of cases/patients; (3) Results are based on a shorter time period than required; (4) Data suppressed by CMS for one or more quarters; (5) Results are not available for this reporting period; (6) Fewer than 100 patients completed the HCAHPS survey; (7) No cases met the criteria for this measure; (8) The lower limit of the confidence interval cannot be calculated if the number of observed infections equals zero; (9) No data are available from the state/territory for this reporting period; (10) The scores shown reflect fewer than 50 completed surveys; (11) There were discrepancies in the data collection process; (12) This measure does not apply to this hospital for this reporting period; (13) Results cannot be calculated for this reporting period; (14) The results for this state are combined with nearby states to protect confidentiality; Please refer to the User's Guide for a full explanation of data.

Measure	Cases	This Hosp.	State Avg.	U.S. Avg.
Combination Abdominal CT Scan	193	5.2%	8.7%	10.5%
Combination Brain/Sinus CT Scan	163	1.2%	2.2%	2.7%
Combination Chest CT Scan	143	2.1%	3.6%	2.7%
Follow-up Mammogram/Ultrasound	316	11.1%	8.2%	8.8%
Lumbar Spine MRI for Low Back Pain[1]	-	-	36.9%	37.2%

Sparrow Clinton Hospital

805 S Oakland
Saint Johns, MI 48879
Phone: 989-224-6881
Fax: 989-227-3347
URL: www.clintonmemorial.org
Type: Critical Access Hospitals
Emergency Services: Yes
Ownership: Proprietary
Beds: 28

Key Personnel:

CEO/President. . . . . Ed Brunn
Radiology. . . . . Michael Buetow
Infection Control. . . . . Ricki Burk
Quality Assurance . . . . Cathy Hallead
Operating Room. . . . . Kathleen McElroy
Chief of Medical Staff . . . . Paul David Minnick
Emergency Room . . . . Diane Simon

Measure	Cases	This Hosp.	State Avg.	U.S. Avg.
Blood Clot Prevention and Treatment				
Anticoagulation Overlap Therapy[2]	14	100%	90%	93%
ICU Venous Thromboembolism Prophylaxis[1,2]	-	-	93%	92%
Incidence of Potentially Preventable VTE[2,7]	-	-	8%	10%
UFH with Dosages/Platelet Monitoring[1,2]	-	-	96%	97%
Venous Thromboembolism Prophylaxis[2]	306	75%	87%	85%
Warfarin Therapy Discharge Instructions[1,2]	-	-	72%	75%
Chest Pain/Possible Heart Attack Care				
Aspirin Given Within 24 Hours of Arrival	29	100%	96%	96%
Fibrinolytic Meds Within 30 Min. of Arrival[7]	-	-	63%	58%
Average Time to ECG (minutes)	30	6	8	7
Average Time to Transfer (minutes)[1]	-	-	53	60
Children's Asthma Care				
Received Home Management Plan of Care	-	-	-	88%
Received Reliever Medication	-	-	-	100%
Received Systemic Corticosteroids	-	-	-	100%
Emergency Department				
Admittance Decision Time (minutes)[2]	542	45	102	98
Head CT Results Within 45 Min. of Arrival[5]	-	-	54%	57%
Patients Who Left ER Before Being Seen[5]	-	-	2%	2%
Time from ER Arrival to Admit. (minutes)[2]	544	230	288	274
Time from ER Arrival to Discharge (minutes)	445	114	128	134
Time in ER Before Being Evaluated (minutes)	472	39	22	26
Time to Pain Meds for Fractures (minutes)[5]	-	-	55	57
Heart Attack Care				
Aspirin Given at Discharge[5]	-	-	99%	99%
Fibrinolytic Meds Within 30 Min. of Arrival[5]	-	-	20%	54%
PCI Within 90 Minutes of Arrival[5]	-	-	95%	96%
Statin Prescribed at Discharge[5]	-	-	98%	98%
Heart Failure Care				
ACE Inhibitor or ARB for LVSD	14	100%	96%	97%
Discharge Instructions Given	34	100%	94%	94%
Evaluation of LVS Function	49	98%	99%	99%
Medicare Spending				
Medicare Spending per Patient (ratio)	-	-	0.96	0.98
Pneumonia Care				
Appropriate Initial Antibiotic Given	24	100%	96%	95%
Blood Culture Timing	34	97%	98%	98%
Pregnancy and Delivery Care				
Newborn Deliveries Scheduled Early[5]	-	-	3%	6%
Preventive Care				
Immunization for Influenza[5]	-	-	89%	90%
Immunization for Pneumonia[5]	-	-	90%	92%
Stroke Care				
Anticoagulation Therapy for Atrial Fibrillation[5]	-	-	92%	95%
Antithrombotic Therapy Timing[5]	-	-	97%	98%
Assessed for Rehabilitation[5]	-	-	97%	97%
Discharged on Antithrombotic Therapy[5]	-	-	99%	99%
Discharged on Statin Medication[5]	-	-	94%	94%
Thrombolytic Therapy Timing[5]	-	-	69%	66%
Venous Thromboembolism Prophylaxis[5]	-	-	94%	94%
Written Stroke Educational Materials Given[5]	-	-	87%	88%
Surgical Care Improvement Project				
Appropriate Beta Blocker Usage	27	100%	98%	98%
Appropriate VTP Within 24 Hours	46	100%	98%	98%
Controlled Postoperative Blood Glucose[7]	-	-	97%	97%
Perioperative Temperature Management	55	100%	100%	100%
Prophylactic Antibiotic Selection	39	97%	99%	99%
Prophylactic Antibiotic Selection (Outpatient)[5]	-	-	97%	98%
Prophylactic Antibiotic Stopped	39	92%	98%	98%
Prophylactic Antibiotic Timing	39	100%	98%	99%
Prophylactic Antibiotic Timing (Outpatient)[5]	-	-	97%	98%
Urinary Catheter Removal	42	98%	97%	97%
Survey of Patients' Hospital Experiences				
Area Around Room 'Always' Quiet at Night	(a)	61%	60%	61%
Doctors 'Always' Communicated Well	(a)	86%	81%	82%
Home Recovery Information Given	(a)	91%	87%	85%
Hospital Given 9 or 10 on 10 Point Scale	(a)	81%	71%	71%
Meds 'Always' Explained Before Given	(a)	68%	64%	64%
Nurses 'Always' Communicated Well	(a)	84%	80%	79%
Pain 'Always' Well Controlled	(a)	71%	71%	71%
Room and Bathroom 'Always' Clean	(a)	77%	73%	73%
Timely Help 'Always' Received	(a)	76%	70%	68%
Would Definitely Recommend Hospital	(a)	80%	71%	71%
Use of Medical Imaging				
Cardiac Imaging Stress Test before Surgery	195	7.7%	5.1%	5.3%
Combination Abdominal CT Scan	404	4.5%	8.7%	10.5%
Combination Brain/Sinus CT Scan[1]	-	-	2.2%	2.7%
Combination Chest CT Scan	157	0.6%	3.6%	2.7%
Follow-up Mammogram/Ultrasound	334	3.9%	8.2%	8.8%
Lumbar Spine MRI for Low Back Pain	53	37.7%	36.9%	37.2%

Lakeland Hospital - Saint Joseph

1234 Napier Avenue
Saint Joseph, MI 49085
Phone: 269-983-8300
Fax: 269-982-4855
URL: www.lakelandhealth.org
Type: Acute Care Hospitals
Emergency Services: Yes
Ownership: Voluntary non-profit - Private
Beds: 254

Key Personnel:

Operating Room. . . . . Gayle Beward
Cardiac Laboratory. . . . . Bart Btrndt
President/CEO. . . . . Loren Hamel, MD
Chief of Medical Staff. . . . . Lowell Hamel, MD
Pediatric In-Patient Care . . . . Fred Johansen, MD
Radiology. . . . . William Leahey, MD
Quality Assurance . . . . Mary Ann Pater
Patient Relations . . . . Eileen Willits

Measure	Cases	This Hosp.	State Avg.	U.S. Avg.
Blood Clot Prevention and Treatment				
Anticoagulation Overlap Therapy[2]	118	70%	90%	93%
ICU Venous Thromboembolism Prophylaxis[2]	36	83%	93%	92%
Incidence of Potentially Preventable VTE[2]	14	7%	8%	10%
UFH with Dosages/Platelet Monitoring[2]	104	95%	96%	97%
Venous Thromboembolism Prophylaxis[2]	343	84%	87%	85%
Warfarin Therapy Discharge Instructions[2]	97	22%	72%	75%
Chest Pain/Possible Heart Attack Care				
Aspirin Given Within 24 Hours of Arrival[1,3]	-	-	96%	96%
Fibrinolytic Meds Within 30 Min. of Arrival[1,3]	-	-	63%	58%
Average Time to ECG (minutes)[1,3]	-	-	8	7
Average Time to Transfer (minutes)[1,3]	-	-	53	60
Children's Asthma Care				
Received Home Management Plan of Care	-	-	-	88%
Received Reliever Medication	-	-	-	100%
Received Systemic Corticosteroids	-	-	-	100%
Emergency Department				
Admittance Decision Time (minutes)[2]	618	90	102	98
Head CT Results Within 45 Min. of Arrival[1]	-	-	54%	57%
Patients Who Left ER Before Being Seen	69,855	3%	2%	2%
Time from ER Arrival to Admit. (minutes)[2]	623	279	288	274
Time from ER Arrival to Discharge (minutes)	359	128	128	134
Time in ER Before Being Evaluated (minutes)	378	18	22	26
Time to Pain Meds for Fractures (minutes)	249	60	55	57
Heart Attack Care				
Aspirin Given at Discharge	301	99%	99%	99%
Fibrinolytic Meds Within 30 Min. of Arrival[1]	-	-	20%	54%
PCI Within 90 Minutes of Arrival	41	93%	95%	96%
Statin Prescribed at Discharge	282	99%	98%	98%
Heart Failure Care				
ACE Inhibitor or ARB for LVSD[2]	100	94%	96%	97%
Discharge Instructions Given[2]	263	93%	94%	94%
Evaluation of LVS Function[2]	318	100%	99%	99%
Medicare Spending				
Medicare Spending per Patient (ratio)	-	0.95	0.96	0.98
Pneumonia Care				
Appropriate Initial Antibiotic Given[2]	75	93%	96%	95%
Blood Culture Timing[2]	137	99%	98%	98%
Pregnancy and Delivery Care				
Newborn Deliveries Scheduled Early[2]	21	0%	3%	6%
Preventive Care				
Immunization for Influenza[2]	532	92%	89%	90%
Immunization for Pneumonia[2]	722	88%	90%	92%
Stroke Care				
Anticoagulation Therapy for Atrial Fibrillation	27	96%	92%	95%
Antithrombotic Therapy Timing	169	99%	97%	98%
Assessed for Rehabilitation	195	100%	97%	97%
Discharged on Antithrombotic Therapy	179	99%	99%	99%
Discharged on Statin Medication	128	98%	94%	94%
Thrombolytic Therapy Timing[1]	-	-	69%	66%
Venous Thromboembolism Prophylaxis	203	97%	94%	94%
Written Stroke Educational Materials Given	107	100%	87%	88%
Surgical Care Improvement Project				
Appropriate Beta Blocker Usage[2]	210	100%	98%	98%
Appropriate VTP Within 24 Hours[2]	352	99%	98%	98%
Controlled Postoperative Blood Glucose[2]	96	98%	97%	97%
Perioperative Temperature Management[2]	485	100%	100%	100%
Prophylactic Antibiotic Selection[2]	424	99%	99%	99%
Prophylactic Antibiotic Selection (Outpatient)	288	99%	97%	98%
Prophylactic Antibiotic Stopped[2]	418	98%	98%	98%
Prophylactic Antibiotic Timing[2]	425	99%	98%	99%
Prophylactic Antibiotic Timing (Outpatient)	284	98%	97%	98%
Urinary Catheter Removal[2]	361	97%	97%	97%
Survey of Patients' Hospital Experiences				
Area Around Room 'Always' Quiet at Night	300+	60%	60%	61%
Doctors 'Always' Communicated Well	300+	81%	81%	82%
Home Recovery Information Given	300+	86%	87%	85%
Hospital Given 9 or 10 on 10 Point Scale	300+	73%	71%	71%
Meds 'Always' Explained Before Given	300+	64%	64%	64%
Nurses 'Always' Communicated Well	300+	79%	80%	79%
Pain 'Always' Well Controlled	300+	71%	71%	71%
Room and Bathroom 'Always' Clean	300+	73%	73%	73%
Timely Help 'Always' Received	300+	65%	70%	68%
Would Definitely Recommend Hospital	300+	70%	71%	71%
Use of Medical Imaging				
Cardiac Imaging Stress Test before Surgery	49	2.0%	5.1%	5.3%
Combination Abdominal CT Scan	1,530	5.1%	8.7%	10.5%
Combination Brain/Sinus CT Scan	1,163	2.1%	2.2%	2.7%
Combination Chest CT Scan	905	1.2%	3.6%	2.7%
Follow-up Mammogram/Ultrasound	3,115	5.0%	8.2%	8.8%
Lumbar Spine MRI for Low Back Pain	248	37.1%	36.9%	37.2%

McKenzie Health System

120 N Delaware Street
Sandusky, MI 48471
Phone: 810-648-3770
Fax: 810-648-4204
URL: www.mckenziehospital.com
Type: Critical Access Hospitals
Emergency Services: Yes
Ownership: Voluntary non-profit - Private
Beds: 25

Key Personnel:

Operating Room. . . . . Sue Abrego, RN
CEO/President. . . . . Steve Barnett
Chief of Medical Staff . . . . M M Elrahman, MD
Patient Relations . . . . Jenny Morzo, RN
Quality Assurance . . . . Jenny Morzo, RN
Infection Control. . . . . Bonnie Powell, RN
Emergency Room . . . . Allen Williams, MD

Measure	Cases	This Hosp.	State Avg.	U.S. Avg.
Blood Clot Prevention and Treatment				
Anticoagulation Overlap Therapy[5]	-	-	90%	93%
ICU Venous Thromboembolism Prophylaxis[5]	-	-	93%	92%
Incidence of Potentially Preventable VTE[5]	-	-	8%	10%
UFH with Dosages/Platelet Monitoring[5]	-	-	96%	97%
Venous Thromboembolism Prophylaxis[5]	-	-	87%	85%

NOTE: Hospital profiles are in alphabetical order by state, then city, then hospital within the city; Rankings exclude hospitals with less than 25 cases except for patient surveys which excludes hospitals with less than 100 cases; (a) 100-299 cases; (1) The number of cases/patients is too few to report; (2) Data submitted were based on a sample of cases/patients; (3) Results are based on a shorter time period than required; (4) Data suppressed by CMS for one or more quarters; (5) Results are not available for this reporting period; (6) Fewer than 100 patients completed the HCAHPS survey; (7) No cases met the criteria for this measure; (8) The lower limit of the confidence interval cannot be calculated if the number of observed infections equals zero; (9) No data are available from the state/territory for this reporting period; (10) The scores shown reflect fewer than 50 completed surveys; (11) There were discrepancies in the data collection process; (12) This measure does not apply to this hospital for this reporting period; (13) Results cannot be calculated for this reporting period; (14) The results for this state are combined with nearby states to protect confidentiality; Please refer to the User's Guide for a full explanation of data.

Measure	Cases	This Hosp.	State Avg.	U.S. Avg.
Warfarin Therapy Discharge Instructions[5]	-	-	72%	75%
Chest Pain/Possible Heart Attack Care				
Aspirin Given Within 24 Hours of Arrival	23	100%	96%	96%
Fibrinolytic Meds Within 30 Min. of Arrival[1,3]	-	-	63%	58%
Average Time to ECG (minutes)	23	5	8	7
Average Time to Transfer (minutes)[1,3]	-	-	53	60
Children's Asthma Care				
Received Home Management Plan of Care	-	-	-	88%
Received Reliever Medication	-	-	-	100%
Received Systemic Corticosteroids	-	-	-	100%
Emergency Department				
Admittance Decision Time (minutes)[5]	-	-	102	98
Head CT Results Within 45 Min. of Arrival[5]	-	-	54%	57%
Patients Who Left ER Before Being Seen[5]	-	-	2%	2%
Time from ER Arrival to Admit. (minutes)[5]	-	-	288	274
Time from ER Arrival to Discharge (minutes)	359	74	128	134
Time in ER Before Being Evaluated (minutes)	385	12	22	26
Time to Pain Meds for Fractures (minutes)[5]	-	-	55	57
Heart Attack Care				
Aspirin Given at Discharge[5]	-	-	99%	99%
Fibrinolytic Meds Within 30 Min. of Arrival[5]	-	-	20%	54%
PCI Within 90 Minutes of Arrival[5]	-	-	95%	96%
Statin Prescribed at Discharge[5]	-	-	98%	98%
Heart Failure Care				
ACE Inhibitor or ARB for LVSD[1]	-	-	96%	97%
Discharge Instructions Given	12	100%	94%	94%
Evaluation of LVS Function	14	100%	99%	99%
Medicare Spending				
Medicare Spending per Patient (ratio)	-	-	0.96	0.98
Pneumonia Care				
Appropriate Initial Antibiotic Given	33	94%	96%	95%
Blood Culture Timing	44	100%	98%	98%
Pregnancy and Delivery Care				
Newborn Deliveries Scheduled Early[5]	-	-	3%	6%
Preventive Care				
Immunization for Influenza[5]	-	-	89%	90%
Immunization for Pneumonia[5]	-	-	90%	92%
Stroke Care				
Anticoagulation Therapy for Atrial Fibrillation[5]	-	-	92%	95%
Antithrombotic Therapy Timing[5]	-	-	97%	98%
Assessed for Rehabilitation[5]	-	-	97%	97%
Discharged on Antithrombotic Therapy[5]	-	-	99%	99%
Discharged on Statin Medication[5]	-	-	94%	94%
Thrombolytic Therapy Timing[5]	-	-	69%	66%
Venous Thromboembolism Prophylaxis[5]	-	-	94%	94%
Written Stroke Educational Materials Given[5]	-	-	87%	88%
Surgical Care Improvement Project				
Appropriate Beta Blocker Usage[1]	-	-	98%	98%
Appropriate VTP Within 24 Hours	12	50%	98%	98%
Controlled Postoperative Blood Glucose[7]	-	-	97%	97%
Perioperative Temperature Management	12	100%	100%	100%
Prophylactic Antibiotic Selection[1]	-	-	99%	99%
Prophylactic Antibiotic Selection (Outpatient)[1]	-	-	97%	98%
Prophylactic Antibiotic Stopped[1]	-	-	98%	98%
Prophylactic Antibiotic Timing[1]	-	-	98%	99%
Prophylactic Antibiotic Timing (Outpatient)[1]	-	-	97%	98%
Urinary Catheter Removal	11	100%	97%	97%
Survey of Patients' Hospital Experiences				
Area Around Room 'Always' Quiet at Night[6]	<100	60%	60%	61%
Doctors 'Always' Communicated Well[6]	<100	82%	81%	82%
Home Recovery Information Given[6]	<100	87%	87%	85%
Hospital Given 9 or 10 on 10 Point Scale[6]	<100	67%	71%	71%
Meds 'Always' Explained Before Given[6]	<100	74%	64%	64%
Nurses 'Always' Communicated Well[6]	<100	79%	80%	79%
Pain 'Always' Well Controlled[6]	<100	76%	71%	71%
Room and Bathroom 'Always' Clean[6]	<100	82%	73%	73%
Timely Help 'Always' Received[6]	<100	77%	70%	68%
Would Definitely Recommend Hospital[6]	<100	70%	71%	71%
Use of Medical Imaging				
Cardiac Imaging Stress Test before Surgery	71	5.6%	5.1%	5.3%
Combination Abdominal CT Scan	204	3.4%	8.7%	10.5%
Combination Brain/Sinus CT Scan[1]	-	-	2.2%	2.7%
Combination Chest CT Scan	97	1.0%	3.6%	2.7%
Follow-up Mammogram/Ultrasound	208	12.5%	8.2%	8.8%
Lumbar Spine MRI for Low Back Pain[7]	-	-	36.9%	37.2%

Chippewa County War Memorial Hospital

500 Osborn Blvd
Sault Sainte Marie, MI 49783
Phone: 906-635-4460
Fax: 906-635-4467
Type: Acute Care Hospitals
Emergency Services: Yes
Ownership: Voluntary non-profit - Private

Key Personnel:
Radiology. . . . . R J Duman
Chief of Medical Staff. . . . . R J Graham
CEO/President. . . . . David Jahn
Emergency Room . . . . Jane McLeod, RN
Quality Assurance . . . . Mitch Zaborowski

Measure	Cases	This Hosp.	State Avg.	U.S. Avg.
Blood Clot Prevention and Treatment				
Anticoagulation Overlap Therapy[2]	20	60%	90%	93%
ICU Venous Thromboembolism Prophylaxis[2]	64	77%	93%	92%
Incidence of Potentially Preventable VTE[1,2]	-	-	8%	10%
UFH with Dosages/Platelet Monitoring[1,2]	-	-	96%	97%
Venous Thromboembolism Prophylaxis[2]	218	91%	87%	85%
Warfarin Therapy Discharge Instructions[2]	13	100%	72%	75%
Chest Pain/Possible Heart Attack Care				
Aspirin Given Within 24 Hours of Arrival	84	96%	96%	96%
Fibrinolytic Meds Within 30 Min. of Arrival	11	55%	63%	58%
Average Time to ECG (minutes)	85	13	8	7
Average Time to Transfer (minutes)[1]	-	-	53	60
Children's Asthma Care				
Received Home Management Plan of Care	-	-	-	88%
Received Reliever Medication	-	-	-	100%
Received Systemic Corticosteroids	-	-	-	100%
Emergency Department				
Admittance Decision Time (minutes)[2]	405	62	102	98
Head CT Results Within 45 Min. of Arrival	12	50%	54%	57%
Patients Who Left ER Before Being Seen	17,121	2%	2%	2%
Time from ER Arrival to Admit. (minutes)[2]	408	240	288	274
Time from ER Arrival to Discharge (minutes)	310	136	128	134
Time in ER Before Being Evaluated (minutes)	280	44	22	26
Time to Pain Meds for Fractures (minutes)	66	63	55	57
Heart Attack Care				
Aspirin Given at Discharge	25	96%	99%	99%
Fibrinolytic Meds Within 30 Min. of Arrival[7]	-	-	20%	54%
PCI Within 90 Minutes of Arrival[7]	-	-	95%	96%
Statin Prescribed at Discharge	20	75%	98%	98%
Heart Failure Care				
ACE Inhibitor or ARB for LVSD	33	94%	96%	97%
Discharge Instructions Given	81	78%	94%	94%
Evaluation of LVS Function	97	98%	99%	99%
Medicare Spending				
Medicare Spending per Patient (ratio)	-	0.90	0.96	0.98
Pneumonia Care				
Appropriate Initial Antibiotic Given	100	90%	96%	95%
Blood Culture Timing	155	96%	98%	98%
Pregnancy and Delivery Care				
Newborn Deliveries Scheduled Early[2]	22	0%	3%	6%
Preventive Care				
Immunization for Influenza[2]	293	73%	89%	90%
Immunization for Pneumonia[2]	373	87%	90%	92%
Stroke Care				
Anticoagulation Therapy for Atrial Fibrillation[1]	-	-	92%	95%
Antithrombotic Therapy Timing	30	90%	97%	98%
Assessed for Rehabilitation	32	81%	97%	97%
Discharged on Antithrombotic Therapy	32	100%	99%	99%
Discharged on Statin Medication	26	73%	94%	94%
Thrombolytic Therapy Timing[1]	-	-	69%	66%
Venous Thromboembolism Prophylaxis	29	97%	94%	94%
Written Stroke Educational Materials Given	21	57%	87%	88%
Surgical Care Improvement Project				
Appropriate Beta Blocker Usage	76	97%	98%	98%
Appropriate VTP Within 24 Hours	198	97%	98%	98%
Controlled Postoperative Blood Glucose[7]	-	-	97%	97%
Perioperative Temperature Management	222	100%	100%	100%
Prophylactic Antibiotic Selection	178	99%	99%	99%
Prophylactic Antibiotic Selection (Outpatient)	16	81%	97%	98%
Prophylactic Antibiotic Stopped	170	96%	98%	98%
Prophylactic Antibiotic Timing	178	100%	98%	99%
Prophylactic Antibiotic Timing (Outpatient)	17	94%	97%	98%
Urinary Catheter Removal	53	91%	97%	97%
Survey of Patients' Hospital Experiences				
Area Around Room 'Always' Quiet at Night	300+	56%	60%	61%
Doctors 'Always' Communicated Well	300+	81%	81%	82%
Home Recovery Information Given	300+	88%	87%	85%
Hospital Given 9 or 10 on 10 Point Scale	300+	73%	71%	71%
Meds 'Always' Explained Before Given	300+	66%	64%	64%
Nurses 'Always' Communicated Well	300+	83%	80%	79%
Pain 'Always' Well Controlled	300+	74%	71%	71%
Room and Bathroom 'Always' Clean	300+	70%	73%	73%
Timely Help 'Always' Received	300+	75%	70%	68%
Would Definitely Recommend Hospital	300+	71%	71%	71%
Use of Medical Imaging				
Cardiac Imaging Stress Test before Surgery	302	3.0%	5.1%	5.3%
Combination Abdominal CT Scan	465	10.3%	8.7%	10.5%
Combination Brain/Sinus CT Scan	429	4.2%	2.2%	2.7%
Combination Chest CT Scan	282	3.5%	3.6%	2.7%
Follow-up Mammogram/Ultrasound	738	5.0%	8.2%	8.8%
Lumbar Spine MRI for Low Back Pain	118	42.4%	36.9%	37.2%

Mercy Health Lakeshore Campus

72 South State Street
Shelby, MI 49455
Phone: 231-861-2156
Type: Critical Access Hospitals
Emergency Services: Yes
Ownership: Voluntary non-profit - Other

Measure	Cases	This Hosp.	State Avg.	U.S. Avg.
Blood Clot Prevention and Treatment				
Anticoagulation Overlap Therapy[1,2]	-	-	90%	93%
ICU Venous Thromboembolism Prophylaxis[1,2]	-	-	93%	92%
Incidence of Potentially Preventable VTE[1,2]	-	-	8%	10%
UFH with Dosages/Platelet Monitoring[1,2]	-	-	96%	97%
Venous Thromboembolism Prophylaxis[2]	69	42%	87%	85%
Warfarin Therapy Discharge Instructions[1,2]	-	-	72%	75%
Chest Pain/Possible Heart Attack Care				
Aspirin Given Within 24 Hours of Arrival	30	77%	96%	96%
Fibrinolytic Meds Within 30 Min. of Arrival[7]	-	-	63%	58%
Average Time to ECG (minutes)	34	14	8	7
Average Time to Transfer (minutes)[1]	-	-	53	60
Children's Asthma Care				
Received Home Management Plan of Care	-	-	-	88%
Received Reliever Medication	-	-	-	100%
Received Systemic Corticosteroids	-	-	-	100%
Emergency Department				
Admittance Decision Time (minutes)[5]	-	-	102	98
Head CT Results Within 45 Min. of Arrival[5]	-	-	54%	57%
Patients Who Left ER Before Being Seen[5]	-	-	2%	2%
Time from ER Arrival to Admit. (minutes)[5]	-	-	288	274
Time from ER Arrival to Discharge (minutes)	355	85	128	134
Time in ER Before Being Evaluated (minutes)	382	8	22	26
Time to Pain Meds for Fractures (minutes)[5]	-	-	55	57
Heart Attack Care				
Aspirin Given at Discharge[1,3]	-	-	99%	99%
Fibrinolytic Meds Within 30 Min. of Arrival[3,7]	-	-	20%	54%
PCI Within 90 Minutes of Arrival[3,7]	-	-	95%	96%
Statin Prescribed at Discharge[1,3]	-	-	98%	98%
Heart Failure Care				
ACE Inhibitor or ARB for LVSD[1]	-	-	96%	97%
Discharge Instructions Given[1]	-	-	94%	94%
Evaluation of LVS Function	12	75%	99%	99%
Medicare Spending				
Medicare Spending per Patient (ratio)	-	-	0.96	0.98
Pneumonia Care				
Appropriate Initial Antibiotic Given	21	90%	96%	95%
Blood Culture Timing	13	92%	98%	98%
Pregnancy and Delivery Care				
Newborn Deliveries Scheduled Early[5]	-	-	3%	6%
Preventive Care				

NOTE: Hospital profiles are in alphabetical order by state, then city, then hospital within the city; Rankings exclude hospitals with less than 25 cases except for patient surveys which excludes hospitals with less than 100 cases; (a) 100-299 cases; (1) The number of cases/patients is too few to report; (2) Data submitted were based on a sample of cases/patients; (3) Results are based on a shorter time period than required; (4) Data suppressed by CMS for one or more quarters; (5) Results are not available for this reporting period; (6) Fewer than 100 patients completed the HCAHPS survey; (7) No cases met the criteria for this measure; (8) The lower limit of the confidence interval cannot be calculated if the number of observed infections equals zero; (9) No data are available from the state/territory for this reporting period; (10) The scores shown reflect fewer than 50 completed surveys; (11) There were discrepancies in the data collection process; (12) This measure does not apply to this hospital for this reporting period; (13) Results cannot be calculated for this reporting period; (14) The results for this state are combined with nearby states to protect confidentiality; Please refer to the User's Guide for a full explanation of data.

Measure	Cases	This Hosp.	State Avg.	U.S. Avg.
Immunization for Influenza[5]	-	-	89%	90%
Immunization for Pneumonia[5]	-	-	90%	92%
Stroke Care				
Anticoagulation Therapy for Atrial Fibrillation[5]	-	-	92%	95%
Antithrombotic Therapy Timing[5]	-	-	97%	98%
Assessed for Rehabilitation[5]	-	-	97%	97%
Discharged on Antithrombotic Therapy[5]	-	-	99%	99%
Discharged on Statin Medication[5]	-	-	94%	94%
Thrombolytic Therapy Timing[5]	-	-	69%	66%
Venous Thromboembolism Prophylaxis[5]	-	-	94%	94%
Written Stroke Educational Materials Given[5]	-	-	87%	88%
Surgical Care Improvement Project				
Appropriate Beta Blocker Usage[1]	-	-	98%	98%
Appropriate VTP Within 24 Hours[1]	-	-	98%	98%
Controlled Postoperative Blood Glucose[7]	-	-	97%	97%
Perioperative Temperature Management	16	75%	100%	100%
Prophylactic Antibiotic Selection[1]	-	-	99%	99%
Prophylactic Antibiotic Selection (Outpatient)[1,3]	-	-	97%	98%
Prophylactic Antibiotic Stopped[1]	-	-	98%	98%
Prophylactic Antibiotic Timing[1]	-	-	98%	99%
Prophylactic Antibiotic Timing (Outpatient)[1,3]	-	-	97%	98%
Urinary Catheter Removal[1]	-	-	97%	97%
Survey of Patients' Hospital Experiences				
Area Around Room 'Always' Quiet at Night[5]	-	-	60%	61%
Doctors 'Always' Communicated Well[5]	-	-	81%	82%
Home Recovery Information Given[5]	-	-	87%	85%
Hospital Given 9 or 10 on 10 Point Scale[5]	-	-	71%	71%
Meds 'Always' Explained Before Given[5]	-	-	64%	64%
Nurses 'Always' Communicated Well[5]	-	-	80%	79%
Pain 'Always' Well Controlled[5]	-	-	71%	71%
Room and Bathroom 'Always' Clean[5]	-	-	73%	73%
Timely Help 'Always' Received[5]	-	-	70%	68%
Would Definitely Recommend Hospital[5]	-	-	71%	71%
Use of Medical Imaging				
Cardiac Imaging Stress Test before Surgery[7]	-	-	5.1%	5.3%
Combination Abdominal CT Scan	153	4.6%	8.7%	10.5%
Combination Brain/Sinus CT Scan[1]	-	-	2.2%	2.7%
Combination Chest CT Scan	71	2.8%	3.6%	2.7%
Follow-up Mammogram/Ultrasound	435	4.8%	8.2%	8.8%
Lumbar Spine MRI for Low Back Pain[1]	-	-	36.9%	37.2%

Sheridan Community Hospital

301 N Main St
Sheridan, MI 48884
Phone: 989-291-3261
Fax: 989-291-3062
URL: www.sheridanhospital.com
Type: Critical Access Hospitals
Emergency Services: No
Ownership: Voluntary non-profit - Other
Beds: 25

Key Personnel:
CEO/President. . . . . Kevin J Cawley
Radiology. . . . . Donna R Moyer
Chief of Medical Staff. . . . . Brian Thwaites

Measure	Cases	This Hosp.	State Avg.	U.S. Avg.
Blood Clot Prevention and Treatment				
Anticoagulation Overlap Therapy[5]	-	-	90%	93%
ICU Venous Thromboembolism Prophylaxis[5]	-	-	93%	92%
Incidence of Potentially Preventable VTE[5]	-	-	8%	10%
UFH with Dosages/Platelet Monitoring[5]	-	-	96%	97%
Venous Thromboembolism Prophylaxis[5]	-	-	87%	85%
Warfarin Therapy Discharge Instructions[5]	-	-	72%	75%
Chest Pain/Possible Heart Attack Care				
Aspirin Given Within 24 Hours of Arrival	16	100%	96%	96%
Fibrinolytic Meds Within 30 Min. of Arrival[3,7]	-	-	63%	58%
Average Time to ECG (minutes)	17	7	8	7
Average Time to Transfer (minutes)[3,7]	-	-	53	60
Children's Asthma Care				
Received Home Management Plan of Care	-	-	-	88%
Received Reliever Medication	-	-	-	100%
Received Systemic Corticosteroids	-	-	-	100%
Emergency Department				
Admittance Decision Time (minutes)[5]	-	-	102	98
Head CT Results Within 45 Min. of Arrival[5]	-	-	54%	57%
Patients Who Left ER Before Being Seen[5]	-	-	2%	2%
Time from ER Arrival to Admit. (minutes)[5]	-	-	288	274
Time from ER Arrival to Discharge (minutes)	1,178	138	128	134
Time in ER Before Being Evaluated (minutes)	1,283	33	22	26
Time to Pain Meds for Fractures (minutes)[5]	-	-	55	57
Heart Attack Care				
Aspirin Given at Discharge[5]	-	-	99%	99%
Fibrinolytic Meds Within 30 Min. of Arrival[5]	-	-	20%	54%
PCI Within 90 Minutes of Arrival[5]	-	-	95%	96%
Statin Prescribed at Discharge[5]	-	-	98%	98%
Heart Failure Care				
ACE Inhibitor or ARB for LVSD[1]	-	-	96%	97%
Discharge Instructions Given[1]	-	-	94%	94%
Evaluation of LVS Function[1]	-	-	99%	99%
Medicare Spending				
Medicare Spending per Patient (ratio)	-	-	0.96	0.98
Pneumonia Care				
Appropriate Initial Antibiotic Given	19	74%	96%	95%
Blood Culture Timing	23	100%	98%	98%
Pregnancy and Delivery Care				
Newborn Deliveries Scheduled Early[5]	-	-	3%	6%
Preventive Care				
Immunization for Influenza[5]	-	-	89%	90%
Immunization for Pneumonia[5]	-	-	90%	92%
Stroke Care				
Anticoagulation Therapy for Atrial Fibrillation[5]	-	-	92%	95%
Antithrombotic Therapy Timing[5]	-	-	97%	98%
Assessed for Rehabilitation[5]	-	-	97%	97%
Discharged on Antithrombotic Therapy[5]	-	-	99%	99%
Discharged on Statin Medication[5]	-	-	94%	94%
Thrombolytic Therapy Timing[5]	-	-	69%	66%
Venous Thromboembolism Prophylaxis[5]	-	-	94%	94%
Written Stroke Educational Materials Given[5]	-	-	87%	88%
Surgical Care Improvement Project				
Appropriate Beta Blocker Usage[5]	-	-	98%	98%
Appropriate VTP Within 24 Hours[5]	-	-	98%	98%
Controlled Postoperative Blood Glucose[5]	-	-	97%	97%
Perioperative Temperature Management[5]	-	-	100%	100%
Prophylactic Antibiotic Selection[5]	-	-	99%	99%
Prophylactic Antibiotic Selection (Outpatient)[5]	-	-	97%	98%
Prophylactic Antibiotic Stopped[5]	-	-	98%	98%
Prophylactic Antibiotic Timing[5]	-	-	98%	99%
Prophylactic Antibiotic Timing (Outpatient)[5]	-	-	97%	98%
Urinary Catheter Removal[5]	-	-	97%	97%
Survey of Patients' Hospital Experiences				
Area Around Room 'Always' Quiet at Night[6]	<100	66%	60%	61%
Doctors 'Always' Communicated Well[6]	<100	92%	81%	82%
Home Recovery Information Given[6]	<100	91%	87%	85%
Hospital Given 9 or 10 on 10 Point Scale[6]	<100	81%	71%	71%
Meds 'Always' Explained Before Given[6]	<100	78%	64%	64%
Nurses 'Always' Communicated Well[6]	<100	86%	80%	79%
Pain 'Always' Well Controlled[6]	<100	88%	71%	71%
Room and Bathroom 'Always' Clean[6]	<100	86%	73%	73%
Timely Help 'Always' Received[6]	<100	86%	70%	68%
Would Definitely Recommend Hospital[6]	<100	79%	71%	71%
Use of Medical Imaging				
Cardiac Imaging Stress Test before Surgery[1]	-	-	5.1%	5.3%
Combination Abdominal CT Scan	97	7.2%	8.7%	10.5%
Combination Brain/Sinus CT Scan	149	0.7%	2.2%	2.7%
Combination Chest CT Scan	57	0.0%	3.6%	2.7%
Follow-up Mammogram/Ultrasound	186	12.4%	8.2%	8.8%
Lumbar Spine MRI for Low Back Pain[7]	-	-	36.9%	37.2%

South Haven Community Hospital

955 S Bailey Ave
South Haven, MI 49090
Phone: 269-637-5271
Fax: 269-639-1208
E-mail: info@shch.org
URL: www.shch.org
Type: Acute Care Hospitals
Emergency Services: Yes
Ownership: Govt - Hospital Dist/Auth
Beds: 82

Key Personnel:
Surgery . . . . Maura Buckhingham, MD
Surgery . . . . Allan Caudill
Radiology. . . . . T Johnson, MD
Pediatrics. . . . . Karen Jonson
Radiology. . . . . E Theodore Ostermann, MD
Quality Assurance . . . . Debbie Smith, RN
CEO/President. . . . . Joanne Urbanski
Emergency Room . . . . Paul Wahby, DO

Measure	Cases	This Hosp.	State Avg.	U.S. Avg.
Blood Clot Prevention and Treatment				
Anticoagulation Overlap Therapy[1,2]	-	-	90%	93%
ICU Venous Thromboembolism Prophylaxis[1,2]	-	-	93%	92%
Incidence of Potentially Preventable VTE[1,2]	-	-	8%	10%
UFH with Dosages/Platelet Monitoring[1,2]	-	-	96%	97%
Venous Thromboembolism Prophylaxis[2]	120	93%	87%	85%
Warfarin Therapy Discharge Instructions[1,2]	-	-	72%	75%
Chest Pain/Possible Heart Attack Care				
Aspirin Given Within 24 Hours of Arrival	78	97%	96%	96%
Fibrinolytic Meds Within 30 Min. of Arrival[1]	-	-	63%	58%
Average Time to ECG (minutes)	82	10	8	7
Average Time to Transfer (minutes)[1]	-	-	53	60
Children's Asthma Care				
Received Home Management Plan of Care	-	-	-	88%
Received Reliever Medication	-	-	-	100%
Received Systemic Corticosteroids	-	-	-	100%
Emergency Department				
Admittance Decision Time (minutes)[2]	277	94	102	98
Head CT Results Within 45 Min. of Arrival[1]	-	-	54%	57%
Patients Who Left ER Before Being Seen	14,363	1%	2%	2%
Time from ER Arrival to Admit. (minutes)[2]	278	325	288	274
Time from ER Arrival to Discharge (minutes)	439	147	128	134
Time in ER Before Being Evaluated (minutes)	522	30	22	26
Time to Pain Meds for Fractures (minutes)	61	47	55	57
Heart Attack Care				
Aspirin Given at Discharge[1,3]	-	-	99%	99%
Fibrinolytic Meds Within 30 Min. of Arrival[3,7]	-	-	20%	54%
PCI Within 90 Minutes of Arrival[3,7]	-	-	95%	96%
Statin Prescribed at Discharge[3,7]	-	-	98%	98%
Heart Failure Care				
ACE Inhibitor or ARB for LVSD[1]	-	-	96%	97%
Discharge Instructions Given	21	86%	94%	94%
Evaluation of LVS Function	28	96%	99%	99%
Medicare Spending				
Medicare Spending per Patient (ratio)	-	0.91	0.96	0.98
Pneumonia Care				
Appropriate Initial Antibiotic Given	39	97%	96%	95%
Blood Culture Timing	55	96%	98%	98%
Pregnancy and Delivery Care				
Newborn Deliveries Scheduled Early[2]	25	8%	3%	6%
Preventive Care				
Immunization for Influenza[2]	266	97%	89%	90%
Immunization for Pneumonia[2]	266	97%	90%	92%
Stroke Care				
Anticoagulation Therapy for Atrial Fibrillation[1]	-	-	92%	95%
Antithrombotic Therapy Timing[1]	-	-	97%	98%
Assessed for Rehabilitation[1]	-	-	97%	97%
Discharged on Antithrombotic Therapy[1]	-	-	99%	99%
Discharged on Statin Medication[1]	-	-	94%	94%
Thrombolytic Therapy Timing[7]	-	-	69%	66%
Venous Thromboembolism Prophylaxis	12	100%	94%	94%
Written Stroke Educational Materials Given[1]	-	-	87%	88%
Surgical Care Improvement Project				
Appropriate Beta Blocker Usage	19	89%	98%	98%
Appropriate VTP Within 24 Hours	63	97%	98%	98%
Controlled Postoperative Blood Glucose[7]	-	-	97%	97%
Perioperative Temperature Management	69	100%	100%	100%
Prophylactic Antibiotic Selection	53	94%	99%	99%
Prophylactic Antibiotic Selection (Outpatient)[1]	-	-	97%	98%
Prophylactic Antibiotic Stopped	53	100%	98%	98%
Prophylactic Antibiotic Timing	53	100%	98%	99%
Prophylactic Antibiotic Timing (Outpatient)[1]	-	-	97%	98%
Urinary Catheter Removal	50	100%	97%	97%
Survey of Patients' Hospital Experiences				
Area Around Room 'Always' Quiet at Night	300+	63%	60%	61%
Doctors 'Always' Communicated Well	300+	83%	81%	82%
Home Recovery Information Given	300+	86%	87%	85%
Hospital Given 9 or 10 on 10 Point Scale	300+	71%	71%	71%
Meds 'Always' Explained Before Given	300+	64%	64%	64%

NOTE: Hospital profiles are in alphabetical order by state, then city, then hospital within the city; Rankings exclude hospitals with less than 25 cases except for patient surveys which excludes hospitals with less than 100 cases; (a) 100-299 cases; (1) The number of cases/patients is too few to report; (2) Data submitted were based on a sample of cases/patients; (3) Results are based on a shorter time period than required; (4) Data suppressed by CMS for one or more quarters; (5) Results are not available for this reporting period; (6) Fewer than 100 patients completed the HCAHPS survey; (7) No cases met the criteria for this measure; (8) The lower limit of the confidence interval cannot be calculated if the number of observed infections equals zero; (9) No data are available from the state/territory for this reporting period; (10) The scores shown reflect fewer than 50 completed surveys; (11) There were discrepancies in the data collection process; (12) This measure does not apply to this hospital for this reporting period; (13) Results cannot be calculated for this reporting period; (14) The results for this state are combined with nearby states to protect confidentiality; Please refer to the User's Guide for a full explanation of data.

Nurses 'Always' Communicated Well	300+	81%	80%	79%
Pain 'Always' Well Controlled	300+	71%	71%	71%
Room and Bathroom 'Always' Clean	300+	72%	73%	73%
Timely Help 'Always' Received	300+	77%	70%	68%
Would Definitely Recommend Hospital	300+	63%	71%	71%
Use of Medical Imaging				
Cardiac Imaging Stress Test before Surgery	114	3.5%	5.1%	5.3%
Combination Abdominal CT Scan	224	6.7%	8.7%	10.5%
Combination Brain/Sinus CT Scan[1]	-	-	2.2%	2.7%
Combination Chest CT Scan	92	1.1%	3.6%	2.7%
Follow-up Mammogram/Ultrasound	420	6.0%	8.2%	8.8%
Lumbar Spine MRI for Low Back Pain[1]	-	-	36.9%	37.2%

Oakland Regional Hospital

22401 Foster Winter Drive
Southfield, MI 48075
Phone: 248-423-5100
URL: www.oaklandregionalhospital.com
Type: Acute Care Hospitals
Emergency Services: No
Ownership: Physician
Key Personnel:
CEO . . . . Dan Babb
Chairman/CEO . . . . Edward Burke
Radiology. . . . . Marianne Chrzanowski

Measure	Cases	This Hosp.	State Avg.	U.S. Avg.
Blood Clot Prevention and Treatment				
Anticoagulation Overlap Therapy[7]	-	-	90%	93%
ICU Venous Thromboembolism Prophylaxis[7]	-	-	93%	92%
Incidence of Potentially Preventable VTE[7]	-	-	8%	10%
UFH with Dosages/Platelet Monitoring[7]	-	-	96%	97%
Venous Thromboembolism Prophylaxis	251	92%	87%	85%
Warfarin Therapy Discharge Instructions[7]	-	-	72%	75%
Chest Pain/Possible Heart Attack Care				
Aspirin Given Within 24 Hours of Arrival[5]	-	-	96%	96%
Fibrinolytic Meds Within 30 Min. of Arrival[5]	-	-	63%	58%
Average Time to ECG (minutes)[5]	-	-	8	7
Average Time to Transfer (minutes)[5]	-	-	53	60
Children's Asthma Care				
Received Home Management Plan of Care	-	-	-	88%
Received Reliever Medication	-	-	-	100%
Received Systemic Corticosteroids	-	-	-	100%
Emergency Department				
Admittance Decision Time (minutes)[7]	-	-	102	98
Head CT Results Within 45 Min. of Arrival[5]	-	-	54%	57%
Patients Who Left ER Before Being Seen[5]	-	-	2%	2%
Time from ER Arrival to Admit. (minutes)[7]	-	-	288	274
Time from ER Arrival to Discharge (minutes)[5]	-	-	128	134
Time in ER Before Being Evaluated (minutes)[5]	-	-	22	26
Time to Pain Meds for Fractures (minutes)[5]	-	-	55	57
Heart Attack Care				
Aspirin Given at Discharge[5]	-	-	99%	99%
Fibrinolytic Meds Within 30 Min. of Arrival[5]	-	-	20%	54%
PCI Within 90 Minutes of Arrival[5]	-	-	95%	96%
Statin Prescribed at Discharge[5]	-	-	98%	98%
Heart Failure Care				
ACE Inhibitor or ARB for LVSD[5]	-	-	96%	97%
Discharge Instructions Given[5]	-	-	94%	94%
Evaluation of LVS Function[5]	-	-	99%	99%
Medicare Spending				
Medicare Spending per Patient (ratio)	-	0.94	0.96	0.98
Pneumonia Care				
Appropriate Initial Antibiotic Given[5]	-	-	96%	95%
Blood Culture Timing[5]	-	-	98%	98%
Pregnancy and Delivery Care				
Newborn Deliveries Scheduled Early[7]	-	-	3%	6%
Preventive Care				
Immunization for Influenza	196	78%	89%	90%
Immunization for Pneumonia	325	84%	90%	92%
Stroke Care				
Anticoagulation Therapy for Atrial Fibrillation[5]	-	-	92%	95%
Antithrombotic Therapy Timing[5]	-	-	97%	98%
Assessed for Rehabilitation[5]	-	-	97%	97%
Discharged on Antithrombotic Therapy[5]	-	-	99%	99%
Discharged on Statin Medication[5]	-	-	94%	94%
Thrombolytic Therapy Timing[5]	-	-	69%	66%
Venous Thromboembolism Prophylaxis[5]	-	-	94%	94%
Written Stroke Educational Materials Given[5]	-	-	87%	88%
Surgical Care Improvement Project				
Appropriate Beta Blocker Usage[1]	-	-	98%	98%
Appropriate VTP Within 24 Hours	52	63%	98%	98%
Controlled Postoperative Blood Glucose[7]	-	-	97%	97%
Perioperative Temperature Management	62	97%	100%	100%
Prophylactic Antibiotic Selection	41	100%	99%	99%
Prophylactic Antibiotic Selection (Outpatient)[5]	-	-	97%	98%
Prophylactic Antibiotic Stopped	41	100%	98%	98%
Prophylactic Antibiotic Timing	41	95%	98%	99%
Prophylactic Antibiotic Timing (Outpatient)[5]	-	-	97%	98%
Urinary Catheter Removal	39	100%	97%	97%
Survey of Patients' Hospital Experiences				
Area Around Room 'Always' Quiet at Night[10]	<100	83%	60%	61%
Doctors 'Always' Communicated Well[10]	<100	85%	81%	82%
Home Recovery Information Given[10]	<100	78%	87%	85%
Hospital Given 9 or 10 on 10 Point Scale[10]	<100	54%	71%	71%
Meds 'Always' Explained Before Given[10]	<100	34%	64%	64%
Nurses 'Always' Communicated Well[10]	<100	63%	80%	79%
Pain 'Always' Well Controlled[10]	<100	65%	71%	71%
Room and Bathroom 'Always' Clean[10]	<100	71%	73%	73%
Timely Help 'Always' Received[10]	<100	51%	70%	68%
Would Definitely Recommend Hospital[10]	<100	53%	71%	71%
Use of Medical Imaging				
Cardiac Imaging Stress Test before Surgery[7]	-	-	5.1%	5.3%
Combination Abdominal CT Scan[1]	-	-	8.7%	10.5%
Combination Brain/Sinus CT Scan[1]	-	-	2.2%	2.7%
Combination Chest CT Scan[1]	-	-	3.6%	2.7%
Follow-up Mammogram/Ultrasound[7]	-	-	8.2%	8.8%
Lumbar Spine MRI for Low Back Pain[1]	-	-	36.9%	37.2%

Providence Hospital & Medical Centers

16001 W Nine Mile Rd
Southfield, MI 48075
Phone: 248-849-3011
Fax: 248-849-3035
URL: www.stjohn.org/providence
Type: Acute Care Hospitals
Emergency Services: Yes
Ownership: Voluntary non-profit - Church
Beds: 459
Key Personnel:
Radiology. . . . . James Karo, MD
Infection Control. . . . . Tom Madhaven, MD
Emergency Room . . . . John McCabe, MD
Anesthesiology. . . . . Gregory Smith
CEO/President. . . . . Michael Wiemann, MD

Measure	Cases	This Hosp.	State Avg.	U.S. Avg.
Blood Clot Prevention and Treatment				
Anticoagulation Overlap Therapy[2]	304	94%	90%	93%
ICU Venous Thromboembolism Prophylaxis[2]	102	98%	93%	92%
Incidence of Potentially Preventable VTE[2]	62	2%	8%	10%
UFH with Dosages/Platelet Monitoring[2]	363	99%	96%	97%
Venous Thromboembolism Prophylaxis[2]	720	95%	87%	85%
Warfarin Therapy Discharge Instructions[2]	226	98%	72%	75%
Chest Pain/Possible Heart Attack Care				
Aspirin Given Within 24 Hours of Arrival	16	88%	96%	96%
Fibrinolytic Meds Within 30 Min. of Arrival[3,7]	-	-	63%	58%
Average Time to ECG (minutes)	16	12	8	7
Average Time to Transfer (minutes)[3,7]	-	-	53	60
Children's Asthma Care				
Received Home Management Plan of Care	-	-	-	88%
Received Reliever Medication	-	-	-	100%
Received Systemic Corticosteroids	-	-	-	100%
Emergency Department				
Admittance Decision Time (minutes)[2]	1,281	127	102	98
Head CT Results Within 45 Min. of Arrival[1]	-	-	54%	57%
Patients Who Left ER Before Being Seen	>100k	1%	2%	2%
Time from ER Arrival to Admit. (minutes)[2]	1,300	321	288	274
Time from ER Arrival to Discharge (minutes)	720	156	128	134
Time in ER Before Being Evaluated (minutes)	822	20	22	26
Time to Pain Meds for Fractures (minutes)	332	45	55	57
Heart Attack Care				
Aspirin Given at Discharge	469	100%	99%	99%
Fibrinolytic Meds Within 30 Min. of Arrival[7]	-	-	20%	54%
PCI Within 90 Minutes of Arrival	71	89%	95%	96%
Statin Prescribed at Discharge	459	99%	98%	98%
Heart Failure Care				
ACE Inhibitor or ARB for LVSD	338	97%	96%	97%
Discharge Instructions Given	893	100%	94%	94%
Evaluation of LVS Function	1,067	100%	99%	99%
Medicare Spending				
Medicare Spending per Patient (ratio)	-	0.98	0.96	0.98
Pneumonia Care				
Appropriate Initial Antibiotic Given	394	98%	96%	95%
Blood Culture Timing	450	100%	98%	98%
Pregnancy and Delivery Care				
Newborn Deliveries Scheduled Early	394	2%	3%	6%
Preventive Care				
Immunization for Influenza[2]	1,113	95%	89%	90%
Immunization for Pneumonia[2]	1,429	94%	90%	92%
Stroke Care				
Anticoagulation Therapy for Atrial Fibrillation	36	89%	92%	95%
Antithrombotic Therapy Timing	303	98%	97%	98%
Assessed for Rehabilitation	422	98%	97%	97%
Discharged on Antithrombotic Therapy	336	99%	99%	99%
Discharged on Statin Medication	247	99%	94%	94%
Thrombolytic Therapy Timing	23	100%	69%	66%
Venous Thromboembolism Prophylaxis	436	99%	94%	94%
Written Stroke Educational Materials Given	236	95%	87%	88%
Surgical Care Improvement Project				
Appropriate Beta Blocker Usage[2]	866	100%	98%	98%
Appropriate VTP Within 24 Hours[2]	2,140	100%	98%	98%
Controlled Postoperative Blood Glucose[2]	175	98%	97%	97%
Perioperative Temperature Management[2]	2,402	100%	100%	100%
Prophylactic Antibiotic Selection[2]	1,856	100%	99%	99%
Prophylactic Antibiotic Selection (Outpatient)	927	100%	97%	98%
Prophylactic Antibiotic Stopped[2]	1,745	99%	98%	98%
Prophylactic Antibiotic Timing[2]	1,856	100%	98%	99%
Prophylactic Antibiotic Timing (Outpatient)	931	98%	97%	98%
Urinary Catheter Removal[2]	1,656	99%	97%	97%
Survey of Patients' Hospital Experiences				
Area Around Room 'Always' Quiet at Night	300+	56%	60%	61%
Doctors 'Always' Communicated Well	300+	79%	81%	82%
Home Recovery Information Given	300+	85%	87%	85%
Hospital Given 9 or 10 on 10 Point Scale	300+	70%	71%	71%
Meds 'Always' Explained Before Given	300+	59%	64%	64%
Nurses 'Always' Communicated Well	300+	76%	80%	79%
Pain 'Always' Well Controlled	300+	67%	71%	71%
Room and Bathroom 'Always' Clean	300+	59%	73%	73%
Timely Help 'Always' Received	300+	61%	70%	68%
Would Definitely Recommend Hospital	300+	72%	71%	71%
Use of Medical Imaging				
Cardiac Imaging Stress Test before Surgery	2,660	4.6%	5.1%	5.3%
Combination Abdominal CT Scan	2,119	4.9%	8.7%	10.5%
Combination Brain/Sinus CT Scan	1,574	1.5%	2.2%	2.7%
Combination Chest CT Scan	1,819	1.1%	3.6%	2.7%
Follow-up Mammogram/Ultrasound	5,415	6.3%	8.2%	8.8%
Lumbar Spine MRI for Low Back Pain	396	37.6%	36.9%	37.2%

Straith Hospital For Special Surgery

23901 Lahser
Southfield, MI 48033
Phone: 248-357-3360
Type: Acute Care Hospitals
Emergency Services: No
Ownership: Voluntary non-profit - Private
Beds: 27
Key Personnel:
CEO/President. . . . . Gregory Hoose

Measure	Cases	This Hosp.	State Avg.	U.S. Avg.
Blood Clot Prevention and Treatment				
Anticoagulation Overlap Therapy[7]	-	-	90%	93%
ICU Venous Thromboembolism Prophylaxis[7]	-	-	93%	92%
Incidence of Potentially Preventable VTE[7]	-	-	8%	10%
UFH with Dosages/Platelet Monitoring[7]	-	-	96%	97%
Venous Thromboembolism Prophylaxis	447	99%	87%	85%
Warfarin Therapy Discharge Instructions[7]	-	-	72%	75%
Chest Pain/Possible Heart Attack Care				
Aspirin Given Within 24 Hours of Arrival[5]	-	-	96%	96%

NOTE: Hospital profiles are in alphabetical order by state, then city, then hospital within the city; Rankings exclude hospitals with less than 25 cases except for patient surveys which excludes hospitals with less than 100 cases; (a) 100-299 cases; (1) The number of cases/patients is too few to report; (2) Data submitted were based on a sample of cases/patients; (3) Results are based on a shorter time period than required; (4) Data suppressed by CMS for one or more quarters; (5) Results are not available for this reporting period; (6) Fewer than 100 patients completed the HCAHPS survey; (7) No cases met the criteria for this measure; (8) The lower limit of the confidence interval cannot be calculated if the number of observed infections equals zero; (9) No data are available from the state/territory for this reporting period; (10) The scores shown reflect fewer than 50 completed surveys; (11) There were discrepancies in the data collection process; (12) This measure does not apply to this hospital for this reporting period; (13) Results cannot be calculated for this reporting period; (14) The results for this state are combined with nearby states to protect confidentiality; Please refer to the User's Guide for a full explanation of data.

Measure	Cases	This Hosp.	State Avg.	U.S. Avg.
Fibrinolytic Meds Within 30 Min. of Arrival[5]	-	-	63%	58%
Average Time to ECG (minutes)[5]	-	-	8	7
Average Time to Transfer (minutes)[5]	-	-	53	60
Children's Asthma Care				
Received Home Management Plan of Care	-	-	-	88%
Received Reliever Medication	-	-	-	100%
Received Systemic Corticosteroids	-	-	-	100%
Emergency Department				
Admittance Decision Time (minutes)[2,7]	-	-	102	98
Head CT Results Within 45 Min. of Arrival[5]	-	-	54%	57%
Patients Who Left ER Before Being Seen[5]	-	-	2%	2%
Time from ER Arrival to Admit. (minutes)[2,7]	-	-	288	274
Time from ER Arrival to Discharge (minutes)[5]	-	-	128	134
Time in ER Before Being Evaluated (minutes)[5]	-	-	22	26
Time to Pain Meds for Fractures (minutes)[5]	-	-	55	57
Heart Attack Care				
Aspirin Given at Discharge[5]	-	-	99%	99%
Fibrinolytic Meds Within 30 Min. of Arrival[5]	-	-	20%	54%
PCI Within 90 Minutes of Arrival[5]	-	-	95%	96%
Statin Prescribed at Discharge[5]	-	-	98%	98%
Heart Failure Care				
ACE Inhibitor or ARB for LVSD[5]	-	-	96%	97%
Discharge Instructions Given[5]	-	-	94%	94%
Evaluation of LVS Function[5]	-	-	99%	99%
Medicare Spending				
Medicare Spending per Patient (ratio)	-	1.11	0.96	0.98
Pneumonia Care				
Appropriate Initial Antibiotic Given[5]	-	-	96%	95%
Blood Culture Timing[5]	-	-	98%	98%
Pregnancy and Delivery Care				
Newborn Deliveries Scheduled Early[7]	-	-	3%	6%
Preventive Care				
Immunization for Influenza[2]	285	98%	89%	90%
Immunization for Pneumonia[2]	562	97%	90%	92%
Stroke Care				
Anticoagulation Therapy for Atrial Fibrillation[5]	-	-	92%	95%
Antithrombotic Therapy Timing[5]	-	-	97%	98%
Assessed for Rehabilitation[5]	-	-	97%	97%
Discharged on Antithrombotic Therapy[5]	-	-	99%	99%
Discharged on Statin Medication[5]	-	-	94%	94%
Thrombolytic Therapy Timing[5]	-	-	69%	66%
Venous Thromboembolism Prophylaxis[5]	-	-	94%	94%
Written Stroke Educational Materials Given[5]	-	-	87%	88%
Surgical Care Improvement Project				
Appropriate Beta Blocker Usage[5]	-	-	98%	98%
Appropriate VTP Within 24 Hours[5]	-	-	98%	98%
Controlled Postoperative Blood Glucose[5]	-	-	97%	97%
Perioperative Temperature Management[5]	-	-	100%	100%
Prophylactic Antibiotic Selection[5]	-	-	99%	99%
Prophylactic Antibiotic Selection (Outpatient)[5]	-	-	97%	98%
Prophylactic Antibiotic Stopped[5]	-	-	98%	98%
Prophylactic Antibiotic Timing[5]	-	-	98%	99%
Prophylactic Antibiotic Timing (Outpatient)[5]	-	-	97%	98%
Urinary Catheter Removal[5]	-	-	97%	97%
Survey of Patients' Hospital Experiences				
Area Around Room 'Always' Quiet at Night[1]	-	-	60%	61%
Doctors 'Always' Communicated Well[1]	-	-	81%	82%
Home Recovery Information Given[1]	-	-	87%	85%
Hospital Given 9 or 10 on 10 Point Scale[1]	-	-	71%	71%
Meds 'Always' Explained Before Given[1]	-	-	64%	64%
Nurses 'Always' Communicated Well[1]	-	-	80%	79%
Pain 'Always' Well Controlled[1]	-	-	71%	71%
Room and Bathroom 'Always' Clean[1]	-	-	73%	73%
Timely Help 'Always' Received[1]	-	-	70%	68%
Would Definitely Recommend Hospital[1]	-	-	71%	71%
Use of Medical Imaging				
Cardiac Imaging Stress Test before Surgery[7]	-	-	5.1%	5.3%
Combination Abdominal CT Scan[7]	-	-	8.7%	10.5%
Combination Brain/Sinus CT Scan[7]	-	-	2.2%	2.7%
Combination Chest CT Scan[7]	-	-	3.6%	2.7%
Follow-up Mammogram/Ultrasound[7]	-	-	8.2%	8.8%
Lumbar Spine MRI for Low Back Pain[7]	-	-	36.9%	37.2%

Saint Mary's Standish Community Hospital

805 W Cedar St
Standish, MI 48658
Phone: 517-846-4521
Fax: 989-846-3549
Type: Critical Access Hospitals
Emergency Services: Yes
Ownership: Voluntary non-profit - Private
Beds: 68

Key Personnel:
Infection Control. . . . . Jean Lohr
Coronary Care . . . . Roxanne Lushnat
Quality Assurance . . . . Joe Nicholl
Chief of Medical Staff. . . . . Gordon Page, MD
CEO/President. . . . . Jeff Probus
Pediatric Ambulatory Care . . . . . . I Shamieh, MD
Pediatric In-Patient Care . . . . I Shamieh, MD
Operating Room. . . . . Kim Szostak, RN

Measure	Cases	This Hosp.	State Avg.	U.S. Avg.
Blood Clot Prevention and Treatment				
Anticoagulation Overlap Therapy[1,2]	-	-	90%	93%
ICU Venous Thromboembolism Prophylaxis[2]	20	65%	93%	92%
Incidence of Potentially Preventable VTE[2,7]	-	-	8%	10%
UFH with Dosages/Platelet Monitoring[1,2]	-	-	96%	97%
Venous Thromboembolism Prophylaxis[2]	82	32%	87%	85%
Warfarin Therapy Discharge Instructions[1,2]	-	-	72%	75%
Chest Pain/Possible Heart Attack Care				
Aspirin Given Within 24 Hours of Arrival	132	95%	96%	96%
Fibrinolytic Meds Within 30 Min. of Arrival[1]	-	-	63%	58%
Average Time to ECG (minutes)	133	20	8	7
Average Time to Transfer (minutes)[1]	-	-	53	60
Children's Asthma Care				
Received Home Management Plan of Care	-	-	-	88%
Received Reliever Medication	-	-	-	100%
Received Systemic Corticosteroids	-	-	-	100%
Emergency Department				
Admittance Decision Time (minutes)[5]	-	-	102	98
Head CT Results Within 45 Min. of Arrival[5]	-	-	54%	57%
Patients Who Left ER Before Being Seen[5]	-	-	2%	2%
Time from ER Arrival to Admit. (minutes)[5]	-	-	288	274
Time from ER Arrival to Discharge (minutes)	371	80	128	134
Time in ER Before Being Evaluated (minutes)	425	23	22	26
Time to Pain Meds for Fractures (minutes)[5]	-	-	55	57
Heart Attack Care				
Aspirin Given at Discharge	18	67%	99%	99%
Fibrinolytic Meds Within 30 Min. of Arrival[7]	-	-	20%	54%
PCI Within 90 Minutes of Arrival[7]	-	-	95%	96%
Statin Prescribed at Discharge	14	36%	98%	98%
Heart Failure Care				
ACE Inhibitor or ARB for LVSD[1]	-	-	96%	97%
Discharge Instructions Given	14	79%	94%	94%
Evaluation of LVS Function	19	74%	99%	99%
Medicare Spending				
Medicare Spending per Patient (ratio)	-	-	0.96	0.98
Pneumonia Care				
Appropriate Initial Antibiotic Given	28	96%	96%	95%
Blood Culture Timing	39	90%	98%	98%
Pregnancy and Delivery Care				
Newborn Deliveries Scheduled Early[5]	-	-	3%	6%
Preventive Care				
Immunization for Influenza[5]	-	-	89%	90%
Immunization for Pneumonia[5]	-	-	90%	92%
Stroke Care				
Anticoagulation Therapy for Atrial Fibrillation[1]	-	-	92%	95%
Antithrombotic Therapy Timing[1]	-	-	97%	98%
Assessed for Rehabilitation[1]	-	-	97%	97%
Discharged on Antithrombotic Therapy[1]	-	-	99%	99%
Discharged on Statin Medication[1]	-	-	94%	94%
Thrombolytic Therapy Timing[1]	-	-	69%	66%
Venous Thromboembolism Prophylaxis[1]	-	-	94%	94%
Written Stroke Educational Materials Given[1]	-	-	87%	88%
Surgical Care Improvement Project				
Appropriate Beta Blocker Usage[3,7]	-	-	98%	98%
Appropriate VTP Within 24 Hours[1,3]	-	-	98%	98%
Controlled Postoperative Blood Glucose[3,7]	-	-	97%	97%
Perioperative Temperature Management[1,3]	-	-	100%	100%
Prophylactic Antibiotic Selection[3,7]	-	-	99%	99%
Prophylactic Antibiotic Selection (Outpatient)[1,3]	-	-	97%	98%
Prophylactic Antibiotic Stopped[3,7]	-	-	98%	98%
Prophylactic Antibiotic Timing[3,7]	-	-	98%	99%
Prophylactic Antibiotic Timing (Outpatient)[1,3]	-	-	97%	98%
Urinary Catheter Removal[1,3]	-	-	97%	97%
Survey of Patients' Hospital Experiences				
Area Around Room 'Always' Quiet at Night	(a)	65%	60%	61%
Doctors 'Always' Communicated Well	(a)	85%	81%	82%
Home Recovery Information Given	(a)	89%	87%	85%
Hospital Given 9 or 10 on 10 Point Scale	(a)	76%	71%	71%
Meds 'Always' Explained Before Given	(a)	68%	64%	64%
Nurses 'Always' Communicated Well	(a)	80%	80%	79%
Pain 'Always' Well Controlled	(a)	76%	71%	71%
Room and Bathroom 'Always' Clean	(a)	69%	73%	73%
Timely Help 'Always' Received	(a)	79%	70%	68%
Would Definitely Recommend Hospital	(a)	67%	71%	71%
Use of Medical Imaging				
Cardiac Imaging Stress Test before Surgery	162	4.9%	5.1%	5.3%
Combination Abdominal CT Scan	445	8.3%	8.7%	10.5%
Combination Brain/Sinus CT Scan	280	0.4%	2.2%	2.7%
Combination Chest CT Scan	208	8.7%	3.6%	2.7%
Follow-up Mammogram/Ultrasound	337	6.8%	8.2%	8.8%
Lumbar Spine MRI for Low Back Pain	67	44.8%	36.9%	37.2%

Sturgis Hospital

916 Myrtle Ave
Sturgis, MI 49091
Phone: 269-651-7824
Fax: 269-659-6713
URL: www.sturgishospital.com
Type: Acute Care Hospitals
Emergency Services: Yes
Ownership: Government - Local
Beds: 94

Key Personnel:
Cardiac Laboratory. . . . . Shirley Betts
Operating Room. . . . . Martha Gillespie
Chief of Medical Staff . . . . Edward Griffin, MD
Infection Control. . . . . Sarah Hagen
Radiology. . . . . John C Kirkpatrick, MD
CEO/President. . . . . John Mayor
Quality Assurance . . . . Shari Ransberger, RN

Measure	Cases	This Hosp.	State Avg.	U.S. Avg.
Blood Clot Prevention and Treatment				
Anticoagulation Overlap Therapy[2]	17	100%	90%	93%
ICU Venous Thromboembolism Prophylaxis[1,2]	-	-	93%	92%
Incidence of Potentially Preventable VTE[2,7]	-	-	8%	10%
UFH with Dosages/Platelet Monitoring[1,2]	-	-	96%	97%
Venous Thromboembolism Prophylaxis[2]	109	80%	87%	85%
Warfarin Therapy Discharge Instructions[2]	15	87%	72%	75%
Chest Pain/Possible Heart Attack Care				
Aspirin Given Within 24 Hours of Arrival	65	91%	96%	96%
Fibrinolytic Meds Within 30 Min. of Arrival[7]	-	-	63%	58%
Average Time to ECG (minutes)	72	0	8	7
Average Time to Transfer (minutes)	14	55	53	60
Children's Asthma Care				
Received Home Management Plan of Care	-	-	-	88%
Received Reliever Medication	-	-	-	100%
Received Systemic Corticosteroids	-	-	-	100%
Emergency Department				
Admittance Decision Time (minutes)[2]	173	50	102	98
Head CT Results Within 45 Min. of Arrival[1]	-	-	54%	57%
Patients Who Left ER Before Being Seen	15,568	1%	2%	2%
Time from ER Arrival to Admit. (minutes)[2]	186	208	288	274
Time from ER Arrival to Discharge (minutes)	332	96	128	134
Time in ER Before Being Evaluated (minutes)	355	23	22	26
Time to Pain Meds for Fractures (minutes)	77	43	55	57
Heart Attack Care				
Aspirin Given at Discharge[1,3]	-	-	99%	99%
Fibrinolytic Meds Within 30 Min. of Arrival[3,7]	-	-	20%	54%
PCI Within 90 Minutes of Arrival[3,7]	-	-	95%	96%
Statin Prescribed at Discharge[1,3]	-	-	98%	98%
Heart Failure Care				
ACE Inhibitor or ARB for LVSD[1]	-	-	96%	97%
Discharge Instructions Given	37	97%	94%	94%
Evaluation of LVS Function	51	96%	99%	99%
Medicare Spending				
Medicare Spending per Patient (ratio)	-	0.95	0.96	0.98
Pneumonia Care				

NOTE: Hospital profiles are in alphabetical order by state, then city, then hospital within the city; Rankings exclude hospitals with less than 25 cases except for patient surveys which excludes hospitals with less than 100 cases; (a) 100-299 cases; (1) The number of cases/patients is too few to report; (2) Data submitted were based on a sample of cases/patients; (3) Results are based on a shorter time period than required; (4) Data suppressed by CMS for one or more quarters; (5) Results are not available for this reporting period; (6) Fewer than 100 patients completed the HCAHPS survey; (7) No cases met the criteria for this measure; (8) The lower limit of the confidence interval cannot be calculated if the number of observed infections equals zero; (9) No data are available from the state/territory for this reporting period; (10) The scores shown reflect fewer than 50 completed surveys; (11) There were discrepancies in the data collection process; (12) This measure does not apply to this hospital for this reporting period; (13) Results cannot be calculated for this reporting period; (14) The results for this state are combined with nearby states to protect confidentiality; Please refer to the User's Guide for a full explanation of data.

Measure	Cases	This Hosp.	State Avg.	U.S. Avg.
Appropriate Initial Antibiotic Given	42	79%	96%	95%
Blood Culture Timing	70	97%	98%	98%
Pregnancy and Delivery Care				
Newborn Deliveries Scheduled Early[2]	38	3%	3%	6%
Preventive Care				
Immunization for Influenza[2]	234	96%	89%	90%
Immunization for Pneumonia[2]	274	99%	90%	92%
Stroke Care				
Anticoagulation Therapy for Atrial Fibrillation[1]	-	-	92%	95%
Antithrombotic Therapy Timing[1]	-	-	97%	98%
Assessed for Rehabilitation[1]	-	-	97%	97%
Discharged on Antithrombotic Therapy[1]	-	-	99%	99%
Discharged on Statin Medication[1]	-	-	94%	94%
Thrombolytic Therapy Timing[1]	-	-	69%	66%
Venous Thromboembolism Prophylaxis[1]	-	-	94%	94%
Written Stroke Educational Materials Given[1]	-	-	87%	88%
Surgical Care Improvement Project				
Appropriate Beta Blocker Usage	25	84%	98%	98%
Appropriate VTP Within 24 Hours	89	100%	98%	98%
Controlled Postoperative Blood Glucose[7]	-	-	97%	97%
Perioperative Temperature Management	105	100%	100%	100%
Prophylactic Antibiotic Selection	73	100%	99%	99%
Prophylactic Antibiotic Selection (Outpatient)	56	96%	97%	98%
Prophylactic Antibiotic Stopped	69	94%	98%	98%
Prophylactic Antibiotic Timing	73	99%	98%	99%
Prophylactic Antibiotic Timing (Outpatient)	53	94%	97%	98%
Urinary Catheter Removal	64	97%	97%	97%
Survey of Patients' Hospital Experiences				
Area Around Room 'Always' Quiet at Night	300+	60%	60%	61%
Doctors 'Always' Communicated Well	300+	82%	81%	82%
Home Recovery Information Given	300+	88%	87%	85%
Hospital Given 9 or 10 on 10 Point Scale	300+	72%	71%	71%
Meds 'Always' Explained Before Given	300+	65%	64%	64%
Nurses 'Always' Communicated Well	300+	82%	80%	79%
Pain 'Always' Well Controlled	300+	76%	71%	71%
Room and Bathroom 'Always' Clean	300+	79%	73%	73%
Timely Help 'Always' Received	300+	70%	70%	68%
Would Definitely Recommend Hospital	300+	67%	71%	71%
Use of Medical Imaging				
Cardiac Imaging Stress Test before Surgery	307	7.5%	5.1%	5.3%
Combination Abdominal CT Scan	368	3.0%	8.7%	10.5%
Combination Brain/Sinus CT Scan[1]	-	-	2.2%	2.7%
Combination Chest CT Scan	214	1.9%	3.6%	2.7%
Follow-up Mammogram/Ultrasound	537	5.4%	8.2%	8.8%
Lumbar Spine MRI for Low Back Pain	49	32.7%	36.9%	37.2%

Tawas Saint Joseph Hospital

200 Hemlock
Tawas City, MI 48764
URL: www.sjhsys.org
Phone: 989-362-9301
Fax: 989-362-9376
Type: Acute Care Hospitals
Ownership: Govt - Hospital Dist/Auth
Emergency Services: Yes
Beds: 49

Key Personnel:
Patient Relations . . . . Martie Hang
Anesthesiology. . . . . Jon Kaliszewski, MD
CEO/President. . . . . Patrick J Murtha
Operating Room. . . . . Pat Visscher

Measure	Cases	This Hosp.	State Avg.	U.S. Avg.
Blood Clot Prevention and Treatment				
Anticoagulation Overlap Therapy[1,2]	-	-	90%	93%
ICU Venous Thromboembolism Prophylaxis[2]	23	100%	93%	92%
Incidence of Potentially Preventable VTE[2,7]	-	-	8%	10%
UFH with Dosages/Platelet Monitoring[1,2]	-	-	96%	97%
Venous Thromboembolism Prophylaxis[2]	95	93%	87%	85%
Warfarin Therapy Discharge Instructions[1,2]	-	-	72%	75%
Chest Pain/Possible Heart Attack Care				
Aspirin Given Within 24 Hours of Arrival	180	97%	96%	96%
Fibrinolytic Meds Within 30 Min. of Arrival	27	59%	63%	58%
Average Time to ECG (minutes)	182	4	8	7
Average Time to Transfer (minutes)[7]	-	-	53	60
Children's Asthma Care				
Received Home Management Plan of Care	-	-	-	88%
Received Reliever Medication	-	-	-	100%
Received Systemic Corticosteroids	-	-	-	100%
Emergency Department				
Admittance Decision Time (minutes)[2]	286	52	102	98
Head CT Results Within 45 Min. of Arrival	11	73%	54%	57%
Patients Who Left ER Before Being Seen	16,843	1%	2%	2%
Time from ER Arrival to Admit. (minutes)[2]	297	213	288	274
Time from ER Arrival to Discharge (minutes)	377	100	128	134
Time in ER Before Being Evaluated (minutes)	411	26	22	26
Time to Pain Meds for Fractures (minutes)	72	47	55	57
Heart Attack Care				
Aspirin Given at Discharge[1,3]	-	-	99%	99%
Fibrinolytic Meds Within 30 Min. of Arrival[3,7]	-	-	20%	54%
PCI Within 90 Minutes of Arrival[3,7]	-	-	95%	96%
Statin Prescribed at Discharge[1,3]	-	-	98%	98%
Heart Failure Care				
ACE Inhibitor or ARB for LVSD	14	93%	96%	97%
Discharge Instructions Given	42	98%	94%	94%
Evaluation of LVS Function	52	98%	99%	99%
Medicare Spending				
Medicare Spending per Patient (ratio)	-	0.91	0.96	0.98
Pneumonia Care				
Appropriate Initial Antibiotic Given	49	98%	96%	95%
Blood Culture Timing	86	98%	98%	98%
Pregnancy and Delivery Care				
Newborn Deliveries Scheduled Early	12	0%	3%	6%
Preventive Care				
Immunization for Influenza[2]	258	98%	89%	90%
Immunization for Pneumonia[2]	305	93%	90%	92%
Stroke Care				
Anticoagulation Therapy for Atrial Fibrillation[1]	-	-	92%	95%
Antithrombotic Therapy Timing[1]	-	-	97%	98%
Assessed for Rehabilitation[1]	-	-	97%	97%
Discharged on Antithrombotic Therapy[1]	-	-	99%	99%
Discharged on Statin Medication[1]	-	-	94%	94%
Thrombolytic Therapy Timing[1]	-	-	69%	66%
Venous Thromboembolism Prophylaxis[1]	-	-	94%	94%
Written Stroke Educational Materials Given[1]	-	-	87%	88%
Surgical Care Improvement Project				
Appropriate Beta Blocker Usage	56	96%	98%	98%
Appropriate VTP Within 24 Hours	140	100%	98%	98%
Controlled Postoperative Blood Glucose[7]	-	-	97%	97%
Perioperative Temperature Management	161	100%	100%	100%
Prophylactic Antibiotic Selection	130	100%	99%	99%
Prophylactic Antibiotic Selection (Outpatient)	36	94%	97%	98%
Prophylactic Antibiotic Stopped	130	98%	98%	98%
Prophylactic Antibiotic Timing	130	100%	98%	99%
Prophylactic Antibiotic Timing (Outpatient)	37	95%	97%	98%
Urinary Catheter Removal	121	99%	97%	97%
Survey of Patients' Hospital Experiences				
Area Around Room 'Always' Quiet at Night	300+	65%	60%	61%
Doctors 'Always' Communicated Well	300+	81%	81%	82%
Home Recovery Information Given	300+	87%	87%	85%
Hospital Given 9 or 10 on 10 Point Scale	300+	69%	71%	71%
Meds 'Always' Explained Before Given	300+	64%	64%	64%
Nurses 'Always' Communicated Well	300+	80%	80%	79%
Pain 'Always' Well Controlled	300+	72%	71%	71%
Room and Bathroom 'Always' Clean	300+	74%	73%	73%
Timely Help 'Always' Received	300+	76%	70%	68%
Would Definitely Recommend Hospital	300+	67%	71%	71%
Use of Medical Imaging				
Cardiac Imaging Stress Test before Surgery	444	4.3%	5.1%	5.3%
Combination Abdominal CT Scan	743	17.5%	8.7%	10.5%
Combination Brain/Sinus CT Scan	621	2.6%	2.2%	2.7%
Combination Chest CT Scan	388	18.8%	3.6%	2.7%
Follow-up Mammogram/Ultrasound	1,216	4.0%	8.2%	8.8%
Lumbar Spine MRI for Low Back Pain	131	47.3%	36.9%	37.2%

Oakwood Hospital - Taylor

10000 Telegraph Road
Taylor, MI 48180
E-mail: leijas@oakwood.org
URL: www.oakwod.org
Phone: 313-295-5253
Fax: 313-295-5085
Type: Acute Care Hospitals
Ownership: Govt - Hospital Dist/Auth
Emergency Services: Yes
Beds: 248

Key Personnel:
President/CEO. . . . . Brain Connolly
Quality Assurance . . . . Maureen D'Agostino
Chief of Medical Staff. . . . . Malcolm Henoch, MD
Coronary Care. . . . . Abil Karamali
Operating Room. . . . . Sameeh Kawar
Quality Assurance . . . . Tina Lowery
Emergency Room . . . . Deb Vogel, RN

Measure	Cases	This Hosp.	State Avg.	U.S. Avg.
Blood Clot Prevention and Treatment				
Anticoagulation Overlap Therapy[2]	54	87%	90%	93%
ICU Venous Thromboembolism Prophylaxis[2]	64	89%	93%	92%
Incidence of Potentially Preventable VTE[1,2]	-	-	8%	10%
UFH with Dosages/Platelet Monitoring[2]	55	100%	96%	97%
Venous Thromboembolism Prophylaxis[2]	320	83%	87%	85%
Warfarin Therapy Discharge Instructions[2]	33	0%	72%	75%
Chest Pain/Possible Heart Attack Care				
Aspirin Given Within 24 Hours of Arrival	59	98%	96%	96%
Fibrinolytic Meds Within 30 Min. of Arrival[7]	-	-	63%	58%
Average Time to ECG (minutes)	60	5	8	7
Average Time to Transfer (minutes)	16	46	53	60
Children's Asthma Care				
Received Home Management Plan of Care	-	-	-	88%
Received Reliever Medication	-	-	-	100%
Received Systemic Corticosteroids	-	-	-	100%
Emergency Department				
Admittance Decision Time (minutes)[2]	593	119	102	98
Head CT Results Within 45 Min. of Arrival[1]	-	-	54%	57%
Patients Who Left ER Before Being Seen	31,654	4%	2%	2%
Time from ER Arrival to Admit. (minutes)[2]	593	351	288	274
Time from ER Arrival to Discharge (minutes)	332	173	128	134
Time in ER Before Being Evaluated (minutes)	362	32	22	26
Time to Pain Meds for Fractures (minutes)	83	60	55	57
Heart Attack Care				
Aspirin Given at Discharge[1]	-	-	99%	99%
Fibrinolytic Meds Within 30 Min. of Arrival[7]	-	-	20%	54%
PCI Within 90 Minutes of Arrival[7]	-	-	95%	96%
Statin Prescribed at Discharge	11	100%	98%	98%
Heart Failure Care				
ACE Inhibitor or ARB for LVSD	51	100%	96%	97%
Discharge Instructions Given	88	94%	94%	94%
Evaluation of LVS Function	141	100%	99%	99%
Medicare Spending				
Medicare Spending per Patient (ratio)	-	1.10	0.96	0.98
Pneumonia Care				
Appropriate Initial Antibiotic Given[2]	81	95%	96%	95%
Blood Culture Timing[2]	171	99%	98%	98%
Pregnancy and Delivery Care				
Newborn Deliveries Scheduled Early[7]	-	-	3%	6%
Preventive Care				
Immunization for Influenza[2]	581	91%	89%	90%
Immunization for Pneumonia[2]	798	95%	90%	92%
Stroke Care				
Anticoagulation Therapy for Atrial Fibrillation[1]	-	-	92%	95%
Antithrombotic Therapy Timing	50	94%	97%	98%
Assessed for Rehabilitation	50	90%	97%	97%
Discharged on Antithrombotic Therapy	49	86%	99%	99%
Discharged on Statin Medication	41	68%	94%	94%
Thrombolytic Therapy Timing[1]	-	-	69%	66%
Venous Thromboembolism Prophylaxis	49	86%	94%	94%
Written Stroke Educational Materials Given	25	32%	87%	88%
Surgical Care Improvement Project				
Appropriate Beta Blocker Usage[2]	102	99%	98%	98%
Appropriate VTP Within 24 Hours[2]	269	100%	98%	98%
Controlled Postoperative Blood Glucose[2,7]	-	-	97%	97%
Perioperative Temperature Management[2]	278	100%	100%	100%
Prophylactic Antibiotic Selection[2]	199	100%	99%	99%

NOTE: Hospital profiles are in alphabetical order by state, then city, then hospital within the city; Rankings exclude hospitals with less than 25 cases except for patient surveys which excludes hospitals with less than 100 cases; (a) 100-299 cases; (1) The number of cases/patients is too few to report; (2) Data submitted were based on a sample of cases/patients; (3) Results are based on a shorter time period than required; (4) Data suppressed by CMS for one or more quarters; (5) Results are not available for this reporting period; (6) Fewer than 100 patients completed the HCAHPS survey; (7) No cases met the criteria for this measure; (8) The lower limit of the confidence interval cannot be calculated if the number of observed infections equals zero; (9) No data are available from the state/territory for this reporting period; (10) The scores shown reflect fewer than 50 completed surveys; (11) There were discrepancies in the data collection process; (12) This measure does not apply to this hospital for this reporting period; (13) Results cannot be calculated for this reporting period; (14) The results for this state are combined with nearby states to protect confidentiality; Please refer to the User's Guide for a full explanation of data.

Measure	Cases	This Hosp.	State Avg.	U.S. Avg.
Prophylactic Antibiotic Selection (Outpatient)	14	86%	97%	98%
Prophylactic Antibiotic Stopped[2]	186	99%	98%	98%
Prophylactic Antibiotic Timing[2]	199	100%	98%	99%
Prophylactic Antibiotic Timing (Outpatient)	14	100%	97%	98%
Urinary Catheter Removal[2]	66	97%	97%	97%
Survey of Patients' Hospital Experiences				
Area Around Room 'Always' Quiet at Night	300+	58%	60%	61%
Doctors 'Always' Communicated Well	300+	80%	81%	82%
Home Recovery Information Given	300+	87%	87%	85%
Hospital Given 9 or 10 on 10 Point Scale	300+	74%	71%	71%
Meds 'Always' Explained Before Given	300+	68%	64%	64%
Nurses 'Always' Communicated Well	300+	84%	80%	79%
Pain 'Always' Well Controlled	300+	76%	71%	71%
Room and Bathroom 'Always' Clean	300+	71%	73%	73%
Timely Help 'Always' Received	300+	75%	70%	68%
Would Definitely Recommend Hospital	300+	73%	71%	71%
Use of Medical Imaging				
Cardiac Imaging Stress Test before Surgery	248	5.2%	5.1%	5.3%
Combination Abdominal CT Scan	449	5.3%	8.7%	10.5%
Combination Brain/Sinus CT Scan[1]	-	-	2.2%	2.7%
Combination Chest CT Scan	267	1.1%	3.6%	2.7%
Follow-up Mammogram/Ultrasound	745	9.3%	8.2%	8.8%
Lumbar Spine MRI for Low Back Pain	51	41.2%	36.9%	37.2%

Promedica Herrick Hospital

500 E Pottawatamie Street
Tecumseh, MI 49286
URL: www.promedica.org/herrick
Type: Critical Access Hospitals
Ownership: Government - Federal

Phone: 517-424-3000
Fax: 517-424-3900

Emergency Services: Yes
Beds: 100

Key Personnel:
Surgery . . . . Emmett Boyle
Anesthesiology. . . . . Cathy Cook, D.O.
Intensive Care Unit. . . . . Christine Mathis
Operating Room. . . . . Marcia Olieman
CEO/President. . . . . Randy Oostra
Chair/CEO . . . . Stephen Staelin, MD
Emergency Room . . . . Rosalie Turek, MD
Quality Assurance . . . . Linda Yielding

Measure	Cases	This Hosp.	State Avg.	U.S. Avg.
Blood Clot Prevention and Treatment				
Anticoagulation Overlap Therapy[1,2]	-	-	90%	93%
ICU Venous Thromboembolism Prophylaxis[2]	25	84%	93%	92%
Incidence of Potentially Preventable VTE[2,7]	-	-	8%	10%
UFH with Dosages/Platelet Monitoring[1,2]	-	-	96%	97%
Venous Thromboembolism Prophylaxis[2]	71	85%	87%	85%
Warfarin Therapy Discharge Instructions[1,2]	-	-	72%	75%
Chest Pain/Possible Heart Attack Care				
Aspirin Given Within 24 Hours of Arrival	70	97%	96%	96%
Fibrinolytic Meds Within 30 Min. of Arrival[1]	-	-	63%	58%
Average Time to ECG (minutes)	74	7	8	7
Average Time to Transfer (minutes)[7]	-	-	53	60
Children's Asthma Care				
Received Home Management Plan of Care	-	-	-	88%
Received Reliever Medication	-	-	-	100%
Received Systemic Corticosteroids	-	-	-	100%
Emergency Department				
Admittance Decision Time (minutes)[2]	419	77	102	98
Head CT Results Within 45 Min. of Arrival[1]	-	-	54%	57%
Patients Who Left ER Before Being Seen[5]	-	-	2%	2%
Time from ER Arrival to Admit. (minutes)[2]	419	217	288	274
Time from ER Arrival to Discharge (minutes)	321	91	128	134
Time in ER Before Being Evaluated (minutes)	384	2	22	26
Time to Pain Meds for Fractures (minutes)	60	40	55	57
Heart Attack Care				
Aspirin Given at Discharge[1]	-	-	99%	99%
Fibrinolytic Meds Within 30 Min. of Arrival[7]	-	-	20%	54%
PCI Within 90 Minutes of Arrival[7]	-	-	95%	96%
Statin Prescribed at Discharge[1]	-	-	98%	98%
Heart Failure Care				
ACE Inhibitor or ARB for LVSD[1]	-	-	96%	97%
Discharge Instructions Given	39	85%	94%	94%
Evaluation of LVS Function	50	100%	99%	99%
Medicare Spending				
Medicare Spending per Patient (ratio)	-	-	0.96	0.98
Pneumonia Care				
Appropriate Initial Antibiotic Given	32	100%	96%	95%
Blood Culture Timing	47	100%	98%	98%
Pregnancy and Delivery Care				
Newborn Deliveries Scheduled Early[5]	-	-	3%	6%
Preventive Care				
Immunization for Influenza[2]	287	95%	89%	90%
Immunization for Pneumonia[2]	466	93%	90%	92%
Stroke Care				
Anticoagulation Therapy for Atrial Fibrillation[7]	-	-	92%	95%
Antithrombotic Therapy Timing	14	100%	97%	98%
Assessed for Rehabilitation	14	100%	97%	97%
Discharged on Antithrombotic Therapy	14	100%	99%	99%
Discharged on Statin Medication	12	83%	94%	94%
Thrombolytic Therapy Timing[7]	-	-	69%	66%
Venous Thromboembolism Prophylaxis	15	93%	94%	94%
Written Stroke Educational Materials Given[1]	-	-	87%	88%
Surgical Care Improvement Project				
Appropriate Beta Blocker Usage[2]	35	100%	98%	98%
Appropriate VTP Within 24 Hours[2]	89	100%	98%	98%
Controlled Postoperative Blood Glucose[2,7]	-	-	97%	97%
Perioperative Temperature Management[2]	101	100%	100%	100%
Prophylactic Antibiotic Selection[2]	72	100%	99%	99%
Prophylactic Antibiotic Selection (Outpatient)	12	83%	97%	98%
Prophylactic Antibiotic Stopped[2]	68	99%	98%	98%
Prophylactic Antibiotic Timing[2]	72	99%	98%	99%
Prophylactic Antibiotic Timing (Outpatient)	13	85%	97%	98%
Urinary Catheter Removal[2]	81	95%	97%	97%
Survey of Patients' Hospital Experiences				
Area Around Room 'Always' Quiet at Night	(a)	65%	60%	61%
Doctors 'Always' Communicated Well	(a)	82%	81%	82%
Home Recovery Information Given	(a)	91%	87%	85%
Hospital Given 9 or 10 on 10 Point Scale	(a)	74%	71%	71%
Meds 'Always' Explained Before Given	(a)	65%	64%	64%
Nurses 'Always' Communicated Well	(a)	82%	80%	79%
Pain 'Always' Well Controlled	(a)	72%	71%	71%
Room and Bathroom 'Always' Clean	(a)	76%	73%	73%
Timely Help 'Always' Received	(a)	71%	70%	68%
Would Definitely Recommend Hospital	(a)	73%	71%	71%
Use of Medical Imaging				
Cardiac Imaging Stress Test before Surgery	177	4.5%	5.1%	5.3%
Combination Abdominal CT Scan	265	4.2%	8.7%	10.5%
Combination Brain/Sinus CT Scan[1]	-	-	2.2%	2.7%
Combination Chest CT Scan	125	0.0%	3.6%	2.7%
Follow-up Mammogram/Ultrasound	1,082	9.9%	8.2%	8.8%
Lumbar Spine MRI for Low Back Pain[7]	-	-	36.9%	37.2%

Three Rivers Health

701 S Health Parkway
Three Rivers, MI 49093
E-mail: info@threerivershealth.org
URL: www.threerivershealth.org
Type: Acute Care Hospitals
Ownership: Govt - Hospital Dist/Auth

Phone: 269-273-9602
Fax: 269-273-9611

Emergency Services: Yes
Beds: 60

Key Personnel:
Radiology. . . . . George J Balogh
Emergency Room . . . . Brian Bowdich, MD
Chairman/CEO . . . . Larry Clark
Operating Room. . . . . Jo Lindsley, RN
Anesthesiology. . . . . Lalitha Mutnal, MD

Measure	Cases	This Hosp.	State Avg.	U.S. Avg.
Blood Clot Prevention and Treatment				
Anticoagulation Overlap Therapy[1,2]	-	-	90%	93%
ICU Venous Thromboembolism Prophylaxis[2]	92	86%	93%	92%
Incidence of Potentially Preventable VTE[1,2]	-	-	8%	10%
UFH with Dosages/Platelet Monitoring[1,2]	-	-	96%	97%
Venous Thromboembolism Prophylaxis[2]	582	90%	87%	85%
Warfarin Therapy Discharge Instructions[1,2]	-	-	72%	75%
Chest Pain/Possible Heart Attack Care				
Aspirin Given Within 24 Hours of Arrival	237	73%	96%	96%
Fibrinolytic Meds Within 30 Min. of Arrival[1]	-	-	63%	58%
Average Time to ECG (minutes)	250	10	8	7
Average Time to Transfer (minutes)	13	54	53	60
Children's Asthma Care				
Received Home Management Plan of Care	-	-	-	88%
Received Reliever Medication	-	-	-	100%
Received Systemic Corticosteroids	-	-	-	100%
Emergency Department				
Admittance Decision Time (minutes)[2]	349	60	102	98
Head CT Results Within 45 Min. of Arrival	14	29%	54%	57%
Patients Who Left ER Before Being Seen	20,605	1%	2%	2%
Time from ER Arrival to Admit. (minutes)[2]	367	232	288	274
Time from ER Arrival to Discharge (minutes)	602	101	128	134
Time in ER Before Being Evaluated (minutes)	682	28	22	26
Time to Pain Meds for Fractures (minutes)	83	40	55	57
Heart Attack Care				
Aspirin Given at Discharge[1,3]	-	-	99%	99%
Fibrinolytic Meds Within 30 Min. of Arrival[3,7]	-	-	20%	54%
PCI Within 90 Minutes of Arrival[3,7]	-	-	95%	96%
Statin Prescribed at Discharge[1,3]	-	-	98%	98%
Heart Failure Care				
ACE Inhibitor or ARB for LVSD	16	88%	96%	97%
Discharge Instructions Given	61	97%	94%	94%
Evaluation of LVS Function	72	97%	99%	99%
Medicare Spending				
Medicare Spending per Patient (ratio)	-	0.95	0.96	0.98
Pneumonia Care				
Appropriate Initial Antibiotic Given	58	91%	96%	95%
Blood Culture Timing	87	93%	98%	98%
Pregnancy and Delivery Care				
Newborn Deliveries Scheduled Early	23	0%	3%	6%
Preventive Care				
Immunization for Influenza[2]	261	84%	89%	90%
Immunization for Pneumonia[2]	389	80%	90%	92%
Stroke Care				
Anticoagulation Therapy for Atrial Fibrillation[1]	-	-	92%	95%
Antithrombotic Therapy Timing	12	92%	97%	98%
Assessed for Rehabilitation	11	91%	97%	97%
Discharged on Antithrombotic Therapy	11	91%	99%	99%
Discharged on Statin Medication[1]	-	-	94%	94%
Thrombolytic Therapy Timing[1]	-	-	69%	66%
Venous Thromboembolism Prophylaxis	13	77%	94%	94%
Written Stroke Educational Materials Given[1]	-	-	87%	88%
Surgical Care Improvement Project				
Appropriate Beta Blocker Usage[1]	-	-	98%	98%
Appropriate VTP Within 24 Hours	20	75%	98%	98%
Controlled Postoperative Blood Glucose[7]	-	-	97%	97%
Perioperative Temperature Management	26	100%	100%	100%
Prophylactic Antibiotic Selection	17	88%	99%	99%
Prophylactic Antibiotic Selection (Outpatient)[3]	23	91%	97%	98%
Prophylactic Antibiotic Stopped	17	100%	98%	98%
Prophylactic Antibiotic Timing	17	94%	98%	99%
Prophylactic Antibiotic Timing (Outpatient)[3]	23	96%	97%	98%
Urinary Catheter Removal	14	79%	97%	97%
Survey of Patients' Hospital Experiences				
Area Around Room 'Always' Quiet at Night	(a)	62%	60%	61%
Doctors 'Always' Communicated Well	(a)	73%	81%	82%
Home Recovery Information Given	(a)	86%	87%	85%
Hospital Given 9 or 10 on 10 Point Scale	(a)	64%	71%	71%
Meds 'Always' Explained Before Given	(a)	62%	64%	64%
Nurses 'Always' Communicated Well	(a)	77%	80%	79%
Pain 'Always' Well Controlled	(a)	72%	71%	71%
Room and Bathroom 'Always' Clean	(a)	77%	73%	73%
Timely Help 'Always' Received	(a)	69%	70%	68%
Would Definitely Recommend Hospital	(a)	60%	71%	71%
Use of Medical Imaging				
Cardiac Imaging Stress Test before Surgery	191	3.1%	5.1%	5.3%
Combination Abdominal CT Scan	338	7.4%	8.7%	10.5%
Combination Brain/Sinus CT Scan[1]	-	-	2.2%	2.7%
Combination Chest CT Scan	185	2.2%	3.6%	2.7%
Follow-up Mammogram/Ultrasound	324	5.2%	8.2%	8.8%
Lumbar Spine MRI for Low Back Pain	53	37.7%	36.9%	37.2%

NOTE: Hospital profiles are in alphabetical order by state, then city, then hospital within the city; Rankings exclude hospitals with less than 25 cases except for patient surveys which excludes hospitals with less than 100 cases; (a) 100-299 cases; (1) The number of cases/patients is too few to report; (2) Data submitted were based on a sample of cases/patients; (3) Results are based on a shorter time period than required; (4) Data suppressed by CMS for one or more quarters; (5) Results are not available for this reporting period; (6) Fewer than 100 patients completed the HCAHPS survey; (7) No cases met the criteria for this measure; (8) The lower limit of the confidence interval cannot be calculated if the number of observed infections equals zero; (9) No data are available from the state/territory for this reporting period; (10) The scores shown reflect fewer than 50 completed surveys; (11) There were discrepancies in the data collection process; (12) This measure does not apply to this hospital for this reporting period; (13) Results cannot be calculated for this reporting period; (14) The results for this state are combined with nearby states to protect confidentiality; Please refer to the User's Guide for a full explanation of data.

Munson Medical Center

1105 Sixth Street
Traverse City, MI 49684
E-mail: contact@mhc.net
URL: www.munsonhealthcare.org
Type: Acute Care Hospitals
Ownership: Voluntary non-profit - Other
Phone: 231-935-5000
Fax: 231-935-6548
Emergency Services: Yes
Beds: 391

Key Personnel:
Chair/CEO . . . . Rex Antinozzi, MD
CEO/President. . . . . K Douglas Deck
Patient Relations . . . . Jim P Fischer
Quality Assurance . . . . Terry Haslinger

Measure	Cases	This Hosp.	State Avg.	U.S. Avg.
Blood Clot Prevention and Treatment				
Anticoagulation Overlap Therapy[2]	112	94%	90%	93%
ICU Venous Thromboembolism Prophylaxis[2]	26	96%	93%	92%
Incidence of Potentially Preventable VTE[2]	24	12%	8%	10%
UFH with Dosages/Platelet Monitoring[2]	84	100%	96%	97%
Venous Thromboembolism Prophylaxis[2]	430	90%	87%	85%
Warfarin Therapy Discharge Instructions[2]	88	33%	72%	75%
Chest Pain/Possible Heart Attack Care				
Aspirin Given Within 24 Hours of Arrival[1,3]	-	-	96%	96%
Fibrinolytic Meds Within 30 Min. of Arrival[5]	-	-	63%	58%
Average Time to ECG (minutes)[1,3]	-	-	8	7
Average Time to Transfer (minutes)[5]	-	-	53	60
Children's Asthma Care				
Received Home Management Plan of Care	-	-	-	88%
Received Reliever Medication	-	-	-	100%
Received Systemic Corticosteroids	-	-	-	100%
Emergency Department				
Admittance Decision Time (minutes)[2]	523	177	102	98
Head CT Results Within 45 Min. of Arrival[1]	-	-	54%	57%
Patients Who Left ER Before Being Seen	25,657	1%	2%	2%
Time from ER Arrival to Admit. (minutes)[2]	532	326	288	274
Time from ER Arrival to Discharge (minutes)	393	159	128	134
Time in ER Before Being Evaluated (minutes)	454	19	22	26
Time to Pain Meds for Fractures (minutes)	146	53	55	57
Heart Attack Care				
Aspirin Given at Discharge[2]	347	100%	99%	99%
Fibrinolytic Meds Within 30 Min. of Arrival[2,7]	-	-	20%	54%
PCI Within 90 Minutes of Arrival[2]	29	97%	95%	96%
Statin Prescribed at Discharge[2]	312	100%	98%	98%
Heart Failure Care				
ACE Inhibitor or ARB for LVSD[2]	90	93%	96%	97%
Discharge Instructions Given[2]	286	97%	94%	94%
Evaluation of LVS Function[2]	330	100%	99%	99%
Medicare Spending				
Medicare Spending per Patient (ratio)	-	0.90	0.96	0.98
Pneumonia Care				
Appropriate Initial Antibiotic Given[2]	114	99%	96%	95%
Blood Culture Timing[2]	201	99%	98%	98%
Pregnancy and Delivery Care				
Newborn Deliveries Scheduled Early[2]	28	0%	3%	6%
Preventive Care				
Immunization for Influenza[2]	605	97%	89%	90%
Immunization for Pneumonia[2]	801	93%	90%	92%
Stroke Care				
Anticoagulation Therapy for Atrial Fibrillation[2]	20	100%	92%	95%
Antithrombotic Therapy Timing[2]	99	100%	97%	98%
Assessed for Rehabilitation[2]	126	98%	97%	97%
Discharged on Antithrombotic Therapy[2]	116	99%	99%	99%
Discharged on Statin Medication[2]	84	100%	94%	94%
Thrombolytic Therapy Timing[2]	23	74%	69%	66%
Venous Thromboembolism Prophylaxis[2]	135	93%	94%	94%
Written Stroke Educational Materials Given[2]	68	93%	87%	88%
Surgical Care Improvement Project				
Appropriate Beta Blocker Usage[2]	333	100%	98%	98%
Appropriate VTP Within 24 Hours[2]	438	100%	98%	98%
Controlled Postoperative Blood Glucose[2]	179	96%	97%	97%
Perioperative Temperature Management[2]	751	100%	100%	100%
Prophylactic Antibiotic Selection[2]	592	99%	99%	99%
Prophylactic Antibiotic Selection (Outpatient)	522	98%	97%	98%
Prophylactic Antibiotic Stopped[2]	563	99%	98%	98%
Prophylactic Antibiotic Timing[2]	592	100%	98%	99%
Prophylactic Antibiotic Timing (Outpatient)	496	97%	97%	98%
Urinary Catheter Removal[2]	308	96%	97%	97%
Survey of Patients' Hospital Experiences				
Area Around Room 'Always' Quiet at Night	300+	58%	60%	61%
Doctors 'Always' Communicated Well	300+	83%	81%	82%
Home Recovery Information Given	300+	87%	87%	85%
Hospital Given 9 or 10 on 10 Point Scale	300+	81%	71%	71%
Meds 'Always' Explained Before Given	300+	66%	64%	64%
Nurses 'Always' Communicated Well	300+	85%	80%	79%
Pain 'Always' Well Controlled	300+	76%	71%	71%
Room and Bathroom 'Always' Clean	300+	75%	73%	73%
Timely Help 'Always' Received	300+	76%	70%	68%
Would Definitely Recommend Hospital	300+	87%	71%	71%
Use of Medical Imaging				
Cardiac Imaging Stress Test before Surgery	2,620	4.7%	5.1%	5.3%
Combination Abdominal CT Scan	1,462	4.4%	8.7%	10.5%
Combination Brain/Sinus CT Scan	1,326	2.0%	2.2%	2.7%
Combination Chest CT Scan	1,043	0.1%	3.6%	2.7%
Follow-up Mammogram/Ultrasound	3,778	9.5%	8.2%	8.8%
Lumbar Spine MRI for Low Back Pain	357	32.8%	36.9%	37.2%

Oakwood Hospital - Southshore

5450 Fort Street
Trenton, MI 48183
URL: www.oakwood.org/oakwood-hospital-southshore
Type: Acute Care Hospitals
Ownership: Govt - Hospital Dist/Auth
Phone: 734-671-3800
Fax: 734-671-3891
Emergency Services: Yes
Beds: 203

Key Personnel:
CEO/President. . . . . Jerry Fitzgerald
Cardiac Laboratory. . . . . D Flood
Chief of Medical Staff . . . . Malcolm Henoch
Intensive Care Unit. . . . . Carol Lampe
Operating Room. . . . . Joanne McKay
Infection Control. . . . . Susan Ottosen
Patient Relations . . . . Jan Sladewski
Anesthesiology. . . . . Eric Suris, DO

Measure	Cases	This Hosp.	State Avg.	U.S. Avg.
Blood Clot Prevention and Treatment				
Anticoagulation Overlap Therapy[2]	98	81%	90%	93%
ICU Venous Thromboembolism Prophylaxis[2]	54	91%	93%	92%
Incidence of Potentially Preventable VTE[2]	17	29%	8%	10%
UFH with Dosages/Platelet Monitoring[2]	107	100%	96%	97%
Venous Thromboembolism Prophylaxis[2]	363	64%	87%	85%
Warfarin Therapy Discharge Instructions[2]	76	3%	72%	75%
Chest Pain/Possible Heart Attack Care				
Aspirin Given Within 24 Hours of Arrival	56	100%	96%	96%
Fibrinolytic Meds Within 30 Min. of Arrival[7]	-	-	63%	58%
Average Time to ECG (minutes)	55	3	8	7
Average Time to Transfer (minutes)[7]	-	-	53	60
Children's Asthma Care				
Received Home Management Plan of Care	-	-	-	88%
Received Reliever Medication	-	-	-	100%
Received Systemic Corticosteroids	-	-	-	100%
Emergency Department				
Admittance Decision Time (minutes)[2]	797	99	102	98
Head CT Results Within 45 Min. of Arrival[1]	-	-	54%	57%
Patients Who Left ER Before Being Seen	30,111	1%	2%	2%
Time from ER Arrival to Admit. (minutes)[2]	797	347	288	274
Time from ER Arrival to Discharge (minutes)	338	198	128	134
Time in ER Before Being Evaluated (minutes)	383	26	22	26
Time to Pain Meds for Fractures (minutes)	98	56	55	57
Heart Attack Care				
Aspirin Given at Discharge	70	97%	99%	99%
Fibrinolytic Meds Within 30 Min. of Arrival[7]	-	-	20%	54%
PCI Within 90 Minutes of Arrival	30	100%	95%	96%
Statin Prescribed at Discharge	68	99%	98%	98%
Heart Failure Care				
ACE Inhibitor or ARB for LVSD[2]	58	100%	96%	97%
Discharge Instructions Given[2]	177	97%	94%	94%
Evaluation of LVS Function[2]	217	100%	99%	99%
Medicare Spending				
Medicare Spending per Patient (ratio)	-	1.02	0.96	0.98
Pneumonia Care				
Appropriate Initial Antibiotic Given[2]	102	97%	96%	95%
Blood Culture Timing[2]	124	97%	98%	98%
Pregnancy and Delivery Care				
Newborn Deliveries Scheduled Early[2]	134	1%	3%	6%
Preventive Care				
Immunization for Influenza[2]	539	97%	89%	90%
Immunization for Pneumonia[2]	762	94%	90%	92%
Stroke Care				
Anticoagulation Therapy for Atrial Fibrillation[2]	12	75%	92%	95%
Antithrombotic Therapy Timing[2]	74	95%	97%	98%
Assessed for Rehabilitation[2]	85	92%	97%	97%
Discharged on Antithrombotic Therapy[2]	78	97%	99%	99%
Discharged on Statin Medication[2]	67	73%	94%	94%
Thrombolytic Therapy Timing[2]	12	58%	69%	66%
Venous Thromboembolism Prophylaxis[2]	89	69%	94%	94%
Written Stroke Educational Materials Given[2]	47	36%	87%	88%
Surgical Care Improvement Project				
Appropriate Beta Blocker Usage[2]	118	94%	98%	98%
Appropriate VTP Within 24 Hours[2]	285	99%	98%	98%
Controlled Postoperative Blood Glucose[2,7]	-	-	97%	97%
Perioperative Temperature Management[2]	354	100%	100%	100%
Prophylactic Antibiotic Selection[2]	240	99%	99%	99%
Prophylactic Antibiotic Selection (Outpatient)	105	98%	97%	98%
Prophylactic Antibiotic Stopped[2]	237	97%	98%	98%
Prophylactic Antibiotic Timing[2]	241	99%	98%	99%
Prophylactic Antibiotic Timing (Outpatient)	103	94%	97%	98%
Urinary Catheter Removal[2]	76	89%	97%	97%
Survey of Patients' Hospital Experiences				
Area Around Room 'Always' Quiet at Night	300+	61%	60%	61%
Doctors 'Always' Communicated Well	300+	81%	81%	82%
Home Recovery Information Given	300+	83%	87%	85%
Hospital Given 9 or 10 on 10 Point Scale	300+	74%	71%	71%
Meds 'Always' Explained Before Given	300+	65%	64%	64%
Nurses 'Always' Communicated Well	300+	81%	80%	79%
Pain 'Always' Well Controlled	300+	73%	71%	71%
Room and Bathroom 'Always' Clean	300+	76%	73%	73%
Timely Help 'Always' Received	300+	71%	70%	68%
Would Definitely Recommend Hospital	300+	75%	71%	71%
Use of Medical Imaging				
Cardiac Imaging Stress Test before Surgery	461	5.6%	5.1%	5.3%
Combination Abdominal CT Scan	768	12.1%	8.7%	10.5%
Combination Brain/Sinus CT Scan[1]	-	-	2.2%	2.7%
Combination Chest CT Scan	546	1.3%	3.6%	2.7%
Follow-up Mammogram/Ultrasound	674	8.9%	8.2%	8.8%
Lumbar Spine MRI for Low Back Pain	98	28.6%	36.9%	37.2%

William Beaumont Hospital - Troy

44201 Dequindre Road
Troy, MI 48085
URL: www.beaumonthospitals.com
Type: Acute Care Hospitals
Ownership: Voluntary non-profit - Other
Phone: 248-964-8800
Fax: 248-964-8842
Emergency Services: Yes
Beds: 226

Key Personnel:
Chief of Medical Staff . . . . Ananias C. Diokno, MD
Operating Room. . . . . Dee Henderson
Quality Assurance . . . . Janna Hoff
Pediatric Ambulatory Care . . . . . . Karen Hufnagle, MD
Pediatric In-Patient Care . . . . Karen Hufnagle, MD
Infection Control. . . . . Doris Neumeyer
Radiology. . . . . Thomas Verhelle, MD
Cardiac Laboratory. . . . . Terry Wagner

Measure	Cases	This Hosp.	State Avg.	U.S. Avg.
Blood Clot Prevention and Treatment				
Anticoagulation Overlap Therapy[2]	227	100%	90%	93%
ICU Venous Thromboembolism Prophylaxis[2]	46	100%	93%	92%
Incidence of Potentially Preventable VTE[2]	31	0%	8%	10%
UFH with Dosages/Platelet Monitoring[2]	256	100%	96%	97%
Venous Thromboembolism Prophylaxis[2]	355	90%	87%	85%
Warfarin Therapy Discharge Instructions[2]	152	99%	72%	75%
Chest Pain/Possible Heart Attack Care				
Aspirin Given Within 24 Hours of Arrival[1]	-	-	96%	96%
Fibrinolytic Meds Within 30 Min. of Arrival[5]	-	-	63%	58%
Average Time to ECG (minutes)[1]	-	-	8	7
Average Time to Transfer (minutes)[5]	-	-	53	60

NOTE: Hospital profiles are in alphabetical order by state, then city, then hospital within the city; Rankings exclude hospitals with less than 25 cases except for patient surveys which excludes hospitals with less than 100 cases; (a) 100-299 cases; (1) The number of cases/patients is too few to report; (2) Data submitted were based on a sample of cases/patients; (3) Results are based on a shorter time period than required; (4) Data suppressed by CMS for one or more quarters; (5) Results are not available for this reporting period; (6) Fewer than 100 patients completed the HCAHPS survey; (7) No cases met the criteria for this measure; (8) The lower limit of the confidence interval cannot be calculated if the number of observed infections equals zero; (9) No data are available from the state/territory for this reporting period; (10) The scores shown reflect fewer than 50 completed surveys; (11) There were discrepancies in the data collection process; (12) This measure does not apply to this hospital for this reporting period; (13) Results cannot be calculated for this reporting period; (14) The results for this state are combined with nearby states to protect confidentiality; Please refer to the User's Guide for a full explanation of data.

Measure	Cases	This Hosp.	State Avg.	U.S. Avg.
Children's Asthma Care				
Received Home Management Plan of Care	-	-	-	88%
Received Reliever Medication	-	-	-	100%
Received Systemic Corticosteroids	-	-	-	100%
Emergency Department				
Admittance Decision Time (minutes)[2]	661	138	102	98
Head CT Results Within 45 Min. of Arrival[1]	-	-	54%	57%
Patients Who Left ER Before Being Seen	79,773	1%	2%	2%
Time from ER Arrival to Admit. (minutes)[2]	664	352	288	274
Time from ER Arrival to Discharge (minutes)	325	174	128	134
Time in ER Before Being Evaluated (minutes)	310	38	22	26
Time to Pain Meds for Fractures (minutes)	185	57	55	57
Heart Attack Care				
Aspirin Given at Discharge	475	100%	99%	99%
Fibrinolytic Meds Within 30 Min. of Arrival[7]	-	-	20%	54%
PCI Within 90 Minutes of Arrival	79	99%	95%	96%
Statin Prescribed at Discharge	464	100%	98%	98%
Heart Failure Care				
ACE Inhibitor or ARB for LVSD	191	100%	96%	97%
Discharge Instructions Given	579	100%	94%	94%
Evaluation of LVS Function	720	100%	99%	99%
Medicare Spending				
Medicare Spending per Patient (ratio)	-	1.01	0.96	0.98
Pneumonia Care				
Appropriate Initial Antibiotic Given[2]	124	100%	96%	95%
Blood Culture Timing[2]	184	100%	98%	98%
Pregnancy and Delivery Care				
Newborn Deliveries Scheduled Early[2]	66	5%	3%	6%
Preventive Care				
Immunization for Influenza[2]	570	96%	89%	90%
Immunization for Pneumonia[2]	759	95%	90%	92%
Stroke Care				
Anticoagulation Therapy for Atrial Fibrillation	36	100%	92%	95%
Antithrombotic Therapy Timing	220	100%	97%	98%
Assessed for Rehabilitation	265	100%	97%	97%
Discharged on Antithrombotic Therapy	246	100%	99%	99%
Discharged on Statin Medication	184	100%	94%	94%
Thrombolytic Therapy Timing	12	83%	69%	66%
Venous Thromboembolism Prophylaxis	252	96%	94%	94%
Written Stroke Educational Materials Given	147	93%	87%	88%
Surgical Care Improvement Project				
Appropriate Beta Blocker Usage[2]	210	100%	98%	98%
Appropriate VTP Within 24 Hours[2]	282	100%	98%	98%
Controlled Postoperative Blood Glucose[2]	119	100%	97%	97%
Perioperative Temperature Management[2]	399	100%	100%	100%
Prophylactic Antibiotic Selection[2]	360	99%	99%	99%
Prophylactic Antibiotic Selection (Outpatient)	452	99%	97%	98%
Prophylactic Antibiotic Stopped[2]	344	100%	98%	98%
Prophylactic Antibiotic Timing[2]	362	99%	98%	99%
Prophylactic Antibiotic Timing (Outpatient)	442	99%	97%	98%
Urinary Catheter Removal[2]	313	99%	97%	97%
Survey of Patients' Hospital Experiences				
Area Around Room 'Always' Quiet at Night	300+	46%	60%	61%
Doctors 'Always' Communicated Well	300+	76%	81%	82%
Home Recovery Information Given	300+	84%	87%	85%
Hospital Given 9 or 10 on 10 Point Scale	300+	71%	71%	71%
Meds 'Always' Explained Before Given	300+	58%	64%	64%
Nurses 'Always' Communicated Well	300+	77%	80%	79%
Pain 'Always' Well Controlled	300+	70%	71%	71%
Room and Bathroom 'Always' Clean	300+	69%	73%	73%
Timely Help 'Always' Received	300+	67%	70%	68%
Would Definitely Recommend Hospital	300+	75%	71%	71%
Use of Medical Imaging				
Cardiac Imaging Stress Test before Surgery	1,206	6.0%	5.1%	5.3%
Combination Abdominal CT Scan	2,747	6.7%	8.7%	10.5%
Combination Brain/Sinus CT Scan	1,623	1.2%	2.2%	2.7%
Combination Chest CT Scan	2,523	2.2%	3.6%	2.7%
Follow-up Mammogram/Ultrasound	5,505	10.2%	8.2%	8.8%
Lumbar Spine MRI for Low Back Pain	535	32.0%	36.9%	37.2%

Henry Ford West Bloomfield Hospital

6777 West Maple Road
W Bloomfield, MI 48322
Phone: 248-325-1000
URL: www.henryford.com
Type: Acute Care Hospitals
Emergency Services: Yes
Ownership: Govt - Hospital Dist/Auth
Beds: 300

Key Personnel:
Chief of Medical Staff .... Betty Chu, MD, MBA
President .... Robert G Ringley
Emergency .... Debbie Spencer
CEO/President..................... Lynn Torossian

Measure	Cases	This Hosp.	State Avg.	U.S. Avg.
Blood Clot Prevention and Treatment				
Anticoagulation Overlap Therapy[2]	119	92%	90%	93%
ICU Venous Thromboembolism Prophylaxis[2]	97	96%	93%	92%
Incidence of Potentially Preventable VTE[2]	35	6%	8%	10%
UFH with Dosages/Platelet Monitoring[2]	139	97%	96%	97%
Venous Thromboembolism Prophylaxis[2]	306	86%	87%	85%
Warfarin Therapy Discharge Instructions[2]	83	77%	72%	75%
Chest Pain/Possible Heart Attack Care				
Aspirin Given Within 24 Hours of Arrival[1,3]	-	-	96%	96%
Fibrinolytic Meds Within 30 Min. of Arrival[5]	-	-	63%	58%
Average Time to ECG (minutes)[1,3]	-	-	8	7
Average Time to Transfer (minutes)[5]	-	-	53	60
Children's Asthma Care				
Received Home Management Plan of Care	-	-	-	88%
Received Reliever Medication	-	-	-	100%
Received Systemic Corticosteroids	-	-	-	100%
Emergency Department				
Admittance Decision Time (minutes)[2]	566	236	102	98
Head CT Results Within 45 Min. of Arrival[1,3]	-	-	54%	57%
Patients Who Left ER Before Being Seen	39,507	1%	2%	2%
Time from ER Arrival to Admit. (minutes)[2]	568	326	288	274
Time from ER Arrival to Discharge (minutes)	382	160	128	134
Time in ER Before Being Evaluated (minutes)	395	27	22	26
Time to Pain Meds for Fractures (minutes)	116	74	55	57
Heart Attack Care				
Aspirin Given at Discharge	135	99%	99%	99%
Fibrinolytic Meds Within 30 Min. of Arrival[7]	-	-	20%	54%
PCI Within 90 Minutes of Arrival	22	95%	95%	96%
Statin Prescribed at Discharge	132	98%	98%	98%
Heart Failure Care				
ACE Inhibitor or ARB for LVSD	64	94%	96%	97%
Discharge Instructions Given	239	99%	94%	94%
Evaluation of LVS Function	324	98%	99%	99%
Medicare Spending				
Medicare Spending per Patient (ratio)	-	1.01	0.96	0.98
Pneumonia Care				
Appropriate Initial Antibiotic Given[2]	71	83%	96%	95%
Blood Culture Timing[2]	192	96%	98%	98%
Pregnancy and Delivery Care				
Newborn Deliveries Scheduled Early	109	1%	3%	6%
Preventive Care				
Immunization for Influenza[2]	525	84%	89%	90%
Immunization for Pneumonia[2]	655	82%	90%	92%
Stroke Care				
Anticoagulation Therapy for Atrial Fibrillation	26	88%	92%	95%
Antithrombotic Therapy Timing	129	94%	97%	98%
Assessed for Rehabilitation	159	97%	97%	97%
Discharged on Antithrombotic Therapy	147	99%	99%	99%
Discharged on Statin Medication	122	95%	94%	94%
Thrombolytic Therapy Timing	19	58%	69%	66%
Venous Thromboembolism Prophylaxis	156	96%	94%	94%
Written Stroke Educational Materials Given	80	84%	87%	88%
Surgical Care Improvement Project				
Appropriate Beta Blocker Usage[2]	120	99%	98%	98%
Appropriate VTP Within 24 Hours[2]	359	98%	98%	98%
Controlled Postoperative Blood Glucose[2,7]	-	-	97%	97%
Perioperative Temperature Management[2]	441	100%	100%	100%
Prophylactic Antibiotic Selection[2]	287	100%	99%	99%
Prophylactic Antibiotic Selection (Outpatient)	271	90%	97%	98%
Prophylactic Antibiotic Stopped[2]	279	99%	98%	98%
Prophylactic Antibiotic Timing[2]	287	95%	98%	99%
Prophylactic Antibiotic Timing (Outpatient)	119	92%	97%	98%
Urinary Catheter Removal[2]	235	96%	97%	97%
Survey of Patients' Hospital Experiences				
Area Around Room 'Always' Quiet at Night	300+	71%	60%	61%
Doctors 'Always' Communicated Well	300+	79%	81%	82%
Home Recovery Information Given	300+	84%	87%	85%
Hospital Given 9 or 10 on 10 Point Scale	300+	80%	71%	71%
Meds 'Always' Explained Before Given	300+	62%	64%	64%
Nurses 'Always' Communicated Well	300+	77%	80%	79%
Pain 'Always' Well Controlled	300+	69%	71%	71%
Room and Bathroom 'Always' Clean	300+	71%	73%	73%
Timely Help 'Always' Received	300+	63%	70%	68%
Would Definitely Recommend Hospital	300+	82%	71%	71%
Use of Medical Imaging				
Cardiac Imaging Stress Test before Surgery	396	5.6%	5.1%	5.3%
Combination Abdominal CT Scan	1,037	4.5%	8.7%	10.5%
Combination Brain/Sinus CT Scan	774	0.1%	2.2%	2.7%
Combination Chest CT Scan	907	3.4%	3.6%	2.7%
Follow-up Mammogram/Ultrasound	1,204	7.5%	8.2%	8.8%
Lumbar Spine MRI for Low Back Pain	121	42.1%	36.9%	37.2%

Saint John Macomb - Oakland Hospital - Macomb Center

11800 East Twelve Mile Road
Warren, MI 48093
Phone: 586-573-5000
Fax: 586-573-5199
URL: www.stjohn.org
Type: Acute Care Hospitals
Emergency Services: Yes
Ownership: Voluntary non-profit - Private
Beds: 535

Key Personnel:
Quality Assurance .... Sue M Carrier-Winzer
Pediatric In-Patient Care .... Mun Kim, MD
CEO/President................. John E Knox
Chief of Medical Staff.......... Suraj Nighoon, MD
Infection Control............... Richard Pokriefka, D.O.
Operating Room............... Suzanne Wassom
Radiology..................... Jay Zeskino, MD

Measure	Cases	This Hosp.	State Avg.	U.S. Avg.
Blood Clot Prevention and Treatment				
Anticoagulation Overlap Therapy[2]	213	87%	90%	93%
ICU Venous Thromboembolism Prophylaxis[2]	49	100%	93%	92%
Incidence of Potentially Preventable VTE[2]	41	0%	8%	10%
UFH with Dosages/Platelet Monitoring[2]	229	100%	96%	97%
Venous Thromboembolism Prophylaxis[2]	401	93%	87%	85%
Warfarin Therapy Discharge Instructions[2]	151	81%	72%	75%
Chest Pain/Possible Heart Attack Care				
Aspirin Given Within 24 Hours of Arrival	65	98%	96%	96%
Fibrinolytic Meds Within 30 Min. of Arrival[7]	-	-	63%	58%
Average Time to ECG (minutes)	67	7	8	7
Average Time to Transfer (minutes)	18	54	53	60
Children's Asthma Care				
Received Home Management Plan of Care	-	-	-	88%
Received Reliever Medication	-	-	-	100%
Received Systemic Corticosteroids	-	-	-	100%
Emergency Department				
Admittance Decision Time (minutes)[2]	840	130	102	98
Head CT Results Within 45 Min. of Arrival	50	40%	54%	57%
Patients Who Left ER Before Being Seen	>100k	2%	2%	2%
Time from ER Arrival to Admit. (minutes)[2]	848	338	288	274
Time from ER Arrival to Discharge (minutes)	357	174	128	134
Time in ER Before Being Evaluated (minutes)	411	26	22	26
Time to Pain Meds for Fractures (minutes)	330	68	55	57
Heart Attack Care				
Aspirin Given at Discharge	359	100%	99%	99%
Fibrinolytic Meds Within 30 Min. of Arrival[7]	-	-	20%	54%
PCI Within 90 Minutes of Arrival	72	100%	95%	96%
Statin Prescribed at Discharge	351	99%	98%	98%
Heart Failure Care				
ACE Inhibitor or ARB for LVSD	272	100%	96%	97%
Discharge Instructions Given	719	100%	94%	94%
Evaluation of LVS Function	878	100%	99%	99%
Medicare Spending				
Medicare Spending per Patient (ratio)	-	1.04	0.96	0.98
Pneumonia Care				
Appropriate Initial Antibiotic Given	417	97%	96%	95%

NOTE: Hospital profiles are in alphabetical order by state, then city, then hospital within the city; Rankings exclude hospitals with less than 25 cases except for patient surveys which excludes hospitals with less than 100 cases; (a) 100-299 cases; (1) The number of cases/patients is too few to report; (2) Data submitted were based on a sample of cases/patients; (3) Results are based on a shorter time period than required; (4) Data suppressed by CMS for one or more quarters; (5) Results are not available for this reporting period; (6) Fewer than 100 patients completed the HCAHPS survey; (7) No cases met the criteria for this measure; (8) The lower limit of the confidence interval cannot be calculated if the number of observed infections equals zero; (9) No data are available from the state/territory for this reporting period; (10) The scores shown reflect fewer than 50 completed surveys; (11) There were discrepancies in the data collection process; (12) This measure does not apply to this hospital for this reporting period; (13) Results cannot be calculated for this reporting period; (14) The results for this state are combined with nearby states to protect confidentiality; Please refer to the User's Guide for a full explanation of data.

Measure	Cases	This Hosp.	State Avg.	U.S. Avg.
Blood Culture Timing	468	100%	98%	98%
Pregnancy and Delivery Care				
Newborn Deliveries Scheduled Early	103	8%	3%	6%
Preventive Care				
Immunization for Influenza[2]	584	93%	89%	90%
Immunization for Pneumonia[2]	862	92%	90%	92%
Stroke Care				
Anticoagulation Therapy for Atrial Fibrillation	31	97%	92%	95%
Antithrombotic Therapy Timing	222	99%	97%	98%
Assessed for Rehabilitation	209	100%	97%	97%
Discharged on Antithrombotic Therapy	204	100%	99%	99%
Discharged on Statin Medication	159	98%	94%	94%
Thrombolytic Therapy Timing[1]	-	-	69%	66%
Venous Thromboembolism Prophylaxis	229	98%	94%	94%
Written Stroke Educational Materials Given	121	95%	87%	88%
Surgical Care Improvement Project				
Appropriate Beta Blocker Usage[2]	431	100%	98%	98%
Appropriate VTP Within 24 Hours[2]	808	99%	98%	98%
Controlled Postoperative Blood Glucose[2]	129	97%	97%	97%
Perioperative Temperature Management[2]	964	100%	100%	100%
Prophylactic Antibiotic Selection[2]	810	99%	99%	99%
Prophylactic Antibiotic Selection (Outpatient)	548	97%	97%	98%
Prophylactic Antibiotic Stopped[2]	783	99%	98%	98%
Prophylactic Antibiotic Timing[2]	811	97%	98%	99%
Prophylactic Antibiotic Timing (Outpatient)	550	98%	97%	98%
Urinary Catheter Removal[2]	713	99%	97%	97%
Survey of Patients' Hospital Experiences				
Area Around Room 'Always' Quiet at Night	300+	46%	60%	61%
Doctors 'Always' Communicated Well	300+	74%	81%	82%
Home Recovery Information Given	300+	82%	87%	85%
Hospital Given 9 or 10 on 10 Point Scale	300+	60%	71%	71%
Meds 'Always' Explained Before Given	300+	56%	64%	64%
Nurses 'Always' Communicated Well	300+	72%	80%	79%
Pain 'Always' Well Controlled	300+	63%	71%	71%
Room and Bathroom 'Always' Clean	300+	63%	73%	73%
Timely Help 'Always' Received	300+	56%	70%	68%
Would Definitely Recommend Hospital	300+	61%	71%	71%
Use of Medical Imaging				
Cardiac Imaging Stress Test before Surgery	1,168	6.3%	5.1%	5.3%
Combination Abdominal CT Scan	1,650	15.7%	8.7%	10.5%
Combination Brain/Sinus CT Scan	1,824	2.9%	2.2%	2.7%
Combination Chest CT Scan	923	7.7%	3.6%	2.7%
Follow-up Mammogram/Ultrasound	2,132	5.8%	8.2%	8.8%
Lumbar Spine MRI for Low Back Pain	197	29.4%	36.9%	37.2%

Southeast Michigan Surgical Hospital

21230 Dequindre Road
Warren, MI 48091
Phone: 586-427-1000
Fax: 586-759-0237
Type: Acute Care Hospitals
Emergency Services: No
Ownership: Voluntary non-profit - Private
Beds: 20

Key Personnel:
CEO/President. . . . . Larry Belenke
Chief of Medical Staff. . . . . John D'Alessandro, DO

Measure	Cases	This Hosp.	State Avg.	U.S. Avg.
Blood Clot Prevention and Treatment				
Anticoagulation Overlap Therapy[7]	-	-	90%	93%
ICU Venous Thromboembolism Prophylaxis[7]	-	-	93%	92%
Incidence of Potentially Preventable VTE[7]	-	-	8%	10%
UFH with Dosages/Platelet Monitoring[7]	-	-	96%	97%
Venous Thromboembolism Prophylaxis	31	97%	87%	85%
Warfarin Therapy Discharge Instructions[7]	-	-	72%	75%
Chest Pain/Possible Heart Attack Care				
Aspirin Given Within 24 Hours of Arrival[5]	-	-	96%	96%
Fibrinolytic Meds Within 30 Min. of Arrival[5]	-	-	63%	58%
Average Time to ECG (minutes)[5]	-	-	8	7
Average Time to Transfer (minutes)[5]	-	-	53	60
Children's Asthma Care				
Received Home Management Plan of Care	-	-	-	88%
Received Reliever Medication	-	-	-	100%
Received Systemic Corticosteroids	-	-	-	100%
Emergency Department				
Admittance Decision Time (minutes)[7]	-	-	102	98
Head CT Results Within 45 Min. of Arrival[5]	-	-	54%	57%
Patients Who Left ER Before Being Seen[5]	-	-	2%	2%
Time from ER Arrival to Admit. (minutes)[7]	-	-	288	274
Time from ER Arrival to Discharge (minutes)[5]	-	-	128	134
Time in ER Before Being Evaluated (minutes)[5]	-	-	22	26
Time to Pain Meds for Fractures (minutes)[5]	-	-	55	57
Heart Attack Care				
Aspirin Given at Discharge[5]	-	-	99%	99%
Fibrinolytic Meds Within 30 Min. of Arrival[5]	-	-	20%	54%
PCI Within 90 Minutes of Arrival[5]	-	-	95%	96%
Statin Prescribed at Discharge[5]	-	-	98%	98%
Heart Failure Care				
ACE Inhibitor or ARB for LVSD[5]	-	-	96%	97%
Discharge Instructions Given[5]	-	-	94%	94%
Evaluation of LVS Function[5]	-	-	99%	99%
Medicare Spending				
Medicare Spending per Patient (ratio)[1]	-	-	0.96	0.98
Pneumonia Care				
Appropriate Initial Antibiotic Given[5]	-	-	96%	95%
Blood Culture Timing[5]	-	-	98%	98%
Pregnancy and Delivery Care				
Newborn Deliveries Scheduled Early[7]	-	-	3%	6%
Preventive Care				
Immunization for Influenza	84	61%	89%	90%
Immunization for Pneumonia	44	75%	90%	92%
Stroke Care				
Anticoagulation Therapy for Atrial Fibrillation[5]	-	-	92%	95%
Antithrombotic Therapy Timing[5]	-	-	97%	98%
Assessed for Rehabilitation[5]	-	-	97%	97%
Discharged on Antithrombotic Therapy[5]	-	-	99%	99%
Discharged on Statin Medication[5]	-	-	94%	94%
Thrombolytic Therapy Timing[5]	-	-	69%	66%
Venous Thromboembolism Prophylaxis[5]	-	-	94%	94%
Written Stroke Educational Materials Given[5]	-	-	87%	88%
Surgical Care Improvement Project				
Appropriate Beta Blocker Usage[5]	-	-	98%	98%
Appropriate VTP Within 24 Hours[5]	-	-	98%	98%
Controlled Postoperative Blood Glucose[5]	-	-	97%	97%
Perioperative Temperature Management[5]	-	-	100%	100%
Prophylactic Antibiotic Selection[5]	-	-	99%	99%
Prophylactic Antibiotic Selection (Outpatient)	23	96%	97%	98%
Prophylactic Antibiotic Stopped[5]	-	-	98%	98%
Prophylactic Antibiotic Timing[5]	-	-	98%	99%
Prophylactic Antibiotic Timing (Outpatient)	23	96%	97%	98%
Urinary Catheter Removal[5]	-	-	97%	97%
Survey of Patients' Hospital Experiences				
Area Around Room 'Always' Quiet at Night[10]	<100	78%	60%	61%
Doctors 'Always' Communicated Well[10]	<100	87%	81%	82%
Home Recovery Information Given[10]	<100	91%	87%	85%
Hospital Given 9 or 10 on 10 Point Scale[10]	<100	89%	71%	71%
Meds 'Always' Explained Before Given[10]	<100	80%	64%	64%
Nurses 'Always' Communicated Well[10]	<100	90%	80%	79%
Pain 'Always' Well Controlled[10]	<100	76%	71%	71%
Room and Bathroom 'Always' Clean[10]	<100	79%	73%	73%
Timely Help 'Always' Received[10]	<100	81%	70%	68%
Would Definitely Recommend Hospital[10]	<100	84%	71%	71%
Use of Medical Imaging				
Cardiac Imaging Stress Test before Surgery[7]	-	-	5.1%	5.3%
Combination Abdominal CT Scan[7]	-	-	8.7%	10.5%
Combination Brain/Sinus CT Scan[7]	-	-	2.2%	2.7%
Combination Chest CT Scan[7]	-	-	3.6%	2.7%
Follow-up Mammogram/Ultrasound[7]	-	-	8.2%	8.8%
Lumbar Spine MRI for Low Back Pain[7]	-	-	36.9%	37.2%

Lakeland Community Hospital - Watervliet

400 Medical Park Dr
Watervliet, MI 49098
Phone: 269-463-3111
Fax: 269-463-3177
URL: www.communityhospitalwatervliet.com
Type: Acute Care Hospitals
Emergency Services: Yes
Ownership: Voluntary non-profit - Private
Beds: 70

Key Personnel:
Cardiac Laboratory. . . . . Donald Brooks
Radiology. . . . . Craig Davis
Emergency Room . . . . Kathy Davis
CEO/President. . . . . Fritz Fahrenbacher
Operating Room. . . . . Edythe Hedman
Infection Control. . . . . Theda Koshar

Measure	Cases	This Hosp.	State Avg.	U.S. Avg.
Blood Clot Prevention and Treatment				
Anticoagulation Overlap Therapy[1,2]	-	-	90%	93%
ICU Venous Thromboembolism Prophylaxis[2,7]	-	-	93%	92%
Incidence of Potentially Preventable VTE[2,7]	-	-	8%	10%
UFH with Dosages/Platelet Monitoring[1,2]	-	-	96%	97%
Venous Thromboembolism Prophylaxis[2]	64	62%	87%	85%
Warfarin Therapy Discharge Instructions[1,2]	-	-	72%	75%
Chest Pain/Possible Heart Attack Care				
Aspirin Given Within 24 Hours of Arrival	25	96%	96%	96%
Fibrinolytic Meds Within 30 Min. of Arrival[1]	-	-	63%	58%
Average Time to ECG (minutes)	25	7	8	7
Average Time to Transfer (minutes)[7]	-	-	53	60
Children's Asthma Care				
Received Home Management Plan of Care	-	-	-	88%
Received Reliever Medication	-	-	-	100%
Received Systemic Corticosteroids	-	-	-	100%
Emergency Department				
Admittance Decision Time (minutes)[2]	282	37	102	98
Head CT Results Within 45 Min. of Arrival[1]	-	-	54%	57%
Patients Who Left ER Before Being Seen	11,542	3%	2%	2%
Time from ER Arrival to Admit. (minutes)[2]	282	210	288	274
Time from ER Arrival to Discharge (minutes)	363	102	128	134
Time in ER Before Being Evaluated (minutes)	386	21	22	26
Time to Pain Meds for Fractures (minutes)	55	50	55	57
Heart Attack Care				
Aspirin Given at Discharge[1]	-	-	99%	99%
Fibrinolytic Meds Within 30 Min. of Arrival[7]	-	-	20%	54%
PCI Within 90 Minutes of Arrival[7]	-	-	95%	96%
Statin Prescribed at Discharge[1]	-	-	98%	98%
Heart Failure Care				
ACE Inhibitor or ARB for LVSD[1]	-	-	96%	97%
Discharge Instructions Given	19	100%	94%	94%
Evaluation of LVS Function	23	100%	99%	99%
Medicare Spending				
Medicare Spending per Patient (ratio)	-	0.96	0.96	0.98
Pneumonia Care				
Appropriate Initial Antibiotic Given	42	95%	96%	95%
Blood Culture Timing	48	96%	98%	98%
Pregnancy and Delivery Care				
Newborn Deliveries Scheduled Early[7]	-	-	3%	6%
Preventive Care				
Immunization for Influenza[2]	254	96%	89%	90%
Immunization for Pneumonia[2]	392	98%	90%	92%
Stroke Care				
Anticoagulation Therapy for Atrial Fibrillation[7]	-	-	92%	95%
Antithrombotic Therapy Timing[1]	-	-	97%	98%
Assessed for Rehabilitation[1]	-	-	97%	97%
Discharged on Antithrombotic Therapy[1]	-	-	99%	99%
Discharged on Statin Medication[1]	-	-	94%	94%
Thrombolytic Therapy Timing[7]	-	-	69%	66%
Venous Thromboembolism Prophylaxis[1]	-	-	94%	94%
Written Stroke Educational Materials Given[1]	-	-	87%	88%
Surgical Care Improvement Project				
Appropriate Beta Blocker Usage	42	95%	98%	98%
Appropriate VTP Within 24 Hours	156	100%	98%	98%
Controlled Postoperative Blood Glucose[7]	-	-	97%	97%
Perioperative Temperature Management	161	100%	100%	100%
Prophylactic Antibiotic Selection	132	100%	99%	99%
Prophylactic Antibiotic Selection (Outpatient)[1,3]	-	-	97%	98%
Prophylactic Antibiotic Stopped	132	100%	98%	98%
Prophylactic Antibiotic Timing	132	100%	98%	99%
Prophylactic Antibiotic Timing (Outpatient)[1,3]	-	-	97%	98%
Urinary Catheter Removal	153	99%	97%	97%
Survey of Patients' Hospital Experiences				
Area Around Room 'Always' Quiet at Night	(a)	66%	60%	61%
Doctors 'Always' Communicated Well	(a)	86%	81%	82%
Home Recovery Information Given	(a)	89%	87%	85%
Hospital Given 9 or 10 on 10 Point Scale	(a)	79%	71%	71%
Meds 'Always' Explained Before Given	(a)	69%	64%	64%

NOTE: Hospital profiles are in alphabetical order by state, then city, then hospital within the city; Rankings exclude hospitals with less than 25 cases except for patient surveys which excludes hospitals with less than 100 cases; (a) 100-299 cases; (1) The number of cases/patients is too few to report; (2) Data submitted were based on a sample of cases/patients; (3) Results are based on a shorter time period than required; (4) Data suppressed by CMS for one or more quarters; (5) Results are not available for this reporting period; (6) Fewer than 100 patients completed the HCAHPS survey; (7) No cases met the criteria for this measure; (8) The lower limit of the confidence interval cannot be calculated if the number of observed infections equals zero; (9) No data are available from the state/territory for this reporting period; (10) The scores shown reflect fewer than 50 completed surveys; (11) There were discrepancies in the data collection process; (12) This measure does not apply to this hospital for this reporting period; (13) Results cannot be calculated for this reporting period; (14) The results for this state are combined with nearby states to protect confidentiality; Please refer to the User's Guide for a full explanation of data.

Nurses 'Always' Communicated Well	(a)	84%	80%	79%
Pain 'Always' Well Controlled	(a)	76%	71%	71%
Room and Bathroom 'Always' Clean	(a)	80%	73%	73%
Timely Help 'Always' Received	(a)	84%	70%	68%
Would Definitely Recommend Hospital	(a)	76%	71%	71%
Use of Medical Imaging				
Cardiac Imaging Stress Test before Surgery[7]	-	-	5.1%	5.3%
Combination Abdominal CT Scan	256	2.7%	8.7%	10.5%
Combination Brain/Sinus CT Scan[1]	-	-	2.2%	2.7%
Combination Chest CT Scan	81	3.7%	3.6%	2.7%
Follow-up Mammogram/Ultrasound	395	9.1%	8.2%	8.8%
Lumbar Spine MRI for Low Back Pain[1]	-	-	36.9%	37.2%

Oakwood Hospital - Wayne

33155 Annapolis Ave
Wayne, MI 48184
Phone: 734-467-4175
Fax: 734-467-4017
E-mail: filekm@oakwood.org
URL: www.oakwood.org
Type: Acute Care Hospitals
Emergency Services: Yes
Ownership: Govt - Hospital Dist/Auth
Beds: 247

Key Personnel:

Operating Room. . . . . Muzammil Ahmed
Emergency Room . . . . Charles Ceeter
President/CEO. . . . . Brain Connolly
Quality Assurance . . . . Maureen D'Agostino
Quality Assurance . . . . Marie Daneil
Chief of Medical Staff. . . . . Malcolm Henoch
Pediatric In-Patient Care . . . . Ben Raju, MD
Anesthesiology. . . . . John Rivard

Measure	Cases	This Hosp.	State Avg.	U.S. Avg.
Blood Clot Prevention and Treatment				
Anticoagulation Overlap Therapy[2]	69	38%	90%	93%
ICU Venous Thromboembolism Prophylaxis[2]	98	85%	93%	92%
Incidence of Potentially Preventable VTE[1,2]	-	-	8%	10%
UFH with Dosages/Platelet Monitoring[2]	81	100%	96%	97%
Venous Thromboembolism Prophylaxis[2]	339	53%	87%	85%
Warfarin Therapy Discharge Instructions[2]	34	65%	72%	75%
Chest Pain/Possible Heart Attack Care				
Aspirin Given Within 24 Hours of Arrival	48	98%	96%	96%
Fibrinolytic Meds Within 30 Min. of Arrival[7]	-	-	63%	58%
Average Time to ECG (minutes)	53	6	8	7
Average Time to Transfer (minutes)[1]	-	-	53	60
Children's Asthma Care				
Received Home Management Plan of Care	-	-	-	88%
Received Reliever Medication	-	-	-	100%
Received Systemic Corticosteroids	-	-	-	100%
Emergency Department				
Admittance Decision Time (minutes)[2]	800	108	102	98
Head CT Results Within 45 Min. of Arrival	12	25%	54%	57%
Patients Who Left ER Before Being Seen	41,400	7%	2%	2%
Time from ER Arrival to Admit. (minutes)[2]	800	352	288	274
Time from ER Arrival to Discharge (minutes)	334	142	128	134
Time in ER Before Being Evaluated (minutes)	381	31	22	26
Time to Pain Meds for Fractures (minutes)	142	57	55	57
Heart Attack Care				
Aspirin Given at Discharge	90	100%	99%	99%
Fibrinolytic Meds Within 30 Min. of Arrival[7]	-	-	20%	54%
PCI Within 90 Minutes of Arrival	32	100%	95%	96%
Statin Prescribed at Discharge	94	97%	98%	98%
Heart Failure Care				
ACE Inhibitor or ARB for LVSD	67	93%	96%	97%
Discharge Instructions Given	156	87%	94%	94%
Evaluation of LVS Function	190	97%	99%	99%
Medicare Spending				
Medicare Spending per Patient (ratio)	-	1.07	0.96	0.98
Pneumonia Care				
Appropriate Initial Antibiotic Given[2]	93	92%	96%	95%
Blood Culture Timing[2]	180	98%	98%	98%
Pregnancy and Delivery Care				
Newborn Deliveries Scheduled Early[2]	168	0%	3%	6%
Preventive Care				
Immunization for Influenza[2]	532	65%	89%	90%
Immunization for Pneumonia[2]	701	89%	90%	92%
Stroke Care				
Anticoagulation Therapy for Atrial Fibrillation[1,2]	-	-	92%	95%
Antithrombotic Therapy Timing[2]	62	92%	97%	98%
Assessed for Rehabilitation[2]	68	94%	97%	97%
Discharged on Antithrombotic Therapy[2]	66	95%	99%	99%
Discharged on Statin Medication[2]	53	81%	94%	94%
Thrombolytic Therapy Timing[1,2]	-	-	69%	66%
Venous Thromboembolism Prophylaxis[2]	68	78%	94%	94%
Written Stroke Educational Materials Given[2]	36	56%	87%	88%
Surgical Care Improvement Project				
Appropriate Beta Blocker Usage[2]	65	98%	98%	98%
Appropriate VTP Within 24 Hours[2]	236	99%	98%	98%
Controlled Postoperative Blood Glucose[2,7]	-	-	97%	97%
Perioperative Temperature Management[2]	261	100%	100%	100%
Prophylactic Antibiotic Selection[2]	160	99%	99%	99%
Prophylactic Antibiotic Selection (Outpatient)	199	99%	97%	98%
Prophylactic Antibiotic Stopped[2]	156	97%	98%	98%
Prophylactic Antibiotic Timing[2]	161	98%	98%	99%
Prophylactic Antibiotic Timing (Outpatient)	170	96%	97%	98%
Urinary Catheter Removal[2]	50	94%	97%	97%
Survey of Patients' Hospital Experiences				
Area Around Room 'Always' Quiet at Night	300+	55%	60%	61%
Doctors 'Always' Communicated Well	300+	75%	81%	82%
Home Recovery Information Given	300+	80%	87%	85%
Hospital Given 9 or 10 on 10 Point Scale	300+	67%	71%	71%
Meds 'Always' Explained Before Given	300+	61%	64%	64%
Nurses 'Always' Communicated Well	300+	80%	80%	79%
Pain 'Always' Well Controlled	300+	71%	71%	71%
Room and Bathroom 'Always' Clean	300+	71%	73%	73%
Timely Help 'Always' Received	300+	68%	70%	68%
Would Definitely Recommend Hospital	300+	65%	71%	71%
Use of Medical Imaging				
Cardiac Imaging Stress Test before Surgery	427	9.6%	5.1%	5.3%
Combination Abdominal CT Scan	783	9.6%	8.7%	10.5%
Combination Brain/Sinus CT Scan	983	3.9%	2.2%	2.7%
Combination Chest CT Scan	499	9.0%	3.6%	2.7%
Follow-up Mammogram/Ultrasound	1,403	13.0%	8.2%	8.8%
Lumbar Spine MRI for Low Back Pain	188	34.6%	36.9%	37.2%

West Branch Regional Medical Center

2463 South M-30
West Branch, MI 48661
Phone: 989-345-6366
Fax: 989-343-3113
URL: www.wbrmc.org
Type: Acute Care Hospitals
Emergency Services: Yes
Ownership: Government - Local
Beds: 88

Key Personnel:

Chief of Medical Staff. . . . . Wilfredo Abesamis, MD
Pediatric Ambulatory Care . . . . . . Wilfredo Abesamis, MD
Pediatric In-Patient Care . . . . Wilfredo Abesamis, MD
Infection Control. . . . . Kathleen DeHaan, RN
Quality Assurance . . . . Edward A Napierala
CEO/President. . . . . Douglas E Pattullo
Operating Room. . . . . Bobbi Simon
Radiology. . . . . Mathew Waack, MD

Measure	Cases	This Hosp.	State Avg.	U.S. Avg.
Blood Clot Prevention and Treatment				
Anticoagulation Overlap Therapy[2]	26	54%	90%	93%
ICU Venous Thromboembolism Prophylaxis[2]	76	62%	93%	92%
Incidence of Potentially Preventable VTE[2,7]	-	-	8%	10%
UFH with Dosages/Platelet Monitoring[1,2]	-	-	96%	97%
Venous Thromboembolism Prophylaxis[2]	130	38%	87%	85%
Warfarin Therapy Discharge Instructions[2]	26	100%	72%	75%
Chest Pain/Possible Heart Attack Care				
Aspirin Given Within 24 Hours of Arrival	79	97%	96%	96%
Fibrinolytic Meds Within 30 Min. of Arrival[1]	-	-	63%	58%
Average Time to ECG (minutes)	81	10	8	7
Average Time to Transfer (minutes)[1]	-	-	53	60
Children's Asthma Care				
Received Home Management Plan of Care	-	-	-	88%
Received Reliever Medication	-	-	-	100%
Received Systemic Corticosteroids	-	-	-	100%
Emergency Department				
Admittance Decision Time (minutes)[2]	174	65	102	98
Head CT Results Within 45 Min. of Arrival	23	39%	54%	57%
Patients Who Left ER Before Being Seen	16,318	4%	2%	2%
Time from ER Arrival to Admit. (minutes)[2]	195	296	288	274
Time from ER Arrival to Discharge (minutes)	377	168	128	134
Time in ER Before Being Evaluated (minutes)	447	30	22	26
Time to Pain Meds for Fractures (minutes)	76	62	55	57
Heart Attack Care				
Aspirin Given at Discharge	23	96%	99%	99%
Fibrinolytic Meds Within 30 Min. of Arrival[7]	-	-	20%	54%
PCI Within 90 Minutes of Arrival[7]	-	-	95%	96%
Statin Prescribed at Discharge	22	100%	98%	98%
Heart Failure Care				
ACE Inhibitor or ARB for LVSD	34	85%	96%	97%
Discharge Instructions Given	83	86%	94%	94%
Evaluation of LVS Function	96	94%	99%	99%
Medicare Spending				
Medicare Spending per Patient (ratio)	-	0.98	0.96	0.98
Pneumonia Care				
Appropriate Initial Antibiotic Given[2]	64	73%	96%	95%
Blood Culture Timing[2]	76	89%	98%	98%
Pregnancy and Delivery Care				
Newborn Deliveries Scheduled Early[7]	-	-	3%	6%
Preventive Care				
Immunization for Influenza[2]	288	66%	89%	90%
Immunization for Pneumonia[2]	475	72%	90%	92%
Stroke Care				
Anticoagulation Therapy for Atrial Fibrillation[1]	-	-	92%	95%
Antithrombotic Therapy Timing[1]	-	-	97%	98%
Assessed for Rehabilitation[1]	-	-	97%	97%
Discharged on Antithrombotic Therapy[1]	-	-	99%	99%
Discharged on Statin Medication[1]	-	-	94%	94%
Thrombolytic Therapy Timing[1]	-	-	69%	66%
Venous Thromboembolism Prophylaxis[1]	-	-	94%	94%
Written Stroke Educational Materials Given[1]	-	-	87%	88%
Surgical Care Improvement Project				
Appropriate Beta Blocker Usage[2]	61	100%	98%	98%
Appropriate VTP Within 24 Hours[2]	175	95%	98%	98%
Controlled Postoperative Blood Glucose[2,7]	-	-	97%	97%
Perioperative Temperature Management[2]	189	99%	100%	100%
Prophylactic Antibiotic Selection[2]	168	50%	99%	99%
Prophylactic Antibiotic Selection (Outpatient)	58	97%	97%	98%
Prophylactic Antibiotic Stopped[2]	160	94%	98%	98%
Prophylactic Antibiotic Timing[2]	169	75%	98%	99%
Prophylactic Antibiotic Timing (Outpatient)	62	90%	97%	98%
Urinary Catheter Removal[2]	173	93%	97%	97%
Survey of Patients' Hospital Experiences				
Area Around Room 'Always' Quiet at Night	300+	61%	60%	61%
Doctors 'Always' Communicated Well	300+	76%	81%	82%
Home Recovery Information Given	300+	88%	87%	85%
Hospital Given 9 or 10 on 10 Point Scale	300+	64%	71%	71%
Meds 'Always' Explained Before Given	300+	60%	64%	64%
Nurses 'Always' Communicated Well	300+	75%	80%	79%
Pain 'Always' Well Controlled	300+	67%	71%	71%
Room and Bathroom 'Always' Clean	300+	72%	73%	73%
Timely Help 'Always' Received	300+	67%	70%	68%
Would Definitely Recommend Hospital	300+	64%	71%	71%
Use of Medical Imaging				
Cardiac Imaging Stress Test before Surgery	643	6.5%	5.1%	5.3%
Combination Abdominal CT Scan	793	23.8%	8.7%	10.5%
Combination Brain/Sinus CT Scan	586	1.7%	2.2%	2.7%
Combination Chest CT Scan	726	26.9%	3.6%	2.7%
Follow-up Mammogram/Ultrasound	874	2.4%	8.2%	8.8%
Lumbar Spine MRI for Low Back Pain	160	53.1%	36.9%	37.2%

Henry Ford Wyandotte Hospital

2333 Biddle Ave
Wyandotte, MI 48192
Phone: 734-246-6000
Fax: 734-246-8795
URL: www.henryfordwyandotte.com
Type: Acute Care Hospitals
Emergency Services: Yes
Ownership: Voluntary non-profit - Private
Beds: 162

Key Personnel:

CEO/President. . . . . Anthony Armada
Radiology. . . . . Manuel Brown
Operating Room. . . . . Pat Egbert
Quality Assurance . . . . Cathy Garrett
Emergency Room . . . . Paula Lane, RN
Patient Relations . . . . Bridget Schenavar

NOTE: Hospital profiles are in alphabetical order by state, then city, then hospital within the city; Rankings exclude hospitals with less than 25 cases except for patient surveys which excludes hospitals with less than 100 cases; (a) 100-299 cases; (1) The number of cases/patients is too few to report; (2) Data submitted were based on a sample of cases/patients; (3) Results are based on a shorter time period than required; (4) Data suppressed by CMS for one or more quarters; (5) Results are not available for this reporting period; (6) Fewer than 100 patients completed the HCAHPS survey; (7) No cases met the criteria for this measure; (8) The lower limit of the confidence interval cannot be calculated if the number of observed infections equals zero; (9) No data are available from the state/territory for this reporting period; (10) The scores shown reflect fewer than 50 completed surveys; (11) There were discrepancies in the data collection process; (12) This measure does not apply to this hospital for this reporting period; (13) Results cannot be calculated for this reporting period; (14) The results for this state are combined with nearby states to protect confidentiality; Please refer to the User's Guide for a full explanation of data.

Chief of Medical Staff. . . . . Malcolm E Williamson, DO

Measure	Cases	This Hosp.	State Avg.	U.S. Avg.
Blood Clot Prevention and Treatment				
Anticoagulation Overlap Therapy[2]	183	93%	90%	93%
ICU Venous Thromboembolism Prophylaxis[2]	64	92%	93%	92%
Incidence of Potentially Preventable VTE[2]	35	6%	8%	10%
UFH with Dosages/Platelet Monitoring[2]	168	100%	96%	97%
Venous Thromboembolism Prophylaxis[2]	365	78%	87%	85%
Warfarin Therapy Discharge Instructions[2]	143	94%	72%	75%
Chest Pain/Possible Heart Attack Care				
Aspirin Given Within 24 Hours of Arrival	105	95%	96%	96%
Fibrinolytic Meds Within 30 Min. of Arrival[7]	-	-	63%	58%
Average Time to ECG (minutes)	107	7	8	7
Average Time to Transfer (minutes)[1]	-	-	53	60
Children's Asthma Care				
Received Home Management Plan of Care	-	-	-	88%
Received Reliever Medication	-	-	-	100%
Received Systemic Corticosteroids	-	-	-	100%
Emergency Department				
Admittance Decision Time (minutes)[2]	738	218	102	98
Head CT Results Within 45 Min. of Arrival	33	67%	54%	57%
Patients Who Left ER Before Being Seen	93,821	0%	2%	2%
Time from ER Arrival to Admit. (minutes)[2]	764	408	288	274
Time from ER Arrival to Discharge (minutes)	376	118	128	134
Time in ER Before Being Evaluated (minutes)	371	42	22	26
Time to Pain Meds for Fractures (minutes)	250	44	55	57
Heart Attack Care				
Aspirin Given at Discharge[2]	192	92%	99%	99%
Fibrinolytic Meds Within 30 Min. of Arrival[2,7]	-	-	20%	54%
PCI Within 90 Minutes of Arrival[2]	29	93%	95%	96%
Statin Prescribed at Discharge[2]	174	90%	98%	98%
Heart Failure Care				
ACE Inhibitor or ARB for LVSD[2]	56	89%	96%	97%
Discharge Instructions Given[2]	248	100%	94%	94%
Evaluation of LVS Function[2]	297	99%	99%	99%
Medicare Spending				
Medicare Spending per Patient (ratio)	-	0.99	0.96	0.98
Pneumonia Care				
Appropriate Initial Antibiotic Given[2]	73	90%	96%	95%
Blood Culture Timing[2]	113	99%	98%	98%
Pregnancy and Delivery Care				
Newborn Deliveries Scheduled Early	146	2%	3%	6%
Preventive Care				
Immunization for Influenza[2]	563	86%	89%	90%
Immunization for Pneumonia[2]	737	82%	90%	92%
Stroke Care				
Anticoagulation Therapy for Atrial Fibrillation[2]	19	89%	92%	95%
Antithrombotic Therapy Timing[2]	102	97%	97%	98%
Assessed for Rehabilitation[2]	116	90%	97%	97%
Discharged on Antithrombotic Therapy[2]	109	92%	99%	99%
Discharged on Statin Medication[2]	91	85%	94%	94%
Thrombolytic Therapy Timing[1,2]	-	-	69%	66%
Venous Thromboembolism Prophylaxis[2]	109	81%	94%	94%
Written Stroke Educational Materials Given[2]	77	92%	87%	88%
Surgical Care Improvement Project				
Appropriate Beta Blocker Usage[2]	138	99%	98%	98%
Appropriate VTP Within 24 Hours[2]	413	100%	98%	98%
Controlled Postoperative Blood Glucose[2,7]	-	-	97%	97%
Perioperative Temperature Management[2]	481	100%	100%	100%
Prophylactic Antibiotic Selection[2]	321	100%	99%	99%
Prophylactic Antibiotic Selection (Outpatient)	333	98%	97%	98%
Prophylactic Antibiotic Stopped[2]	314	98%	98%	98%
Prophylactic Antibiotic Timing[2]	322	98%	98%	99%
Prophylactic Antibiotic Timing (Outpatient)	332	98%	97%	98%
Urinary Catheter Removal[2]	139	85%	97%	97%
Survey of Patients' Hospital Experiences				
Area Around Room 'Always' Quiet at Night	300+	42%	60%	61%
Doctors 'Always' Communicated Well	300+	75%	81%	82%
Home Recovery Information Given	300+	84%	87%	85%
Hospital Given 9 or 10 on 10 Point Scale	300+	66%	71%	71%
Meds 'Always' Explained Before Given	300+	58%	64%	64%
Nurses 'Always' Communicated Well	300+	75%	80%	79%
Pain 'Always' Well Controlled	300+	67%	71%	71%
Room and Bathroom 'Always' Clean	300+	64%	73%	73%
Timely Help 'Always' Received	300+	62%	70%	68%
Would Definitely Recommend Hospital	300+	65%	71%	71%
Use of Medical Imaging				
Cardiac Imaging Stress Test before Surgery	630	6.2%	5.1%	5.3%
Combination Abdominal CT Scan	1,316	3.6%	8.7%	10.5%
Combination Brain/Sinus CT Scan	997	2.3%	2.2%	2.7%
Combination Chest CT Scan	1,007	0.1%	3.6%	2.7%
Follow-up Mammogram/Ultrasound	1,608	10.4%	8.2%	8.8%
Lumbar Spine MRI for Low Back Pain	249	32.5%	36.9%	37.2%

Metro Health Hospital

5900 Byron Center Avenue, Sw
Wyoming, MI 49519
Phone: 616-252-7200
Fax: 616-252-7478
URL: www.metrohealth.net
Type: Acute Care Hospitals
Emergency Services: Yes
Ownership: Voluntary non-profit - Private
Beds: 208
Key Personnel:
Radiology. . . . . Farid Aladham
Operating Room. . . . . Robert Cali
Chief of Medical Staff. . . . . William Cunningham, MD
CEO/President. . . . . Michael Faas
Intensive Care Unit. . . . . Ann Glass
Quality Assurance . . . . Christine Lawrence
Ambulatory Care . . . . Daryl Lawrence-Fried
Infection Control. . . . . Deborah Paul-Cheadle

Measure	Cases	This Hosp.	State Avg.	U.S. Avg.
Blood Clot Prevention and Treatment				
Anticoagulation Overlap Therapy[2]	64	86%	90%	93%
ICU Venous Thromboembolism Prophylaxis[2]	52	96%	93%	92%
Incidence of Potentially Preventable VTE[2]	11	0%	8%	10%
UFH with Dosages/Platelet Monitoring[2]	59	100%	96%	97%
Venous Thromboembolism Prophylaxis[2]	328	92%	87%	85%
Warfarin Therapy Discharge Instructions[2]	55	29%	72%	75%
Chest Pain/Possible Heart Attack Care				
Aspirin Given Within 24 Hours of Arrival[1,3]	-	-	96%	96%
Fibrinolytic Meds Within 30 Min. of Arrival[3,7]	-	-	63%	58%
Average Time to ECG (minutes)[1,3]	-	-	8	7
Average Time to Transfer (minutes)[3,7]	-	-	53	60
Children's Asthma Care				
Received Home Management Plan of Care	-	-	-	88%
Received Reliever Medication	-	-	-	100%
Received Systemic Corticosteroids	-	-	-	100%
Emergency Department				
Admittance Decision Time (minutes)[2]	585	52	102	98
Head CT Results Within 45 Min. of Arrival[1,3]	-	-	54%	57%
Patients Who Left ER Before Being Seen	32,356	3%	2%	2%
Time from ER Arrival to Admit. (minutes)[2]	637	195	288	274
Time from ER Arrival to Discharge (minutes)	465	111	128	134
Time in ER Before Being Evaluated (minutes)	365	6	22	26
Time to Pain Meds for Fractures (minutes)	253	43	55	57
Heart Attack Care				
Aspirin Given at Discharge	135	100%	99%	99%
Fibrinolytic Meds Within 30 Min. of Arrival[7]	-	-	20%	54%
PCI Within 90 Minutes of Arrival	39	97%	95%	96%
Statin Prescribed at Discharge	130	100%	98%	98%
Heart Failure Care				
ACE Inhibitor or ARB for LVSD	52	100%	96%	97%
Discharge Instructions Given	175	97%	94%	94%
Evaluation of LVS Function	209	100%	99%	99%
Medicare Spending				
Medicare Spending per Patient (ratio)	-	0.93	0.96	0.98
Pneumonia Care				
Appropriate Initial Antibiotic Given[2]	101	99%	96%	95%
Blood Culture Timing[2]	223	97%	98%	98%
Pregnancy and Delivery Care				
Newborn Deliveries Scheduled Early	122	4%	3%	6%
Preventive Care				
Immunization for Influenza[2]	536	94%	89%	90%
Immunization for Pneumonia[2]	552	93%	90%	92%
Stroke Care				
Anticoagulation Therapy for Atrial Fibrillation	13	100%	92%	95%
Antithrombotic Therapy Timing	84	100%	97%	98%
Assessed for Rehabilitation	120	99%	97%	97%
Discharged on Antithrombotic Therapy	103	100%	99%	99%
Discharged on Statin Medication	81	94%	94%	94%
Thrombolytic Therapy Timing	25	48%	69%	66%
Venous Thromboembolism Prophylaxis	105	99%	94%	94%
Written Stroke Educational Materials Given	82	96%	87%	88%
Surgical Care Improvement Project				
Appropriate Beta Blocker Usage[2]	100	98%	98%	98%
Appropriate VTP Within 24 Hours[2]	326	99%	98%	98%
Controlled Postoperative Blood Glucose[2,7]	-	-	97%	97%
Perioperative Temperature Management[2]	398	100%	100%	100%
Prophylactic Antibiotic Selection[2]	239	99%	99%	99%
Prophylactic Antibiotic Selection (Outpatient)	724	99%	97%	98%
Prophylactic Antibiotic Stopped[2]	235	97%	98%	98%
Prophylactic Antibiotic Timing[2]	239	98%	98%	99%
Prophylactic Antibiotic Timing (Outpatient)	726	99%	97%	98%
Urinary Catheter Removal[2]	253	98%	97%	97%
Survey of Patients' Hospital Experiences				
Area Around Room 'Always' Quiet at Night	300+	64%	60%	61%
Doctors 'Always' Communicated Well	300+	82%	81%	82%
Home Recovery Information Given	300+	92%	87%	85%
Hospital Given 9 or 10 on 10 Point Scale	300+	83%	71%	71%
Meds 'Always' Explained Before Given	300+	66%	64%	64%
Nurses 'Always' Communicated Well	300+	80%	80%	79%
Pain 'Always' Well Controlled	300+	72%	71%	71%
Room and Bathroom 'Always' Clean	300+	75%	73%	73%
Timely Help 'Always' Received	300+	68%	70%	68%
Would Definitely Recommend Hospital	300+	82%	71%	71%
Use of Medical Imaging				
Cardiac Imaging Stress Test before Surgery	698	5.6%	5.1%	5.3%
Combination Abdominal CT Scan	882	7.5%	8.7%	10.5%
Combination Brain/Sinus CT Scan	704	2.0%	2.2%	2.7%
Combination Chest CT Scan	516	5.0%	3.6%	2.7%
Follow-up Mammogram/Ultrasound	1,167	13.2%	8.2%	8.8%
Lumbar Spine MRI for Low Back Pain	147	40.8%	36.9%	37.2%

Spectrum Health Zeeland Community Hospital

8333 Felch St
Zeeland, MI 49464
Phone: 616-772-4644
Fax: 616-748-2828
E-mail: parnoldink@zch.org
URL: www.zch.org
Type: Acute Care Hospitals
Emergency Services: Yes
Ownership: Voluntary non-profit - Private
Beds: 57
Key Personnel:
Pediatric Ambulatory Care . . . . . . Julianne Carey
Pediatric In-Patient Care . . . . Julianne Carey
Operating Room. . . . . Marlene Holstine
Quality Assurance . . . . Carrie Miedema
Chief of Medical Staff. . . . . Richard Strabbing, DO
Infection Control. . . . . Pat VanOmen, RN
CEO/President. . . . . Henry A Veenstra
Radiology. . . . . Scott Weenum

Measure	Cases	This Hosp.	State Avg.	U.S. Avg.
Blood Clot Prevention and Treatment				
Anticoagulation Overlap Therapy[2]	31	100%	90%	93%
ICU Venous Thromboembolism Prophylaxis[2]	15	100%	93%	92%
Incidence of Potentially Preventable VTE[1,2]	-	-	8%	10%
UFH with Dosages/Platelet Monitoring[2]	19	100%	96%	97%
Venous Thromboembolism Prophylaxis[2]	160	95%	87%	85%
Warfarin Therapy Discharge Instructions[2]	24	62%	72%	75%
Chest Pain/Possible Heart Attack Care				
Aspirin Given Within 24 Hours of Arrival	78	100%	96%	96%
Fibrinolytic Meds Within 30 Min. of Arrival[7]	-	-	63%	58%
Average Time to ECG (minutes)	80	9	8	7
Average Time to Transfer (minutes)	13	59	53	60
Children's Asthma Care				
Received Home Management Plan of Care	-	-	-	88%
Received Reliever Medication	-	-	-	100%
Received Systemic Corticosteroids	-	-	-	100%
Emergency Department				
Admittance Decision Time (minutes)[2]	224	102	102	98
Head CT Results Within 45 Min. of Arrival[1]	-	-	54%	57%
Patients Who Left ER Before Being Seen	22,256	0%	2%	2%

NOTE: Hospital profiles are in alphabetical order by state, then city, then hospital within the city; Rankings exclude hospitals with less than 25 cases except for patient surveys which excludes hospitals with less than 100 cases; (a) 100-299 cases; (1) The number of cases/patients is too few to report; (2) Data submitted were based on a sample of cases/patients; (3) Results are based on a shorter time period than required; (4) Data suppressed by CMS for one or more quarters; (5) Results are not available for this reporting period; (6) Fewer than 100 patients completed the HCAHPS survey; (7) No cases met the criteria for this measure; (8) The lower limit of the confidence interval cannot be calculated if the number of observed infections equals zero; (9) No data are available from the state/territory for this reporting period; (10) The scores shown reflect fewer than 50 completed surveys; (11) There were discrepancies in the data collection process; (12) This measure does not apply to this hospital for this reporting period; (13) Results cannot be calculated for this reporting period; (14) The results for this state are combined with nearby states to protect confidentiality; Please refer to the User's Guide for a full explanation of data.

Time from ER Arrival to Admit. (minutes)[2]	229	263	288	274
Time from ER Arrival to Discharge (minutes)	354	106	128	134
Time in ER Before Being Evaluated (minutes)	246	18	22	26
Time to Pain Meds for Fractures (minutes)	88	40	55	57
Heart Attack Care				
Aspirin Given at Discharge[1,3]	-	-	99%	99%
Fibrinolytic Meds Within 30 Min. of Arrival[3,7]	-	-	20%	54%
PCI Within 90 Minutes of Arrival[3,7]	-	-	95%	96%
Statin Prescribed at Discharge[1,3]	-	-	98%	98%
Heart Failure Care				
ACE Inhibitor or ARB for LVSD	18	100%	96%	97%
Discharge Instructions Given	56	93%	94%	94%
Evaluation of LVS Function	70	100%	99%	99%
Medicare Spending				
Medicare Spending per Patient (ratio)	-	0.91	0.96	0.98
Pneumonia Care				
Appropriate Initial Antibiotic Given	74	99%	96%	95%
Blood Culture Timing	133	95%	98%	98%
Pregnancy and Delivery Care				
Newborn Deliveries Scheduled Early[2]	35	3%	3%	6%
Preventive Care				
Immunization for Influenza[2]	224	96%	89%	90%
Immunization for Pneumonia[2]	265	97%	90%	92%
Stroke Care				
Anticoagulation Therapy for Atrial Fibrillation[1]	-	-	92%	95%
Antithrombotic Therapy Timing	20	100%	97%	98%
Assessed for Rehabilitation	23	100%	97%	97%
Discharged on Antithrombotic Therapy	22	100%	99%	99%
Discharged on Statin Medication	15	93%	94%	94%
Thrombolytic Therapy Timing[1]	-	-	69%	66%
Venous Thromboembolism Prophylaxis	17	100%	94%	94%
Written Stroke Educational Materials Given	15	93%	87%	88%
Surgical Care Improvement Project				
Appropriate Beta Blocker Usage	69	96%	98%	98%
Appropriate VTP Within 24 Hours	166	100%	98%	98%
Controlled Postoperative Blood Glucose[7]	-	-	97%	97%
Perioperative Temperature Management	222	100%	100%	100%
Prophylactic Antibiotic Selection	151	100%	99%	99%
Prophylactic Antibiotic Selection (Outpatient)	12	100%	97%	98%
Prophylactic Antibiotic Stopped	150	99%	98%	98%
Prophylactic Antibiotic Timing	151	99%	98%	99%
Prophylactic Antibiotic Timing (Outpatient)	12	100%	97%	98%
Urinary Catheter Removal	40	100%	97%	97%
Survey of Patients' Hospital Experiences				
Area Around Room 'Always' Quiet at Night	300+	70%	60%	61%
Doctors 'Always' Communicated Well	300+	86%	81%	82%
Home Recovery Information Given	300+	91%	87%	85%
Hospital Given 9 or 10 on 10 Point Scale	300+	83%	71%	71%
Meds 'Always' Explained Before Given	300+	68%	64%	64%
Nurses 'Always' Communicated Well	300+	86%	80%	79%
Pain 'Always' Well Controlled	300+	73%	71%	71%
Room and Bathroom 'Always' Clean	300+	85%	73%	73%
Timely Help 'Always' Received	300+	73%	70%	68%
Would Definitely Recommend Hospital	300+	84%	71%	71%
Use of Medical Imaging				
Cardiac Imaging Stress Test before Surgery	56	5.4%	5.1%	5.3%
Combination Abdominal CT Scan	195	4.1%	8.7%	10.5%
Combination Brain/Sinus CT Scan[1]	-	-	2.2%	2.7%
Combination Chest CT Scan	77	3.9%	3.6%	2.7%
Follow-up Mammogram/Ultrasound	350	2.9%	8.2%	8.8%
Lumbar Spine MRI for Low Back Pain[1]	-	-	36.9%	37.2%

NOTE: Hospital profiles are in alphabetical order by state, then city, then hospital within the city; Rankings exclude hospitals with less than 25 cases except for patient surveys which excludes hospitals with less than 100 cases; (a) 100-299 cases; (1) The number of cases/patients is too few to report; (2) Data submitted were based on a sample of cases/patients; (3) Results are based on a shorter time period than required; (4) Data suppressed by CMS for one or more quarters; (5) Results are not available for this reporting period; (6) Fewer than 100 patients completed the HCAHPS survey; (7) No cases met the criteria for this measure; (8) The lower limit of the confidence interval cannot be calculated if the number of observed infections equals zero; (9) No data are available from the state/territory for this reporting period; (10) The scores shown reflect fewer than 50 completed surveys; (11) There were discrepancies in the data collection process; (12) This measure does not apply to this hospital for this reporting period; (13) Results cannot be calculated for this reporting period; (14) The results for this state are combined with nearby states to protect confidentiality; Please refer to the User's Guide for a full explanation of data.

Blood Clot Prevention and Treatment

Anticoagulation Overlap Therapy

Hospital Name	City	Rate	Cases
Buffalo Hospital[2]	Buffalo	100%	27
Fairview Lakes Medical Center[2]	Wyoming	100%	27
Fairview Southdale Hospital[2]	Edina	100%	156
Lakeview Memorial Hospital[2]	Stillwater	100%	26
Maple Grove Hospital[2]	Maple Grove	100%	47
Saint Francis Regional Medical Center[2]	Shakopee	100%	28
Abbott Northwestern Hospital[2]	Minneapolis	99%	221
Healtheast Saint John's Hospital[2]	Maplewood	99%	83
Mayo Clinic Health System - Mankato[2]	Mankato	99%	104
Mayo Clinic Hospital Rochester[2]	Rochester	99%	297
Mercy Hospital[2]	Coon Rapids	99%	142
North Memorial Medical Center[2]	Robbinsdale	99%	170
Essentia Health St Joseph's Med Ctr[2]	Brainerd	98%	41
Essentia Health St Mary's Med Ctr[2]	Duluth	98%	95
Fairview Ridges Hospital[2]	Burnsville	98%	114
Park Nicollet Methodist Hospital[2]	Saint Louis Park	98%	208
United Hospital[2]	Saint Paul	98%	170
Healtheast Woodwinds Hospital[2]	Woodbury	97%	59
Mayo Clinic Methodist- Hospital[2]	Rochester	97%	38
Regions Hospital[2]	Saint Paul	97%	126
Univ of Minnesota Med Ctr, Fairview[2]	Minneapolis	97%	124
Saint Luke's Hospital[2]	Duluth	96%	57
Hennepin County Medical Center[2]	Minneapolis	94%	88
Unity Hospital[2]	Fridley	94%	93
Saint Joseph's Hospital[2]	Saint Paul	92%	72
Saint Cloud Hospital[2]	Saint Cloud	88%	214
Ridgeview Medical Center[2]	Waconia	86%	50

ICU Venous Thromboembolism Prophylaxis

Hospital Name	City	Rate	Cases
Fairview Northland Regional Hospital[2]	Princeton	100%	27
Fairview Southdale Hospital[2]	Edina	100%	59
Mayo Clinic Health System - Albert Lea[2]	Albert Lea	100%	61
Mayo Clinic Health System - Red Wing[2]	Red Wing	100%	25
Mayo Clinic Methodist- Hospital[2]	Rochester	100%	27
Mercy Hospital[2]	Coon Rapids	100%	49
Douglas County Hospital[2]	Alexandria	98%	59
Fairview Lakes Medical Center[2]	Wyoming	98%	44
Mayo Clinic Hospital Rochester[2]	Rochester	98%	110
United Hospital[2]	Saint Paul	98%	56
Univ Med Ctr-Mesabi/Mesaba Clinics[2]	Hibbing	98%	42
Hutchinson Health[2]	Hutchinson	97%	29
Mayo Clinic Health System - Mankato[2]	Mankato	97%	29
Regions Hospital[2]	Saint Paul	97%	87
Olmsted Medical Center	Rochester	96%	73
Unity Hospital[2]	Fridley	96%	49
Lake Region Healthcare Corporation[2]	Fergus Falls	95%	40
Saint Joseph's Hospital[2]	Saint Paul	95%	131
Essentia Health Virginia[2]	Virginia	94%	34
Healtheast Saint John's Hospital[2]	Maplewood	93%	60
Abbott Northwestern Hospital[2]	Minneapolis	92%	80
Essentia Health Saint Marys[2]	Detroit Lakes	91%	56
Lakeview Memorial Hospital[2]	Stillwater	91%	44
Saint Luke's Hospital[2]	Duluth	91%	77
Univ of Minnesota Med Ctr, Fairview[2]	Minneapolis	91%	81
Essentia Health St Joseph's Med Ctr[2]	Brainerd	90%	30
Hennepin County Medical Center[2]	Minneapolis	90%	73
North Memorial Medical Center[2]	Robbinsdale	90%	102
Saint Cloud Hospital[2]	Saint Cloud	90%	41
Healtheast Woodwinds Hospital[2]	Woodbury	87%	31
Fairview Ridges Hospital[2]	Burnsville	85%	62
Rice Memorial Hospital[2]	Willmar	82%	50
Ridgeview Medical Center[2]	Waconia	77%	35
Sanford Bemidji Medical Center[2]	Bemidji	77%	92
Essentia Health St Mary's Med Ctr[2]	Duluth	76%	38
Winona Health Services[2]	Winona	70%	77
Mayo Clinic Health System - Fairmont[2]	Fairmont	67%	27

Incidence of Potentially Preventable VTE

Hospital Name	City	Rate	Cases
Mayo Clinic Hospital Rochester[2]	Rochester	0%	75
Mayo Clinic Methodist- Hospital[2]	Rochester	0%	28
North Memorial Medical Center[2]	Robbinsdale	5%	37
Hennepin County Medical Center[2]	Minneapolis	8%	25
Park Nicollet Methodist Hospital[2]	Saint Louis Park	8%	25
Abbott Northwestern Hospital[2]	Minneapolis	13%	38
Regions Hospital[2]	Saint Paul	23%	48

UFH with Dosages/Platelet Count Monitoring

Hospital Name	City	Rate	Cases
Abbott Northwestern Hospital[2]	Minneapolis	100%	217
Essentia Health St Mary's Med Ctr[2]	Duluth	100%	82
Fairview Ridges Hospital[2]	Burnsville	100%	88
Fairview Southdale Hospital[2]	Edina	100%	147
Healtheast Woodwinds Hospital[2]	Woodbury	100%	25
Maple Grove Hospital[2]	Maple Grove	100%	37
Mayo Clinic Hospital Rochester[2]	Rochester	100%	329
Mayo Clinic Methodist- Hospital[2]	Rochester	100%	65
Regions Hospital[2]	Saint Paul	100%	115
Ridgeview Medical Center[2]	Waconia	100%	37
Saint Cloud Hospital[2]	Saint Cloud	100%	193
Saint Luke's Hospital[2]	Duluth	100%	38
Unity Hospital[2]	Fridley	100%	82
Mayo Clinic Health System - Mankato[2]	Mankato	99%	87
North Memorial Medical Center[2]	Robbinsdale	99%	148
United Hospital[2]	Saint Paul	99%	152
Saint Joseph's Hospital[2]	Saint Paul	98%	46
Hennepin County Medical Center[2]	Minneapolis	97%	64
Univ of Minnesota Med Ctr, Fairview[2]	Minneapolis	97%	130
Healtheast Saint John's Hospital[2]	Maplewood	96%	53
Mercy Hospital[2]	Coon Rapids	96%	128
Park Nicollet Methodist Hospital[2]	Saint Louis Park	86%	116

Venous Thromboembolism Prophylaxis

Hospital Name	City	Rate	Cases
Bigfork Valley Hospital[2]	Bigfork	99%	110
Fairview Northland Regional Hospital[2]	Princeton	99%	95
Hutchinson Health[2]	Hutchinson	99%	84
Mayo Clinic Hospital Rochester[2]	Rochester	99%	307
Regina Hospital[2]	Hastings	99%	158
Fairview Southdale Hospital[2]	Edina	98%	327
Mercy Hospital[2]	Moose Lake	98%	223
Fairview Lakes Medical Center[2]	Wyoming	97%	204
Mayo Clinic Health System - Albert Lea[2]	Albert Lea	97%	164
Buffalo Hospital[2]	Buffalo	96%	114
Cambridge Medical Center[2]	Cambridge	96%	153
Douglas County Hospital[2]	Alexandria	96%	234
Olmsted Medical Center	Rochester	96%	254
Mayo Clinic Methodist- Hospital[2]	Rochester	95%	252
Lake Region Healthcare Corporation[2]	Fergus Falls	94%	143
Mayo Clinic Health System - Red Wing[2]	Red Wing	94%	100
New Ulm Medical Center[2]	New Ulm	93%	123
Unity Hospital[2]	Fridley	93%	268
Lakeview Memorial Hospital[2]	Stillwater	92%	178
Mayo Clinic Health System - Mankato[2]	Mankato	92%	276
Saint Francis Regional Medical Center[2]	Shakopee	92%	291
Owatonna Hospital[2]	Owatonna	91%	163
Regions Hospital[2]	Saint Paul	91%	341
Saint Cloud Hospital[2]	Saint Cloud	91%	333
Essentia Health Saint Marys[2]	Detroit Lakes	90%	90
Mercy Hospital[2]	Coon Rapids	90%	260
District One Hospital[2]	Faribault	89%	93
United Hospital[2]	Saint Paul	89%	280
Essentia Health St Joseph's Med Ctr[2]	Brainerd	87%	276
Abbott Northwestern Hospital[2]	Minneapolis	86%	258
Healtheast Woodwinds Hospital[2]	Woodbury	86%	230
Red Lake Hospital	Redlake	86%	110
Univ Med Ctr-Mesabi/Mesaba Clinics[2]	Hibbing	86%	159
Essentia Health Virginia[2]	Virginia	85%	122
Winona Health Services[2]	Winona	85%	118
Fairview Ridges Hospital[2]	Burnsville	83%	318
Grand Itasca Clinic & Hospital[2]	Grand Rapids	83%	125
Rice Memorial Hospital[2]	Willmar	83%	154
Essentia Health Duluth[2]	Duluth	82%	121
North Memorial Medical Center[2]	Robbinsdale	82%	269
Saint Luke's Hospital[2]	Duluth	82%	305
Maple Grove Hospital[2]	Maple Grove	81%	283
Mayo Clinic Health System - Fairmont[2]	Fairmont	81%	146
Sanford Bemidji Medical Center[2]	Bemidji	81%	274
Essentia Health St Mary's Med Ctr[2]	Duluth	79%	340
Healtheast Saint John's Hospital[2]	Maplewood	79%	307
Hennepin County Medical Center[2]	Minneapolis	74%	311
Northfield Hospital[2]	Northfield	74%	112
Saint Joseph's Hospital[2]	Saint Paul	71%	261
Park Nicollet Methodist Hospital[2]	Saint Louis Park	69%	340
Univ of Minnesota Med Ctr, Fairview[2]	Minneapolis	68%	330
Sanford Worthington Medical Center[2]	Worthington	66%	140
Ridgeview Medical Center[2]	Waconia	53%	311

Warfarin Therapy Discharge Instructions

Hospital Name	City	Rate	Cases
Fairview Lakes Medical Center[2]	Wyoming	100%	28
Fairview Southdale Hospital[2]	Edina	99%	109
Maple Grove Hospital[2]	Maple Grove	98%	41
Mayo Clinic Hospital Rochester[2]	Rochester	97%	210
Park Nicollet Methodist Hospital[2]	Saint Louis Park	95%	153
Essentia Health St Mary's Med Ctr[2]	Duluth	92%	84
Mayo Clinic Methodist- Hospital[2]	Rochester	90%	30
Unity Hospital[2]	Fridley	89%	79
Saint Luke's Hospital[2]	Duluth	82%	44
Mercy Hospital[2]	Coon Rapids	77%	124
Regions Hospital[2]	Saint Paul	67%	90
North Memorial Medical Center[2]	Robbinsdale	66%	135
Healtheast Saint John's Hospital[2]	Maplewood	57%	67
Fairview Ridges Hospital[2]	Burnsville	54%	96
Healtheast Woodwinds Hospital[2]	Woodbury	49%	55
Saint Cloud Hospital[2]	Saint Cloud	49%	171
Saint Francis Regional Medical Center[2]	Shakopee	44%	25
Essentia Health St Joseph's Med Ctr[2]	Brainerd	43%	35
Ridgeview Medical Center[2]	Waconia	43%	37
United Hospital[2]	Saint Paul	32%	130
Hennepin County Medical Center[2]	Minneapolis	28%	58
Mayo Clinic Health System - Mankato[2]	Mankato	28%	78
Saint Joseph's Hospital[2]	Saint Paul	22%	51
Univ of Minnesota Med Ctr, Fairview[2]	Minneapolis	22%	86
Abbott Northwestern Hospital[2]	Minneapolis	11%	165

Chest Pain/Possible Heart Attack Care

Aspirin Given Within 24 Hours of Arrival

Hospital Name	City	Rate	Cases
Avera Marshall Regional Medical Center	Marshall	100%	29
Community Memorial Hospital	Cloquet	100%	44
Cuyuna Regional Medical Center	Crosby	100%	34
Essentia Health N Pines Med Ctr[3]	Aurora	100%	26
Essentia Health St Joseph's Med Ctr	Brainerd	100%	57
Fairview Lakes Medical Center	Wyoming	100%	140
Fairview Ridges Hospital	Burnsville	100%	63
Healtheast Woodwinds Hospital	Woodbury	100%	47
Hutchinson Health	Hutchinson	100%	52
Lake Region Healthcare Corporation	Fergus Falls	100%	56
Mayo Clinic Health System - New Prague	New Prague	100%	39
Mayo Clinic Health System - Red Wing	Red Wing	100%	68
Mille Lacs Health System	Onamia	100%	32
New Ulm Medical Center	New Ulm	100%	40
Olmsted Medical Center	Rochester	100%	40
Owatonna Hospital	Owatonna	100%	72
Perham Health	Perham	100%	47
Redwood Area Hospital	Redwood Falls	100%	31
Saint Joseph's Area Health Services	Park Rapids	100%	77
Sanford Medical Center Thief River Falls	Thief River Falls	100%	31
Tri County Hospital	Wadena	100%	38
Unity Hospital	Fridley	100%	71
Buffalo Hospital	Buffalo	99%	72
Essentia Health Saint Marys	Detroit Lakes	99%	73
Fairview Northland Regional Hospital	Princeton	99%	90
Grand Itasca Clinic & Hospital	Grand Rapids	99%	77
Maple Grove Hospital	Maple Grove	99%	86
Winona Health Services	Winona	99%	68
Centracare Health - Monticello	Monticello	98%	65
Firstlight Health System	Mora	98%	51
Lifecare Medical Center	Roseau	98%	56
Regina Hospital	Hastings	98%	54
Saint Francis Regional Medical Center	Shakopee	98%	83
Univ Med Ctr-Mesabi/Mesaba Clinics	Hibbing	98%	59
Cambridge Medical Center	Cambridge	97%	65
District One Hospital	Faribault	97%	86
Douglas County Hospital	Alexandria	97%	125
Mayo Clinic Health System - Waseca	Waseca	97%	34
Rice Memorial Hospital	Willmar	97%	66
Sanford Worthington Medical Center	Worthington	97%	37
Chippewa County Hospital	Montevideo	96%	25
Healtheast Saint John's Hospital	Maplewood	96%	52
Mayo Clinic Health System - Fairmont	Fairmont	96%	45
Mercy Hospital	Moose Lake	96%	27
Ridgeview Medical Center	Waconia	96%	132
Lake View Memorial Hospital	Two Harbors	95%	44
Lakeview Memorial Hospital	Stillwater	95%	40
Northfield Hospital	Northfield	95%	79
United Hospital District	Blue Earth	94%	32
Essentia Health Virginia	Virginia	93%	81
Saint Gabriels Hospital	Little Falls	93%	46
Mayo Clinic Health System - Albert Lea	Albert Lea	92%	98
Essentia Health Sandstone	Sandstone	91%	34
Rainy Lake Medical Center	Int'l Falls	89%	54

Average Time to ECG (minutes)

Hospital Name	City	Min.	Cases
Lake Region Healthcare Corporation	Fergus Falls	2	59
Mercy Hospital	Moose Lake	3	29
New Ulm Medical Center	New Ulm	3	40
Maple Grove Hospital	Maple Grove	4	89
Unity Hospital	Fridley	4	71
Univ Med Ctr-Mesabi/Mesaba Clinics	Hibbing	4	61
Winona Health Services	Winona	4	68
Douglas County Hospital	Alexandria	5	128
Hutchinson Health	Hutchinson	5	53
Lake View Memorial Hospital	Two Harbors	5	44
United Hospital District	Blue Earth	5	33
Centracare Health - Monticello	Monticello	6	70
District One Hospital	Faribault	6	91
Lifecare Medical Center	Roseau	6	56
Mayo Clinic Health System - Red Wing	Red Wing	6	69
Mille Lacs Health System	Onamia	6	33
Owatonna Hospital	Owatonna	6	75

NOTE: Hospital profiles are in alphabetical order by state, then city, then hospital within the city; Rankings exclude hospitals with less than 25 cases except for patient surveys which excludes hospitals with less than 100 cases; (a) 100-299 cases; (1) The number of cases/patients is too few to report; (2) Data submitted were based on a sample of cases/patients; (3) Results are based on a shorter time period than required; (4) Data suppressed by CMS for one or more quarters; (5) Results are not available for this reporting period; (6) Fewer than 100 patients completed the HCAHPS survey; (7) No cases met the criteria for this measure; (8) The lower limit of the confidence interval cannot be calculated if the number of observed infections equals zero; (9) No data are available from the state/territory for this reporting period; (10) The scores shown reflect fewer than 50 completed surveys; (11) There were discrepancies in the data collection process; (12) This measure does not apply to this hospital for this reporting period; (13) Results cannot be calculated for this reporting period; (14) The results for this state are combined with nearby states to protect confidentiality; Please refer to the User's Guide for a full explanation of data.

Hospital Name	City	Min.	Cases
Avera Marshall Regional Medical Center	Marshall	7	29
Buffalo Hospital	Buffalo	7	73
Community Memorial Hospital	Cloquet	7	48
Fairview Northland Regional Hospital	Princeton	7	90
Fairview Ridges Hospital	Burnsville	7	64
Grand Itasca Clinic & Hospital	Grand Rapids	7	75
Lakeview Memorial Hospital	Stillwater	7	42
Mayo Clinic Health System - Fairmont	Fairmont	7	44
Mayo Clinic Health System - New Prague	New Prague	7	40
Northfield Hospital	Northfield	7	83
Saint Gabriels Hospital	Little Falls	7	46
Cambridge Medical Center	Cambridge	8	68
Essentia Health Saint Marys	Detroit Lakes	8	74
Healtheast Woodwinds Hospital	Woodbury	8	48
Mayo Clinic Health System - Waseca	Waseca	8	35
Perham Health	Perham	8	43
Rainy Lake Medical Center	Int'l Falls	8	48
Regina Hospital	Hastings	8	56
Saint Francis Regional Medical Center	Shakopee	8	85
Tri County Hospital	Wadena	8	41
Fairview Lakes Medical Center	Wyoming	9	148
Healtheast Saint John's Hospital	Maplewood	9	53
Mayo Clinic Health System - Albert Lea	Albert Lea	9	104
Ridgeview Medical Center	Waconia	9	138
Essentia Health N Pines Med Ctr[3]	Aurora	10	25
Essentia Health St Joseph's Med Ctr	Brainerd	10	57
Firstlight Health System	Mora	10	52
Redwood Area Hospital	Redwood Falls	10	33
Rice Memorial Hospital	Willmar	10	65
Essentia Health Sandstone	Sandstone	12	35
Cuyuna Regional Medical Center	Crosby	13	35
Essentia Health Virginia	Virginia	13	83
Sanford Medical Center Thief River Falls	Thief River Falls	13	30
Sanford Worthington Medical Center	Worthington	13	38
Saint Joseph's Area Health Services	Park Rapids	15	77
Olmsted Medical Center	Rochester	18	39

Average Time to Transfer (minutes)

Hospital Name	City	Min.	Cases
Fairview Ridges Hospital	Burnsville	43	25

Children's Asthma Care

Received Home Management Plan of Care

Hospital Name	City	Rate	Cases
Hennepin County Medical Center[2]	Minneapolis	95%	39
Children's Hosps & Clinics of MN[2]	Minneapolis	84%	285
Univ of Minnesota Med Ctr, Fairview	Minneapolis	75%	28

Received Reliever Medication

Hospital Name	City	Rate	Cases
Children's Hosps & Clinics of MN[2]	Minneapolis	100%	285
Hennepin County Medical Center	Minneapolis	100%	39
Univ of Minnesota Med Ctr, Fairview	Minneapolis	100%	28

Received Systemic Corticosteroids

Hospital Name	City	Rate	Cases
Children's Hosps & Clinics of MN[2]	Minneapolis	100%	285
Hennepin County Medical Center	Minneapolis	100%	39
Univ of Minnesota Med Ctr, Fairview	Minneapolis	100%	28

Emergency Department

Admittance Decision Time (minutes)

Hospital Name	City	Min.	Cases
Albany Area Hospital[2,3]	Albany	0	37
Appleton Municipal Hospital	Appleton	0	36
Centra Care Health Paynesville	Paynesville	0	134
Centracare Health Sys-Melrose Hosp[2]	Melrose	0	215
Cook Hospital	Cook	0	165
Essentia Health Holy Trinity Hospital	Graceville	0	39
Hendricks Community Hospital	Hendricks	0	56
Lake View Memorial Hospital	Two Harbors	0	76
Murray County Memorial Hospital[2]	Slayton	0	78
Ortonville Area Health Services	Ortonville	0	88
Swift County Benson Hospital	Benson	0	66
Tyler Healthcare Center[3]	Tyler	0	37
United Hospital District	Blue Earth	0	315
Ridgeview Sibley Medical Center	Arlington	1	71
Centracare Health System - Sauk Centre	Sauk Centre	5	91
Madelia Community Hospital	Madelia	5	42
Rainy Lake Medical Center	Int'l Falls	5	83
Johnson Memorial Hospital	Dawson	10	55
Sanford Luverne Medical Center[2]	Luverne	10	178
Sleepy Eye Municipal Hospital[3]	Sleepy Eye	10	81
Bigfork Valley Hospital	Bigfork	11	86
Windom Area Hospital[2]	Windom	12	32
Mayo Clinic Health System - Saint James	Saint James	14	52
Mayo Clinic Health System - Springfield	Springfield	14	31
Lakewood Health Center[2]	Baudette	15	50
Municipal Hospital & Granite Manor	Granite Falls	15	153
North Valley Health Center	Warren	15	57
Perham Health[2]	Perham	15	89
Essentia Health Sandstone[2]	Sandstone	16	106
Sanford Medical Center Thief River Falls[2]	Thief River Falls	18	166
Essentia Health N Pines Med Ctr[2,3]	Aurora	19	56
Saint Elizabeth Medical Center	Wabasha	20	70
Sanford Bagley Medical Center	Bagley	20	93
Winona Health Services[2]	Winona	21	307
Sanford Worthington Medical Center[2]	Worthington	22	170
Ely Bloomenson Community Hospital	Ely	23	149
Saint Francis Medical Center[2]	Breckenridge	24	174
Deer River Healthcare Center[2]	Deer River	25	124
Glacial Ridge Hospital[2]	Glenwood	25	260
Stevens Community Medical Center[2]	Morris	25	135
Lifecare Medical Center[2]	Roseau	26	330
Glencoe Regional Health Services[2]	Glencoe	30	177
Lakewood Health System[2]	Staples	30	183
Redwood Area Hospital[2]	Redwood Falls	30	124
Saint Gabriels Hospital[2]	Little Falls	35	240
Lake Region Healthcare Corporation[2]	Fergus Falls	36	130
Essentia Health St Joseph's Med Ctr[2]	Brainerd	37	594
Mille Lacs Health System[2]	Onamia	37	349
Riverview Hospital[2]	Crookston	37	259
Firstlight Health System[2]	Mora	38	396
Mayo Clinic Health System - Fairmont[2]	Fairmont	38	268
Centracare Health - Monticello[2]	Monticello	40	462
Mayo Clinic Health System - New Prague[2]	New Prague	40	173
Mayo Clinic Health System - Red Wing[2]	Red Wing	40	210
Hutchinson Health[2]	Hutchinson	41	196
Mayo Clinic Health System - Waseca	Waseca	41	81
Avera Marshall Regional Medical Center[2]	Marshall	42	166
Meeker Memorial Hospital[2]	Litchfield	42	121
Community Memorial Hospital[2]	Cloquet	43	395
Mayo Clinic Health System - Albert Lea[2]	Albert Lea	43	266
Tri County Hospital[2]	Wadena	43	308
Mayo Clinic Health System - Cannon Falls	Cannon Falls	44	92
River's Edge Hospital & Clinic[2]	Saint Peter	44	137
Sanford Tracy[2]	Tracy	44	29
Essentia Health Virginia[2]	Virginia	48	173
Douglas County Hospital[2]	Alexandria	50	318
Mercy Hospital[2]	Moose Lake	51	218
Lakeview Memorial Hospital[2]	Stillwater	52	196
Regina Hospital[2]	Hastings	52	269
District One Hospital[2]	Faribault	55	221
Sanford Bemidji Medical Center[2]	Bemidji	55	347
Maple Grove Hospital[2]	Maple Grove	56	298
Saint Joseph's Area Health Services[2]	Park Rapids	58	231
Univ Med Ctr-Mesabi/Mesaba Clinics[2]	Hibbing	60	249
Healtheast Saint John's Hospital[2]	Maplewood	63	481
Mayo Clinic Hospital Rochester[2]	Rochester	64	457
Essentia Health Saint Marys[2]	Detroit Lakes	67	234
Ridgeview Medical Center[2]	Waconia	67	383
Northfield Hospital[2]	Northfield	68	107
Saint Joseph's Hospital[2]	Saint Paul	69	472
Grand Itasca Clinic & Hospital[2]	Grand Rapids	73	308
Healtheast Woodwinds Hospital[2]	Woodbury	74	404
Red Lake Hospital	Redlake	76	241
Rice Memorial Hospital[2]	Willmar	78	126
Saint Cloud Hospital[2]	Saint Cloud	84	374
Saint Luke's Hospital[2]	Duluth	84	451
Olmsted Medical Center	Rochester	85	250
Fairview Lakes Medical Center[2]	Wyoming	89	420
Cuyuna Regional Medical Center[2]	Crosby	90	278
Fairview Northland Regional Hospital[2]	Princeton	92	277
Fairview Ridges Hospital[2]	Burnsville	95	571
Fairview Southdale Hospital[2]	Edina	98	478
Owatonna Hospital[2]	Owatonna	99	238
Cambridge Medical Center[2]	Cambridge	102	324
Park Nicollet Methodist Hospital[2]	Saint Louis Park	103	590
Univ of Minnesota Med Ctr, Fairview[2]	Minneapolis	107	429
New Ulm Medical Center[2]	New Ulm	110	308
Mayo Clinic Health System - Mankato[2]	Mankato	113	317
North Memorial Medical Center[2]	Robbinsdale	116	732
Essentia Health St Mary's Med Ctr[2]	Duluth	117	466
Saint Francis Regional Medical Center[2]	Shakopee	119	576
Regions Hospital[2]	Saint Paul	124	542
United Hospital[2]	Saint Paul	129	456
Abbott Northwestern Hospital[2]	Minneapolis	134	315
Buffalo Hospital[2]	Buffalo	134	238
Hennepin County Medical Center[2]	Minneapolis	196	468
Mercy Hospital[2]	Coon Rapids	202	676
Unity Hospital[2]	Fridley	210	652

Head CT Results Within 45 Minutes of Arrival

Hospital Name	City	Rate	Cases
Ridgeview Medical Center	Waconia	30%	40

Patients Who Left ER Before Being Seen

Hospital Name	City	Rate	Cases
Buffalo Hospital	Buffalo	0%	18779
Cambridge Medical Center	Cambridge	0%	16285
Centra Care Health Paynesville	Paynesville	0%	3192
Centracare Health - Monticello	Monticello	0%	126220
Essentia Health N Pines Med Ctr	Aurora	0%	1867
Fairview Northland Regional Hospital	Princeton	0%	16588
Glencoe Regional Health Services	Glencoe	0%	3777
Lakeview Memorial Hospital	Stillwater	0%	9971
Lifecare Medical Center	Roseau	0%	9273
Maple Grove Hospital	Maple Grove	0%	32216
Mayo Clinic Health System - Fairmont	Fairmont	0%	8857
Mayo Clinic Health System - Mankato	Mankato	0%	22282
Mayo Clinic Health System - New Prague	New Prague	0%	6494
Mayo Clinic Health System - Saint James	Saint James	0%	2301
Mayo Clinic Health System - Springfield	Springfield	0%	1365
Mayo Clinic Health System - Waseca	Waseca	0%	4199
Northfield Hospital	Northfield	0%	10104
Ridgeview Medical Center	Waconia	0%	49551
Saint Francis Medical Center	Breckenridge	0%	5106
Sanford Bemidji Medical Center	Bemidji	0%	27893
Sanford Worthington Medical Center	Worthington	0%	5767
Sleepy Eye Municipal Hospital	Sleepy Eye	0%	1093
Winona Health Services	Winona	0%	17766
District One Hospital	Faribault	1%	14553
Douglas County Hospital	Alexandria	1%	15141
Essentia Health St Joseph's Med Ctr	Brainerd	1%	24928
Fairview Lakes Medical Center	Wyoming	1%	27073
Fairview Ridges Hospital	Burnsville	1%	51980
Grand Itasca Clinic & Hospital	Grand Rapids	1%	16231
Healtheast Woodwinds Hospital	Woodbury	1%	26395
Hutchinson Health	Hutchinson	1%	7901
Lake Region Healthcare Corporation	Fergus Falls	1%	12396
Mayo Clinic Health System - Red Wing	Red Wing	1%	10855
New Ulm Medical Center	New Ulm	1%	11382
Olmsted Medical Center	Rochester	1%	16268
Owatonna Hospital	Owatonna	1%	13677
Park Nicollet Methodist Hospital	Saint Louis Park	1%	49285
River's Edge Hospital & Clinic	Saint Peter	1%	6369
Saint Cloud Hospital	Saint Cloud	1%	58327
Saint Francis Regional Medical Center	Shakopee	1%	28139
Sanford Medical Center Thief River Falls	Thief River Falls	1%	6725
Unity Hospital	Fridley	1%	51846
Univ of Minnesota Med Ctr, Fairview	Minneapolis	1%	57244
Abbott Northwestern Hospital	Minneapolis	2%	49073
Essentia Health St Mary's Med Ctr	Duluth	2%	43604
Essentia Health Sandstone	Sandstone	2%	5403
Mayo Clinic Hospital Rochester	Rochester	2%	73006
Mercy Hospital	Coon Rapids	2%	58737
Regina Hospital	Hastings	2%	11108
Regions Hospital	Saint Paul	2%	38689
Rice Memorial Hospital	Willmar	2%	13062
Saint Luke's Hospital	Duluth	2%	27471
United Hospital	Saint Paul	2%	52750
Univ Med Ctr-Mesabi/Mesaba Clinics	Hibbing	2%	13545
Essentia Health Saint Marys	Detroit Lakes	3%	11470
Essentia Health Virginia	Virginia	3%	12117
Fairview Southdale Hospital	Edina	3%	44431
Healtheast Saint John's Hospital	Maplewood	3%	36449
Mayo Clinic Health System - Albert Lea	Albert Lea	3%	13721
North Memorial Medical Center	Robbinsdale	3%	76640
Saint Joseph's Hospital	Saint Paul	3%	22628
Hennepin County Medical Center	Minneapolis	6%	111811

Time from ER Arrival to Being Admitted (minutes)

Hospital Name	City	Min.	Cases
Stevens Community Medical Center[2]	Morris	70	149
Sanford Canby Medical Center[2]	Canby	83	98
Tyler Healthcare Center[3]	Tyler	83	37
Madison Hospital[3]	Madison	88	157
Essentia Health Holy Trinity Hospital	Graceville	91	39
Sleepy Eye Municipal Hospital[3]	Sleepy Eye	93	91
Sanford Tracy[2]	Tracy	94	76
Johnson Memorial Hospital	Dawson	95	57
Swift County Benson Hospital	Benson	103	72
Lakewood Health Center[2]	Baudette	104	75
Bigfork Valley Hospital	Bigfork	105	138
Murray County Memorial Hospital[2]	Slayton	106	78
Glacial Ridge Hospital[2]	Glenwood	108	290
North Valley Health Center	Warren	108	98
Madelia Community Hospital	Madelia	110	54
Sanford Westbrook Medical Center	Westbrook	110	32
Ely Bloomenson Community Hospital	Ely	112	191
Perham Health[2]	Perham	112	152
Centracare Health Sys-Melrose Hosp[2]	Melrose	115	215
Mayo Clinic Health System - Springfield	Springfield	116	68
Sanford Jackson Medical Center	Jackson	117	51
Appleton Municipal Hospital	Appleton	118	51
Municipal Hospital & Granite Manor	Granite Falls	120	166

NOTE: Hospital profiles are in alphabetical order by state, then city, then hospital within the city; Rankings exclude hospitals with less than 25 cases except for patient surveys which excludes hospitals with less than 100 cases; (a) 100-299 cases; (1) The number of cases/patients is too few to report; (2) Data submitted were based on a sample of cases/patients; (3) Results are based on a shorter time period than required; (4) Data suppressed by CMS for one or more quarters; (5) Results are not available for this reporting period; (6) Fewer than 100 patients completed the HCAHPS survey; (7) No cases met the criteria for this measure; (8) The lower limit of the confidence interval cannot be calculated if the number of observed infections equals zero; (9) No data are available from the state/territory for this reporting period; (10) The scores shown reflect fewer than 50 completed surveys; (11) There were discrepancies in the data collection process; (12) This measure does not apply to this hospital for this reporting period; (13) Results cannot be calculated for this reporting period; (14) The results for this state are combined with nearby states to protect confidentiality; Please refer to the User's Guide for a full explanation of data.

Centra Care Health Paynesville	Paynesville	122	139
Centracare Health System - Sauk Centre	Sauk Centre	122	189
Sanford Bagley Medical Center	Bagley	124	96
Hendricks Community Hospital	Hendricks	125	56
Ortonville Area Health Services	Ortonville	126	88
Essentia Health N Pines Med Ctr[2,3]	Aurora	128	64
Sanford Luverne Medical Center[2]	Luverne	132	268
Mayo Clinic Health System - Lake City[2]	Lake City	134	112
Windom Area Hospital[2]	Windom	134	148
Ridgeview Sibley Medical Center	Arlington	135	71
Albany Area Hospital[2,3]	Albany	138	38
Winona Health Services[2]	Winona	138	323
Mayo Clinic Health System - Saint James	Saint James	139	79
Cook Hospital	Cook	143	165
Mayo Clinic Health System - Fairmont[2]	Fairmont	144	289
Saint Elizabeth Medical Center	Wabasha	145	134
Meeker Memorial Hospital[2]	Litchfield	150	236
Lake View Memorial Hospital	Two Harbors	154	90
Pipestone County Medical Center[2]	Pipestone	154	102
Saint Francis Medical Center[2]	Breckenridge	155	204
Deer River Healthcare Center[2]	Deer River	156	128
Essentia Health St Joseph's Med Ctr[2]	Brainerd	160	595
Redwood Area Hospital[2]	Redwood Falls	161	129
Riverwood Healthcare Center[2,3]	Aitkin	163	25
Mayo Clinic Health System - Cannon Falls	Cannon Falls	165	143
Lake Region Healthcare Corporation[2]	Fergus Falls	166	204
Lifecare Medical Center[2]	Roseau	166	334
United Hospital District	Blue Earth	168	316
Mercy Hospital[2]	Moose Lake	169	219
Rainy Lake Medical Center	Int'l Falls	170	226
Sanford Worthington Medical Center[2]	Worthington	171	264
Avera Marshall Regional Medical Center[2]	Marshall	174	166
Mayo Clinic Health System - Waseca	Waseca	178	97
Mille Lacs Health System[2]	Onamia	180	357
Sanford Medical Center Thief River Falls[2]	Thief River Falls	180	188
Glencoe Regional Health Services[2]	Glencoe	181	177
Riverview Hospital[2]	Crookston	181	292
Essentia Health Sandstone[2]	Sandstone	182	144
Essentia Health Virginia[2]	Virginia	182	217
Northfield Hospital[2]	Northfield	182	132
Centracare Health - Monticello[2]	Monticello	186	470
Lakewood Health System[2]	Staples	186	269
Regina Hospital[2]	Hastings	187	280
Mayo Clinic Health System - Red Wing[2]	Red Wing	189	211
River's Edge Hospital & Clinic[2]	Saint Peter	189	172
Saint Luke's Hospital[2]	Duluth	190	451
Mayo Clinic Health System - New Prague[2]	New Prague	192	197
Tri County Hospital[2]	Wadena	192	308
Douglas County Hospital[2]	Alexandria	195	378
Lakeview Memorial Hospital[2]	Stillwater	197	207
New Ulm Medical Center[2]	New Ulm	198	326
Maple Grove Hospital[2]	Maple Grove	202	298
Saint Francis Regional Medical Center[2]	Shakopee	203	579
Mayo Clinic Health System - Albert Lea[2]	Albert Lea	204	320
Saint Cloud Hospital[2]	Saint Cloud	205	397
Rice Memorial Hospital[2]	Willmar	206	146
Sanford Bemidji Medical Center[2]	Bemidji	206	398
Mayo Clinic Health System - Mankato[2]	Mankato	207	366
Cuyuna Regional Medical Center[2]	Crosby	208	278
Hutchinson Health[2]	Hutchinson	208	248
Firstlight Health System[2]	Mora	210	401
Community Memorial Hospital[2]	Cloquet	211	403
Buffalo Hospital[2]	Buffalo	214	240
Essentia Health Saint Marys[2]	Detroit Lakes	215	237
Owatonna Hospital[2]	Owatonna	219	239
North Memorial Medical Center[2]	Robbinsdale	220	732
Red Lake Hospital	Redlake	220	245
Saint Gabriels Hospital[2]	Little Falls	222	244
Ridgeview Medical Center[2]	Waconia	223	440
Cambridge Medical Center[2]	Cambridge	224	328
District One Hospital[2]	Faribault	225	257
Saint Joseph's Hospital[2]	Saint Paul	229	509
Mayo Clinic Hospital Rochester[2]	Rochester	230	494
Saint Joseph's Area Health Services[2]	Park Rapids	230	240
Univ Med Ctr-Mesabi/Mesaba Clinics[2]	Hibbing	233	261
Healtheast Woodwinds Hospital[2]	Woodbury	234	409
Essentia Health St Mary's Med Ctr[2]	Duluth	236	480
Healtheast Saint John's Hospital[2]	Maplewood	245	521
Fairview Southdale Hospital[2]	Edina	247	478
Park Nicollet Methodist Hospital[2]	Saint Louis Park	247	605
Abbott Northwestern Hospital[2]	Minneapolis	248	318
Grand Itasca Clinic & Hospital[2]	Grand Rapids	249	325
Fairview Northland Regional Hospital[2]	Princeton	252	281
United Hospital[2]	Saint Paul	257	458
Unity Hospital[2]	Fridley	258	653
Fairview Ridges Hospital[2]	Burnsville	261	572
Univ of Minnesota Med Ctr, Fairview[2]	Minneapolis	265	443
Olmsted Medical Center	Rochester	266	375
Mercy Hospital[2]	Coon Rapids	270	680
Fairview Lakes Medical Center[2]	Wyoming	276	420
Hennepin County Medical Center[2]	Minneapolis	282	469
Regions Hospital[2]	Saint Paul	293	549

Time from ER Arrival to Discharge (minutes)

Hospital Name	City	Min.	Cases
Cook County Northshore Hospital[3]	Grand Marais	76	87
Riverview Hospital[3]	Crookston	84	180
Winona Health Services	Winona	85	335
Albany Area Hospital[3]	Albany	86	113
Riverwood Healthcare Center[3]	Aitkin	86	209
Bigfork Valley Hospital	Bigfork	89	119
Lake Region Healthcare Corporation	Fergus Falls	89	399
New Ulm Medical Center	New Ulm	89	373
Mayo Clinic Health System - Fairmont	Fairmont	92	367
Mayo Clinic Health System - Red Wing	Red Wing	97	343
Centra Care Health Paynesville	Paynesville	98	290
Mercy Hospital	Moose Lake	98	257
Saint Gabriels Hospital	Little Falls	100	359
Northfield Hospital	Northfield	102	428
Sanford Worthington Medical Center	Worthington	103	430
District One Hospital	Faribault	105	339
Sanford Bemidji Medical Center	Bemidji	107	456
Douglas County Hospital	Alexandria	108	868
Sanford Medical Center Wheaton[3]	Wheaton	110	96
Buffalo Hospital	Buffalo	112	372
Essentia Health St Joseph's Med Ctr	Brainerd	112	366
Hutchinson Health	Hutchinson	112	367
Maple Grove Hospital	Maple Grove	112	374
Owatonna Hospital	Owatonna	115	349
Rice Memorial Hospital	Willmar	116	605
Regina Hospital	Hastings	117	367
Saint Francis Regional Medical Center	Shakopee	118	351
Essentia Health Saint Marys	Detroit Lakes	119	351
Olmsted Medical Center	Rochester	122	17467
Cambridge Medical Center	Cambridge	123	488
Lakeview Memorial Hospital	Stillwater	124	409
Fairview Northland Regional Hospital	Princeton	126	358
Essentia Health Sandstone	Sandstone	128	217
Essentia Health Virginia	Virginia	128	383
Grand Itasca Clinic & Hospital	Grand Rapids	128	348
Mayo Clinic Health System - Mankato	Mankato	128	380
Mayo Clinic Health System - Albert Lea	Albert Lea	134	439
North Memorial Medical Center	Robbinsdale	137	368
Unity Hospital	Fridley	143	387
Ridgeview Medical Center	Waconia	144	371
Univ of Minnesota Med Ctr, Fairview	Minneapolis	145	421
Ridgeview Sibley Medical Center	Arlington	147	86
Saint Luke's Hospital	Duluth	150	450
Healtheast Woodwinds Hospital	Woodbury	151	389
Fairview Lakes Medical Center	Wyoming	156	343
Fairview Ridges Hospital	Burnsville	157	365
Mercy Hospital	Coon Rapids	160	385
Essentia Health St Mary's Med Ctr	Duluth	161	329
Saint Cloud Hospital	Saint Cloud	163	343
United Hospital	Saint Paul	165	413
Mayo Clinic Hospital Rochester	Rochester	166	372
Abbott Northwestern Hospital	Minneapolis	171	423
Univ Med Ctr-Mesabi/Mesaba Clinics	Hibbing	172	300
Park Nicollet Methodist Hospital	Saint Louis Park	175	373
Saint Joseph's Hospital	Saint Paul	185	360
Fairview Southdale Hospital	Edina	186	418
Healtheast Saint John's Hospital	Maplewood	186	378
Regions Hospital	Saint Paul	186	320
Hennepin County Medical Center	Minneapolis	230	338

Time in ER Before Being Evaluated (minutes)

Hospital Name	City	Min.	Cases
Buffalo Hospital	Buffalo	7	427
Maple Grove Hospital	Maple Grove	9	403
Ridgeview Sibley Medical Center	Arlington	9	101
Riverwood Healthcare Center[3]	Aitkin	9	156
Bigfork Valley Hospital	Bigfork	10	230
Saint Francis Regional Medical Center	Shakopee	10	385
Cambridge Medical Center	Cambridge	12	544
Mayo Clinic Health System - Fairmont	Fairmont	12	400
Owatonna Hospital	Owatonna	12	398
Riverview Hospital[3]	Crookston	12	198
Hutchinson Health	Hutchinson	13	375
Mayo Clinic Health System - Mankato	Mankato	13	426
United Hospital	Saint Paul	13	468
Centra Care Health Paynesville	Paynesville	14	302
Essentia Health Sandstone	Sandstone	14	183
Winona Health Services	Winona	14	291
Albany Area Hospital[3]	Albany	15	97
Sanford Worthington Medical Center	Worthington	15	273
Lake Region Healthcare Corporation	Fergus Falls	16	379
Fairview Ridges Hospital	Burnsville	17	408
Lakeview Memorial Hospital	Stillwater	17	221
Mercy Hospital	Moose Lake	17	378
North Memorial Medical Center	Robbinsdale	18	408
Fairview Lakes Medical Center	Wyoming	19	382
Northfield Hospital	Northfield	19	483
District One Hospital	Faribault	20	285
New Ulm Medical Center	New Ulm	20	409
Unity Hospital	Fridley	20	417
Douglas County Hospital	Alexandria	21	604
Essentia Health St Joseph's Med Ctr	Brainerd	21	128
Mayo Clinic Hospital Rochester	Rochester	21	400
Sanford Bemidji Medical Center	Bemidji	21	149
Abbott Northwestern Hospital	Minneapolis	22	490
Cook County Northshore Hospital[3]	Grand Marais	22	66
Essentia Health Saint Marys	Detroit Lakes	22	112
Ridgeview Medical Center	Waconia	22	380
Univ of Minnesota Med Ctr, Fairview	Minneapolis	22	465
Regions Hospital	Saint Paul	23	426
Fairview Northland Regional Hospital	Princeton	24	384
Regina Hospital	Hastings	25	400
Saint Gabriels Hospital	Little Falls	25	205
Sanford Medical Center Wheaton[3]	Wheaton	25	123
Hennepin County Medical Center	Minneapolis	26	337
Mayo Clinic Health System - Red Wing	Red Wing	26	370
Healtheast Woodwinds Hospital	Woodbury	27	391
Mayo Clinic Health System - Albert Lea	Albert Lea	27	494
Mercy Hospital	Coon Rapids	28	436
Essentia Health St Mary's Med Ctr	Duluth	30	116
Essentia Health Virginia	Virginia	30	260
Rice Memorial Hospital	Willmar	30	561
Grand Itasca Clinic & Hospital	Grand Rapids	31	372
Univ Med Ctr-Mesabi/Mesaba Clinics	Hibbing	32	309
Fairview Southdale Hospital	Edina	33	439
Saint Cloud Hospital	Saint Cloud	36	367
Saint Luke's Hospital	Duluth	40	484
Park Nicollet Methodist Hospital	Saint Louis Park	44	344
Olmsted Medical Center	Rochester	45	14960
Saint Joseph's Hospital	Saint Paul	46	401
Healtheast Saint John's Hospital	Maplewood	50	397

Time to Pain Meds for Bone Fractures (minutes)

Hospital Name	City	Min.	Cases
Mille Lacs Health System	Onamia	24	26
Hutchinson Health	Hutchinson	26	30
Winona Health Services	Winona	27	54
Univ Med Ctr-Mesabi/Mesaba Clinics	Hibbing	29	35
Lake Region Healthcare Corporation	Fergus Falls	30	41
Lakeview Memorial Hospital	Stillwater	30	44
New Ulm Medical Center	New Ulm	30	37
Rice Memorial Hospital	Willmar	30	82
Saint Francis Regional Medical Center	Shakopee	30	100
Buffalo Hospital	Buffalo	33	82
Maple Grove Hospital	Maple Grove	33	185
Fairview Ridges Hospital	Burnsville	34	256
District One Hospital	Faribault	35	87
Owatonna Hospital	Owatonna	35	49
Mayo Clinic Health System - Mankato	Mankato	36	105
Ridgeview Medical Center	Waconia	36	198
Essentia Health St Joseph's Med Ctr	Brainerd	37	101
Mayo Clinic Health System - Fairmont	Fairmont	37	31
Essentia Health Saint Marys	Detroit Lakes	38	60
Healtheast Woodwinds Hospital	Woodbury	38	123
Sanford Worthington Medical Center	Worthington	39	60
Grand Itasca Clinic & Hospital	Grand Rapids	40	46
Cambridge Medical Center	Cambridge	42	50
Fairview Lakes Medical Center	Wyoming	42	125
Unity Hospital	Fridley	42	157
Hennepin County Medical Center	Minneapolis	43	95
Fairview Northland Regional Hospital	Princeton	44	74
Abbott Northwestern Hospital	Minneapolis	46	81
North Memorial Medical Center	Robbinsdale	46	146
Regina Hospital	Hastings	47	59
Northfield Hospital	Northfield	48	34
Univ of Minnesota Med Ctr, Fairview	Minneapolis	49	131
Mayo Clinic Health System - Albert Lea	Albert Lea	50	41
Mercy Hospital	Coon Rapids	50	177
United Hospital	Saint Paul	50	56
Douglas County Hospital	Alexandria	51	78
Essentia Health St Mary's Med Ctr	Duluth	51	154
Mayo Clinic Hospital Rochester	Rochester	51	325
Regions Hospital	Saint Paul	51	129
Essentia Health Virginia	Virginia	54	64
Fairview Southdale Hospital	Edina	54	191
Saint Cloud Hospital	Saint Cloud	54	177
Saint Joseph's Hospital	Saint Paul	55	38
Sanford Bemidji Medical Center	Bemidji	57	109
Mayo Clinic Health System - Red Wing	Red Wing	58	32
Saint Luke's Hospital	Duluth	66	62
Park Nicollet Methodist Hospital	Saint Louis Park	70	154
Healtheast Saint John's Hospital	Maplewood	71	136
Olmsted Medical Center	Rochester	79	86

NOTE: Hospital profiles are in alphabetical order by state, then city, then hospital within the city; Rankings exclude hospitals with less than 25 cases except for patient surveys which excludes hospitals with less than 100 cases; (a) 100-299 cases; (1) The number of cases/patients is too few to report; (2) Data submitted were based on a sample of cases/patients; (3) Results are based on a shorter time period than required; (4) Data suppressed by CMS for one or more quarters; (5) Results are not available for this reporting period; (6) Fewer than 100 patients completed the HCAHPS survey; (7) No cases met the criteria for this measure; (8) The lower limit of the confidence interval cannot be calculated if the number of observed infections equals zero; (9) No data are available from the state/territory for this reporting period; (10) The scores shown reflect fewer than 50 completed surveys; (11) There were discrepancies in the data collection process; (12) This measure does not apply to this hospital for this reporting period; (13) Results cannot be calculated for this reporting period; (14) The results for this state are combined with nearby states to protect confidentiality; Please refer to the User's Guide for a full explanation of data.

Heart Attack Care

Aspirin Given at Discharge

Hospital Name	City	Rate	Cases
Abbott Northwestern Hospital	Minneapolis	100%	904
Fairview Ridges Hospital	Burnsville	100%	113
Fairview Southdale Hospital[2]	Edina	100%	342
Hennepin County Medical Center	Minneapolis	100%	152
Mayo Clinic Health System - Albert Lea	Albert Lea	100%	27
Mayo Clinic Hospital Rochester[2]	Rochester	100%	307
Mercy Hospital	Coon Rapids	100%	483
Minneapolis VA Medical Center	Minneapolis	100%	107
Regions Hospital	Saint Paul	100%	488
Saint Cloud Hospital	Saint Cloud	100%	738
United Hospital	Saint Paul	100%	471
Univ of Minnesota Med Ctr, Fairview	Minneapolis	100%	208
Essentia Health St Mary's Med Ctr[2]	Duluth	99%	356
Mayo Clinic Health System - Mankato	Mankato	99%	220
North Memorial Medical Center[2]	Robbinsdale	99%	301
Park Nicollet Methodist Hospital	Saint Louis Park	99%	326
Saint Joseph's Hospital	Saint Paul	99%	325
Saint Luke's Hospital	Duluth	99%	228
Ridgeview Medical Center	Waconia	97%	39
Sanford Bemidji Medical Center	Bemidji	97%	96
Essentia Health St Joseph's Med Ctr	Brainerd	94%	85

PCI Within 90 Minutes of Arrival

Hospital Name	City	Rate	Cases
Fairview Southdale Hospital[2]	Edina	100%	60
Saint Luke's Hospital	Duluth	100%	25
North Memorial Medical Center[2]	Robbinsdale	99%	73
Saint Joseph's Hospital	Saint Paul	98%	43
Abbott Northwestern Hospital	Minneapolis	96%	50
Park Nicollet Methodist Hospital	Saint Louis Park	96%	51
Regions Hospital	Saint Paul	96%	77
Saint Cloud Hospital	Saint Cloud	96%	68
Mercy Hospital	Coon Rapids	93%	61
United Hospital	Saint Paul	93%	43
Hennepin County Medical Center	Minneapolis	92%	38

Statin Prescribed at Discharge

Hospital Name	City	Rate	Cases
Abbott Northwestern Hospital	Minneapolis	100%	868
Essentia Health St Mary's Med Ctr[2]	Duluth	100%	335
Fairview Ridges Hospital	Burnsville	100%	112
Fairview Southdale Hospital[2]	Edina	100%	351
Hennepin County Medical Center	Minneapolis	100%	149
Mayo Clinic Hospital Rochester[2]	Rochester	100%	304
Mercy Hospital	Coon Rapids	100%	480
Regions Hospital	Saint Paul	100%	476
Saint Cloud Hospital	Saint Cloud	100%	698
Saint Luke's Hospital	Duluth	100%	223
Univ of Minnesota Med Ctr, Fairview	Minneapolis	100%	201
Minneapolis VA Medical Center	Minneapolis	99%	109
Park Nicollet Methodist Hospital	Saint Louis Park	99%	323
Saint Joseph's Hospital	Saint Paul	99%	328
United Hospital	Saint Paul	99%	451
Mayo Clinic Health System - Mankato	Mankato	98%	212
North Memorial Medical Center[2]	Robbinsdale	98%	292
Essentia Health St Joseph's Med Ctr	Brainerd	95%	85
Sanford Bemidji Medical Center	Bemidji	95%	94
Mayo Clinic Health System - Albert Lea	Albert Lea	93%	28
Ridgeview Medical Center	Waconia	92%	37

Heart Failure Care

ACE Inhibitor or ARB for LVSD

Hospital Name	City	Rate	Cases
Essentia Health St Mary's Med Ctr[2]	Duluth	100%	97
Fairview Southdale Hospital[2]	Edina	100%	80
Healtheast Saint John's Hospital	Maplewood	100%	61
Mercy Hospital	Coon Rapids	100%	109
Ridgeview Medical Center	Waconia	100%	30
Sanford Bemidji Medical Center	Bemidji	100%	31
Unity Hospital	Fridley	100%	45
Hennepin County Medical Center[2]	Minneapolis	99%	111
Saint Cloud Hospital	Saint Cloud	99%	159
Saint Joseph's Hospital	Saint Paul	99%	103
Univ of Minnesota Med Ctr, Fairview	Minneapolis	99%	156
Fairview Ridges Hospital	Burnsville	98%	62
Minneapolis VA Medical Center	Minneapolis	98%	63
Regions Hospital	Saint Paul	98%	98
Park Nicollet Methodist Hospital	Saint Louis Park	97%	119
United Hospital	Saint Paul	97%	135
Saint Luke's Hospital	Duluth	96%	52
Abbott Northwestern Hospital	Minneapolis	93%	234
North Memorial Medical Center[2]	Robbinsdale	93%	69
Mayo Clinic Hospital Rochester[2]	Rochester	92%	72
Mayo Clinic Health System - Mankato	Mankato	90%	58
Essentia Health St Joseph's Med Ctr	Brainerd	87%	52
Mayo Clinic Health System - Fairmont	Fairmont	84%	31

Discharge Instructions Given

Hospital Name	City	Rate	Cases
Fairview Southdale Hospital[2]	Edina	100%	221
Maple Grove Hospital	Maple Grove	100%	78
Mayo Clinic Health System - Red Wing	Red Wing	100%	39
Regions Hospital	Saint Paul	100%	286
Tri County Hospital	Wadena	100%	34
Univ of Minnesota Med Ctr, Fairview	Minneapolis	100%	358
Abbott Northwestern Hospital	Minneapolis	99%	609
Mercy Hospital	Coon Rapids	99%	363
Saint Francis Regional Medical Center	Shakopee	99%	88
Unity Hospital	Fridley	99%	132
Buffalo Hospital	Buffalo	98%	56
Cambridge Medical Center	Cambridge	98%	59
Fairview Lakes Medical Center	Wyoming	98%	46
Fairview Ridges Hospital	Burnsville	98%	199
New Ulm Medical Center	New Ulm	98%	47
North Memorial Medical Center[2]	Robbinsdale	98%	220
United Hospital	Saint Paul	98%	331
Winona Health Services	Winona	98%	49
Centracare Health - Monticello	Monticello	97%	30
District One Hospital	Faribault	97%	29
Healtheast Saint John's Hospital	Maplewood	97%	174
Mille Lacs Health System[2]	Onamia	97%	30
Minneapolis VA Medical Center	Minneapolis	97%	185
Saint Cloud Hospital	Saint Cloud	97%	527
Essentia Health Saint Marys	Detroit Lakes	96%	28
Fairview Northland Regional Hospital	Princeton	96%	25
Healtheast Woodwinds Hospital	Woodbury	96%	70
Mayo Clinic Hospital Rochester[2]	Rochester	96%	261
Owatonna Hospital	Owatonna	96%	47
Park Nicollet Methodist Hospital	Saint Louis Park	96%	345
Douglas County Hospital	Alexandria	95%	58
Hennepin County Medical Center[2]	Minneapolis	95%	235
Ridgeview Medical Center	Waconia	94%	88
Essentia Health St Mary's Med Ctr[2]	Duluth	93%	227
Saint Joseph's Hospital	Saint Paul	93%	228
Saint Luke's Hospital	Duluth	93%	101
Mayo Clinic Health System - Albert Lea	Albert Lea	92%	73
Regina Hospital	Hastings	92%	52
Rice Memorial Hospital	Willmar	92%	60
Grand Itasca Clinic & Hospital	Grand Rapids	91%	43
Essentia Health St Joseph's Med Ctr	Brainerd	89%	178
Univ Med Ctr-Mesabi/Mesaba Clinics	Hibbing	88%	34
Lake Region Healthcare Corporation	Fergus Falls	85%	33
Lakeview Memorial Hospital	Stillwater	85%	41
Mayo Clinic Health System - Fairmont	Fairmont	81%	67
Mayo Clinic Health System - Mankato	Mankato	80%	188
Sanford Bemidji Medical Center	Bemidji	77%	95
Cuyuna Regional Medical Center	Crosby	76%	33
Essentia Health Virginia	Virginia	73%	41
Northfield Hospital	Northfield	54%	26
Firstlight Health System	Mora	52%	27
Stevens Community Medical Center	Morris	0%	29

Evaluation of LVS Function

Hospital Name	City	Rate	Cases
Abbott Northwestern Hospital	Minneapolis	100%	752
Buffalo Hospital	Buffalo	100%	77
Cambridge Medical Center	Cambridge	100%	68
Centracare Health - Monticello	Monticello	100%	43
Cuyuna Regional Medical Center	Crosby	100%	44
District One Hospital	Faribault	100%	38
Douglas County Hospital	Alexandria	100%	101
Essentia Health St Joseph's Med Ctr	Brainerd	100%	212
Essentia Health St Mary's Med Ctr[2]	Duluth	100%	285
Essentia Health Saint Marys	Detroit Lakes	100%	44
Fairview Lakes Medical Center	Wyoming	100%	60
Fairview Northland Regional Hospital	Princeton	100%	46
Fairview Ridges Hospital	Burnsville	100%	256
Fairview Southdale Hospital[2]	Edina	100%	352
Glacial Ridge Hospital[2]	Glenwood	100%	29
Glencoe Regional Health Services	Glencoe	100%	30
Hennepin County Medical Center[2]	Minneapolis	100%	278
Hutchinson Health	Hutchinson	100%	47
Maple Grove Hospital	Maple Grove	100%	95
Mayo Clinic Health System - Mankato	Mankato	100%	231
Mayo Clinic Health System - Red Wing	Red Wing	100%	55
Mayo Clinic Hospital Rochester[2]	Rochester	100%	321
Mercy Hospital	Coon Rapids	100%	445
Minneapolis VA Medical Center	Minneapolis	100%	227
North Memorial Medical Center[2]	Robbinsdale	100%	289
Owatonna Hospital	Owatonna	100%	76
Park Nicollet Methodist Hospital	Saint Louis Park	100%	448
Regina Hospital	Hastings	100%	69
Regions Hospital	Saint Paul	100%	382
Rice Memorial Hospital	Willmar	100%	91
Saint Cloud Hospital	Saint Cloud	100%	731
Saint Francis Regional Medical Center	Shakopee	100%	120
United Hospital	Saint Paul	100%	428
Unity Hospital	Fridley	100%	176
Univ of Minnesota Med Ctr, Fairview	Minneapolis	100%	431
Healtheast Saint John's Hospital	Maplewood	99%	229
Healtheast Woodwinds Hospital	Woodbury	99%	92
Mayo Clinic Health System - Albert Lea	Albert Lea	99%	102
New Ulm Medical Center	New Ulm	99%	67
Ridgeview Medical Center	Waconia	99%	124
Saint Joseph's Hospital	Saint Paul	99%	279
Saint Luke's Hospital	Duluth	99%	149
Lake Region Healthcare Corporation	Fergus Falls	98%	61
Lakeview Memorial Hospital	Stillwater	98%	59
Sanford Bemidji Medical Center	Bemidji	98%	122
Tri County Hospital	Wadena	98%	42
Univ Med Ctr-Mesabi/Mesaba Clinics	Hibbing	98%	46
Firstlight Health System	Mora	97%	32
Mille Lacs Health System[2]	Onamia	97%	35
Saint Francis Medical Center[2]	Breckenridge	97%	31
Grand Itasca Clinic & Hospital	Grand Rapids	96%	57
Mayo Clinic Health System - Fairmont	Fairmont	96%	101
Northfield Hospital	Northfield	96%	46
Essentia Health Virginia	Virginia	95%	60
Winona Health Services	Winona	94%	65
Sanford Medical Center Thief River Falls	Thief River Falls	91%	32
Lifecare Medical Center	Roseau	88%	26
Stevens Community Medical Center	Morris	82%	39
Sanford Worthington Medical Center[2]	Worthington	78%	27
Perham Health	Perham	47%	34

Medicare Spending

Medicare Spending per Patient (ratio)

Hospital Name	City	Ratio	Cases
Red Lake Hospital	Redlake	0.75	-
Phillips Eye Institute	Minneapolis	0.77	-
Northfield Hospital	Northfield	0.81	-
District One Hospital	Faribault	0.82	-
Mayo Clinic Health System - Fairmont	Fairmont	0.82	-
Mayo Clinic Health System - Red Wing	Red Wing	0.83	-
Sanford Worthington Medical Center	Worthington	0.84	-
Essentia Health St Joseph's Med Ctr	Brainerd	0.85	-
Fairview Northland Regional Hospital	Princeton	0.86	-
Hutchinson Health	Hutchinson	0.86	-
Winona Health Services	Winona	0.86	-
Essentia Health Virginia	Virginia	0.87	-
Fairview Lakes Medical Center	Wyoming	0.87	-
Grand Itasca Clinic & Hospital	Grand Rapids	0.87	-
Healtheast Woodwinds Hospital	Woodbury	0.87	-
Owatonna Hospital	Owatonna	0.87	-
Buffalo Hospital	Buffalo	0.88	-
Cambridge Medical Center	Cambridge	0.88	-
Maple Grove Hospital	Maple Grove	0.88	-
Regina Hospital	Hastings	0.88	-
Sanford Bemidji Medical Center	Bemidji	0.88	-
Univ Med Ctr-Mesabi/Mesaba Clinics	Hibbing	0.88	-
Lakeview Memorial Hospital	Stillwater	0.89	-
Olmsted Medical Center	Rochester	0.89	-
Saint Cloud Hospital	Saint Cloud	0.89	-
Mayo Clinic Health System - Albert Lea	Albert Lea	0.90	-
Mayo Clinic Health System - Mankato	Mankato	0.90	-
Healtheast Saint John's Hospital	Maplewood	0.91	-
Rice Memorial Hospital	Willmar	0.91	-
Hennepin County Medical Center	Minneapolis	0.92	-
Mayo Clinic Methodist- Hospital	Rochester	0.92	-
Mercy Hospital	Coon Rapids	0.92	-
Park Nicollet Methodist Hospital	Saint Louis Park	0.92	-
Abbott Northwestern Hospital	Minneapolis	0.93	-
North Memorial Medical Center	Robbinsdale	0.93	-
Douglas County Hospital	Alexandria	0.94	-
Essentia Health Saint Marys	Detroit Lakes	0.94	-
Fairview Ridges Hospital	Burnsville	0.94	-
Mayo Clinic Hospital Rochester	Rochester	0.94	-
Regions Hospital	Saint Paul	0.94	-
Ridgeview Medical Center	Waconia	0.94	-
Unity Hospital	Fridley	0.94	-
Saint Francis Regional Medical Center	Shakopee	0.95	-
Essentia Health Duluth	Duluth	0.96	-
Lake Region Healthcare Corporation	Fergus Falls	0.96	-
United Hospital	Saint Paul	0.96	-
Essentia Health St Mary's Med Ctr	Duluth	0.97	-
Fairview Southdale Hospital	Edina	0.97	-
Saint Joseph's Hospital	Saint Paul	0.97	-
Univ of Minnesota Med Ctr, Fairview	Minneapolis	0.97	-
Saint Luke's Hospital	Duluth	0.98	-

NOTE: Hospital profiles are in alphabetical order by state, then city, then hospital within the city; Rankings exclude hospitals with less than 25 cases except for patient surveys which excludes hospitals with less than 100 cases; (a) 100-299 cases; (1) The number of cases/patients is too few to report; (2) Data submitted were based on a sample of cases/patients; (3) Results are based on a shorter time period than required; (4) Data suppressed by CMS for one or more quarters; (5) Results are not available for this reporting period; (6) Fewer than 100 patients completed the HCAHPS survey; (7) No cases met the criteria for this measure; (8) The lower limit of the confidence interval cannot be calculated if the number of observed infections equals zero; (9) No data are available from the state/territory for this reporting period; (10) The scores shown reflect fewer than 50 completed surveys; (11) There were discrepancies in the data collection process; (12) This measure does not apply to this hospital for this reporting period; (13) Results cannot be calculated for this reporting period; (14) The results for this state are combined with nearby states to protect confidentiality; Please refer to the User's Guide for a full explanation of data.

Pneumonia Care

Appropriate Initial Antibiotic Given

Hospital Name	City	Rate	Cases
Avera Marshall Regional Medical Center	Marshall	100%	26
Cambridge Medical Center	Cambridge	100%	68
Hutchinson Health	Hutchinson	100%	33
Mayo Clinic Health System - Fairmont	Fairmont	100%	40
New Ulm Medical Center	New Ulm	100%	26
Rice Memorial Hospital	Willmar	100%	58
Sanford Bemidji Medical Center	Bemidji	100%	66
Fairview Ridges Hospital	Burnsville	99%	150
Fairview Southdale Hospital	Edina	99%	199
Healtheast Saint John's Hospital[2]	Maplewood	99%	117
Healtheast Woodwinds Hospital[2]	Woodbury	99%	71
Maple Grove Hospital	Maple Grove	99%	119
Saint Francis Regional Medical Center	Shakopee	99%	70
Unity Hospital	Fridley	99%	185
Buffalo Hospital	Buffalo	98%	42
Fairview Lakes Medical Center	Wyoming	98%	45
Fairview Northland Regional Hospital	Princeton	98%	52
Grand Itasca Clinic & Hospital	Grand Rapids	98%	66
Hennepin County Medical Center[2]	Minneapolis	98%	49
Lake Region Healthcare Corporation	Fergus Falls	98%	49
Mayo Clinic Health System - Mankato	Mankato	98%	84
Minneapolis VA Medical Center	Minneapolis	98%	40
Owatonna Hospital	Owatonna	98%	43
Saint Francis Medical Center[2]	Breckenridge	98%	42
United Hospital	Saint Paul	98%	161
Abbott Northwestern Hospital	Minneapolis	97%	133
Community Memorial Hospital	Cloquet	97%	34
Cuyuna Regional Medical Center	Crosby	97%	31
Essentia Health St Joseph's Med Ctr	Brainerd	97%	92
Lakeview Memorial Hospital	Stillwater	97%	37
Mercy Hospital	Coon Rapids	97%	193
Regions Hospital	Saint Paul	97%	199
Univ of Minnesota Med Ctr, Fairview	Minneapolis	97%	79
Lifecare Medical Center	Roseau	96%	25
Saint Joseph's Hospital[2]	Saint Paul	96%	82
Essentia Health Saint Marys	Detroit Lakes	95%	37
Firstlight Health System	Mora	95%	41
Mayo Clinic Health System - Albert Lea	Albert Lea	95%	78
Mayo Clinic Health System - Red Wing	Red Wing	95%	38
Univ Med Ctr-Mesabi/Mesaba Clinics	Hibbing	95%	63
Winona Health Services	Winona	95%	59
Ridgeview Medical Center	Waconia	94%	88
Saint Cloud Hospital	Saint Cloud	94%	216
North Memorial Medical Center[2]	Robbinsdale	93%	72
Regina Hospital	Hastings	93%	56
Saint Luke's Hospital[2]	Duluth	93%	72
Park Nicollet Methodist Hospital	Saint Louis Park	92%	310
Saint Gabriels Hospital	Little Falls	92%	37
Tri County Hospital	Wadena	92%	38
District One Hospital	Faribault	91%	67
Essentia Health Virginia	Virginia	91%	33
Perham Health	Perham	91%	32
Essentia Health St Mary's Med Ctr[2]	Duluth	90%	68
Douglas County Hospital	Alexandria	88%	66
Mille Lacs Health System	Onamia	88%	25
Olmsted Medical Center	Rochester	88%	34
Mayo Clinic Hospital Rochester[2]	Rochester	84%	31
Sanford Worthington Medical Center[2]	Worthington	83%	29
Lakewood Health System[2]	Staples	80%	30
Sanford Medical Center Thief River Falls	Thief River Falls	77%	31
Stevens Community Medical Center	Morris	75%	32

Blood Culture Timing

Hospital Name	City	Rate	Cases
Avera Marshall Regional Medical Center	Marshall	100%	35
Centracare Health - Monticello[2]	Monticello	100%	34
District One Hospital	Faribault	100%	71
Fairview Ridges Hospital	Burnsville	100%	251
Hennepin County Medical Center[2]	Minneapolis	100%	54
Hutchinson Health	Hutchinson	100%	53
Mayo Clinic Health System - Fairmont	Fairmont	100%	44
Mayo Clinic Health System - Red Wing	Red Wing	100%	45
New Ulm Medical Center	New Ulm	100%	54
Saint Francis Medical Center[2]	Breckenridge	100%	25
Saint Francis Regional Medical Center	Shakopee	100%	63
Tri County Hospital	Wadena	100%	30
Douglas County Hospital	Alexandria	99%	125
Essentia Health St Joseph's Med Ctr	Brainerd	99%	135
Fairview Northland Regional Hospital	Princeton	99%	110
Fairview Southdale Hospital	Edina	99%	364
Maple Grove Hospital	Maple Grove	99%	148
Minneapolis VA Medical Center	Minneapolis	99%	119
North Memorial Medical Center[2]	Robbinsdale	99%	105
Regions Hospital	Saint Paul	99%	237
Rice Memorial Hospital	Willmar	99%	78
Saint Luke's Hospital[2]	Duluth	99%	149
Univ of Minnesota Med Ctr, Fairview	Minneapolis	99%	262
Winona Health Services	Winona	99%	108
Abbott Northwestern Hospital	Minneapolis	98%	230
Cambridge Medical Center	Cambridge	98%	103
Fairview Lakes Medical Center	Wyoming	98%	102
Healtheast Saint John's Hospital[2]	Maplewood	98%	186
Lake Region Healthcare Corporation	Fergus Falls	98%	81
Mercy Hospital	Coon Rapids	98%	182
Regina Hospital	Hastings	98%	60
Saint Cloud Hospital	Saint Cloud	98%	359
Saint Joseph's Hospital[2]	Saint Paul	98%	128
United Hospital	Saint Paul	98%	246
Unity Hospital	Fridley	98%	309
Healtheast Woodwinds Hospital[2]	Woodbury	97%	118
Mayo Clinic Health System - Albert Lea	Albert Lea	97%	121
Mayo Clinic Health System - Mankato	Mankato	97%	156
Owatonna Hospital	Owatonna	97%	36
Ridgeview Medical Center	Waconia	97%	168
Sanford Worthington Medical Center[2]	Worthington	97%	38
Univ Med Ctr-Mesabi/Mesaba Clinics	Hibbing	97%	65
Essentia Health St Mary's Med Ctr[2]	Duluth	96%	85
Lakeview Memorial Hospital	Stillwater	96%	26
Mayo Clinic Hospital Rochester[2]	Rochester	96%	81
Park Nicollet Methodist Hospital	Saint Louis Park	96%	382
Community Memorial Hospital	Cloquet	95%	44
Sanford Bemidji Medical Center	Bemidji	95%	113
Buffalo Hospital	Buffalo	94%	47
Cuyuna Regional Medical Center	Crosby	94%	48
Essentia Health Saint Marys	Detroit Lakes	94%	52
Firstlight Health System	Mora	94%	33
Olmsted Medical Center	Rochester	94%	53
Saint Gabriels Hospital	Little Falls	93%	56
Essentia Health Virginia	Virginia	91%	43
Mille Lacs Health System	Onamia	91%	33
Grand Itasca Clinic & Hospital	Grand Rapids	89%	97

Pregnancy and Delivery Care

Newborns whose Deliveries were Scheduled Early

Hospital Name	City	Rate	Cases
Abbott Northwestern Hospital[2]	Minneapolis	0%	64
Essentia Health Virginia	Virginia	0%	29
Fairview Lakes Medical Center	Wyoming	0%	130
Healtheast Woodwinds Hospital[2]	Woodbury	0%	35
Hennepin County Medical Center	Minneapolis	0%	59
Hutchinson Health	Hutchinson	0%	27
Olmsted Medical Center	Rochester	0%	101
Saint Joseph's Hospital[2]	Saint Paul	0%	28
Saint Luke's Hospital[2]	Duluth	0%	35
Sanford Worthington Medical Center	Worthington	0%	75
Univ of Minnesota Med Ctr, Fairview[2]	Minneapolis	0%	26
Essentia Health St Mary's Med Ctr	Duluth	1%	80
Sanford Bemidji Medical Center	Bemidji	1%	90
Essentia Health Saint Marys	Detroit Lakes	2%	63
Fairview Southdale Hospital[2]	Edina	2%	43
Maple Grove Hospital[2]	Maple Grove	2%	103
Mercy Hospital[2]	Coon Rapids	2%	45
Regions Hospital	Saint Paul	2%	171
Douglas County Hospital	Alexandria	3%	58
Healtheast Saint John's Hospital[2]	Maplewood	3%	58
Ridgeview Medical Center[2]	Waconia	3%	29
Saint Francis Regional Medical Center[2]	Shakopee	3%	35
Essentia Health St Joseph's Med Ctr	Brainerd	4%	28
Fairview Northland Regional Hospital	Princeton	4%	25
Park Nicollet Methodist Hospital	Saint Louis Park	4%	204
United Hospital[2]	Saint Paul	4%	51
Winona Health Services[2]	Winona	4%	28
Mayo Clinic Health System - Albert Lea	Albert Lea	5%	40
Saint Cloud Hospital[2]	Saint Cloud	5%	375
Northfield Hospital[2]	Northfield	6%	34
Unity Hospital[2]	Fridley	6%	33
Mayo Clinic Health System - Mankato	Mankato	8%	130
Buffalo Hospital[2]	Buffalo	10%	41
District One Hospital	Faribault	10%	58
Owatonna Hospital[2]	Owatonna	10%	40
Grand Itasca Clinic & Hospital	Grand Rapids	11%	36
Univ Med Ctr-Mesabi/Mesaba Clinics[2]	Hibbing	15%	34
Fairview Ridges Hospital[2]	Burnsville	17%	30
Lake Region Healthcare Corporation	Fergus Falls	31%	48

Preventive Care

Immunization for Influenza

Hospital Name	City	Rate	Cases
Mayo Clinic Health System - Saint James	Saint James	100%	90
Olmsted Medical Center	Rochester	100%	860
Ortonville Area Health Services	Ortonville	100%	29
Avera Marshall Regional Medical Center[2]	Marshall	99%	236
Essentia Health St Joseph's Med Ctr[2]	Brainerd	99%	536
Fairview Lakes Medical Center[2]	Wyoming	99%	326
Fairview Northland Regional Hospital[2]	Princeton	99%	235
Mayo Clinic Health System - Waseca	Waseca	99%	159
Buffalo Hospital[2]	Buffalo	98%	253
Cambridge Medical Center[2]	Cambridge	98%	298
Essentia Health N Pines Med Ctr[2,3]	Aurora	98%	45
Hutchinson Health[2]	Hutchinson	98%	252
Redwood Area Hospital[2]	Redwood Falls	98%	113
Saint Luke's Hospital[2]	Duluth	98%	588
Tri County Hospital[2]	Wadena	98%	292
Regions Hospital[2]	Saint Paul	97%	556
Saint Cloud Hospital[2]	Saint Cloud	97%	520
Saint Francis Regional Medical Center[2]	Shakopee	97%	542
Saint Joseph's Area Health Services[2]	Park Rapids	97%	274
Unity Hospital[2]	Fridley	97%	553
Centracare Health System - Sauk Centre	Sauk Centre	96%	192
District One Hospital[2]	Faribault	96%	246
Essentia Health Sandstone[2]	Sandstone	96%	108
Maple Grove Hospital[2]	Maple Grove	96%	413
Saint Gabriels Hospital[2]	Little Falls	96%	265
Abbott Northwestern Hospital[2]	Minneapolis	95%	566
Mayo Clinic Health System - Red Wing[2]	Red Wing	95%	256
Mercy Hospital[2]	Moose Lake	95%	257
Phillips Eye Institute	Minneapolis	95%	55
Rice Memorial Hospital[2]	Willmar	95%	327
Sanford Luverne Medical Center	Luverne	95%	236
Healtheast Saint John's Hospital[2]	Maplewood	94%	503
Mayo Clinic Health System - Springfield	Springfield	94%	71
Saint Joseph's Hospital[2]	Saint Paul	94%	557
Sanford Bemidji Medical Center[2]	Bemidji	94%	505
Sanford Canby Medical Center	Canby	94%	149
Essentia Health Virginia[2]	Virginia	93%	252
Fairview Southdale Hospital[2]	Edina	93%	565
Lake Region Healthcare Corporation[2]	Fergus Falls	93%	282
Mayo Clinic Health System - Cannon Falls	Cannon Falls	93%	107
Mayo Clinic Health System - Fairmont[2]	Fairmont	93%	270
North Memorial Medical Center[2]	Robbinsdale	93%	572
Park Nicollet Methodist Hospital[2]	Saint Louis Park	93%	563
Bigfork Valley Hospital	Bigfork	92%	148
Essentia Health St Mary's Med Ctr[2]	Duluth	92%	568
Mayo Clinic Health System - Albert Lea[2]	Albert Lea	92%	312
Mayo Clinic Health System - Mankato[2]	Mankato	92%	532
Mayo Clinic Methodist- Hospital[2]	Rochester	92%	555
Mercy Hospital[2]	Coon Rapids	92%	592
New Ulm Medical Center[2]	New Ulm	92%	253
Pipestone County Medical Center[2]	Pipestone	92%	142
Cuyuna Regional Medical Center[2]	Crosby	91%	256
Ridgeview Medical Center[2]	Waconia	91%	513
Sanford Worthington Medical Center[2]	Worthington	91%	380
United Hospital[2]	Saint Paul	91%	570
Firstlight Health System[2]	Mora	90%	267
Glencoe Regional Health Services[2]	Glencoe	90%	234
Northfield Hospital[2]	Northfield	90%	257
Douglas County Hospital[2]	Alexandria	89%	390
Grand Itasca Clinic & Hospital[2]	Grand Rapids	89%	257
Mayo Clinic Health System - Lake City[2]	Lake City	89%	214
Mayo Clinic Hospital Rochester[2]	Rochester	89%	617
Murray County Memorial Hospital	Slayton	89%	123
Owatonna Hospital[2]	Owatonna	89%	242
Saint Francis Medical Center[2]	Breckenridge	89%	246
Centracare Health Sys-Melrose Hosp	Melrose	88%	269
Healtheast Woodwinds Hospital[2]	Woodbury	88%	504
Johnson Memorial Hospital[2]	Dawson	88%	56
River's Edge Hospital & Clinic	Saint Peter	88%	161
Univ of Minnesota Med Ctr, Fairview[2]	Minneapolis	88%	556
Fairview Ridges Hospital[2]	Burnsville	87%	495
Glacial Ridge Hospital[2]	Glenwood	87%	257
Municipal Hospital & Granite Manor	Granite Falls	87%	161
Sanford Westbrook Medical Center[2]	Westbrook	87%	38
United Hospital District	Blue Earth	87%	260
Univ Med Ctr-Mesabi/Mesaba Clinics[2]	Hibbing	87%	277
Essentia Health Duluth[2]	Duluth	86%	340
Regina Hospital[2]	Hastings	86%	277
Centracare Health - Monticello[2]	Monticello	84%	283
Hennepin County Medical Center[2]	Minneapolis	84%	506
Lakeview Memorial Hospital[2]	Stillwater	84%	393
Lakewood Health Center[2]	Baudette	84%	56
Saint Elizabeth Medical Center	Wabasha	84%	167
Sanford Tracy	Tracy	84%	79
Windom Area Hospital	Windom	84%	187
Madelia Community Hospital	Madelia	83%	52
Mille Lacs Health System[2]	Onamia	83%	190
Renville County Hospital & Clinics	Olivia	83%	72
Lifecare Medical Center	Roseau	82%	312
Sanford Bagley Medical Center	Bagley	82%	77
Sleepy Eye Municipal Hospital	Sleepy Eye	82%	153
Tyler Healthcare Center	Tyler	82%	34
Centra Care Health Paynesville	Paynesville	80%	213
Sanford Medical Center Thief River Falls[2]	Thief River Falls	80%	286
Lake View Memorial Hospital[2]	Two Harbors	79%	68
Winona Health Services[2]	Winona	79%	272
Essentia Health Saint Marys[2]	Detroit Lakes	78%	252

NOTE: Hospital profiles are in alphabetical order by state, then city, then hospital within the city; Rankings exclude hospitals with less than 25 cases except for patient surveys which excludes hospitals with less than 100 cases; (a) 100-299 cases; (1) The number of cases/patients is too few to report; (2) Data submitted were based on a sample of cases/patients; (3) Results are based on a shorter time period than required; (4) Data suppressed by CMS for one or more quarters; (5) Results are not available for this reporting period; (6) Fewer than 100 patients completed the HCAHPS survey; (7) No cases met the criteria for this measure; (8) The lower limit of the confidence interval cannot be calculated if the number of observed infections equals zero; (9) No data are available from the state/territory for this reporting period; (10) The scores shown reflect fewer than 50 completed surveys; (11) There were discrepancies in the data collection process; (12) This measure does not apply to this hospital for this reporting period; (13) Results cannot be calculated for this reporting period; (14) The results for this state are combined with nearby states to protect confidentiality; Please refer to the User's Guide for a full explanation of data.

Hospital Name	City	Rate	Cases
North Valley Health Center	Warren	78%	100
Appleton Municipal Hospital	Appleton	76%	37
Community Memorial Hospital[2]	Cloquet	76%	289
Mayo Clinic Health System - New Prague[2]	New Prague	76%	240
Ridgeview Sibley Medical Center	Arlington	75%	65
Essentia Health Holy Trinity Hospital	Graceville	74%	34
Hendricks Community Hospital	Hendricks	73%	37
Ely Bloomenson Community Hospital	Ely	72%	129
Red Lake Hospital	Redlake	72%	170
Saint Cloud VA Medical Center[2,3]	Saint Cloud	71%	95
Stevens Community Medical Center[2]	Morris	69%	264
Cook Hospital	Cook	66%	105
Meeker Memorial Hospital[2]	Litchfield	66%	252
Perham Health[2]	Perham	66%	176
Swift County Benson Hospital	Benson	66%	134
Centracare Health System - Long Prairie[2]	Long Prairie	60%	163
Deer River Healthcare Center	Deer River	57%	228
Rainy Lake Medical Center	Int'l Falls	56%	171
Riverview Hospital	Crookston	56%	162
Chippewa County Hospital[2,3]	Montevideo	48%	137
Lakewood Health System[2]	Staples	16%	282

Immunization for Pneumonia

Hospital Name	City	Rate	Cases
Sanford Jackson Medical Center	Jackson	100%	39
District One Hospital[2]	Faribault	99%	241
Essentia Health N Pines Med Ctr[2,3]	Aurora	99%	114
Essentia Health St Joseph's Med Ctr[2]	Brainerd	99%	673
Saint Cloud VA Medical Center[2,3]	Saint Cloud	99%	92
Essentia Health St Mary's Med Ctr[2]	Duluth	98%	660
Fairview Northland Regional Hospital[2]	Princeton	98%	247
Mayo Clinic Health System - Cannon Falls	Cannon Falls	98%	168
Mayo Clinic Health System - Waseca	Waseca	98%	260
Saint Elizabeth Medical Center	Wabasha	98%	212
Saint Luke's Hospital[2]	Duluth	98%	678
Essentia Health Sandstone[2]	Sandstone	97%	150
Fairview Lakes Medical Center[2]	Wyoming	97%	343
Mayo Clinic Health System - Saint James	Saint James	97%	151
Mayo Clinic Health System - Springfield	Springfield	97%	123
Olmsted Medical Center	Rochester	97%	643
Phillips Eye Institute	Minneapolis	97%	87
Saint Cloud Hospital[2]	Saint Cloud	97%	587
Saint Gabriels Hospital[2]	Little Falls	97%	309
Sanford Luverne Medical Center[2]	Luverne	97%	266
Unity Hospital[2]	Fridley	97%	628
Hutchinson Health[2]	Hutchinson	96%	283
Johnson Memorial Hospital[2]	Dawson	96%	96
Mayo Clinic Health System - Red Wing[2]	Red Wing	96%	293
Redwood Area Hospital[2]	Redwood Falls	96%	145
Saint Francis Regional Medical Center[2]	Shakopee	96%	548
Tri County Hospital[2]	Wadena	96%	355
Essentia Health Saint Marys[2]	Detroit Lakes	95%	242
Mayo Clinic Health System - Albert Lea[2]	Albert Lea	95%	413
New Ulm Medical Center[2]	New Ulm	95%	323
Regions Hospital[2]	Saint Paul	95%	575
Ridgeview Medical Center[2]	Waconia	95%	547
Sanford Westbrook Medical Center[2]	Westbrook	95%	64
Avera Marshall Regional Medical Center[2]	Marshall	94%	211
Cambridge Medical Center[2]	Cambridge	94%	292
Essentia Health Duluth[2]	Duluth	94%	258
Lake Region Healthcare Corporation[2]	Fergus Falls	94%	335
Maple Grove Hospital[2]	Maple Grove	94%	240
Owatonna Hospital[2]	Owatonna	94%	224
Red Lake Hospital	Redlake	94%	186
Abbott Northwestern Hospital[2]	Minneapolis	93%	615
Buffalo Hospital[2]	Buffalo	93%	231
Healtheast Saint John's Hospital[2]	Maplewood	93%	547
Mayo Clinic Health System - Fairmont[2]	Fairmont	93%	358
Mayo Clinic Health System - Lake City[2]	Lake City	93%	276
Mercy Hospital[2]	Coon Rapids	93%	681
Ortonville Area Health Services	Ortonville	93%	111
Sanford Bemidji Medical Center[2]	Bemidji	93%	590
Centracare Health Sys-Melrose Hosp	Melrose	92%	265
Centracare Health System - Sauk Centre	Sauk Centre	92%	222
Douglas County Hospital[2]	Alexandria	92%	478
Mercy Hospital[2]	Moose Lake	92%	288
Northfield Hospital[2]	Northfield	92%	225
Pipestone County Medical Center[2]	Pipestone	92%	169
Saint Francis Medical Center[2]	Breckenridge	92%	295
Fairview Southdale Hospital[2]	Edina	91%	629
Firstlight Health System[2]	Mora	91%	326
Park Nicollet Methodist Hospital[2]	Saint Louis Park	91%	707
Saint Joseph's Hospital[2]	Saint Paul	91%	739
United Hospital[2]	Saint Paul	91%	612
Univ Med Ctr-Mesabi/Mesaba Clinics[2]	Hibbing	91%	297
Grand Itasca Clinic & Hospital[2]	Grand Rapids	90%	320
Mayo Clinic Methodist- Hospital[2]	Rochester	90%	499
Mille Lacs Health System[2]	Onamia	90%	229
North Memorial Medical Center[2]	Robbinsdale	90%	719
Saint Joseph's Area Health Services[2]	Park Rapids	90%	311
Bigfork Valley Hospital	Bigfork	89%	219
Hennepin County Medical Center[2]	Minneapolis	89%	483
Lakeview Memorial Hospital[2]	Stillwater	89%	430
Lifecare Medical Center	Roseau	89%	340
Mayo Clinic Health System - Mankato[2]	Mankato	89%	642
Mayo Clinic Hospital Rochester[2]	Rochester	89%	746
Ridgeview Sibley Medical Center[2]	Arlington	89%	89
Centracare Health - Monticello[2]	Monticello	88%	395
Cuyuna Regional Medical Center[2]	Crosby	88%	289
Sanford Canby Medical Center	Canby	88%	164
Sanford Medical Center Thief River Falls[2]	Thief River Falls	88%	291
Sanford Tracy	Tracy	88%	130
Centra Care Health Paynesville	Paynesville	87%	248
Healtheast Woodwinds Hospital[2]	Woodbury	87%	460
Murray County Memorial Hospital	Slayton	87%	171
Regina Hospital[2]	Hastings	87%	350
River's Edge Hospital & Clinic	Saint Peter	87%	239
Mayo Clinic Health System - New Prague[2]	New Prague	86%	324
Univ of Minnesota Med Ctr, Fairview[2]	Minneapolis	86%	499
Winona Health Services[2]	Winona	86%	314
Glencoe Regional Health Services[2]	Glencoe	85%	286
United Hospital District	Blue Earth	85%	335
Glacial Ridge Hospital[2]	Glenwood	84%	340
Community Memorial Hospital[2]	Cloquet	83%	412
Fairview Ridges Hospital[2]	Burnsville	83%	467
Sleepy Eye Municipal Hospital[3]	Sleepy Eye	83%	116
Municipal Hospital & Granite Manor	Granite Falls	82%	271
Riverwood Healthcare Center[2,3]	Aitkin	82%	73
Sanford Worthington Medical Center[2]	Worthington	82%	340
Albany Area Hospital[2,3]	Albany	81%	52
Hendricks Community Hospital	Hendricks	81%	79
Windom Area Hospital	Windom	81%	172
Essentia Health Virginia[2]	Virginia	80%	316
Rice Memorial Hospital[2]	Willmar	80%	326
Swift County Benson Hospital	Benson	80%	198
Essentia Health Holy Trinity Hospital	Graceville	79%	61
Lakewood Health Center[2]	Baudette	79%	89
Perham Health[2]	Perham	79%	386
Renville County Hospital & Clinics	Olivia	79%	101
North Valley Health Center	Warren	77%	151
Sanford Bagley Medical Center	Bagley	77%	115
Centracare Health System - Long Prairie[2]	Long Prairie	76%	213
Lake View Memorial Hospital[2]	Two Harbors	76%	109
Madelia Community Hospital[2]	Madelia	75%	91
Sanford Medical Center Wheaton[3]	Wheaton	73%	44
Tyler Healthcare Center[2]	Tyler	73%	73
Ely Bloomenson Community Hospital	Ely	71%	164
Rainy Lake Medical Center	Int'l Falls	71%	231
Riverview Hospital	Crookston	71%	318
Cook Hospital	Cook	70%	105
Stevens Community Medical Center[2]	Morris	68%	351
Appleton Municipal Hospital	Appleton	64%	66
Meeker Memorial Hospital[2]	Litchfield	63%	282
Deer River Healthcare Center[2]	Deer River	59%	266
Chippewa County Hospital[2,3]	Montevideo	53%	269
Essentia Health Ada	Ada	47%	32
Madison Hospital[3]	Madison	38%	42
Lakewood Health System[2]	Staples	23%	224

Stroke Care

Anticoagulation Therapy for Atrial Fibrillation

Hospital Name	City	Rate	Cases
Fairview Southdale Hospital	Edina	100%	32
Mayo Clinic Hospital Rochester	Rochester	100%	72
North Memorial Medical Center	Robbinsdale	100%	65
Park Nicollet Methodist Hospital	Saint Louis Park	100%	39
Saint Joseph's Hospital[2]	Saint Paul	100%	32
United Hospital	Saint Paul	98%	50
Abbott Northwestern Hospital	Minneapolis	97%	91
Essentia Health St Mary's Med Ctr	Duluth	96%	27
Mercy Hospital	Coon Rapids	95%	37
Saint Cloud Hospital	Saint Cloud	92%	65
Regions Hospital	Saint Paul	87%	30

Antithrombotic Therapy Timing

Hospital Name	City	Rate	Cases
Fairview Ridges Hospital	Burnsville	100%	63
Fairview Southdale Hospital	Edina	100%	213
Ridgeview Medical Center	Waconia	100%	40
Unity Hospital	Fridley	100%	70
Essentia Health St Mary's Med Ctr	Duluth	99%	141
Mayo Clinic Health System - Mankato	Mankato	99%	71
Park Nicollet Methodist Hospital	Saint Louis Park	99%	170
Saint Cloud Hospital	Saint Cloud	99%	216
Univ of Minnesota Med Ctr, Fairview	Minneapolis	99%	84
Abbott Northwestern Hospital	Minneapolis	98%	242
Essentia Health St Joseph's Med Ctr	Brainerd	98%	47
Mercy Hospital	Coon Rapids	98%	151
Regions Hospital	Saint Paul	98%	159
Sanford Bemidji Medical Center	Bemidji	98%	43
United Hospital	Saint Paul	98%	177
Healtheast Saint John's Hospital	Maplewood	97%	103
North Memorial Medical Center	Robbinsdale	97%	233
Saint Francis Regional Medical Center	Shakopee	97%	32
Healtheast Woodwinds Hospital	Woodbury	96%	28
Mayo Clinic Hospital Rochester	Rochester	96%	273
Saint Joseph's Hospital[2]	Saint Paul	96%	106
Saint Luke's Hospital	Duluth	96%	76
Hennepin County Medical Center[2]	Minneapolis	94%	63

Assessed for Rehabilitation

Hospital Name	City	Rate	Cases
Fairview Southdale Hospital	Edina	100%	274
Grand Itasca Clinic & Hospital	Grand Rapids	100%	26
Healtheast Woodwinds Hospital	Woodbury	100%	47
Hennepin County Medical Center[2]	Minneapolis	100%	105
Lake Region Healthcare Corporation	Fergus Falls	100%	25
Saint Francis Regional Medical Center	Shakopee	100%	40
United Hospital	Saint Paul	100%	285
Unity Hospital	Fridley	100%	81
Abbott Northwestern Hospital	Minneapolis	99%	425
Saint Cloud Hospital	Saint Cloud	99%	376
Essentia Health St Mary's Med Ctr	Duluth	98%	218
North Memorial Medical Center	Robbinsdale	98%	354
Saint Joseph's Hospital[2]	Saint Paul	98%	191
Saint Luke's Hospital	Duluth	98%	92
Healtheast Saint John's Hospital	Maplewood	97%	123
Mayo Clinic Hospital Rochester	Rochester	97%	499
Mercy Hospital	Coon Rapids	97%	215
Park Nicollet Methodist Hospital	Saint Louis Park	97%	248
Regions Hospital	Saint Paul	97%	267
Fairview Ridges Hospital	Burnsville	96%	67
Univ of Minnesota Med Ctr, Fairview	Minneapolis	96%	166
Mayo Clinic Health System - Mankato	Mankato	94%	84
Sanford Bemidji Medical Center	Bemidji	94%	50
Essentia Health St Joseph's Med Ctr	Brainerd	92%	61
Ridgeview Medical Center	Waconia	91%	45

Discharged on Antithrombotic Therapy

Hospital Name	City	Rate	Cases
Abbott Northwestern Hospital	Minneapolis	100%	344
Essentia Health St Joseph's Med Ctr	Brainerd	100%	61
Fairview Southdale Hospital	Edina	100%	251
Grand Itasca Clinic & Hospital	Grand Rapids	100%	26
Healtheast Saint John's Hospital	Maplewood	100%	119
Healtheast Woodwinds Hospital	Woodbury	100%	46
Hennepin County Medical Center[2]	Minneapolis	100%	79
Mayo Clinic Hospital Rochester	Rochester	100%	393
Mercy Hospital	Coon Rapids	100%	188
Park Nicollet Methodist Hospital	Saint Louis Park	100%	223
Regions Hospital	Saint Paul	100%	204
Saint Francis Regional Medical Center	Shakopee	100%	39
Saint Luke's Hospital	Duluth	100%	86
Unity Hospital	Fridley	100%	77
Univ of Minnesota Med Ctr, Fairview	Minneapolis	100%	113
Mayo Clinic Health System - Mankato	Mankato	99%	79
North Memorial Medical Center	Robbinsdale	99%	317
Saint Joseph's Hospital[2]	Saint Paul	99%	143
United Hospital	Saint Paul	99%	247
Essentia Health St Mary's Med Ctr	Duluth	98%	182
Fairview Ridges Hospital	Burnsville	98%	65
Ridgeview Medical Center	Waconia	98%	40
Saint Cloud Hospital	Saint Cloud	98%	330
Sanford Bemidji Medical Center	Bemidji	88%	43

Discharged on Statin Medication

Hospital Name	City	Rate	Cases
United Hospital	Saint Paul	100%	205
Abbott Northwestern Hospital	Minneapolis	99%	278
Essentia Health St Mary's Med Ctr	Duluth	98%	131
Fairview Ridges Hospital	Burnsville	98%	52
Fairview Southdale Hospital	Edina	98%	193
Mayo Clinic Hospital Rochester	Rochester	98%	289
Mercy Hospital	Coon Rapids	98%	147
Park Nicollet Methodist Hospital	Saint Louis Park	98%	149
Unity Hospital	Fridley	98%	60
Healtheast Woodwinds Hospital	Woodbury	97%	37
Regions Hospital	Saint Paul	97%	161
Saint Francis Regional Medical Center	Shakopee	97%	33
Saint Joseph's Hospital[2]	Saint Paul	97%	109
Saint Cloud Hospital	Saint Cloud	96%	266
Saint Luke's Hospital	Duluth	96%	70
Univ of Minnesota Med Ctr, Fairview	Minneapolis	95%	79
Hennepin County Medical Center[2]	Minneapolis	94%	52
Mayo Clinic Health System - Mankato	Mankato	94%	65
North Memorial Medical Center	Robbinsdale	93%	257
Grand Itasca Clinic & Hospital	Grand Rapids	92%	25
Healtheast Saint John's Hospital	Maplewood	92%	102
Essentia Health St Joseph's Med Ctr	Brainerd	88%	51
Sanford Bemidji Medical Center	Bemidji	71%	34

NOTE: Hospital profiles are in alphabetical order by state, then city, then hospital within the city; Rankings exclude hospitals with less than 25 cases except for patient surveys which excludes hospitals with less than 100 cases; (a) 100-299 cases; (1) The number of cases/patients is too few to report; (2) Data submitted were based on a sample of cases/patients; (3) Results are based on a shorter time period than required; (4) Data suppressed by CMS for one or more quarters; (5) Results are not available for this reporting period; (6) Fewer than 100 patients completed the HCAHPS survey; (7) No cases met the criteria for this measure; (8) The lower limit of the confidence interval cannot be calculated if the number of observed infections equals zero; (9) No data are available from the state/territory for this reporting period; (10) The scores shown reflect fewer than 50 completed surveys; (11) There were discrepancies in the data collection process; (12) This measure does not apply to this hospital for this reporting period; (13) Results cannot be calculated for this reporting period; (14) The results for this state are combined with nearby states to protect confidentiality; Please refer to the User's Guide for a full explanation of data.

Hospital Name	City	Rate	Cases
Ridgeview Medical Center	Waconia	69%	36

Thrombolytic Therapy Timing

Hospital Name	City	Rate	Cases
Fairview Southdale Hospital	Edina	100%	26
North Memorial Medical Center	Robbinsdale	97%	30
United Hospital	Saint Paul	96%	46
Mayo Clinic Hospital Rochester	Rochester	92%	25
Abbott Northwestern Hospital	Minneapolis	86%	28
Saint Cloud Hospital	Saint Cloud	79%	34
Park Nicollet Methodist Hospital	Saint Louis Park	38%	66

Venous Thromboembolism (VTE) Prophylaxis

Hospital Name	City	Rate	Cases
Fairview Southdale Hospital	Edina	100%	276
Mayo Clinic Hospital Rochester	Rochester	100%	472
Saint Francis Regional Medical Center	Shakopee	100%	36
Unity Hospital	Fridley	100%	74
Mercy Hospital	Coon Rapids	99%	204
Saint Cloud Hospital	Saint Cloud	99%	338
Fairview Ridges Hospital	Burnsville	98%	59
Univ of Minnesota Med Ctr, Fairview	Minneapolis	98%	161
North Memorial Medical Center	Robbinsdale	97%	315
Saint Joseph's Hospital[2]	Saint Paul	97%	199
Essentia Health St Mary's Med Ctr	Duluth	96%	220
Abbott Northwestern Hospital	Minneapolis	95%	419
Healtheast Woodwinds Hospital	Woodbury	95%	38
United Hospital	Saint Paul	95%	283
Essentia Health St Joseph's Med Ctr	Brainerd	94%	47
Mayo Clinic Health System - Mankato	Mankato	92%	79
Park Nicollet Methodist Hospital	Saint Louis Park	91%	226
Hennepin County Medical Center[2]	Minneapolis	88%	117
Regions Hospital	Saint Paul	88%	249
Sanford Bemidji Medical Center	Bemidji	86%	49
Saint Luke's Hospital	Duluth	81%	91
Healtheast Saint John's Hospital	Maplewood	80%	115
Ridgeview Medical Center	Waconia	50%	42

Written Stroke Educational Materials Given

Hospital Name	City	Rate	Cases
Saint Francis Regional Medical Center	Shakopee	100%	28
United Hospital	Saint Paul	100%	152
Abbott Northwestern Hospital	Minneapolis	99%	239
Mercy Hospital	Coon Rapids	98%	127
Essentia Health St Mary's Med Ctr	Duluth	96%	113
Hennepin County Medical Center[2]	Minneapolis	96%	48
Saint Cloud Hospital	Saint Cloud	96%	203
Unity Hospital	Fridley	96%	49
Fairview Ridges Hospital	Burnsville	95%	44
Fairview Southdale Hospital	Edina	95%	139
Saint Luke's Hospital	Duluth	94%	32
Regions Hospital	Saint Paul	89%	132
Healtheast Woodwinds Hospital	Woodbury	88%	25
Mayo Clinic Hospital Rochester	Rochester	87%	251
North Memorial Medical Center	Robbinsdale	84%	186
Univ of Minnesota Med Ctr, Fairview	Minneapolis	83%	88
Essentia Health St Joseph's Med Ctr	Brainerd	80%	40
Park Nicollet Methodist Hospital	Saint Louis Park	80%	142
Healtheast Saint John's Hospital	Maplewood	76%	75
Saint Joseph's Hospital[2]	Saint Paul	75%	96
Mayo Clinic Health System - Mankato	Mankato	69%	45

Surgical Care Improvement Project

Appropriate Beta Blocker Usage

Hospital Name	City	Rate	Cases
Abbott Northwestern Hospital[2]	Minneapolis	100%	266
Avera Marshall Regional Medical Center	Marshall	100%	32
Cambridge Medical Center	Cambridge	100%	57
Fairview Lakes Medical Center[2]	Wyoming	100%	94
Fairview Ridges Hospital[2]	Burnsville	100%	249
Fairview Southdale Hospital[2]	Edina	100%	458
Hennepin County Medical Center[2]	Minneapolis	100%	86
Lake Region Healthcare Corporation	Fergus Falls	100%	82
Mayo Clinic Hospital Rochester[2]	Rochester	100%	333
Mayo Clinic Methodist- Hospital[2]	Rochester	100%	194
New Ulm Medical Center	New Ulm	100%	50
Park Nicollet Methodist Hospital[2]	Saint Louis Park	100%	389
Ridgeview Medical Center[2]	Waconia	100%	100
Saint Francis Regional Medical Center[2]	Shakopee	100%	165
Saint Joseph's Hospital[2]	Saint Paul	100%	304
Saint Luke's Hospital[2]	Duluth	100%	174
United Hospital[2]	Saint Paul	100%	244
Unity Hospital[2]	Fridley	100%	143
Univ of Minnesota Med Ctr, Fairview[2]	Minneapolis	100%	515
Buffalo Hospital	Buffalo	99%	68
Douglas County Hospital[2]	Alexandria	99%	150
Essentia Health St Mary's Med Ctr[2]	Duluth	99%	247
Healtheast Woodwinds Hospital[2]	Woodbury	99%	92
Maple Grove Hospital	Maple Grove	99%	167
Mayo Clinic Health System - Albert Lea	Albert Lea	99%	90
Mayo Clinic Health System - Mankato[2]	Mankato	99%	156
Mercy Hospital[2]	Coon Rapids	99%	324
Minneapolis VA Medical Center[2]	Minneapolis	99%	256
Olmsted Medical Center	Rochester	99%	97
Saint Cloud Hospital[2]	Saint Cloud	99%	285
Cuyuna Regional Medical Center	Crosby	98%	89
Essentia Health Virginia	Virginia	98%	61
Healtheast Saint John's Hospital[2]	Maplewood	98%	163
Hutchinson Health	Hutchinson	98%	55
Lakeview Memorial Hospital[2]	Stillwater	98%	105
Mayo Clinic Health System - Fairmont	Fairmont	98%	56
Mayo Clinic Health System - Red Wing[2]	Red Wing	98%	52
Owatonna Hospital[2]	Owatonna	98%	65
Regina Hospital[2]	Hastings	98%	52
Regions Hospital[2]	Saint Paul	98%	311
Saint Gabriels Hospital[2]	Little Falls	98%	62
District One Hospital	Faribault	97%	58
North Memorial Medical Center[2]	Robbinsdale	97%	223
Sanford Bemidji Medical Center	Bemidji	97%	182
Sanford Medical Center Thief River Falls	Thief River Falls	97%	33
Univ Med Ctr-Mesabi/Mesaba Clinics[2]	Hibbing	97%	30
Essentia Health St Joseph's Med Ctr[2]	Brainerd	96%	90
Essentia Health Saint Marys	Detroit Lakes	95%	103
Winona Health Services	Winona	95%	62
Northfield Hospital	Northfield	94%	48
Community Memorial Hospital	Cloquet	93%	28
Firstlight Health System	Mora	93%	28
Grand Itasca Clinic & Hospital	Grand Rapids	93%	58
Mayo Clinic Health System - New Prague	New Prague	93%	27
Rice Memorial Hospital[2]	Willmar	89%	79
Riverwood Healthcare Center	Aitkin	89%	35

Appropriate VTP Within 24 Hours

Hospital Name	City	Rate	Cases
Abbott Northwestern Hospital[2]	Minneapolis	100%	467
Avera Marshall Regional Medical Center	Marshall	100%	113
Bigfork Valley Hospital	Bigfork	100%	73
Cambridge Medical Center	Cambridge	100%	174
Centra Care Health Paynesville	Paynesville	100%	45
Cuyuna Regional Medical Center	Crosby	100%	205
Deer River Healthcare Center	Deer River	100%	30
Essentia Health Duluth[2]	Duluth	100%	36
Essentia Health St Joseph's Med Ctr[2]	Brainerd	100%	291
Fairview Lakes Medical Center[2]	Wyoming	100%	264
Fairview Southdale Hospital[2]	Edina	100%	900
Firstlight Health System	Mora	100%	80
Glencoe Regional Health Services	Glencoe	100%	35
Healtheast Saint John's Hospital[2]	Maplewood	100%	448
Healtheast Woodwinds Hospital[2]	Woodbury	100%	331
Hennepin County Medical Center[2]	Minneapolis	100%	258
Mayo Clinic Health System - Albert Lea	Albert Lea	100%	230
Mayo Clinic Health System - Cannon Falls	Cannon Falls	100%	28
Mayo Clinic Health System - Lake City	Lake City	100%	34
Mayo Clinic Health System - Mankato[2]	Mankato	100%	445
Mayo Clinic Hospital Rochester[2]	Rochester	100%	301
Mayo Clinic Methodist- Hospital[2]	Rochester	100%	624
Meeker Memorial Hospital	Litchfield	100%	51
Minneapolis VA Medical Center[2]	Minneapolis	100%	306
Regions Hospital[2]	Saint Paul	100%	495
Ridgeview Medical Center[2]	Waconia	100%	341
River's Edge Hospital & Clinic	Saint Peter	100%	42
Saint Elizabeth Medical Center	Wabasha	100%	40
Saint Francis Regional Medical Center[2]	Shakopee	100%	458
Tri County Hospital	Wadena	100%	28
Univ of Minnesota Med Ctr, Fairview[2]	Minneapolis	100%	1741
Buffalo Hospital	Buffalo	99%	161
Douglas County Hospital[2]	Alexandria	99%	394
Fairview Northland Regional Hospital	Princeton	99%	76
Fairview Ridges Hospital[2]	Burnsville	99%	744
Hutchinson Health	Hutchinson	99%	135
Maple Grove Hospital	Maple Grove	99%	572
Mayo Clinic Health System - Red Wing[2]	Red Wing	99%	175
Mercy Hospital[2]	Coon Rapids	99%	394
New Ulm Medical Center	New Ulm	99%	135
North Memorial Medical Center[2]	Robbinsdale	99%	341
Owatonna Hospital[2]	Owatonna	99%	160
Regina Hospital[2]	Hastings	99%	158
Saint Cloud Hospital[2]	Saint Cloud	99%	345
Saint Joseph's Area Health Services	Park Rapids	99%	135
Saint Joseph's Hospital[2]	Saint Paul	99%	337
Sanford Worthington Medical Center[2]	Worthington	99%	83
Unity Hospital[2]	Fridley	99%	351
Winona Health Services	Winona	99%	135
Community Memorial Hospital	Cloquet	98%	95
Essentia Health Saint Marys	Detroit Lakes	98%	262
Grand Itasca Clinic & Hospital	Grand Rapids	98%	121
Lake Region Healthcare Corporation	Fergus Falls	98%	223
Mayo Clinic Health System - Fairmont	Fairmont	98%	112
Park Nicollet Methodist Hospital[2]	Saint Louis Park	98%	572
Riverwood Healthcare Center	Aitkin	98%	98
Saint Gabriels Hospital[2]	Little Falls	98%	196
Saint Luke's Hospital[2]	Duluth	98%	320
United Hospital[2]	Saint Paul	98%	386
Essentia Health St Mary's Med Ctr[2]	Duluth	97%	320
Lakeview Memorial Hospital[2]	Stillwater	97%	299
Mayo Clinic Health System - New Prague	New Prague	97%	77
Northfield Hospital	Northfield	97%	175
Rice Memorial Hospital[2]	Willmar	97%	246
Sanford Medical Center Thief River Falls	Thief River Falls	97%	112
Essentia Health Virginia	Virginia	96%	128
Olmsted Medical Center	Rochester	96%	224
Univ Med Ctr-Mesabi/Mesaba Clinics[2]	Hibbing	96%	105
District One Hospital	Faribault	95%	131
Sanford Bemidji Medical Center	Bemidji	95%	483
Saint Francis Medical Center	Breckenridge	90%	48
United Hospital District	Blue Earth	89%	53
Mercy Hospital[2]	Moose Lake	83%	42
Lakewood Health System[2]	Staples	81%	67
Riverview Hospital	Crookston	81%	48
Stevens Community Medical Center	Morris	68%	65

Controlled Postoperative Blood Glucose

Hospital Name	City	Rate	Cases
Hennepin County Medical Center[2]	Minneapolis	100%	44
Regions Hospital[2]	Saint Paul	100%	208
Fairview Southdale Hospital[2]	Edina	99%	232
Park Nicollet Methodist Hospital[2]	Saint Louis Park	98%	180
Saint Joseph's Hospital[2]	Saint Paul	98%	204
Saint Luke's Hospital[2]	Duluth	98%	132
United Hospital[2]	Saint Paul	98%	123
Mercy Hospital[2]	Coon Rapids	97%	156
Abbott Northwestern Hospital[2]	Minneapolis	96%	137
Essentia Health St Mary's Med Ctr[2]	Duluth	96%	121
Minneapolis VA Medical Center[2]	Minneapolis	96%	189
Univ of Minnesota Med Ctr, Fairview[2]	Minneapolis	96%	196
Mayo Clinic Hospital Rochester[2]	Rochester	94%	253
North Memorial Medical Center[2]	Robbinsdale	94%	144
Saint Cloud Hospital[2]	Saint Cloud	91%	139

Perioperative Temperature Management

Hospital Name	City	Rate	Cases
Abbott Northwestern Hospital[2]	Minneapolis	100%	632
Bigfork Valley Hospital	Bigfork	100%	79
Buffalo Hospital	Buffalo	100%	209
Cambridge Medical Center	Cambridge	100%	211
Community Memorial Hospital	Cloquet	100%	113
Cuyuna Regional Medical Center	Crosby	100%	266
Essentia Health Duluth[2]	Duluth	100%	83
Essentia Health St Joseph's Med Ctr[2]	Brainerd	100%	321
Essentia Health St Mary's Med Ctr[2]	Duluth	100%	463
Essentia Health Saint Marys	Detroit Lakes	100%	301
Essentia Health Virginia	Virginia	100%	143
Fairview Lakes Medical Center[2]	Wyoming	100%	326
Fairview Northland Regional Hospital	Princeton	100%	85
Fairview Ridges Hospital[2]	Burnsville	100%	854
Fairview Southdale Hospital[2]	Edina	100%	1083
Glencoe Regional Health Services	Glencoe	100%	39
Healtheast Saint John's Hospital[2]	Maplewood	100%	581
Healtheast Woodwinds Hospital[2]	Woodbury	100%	426
Hutchinson Health	Hutchinson	100%	161
Lake Region Healthcare Corporation	Fergus Falls	100%	273
Maple Grove Hospital	Maple Grove	100%	634
Mayo Clinic Health System - Cannon Falls	Cannon Falls	100%	29
Mayo Clinic Health System - Fairmont	Fairmont	100%	134
Mayo Clinic Health System - Lake City	Lake City	100%	33
Mayo Clinic Health System - Mankato[2]	Mankato	100%	499
Mayo Clinic Health System - Red Wing[2]	Red Wing	100%	206
Mayo Clinic Hospital Rochester[2]	Rochester	100%	491
Mayo Clinic Methodist- Hospital[2]	Rochester	100%	717
Meeker Memorial Hospital	Litchfield	100%	56
Mercy Hospital[2]	Coon Rapids	100%	588
North Memorial Medical Center[2]	Robbinsdale	100%	451
Olmsted Medical Center	Rochester	100%	259
Owatonna Hospital[2]	Owatonna	100%	192
Park Nicollet Methodist Hospital[2]	Saint Louis Park	100%	783
Regions Hospital[2]	Saint Paul	100%	609
Ridgeview Medical Center[2]	Waconia	100%	405
River's Edge Hospital & Clinic	Saint Peter	100%	44
Riverwood Healthcare Center	Aitkin	100%	107
Saint Cloud Hospital[2]	Saint Cloud	100%	487
Saint Elizabeth Medical Center	Wabasha	100%	42
Saint Francis Medical Center	Breckenridge	100%	54
Saint Francis Regional Medical Center[2]	Shakopee	100%	564
Saint Gabriels Hospital[2]	Little Falls	100%	216
Saint Joseph's Area Health Services	Park Rapids	100%	149
Saint Joseph's Hospital[2]	Saint Paul	100%	429
Sanford Medical Center Thief River Falls	Thief River Falls	100%	131
Tri County Hospital	Wadena	100%	33
United Hospital[2]	Saint Paul	100%	508

NOTE: Hospital profiles are in alphabetical order by state, then city, then hospital within the city; Rankings exclude hospitals with less than 25 cases except for patient surveys which excludes hospitals with less than 100 cases; (a) 100-299 cases; (1) The number of cases/patients is too few to report; (2) Data submitted were based on a sample of cases/patients; (3) Results are based on a shorter time period than required; (4) Data suppressed by CMS for one or more quarters; (5) Results are not available for this reporting period; (6) Fewer than 100 patients completed the HCAHPS survey; (7) No cases met the criteria for this measure; (8) The lower limit of the confidence interval cannot be calculated if the number of observed infections equals zero; (9) No data are available from the state/territory for this reporting period; (10) The scores shown reflect fewer than 50 completed surveys; (11) There were discrepancies in the data collection process; (12) This measure does not apply to this hospital for this reporting period; (13) Results cannot be calculated for this reporting period; (14) The results for this state are combined with nearby states to protect confidentiality; Please refer to the User's Guide for a full explanation of data.

Hospital Name	City	Rate	Cases
United Hospital District	Blue Earth	100%	55
Unity Hospital[2]	Fridley	100%	395
Univ Med Ctr-Mesabi/Mesaba Clinics[2]	Hibbing	100%	117
Univ of Minnesota Med Ctr, Fairview[2]	Minneapolis	100%	2100
Winona Health Services	Winona	100%	178
Avera Marshall Regional Medical Center	Marshall	99%	137
District One Hospital	Faribault	99%	151
Grand Itasca Clinic & Hospital	Grand Rapids	99%	139
Hennepin County Medical Center[2]	Minneapolis	99%	321
Lakeview Memorial Hospital[2]	Stillwater	99%	375
Mayo Clinic Health System - Albert Lea	Albert Lea	99%	264
Mayo Clinic Health System - New Prague	New Prague	99%	85
New Ulm Medical Center	New Ulm	99%	146
Northfield Hospital	Northfield	99%	185
Rice Memorial Hospital[2]	Willmar	99%	273
Saint Luke's Hospital[2]	Duluth	99%	391
Sanford Bemidji Medical Center	Bemidji	99%	595
Centra Care Health Paynesville	Paynesville	98%	50
Deer River Healthcare Center	Deer River	98%	42
Mercy Hospital[2]	Moose Lake	98%	57
Minneapolis VA Medical Center[2]	Minneapolis	98%	371
Regina Hospital[2]	Hastings	98%	223
Riverview Hospital	Crookston	98%	60
Sanford Worthington Medical Center[2]	Worthington	98%	94
Glacial Ridge Hospital[2]	Glenwood	97%	31
Lakewood Health System[2]	Staples	97%	79
Firstlight Health System	Mora	96%	104
Douglas County Hospital[2]	Alexandria	92%	423
Chippewa County Hospital[2]	Montevideo	77%	26
Stevens Community Medical Center	Morris	77%	79

Prophylactic Antibiotic Selection

Hospital Name	City	Rate	Cases
Abbott Northwestern Hospital[2]	Minneapolis	100%	492
Bigfork Valley Hospital	Bigfork	100%	77
Buffalo Hospital	Buffalo	100%	139
Cuyuna Regional Medical Center	Crosby	100%	210
Deer River Healthcare Center	Deer River	100%	39
Essentia Health Duluth[2]	Duluth	100%	75
Essentia Health Saint Marys	Detroit Lakes	100%	245
Essentia Health Virginia	Virginia	100%	102
Fairview Lakes Medical Center[2]	Wyoming	100%	275
Fairview Ridges Hospital[2]	Burnsville	100%	678
Firstlight Health System	Mora	100%	88
Glencoe Regional Health Services	Glencoe	100%	27
Hennepin County Medical Center[2]	Minneapolis	100%	233
Lake Region Healthcare Corporation	Fergus Falls	100%	173
Maple Grove Hospital	Maple Grove	100%	536
Mayo Clinic Health System - Albert Lea	Albert Lea	100%	196
Mayo Clinic Health System - Cannon Falls	Cannon Falls	100%	25
Mayo Clinic Health System - Fairmont	Fairmont	100%	100
Mayo Clinic Health System - Lake City	Lake City	100%	30
Mayo Clinic Health System - Mankato[2]	Mankato	100%	283
Mayo Clinic Health System - New Prague	New Prague	100%	70
Mayo Clinic Health System - Red Wing[2]	Red Wing	100%	145
Mayo Clinic Hospital Rochester[2]	Rochester	100%	378
Mayo Clinic Methodist- Hospital[2]	Rochester	100%	406
Meeker Memorial Hospital	Litchfield	100%	39
Mercy Hospital[2]	Coon Rapids	100%	473
Mercy Hospital[2]	Moose Lake	100%	48
New Ulm Medical Center	New Ulm	100%	117
North Memorial Medical Center[2]	Robbinsdale	100%	411
Owatonna Hospital[2]	Owatonna	100%	145
Ridgeview Medical Center[2]	Waconia	100%	272
River's Edge Hospital & Clinic	Saint Peter	100%	44
Saint Elizabeth Medical Center	Wabasha	100%	39
Saint Francis Medical Center	Breckenridge	100%	29
Saint Francis Regional Medical Center[2]	Shakopee	100%	388
Saint Joseph's Hospital[2]	Saint Paul	100%	451
Sanford Worthington Medical Center[2]	Worthington	100%	80
United Hospital[2]	Saint Paul	100%	416
United Hospital District	Blue Earth	100%	39
Avera Marshall Regional Medical Center	Marshall	99%	115
Cambridge Medical Center	Cambridge	99%	144
Community Memorial Hospital	Cloquet	99%	94
District One Hospital	Faribault	99%	127
Douglas County Hospital[2]	Alexandria	99%	326
Essentia Health St Joseph's Med Ctr[2]	Brainerd	99%	203
Essentia Health St Mary's Med Ctr[2]	Duluth	99%	432
Fairview Southdale Hospital[2]	Edina	99%	1040
Healtheast Saint John's Hospital[2]	Maplewood	99%	376
Healtheast Woodwinds Hospital[2]	Woodbury	99%	294
Hutchinson Health	Hutchinson	99%	121
Lakeview Memorial Hospital[2]	Stillwater	99%	248
Minneapolis VA Medical Center	Minneapolis	99%	401
Northfield Hospital	Northfield	99%	153
Olmsted Medical Center	Rochester	99%	224
Park Nicollet Methodist Hospital[2]	Saint Louis Park	99%	706
Regina Hospital[2]	Hastings	99%	161
Rice Memorial Hospital[2]	Willmar	99%	181
Riverwood Healthcare Center	Aitkin	99%	102
Saint Cloud Hospital[2]	Saint Cloud	99%	431
Saint Gabriels Hospital[2]	Little Falls	99%	183
Saint Luke's Hospital[2]	Duluth	99%	361
Unity Hospital[2]	Fridley	99%	213
Univ of Minnesota Med Ctr, Fairview[2]	Minneapolis	99%	1099
Fairview Northland Regional Hospital	Princeton	98%	63
Grand Itasca Clinic & Hospital	Grand Rapids	98%	100
Regions Hospital[2]	Saint Paul	98%	600
Stevens Community Medical Center	Morris	98%	60
Lakewood Health System[2]	Staples	97%	33
Winona Health Services	Winona	97%	122
Sanford Medical Center Thief River Falls	Thief River Falls	96%	95
Univ Med Ctr-Mesabi/Mesaba Clinics[2]	Hibbing	96%	75
Centra Care Health Paynesville	Paynesville	95%	43
Sanford Bemidji Medical Center	Bemidji	95%	476
Riverview Hospital	Crookston	88%	42

Prophylactic Antibiotic Selection (Outpatient)

Hospital Name	City	Rate	Cases
Cambridge Medical Center	Cambridge	100%	41
District One Hospital	Faribault	100%	33
Fairview Northland Regional Hospital	Princeton	100%	66
Lakeview Memorial Hospital	Stillwater	100%	237
Maple Grove Hospital	Maple Grove	100%	287
Mayo Clinic Health System - Albert Lea	Albert Lea	100%	60
Mayo Clinic Methodist- Hospital	Rochester	100%	643
New Ulm Medical Center	New Ulm	100%	27
North Memorial Medical Center	Robbinsdale	100%	332
Prairie Ridge Hospital & Health Services[3]	Elbow Lake	100%	29
Riverview Hospital	Crookston	100%	53
Saint Cloud Hospital	Saint Cloud	100%	1022
Saint Francis Regional Medical Center	Shakopee	100%	121
Saint Joseph's Hospital	Saint Paul	100%	274
Saint Luke's Hospital	Duluth	100%	572
Abbott Northwestern Hospital	Minneapolis	99%	685
Fairview Lakes Medical Center	Wyoming	99%	73
Fairview Ridges Hospital	Burnsville	99%	319
Healtheast Saint John's Hospital	Maplewood	99%	286
Healtheast Woodwinds Hospital	Woodbury	99%	164
Hennepin County Medical Center	Minneapolis	99%	167
Mayo Clinic Hospital Rochester	Rochester	99%	697
Park Nicollet Methodist Hospital	Saint Louis Park	99%	1000
Ridgeview Medical Center	Waconia	99%	121
Essentia Health St Mary's Med Ctr	Duluth	98%	493
Fairview Southdale Hospital	Edina	98%	650
Hutchinson Health	Hutchinson	98%	51
Lake Region Healthcare Corporation	Fergus Falls	98%	82
Mercy Hospital	Coon Rapids	98%	380
Owatonna Hospital	Owatonna	98%	108
Regions Hospital	Saint Paul	98%	376
Rice Memorial Hospital	Willmar	98%	54
Sanford Bemidji Medical Center	Bemidji	98%	60
Unity Hospital	Fridley	98%	180
Grand Itasca Clinic & Hospital	Grand Rapids	97%	107
Tri County Hospital	Wadena	97%	38
Buffalo Hospital	Buffalo	96%	185
Lakewood Health System	Staples	96%	68
United Hospital	Saint Paul	96%	510
Mayo Clinic Health System - Fairmont	Fairmont	95%	59
Winona Health Services	Winona	95%	58
Mayo Clinic Health System - Mankato	Mankato	94%	320
Olmsted Medical Center	Rochester	94%	54
Douglas County Hospital	Alexandria	93%	214
Essentia Health St Joseph's Med Ctr	Brainerd	92%	163
Regina Hospital	Hastings	92%	26
Univ of Minnesota Med Ctr, Fairview	Minneapolis	91%	581
Cuyuna Regional Medical Center	Crosby	90%	68
Essentia Health Duluth	Duluth	84%	318
Firstlight Health System	Mora	76%	25

Prophylactic Antibiotic Stopped

Hospital Name	City	Rate	Cases
Bigfork Valley Hospital	Bigfork	100%	76
Cambridge Medical Center	Cambridge	100%	140
Deer River Healthcare Center	Deer River	100%	39
Fairview Lakes Medical Center[2]	Wyoming	100%	272
Fairview Southdale Hospital[2]	Edina	100%	1012
Glencoe Regional Health Services	Glencoe	100%	27
Maple Grove Hospital	Maple Grove	100%	534
Mayo Clinic Health System - Cannon Falls	Cannon Falls	100%	25
Mayo Clinic Health System - Fairmont	Fairmont	100%	99
Mayo Clinic Health System - Lake City	Lake City	100%	30
Meeker Memorial Hospital	Litchfield	100%	39
New Ulm Medical Center	New Ulm	100%	116
Regina Hospital[2]	Hastings	100%	160
Ridgeview Medical Center[2]	Waconia	100%	268
Riverwood Healthcare Center	Aitkin	100%	102
Saint Francis Regional Medical Center[2]	Shakopee	100%	386
Stevens Community Medical Center	Morris	100%	60
Abbott Northwestern Hospital[2]	Minneapolis	99%	472
Avera Marshall Regional Medical Center	Marshall	99%	113
Buffalo Hospital	Buffalo	99%	137
Cuyuna Regional Medical Center	Crosby	99%	209
Douglas County Hospital[2]	Alexandria	99%	322
Fairview Ridges Hospital[2]	Burnsville	99%	671
Firstlight Health System	Mora	99%	87
Healtheast Saint John's Hospital[2]	Maplewood	99%	361
Healtheast Woodwinds Hospital[2]	Woodbury	99%	290
Hennepin County Medical Center[2]	Minneapolis	99%	225
Lake Region Healthcare Corporation	Fergus Falls	99%	171
Lakeview Memorial Hospital[2]	Stillwater	99%	248
Mayo Clinic Health System - Albert Lea	Albert Lea	99%	192
Mayo Clinic Health System - New Prague	New Prague	99%	69
Mayo Clinic Health System - Red Wing[2]	Red Wing	99%	143
Mayo Clinic Methodist- Hospital[2]	Rochester	99%	395
Mercy Hospital[2]	Coon Rapids	99%	460
Minneapolis VA Medical Center	Minneapolis	99%	398
North Memorial Medical Center[2]	Robbinsdale	99%	410
Regions Hospital[2]	Saint Paul	99%	577
Saint Cloud Hospital[2]	Saint Cloud	99%	426
Saint Gabriels Hospital[2]	Little Falls	99%	183
Saint Luke's Hospital[2]	Duluth	99%	356
Sanford Worthington Medical Center[2]	Worthington	99%	80
Univ of Minnesota Med Ctr, Fairview[2]	Minneapolis	99%	1085
Community Memorial Hospital	Cloquet	98%	93
District One Hospital	Faribault	98%	127
Essentia Health St Joseph's Med Ctr[2]	Brainerd	98%	201
Fairview Northland Regional Hospital	Princeton	98%	63
Grand Itasca Clinic & Hospital	Grand Rapids	98%	96
Mayo Clinic Health System - Mankato[2]	Mankato	98%	276
Olmsted Medical Center	Rochester	98%	219
Owatonna Hospital[2]	Owatonna	98%	140
Park Nicollet Methodist Hospital[2]	Saint Louis Park	98%	687
Rice Memorial Hospital[2]	Willmar	98%	180
Riverview Hospital	Crookston	98%	40
Saint Joseph's Hospital[2]	Saint Paul	98%	431
United Hospital[2]	Saint Paul	98%	403
Unity Hospital[2]	Fridley	98%	211
Essentia Health Duluth[2]	Duluth	97%	75
Essentia Health St Mary's Med Ctr[2]	Duluth	97%	414
Essentia Health Saint Marys	Detroit Lakes	97%	241
Mayo Clinic Hospital Rochester[2]	Rochester	97%	371
Northfield Hospital	Northfield	97%	151
Winona Health Services	Winona	97%	119
Essentia Health Virginia	Virginia	96%	100
Hutchinson Health	Hutchinson	96%	119
Saint Francis Medical Center	Breckenridge	96%	27
Sanford Bemidji Medical Center	Bemidji	96%	463
Univ Med Ctr-Mesabi/Mesaba Clinics[2]	Hibbing	96%	68
River's Edge Hospital & Clinic	Saint Peter	95%	44
Saint Elizabeth Medical Center	Wabasha	95%	38
Lakewood Health System[2]	Staples	94%	32
Mercy Hospital[2]	Moose Lake	94%	48
Centra Care Health Paynesville	Paynesville	93%	43
Sanford Medical Center Thief River Falls	Thief River Falls	93%	94
United Hospital District	Blue Earth	82%	39

Prophylactic Antibiotic Timing

Hospital Name	City	Rate	Cases
Buffalo Hospital	Buffalo	100%	139
Essentia Health Duluth[2]	Duluth	100%	75
Essentia Health Saint Marys	Detroit Lakes	100%	246
Fairview Northland Regional Hospital	Princeton	100%	63
Fairview Ridges Hospital[2]	Burnsville	100%	679
Fairview Southdale Hospital[2]	Edina	100%	1045
Hennepin County Medical Center[2]	Minneapolis	100%	234
Mayo Clinic Health System - Cannon Falls	Cannon Falls	100%	25
Mayo Clinic Health System - Red Wing[2]	Red Wing	100%	145
Mayo Clinic Methodist- Hospital[2]	Rochester	100%	406
Mercy Hospital[2]	Coon Rapids	100%	473
Mercy Hospital[2]	Moose Lake	100%	48
Abbott Northwestern Hospital[2]	Minneapolis	99%	493
Avera Marshall Regional Medical Center	Marshall	99%	115
Cambridge Medical Center	Cambridge	99%	144
Cuyuna Regional Medical Center	Crosby	99%	210
Douglas County Hospital[2]	Alexandria	99%	327
Essentia Health St Joseph's Med Ctr[2]	Brainerd	99%	204
Essentia Health Virginia	Virginia	99%	102
Fairview Lakes Medical Center[2]	Wyoming	99%	275
Grand Itasca Clinic & Hospital	Grand Rapids	99%	100
Healtheast Saint John's Hospital[2]	Maplewood	99%	376
Healtheast Woodwinds Hospital[2]	Woodbury	99%	294
Hutchinson Health	Hutchinson	99%	121
Maple Grove Hospital	Maple Grove	99%	536
Mayo Clinic Health System - Albert Lea	Albert Lea	99%	196
Mayo Clinic Health System - Mankato[2]	Mankato	99%	284
Mayo Clinic Hospital Rochester[2]	Rochester	99%	380
Minneapolis VA Medical Center	Minneapolis	99%	401
New Ulm Medical Center	New Ulm	99%	117
North Memorial Medical Center[2]	Robbinsdale	99%	412
Northfield Hospital	Northfield	99%	153

NOTE: Hospital profiles are in alphabetical order by state, then city, then hospital within the city; Rankings exclude hospitals with less than 25 cases except for patient surveys which excludes hospitals with less than 100 cases; (a) 100-299 cases; (1) The number of cases/patients is too few to report; (2) Data submitted were based on a sample of cases/patients; (3) Results are based on a shorter time period than required; (4) Data suppressed by CMS for one or more quarters; (5) Results are not available for this reporting period; (6) Fewer than 100 patients completed the HCAHPS survey; (7) No cases met the criteria for this measure; (8) The lower limit of the confidence interval cannot be calculated if the number of observed infections equals zero; (9) No data are available from the state/territory for this reporting period; (10) The scores shown reflect fewer than 50 completed surveys; (11) There were discrepancies in the data collection process; (12) This measure does not apply to this hospital for this reporting period; (13) Results cannot be calculated for this reporting period; (14) The results for this state are combined with nearby states to protect confidentiality; Please refer to the User's Guide for a full explanation of data.

Hospital Name	City	Rate	Cases
Owatonna Hospital[2]	Owatonna	99%	145
Regina Hospital[2]	Hastings	99%	161
Regions Hospital[2]	Saint Paul	99%	601
Rice Memorial Hospital[2]	Willmar	99%	181
Ridgeview Medical Center[2]	Waconia	99%	272
Saint Francis Regional Medical Center[2]	Shakopee	99%	388
Saint Joseph's Hospital[2]	Saint Paul	99%	451
Sanford Worthington Medical Center[2]	Worthington	99%	80
Unity Hospital[2]	Fridley	99%	214
Univ of Minnesota Med Ctr, Fairview[2]	Minneapolis	99%	1101
Winona Health Services	Winona	99%	122
Essentia Health St Mary's Med Ctr[2]	Duluth	98%	435
Firstlight Health System	Mora	98%	89
Lake Region Healthcare Corporation	Fergus Falls	98%	173
Lakeview Memorial Hospital[2]	Stillwater	98%	248
Mayo Clinic Health System - Fairmont	Fairmont	98%	100
Park Nicollet Methodist Hospital[2]	Saint Louis Park	98%	707
Saint Cloud Hospital[2]	Saint Cloud	98%	431
Saint Gabriels Hospital[2]	Little Falls	98%	184
Saint Luke's Hospital[2]	Duluth	98%	362
Sanford Bemidji Medical Center	Bemidji	98%	476
United Hospital[2]	Saint Paul	98%	417
District One Hospital	Faribault	97%	127
Lakewood Health System[2]	Staples	97%	33
Olmsted Medical Center	Rochester	97%	227
Riverwood Healthcare Center	Aitkin	97%	102
Saint Elizabeth Medical Center	Wabasha	97%	39
Saint Francis Medical Center	Breckenridge	97%	29
Univ Med Ctr-Mesabi/Mesaba Clinics[2]	Hibbing	97%	75
Community Memorial Hospital	Cloquet	96%	94
Glencoe Regional Health Services	Glencoe	96%	27
Bigfork Valley Hospital	Bigfork	95%	77
Centra Care Health Paynesville	Paynesville	95%	43
Sanford Medical Center Thief River Falls	Thief River Falls	95%	95
Mayo Clinic Health System - New Prague	New Prague	94%	70
Mayo Clinic Health System - Lake City	Lake City	90%	30
River's Edge Hospital & Clinic	Saint Peter	89%	44
Meeker Memorial Hospital	Litchfield	87%	39
Stevens Community Medical Center	Morris	84%	61
Deer River Healthcare Center	Deer River	79%	39
United Hospital District	Blue Earth	77%	39
Riverview Hospital	Crookston	76%	42

Prophylactic Antibiotic Timing (Outpatient)

Hospital Name	City	Rate	Cases
Healtheast Saint John's Hospital	Maplewood	100%	287
Maple Grove Hospital	Maple Grove	100%	287
New Ulm Medical Center	New Ulm	100%	27
Prairie Ridge Hospital & Health Services[3]	Elbow Lake	100%	29
Abbott Northwestern Hospital	Minneapolis	99%	686
Essentia Health St Mary's Med Ctr	Duluth	99%	493
Healtheast Woodwinds Hospital	Woodbury	99%	164
Ridgeview Medical Center	Waconia	99%	122
Saint Francis Regional Medical Center	Shakopee	99%	121
Saint Joseph's Hospital	Saint Paul	99%	274
Buffalo Hospital	Buffalo	98%	186
Essentia Health Duluth	Duluth	98%	175
Fairview Northland Regional Hospital	Princeton	98%	66
Fairview Ridges Hospital	Burnsville	98%	319
Fairview Southdale Hospital	Edina	98%	647
Mayo Clinic Health System - Albert Lea	Albert Lea	98%	41
Mayo Clinic Methodist- Hospital	Rochester	98%	508
Mercy Hospital	Coon Rapids	98%	382
North Memorial Medical Center	Robbinsdale	98%	328
Park Nicollet Methodist Hospital	Saint Louis Park	98%	1003
Saint Cloud Hospital	Saint Cloud	98%	1029
Saint Luke's Hospital	Duluth	98%	574
Unity Hospital	Fridley	98%	180
Winona Health Services	Winona	98%	43
District One Hospital	Faribault	97%	33
Douglas County Hospital	Alexandria	97%	216
Grand Itasca Clinic & Hospital	Grand Rapids	97%	101
Lakeview Memorial Hospital	Stillwater	97%	240
Lakewood Health System	Staples	97%	70
Regions Hospital	Saint Paul	97%	383
United Hospital	Saint Paul	97%	513
Fairview Lakes Medical Center	Wyoming	96%	72
Mayo Clinic Health System - Mankato	Mankato	96%	320
Mayo Clinic Hospital Rochester	Rochester	96%	707
Hutchinson Health	Hutchinson	95%	41
Owatonna Hospital	Owatonna	95%	108
Hennepin County Medical Center	Minneapolis	94%	125
Cambridge Medical Center	Cambridge	93%	44
Mayo Clinic Health System - Fairmont	Fairmont	93%	29
Olmsted Medical Center	Rochester	93%	55
Regina Hospital	Hastings	93%	27
Cuyuna Regional Medical Center	Crosby	91%	74
Univ of Minnesota Med Ctr, Fairview	Minneapolis	90%	531
Rice Memorial Hospital	Willmar	88%	60
Essentia Health St Joseph's Med Ctr	Brainerd	87%	115
Sanford Bemidji Medical Center	Bemidji	85%	53
Riverview Hospital	Crookston	77%	60
Lake Region Healthcare Corporation	Fergus Falls	52%	69

Urinary Catheter Removal

Hospital Name	City	Rate	Cases
Bigfork Valley Hospital	Bigfork	100%	75
Buffalo Hospital	Buffalo	100%	170
District One Hospital	Faribault	100%	54
Essentia Health Saint Marys	Detroit Lakes	100%	203
Fairview Lakes Medical Center[2]	Wyoming	100%	177
Fairview Northland Regional Hospital	Princeton	100%	34
Fairview Ridges Hospital[2]	Burnsville	100%	586
Hennepin County Medical Center[2]	Minneapolis	100%	207
Maple Grove Hospital	Maple Grove	100%	379
Mayo Clinic Health System - Albert Lea	Albert Lea	100%	218
Mayo Clinic Health System - Cannon Falls	Cannon Falls	100%	29
Mayo Clinic Health System - Red Wing[2]	Red Wing	100%	170
Mayo Clinic Methodist- Hospital[2]	Rochester	100%	178
Minneapolis VA Medical Center[2]	Minneapolis	100%	243
New Ulm Medical Center	New Ulm	100%	56
Regina Hospital[2]	Hastings	100%	28
Saint Elizabeth Medical Center	Wabasha	100%	35
Saint Francis Medical Center	Breckenridge	100%	37
Saint Francis Regional Medical Center[2]	Shakopee	100%	239
Saint Gabriels Hospital[2]	Little Falls	100%	97
Cambridge Medical Center	Cambridge	99%	132
Community Memorial Hospital	Cloquet	99%	77
Fairview Southdale Hospital[2]	Edina	99%	754
Lakeview Memorial Hospital[2]	Stillwater	99%	257
Mayo Clinic Health System - New Prague	New Prague	99%	68
Mayo Clinic Hospital Rochester[2]	Rochester	99%	489
Northfield Hospital	Northfield	99%	121
Olmsted Medical Center	Rochester	99%	207
Owatonna Hospital[2]	Owatonna	99%	134
Regions Hospital[2]	Saint Paul	99%	579
Univ of Minnesota Med Ctr, Fairview[2]	Minneapolis	99%	1302
Avera Marshall Regional Medical Center	Marshall	98%	80
Grand Itasca Clinic & Hospital	Grand Rapids	98%	60
Healtheast Woodwinds Hospital[2]	Woodbury	98%	220
Mercy Hospital[2]	Coon Rapids	98%	296
Abbott Northwestern Hospital[2]	Minneapolis	97%	458
Centra Care Health Paynesville	Paynesville	97%	32
Essentia Health St Joseph's Med Ctr[2]	Brainerd	97%	93
Healtheast Saint John's Hospital[2]	Maplewood	97%	273
Hutchinson Health	Hutchinson	97%	37
Mayo Clinic Health System - Lake City	Lake City	97%	31
United Hospital[2]	Saint Paul	97%	327
Unity Hospital[2]	Fridley	97%	76
Univ Med Ctr-Mesabi/Mesaba Clinics[2]	Hibbing	97%	35
Firstlight Health System	Mora	96%	52
Lake Region Healthcare Corporation	Fergus Falls	96%	51
North Memorial Medical Center[2]	Robbinsdale	96%	357
Park Nicollet Methodist Hospital[2]	Saint Louis Park	96%	393
Stevens Community Medical Center	Morris	96%	52
Mayo Clinic Health System - Fairmont	Fairmont	95%	107
Saint Cloud Hospital[2]	Saint Cloud	95%	279
Saint Joseph's Hospital[2]	Saint Paul	95%	397
Saint Luke's Hospital[2]	Duluth	94%	208
Sanford Bemidji Medical Center	Bemidji	94%	309
Winona Health Services	Winona	94%	102
Essentia Health St Mary's Med Ctr[2]	Duluth	93%	212
Rice Memorial Hospital[2]	Willmar	93%	196
Saint Joseph's Area Health Services	Park Rapids	93%	97
Sanford Medical Center Thief River Falls	Thief River Falls	93%	96
Douglas County Hospital[2]	Alexandria	92%	359
Mayo Clinic Health System - Mankato[2]	Mankato	92%	156
Essentia Health Virginia	Virginia	90%	88
Ridgeview Medical Center[2]	Waconia	90%	105
Sanford Worthington Medical Center[2]	Worthington	87%	54
Cuyuna Regional Medical Center	Crosby	84%	31
Riverview Hospital	Crookston	84%	25

Survey of Patients' Hospital Experiences

Area Around Room 'Always' Quiet at Night

Hospital Name	City	Rate	Cases
Redwood Area Hospital[11]	Redwood Falls	81%	(a)
Centracare Health - Monticello	Monticello	80%	(a)
Meeker Memorial Hospital	Litchfield	78%	(a)
Centra Care Health Paynesville	Paynesville	76%	(a)
Chippewa County Hospital[11]	Montevideo	76%	(a)
United Hospital District	Blue Earth	75%	(a)
Bigfork Valley Hospital[11]	Bigfork	74%	(a)
Regina Hospital	Hastings	74%	300+
Perham Health	Perham	73%	(a)
Riverwood Healthcare Center	Aitkin	73%	300+
Lakeview Memorial Hospital	Stillwater	72%	300+
Riverview Hospital	Crookston	72%	(a)
Healtheast Woodwinds Hospital	Woodbury	71%	300+
Community Memorial Hospital	Cloquet	70%	(a)
District One Hospital	Faribault	70%	300+
Douglas County Hospital	Alexandria	70%	300+
Hutchinson Health	Hutchinson	70%	300+
Lakewood Health System	Staples	70%	300+
Sanford Luverne Medical Center	Luverne	70%	(a)
Stevens Community Medical Center	Morris	70%	(a)
Mayo Clinic Methodist- Hospital[11]	Rochester	69%	300+
Rice Memorial Hospital	Willmar	69%	300+
Ridgeview Medical Center	Waconia	69%	300+
Maple Grove Hospital	Maple Grove	68%	300+
Mayo Clinic Health System - New Prague	New Prague	68%	(a)
Saint Francis Regional Medical Center	Shakopee	68%	300+
Saint Gabriels Hospital	Little Falls	68%	(a)
Swift County Benson Hospital[11]	Benson	68%	(a)
Glacial Ridge Hospital	Glenwood	67%	(a)
Saint Cloud Hospital	Saint Cloud	67%	300+
Glencoe Regional Health Services	Glencoe	66%	(a)
Murray County Memorial Hospital[11]	Slayton	66%	(a)
Saint Joseph's Area Health Services	Park Rapids	66%	(a)
Mayo Clinic Health System - Red Wing	Red Wing	65%	300+
Mercy Hospital	Moose Lake	65%	(a)
Regions Hospital	Saint Paul	65%	300+
Sanford Medical Center Thief River Falls	Thief River Falls	65%	300+
Cambridge Medical Center	Cambridge	64%	300+
Mille Lacs Health System	Onamia	64%	(a)
Grand Itasca Clinic & Hospital	Grand Rapids	63%	300+
New Ulm Medical Center	New Ulm	63%	300+
Saint Elizabeth Medical Center	Wabasha	63%	(a)
Univ Med Ctr-Mesabi/Mesaba Clinics	Hibbing	63%	300+
Winona Health Services	Winona	63%	300+
Essentia Health St Joseph's Med Ctr	Brainerd	62%	300+
Mayo Clinic Hospital Rochester[11]	Rochester	62%	300+
Saint Joseph's Hospital	Saint Paul	62%	300+
Essentia Health Saint Marys	Detroit Lakes	61%	300+
Fairview Lakes Medical Center	Wyoming	61%	300+
Fairview Northland Regional Hospital	Princeton	61%	300+
Lake Region Healthcare Corporation	Fergus Falls	61%	300+
Northfield Hospital	Northfield	61%	300+
Saint Francis Medical Center	Breckenridge	61%	(a)
Sanford Worthington Medical Center	Worthington	61%	300+
Tri County Hospital	Wadena	61%	300+
Cuyuna Regional Medical Center	Crosby	60%	300+
Fairview Ridges Hospital	Burnsville	60%	300+
Firstlight Health System	Mora	60%	300+
Lifecare Medical Center	Roseau	60%	(a)
Olmsted Medical Center	Rochester	60%	(a)
Owatonna Hospital	Owatonna	60%	300+
Windom Area Hospital	Windom	60%	(a)
Buffalo Hospital	Buffalo	59%	300+
Avera Marshall Regional Medical Center	Marshall	58%	300+
North Memorial Medical Center	Robbinsdale	58%	300+
Healtheast Saint John's Hospital	Maplewood	57%	300+
Mayo Clinic Health System - Albert Lea	Albert Lea	56%	300+
Mercy Hospital	Coon Rapids	56%	300+
Hennepin County Medical Center	Minneapolis	55%	300+
Mayo Clinic Health System - Fairmont	Fairmont	55%	300+
Sanford Bemidji Medical Center	Bemidji	55%	300+
Fairview Southdale Hospital	Edina	54%	300+
Unity Hospital	Fridley	54%	300+
Abbott Northwestern Hospital	Minneapolis	53%	300+
Essentia Health Duluth	Duluth	53%	300+
United Hospital	Saint Paul	52%	300+
Essentia Health Virginia	Virginia	50%	300+
Park Nicollet Methodist Hospital	Saint Louis Park	49%	300+
Saint Luke's Hospital	Duluth	49%	300+
Essentia Health St Mary's Med Ctr	Duluth	47%	300+
Univ of Minnesota Med Ctr, Fairview[11]	Minneapolis	47%	300+
Mayo Clinic Health System - Mankato	Mankato	46%	300+

Doctors 'Always' Communicated Well

Hospital Name	City	Rate	Cases
Bigfork Valley Hospital[11]	Bigfork	93%	(a)
Mille Lacs Health System	Onamia	93%	(a)
Sanford Luverne Medical Center	Luverne	91%	(a)
United Hospital District	Blue Earth	91%	(a)
Cuyuna Regional Medical Center	Crosby	89%	300+
Chippewa County Hospital[11]	Montevideo	88%	(a)
Glacial Ridge Hospital	Glenwood	88%	(a)
Meeker Memorial Hospital	Litchfield	88%	(a)
Murray County Memorial Hospital[11]	Slayton	88%	(a)
New Ulm Medical Center	New Ulm	88%	300+
Hutchinson Health	Hutchinson	87%	300+
Lakewood Health System	Staples	87%	300+
Regina Hospital	Hastings	87%	300+
Saint Francis Medical Center	Breckenridge	87%	(a)
Saint Joseph's Area Health Services	Park Rapids	87%	(a)
Riverview Hospital	Crookston	86%	(a)
Riverwood Healthcare Center	Aitkin	86%	300+
Swift County Benson Hospital[11]	Benson	86%	(a)
Windom Area Hospital	Windom	86%	(a)
Fairview Northland Regional Hospital	Princeton	85%	300+

NOTE: Hospital profiles are in alphabetical order by state, then city, then hospital within the city; Rankings exclude hospitals with less than 25 cases except for patient surveys which excludes hospitals with less than 100 cases; (a) 100-299 cases; (1) The number of cases/patients is too few to report; (2) Data submitted were based on a sample of cases/patients; (3) Results are based on a shorter time period than required; (4) Data suppressed by CMS for one or more quarters; (5) Results are not available for this reporting period; (6) Fewer than 100 patients completed the HCAHPS survey; (7) No cases met the criteria for this measure; (8) The lower limit of the confidence interval cannot be calculated if the number of observed infections equals zero; (9) No data are available from the state/territory for this reporting period; (10) The scores shown reflect fewer than 50 completed surveys; (11) There were discrepancies in the data collection process; (12) This measure does not apply to this hospital for this reporting period; (13) Results cannot be calculated for this reporting period; (14) The results for this state are combined with nearby states to protect confidentiality; Please refer to the User's Guide for a full explanation of data.

Hospital Name	City	Rate	Cases
Grand Itasca Clinic & Hospital	Grand Rapids	85%	300+
Lakeview Memorial Hospital	Stillwater	85%	300+
Mayo Clinic Health System - New Prague	New Prague	85%	(a)
Northfield Hospital	Northfield	85%	300+
Redwood Area Hospital[11]	Redwood Falls	85%	(a)
Ridgeview Medical Center	Waconia	85%	300+
Saint Gabriels Hospital	Little Falls	85%	(a)
Stevens Community Medical Center	Morris	85%	(a)
Essentia Health Duluth	Duluth	84%	300+
Glencoe Regional Health Services	Glencoe	84%	(a)
Lifecare Medical Center	Roseau	84%	(a)
Mayo Clinic Health System - Red Wing	Red Wing	84%	300+
Mayo Clinic Methodist- Hospital[11]	Rochester	84%	300+
Mercy Hospital	Moose Lake	84%	(a)
Saint Elizabeth Medical Center	Wabasha	84%	(a)
Univ Med Ctr-Mesabi/Mesaba Clinics	Hibbing	84%	300+
Avera Marshall Regional Medical Center	Marshall	83%	300+
Buffalo Hospital	Buffalo	83%	300+
Cambridge Medical Center	Cambridge	83%	300+
Centra Care Health Paynesville	Paynesville	83%	(a)
District One Hospital	Faribault	83%	300+
Firstlight Health System	Mora	83%	300+
Healtheast Woodwinds Hospital	Woodbury	83%	300+
Mayo Clinic Hospital Rochester[11]	Rochester	83%	300+
Owatonna Hospital	Owatonna	83%	300+
Perham Health	Perham	83%	(a)
Rice Memorial Hospital	Willmar	83%	300+
Tri County Hospital	Wadena	83%	300+
Centracare Health - Monticello	Monticello	82%	(a)
Essentia Health St Joseph's Med Ctr	Brainerd	82%	300+
Fairview Southdale Hospital	Edina	82%	300+
Saint Cloud Hospital	Saint Cloud	82%	300+
Saint Francis Regional Medical Center	Shakopee	82%	300+
Saint Luke's Hospital	Duluth	82%	300+
Essentia Health Saint Marys	Detroit Lakes	81%	300+
Mayo Clinic Health System - Albert Lea	Albert Lea	81%	300+
Abbott Northwestern Hospital	Minneapolis	80%	300+
Douglas County Hospital	Alexandria	80%	300+
Essentia Health St Mary's Med Ctr	Duluth	80%	300+
Olmsted Medical Center	Rochester	80%	(a)
Park Nicollet Methodist Hospital	Saint Louis Park	80%	300+
Fairview Ridges Hospital	Burnsville	79%	300+
Lake Region Healthcare Corporation	Fergus Falls	79%	300+
Mercy Hospital	Coon Rapids	79%	300+
Regions Hospital	Saint Paul	79%	300+
Sanford Bemidji Medical Center	Bemidji	79%	300+
Sanford Medical Center Thief River Falls	Thief River Falls	79%	300+
Winona Health Services	Winona	79%	300+
Saint Joseph's Hospital	Saint Paul	78%	300+
Unity Hospital	Fridley	78%	300+
Community Memorial Hospital	Cloquet	77%	(a)
Fairview Lakes Medical Center	Wyoming	77%	300+
Maple Grove Hospital	Maple Grove	77%	300+
Mayo Clinic Health System - Mankato	Mankato	77%	300+
Sanford Worthington Medical Center	Worthington	77%	300+
United Hospital	Saint Paul	77%	300+
Univ of Minnesota Med Ctr, Fairview[11]	Minneapolis	77%	300+
Healtheast Saint John's Hospital	Maplewood	76%	300+
North Memorial Medical Center	Robbinsdale	75%	300+
Essentia Health Virginia	Virginia	74%	300+
Hennepin County Medical Center	Minneapolis	73%	300+
Mayo Clinic Health System - Fairmont	Fairmont	73%	300+

Home Recovery Information Given

Hospital Name	City	Rate	Cases
Bigfork Valley Hospital[11]	Bigfork	95%	(a)
Mille Lacs Health System	Onamia	94%	(a)
Sanford Luverne Medical Center	Luverne	94%	(a)
Redwood Area Hospital[11]	Redwood Falls	93%	(a)
Lake Region Healthcare Corporation	Fergus Falls	92%	300+
Mayo Clinic Health System - New Prague	New Prague	92%	(a)
Mayo Clinic Methodist- Hospital[11]	Rochester	92%	300+
Saint Elizabeth Medical Center	Wabasha	92%	(a)
Univ Med Ctr-Mesabi/Mesaba Clinics	Hibbing	92%	300+
Buffalo Hospital	Buffalo	91%	300+
Essentia Health St Joseph's Med Ctr	Brainerd	91%	300+
Lakeview Memorial Hospital	Stillwater	91%	300+
Olmsted Medical Center	Rochester	91%	(a)
Ridgeview Medical Center	Waconia	91%	300+
Avera Marshall Regional Medical Center	Marshall	90%	300+
Centracare Health - Monticello	Monticello	90%	(a)
Glencoe Regional Health Services	Glencoe	90%	(a)
Healtheast Woodwinds Hospital	Woodbury	90%	300+
Lifecare Medical Center	Roseau	90%	(a)
Mayo Clinic Hospital Rochester[11]	Rochester	90%	300+
Murray County Memorial Hospital[11]	Slayton	90%	(a)
Regina Hospital	Hastings	90%	300+
Riverview Hospital	Crookston	90%	(a)
Saint Francis Medical Center	Breckenridge	90%	(a)
Saint Joseph's Area Health Services	Park Rapids	90%	(a)
Saint Luke's Hospital	Duluth	90%	300+
Fairview Northland Regional Hospital	Princeton	89%	300+
Firstlight Health System	Mora	89%	300+
Glacial Ridge Hospital	Glenwood	89%	(a)
Lakewood Health System	Staples	89%	300+
Regions Hospital	Saint Paul	89%	300+
Saint Francis Regional Medical Center	Shakopee	89%	300+
Saint Gabriels Hospital	Little Falls	89%	(a)
Saint Joseph's Hospital	Saint Paul	89%	300+
Abbott Northwestern Hospital	Minneapolis	88%	300+
Cambridge Medical Center	Cambridge	88%	300+
Cuyuna Regional Medical Center	Crosby	88%	300+
Douglas County Hospital	Alexandria	88%	300+
Essentia Health Duluth	Duluth	88%	300+
Essentia Health St Mary's Med Ctr	Duluth	88%	300+
Essentia Health Saint Marys	Detroit Lakes	88%	300+
Hutchinson Health	Hutchinson	88%	300+
Maple Grove Hospital	Maple Grove	88%	300+
Mercy Hospital	Coon Rapids	88%	300+
New Ulm Medical Center	New Ulm	88%	300+
Rice Memorial Hospital	Willmar	88%	300+
Riverwood Healthcare Center	Aitkin	88%	300+
Swift County Benson Hospital[11]	Benson	88%	(a)
Tri County Hospital	Wadena	88%	300+
Fairview Ridges Hospital	Burnsville	87%	300+
Fairview Southdale Hospital	Edina	87%	300+
Healtheast Saint John's Hospital	Maplewood	87%	300+
Mayo Clinic Health System - Red Wing	Red Wing	87%	300+
Northfield Hospital	Northfield	87%	300+
Owatonna Hospital	Owatonna	87%	300+
Saint Cloud Hospital	Saint Cloud	87%	300+
Sanford Worthington Medical Center	Worthington	87%	300+
Unity Hospital	Fridley	87%	300+
Univ of Minnesota Med Ctr, Fairview[11]	Minneapolis	87%	300+
Windom Area Hospital	Windom	87%	(a)
Winona Health Services	Winona	87%	300+
Chippewa County Hospital[11]	Montevideo	86%	(a)
District One Hospital	Faribault	86%	300+
Fairview Lakes Medical Center	Wyoming	86%	300+
Mayo Clinic Health System - Albert Lea	Albert Lea	86%	300+
North Memorial Medical Center	Robbinsdale	86%	300+
United Hospital	Saint Paul	86%	300+
Centra Care Health Paynesville	Paynesville	85%	(a)
Grand Itasca Clinic & Hospital	Grand Rapids	85%	300+
Mayo Clinic Health System - Fairmont	Fairmont	85%	300+
Park Nicollet Methodist Hospital	Saint Louis Park	85%	300+
Perham Health	Perham	85%	(a)
Stevens Community Medical Center	Morris	85%	(a)
Essentia Health Virginia	Virginia	84%	300+
Mayo Clinic Health System - Mankato	Mankato	84%	300+
Mercy Hospital	Moose Lake	84%	(a)
Hennepin County Medical Center	Minneapolis	83%	300+
Sanford Medical Center Thief River Falls	Thief River Falls	82%	300+
United Hospital District	Blue Earth	82%	(a)
Community Memorial Hospital	Cloquet	81%	(a)
Meeker Memorial Hospital	Litchfield	81%	(a)
Sanford Bemidji Medical Center	Bemidji	81%	300+

Hospital Given 9 or 10 on 10 Point Scale

Hospital Name	City	Rate	Cases
Bigfork Valley Hospital[11]	Bigfork	89%	(a)
Mayo Clinic Hospital Rochester[11]	Rochester	86%	300+
Mayo Clinic Methodist- Hospital[11]	Rochester	86%	300+
Healtheast Woodwinds Hospital	Woodbury	85%	300+
Maple Grove Hospital	Maple Grove	85%	300+
Centra Care Health Paynesville	Paynesville	84%	(a)
Cuyuna Regional Medical Center	Crosby	84%	300+
Lakewood Health System	Staples	84%	300+
Meeker Memorial Hospital	Litchfield	84%	(a)
Redwood Area Hospital[11]	Redwood Falls	84%	(a)
Sanford Luverne Medical Center	Luverne	84%	(a)
Lakeview Memorial Hospital	Stillwater	83%	300+
Mayo Clinic Health System - New Prague	New Prague	83%	(a)
Olmsted Medical Center	Rochester	83%	(a)
Perham Health	Perham	82%	(a)
Glacial Ridge Hospital	Glenwood	81%	(a)
Ridgeview Medical Center	Waconia	81%	300+
Saint Joseph's Area Health Services	Park Rapids	79%	(a)
Fairview Northland Regional Hospital	Princeton	78%	300+
Regina Hospital	Hastings	78%	300+
Riverwood Healthcare Center	Aitkin	78%	300+
Saint Gabriels Hospital	Little Falls	78%	(a)
Lifecare Medical Center	Roseau	77%	(a)
Mille Lacs Health System	Onamia	77%	(a)
Murray County Memorial Hospital[11]	Slayton	77%	(a)
Northfield Hospital	Northfield	77%	300+
Saint Cloud Hospital	Saint Cloud	77%	300+
Saint Francis Regional Medical Center	Shakopee	77%	300+
Saint Joseph's Hospital	Saint Paul	77%	300+
Community Memorial Hospital	Cloquet	76%	(a)
Mayo Clinic Health System - Red Wing	Red Wing	76%	300+
United Hospital District	Blue Earth	76%	(a)

Hospital Name	City	Rate	Cases
Cambridge Medical Center	Cambridge	75%	300+
Centracare Health - Monticello	Monticello	75%	(a)
Essentia Health St Joseph's Med Ctr	Brainerd	75%	300+
New Ulm Medical Center	New Ulm	75%	300+
Stevens Community Medical Center	Morris	75%	(a)
Tri County Hospital	Wadena	75%	300+
Abbott Northwestern Hospital	Minneapolis	74%	300+
Riverview Hospital	Crookston	74%	(a)
Mercy Hospital	Coon Rapids	73%	300+
Owatonna Hospital	Owatonna	73%	300+
Saint Elizabeth Medical Center	Wabasha	73%	(a)
Saint Luke's Hospital	Duluth	73%	300+
Windom Area Hospital	Windom	73%	(a)
Buffalo Hospital	Buffalo	72%	300+
District One Hospital	Faribault	72%	300+
Essentia Health Saint Marys	Detroit Lakes	72%	300+
Mayo Clinic Health System - Albert Lea	Albert Lea	72%	300+
Regions Hospital	Saint Paul	72%	300+
Saint Francis Medical Center	Breckenridge	72%	(a)
Swift County Benson Hospital[11]	Benson	72%	(a)
Avera Marshall Regional Medical Center	Marshall	71%	300+
Douglas County Hospital	Alexandria	71%	300+
Fairview Southdale Hospital	Edina	71%	300+
Grand Itasca Clinic & Hospital	Grand Rapids	71%	300+
Mercy Hospital	Moose Lake	71%	(a)
Rice Memorial Hospital	Willmar	71%	300+
Healtheast Saint John's Hospital	Maplewood	70%	300+
Hutchinson Health	Hutchinson	70%	300+
Chippewa County Hospital[11]	Montevideo	69%	(a)
Fairview Lakes Medical Center	Wyoming	69%	300+
Lake Region Healthcare Corporation	Fergus Falls	69%	300+
Essentia Health St Mary's Med Ctr	Duluth	68%	300+
Firstlight Health System	Mora	68%	300+
Sanford Worthington Medical Center	Worthington	68%	300+
United Hospital	Saint Paul	68%	300+
Univ of Minnesota Med Ctr, Fairview[11]	Minneapolis	68%	300+
Essentia Health Duluth	Duluth	67%	300+
Fairview Ridges Hospital	Burnsville	67%	300+
North Memorial Medical Center	Robbinsdale	67%	300+
Park Nicollet Methodist Hospital	Saint Louis Park	67%	300+
Univ Med Ctr-Mesabi/Mesaba Clinics	Hibbing	67%	300+
Glencoe Regional Health Services	Glencoe	66%	(a)
Unity Hospital	Fridley	66%	300+
Winona Health Services	Winona	66%	300+
Mayo Clinic Health System - Fairmont	Fairmont	65%	300+
Mayo Clinic Health System - Mankato	Mankato	62%	300+
Essentia Health Virginia	Virginia	59%	300+
Hennepin County Medical Center	Minneapolis	59%	300+
Sanford Bemidji Medical Center	Bemidji	59%	300+
Sanford Medical Center Thief River Falls	Thief River Falls	59%	300+

Meds 'Always' Explained Before Given

Hospital Name	City	Rate	Cases
Bigfork Valley Hospital[11]	Bigfork	81%	(a)
Mille Lacs Health System	Onamia	76%	(a)
Glacial Ridge Hospital	Glenwood	73%	(a)
Centra Care Health Paynesville	Paynesville	72%	(a)
Cuyuna Regional Medical Center	Crosby	72%	300+
Lakeview Memorial Hospital	Stillwater	72%	300+
Meeker Memorial Hospital	Litchfield	72%	(a)
Riverwood Healthcare Center	Aitkin	72%	300+
Swift County Benson Hospital[11]	Benson	72%	(a)
Regina Hospital	Hastings	71%	300+
Saint Elizabeth Medical Center	Wabasha	71%	(a)
Fairview Northland Regional Hospital	Princeton	70%	300+
Mayo Clinic Health System - New Prague	New Prague	70%	(a)
Murray County Memorial Hospital[11]	Slayton	70%	(a)
Riverview Hospital	Crookston	70%	(a)
Saint Francis Medical Center	Breckenridge	70%	(a)
Windom Area Hospital	Windom	70%	(a)
Healtheast Woodwinds Hospital	Woodbury	69%	300+
Grand Itasca Clinic & Hospital	Grand Rapids	68%	300+
Lakewood Health System	Staples	68%	300+
Mayo Clinic Health System - Red Wing	Red Wing	68%	300+
Mayo Clinic Hospital Rochester[11]	Rochester	68%	300+
Mayo Clinic Methodist- Hospital[11]	Rochester	68%	300+
Rice Memorial Hospital	Willmar	68%	300+
Saint Francis Regional Medical Center	Shakopee	68%	300+
Essentia Health St Joseph's Med Ctr	Brainerd	67%	300+
Fairview Lakes Medical Center	Wyoming	67%	300+
Perham Health	Perham	67%	(a)
Redwood Area Hospital[11]	Redwood Falls	67%	(a)
Saint Cloud Hospital	Saint Cloud	67%	300+
Tri County Hospital	Wadena	67%	300+
Buffalo Hospital	Buffalo	66%	300+
Cambridge Medical Center	Cambridge	66%	300+
Hutchinson Health	Hutchinson	66%	300+
Saint Joseph's Area Health Services	Park Rapids	66%	(a)
Sanford Worthington Medical Center	Worthington	66%	300+
District One Hospital	Faribault	65%	300+
Lake Region Healthcare Corporation	Fergus Falls	65%	300+

NOTE: Hospital profiles are in alphabetical order by state, then city, then hospital within the city; Rankings exclude hospitals with less than 25 cases except for patient surveys which excludes hospitals with less than 100 cases; (a) 100-299 cases; (1) The number of cases/patients is too few to report; (2) Data submitted were based on a sample of cases/patients; (3) Results are based on a shorter time period than required; (4) Data suppressed by CMS for one or more quarters; (5) Results are not available for this reporting period; (6) Fewer than 100 patients completed the HCAHPS survey; (7) No cases met the criteria for this measure; (8) The lower limit of the confidence interval cannot be calculated if the number of observed infections equals zero; (9) No data are available from the state/territory for this reporting period; (10) The scores shown reflect fewer than 50 completed surveys; (11) There were discrepancies in the data collection process; (12) This measure does not apply to this hospital for this reporting period; (13) Results cannot be calculated for this reporting period; (14) The results for this state are combined with nearby states to protect confidentiality; Please refer to the User's Guide for a full explanation of data.

Hospital Name	City	Rate	Cases
Mayo Clinic Health System - Albert Lea	Albert Lea	65%	300+
New Ulm Medical Center	New Ulm	65%	300+
Olmsted Medical Center	Rochester	65%	(a)
Ridgeview Medical Center	Waconia	65%	300+
Sanford Luverne Medical Center	Luverne	65%	(a)
Avera Marshall Regional Medical Center	Marshall	64%	300+
Community Memorial Hospital	Cloquet	64%	(a)
Essentia Health St Mary's Med Ctr	Duluth	64%	300+
Firstlight Health System	Mora	64%	300+
Mercy Hospital	Coon Rapids	64%	300+
Essentia Health Duluth	Duluth	63%	300+
Essentia Health Virginia	Virginia	63%	300+
Mayo Clinic Health System - Fairmont	Fairmont	63%	300+
Northfield Hospital	Northfield	63%	300+
Saint Gabriels Hospital	Little Falls	63%	(a)
Sanford Medical Center Thief River Falls	Thief River Falls	63%	300+
Stevens Community Medical Center	Morris	63%	(a)
United Hospital District	Blue Earth	63%	(a)
Univ Med Ctr-Mesabi/Mesaba Clinics	Hibbing	63%	300+
Essentia Health Saint Marys	Detroit Lakes	62%	300+
Lifecare Medical Center	Roseau	62%	(a)
Mayo Clinic Health System - Mankato	Mankato	62%	300+
Owatonna Hospital	Owatonna	62%	300+
Abbott Northwestern Hospital	Minneapolis	61%	300+
Centracare Health - Monticello	Monticello	61%	(a)
Mercy Hospital	Moose Lake	61%	(a)
Saint Luke's Hospital	Duluth	61%	300+
Winona Health Services	Winona	61%	300+
Fairview Ridges Hospital	Burnsville	60%	300+
Fairview Southdale Hospital	Edina	60%	300+
North Memorial Medical Center	Robbinsdale	60%	300+
Park Nicollet Methodist Hospital	Saint Louis Park	60%	300+
Regions Hospital	Saint Paul	60%	300+
Saint Joseph's Hospital	Saint Paul	60%	300+
United Hospital	Saint Paul	60%	300+
Unity Hospital	Fridley	60%	300+
Univ of Minnesota Med Ctr, Fairview[11]	Minneapolis	60%	300+
Douglas County Hospital	Alexandria	59%	300+
Glencoe Regional Health Services	Glencoe	59%	(a)
Healtheast Saint John's Hospital	Maplewood	59%	300+
Maple Grove Hospital	Maple Grove	59%	300+
Sanford Bemidji Medical Center	Bemidji	57%	300+
Chippewa County Hospital[11]	Montevideo	55%	(a)
Hennepin County Medical Center	Minneapolis	52%	300+

Nurses 'Always' Communicated Well

Hospital Name	City	Rate	Cases
Bigfork Valley Hospital[11]	Bigfork	93%	(a)
Centra Care Health Paynesville	Paynesville	89%	(a)
Mille Lacs Health System	Onamia	87%	(a)
Glacial Ridge Hospital	Glenwood	86%	(a)
Healtheast Woodwinds Hospital	Woodbury	86%	300+
Lakeview Memorial Hospital	Stillwater	86%	300+
Windom Area Hospital	Windom	86%	(a)
Cuyuna Regional Medical Center	Crosby	85%	300+
Ridgeview Medical Center	Waconia	85%	300+
Riverwood Healthcare Center	Aitkin	85%	300+
Saint Elizabeth Medical Center	Wabasha	85%	(a)
Hutchinson Health	Hutchinson	84%	300+
Lakewood Health System	Staples	84%	300+
Mayo Clinic Health System - New Prague	New Prague	84%	(a)
Mayo Clinic Methodist- Hospital[11]	Rochester	84%	300+
Redwood Area Hospital[11]	Redwood Falls	84%	(a)
United Hospital District	Blue Earth	84%	(a)
Mayo Clinic Hospital Rochester[11]	Rochester	83%	300+
Olmsted Medical Center	Rochester	83%	(a)
Perham Health	Perham	83%	(a)
Riverview Hospital	Crookston	83%	(a)
Saint Cloud Hospital	Saint Cloud	83%	300+
Saint Joseph's Area Health Services	Park Rapids	83%	(a)
Sanford Luverne Medical Center	Luverne	83%	(a)
Essentia Health St Joseph's Med Ctr	Brainerd	82%	300+
Fairview Northland Regional Hospital	Princeton	82%	300+
Mayo Clinic Health System - Red Wing	Red Wing	82%	300+
Murray County Memorial Hospital[11]	Slayton	82%	(a)
Regina Hospital	Hastings	82%	300+
Univ Med Ctr-Mesabi/Mesaba Clinics	Hibbing	82%	300+
Buffalo Hospital	Buffalo	81%	300+
Cambridge Medical Center	Cambridge	81%	300+
Grand Itasca Clinic & Hospital	Grand Rapids	81%	300+
New Ulm Medical Center	New Ulm	81%	300+
Northfield Hospital	Northfield	81%	300+
Saint Gabriels Hospital	Little Falls	81%	(a)
Avera Marshall Regional Medical Center	Marshall	80%	300+
District One Hospital	Faribault	80%	300+
Lifecare Medical Center	Roseau	80%	(a)
Maple Grove Hospital	Maple Grove	80%	300+
Mayo Clinic Health System - Albert Lea	Albert Lea	80%	300+
Meeker Memorial Hospital	Litchfield	80%	(a)
Mercy Hospital	Moose Lake	80%	(a)
Rice Memorial Hospital	Willmar	80%	300+
Saint Francis Regional Medical Center	Shakopee	80%	300+
Swift County Benson Hospital[11]	Benson	80%	(a)
Tri County Hospital	Wadena	80%	300+
Winona Health Services	Winona	80%	300+
Centracare Health - Monticello	Monticello	79%	(a)
Community Memorial Hospital	Cloquet	79%	(a)
Essentia Health Saint Marys	Detroit Lakes	79%	300+
Owatonna Hospital	Owatonna	79%	300+
Sanford Worthington Medical Center	Worthington	79%	300+
Stevens Community Medical Center	Morris	79%	(a)
Fairview Lakes Medical Center	Wyoming	78%	300+
Fairview Southdale Hospital	Edina	78%	300+
Mercy Hospital	Coon Rapids	78%	300+
Saint Francis Medical Center	Breckenridge	78%	(a)
Saint Joseph's Hospital	Saint Paul	78%	300+
Sanford Medical Center Thief River Falls	Thief River Falls	78%	300+
Essentia Health St Mary's Med Ctr	Duluth	77%	300+
Firstlight Health System	Mora	77%	300+
Lake Region Healthcare Corporation	Fergus Falls	77%	300+
Mayo Clinic Health System - Fairmont	Fairmont	77%	300+
Abbott Northwestern Hospital	Minneapolis	76%	300+
Essentia Health Virginia	Virginia	76%	300+
Fairview Ridges Hospital	Burnsville	76%	300+
Glencoe Regional Health Services	Glencoe	76%	(a)
Healtheast Saint John's Hospital	Maplewood	76%	300+
Saint Luke's Hospital	Duluth	76%	300+
Essentia Health Duluth	Duluth	75%	300+
Mayo Clinic Health System - Mankato	Mankato	75%	300+
United Hospital	Saint Paul	75%	300+
Douglas County Hospital	Alexandria	74%	300+
Park Nicollet Methodist Hospital	Saint Louis Park	74%	300+
Regions Hospital	Saint Paul	74%	300+
Unity Hospital	Fridley	74%	300+
Univ of Minnesota Med Ctr, Fairview[11]	Minneapolis	74%	300+
Chippewa County Hospital[11]	Montevideo	73%	(a)
North Memorial Medical Center	Robbinsdale	72%	300+
Sanford Bemidji Medical Center	Bemidji	72%	300+
Hennepin County Medical Center	Minneapolis	69%	300+

Pain 'Always' Well Controlled

Hospital Name	City	Rate	Cases
Bigfork Valley Hospital[11]	Bigfork	85%	(a)
Mayo Clinic Health System - New Prague	New Prague	79%	(a)
Glacial Ridge Hospital	Glenwood	77%	(a)
Lakeview Memorial Hospital	Stillwater	77%	300+
United Hospital District	Blue Earth	77%	(a)
Buffalo Hospital	Buffalo	76%	300+
Cuyuna Regional Medical Center	Crosby	76%	300+
Fairview Northland Regional Hospital	Princeton	76%	300+
Meeker Memorial Hospital	Litchfield	76%	(a)
Mille Lacs Health System	Onamia	76%	(a)
Saint Joseph's Area Health Services	Park Rapids	76%	(a)
Sanford Luverne Medical Center	Luverne	76%	(a)
Essentia Health St Joseph's Med Ctr	Brainerd	75%	300+
Maple Grove Hospital	Maple Grove	75%	300+
Riverwood Healthcare Center	Aitkin	75%	300+
Grand Itasca Clinic & Hospital	Grand Rapids	74%	300+
Lakewood Health System	Staples	74%	300+
Mayo Clinic Methodist- Hospital[11]	Rochester	74%	300+
New Ulm Medical Center	New Ulm	74%	300+
Regina Hospital	Hastings	74%	300+
Saint Cloud Hospital	Saint Cloud	74%	300+
Centracare Health - Monticello	Monticello	73%	(a)
Chippewa County Hospital[11]	Montevideo	73%	(a)
District One Hospital	Faribault	73%	300+
Healtheast Woodwinds Hospital	Woodbury	73%	300+
Redwood Area Hospital[11]	Redwood Falls	73%	(a)
Ridgeview Medical Center	Waconia	73%	300+
Saint Francis Medical Center	Breckenridge	73%	(a)
Saint Francis Regional Medical Center	Shakopee	73%	300+
Univ Med Ctr-Mesabi/Mesaba Clinics	Hibbing	73%	300+
Windom Area Hospital	Windom	73%	(a)
Douglas County Hospital	Alexandria	72%	300+
Fairview Southdale Hospital	Edina	72%	300+
Hutchinson Health	Hutchinson	72%	300+
Olmsted Medical Center	Rochester	72%	(a)
Owatonna Hospital	Owatonna	72%	300+
Saint Joseph's Hospital	Saint Paul	72%	300+
Sanford Worthington Medical Center	Worthington	72%	300+
Swift County Benson Hospital[11]	Benson	72%	(a)
Cambridge Medical Center	Cambridge	71%	300+
Community Memorial Hospital	Cloquet	71%	(a)
Fairview Ridges Hospital	Burnsville	71%	300+
Mayo Clinic Hospital Rochester[11]	Rochester	71%	300+
Mercy Hospital	Moose Lake	71%	(a)
Northfield Hospital	Northfield	71%	300+
Saint Gabriels Hospital	Little Falls	71%	(a)
Firstlight Health System	Mora	70%	300+
Mayo Clinic Health System - Albert Lea	Albert Lea	70%	300+
Mayo Clinic Health System - Red Wing	Red Wing	70%	300+
Mercy Hospital	Coon Rapids	70%	300+
Saint Luke's Hospital	Duluth	70%	300+
Sanford Medical Center Thief River Falls	Thief River Falls	70%	300+
Abbott Northwestern Hospital	Minneapolis	69%	300+
Fairview Lakes Medical Center	Wyoming	69%	300+
Glencoe Regional Health Services	Glencoe	69%	(a)
Lake Region Healthcare Corporation	Fergus Falls	69%	300+
Mayo Clinic Health System - Fairmont	Fairmont	69%	300+
North Memorial Medical Center	Robbinsdale	69%	300+
Riverview Hospital	Crookston	69%	(a)
Saint Elizabeth Medical Center	Wabasha	69%	(a)
Tri County Hospital	Wadena	69%	300+
United Hospital	Saint Paul	69%	300+
Avera Marshall Regional Medical Center	Marshall	68%	300+
Centra Care Health Paynesville	Paynesville	68%	(a)
Essentia Health Saint Marys	Detroit Lakes	68%	300+
Mayo Clinic Health System - Mankato	Mankato	68%	300+
Regions Hospital	Saint Paul	68%	300+
Essentia Health Duluth	Duluth	67%	300+
Essentia Health St Mary's Med Ctr	Duluth	67%	300+
Healtheast Saint John's Hospital	Maplewood	67%	300+
Park Nicollet Methodist Hospital	Saint Louis Park	67%	300+
Stevens Community Medical Center	Morris	67%	(a)
Unity Hospital	Fridley	67%	300+
Winona Health Services	Winona	67%	300+
Lifecare Medical Center	Roseau	66%	(a)
Perham Health	Perham	66%	(a)
Rice Memorial Hospital	Willmar	66%	300+
Sanford Bemidji Medical Center	Bemidji	66%	300+
Essentia Health Virginia	Virginia	65%	300+
Univ of Minnesota Med Ctr, Fairview[11]	Minneapolis	65%	300+
Murray County Memorial Hospital[11]	Slayton	64%	(a)
Hennepin County Medical Center	Minneapolis	62%	300+

Room and Bathroom 'Always' Clean

Hospital Name	City	Rate	Cases
Sanford Luverne Medical Center	Luverne	92%	(a)
Bigfork Valley Hospital[11]	Bigfork	91%	(a)
Stevens Community Medical Center	Morris	89%	(a)
Lakewood Health System	Staples	87%	300+
Glacial Ridge Hospital	Glenwood	86%	(a)
Meeker Memorial Hospital	Litchfield	86%	(a)
Murray County Memorial Hospital[11]	Slayton	85%	(a)
Perham Health	Perham	85%	(a)
Saint Elizabeth Medical Center	Wabasha	85%	(a)
United Hospital District	Blue Earth	85%	(a)
Centra Care Health Paynesville	Paynesville	84%	(a)
Lakeview Memorial Hospital	Stillwater	84%	300+
Mayo Clinic Health System - New Prague	New Prague	84%	(a)
Mille Lacs Health System	Onamia	84%	(a)
Redwood Area Hospital[11]	Redwood Falls	84%	(a)
Riverwood Healthcare Center	Aitkin	84%	300+
Community Memorial Hospital	Cloquet	83%	(a)
New Ulm Medical Center	New Ulm	83%	300+
Ridgeview Medical Center	Waconia	82%	300+
Tri County Hospital	Wadena	82%	300+
Windom Area Hospital	Windom	82%	(a)
Centracare Health - Monticello	Monticello	81%	(a)
Swift County Benson Hospital[11]	Benson	81%	(a)
Cuyuna Regional Medical Center	Crosby	80%	300+
Fairview Lakes Medical Center	Wyoming	80%	300+
Mayo Clinic Health System - Fairmont	Fairmont	80%	300+
Sanford Worthington Medical Center	Worthington	80%	300+
Douglas County Hospital	Alexandria	79%	300+
Fairview Northland Regional Hospital	Princeton	79%	300+
Mayo Clinic Hospital Rochester[11]	Rochester	79%	300+
Saint Cloud Hospital	Saint Cloud	79%	300+
Univ Med Ctr-Mesabi/Mesaba Clinics	Hibbing	79%	300+
Buffalo Hospital	Buffalo	78%	300+
Healtheast Woodwinds Hospital	Woodbury	78%	300+
Hutchinson Health	Hutchinson	78%	300+
Regina Hospital	Hastings	78%	300+
Essentia Health St Joseph's Med Ctr	Brainerd	77%	300+
Lifecare Medical Center	Roseau	77%	(a)
Mayo Clinic Health System - Albert Lea	Albert Lea	77%	300+
Mayo Clinic Methodist- Hospital[11]	Rochester	77%	300+
Mercy Hospital	Moose Lake	77%	(a)
Owatonna Hospital	Owatonna	77%	300+
Saint Joseph's Hospital	Saint Paul	77%	300+
Chippewa County Hospital[11]	Montevideo	76%	(a)
Firstlight Health System	Mora	76%	300+
Mayo Clinic Health System - Red Wing	Red Wing	76%	300+
Olmsted Medical Center	Rochester	76%	(a)
Saint Francis Medical Center	Breckenridge	76%	(a)
Saint Gabriels Hospital	Little Falls	76%	(a)
Saint Joseph's Area Health Services	Park Rapids	76%	(a)
Winona Health Services	Winona	76%	300+
Avera Marshall Regional Medical Center	Marshall	75%	300+
Saint Francis Regional Medical Center	Shakopee	75%	300+
Cambridge Medical Center	Cambridge	74%	300+
District One Hospital	Faribault	74%	300+
Mercy Hospital	Coon Rapids	74%	300+

NOTE: Hospital profiles are in alphabetical order by state, then city, then hospital within the city; Rankings exclude hospitals with less than 25 cases except for patient surveys which excludes hospitals with less than 100 cases; (a) 100-299 cases; (1) The number of cases/patients is too few to report; (2) Data submitted were based on a sample of cases/patients; (3) Results are based on a shorter time period than required; (4) Data suppressed by CMS for one or more quarters; (5) Results are not available for this reporting period; (6) Fewer than 100 patients completed the HCAHPS survey; (7) No cases met the criteria for this measure; (8) The lower limit of the confidence interval cannot be calculated if the number of observed infections equals zero; (9) No data are available from the state/territory for this reporting period; (10) The scores shown reflect fewer than 50 completed surveys; (11) There were discrepancies in the data collection process; (12) This measure does not apply to this hospital for this reporting period; (13) Results cannot be calculated for this reporting period; (14) The results for this state are combined with nearby states to protect confidentiality; Please refer to the User's Guide for a full explanation of data.

Hospital Name	City	Rate	Cases
Northfield Hospital	Northfield	74%	300+
Sanford Medical Center Thief River Falls	Thief River Falls	74%	300+
Glencoe Regional Health Services	Glencoe	73%	(a)
Healtheast Saint John's Hospital	Maplewood	73%	300+
Lake Region Healthcare Corporation	Fergus Falls	73%	300+
Rice Memorial Hospital	Willmar	73%	300+
Riverview Hospital	Crookston	73%	(a)
Regions Hospital	Saint Paul	72%	300+
Essentia Health Saint Marys	Detroit Lakes	71%	300+
Grand Itasca Clinic & Hospital	Grand Rapids	71%	300+
Mayo Clinic Health System - Mankato	Mankato	71%	300+
Abbott Northwestern Hospital	Minneapolis	70%	300+
Fairview Ridges Hospital	Burnsville	70%	300+
Saint Luke's Hospital	Duluth	70%	300+
United Hospital	Saint Paul	70%	300+
Essentia Health Duluth	Duluth	69%	300+
Fairview Southdale Hospital	Edina	69%	300+
Unity Hospital	Fridley	69%	300+
Maple Grove Hospital	Maple Grove	67%	300+
North Memorial Medical Center	Robbinsdale	67%	300+
Essentia Health Virginia	Virginia	66%	300+
Sanford Bemidji Medical Center	Bemidji	66%	300+
Essentia Health St Mary's Med Ctr	Duluth	65%	300+
Park Nicollet Methodist Hospital	Saint Louis Park	64%	300+
Univ of Minnesota Med Ctr, Fairview[11]	Minneapolis	64%	300+
Hennepin County Medical Center	Minneapolis	63%	300+

Timely Help 'Always' Received

Hospital Name	City	Rate	Cases
Bigfork Valley Hospital[11]	Bigfork	95%	(a)
Centra Care Health Paynesville	Paynesville	84%	(a)
Murray County Memorial Hospital[11]	Slayton	83%	(a)
Riverwood Healthcare Center	Aitkin	83%	300+
Stevens Community Medical Center	Morris	83%	(a)
Swift County Benson Hospital[11]	Benson	83%	(a)
Mayo Clinic Health System - New Prague	New Prague	82%	(a)
Lakeview Memorial Hospital	Stillwater	81%	300+
Regina Hospital	Hastings	81%	300+
Cambridge Medical Center	Cambridge	80%	300+
Community Memorial Hospital	Cloquet	80%	(a)
Glacial Ridge Hospital	Glenwood	80%	(a)
Meeker Memorial Hospital	Litchfield	80%	(a)
Saint Elizabeth Medical Center	Wabasha	80%	(a)
Mercy Hospital	Moose Lake	79%	(a)
Olmsted Medical Center	Rochester	78%	(a)
Redwood Area Hospital[11]	Redwood Falls	78%	(a)
District One Hospital	Faribault	77%	300+
Hutchinson Health	Hutchinson	77%	300+
Mayo Clinic Health System - Red Wing	Red Wing	77%	300+
Mille Lacs Health System	Onamia	77%	(a)
Perham Health	Perham	77%	(a)
Windom Area Hospital	Windom	77%	(a)
Cuyuna Regional Medical Center	Crosby	76%	300+
Riverview Hospital	Crookston	76%	(a)
Saint Joseph's Area Health Services	Park Rapids	76%	(a)
Sanford Worthington Medical Center	Worthington	76%	300+
Essentia Health Virginia	Virginia	75%	300+
Fairview Northland Regional Hospital	Princeton	75%	300+
Grand Itasca Clinic & Hospital	Grand Rapids	75%	300+
Healtheast Woodwinds Hospital	Woodbury	75%	300+
Lakewood Health System	Staples	75%	300+
Northfield Hospital	Northfield	75%	300+
Fairview Lakes Medical Center	Wyoming	74%	300+
Glencoe Regional Health Services	Glencoe	74%	(a)
Mayo Clinic Methodist- Hospital[11]	Rochester	74%	300+
New Ulm Medical Center	New Ulm	74%	300+
Ridgeview Medical Center	Waconia	74%	300+
Saint Cloud Hospital	Saint Cloud	74%	300+
Sanford Luverne Medical Center	Luverne	74%	(a)
Tri County Hospital	Wadena	74%	300+
United Hospital District	Blue Earth	74%	(a)
Univ Med Ctr-Mesabi/Mesaba Clinics	Hibbing	74%	300+
Centracare Health - Monticello	Monticello	73%	(a)
Essentia Health St Joseph's Med Ctr	Brainerd	73%	300+
Essentia Health Saint Marys	Detroit Lakes	73%	300+
Mayo Clinic Hospital Rochester[11]	Rochester	73%	300+
Owatonna Hospital	Owatonna	73%	300+
Saint Gabriels Hospital	Little Falls	73%	(a)
Saint Francis Medical Center	Breckenridge	72%	(a)
Buffalo Hospital	Buffalo	71%	300+
Lifecare Medical Center	Roseau	71%	(a)
Chippewa County Hospital[11]	Montevideo	70%	(a)
Firstlight Health System	Mora	70%	300+
Rice Memorial Hospital	Willmar	70%	300+
Mayo Clinic Health System - Albert Lea	Albert Lea	69%	300+
Winona Health Services	Winona	69%	300+
Saint Francis Regional Medical Center	Shakopee	68%	300+
Saint Joseph's Hospital	Saint Paul	68%	300+
Douglas County Hospital	Alexandria	67%	300+
Sanford Medical Center Thief River Falls	Thief River Falls	67%	300+
Essentia Health St Mary's Med Ctr	Duluth	66%	300+

Hospital Name	City	Rate	Cases
Fairview Ridges Hospital	Burnsville	66%	300+
Maple Grove Hospital	Maple Grove	66%	300+
Abbott Northwestern Hospital	Minneapolis	65%	300+
Essentia Health Duluth	Duluth	65%	300+
Fairview Southdale Hospital	Edina	65%	300+
Park Nicollet Methodist Hospital	Saint Louis Park	65%	300+
Mercy Hospital	Coon Rapids	64%	300+
Avera Marshall Regional Medical Center	Marshall	63%	300+
Lake Region Healthcare Corporation	Fergus Falls	63%	300+
Mayo Clinic Health System - Fairmont	Fairmont	63%	300+
Mayo Clinic Health System - Mankato	Mankato	63%	300+
Regions Hospital	Saint Paul	63%	300+
United Hospital	Saint Paul	63%	300+
Healtheast Saint John's Hospital	Maplewood	62%	300+
Unity Hospital	Fridley	62%	300+
Saint Luke's Hospital	Duluth	61%	300+
Sanford Bemidji Medical Center	Bemidji	61%	300+
North Memorial Medical Center	Robbinsdale	60%	300+
Univ of Minnesota Med Ctr, Fairview[11]	Minneapolis	59%	300+
Hennepin County Medical Center	Minneapolis	52%	300+

Would Definitely Recommend Hospital

Hospital Name	City	Rate	Cases
Mayo Clinic Methodist- Hospital[11]	Rochester	90%	300+
Mayo Clinic Hospital Rochester[11]	Rochester	89%	300+
Cuyuna Regional Medical Center	Crosby	88%	300+
Olmsted Medical Center	Rochester	87%	(a)
Ridgeview Medical Center	Waconia	87%	300+
Lakeview Memorial Hospital	Stillwater	86%	300+
Lakewood Health System	Staples	85%	300+
Maple Grove Hospital	Maple Grove	85%	300+
Healtheast Woodwinds Hospital	Woodbury	84%	300+
Glacial Ridge Hospital	Glenwood	83%	(a)
Perham Health	Perham	83%	(a)
Saint Cloud Hospital	Saint Cloud	82%	300+
Sanford Luverne Medical Center	Luverne	82%	(a)
Mayo Clinic Health System - New Prague	New Prague	81%	(a)
Centra Care Health Paynesville	Paynesville	80%	(a)
Riverwood Healthcare Center	Aitkin	80%	300+
Abbott Northwestern Hospital	Minneapolis	79%	300+
Meeker Memorial Hospital	Litchfield	79%	(a)
Northfield Hospital	Northfield	78%	300+
Saint Elizabeth Medical Center	Wabasha	78%	(a)
Saint Francis Regional Medical Center	Shakopee	78%	300+
Saint Joseph's Area Health Services	Park Rapids	78%	(a)
Saint Joseph's Hospital	Saint Paul	78%	300+
Riverview Hospital	Crookston	77%	(a)
Saint Luke's Hospital	Duluth	77%	300+
Community Memorial Hospital	Cloquet	76%	(a)
Mille Lacs Health System	Onamia	76%	(a)
New Ulm Medical Center	New Ulm	75%	300+
Douglas County Hospital	Alexandria	74%	300+
Essentia Health Duluth	Duluth	74%	300+
Essentia Health St Joseph's Med Ctr	Brainerd	74%	300+
Fairview Southdale Hospital	Edina	74%	300+
Mercy Hospital	Coon Rapids	74%	300+
Owatonna Hospital	Owatonna	74%	300+
Regions Hospital	Saint Paul	74%	300+
Univ of Minnesota Med Ctr, Fairview[11]	Minneapolis	74%	300+
Windom Area Hospital	Windom	74%	(a)
Avera Marshall Regional Medical Center	Marshall	73%	300+
Buffalo Hospital	Buffalo	73%	300+
Essentia Health St Mary's Med Ctr	Duluth	73%	300+
Mayo Clinic Health System - Red Wing	Red Wing	73%	300+
Park Nicollet Methodist Hospital	Saint Louis Park	73%	300+
Saint Gabriels Hospital	Little Falls	73%	(a)
Stevens Community Medical Center	Morris	73%	(a)
Tri County Hospital	Wadena	73%	300+
Fairview Northland Regional Hospital	Princeton	72%	300+
Glencoe Regional Health Services	Glencoe	72%	(a)
Healtheast Saint John's Hospital	Maplewood	72%	300+
Regina Hospital	Hastings	72%	300+
Hutchinson Health	Hutchinson	71%	300+
United Hospital	Saint Paul	71%	300+
United Hospital District	Blue Earth	71%	(a)
Cambridge Medical Center	Cambridge	70%	300+
Fairview Ridges Hospital	Burnsville	70%	300+
Lake Region Healthcare Corporation	Fergus Falls	70%	300+
North Memorial Medical Center	Robbinsdale	70%	300+
Rice Memorial Hospital	Willmar	70%	300+
District One Hospital	Faribault	69%	300+
Fairview Lakes Medical Center	Wyoming	69%	300+
Lifecare Medical Center	Roseau	69%	(a)
Mercy Hospital	Moose Lake	69%	(a)
Saint Francis Medical Center	Breckenridge	69%	(a)
Grand Itasca Clinic & Hospital	Grand Rapids	68%	300+
Essentia Health Saint Marys	Detroit Lakes	67%	300+
Mayo Clinic Health System - Albert Lea	Albert Lea	67%	300+
Unity Hospital	Fridley	66%	300+
Sanford Worthington Medical Center	Worthington	65%	300+
Univ Med Ctr-Mesabi/Mesaba Clinics	Hibbing	65%	300+

Hospital Name	City	Rate	Cases
Centracare Health - Monticello	Monticello	64%	(a)
Hennepin County Medical Center	Minneapolis	64%	300+
Firstlight Health System	Mora	63%	300+
Mayo Clinic Health System - Mankato	Mankato	63%	300+
Bigfork Valley Hospital[11]	Bigfork	62%	(a)
Sanford Bemidji Medical Center	Bemidji	62%	300+
Winona Health Services	Winona	62%	300+
Essentia Health Virginia	Virginia	58%	300+
Mayo Clinic Health System - Fairmont	Fairmont	58%	300+
Sanford Medical Center Thief River Falls	Thief River Falls	55%	300+
Murray County Memorial Hospital[11]	Slayton	50%	(a)
Swift County Benson Hospital[11]	Benson	48%	(a)
Chippewa County Hospital[11]	Montevideo	46%	(a)
Redwood Area Hospital[11]	Redwood Falls	44%	(a)

Use of Medical Imaging

Cardiac Imaging Stress Test before OP Surgery

Hospital Name	City	Rate	Cases
Essentia Health Virginia	Virginia	1.4%	72
District One Hospital	Faribault	1.8%	55
Olmsted Medical Center	Rochester	1.8%	57
Regina Hospital	Hastings	1.8%	56
Ortonville Area Health Services	Ortonville	2.1%	47
Murray County Memorial Hospital	Slayton	2.2%	45
Douglas County Hospital	Alexandria	2.5%	119
Lakeview Memorial Hospital	Stillwater	2.7%	111
Sanford Bemidji Medical Center	Bemidji	3.0%	198
Abbott Northwestern Hospital	Minneapolis	3.6%	335
Sanford Medical Center Thief River Falls	Thief River Falls	3.9%	77
Hutchinson Health	Hutchinson	4.0%	50
Fairview Lakes Medical Center	Wyoming	4.3%	161
Fairview Southdale Hospital	Edina	4.3%	670
Lake Region Healthcare Corporation	Fergus Falls	4.3%	69
Ridgeview Medical Center	Waconia	4.3%	117
Saint Cloud Hospital	Saint Cloud	4.5%	508
United Hospital	Saint Paul	4.6%	636
Saint Luke's Hospital	Duluth	4.7%	360
Healtheast Saint John's Hospital	Maplewood	4.9%	366
Mercy Hospital	Coon Rapids	4.9%	474
Essentia Health St Mary's Med Ctr	Duluth	5.0%	820
Park Nicollet Methodist Hospital	Saint Louis Park	5.0%	784
North Memorial Medical Center	Robbinsdale	5.1%	451
Mayo Clinic Health System - Albert Lea	Albert Lea	5.2%	97
Regions Hospital	Saint Paul	5.2%	386
New Ulm Medical Center	New Ulm	5.3%	133
Unity Hospital	Fridley	5.4%	204
Buffalo Hospital	Buffalo	5.6%	90
Fairview Ridges Hospital	Burnsville	5.6%	284
Grand Itasca Clinic & Hospital	Grand Rapids	5.6%	71
Mayo Clinic Health System - Mankato	Mankato	5.8%	243
Saint Francis Regional Medical Center	Shakopee	6.1%	179
Saint Joseph's Hospital	Saint Paul	6.4%	218
Cambridge Medical Center	Cambridge	6.5%	123
Mayo Clinic Health System - Red Wing	Red Wing	6.6%	61
Sanford Worthington Medical Center	Worthington	6.6%	122
Firstlight Health System	Mora	7.1%	70
Essentia Health St Joseph's Med Ctr	Brainerd	7.2%	221
Healtheast Woodwinds Hospital	Woodbury	7.3%	179
Riverview Hospital	Crookston	7.3%	82
Fairview Northland Regional Hospital	Princeton	7.9%	76
Riverwood Healthcare Center	Aitkin	7.9%	63
Hennepin County Medical Center	Minneapolis	8.0%	237
Mayo Clinic Hospital Rochester	Rochester	8.2%	243
Saint Joseph's Area Health Services	Park Rapids	8.2%	97
Rice Memorial Hospital	Willmar	8.9%	79
Cuyuna Regional Medical Center	Crosby	9.6%	83
Univ Med Ctr-Mesabi/Mesaba Clinics	Hibbing	9.7%	124
Univ of Minnesota Med Ctr, Fairview	Minneapolis	9.7%	424
Mayo Clinic Methodist- Hospital	Rochester	11.3%	2221

Combination Abdominal CT Scan

Hospital Name	City	Rate	Cases
Maple Grove Hospital	Maple Grove	0.6%	164
Unity Hospital	Fridley	0.8%	396
Hutchinson Health	Hutchinson	1.1%	188
Sanford Medical Center Thief River Falls	Thief River Falls	1.4%	144
Mille Lacs Health System	Onamia	1.6%	63
Essentia Health Fosston	Fosston	1.7%	60
Avera Marshall Regional Medical Center	Marshall	2.0%	152
Centracare Health System - Long Prairie	Long Prairie	2.0%	50
Regina Hospital	Hastings	2.0%	197
River's Edge Hospital & Clinic	Saint Peter	2.0%	51
Mercy Hospital	Coon Rapids	2.2%	632
Saint Joseph's Hospital	Saint Paul	2.2%	319
Tri County Hospital	Wadena	2.2%	135
Univ of Minnesota Med Ctr, Fairview	Minneapolis	2.2%	1065
Cambridge Medical Center	Cambridge	2.4%	253
Healtheast Woodwinds Hospital	Woodbury	2.4%	457
Mayo Clinic Health System - Albert Lea	Albert Lea	2.4%	334

NOTE: Hospital profiles are in alphabetical order by state, then city, then hospital within the city; Rankings exclude hospitals with less than 25 cases except for patient surveys which excludes hospitals with less than 100 cases; (a) 100-299 cases; (1) The number of cases/patients is too few to report; (2) Data submitted were based on a sample of cases/patients; (3) Results are based on a shorter time period than required; (4) Data suppressed by CMS for one or more quarters; (5) Results are not available for this reporting period; (6) Fewer than 100 patients completed the HCAHPS survey; (7) No cases met the criteria for this measure; (8) The lower limit of the confidence interval cannot be calculated if the number of observed infections equals zero; (9) No data are available from the state/territory for this reporting period; (10) The scores shown reflect fewer than 50 completed surveys; (11) There were discrepancies in the data collection process; (12) This measure does not apply to this hospital for this reporting period; (13) Results cannot be calculated for this reporting period; (14) The results for this state are combined with nearby states to protect confidentiality; Please refer to the User's Guide for a full explanation of data.

Hospital Name	City	Rate	Cases
Sleepy Eye Municipal Hospital	Sleepy Eye	2.4%	85
Fairview Lakes Medical Center	Wyoming	2.5%	359
Park Nicollet Methodist Hospital	Saint Louis Park	2.5%	1047
United Hospital District	Blue Earth	2.6%	76
Centra Care Health Paynesville	Paynesville	2.7%	73
Northfield Hospital	Northfield	2.7%	112
Fairview Southdale Hospital	Edina	2.8%	603
Healtheast Saint John's Hospital	Maplewood	2.8%	576
Saint Cloud Hospital	Saint Cloud	2.8%	993
Sanford Luverne Medical Center	Luverne	2.8%	71
Mayo Clinic Health System - Lake City	Lake City	3.0%	66
Ridgeview Medical Center	Waconia	3.0%	371
Saint Gabriels Hospital	Little Falls	3.0%	165
Fairview Ridges Hospital	Burnsville	3.1%	586
United Hospital	Saint Paul	3.1%	635
Mayo Clinic Health System - Red Wing	Red Wing	3.3%	153
Municipal Hospital & Granite Manor	Granite Falls	3.6%	56
Riverwood Healthcare Center	Aitkin	3.6%	139
Buffalo Hospital	Buffalo	3.8%	313
District One Hospital	Faribault	3.8%	213
North Memorial Medical Center	Robbinsdale	3.9%	665
Essentia Health Saint Marys	Detroit Lakes	4.0%	124
Saint Joseph's Area Health Services	Park Rapids	4.0%	198
Lake Region Healthcare Corporation	Fergus Falls	4.1%	194
Riverview Hospital	Crookston	4.1%	123
Saint Francis Regional Medical Center	Shakopee	4.1%	267
Stevens Community Medical Center	Morris	4.1%	148
Mayo Clinic Hospital Rochester	Rochester	4.2%	803
Glencoe Regional Health Services	Glencoe	4.3%	93
Rice Memorial Hospital	Willmar	4.3%	210
Windom Area Hospital	Windom	4.3%	92
Centracare Health - Monticello	Monticello	4.9%	122
Fairview Northland Regional Hospital	Princeton	4.9%	204
Univ Med Ctr-Mesabi/Mesaba Clinics	Hibbing	5.0%	301
Essentia Health Virginia	Virginia	5.1%	296
Owatonna Hospital	Owatonna	5.1%	136
Firstlight Health System	Mora	5.2%	212
Mayo Clinic Health System - Fairmont	Fairmont	5.2%	251
Saint Elizabeth Medical Center	Wabasha	5.2%	58
Abbott Northwestern Hospital	Minneapolis	5.3%	1110
Mayo Clinic Methodist- Hospital	Rochester	5.3%	190
Hennepin County Medical Center	Minneapolis	5.4%	427
Lakeview Memorial Hospital	Stillwater	5.5%	308
Mercy Hospital	Moose Lake	5.6%	71
Essentia Health St Joseph's Med Ctr	Brainerd	5.8%	431
Redwood Area Hospital	Redwood Falls	5.8%	103
Regions Hospital	Saint Paul	6.0%	714
New Ulm Medical Center	New Ulm	6.1%	247
Essentia Health Duluth	Duluth	6.2%	532
Rainy Lake Medical Center	Int'l Falls	6.2%	129
Saint Francis Medical Center	Breckenridge	6.5%	139
Sanford Worthington Medical Center	Worthington	6.8%	176
Winona Health Services	Winona	6.8%	251
Lakewood Health System	Staples	6.9%	145
Sanford Bemidji Medical Center	Bemidji	7.1%	595
Grand Itasca Clinic & Hospital	Grand Rapids	7.7%	246
Cuyuna Regional Medical Center	Crosby	7.9%	215
Douglas County Hospital	Alexandria	8.3%	327
Perham Health	Perham	8.5%	82
Deer River Healthcare Center	Deer River	9.0%	67
Community Memorial Hospital	Cloquet	9.1%	143
Olmsted Medical Center	Rochester	10.6%	189
Saint Luke's Hospital	Duluth	10.6%	691
Essentia Health St Mary's Med Ctr	Duluth	11.7%	532
Pipestone County Medical Center	Pipestone	12.1%	107
Murray County Memorial Hospital	Slayton	13.7%	95
Mayo Clinic Health System - New Prague	New Prague	14.9%	134
Mayo Clinic Health System - Mankato	Mankato	15.7%	471
Mayo Clinic Health System - Waseca	Waseca	17.1%	70
Lake View Memorial Hospital	Two Harbors	21.0%	62
Mayo Clinic Health System - Saint James	Saint James	21.9%	64
Renville County Hospital & Clinics	Olivia	59.1%	44
Chippewa County Hospital	Montevideo	75.5%	98
Ortonville Area Health Services	Ortonville	81.5%	81

Combination Brain/Sinus CT Scan

Hospital Name	City	Rate	Cases
Appleton Municipal Hospital	Appleton	0.0%	35
Centracare Health System - Long Prairie	Long Prairie	0.0%	37
Centracare Health Sys-Melrose Hosp	Melrose	0.0%	33
Essentia Health Duluth	Duluth	0.0%	60
Essentia Health Fosston	Fosston	0.0%	40
Essentia Health Holy Trinity Hospital	Graceville	0.0%	33
Hendricks Community Hospital	Hendricks	0.0%	34
Mayo Clinic Health System - Cannon Falls	Cannon Falls	0.0%	52
Mayo Clinic Health System - Lake City	Lake City	0.0%	61
Mayo Clinic Health System - Springfield	Springfield	0.0%	46
Mayo Clinic Health System - Waseca	Waseca	0.0%	53
Meeker Memorial Hospital	Litchfield	0.0%	33
Mille Lacs Health System	Onamia	0.0%	79
Renville County Hospital & Clinics	Olivia	0.0%	68
Ridgeview Sibley Medical Center	Arlington	0.0%	44
Saint Francis Medical Center	Breckenridge	0.0%	162
Sanford Luverne Medical Center	Luverne	0.0%	87
Sanford Tracy	Tracy	0.0%	58
Sanford Westbrook Medical Center	Westbrook	0.0%	30
Swift County Benson Hospital	Benson	0.0%	34
Lakeview Memorial Hospital	Stillwater	0.6%	177
Hennepin County Medical Center	Minneapolis	0.8%	378
Mayo Clinic Health System - Albert Lea	Albert Lea	1.0%	299
Mayo Clinic Health System - Fairmont	Fairmont	1.0%	202
Regions Hospital	Saint Paul	1.0%	388
Univ of Minnesota Med Ctr, Fairview	Minneapolis	1.2%	260
Fairview Southdale Hospital	Edina	1.3%	543
Mercy Hospital	Coon Rapids	1.4%	428
Mayo Clinic Health System - Mankato	Mankato	1.5%	335
Park Nicollet Methodist Hospital	Saint Louis Park	1.5%	604
Fairview Ridges Hospital	Burnsville	1.6%	495
North Memorial Medical Center	Robbinsdale	2.2%	418
Mayo Clinic Hospital Rochester	Rochester	2.3%	814
Essentia Health St Mary's Med Ctr	Duluth	2.5%	511
Saint Cloud Hospital	Saint Cloud	2.5%	517
United Hospital	Saint Paul	2.7%	552
Abbott Northwestern Hospital	Minneapolis	4.1%	465
Healtheast Woodwinds Hospital	Woodbury	5.2%	229
Unity Hospital	Fridley	5.3%	303
Cambridge Medical Center	Cambridge	6.7%	150
Lakewood Health System	Staples	9.1%	88
Sanford Jackson Medical Center	Jackson	9.4%	53

Combination Chest CT Scan

Hospital Name	City	Rate	Cases
Buffalo Hospital	Buffalo	0.0%	182
Cambridge Medical Center	Cambridge	0.0%	193
Centra Care Health Paynesville	Paynesville	0.0%	67
Centracare Health - Monticello	Monticello	0.0%	80
Cuyuna Regional Medical Center	Crosby	0.0%	190
District One Hospital	Faribault	0.0%	184
Essentia Health Duluth	Duluth	0.0%	541
Essentia Health St Joseph's Med Ctr	Brainerd	0.0%	319
Essentia Health Saint Marys	Detroit Lakes	0.0%	136
Essentia Health Virginia	Virginia	0.0%	181
Fairview Lakes Medical Center	Wyoming	0.0%	315
Fairview Northland Regional Hospital	Princeton	0.0%	152
Healtheast Saint John's Hospital	Maplewood	0.0%	313
Healtheast Woodwinds Hospital	Woodbury	0.0%	196
Lake Region Healthcare Corporation	Fergus Falls	0.0%	114
Lakeview Memorial Hospital	Stillwater	0.0%	190
Mayo Clinic Health System - Albert Lea	Albert Lea	0.0%	183
Mayo Clinic Health System - New Prague	New Prague	0.0%	66
Mayo Clinic Health System - Red Wing	Red Wing	0.0%	124
Mayo Clinic Hospital Rochester	Rochester	0.0%	89
Mayo Clinic Methodist- Hospital	Rochester	0.0%	162
Perham Health	Perham	0.0%	50
Redwood Area Hospital	Redwood Falls	0.0%	78
Regions Hospital	Saint Paul	0.0%	473
Ridgeview Medical Center	Waconia	0.0%	218
Riverview Hospital	Crookston	0.0%	56
Riverwood Healthcare Center	Aitkin	0.0%	107
Saint Francis Regional Medical Center	Shakopee	0.0%	194
Saint Gabriels Hospital	Little Falls	0.0%	113
Saint Luke's Hospital	Duluth	0.0%	575
Sanford Luverne Medical Center	Luverne	0.0%	52
Sanford Medical Center Thief River Falls	Thief River Falls	0.0%	95
Sanford Worthington Medical Center	Worthington	0.0%	89
Univ Med Ctr-Mesabi/Mesaba Clinics	Hibbing	0.0%	177
Hennepin County Medical Center	Minneapolis	0.2%	409
Sanford Bemidji Medical Center	Bemidji	0.2%	413
Abbott Northwestern Hospital	Minneapolis	0.3%	1100
United Hospital	Saint Paul	0.3%	371
Douglas County Hospital	Alexandria	0.4%	267
Mercy Hospital	Coon Rapids	0.4%	524
Saint Cloud Hospital	Saint Cloud	0.4%	1003
Univ of Minnesota Med Ctr, Fairview	Minneapolis	0.4%	1126
Fairview Ridges Hospital	Burnsville	0.5%	441
New Ulm Medical Center	New Ulm	0.5%	187
Mayo Clinic Health System - Mankato	Mankato	0.6%	324
Unity Hospital	Fridley	0.6%	312
Rice Memorial Hospital	Willmar	0.7%	143
Essentia Health St Mary's Med Ctr	Duluth	0.9%	319
Fairview Southdale Hospital	Edina	0.9%	542
Firstlight Health System	Mora	0.9%	115
Saint Joseph's Area Health Services	Park Rapids	0.9%	112
Northfield Hospital	Northfield	1.0%	101
Owatonna Hospital	Owatonna	1.0%	104
Community Memorial Hospital	Cloquet	1.5%	65
Lakewood Health System	Staples	1.5%	67
Grand Itasca Clinic & Hospital	Grand Rapids	1.6%	182
Mercy Hospital	Moose Lake	1.7%	59
Stevens Community Medical Center	Morris	1.8%	57
Winona Health Services	Winona	2.1%	146
Hutchinson Health	Hutchinson	2.4%	125
Avera Marshall Regional Medical Center	Marshall	2.6%	78
Mayo Clinic Health System - Fairmont	Fairmont	2.8%	145
North Memorial Medical Center	Robbinsdale	3.2%	471
Tri County Hospital	Wadena	3.5%	57
Murray County Memorial Hospital	Slayton	3.9%	51
Pipestone County Medical Center	Pipestone	4.2%	48
Regina Hospital	Hastings	4.5%	132
Saint Francis Medical Center	Breckenridge	4.6%	65
Rainy Lake Medical Center	Int'l Falls	4.9%	82
Olmsted Medical Center	Rochester	5.4%	93
Park Nicollet Methodist Hospital	Saint Louis Park	22.3%	970

Follow-up Mammogram/Ultrasound

A follow-up rate near zero may indicate missed cancer; a rate higher than 14% may mean there is unnecessary follow up.

Hospital Name	City	Rate	Cases
Sanford Medical Center Thief River Falls	Thief River Falls	1.1%	380
Essentia Health Sandstone	Sandstone	1.5%	68
Sanford Canby Medical Center	Canby	1.8%	166
Hendricks Community Hospital	Hendricks	2.6%	76
Cook County Northshore Hospital	Grand Marais	2.9%	103
Centracare Health - Monticello	Monticello	3.0%	67
Healtheast Saint John's Hospital	Maplewood	3.3%	1260
Riverview Hospital	Crookston	3.4%	296
Sanford Medical Center Wheaton	Wheaton	3.7%	108
River's Edge Hospital & Clinic	Saint Peter	3.8%	159
Lakewood Health Center	Baudette	3.9%	76
Saint Francis Regional Medical Center	Shakopee	3.9%	487
Hennepin County Medical Center	Minneapolis	4.2%	596
Cambridge Medical Center	Cambridge	4.3%	507
Essentia Health Ada	Ada	4.3%	46
Ortonville Area Health Services	Ortonville	4.4%	203
Sanford Luverne Medical Center	Luverne	4.4%	227
United Hospital District	Blue Earth	4.5%	154
Fairview Lakes Medical Center	Wyoming	4.6%	350
Lake View Memorial Hospital	Two Harbors	4.6%	151
Essentia Health Virginia	Virginia	4.7%	211
Hutchinson Health	Hutchinson	4.7%	274
Renville County Hospital & Clinics	Olivia	4.7%	149
Sleepy Eye Municipal Hospital	Sleepy Eye	4.7%	86
Fairview Southdale Hospital	Edina	4.9%	1213
Grand Itasca Clinic & Hospital	Grand Rapids	4.9%	631
Lakeview Memorial Hospital	Stillwater	4.9%	675
North Memorial Medical Center	Robbinsdale	5.0%	503
Essentia Health Saint Marys	Detroit Lakes	5.1%	276
Mayo Clinic Health System - Cannon Falls	Cannon Falls	5.1%	78
Deer River Healthcare Center	Deer River	5.2%	173
Meeker Memorial Hospital	Litchfield	5.2%	153
Saint Luke's Hospital	Duluth	5.2%	1160
Glencoe Regional Health Services	Glencoe	5.3%	190
New Ulm Medical Center	New Ulm	5.4%	572
Olmsted Medical Center	Rochester	5.4%	878
Saint Cloud Hospital	Saint Cloud	5.4%	1202
Essentia Health Duluth	Duluth	5.5%	1598
Mayo Clinic Health System - Saint James	Saint James	5.5%	182
Prairie Ridge Hospital & Health Services	Elbow Lake	5.5%	145
Univ of Minnesota Med Ctr, Fairview	Minneapolis	5.5%	598
Buffalo Hospital	Buffalo	5.6%	233
Municipal Hospital & Granite Manor	Granite Falls	5.6%	124
Saint Joseph's Hospital	Saint Paul	5.7%	296
Chippewa County Hospital	Montevideo	5.8%	226
Essentia Health Fosston	Fosston	5.8%	86
Essentia Health St Joseph's Med Ctr	Brainerd	6.0%	1105
United Hospital	Saint Paul	6.0%	884
Healtheast Woodwinds Hospital	Woodbury	6.1%	718
Regions Hospital	Saint Paul	6.2%	773
Regina Hospital	Hastings	6.4%	377
Perham Health	Perham	6.5%	217
Ridgeview Medical Center	Waconia	6.7%	253
Firstlight Health System	Mora	6.8%	250
Abbott Northwestern Hospital	Minneapolis	6.9%	1576
Lake Region Healthcare Corporation	Fergus Falls	6.9%	364
Avera Marshall Regional Medical Center	Marshall	7.0%	100
Swift County Benson Hospital	Benson	7.0%	100
Community Memorial Hospital	Cloquet	7.1%	267
Mayo Clinic Health System - Albert Lea	Albert Lea	7.2%	667
Fairview Ridges Hospital	Burnsville	7.3%	579
Mayo Clinic Health System - Springfield	Springfield	7.3%	137
Sanford Worthington Medical Center	Worthington	7.3%	165
Mayo Clinic Health System - Fairmont	Fairmont	7.5%	530
Riverwood Healthcare Center	Aitkin	7.5%	373
Saint Joseph's Area Health Services	Park Rapids	7.5%	358
Centracare Health System - Sauk Centre	Sauk Centre	7.6%	132
Saint Elizabeth Medical Center	Wabasha	7.6%	249
Tri County Hospital	Wadena	7.6%	172
Kittson Memorial Hospital	Hallock	7.7%	78
Glacial Ridge Hospital	Glenwood	7.8%	141
Lakewood Health System	Staples	7.9%	215
Mayo Clinic Health System - Waseca	Waseca	8.0%	125
Univ Med Ctr-Mesabi/Mesaba Clinics	Hibbing	8.1%	307
Mayo Clinic Health System - Red Wing	Red Wing	8.2%	401

NOTE: Hospital profiles are in alphabetical order by state, then city, then hospital within the city; Rankings exclude hospitals with less than 25 cases except for patient surveys which excludes hospitals with less than 100 cases; (a) 100-299 cases; (1) The number of cases/patients is too few to report; (2) Data submitted were based on a sample of cases/patients; (3) Results are based on a shorter time period than required; (4) Data suppressed by CMS for one or more quarters; (5) Results are not available for this reporting period; (6) Fewer than 100 patients completed the HCAHPS survey; (7) No cases met the criteria for this measure; (8) The lower limit of the confidence interval cannot be calculated if the number of observed infections equals zero; (9) No data are available from the state/territory for this reporting period; (10) The scores shown reflect fewer than 50 completed surveys; (11) There were discrepancies in the data collection process; (12) This measure does not apply to this hospital for this reporting period; (13) Results cannot be calculated for this reporting period; (14) The results for this state are combined with nearby states to protect confidentiality; Please refer to the User's Guide for a full explanation of data.

Cuyuna Regional Medical Center	Crosby	8.3%	387
Centra Care Health Paynesville	Paynesville	8.6%	198
Fairview Northland Regional Hospital	Princeton	8.7%	218
Mayo Clinic Health System - New Prague	New Prague	8.8%	182
Mercy Hospital	Moose Lake	8.8%	159
Mayo Clinic Health System - Lake City	Lake City	9.2%	152
Minnesota Valley Health Center	Le Sueur	9.2%	87
Mille Lacs Health System	Onamia	9.3%	118
Sanford Jackson Medical Center	Jackson	9.3%	150
District One Hospital	Faribault	9.5%	274
Bigfork Valley Hospital	Bigfork	9.7%	72
Saint Gabriels Hospital	Little Falls	9.7%	299
Murray County Memorial Hospital	Slayton	9.8%	132
Centracare Health Sys-Melrose Hosp	Melrose	10.1%	119
Lifecare Medical Center	Roseau	10.7%	121
Saint Francis Medical Center	Breckenridge	10.7%	112
Douglas County Hospital	Alexandria	11.1%	506
Windom Area Hospital	Windom	11.7%	111
Sanford Westbrook Medical Center	Westbrook	12.5%	72
Northfield Hospital	Northfield	12.6%	151
Pipestone County Medical Center	Pipestone	12.7%	220
Tyler Healthcare Center	Tyler	12.9%	70
Winona Health Services	Winona	13.4%	635
Stevens Community Medical Center	Morris	14.3%	112
Rainy Lake Medical Center	Int'l Falls	14.4%	139
Sanford Tracy	Tracy	14.5%	83

Lumbar Spine MRI for Low Back Pain

Hospital Name	City	Rate	Cases
New Ulm Medical Center	New Ulm	25.4%	71
Douglas County Hospital	Alexandria	29.8%	124
Park Nicollet Methodist Hospital	Saint Louis Park	31.5%	111
United Hospital	Saint Paul	32.6%	86
Healtheast Saint John's Hospital	Maplewood	32.8%	58
Fairview Lakes Medical Center	Wyoming	32.9%	76
Essentia Health St Joseph's Med Ctr	Brainerd	33.3%	81
Essentia Health Virginia	Virginia	33.3%	51
Essentia Health Duluth	Duluth	33.8%	80
Sanford Bemidji Medical Center	Bemidji	34.0%	100
Fairview Northland Regional Hospital	Princeton	36.0%	50
Saint Cloud Hospital	Saint Cloud	37.9%	87
Healtheast Woodwinds Hospital	Woodbury	38.2%	55
Saint Francis Regional Medical Center	Shakopee	38.2%	55
Abbott Northwestern Hospital	Minneapolis	40.7%	123
Regions Hospital	Saint Paul	41.3%	121
Grand Itasca Clinic & Hospital	Grand Rapids	41.9%	62
Ridgeview Medical Center	Waconia	42.6%	47
Fairview Southdale Hospital	Edina	43.2%	37
Univ of Minnesota Med Ctr, Fairview	Minneapolis	43.4%	53
Cuyuna Regional Medical Center	Crosby	43.9%	41
Cambridge Medical Center	Cambridge	45.0%	40
Saint Joseph's Area Health Services	Park Rapids	45.8%	48
Firstlight Health System	Mora	45.9%	37
Lakeview Memorial Hospital	Stillwater	47.5%	40
Fairview Ridges Hospital	Burnsville	48.3%	60
Hutchinson Health	Hutchinson	50.0%	38
Univ Med Ctr-Mesabi/Mesaba Clinics	Hibbing	50.7%	67
North Memorial Medical Center	Robbinsdale	51.3%	76
Tri County Hospital	Wadena	60.0%	40

NOTE: Hospital profiles are in alphabetical order by state, then city, then hospital within the city; Rankings exclude hospitals with less than 25 cases except for patient surveys which excludes hospitals with less than 100 cases; (a) 100-299 cases; (1) The number of cases/patients is too few to report; (2) Data submitted were based on a sample of cases/patients; (3) Results are based on a shorter time period than required; (4) Data suppressed by CMS for one or more quarters; (5) Results are not available for this reporting period; (6) Fewer than 100 patients completed the HCAHPS survey; (7) No cases met the criteria for this measure; (8) The lower limit of the confidence interval cannot be calculated if the number of observed infections equals zero; (9) No data are available from the state/territory for this reporting period; (10) The scores shown reflect fewer than 50 completed surveys; (11) There were discrepancies in the data collection process; (12) This measure does not apply to this hospital for this reporting period; (13) Results cannot be calculated for this reporting period; (14) The results for this state are combined with nearby states to protect confidentiality; Please refer to the User's Guide for a full explanation of data.

Essentia Health Ada

201 9th Street West
Ada, MN 56510
Phone: 218-784-5000
Fax: 218-784-3753
Type: Critical Access Hospitals
Emergency Services: Yes
Ownership: Voluntary non-profit - Private
Beds: 63

Key Personnel:

Chair/CEO . . . . Richard Blair
CEO/President. . . . . Peter Person, MD
Chief of Medical Staff . . . . Patrick Twomey, MD

Measure	Cases	This Hosp.	State Avg.	U.S. Avg.
Blood Clot Prevention and Treatment				
Anticoagulation Overlap Therapy[5]	-	-	96%	93%
ICU Venous Thromboembolism Prophylaxis[5]	-	-	91%	92%
Incidence of Potentially Preventable VTE[5]	-	-	9%	10%
UFH with Dosages/Platelet Monitoring[5]	-	-	98%	97%
Venous Thromboembolism Prophylaxis[5]	-	-	86%	85%
Warfarin Therapy Discharge Instructions[5]	-	-	63%	75%
Chest Pain/Possible Heart Attack Care				
Aspirin Given Within 24 Hours of Arrival[1,3]	-	-	97%	96%
Fibrinolytic Meds Within 30 Min. of Arrival[3,7]	-	-	48%	58%
Average Time to ECG (minutes)[3,7]	-	-	7	7
Average Time to Transfer (minutes)[3,7]	-	-	54	60
Children's Asthma Care				
Received Home Management Plan of Care	-	-	-	88%
Received Reliever Medication	-	-	-	100%
Received Systemic Corticosteroids	-	-	-	100%
Emergency Department				
Admittance Decision Time (minutes)[3]	22	0	62	98
Head CT Results Within 45 Min. of Arrival[5]	-	-	54%	57%
Patients Who Left ER Before Being Seen[5]	-	-	2%	2%
Time from ER Arrival to Admit. (minutes)[3]	22	90	199	274
Time from ER Arrival to Discharge (minutes)[5]	-	-	125	134
Time in ER Before Being Evaluated (minutes)[5]	-	-	31	26
Time to Pain Meds for Fractures (minutes)[5]	-	-	45	57
Heart Attack Care				
Aspirin Given at Discharge[5]	-	-	99%	99%
Fibrinolytic Meds Within 30 Min. of Arrival[5]	-	-	-	54%
PCI Within 90 Minutes of Arrival[5]	-	-	96%	96%
Statin Prescribed at Discharge[5]	-	-	99%	98%
Heart Failure Care				
ACE Inhibitor or ARB for LVSD[3,7]	-	-	96%	97%
Discharge Instructions Given[1,3]	-	-	93%	94%
Evaluation of LVS Function[1,3]	-	-	97%	99%
Medicare Spending				
Medicare Spending per Patient (ratio)	-	-	0.9	0.98
Pneumonia Care				
Appropriate Initial Antibiotic Given	13	92%	94%	95%
Blood Culture Timing[1]	-	-	97%	98%
Pregnancy and Delivery Care				
Newborn Deliveries Scheduled Early[5]	-	-	5%	6%
Preventive Care				
Immunization for Influenza	18	56%	89%	90%
Immunization for Pneumonia	32	47%	89%	92%
Stroke Care				
Anticoagulation Therapy for Atrial Fibrillation[5]	-	-	96%	95%
Antithrombotic Therapy Timing[5]	-	-	98%	98%
Assessed for Rehabilitation[5]	-	-	98%	97%
Discharged on Antithrombotic Therapy[5]	-	-	99%	99%
Discharged on Statin Medication[5]	-	-	95%	94%
Thrombolytic Therapy Timing[5]	-	-	74%	66%
Venous Thromboembolism Prophylaxis[5]	-	-	95%	94%
Written Stroke Educational Materials Given[5]	-	-	88%	88%
Surgical Care Improvement Project				
Appropriate Beta Blocker Usage[5]	-	-	98%	98%
Appropriate VTP Within 24 Hours[5]	-	-	98%	98%
Controlled Postoperative Blood Glucose[5]	-	-	97%	97%
Perioperative Temperature Management[5]	-	-	99%	100%
Prophylactic Antibiotic Selection[5]	-	-	99%	99%
Prophylactic Antibiotic Selection (Outpatient)[5]	-	-	98%	98%
Prophylactic Antibiotic Stopped[5]	-	-	99%	98%
Prophylactic Antibiotic Timing[5]	-	-	98%	99%
Prophylactic Antibiotic Timing (Outpatient)[5]	-	-	97%	98%
Urinary Catheter Removal[5]	-	-	97%	97%
Survey of Patients' Hospital Experiences				
Area Around Room 'Always' Quiet at Night[5]	-	-	65%	61%
Doctors 'Always' Communicated Well[5]	-	-	84%	82%
Home Recovery Information Given[5]	-	-	88%	85%
Hospital Given 9 or 10 on 10 Point Scale[5]	-	-	74%	71%
Meds 'Always' Explained Before Given[5]	-	-	67%	64%
Nurses 'Always' Communicated Well[5]	-	-	81%	79%
Pain 'Always' Well Controlled[5]	-	-	72%	71%
Room and Bathroom 'Always' Clean[5]	-	-	78%	73%
Timely Help 'Always' Received[5]	-	-	74%	68%
Would Definitely Recommend Hospital[5]	-	-	71%	71%
Use of Medical Imaging				
Cardiac Imaging Stress Test before Surgery[7]	-	-	6.3%	5.3%
Combination Abdominal CT Scan[1]	-	-	5.7%	10.5%
Combination Brain/Sinus CT Scan[1]	-	-	2.3%	2.7%
Combination Chest CT Scan[1]	-	-	1.9%	2.7%
Follow-up Mammogram/Ultrasound	46	4.3%	6.3%	8.8%
Lumbar Spine MRI for Low Back Pain[1]	-	-	37.6%	37.2%

Riverwood Healthcare Center

200 Bunker Hill Drive
Aitkin, MN 56431
Phone: 218-927-5501
Fax: 218-927-5575
URL: www.riverwoodhealthcare.com
Type: Critical Access Hospitals
Emergency Services: Yes
Ownership: Voluntary non-profit - Private
Beds: 36

Key Personnel:

Quality Assurance . . . . Jayme Anderson
Infection Control. . . . . Linda Chantland, RN
CEO/President. . . . . Michael Hagen
Chief of Medical Staff. . . . . James Harris, MD
Emergency Room . . . . James Harris

Measure	Cases	This Hosp.	State Avg.	U.S. Avg.
Blood Clot Prevention and Treatment				
Anticoagulation Overlap Therapy[5]	-	-	96%	93%
ICU Venous Thromboembolism Prophylaxis[5]	-	-	91%	92%
Incidence of Potentially Preventable VTE[5]	-	-	9%	10%
UFH with Dosages/Platelet Monitoring[5]	-	-	98%	97%
Venous Thromboembolism Prophylaxis[5]	-	-	86%	85%
Warfarin Therapy Discharge Instructions[5]	-	-	63%	75%
Chest Pain/Possible Heart Attack Care				
Aspirin Given Within 24 Hours of Arrival[1,3]	-	-	97%	96%
Fibrinolytic Meds Within 30 Min. of Arrival[5]	-	-	48%	58%
Average Time to ECG (minutes)[1,3]	-	-	7	7
Average Time to Transfer (minutes)[5]	-	-	54	60
Children's Asthma Care				
Received Home Management Plan of Care	-	-	-	88%
Received Reliever Medication	-	-	-	100%
Received Systemic Corticosteroids	-	-	-	100%
Emergency Department				
Admittance Decision Time (minutes)[2,3]	21	47	62	98
Head CT Results Within 45 Min. of Arrival[5]	-	-	54%	57%
Patients Who Left ER Before Being Seen[5]	-	-	2%	2%
Time from ER Arrival to Admit. (minutes)[2,3]	25	163	199	274
Time from ER Arrival to Discharge (minutes)[3]	209	86	125	134
Time in ER Before Being Evaluated (minutes)[3]	156	9	31	26
Time to Pain Meds for Fractures (minutes)[5]	-	-	45	57
Heart Attack Care				
Aspirin Given at Discharge[1,3]	-	-	99%	99%
Fibrinolytic Meds Within 30 Min. of Arrival[3,7]	-	-	-	54%
PCI Within 90 Minutes of Arrival[3,7]	-	-	96%	96%
Statin Prescribed at Discharge[1,3]	-	-	99%	98%
Heart Failure Care				
ACE Inhibitor or ARB for LVSD[7]	-	-	96%	97%
Discharge Instructions Given[1]	-	-	93%	94%
Evaluation of LVS Function[1]	-	-	97%	99%
Medicare Spending				
Medicare Spending per Patient (ratio)	-	-	0.9	0.98
Pneumonia Care				
Appropriate Initial Antibiotic Given	23	74%	94%	95%
Blood Culture Timing	23	87%	97%	98%
Pregnancy and Delivery Care				
Newborn Deliveries Scheduled Early[5]	-	-	5%	6%
Preventive Care				
Immunization for Influenza[5]	-	-	89%	90%
Immunization for Pneumonia[2,3]	73	82%	89%	92%
Stroke Care				
Anticoagulation Therapy for Atrial Fibrillation[5]	-	-	96%	95%
Antithrombotic Therapy Timing[5]	-	-	98%	98%
Assessed for Rehabilitation[5]	-	-	98%	97%
Discharged on Antithrombotic Therapy[5]	-	-	99%	99%
Discharged on Statin Medication[5]	-	-	95%	94%
Thrombolytic Therapy Timing[5]	-	-	74%	66%
Venous Thromboembolism Prophylaxis[5]	-	-	95%	94%
Written Stroke Educational Materials Given[5]	-	-	88%	88%
Surgical Care Improvement Project				
Appropriate Beta Blocker Usage	35	89%	98%	98%
Appropriate VTP Within 24 Hours	98	98%	98%	98%
Controlled Postoperative Blood Glucose[7]	-	-	97%	97%
Perioperative Temperature Management	107	100%	99%	100%
Prophylactic Antibiotic Selection	102	99%	99%	99%
Prophylactic Antibiotic Selection (Outpatient)[1,3]	-	-	98%	98%
Prophylactic Antibiotic Stopped	102	100%	99%	98%
Prophylactic Antibiotic Timing	102	97%	98%	99%
Prophylactic Antibiotic Timing (Outpatient)[1,3]	-	-	97%	98%
Urinary Catheter Removal	15	73%	97%	97%
Survey of Patients' Hospital Experiences				
Area Around Room 'Always' Quiet at Night	300+	73%	65%	61%
Doctors 'Always' Communicated Well	300+	86%	84%	82%
Home Recovery Information Given	300+	88%	88%	85%
Hospital Given 9 or 10 on 10 Point Scale	300+	78%	74%	71%
Meds 'Always' Explained Before Given	300+	72%	67%	64%
Nurses 'Always' Communicated Well	300+	85%	81%	79%
Pain 'Always' Well Controlled	300+	75%	72%	71%
Room and Bathroom 'Always' Clean	300+	84%	78%	73%
Timely Help 'Always' Received	300+	83%	74%	68%
Would Definitely Recommend Hospital	300+	80%	71%	71%
Use of Medical Imaging				
Cardiac Imaging Stress Test before Surgery	63	7.9%	6.3%	5.3%
Combination Abdominal CT Scan	139	3.6%	5.7%	10.5%
Combination Brain/Sinus CT Scan[1]	-	-	2.3%	2.7%
Combination Chest CT Scan	107	0.0%	1.9%	2.7%
Follow-up Mammogram/Ultrasound	373	7.5%	6.3%	8.8%
Lumbar Spine MRI for Low Back Pain[1]	-	-	37.6%	37.2%

Albany Area Hospital

300 Third Avenue
Albany, MN 56307
Phone: 320-845-2121
Fax: 320-845-4707
E-mail: mgoebel@means.net
URL: www.albanyareahospital.com
Type: Critical Access Hospitals
Emergency Services: Yes
Ownership: Voluntary non-profit - Private
Beds: 17

Key Personnel:

Emergency Room . . . . Josh Arickx, PA-C
Radiology. . . . . Mohammad Dogar
Chief of Medical Staff . . . . Daron Gersch
Infection Control . . . . Bernita Hinnenkamp
Anesthesiology. . . . . Mark Janorschke, CRNA

Measure	Cases	This Hosp.	State Avg.	U.S. Avg.
Blood Clot Prevention and Treatment				
Anticoagulation Overlap Therapy[5]	-	-	96%	93%
ICU Venous Thromboembolism Prophylaxis[5]	-	-	91%	92%
Incidence of Potentially Preventable VTE[5]	-	-	9%	10%
UFH with Dosages/Platelet Monitoring[5]	-	-	98%	97%
Venous Thromboembolism Prophylaxis[5]	-	-	86%	85%
Warfarin Therapy Discharge Instructions[5]	-	-	63%	75%
Chest Pain/Possible Heart Attack Care				
Aspirin Given Within 24 Hours of Arrival[1,3]	-	-	97%	96%
Fibrinolytic Meds Within 30 Min. of Arrival[3,7]	-	-	48%	58%
Average Time to ECG (minutes)[1,3]	-	-	7	7
Average Time to Transfer (minutes)[3,7]	-	-	54	60
Children's Asthma Care				
Received Home Management Plan of Care	-	-	-	88%
Received Reliever Medication	-	-	-	100%
Received Systemic Corticosteroids	-	-	-	100%
Emergency Department				
Admittance Decision Time (minutes)[2,3]	37	0	62	98
Head CT Results Within 45 Min. of Arrival[5]	-	-	54%	57%
Patients Who Left ER Before Being Seen[5]	-	-	2%	2%

NOTE: Hospital profiles are in alphabetical order by state, then city, then hospital within the city; Rankings exclude hospitals with less than 25 cases except for patient surveys which excludes hospitals with less than 100 cases; (a) 100-299 cases; (1) The number of cases/patients is too few to report; (2) Data submitted were based on a sample of cases/patients; (3) Results are based on a shorter time period than required; (4) Data suppressed by CMS for one or more quarters; (5) Results are not available for this reporting period; (6) Fewer than 100 patients completed the HCAHPS survey; (7) No cases met the criteria for this measure; (8) The lower limit of the confidence interval cannot be calculated if the number of observed infections equals zero; (9) No data are available from the state/territory for this reporting period; (10) The scores shown reflect fewer than 50 completed surveys; (11) There were discrepancies in the data collection process; (12) This measure does not apply to this hospital for this reporting period; (13) Results cannot be calculated for this reporting period; (14) The results for this state are combined with nearby states to protect confidentiality; Please refer to the User's Guide for a full explanation of data.

Measure	Cases	This Hosp.	State Avg.	U.S. Avg.
Time from ER Arrival to Admit. (minutes)[2,3]	38	138	199	274
Time from ER Arrival to Discharge (minutes)[3]	113	86	125	134
Time in ER Before Being Evaluated (minutes)[3]	97	15	31	26
Time to Pain Meds for Fractures (minutes)[1,3]	-	-	45	57
Heart Attack Care				
Aspirin Given at Discharge[1,3]	-	-	99%	99%
Fibrinolytic Meds Within 30 Min. of Arrival[3,7]	-	-	-	54%
PCI Within 90 Minutes of Arrival[3,7]	-	-	96%	96%
Statin Prescribed at Discharge[1,3]	-	-	99%	98%
Heart Failure Care				
ACE Inhibitor or ARB for LVSD[1,3]	-	-	96%	97%
Discharge Instructions Given[1,3]	-	-	93%	94%
Evaluation of LVS Function[1,3]	-	-	97%	99%
Medicare Spending				
Medicare Spending per Patient (ratio)	-	-	0.9	0.98
Pneumonia Care				
Appropriate Initial Antibiotic Given[1]	-	-	94%	95%
Blood Culture Timing[1]	-	-	97%	98%
Pregnancy and Delivery Care				
Newborn Deliveries Scheduled Early[5]	-	-	5%	6%
Preventive Care				
Immunization for Influenza[5]	-	-	89%	90%
Immunization for Pneumonia[2,3]	52	81%	89%	92%
Stroke Care				
Anticoagulation Therapy for Atrial Fibrillation[5]	-	-	96%	95%
Antithrombotic Therapy Timing[5]	-	-	98%	98%
Assessed for Rehabilitation[5]	-	-	98%	97%
Discharged on Antithrombotic Therapy[5]	-	-	99%	99%
Discharged on Statin Medication[5]	-	-	95%	94%
Thrombolytic Therapy Timing[5]	-	-	74%	66%
Venous Thromboembolism Prophylaxis[5]	-	-	95%	94%
Written Stroke Educational Materials Given[5]	-	-	88%	88%
Surgical Care Improvement Project				
Appropriate Beta Blocker Usage[3,7]	-	-	98%	98%
Appropriate VTP Within 24 Hours[1,3]	-	-	98%	98%
Controlled Postoperative Blood Glucose[3,7]	-	-	97%	97%
Perioperative Temperature Management[1,3]	-	-	99%	100%
Prophylactic Antibiotic Selection[1,3]	-	-	99%	99%
Prophylactic Antibiotic Selection (Outpatient)[5]	-	-	98%	98%
Prophylactic Antibiotic Stopped[1,3]	-	-	99%	98%
Prophylactic Antibiotic Timing[1,3]	-	-	98%	99%
Prophylactic Antibiotic Timing (Outpatient)[5]	-	-	97%	98%
Urinary Catheter Removal[1,3]	-	-	97%	97%
Survey of Patients' Hospital Experiences				
Area Around Room 'Always' Quiet at Night[10]	<100	79%	65%	61%
Doctors 'Always' Communicated Well[10]	<100	87%	84%	82%
Home Recovery Information Given[10]	<100	91%	88%	85%
Hospital Given 9 or 10 on 10 Point Scale[10]	<100	83%	74%	71%
Meds 'Always' Explained Before Given[10]	<100	77%	67%	64%
Nurses 'Always' Communicated Well[10]	<100	86%	81%	79%
Pain 'Always' Well Controlled[10]	<100	63%	72%	71%
Room and Bathroom 'Always' Clean[10]	<100	77%	78%	73%
Timely Help 'Always' Received[10]	<100	74%	74%	68%
Would Definitely Recommend Hospital[10]	<100	74%	71%	71%
Use of Medical Imaging				
Cardiac Imaging Stress Test before Surgery[1]	-	-	6.3%	5.3%
Combination Abdominal CT Scan[1]	-	-	5.7%	10.5%
Combination Brain/Sinus CT Scan[1]	-	-	2.3%	2.7%
Combination Chest CT Scan[1]	-	-	1.9%	2.7%
Follow-up Mammogram/Ultrasound[1]	-	-	6.3%	8.8%
Lumbar Spine MRI for Low Back Pain[1]	-	-	37.6%	37.2%

Mayo Clinic Health System - Albert Lea

404 West Fountain Street
Albert Lea, MN 56007
Phone: 507-373-2384
Fax: 507-377-6248
URL: www.mayoclinichealthsystem.org
Type: Acute Care Hospitals
Emergency Services: Yes
Ownership: Voluntary non-profit - Private
Beds: 119

Key Personnel:

Operating Room. . . . . Jill Berg
Intensive Care Unit. . . . . Nancy Christensen
CEO/President. . . . . Mark Ciota, MD
Chief of Medical Staff. . . . . John Grzybowski, MD
Patient Relations . . . . Jane Killpack
Quality Assurance . . . . Toni Lauer
Radiology. . . . . Lisa Routh
Infection Control. . . . . Tammy Williams

Measure	Cases	This Hosp.	State Avg.	U.S. Avg.
Blood Clot Prevention and Treatment				
Anticoagulation Overlap Therapy[2]	21	100%	96%	93%
ICU Venous Thromboembolism Prophylaxis[2]	61	100%	91%	92%
Incidence of Potentially Preventable VTE[1,2]	-	-	9%	10%
UFH with Dosages/Platelet Monitoring[2]	16	100%	98%	97%
Venous Thromboembolism Prophylaxis[2]	164	97%	86%	85%
Warfarin Therapy Discharge Instructions[2]	15	87%	63%	75%
Chest Pain/Possible Heart Attack Care				
Aspirin Given Within 24 Hours of Arrival	98	92%	97%	96%
Fibrinolytic Meds Within 30 Min. of Arrival[1]	-	-	48%	58%
Average Time to ECG (minutes)	104	9	7	7
Average Time to Transfer (minutes)	17	85	54	60
Children's Asthma Care				
Received Home Management Plan of Care	-	-	-	88%
Received Reliever Medication	-	-	-	100%
Received Systemic Corticosteroids	-	-	-	100%
Emergency Department				
Admittance Decision Time (minutes)[2]	266	43	62	98
Head CT Results Within 45 Min. of Arrival	19	74%	54%	57%
Patients Who Left ER Before Being Seen	13,721	3%	2%	2%
Time from ER Arrival to Admit. (minutes)[2]	320	204	199	274
Time from ER Arrival to Discharge (minutes)	439	134	125	134
Time in ER Before Being Evaluated (minutes)	494	27	31	26
Time to Pain Meds for Fractures (minutes)	41	50	45	57
Heart Attack Care				
Aspirin Given at Discharge	27	100%	99%	99%
Fibrinolytic Meds Within 30 Min. of Arrival[7]	-	-	-	54%
PCI Within 90 Minutes of Arrival[7]	-	-	96%	96%
Statin Prescribed at Discharge	28	93%	99%	98%
Heart Failure Care				
ACE Inhibitor or ARB for LVSD	24	96%	96%	97%
Discharge Instructions Given	73	92%	93%	94%
Evaluation of LVS Function	102	99%	97%	99%
Medicare Spending				
Medicare Spending per Patient (ratio)	-	0.90	0.9	0.98
Pneumonia Care				
Appropriate Initial Antibiotic Given	78	95%	94%	95%
Blood Culture Timing	121	97%	97%	98%
Pregnancy and Delivery Care				
Newborn Deliveries Scheduled Early	40	5%	5%	6%
Preventive Care				
Immunization for Influenza[2]	312	92%	89%	90%
Immunization for Pneumonia[2]	413	95%	89%	92%
Stroke Care				
Anticoagulation Therapy for Atrial Fibrillation[1]	-	-	96%	95%
Antithrombotic Therapy Timing	15	53%	98%	98%
Assessed for Rehabilitation	17	71%	98%	97%
Discharged on Antithrombotic Therapy	11	100%	99%	99%
Discharged on Statin Medication	12	100%	95%	94%
Thrombolytic Therapy Timing[1]	-	-	74%	66%
Venous Thromboembolism Prophylaxis	24	88%	95%	94%
Written Stroke Educational Materials Given[1]	-	-	88%	88%
Surgical Care Improvement Project				
Appropriate Beta Blocker Usage	90	99%	98%	98%
Appropriate VTP Within 24 Hours	230	100%	98%	98%
Controlled Postoperative Blood Glucose[7]	-	-	97%	97%
Perioperative Temperature Management	264	99%	99%	100%
Prophylactic Antibiotic Selection	196	100%	99%	99%
Prophylactic Antibiotic Selection (Outpatient)	60	100%	98%	98%
Prophylactic Antibiotic Stopped	192	99%	99%	98%
Prophylactic Antibiotic Timing	196	99%	98%	99%
Prophylactic Antibiotic Timing (Outpatient)	41	98%	97%	98%
Urinary Catheter Removal	218	100%	97%	97%
Survey of Patients' Hospital Experiences				
Area Around Room 'Always' Quiet at Night	300+	56%	65%	61%
Doctors 'Always' Communicated Well	300+	81%	84%	82%
Home Recovery Information Given	300+	86%	88%	85%
Hospital Given 9 or 10 on 10 Point Scale	300+	72%	74%	71%
Meds 'Always' Explained Before Given	300+	65%	67%	64%
Nurses 'Always' Communicated Well	300+	80%	81%	79%
Pain 'Always' Well Controlled	300+	70%	72%	71%
Room and Bathroom 'Always' Clean	300+	77%	78%	73%
Timely Help 'Always' Received	300+	69%	74%	68%
Would Definitely Recommend Hospital	300+	67%	71%	71%
Use of Medical Imaging				
Cardiac Imaging Stress Test before Surgery	97	5.2%	6.3%	5.3%
Combination Abdominal CT Scan	334	2.4%	5.7%	10.5%
Combination Brain/Sinus CT Scan	299	1.0%	2.3%	2.7%
Combination Chest CT Scan	183	0.0%	1.9%	2.7%
Follow-up Mammogram/Ultrasound	667	7.2%	6.3%	8.8%
Lumbar Spine MRI for Low Back Pain[1]	-	-	37.6%	37.2%

Douglas County Hospital

111 17th Avenue East
Alexandria, MN 56308
Phone: 320-762-1511
Fax: 320-762-6034
E-mail: hr@dchospital.com
URL: www.dchospital.com
Type: Acute Care Hospitals
Emergency Services: Yes
Ownership: Government - Local
Beds: 127

Key Personnel:

Radiology. . . . . Richard D Eiser
Infection Control. . . . . Bonnie Freudenberg
Operating Room. . . . . Billie Glade
Quality Assurance . . . . Doug Leinhart
Intensive Care Unit. . . . . Lois Nelson, RN
CEO . . . . Carl Vaagenes
Emergency Room . . . . Kevin Wedman, RN
Chief of Medical Staff. . . . . Bruce Wymore

Measure	Cases	This Hosp.	State Avg.	U.S. Avg.
Blood Clot Prevention and Treatment				
Anticoagulation Overlap Therapy[2]	20	100%	96%	93%
ICU Venous Thromboembolism Prophylaxis[2]	59	98%	91%	92%
Incidence of Potentially Preventable VTE[1,2]	-	-	9%	10%
UFH with Dosages/Platelet Monitoring[1,2]	-	-	98%	97%
Venous Thromboembolism Prophylaxis[2]	234	96%	86%	85%
Warfarin Therapy Discharge Instructions[2]	13	100%	63%	75%
Chest Pain/Possible Heart Attack Care				
Aspirin Given Within 24 Hours of Arrival	125	97%	97%	96%
Fibrinolytic Meds Within 30 Min. of Arrival[7]	-	-	48%	58%
Average Time to ECG (minutes)	128	5	7	7
Average Time to Transfer (minutes)	20	40	54	60
Children's Asthma Care				
Received Home Management Plan of Care	-	-	-	88%
Received Reliever Medication	-	-	-	100%
Received Systemic Corticosteroids	-	-	-	100%
Emergency Department				
Admittance Decision Time (minutes)[2]	318	50	62	98
Head CT Results Within 45 Min. of Arrival	20	65%	54%	57%
Patients Who Left ER Before Being Seen	15,141	1%	2%	2%
Time from ER Arrival to Admit. (minutes)[2]	378	195	199	274
Time from ER Arrival to Discharge (minutes)	868	108	125	134
Time in ER Before Being Evaluated (minutes)	604	21	31	26
Time to Pain Meds for Fractures (minutes)	78	51	45	57
Heart Attack Care				
Aspirin Given at Discharge[1]	-	-	99%	99%
Fibrinolytic Meds Within 30 Min. of Arrival[7]	-	-	-	54%
PCI Within 90 Minutes of Arrival[7]	-	-	96%	96%
Statin Prescribed at Discharge[1]	-	-	99%	98%
Heart Failure Care				
ACE Inhibitor or ARB for LVSD	22	100%	96%	97%
Discharge Instructions Given	58	95%	93%	94%
Evaluation of LVS Function	101	100%	97%	99%
Medicare Spending				
Medicare Spending per Patient (ratio)	-	0.94	0.9	0.98
Pneumonia Care				
Appropriate Initial Antibiotic Given	66	88%	94%	95%
Blood Culture Timing	125	99%	97%	98%
Pregnancy and Delivery Care				
Newborn Deliveries Scheduled Early	58	3%	5%	6%
Preventive Care				
Immunization for Influenza[2]	390	89%	89%	90%
Immunization for Pneumonia[2]	478	92%	89%	92%
Stroke Care				

NOTE: Hospital profiles are in alphabetical order by state, then city, then hospital within the city; Rankings exclude hospitals with less than 25 cases except for patient surveys which excludes hospitals with less than 100 cases; (a) 100-299 cases; (1) The number of cases/patients is too few to report; (2) Data submitted were based on a sample of cases/patients; (3) Results are based on a shorter time period than required; (4) Data suppressed by CMS for one or more quarters; (5) Results are not available for this reporting period; (6) Fewer than 100 patients completed the HCAHPS survey; (7) No cases met the criteria for this measure; (8) The lower limit of the confidence interval cannot be calculated if the number of observed infections equals zero; (9) No data are available from the state/territory for this reporting period; (10) The scores shown reflect fewer than 50 completed surveys; (11) There were discrepancies in the data collection process; (12) This measure does not apply to this hospital for this reporting period; (13) Results cannot be calculated for this reporting period; (14) The results for this state are combined with nearby states to protect confidentiality; Please refer to the User's Guide for a full explanation of data.

Measure	Cases	This Hosp.	State Avg.	U.S. Avg.
Anticoagulation Therapy for Atrial Fibrillation[1]	-	-	96%	95%
Antithrombotic Therapy Timing	17	100%	98%	98%
Assessed for Rehabilitation	18	100%	98%	97%
Discharged on Antithrombotic Therapy	17	100%	99%	99%
Discharged on Statin Medication	13	100%	95%	94%
Thrombolytic Therapy Timing[1]	-	-	74%	66%
Venous Thromboembolism Prophylaxis	20	90%	95%	94%
Written Stroke Educational Materials Given[1]	-	-	88%	88%
Surgical Care Improvement Project				
Appropriate Beta Blocker Usage[2]	150	99%	98%	98%
Appropriate VTP Within 24 Hours[2]	394	99%	98%	98%
Controlled Postoperative Blood Glucose[2,7]	-	-	97%	97%
Perioperative Temperature Management[2]	423	92%	99%	100%
Prophylactic Antibiotic Selection[2]	326	99%	99%	99%
Prophylactic Antibiotic Selection (Outpatient)	214	93%	98%	98%
Prophylactic Antibiotic Stopped[2]	322	99%	99%	98%
Prophylactic Antibiotic Timing[2]	327	99%	98%	99%
Prophylactic Antibiotic Timing (Outpatient)	216	97%	97%	98%
Urinary Catheter Removal[2]	359	92%	97%	97%
Survey of Patients' Hospital Experiences				
Area Around Room 'Always' Quiet at Night	300+	70%	65%	61%
Doctors 'Always' Communicated Well	300+	80%	84%	82%
Home Recovery Information Given	300+	88%	88%	85%
Hospital Given 9 or 10 on 10 Point Scale	300+	71%	74%	71%
Meds 'Always' Explained Before Given	300+	59%	67%	64%
Nurses 'Always' Communicated Well	300+	74%	81%	79%
Pain 'Always' Well Controlled	300+	72%	72%	71%
Room and Bathroom 'Always' Clean	300+	79%	78%	73%
Timely Help 'Always' Received	300+	67%	74%	68%
Would Definitely Recommend Hospital	300+	74%	71%	71%
Use of Medical Imaging				
Cardiac Imaging Stress Test before Surgery	119	2.5%	6.3%	5.3%
Combination Abdominal CT Scan	327	8.3%	5.7%	10.5%
Combination Brain/Sinus CT Scan[1]	-	-	2.3%	2.7%
Combination Chest CT Scan	267	0.4%	1.9%	2.7%
Follow-up Mammogram/Ultrasound	506	11.1%	6.3%	8.8%
Lumbar Spine MRI for Low Back Pain	124	29.8%	37.6%	37.2%

Appleton Municipal Hospital

30 South Behl Street
Appleton, MN 56208
Type: Critical Access Hospitals
Ownership: Government - Local
Phone: 320-289-1580
Fax: 320-289-1797
Emergency Services: Yes
Beds: 131

Key Personnel:
Emergency Room . . . . Limpi Ado, MD
CEO/President. . . . . Daniel Swenson

Measure	Cases	This Hosp.	State Avg.	U.S. Avg.
Blood Clot Prevention and Treatment				
Anticoagulation Overlap Therapy[1,3]	-	-	96%	93%
ICU Venous Thromboembolism Prophylaxis[3,7]	-	-	91%	92%
Incidence of Potentially Preventable VTE[3,7]	-	-	9%	10%
UFH with Dosages/Platelet Monitoring[1,3]	-	-	98%	97%
Venous Thromboembolism Prophylaxis[3,7]	-	-	86%	85%
Warfarin Therapy Discharge Instructions[1,3]	-	-	63%	75%
Chest Pain/Possible Heart Attack Care				
Aspirin Given Within 24 Hours of Arrival[1,3]	-	-	97%	96%
Fibrinolytic Meds Within 30 Min. of Arrival[5]	-	-	48%	58%
Average Time to ECG (minutes)[1,3]	-	-	7	7
Average Time to Transfer (minutes)[5]	-	-	54	60
Children's Asthma Care				
Received Home Management Plan of Care	-	-	-	88%
Received Reliever Medication	-	-	-	100%
Received Systemic Corticosteroids	-	-	-	100%
Emergency Department				
Admittance Decision Time (minutes)	36	0	62	98
Head CT Results Within 45 Min. of Arrival[1,3]	-	-	54%	57%
Patients Who Left ER Before Being Seen[5]	-	-	2%	2%
Time from ER Arrival to Admit. (minutes)	51	118	199	274
Time from ER Arrival to Discharge (minutes)[5]	-	-	125	134
Time in ER Before Being Evaluated (minutes)[5]	-	-	31	26
Time to Pain Meds for Fractures (minutes)[1,3]	-	-	45	57
Heart Attack Care				
Aspirin Given at Discharge[5]	-	-	99%	99%
Fibrinolytic Meds Within 30 Min. of Arrival[5]	-	-	-	54%
PCI Within 90 Minutes of Arrival[5]	-	-	96%	96%
Statin Prescribed at Discharge[5]	-	-	99%	98%
Heart Failure Care				
ACE Inhibitor or ARB for LVSD[1]	-	-	96%	97%
Discharge Instructions Given[1]	-	-	93%	94%
Evaluation of LVS Function	13	69%	97%	99%
Medicare Spending				
Medicare Spending per Patient (ratio)	-	-	0.9	0.98
Pneumonia Care				
Appropriate Initial Antibiotic Given[1]	-	-	94%	95%
Blood Culture Timing[7]	-	-	97%	98%
Pregnancy and Delivery Care				
Newborn Deliveries Scheduled Early[5]	-	-	5%	6%
Preventive Care				
Immunization for Influenza	37	76%	89%	90%
Immunization for Pneumonia	66	64%	89%	92%
Stroke Care				
Anticoagulation Therapy for Atrial Fibrillation[1,3]	-	-	96%	95%
Antithrombotic Therapy Timing[1,3]	-	-	98%	98%
Assessed for Rehabilitation[1,3]	-	-	98%	97%
Discharged on Antithrombotic Therapy[1,3]	-	-	99%	99%
Discharged on Statin Medication[1,3]	-	-	95%	94%
Thrombolytic Therapy Timing[1,3]	-	-	74%	66%
Venous Thromboembolism Prophylaxis[1,3]	-	-	95%	94%
Written Stroke Educational Materials Given[3,7]	-	-	88%	88%
Surgical Care Improvement Project				
Appropriate Beta Blocker Usage[5]	-	-	98%	98%
Appropriate VTP Within 24 Hours[5]	-	-	98%	98%
Controlled Postoperative Blood Glucose[5]	-	-	97%	97%
Perioperative Temperature Management[5]	-	-	99%	100%
Prophylactic Antibiotic Selection[5]	-	-	99%	99%
Prophylactic Antibiotic Selection (Outpatient)[3,7]	-	-	98%	98%
Prophylactic Antibiotic Stopped[5]	-	-	99%	98%
Prophylactic Antibiotic Timing[5]	-	-	98%	99%
Prophylactic Antibiotic Timing (Outpatient)[1,3]	-	-	97%	98%
Urinary Catheter Removal[5]	-	-	97%	97%
Survey of Patients' Hospital Experiences				
Area Around Room 'Always' Quiet at Night[10,11]	<100	71%	65%	61%
Doctors 'Always' Communicated Well[10,11]	<100	92%	84%	82%
Home Recovery Information Given[10,11]	<100	81%	88%	85%
Hospital Given 9 or 10 on 10 Point Scale[10,11]	<100	80%	74%	71%
Meds 'Always' Explained Before Given[10,11]	<100	88%	67%	64%
Nurses 'Always' Communicated Well[10,11]	<100	82%	81%	79%
Pain 'Always' Well Controlled[10,11]	<100	76%	72%	71%
Room and Bathroom 'Always' Clean[10,11]	<100	91%	78%	73%
Timely Help 'Always' Received[10,11]	<100	88%	74%	68%
Would Definitely Recommend Hospital[10,11]	<100	68%	71%	71%
Use of Medical Imaging				
Cardiac Imaging Stress Test before Surgery[1]	-	-	6.3%	5.3%
Combination Abdominal CT Scan[1]	-	-	5.7%	10.5%
Combination Brain/Sinus CT Scan	35	0.0%	2.3%	2.7%
Combination Chest CT Scan[1]	-	-	1.9%	2.7%
Follow-up Mammogram/Ultrasound[1]	-	-	6.3%	8.8%
Lumbar Spine MRI for Low Back Pain[1]	-	-	37.6%	37.2%

Ridgeview Sibley Medical Center

601 West Chandler
Arlington, MN 55307
E-mail: anhhosp@frontiernet.net
URL: www.sibleymedical.com
Type: Critical Access Hospitals
Ownership: Government - Local
Phone: 507-964-2271
Fax: 507-964-5898
Emergency Services: Yes
Beds: 20

Key Personnel:
Chief of Medical Staff. . . . . Dean Bergersen
Operating Room. . . . . Beth Miller, RN
CEO . . . . Todd Sandberg

Measure	Cases	This Hosp.	State Avg.	U.S. Avg.
Blood Clot Prevention and Treatment				
Anticoagulation Overlap Therapy[5]	-	-	96%	93%
ICU Venous Thromboembolism Prophylaxis[5]	-	-	91%	92%
Incidence of Potentially Preventable VTE[5]	-	-	9%	10%
UFH with Dosages/Platelet Monitoring[5]	-	-	98%	97%
Venous Thromboembolism Prophylaxis[5]	-	-	86%	85%
Warfarin Therapy Discharge Instructions[5]	-	-	63%	75%
Chest Pain/Possible Heart Attack Care				
Aspirin Given Within 24 Hours of Arrival	11	82%	97%	96%
Fibrinolytic Meds Within 30 Min. of Arrival[1]	-	-	48%	58%
Average Time to ECG (minutes)	12	12	7	7
Average Time to Transfer (minutes)[1]	-	-	54	60
Children's Asthma Care				
Received Home Management Plan of Care	-	-	-	88%
Received Reliever Medication	-	-	-	100%
Received Systemic Corticosteroids	-	-	-	100%
Emergency Department				
Admittance Decision Time (minutes)	71	1	62	98
Head CT Results Within 45 Min. of Arrival[5]	-	-	54%	57%
Patients Who Left ER Before Being Seen[5]	-	-	2%	2%
Time from ER Arrival to Admit. (minutes)	71	135	199	274
Time from ER Arrival to Discharge (minutes)	86	147	125	134
Time in ER Before Being Evaluated (minutes)	101	9	31	26
Time to Pain Meds for Fractures (minutes)[5]	-	-	45	57
Heart Attack Care				
Aspirin Given at Discharge[1,3]	-	-	99%	99%
Fibrinolytic Meds Within 30 Min. of Arrival[3,7]	-	-	-	54%
PCI Within 90 Minutes of Arrival[3,7]	-	-	96%	96%
Statin Prescribed at Discharge[1,3]	-	-	99%	98%
Heart Failure Care				
ACE Inhibitor or ARB for LVSD[1]	-	-	96%	97%
Discharge Instructions Given[1]	-	-	93%	94%
Evaluation of LVS Function[1]	-	-	97%	99%
Medicare Spending				
Medicare Spending per Patient (ratio)	-	-	0.9	0.98
Pneumonia Care				
Appropriate Initial Antibiotic Given	13	85%	94%	95%
Blood Culture Timing[1]	-	-	97%	98%
Pregnancy and Delivery Care				
Newborn Deliveries Scheduled Early[5]	-	-	5%	6%
Preventive Care				
Immunization for Influenza	65	75%	89%	90%
Immunization for Pneumonia[2]	89	89%	89%	92%
Stroke Care				
Anticoagulation Therapy for Atrial Fibrillation[5]	-	-	96%	95%
Antithrombotic Therapy Timing[5]	-	-	98%	98%
Assessed for Rehabilitation[5]	-	-	98%	97%
Discharged on Antithrombotic Therapy[5]	-	-	99%	99%
Discharged on Statin Medication[5]	-	-	95%	94%
Thrombolytic Therapy Timing[5]	-	-	74%	66%
Venous Thromboembolism Prophylaxis[5]	-	-	95%	94%
Written Stroke Educational Materials Given[5]	-	-	88%	88%
Surgical Care Improvement Project				
Appropriate Beta Blocker Usage[5]	-	-	98%	98%
Appropriate VTP Within 24 Hours[5]	-	-	98%	98%
Controlled Postoperative Blood Glucose[5]	-	-	97%	97%
Perioperative Temperature Management[5]	-	-	99%	100%
Prophylactic Antibiotic Selection[5]	-	-	99%	99%
Prophylactic Antibiotic Selection (Outpatient)[5]	-	-	98%	98%
Prophylactic Antibiotic Stopped[5]	-	-	99%	98%
Prophylactic Antibiotic Timing[5]	-	-	98%	99%
Prophylactic Antibiotic Timing (Outpatient)[5]	-	-	97%	98%
Urinary Catheter Removal[5]	-	-	97%	97%
Survey of Patients' Hospital Experiences				
Area Around Room 'Always' Quiet at Night[5]	-	-	65%	61%
Doctors 'Always' Communicated Well[5]	-	-	84%	82%
Home Recovery Information Given[5]	-	-	88%	85%
Hospital Given 9 or 10 on 10 Point Scale[5]	-	-	74%	71%
Meds 'Always' Explained Before Given[5]	-	-	67%	64%
Nurses 'Always' Communicated Well[5]	-	-	81%	79%
Pain 'Always' Well Controlled[5]	-	-	72%	71%
Room and Bathroom 'Always' Clean[5]	-	-	78%	73%
Timely Help 'Always' Received[5]	-	-	74%	68%
Would Definitely Recommend Hospital[5]	-	-	71%	71%
Use of Medical Imaging				
Cardiac Imaging Stress Test before Surgery[1]	-	-	6.3%	5.3%
Combination Abdominal CT Scan[1]	-	-	5.7%	10.5%

NOTE: Hospital profiles are in alphabetical order by state, then city, then hospital within the city; Rankings exclude hospitals with less than 25 cases except for patient surveys which excludes hospitals with less than 100 cases; (a) 100-299 cases; (1) The number of cases/patients is too few to report; (2) Data submitted were based on a sample of cases/patients; (3) Results are based on a shorter time period than required; (4) Data suppressed by CMS for one or more quarters; (5) Results are not available for this reporting period; (6) Fewer than 100 patients completed the HCAHPS survey; (7) No cases met the criteria for this measure; (8) The lower limit of the confidence interval cannot be calculated if the number of observed infections equals zero; (9) No data are available from the state/territory for this reporting period; (10) The scores shown reflect fewer than 50 completed surveys; (11) There were discrepancies in the data collection process; (12) This measure does not apply to this hospital for this reporting period; (13) Results cannot be calculated for this reporting period; (14) The results for this state are combined with nearby states to protect confidentiality; Please refer to the User's Guide for a full explanation of data.

Combination Brain/Sinus CT Scan	44	0.0%	2.3%	2.7%
Combination Chest CT Scan[1]	-	-	1.9%	2.7%
Follow-up Mammogram/Ultrasound[1]	-	-	6.3%	8.8%
Lumbar Spine MRI for Low Back Pain[1]	-	-	37.6%	37.2%

Essentia Health Northern Pines Medical Center

5211 Highway 110
Aurora, MN 55705
Phone: 218-229-2211
Fax: 218-229-2042
E-mail: info@whitetech.org
URL: www.whitetech.org

Type: Critical Access Hospitals
Emergency Services: No
Ownership: Voluntary non-profit - Private
Beds: 85

Key Personnel:
Infection Control. . . . . Randi Dix, RN
CEO/President. . . . . Paula Schaefbaurer
Quality Assurance . . . . Paula Schaefbaurer
Chief of Medical Staff. . . . . Christopher Whiting, MD

Measure	Cases	This Hosp.	State Avg.	U.S. Avg.
Blood Clot Prevention and Treatment				
Anticoagulation Overlap Therapy[5]	-	-	96%	93%
ICU Venous Thromboembolism Prophylaxis[5]	-	-	91%	92%
Incidence of Potentially Preventable VTE[5]	-	-	9%	10%
UFH with Dosages/Platelet Monitoring[5]	-	-	98%	97%
Venous Thromboembolism Prophylaxis[5]	-	-	86%	85%
Warfarin Therapy Discharge Instructions[5]	-	-	63%	75%
Chest Pain/Possible Heart Attack Care				
Aspirin Given Within 24 Hours of Arrival[3]	26	100%	97%	96%
Fibrinolytic Meds Within 30 Min. of Arrival[1,3]	-	-	48%	58%
Average Time to ECG (minutes)[3]	25	10	7	7
Average Time to Transfer (minutes)[1,3]	-	-	54	60
Children's Asthma Care				
Received Home Management Plan of Care	-	-	-	88%
Received Reliever Medication	-	-	-	100%
Received Systemic Corticosteroids	-	-	-	100%
Emergency Department				
Admittance Decision Time (minutes)[2,3]	56	19	62	98
Head CT Results Within 45 Min. of Arrival[5]	-	-	54%	57%
Patients Who Left ER Before Being Seen	1,867	0%	2%	2%
Time from ER Arrival to Admit. (minutes)[2,3]	64	128	199	274
Time from ER Arrival to Discharge (minutes)[5]	-	-	125	134
Time in ER Before Being Evaluated (minutes)[5]	-	-	31	26
Time to Pain Meds for Fractures (minutes)[5]	-	-	45	57
Heart Attack Care				
Aspirin Given at Discharge[5]	-	-	99%	99%
Fibrinolytic Meds Within 30 Min. of Arrival[5]	-	-	-	54%
PCI Within 90 Minutes of Arrival[5]	-	-	96%	96%
Statin Prescribed at Discharge[5]	-	-	99%	98%
Heart Failure Care				
ACE Inhibitor or ARB for LVSD[1,2]	-	-	96%	97%
Discharge Instructions Given[1,2]	-	-	93%	94%
Evaluation of LVS Function[1,2]	-	-	97%	99%
Medicare Spending				
Medicare Spending per Patient (ratio)	-	-	0.9	0.98
Pneumonia Care				
Appropriate Initial Antibiotic Given[1,2]	-	-	94%	95%
Blood Culture Timing[1,2]	-	-	97%	98%
Pregnancy and Delivery Care				
Newborn Deliveries Scheduled Early[5]	-	-	5%	6%
Preventive Care				
Immunization for Influenza[2,3]	45	98%	89%	90%
Immunization for Pneumonia[2,3]	114	99%	89%	92%
Stroke Care				
Anticoagulation Therapy for Atrial Fibrillation[5]	-	-	96%	95%
Antithrombotic Therapy Timing[5]	-	-	98%	98%
Assessed for Rehabilitation[5]	-	-	98%	97%
Discharged on Antithrombotic Therapy[5]	-	-	99%	99%
Discharged on Statin Medication[5]	-	-	95%	94%
Thrombolytic Therapy Timing[5]	-	-	74%	66%
Venous Thromboembolism Prophylaxis[5]	-	-	95%	94%
Written Stroke Educational Materials Given[5]	-	-	88%	88%
Surgical Care Improvement Project				
Appropriate Beta Blocker Usage[5]	-	-	98%	98%
Appropriate VTP Within 24 Hours[5]	-	-	98%	98%
Controlled Postoperative Blood Glucose[5]	-	-	97%	97%
Perioperative Temperature Management[5]	-	-	99%	100%
Prophylactic Antibiotic Selection[5]	-	-	99%	99%
Prophylactic Antibiotic Selection (Outpatient)[5]	-	-	98%	98%
Prophylactic Antibiotic Stopped[5]	-	-	99%	98%
Prophylactic Antibiotic Timing[5]	-	-	98%	99%
Prophylactic Antibiotic Timing (Outpatient)[5]	-	-	97%	98%
Urinary Catheter Removal[5]	-	-	97%	97%
Survey of Patients' Hospital Experiences				
Area Around Room 'Always' Quiet at Night[5]	-	-	65%	61%
Doctors 'Always' Communicated Well[5]	-	-	84%	82%
Home Recovery Information Given[5]	-	-	88%	85%
Hospital Given 9 or 10 on 10 Point Scale[5]	-	-	74%	71%
Meds 'Always' Explained Before Given[5]	-	-	67%	64%
Nurses 'Always' Communicated Well[5]	-	-	81%	79%
Pain 'Always' Well Controlled[5]	-	-	72%	71%
Room and Bathroom 'Always' Clean[5]	-	-	78%	73%
Timely Help 'Always' Received[5]	-	-	74%	68%
Would Definitely Recommend Hospital[5]	-	-	71%	71%
Use of Medical Imaging				
Cardiac Imaging Stress Test before Surgery[7]	-	-	6.3%	5.3%
Combination Abdominal CT Scan[1]	-	-	5.7%	10.5%
Combination Brain/Sinus CT Scan[1]	-	-	2.3%	2.7%
Combination Chest CT Scan[1]	-	-	1.9%	2.7%
Follow-up Mammogram/Ultrasound[7]	-	-	6.3%	8.8%
Lumbar Spine MRI for Low Back Pain[7]	-	-	37.6%	37.2%

Sanford Bagley Medical Center

203 4th Street Northwest
Bagley, MN 56621
Phone: 218-694-6501
Fax: 218-694-3528
E-mail: ccmh@bagley.means.net
URL: www.clearwaterhs.com

Type: Critical Access Hospitals
Emergency Services: Yes
Ownership: Voluntary non-profit - Private
Beds: 77

Key Personnel:
Chief of Medical Staff. . . . . Francis Abraham, MD
Emergency Room . . . . Rick Ames
Operating Room. . . . . Rick Ames
Infection Control. . . . . Bruce Muckala
Quality Assurance . . . . Bruce Muckala

Measure	Cases	This Hosp.	State Avg.	U.S. Avg.
Blood Clot Prevention and Treatment				
Anticoagulation Overlap Therapy[5]	-	-	96%	93%
ICU Venous Thromboembolism Prophylaxis[5]	-	-	91%	92%
Incidence of Potentially Preventable VTE[5]	-	-	9%	10%
UFH with Dosages/Platelet Monitoring[5]	-	-	98%	97%
Venous Thromboembolism Prophylaxis[5]	-	-	86%	85%
Warfarin Therapy Discharge Instructions[5]	-	-	63%	75%
Chest Pain/Possible Heart Attack Care				
Aspirin Given Within 24 Hours of Arrival	-	-	97%	96%
Fibrinolytic Meds Within 30 Min. of Arrival	-	-	48%	58%
Average Time to ECG (minutes)	-	-	7	7
Average Time to Transfer (minutes)	-	-	54	60
Children's Asthma Care				
Received Home Management Plan of Care	-	-	-	88%
Received Reliever Medication	-	-	-	100%
Received Systemic Corticosteroids	-	-	-	100%
Emergency Department				
Admittance Decision Time (minutes)	93	20	62	98
Head CT Results Within 45 Min. of Arrival	-	-	54%	57%
Patients Who Left ER Before Being Seen	-	-	2%	2%
Time from ER Arrival to Admit. (minutes)	96	124	199	274
Time from ER Arrival to Discharge (minutes)	-	-	125	134
Time in ER Before Being Evaluated (minutes)	-	-	31	26
Time to Pain Meds for Fractures (minutes)	-	-	45	57
Heart Attack Care				
Aspirin Given at Discharge[5]	-	-	99%	99%
Fibrinolytic Meds Within 30 Min. of Arrival[5]	-	-	-	54%
PCI Within 90 Minutes of Arrival[5]	-	-	96%	96%
Statin Prescribed at Discharge[5]	-	-	99%	98%
Heart Failure Care				
ACE Inhibitor or ARB for LVSD[7]	-	-	96%	97%
Discharge Instructions Given[1]	-	-	93%	94%
Evaluation of LVS Function	12	0%	97%	99%
Medicare Spending				
Medicare Spending per Patient (ratio)	-	-	0.9	0.98
Pneumonia Care				
Appropriate Initial Antibiotic Given[1]	-	-	94%	95%
Blood Culture Timing[1]	-	-	97%	98%
Pregnancy and Delivery Care				
Newborn Deliveries Scheduled Early[5]	-	-	5%	6%
Preventive Care				
Immunization for Influenza	77	82%	89%	90%
Immunization for Pneumonia	115	77%	89%	92%
Stroke Care				
Anticoagulation Therapy for Atrial Fibrillation[5]	-	-	96%	95%
Antithrombotic Therapy Timing[5]	-	-	98%	98%
Assessed for Rehabilitation[5]	-	-	98%	97%
Discharged on Antithrombotic Therapy[5]	-	-	99%	99%
Discharged on Statin Medication[5]	-	-	95%	94%
Thrombolytic Therapy Timing[5]	-	-	74%	66%
Venous Thromboembolism Prophylaxis[5]	-	-	95%	94%
Written Stroke Educational Materials Given[5]	-	-	88%	88%
Surgical Care Improvement Project				
Appropriate Beta Blocker Usage[5]	-	-	98%	98%
Appropriate VTP Within 24 Hours[5]	-	-	98%	98%
Controlled Postoperative Blood Glucose[5]	-	-	97%	97%
Perioperative Temperature Management[5]	-	-	99%	100%
Prophylactic Antibiotic Selection[5]	-	-	99%	99%
Prophylactic Antibiotic Selection (Outpatient)	-	-	98%	98%
Prophylactic Antibiotic Stopped[5]	-	-	99%	98%
Prophylactic Antibiotic Timing[5]	-	-	98%	99%
Prophylactic Antibiotic Timing (Outpatient)	-	-	97%	98%
Urinary Catheter Removal[5]	-	-	97%	97%
Survey of Patients' Hospital Experiences				
Area Around Room 'Always' Quiet at Night[5]	-	-	65%	61%
Doctors 'Always' Communicated Well[5]	-	-	84%	82%
Home Recovery Information Given[5]	-	-	88%	85%
Hospital Given 9 or 10 on 10 Point Scale[5]	-	-	74%	71%
Meds 'Always' Explained Before Given[5]	-	-	67%	64%
Nurses 'Always' Communicated Well[5]	-	-	81%	79%
Pain 'Always' Well Controlled[5]	-	-	72%	71%
Room and Bathroom 'Always' Clean[5]	-	-	78%	73%
Timely Help 'Always' Received[5]	-	-	74%	68%
Would Definitely Recommend Hospital[5]	-	-	71%	71%
Use of Medical Imaging				
Cardiac Imaging Stress Test before Surgery	-	-	6.3%	5.3%
Combination Abdominal CT Scan	-	-	5.7%	10.5%
Combination Brain/Sinus CT Scan	-	-	2.3%	2.7%
Combination Chest CT Scan	-	-	1.9%	2.7%
Follow-up Mammogram/Ultrasound	-	-	6.3%	8.8%
Lumbar Spine MRI for Low Back Pain	-	-	37.6%	37.2%

Lakewood Health Center

600 Main Ave S
Baudette, MN 56623
Phone: 218-634-2120
Fax: 218-634-1307

Type: Critical Access Hospitals
Emergency Services: Yes
Ownership: Voluntary non-profit - Church
Beds: 15

Key Personnel:
CEO/President. . . . . SharRay Feickert
Quality Assurance . . . . Tom Mio
Chief of Medical Staff. . . . . Robert Rayer, MD

Measure	Cases	This Hosp.	State Avg.	U.S. Avg.
Blood Clot Prevention and Treatment				
Anticoagulation Overlap Therapy[5]	-	-	96%	93%
ICU Venous Thromboembolism Prophylaxis[5]	-	-	91%	92%
Incidence of Potentially Preventable VTE[5]	-	-	9%	10%
UFH with Dosages/Platelet Monitoring[5]	-	-	98%	97%
Venous Thromboembolism Prophylaxis[5]	-	-	86%	85%
Warfarin Therapy Discharge Instructions[5]	-	-	63%	75%
Chest Pain/Possible Heart Attack Care				
Aspirin Given Within 24 Hours of Arrival[1,3]	-	-	97%	96%
Fibrinolytic Meds Within 30 Min. of Arrival[3,7]	-	-	48%	58%
Average Time to ECG (minutes)[1,3]	-	-	7	7
Average Time to Transfer (minutes)[3,7]	-	-	54	60
Children's Asthma Care				
Received Home Management Plan of Care	-	-	-	88%
Received Reliever Medication	-	-	-	100%

NOTE: Hospital profiles are in alphabetical order by state, then city, then hospital within the city; Rankings exclude hospitals with less than 25 cases except for patient surveys which excludes hospitals with less than 100 cases; (a) 100-299 cases; (1) The number of cases/patients is too few to report; (2) Data submitted were based on a sample of cases/patients; (3) Results are based on a shorter time period than required; (4) Data suppressed by CMS for one or more quarters; (5) Results are not available for this reporting period; (6) Fewer than 100 patients completed the HCAHPS survey; (7) No cases met the criteria for this measure; (8) The lower limit of the confidence interval cannot be calculated if the number of observed infections equals zero; (9) No data are available from the state/territory for this reporting period; (10) The scores shown reflect fewer than 50 completed surveys; (11) There were discrepancies in the data collection process; (12) This measure does not apply to this hospital for this reporting period; (13) Results cannot be calculated for this reporting period; (14) The results for this state are combined with nearby states to protect confidentiality; Please refer to the User's Guide for a full explanation of data.

Measure	Cases	This Hosp.	State Avg.	U.S. Avg.
Received Systemic Corticosteroids	-	-	-	100%
Emergency Department				
Admittance Decision Time (minutes)[2]	50	15	62	98
Head CT Results Within 45 Min. of Arrival[5]	-	-	54%	57%
Patients Who Left ER Before Being Seen[5]	-	-	2%	2%
Time from ER Arrival to Admit. (minutes)[2]	75	104	199	274
Time from ER Arrival to Discharge (minutes)[5]	-	-	125	134
Time in ER Before Being Evaluated (minutes)[5]	-	-	31	26
Time to Pain Meds for Fractures (minutes)[5]	-	-	45	57
Heart Attack Care				
Aspirin Given at Discharge[1,3]	-	-	99%	99%
Fibrinolytic Meds Within 30 Min. of Arrival[1,3]	-	-	-	54%
PCI Within 90 Minutes of Arrival[3,7]	-	-	96%	96%
Statin Prescribed at Discharge[1,3]	-	-	99%	98%
Heart Failure Care				
ACE Inhibitor or ARB for LVSD[1]	-	-	96%	97%
Discharge Instructions Given[1]	-	-	93%	94%
Evaluation of LVS Function	14	86%	97%	99%
Medicare Spending				
Medicare Spending per Patient (ratio)	-	-	0.9	0.98
Pneumonia Care				
Appropriate Initial Antibiotic Given[7]	-	-	94%	95%
Blood Culture Timing[7]	-	-	97%	98%
Pregnancy and Delivery Care				
Newborn Deliveries Scheduled Early[5]	-	-	5%	6%
Preventive Care				
Immunization for Influenza[2]	56	84%	89%	90%
Immunization for Pneumonia[2]	89	79%	89%	92%
Stroke Care				
Anticoagulation Therapy for Atrial Fibrillation[5]	-	-	96%	95%
Antithrombotic Therapy Timing[5]	-	-	98%	98%
Assessed for Rehabilitation[5]	-	-	98%	97%
Discharged on Antithrombotic Therapy[5]	-	-	99%	99%
Discharged on Statin Medication[5]	-	-	95%	94%
Thrombolytic Therapy Timing[5]	-	-	74%	66%
Venous Thromboembolism Prophylaxis[5]	-	-	95%	94%
Written Stroke Educational Materials Given[5]	-	-	88%	88%
Surgical Care Improvement Project				
Appropriate Beta Blocker Usage[5]	-	-	98%	98%
Appropriate VTP Within 24 Hours[5]	-	-	98%	98%
Controlled Postoperative Blood Glucose[5]	-	-	97%	97%
Perioperative Temperature Management[5]	-	-	99%	100%
Prophylactic Antibiotic Selection[5]	-	-	99%	99%
Prophylactic Antibiotic Selection (Outpatient)[5]	-	-	98%	98%
Prophylactic Antibiotic Stopped[5]	-	-	99%	98%
Prophylactic Antibiotic Timing[5]	-	-	98%	99%
Prophylactic Antibiotic Timing (Outpatient)[5]	-	-	97%	98%
Urinary Catheter Removal[5]	-	-	97%	97%
Survey of Patients' Hospital Experiences				
Area Around Room 'Always' Quiet at Night[10]	<100	77%	65%	61%
Doctors 'Always' Communicated Well[10]	<100	87%	84%	82%
Home Recovery Information Given[10]	<100	98%	88%	85%
Hospital Given 9 or 10 on 10 Point Scale[10]	<100	89%	74%	71%
Meds 'Always' Explained Before Given[10]	<100	99%	67%	64%
Nurses 'Always' Communicated Well[10]	<100	87%	81%	79%
Pain 'Always' Well Controlled[10]	<100	92%	72%	71%
Room and Bathroom 'Always' Clean[10]	<100	90%	78%	73%
Timely Help 'Always' Received[10]	<100	90%	74%	68%
Would Definitely Recommend Hospital[10]	<100	87%	71%	71%
Use of Medical Imaging				
Cardiac Imaging Stress Test before Surgery[1]	-	-	6.3%	5.3%
Combination Abdominal CT Scan[1]	-	-	5.7%	10.5%
Combination Brain/Sinus CT Scan[1]	-	-	2.3%	2.7%
Combination Chest CT Scan[1]	-	-	1.9%	2.7%
Follow-up Mammogram/Ultrasound	76	3.9%	6.3%	8.8%
Lumbar Spine MRI for Low Back Pain[1]	-	-	37.6%	37.2%

Sanford Bemidji Medical Center

1300 Anne Saint Nw
Bemidji, MN 56601
Phone: 218-751-5430
Fax: 218-333-5880
URL: www.nchs.com
Type: Acute Care Hospitals
Emergency Services: Yes
Ownership: Voluntary non-profit - Private
Beds: 184

Key Personnel:
Chief of Medical Staff.......... Daniel P DeKrey
Coronary Care............... Kathryn Edwards-Olson
Infection Control............. Wendy Gullicksrad
Quality Assurance .... Wendy Gullicksrad
Radiology.................. Ravishankar Konchada
CEO/President............... Kelby K. Krabbenhoft
Pediatric In-Patient Care .... Shannon Rankin, RN

Measure	Cases	This Hosp.	State Avg.	U.S. Avg.
Blood Clot Prevention and Treatment				
Anticoagulation Overlap Therapy[2]	16	100%	96%	93%
ICU Venous Thromboembolism Prophylaxis[2]	92	77%	91%	92%
Incidence of Potentially Preventable VTE[1,2]	-	-	9%	10%
UFH with Dosages/Platelet Monitoring[1,2]	-	-	98%	97%
Venous Thromboembolism Prophylaxis[2]	274	81%	86%	85%
Warfarin Therapy Discharge Instructions[2]	15	33%	63%	75%
Chest Pain/Possible Heart Attack Care				
Aspirin Given Within 24 Hours of Arrival[3]	19	100%	97%	96%
Fibrinolytic Meds Within 30 Min. of Arrival[3,7]	-	-	48%	58%
Average Time to ECG (minutes)[3]	18	8	7	7
Average Time to Transfer (minutes)[1,3]	-	-	54	60
Children's Asthma Care				
Received Home Management Plan of Care	-	-	-	88%
Received Reliever Medication	-	-	-	100%
Received Systemic Corticosteroids	-	-	-	100%
Emergency Department				
Admittance Decision Time (minutes)[2]	347	55	62	98
Head CT Results Within 45 Min. of Arrival[1]	-	-	54%	57%
Patients Who Left ER Before Being Seen	27,893	0%	2%	2%
Time from ER Arrival to Admit. (minutes)[2]	398	206	199	274
Time from ER Arrival to Discharge (minutes)	456	107	125	134
Time in ER Before Being Evaluated (minutes)	149	21	31	26
Time to Pain Meds for Fractures (minutes)	109	57	45	57
Heart Attack Care				
Aspirin Given at Discharge	96	97%	99%	99%
Fibrinolytic Meds Within 30 Min. of Arrival[7]	-	-	-	54%
PCI Within 90 Minutes of Arrival	11	73%	96%	96%
Statin Prescribed at Discharge	94	95%	99%	98%
Heart Failure Care				
ACE Inhibitor or ARB for LVSD	31	100%	96%	97%
Discharge Instructions Given	95	77%	93%	94%
Evaluation of LVS Function	122	98%	97%	99%
Medicare Spending				
Medicare Spending per Patient (ratio)	-	0.88	0.9	0.98
Pneumonia Care				
Appropriate Initial Antibiotic Given	66	100%	94%	95%
Blood Culture Timing	113	95%	97%	98%
Pregnancy and Delivery Care				
Newborn Deliveries Scheduled Early	90	1%	5%	6%
Preventive Care				
Immunization for Influenza[2]	505	94%	89%	90%
Immunization for Pneumonia[2]	590	93%	89%	92%
Stroke Care				
Anticoagulation Therapy for Atrial Fibrillation[1]	-	-	96%	95%
Antithrombotic Therapy Timing	43	98%	98%	98%
Assessed for Rehabilitation	50	94%	98%	97%
Discharged on Antithrombotic Therapy	43	88%	99%	99%
Discharged on Statin Medication	34	71%	95%	94%
Thrombolytic Therapy Timing[1]	-	-	74%	66%
Venous Thromboembolism Prophylaxis	49	86%	95%	94%
Written Stroke Educational Materials Given	20	0%	88%	88%
Surgical Care Improvement Project				
Appropriate Beta Blocker Usage	182	97%	98%	98%
Appropriate VTP Within 24 Hours	483	95%	98%	98%
Controlled Postoperative Blood Glucose[7]	-	-	97%	97%
Perioperative Temperature Management	595	99%	99%	100%
Prophylactic Antibiotic Selection	476	95%	99%	99%
Prophylactic Antibiotic Selection (Outpatient)	60	98%	98%	98%
Prophylactic Antibiotic Stopped	463	96%	99%	98%
Prophylactic Antibiotic Timing	476	98%	98%	99%
Prophylactic Antibiotic Timing (Outpatient)	53	85%	97%	98%
Urinary Catheter Removal	309	94%	97%	97%
Survey of Patients' Hospital Experiences				
Area Around Room 'Always' Quiet at Night	300+	55%	65%	61%
Doctors 'Always' Communicated Well	300+	79%	84%	82%
Home Recovery Information Given	300+	81%	88%	85%
Hospital Given 9 or 10 on 10 Point Scale	300+	59%	74%	71%
Meds 'Always' Explained Before Given	300+	57%	67%	64%
Nurses 'Always' Communicated Well	300+	72%	81%	79%
Pain 'Always' Well Controlled	300+	66%	72%	71%
Room and Bathroom 'Always' Clean	300+	66%	78%	73%
Timely Help 'Always' Received	300+	61%	74%	68%
Would Definitely Recommend Hospital	300+	62%	71%	71%
Use of Medical Imaging				
Cardiac Imaging Stress Test before Surgery	198	3.0%	6.3%	5.3%
Combination Abdominal CT Scan	595	7.1%	5.7%	10.5%
Combination Brain/Sinus CT Scan[1]	-	-	2.3%	2.7%
Combination Chest CT Scan	413	0.2%	1.9%	2.7%
Follow-up Mammogram/Ultrasound[1]	-	-	6.3%	8.8%
Lumbar Spine MRI for Low Back Pain	100	34.0%	37.6%	37.2%

Swift County Benson Hospital

1815 Wisconsin Avenue
Benson, MN 56215
Phone: 320-843-4232
Fax: 320-843-4172
URL: www.scbh.org
Type: Critical Access Hospitals
Emergency Services: Yes
Ownership: Govt - Hospital Dist/Auth
Beds: 31

Key Personnel:
Emergency Room .... Roberta Carter
Operating Room.............. Helan Clauseen, RN
Quality Assurance .... Stella Kalthoff
CEO .... Frank Lawatsch
Infection Control.............. Holly Rodahl, RN

Measure	Cases	This Hosp.	State Avg.	U.S. Avg.
Blood Clot Prevention and Treatment				
Anticoagulation Overlap Therapy[5]	-	-	96%	93%
ICU Venous Thromboembolism Prophylaxis[5]	-	-	91%	92%
Incidence of Potentially Preventable VTE[5]	-	-	9%	10%
UFH with Dosages/Platelet Monitoring[5]	-	-	98%	97%
Venous Thromboembolism Prophylaxis[5]	-	-	86%	85%
Warfarin Therapy Discharge Instructions[5]	-	-	63%	75%
Chest Pain/Possible Heart Attack Care				
Aspirin Given Within 24 Hours of Arrival	12	100%	97%	96%
Fibrinolytic Meds Within 30 Min. of Arrival[3,7]	-	-	48%	58%
Average Time to ECG (minutes)	13	5	7	7
Average Time to Transfer (minutes)[3,7]	-	-	54	60
Children's Asthma Care				
Received Home Management Plan of Care	-	-	-	88%
Received Reliever Medication	-	-	-	100%
Received Systemic Corticosteroids	-	-	-	100%
Emergency Department				
Admittance Decision Time (minutes)	66	0	62	98
Head CT Results Within 45 Min. of Arrival[5]	-	-	54%	57%
Patients Who Left ER Before Being Seen[5]	-	-	2%	2%
Time from ER Arrival to Admit. (minutes)	72	103	199	274
Time from ER Arrival to Discharge (minutes)[5]	-	-	125	134
Time in ER Before Being Evaluated (minutes)[5]	-	-	31	26
Time to Pain Meds for Fractures (minutes)[5]	-	-	45	57
Heart Attack Care				
Aspirin Given at Discharge[1,3]	-	-	99%	99%
Fibrinolytic Meds Within 30 Min. of Arrival[3,7]	-	-	-	54%
PCI Within 90 Minutes of Arrival[3,7]	-	-	96%	96%
Statin Prescribed at Discharge[1,3]	-	-	99%	98%
Heart Failure Care				
ACE Inhibitor or ARB for LVSD[1]	-	-	96%	97%
Discharge Instructions Given[1]	-	-	93%	94%
Evaluation of LVS Function	14	36%	97%	99%
Medicare Spending				
Medicare Spending per Patient (ratio)	-	-	0.9	0.98
Pneumonia Care				
Appropriate Initial Antibiotic Given[1]	-	-	94%	95%

NOTE: Hospital profiles are in alphabetical order by state, then city, then hospital within the city; Rankings exclude hospitals with less than 25 cases except for patient surveys which excludes hospitals with less than 100 cases; (a) 100-299 cases; (1) The number of cases/patients is too few to report; (2) Data submitted were based on a sample of cases/patients; (3) Results are based on a shorter time period than required; (4) Data suppressed by CMS for one or more quarters; (5) Results are not available for this reporting period; (6) Fewer than 100 patients completed the HCAHPS survey; (7) No cases met the criteria for this measure; (8) The lower limit of the confidence interval cannot be calculated if the number of observed infections equals zero; (9) No data are available from the state/territory for this reporting period; (10) The scores shown reflect fewer than 50 completed surveys; (11) There were discrepancies in the data collection process; (12) This measure does not apply to this hospital for this reporting period; (13) Results cannot be calculated for this reporting period; (14) The results for this state are combined with nearby states to protect confidentiality; Please refer to the User's Guide for a full explanation of data.

Blood Culture Timing[1]	-	-	97%	98%
Pregnancy and Delivery Care				
Newborn Deliveries Scheduled Early[5]	-	-	5%	6%
Preventive Care				
Immunization for Influenza	134	66%	89%	90%
Immunization for Pneumonia	198	80%	89%	92%
Stroke Care				
Anticoagulation Therapy for Atrial Fibrillation[5]	-	-	96%	95%
Antithrombotic Therapy Timing[5]	-	-	98%	98%
Assessed for Rehabilitation[5]	-	-	98%	97%
Discharged on Antithrombotic Therapy[5]	-	-	99%	99%
Discharged on Statin Medication[5]	-	-	95%	94%
Thrombolytic Therapy Timing[5]	-	-	74%	66%
Venous Thromboembolism Prophylaxis[5]	-	-	95%	94%
Written Stroke Educational Materials Given[5]	-	-	88%	88%
Surgical Care Improvement Project				
Appropriate Beta Blocker Usage[1]	-	-	98%	98%
Appropriate VTP Within 24 Hours	20	100%	98%	98%
Controlled Postoperative Blood Glucose[7]	-	-	97%	97%
Perioperative Temperature Management[1]	-	-	99%	100%
Prophylactic Antibiotic Selection	20	100%	99%	99%
Prophylactic Antibiotic Selection (Outpatient)[5]	-	-	98%	98%
Prophylactic Antibiotic Stopped	20	100%	99%	98%
Prophylactic Antibiotic Timing	20	100%	98%	99%
Prophylactic Antibiotic Timing (Outpatient)[5]	-	-	97%	98%
Urinary Catheter Removal	20	100%	97%	97%
Survey of Patients' Hospital Experiences				
Area Around Room 'Always' Quiet at Night[11]	(a)	68%	65%	61%
Doctors 'Always' Communicated Well[11]	(a)	86%	84%	82%
Home Recovery Information Given[11]	(a)	88%	88%	85%
Hospital Given 9 or 10 on 10 Point Scale[11]	(a)	72%	74%	71%
Meds 'Always' Explained Before Given[11]	(a)	72%	67%	64%
Nurses 'Always' Communicated Well[11]	(a)	80%	81%	79%
Pain 'Always' Well Controlled[11]	(a)	72%	72%	71%
Room and Bathroom 'Always' Clean[11]	(a)	81%	78%	73%
Timely Help 'Always' Received[11]	(a)	83%	74%	68%
Would Definitely Recommend Hospital[11]	(a)	48%	71%	71%
Use of Medical Imaging				
Cardiac Imaging Stress Test before Surgery[1]	-	-	6.3%	5.3%
Combination Abdominal CT Scan[1]	-	-	5.7%	10.5%
Combination Brain/Sinus CT Scan	34	0.0%	2.3%	2.7%
Combination Chest CT Scan[1]	-	-	1.9%	2.7%
Follow-up Mammogram/Ultrasound	100	7.0%	6.3%	8.8%
Lumbar Spine MRI for Low Back Pain[1]	-	-	37.6%	37.2%

Bigfork Valley Hospital

258 Pine Tree Drive PO Box 258
Bigfork, MN 56628
Phone: 218-743-3177
Fax: 218-743-3559
E-mail: wecare@bigforkvalley.org
URL: www.bigforkvalley.org
Type: Critical Access Hospitals
Emergency Services: Yes
Ownership: Govt - Hospital Dist/Auth
Beds: 20

Key Personnel:
CEO . . . . Dan Odegaard
Chief of Medical Staff . . . . George Rounds

Measure	Cases	This Hosp.	State Avg.	U.S. Avg.
Blood Clot Prevention and Treatment				
Anticoagulation Overlap Therapy[1,2]	-	-	96%	93%
ICU Venous Thromboembolism Prophylaxis[2,7]	-	-	91%	92%
Incidence of Potentially Preventable VTE[2,7]	-	-	9%	10%
UFH with Dosages/Platelet Monitoring[1,2]	-	-	98%	97%
Venous Thromboembolism Prophylaxis[2]	110	99%	86%	85%
Warfarin Therapy Discharge Instructions[2,7]	-	-	63%	75%
Chest Pain/Possible Heart Attack Care				
Aspirin Given Within 24 Hours of Arrival	23	100%	97%	96%
Fibrinolytic Meds Within 30 Min. of Arrival[1,3]	-	-	48%	58%
Average Time to ECG (minutes)	24	10	7	7
Average Time to Transfer (minutes)[3,7]	-	-	54	60
Children's Asthma Care				
Received Home Management Plan of Care	-	-	-	88%
Received Reliever Medication	-	-	-	100%
Received Systemic Corticosteroids	-	-	-	100%
Emergency Department				
Admittance Decision Time (minutes)	86	11	62	98
Head CT Results Within 45 Min. of Arrival[3,7]	-	-	54%	57%
Patients Who Left ER Before Being Seen[5]	-	-	2%	2%
Time from ER Arrival to Admit. (minutes)	138	105	199	274
Time from ER Arrival to Discharge (minutes)	119	89	125	134
Time in ER Before Being Evaluated (minutes)	230	10	31	26
Time to Pain Meds for Fractures (minutes)[1,3]	-	-	45	57
Heart Attack Care				
Aspirin Given at Discharge[1,3]	-	-	99%	99%
Fibrinolytic Meds Within 30 Min. of Arrival[3,7]	-	-	-	54%
PCI Within 90 Minutes of Arrival[5]	-	-	96%	96%
Statin Prescribed at Discharge[1,3]	-	-	99%	98%
Heart Failure Care				
ACE Inhibitor or ARB for LVSD[1]	-	-	96%	97%
Discharge Instructions Given[1]	-	-	93%	94%
Evaluation of LVS Function[1]	-	-	97%	99%
Medicare Spending				
Medicare Spending per Patient (ratio)	-	-	0.9	0.98
Pneumonia Care				
Appropriate Initial Antibiotic Given	12	92%	94%	95%
Blood Culture Timing[1]	-	-	97%	98%
Pregnancy and Delivery Care				
Newborn Deliveries Scheduled Early[5]	-	-	5%	6%
Preventive Care				
Immunization for Influenza	148	92%	89%	90%
Immunization for Pneumonia	219	89%	89%	92%
Stroke Care				
Anticoagulation Therapy for Atrial Fibrillation[5]	-	-	96%	95%
Antithrombotic Therapy Timing[5]	-	-	98%	98%
Assessed for Rehabilitation[5]	-	-	98%	97%
Discharged on Antithrombotic Therapy[5]	-	-	99%	99%
Discharged on Statin Medication[5]	-	-	95%	94%
Thrombolytic Therapy Timing[5]	-	-	74%	66%
Venous Thromboembolism Prophylaxis[5]	-	-	95%	94%
Written Stroke Educational Materials Given[5]	-	-	88%	88%
Surgical Care Improvement Project				
Appropriate Beta Blocker Usage	20	90%	98%	98%
Appropriate VTP Within 24 Hours	73	100%	98%	98%
Controlled Postoperative Blood Glucose[3,7]	-	-	97%	97%
Perioperative Temperature Management	79	100%	99%	100%
Prophylactic Antibiotic Selection	77	100%	99%	99%
Prophylactic Antibiotic Selection (Outpatient)[5]	-	-	98%	98%
Prophylactic Antibiotic Stopped	76	100%	99%	98%
Prophylactic Antibiotic Timing	77	95%	98%	99%
Prophylactic Antibiotic Timing (Outpatient)[5]	-	-	97%	98%
Urinary Catheter Removal	75	100%	97%	97%
Survey of Patients' Hospital Experiences				
Area Around Room 'Always' Quiet at Night[11]	(a)	74%	65%	61%
Doctors 'Always' Communicated Well[11]	(a)	93%	84%	82%
Home Recovery Information Given[11]	(a)	95%	88%	85%
Hospital Given 9 or 10 on 10 Point Scale[11]	(a)	89%	74%	71%
Meds 'Always' Explained Before Given[11]	(a)	81%	67%	64%
Nurses 'Always' Communicated Well[11]	(a)	93%	81%	79%
Pain 'Always' Well Controlled[11]	(a)	85%	72%	71%
Room and Bathroom 'Always' Clean[11]	(a)	91%	78%	73%
Timely Help 'Always' Received[11]	(a)	95%	74%	68%
Would Definitely Recommend Hospital[11]	(a)	62%	71%	71%
Use of Medical Imaging				
Cardiac Imaging Stress Test before Surgery[7]	-	-	6.3%	5.3%
Combination Abdominal CT Scan[1]	-	-	5.7%	10.5%
Combination Brain/Sinus CT Scan[1]	-	-	2.3%	2.7%
Combination Chest CT Scan[1]	-	-	1.9%	2.7%
Follow-up Mammogram/Ultrasound	72	9.7%	6.3%	8.8%
Lumbar Spine MRI for Low Back Pain[1]	-	-	37.6%	37.2%

United Hospital District

515 South Moore Street, PO Box 160
Blue Earth, MN 56013
Phone: 507-526-3273
Fax: 507-526-3621
URL: www.uhd.org
Type: Critical Access Hospitals
Emergency Services: Yes
Ownership: Govt - Hospital Dist/Auth
Beds: 43

Key Personnel:
Chief of Medical Staff . . . . Kevin Kimm, DO
Infection Control . . . . Pam Manzke
Quality Assurance . . . . Pam Manzle
Operating Room. . . . . Melissa Storbeck
Surgery . . . . Alex Wong, MD

Measure	Cases	This Hosp.	State Avg.	U.S. Avg.
Blood Clot Prevention and Treatment				
Anticoagulation Overlap Therapy[5]	-	-	96%	93%
ICU Venous Thromboembolism Prophylaxis[5]	-	-	91%	92%
Incidence of Potentially Preventable VTE[5]	-	-	9%	10%
UFH with Dosages/Platelet Monitoring[5]	-	-	98%	97%
Venous Thromboembolism Prophylaxis[5]	-	-	86%	85%
Warfarin Therapy Discharge Instructions[5]	-	-	63%	75%
Chest Pain/Possible Heart Attack Care				
Aspirin Given Within 24 Hours of Arrival	32	94%	97%	96%
Fibrinolytic Meds Within 30 Min. of Arrival[1]	-	-	48%	58%
Average Time to ECG (minutes)	33	5	7	7
Average Time to Transfer (minutes)[7]	-	-	54	60
Children's Asthma Care				
Received Home Management Plan of Care	-	-	-	88%
Received Reliever Medication	-	-	-	100%
Received Systemic Corticosteroids	-	-	-	100%
Emergency Department				
Admittance Decision Time (minutes)	315	0	62	98
Head CT Results Within 45 Min. of Arrival[5]	-	-	54%	57%
Patients Who Left ER Before Being Seen[5]	-	-	2%	2%
Time from ER Arrival to Admit. (minutes)	316	168	199	274
Time from ER Arrival to Discharge (minutes)[5]	-	-	125	134
Time in ER Before Being Evaluated (minutes)[5]	-	-	31	26
Time to Pain Meds for Fractures (minutes)[5]	-	-	45	57
Heart Attack Care				
Aspirin Given at Discharge[1,3]	-	-	99%	99%
Fibrinolytic Meds Within 30 Min. of Arrival[3,7]	-	-	-	54%
PCI Within 90 Minutes of Arrival[3,7]	-	-	96%	96%
Statin Prescribed at Discharge[1,3]	-	-	99%	98%
Heart Failure Care				
ACE Inhibitor or ARB for LVSD[1]	-	-	96%	97%
Discharge Instructions Given[1]	-	-	93%	94%
Evaluation of LVS Function	16	88%	97%	99%
Medicare Spending				
Medicare Spending per Patient (ratio)	-	-	0.9	0.98
Pneumonia Care				
Appropriate Initial Antibiotic Given[1,3]	-	-	94%	95%
Blood Culture Timing	17	94%	97%	98%
Pregnancy and Delivery Care				
Newborn Deliveries Scheduled Early[1]	-	-	5%	6%
Preventive Care				
Immunization for Influenza	260	87%	89%	90%
Immunization for Pneumonia	335	85%	89%	92%
Stroke Care				
Anticoagulation Therapy for Atrial Fibrillation[5]	-	-	96%	95%
Antithrombotic Therapy Timing[5]	-	-	98%	98%
Assessed for Rehabilitation[5]	-	-	98%	97%
Discharged on Antithrombotic Therapy[5]	-	-	99%	99%
Discharged on Statin Medication[5]	-	-	95%	94%
Thrombolytic Therapy Timing[5]	-	-	74%	66%
Venous Thromboembolism Prophylaxis[5]	-	-	95%	94%
Written Stroke Educational Materials Given[5]	-	-	88%	88%
Surgical Care Improvement Project				
Appropriate Beta Blocker Usage	17	94%	98%	98%
Appropriate VTP Within 24 Hours	53	89%	98%	98%
Controlled Postoperative Blood Glucose[3,7]	-	-	97%	97%
Perioperative Temperature Management	55	100%	99%	100%
Prophylactic Antibiotic Selection	39	100%	99%	99%
Prophylactic Antibiotic Selection (Outpatient)[1,3]	-	-	98%	98%
Prophylactic Antibiotic Stopped	39	82%	99%	98%
Prophylactic Antibiotic Timing	39	77%	98%	99%
Prophylactic Antibiotic Timing (Outpatient)[1,3]	-	-	97%	98%
Urinary Catheter Removal	19	89%	97%	97%
Survey of Patients' Hospital Experiences				
Area Around Room 'Always' Quiet at Night	(a)	75%	65%	61%
Doctors 'Always' Communicated Well	(a)	91%	84%	82%
Home Recovery Information Given	(a)	82%	88%	85%
Hospital Given 9 or 10 on 10 Point Scale	(a)	76%	74%	71%

NOTE: Hospital profiles are in alphabetical order by state, then city, then hospital within the city; Rankings exclude hospitals with less than 25 cases except for patient surveys which excludes hospitals with less than 100 cases; (a) 100-299 cases; (1) The number of cases/patients is too few to report; (2) Data submitted were based on a sample of cases/patients; (3) Results are based on a shorter time period than required; (4) Data suppressed by CMS for one or more quarters; (5) Results are not available for this reporting period; (6) Fewer than 100 patients completed the HCAHPS survey; (7) No cases met the criteria for this measure; (8) The lower limit of the confidence interval cannot be calculated if the number of observed infections equals zero; (9) No data are available from the state/territory for this reporting period; (10) The scores shown reflect fewer than 50 completed surveys; (11) There were discrepancies in the data collection process; (12) This measure does not apply to this hospital for this reporting period; (13) Results cannot be calculated for this reporting period; (14) The results for this state are combined with nearby states to protect confidentiality; Please refer to the User's Guide for a full explanation of data.

Measure	Cases	This Hosp.	State Avg.	U.S. Avg.
Meds 'Always' Explained Before Given	(a)	63%	67%	64%
Nurses 'Always' Communicated Well	(a)	84%	81%	79%
Pain 'Always' Well Controlled	(a)	77%	72%	71%
Room and Bathroom 'Always' Clean	(a)	85%	78%	73%
Timely Help 'Always' Received	(a)	74%	74%	68%
Would Definitely Recommend Hospital	(a)	71%	71%	71%
Use of Medical Imaging				
Cardiac Imaging Stress Test before Surgery[1]	-	-	6.3%	5.3%
Combination Abdominal CT Scan	76	2.6%	5.7%	10.5%
Combination Brain/Sinus CT Scan[1]	-	-	2.3%	2.7%
Combination Chest CT Scan[1]	-	-	1.9%	2.7%
Follow-up Mammogram/Ultrasound	154	4.5%	6.3%	8.8%
Lumbar Spine MRI for Low Back Pain[1]	-	-	37.6%	37.2%

Essentia Health Saint Joseph's Medical Center

523 North 3rd Street
Brainerd, MN 56401
Phone: 218-829-2861
Fax: 218-828-3103
URL: www.sjmcmn.org
Type: Acute Care Hospitals
Emergency Services: Yes
Ownership: Voluntary non-profit - Church
Beds: 162

Key Personnel:
Quality Assurance . . . . Dennis A Acrea
Radiology. . . . . Charles A Benson
Chief of Medical Staff. . . . . Nicholas Bernier
CEO . . . . Peter Person
CEO/President. . . . . Jani Wiebolt

Measure	Cases	This Hosp.	State Avg.	U.S. Avg.
Blood Clot Prevention and Treatment				
Anticoagulation Overlap Therapy[2]	41	98%	96%	93%
ICU Venous Thromboembolism Prophylaxis[2]	30	90%	91%	92%
Incidence of Potentially Preventable VTE[1,2]	-	-	9%	10%
UFH with Dosages/Platelet Monitoring[2]	15	100%	98%	97%
Venous Thromboembolism Prophylaxis[2]	276	87%	86%	85%
Warfarin Therapy Discharge Instructions[2]	35	43%	63%	75%
Chest Pain/Possible Heart Attack Care				
Aspirin Given Within 24 Hours of Arrival	57	100%	97%	96%
Fibrinolytic Meds Within 30 Min. of Arrival[7]	-	-	48%	58%
Average Time to ECG (minutes)	57	10	7	7
Average Time to Transfer (minutes)[1]	-	-	54	60
Children's Asthma Care				
Received Home Management Plan of Care	-	-	-	88%
Received Reliever Medication	-	-	-	100%
Received Systemic Corticosteroids	-	-	-	100%
Emergency Department				
Admittance Decision Time (minutes)[2]	594	37	62	98
Head CT Results Within 45 Min. of Arrival	19	37%	54%	57%
Patients Who Left ER Before Being Seen	24,928	1%	2%	2%
Time from ER Arrival to Admit. (minutes)[2]	595	160	199	274
Time from ER Arrival to Discharge (minutes)	366	112	125	134
Time in ER Before Being Evaluated (minutes)	128	21	31	26
Time to Pain Meds for Fractures (minutes)	101	37	45	57
Heart Attack Care				
Aspirin Given at Discharge	85	94%	99%	99%
Fibrinolytic Meds Within 30 Min. of Arrival[7]	-	-	-	54%
PCI Within 90 Minutes of Arrival[1]	-	-	96%	96%
Statin Prescribed at Discharge	85	95%	99%	98%
Heart Failure Care				
ACE Inhibitor or ARB for LVSD	52	87%	96%	97%
Discharge Instructions Given	178	89%	93%	94%
Evaluation of LVS Function	212	100%	97%	99%
Medicare Spending				
Medicare Spending per Patient (ratio)	-	0.85	0.9	0.98
Pneumonia Care				
Appropriate Initial Antibiotic Given	92	97%	94%	95%
Blood Culture Timing	135	99%	97%	98%
Pregnancy and Delivery Care				
Newborn Deliveries Scheduled Early	28	4%	5%	6%
Preventive Care				
Immunization for Influenza[2]	536	99%	89%	90%
Immunization for Pneumonia[2]	673	99%	89%	92%
Stroke Care				
Anticoagulation Therapy for Atrial Fibrillation	15	100%	96%	95%
Antithrombotic Therapy Timing	47	98%	98%	98%
Assessed for Rehabilitation	61	92%	98%	97%
Discharged on Antithrombotic Therapy	61	100%	99%	99%
Discharged on Statin Medication	51	88%	95%	94%
Thrombolytic Therapy Timing[1]	-	-	74%	66%
Venous Thromboembolism Prophylaxis	47	94%	95%	94%
Written Stroke Educational Materials Given	40	80%	88%	88%
Surgical Care Improvement Project				
Appropriate Beta Blocker Usage[2]	90	96%	98%	98%
Appropriate VTP Within 24 Hours[2]	291	100%	98%	98%
Controlled Postoperative Blood Glucose[2,7]	-	-	97%	97%
Perioperative Temperature Management[2]	321	100%	99%	100%
Prophylactic Antibiotic Selection[2]	203	99%	99%	99%
Prophylactic Antibiotic Selection (Outpatient)	163	92%	98%	98%
Prophylactic Antibiotic Stopped[2]	201	98%	99%	98%
Prophylactic Antibiotic Timing[2]	204	99%	98%	99%
Prophylactic Antibiotic Timing (Outpatient)	115	87%	97%	98%
Urinary Catheter Removal[2]	93	97%	97%	97%
Survey of Patients' Hospital Experiences				
Area Around Room 'Always' Quiet at Night	300+	62%	65%	61%
Doctors 'Always' Communicated Well	300+	82%	84%	82%
Home Recovery Information Given	300+	91%	88%	85%
Hospital Given 9 or 10 on 10 Point Scale	300+	75%	74%	71%
Meds 'Always' Explained Before Given	300+	67%	67%	64%
Nurses 'Always' Communicated Well	300+	82%	81%	79%
Pain 'Always' Well Controlled	300+	75%	72%	71%
Room and Bathroom 'Always' Clean	300+	77%	78%	73%
Timely Help 'Always' Received	300+	73%	74%	68%
Would Definitely Recommend Hospital	300+	74%	71%	71%
Use of Medical Imaging				
Cardiac Imaging Stress Test before Surgery	221	7.2%	6.3%	5.3%
Combination Abdominal CT Scan	431	5.8%	5.7%	10.5%
Combination Brain/Sinus CT Scan[1]	-	-	2.3%	2.7%
Combination Chest CT Scan	319	0.0%	1.9%	2.7%
Follow-up Mammogram/Ultrasound	1,105	6.0%	6.3%	8.8%
Lumbar Spine MRI for Low Back Pain	81	33.3%	37.6%	37.2%

Saint Francis Medical Center

2400 Saint Francis Drive
Breckenridge, MN 56520
Phone: 218-643-3000
Fax: 218-643-7502
URL: www.sfcare.org
Type: Critical Access Hospitals
Emergency Services: Yes
Ownership: Voluntary non-profit - Church
Beds: 42

Key Personnel:
Quality Assurance . . . . Mary Helland
Radiology. . . . . Lawrence Licht, MD
CEO/President. . . . . David Nelson

Measure	Cases	This Hosp.	State Avg.	U.S. Avg.
Blood Clot Prevention and Treatment				
Anticoagulation Overlap Therapy[5]	-	-	96%	93%
ICU Venous Thromboembolism Prophylaxis[5]	-	-	91%	92%
Incidence of Potentially Preventable VTE[5]	-	-	9%	10%
UFH with Dosages/Platelet Monitoring[5]	-	-	98%	97%
Venous Thromboembolism Prophylaxis[5]	-	-	86%	85%
Warfarin Therapy Discharge Instructions[5]	-	-	63%	75%
Chest Pain/Possible Heart Attack Care				
Aspirin Given Within 24 Hours of Arrival	15	100%	97%	96%
Fibrinolytic Meds Within 30 Min. of Arrival[7]	-	-	48%	58%
Average Time to ECG (minutes)	17	8	7	7
Average Time to Transfer (minutes)[1]	-	-	54	60
Children's Asthma Care				
Received Home Management Plan of Care	-	-	-	88%
Received Reliever Medication	-	-	-	100%
Received Systemic Corticosteroids	-	-	-	100%
Emergency Department				
Admittance Decision Time (minutes)[2]	174	24	62	98
Head CT Results Within 45 Min. of Arrival[5]	-	-	54%	57%
Patients Who Left ER Before Being Seen	5,106	0%	2%	2%
Time from ER Arrival to Admit. (minutes)[2]	204	155	199	274
Time from ER Arrival to Discharge (minutes)[5]	-	-	125	134
Time in ER Before Being Evaluated (minutes)[5]	-	-	31	26
Time to Pain Meds for Fractures (minutes)[5]	-	-	45	57
Heart Attack Care				
Aspirin Given at Discharge[1]	-	-	99%	99%
Fibrinolytic Meds Within 30 Min. of Arrival[7]	-	-	-	54%
PCI Within 90 Minutes of Arrival[7]	-	-	96%	96%
Statin Prescribed at Discharge[1]	-	-	99%	98%
Heart Failure Care				
ACE Inhibitor or ARB for LVSD[1,2]	-	-	96%	97%
Discharge Instructions Given[2]	20	95%	93%	94%
Evaluation of LVS Function[2]	31	97%	97%	99%
Medicare Spending				
Medicare Spending per Patient (ratio)	-	-	0.9	0.98
Pneumonia Care				
Appropriate Initial Antibiotic Given[2]	42	98%	94%	95%
Blood Culture Timing[2]	25	100%	97%	98%
Pregnancy and Delivery Care				
Newborn Deliveries Scheduled Early[5]	-	-	5%	6%
Preventive Care				
Immunization for Influenza[2]	246	89%	89%	90%
Immunization for Pneumonia[2]	295	92%	89%	92%
Stroke Care				
Anticoagulation Therapy for Atrial Fibrillation[5]	-	-	96%	95%
Antithrombotic Therapy Timing[5]	-	-	98%	98%
Assessed for Rehabilitation[5]	-	-	98%	97%
Discharged on Antithrombotic Therapy[5]	-	-	99%	99%
Discharged on Statin Medication[5]	-	-	95%	94%
Thrombolytic Therapy Timing[5]	-	-	74%	66%
Venous Thromboembolism Prophylaxis[5]	-	-	95%	94%
Written Stroke Educational Materials Given[5]	-	-	88%	88%
Surgical Care Improvement Project				
Appropriate Beta Blocker Usage	16	81%	98%	98%
Appropriate VTP Within 24 Hours	48	90%	98%	98%
Controlled Postoperative Blood Glucose[7]	-	-	97%	97%
Perioperative Temperature Management	54	100%	99%	100%
Prophylactic Antibiotic Selection	29	100%	99%	99%
Prophylactic Antibiotic Selection (Outpatient)[5]	-	-	98%	98%
Prophylactic Antibiotic Stopped	27	96%	99%	98%
Prophylactic Antibiotic Timing	29	97%	98%	99%
Prophylactic Antibiotic Timing (Outpatient)[5]	-	-	97%	98%
Urinary Catheter Removal	37	100%	97%	97%
Survey of Patients' Hospital Experiences				
Area Around Room 'Always' Quiet at Night	(a)	61%	65%	61%
Doctors 'Always' Communicated Well	(a)	87%	84%	82%
Home Recovery Information Given	(a)	90%	88%	85%
Hospital Given 9 or 10 on 10 Point Scale	(a)	72%	74%	71%
Meds 'Always' Explained Before Given	(a)	70%	67%	64%
Nurses 'Always' Communicated Well	(a)	78%	81%	79%
Pain 'Always' Well Controlled	(a)	73%	72%	71%
Room and Bathroom 'Always' Clean	(a)	76%	78%	73%
Timely Help 'Always' Received	(a)	72%	74%	68%
Would Definitely Recommend Hospital	(a)	69%	71%	71%
Use of Medical Imaging				
Cardiac Imaging Stress Test before Surgery[7]	-	-	6.3%	5.3%
Combination Abdominal CT Scan	139	6.5%	5.7%	10.5%
Combination Brain/Sinus CT Scan	162	0.0%	2.3%	2.7%
Combination Chest CT Scan	65	4.6%	1.9%	2.7%
Follow-up Mammogram/Ultrasound	112	10.7%	6.3%	8.8%
Lumbar Spine MRI for Low Back Pain[1]	-	-	37.6%	37.2%

Buffalo Hospital

303 Catlin St
Buffalo, MN 55313
Phone: 763-684-1212
Fax: 763-684-7104
URL: www.buffalohospital.org
Type: Acute Care Hospitals
Emergency Services: Yes
Ownership: Voluntary non-profit - Other
Beds: 65

Key Personnel:
Patient Relations . . . . Linda Auleciems
Intensive Care Unit. . . . . Gretchen Frederick
Quality Assurance . . . . Gretchen Frederick
CEO/President. . . . . Steve Hatkin
Emergency Room . . . . Charles Lick
Radiology. . . . . Kurt Scheurer, MD
Operating Room. . . . . Julianne Wagner
Chief of Medical Staff. . . . . Dr Charles Yancey

Measure	Cases	This Hosp.	State Avg.	U.S. Avg.
Blood Clot Prevention and Treatment				
Anticoagulation Overlap Therapy[2]	27	100%	96%	93%
ICU Venous Thromboembolism Prophylaxis[1,2]	-	-	91%	92%

NOTE: Hospital profiles are in alphabetical order by state, then city, then hospital within the city; Rankings exclude hospitals with less than 25 cases except for patient surveys which excludes hospitals with less than 100 cases; (a) 100-299 cases; (1) The number of cases/patients is too few to report; (2) Data submitted were based on a sample of cases/patients; (3) Results are based on a shorter time period than required; (4) Data suppressed by CMS for one or more quarters; (5) Results are not available for this reporting period; (6) Fewer than 100 patients completed the HCAHPS survey; (7) No cases met the criteria for this measure; (8) The lower limit of the confidence interval cannot be calculated if the number of observed infections equals zero; (9) No data are available from the state/territory for this reporting period; (10) The scores shown reflect fewer than 50 completed surveys; (11) There were discrepancies in the data collection process; (12) This measure does not apply to this hospital for this reporting period; (13) Results cannot be calculated for this reporting period; (14) The results for this state are combined with nearby states to protect confidentiality; Please refer to the User's Guide for a full explanation of data.

Incidence of Potentially Preventable VTE[2,7]	-	-	9%	10%
UFH with Dosages/Platelet Monitoring[2]	12	92%	98%	97%
Venous Thromboembolism Prophylaxis[2]	114	96%	86%	85%
Warfarin Therapy Discharge Instructions[2]	23	61%	63%	75%
Chest Pain/Possible Heart Attack Care				
Aspirin Given Within 24 Hours of Arrival	72	99%	97%	96%
Fibrinolytic Meds Within 30 Min. of Arrival[7]	-	-	48%	58%
Average Time to ECG (minutes)	73	7	7	7
Average Time to Transfer (minutes)[1]	-	-	54	60
Children's Asthma Care				
Received Home Management Plan of Care	-	-	-	88%
Received Reliever Medication	-	-	-	100%
Received Systemic Corticosteroids	-	-	-	100%
Emergency Department				
Admittance Decision Time (minutes)[2]	238	134	62	98
Head CT Results Within 45 Min. of Arrival	13	62%	54%	57%
Patients Who Left ER Before Being Seen	18,779	0%	2%	2%
Time from ER Arrival to Admit. (minutes)[2]	240	214	199	274
Time from ER Arrival to Discharge (minutes)	372	112	125	134
Time in ER Before Being Evaluated (minutes)	427	7	31	26
Time to Pain Meds for Fractures (minutes)	82	33	45	57
Heart Attack Care				
Aspirin Given at Discharge[3,7]	-	-	99%	99%
Fibrinolytic Meds Within 30 Min. of Arrival[3,7]	-	-	-	54%
PCI Within 90 Minutes of Arrival[3,7]	-	-	96%	96%
Statin Prescribed at Discharge[3,7]	-	-	99%	98%
Heart Failure Care				
ACE Inhibitor or ARB for LVSD	17	100%	96%	97%
Discharge Instructions Given	56	98%	93%	94%
Evaluation of LVS Function	77	100%	97%	99%
Medicare Spending				
Medicare Spending per Patient (ratio)	-	0.88	0.9	0.98
Pneumonia Care				
Appropriate Initial Antibiotic Given	42	98%	94%	95%
Blood Culture Timing	47	94%	97%	98%
Pregnancy and Delivery Care				
Newborn Deliveries Scheduled Early[2]	41	10%	5%	6%
Preventive Care				
Immunization for Influenza[2]	253	98%	89%	90%
Immunization for Pneumonia[2]	231	93%	89%	92%
Stroke Care				
Anticoagulation Therapy for Atrial Fibrillation[7]	-	-	96%	95%
Antithrombotic Therapy Timing[1]	-	-	98%	98%
Assessed for Rehabilitation[1]	-	-	98%	97%
Discharged on Antithrombotic Therapy[1]	-	-	99%	99%
Discharged on Statin Medication[1]	-	-	95%	94%
Thrombolytic Therapy Timing[1]	-	-	74%	66%
Venous Thromboembolism Prophylaxis[1]	-	-	95%	94%
Written Stroke Educational Materials Given[1]	-	-	88%	88%
Surgical Care Improvement Project				
Appropriate Beta Blocker Usage	68	99%	98%	98%
Appropriate VTP Within 24 Hours	161	99%	98%	98%
Controlled Postoperative Blood Glucose[7]	-	-	97%	97%
Perioperative Temperature Management	209	100%	99%	100%
Prophylactic Antibiotic Selection	139	100%	99%	99%
Prophylactic Antibiotic Selection (Outpatient)	185	96%	98%	98%
Prophylactic Antibiotic Stopped	137	99%	99%	98%
Prophylactic Antibiotic Timing	139	100%	98%	99%
Prophylactic Antibiotic Timing (Outpatient)	186	98%	97%	98%
Urinary Catheter Removal	170	100%	97%	97%
Survey of Patients' Hospital Experiences				
Area Around Room 'Always' Quiet at Night	300+	59%	65%	61%
Doctors 'Always' Communicated Well	300+	83%	84%	82%
Home Recovery Information Given	300+	91%	88%	85%
Hospital Given 9 or 10 on 10 Point Scale	300+	72%	74%	71%
Meds 'Always' Explained Before Given	300+	66%	67%	64%
Nurses 'Always' Communicated Well	300+	81%	81%	79%
Pain 'Always' Well Controlled	300+	76%	72%	71%
Room and Bathroom 'Always' Clean	300+	78%	78%	73%
Timely Help 'Always' Received	300+	71%	74%	68%
Would Definitely Recommend Hospital	300+	73%	71%	71%
Use of Medical Imaging				
Cardiac Imaging Stress Test before Surgery	90	5.6%	6.3%	5.3%
Combination Abdominal CT Scan	313	3.8%	5.7%	10.5%
Combination Brain/Sinus CT Scan[1]	-	-	2.3%	2.7%
Combination Chest CT Scan	182	0.0%	1.9%	2.7%
Follow-up Mammogram/Ultrasound	233	5.6%	6.3%	8.8%
Lumbar Spine MRI for Low Back Pain[1]	-	-	37.6%	37.2%

Fairview Ridges Hospital

201 East Nicollet Boulevard
Burnsville, MN 55337
Phone: 952-892-2000
Fax: 952-892-2107
URL: www.fairview.org
Type: Acute Care Hospitals
Emergency Services: Yes
Ownership: Voluntary non-profit - Church
Beds: 150

Key Personnel:
CEO/President. . . . . Beth Krehbiel
Chief of Medical Staff. . . . . Lois A Lenarz
Patient Relations . . . . Helen Strike

Measure	Cases	This Hosp.	State Avg.	U.S. Avg.
Blood Clot Prevention and Treatment				
Anticoagulation Overlap Therapy[2]	114	98%	96%	93%
ICU Venous Thromboembolism Prophylaxis[2]	62	85%	91%	92%
Incidence of Potentially Preventable VTE[1,2]	-	-	9%	10%
UFH with Dosages/Platelet Monitoring[2]	88	100%	98%	97%
Venous Thromboembolism Prophylaxis[2]	318	83%	86%	85%
Warfarin Therapy Discharge Instructions[2]	96	54%	63%	75%
Chest Pain/Possible Heart Attack Care				
Aspirin Given Within 24 Hours of Arrival	63	100%	97%	96%
Fibrinolytic Meds Within 30 Min. of Arrival[7]	-	-	48%	58%
Average Time to ECG (minutes)	64	7	7	7
Average Time to Transfer (minutes)	25	43	54	60
Children's Asthma Care				
Received Home Management Plan of Care	-	-	-	88%
Received Reliever Medication	-	-	-	100%
Received Systemic Corticosteroids	-	-	-	100%
Emergency Department				
Admittance Decision Time (minutes)[2]	571	95	62	98
Head CT Results Within 45 Min. of Arrival	16	25%	54%	57%
Patients Who Left ER Before Being Seen	51,980	1%	2%	2%
Time from ER Arrival to Admit. (minutes)[2]	572	261	199	274
Time from ER Arrival to Discharge (minutes)	365	157	125	134
Time in ER Before Being Evaluated (minutes)	408	17	31	26
Time to Pain Meds for Fractures (minutes)	256	34	45	57
Heart Attack Care				
Aspirin Given at Discharge	113	100%	99%	99%
Fibrinolytic Meds Within 30 Min. of Arrival[7]	-	-	-	54%
PCI Within 90 Minutes of Arrival	14	100%	96%	96%
Statin Prescribed at Discharge	112	100%	99%	98%
Heart Failure Care				
ACE Inhibitor or ARB for LVSD	62	98%	96%	97%
Discharge Instructions Given	199	98%	93%	94%
Evaluation of LVS Function	256	100%	97%	99%
Medicare Spending				
Medicare Spending per Patient (ratio)	-	0.94	0.9	0.98
Pneumonia Care				
Appropriate Initial Antibiotic Given	150	99%	94%	95%
Blood Culture Timing	251	100%	97%	98%
Pregnancy and Delivery Care				
Newborn Deliveries Scheduled Early[2]	30	17%	5%	6%
Preventive Care				
Immunization for Influenza[2]	495	87%	89%	90%
Immunization for Pneumonia[2]	467	83%	89%	92%
Stroke Care				
Anticoagulation Therapy for Atrial Fibrillation	12	100%	96%	95%
Antithrombotic Therapy Timing	63	100%	98%	98%
Assessed for Rehabilitation	67	96%	98%	97%
Discharged on Antithrombotic Therapy	65	98%	99%	99%
Discharged on Statin Medication	52	98%	95%	94%
Thrombolytic Therapy Timing[1]	-	-	74%	66%
Venous Thromboembolism Prophylaxis	59	98%	95%	94%
Written Stroke Educational Materials Given	44	95%	88%	88%
Surgical Care Improvement Project				
Appropriate Beta Blocker Usage[2]	249	100%	98%	98%
Appropriate VTP Within 24 Hours[2]	744	99%	98%	98%
Controlled Postoperative Blood Glucose[2,7]	-	-	97%	97%
Perioperative Temperature Management[2]	854	100%	99%	100%
Prophylactic Antibiotic Selection[2]	678	100%	99%	99%
Prophylactic Antibiotic Selection (Outpatient)	319	99%	98%	98%
Prophylactic Antibiotic Stopped[2]	671	99%	99%	98%
Prophylactic Antibiotic Timing[2]	679	100%	98%	99%
Prophylactic Antibiotic Timing (Outpatient)	319	98%	97%	98%
Urinary Catheter Removal[2]	586	100%	97%	97%
Survey of Patients' Hospital Experiences				
Area Around Room 'Always' Quiet at Night	300+	60%	65%	61%
Doctors 'Always' Communicated Well	300+	79%	84%	82%
Home Recovery Information Given	300+	87%	88%	85%
Hospital Given 9 or 10 on 10 Point Scale	300+	67%	74%	71%
Meds 'Always' Explained Before Given	300+	60%	67%	64%
Nurses 'Always' Communicated Well	300+	76%	81%	79%
Pain 'Always' Well Controlled	300+	71%	72%	71%
Room and Bathroom 'Always' Clean	300+	70%	78%	73%
Timely Help 'Always' Received	300+	66%	74%	68%
Would Definitely Recommend Hospital	300+	70%	71%	71%
Use of Medical Imaging				
Cardiac Imaging Stress Test before Surgery	284	5.6%	6.3%	5.3%
Combination Abdominal CT Scan	586	3.1%	5.7%	10.5%
Combination Brain/Sinus CT Scan	495	1.6%	2.3%	2.7%
Combination Chest CT Scan	441	0.5%	1.9%	2.7%
Follow-up Mammogram/Ultrasound	579	7.3%	6.3%	8.8%
Lumbar Spine MRI for Low Back Pain	60	48.3%	37.6%	37.2%

Cambridge Medical Center

701 South Dellwood Avenue
Cambridge, MN 55008
Phone: 763-689-7700
Type: Acute Care Hospitals
Emergency Services: Yes
Ownership: Voluntary non-profit - Private

Key Personnel:
Chief of Medical Staff. . . . . Robert Callen, MD
CEO/President. . . . . Dennis Doran

Measure	Cases	This Hosp.	State Avg.	U.S. Avg.
Blood Clot Prevention and Treatment				
Anticoagulation Overlap Therapy[2]	22	100%	96%	93%
ICU Venous Thromboembolism Prophylaxis[2,7]	-	-	91%	92%
Incidence of Potentially Preventable VTE[1,2]	-	-	9%	10%
UFH with Dosages/Platelet Monitoring[2]	12	100%	98%	97%
Venous Thromboembolism Prophylaxis[2]	153	96%	86%	85%
Warfarin Therapy Discharge Instructions[2]	16	56%	63%	75%
Chest Pain/Possible Heart Attack Care				
Aspirin Given Within 24 Hours of Arrival	65	97%	97%	96%
Fibrinolytic Meds Within 30 Min. of Arrival[1]	-	-	48%	58%
Average Time to ECG (minutes)	68	8	7	7
Average Time to Transfer (minutes)[1]	-	-	54	60
Children's Asthma Care				
Received Home Management Plan of Care	-	-	-	88%
Received Reliever Medication	-	-	-	100%
Received Systemic Corticosteroids	-	-	-	100%
Emergency Department				
Admittance Decision Time (minutes)[2]	324	102	62	98
Head CT Results Within 45 Min. of Arrival[1]	-	-	54%	57%
Patients Who Left ER Before Being Seen	16,285	0%	2%	2%
Time from ER Arrival to Admit. (minutes)[2]	328	224	199	274
Time from ER Arrival to Discharge (minutes)	488	123	125	134
Time in ER Before Being Evaluated (minutes)	544	12	31	26
Time to Pain Meds for Fractures (minutes)	50	42	45	57
Heart Attack Care				
Aspirin Given at Discharge[1]	-	-	99%	99%
Fibrinolytic Meds Within 30 Min. of Arrival[7]	-	-	-	54%
PCI Within 90 Minutes of Arrival[7]	-	-	96%	96%
Statin Prescribed at Discharge[1]	-	-	99%	98%
Heart Failure Care				
ACE Inhibitor or ARB for LVSD[1]	-	-	96%	97%
Discharge Instructions Given	59	98%	93%	94%
Evaluation of LVS Function	68	100%	97%	99%
Medicare Spending				
Medicare Spending per Patient (ratio)	-	0.88	0.9	0.98
Pneumonia Care				
Appropriate Initial Antibiotic Given	68	100%	94%	95%

NOTE: Hospital profiles are in alphabetical order by state, then city, then hospital within the city; Rankings exclude hospitals with less than 25 cases except for patient surveys which excludes hospitals with less than 100 cases; (a) 100-299 cases; (1) The number of cases/patients is too few to report; (2) Data submitted were based on a sample of cases/patients; (3) Results are based on a shorter time period than required; (4) Data suppressed by CMS for one or more quarters; (5) Results are not available for this reporting period; (6) Fewer than 100 patients completed the HCAHPS survey; (7) No cases met the criteria for this measure; (8) The lower limit of the confidence interval cannot be calculated if the number of observed infections equals zero; (9) No data are available from the state/territory for this reporting period; (10) The scores shown reflect fewer than 50 completed surveys; (11) There were discrepancies in the data collection process; (12) This measure does not apply to this hospital for this reporting period; (13) Results cannot be calculated for this reporting period; (14) The results for this state are combined with nearby states to protect confidentiality; Please refer to the User's Guide for a full explanation of data.

Measure	Cases	This Hosp.	State Avg.	U.S. Avg.
Blood Culture Timing	103	98%	97%	98%
Pregnancy and Delivery Care				
Newborn Deliveries Scheduled Early[2]	24	8%	5%	6%
Preventive Care				
Immunization for Influenza[2]	298	98%	89%	90%
Immunization for Pneumonia[2]	292	94%	89%	92%
Stroke Care				
Anticoagulation Therapy for Atrial Fibrillation[1]	-	-	96%	95%
Antithrombotic Therapy Timing	14	100%	98%	98%
Assessed for Rehabilitation	21	100%	98%	97%
Discharged on Antithrombotic Therapy	21	100%	99%	99%
Discharged on Statin Medication	15	100%	95%	94%
Thrombolytic Therapy Timing[7]	-	-	74%	66%
Venous Thromboembolism Prophylaxis	14	100%	95%	94%
Written Stroke Educational Materials Given	16	94%	88%	88%
Surgical Care Improvement Project				
Appropriate Beta Blocker Usage	57	100%	98%	98%
Appropriate VTP Within 24 Hours	174	100%	98%	98%
Controlled Postoperative Blood Glucose[7]	-	-	97%	97%
Perioperative Temperature Management	211	100%	99%	100%
Prophylactic Antibiotic Selection	144	99%	99%	99%
Prophylactic Antibiotic Selection (Outpatient)	41	100%	98%	98%
Prophylactic Antibiotic Stopped	140	100%	99%	98%
Prophylactic Antibiotic Timing	144	99%	98%	99%
Prophylactic Antibiotic Timing (Outpatient)	44	93%	97%	98%
Urinary Catheter Removal	132	99%	97%	97%
Survey of Patients' Hospital Experiences				
Area Around Room 'Always' Quiet at Night	300+	64%	65%	61%
Doctors 'Always' Communicated Well	300+	83%	84%	82%
Home Recovery Information Given	300+	88%	88%	85%
Hospital Given 9 or 10 on 10 Point Scale	300+	75%	74%	71%
Meds 'Always' Explained Before Given	300+	66%	67%	64%
Nurses 'Always' Communicated Well	300+	81%	81%	79%
Pain 'Always' Well Controlled	300+	71%	72%	71%
Room and Bathroom 'Always' Clean	300+	74%	78%	73%
Timely Help 'Always' Received	300+	80%	74%	68%
Would Definitely Recommend Hospital	300+	70%	71%	71%
Use of Medical Imaging				
Cardiac Imaging Stress Test before Surgery	123	6.5%	6.3%	5.3%
Combination Abdominal CT Scan	253	2.4%	5.7%	10.5%
Combination Brain/Sinus CT Scan	150	6.7%	2.3%	2.7%
Combination Chest CT Scan	193	0.0%	1.9%	2.7%
Follow-up Mammogram/Ultrasound	507	4.3%	6.3%	8.8%
Lumbar Spine MRI for Low Back Pain	40	45.0%	37.6%	37.2%

Sanford Canby Medical Center

112 Saint Olaf Avenue South
Canby, MN 56220
E-mail: info@siouxvalleycanbycampus.org
URL: www.siouxvalleycanbycampus.org
Phone: 507-223-7277
Fax: 507-223-7465
Type: Critical Access Hospitals
Ownership: Govt - Hospital Dist/Auth
Emergency Services: Yes
Beds: 102
Key Personnel:
CEO/President. . . . . Robert Foreman
Quality Assurance . . . . Sally Vogt

Measure	Cases	This Hosp.	State Avg.	U.S. Avg.
Blood Clot Prevention and Treatment				
Anticoagulation Overlap Therapy[5]	-	-	96%	93%
ICU Venous Thromboembolism Prophylaxis[5]	-	-	91%	92%
Incidence of Potentially Preventable VTE[5]	-	-	9%	10%
UFH with Dosages/Platelet Monitoring[5]	-	-	98%	97%
Venous Thromboembolism Prophylaxis[5]	-	-	86%	85%
Warfarin Therapy Discharge Instructions[5]	-	-	63%	75%
Chest Pain/Possible Heart Attack Care				
Aspirin Given Within 24 Hours of Arrival[1,3]	-	-	97%	96%
Fibrinolytic Meds Within 30 Min. of Arrival[1,3]	-	-	48%	58%
Average Time to ECG (minutes)[1,3]	-	-	7	7
Average Time to Transfer (minutes)[3,7]	-	-	54	60
Children's Asthma Care				
Received Home Management Plan of Care	-	-	-	88%
Received Reliever Medication	-	-	-	100%
Received Systemic Corticosteroids	-	-	-	100%
Emergency Department				
Admittance Decision Time (minutes)[1,2]	-	-	62	98
Head CT Results Within 45 Min. of Arrival[3,7]	-	-	54%	57%
Patients Who Left ER Before Being Seen[5]	-	-	2%	2%
Time from ER Arrival to Admit. (minutes)[2]	98	83	199	274
Time from ER Arrival to Discharge (minutes)[5]	-	-	125	134
Time in ER Before Being Evaluated (minutes)[5]	-	-	31	26
Time to Pain Meds for Fractures (minutes)[5]	-	-	45	57
Heart Attack Care				
Aspirin Given at Discharge[1,3]	-	-	99%	99%
Fibrinolytic Meds Within 30 Min. of Arrival[3,7]	-	-	-	54%
PCI Within 90 Minutes of Arrival[3,7]	-	-	96%	96%
Statin Prescribed at Discharge[1,3]	-	-	99%	98%
Heart Failure Care				
ACE Inhibitor or ARB for LVSD[1,3]	-	-	96%	97%
Discharge Instructions Given[1,3]	-	-	93%	94%
Evaluation of LVS Function[1,3]	-	-	97%	99%
Medicare Spending				
Medicare Spending per Patient (ratio)	-	-	0.9	0.98
Pneumonia Care				
Appropriate Initial Antibiotic Given	17	94%	94%	95%
Blood Culture Timing[1]	-	-	97%	98%
Pregnancy and Delivery Care				
Newborn Deliveries Scheduled Early[5]	-	-	5%	6%
Preventive Care				
Immunization for Influenza	149	94%	89%	90%
Immunization for Pneumonia	164	88%	89%	92%
Stroke Care				
Anticoagulation Therapy for Atrial Fibrillation[3,7]	-	-	96%	95%
Antithrombotic Therapy Timing[1,3]	-	-	98%	98%
Assessed for Rehabilitation[1,3]	-	-	98%	97%
Discharged on Antithrombotic Therapy[1,3]	-	-	99%	99%
Discharged on Statin Medication[1,3]	-	-	95%	94%
Thrombolytic Therapy Timing[3,7]	-	-	74%	66%
Venous Thromboembolism Prophylaxis[1,3]	-	-	95%	94%
Written Stroke Educational Materials Given[3,7]	-	-	88%	88%
Surgical Care Improvement Project				
Appropriate Beta Blocker Usage[1,3]	-	-	98%	98%
Appropriate VTP Within 24 Hours[1,3]	-	-	98%	98%
Controlled Postoperative Blood Glucose[3,7]	-	-	97%	97%
Perioperative Temperature Management[1,3]	-	-	99%	100%
Prophylactic Antibiotic Selection[1,3]	-	-	99%	99%
Prophylactic Antibiotic Selection (Outpatient)[1]	-	-	98%	98%
Prophylactic Antibiotic Stopped[1,3]	-	-	99%	98%
Prophylactic Antibiotic Timing[1,3]	-	-	98%	99%
Prophylactic Antibiotic Timing (Outpatient)[1]	-	-	97%	98%
Urinary Catheter Removal[1,3]	-	-	97%	97%
Survey of Patients' Hospital Experiences				
Area Around Room 'Always' Quiet at Night[6]	<100	64%	65%	61%
Doctors 'Always' Communicated Well[6]	<100	81%	84%	82%
Home Recovery Information Given[6]	<100	93%	88%	85%
Hospital Given 9 or 10 on 10 Point Scale[6]	<100	74%	74%	71%
Meds 'Always' Explained Before Given[6]	<100	73%	67%	64%
Nurses 'Always' Communicated Well[6]	<100	82%	81%	79%
Pain 'Always' Well Controlled[6]	<100	68%	72%	71%
Room and Bathroom 'Always' Clean[6]	<100	68%	78%	73%
Timely Help 'Always' Received[6]	<100	71%	74%	68%
Would Definitely Recommend Hospital[6]	<100	75%	71%	71%
Use of Medical Imaging				
Cardiac Imaging Stress Test before Surgery[1]	-	-	6.3%	5.3%
Combination Abdominal CT Scan[1]	-	-	5.7%	10.5%
Combination Brain/Sinus CT Scan[1]	-	-	2.3%	2.7%
Combination Chest CT Scan[1]	-	-	1.9%	2.7%
Follow-up Mammogram/Ultrasound	166	1.8%	6.3%	8.8%
Lumbar Spine MRI for Low Back Pain[1]	-	-	37.6%	37.2%

Mayo Clinic Health System - Cannon Falls

1116 West Mill Street
Cannon Falls, MN 55009
Phone: 507-263-4221
Fax: 507-263-0221
Type: Critical Access Hospitals
Ownership: Voluntary non-profit - Private
Emergency Services: Yes
Beds: 21
Key Personnel:
CEO/President. . . . . Glenn Christian

Measure	Cases	This Hosp.	State Avg.	U.S. Avg.
Blood Clot Prevention and Treatment				
Anticoagulation Overlap Therapy[5]	-	-	96%	93%
ICU Venous Thromboembolism Prophylaxis[5]	-	-	91%	92%
Incidence of Potentially Preventable VTE[5]	-	-	9%	10%
UFH with Dosages/Platelet Monitoring[5]	-	-	98%	97%
Venous Thromboembolism Prophylaxis[5]	-	-	86%	85%
Warfarin Therapy Discharge Instructions[5]	-	-	63%	75%
Chest Pain/Possible Heart Attack Care				
Aspirin Given Within 24 Hours of Arrival	20	100%	97%	96%
Fibrinolytic Meds Within 30 Min. of Arrival[1]	-	-	48%	58%
Average Time to ECG (minutes)	20	9	7	7
Average Time to Transfer (minutes)[1]	-	-	54	60
Children's Asthma Care				
Received Home Management Plan of Care	-	-	-	88%
Received Reliever Medication	-	-	-	100%
Received Systemic Corticosteroids	-	-	-	100%
Emergency Department				
Admittance Decision Time (minutes)	92	44	62	98
Head CT Results Within 45 Min. of Arrival[5]	-	-	54%	57%
Patients Who Left ER Before Being Seen[5]	-	-	2%	2%
Time from ER Arrival to Admit. (minutes)	143	165	199	274
Time from ER Arrival to Discharge (minutes)[5]	-	-	125	134
Time in ER Before Being Evaluated (minutes)[5]	-	-	31	26
Time to Pain Meds for Fractures (minutes)[5]	-	-	45	57
Heart Attack Care				
Aspirin Given at Discharge[5]	-	-	99%	99%
Fibrinolytic Meds Within 30 Min. of Arrival[5]	-	-	-	54%
PCI Within 90 Minutes of Arrival[5]	-	-	96%	96%
Statin Prescribed at Discharge[5]	-	-	99%	98%
Heart Failure Care				
ACE Inhibitor or ARB for LVSD[1]	-	-	96%	97%
Discharge Instructions Given[1]	-	-	93%	94%
Evaluation of LVS Function	12	100%	97%	99%
Medicare Spending				
Medicare Spending per Patient (ratio)	-	-	0.9	0.98
Pneumonia Care				
Appropriate Initial Antibiotic Given	12	92%	94%	95%
Blood Culture Timing	15	100%	97%	98%
Pregnancy and Delivery Care				
Newborn Deliveries Scheduled Early[5]	-	-	5%	6%
Preventive Care				
Immunization for Influenza	107	93%	89%	90%
Immunization for Pneumonia	168	98%	89%	92%
Stroke Care				
Anticoagulation Therapy for Atrial Fibrillation[5]	-	-	96%	95%
Antithrombotic Therapy Timing[5]	-	-	98%	98%
Assessed for Rehabilitation[5]	-	-	98%	97%
Discharged on Antithrombotic Therapy[5]	-	-	99%	99%
Discharged on Statin Medication[5]	-	-	95%	94%
Thrombolytic Therapy Timing[5]	-	-	74%	66%
Venous Thromboembolism Prophylaxis[5]	-	-	95%	94%
Written Stroke Educational Materials Given[5]	-	-	88%	88%
Surgical Care Improvement Project				
Appropriate Beta Blocker Usage[1]	-	-	98%	98%
Appropriate VTP Within 24 Hours	28	100%	98%	98%
Controlled Postoperative Blood Glucose[7]	-	-	97%	97%
Perioperative Temperature Management	29	100%	99%	100%
Prophylactic Antibiotic Selection	25	100%	99%	99%
Prophylactic Antibiotic Selection (Outpatient)[5]	-	-	98%	98%
Prophylactic Antibiotic Stopped	25	100%	99%	98%
Prophylactic Antibiotic Timing	25	100%	98%	99%
Prophylactic Antibiotic Timing (Outpatient)[5]	-	-	97%	98%
Urinary Catheter Removal	29	100%	97%	97%
Survey of Patients' Hospital Experiences				
Area Around Room 'Always' Quiet at Night[5]	-	-	65%	61%
Doctors 'Always' Communicated Well[5]	-	-	84%	82%
Home Recovery Information Given[5]	-	-	88%	85%
Hospital Given 9 or 10 on 10 Point Scale[5]	-	-	74%	71%
Meds 'Always' Explained Before Given[5]	-	-	67%	64%
Nurses 'Always' Communicated Well[5]	-	-	81%	79%
Pain 'Always' Well Controlled[5]	-	-	72%	71%

NOTE: Hospital profiles are in alphabetical order by state, then city, then hospital within the city; Rankings exclude hospitals with less than 25 cases except for patient surveys which excludes hospitals with less than 100 cases; (a) 100-299 cases; (1) The number of cases/patients is too few to report; (2) Data submitted were based on a sample of cases/patients; (3) Results are based on a shorter time period than required; (4) Data suppressed by CMS for one or more quarters; (5) Results are not available for this reporting period; (6) Fewer than 100 patients completed the HCAHPS survey; (7) No cases met the criteria for this measure; (8) The lower limit of the confidence interval cannot be calculated if the number of observed infections equals zero; (9) No data are available from the state/territory for this reporting period; (10) The scores shown reflect fewer than 50 completed surveys; (11) There were discrepancies in the data collection process; (12) This measure does not apply to this hospital for this reporting period; (13) Results cannot be calculated for this reporting period; (14) The results for this state are combined with nearby states to protect confidentiality; Please refer to the User's Guide for a full explanation of data.

Measure	Cases	This Hosp.	State Avg.	U.S. Avg.
Room and Bathroom 'Always' Clean[5]	-	-	78%	73%
Timely Help 'Always' Received[5]	-	-	74%	68%
Would Definitely Recommend Hospital[5]	-	-	71%	71%
Use of Medical Imaging				
Cardiac Imaging Stress Test before Surgery[1]	-	-	6.3%	5.3%
Combination Abdominal CT Scan[1]	-	-	5.7%	10.5%
Combination Brain/Sinus CT Scan	52	0.0%	2.3%	2.7%
Combination Chest CT Scan[1]	-	-	1.9%	2.7%
Follow-up Mammogram/Ultrasound	78	5.1%	6.3%	8.8%
Lumbar Spine MRI for Low Back Pain[1]	-	-	37.6%	37.2%

Cass Lake Indian Health Services Hospital

425 7th Street Nw — Phone: 218-335-3200
Cass Lake, MN 56633
Type: Critical Access Hospitals — Emergency Services: Yes
Ownership: Government - Federal

Measure	Cases	This Hosp.	State Avg.	U.S. Avg.
Blood Clot Prevention and Treatment				
Anticoagulation Overlap Therapy	-	-	96%	93%
ICU Venous Thromboembolism Prophylaxis	-	-	91%	92%
Incidence of Potentially Preventable VTE	-	-	9%	10%
UFH with Dosages/Platelet Monitoring	-	-	98%	97%
Venous Thromboembolism Prophylaxis	-	-	86%	85%
Warfarin Therapy Discharge Instructions	-	-	63%	75%
Chest Pain/Possible Heart Attack Care				
Aspirin Given Within 24 Hours of Arrival[5]	-	-	97%	96%
Fibrinolytic Meds Within 30 Min. of Arrival[5]	-	-	48%	58%
Average Time to ECG (minutes)[5]	-	-	7	7
Average Time to Transfer (minutes)[5]	-	-	54	60
Children's Asthma Care				
Received Home Management Plan of Care	-	-	-	88%
Received Reliever Medication	-	-	-	100%
Received Systemic Corticosteroids	-	-	-	100%
Emergency Department				
Admittance Decision Time (minutes)	-	-	62	98
Head CT Results Within 45 Min. of Arrival[5]	-	-	54%	57%
Patients Who Left ER Before Being Seen[5]	-	-	2%	2%
Time from ER Arrival to Admit. (minutes)	-	-	199	274
Time from ER Arrival to Discharge (minutes)[5]	-	-	125	134
Time in ER Before Being Evaluated (minutes)[5]	-	-	31	26
Time to Pain Meds for Fractures (minutes)[5]	-	-	45	57
Heart Attack Care				
Aspirin Given at Discharge	-	-	99%	99%
Fibrinolytic Meds Within 30 Min. of Arrival	-	-	-	54%
PCI Within 90 Minutes of Arrival	-	-	96%	96%
Statin Prescribed at Discharge	-	-	99%	98%
Heart Failure Care				
ACE Inhibitor or ARB for LVSD	-	-	96%	97%
Discharge Instructions Given	-	-	93%	94%
Evaluation of LVS Function	-	-	97%	99%
Medicare Spending				
Medicare Spending per Patient (ratio)	-	-	0.9	0.98
Pneumonia Care				
Appropriate Initial Antibiotic Given	-	-	94%	95%
Blood Culture Timing	-	-	97%	98%
Pregnancy and Delivery Care				
Newborn Deliveries Scheduled Early	-	-	5%	6%
Preventive Care				
Immunization for Influenza	-	-	89%	90%
Immunization for Pneumonia	-	-	89%	92%
Stroke Care				
Anticoagulation Therapy for Atrial Fibrillation	-	-	96%	95%
Antithrombotic Therapy Timing	-	-	98%	98%
Assessed for Rehabilitation	-	-	98%	97%
Discharged on Antithrombotic Therapy	-	-	99%	99%
Discharged on Statin Medication	-	-	95%	94%
Thrombolytic Therapy Timing	-	-	74%	66%
Venous Thromboembolism Prophylaxis	-	-	95%	94%
Written Stroke Educational Materials Given	-	-	88%	88%
Surgical Care Improvement Project				
Appropriate Beta Blocker Usage	-	-	98%	98%
Appropriate VTP Within 24 Hours	-	-	98%	98%
Controlled Postoperative Blood Glucose	-	-	97%	97%
Perioperative Temperature Management	-	-	99%	100%
Prophylactic Antibiotic Selection	-	-	99%	99%
Prophylactic Antibiotic Selection (Outpatient)[5]	-	-	98%	98%
Prophylactic Antibiotic Stopped	-	-	99%	98%
Prophylactic Antibiotic Timing	-	-	98%	99%
Prophylactic Antibiotic Timing (Outpatient)[5]	-	-	97%	98%
Urinary Catheter Removal	-	-	97%	97%
Survey of Patients' Hospital Experiences				
Area Around Room 'Always' Quiet at Night	-	-	65%	61%
Doctors 'Always' Communicated Well	-	-	84%	82%
Home Recovery Information Given	-	-	88%	85%
Hospital Given 9 or 10 on 10 Point Scale	-	-	74%	71%
Meds 'Always' Explained Before Given	-	-	67%	64%
Nurses 'Always' Communicated Well	-	-	81%	79%
Pain 'Always' Well Controlled	-	-	72%	71%
Room and Bathroom 'Always' Clean	-	-	78%	73%
Timely Help 'Always' Received	-	-	74%	68%
Would Definitely Recommend Hospital	-	-	71%	71%
Use of Medical Imaging				
Cardiac Imaging Stress Test before Surgery[7]	-	-	6.3%	5.3%
Combination Abdominal CT Scan[7]	-	-	5.7%	10.5%
Combination Brain/Sinus CT Scan[7]	-	-	2.3%	2.7%
Combination Chest CT Scan[7]	-	-	1.9%	2.7%
Follow-up Mammogram/Ultrasound[7]	-	-	6.3%	8.8%
Lumbar Spine MRI for Low Back Pain[7]	-	-	37.6%	37.2%

Community Memorial Hospital

512 Skyline Boulevard — Phone: 218-879-4641
Cloquet, MN 55720 — Fax: 218-879-9167
URL: www.cloquethospital.com
Type: Critical Access Hospitals — Emergency Services: Yes
Ownership: Voluntary non-profit - Private — Beds: 124
Key Personnel:
Chief of Medical Staff.......... Vickie L Anderson, MD
Quality Assurance .... Margo Binsfield
Administrator .... Rick Breuer
Infection Control............. Andrea Peterson
Pediatric Ambulatory Care ...... Lee E Riess, MD
Emergency Room .... Kenneth Ripp, MD
Cardiac Laboratory............ Linda Vittperner
Operating Room............. Steven Vopat, MD

Measure	Cases	This Hosp.	State Avg.	U.S. Avg.
Blood Clot Prevention and Treatment				
Anticoagulation Overlap Therapy[5]	-	-	96%	93%
ICU Venous Thromboembolism Prophylaxis[5]	-	-	91%	92%
Incidence of Potentially Preventable VTE[5]	-	-	9%	10%
UFH with Dosages/Platelet Monitoring[5]	-	-	98%	97%
Venous Thromboembolism Prophylaxis[5]	-	-	86%	85%
Warfarin Therapy Discharge Instructions[5]	-	-	63%	75%
Chest Pain/Possible Heart Attack Care				
Aspirin Given Within 24 Hours of Arrival	44	100%	97%	96%
Fibrinolytic Meds Within 30 Min. of Arrival[7]	-	-	48%	58%
Average Time to ECG (minutes)	48	7	7	7
Average Time to Transfer (minutes)	17	33	54	60
Children's Asthma Care				
Received Home Management Plan of Care	-	-	-	88%
Received Reliever Medication	-	-	-	100%
Received Systemic Corticosteroids	-	-	-	100%
Emergency Department				
Admittance Decision Time (minutes)[2]	395	43	62	98
Head CT Results Within 45 Min. of Arrival[5]	-	-	54%	57%
Patients Who Left ER Before Being Seen[5]	-	-	2%	2%
Time from ER Arrival to Admit. (minutes)[2]	403	211	199	274
Time from ER Arrival to Discharge (minutes)[5]	-	-	125	134
Time in ER Before Being Evaluated (minutes)[5]	-	-	31	26
Time to Pain Meds for Fractures (minutes)[5]	-	-	45	57
Heart Attack Care				
Aspirin Given at Discharge[1]	-	-	99%	99%
Fibrinolytic Meds Within 30 Min. of Arrival[7]	-	-	-	54%
PCI Within 90 Minutes of Arrival[3,7]	-	-	96%	96%
Statin Prescribed at Discharge[1]	-	-	99%	98%
Heart Failure Care				
ACE Inhibitor or ARB for LVSD[1,2]	-	-	96%	97%
Discharge Instructions Given[1,2]	-	-	93%	94%
Evaluation of LVS Function[2]	21	100%	97%	99%
Medicare Spending				
Medicare Spending per Patient (ratio)	-	-	0.9	0.98
Pneumonia Care				
Appropriate Initial Antibiotic Given	34	97%	94%	95%
Blood Culture Timing	44	95%	97%	98%
Pregnancy and Delivery Care				
Newborn Deliveries Scheduled Early[5]	-	-	5%	6%
Preventive Care				
Immunization for Influenza[2]	289	76%	89%	90%
Immunization for Pneumonia[2]	412	83%	89%	92%
Stroke Care				
Anticoagulation Therapy for Atrial Fibrillation[5]	-	-	96%	95%
Antithrombotic Therapy Timing[5]	-	-	98%	98%
Assessed for Rehabilitation[5]	-	-	98%	97%
Discharged on Antithrombotic Therapy[5]	-	-	99%	99%
Discharged on Statin Medication[5]	-	-	95%	94%
Thrombolytic Therapy Timing[5]	-	-	74%	66%
Venous Thromboembolism Prophylaxis[5]	-	-	95%	94%
Written Stroke Educational Materials Given[5]	-	-	88%	88%
Surgical Care Improvement Project				
Appropriate Beta Blocker Usage	28	93%	98%	98%
Appropriate VTP Within 24 Hours	95	98%	98%	98%
Controlled Postoperative Blood Glucose[3,7]	-	-	97%	97%
Perioperative Temperature Management	113	100%	99%	100%
Prophylactic Antibiotic Selection	94	99%	99%	99%
Prophylactic Antibiotic Selection (Outpatient)[1]	-	-	98%	98%
Prophylactic Antibiotic Stopped	93	98%	99%	98%
Prophylactic Antibiotic Timing	94	96%	98%	99%
Prophylactic Antibiotic Timing (Outpatient)[1]	-	-	97%	98%
Urinary Catheter Removal	77	99%	97%	97%
Survey of Patients' Hospital Experiences				
Area Around Room 'Always' Quiet at Night	(a)	70%	65%	61%
Doctors 'Always' Communicated Well	(a)	77%	84%	82%
Home Recovery Information Given	(a)	81%	88%	85%
Hospital Given 9 or 10 on 10 Point Scale	(a)	76%	74%	71%
Meds 'Always' Explained Before Given	(a)	64%	67%	64%
Nurses 'Always' Communicated Well	(a)	79%	81%	79%
Pain 'Always' Well Controlled	(a)	71%	72%	71%
Room and Bathroom 'Always' Clean	(a)	83%	78%	73%
Timely Help 'Always' Received	(a)	80%	74%	68%
Would Definitely Recommend Hospital	(a)	76%	71%	71%
Use of Medical Imaging				
Cardiac Imaging Stress Test before Surgery[1]	-	-	6.3%	5.3%
Combination Abdominal CT Scan	143	9.1%	5.7%	10.5%
Combination Brain/Sinus CT Scan[1]	-	-	2.3%	2.7%
Combination Chest CT Scan	65	1.5%	1.9%	2.7%
Follow-up Mammogram/Ultrasound	267	7.1%	6.3%	8.8%
Lumbar Spine MRI for Low Back Pain[1]	-	-	37.6%	37.2%

Cook Hospital

10 Se Fifth St — Phone: 218-666-5945
Cook, MN 55723 — Fax: 218-666-6239
Type: Critical Access Hospitals — Emergency Services: Yes
Ownership: Govt - Hospital Dist/Auth — Beds: 14
Key Personnel:
Radiology.................... Dan Courneya
Infection Control.............. Teresa Debevecn
Quality Assurance .... Karen Hollanitsch
Chief of Medical Staff.......... Harold Johnston, MD

Measure	Cases	This Hosp.	State Avg.	U.S. Avg.
Blood Clot Prevention and Treatment				
Anticoagulation Overlap Therapy[5]	-	-	96%	93%
ICU Venous Thromboembolism Prophylaxis[5]	-	-	91%	92%
Incidence of Potentially Preventable VTE[5]	-	-	9%	10%
UFH with Dosages/Platelet Monitoring[5]	-	-	98%	97%
Venous Thromboembolism Prophylaxis[5]	-	-	86%	85%
Warfarin Therapy Discharge Instructions[5]	-	-	63%	75%
Chest Pain/Possible Heart Attack Care				
Aspirin Given Within 24 Hours of Arrival	11	91%	97%	96%
Fibrinolytic Meds Within 30 Min. of Arrival[1]	-	-	48%	58%
Average Time to ECG (minutes)	12	10	7	7

NOTE: Hospital profiles are in alphabetical order by state, then city, then hospital within the city; Rankings exclude hospitals with less than 25 cases except for patient surveys which excludes hospitals with less than 100 cases; (a) 100-299 cases; (1) The number of cases/patients is too few to report; (2) Data submitted were based on a sample of cases/patients; (3) Results are based on a shorter time period than required; (4) Data suppressed by CMS for one or more quarters; (5) Results are not available for this reporting period; (6) Fewer than 100 patients completed the HCAHPS survey; (7) No cases met the criteria for this measure; (8) The lower limit of the confidence interval cannot be calculated if the number of observed infections equals zero; (9) No data are available from the state/territory for this reporting period; (10) The scores shown reflect fewer than 50 completed surveys; (11) There were discrepancies in the data collection process; (12) This measure does not apply to this hospital for this reporting period; (13) Results cannot be calculated for this reporting period; (14) The results for this state are combined with nearby states to protect confidentiality; Please refer to the User's Guide for a full explanation of data.

Measure	Cases	This Hosp.	State Avg.	U.S. Avg.
Average Time to Transfer (minutes)[1]	-	-	54	60
Children's Asthma Care				
Received Home Management Plan of Care	-	-	-	88%
Received Reliever Medication	-	-	-	100%
Received Systemic Corticosteroids	-	-	-	100%
Emergency Department				
Admittance Decision Time (minutes)	165	0	62	98
Head CT Results Within 45 Min. of Arrival[5]	-	-	54%	57%
Patients Who Left ER Before Being Seen[5]	-	-	2%	2%
Time from ER Arrival to Admit. (minutes)	165	143	199	274
Time from ER Arrival to Discharge (minutes)[5]	-	-	125	134
Time in ER Before Being Evaluated (minutes)[5]	-	-	31	26
Time to Pain Meds for Fractures (minutes)[5]	-	-	45	57
Heart Attack Care				
Aspirin Given at Discharge[3,7]	-	-	99%	99%
Fibrinolytic Meds Within 30 Min. of Arrival[3,7]	-	-	-	54%
PCI Within 90 Minutes of Arrival[3,7]	-	-	96%	96%
Statin Prescribed at Discharge[3,7]	-	-	99%	98%
Heart Failure Care				
ACE Inhibitor or ARB for LVSD[1,3]	-	-	96%	97%
Discharge Instructions Given[1,3]	-	-	93%	94%
Evaluation of LVS Function[1,3]	-	-	97%	99%
Medicare Spending				
Medicare Spending per Patient (ratio)	-	-	0.9	0.98
Pneumonia Care				
Appropriate Initial Antibiotic Given[1,3]	-	-	94%	95%
Blood Culture Timing[1,3]	-	-	97%	98%
Pregnancy and Delivery Care				
Newborn Deliveries Scheduled Early[5]	-	-	5%	6%
Preventive Care				
Immunization for Influenza	105	66%	89%	90%
Immunization for Pneumonia	105	70%	89%	92%
Stroke Care				
Anticoagulation Therapy for Atrial Fibrillation[5]	-	-	96%	95%
Antithrombotic Therapy Timing[5]	-	-	98%	98%
Assessed for Rehabilitation[5]	-	-	98%	97%
Discharged on Antithrombotic Therapy[5]	-	-	99%	99%
Discharged on Statin Medication[5]	-	-	95%	94%
Thrombolytic Therapy Timing[5]	-	-	74%	66%
Venous Thromboembolism Prophylaxis[5]	-	-	95%	94%
Written Stroke Educational Materials Given[5]	-	-	88%	88%
Surgical Care Improvement Project				
Appropriate Beta Blocker Usage[5]	-	-	98%	98%
Appropriate VTP Within 24 Hours[5]	-	-	98%	98%
Controlled Postoperative Blood Glucose[5]	-	-	97%	97%
Perioperative Temperature Management[5]	-	-	99%	100%
Prophylactic Antibiotic Selection[5]	-	-	99%	99%
Prophylactic Antibiotic Selection (Outpatient)[5]	-	-	98%	98%
Prophylactic Antibiotic Stopped[5]	-	-	99%	98%
Prophylactic Antibiotic Timing[5]	-	-	98%	99%
Prophylactic Antibiotic Timing (Outpatient)[5]	-	-	97%	98%
Urinary Catheter Removal[5]	-	-	97%	97%
Survey of Patients' Hospital Experiences				
Area Around Room 'Always' Quiet at Night[5]	-	-	65%	61%
Doctors 'Always' Communicated Well[5]	-	-	84%	82%
Home Recovery Information Given[5]	-	-	88%	85%
Hospital Given 9 or 10 on 10 Point Scale[5]	-	-	74%	71%
Meds 'Always' Explained Before Given[5]	-	-	67%	64%
Nurses 'Always' Communicated Well[5]	-	-	81%	79%
Pain 'Always' Well Controlled[5]	-	-	72%	71%
Room and Bathroom 'Always' Clean[5]	-	-	78%	73%
Timely Help 'Always' Received[5]	-	-	74%	68%
Would Definitely Recommend Hospital[5]	-	-	71%	71%
Use of Medical Imaging				
Cardiac Imaging Stress Test before Surgery[7]	-	-	6.3%	5.3%
Combination Abdominal CT Scan[1]	-	-	5.7%	10.5%
Combination Brain/Sinus CT Scan[1]	-	-	2.3%	2.7%
Combination Chest CT Scan[1]	-	-	1.9%	2.7%
Follow-up Mammogram/Ultrasound[1]	-	-	6.3%	8.8%
Lumbar Spine MRI for Low Back Pain[1]	-	-	37.6%	37.2%

Mercy Hospital

4050 Coon Rapids Blvd
Coon Rapids, MN 55433
Phone: 763-236-8205
Fax: 763-236-8124
URL: www.allinamercy.org
Type: Acute Care Hospitals
Emergency Services: Yes
Ownership: Voluntary non-profit - Private
Beds: 271

Key Personnel:

Chief of Medical Staff.......... Donald Collins
CEO/President............... Sara Criger
Emergency Room .... Allen Fuller
Cardiac Laboratory............ Steven Remole

Measure	Cases	This Hosp.	State Avg.	U.S. Avg.
Blood Clot Prevention and Treatment				
Anticoagulation Overlap Therapy[2]	142	99%	96%	93%
ICU Venous Thromboembolism Prophylaxis[2]	49	100%	91%	92%
Incidence of Potentially Preventable VTE[2]	11	0%	9%	10%
UFH with Dosages/Platelet Monitoring[2]	128	96%	98%	97%
Venous Thromboembolism Prophylaxis[2]	260	90%	86%	85%
Warfarin Therapy Discharge Instructions[2]	124	77%	63%	75%
Chest Pain/Possible Heart Attack Care				
Aspirin Given Within 24 Hours of Arrival	14	93%	97%	96%
Fibrinolytic Meds Within 30 Min. of Arrival[3,7]	-	-	48%	58%
Average Time to ECG (minutes)	15	6	7	7
Average Time to Transfer (minutes)[3,7]	-	-	54	60
Children's Asthma Care				
Received Home Management Plan of Care	-	-	-	88%
Received Reliever Medication	-	-	-	100%
Received Systemic Corticosteroids	-	-	-	100%
Emergency Department				
Admittance Decision Time (minutes)[2]	676	202	62	98
Head CT Results Within 45 Min. of Arrival	16	81%	54%	57%
Patients Who Left ER Before Being Seen	58,737	2%	2%	2%
Time from ER Arrival to Admit. (minutes)[2]	680	270	199	274
Time from ER Arrival to Discharge (minutes)	385	160	125	134
Time in ER Before Being Evaluated (minutes)	436	28	31	26
Time to Pain Meds for Fractures (minutes)	177	50	45	57
Heart Attack Care				
Aspirin Given at Discharge	483	100%	99%	99%
Fibrinolytic Meds Within 30 Min. of Arrival[7]	-	-	-	54%
PCI Within 90 Minutes of Arrival	61	93%	96%	96%
Statin Prescribed at Discharge	480	100%	99%	98%
Heart Failure Care				
ACE Inhibitor or ARB for LVSD	109	100%	96%	97%
Discharge Instructions Given	363	99%	93%	94%
Evaluation of LVS Function	445	100%	97%	99%
Medicare Spending				
Medicare Spending per Patient (ratio)	-	0.92	0.9	0.98
Pneumonia Care				
Appropriate Initial Antibiotic Given	193	97%	94%	95%
Blood Culture Timing	182	98%	97%	98%
Pregnancy and Delivery Care				
Newborn Deliveries Scheduled Early[2]	45	2%	5%	6%
Preventive Care				
Immunization for Influenza[2]	592	92%	89%	90%
Immunization for Pneumonia[2]	681	93%	89%	92%
Stroke Care				
Anticoagulation Therapy for Atrial Fibrillation	37	95%	96%	95%
Antithrombotic Therapy Timing	151	98%	98%	98%
Assessed for Rehabilitation	215	97%	98%	97%
Discharged on Antithrombotic Therapy	188	100%	99%	99%
Discharged on Statin Medication	147	98%	95%	94%
Thrombolytic Therapy Timing	19	89%	74%	66%
Venous Thromboembolism Prophylaxis	204	99%	95%	94%
Written Stroke Educational Materials Given	127	98%	88%	88%
Surgical Care Improvement Project				
Appropriate Beta Blocker Usage[2]	324	99%	98%	98%
Appropriate VTP Within 24 Hours[2]	394	99%	98%	98%
Controlled Postoperative Blood Glucose[2]	156	97%	97%	97%
Perioperative Temperature Management[2]	588	100%	99%	100%
Prophylactic Antibiotic Selection[2]	473	100%	99%	99%
Prophylactic Antibiotic Selection (Outpatient)	380	98%	98%	98%
Prophylactic Antibiotic Stopped[2]	460	99%	99%	98%
Prophylactic Antibiotic Timing[2]	473	100%	98%	99%
Prophylactic Antibiotic Timing (Outpatient)	382	98%	97%	98%
Urinary Catheter Removal[2]	296	98%	97%	97%
Survey of Patients' Hospital Experiences				
Area Around Room 'Always' Quiet at Night	300+	56%	65%	61%
Doctors 'Always' Communicated Well	300+	79%	84%	82%
Home Recovery Information Given	300+	88%	88%	85%
Hospital Given 9 or 10 on 10 Point Scale	300+	73%	74%	71%
Meds 'Always' Explained Before Given	300+	64%	67%	64%
Nurses 'Always' Communicated Well	300+	78%	81%	79%
Pain 'Always' Well Controlled	300+	70%	72%	71%
Room and Bathroom 'Always' Clean	300+	74%	78%	73%
Timely Help 'Always' Received	300+	64%	74%	68%
Would Definitely Recommend Hospital	300+	74%	71%	71%
Use of Medical Imaging				
Cardiac Imaging Stress Test before Surgery	474	4.9%	6.3%	5.3%
Combination Abdominal CT Scan	632	2.2%	5.7%	10.5%
Combination Brain/Sinus CT Scan	428	1.4%	2.3%	2.7%
Combination Chest CT Scan	524	0.4%	1.9%	2.7%
Follow-up Mammogram/Ultrasound[7]	-	-	6.3%	8.8%
Lumbar Spine MRI for Low Back Pain[1]	-	-	37.6%	37.2%

Riverview Hospital

323 South Minnesota
Crookston, MN 56716
Phone: 218-281-9200
Fax: 218-281-9222
URL: www.riverviewhealth.org
Type: Critical Access Hospitals
Emergency Services: Yes
Ownership: Voluntary non-profit - Private
Beds: 49

Key Personnel:

Operating Room.............. Idatonye Afonya
Radiology.................. Hilton Bakker
Quality Assurance .... Robynn Coavette
Chief of Medical Staff.......... Dr Erik Kanten, MD
Patient Relations .... Nancy Lankow
CEO/President.............. Carrie Michalski
Emergency Room .... Mary Pufall
Infection Control.............. Dee Dee Wielsma

Measure	Cases	This Hosp.	State Avg.	U.S. Avg.
Blood Clot Prevention and Treatment				
Anticoagulation Overlap Therapy[5]	-	-	96%	93%
ICU Venous Thromboembolism Prophylaxis[5]	-	-	91%	92%
Incidence of Potentially Preventable VTE[5]	-	-	9%	10%
UFH with Dosages/Platelet Monitoring[5]	-	-	98%	97%
Venous Thromboembolism Prophylaxis[5]	-	-	86%	85%
Warfarin Therapy Discharge Instructions[5]	-	-	63%	75%
Chest Pain/Possible Heart Attack Care				
Aspirin Given Within 24 Hours of Arrival	18	89%	97%	96%
Fibrinolytic Meds Within 30 Min. of Arrival[7]	-	-	48%	58%
Average Time to ECG (minutes)	19	14	7	7
Average Time to Transfer (minutes)[1]	-	-	54	60
Children's Asthma Care				
Received Home Management Plan of Care	-	-	-	88%
Received Reliever Medication	-	-	-	100%
Received Systemic Corticosteroids	-	-	-	100%
Emergency Department				
Admittance Decision Time (minutes)[2]	259	37	62	98
Head CT Results Within 45 Min. of Arrival[1,3]	-	-	54%	57%
Patients Who Left ER Before Being Seen[5]	-	-	2%	2%
Time from ER Arrival to Admit. (minutes)[2]	292	181	199	274
Time from ER Arrival to Discharge (minutes)[3]	180	84	125	134
Time in ER Before Being Evaluated (minutes)[3]	198	12	31	26
Time to Pain Meds for Fractures (minutes)[3]	11	61	45	57
Heart Attack Care				
Aspirin Given at Discharge[1,3]	-	-	99%	99%
Fibrinolytic Meds Within 30 Min. of Arrival[3,7]	-	-	-	54%
PCI Within 90 Minutes of Arrival[3,7]	-	-	96%	96%
Statin Prescribed at Discharge[1,3]	-	-	99%	98%
Heart Failure Care				
ACE Inhibitor or ARB for LVSD[1]	-	-	96%	97%
Discharge Instructions Given	11	82%	93%	94%
Evaluation of LVS Function	20	40%	97%	99%
Medicare Spending				
Medicare Spending per Patient (ratio)	-	-	0.9	0.98
Pneumonia Care				
Appropriate Initial Antibiotic Given	21	90%	94%	95%

NOTE: Hospital profiles are in alphabetical order by state, then city, then hospital within the city; Rankings exclude hospitals with less than 25 cases except for patient surveys which excludes hospitals with less than 100 cases; (a) 100-299 cases; (1) The number of cases/patients is too few to report; (2) Data submitted were based on a sample of cases/patients; (3) Results are based on a shorter time period than required; (4) Data suppressed by CMS for one or more quarters; (5) Results are not available for this reporting period; (6) Fewer than 100 patients completed the HCAHPS survey; (7) No cases met the criteria for this measure; (8) The lower limit of the confidence interval cannot be calculated if the number of observed infections equals zero; (9) No data are available from the state/territory for this reporting period; (10) The scores shown reflect fewer than 50 completed surveys; (11) There were discrepancies in the data collection process; (12) This measure does not apply to this hospital for this reporting period; (13) Results cannot be calculated for this reporting period; (14) The results for this state are combined with nearby states to protect confidentiality; Please refer to the User's Guide for a full explanation of data.

Measure	Cases	This Hosp.	State Avg.	U.S. Avg.
Blood Culture Timing	20	95%	97%	98%
Pregnancy and Delivery Care				
Newborn Deliveries Scheduled Early[5]	-	-	5%	6%
Preventive Care				
Immunization for Influenza	162	56%	89%	90%
Immunization for Pneumonia	318	71%	89%	92%
Stroke Care				
Anticoagulation Therapy for Atrial Fibrillation[5]	-	-	96%	95%
Antithrombotic Therapy Timing[5]	-	-	98%	98%
Assessed for Rehabilitation[5]	-	-	98%	97%
Discharged on Antithrombotic Therapy[5]	-	-	99%	99%
Discharged on Statin Medication[5]	-	-	95%	94%
Thrombolytic Therapy Timing[5]	-	-	74%	66%
Venous Thromboembolism Prophylaxis[5]	-	-	95%	94%
Written Stroke Educational Materials Given[5]	-	-	88%	88%
Surgical Care Improvement Project				
Appropriate Beta Blocker Usage	14	93%	98%	98%
Appropriate VTP Within 24 Hours	48	81%	98%	98%
Controlled Postoperative Blood Glucose[7]	-	-	97%	97%
Perioperative Temperature Management	60	98%	99%	100%
Prophylactic Antibiotic Selection	42	88%	99%	99%
Prophylactic Antibiotic Selection (Outpatient)	53	100%	98%	98%
Prophylactic Antibiotic Stopped	40	98%	99%	98%
Prophylactic Antibiotic Timing	42	76%	98%	99%
Prophylactic Antibiotic Timing (Outpatient)	60	77%	97%	98%
Urinary Catheter Removal	25	84%	97%	97%
Survey of Patients' Hospital Experiences				
Area Around Room 'Always' Quiet at Night	(a)	72%	65%	61%
Doctors 'Always' Communicated Well	(a)	86%	84%	82%
Home Recovery Information Given	(a)	90%	88%	85%
Hospital Given 9 or 10 on 10 Point Scale	(a)	74%	74%	71%
Meds 'Always' Explained Before Given	(a)	70%	67%	64%
Nurses 'Always' Communicated Well	(a)	83%	81%	79%
Pain 'Always' Well Controlled	(a)	69%	72%	71%
Room and Bathroom 'Always' Clean	(a)	73%	78%	73%
Timely Help 'Always' Received	(a)	76%	74%	68%
Would Definitely Recommend Hospital	(a)	77%	71%	71%
Use of Medical Imaging				
Cardiac Imaging Stress Test before Surgery	82	7.3%	6.3%	5.3%
Combination Abdominal CT Scan	123	4.1%	5.7%	10.5%
Combination Brain/Sinus CT Scan[1]	-	-	2.3%	2.7%
Combination Chest CT Scan	56	0.0%	1.9%	2.7%
Follow-up Mammogram/Ultrasound	296	3.4%	6.3%	8.8%
Lumbar Spine MRI for Low Back Pain[1]	-	-	37.6%	37.2%

Cuyuna Regional Medical Center

320 East Main Street
Crosby, MN 56441
Phone: 218-546-7000
Fax: 218-546-6091
URL: www.cuyunamed.org
Type: Critical Access Hospitals
Emergency Services: Yes
Ownership: Govt - Hospital Dist/Auth
Beds: 42

Key Personnel:
Infection Control . . . . Brian Blom
Operating Room. . . . . Dennis Bowles
Radiology. . . . . Bryan Brindley, MD
Quality Assurance . . . . Maxine Ehlers
Emergency Room . . . . Tom Lorenz, MD
CEO/President. . . . . John Solheim
Hemotology Center . . . . Gail Temple, RN
Chief of Medical Staff. . . . . Dr. Robert Westin

Measure	Cases	This Hosp.	State Avg.	U.S. Avg.
Blood Clot Prevention and Treatment				
Anticoagulation Overlap Therapy[5]	-	-	96%	93%
ICU Venous Thromboembolism Prophylaxis[5]	-	-	91%	92%
Incidence of Potentially Preventable VTE[5]	-	-	9%	10%
UFH with Dosages/Platelet Monitoring[5]	-	-	98%	97%
Venous Thromboembolism Prophylaxis[5]	-	-	86%	85%
Warfarin Therapy Discharge Instructions[5]	-	-	63%	75%
Chest Pain/Possible Heart Attack Care				
Aspirin Given Within 24 Hours of Arrival	34	100%	97%	96%
Fibrinolytic Meds Within 30 Min. of Arrival[1]	-	-	48%	58%
Average Time to ECG (minutes)	35	13	7	7
Average Time to Transfer (minutes)[1]	-	-	54	60
Children's Asthma Care				
Received Home Management Plan of Care	-	-	-	88%
Received Reliever Medication	-	-	-	100%
Received Systemic Corticosteroids	-	-	-	100%
Emergency Department				
Admittance Decision Time (minutes)[2]	278	90	62	98
Head CT Results Within 45 Min. of Arrival[5]	-	-	54%	57%
Patients Who Left ER Before Being Seen[5]	-	-	2%	2%
Time from ER Arrival to Admit. (minutes)[2]	278	208	199	274
Time from ER Arrival to Discharge (minutes)[5]	-	-	125	134
Time in ER Before Being Evaluated (minutes)[5]	-	-	31	26
Time to Pain Meds for Fractures (minutes)[5]	-	-	45	57
Heart Attack Care				
Aspirin Given at Discharge[1,3]	-	-	99%	99%
Fibrinolytic Meds Within 30 Min. of Arrival[3,7]	-	-	-	54%
PCI Within 90 Minutes of Arrival[3,7]	-	-	96%	96%
Statin Prescribed at Discharge[1,3]	-	-	99%	98%
Heart Failure Care				
ACE Inhibitor or ARB for LVSD[1]	-	-	96%	97%
Discharge Instructions Given	33	76%	93%	94%
Evaluation of LVS Function	44	100%	97%	99%
Medicare Spending				
Medicare Spending per Patient (ratio)	-	-	0.9	0.98
Pneumonia Care				
Appropriate Initial Antibiotic Given	31	97%	94%	95%
Blood Culture Timing	48	94%	97%	98%
Pregnancy and Delivery Care				
Newborn Deliveries Scheduled Early[5]	-	-	5%	6%
Preventive Care				
Immunization for Influenza[2]	256	91%	89%	90%
Immunization for Pneumonia[2]	289	88%	89%	92%
Stroke Care				
Anticoagulation Therapy for Atrial Fibrillation[5]	-	-	96%	95%
Antithrombotic Therapy Timing[5]	-	-	98%	98%
Assessed for Rehabilitation[5]	-	-	98%	97%
Discharged on Antithrombotic Therapy[5]	-	-	99%	99%
Discharged on Statin Medication[5]	-	-	95%	94%
Thrombolytic Therapy Timing[5]	-	-	74%	66%
Venous Thromboembolism Prophylaxis[5]	-	-	95%	94%
Written Stroke Educational Materials Given[5]	-	-	88%	88%
Surgical Care Improvement Project				
Appropriate Beta Blocker Usage	89	98%	98%	98%
Appropriate VTP Within 24 Hours	205	100%	98%	98%
Controlled Postoperative Blood Glucose[7]	-	-	97%	97%
Perioperative Temperature Management	266	100%	99%	100%
Prophylactic Antibiotic Selection	210	100%	99%	99%
Prophylactic Antibiotic Selection (Outpatient)	68	90%	98%	98%
Prophylactic Antibiotic Stopped	209	99%	99%	98%
Prophylactic Antibiotic Timing	210	99%	98%	99%
Prophylactic Antibiotic Timing (Outpatient)	74	91%	97%	98%
Urinary Catheter Removal	31	84%	97%	97%
Survey of Patients' Hospital Experiences				
Area Around Room 'Always' Quiet at Night	300+	60%	65%	61%
Doctors 'Always' Communicated Well	300+	89%	84%	82%
Home Recovery Information Given	300+	88%	88%	85%
Hospital Given 9 or 10 on 10 Point Scale	300+	84%	74%	71%
Meds 'Always' Explained Before Given	300+	72%	67%	64%
Nurses 'Always' Communicated Well	300+	85%	81%	79%
Pain 'Always' Well Controlled	300+	76%	72%	71%
Room and Bathroom 'Always' Clean	300+	80%	78%	73%
Timely Help 'Always' Received	300+	76%	74%	68%
Would Definitely Recommend Hospital	300+	88%	71%	71%
Use of Medical Imaging				
Cardiac Imaging Stress Test before Surgery	83	9.6%	6.3%	5.3%
Combination Abdominal CT Scan	215	7.9%	5.7%	10.5%
Combination Brain/Sinus CT Scan[1]	-	-	2.3%	2.7%
Combination Chest CT Scan	190	0.0%	1.9%	2.7%
Follow-up Mammogram/Ultrasound	387	8.3%	6.3%	8.8%
Lumbar Spine MRI for Low Back Pain	41	43.9%	37.6%	37.2%

Johnson Memorial Hospital

1282 Walnut Street
Dawson, MN 56232
Phone: 320-769-4323
Fax: 320-769-4576
URL: www.jmhsdawson.com
Type: Critical Access Hospitals
Emergency Services: Yes
Ownership: Govt - Hospital Dist/Auth
Beds: 94

Key Personnel:
Quality Assurance . . . . Laura Dahl
Chair/CEO . . . . Dan Fondell
Chief of Medical Staff . . . . Ralph Gerbig, MD
Emergency Room . . . . Sue Johnson

Measure	Cases	This Hosp.	State Avg.	U.S. Avg.
Blood Clot Prevention and Treatment				
Anticoagulation Overlap Therapy[1,3]	-	-	96%	93%
ICU Venous Thromboembolism Prophylaxis[3,7]	-	-	91%	92%
Incidence of Potentially Preventable VTE[3,7]	-	-	9%	10%
UFH with Dosages/Platelet Monitoring[1,3]	-	-	98%	97%
Venous Thromboembolism Prophylaxis[3,7]	-	-	86%	85%
Warfarin Therapy Discharge Instructions[1,3]	-	-	63%	75%
Chest Pain/Possible Heart Attack Care				
Aspirin Given Within 24 Hours of Arrival[1,3]	-	-	97%	96%
Fibrinolytic Meds Within 30 Min. of Arrival[3,7]	-	-	48%	58%
Average Time to ECG (minutes)[1,3]	-	-	7	7
Average Time to Transfer (minutes)[1,3]	-	-	54	60
Children's Asthma Care				
Received Home Management Plan of Care	-	-	-	88%
Received Reliever Medication	-	-	-	100%
Received Systemic Corticosteroids	-	-	-	100%
Emergency Department				
Admittance Decision Time (minutes)	55	10	62	98
Head CT Results Within 45 Min. of Arrival[5]	-	-	54%	57%
Patients Who Left ER Before Being Seen[5]	-	-	2%	2%
Time from ER Arrival to Admit. (minutes)	57	95	199	274
Time from ER Arrival to Discharge (minutes)[5]	-	-	125	134
Time in ER Before Being Evaluated (minutes)[5]	-	-	31	26
Time to Pain Meds for Fractures (minutes)[5]	-	-	45	57
Heart Attack Care				
Aspirin Given at Discharge[1,3]	-	-	99%	99%
Fibrinolytic Meds Within 30 Min. of Arrival[3,7]	-	-	-	54%
PCI Within 90 Minutes of Arrival[3,7]	-	-	96%	96%
Statin Prescribed at Discharge[1,3]	-	-	99%	98%
Heart Failure Care				
ACE Inhibitor or ARB for LVSD[1,3]	-	-	96%	97%
Discharge Instructions Given[1,3]	-	-	93%	94%
Evaluation of LVS Function[1,3]	-	-	97%	99%
Medicare Spending				
Medicare Spending per Patient (ratio)	-	-	0.9	0.98
Pneumonia Care				
Appropriate Initial Antibiotic Given	12	100%	94%	95%
Blood Culture Timing[1]	-	-	97%	98%
Pregnancy and Delivery Care				
Newborn Deliveries Scheduled Early[5]	-	-	5%	6%
Preventive Care				
Immunization for Influenza[2]	56	88%	89%	90%
Immunization for Pneumonia[2]	96	96%	89%	92%
Stroke Care				
Anticoagulation Therapy for Atrial Fibrillation[5]	-	-	96%	95%
Antithrombotic Therapy Timing[5]	-	-	98%	98%
Assessed for Rehabilitation[5]	-	-	98%	97%
Discharged on Antithrombotic Therapy[5]	-	-	99%	99%
Discharged on Statin Medication[5]	-	-	95%	94%
Thrombolytic Therapy Timing[5]	-	-	74%	66%
Venous Thromboembolism Prophylaxis[5]	-	-	95%	94%
Written Stroke Educational Materials Given[5]	-	-	88%	88%
Surgical Care Improvement Project				
Appropriate Beta Blocker Usage[5]	-	-	98%	98%
Appropriate VTP Within 24 Hours[5]	-	-	98%	98%
Controlled Postoperative Blood Glucose[5]	-	-	97%	97%
Perioperative Temperature Management[5]	-	-	99%	100%
Prophylactic Antibiotic Selection[5]	-	-	99%	99%
Prophylactic Antibiotic Selection (Outpatient)[1,3]	-	-	98%	98%
Prophylactic Antibiotic Stopped[5]	-	-	99%	98%
Prophylactic Antibiotic Timing[5]	-	-	98%	99%

NOTE: Hospital profiles are in alphabetical order by state, then city, then hospital within the city; Rankings exclude hospitals with less than 25 cases except for patient surveys which excludes hospitals with less than 100 cases; (a) 100-299 cases; (1) The number of cases/patients is too few to report; (2) Data submitted were based on a sample of cases/patients; (3) Results are based on a shorter time period than required; (4) Data suppressed by CMS for one or more quarters; (5) Results are not available for this reporting period; (6) Fewer than 100 patients completed the HCAHPS survey; (7) No cases met the criteria for this measure; (8) The lower limit of the confidence interval cannot be calculated if the number of observed infections equals zero; (9) No data are available from the state/territory for this reporting period; (10) The scores shown reflect fewer than 50 completed surveys; (11) There were discrepancies in the data collection process; (12) This measure does not apply to this hospital for this reporting period; (13) Results cannot be calculated for this reporting period; (14) The results for this state are combined with nearby states to protect confidentiality; Please refer to the User's Guide for a full explanation of data.

Measure	Cases	This Hosp.	State Avg.	U.S. Avg.
Prophylactic Antibiotic Timing (Outpatient)[1,3]	-	-	97%	98%
Urinary Catheter Removal[5]	-	-	97%	97%
Survey of Patients' Hospital Experiences				
Area Around Room 'Always' Quiet at Night[10,11]	<100	84%	65%	61%
Doctors 'Always' Communicated Well[10,11]	<100	83%	84%	82%
Home Recovery Information Given[10,11]	<100	92%	88%	85%
Hospital Given 9 or 10 on 10 Point Scale[10,11]	<100	91%	74%	71%
Meds 'Always' Explained Before Given[10,11]	<100	91%	67%	64%
Nurses 'Always' Communicated Well[10,11]	<100	91%	81%	79%
Pain 'Always' Well Controlled[10,11]	<100	88%	72%	71%
Room and Bathroom 'Always' Clean[10,11]	<100	83%	78%	73%
Timely Help 'Always' Received[10,11]	<100	88%	74%	68%
Would Definitely Recommend Hospital[10,11]	<100	53%	71%	71%
Use of Medical Imaging				
Cardiac Imaging Stress Test before Surgery[1]	-	-	6.3%	5.3%
Combination Abdominal CT Scan[1]	-	-	5.7%	10.5%
Combination Brain/Sinus CT Scan[1]	-	-	2.3%	2.7%
Combination Chest CT Scan[1]	-	-	1.9%	2.7%
Follow-up Mammogram/Ultrasound[1]	-	-	6.3%	8.8%
Lumbar Spine MRI for Low Back Pain[1]	-	-	37.6%	37.2%

Deer River Healthcare Center

115 10th Avenue Northeast
Deer River, MN 56636
URL: www.drhc.org
Phone: 218-246-2900
Fax: 218-246-3013
Type: Critical Access Hospitals
Emergency Services: Yes
Ownership: Voluntary non-profit - Private
Beds: 20

Key Personnel:
Infection Control. . . . . Christine Adams
Chief of Medical Staff. . . . . David Goodall, MD
Radiology. . . . . Abe Latvala
Patient Relations . . . . Angela Olson
Cardiac Laboratory. . . . . Angie Olson, RN
Emergency Room . . . . Kelly Skelly, RN
CEO/President. . . . . Jeffrey Stampohar

Measure	Cases	This Hosp.	State Avg.	U.S. Avg.
Blood Clot Prevention and Treatment				
Anticoagulation Overlap Therapy[1,2]	-	-	96%	93%
ICU Venous Thromboembolism Prophylaxis[2,3]	-	-	91%	92%
Incidence of Potentially Preventable VTE[2,3]	-	-	9%	10%
UFH with Dosages/Platelet Monitoring[1,2]	-	-	98%	97%
Venous Thromboembolism Prophylaxis[2,3]	-	-	86%	85%
Warfarin Therapy Discharge Instructions[1,2]	-	-	63%	75%
Chest Pain/Possible Heart Attack Care				
Aspirin Given Within 24 Hours of Arrival	13	100%	97%	96%
Fibrinolytic Meds Within 30 Min. of Arrival[1]	-	-	48%	58%
Average Time to ECG (minutes)	12	7	7	7
Average Time to Transfer (minutes)[1]	-	-	54	60
Children's Asthma Care				
Received Home Management Plan of Care	-	-	-	88%
Received Reliever Medication	-	-	-	100%
Received Systemic Corticosteroids	-	-	-	100%
Emergency Department				
Admittance Decision Time (minutes)[2]	124	25	62	98
Head CT Results Within 45 Min. of Arrival[1,3]	-	-	54%	57%
Patients Who Left ER Before Being Seen[5]	-	-	2%	2%
Time from ER Arrival to Admit. (minutes)[2]	128	156	199	274
Time from ER Arrival to Discharge (minutes)[1,3]	-	-	125	134
Time in ER Before Being Evaluated (minutes)[1,3]	-	-	31	26
Time to Pain Meds for Fractures (minutes)[1,3]	-	-	45	57
Heart Attack Care				
Aspirin Given at Discharge[1,3]	-	-	99%	99%
Fibrinolytic Meds Within 30 Min. of Arrival[3,7]	-	-	-	54%
PCI Within 90 Minutes of Arrival[3,7]	-	-	96%	96%
Statin Prescribed at Discharge[1,3]	-	-	99%	98%
Heart Failure Care				
ACE Inhibitor or ARB for LVSD[1]	-	-	96%	97%
Discharge Instructions Given	13	54%	93%	94%
Evaluation of LVS Function	15	47%	97%	99%
Medicare Spending				
Medicare Spending per Patient (ratio)	-	-	0.9	0.98
Pneumonia Care				
Appropriate Initial Antibiotic Given[1]	-	-	94%	95%
Blood Culture Timing	12	92%	97%	98%
Pregnancy and Delivery Care				
Newborn Deliveries Scheduled Early[5]	-	-	5%	6%
Preventive Care				
Immunization for Influenza	228	57%	89%	90%
Immunization for Pneumonia[2]	266	59%	89%	92%
Stroke Care				
Anticoagulation Therapy for Atrial Fibrillation[3,7]	-	-	96%	95%
Antithrombotic Therapy Timing[1,3]	-	-	98%	98%
Assessed for Rehabilitation[1,3]	-	-	98%	97%
Discharged on Antithrombotic Therapy[1,3]	-	-	99%	99%
Discharged on Statin Medication[1,3]	-	-	95%	94%
Thrombolytic Therapy Timing[1,3]	-	-	74%	66%
Venous Thromboembolism Prophylaxis[1,3]	-	-	95%	94%
Written Stroke Educational Materials Given[1,3]	-	-	88%	88%
Surgical Care Improvement Project				
Appropriate Beta Blocker Usage	14	64%	98%	98%
Appropriate VTP Within 24 Hours	30	100%	98%	98%
Controlled Postoperative Blood Glucose[7]	-	-	97%	97%
Perioperative Temperature Management	42	98%	99%	100%
Prophylactic Antibiotic Selection	39	100%	99%	99%
Prophylactic Antibiotic Selection (Outpatient)[1,3]	-	-	98%	98%
Prophylactic Antibiotic Stopped	39	100%	99%	98%
Prophylactic Antibiotic Timing	39	79%	98%	99%
Prophylactic Antibiotic Timing (Outpatient)[1,3]	-	-	97%	98%
Urinary Catheter Removal[1]	-	-	97%	97%
Survey of Patients' Hospital Experiences				
Area Around Room 'Always' Quiet at Night[5]	-	-	65%	61%
Doctors 'Always' Communicated Well[5]	-	-	84%	82%
Home Recovery Information Given[5]	-	-	88%	85%
Hospital Given 9 or 10 on 10 Point Scale[5]	-	-	74%	71%
Meds 'Always' Explained Before Given[5]	-	-	67%	64%
Nurses 'Always' Communicated Well[5]	-	-	81%	79%
Pain 'Always' Well Controlled[5]	-	-	72%	71%
Room and Bathroom 'Always' Clean[5]	-	-	78%	73%
Timely Help 'Always' Received[5]	-	-	74%	68%
Would Definitely Recommend Hospital[5]	-	-	71%	71%
Use of Medical Imaging				
Cardiac Imaging Stress Test before Surgery[1]	-	-	6.3%	5.3%
Combination Abdominal CT Scan	67	9.0%	5.7%	10.5%
Combination Brain/Sinus CT Scan[1]	-	-	2.3%	2.7%
Combination Chest CT Scan[1]	-	-	1.9%	2.7%
Follow-up Mammogram/Ultrasound	173	5.2%	6.3%	8.8%
Lumbar Spine MRI for Low Back Pain[1]	-	-	37.6%	37.2%

Essentia Health Saint Marys

1027 Washington Ave
Detroit Lakes, MN 56501
URL: www.smrhc.com
Phone: 218-847-0852
Fax: 218-847-7674
Type: Acute Care Hospitals
Emergency Services: Yes
Ownership: Voluntary non-profit - Church
Beds: 187

Key Personnel:
Quality Assurance . . . . Dennis A Acrea
Radiology. . . . . A Douglas Landers, MD
Infection Control. . . . . Jackie Nordick
Operating Room. . . . . Marcia Rogers
Intensive Care Unit. . . . . Peg Severson
CEO/President. . . . . Thomas R Thompson
Chief of Medical Staff. . . . . Knute Thorsgard, MD
Patient Relations . . . . Jane Wasvick

Measure	Cases	This Hosp.	State Avg.	U.S. Avg.
Blood Clot Prevention and Treatment				
Anticoagulation Overlap Therapy[1,2]	-	-	96%	93%
ICU Venous Thromboembolism Prophylaxis[2]	56	91%	91%	92%
Incidence of Potentially Preventable VTE[1,2]	-	-	9%	10%
UFH with Dosages/Platelet Monitoring[1,2]	-	-	98%	97%
Venous Thromboembolism Prophylaxis[2]	90	90%	86%	85%
Warfarin Therapy Discharge Instructions[1,2]	-	-	63%	75%
Chest Pain/Possible Heart Attack Care				
Aspirin Given Within 24 Hours of Arrival	73	99%	97%	96%
Fibrinolytic Meds Within 30 Min. of Arrival[1]	-	-	48%	58%
Average Time to ECG (minutes)	74	8	7	7
Average Time to Transfer (minutes)	11	50	54	60
Children's Asthma Care				
Received Home Management Plan of Care	-	-	-	88%
Received Reliever Medication	-	-	-	100%
Received Systemic Corticosteroids	-	-	-	100%
Emergency Department				
Admittance Decision Time (minutes)[2]	234	67	62	98
Head CT Results Within 45 Min. of Arrival[1]	-	-	54%	57%
Patients Who Left ER Before Being Seen	11,470	3%	2%	2%
Time from ER Arrival to Admit. (minutes)[2]	237	215	199	274
Time from ER Arrival to Discharge (minutes)	351	119	125	134
Time in ER Before Being Evaluated (minutes)	112	22	31	26
Time to Pain Meds for Fractures (minutes)	60	38	45	57
Heart Attack Care				
Aspirin Given at Discharge[1]	-	-	99%	99%
Fibrinolytic Meds Within 30 Min. of Arrival[7]	-	-	-	54%
PCI Within 90 Minutes of Arrival[7]	-	-	96%	96%
Statin Prescribed at Discharge[1]	-	-	99%	98%
Heart Failure Care				
ACE Inhibitor or ARB for LVSD	15	100%	96%	97%
Discharge Instructions Given	28	96%	93%	94%
Evaluation of LVS Function	44	100%	97%	99%
Medicare Spending				
Medicare Spending per Patient (ratio)	-	0.94	0.9	0.98
Pneumonia Care				
Appropriate Initial Antibiotic Given	37	95%	94%	95%
Blood Culture Timing	52	94%	97%	98%
Pregnancy and Delivery Care				
Newborn Deliveries Scheduled Early	63	2%	5%	6%
Preventive Care				
Immunization for Influenza[2]	252	78%	89%	90%
Immunization for Pneumonia[2]	242	95%	89%	92%
Stroke Care				
Anticoagulation Therapy for Atrial Fibrillation[1]	-	-	96%	95%
Antithrombotic Therapy Timing[1]	-	-	98%	98%
Assessed for Rehabilitation[1]	-	-	98%	97%
Discharged on Antithrombotic Therapy[1]	-	-	99%	99%
Discharged on Statin Medication[1]	-	-	95%	94%
Thrombolytic Therapy Timing[7]	-	-	74%	66%
Venous Thromboembolism Prophylaxis[1]	-	-	95%	94%
Written Stroke Educational Materials Given[1]	-	-	88%	88%
Surgical Care Improvement Project				
Appropriate Beta Blocker Usage	103	95%	98%	98%
Appropriate VTP Within 24 Hours	262	98%	98%	98%
Controlled Postoperative Blood Glucose[7]	-	-	97%	97%
Perioperative Temperature Management	301	100%	99%	100%
Prophylactic Antibiotic Selection	245	100%	99%	99%
Prophylactic Antibiotic Selection (Outpatient)	16	94%	98%	98%
Prophylactic Antibiotic Stopped	241	97%	99%	98%
Prophylactic Antibiotic Timing	246	100%	98%	99%
Prophylactic Antibiotic Timing (Outpatient)[1]	-	-	97%	98%
Urinary Catheter Removal	203	100%	97%	97%
Survey of Patients' Hospital Experiences				
Area Around Room 'Always' Quiet at Night	300+	61%	65%	61%
Doctors 'Always' Communicated Well	300+	81%	84%	82%
Home Recovery Information Given	300+	88%	88%	85%
Hospital Given 9 or 10 on 10 Point Scale	300+	72%	74%	71%
Meds 'Always' Explained Before Given	300+	62%	67%	64%
Nurses 'Always' Communicated Well	300+	79%	81%	79%
Pain 'Always' Well Controlled	300+	68%	72%	71%
Room and Bathroom 'Always' Clean	300+	71%	78%	73%
Timely Help 'Always' Received	300+	73%	74%	68%
Would Definitely Recommend Hospital	300+	67%	71%	71%
Use of Medical Imaging				
Cardiac Imaging Stress Test before Surgery[1]	-	-	6.3%	5.3%
Combination Abdominal CT Scan	124	4.0%	5.7%	10.5%
Combination Brain/Sinus CT Scan[1]	-	-	2.3%	2.7%
Combination Chest CT Scan	136	0.0%	1.9%	2.7%
Follow-up Mammogram/Ultrasound	276	5.1%	6.3%	8.8%
Lumbar Spine MRI for Low Back Pain[1]	-	-	37.6%	37.2%

NOTE: Hospital profiles are in alphabetical order by state, then city, then hospital within the city; Rankings exclude hospitals with less than 25 cases except for patient surveys which excludes hospitals with less than 100 cases; (a) 100-299 cases; (1) The number of cases/patients is too few to report; (2) Data submitted were based on a sample of cases/patients; (3) Results are based on a shorter time period than required; (4) Data suppressed by CMS for one or more quarters; (5) Results are not available for this reporting period; (6) Fewer than 100 patients completed the HCAHPS survey; (7) No cases met the criteria for this measure; (8) The lower limit of the confidence interval cannot be calculated if the number of observed infections equals zero; (9) No data are available from the state/territory for this reporting period; (10) The scores shown reflect fewer than 50 completed surveys; (11) There were discrepancies in the data collection process; (12) This measure does not apply to this hospital for this reporting period; (13) Results cannot be calculated for this reporting period; (14) The results for this state are combined with nearby states to protect confidentiality; Please refer to the User's Guide for a full explanation of data.

Essentia Health Duluth

502 East Second Street
Duluth, MN 55805
Phone: 218-786-2646
Type: Acute Care Hospitals
Emergency Services: No
Ownership: Voluntary non-profit - Private

Key Personnel:

Ambulatory Care .... Michael C Metcalf
Chief of Medical Staff .... Thomas G Patnoe, MD
CEO .... Peter Person, MD
Patient Relations .... Terri Ruberg

Measure	Cases	This Hosp.	State Avg.	U.S. Avg.
Blood Clot Prevention and Treatment				
Anticoagulation Overlap Therapy[1,2]	-	-	96%	93%
ICU Venous Thromboembolism Prophylaxis[1,2]	-	-	91%	92%
Incidence of Potentially Preventable VTE[1,2]	-	-	9%	10%
UFH with Dosages/Platelet Monitoring[1,2]	-	-	98%	97%
Venous Thromboembolism Prophylaxis[2]	121	82%	86%	85%
Warfarin Therapy Discharge Instructions[1,2]	-	-	63%	75%
Chest Pain/Possible Heart Attack Care				
Aspirin Given Within 24 Hours of Arrival[5]	-	-	97%	96%
Fibrinolytic Meds Within 30 Min. of Arrival[5]	-	-	48%	58%
Average Time to ECG (minutes)[5]	-	-	7	7
Average Time to Transfer (minutes)[5]	-	-	54	60
Children's Asthma Care				
Received Home Management Plan of Care	-	-	-	88%
Received Reliever Medication	-	-	-	100%
Received Systemic Corticosteroids	-	-	-	100%
Emergency Department				
Admittance Decision Time (minutes)[1,2]	-	-	62	98
Head CT Results Within 45 Min. of Arrival[5]	-	-	54%	57%
Patients Who Left ER Before Being Seen[5]	-	-	2%	2%
Time from ER Arrival to Admit. (minutes)[1,2]	-	-	199	274
Time from ER Arrival to Discharge (minutes)[5]	-	-	125	134
Time in ER Before Being Evaluated (minutes)[5]	-	-	31	26
Time to Pain Meds for Fractures (minutes)[5]	-	-	45	57
Heart Attack Care				
Aspirin Given at Discharge[1,3]	-	-	99%	99%
Fibrinolytic Meds Within 30 Min. of Arrival[3,7]	-	-	-	54%
PCI Within 90 Minutes of Arrival[3,7]	-	-	96%	96%
Statin Prescribed at Discharge[1,3]	-	-	99%	98%
Heart Failure Care				
ACE Inhibitor or ARB for LVSD[3,7]	-	-	96%	97%
Discharge Instructions Given[1,3]	-	-	93%	94%
Evaluation of LVS Function[1,3]	-	-	97%	99%
Medicare Spending				
Medicare Spending per Patient (ratio)	-	0.96	0.9	0.98
Pneumonia Care				
Appropriate Initial Antibiotic Given[1]	-	-	94%	95%
Blood Culture Timing[7]	-	-	97%	98%
Pregnancy and Delivery Care				
Newborn Deliveries Scheduled Early[7]	-	-	5%	6%
Preventive Care				
Immunization for Influenza[2]	340	86%	89%	90%
Immunization for Pneumonia[2]	258	94%	89%	92%
Stroke Care				
Anticoagulation Therapy for Atrial Fibrillation[7]	-	-	96%	95%
Antithrombotic Therapy Timing[1]	-	-	98%	98%
Assessed for Rehabilitation[1]	-	-	98%	97%
Discharged on Antithrombotic Therapy[1]	-	-	99%	99%
Discharged on Statin Medication[1]	-	-	95%	94%
Thrombolytic Therapy Timing[7]	-	-	74%	66%
Venous Thromboembolism Prophylaxis[1]	-	-	95%	94%
Written Stroke Educational Materials Given[1]	-	-	88%	88%
Surgical Care Improvement Project				
Appropriate Beta Blocker Usage[2]	13	100%	98%	98%
Appropriate VTP Within 24 Hours[2]	36	100%	98%	98%
Controlled Postoperative Blood Glucose[2,7]	-	-	97%	97%
Perioperative Temperature Management[2]	83	100%	99%	100%
Prophylactic Antibiotic Selection[2]	75	100%	99%	99%
Prophylactic Antibiotic Selection (Outpatient)	318	84%	98%	98%
Prophylactic Antibiotic Stopped[2]	75	97%	99%	98%
Prophylactic Antibiotic Timing[2]	75	100%	98%	99%
Prophylactic Antibiotic Timing (Outpatient)	175	98%	97%	98%
Urinary Catheter Removal[2,7]	-	-	97%	97%
Survey of Patients' Hospital Experiences				
Area Around Room 'Always' Quiet at Night	300+	53%	65%	61%
Doctors 'Always' Communicated Well	300+	84%	84%	82%
Home Recovery Information Given	300+	88%	88%	85%
Hospital Given 9 or 10 on 10 Point Scale	300+	67%	74%	71%
Meds 'Always' Explained Before Given	300+	63%	67%	64%
Nurses 'Always' Communicated Well	300+	75%	81%	79%
Pain 'Always' Well Controlled	300+	67%	72%	71%
Room and Bathroom 'Always' Clean	300+	69%	78%	73%
Timely Help 'Always' Received	300+	65%	74%	68%
Would Definitely Recommend Hospital	300+	74%	71%	71%
Use of Medical Imaging				
Cardiac Imaging Stress Test before Surgery[7]	-	-	6.3%	5.3%
Combination Abdominal CT Scan	532	6.2%	5.7%	10.5%
Combination Brain/Sinus CT Scan	60	0.0%	2.3%	2.7%
Combination Chest CT Scan	541	0.0%	1.9%	2.7%
Follow-up Mammogram/Ultrasound	1,598	5.5%	6.3%	8.8%
Lumbar Spine MRI for Low Back Pain	80	33.8%	37.6%	37.2%

Essentia Health Saint Mary's Medical Center

407 East Third Street
Duluth, MN 55805
URL: www.smdc.org
Phone: 218-786-4000
Fax: 218-727-7258
Type: Acute Care Hospitals
Emergency Services: Yes
Ownership: Voluntary non-profit - Private
Beds: 690

Key Personnel:

Operating Room.............. Thurza Bender
CEO/President............... Peter E Person, MD
Patient Relations .... Suzanne Rozinka
Quality Assurance .... Suzanne Rozinka
Pediatric Ambulatory Care ...... Cindy Sorenson
Chief of Medical Staff.......... Patrick Twomey, MD
Emergency Room .... Linda Waigh
Infection Control.............. Cindi Welch

Measure	Cases	This Hosp.	State Avg.	U.S. Avg.
Blood Clot Prevention and Treatment				
Anticoagulation Overlap Therapy[2]	95	98%	96%	93%
ICU Venous Thromboembolism Prophylaxis[2]	38	76%	91%	92%
Incidence of Potentially Preventable VTE[2]	15	7%	9%	10%
UFH with Dosages/Platelet Monitoring[2]	82	100%	98%	97%
Venous Thromboembolism Prophylaxis[2]	340	79%	86%	85%
Warfarin Therapy Discharge Instructions[2]	84	92%	63%	75%
Chest Pain/Possible Heart Attack Care				
Aspirin Given Within 24 Hours of Arrival[1]	-	-	97%	96%
Fibrinolytic Meds Within 30 Min. of Arrival[5]	-	-	48%	58%
Average Time to ECG (minutes)[1]	-	-	7	7
Average Time to Transfer (minutes)[5]	-	-	54	60
Children's Asthma Care				
Received Home Management Plan of Care	-	-	-	88%
Received Reliever Medication	-	-	-	100%
Received Systemic Corticosteroids	-	-	-	100%
Emergency Department				
Admittance Decision Time (minutes)[2]	466	117	62	98
Head CT Results Within 45 Min. of Arrival[1]	-	-	54%	57%
Patients Who Left ER Before Being Seen	43,604	2%	2%	2%
Time from ER Arrival to Admit. (minutes)[2]	480	236	199	274
Time from ER Arrival to Discharge (minutes)	329	161	125	134
Time in ER Before Being Evaluated (minutes)	116	30	31	26
Time to Pain Meds for Fractures (minutes)	154	51	45	57
Heart Attack Care				
Aspirin Given at Discharge[2]	356	99%	99%	99%
Fibrinolytic Meds Within 30 Min. of Arrival[2,7]	-	-	-	54%
PCI Within 90 Minutes of Arrival[2]	11	82%	96%	96%
Statin Prescribed at Discharge[2]	335	100%	99%	98%
Heart Failure Care				
ACE Inhibitor or ARB for LVSD[2]	97	100%	96%	97%
Discharge Instructions Given[2]	227	93%	93%	94%
Evaluation of LVS Function[2]	285	100%	97%	99%
Medicare Spending				
Medicare Spending per Patient (ratio)	-	0.97	0.9	0.98
Pneumonia Care				
Appropriate Initial Antibiotic Given[2]	68	90%	94%	95%
Blood Culture Timing[2]	85	96%	97%	98%
Pregnancy and Delivery Care				
Newborn Deliveries Scheduled Early	80	1%	5%	6%
Preventive Care				
Immunization for Influenza[2]	568	92%	89%	90%
Immunization for Pneumonia[2]	660	98%	89%	92%
Stroke Care				
Anticoagulation Therapy for Atrial Fibrillation	27	96%	96%	95%
Antithrombotic Therapy Timing	141	99%	98%	98%
Assessed for Rehabilitation	218	98%	98%	97%
Discharged on Antithrombotic Therapy	182	98%	99%	99%
Discharged on Statin Medication	131	98%	95%	94%
Thrombolytic Therapy Timing	21	86%	74%	66%
Venous Thromboembolism Prophylaxis	220	96%	95%	94%
Written Stroke Educational Materials Given	113	96%	88%	88%
Surgical Care Improvement Project				
Appropriate Beta Blocker Usage[2]	247	99%	98%	98%
Appropriate VTP Within 24 Hours[2]	320	97%	98%	98%
Controlled Postoperative Blood Glucose[2]	121	96%	97%	97%
Perioperative Temperature Management[2]	463	100%	99%	100%
Prophylactic Antibiotic Selection[2]	432	99%	99%	99%
Prophylactic Antibiotic Selection (Outpatient)	493	98%	98%	98%
Prophylactic Antibiotic Stopped[2]	414	97%	99%	98%
Prophylactic Antibiotic Timing[2]	435	98%	98%	99%
Prophylactic Antibiotic Timing (Outpatient)	493	99%	97%	98%
Urinary Catheter Removal[2]	212	93%	97%	97%
Survey of Patients' Hospital Experiences				
Area Around Room 'Always' Quiet at Night	300+	47%	65%	61%
Doctors 'Always' Communicated Well	300+	80%	84%	82%
Home Recovery Information Given	300+	88%	88%	85%
Hospital Given 9 or 10 on 10 Point Scale	300+	68%	74%	71%
Meds 'Always' Explained Before Given	300+	64%	67%	64%
Nurses 'Always' Communicated Well	300+	77%	81%	79%
Pain 'Always' Well Controlled	300+	67%	72%	71%
Room and Bathroom 'Always' Clean	300+	65%	78%	73%
Timely Help 'Always' Received	300+	66%	74%	68%
Would Definitely Recommend Hospital	300+	73%	71%	71%
Use of Medical Imaging				
Cardiac Imaging Stress Test before Surgery	820	5.0%	6.3%	5.3%
Combination Abdominal CT Scan	532	11.7%	5.7%	10.5%
Combination Brain/Sinus CT Scan	511	2.5%	2.3%	2.7%
Combination Chest CT Scan	319	0.9%	1.9%	2.7%
Follow-up Mammogram/Ultrasound[7]	-	-	6.3%	8.8%
Lumbar Spine MRI for Low Back Pain[1]	-	-	37.6%	37.2%

Saint Luke's Hospital

915 East 1st Street
Duluth, MN 55805
URL: www.slhduluth.com
Phone: 218-249-5555
Type: Acute Care Hospitals
Emergency Services: Yes
Ownership: Voluntary non-profit - Private
Beds: 267

Key Personnel:

Chair/CEO.................. Dale Moe
CEO/President................ John Strange

Measure	Cases	This Hosp.	State Avg.	U.S. Avg.
Blood Clot Prevention and Treatment				
Anticoagulation Overlap Therapy[2]	57	96%	96%	93%
ICU Venous Thromboembolism Prophylaxis[2]	77	91%	91%	92%
Incidence of Potentially Preventable VTE[1,2]	-	-	9%	10%
UFH with Dosages/Platelet Monitoring[2]	38	100%	98%	97%
Venous Thromboembolism Prophylaxis[2]	305	82%	86%	85%
Warfarin Therapy Discharge Instructions[2]	44	82%	63%	75%
Chest Pain/Possible Heart Attack Care				
Aspirin Given Within 24 Hours of Arrival[1,3]	-	-	97%	96%
Fibrinolytic Meds Within 30 Min. of Arrival[3,7]	-	-	48%	58%
Average Time to ECG (minutes)[1,3]	-	-	7	7
Average Time to Transfer (minutes)[3,7]	-	-	54	60
Children's Asthma Care				
Received Home Management Plan of Care	-	-	-	88%
Received Reliever Medication	-	-	-	100%
Received Systemic Corticosteroids	-	-	-	100%
Emergency Department				
Admittance Decision Time (minutes)[2]	451	84	62	98
Head CT Results Within 45 Min. of Arrival[1]	-	-	54%	57%

NOTE: Hospital profiles are in alphabetical order by state, then city, then hospital within the city; Rankings exclude hospitals with less than 25 cases except for patient surveys which excludes hospitals with less than 100 cases; (a) 100-299 cases; (1) The number of cases/patients is too few to report; (2) Data submitted were based on a sample of cases/patients; (3) Results are based on a shorter time period than required; (4) Data suppressed by CMS for one or more quarters; (5) Results are not available for this reporting period; (6) Fewer than 100 patients completed the HCAHPS survey; (7) No cases met the criteria for this measure; (8) The lower limit of the confidence interval cannot be calculated if the number of observed infections equals zero; (9) No data are available from the state/territory for this reporting period; (10) The scores shown reflect fewer than 50 completed surveys; (11) There were discrepancies in the data collection process; (12) This measure does not apply to this hospital for this reporting period; (13) Results cannot be calculated for this reporting period; (14) The results for this state are combined with nearby states to protect confidentiality; Please refer to the User's Guide for a full explanation of data.

Patients Who Left ER Before Being Seen	27,471	2%	2%	2%
Time from ER Arrival to Admit. (minutes)[2]	451	190	199	274
Time from ER Arrival to Discharge (minutes)	450	150	125	134
Time in ER Before Being Evaluated (minutes)	484	40	31	26
Time to Pain Meds for Fractures (minutes)	62	66	45	57
Heart Attack Care				
Aspirin Given at Discharge	228	99%	99%	99%
Fibrinolytic Meds Within 30 Min. of Arrival[7]	-	-	-	54%
PCI Within 90 Minutes of Arrival	25	100%	96%	96%
Statin Prescribed at Discharge	223	100%	99%	98%
Heart Failure Care				
ACE Inhibitor or ARB for LVSD	52	96%	96%	97%
Discharge Instructions Given	101	93%	93%	94%
Evaluation of LVS Function	149	99%	97%	99%
Medicare Spending				
Medicare Spending per Patient (ratio)	-	0.98	0.9	0.98
Pneumonia Care				
Appropriate Initial Antibiotic Given[2]	72	93%	94%	95%
Blood Culture Timing[2]	149	99%	97%	98%
Pregnancy and Delivery Care				
Newborn Deliveries Scheduled Early[2]	35	0%	5%	6%
Preventive Care				
Immunization for Influenza[2]	588	98%	89%	90%
Immunization for Pneumonia[2]	678	98%	89%	92%
Stroke Care				
Anticoagulation Therapy for Atrial Fibrillation[1]	-	-	96%	95%
Antithrombotic Therapy Timing	76	96%	98%	98%
Assessed for Rehabilitation	92	98%	98%	97%
Discharged on Antithrombotic Therapy	86	100%	99%	99%
Discharged on Statin Medication	70	96%	95%	94%
Thrombolytic Therapy Timing[1]	-	-	74%	66%
Venous Thromboembolism Prophylaxis	91	81%	95%	94%
Written Stroke Educational Materials Given	32	94%	88%	88%
Surgical Care Improvement Project				
Appropriate Beta Blocker Usage[2]	174	100%	98%	98%
Appropriate VTP Within 24 Hours[2]	320	98%	98%	98%
Controlled Postoperative Blood Glucose[2]	132	98%	97%	97%
Perioperative Temperature Management[2]	391	99%	99%	100%
Prophylactic Antibiotic Selection[2]	361	99%	99%	99%
Prophylactic Antibiotic Selection (Outpatient)	572	100%	98%	98%
Prophylactic Antibiotic Stopped[2]	356	99%	99%	98%
Prophylactic Antibiotic Timing[2]	362	98%	98%	99%
Prophylactic Antibiotic Timing (Outpatient)	574	98%	97%	98%
Urinary Catheter Removal[2]	208	94%	97%	97%
Survey of Patients' Hospital Experiences				
Area Around Room 'Always' Quiet at Night	300+	49%	65%	61%
Doctors 'Always' Communicated Well	300+	82%	84%	82%
Home Recovery Information Given	300+	90%	88%	85%
Hospital Given 9 or 10 on 10 Point Scale	300+	73%	74%	71%
Meds 'Always' Explained Before Given	300+	61%	67%	64%
Nurses 'Always' Communicated Well	300+	76%	81%	79%
Pain 'Always' Well Controlled	300+	70%	72%	71%
Room and Bathroom 'Always' Clean	300+	70%	78%	73%
Timely Help 'Always' Received	300+	61%	74%	68%
Would Definitely Recommend Hospital	300+	77%	71%	71%
Use of Medical Imaging				
Cardiac Imaging Stress Test before Surgery	360	4.7%	6.3%	5.3%
Combination Abdominal CT Scan	691	10.6%	5.7%	10.5%
Combination Brain/Sinus CT Scan[1]	-	-	2.3%	2.7%
Combination Chest CT Scan	575	0.0%	1.9%	2.7%
Follow-up Mammogram/Ultrasound	1,160	5.2%	6.3%	8.8%
Lumbar Spine MRI for Low Back Pain[7]	-	-	37.6%	37.2%

Fairview Southdale Hospital

6401 France Avenue South
Edina, MN 55435
URL: www.fairview.org
Type: Acute Care Hospitals
Ownership: Voluntary non-profit - Other
Phone: 952-924-5000
Fax: 952-924-5970
Emergency Services: Yes
Beds: 390

Key Personnel:
Coronary Care . . . . Kaysie Banton, MD
Chief of Medical Staff . . . . James Bishop, MD
Cardiac Laboratory . . . . Norman Chapel, MD, FACC
Quality Assurance . . . . Laura Deneui
Operating Room . . . . Bonnie Herda
Infection Control . . . . Terese Paulson, MD
Radiology . . . . Judy Sager
CEO/President . . . . Rulon F. Stacey, PhD, FACHE

Measure	Cases	This Hosp.	State Avg.	U.S. Avg.
Blood Clot Prevention and Treatment				
Anticoagulation Overlap Therapy[2]	156	100%	96%	93%
ICU Venous Thromboembolism Prophylaxis[2]	59	100%	91%	92%
Incidence of Potentially Preventable VTE[2]	20	5%	9%	10%
UFH with Dosages/Platelet Monitoring[2]	147	100%	98%	97%
Venous Thromboembolism Prophylaxis[2]	327	98%	86%	85%
Warfarin Therapy Discharge Instructions[2]	109	99%	63%	75%
Chest Pain/Possible Heart Attack Care				
Aspirin Given Within 24 Hours of Arrival[1,3]	-	-	97%	96%
Fibrinolytic Meds Within 30 Min. of Arrival[5]	-	-	48%	58%
Average Time to ECG (minutes)[1,3]	-	-	7	7
Average Time to Transfer (minutes)[5]	-	-	54	60
Children's Asthma Care				
Received Home Management Plan of Care	-	-	-	88%
Received Reliever Medication	-	-	-	100%
Received Systemic Corticosteroids	-	-	-	100%
Emergency Department				
Admittance Decision Time (minutes)[2]	478	98	62	98
Head CT Results Within 45 Min. of Arrival[1]	-	-	54%	57%
Patients Who Left ER Before Being Seen	44,431	3%	2%	2%
Time from ER Arrival to Admit. (minutes)[2]	478	247	199	274
Time from ER Arrival to Discharge (minutes)	418	186	125	134
Time in ER Before Being Evaluated (minutes)	439	33	31	26
Time to Pain Meds for Fractures (minutes)	191	54	45	57
Heart Attack Care				
Aspirin Given at Discharge[2]	342	100%	99%	99%
Fibrinolytic Meds Within 30 Min. of Arrival[2,7]	-	-	-	54%
PCI Within 90 Minutes of Arrival[2]	60	100%	96%	96%
Statin Prescribed at Discharge[2]	351	100%	99%	98%
Heart Failure Care				
ACE Inhibitor or ARB for LVSD[2]	80	100%	96%	97%
Discharge Instructions Given[2]	221	100%	93%	94%
Evaluation of LVS Function[2]	352	100%	97%	99%
Medicare Spending				
Medicare Spending per Patient (ratio)	-	0.97	0.9	0.98
Pneumonia Care				
Appropriate Initial Antibiotic Given	199	99%	94%	95%
Blood Culture Timing	364	99%	97%	98%
Pregnancy and Delivery Care				
Newborn Deliveries Scheduled Early[2]	43	2%	5%	6%
Preventive Care				
Immunization for Influenza[2]	565	93%	89%	90%
Immunization for Pneumonia[2]	629	91%	89%	92%
Stroke Care				
Anticoagulation Therapy for Atrial Fibrillation	32	100%	96%	95%
Antithrombotic Therapy Timing	213	100%	98%	98%
Assessed for Rehabilitation	274	100%	98%	97%
Discharged on Antithrombotic Therapy	251	100%	99%	99%
Discharged on Statin Medication	193	98%	95%	94%
Thrombolytic Therapy Timing	26	100%	74%	66%
Venous Thromboembolism Prophylaxis	276	100%	95%	94%
Written Stroke Educational Materials Given	139	95%	88%	88%
Surgical Care Improvement Project				
Appropriate Beta Blocker Usage[2]	458	100%	98%	98%
Appropriate VTP Within 24 Hours[2]	900	100%	98%	98%
Controlled Postoperative Blood Glucose[2]	232	99%	97%	97%
Perioperative Temperature Management[2]	1,083	100%	99%	100%
Prophylactic Antibiotic Selection[2]	1,040	99%	99%	99%
Prophylactic Antibiotic Selection (Outpatient)	650	98%	98%	98%
Prophylactic Antibiotic Stopped[2]	1,012	100%	99%	98%
Prophylactic Antibiotic Timing[2]	1,045	100%	98%	99%
Prophylactic Antibiotic Timing (Outpatient)	647	98%	97%	98%
Urinary Catheter Removal[2]	754	99%	97%	97%
Survey of Patients' Hospital Experiences				
Area Around Room 'Always' Quiet at Night	300+	54%	65%	61%
Doctors 'Always' Communicated Well	300+	82%	84%	82%
Home Recovery Information Given	300+	87%	88%	85%
Hospital Given 9 or 10 on 10 Point Scale	300+	71%	74%	71%
Meds 'Always' Explained Before Given	300+	60%	67%	64%
Nurses 'Always' Communicated Well	300+	78%	81%	79%
Pain 'Always' Well Controlled	300+	72%	72%	71%
Room and Bathroom 'Always' Clean	300+	69%	78%	73%
Timely Help 'Always' Received	300+	65%	74%	68%
Would Definitely Recommend Hospital	300+	74%	71%	71%
Use of Medical Imaging				
Cardiac Imaging Stress Test before Surgery	670	4.3%	6.3%	5.3%
Combination Abdominal CT Scan	603	2.8%	5.7%	10.5%
Combination Brain/Sinus CT Scan	543	1.3%	2.3%	2.7%
Combination Chest CT Scan	542	0.9%	1.9%	2.7%
Follow-up Mammogram/Ultrasound	1,213	4.9%	6.3%	8.8%
Lumbar Spine MRI for Low Back Pain	37	43.2%	37.6%	37.2%

Prairie Ridge Hospital & Health Services

930 First Street Northeast
Elbow Lake, MN 56531
E-mail: nleavitt@eleahmed.org
URL: www.eleahmed.org
Type: Critical Access Hospitals
Ownership: Voluntary non-profit - Private
Phone: 218-685-4461
Fax: 218-685-4240
Emergency Services: Yes
Beds: 20

Key Personnel:
CEO/President . . . . Larry Rapp

Measure	Cases	This Hosp.	State Avg.	U.S. Avg.
Blood Clot Prevention and Treatment				
Anticoagulation Overlap Therapy[5]	-	-	96%	93%
ICU Venous Thromboembolism Prophylaxis[5]	-	-	91%	92%
Incidence of Potentially Preventable VTE[5]	-	-	9%	10%
UFH with Dosages/Platelet Monitoring[5]	-	-	98%	97%
Venous Thromboembolism Prophylaxis[5]	-	-	86%	85%
Warfarin Therapy Discharge Instructions[5]	-	-	63%	75%
Chest Pain/Possible Heart Attack Care				
Aspirin Given Within 24 Hours of Arrival[1,3]	-	-	97%	96%
Fibrinolytic Meds Within 30 Min. of Arrival[1,3]	-	-	48%	58%
Average Time to ECG (minutes)[1,3]	-	-	7	7
Average Time to Transfer (minutes)[3,7]	-	-	54	60
Children's Asthma Care				
Received Home Management Plan of Care	-	-	-	88%
Received Reliever Medication	-	-	-	100%
Received Systemic Corticosteroids	-	-	-	100%
Emergency Department				
Admittance Decision Time (minutes)[5]	-	-	62	98
Head CT Results Within 45 Min. of Arrival[5]	-	-	54%	57%
Patients Who Left ER Before Being Seen[5]	-	-	2%	2%
Time from ER Arrival to Admit. (minutes)[5]	-	-	199	274
Time from ER Arrival to Discharge (minutes)[5]	-	-	125	134
Time in ER Before Being Evaluated (minutes)[5]	-	-	31	26
Time to Pain Meds for Fractures (minutes)[1,3]	-	-	45	57
Heart Attack Care				
Aspirin Given at Discharge[5]	-	-	99%	99%
Fibrinolytic Meds Within 30 Min. of Arrival[5]	-	-	-	54%
PCI Within 90 Minutes of Arrival[5]	-	-	96%	96%
Statin Prescribed at Discharge[5]	-	-	99%	98%
Heart Failure Care				
ACE Inhibitor or ARB for LVSD[1,2]	-	-	96%	97%
Discharge Instructions Given[2]	11	45%	93%	94%
Evaluation of LVS Function[2]	11	55%	97%	99%
Medicare Spending				
Medicare Spending per Patient (ratio)	-	-	0.9	0.98
Pneumonia Care				
Appropriate Initial Antibiotic Given[1]	-	-	94%	95%
Blood Culture Timing[1]	-	-	97%	98%
Pregnancy and Delivery Care				
Newborn Deliveries Scheduled Early[5]	-	-	5%	6%
Preventive Care				
Immunization for Influenza[5]	-	-	89%	90%
Immunization for Pneumonia[5]	-	-	89%	92%
Stroke Care				
Anticoagulation Therapy for Atrial Fibrillation[5]	-	-	96%	95%
Antithrombotic Therapy Timing[5]	-	-	98%	98%
Assessed for Rehabilitation[5]	-	-	98%	97%
Discharged on Antithrombotic Therapy[5]	-	-	99%	99%
Discharged on Statin Medication[5]	-	-	95%	94%

NOTE: Hospital profiles are in alphabetical order by state, then city, then hospital within the city; Rankings exclude hospitals with less than 25 cases except for patient surveys which excludes hospitals with less than 100 cases; (a) 100-299 cases; (1) The number of cases/patients is too few to report; (2) Data submitted were based on a sample of cases/patients; (3) Results are based on a shorter time period than required; (4) Data suppressed by CMS for one or more quarters; (5) Results are not available for this reporting period; (6) Fewer than 100 patients completed the HCAHPS survey; (7) No cases met the criteria for this measure; (8) The lower limit of the confidence interval cannot be calculated if the number of observed infections equals zero; (9) No data are available from the state/territory for this reporting period; (10) The scores shown reflect fewer than 50 completed surveys; (11) There were discrepancies in the data collection process; (12) This measure does not apply to this hospital for this reporting period; (13) Results cannot be calculated for this reporting period; (14) The results for this state are combined with nearby states to protect confidentiality; Please refer to the User's Guide for a full explanation of data.

Measure	Cases	This Hosp.	State Avg.	U.S. Avg.
Thrombolytic Therapy Timing[5]	-	-	74%	66%
Venous Thromboembolism Prophylaxis[5]	-	-	95%	94%
Written Stroke Educational Materials Given[5]	-	-	88%	88%
Surgical Care Improvement Project				
Appropriate Beta Blocker Usage[5]	-	-	98%	98%
Appropriate VTP Within 24 Hours[5]	-	-	98%	98%
Controlled Postoperative Blood Glucose[5]	-	-	97%	97%
Perioperative Temperature Management[5]	-	-	99%	100%
Prophylactic Antibiotic Selection[5]	-	-	99%	99%
Prophylactic Antibiotic Selection (Outpatient)[3]	29	100%	98%	98%
Prophylactic Antibiotic Stopped[5]	-	-	99%	98%
Prophylactic Antibiotic Timing[5]	-	-	98%	99%
Prophylactic Antibiotic Timing (Outpatient)[3]	29	100%	97%	98%
Urinary Catheter Removal[5]	-	-	97%	97%
Survey of Patients' Hospital Experiences				
Area Around Room 'Always' Quiet at Night[5]	-	-	65%	61%
Doctors 'Always' Communicated Well[5]	-	-	84%	82%
Home Recovery Information Given[5]	-	-	88%	85%
Hospital Given 9 or 10 on 10 Point Scale[5]	-	-	74%	71%
Meds 'Always' Explained Before Given[5]	-	-	67%	64%
Nurses 'Always' Communicated Well[5]	-	-	81%	79%
Pain 'Always' Well Controlled[5]	-	-	72%	71%
Room and Bathroom 'Always' Clean[5]	-	-	78%	73%
Timely Help 'Always' Received[5]	-	-	74%	68%
Would Definitely Recommend Hospital[5]	-	-	71%	71%
Use of Medical Imaging				
Cardiac Imaging Stress Test before Surgery[1]	-	-	6.3%	5.3%
Combination Abdominal CT Scan[1]	-	-	5.7%	10.5%
Combination Brain/Sinus CT Scan[1]	-	-	2.3%	2.7%
Combination Chest CT Scan[1]	-	-	1.9%	2.7%
Follow-up Mammogram/Ultrasound	145	5.5%	6.3%	8.8%
Lumbar Spine MRI for Low Back Pain[1]	-	-	37.6%	37.2%

Ely Bloomenson Community Hospital

328 West Conan Street
Ely, MN 55731
Phone: 218-365-3271
Fax: 218-365-8777
URL: www.ebch.org
Type: Critical Access Hospitals
Emergency Services: Yes
Ownership: Voluntary non-profit - Private
Beds: 32

Key Personnel:

Quality Assurance . . . . Nancy Andreae
Chief of Medical Staff. . . . . Mary Bianco
CEO . . . . John Fossum
Anesthesiology. . . . . Bruce Kuam
Radiology. . . . . Mike Pechek
Infection Control. . . . . Mary Ann Smith, RN
Operating Room. . . . . Kyle Westrick, RN

Measure	Cases	This Hosp.	State Avg.	U.S. Avg.
Blood Clot Prevention and Treatment				
Anticoagulation Overlap Therapy[5]	-	-	96%	93%
ICU Venous Thromboembolism Prophylaxis[5]	-	-	91%	92%
Incidence of Potentially Preventable VTE[5]	-	-	9%	10%
UFH with Dosages/Platelet Monitoring[5]	-	-	98%	97%
Venous Thromboembolism Prophylaxis[5]	-	-	86%	85%
Warfarin Therapy Discharge Instructions[5]	-	-	63%	75%
Chest Pain/Possible Heart Attack Care				
Aspirin Given Within 24 Hours of Arrival	-	-	97%	96%
Fibrinolytic Meds Within 30 Min. of Arrival	-	-	48%	58%
Average Time to ECG (minutes)	-	-	7	7
Average Time to Transfer (minutes)	-	-	54	60
Children's Asthma Care				
Received Home Management Plan of Care	-	-	-	88%
Received Reliever Medication	-	-	-	100%
Received Systemic Corticosteroids	-	-	-	100%
Emergency Department				
Admittance Decision Time (minutes)	149	23	62	98
Head CT Results Within 45 Min. of Arrival	-	-	54%	57%
Patients Who Left ER Before Being Seen	-	-	2%	2%
Time from ER Arrival to Admit. (minutes)	191	112	199	274
Time from ER Arrival to Discharge (minutes)	-	-	125	134
Time in ER Before Being Evaluated (minutes)	-	-	31	26
Time to Pain Meds for Fractures (minutes)	-	-	45	57
Heart Attack Care				
Aspirin Given at Discharge[1,3]	-	-	99%	99%
Fibrinolytic Meds Within 30 Min. of Arrival[3,7]	-	-	-	54%
PCI Within 90 Minutes of Arrival[3,7]	-	-	96%	96%
Statin Prescribed at Discharge[1,3]	-	-	99%	98%
Heart Failure Care				
ACE Inhibitor or ARB for LVSD[1]	-	-	96%	97%
Discharge Instructions Given[1]	-	-	93%	94%
Evaluation of LVS Function[1]	-	-	97%	99%
Medicare Spending				
Medicare Spending per Patient (ratio)	-	-	0.9	0.98
Pneumonia Care				
Appropriate Initial Antibiotic Given[1]	-	-	94%	95%
Blood Culture Timing[1]	-	-	97%	98%
Pregnancy and Delivery Care				
Newborn Deliveries Scheduled Early[5]	-	-	5%	6%
Preventive Care				
Immunization for Influenza	129	72%	89%	90%
Immunization for Pneumonia	164	71%	89%	92%
Stroke Care				
Anticoagulation Therapy for Atrial Fibrillation[5]	-	-	96%	95%
Antithrombotic Therapy Timing[5]	-	-	98%	98%
Assessed for Rehabilitation[5]	-	-	98%	97%
Discharged on Antithrombotic Therapy[5]	-	-	99%	99%
Discharged on Statin Medication[5]	-	-	95%	94%
Thrombolytic Therapy Timing[5]	-	-	74%	66%
Venous Thromboembolism Prophylaxis[5]	-	-	95%	94%
Written Stroke Educational Materials Given[5]	-	-	88%	88%
Surgical Care Improvement Project				
Appropriate Beta Blocker Usage[5]	-	-	98%	98%
Appropriate VTP Within 24 Hours[5]	-	-	98%	98%
Controlled Postoperative Blood Glucose[5]	-	-	97%	97%
Perioperative Temperature Management[5]	-	-	99%	100%
Prophylactic Antibiotic Selection[5]	-	-	99%	99%
Prophylactic Antibiotic Selection (Outpatient)	-	-	98%	98%
Prophylactic Antibiotic Stopped[5]	-	-	99%	98%
Prophylactic Antibiotic Timing[5]	-	-	98%	99%
Prophylactic Antibiotic Timing (Outpatient)	-	-	97%	98%
Urinary Catheter Removal[5]	-	-	97%	97%
Survey of Patients' Hospital Experiences				
Area Around Room 'Always' Quiet at Night[5]	-	-	65%	61%
Doctors 'Always' Communicated Well[5]	-	-	84%	82%
Home Recovery Information Given[5]	-	-	88%	85%
Hospital Given 9 or 10 on 10 Point Scale[5]	-	-	74%	71%
Meds 'Always' Explained Before Given[5]	-	-	67%	64%
Nurses 'Always' Communicated Well[5]	-	-	81%	79%
Pain 'Always' Well Controlled[5]	-	-	72%	71%
Room and Bathroom 'Always' Clean[5]	-	-	78%	73%
Timely Help 'Always' Received[5]	-	-	74%	68%
Would Definitely Recommend Hospital[5]	-	-	71%	71%
Use of Medical Imaging				
Cardiac Imaging Stress Test before Surgery	-	-	6.3%	5.3%
Combination Abdominal CT Scan	-	-	5.7%	10.5%
Combination Brain/Sinus CT Scan	-	-	2.3%	2.7%
Combination Chest CT Scan	-	-	1.9%	2.7%
Follow-up Mammogram/Ultrasound	-	-	6.3%	8.8%
Lumbar Spine MRI for Low Back Pain	-	-	37.6%	37.2%

Mayo Clinic Health System - Fairmont

800 Medical Center Drive, PO Box 800
Fairmont, MN 56031
Phone: 507-238-8101
Fax: 507-238-8686
URL: www.fairmontmedicalcenter.org
Type: Acute Care Hospitals
Emergency Services: Yes
Ownership: Voluntary non-profit - Private
Beds: 94

Key Personnel:

CEO/President. . . . . Barbara Allen, MD
Chief of Medical Staff. . . . . Timothy Bachenberg
Infection Control. . . . . Roger Drahota
Radiology. . . . . Rufus Rodriguez
Emergency Room . . . . Carol Shukla
Intensive Care Unit. . . . . Carol Shukla
Operating Room. . . . . Marti Walter

Measure	Cases	This Hosp.	State Avg.	U.S. Avg.
Blood Clot Prevention and Treatment				
Anticoagulation Overlap Therapy[1,2]	-	-	96%	93%
ICU Venous Thromboembolism Prophylaxis[2]	27	67%	91%	92%
Incidence of Potentially Preventable VTE[1,2]	-	-	9%	10%
UFH with Dosages/Platelet Monitoring[1,2]	-	-	98%	97%
Venous Thromboembolism Prophylaxis[2]	146	81%	86%	85%
Warfarin Therapy Discharge Instructions[1,2]	-	-	63%	75%
Chest Pain/Possible Heart Attack Care				
Aspirin Given Within 24 Hours of Arrival	45	96%	97%	96%
Fibrinolytic Meds Within 30 Min. of Arrival[1]	-	-	48%	58%
Average Time to ECG (minutes)	44	7	7	7
Average Time to Transfer (minutes)[1]	-	-	54	60
Children's Asthma Care				
Received Home Management Plan of Care	-	-	-	88%
Received Reliever Medication	-	-	-	100%
Received Systemic Corticosteroids	-	-	-	100%
Emergency Department				
Admittance Decision Time (minutes)[2]	268	38	62	98
Head CT Results Within 45 Min. of Arrival[1]	-	-	54%	57%
Patients Who Left ER Before Being Seen	8,857	0%	2%	2%
Time from ER Arrival to Admit. (minutes)[2]	289	144	199	274
Time from ER Arrival to Discharge (minutes)	367	92	125	134
Time in ER Before Being Evaluated (minutes)	400	12	31	26
Time to Pain Meds for Fractures (minutes)	31	37	45	57
Heart Attack Care				
Aspirin Given at Discharge	14	86%	99%	99%
Fibrinolytic Meds Within 30 Min. of Arrival[7]	-	-	-	54%
PCI Within 90 Minutes of Arrival[7]	-	-	96%	96%
Statin Prescribed at Discharge	15	67%	99%	98%
Heart Failure Care				
ACE Inhibitor or ARB for LVSD	31	84%	96%	97%
Discharge Instructions Given	67	81%	93%	94%
Evaluation of LVS Function	101	96%	97%	99%
Medicare Spending				
Medicare Spending per Patient (ratio)	-	0.82	0.9	0.98
Pneumonia Care				
Appropriate Initial Antibiotic Given	40	100%	94%	95%
Blood Culture Timing	44	100%	97%	98%
Pregnancy and Delivery Care				
Newborn Deliveries Scheduled Early	19	26%	5%	6%
Preventive Care				
Immunization for Influenza[2]	270	93%	89%	90%
Immunization for Pneumonia[2]	358	93%	89%	92%
Stroke Care				
Anticoagulation Therapy for Atrial Fibrillation[7]	-	-	96%	95%
Antithrombotic Therapy Timing[1]	-	-	98%	98%
Assessed for Rehabilitation[1]	-	-	98%	97%
Discharged on Antithrombotic Therapy[1]	-	-	99%	99%
Discharged on Statin Medication[1]	-	-	95%	94%
Thrombolytic Therapy Timing[7]	-	-	74%	66%
Venous Thromboembolism Prophylaxis[1]	-	-	95%	94%
Written Stroke Educational Materials Given[1]	-	-	88%	88%
Surgical Care Improvement Project				
Appropriate Beta Blocker Usage	56	98%	98%	98%
Appropriate VTP Within 24 Hours	112	98%	98%	98%
Controlled Postoperative Blood Glucose[7]	-	-	97%	97%
Perioperative Temperature Management	134	100%	99%	100%
Prophylactic Antibiotic Selection	100	100%	99%	99%
Prophylactic Antibiotic Selection (Outpatient)	59	95%	98%	98%
Prophylactic Antibiotic Stopped	99	100%	99%	98%
Prophylactic Antibiotic Timing	100	98%	98%	99%
Prophylactic Antibiotic Timing (Outpatient)	29	93%	97%	98%
Urinary Catheter Removal	107	95%	97%	97%
Survey of Patients' Hospital Experiences				
Area Around Room 'Always' Quiet at Night	300+	55%	65%	61%
Doctors 'Always' Communicated Well	300+	73%	84%	82%
Home Recovery Information Given	300+	85%	88%	85%
Hospital Given 9 or 10 on 10 Point Scale	300+	65%	74%	71%
Meds 'Always' Explained Before Given	300+	63%	67%	64%
Nurses 'Always' Communicated Well	300+	77%	81%	79%
Pain 'Always' Well Controlled	300+	69%	72%	71%
Room and Bathroom 'Always' Clean	300+	80%	78%	73%
Timely Help 'Always' Received	300+	63%	74%	68%
Would Definitely Recommend Hospital	300+	58%	71%	71%
Use of Medical Imaging				

NOTE: Hospital profiles are in alphabetical order by state, then city, then hospital within the city; Rankings exclude hospitals with less than 25 cases except for patient surveys which excludes hospitals with less than 100 cases; (a) 100-299 cases; (1) The number of cases/patients is too few to report; (2) Data submitted were based on a sample of cases/patients; (3) Results are based on a shorter time period than required; (4) Data suppressed by CMS for one or more quarters; (5) Results are not available for this reporting period; (6) Fewer than 100 patients completed the HCAHPS survey; (7) No cases met the criteria for this measure; (8) The lower limit of the confidence interval cannot be calculated if the number of observed infections equals zero; (9) No data are available from the state/territory for this reporting period; (10) The scores shown reflect fewer than 50 completed surveys; (11) There were discrepancies in the data collection process; (12) This measure does not apply to this hospital for this reporting period; (13) Results cannot be calculated for this reporting period; (14) The results for this state are combined with nearby states to protect confidentiality; Please refer to the User's Guide for a full explanation of data.

Measure	Cases	This Hosp.	State Avg.	U.S. Avg.
Cardiac Imaging Stress Test before Surgery[1]	-	-	6.3%	5.3%
Combination Abdominal CT Scan	251	5.2%	5.7%	10.5%
Combination Brain/Sinus CT Scan	202	1.0%	2.3%	2.7%
Combination Chest CT Scan	145	2.8%	1.9%	2.7%
Follow-up Mammogram/Ultrasound	530	7.5%	6.3%	8.8%
Lumbar Spine MRI for Low Back Pain[1]	-	-	37.6%	37.2%

District One Hospital

200 State Avenue
Faribault, MN 55021
Phone: 507-334-6451
Fax: 507-332-4848
E-mail: doh@districtonehospital.com
URL: www.districtonehospital.com
Type: Acute Care Hospitals
Emergency Services: Yes
Ownership: Govt - Hospital Dist/Auth
Beds: 99

Key Personnel:

Emergency Room . . . . Melissa Appel
Operating Room. . . . . Kris Bauer
Anesthesiology. . . . . Charles Boyle, CRNA
Patient Relations . . . . Joan Boysen
Intensive Care Unit. . . . . Mary Campbell
Quality Assurance . . . . Rhonda Mulder
Infection Control. . . . . Rae Ormsby
CEO/President. . . . . James Wolf

Measure	Cases	This Hosp.	State Avg.	U.S. Avg.
Blood Clot Prevention and Treatment				
Anticoagulation Overlap Therapy[2]	16	75%	96%	93%
ICU Venous Thromboembolism Prophylaxis[2]	14	79%	91%	92%
Incidence of Potentially Preventable VTE[1,2]	-	-	9%	10%
UFH with Dosages/Platelet Monitoring[2]	15	100%	98%	97%
Venous Thromboembolism Prophylaxis[2]	93	89%	86%	85%
Warfarin Therapy Discharge Instructions[2]	15	33%	63%	75%
Chest Pain/Possible Heart Attack Care				
Aspirin Given Within 24 Hours of Arrival	86	97%	97%	96%
Fibrinolytic Meds Within 30 Min. of Arrival[7]	-	-	48%	58%
Average Time to ECG (minutes)	91	6	7	7
Average Time to Transfer (minutes)[1]	-	-	54	60
Children's Asthma Care				
Received Home Management Plan of Care	-	-	-	88%
Received Reliever Medication	-	-	-	100%
Received Systemic Corticosteroids	-	-	-	100%
Emergency Department				
Admittance Decision Time (minutes)[2]	221	55	62	98
Head CT Results Within 45 Min. of Arrival	13	31%	54%	57%
Patients Who Left ER Before Being Seen	14,553	1%	2%	2%
Time from ER Arrival to Admit. (minutes)[2]	257	225	199	274
Time from ER Arrival to Discharge (minutes)	339	105	125	134
Time in ER Before Being Evaluated (minutes)	285	20	31	26
Time to Pain Meds for Fractures (minutes)	87	35	45	57
Heart Attack Care				
Aspirin Given at Discharge[1,3]	-	-	99%	99%
Fibrinolytic Meds Within 30 Min. of Arrival[3,7]	-	-	-	54%
PCI Within 90 Minutes of Arrival[3,7]	-	-	96%	96%
Statin Prescribed at Discharge[1,3]	-	-	99%	98%
Heart Failure Care				
ACE Inhibitor or ARB for LVSD[1]	-	-	96%	97%
Discharge Instructions Given	29	97%	93%	94%
Evaluation of LVS Function	38	100%	97%	99%
Medicare Spending				
Medicare Spending per Patient (ratio)	-	0.82	0.9	0.98
Pneumonia Care				
Appropriate Initial Antibiotic Given	67	91%	94%	95%
Blood Culture Timing	71	100%	97%	98%
Pregnancy and Delivery Care				
Newborn Deliveries Scheduled Early	58	10%	5%	6%
Preventive Care				
Immunization for Influenza[2]	246	96%	89%	90%
Immunization for Pneumonia[2]	241	99%	89%	92%
Stroke Care				
Anticoagulation Therapy for Atrial Fibrillation[1]	-	-	96%	95%
Antithrombotic Therapy Timing[1]	-	-	98%	98%
Assessed for Rehabilitation	13	85%	98%	97%
Discharged on Antithrombotic Therapy	13	100%	99%	99%
Discharged on Statin Medication	11	45%	95%	94%
Thrombolytic Therapy Timing[7]	-	-	74%	66%
Venous Thromboembolism Prophylaxis	11	82%	95%	94%
Written Stroke Educational Materials Given[1]	-	-	88%	88%
Surgical Care Improvement Project				
Appropriate Beta Blocker Usage	58	97%	98%	98%
Appropriate VTP Within 24 Hours	131	95%	98%	98%
Controlled Postoperative Blood Glucose[7]	-	-	97%	97%
Perioperative Temperature Management	151	99%	99%	100%
Prophylactic Antibiotic Selection	127	99%	99%	99%
Prophylactic Antibiotic Selection (Outpatient)	33	100%	98%	98%
Prophylactic Antibiotic Stopped	127	98%	99%	98%
Prophylactic Antibiotic Timing	127	97%	98%	99%
Prophylactic Antibiotic Timing (Outpatient)	33	97%	97%	98%
Urinary Catheter Removal	54	100%	97%	97%
Survey of Patients' Hospital Experiences				
Area Around Room 'Always' Quiet at Night	300+	70%	65%	61%
Doctors 'Always' Communicated Well	300+	83%	84%	82%
Home Recovery Information Given	300+	86%	88%	85%
Hospital Given 9 or 10 on 10 Point Scale	300+	72%	74%	71%
Meds 'Always' Explained Before Given	300+	65%	67%	64%
Nurses 'Always' Communicated Well	300+	80%	81%	79%
Pain 'Always' Well Controlled	300+	73%	72%	71%
Room and Bathroom 'Always' Clean	300+	74%	78%	73%
Timely Help 'Always' Received	300+	77%	74%	68%
Would Definitely Recommend Hospital	300+	69%	71%	71%
Use of Medical Imaging				
Cardiac Imaging Stress Test before Surgery	55	1.8%	6.3%	5.3%
Combination Abdominal CT Scan	213	3.8%	5.7%	10.5%
Combination Brain/Sinus CT Scan[1]	-	-	2.3%	2.7%
Combination Chest CT Scan	184	0.0%	1.9%	2.7%
Follow-up Mammogram/Ultrasound	274	9.5%	6.3%	8.8%
Lumbar Spine MRI for Low Back Pain[1]	-	-	37.6%	37.2%

Lake Region Healthcare Corporation

712 South Cascade
Fergus Falls, MN 56537
Phone: 218-736-8000
Fax: 218-736-8765
URL: www.lrhc.org
Type: Acute Care Hospitals
Emergency Services: Yes
Ownership: Voluntary non-profit - Private
Beds: 108

Key Personnel:

Infection Control. . . . . JoAnn Bowman, RN
Coronary Care . . . . Rick Dean
Intensive Care Unit. . . . . Rick Dean
Hemotology Center . . . . Paul Etzell
Operating Room. . . . . Angelo Griego
Radiology. . . . . Tom Larson
CEO/President. . . . . Ed Mehl
Chief of Medical Staff. . . . . D Traiser, MD

Measure	Cases	This Hosp.	State Avg.	U.S. Avg.
Blood Clot Prevention and Treatment				
Anticoagulation Overlap Therapy[2]	21	100%	96%	93%
ICU Venous Thromboembolism Prophylaxis[2]	40	95%	91%	92%
Incidence of Potentially Preventable VTE[1,2]	-	-	9%	10%
UFH with Dosages/Platelet Monitoring[2]	17	76%	98%	97%
Venous Thromboembolism Prophylaxis[2]	143	94%	86%	85%
Warfarin Therapy Discharge Instructions[2]	11	55%	63%	75%
Chest Pain/Possible Heart Attack Care				
Aspirin Given Within 24 Hours of Arrival	56	100%	97%	96%
Fibrinolytic Meds Within 30 Min. of Arrival[7]	-	-	48%	58%
Average Time to ECG (minutes)	59	2	7	7
Average Time to Transfer (minutes)[1]	-	-	54	60
Children's Asthma Care				
Received Home Management Plan of Care	-	-	-	88%
Received Reliever Medication	-	-	-	100%
Received Systemic Corticosteroids	-	-	-	100%
Emergency Department				
Admittance Decision Time (minutes)[2]	130	36	62	98
Head CT Results Within 45 Min. of Arrival[1]	-	-	54%	57%
Patients Who Left ER Before Being Seen	12,396	1%	2%	2%
Time from ER Arrival to Admit. (minutes)[2]	204	166	199	274
Time from ER Arrival to Discharge (minutes)	399	89	125	134
Time in ER Before Being Evaluated (minutes)	379	16	31	26
Time to Pain Meds for Fractures (minutes)	41	30	45	57
Heart Attack Care				
Aspirin Given at Discharge	17	100%	99%	99%
Fibrinolytic Meds Within 30 Min. of Arrival[7]	-	-	-	54%
PCI Within 90 Minutes of Arrival[7]	-	-	96%	96%
Statin Prescribed at Discharge	16	94%	99%	98%
Heart Failure Care				
ACE Inhibitor or ARB for LVSD	18	100%	96%	97%
Discharge Instructions Given	33	85%	93%	94%
Evaluation of LVS Function	61	98%	97%	99%
Medicare Spending				
Medicare Spending per Patient (ratio)	-	0.96	0.9	0.98
Pneumonia Care				
Appropriate Initial Antibiotic Given	49	98%	94%	95%
Blood Culture Timing	81	98%	97%	98%
Pregnancy and Delivery Care				
Newborn Deliveries Scheduled Early	48	31%	5%	6%
Preventive Care				
Immunization for Influenza[2]	282	93%	89%	90%
Immunization for Pneumonia[2]	335	94%	89%	92%
Stroke Care				
Anticoagulation Therapy for Atrial Fibrillation[1]	-	-	96%	95%
Antithrombotic Therapy Timing	17	100%	98%	98%
Assessed for Rehabilitation	25	100%	98%	97%
Discharged on Antithrombotic Therapy	24	100%	99%	99%
Discharged on Statin Medication	19	79%	95%	94%
Thrombolytic Therapy Timing[1]	-	-	74%	66%
Venous Thromboembolism Prophylaxis	21	100%	95%	94%
Written Stroke Educational Materials Given[1]	-	-	88%	88%
Surgical Care Improvement Project				
Appropriate Beta Blocker Usage	82	100%	98%	98%
Appropriate VTP Within 24 Hours	223	98%	98%	98%
Controlled Postoperative Blood Glucose[7]	-	-	97%	97%
Perioperative Temperature Management	273	100%	99%	100%
Prophylactic Antibiotic Selection	173	100%	99%	99%
Prophylactic Antibiotic Selection (Outpatient)	82	98%	98%	98%
Prophylactic Antibiotic Stopped	171	99%	99%	98%
Prophylactic Antibiotic Timing	173	98%	98%	99%
Prophylactic Antibiotic Timing (Outpatient)	69	52%	97%	98%
Urinary Catheter Removal	51	96%	97%	97%
Survey of Patients' Hospital Experiences				
Area Around Room 'Always' Quiet at Night	300+	61%	65%	61%
Doctors 'Always' Communicated Well	300+	79%	84%	82%
Home Recovery Information Given	300+	92%	88%	85%
Hospital Given 9 or 10 on 10 Point Scale	300+	69%	74%	71%
Meds 'Always' Explained Before Given	300+	65%	67%	64%
Nurses 'Always' Communicated Well	300+	77%	81%	79%
Pain 'Always' Well Controlled	300+	69%	72%	71%
Room and Bathroom 'Always' Clean	300+	73%	78%	73%
Timely Help 'Always' Received	300+	63%	74%	68%
Would Definitely Recommend Hospital	300+	70%	71%	71%
Use of Medical Imaging				
Cardiac Imaging Stress Test before Surgery	69	4.3%	6.3%	5.3%
Combination Abdominal CT Scan	194	4.1%	5.7%	10.5%
Combination Brain/Sinus CT Scan[1]	-	-	2.3%	2.7%
Combination Chest CT Scan	114	0.0%	1.9%	2.7%
Follow-up Mammogram/Ultrasound	364	6.9%	6.3%	8.8%
Lumbar Spine MRI for Low Back Pain[1]	-	-	37.6%	37.2%

Essentia Health Fosston

900 Hilligoss Boulevard Se
Fosston, MN 56542
Phone: 218-435-1133
URL: www.firstcare.org
Type: Critical Access Hospitals
Emergency Services: Yes
Ownership: Voluntary non-profit - Private

Key Personnel:

President . . . . Patricia Wangler

Measure	Cases	This Hosp.	State Avg.	U.S. Avg.
Blood Clot Prevention and Treatment				
Anticoagulation Overlap Therapy[5]	-	-	96%	93%
ICU Venous Thromboembolism Prophylaxis[5]	-	-	91%	92%
Incidence of Potentially Preventable VTE[5]	-	-	9%	10%
UFH with Dosages/Platelet Monitoring[5]	-	-	98%	97%
Venous Thromboembolism Prophylaxis[5]	-	-	86%	85%
Warfarin Therapy Discharge Instructions[5]	-	-	63%	75%
Chest Pain/Possible Heart Attack Care				

NOTE: Hospital profiles are in alphabetical order by state, then city, then hospital within the city; Rankings exclude hospitals with less than 25 cases except for patient surveys which excludes hospitals with less than 100 cases; (a) 100-299 cases; (1) The number of cases/patients is too few to report; (2) Data submitted were based on a sample of cases/patients; (3) Results are based on a shorter time period than required; (4) Data suppressed by CMS for one or more quarters; (5) Results are not available for this reporting period; (6) Fewer than 100 patients completed the HCAHPS survey; (7) No cases met the criteria for this measure; (8) The lower limit of the confidence interval cannot be calculated if the number of observed infections equals zero; (9) No data are available from the state/territory for this reporting period; (10) The scores shown reflect fewer than 50 completed surveys; (11) There were discrepancies in the data collection process; (12) This measure does not apply to this hospital for this reporting period; (13) Results cannot be calculated for this reporting period; (14) The results for this state are combined with nearby states to protect confidentiality; Please refer to the User's Guide for a full explanation of data.

Measure	Cases	This Hosp.	State Avg.	U.S. Avg.
Aspirin Given Within 24 Hours of Arrival[5]	-	-	97%	96%
Fibrinolytic Meds Within 30 Min. of Arrival[5]	-	-	48%	58%
Average Time to ECG (minutes)[5]	-	-	7	7
Average Time to Transfer (minutes)[5]	-	-	54	60
Children's Asthma Care				
Received Home Management Plan of Care	-	-	-	88%
Received Reliever Medication	-	-	-	100%
Received Systemic Corticosteroids	-	-	-	100%
Emergency Department				
Admittance Decision Time (minutes)[5]	-	-	62	98
Head CT Results Within 45 Min. of Arrival[5]	-	-	54%	57%
Patients Who Left ER Before Being Seen[5]	-	-	2%	2%
Time from ER Arrival to Admit. (minutes)[5]	-	-	199	274
Time from ER Arrival to Discharge (minutes)[5]	-	-	125	134
Time in ER Before Being Evaluated (minutes)[5]	-	-	31	26
Time to Pain Meds for Fractures (minutes)[5]	-	-	45	57
Heart Attack Care				
Aspirin Given at Discharge[1,3]	-	-	99%	99%
Fibrinolytic Meds Within 30 Min. of Arrival[3,7]	-	-	-	54%
PCI Within 90 Minutes of Arrival[3,7]	-	-	96%	96%
Statin Prescribed at Discharge[1,3]	-	-	99%	98%
Heart Failure Care				
ACE Inhibitor or ARB for LVSD[1,3]	-	-	96%	97%
Discharge Instructions Given[3]	12	100%	93%	94%
Evaluation of LVS Function[3]	16	100%	97%	99%
Medicare Spending				
Medicare Spending per Patient (ratio)	-	-	0.9	0.98
Pneumonia Care				
Appropriate Initial Antibiotic Given[2,3]	16	100%	94%	95%
Blood Culture Timing[1,2]	-	-	97%	98%
Pregnancy and Delivery Care				
Newborn Deliveries Scheduled Early[5]	-	-	5%	6%
Preventive Care				
Immunization for Influenza[5]	-	-	89%	90%
Immunization for Pneumonia[3]	19	100%	89%	92%
Stroke Care				
Anticoagulation Therapy for Atrial Fibrillation[5]	-	-	96%	95%
Antithrombotic Therapy Timing[5]	-	-	98%	98%
Assessed for Rehabilitation[5]	-	-	98%	97%
Discharged on Antithrombotic Therapy[5]	-	-	99%	99%
Discharged on Statin Medication[5]	-	-	95%	94%
Thrombolytic Therapy Timing[5]	-	-	74%	66%
Venous Thromboembolism Prophylaxis[5]	-	-	95%	94%
Written Stroke Educational Materials Given[5]	-	-	88%	88%
Surgical Care Improvement Project				
Appropriate Beta Blocker Usage[1]	-	-	98%	98%
Appropriate VTP Within 24 Hours	18	100%	98%	98%
Controlled Postoperative Blood Glucose[7]	-	-	97%	97%
Perioperative Temperature Management	20	100%	99%	100%
Prophylactic Antibiotic Selection	17	100%	99%	99%
Prophylactic Antibiotic Selection (Outpatient)	17	100%	98%	98%
Prophylactic Antibiotic Stopped	17	100%	99%	98%
Prophylactic Antibiotic Timing	17	100%	98%	99%
Prophylactic Antibiotic Timing (Outpatient)	17	100%	97%	98%
Urinary Catheter Removal[1]	-	-	97%	97%
Survey of Patients' Hospital Experiences				
Area Around Room 'Always' Quiet at Night[6]	<100	66%	65%	61%
Doctors 'Always' Communicated Well[6]	<100	87%	84%	82%
Home Recovery Information Given[6]	<100	90%	88%	85%
Hospital Given 9 or 10 on 10 Point Scale[6]	<100	78%	74%	71%
Meds 'Always' Explained Before Given[6]	<100	66%	67%	64%
Nurses 'Always' Communicated Well[6]	<100	77%	81%	79%
Pain 'Always' Well Controlled[6]	<100	71%	72%	71%
Room and Bathroom 'Always' Clean[6]	<100	84%	78%	73%
Timely Help 'Always' Received[6]	<100	70%	74%	68%
Would Definitely Recommend Hospital[6]	<100	76%	71%	71%
Use of Medical Imaging				
Cardiac Imaging Stress Test before Surgery[1]	-	-	6.3%	5.3%
Combination Abdominal CT Scan	60	1.7%	5.7%	10.5%
Combination Brain/Sinus CT Scan	40	0.0%	2.3%	2.7%
Combination Chest CT Scan[1]	-	-	1.9%	2.7%
Follow-up Mammogram/Ultrasound	86	5.8%	6.3%	8.8%
Lumbar Spine MRI for Low Back Pain[1]	-	-	37.6%	37.2%

Unity Hospital

550 Osborne Road
Fridley, MN 55432
Phone: 763-236-5000
Fax: 763-236-3516
URL: www.mercyunity.com
Type: Acute Care Hospitals
Emergency Services: Yes
Ownership: Voluntary non-profit - Other
Beds: 200

Key Personnel:
Radiology. . . . . Ellen L Abeln
CEO/President. . . . . Venetia H M Kudrle

Measure	Cases	This Hosp.	State Avg.	U.S. Avg.
Blood Clot Prevention and Treatment				
Anticoagulation Overlap Therapy[2]	93	94%	96%	93%
ICU Venous Thromboembolism Prophylaxis[2]	49	96%	91%	92%
Incidence of Potentially Preventable VTE[1,2]	-	-	9%	10%
UFH with Dosages/Platelet Monitoring[2]	82	100%	98%	97%
Venous Thromboembolism Prophylaxis[2]	268	93%	86%	85%
Warfarin Therapy Discharge Instructions[2]	79	89%	63%	75%
Chest Pain/Possible Heart Attack Care				
Aspirin Given Within 24 Hours of Arrival	71	100%	97%	96%
Fibrinolytic Meds Within 30 Min. of Arrival[7]	-	-	48%	58%
Average Time to ECG (minutes)	71	4	7	7
Average Time to Transfer (minutes)	13	39	54	60
Children's Asthma Care				
Received Home Management Plan of Care	-	-	-	88%
Received Reliever Medication	-	-	-	100%
Received Systemic Corticosteroids	-	-	-	100%
Emergency Department				
Admittance Decision Time (minutes)[2]	652	210	62	98
Head CT Results Within 45 Min. of Arrival[1]	-	-	54%	57%
Patients Who Left ER Before Being Seen	51,846	1%	2%	2%
Time from ER Arrival to Admit. (minutes)[2]	653	258	199	274
Time from ER Arrival to Discharge (minutes)	387	143	125	134
Time in ER Before Being Evaluated (minutes)	417	20	31	26
Time to Pain Meds for Fractures (minutes)	157	42	45	57
Heart Attack Care				
Aspirin Given at Discharge	23	100%	99%	99%
Fibrinolytic Meds Within 30 Min. of Arrival[7]	-	-	-	54%
PCI Within 90 Minutes of Arrival[7]	-	-	96%	96%
Statin Prescribed at Discharge	19	100%	99%	98%
Heart Failure Care				
ACE Inhibitor or ARB for LVSD	45	100%	96%	97%
Discharge Instructions Given	132	99%	93%	94%
Evaluation of LVS Function	176	100%	97%	99%
Medicare Spending				
Medicare Spending per Patient (ratio)	-	0.94	0.9	0.98
Pneumonia Care				
Appropriate Initial Antibiotic Given	185	99%	94%	95%
Blood Culture Timing	309	98%	97%	98%
Pregnancy and Delivery Care				
Newborn Deliveries Scheduled Early[2]	33	6%	5%	6%
Preventive Care				
Immunization for Influenza[2]	553	97%	89%	90%
Immunization for Pneumonia[2]	628	97%	89%	92%
Stroke Care				
Anticoagulation Therapy for Atrial Fibrillation	13	92%	96%	95%
Antithrombotic Therapy Timing	70	100%	98%	98%
Assessed for Rehabilitation	81	100%	98%	97%
Discharged on Antithrombotic Therapy	77	100%	99%	99%
Discharged on Statin Medication	60	98%	95%	94%
Thrombolytic Therapy Timing[1]	-	-	74%	66%
Venous Thromboembolism Prophylaxis	74	100%	95%	94%
Written Stroke Educational Materials Given	49	96%	88%	88%
Surgical Care Improvement Project				
Appropriate Beta Blocker Usage[2]	143	100%	98%	98%
Appropriate VTP Within 24 Hours[2]	351	99%	98%	98%
Controlled Postoperative Blood Glucose[2,7]	-	-	97%	97%
Perioperative Temperature Management[2]	395	100%	99%	100%
Prophylactic Antibiotic Selection[2]	213	99%	99%	99%
Prophylactic Antibiotic Selection (Outpatient)	180	98%	98%	98%
Prophylactic Antibiotic Stopped[2]	211	98%	99%	98%
Prophylactic Antibiotic Timing[2]	214	99%	98%	99%
Prophylactic Antibiotic Timing (Outpatient)	180	98%	97%	98%
Urinary Catheter Removal[2]	76	97%	97%	97%
Survey of Patients' Hospital Experiences				
Area Around Room 'Always' Quiet at Night	300+	54%	65%	61%
Doctors 'Always' Communicated Well	300+	78%	84%	82%
Home Recovery Information Given	300+	87%	88%	85%
Hospital Given 9 or 10 on 10 Point Scale	300+	66%	74%	71%
Meds 'Always' Explained Before Given	300+	60%	67%	64%
Nurses 'Always' Communicated Well	300+	74%	81%	79%
Pain 'Always' Well Controlled	300+	67%	72%	71%
Room and Bathroom 'Always' Clean	300+	69%	78%	73%
Timely Help 'Always' Received	300+	62%	74%	68%
Would Definitely Recommend Hospital	300+	66%	71%	71%
Use of Medical Imaging				
Cardiac Imaging Stress Test before Surgery	204	5.4%	6.3%	5.3%
Combination Abdominal CT Scan	396	0.8%	5.7%	10.5%
Combination Brain/Sinus CT Scan	303	5.3%	2.3%	2.7%
Combination Chest CT Scan	312	0.6%	1.9%	2.7%
Follow-up Mammogram/Ultrasound[7]	-	-	6.3%	8.8%
Lumbar Spine MRI for Low Back Pain[1]	-	-	37.6%	37.2%

Glencoe Regional Health Services

1805 Hennepin Avenue North
Glencoe, MN 55336
Phone: 320-864-3121
Fax: 320-864-7887
URL: www.grhsonline.org
Type: Critical Access Hospitals
Emergency Services: Yes
Ownership: Voluntary non-profit - Private
Beds: 25

Key Personnel:
Operating Room. . . . . John Bergseng, RN
CEO/President. . . . . John D Braband
Infection Control. . . . . Rhonda Buerkle
Chief of Medical Staff . . . . Dennis Jacobson, MD
Anesthesiology. . . . . Bob Larter
Intensive Care Unit. . . . . Barb Magnuson, RN
Emergency Room . . . . Bryan Petersen, RN
Quality Assurance . . . . Ann Ripley

Measure	Cases	This Hosp.	State Avg.	U.S. Avg.
Blood Clot Prevention and Treatment				
Anticoagulation Overlap Therapy[5]	-	-	96%	93%
ICU Venous Thromboembolism Prophylaxis[5]	-	-	91%	92%
Incidence of Potentially Preventable VTE[5]	-	-	9%	10%
UFH with Dosages/Platelet Monitoring[5]	-	-	98%	97%
Venous Thromboembolism Prophylaxis[5]	-	-	86%	85%
Warfarin Therapy Discharge Instructions[5]	-	-	63%	75%
Chest Pain/Possible Heart Attack Care				
Aspirin Given Within 24 Hours of Arrival[1]	-	-	97%	96%
Fibrinolytic Meds Within 30 Min. of Arrival[3,7]	-	-	48%	58%
Average Time to ECG (minutes)[1]	-	-	7	7
Average Time to Transfer (minutes)[1,3]	-	-	54	60
Children's Asthma Care				
Received Home Management Plan of Care	-	-	-	88%
Received Reliever Medication	-	-	-	100%
Received Systemic Corticosteroids	-	-	-	100%
Emergency Department				
Admittance Decision Time (minutes)[2]	177	30	62	98
Head CT Results Within 45 Min. of Arrival[5]	-	-	54%	57%
Patients Who Left ER Before Being Seen	3,777	0%	2%	2%
Time from ER Arrival to Admit. (minutes)[2]	177	181	199	274
Time from ER Arrival to Discharge (minutes)[5]	-	-	125	134
Time in ER Before Being Evaluated (minutes)[5]	-	-	31	26
Time to Pain Meds for Fractures (minutes)[5]	-	-	45	57
Heart Attack Care				
Aspirin Given at Discharge[5]	-	-	99%	99%
Fibrinolytic Meds Within 30 Min. of Arrival[5]	-	-	-	54%
PCI Within 90 Minutes of Arrival[5]	-	-	96%	96%
Statin Prescribed at Discharge[5]	-	-	99%	98%
Heart Failure Care				
ACE Inhibitor or ARB for LVSD	11	91%	96%	97%
Discharge Instructions Given	12	92%	93%	94%
Evaluation of LVS Function	30	100%	97%	99%
Medicare Spending				
Medicare Spending per Patient (ratio)	-	-	0.9	0.98
Pneumonia Care				
Appropriate Initial Antibiotic Given	24	100%	94%	95%

NOTE: Hospital profiles are in alphabetical order by state, then city, then hospital within the city; Rankings exclude hospitals with less than 25 cases except for patient surveys which excludes hospitals with less than 100 cases; (a) 100-299 cases; (1) The number of cases/patients is too few to report; (2) Data submitted were based on a sample of cases/patients; (3) Results are based on a shorter time period than required; (4) Data suppressed by CMS for one or more quarters; (5) Results are not available for this reporting period; (6) Fewer than 100 patients completed the HCAHPS survey; (7) No cases met the criteria for this measure; (8) The lower limit of the confidence interval cannot be calculated if the number of observed infections equals zero; (9) No data are available from the state/territory for this reporting period; (10) The scores shown reflect fewer than 50 completed surveys; (11) There were discrepancies in the data collection process; (12) This measure does not apply to this hospital for this reporting period; (13) Results cannot be calculated for this reporting period; (14) The results for this state are combined with nearby states to protect confidentiality; Please refer to the User's Guide for a full explanation of data.

Measure	Cases	This Hosp.	State Avg.	U.S. Avg.
Blood Culture Timing[1]	-	-	97%	98%
Pregnancy and Delivery Care				
Newborn Deliveries Scheduled Early[5]	-	-	5%	6%
Preventive Care				
Immunization for Influenza[2]	234	90%	89%	90%
Immunization for Pneumonia[2]	286	85%	89%	92%
Stroke Care				
Anticoagulation Therapy for Atrial Fibrillation[5]	-	-	96%	95%
Antithrombotic Therapy Timing[5]	-	-	98%	98%
Assessed for Rehabilitation[5]	-	-	98%	97%
Discharged on Antithrombotic Therapy[5]	-	-	99%	99%
Discharged on Statin Medication[5]	-	-	95%	94%
Thrombolytic Therapy Timing[5]	-	-	74%	66%
Venous Thromboembolism Prophylaxis[5]	-	-	95%	94%
Written Stroke Educational Materials Given[5]	-	-	88%	88%
Surgical Care Improvement Project				
Appropriate Beta Blocker Usage	11	100%	98%	98%
Appropriate VTP Within 24 Hours	35	100%	98%	98%
Controlled Postoperative Blood Glucose[7]	-	-	97%	97%
Perioperative Temperature Management	39	100%	99%	100%
Prophylactic Antibiotic Selection	27	100%	99%	99%
Prophylactic Antibiotic Selection (Outpatient)[1]	-	-	98%	98%
Prophylactic Antibiotic Stopped	27	100%	99%	98%
Prophylactic Antibiotic Timing	27	96%	98%	99%
Prophylactic Antibiotic Timing (Outpatient)[1]	-	-	97%	98%
Urinary Catheter Removal	19	95%	97%	97%
Survey of Patients' Hospital Experiences				
Area Around Room 'Always' Quiet at Night	(a)	66%	65%	61%
Doctors 'Always' Communicated Well	(a)	84%	84%	82%
Home Recovery Information Given	(a)	90%	88%	85%
Hospital Given 9 or 10 on 10 Point Scale	(a)	66%	74%	71%
Meds 'Always' Explained Before Given	(a)	59%	67%	64%
Nurses 'Always' Communicated Well	(a)	76%	81%	79%
Pain 'Always' Well Controlled	(a)	69%	72%	71%
Room and Bathroom 'Always' Clean	(a)	73%	78%	73%
Timely Help 'Always' Received	(a)	74%	74%	68%
Would Definitely Recommend Hospital	(a)	72%	71%	71%
Use of Medical Imaging				
Cardiac Imaging Stress Test before Surgery[1]	-	-	6.3%	5.3%
Combination Abdominal CT Scan	93	4.3%	5.7%	10.5%
Combination Brain/Sinus CT Scan[1]	-	-	2.3%	2.7%
Combination Chest CT Scan[1]	-	-	1.9%	2.7%
Follow-up Mammogram/Ultrasound	190	5.3%	6.3%	8.8%
Lumbar Spine MRI for Low Back Pain[1]	-	-	37.6%	37.2%

Glacial Ridge Hospital

10 4th Avenue Southeast
Glenwood, MN 56334
URL: www.glacialridge.org
Type: Critical Access Hospitals
Ownership: Govt - Hospital Dist/Auth

Phone: 320-634-2208
Fax: 320-634-2253
Emergency Services: Yes
Beds: 19

Key Personnel:
Infection Control. . . . . Lynn Flesner
Operating Room. . . . . Lynn Flesner
CEO/President. . . . . Kirk Stensrud
Chief of Medical Staff. . . . . D Eric Westberg, MD
Emergency Room . . . . D Eric Westberg, MD

Measure	Cases	This Hosp.	State Avg.	U.S. Avg.
Blood Clot Prevention and Treatment				
Anticoagulation Overlap Therapy[5]	-	-	96%	93%
ICU Venous Thromboembolism Prophylaxis[5]	-	-	91%	92%
Incidence of Potentially Preventable VTE[5]	-	-	9%	10%
UFH with Dosages/Platelet Monitoring[5]	-	-	98%	97%
Venous Thromboembolism Prophylaxis[5]	-	-	86%	85%
Warfarin Therapy Discharge Instructions[5]	-	-	63%	75%
Chest Pain/Possible Heart Attack Care				
Aspirin Given Within 24 Hours of Arrival	17	94%	97%	96%
Fibrinolytic Meds Within 30 Min. of Arrival[7]	-	-	48%	58%
Average Time to ECG (minutes)	17	10	7	7
Average Time to Transfer (minutes)[1]	-	-	54	60
Children's Asthma Care				
Received Home Management Plan of Care	-	-	-	88%
Received Reliever Medication	-	-	-	100%
Received Systemic Corticosteroids	-	-	-	100%
Emergency Department				
Admittance Decision Time (minutes)[2]	260	25	62	98
Head CT Results Within 45 Min. of Arrival[5]	-	-	54%	57%
Patients Who Left ER Before Being Seen[5]	-	-	2%	2%
Time from ER Arrival to Admit. (minutes)[2]	290	108	199	274
Time from ER Arrival to Discharge (minutes)[5]	-	-	125	134
Time in ER Before Being Evaluated (minutes)[5]	-	-	31	26
Time to Pain Meds for Fractures (minutes)[5]	-	-	45	57
Heart Attack Care				
Aspirin Given at Discharge[1,2]	-	-	99%	99%
Fibrinolytic Meds Within 30 Min. of Arrival[2,3]	-	-	-	54%
PCI Within 90 Minutes of Arrival[2,3]	-	-	96%	96%
Statin Prescribed at Discharge[1,2]	-	-	99%	98%
Heart Failure Care				
ACE Inhibitor or ARB for LVSD[1,2]	-	-	96%	97%
Discharge Instructions Given[2]	14	86%	93%	94%
Evaluation of LVS Function[2]	29	100%	97%	99%
Medicare Spending				
Medicare Spending per Patient (ratio)	-	-	0.9	0.98
Pneumonia Care				
Appropriate Initial Antibiotic Given[2]	11	100%	94%	95%
Blood Culture Timing[1,2]	-	-	97%	98%
Pregnancy and Delivery Care				
Newborn Deliveries Scheduled Early[5]	-	-	5%	6%
Preventive Care				
Immunization for Influenza[2]	257	87%	89%	90%
Immunization for Pneumonia[2]	340	84%	89%	92%
Stroke Care				
Anticoagulation Therapy for Atrial Fibrillation[5]	-	-	96%	95%
Antithrombotic Therapy Timing[5]	-	-	98%	98%
Assessed for Rehabilitation[5]	-	-	98%	97%
Discharged on Antithrombotic Therapy[5]	-	-	99%	99%
Discharged on Statin Medication[5]	-	-	95%	94%
Thrombolytic Therapy Timing[5]	-	-	74%	66%
Venous Thromboembolism Prophylaxis[5]	-	-	95%	94%
Written Stroke Educational Materials Given[5]	-	-	88%	88%
Surgical Care Improvement Project				
Appropriate Beta Blocker Usage[2,7]	-	-	98%	98%
Appropriate VTP Within 24 Hours[2]	23	87%	98%	98%
Controlled Postoperative Blood Glucose[2,7]	-	-	97%	97%
Perioperative Temperature Management[2]	31	97%	99%	100%
Prophylactic Antibiotic Selection[1,2]	-	-	99%	99%
Prophylactic Antibiotic Selection (Outpatient)[1,3]	-	-	98%	98%
Prophylactic Antibiotic Stopped[1,2]	-	-	99%	98%
Prophylactic Antibiotic Timing[1,2]	-	-	98%	99%
Prophylactic Antibiotic Timing (Outpatient)[1,3]	-	-	97%	98%
Urinary Catheter Removal[2]	20	100%	97%	97%
Survey of Patients' Hospital Experiences				
Area Around Room 'Always' Quiet at Night	(a)	67%	65%	61%
Doctors 'Always' Communicated Well	(a)	88%	84%	82%
Home Recovery Information Given	(a)	89%	88%	85%
Hospital Given 9 or 10 on 10 Point Scale	(a)	81%	74%	71%
Meds 'Always' Explained Before Given	(a)	73%	67%	64%
Nurses 'Always' Communicated Well	(a)	86%	81%	79%
Pain 'Always' Well Controlled	(a)	77%	72%	71%
Room and Bathroom 'Always' Clean	(a)	86%	78%	73%
Timely Help 'Always' Received	(a)	80%	74%	68%
Would Definitely Recommend Hospital	(a)	83%	71%	71%
Use of Medical Imaging				
Cardiac Imaging Stress Test before Surgery[1]	-	-	6.3%	5.3%
Combination Abdominal CT Scan[1]	-	-	5.7%	10.5%
Combination Brain/Sinus CT Scan[1]	-	-	2.3%	2.7%
Combination Chest CT Scan[1]	-	-	1.9%	2.7%
Follow-up Mammogram/Ultrasound	141	7.8%	6.3%	8.8%
Lumbar Spine MRI for Low Back Pain[1]	-	-	37.6%	37.2%

Essentia Health Holy Trinity Hospital

115 Second Street West, Box 157
Graceville, MN 56240
Type: Critical Access Hospitals
Ownership: Voluntary non-profit - Private

Phone: 320-748-8200
Fax: 320-748-7225
Emergency Services: Yes
Beds: 32

Key Personnel:
Operating Room. . . . . Joanne Abel, RN
Quality Assurance . . . . Carol Lee Brinkman
Chief of Medical Staff . . . . Stan Gallagher, MD
Infection Control. . . . . Becky Pansch

Measure	Cases	This Hosp.	State Avg.	U.S. Avg.
Blood Clot Prevention and Treatment				
Anticoagulation Overlap Therapy[5]	-	-	96%	93%
ICU Venous Thromboembolism Prophylaxis[5]	-	-	91%	92%
Incidence of Potentially Preventable VTE[5]	-	-	9%	10%
UFH with Dosages/Platelet Monitoring[5]	-	-	98%	97%
Venous Thromboembolism Prophylaxis[5]	-	-	86%	85%
Warfarin Therapy Discharge Instructions[5]	-	-	63%	75%
Chest Pain/Possible Heart Attack Care				
Aspirin Given Within 24 Hours of Arrival[1,3]	-	-	97%	96%
Fibrinolytic Meds Within 30 Min. of Arrival[3,7]	-	-	48%	58%
Average Time to ECG (minutes)[1,3]	-	-	7	7
Average Time to Transfer (minutes)[1,3]	-	-	54	60
Children's Asthma Care				
Received Home Management Plan of Care	-	-	-	88%
Received Reliever Medication	-	-	-	100%
Received Systemic Corticosteroids	-	-	-	100%
Emergency Department				
Admittance Decision Time (minutes)	39	0	62	98
Head CT Results Within 45 Min. of Arrival[3,7]	-	-	54%	57%
Patients Who Left ER Before Being Seen[5]	-	-	2%	2%
Time from ER Arrival to Admit. (minutes)	39	91	199	274
Time from ER Arrival to Discharge (minutes)[3,7]	-	-	125	134
Time in ER Before Being Evaluated (minutes)[1,3]	-	-	31	26
Time to Pain Meds for Fractures (minutes)[1,3]	-	-	45	57
Heart Attack Care				
Aspirin Given at Discharge[1,3]	-	-	99%	99%
Fibrinolytic Meds Within 30 Min. of Arrival[3,7]	-	-	-	54%
PCI Within 90 Minutes of Arrival[3,7]	-	-	96%	96%
Statin Prescribed at Discharge[1,3]	-	-	99%	98%
Heart Failure Care				
ACE Inhibitor or ARB for LVSD[1]	-	-	96%	97%
Discharge Instructions Given[1]	-	-	93%	94%
Evaluation of LVS Function[1]	-	-	97%	99%
Medicare Spending				
Medicare Spending per Patient (ratio)	-	-	0.9	0.98
Pneumonia Care				
Appropriate Initial Antibiotic Given[1]	-	-	94%	95%
Blood Culture Timing[1]	-	-	97%	98%
Pregnancy and Delivery Care				
Newborn Deliveries Scheduled Early[5]	-	-	5%	6%
Preventive Care				
Immunization for Influenza	34	74%	89%	90%
Immunization for Pneumonia	61	79%	89%	92%
Stroke Care				
Anticoagulation Therapy for Atrial Fibrillation[5]	-	-	96%	95%
Antithrombotic Therapy Timing[5]	-	-	98%	98%
Assessed for Rehabilitation[5]	-	-	98%	97%
Discharged on Antithrombotic Therapy[5]	-	-	99%	99%
Discharged on Statin Medication[5]	-	-	95%	94%
Thrombolytic Therapy Timing[5]	-	-	74%	66%
Venous Thromboembolism Prophylaxis[5]	-	-	95%	94%
Written Stroke Educational Materials Given[5]	-	-	88%	88%
Surgical Care Improvement Project				
Appropriate Beta Blocker Usage[5]	-	-	98%	98%
Appropriate VTP Within 24 Hours[5]	-	-	98%	98%
Controlled Postoperative Blood Glucose[5]	-	-	97%	97%
Perioperative Temperature Management[5]	-	-	99%	100%
Prophylactic Antibiotic Selection[5]	-	-	99%	99%
Prophylactic Antibiotic Selection (Outpatient)[1,3]	-	-	98%	98%
Prophylactic Antibiotic Stopped[5]	-	-	99%	98%
Prophylactic Antibiotic Timing[5]	-	-	98%	99%
Prophylactic Antibiotic Timing (Outpatient)[1,3]	-	-	97%	98%
Urinary Catheter Removal[5]	-	-	97%	97%
Survey of Patients' Hospital Experiences				
Area Around Room 'Always' Quiet at Night[5]	-	-	65%	61%
Doctors 'Always' Communicated Well[5]	-	-	84%	82%
Home Recovery Information Given[5]	-	-	88%	85%

NOTE: Hospital profiles are in alphabetical order by state, then city, then hospital within the city; Rankings exclude hospitals with less than 25 cases except for patient surveys which excludes hospitals with less than 100 cases; (a) 100-299 cases; (1) The number of cases/patients is too few to report; (2) Data submitted were based on a sample of cases/patients; (3) Results are based on a shorter time period than required; (4) Data suppressed by CMS for one or more quarters; (5) Results are not available for this reporting period; (6) Fewer than 100 patients completed the HCAHPS survey; (7) No cases met the criteria for this measure; (8) The lower limit of the confidence interval cannot be calculated if the number of observed infections equals zero; (9) No data are available from the state/territory for this reporting period; (10) The scores shown reflect fewer than 50 completed surveys; (11) There were discrepancies in the data collection process; (12) This measure does not apply to this hospital for this reporting period; (13) Results cannot be calculated for this reporting period; (14) The results for this state are combined with nearby states to protect confidentiality; Please refer to the User's Guide for a full explanation of data.

Measure	Cases	This Hosp.	State Avg.	U.S. Avg.
Hospital Given 9 or 10 on 10 Point Scale[5]	-	-	74%	71%
Meds 'Always' Explained Before Given[5]	-	-	67%	64%
Nurses 'Always' Communicated Well[5]	-	-	81%	79%
Pain 'Always' Well Controlled[5]	-	-	72%	71%
Room and Bathroom 'Always' Clean[5]	-	-	78%	73%
Timely Help 'Always' Received[5]	-	-	74%	68%
Would Definitely Recommend Hospital[5]	-	-	71%	71%
Use of Medical Imaging				
Cardiac Imaging Stress Test before Surgery[1]	-	-	6.3%	5.3%
Combination Abdominal CT Scan[1]	-	-	5.7%	10.5%
Combination Brain/Sinus CT Scan	33	0.0%	2.3%	2.7%
Combination Chest CT Scan[1]	-	-	1.9%	2.7%
Follow-up Mammogram/Ultrasound[1]	-	-	6.3%	8.8%
Lumbar Spine MRI for Low Back Pain[1]	-	-	37.6%	37.2%

Cook County Northshore Hospital

515 5th Ave West
Grand Marais, MN 55604
Phone: 218-387-3040
URL: www.nshorehospital.com
Type: Critical Access Hospitals
Emergency Services: Yes
Ownership: Govt - Hospital Dist/Auth
Beds: 16
Key Personnel:
Radiology. . . . . Caroline Hanford
Administrator . . . . Kimber L Wraalstad

Measure	Cases	This Hosp.	State Avg.	U.S. Avg.
Blood Clot Prevention and Treatment				
Anticoagulation Overlap Therapy[1,3]	-	-	96%	93%
ICU Venous Thromboembolism Prophylaxis[3,7]	-	-	91%	92%
Incidence of Potentially Preventable VTE[3,7]	-	-	9%	10%
UFH with Dosages/Platelet Monitoring[3,7]	-	-	98%	97%
Venous Thromboembolism Prophylaxis[3,7]	-	-	86%	85%
Warfarin Therapy Discharge Instructions[1,3]	-	-	63%	75%
Chest Pain/Possible Heart Attack Care				
Aspirin Given Within 24 Hours of Arrival[1,3]	-	-	97%	96%
Fibrinolytic Meds Within 30 Min. of Arrival[3,7]	-	-	48%	58%
Average Time to ECG (minutes)[1,3]	-	-	7	7
Average Time to Transfer (minutes)[3,7]	-	-	54	60
Children's Asthma Care				
Received Home Management Plan of Care	-	-	-	88%
Received Reliever Medication	-	-	-	100%
Received Systemic Corticosteroids	-	-	-	100%
Emergency Department				
Admittance Decision Time (minutes)[5]	-	-	62	98
Head CT Results Within 45 Min. of Arrival[1,3]	-	-	54%	57%
Patients Who Left ER Before Being Seen[5]	-	-	2%	2%
Time from ER Arrival to Admit. (minutes)[5]	-	-	199	274
Time from ER Arrival to Discharge (minutes)[3]	87	76	125	134
Time in ER Before Being Evaluated (minutes)[3]	66	22	31	26
Time to Pain Meds for Fractures (minutes)[1,3]	-	-	45	57
Heart Attack Care				
Aspirin Given at Discharge[1,3]	-	-	99%	99%
Fibrinolytic Meds Within 30 Min. of Arrival[3,7]	-	-	-	54%
PCI Within 90 Minutes of Arrival[3,7]	-	-	96%	96%
Statin Prescribed at Discharge[1,3]	-	-	99%	98%
Heart Failure Care				
ACE Inhibitor or ARB for LVSD[7]	-	-	96%	97%
Discharge Instructions Given[1]	-	-	93%	94%
Evaluation of LVS Function[1]	-	-	97%	99%
Medicare Spending				
Medicare Spending per Patient (ratio)	-	-	0.9	0.98
Pneumonia Care				
Appropriate Initial Antibiotic Given[1]	-	-	94%	95%
Blood Culture Timing[1]	-	-	97%	98%
Pregnancy and Delivery Care				
Newborn Deliveries Scheduled Early[5]	-	-	5%	6%
Preventive Care				
Immunization for Influenza[5]	-	-	89%	90%
Immunization for Pneumonia[5]	-	-	89%	92%
Stroke Care				
Anticoagulation Therapy for Atrial Fibrillation[1]	-	-	96%	95%
Antithrombotic Therapy Timing[1]	-	-	98%	98%
Assessed for Rehabilitation[1]	-	-	98%	97%
Discharged on Antithrombotic Therapy[1]	-	-	99%	99%
Discharged on Statin Medication[1]	-	-	95%	94%
Thrombolytic Therapy Timing[7]	-	-	74%	66%
Venous Thromboembolism Prophylaxis[1]	-	-	95%	94%
Written Stroke Educational Materials Given[1]	-	-	88%	88%
Surgical Care Improvement Project				
Appropriate Beta Blocker Usage[5]	-	-	98%	98%
Appropriate VTP Within 24 Hours[5]	-	-	98%	98%
Controlled Postoperative Blood Glucose[5]	-	-	97%	97%
Perioperative Temperature Management[5]	-	-	99%	100%
Prophylactic Antibiotic Selection[5]	-	-	99%	99%
Prophylactic Antibiotic Selection (Outpatient)[5]	-	-	98%	98%
Prophylactic Antibiotic Stopped[5]	-	-	99%	98%
Prophylactic Antibiotic Timing[5]	-	-	98%	99%
Prophylactic Antibiotic Timing (Outpatient)[5]	-	-	97%	98%
Urinary Catheter Removal[5]	-	-	97%	97%
Survey of Patients' Hospital Experiences				
Area Around Room 'Always' Quiet at Night[5]	-	-	65%	61%
Doctors 'Always' Communicated Well[5]	-	-	84%	82%
Home Recovery Information Given[5]	-	-	88%	85%
Hospital Given 9 or 10 on 10 Point Scale[5]	-	-	74%	71%
Meds 'Always' Explained Before Given[5]	-	-	67%	64%
Nurses 'Always' Communicated Well[5]	-	-	81%	79%
Pain 'Always' Well Controlled[5]	-	-	72%	71%
Room and Bathroom 'Always' Clean[5]	-	-	78%	73%
Timely Help 'Always' Received[5]	-	-	74%	68%
Would Definitely Recommend Hospital[5]	-	-	71%	71%
Use of Medical Imaging				
Cardiac Imaging Stress Test before Surgery[7]	-	-	6.3%	5.3%
Combination Abdominal CT Scan[1]	-	-	5.7%	10.5%
Combination Brain/Sinus CT Scan[1]	-	-	2.3%	2.7%
Combination Chest CT Scan[1]	-	-	1.9%	2.7%
Follow-up Mammogram/Ultrasound	103	2.9%	6.3%	8.8%
Lumbar Spine MRI for Low Back Pain[7]	-	-	37.6%	37.2%

Grand Itasca Clinic & Hospital

1601 Golf Course Road
Grand Rapids, MN 55744
Phone: 218-326-3401
Fax: 218-999-1514
E-mail: info@granditasca.org
URL: www.granditasca.org
Type: Acute Care Hospitals
Emergency Services: Yes
Ownership: Voluntary non-profit - Private
Beds: 60
Key Personnel:
Chief of Medical Staff. . . . . Jack Carlisle
Radiology. . . . . Steve Haugen, MD
Emergency Room . . . . Michael Johnson, MD
Operating Room. . . . . John Kole, MD
CEO/President. . . . . John Kutch
Anesthesiology. . . . . Jeffrey Lunn, MD
Chair/CEO. . . . . Elizabeth Miskovich

Measure	Cases	This Hosp.	State Avg.	U.S. Avg.
Blood Clot Prevention and Treatment				
Anticoagulation Overlap Therapy[2]	12	100%	96%	93%
ICU Venous Thromboembolism Prophylaxis[2]	22	91%	91%	92%
Incidence of Potentially Preventable VTE[1,2]	-	-	9%	10%
UFH with Dosages/Platelet Monitoring[1,2]	-	-	98%	97%
Venous Thromboembolism Prophylaxis[2]	125	83%	86%	85%
Warfarin Therapy Discharge Instructions[1,2]	-	-	63%	75%
Chest Pain/Possible Heart Attack Care				
Aspirin Given Within 24 Hours of Arrival	77	99%	97%	96%
Fibrinolytic Meds Within 30 Min. of Arrival[1]	-	-	48%	58%
Average Time to ECG (minutes)	75	7	7	7
Average Time to Transfer (minutes)[1]	-	-	54	60
Children's Asthma Care				
Received Home Management Plan of Care	-	-	-	88%
Received Reliever Medication	-	-	-	100%
Received Systemic Corticosteroids	-	-	-	100%
Emergency Department				
Admittance Decision Time (minutes)[2]	308	73	62	98
Head CT Results Within 45 Min. of Arrival[1]	-	-	54%	57%
Patients Who Left ER Before Being Seen	16,231	1%	2%	2%
Time from ER Arrival to Admit. (minutes)[2]	325	249	199	274
Time from ER Arrival to Discharge (minutes)	348	128	125	134
Time in ER Before Being Evaluated (minutes)	372	31	31	26
Time to Pain Meds for Fractures (minutes)	46	40	45	57
Heart Attack Care				
Aspirin Given at Discharge[1]	-	-	99%	99%
Fibrinolytic Meds Within 30 Min. of Arrival[7]	-	-	-	54%
PCI Within 90 Minutes of Arrival[7]	-	-	96%	96%
Statin Prescribed at Discharge[1]	-	-	99%	98%
Heart Failure Care				
ACE Inhibitor or ARB for LVSD	17	94%	96%	97%
Discharge Instructions Given	43	91%	93%	94%
Evaluation of LVS Function	57	96%	97%	99%
Medicare Spending				
Medicare Spending per Patient (ratio)	-	0.87	0.9	0.98
Pneumonia Care				
Appropriate Initial Antibiotic Given	66	98%	94%	95%
Blood Culture Timing	97	89%	97%	98%
Pregnancy and Delivery Care				
Newborn Deliveries Scheduled Early	36	11%	5%	6%
Preventive Care				
Immunization for Influenza[2]	257	89%	89%	90%
Immunization for Pneumonia[2]	320	90%	89%	92%
Stroke Care				
Anticoagulation Therapy for Atrial Fibrillation[1]	-	-	96%	95%
Antithrombotic Therapy Timing	20	100%	98%	98%
Assessed for Rehabilitation	26	100%	98%	97%
Discharged on Antithrombotic Therapy	26	100%	99%	99%
Discharged on Statin Medication	25	92%	95%	94%
Thrombolytic Therapy Timing[1]	-	-	74%	66%
Venous Thromboembolism Prophylaxis	20	90%	95%	94%
Written Stroke Educational Materials Given	12	33%	88%	88%
Surgical Care Improvement Project				
Appropriate Beta Blocker Usage	58	93%	98%	98%
Appropriate VTP Within 24 Hours	121	98%	98%	98%
Controlled Postoperative Blood Glucose[7]	-	-	97%	97%
Perioperative Temperature Management	139	99%	99%	100%
Prophylactic Antibiotic Selection	100	98%	99%	99%
Prophylactic Antibiotic Selection (Outpatient)	107	97%	98%	98%
Prophylactic Antibiotic Stopped	96	98%	99%	98%
Prophylactic Antibiotic Timing	100	99%	98%	99%
Prophylactic Antibiotic Timing (Outpatient)	101	97%	97%	98%
Urinary Catheter Removal	60	98%	97%	97%
Survey of Patients' Hospital Experiences				
Area Around Room 'Always' Quiet at Night	300+	63%	65%	61%
Doctors 'Always' Communicated Well	300+	85%	84%	82%
Home Recovery Information Given	300+	85%	88%	85%
Hospital Given 9 or 10 on 10 Point Scale	300+	71%	74%	71%
Meds 'Always' Explained Before Given	300+	68%	67%	64%
Nurses 'Always' Communicated Well	300+	81%	81%	79%
Pain 'Always' Well Controlled	300+	74%	72%	71%
Room and Bathroom 'Always' Clean	300+	71%	78%	73%
Timely Help 'Always' Received	300+	75%	74%	68%
Would Definitely Recommend Hospital	300+	68%	71%	71%
Use of Medical Imaging				
Cardiac Imaging Stress Test before Surgery	71	5.6%	6.3%	5.3%
Combination Abdominal CT Scan	246	7.7%	5.7%	10.5%
Combination Brain/Sinus CT Scan[1]	-	-	2.3%	2.7%
Combination Chest CT Scan	182	1.6%	1.9%	2.7%
Follow-up Mammogram/Ultrasound	631	4.9%	6.3%	8.8%
Lumbar Spine MRI for Low Back Pain	62	41.9%	37.6%	37.2%

Municipal Hospital & Granite Manor

345 Tenth Avenue
Granite Falls, MN 56241
Phone: 320-564-3111
URL: www.gfmhm.com
Type: Critical Access Hospitals
Emergency Services: Yes
Ownership: Government - Local
Key Personnel:
Infection Control. . . . . Patti Anderson
Operating Room. . . . . Lucy Balfany
Cardiac Laboratory. . . . . Dennis Baumann
CEO/President. . . . . George Gerlach
Anesthesiology. . . . . Greg Gill
Ambulatory Care . . . . Gene Hughes
Radiology. . . . . Shannon Sander

Measure	Cases	This Hosp.	State Avg.	U.S. Avg.
Blood Clot Prevention and Treatment				

NOTE: Hospital profiles are in alphabetical order by state, then city, then hospital within the city; Rankings exclude hospitals with less than 25 cases except for patient surveys which excludes hospitals with less than 100 cases; (a) 100-299 cases; (1) The number of cases/patients is too few to report; (2) Data submitted were based on a sample of cases/patients; (3) Results are based on a shorter time period than required; (4) Data suppressed by CMS for one or more quarters; (5) Results are not available for this reporting period; (6) Fewer than 100 patients completed the HCAHPS survey; (7) No cases met the criteria for this measure; (8) The lower limit of the confidence interval cannot be calculated if the number of observed infections equals zero; (9) No data are available from the state/territory for this reporting period; (10) The scores shown reflect fewer than 50 completed surveys; (11) There were discrepancies in the data collection process; (12) This measure does not apply to this hospital for this reporting period; (13) Results cannot be calculated for this reporting period; (14) The results for this state are combined with nearby states to protect confidentiality; Please refer to the User's Guide for a full explanation of data.

Measure	Cases	This Hosp.	State Avg.	U.S. Avg.
Anticoagulation Overlap Therapy[5]	-	-	96%	93%
ICU Venous Thromboembolism Prophylaxis[5]	-	-	91%	92%
Incidence of Potentially Preventable VTE[5]	-	-	9%	10%
UFH with Dosages/Platelet Monitoring[5]	-	-	98%	97%
Venous Thromboembolism Prophylaxis[5]	-	-	86%	85%
Warfarin Therapy Discharge Instructions[5]	-	-	63%	75%
Chest Pain/Possible Heart Attack Care				
Aspirin Given Within 24 Hours of Arrival	16	100%	97%	96%
Fibrinolytic Meds Within 30 Min. of Arrival[7]	-	-	48%	58%
Average Time to ECG (minutes)	16	16	7	7
Average Time to Transfer (minutes)[1]	-	-	54	60
Children's Asthma Care				
Received Home Management Plan of Care	-	-	-	88%
Received Reliever Medication	-	-	-	100%
Received Systemic Corticosteroids	-	-	-	100%
Emergency Department				
Admittance Decision Time (minutes)	153	15	62	98
Head CT Results Within 45 Min. of Arrival[1]	-	-	54%	57%
Patients Who Left ER Before Being Seen[5]	-	-	2%	2%
Time from ER Arrival to Admit. (minutes)	166	120	199	274
Time from ER Arrival to Discharge (minutes)[5]	-	-	125	134
Time in ER Before Being Evaluated (minutes)[5]	-	-	31	26
Time to Pain Meds for Fractures (minutes)	18	34	45	57
Heart Attack Care				
Aspirin Given at Discharge[5]	-	-	99%	99%
Fibrinolytic Meds Within 30 Min. of Arrival[5]	-	-	-	54%
PCI Within 90 Minutes of Arrival[5]	-	-	96%	96%
Statin Prescribed at Discharge[5]	-	-	99%	98%
Heart Failure Care				
ACE Inhibitor or ARB for LVSD[1]	-	-	96%	97%
Discharge Instructions Given[1]	-	-	93%	94%
Evaluation of LVS Function	15	80%	97%	99%
Medicare Spending				
Medicare Spending per Patient (ratio)	-	-	0.9	0.98
Pneumonia Care				
Appropriate Initial Antibiotic Given	21	81%	94%	95%
Blood Culture Timing[1]	-	-	97%	98%
Pregnancy and Delivery Care				
Newborn Deliveries Scheduled Early[1,3]	-	-	5%	6%
Preventive Care				
Immunization for Influenza	161	87%	89%	90%
Immunization for Pneumonia	271	82%	89%	92%
Stroke Care				
Anticoagulation Therapy for Atrial Fibrillation[7]	-	-	96%	95%
Antithrombotic Therapy Timing[1]	-	-	98%	98%
Assessed for Rehabilitation[1]	-	-	98%	97%
Discharged on Antithrombotic Therapy[1]	-	-	99%	99%
Discharged on Statin Medication[1]	-	-	95%	94%
Thrombolytic Therapy Timing[7]	-	-	74%	66%
Venous Thromboembolism Prophylaxis[1]	-	-	95%	94%
Written Stroke Educational Materials Given[1]	-	-	88%	88%
Surgical Care Improvement Project				
Appropriate Beta Blocker Usage[5]	-	-	98%	98%
Appropriate VTP Within 24 Hours[5]	-	-	98%	98%
Controlled Postoperative Blood Glucose[5]	-	-	97%	97%
Perioperative Temperature Management[5]	-	-	99%	100%
Prophylactic Antibiotic Selection[5]	-	-	99%	99%
Prophylactic Antibiotic Selection (Outpatient)[3,7]	-	-	98%	98%
Prophylactic Antibiotic Stopped[5]	-	-	99%	98%
Prophylactic Antibiotic Timing[5]	-	-	98%	99%
Prophylactic Antibiotic Timing (Outpatient)[1,3]	-	-	97%	98%
Urinary Catheter Removal[5]	-	-	97%	97%
Survey of Patients' Hospital Experiences				
Area Around Room 'Always' Quiet at Night[6,11]	<100	63%	65%	61%
Doctors 'Always' Communicated Well[6,11]	<100	83%	84%	82%
Home Recovery Information Given[6,11]	<100	83%	88%	85%
Hospital Given 9 or 10 on 10 Point Scale[6,11]	<100	70%	74%	71%
Meds 'Always' Explained Before Given[6,11]	<100	71%	67%	64%
Nurses 'Always' Communicated Well[6,11]	<100	84%	81%	79%
Pain 'Always' Well Controlled[6,11]	<100	74%	72%	71%
Room and Bathroom 'Always' Clean[6,11]	<100	80%	78%	73%
Timely Help 'Always' Received[6,11]	<100	80%	74%	68%
Would Definitely Recommend Hospital[6,11]	<100	48%	71%	71%
Use of Medical Imaging				
Cardiac Imaging Stress Test before Surgery[1]	-	-	6.3%	5.3%
Combination Abdominal CT Scan	56	3.6%	5.7%	10.5%
Combination Brain/Sinus CT Scan[1]	-	-	2.3%	2.7%
Combination Chest CT Scan[1]	-	-	1.9%	2.7%
Follow-up Mammogram/Ultrasound	124	5.6%	6.3%	8.8%
Lumbar Spine MRI for Low Back Pain[1]	-	-	37.6%	37.2%

Kittson Memorial Hospital

1010 South Birch
Hallock, MN 56728
Phone: 218-843-3612
Fax: 218-843-2311
Type: Critical Access Hospitals
Emergency Services: Yes
Ownership: Voluntary non-profit - Other
Beds: 20

Key Personnel:
Quality Assurance . . . . Joelle Klegstad, RN
Chief of Medical Staff. . . . . Roland Larter, MD
Emergency Room . . . . Ginger Ledoux

Measure	Cases	This Hosp.	State Avg.	U.S. Avg.
Blood Clot Prevention and Treatment				
Anticoagulation Overlap Therapy[5]	-	-	96%	93%
ICU Venous Thromboembolism Prophylaxis[5]	-	-	91%	92%
Incidence of Potentially Preventable VTE[5]	-	-	9%	10%
UFH with Dosages/Platelet Monitoring[5]	-	-	98%	97%
Venous Thromboembolism Prophylaxis[5]	-	-	86%	85%
Warfarin Therapy Discharge Instructions[5]	-	-	63%	75%
Chest Pain/Possible Heart Attack Care				
Aspirin Given Within 24 Hours of Arrival[1]	-	-	97%	96%
Fibrinolytic Meds Within 30 Min. of Arrival[1,3]	-	-	48%	58%
Average Time to ECG (minutes)[1]	-	-	7	7
Average Time to Transfer (minutes)[3,7]	-	-	54	60
Children's Asthma Care				
Received Home Management Plan of Care	-	-	-	88%
Received Reliever Medication	-	-	-	100%
Received Systemic Corticosteroids	-	-	-	100%
Emergency Department				
Admittance Decision Time (minutes)[2,3]	-	-	62	98
Head CT Results Within 45 Min. of Arrival[5]	-	-	54%	57%
Patients Who Left ER Before Being Seen[5]	-	-	2%	2%
Time from ER Arrival to Admit. (minutes)[2,3]	-	-	199	274
Time from ER Arrival to Discharge (minutes)[5]	-	-	125	134
Time in ER Before Being Evaluated (minutes)[5]	-	-	31	26
Time to Pain Meds for Fractures (minutes)[5]	-	-	45	57
Heart Attack Care				
Aspirin Given at Discharge[5]	-	-	99%	99%
Fibrinolytic Meds Within 30 Min. of Arrival[5]	-	-	-	54%
PCI Within 90 Minutes of Arrival[5]	-	-	96%	96%
Statin Prescribed at Discharge[5]	-	-	99%	98%
Heart Failure Care				
ACE Inhibitor or ARB for LVSD[1,2]	-	-	96%	97%
Discharge Instructions Given[1,2]	-	-	93%	94%
Evaluation of LVS Function[2]	14	21%	97%	99%
Medicare Spending				
Medicare Spending per Patient (ratio)	-	-	0.9	0.98
Pneumonia Care				
Appropriate Initial Antibiotic Given[1,2]	-	-	94%	95%
Blood Culture Timing[2,7]	-	-	97%	98%
Pregnancy and Delivery Care				
Newborn Deliveries Scheduled Early[5]	-	-	5%	6%
Preventive Care				
Immunization for Influenza[5]	-	-	89%	90%
Immunization for Pneumonia[5]	-	-	89%	92%
Stroke Care				
Anticoagulation Therapy for Atrial Fibrillation[5]	-	-	96%	95%
Antithrombotic Therapy Timing[5]	-	-	98%	98%
Assessed for Rehabilitation[5]	-	-	98%	97%
Discharged on Antithrombotic Therapy[5]	-	-	99%	99%
Discharged on Statin Medication[5]	-	-	95%	94%
Thrombolytic Therapy Timing[5]	-	-	74%	66%
Venous Thromboembolism Prophylaxis[5]	-	-	95%	94%
Written Stroke Educational Materials Given[5]	-	-	88%	88%
Surgical Care Improvement Project				
Appropriate Beta Blocker Usage[5]	-	-	98%	98%
Appropriate VTP Within 24 Hours[5]	-	-	98%	98%
Controlled Postoperative Blood Glucose[5]	-	-	97%	97%
Perioperative Temperature Management[5]	-	-	99%	100%
Prophylactic Antibiotic Selection[5]	-	-	99%	99%
Prophylactic Antibiotic Selection (Outpatient)[5]	-	-	98%	98%
Prophylactic Antibiotic Stopped[5]	-	-	99%	98%
Prophylactic Antibiotic Timing[5]	-	-	98%	99%
Prophylactic Antibiotic Timing (Outpatient)[5]	-	-	97%	98%
Urinary Catheter Removal[5]	-	-	97%	97%
Survey of Patients' Hospital Experiences				
Area Around Room 'Always' Quiet at Night[5]	-	-	65%	61%
Doctors 'Always' Communicated Well[5]	-	-	84%	82%
Home Recovery Information Given[5]	-	-	88%	85%
Hospital Given 9 or 10 on 10 Point Scale[5]	-	-	74%	71%
Meds 'Always' Explained Before Given[5]	-	-	67%	64%
Nurses 'Always' Communicated Well[5]	-	-	81%	79%
Pain 'Always' Well Controlled[5]	-	-	72%	71%
Room and Bathroom 'Always' Clean[5]	-	-	78%	73%
Timely Help 'Always' Received[5]	-	-	74%	68%
Would Definitely Recommend Hospital[5]	-	-	71%	71%
Use of Medical Imaging				
Cardiac Imaging Stress Test before Surgery[7]	-	-	6.3%	5.3%
Combination Abdominal CT Scan[1]	-	-	5.7%	10.5%
Combination Brain/Sinus CT Scan[1]	-	-	2.3%	2.7%
Combination Chest CT Scan[1]	-	-	1.9%	2.7%
Follow-up Mammogram/Ultrasound	78	7.7%	6.3%	8.8%
Lumbar Spine MRI for Low Back Pain[1]	-	-	37.6%	37.2%

Regina Hospital

1175 Nininger Road
Hastings, MN 55033
Phone: 651-480-4100
Fax: 651-480-4212
URL: www.reginamedical.org
Type: Acute Care Hospitals
Emergency Services: Yes
Ownership: Voluntary non-profit - Church
Beds: 57

Key Personnel:
Patient Relations . . . . Solveig Dittmann
Emergency Room . . . . Lawrence Erickson
CEO/President. . . . . Ty Erickson
Operating Room. . . . . Barb Kendall
Chief of Medical Staff . . . . James Noreen, MD

Measure	Cases	This Hosp.	State Avg.	U.S. Avg.
Blood Clot Prevention and Treatment				
Anticoagulation Overlap Therapy[1,2]	-	-	96%	93%
ICU Venous Thromboembolism Prophylaxis[2,7]	-	-	91%	92%
Incidence of Potentially Preventable VTE[1,2]	-	-	9%	10%
UFH with Dosages/Platelet Monitoring[1,2]	-	-	98%	97%
Venous Thromboembolism Prophylaxis[2]	158	99%	86%	85%
Warfarin Therapy Discharge Instructions[1,2]	-	-	63%	75%
Chest Pain/Possible Heart Attack Care				
Aspirin Given Within 24 Hours of Arrival	54	98%	97%	96%
Fibrinolytic Meds Within 30 Min. of Arrival[7]	-	-	48%	58%
Average Time to ECG (minutes)	56	8	7	7
Average Time to Transfer (minutes)[1]	-	-	54	60
Children's Asthma Care				
Received Home Management Plan of Care	-	-	-	88%
Received Reliever Medication	-	-	-	100%
Received Systemic Corticosteroids	-	-	-	100%
Emergency Department				
Admittance Decision Time (minutes)[2]	269	52	62	98
Head CT Results Within 45 Min. of Arrival[1]	-	-	54%	57%
Patients Who Left ER Before Being Seen	11,108	2%	2%	2%
Time from ER Arrival to Admit. (minutes)[2]	280	187	199	274
Time from ER Arrival to Discharge (minutes)	367	117	125	134
Time in ER Before Being Evaluated (minutes)	400	25	31	26
Time to Pain Meds for Fractures (minutes)	59	47	45	57
Heart Attack Care				
Aspirin Given at Discharge[1]	-	-	99%	99%
Fibrinolytic Meds Within 30 Min. of Arrival[7]	-	-	-	54%
PCI Within 90 Minutes of Arrival[7]	-	-	96%	96%
Statin Prescribed at Discharge[1]	-	-	99%	98%
Heart Failure Care				
ACE Inhibitor or ARB for LVSD	21	100%	96%	97%
Discharge Instructions Given	52	92%	93%	94%

NOTE: Hospital profiles are in alphabetical order by state, then city, then hospital within the city; Rankings exclude hospitals with less than 25 cases except for patient surveys which excludes hospitals with less than 100 cases; (a) 100-299 cases; (1) The number of cases/patients is too few to report; (2) Data submitted were based on a sample of cases/patients; (3) Results are based on a shorter time period than required; (4) Data suppressed by CMS for one or more quarters; (5) Results are not available for this reporting period; (6) Fewer than 100 patients completed the HCAHPS survey; (7) No cases met the criteria for this measure; (8) The lower limit of the confidence interval cannot be calculated if the number of observed infections equals zero; (9) No data are available from the state/territory for this reporting period; (10) The scores shown reflect fewer than 50 completed surveys; (11) There were discrepancies in the data collection process; (12) This measure does not apply to this hospital for this reporting period; (13) Results cannot be calculated for this reporting period; (14) The results for this state are combined with nearby states to protect confidentiality; Please refer to the User's Guide for a full explanation of data.

Evaluation of LVS Function	69	100%	97%	99%
Medicare Spending				
Medicare Spending per Patient (ratio)	-	0.88	0.9	0.98
Pneumonia Care				
Appropriate Initial Antibiotic Given	56	93%	94%	95%
Blood Culture Timing	60	98%	97%	98%
Pregnancy and Delivery Care				
Newborn Deliveries Scheduled Early[2]	21	38%	5%	6%
Preventive Care				
Immunization for Influenza[2]	277	86%	89%	90%
Immunization for Pneumonia[2]	350	87%	89%	92%
Stroke Care				
Anticoagulation Therapy for Atrial Fibrillation[1]	-	-	96%	95%
Antithrombotic Therapy Timing[1]	-	-	98%	98%
Assessed for Rehabilitation[1]	-	-	98%	97%
Discharged on Antithrombotic Therapy[1]	-	-	99%	99%
Discharged on Statin Medication[1]	-	-	95%	94%
Thrombolytic Therapy Timing[7]	-	-	74%	66%
Venous Thromboembolism Prophylaxis[1]	-	-	95%	94%
Written Stroke Educational Materials Given[1]	-	-	88%	88%
Surgical Care Improvement Project				
Appropriate Beta Blocker Usage[2]	52	98%	98%	98%
Appropriate VTP Within 24 Hours[2]	158	99%	98%	98%
Controlled Postoperative Blood Glucose[2,7]	-	-	97%	97%
Perioperative Temperature Management[2]	223	98%	99%	100%
Prophylactic Antibiotic Selection[2]	161	99%	99%	99%
Prophylactic Antibiotic Selection (Outpatient)	26	92%	98%	98%
Prophylactic Antibiotic Stopped[2]	160	100%	99%	98%
Prophylactic Antibiotic Timing[2]	161	99%	98%	99%
Prophylactic Antibiotic Timing (Outpatient)	27	93%	97%	98%
Urinary Catheter Removal[2]	28	100%	97%	97%
Survey of Patients' Hospital Experiences				
Area Around Room 'Always' Quiet at Night	300+	74%	65%	61%
Doctors 'Always' Communicated Well	300+	87%	84%	82%
Home Recovery Information Given	300+	90%	88%	85%
Hospital Given 9 or 10 on 10 Point Scale	300+	78%	74%	71%
Meds 'Always' Explained Before Given	300+	71%	67%	64%
Nurses 'Always' Communicated Well	300+	82%	81%	79%
Pain 'Always' Well Controlled	300+	74%	72%	71%
Room and Bathroom 'Always' Clean	300+	78%	78%	73%
Timely Help 'Always' Received	300+	81%	74%	68%
Would Definitely Recommend Hospital	300+	72%	71%	71%
Use of Medical Imaging				
Cardiac Imaging Stress Test before Surgery	56	1.8%	6.3%	5.3%
Combination Abdominal CT Scan	197	2.0%	5.7%	10.5%
Combination Brain/Sinus CT Scan[1]	-	-	2.3%	2.7%
Combination Chest CT Scan	132	4.5%	1.9%	2.7%
Follow-up Mammogram/Ultrasound	377	6.4%	6.3%	8.8%
Lumbar Spine MRI for Low Back Pain[1]	-	-	37.6%	37.2%

Hendricks Community Hospital

503 E Lincoln Street
Hendricks, MN 56136
URL: www.hendrickshosp.org
Type: Critical Access Hospitals
Ownership: Voluntary non-profit - Private
Phone: 507-275-3134
Fax: 507-275-3104
Emergency Services: Yes
Beds: 26

Measure	Cases	This Hosp.	State Avg.	U.S. Avg.
Blood Clot Prevention and Treatment				
Anticoagulation Overlap Therapy[5]	-	-	96%	93%
ICU Venous Thromboembolism Prophylaxis[5]	-	-	91%	92%
Incidence of Potentially Preventable VTE[5]	-	-	9%	10%
UFH with Dosages/Platelet Monitoring[5]	-	-	98%	97%
Venous Thromboembolism Prophylaxis[5]	-	-	86%	85%
Warfarin Therapy Discharge Instructions[5]	-	-	63%	75%
Chest Pain/Possible Heart Attack Care				
Aspirin Given Within 24 Hours of Arrival[1,3]	-	-	97%	96%
Fibrinolytic Meds Within 30 Min. of Arrival[1,3]	-	-	48%	58%
Average Time to ECG (minutes)[1,3]	-	-	7	7
Average Time to Transfer (minutes)[3,7]	-	-	54	60
Children's Asthma Care				
Received Home Management Plan of Care	-	-	-	88%
Received Reliever Medication	-	-	-	100%
Received Systemic Corticosteroids	-	-	-	100%
Emergency Department				
Admittance Decision Time (minutes)	56	0	62	98
Head CT Results Within 45 Min. of Arrival[5]	-	-	54%	57%
Patients Who Left ER Before Being Seen[5]	-	-	2%	2%
Time from ER Arrival to Admit. (minutes)	56	125	199	274
Time from ER Arrival to Discharge (minutes)[5]	-	-	125	134
Time in ER Before Being Evaluated (minutes)[5]	-	-	31	26
Time to Pain Meds for Fractures (minutes)[5]	-	-	45	57
Heart Attack Care				
Aspirin Given at Discharge[5]	-	-	99%	99%
Fibrinolytic Meds Within 30 Min. of Arrival[5]	-	-	-	54%
PCI Within 90 Minutes of Arrival[5]	-	-	96%	96%
Statin Prescribed at Discharge[5]	-	-	99%	98%
Heart Failure Care				
ACE Inhibitor or ARB for LVSD[1,3]	-	-	96%	97%
Discharge Instructions Given[1,3]	-	-	93%	94%
Evaluation of LVS Function[1,3]	-	-	97%	99%
Medicare Spending				
Medicare Spending per Patient (ratio)	-	-	0.9	0.98
Pneumonia Care				
Appropriate Initial Antibiotic Given[1,3]	-	-	94%	95%
Blood Culture Timing[3,7]	-	-	97%	98%
Pregnancy and Delivery Care				
Newborn Deliveries Scheduled Early[5]	-	-	5%	6%
Preventive Care				
Immunization for Influenza	37	73%	89%	90%
Immunization for Pneumonia	79	81%	89%	92%
Stroke Care				
Anticoagulation Therapy for Atrial Fibrillation[5]	-	-	96%	95%
Antithrombotic Therapy Timing[5]	-	-	98%	98%
Assessed for Rehabilitation[5]	-	-	98%	97%
Discharged on Antithrombotic Therapy[5]	-	-	99%	99%
Discharged on Statin Medication[5]	-	-	95%	94%
Thrombolytic Therapy Timing[5]	-	-	74%	66%
Venous Thromboembolism Prophylaxis[5]	-	-	95%	94%
Written Stroke Educational Materials Given[5]	-	-	88%	88%
Surgical Care Improvement Project				
Appropriate Beta Blocker Usage[7]	-	-	98%	98%
Appropriate VTP Within 24 Hours	11	100%	98%	98%
Controlled Postoperative Blood Glucose[7]	-	-	97%	97%
Perioperative Temperature Management	11	82%	99%	100%
Prophylactic Antibiotic Selection[1]	-	-	99%	99%
Prophylactic Antibiotic Selection (Outpatient)[5]	-	-	98%	98%
Prophylactic Antibiotic Stopped[1]	-	-	99%	98%
Prophylactic Antibiotic Timing[1]	-	-	98%	99%
Prophylactic Antibiotic Timing (Outpatient)[5]	-	-	97%	98%
Urinary Catheter Removal[1]	-	-	97%	97%
Survey of Patients' Hospital Experiences				
Area Around Room 'Always' Quiet at Night[5]	-	-	65%	61%
Doctors 'Always' Communicated Well[5]	-	-	84%	82%
Home Recovery Information Given[5]	-	-	88%	85%
Hospital Given 9 or 10 on 10 Point Scale[5]	-	-	74%	71%
Meds 'Always' Explained Before Given[5]	-	-	67%	64%
Nurses 'Always' Communicated Well[5]	-	-	81%	79%
Pain 'Always' Well Controlled[5]	-	-	72%	71%
Room and Bathroom 'Always' Clean[5]	-	-	78%	73%
Timely Help 'Always' Received[5]	-	-	74%	68%
Would Definitely Recommend Hospital[5]	-	-	71%	71%
Use of Medical Imaging				
Cardiac Imaging Stress Test before Surgery[1]	-	-	6.3%	5.3%
Combination Abdominal CT Scan[1]	-	-	5.7%	10.5%
Combination Brain/Sinus CT Scan	34	0.0%	2.3%	2.7%
Combination Chest CT Scan[1]	-	-	1.9%	2.7%
Follow-up Mammogram/Ultrasound	76	2.6%	6.3%	8.8%
Lumbar Spine MRI for Low Back Pain[1]	-	-	37.6%	37.2%

University Medical Center - Mesabi/Mesaba Clinics

750 East 34th St
Hibbing, MN 55746
Type: Acute Care Hospitals
Ownership: Voluntary non-profit - Other
Phone: 218-362-6659
Fax: 218-362-6619
Emergency Services: Yes
Beds: 175

Key Personnel:
Quality Assurance . . . . Carol Beck
Pediatric Ambulatory Care . . . . . . Joel Cassingham, MD
Pediatric In-Patient Care . . . . Joel Cassingham, MD
Radiology. . . . . Daniel Courneya, MD
Operating Room. . . . . Brenda McIntyre
CEO/President. . . . . Larry Pfaff
Infection Control. . . . . Char Pulling
Chief of Medical Staff . . . . Ann Steciw, MD

Measure	Cases	This Hosp.	State Avg.	U.S. Avg.
Blood Clot Prevention and Treatment				
Anticoagulation Overlap Therapy[2]	15	80%	96%	93%
ICU Venous Thromboembolism Prophylaxis[2]	42	98%	91%	92%
Incidence of Potentially Preventable VTE[2,7]	-	-	9%	10%
UFH with Dosages/Platelet Monitoring[1,2]	-	-	98%	97%
Venous Thromboembolism Prophylaxis[2]	159	86%	86%	85%
Warfarin Therapy Discharge Instructions[2]	11	91%	63%	75%
Chest Pain/Possible Heart Attack Care				
Aspirin Given Within 24 Hours of Arrival	59	98%	97%	96%
Fibrinolytic Meds Within 30 Min. of Arrival[1]	-	-	48%	58%
Average Time to ECG (minutes)	61	4	7	7
Average Time to Transfer (minutes)	12	72	54	60
Children's Asthma Care				
Received Home Management Plan of Care	-	-	-	88%
Received Reliever Medication	-	-	-	100%
Received Systemic Corticosteroids	-	-	-	100%
Emergency Department				
Admittance Decision Time (minutes)[2]	249	60	62	98
Head CT Results Within 45 Min. of Arrival[1]	-	-	54%	57%
Patients Who Left ER Before Being Seen	13,545	2%	2%	2%
Time from ER Arrival to Admit. (minutes)[2]	261	233	199	274
Time from ER Arrival to Discharge (minutes)	300	172	125	134
Time in ER Before Being Evaluated (minutes)	309	32	31	26
Time to Pain Meds for Fractures (minutes)	35	29	45	57
Heart Attack Care				
Aspirin Given at Discharge[1]	-	-	99%	99%
Fibrinolytic Meds Within 30 Min. of Arrival[7]	-	-	-	54%
PCI Within 90 Minutes of Arrival[7]	-	-	96%	96%
Statin Prescribed at Discharge[1]	-	-	99%	98%
Heart Failure Care				
ACE Inhibitor or ARB for LVSD	13	100%	96%	97%
Discharge Instructions Given	34	88%	93%	94%
Evaluation of LVS Function	46	98%	97%	99%
Medicare Spending				
Medicare Spending per Patient (ratio)	-	0.88	0.9	0.98
Pneumonia Care				
Appropriate Initial Antibiotic Given	63	95%	94%	95%
Blood Culture Timing	65	97%	97%	98%
Pregnancy and Delivery Care				
Newborn Deliveries Scheduled Early[2]	34	15%	5%	6%
Preventive Care				
Immunization for Influenza[2]	277	87%	89%	90%
Immunization for Pneumonia[2]	297	91%	89%	92%
Stroke Care				
Anticoagulation Therapy for Atrial Fibrillation[7]	-	-	96%	95%
Antithrombotic Therapy Timing	11	82%	98%	98%
Assessed for Rehabilitation	12	100%	98%	97%
Discharged on Antithrombotic Therapy	12	100%	99%	99%
Discharged on Statin Medication[1]	-	-	95%	94%
Thrombolytic Therapy Timing[7]	-	-	74%	66%
Venous Thromboembolism Prophylaxis	11	82%	95%	94%
Written Stroke Educational Materials Given[1]	-	-	88%	88%
Surgical Care Improvement Project				
Appropriate Beta Blocker Usage[2]	30	97%	98%	98%
Appropriate VTP Within 24 Hours[2]	105	96%	98%	98%
Controlled Postoperative Blood Glucose[2,7]	-	-	97%	97%
Perioperative Temperature Management[2]	117	100%	99%	100%
Prophylactic Antibiotic Selection[2]	75	96%	99%	99%
Prophylactic Antibiotic Selection (Outpatient)	21	90%	98%	98%
Prophylactic Antibiotic Stopped[2]	68	96%	99%	98%
Prophylactic Antibiotic Timing[2]	75	97%	98%	99%
Prophylactic Antibiotic Timing (Outpatient)	15	93%	97%	98%
Urinary Catheter Removal[2]	35	97%	97%	97%
Survey of Patients' Hospital Experiences				
Area Around Room 'Always' Quiet at Night	300+	63%	65%	61%

NOTE: Hospital profiles are in alphabetical order by state, then city, then hospital within the city; Rankings exclude hospitals with less than 25 cases except for patient surveys which excludes hospitals with less than 100 cases; (a) 100-299 cases; (1) The number of cases/patients is too few to report; (2) Data submitted were based on a sample of cases/patients; (3) Results are based on a shorter time period than required; (4) Data suppressed by CMS for one or more quarters; (5) Results are not available for this reporting period; (6) Fewer than 100 patients completed the HCAHPS survey; (7) No cases met the criteria for this measure; (8) The lower limit of the confidence interval cannot be calculated if the number of observed infections equals zero; (9) No data are available from the state/territory for this reporting period; (10) The scores shown reflect fewer than 50 completed surveys; (11) There were discrepancies in the data collection process; (12) This measure does not apply to this hospital for this reporting period; (13) Results cannot be calculated for this reporting period; (14) The results for this state are combined with nearby states to protect confidentiality; Please refer to the User's Guide for a full explanation of data.

Measure	Cases	This Hosp.	State Avg.	U.S. Avg.
Doctors 'Always' Communicated Well	300+	84%	84%	82%
Home Recovery Information Given	300+	92%	88%	85%
Hospital Given 9 or 10 on 10 Point Scale	300+	67%	74%	71%
Meds 'Always' Explained Before Given	300+	63%	67%	64%
Nurses 'Always' Communicated Well	300+	82%	81%	79%
Pain 'Always' Well Controlled	300+	73%	72%	71%
Room and Bathroom 'Always' Clean	300+	79%	78%	73%
Timely Help 'Always' Received	300+	74%	74%	68%
Would Definitely Recommend Hospital	300+	65%	71%	71%
Use of Medical Imaging				
Cardiac Imaging Stress Test before Surgery	124	9.7%	6.3%	5.3%
Combination Abdominal CT Scan	301	5.0%	5.7%	10.5%
Combination Brain/Sinus CT Scan[1]	-	-	2.3%	2.7%
Combination Chest CT Scan	177	0.0%	1.9%	2.7%
Follow-up Mammogram/Ultrasound	307	8.1%	6.3%	8.8%
Lumbar Spine MRI for Low Back Pain	67	50.7%	37.6%	37.2%

Hutchinson Health

1095 Highway 15 South
Hutchinson, MN 55350
Phone: 320-234-5000
Fax: 320-587-3340
URL: www.hahc-hmc.com
Type: Acute Care Hospitals
Emergency Services: Yes
Ownership: Voluntary non-profit - Private
Beds: 66

Key Personnel:
Quality Assurance . . . . Corrine Almundson
Radiology. . . . . Daniel S Beggs
Emergency Room . . . . George Gordon
Operating Room. . . . . Barb Keller
Infection Control. . . . . Linette Wendlandt

Measure	Cases	This Hosp.	State Avg.	U.S. Avg.
Blood Clot Prevention and Treatment				
Anticoagulation Overlap Therapy[2]	11	100%	96%	93%
ICU Venous Thromboembolism Prophylaxis[2]	29	97%	91%	92%
Incidence of Potentially Preventable VTE[1,2]	-	-	9%	10%
UFH with Dosages/Platelet Monitoring[1,2]	-	-	98%	97%
Venous Thromboembolism Prophylaxis[2]	84	99%	86%	85%
Warfarin Therapy Discharge Instructions[1,2]	-	-	63%	75%
Chest Pain/Possible Heart Attack Care				
Aspirin Given Within 24 Hours of Arrival	52	100%	97%	96%
Fibrinolytic Meds Within 30 Min. of Arrival[7]	-	-	48%	58%
Average Time to ECG (minutes)	53	5	7	7
Average Time to Transfer (minutes)[1]	-	-	54	60
Children's Asthma Care				
Received Home Management Plan of Care	-	-	-	88%
Received Reliever Medication	-	-	-	100%
Received Systemic Corticosteroids	-	-	-	100%
Emergency Department				
Admittance Decision Time (minutes)[2]	196	41	62	98
Head CT Results Within 45 Min. of Arrival[1]	-	-	54%	57%
Patients Who Left ER Before Being Seen	7,901	1%	2%	2%
Time from ER Arrival to Admit. (minutes)[2]	248	208	199	274
Time from ER Arrival to Discharge (minutes)	367	112	125	134
Time in ER Before Being Evaluated (minutes)	375	13	31	26
Time to Pain Meds for Fractures (minutes)	30	26	45	57
Heart Attack Care				
Aspirin Given at Discharge[1]	-	-	99%	99%
Fibrinolytic Meds Within 30 Min. of Arrival[7]	-	-	-	54%
PCI Within 90 Minutes of Arrival[7]	-	-	96%	96%
Statin Prescribed at Discharge[1]	-	-	99%	98%
Heart Failure Care				
ACE Inhibitor or ARB for LVSD[1]	-	-	96%	97%
Discharge Instructions Given	22	91%	93%	94%
Evaluation of LVS Function	47	100%	97%	99%
Medicare Spending				
Medicare Spending per Patient (ratio)	-	0.86	0.9	0.98
Pneumonia Care				
Appropriate Initial Antibiotic Given	33	100%	94%	95%
Blood Culture Timing	53	100%	97%	98%
Pregnancy and Delivery Care				
Newborn Deliveries Scheduled Early	27	0%	5%	6%
Preventive Care				
Immunization for Influenza[2]	252	98%	89%	90%
Immunization for Pneumonia[2]	283	96%	89%	92%
Stroke Care				
Anticoagulation Therapy for Atrial Fibrillation[7]	-	-	96%	95%
Antithrombotic Therapy Timing[1]	-	-	98%	98%
Assessed for Rehabilitation[1]	-	-	98%	97%
Discharged on Antithrombotic Therapy[1]	-	-	99%	99%
Discharged on Statin Medication[1]	-	-	95%	94%
Thrombolytic Therapy Timing[7]	-	-	74%	66%
Venous Thromboembolism Prophylaxis[1]	-	-	95%	94%
Written Stroke Educational Materials Given[1]	-	-	88%	88%
Surgical Care Improvement Project				
Appropriate Beta Blocker Usage	55	98%	98%	98%
Appropriate VTP Within 24 Hours	135	99%	98%	98%
Controlled Postoperative Blood Glucose[7]	-	-	97%	97%
Perioperative Temperature Management	161	100%	99%	100%
Prophylactic Antibiotic Selection	121	99%	99%	99%
Prophylactic Antibiotic Selection (Outpatient)	51	98%	98%	98%
Prophylactic Antibiotic Stopped	119	96%	99%	98%
Prophylactic Antibiotic Timing	121	99%	98%	99%
Prophylactic Antibiotic Timing (Outpatient)	41	95%	97%	98%
Urinary Catheter Removal	37	97%	97%	97%
Survey of Patients' Hospital Experiences				
Area Around Room 'Always' Quiet at Night	300+	70%	65%	61%
Doctors 'Always' Communicated Well	300+	87%	84%	82%
Home Recovery Information Given	300+	88%	88%	85%
Hospital Given 9 or 10 on 10 Point Scale	300+	70%	74%	71%
Meds 'Always' Explained Before Given	300+	66%	67%	64%
Nurses 'Always' Communicated Well	300+	84%	81%	79%
Pain 'Always' Well Controlled	300+	72%	72%	71%
Room and Bathroom 'Always' Clean	300+	78%	78%	73%
Timely Help 'Always' Received	300+	77%	74%	68%
Would Definitely Recommend Hospital	300+	71%	71%	71%
Use of Medical Imaging				
Cardiac Imaging Stress Test before Surgery	50	4.0%	6.3%	5.3%
Combination Abdominal CT Scan	188	1.1%	5.7%	10.5%
Combination Brain/Sinus CT Scan[1]	-	-	2.3%	2.7%
Combination Chest CT Scan	125	2.4%	1.9%	2.7%
Follow-up Mammogram/Ultrasound	274	4.7%	6.3%	8.8%
Lumbar Spine MRI for Low Back Pain	38	50.0%	37.6%	37.2%

Rainy Lake Medical Center

1400 Highway 71
International Falls, MN 56649
Phone: 218-283-5400
Fax: 218-283-2281
URL: www.fmh-mn.com
Type: Critical Access Hospitals
Emergency Services: Yes
Ownership: Voluntary non-profit - Private
Beds: 25

Key Personnel:
Operating Room. . . . . Lori Constantine
Radiology. . . . . Daniel Courneya, MD
Infection Control. . . . . Douglas Johnson, MD
Emergency Room . . . . Jay Knaak, MD
CEO/President. . . . . Brian Long
Chief of Medical Staff. . . . . Anthony Stone, MD
Quality Assurance . . . . Laurie Whitefield

Measure	Cases	This Hosp.	State Avg.	U.S. Avg.
Blood Clot Prevention and Treatment				
Anticoagulation Overlap Therapy[5]	-	-	96%	93%
ICU Venous Thromboembolism Prophylaxis[5]	-	-	91%	92%
Incidence of Potentially Preventable VTE[5]	-	-	9%	10%
UFH with Dosages/Platelet Monitoring[5]	-	-	98%	97%
Venous Thromboembolism Prophylaxis[5]	-	-	86%	85%
Warfarin Therapy Discharge Instructions[5]	-	-	63%	75%
Chest Pain/Possible Heart Attack Care				
Aspirin Given Within 24 Hours of Arrival	54	89%	97%	96%
Fibrinolytic Meds Within 30 Min. of Arrival[1]	-	-	48%	58%
Average Time to ECG (minutes)	48	8	7	7
Average Time to Transfer (minutes)[7]	-	-	54	60
Children's Asthma Care				
Received Home Management Plan of Care	-	-	-	88%
Received Reliever Medication	-	-	-	100%
Received Systemic Corticosteroids	-	-	-	100%
Emergency Department				
Admittance Decision Time (minutes)	83	5	62	98
Head CT Results Within 45 Min. of Arrival[5]	-	-	54%	57%
Patients Who Left ER Before Being Seen[5]	-	-	2%	2%
Time from ER Arrival to Admit. (minutes)	226	170	199	274
Time from ER Arrival to Discharge (minutes)[5]	-	-	125	134
Time in ER Before Being Evaluated (minutes)[5]	-	-	31	26
Time to Pain Meds for Fractures (minutes)[5]	-	-	45	57
Heart Attack Care				
Aspirin Given at Discharge[1,3]	-	-	99%	99%
Fibrinolytic Meds Within 30 Min. of Arrival[3,7]	-	-	-	54%
PCI Within 90 Minutes of Arrival[3,7]	-	-	96%	96%
Statin Prescribed at Discharge[1,3]	-	-	99%	98%
Heart Failure Care				
ACE Inhibitor or ARB for LVSD[1]	-	-	96%	97%
Discharge Instructions Given	19	42%	93%	94%
Evaluation of LVS Function	24	50%	97%	99%
Medicare Spending				
Medicare Spending per Patient (ratio)	-	-	0.9	0.98
Pneumonia Care				
Appropriate Initial Antibiotic Given	11	91%	94%	95%
Blood Culture Timing[1]	-	-	97%	98%
Pregnancy and Delivery Care				
Newborn Deliveries Scheduled Early[5]	-	-	5%	6%
Preventive Care				
Immunization for Influenza	171	56%	89%	90%
Immunization for Pneumonia	231	71%	89%	92%
Stroke Care				
Anticoagulation Therapy for Atrial Fibrillation[5]	-	-	96%	95%
Antithrombotic Therapy Timing[5]	-	-	98%	98%
Assessed for Rehabilitation[5]	-	-	98%	97%
Discharged on Antithrombotic Therapy[5]	-	-	99%	99%
Discharged on Statin Medication[5]	-	-	95%	94%
Thrombolytic Therapy Timing[5]	-	-	74%	66%
Venous Thromboembolism Prophylaxis[5]	-	-	95%	94%
Written Stroke Educational Materials Given[5]	-	-	88%	88%
Surgical Care Improvement Project				
Appropriate Beta Blocker Usage[1]	-	-	98%	98%
Appropriate VTP Within 24 Hours[1]	-	-	98%	98%
Controlled Postoperative Blood Glucose[3,7]	-	-	97%	97%
Perioperative Temperature Management[1]	-	-	99%	100%
Prophylactic Antibiotic Selection[1]	-	-	99%	99%
Prophylactic Antibiotic Selection (Outpatient)[1]	-	-	98%	98%
Prophylactic Antibiotic Stopped[1]	-	-	99%	98%
Prophylactic Antibiotic Timing[1]	-	-	98%	99%
Prophylactic Antibiotic Timing (Outpatient)[1]	-	-	97%	98%
Urinary Catheter Removal[1]	-	-	97%	97%
Survey of Patients' Hospital Experiences				
Area Around Room 'Always' Quiet at Night[6]	<100	65%	65%	61%
Doctors 'Always' Communicated Well[6]	<100	83%	84%	82%
Home Recovery Information Given[6]	<100	86%	88%	85%
Hospital Given 9 or 10 on 10 Point Scale[6]	<100	55%	74%	71%
Meds 'Always' Explained Before Given[6]	<100	64%	67%	64%
Nurses 'Always' Communicated Well[6]	<100	77%	81%	79%
Pain 'Always' Well Controlled[6]	<100	73%	72%	71%
Room and Bathroom 'Always' Clean[6]	<100	66%	78%	73%
Timely Help 'Always' Received[6]	<100	78%	74%	68%
Would Definitely Recommend Hospital[6]	<100	50%	71%	71%
Use of Medical Imaging				
Cardiac Imaging Stress Test before Surgery[1]	-	-	6.3%	5.3%
Combination Abdominal CT Scan	129	6.2%	5.7%	10.5%
Combination Brain/Sinus CT Scan[1]	-	-	2.3%	2.7%
Combination Chest CT Scan	82	4.9%	1.9%	2.7%
Follow-up Mammogram/Ultrasound	139	14.4%	6.3%	8.8%
Lumbar Spine MRI for Low Back Pain[1]	-	-	37.6%	37.2%

Sanford Jackson Medical Center

1430 North Highway
Jackson, MN 56143
Phone: 507-847-2420
Fax: 507-847-3728
E-mail: pederson@sanfordhealth.org
URL: www.sanfordjackson.org
Type: Critical Access Hospitals
Emergency Services: Yes
Ownership: Voluntary non-profit - Other
Beds: 20

Key Personnel:
Quality Assurance . . . . Karen Anderson
Operating Room. . . . . Leroy Hodge
Chief of Medical Staff . . . . Marie Paul Lockerd, DO
Hemotology Center . . . . Dr Michael McHale
CEO/President. . . . . Mary Ruyter
Radiology. . . . . Jeffrey Willis

NOTE: Hospital profiles are in alphabetical order by state, then city, then hospital within the city; Rankings exclude hospitals with less than 25 cases except for patient surveys which excludes hospitals with less than 100 cases; (a) 100-299 cases; (1) The number of cases/patients is too few to report; (2) Data submitted were based on a sample of cases/patients; (3) Results are based on a shorter time period than required; (4) Data suppressed by CMS for one or more quarters; (5) Results are not available for this reporting period; (6) Fewer than 100 patients completed the HCAHPS survey; (7) No cases met the criteria for this measure; (8) The lower limit of the confidence interval cannot be calculated if the number of observed infections equals zero; (9) No data are available from the state/territory for this reporting period; (10) The scores shown reflect fewer than 50 completed surveys; (11) There were discrepancies in the data collection process; (12) This measure does not apply to this hospital for this reporting period; (13) Results cannot be calculated for this reporting period; (14) The results for this state are combined with nearby states to protect confidentiality; Please refer to the User's Guide for a full explanation of data.

Measure	Cases	This Hosp.	State Avg.	U.S. Avg.
Blood Clot Prevention and Treatment				
Anticoagulation Overlap Therapy[5]	-	-	96%	93%
ICU Venous Thromboembolism Prophylaxis[5]	-	-	91%	92%
Incidence of Potentially Preventable VTE[5]	-	-	9%	10%
UFH with Dosages/Platelet Monitoring[5]	-	-	98%	97%
Venous Thromboembolism Prophylaxis[5]	-	-	86%	85%
Warfarin Therapy Discharge Instructions[5]	-	-	63%	75%
Chest Pain/Possible Heart Attack Care				
Aspirin Given Within 24 Hours of Arrival[1,3]	-	-	97%	96%
Fibrinolytic Meds Within 30 Min. of Arrival[1,3]	-	-	48%	58%
Average Time to ECG (minutes)[1,3]	-	-	7	7
Average Time to Transfer (minutes)[3,7]	-	-	54	60
Children's Asthma Care				
Received Home Management Plan of Care	-	-	-	88%
Received Reliever Medication	-	-	-	100%
Received Systemic Corticosteroids	-	-	-	100%
Emergency Department				
Admittance Decision Time (minutes)[1]	-	-	62	98
Head CT Results Within 45 Min. of Arrival[1,3]	-	-	54%	57%
Patients Who Left ER Before Being Seen[5]	-	-	2%	2%
Time from ER Arrival to Admit. (minutes)	51	117	199	274
Time from ER Arrival to Discharge (minutes)[5]	-	-	125	134
Time in ER Before Being Evaluated (minutes)[5]	-	-	31	26
Time to Pain Meds for Fractures (minutes)[5]	-	-	45	57
Heart Attack Care				
Aspirin Given at Discharge[3,7]	-	-	99%	99%
Fibrinolytic Meds Within 30 Min. of Arrival[3,7]	-	-	-	54%
PCI Within 90 Minutes of Arrival[3,7]	-	-	96%	96%
Statin Prescribed at Discharge[3,7]	-	-	99%	98%
Heart Failure Care				
ACE Inhibitor or ARB for LVSD[3,7]	-	-	96%	97%
Discharge Instructions Given[1,3]	-	-	93%	94%
Evaluation of LVS Function[1,3]	-	-	97%	99%
Medicare Spending				
Medicare Spending per Patient (ratio)	-	-	0.9	0.98
Pneumonia Care				
Appropriate Initial Antibiotic Given[1]	-	-	94%	95%
Blood Culture Timing[1]	-	-	97%	98%
Pregnancy and Delivery Care				
Newborn Deliveries Scheduled Early[5]	-	-	5%	6%
Preventive Care				
Immunization for Influenza	21	100%	89%	90%
Immunization for Pneumonia	39	100%	89%	92%
Stroke Care				
Anticoagulation Therapy for Atrial Fibrillation[3,7]	-	-	96%	95%
Antithrombotic Therapy Timing[1,3]	-	-	98%	98%
Assessed for Rehabilitation[1,3]	-	-	98%	97%
Discharged on Antithrombotic Therapy[1,3]	-	-	99%	99%
Discharged on Statin Medication[1,3]	-	-	95%	94%
Thrombolytic Therapy Timing[3,7]	-	-	74%	66%
Venous Thromboembolism Prophylaxis[1,3]	-	-	95%	94%
Written Stroke Educational Materials Given[1,3]	-	-	88%	88%
Surgical Care Improvement Project				
Appropriate Beta Blocker Usage[5]	-	-	98%	98%
Appropriate VTP Within 24 Hours[5]	-	-	98%	98%
Controlled Postoperative Blood Glucose[5]	-	-	97%	97%
Perioperative Temperature Management[5]	-	-	99%	100%
Prophylactic Antibiotic Selection[5]	-	-	99%	99%
Prophylactic Antibiotic Selection (Outpatient)[5]	-	-	98%	98%
Prophylactic Antibiotic Stopped[5]	-	-	99%	98%
Prophylactic Antibiotic Timing[5]	-	-	98%	99%
Prophylactic Antibiotic Timing (Outpatient)[5]	-	-	97%	98%
Urinary Catheter Removal[5]	-	-	97%	97%
Survey of Patients' Hospital Experiences				
Area Around Room 'Always' Quiet at Night[10]	<100	65%	65%	61%
Doctors 'Always' Communicated Well[10]	<100	72%	84%	82%
Home Recovery Information Given[10]	<100	65%	88%	85%
Hospital Given 9 or 10 on 10 Point Scale[10]	<100	60%	74%	71%
Meds 'Always' Explained Before Given[10]	<100	68%	67%	64%
Nurses 'Always' Communicated Well[10]	<100	80%	81%	79%
Pain 'Always' Well Controlled[10]	<100	56%	72%	71%
Room and Bathroom 'Always' Clean[10]	<100	89%	78%	73%
Timely Help 'Always' Received[10]	<100	60%	74%	68%
Would Definitely Recommend Hospital[10]	<100	42%	71%	71%
Use of Medical Imaging				
Cardiac Imaging Stress Test before Surgery[1]	-	-	6.3%	5.3%
Combination Abdominal CT Scan[1]	-	-	5.7%	10.5%
Combination Brain/Sinus CT Scan	53	9.4%	2.3%	2.7%
Combination Chest CT Scan[1]	-	-	1.9%	2.7%
Follow-up Mammogram/Ultrasound	150	9.3%	6.3%	8.8%
Lumbar Spine MRI for Low Back Pain[1]	-	-	37.6%	37.2%

Mayo Clinic Health System - Lake City

500 West Grant Street
Lake City, MN 55041
Phone: 651-345-1114
Type: Critical Access Hospitals
Emergency Services: Yes
Ownership: Voluntary non-profit - Private
Key Personnel:
CEO/President. . . . . Thomas Witt

Measure	Cases	This Hosp.	State Avg.	U.S. Avg.
Blood Clot Prevention and Treatment				
Anticoagulation Overlap Therapy[5]	-	-	96%	93%
ICU Venous Thromboembolism Prophylaxis[5]	-	-	91%	92%
Incidence of Potentially Preventable VTE[5]	-	-	9%	10%
UFH with Dosages/Platelet Monitoring[5]	-	-	98%	97%
Venous Thromboembolism Prophylaxis[5]	-	-	86%	85%
Warfarin Therapy Discharge Instructions[5]	-	-	63%	75%
Chest Pain/Possible Heart Attack Care				
Aspirin Given Within 24 Hours of Arrival	15	100%	97%	96%
Fibrinolytic Meds Within 30 Min. of Arrival[1]	-	-	48%	58%
Average Time to ECG (minutes)	16	2	7	7
Average Time to Transfer (minutes)[1]	-	-	54	60
Children's Asthma Care				
Received Home Management Plan of Care	-	-	-	88%
Received Reliever Medication	-	-	-	100%
Received Systemic Corticosteroids	-	-	-	100%
Emergency Department				
Admittance Decision Time (minutes)[1,2]	-	-	62	98
Head CT Results Within 45 Min. of Arrival[5]	-	-	54%	57%
Patients Who Left ER Before Being Seen[5]	-	-	2%	2%
Time from ER Arrival to Admit. (minutes)[2]	112	134	199	274
Time from ER Arrival to Discharge (minutes)[5]	-	-	125	134
Time in ER Before Being Evaluated (minutes)[5]	-	-	31	26
Time to Pain Meds for Fractures (minutes)[5]	-	-	45	57
Heart Attack Care				
Aspirin Given at Discharge[1,3]	-	-	99%	99%
Fibrinolytic Meds Within 30 Min. of Arrival[3,7]	-	-	-	54%
PCI Within 90 Minutes of Arrival[3,7]	-	-	96%	96%
Statin Prescribed at Discharge[1,3]	-	-	99%	98%
Heart Failure Care				
ACE Inhibitor or ARB for LVSD[1]	-	-	96%	97%
Discharge Instructions Given	11	91%	93%	94%
Evaluation of LVS Function	18	100%	97%	99%
Medicare Spending				
Medicare Spending per Patient (ratio)	-	-	0.9	0.98
Pneumonia Care				
Appropriate Initial Antibiotic Given	11	100%	94%	95%
Blood Culture Timing[1]	-	-	97%	98%
Pregnancy and Delivery Care				
Newborn Deliveries Scheduled Early[5]	-	-	5%	6%
Preventive Care				
Immunization for Influenza[2]	214	89%	89%	90%
Immunization for Pneumonia[2]	276	93%	89%	92%
Stroke Care				
Anticoagulation Therapy for Atrial Fibrillation[5]	-	-	96%	95%
Antithrombotic Therapy Timing[5]	-	-	98%	98%
Assessed for Rehabilitation[5]	-	-	98%	97%
Discharged on Antithrombotic Therapy[5]	-	-	99%	99%
Discharged on Statin Medication[5]	-	-	95%	94%
Thrombolytic Therapy Timing[5]	-	-	74%	66%
Venous Thromboembolism Prophylaxis[5]	-	-	95%	94%
Written Stroke Educational Materials Given[5]	-	-	88%	88%
Surgical Care Improvement Project				
Appropriate Beta Blocker Usage[1]	-	-	98%	98%
Appropriate VTP Within 24 Hours	34	100%	98%	98%
Controlled Postoperative Blood Glucose[7]	-	-	97%	97%
Perioperative Temperature Management	33	100%	99%	100%
Prophylactic Antibiotic Selection	30	100%	99%	99%
Prophylactic Antibiotic Selection (Outpatient)[5]	-	-	98%	98%
Prophylactic Antibiotic Stopped	30	100%	99%	98%
Prophylactic Antibiotic Timing	30	90%	98%	99%
Prophylactic Antibiotic Timing (Outpatient)[5]	-	-	97%	98%
Urinary Catheter Removal	31	97%	97%	97%
Survey of Patients' Hospital Experiences				
Area Around Room 'Always' Quiet at Night[6]	<100	56%	65%	61%
Doctors 'Always' Communicated Well[6]	<100	84%	84%	82%
Home Recovery Information Given[6]	<100	84%	88%	85%
Hospital Given 9 or 10 on 10 Point Scale[6]	<100	75%	74%	71%
Meds 'Always' Explained Before Given[6]	<100	59%	67%	64%
Nurses 'Always' Communicated Well[6]	<100	77%	81%	79%
Pain 'Always' Well Controlled[6]	<100	61%	72%	71%
Room and Bathroom 'Always' Clean[6]	<100	74%	78%	73%
Timely Help 'Always' Received[6]	<100	70%	74%	68%
Would Definitely Recommend Hospital[6]	<100	76%	71%	71%
Use of Medical Imaging				
Cardiac Imaging Stress Test before Surgery[1]	-	-	6.3%	5.3%
Combination Abdominal CT Scan	66	3.0%	5.7%	10.5%
Combination Brain/Sinus CT Scan	61	0.0%	2.3%	2.7%
Combination Chest CT Scan[1]	-	-	1.9%	2.7%
Follow-up Mammogram/Ultrasound	152	9.2%	6.3%	8.8%
Lumbar Spine MRI for Low Back Pain[1]	-	-	37.6%	37.2%

Minnesota Valley Health Center

621 South Fourth Street
Le Sueur, MN 56058
Phone: 507-665-3375
Fax: 507-665-2191
E-mail: mvhc@mnic.net
Type: Critical Access Hospitals
Emergency Services: Yes
Ownership: Voluntary non-profit - Private
Beds: 109
Key Personnel:
Cardiac Laboratory. . . . . John Bernhardson
Chief of Medical Staff. . . . . John N Taylor
Emergency Room . . . . Pam William

Measure	Cases	This Hosp.	State Avg.	U.S. Avg.
Blood Clot Prevention and Treatment				
Anticoagulation Overlap Therapy[5]	-	-	96%	93%
ICU Venous Thromboembolism Prophylaxis[5]	-	-	91%	92%
Incidence of Potentially Preventable VTE[5]	-	-	9%	10%
UFH with Dosages/Platelet Monitoring[5]	-	-	98%	97%
Venous Thromboembolism Prophylaxis[5]	-	-	86%	85%
Warfarin Therapy Discharge Instructions[5]	-	-	63%	75%
Chest Pain/Possible Heart Attack Care				
Aspirin Given Within 24 Hours of Arrival[1,3]	-	-	97%	96%
Fibrinolytic Meds Within 30 Min. of Arrival[3,7]	-	-	48%	58%
Average Time to ECG (minutes)[1,3]	-	-	7	7
Average Time to Transfer (minutes)[1,3]	-	-	54	60
Children's Asthma Care				
Received Home Management Plan of Care	-	-	-	88%
Received Reliever Medication	-	-	-	100%
Received Systemic Corticosteroids	-	-	-	100%
Emergency Department				
Admittance Decision Time (minutes)[3]	12	0	62	98
Head CT Results Within 45 Min. of Arrival[5]	-	-	54%	57%
Patients Who Left ER Before Being Seen[5]	-	-	2%	2%
Time from ER Arrival to Admit. (minutes)[3]	12	130	199	274
Time from ER Arrival to Discharge (minutes)[5]	-	-	125	134
Time in ER Before Being Evaluated (minutes)[5]	-	-	31	26
Time to Pain Meds for Fractures (minutes)[5]	-	-	45	57
Heart Attack Care				
Aspirin Given at Discharge[5]	-	-	99%	99%
Fibrinolytic Meds Within 30 Min. of Arrival[5]	-	-	-	54%
PCI Within 90 Minutes of Arrival[5]	-	-	96%	96%
Statin Prescribed at Discharge[5]	-	-	99%	98%
Heart Failure Care				
ACE Inhibitor or ARB for LVSD[3,7]	-	-	96%	97%
Discharge Instructions Given[1,3]	-	-	93%	94%
Evaluation of LVS Function[1,3]	-	-	97%	99%
Medicare Spending				

NOTE: Hospital profiles are in alphabetical order by state, then city, then hospital within the city; Rankings exclude hospitals with less than 25 cases except for patient surveys which excludes hospitals with less than 100 cases; (a) 100-299 cases; (1) The number of cases/patients is too few to report; (2) Data submitted were based on a sample of cases/patients; (3) Results are based on a shorter time period than required; (4) Data suppressed by CMS for one or more quarters; (5) Results are not available for this reporting period; (6) Fewer than 100 patients completed the HCAHPS survey; (7) No cases met the criteria for this measure; (8) The lower limit of the confidence interval cannot be calculated if the number of observed infections equals zero; (9) No data are available from the state/territory for this reporting period; (10) The scores shown reflect fewer than 50 completed surveys; (11) There were discrepancies in the data collection process; (12) This measure does not apply to this hospital for this reporting period; (13) Results cannot be calculated for this reporting period; (14) The results for this state are combined with nearby states to protect confidentiality; Please refer to the User's Guide for a full explanation of data.

Measure	Cases	This Hosp.	State Avg.	U.S. Avg.
Medicare Spending per Patient (ratio)	-	-	0.9	0.98
Pneumonia Care				
Appropriate Initial Antibiotic Given[1,3]	-	-	94%	95%
Blood Culture Timing[1,3]	-	-	97%	98%
Pregnancy and Delivery Care				
Newborn Deliveries Scheduled Early[5]	-	-	5%	6%
Preventive Care				
Immunization for Influenza[1]	-	-	89%	90%
Immunization for Pneumonia	13	85%	89%	92%
Stroke Care				
Anticoagulation Therapy for Atrial Fibrillation[5]	-	-	96%	95%
Antithrombotic Therapy Timing[5]	-	-	98%	98%
Assessed for Rehabilitation[5]	-	-	98%	97%
Discharged on Antithrombotic Therapy[5]	-	-	99%	99%
Discharged on Statin Medication[5]	-	-	95%	94%
Thrombolytic Therapy Timing[5]	-	-	74%	66%
Venous Thromboembolism Prophylaxis[5]	-	-	95%	94%
Written Stroke Educational Materials Given[5]	-	-	88%	88%
Surgical Care Improvement Project				
Appropriate Beta Blocker Usage[5]	-	-	98%	98%
Appropriate VTP Within 24 Hours[5]	-	-	98%	98%
Controlled Postoperative Blood Glucose[5]	-	-	97%	97%
Perioperative Temperature Management[5]	-	-	99%	100%
Prophylactic Antibiotic Selection[5]	-	-	99%	99%
Prophylactic Antibiotic Selection (Outpatient)[5]	-	-	98%	98%
Prophylactic Antibiotic Stopped[5]	-	-	99%	98%
Prophylactic Antibiotic Timing[5]	-	-	98%	99%
Prophylactic Antibiotic Timing (Outpatient)[5]	-	-	97%	98%
Urinary Catheter Removal[5]	-	-	97%	97%
Survey of Patients' Hospital Experiences				
Area Around Room 'Always' Quiet at Night[5]	-	-	65%	61%
Doctors 'Always' Communicated Well[5]	-	-	84%	82%
Home Recovery Information Given[5]	-	-	88%	85%
Hospital Given 9 or 10 on 10 Point Scale[5]	-	-	74%	71%
Meds 'Always' Explained Before Given[5]	-	-	67%	64%
Nurses 'Always' Communicated Well[5]	-	-	81%	79%
Pain 'Always' Well Controlled[5]	-	-	72%	71%
Room and Bathroom 'Always' Clean[5]	-	-	78%	73%
Timely Help 'Always' Received[5]	-	-	74%	68%
Would Definitely Recommend Hospital[5]	-	-	71%	71%
Use of Medical Imaging				
Cardiac Imaging Stress Test before Surgery[7]	-	-	6.3%	5.3%
Combination Abdominal CT Scan[1]	-	-	5.7%	10.5%
Combination Brain/Sinus CT Scan[1]	-	-	2.3%	2.7%
Combination Chest CT Scan[1]	-	-	1.9%	2.7%
Follow-up Mammogram/Ultrasound	87	9.2%	6.3%	8.8%
Lumbar Spine MRI for Low Back Pain[1]	-	-	37.6%	37.2%

Meeker Memorial Hospital

612 South Sibley Avenue
Litchfield, MN 55355
Phone: 320-693-3242
Fax: 320-693-4567
URL: www.meekermemorial.org
Type: Critical Access Hospitals
Emergency Services: Yes
Ownership: Proprietary
Beds: 40

Key Personnel:

Operating Room. . . . . Tammy Birr, RN
Infection Control. . . . . Joyce Carlson, RN
Intensive Care Unit. . . . . Angie Dietel
Quality Assurance . . . . Ann Lien, DON
Emergency Room . . . . David Ross
Chief of Medical Staff. . . . . David M Ross, MD
CEO/President. . . . . Michael Schramm
Hemotology Center . . . . Jeanne Westphal, RN

Measure	Cases	This Hosp.	State Avg.	U.S. Avg.
Blood Clot Prevention and Treatment				
Anticoagulation Overlap Therapy[5]	-	-	96%	93%
ICU Venous Thromboembolism Prophylaxis[5]	-	-	91%	92%
Incidence of Potentially Preventable VTE[5]	-	-	9%	10%
UFH with Dosages/Platelet Monitoring[5]	-	-	98%	97%
Venous Thromboembolism Prophylaxis[5]	-	-	86%	85%
Warfarin Therapy Discharge Instructions[5]	-	-	63%	75%
Chest Pain/Possible Heart Attack Care				
Aspirin Given Within 24 Hours of Arrival	19	74%	97%	96%
Fibrinolytic Meds Within 30 Min. of Arrival[3,7]	-	-	48%	58%
Average Time to ECG (minutes)	19	8	7	7
Average Time to Transfer (minutes)[1,3]	-	-	54	60
Children's Asthma Care				
Received Home Management Plan of Care	-	-	-	88%
Received Reliever Medication	-	-	-	100%
Received Systemic Corticosteroids	-	-	-	100%
Emergency Department				
Admittance Decision Time (minutes)[2]	121	42	62	98
Head CT Results Within 45 Min. of Arrival[5]	-	-	54%	57%
Patients Who Left ER Before Being Seen[5]	-	-	2%	2%
Time from ER Arrival to Admit. (minutes)[2]	236	150	199	274
Time from ER Arrival to Discharge (minutes)[5]	-	-	125	134
Time in ER Before Being Evaluated (minutes)[5]	-	-	31	26
Time to Pain Meds for Fractures (minutes)[5]	-	-	45	57
Heart Attack Care				
Aspirin Given at Discharge[3,7]	-	-	99%	99%
Fibrinolytic Meds Within 30 Min. of Arrival[3,7]	-	-	-	54%
PCI Within 90 Minutes of Arrival[3,7]	-	-	96%	96%
Statin Prescribed at Discharge[3,7]	-	-	99%	98%
Heart Failure Care				
ACE Inhibitor or ARB for LVSD[1]	-	-	96%	97%
Discharge Instructions Given	16	50%	93%	94%
Evaluation of LVS Function	24	79%	97%	99%
Medicare Spending				
Medicare Spending per Patient (ratio)	-	-	0.9	0.98
Pneumonia Care				
Appropriate Initial Antibiotic Given	14	100%	94%	95%
Blood Culture Timing[1]	-	-	97%	98%
Pregnancy and Delivery Care				
Newborn Deliveries Scheduled Early[5]	-	-	5%	6%
Preventive Care				
Immunization for Influenza[2]	252	66%	89%	90%
Immunization for Pneumonia[2]	282	63%	89%	92%
Stroke Care				
Anticoagulation Therapy for Atrial Fibrillation[5]	-	-	96%	95%
Antithrombotic Therapy Timing[5]	-	-	98%	98%
Assessed for Rehabilitation[5]	-	-	98%	97%
Discharged on Antithrombotic Therapy[5]	-	-	99%	99%
Discharged on Statin Medication[5]	-	-	95%	94%
Thrombolytic Therapy Timing[5]	-	-	74%	66%
Venous Thromboembolism Prophylaxis[5]	-	-	95%	94%
Written Stroke Educational Materials Given[5]	-	-	88%	88%
Surgical Care Improvement Project				
Appropriate Beta Blocker Usage	16	94%	98%	98%
Appropriate VTP Within 24 Hours	51	100%	98%	98%
Controlled Postoperative Blood Glucose[3,7]	-	-	97%	97%
Perioperative Temperature Management	56	100%	99%	100%
Prophylactic Antibiotic Selection	39	100%	99%	99%
Prophylactic Antibiotic Selection (Outpatient)[1,3]	-	-	98%	98%
Prophylactic Antibiotic Stopped	39	100%	99%	98%
Prophylactic Antibiotic Timing	39	87%	98%	99%
Prophylactic Antibiotic Timing (Outpatient)[1,3]	-	-	97%	98%
Urinary Catheter Removal	17	88%	97%	97%
Survey of Patients' Hospital Experiences				
Area Around Room 'Always' Quiet at Night	(a)	78%	65%	61%
Doctors 'Always' Communicated Well	(a)	88%	84%	82%
Home Recovery Information Given	(a)	81%	88%	85%
Hospital Given 9 or 10 on 10 Point Scale	(a)	84%	74%	71%
Meds 'Always' Explained Before Given	(a)	72%	67%	64%
Nurses 'Always' Communicated Well	(a)	80%	81%	79%
Pain 'Always' Well Controlled	(a)	76%	72%	71%
Room and Bathroom 'Always' Clean	(a)	86%	78%	73%
Timely Help 'Always' Received	(a)	80%	74%	68%
Would Definitely Recommend Hospital	(a)	79%	71%	71%
Use of Medical Imaging				
Cardiac Imaging Stress Test before Surgery[1]	-	-	6.3%	5.3%
Combination Abdominal CT Scan[1]	-	-	5.7%	10.5%
Combination Brain/Sinus CT Scan	33	0.0%	2.3%	2.7%
Combination Chest CT Scan[1]	-	-	1.9%	2.7%
Follow-up Mammogram/Ultrasound	153	5.2%	6.3%	8.8%
Lumbar Spine MRI for Low Back Pain[1]	-	-	37.6%	37.2%

Saint Gabriels Hospital

815 Southeast Second Street
Little Falls, MN 56345
Phone: 320-632-5441
Fax: 320-632-1190
URL: www.stgabriels.com
Type: Critical Access Hospitals
Emergency Services: Yes
Ownership: Voluntary non-profit - Private
Beds: 49

Key Personnel:

Operating Room. . . . . Mary Bauer
Chief of Medical Staff . . . . Heide Gunn
Emergency Room . . . . Heide Gunn
Quality Assurance . . . . Peggy Martin
Infection Control. . . . . Susan Newkirk
Coronary Care . . . . Jane Smalley
Intensive Care Unit. . . . . Jane Smalley
CEO/President. . . . . Carl Vaagenes

Measure	Cases	This Hosp.	State Avg.	U.S. Avg.
Blood Clot Prevention and Treatment				
Anticoagulation Overlap Therapy[5]	-	-	96%	93%
ICU Venous Thromboembolism Prophylaxis[5]	-	-	91%	92%
Incidence of Potentially Preventable VTE[5]	-	-	9%	10%
UFH with Dosages/Platelet Monitoring[5]	-	-	98%	97%
Venous Thromboembolism Prophylaxis[5]	-	-	86%	85%
Warfarin Therapy Discharge Instructions[5]	-	-	63%	75%
Chest Pain/Possible Heart Attack Care				
Aspirin Given Within 24 Hours of Arrival	46	93%	97%	96%
Fibrinolytic Meds Within 30 Min. of Arrival[7]	-	-	48%	58%
Average Time to ECG (minutes)	46	7	7	7
Average Time to Transfer (minutes)[1]	-	-	54	60
Children's Asthma Care				
Received Home Management Plan of Care	-	-	-	88%
Received Reliever Medication	-	-	-	100%
Received Systemic Corticosteroids	-	-	-	100%
Emergency Department				
Admittance Decision Time (minutes)[2]	240	35	62	98
Head CT Results Within 45 Min. of Arrival[5]	-	-	54%	57%
Patients Who Left ER Before Being Seen[5]	-	-	2%	2%
Time from ER Arrival to Admit. (minutes)[2]	244	222	199	274
Time from ER Arrival to Discharge (minutes)	359	100	125	134
Time in ER Before Being Evaluated (minutes)	205	25	31	26
Time to Pain Meds for Fractures (minutes)[5]	-	-	45	57
Heart Attack Care				
Aspirin Given at Discharge[1]	-	-	99%	99%
Fibrinolytic Meds Within 30 Min. of Arrival[7]	-	-	-	54%
PCI Within 90 Minutes of Arrival[7]	-	-	96%	96%
Statin Prescribed at Discharge[1]	-	-	99%	98%
Heart Failure Care				
ACE Inhibitor or ARB for LVSD[1]	-	-	96%	97%
Discharge Instructions Given	21	86%	93%	94%
Evaluation of LVS Function	24	96%	97%	99%
Medicare Spending				
Medicare Spending per Patient (ratio)	-	-	0.9	0.98
Pneumonia Care				
Appropriate Initial Antibiotic Given	37	92%	94%	95%
Blood Culture Timing	56	93%	97%	98%
Pregnancy and Delivery Care				
Newborn Deliveries Scheduled Early[3]	20	55%	5%	6%
Preventive Care				
Immunization for Influenza[2]	265	96%	89%	90%
Immunization for Pneumonia[2]	309	97%	89%	92%
Stroke Care				
Anticoagulation Therapy for Atrial Fibrillation[5]	-	-	96%	95%
Antithrombotic Therapy Timing[5]	-	-	98%	98%
Assessed for Rehabilitation[5]	-	-	98%	97%
Discharged on Antithrombotic Therapy[5]	-	-	99%	99%
Discharged on Statin Medication[5]	-	-	95%	94%
Thrombolytic Therapy Timing[5]	-	-	74%	66%
Venous Thromboembolism Prophylaxis[5]	-	-	95%	94%
Written Stroke Educational Materials Given[5]	-	-	88%	88%
Surgical Care Improvement Project				
Appropriate Beta Blocker Usage[2]	62	98%	98%	98%
Appropriate VTP Within 24 Hours[2]	196	98%	98%	98%
Controlled Postoperative Blood Glucose[2,7]	-	-	97%	97%
Perioperative Temperature Management[2]	216	100%	99%	100%
Prophylactic Antibiotic Selection[2]	183	99%	99%	99%

NOTE: Hospital profiles are in alphabetical order by state, then city, then hospital within the city; Rankings exclude hospitals with less than 25 cases except for patient surveys which excludes hospitals with less than 100 cases; (a) 100-299 cases; (1) The number of cases/patients is too few to report; (2) Data submitted were based on a sample of cases/patients; (3) Results are based on a shorter time period than required; (4) Data suppressed by CMS for one or more quarters; (5) Results are not available for this reporting period; (6) Fewer than 100 patients completed the HCAHPS survey; (7) No cases met the criteria for this measure; (8) The lower limit of the confidence interval cannot be calculated if the number of observed infections equals zero; (9) No data are available from the state/territory for this reporting period; (10) The scores shown reflect fewer than 50 completed surveys; (11) There were discrepancies in the data collection process; (12) This measure does not apply to this hospital for this reporting period; (13) Results cannot be calculated for this reporting period; (14) The results for this state are combined with nearby states to protect confidentiality; Please refer to the User's Guide for a full explanation of data.

Prophylactic Antibiotic Selection (Outpatient)	19	95%	98%	98%
Prophylactic Antibiotic Stopped[2]	183	99%	99%	98%
Prophylactic Antibiotic Timing[2]	184	98%	98%	99%
Prophylactic Antibiotic Timing (Outpatient)	20	90%	97%	98%
Urinary Catheter Removal[2]	97	100%	97%	97%
Survey of Patients' Hospital Experiences				
Area Around Room 'Always' Quiet at Night	(a)	68%	65%	61%
Doctors 'Always' Communicated Well	(a)	85%	84%	82%
Home Recovery Information Given	(a)	89%	88%	85%
Hospital Given 9 or 10 on 10 Point Scale	(a)	78%	74%	71%
Meds 'Always' Explained Before Given	(a)	63%	67%	64%
Nurses 'Always' Communicated Well	(a)	81%	81%	79%
Pain 'Always' Well Controlled	(a)	71%	72%	71%
Room and Bathroom 'Always' Clean	(a)	76%	78%	73%
Timely Help 'Always' Received	(a)	73%	74%	68%
Would Definitely Recommend Hospital	(a)	73%	71%	71%
Use of Medical Imaging				
Cardiac Imaging Stress Test before Surgery[1]	-	-	6.3%	5.3%
Combination Abdominal CT Scan	165	3.0%	5.7%	10.5%
Combination Brain/Sinus CT Scan[1]	-	-	2.3%	2.7%
Combination Chest CT Scan	113	0.0%	1.9%	2.7%
Follow-up Mammogram/Ultrasound	299	9.7%	6.3%	8.8%
Lumbar Spine MRI for Low Back Pain[1]	-	-	37.6%	37.2%

Centracare Health System - Long Prairie

20 Ninth Street Southeast
Long Prairie, MN 56347
Phone: 320-732-7210
Fax: 320-732-3802
E-mail: lpm@centracare.com
URL: www.centracare.com
Type: Critical Access Hospitals
Emergency Services: Yes
Ownership: Proprietary
Beds: 34

Key Personnel:
Radiology. . . . . Jody A Bolton
Chief of Medical Staff. . . . . Rene Eldidy, Jr
Operating Room. . . . . Marie Katterhagen
Quality Assurance . . . . Kathy Konetzko
President . . . . Terence Pladson, MD, MBA, FACPE
Administrator . . . . Dan Swenson

Measure	Cases	This Hosp.	State Avg.	U.S. Avg.
Blood Clot Prevention and Treatment				
Anticoagulation Overlap Therapy[5]	-	-	96%	93%
ICU Venous Thromboembolism Prophylaxis[5]	-	-	91%	92%
Incidence of Potentially Preventable VTE[5]	-	-	9%	10%
UFH with Dosages/Platelet Monitoring[5]	-	-	98%	97%
Venous Thromboembolism Prophylaxis[5]	-	-	86%	85%
Warfarin Therapy Discharge Instructions[5]	-	-	63%	75%
Chest Pain/Possible Heart Attack Care				
Aspirin Given Within 24 Hours of Arrival	12	100%	97%	96%
Fibrinolytic Meds Within 30 Min. of Arrival[3,7]	-	-	48%	58%
Average Time to ECG (minutes)	12	7	7	7
Average Time to Transfer (minutes)[1,3]	-	-	54	60
Children's Asthma Care				
Received Home Management Plan of Care	-	-	-	88%
Received Reliever Medication	-	-	-	100%
Received Systemic Corticosteroids	-	-	-	100%
Emergency Department				
Admittance Decision Time (minutes)[5]	-	-	62	98
Head CT Results Within 45 Min. of Arrival[5]	-	-	54%	57%
Patients Who Left ER Before Being Seen[5]	-	-	2%	2%
Time from ER Arrival to Admit. (minutes)[5]	-	-	199	274
Time from ER Arrival to Discharge (minutes)[5]	-	-	125	134
Time in ER Before Being Evaluated (minutes)[5]	-	-	31	26
Time to Pain Meds for Fractures (minutes)[5]	-	-	45	57
Heart Attack Care				
Aspirin Given at Discharge[3,7]	-	-	99%	99%
Fibrinolytic Meds Within 30 Min. of Arrival[3,7]	-	-	-	54%
PCI Within 90 Minutes of Arrival[3,7]	-	-	96%	96%
Statin Prescribed at Discharge[3,7]	-	-	99%	98%
Heart Failure Care				
ACE Inhibitor or ARB for LVSD[1]	-	-	96%	97%
Discharge Instructions Given	13	8%	93%	94%
Evaluation of LVS Function	15	47%	97%	99%
Medicare Spending				
Medicare Spending per Patient (ratio)	-	-	0.9	0.98
Pneumonia Care				
Appropriate Initial Antibiotic Given[1,2]	-	-	94%	95%
Blood Culture Timing[1,2]	-	-	97%	98%
Pregnancy and Delivery Care				
Newborn Deliveries Scheduled Early[5]	-	-	5%	6%
Preventive Care				
Immunization for Influenza[2]	163	60%	89%	90%
Immunization for Pneumonia[2]	213	76%	89%	92%
Stroke Care				
Anticoagulation Therapy for Atrial Fibrillation[5]	-	-	96%	95%
Antithrombotic Therapy Timing[5]	-	-	98%	98%
Assessed for Rehabilitation[5]	-	-	98%	97%
Discharged on Antithrombotic Therapy[5]	-	-	99%	99%
Discharged on Statin Medication[5]	-	-	95%	94%
Thrombolytic Therapy Timing[5]	-	-	74%	66%
Venous Thromboembolism Prophylaxis[5]	-	-	95%	94%
Written Stroke Educational Materials Given[5]	-	-	88%	88%
Surgical Care Improvement Project				
Appropriate Beta Blocker Usage[1]	-	-	98%	98%
Appropriate VTP Within 24 Hours[1]	-	-	98%	98%
Controlled Postoperative Blood Glucose[7]	-	-	97%	97%
Perioperative Temperature Management	12	92%	99%	100%
Prophylactic Antibiotic Selection[1]	-	-	99%	99%
Prophylactic Antibiotic Selection (Outpatient)[1,3]	-	-	98%	98%
Prophylactic Antibiotic Stopped[1]	-	-	99%	98%
Prophylactic Antibiotic Timing[1]	-	-	98%	99%
Prophylactic Antibiotic Timing (Outpatient)[1,3]	-	-	97%	98%
Urinary Catheter Removal[1]	-	-	97%	97%
Survey of Patients' Hospital Experiences				
Area Around Room 'Always' Quiet at Night[5]	-	-	65%	61%
Doctors 'Always' Communicated Well[5]	-	-	84%	82%
Home Recovery Information Given[5]	-	-	88%	85%
Hospital Given 9 or 10 on 10 Point Scale[5]	-	-	74%	71%
Meds 'Always' Explained Before Given[5]	-	-	67%	64%
Nurses 'Always' Communicated Well[5]	-	-	81%	79%
Pain 'Always' Well Controlled[5]	-	-	72%	71%
Room and Bathroom 'Always' Clean[5]	-	-	78%	73%
Timely Help 'Always' Received[5]	-	-	74%	68%
Would Definitely Recommend Hospital[5]	-	-	71%	71%
Use of Medical Imaging				
Cardiac Imaging Stress Test before Surgery[1]	-	-	6.3%	5.3%
Combination Abdominal CT Scan	50	2.0%	5.7%	10.5%
Combination Brain/Sinus CT Scan	37	0.0%	2.3%	2.7%
Combination Chest CT Scan[1]	-	-	1.9%	2.7%
Follow-up Mammogram/Ultrasound[1]	-	-	6.3%	8.8%
Lumbar Spine MRI for Low Back Pain[1]	-	-	37.6%	37.2%

Sanford Luverne Medical Center

1600 North Kniss Avenue PO Box 1019
Luverne, MN 56156
Phone: 507-283-2321
Fax: 507-283-2091
E-mail: info@sanfordluverne.org
URL: www.sanfordluverne.org
Type: Critical Access Hospitals
Emergency Services: Yes
Ownership: Voluntary non-profit - Private
Beds: 28

Key Personnel:
Emergency Room . . . . Lynn DeBerg, RN
Quality Assurance . . . . Nancy Drenth, RN
CEO/President. . . . . Mark A Henke
Anesthesiology. . . . . Dave Knips, CRNA
Chief of Medical Staff. . . . . Richard Morgan, MD
Infection Control. . . . . Kristin Peterson
Operating Room. . . . . Tom Rolfs, RN
Patient Relations . . . . Sue Sandbulte

Measure	Cases	This Hosp.	State Avg.	U.S. Avg.
Blood Clot Prevention and Treatment				
Anticoagulation Overlap Therapy[5]	-	-	96%	93%
ICU Venous Thromboembolism Prophylaxis[5]	-	-	91%	92%
Incidence of Potentially Preventable VTE[5]	-	-	9%	10%
UFH with Dosages/Platelet Monitoring[5]	-	-	98%	97%
Venous Thromboembolism Prophylaxis[5]	-	-	86%	85%
Warfarin Therapy Discharge Instructions[5]	-	-	63%	75%
Chest Pain/Possible Heart Attack Care				
Aspirin Given Within 24 Hours of Arrival	20	95%	97%	96%
Fibrinolytic Meds Within 30 Min. of Arrival[1]	-	-	48%	58%
Average Time to ECG (minutes)	22	8	7	7
Average Time to Transfer (minutes)[1]	-	-	54	60
Children's Asthma Care				
Received Home Management Plan of Care	-	-	-	88%
Received Reliever Medication	-	-	-	100%
Received Systemic Corticosteroids	-	-	-	100%
Emergency Department				
Admittance Decision Time (minutes)[2]	178	10	62	98
Head CT Results Within 45 Min. of Arrival[5]	-	-	54%	57%
Patients Who Left ER Before Being Seen[5]	-	-	2%	2%
Time from ER Arrival to Admit. (minutes)[2]	268	132	199	274
Time from ER Arrival to Discharge (minutes)[5]	-	-	125	134
Time in ER Before Being Evaluated (minutes)[5]	-	-	31	26
Time to Pain Meds for Fractures (minutes)[5]	-	-	45	57
Heart Attack Care				
Aspirin Given at Discharge[3,7]	-	-	99%	99%
Fibrinolytic Meds Within 30 Min. of Arrival[3,7]	-	-	-	54%
PCI Within 90 Minutes of Arrival[3,7]	-	-	96%	96%
Statin Prescribed at Discharge[3,7]	-	-	99%	98%
Heart Failure Care				
ACE Inhibitor or ARB for LVSD[1]	-	-	96%	97%
Discharge Instructions Given[1]	-	-	93%	94%
Evaluation of LVS Function	13	100%	97%	99%
Medicare Spending				
Medicare Spending per Patient (ratio)	-	-	0.9	0.98
Pneumonia Care				
Appropriate Initial Antibiotic Given	14	100%	94%	95%
Blood Culture Timing	19	100%	97%	98%
Pregnancy and Delivery Care				
Newborn Deliveries Scheduled Early[5]	-	-	5%	6%
Preventive Care				
Immunization for Influenza	236	95%	89%	90%
Immunization for Pneumonia[2]	266	97%	89%	92%
Stroke Care				
Anticoagulation Therapy for Atrial Fibrillation[5]	-	-	96%	95%
Antithrombotic Therapy Timing[5]	-	-	98%	98%
Assessed for Rehabilitation[5]	-	-	98%	97%
Discharged on Antithrombotic Therapy[5]	-	-	99%	99%
Discharged on Statin Medication[5]	-	-	95%	94%
Thrombolytic Therapy Timing[5]	-	-	74%	66%
Venous Thromboembolism Prophylaxis[5]	-	-	95%	94%
Written Stroke Educational Materials Given[5]	-	-	88%	88%
Surgical Care Improvement Project				
Appropriate Beta Blocker Usage[1,3]	-	-	98%	98%
Appropriate VTP Within 24 Hours[1,3]	-	-	98%	98%
Controlled Postoperative Blood Glucose[3,7]	-	-	97%	97%
Perioperative Temperature Management[1,3]	-	-	99%	100%
Prophylactic Antibiotic Selection[1,3]	-	-	99%	99%
Prophylactic Antibiotic Selection (Outpatient)[1,3]	-	-	98%	98%
Prophylactic Antibiotic Stopped[1,3]	-	-	99%	98%
Prophylactic Antibiotic Timing[1,3]	-	-	98%	99%
Prophylactic Antibiotic Timing (Outpatient)[1,3]	-	-	97%	98%
Urinary Catheter Removal[1,3]	-	-	97%	97%
Survey of Patients' Hospital Experiences				
Area Around Room 'Always' Quiet at Night	(a)	70%	65%	61%
Doctors 'Always' Communicated Well	(a)	91%	84%	82%
Home Recovery Information Given	(a)	94%	88%	85%
Hospital Given 9 or 10 on 10 Point Scale	(a)	84%	74%	71%
Meds 'Always' Explained Before Given	(a)	65%	67%	64%
Nurses 'Always' Communicated Well	(a)	83%	81%	79%
Pain 'Always' Well Controlled	(a)	76%	72%	71%
Room and Bathroom 'Always' Clean	(a)	92%	78%	73%
Timely Help 'Always' Received	(a)	74%	74%	68%
Would Definitely Recommend Hospital	(a)	82%	71%	71%
Use of Medical Imaging				
Cardiac Imaging Stress Test before Surgery[1]	-	-	6.3%	5.3%
Combination Abdominal CT Scan	71	2.8%	5.7%	10.5%
Combination Brain/Sinus CT Scan	87	0.0%	2.3%	2.7%
Combination Chest CT Scan	52	0.0%	1.9%	2.7%
Follow-up Mammogram/Ultrasound	227	4.4%	6.3%	8.8%
Lumbar Spine MRI for Low Back Pain[1]	-	-	37.6%	37.2%

NOTE: Hospital profiles are in alphabetical order by state, then city, then hospital within the city; Rankings exclude hospitals with less than 25 cases except for patient surveys which excludes hospitals with less than 100 cases; (a) 100-299 cases; (1) The number of cases/patients is too few to report; (2) Data submitted were based on a sample of cases/patients; (3) Results are based on a shorter time period than required; (4) Data suppressed by CMS for one or more quarters; (5) Results are not available for this reporting period; (6) Fewer than 100 patients completed the HCAHPS survey; (7) No cases met the criteria for this measure; (8) The lower limit of the confidence interval cannot be calculated if the number of observed infections equals zero; (9) No data are available from the state/territory for this reporting period; (10) The scores shown reflect fewer than 50 completed surveys; (11) There were discrepancies in the data collection process; (12) This measure does not apply to this hospital for this reporting period; (13) Results cannot be calculated for this reporting period; (14) The results for this state are combined with nearby states to protect confidentiality; Please refer to the User's Guide for a full explanation of data.

Madelia Community Hospital

121 Drew Avenue Southeast
Madelia, MN 56062
URL: www.mchospital.org
Type: Critical Access Hospitals
Ownership: Voluntary non-profit - Other

Phone: 507-642-3255
Fax: 507-642-8516
Emergency Services: Yes
Beds: 25

Key Personnel:
Infection Control. . . . . Terri Baumgartner
CEO/President. . . . . Candace Fenske
Coronary Care . . . . Deidre Hruby
Intensive Care Unit. . . . . Deidre Hruby
Radiology. . . . . Melissa Hunt
Chief of Medical Staff. . . . . Jennifer Longbehn, DO
Operating Room. . . . . Jennifer McLaughlin
Emergency Room . . . . Jennifer McLoughlin

Measure	Cases	This Hosp.	State Avg.	U.S. Avg.
Blood Clot Prevention and Treatment				
Anticoagulation Overlap Therapy[5]	-	-	96%	93%
ICU Venous Thromboembolism Prophylaxis[5]	-	-	91%	92%
Incidence of Potentially Preventable VTE[5]	-	-	9%	10%
UFH with Dosages/Platelet Monitoring[5]	-	-	98%	97%
Venous Thromboembolism Prophylaxis[5]	-	-	86%	85%
Warfarin Therapy Discharge Instructions[5]	-	-	63%	75%
Chest Pain/Possible Heart Attack Care				
Aspirin Given Within 24 Hours of Arrival	-	-	97%	96%
Fibrinolytic Meds Within 30 Min. of Arrival	-	-	48%	58%
Average Time to ECG (minutes)	-	-	7	7
Average Time to Transfer (minutes)	-	-	54	60
Children's Asthma Care				
Received Home Management Plan of Care	-	-	-	88%
Received Reliever Medication	-	-	-	100%
Received Systemic Corticosteroids	-	-	-	100%
Emergency Department				
Admittance Decision Time (minutes)	42	5	62	98
Head CT Results Within 45 Min. of Arrival	-	-	54%	57%
Patients Who Left ER Before Being Seen	-	-	2%	2%
Time from ER Arrival to Admit. (minutes)	54	110	199	274
Time from ER Arrival to Discharge (minutes)	-	-	125	134
Time in ER Before Being Evaluated (minutes)	-	-	31	26
Time to Pain Meds for Fractures (minutes)	-	-	45	57
Heart Attack Care				
Aspirin Given at Discharge[5]	-	-	99%	99%
Fibrinolytic Meds Within 30 Min. of Arrival[5]	-	-	-	54%
PCI Within 90 Minutes of Arrival[5]	-	-	96%	96%
Statin Prescribed at Discharge[5]	-	-	99%	98%
Heart Failure Care				
ACE Inhibitor or ARB for LVSD[7]	-	-	96%	97%
Discharge Instructions Given[1]	-	-	93%	94%
Evaluation of LVS Function[1]	-	-	97%	99%
Medicare Spending				
Medicare Spending per Patient (ratio)	-	-	0.9	0.98
Pneumonia Care				
Appropriate Initial Antibiotic Given[1]	-	-	94%	95%
Blood Culture Timing[1]	-	-	97%	98%
Pregnancy and Delivery Care				
Newborn Deliveries Scheduled Early[5]	-	-	5%	6%
Preventive Care				
Immunization for Influenza	52	83%	89%	90%
Immunization for Pneumonia[2]	91	75%	89%	92%
Stroke Care				
Anticoagulation Therapy for Atrial Fibrillation[5]	-	-	96%	95%
Antithrombotic Therapy Timing[5]	-	-	98%	98%
Assessed for Rehabilitation[5]	-	-	98%	97%
Discharged on Antithrombotic Therapy[5]	-	-	99%	99%
Discharged on Statin Medication[5]	-	-	95%	94%
Thrombolytic Therapy Timing[5]	-	-	74%	66%
Venous Thromboembolism Prophylaxis[5]	-	-	95%	94%
Written Stroke Educational Materials Given[5]	-	-	88%	88%
Surgical Care Improvement Project				
Appropriate Beta Blocker Usage[5]	-	-	98%	98%
Appropriate VTP Within 24 Hours[5]	-	-	98%	98%
Controlled Postoperative Blood Glucose[5]	-	-	97%	97%
Perioperative Temperature Management[5]	-	-	99%	100%
Prophylactic Antibiotic Selection[5]	-	-	99%	99%
Prophylactic Antibiotic Selection (Outpatient)	-	-	98%	98%
Prophylactic Antibiotic Stopped[5]	-	-	99%	98%
Prophylactic Antibiotic Timing[5]	-	-	98%	99%
Prophylactic Antibiotic Timing (Outpatient)	-	-	97%	98%
Urinary Catheter Removal[5]	-	-	97%	97%
Survey of Patients' Hospital Experiences				
Area Around Room 'Always' Quiet at Night[5]	-	-	65%	61%
Doctors 'Always' Communicated Well[5]	-	-	84%	82%
Home Recovery Information Given[5]	-	-	88%	85%
Hospital Given 9 or 10 on 10 Point Scale[5]	-	-	74%	71%
Meds 'Always' Explained Before Given[5]	-	-	67%	64%
Nurses 'Always' Communicated Well[5]	-	-	81%	79%
Pain 'Always' Well Controlled[5]	-	-	72%	71%
Room and Bathroom 'Always' Clean[5]	-	-	78%	73%
Timely Help 'Always' Received[5]	-	-	74%	68%
Would Definitely Recommend Hospital[5]	-	-	71%	71%
Use of Medical Imaging				
Cardiac Imaging Stress Test before Surgery	-	-	6.3%	5.3%
Combination Abdominal CT Scan	-	-	5.7%	10.5%
Combination Brain/Sinus CT Scan	-	-	2.3%	2.7%
Combination Chest CT Scan	-	-	1.9%	2.7%
Follow-up Mammogram/Ultrasound	-	-	6.3%	8.8%
Lumbar Spine MRI for Low Back Pain	-	-	37.6%	37.2%

Madison Hospital

820 Third Avenue
Madison, MN 56256
URL: www.madisonlutheranhome.com
Type: Critical Access Hospitals
Ownership: Proprietary

Phone: 320-598-7536
Fax: 320-598-3923
Emergency Services: Yes
Beds: 21

Key Personnel:
Chief of Medical Staff . . . . Larry Grong, MD
CEO/President. . . . . Scott Larson
Infection Control. . . . . Mary Woodrich

Measure	Cases	This Hosp.	State Avg.	U.S. Avg.
Blood Clot Prevention and Treatment				
Anticoagulation Overlap Therapy[5]	-	-	96%	93%
ICU Venous Thromboembolism Prophylaxis[5]	-	-	91%	92%
Incidence of Potentially Preventable VTE[5]	-	-	9%	10%
UFH with Dosages/Platelet Monitoring[5]	-	-	98%	97%
Venous Thromboembolism Prophylaxis[5]	-	-	86%	85%
Warfarin Therapy Discharge Instructions[5]	-	-	63%	75%
Chest Pain/Possible Heart Attack Care				
Aspirin Given Within 24 Hours of Arrival[5]	-	-	97%	96%
Fibrinolytic Meds Within 30 Min. of Arrival[5]	-	-	48%	58%
Average Time to ECG (minutes)[5]	-	-	7	7
Average Time to Transfer (minutes)[5]	-	-	54	60
Children's Asthma Care				
Received Home Management Plan of Care	-	-	-	88%
Received Reliever Medication	-	-	-	100%
Received Systemic Corticosteroids	-	-	-	100%
Emergency Department				
Admittance Decision Time (minutes)[1,3]	-	-	62	98
Head CT Results Within 45 Min. of Arrival[5]	-	-	54%	57%
Patients Who Left ER Before Being Seen[5]	-	-	2%	2%
Time from ER Arrival to Admit. (minutes)[3]	157	88	199	274
Time from ER Arrival to Discharge (minutes)[5]	-	-	125	134
Time in ER Before Being Evaluated (minutes)[5]	-	-	31	26
Time to Pain Meds for Fractures (minutes)[5]	-	-	45	57
Heart Attack Care				
Aspirin Given at Discharge[5]	-	-	99%	99%
Fibrinolytic Meds Within 30 Min. of Arrival[5]	-	-	-	54%
PCI Within 90 Minutes of Arrival[5]	-	-	96%	96%
Statin Prescribed at Discharge[5]	-	-	99%	98%
Heart Failure Care				
ACE Inhibitor or ARB for LVSD[3,7]	-	-	96%	97%
Discharge Instructions Given[1,3]	-	-	93%	94%
Evaluation of LVS Function[1,3]	-	-	97%	99%
Medicare Spending				
Medicare Spending per Patient (ratio)	-	-	0.9	0.98
Pneumonia Care				
Appropriate Initial Antibiotic Given[1,3]	-	-	94%	95%
Blood Culture Timing[3,7]	-	-	97%	98%
Pregnancy and Delivery Care				
Newborn Deliveries Scheduled Early[5]	-	-	5%	6%
Preventive Care				
Immunization for Influenza[5]	-	-	89%	90%
Immunization for Pneumonia[3]	42	38%	89%	92%
Stroke Care				
Anticoagulation Therapy for Atrial Fibrillation[3,7]	-	-	96%	95%
Antithrombotic Therapy Timing[1,3]	-	-	98%	98%
Assessed for Rehabilitation[1,3]	-	-	98%	97%
Discharged on Antithrombotic Therapy[1,3]	-	-	99%	99%
Discharged on Statin Medication[1,3]	-	-	95%	94%
Thrombolytic Therapy Timing[3,7]	-	-	74%	66%
Venous Thromboembolism Prophylaxis[1,3]	-	-	95%	94%
Written Stroke Educational Materials Given[3,7]	-	-	88%	88%
Surgical Care Improvement Project				
Appropriate Beta Blocker Usage[5]	-	-	98%	98%
Appropriate VTP Within 24 Hours[5]	-	-	98%	98%
Controlled Postoperative Blood Glucose[5]	-	-	97%	97%
Perioperative Temperature Management[5]	-	-	99%	100%
Prophylactic Antibiotic Selection[5]	-	-	99%	99%
Prophylactic Antibiotic Selection (Outpatient)[5]	-	-	98%	98%
Prophylactic Antibiotic Stopped[5]	-	-	99%	98%
Prophylactic Antibiotic Timing[5]	-	-	98%	99%
Prophylactic Antibiotic Timing (Outpatient)[5]	-	-	97%	98%
Urinary Catheter Removal[5]	-	-	97%	97%
Survey of Patients' Hospital Experiences				
Area Around Room 'Always' Quiet at Night[6,11]	<100	69%	65%	61%
Doctors 'Always' Communicated Well[6,11]	<100	88%	84%	82%
Home Recovery Information Given[6,11]	<100	82%	88%	85%
Hospital Given 9 or 10 on 10 Point Scale[6,11]	<100	83%	74%	71%
Meds 'Always' Explained Before Given[6,11]	<100	67%	67%	64%
Nurses 'Always' Communicated Well[6,11]	<100	84%	81%	79%
Pain 'Always' Well Controlled[6,11]	<100	79%	72%	71%
Room and Bathroom 'Always' Clean[6,11]	<100	75%	78%	73%
Timely Help 'Always' Received[6,11]	<100	84%	74%	68%
Would Definitely Recommend Hospital[6,11]	<100	64%	71%	71%
Use of Medical Imaging				
Cardiac Imaging Stress Test before Surgery[1]	-	-	6.3%	5.3%
Combination Abdominal CT Scan[1]	-	-	5.7%	10.5%
Combination Brain/Sinus CT Scan[1]	-	-	2.3%	2.7%
Combination Chest CT Scan[1]	-	-	1.9%	2.7%
Follow-up Mammogram/Ultrasound[1]	-	-	6.3%	8.8%
Lumbar Spine MRI for Low Back Pain[1]	-	-	37.6%	37.2%

Mahnomen Health Center

414 W Jefferson PO Box 396
Mahnomen, MN 56557
URL: www.mahnomenhealthcenter.com
Type: Critical Access Hospitals
Ownership: Voluntary non-profit - Other

Phone: 218-935-2511
Fax: 218-935-2370
Emergency Services: Yes
Beds: 63

Key Personnel:
Chairman/CEO . . . . Karen Ahmann
Emergency Room . . . . Mike Bunker
Quality Assurance . . . . Bob Crawford
Chief of Medical Staff. . . . . Dr Sanjit Dutta
Cardiac Laboratory. . . . . Barbara Fluellen
CEO/President. . . . . Sue Klassen
Radiology. . . . . Richard Marsden

Measure	Cases	This Hosp.	State Avg.	U.S. Avg.
Blood Clot Prevention and Treatment				
Anticoagulation Overlap Therapy[5]	-	-	96%	93%
ICU Venous Thromboembolism Prophylaxis[5]	-	-	91%	92%
Incidence of Potentially Preventable VTE[5]	-	-	9%	10%
UFH with Dosages/Platelet Monitoring[5]	-	-	98%	97%
Venous Thromboembolism Prophylaxis[5]	-	-	86%	85%
Warfarin Therapy Discharge Instructions[5]	-	-	63%	75%
Chest Pain/Possible Heart Attack Care				
Aspirin Given Within 24 Hours of Arrival[3,7]	-	-	97%	96%
Fibrinolytic Meds Within 30 Min. of Arrival[5]	-	-	48%	58%
Average Time to ECG (minutes)[3,7]	-	-	7	7
Average Time to Transfer (minutes)[5]	-	-	54	60
Children's Asthma Care				
Received Home Management Plan of Care	-	-	-	88%
Received Reliever Medication	-	-	-	100%

NOTE: Hospital profiles are in alphabetical order by state, then city, then hospital within the city; Rankings exclude hospitals with less than 25 cases except for patient surveys which excludes hospitals with less than 100 cases; (a) 100-299 cases; (1) The number of cases/patients is too few to report; (2) Data submitted were based on a sample of cases/patients; (3) Results are based on a shorter time period than required; (4) Data suppressed by CMS for one or more quarters; (5) Results are not available for this reporting period; (6) Fewer than 100 patients completed the HCAHPS survey; (7) No cases met the criteria for this measure; (8) The lower limit of the confidence interval cannot be calculated if the number of observed infections equals zero; (9) No data are available from the state/territory for this reporting period; (10) The scores shown reflect fewer than 50 completed surveys; (11) There were discrepancies in the data collection process; (12) This measure does not apply to this hospital for this reporting period; (13) Results cannot be calculated for this reporting period; (14) The results for this state are combined with nearby states to protect confidentiality; Please refer to the User's Guide for a full explanation of data.

Measure	Cases	This Hosp.	State Avg.	U.S. Avg.
Received Systemic Corticosteroids	-	-	-	100%
Emergency Department				
Admittance Decision Time (minutes)[5]	-	-	62	98
Head CT Results Within 45 Min. of Arrival[5]	-	-	54%	57%
Patients Who Left ER Before Being Seen[5]	-	-	2%	2%
Time from ER Arrival to Admit. (minutes)[5]	-	-	199	274
Time from ER Arrival to Discharge (minutes)[5]	-	-	125	134
Time in ER Before Being Evaluated (minutes)[5]	-	-	31	26
Time to Pain Meds for Fractures (minutes)[5]	-	-	45	57
Heart Attack Care				
Aspirin Given at Discharge[5]	-	-	99%	99%
Fibrinolytic Meds Within 30 Min. of Arrival[5]	-	-	-	54%
PCI Within 90 Minutes of Arrival[5]	-	-	96%	96%
Statin Prescribed at Discharge[5]	-	-	99%	98%
Heart Failure Care				
ACE Inhibitor or ARB for LVSD[5]	-	-	96%	97%
Discharge Instructions Given[5]	-	-	93%	94%
Evaluation of LVS Function[5]	-	-	97%	99%
Medicare Spending				
Medicare Spending per Patient (ratio)	-	-	0.9	0.98
Pneumonia Care				
Appropriate Initial Antibiotic Given[3,7]	-	-	94%	95%
Blood Culture Timing[3,7]	-	-	97%	98%
Pregnancy and Delivery Care				
Newborn Deliveries Scheduled Early[5]	-	-	5%	6%
Preventive Care				
Immunization for Influenza[5]	-	-	89%	90%
Immunization for Pneumonia[5]	-	-	89%	92%
Stroke Care				
Anticoagulation Therapy for Atrial Fibrillation[5]	-	-	96%	95%
Antithrombotic Therapy Timing[5]	-	-	98%	98%
Assessed for Rehabilitation[5]	-	-	98%	97%
Discharged on Antithrombotic Therapy[5]	-	-	99%	99%
Discharged on Statin Medication[5]	-	-	95%	94%
Thrombolytic Therapy Timing[5]	-	-	74%	66%
Venous Thromboembolism Prophylaxis[5]	-	-	95%	94%
Written Stroke Educational Materials Given[5]	-	-	88%	88%
Surgical Care Improvement Project				
Appropriate Beta Blocker Usage[5]	-	-	98%	98%
Appropriate VTP Within 24 Hours[5]	-	-	98%	98%
Controlled Postoperative Blood Glucose[5]	-	-	97%	97%
Perioperative Temperature Management[5]	-	-	99%	100%
Prophylactic Antibiotic Selection[5]	-	-	99%	99%
Prophylactic Antibiotic Selection (Outpatient)[5]	-	-	98%	98%
Prophylactic Antibiotic Stopped[5]	-	-	99%	98%
Prophylactic Antibiotic Timing[5]	-	-	98%	99%
Prophylactic Antibiotic Timing (Outpatient)[5]	-	-	97%	98%
Urinary Catheter Removal[5]	-	-	97%	97%
Survey of Patients' Hospital Experiences				
Area Around Room 'Always' Quiet at Night[5]	-	-	65%	61%
Doctors 'Always' Communicated Well[5]	-	-	84%	82%
Home Recovery Information Given[5]	-	-	88%	85%
Hospital Given 9 or 10 on 10 Point Scale[5]	-	-	74%	71%
Meds 'Always' Explained Before Given[5]	-	-	67%	64%
Nurses 'Always' Communicated Well[5]	-	-	81%	79%
Pain 'Always' Well Controlled[5]	-	-	72%	71%
Room and Bathroom 'Always' Clean[5]	-	-	78%	73%
Timely Help 'Always' Received[5]	-	-	74%	68%
Would Definitely Recommend Hospital[5]	-	-	71%	71%
Use of Medical Imaging				
Cardiac Imaging Stress Test before Surgery[7]	-	-	6.3%	5.3%
Combination Abdominal CT Scan[1]	-	-	5.7%	10.5%
Combination Brain/Sinus CT Scan[1]	-	-	2.3%	2.7%
Combination Chest CT Scan[1]	-	-	1.9%	2.7%
Follow-up Mammogram/Ultrasound[1]	-	-	6.3%	8.8%
Lumbar Spine MRI for Low Back Pain[1]	-	-	37.6%	37.2%

Mayo Clinic Health System - Mankato

1025 Marsh Street Box 8673
Mankato, MN 56001
E-mail: isjinfo@mayo.edu
URL: www.isj-mhs.org
Phone: 507-625-4031
Fax: 507-385-2908
Type: Acute Care Hospitals
Emergency Services: Yes
Ownership: Voluntary non-profit - Private
Beds: 272

Key Personnel:
Surgery . . . . Don Beitzel, P.A.-C.
Operating Room. . . . . Colette Brust
Radiology. . . . . Anne Chapman
CEO/President. . . . . Greg Kutcher, MD
Patient Relations . . . . Theresa Mees
Quality Assurance . . . . Theresa Mees
Infection Control. . . . . Judy Webber, RN
Chief of Medical Staff . . . . Michael Wolf, MD

Measure	Cases	This Hosp.	State Avg.	U.S. Avg.
Blood Clot Prevention and Treatment				
Anticoagulation Overlap Therapy[2]	104	99%	96%	93%
ICU Venous Thromboembolism Prophylaxis[2]	29	97%	91%	92%
Incidence of Potentially Preventable VTE[2]	19	26%	9%	10%
UFH with Dosages/Platelet Monitoring[2]	87	99%	98%	97%
Venous Thromboembolism Prophylaxis[2]	276	92%	86%	85%
Warfarin Therapy Discharge Instructions[2]	78	28%	63%	75%
Chest Pain/Possible Heart Attack Care				
Aspirin Given Within 24 Hours of Arrival[1]	-	-	97%	96%
Fibrinolytic Meds Within 30 Min. of Arrival[3,7]	-	-	48%	58%
Average Time to ECG (minutes)[1]	-	-	7	7
Average Time to Transfer (minutes)[3,7]	-	-	54	60
Children's Asthma Care				
Received Home Management Plan of Care	-	-	-	88%
Received Reliever Medication	-	-	-	100%
Received Systemic Corticosteroids	-	-	-	100%
Emergency Department				
Admittance Decision Time (minutes)[2]	317	113	62	98
Head CT Results Within 45 Min. of Arrival[1]	-	-	54%	57%
Patients Who Left ER Before Being Seen	22,282	0%	2%	2%
Time from ER Arrival to Admit. (minutes)[2]	366	207	199	274
Time from ER Arrival to Discharge (minutes)	380	128	125	134
Time in ER Before Being Evaluated (minutes)	426	13	31	26
Time to Pain Meds for Fractures (minutes)	105	36	45	57
Heart Attack Care				
Aspirin Given at Discharge	220	99%	99%	99%
Fibrinolytic Meds Within 30 Min. of Arrival[7]	-	-	-	54%
PCI Within 90 Minutes of Arrival	18	100%	96%	96%
Statin Prescribed at Discharge	212	98%	99%	98%
Heart Failure Care				
ACE Inhibitor or ARB for LVSD	58	90%	96%	97%
Discharge Instructions Given	188	80%	93%	94%
Evaluation of LVS Function	231	100%	97%	99%
Medicare Spending				
Medicare Spending per Patient (ratio)	-	0.90	0.9	0.98
Pneumonia Care				
Appropriate Initial Antibiotic Given	84	98%	94%	95%
Blood Culture Timing	156	97%	97%	98%
Pregnancy and Delivery Care				
Newborn Deliveries Scheduled Early	130	8%	5%	6%
Preventive Care				
Immunization for Influenza[2]	532	92%	89%	90%
Immunization for Pneumonia[2]	642	89%	89%	92%
Stroke Care				
Anticoagulation Therapy for Atrial Fibrillation	14	93%	96%	95%
Antithrombotic Therapy Timing	71	99%	98%	98%
Assessed for Rehabilitation	84	94%	98%	97%
Discharged on Antithrombotic Therapy	79	99%	99%	99%
Discharged on Statin Medication	65	94%	95%	94%
Thrombolytic Therapy Timing[1]	-	-	74%	66%
Venous Thromboembolism Prophylaxis	79	92%	95%	94%
Written Stroke Educational Materials Given	45	69%	88%	88%
Surgical Care Improvement Project				
Appropriate Beta Blocker Usage[2]	156	99%	98%	98%
Appropriate VTP Within 24 Hours[2]	445	100%	98%	98%
Controlled Postoperative Blood Glucose[2,7]	-	-	97%	97%
Perioperative Temperature Management[2]	499	100%	99%	100%
Prophylactic Antibiotic Selection[2]	283	100%	99%	99%
Prophylactic Antibiotic Selection (Outpatient)	320	94%	98%	98%
Prophylactic Antibiotic Stopped[2]	276	98%	99%	98%
Prophylactic Antibiotic Timing[2]	284	99%	98%	99%
Prophylactic Antibiotic Timing (Outpatient)	320	96%	97%	98%
Urinary Catheter Removal[2]	156	92%	97%	97%
Survey of Patients' Hospital Experiences				
Area Around Room 'Always' Quiet at Night	300+	46%	65%	61%
Doctors 'Always' Communicated Well	300+	77%	84%	82%
Home Recovery Information Given	300+	84%	88%	85%
Hospital Given 9 or 10 on 10 Point Scale	300+	62%	74%	71%
Meds 'Always' Explained Before Given	300+	62%	67%	64%
Nurses 'Always' Communicated Well	300+	75%	81%	79%
Pain 'Always' Well Controlled	300+	68%	72%	71%
Room and Bathroom 'Always' Clean	300+	71%	78%	73%
Timely Help 'Always' Received	300+	63%	74%	68%
Would Definitely Recommend Hospital	300+	63%	71%	71%
Use of Medical Imaging				
Cardiac Imaging Stress Test before Surgery	243	5.8%	6.3%	5.3%
Combination Abdominal CT Scan	471	15.7%	5.7%	10.5%
Combination Brain/Sinus CT Scan	335	1.5%	2.3%	2.7%
Combination Chest CT Scan	324	0.6%	1.9%	2.7%
Follow-up Mammogram/Ultrasound[7]	-	-	6.3%	8.8%
Lumbar Spine MRI for Low Back Pain[1]	-	-	37.6%	37.2%

Maple Grove Hospital

9875 Hospital Drive
Maple Grove, MN 55369
URL: www.maplegrove.org
Phone: 763-581-1000
Type: Acute Care Hospitals
Emergency Services: Yes
Ownership: Voluntary non-profit - Private
Beds: 119

Key Personnel:
CEO . . . . Andrew S Cochrane
Chief of Medical Staff . . . . Jill Hallstrom
Chair/CEO . . . . Loren L. Taylor

Measure	Cases	This Hosp.	State Avg.	U.S. Avg.
Blood Clot Prevention and Treatment				
Anticoagulation Overlap Therapy[2]	47	100%	96%	93%
ICU Venous Thromboembolism Prophylaxis[2]	24	92%	91%	92%
Incidence of Potentially Preventable VTE[1,2]	-	-	9%	10%
UFH with Dosages/Platelet Monitoring[2]	37	100%	98%	97%
Venous Thromboembolism Prophylaxis[2]	283	81%	86%	85%
Warfarin Therapy Discharge Instructions[2]	41	98%	63%	75%
Chest Pain/Possible Heart Attack Care				
Aspirin Given Within 24 Hours of Arrival	86	99%	97%	96%
Fibrinolytic Meds Within 30 Min. of Arrival[7]	-	-	48%	58%
Average Time to ECG (minutes)	89	4	7	7
Average Time to Transfer (minutes)	20	38	54	60
Children's Asthma Care				
Received Home Management Plan of Care	-	-	-	88%
Received Reliever Medication	-	-	-	100%
Received Systemic Corticosteroids	-	-	-	100%
Emergency Department				
Admittance Decision Time (minutes)[2]	298	56	62	98
Head CT Results Within 45 Min. of Arrival[1]	-	-	54%	57%
Patients Who Left ER Before Being Seen	32,216	0%	2%	2%
Time from ER Arrival to Admit. (minutes)[2]	298	202	199	274
Time from ER Arrival to Discharge (minutes)	374	112	125	134
Time in ER Before Being Evaluated (minutes)	403	9	31	26
Time to Pain Meds for Fractures (minutes)	185	33	45	57
Heart Attack Care				
Aspirin Given at Discharge[1,3]	-	-	99%	99%
Fibrinolytic Meds Within 30 Min. of Arrival[3,7]	-	-	-	54%
PCI Within 90 Minutes of Arrival[3,7]	-	-	96%	96%
Statin Prescribed at Discharge[1,3]	-	-	99%	98%
Heart Failure Care				
ACE Inhibitor or ARB for LVSD	19	95%	96%	97%
Discharge Instructions Given	78	100%	93%	94%
Evaluation of LVS Function	95	100%	97%	99%
Medicare Spending				
Medicare Spending per Patient (ratio)	-	0.88	0.9	0.98
Pneumonia Care				
Appropriate Initial Antibiotic Given	119	99%	94%	95%

NOTE: Hospital profiles are in alphabetical order by state, then city, then hospital within the city; Rankings exclude hospitals with less than 25 cases except for patient surveys which excludes hospitals with less than 100 cases; (a) 100-299 cases; (1) The number of cases/patients is too few to report; (2) Data submitted were based on a sample of cases/patients; (3) Results are based on a shorter time period than required; (4) Data suppressed by CMS for one or more quarters; (5) Results are not available for this reporting period; (6) Fewer than 100 patients completed the HCAHPS survey; (7) No cases met the criteria for this measure; (8) The lower limit of the confidence interval cannot be calculated if the number of observed infections equals zero; (9) No data are available from the state/territory for this reporting period; (10) The scores shown reflect fewer than 50 completed surveys; (11) There were discrepancies in the data collection process; (12) This measure does not apply to this hospital for this reporting period; (13) Results cannot be calculated for this reporting period; (14) The results for this state are combined with nearby states to protect confidentiality; Please refer to the User's Guide for a full explanation of data.

Measure	Cases	This Hosp.	State Avg.	U.S. Avg.
Blood Culture Timing	148	99%	97%	98%
Pregnancy and Delivery Care				
Newborn Deliveries Scheduled Early[2]	103	2%	5%	6%
Preventive Care				
Immunization for Influenza[2]	413	96%	89%	90%
Immunization for Pneumonia[2]	240	94%	89%	92%
Stroke Care				
Anticoagulation Therapy for Atrial Fibrillation[5]	-	-	96%	95%
Antithrombotic Therapy Timing[5]	-	-	98%	98%
Assessed for Rehabilitation[5]	-	-	98%	97%
Discharged on Antithrombotic Therapy[5]	-	-	99%	99%
Discharged on Statin Medication[5]	-	-	95%	94%
Thrombolytic Therapy Timing[5]	-	-	74%	66%
Venous Thromboembolism Prophylaxis[5]	-	-	95%	94%
Written Stroke Educational Materials Given[5]	-	-	88%	88%
Surgical Care Improvement Project				
Appropriate Beta Blocker Usage	167	99%	98%	98%
Appropriate VTP Within 24 Hours	572	99%	98%	98%
Controlled Postoperative Blood Glucose[7]	-	-	97%	97%
Perioperative Temperature Management	634	100%	99%	100%
Prophylactic Antibiotic Selection	536	100%	99%	99%
Prophylactic Antibiotic Selection (Outpatient)	287	100%	98%	98%
Prophylactic Antibiotic Stopped	534	100%	99%	98%
Prophylactic Antibiotic Timing	536	99%	98%	99%
Prophylactic Antibiotic Timing (Outpatient)	287	100%	97%	98%
Urinary Catheter Removal	379	100%	97%	97%
Survey of Patients' Hospital Experiences				
Area Around Room 'Always' Quiet at Night	300+	68%	65%	61%
Doctors 'Always' Communicated Well	300+	77%	84%	82%
Home Recovery Information Given	300+	88%	88%	85%
Hospital Given 9 or 10 on 10 Point Scale	300+	85%	74%	71%
Meds 'Always' Explained Before Given	300+	59%	67%	64%
Nurses 'Always' Communicated Well	300+	80%	81%	79%
Pain 'Always' Well Controlled	300+	75%	72%	71%
Room and Bathroom 'Always' Clean	300+	67%	78%	73%
Timely Help 'Always' Received	300+	66%	74%	68%
Would Definitely Recommend Hospital	300+	85%	71%	71%
Use of Medical Imaging				
Cardiac Imaging Stress Test before Surgery[1]	-	-	6.3%	5.3%
Combination Abdominal CT Scan	164	0.6%	5.7%	10.5%
Combination Brain/Sinus CT Scan[1]	-	-	2.3%	2.7%
Combination Chest CT Scan[1]	-	-	1.9%	2.7%
Follow-up Mammogram/Ultrasound[7]	-	-	6.3%	8.8%
Lumbar Spine MRI for Low Back Pain[1]	-	-	37.6%	37.2%

Healtheast Saint John's Hospital

1575 Beam Avenue
Maplewood, MN 55109
Phone: 651-232-7000
Fax: 651-232-7240
URL: www.stjohnshospital-mn.org
Type: Acute Care Hospitals
Emergency Services: Yes
Ownership: Voluntary non-profit - Private
Beds: 184

Key Personnel:

President/CEO. . . . . Kathryn Correia
Operating Room. . . . . Jan Edwards
Chief of Medical Staff. . . . . Steve Kolar, MD
Infection Control. . . . . Kathy Miller, RN
Pediatric Ambulatory Care . . . . . . James Prall, MD
Pediatric In-Patient Care . . . . James Prall, MD
Quality Assurance . . . . Jan Weidner

Measure	Cases	This Hosp.	State Avg.	U.S. Avg.
Blood Clot Prevention and Treatment				
Anticoagulation Overlap Therapy[2]	83	99%	96%	93%
ICU Venous Thromboembolism Prophylaxis[2]	60	93%	91%	92%
Incidence of Potentially Preventable VTE[1,2]	-	-	9%	10%
UFH with Dosages/Platelet Monitoring[2]	53	96%	98%	97%
Venous Thromboembolism Prophylaxis[2]	307	79%	86%	85%
Warfarin Therapy Discharge Instructions[2]	67	57%	63%	75%
Chest Pain/Possible Heart Attack Care				
Aspirin Given Within 24 Hours of Arrival	52	96%	97%	96%
Fibrinolytic Meds Within 30 Min. of Arrival[7]	-	-	48%	58%
Average Time to ECG (minutes)	53	9	7	7
Average Time to Transfer (minutes)[1]	-	-	54	60
Children's Asthma Care				
Received Home Management Plan of Care	-	-	-	88%
Received Reliever Medication	-	-	-	100%
Received Systemic Corticosteroids	-	-	-	100%
Emergency Department				
Admittance Decision Time (minutes)[2]	481	63	62	98
Head CT Results Within 45 Min. of Arrival	11	36%	54%	57%
Patients Who Left ER Before Being Seen	36,449	3%	2%	2%
Time from ER Arrival to Admit. (minutes)[2]	521	245	199	274
Time from ER Arrival to Discharge (minutes)	378	186	125	134
Time in ER Before Being Evaluated (minutes)	397	50	31	26
Time to Pain Meds for Fractures (minutes)	136	71	45	57
Heart Attack Care				
Aspirin Given at Discharge	18	100%	99%	99%
Fibrinolytic Meds Within 30 Min. of Arrival[7]	-	-	-	54%
PCI Within 90 Minutes of Arrival[7]	-	-	96%	96%
Statin Prescribed at Discharge	19	84%	99%	98%
Heart Failure Care				
ACE Inhibitor or ARB for LVSD	61	100%	96%	97%
Discharge Instructions Given	174	97%	93%	94%
Evaluation of LVS Function	229	99%	97%	99%
Medicare Spending				
Medicare Spending per Patient (ratio)	-	0.91	0.9	0.98
Pneumonia Care				
Appropriate Initial Antibiotic Given[2]	117	99%	94%	95%
Blood Culture Timing[2]	186	98%	97%	98%
Pregnancy and Delivery Care				
Newborn Deliveries Scheduled Early[2]	58	3%	5%	6%
Preventive Care				
Immunization for Influenza[2]	503	94%	89%	90%
Immunization for Pneumonia[2]	547	93%	89%	92%
Stroke Care				
Anticoagulation Therapy for Atrial Fibrillation	16	94%	96%	95%
Antithrombotic Therapy Timing	103	97%	98%	98%
Assessed for Rehabilitation	123	97%	98%	97%
Discharged on Antithrombotic Therapy	119	100%	99%	99%
Discharged on Statin Medication	102	92%	95%	94%
Thrombolytic Therapy Timing	11	82%	74%	66%
Venous Thromboembolism Prophylaxis	115	80%	95%	94%
Written Stroke Educational Materials Given	75	76%	88%	88%
Surgical Care Improvement Project				
Appropriate Beta Blocker Usage[2]	163	98%	98%	98%
Appropriate VTP Within 24 Hours[2]	448	100%	98%	98%
Controlled Postoperative Blood Glucose[2,7]	-	-	97%	97%
Perioperative Temperature Management[2]	581	100%	99%	100%
Prophylactic Antibiotic Selection[2]	376	99%	99%	99%
Prophylactic Antibiotic Selection (Outpatient)	286	99%	98%	98%
Prophylactic Antibiotic Stopped[2]	361	99%	99%	98%
Prophylactic Antibiotic Timing[2]	376	99%	98%	99%
Prophylactic Antibiotic Timing (Outpatient)	287	100%	97%	98%
Urinary Catheter Removal[2]	273	97%	97%	97%
Survey of Patients' Hospital Experiences				
Area Around Room 'Always' Quiet at Night	300+	57%	65%	61%
Doctors 'Always' Communicated Well	300+	76%	84%	82%
Home Recovery Information Given	300+	87%	88%	85%
Hospital Given 9 or 10 on 10 Point Scale	300+	70%	74%	71%
Meds 'Always' Explained Before Given	300+	59%	67%	64%
Nurses 'Always' Communicated Well	300+	76%	81%	79%
Pain 'Always' Well Controlled	300+	67%	72%	71%
Room and Bathroom 'Always' Clean	300+	73%	78%	73%
Timely Help 'Always' Received	300+	62%	74%	68%
Would Definitely Recommend Hospital	300+	72%	71%	71%
Use of Medical Imaging				
Cardiac Imaging Stress Test before Surgery	366	4.9%	6.3%	5.3%
Combination Abdominal CT Scan	576	2.8%	5.7%	10.5%
Combination Brain/Sinus CT Scan[1]	-	-	2.3%	2.7%
Combination Chest CT Scan	313	0.0%	1.9%	2.7%
Follow-up Mammogram/Ultrasound	1,260	3.3%	6.3%	8.8%
Lumbar Spine MRI for Low Back Pain	58	32.8%	37.6%	37.2%

Avera Marshall Regional Medical Center

300 South Bruce Street
Marshall, MN 56258
Phone: 507-537-9661
Fax: 507-537-9053
E-mail: info@averamarshall.org
URL: www.averamarshall.org
Type: Critical Access Hospitals
Emergency Services: Yes
Ownership: Voluntary non-profit - Private
Beds: 49

Key Personnel:

CEO/President. . . . . M Burmam
Infection Control. . . . . Jo Coover
Operating Room. . . . . Donna Erbes
Chair/CEO . . . . James Fuhrmann
Anesthesiology. . . . . Gene Larson, CRNA
Emergency Room . . . . T Odland, MD
Cardiac Laboratory. . . . . Monica Senden
Chief of Medical Staff . . . . Joe Willett

Measure	Cases	This Hosp.	State Avg.	U.S. Avg.
Blood Clot Prevention and Treatment				
Anticoagulation Overlap Therapy[5]	-	-	96%	93%
ICU Venous Thromboembolism Prophylaxis[5]	-	-	91%	92%
Incidence of Potentially Preventable VTE[5]	-	-	9%	10%
UFH with Dosages/Platelet Monitoring[5]	-	-	98%	97%
Venous Thromboembolism Prophylaxis[5]	-	-	86%	85%
Warfarin Therapy Discharge Instructions[5]	-	-	63%	75%
Chest Pain/Possible Heart Attack Care				
Aspirin Given Within 24 Hours of Arrival	29	100%	97%	96%
Fibrinolytic Meds Within 30 Min. of Arrival[1]	-	-	48%	58%
Average Time to ECG (minutes)	29	7	7	7
Average Time to Transfer (minutes)[7]	-	-	54	60
Children's Asthma Care				
Received Home Management Plan of Care	-	-	-	88%
Received Reliever Medication	-	-	-	100%
Received Systemic Corticosteroids	-	-	-	100%
Emergency Department				
Admittance Decision Time (minutes)[2]	166	42	62	98
Head CT Results Within 45 Min. of Arrival[5]	-	-	54%	57%
Patients Who Left ER Before Being Seen[5]	-	-	2%	2%
Time from ER Arrival to Admit. (minutes)[2]	166	174	199	274
Time from ER Arrival to Discharge (minutes)[5]	-	-	125	134
Time in ER Before Being Evaluated (minutes)[5]	-	-	31	26
Time to Pain Meds for Fractures (minutes)[5]	-	-	45	57
Heart Attack Care				
Aspirin Given at Discharge[1,3]	-	-	99%	99%
Fibrinolytic Meds Within 30 Min. of Arrival[3,7]	-	-	-	54%
PCI Within 90 Minutes of Arrival[3,7]	-	-	96%	96%
Statin Prescribed at Discharge[1,3]	-	-	99%	98%
Heart Failure Care				
ACE Inhibitor or ARB for LVSD[1]	-	-	96%	97%
Discharge Instructions Given	14	93%	93%	94%
Evaluation of LVS Function	19	100%	97%	99%
Medicare Spending				
Medicare Spending per Patient (ratio)	-	-	0.9	0.98
Pneumonia Care				
Appropriate Initial Antibiotic Given	26	100%	94%	95%
Blood Culture Timing	35	100%	97%	98%
Pregnancy and Delivery Care				
Newborn Deliveries Scheduled Early[5]	-	-	5%	6%
Preventive Care				
Immunization for Influenza[2]	236	99%	89%	90%
Immunization for Pneumonia[2]	211	94%	89%	92%
Stroke Care				
Anticoagulation Therapy for Atrial Fibrillation[5]	-	-	96%	95%
Antithrombotic Therapy Timing[5]	-	-	98%	98%
Assessed for Rehabilitation[5]	-	-	98%	97%
Discharged on Antithrombotic Therapy[5]	-	-	99%	99%
Discharged on Statin Medication[5]	-	-	95%	94%
Thrombolytic Therapy Timing[5]	-	-	74%	66%
Venous Thromboembolism Prophylaxis[5]	-	-	95%	94%
Written Stroke Educational Materials Given[5]	-	-	88%	88%
Surgical Care Improvement Project				
Appropriate Beta Blocker Usage	32	100%	98%	98%
Appropriate VTP Within 24 Hours	113	100%	98%	98%
Controlled Postoperative Blood Glucose[3,7]	-	-	97%	97%
Perioperative Temperature Management	137	99%	99%	100%

NOTE: Hospital profiles are in alphabetical order by state, then city, then hospital within the city; Rankings exclude hospitals with less than 25 cases except for patient surveys which excludes hospitals with less than 100 cases; (a) 100-299 cases; (1) The number of cases/patients is too few to report; (2) Data submitted were based on a sample of cases/patients; (3) Results are based on a shorter time period than required; (4) Data suppressed by CMS for one or more quarters; (5) Results are not available for this reporting period; (6) Fewer than 100 patients completed the HCAHPS survey; (7) No cases met the criteria for this measure; (8) The lower limit of the confidence interval cannot be calculated if the number of observed infections equals zero; (9) No data are available from the state/territory for this reporting period; (10) The scores shown reflect fewer than 50 completed surveys; (11) There were discrepancies in the data collection process; (12) This measure does not apply to this hospital for this reporting period; (13) Results cannot be calculated for this reporting period; (14) The results for this state are combined with nearby states to protect confidentiality; Please refer to the User's Guide for a full explanation of data.

Measure	Cases	This Hosp.	State Avg.	U.S. Avg.
Prophylactic Antibiotic Selection	115	99%	99%	99%
Prophylactic Antibiotic Selection (Outpatient)	16	100%	98%	98%
Prophylactic Antibiotic Stopped	113	99%	99%	98%
Prophylactic Antibiotic Timing	115	99%	98%	99%
Prophylactic Antibiotic Timing (Outpatient)	16	100%	97%	98%
Urinary Catheter Removal	80	98%	97%	97%
Survey of Patients' Hospital Experiences				
Area Around Room 'Always' Quiet at Night	300+	58%	65%	61%
Doctors 'Always' Communicated Well	300+	83%	84%	82%
Home Recovery Information Given	300+	90%	88%	85%
Hospital Given 9 or 10 on 10 Point Scale	300+	71%	74%	71%
Meds 'Always' Explained Before Given	300+	64%	67%	64%
Nurses 'Always' Communicated Well	300+	80%	81%	79%
Pain 'Always' Well Controlled	300+	68%	72%	71%
Room and Bathroom 'Always' Clean	300+	75%	78%	73%
Timely Help 'Always' Received	300+	63%	74%	68%
Would Definitely Recommend Hospital	300+	73%	71%	71%
Use of Medical Imaging				
Cardiac Imaging Stress Test before Surgery[1]	-	-	6.3%	5.3%
Combination Abdominal CT Scan	152	2.0%	5.7%	10.5%
Combination Brain/Sinus CT Scan[1]	-	-	2.3%	2.7%
Combination Chest CT Scan	78	2.6%	1.9%	2.7%
Follow-up Mammogram/Ultrasound	100	7.0%	6.3%	8.8%
Lumbar Spine MRI for Low Back Pain[1]	-	-	37.6%	37.2%

Centracare Health System - Melrose Hospital

525 West Main Street — Phone: 320-256-4231
Melrose, MN 56352 — Fax: 320-256-4949
E-mail: melrosehospital@centracare.com
URL: www.centracare.com/melrose
Type: Critical Access Hospitals — Emergency Services: Yes
Ownership: Voluntary non-profit - Private — Beds: 28

Key Personnel:
Chief of Medical Staff . . . . Darte C Beretta, MD
CEO/President . . . . Gerry Gilbertson, CEO
Ambulatory Care . . . . Keri Wimmer, RN

Measure	Cases	This Hosp.	State Avg.	U.S. Avg.
Blood Clot Prevention and Treatment				
Anticoagulation Overlap Therapy[5]	-	-	96%	93%
ICU Venous Thromboembolism Prophylaxis[5]	-	-	91%	92%
Incidence of Potentially Preventable VTE[5]	-	-	9%	10%
UFH with Dosages/Platelet Monitoring[5]	-	-	98%	97%
Venous Thromboembolism Prophylaxis[5]	-	-	86%	85%
Warfarin Therapy Discharge Instructions[5]	-	-	63%	75%
Chest Pain/Possible Heart Attack Care				
Aspirin Given Within 24 Hours of Arrival[1,3]	-	-	97%	96%
Fibrinolytic Meds Within 30 Min. of Arrival[3,7]	-	-	48%	58%
Average Time to ECG (minutes)[1,3]	-	-	7	7
Average Time to Transfer (minutes)[1,3]	-	-	54	60
Children's Asthma Care				
Received Home Management Plan of Care	-	-	-	88%
Received Reliever Medication	-	-	-	100%
Received Systemic Corticosteroids	-	-	-	100%
Emergency Department				
Admittance Decision Time (minutes)[2]	215	0	62	98
Head CT Results Within 45 Min. of Arrival[1,3]	-	-	54%	57%
Patients Who Left ER Before Being Seen[5]	-	-	2%	2%
Time from ER Arrival to Admit. (minutes)[2]	215	115	199	274
Time from ER Arrival to Discharge (minutes)[5]	-	-	125	134
Time in ER Before Being Evaluated (minutes)[5]	-	-	31	26
Time to Pain Meds for Fractures (minutes)[5]	-	-	45	57
Heart Attack Care				
Aspirin Given at Discharge[3,7]	-	-	99%	99%
Fibrinolytic Meds Within 30 Min. of Arrival[3,7]	-	-	-	54%
PCI Within 90 Minutes of Arrival[3,7]	-	-	96%	96%
Statin Prescribed at Discharge[3,7]	-	-	99%	98%
Heart Failure Care				
ACE Inhibitor or ARB for LVSD[1,2]	-	-	96%	97%
Discharge Instructions Given[1,2]	-	-	93%	94%
Evaluation of LVS Function[2]	17	88%	97%	99%
Medicare Spending				
Medicare Spending per Patient (ratio)	-	-	0.9	0.98
Pneumonia Care				
Appropriate Initial Antibiotic Given	14	93%	94%	95%
Blood Culture Timing	14	86%	97%	98%
Pregnancy and Delivery Care				
Newborn Deliveries Scheduled Early[5]	-	-	5%	6%
Preventive Care				
Immunization for Influenza	269	88%	89%	90%
Immunization for Pneumonia	265	92%	89%	92%
Stroke Care				
Anticoagulation Therapy for Atrial Fibrillation[5]	-	-	96%	95%
Antithrombotic Therapy Timing[5]	-	-	98%	98%
Assessed for Rehabilitation[5]	-	-	98%	97%
Discharged on Antithrombotic Therapy[5]	-	-	99%	99%
Discharged on Statin Medication[5]	-	-	95%	94%
Thrombolytic Therapy Timing[5]	-	-	74%	66%
Venous Thromboembolism Prophylaxis[5]	-	-	95%	94%
Written Stroke Educational Materials Given[5]	-	-	88%	88%
Surgical Care Improvement Project				
Appropriate Beta Blocker Usage[1,3]	-	-	98%	98%
Appropriate VTP Within 24 Hours[1,3]	-	-	98%	98%
Controlled Postoperative Blood Glucose[3,7]	-	-	97%	97%
Perioperative Temperature Management[1,3]	-	-	99%	100%
Prophylactic Antibiotic Selection[1,3]	-	-	99%	99%
Prophylactic Antibiotic Selection (Outpatient)	15	100%	98%	98%
Prophylactic Antibiotic Stopped[1,3]	-	-	99%	98%
Prophylactic Antibiotic Timing[1,3]	-	-	98%	99%
Prophylactic Antibiotic Timing (Outpatient)	11	100%	97%	98%
Urinary Catheter Removal[1,3]	-	-	97%	97%
Survey of Patients' Hospital Experiences				
Area Around Room 'Always' Quiet at Night[5]	-	-	65%	61%
Doctors 'Always' Communicated Well[5]	-	-	84%	82%
Home Recovery Information Given[5]	-	-	88%	85%
Hospital Given 9 or 10 on 10 Point Scale[5]	-	-	74%	71%
Meds 'Always' Explained Before Given[5]	-	-	67%	64%
Nurses 'Always' Communicated Well[5]	-	-	81%	79%
Pain 'Always' Well Controlled[5]	-	-	72%	71%
Room and Bathroom 'Always' Clean[5]	-	-	78%	73%
Timely Help 'Always' Received[5]	-	-	74%	68%
Would Definitely Recommend Hospital[5]	-	-	71%	71%
Use of Medical Imaging				
Cardiac Imaging Stress Test before Surgery[1]	-	-	6.3%	5.3%
Combination Abdominal CT Scan[1]	-	-	5.7%	10.5%
Combination Brain/Sinus CT Scan	33	0.0%	2.3%	2.7%
Combination Chest CT Scan[1]	-	-	1.9%	2.7%
Follow-up Mammogram/Ultrasound	119	10.1%	6.3%	8.8%
Lumbar Spine MRI for Low Back Pain[1]	-	-	37.6%	37.2%

Abbott Northwestern Hospital

800 East 28th Street — Phone: 612-863-4509
Minneapolis, MN 55407 — Fax: 612-863-5667
URL: www.abbottnorthwestern.com
Type: Acute Care Hospitals — Emergency Services: Yes
Ownership: Voluntary non-profit - Private — Beds: 926

Key Personnel:
President . . . . Ben Bache-Wiig, MD
Cardiac Laboratory . . . . Robert Hauser, MD
Surgery . . . . Dawn Johnson, MD
Operating Room . . . . Mark Migliori, MD
Anesthesiology . . . . John Mrachek, MD
CEO . . . . Kenneth H. Paulus
Radiology . . . . Lisa Schneider, MD
Chief of Medical Staff . . . . Michael Tedford, MD

Measure	Cases	This Hosp.	State Avg.	U.S. Avg.
Blood Clot Prevention and Treatment				
Anticoagulation Overlap Therapy[2]	221	99%	96%	93%
ICU Venous Thromboembolism Prophylaxis[2]	80	92%	91%	92%
Incidence of Potentially Preventable VTE[2]	38	13%	9%	10%
UFH with Dosages/Platelet Monitoring[2]	217	100%	98%	97%
Venous Thromboembolism Prophylaxis[2]	258	86%	86%	85%
Warfarin Therapy Discharge Instructions[2]	165	11%	63%	75%
Chest Pain/Possible Heart Attack Care				
Aspirin Given Within 24 Hours of Arrival	12	92%	97%	96%
Fibrinolytic Meds Within 30 Min. of Arrival[3,7]	-	-	48%	58%
Average Time to ECG (minutes)	13	6	7	7
Average Time to Transfer (minutes)[1,3]	-	-	54	60
Children's Asthma Care				
Received Home Management Plan of Care	-	-	-	88%
Received Reliever Medication	-	-	-	100%
Received Systemic Corticosteroids	-	-	-	100%
Emergency Department				
Admittance Decision Time (minutes)[2]	315	134	62	98
Head CT Results Within 45 Min. of Arrival[7]	-	-	54%	57%
Patients Who Left ER Before Being Seen	49,073	2%	2%	2%
Time from ER Arrival to Admit. (minutes)[2]	318	248	199	274
Time from ER Arrival to Discharge (minutes)	423	171	125	134
Time in ER Before Being Evaluated (minutes)	490	22	31	26
Time to Pain Meds for Fractures (minutes)	81	46	45	57
Heart Attack Care				
Aspirin Given at Discharge	904	100%	99%	99%
Fibrinolytic Meds Within 30 Min. of Arrival[7]	-	-	-	54%
PCI Within 90 Minutes of Arrival	50	96%	96%	96%
Statin Prescribed at Discharge	868	100%	99%	98%
Heart Failure Care				
ACE Inhibitor or ARB for LVSD	234	93%	96%	97%
Discharge Instructions Given	609	99%	93%	94%
Evaluation of LVS Function	752	100%	97%	99%
Medicare Spending				
Medicare Spending per Patient (ratio)	-	0.93	0.9	0.98
Pneumonia Care				
Appropriate Initial Antibiotic Given	133	97%	94%	95%
Blood Culture Timing	230	98%	97%	98%
Pregnancy and Delivery Care				
Newborn Deliveries Scheduled Early[2]	64	0%	5%	6%
Preventive Care				
Immunization for Influenza[2]	566	95%	89%	90%
Immunization for Pneumonia[2]	615	93%	89%	92%
Stroke Care				
Anticoagulation Therapy for Atrial Fibrillation	91	97%	96%	95%
Antithrombotic Therapy Timing	242	98%	98%	98%
Assessed for Rehabilitation	425	99%	98%	97%
Discharged on Antithrombotic Therapy	344	100%	99%	99%
Discharged on Statin Medication	278	99%	95%	94%
Thrombolytic Therapy Timing	28	86%	74%	66%
Venous Thromboembolism Prophylaxis	419	95%	95%	94%
Written Stroke Educational Materials Given	239	99%	88%	88%
Surgical Care Improvement Project				
Appropriate Beta Blocker Usage[2]	266	100%	98%	98%
Appropriate VTP Within 24 Hours[2]	467	100%	98%	98%
Controlled Postoperative Blood Glucose[2]	137	96%	97%	97%
Perioperative Temperature Management[2]	632	100%	99%	100%
Prophylactic Antibiotic Selection[2]	492	100%	99%	99%
Prophylactic Antibiotic Selection (Outpatient)	685	99%	98%	98%
Prophylactic Antibiotic Stopped[2]	472	99%	99%	98%
Prophylactic Antibiotic Timing[2]	493	99%	98%	99%
Prophylactic Antibiotic Timing (Outpatient)	686	99%	97%	98%
Urinary Catheter Removal[2]	458	97%	97%	97%
Survey of Patients' Hospital Experiences				
Area Around Room 'Always' Quiet at Night	300+	53%	65%	61%
Doctors 'Always' Communicated Well	300+	80%	84%	82%
Home Recovery Information Given	300+	88%	88%	85%
Hospital Given 9 or 10 on 10 Point Scale	300+	74%	74%	71%
Meds 'Always' Explained Before Given	300+	61%	67%	64%
Nurses 'Always' Communicated Well	300+	76%	81%	79%
Pain 'Always' Well Controlled	300+	69%	72%	71%
Room and Bathroom 'Always' Clean	300+	70%	78%	73%
Timely Help 'Always' Received	300+	65%	74%	68%
Would Definitely Recommend Hospital	300+	79%	71%	71%
Use of Medical Imaging				
Cardiac Imaging Stress Test before Surgery	335	3.6%	6.3%	5.3%
Combination Abdominal CT Scan	1,110	5.3%	5.7%	10.5%
Combination Brain/Sinus CT Scan	465	4.1%	2.3%	2.7%
Combination Chest CT Scan	1,100	0.3%	1.9%	2.7%
Follow-up Mammogram/Ultrasound	1,576	6.9%	6.3%	8.8%
Lumbar Spine MRI for Low Back Pain	123	40.7%	37.6%	37.2%

NOTE: Hospital profiles are in alphabetical order by state, then city, then hospital within the city; Rankings exclude hospitals with less than 25 cases except for patient surveys which excludes hospitals with less than 100 cases; (a) 100-299 cases; (1) The number of cases/patients is too few to report; (2) Data submitted were based on a sample of cases/patients; (3) Results are based on a shorter time period than required; (4) Data suppressed by CMS for one or more quarters; (5) Results are not available for this reporting period; (6) Fewer than 100 patients completed the HCAHPS survey; (7) No cases met the criteria for this measure; (8) The lower limit of the confidence interval cannot be calculated if the number of observed infections equals zero; (9) No data are available from the state/territory for this reporting period; (10) The scores shown reflect fewer than 50 completed surveys; (11) There were discrepancies in the data collection process; (12) This measure does not apply to this hospital for this reporting period; (13) Results cannot be calculated for this reporting period; (14) The results for this state are combined with nearby states to protect confidentiality; Please refer to the User's Guide for a full explanation of data.

Children's Hospitals & Clinics of Minnesota

2525 Chicago Avenue South Phone: 612-813-6112
Minneapolis, MN 55404
URL: www.childrensmn.org
Type: Childrens Emergency Services: Yes
Ownership: Voluntary non-profit - Private Beds: 340

Key Personnel:
Chair/CEO . . . . Russ Becker
President/CEO. . . . . Alan L Goldbloom, MD
Chief of Medical Staff. . . . . Phillip Kibort, MD, MBA

Measure	Cases	This Hosp.	State Avg.	U.S. Avg.
Blood Clot Prevention and Treatment				
Anticoagulation Overlap Therapy[5]	-	-	96%	93%
ICU Venous Thromboembolism Prophylaxis[5]	-	-	91%	92%
Incidence of Potentially Preventable VTE[5]	-	-	9%	10%
UFH with Dosages/Platelet Monitoring[5]	-	-	98%	97%
Venous Thromboembolism Prophylaxis[5]	-	-	86%	85%
Warfarin Therapy Discharge Instructions[5]	-	-	63%	75%
Chest Pain/Possible Heart Attack Care				
Aspirin Given Within 24 Hours of Arrival	-	-	97%	96%
Fibrinolytic Meds Within 30 Min. of Arrival	-	-	48%	58%
Average Time to ECG (minutes)	-	-	7	7
Average Time to Transfer (minutes)	-	-	54	60
Children's Asthma Care				
Received Home Management Plan of Care[2]	285	84%	-	88%
Received Reliever Medication[2]	285	100%	-	100%
Received Systemic Corticosteroids[2]	285	100%	-	100%
Emergency Department				
Admittance Decision Time (minutes)[5]	-	-	62	98
Head CT Results Within 45 Min. of Arrival	-	-	54%	57%
Patients Who Left ER Before Being Seen	-	-	2%	2%
Time from ER Arrival to Admit. (minutes)[5]	-	-	199	274
Time from ER Arrival to Discharge (minutes)	-	-	125	134
Time in ER Before Being Evaluated (minutes)	-	-	31	26
Time to Pain Meds for Fractures (minutes)	-	-	45	57
Heart Attack Care				
Aspirin Given at Discharge[5]	-	-	99%	99%
Fibrinolytic Meds Within 30 Min. of Arrival[5]	-	-	-	54%
PCI Within 90 Minutes of Arrival[5]	-	-	96%	96%
Statin Prescribed at Discharge[5]	-	-	99%	98%
Heart Failure Care				
ACE Inhibitor or ARB for LVSD[5]	-	-	96%	97%
Discharge Instructions Given[5]	-	-	93%	94%
Evaluation of LVS Function[5]	-	-	97%	99%
Medicare Spending				
Medicare Spending per Patient (ratio)	-	-	0.9	0.98
Pneumonia Care				
Appropriate Initial Antibiotic Given[5]	-	-	94%	95%
Blood Culture Timing[5]	-	-	97%	98%
Pregnancy and Delivery Care				
Newborn Deliveries Scheduled Early[5]	-	-	5%	6%
Preventive Care				
Immunization for Influenza[5]	-	-	89%	90%
Immunization for Pneumonia[5]	-	-	89%	92%
Stroke Care				
Anticoagulation Therapy for Atrial Fibrillation[5]	-	-	96%	95%
Antithrombotic Therapy Timing[5]	-	-	98%	98%
Assessed for Rehabilitation[5]	-	-	98%	97%
Discharged on Antithrombotic Therapy[5]	-	-	99%	99%
Discharged on Statin Medication[5]	-	-	95%	94%
Thrombolytic Therapy Timing[5]	-	-	74%	66%
Venous Thromboembolism Prophylaxis[5]	-	-	95%	94%
Written Stroke Educational Materials Given[5]	-	-	88%	88%
Surgical Care Improvement Project				
Appropriate Beta Blocker Usage[5]	-	-	98%	98%
Appropriate VTP Within 24 Hours[5]	-	-	98%	98%
Controlled Postoperative Blood Glucose[5]	-	-	97%	97%
Perioperative Temperature Management[5]	-	-	99%	100%
Prophylactic Antibiotic Selection[5]	-	-	99%	99%
Prophylactic Antibiotic Selection (Outpatient)	-	-	98%	98%
Prophylactic Antibiotic Stopped[5]	-	-	99%	98%
Prophylactic Antibiotic Timing[5]	-	-	98%	99%
Prophylactic Antibiotic Timing (Outpatient)	-	-	97%	98%
Urinary Catheter Removal[5]	-	-	97%	97%
Survey of Patients' Hospital Experiences				
Area Around Room 'Always' Quiet at Night[5]	-	-	65%	61%
Doctors 'Always' Communicated Well[5]	-	-	84%	82%
Home Recovery Information Given[5]	-	-	88%	85%
Hospital Given 9 or 10 on 10 Point Scale[5]	-	-	74%	71%
Meds 'Always' Explained Before Given[5]	-	-	67%	64%
Nurses 'Always' Communicated Well[5]	-	-	81%	79%
Pain 'Always' Well Controlled[5]	-	-	72%	71%
Room and Bathroom 'Always' Clean[5]	-	-	78%	73%
Timely Help 'Always' Received[5]	-	-	74%	68%
Would Definitely Recommend Hospital[5]	-	-	71%	71%
Use of Medical Imaging				
Cardiac Imaging Stress Test before Surgery	-	-	6.3%	5.3%
Combination Abdominal CT Scan	-	-	5.7%	10.5%
Combination Brain/Sinus CT Scan	-	-	2.3%	2.7%
Combination Chest CT Scan	-	-	1.9%	2.7%
Follow-up Mammogram/Ultrasound	-	-	6.3%	8.8%
Lumbar Spine MRI for Low Back Pain	-	-	37.6%	37.2%

Hennepin County Medical Center

701 Park Avenue Phone: 612-873-3000
Minneapolis, MN 55415 Fax: 612-904-4214
URL: www.hcmc.org
Type: Acute Care Hospitals Emergency Services: Yes
Ownership: Government - Local Beds: 910

Key Personnel:
CEO/President. . . . . Lynn Abrahamsen MHA
Chief of Medical Staff . . . . Michael B Belzer, MD
Chair/CEO . . . . Mike Opat
CEO . . . . Jon L. Pryor, MD, MBA

Measure	Cases	This Hosp.	State Avg.	U.S. Avg.
Blood Clot Prevention and Treatment				
Anticoagulation Overlap Therapy[2]	88	94%	96%	93%
ICU Venous Thromboembolism Prophylaxis[2]	73	90%	91%	92%
Incidence of Potentially Preventable VTE[2]	25	8%	9%	10%
UFH with Dosages/Platelet Monitoring[2]	64	97%	98%	97%
Venous Thromboembolism Prophylaxis[2]	311	74%	86%	85%
Warfarin Therapy Discharge Instructions[2]	58	28%	63%	75%
Chest Pain/Possible Heart Attack Care				
Aspirin Given Within 24 Hours of Arrival[5]	-	-	97%	96%
Fibrinolytic Meds Within 30 Min. of Arrival[5]	-	-	48%	58%
Average Time to ECG (minutes)[5]	-	-	7	7
Average Time to Transfer (minutes)[5]	-	-	54	60
Children's Asthma Care				
Received Home Management Plan of Care[2]	39	95%	-	88%
Received Reliever Medication	39	100%	-	100%
Received Systemic Corticosteroids	39	100%	-	100%
Emergency Department				
Admittance Decision Time (minutes)[2]	468	196	62	98
Head CT Results Within 45 Min. of Arrival[3,7]	-	-	54%	57%
Patients Who Left ER Before Being Seen	>100k	6%	2%	2%
Time from ER Arrival to Admit. (minutes)[2]	469	282	199	274
Time from ER Arrival to Discharge (minutes)	338	230	125	134
Time in ER Before Being Evaluated (minutes)	337	26	31	26
Time to Pain Meds for Fractures (minutes)	95	43	45	57
Heart Attack Care				
Aspirin Given at Discharge	152	100%	99%	99%
Fibrinolytic Meds Within 30 Min. of Arrival[7]	-	-	-	54%
PCI Within 90 Minutes of Arrival	38	92%	96%	96%
Statin Prescribed at Discharge	149	100%	99%	98%
Heart Failure Care				
ACE Inhibitor or ARB for LVSD[2]	111	99%	96%	97%
Discharge Instructions Given[2]	235	95%	93%	94%
Evaluation of LVS Function[2]	278	100%	97%	99%
Medicare Spending				
Medicare Spending per Patient (ratio)	-	0.92	0.9	0.98
Pneumonia Care				
Appropriate Initial Antibiotic Given[2]	49	98%	94%	95%
Blood Culture Timing[2]	54	100%	97%	98%
Pregnancy and Delivery Care				
Newborn Deliveries Scheduled Early	59	0%	5%	6%
Preventive Care				
Immunization for Influenza[2]	506	84%	89%	90%
Immunization for Pneumonia[2]	483	89%	89%	92%
Stroke Care				
Anticoagulation Therapy for Atrial Fibrillation[1,2]	-	-	96%	95%
Antithrombotic Therapy Timing[2]	63	94%	98%	98%
Assessed for Rehabilitation[2]	105	100%	98%	97%
Discharged on Antithrombotic Therapy[2]	79	100%	99%	99%
Discharged on Statin Medication[2]	52	94%	95%	94%
Thrombolytic Therapy Timing[2]	11	91%	74%	66%
Venous Thromboembolism Prophylaxis[2]	117	88%	95%	94%
Written Stroke Educational Materials Given[2]	48	96%	88%	88%
Surgical Care Improvement Project				
Appropriate Beta Blocker Usage[2]	86	100%	98%	98%
Appropriate VTP Within 24 Hours[2]	258	100%	98%	98%
Controlled Postoperative Blood Glucose[2]	44	100%	97%	97%
Perioperative Temperature Management[2]	321	99%	99%	100%
Prophylactic Antibiotic Selection[2]	233	100%	99%	99%
Prophylactic Antibiotic Selection (Outpatient)	167	99%	98%	98%
Prophylactic Antibiotic Stopped[2]	225	99%	99%	98%
Prophylactic Antibiotic Timing[2]	234	100%	98%	99%
Prophylactic Antibiotic Timing (Outpatient)	125	94%	97%	98%
Urinary Catheter Removal[2]	207	100%	97%	97%
Survey of Patients' Hospital Experiences				
Area Around Room 'Always' Quiet at Night	300+	55%	65%	61%
Doctors 'Always' Communicated Well	300+	73%	84%	82%
Home Recovery Information Given	300+	83%	88%	85%
Hospital Given 9 or 10 on 10 Point Scale	300+	59%	74%	71%
Meds 'Always' Explained Before Given	300+	52%	67%	64%
Nurses 'Always' Communicated Well	300+	69%	81%	79%
Pain 'Always' Well Controlled	300+	62%	72%	71%
Room and Bathroom 'Always' Clean	300+	63%	78%	73%
Timely Help 'Always' Received	300+	52%	74%	68%
Would Definitely Recommend Hospital	300+	64%	71%	71%
Use of Medical Imaging				
Cardiac Imaging Stress Test before Surgery	237	8.0%	6.3%	5.3%
Combination Abdominal CT Scan	427	5.4%	5.7%	10.5%
Combination Brain/Sinus CT Scan	378	0.8%	2.3%	2.7%
Combination Chest CT Scan	409	0.2%	1.9%	2.7%
Follow-up Mammogram/Ultrasound	596	4.2%	6.3%	8.8%
Lumbar Spine MRI for Low Back Pain[1]	-	-	37.6%	37.2%

Minneapolis VA Medical Center

One Veterans Drive Phone: 612-725-2000
Minneapolis, MN 55417 Fax: 612-725-2049
URL: www1.va.gov/minneapolis
Type: Acute Care - VA Emergency Services: No
Ownership: Government Federal Beds: 341

Key Personnel:
Radiology. . . . . Howard Ansel, MD
Emergency Room . . . . Dale Berg, MD
Anesthesiology. . . . . Shep Cohen, MD
Chief of Medical Staff . . . . Kent Crossley, MD, MHA
Quality Assurance . . . . Linda Duffy
Hemotology Center . . . . Sharon Luikart, MD
Infection Control. . . . . Joseph Thurn, MD

Measure	Cases	This Hosp.	State Avg.	U.S. Avg.
Blood Clot Prevention and Treatment				
Anticoagulation Overlap Therapy	-	-	96%	93%
ICU Venous Thromboembolism Prophylaxis	-	-	91%	92%
Incidence of Potentially Preventable VTE	-	-	9%	10%
UFH with Dosages/Platelet Monitoring	-	-	98%	97%
Venous Thromboembolism Prophylaxis	-	-	86%	85%
Warfarin Therapy Discharge Instructions	-	-	63%	75%
Chest Pain/Possible Heart Attack Care				
Aspirin Given Within 24 Hours of Arrival	-	-	97%	96%
Fibrinolytic Meds Within 30 Min. of Arrival	-	-	48%	58%
Average Time to ECG (minutes)	-	-	7	7
Average Time to Transfer (minutes)	-	-	54	60
Children's Asthma Care				
Received Home Management Plan of Care	-	-	-	88%
Received Reliever Medication	-	-	-	100%
Received Systemic Corticosteroids	-	-	-	100%
Emergency Department				
Admittance Decision Time (minutes)	-	-	62	98

NOTE: Hospital profiles are in alphabetical order by state, then city, then hospital within the city; Rankings exclude hospitals with less than 25 cases except for patient surveys which excludes hospitals with less than 100 cases; (a) 100-299 cases; (1) The number of cases/patients is too few to report; (2) Data submitted were based on a sample of cases/patients; (3) Results are based on a shorter time period than required; (4) Data suppressed by CMS for one or more quarters; (5) Results are not available for this reporting period; (6) Fewer than 100 patients completed the HCAHPS survey; (7) No cases met the criteria for this measure; (8) The lower limit of the confidence interval cannot be calculated if the number of observed infections equals zero; (9) No data are available from the state/territory for this reporting period; (10) The scores shown reflect fewer than 50 completed surveys; (11) There were discrepancies in the data collection process; (12) This measure does not apply to this hospital for this reporting period; (13) Results cannot be calculated for this reporting period; (14) The results for this state are combined with nearby states to protect confidentiality; Please refer to the User's Guide for a full explanation of data.

Measure	Cases	This Hosp.	State Avg.	U.S. Avg.
Head CT Results Within 45 Min. of Arrival	-	-	54%	57%
Patients Who Left ER Before Being Seen	-	-	2%	2%
Time from ER Arrival to Admit. (minutes)	-	-	199	274
Time from ER Arrival to Discharge (minutes)	-	-	125	134
Time in ER Before Being Evaluated (minutes)	-	-	31	26
Time to Pain Meds for Fractures (minutes)	-	-	45	57
Heart Attack Care				
Aspirin Given at Discharge	107	100%	99%	99%
Fibrinolytic Meds Within 30 Min. of Arrival[5]	-	-	-	54%
PCI Within 90 Minutes of Arrival[1]	11	73%	96%	96%
Statin Prescribed at Discharge	109	99%	99%	98%
Heart Failure Care				
ACE Inhibitor or ARB for LVSD	63	98%	96%	97%
Discharge Instructions Given	185	97%	93%	94%
Evaluation of LVS Function	227	100%	97%	99%
Medicare Spending				
Medicare Spending per Patient (ratio)	-	-	0.9	0.98
Pneumonia Care				
Appropriate Initial Antibiotic Given	40	98%	94%	95%
Blood Culture Timing	119	99%	97%	98%
Pregnancy and Delivery Care				
Newborn Deliveries Scheduled Early	-	-	5%	6%
Preventive Care				
Immunization for Influenza[5]	-	-	89%	90%
Immunization for Pneumonia[5]	-	-	89%	92%
Stroke Care				
Anticoagulation Therapy for Atrial Fibrillation	-	-	96%	95%
Antithrombotic Therapy Timing	-	-	98%	98%
Assessed for Rehabilitation	-	-	98%	97%
Discharged on Antithrombotic Therapy	-	-	99%	99%
Discharged on Statin Medication	-	-	95%	94%
Thrombolytic Therapy Timing	-	-	74%	66%
Venous Thromboembolism Prophylaxis	-	-	95%	94%
Written Stroke Educational Materials Given	-	-	88%	88%
Surgical Care Improvement Project				
Appropriate Beta Blocker Usage[2]	256	99%	98%	98%
Appropriate VTP Within 24 Hours[2]	306	100%	98%	98%
Controlled Postoperative Blood Glucose[2]	189	96%	97%	97%
Perioperative Temperature Management[2]	371	98%	99%	100%
Prophylactic Antibiotic Selection	401	99%	99%	99%
Prophylactic Antibiotic Selection (Outpatient)	-	-	98%	98%
Prophylactic Antibiotic Stopped	398	99%	99%	98%
Prophylactic Antibiotic Timing	401	99%	98%	99%
Prophylactic Antibiotic Timing (Outpatient)	-	-	97%	98%
Urinary Catheter Removal[2]	243	100%	97%	97%
Survey of Patients' Hospital Experiences				
Area Around Room 'Always' Quiet at Night	-	-	65%	61%
Doctors 'Always' Communicated Well	-	-	84%	82%
Home Recovery Information Given	-	-	88%	85%
Hospital Given 9 or 10 on 10 Point Scale	-	-	74%	71%
Meds 'Always' Explained Before Given	-	-	67%	64%
Nurses 'Always' Communicated Well	-	-	81%	79%
Pain 'Always' Well Controlled	-	-	72%	71%
Room and Bathroom 'Always' Clean	-	-	78%	73%
Timely Help 'Always' Received	-	-	74%	68%
Would Definitely Recommend Hospital	-	-	71%	71%
Use of Medical Imaging				
Cardiac Imaging Stress Test before Surgery	-	-	6.3%	5.3%
Combination Abdominal CT Scan	-	-	5.7%	10.5%
Combination Brain/Sinus CT Scan	-	-	2.3%	2.7%
Combination Chest CT Scan	-	-	1.9%	2.7%
Follow-up Mammogram/Ultrasound	-	-	6.3%	8.8%
Lumbar Spine MRI for Low Back Pain	-	-	37.6%	37.2%

Phillips Eye Institute

2215 Park Avenue South
Minneapolis, MN 55404
Phone: 612-775-8815
URL: www.allina.com/ahs/pei.nsf
Type: Acute Care Hospitals
Emergency Services: No
Ownership: Government - Federal

Measure	Cases	This Hosp.	State Avg.	U.S. Avg.
Blood Clot Prevention and Treatment				
Anticoagulation Overlap Therapy[7]	-	-	96%	93%
ICU Venous Thromboembolism Prophylaxis[7]	-	-	91%	92%
Incidence of Potentially Preventable VTE[7]	-	-	9%	10%
UFH with Dosages/Platelet Monitoring[7]	-	-	98%	97%
Venous Thromboembolism Prophylaxis[1]	-	-	86%	85%
Warfarin Therapy Discharge Instructions[7]	-	-	63%	75%
Chest Pain/Possible Heart Attack Care				
Aspirin Given Within 24 Hours of Arrival[5]	-	-	97%	96%
Fibrinolytic Meds Within 30 Min. of Arrival[5]	-	-	48%	58%
Average Time to ECG (minutes)[5]	-	-	7	7
Average Time to Transfer (minutes)[5]	-	-	54	60
Children's Asthma Care				
Received Home Management Plan of Care	-	-	-	88%
Received Reliever Medication	-	-	-	100%
Received Systemic Corticosteroids	-	-	-	100%
Emergency Department				
Admittance Decision Time (minutes)[7]	-	-	62	98
Head CT Results Within 45 Min. of Arrival[5]	-	-	54%	57%
Patients Who Left ER Before Being Seen[5]	-	-	2%	2%
Time from ER Arrival to Admit. (minutes)[7]	-	-	199	274
Time from ER Arrival to Discharge (minutes)[5]	-	-	125	134
Time in ER Before Being Evaluated (minutes)[5]	-	-	31	26
Time to Pain Meds for Fractures (minutes)[5]	-	-	45	57
Heart Attack Care				
Aspirin Given at Discharge[5]	-	-	99%	99%
Fibrinolytic Meds Within 30 Min. of Arrival[5]	-	-	-	54%
PCI Within 90 Minutes of Arrival[5]	-	-	96%	96%
Statin Prescribed at Discharge[5]	-	-	99%	98%
Heart Failure Care				
ACE Inhibitor or ARB for LVSD[5]	-	-	96%	97%
Discharge Instructions Given[5]	-	-	93%	94%
Evaluation of LVS Function[5]	-	-	97%	99%
Medicare Spending				
Medicare Spending per Patient (ratio)	-	0.77	0.9	0.98
Pneumonia Care				
Appropriate Initial Antibiotic Given[5]	-	-	94%	95%
Blood Culture Timing[5]	-	-	97%	98%
Pregnancy and Delivery Care				
Newborn Deliveries Scheduled Early[7]	-	-	5%	6%
Preventive Care				
Immunization for Influenza	55	95%	89%	90%
Immunization for Pneumonia	87	97%	89%	92%
Stroke Care				
Anticoagulation Therapy for Atrial Fibrillation[5]	-	-	96%	95%
Antithrombotic Therapy Timing[5]	-	-	98%	98%
Assessed for Rehabilitation[5]	-	-	98%	97%
Discharged on Antithrombotic Therapy[5]	-	-	99%	99%
Discharged on Statin Medication[5]	-	-	95%	94%
Thrombolytic Therapy Timing[5]	-	-	74%	66%
Venous Thromboembolism Prophylaxis[5]	-	-	95%	94%
Written Stroke Educational Materials Given[5]	-	-	88%	88%
Surgical Care Improvement Project				
Appropriate Beta Blocker Usage[5]	-	-	98%	98%
Appropriate VTP Within 24 Hours[5]	-	-	98%	98%
Controlled Postoperative Blood Glucose[5]	-	-	97%	97%
Perioperative Temperature Management[5]	-	-	99%	100%
Prophylactic Antibiotic Selection[5]	-	-	99%	99%
Prophylactic Antibiotic Selection (Outpatient)[5]	-	-	98%	98%
Prophylactic Antibiotic Stopped[5]	-	-	99%	98%
Prophylactic Antibiotic Timing[5]	-	-	98%	99%
Prophylactic Antibiotic Timing (Outpatient)[5]	-	-	97%	98%
Urinary Catheter Removal[5]	-	-	97%	97%
Survey of Patients' Hospital Experiences				
Area Around Room 'Always' Quiet at Night[10]	<100	80%	65%	61%
Doctors 'Always' Communicated Well[10]	<100	89%	84%	82%
Home Recovery Information Given[10]	<100	87%	88%	85%
Hospital Given 9 or 10 on 10 Point Scale[10]	<100	81%	74%	71%
Meds 'Always' Explained Before Given[10]	<100	89%	67%	64%
Nurses 'Always' Communicated Well[10]	<100	91%	81%	79%
Pain 'Always' Well Controlled[10]	<100	89%	72%	71%
Room and Bathroom 'Always' Clean[10]	<100	87%	78%	73%
Timely Help 'Always' Received[10]	<100	95%	74%	68%
Would Definitely Recommend Hospital[10]	<100	86%	71%	71%
Use of Medical Imaging				
Cardiac Imaging Stress Test before Surgery[7]	-	-	6.3%	5.3%
Combination Abdominal CT Scan[7]	-	-	5.7%	10.5%
Combination Brain/Sinus CT Scan[7]	-	-	2.3%	2.7%
Combination Chest CT Scan[7]	-	-	1.9%	2.7%
Follow-up Mammogram/Ultrasound[7]	-	-	6.3%	8.8%
Lumbar Spine MRI for Low Back Pain[7]	-	-	37.6%	37.2%

University of Minnesota Medical Center - Fairview

2450 Riverside Avenue
Minneapolis, MN 55454
Phone: 612-273-3000
Fax: 612-672-7186
URL: www.uofmmedicalcenter.org
Type: Acute Care Hospitals
Emergency Services: Yes
Ownership: Voluntary non-profit - Private
Beds: 1,868

Key Personnel:
CEO/President. . . . . Mark A Eustis
Quality Assurance . . . . Sally Huntington
Pediatric Ambulatory Care . . . . . . Alfred Michael, MD
Pediatric In-Patient Care . . . . Alfred Michael, MD
Infection Control. . . . . Frank Rhame, MD
Radiology. . . . . William Thompson, MD
Operating Room. . . . . Cheryl Vogel

Measure	Cases	This Hosp.	State Avg.	U.S. Avg.
Blood Clot Prevention and Treatment				
Anticoagulation Overlap Therapy[2]	124	97%	96%	93%
ICU Venous Thromboembolism Prophylaxis[2]	81	91%	91%	92%
Incidence of Potentially Preventable VTE[2]	21	5%	9%	10%
UFH with Dosages/Platelet Monitoring[2]	130	97%	98%	97%
Venous Thromboembolism Prophylaxis[2]	330	68%	86%	85%
Warfarin Therapy Discharge Instructions[2]	86	22%	63%	75%
Chest Pain/Possible Heart Attack Care				
Aspirin Given Within 24 Hours of Arrival[5]	-	-	97%	96%
Fibrinolytic Meds Within 30 Min. of Arrival[5]	-	-	48%	58%
Average Time to ECG (minutes)[5]	-	-	7	7
Average Time to Transfer (minutes)[5]	-	-	54	60
Children's Asthma Care				
Received Home Management Plan of Care	28	75%	-	88%
Received Reliever Medication	28	100%	-	100%
Received Systemic Corticosteroids	28	100%	-	100%
Emergency Department				
Admittance Decision Time (minutes)[2]	429	107	62	98
Head CT Results Within 45 Min. of Arrival[3,7]	-	-	54%	57%
Patients Who Left ER Before Being Seen	57,244	1%	2%	2%
Time from ER Arrival to Admit. (minutes)[2]	443	265	199	274
Time from ER Arrival to Discharge (minutes)	421	145	125	134
Time in ER Before Being Evaluated (minutes)	465	22	31	26
Time to Pain Meds for Fractures (minutes)	131	49	45	57
Heart Attack Care				
Aspirin Given at Discharge	208	100%	99%	99%
Fibrinolytic Meds Within 30 Min. of Arrival[7]	-	-	-	54%
PCI Within 90 Minutes of Arrival	13	100%	96%	96%
Statin Prescribed at Discharge	201	100%	99%	98%
Heart Failure Care				
ACE Inhibitor or ARB for LVSD	156	99%	96%	97%
Discharge Instructions Given	358	100%	93%	94%
Evaluation of LVS Function	431	100%	97%	99%
Medicare Spending				
Medicare Spending per Patient (ratio)	-	0.97	0.9	0.98
Pneumonia Care				
Appropriate Initial Antibiotic Given	79	97%	94%	95%
Blood Culture Timing	262	99%	97%	98%
Pregnancy and Delivery Care				
Newborn Deliveries Scheduled Early[2]	26	0%	5%	6%
Preventive Care				
Immunization for Influenza[2]	556	88%	89%	90%
Immunization for Pneumonia[2]	499	86%	89%	92%
Stroke Care				
Anticoagulation Therapy for Atrial Fibrillation	13	100%	96%	95%
Antithrombotic Therapy Timing	84	99%	98%	98%
Assessed for Rehabilitation	166	96%	98%	97%
Discharged on Antithrombotic Therapy	113	100%	99%	99%
Discharged on Statin Medication	79	95%	95%	94%
Thrombolytic Therapy Timing[1]	-	-	74%	66%

NOTE: Hospital profiles are in alphabetical order by state, then city, then hospital within the city; Rankings exclude hospitals with less than 25 cases except for patient surveys which excludes hospitals with less than 100 cases; (a) 100-299 cases; (1) The number of cases/patients is too few to report; (2) Data submitted were based on a sample of cases/patients; (3) Results are based on a shorter time period than required; (4) Data suppressed by CMS for one or more quarters; (5) Results are not available for this reporting period; (6) Fewer than 100 patients completed the HCAHPS survey; (7) No cases met the criteria for this measure; (8) The lower limit of the confidence interval cannot be calculated if the number of observed infections equals zero; (9) No data are available from the state/territory for this reporting period; (10) The scores shown reflect fewer than 50 completed surveys; (11) There were discrepancies in the data collection process; (12) This measure does not apply to this hospital for this reporting period; (13) Results cannot be calculated for this reporting period; (14) The results for this state are combined with nearby states to protect confidentiality; Please refer to the User's Guide for a full explanation of data.

Measure	Cases	This Hosp.	State Avg.	U.S. Avg.
Venous Thromboembolism Prophylaxis	161	98%	95%	94%
Written Stroke Educational Materials Given	88	83%	88%	88%
Surgical Care Improvement Project				
Appropriate Beta Blocker Usage[2]	515	100%	98%	98%
Appropriate VTP Within 24 Hours[2]	1,741	100%	98%	98%
Controlled Postoperative Blood Glucose[2]	196	96%	97%	97%
Perioperative Temperature Management[2]	2,100	100%	99%	100%
Prophylactic Antibiotic Selection[2]	1,099	99%	99%	99%
Prophylactic Antibiotic Selection (Outpatient)	581	91%	98%	98%
Prophylactic Antibiotic Stopped[2]	1,085	99%	99%	98%
Prophylactic Antibiotic Timing[2]	1,101	99%	98%	99%
Prophylactic Antibiotic Timing (Outpatient)	531	90%	97%	98%
Urinary Catheter Removal[2]	1,302	99%	97%	97%
Survey of Patients' Hospital Experiences				
Area Around Room 'Always' Quiet at Night[11]	300+	47%	65%	61%
Doctors 'Always' Communicated Well[11]	300+	77%	84%	82%
Home Recovery Information Given[11]	300+	87%	88%	85%
Hospital Given 9 or 10 on 10 Point Scale[11]	300+	68%	74%	71%
Meds 'Always' Explained Before Given[11]	300+	60%	67%	64%
Nurses 'Always' Communicated Well[11]	300+	74%	81%	79%
Pain 'Always' Well Controlled[11]	300+	65%	72%	71%
Room and Bathroom 'Always' Clean[11]	300+	64%	78%	73%
Timely Help 'Always' Received[11]	300+	59%	74%	68%
Would Definitely Recommend Hospital[11]	300+	74%	71%	71%
Use of Medical Imaging				
Cardiac Imaging Stress Test before Surgery	424	9.7%	6.3%	5.3%
Combination Abdominal CT Scan	1,065	2.2%	5.7%	10.5%
Combination Brain/Sinus CT Scan	260	1.2%	2.3%	2.7%
Combination Chest CT Scan	1,126	0.4%	1.9%	2.7%
Follow-up Mammogram/Ultrasound	598	5.5%	6.3%	8.8%
Lumbar Spine MRI for Low Back Pain	53	43.4%	37.6%	37.2%

Chippewa County Hospital

824 North 11th Street
Montevideo, MN 56265
Phone: 320-321-8100
Fax: 320-269-8186
Type: Critical Access Hospitals
Emergency Services: Yes
Ownership: Voluntary non-profit - Other
Beds: 35

Key Personnel:
Chief of Medical Staff . . . . Eleazar Briones, MD
CEO/President . . . . Mark Paulson
Hemotology Center . . . . Harold Windschitl, MD

Measure	Cases	This Hosp.	State Avg.	U.S. Avg.
Blood Clot Prevention and Treatment				
Anticoagulation Overlap Therapy[5]	-	-	96%	93%
ICU Venous Thromboembolism Prophylaxis[5]	-	-	91%	92%
Incidence of Potentially Preventable VTE[5]	-	-	9%	10%
UFH with Dosages/Platelet Monitoring[5]	-	-	98%	97%
Venous Thromboembolism Prophylaxis[5]	-	-	86%	85%
Warfarin Therapy Discharge Instructions[5]	-	-	63%	75%
Chest Pain/Possible Heart Attack Care				
Aspirin Given Within 24 Hours of Arrival	25	96%	97%	96%
Fibrinolytic Meds Within 30 Min. of Arrival[1]	-	-	48%	58%
Average Time to ECG (minutes)	21	8	7	7
Average Time to Transfer (minutes)[1]	-	-	54	60
Children's Asthma Care				
Received Home Management Plan of Care	-	-	-	88%
Received Reliever Medication	-	-	-	100%
Received Systemic Corticosteroids	-	-	-	100%
Emergency Department				
Admittance Decision Time (minutes)[5]	-	-	62	98
Head CT Results Within 45 Min. of Arrival[5]	-	-	54%	57%
Patients Who Left ER Before Being Seen[5]	-	-	2%	2%
Time from ER Arrival to Admit. (minutes)[5]	-	-	199	274
Time from ER Arrival to Discharge (minutes)[5]	-	-	125	134
Time in ER Before Being Evaluated (minutes)[5]	-	-	31	26
Time to Pain Meds for Fractures (minutes)[5]	-	-	45	57
Heart Attack Care				
Aspirin Given at Discharge[1,2]	-	-	99%	99%
Fibrinolytic Meds Within 30 Min. of Arrival[2,7]	-	-	-	54%
PCI Within 90 Minutes of Arrival[2,7]	-	-	96%	96%
Statin Prescribed at Discharge[1,2]	-	-	99%	98%
Heart Failure Care				
ACE Inhibitor or ARB for LVSD[1,2]	-	-	96%	97%
Discharge Instructions Given[2]	19	26%	93%	94%
Evaluation of LVS Function[2]	23	57%	97%	99%
Medicare Spending				
Medicare Spending per Patient (ratio)	-	-	0.9	0.98
Pneumonia Care				
Appropriate Initial Antibiotic Given[2]	21	81%	94%	95%
Blood Culture Timing[2]	18	94%	97%	98%
Pregnancy and Delivery Care				
Newborn Deliveries Scheduled Early[5]	-	-	5%	6%
Preventive Care				
Immunization for Influenza[2,3]	137	48%	89%	90%
Immunization for Pneumonia[2,3]	269	53%	89%	92%
Stroke Care				
Anticoagulation Therapy for Atrial Fibrillation[5]	-	-	96%	95%
Antithrombotic Therapy Timing[5]	-	-	98%	98%
Assessed for Rehabilitation[5]	-	-	98%	97%
Discharged on Antithrombotic Therapy[5]	-	-	99%	99%
Discharged on Statin Medication[5]	-	-	95%	94%
Thrombolytic Therapy Timing[5]	-	-	74%	66%
Venous Thromboembolism Prophylaxis[5]	-	-	95%	94%
Written Stroke Educational Materials Given[5]	-	-	88%	88%
Surgical Care Improvement Project				
Appropriate Beta Blocker Usage[1,2]	-	-	98%	98%
Appropriate VTP Within 24 Hours[2]	17	94%	98%	98%
Controlled Postoperative Blood Glucose[2,7]	-	-	97%	97%
Perioperative Temperature Management[2]	26	77%	99%	100%
Prophylactic Antibiotic Selection[2]	13	100%	99%	99%
Prophylactic Antibiotic Selection (Outpatient)[1,3]	-	-	98%	98%
Prophylactic Antibiotic Stopped[2]	13	100%	99%	98%
Prophylactic Antibiotic Timing[2]	13	85%	98%	99%
Prophylactic Antibiotic Timing (Outpatient)[1,3]	-	-	97%	98%
Urinary Catheter Removal[2]	12	92%	97%	97%
Survey of Patients' Hospital Experiences				
Area Around Room 'Always' Quiet at Night[11]	(a)	76%	65%	61%
Doctors 'Always' Communicated Well[11]	(a)	88%	84%	82%
Home Recovery Information Given[11]	(a)	86%	88%	85%
Hospital Given 9 or 10 on 10 Point Scale[11]	(a)	69%	74%	71%
Meds 'Always' Explained Before Given[11]	(a)	55%	67%	64%
Nurses 'Always' Communicated Well[11]	(a)	73%	81%	79%
Pain 'Always' Well Controlled[11]	(a)	73%	72%	71%
Room and Bathroom 'Always' Clean[11]	(a)	76%	78%	73%
Timely Help 'Always' Received[11]	(a)	70%	74%	68%
Would Definitely Recommend Hospital[11]	(a)	46%	71%	71%
Use of Medical Imaging				
Cardiac Imaging Stress Test before Surgery[1]	-	-	6.3%	5.3%
Combination Abdominal CT Scan	98	75.5%	5.7%	10.5%
Combination Brain/Sinus CT Scan[1]	-	-	2.3%	2.7%
Combination Chest CT Scan[1]	-	-	1.9%	2.7%
Follow-up Mammogram/Ultrasound	226	5.8%	6.3%	8.8%
Lumbar Spine MRI for Low Back Pain[1]	-	-	37.6%	37.2%

Centracare Health - Monticello

1013 Hart Boulevard
Monticello, MN 55362
Phone: 763-295-2945
Fax: 763-295-4593
URL: www.mblch.com
Type: Critical Access Hospitals
Emergency Services: Yes
Ownership: Govt - Hospital Dist/Auth
Beds: 25

Key Personnel:
Surgery . . . . Adrianne Bowen, MD
Administrator . . . . Mary Ellen Wells
Chief of Medical Staff . . . . Dr. Allen Horn
Radiology . . . . Robert Pollock

Measure	Cases	This Hosp.	State Avg.	U.S. Avg.
Blood Clot Prevention and Treatment				
Anticoagulation Overlap Therapy[5]	-	-	96%	93%
ICU Venous Thromboembolism Prophylaxis[5]	-	-	91%	92%
Incidence of Potentially Preventable VTE[5]	-	-	9%	10%
UFH with Dosages/Platelet Monitoring[5]	-	-	98%	97%
Venous Thromboembolism Prophylaxis[5]	-	-	86%	85%
Warfarin Therapy Discharge Instructions[5]	-	-	63%	75%
Chest Pain/Possible Heart Attack Care				
Aspirin Given Within 24 Hours of Arrival	65	98%	97%	96%
Fibrinolytic Meds Within 30 Min. of Arrival[7]	-	-	48%	58%
Average Time to ECG (minutes)	70	6	7	7
Average Time to Transfer (minutes)	12	55	54	60
Children's Asthma Care				
Received Home Management Plan of Care	-	-	-	88%
Received Reliever Medication	-	-	-	100%
Received Systemic Corticosteroids	-	-	-	100%
Emergency Department				
Admittance Decision Time (minutes)[2]	462	40	62	98
Head CT Results Within 45 Min. of Arrival[5]	-	-	54%	57%
Patients Who Left ER Before Being Seen	>100k	0%	2%	2%
Time from ER Arrival to Admit. (minutes)[2]	470	186	199	274
Time from ER Arrival to Discharge (minutes)[5]	-	-	125	134
Time in ER Before Being Evaluated (minutes)[5]	-	-	31	26
Time to Pain Meds for Fractures (minutes)[5]	-	-	45	57
Heart Attack Care				
Aspirin Given at Discharge[2,3]	-	-	99%	99%
Fibrinolytic Meds Within 30 Min. of Arrival[2,3]	-	-	-	54%
PCI Within 90 Minutes of Arrival[2,3]	-	-	96%	96%
Statin Prescribed at Discharge[2,3]	-	-	99%	98%
Heart Failure Care				
ACE Inhibitor or ARB for LVSD[1]	-	-	96%	97%
Discharge Instructions Given	30	97%	93%	94%
Evaluation of LVS Function	43	100%	97%	99%
Medicare Spending				
Medicare Spending per Patient (ratio)	-	-	0.9	0.98
Pneumonia Care				
Appropriate Initial Antibiotic Given[2]	19	95%	94%	95%
Blood Culture Timing[2]	34	100%	97%	98%
Pregnancy and Delivery Care				
Newborn Deliveries Scheduled Early[2,3]	-	-	5%	6%
Preventive Care				
Immunization for Influenza[2]	283	84%	89%	90%
Immunization for Pneumonia[2]	395	88%	89%	92%
Stroke Care				
Anticoagulation Therapy for Atrial Fibrillation[5]	-	-	96%	95%
Antithrombotic Therapy Timing[5]	-	-	98%	98%
Assessed for Rehabilitation[5]	-	-	98%	97%
Discharged on Antithrombotic Therapy[5]	-	-	99%	99%
Discharged on Statin Medication[5]	-	-	95%	94%
Thrombolytic Therapy Timing[5]	-	-	74%	66%
Venous Thromboembolism Prophylaxis[5]	-	-	95%	94%
Written Stroke Educational Materials Given[5]	-	-	88%	88%
Surgical Care Improvement Project				
Appropriate Beta Blocker Usage[1,2]	-	-	98%	98%
Appropriate VTP Within 24 Hours[1,2]	-	-	98%	98%
Controlled Postoperative Blood Glucose[2,7]	-	-	97%	97%
Perioperative Temperature Management[2]	13	100%	99%	100%
Prophylactic Antibiotic Selection[1,2]	-	-	99%	99%
Prophylactic Antibiotic Selection (Outpatient)[1,3]	-	-	98%	98%
Prophylactic Antibiotic Stopped[1,2]	-	-	99%	98%
Prophylactic Antibiotic Timing[1,2]	-	-	98%	99%
Prophylactic Antibiotic Timing (Outpatient)[1,3]	-	-	97%	98%
Urinary Catheter Removal[1,2]	-	-	97%	97%
Survey of Patients' Hospital Experiences				
Area Around Room 'Always' Quiet at Night	(a)	80%	65%	61%
Doctors 'Always' Communicated Well	(a)	82%	84%	82%
Home Recovery Information Given	(a)	90%	88%	85%
Hospital Given 9 or 10 on 10 Point Scale	(a)	75%	74%	71%
Meds 'Always' Explained Before Given	(a)	61%	67%	64%
Nurses 'Always' Communicated Well	(a)	79%	81%	79%
Pain 'Always' Well Controlled	(a)	73%	72%	71%
Room and Bathroom 'Always' Clean	(a)	81%	78%	73%
Timely Help 'Always' Received	(a)	73%	74%	68%
Would Definitely Recommend Hospital	(a)	64%	71%	71%
Use of Medical Imaging				
Cardiac Imaging Stress Test before Surgery[1]	-	-	6.3%	5.3%
Combination Abdominal CT Scan	122	4.9%	5.7%	10.5%
Combination Brain/Sinus CT Scan[1]	-	-	2.3%	2.7%
Combination Chest CT Scan	80	0.0%	1.9%	2.7%
Follow-up Mammogram/Ultrasound	67	3.0%	6.3%	8.8%
Lumbar Spine MRI for Low Back Pain[1]	-	-	37.6%	37.2%

NOTE: Hospital profiles are in alphabetical order by state, then city, then hospital within the city; Rankings exclude hospitals with less than 25 cases except for patient surveys which excludes hospitals with less than 100 cases; (a) 100-299 cases; (1) The number of cases/patients is too few to report; (2) Data submitted were based on a sample of cases/patients; (3) Results are based on a shorter time period than required; (4) Data suppressed by CMS for one or more quarters; (5) Results are not available for this reporting period; (6) Fewer than 100 patients completed the HCAHPS survey; (7) No cases met the criteria for this measure; (8) The lower limit of the confidence interval cannot be calculated if the number of observed infections equals zero; (9) No data are available from the state/territory for this reporting period; (10) The scores shown reflect fewer than 50 completed surveys; (11) There were discrepancies in the data collection process; (12) This measure does not apply to this hospital for this reporting period; (13) Results cannot be calculated for this reporting period; (14) The results for this state are combined with nearby states to protect confidentiality; Please refer to the User's Guide for a full explanation of data.

Mercy Hospital

710 Kenwood Avenue South
Moose Lake, MN 55767
Phone: 218-485-4481
Fax: 218-485-5855
URL: www.mercymooselake.org
Type: Critical Access Hospitals
Emergency Services: Yes
Ownership: Govt - Hospital Dist/Auth
Beds: 25

Key Personnel:
Infection Control. . . . . Sally Behn
Radiology. . . . . Daniel Courneya, MD
CEO . . . . Michael Delfs
Patient Relations . . . . Linda Johnson
Quality Assurance . . . . Trina Lower
Chief of Medical Staff. . . . . Barbara Reed

Measure	Cases	This Hosp.	State Avg.	U.S. Avg.
Blood Clot Prevention and Treatment				
Anticoagulation Overlap Therapy[1,2]	-	-	96%	93%
ICU Venous Thromboembolism Prophylaxis[1,2]	-	-	91%	92%
Incidence of Potentially Preventable VTE[2,7]	-	-	9%	10%
UFH with Dosages/Platelet Monitoring[2,7]	-	-	98%	97%
Venous Thromboembolism Prophylaxis[2]	223	98%	86%	85%
Warfarin Therapy Discharge Instructions[1,2]	-	-	63%	75%
Chest Pain/Possible Heart Attack Care				
Aspirin Given Within 24 Hours of Arrival	27	96%	97%	96%
Fibrinolytic Meds Within 30 Min. of Arrival[1]	-	-	48%	58%
Average Time to ECG (minutes)	29	3	7	7
Average Time to Transfer (minutes)[1]	-	-	54	60
Children's Asthma Care				
Received Home Management Plan of Care	-	-	-	88%
Received Reliever Medication	-	-	-	100%
Received Systemic Corticosteroids	-	-	-	100%
Emergency Department				
Admittance Decision Time (minutes)[2]	218	51	62	98
Head CT Results Within 45 Min. of Arrival[1]	-	-	54%	57%
Patients Who Left ER Before Being Seen[5]	-	-	2%	2%
Time from ER Arrival to Admit. (minutes)[2]	219	169	199	274
Time from ER Arrival to Discharge (minutes)	257	98	125	134
Time in ER Before Being Evaluated (minutes)	378	17	31	26
Time to Pain Meds for Fractures (minutes)	17	27	45	57
Heart Attack Care				
Aspirin Given at Discharge[1,2]	-	-	99%	99%
Fibrinolytic Meds Within 30 Min. of Arrival[2,7]	-	-	-	54%
PCI Within 90 Minutes of Arrival[2,7]	-	-	96%	96%
Statin Prescribed at Discharge[2,7]	-	-	99%	98%
Heart Failure Care				
ACE Inhibitor or ARB for LVSD[2,7]	-	-	96%	97%
Discharge Instructions Given[1,2]	-	-	93%	94%
Evaluation of LVS Function[1,2]	-	-	97%	99%
Medicare Spending				
Medicare Spending per Patient (ratio)	-	-	0.9	0.98
Pneumonia Care				
Appropriate Initial Antibiotic Given[2]	16	100%	94%	95%
Blood Culture Timing[2]	21	100%	97%	98%
Pregnancy and Delivery Care				
Newborn Deliveries Scheduled Early[5]	-	-	5%	6%
Preventive Care				
Immunization for Influenza[2]	257	95%	89%	90%
Immunization for Pneumonia[2]	288	92%	89%	92%
Stroke Care				
Anticoagulation Therapy for Atrial Fibrillation[2,3]	-	-	96%	95%
Antithrombotic Therapy Timing[1,2]	-	-	98%	98%
Assessed for Rehabilitation[1,2]	-	-	98%	97%
Discharged on Antithrombotic Therapy[1,2]	-	-	99%	99%
Discharged on Statin Medication[1,2]	-	-	95%	94%
Thrombolytic Therapy Timing[1,2]	-	-	74%	66%
Venous Thromboembolism Prophylaxis[1,2]	-	-	95%	94%
Written Stroke Educational Materials Given[1,2]	-	-	88%	88%
Surgical Care Improvement Project				
Appropriate Beta Blocker Usage[2]	13	100%	98%	98%
Appropriate VTP Within 24 Hours[2]	42	83%	98%	98%
Controlled Postoperative Blood Glucose[2,7]	-	-	97%	97%
Perioperative Temperature Management[2]	57	98%	99%	100%
Prophylactic Antibiotic Selection[2]	48	100%	99%	99%
Prophylactic Antibiotic Selection (Outpatient)	17	82%	98%	98%
Prophylactic Antibiotic Stopped[2]	48	94%	99%	98%
Prophylactic Antibiotic Timing[2]	48	100%	98%	99%
Prophylactic Antibiotic Timing (Outpatient)	23	61%	97%	98%
Urinary Catheter Removal[2]	23	61%	97%	97%
Survey of Patients' Hospital Experiences				
Area Around Room 'Always' Quiet at Night	(a)	65%	65%	61%
Doctors 'Always' Communicated Well	(a)	84%	84%	82%
Home Recovery Information Given	(a)	84%	88%	85%
Hospital Given 9 or 10 on 10 Point Scale	(a)	71%	74%	71%
Meds 'Always' Explained Before Given	(a)	61%	67%	64%
Nurses 'Always' Communicated Well	(a)	80%	81%	79%
Pain 'Always' Well Controlled	(a)	71%	72%	71%
Room and Bathroom 'Always' Clean	(a)	77%	78%	73%
Timely Help 'Always' Received	(a)	79%	74%	68%
Would Definitely Recommend Hospital	(a)	69%	71%	71%
Use of Medical Imaging				
Cardiac Imaging Stress Test before Surgery[1]	-	-	6.3%	5.3%
Combination Abdominal CT Scan	71	5.6%	5.7%	10.5%
Combination Brain/Sinus CT Scan[1]	-	-	2.3%	2.7%
Combination Chest CT Scan	59	1.7%	1.9%	2.7%
Follow-up Mammogram/Ultrasound	159	8.8%	6.3%	8.8%
Lumbar Spine MRI for Low Back Pain[1]	-	-	37.6%	37.2%

Firstlight Health System

301 South Highway 65
Mora, MN 55051
Phone: 320-225-3315
Fax: 320-225-3613
Type: Critical Access Hospitals
Emergency Services: Yes
Ownership: Government - Local
Beds: 49

Key Personnel:
Chief of Medical Staff. . . . . Randy Bostrom, MD
Operating Room. . . . . Mary Jo Henk-Buckley
Emergency Room . . . . Dorothy Kohl, RN
Anesthesiology. . . . . Dustin Paulson
Patient Relations . . . . Diane Saari
Quality Assurance . . . . Diane Saari
CEO/President. . . . . Randy Ulseth
Infection Control. . . . . Barry Vermilyea

Measure	Cases	This Hosp.	State Avg.	U.S. Avg.
Blood Clot Prevention and Treatment				
Anticoagulation Overlap Therapy[5]	-	-	96%	93%
ICU Venous Thromboembolism Prophylaxis[5]	-	-	91%	92%
Incidence of Potentially Preventable VTE[5]	-	-	9%	10%
UFH with Dosages/Platelet Monitoring[5]	-	-	98%	97%
Venous Thromboembolism Prophylaxis[5]	-	-	86%	85%
Warfarin Therapy Discharge Instructions[5]	-	-	63%	75%
Chest Pain/Possible Heart Attack Care				
Aspirin Given Within 24 Hours of Arrival	51	98%	97%	96%
Fibrinolytic Meds Within 30 Min. of Arrival[1]	-	-	48%	58%
Average Time to ECG (minutes)	52	10	7	7
Average Time to Transfer (minutes)[1]	-	-	54	60
Children's Asthma Care				
Received Home Management Plan of Care	-	-	-	88%
Received Reliever Medication	-	-	-	100%
Received Systemic Corticosteroids	-	-	-	100%
Emergency Department				
Admittance Decision Time (minutes)[2]	396	38	62	98
Head CT Results Within 45 Min. of Arrival[5]	-	-	54%	57%
Patients Who Left ER Before Being Seen[5]	-	-	2%	2%
Time from ER Arrival to Admit. (minutes)[2]	401	210	199	274
Time from ER Arrival to Discharge (minutes)[5]	-	-	125	134
Time in ER Before Being Evaluated (minutes)[5]	-	-	31	26
Time to Pain Meds for Fractures (minutes)[5]	-	-	45	57
Heart Attack Care				
Aspirin Given at Discharge[1,3]	-	-	99%	99%
Fibrinolytic Meds Within 30 Min. of Arrival[3,7]	-	-	-	54%
PCI Within 90 Minutes of Arrival[3,7]	-	-	96%	96%
Statin Prescribed at Discharge[1,3]	-	-	99%	98%
Heart Failure Care				
ACE Inhibitor or ARB for LVSD[1]	-	-	96%	97%
Discharge Instructions Given	27	52%	93%	94%
Evaluation of LVS Function	32	97%	97%	99%
Medicare Spending				
Medicare Spending per Patient (ratio)	-	-	0.9	0.98
Pneumonia Care				
Appropriate Initial Antibiotic Given	41	95%	94%	95%
Blood Culture Timing	33	94%	97%	98%
Pregnancy and Delivery Care				
Newborn Deliveries Scheduled Early[5]	-	-	5%	6%
Preventive Care				
Immunization for Influenza[2]	267	90%	89%	90%
Immunization for Pneumonia[2]	326	91%	89%	92%
Stroke Care				
Anticoagulation Therapy for Atrial Fibrillation[5]	-	-	96%	95%
Antithrombotic Therapy Timing[5]	-	-	98%	98%
Assessed for Rehabilitation[5]	-	-	98%	97%
Discharged on Antithrombotic Therapy[5]	-	-	99%	99%
Discharged on Statin Medication[5]	-	-	95%	94%
Thrombolytic Therapy Timing[5]	-	-	74%	66%
Venous Thromboembolism Prophylaxis[5]	-	-	95%	94%
Written Stroke Educational Materials Given[5]	-	-	88%	88%
Surgical Care Improvement Project				
Appropriate Beta Blocker Usage	28	93%	98%	98%
Appropriate VTP Within 24 Hours	80	100%	98%	98%
Controlled Postoperative Blood Glucose[7]	-	-	97%	97%
Perioperative Temperature Management	104	96%	99%	100%
Prophylactic Antibiotic Selection	88	100%	99%	99%
Prophylactic Antibiotic Selection (Outpatient)	25	76%	98%	98%
Prophylactic Antibiotic Stopped	87	99%	99%	98%
Prophylactic Antibiotic Timing	89	98%	98%	99%
Prophylactic Antibiotic Timing (Outpatient)[1]	-	-	97%	98%
Urinary Catheter Removal	52	96%	97%	97%
Survey of Patients' Hospital Experiences				
Area Around Room 'Always' Quiet at Night	300+	60%	65%	61%
Doctors 'Always' Communicated Well	300+	83%	84%	82%
Home Recovery Information Given	300+	89%	88%	85%
Hospital Given 9 or 10 on 10 Point Scale	300+	68%	74%	71%
Meds 'Always' Explained Before Given	300+	64%	67%	64%
Nurses 'Always' Communicated Well	300+	77%	81%	79%
Pain 'Always' Well Controlled	300+	70%	72%	71%
Room and Bathroom 'Always' Clean	300+	76%	78%	73%
Timely Help 'Always' Received	300+	70%	74%	68%
Would Definitely Recommend Hospital	300+	63%	71%	71%
Use of Medical Imaging				
Cardiac Imaging Stress Test before Surgery	70	7.1%	6.3%	5.3%
Combination Abdominal CT Scan	212	5.2%	5.7%	10.5%
Combination Brain/Sinus CT Scan[1]	-	-	2.3%	2.7%
Combination Chest CT Scan	115	0.9%	1.9%	2.7%
Follow-up Mammogram/Ultrasound	250	6.8%	6.3%	8.8%
Lumbar Spine MRI for Low Back Pain	37	45.9%	37.6%	37.2%

Stevens Community Medical Center

400 East First Street, PO Box 660
Morris, MN 56267
Phone: 320-589-1313
Fax: 320-589-1065
URL: www.scmcmorris.com
Type: Critical Access Hospitals
Emergency Services: Yes
Ownership: Voluntary non-profit - Private
Beds: 54

Key Personnel:
Emergency Room . . . . Gaither Bynum, MD
Quality Assurance . . . . Suzie Erlund, RN
Radiology. . . . . Andrea Giambi
Infection Control. . . . . Bev Larson, RN
CEO/President. . . . . John Rau
Chief of Medical Staff. . . . . Olyn Wernsing, MD

Measure	Cases	This Hosp.	State Avg.	U.S. Avg.
Blood Clot Prevention and Treatment				
Anticoagulation Overlap Therapy[5]	-	-	96%	93%
ICU Venous Thromboembolism Prophylaxis[5]	-	-	91%	92%
Incidence of Potentially Preventable VTE[5]	-	-	9%	10%
UFH with Dosages/Platelet Monitoring[5]	-	-	98%	97%
Venous Thromboembolism Prophylaxis[5]	-	-	86%	85%
Warfarin Therapy Discharge Instructions[5]	-	-	63%	75%
Chest Pain/Possible Heart Attack Care				
Aspirin Given Within 24 Hours of Arrival[1]	-	-	97%	96%
Fibrinolytic Meds Within 30 Min. of Arrival[1]	-	-	48%	58%
Average Time to ECG (minutes)[1]	-	-	7	7
Average Time to Transfer (minutes)[1]	-	-	54	60
Children's Asthma Care				
Received Home Management Plan of Care	-	-	-	88%
Received Reliever Medication	-	-	-	100%

NOTE: Hospital profiles are in alphabetical order by state, then city, then hospital within the city; Rankings exclude hospitals with less than 25 cases except for patient surveys which excludes hospitals with less than 100 cases; (a) 100-299 cases; (1) The number of cases/patients is too few to report; (2) Data submitted were based on a sample of cases/patients; (3) Results are based on a shorter time period than required; (4) Data suppressed by CMS for one or more quarters; (5) Results are not available for this reporting period; (6) Fewer than 100 patients completed the HCAHPS survey; (7) No cases met the criteria for this measure; (8) The lower limit of the confidence interval cannot be calculated if the number of observed infections equals zero; (9) No data are available from the state/territory for this reporting period; (10) The scores shown reflect fewer than 50 completed surveys; (11) There were discrepancies in the data collection process; (12) This measure does not apply to this hospital for this reporting period; (13) Results cannot be calculated for this reporting period; (14) The results for this state are combined with nearby states to protect confidentiality; Please refer to the User's Guide for a full explanation of data.

Measure	Cases	This Hosp.	State Avg.	U.S. Avg.
Received Systemic Corticosteroids	-	-	-	100%
Emergency Department				
Admittance Decision Time (minutes)[2]	135	25	62	98
Head CT Results Within 45 Min. of Arrival[5]	-	-	54%	57%
Patients Who Left ER Before Being Seen[5]	-	-	2%	2%
Time from ER Arrival to Admit. (minutes)[2]	149	70	199	274
Time from ER Arrival to Discharge (minutes)[5]	-	-	125	134
Time in ER Before Being Evaluated (minutes)[5]	-	-	31	26
Time to Pain Meds for Fractures (minutes)[5]	-	-	45	57
Heart Attack Care				
Aspirin Given at Discharge[1]	-	-	99%	99%
Fibrinolytic Meds Within 30 Min. of Arrival[7]	-	-	-	54%
PCI Within 90 Minutes of Arrival[7]	-	-	96%	96%
Statin Prescribed at Discharge[1]	-	-	99%	98%
Heart Failure Care				
ACE Inhibitor or ARB for LVSD	11	73%	96%	97%
Discharge Instructions Given	29	0%	93%	94%
Evaluation of LVS Function	39	82%	97%	99%
Medicare Spending				
Medicare Spending per Patient (ratio)	-	-	0.9	0.98
Pneumonia Care				
Appropriate Initial Antibiotic Given	32	75%	94%	95%
Blood Culture Timing	16	75%	97%	98%
Pregnancy and Delivery Care				
Newborn Deliveries Scheduled Early[5]	-	-	5%	6%
Preventive Care				
Immunization for Influenza[2]	264	69%	89%	90%
Immunization for Pneumonia[2]	351	68%	89%	92%
Stroke Care				
Anticoagulation Therapy for Atrial Fibrillation[5]	-	-	96%	95%
Antithrombotic Therapy Timing[5]	-	-	98%	98%
Assessed for Rehabilitation[5]	-	-	98%	97%
Discharged on Antithrombotic Therapy[5]	-	-	99%	99%
Discharged on Statin Medication[5]	-	-	95%	94%
Thrombolytic Therapy Timing[5]	-	-	74%	66%
Venous Thromboembolism Prophylaxis[5]	-	-	95%	94%
Written Stroke Educational Materials Given[5]	-	-	88%	88%
Surgical Care Improvement Project				
Appropriate Beta Blocker Usage	18	94%	98%	98%
Appropriate VTP Within 24 Hours	65	68%	98%	98%
Controlled Postoperative Blood Glucose[7]	-	-	97%	97%
Perioperative Temperature Management	79	77%	99%	100%
Prophylactic Antibiotic Selection	60	98%	99%	99%
Prophylactic Antibiotic Selection (Outpatient)[5]	-	-	98%	98%
Prophylactic Antibiotic Stopped	60	100%	99%	98%
Prophylactic Antibiotic Timing	61	84%	98%	99%
Prophylactic Antibiotic Timing (Outpatient)[5]	-	-	97%	98%
Urinary Catheter Removal	52	96%	97%	97%
Survey of Patients' Hospital Experiences				
Area Around Room 'Always' Quiet at Night	(a)	70%	65%	61%
Doctors 'Always' Communicated Well	(a)	85%	84%	82%
Home Recovery Information Given	(a)	85%	88%	85%
Hospital Given 9 or 10 on 10 Point Scale	(a)	75%	74%	71%
Meds 'Always' Explained Before Given	(a)	63%	67%	64%
Nurses 'Always' Communicated Well	(a)	79%	81%	79%
Pain 'Always' Well Controlled	(a)	67%	72%	71%
Room and Bathroom 'Always' Clean	(a)	89%	78%	73%
Timely Help 'Always' Received	(a)	83%	74%	68%
Would Definitely Recommend Hospital	(a)	73%	71%	71%
Use of Medical Imaging				
Cardiac Imaging Stress Test before Surgery[1]	-	-	6.3%	5.3%
Combination Abdominal CT Scan	148	4.1%	5.7%	10.5%
Combination Brain/Sinus CT Scan[1]	-	-	2.3%	2.7%
Combination Chest CT Scan	57	1.8%	1.9%	2.7%
Follow-up Mammogram/Ultrasound	112	14.3%	6.3%	8.8%
Lumbar Spine MRI for Low Back Pain[1]	-	-	37.6%	37.2%

Mayo Clinic Health System - New Prague

301 2nd Street Northeast
New Prague, MN 56071
E-mail: info@qofp.org
URL: www.queenofpeacehospital.com
Phone: 952-758-8101
Fax: 952-758-5009
Type: Critical Access Hospitals
Emergency Services: Yes
Ownership: Voluntary non-profit - Private
Beds: 25

Key Personnel:
Emergency Room .... Kelly Ashley, RN
Coronary Care .... Diann Kelly, RN
Administrator .... Mary Klimp
Operating Room.............. Karen Neis, RN
Quality Assurance .... Mark Powell
Patient Relations .... Peggy Sullivan

Measure	Cases	This Hosp.	State Avg.	U.S. Avg.
Blood Clot Prevention and Treatment				
Anticoagulation Overlap Therapy[5]	-	-	96%	93%
ICU Venous Thromboembolism Prophylaxis[5]	-	-	91%	92%
Incidence of Potentially Preventable VTE[5]	-	-	9%	10%
UFH with Dosages/Platelet Monitoring[5]	-	-	98%	97%
Venous Thromboembolism Prophylaxis[5]	-	-	86%	85%
Warfarin Therapy Discharge Instructions[5]	-	-	63%	75%
Chest Pain/Possible Heart Attack Care				
Aspirin Given Within 24 Hours of Arrival	39	100%	97%	96%
Fibrinolytic Meds Within 30 Min. of Arrival[1]	-	-	48%	58%
Average Time to ECG (minutes)	40	7	7	7
Average Time to Transfer (minutes)[1]	-	-	54	60
Children's Asthma Care				
Received Home Management Plan of Care	-	-	-	88%
Received Reliever Medication	-	-	-	100%
Received Systemic Corticosteroids	-	-	-	100%
Emergency Department				
Admittance Decision Time (minutes)[2]	173	40	62	98
Head CT Results Within 45 Min. of Arrival[5]	-	-	54%	57%
Patients Who Left ER Before Being Seen	6,494	0%	2%	2%
Time from ER Arrival to Admit. (minutes)[2]	197	192	199	274
Time from ER Arrival to Discharge (minutes)[5]	-	-	125	134
Time in ER Before Being Evaluated (minutes)[5]	-	-	31	26
Time to Pain Meds for Fractures (minutes)[5]	-	-	45	57
Heart Attack Care				
Aspirin Given at Discharge[1]	-	-	99%	99%
Fibrinolytic Meds Within 30 Min. of Arrival[7]	-	-	-	54%
PCI Within 90 Minutes of Arrival[7]	-	-	96%	96%
Statin Prescribed at Discharge[1]	-	-	99%	98%
Heart Failure Care				
ACE Inhibitor or ARB for LVSD[1]	-	-	96%	97%
Discharge Instructions Given	16	88%	93%	94%
Evaluation of LVS Function	23	91%	97%	99%
Medicare Spending				
Medicare Spending per Patient (ratio)	-	-	0.9	0.98
Pneumonia Care				
Appropriate Initial Antibiotic Given[1]	-	-	94%	95%
Blood Culture Timing[1]	-	-	97%	98%
Pregnancy and Delivery Care				
Newborn Deliveries Scheduled Early[5]	-	-	5%	6%
Preventive Care				
Immunization for Influenza[2]	240	76%	89%	90%
Immunization for Pneumonia[2]	324	86%	89%	92%
Stroke Care				
Anticoagulation Therapy for Atrial Fibrillation[5]	-	-	96%	95%
Antithrombotic Therapy Timing[5]	-	-	98%	98%
Assessed for Rehabilitation[5]	-	-	98%	97%
Discharged on Antithrombotic Therapy[5]	-	-	99%	99%
Discharged on Statin Medication[5]	-	-	95%	94%
Thrombolytic Therapy Timing[5]	-	-	74%	66%
Venous Thromboembolism Prophylaxis[5]	-	-	95%	94%
Written Stroke Educational Materials Given[5]	-	-	88%	88%
Surgical Care Improvement Project				
Appropriate Beta Blocker Usage	27	93%	98%	98%
Appropriate VTP Within 24 Hours	77	97%	98%	98%
Controlled Postoperative Blood Glucose[7]	-	-	97%	97%
Perioperative Temperature Management	85	99%	99%	100%
Prophylactic Antibiotic Selection	70	100%	99%	99%
Prophylactic Antibiotic Selection (Outpatient)	19	95%	98%	98%
Prophylactic Antibiotic Stopped	69	99%	99%	98%
Prophylactic Antibiotic Timing	70	94%	98%	99%
Prophylactic Antibiotic Timing (Outpatient)[1]	-	-	97%	98%
Urinary Catheter Removal	68	99%	97%	97%
Survey of Patients' Hospital Experiences				
Area Around Room 'Always' Quiet at Night	(a)	68%	65%	61%
Doctors 'Always' Communicated Well	(a)	85%	84%	82%
Home Recovery Information Given	(a)	92%	88%	85%
Hospital Given 9 or 10 on 10 Point Scale	(a)	83%	74%	71%
Meds 'Always' Explained Before Given	(a)	70%	67%	64%
Nurses 'Always' Communicated Well	(a)	84%	81%	79%
Pain 'Always' Well Controlled	(a)	79%	72%	71%
Room and Bathroom 'Always' Clean	(a)	84%	78%	73%
Timely Help 'Always' Received	(a)	82%	74%	68%
Would Definitely Recommend Hospital	(a)	81%	71%	71%
Use of Medical Imaging				
Cardiac Imaging Stress Test before Surgery[1]	-	-	6.3%	5.3%
Combination Abdominal CT Scan	134	14.9%	5.7%	10.5%
Combination Brain/Sinus CT Scan[1]	-	-	2.3%	2.7%
Combination Chest CT Scan	66	0.0%	1.9%	2.7%
Follow-up Mammogram/Ultrasound	182	8.8%	6.3%	8.8%
Lumbar Spine MRI for Low Back Pain[1]	-	-	37.6%	37.2%

New Ulm Medical Center

1324 Fifth North Street
New Ulm, MN 56073
URL: www.newulmmedicalcenter.com
Phone: 507-233-1000
Fax: 507-233-1552
Type: Critical Access Hospitals
Emergency Services: Yes
Ownership: Voluntary non-profit - Private
Beds: 62

Key Personnel:
Radiology.................. Kathleen Bauer
Intensive Care Unit........... Chris Goplin
Emergency Room .... Joan Krikava
Chief of Medical Staff.......... John Krikavar, MD
Hemotology Center .... Brenda Nielsen
Infection Control............... Connie Thompson
Quality Assurance .... Kathy Thompson

Measure	Cases	This Hosp.	State Avg.	U.S. Avg.
Blood Clot Prevention and Treatment				
Anticoagulation Overlap Therapy[2]	17	88%	96%	93%
ICU Venous Thromboembolism Prophylaxis[2,7]	-	-	91%	92%
Incidence of Potentially Preventable VTE[1,2]	-	-	9%	10%
UFH with Dosages/Platelet Monitoring[2]	13	100%	98%	97%
Venous Thromboembolism Prophylaxis[2]	123	93%	86%	85%
Warfarin Therapy Discharge Instructions[2]	12	58%	63%	75%
Chest Pain/Possible Heart Attack Care				
Aspirin Given Within 24 Hours of Arrival	40	100%	97%	96%
Fibrinolytic Meds Within 30 Min. of Arrival[1]	-	-	48%	58%
Average Time to ECG (minutes)	40	3	7	7
Average Time to Transfer (minutes)[1]	-	-	54	60
Children's Asthma Care				
Received Home Management Plan of Care	-	-	-	88%
Received Reliever Medication	-	-	-	100%
Received Systemic Corticosteroids	-	-	-	100%
Emergency Department				
Admittance Decision Time (minutes)[2]	308	110	62	98
Head CT Results Within 45 Min. of Arrival[1]	-	-	54%	57%
Patients Who Left ER Before Being Seen	11,382	1%	2%	2%
Time from ER Arrival to Admit. (minutes)[2]	326	198	199	274
Time from ER Arrival to Discharge (minutes)	373	89	125	134
Time in ER Before Being Evaluated (minutes)	409	20	31	26
Time to Pain Meds for Fractures (minutes)	37	30	45	57
Heart Attack Care				
Aspirin Given at Discharge[1]	-	-	99%	99%
Fibrinolytic Meds Within 30 Min. of Arrival[7]	-	-	-	54%
PCI Within 90 Minutes of Arrival[7]	-	-	96%	96%
Statin Prescribed at Discharge[1]	-	-	99%	98%
Heart Failure Care				
ACE Inhibitor or ARB for LVSD[1]	-	-	96%	97%
Discharge Instructions Given	47	98%	93%	94%
Evaluation of LVS Function	67	99%	97%	99%
Medicare Spending				
Medicare Spending per Patient (ratio)	-	-	0.9	0.98
Pneumonia Care				

NOTE: Hospital profiles are in alphabetical order by state, then city, then hospital within the city; Rankings exclude hospitals with less than 25 cases except for patient surveys which excludes hospitals with less than 100 cases; (a) 100-299 cases; (1) The number of cases/patients is too few to report; (2) Data submitted were based on a sample of cases/patients; (3) Results are based on a shorter time period than required; (4) Data suppressed by CMS for one or more quarters; (5) Results are not available for this reporting period; (6) Fewer than 100 patients completed the HCAHPS survey; (7) No cases met the criteria for this measure; (8) The lower limit of the confidence interval cannot be calculated if the number of observed infections equals zero; (9) No data are available from the state/territory for this reporting period; (10) The scores shown reflect fewer than 50 completed surveys; (11) There were discrepancies in the data collection process; (12) This measure does not apply to this hospital for this reporting period; (13) Results cannot be calculated for this reporting period; (14) The results for this state are combined with nearby states to protect confidentiality; Please refer to the User's Guide for a full explanation of data.

Measure	Cases	This Hosp.	State Avg.	U.S. Avg.
Appropriate Initial Antibiotic Given	26	100%	94%	95%
Blood Culture Timing	54	100%	97%	98%
Pregnancy and Delivery Care				
Newborn Deliveries Scheduled Early[2]	22	5%	5%	6%
Preventive Care				
Immunization for Influenza[2]	253	92%	89%	90%
Immunization for Pneumonia[2]	323	95%	89%	92%
Stroke Care				
Anticoagulation Therapy for Atrial Fibrillation[1]	-	-	96%	95%
Antithrombotic Therapy Timing[1]	-	-	98%	98%
Assessed for Rehabilitation	13	100%	98%	97%
Discharged on Antithrombotic Therapy	12	100%	99%	99%
Discharged on Statin Medication[1]	-	-	95%	94%
Thrombolytic Therapy Timing[7]	-	-	74%	66%
Venous Thromboembolism Prophylaxis[1]	-	-	95%	94%
Written Stroke Educational Materials Given[1]	-	-	88%	88%
Surgical Care Improvement Project				
Appropriate Beta Blocker Usage	50	100%	98%	98%
Appropriate VTP Within 24 Hours	135	99%	98%	98%
Controlled Postoperative Blood Glucose[7]	-	-	97%	97%
Perioperative Temperature Management	146	99%	99%	100%
Prophylactic Antibiotic Selection	117	100%	99%	99%
Prophylactic Antibiotic Selection (Outpatient)	27	100%	98%	98%
Prophylactic Antibiotic Stopped	116	100%	99%	98%
Prophylactic Antibiotic Timing	117	99%	98%	99%
Prophylactic Antibiotic Timing (Outpatient)	27	100%	97%	98%
Urinary Catheter Removal	56	100%	97%	97%
Survey of Patients' Hospital Experiences				
Area Around Room 'Always' Quiet at Night	300+	63%	65%	61%
Doctors 'Always' Communicated Well	300+	88%	84%	82%
Home Recovery Information Given	300+	88%	88%	85%
Hospital Given 9 or 10 on 10 Point Scale	300+	75%	74%	71%
Meds 'Always' Explained Before Given	300+	65%	67%	64%
Nurses 'Always' Communicated Well	300+	81%	81%	79%
Pain 'Always' Well Controlled	300+	74%	72%	71%
Room and Bathroom 'Always' Clean	300+	83%	78%	73%
Timely Help 'Always' Received	300+	74%	74%	68%
Would Definitely Recommend Hospital	300+	75%	71%	71%
Use of Medical Imaging				
Cardiac Imaging Stress Test before Surgery	133	5.3%	6.3%	5.3%
Combination Abdominal CT Scan	247	6.1%	5.7%	10.5%
Combination Brain/Sinus CT Scan[1]	-	-	2.3%	2.7%
Combination Chest CT Scan	187	0.5%	1.9%	2.7%
Follow-up Mammogram/Ultrasound	572	5.4%	6.3%	8.8%
Lumbar Spine MRI for Low Back Pain	71	25.4%	37.6%	37.2%

Northfield Hospital

2000 North Avenue
Northfield, MN 55057
Phone: 507-646-1001
Fax: 507-646-1392
E-mail: richardsons@northfieldhospital.org
URL: www.northfieldhospital.org
Type: Acute Care Hospitals
Emergency Services: Yes
Ownership: Government - Local
Beds: 37

Key Personnel:

Radiology. . . . . Charles Donovan
Emergency Room . . . . Doris Ertekeson
Operating Room. . . . . Karen Geiger
Coronary Care . . . . Margi Henry
Anesthesiology. . . . . Dan Olson
Quality Assurance . . . . Laura Peterson
Infection Control. . . . . Bernice Pulja
CEO/President. . . . . Steve Underdahl

Measure	Cases	This Hosp.	State Avg.	U.S. Avg.
Blood Clot Prevention and Treatment				
Anticoagulation Overlap Therapy[1,2]	-	-	96%	93%
ICU Venous Thromboembolism Prophylaxis[2,7]	-	-	91%	92%
Incidence of Potentially Preventable VTE[2,7]	-	-	9%	10%
UFH with Dosages/Platelet Monitoring[2,7]	-	-	98%	97%
Venous Thromboembolism Prophylaxis[2]	112	74%	86%	85%
Warfarin Therapy Discharge Instructions[1,2]	-	-	63%	75%
Chest Pain/Possible Heart Attack Care				
Aspirin Given Within 24 Hours of Arrival	79	95%	97%	96%
Fibrinolytic Meds Within 30 Min. of Arrival[1]	-	-	48%	58%
Average Time to ECG (minutes)	83	7	7	7
Average Time to Transfer (minutes)[1]	-	-	54	60
Children's Asthma Care				
Received Home Management Plan of Care	-	-	-	88%
Received Reliever Medication	-	-	-	100%
Received Systemic Corticosteroids	-	-	-	100%
Emergency Department				
Admittance Decision Time (minutes)[2]	107	68	62	98
Head CT Results Within 45 Min. of Arrival[1]	-	-	54%	57%
Patients Who Left ER Before Being Seen	10,104	0%	2%	2%
Time from ER Arrival to Admit. (minutes)[2]	132	182	199	274
Time from ER Arrival to Discharge (minutes)	428	102	125	134
Time in ER Before Being Evaluated (minutes)	483	19	31	26
Time to Pain Meds for Fractures (minutes)	34	48	45	57
Heart Attack Care				
Aspirin Given at Discharge[1,3]	-	-	99%	99%
Fibrinolytic Meds Within 30 Min. of Arrival[3,7]	-	-	-	54%
PCI Within 90 Minutes of Arrival[3,7]	-	-	96%	96%
Statin Prescribed at Discharge[1,3]	-	-	99%	98%
Heart Failure Care				
ACE Inhibitor or ARB for LVSD[1]	-	-	96%	97%
Discharge Instructions Given	26	54%	93%	94%
Evaluation of LVS Function	46	96%	97%	99%
Medicare Spending				
Medicare Spending per Patient (ratio)	-	0.81	0.9	0.98
Pneumonia Care				
Appropriate Initial Antibiotic Given	24	92%	94%	95%
Blood Culture Timing	22	100%	97%	98%
Pregnancy and Delivery Care				
Newborn Deliveries Scheduled Early[2]	34	6%	5%	6%
Preventive Care				
Immunization for Influenza[2]	257	90%	89%	90%
Immunization for Pneumonia[2]	225	92%	89%	92%
Stroke Care				
Anticoagulation Therapy for Atrial Fibrillation[1]	-	-	96%	95%
Antithrombotic Therapy Timing[1]	-	-	98%	98%
Assessed for Rehabilitation[1]	-	-	98%	97%
Discharged on Antithrombotic Therapy[1]	-	-	99%	99%
Discharged on Statin Medication[1]	-	-	95%	94%
Thrombolytic Therapy Timing[7]	-	-	74%	66%
Venous Thromboembolism Prophylaxis[1]	-	-	95%	94%
Written Stroke Educational Materials Given[1]	-	-	88%	88%
Surgical Care Improvement Project				
Appropriate Beta Blocker Usage	48	94%	98%	98%
Appropriate VTP Within 24 Hours	175	97%	98%	98%
Controlled Postoperative Blood Glucose[7]	-	-	97%	97%
Perioperative Temperature Management	185	99%	99%	100%
Prophylactic Antibiotic Selection	153	99%	99%	99%
Prophylactic Antibiotic Selection (Outpatient)	24	100%	98%	98%
Prophylactic Antibiotic Stopped	151	97%	99%	98%
Prophylactic Antibiotic Timing	153	99%	98%	99%
Prophylactic Antibiotic Timing (Outpatient)	24	100%	97%	98%
Urinary Catheter Removal	121	99%	97%	97%
Survey of Patients' Hospital Experiences				
Area Around Room 'Always' Quiet at Night	300+	61%	65%	61%
Doctors 'Always' Communicated Well	300+	85%	84%	82%
Home Recovery Information Given	300+	87%	88%	85%
Hospital Given 9 or 10 on 10 Point Scale	300+	77%	74%	71%
Meds 'Always' Explained Before Given	300+	63%	67%	64%
Nurses 'Always' Communicated Well	300+	81%	81%	79%
Pain 'Always' Well Controlled	300+	71%	72%	71%
Room and Bathroom 'Always' Clean	300+	74%	78%	73%
Timely Help 'Always' Received	300+	75%	74%	68%
Would Definitely Recommend Hospital	300+	78%	71%	71%
Use of Medical Imaging				
Cardiac Imaging Stress Test before Surgery[1]	-	-	6.3%	5.3%
Combination Abdominal CT Scan	112	2.7%	5.7%	10.5%
Combination Brain/Sinus CT Scan[1]	-	-	2.3%	2.7%
Combination Chest CT Scan	101	1.0%	1.9%	2.7%
Follow-up Mammogram/Ultrasound	151	12.6%	6.3%	8.8%
Lumbar Spine MRI for Low Back Pain[1]	-	-	37.6%	37.2%

Renville County Hospital & Clinics

611 East Fairview
Olivia, MN 56277
Phone: 320-523-1261
Fax: 320-523-3490
E-mail: mahers@rchospital.com
URL: www.renvillecountyhospital.org
Type: Critical Access Hospitals
Emergency Services: Yes
Ownership: Voluntary non-profit - Other
Beds: 41

Key Personnel:

CEO/President. . . . . Glenn Haugo
Chief of Medical Staff . . . . Paul E Thompson

Measure	Cases	This Hosp.	State Avg.	U.S. Avg.
Blood Clot Prevention and Treatment				
Anticoagulation Overlap Therapy[5]	-	-	96%	93%
ICU Venous Thromboembolism Prophylaxis[5]	-	-	91%	92%
Incidence of Potentially Preventable VTE[5]	-	-	9%	10%
UFH with Dosages/Platelet Monitoring[5]	-	-	98%	97%
Venous Thromboembolism Prophylaxis[5]	-	-	86%	85%
Warfarin Therapy Discharge Instructions[5]	-	-	63%	75%
Chest Pain/Possible Heart Attack Care				
Aspirin Given Within 24 Hours of Arrival	11	91%	97%	96%
Fibrinolytic Meds Within 30 Min. of Arrival[7]	-	-	48%	58%
Average Time to ECG (minutes)[1]	-	-	7	7
Average Time to Transfer (minutes)[7]	-	-	54	60
Children's Asthma Care				
Received Home Management Plan of Care	-	-	-	88%
Received Reliever Medication	-	-	-	100%
Received Systemic Corticosteroids	-	-	-	100%
Emergency Department				
Admittance Decision Time (minutes)	11	0	62	98
Head CT Results Within 45 Min. of Arrival[5]	-	-	54%	57%
Patients Who Left ER Before Being Seen[5]	-	-	2%	2%
Time from ER Arrival to Admit. (minutes)	17	107	199	274
Time from ER Arrival to Discharge (minutes)[5]	-	-	125	134
Time in ER Before Being Evaluated (minutes)[5]	-	-	31	26
Time to Pain Meds for Fractures (minutes)[5]	-	-	45	57
Heart Attack Care				
Aspirin Given at Discharge[1,3]	-	-	99%	99%
Fibrinolytic Meds Within 30 Min. of Arrival[3,7]	-	-	-	54%
PCI Within 90 Minutes of Arrival[3,7]	-	-	96%	96%
Statin Prescribed at Discharge[1,3]	-	-	99%	98%
Heart Failure Care				
ACE Inhibitor or ARB for LVSD[1,3]	-	-	96%	97%
Discharge Instructions Given[1,3]	-	-	93%	94%
Evaluation of LVS Function[1,3]	-	-	97%	99%
Medicare Spending				
Medicare Spending per Patient (ratio)	-	-	0.9	0.98
Pneumonia Care				
Appropriate Initial Antibiotic Given[1,3]	-	-	94%	95%
Blood Culture Timing[3,7]	-	-	97%	98%
Pregnancy and Delivery Care				
Newborn Deliveries Scheduled Early[5]	-	-	5%	6%
Preventive Care				
Immunization for Influenza	72	83%	89%	90%
Immunization for Pneumonia	101	79%	89%	92%
Stroke Care				
Anticoagulation Therapy for Atrial Fibrillation[5]	-	-	96%	95%
Antithrombotic Therapy Timing[5]	-	-	98%	98%
Assessed for Rehabilitation[5]	-	-	98%	97%
Discharged on Antithrombotic Therapy[5]	-	-	99%	99%
Discharged on Statin Medication[5]	-	-	95%	94%
Thrombolytic Therapy Timing[5]	-	-	74%	66%
Venous Thromboembolism Prophylaxis[5]	-	-	95%	94%
Written Stroke Educational Materials Given[5]	-	-	88%	88%
Surgical Care Improvement Project				
Appropriate Beta Blocker Usage[5]	-	-	98%	98%
Appropriate VTP Within 24 Hours[5]	-	-	98%	98%
Controlled Postoperative Blood Glucose[5]	-	-	97%	97%
Perioperative Temperature Management[5]	-	-	99%	100%
Prophylactic Antibiotic Selection[5]	-	-	99%	99%
Prophylactic Antibiotic Selection (Outpatient)[5]	-	-	98%	98%
Prophylactic Antibiotic Stopped[5]	-	-	99%	98%
Prophylactic Antibiotic Timing[5]	-	-	98%	99%
Prophylactic Antibiotic Timing (Outpatient)[5]	-	-	97%	98%

NOTE: Hospital profiles are in alphabetical order by state, then city, then hospital within the city; Rankings exclude hospitals with less than 25 cases except for patient surveys which excludes hospitals with less than 100 cases; (a) 100-299 cases; (1) The number of cases/patients is too few to report; (2) Data submitted were based on a sample of cases/patients; (3) Results are based on a shorter time period than required; (4) Data suppressed by CMS for one or more quarters; (5) Results are not available for this reporting period; (6) Fewer than 100 patients completed the HCAHPS survey; (7) No cases met the criteria for this measure; (8) The lower limit of the confidence interval cannot be calculated if the number of observed infections equals zero; (9) No data are available from the state/territory for this reporting period; (10) The scores shown reflect fewer than 50 completed surveys; (11) There were discrepancies in the data collection process; (12) This measure does not apply to this hospital for this reporting period; (13) Results cannot be calculated for this reporting period; (14) The results for this state are combined with nearby states to protect confidentiality; Please refer to the User's Guide for a full explanation of data.

Measure	Cases	This Hosp.	State Avg.	U.S. Avg.
Urinary Catheter Removal[5]	-	-	97%	97%
Survey of Patients' Hospital Experiences				
Area Around Room 'Always' Quiet at Night[6,11]	<100	69%	65%	61%
Doctors 'Always' Communicated Well[6,11]	<100	82%	84%	82%
Home Recovery Information Given[6,11]	<100	89%	88%	85%
Hospital Given 9 or 10 on 10 Point Scale[6,11]	<100	69%	74%	71%
Meds 'Always' Explained Before Given[6,11]	<100	54%	67%	64%
Nurses 'Always' Communicated Well[6,11]	<100	78%	81%	79%
Pain 'Always' Well Controlled[6,11]	<100	58%	72%	71%
Room and Bathroom 'Always' Clean[6,11]	<100	88%	78%	73%
Timely Help 'Always' Received[6,11]	<100	77%	74%	68%
Would Definitely Recommend Hospital[6,11]	<100	44%	71%	71%
Use of Medical Imaging				
Cardiac Imaging Stress Test before Surgery[1]	-	-	6.3%	5.3%
Combination Abdominal CT Scan	44	59.1%	5.7%	10.5%
Combination Brain/Sinus CT Scan	68	0.0%	2.3%	2.7%
Combination Chest CT Scan[1]	-	-	1.9%	2.7%
Follow-up Mammogram/Ultrasound	149	4.7%	6.3%	8.8%
Lumbar Spine MRI for Low Back Pain[1]	-	-	37.6%	37.2%

Mille Lacs Health System

200 North Elm Street
Onamia, MN 56359
Phone: 320-532-8020
Fax: 320-532-3111
Type: Critical Access Hospitals
Emergency Services: Yes
Ownership: Voluntary non-profit - Private
Beds: 108

Key Personnel:
Cardiology . . . . Richard Aplin, MD
Cardiology . . . . Richard Backes, MD
Radiology. . . . . Andrew Burnside
Operating Room. . . . . Linda Heinrich
Surgery . . . . Richard Kubicka, MD
CEO . . . . Bill Nelson
Surgery . . . . Joseph Pietrafitta, MD
Chief of Medical Staff. . . . . Arden Virnig, MD

Measure	Cases	This Hosp.	State Avg.	U.S. Avg.
Blood Clot Prevention and Treatment				
Anticoagulation Overlap Therapy[3,7]	-	-	96%	93%
ICU Venous Thromboembolism Prophylaxis[3,7]	-	-	91%	92%
Incidence of Potentially Preventable VTE[3,7]	-	-	9%	10%
UFH with Dosages/Platelet Monitoring[3,7]	-	-	98%	97%
Venous Thromboembolism Prophylaxis[1,3]	-	-	86%	85%
Warfarin Therapy Discharge Instructions[3,7]	-	-	63%	75%
Chest Pain/Possible Heart Attack Care				
Aspirin Given Within 24 Hours of Arrival	32	100%	97%	96%
Fibrinolytic Meds Within 30 Min. of Arrival[3,7]	-	-	48%	58%
Average Time to ECG (minutes)	33	6	7	7
Average Time to Transfer (minutes)[3,7]	-	-	54	60
Children's Asthma Care				
Received Home Management Plan of Care	-	-	-	88%
Received Reliever Medication	-	-	-	100%
Received Systemic Corticosteroids	-	-	-	100%
Emergency Department				
Admittance Decision Time (minutes)[2]	349	37	62	98
Head CT Results Within 45 Min. of Arrival[1]	-	-	54%	57%
Patients Who Left ER Before Being Seen[5]	-	-	2%	2%
Time from ER Arrival to Admit. (minutes)[2]	357	180	199	274
Time from ER Arrival to Discharge (minutes)[5]	-	-	125	134
Time in ER Before Being Evaluated (minutes)[5]	-	-	31	26
Time to Pain Meds for Fractures (minutes)	26	24	45	57
Heart Attack Care				
Aspirin Given at Discharge[1,3]	-	-	99%	99%
Fibrinolytic Meds Within 30 Min. of Arrival[3,7]	-	-	-	54%
PCI Within 90 Minutes of Arrival[3,7]	-	-	96%	96%
Statin Prescribed at Discharge[1,3]	-	-	99%	98%
Heart Failure Care				
ACE Inhibitor or ARB for LVSD[1,2]	-	-	96%	97%
Discharge Instructions Given[2]	30	97%	93%	94%
Evaluation of LVS Function[2]	35	97%	97%	99%
Medicare Spending				
Medicare Spending per Patient (ratio)	-	-	0.9	0.98
Pneumonia Care				
Appropriate Initial Antibiotic Given	25	88%	94%	95%
Blood Culture Timing	33	91%	97%	98%
Pregnancy and Delivery Care				
Newborn Deliveries Scheduled Early[5]	-	-	5%	6%
Preventive Care				
Immunization for Influenza[2]	190	83%	89%	90%
Immunization for Pneumonia[2]	229	90%	89%	92%
Stroke Care				
Anticoagulation Therapy for Atrial Fibrillation[5]	-	-	96%	95%
Antithrombotic Therapy Timing[5]	-	-	98%	98%
Assessed for Rehabilitation[5]	-	-	98%	97%
Discharged on Antithrombotic Therapy[5]	-	-	99%	99%
Discharged on Statin Medication[5]	-	-	95%	94%
Thrombolytic Therapy Timing[5]	-	-	74%	66%
Venous Thromboembolism Prophylaxis[5]	-	-	95%	94%
Written Stroke Educational Materials Given[5]	-	-	88%	88%
Surgical Care Improvement Project				
Appropriate Beta Blocker Usage[1,3]	-	-	98%	98%
Appropriate VTP Within 24 Hours[1,3]	-	-	98%	98%
Controlled Postoperative Blood Glucose[3,7]	-	-	97%	97%
Perioperative Temperature Management[1,3]	-	-	99%	100%
Prophylactic Antibiotic Selection[1,3]	-	-	99%	99%
Prophylactic Antibiotic Selection (Outpatient)[1,3]	-	-	98%	98%
Prophylactic Antibiotic Stopped[1,3]	-	-	99%	98%
Prophylactic Antibiotic Timing[1,3]	-	-	98%	99%
Prophylactic Antibiotic Timing (Outpatient)[1,3]	-	-	97%	98%
Urinary Catheter Removal[3,7]	-	-	97%	97%
Survey of Patients' Hospital Experiences				
Area Around Room 'Always' Quiet at Night	(a)	64%	65%	61%
Doctors 'Always' Communicated Well	(a)	93%	84%	82%
Home Recovery Information Given	(a)	94%	88%	85%
Hospital Given 9 or 10 on 10 Point Scale	(a)	77%	74%	71%
Meds 'Always' Explained Before Given	(a)	76%	67%	64%
Nurses 'Always' Communicated Well	(a)	87%	81%	79%
Pain 'Always' Well Controlled	(a)	76%	72%	71%
Room and Bathroom 'Always' Clean	(a)	84%	78%	73%
Timely Help 'Always' Received	(a)	77%	74%	68%
Would Definitely Recommend Hospital	(a)	76%	71%	71%
Use of Medical Imaging				
Cardiac Imaging Stress Test before Surgery[1]	-	-	6.3%	5.3%
Combination Abdominal CT Scan	63	1.6%	5.7%	10.5%
Combination Brain/Sinus CT Scan	79	0.0%	2.3%	2.7%
Combination Chest CT Scan[1]	-	-	1.9%	2.7%
Follow-up Mammogram/Ultrasound	118	9.3%	6.3%	8.8%
Lumbar Spine MRI for Low Back Pain[1]	-	-	37.6%	37.2%

Ortonville Area Health Services

450 Eastvold Ave
Ortonville, MN 56278
Phone: 320-839-2502
Fax: 320-839-4107
E-mail: lillehak@oahs.us
URL: www.oahs.us
Type: Critical Access Hospitals
Emergency Services: Yes
Ownership: Government - Local
Beds: 105

Key Personnel:
CEO/President. . . . . Richard Ash
Chief of Medical Staff. . . . . Bryan S Delage, MD
Quality Assurance . . . . Jeanette Felton, RN
Infection Control. . . . . Kristine Meyer
Operating Room. . . . . Ranet Schmeichel
Emergency Room . . . . Linda Sis
Anesthesiology. . . . . John Sovell

Measure	Cases	This Hosp.	State Avg.	U.S. Avg.
Blood Clot Prevention and Treatment				
Anticoagulation Overlap Therapy[5]	-	-	96%	93%
ICU Venous Thromboembolism Prophylaxis[5]	-	-	91%	92%
Incidence of Potentially Preventable VTE[5]	-	-	9%	10%
UFH with Dosages/Platelet Monitoring[5]	-	-	98%	97%
Venous Thromboembolism Prophylaxis[5]	-	-	86%	85%
Warfarin Therapy Discharge Instructions[5]	-	-	63%	75%
Chest Pain/Possible Heart Attack Care				
Aspirin Given Within 24 Hours of Arrival[1]	-	-	97%	96%
Fibrinolytic Meds Within 30 Min. of Arrival[1]	-	-	48%	58%
Average Time to ECG (minutes)[1]	-	-	7	7
Average Time to Transfer (minutes)[1]	-	-	54	60
Children's Asthma Care				
Received Home Management Plan of Care	-	-	-	88%
Received Reliever Medication	-	-	-	100%
Received Systemic Corticosteroids	-	-	-	100%
Emergency Department				
Admittance Decision Time (minutes)	88	0	62	98
Head CT Results Within 45 Min. of Arrival[5]	-	-	54%	57%
Patients Who Left ER Before Being Seen[5]	-	-	2%	2%
Time from ER Arrival to Admit. (minutes)	88	126	199	274
Time from ER Arrival to Discharge (minutes)[5]	-	-	125	134
Time in ER Before Being Evaluated (minutes)[5]	-	-	31	26
Time to Pain Meds for Fractures (minutes)[5]	-	-	45	57
Heart Attack Care				
Aspirin Given at Discharge[1,3]	-	-	99%	99%
Fibrinolytic Meds Within 30 Min. of Arrival[3,7]	-	-	-	54%
PCI Within 90 Minutes of Arrival[3,7]	-	-	96%	96%
Statin Prescribed at Discharge[1,3]	-	-	99%	98%
Heart Failure Care				
ACE Inhibitor or ARB for LVSD[3,7]	-	-	96%	97%
Discharge Instructions Given[1,3]	-	-	93%	94%
Evaluation of LVS Function[1,3]	-	-	97%	99%
Medicare Spending				
Medicare Spending per Patient (ratio)	-	-	0.9	0.98
Pneumonia Care				
Appropriate Initial Antibiotic Given[1,3]	-	-	94%	95%
Blood Culture Timing[3,7]	-	-	97%	98%
Pregnancy and Delivery Care				
Newborn Deliveries Scheduled Early[5]	-	-	5%	6%
Preventive Care				
Immunization for Influenza	29	100%	89%	90%
Immunization for Pneumonia	111	93%	89%	92%
Stroke Care				
Anticoagulation Therapy for Atrial Fibrillation[5]	-	-	96%	95%
Antithrombotic Therapy Timing[5]	-	-	98%	98%
Assessed for Rehabilitation[5]	-	-	98%	97%
Discharged on Antithrombotic Therapy[5]	-	-	99%	99%
Discharged on Statin Medication[5]	-	-	95%	94%
Thrombolytic Therapy Timing[5]	-	-	74%	66%
Venous Thromboembolism Prophylaxis[5]	-	-	95%	94%
Written Stroke Educational Materials Given[5]	-	-	88%	88%
Surgical Care Improvement Project				
Appropriate Beta Blocker Usage[3,7]	-	-	98%	98%
Appropriate VTP Within 24 Hours[1,3]	-	-	98%	98%
Controlled Postoperative Blood Glucose[3,7]	-	-	97%	97%
Perioperative Temperature Management[1,3]	-	-	99%	100%
Prophylactic Antibiotic Selection[1,3]	-	-	99%	99%
Prophylactic Antibiotic Selection (Outpatient)[1,3]	-	-	98%	98%
Prophylactic Antibiotic Stopped[1,3]	-	-	99%	98%
Prophylactic Antibiotic Timing[1,3]	-	-	98%	99%
Prophylactic Antibiotic Timing (Outpatient)[1,3]	-	-	97%	98%
Urinary Catheter Removal[1,3]	-	-	97%	97%
Survey of Patients' Hospital Experiences				
Area Around Room 'Always' Quiet at Night[6]	<100	74%	65%	61%
Doctors 'Always' Communicated Well[6]	<100	88%	84%	82%
Home Recovery Information Given[6]	<100	86%	88%	85%
Hospital Given 9 or 10 on 10 Point Scale[6]	<100	82%	74%	71%
Meds 'Always' Explained Before Given[6]	<100	54%	67%	64%
Nurses 'Always' Communicated Well[6]	<100	79%	81%	79%
Pain 'Always' Well Controlled[6]	<100	69%	72%	71%
Room and Bathroom 'Always' Clean[6]	<100	82%	78%	73%
Timely Help 'Always' Received[6]	<100	83%	74%	68%
Would Definitely Recommend Hospital[6]	<100	84%	71%	71%
Use of Medical Imaging				
Cardiac Imaging Stress Test before Surgery	47	2.1%	6.3%	5.3%
Combination Abdominal CT Scan	81	81.5%	5.7%	10.5%
Combination Brain/Sinus CT Scan[1]	-	-	2.3%	2.7%
Combination Chest CT Scan[1]	-	-	1.9%	2.7%
Follow-up Mammogram/Ultrasound	203	4.4%	6.3%	8.8%
Lumbar Spine MRI for Low Back Pain[1]	-	-	37.6%	37.2%

NOTE: Hospital profiles are in alphabetical order by state, then city, then hospital within the city; Rankings exclude hospitals with less than 25 cases except for patient surveys which excludes hospitals with less than 100 cases; (a) 100-299 cases; (1) The number of cases/patients is too few to report; (2) Data submitted were based on a sample of cases/patients; (3) Results are based on a shorter time period than required; (4) Data suppressed by CMS for one or more quarters; (5) Results are not available for this reporting period; (6) Fewer than 100 patients completed the HCAHPS survey; (7) No cases met the criteria for this measure; (8) The lower limit of the confidence interval cannot be calculated if the number of observed infections equals zero; (9) No data are available from the state/territory for this reporting period; (10) The scores shown reflect fewer than 50 completed surveys; (11) There were discrepancies in the data collection process; (12) This measure does not apply to this hospital for this reporting period; (13) Results cannot be calculated for this reporting period; (14) The results for this state are combined with nearby states to protect confidentiality; Please refer to the User's Guide for a full explanation of data.

Owatonna Hospital

2250 26th Street Northwest
Owatonna, MN 55060
URL: www.owatonnahospital.com
Type: Acute Care Hospitals
Ownership: Voluntary non-profit - Other
Phone: 507-451-3850
Fax: 507-444-6053
Emergency Services: Yes
Beds: 77

Key Personnel:
Radiology.................. Joseph Accurso
CEO/President............... David Albrecht
Chief of Medical Staff.......... Michael Baker, MD
Quality Assurance .... Becky Christensen
Coronary Care .... Sharon Kopp
Infection Control............. Pam Schultz

Measure	Cases	This Hosp.	State Avg.	U.S. Avg.
Blood Clot Prevention and Treatment				
Anticoagulation Overlap Therapy[2]	19	84%	96%	93%
ICU Venous Thromboembolism Prophylaxis[2,7]	-	-	91%	92%
Incidence of Potentially Preventable VTE[1,2]	-	-	9%	10%
UFH with Dosages/Platelet Monitoring[1,2]	-	-	98%	97%
Venous Thromboembolism Prophylaxis[2]	163	91%	86%	85%
Warfarin Therapy Discharge Instructions[2]	14	50%	63%	75%
Chest Pain/Possible Heart Attack Care				
Aspirin Given Within 24 Hours of Arrival	72	100%	97%	96%
Fibrinolytic Meds Within 30 Min. of Arrival[1]	-	-	48%	58%
Average Time to ECG (minutes)	75	6	7	7
Average Time to Transfer (minutes)[1]	-	-	54	60
Children's Asthma Care				
Received Home Management Plan of Care	-	-	-	88%
Received Reliever Medication	-	-	-	100%
Received Systemic Corticosteroids	-	-	-	100%
Emergency Department				
Admittance Decision Time (minutes)[2]	238	99	62	98
Head CT Results Within 45 Min. of Arrival[1]	-	-	54%	57%
Patients Who Left ER Before Being Seen	13,677	1%	2%	2%
Time from ER Arrival to Admit. (minutes)[2]	239	219	199	274
Time from ER Arrival to Discharge (minutes)	349	115	125	134
Time in ER Before Being Evaluated (minutes)	398	12	31	26
Time to Pain Meds for Fractures (minutes)	49	35	45	57
Heart Attack Care				
Aspirin Given at Discharge	16	100%	99%	99%
Fibrinolytic Meds Within 30 Min. of Arrival[7]	-	-	-	54%
PCI Within 90 Minutes of Arrival[7]	-	-	96%	96%
Statin Prescribed at Discharge	17	88%	99%	98%
Heart Failure Care				
ACE Inhibitor or ARB for LVSD	11	100%	96%	97%
Discharge Instructions Given	47	96%	93%	94%
Evaluation of LVS Function	76	100%	97%	99%
Medicare Spending				
Medicare Spending per Patient (ratio)	-	0.87	0.9	0.98
Pneumonia Care				
Appropriate Initial Antibiotic Given	43	98%	94%	95%
Blood Culture Timing	36	97%	97%	98%
Pregnancy and Delivery Care				
Newborn Deliveries Scheduled Early[2]	40	10%	5%	6%
Preventive Care				
Immunization for Influenza[2]	242	89%	89%	90%
Immunization for Pneumonia[2]	224	94%	89%	92%
Stroke Care				
Anticoagulation Therapy for Atrial Fibrillation[1]	-	-	96%	95%
Antithrombotic Therapy Timing[1]	-	-	98%	98%
Assessed for Rehabilitation[1]	-	-	98%	97%
Discharged on Antithrombotic Therapy[1]	-	-	99%	99%
Discharged on Statin Medication[1]	-	-	95%	94%
Thrombolytic Therapy Timing[7]	-	-	74%	66%
Venous Thromboembolism Prophylaxis[1]	-	-	95%	94%
Written Stroke Educational Materials Given[1]	-	-	88%	88%
Surgical Care Improvement Project				
Appropriate Beta Blocker Usage[2]	65	98%	98%	98%
Appropriate VTP Within 24 Hours[2]	160	99%	98%	98%
Controlled Postoperative Blood Glucose[2,7]	-	-	97%	97%
Perioperative Temperature Management[2]	192	100%	99%	100%
Prophylactic Antibiotic Selection[2]	145	100%	99%	99%
Prophylactic Antibiotic Selection (Outpatient)	108	98%	98%	98%
Prophylactic Antibiotic Stopped[2]	140	98%	99%	98%
Prophylactic Antibiotic Timing[2]	145	99%	98%	99%
Prophylactic Antibiotic Timing (Outpatient)	108	95%	97%	98%
Urinary Catheter Removal[2]	134	99%	97%	97%
Survey of Patients' Hospital Experiences				
Area Around Room 'Always' Quiet at Night	300+	60%	65%	61%
Doctors 'Always' Communicated Well	300+	83%	84%	82%
Home Recovery Information Given	300+	87%	88%	85%
Hospital Given 9 or 10 on 10 Point Scale	300+	73%	74%	71%
Meds 'Always' Explained Before Given	300+	62%	67%	64%
Nurses 'Always' Communicated Well	300+	79%	81%	79%
Pain 'Always' Well Controlled	300+	72%	72%	71%
Room and Bathroom 'Always' Clean	300+	77%	78%	73%
Timely Help 'Always' Received	300+	73%	74%	68%
Would Definitely Recommend Hospital	300+	74%	71%	71%
Use of Medical Imaging				
Cardiac Imaging Stress Test before Surgery[7]	-	-	6.3%	5.3%
Combination Abdominal CT Scan	136	5.1%	5.7%	10.5%
Combination Brain/Sinus CT Scan[1]	-	-	2.3%	2.7%
Combination Chest CT Scan	104	1.0%	1.9%	2.7%
Follow-up Mammogram/Ultrasound[7]	-	-	6.3%	8.8%
Lumbar Spine MRI for Low Back Pain[7]	-	-	37.6%	37.2%

Saint Joseph's Area Health Services

600 Pleasant Avenue
Park Rapids, MN 56470
URL: www.sjahs.org
Type: Critical Access Hospitals
Ownership: Voluntary non-profit - Private
Phone: 218-732-3311
Fax: 218-732-1368
Emergency Services: Yes
Beds: 50

Key Personnel:
Emergency Room .... Darryl A Beehler
Radiology................ Donald G Douglas
Operating Room............ Paulette Goldammer
Patient Relations .... Nancy Hall
CEO/President.............. Ben Koppelman
Intensive Care Unit........... Bob Sauser
Quality Assurance .... Laurie Skare
Ambulatory Care .... Judy Thompson

Measure	Cases	This Hosp.	State Avg.	U.S. Avg.
Blood Clot Prevention and Treatment				
Anticoagulation Overlap Therapy[5]	-	-	96%	93%
ICU Venous Thromboembolism Prophylaxis[5]	-	-	91%	92%
Incidence of Potentially Preventable VTE[5]	-	-	9%	10%
UFH with Dosages/Platelet Monitoring[5]	-	-	98%	97%
Venous Thromboembolism Prophylaxis[5]	-	-	86%	85%
Warfarin Therapy Discharge Instructions[5]	-	-	63%	75%
Chest Pain/Possible Heart Attack Care				
Aspirin Given Within 24 Hours of Arrival	77	100%	97%	96%
Fibrinolytic Meds Within 30 Min. of Arrival[1]	-	-	48%	58%
Average Time to ECG (minutes)	77	15	7	7
Average Time to Transfer (minutes)	13	55	54	60
Children's Asthma Care				
Received Home Management Plan of Care	-	-	-	88%
Received Reliever Medication	-	-	-	100%
Received Systemic Corticosteroids	-	-	-	100%
Emergency Department				
Admittance Decision Time (minutes)[2]	231	58	62	98
Head CT Results Within 45 Min. of Arrival[5]	-	-	54%	57%
Patients Who Left ER Before Being Seen[5]	-	-	2%	2%
Time from ER Arrival to Admit. (minutes)[2]	240	230	199	274
Time from ER Arrival to Discharge (minutes)[5]	-	-	125	134
Time in ER Before Being Evaluated (minutes)[5]	-	-	31	26
Time to Pain Meds for Fractures (minutes)[5]	-	-	45	57
Heart Attack Care				
Aspirin Given at Discharge[1,3]	-	-	99%	99%
Fibrinolytic Meds Within 30 Min. of Arrival[3,7]	-	-	-	54%
PCI Within 90 Minutes of Arrival[3,7]	-	-	96%	96%
Statin Prescribed at Discharge[1,3]	-	-	99%	98%
Heart Failure Care				
ACE Inhibitor or ARB for LVSD[1]	-	-	96%	97%
Discharge Instructions Given	20	90%	93%	94%
Evaluation of LVS Function	23	96%	97%	99%
Medicare Spending				
Medicare Spending per Patient (ratio)	-	-	0.9	0.98
Pneumonia Care				
Appropriate Initial Antibiotic Given	20	90%	94%	95%
Blood Culture Timing	23	96%	97%	98%
Pregnancy and Delivery Care				
Newborn Deliveries Scheduled Early[5]	-	-	5%	6%
Preventive Care				
Immunization for Influenza[2]	274	97%	89%	90%
Immunization for Pneumonia[2]	311	90%	89%	92%
Stroke Care				
Anticoagulation Therapy for Atrial Fibrillation[5]	-	-	96%	95%
Antithrombotic Therapy Timing[5]	-	-	98%	98%
Assessed for Rehabilitation[5]	-	-	98%	97%
Discharged on Antithrombotic Therapy[5]	-	-	99%	99%
Discharged on Statin Medication[5]	-	-	95%	94%
Thrombolytic Therapy Timing[5]	-	-	74%	66%
Venous Thromboembolism Prophylaxis[5]	-	-	95%	94%
Written Stroke Educational Materials Given[5]	-	-	88%	88%
Surgical Care Improvement Project				
Appropriate Beta Blocker Usage[1]	-	-	98%	98%
Appropriate VTP Within 24 Hours	135	99%	98%	98%
Controlled Postoperative Blood Glucose[7]	-	-	97%	97%
Perioperative Temperature Management	149	100%	99%	100%
Prophylactic Antibiotic Selection	20	90%	99%	99%
Prophylactic Antibiotic Selection (Outpatient)[1]	-	-	98%	98%
Prophylactic Antibiotic Stopped	19	95%	99%	98%
Prophylactic Antibiotic Timing	20	95%	98%	99%
Prophylactic Antibiotic Timing (Outpatient)[1]	-	-	97%	98%
Urinary Catheter Removal	97	93%	97%	97%
Survey of Patients' Hospital Experiences				
Area Around Room 'Always' Quiet at Night	(a)	66%	65%	61%
Doctors 'Always' Communicated Well	(a)	87%	84%	82%
Home Recovery Information Given	(a)	90%	88%	85%
Hospital Given 9 or 10 on 10 Point Scale	(a)	79%	74%	71%
Meds 'Always' Explained Before Given	(a)	66%	67%	64%
Nurses 'Always' Communicated Well	(a)	83%	81%	79%
Pain 'Always' Well Controlled	(a)	76%	72%	71%
Room and Bathroom 'Always' Clean	(a)	76%	78%	73%
Timely Help 'Always' Received	(a)	76%	74%	68%
Would Definitely Recommend Hospital	(a)	78%	71%	71%
Use of Medical Imaging				
Cardiac Imaging Stress Test before Surgery	97	8.2%	6.3%	5.3%
Combination Abdominal CT Scan	198	4.0%	5.7%	10.5%
Combination Brain/Sinus CT Scan[1]	-	-	2.3%	2.7%
Combination Chest CT Scan	112	0.9%	1.9%	2.7%
Follow-up Mammogram/Ultrasound	358	7.5%	6.3%	8.8%
Lumbar Spine MRI for Low Back Pain	48	45.8%	37.6%	37.2%

Centra Care Health Paynesville

200 1st Street West
Paynesville, MN 56362
URL: www.pahcs.com
Type: Critical Access Hospitals
Ownership: Govt - Hospital Dist/Auth
Phone: 320-243-3767
Fax: 320-243-6707
Emergency Services: Yes
Beds: 94

Key Personnel:
Radiology.................. Mark Dingmann
Infection Control............. Tami Stanger
CEO/President............... Bobbe Teigen

Measure	Cases	This Hosp.	State Avg.	U.S. Avg.
Blood Clot Prevention and Treatment				
Anticoagulation Overlap Therapy[5]	-	-	96%	93%
ICU Venous Thromboembolism Prophylaxis[5]	-	-	91%	92%
Incidence of Potentially Preventable VTE[5]	-	-	9%	10%
UFH with Dosages/Platelet Monitoring[5]	-	-	98%	97%
Venous Thromboembolism Prophylaxis[5]	-	-	86%	85%
Warfarin Therapy Discharge Instructions[5]	-	-	63%	75%
Chest Pain/Possible Heart Attack Care				
Aspirin Given Within 24 Hours of Arrival	17	100%	97%	96%
Fibrinolytic Meds Within 30 Min. of Arrival[7]	-	-	48%	58%
Average Time to ECG (minutes)	16	4	7	7
Average Time to Transfer (minutes)[1]	-	-	54	60
Children's Asthma Care				
Received Home Management Plan of Care	-	-	-	88%
Received Reliever Medication	-	-	-	100%
Received Systemic Corticosteroids	-	-	-	100%

NOTE: Hospital profiles are in alphabetical order by state, then city, then hospital within the city; Rankings exclude hospitals with less than 25 cases except for patient surveys which excludes hospitals with less than 100 cases; (a) 100-299 cases; (1) The number of cases/patients is too few to report; (2) Data submitted were based on a sample of cases/patients; (3) Results are based on a shorter time period than required; (4) Data suppressed by CMS for one or more quarters; (5) Results are not available for this reporting period; (6) Fewer than 100 patients completed the HCAHPS survey; (7) No cases met the criteria for this measure; (8) The lower limit of the confidence interval cannot be calculated if the number of observed infections equals zero; (9) No data are available from the state/territory for this reporting period; (10) The scores shown reflect fewer than 50 completed surveys; (11) There were discrepancies in the data collection process; (12) This measure does not apply to this hospital for this reporting period; (13) Results cannot be calculated for this reporting period; (14) The results for this state are combined with nearby states to protect confidentiality; Please refer to the User's Guide for a full explanation of data.

Measure	Cases	This Hosp.	State Avg.	U.S. Avg.
Emergency Department				
Admittance Decision Time (minutes)	134	0	62	98
Head CT Results Within 45 Min. of Arrival[5]	-	-	54%	57%
Patients Who Left ER Before Being Seen	3,192	0%	2%	2%
Time from ER Arrival to Admit. (minutes)	139	122	199	274
Time from ER Arrival to Discharge (minutes)	290	98	125	134
Time in ER Before Being Evaluated (minutes)	302	14	31	26
Time to Pain Meds for Fractures (minutes)[5]	-	-	45	57
Heart Attack Care				
Aspirin Given at Discharge[1]	-	-	99%	99%
Fibrinolytic Meds Within 30 Min. of Arrival[7]	-	-	-	54%
PCI Within 90 Minutes of Arrival[7]	-	-	96%	96%
Statin Prescribed at Discharge[1]	-	-	99%	98%
Heart Failure Care				
ACE Inhibitor or ARB for LVSD[1]	-	-	96%	97%
Discharge Instructions Given[1]	-	-	93%	94%
Evaluation of LVS Function[1]	-	-	97%	99%
Medicare Spending				
Medicare Spending per Patient (ratio)	-	-	0.9	0.98
Pneumonia Care				
Appropriate Initial Antibiotic Given[1]	-	-	94%	95%
Blood Culture Timing[7]	-	-	97%	98%
Pregnancy and Delivery Care				
Newborn Deliveries Scheduled Early[5]	-	-	5%	6%
Preventive Care				
Immunization for Influenza	213	80%	89%	90%
Immunization for Pneumonia	248	87%	89%	92%
Stroke Care				
Anticoagulation Therapy for Atrial Fibrillation[5]	-	-	96%	95%
Antithrombotic Therapy Timing[5]	-	-	98%	98%
Assessed for Rehabilitation[5]	-	-	98%	97%
Discharged on Antithrombotic Therapy[5]	-	-	99%	99%
Discharged on Statin Medication[5]	-	-	95%	94%
Thrombolytic Therapy Timing[5]	-	-	74%	66%
Venous Thromboembolism Prophylaxis[5]	-	-	95%	94%
Written Stroke Educational Materials Given[5]	-	-	88%	88%
Surgical Care Improvement Project				
Appropriate Beta Blocker Usage	12	75%	98%	98%
Appropriate VTP Within 24 Hours	45	100%	98%	98%
Controlled Postoperative Blood Glucose[7]	-	-	97%	97%
Perioperative Temperature Management	50	98%	99%	100%
Prophylactic Antibiotic Selection	43	95%	99%	99%
Prophylactic Antibiotic Selection (Outpatient)	11	100%	98%	98%
Prophylactic Antibiotic Stopped	43	93%	99%	98%
Prophylactic Antibiotic Timing	43	95%	98%	99%
Prophylactic Antibiotic Timing (Outpatient)	12	58%	97%	98%
Urinary Catheter Removal	32	97%	97%	97%
Survey of Patients' Hospital Experiences				
Area Around Room 'Always' Quiet at Night	(a)	76%	65%	61%
Doctors 'Always' Communicated Well	(a)	83%	84%	82%
Home Recovery Information Given	(a)	85%	88%	85%
Hospital Given 9 or 10 on 10 Point Scale	(a)	84%	74%	71%
Meds 'Always' Explained Before Given	(a)	72%	67%	64%
Nurses 'Always' Communicated Well	(a)	89%	81%	79%
Pain 'Always' Well Controlled	(a)	68%	72%	71%
Room and Bathroom 'Always' Clean	(a)	84%	78%	73%
Timely Help 'Always' Received	(a)	84%	74%	68%
Would Definitely Recommend Hospital	(a)	80%	71%	71%
Use of Medical Imaging				
Cardiac Imaging Stress Test before Surgery[1]	-	-	6.3%	5.3%
Combination Abdominal CT Scan	73	2.7%	5.7%	10.5%
Combination Brain/Sinus CT Scan[1]	-	-	2.3%	2.7%
Combination Chest CT Scan	67	0.0%	1.9%	2.7%
Follow-up Mammogram/Ultrasound	198	8.6%	6.3%	8.8%
Lumbar Spine MRI for Low Back Pain[1]	-	-	37.6%	37.2%

Perham Health

1000 Coney Street West
Perham, MN 56573
E-mail: information@pmhh.com
URL: www.pmhh.com
Phone: 218-347-4500
Fax: 218-346-4540
Type: Critical Access Hospitals
Ownership: Govt - Hospital Dist/Auth
Emergency Services: Yes
Beds: 25

Key Personnel:

Infection Control. . . . . Nancy Fehrenbach
Quality Assurance . . . . Nancy Fehrenbach
CEO/President. . . . . Roger Gilbertson
Radiology. . . . . Richard Marsden
Operating Room. . . . . Mary Peeters
Chief of Medical Staff. . . . . Timothy J Studer, MD

Measure	Cases	This Hosp.	State Avg.	U.S. Avg.
Blood Clot Prevention and Treatment				
Anticoagulation Overlap Therapy[1,3]	-	-	96%	93%
ICU Venous Thromboembolism Prophylaxis[3,7]	-	-	91%	92%
Incidence of Potentially Preventable VTE[3,7]	-	-	9%	10%
UFH with Dosages/Platelet Monitoring[1,3]	-	-	98%	97%
Venous Thromboembolism Prophylaxis[1,3]	-	-	86%	85%
Warfarin Therapy Discharge Instructions[1,3]	-	-	63%	75%
Chest Pain/Possible Heart Attack Care				
Aspirin Given Within 24 Hours of Arrival	47	100%	97%	96%
Fibrinolytic Meds Within 30 Min. of Arrival[7]	-	-	48%	58%
Average Time to ECG (minutes)	43	8	7	7
Average Time to Transfer (minutes)[1]	-	-	54	60
Children's Asthma Care				
Received Home Management Plan of Care	-	-	-	88%
Received Reliever Medication	-	-	-	100%
Received Systemic Corticosteroids	-	-	-	100%
Emergency Department				
Admittance Decision Time (minutes)[2]	89	15	62	98
Head CT Results Within 45 Min. of Arrival[1]	-	-	54%	57%
Patients Who Left ER Before Being Seen[5]	-	-	2%	2%
Time from ER Arrival to Admit. (minutes)[2]	152	112	199	274
Time from ER Arrival to Discharge (minutes)[5]	-	-	125	134
Time in ER Before Being Evaluated (minutes)[5]	-	-	31	26
Time to Pain Meds for Fractures (minutes)	24	30	45	57
Heart Attack Care				
Aspirin Given at Discharge[1]	-	-	99%	99%
Fibrinolytic Meds Within 30 Min. of Arrival[7]	-	-	-	54%
PCI Within 90 Minutes of Arrival[7]	-	-	96%	96%
Statin Prescribed at Discharge[1]	-	-	99%	98%
Heart Failure Care				
ACE Inhibitor or ARB for LVSD[1]	-	-	96%	97%
Discharge Instructions Given	22	45%	93%	94%
Evaluation of LVS Function	34	47%	97%	99%
Medicare Spending				
Medicare Spending per Patient (ratio)	-	-	0.9	0.98
Pneumonia Care				
Appropriate Initial Antibiotic Given	32	91%	94%	95%
Blood Culture Timing[1]	-	-	97%	98%
Pregnancy and Delivery Care				
Newborn Deliveries Scheduled Early[5]	-	-	5%	6%
Preventive Care				
Immunization for Influenza[2]	176	66%	89%	90%
Immunization for Pneumonia[2]	386	79%	89%	92%
Stroke Care				
Anticoagulation Therapy for Atrial Fibrillation[7]	-	-	96%	95%
Antithrombotic Therapy Timing[1]	-	-	98%	98%
Assessed for Rehabilitation[1]	-	-	98%	97%
Discharged on Antithrombotic Therapy[1]	-	-	99%	99%
Discharged on Statin Medication[1]	-	-	95%	94%
Thrombolytic Therapy Timing[1]	-	-	74%	66%
Venous Thromboembolism Prophylaxis[1]	-	-	95%	94%
Written Stroke Educational Materials Given[1]	-	-	88%	88%
Surgical Care Improvement Project				
Appropriate Beta Blocker Usage[1]	-	-	98%	98%
Appropriate VTP Within 24 Hours[1]	-	-	98%	98%
Controlled Postoperative Blood Glucose[7]	-	-	97%	97%
Perioperative Temperature Management[1]	-	-	99%	100%
Prophylactic Antibiotic Selection[1]	-	-	99%	99%
Prophylactic Antibiotic Selection (Outpatient)[1,3]	-	-	98%	98%
Prophylactic Antibiotic Stopped[1]	-	-	99%	98%
Prophylactic Antibiotic Timing[1]	-	-	98%	99%
Prophylactic Antibiotic Timing (Outpatient)[1,3]	-	-	97%	98%
Urinary Catheter Removal[1]	-	-	97%	97%
Survey of Patients' Hospital Experiences				
Area Around Room 'Always' Quiet at Night	(a)	73%	65%	61%
Doctors 'Always' Communicated Well	(a)	83%	84%	82%
Home Recovery Information Given	(a)	85%	88%	85%
Hospital Given 9 or 10 on 10 Point Scale	(a)	82%	74%	71%
Meds 'Always' Explained Before Given	(a)	67%	67%	64%
Nurses 'Always' Communicated Well	(a)	83%	81%	79%
Pain 'Always' Well Controlled	(a)	66%	72%	71%
Room and Bathroom 'Always' Clean	(a)	85%	78%	73%
Timely Help 'Always' Received	(a)	77%	74%	68%
Would Definitely Recommend Hospital	(a)	83%	71%	71%
Use of Medical Imaging				
Cardiac Imaging Stress Test before Surgery[1]	-	-	6.3%	5.3%
Combination Abdominal CT Scan	82	8.5%	5.7%	10.5%
Combination Brain/Sinus CT Scan[1]	-	-	2.3%	2.7%
Combination Chest CT Scan	50	0.0%	1.9%	2.7%
Follow-up Mammogram/Ultrasound	217	6.5%	6.3%	8.8%
Lumbar Spine MRI for Low Back Pain[1]	-	-	37.6%	37.2%

Pipestone County Medical Center

916 4th Avenue Southwest
Pipestone, MN 56164
URL: www.pcmchealth.org
Phone: 507-825-5811
Fax: 507-825-5733
Type: Critical Access Hospitals
Ownership: Government - Local
Emergency Services: Yes
Beds: 84

Key Personnel:

Operating Room. . . . . Susan Borman
Infection Control. . . . . Nancy Johnson
Quality Assurance . . . . Nancy Johnson, RN
Radiology. . . . . Wayne P Panning

Measure	Cases	This Hosp.	State Avg.	U.S. Avg.
Blood Clot Prevention and Treatment				
Anticoagulation Overlap Therapy[5]	-	-	96%	93%
ICU Venous Thromboembolism Prophylaxis[5]	-	-	91%	92%
Incidence of Potentially Preventable VTE[5]	-	-	9%	10%
UFH with Dosages/Platelet Monitoring[5]	-	-	98%	97%
Venous Thromboembolism Prophylaxis[5]	-	-	86%	85%
Warfarin Therapy Discharge Instructions[5]	-	-	63%	75%
Chest Pain/Possible Heart Attack Care				
Aspirin Given Within 24 Hours of Arrival[1]	-	-	97%	96%
Fibrinolytic Meds Within 30 Min. of Arrival[1,3]	-	-	48%	58%
Average Time to ECG (minutes)[1]	-	-	7	7
Average Time to Transfer (minutes)[1,3]	-	-	54	60
Children's Asthma Care				
Received Home Management Plan of Care	-	-	-	88%
Received Reliever Medication	-	-	-	100%
Received Systemic Corticosteroids	-	-	-	100%
Emergency Department				
Admittance Decision Time (minutes)[2,7]	-	-	62	98
Head CT Results Within 45 Min. of Arrival[5]	-	-	54%	57%
Patients Who Left ER Before Being Seen[5]	-	-	2%	2%
Time from ER Arrival to Admit. (minutes)[2]	102	154	199	274
Time from ER Arrival to Discharge (minutes)[5]	-	-	125	134
Time in ER Before Being Evaluated (minutes)[5]	-	-	31	26
Time to Pain Meds for Fractures (minutes)[5]	-	-	45	57
Heart Attack Care				
Aspirin Given at Discharge[3,7]	-	-	99%	99%
Fibrinolytic Meds Within 30 Min. of Arrival[3,7]	-	-	-	54%
PCI Within 90 Minutes of Arrival[3,7]	-	-	96%	96%
Statin Prescribed at Discharge[3,7]	-	-	99%	98%
Heart Failure Care				
ACE Inhibitor or ARB for LVSD[7]	-	-	96%	97%
Discharge Instructions Given[1]	-	-	93%	94%
Evaluation of LVS Function[1]	-	-	97%	99%
Medicare Spending				
Medicare Spending per Patient (ratio)	-	-	0.9	0.98
Pneumonia Care				
Appropriate Initial Antibiotic Given	13	100%	94%	95%
Blood Culture Timing[1]	-	-	97%	98%

NOTE: Hospital profiles are in alphabetical order by state, then city, then hospital within the city; Rankings exclude hospitals with less than 25 cases except for patient surveys which excludes hospitals with less than 100 cases; (a) 100-299 cases; (1) The number of cases/patients is too few to report; (2) Data submitted were based on a sample of cases/patients; (3) Results are based on a shorter time period than required; (4) Data suppressed by CMS for one or more quarters; (5) Results are not available for this reporting period; (6) Fewer than 100 patients completed the HCAHPS survey; (7) No cases met the criteria for this measure; (8) The lower limit of the confidence interval cannot be calculated if the number of observed infections equals zero; (9) No data are available from the state/territory for this reporting period; (10) The scores shown reflect fewer than 50 completed surveys; (11) There were discrepancies in the data collection process; (12) This measure does not apply to this hospital for this reporting period; (13) Results cannot be calculated for this reporting period; (14) The results for this state are combined with nearby states to protect confidentiality; Please refer to the User's Guide for a full explanation of data.

Measure	Cases	This Hosp.	State Avg.	U.S. Avg.
Pregnancy and Delivery Care				
Newborn Deliveries Scheduled Early[5]	-	-	5%	6%
Preventive Care				
Immunization for Influenza[2]	142	92%	89%	90%
Immunization for Pneumonia[2]	169	92%	89%	92%
Stroke Care				
Anticoagulation Therapy for Atrial Fibrillation[5]	-	-	96%	95%
Antithrombotic Therapy Timing[5]	-	-	98%	98%
Assessed for Rehabilitation[5]	-	-	98%	97%
Discharged on Antithrombotic Therapy[5]	-	-	99%	99%
Discharged on Statin Medication[5]	-	-	95%	94%
Thrombolytic Therapy Timing[5]	-	-	74%	66%
Venous Thromboembolism Prophylaxis[5]	-	-	95%	94%
Written Stroke Educational Materials Given[5]	-	-	88%	88%
Surgical Care Improvement Project				
Appropriate Beta Blocker Usage[1]	-	-	98%	98%
Appropriate VTP Within 24 Hours	13	85%	98%	98%
Controlled Postoperative Blood Glucose[3,7]	-	-	97%	97%
Perioperative Temperature Management	13	100%	99%	100%
Prophylactic Antibiotic Selection[1]	-	-	99%	99%
Prophylactic Antibiotic Selection (Outpatient)[5]	-	-	98%	98%
Prophylactic Antibiotic Stopped[1]	-	-	99%	98%
Prophylactic Antibiotic Timing[1]	-	-	98%	99%
Prophylactic Antibiotic Timing (Outpatient)[5]	-	-	97%	98%
Urinary Catheter Removal[1]	-	-	97%	97%
Survey of Patients' Hospital Experiences				
Area Around Room 'Always' Quiet at Night[6]	<100	67%	65%	61%
Doctors 'Always' Communicated Well[6]	<100	90%	84%	82%
Home Recovery Information Given[6]	<100	92%	88%	85%
Hospital Given 9 or 10 on 10 Point Scale[6]	<100	79%	74%	71%
Meds 'Always' Explained Before Given[6]	<100	69%	67%	64%
Nurses 'Always' Communicated Well[6]	<100	84%	81%	79%
Pain 'Always' Well Controlled[6]	<100	78%	72%	71%
Room and Bathroom 'Always' Clean[6]	<100	80%	78%	73%
Timely Help 'Always' Received[6]	<100	76%	74%	68%
Would Definitely Recommend Hospital[6]	<100	81%	71%	71%
Use of Medical Imaging				
Cardiac Imaging Stress Test before Surgery[1]	-	-	6.3%	5.3%
Combination Abdominal CT Scan	107	12.1%	5.7%	10.5%
Combination Brain/Sinus CT Scan[1]	-	-	2.3%	2.7%
Combination Chest CT Scan	48	4.2%	1.9%	2.7%
Follow-up Mammogram/Ultrasound	220	12.7%	6.3%	8.8%
Lumbar Spine MRI for Low Back Pain[1]	-	-	37.6%	37.2%

Fairview Northland Regional Hospital

911 Northland Dr
Princeton, MN 55371
Phone: 763-389-1313
Fax: 763-389-6306
Type: Acute Care Hospitals
Emergency Services: Yes
Ownership: Voluntary non-profit - Other
Beds: 41

Key Personnel:
Emergency Room . . . . David Anderson, MD
Radiology. . . . . Manfred Benson, MD
Cardiology . . . . Alan Berger, MD
CEO/President. . . . . Jon R Campbell
Surgery . . . . Timothy F. Deaconson, MD
Pediatrics. . . . . Amy Fair, MD
Hemotology Center . . . . L. Lisa Ge, MD

Measure	Cases	This Hosp.	State Avg.	U.S. Avg.
Blood Clot Prevention and Treatment				
Anticoagulation Overlap Therapy[2]	14	100%	96%	93%
ICU Venous Thromboembolism Prophylaxis[2]	27	100%	91%	92%
Incidence of Potentially Preventable VTE[2,7]	-	-	9%	10%
UFH with Dosages/Platelet Monitoring[1,2]	-	-	98%	97%
Venous Thromboembolism Prophylaxis[2]	95	99%	86%	85%
Warfarin Therapy Discharge Instructions[2]	11	100%	63%	75%
Chest Pain/Possible Heart Attack Care				
Aspirin Given Within 24 Hours of Arrival	90	99%	97%	96%
Fibrinolytic Meds Within 30 Min. of Arrival[7]	-	-	48%	58%
Average Time to ECG (minutes)	90	7	7	7
Average Time to Transfer (minutes)	16	53	54	60
Children's Asthma Care				
Received Home Management Plan of Care	-	-	-	88%
Received Reliever Medication	-	-	-	100%
Received Systemic Corticosteroids	-	-	-	100%
Emergency Department				
Admittance Decision Time (minutes)[2]	277	92	62	98
Head CT Results Within 45 Min. of Arrival[1]	-	-	54%	57%
Patients Who Left ER Before Being Seen	16,588	0%	2%	2%
Time from ER Arrival to Admit. (minutes)[2]	281	252	199	274
Time from ER Arrival to Discharge (minutes)	358	126	125	134
Time in ER Before Being Evaluated (minutes)	384	24	31	26
Time to Pain Meds for Fractures (minutes)	74	44	45	57
Heart Attack Care				
Aspirin Given at Discharge[1]	-	-	99%	99%
Fibrinolytic Meds Within 30 Min. of Arrival[7]	-	-	-	54%
PCI Within 90 Minutes of Arrival[7]	-	-	96%	96%
Statin Prescribed at Discharge[1]	-	-	99%	98%
Heart Failure Care				
ACE Inhibitor or ARB for LVSD	19	100%	96%	97%
Discharge Instructions Given	25	96%	93%	94%
Evaluation of LVS Function	46	100%	97%	99%
Medicare Spending				
Medicare Spending per Patient (ratio)	-	0.86	0.9	0.98
Pneumonia Care				
Appropriate Initial Antibiotic Given	52	98%	94%	95%
Blood Culture Timing	110	99%	97%	98%
Pregnancy and Delivery Care				
Newborn Deliveries Scheduled Early	25	4%	5%	6%
Preventive Care				
Immunization for Influenza[2]	235	99%	89%	90%
Immunization for Pneumonia[2]	247	98%	89%	92%
Stroke Care				
Anticoagulation Therapy for Atrial Fibrillation[1]	-	-	96%	95%
Antithrombotic Therapy Timing	11	100%	98%	98%
Assessed for Rehabilitation	14	100%	98%	97%
Discharged on Antithrombotic Therapy	14	100%	99%	99%
Discharged on Statin Medication[1]	-	-	95%	94%
Thrombolytic Therapy Timing[7]	-	-	74%	66%
Venous Thromboembolism Prophylaxis[1]	-	-	95%	94%
Written Stroke Educational Materials Given[1]	-	-	88%	88%
Surgical Care Improvement Project				
Appropriate Beta Blocker Usage	22	100%	98%	98%
Appropriate VTP Within 24 Hours	76	99%	98%	98%
Controlled Postoperative Blood Glucose[7]	-	-	97%	97%
Perioperative Temperature Management	85	100%	99%	100%
Prophylactic Antibiotic Selection	63	98%	99%	99%
Prophylactic Antibiotic Selection (Outpatient)	66	100%	98%	98%
Prophylactic Antibiotic Stopped	63	98%	99%	98%
Prophylactic Antibiotic Timing	63	100%	98%	99%
Prophylactic Antibiotic Timing (Outpatient)	66	98%	97%	98%
Urinary Catheter Removal	34	100%	97%	97%
Survey of Patients' Hospital Experiences				
Area Around Room 'Always' Quiet at Night	300+	61%	65%	61%
Doctors 'Always' Communicated Well	300+	85%	84%	82%
Home Recovery Information Given	300+	89%	88%	85%
Hospital Given 9 or 10 on 10 Point Scale	300+	78%	74%	71%
Meds 'Always' Explained Before Given	300+	70%	67%	64%
Nurses 'Always' Communicated Well	300+	82%	81%	79%
Pain 'Always' Well Controlled	300+	76%	72%	71%
Room and Bathroom 'Always' Clean	300+	79%	78%	73%
Timely Help 'Always' Received	300+	75%	74%	68%
Would Definitely Recommend Hospital	300+	72%	71%	71%
Use of Medical Imaging				
Cardiac Imaging Stress Test before Surgery	76	7.9%	6.3%	5.3%
Combination Abdominal CT Scan	204	4.9%	5.7%	10.5%
Combination Brain/Sinus CT Scan[1]	-	-	2.3%	2.7%
Combination Chest CT Scan	152	0.0%	1.9%	2.7%
Follow-up Mammogram/Ultrasound	218	8.7%	6.3%	8.8%
Lumbar Spine MRI for Low Back Pain	50	36.0%	37.6%	37.2%

Mayo Clinic Health System - Red Wing

701 Hewitt Boulevard, PO Box 95
Red Wing, MN 55066
Phone: 651-267-5000
Fax: 651-385-3304
URL: www.redwing.fairview.org
Type: Acute Care Hospitals
Emergency Services: Yes
Ownership: Voluntary non-profit - Private
Beds: 96

Key Personnel:
Chief of Medical Staff . . . . Jack Alexander
Anesthesiology. . . . . Shelly Bakker
Emergency Room . . . . Jane Gisslen
Operating Room. . . . . Cheryl Luettinger
Intensive Care Unit. . . . . Helen McKay
Quality Assurance . . . . Dawn Ulveness

Measure	Cases	This Hosp.	State Avg.	U.S. Avg.
Blood Clot Prevention and Treatment				
Anticoagulation Overlap Therapy[2]	13	100%	96%	93%
ICU Venous Thromboembolism Prophylaxis[2]	25	100%	91%	92%
Incidence of Potentially Preventable VTE[1,2]	-	-	9%	10%
UFH with Dosages/Platelet Monitoring[1,2]	-	-	98%	97%
Venous Thromboembolism Prophylaxis[2]	100	94%	86%	85%
Warfarin Therapy Discharge Instructions[2]	13	100%	63%	75%
Chest Pain/Possible Heart Attack Care				
Aspirin Given Within 24 Hours of Arrival	68	100%	97%	96%
Fibrinolytic Meds Within 30 Min. of Arrival[7]	-	-	48%	58%
Average Time to ECG (minutes)	69	6	7	7
Average Time to Transfer (minutes)[1]	-	-	54	60
Children's Asthma Care				
Received Home Management Plan of Care	-	-	-	88%
Received Reliever Medication	-	-	-	100%
Received Systemic Corticosteroids	-	-	-	100%
Emergency Department				
Admittance Decision Time (minutes)[2]	210	40	62	98
Head CT Results Within 45 Min. of Arrival	12	67%	54%	57%
Patients Who Left ER Before Being Seen	10,855	1%	2%	2%
Time from ER Arrival to Admit. (minutes)[2]	211	189	199	274
Time from ER Arrival to Discharge (minutes)	343	97	125	134
Time in ER Before Being Evaluated (minutes)	370	26	31	26
Time to Pain Meds for Fractures (minutes)	32	58	45	57
Heart Attack Care				
Aspirin Given at Discharge[1]	-	-	99%	99%
Fibrinolytic Meds Within 30 Min. of Arrival[7]	-	-	-	54%
PCI Within 90 Minutes of Arrival[7]	-	-	96%	96%
Statin Prescribed at Discharge[1]	-	-	99%	98%
Heart Failure Care				
ACE Inhibitor or ARB for LVSD	15	100%	96%	97%
Discharge Instructions Given	39	100%	93%	94%
Evaluation of LVS Function	55	100%	97%	99%
Medicare Spending				
Medicare Spending per Patient (ratio)	-	0.83	0.9	0.98
Pneumonia Care				
Appropriate Initial Antibiotic Given	38	95%	94%	95%
Blood Culture Timing	45	100%	97%	98%
Pregnancy and Delivery Care				
Newborn Deliveries Scheduled Early	12	0%	5%	6%
Preventive Care				
Immunization for Influenza[2]	256	95%	89%	90%
Immunization for Pneumonia[2]	293	96%	89%	92%
Stroke Care				
Anticoagulation Therapy for Atrial Fibrillation[1]	-	-	96%	95%
Antithrombotic Therapy Timing	12	100%	98%	98%
Assessed for Rehabilitation	15	93%	98%	97%
Discharged on Antithrombotic Therapy	13	92%	99%	99%
Discharged on Statin Medication	11	91%	95%	94%
Thrombolytic Therapy Timing[1]	-	-	74%	66%
Venous Thromboembolism Prophylaxis	14	100%	95%	94%
Written Stroke Educational Materials Given[1]	-	-	88%	88%
Surgical Care Improvement Project				
Appropriate Beta Blocker Usage[2]	52	98%	98%	98%
Appropriate VTP Within 24 Hours[2]	175	99%	98%	98%
Controlled Postoperative Blood Glucose[2,7]	-	-	97%	97%
Perioperative Temperature Management[2]	206	100%	99%	100%
Prophylactic Antibiotic Selection[2]	145	100%	99%	99%
Prophylactic Antibiotic Selection (Outpatient)	19	95%	98%	98%
Prophylactic Antibiotic Stopped[2]	143	99%	99%	98%
Prophylactic Antibiotic Timing[2]	145	100%	98%	99%
Prophylactic Antibiotic Timing (Outpatient)	12	100%	97%	98%
Urinary Catheter Removal[2]	170	100%	97%	97%
Survey of Patients' Hospital Experiences				
Area Around Room 'Always' Quiet at Night	300+	65%	65%	61%
Doctors 'Always' Communicated Well	300+	84%	84%	82%

NOTE: Hospital profiles are in alphabetical order by state, then city, then hospital within the city; Rankings exclude hospitals with less than 25 cases except for patient surveys which excludes hospitals with less than 100 cases; (a) 100-299 cases; (1) The number of cases/patients is too few to report; (2) Data submitted were based on a sample of cases/patients; (3) Results are based on a shorter time period than required; (4) Data suppressed by CMS for one or more quarters; (5) Results are not available for this reporting period; (6) Fewer than 100 patients completed the HCAHPS survey; (7) No cases met the criteria for this measure; (8) The lower limit of the confidence interval cannot be calculated if the number of observed infections equals zero; (9) No data are available from the state/territory for this reporting period; (10) The scores shown reflect fewer than 50 completed surveys; (11) There were discrepancies in the data collection process; (12) This measure does not apply to this hospital for this reporting period; (13) Results cannot be calculated for this reporting period; (14) The results for this state are combined with nearby states to protect confidentiality; Please refer to the User's Guide for a full explanation of data.

Measure	Cases	This Hosp.	State Avg.	U.S. Avg.
Home Recovery Information Given	300+	87%	88%	85%
Hospital Given 9 or 10 on 10 Point Scale	300+	76%	74%	71%
Meds 'Always' Explained Before Given	300+	68%	67%	64%
Nurses 'Always' Communicated Well	300+	82%	81%	79%
Pain 'Always' Well Controlled	300+	70%	72%	71%
Room and Bathroom 'Always' Clean	300+	76%	78%	73%
Timely Help 'Always' Received	300+	77%	74%	68%
Would Definitely Recommend Hospital	300+	73%	71%	71%
Use of Medical Imaging				
Cardiac Imaging Stress Test before Surgery	61	6.6%	6.3%	5.3%
Combination Abdominal CT Scan	153	3.3%	5.7%	10.5%
Combination Brain/Sinus CT Scan[1]	-	-	2.3%	2.7%
Combination Chest CT Scan	124	0.0%	1.9%	2.7%
Follow-up Mammogram/Ultrasound	401	8.2%	6.3%	8.8%
Lumbar Spine MRI for Low Back Pain[1]	-	-	37.6%	37.2%

Red Lake Hospital

PO Box 497
Redlake, MN 56671
Phone: 218-679-3912
Fax: 218-679-3990
Type: Acute Care Hospitals
Emergency Services: Yes
Ownership: Government - Federal
Beds: 23

Key Personnel:
CEO/President. . . . . Tony James
Emergency Room . . . . Joyce Kennedy
Chief of Medical Staff . . . . John Robinson
Quality Assurance . . . . Bonnie Smprud

Measure	Cases	This Hosp.	State Avg.	U.S. Avg.
Blood Clot Prevention and Treatment				
Anticoagulation Overlap Therapy[7]	-	-	96%	93%
ICU Venous Thromboembolism Prophylaxis[7]	-	-	91%	92%
Incidence of Potentially Preventable VTE[7]	-	-	9%	10%
UFH with Dosages/Platelet Monitoring[7]	-	-	98%	97%
Venous Thromboembolism Prophylaxis	110	86%	86%	85%
Warfarin Therapy Discharge Instructions[7]	-	-	63%	75%
Chest Pain/Possible Heart Attack Care				
Aspirin Given Within 24 Hours of Arrival	-	-	97%	96%
Fibrinolytic Meds Within 30 Min. of Arrival	-	-	48%	58%
Average Time to ECG (minutes)	-	-	7	7
Average Time to Transfer (minutes)	-	-	54	60
Children's Asthma Care				
Received Home Management Plan of Care	-	-	-	88%
Received Reliever Medication	-	-	-	100%
Received Systemic Corticosteroids	-	-	-	100%
Emergency Department				
Admittance Decision Time (minutes)	241	76	62	98
Head CT Results Within 45 Min. of Arrival	-	-	54%	57%
Patients Who Left ER Before Being Seen	-	-	2%	2%
Time from ER Arrival to Admit. (minutes)	245	220	199	274
Time from ER Arrival to Discharge (minutes)	-	-	125	134
Time in ER Before Being Evaluated (minutes)	-	-	31	26
Time to Pain Meds for Fractures (minutes)	-	-	45	57
Heart Attack Care				
Aspirin Given at Discharge[3,7]	-	-	99%	99%
Fibrinolytic Meds Within 30 Min. of Arrival[3,7]	-	-	-	54%
PCI Within 90 Minutes of Arrival[3,7]	-	-	96%	96%
Statin Prescribed at Discharge[3,7]	-	-	99%	98%
Heart Failure Care				
ACE Inhibitor or ARB for LVSD[1]	-	-	96%	97%
Discharge Instructions Given	11	73%	93%	94%
Evaluation of LVS Function	12	92%	97%	99%
Medicare Spending				
Medicare Spending per Patient (ratio)	-	0.75	0.9	0.98
Pneumonia Care				
Appropriate Initial Antibiotic Given	14	50%	94%	95%
Blood Culture Timing	11	82%	97%	98%
Pregnancy and Delivery Care				
Newborn Deliveries Scheduled Early[7]	-	-	5%	6%
Preventive Care				
Immunization for Influenza	170	72%	89%	90%
Immunization for Pneumonia	186	94%	89%	92%
Stroke Care				
Anticoagulation Therapy for Atrial Fibrillation[3,7]	-	-	96%	95%
Antithrombotic Therapy Timing[3,7]	-	-	98%	98%
Assessed for Rehabilitation[3,7]	-	-	98%	97%
Discharged on Antithrombotic Therapy[3,7]	-	-	99%	99%
Discharged on Statin Medication[3,7]	-	-	95%	94%
Thrombolytic Therapy Timing[3,7]	-	-	74%	66%
Venous Thromboembolism Prophylaxis[1,3]	-	-	95%	94%
Written Stroke Educational Materials Given[3,7]	-	-	88%	88%
Surgical Care Improvement Project				
Appropriate Beta Blocker Usage[5]	-	-	98%	98%
Appropriate VTP Within 24 Hours[5]	-	-	98%	98%
Controlled Postoperative Blood Glucose[5]	-	-	97%	97%
Perioperative Temperature Management[5]	-	-	99%	100%
Prophylactic Antibiotic Selection[5]	-	-	99%	99%
Prophylactic Antibiotic Selection (Outpatient)	-	-	98%	98%
Prophylactic Antibiotic Stopped[5]	-	-	99%	98%
Prophylactic Antibiotic Timing[5]	-	-	98%	99%
Prophylactic Antibiotic Timing (Outpatient)	-	-	97%	98%
Urinary Catheter Removal[5]	-	-	97%	97%
Survey of Patients' Hospital Experiences				
Area Around Room 'Always' Quiet at Night[10]	<100	82%	65%	61%
Doctors 'Always' Communicated Well[10]	<100	94%	84%	82%
Home Recovery Information Given[10]	<100	76%	88%	85%
Hospital Given 9 or 10 on 10 Point Scale[10]	<100	76%	74%	71%
Meds 'Always' Explained Before Given[10]	<100	68%	67%	64%
Nurses 'Always' Communicated Well[10]	<100	89%	81%	79%
Pain 'Always' Well Controlled[10]	<100	100%	72%	71%
Room and Bathroom 'Always' Clean[10]	<100	88%	78%	73%
Timely Help 'Always' Received[10]	<100	84%	74%	68%
Would Definitely Recommend Hospital[10]	<100	36%	71%	71%
Use of Medical Imaging				
Cardiac Imaging Stress Test before Surgery	-	-	6.3%	5.3%
Combination Abdominal CT Scan	-	-	5.7%	10.5%
Combination Brain/Sinus CT Scan	-	-	2.3%	2.7%
Combination Chest CT Scan	-	-	1.9%	2.7%
Follow-up Mammogram/Ultrasound	-	-	6.3%	8.8%
Lumbar Spine MRI for Low Back Pain	-	-	37.6%	37.2%

Redwood Area Hospital

100 Fallwood Road
Redwood Falls, MN 56283
Phone: 507-637-4500
Fax: 507-697-6000
URL: www.redwoodareahospital.org
Type: Critical Access Hospitals
Emergency Services: Yes
Ownership: Government - Local
Beds: 25

Key Personnel:
Emergency Room . . . . Wayne Belling, DO
Infection Control. . . . . Julie Fiala, RN
Chief of Medical Staff. . . . . Cindi Gronan
Cardiac Laboratory. . . . . Lori Highty
Anesthesiology. . . . . Loretta Krahn
Quality Assurance . . . . Gloria Lothert, RN
Operating Room. . . . . Julie Salmon
CEO/President. . . . . James E Schulte

Measure	Cases	This Hosp.	State Avg.	U.S. Avg.
Blood Clot Prevention and Treatment				
Anticoagulation Overlap Therapy[5]	-	-	96%	93%
ICU Venous Thromboembolism Prophylaxis[5]	-	-	91%	92%
Incidence of Potentially Preventable VTE[5]	-	-	9%	10%
UFH with Dosages/Platelet Monitoring[5]	-	-	98%	97%
Venous Thromboembolism Prophylaxis[5]	-	-	86%	85%
Warfarin Therapy Discharge Instructions[5]	-	-	63%	75%
Chest Pain/Possible Heart Attack Care				
Aspirin Given Within 24 Hours of Arrival	31	100%	97%	96%
Fibrinolytic Meds Within 30 Min. of Arrival[1]	-	-	48%	58%
Average Time to ECG (minutes)	33	10	7	7
Average Time to Transfer (minutes)[1]	-	-	54	60
Children's Asthma Care				
Received Home Management Plan of Care	-	-	-	88%
Received Reliever Medication	-	-	-	100%
Received Systemic Corticosteroids	-	-	-	100%
Emergency Department				
Admittance Decision Time (minutes)[2]	124	30	62	98
Head CT Results Within 45 Min. of Arrival[5]	-	-	54%	57%
Patients Who Left ER Before Being Seen[5]	-	-	2%	2%
Time from ER Arrival to Admit. (minutes)[2]	129	161	199	274
Time from ER Arrival to Discharge (minutes)[5]	-	-	125	134
Time in ER Before Being Evaluated (minutes)[5]	-	-	31	26
Time to Pain Meds for Fractures (minutes)[5]	-	-	45	57
Heart Attack Care				
Aspirin Given at Discharge[1,3]	-	-	99%	99%
Fibrinolytic Meds Within 30 Min. of Arrival[3,7]	-	-	-	54%
PCI Within 90 Minutes of Arrival[3,7]	-	-	96%	96%
Statin Prescribed at Discharge[1,3]	-	-	99%	98%
Heart Failure Care				
ACE Inhibitor or ARB for LVSD[1]	-	-	96%	97%
Discharge Instructions Given	16	100%	93%	94%
Evaluation of LVS Function	21	90%	97%	99%
Medicare Spending				
Medicare Spending per Patient (ratio)	-	-	0.9	0.98
Pneumonia Care				
Appropriate Initial Antibiotic Given	12	100%	94%	95%
Blood Culture Timing	21	100%	97%	98%
Pregnancy and Delivery Care				
Newborn Deliveries Scheduled Early[5]	-	-	5%	6%
Preventive Care				
Immunization for Influenza[2]	113	98%	89%	90%
Immunization for Pneumonia[2]	145	96%	89%	92%
Stroke Care				
Anticoagulation Therapy for Atrial Fibrillation[5]	-	-	96%	95%
Antithrombotic Therapy Timing[5]	-	-	98%	98%
Assessed for Rehabilitation[5]	-	-	98%	97%
Discharged on Antithrombotic Therapy[5]	-	-	99%	99%
Discharged on Statin Medication[5]	-	-	95%	94%
Thrombolytic Therapy Timing[5]	-	-	74%	66%
Venous Thromboembolism Prophylaxis[5]	-	-	95%	94%
Written Stroke Educational Materials Given[5]	-	-	88%	88%
Surgical Care Improvement Project				
Appropriate Beta Blocker Usage[5]	-	-	98%	98%
Appropriate VTP Within 24 Hours[5]	-	-	98%	98%
Controlled Postoperative Blood Glucose[5]	-	-	97%	97%
Perioperative Temperature Management[5]	-	-	99%	100%
Prophylactic Antibiotic Selection[5]	-	-	99%	99%
Prophylactic Antibiotic Selection (Outpatient)[5]	-	-	98%	98%
Prophylactic Antibiotic Stopped[5]	-	-	99%	98%
Prophylactic Antibiotic Timing[5]	-	-	98%	99%
Prophylactic Antibiotic Timing (Outpatient)[5]	-	-	97%	98%
Urinary Catheter Removal[5]	-	-	97%	97%
Survey of Patients' Hospital Experiences				
Area Around Room 'Always' Quiet at Night[11]	(a)	81%	65%	61%
Doctors 'Always' Communicated Well[11]	(a)	85%	84%	82%
Home Recovery Information Given[11]	(a)	93%	88%	85%
Hospital Given 9 or 10 on 10 Point Scale[11]	(a)	84%	74%	71%
Meds 'Always' Explained Before Given[11]	(a)	67%	67%	64%
Nurses 'Always' Communicated Well[11]	(a)	84%	81%	79%
Pain 'Always' Well Controlled[11]	(a)	73%	72%	71%
Room and Bathroom 'Always' Clean[11]	(a)	84%	78%	73%
Timely Help 'Always' Received[11]	(a)	78%	74%	68%
Would Definitely Recommend Hospital[11]	(a)	44%	71%	71%
Use of Medical Imaging				
Cardiac Imaging Stress Test before Surgery[1]	-	-	6.3%	5.3%
Combination Abdominal CT Scan	103	5.8%	5.7%	10.5%
Combination Brain/Sinus CT Scan[1]	-	-	2.3%	2.7%
Combination Chest CT Scan	78	0.0%	1.9%	2.7%
Follow-up Mammogram/Ultrasound[7]	-	-	6.3%	8.8%
Lumbar Spine MRI for Low Back Pain[1]	-	-	37.6%	37.2%

North Memorial Medical Center

3300 Oakdale North
Robbinsdale, MN 55422
Phone: 763-520-5200
Fax: 763-520-5006
URL: www.northmemorial.com
Type: Acute Care Hospitals
Emergency Services: Yes
Ownership: Voluntary non-profit - Private
Beds: 518

Key Personnel:
Operating Room. . . . . Lois Bergquist
CEO/President. . . . . David Cress
Chief of Medical Staff. . . . . J. Kevin Croston, MD, FACS
CEO . . . . Loren Larry Taylor
Pediatric Ambulatory Care . . . . . . Diane Meier, MD
Pediatric In-Patient Care . . . . Diane Meier, MD
Infection Control. . . . . CG Schrock, MD
Radiology. . . . . Tony Werner

NOTE: Hospital profiles are in alphabetical order by state, then city, then hospital within the city; Rankings exclude hospitals with less than 25 cases except for patient surveys which excludes hospitals with less than 100 cases; (a) 100-299 cases; (1) The number of cases/patients is too few to report; (2) Data submitted were based on a sample of cases/patients; (3) Results are based on a shorter time period than required; (4) Data suppressed by CMS for one or more quarters; (5) Results are not available for this reporting period; (6) Fewer than 100 patients completed the HCAHPS survey; (7) No cases met the criteria for this measure; (8) The lower limit of the confidence interval cannot be calculated if the number of observed infections equals zero; (9) No data are available from the state/territory for this reporting period; (10) The scores shown reflect fewer than 50 completed surveys; (11) There were discrepancies in the data collection process; (12) This measure does not apply to this hospital for this reporting period; (13) Results cannot be calculated for this reporting period; (14) The results for this state are combined with nearby states to protect confidentiality; Please refer to the User's Guide for a full explanation of data.

Measure	Cases	This Hosp.	State Avg.	U.S. Avg.
Blood Clot Prevention and Treatment				
Anticoagulation Overlap Therapy[2]	170	99%	96%	93%
ICU Venous Thromboembolism Prophylaxis[2]	102	90%	91%	92%
Incidence of Potentially Preventable VTE[2]	37	5%	9%	10%
UFH with Dosages/Platelet Monitoring[2]	148	99%	98%	97%
Venous Thromboembolism Prophylaxis[2]	269	82%	86%	85%
Warfarin Therapy Discharge Instructions[2]	135	66%	63%	75%
Chest Pain/Possible Heart Attack Care				
Aspirin Given Within 24 Hours of Arrival[3,7]	-	-	97%	96%
Fibrinolytic Meds Within 30 Min. of Arrival[5]	-	-	48%	58%
Average Time to ECG (minutes)[1,3]	-	-	7	7
Average Time to Transfer (minutes)[5]	-	-	54	60
Children's Asthma Care				
Received Home Management Plan of Care	-	-	-	88%
Received Reliever Medication	-	-	-	100%
Received Systemic Corticosteroids	-	-	-	100%
Emergency Department				
Admittance Decision Time (minutes)[2]	732	116	62	98
Head CT Results Within 45 Min. of Arrival[1,3]	-	-	54%	57%
Patients Who Left ER Before Being Seen	76,640	3%	2%	2%
Time from ER Arrival to Admit. (minutes)[2]	732	220	199	274
Time from ER Arrival to Discharge (minutes)	368	137	125	134
Time in ER Before Being Evaluated (minutes)	408	18	31	26
Time to Pain Meds for Fractures (minutes)	146	46	45	57
Heart Attack Care				
Aspirin Given at Discharge[2]	301	99%	99%	99%
Fibrinolytic Meds Within 30 Min. of Arrival[2,7]	-	-	-	54%
PCI Within 90 Minutes of Arrival[2]	73	99%	96%	96%
Statin Prescribed at Discharge[2]	292	98%	99%	98%
Heart Failure Care				
ACE Inhibitor or ARB for LVSD[2]	69	93%	96%	97%
Discharge Instructions Given[2]	220	98%	93%	94%
Evaluation of LVS Function[2]	289	100%	97%	99%
Medicare Spending				
Medicare Spending per Patient (ratio)	-	0.93	0.9	0.98
Pneumonia Care				
Appropriate Initial Antibiotic Given[2]	72	93%	94%	95%
Blood Culture Timing[2]	105	99%	97%	98%
Pregnancy and Delivery Care				
Newborn Deliveries Scheduled Early[2]	23	4%	5%	6%
Preventive Care				
Immunization for Influenza[2]	572	93%	89%	90%
Immunization for Pneumonia[2]	719	90%	89%	92%
Stroke Care				
Anticoagulation Therapy for Atrial Fibrillation	65	100%	96%	95%
Antithrombotic Therapy Timing	233	97%	98%	98%
Assessed for Rehabilitation	354	98%	98%	97%
Discharged on Antithrombotic Therapy	317	99%	99%	99%
Discharged on Statin Medication	257	93%	95%	94%
Thrombolytic Therapy Timing	30	97%	74%	66%
Venous Thromboembolism Prophylaxis	315	97%	95%	94%
Written Stroke Educational Materials Given	186	84%	88%	88%
Surgical Care Improvement Project				
Appropriate Beta Blocker Usage[2]	223	97%	98%	98%
Appropriate VTP Within 24 Hours[2]	341	99%	98%	98%
Controlled Postoperative Blood Glucose[2]	144	94%	97%	97%
Perioperative Temperature Management[2]	451	100%	99%	100%
Prophylactic Antibiotic Selection[2]	411	100%	99%	99%
Prophylactic Antibiotic Selection (Outpatient)	332	100%	98%	98%
Prophylactic Antibiotic Stopped[2]	410	99%	99%	98%
Prophylactic Antibiotic Timing[2]	412	99%	98%	99%
Prophylactic Antibiotic Timing (Outpatient)	328	98%	97%	98%
Urinary Catheter Removal[2]	357	96%	97%	97%
Survey of Patients' Hospital Experiences				
Area Around Room 'Always' Quiet at Night	300+	58%	65%	61%
Doctors 'Always' Communicated Well	300+	75%	84%	82%
Home Recovery Information Given	300+	86%	88%	85%
Hospital Given 9 or 10 on 10 Point Scale	300+	67%	74%	71%
Meds 'Always' Explained Before Given	300+	60%	67%	64%
Nurses 'Always' Communicated Well	300+	72%	81%	79%
Pain 'Always' Well Controlled	300+	69%	72%	71%
Room and Bathroom 'Always' Clean	300+	67%	78%	73%
Timely Help 'Always' Received	300+	60%	74%	68%
Would Definitely Recommend Hospital	300+	70%	71%	71%
Use of Medical Imaging				
Cardiac Imaging Stress Test before Surgery	451	5.1%	6.3%	5.3%
Combination Abdominal CT Scan	665	3.9%	5.7%	10.5%
Combination Brain/Sinus CT Scan	418	2.2%	2.3%	2.7%
Combination Chest CT Scan	471	3.2%	1.9%	2.7%
Follow-up Mammogram/Ultrasound	503	5.0%	6.3%	8.8%
Lumbar Spine MRI for Low Back Pain	76	51.3%	37.6%	37.2%

Mayo Clinic Hospital Rochester

1216 Second Street Southwest
Rochester, MN 55902
Phone: 507-255-5123
URL: www.mayoclinic.org/saintmaryshospital
Type: Acute Care Hospitals
Ownership: Voluntary non-profit - Church
Emergency Services: Yes
Beds: 1,157

Measure	Cases	This Hosp.	State Avg.	U.S. Avg.
Blood Clot Prevention and Treatment				
Anticoagulation Overlap Therapy[2]	297	99%	96%	93%
ICU Venous Thromboembolism Prophylaxis[2]	110	98%	91%	92%
Incidence of Potentially Preventable VTE[2]	75	0%	9%	10%
UFH with Dosages/Platelet Monitoring[2]	329	100%	98%	97%
Venous Thromboembolism Prophylaxis[2]	307	99%	86%	85%
Warfarin Therapy Discharge Instructions[2]	210	97%	63%	75%
Chest Pain/Possible Heart Attack Care				
Aspirin Given Within 24 Hours of Arrival[1]	-	-	97%	96%
Fibrinolytic Meds Within 30 Min. of Arrival[5]	-	-	48%	58%
Average Time to ECG (minutes)[1]	-	-	7	7
Average Time to Transfer (minutes)[5]	-	-	54	60
Children's Asthma Care				
Received Home Management Plan of Care	-	-	-	88%
Received Reliever Medication	-	-	-	100%
Received Systemic Corticosteroids	-	-	-	100%
Emergency Department				
Admittance Decision Time (minutes)[2]	457	64	62	98
Head CT Results Within 45 Min. of Arrival[1]	-	-	54%	57%
Patients Who Left ER Before Being Seen	73,006	2%	2%	2%
Time from ER Arrival to Admit. (minutes)[2]	494	230	199	274
Time from ER Arrival to Discharge (minutes)	372	166	125	134
Time in ER Before Being Evaluated (minutes)	400	21	31	26
Time to Pain Meds for Fractures (minutes)	325	51	45	57
Heart Attack Care				
Aspirin Given at Discharge[2]	307	100%	99%	99%
Fibrinolytic Meds Within 30 Min. of Arrival[2,7]	-	-	-	54%
PCI Within 90 Minutes of Arrival[2]	17	94%	96%	96%
Statin Prescribed at Discharge[2]	304	100%	99%	98%
Heart Failure Care				
ACE Inhibitor or ARB for LVSD[2]	72	92%	96%	97%
Discharge Instructions Given[2]	261	96%	93%	94%
Evaluation of LVS Function[2]	321	100%	97%	99%
Medicare Spending				
Medicare Spending per Patient (ratio)	-	0.94	0.9	0.98
Pneumonia Care				
Appropriate Initial Antibiotic Given[2]	31	84%	94%	95%
Blood Culture Timing[2]	81	96%	97%	98%
Pregnancy and Delivery Care				
Newborn Deliveries Scheduled Early[7]	-	-	5%	6%
Preventive Care				
Immunization for Influenza[2]	617	89%	89%	90%
Immunization for Pneumonia[2]	746	89%	89%	92%
Stroke Care				
Anticoagulation Therapy for Atrial Fibrillation	72	100%	96%	95%
Antithrombotic Therapy Timing	273	96%	98%	98%
Assessed for Rehabilitation	499	97%	98%	97%
Discharged on Antithrombotic Therapy	393	100%	99%	99%
Discharged on Statin Medication	289	98%	95%	94%
Thrombolytic Therapy Timing	25	92%	74%	66%
Venous Thromboembolism Prophylaxis	472	100%	95%	94%
Written Stroke Educational Materials Given	251	87%	88%	88%
Surgical Care Improvement Project				
Appropriate Beta Blocker Usage[2]	333	100%	98%	98%
Appropriate VTP Within 24 Hours[2]	301	100%	98%	98%
Controlled Postoperative Blood Glucose[2]	253	94%	97%	97%
Perioperative Temperature Management[2]	491	100%	99%	100%
Prophylactic Antibiotic Selection[2]	378	100%	99%	99%
Prophylactic Antibiotic Selection (Outpatient)	697	99%	98%	98%
Prophylactic Antibiotic Stopped[2]	371	97%	99%	98%
Prophylactic Antibiotic Timing[2]	380	99%	98%	99%
Prophylactic Antibiotic Timing (Outpatient)	707	96%	97%	98%
Urinary Catheter Removal[2]	489	99%	97%	97%
Survey of Patients' Hospital Experiences				
Area Around Room 'Always' Quiet at Night[11]	300+	62%	65%	61%
Doctors 'Always' Communicated Well[11]	300+	83%	84%	82%
Home Recovery Information Given[11]	300+	90%	88%	85%
Hospital Given 9 or 10 on 10 Point Scale[11]	300+	86%	74%	71%
Meds 'Always' Explained Before Given[11]	300+	68%	67%	64%
Nurses 'Always' Communicated Well[11]	300+	83%	81%	79%
Pain 'Always' Well Controlled[11]	300+	71%	72%	71%
Room and Bathroom 'Always' Clean[11]	300+	79%	78%	73%
Timely Help 'Always' Received[11]	300+	73%	74%	68%
Would Definitely Recommend Hospital[11]	300+	89%	71%	71%
Use of Medical Imaging				
Cardiac Imaging Stress Test before Surgery	243	8.2%	6.3%	5.3%
Combination Abdominal CT Scan	803	4.2%	5.7%	10.5%
Combination Brain/Sinus CT Scan	814	2.3%	2.3%	2.7%
Combination Chest CT Scan	89	0.0%	1.9%	2.7%
Follow-up Mammogram/Ultrasound[7]	-	-	6.3%	8.8%
Lumbar Spine MRI for Low Back Pain[1]	-	-	37.6%	37.2%

Mayo Clinic Methodist- Hospital

201 West Center Street
Rochester, MN 55902
Phone: 507-266-7890
Fax: 507-284-0161
URL: www.mayoclinic.org/methodisthospital
Type: Acute Care Hospitals
Ownership: Voluntary non-profit - Other
Emergency Services: Yes
Beds: 794

Key Personnel:

Intensive Care Unit. . . . . Malcolm R Bell, MD
Hemotology Center . . . . Robert B Diasio, MD
Operating Room. . . . . Doreen Frusti
CEO/President. . . . . John H. Noseworhty, MD
Anesthesiology. . . . . Duane K Rorie, MD
Cardiac Laboratory. . . . . Randal J Thomas, MD, MS
Infection Control. . . . . Rodney Thompson, MD

Measure	Cases	This Hosp.	State Avg.	U.S. Avg.
Blood Clot Prevention and Treatment				
Anticoagulation Overlap Therapy[2]	38	97%	96%	93%
ICU Venous Thromboembolism Prophylaxis[2]	27	100%	91%	92%
Incidence of Potentially Preventable VTE[2]	28	0%	9%	10%
UFH with Dosages/Platelet Monitoring[2]	65	100%	98%	97%
Venous Thromboembolism Prophylaxis[2]	252	95%	86%	85%
Warfarin Therapy Discharge Instructions[2]	30	90%	63%	75%
Chest Pain/Possible Heart Attack Care				
Aspirin Given Within 24 Hours of Arrival[5]	-	-	97%	96%
Fibrinolytic Meds Within 30 Min. of Arrival[5]	-	-	48%	58%
Average Time to ECG (minutes)[5]	-	-	7	7
Average Time to Transfer (minutes)[5]	-	-	54	60
Children's Asthma Care				
Received Home Management Plan of Care	-	-	-	88%
Received Reliever Medication	-	-	-	100%
Received Systemic Corticosteroids	-	-	-	100%
Emergency Department				
Admittance Decision Time (minutes)[1,2]	-	-	62	98
Head CT Results Within 45 Min. of Arrival[5]	-	-	54%	57%
Patients Who Left ER Before Being Seen[5]	-	-	2%	2%
Time from ER Arrival to Admit. (minutes)[1,2]	-	-	199	274
Time from ER Arrival to Discharge (minutes)[5]	-	-	125	134
Time in ER Before Being Evaluated (minutes)[5]	-	-	31	26
Time to Pain Meds for Fractures (minutes)[5]	-	-	45	57
Heart Attack Care				
Aspirin Given at Discharge[5]	-	-	99%	99%
Fibrinolytic Meds Within 30 Min. of Arrival[5]	-	-	-	54%
PCI Within 90 Minutes of Arrival[5]	-	-	96%	96%
Statin Prescribed at Discharge[5]	-	-	99%	98%
Heart Failure Care				
ACE Inhibitor or ARB for LVSD[1]	-	-	96%	97%

NOTE: Hospital profiles are in alphabetical order by state, then city, then hospital within the city; Rankings exclude hospitals with less than 25 cases except for patient surveys which excludes hospitals with less than 100 cases; (a) 100-299 cases; (1) The number of cases/patients is too few to report; (2) Data submitted were based on a sample of cases/patients; (3) Results are based on a shorter time period than required; (4) Data suppressed by CMS for one or more quarters; (5) Results are not available for this reporting period; (6) Fewer than 100 patients completed the HCAHPS survey; (7) No cases met the criteria for this measure; (8) The lower limit of the confidence interval cannot be calculated if the number of observed infections equals zero; (9) No data are available from the state/territory for this reporting period; (10) The scores shown reflect fewer than 50 completed surveys; (11) There were discrepancies in the data collection process; (12) This measure does not apply to this hospital for this reporting period; (13) Results cannot be calculated for this reporting period; (14) The results for this state are combined with nearby states to protect confidentiality; Please refer to the User's Guide for a full explanation of data.

Measure	Cases	This Hosp.	State Avg.	U.S. Avg.
Discharge Instructions Given	23	78%	93%	94%
Evaluation of LVS Function	23	96%	97%	99%
Medicare Spending				
Medicare Spending per Patient (ratio)	-	0.92	0.9	0.98
Pneumonia Care				
Appropriate Initial Antibiotic Given[1]	-	-	94%	95%
Blood Culture Timing[7]	-	-	97%	98%
Pregnancy and Delivery Care				
Newborn Deliveries Scheduled Early[2]	17	0%	5%	6%
Preventive Care				
Immunization for Influenza[2]	555	92%	89%	90%
Immunization for Pneumonia[2]	499	90%	89%	92%
Stroke Care				
Anticoagulation Therapy for Atrial Fibrillation[7]	-	-	96%	95%
Antithrombotic Therapy Timing[1]	-	-	98%	98%
Assessed for Rehabilitation[1]	-	-	98%	97%
Discharged on Antithrombotic Therapy[1]	-	-	99%	99%
Discharged on Statin Medication[1]	-	-	95%	94%
Thrombolytic Therapy Timing[7]	-	-	74%	66%
Venous Thromboembolism Prophylaxis[1]	-	-	95%	94%
Written Stroke Educational Materials Given[1]	-	-	88%	88%
Surgical Care Improvement Project				
Appropriate Beta Blocker Usage[2]	194	100%	98%	98%
Appropriate VTP Within 24 Hours[2]	624	100%	98%	98%
Controlled Postoperative Blood Glucose[2,7]	-	-	97%	97%
Perioperative Temperature Management[2]	717	100%	99%	100%
Prophylactic Antibiotic Selection[2]	406	100%	99%	99%
Prophylactic Antibiotic Selection (Outpatient)	643	100%	98%	98%
Prophylactic Antibiotic Stopped[2]	395	99%	99%	98%
Prophylactic Antibiotic Timing[2]	406	100%	98%	99%
Prophylactic Antibiotic Timing (Outpatient)	508	98%	97%	98%
Urinary Catheter Removal[2]	178	100%	97%	97%
Survey of Patients' Hospital Experiences				
Area Around Room 'Always' Quiet at Night[11]	300+	69%	65%	61%
Doctors 'Always' Communicated Well[11]	300+	84%	84%	82%
Home Recovery Information Given[11]	300+	92%	88%	85%
Hospital Given 9 or 10 on 10 Point Scale[11]	300+	86%	74%	71%
Meds 'Always' Explained Before Given[11]	300+	68%	67%	64%
Nurses 'Always' Communicated Well[11]	300+	84%	81%	79%
Pain 'Always' Well Controlled[11]	300+	74%	72%	71%
Room and Bathroom 'Always' Clean[11]	300+	77%	78%	73%
Timely Help 'Always' Received[11]	300+	74%	74%	68%
Would Definitely Recommend Hospital[11]	300+	90%	71%	71%
Use of Medical Imaging				
Cardiac Imaging Stress Test before Surgery	2,221	11.3%	6.3%	5.3%
Combination Abdominal CT Scan	190	5.3%	5.7%	10.5%
Combination Brain/Sinus CT Scan[1]	-	-	2.3%	2.7%
Combination Chest CT Scan	162	0.0%	1.9%	2.7%
Follow-up Mammogram/Ultrasound[1]	-	-	6.3%	8.8%
Lumbar Spine MRI for Low Back Pain[1]	-	-	37.6%	37.2%

Olmsted Medical Center

1650 Fourth Street Southeast
Rochester, MN 55904
Phone: 507-287-2761
Fax: 507-529-6622
URL: www.olmsteadmedicalcenter.org
Type: Acute Care Hospitals
Emergency Services: Yes
Ownership: Voluntary non-profit - Private
Beds: 61

Key Personnel:

Quality Assurance . . . . Sue Klenner
CEO/President. . . . . Kathryn Lombardo, MD
Emergency Room . . . . Jay Myers
Radiology. . . . . Diya Odeh
Operating Room. . . . . Ben Riker
Infection Control. . . . . Vicky Shultz
CEO . . . . Tim W. Weir, FACHE
Chief of Medical Staff . . . . David Westgard, MD

Measure	Cases	This Hosp.	State Avg.	U.S. Avg.
Blood Clot Prevention and Treatment				
Anticoagulation Overlap Therapy[1]	-	-	96%	93%
ICU Venous Thromboembolism Prophylaxis	73	96%	91%	92%
Incidence of Potentially Preventable VTE[1]	-	-	9%	10%
UFH with Dosages/Platelet Monitoring[1]	-	-	98%	97%
Venous Thromboembolism Prophylaxis	254	96%	86%	85%
Warfarin Therapy Discharge Instructions[1]	-	-	63%	75%
Chest Pain/Possible Heart Attack Care				
Aspirin Given Within 24 Hours of Arrival	40	100%	97%	96%
Fibrinolytic Meds Within 30 Min. of Arrival[7]	-	-	48%	58%
Average Time to ECG (minutes)	39	18	7	7
Average Time to Transfer (minutes)[7]	-	-	54	60
Children's Asthma Care				
Received Home Management Plan of Care	-	-	-	88%
Received Reliever Medication	-	-	-	100%
Received Systemic Corticosteroids	-	-	-	100%
Emergency Department				
Admittance Decision Time (minutes)	250	85	62	98
Head CT Results Within 45 Min. of Arrival[1]	-	-	54%	57%
Patients Who Left ER Before Being Seen	16,268	1%	2%	2%
Time from ER Arrival to Admit. (minutes)	375	266	199	274
Time from ER Arrival to Discharge (minutes)	17,467	122	125	134
Time in ER Before Being Evaluated (minutes)	14,960	45	31	26
Time to Pain Meds for Fractures (minutes)	86	79	45	57
Heart Attack Care				
Aspirin Given at Discharge[3,7]	-	-	99%	99%
Fibrinolytic Meds Within 30 Min. of Arrival[3,7]	-	-	-	54%
PCI Within 90 Minutes of Arrival[3,7]	-	-	96%	96%
Statin Prescribed at Discharge[3,7]	-	-	99%	98%
Heart Failure Care				
ACE Inhibitor or ARB for LVSD[1]	-	-	96%	97%
Discharge Instructions Given	16	100%	93%	94%
Evaluation of LVS Function	23	100%	97%	99%
Medicare Spending				
Medicare Spending per Patient (ratio)	-	0.89	0.9	0.98
Pneumonia Care				
Appropriate Initial Antibiotic Given	34	88%	94%	95%
Blood Culture Timing	53	94%	97%	98%
Pregnancy and Delivery Care				
Newborn Deliveries Scheduled Early	101	0%	5%	6%
Preventive Care				
Immunization for Influenza	860	100%	89%	90%
Immunization for Pneumonia	643	97%	89%	92%
Stroke Care				
Anticoagulation Therapy for Atrial Fibrillation[3,7]	-	-	96%	95%
Antithrombotic Therapy Timing[3,7]	-	-	98%	98%
Assessed for Rehabilitation[1,3]	-	-	98%	97%
Discharged on Antithrombotic Therapy[1,3]	-	-	99%	99%
Discharged on Statin Medication[3,7]	-	-	95%	94%
Thrombolytic Therapy Timing[3,7]	-	-	74%	66%
Venous Thromboembolism Prophylaxis[1,3]	-	-	95%	94%
Written Stroke Educational Materials Given[3,7]	-	-	88%	88%
Surgical Care Improvement Project				
Appropriate Beta Blocker Usage	97	99%	98%	98%
Appropriate VTP Within 24 Hours	224	96%	98%	98%
Controlled Postoperative Blood Glucose[7]	-	-	97%	97%
Perioperative Temperature Management	259	100%	99%	100%
Prophylactic Antibiotic Selection	224	99%	99%	99%
Prophylactic Antibiotic Selection (Outpatient)	54	94%	98%	98%
Prophylactic Antibiotic Stopped	219	98%	99%	98%
Prophylactic Antibiotic Timing	227	97%	98%	99%
Prophylactic Antibiotic Timing (Outpatient)	55	93%	97%	98%
Urinary Catheter Removal	207	99%	97%	97%
Survey of Patients' Hospital Experiences				
Area Around Room 'Always' Quiet at Night	(a)	60%	65%	61%
Doctors 'Always' Communicated Well	(a)	80%	84%	82%
Home Recovery Information Given	(a)	91%	88%	85%
Hospital Given 9 or 10 on 10 Point Scale	(a)	83%	74%	71%
Meds 'Always' Explained Before Given	(a)	65%	67%	64%
Nurses 'Always' Communicated Well	(a)	83%	81%	79%
Pain 'Always' Well Controlled	(a)	72%	72%	71%
Room and Bathroom 'Always' Clean	(a)	76%	78%	73%
Timely Help 'Always' Received	(a)	78%	74%	68%
Would Definitely Recommend Hospital	(a)	87%	71%	71%
Use of Medical Imaging				
Cardiac Imaging Stress Test before Surgery	57	1.8%	6.3%	5.3%
Combination Abdominal CT Scan	189	10.6%	5.7%	10.5%
Combination Brain/Sinus CT Scan[1]	-	-	2.3%	2.7%
Combination Chest CT Scan	93	5.4%	1.9%	2.7%
Follow-up Mammogram/Ultrasound	878	5.4%	6.3%	8.8%
Lumbar Spine MRI for Low Back Pain[1]	-	-	37.6%	37.2%

Lifecare Medical Center

715 Delmore Drive
Roseau, MN 56751
Phone: 218-463-2500
Fax: 218-463-1266
URL: www.lifecaremedicalcenter.org
Type: Critical Access Hospitals
Emergency Services: Yes
Ownership: Voluntary non-profit - Private
Beds: 25

Key Personnel:

Chief of Medical Staff . . . . Robert Anderson, MD
Pulmonology . . . . Chris Berger
Emergency Room . . . . Ronald Brummer, MD
Infection Control. . . . . Jane Hirst, RN
Quality Assurance . . . . Kelly Hulst, RN
Patient Relations . . . . Sue Lisell
CEO/President. . . . . Keith Okeson
Radiology. . . . . Sharlene Peterson

Measure	Cases	This Hosp.	State Avg.	U.S. Avg.
Blood Clot Prevention and Treatment				
Anticoagulation Overlap Therapy[5]	-	-	96%	93%
ICU Venous Thromboembolism Prophylaxis[5]	-	-	91%	92%
Incidence of Potentially Preventable VTE[5]	-	-	9%	10%
UFH with Dosages/Platelet Monitoring[5]	-	-	98%	97%
Venous Thromboembolism Prophylaxis[5]	-	-	86%	85%
Warfarin Therapy Discharge Instructions[5]	-	-	63%	75%
Chest Pain/Possible Heart Attack Care				
Aspirin Given Within 24 Hours of Arrival	56	98%	97%	96%
Fibrinolytic Meds Within 30 Min. of Arrival[1]	-	-	48%	58%
Average Time to ECG (minutes)	56	6	7	7
Average Time to Transfer (minutes)[1]	-	-	54	60
Children's Asthma Care				
Received Home Management Plan of Care	-	-	-	88%
Received Reliever Medication	-	-	-	100%
Received Systemic Corticosteroids	-	-	-	100%
Emergency Department				
Admittance Decision Time (minutes)[2]	330	26	62	98
Head CT Results Within 45 Min. of Arrival[5]	-	-	54%	57%
Patients Who Left ER Before Being Seen	9,273	0%	2%	2%
Time from ER Arrival to Admit. (minutes)[2]	334	166	199	274
Time from ER Arrival to Discharge (minutes)[5]	-	-	125	134
Time in ER Before Being Evaluated (minutes)[5]	-	-	31	26
Time to Pain Meds for Fractures (minutes)[5]	-	-	45	57
Heart Attack Care				
Aspirin Given at Discharge[1,3]	-	-	99%	99%
Fibrinolytic Meds Within 30 Min. of Arrival[3,7]	-	-	-	54%
PCI Within 90 Minutes of Arrival[3,7]	-	-	96%	96%
Statin Prescribed at Discharge[1,3]	-	-	99%	98%
Heart Failure Care				
ACE Inhibitor or ARB for LVSD[1]	-	-	96%	97%
Discharge Instructions Given	17	76%	93%	94%
Evaluation of LVS Function	26	88%	97%	99%
Medicare Spending				
Medicare Spending per Patient (ratio)	-	-	0.9	0.98
Pneumonia Care				
Appropriate Initial Antibiotic Given	25	96%	94%	95%
Blood Culture Timing	20	100%	97%	98%
Pregnancy and Delivery Care				
Newborn Deliveries Scheduled Early[5]	-	-	5%	6%
Preventive Care				
Immunization for Influenza	312	82%	89%	90%
Immunization for Pneumonia	340	89%	89%	92%
Stroke Care				
Anticoagulation Therapy for Atrial Fibrillation[5]	-	-	96%	95%
Antithrombotic Therapy Timing[5]	-	-	98%	98%
Assessed for Rehabilitation[5]	-	-	98%	97%
Discharged on Antithrombotic Therapy[5]	-	-	99%	99%
Discharged on Statin Medication[5]	-	-	95%	94%
Thrombolytic Therapy Timing[5]	-	-	74%	66%
Venous Thromboembolism Prophylaxis[5]	-	-	95%	94%
Written Stroke Educational Materials Given[5]	-	-	88%	88%
Surgical Care Improvement Project				
Appropriate Beta Blocker Usage[7]	-	-	98%	98%
Appropriate VTP Within 24 Hours[1]	-	-	98%	98%

NOTE: Hospital profiles are in alphabetical order by state, then city, then hospital within the city; Rankings exclude hospitals with less than 25 cases except for patient surveys which excludes hospitals with less than 100 cases; (a) 100-299 cases; (1) The number of cases/patients is too few to report; (2) Data submitted were based on a sample of cases/patients; (3) Results are based on a shorter time period than required; (4) Data suppressed by CMS for one or more quarters; (5) Results are not available for this reporting period; (6) Fewer than 100 patients completed the HCAHPS survey; (7) No cases met the criteria for this measure; (8) The lower limit of the confidence interval cannot be calculated if the number of observed infections equals zero; (9) No data are available from the state/territory for this reporting period; (10) The scores shown reflect fewer than 50 completed surveys; (11) There were discrepancies in the data collection process; (12) This measure does not apply to this hospital for this reporting period; (13) Results cannot be calculated for this reporting period; (14) The results for this state are combined with nearby states to protect confidentiality; Please refer to the User's Guide for a full explanation of data.

Measure	Cases	This Hosp.	State Avg.	U.S. Avg.
Controlled Postoperative Blood Glucose[7]	-	-	97%	97%
Perioperative Temperature Management[1]	-	-	99%	100%
Prophylactic Antibiotic Selection[1]	-	-	99%	99%
Prophylactic Antibiotic Selection (Outpatient)[1,3]	-	-	98%	98%
Prophylactic Antibiotic Stopped[1]	-	-	99%	98%
Prophylactic Antibiotic Timing[1]	-	-	98%	99%
Prophylactic Antibiotic Timing (Outpatient)[1,3]	-	-	97%	98%
Urinary Catheter Removal[1]	-	-	97%	97%
Survey of Patients' Hospital Experiences				
Area Around Room 'Always' Quiet at Night	(a)	60%	65%	61%
Doctors 'Always' Communicated Well	(a)	84%	84%	82%
Home Recovery Information Given	(a)	90%	88%	85%
Hospital Given 9 or 10 on 10 Point Scale	(a)	77%	74%	71%
Meds 'Always' Explained Before Given	(a)	62%	67%	64%
Nurses 'Always' Communicated Well	(a)	80%	81%	79%
Pain 'Always' Well Controlled	(a)	66%	72%	71%
Room and Bathroom 'Always' Clean	(a)	77%	78%	73%
Timely Help 'Always' Received	(a)	71%	74%	68%
Would Definitely Recommend Hospital	(a)	69%	71%	71%
Use of Medical Imaging				
Cardiac Imaging Stress Test before Surgery[1]	-	-	6.3%	5.3%
Combination Abdominal CT Scan[1]	-	-	5.7%	10.5%
Combination Brain/Sinus CT Scan[1]	-	-	2.3%	2.7%
Combination Chest CT Scan[1]	-	-	1.9%	2.7%
Follow-up Mammogram/Ultrasound	121	10.7%	6.3%	8.8%
Lumbar Spine MRI for Low Back Pain[1]	-	-	37.6%	37.2%

Saint Cloud Hospital

1406 6th Ave North
Saint Cloud, MN 56303
URL: www.centracare.com
Type: Acute Care Hospitals
Ownership: Voluntary non-profit - Private
Phone: 320-251-2700
Fax: 320-255-5711
Emergency Services: Yes
Beds: 489

Key Personnel:
Operating Room.............. Larry Asplin
CEO/President.............. Craig Broman
Chief of Medical Staff.......... Richard Jolkovsky, MD
Pediatric Ambulatory Care...... Tom Schrup, MD
Pediatric In-Patient Care....... Tom Schrup, MD
Emergency Room............ Jack Stinolgel DO
Radiology.................. Mary Super

Measure	Cases	This Hosp.	State Avg.	U.S. Avg.
Blood Clot Prevention and Treatment				
Anticoagulation Overlap Therapy[2]	214	88%	96%	93%
ICU Venous Thromboembolism Prophylaxis[2]	41	90%	91%	92%
Incidence of Potentially Preventable VTE[2]	22	0%	9%	10%
UFH with Dosages/Platelet Monitoring[2]	193	100%	98%	97%
Venous Thromboembolism Prophylaxis[2]	333	91%	86%	85%
Warfarin Therapy Discharge Instructions[2]	171	49%	63%	75%
Chest Pain/Possible Heart Attack Care				
Aspirin Given Within 24 Hours of Arrival[3,7]	-	-	97%	96%
Fibrinolytic Meds Within 30 Min. of Arrival[5]	-	-	48%	58%
Average Time to ECG (minutes)[3,7]	-	-	7	7
Average Time to Transfer (minutes)[5]	-	-	54	60
Children's Asthma Care				
Received Home Management Plan of Care	-	-	-	88%
Received Reliever Medication	-	-	-	100%
Received Systemic Corticosteroids	-	-	-	100%
Emergency Department				
Admittance Decision Time (minutes)[2]	374	84	62	98
Head CT Results Within 45 Min. of Arrival[1,3]	-	-	54%	57%
Patients Who Left ER Before Being Seen	58,327	1%	2%	2%
Time from ER Arrival to Admit. (minutes)[2]	397	205	199	274
Time from ER Arrival to Discharge (minutes)	343	163	125	134
Time in ER Before Being Evaluated (minutes)	367	36	31	26
Time to Pain Meds for Fractures (minutes)	177	54	45	57
Heart Attack Care				
Aspirin Given at Discharge	738	100%	99%	99%
Fibrinolytic Meds Within 30 Min. of Arrival[7]	-	-	-	54%
PCI Within 90 Minutes of Arrival	68	96%	96%	96%
Statin Prescribed at Discharge	698	100%	99%	98%
Heart Failure Care				
ACE Inhibitor or ARB for LVSD	159	99%	96%	97%
Discharge Instructions Given	527	97%	93%	94%
Evaluation of LVS Function	731	100%	97%	99%
Medicare Spending				
Medicare Spending per Patient (ratio)	-	0.89	0.9	0.98
Pneumonia Care				
Appropriate Initial Antibiotic Given	216	94%	94%	95%
Blood Culture Timing	359	98%	97%	98%
Pregnancy and Delivery Care				
Newborn Deliveries Scheduled Early[2]	375	5%	5%	6%
Preventive Care				
Immunization for Influenza[2]	520	97%	89%	90%
Immunization for Pneumonia[2]	587	97%	89%	92%
Stroke Care				
Anticoagulation Therapy for Atrial Fibrillation	65	92%	96%	95%
Antithrombotic Therapy Timing	216	99%	98%	98%
Assessed for Rehabilitation	376	99%	98%	97%
Discharged on Antithrombotic Therapy	330	98%	99%	99%
Discharged on Statin Medication	266	96%	95%	94%
Thrombolytic Therapy Timing	34	79%	74%	66%
Venous Thromboembolism Prophylaxis	338	99%	95%	94%
Written Stroke Educational Materials Given	203	96%	88%	88%
Surgical Care Improvement Project				
Appropriate Beta Blocker Usage[2]	285	99%	98%	98%
Appropriate VTP Within 24 Hours[2]	345	99%	98%	98%
Controlled Postoperative Blood Glucose[2]	139	91%	97%	97%
Perioperative Temperature Management[2]	487	100%	99%	100%
Prophylactic Antibiotic Selection[2]	431	99%	99%	99%
Prophylactic Antibiotic Selection (Outpatient)	1,022	100%	98%	98%
Prophylactic Antibiotic Stopped[2]	426	99%	99%	98%
Prophylactic Antibiotic Timing[2]	431	98%	98%	99%
Prophylactic Antibiotic Timing (Outpatient)	1,029	98%	97%	98%
Urinary Catheter Removal[2]	279	95%	97%	97%
Survey of Patients' Hospital Experiences				
Area Around Room 'Always' Quiet at Night	300+	67%	65%	61%
Doctors 'Always' Communicated Well	300+	82%	84%	82%
Home Recovery Information Given	300+	87%	88%	85%
Hospital Given 9 or 10 on 10 Point Scale	300+	77%	74%	71%
Meds 'Always' Explained Before Given	300+	67%	67%	64%
Nurses 'Always' Communicated Well	300+	83%	81%	79%
Pain 'Always' Well Controlled	300+	74%	72%	71%
Room and Bathroom 'Always' Clean	300+	79%	78%	73%
Timely Help 'Always' Received	300+	74%	74%	68%
Would Definitely Recommend Hospital	300+	82%	71%	71%
Use of Medical Imaging				
Cardiac Imaging Stress Test before Surgery	508	4.5%	6.3%	5.3%
Combination Abdominal CT Scan	993	2.8%	5.7%	10.5%
Combination Brain/Sinus CT Scan	517	2.5%	2.3%	2.7%
Combination Chest CT Scan	1,003	0.4%	1.9%	2.7%
Follow-up Mammogram/Ultrasound	1,202	5.4%	6.3%	8.8%
Lumbar Spine MRI for Low Back Pain	87	37.9%	37.6%	37.2%

Saint Cloud VA Medical Center

4801 8th Street N
Saint Cloud, MN 56303
Type: Acute Care - VA
Ownership: Government Federal
Phone: 320-252-1670
Fax: 320-255-6426
Emergency Services: No
Beds: 408

Key Personnel:
Radiology.................. Marilyn Crandell
Ambulatory Care............ George Feyda, MD
Chief of Medical Staff.......... Susan M. Markstrom, MD
Patient Relations............ Barry Venable

Measure	Cases	This Hosp.	State Avg.	U.S. Avg.
Blood Clot Prevention and Treatment				
Anticoagulation Overlap Therapy	-	-	96%	93%
ICU Venous Thromboembolism Prophylaxis	-	-	91%	92%
Incidence of Potentially Preventable VTE	-	-	9%	10%
UFH with Dosages/Platelet Monitoring	-	-	98%	97%
Venous Thromboembolism Prophylaxis	-	-	86%	85%
Warfarin Therapy Discharge Instructions	-	-	63%	75%
Chest Pain/Possible Heart Attack Care				
Aspirin Given Within 24 Hours of Arrival	-	-	97%	96%
Fibrinolytic Meds Within 30 Min. of Arrival	-	-	48%	58%
Average Time to ECG (minutes)	-	-	7	7
Average Time to Transfer (minutes)	-	-	54	60
Children's Asthma Care				
Received Home Management Plan of Care	-	-	-	88%
Received Reliever Medication	-	-	-	100%
Received Systemic Corticosteroids	-	-	-	100%
Emergency Department				
Admittance Decision Time (minutes)	-	-	62	98
Head CT Results Within 45 Min. of Arrival	-	-	54%	57%
Patients Who Left ER Before Being Seen	-	-	2%	2%
Time from ER Arrival to Admit. (minutes)	-	-	199	274
Time from ER Arrival to Discharge (minutes)	-	-	125	134
Time in ER Before Being Evaluated (minutes)	-	-	31	26
Time to Pain Meds for Fractures (minutes)	-	-	45	57
Heart Attack Care				
Aspirin Given at Discharge[5]	-	-	99%	99%
Fibrinolytic Meds Within 30 Min. of Arrival[5]	-	-	-	54%
PCI Within 90 Minutes of Arrival[5]	-	-	96%	96%
Statin Prescribed at Discharge[5]	-	-	99%	98%
Heart Failure Care				
ACE Inhibitor or ARB for LVSD[5]	-	-	96%	97%
Discharge Instructions Given[5]	-	-	93%	94%
Evaluation of LVS Function[5]	-	-	97%	99%
Medicare Spending				
Medicare Spending per Patient (ratio)	-	-	0.9	0.98
Pneumonia Care				
Appropriate Initial Antibiotic Given[5]	-	-	94%	95%
Blood Culture Timing[5]	-	-	97%	98%
Pregnancy and Delivery Care				
Newborn Deliveries Scheduled Early	-	-	5%	6%
Preventive Care				
Immunization for Influenza[2,3]	95	71%	89%	90%
Immunization for Pneumonia[2,3]	92	99%	89%	92%
Stroke Care				
Anticoagulation Therapy for Atrial Fibrillation	-	-	96%	95%
Antithrombotic Therapy Timing	-	-	98%	98%
Assessed for Rehabilitation	-	-	98%	97%
Discharged on Antithrombotic Therapy	-	-	99%	99%
Discharged on Statin Medication	-	-	95%	94%
Thrombolytic Therapy Timing	-	-	74%	66%
Venous Thromboembolism Prophylaxis	-	-	95%	94%
Written Stroke Educational Materials Given	-	-	88%	88%
Surgical Care Improvement Project				
Appropriate Beta Blocker Usage[5]	-	-	98%	98%
Appropriate VTP Within 24 Hours[5]	-	-	98%	98%
Controlled Postoperative Blood Glucose[5]	-	-	97%	97%
Perioperative Temperature Management[5]	-	-	99%	100%
Prophylactic Antibiotic Selection[5]	-	-	99%	99%
Prophylactic Antibiotic Selection (Outpatient)	-	-	98%	98%
Prophylactic Antibiotic Stopped[5]	-	-	99%	98%
Prophylactic Antibiotic Timing[5]	-	-	98%	99%
Prophylactic Antibiotic Timing (Outpatient)	-	-	97%	98%
Urinary Catheter Removal[5]	-	-	97%	97%
Survey of Patients' Hospital Experiences				
Area Around Room 'Always' Quiet at Night	-	-	65%	61%
Doctors 'Always' Communicated Well	-	-	84%	82%
Home Recovery Information Given	-	-	88%	85%
Hospital Given 9 or 10 on 10 Point Scale	-	-	74%	71%
Meds 'Always' Explained Before Given	-	-	67%	64%
Nurses 'Always' Communicated Well	-	-	81%	79%
Pain 'Always' Well Controlled	-	-	72%	71%
Room and Bathroom 'Always' Clean	-	-	78%	73%
Timely Help 'Always' Received	-	-	74%	68%
Would Definitely Recommend Hospital	-	-	71%	71%
Use of Medical Imaging				
Cardiac Imaging Stress Test before Surgery	-	-	6.3%	5.3%
Combination Abdominal CT Scan	-	-	5.7%	10.5%
Combination Brain/Sinus CT Scan	-	-	2.3%	2.7%
Combination Chest CT Scan	-	-	1.9%	2.7%
Follow-up Mammogram/Ultrasound	-	-	6.3%	8.8%
Lumbar Spine MRI for Low Back Pain	-	-	37.6%	37.2%

NOTE: Hospital profiles are in alphabetical order by state, then city, then hospital within the city; Rankings exclude hospitals with less than 25 cases except for patient surveys which excludes hospitals with less than 100 cases; (a) 100-299 cases; (1) The number of cases/patients is too few to report; (2) Data submitted were based on a sample of cases/patients; (3) Results are based on a shorter time period than required; (4) Data suppressed by CMS for one or more quarters; (5) Results are not available for this reporting period; (6) Fewer than 100 patients completed the HCAHPS survey; (7) No cases met the criteria for this measure; (8) The lower limit of the confidence interval cannot be calculated if the number of observed infections equals zero; (9) No data are available from the state/territory for this reporting period; (10) The scores shown reflect fewer than 50 completed surveys; (11) There were discrepancies in the data collection process; (12) This measure does not apply to this hospital for this reporting period; (13) Results cannot be calculated for this reporting period; (14) The results for this state are combined with nearby states to protect confidentiality; Please refer to the User's Guide for a full explanation of data.

Mayo Clinic Health System - Saint James

1101 Moulton & Parsons Drive
Saint James, MN 56081
Phone: 507-375-3261
Fax: 507-375-8605
URL: www.stjmc.org
Type: Critical Access Hospitals
Emergency Services: Yes
Ownership: Voluntary non-profit - Other
Beds: 31

Key Personnel:
Quality Assurance . . . . Doug Holz
CEO/President. . . . . John H Noseworthy, MD
Infection Control. . . . . Sue Piper
Emergency Room . . . . Linda Winkleman
Operating Room. . . . . Linda Winkleman

Measure	Cases	This Hosp.	State Avg.	U.S. Avg.
Blood Clot Prevention and Treatment				
Anticoagulation Overlap Therapy[5]	-	-	96%	93%
ICU Venous Thromboembolism Prophylaxis[5]	-	-	91%	92%
Incidence of Potentially Preventable VTE[5]	-	-	9%	10%
UFH with Dosages/Platelet Monitoring[5]	-	-	98%	97%
Venous Thromboembolism Prophylaxis[5]	-	-	86%	85%
Warfarin Therapy Discharge Instructions[5]	-	-	63%	75%
Chest Pain/Possible Heart Attack Care				
Aspirin Given Within 24 Hours of Arrival[3]	15	93%	97%	96%
Fibrinolytic Meds Within 30 Min. of Arrival[3,7]	-	-	48%	58%
Average Time to ECG (minutes)[3]	15	7	7	7
Average Time to Transfer (minutes)[1,3]	-	-	54	60
Children's Asthma Care				
Received Home Management Plan of Care	-	-	-	88%
Received Reliever Medication	-	-	-	100%
Received Systemic Corticosteroids	-	-	-	100%
Emergency Department				
Admittance Decision Time (minutes)	52	14	62	98
Head CT Results Within 45 Min. of Arrival[5]	-	-	54%	57%
Patients Who Left ER Before Being Seen	2,301	0%	2%	2%
Time from ER Arrival to Admit. (minutes)	79	139	199	274
Time from ER Arrival to Discharge (minutes)[5]	-	-	125	134
Time in ER Before Being Evaluated (minutes)[5]	-	-	31	26
Time to Pain Meds for Fractures (minutes)[5]	-	-	45	57
Heart Attack Care				
Aspirin Given at Discharge[3,7]	-	-	99%	99%
Fibrinolytic Meds Within 30 Min. of Arrival[3,7]	-	-	-	54%
PCI Within 90 Minutes of Arrival[3,7]	-	-	96%	96%
Statin Prescribed at Discharge[3,7]	-	-	99%	98%
Heart Failure Care				
ACE Inhibitor or ARB for LVSD[1]	-	-	96%	97%
Discharge Instructions Given[1]	-	-	93%	94%
Evaluation of LVS Function[1]	-	-	97%	99%
Medicare Spending				
Medicare Spending per Patient (ratio)	-	-	0.9	0.98
Pneumonia Care				
Appropriate Initial Antibiotic Given[1]	-	-	94%	95%
Blood Culture Timing[1]	-	-	97%	98%
Pregnancy and Delivery Care				
Newborn Deliveries Scheduled Early[3,7]	-	-	5%	6%
Preventive Care				
Immunization for Influenza	90	100%	89%	90%
Immunization for Pneumonia	151	97%	89%	92%
Stroke Care				
Anticoagulation Therapy for Atrial Fibrillation[5]	-	-	96%	95%
Antithrombotic Therapy Timing[5]	-	-	98%	98%
Assessed for Rehabilitation[5]	-	-	98%	97%
Discharged on Antithrombotic Therapy[5]	-	-	99%	99%
Discharged on Statin Medication[5]	-	-	95%	94%
Thrombolytic Therapy Timing[5]	-	-	74%	66%
Venous Thromboembolism Prophylaxis[5]	-	-	95%	94%
Written Stroke Educational Materials Given[5]	-	-	88%	88%
Surgical Care Improvement Project				
Appropriate Beta Blocker Usage[5]	-	-	98%	98%
Appropriate VTP Within 24 Hours[5]	-	-	98%	98%
Controlled Postoperative Blood Glucose[5]	-	-	97%	97%
Perioperative Temperature Management[5]	-	-	99%	100%
Prophylactic Antibiotic Selection[5]	-	-	99%	99%
Prophylactic Antibiotic Selection (Outpatient)[5]	-	-	98%	98%
Prophylactic Antibiotic Stopped[5]	-	-	99%	98%
Prophylactic Antibiotic Timing[5]	-	-	98%	99%
Prophylactic Antibiotic Timing (Outpatient)[5]	-	-	97%	98%
Urinary Catheter Removal[5]	-	-	97%	97%
Survey of Patients' Hospital Experiences				
Area Around Room 'Always' Quiet at Night[10]	<100	67%	65%	61%
Doctors 'Always' Communicated Well[10]	<100	84%	84%	82%
Home Recovery Information Given[10]	<100	87%	88%	85%
Hospital Given 9 or 10 on 10 Point Scale[10]	<100	63%	74%	71%
Meds 'Always' Explained Before Given[10]	<100	63%	67%	64%
Nurses 'Always' Communicated Well[10]	<100	75%	81%	79%
Pain 'Always' Well Controlled[10]	<100	59%	72%	71%
Room and Bathroom 'Always' Clean[10]	<100	79%	78%	73%
Timely Help 'Always' Received[10]	<100	61%	74%	68%
Would Definitely Recommend Hospital[10]	<100	66%	71%	71%
Use of Medical Imaging				
Cardiac Imaging Stress Test before Surgery[7]	-	-	6.3%	5.3%
Combination Abdominal CT Scan	64	21.9%	5.7%	10.5%
Combination Brain/Sinus CT Scan[1]	-	-	2.3%	2.7%
Combination Chest CT Scan[1]	-	-	1.9%	2.7%
Follow-up Mammogram/Ultrasound	182	5.5%	6.3%	8.8%
Lumbar Spine MRI for Low Back Pain[1]	-	-	37.6%	37.2%

Park Nicollet Methodist Hospital

6500 Excelsior Blvd
Saint Louis Park, MN 55426
Phone: 952-993-5000
Fax: 952-993-5936
URL: www.parknicollet.com/methodist
Type: Acute Care Hospitals
Emergency Services: Yes
Ownership: Voluntary non-profit - Private
Beds: 426

Key Personnel:
Chief of Medical Staff . . . . Curt Boehm, MD
Emergency Room . . . . Rebecca Bryson
Pediatric In-Patient Care . . . . Anne Edwards, MD
Operating Room. . . . . Kevin Ose, MD
Radiology. . . . . Kurt Simpson, MD
Anesthesiology. . . . . Beverlee Smiley
Quality Assurance . . . . Victoria Wayne
Hemotology Center . . . . Mark Wilkowske

Measure	Cases	This Hosp.	State Avg.	U.S. Avg.
Blood Clot Prevention and Treatment				
Anticoagulation Overlap Therapy[2]	208	98%	96%	93%
ICU Venous Thromboembolism Prophylaxis[2]	22	86%	91%	92%
Incidence of Potentially Preventable VTE[2]	25	8%	9%	10%
UFH with Dosages/Platelet Monitoring[2]	116	86%	98%	97%
Venous Thromboembolism Prophylaxis[2]	340	69%	86%	85%
Warfarin Therapy Discharge Instructions[2]	153	95%	63%	75%
Chest Pain/Possible Heart Attack Care				
Aspirin Given Within 24 Hours of Arrival[5]	-	-	97%	96%
Fibrinolytic Meds Within 30 Min. of Arrival[5]	-	-	48%	58%
Average Time to ECG (minutes)[5]	-	-	7	7
Average Time to Transfer (minutes)[5]	-	-	54	60
Children's Asthma Care				
Received Home Management Plan of Care	-	-	-	88%
Received Reliever Medication	-	-	-	100%
Received Systemic Corticosteroids	-	-	-	100%
Emergency Department				
Admittance Decision Time (minutes)[2]	590	103	62	98
Head CT Results Within 45 Min. of Arrival[3,7]	-	-	54%	57%
Patients Who Left ER Before Being Seen	49,285	1%	2%	2%
Time from ER Arrival to Admit. (minutes)[2]	605	247	199	274
Time from ER Arrival to Discharge (minutes)	373	175	125	134
Time in ER Before Being Evaluated (minutes)	344	44	31	26
Time to Pain Meds for Fractures (minutes)	154	70	45	57
Heart Attack Care				
Aspirin Given at Discharge	326	99%	99%	99%
Fibrinolytic Meds Within 30 Min. of Arrival[7]	-	-	-	54%
PCI Within 90 Minutes of Arrival	51	96%	96%	96%
Statin Prescribed at Discharge	323	99%	99%	98%
Heart Failure Care				
ACE Inhibitor or ARB for LVSD	119	97%	96%	97%
Discharge Instructions Given	345	96%	93%	94%
Evaluation of LVS Function	448	100%	97%	99%
Medicare Spending				
Medicare Spending per Patient (ratio)	-	0.92	0.9	0.98
Pneumonia Care				
Appropriate Initial Antibiotic Given	310	92%	94%	95%
Blood Culture Timing	382	96%	97%	98%
Pregnancy and Delivery Care				
Newborn Deliveries Scheduled Early	204	4%	5%	6%
Preventive Care				
Immunization for Influenza[2]	563	93%	89%	90%
Immunization for Pneumonia[2]	707	91%	89%	92%
Stroke Care				
Anticoagulation Therapy for Atrial Fibrillation	39	100%	96%	95%
Antithrombotic Therapy Timing	170	99%	98%	98%
Assessed for Rehabilitation	248	97%	98%	97%
Discharged on Antithrombotic Therapy	223	100%	99%	99%
Discharged on Statin Medication	149	98%	95%	94%
Thrombolytic Therapy Timing	66	38%	74%	66%
Venous Thromboembolism Prophylaxis	226	91%	95%	94%
Written Stroke Educational Materials Given	142	80%	88%	88%
Surgical Care Improvement Project				
Appropriate Beta Blocker Usage[2]	389	100%	98%	98%
Appropriate VTP Within 24 Hours[2]	572	98%	98%	98%
Controlled Postoperative Blood Glucose[2]	180	98%	97%	97%
Perioperative Temperature Management[2]	783	100%	99%	100%
Prophylactic Antibiotic Selection[2]	706	99%	99%	99%
Prophylactic Antibiotic Selection (Outpatient)	1,000	99%	98%	98%
Prophylactic Antibiotic Stopped[2]	687	98%	99%	98%
Prophylactic Antibiotic Timing[2]	707	98%	98%	99%
Prophylactic Antibiotic Timing (Outpatient)	1,003	98%	97%	98%
Urinary Catheter Removal[2]	393	96%	97%	97%
Survey of Patients' Hospital Experiences				
Area Around Room 'Always' Quiet at Night	300+	49%	65%	61%
Doctors 'Always' Communicated Well	300+	80%	84%	82%
Home Recovery Information Given	300+	85%	88%	85%
Hospital Given 9 or 10 on 10 Point Scale	300+	67%	74%	71%
Meds 'Always' Explained Before Given	300+	60%	67%	64%
Nurses 'Always' Communicated Well	300+	74%	81%	79%
Pain 'Always' Well Controlled	300+	67%	72%	71%
Room and Bathroom 'Always' Clean	300+	64%	78%	73%
Timely Help 'Always' Received	300+	65%	74%	68%
Would Definitely Recommend Hospital	300+	73%	71%	71%
Use of Medical Imaging				
Cardiac Imaging Stress Test before Surgery	784	5.0%	6.3%	5.3%
Combination Abdominal CT Scan	1,047	2.5%	5.7%	10.5%
Combination Brain/Sinus CT Scan	604	1.5%	2.3%	2.7%
Combination Chest CT Scan	970	22.3%	1.9%	2.7%
Follow-up Mammogram/Ultrasound[7]	-	-	6.3%	8.8%
Lumbar Spine MRI for Low Back Pain	111	31.5%	37.6%	37.2%

Regions Hospital

640 Jackson Street
Saint Paul, MN 55101
Phone: 651-254-0975
Fax: 651-254-2836
URL: www.regionshospital.com
Type: Acute Care Hospitals
Emergency Services: Yes
Ownership: Voluntary non-profit - Private
Beds: 427

Key Personnel:
Chief of Medical Staff . . . . Sue Freeman, MD
Anesthesiology. . . . . Greg Garbim, MD
Emergency Room . . . . Wayne Hass, MD
Intensive Care Unit. . . . . Shirley Hubenette
Pediatric Ambulatory Care . . . . . . Thomas Rolewicz, MD
Pediatric In-Patient Care . . . . Thomas Rolewicz, MD
Operating Room. . . . . Emily Svendsen
Radiology. . . . . Joseph Tashjiam, MD

Measure	Cases	This Hosp.	State Avg.	U.S. Avg.
Blood Clot Prevention and Treatment				
Anticoagulation Overlap Therapy[2]	126	97%	96%	93%
ICU Venous Thromboembolism Prophylaxis[2]	87	97%	91%	92%
Incidence of Potentially Preventable VTE[2]	48	23%	9%	10%
UFH with Dosages/Platelet Monitoring[2]	115	100%	98%	97%
Venous Thromboembolism Prophylaxis[2]	341	91%	86%	85%
Warfarin Therapy Discharge Instructions[2]	90	67%	63%	75%
Chest Pain/Possible Heart Attack Care				
Aspirin Given Within 24 Hours of Arrival[1,3]	-	-	97%	96%
Fibrinolytic Meds Within 30 Min. of Arrival[3,7]	-	-	48%	58%
Average Time to ECG (minutes)[1,3]	-	-	7	7
Average Time to Transfer (minutes)[1,3]	-	-	54	60

NOTE: Hospital profiles are in alphabetical order by state, then city, then hospital within the city; Rankings exclude hospitals with less than 25 cases except for patient surveys which excludes hospitals with less than 100 cases; (a) 100-299 cases; (1) The number of cases/patients is too few to report; (2) Data submitted were based on a sample of cases/patients; (3) Results are based on a shorter time period than required; (4) Data suppressed by CMS for one or more quarters; (5) Results are not available for this reporting period; (6) Fewer than 100 patients completed the HCAHPS survey; (7) No cases met the criteria for this measure; (8) The lower limit of the confidence interval cannot be calculated if the number of observed infections equals zero; (9) No data are available from the state/territory for this reporting period; (10) The scores shown reflect fewer than 50 completed surveys; (11) There were discrepancies in the data collection process; (12) This measure does not apply to this hospital for this reporting period; (13) Results cannot be calculated for this reporting period; (14) The results for this state are combined with nearby states to protect confidentiality; Please refer to the User's Guide for a full explanation of data.

Measure	Cases	This Hosp.	State Avg.	U.S. Avg.
Children's Asthma Care				
Received Home Management Plan of Care	-	-	-	88%
Received Reliever Medication	-	-	-	100%
Received Systemic Corticosteroids	-	-	-	100%
Emergency Department				
Admittance Decision Time (minutes)[2]	542	124	62	98
Head CT Results Within 45 Min. of Arrival[1]	-	-	54%	57%
Patients Who Left ER Before Being Seen	38,689	2%	2%	2%
Time from ER Arrival to Admit. (minutes)[2]	549	293	199	274
Time from ER Arrival to Discharge (minutes)	320	186	125	134
Time in ER Before Being Evaluated (minutes)	426	23	31	26
Time to Pain Meds for Fractures (minutes)	129	51	45	57
Heart Attack Care				
Aspirin Given at Discharge	488	100%	99%	99%
Fibrinolytic Meds Within 30 Min. of Arrival[7]	-	-	-	54%
PCI Within 90 Minutes of Arrival	77	96%	96%	96%
Statin Prescribed at Discharge	476	100%	99%	98%
Heart Failure Care				
ACE Inhibitor or ARB for LVSD	98	98%	96%	97%
Discharge Instructions Given	286	100%	93%	94%
Evaluation of LVS Function	382	100%	97%	99%
Medicare Spending				
Medicare Spending per Patient (ratio)	-	0.94	0.9	0.98
Pneumonia Care				
Appropriate Initial Antibiotic Given	199	97%	94%	95%
Blood Culture Timing	237	99%	97%	98%
Pregnancy and Delivery Care				
Newborn Deliveries Scheduled Early	171	2%	5%	6%
Preventive Care				
Immunization for Influenza[2]	556	97%	89%	90%
Immunization for Pneumonia[2]	575	95%	89%	92%
Stroke Care				
Anticoagulation Therapy for Atrial Fibrillation	30	87%	96%	95%
Antithrombotic Therapy Timing	159	98%	98%	98%
Assessed for Rehabilitation	267	97%	98%	97%
Discharged on Antithrombotic Therapy	204	100%	99%	99%
Discharged on Statin Medication	161	97%	95%	94%
Thrombolytic Therapy Timing	15	87%	74%	66%
Venous Thromboembolism Prophylaxis	249	88%	95%	94%
Written Stroke Educational Materials Given	132	89%	88%	88%
Surgical Care Improvement Project				
Appropriate Beta Blocker Usage[2]	311	98%	98%	98%
Appropriate VTP Within 24 Hours[2]	495	100%	98%	98%
Controlled Postoperative Blood Glucose[2]	208	100%	97%	97%
Perioperative Temperature Management[2]	609	100%	99%	100%
Prophylactic Antibiotic Selection[2]	600	98%	99%	99%
Prophylactic Antibiotic Selection (Outpatient)	376	98%	98%	98%
Prophylactic Antibiotic Stopped[2]	577	99%	99%	98%
Prophylactic Antibiotic Timing[2]	601	99%	98%	99%
Prophylactic Antibiotic Timing (Outpatient)	383	97%	97%	98%
Urinary Catheter Removal[2]	579	99%	97%	97%
Survey of Patients' Hospital Experiences				
Area Around Room 'Always' Quiet at Night	300+	65%	65%	61%
Doctors 'Always' Communicated Well	300+	79%	84%	82%
Home Recovery Information Given	300+	89%	88%	85%
Hospital Given 9 or 10 on 10 Point Scale	300+	72%	74%	71%
Meds 'Always' Explained Before Given	300+	60%	67%	64%
Nurses 'Always' Communicated Well	300+	74%	81%	79%
Pain 'Always' Well Controlled	300+	68%	72%	71%
Room and Bathroom 'Always' Clean	300+	72%	78%	73%
Timely Help 'Always' Received	300+	63%	74%	68%
Would Definitely Recommend Hospital	300+	74%	71%	71%
Use of Medical Imaging				
Cardiac Imaging Stress Test before Surgery	386	5.2%	6.3%	5.3%
Combination Abdominal CT Scan	714	6.0%	5.7%	10.5%
Combination Brain/Sinus CT Scan	388	1.0%	2.3%	2.7%
Combination Chest CT Scan	473	0.0%	1.9%	2.7%
Follow-up Mammogram/Ultrasound	773	6.2%	6.3%	8.8%
Lumbar Spine MRI for Low Back Pain	121	41.3%	37.6%	37.2%

Saint Joseph's Hospital

45 West 10th Street
Saint Paul, MN 55102
URL: www.stjosephs-stpaul.org
Type: Acute Care Hospitals
Ownership: Voluntary non-profit - Private
Phone: 651-232-7707
Fax: 651-232-3601
Emergency Services: Yes
Beds: 401

Key Personnel:
Operating Room. . . . . Mary Jo Harrington, RN
Chief of Medical Staff . . . . John Kvasnicka, MD
CEO/President. . . . . Scott L. North
Pediatric In-Patient Care . . . . James Prall, MD
Infection Control. . . . . Luis Villar, MD
Quality Assurance . . . . Bryan Weinzierl
Radiology. . . . . Duane Ytredal, MD

Measure	Cases	This Hosp.	State Avg.	U.S. Avg.
Blood Clot Prevention and Treatment				
Anticoagulation Overlap Therapy[2]	72	92%	96%	93%
ICU Venous Thromboembolism Prophylaxis[2]	131	95%	91%	92%
Incidence of Potentially Preventable VTE[2]	14	14%	9%	10%
UFH with Dosages/Platelet Monitoring[2]	46	98%	98%	97%
Venous Thromboembolism Prophylaxis[2]	261	71%	86%	85%
Warfarin Therapy Discharge Instructions[2]	51	22%	63%	75%
Chest Pain/Possible Heart Attack Care				
Aspirin Given Within 24 Hours of Arrival[1,3]	-	-	97%	96%
Fibrinolytic Meds Within 30 Min. of Arrival[5]	-	-	48%	58%
Average Time to ECG (minutes)[1,3]	-	-	7	7
Average Time to Transfer (minutes)[5]	-	-	54	60
Children's Asthma Care				
Received Home Management Plan of Care	-	-	-	88%
Received Reliever Medication	-	-	-	100%
Received Systemic Corticosteroids	-	-	-	100%
Emergency Department				
Admittance Decision Time (minutes)[2]	472	69	62	98
Head CT Results Within 45 Min. of Arrival[7]	-	-	54%	57%
Patients Who Left ER Before Being Seen	22,628	3%	2%	2%
Time from ER Arrival to Admit. (minutes)[2]	509	229	199	274
Time from ER Arrival to Discharge (minutes)	360	185	125	134
Time in ER Before Being Evaluated (minutes)	401	46	31	26
Time to Pain Meds for Fractures (minutes)	38	55	45	57
Heart Attack Care				
Aspirin Given at Discharge	325	99%	99%	99%
Fibrinolytic Meds Within 30 Min. of Arrival[7]	-	-	-	54%
PCI Within 90 Minutes of Arrival	43	98%	96%	96%
Statin Prescribed at Discharge	328	99%	99%	98%
Heart Failure Care				
ACE Inhibitor or ARB for LVSD	103	99%	96%	97%
Discharge Instructions Given	228	93%	93%	94%
Evaluation of LVS Function	279	99%	97%	99%
Medicare Spending				
Medicare Spending per Patient (ratio)	-	0.97	0.9	0.98
Pneumonia Care				
Appropriate Initial Antibiotic Given[2]	82	96%	94%	95%
Blood Culture Timing[2]	128	98%	97%	98%
Pregnancy and Delivery Care				
Newborn Deliveries Scheduled Early[2]	28	0%	5%	6%
Preventive Care				
Immunization for Influenza[2]	557	94%	89%	90%
Immunization for Pneumonia[2]	739	91%	89%	92%
Stroke Care				
Anticoagulation Therapy for Atrial Fibrillation[2]	32	100%	96%	95%
Antithrombotic Therapy Timing[2]	106	96%	98%	98%
Assessed for Rehabilitation[2]	191	98%	98%	97%
Discharged on Antithrombotic Therapy[2]	143	99%	99%	99%
Discharged on Statin Medication[2]	109	97%	95%	94%
Thrombolytic Therapy Timing[2]	19	89%	74%	66%
Venous Thromboembolism Prophylaxis[2]	199	97%	95%	94%
Written Stroke Educational Materials Given[2]	96	75%	88%	88%
Surgical Care Improvement Project				
Appropriate Beta Blocker Usage[2]	304	100%	98%	98%
Appropriate VTP Within 24 Hours[2]	337	99%	98%	98%
Controlled Postoperative Blood Glucose[2]	204	98%	97%	97%
Perioperative Temperature Management[2]	429	100%	99%	100%
Prophylactic Antibiotic Selection[2]	451	100%	99%	99%
Prophylactic Antibiotic Selection (Outpatient)	274	100%	98%	98%
Prophylactic Antibiotic Stopped[2]	431	98%	99%	98%
Prophylactic Antibiotic Timing[2]	451	99%	98%	99%
Prophylactic Antibiotic Timing (Outpatient)	274	99%	97%	98%
Urinary Catheter Removal[2]	397	95%	97%	97%
Survey of Patients' Hospital Experiences				
Area Around Room 'Always' Quiet at Night	300+	62%	65%	61%
Doctors 'Always' Communicated Well	300+	78%	84%	82%
Home Recovery Information Given	300+	89%	88%	85%
Hospital Given 9 or 10 on 10 Point Scale	300+	77%	74%	71%
Meds 'Always' Explained Before Given	300+	60%	67%	64%
Nurses 'Always' Communicated Well	300+	78%	81%	79%
Pain 'Always' Well Controlled	300+	72%	72%	71%
Room and Bathroom 'Always' Clean	300+	77%	78%	73%
Timely Help 'Always' Received	300+	68%	74%	68%
Would Definitely Recommend Hospital	300+	78%	71%	71%
Use of Medical Imaging				
Cardiac Imaging Stress Test before Surgery	218	6.4%	6.3%	5.3%
Combination Abdominal CT Scan	319	2.2%	5.7%	10.5%
Combination Brain/Sinus CT Scan[1]	-	-	2.3%	2.7%
Combination Chest CT Scan[1]	-	-	1.9%	2.7%
Follow-up Mammogram/Ultrasound	296	5.7%	6.3%	8.8%
Lumbar Spine MRI for Low Back Pain[1]	-	-	37.6%	37.2%

United Hospital

333 North Smith Avenue
Saint Paul, MN 55102
URL: www.allinahealth.org/ahs/united.nsf
Type: Acute Care Hospitals
Ownership: Voluntary non-profit - Private
Phone: 651-241-8802
Fax: 651-241-8118
Emergency Services: Yes
Beds: 572

Key Personnel:
Intensive Care Unit. . . . . Julianne Deutsch
Chief of Medical Staff . . . . Daniel Foley, MD
Operating Room. . . . . Marnie Halligan
CEO/President. . . . . Mark Mishek
Infection Control. . . . . Anita Romani
Quality Assurance . . . . Laura Rutledge
Hemotology Center . . . . Carol Wilcox

Measure	Cases	This Hosp.	State Avg.	U.S. Avg.
Blood Clot Prevention and Treatment				
Anticoagulation Overlap Therapy[2]	170	98%	96%	93%
ICU Venous Thromboembolism Prophylaxis[2]	56	98%	91%	92%
Incidence of Potentially Preventable VTE[2]	20	20%	9%	10%
UFH with Dosages/Platelet Monitoring[2]	152	99%	98%	97%
Venous Thromboembolism Prophylaxis[2]	280	89%	86%	85%
Warfarin Therapy Discharge Instructions[2]	130	32%	63%	75%
Chest Pain/Possible Heart Attack Care				
Aspirin Given Within 24 Hours of Arrival[1,3]	-	-	97%	96%
Fibrinolytic Meds Within 30 Min. of Arrival[3,7]	-	-	48%	58%
Average Time to ECG (minutes)[1,3]	-	-	7	7
Average Time to Transfer (minutes)[3,7]	-	-	54	60
Children's Asthma Care				
Received Home Management Plan of Care	-	-	-	88%
Received Reliever Medication	-	-	-	100%
Received Systemic Corticosteroids	-	-	-	100%
Emergency Department				
Admittance Decision Time (minutes)[2]	456	129	62	98
Head CT Results Within 45 Min. of Arrival[7]	-	-	54%	57%
Patients Who Left ER Before Being Seen	52,750	2%	2%	2%
Time from ER Arrival to Admit. (minutes)[2]	458	257	199	274
Time from ER Arrival to Discharge (minutes)	413	165	125	134
Time in ER Before Being Evaluated (minutes)	468	13	31	26
Time to Pain Meds for Fractures (minutes)	56	50	45	57
Heart Attack Care				
Aspirin Given at Discharge	471	100%	99%	99%
Fibrinolytic Meds Within 30 Min. of Arrival[7]	-	-	-	54%
PCI Within 90 Minutes of Arrival	43	93%	96%	96%
Statin Prescribed at Discharge	451	99%	99%	98%
Heart Failure Care				
ACE Inhibitor or ARB for LVSD	135	97%	96%	97%
Discharge Instructions Given	331	98%	93%	94%
Evaluation of LVS Function	428	100%	97%	99%
Medicare Spending				
Medicare Spending per Patient (ratio)	-	0.96	0.9	0.98
Pneumonia Care				

NOTE: Hospital profiles are in alphabetical order by state, then city, then hospital within the city; Rankings exclude hospitals with less than 25 cases except for patient surveys which excludes hospitals with less than 100 cases; (a) 100-299 cases; (1) The number of cases/patients is too few to report; (2) Data submitted were based on a sample of cases/patients; (3) Results are based on a shorter time period than required; (4) Data suppressed by CMS for one or more quarters; (5) Results are not available for this reporting period; (6) Fewer than 100 patients completed the HCAHPS survey; (7) No cases met the criteria for this measure; (8) The lower limit of the confidence interval cannot be calculated if the number of observed infections equals zero; (9) No data are available from the state/territory for this reporting period; (10) The scores shown reflect fewer than 50 completed surveys; (11) There were discrepancies in the data collection process; (12) This measure does not apply to this hospital for this reporting period; (13) Results cannot be calculated for this reporting period; (14) The results for this state are combined with nearby states to protect confidentiality; Please refer to the User's Guide for a full explanation of data.

Measure	Cases	This Hosp.	State Avg.	U.S. Avg.
Appropriate Initial Antibiotic Given	161	98%	94%	95%
Blood Culture Timing	246	98%	97%	98%
Pregnancy and Delivery Care				
Newborn Deliveries Scheduled Early[2]	51	4%	5%	6%
Preventive Care				
Immunization for Influenza[2]	570	91%	89%	90%
Immunization for Pneumonia[2]	612	91%	89%	92%
Stroke Care				
Anticoagulation Therapy for Atrial Fibrillation	50	98%	96%	95%
Antithrombotic Therapy Timing	177	98%	98%	98%
Assessed for Rehabilitation	285	100%	98%	97%
Discharged on Antithrombotic Therapy	247	99%	99%	99%
Discharged on Statin Medication	205	100%	95%	94%
Thrombolytic Therapy Timing	46	96%	74%	66%
Venous Thromboembolism Prophylaxis	283	95%	95%	94%
Written Stroke Educational Materials Given	152	100%	88%	88%
Surgical Care Improvement Project				
Appropriate Beta Blocker Usage[2]	244	100%	98%	98%
Appropriate VTP Within 24 Hours[2]	386	98%	98%	98%
Controlled Postoperative Blood Glucose[2]	123	98%	97%	97%
Perioperative Temperature Management[2]	508	100%	99%	100%
Prophylactic Antibiotic Selection[2]	416	100%	99%	99%
Prophylactic Antibiotic Selection (Outpatient)	510	96%	98%	98%
Prophylactic Antibiotic Stopped[2]	403	98%	99%	98%
Prophylactic Antibiotic Timing[2]	417	98%	98%	99%
Prophylactic Antibiotic Timing (Outpatient)	513	97%	97%	98%
Urinary Catheter Removal[2]	327	97%	97%	97%
Survey of Patients' Hospital Experiences				
Area Around Room 'Always' Quiet at Night	300+	52%	65%	61%
Doctors 'Always' Communicated Well	300+	77%	84%	82%
Home Recovery Information Given	300+	86%	88%	85%
Hospital Given 9 or 10 on 10 Point Scale	300+	68%	74%	71%
Meds 'Always' Explained Before Given	300+	60%	67%	64%
Nurses 'Always' Communicated Well	300+	75%	81%	79%
Pain 'Always' Well Controlled	300+	69%	72%	71%
Room and Bathroom 'Always' Clean	300+	70%	78%	73%
Timely Help 'Always' Received	300+	63%	74%	68%
Would Definitely Recommend Hospital	300+	71%	71%	71%
Use of Medical Imaging				
Cardiac Imaging Stress Test before Surgery	636	4.6%	6.3%	5.3%
Combination Abdominal CT Scan	635	3.1%	5.7%	10.5%
Combination Brain/Sinus CT Scan	552	2.7%	2.3%	2.7%
Combination Chest CT Scan	371	0.3%	1.9%	2.7%
Follow-up Mammogram/Ultrasound	884	6.0%	6.3%	8.8%
Lumbar Spine MRI for Low Back Pain	86	32.6%	37.6%	37.2%

River's Edge Hospital & Clinic

1900 North Sunrise Drive
Saint Peter, MN 56082
Phone: 507-934-7602
Fax: 507-934-7651
URL: www.stpeterhealth.org
Type: Critical Access Hospitals
Emergency Services: Yes
Ownership: Government - Local
Beds: 70

Key Personnel:

Intensive Care Unit. . . . . Mary Hirn
Operating Room. . . . . Joanne Hohenstein
CEO/President. . . . . Jeanne Johnson
Chief of Medical Staff. . . . . Paulette Redman
Infection Control. . . . . Jan Wimpsett
Quality Assurance . . . . Jan Wimpsett

Measure	Cases	This Hosp.	State Avg.	U.S. Avg.
Blood Clot Prevention and Treatment				
Anticoagulation Overlap Therapy[5]	-	-	96%	93%
ICU Venous Thromboembolism Prophylaxis[5]	-	-	91%	92%
Incidence of Potentially Preventable VTE[5]	-	-	9%	10%
UFH with Dosages/Platelet Monitoring[5]	-	-	98%	97%
Venous Thromboembolism Prophylaxis[5]	-	-	86%	85%
Warfarin Therapy Discharge Instructions[5]	-	-	63%	75%
Chest Pain/Possible Heart Attack Care				
Aspirin Given Within 24 Hours of Arrival	22	100%	97%	96%
Fibrinolytic Meds Within 30 Min. of Arrival[1]	-	-	48%	58%
Average Time to ECG (minutes)	22	4	7	7
Average Time to Transfer (minutes)[1]	-	-	54	60
Children's Asthma Care				
Received Home Management Plan of Care	-	-	-	88%
Received Reliever Medication	-	-	-	100%
Received Systemic Corticosteroids	-	-	-	100%
Emergency Department				
Admittance Decision Time (minutes)[2]	137	44	62	98
Head CT Results Within 45 Min. of Arrival[5]	-	-	54%	57%
Patients Who Left ER Before Being Seen	6,369	1%	2%	2%
Time from ER Arrival to Admit. (minutes)[2]	172	189	199	274
Time from ER Arrival to Discharge (minutes)[5]	-	-	125	134
Time in ER Before Being Evaluated (minutes)[5]	-	-	31	26
Time to Pain Meds for Fractures (minutes)[5]	-	-	45	57
Heart Attack Care				
Aspirin Given at Discharge[1]	-	-	99%	99%
Fibrinolytic Meds Within 30 Min. of Arrival[7]	-	-	-	54%
PCI Within 90 Minutes of Arrival[7]	-	-	96%	96%
Statin Prescribed at Discharge[1]	-	-	99%	98%
Heart Failure Care				
ACE Inhibitor or ARB for LVSD[1]	-	-	96%	97%
Discharge Instructions Given[1]	-	-	93%	94%
Evaluation of LVS Function[1]	-	-	97%	99%
Medicare Spending				
Medicare Spending per Patient (ratio)	-	-	0.9	0.98
Pneumonia Care				
Appropriate Initial Antibiotic Given	20	100%	94%	95%
Blood Culture Timing	15	100%	97%	98%
Pregnancy and Delivery Care				
Newborn Deliveries Scheduled Early[5]	-	-	5%	6%
Preventive Care				
Immunization for Influenza	161	88%	89%	90%
Immunization for Pneumonia	239	87%	89%	92%
Stroke Care				
Anticoagulation Therapy for Atrial Fibrillation[5]	-	-	96%	95%
Antithrombotic Therapy Timing[5]	-	-	98%	98%
Assessed for Rehabilitation[5]	-	-	98%	97%
Discharged on Antithrombotic Therapy[5]	-	-	99%	99%
Discharged on Statin Medication[5]	-	-	95%	94%
Thrombolytic Therapy Timing[5]	-	-	74%	66%
Venous Thromboembolism Prophylaxis[5]	-	-	95%	94%
Written Stroke Educational Materials Given[5]	-	-	88%	88%
Surgical Care Improvement Project				
Appropriate Beta Blocker Usage[1]	-	-	98%	98%
Appropriate VTP Within 24 Hours	42	100%	98%	98%
Controlled Postoperative Blood Glucose[7]	-	-	97%	97%
Perioperative Temperature Management	44	100%	99%	100%
Prophylactic Antibiotic Selection	44	100%	99%	99%
Prophylactic Antibiotic Selection (Outpatient)[5]	-	-	98%	98%
Prophylactic Antibiotic Stopped	44	95%	99%	98%
Prophylactic Antibiotic Timing	44	89%	98%	99%
Prophylactic Antibiotic Timing (Outpatient)[5]	-	-	97%	98%
Urinary Catheter Removal[1]	-	-	97%	97%
Survey of Patients' Hospital Experiences				
Area Around Room 'Always' Quiet at Night[6]	<100	75%	65%	61%
Doctors 'Always' Communicated Well[6]	<100	85%	84%	82%
Home Recovery Information Given[6]	<100	92%	88%	85%
Hospital Given 9 or 10 on 10 Point Scale[6]	<100	78%	74%	71%
Meds 'Always' Explained Before Given[6]	<100	71%	67%	64%
Nurses 'Always' Communicated Well[6]	<100	84%	81%	79%
Pain 'Always' Well Controlled[6]	<100	72%	72%	71%
Room and Bathroom 'Always' Clean[6]	<100	93%	78%	73%
Timely Help 'Always' Received[6]	<100	87%	74%	68%
Would Definitely Recommend Hospital[6]	<100	81%	71%	71%
Use of Medical Imaging				
Cardiac Imaging Stress Test before Surgery[7]	-	-	6.3%	5.3%
Combination Abdominal CT Scan	51	2.0%	5.7%	10.5%
Combination Brain/Sinus CT Scan[1]	-	-	2.3%	2.7%
Combination Chest CT Scan[1]	-	-	1.9%	2.7%
Follow-up Mammogram/Ultrasound	159	3.8%	6.3%	8.8%
Lumbar Spine MRI for Low Back Pain[1]	-	-	37.6%	37.2%

Essentia Health Sandstone

109 Court Ave South
Sandstone, MN 55072
Phone: 320-245-5601
Fax: 320-245-2359
URL: www.smdc.org
Type: Critical Access Hospitals
Emergency Services: Yes
Ownership: Govt - Hospital Dist/Auth
Beds: 30

Key Personnel:

Emergency Room . . . . Kathy Barkhardt, RN
Chief of Medical Staff. . . . . Brian Barstad, MD
Patient Relations . . . . Teresa Fisher, RN
CEO/President. . . . . Michael Hendrix
Operating Room. . . . . Mike Monzel, CRNA
Quality Assurance . . . . Katie Runquist

Measure	Cases	This Hosp.	State Avg.	U.S. Avg.
Blood Clot Prevention and Treatment				
Anticoagulation Overlap Therapy[5]	-	-	96%	93%
ICU Venous Thromboembolism Prophylaxis[5]	-	-	91%	92%
Incidence of Potentially Preventable VTE[5]	-	-	9%	10%
UFH with Dosages/Platelet Monitoring[5]	-	-	98%	97%
Venous Thromboembolism Prophylaxis[5]	-	-	86%	85%
Warfarin Therapy Discharge Instructions[5]	-	-	63%	75%
Chest Pain/Possible Heart Attack Care				
Aspirin Given Within 24 Hours of Arrival	34	91%	97%	96%
Fibrinolytic Meds Within 30 Min. of Arrival[1]	-	-	48%	58%
Average Time to ECG (minutes)	35	12	7	7
Average Time to Transfer (minutes)[1]	-	-	54	60
Children's Asthma Care				
Received Home Management Plan of Care	-	-	-	88%
Received Reliever Medication	-	-	-	100%
Received Systemic Corticosteroids	-	-	-	100%
Emergency Department				
Admittance Decision Time (minutes)[2]	106	16	62	98
Head CT Results Within 45 Min. of Arrival[1]	-	-	54%	57%
Patients Who Left ER Before Being Seen	5,403	2%	2%	2%
Time from ER Arrival to Admit. (minutes)[2]	144	182	199	274
Time from ER Arrival to Discharge (minutes)	217	128	125	134
Time in ER Before Being Evaluated (minutes)	183	14	31	26
Time to Pain Meds for Fractures (minutes)	16	40	45	57
Heart Attack Care				
Aspirin Given at Discharge[1,3]	-	-	99%	99%
Fibrinolytic Meds Within 30 Min. of Arrival[3,7]	-	-	-	54%
PCI Within 90 Minutes of Arrival[3,7]	-	-	96%	96%
Statin Prescribed at Discharge[1,3]	-	-	99%	98%
Heart Failure Care				
ACE Inhibitor or ARB for LVSD[1]	-	-	96%	97%
Discharge Instructions Given[1]	-	-	93%	94%
Evaluation of LVS Function	11	91%	97%	99%
Medicare Spending				
Medicare Spending per Patient (ratio)	-	-	0.9	0.98
Pneumonia Care				
Appropriate Initial Antibiotic Given	12	92%	94%	95%
Blood Culture Timing[1]	-	-	97%	98%
Pregnancy and Delivery Care				
Newborn Deliveries Scheduled Early[5]	-	-	5%	6%
Preventive Care				
Immunization for Influenza[2]	108	96%	89%	90%
Immunization for Pneumonia[2]	150	97%	89%	92%
Stroke Care				
Anticoagulation Therapy for Atrial Fibrillation[5]	-	-	96%	95%
Antithrombotic Therapy Timing[5]	-	-	98%	98%
Assessed for Rehabilitation[5]	-	-	98%	97%
Discharged on Antithrombotic Therapy[5]	-	-	99%	99%
Discharged on Statin Medication[5]	-	-	95%	94%
Thrombolytic Therapy Timing[5]	-	-	74%	66%
Venous Thromboembolism Prophylaxis[5]	-	-	95%	94%
Written Stroke Educational Materials Given[5]	-	-	88%	88%
Surgical Care Improvement Project				
Appropriate Beta Blocker Usage[5]	-	-	98%	98%
Appropriate VTP Within 24 Hours[5]	-	-	98%	98%
Controlled Postoperative Blood Glucose[5]	-	-	97%	97%
Perioperative Temperature Management[5]	-	-	99%	100%
Prophylactic Antibiotic Selection[5]	-	-	99%	99%
Prophylactic Antibiotic Selection (Outpatient)[3,7]	-	-	98%	98%
Prophylactic Antibiotic Stopped[5]	-	-	99%	98%

NOTE: Hospital profiles are in alphabetical order by state, then city, then hospital within the city; Rankings exclude hospitals with less than 25 cases except for patient surveys which excludes hospitals with less than 100 cases; (a) 100-299 cases; (1) The number of cases/patients is too few to report; (2) Data submitted were based on a sample of cases/patients; (3) Results are based on a shorter time period than required; (4) Data suppressed by CMS for one or more quarters; (5) Results are not available for this reporting period; (6) Fewer than 100 patients completed the HCAHPS survey; (7) No cases met the criteria for this measure; (8) The lower limit of the confidence interval cannot be calculated if the number of observed infections equals zero; (9) No data are available from the state/territory for this reporting period; (10) The scores shown reflect fewer than 50 completed surveys; (11) There were discrepancies in the data collection process; (12) This measure does not apply to this hospital for this reporting period; (13) Results cannot be calculated for this reporting period; (14) The results for this state are combined with nearby states to protect confidentiality; Please refer to the User's Guide for a full explanation of data.

Prophylactic Antibiotic Timing[5]	-	-	98%	99%
Prophylactic Antibiotic Timing (Outpatient)[1,3]	-	-	97%	98%
Urinary Catheter Removal[5]	-	-	97%	97%
Survey of Patients' Hospital Experiences				
Area Around Room 'Always' Quiet at Night[10]	<100	65%	65%	61%
Doctors 'Always' Communicated Well[10]	<100	88%	84%	82%
Home Recovery Information Given[10]	<100	84%	88%	85%
Hospital Given 9 or 10 on 10 Point Scale[10]	<100	68%	74%	71%
Meds 'Always' Explained Before Given[10]	<100	60%	67%	64%
Nurses 'Always' Communicated Well[10]	<100	78%	81%	79%
Pain 'Always' Well Controlled[10]	<100	67%	72%	71%
Room and Bathroom 'Always' Clean[10]	<100	56%	78%	73%
Timely Help 'Always' Received[10]	<100	56%	74%	68%
Would Definitely Recommend Hospital[10]	<100	62%	71%	71%
Use of Medical Imaging				
Cardiac Imaging Stress Test before Surgery[1]	-	-	6.3%	5.3%
Combination Abdominal CT Scan[1]	-	-	5.7%	10.5%
Combination Brain/Sinus CT Scan[1]	-	-	2.3%	2.7%
Combination Chest CT Scan[1]	-	-	1.9%	2.7%
Follow-up Mammogram/Ultrasound	68	1.5%	6.3%	8.8%
Lumbar Spine MRI for Low Back Pain[1]	-	-	37.6%	37.2%

Centracare Health System - Sauk Centre

425 North Elm Street
Sauk Centre, MN 56378
Phone: 320-352-2221
Fax: 320-352-5150
E-mail: andreaf@stmichaelshospital.org
URL: www.stmichaelshospital.org
Type: Critical Access Hospitals
Emergency Services: Yes
Ownership: Voluntary non-profit - Private
Beds: 28

Key Personnel:
CEO/President. . . . . Del Christianson
Radiology. . . . . Marie George
Chief of Medical Staff . . . . Keith Olson, MD

Measure	Cases	This Hosp.	State Avg.	U.S. Avg.
Blood Clot Prevention and Treatment				
Anticoagulation Overlap Therapy[5]	-	-	96%	93%
ICU Venous Thromboembolism Prophylaxis[5]	-	-	91%	92%
Incidence of Potentially Preventable VTE[5]	-	-	9%	10%
UFH with Dosages/Platelet Monitoring[5]	-	-	98%	97%
Venous Thromboembolism Prophylaxis[5]	-	-	86%	85%
Warfarin Therapy Discharge Instructions[5]	-	-	63%	75%
Chest Pain/Possible Heart Attack Care				
Aspirin Given Within 24 Hours of Arrival[1,3]	-	-	97%	96%
Fibrinolytic Meds Within 30 Min. of Arrival[3,7]	-	-	48%	58%
Average Time to ECG (minutes)[1,3]	-	-	7	7
Average Time to Transfer (minutes)[1,3]	-	-	54	60
Children's Asthma Care				
Received Home Management Plan of Care	-	-	-	88%
Received Reliever Medication	-	-	-	100%
Received Systemic Corticosteroids	-	-	-	100%
Emergency Department				
Admittance Decision Time (minutes)	91	5	62	98
Head CT Results Within 45 Min. of Arrival[5]	-	-	54%	57%
Patients Who Left ER Before Being Seen[5]	-	-	2%	2%
Time from ER Arrival to Admit. (minutes)	189	122	199	274
Time from ER Arrival to Discharge (minutes)[5]	-	-	125	134
Time in ER Before Being Evaluated (minutes)[5]	-	-	31	26
Time to Pain Meds for Fractures (minutes)[5]	-	-	45	57
Heart Attack Care				
Aspirin Given at Discharge[3,7]	-	-	99%	99%
Fibrinolytic Meds Within 30 Min. of Arrival[3,7]	-	-	-	54%
PCI Within 90 Minutes of Arrival[3,7]	-	-	96%	96%
Statin Prescribed at Discharge[3,7]	-	-	99%	98%
Heart Failure Care				
ACE Inhibitor or ARB for LVSD[1]	-	-	96%	97%
Discharge Instructions Given	13	85%	93%	94%
Evaluation of LVS Function	15	53%	97%	99%
Medicare Spending				
Medicare Spending per Patient (ratio)	-	-	0.9	0.98
Pneumonia Care				
Appropriate Initial Antibiotic Given	15	100%	94%	95%
Blood Culture Timing[1]	-	-	97%	98%
Pregnancy and Delivery Care				
Newborn Deliveries Scheduled Early[5]	-	-	5%	6%
Preventive Care				
Immunization for Influenza	192	96%	89%	90%
Immunization for Pneumonia	222	92%	89%	92%
Stroke Care				
Anticoagulation Therapy for Atrial Fibrillation[5]	-	-	96%	95%
Antithrombotic Therapy Timing[5]	-	-	98%	98%
Assessed for Rehabilitation[5]	-	-	98%	97%
Discharged on Antithrombotic Therapy[5]	-	-	99%	99%
Discharged on Statin Medication[5]	-	-	95%	94%
Thrombolytic Therapy Timing[5]	-	-	74%	66%
Venous Thromboembolism Prophylaxis[5]	-	-	95%	94%
Written Stroke Educational Materials Given[5]	-	-	88%	88%
Surgical Care Improvement Project				
Appropriate Beta Blocker Usage[1,3]	-	-	98%	98%
Appropriate VTP Within 24 Hours[3]	12	100%	98%	98%
Controlled Postoperative Blood Glucose[3,7]	-	-	97%	97%
Perioperative Temperature Management[3]	17	100%	99%	100%
Prophylactic Antibiotic Selection[3]	16	100%	99%	99%
Prophylactic Antibiotic Selection (Outpatient)[3,7]	-	-	98%	98%
Prophylactic Antibiotic Stopped[3]	16	100%	99%	98%
Prophylactic Antibiotic Timing[3]	16	88%	98%	99%
Prophylactic Antibiotic Timing (Outpatient)[1,3]	-	-	97%	98%
Urinary Catheter Removal[1,3]	-	-	97%	97%
Survey of Patients' Hospital Experiences				
Area Around Room 'Always' Quiet at Night[5]	-	-	65%	61%
Doctors 'Always' Communicated Well[5]	-	-	84%	82%
Home Recovery Information Given[5]	-	-	88%	85%
Hospital Given 9 or 10 on 10 Point Scale[5]	-	-	74%	71%
Meds 'Always' Explained Before Given[5]	-	-	67%	64%
Nurses 'Always' Communicated Well[5]	-	-	81%	79%
Pain 'Always' Well Controlled[5]	-	-	72%	71%
Room and Bathroom 'Always' Clean[5]	-	-	78%	73%
Timely Help 'Always' Received[5]	-	-	74%	68%
Would Definitely Recommend Hospital[5]	-	-	71%	71%
Use of Medical Imaging				
Cardiac Imaging Stress Test before Surgery[1]	-	-	6.3%	5.3%
Combination Abdominal CT Scan[1]	-	-	5.7%	10.5%
Combination Brain/Sinus CT Scan[1]	-	-	2.3%	2.7%
Combination Chest CT Scan[1]	-	-	1.9%	2.7%
Follow-up Mammogram/Ultrasound	132	7.6%	6.3%	8.8%
Lumbar Spine MRI for Low Back Pain[1]	-	-	37.6%	37.2%

Saint Francis Regional Medical Center

1455 Saint Francis Avenue
Shakopee, MN 55379
Phone: 952-403-3000
Fax: 952-403-2767
URL: www.stfrancis-shakopee.com
Type: Acute Care Hospitals
Emergency Services: Yes
Ownership: Voluntary non-profit - Church
Beds: 70

Key Personnel:
Radiology. Norman Arslanian
President . . . . Mike McMahan
Chief of Medical Staff . . . . Matt Risken
Emergency Room . . . . Matt Risken

Measure	Cases	This Hosp.	State Avg.	U.S. Avg.
Blood Clot Prevention and Treatment				
Anticoagulation Overlap Therapy[2]	28	100%	96%	93%
ICU Venous Thromboembolism Prophylaxis[1,2]	-	-	91%	92%
Incidence of Potentially Preventable VTE[1,2]	-	-	9%	10%
UFH with Dosages/Platelet Monitoring[2]	18	100%	98%	97%
Venous Thromboembolism Prophylaxis[2]	291	92%	86%	85%
Warfarin Therapy Discharge Instructions[2]	25	44%	63%	75%
Chest Pain/Possible Heart Attack Care				
Aspirin Given Within 24 Hours of Arrival	83	98%	97%	96%
Fibrinolytic Meds Within 30 Min. of Arrival[7]	-	-	48%	58%
Average Time to ECG (minutes)	85	8	7	7
Average Time to Transfer (minutes)[1]	-	-	54	60
Children's Asthma Care				
Received Home Management Plan of Care	-	-	-	88%
Received Reliever Medication	-	-	-	100%
Received Systemic Corticosteroids	-	-	-	100%
Emergency Department				
Admittance Decision Time (minutes)[2]	576	119	62	98
Head CT Results Within 45 Min. of Arrival	12	58%	54%	57%
Patients Who Left ER Before Being Seen	28,139	1%	2%	2%
Time from ER Arrival to Admit. (minutes)[2]	579	203	199	274
Time from ER Arrival to Discharge (minutes)	351	118	125	134
Time in ER Before Being Evaluated (minutes)	385	10	31	26
Time to Pain Meds for Fractures (minutes)	100	30	45	57
Heart Attack Care				
Aspirin Given at Discharge[1]	-	-	99%	99%
Fibrinolytic Meds Within 30 Min. of Arrival[7]	-	-	-	54%
PCI Within 90 Minutes of Arrival[7]	-	-	96%	96%
Statin Prescribed at Discharge[1]	-	-	99%	98%
Heart Failure Care				
ACE Inhibitor or ARB for LVSD	24	100%	96%	97%
Discharge Instructions Given	88	99%	93%	94%
Evaluation of LVS Function	120	100%	97%	99%
Medicare Spending				
Medicare Spending per Patient (ratio)	-	0.95	0.9	0.98
Pneumonia Care				
Appropriate Initial Antibiotic Given	70	99%	94%	95%
Blood Culture Timing	63	100%	97%	98%
Pregnancy and Delivery Care				
Newborn Deliveries Scheduled Early[2]	35	3%	5%	6%
Preventive Care				
Immunization for Influenza[2]	542	97%	89%	90%
Immunization for Pneumonia[2]	548	96%	89%	92%
Stroke Care				
Anticoagulation Therapy for Atrial Fibrillation[1]	-	-	96%	95%
Antithrombotic Therapy Timing	32	97%	98%	98%
Assessed for Rehabilitation	40	100%	98%	97%
Discharged on Antithrombotic Therapy	39	100%	99%	99%
Discharged on Statin Medication	33	97%	95%	94%
Thrombolytic Therapy Timing[1]	-	-	74%	66%
Venous Thromboembolism Prophylaxis	36	100%	95%	94%
Written Stroke Educational Materials Given	28	100%	88%	88%
Surgical Care Improvement Project				
Appropriate Beta Blocker Usage[2]	165	100%	98%	98%
Appropriate VTP Within 24 Hours[2]	458	100%	98%	98%
Controlled Postoperative Blood Glucose[2,7]	-	-	97%	97%
Perioperative Temperature Management[2]	564	100%	99%	100%
Prophylactic Antibiotic Selection[2]	388	100%	99%	99%
Prophylactic Antibiotic Selection (Outpatient)	121	100%	98%	98%
Prophylactic Antibiotic Stopped[2]	386	100%	99%	98%
Prophylactic Antibiotic Timing[2]	388	99%	98%	99%
Prophylactic Antibiotic Timing (Outpatient)	121	99%	97%	98%
Urinary Catheter Removal[2]	239	100%	97%	97%
Survey of Patients' Hospital Experiences				
Area Around Room 'Always' Quiet at Night	300+	68%	65%	61%
Doctors 'Always' Communicated Well	300+	82%	84%	82%
Home Recovery Information Given	300+	89%	88%	85%
Hospital Given 9 or 10 on 10 Point Scale	300+	77%	74%	71%
Meds 'Always' Explained Before Given	300+	68%	67%	64%
Nurses 'Always' Communicated Well	300+	80%	81%	79%
Pain 'Always' Well Controlled	300+	73%	72%	71%
Room and Bathroom 'Always' Clean	300+	75%	78%	73%
Timely Help 'Always' Received	300+	68%	74%	68%
Would Definitely Recommend Hospital	300+	78%	71%	71%
Use of Medical Imaging				
Cardiac Imaging Stress Test before Surgery	179	6.1%	6.3%	5.3%
Combination Abdominal CT Scan	267	4.1%	5.7%	10.5%
Combination Brain/Sinus CT Scan[1]	-	-	2.3%	2.7%
Combination Chest CT Scan	194	0.0%	1.9%	2.7%
Follow-up Mammogram/Ultrasound	487	3.9%	6.3%	8.8%
Lumbar Spine MRI for Low Back Pain	55	38.2%	37.6%	37.2%

Murray County Memorial Hospital

2042 Juniper Avenue
Slayton, MN 56172
Phone: 507-836-1277
Fax: 507-836-6700
URL: www.murraycountymed.org
Type: Critical Access Hospitals
Emergency Services: Yes
Ownership: Government - Local
Beds: 25

Key Personnel:
Intensive Care Unit. . . . . Shari Achterhoff, RN CNO
Emergency Room . . . . Barb Bergman, RN, CNO
Quality Assurance . . . . Karen Honermann

NOTE: Hospital profiles are in alphabetical order by state, then city, then hospital within the city; Rankings exclude hospitals with less than 25 cases except for patient surveys which excludes hospitals with less than 100 cases; (a) 100-299 cases; (1) The number of cases/patients is too few to report; (2) Data submitted were based on a sample of cases/patients; (3) Results are based on a shorter time period than required; (4) Data suppressed by CMS for one or more quarters; (5) Results are not available for this reporting period; (6) Fewer than 100 patients completed the HCAHPS survey; (7) No cases met the criteria for this measure; (8) The lower limit of the confidence interval cannot be calculated if the number of observed infections equals zero; (9) No data are available from the state/territory for this reporting period; (10) The scores shown reflect fewer than 50 completed surveys; (11) There were discrepancies in the data collection process; (12) This measure does not apply to this hospital for this reporting period; (13) Results cannot be calculated for this reporting period; (14) The results for this state are combined with nearby states to protect confidentiality; Please refer to the User's Guide for a full explanation of data.

Radiology. . . . . Nicole Johnson
Chief of Medical Staff . . . . Carol Lang, DO
Infection Control. . . . . Darlene Mechtenberg
Operating Room. . . . . Ryan Tjeerdsma, RN

Measure	Cases	This Hosp.	State Avg.	U.S. Avg.
Blood Clot Prevention and Treatment				
Anticoagulation Overlap Therapy[5]	-	-	96%	93%
ICU Venous Thromboembolism Prophylaxis[5]	-	-	91%	92%
Incidence of Potentially Preventable VTE[5]	-	-	9%	10%
UFH with Dosages/Platelet Monitoring[5]	-	-	98%	97%
Venous Thromboembolism Prophylaxis[5]	-	-	86%	85%
Warfarin Therapy Discharge Instructions[5]	-	-	63%	75%
Chest Pain/Possible Heart Attack Care				
Aspirin Given Within 24 Hours of Arrival[1]	-	-	97%	96%
Fibrinolytic Meds Within 30 Min. of Arrival[1,3]	-	-	48%	58%
Average Time to ECG (minutes)[1]	-	-	7	7
Average Time to Transfer (minutes)[3,7]	-	-	54	60
Children's Asthma Care				
Received Home Management Plan of Care	-	-	-	88%
Received Reliever Medication	-	-	-	100%
Received Systemic Corticosteroids	-	-	-	100%
Emergency Department				
Admittance Decision Time (minutes)[2]	78	0	62	98
Head CT Results Within 45 Min. of Arrival[5]	-	-	54%	57%
Patients Who Left ER Before Being Seen[5]	-	-	2%	2%
Time from ER Arrival to Admit. (minutes)[2]	78	106	199	274
Time from ER Arrival to Discharge (minutes)[5]	-	-	125	134
Time in ER Before Being Evaluated (minutes)[5]	-	-	31	26
Time to Pain Meds for Fractures (minutes)[5]	-	-	45	57
Heart Attack Care				
Aspirin Given at Discharge[1,3]	-	-	99%	99%
Fibrinolytic Meds Within 30 Min. of Arrival[3,7]	-	-	-	54%
PCI Within 90 Minutes of Arrival[3,7]	-	-	96%	96%
Statin Prescribed at Discharge[1,3]	-	-	99%	98%
Heart Failure Care				
ACE Inhibitor or ARB for LVSD[1]	-	-	96%	97%
Discharge Instructions Given[1]	-	-	93%	94%
Evaluation of LVS Function[1]	-	-	97%	99%
Medicare Spending				
Medicare Spending per Patient (ratio)	-	-	0.9	0.98
Pneumonia Care				
Appropriate Initial Antibiotic Given[1,3]	-	-	94%	95%
Blood Culture Timing[1,3]	-	-	97%	98%
Pregnancy and Delivery Care				
Newborn Deliveries Scheduled Early[5]	-	-	5%	6%
Preventive Care				
Immunization for Influenza	123	89%	89%	90%
Immunization for Pneumonia	171	87%	89%	92%
Stroke Care				
Anticoagulation Therapy for Atrial Fibrillation[5]	-	-	96%	95%
Antithrombotic Therapy Timing[5]	-	-	98%	98%
Assessed for Rehabilitation[5]	-	-	98%	97%
Discharged on Antithrombotic Therapy[5]	-	-	99%	99%
Discharged on Statin Medication[5]	-	-	95%	94%
Thrombolytic Therapy Timing[5]	-	-	74%	66%
Venous Thromboembolism Prophylaxis[5]	-	-	95%	94%
Written Stroke Educational Materials Given[5]	-	-	88%	88%
Surgical Care Improvement Project				
Appropriate Beta Blocker Usage[1]	-	-	98%	98%
Appropriate VTP Within 24 Hours	20	95%	98%	98%
Controlled Postoperative Blood Glucose[7]	-	-	97%	97%
Perioperative Temperature Management	21	90%	99%	100%
Prophylactic Antibiotic Selection	16	88%	99%	99%
Prophylactic Antibiotic Selection (Outpatient)[5]	-	-	98%	98%
Prophylactic Antibiotic Stopped	16	94%	99%	98%
Prophylactic Antibiotic Timing	16	94%	98%	99%
Prophylactic Antibiotic Timing (Outpatient)[5]	-	-	97%	98%
Urinary Catheter Removal	19	100%	97%	97%
Survey of Patients' Hospital Experiences				
Area Around Room 'Always' Quiet at Night[11]	(a)	66%	65%	61%
Doctors 'Always' Communicated Well[11]	(a)	88%	84%	82%
Home Recovery Information Given[11]	(a)	90%	88%	85%
Hospital Given 9 or 10 on 10 Point Scale[11]	(a)	77%	74%	71%
Meds 'Always' Explained Before Given[11]	(a)	70%	67%	64%
Nurses 'Always' Communicated Well[11]	(a)	82%	81%	79%
Pain 'Always' Well Controlled[11]	(a)	64%	72%	71%
Room and Bathroom 'Always' Clean[11]	(a)	85%	78%	73%
Timely Help 'Always' Received[11]	(a)	83%	74%	68%
Would Definitely Recommend Hospital[11]	(a)	50%	71%	71%
Use of Medical Imaging				
Cardiac Imaging Stress Test before Surgery	45	2.2%	6.3%	5.3%
Combination Abdominal CT Scan	95	13.7%	5.7%	10.5%
Combination Brain/Sinus CT Scan[1]	-	-	2.3%	2.7%
Combination Chest CT Scan	51	3.9%	1.9%	2.7%
Follow-up Mammogram/Ultrasound	132	9.8%	6.3%	8.8%
Lumbar Spine MRI for Low Back Pain[1]	-	-	37.6%	37.2%

Sleepy Eye Municipal Hospital

400 Fourth Avenue Northwest
Sleepy Eye, MN 56085
Type: Critical Access Hospitals
Ownership: Government - Local
Phone: 507-794-8440
Fax: 507-794-5460
Emergency Services: Yes
Beds: 25

Key Personnel:
Infection Control. . . . . Sandy Domeier
Operating Room. . . . . Venkata K Murthy
Quality Assurance . . . . Cheryl Reniger

Measure	Cases	This Hosp.	State Avg.	U.S. Avg.
Blood Clot Prevention and Treatment				
Anticoagulation Overlap Therapy[5]	-	-	96%	93%
ICU Venous Thromboembolism Prophylaxis[5]	-	-	91%	92%
Incidence of Potentially Preventable VTE[5]	-	-	9%	10%
UFH with Dosages/Platelet Monitoring[5]	-	-	98%	97%
Venous Thromboembolism Prophylaxis[5]	-	-	86%	85%
Warfarin Therapy Discharge Instructions[5]	-	-	63%	75%
Chest Pain/Possible Heart Attack Care				
Aspirin Given Within 24 Hours of Arrival	17	94%	97%	96%
Fibrinolytic Meds Within 30 Min. of Arrival[1]	-	-	48%	58%
Average Time to ECG (minutes)	16	8	7	7
Average Time to Transfer (minutes)[1]	-	-	54	60
Children's Asthma Care				
Received Home Management Plan of Care	-	-	-	88%
Received Reliever Medication	-	-	-	100%
Received Systemic Corticosteroids	-	-	-	100%
Emergency Department				
Admittance Decision Time (minutes)[3]	81	10	62	98
Head CT Results Within 45 Min. of Arrival[5]	-	-	54%	57%
Patients Who Left ER Before Being Seen	1,093	0%	2%	2%
Time from ER Arrival to Admit. (minutes)[3]	91	93	199	274
Time from ER Arrival to Discharge (minutes)[5]	-	-	125	134
Time in ER Before Being Evaluated (minutes)[5]	-	-	31	26
Time to Pain Meds for Fractures (minutes)[5]	-	-	45	57
Heart Attack Care				
Aspirin Given at Discharge[3,7]	-	-	99%	99%
Fibrinolytic Meds Within 30 Min. of Arrival[3,7]	-	-	-	54%
PCI Within 90 Minutes of Arrival[3,7]	-	-	96%	96%
Statin Prescribed at Discharge[3,7]	-	-	99%	98%
Heart Failure Care				
ACE Inhibitor or ARB for LVSD[1]	-	-	96%	97%
Discharge Instructions Given	13	77%	93%	94%
Evaluation of LVS Function	20	70%	97%	99%
Medicare Spending				
Medicare Spending per Patient (ratio)	-	-	0.9	0.98
Pneumonia Care				
Appropriate Initial Antibiotic Given	12	75%	94%	95%
Blood Culture Timing[1]	-	-	97%	98%
Pregnancy and Delivery Care				
Newborn Deliveries Scheduled Early[5]	-	-	5%	6%
Preventive Care				
Immunization for Influenza	153	82%	89%	90%
Immunization for Pneumonia[3]	116	83%	89%	92%
Stroke Care				
Anticoagulation Therapy for Atrial Fibrillation[5]	-	-	96%	95%
Antithrombotic Therapy Timing[5]	-	-	98%	98%
Assessed for Rehabilitation[5]	-	-	98%	97%
Discharged on Antithrombotic Therapy[5]	-	-	99%	99%
Discharged on Statin Medication[5]	-	-	95%	94%
Thrombolytic Therapy Timing[5]	-	-	74%	66%
Venous Thromboembolism Prophylaxis[5]	-	-	95%	94%
Written Stroke Educational Materials Given[5]	-	-	88%	88%
Surgical Care Improvement Project				
Appropriate Beta Blocker Usage[1,3]	-	-	98%	98%
Appropriate VTP Within 24 Hours[1,3]	-	-	98%	98%
Controlled Postoperative Blood Glucose[3,7]	-	-	97%	97%
Perioperative Temperature Management[1,3]	-	-	99%	100%
Prophylactic Antibiotic Selection[1,3]	-	-	99%	99%
Prophylactic Antibiotic Selection (Outpatient)[5]	-	-	98%	98%
Prophylactic Antibiotic Stopped[1,3]	-	-	99%	98%
Prophylactic Antibiotic Timing[1,3]	-	-	98%	99%
Prophylactic Antibiotic Timing (Outpatient)[5]	-	-	97%	98%
Urinary Catheter Removal[1,3]	-	-	97%	97%
Survey of Patients' Hospital Experiences				
Area Around Room 'Always' Quiet at Night[5]	-	-	65%	61%
Doctors 'Always' Communicated Well[5]	-	-	84%	82%
Home Recovery Information Given[5]	-	-	88%	85%
Hospital Given 9 or 10 on 10 Point Scale[5]	-	-	74%	71%
Meds 'Always' Explained Before Given[5]	-	-	67%	64%
Nurses 'Always' Communicated Well[5]	-	-	81%	79%
Pain 'Always' Well Controlled[5]	-	-	72%	71%
Room and Bathroom 'Always' Clean[5]	-	-	78%	73%
Timely Help 'Always' Received[5]	-	-	74%	68%
Would Definitely Recommend Hospital[5]	-	-	71%	71%
Use of Medical Imaging				
Cardiac Imaging Stress Test before Surgery[1]	-	-	6.3%	5.3%
Combination Abdominal CT Scan	85	2.4%	5.7%	10.5%
Combination Brain/Sinus CT Scan[1]	-	-	2.3%	2.7%
Combination Chest CT Scan[1]	-	-	1.9%	2.7%
Follow-up Mammogram/Ultrasound	86	4.7%	6.3%	8.8%
Lumbar Spine MRI for Low Back Pain[1]	-	-	37.6%	37.2%

Mayo Clinic Health System - Springfield

625 North Jackson Street
Springfield, MN 56087
URL: www.mayohealthsystem.org
Type: Critical Access Hospitals
Ownership: Voluntary non-profit - Private
Phone: 507-723-6201
Fax: 507-723-6447
Emergency Services: Yes
Beds: 24

Key Personnel:
Radiology. . . . . David W Johnson
Operating Room. . . . . Diane Kruse, RN
Quality Assurance . . . . Diane Kruse, RN
Anesthesiology. . . . . Fred Probe
Infection Control. . . . . Janet Redman
Chief of Medical Staff . . . . Margo Woodford
Emergency Room . . . . Margo Woodford, RN

Measure	Cases	This Hosp.	State Avg.	U.S. Avg.
Blood Clot Prevention and Treatment				
Anticoagulation Overlap Therapy[5]	-	-	96%	93%
ICU Venous Thromboembolism Prophylaxis[5]	-	-	91%	92%
Incidence of Potentially Preventable VTE[5]	-	-	9%	10%
UFH with Dosages/Platelet Monitoring[5]	-	-	98%	97%
Venous Thromboembolism Prophylaxis[5]	-	-	86%	85%
Warfarin Therapy Discharge Instructions[5]	-	-	63%	75%
Chest Pain/Possible Heart Attack Care				
Aspirin Given Within 24 Hours of Arrival[1]	-	-	97%	96%
Fibrinolytic Meds Within 30 Min. of Arrival[1,3]	-	-	48%	58%
Average Time to ECG (minutes)[1]	-	-	7	7
Average Time to Transfer (minutes)[1,3]	-	-	54	60
Children's Asthma Care				
Received Home Management Plan of Care	-	-	-	88%
Received Reliever Medication	-	-	-	100%
Received Systemic Corticosteroids	-	-	-	100%
Emergency Department				
Admittance Decision Time (minutes)	31	14	62	98
Head CT Results Within 45 Min. of Arrival[5]	-	-	54%	57%
Patients Who Left ER Before Being Seen	1,365	0%	2%	2%
Time from ER Arrival to Admit. (minutes)	68	116	199	274
Time from ER Arrival to Discharge (minutes)[5]	-	-	125	134
Time in ER Before Being Evaluated (minutes)[5]	-	-	31	26
Time to Pain Meds for Fractures (minutes)[5]	-	-	45	57
Heart Attack Care				

NOTE: Hospital profiles are in alphabetical order by state, then city, then hospital within the city; Rankings exclude hospitals with less than 25 cases except for patient surveys which excludes hospitals with less than 100 cases; (a) 100-299 cases; (1) The number of cases/patients is too few to report; (2) Data submitted were based on a sample of cases/patients; (3) Results are based on a shorter time period than required; (4) Data suppressed by CMS for one or more quarters; (5) Results are not available for this reporting period; (6) Fewer than 100 patients completed the HCAHPS survey; (7) No cases met the criteria for this measure; (8) The lower limit of the confidence interval cannot be calculated if the number of observed infections equals zero; (9) No data are available from the state/territory for this reporting period; (10) The scores shown reflect fewer than 50 completed surveys; (11) There were discrepancies in the data collection process; (12) This measure does not apply to this hospital for this reporting period; (13) Results cannot be calculated for this reporting period; (14) The results for this state are combined with nearby states to protect confidentiality; Please refer to the User's Guide for a full explanation of data.

Measure	Cases	This Hosp.	State Avg.	U.S. Avg.
Aspirin Given at Discharge[1,3]	-	-	99%	99%
Fibrinolytic Meds Within 30 Min. of Arrival[3,7]	-	-	-	54%
PCI Within 90 Minutes of Arrival[3,7]	-	-	96%	96%
Statin Prescribed at Discharge[1,3]	-	-	99%	98%
Heart Failure Care				
ACE Inhibitor or ARB for LVSD[1]	-	-	96%	97%
Discharge Instructions Given[1]	-	-	93%	94%
Evaluation of LVS Function[1]	-	-	97%	99%
Medicare Spending				
Medicare Spending per Patient (ratio)	-	-	0.9	0.98
Pneumonia Care				
Appropriate Initial Antibiotic Given[1]	-	-	94%	95%
Blood Culture Timing[1]	-	-	97%	98%
Pregnancy and Delivery Care				
Newborn Deliveries Scheduled Early[3,7]	-	-	5%	6%
Preventive Care				
Immunization for Influenza	71	94%	89%	90%
Immunization for Pneumonia	123	97%	89%	92%
Stroke Care				
Anticoagulation Therapy for Atrial Fibrillation[5]	-	-	96%	95%
Antithrombotic Therapy Timing[5]	-	-	98%	98%
Assessed for Rehabilitation[5]	-	-	98%	97%
Discharged on Antithrombotic Therapy[5]	-	-	99%	99%
Discharged on Statin Medication[5]	-	-	95%	94%
Thrombolytic Therapy Timing[5]	-	-	74%	66%
Venous Thromboembolism Prophylaxis[5]	-	-	95%	94%
Written Stroke Educational Materials Given[5]	-	-	88%	88%
Surgical Care Improvement Project				
Appropriate Beta Blocker Usage[5]	-	-	98%	98%
Appropriate VTP Within 24 Hours[5]	-	-	98%	98%
Controlled Postoperative Blood Glucose[5]	-	-	97%	97%
Perioperative Temperature Management[5]	-	-	99%	100%
Prophylactic Antibiotic Selection[5]	-	-	99%	99%
Prophylactic Antibiotic Selection (Outpatient)[5]	-	-	98%	98%
Prophylactic Antibiotic Stopped[5]	-	-	99%	98%
Prophylactic Antibiotic Timing[5]	-	-	98%	99%
Prophylactic Antibiotic Timing (Outpatient)[5]	-	-	97%	98%
Urinary Catheter Removal[5]	-	-	97%	97%
Survey of Patients' Hospital Experiences				
Area Around Room 'Always' Quiet at Night[10]	<100	91%	65%	61%
Doctors 'Always' Communicated Well[10]	<100	84%	84%	82%
Home Recovery Information Given[10]	<100	92%	88%	85%
Hospital Given 9 or 10 on 10 Point Scale[10]	<100	78%	74%	71%
Meds 'Always' Explained Before Given[10]	<100	85%	67%	64%
Nurses 'Always' Communicated Well[10]	<100	96%	81%	79%
Pain 'Always' Well Controlled[10]	<100	89%	72%	71%
Room and Bathroom 'Always' Clean[10]	<100	99%	78%	73%
Timely Help 'Always' Received[10]	<100	91%	74%	68%
Would Definitely Recommend Hospital[10]	<100	67%	71%	71%
Use of Medical Imaging				
Cardiac Imaging Stress Test before Surgery[7]	-	-	6.3%	5.3%
Combination Abdominal CT Scan[1]	-	-	5.7%	10.5%
Combination Brain/Sinus CT Scan	46	0.0%	2.3%	2.7%
Combination Chest CT Scan[1]	-	-	1.9%	2.7%
Follow-up Mammogram/Ultrasound	137	7.3%	6.3%	8.8%
Lumbar Spine MRI for Low Back Pain[1]	-	-	37.6%	37.2%

Lakewood Health System

49725 County Road 83
Staples, MN 56479
Phone: 218-894-1515
Fax: 218-894-8355
URL: www.lakewoodhealthsystem.com
Type: Critical Access Hospitals
Emergency Services: Yes
Ownership: Voluntary non-profit - Private
Beds: 140

Key Personnel:
Emergency Room . . . . Laurie Bach, MD
Pediatrics. . . . . Neil Bratney
Quality Assurance . . . . Cindy Denning
Anesthesiology. . . . . Patricia Gordon, MD
Chief of Medical Staff. . . . . John Halfen, MD
Surgery . . . . Jay Lenz, MD
CEO/President. . . . . Tim Rice

Measure	Cases	This Hosp.	State Avg.	U.S. Avg.
Blood Clot Prevention and Treatment				
Anticoagulation Overlap Therapy[5]	-	-	96%	93%
ICU Venous Thromboembolism Prophylaxis[5]	-	-	91%	92%
Incidence of Potentially Preventable VTE[5]	-	-	9%	10%
UFH with Dosages/Platelet Monitoring[5]	-	-	98%	97%
Venous Thromboembolism Prophylaxis[5]	-	-	86%	85%
Warfarin Therapy Discharge Instructions[5]	-	-	63%	75%
Chest Pain/Possible Heart Attack Care				
Aspirin Given Within 24 Hours of Arrival[5]	-	-	97%	96%
Fibrinolytic Meds Within 30 Min. of Arrival[5]	-	-	48%	58%
Average Time to ECG (minutes)[5]	-	-	7	7
Average Time to Transfer (minutes)[5]	-	-	54	60
Children's Asthma Care				
Received Home Management Plan of Care	-	-	-	88%
Received Reliever Medication	-	-	-	100%
Received Systemic Corticosteroids	-	-	-	100%
Emergency Department				
Admittance Decision Time (minutes)[2]	183	30	62	98
Head CT Results Within 45 Min. of Arrival[5]	-	-	54%	57%
Patients Who Left ER Before Being Seen[5]	-	-	2%	2%
Time from ER Arrival to Admit. (minutes)[2]	269	186	199	274
Time from ER Arrival to Discharge (minutes)[5]	-	-	125	134
Time in ER Before Being Evaluated (minutes)[5]	-	-	31	26
Time to Pain Meds for Fractures (minutes)[5]	-	-	45	57
Heart Attack Care				
Aspirin Given at Discharge[3,7]	-	-	99%	99%
Fibrinolytic Meds Within 30 Min. of Arrival[3,7]	-	-	-	54%
PCI Within 90 Minutes of Arrival[3,7]	-	-	96%	96%
Statin Prescribed at Discharge[3,7]	-	-	99%	98%
Heart Failure Care				
ACE Inhibitor or ARB for LVSD[1,2]	-	-	96%	97%
Discharge Instructions Given[1,2]	-	-	93%	94%
Evaluation of LVS Function[1,2]	-	-	97%	99%
Medicare Spending				
Medicare Spending per Patient (ratio)	-	-	0.9	0.98
Pneumonia Care				
Appropriate Initial Antibiotic Given[2]	30	80%	94%	95%
Blood Culture Timing[2]	16	94%	97%	98%
Pregnancy and Delivery Care				
Newborn Deliveries Scheduled Early[5]	-	-	5%	6%
Preventive Care				
Immunization for Influenza[2]	282	16%	89%	90%
Immunization for Pneumonia[2]	224	23%	89%	92%
Stroke Care				
Anticoagulation Therapy for Atrial Fibrillation[5]	-	-	96%	95%
Antithrombotic Therapy Timing[5]	-	-	98%	98%
Assessed for Rehabilitation[5]	-	-	98%	97%
Discharged on Antithrombotic Therapy[5]	-	-	99%	99%
Discharged on Statin Medication[5]	-	-	95%	94%
Thrombolytic Therapy Timing[5]	-	-	74%	66%
Venous Thromboembolism Prophylaxis[5]	-	-	95%	94%
Written Stroke Educational Materials Given[5]	-	-	88%	88%
Surgical Care Improvement Project				
Appropriate Beta Blocker Usage[2]	18	83%	98%	98%
Appropriate VTP Within 24 Hours[2]	67	81%	98%	98%
Controlled Postoperative Blood Glucose[2,7]	-	-	97%	97%
Perioperative Temperature Management[2]	79	97%	99%	100%
Prophylactic Antibiotic Selection[2]	33	97%	99%	99%
Prophylactic Antibiotic Selection (Outpatient)	68	96%	98%	98%
Prophylactic Antibiotic Stopped[2]	32	94%	99%	98%
Prophylactic Antibiotic Timing[2]	33	97%	98%	99%
Prophylactic Antibiotic Timing (Outpatient)	70	97%	97%	98%
Urinary Catheter Removal[1,2]	-	-	97%	97%
Survey of Patients' Hospital Experiences				
Area Around Room 'Always' Quiet at Night	300+	70%	65%	61%
Doctors 'Always' Communicated Well	300+	87%	84%	82%
Home Recovery Information Given	300+	89%	88%	85%
Hospital Given 9 or 10 on 10 Point Scale	300+	84%	74%	71%
Meds 'Always' Explained Before Given	300+	68%	67%	64%
Nurses 'Always' Communicated Well	300+	84%	81%	79%
Pain 'Always' Well Controlled	300+	74%	72%	71%
Room and Bathroom 'Always' Clean	300+	87%	78%	73%
Timely Help 'Always' Received	300+	75%	74%	68%
Would Definitely Recommend Hospital	300+	85%	71%	71%
Use of Medical Imaging				
Cardiac Imaging Stress Test before Surgery[1]	-	-	6.3%	5.3%
Combination Abdominal CT Scan	145	6.9%	5.7%	10.5%
Combination Brain/Sinus CT Scan	88	9.1%	2.3%	2.7%
Combination Chest CT Scan	67	1.5%	1.9%	2.7%
Follow-up Mammogram/Ultrasound	215	7.9%	6.3%	8.8%
Lumbar Spine MRI for Low Back Pain[1]	-	-	37.6%	37.2%

Lakeview Memorial Hospital

927 West Churchill Street
Stillwater, MN 55082
Phone: 651-439-5330
Fax: 651-430-4528
URL: www.lakeview.org
Type: Acute Care Hospitals
Emergency Services: Yes
Ownership: Voluntary non-profit - Private
Beds: 98

Key Personnel:
Emergency Room . . . . Di Anne, RN
Quality Assurance . . . . Judy Bakke
Chief of Medical Staff. . . . . Charles W Bransford, MD
CEO/President. . . . . Doug Johnson
Radiology. . . . . Steven D Johnson

Measure	Cases	This Hosp.	State Avg.	U.S. Avg.
Blood Clot Prevention and Treatment				
Anticoagulation Overlap Therapy[2]	26	100%	96%	93%
ICU Venous Thromboembolism Prophylaxis[2]	44	91%	91%	92%
Incidence of Potentially Preventable VTE[1,2]	-	-	9%	10%
UFH with Dosages/Platelet Monitoring[1,2]	-	-	98%	97%
Venous Thromboembolism Prophylaxis[2]	178	92%	86%	85%
Warfarin Therapy Discharge Instructions[2]	23	48%	63%	75%
Chest Pain/Possible Heart Attack Care				
Aspirin Given Within 24 Hours of Arrival	40	95%	97%	96%
Fibrinolytic Meds Within 30 Min. of Arrival[7]	-	-	48%	58%
Average Time to ECG (minutes)	42	7	7	7
Average Time to Transfer (minutes)[1]	-	-	54	60
Children's Asthma Care				
Received Home Management Plan of Care	-	-	-	88%
Received Reliever Medication	-	-	-	100%
Received Systemic Corticosteroids	-	-	-	100%
Emergency Department				
Admittance Decision Time (minutes)[2]	196	52	62	98
Head CT Results Within 45 Min. of Arrival[1]	-	-	54%	57%
Patients Who Left ER Before Being Seen	9,971	0%	2%	2%
Time from ER Arrival to Admit. (minutes)[2]	207	197	199	274
Time from ER Arrival to Discharge (minutes)	409	124	125	134
Time in ER Before Being Evaluated (minutes)	221	17	31	26
Time to Pain Meds for Fractures (minutes)	44	30	45	57
Heart Attack Care				
Aspirin Given at Discharge[1,3]	-	-	99%	99%
Fibrinolytic Meds Within 30 Min. of Arrival[3,7]	-	-	-	54%
PCI Within 90 Minutes of Arrival[3,7]	-	-	96%	96%
Statin Prescribed at Discharge[1,3]	-	-	99%	98%
Heart Failure Care				
ACE Inhibitor or ARB for LVSD[1]	-	-	96%	97%
Discharge Instructions Given	41	85%	93%	94%
Evaluation of LVS Function	59	98%	97%	99%
Medicare Spending				
Medicare Spending per Patient (ratio)	-	0.89	0.9	0.98
Pneumonia Care				
Appropriate Initial Antibiotic Given	37	97%	94%	95%
Blood Culture Timing	26	96%	97%	98%
Pregnancy and Delivery Care				
Newborn Deliveries Scheduled Early[2]	14	0%	5%	6%
Preventive Care				
Immunization for Influenza[2]	393	84%	89%	90%
Immunization for Pneumonia[2]	430	89%	89%	92%
Stroke Care				
Anticoagulation Therapy for Atrial Fibrillation[1]	-	-	96%	95%
Antithrombotic Therapy Timing[1]	-	-	98%	98%
Assessed for Rehabilitation	11	100%	98%	97%
Discharged on Antithrombotic Therapy	11	100%	99%	99%
Discharged on Statin Medication[1]	-	-	95%	94%
Thrombolytic Therapy Timing[7]	-	-	74%	66%
Venous Thromboembolism Prophylaxis[1]	-	-	95%	94%
Written Stroke Educational Materials Given[1]	-	-	88%	88%
Surgical Care Improvement Project				

NOTE: Hospital profiles are in alphabetical order by state, then city, then hospital within the city; Rankings exclude hospitals with less than 25 cases except for patient surveys which excludes hospitals with less than 100 cases; (a) 100-299 cases; (1) The number of cases/patients is too few to report; (2) Data submitted were based on a sample of cases/patients; (3) Results are based on a shorter time period than required; (4) Data suppressed by CMS for one or more quarters; (5) Results are not available for this reporting period; (6) Fewer than 100 patients completed the HCAHPS survey; (7) No cases met the criteria for this measure; (8) The lower limit of the confidence interval cannot be calculated if the number of observed infections equals zero; (9) No data are available from the state/territory for this reporting period; (10) The scores shown reflect fewer than 50 completed surveys; (11) There were discrepancies in the data collection process; (12) This measure does not apply to this hospital for this reporting period; (13) Results cannot be calculated for this reporting period; (14) The results for this state are combined with nearby states to protect confidentiality; Please refer to the User's Guide for a full explanation of data.

Appropriate Beta Blocker Usage[2]	105	98%	98%	98%
Appropriate VTP Within 24 Hours[2]	299	97%	98%	98%
Controlled Postoperative Blood Glucose[2,7]	-	-	97%	97%
Perioperative Temperature Management[2]	375	99%	99%	100%
Prophylactic Antibiotic Selection[2]	248	99%	99%	99%
Prophylactic Antibiotic Selection (Outpatient)	237	100%	98%	98%
Prophylactic Antibiotic Stopped[2]	248	99%	99%	98%
Prophylactic Antibiotic Timing[2]	248	98%	98%	99%
Prophylactic Antibiotic Timing (Outpatient)	240	97%	97%	98%
Urinary Catheter Removal[2]	257	99%	97%	97%
Survey of Patients' Hospital Experiences				
Area Around Room 'Always' Quiet at Night	300+	72%	65%	61%
Doctors 'Always' Communicated Well	300+	85%	84%	82%
Home Recovery Information Given	300+	91%	88%	85%
Hospital Given 9 or 10 on 10 Point Scale	300+	83%	74%	71%
Meds 'Always' Explained Before Given	300+	72%	67%	64%
Nurses 'Always' Communicated Well	300+	86%	81%	79%
Pain 'Always' Well Controlled	300+	77%	72%	71%
Room and Bathroom 'Always' Clean	300+	84%	78%	73%
Timely Help 'Always' Received	300+	81%	74%	68%
Would Definitely Recommend Hospital	300+	86%	71%	71%
Use of Medical Imaging				
Cardiac Imaging Stress Test before Surgery	111	2.7%	6.3%	5.3%
Combination Abdominal CT Scan	308	5.5%	5.7%	10.5%
Combination Brain/Sinus CT Scan	177	0.6%	2.3%	2.7%
Combination Chest CT Scan	190	0.0%	1.9%	2.7%
Follow-up Mammogram/Ultrasound	675	4.9%	6.3%	8.8%
Lumbar Spine MRI for Low Back Pain	40	47.5%	37.6%	37.2%

Sanford Medical Center Thief River Falls

120 Labree Avenue South
Thief River Falls, MN 56701
Phone: 218-681-4240
Fax: 218-681-5614
E-mail: nwmc@nwmc.org
URL: www.nwmc.org
Type: Critical Access Hospitals
Emergency Services: Yes
Ownership: Voluntary non-profit - Private
Beds: 99

Key Personnel:
CEO/President. . . . . Christine Harff
Infection Control. . . . . Sharon Jorde, RN
Chief of Medical Staff . . . . Jaward Khan
Operating Room. . . . . Susie Koland, RN
Quality Assurance . . . . Tracy Spry

Measure	Cases	This Hosp.	State Avg.	U.S. Avg.
Blood Clot Prevention and Treatment				
Anticoagulation Overlap Therapy[5]	-	-	96%	93%
ICU Venous Thromboembolism Prophylaxis[5]	-	-	91%	92%
Incidence of Potentially Preventable VTE[5]	-	-	9%	10%
UFH with Dosages/Platelet Monitoring[5]	-	-	98%	97%
Venous Thromboembolism Prophylaxis[5]	-	-	86%	85%
Warfarin Therapy Discharge Instructions[5]	-	-	63%	75%
Chest Pain/Possible Heart Attack Care				
Aspirin Given Within 24 Hours of Arrival	31	100%	97%	96%
Fibrinolytic Meds Within 30 Min. of Arrival[1]	-	-	48%	58%
Average Time to ECG (minutes)	30	13	7	7
Average Time to Transfer (minutes)[1]	-	-	54	60
Children's Asthma Care				
Received Home Management Plan of Care	-	-	-	88%
Received Reliever Medication	-	-	-	100%
Received Systemic Corticosteroids	-	-	-	100%
Emergency Department				
Admittance Decision Time (minutes)[2]	166	18	62	98
Head CT Results Within 45 Min. of Arrival[5]	-	-	54%	57%
Patients Who Left ER Before Being Seen	6,725	1%	2%	2%
Time from ER Arrival to Admit. (minutes)[2]	188	180	199	274
Time from ER Arrival to Discharge (minutes)[5]	-	-	125	134
Time in ER Before Being Evaluated (minutes)[5]	-	-	31	26
Time to Pain Meds for Fractures (minutes)[5]	-	-	45	57
Heart Attack Care				
Aspirin Given at Discharge[1]	-	-	99%	99%
Fibrinolytic Meds Within 30 Min. of Arrival[7]	-	-	-	54%
PCI Within 90 Minutes of Arrival[7]	-	-	96%	96%
Statin Prescribed at Discharge[1]	-	-	99%	98%
Heart Failure Care				
ACE Inhibitor or ARB for LVSD[1]	-	-	96%	97%
Discharge Instructions Given	23	35%	93%	94%
Evaluation of LVS Function	32	91%	97%	99%
Medicare Spending				
Medicare Spending per Patient (ratio)	-	-	0.9	0.98
Pneumonia Care				
Appropriate Initial Antibiotic Given	31	77%	94%	95%
Blood Culture Timing	22	82%	97%	98%
Pregnancy and Delivery Care				
Newborn Deliveries Scheduled Early[5]	-	-	5%	6%
Preventive Care				
Immunization for Influenza[2]	286	80%	89%	90%
Immunization for Pneumonia[2]	291	88%	89%	92%
Stroke Care				
Anticoagulation Therapy for Atrial Fibrillation[5]	-	-	96%	95%
Antithrombotic Therapy Timing[5]	-	-	98%	98%
Assessed for Rehabilitation[5]	-	-	98%	97%
Discharged on Antithrombotic Therapy[5]	-	-	99%	99%
Discharged on Statin Medication[5]	-	-	95%	94%
Thrombolytic Therapy Timing[5]	-	-	74%	66%
Venous Thromboembolism Prophylaxis[5]	-	-	95%	94%
Written Stroke Educational Materials Given[5]	-	-	88%	88%
Surgical Care Improvement Project				
Appropriate Beta Blocker Usage	33	97%	98%	98%
Appropriate VTP Within 24 Hours	112	97%	98%	98%
Controlled Postoperative Blood Glucose[7]	-	-	97%	97%
Perioperative Temperature Management	131	100%	99%	100%
Prophylactic Antibiotic Selection	95	96%	99%	99%
Prophylactic Antibiotic Selection (Outpatient)[1,3]	-	-	98%	98%
Prophylactic Antibiotic Stopped	94	93%	99%	98%
Prophylactic Antibiotic Timing	95	95%	98%	99%
Prophylactic Antibiotic Timing (Outpatient)[1,3]	-	-	97%	98%
Urinary Catheter Removal	96	93%	97%	97%
Survey of Patients' Hospital Experiences				
Area Around Room 'Always' Quiet at Night	300+	65%	65%	61%
Doctors 'Always' Communicated Well	300+	79%	84%	82%
Home Recovery Information Given	300+	82%	88%	85%
Hospital Given 9 or 10 on 10 Point Scale	300+	59%	74%	71%
Meds 'Always' Explained Before Given	300+	63%	67%	64%
Nurses 'Always' Communicated Well	300+	78%	81%	79%
Pain 'Always' Well Controlled	300+	70%	72%	71%
Room and Bathroom 'Always' Clean	300+	74%	78%	73%
Timely Help 'Always' Received	300+	67%	74%	68%
Would Definitely Recommend Hospital	300+	55%	71%	71%
Use of Medical Imaging				
Cardiac Imaging Stress Test before Surgery	77	3.9%	6.3%	5.3%
Combination Abdominal CT Scan	144	1.4%	5.7%	10.5%
Combination Brain/Sinus CT Scan[1]	-	-	2.3%	2.7%
Combination Chest CT Scan	95	0.0%	1.9%	2.7%
Follow-up Mammogram/Ultrasound	380	1.1%	6.3%	8.8%
Lumbar Spine MRI for Low Back Pain[1]	-	-	37.6%	37.2%

Sanford Tracy

251 Fifth Street East
Tracy, MN 56175
Phone: 507-629-3200
Fax: 507-629-3202
Type: Critical Access Hospitals
Emergency Services: Yes
Ownership: Voluntary non-profit - Private
Beds: 37

Key Personnel:
Chief of Medical Staff. . . . . Jared Fazal, MD
Operating Room. . . . . Maggie Harp, RN
Emergency Room . . . . Becky Iverson, RN
CEO/President. . . . . Rick Nordahl
Infection Control. . . . . Sue Swan, RN

Measure	Cases	This Hosp.	State Avg.	U.S. Avg.
Blood Clot Prevention and Treatment				
Anticoagulation Overlap Therapy[5]	-	-	96%	93%
ICU Venous Thromboembolism Prophylaxis[5]	-	-	91%	92%
Incidence of Potentially Preventable VTE[5]	-	-	9%	10%
UFH with Dosages/Platelet Monitoring[5]	-	-	98%	97%
Venous Thromboembolism Prophylaxis[5]	-	-	86%	85%
Warfarin Therapy Discharge Instructions[5]	-	-	63%	75%
Chest Pain/Possible Heart Attack Care				
Aspirin Given Within 24 Hours of Arrival[1,3]	-	-	97%	96%
Fibrinolytic Meds Within 30 Min. of Arrival[3,7]	-	-	48%	58%
Average Time to ECG (minutes)[1,3]	-	-	7	7
Average Time to Transfer (minutes)[1,3]	-	-	54	60
Children's Asthma Care				
Received Home Management Plan of Care	-	-	-	88%
Received Reliever Medication	-	-	-	100%
Received Systemic Corticosteroids	-	-	-	100%
Emergency Department				
Admittance Decision Time (minutes)[2]	29	44	62	98
Head CT Results Within 45 Min. of Arrival[5]	-	-	54%	57%
Patients Who Left ER Before Being Seen[5]	-	-	2%	2%
Time from ER Arrival to Admit. (minutes)[2]	76	94	199	274
Time from ER Arrival to Discharge (minutes)[5]	-	-	125	134
Time in ER Before Being Evaluated (minutes)[5]	-	-	31	26
Time to Pain Meds for Fractures (minutes)[5]	-	-	45	57
Heart Attack Care				
Aspirin Given at Discharge[5]	-	-	99%	99%
Fibrinolytic Meds Within 30 Min. of Arrival[5]	-	-	-	54%
PCI Within 90 Minutes of Arrival[5]	-	-	96%	96%
Statin Prescribed at Discharge[5]	-	-	99%	98%
Heart Failure Care				
ACE Inhibitor or ARB for LVSD[1]	-	-	96%	97%
Discharge Instructions Given[1]	-	-	93%	94%
Evaluation of LVS Function	11	91%	97%	99%
Medicare Spending				
Medicare Spending per Patient (ratio)	-	-	0.9	0.98
Pneumonia Care				
Appropriate Initial Antibiotic Given[1]	-	-	94%	95%
Blood Culture Timing[1]	-	-	97%	98%
Pregnancy and Delivery Care				
Newborn Deliveries Scheduled Early[5]	-	-	5%	6%
Preventive Care				
Immunization for Influenza	79	84%	89%	90%
Immunization for Pneumonia	130	88%	89%	92%
Stroke Care				
Anticoagulation Therapy for Atrial Fibrillation[5]	-	-	96%	95%
Antithrombotic Therapy Timing[5]	-	-	98%	98%
Assessed for Rehabilitation[5]	-	-	98%	97%
Discharged on Antithrombotic Therapy[5]	-	-	99%	99%
Discharged on Statin Medication[5]	-	-	95%	94%
Thrombolytic Therapy Timing[5]	-	-	74%	66%
Venous Thromboembolism Prophylaxis[5]	-	-	95%	94%
Written Stroke Educational Materials Given[5]	-	-	88%	88%
Surgical Care Improvement Project				
Appropriate Beta Blocker Usage[5]	-	-	98%	98%
Appropriate VTP Within 24 Hours[5]	-	-	98%	98%
Controlled Postoperative Blood Glucose[5]	-	-	97%	97%
Perioperative Temperature Management[5]	-	-	99%	100%
Prophylactic Antibiotic Selection[5]	-	-	99%	99%
Prophylactic Antibiotic Selection (Outpatient)[1,3]	-	-	98%	98%
Prophylactic Antibiotic Stopped[5]	-	-	99%	98%
Prophylactic Antibiotic Timing[5]	-	-	98%	99%
Prophylactic Antibiotic Timing (Outpatient)[1,3]	-	-	97%	98%
Urinary Catheter Removal[5]	-	-	97%	97%
Survey of Patients' Hospital Experiences				
Area Around Room 'Always' Quiet at Night[10]	<100	60%	65%	61%
Doctors 'Always' Communicated Well[10]	<100	91%	84%	82%
Home Recovery Information Given[10]	<100	93%	88%	85%
Hospital Given 9 or 10 on 10 Point Scale[10]	<100	76%	74%	71%
Meds 'Always' Explained Before Given[10]	<100	81%	67%	64%
Nurses 'Always' Communicated Well[10]	<100	90%	81%	79%
Pain 'Always' Well Controlled[10]	<100	72%	72%	71%
Room and Bathroom 'Always' Clean[10]	<100	85%	78%	73%
Timely Help 'Always' Received[10]	<100	87%	74%	68%
Would Definitely Recommend Hospital[10]	<100	77%	71%	71%
Use of Medical Imaging				
Cardiac Imaging Stress Test before Surgery[1]	-	-	6.3%	5.3%
Combination Abdominal CT Scan[1]	-	-	5.7%	10.5%
Combination Brain/Sinus CT Scan	58	0.0%	2.3%	2.7%
Combination Chest CT Scan[1]	-	-	1.9%	2.7%
Follow-up Mammogram/Ultrasound	83	14.5%	6.3%	8.8%
Lumbar Spine MRI for Low Back Pain[1]	-	-	37.6%	37.2%

NOTE: Hospital profiles are in alphabetical order by state, then city, then hospital within the city; Rankings exclude hospitals with less than 25 cases except for patient surveys which excludes hospitals with less than 100 cases; (a) 100-299 cases; (1) The number of cases/patients is too few to report; (2) Data submitted were based on a sample of cases/patients; (3) Results are based on a shorter time period than required; (4) Data suppressed by CMS for one or more quarters; (5) Results are not available for this reporting period; (6) Fewer than 100 patients completed the HCAHPS survey; (7) No cases met the criteria for this measure; (8) The lower limit of the confidence interval cannot be calculated if the number of observed infections equals zero; (9) No data are available from the state/territory for this reporting period; (10) The scores shown reflect fewer than 50 completed surveys; (11) There were discrepancies in the data collection process; (12) This measure does not apply to this hospital for this reporting period; (13) Results cannot be calculated for this reporting period; (14) The results for this state are combined with nearby states to protect confidentiality; Please refer to the User's Guide for a full explanation of data.

Lake View Memorial Hospital

325 Eleventh Ave
Two Harbors, MN 55616
Phone: 218-834-7300
Fax: 218-834-7388
Type: Critical Access Hospitals
Emergency Services: Yes
Ownership: Voluntary non-profit - Private
Beds: 80

Key Personnel:
CEO/President. . . . . Brian Carlson
Chief of Medical Staff . . . . Howard Josephs
Radiology. . . . . Terri McDannold

Measure	Cases	This Hosp.	State Avg.	U.S. Avg.
Blood Clot Prevention and Treatment				
Anticoagulation Overlap Therapy[5]	-	-	96%	93%
ICU Venous Thromboembolism Prophylaxis[5]	-	-	91%	92%
Incidence of Potentially Preventable VTE[5]	-	-	9%	10%
UFH with Dosages/Platelet Monitoring[5]	-	-	98%	97%
Venous Thromboembolism Prophylaxis[5]	-	-	86%	85%
Warfarin Therapy Discharge Instructions[5]	-	-	63%	75%
Chest Pain/Possible Heart Attack Care				
Aspirin Given Within 24 Hours of Arrival	44	95%	97%	96%
Fibrinolytic Meds Within 30 Min. of Arrival[7]	-	-	48%	58%
Average Time to ECG (minutes)	44	5	7	7
Average Time to Transfer (minutes)[1]	-	-	54	60
Children's Asthma Care				
Received Home Management Plan of Care	-	-	-	88%
Received Reliever Medication	-	-	-	100%
Received Systemic Corticosteroids	-	-	-	100%
Emergency Department				
Admittance Decision Time (minutes)	76	0	62	98
Head CT Results Within 45 Min. of Arrival[5]	-	-	54%	57%
Patients Who Left ER Before Being Seen[5]	-	-	2%	2%
Time from ER Arrival to Admit. (minutes)	90	154	199	274
Time from ER Arrival to Discharge (minutes)[5]	-	-	125	134
Time in ER Before Being Evaluated (minutes)[5]	-	-	31	26
Time to Pain Meds for Fractures (minutes)[5]	-	-	45	57
Heart Attack Care				
Aspirin Given at Discharge[1,3]	-	-	99%	99%
Fibrinolytic Meds Within 30 Min. of Arrival[3,7]	-	-	-	54%
PCI Within 90 Minutes of Arrival[3,7]	-	-	96%	96%
Statin Prescribed at Discharge[1,3]	-	-	99%	98%
Heart Failure Care				
ACE Inhibitor or ARB for LVSD[3,7]	-	-	96%	97%
Discharge Instructions Given[1,3]	-	-	93%	94%
Evaluation of LVS Function[1,3]	-	-	97%	99%
Medicare Spending				
Medicare Spending per Patient (ratio)	-	-	0.9	0.98
Pneumonia Care				
Appropriate Initial Antibiotic Given[1,2]	-	-	94%	95%
Blood Culture Timing[1,2]	-	-	97%	98%
Pregnancy and Delivery Care				
Newborn Deliveries Scheduled Early[5]	-	-	5%	6%
Preventive Care				
Immunization for Influenza[2]	68	79%	89%	90%
Immunization for Pneumonia[2]	109	76%	89%	92%
Stroke Care				
Anticoagulation Therapy for Atrial Fibrillation[5]	-	-	96%	95%
Antithrombotic Therapy Timing[5]	-	-	98%	98%
Assessed for Rehabilitation[5]	-	-	98%	97%
Discharged on Antithrombotic Therapy[5]	-	-	99%	99%
Discharged on Statin Medication[5]	-	-	95%	94%
Thrombolytic Therapy Timing[5]	-	-	74%	66%
Venous Thromboembolism Prophylaxis[5]	-	-	95%	94%
Written Stroke Educational Materials Given[5]	-	-	88%	88%
Surgical Care Improvement Project				
Appropriate Beta Blocker Usage[5]	-	-	98%	98%
Appropriate VTP Within 24 Hours[5]	-	-	98%	98%
Controlled Postoperative Blood Glucose[5]	-	-	97%	97%
Perioperative Temperature Management[5]	-	-	99%	100%
Prophylactic Antibiotic Selection[5]	-	-	99%	99%
Prophylactic Antibiotic Selection (Outpatient)[5]	-	-	98%	98%
Prophylactic Antibiotic Stopped[5]	-	-	99%	98%
Prophylactic Antibiotic Timing[5]	-	-	98%	99%
Prophylactic Antibiotic Timing (Outpatient)[5]	-	-	97%	98%
Urinary Catheter Removal[5]	-	-	97%	97%
Survey of Patients' Hospital Experiences				
Area Around Room 'Always' Quiet at Night[5]	-	-	65%	61%
Doctors 'Always' Communicated Well[5]	-	-	84%	82%
Home Recovery Information Given[5]	-	-	88%	85%
Hospital Given 9 or 10 on 10 Point Scale[5]	-	-	74%	71%
Meds 'Always' Explained Before Given[5]	-	-	67%	64%
Nurses 'Always' Communicated Well[5]	-	-	81%	79%
Pain 'Always' Well Controlled[5]	-	-	72%	71%
Room and Bathroom 'Always' Clean[5]	-	-	78%	73%
Timely Help 'Always' Received[5]	-	-	74%	68%
Would Definitely Recommend Hospital[5]	-	-	71%	71%
Use of Medical Imaging				
Cardiac Imaging Stress Test before Surgery[7]	-	-	6.3%	5.3%
Combination Abdominal CT Scan	62	21.0%	5.7%	10.5%
Combination Brain/Sinus CT Scan[1]	-	-	2.3%	2.7%
Combination Chest CT Scan[1]	-	-	1.9%	2.7%
Follow-up Mammogram/Ultrasound	151	4.6%	6.3%	8.8%
Lumbar Spine MRI for Low Back Pain[1]	-	-	37.6%	37.2%

Tyler Healthcare Center

240 Willow Street
Tyler, MN 56178
Phone: 507-247-5521
Fax: 507-247-5972
URL: www.averamckennan.org
Type: Critical Access Hospitals
Emergency Services: Yes
Ownership: Voluntary non-profit - Private
Beds: 20

Key Personnel:
Chief of Medical Staff. . . . . Ranilo Asuncion, MD
Emergency Room . . . . Ranilo Asuncion, RN
Infection Control. . . . . Stacy Fritz
Quality Assurance . . . . Laurie Johansen, RN
CEO/President. . . . . Dale Kruger
Patient Relations . . . . Kathe Miranowski

Measure	Cases	This Hosp.	State Avg.	U.S. Avg.
Blood Clot Prevention and Treatment				
Anticoagulation Overlap Therapy[5]	-	-	96%	93%
ICU Venous Thromboembolism Prophylaxis[5]	-	-	91%	92%
Incidence of Potentially Preventable VTE[5]	-	-	9%	10%
UFH with Dosages/Platelet Monitoring[5]	-	-	98%	97%
Venous Thromboembolism Prophylaxis[5]	-	-	86%	85%
Warfarin Therapy Discharge Instructions[5]	-	-	63%	75%
Chest Pain/Possible Heart Attack Care				
Aspirin Given Within 24 Hours of Arrival[1,3]	-	-	97%	96%
Fibrinolytic Meds Within 30 Min. of Arrival[3,7]	-	-	48%	58%
Average Time to ECG (minutes)[1,3]	-	-	7	7
Average Time to Transfer (minutes)[3,7]	-	-	54	60
Children's Asthma Care				
Received Home Management Plan of Care	-	-	-	88%
Received Reliever Medication	-	-	-	100%
Received Systemic Corticosteroids	-	-	-	100%
Emergency Department				
Admittance Decision Time (minutes)[3]	37	0	62	98
Head CT Results Within 45 Min. of Arrival[5]	-	-	54%	57%
Patients Who Left ER Before Being Seen[5]	-	-	2%	2%
Time from ER Arrival to Admit. (minutes)[3]	37	83	199	274
Time from ER Arrival to Discharge (minutes)[5]	-	-	125	134
Time in ER Before Being Evaluated (minutes)[5]	-	-	31	26
Time to Pain Meds for Fractures (minutes)[5]	-	-	45	57
Heart Attack Care				
Aspirin Given at Discharge[5]	-	-	99%	99%
Fibrinolytic Meds Within 30 Min. of Arrival[5]	-	-	-	54%
PCI Within 90 Minutes of Arrival[5]	-	-	96%	96%
Statin Prescribed at Discharge[5]	-	-	99%	98%
Heart Failure Care				
ACE Inhibitor or ARB for LVSD[2,3]	-	-	96%	97%
Discharge Instructions Given[2,3]	-	-	93%	94%
Evaluation of LVS Function[2,3]	-	-	97%	99%
Medicare Spending				
Medicare Spending per Patient (ratio)	-	-	0.9	0.98
Pneumonia Care				
Appropriate Initial Antibiotic Given[1]	-	-	94%	95%
Blood Culture Timing[1]	-	-	97%	98%
Pregnancy and Delivery Care				
Newborn Deliveries Scheduled Early[5]	-	-	5%	6%
Preventive Care				
Immunization for Influenza	34	82%	89%	90%
Immunization for Pneumonia[2]	73	73%	89%	92%
Stroke Care				
Anticoagulation Therapy for Atrial Fibrillation[5]	-	-	96%	95%
Antithrombotic Therapy Timing[5]	-	-	98%	98%
Assessed for Rehabilitation[5]	-	-	98%	97%
Discharged on Antithrombotic Therapy[5]	-	-	99%	99%
Discharged on Statin Medication[5]	-	-	95%	94%
Thrombolytic Therapy Timing[5]	-	-	74%	66%
Venous Thromboembolism Prophylaxis[5]	-	-	95%	94%
Written Stroke Educational Materials Given[5]	-	-	88%	88%
Surgical Care Improvement Project				
Appropriate Beta Blocker Usage[5]	-	-	98%	98%
Appropriate VTP Within 24 Hours[5]	-	-	98%	98%
Controlled Postoperative Blood Glucose[5]	-	-	97%	97%
Perioperative Temperature Management[5]	-	-	99%	100%
Prophylactic Antibiotic Selection[5]	-	-	99%	99%
Prophylactic Antibiotic Selection (Outpatient)[5]	-	-	98%	98%
Prophylactic Antibiotic Stopped[5]	-	-	99%	98%
Prophylactic Antibiotic Timing[5]	-	-	98%	99%
Prophylactic Antibiotic Timing (Outpatient)[5]	-	-	97%	98%
Urinary Catheter Removal[5]	-	-	97%	97%
Survey of Patients' Hospital Experiences				
Area Around Room 'Always' Quiet at Night[10]	<100	62%	65%	61%
Doctors 'Always' Communicated Well[10]	<100	91%	84%	82%
Home Recovery Information Given[10]	<100	73%	88%	85%
Hospital Given 9 or 10 on 10 Point Scale[10]	<100	87%	74%	71%
Meds 'Always' Explained Before Given[10]	<100	64%	67%	64%
Nurses 'Always' Communicated Well[10]	<100	88%	81%	79%
Pain 'Always' Well Controlled[10]	<100	66%	72%	71%
Room and Bathroom 'Always' Clean[10]	<100	89%	78%	73%
Timely Help 'Always' Received[10]	<100	76%	74%	68%
Would Definitely Recommend Hospital[10]	<100	91%	71%	71%
Use of Medical Imaging				
Cardiac Imaging Stress Test before Surgery[1]	-	-	6.3%	5.3%
Combination Abdominal CT Scan[1]	-	-	5.7%	10.5%
Combination Brain/Sinus CT Scan[1]	-	-	2.3%	2.7%
Combination Chest CT Scan[1]	-	-	1.9%	2.7%
Follow-up Mammogram/Ultrasound	70	12.9%	6.3%	8.8%
Lumbar Spine MRI for Low Back Pain[1]	-	-	37.6%	37.2%

Essentia Health Virginia

901 9th Street North
Virginia, MN 55792
Phone: 218-741-3340
Fax: 218-749-9448
E-mail: marketing@vrmc.org
URL: www.vrmc.org
Type: Acute Care Hospitals
Emergency Services: No
Ownership: Government - Local
Beds: 83

Key Personnel:
Radiology. . . . . William W Chuang
Infection Control. . . . . Jan Jonassen
Anesthesiology. . . . . Ken Klos
Cardiac Laboratory. . . . . Heather Parenteau
Operating Room. . . . . Linda Pogorelic

Measure	Cases	This Hosp.	State Avg.	U.S. Avg.
Blood Clot Prevention and Treatment				
Anticoagulation Overlap Therapy[1,2]	-	-	96%	93%
ICU Venous Thromboembolism Prophylaxis[2]	34	94%	91%	92%
Incidence of Potentially Preventable VTE[2,7]	-	-	9%	10%
UFH with Dosages/Platelet Monitoring[1,2]	-	-	98%	97%
Venous Thromboembolism Prophylaxis[2]	122	85%	86%	85%
Warfarin Therapy Discharge Instructions[1,2]	-	-	63%	75%
Chest Pain/Possible Heart Attack Care				
Aspirin Given Within 24 Hours of Arrival	81	93%	97%	96%
Fibrinolytic Meds Within 30 Min. of Arrival[1]	-	-	48%	58%
Average Time to ECG (minutes)	83	13	7	7
Average Time to Transfer (minutes)[1]	-	-	54	60
Children's Asthma Care				
Received Home Management Plan of Care	-	-	-	88%
Received Reliever Medication	-	-	-	100%
Received Systemic Corticosteroids	-	-	-	100%
Emergency Department				
Admittance Decision Time (minutes)[2]	173	48	62	98
Head CT Results Within 45 Min. of Arrival	12	67%	54%	57%

NOTE: Hospital profiles are in alphabetical order by state, then city, then hospital within the city; Rankings exclude hospitals with less than 25 cases except for patient surveys which excludes hospitals with less than 100 cases; (a) 100-299 cases; (1) The number of cases/patients is too few to report; (2) Data submitted were based on a sample of cases/patients; (3) Results are based on a shorter time period than required; (4) Data suppressed by CMS for one or more quarters; (5) Results are not available for this reporting period; (6) Fewer than 100 patients completed the HCAHPS survey; (7) No cases met the criteria for this measure; (8) The lower limit of the confidence interval cannot be calculated if the number of observed infections equals zero; (9) No data are available from the state/territory for this reporting period; (10) The scores shown reflect fewer than 50 completed surveys; (11) There were discrepancies in the data collection process; (12) This measure does not apply to this hospital for this reporting period; (13) Results cannot be calculated for this reporting period; (14) The results for this state are combined with nearby states to protect confidentiality; Please refer to the User's Guide for a full explanation of data.

Measure	Cases	This Hosp.	State Avg.	U.S. Avg.
Patients Who Left ER Before Being Seen	12,117	3%	2%	2%
Time from ER Arrival to Admit. (minutes)[2]	217	182	199	274
Time from ER Arrival to Discharge (minutes)	383	128	125	134
Time in ER Before Being Evaluated (minutes)	260	30	31	26
Time to Pain Meds for Fractures (minutes)	64	54	45	57
Heart Attack Care				
Aspirin Given at Discharge	15	87%	99%	99%
Fibrinolytic Meds Within 30 Min. of Arrival[7]	-	-	-	54%
PCI Within 90 Minutes of Arrival[7]	-	-	96%	96%
Statin Prescribed at Discharge	12	75%	99%	98%
Heart Failure Care				
ACE Inhibitor or ARB for LVSD	16	94%	96%	97%
Discharge Instructions Given	41	73%	93%	94%
Evaluation of LVS Function	60	95%	97%	99%
Medicare Spending				
Medicare Spending per Patient (ratio)	-	0.87	0.9	0.98
Pneumonia Care				
Appropriate Initial Antibiotic Given	33	91%	94%	95%
Blood Culture Timing	43	91%	97%	98%
Pregnancy and Delivery Care				
Newborn Deliveries Scheduled Early	29	0%	5%	6%
Preventive Care				
Immunization for Influenza[2]	252	93%	89%	90%
Immunization for Pneumonia[2]	316	80%	89%	92%
Stroke Care				
Anticoagulation Therapy for Atrial Fibrillation[1]	-	-	96%	95%
Antithrombotic Therapy Timing	16	94%	98%	98%
Assessed for Rehabilitation	17	94%	98%	97%
Discharged on Antithrombotic Therapy	17	82%	99%	99%
Discharged on Statin Medication	13	69%	95%	94%
Thrombolytic Therapy Timing[1]	-	-	74%	66%
Venous Thromboembolism Prophylaxis	14	93%	95%	94%
Written Stroke Educational Materials Given[1]	-	-	88%	88%
Surgical Care Improvement Project				
Appropriate Beta Blocker Usage	61	98%	98%	98%
Appropriate VTP Within 24 Hours	128	96%	98%	98%
Controlled Postoperative Blood Glucose[7]	-	-	97%	97%
Perioperative Temperature Management	143	100%	99%	100%
Prophylactic Antibiotic Selection	102	100%	99%	99%
Prophylactic Antibiotic Selection (Outpatient)	17	94%	98%	98%
Prophylactic Antibiotic Stopped	100	96%	99%	98%
Prophylactic Antibiotic Timing	102	99%	98%	99%
Prophylactic Antibiotic Timing (Outpatient)[1]	-	-	97%	98%
Urinary Catheter Removal	88	90%	97%	97%
Survey of Patients' Hospital Experiences				
Area Around Room 'Always' Quiet at Night	300+	50%	65%	61%
Doctors 'Always' Communicated Well	300+	74%	84%	82%
Home Recovery Information Given	300+	84%	88%	85%
Hospital Given 9 or 10 on 10 Point Scale	300+	59%	74%	71%
Meds 'Always' Explained Before Given	300+	63%	67%	64%
Nurses 'Always' Communicated Well	300+	76%	81%	79%
Pain 'Always' Well Controlled	300+	65%	72%	71%
Room and Bathroom 'Always' Clean	300+	66%	78%	73%
Timely Help 'Always' Received	300+	75%	74%	68%
Would Definitely Recommend Hospital	300+	58%	71%	71%
Use of Medical Imaging				
Cardiac Imaging Stress Test before Surgery	72	1.4%	6.3%	5.3%
Combination Abdominal CT Scan	296	5.1%	5.7%	10.5%
Combination Brain/Sinus CT Scan[1]	-	-	2.3%	2.7%
Combination Chest CT Scan	181	0.0%	1.9%	2.7%
Follow-up Mammogram/Ultrasound	211	4.7%	6.3%	8.8%
Lumbar Spine MRI for Low Back Pain	51	33.3%	37.6%	37.2%

Saint Elizabeth Medical Center

1200 Grant Blvd W
Wabasha, MN 55981
URL: www.stelizabethswabasha.org
Phone: 651-565-4531
Fax: 651-565-2482
Type: Critical Access Hospitals
Emergency Services: Yes
Ownership: Voluntary non-profit - Private
Beds: 31

Key Personnel:

CEO/President. . . . . Tom Crowley
Emergency Room . . . . Meresa Hager
Quality Assurance . . . . Tracy Henn
Chief of Medical Staff. . . . . Rob Taylor, DO
Operating Room. . . . . Jan Wise

Measure	Cases	This Hosp.	State Avg.	U.S. Avg.
Blood Clot Prevention and Treatment				
Anticoagulation Overlap Therapy[5]	-	-	96%	93%
ICU Venous Thromboembolism Prophylaxis[5]	-	-	91%	92%
Incidence of Potentially Preventable VTE[5]	-	-	9%	10%
UFH with Dosages/Platelet Monitoring[5]	-	-	98%	97%
Venous Thromboembolism Prophylaxis[5]	-	-	86%	85%
Warfarin Therapy Discharge Instructions[5]	-	-	63%	75%
Chest Pain/Possible Heart Attack Care				
Aspirin Given Within 24 Hours of Arrival	17	100%	97%	96%
Fibrinolytic Meds Within 30 Min. of Arrival[1,3]	-	-	48%	58%
Average Time to ECG (minutes)	18	9	7	7
Average Time to Transfer (minutes)[3,7]	-	-	54	60
Children's Asthma Care				
Received Home Management Plan of Care	-	-	-	88%
Received Reliever Medication	-	-	-	100%
Received Systemic Corticosteroids	-	-	-	100%
Emergency Department				
Admittance Decision Time (minutes)	70	20	62	98
Head CT Results Within 45 Min. of Arrival[5]	-	-	54%	57%
Patients Who Left ER Before Being Seen[5]	-	-	2%	2%
Time from ER Arrival to Admit. (minutes)	134	145	199	274
Time from ER Arrival to Discharge (minutes)[5]	-	-	125	134
Time in ER Before Being Evaluated (minutes)[5]	-	-	31	26
Time to Pain Meds for Fractures (minutes)[5]	-	-	45	57
Heart Attack Care				
Aspirin Given at Discharge[1,3]	-	-	99%	99%
Fibrinolytic Meds Within 30 Min. of Arrival[3,7]	-	-	-	54%
PCI Within 90 Minutes of Arrival[3,7]	-	-	96%	96%
Statin Prescribed at Discharge[1,3]	-	-	99%	98%
Heart Failure Care				
ACE Inhibitor or ARB for LVSD[1]	-	-	96%	97%
Discharge Instructions Given[1]	-	-	93%	94%
Evaluation of LVS Function[1]	-	-	97%	99%
Medicare Spending				
Medicare Spending per Patient (ratio)	-	-	0.9	0.98
Pneumonia Care				
Appropriate Initial Antibiotic Given[1]	-	-	94%	95%
Blood Culture Timing[1]	-	-	97%	98%
Pregnancy and Delivery Care				
Newborn Deliveries Scheduled Early[5]	-	-	5%	6%
Preventive Care				
Immunization for Influenza	167	84%	89%	90%
Immunization for Pneumonia	212	98%	89%	92%
Stroke Care				
Anticoagulation Therapy for Atrial Fibrillation[5]	-	-	96%	95%
Antithrombotic Therapy Timing[5]	-	-	98%	98%
Assessed for Rehabilitation[5]	-	-	98%	97%
Discharged on Antithrombotic Therapy[5]	-	-	99%	99%
Discharged on Statin Medication[5]	-	-	95%	94%
Thrombolytic Therapy Timing[5]	-	-	74%	66%
Venous Thromboembolism Prophylaxis[5]	-	-	95%	94%
Written Stroke Educational Materials Given[5]	-	-	88%	88%
Surgical Care Improvement Project				
Appropriate Beta Blocker Usage	15	100%	98%	98%
Appropriate VTP Within 24 Hours	40	100%	98%	98%
Controlled Postoperative Blood Glucose[7]	-	-	97%	97%
Perioperative Temperature Management	42	100%	99%	100%
Prophylactic Antibiotic Selection	39	100%	99%	99%
Prophylactic Antibiotic Selection (Outpatient)[1,3]	-	-	98%	98%
Prophylactic Antibiotic Stopped	38	95%	99%	98%
Prophylactic Antibiotic Timing	39	97%	98%	99%
Prophylactic Antibiotic Timing (Outpatient)[1,3]	-	-	97%	98%
Urinary Catheter Removal	35	100%	97%	97%
Survey of Patients' Hospital Experiences				
Area Around Room 'Always' Quiet at Night	(a)	63%	65%	61%
Doctors 'Always' Communicated Well	(a)	84%	84%	82%
Home Recovery Information Given	(a)	92%	88%	85%
Hospital Given 9 or 10 on 10 Point Scale	(a)	73%	74%	71%
Meds 'Always' Explained Before Given	(a)	71%	67%	64%
Nurses 'Always' Communicated Well	(a)	85%	81%	79%
Pain 'Always' Well Controlled	(a)	69%	72%	71%
Room and Bathroom 'Always' Clean	(a)	85%	78%	73%
Timely Help 'Always' Received	(a)	80%	74%	68%
Would Definitely Recommend Hospital	(a)	78%	71%	71%
Use of Medical Imaging				
Cardiac Imaging Stress Test before Surgery[7]	-	-	6.3%	5.3%
Combination Abdominal CT Scan	58	5.2%	5.7%	10.5%
Combination Brain/Sinus CT Scan[1]	-	-	2.3%	2.7%
Combination Chest CT Scan[1]	-	-	1.9%	2.7%
Follow-up Mammogram/Ultrasound	249	7.6%	6.3%	8.8%
Lumbar Spine MRI for Low Back Pain[1]	-	-	37.6%	37.2%

Ridgeview Medical Center

500 South Maple Street
Waconia, MN 55387
Phone: 952-442-2191
Fax: 952-442-6529
E-mail: info@ridgeviewmedical.org
URL: www.ridgeviewmedical.org
Type: Acute Care Hospitals
Emergency Services: Yes
Ownership: Voluntary non-profit - Private
Beds: 109

Key Personnel:

Chief of Medical Staff. . . . . Charles F Barer
Emergency Room . . . . Elizabeth Boyum
Radiology. . . . . Geoffrey D Raile
CEO/President. . . . . Robert Stevens

Measure	Cases	This Hosp.	State Avg.	U.S. Avg.
Blood Clot Prevention and Treatment				
Anticoagulation Overlap Therapy[2]	50	86%	96%	93%
ICU Venous Thromboembolism Prophylaxis[2]	35	77%	91%	92%
Incidence of Potentially Preventable VTE[1,2]	-	-	9%	10%
UFH with Dosages/Platelet Monitoring[2]	37	100%	98%	97%
Venous Thromboembolism Prophylaxis[2]	311	53%	86%	85%
Warfarin Therapy Discharge Instructions[2]	37	43%	63%	75%
Chest Pain/Possible Heart Attack Care				
Aspirin Given Within 24 Hours of Arrival	132	96%	97%	96%
Fibrinolytic Meds Within 30 Min. of Arrival[7]	-	-	48%	58%
Average Time to ECG (minutes)	138	9	7	7
Average Time to Transfer (minutes)[1]	-	-	54	60
Children's Asthma Care				
Received Home Management Plan of Care	-	-	-	88%
Received Reliever Medication	-	-	-	100%
Received Systemic Corticosteroids	-	-	-	100%
Emergency Department				
Admittance Decision Time (minutes)[2]	383	67	62	98
Head CT Results Within 45 Min. of Arrival	40	30%	54%	57%
Patients Who Left ER Before Being Seen	49,551	0%	2%	2%
Time from ER Arrival to Admit. (minutes)[2]	440	223	199	274
Time from ER Arrival to Discharge (minutes)	371	144	125	134
Time in ER Before Being Evaluated (minutes)	380	22	31	26
Time to Pain Meds for Fractures (minutes)	198	36	45	57
Heart Attack Care				
Aspirin Given at Discharge	39	97%	99%	99%
Fibrinolytic Meds Within 30 Min. of Arrival[7]	-	-	-	54%
PCI Within 90 Minutes of Arrival[7]	-	-	96%	96%
Statin Prescribed at Discharge	37	92%	99%	98%
Heart Failure Care				
ACE Inhibitor or ARB for LVSD	30	100%	96%	97%
Discharge Instructions Given	88	94%	93%	94%
Evaluation of LVS Function	124	99%	97%	99%
Medicare Spending				
Medicare Spending per Patient (ratio)	-	0.94	0.9	0.98
Pneumonia Care				
Appropriate Initial Antibiotic Given	88	94%	94%	95%
Blood Culture Timing	168	97%	97%	98%
Pregnancy and Delivery Care				
Newborn Deliveries Scheduled Early[2]	29	3%	5%	6%
Preventive Care				
Immunization for Influenza[2]	513	91%	89%	90%
Immunization for Pneumonia[2]	547	95%	89%	92%
Stroke Care				
Anticoagulation Therapy for Atrial Fibrillation[1]	-	-	96%	95%
Antithrombotic Therapy Timing	40	100%	98%	98%
Assessed for Rehabilitation	45	91%	98%	97%
Discharged on Antithrombotic Therapy	40	98%	99%	99%
Discharged on Statin Medication	36	69%	95%	94%
Thrombolytic Therapy Timing[1]	-	-	74%	66%

NOTE: Hospital profiles are in alphabetical order by state, then city, then hospital within the city; Rankings exclude hospitals with less than 25 cases except for patient surveys which excludes hospitals with less than 100 cases; (a) 100-299 cases; (1) The number of cases/patients is too few to report; (2) Data submitted were based on a sample of cases/patients; (3) Results are based on a shorter time period than required; (4) Data suppressed by CMS for one or more quarters; (5) Results are not available for this reporting period; (6) Fewer than 100 patients completed the HCAHPS survey; (7) No cases met the criteria for this measure; (8) The lower limit of the confidence interval cannot be calculated if the number of observed infections equals zero; (9) No data are available from the state/territory for this reporting period; (10) The scores shown reflect fewer than 50 completed surveys; (11) There were discrepancies in the data collection process; (12) This measure does not apply to this hospital for this reporting period; (13) Results cannot be calculated for this reporting period; (14) The results for this state are combined with nearby states to protect confidentiality; Please refer to the User's Guide for a full explanation of data.

Measure	Cases	This Hosp.	State Avg.	U.S. Avg.
Venous Thromboembolism Prophylaxis	42	50%	95%	94%
Written Stroke Educational Materials Given	24	54%	88%	88%
Surgical Care Improvement Project				
Appropriate Beta Blocker Usage[2]	100	100%	98%	98%
Appropriate VTP Within 24 Hours[2]	341	100%	98%	98%
Controlled Postoperative Blood Glucose[2,7]	-	-	97%	97%
Perioperative Temperature Management[2]	405	100%	99%	100%
Prophylactic Antibiotic Selection[2]	272	100%	99%	99%
Prophylactic Antibiotic Selection (Outpatient)	121	99%	98%	98%
Prophylactic Antibiotic Stopped[2]	268	100%	99%	98%
Prophylactic Antibiotic Timing[2]	272	99%	98%	99%
Prophylactic Antibiotic Timing (Outpatient)	122	99%	97%	98%
Urinary Catheter Removal[2]	105	90%	97%	97%
Survey of Patients' Hospital Experiences				
Area Around Room 'Always' Quiet at Night	300+	69%	65%	61%
Doctors 'Always' Communicated Well	300+	85%	84%	82%
Home Recovery Information Given	300+	91%	88%	85%
Hospital Given 9 or 10 on 10 Point Scale	300+	81%	74%	71%
Meds 'Always' Explained Before Given	300+	65%	67%	64%
Nurses 'Always' Communicated Well	300+	85%	81%	79%
Pain 'Always' Well Controlled	300+	73%	72%	71%
Room and Bathroom 'Always' Clean	300+	82%	78%	73%
Timely Help 'Always' Received	300+	74%	74%	68%
Would Definitely Recommend Hospital	300+	87%	71%	71%
Use of Medical Imaging				
Cardiac Imaging Stress Test before Surgery	117	4.3%	6.3%	5.3%
Combination Abdominal CT Scan	371	3.0%	5.7%	10.5%
Combination Brain/Sinus CT Scan[1]	-	-	2.3%	2.7%
Combination Chest CT Scan	218	0.0%	1.9%	2.7%
Follow-up Mammogram/Ultrasound	253	6.7%	6.3%	8.8%
Lumbar Spine MRI for Low Back Pain	47	42.6%	37.6%	37.2%

Tri County Hospital

415 Jefferson Street North
Wadena, MN 56482
Phone: 218-631-3510
Fax: 218-631-7496
E-mail: contact@tricountyhospital.org
URL: www.tricountyhospital.org
Type: Critical Access Hospitals
Emergency Services: Yes
Ownership: Voluntary non-profit - Other
Beds: 49

Key Personnel:

Quality Assurance . . . . Kris Anderson
Operating Room. . . . . Lois Lawson
Radiology. . . . . Gerald McCullough
CEO/President. . . . . Dennis Miley
Cardiac Laboratory. . . . . Lois Miller
Infection Control. . . . . Corinne Neisess
Chair/CEO . . . . David Quincer
Chief of Medical Staff . . . . Shaneen Schmidt, MD

Measure	Cases	This Hosp.	State Avg.	U.S. Avg.
Blood Clot Prevention and Treatment				
Anticoagulation Overlap Therapy[5]	-	-	96%	93%
ICU Venous Thromboembolism Prophylaxis[5]	-	-	91%	92%
Incidence of Potentially Preventable VTE[5]	-	-	9%	10%
UFH with Dosages/Platelet Monitoring[5]	-	-	98%	97%
Venous Thromboembolism Prophylaxis[5]	-	-	86%	85%
Warfarin Therapy Discharge Instructions[5]	-	-	63%	75%
Chest Pain/Possible Heart Attack Care				
Aspirin Given Within 24 Hours of Arrival	38	100%	97%	96%
Fibrinolytic Meds Within 30 Min. of Arrival[7]	-	-	48%	58%
Average Time to ECG (minutes)	41	8	7	7
Average Time to Transfer (minutes)	12	58	54	60
Children's Asthma Care				
Received Home Management Plan of Care	-	-	-	88%
Received Reliever Medication	-	-	-	100%
Received Systemic Corticosteroids	-	-	-	100%
Emergency Department				
Admittance Decision Time (minutes)[2]	308	43	62	98
Head CT Results Within 45 Min. of Arrival[5]	-	-	54%	57%
Patients Who Left ER Before Being Seen[5]	-	-	2%	2%
Time from ER Arrival to Admit. (minutes)[2]	308	192	199	274
Time from ER Arrival to Discharge (minutes)[5]	-	-	125	134
Time in ER Before Being Evaluated (minutes)[5]	-	-	31	26
Time to Pain Meds for Fractures (minutes)[5]	-	-	45	57
Heart Attack Care				
Aspirin Given at Discharge[1]	-	-	99%	99%
Fibrinolytic Meds Within 30 Min. of Arrival[7]	-	-	-	54%
PCI Within 90 Minutes of Arrival[3,7]	-	-	96%	96%
Statin Prescribed at Discharge[1]	-	-	99%	98%
Heart Failure Care				
ACE Inhibitor or ARB for LVSD[1]	-	-	96%	97%
Discharge Instructions Given	34	100%	93%	94%
Evaluation of LVS Function	42	98%	97%	99%
Medicare Spending				
Medicare Spending per Patient (ratio)	-	-	0.9	0.98
Pneumonia Care				
Appropriate Initial Antibiotic Given	38	92%	94%	95%
Blood Culture Timing	30	100%	97%	98%
Pregnancy and Delivery Care				
Newborn Deliveries Scheduled Early[5]	-	-	5%	6%
Preventive Care				
Immunization for Influenza[2]	292	98%	89%	90%
Immunization for Pneumonia[2]	355	96%	89%	92%
Stroke Care				
Anticoagulation Therapy for Atrial Fibrillation[5]	-	-	96%	95%
Antithrombotic Therapy Timing[5]	-	-	98%	98%
Assessed for Rehabilitation[5]	-	-	98%	97%
Discharged on Antithrombotic Therapy[5]	-	-	99%	99%
Discharged on Statin Medication[5]	-	-	95%	94%
Thrombolytic Therapy Timing[5]	-	-	74%	66%
Venous Thromboembolism Prophylaxis[5]	-	-	95%	94%
Written Stroke Educational Materials Given[5]	-	-	88%	88%
Surgical Care Improvement Project				
Appropriate Beta Blocker Usage	14	93%	98%	98%
Appropriate VTP Within 24 Hours	28	100%	98%	98%
Controlled Postoperative Blood Glucose[3,7]	-	-	97%	97%
Perioperative Temperature Management	33	100%	99%	100%
Prophylactic Antibiotic Selection	12	92%	99%	99%
Prophylactic Antibiotic Selection (Outpatient)	38	97%	98%	98%
Prophylactic Antibiotic Stopped[1]	-	-	99%	98%
Prophylactic Antibiotic Timing	12	92%	98%	99%
Prophylactic Antibiotic Timing (Outpatient)	21	90%	97%	98%
Urinary Catheter Removal	13	100%	97%	97%
Survey of Patients' Hospital Experiences				
Area Around Room 'Always' Quiet at Night	300+	61%	65%	61%
Doctors 'Always' Communicated Well	300+	83%	84%	82%
Home Recovery Information Given	300+	88%	88%	85%
Hospital Given 9 or 10 on 10 Point Scale	300+	75%	74%	71%
Meds 'Always' Explained Before Given	300+	67%	67%	64%
Nurses 'Always' Communicated Well	300+	80%	81%	79%
Pain 'Always' Well Controlled	300+	69%	72%	71%
Room and Bathroom 'Always' Clean	300+	82%	78%	73%
Timely Help 'Always' Received	300+	74%	74%	68%
Would Definitely Recommend Hospital	300+	73%	71%	71%
Use of Medical Imaging				
Cardiac Imaging Stress Test before Surgery[1]	-	-	6.3%	5.3%
Combination Abdominal CT Scan	135	2.2%	5.7%	10.5%
Combination Brain/Sinus CT Scan[1]	-	-	2.3%	2.7%
Combination Chest CT Scan	57	3.5%	1.9%	2.7%
Follow-up Mammogram/Ultrasound	172	7.6%	6.3%	8.8%
Lumbar Spine MRI for Low Back Pain	40	60.0%	37.6%	37.2%

North Valley Health Center

300 West Good Samaritan Drive
Warren, MN 56762
Phone: 218-745-4211
Fax: 218-745-4215
Type: Critical Access Hospitals
Emergency Services: Yes
Ownership: Voluntary non-profit - Private
Beds: 20

Key Personnel:

Radiology. . . . . Robin Bottem
Chief of Medical Staff . . . . Judith Campbell, MD
CEO . . . . Ashley King
President . . . . Tim Sedlacek

Measure	Cases	This Hosp.	State Avg.	U.S. Avg.
Blood Clot Prevention and Treatment				
Anticoagulation Overlap Therapy[5]	-	-	96%	93%
ICU Venous Thromboembolism Prophylaxis[5]	-	-	91%	92%
Incidence of Potentially Preventable VTE[5]	-	-	9%	10%
UFH with Dosages/Platelet Monitoring[5]	-	-	98%	97%
Venous Thromboembolism Prophylaxis[5]	-	-	86%	85%
Warfarin Therapy Discharge Instructions[5]	-	-	63%	75%
Chest Pain/Possible Heart Attack Care				
Aspirin Given Within 24 Hours of Arrival	-	-	97%	96%
Fibrinolytic Meds Within 30 Min. of Arrival	-	-	48%	58%
Average Time to ECG (minutes)	-	-	7	7
Average Time to Transfer (minutes)	-	-	54	60
Children's Asthma Care				
Received Home Management Plan of Care	-	-	-	88%
Received Reliever Medication	-	-	-	100%
Received Systemic Corticosteroids	-	-	-	100%
Emergency Department				
Admittance Decision Time (minutes)	57	15	62	98
Head CT Results Within 45 Min. of Arrival	-	-	54%	57%
Patients Who Left ER Before Being Seen	-	-	2%	2%
Time from ER Arrival to Admit. (minutes)	98	108	199	274
Time from ER Arrival to Discharge (minutes)	-	-	125	134
Time in ER Before Being Evaluated (minutes)	-	-	31	26
Time to Pain Meds for Fractures (minutes)	-	-	45	57
Heart Attack Care				
Aspirin Given at Discharge[1,3]	-	-	99%	99%
Fibrinolytic Meds Within 30 Min. of Arrival[3,7]	-	-	-	54%
PCI Within 90 Minutes of Arrival[3,7]	-	-	96%	96%
Statin Prescribed at Discharge[1,3]	-	-	99%	98%
Heart Failure Care				
ACE Inhibitor or ARB for LVSD[1]	-	-	96%	97%
Discharge Instructions Given[1]	-	-	93%	94%
Evaluation of LVS Function[1]	-	-	97%	99%
Medicare Spending				
Medicare Spending per Patient (ratio)	-	-	0.9	0.98
Pneumonia Care				
Appropriate Initial Antibiotic Given[1]	-	-	94%	95%
Blood Culture Timing[1]	-	-	97%	98%
Pregnancy and Delivery Care				
Newborn Deliveries Scheduled Early[5]	-	-	5%	6%
Preventive Care				
Immunization for Influenza	100	78%	89%	90%
Immunization for Pneumonia	151	77%	89%	92%
Stroke Care				
Anticoagulation Therapy for Atrial Fibrillation[5]	-	-	96%	95%
Antithrombotic Therapy Timing[5]	-	-	98%	98%
Assessed for Rehabilitation[5]	-	-	98%	97%
Discharged on Antithrombotic Therapy[5]	-	-	99%	99%
Discharged on Statin Medication[5]	-	-	95%	94%
Thrombolytic Therapy Timing[5]	-	-	74%	66%
Venous Thromboembolism Prophylaxis[5]	-	-	95%	94%
Written Stroke Educational Materials Given[5]	-	-	88%	88%
Surgical Care Improvement Project				
Appropriate Beta Blocker Usage[5]	-	-	98%	98%
Appropriate VTP Within 24 Hours[5]	-	-	98%	98%
Controlled Postoperative Blood Glucose[5]	-	-	97%	97%
Perioperative Temperature Management[5]	-	-	99%	100%
Prophylactic Antibiotic Selection[5]	-	-	99%	99%
Prophylactic Antibiotic Selection (Outpatient)	-	-	98%	98%
Prophylactic Antibiotic Stopped[5]	-	-	99%	98%
Prophylactic Antibiotic Timing[5]	-	-	98%	99%
Prophylactic Antibiotic Timing (Outpatient)	-	-	97%	98%
Urinary Catheter Removal[5]	-	-	97%	97%
Survey of Patients' Hospital Experiences				
Area Around Room 'Always' Quiet at Night[5]	-	-	65%	61%
Doctors 'Always' Communicated Well[5]	-	-	84%	82%
Home Recovery Information Given[5]	-	-	88%	85%
Hospital Given 9 or 10 on 10 Point Scale[5]	-	-	74%	71%
Meds 'Always' Explained Before Given[5]	-	-	67%	64%
Nurses 'Always' Communicated Well[5]	-	-	81%	79%
Pain 'Always' Well Controlled[5]	-	-	72%	71%
Room and Bathroom 'Always' Clean[5]	-	-	78%	73%
Timely Help 'Always' Received[5]	-	-	74%	68%
Would Definitely Recommend Hospital[5]	-	-	71%	71%
Use of Medical Imaging				
Cardiac Imaging Stress Test before Surgery	-	-	6.3%	5.3%
Combination Abdominal CT Scan	-	-	5.7%	10.5%

NOTE: Hospital profiles are in alphabetical order by state, then city, then hospital within the city; Rankings exclude hospitals with less than 25 cases except for patient surveys which excludes hospitals with less than 100 cases; (a) 100-299 cases; (1) The number of cases/patients is too few to report; (2) Data submitted were based on a sample of cases/patients; (3) Results are based on a shorter time period than required; (4) Data suppressed by CMS for one or more quarters; (5) Results are not available for this reporting period; (6) Fewer than 100 patients completed the HCAHPS survey; (7) No cases met the criteria for this measure; (8) The lower limit of the confidence interval cannot be calculated if the number of observed infections equals zero; (9) No data are available from the state/territory for this reporting period; (10) The scores shown reflect fewer than 50 completed surveys; (11) There were discrepancies in the data collection process; (12) This measure does not apply to this hospital for this reporting period; (13) Results cannot be calculated for this reporting period; (14) The results for this state are combined with nearby states to protect confidentiality; Please refer to the User's Guide for a full explanation of data.

Measure	Cases	This Hosp.	State Avg.	U.S. Avg.
Combination Brain/Sinus CT Scan	-	-	2.3%	2.7%
Combination Chest CT Scan	-	-	1.9%	2.7%
Follow-up Mammogram/Ultrasound	-	-	6.3%	8.8%
Lumbar Spine MRI for Low Back Pain	-	-	37.6%	37.2%

Mayo Clinic Health System - Waseca

501 North State Street
Waseca, MN 56093
Phone: 507-835-1210
Fax: 507-837-4280
Type: Critical Access Hospitals
Emergency Services: Yes
Ownership: Voluntary non-profit - Private
Beds: 35

Key Personnel:
Operating Room. . . . . Marian Keller

Measure	Cases	This Hosp.	State Avg.	U.S. Avg.
Blood Clot Prevention and Treatment				
Anticoagulation Overlap Therapy[5]	-	-	96%	93%
ICU Venous Thromboembolism Prophylaxis[5]	-	-	91%	92%
Incidence of Potentially Preventable VTE[5]	-	-	9%	10%
UFH with Dosages/Platelet Monitoring[5]	-	-	98%	97%
Venous Thromboembolism Prophylaxis[5]	-	-	86%	85%
Warfarin Therapy Discharge Instructions[5]	-	-	63%	75%
Chest Pain/Possible Heart Attack Care				
Aspirin Given Within 24 Hours of Arrival	34	97%	97%	96%
Fibrinolytic Meds Within 30 Min. of Arrival[1]	-	-	48%	58%
Average Time to ECG (minutes)	35	8	7	7
Average Time to Transfer (minutes)[1]	-	-	54	60
Children's Asthma Care				
Received Home Management Plan of Care	-	-	-	88%
Received Reliever Medication	-	-	-	100%
Received Systemic Corticosteroids	-	-	-	100%
Emergency Department				
Admittance Decision Time (minutes)	81	41	62	98
Head CT Results Within 45 Min. of Arrival[5]	-	-	54%	57%
Patients Who Left ER Before Being Seen	4,199	0%	2%	2%
Time from ER Arrival to Admit. (minutes)	97	178	199	274
Time from ER Arrival to Discharge (minutes)[5]	-	-	125	134
Time in ER Before Being Evaluated (minutes)[5]	-	-	31	26
Time to Pain Meds for Fractures (minutes)[5]	-	-	45	57
Heart Attack Care				
Aspirin Given at Discharge[3,7]	-	-	99%	99%
Fibrinolytic Meds Within 30 Min. of Arrival[3,7]	-	-	-	54%
PCI Within 90 Minutes of Arrival[3,7]	-	-	96%	96%
Statin Prescribed at Discharge[3,7]	-	-	99%	98%
Heart Failure Care				
ACE Inhibitor or ARB for LVSD[1]	-	-	96%	97%
Discharge Instructions Given[1]	-	-	93%	94%
Evaluation of LVS Function	12	100%	97%	99%
Medicare Spending				
Medicare Spending per Patient (ratio)	-	-	0.9	0.98
Pneumonia Care				
Appropriate Initial Antibiotic Given[1]	-	-	94%	95%
Blood Culture Timing[1]	-	-	97%	98%
Pregnancy and Delivery Care				
Newborn Deliveries Scheduled Early[3,7]	-	-	5%	6%
Preventive Care				
Immunization for Influenza	159	99%	89%	90%
Immunization for Pneumonia	260	98%	89%	92%
Stroke Care				
Anticoagulation Therapy for Atrial Fibrillation[5]	-	-	96%	95%
Antithrombotic Therapy Timing[5]	-	-	98%	98%
Assessed for Rehabilitation[5]	-	-	98%	97%
Discharged on Antithrombotic Therapy[5]	-	-	99%	99%
Discharged on Statin Medication[5]	-	-	95%	94%
Thrombolytic Therapy Timing[5]	-	-	74%	66%
Venous Thromboembolism Prophylaxis[5]	-	-	95%	94%
Written Stroke Educational Materials Given[5]	-	-	88%	88%
Surgical Care Improvement Project				
Appropriate Beta Blocker Usage[5]	-	-	98%	98%
Appropriate VTP Within 24 Hours[5]	-	-	98%	98%
Controlled Postoperative Blood Glucose[5]	-	-	97%	97%
Perioperative Temperature Management[5]	-	-	99%	100%
Prophylactic Antibiotic Selection[5]	-	-	99%	99%
Prophylactic Antibiotic Selection (Outpatient)[5]	-	-	98%	98%
Prophylactic Antibiotic Stopped[5]	-	-	99%	98%
Prophylactic Antibiotic Timing[5]	-	-	98%	99%
Prophylactic Antibiotic Timing (Outpatient)[5]	-	-	97%	98%
Urinary Catheter Removal[5]	-	-	97%	97%
Survey of Patients' Hospital Experiences				
Area Around Room 'Always' Quiet at Night[10]	<100	76%	65%	61%
Doctors 'Always' Communicated Well[10]	<100	84%	84%	82%
Home Recovery Information Given[10]	<100	90%	88%	85%
Hospital Given 9 or 10 on 10 Point Scale[10]	<100	69%	74%	71%
Meds 'Always' Explained Before Given[10]	<100	64%	67%	64%
Nurses 'Always' Communicated Well[10]	<100	75%	81%	79%
Pain 'Always' Well Controlled[10]	<100	64%	72%	71%
Room and Bathroom 'Always' Clean[10]	<100	86%	78%	73%
Timely Help 'Always' Received[10]	<100	66%	74%	68%
Would Definitely Recommend Hospital[10]	<100	70%	71%	71%
Use of Medical Imaging				
Cardiac Imaging Stress Test before Surgery[1]	-	-	6.3%	5.3%
Combination Abdominal CT Scan	70	17.1%	5.7%	10.5%
Combination Brain/Sinus CT Scan	53	0.0%	2.3%	2.7%
Combination Chest CT Scan[1]	-	-	1.9%	2.7%
Follow-up Mammogram/Ultrasound	125	8.0%	6.3%	8.8%
Lumbar Spine MRI for Low Back Pain[1]	-	-	37.6%	37.2%

Sanford Westbrook Medical Center

920 Bell Avenue PO Box 188
Westbrook, MN 56183
Phone: 507-274-6121
Fax: 507-274-5671
Type: Critical Access Hospitals
Emergency Services: Yes
Ownership: Voluntary non-profit - Private
Beds: 13

Key Personnel:
Chief of Medical Staff. . . . . JC Cassel, MD
Emergency Room . . . . Priscilla Comnick
Infection Control. . . . . Karen Fay
CEO/President. . . . . Kelby K. Krabbenhoft
Operating Room. . . . . Marna Wahl
Quality Assurance . . . . Diana Williams, RN

Measure	Cases	This Hosp.	State Avg.	U.S. Avg.
Blood Clot Prevention and Treatment				
Anticoagulation Overlap Therapy[5]	-	-	96%	93%
ICU Venous Thromboembolism Prophylaxis[5]	-	-	91%	92%
Incidence of Potentially Preventable VTE[5]	-	-	9%	10%
UFH with Dosages/Platelet Monitoring[5]	-	-	98%	97%
Venous Thromboembolism Prophylaxis[5]	-	-	86%	85%
Warfarin Therapy Discharge Instructions[5]	-	-	63%	75%
Chest Pain/Possible Heart Attack Care				
Aspirin Given Within 24 Hours of Arrival[1,3]	-	-	97%	96%
Fibrinolytic Meds Within 30 Min. of Arrival[3,7]	-	-	48%	58%
Average Time to ECG (minutes)[1,3]	-	-	7	7
Average Time to Transfer (minutes)[1,3]	-	-	54	60
Children's Asthma Care				
Received Home Management Plan of Care	-	-	-	88%
Received Reliever Medication	-	-	-	100%
Received Systemic Corticosteroids	-	-	-	100%
Emergency Department				
Admittance Decision Time (minutes)	21	64	62	98
Head CT Results Within 45 Min. of Arrival[5]	-	-	54%	57%
Patients Who Left ER Before Being Seen[5]	-	-	2%	2%
Time from ER Arrival to Admit. (minutes)	32	110	199	274
Time from ER Arrival to Discharge (minutes)[5]	-	-	125	134
Time in ER Before Being Evaluated (minutes)[5]	-	-	31	26
Time to Pain Meds for Fractures (minutes)[5]	-	-	45	57
Heart Attack Care				
Aspirin Given at Discharge[5]	-	-	99%	99%
Fibrinolytic Meds Within 30 Min. of Arrival[5]	-	-	-	54%
PCI Within 90 Minutes of Arrival[5]	-	-	96%	96%
Statin Prescribed at Discharge[5]	-	-	99%	98%
Heart Failure Care				
ACE Inhibitor or ARB for LVSD[3,7]	-	-	96%	97%
Discharge Instructions Given[1,3]	-	-	93%	94%
Evaluation of LVS Function[1,3]	-	-	97%	99%
Medicare Spending				
Medicare Spending per Patient (ratio)	-	-	0.9	0.98
Pneumonia Care				
Appropriate Initial Antibiotic Given[1,3]	-	-	94%	95%
Blood Culture Timing[1,3]	-	-	97%	98%
Pregnancy and Delivery Care				
Newborn Deliveries Scheduled Early[5]	-	-	5%	6%
Preventive Care				
Immunization for Influenza[2]	38	87%	89%	90%
Immunization for Pneumonia[2]	64	95%	89%	92%
Stroke Care				
Anticoagulation Therapy for Atrial Fibrillation[5]	-	-	96%	95%
Antithrombotic Therapy Timing[5]	-	-	98%	98%
Assessed for Rehabilitation[5]	-	-	98%	97%
Discharged on Antithrombotic Therapy[5]	-	-	99%	99%
Discharged on Statin Medication[5]	-	-	95%	94%
Thrombolytic Therapy Timing[5]	-	-	74%	66%
Venous Thromboembolism Prophylaxis[5]	-	-	95%	94%
Written Stroke Educational Materials Given[5]	-	-	88%	88%
Surgical Care Improvement Project				
Appropriate Beta Blocker Usage[5]	-	-	98%	98%
Appropriate VTP Within 24 Hours[5]	-	-	98%	98%
Controlled Postoperative Blood Glucose[5]	-	-	97%	97%
Perioperative Temperature Management[5]	-	-	99%	100%
Prophylactic Antibiotic Selection[5]	-	-	99%	99%
Prophylactic Antibiotic Selection (Outpatient)[5]	-	-	98%	98%
Prophylactic Antibiotic Stopped[5]	-	-	99%	98%
Prophylactic Antibiotic Timing[5]	-	-	98%	99%
Prophylactic Antibiotic Timing (Outpatient)[5]	-	-	97%	98%
Urinary Catheter Removal[5]	-	-	97%	97%
Survey of Patients' Hospital Experiences				
Area Around Room 'Always' Quiet at Night[10]	<100	75%	65%	61%
Doctors 'Always' Communicated Well[10]	<100	100%	84%	82%
Home Recovery Information Given[10]	<100	96%	88%	85%
Hospital Given 9 or 10 on 10 Point Scale[10]	<100	74%	74%	71%
Meds 'Always' Explained Before Given[10]	<100	90%	67%	64%
Nurses 'Always' Communicated Well[10]	<100	99%	81%	79%
Pain 'Always' Well Controlled[10]	<100	92%	72%	71%
Room and Bathroom 'Always' Clean[10]	<100	91%	78%	73%
Timely Help 'Always' Received[10]	<100	100%	74%	68%
Would Definitely Recommend Hospital[10]	<100	83%	71%	71%
Use of Medical Imaging				
Cardiac Imaging Stress Test before Surgery[1]	-	-	6.3%	5.3%
Combination Abdominal CT Scan[1]	-	-	5.7%	10.5%
Combination Brain/Sinus CT Scan	30	0.0%	2.3%	2.7%
Combination Chest CT Scan[1]	-	-	1.9%	2.7%
Follow-up Mammogram/Ultrasound	72	12.5%	6.3%	8.8%
Lumbar Spine MRI for Low Back Pain[1]	-	-	37.6%	37.2%

Sanford Medical Center Wheaton

401 12th Street North
Wheaton, MN 56296
Phone: 320-563-8226
Fax: 320-563-8012
URL: www.wheatonhealthcare.org
Type: Critical Access Hospitals
Emergency Services: Yes
Ownership: Voluntary non-profit - Private
Beds: 25

Key Personnel:
Radiology. . . . . Anthony Aukes
Cardiac Laboratory. . . . . Jo Ann Foltz
Ambulatory Care . . . . Joann Foltz
CEO/President. . . . . Kelby K. Krabbenhoft
Chief of Medical Staff . . . . George Kuzma
Infection Control. . . . . Morgan Rinke
Emergency Room . . . . Donna Wahl

Measure	Cases	This Hosp.	State Avg.	U.S. Avg.
Blood Clot Prevention and Treatment				
Anticoagulation Overlap Therapy[5]	-	-	96%	93%
ICU Venous Thromboembolism Prophylaxis[5]	-	-	91%	92%
Incidence of Potentially Preventable VTE[5]	-	-	9%	10%
UFH with Dosages/Platelet Monitoring[5]	-	-	98%	97%
Venous Thromboembolism Prophylaxis[5]	-	-	86%	85%
Warfarin Therapy Discharge Instructions[5]	-	-	63%	75%
Chest Pain/Possible Heart Attack Care				
Aspirin Given Within 24 Hours of Arrival[1,3]	-	-	97%	96%
Fibrinolytic Meds Within 30 Min. of Arrival[3,7]	-	-	48%	58%
Average Time to ECG (minutes)[1,3]	-	-	7	7
Average Time to Transfer (minutes)[1,3]	-	-	54	60
Children's Asthma Care				
Received Home Management Plan of Care	-	-	-	88%
Received Reliever Medication	-	-	-	100%
Received Systemic Corticosteroids	-	-	-	100%

NOTE: Hospital profiles are in alphabetical order by state, then city, then hospital within the city; Rankings exclude hospitals with less than 25 cases except for patient surveys which excludes hospitals with less than 100 cases; (a) 100-299 cases; (1) The number of cases/patients is too few to report; (2) Data submitted were based on a sample of cases/patients; (3) Results are based on a shorter time period than required; (4) Data suppressed by CMS for one or more quarters; (5) Results are not available for this reporting period; (6) Fewer than 100 patients completed the HCAHPS survey; (7) No cases met the criteria for this measure; (8) The lower limit of the confidence interval cannot be calculated if the number of observed infections equals zero; (9) No data are available from the state/territory for this reporting period; (10) The scores shown reflect fewer than 50 completed surveys; (11) There were discrepancies in the data collection process; (12) This measure does not apply to this hospital for this reporting period; (13) Results cannot be calculated for this reporting period; (14) The results for this state are combined with nearby states to protect confidentiality; Please refer to the User's Guide for a full explanation of data.

Measure	Cases	This Hosp.	State Avg.	U.S. Avg.
Emergency Department				
Admittance Decision Time (minutes)[3]	21	29	62	98
Head CT Results Within 45 Min. of Arrival[5]	-	-	54%	57%
Patients Who Left ER Before Being Seen[5]	-	-	2%	2%
Time from ER Arrival to Admit. (minutes)[3]	21	188	199	274
Time from ER Arrival to Discharge (minutes)[3]	96	110	125	134
Time in ER Before Being Evaluated (minutes)[3]	123	25	31	26
Time to Pain Meds for Fractures (minutes)[5]	-	-	45	57
Heart Attack Care				
Aspirin Given at Discharge[1,3]	-	-	99%	99%
Fibrinolytic Meds Within 30 Min. of Arrival[3,7]	-	-	-	54%
PCI Within 90 Minutes of Arrival[3,7]	-	-	96%	96%
Statin Prescribed at Discharge[1,3]	-	-	99%	98%
Heart Failure Care				
ACE Inhibitor or ARB for LVSD[1]	-	-	96%	97%
Discharge Instructions Given[1]	-	-	93%	94%
Evaluation of LVS Function[1]	-	-	97%	99%
Medicare Spending				
Medicare Spending per Patient (ratio)	-	-	0.9	0.98
Pneumonia Care				
Appropriate Initial Antibiotic Given[1]	-	-	94%	95%
Blood Culture Timing[1]	-	-	97%	98%
Pregnancy and Delivery Care				
Newborn Deliveries Scheduled Early[5]	-	-	5%	6%
Preventive Care				
Immunization for Influenza[3]	24	83%	89%	90%
Immunization for Pneumonia[3]	44	73%	89%	92%
Stroke Care				
Anticoagulation Therapy for Atrial Fibrillation[5]	-	-	96%	95%
Antithrombotic Therapy Timing[5]	-	-	98%	98%
Assessed for Rehabilitation[5]	-	-	98%	97%
Discharged on Antithrombotic Therapy[5]	-	-	99%	99%
Discharged on Statin Medication[5]	-	-	95%	94%
Thrombolytic Therapy Timing[5]	-	-	74%	66%
Venous Thromboembolism Prophylaxis[5]	-	-	95%	94%
Written Stroke Educational Materials Given[5]	-	-	88%	88%
Surgical Care Improvement Project				
Appropriate Beta Blocker Usage[1,3]	-	-	98%	98%
Appropriate VTP Within 24 Hours[1,3]	-	-	98%	98%
Controlled Postoperative Blood Glucose[3,7]	-	-	97%	97%
Perioperative Temperature Management[1,3]	-	-	99%	100%
Prophylactic Antibiotic Selection[3,7]	-	-	99%	99%
Prophylactic Antibiotic Selection (Outpatient)[5]	-	-	98%	98%
Prophylactic Antibiotic Stopped[3,7]	-	-	99%	98%
Prophylactic Antibiotic Timing[3,7]	-	-	98%	99%
Prophylactic Antibiotic Timing (Outpatient)[5]	-	-	97%	98%
Urinary Catheter Removal[3,7]	-	-	97%	97%
Survey of Patients' Hospital Experiences				
Area Around Room 'Always' Quiet at Night[5]	-	-	65%	61%
Doctors 'Always' Communicated Well[5]	-	-	84%	82%
Home Recovery Information Given[5]	-	-	88%	85%
Hospital Given 9 or 10 on 10 Point Scale[5]	-	-	74%	71%
Meds 'Always' Explained Before Given[5]	-	-	67%	64%
Nurses 'Always' Communicated Well[5]	-	-	81%	79%
Pain 'Always' Well Controlled[5]	-	-	72%	71%
Room and Bathroom 'Always' Clean[5]	-	-	78%	73%
Timely Help 'Always' Received[5]	-	-	74%	68%
Would Definitely Recommend Hospital[5]	-	-	71%	71%
Use of Medical Imaging				
Cardiac Imaging Stress Test before Surgery[1]	-	-	6.3%	5.3%
Combination Abdominal CT Scan[1]	-	-	5.7%	10.5%
Combination Brain/Sinus CT Scan[1]	-	-	2.3%	2.7%
Combination Chest CT Scan[1]	-	-	1.9%	2.7%
Follow-up Mammogram/Ultrasound	108	3.7%	6.3%	8.8%
Lumbar Spine MRI for Low Back Pain[1]	-	-	37.6%	37.2%

Rice Memorial Hospital

301 Becker Ave Sw
Willmar, MN 56201
Phone: 320-231-4227
Fax: 320-231-4869
E-mail: nski@rice.willmar.mn.us
URL: www.ricememorial.com
Type: Acute Care Hospitals
Emergency Services: Yes
Ownership: Government - Local
Beds: 136

Key Personnel:
Intensive Care Unit. . . . . Kathy Dillox, RN
Pediatric Ambulatory Care . . . . . . MJ Hodapp
Chief of Medical Staff . . . . Dr. Fred Hund, MD
CEO/President. . . . . Lawrence J Massa
Radiology. . . . . DB Nguyen, MD
Infection Control. . . . . Barb Piasecki
Operating Room. . . . . Ruth Rand
Quality Assurance . . . . Peggy Sietsema, RN

Measure	Cases	This Hosp.	State Avg.	U.S. Avg.
Blood Clot Prevention and Treatment				
Anticoagulation Overlap Therapy[2]	15	100%	96%	93%
ICU Venous Thromboembolism Prophylaxis[2]	50	82%	91%	92%
Incidence of Potentially Preventable VTE[1,2]	-	-	9%	10%
UFH with Dosages/Platelet Monitoring[1,2]	-	-	98%	97%
Venous Thromboembolism Prophylaxis[2]	154	83%	86%	85%
Warfarin Therapy Discharge Instructions[1,2]	-	-	63%	75%
Chest Pain/Possible Heart Attack Care				
Aspirin Given Within 24 Hours of Arrival	66	97%	97%	96%
Fibrinolytic Meds Within 30 Min. of Arrival[7]	-	-	48%	58%
Average Time to ECG (minutes)	65	10	7	7
Average Time to Transfer (minutes)	11	54	54	60
Children's Asthma Care				
Received Home Management Plan of Care	-	-	-	88%
Received Reliever Medication	-	-	-	100%
Received Systemic Corticosteroids	-	-	-	100%
Emergency Department				
Admittance Decision Time (minutes)[2]	126	78	62	98
Head CT Results Within 45 Min. of Arrival[1]	-	-	54%	57%
Patients Who Left ER Before Being Seen	13,062	2%	2%	2%
Time from ER Arrival to Admit. (minutes)[2]	146	206	199	274
Time from ER Arrival to Discharge (minutes)	605	116	125	134
Time in ER Before Being Evaluated (minutes)	561	30	31	26
Time to Pain Meds for Fractures (minutes)	82	30	45	57
Heart Attack Care				
Aspirin Given at Discharge[1]	-	-	99%	99%
Fibrinolytic Meds Within 30 Min. of Arrival[7]	-	-	-	54%
PCI Within 90 Minutes of Arrival[7]	-	-	96%	96%
Statin Prescribed at Discharge	11	100%	99%	98%
Heart Failure Care				
ACE Inhibitor or ARB for LVSD	22	91%	96%	97%
Discharge Instructions Given	60	92%	93%	94%
Evaluation of LVS Function	91	100%	97%	99%
Medicare Spending				
Medicare Spending per Patient (ratio)	-	0.91	0.9	0.98
Pneumonia Care				
Appropriate Initial Antibiotic Given	58	100%	94%	95%
Blood Culture Timing	78	99%	97%	98%
Pregnancy and Delivery Care				
Newborn Deliveries Scheduled Early[2]	17	6%	5%	6%
Preventive Care				
Immunization for Influenza[2]	327	95%	89%	90%
Immunization for Pneumonia[2]	326	80%	89%	92%
Stroke Care				
Anticoagulation Therapy for Atrial Fibrillation[1]	-	-	96%	95%
Antithrombotic Therapy Timing	20	100%	98%	98%
Assessed for Rehabilitation	24	100%	98%	97%
Discharged on Antithrombotic Therapy	22	100%	99%	99%
Discharged on Statin Medication	18	83%	95%	94%
Thrombolytic Therapy Timing[1]	-	-	74%	66%
Venous Thromboembolism Prophylaxis	22	86%	95%	94%
Written Stroke Educational Materials Given	15	93%	88%	88%
Surgical Care Improvement Project				
Appropriate Beta Blocker Usage[2]	79	89%	98%	98%
Appropriate VTP Within 24 Hours[2]	246	97%	98%	98%
Controlled Postoperative Blood Glucose[2,7]	-	-	97%	97%
Perioperative Temperature Management[2]	273	99%	99%	100%
Prophylactic Antibiotic Selection[2]	181	99%	99%	99%
Prophylactic Antibiotic Selection (Outpatient)	54	98%	98%	98%
Prophylactic Antibiotic Stopped[2]	180	98%	99%	98%
Prophylactic Antibiotic Timing[2]	181	99%	98%	99%
Prophylactic Antibiotic Timing (Outpatient)	60	88%	97%	98%
Urinary Catheter Removal[2]	196	93%	97%	97%
Survey of Patients' Hospital Experiences				
Area Around Room 'Always' Quiet at Night	300+	69%	65%	61%
Doctors 'Always' Communicated Well	300+	83%	84%	82%
Home Recovery Information Given	300+	88%	88%	85%
Hospital Given 9 or 10 on 10 Point Scale	300+	71%	74%	71%
Meds 'Always' Explained Before Given	300+	68%	67%	64%
Nurses 'Always' Communicated Well	300+	80%	81%	79%
Pain 'Always' Well Controlled	300+	66%	72%	71%
Room and Bathroom 'Always' Clean	300+	73%	78%	73%
Timely Help 'Always' Received	300+	70%	74%	68%
Would Definitely Recommend Hospital	300+	70%	71%	71%
Use of Medical Imaging				
Cardiac Imaging Stress Test before Surgery	79	8.9%	6.3%	5.3%
Combination Abdominal CT Scan	210	4.3%	5.7%	10.5%
Combination Brain/Sinus CT Scan[1]	-	-	2.3%	2.7%
Combination Chest CT Scan	143	0.7%	1.9%	2.7%
Follow-up Mammogram/Ultrasound[7]	-	-	6.3%	8.8%
Lumbar Spine MRI for Low Back Pain[1]	-	-	37.6%	37.2%

Windom Area Hospital

2150 Hospital Drive, PO Box 339
Windom, MN 56101
Phone: 507-831-2400
Fax: 507-831-5749
E-mail: contactus@windomareahospital.com
URL: www.windomareahospital.com
Type: Critical Access Hospitals
Emergency Services: Yes
Ownership: Government - Local
Beds: 35

Key Personnel:
CEO/President. . . . . Gerri Burmeister
Chief of Medical Staff . . . . Rod Dynes, MD
Infection Control. . . . . Marcia Fast, RN
Quality Assurance . . . . Marcia Fast, RN
Operating Room. . . . . Nancy Jenson, RN
Anesthesiology. . . . . Loretta Krahn, CRNA
Emergency Room . . . . Jeffery Taber, RN

Measure	Cases	This Hosp.	State Avg.	U.S. Avg.
Blood Clot Prevention and Treatment				
Anticoagulation Overlap Therapy[5]	-	-	96%	93%
ICU Venous Thromboembolism Prophylaxis[5]	-	-	91%	92%
Incidence of Potentially Preventable VTE[5]	-	-	9%	10%
UFH with Dosages/Platelet Monitoring[5]	-	-	98%	97%
Venous Thromboembolism Prophylaxis[5]	-	-	86%	85%
Warfarin Therapy Discharge Instructions[5]	-	-	63%	75%
Chest Pain/Possible Heart Attack Care				
Aspirin Given Within 24 Hours of Arrival	21	90%	97%	96%
Fibrinolytic Meds Within 30 Min. of Arrival[1,3]	-	-	48%	58%
Average Time to ECG (minutes)	22	11	7	7
Average Time to Transfer (minutes)[3,7]	-	-	54	60
Children's Asthma Care				
Received Home Management Plan of Care	-	-	-	88%
Received Reliever Medication	-	-	-	100%
Received Systemic Corticosteroids	-	-	-	100%
Emergency Department				
Admittance Decision Time (minutes)[2]	32	12	62	98
Head CT Results Within 45 Min. of Arrival[1,3]	-	-	54%	57%
Patients Who Left ER Before Being Seen[5]	-	-	2%	2%
Time from ER Arrival to Admit. (minutes)[2]	148	134	199	274
Time from ER Arrival to Discharge (minutes)[5]	-	-	125	134
Time in ER Before Being Evaluated (minutes)[5]	-	-	31	26
Time to Pain Meds for Fractures (minutes)	16	46	45	57
Heart Attack Care				
Aspirin Given at Discharge[1,3]	-	-	99%	99%
Fibrinolytic Meds Within 30 Min. of Arrival[3,7]	-	-	-	54%
PCI Within 90 Minutes of Arrival[3,7]	-	-	96%	96%
Statin Prescribed at Discharge[1,3]	-	-	99%	98%
Heart Failure Care				
ACE Inhibitor or ARB for LVSD[1]	-	-	96%	97%
Discharge Instructions Given	13	62%	93%	94%
Evaluation of LVS Function	16	88%	97%	99%

NOTE: Hospital profiles are in alphabetical order by state, then city, then hospital within the city; Rankings exclude hospitals with less than 25 cases except for patient surveys which excludes hospitals with less than 100 cases; (a) 100-299 cases; (1) The number of cases/patients is too few to report; (2) Data submitted were based on a sample of cases/patients; (3) Results are based on a shorter time period than required; (4) Data suppressed by CMS for one or more quarters; (5) Results are not available for this reporting period; (6) Fewer than 100 patients completed the HCAHPS survey; (7) No cases met the criteria for this measure; (8) The lower limit of the confidence interval cannot be calculated if the number of observed infections equals zero; (9) No data are available from the state/territory for this reporting period; (10) The scores shown reflect fewer than 50 completed surveys; (11) There were discrepancies in the data collection process; (12) This measure does not apply to this hospital for this reporting period; (13) Results cannot be calculated for this reporting period; (14) The results for this state are combined with nearby states to protect confidentiality; Please refer to the User's Guide for a full explanation of data.

Measure	Cases	This Hosp.	State Avg.	U.S. Avg.
Medicare Spending				
Medicare Spending per Patient (ratio)	-	-	0.9	0.98
Pneumonia Care				
Appropriate Initial Antibiotic Given	14	86%	94%	95%
Blood Culture Timing	13	92%	97%	98%
Pregnancy and Delivery Care				
Newborn Deliveries Scheduled Early[5]	-	-	5%	6%
Preventive Care				
Immunization for Influenza	187	84%	89%	90%
Immunization for Pneumonia	172	81%	89%	92%
Stroke Care				
Anticoagulation Therapy for Atrial Fibrillation[5]	-	-	96%	95%
Antithrombotic Therapy Timing[5]	-	-	98%	98%
Assessed for Rehabilitation[5]	-	-	98%	97%
Discharged on Antithrombotic Therapy[5]	-	-	99%	99%
Discharged on Statin Medication[5]	-	-	95%	94%
Thrombolytic Therapy Timing[5]	-	-	74%	66%
Venous Thromboembolism Prophylaxis[5]	-	-	95%	94%
Written Stroke Educational Materials Given[5]	-	-	88%	88%
Surgical Care Improvement Project				
Appropriate Beta Blocker Usage[5]	-	-	98%	98%
Appropriate VTP Within 24 Hours[5]	-	-	98%	98%
Controlled Postoperative Blood Glucose[5]	-	-	97%	97%
Perioperative Temperature Management[5]	-	-	99%	100%
Prophylactic Antibiotic Selection[5]	-	-	99%	99%
Prophylactic Antibiotic Selection (Outpatient)[5]	-	-	98%	98%
Prophylactic Antibiotic Stopped[5]	-	-	99%	98%
Prophylactic Antibiotic Timing[5]	-	-	98%	99%
Prophylactic Antibiotic Timing (Outpatient)[5]	-	-	97%	98%
Urinary Catheter Removal[5]	-	-	97%	97%
Survey of Patients' Hospital Experiences				
Area Around Room 'Always' Quiet at Night	(a)	60%	65%	61%
Doctors 'Always' Communicated Well	(a)	86%	84%	82%
Home Recovery Information Given	(a)	87%	88%	85%
Hospital Given 9 or 10 on 10 Point Scale	(a)	73%	74%	71%
Meds 'Always' Explained Before Given	(a)	70%	67%	64%
Nurses 'Always' Communicated Well	(a)	86%	81%	79%
Pain 'Always' Well Controlled	(a)	73%	72%	71%
Room and Bathroom 'Always' Clean	(a)	82%	78%	73%
Timely Help 'Always' Received	(a)	77%	74%	68%
Would Definitely Recommend Hospital	(a)	74%	71%	71%
Use of Medical Imaging				
Cardiac Imaging Stress Test before Surgery[1]	-	-	6.3%	5.3%
Combination Abdominal CT Scan	92	4.3%	5.7%	10.5%
Combination Brain/Sinus CT Scan[1]	-	-	2.3%	2.7%
Combination Chest CT Scan[1]	-	-	1.9%	2.7%
Follow-up Mammogram/Ultrasound	111	11.7%	6.3%	8.8%
Lumbar Spine MRI for Low Back Pain[1]	-	-	37.6%	37.2%

Winona Health Services

855 Mankato Avenue
Winona, MN 55987
Phone: 507-454-3650
Fax: 507-457-4413
URL: www.winonahealth.org
Type: Acute Care Hospitals
Emergency Services: Yes
Ownership: Voluntary non-profit - Private
Beds: 99

Key Personnel:
Coronary Care.............. Kathleen Lanik
Quality Assurance.............. Kathleen Lanik
Radiology.................. Laurel Littrell, MD
Infection Control.............. Linda Pozanc
CEO/President.............. Rachelle Schultz
Chief of Medical Staff.......... Charles Shepard

Measure	Cases	This Hosp.	State Avg.	U.S. Avg.
Blood Clot Prevention and Treatment				
Anticoagulation Overlap Therapy[2]	17	82%	96%	93%
ICU Venous Thromboembolism Prophylaxis[2]	77	70%	91%	92%
Incidence of Potentially Preventable VTE[1,2]	-	-	9%	10%
UFH with Dosages/Platelet Monitoring[2]	11	100%	98%	97%
Venous Thromboembolism Prophylaxis[2]	118	85%	86%	85%
Warfarin Therapy Discharge Instructions[2]	12	100%	63%	75%
Chest Pain/Possible Heart Attack Care				
Aspirin Given Within 24 Hours of Arrival	68	99%	97%	96%
Fibrinolytic Meds Within 30 Min. of Arrival[7]	-	-	48%	58%
Average Time to ECG (minutes)	68	4	7	7
Average Time to Transfer (minutes)[7]	-	-	54	60
Children's Asthma Care				
Received Home Management Plan of Care	-	-	-	88%
Received Reliever Medication	-	-	-	100%
Received Systemic Corticosteroids	-	-	-	100%
Emergency Department				
Admittance Decision Time (minutes)[2]	307	21	62	98
Head CT Results Within 45 Min. of Arrival	11	18%	54%	57%
Patients Who Left ER Before Being Seen	17,766	0%	2%	2%
Time from ER Arrival to Admit. (minutes)[2]	323	138	199	274
Time from ER Arrival to Discharge (minutes)	335	85	125	134
Time in ER Before Being Evaluated (minutes)	291	14	31	26
Time to Pain Meds for Fractures (minutes)	54	27	45	57
Heart Attack Care				
Aspirin Given at Discharge	17	94%	99%	99%
Fibrinolytic Meds Within 30 Min. of Arrival[7]	-	-	-	54%
PCI Within 90 Minutes of Arrival[7]	-	-	96%	96%
Statin Prescribed at Discharge	16	100%	99%	98%
Heart Failure Care				
ACE Inhibitor or ARB for LVSD	17	100%	96%	97%
Discharge Instructions Given	49	98%	93%	94%
Evaluation of LVS Function	65	94%	97%	99%
Medicare Spending				
Medicare Spending per Patient (ratio)	-	0.86	0.9	0.98
Pneumonia Care				
Appropriate Initial Antibiotic Given	59	95%	94%	95%
Blood Culture Timing	108	99%	97%	98%
Pregnancy and Delivery Care				
Newborn Deliveries Scheduled Early[2]	28	4%	5%	6%
Preventive Care				
Immunization for Influenza[2]	272	79%	89%	90%
Immunization for Pneumonia[2]	314	86%	89%	92%
Stroke Care				
Anticoagulation Therapy for Atrial Fibrillation[1,2]	-	-	96%	95%
Antithrombotic Therapy Timing[2]	14	93%	98%	98%
Assessed for Rehabilitation[2]	19	100%	98%	97%
Discharged on Antithrombotic Therapy[2]	18	100%	99%	99%
Discharged on Statin Medication[2]	13	100%	95%	94%
Thrombolytic Therapy Timing[1,2]	-	-	74%	66%
Venous Thromboembolism Prophylaxis[2]	17	100%	95%	94%
Written Stroke Educational Materials Given[1,2]	-	-	88%	88%
Surgical Care Improvement Project				
Appropriate Beta Blocker Usage	62	95%	98%	98%
Appropriate VTP Within 24 Hours	135	99%	98%	98%
Controlled Postoperative Blood Glucose[7]	-	-	97%	97%
Perioperative Temperature Management	178	100%	99%	100%
Prophylactic Antibiotic Selection	122	97%	99%	99%
Prophylactic Antibiotic Selection (Outpatient)	58	95%	98%	98%
Prophylactic Antibiotic Stopped	119	97%	99%	98%
Prophylactic Antibiotic Timing	122	99%	98%	99%
Prophylactic Antibiotic Timing (Outpatient)	43	98%	97%	98%
Urinary Catheter Removal	102	94%	97%	97%
Survey of Patients' Hospital Experiences				
Area Around Room 'Always' Quiet at Night	300+	63%	65%	61%
Doctors 'Always' Communicated Well	300+	79%	84%	82%
Home Recovery Information Given	300+	87%	88%	85%
Hospital Given 9 or 10 on 10 Point Scale	300+	66%	74%	71%
Meds 'Always' Explained Before Given	300+	61%	67%	64%
Nurses 'Always' Communicated Well	300+	80%	81%	79%
Pain 'Always' Well Controlled	300+	67%	72%	71%
Room and Bathroom 'Always' Clean	300+	76%	78%	73%
Timely Help 'Always' Received	300+	69%	74%	68%
Would Definitely Recommend Hospital	300+	62%	71%	71%
Use of Medical Imaging				
Cardiac Imaging Stress Test before Surgery[1]	-	-	6.3%	5.3%
Combination Abdominal CT Scan	251	6.8%	5.7%	10.5%
Combination Brain/Sinus CT Scan[1]	-	-	2.3%	2.7%
Combination Chest CT Scan	146	2.1%	1.9%	2.7%
Follow-up Mammogram/Ultrasound	635	13.4%	6.3%	8.8%
Lumbar Spine MRI for Low Back Pain[1]	-	-	37.6%	37.2%

Healtheast Woodwinds Hospital

1925 Woodwinds Drive
Woodbury, MN 55125
Phone: 651-232-6880
Fax: 651-232-2551
URL: www.woodwinds.org
Type: Acute Care Hospitals
Emergency Services: No
Ownership: Voluntary non-profit - Private
Beds: 78

Key Personnel:
Cardiology.................. Stuart W Adler
Anesthesiology.............. Donald Anderson
Anesthesiology.............. James V Anderson
Cardiology.................. Steven L Benton, MD
Anesthesiology.............. Faisal M Choudhary
CEO/President............... Julie Schmidt

Measure	Cases	This Hosp.	State Avg.	U.S. Avg.
Blood Clot Prevention and Treatment				
Anticoagulation Overlap Therapy[2]	59	97%	96%	93%
ICU Venous Thromboembolism Prophylaxis[2]	31	87%	91%	92%
Incidence of Potentially Preventable VTE[1,2]	-	-	9%	10%
UFH with Dosages/Platelet Monitoring[2]	25	100%	98%	97%
Venous Thromboembolism Prophylaxis[2]	230	86%	86%	85%
Warfarin Therapy Discharge Instructions[2]	55	49%	63%	75%
Chest Pain/Possible Heart Attack Care				
Aspirin Given Within 24 Hours of Arrival	47	100%	97%	96%
Fibrinolytic Meds Within 30 Min. of Arrival[7]	-	-	48%	58%
Average Time to ECG (minutes)	48	8	7	7
Average Time to Transfer (minutes)[7]	-	-	54	60
Children's Asthma Care				
Received Home Management Plan of Care	-	-	-	88%
Received Reliever Medication	-	-	-	100%
Received Systemic Corticosteroids	-	-	-	100%
Emergency Department				
Admittance Decision Time (minutes)[2]	404	74	62	98
Head CT Results Within 45 Min. of Arrival[1]	-	-	54%	57%
Patients Who Left ER Before Being Seen	26,395	1%	2%	2%
Time from ER Arrival to Admit. (minutes)[2]	409	234	199	274
Time from ER Arrival to Discharge (minutes)	389	151	125	134
Time in ER Before Being Evaluated (minutes)	391	27	31	26
Time to Pain Meds for Fractures (minutes)	123	38	45	57
Heart Attack Care				
Aspirin Given at Discharge[1]	-	-	99%	99%
Fibrinolytic Meds Within 30 Min. of Arrival[7]	-	-	-	54%
PCI Within 90 Minutes of Arrival[7]	-	-	96%	96%
Statin Prescribed at Discharge[1]	-	-	99%	98%
Heart Failure Care				
ACE Inhibitor or ARB for LVSD	19	100%	96%	97%
Discharge Instructions Given	70	96%	93%	94%
Evaluation of LVS Function	92	99%	97%	99%
Medicare Spending				
Medicare Spending per Patient (ratio)	-	0.87	0.9	0.98
Pneumonia Care				
Appropriate Initial Antibiotic Given[2]	71	99%	94%	95%
Blood Culture Timing[2]	118	97%	97%	98%
Pregnancy and Delivery Care				
Newborn Deliveries Scheduled Early[2]	35	0%	5%	6%
Preventive Care				
Immunization for Influenza[2]	504	88%	89%	90%
Immunization for Pneumonia[2]	460	87%	89%	92%
Stroke Care				
Anticoagulation Therapy for Atrial Fibrillation[1]	-	-	96%	95%
Antithrombotic Therapy Timing	28	96%	98%	98%
Assessed for Rehabilitation	47	100%	98%	97%
Discharged on Antithrombotic Therapy	46	100%	99%	99%
Discharged on Statin Medication	37	97%	95%	94%
Thrombolytic Therapy Timing[1]	-	-	74%	66%
Venous Thromboembolism Prophylaxis	38	95%	95%	94%
Written Stroke Educational Materials Given	25	88%	88%	88%
Surgical Care Improvement Project				
Appropriate Beta Blocker Usage[2]	92	99%	98%	98%
Appropriate VTP Within 24 Hours[2]	331	100%	98%	98%
Controlled Postoperative Blood Glucose[2,7]	-	-	97%	97%
Perioperative Temperature Management[2]	426	100%	99%	100%
Prophylactic Antibiotic Selection[2]	294	99%	99%	99%
Prophylactic Antibiotic Selection (Outpatient)	164	99%	98%	98%
Prophylactic Antibiotic Stopped[2]	290	99%	99%	98%

NOTE: Hospital profiles are in alphabetical order by state, then city, then hospital within the city; Rankings exclude hospitals with less than 25 cases except for patient surveys which excludes hospitals with less than 100 cases; (a) 100-299 cases; (1) The number of cases/patients is too few to report; (2) Data submitted were based on a sample of cases/patients; (3) Results are based on a shorter time period than required; (4) Data suppressed by CMS for one or more quarters; (5) Results are not available for this reporting period; (6) Fewer than 100 patients completed the HCAHPS survey; (7) No cases met the criteria for this measure; (8) The lower limit of the confidence interval cannot be calculated if the number of observed infections equals zero; (9) No data are available from the state/territory for this reporting period; (10) The scores shown reflect fewer than 50 completed surveys; (11) There were discrepancies in the data collection process; (12) This measure does not apply to this hospital for this reporting period; (13) Results cannot be calculated for this reporting period; (14) The results for this state are combined with nearby states to protect confidentiality; Please refer to the User's Guide for a full explanation of data.

Measure	Cases	This Hosp.	State Avg.	U.S. Avg.
Prophylactic Antibiotic Timing[2]	294	99%	98%	99%
Prophylactic Antibiotic Timing (Outpatient)	164	99%	97%	98%
Urinary Catheter Removal[2]	220	98%	97%	97%
Survey of Patients' Hospital Experiences				
Area Around Room 'Always' Quiet at Night	300+	71%	65%	61%
Doctors 'Always' Communicated Well	300+	83%	84%	82%
Home Recovery Information Given	300+	90%	88%	85%
Hospital Given 9 or 10 on 10 Point Scale	300+	85%	74%	71%
Meds 'Always' Explained Before Given	300+	69%	67%	64%
Nurses 'Always' Communicated Well	300+	86%	81%	79%
Pain 'Always' Well Controlled	300+	73%	72%	71%
Room and Bathroom 'Always' Clean	300+	78%	78%	73%
Timely Help 'Always' Received	300+	75%	74%	68%
Would Definitely Recommend Hospital	300+	84%	71%	71%
Use of Medical Imaging				
Cardiac Imaging Stress Test before Surgery	179	7.3%	6.3%	5.3%
Combination Abdominal CT Scan	457	2.4%	5.7%	10.5%
Combination Brain/Sinus CT Scan	229	5.2%	2.3%	2.7%
Combination Chest CT Scan	196	0.0%	1.9%	2.7%
Follow-up Mammogram/Ultrasound	718	6.1%	6.3%	8.8%
Lumbar Spine MRI for Low Back Pain	55	38.2%	37.6%	37.2%

Sanford Worthington Medical Center

1018 Sixth Avenue PO Box 997 Phone: 507-372-2941
Worthington, MN 56187 Fax: 507-372-7686
URL: www.worthingtonhospital.com
Type: Acute Care Hospitals Emergency Services: Yes
Ownership: Voluntary non-profit - Private Beds: 66

Key Personnel:
Operating Room. . . . . Paula Ausham
Emergency Room . . . . Charles Fitch, MD
Infection Control. . . . . LaVonne Foss
Quality Assurance . . . . LaVonne Foss
Radiology. . . . . Jim I Myerly
Intensive Care Unit. . . . . Diane Zandstra

Measure	Cases	This Hosp.	State Avg.	U.S. Avg.
Blood Clot Prevention and Treatment				
Anticoagulation Overlap Therapy[1,2]	-	-	96%	93%
ICU Venous Thromboembolism Prophylaxis[2]	17	88%	91%	92%
Incidence of Potentially Preventable VTE[1,2]	-	-	9%	10%
UFH with Dosages/Platelet Monitoring[1,2]	-	-	98%	97%
Venous Thromboembolism Prophylaxis[2]	140	66%	86%	85%
Warfarin Therapy Discharge Instructions[1,2]	-	-	63%	75%
Chest Pain/Possible Heart Attack Care				
Aspirin Given Within 24 Hours of Arrival	37	97%	97%	96%
Fibrinolytic Meds Within 30 Min. of Arrival[1]	-	-	48%	58%
Average Time to ECG (minutes)	38	13	7	7
Average Time to Transfer (minutes)[7]	-	-	54	60
Children's Asthma Care				
Received Home Management Plan of Care	-	-	-	88%
Received Reliever Medication	-	-	-	100%
Received Systemic Corticosteroids	-	-	-	100%
Emergency Department				
Admittance Decision Time (minutes)[2]	170	22	62	98
Head CT Results Within 45 Min. of Arrival[1]	-	-	54%	57%
Patients Who Left ER Before Being Seen	5,767	0%	2%	2%
Time from ER Arrival to Admit. (minutes)[2]	264	171	199	274
Time from ER Arrival to Discharge (minutes)	430	103	125	134
Time in ER Before Being Evaluated (minutes)	273	15	31	26
Time to Pain Meds for Fractures (minutes)	60	39	45	57
Heart Attack Care				
Aspirin Given at Discharge[1,3]	-	-	99%	99%
Fibrinolytic Meds Within 30 Min. of Arrival[3,7]	-	-	-	54%
PCI Within 90 Minutes of Arrival[3,7]	-	-	96%	96%
Statin Prescribed at Discharge[1,3]	-	-	99%	98%
Heart Failure Care				
ACE Inhibitor or ARB for LVSD[1,2]	-	-	96%	97%
Discharge Instructions Given[2]	15	93%	93%	94%
Evaluation of LVS Function[2]	27	78%	97%	99%
Medicare Spending				
Medicare Spending per Patient (ratio)	-	0.84	0.9	0.98
Pneumonia Care				
Appropriate Initial Antibiotic Given[2]	29	83%	94%	95%
Blood Culture Timing[2]	38	97%	97%	98%
Pregnancy and Delivery Care				
Newborn Deliveries Scheduled Early	75	0%	5%	6%
Preventive Care				
Immunization for Influenza[2]	380	91%	89%	90%
Immunization for Pneumonia[2]	340	82%	89%	92%
Stroke Care				
Anticoagulation Therapy for Atrial Fibrillation[1,3]	-	-	96%	95%
Antithrombotic Therapy Timing[1,3]	-	-	98%	98%
Assessed for Rehabilitation[1,3]	-	-	98%	97%
Discharged on Antithrombotic Therapy[1,3]	-	-	99%	99%
Discharged on Statin Medication[1,3]	-	-	95%	94%
Thrombolytic Therapy Timing[3,7]	-	-	74%	66%
Venous Thromboembolism Prophylaxis[1,3]	-	-	95%	94%
Written Stroke Educational Materials Given[3,7]	-	-	88%	88%
Surgical Care Improvement Project				
Appropriate Beta Blocker Usage[2]	13	100%	98%	98%
Appropriate VTP Within 24 Hours[2]	83	99%	98%	98%
Controlled Postoperative Blood Glucose[2,7]	-	-	97%	97%
Perioperative Temperature Management[2]	94	98%	99%	100%
Prophylactic Antibiotic Selection[2]	80	100%	99%	99%
Prophylactic Antibiotic Selection (Outpatient)	12	83%	98%	98%
Prophylactic Antibiotic Stopped[2]	80	99%	99%	98%
Prophylactic Antibiotic Timing[2]	80	99%	98%	99%
Prophylactic Antibiotic Timing (Outpatient)	12	100%	97%	98%
Urinary Catheter Removal[2]	54	87%	97%	97%
Survey of Patients' Hospital Experiences				
Area Around Room 'Always' Quiet at Night	300+	61%	65%	61%
Doctors 'Always' Communicated Well	300+	77%	84%	82%
Home Recovery Information Given	300+	87%	88%	85%
Hospital Given 9 or 10 on 10 Point Scale	300+	68%	74%	71%
Meds 'Always' Explained Before Given	300+	66%	67%	64%
Nurses 'Always' Communicated Well	300+	79%	81%	79%
Pain 'Always' Well Controlled	300+	72%	72%	71%
Room and Bathroom 'Always' Clean	300+	80%	78%	73%
Timely Help 'Always' Received	300+	76%	74%	68%
Would Definitely Recommend Hospital	300+	65%	71%	71%
Use of Medical Imaging				
Cardiac Imaging Stress Test before Surgery	122	6.6%	6.3%	5.3%
Combination Abdominal CT Scan	176	6.8%	5.7%	10.5%
Combination Brain/Sinus CT Scan[1]	-	-	2.3%	2.7%
Combination Chest CT Scan	89	0.0%	1.9%	2.7%
Follow-up Mammogram/Ultrasound	165	7.3%	6.3%	8.8%
Lumbar Spine MRI for Low Back Pain[1]	-	-	37.6%	37.2%

Fairview Lakes Medical Center

5200 Fairview Boulevard Phone: 651-982-7104
Wyoming, MN 55092 Fax: 651-982-7298
URL: www.lakes.fairview.org
Type: Acute Care Hospitals Emergency Services: Yes
Ownership: Voluntary non-profit - Private Beds: 59

Key Personnel:
Emergency Room . . . . Joseph Alfano, MD
Pediatrics. . . . . Catherine Berry, MD, PhD
Surgery . . . . James M. Cain, MD, FACS
Cardiology . . . . Norman Chapel, MD, FACC
Hemotology Center . . . . L. Lisa Ge, MD
Chief of Medical Staff . . . . Lois A Lenarz, MD, AAFP
Infection Control. . . . . Dipi Sharma, MD
CEO/President. . . . . Rulon F. Stacey, PhD, FACHE

Measure	Cases	This Hosp.	State Avg.	U.S. Avg.
Blood Clot Prevention and Treatment				
Anticoagulation Overlap Therapy[2]	27	100%	96%	93%
ICU Venous Thromboembolism Prophylaxis[2]	44	98%	91%	92%
Incidence of Potentially Preventable VTE[1,2]	-	-	9%	10%
UFH with Dosages/Platelet Monitoring[1,2]	-	-	98%	97%
Venous Thromboembolism Prophylaxis[2]	204	97%	86%	85%
Warfarin Therapy Discharge Instructions[2]	28	100%	63%	75%
Chest Pain/Possible Heart Attack Care				
Aspirin Given Within 24 Hours of Arrival	140	100%	97%	96%
Fibrinolytic Meds Within 30 Min. of Arrival[7]	-	-	48%	58%
Average Time to ECG (minutes)	148	9	7	7
Average Time to Transfer (minutes)	14	49	54	60
Children's Asthma Care				
Received Home Management Plan of Care	-	-	-	88%
Received Reliever Medication	-	-	-	100%
Received Systemic Corticosteroids	-	-	-	100%
Emergency Department				
Admittance Decision Time (minutes)[2]	420	89	62	98
Head CT Results Within 45 Min. of Arrival	22	41%	54%	57%
Patients Who Left ER Before Being Seen	27,073	1%	2%	2%
Time from ER Arrival to Admit. (minutes)[2]	420	276	199	274
Time from ER Arrival to Discharge (minutes)	343	156	125	134
Time in ER Before Being Evaluated (minutes)	382	19	31	26
Time to Pain Meds for Fractures (minutes)	125	42	45	57
Heart Attack Care				
Aspirin Given at Discharge[1,3]	-	-	99%	99%
Fibrinolytic Meds Within 30 Min. of Arrival[3,7]	-	-	-	54%
PCI Within 90 Minutes of Arrival[3,7]	-	-	96%	96%
Statin Prescribed at Discharge[1,3]	-	-	99%	98%
Heart Failure Care				
ACE Inhibitor or ARB for LVSD	14	100%	96%	97%
Discharge Instructions Given	46	98%	93%	94%
Evaluation of LVS Function	60	100%	97%	99%
Medicare Spending				
Medicare Spending per Patient (ratio)	-	0.87	0.9	0.98
Pneumonia Care				
Appropriate Initial Antibiotic Given	45	98%	94%	95%
Blood Culture Timing	102	98%	97%	98%
Pregnancy and Delivery Care				
Newborn Deliveries Scheduled Early	130	0%	5%	6%
Preventive Care				
Immunization for Influenza[2]	326	99%	89%	90%
Immunization for Pneumonia[2]	343	97%	89%	92%
Stroke Care				
Anticoagulation Therapy for Atrial Fibrillation[1]	-	-	96%	95%
Antithrombotic Therapy Timing	13	100%	98%	98%
Assessed for Rehabilitation	15	100%	98%	97%
Discharged on Antithrombotic Therapy	11	100%	99%	99%
Discharged on Statin Medication	13	100%	95%	94%
Thrombolytic Therapy Timing[7]	-	-	74%	66%
Venous Thromboembolism Prophylaxis	15	100%	95%	94%
Written Stroke Educational Materials Given[1]	-	-	88%	88%
Surgical Care Improvement Project				
Appropriate Beta Blocker Usage[2]	94	100%	98%	98%
Appropriate VTP Within 24 Hours[2]	264	100%	98%	98%
Controlled Postoperative Blood Glucose[2,7]	-	-	97%	97%
Perioperative Temperature Management[2]	326	100%	99%	100%
Prophylactic Antibiotic Selection[2]	275	100%	99%	99%
Prophylactic Antibiotic Selection (Outpatient)	73	99%	98%	98%
Prophylactic Antibiotic Stopped[2]	272	100%	99%	98%
Prophylactic Antibiotic Timing[2]	275	99%	98%	99%
Prophylactic Antibiotic Timing (Outpatient)	72	96%	97%	98%
Urinary Catheter Removal[2]	177	100%	97%	97%
Survey of Patients' Hospital Experiences				
Area Around Room 'Always' Quiet at Night	300+	61%	65%	61%
Doctors 'Always' Communicated Well	300+	77%	84%	82%
Home Recovery Information Given	300+	86%	88%	85%
Hospital Given 9 or 10 on 10 Point Scale	300+	69%	74%	71%
Meds 'Always' Explained Before Given	300+	67%	67%	64%
Nurses 'Always' Communicated Well	300+	78%	81%	79%
Pain 'Always' Well Controlled	300+	69%	72%	71%
Room and Bathroom 'Always' Clean	300+	80%	78%	73%
Timely Help 'Always' Received	300+	74%	74%	68%
Would Definitely Recommend Hospital	300+	69%	71%	71%
Use of Medical Imaging				
Cardiac Imaging Stress Test before Surgery	161	4.3%	6.3%	5.3%
Combination Abdominal CT Scan	359	2.5%	5.7%	10.5%
Combination Brain/Sinus CT Scan[1]	-	-	2.3%	2.7%
Combination Chest CT Scan	315	0.0%	1.9%	2.7%
Follow-up Mammogram/Ultrasound	350	4.6%	6.3%	8.8%
Lumbar Spine MRI for Low Back Pain	76	32.9%	37.6%	37.2%

NOTE: Hospital profiles are in alphabetical order by state, then city, then hospital within the city; Rankings exclude hospitals with less than 25 cases except for patient surveys which excludes hospitals with less than 100 cases; (a) 100-299 cases; (1) The number of cases/patients is too few to report; (2) Data submitted were based on a sample of cases/patients; (3) Results are based on a shorter time period than required; (4) Data suppressed by CMS for one or more quarters; (5) Results are not available for this reporting period; (6) Fewer than 100 patients completed the HCAHPS survey; (7) No cases met the criteria for this measure; (8) The lower limit of the confidence interval cannot be calculated if the number of observed infections equals zero; (9) No data are available from the state/territory for this reporting period; (10) The scores shown reflect fewer than 50 completed surveys; (11) There were discrepancies in the data collection process; (12) This measure does not apply to this hospital for this reporting period; (13) Results cannot be calculated for this reporting period; (14) The results for this state are combined with nearby states to protect confidentiality; Please refer to the User's Guide for a full explanation of data.

Blood Clot Prevention and Treatment

Anticoagulation Overlap Therapy

Hospital Name	City	Rate	Cases
Centerpoint Medical Center[2]	Independence	100%	104
Freeman Health System - Freeman West[2]	Joplin	100%	84
Saint Luke's East Lee's Summit Hospital[2]	Lees Summit	100%	59
Saint Luke's Northland Hospital[2]	Kansas City	100%	29
Saint Mary's Health Center[2]	Jefferson City	100%	38
Saint Mary's Medical Center[2]	Blue Springs	100%	48
Truman Medical Center Hospital Hill[2]	Kansas City	100%	58
Heartland Regional Medical Center[2]	Saint Joseph	99%	102
Mercy Hospital Saint Louis[2]	Saint Louis	98%	171
Poplar Bluff Regional Medical Center[2]	Poplar Bluff	98%	85
Saint Francis Medical Center[2]	Cape Girardeau	98%	45
Saint Joseph Medical Center[2]	Kansas City	98%	89
Saint Luke's Hospital[2]	Chesterfield	98%	140
University of Missouri Health Care[2]	Columbia	98%	111
Barnes-Jewish Hospital[2]	Saint Louis	97%	310
Barnes-Jewish Saint Peters Hospital[2]	Saint Peters	97%	64
Boone Hospital Center[2]	Columbia	97%	95
Capital Region Medical Center[2]	Jefferson City	97%	29
Cox Medical Center Branson[2]	Branson	97%	68
Research Medical Center[2]	Kansas City	97%	105
Saint Luke's Hospital of Kansas City[2]	Kansas City	97%	152
Christian Hospital Northeast - Northwest[2]	Saint Louis	95%	150
SSM Saint Clare Health Center[2]	Fenton	95%	63
SSM Saint Joseph Health Center[2]	Saint Charles	95%	57
Mercy Hospital Jefferson[2]	Crystal City	94%	66
Mercy Hospital Springfield[2]	Springfield	94%	242
Missouri Baptist Medical Center[2]	Town & Country	94%	47
North Kansas City Hospital[2]	N Kansas City	94%	160
SSM Saint Marys Health Center[2]	Richmond Hghts	93%	97
Mercy Hospital Joplin[2]	Joplin	92%	52
Saint Anthony's Medical Center[2]	Saint Louis	92%	150
SSM Depaul Health Center[2]	Bridgeton	92%	145
Des Peres Hospital[2]	Saint Louis	91%	32
SSM Saint Joseph Hospital West[2]	Lake Saint Louis	91%	57
Cox Medical Center[2]	Springfield	89%	159
Liberty Hospital[2]	Liberty	89%	80
Saint Louis University Hospital[2]	Saint Louis	89%	105
Mercy Hospital Washington[2]	Washington	88%	33
Southeast Missouri Hospital[2]	Cape Girardeau	83%	53
Ozarks Medical Center[2]	West Plains	80%	35
Hannibal Regional Hospital[2]	Hannibal	74%	42

ICU Venous Thromboembolism Prophylaxis

Hospital Name	City	Rate	Cases
Belton Regional Medical Center[2]	Belton	100%	43
Boone Hospital Center[2]	Columbia	100%	69
Centerpoint Medical Center[2]	Independence	100%	72
Lee's Summit Medical Center[2]	Lees Summit	100%	93
Missouri Baptist Medical Center[2]	Town & Country	100%	40
Moberly Regional Medical Center[2]	Moberly	100%	71
Northeast Regional Medical Center[2]	Kirksville	100%	100
Saint Anthony's Medical Center[2]	Saint Louis	100%	69
Saint Joseph Medical Center[2]	Kansas City	100%	78
Saint Mary's Health Center[2]	Jefferson City	100%	70
Saint Mary's Medical Center[2]	Blue Springs	100%	62
SSM Depaul Health Center[2]	Bridgeton	100%	48
SSM Saint Marys Health Center[2]	Richmond Hghts	100%	54
Des Peres Hospital[2]	Saint Louis	99%	76
Liberty Hospital[2]	Liberty	99%	100
Mercy Hospital Saint Louis[2]	Saint Louis	99%	84
Barnes-Jewish Hospital[2]	Saint Louis	98%	65
Barnes-Jewish Saint Peters Hospital[2]	Saint Peters	98%	50
Research Medical Center[2]	Kansas City	98%	90
University of Missouri Health Care[2]	Columbia	98%	140
Capital Region Medical Center[2]	Jefferson City	97%	70
Lake Regional Health System[2]	Osage Beach	97%	122
Mercy Hospital Springfield[2]	Springfield	97%	73
Missouri Delta Medical Center[2]	Sikeston	97%	91
Saint Louis University Hospital[2]	Saint Louis	97%	155
Truman Medical Center Hospital Hill[2]	Kansas City	97%	68
Freeman Health System - Freeman West[2]	Joplin	96%	93
Heartland Regional Medical Center[2]	Saint Joseph	96%	56
SSM Saint Joseph Hospital West[2]	Lake Saint Louis	96%	51
Golden Valley Memorial Hospital[2]	Clinton	95%	37
Saint Luke's Hospital[2]	Chesterfield	95%	65
SSM Saint Joseph Health Center[2]	Saint Charles	95%	56
Twin Rivers Regional Medical Center[2]	Kennett	95%	41
Bates County Memorial Hospital[2]	Butler	94%	35
Mercy Hospital Lebanon[2]	Lebanon	94%	54
Poplar Bluff Regional Medical Center[2]	Poplar Bluff	94%	94
Progress West Hospital[2]	O Fallon	94%	32
SSM Saint Clare Health Center[2]	Fenton	94%	78
Texas County Memorial Hospital[2]	Houston	94%	31
Mercy Hospital Washington[2]	Washington	93%	69
Truman Medical Center Lakewood[2]	Kansas City	93%	28
Mercy Hospital Joplin[2]	Joplin	92%	64
Saint Luke's Hospital of Kansas City[2]	Kansas City	92%	118
Mineral Area Regional Medical Center[2]	Farmington	91%	43
Phelps County Regional Medical Center[2]	Rolla	91%	88
Christian Hospital Northeast - Northwest[2]	Saint Louis	90%	29
Cox Medical Center[2]	Springfield	89%	85
Cox Medical Center Branson[2]	Branson	89%	113
Mercy Hospital Jefferson[2]	Crystal City	89%	72
Ozarks Medical Center[2]	West Plains	89%	379
North Kansas City Hospital[2]	N Kansas City	86%	74
Southeast Missouri Hospital[2]	Cape Girardeau	86%	85
Lincoln County Medical Center	Troy	85%	124
Saint Alexius Hospital[2]	Saint Louis	85%	53
Parkland Health Center[2]	Farmington	84%	50
Audrain Medical Center[2]	Mexico	82%	44
Saint Luke's East Lee's Summit Hospital[2]	Lees Summit	82%	61
Western Missouri Medical Center[2]	Warrensburg	82%	55
Saint Francis Medical Center[2]	Cape Girardeau	80%	109
Saint Luke's Northland Hospital[2]	Kansas City	79%	66
Citizens Memorial Hospital[2]	Bolivar	78%	63
Hannibal Regional Hospital[2]	Hannibal	72%	88
Cameron Regional Medical Center[2]	Cameron	67%	55
Southeasthealth Center of Stoddard County[2]	Dexter	67%	36
Nevada Regional Medical Center[2]	Nevada	49%	51
Bothwell Regional Health Center[2]	Sedalia	44%	39
Pemiscot County Memorial Hospital[2]	Hayti	40%	48

Incidence of Potentially Preventable VTE

Hospital Name	City	Rate	Cases
Research Medical Center[2]	Kansas City	0%	28
University of Missouri Health Care[2]	Columbia	0%	31
Saint Louis University Hospital[2]	Saint Louis	2%	49
Barnes-Jewish Hospital[2]	Saint Louis	4%	191
Missouri Baptist Medical Center[2]	Town & Country	4%	26
Saint Joseph Medical Center[2]	Kansas City	4%	25
Boone Hospital Center[2]	Columbia	7%	45
Saint Anthony's Medical Center[2]	Saint Louis	8%	37
Saint Luke's Hospital of Kansas City[2]	Kansas City	9%	32
Mercy Hospital Saint Louis[2]	Saint Louis	10%	41
Mercy Hospital Springfield[2]	Springfield	10%	51
Saint Luke's Hospital[2]	Chesterfield	17%	36
Cox Medical Center[2]	Springfield	19%	27

UFH with Dosages/Platelet Count Monitoring

Hospital Name	City	Rate	Cases
Barnes-Jewish Hospital[2]	Saint Louis	100%	410
Centerpoint Medical Center[2]	Independence	100%	25
Christian Hospital Northeast - Northwest[2]	Saint Louis	100%	55
Cox Medical Center Branson[2]	Branson	100%	65
Freeman Health System - Freeman West[2]	Joplin	100%	100
Heartland Regional Medical Center[2]	Saint Joseph	100%	61
Liberty Hospital[2]	Liberty	100%	45
Mercy Hospital Jefferson[2]	Crystal City	100%	27
Mercy Hospital Joplin[2]	Joplin	100%	44
Mercy Hospital Saint Louis[2]	Saint Louis	100%	64
Mercy Hospital Springfield[2]	Springfield	100%	152
Poplar Bluff Regional Medical Center[2]	Poplar Bluff	100%	82
Saint Anthony's Medical Center[2]	Saint Louis	100%	110
Saint Joseph Medical Center[2]	Kansas City	100%	44
Saint Mary's Medical Center[2]	Blue Springs	100%	26
Truman Medical Center Hospital Hill[2]	Kansas City	100%	46
University of Missouri Health Care[2]	Columbia	100%	82
Saint Luke's East Lee's Summit Hospital[2]	Lees Summit	99%	70
Saint Luke's Hospital[2]	Chesterfield	99%	81
North Kansas City Hospital[2]	N Kansas City	98%	116
Research Medical Center[2]	Kansas City	98%	50
Saint Luke's Hospital of Kansas City[2]	Kansas City	98%	128
Missouri Baptist Medical Center[2]	Town & Country	97%	36
Saint Louis University Hospital[2]	Saint Louis	97%	61
Southeast Missouri Hospital[2]	Cape Girardeau	94%	32
SSM Depaul Health Center[2]	Bridgeton	88%	80
SSM Saint Marys Health Center[2]	Richmond Hghts	81%	48
SSM Saint Clare Health Center[2]	Fenton	76%	34
Cox Medical Center[2]	Springfield	28%	82

Venous Thromboembolism Prophylaxis

Hospital Name	City	Rate	Cases
Belton Regional Medical Center[2]	Belton	100%	184
Lafayette Regional Health Center[2]	Lexington	100%	122
Lee's Summit Medical Center[2]	Lees Summit	100%	271
Moberly Regional Medical Center[2]	Moberly	100%	200
Northeast Regional Medical Center[2]	Kirksville	100%	150
Saint Mary's Medical Center[2]	Blue Springs	100%	328
Centerpoint Medical Center[2]	Independence	99%	346
Missouri Baptist Medical Center[2]	Town & Country	99%	340
Research Medical Center[2]	Kansas City	99%	321
Saint Joseph Medical Center[2]	Kansas City	98%	339
Barnes-Jewish West County Hospital[2]	Creve Coeur	97%	123
Boone Hospital Center[2]	Columbia	97%	280
Capital Region Medical Center[2]	Jefferson City	97%	323
Saint Mary's Health Center[2]	Jefferson City	97%	282
Heartland Regional Medical Center[2]	Saint Joseph	96%	296
Missouri Baptist Sullivan Hospital[2]	Sullivan	96%	112
Progress West Hospital[2]	O Fallon	96%	186
Bates County Memorial Hospital[2]	Butler	95%	183
Mercy Hospital Lebanon[2]	Lebanon	95%	165
SSM Saint Joseph Hospital West[2]	Lake Saint Louis	95%	321
Truman Medical Center Hospital Hill[2]	Kansas City	95%	314
Barnes-Jewish Hospital[2]	Saint Louis	94%	300
Christian Hospital Northeast - Northwest[2]	Saint Louis	94%	387
Des Peres Hospital[2]	Saint Louis	94%	323
Liberty Hospital[2]	Liberty	94%	494
Missouri Delta Medical Center[2]	Sikeston	94%	282
Scotland County Hospital[2]	Memphis	94%	217
Barnes-Jewish Saint Peters Hospital[2]	Saint Peters	93%	334
Lake Regional Health System[2]	Osage Beach	93%	481
Twin Rivers Regional Medical Center[2]	Kennett	93%	91
Mineral Area Regional Medical Center[2]	Farmington	92%	154
SSM Saint Marys Health Center[2]	Richmond Hghts	92%	333
Mercy Hospital Saint Louis[2]	Saint Louis	90%	287
Mercy Mccune Brooks Hospital[2,3]	Carthage	90%	29
Poplar Bluff Regional Medical Center[2]	Poplar Bluff	90%	623
Saint Francis Hospital & Health Services	Maryville	90%	183
University of Missouri Health Care[2]	Columbia	90%	277
Cox Medical Center Branson[2]	Branson	89%	329
Freeman Health System - Freeman West[2]	Joplin	89%	267
Mercy Hospital Jefferson[2]	Crystal City	89%	347
Ozarks Medical Center[2]	West Plains	89%	618
Saint Louis University Hospital[2]	Saint Louis	89%	284
Truman Medical Center Lakewood[2]	Kansas City	89%	178
Wright Memorial Hospital[2,3]	Trenton	89%	141
Parkland Health Center[2]	Farmington	87%	246
Cox Medical Center[2]	Springfield	85%	288
Mercy Hospital Joplin[2]	Joplin	85%	248
SSM Depaul Health Center[2]	Bridgeton	85%	296
SSM Saint Clare Health Center[2]	Fenton	85%	297
SSM Saint Joseph Health Center[2]	Saint Charles	85%	373
Citizens Memorial Hospital[2]	Bolivar	84%	129
Mercy Hospital Springfield[2]	Springfield	83%	299
Mercy Hospital Washington[2]	Washington	83%	305
Saint Anthony's Medical Center[2]	Saint Louis	82%	312
Southeast Missouri Hospital[2]	Cape Girardeau	82%	311
Texas County Memorial Hospital[2]	Houston	82%	125
Cooper County Memorial Hospital	Boonville	81%	93
Phelps County Regional Medical Center[2]	Rolla	80%	291
Saint Luke's Hospital[2]	Chesterfield	80%	348
Saint Francis Medical Center[2]	Cape Girardeau	79%	322
Fitzgibbon Hospital[2]	Marshall	78%	168
Saint Alexius Hospital[2]	Saint Louis	78%	148
Saint Luke's Northland Hospital[2]	Kansas City	78%	351
Lincoln County Medical Center	Troy	77%	293
Audrain Medical Center[2]	Mexico	76%	178
Golden Valley Memorial Hospital[2]	Clinton	75%	201
North Kansas City Hospital[2]	N Kansas City	74%	321
Callaway Community Hospital[2]	Fulton	73%	124
Southeasthealth Center of Stoddard County[2]	Dexter	73%	417
Saint Luke's East Lee's Summit Hospital[2]	Lees Summit	72%	316
Saint Luke's Hospital of Kansas City[2]	Kansas City	70%	328
Hannibal Regional Hospital[2]	Hannibal	67%	326
Western Missouri Medical Center[2]	Warrensburg	61%	234
Hedrick Medical Center[2,3]	Chillicothe	60%	45
Southeast Health Center of Ripley County	Doniphan	56%	160
Cameron Regional Medical Center[2]	Cameron	47%	200
Nevada Regional Medical Center[2]	Nevada	47%	154
Black River Community Medical Center[2]	Poplar Bluff	42%	144
Bothwell Regional Health Center[2]	Sedalia	40%	374
Ozarks Community Hospital[2]	Springfield	22%	103
Sac-Osage Hospital[2]	Osceola	9%	123
Pemiscot County Memorial Hospital[2]	Hayti	8%	104

Warfarin Therapy Discharge Instructions

Hospital Name	City	Rate	Cases
Boone Hospital Center[2]	Columbia	100%	64
Centerpoint Medical Center[2]	Independence	100%	78
Heartland Regional Medical Center[2]	Saint Joseph	100%	81
Research Medical Center[2]	Kansas City	100%	64
Saint Louis University Hospital[2]	Saint Louis	99%	74
Cox Medical Center Branson[2]	Branson	98%	48
Mercy Hospital Jefferson[2]	Crystal City	98%	41
Saint Mary's Medical Center[2]	Blue Springs	98%	41
Missouri Baptist Medical Center[2]	Town & Country	96%	26
Truman Medical Center Hospital Hill[2]	Kansas City	96%	56
Barnes-Jewish Hospital[2]	Saint Louis	95%	208
Ozarks Medical Center[2]	West Plains	89%	27
Christian Hospital Northeast - Northwest[2]	Saint Louis	87%	113
Liberty Hospital[2]	Liberty	87%	62
Poplar Bluff Regional Medical Center[2]	Poplar Bluff	87%	68
Saint Mary's Health Center[2]	Jefferson City	87%	31
Barnes-Jewish Saint Peters Hospital[2]	Saint Peters	86%	51
Saint Luke's Hospital[2]	Chesterfield	84%	88
North Kansas City Hospital[2]	N Kansas City	79%	113
Saint Francis Medical Center[2]	Cape Girardeau	79%	38

NOTE: Hospital profiles are in alphabetical order by state, then city, then hospital within the city; Rankings exclude hospitals with less than 25 cases except for patient surveys which excludes hospitals with less than 100 cases; (a) 100-299 cases; (1) The number of cases/patients is too few to report; (2) Data submitted were based on a sample of cases/patients; (3) Results are based on a shorter time period than required; (4) Data suppressed by CMS for one or more quarters; (5) Results are not available for this reporting period; (6) Fewer than 100 patients completed the HCAHPS survey; (7) No cases met the criteria for this measure; (8) The lower limit of the confidence interval cannot be calculated if the number of observed infections equals zero; (9) No data are available from the state/territory for this reporting period; (10) The scores shown reflect fewer than 50 completed surveys; (11) There were discrepancies in the data collection process; (12) This measure does not apply to this hospital for this reporting period; (13) Results cannot be calculated for this reporting period; (14) The results for this state are combined with nearby states to protect confidentiality; Please refer to the User's Guide for a full explanation of data.

Hospital Name	City	Rate	Cases
SSM Saint Marys Health Center[2]	Richmond Hghts	79%	67
Mercy Hospital Springfield[2]	Springfield	78%	185
University of Missouri Health Care[2]	Columbia	77%	81
Southeast Missouri Hospital[2]	Cape Girardeau	75%	36
Cox Medical Center[2]	Springfield	74%	121
Mercy Hospital Joplin[2]	Joplin	65%	43
SSM Saint Joseph Hospital West[2]	Lake Saint Louis	65%	49
Saint Luke's East Lee's Summit Hospital[2]	Lees Summit	63%	38
Hannibal Regional Hospital[2]	Hannibal	62%	29
Freeman Health System - Freeman West[2]	Joplin	61%	41
SSM Saint Joseph Health Center[2]	Saint Charles	59%	49
Saint Luke's Hospital of Kansas City[2]	Kansas City	55%	108
Mercy Hospital Saint Louis[2]	Saint Louis	47%	137
SSM Saint Clare Health Center[2]	Fenton	47%	53
Mercy Hospital Washington[2]	Washington	41%	27
Saint Joseph Medical Center[2]	Kansas City	39%	57
Saint Anthony's Medical Center[2]	Saint Louis	35%	110
SSM Depaul Health Center[2]	Bridgeton	35%	115

Chest Pain/Possible Heart Attack Care

Aspirin Given Within 24 Hours of Arrival

Hospital Name	City	Rate	Cases
Belton Regional Medical Center	Belton	100%	38
Citizens Memorial Hospital	Bolivar	100%	39
Mercy Mccune Brooks Hospital[3]	Carthage	100%	33
Mineral Area Regional Medical Center	Farmington	100%	60
Nevada Regional Medical Center	Nevada	100%	31
Northeast Regional Medical Center	Kirksville	100%	81
Saint Francis Hospital & Health Services	Maryville	100%	29
Poplar Bluff Regional Medical Center	Poplar Bluff	99%	75
Western Missouri Medical Center	Warrensburg	99%	83
Fitzgibbon Hospital	Marshall	98%	51
Mercy Hospital Lebanon	Lebanon	98%	138
Phelps County Regional Medical Center	Rolla	98%	132
Parkland Health Center	Farmington	97%	219
Southeasthealth Center of Stoddard County	Dexter	97%	75
Truman Medical Center Hospital Hill	Kansas City	97%	119
Twin Rivers Regional Medical Center	Kennett	97%	105
Bates County Memorial Hospital	Butler	96%	26
Callaway Community Hospital	Fulton	96%	25
Cameron Regional Medical Center	Cameron	96%	49
Golden Valley Memorial Hospital	Clinton	96%	109
Missouri Baptist Sullivan Hospital	Sullivan	96%	104
Texas County Memorial Hospital	Houston	96%	101
Barnes-Jewish West County Hospital	Creve Coeur	95%	42
Black River Community Medical Center[3]	Poplar Bluff	94%	33
SSM Saint Joseph Hospital West	Lake Saint Louis	94%	34
Truman Medical Center Lakewood	Kansas City	93%	57
Southeast Health Center of Ripley County	Doniphan	91%	32
Missouri Delta Medical Center	Sikeston	89%	95
Bothwell Regional Health Center	Sedalia	88%	121
Wright Memorial Hospital	Trenton	81%	36

Average Time to ECG (minutes)

Hospital Name	City	Min.	Cases
Twin Rivers Regional Medical Center	Kennett	0	110
Golden Valley Memorial Hospital	Clinton	2	116
Truman Medical Center Lakewood	Kansas City	2	54
Northeast Regional Medical Center	Kirksville	3	82
Parkland Health Center	Farmington	3	232
Saint Francis Hospital & Health Services	Maryville	4	31
Mercy Mccune Brooks Hospital[3]	Carthage	5	33
Mineral Area Regional Medical Center	Farmington	5	61
Citizens Memorial Hospital	Bolivar	6	39
Missouri Baptist Sullivan Hospital	Sullivan	6	108
Southeast Health Center of Ripley County	Doniphan	6	34
Black River Community Medical Center[3]	Poplar Bluff	7	33
Western Missouri Medical Center	Warrensburg	7	88
Bates County Memorial Hospital	Butler	8	28
Cameron Regional Medical Center	Cameron	8	49
Nevada Regional Medical Center	Nevada	8	30
Phelps County Regional Medical Center	Rolla	8	139
SSM Saint Joseph Hospital West	Lake Saint Louis	8	36
Truman Medical Center Hospital Hill	Kansas City	8	111
Belton Regional Medical Center	Belton	9	42
Bothwell Regional Health Center	Sedalia	9	123
Southeasthealth Center of Stoddard County	Dexter	9	79
Barnes-Jewish West County Hospital	Creve Coeur	10	42
Callaway Community Hospital	Fulton	10	26
Mercy Hospital Lebanon	Lebanon	10	140
Missouri Delta Medical Center	Sikeston	10	97
Poplar Bluff Regional Medical Center	Poplar Bluff	10	78
Texas County Memorial Hospital	Houston	10	103
Wright Memorial Hospital	Trenton	10	40
Fitzgibbon Hospital	Marshall	24	54

Children's Asthma Care

Received Home Management Plan of Care

Hospital Name	City	Rate	Cases
SSM Saint Marys Health Center[2]	Richmond Hghts	98%	240
Mercy Hospital Saint Louis	Saint Louis	93%	177
Childrens Mercy Hospital[2]	Kansas City	90%	323

Received Reliever Medication

Hospital Name	City	Rate	Cases
Childrens Mercy Hospital[2]	Kansas City	100%	323
Mercy Hospital Saint Louis	Saint Louis	100%	177
SSM Saint Marys Health Center[2]	Richmond Hghts	100%	239

Received Systemic Corticosteroids

Hospital Name	City	Rate	Cases
Mercy Hospital Saint Louis	Saint Louis	100%	177
SSM Saint Marys Health Center[2]	Richmond Hghts	100%	240
Childrens Mercy Hospital[2]	Kansas City	99%	318

Emergency Department

Admittance Decision Time (minutes)

Hospital Name	City	Min.	Cases
Fitzgibbon Hospital[2]	Marshall	28	390
Cooper County Memorial Hospital	Boonville	30	143
Black River Community Medical Center[2,3]	Poplar Bluff	34	88
Carroll County Memorial Hospital	Carrollton	34	91
Mercy Saint Francis Hospital	Mountain View	36	221
Bates County Memorial Hospital[2]	Butler	37	214
Wright Memorial Hospital[2]	Trenton	37	229
Saint Francis Hospital & Health Services	Maryville	39	126
Missouri Baptist Sullivan Hospital[2]	Sullivan	41	209
Texas County Memorial Hospital[2]	Houston	44	353
Moberly Regional Medical Center[2]	Moberly	45	338
Sac-Osage Hospital[2]	Osceola	45	170
Mercy Hospital Cassville	Cassville	48	196
Northeast Regional Medical Center[2]	Kirksville	49	359
Barnes-Jewish West County Hospital[2]	Creve Coeur	50	104
Cameron Regional Medical Center[2]	Cameron	50	401
Scotland County Hospital[2]	Memphis	50	372
Progress West Hospital[2]	O Fallon	52	305
Mercy Mccune Brooks Hospital[2,3]	Carthage	53	50
Liberty Hospital[2]	Liberty	55	492
Mercy Hospital Aurora[2]	Aurora	55	200
Southeasthealth Center of Stoddard County	Dexter	55	592
Ozarks Community Hospital	Springfield	58	346
Southeast Missouri Hospital[2]	Cape Girardeau	58	478
Boone Hospital Center[2]	Columbia	59	217
Golden Valley Memorial Hospital[2]	Clinton	59	280
Lee's Summit Medical Center[2]	Lees Summit	59	361
Audrain Medical Center[2]	Mexico	60	219
Bothwell Regional Health Center[2]	Sedalia	60	540
Callaway Community Hospital	Fulton	60	215
Missouri Delta Medical Center[2]	Sikeston	60	337
Nevada Regional Medical Center[2]	Nevada	60	176
Pemiscot County Memorial Hospital[2]	Hayti	60	236
Twin Rivers Regional Medical Center[2]	Kennett	62	253
Freeman Neosho Hospital[2,3]	Neosho	65	319
Parkland Health Center[2]	Farmington	65	332
Saint Francis Medical Center[2]	Cape Girardeau	65	406
Barnes-Jewish Saint Peters Hospital[2]	Saint Peters	66	711
Heartland Regional Medical Center[2]	Saint Joseph	66	473
Missouri Baptist Medical Center[2]	Town & Country	69	460
Hannibal Regional Hospital[2]	Hannibal	71	427
Phelps County Regional Medical Center[2]	Rolla	72	385
Saint Mary's Health Center[2]	Jefferson City	72	516
Western Missouri Medical Center[2]	Warrensburg	75	215
Lafayette Regional Health Center[2]	Lexington	76	408
University of Missouri Health Care[2]	Columbia	76	337
Mercy Hospital Jefferson[2]	Crystal City	78	748
Saint Luke's Hospital of Kansas City[2]	Kansas City	78	450
Saint Luke's Hospital[2]	Chesterfield	82	646
Lake Regional Health System[2]	Osage Beach	83	690
Centerpoint Medical Center[2]	Independence	84	825
Belton Regional Medical Center[2]	Belton	85	344
Southeast Health Center of Ripley County[2]	Doniphan	85	163
Mercy Hospital Springfield[2]	Springfield	86	402
Saint Alexius Hospital[2]	Saint Louis	86	225
Capital Region Medical Center[2]	Jefferson City	87	515
Citizens Memorial Hospital[2]	Bolivar	88	288
Des Peres Hospital[2]	Saint Louis	88	481
Mercy Hospital Lebanon[2]	Lebanon	88	222
Saint Luke's Northland Hospital[2]	Kansas City	94	505
Truman Medical Center Lakewood[2]	Kansas City	94	263
Research Medical Center[2]	Kansas City	98	556
Mercy Hospital Washington[2]	Washington	99	477
Mineral Area Regional Medical Center[2]	Farmington	101	380
Mercy Hospital Joplin[2,3]	Joplin	103	273
SSM Saint Joseph Hospital West[2]	Lake Saint Louis	103	429
North Kansas City Hospital[2]	N Kansas City	104	458
Saint Joseph Medical Center[2]	Kansas City	106	605
Saint Mary's Medical Center[2]	Blue Springs	110	630
Ozarks Medical Center[2]	West Plains	113	1182
Mercy Hospital Saint Louis[2]	Saint Louis	115	377
Cox Medical Center[2]	Springfield	124	479
SSM Saint Marys Health Center[2]	Richmond Hghts	124	421
Christian Hospital Northeast - Northwest[2]	Saint Louis	127	707
Cox Medical Center Branson[2]	Branson	133	695
Saint Luke's East Lee's Summit Hospital[2]	Lees Summit	134	490
SSM Saint Joseph Health Center[2]	Saint Charles	139	503
Saint Anthony's Medical Center[2]	Saint Louis	143	728
Poplar Bluff Regional Medical Center[2]	Poplar Bluff	144	504
Truman Medical Center Hospital Hill[2]	Kansas City	161	539
SSM Depaul Health Center[2]	Bridgeton	162	353
SSM Saint Clare Health Center[2]	Fenton	166	486
Barnes-Jewish Hospital[2]	Saint Louis	169	351
Freeman Health System - Freeman West[2]	Joplin	188	351
Saint Louis University Hospital[2]	Saint Louis	192	484

Head CT Results Within 45 Minutes of Arrival

Hospital Name	City	Rate	Cases
Capital Region Medical Center	Jefferson City	88%	25
Christian Hospital Northeast - Northwest	Saint Louis	78%	32

Patients Who Left ER Before Being Seen

Hospital Name	City	Rate	Cases
Audrain Medical Center	Mexico	0%	141450
Bates County Memorial Hospital	Butler	0%	8322
Cameron Regional Medical Center	Cameron	0%	9256
Lee's Summit Medical Center	Lees Summit	0%	16699
Mercy Hospital Washington	Washington	0%	35005
Mineral Area Regional Medical Center	Farmington	0%	18793
Saint Luke's Hospital	Chesterfield	0%	30287
SSM Saint Joseph Hospital West	Lake Saint Louis	0%	41416
Barnes-Jewish Saint Peters Hospital	Saint Peters	1%	29998
Bothwell Regional Health Center	Sedalia	1%	24868
Callaway Community Hospital	Fulton	1%	10380
Capital Region Medical Center	Jefferson City	1%	32866
Centerpoint Medical Center	Independence	1%	62216
Christian Hospital Northeast - Northwest	Saint Louis	1%	114388
Cooper County Memorial Hospital	Boonville	1%	7272
Cox Medical Center Branson	Branson	1%	35423
Des Peres Hospital	Saint Louis	1%	9601
Heartland Regional Medical Center	Saint Joseph	1%	60378
Lafayette Regional Health Center	Lexington	1%	9175
Lake Regional Health System	Osage Beach	1%	36778
Mercy Hospital Jefferson	Crystal City	1%	32695
Mercy Hospital Joplin	Joplin	1%	28446
Mercy Hospital Lebanon	Lebanon	1%	29143
Mercy Hospital Saint Louis	Saint Louis	1%	81500
Mercy Mccune Brooks Hospital	Carthage	1%	19056
Missouri Baptist Medical Center	Town & Country	1%	42542
North Kansas City Hospital	N Kansas City	1%	63178
Northeast Regional Medical Center	Kirksville	1%	12615
Ozarks Medical Center	West Plains	1%	26498
Phelps County Regional Medical Center	Rolla	1%	37357
Sac-Osage Hospital	Osceola	1%	2014
Saint Francis Hospital & Health Services	Maryville	1%	7719
SSM Depaul Health Center	Bridgeton	1%	65703
SSM Saint Clare Health Center	Fenton	1%	43462
SSM Saint Joseph Health Center	Saint Charles	1%	40645
SSM Saint Marys Health Center	Richmond Hghts	1%	54056
Barnes-Jewish West County Hospital	Creve Coeur	2%	12021
Belton Regional Medical Center	Belton	2%	19595
Boone Hospital Center	Columbia	2%	31987
Citizens Memorial Hospital	Bolivar	2%	19357
Golden Valley Memorial Hospital	Clinton	2%	14965
Hannibal Regional Hospital	Hannibal	2%	19937
Liberty Hospital	Liberty	2%	37895
Missouri Baptist Sullivan Hospital	Sullivan	2%	22367
Moberly Regional Medical Center	Moberly	2%	14776
Nevada Regional Medical Center	Nevada	2%	9893
Progress West Hospital	O Fallon	2%	24586
Saint Francis Medical Center	Cape Girardeau	2%	39137
Saint Joseph Medical Center	Kansas City	2%	34064
Saint Luke's East Lee's Summit Hospital	Lees Summit	2%	38727
Saint Luke's Northland Hospital	Kansas City	2%	33308
Saint Mary's Health Center	Jefferson City	2%	34388
Saint Mary's Medical Center	Blue Springs	2%	29376
Southeast Health Center of Ripley County	Doniphan	2%	6202
Twin Rivers Regional Medical Center	Kennett	2%	23434
Western Missouri Medical Center	Warrensburg	2%	20098
Fitzgibbon Hospital	Marshall	3%	10851
Ozarks Community Hospital	Springfield	3%	19052
Parkland Health Center	Farmington	3%	26144
Saint Anthony's Medical Center	Saint Louis	3%	72325
Saint Louis University Hospital	Saint Louis	3%	39404
Saint Luke's Hospital of Kansas City	Kansas City	3%	36698

NOTE: Hospital profiles are in alphabetical order by state, then city, then hospital within the city; Rankings exclude hospitals with less than 25 cases except for patient surveys which excludes hospitals with less than 100 cases; (a) 100-299 cases; (1) The number of cases/patients is too few to report; (2) Data submitted were based on a sample of cases/patients; (3) Results are based on a shorter time period than required; (4) Data suppressed by CMS for one or more quarters; (5) Results are not available for this reporting period; (6) Fewer than 100 patients completed the HCAHPS survey; (7) No cases met the criteria for this measure; (8) The lower limit of the confidence interval cannot be calculated if the number of observed infections equals zero; (9) No data are available from the state/territory for this reporting period; (10) The scores shown reflect fewer than 50 completed surveys; (11) There were discrepancies in the data collection process; (12) This measure does not apply to this hospital for this reporting period; (13) Results cannot be calculated for this reporting period; (14) The results for this state are combined with nearby states to protect confidentiality; Please refer to the User's Guide for a full explanation of data.

University of Missouri Health Care	Columbia	3%	56099
Cox Medical Center	Springfield	4%	109895
Poplar Bluff Regional Medical Center	Poplar Bluff	4%	33095
Research Medical Center	Kansas City	4%	65857
Southeast Missouri Hospital	Cape Girardeau	4%	40379
Texas County Memorial Hospital	Houston	4%	12438
Mercy Hospital Springfield	Springfield	5%	96706
Black River Community Medical Center	Poplar Bluff	6%	4338
Truman Medical Center Lakewood	Kansas City	6%	33486
Pemiscot County Memorial Hospital	Hayti	7%	8641
Southeasthealth Center of Stoddard County	Dexter	7%	10989
Barnes-Jewish Hospital	Saint Louis	8%	98239
Freeman Health System - Freeman West	Joplin	8%	50971
Missouri Delta Medical Center	Sikeston	9%	17251
Saint Alexius Hospital	Saint Louis	14%	19217
Truman Medical Center Hospital Hill	Kansas City	14%	67130

Time from ER Arrival to Being Admitted (minutes)

Hospital Name	City	Min.	Cases
Carroll County Memorial Hospital	Carrollton	125	95
Fitzgibbon Hospital[2]	Marshall	136	410
Cameron Regional Medical Center[2]	Cameron	140	474
Bates County Memorial Hospital[2]	Butler	159	287
Lafayette Regional Health Center[2]	Lexington	162	410
Mercy Mccune Brooks Hospital[2,3]	Carthage	170	50
Nevada Regional Medical Center[2]	Nevada	171	201
Black River Community Medical Center[2,3]	Poplar Bluff	173	89
Sac-Osage Hospital[2]	Osceola	174	176
Audrain Medical Center[2]	Mexico	181	262
Northeast Regional Medical Center[2]	Kirksville	181	359
Wright Memorial Hospital[2]	Trenton	181	301
Mercy Saint Francis Hospital	Mountain View	184	229
Cooper County Memorial Hospital	Boonville	185	157
Bothwell Regional Health Center[2]	Sedalia	187	558
Lee's Summit Medical Center[2]	Lees Summit	188	422
Moberly Regional Medical Center[2]	Moberly	189	347
Southeasthealth Center of Stoddard County	Dexter	191	630
Boone Hospital Center[2]	Columbia	194	300
Saint Francis Hospital & Health Services	Maryville	197	129
Golden Valley Memorial Hospital[2]	Clinton	198	289
Heartland Regional Medical Center[2]	Saint Joseph	203	477
Callaway Community Hospital	Fulton	204	222
Freeman Neosho Hospital[2,3]	Neosho	208	341
Twin Rivers Regional Medical Center[2]	Kennett	208	253
Progress West Hospital[2]	O Fallon	209	335
Scotland County Hospital[2]	Memphis	210	394
North Kansas City Hospital[2]	N Kansas City	212	479
Saint Francis Medical Center[2]	Cape Girardeau	212	430
Des Peres Hospital[2]	Saint Louis	218	481
Citizens Memorial Hospital[2]	Bolivar	219	299
SSM Saint Joseph Hospital West[2]	Lake Saint Louis	220	502
Saint Luke's Hospital[2]	Chesterfield	221	652
Southeast Health Center of Ripley County[2]	Doniphan	222	197
SSM Saint Joseph Health Center[2]	Saint Charles	224	552
Barnes-Jewish West County Hospital[2]	Creve Coeur	226	106
Capital Region Medical Center[2]	Jefferson City	227	540
Liberty Hospital[2]	Liberty	232	565
Lake Regional Health System[2]	Osage Beach	233	765
Barnes-Jewish Saint Peters Hospital[2]	Saint Peters	234	729
Research Medical Center[2]	Kansas City	234	556
Saint Luke's Hospital of Kansas City[2]	Kansas City	234	467
Mercy Hospital Springfield[2]	Springfield	235	445
Texas County Memorial Hospital[2]	Houston	235	353
Mercy Hospital Aurora[2]	Aurora	236	205
Western Missouri Medical Center[2]	Warrensburg	238	247
Southeast Missouri Hospital[2]	Cape Girardeau	240	481
Mercy Hospital Washington[2]	Washington	242	512
Mercy Hospital Saint Louis[2]	Saint Louis	243	398
Mercy Hospital Cassville	Cassville	246	202
Belton Regional Medical Center[2]	Belton	248	367
Parkland Health Center[2]	Farmington	248	361
Saint Luke's Northland Hospital[2]	Kansas City	248	506
Phelps County Regional Medical Center[2]	Rolla	249	421
Mercy Hospital Lebanon[2]	Lebanon	250	231
Missouri Baptist Sullivan Hospital[2]	Sullivan	251	210
Mercy Hospital Joplin[2,3]	Joplin	252	288
Pemiscot County Memorial Hospital[2]	Hayti	252	294
Centerpoint Medical Center[2]	Independence	253	825
Mineral Area Regional Medical Center[2]	Farmington	253	380
Saint Anthony's Medical Center[2]	Saint Louis	254	747
University of Missouri Health Care[2]	Columbia	254	366
Saint Joseph Medical Center[2]	Kansas City	255	608
Saint Mary's Health Center[2]	Jefferson City	258	525
Saint Mary's Medical Center[2]	Blue Springs	258	639
Ozarks Community Hospital	Springfield	260	407
Saint Luke's East Lee's Summit Hospital[2]	Lees Summit	266	491
Cox Medical Center Branson[2]	Branson	267	696
SSM Saint Marys Health Center[2]	Richmond Hghts	267	457
Mercy Hospital Jefferson[2]	Crystal City	270	753
Truman Medical Center Lakewood[2]	Kansas City	272	284
Saint Louis University Hospital[2]	Saint Louis	273	503
Missouri Delta Medical Center[2]	Sikeston	274	372
SSM Saint Clare Health Center[2]	Fenton	276	530
Missouri Baptist Medical Center[2]	Town & Country	278	463
Hannibal Regional Hospital[2]	Hannibal	288	445
Ozarks Medical Center[2]	West Plains	289	1270
Cox Medical Center[2]	Springfield	296	481
SSM Depaul Health Center[2]	Bridgeton	302	403
Christian Hospital Northeast - Northwest[2]	Saint Louis	308	720
Poplar Bluff Regional Medical Center[2]	Poplar Bluff	321	504
Freeman Health System - Freeman West[2]	Joplin	343	365
Saint Alexius Hospital[2]	Saint Louis	377	240
Barnes-Jewish Hospital[2]	Saint Louis	394	352
Truman Medical Center Hospital Hill[2]	Kansas City	451	546

Time from ER Arrival to Discharge (minutes)

Hospital Name	City	Min.	Cases
Sullivan County Memorial Hospital[3]	Milan	60	78
Cameron Regional Medical Center	Cameron	70	452
Nevada Regional Medical Center	Nevada	75	448
Ozarks Community Hospital	Springfield	86	362
Lafayette Regional Health Center	Lexington	87	410
Callaway Community Hospital	Fulton	88	435
Cox Medical Center Branson	Branson	89	448
Cooper County Memorial Hospital	Boonville	93	359
Research Medical Center	Kansas City	94	465
Mercy Mccune Brooks Hospital[3]	Carthage	97	264
Bates County Memorial Hospital	Butler	98	386
Fitzgibbon Hospital	Marshall	98	396
Southeasthealth Center of Stoddard County	Dexter	99	404
Saint Francis Hospital & Health Services	Maryville	100	338
Audrain Medical Center	Mexico	102	371
Black River Community Medical Center[3]	Poplar Bluff	103	291
Southeast Health Center of Ripley County	Doniphan	107	452
Mineral Area Regional Medical Center	Farmington	108	385
Lake Regional Health System	Osage Beach	111	667
Lee's Summit Medical Center	Lees Summit	112	428
Saint Mary's Medical Center	Blue Springs	114	358
Twin Rivers Regional Medical Center	Kennett	114	329
Sac-Osage Hospital	Osceola	115	210
Mercy Hospital Washington	Washington	116	368
Northeast Regional Medical Center	Kirksville	116	362
Golden Valley Memorial Hospital	Clinton	117	385
Moberly Regional Medical Center	Moberly	117	375
Belton Regional Medical Center	Belton	118	432
Heartland Regional Medical Center	Saint Joseph	119	357
SSM Saint Marys Health Center	Richmond Hghts	124	372
Missouri Baptist Sullivan Hospital	Sullivan	127	757
Bothwell Regional Health Center	Sedalia	128	419
North Kansas City Hospital	N Kansas City	128	1312
Capital Region Medical Center	Jefferson City	130	384
Parkland Health Center	Farmington	130	728
Saint Luke's Northland Hospital	Kansas City	132	380
Centerpoint Medical Center	Independence	135	493
SSM Saint Joseph Health Center	Saint Charles	136	346
Des Peres Hospital	Saint Louis	137	421
Progress West Hospital	O Fallon	138	793
Mercy Hospital Lebanon	Lebanon	139	338
Barnes-Jewish Saint Peters Hospital	Saint Peters	142	791
Barnes-Jewish West County Hospital	Creve Coeur	142	633
Citizens Memorial Hospital	Bolivar	142	1091
Cox Medical Center	Springfield	142	363
Saint Luke's East Lee's Summit Hospital	Lees Summit	144	353
Texas County Memorial Hospital	Houston	144	286
Saint Joseph Medical Center	Kansas City	145	353
Christian Hospital Northeast - Northwest	Saint Louis	147	783
Mercy Hospital Joplin[3]	Joplin	149	281
Boone Hospital Center	Columbia	150	613
Saint Mary's Health Center	Jefferson City	150	371
University of Missouri Health Care	Columbia	152	454
Western Missouri Medical Center	Warrensburg	152	388
SSM Saint Joseph Hospital West	Lake Saint Louis	155	377
Poplar Bluff Regional Medical Center	Poplar Bluff	156	336
Saint Luke's Hospital	Chesterfield	159	683
Mercy Hospital Jefferson	Crystal City	162	382
Saint Francis Medical Center	Cape Girardeau	163	365
Mercy Hospital Saint Louis	Saint Louis	164	349
Missouri Delta Medical Center	Sikeston	166	381
Ozarks Medical Center	West Plains	166	676
Saint Louis University Hospital	Saint Louis	168	398
Phelps County Regional Medical Center	Rolla	169	171
Truman Medical Center Lakewood	Kansas City	169	379
Liberty Hospital	Liberty	176	631
SSM Depaul Health Center	Bridgeton	178	341
Saint Anthony's Medical Center	Saint Louis	182	382
Pemiscot County Memorial Hospital	Hayti	184	268
Saint Luke's Hospital of Kansas City	Kansas City	186	435
SSM Saint Clare Health Center	Fenton	187	365
Mercy Hospital Springfield	Springfield	189	351
Hannibal Regional Hospital	Hannibal	190	1837
Missouri Baptist Medical Center	Town & Country	192	800
Southeast Missouri Hospital	Cape Girardeau	205	558
Saint Alexius Hospital	Saint Louis	206	286
Freeman Health System - Freeman West	Joplin	208	342
Truman Medical Center Hospital Hill	Kansas City	257	376
Barnes-Jewish Hospital	Saint Louis	262	744

Time in ER Before Being Evaluated (minutes)

Hospital Name	City	Min.	Cases
Lafayette Regional Health Center	Lexington	9	469
Lake Regional Health System	Osage Beach	9	743
Cameron Regional Medical Center	Cameron	10	512
Lee's Summit Medical Center	Lees Summit	13	478
Mercy Hospital Washington	Washington	13	393
Saint Joseph Medical Center	Kansas City	13	384
Mercy Hospital Lebanon	Lebanon	14	394
Mercy Hospital Springfield	Springfield	14	391
Golden Valley Memorial Hospital	Clinton	15	443
Northeast Regional Medical Center	Kirksville	15	423
Research Medical Center	Kansas City	15	503
Sullivan County Memorial Hospital[3]	Milan	15	97
Audrain Medical Center	Mexico	16	383
Heartland Regional Medical Center	Saint Joseph	16	336
Southeast Health Center of Ripley County	Doniphan	16	709
Twin Rivers Regional Medical Center	Kennett	16	385
Bates County Memorial Hospital	Butler	17	409
Belton Regional Medical Center	Belton	17	475
Capital Region Medical Center	Jefferson City	17	402
Centerpoint Medical Center	Independence	17	521
Phelps County Regional Medical Center	Rolla	17	418
Poplar Bluff Regional Medical Center	Poplar Bluff	17	383
Saint Mary's Medical Center	Blue Springs	17	383
Mercy Mccune Brooks Hospital[3]	Carthage	18	291
Mineral Area Regional Medical Center	Farmington	18	433
Nevada Regional Medical Center	Nevada	19	497
Saint Francis Hospital & Health Services	Maryville	19	404
Bothwell Regional Health Center	Sedalia	20	460
Cooper County Memorial Hospital	Boonville	20	407
Moberly Regional Medical Center	Moberly	20	422
North Kansas City Hospital	N Kansas City	20	1483
Texas County Memorial Hospital	Houston	20	425
Des Peres Hospital	Saint Louis	21	459
Sac-Osage Hospital	Osceola	22	244
SSM Saint Joseph Health Center	Saint Charles	22	404
Callaway Community Hospital	Fulton	23	451
Saint Mary's Health Center	Jefferson City	23	206
University of Missouri Health Care	Columbia	23	437
Fitzgibbon Hospital	Marshall	24	469
Mercy Hospital Saint Louis	Saint Louis	24	406
Black River Community Medical Center[3]	Poplar Bluff	25	337
Citizens Memorial Hospital	Bolivar	26	1196
Cox Medical Center	Springfield	27	455
Mercy Hospital Joplin[3]	Joplin	27	294
Missouri Baptist Medical Center	Town & Country	27	812
Saint Louis University Hospital	Saint Louis	27	447
Saint Luke's Hospital	Chesterfield	28	722
SSM Saint Joseph Hospital West	Lake Saint Louis	28	406
Cox Medical Center Branson	Branson	29	490
Ozarks Medical Center	West Plains	29	618
Pemiscot County Memorial Hospital	Hayti	29	220
Missouri Baptist Sullivan Hospital	Sullivan	30	654
Saint Luke's East Lee's Summit Hospital	Lees Summit	30	317
SSM Saint Marys Health Center	Richmond Hghts	32	402
Saint Luke's Northland Hospital	Kansas City	33	296
Saint Anthony's Medical Center	Saint Louis	35	236
Western Missouri Medical Center	Warrensburg	37	392
Freeman Health System - Freeman West	Joplin	39	375
Liberty Hospital	Liberty	39	743
Hannibal Regional Hospital	Hannibal	40	1129
Ozarks Community Hospital	Springfield	40	385
Saint Francis Medical Center	Cape Girardeau	40	396
Saint Luke's Hospital of Kansas City	Kansas City	43	363
SSM Saint Clare Health Center	Fenton	45	407
Parkland Health Center	Farmington	46	740
Southeasthealth Center of Stoddard County	Dexter	46	369
SSM Depaul Health Center	Bridgeton	46	402
Barnes-Jewish West County Hospital	Creve Coeur	48	546
Barnes-Jewish Saint Peters Hospital	Saint Peters	50	798
Progress West Hospital	O Fallon	50	763
Missouri Delta Medical Center	Sikeston	51	444
Boone Hospital Center	Columbia	59	301
Mercy Hospital Jefferson	Crystal City	61	398
Christian Hospital Northeast - Northwest	Saint Louis	64	779
Saint Alexius Hospital	Saint Louis	81	314
Southeast Missouri Hospital	Cape Girardeau	81	551
Truman Medical Center Lakewood	Kansas City	90	41
Truman Medical Center Hospital Hill	Kansas City	94	357
Barnes-Jewish Hospital	Saint Louis	131	825

Time to Pain Meds for Bone Fractures (minutes)

Hospital Name	City	Min.	Cases
SSM Saint Marys Health Center	Richmond Hghts	27	133

NOTE: Hospital profiles are in alphabetical order by state, then city, then hospital within the city; Rankings exclude hospitals with less than 25 cases except for patient surveys which excludes hospitals with less than 100 cases; (a) 100-299 cases; (1) The number of cases/patients is too few to report; (2) Data submitted were based on a sample of cases/patients; (3) Results are based on a shorter time period than required; (4) Data suppressed by CMS for one or more quarters; (5) Results are not available for this reporting period; (6) Fewer than 100 patients completed the HCAHPS survey; (7) No cases met the criteria for this measure; (8) The lower limit of the confidence interval cannot be calculated if the number of observed infections equals zero; (9) No data are available from the state/territory for this reporting period; (10) The scores shown reflect fewer than 50 completed surveys; (11) There were discrepancies in the data collection process; (12) This measure does not apply to this hospital for this reporting period; (13) Results cannot be calculated for this reporting period; (14) The results for this state are combined with nearby states to protect confidentiality; Please refer to the User's Guide for a full explanation of data.

Cameron Regional Medical Center	Cameron	28	32
Mercy Hospital Saint Louis	Saint Louis	29	235
Moberly Regional Medical Center	Moberly	31	61
Heartland Regional Medical Center	Saint Joseph	32	192
Bates County Memorial Hospital	Butler	33	25
SSM Saint Joseph Health Center	Saint Charles	33	45
Missouri Baptist Medical Center	Town & Country	34	237
SSM Saint Joseph Hospital West	Lake Saint Louis	34	92
Progress West Hospital	O Fallon	36	198
Lafayette Regional Health Center	Lexington	37	37
Barnes-Jewish Saint Peters Hospital	Saint Peters	38	171
Nevada Regional Medical Center	Nevada	38	42
Callaway Community Hospital	Fulton	39	45
Saint Mary's Health Center	Jefferson City	39	112
SSM Saint Clare Health Center	Fenton	39	70
Audrain Medical Center	Mexico	40	82
Lee's Summit Medical Center	Lees Summit	40	70
Saint Louis University Hospital	Saint Louis	41	47
Cooper County Memorial Hospital	Boonville	42	38
Mercy Hospital Washington	Washington	42	76
Saint Joseph Medical Center	Kansas City	42	113
Mercy Hospital Lebanon	Lebanon	44	56
Saint Mary's Medical Center	Blue Springs	44	106
Twin Rivers Regional Medical Center	Kennett	44	31
Missouri Baptist Sullivan Hospital	Sullivan	45	99
Saint Anthony's Medical Center	Saint Louis	46	258
Wright Memorial Hospital	Trenton	47	51
Mercy Hospital Springfield	Springfield	48	128
Belton Regional Medical Center	Belton	49	65
Mineral Area Regional Medical Center	Farmington	49	52
Golden Valley Memorial Hospital	Clinton	50	51
North Kansas City Hospital	N Kansas City	50	156
Northeast Regional Medical Center	Kirksville	51	61
Saint Luke's Northland Hospital	Kansas City	51	88
Saint Francis Hospital & Health Services	Maryville	52	43
Southeast Health Center of Ripley County	Doniphan	52	30
Southeasthealth Center of Stoddard County	Dexter	53	57
Lake Regional Health System	Osage Beach	54	203
Research Medical Center	Kansas City	54	72
Capital Region Medical Center	Jefferson City	55	131
Christian Hospital Northeast - Northwest	Saint Louis	55	77
Citizens Memorial Hospital	Bolivar	56	87
Saint Luke's East Lee's Summit Hospital	Lees Summit	56	123
University of Missouri Health Care	Columbia	56	162
Des Peres Hospital	Saint Louis	57	28
Mercy Hospital Jefferson	Crystal City	57	123
Ozarks Community Hospital	Springfield	57	27
Poplar Bluff Regional Medical Center	Poplar Bluff	57	90
Mercy Mccune Brooks Hospital[3]	Carthage	58	36
Saint Luke's Hospital of Kansas City	Kansas City	58	67
Fitzgibbon Hospital	Marshall	59	53
Phelps County Regional Medical Center	Rolla	59	93
Cox Medical Center	Springfield	61	331
Ozarks Medical Center	West Plains	61	125
Saint Luke's Hospital	Chesterfield	61	111
Parkland Health Center	Farmington	62	95
Centerpoint Medical Center	Independence	64	148
Saint Francis Medical Center	Cape Girardeau	64	130
Boone Hospital Center	Columbia	66	116
Bothwell Regional Health Center	Sedalia	66	85
Cox Medical Center Branson	Branson	66	82
Mercy Hospital Joplin[3]	Joplin	66	38
Hannibal Regional Hospital	Hannibal	72	106
Western Missouri Medical Center	Warrensburg	72	72
Barnes-Jewish West County Hospital	Creve Coeur	73	26
Texas County Memorial Hospital	Houston	75	49
Black River Community Medical Center[3]	Poplar Bluff	76	25
Freeman Health System - Freeman West	Joplin	76	221
Liberty Hospital	Liberty	82	118
SSM Depaul Health Center	Bridgeton	83	50
Barnes-Jewish Hospital	Saint Louis	84	155
Missouri Delta Medical Center	Sikeston	84	69
Truman Medical Center Lakewood	Kansas City	88	28
Saint Alexius Hospital	Saint Louis	91	32
Southeast Missouri Hospital	Cape Girardeau	92	80
Truman Medical Center Hospital Hill	Kansas City	92	109

Heart Attack Care

Aspirin Given at Discharge

Hospital Name	City	Rate	Cases
Audrain Medical Center	Mexico	100%	56
Barnes-Jewish Hospital	Saint Louis	100%	545
Barnes-Jewish Saint Peters Hospital	Saint Peters	100%	91
Boone Hospital Center	Columbia	100%	378
Capital Region Medical Center	Jefferson City	100%	139
Centerpoint Medical Center	Independence	100%	284
Columbia MO VA Medical Center	Columbia	100%	44
Cox Medical Center Branson	Branson	100%	181
Des Peres Hospital	Saint Louis	100%	103
Freeman Health System - Freeman West	Joplin	100%	538
Heartland Regional Medical Center	Saint Joseph	100%	321
Lee's Summit Medical Center	Lees Summit	100%	93
Mercy Hospital Saint Louis[2]	Saint Louis	100%	262
Mercy Hospital Springfield[2]	Springfield	100%	281
Mercy Hospital Washington	Washington	100%	151
Missouri Baptist Medical Center	Town & Country	100%	494
Moberly Regional Medical Center	Moberly	100%	45
North Kansas City Hospital[2]	N Kansas City	100%	296
Poplar Bluff Regional Medical Center	Poplar Bluff	100%	171
Progress West Hospital	O Fallon	100%	71
Research Medical Center	Kansas City	100%	187
Saint Francis Medical Center	Cape Girardeau	100%	185
St Louis-John Cochran VA Med Ctr	Saint Louis	100%	81
Saint Louis University Hospital	Saint Louis	100%	168
Saint Luke's East Lee's Summit Hospital	Lees Summit	100%	164
Saint Luke's Hospital	Chesterfield	100%	285
Saint Luke's Hospital of Kansas City	Kansas City	100%	348
Saint Luke's Northland Hospital	Kansas City	100%	127
Saint Mary's Health Center	Jefferson City	100%	112
Saint Mary's Medical Center	Blue Springs	100%	127
Southeast Missouri Hospital	Cape Girardeau	100%	205
SSM Depaul Health Center	Bridgeton	100%	273
SSM Saint Clare Health Center	Fenton	100%	307
SSM Saint Joseph Health Center	Saint Charles	100%	231
SSM Saint Joseph Hospital West	Lake Saint Louis	100%	249
SSM Saint Marys Health Center	Richmond Hghts	100%	209
Truman Medical Center Hospital Hill	Kansas City	100%	167
University of Missouri Health Care	Columbia	100%	284
Christian Hospital Northeast - Northwest	Saint Louis	99%	330
Cox Medical Center[2]	Springfield	99%	385
Hannibal Regional Hospital	Hannibal	99%	80
Liberty Hospital	Liberty	99%	168
Saint Anthony's Medical Center[2]	Saint Louis	99%	304
Saint Joseph Medical Center	Kansas City	99%	266
Citizens Memorial Hospital	Bolivar	98%	52
Lake Regional Health System	Osage Beach	98%	237
Mercy Hospital Joplin[3]	Joplin	98%	126
Mercy Hospital Jefferson[2]	Crystal City	97%	289
Ozarks Medical Center	West Plains	97%	155
Phelps County Regional Medical Center	Rolla	94%	49
Bothwell Regional Health Center	Sedalia	88%	26

PCI Within 90 Minutes of Arrival

Hospital Name	City	Rate	Cases
Barnes-Jewish Hospital	Saint Louis	100%	27
Capital Region Medical Center	Jefferson City	100%	29
Cox Medical Center Branson	Branson	100%	37
Freeman Health System - Freeman West	Joplin	100%	69
Lake Regional Health System	Osage Beach	100%	45
Mercy Hospital Joplin[3]	Joplin	100%	25
Mercy Hospital Springfield[2]	Springfield	100%	44
Missouri Baptist Medical Center	Town & Country	100%	37
Saint Luke's Hospital	Chesterfield	100%	45
Saint Mary's Health Center	Jefferson City	100%	27
Southeast Missouri Hospital	Cape Girardeau	100%	32
SSM Depaul Health Center	Bridgeton	100%	56
SSM Saint Clare Health Center	Fenton	100%	62
SSM Saint Joseph Health Center	Saint Charles	100%	26
SSM Saint Joseph Hospital West	Lake Saint Louis	100%	33
University of Missouri Health Care	Columbia	100%	39
Barnes-Jewish Saint Peters Hospital	Saint Peters	98%	54
Boone Hospital Center	Columbia	98%	44
Heartland Regional Medical Center	Saint Joseph	98%	49
Saint Anthony's Medical Center[2]	Saint Louis	98%	81
Saint Louis University Hospital	Saint Louis	98%	40
Poplar Bluff Regional Medical Center	Poplar Bluff	97%	35
Research Medical Center	Kansas City	97%	29
Saint Francis Medical Center	Cape Girardeau	97%	36
Saint Luke's East Lee's Summit Hospital	Lees Summit	97%	36
Saint Luke's Northland Hospital	Kansas City	97%	31
Saint Mary's Medical Center	Blue Springs	97%	37
Mercy Hospital Jefferson[2]	Crystal City	96%	55
Progress West Hospital	O Fallon	96%	25
Centerpoint Medical Center	Independence	95%	66
Mercy Hospital Saint Louis[2]	Saint Louis	95%	37
Christian Hospital Northeast - Northwest	Saint Louis	94%	31
North Kansas City Hospital[2]	N Kansas City	94%	67
Cox Medical Center[2]	Springfield	93%	70
Mercy Hospital Washington	Washington	93%	29
Saint Joseph Medical Center	Kansas City	92%	39
Liberty Hospital	Liberty	91%	34
Audrain Medical Center	Mexico	88%	25
Hannibal Regional Hospital	Hannibal	87%	30

Statin Prescribed at Discharge

Hospital Name	City	Rate	Cases
Barnes-Jewish Hospital	Saint Louis	100%	509
Barnes-Jewish Saint Peters Hospital	Saint Peters	100%	91
Boone Hospital Center	Columbia	100%	369
Capital Region Medical Center	Jefferson City	100%	140
Centerpoint Medical Center	Independence	100%	281
Des Peres Hospital	Saint Louis	100%	101
Freeman Health System - Freeman West	Joplin	100%	489
Heartland Regional Medical Center	Saint Joseph	100%	314
Lee's Summit Medical Center	Lees Summit	100%	92
Missouri Baptist Medical Center	Town & Country	100%	477
Moberly Regional Medical Center	Moberly	100%	44
North Kansas City Hospital[2]	N Kansas City	100%	284
Research Medical Center	Kansas City	100%	182
St Louis-John Cochran VA Med Ctr	Saint Louis	100%	78
Saint Luke's East Lee's Summit Hospital	Lees Summit	100%	164
Saint Mary's Health Center	Jefferson City	100%	105
SSM Depaul Health Center	Bridgeton	100%	267
SSM Saint Clare Health Center	Fenton	100%	299
SSM Saint Joseph Health Center	Saint Charles	100%	231
SSM Saint Joseph Hospital West	Lake Saint Louis	100%	247
SSM Saint Marys Health Center	Richmond Hghts	100%	208
Truman Medical Center Hospital Hill	Kansas City	100%	161
Christian Hospital Northeast - Northwest	Saint Louis	99%	299
Saint Joseph Medical Center	Kansas City	99%	263
Saint Louis University Hospital	Saint Louis	99%	165
Saint Luke's Hospital of Kansas City	Kansas City	99%	345
Saint Luke's Northland Hospital	Kansas City	99%	122
Southeast Missouri Hospital	Cape Girardeau	99%	202
University of Missouri Health Care	Columbia	99%	284
Columbia MO VA Medical Center	Columbia	98%	44
Cox Medical Center Branson	Branson	98%	172
Lake Regional Health System	Osage Beach	98%	220
Mercy Hospital Jefferson[2]	Crystal City	98%	278
Mercy Hospital Saint Louis[2]	Saint Louis	98%	264
Mercy Hospital Washington	Washington	98%	145
Poplar Bluff Regional Medical Center	Poplar Bluff	98%	169
Saint Anthony's Medical Center[2]	Saint Louis	98%	291
Saint Francis Medical Center	Cape Girardeau	98%	178
Saint Mary's Medical Center	Blue Springs	98%	124
Hannibal Regional Hospital	Hannibal	97%	78
Liberty Hospital	Liberty	97%	158
Mercy Hospital Springfield[2]	Springfield	97%	268
Progress West Hospital	O Fallon	97%	70
Saint Luke's Hospital	Chesterfield	97%	282
Mercy Hospital Joplin[3]	Joplin	96%	127
Cox Medical Center[2]	Springfield	94%	374
Audrain Medical Center	Mexico	93%	54
Ozarks Medical Center	West Plains	89%	148
Citizens Memorial Hospital	Bolivar	83%	52
Phelps County Regional Medical Center	Rolla	80%	51

Heart Failure Care

ACE Inhibitor or ARB for LVSD

Hospital Name	City	Rate	Cases
Capital Region Medical Center	Jefferson City	100%	51
Centerpoint Medical Center	Independence	100%	109
Des Peres Hospital	Saint Louis	100%	36
Heartland Regional Medical Center	Saint Joseph	100%	71
Kansas City VA Medical Center	Kansas City	100%	77
Lee's Summit Medical Center	Lees Summit	100%	34
Mercy Hospital Washington[2]	Washington	100%	59
Missouri Delta Medical Center	Sikeston	100%	69
Poplar Bluff Regional Medical Center	Poplar Bluff	100%	96
Research Medical Center	Kansas City	100%	112
Saint Luke's East Lee's Summit Hospital	Lees Summit	100%	78
Saint Luke's Hospital[2]	Chesterfield	100%	78
Saint Luke's Hospital of Kansas City	Kansas City	100%	237
Saint Luke's Northland Hospital	Kansas City	100%	38
Saint Mary's Health Center	Jefferson City	100%	92
Southeast Missouri Hospital	Cape Girardeau	100%	75
SSM Depaul Health Center[2]	Bridgeton	100%	79
SSM Saint Clare Health Center[2]	Fenton	100%	58
SSM Saint Joseph Health Center[2]	Saint Charles	100%	75
SSM Saint Joseph Hospital West[2]	Lake Saint Louis	100%	50
SSM Saint Marys Health Center[2]	Richmond Hghts	100%	66
Truman Medical Center Hospital Hill	Kansas City	100%	196
Truman Medical Center Lakewood	Kansas City	100%	28
Barnes-Jewish Hospital[2]	Saint Louis	99%	276
Boone Hospital Center[2]	Columbia	99%	133
Mercy Hospital Saint Louis[2]	Saint Louis	99%	74
St Louis-John Cochran VA Med Ctr	Saint Louis	99%	154
Saint Louis University Hospital	Saint Louis	99%	165
Barnes-Jewish Saint Peters Hospital[2]	Saint Peters	98%	47
Columbia MO VA Medical Center	Columbia	98%	50
Freeman Health System - Freeman West	Joplin	98%	90
Missouri Baptist Medical Center[2]	Town & Country	98%	114
North Kansas City Hospital[2]	N Kansas City	98%	137
Saint Joseph Medical Center	Kansas City	98%	106
Christian Hospital Northeast - Northwest[2]	Saint Louis	97%	159
Cox Medical Center Branson	Branson	97%	58
Lake Regional Health System	Osage Beach	97%	64
Mercy Hospital Springfield[2]	Springfield	97%	90

NOTE: Hospital profiles are in alphabetical order by state, then city, then hospital within the city; Rankings exclude hospitals with less than 25 cases except for patient surveys which excludes hospitals with less than 100 cases; (a) 100-299 cases; (1) The number of cases/patients is too few to report; (2) Data submitted were based on a sample of cases/patients; (3) Results are based on a shorter time period than required; (4) Data suppressed by CMS for one or more quarters; (5) Results are not available for this reporting period; (6) Fewer than 100 patients completed the HCAHPS survey; (7) No cases met the criteria for this measure; (8) The lower limit of the confidence interval cannot be calculated if the number of observed infections equals zero; (9) No data are available from the state/territory for this reporting period; (10) The scores shown reflect fewer than 50 completed surveys; (11) There were discrepancies in the data collection process; (12) This measure does not apply to this hospital for this reporting period; (13) Results cannot be calculated for this reporting period; (14) The results for this state are combined with nearby states to protect confidentiality; Please refer to the User's Guide for a full explanation of data.

Hospital Name	City	Rate	Cases
Ozarks Medical Center	West Plains	97%	37
Hannibal Regional Hospital	Hannibal	96%	52
Mercy Hospital Jefferson[2]	Crystal City	96%	72
Saint Anthony's Medical Center[2]	Saint Louis	96%	82
University of Missouri Health Care	Columbia	96%	94
Saint Francis Medical Center	Cape Girardeau	95%	103
Phelps County Regional Medical Center	Rolla	94%	54
Mercy Hospital Joplin[3]	Joplin	92%	52
Golden Valley Memorial Hospital	Clinton	90%	31
Audrain Medical Center	Mexico	89%	37
Mercy Hospital Lebanon	Lebanon	88%	40
Saint Mary's Medical Center	Blue Springs	88%	26
Cox Medical Center[2]	Springfield	86%	104
Liberty Hospital	Liberty	86%	58
Parkland Health Center	Farmington	82%	33
Bothwell Regional Health Center	Sedalia	72%	64

Discharge Instructions Given

Hospital Name	City	Rate	Cases
Barnes-Jewish West County Hospital	Creve Coeur	100%	37
Belton Regional Medical Center	Belton	100%	37
Centerpoint Medical Center	Independence	100%	269
Cox Medical Center[2]	Springfield	100%	334
Fitzgibbon Hospital	Marshall	100%	64
Missouri Baptist Medical Center[2]	Town & Country	100%	412
Missouri Baptist Sullivan Hospital	Sullivan	100%	44
Missouri Delta Medical Center	Sikeston	100%	126
Northeast Regional Medical Center	Kirksville	100%	49
Pike County Memorial Hospital[2]	Louisiana	100%	38
Poplar Bluff VA Medical Center	Poplar Bluff	100%	72
Research Medical Center	Kansas City	100%	278
Saint Mary's Health Center	Jefferson City	100%	210
SSM Depaul Health Center[2]	Bridgeton	100%	215
SSM Saint Marys Health Center[2]	Richmond Hghts	100%	261
Barnes-Jewish Hospital[2]	Saint Louis	99%	506
Boone Hospital Center[2]	Columbia	99%	346
Heartland Regional Medical Center	Saint Joseph	99%	238
Lee's Summit Medical Center	Lees Summit	99%	90
Poplar Bluff Regional Medical Center	Poplar Bluff	99%	264
SSM Saint Clare Health Center[2]	Fenton	99%	199
SSM Saint Joseph Hospital West[2]	Lake Saint Louis	99%	198
University of Missouri Health Care	Columbia	99%	172
Cass Regional Medical Center	Harrisonville	98%	43
Christian Hospital Northeast - Northwest[2]	Saint Louis	98%	443
Progress West Hospital	O Fallon	98%	47
Saint Luke's Hospital[2]	Chesterfield	98%	280
SSM Saint Joseph Health Center[2]	Saint Charles	98%	219
Barnes-Jewish Saint Peters Hospital[2]	Saint Peters	97%	159
Cox Medical Center Branson	Branson	97%	182
Des Peres Hospital	Saint Louis	97%	113
Saint Louis University Hospital	Saint Louis	97%	266
Truman Medical Center Hospital Hill	Kansas City	97%	313
Washington County Memorial Hospital	Potosi	97%	30
Capital Region Medical Center	Jefferson City	96%	139
Mercy Hospital Springfield[2]	Springfield	96%	203
Moberly Regional Medical Center	Moberly	96%	52
Phelps County Regional Medical Center	Rolla	96%	91
Saint Luke's East Lee's Summit Hospital	Lees Summit	96%	239
Golden Valley Memorial Hospital	Clinton	95%	56
Mercy Hospital Lebanon	Lebanon	95%	95
Mercy Hospital Saint Louis[2]	Saint Louis	95%	244
Wright Memorial Hospital	Trenton	95%	38
Citizens Memorial Hospital	Bolivar	94%	36
Mercy Hospital Joplin[3]	Joplin	94%	100
North Kansas City Hospital[2]	N Kansas City	94%	358
Audrain Medical Center	Mexico	93%	89
Lake Regional Health System	Osage Beach	93%	148
Mercy Hospital Washington[2]	Washington	93%	180
Mercy Hospital Jefferson[2]	Crystal City	92%	229
Saint Luke's Hospital of Kansas City	Kansas City	92%	590
Kansas City VA Medical Center	Kansas City	91%	139
Saint Anthony's Medical Center[2]	Saint Louis	91%	218
Saint Francis Medical Center	Cape Girardeau	91%	279
Columbia MO VA Medical Center	Columbia	90%	118
Saint Luke's Northland Hospital	Kansas City	90%	120
Salem Memorial District Hospital	Salem	90%	31
Bothwell Regional Health Center	Sedalia	89%	123
Freeman Health System - Freeman West	Joplin	89%	227
Freeman Neosho Hospital	Neosho	89%	28
Ozarks Medical Center	West Plains	89%	73
Parkland Health Center	Farmington	89%	92
St Louis-John Cochran VA Med Ctr	Saint Louis	88%	349
Twin Rivers Regional Medical Center	Kennett	88%	43
Liberty Hospital	Liberty	87%	172
Truman Medical Center Lakewood	Kansas City	87%	53
Mineral Area Regional Medical Center	Farmington	86%	29
Southeast Missouri Hospital	Cape Girardeau	79%	176
Saint Joseph Medical Center	Kansas City	77%	229
Western Missouri Medical Center	Warrensburg	77%	31
Saint Mary's Medical Center	Blue Springs	74%	81
Hannibal Regional Hospital	Hannibal	67%	118

Hospital Name	City	Rate	Cases
Nevada Regional Medical Center	Nevada	65%	26
Southeasthealth Center of Stoddard County	Dexter	45%	29
Saint Alexius Hospital	Saint Louis	40%	52
Pemiscot County Memorial Hospital[2]	Hayti	23%	86

Evaluation of LVS Function

Hospital Name	City	Rate	Cases
Barnes-Jewish Hospital[2]	Saint Louis	100%	570
Barnes-Jewish Saint Peters Hospital[2]	Saint Peters	100%	190
Barnes-Jewish West County Hospital	Creve Coeur	100%	42
Belton Regional Medical Center	Belton	100%	50
Boone Hospital Center[2]	Columbia	100%	406
Capital Region Medical Center	Jefferson City	100%	170
Cass Regional Medical Center	Harrisonville	100%	75
Centerpoint Medical Center	Independence	100%	368
Christian Hospital Northeast - Northwest[2]	Saint Louis	100%	523
Citizens Memorial Hospital	Bolivar	100%	43
Columbia MO VA Medical Center	Columbia	100%	133
Cox Medical Center[2]	Springfield	100%	401
Cox Medical Center Branson	Branson	100%	199
Freeman Health System - Freeman West	Joplin	100%	290
Freeman Neosho Hospital	Neosho	100%	49
Heartland Regional Medical Center	Saint Joseph	100%	332
Kansas City VA Medical Center	Kansas City	100%	167
Lee's Summit Medical Center	Lees Summit	100%	127
Liberty Hospital	Liberty	100%	214
Mercy Hospital Jefferson[2]	Crystal City	100%	302
Mercy Hospital Joplin[3]	Joplin	100%	141
Mercy Hospital Lebanon	Lebanon	100%	118
Mercy Hospital Saint Louis[2]	Saint Louis	100%	300
Mercy Hospital Springfield[2]	Springfield	100%	272
Mercy Hospital Washington[2]	Washington	100%	224
Mercy Mccune Brooks Hospital[3]	Carthage	100%	32
Missouri Baptist Medical Center[2]	Town & Country	100%	510
Missouri Baptist Sullivan Hospital	Sullivan	100%	72
Missouri Delta Medical Center	Sikeston	100%	159
Moberly Regional Medical Center	Moberly	100%	85
North Kansas City Hospital[2]	N Kansas City	100%	409
Northeast Regional Medical Center	Kirksville	100%	71
Parkland Health Center	Farmington	100%	134
Pike County Memorial Hospital[2]	Louisiana	100%	50
Poplar Bluff Regional Medical Center	Poplar Bluff	100%	316
Poplar Bluff VA Medical Center	Poplar Bluff	100%	75
Progress West Hospital	O Fallon	100%	61
Research Medical Center	Kansas City	100%	326
Saint Alexius Hospital	Saint Louis	100%	67
Saint Anthony's Medical Center[2]	Saint Louis	100%	307
Saint Joseph Medical Center	Kansas City	100%	312
Saint Louis University Hospital	Saint Louis	100%	298
Saint Luke's East Lee's Summit Hospital	Lees Summit	100%	305
Saint Luke's Hospital[2]	Chesterfield	100%	374
Saint Luke's Hospital of Kansas City	Kansas City	100%	692
Saint Luke's Northland Hospital	Kansas City	100%	160
Saint Mary's Health Center	Jefferson City	100%	233
Saint Mary's Medical Center	Blue Springs	100%	106
Sainte Genevieve County Memorial Hospital	Ste Genevieve	100%	36
SSM Depaul Health Center[2]	Bridgeton	100%	287
SSM Saint Clare Health Center[2]	Fenton	100%	240
SSM Saint Joseph Health Center[2]	Saint Charles	100%	253
SSM Saint Joseph Hospital West[2]	Lake Saint Louis	100%	265
SSM Saint Marys Health Center[2]	Richmond Hghts	100%	297
Truman Medical Center Hospital Hill	Kansas City	100%	338
Twin Rivers Regional Medical Center	Kennett	100%	66
University of Missouri Health Care	Columbia	100%	231
Audrain Medical Center	Mexico	99%	128
Bothwell Regional Health Center	Sedalia	99%	159
Des Peres Hospital	Saint Louis	99%	149
Lake Regional Health System	Osage Beach	99%	184
Phelps County Regional Medical Center	Rolla	99%	127
Saint Francis Medical Center	Cape Girardeau	99%	338
St Louis-John Cochran VA Med Ctr	Saint Louis	99%	395
Southeast Missouri Hospital	Cape Girardeau	99%	230
Bates County Memorial Hospital	Butler	98%	40
Fitzgibbon Hospital	Marshall	98%	95
Mineral Area Regional Medical Center	Farmington	98%	49
Ozarks Medical Center	West Plains	98%	107
Truman Medical Center Lakewood	Kansas City	98%	63
Wright Memorial Hospital	Trenton	98%	52
Texas County Memorial Hospital	Houston	97%	36
Cameron Regional Medical Center	Cameron	96%	47
Hannibal Regional Hospital	Hannibal	96%	167
Western Missouri Medical Center	Warrensburg	96%	53
Golden Valley Memorial Hospital	Clinton	95%	94
Nevada Regional Medical Center	Nevada	90%	30
Washington County Memorial Hospital	Potosi	86%	43
Barton County Memorial Hospital	Lamar	82%	34
Southeasthealth Center of Stoddard County	Dexter	76%	50
Salem Memorial District Hospital	Salem	66%	35
Pemiscot County Memorial Hospital[2]	Hayti	53%	100
Pershing Memorial Hospital[3]	Brookfield	19%	37

Medicare Spending

Medicare Spending per Patient (ratio)

Hospital Name	City	Ratio	Cases
Sac-Osage Hospital	Osceola	0.84	-
Bothwell Regional Health Center	Sedalia	0.85	-
Cooper County Memorial Hospital	Boonville	0.85	-
Callaway Community Hospital	Fulton	0.87	-
Nevada Regional Medical Center	Nevada	0.87	-
Pemiscot County Memorial Hospital	Hayti	0.87	-
Barnes-Jewish West County Hospital	Creve Coeur	0.88	-
Northeast Regional Medical Center	Kirksville	0.88	-
Mercy Hospital Lebanon	Lebanon	0.89	-
Texas County Memorial Hospital	Houston	0.89	-
Truman Medical Center Lakewood	Kansas City	0.89	-
Fitzgibbon Hospital	Marshall	0.90	-
Ozarks Medical Center	West Plains	0.90	-
Parkland Health Center	Farmington	0.90	-
Mineral Area Regional Medical Center	Farmington	0.91	-
Audrain Medical Center	Mexico	0.92	-
Lake Regional Health System	Osage Beach	0.92	-
Saint Mary's Health Center	Jefferson City	0.92	-
Western Missouri Medical Center	Warrensburg	0.92	-
Boone Hospital Center	Columbia	0.93	-
Citizens Memorial Hospital	Bolivar	0.93	-
Hannibal Regional Hospital	Hannibal	0.93	-
Mercy Hospital Joplin	Joplin	0.93	-
Mercy Hospital Washington	Washington	0.93	-
Moberly Regional Medical Center	Moberly	0.93	-
Progress West Hospital	O Fallon	0.93	-
Truman Medical Center Hospital Hill	Kansas City	0.93	-
Barnes-Jewish Saint Peters Hospital	Saint Peters	0.94	-
Bates County Memorial Hospital	Butler	0.94	-
Capital Region Medical Center	Jefferson City	0.94	-
Cox Medical Center	Springfield	0.94	-
Freeman Health System - Freeman West	Joplin	0.94	-
Golden Valley Memorial Hospital	Clinton	0.94	-
Poplar Bluff Regional Medical Center	Poplar Bluff	0.94	-
SSM Saint Joseph Hospital West	Lake Saint Louis	0.94	-
Belton Regional Medical Center	Belton	0.95	-
Cox Medical Center Branson	Branson	0.95	-
Heartland Regional Medical Center	Saint Joseph	0.95	-
Mercy Hospital Springfield	Springfield	0.95	-
Missouri Baptist Medical Center	Town & Country	0.95	-
North Kansas City Hospital	N Kansas City	0.95	-
Saint Luke's Hospital	Chesterfield	0.95	-
Southeast Missouri Hospital	Cape Girardeau	0.95	-
Twin Rivers Regional Medical Center	Kennett	0.95	-
Saint Francis Hospital & Health Services	Maryville	0.97	-
SSM Saint Clare Health Center	Fenton	0.97	-
University of Missouri Health Care	Columbia	0.97	-
Barnes-Jewish Hospital	Saint Louis	0.98	-
Cameron Regional Medical Center	Cameron	0.98	-
Mercy Hospital Saint Louis	Saint Louis	0.98	-
Phelps County Regional Medical Center	Rolla	0.98	-
Saint Anthony's Medical Center	Saint Louis	0.98	-
Saint Luke's Northland Hospital	Kansas City	0.98	-
SSM Saint Marys Health Center	Richmond Hghts	0.98	-
Des Peres Hospital	Saint Louis	0.99	-
Liberty Hospital	Liberty	0.99	-
Saint Luke's East Lee's Summit Hospital	Lees Summit	0.99	-
Southeasthealth Center of Stoddard County	Dexter	0.99	-
SSM Saint Joseph Health Center	Saint Charles	0.99	-
Christian Hospital Northeast - Northwest	Saint Louis	1.00	-
Mercy Hospital Jefferson	Crystal City	1.00	-
Missouri Delta Medical Center	Sikeston	1.00	-
Saint Luke's Hospital of Kansas City	Kansas City	1.00	-
SSM Depaul Health Center	Bridgeton	1.00	-
Centerpoint Medical Center	Independence	1.01	-
Lee's Summit Medical Center	Lees Summit	1.01	-
Southeast Health Center of Ripley County	Doniphan	1.01	-
Research Medical Center	Kansas City	1.02	-
Saint Francis Medical Center	Cape Girardeau	1.02	-
Saint Mary's Medical Center	Blue Springs	1.02	-
Saint Louis University Hospital	Saint Louis	1.03	-
Saint Alexius Hospital	Saint Louis	1.04	-
Ozarks Community Hospital	Springfield	1.06	-
Saint Joseph Medical Center	Kansas City	1.06	-

Pneumonia Care

Appropriate Initial Antibiotic Given

Hospital Name	City	Rate	Cases
Belton Regional Medical Center	Belton	100%	36
Lee's Summit Medical Center	Lees Summit	100%	41
Moberly Regional Medical Center	Moberly	100%	48
Northeast Regional Medical Center	Kirksville	100%	33
Progress West Hospital	O Fallon	100%	63
Saint Luke's Northland Hospital	Kansas City	100%	87
SSM Depaul Health Center[2]	Bridgeton	100%	61

NOTE: Hospital profiles are in alphabetical order by state, then city, then hospital within the city; Rankings exclude hospitals with less than 25 cases except for patient surveys which excludes hospitals with less than 100 cases; (a) 100-299 cases; (1) The number of cases/patients is too few to report; (2) Data submitted were based on a sample of cases/patients; (3) Results are based on a shorter time period than required; (4) Data suppressed by CMS for one or more quarters; (5) Results are not available for this reporting period; (6) Fewer than 100 patients completed the HCAHPS survey; (7) No cases met the criteria for this measure; (8) The lower limit of the confidence interval cannot be calculated if the number of observed infections equals zero; (9) No data are available from the state/territory for this reporting period; (10) The scores shown reflect fewer than 50 completed surveys; (11) There were discrepancies in the data collection process; (12) This measure does not apply to this hospital for this reporting period; (13) Results cannot be calculated for this reporting period; (14) The results for this state are combined with nearby states to protect confidentiality; Please refer to the User's Guide for a full explanation of data.

Hospital Name	City	Rate	Cases
Audrain Medical Center	Mexico	99%	74
Centerpoint Medical Center	Independence	99%	221
Heartland Regional Medical Center	Saint Joseph	99%	338
Mercy Hospital Lebanon[2]	Lebanon	99%	67
Research Medical Center	Kansas City	99%	104
Southeast Missouri Hospital	Cape Girardeau	99%	222
SSM Saint Clare Health Center[2]	Fenton	99%	93
SSM Saint Marys Health Center[2]	Richmond Hghts	99%	75
Texas County Memorial Hospital	Houston	99%	82
Truman Medical Center Hospital Hill	Kansas City	99%	111
Barnes-Jewish Hospital[2]	Saint Louis	98%	80
Barnes-Jewish Saint Peters Hospital[2]	Saint Peters	98%	108
Christian Hospital Northeast - Northwest[2]	Saint Louis	98%	115
Cox Medical Center Branson[2]	Branson	98%	105
Fitzgibbon Hospital	Marshall	98%	45
Freeman Neosho Hospital	Neosho	98%	62
Golden Valley Memorial Hospital	Clinton	98%	81
Mercy Hospital Joplin[2,3]	Joplin	98%	40
Poplar Bluff Regional Medical Center	Poplar Bluff	98%	186
Poplar Bluff VA Medical Center	Poplar Bluff	98%	52
Saint Anthony's Medical Center[2]	Saint Louis	98%	90
Saint Luke's East Lee's Summit Hospital	Lees Summit	98%	169
Saint Mary's Medical Center	Blue Springs	98%	139
Capital Region Medical Center	Jefferson City	97%	109
Des Peres Hospital	Saint Louis	97%	59
Mercy Hospital Jefferson[2]	Crystal City	97%	116
Mercy Hospital Washington[2]	Washington	97%	75
Missouri Baptist Medical Center[2]	Town & Country	97%	129
North Kansas City Hospital[2]	N Kansas City	97%	152
St Louis-John Cochran VA Med Ctr	Saint Louis	97%	37
Saint Louis University Hospital[2]	Saint Louis	97%	73
SSM Saint Joseph Health Center[2]	Saint Charles	97%	67
Truman Medical Center Lakewood	Kansas City	97%	71
Twin Rivers Regional Medical Center	Kennett	97%	61
Lake Regional Health System	Osage Beach	96%	150
Liberty Hospital	Liberty	96%	209
Mineral Area Regional Medical Center	Farmington	96%	55
Missouri Delta Medical Center	Sikeston	96%	82
Phelps County Regional Medical Center	Rolla	96%	116
Saint Joseph Medical Center	Kansas City	96%	145
Saint Luke's Hospital[2]	Chesterfield	96%	102
Cox Medical Center[2]	Springfield	95%	111
Freeman Health System - Freeman West[2]	Joplin	95%	57
Mercy Hospital Saint Louis[2]	Saint Louis	95%	64
Missouri Baptist Sullivan Hospital	Sullivan	95%	40
SSM Saint Joseph Hospital West[2]	Lake Saint Louis	95%	80
Boone Hospital Center[2]	Columbia	94%	144
Mercy Mccune Brooks Hospital[3]	Carthage	94%	36
Mercy Saint Francis Hospital	Mountain View	94%	31
Parkland Health Center[2]	Farmington	94%	107
Saint Luke's Hospital of Kansas City	Kansas City	94%	104
Cass Regional Medical Center	Harrisonville	93%	67
Citizens Memorial Hospital	Bolivar	93%	70
Hedrick Medical Center	Chillicothe	93%	29
Mercy Hospital Springfield[2]	Springfield	93%	75
Ozarks Medical Center	West Plains	93%	129
Bates County Memorial Hospital	Butler	92%	59
Kansas City VA Medical Center	Kansas City	92%	73
Bothwell Regional Health Center	Sedalia	91%	100
Columbia MO VA Medical Center	Columbia	91%	33
Cox Monett Hospital	Monett	91%	46
Ozarks Community Hospital	Springfield	91%	33
Pike County Memorial Hospital[2]	Louisiana	91%	33
Saint Francis Medical Center	Cape Girardeau	91%	220
Western Missouri Medical Center	Warrensburg	91%	76
Hannibal Regional Hospital	Hannibal	90%	115
Nevada Regional Medical Center	Nevada	89%	27
Barton County Memorial Hospital	Lamar	88%	60
Mercy Hospital Aurora	Aurora	88%	25
Saint Alexius Hospital	Saint Louis	88%	50
Washington County Memorial Hospital	Potosi	88%	60
Carroll County Memorial Hospital	Carrollton	87%	30
University of Missouri Health Care	Columbia	87%	68
Cameron Regional Medical Center	Cameron	86%	50
Sainte Genevieve County Memorial Hospital	Ste Genevieve	85%	26
Lincoln County Medical Center	Troy	84%	25
Southeasthealth Center of Stoddard County	Dexter	81%	59
Salem Memorial District Hospital	Salem	79%	42
Southeast Health Center of Ripley County	Doniphan	71%	38
Pershing Memorial Hospital	Brookfield	44%	25

Blood Culture Timing

Hospital Name	City	Rate	Cases
Barnes-Jewish Saint Peters Hospital[2]	Saint Peters	100%	238
Cameron Regional Medical Center	Cameron	100%	54
Centerpoint Medical Center	Independence	100%	416
Columbia MO VA Medical Center	Columbia	100%	62
Cox Medical Center[2]	Springfield	100%	243
Des Peres Hospital	Saint Louis	100%	136
Heartland Regional Medical Center	Saint Joseph	100%	567
Kansas City VA Medical Center	Kansas City	100%	139
Lafayette Regional Health Center	Lexington	100%	43
Lee's Summit Medical Center	Lees Summit	100%	75
Mercy Saint Francis Hospital	Mountain View	100%	25
Missouri Baptist Sullivan Hospital	Sullivan	100%	61
Moberly Regional Medical Center	Moberly	100%	95
Northeast Regional Medical Center	Kirksville	100%	117
Parkland Health Center[2]	Farmington	100%	182
Perry County Memorial Hospital[2]	Perryville	100%	61
Research Medical Center	Kansas City	100%	238
Saint Luke's East Lee's Summit Hospital	Lees Summit	100%	285
Saint Luke's Hospital[2]	Chesterfield	100%	129
Sainte Genevieve County Memorial Hospital	Ste Genevieve	100%	40
Salem Memorial District Hospital	Salem	100%	55
Scotland County Hospital	Memphis	100%	31
SSM Saint Marys Health Center[2]	Richmond Hghts	100%	136
Twin Rivers Regional Medical Center	Kennett	100%	131
Wright Memorial Hospital	Trenton	100%	34
Audrain Medical Center	Mexico	99%	114
Barnes-Jewish Hospital[2]	Saint Louis	99%	112
Boone Hospital Center[2]	Columbia	99%	188
Cox Medical Center Branson[2]	Branson	99%	166
Freeman Neosho Hospital	Neosho	99%	109
Lake Regional Health System	Osage Beach	99%	225
Mercy Hospital Jefferson[2]	Crystal City	99%	161
Mercy Hospital Joplin[2,3]	Joplin	99%	83
Mercy Hospital Lebanon[2]	Lebanon	99%	101
Mercy Hospital Saint Louis[2]	Saint Louis	99%	106
Mercy Hospital Springfield[2]	Springfield	99%	164
Mercy Hospital Washington[2]	Washington	99%	93
Mineral Area Regional Medical Center	Farmington	99%	104
Missouri Baptist Medical Center[2]	Town & Country	99%	289
Missouri Delta Medical Center	Sikeston	99%	107
North Kansas City Hospital[2]	N Kansas City	99%	162
Progress West Hospital	O Fallon	99%	86
Saint Alexius Hospital	Saint Louis	99%	73
Saint Luke's Northland Hospital	Kansas City	99%	106
Saint Mary's Health Center	Jefferson City	99%	151
Southeast Missouri Hospital	Cape Girardeau	99%	371
SSM Saint Joseph Health Center[2]	Saint Charles	99%	131
Western Missouri Medical Center	Warrensburg	99%	94
Belton Regional Medical Center	Belton	98%	45
Capital Region Medical Center	Jefferson City	98%	179
Cass Regional Medical Center	Harrisonville	98%	91
Christian Hospital Northeast - Northwest[2]	Saint Louis	98%	253
Fitzgibbon Hospital	Marshall	98%	65
Liberty Hospital	Liberty	98%	234
Ozarks Community Hospital	Springfield	98%	41
Ozarks Medical Center	West Plains	98%	234
Saint Anthony's Medical Center[2]	Saint Louis	98%	179
Saint Francis Medical Center	Cape Girardeau	98%	439
Saint Louis University Hospital[2]	Saint Louis	98%	104
Saint Mary's Medical Center	Blue Springs	98%	190
SSM Depaul Health Center[2]	Bridgeton	98%	117
SSM Saint Clare Health Center[2]	Fenton	98%	129
University of Missouri Health Care	Columbia	98%	125
Citizens Memorial Hospital	Bolivar	97%	119
Freeman Health System - Freeman West[2]	Joplin	97%	117
Hedrick Medical Center	Chillicothe	97%	33
Mercy Mccune Brooks Hospital[3]	Carthage	97%	65
Nevada Regional Medical Center	Nevada	97%	36
Poplar Bluff Regional Medical Center	Poplar Bluff	97%	274
Saint Joseph Medical Center	Kansas City	97%	256
Saint Luke's Hospital of Kansas City	Kansas City	97%	188
SSM Saint Joseph Hospital West[2]	Lake Saint Louis	97%	111
Texas County Memorial Hospital	Houston	97%	133
Truman Medical Center Hospital Hill	Kansas City	97%	175
Truman Medical Center Lakewood	Kansas City	97%	97
Bothwell Regional Health Center	Sedalia	96%	78
Hannibal Regional Hospital	Hannibal	96%	155
Lincoln County Medical Center	Troy	96%	73
Southeasthealth Center of Stoddard County	Dexter	96%	57
Bates County Memorial Hospital	Butler	95%	75
Phelps County Regional Medical Center	Rolla	95%	179
Cox Monett Hospital	Monett	94%	69
Golden Valley Memorial Hospital	Clinton	94%	101
Mercy Hospital Aurora	Aurora	94%	33
St Louis-John Cochran VA Med Ctr	Saint Louis	94%	62
Southeast Health Center of Ripley County	Doniphan	94%	49
Barton County Memorial Hospital	Lamar	93%	43
Cooper County Memorial Hospital	Boonville	93%	28
Washington County Memorial Hospital	Potosi	93%	75
Pike County Memorial Hospital[2]	Louisiana	92%	50

Pregnancy and Delivery Care

Newborns whose Deliveries were Scheduled Early

Hospital Name	City	Rate	Cases
Barnes-Jewish Hospital[2]	Saint Louis	0%	30
Bothwell Regional Health Center	Sedalia	0%	34
Cox Medical Center Branson[2]	Branson	0%	77
Liberty Hospital[2]	Liberty	0%	45
Mercy Hospital Saint Louis[2]	Saint Louis	0%	102
Mercy Hospital Springfield[2]	Springfield	0%	47
Northeast Regional Medical Center[2]	Kirksville	0%	36
Saint Luke's East Lee's Summit Hospital[2]	Lees Summit	0%	26
Saint Luke's Hospital[2]	Chesterfield	0%	73
SSM Saint Marys Health Center[2]	Richmond Hghts	0%	41
Southeast Missouri Hospital	Cape Girardeau	1%	71
Freeman Health System - Freeman West[2]	Joplin	2%	47
Missouri Baptist Medical Center[2]	Town & Country	2%	64
Boone Hospital Center[2]	Columbia	3%	34
Golden Valley Memorial Hospital	Clinton	3%	59
Hannibal Regional Hospital[2]	Hannibal	3%	33
Lake Regional Health System[2]	Osage Beach	3%	67
Mercy Hospital Jefferson	Crystal City	3%	31
Research Medical Center[2]	Kansas City	3%	30
Saint Mary's Health Center[2]	Jefferson City	3%	39
Citizens Memorial Hospital	Bolivar	4%	49
Mercy Hospital Joplin[2]	Joplin	4%	27
Mercy Hospital Lebanon[2]	Lebanon	4%	26
North Kansas City Hospital	N Kansas City	4%	121
SSM Saint Joseph Hospital West[2]	Lake Saint Louis	4%	26
Twin Rivers Regional Medical Center	Kennett	4%	95
Western Missouri Medical Center[2]	Warrensburg	4%	26
Saint Anthony's Medical Center	Saint Louis	5%	128
Saint Luke's Northland Hospital[2]	Kansas City	5%	40
Missouri Delta Medical Center[2]	Sikeston	6%	48
Texas County Memorial Hospital	Houston	6%	50
Mineral Area Regional Medical Center[2]	Farmington	7%	28
SSM Saint Clare Health Center[2]	Fenton	7%	30
Fitzgibbon Hospital	Marshall	8%	40
Missouri Baptist Sullivan Hospital[2]	Sullivan	8%	37
Saint Joseph Medical Center[2]	Kansas City	8%	25
Cox Medical Center[2]	Springfield	9%	54
Saint Francis Medical Center	Cape Girardeau	9%	101
Saint Luke's Hospital of Kansas City[2]	Kansas City	9%	45
Capital Region Medical Center	Jefferson City	13%	86
SSM Depaul Health Center[2]	Bridgeton	13%	31
SSM Saint Joseph Health Center[2]	Saint Charles	17%	29
Saint Francis Hospital & Health Services	Maryville	19%	36
Parkland Health Center[2]	Farmington	23%	26
Poplar Bluff Regional Medical Center[2]	Poplar Bluff	27%	84

Preventive Care

Immunization for Influenza

Hospital Name	City	Rate	Cases
Belton Regional Medical Center[2]	Belton	100%	307
Centerpoint Medical Center[2]	Independence	100%	634
Hedrick Medical Center[2,3]	Chillicothe	100%	144
Lafayette Regional Health Center[2]	Lexington	100%	301
Lee's Summit Medical Center[2]	Lees Summit	100%	425
Moberly Regional Medical Center[2]	Moberly	100%	297
Northeast Regional Medical Center[2]	Kirksville	100%	315
Research Medical Center[2]	Kansas City	100%	630
Saint Mary's Health Center[2]	Jefferson City	100%	545
Bates County Memorial Hospital[2]	Butler	99%	321
Christian Hospital Northeast - Northwest[2]	Saint Louis	99%	584
Des Peres Hospital[2]	Saint Louis	99%	600
Missouri Baptist Medical Center[2]	Town & Country	99%	490
North Kansas City Hospital[2]	N Kansas City	99%	559
SSM Depaul Health Center[2]	Bridgeton	99%	567
SSM Saint Joseph Health Center[2]	Saint Charles	99%	563
SSM Saint Joseph Hospital West[2]	Lake Saint Louis	99%	520
Twin Rivers Regional Medical Center[2]	Kennett	99%	327
Capital Region Medical Center[2]	Jefferson City	98%	505
Heartland Regional Medical Center[2]	Saint Joseph	98%	528
Ozarks Community Hospital	Springfield	98%	276
Poplar Bluff VA Medical Center[2,3]	Poplar Bluff	98%	123
Saint Louis University Hospital[2]	Saint Louis	98%	630
SSM Saint Clare Health Center[2]	Fenton	98%	576
SSM Saint Marys Health Center[2]	Richmond Hghts	98%	543
Mercy Hospital Cassville	Cassville	97%	130
Mercy Hospital Washington[2]	Washington	97%	520
Mineral Area Regional Medical Center[2]	Farmington	97%	452
Missouri Baptist Sullivan Hospital[2]	Sullivan	97%	253
Saint Luke's East Lee's Summit Hospital[2]	Lees Summit	97%	512
Boone Hospital Center[2]	Columbia	96%	517
Ozarks Medical Center[2]	West Plains	96%	978
Truman Medical Center Lakewood[2]	Kansas City	96%	371
Cox Medical Center Branson[2]	Branson	95%	516
Liberty Hospital[2]	Liberty	95%	701
Mercy Hospital Jefferson[2]	Crystal City	95%	578
Poplar Bluff Regional Medical Center[2]	Poplar Bluff	95%	503
Saint Mary's Medical Center[2]	Blue Springs	95%	474
Southeast Health Center of Ripley County[2]	Doniphan	95%	146
Audrain Medical Center[2]	Mexico	94%	261
Freeman Health System - Freeman West[2]	Joplin	94%	525
Lake Regional Health System[2]	Osage Beach	94%	600
Mercy Hospital Joplin[2,3]	Joplin	94%	279

NOTE: Hospital profiles are in alphabetical order by state, then city, then hospital within the city; Rankings exclude hospitals with less than 25 cases except for patient surveys which excludes hospitals with less than 100 cases; (a) 100-299 cases; (1) The number of cases/patients is too few to report; (2) Data submitted were based on a sample of cases/patients; (3) Results are based on a shorter time period than required; (4) Data suppressed by CMS for one or more quarters; (5) Results are not available for this reporting period; (6) Fewer than 100 patients completed the HCAHPS survey; (7) No cases met the criteria for this measure; (8) The lower limit of the confidence interval cannot be calculated if the number of observed infections equals zero; (9) No data are available from the state/territory for this reporting period; (10) The scores shown reflect fewer than 50 completed surveys; (11) There were discrepancies in the data collection process; (12) This measure does not apply to this hospital for this reporting period; (13) Results cannot be calculated for this reporting period; (14) The results for this state are combined with nearby states to protect confidentiality; Please refer to the User's Guide for a full explanation of data.

Hospital Name	City	Rate	Cases
Parkland Health Center[2]	Farmington	94%	331
Phelps County Regional Medical Center[2]	Rolla	94%	416
Saint Francis Hospital & Health Services	Maryville	94%	389
Saint Luke's Hospital[2]	Chesterfield	94%	564
Barnes-Jewish Saint Peters Hospital[2]	Saint Peters	93%	546
Barnes-Jewish West County Hospital[2]	Creve Coeur	93%	306
Missouri Delta Medical Center[2]	Sikeston	93%	381
University of Missouri Health Care[2]	Columbia	93%	658
Nevada Regional Medical Center[2]	Nevada	92%	329
Saint Joseph Medical Center[2]	Kansas City	92%	526
Saint Luke's Northland Hospital[2]	Kansas City	92%	483
Southeast Missouri Hospital[2]	Cape Girardeau	92%	602
Cameron Regional Medical Center[2]	Cameron	91%	329
Progress West Hospital[2]	O Fallon	91%	297
Truman Medical Center Hospital Hill[2]	Kansas City	91%	481
Fitzgibbon Hospital[2]	Marshall	90%	280
Mercy Hospital Saint Louis[2]	Saint Louis	90%	492
Mercy Hospital Springfield[2]	Springfield	90%	535
Saint Anthony's Medical Center[2]	Saint Louis	90%	578
Barnes-Jewish Hospital[2]	Saint Louis	89%	553
Golden Valley Memorial Hospital[2]	Clinton	89%	284
Mercy Hospital Lebanon[2]	Lebanon	89%	271
Bothwell Regional Health Center[2]	Sedalia	88%	502
Cox Medical Center[2]	Springfield	88%	549
Saint Francis Medical Center[2]	Cape Girardeau	87%	570
Wright Memorial Hospital[2]	Trenton	87%	296
Citizens Memorial Hospital[2]	Bolivar	86%	292
Hannibal Regional Hospital[2]	Hannibal	86%	484
Texas County Memorial Hospital[2]	Houston	86%	243
Western Missouri Medical Center[2]	Warrensburg	85%	320
Callaway Community Hospital	Fulton	84%	159
Mercy Hospital Aurora[2]	Aurora	82%	310
Mercy Saint Francis Hospital	Mountain View	82%	171
Saint Luke's Hospital of Kansas City[2]	Kansas City	82%	570
Scotland County Hospital[2]	Memphis	82%	260
Southeasthealth Center of Stoddard County[2]	Dexter	77%	409
Cooper County Memorial Hospital	Boonville	76%	106
Carroll County Memorial Hospital	Carrollton	64%	140
Black River Community Medical Center[2,3]	Poplar Bluff	63%	63
Sac-Osage Hospital[2]	Osceola	54%	134
Saint Alexius Hospital[2]	Saint Louis	49%	439
Pemiscot County Memorial Hospital[2]	Hayti	16%	291

Immunization for Pneumonia

Hospital Name	City	Rate	Cases
Belton Regional Medical Center[2]	Belton	100%	463
Centerpoint Medical Center[2]	Independence	100%	817
Hedrick Medical Center[2,3]	Chillicothe	100%	89
Lafayette Regional Health Center[2]	Lexington	100%	435
Moberly Regional Medical Center[2]	Moberly	100%	398
Northeast Regional Medical Center[2]	Kirksville	100%	350
Research Medical Center[2]	Kansas City	100%	798
Saint Mary's Health Center[2]	Jefferson City	100%	617
SSM Saint Joseph Hospital West[2]	Lake Saint Louis	100%	628
Des Peres Hospital[2]	Saint Louis	99%	857
Lee's Summit Medical Center[2]	Lees Summit	99%	632
Mercy Hospital Lebanon[2]	Lebanon	99%	354
Missouri Baptist Sullivan Hospital[2]	Sullivan	99%	228
North Kansas City Hospital[2]	N Kansas City	99%	761
Poplar Bluff VA Medical Center[2,3]	Poplar Bluff	99%	303
Bates County Memorial Hospital[2]	Butler	98%	498
Bothwell Regional Health Center[2]	Sedalia	98%	666
Capital Region Medical Center[2]	Jefferson City	98%	605
Christian Hospital Northeast - Northwest[2]	Saint Louis	98%	828
Cox Medical Center Branson[2]	Branson	98%	743
Mineral Area Regional Medical Center[2]	Farmington	98%	351
Missouri Baptist Medical Center[2]	Town & Country	98%	612
SSM Depaul Health Center[2]	Bridgeton	98%	757
SSM Saint Joseph Health Center[2]	Saint Charles	98%	764
Twin Rivers Regional Medical Center[2]	Kennett	98%	274
Audrain Medical Center[2]	Mexico	97%	387
Heartland Regional Medical Center[2]	Saint Joseph	97%	622
Mercy Hospital Aurora[2]	Aurora	97%	259
Mercy Hospital Jefferson[2]	Crystal City	97%	813
Mercy Hospital Washington[2]	Washington	97%	685
Poplar Bluff Regional Medical Center[2]	Poplar Bluff	97%	567
Saint Louis University Hospital[2]	Saint Louis	97%	737
Saint Luke's East Lee's Summit Hospital[2]	Lees Summit	97%	608
Southeast Health Center of Ripley County[2]	Doniphan	97%	194
SSM Saint Clare Health Center[2]	Fenton	97%	702
SSM Saint Marys Health Center[2]	Richmond Hghts	97%	446
Fitzgibbon Hospital[2]	Marshall	96%	395
Golden Valley Memorial Hospital[2]	Clinton	96%	365
Liberty Hospital[2]	Liberty	96%	859
Mercy Hospital Cassville	Cassville	96%	194
Progress West Hospital[2]	O Fallon	96%	313
Saint Mary's Medical Center[2]	Blue Springs	96%	582
Boone Hospital Center[2]	Columbia	95%	639
Ozarks Community Hospital	Springfield	95%	440
Phelps County Regional Medical Center[2]	Rolla	95%	533
Saint Luke's Hospital[2]	Chesterfield	95%	749
Barnes-Jewish Saint Peters Hospital[2]	Saint Peters	94%	754
Cameron Regional Medical Center[2]	Cameron	94%	463
Mercy Hospital Joplin[2,3]	Joplin	94%	517
Saint Francis Hospital & Health Services	Maryville	94%	303
Saint Francis Medical Center[2]	Cape Girardeau	93%	762
Saint Joseph Medical Center[2]	Kansas City	93%	715
Saint Luke's Northland Hospital[2]	Kansas City	93%	524
Truman Medical Center Lakewood[2]	Kansas City	93%	241
University of Missouri Health Care[2]	Columbia	93%	600
Barnes-Jewish West County Hospital[2]	Creve Coeur	92%	336
Mercy Hospital Saint Louis[2]	Saint Louis	92%	436
Ozarks Medical Center[2]	West Plains	92%	1425
Freeman Health System - Freeman West[2]	Joplin	91%	602
Lake Regional Health System[2]	Osage Beach	91%	770
Mercy Hospital Springfield[2]	Springfield	91%	660
Mercy Saint Francis Hospital	Mountain View	91%	254
Parkland Health Center[2]	Farmington	91%	439
Saint Anthony's Medical Center[2]	Saint Louis	91%	823
Wright Memorial Hospital[2]	Trenton	91%	317
Citizens Memorial Hospital[2]	Bolivar	90%	365
Cooper County Memorial Hospital	Boonville	90%	164
Missouri Delta Medical Center[2]	Sikeston	90%	456
Texas County Memorial Hospital[2]	Houston	90%	293
Western Missouri Medical Center[2]	Warrensburg	90%	327
Saint Luke's Hospital of Kansas City[2]	Kansas City	89%	705
Truman Medical Center Hospital Hill[2]	Kansas City	89%	458
Barnes-Jewish Hospital[2]	Saint Louis	88%	652
Mercy Mccune Brooks Hospital[2,3]	Carthage	88%	68
Southeasthealth Center of Stoddard County[2]	Dexter	87%	639
Cox Medical Center[2]	Springfield	86%	600
Hannibal Regional Hospital[2]	Hannibal	85%	640
Nevada Regional Medical Center[2]	Nevada	83%	317
Carroll County Memorial Hospital	Carrollton	82%	193
Scotland County Hospital[2]	Memphis	82%	376
Callaway Community Hospital	Fulton	78%	236
Southeast Missouri Hospital[2]	Cape Girardeau	75%	730
Black River Community Medical Center[2,3]	Poplar Bluff	74%	141
Sac-Osage Hospital[2]	Osceola	60%	193
Saint Alexius Hospital[2]	Saint Louis	57%	487
Pemiscot County Memorial Hospital[2]	Hayti	14%	567
SSM Saint Marys Health Center	Richmond Hghts	98%	125
Hannibal Regional Hospital	Hannibal	97%	31
Lake Regional Health System	Osage Beach	97%	66
Mercy Hospital Joplin[2]	Joplin	97%	62
Mercy Hospital Springfield	Springfield	97%	394
Mercy Hospital Washington	Washington	97%	72
North Kansas City Hospital	N Kansas City	97%	146
Saint Anthony's Medical Center	Saint Louis	97%	266
Saint Luke's East Lee's Summit Hospital	Lees Summit	97%	77
Bothwell Regional Health Center	Sedalia	96%	46
Liberty Hospital[2]	Liberty	95%	83
University of Missouri Health Care	Columbia	94%	158
Saint Mary's Health Center	Jefferson City	93%	45
Truman Medical Center Hospital Hill	Kansas City	88%	25

Stroke Care

Anticoagulation Therapy for Atrial Fibrillation

Hospital Name	City	Rate	Cases
Barnes-Jewish Hospital[2]	Saint Louis	100%	92
Boone Hospital Center[2]	Columbia	97%	29
Freeman Health System - Freeman West	Joplin	97%	33
Missouri Baptist Medical Center	Town & Country	97%	35
Saint Luke's Hospital	Chesterfield	97%	32
Saint Luke's Hospital of Kansas City	Kansas City	97%	86
Saint Louis University Hospital[2]	Saint Louis	92%	25
SSM Depaul Health Center	Bridgeton	92%	38
Mercy Hospital Saint Louis	Saint Louis	91%	47
Saint Anthony's Medical Center	Saint Louis	90%	60
Mercy Hospital Springfield	Springfield	89%	76
SSM Saint Clare Health Center	Fenton	88%	34

Antithrombotic Therapy Timing

Hospital Name	City	Rate	Cases
Barnes-Jewish Saint Peters Hospital[2]	Saint Peters	100%	62
Christian Hospital Northeast - Northwest[2]	Saint Louis	100%	177
Cox Medical Center Branson	Branson	100%	59
Heartland Regional Medical Center	Saint Joseph	100%	123
Lee's Summit Medical Center	Lees Summit	100%	38
Mercy Hospital Jefferson	Crystal City	100%	98
Mercy Hospital Saint Louis	Saint Louis	100%	217
Missouri Baptist Medical Center	Town & Country	100%	163
Ozarks Medical Center	West Plains	100%	41
Phelps County Regional Medical Center	Rolla	100%	33
Research Medical Center[2]	Kansas City	100%	73
Saint Joseph Medical Center	Kansas City	100%	73
Saint Luke's Hospital	Chesterfield	100%	122
Saint Mary's Medical Center	Blue Springs	100%	34
Barnes-Jewish Hospital[2]	Saint Louis	99%	412
Boone Hospital Center[2]	Columbia	99%	166
Centerpoint Medical Center[2]	Independence	99%	74
Poplar Bluff Regional Medical Center	Poplar Bluff	99%	96
Saint Francis Medical Center	Cape Girardeau	99%	156
SSM Depaul Health Center	Bridgeton	99%	217
SSM Saint Joseph Hospital West	Lake Saint Louis	99%	88
Capital Region Medical Center	Jefferson City	98%	42
Cox Medical Center[2]	Springfield	98%	87
Freeman Health System - Freeman West	Joplin	98%	172
Saint Louis University Hospital[2]	Saint Louis	98%	129
Saint Luke's Hospital of Kansas City	Kansas City	98%	399
Saint Luke's Northland Hospital	Kansas City	98%	53
Southeast Missouri Hospital	Cape Girardeau	98%	125
SSM Saint Clare Health Center	Fenton	98%	156
SSM Saint Joseph Health Center	Saint Charles	98%	87

Assessed for Rehabilitation

Hospital Name	City	Rate	Cases
Centerpoint Medical Center[2]	Independence	100%	106
Cox Medical Center Branson	Branson	100%	58
Lee's Summit Medical Center	Lees Summit	100%	43
Research Medical Center[2]	Kansas City	100%	106
Saint Francis Medical Center	Cape Girardeau	100%	182
Saint Joseph Medical Center	Kansas City	100%	101
Saint Louis University Hospital[2]	Saint Louis	100%	251
Saint Luke's East Lee's Summit Hospital	Lees Summit	100%	109
Saint Mary's Health Center	Jefferson City	100%	42
SSM Saint Clare Health Center	Fenton	100%	203
SSM Saint Joseph Hospital West	Lake Saint Louis	100%	103
Barnes-Jewish Hospital[2]	Saint Louis	99%	732
Christian Hospital Northeast - Northwest[2]	Saint Louis	99%	179
Heartland Regional Medical Center	Saint Joseph	99%	147
Mercy Hospital Washington	Washington	99%	79
Missouri Baptist Medical Center	Town & Country	99%	210
Saint Luke's Hospital	Chesterfield	99%	164
SSM Depaul Health Center	Bridgeton	99%	338
SSM Saint Marys Health Center	Richmond Hghts	99%	138
Boone Hospital Center[2]	Columbia	98%	228
Cox Medical Center[2]	Springfield	98%	123
Mercy Hospital Saint Louis	Saint Louis	98%	334
Mercy Hospital Springfield	Springfield	98%	571
Ozarks Medical Center	West Plains	98%	62
Phelps County Regional Medical Center	Rolla	98%	45
Saint Anthony's Medical Center	Saint Louis	98%	365
Saint Luke's Hospital of Kansas City	Kansas City	98%	643
Saint Luke's Northland Hospital	Kansas City	98%	61
SSM Saint Joseph Health Center	Saint Charles	98%	106
Hannibal Regional Hospital	Hannibal	97%	33
Mercy Hospital Jefferson	Crystal City	97%	101
Poplar Bluff Regional Medical Center	Poplar Bluff	97%	89
Saint Mary's Medical Center	Blue Springs	97%	37
University of Missouri Health Care	Columbia	97%	255
Lake Regional Health System	Osage Beach	96%	74
Southeast Missouri Hospital	Cape Girardeau	96%	157
Barnes-Jewish Saint Peters Hospital[2]	Saint Peters	95%	83
Truman Medical Center Hospital Hill	Kansas City	95%	39
Freeman Health System - Freeman West	Joplin	94%	201
Mercy Hospital Joplin[2]	Joplin	94%	81
North Kansas City Hospital	N Kansas City	92%	171
Liberty Hospital[2]	Liberty	91%	89
Capital Region Medical Center	Jefferson City	88%	48
Citizens Memorial Hospital	Bolivar	88%	26
Bothwell Regional Health Center	Sedalia	80%	46

Discharged on Antithrombotic Therapy

Hospital Name	City	Rate	Cases
Barnes-Jewish Hospital[2]	Saint Louis	100%	545
Boone Hospital Center[2]	Columbia	100%	197
Capital Region Medical Center	Jefferson City	100%	47
Centerpoint Medical Center[2]	Independence	100%	88
Christian Hospital Northeast - Northwest[2]	Saint Louis	100%	176
Cox Medical Center Branson	Branson	100%	57
Freeman Health System - Freeman West	Joplin	100%	182
Hannibal Regional Hospital	Hannibal	100%	32
Heartland Regional Medical Center	Saint Joseph	100%	129
Lee's Summit Medical Center	Lees Summit	100%	43
Mercy Hospital Jefferson	Crystal City	100%	96
Mercy Hospital Saint Louis	Saint Louis	100%	274
Missouri Baptist Medical Center	Town & Country	100%	191
Research Medical Center[2]	Kansas City	100%	89
Saint Joseph Medical Center	Kansas City	100%	88
Saint Louis University Hospital[2]	Saint Louis	100%	173
Saint Luke's East Lee's Summit Hospital	Lees Summit	100%	106
Saint Luke's Hospital	Chesterfield	100%	148
Saint Luke's Northland Hospital	Kansas City	100%	59
Saint Mary's Health Center	Jefferson City	100%	41
Saint Mary's Medical Center	Blue Springs	100%	34
Southeast Missouri Hospital	Cape Girardeau	100%	131
SSM Depaul Health Center	Bridgeton	100%	295
SSM Saint Clare Health Center	Fenton	100%	182
SSM Saint Joseph Health Center	Saint Charles	100%	92

NOTE: Hospital profiles are in alphabetical order by state, then city, then hospital within the city; Rankings exclude hospitals with less than 25 cases except for patient surveys which excludes hospitals with less than 100 cases; (a) 100-299 cases; (1) The number of cases/patients is too few to report; (2) Data submitted were based on a sample of cases/patients; (3) Results are based on a shorter time period than required; (4) Data suppressed by CMS for one or more quarters; (5) Results are not available for this reporting period; (6) Fewer than 100 patients completed the HCAHPS survey; (7) No cases met the criteria for this measure; (8) The lower limit of the confidence interval cannot be calculated if the number of observed infections equals zero; (9) No data are available from the state/territory for this reporting period; (10) The scores shown reflect fewer than 50 completed surveys; (11) There were discrepancies in the data collection process; (12) This measure does not apply to this hospital for this reporting period; (13) Results cannot be calculated for this reporting period; (14) The results for this state are combined with nearby states to protect confidentiality; Please refer to the User's Guide for a full explanation of data.

Hospital Name	City	Rate	Cases
SSM Saint Marys Health Center	Richmond Hghts	100%	130
University of Missouri Health Care	Columbia	100%	208
Barnes-Jewish Saint Peters Hospital[2]	Saint Peters	99%	81
Lake Regional Health System	Osage Beach	99%	73
Liberty Hospital[2]	Liberty	99%	80
Mercy Hospital Springfield	Springfield	99%	463
Mercy Hospital Washington	Washington	99%	79
North Kansas City Hospital	N Kansas City	99%	152
Poplar Bluff Regional Medical Center	Poplar Bluff	99%	87
Saint Anthony's Medical Center	Saint Louis	99%	329
Saint Francis Medical Center	Cape Girardeau	99%	157
Saint Luke's Hospital of Kansas City	Kansas City	99%	497
SSM Saint Joseph Hospital West	Lake Saint Louis	99%	100
Cox Medical Center[2]	Springfield	98%	102
Ozarks Medical Center	West Plains	98%	57
Phelps County Regional Medical Center	Rolla	98%	43
Bothwell Regional Health Center	Sedalia	96%	46
Mercy Hospital Joplin[2]	Joplin	93%	76
Truman Medical Center Hospital Hill	Kansas City	91%	32

Discharged on Statin Medication

Hospital Name	City	Rate	Cases
Cox Medical Center Branson	Branson	100%	43
Heartland Regional Medical Center	Saint Joseph	100%	109
Lee's Summit Medical Center	Lees Summit	100%	30
Research Medical Center[2]	Kansas City	100%	71
Saint Joseph Medical Center	Kansas City	100%	60
Saint Mary's Health Center	Jefferson City	100%	31
Saint Mary's Medical Center	Blue Springs	100%	25
Barnes-Jewish Hospital[2]	Saint Louis	99%	371
Centerpoint Medical Center[2]	Independence	99%	68
Mercy Hospital Saint Louis	Saint Louis	99%	199
Missouri Baptist Medical Center	Town & Country	99%	149
Saint Louis University Hospital[2]	Saint Louis	99%	131
Saint Luke's East Lee's Summit Hospital	Lees Summit	99%	76
SSM Depaul Health Center	Bridgeton	99%	220
SSM Saint Joseph Hospital West	Lake Saint Louis	99%	77
SSM Saint Marys Health Center	Richmond Hghts	99%	98
Mercy Hospital Jefferson	Crystal City	98%	89
Saint Francis Medical Center	Cape Girardeau	98%	127
Christian Hospital Northeast - Northwest[2]	Saint Louis	97%	143
SSM Saint Joseph Health Center	Saint Charles	97%	71
Cox Medical Center[2]	Springfield	96%	92
Saint Luke's Hospital of Kansas City	Kansas City	96%	367
Southeast Missouri Hospital	Cape Girardeau	96%	115
SSM Saint Clare Health Center	Fenton	96%	128
University of Missouri Health Care	Columbia	96%	156
Barnes-Jewish Saint Peters Hospital[2]	Saint Peters	95%	60
Mercy Hospital Springfield	Springfield	95%	355
Boone Hospital Center[2]	Columbia	94%	158
Saint Anthony's Medical Center	Saint Louis	93%	260
Freeman Health System - Freeman West	Joplin	92%	133
Saint Luke's Hospital	Chesterfield	92%	121
Saint Luke's Northland Hospital	Kansas City	92%	50
Mercy Hospital Washington	Washington	91%	65
Truman Medical Center Hospital Hill	Kansas City	91%	33
North Kansas City Hospital	N Kansas City	90%	122
Lake Regional Health System	Osage Beach	89%	55
Phelps County Regional Medical Center	Rolla	89%	35
Capital Region Medical Center	Jefferson City	87%	39
Liberty Hospital[2]	Liberty	86%	66
Mercy Hospital Joplin[2]	Joplin	86%	56
Ozarks Medical Center	West Plains	86%	43
Hannibal Regional Hospital	Hannibal	81%	27
Poplar Bluff Regional Medical Center	Poplar Bluff	81%	62
Bothwell Regional Health Center	Sedalia	58%	43

Thrombolytic Therapy Timing

Hospital Name	City	Rate	Cases
SSM Depaul Health Center	Bridgeton	97%	33
Saint Luke's Hospital of Kansas City	Kansas City	88%	48
Mercy Hospital Springfield	Springfield	47%	60

Venous Thromboembolism (VTE) Prophylaxis

Hospital Name	City	Rate	Cases
Capital Region Medical Center	Jefferson City	100%	37
Lee's Summit Medical Center	Lees Summit	100%	36
Missouri Baptist Medical Center	Town & Country	100%	184
Research Medical Center[2]	Kansas City	100%	117
Saint Mary's Medical Center	Blue Springs	100%	38
SSM Depaul Health Center	Bridgeton	100%	321
SSM Saint Joseph Hospital West	Lake Saint Louis	100%	93
Centerpoint Medical Center[2]	Independence	99%	107
Christian Hospital Northeast - Northwest[2]	Saint Louis	99%	189
Heartland Regional Medical Center	Saint Joseph	99%	150
SSM Saint Marys Health Center	Richmond Hghts	99%	134
Barnes-Jewish Hospital[2]	Saint Louis	98%	680
Boone Hospital Center[2]	Columbia	98%	223
Cox Medical Center Branson	Branson	98%	61
Saint Joseph Medical Center	Kansas City	98%	103
Saint Louis University Hospital[2]	Saint Louis	98%	260
SSM Saint Clare Health Center	Fenton	98%	204
SSM Saint Joseph Health Center	Saint Charles	98%	111
University of Missouri Health Care	Columbia	98%	265
Cox Medical Center[2]	Springfield	97%	116
Mercy Hospital Jefferson	Crystal City	97%	106
Mercy Hospital Saint Louis	Saint Louis	97%	313
Saint Luke's Hospital of Kansas City	Kansas City	97%	671
Southeast Missouri Hospital	Cape Girardeau	97%	152
Mercy Hospital Springfield	Springfield	96%	580
Saint Francis Medical Center	Cape Girardeau	96%	187
Saint Luke's East Lee's Summit Hospital	Lees Summit	96%	82
Lake Regional Health System	Osage Beach	95%	75
Truman Medical Center Hospital Hill	Kansas City	95%	43
Saint Anthony's Medical Center	Saint Louis	94%	325
Poplar Bluff Regional Medical Center	Poplar Bluff	92%	102
Saint Luke's Northland Hospital	Kansas City	92%	52
Barnes-Jewish Saint Peters Hospital[2]	Saint Peters	91%	79
Mercy Hospital Washington	Washington	91%	79
Liberty Hospital[2]	Liberty	90%	86
Saint Mary's Health Center	Jefferson City	90%	51
Freeman Health System - Freeman West	Joplin	89%	217
Saint Luke's Hospital	Chesterfield	89%	152
Ozarks Medical Center	West Plains	88%	58
Phelps County Regional Medical Center	Rolla	83%	42
Mercy Hospital Joplin[2]	Joplin	78%	73
Hannibal Regional Hospital	Hannibal	67%	33
Bothwell Regional Health Center	Sedalia	58%	48
North Kansas City Hospital	N Kansas City	57%	168

Written Stroke Educational Materials Given

Hospital Name	City	Rate	Cases
Boone Hospital Center[2]	Columbia	100%	132
Capital Region Medical Center	Jefferson City	100%	33
Centerpoint Medical Center[2]	Independence	100%	58
Cox Medical Center Branson	Branson	100%	36
Heartland Regional Medical Center	Saint Joseph	100%	78
Missouri Baptist Medical Center	Town & Country	100%	113
Saint Joseph Medical Center	Kansas City	100%	42
SSM Saint Marys Health Center	Richmond Hghts	100%	53
Barnes-Jewish Hospital[2]	Saint Louis	99%	332
Barnes-Jewish Saint Peters Hospital[2]	Saint Peters	98%	54
Christian Hospital Northeast - Northwest[2]	Saint Louis	98%	97
Poplar Bluff Regional Medical Center	Poplar Bluff	98%	45
Saint Louis University Hospital[2]	Saint Louis	98%	130
SSM Depaul Health Center	Bridgeton	98%	165
SSM Saint Clare Health Center	Fenton	98%	103
SSM Saint Joseph Health Center	Saint Charles	98%	55
Mercy Hospital Jefferson	Crystal City	97%	58
SSM Saint Joseph Hospital West	Lake Saint Louis	97%	61
Mercy Hospital Springfield	Springfield	96%	329
Mercy Hospital Saint Louis	Saint Louis	94%	183
Saint Francis Medical Center	Cape Girardeau	94%	77
Truman Medical Center Hospital Hill	Kansas City	92%	25
Research Medical Center[2]	Kansas City	91%	46
Cox Medical Center[2]	Springfield	90%	70
Saint Luke's Hospital of Kansas City	Kansas City	89%	340
Saint Luke's Hospital	Chesterfield	87%	95
Mercy Hospital Washington	Washington	86%	42
University of Missouri Health Care	Columbia	85%	123
Saint Luke's East Lee's Summit Hospital	Lees Summit	83%	69
Lake Regional Health System	Osage Beach	81%	48
Liberty Hospital[2]	Liberty	79%	61
Ozarks Medical Center	West Plains	79%	39
Saint Anthony's Medical Center	Saint Louis	79%	191
Southeast Missouri Hospital	Cape Girardeau	76%	88
North Kansas City Hospital	N Kansas City	58%	99
Saint Mary's Health Center	Jefferson City	56%	27
Saint Luke's Northland Hospital	Kansas City	55%	40
Freeman Health System - Freeman West	Joplin	43%	110
Mercy Hospital Joplin[2]	Joplin	43%	51

Surgical Care Improvement Project

Appropriate Beta Blocker Usage

Hospital Name	City	Rate	Cases
Belton Regional Medical Center	Belton	100%	49
Cass Regional Medical Center	Harrisonville	100%	29
Christian Hospital Northeast - Northwest[2]	Saint Louis	100%	201
Heartland Regional Medical Center[2]	Saint Joseph	100%	434
Lee's Summit Medical Center	Lees Summit	100%	88
Missouri Delta Medical Center	Sikeston	100%	60
Northeast Regional Medical Center	Kirksville	100%	74
Progress West Hospital[2]	O Fallon	100%	80
Research Medical Center[2]	Kansas City	100%	215
Saint Luke's Hospital of Kansas City[2]	Kansas City	100%	566
Saint Mary's Health Center[2]	Jefferson City	100%	149
Saint Mary's Medical Center[2]	Blue Springs	100%	63
SSM Saint Joseph Health Center[2]	Saint Charles	100%	210
Truman Medical Center Lakewood	Kansas City	100%	49
University of Missouri Health Care[2]	Columbia	100%	302
Barnes-Jewish Hospital[2]	Saint Louis	99%	236
Barnes-Jewish Saint Peters Hospital[2]	Saint Peters	99%	103
Barnes-Jewish West County Hospital[2]	Creve Coeur	99%	107
Capital Region Medical Center[2]	Jefferson City	99%	169
Centerpoint Medical Center[2]	Independence	99%	173
Golden Valley Memorial Hospital	Clinton	99%	72
Lake Regional Health System	Osage Beach	99%	122
Mercy Hospital Joplin[2,3]	Joplin	99%	109
Mercy Hospital Saint Louis[2]	Saint Louis	99%	224
Missouri Baptist Medical Center[2]	Town & Country	99%	206
North Kansas City Hospital[2]	N Kansas City	99%	298
St Louis-John Cochran VA Med Ctr[2]	Saint Louis	99%	93
Saint Louis University Hospital[2]	Saint Louis	99%	139
Saint Luke's East Lee's Summit Hospital	Lees Summit	99%	158
Saint Luke's Hospital[2]	Chesterfield	99%	308
SSM Depaul Health Center[2]	Bridgeton	99%	260
SSM Saint Clare Health Center[2]	Fenton	99%	186
SSM Saint Marys Health Center[2]	Richmond Hghts	99%	172
Cox Medical Center Branson[2]	Branson	98%	80
Freeman Health System - Freeman West[2]	Joplin	98%	314
Mercy Hospital Lebanon[2]	Lebanon	98%	52
Mercy Hospital Springfield[2]	Springfield	98%	247
Mercy Mccune Brooks Hospital[2,3]	Carthage	98%	47
Ozarks Medical Center	West Plains	98%	63
Poplar Bluff Regional Medical Center	Poplar Bluff	98%	167
Saint Anthony's Medical Center[2]	Saint Louis	98%	221
Boone Hospital Center[2]	Columbia	97%	220
Columbia MO VA Medical Center[2]	Columbia	97%	180
Liberty Hospital	Liberty	97%	249
Mercy Hospital Washington[2]	Washington	97%	100
SSM Saint Joseph Hospital West[2]	Lake Saint Louis	97%	98
Mercy Hospital Jefferson	Crystal City	96%	194
Saint Francis Medical Center	Cape Girardeau	96%	400
Saint Joseph Medical Center[2]	Kansas City	96%	153
Southeast Missouri Hospital[2]	Cape Girardeau	96%	241
Cox Medical Center[2]	Springfield	95%	210
Truman Medical Center Hospital Hill[2]	Kansas City	95%	77
Cameron Regional Medical Center	Cameron	94%	33
Des Peres Hospital[2]	Saint Louis	94%	144
Saint Luke's Northland Hospital	Kansas City	94%	88
Hannibal Regional Hospital	Hannibal	93%	222
Phelps County Regional Medical Center	Rolla	93%	107
Western Missouri Medical Center	Warrensburg	93%	57
Audrain Medical Center	Mexico	92%	38
Citizens Memorial Hospital	Bolivar	92%	60
Kansas City VA Medical Center[2]	Kansas City	88%	60
Mineral Area Regional Medical Center	Farmington	82%	38
Bothwell Regional Health Center	Sedalia	79%	100

Appropriate VTP Within 24 Hours

Hospital Name	City	Rate	Cases
Barnes-Jewish West County Hospital[2]	Creve Coeur	100%	457
Belton Regional Medical Center	Belton	100%	287
Boone Hospital Center[2]	Columbia	100%	427
Fitzgibbon Hospital	Marshall	100%	54
Heartland Regional Medical Center[2]	Saint Joseph	100%	704
Lake Regional Health System	Osage Beach	100%	261
Lee's Summit Medical Center	Lees Summit	100%	273
Mercy Hospital Saint Louis[2]	Saint Louis	100%	364
Mercy Mccune Brooks Hospital[2,3]	Carthage	100%	143
Mineral Area Regional Medical Center	Farmington	100%	107
Missouri Baptist Medical Center[2]	Town & Country	100%	437
Missouri Delta Medical Center	Sikeston	100%	162
Moberly Regional Medical Center	Moberly	100%	67
Northeast Regional Medical Center	Kirksville	100%	165
Parkland Health Center	Farmington	100%	66
Perry County Memorial Hospital	Perryville	100%	65
Saint Francis Hospital & Health Services	Maryville	100%	77
Saint Louis University Hospital[2]	Saint Louis	100%	249
Saint Luke's East Lee's Summit Hospital	Lees Summit	100%	503
SSM Saint Joseph Hospital West[2]	Lake Saint Louis	100%	307
Twin Rivers Regional Medical Center	Kennett	100%	80
University of Missouri Health Care[2]	Columbia	100%	606
Barnes-Jewish Hospital[2]	Saint Louis	99%	452
Capital Region Medical Center[2]	Jefferson City	99%	316
Cass Regional Medical Center	Harrisonville	99%	88
Centerpoint Medical Center[2]	Independence	99%	423
Cox Medical Center Branson[2]	Branson	99%	223
Liberty Hospital	Liberty	99%	635
Mercy Hospital Jefferson	Crystal City	99%	400
Phelps County Regional Medical Center	Rolla	99%	344
Progress West Hospital[2]	O Fallon	99%	262
Saint Mary's Health Center[2]	Jefferson City	99%	422
Saint Mary's Medical Center[2]	Blue Springs	99%	234
SSM Depaul Health Center[2]	Bridgeton	99%	446
SSM Saint Joseph Health Center[2]	Saint Charles	99%	350
SSM Saint Marys Health Center[2]	Richmond Hghts	99%	386
Audrain Medical Center	Mexico	98%	97
Barnes-Jewish Saint Peters Hospital[2]	Saint Peters	98%	342
Des Peres Hospital[2]	Saint Louis	98%	293

NOTE: Hospital profiles are in alphabetical order by state, then city, then hospital within the city; Rankings exclude hospitals with less than 25 cases except for patient surveys which excludes hospitals with less than 100 cases; (a) 100-299 cases; (1) The number of cases/patients is too few to report; (2) Data submitted were based on a sample of cases/patients; (3) Results are based on a shorter time period than required; (4) Data suppressed by CMS for one or more quarters; (5) Results are not available for this reporting period; (6) Fewer than 100 patients completed the HCAHPS survey; (7) No cases met the criteria for this measure; (8) The lower limit of the confidence interval cannot be calculated if the number of observed infections equals zero; (9) No data are available from the state/territory for this reporting period; (10) The scores shown reflect fewer than 50 completed surveys; (11) There were discrepancies in the data collection process; (12) This measure does not apply to this hospital for this reporting period; (13) Results cannot be calculated for this reporting period; (14) The results for this state are combined with nearby states to protect confidentiality; Please refer to the User's Guide for a full explanation of data.

Hospital Name	City	Rate	Cases
Freeman Health System - Freeman West[2]	Joplin	98%	601
Golden Valley Memorial Hospital	Clinton	98%	258
Mercy Hospital Lebanon[2]	Lebanon	98%	153
Mercy Hospital Springfield[2]	Springfield	98%	385
Mercy Hospital Washington[2]	Washington	98%	299
Research Medical Center[2]	Kansas City	98%	420
Saint Anthony's Medical Center[2]	Saint Louis	98%	443
Saint Luke's Hospital[2]	Chesterfield	98%	634
Saint Luke's Hospital of Kansas City[2]	Kansas City	98%	551
SSM Saint Clare Health Center[2]	Fenton	98%	366
Western Missouri Medical Center	Warrensburg	98%	171
Christian Hospital Northeast - Northwest[2]	Saint Louis	97%	308
Citizens Memorial Hospital	Bolivar	97%	202
Cox Medical Center[2]	Springfield	97%	379
Lincoln County Medical Center	Troy	97%	29
Mercy Hospital Joplin[2,3]	Joplin	97%	147
North Kansas City Hospital[2]	N Kansas City	97%	514
Poplar Bluff Regional Medical Center	Poplar Bluff	97%	303
Saint Joseph Medical Center[2]	Kansas City	97%	301
Truman Medical Center Hospital Hill[2]	Kansas City	97%	287
Truman Medical Center Lakewood	Kansas City	97%	154
Bates County Memorial Hospital	Butler	96%	26
Columbia MO VA Medical Center[2]	Columbia	96%	171
Kansas City VA Medical Center[2]	Kansas City	96%	192
St Louis-John Cochran VA Med Ctr[2]	Saint Louis	96%	348
Southeast Missouri Hospital[2]	Cape Girardeau	95%	374
Ozarks Medical Center	West Plains	94%	129
Saint Luke's Northland Hospital	Kansas City	94%	267
Hannibal Regional Hospital	Hannibal	93%	443
Saint Francis Medical Center	Cape Girardeau	93%	926
Bothwell Regional Health Center	Sedalia	92%	320
Cameron Regional Medical Center	Cameron	92%	101
Saint Alexius Hospital	Saint Louis	92%	49
Ozarks Community Hospital	Springfield	83%	58

Controlled Postoperative Blood Glucose

Hospital Name	City	Rate	Cases
Missouri Baptist Medical Center[2]	Town & Country	100%	151
Saint Anthony's Medical Center[2]	Saint Louis	100%	136
SSM Saint Joseph Health Center[2]	Saint Charles	100%	95
Cox Medical Center[2]	Springfield	99%	152
Liberty Hospital	Liberty	99%	83
Saint Luke's Hospital of Kansas City[2]	Kansas City	99%	414
Southeast Missouri Hospital[2]	Cape Girardeau	99%	106
SSM Depaul Health Center[2]	Bridgeton	99%	148
SSM Saint Marys Health Center[2]	Richmond Hghts	99%	77
Christian Hospital Northeast - Northwest[2]	Saint Louis	98%	167
North Kansas City Hospital[2]	N Kansas City	98%	157
Poplar Bluff Regional Medical Center	Poplar Bluff	98%	80
Research Medical Center[2]	Kansas City	98%	114
Saint Mary's Health Center[2]	Jefferson City	98%	40
University of Missouri Health Care[2]	Columbia	98%	147
Columbia MO VA Medical Center[2]	Columbia	97%	153
Freeman Health System - Freeman West[2]	Joplin	97%	186
Heartland Regional Medical Center[2]	Saint Joseph	97%	218
Mercy Hospital Saint Louis[2]	Saint Louis	97%	136
Saint Luke's Hospital[2]	Chesterfield	97%	202
SSM Saint Clare Health Center[2]	Fenton	97%	112
Boone Hospital Center[2]	Columbia	96%	138
Mercy Hospital Springfield[2]	Springfield	96%	147
Centerpoint Medical Center[2]	Independence	95%	94
Saint Francis Medical Center	Cape Girardeau	94%	214
Saint Joseph Medical Center[2]	Kansas City	93%	98
Des Peres Hospital[2]	Saint Louis	92%	53
Lake Regional Health System	Osage Beach	92%	39
Mercy Hospital Joplin[2,3]	Joplin	91%	81
Barnes-Jewish Hospital[2]	Saint Louis	90%	125
Capital Region Medical Center[2]	Jefferson City	90%	63
Saint Louis University Hospital[2]	Saint Louis	90%	62
Mercy Hospital Jefferson	Crystal City	87%	52

Perioperative Temperature Management

Hospital Name	City	Rate	Cases
Barnes-Jewish Hospital[2]	Saint Louis	100%	650
Barnes-Jewish Saint Peters Hospital[2]	Saint Peters	100%	370
Barnes-Jewish West County Hospital[2]	Creve Coeur	100%	640
Barton County Memorial Hospital	Lamar	100%	46
Belton Regional Medical Center	Belton	100%	303
Boone Hospital Center[2]	Columbia	100%	563
Cameron Regional Medical Center	Cameron	100%	120
Capital Region Medical Center[2]	Jefferson City	100%	414
Cass Regional Medical Center	Harrisonville	100%	96
Centerpoint Medical Center[2]	Independence	100%	492
Christian Hospital Northeast - Northwest[2]	Saint Louis	100%	407
Citizens Memorial Hospital	Bolivar	100%	218
Columbia MO VA Medical Center[2]	Columbia	100%	202
Cox Medical Center[2]	Springfield	100%	518
Cox Medical Center Branson[2]	Branson	100%	243
Des Peres Hospital[2]	Saint Louis	100%	333
Fitzgibbon Hospital	Marshall	100%	57
Freeman Health System - Freeman West[2]	Joplin	100%	733
Golden Valley Memorial Hospital	Clinton	100%	274
Hannibal Regional Hospital	Hannibal	100%	596
Heartland Regional Medical Center[2]	Saint Joseph	100%	799
Lake Regional Health System	Osage Beach	100%	303
Lee's Summit Medical Center	Lees Summit	100%	316
Liberty Hospital	Liberty	100%	723
Lincoln County Medical Center	Troy	100%	30
Mercy Hospital Jefferson	Crystal City	100%	472
Mercy Hospital Saint Louis[2]	Saint Louis	100%	503
Mercy Hospital Washington[2]	Washington	100%	349
Mercy Mccune Brooks Hospital[2,3]	Carthage	100%	165
Mineral Area Regional Medical Center	Farmington	100%	119
Missouri Baptist Medical Center[2]	Town & Country	100%	576
Missouri Baptist Sullivan Hospital	Sullivan	100%	33
Missouri Delta Medical Center	Sikeston	100%	185
Moberly Regional Medical Center	Moberly	100%	73
North Kansas City Hospital[2]	N Kansas City	100%	614
Northeast Regional Medical Center	Kirksville	100%	194
Ozarks Community Hospital	Springfield	100%	64
Perry County Memorial Hospital	Perryville	100%	73
Phelps County Regional Medical Center	Rolla	100%	385
Poplar Bluff Regional Medical Center	Poplar Bluff	100%	422
Progress West Hospital[2]	O Fallon	100%	273
Research Medical Center[2]	Kansas City	100%	534
Saint Alexius Hospital	Saint Louis	100%	62
Saint Anthony's Medical Center[2]	Saint Louis	100%	574
Saint Francis Hospital & Health Services	Maryville	100%	83
Saint Francis Medical Center	Cape Girardeau	100%	1090
Saint Joseph Medical Center[2]	Kansas City	100%	354
Saint Luke's East Lee's Summit Hospital	Lees Summit	100%	594
Saint Luke's Hospital of Kansas City[2]	Kansas City	100%	696
Saint Mary's Health Center[2]	Jefferson City	100%	455
Saint Mary's Medical Center[2]	Blue Springs	100%	265
Sainte Genevieve County Memorial Hospital	Ste Genevieve	100%	42
Scotland County Hospital	Memphis	100%	29
Southeast Missouri Hospital[2]	Cape Girardeau	100%	529
SSM Depaul Health Center[2]	Bridgeton	100%	527
SSM Saint Clare Health Center[2]	Fenton	100%	462
SSM Saint Joseph Health Center[2]	Saint Charles	100%	435
SSM Saint Joseph Hospital West[2]	Lake Saint Louis	100%	334
SSM Saint Marys Health Center[2]	Richmond Hghts	100%	500
Truman Medical Center Hospital Hill[2]	Kansas City	100%	350
Truman Medical Center Lakewood	Kansas City	100%	223
Twin Rivers Regional Medical Center	Kennett	100%	83
University of Missouri Health Care[2]	Columbia	100%	755
Western Missouri Medical Center	Warrensburg	100%	199
Bothwell Regional Health Center	Sedalia	99%	368
Kansas City VA Medical Center[2]	Kansas City	99%	215
Mercy Hospital Joplin[2,3]	Joplin	99%	211
Mercy Hospital Springfield[2]	Springfield	99%	540
Parkland Health Center	Farmington	99%	74
St Louis-John Cochran VA Med Ctr[2]	Saint Louis	99%	374
Saint Louis University Hospital[2]	Saint Louis	99%	301
Mercy Hospital Lebanon[2]	Lebanon	98%	168
Ozarks Medical Center	West Plains	98%	170
Saint Luke's Hospital[2]	Chesterfield	98%	842
Bates County Memorial Hospital	Butler	96%	28
Audrain Medical Center	Mexico	95%	131
Saint Luke's Northland Hospital	Kansas City	94%	298

Prophylactic Antibiotic Selection

Hospital Name	City	Rate	Cases
Barnes-Jewish West County Hospital[2]	Creve Coeur	100%	437
Bates County Memorial Hospital	Butler	100%	26
Belton Regional Medical Center	Belton	100%	255
Boone Hospital Center[2]	Columbia	100%	536
Cass Regional Medical Center	Harrisonville	100%	79
Columbia MO VA Medical Center	Columbia	100%	264
Des Peres Hospital[2]	Saint Louis	100%	231
Fitzgibbon Hospital	Marshall	100%	52
Freeman Health System - Freeman West[2]	Joplin	100%	656
Heartland Regional Medical Center[2]	Saint Joseph	100%	792
Kansas City VA Medical Center	Kansas City	100%	116
Lake Regional Health System	Osage Beach	100%	222
Lee's Summit Medical Center	Lees Summit	100%	220
Liberty Hospital	Liberty	100%	501
Mercy Hospital Lebanon[2]	Lebanon	100%	134
Mercy Hospital Saint Louis[2]	Saint Louis	100%	442
Mercy Hospital Springfield[2]	Springfield	100%	478
Mercy Hospital Washington[2]	Washington	100%	203
Moberly Regional Medical Center	Moberly	100%	47
North Kansas City Hospital[2]	N Kansas City	100%	524
Northeast Regional Medical Center	Kirksville	100%	120
Perry County Memorial Hospital	Perryville	100%	62
Poplar Bluff Regional Medical Center	Poplar Bluff	100%	316
Progress West Hospital[2]	O Fallon	100%	222
Research Medical Center[2]	Kansas City	100%	432
Saint Anthony's Medical Center[2]	Saint Louis	100%	513
Saint Francis Hospital & Health Services	Maryville	100%	66
Saint Luke's Hospital[2]	Chesterfield	100%	703
Saint Luke's Northland Hospital	Kansas City	100%	186
Saint Mary's Health Center[2]	Jefferson City	100%	354
Sainte Genevieve County Memorial Hospital	Ste Genevieve	100%	34
SSM Saint Clare Health Center[2]	Fenton	100%	356
SSM Saint Joseph Health Center[2]	Saint Charles	100%	328
SSM Saint Joseph Hospital West[2]	Lake Saint Louis	100%	191
Truman Medical Center Hospital Hill[2]	Kansas City	100%	238
Twin Rivers Regional Medical Center	Kennett	100%	55
University of Missouri Health Care[2]	Columbia	100%	571
Audrain Medical Center	Mexico	99%	101
Barnes-Jewish Hospital[2]	Saint Louis	99%	416
Barnes-Jewish Saint Peters Hospital[2]	Saint Peters	99%	237
Centerpoint Medical Center[2]	Independence	99%	364
Christian Hospital Northeast - Northwest[2]	Saint Louis	99%	336
Citizens Memorial Hospital	Bolivar	99%	184
Cox Medical Center[2]	Springfield	99%	490
Cox Medical Center Branson[2]	Branson	99%	174
Golden Valley Memorial Hospital	Clinton	99%	210
Hannibal Regional Hospital	Hannibal	99%	470
Mercy Hospital Jefferson	Crystal City	99%	333
Missouri Baptist Medical Center[2]	Town & Country	99%	522
Phelps County Regional Medical Center	Rolla	99%	267
St Louis-John Cochran VA Med Ctr	Saint Louis	99%	249
Saint Louis University Hospital[2]	Saint Louis	99%	129
Saint Luke's East Lee's Summit Hospital	Lees Summit	99%	344
Saint Luke's Hospital of Kansas City[2]	Kansas City	99%	788
Southeast Missouri Hospital[2]	Cape Girardeau	99%	396
SSM Depaul Health Center[2]	Bridgeton	99%	472
SSM Saint Marys Health Center[2]	Richmond Hghts	99%	385
Truman Medical Center Lakewood	Kansas City	99%	169
Capital Region Medical Center[2]	Jefferson City	98%	320
Mercy Hospital Joplin[2,3]	Joplin	98%	181
Mercy Mccune Brooks Hospital[2,3]	Carthage	98%	122
Mineral Area Regional Medical Center	Farmington	98%	81
Missouri Delta Medical Center	Sikeston	98%	116
Ozarks Community Hospital	Springfield	98%	53
Ozarks Medical Center	West Plains	98%	122
Parkland Health Center	Farmington	98%	65
Saint Francis Medical Center	Cape Girardeau	98%	866
Saint Joseph Medical Center[2]	Kansas City	98%	318
Saint Mary's Medical Center[2]	Blue Springs	97%	175
Saint Alexius Hospital	Saint Louis	94%	36
Western Missouri Medical Center	Warrensburg	90%	155
Bothwell Regional Health Center	Sedalia	89%	250
Cameron Regional Medical Center	Cameron	86%	85

Prophylactic Antibiotic Selection (Outpatient)

Hospital Name	City	Rate	Cases
Belton Regional Medical Center	Belton	100%	55
Mercy Hospital Washington	Washington	100%	271
Missouri Delta Medical Center	Sikeston	100%	86
Nevada Regional Medical Center	Nevada	100%	38
SSM Saint Joseph Health Center	Saint Charles	100%	446
Audrain Medical Center	Mexico	99%	182
Barnes-Jewish Hospital	Saint Louis	99%	766
Barnes-Jewish West County Hospital	Creve Coeur	99%	282
Boone Hospital Center	Columbia	99%	729
Centerpoint Medical Center	Independence	99%	395
Christian Hospital Northeast - Northwest	Saint Louis	99%	377
Des Peres Hospital	Saint Louis	99%	422
Freeman Health System - Freeman West	Joplin	99%	581
Heartland Regional Medical Center	Saint Joseph	99%	568
Lee's Summit Medical Center	Lees Summit	99%	142
Mercy Hospital Jefferson	Crystal City	99%	128
Mercy Hospital Joplin[3]	Joplin	99%	188
Mercy Hospital Saint Louis	Saint Louis	99%	888
Mercy Hospital Springfield	Springfield	99%	756
Missouri Baptist Sullivan Hospital	Sullivan	99%	80
Moberly Regional Medical Center	Moberly	99%	102
Northeast Regional Medical Center	Kirksville	99%	113
Research Medical Center	Kansas City	99%	539
Saint Louis University Hospital	Saint Louis	99%	170
Saint Luke's East Lee's Summit Hospital	Lees Summit	99%	299
Saint Luke's Hospital	Chesterfield	99%	924
Saint Luke's Hospital of Kansas City	Kansas City	99%	578
Saint Mary's Health Center	Jefferson City	99%	285
SSM Depaul Health Center	Bridgeton	99%	461
SSM Saint Clare Health Center	Fenton	99%	422
SSM Saint Joseph Hospital West	Lake Saint Louis	99%	236
SSM Saint Marys Health Center	Richmond Hghts	99%	493
University of Missouri Health Care	Columbia	99%	592
Cox Medical Center	Springfield	98%	794
Cox Medical Center Branson	Branson	98%	122
Hannibal Regional Hospital	Hannibal	98%	98
Lake Regional Health System	Osage Beach	98%	177
Liberty Hospital	Liberty	98%	295
Mercy Hospital Lebanon	Lebanon	98%	45
Missouri Baptist Medical Center	Town & Country	98%	633
North Kansas City Hospital	N Kansas City	98%	641
Phelps County Regional Medical Center	Rolla	98%	170
Progress West Hospital	O Fallon	98%	40

NOTE: Hospital profiles are in alphabetical order by state, then city, then hospital within the city; Rankings exclude hospitals with less than 25 cases except for patient surveys which excludes hospitals with less than 100 cases; (a) 100-299 cases; (1) The number of cases/patients is too few to report; (2) Data submitted were based on a sample of cases/patients; (3) Results are based on a shorter time period than required; (4) Data suppressed by CMS for one or more quarters; (5) Results are not available for this reporting period; (6) Fewer than 100 patients completed the HCAHPS survey; (7) No cases met the criteria for this measure; (8) The lower limit of the confidence interval cannot be calculated if the number of observed infections equals zero; (9) No data are available from the state/territory for this reporting period; (10) The scores shown reflect fewer than 50 completed surveys; (11) There were discrepancies in the data collection process; (12) This measure does not apply to this hospital for this reporting period; (13) Results cannot be calculated for this reporting period; (14) The results for this state are combined with nearby states to protect confidentiality; Please refer to the User's Guide for a full explanation of data.

Hospital Name	City	Rate	Cases
Saint Anthony's Medical Center	Saint Louis	98%	685
Southeast Missouri Hospital	Cape Girardeau	98%	555
Western Missouri Medical Center	Warrensburg	98%	53
Capital Region Medical Center	Jefferson City	97%	219
Citizens Memorial Hospital	Bolivar	97%	149
Parkland Health Center	Farmington	97%	60
Truman Medical Center Hospital Hill	Kansas City	97%	187
Mineral Area Regional Medical Center	Farmington	96%	26
Poplar Bluff Regional Medical Center	Poplar Bluff	96%	312
Saint Francis Medical Center	Cape Girardeau	96%	670
Saint Joseph Medical Center	Kansas City	96%	320
Saint Francis Hospital & Health Services	Maryville	95%	38
Ozarks Community Hospital	Springfield	94%	52
Saint Luke's Northland Hospital	Kansas City	94%	53
Barnes-Jewish Saint Peters Hospital	Saint Peters	92%	100
Ozarks Medical Center	West Plains	89%	183
Bothwell Regional Health Center	Sedalia	88%	156
Mercy Mccune Brooks Hospital[3]	Carthage	88%	51
Saint Alexius Hospital	Saint Louis	87%	45

Prophylactic Antibiotic Stopped

Hospital Name	City	Rate	Cases
Barnes-Jewish Hospital[2]	Saint Louis	100%	400
Barnes-Jewish West County Hospital[2]	Creve Coeur	100%	433
Belton Regional Medical Center	Belton	100%	254
Heartland Regional Medical Center[2]	Saint Joseph	100%	749
Lee's Summit Medical Center	Lees Summit	100%	215
Missouri Baptist Medical Center[2]	Town & Country	100%	506
Ozarks Community Hospital	Springfield	100%	53
Perry County Memorial Hospital	Perryville	100%	61
Saint Luke's East Lee's Summit Hospital	Lees Summit	100%	335
Sainte Genevieve County Memorial Hospital	Ste Genevieve	100%	33
SSM Saint Joseph Hospital West[2]	Lake Saint Louis	100%	187
Truman Medical Center Lakewood	Kansas City	100%	169
Barnes-Jewish Saint Peters Hospital[2]	Saint Peters	99%	232
Cass Regional Medical Center	Harrisonville	99%	78
Centerpoint Medical Center[2]	Independence	99%	349
Citizens Memorial Hospital	Bolivar	99%	182
Columbia MO VA Medical Center	Columbia	99%	264
Cox Medical Center Branson[2]	Branson	99%	167
Freeman Health System - Freeman West[2]	Joplin	99%	637
Mercy Hospital Springfield[2]	Springfield	99%	464
Missouri Delta Medical Center	Sikeston	99%	107
Saint Anthony's Medical Center[2]	Saint Louis	99%	505
Saint Luke's Northland Hospital	Kansas City	99%	181
Saint Mary's Health Center[2]	Jefferson City	99%	345
Saint Mary's Medical Center[2]	Blue Springs	99%	175
SSM Depaul Health Center[2]	Bridgeton	99%	454
SSM Saint Clare Health Center[2]	Fenton	99%	344
SSM Saint Joseph Health Center[2]	Saint Charles	99%	312
Truman Medical Center Hospital Hill[2]	Kansas City	99%	234
University of Missouri Health Care[2]	Columbia	99%	547
Western Missouri Medical Center	Warrensburg	99%	149
Boone Hospital Center[2]	Columbia	98%	534
Christian Hospital Northeast - Northwest[2]	Saint Louis	98%	303
Golden Valley Memorial Hospital	Clinton	98%	207
Liberty Hospital	Liberty	98%	489
Mercy Hospital Joplin[2,3]	Joplin	98%	171
Mercy Hospital Saint Louis[2]	Saint Louis	98%	431
Mercy Hospital Washington[2]	Washington	98%	196
Moberly Regional Medical Center	Moberly	98%	44
North Kansas City Hospital[2]	N Kansas City	98%	500
Poplar Bluff Regional Medical Center	Poplar Bluff	98%	286
Research Medical Center[2]	Kansas City	98%	404
Saint Louis University Hospital[2]	Saint Louis	98%	115
Saint Luke's Hospital of Kansas City[2]	Kansas City	98%	770
SSM Saint Marys Health Center[2]	Richmond Hghts	98%	369
Twin Rivers Regional Medical Center	Kennett	98%	53
Bothwell Regional Health Center	Sedalia	97%	246
Capital Region Medical Center[2]	Jefferson City	97%	307
Cox Medical Center[2]	Springfield	97%	485
Des Peres Hospital[2]	Saint Louis	97%	212
Hannibal Regional Hospital	Hannibal	97%	461
Mercy Hospital Lebanon[2]	Lebanon	97%	134
Phelps County Regional Medical Center	Rolla	97%	261
Progress West Hospital[2]	O Fallon	97%	215
Saint Francis Medical Center	Cape Girardeau	97%	853
Southeast Missouri Hospital[2]	Cape Girardeau	97%	386
Fitzgibbon Hospital	Marshall	96%	49
Kansas City VA Medical Center	Kansas City	96%	114
Mercy Hospital Jefferson	Crystal City	96%	313
Northeast Regional Medical Center	Kirksville	96%	105
Saint Joseph Medical Center[2]	Kansas City	96%	312
Saint Luke's Hospital[2]	Chesterfield	96%	684
Saint Francis Hospital & Health Services	Maryville	95%	65
St Louis-John Cochran VA Med Ctr	Saint Louis	95%	248
Lake Regional Health System	Osage Beach	94%	212
Mineral Area Regional Medical Center	Farmington	94%	79
Ozarks Medical Center	West Plains	94%	117
Cameron Regional Medical Center	Cameron	93%	82
Parkland Health Center	Farmington	93%	61
Bates County Memorial Hospital	Butler	92%	25
Mercy Mccune Brooks Hospital[2,3]	Carthage	91%	120
Saint Alexius Hospital	Saint Louis	88%	32
Audrain Medical Center	Mexico	87%	99

Prophylactic Antibiotic Timing

Hospital Name	City	Rate	Cases
Belton Regional Medical Center	Belton	100%	255
Bothwell Regional Health Center	Sedalia	100%	250
Capital Region Medical Center[2]	Jefferson City	100%	320
Cass Regional Medical Center	Harrisonville	100%	79
Centerpoint Medical Center[2]	Independence	100%	364
Cox Medical Center Branson[2]	Branson	100%	174
Heartland Regional Medical Center[2]	Saint Joseph	100%	795
Lee's Summit Medical Center	Lees Summit	100%	220
Mercy Hospital Jefferson	Crystal City	100%	333
Mercy Hospital Springfield[2]	Springfield	100%	479
Missouri Delta Medical Center	Sikeston	100%	116
Moberly Regional Medical Center	Moberly	100%	47
North Kansas City Hospital[2]	N Kansas City	100%	525
Northeast Regional Medical Center	Kirksville	100%	120
Perry County Memorial Hospital	Perryville	100%	62
Progress West Hospital[2]	O Fallon	100%	222
Research Medical Center[2]	Kansas City	100%	433
Saint Luke's East Lee's Summit Hospital	Lees Summit	100%	344
Saint Luke's Hospital of Kansas City[2]	Kansas City	100%	788
Saint Mary's Health Center[2]	Jefferson City	100%	354
Sainte Genevieve County Memorial Hospital	Ste Genevieve	100%	34
SSM Saint Joseph Hospital West[2]	Lake Saint Louis	100%	192
SSM Saint Marys Health Center[2]	Richmond Hghts	100%	385
Truman Medical Center Hospital Hill[2]	Kansas City	100%	239
Barnes-Jewish West County Hospital[2]	Creve Coeur	99%	437
Boone Hospital Center[2]	Columbia	99%	536
Cameron Regional Medical Center	Cameron	99%	85
Christian Hospital Northeast - Northwest[2]	Saint Louis	99%	336
Des Peres Hospital[2]	Saint Louis	99%	231
Freeman Health System - Freeman West[2]	Joplin	99%	656
Golden Valley Memorial Hospital	Clinton	99%	211
Kansas City VA Medical Center	Kansas City	99%	116
Lake Regional Health System	Osage Beach	99%	222
Mercy Hospital Lebanon[2]	Lebanon	99%	134
Mercy Hospital Saint Louis[2]	Saint Louis	99%	443
Mercy Hospital Washington[2]	Washington	99%	203
Mineral Area Regional Medical Center	Farmington	99%	81
Phelps County Regional Medical Center	Rolla	99%	267
Saint Anthony's Medical Center[2]	Saint Louis	99%	515
Saint Joseph Medical Center[2]	Kansas City	99%	318
Saint Louis University Hospital[2]	Saint Louis	99%	130
Saint Luke's Hospital[2]	Chesterfield	99%	704
Saint Mary's Medical Center[2]	Blue Springs	99%	176
SSM Saint Clare Health Center[2]	Fenton	99%	358
SSM Saint Joseph Health Center[2]	Saint Charles	99%	328
Truman Medical Center Lakewood	Kansas City	99%	169
University of Missouri Health Care[2]	Columbia	99%	572
Audrain Medical Center	Mexico	98%	101
Citizens Memorial Hospital	Bolivar	98%	184
Columbia MO VA Medical Center	Columbia	98%	265
Cox Medical Center[2]	Springfield	98%	492
Hannibal Regional Hospital	Hannibal	98%	470
Missouri Baptist Medical Center[2]	Town & Country	98%	522
Ozarks Medical Center	West Plains	98%	122
Saint Francis Medical Center	Cape Girardeau	98%	867
Saint Luke's Northland Hospital	Kansas City	98%	186
SSM Depaul Health Center[2]	Bridgeton	98%	472
Twin Rivers Regional Medical Center	Kennett	98%	55
Barnes-Jewish Hospital[2]	Saint Louis	97%	419
Barnes-Jewish Saint Peters Hospital[2]	Saint Peters	97%	238
Liberty Hospital	Liberty	97%	501
Poplar Bluff Regional Medical Center	Poplar Bluff	97%	319
Southeast Missouri Hospital[2]	Cape Girardeau	97%	402
Bates County Memorial Hospital	Butler	96%	26
St Louis-John Cochran VA Med Ctr	Saint Louis	96%	254
Western Missouri Medical Center	Warrensburg	96%	157
Parkland Health Center	Farmington	95%	65
Mercy Hospital Joplin[2,3]	Joplin	94%	183
Saint Alexius Hospital	Saint Louis	94%	36
Saint Francis Hospital & Health Services	Maryville	92%	66
Ozarks Community Hospital	Springfield	91%	53
Fitzgibbon Hospital	Marshall	88%	52
Mercy Mccune Brooks Hospital[2,3]	Carthage	88%	123

Prophylactic Antibiotic Timing (Outpatient)

Hospital Name	City	Rate	Cases
Belton Regional Medical Center	Belton	100%	55
Boone Hospital Center	Columbia	100%	729
Centerpoint Medical Center	Independence	100%	395
Heartland Regional Medical Center	Saint Joseph	100%	569
Mercy Hospital Jefferson	Crystal City	100%	128
Mineral Area Regional Medical Center	Farmington	100%	26
Missouri Delta Medical Center	Sikeston	100%	86
Northeast Regional Medical Center	Kirksville	100%	97
Ozarks Community Hospital	Springfield	100%	52
Progress West Hospital	O Fallon	100%	40
Saint Luke's East Lee's Summit Hospital	Lees Summit	100%	299
Saint Mary's Health Center	Jefferson City	100%	285
SSM Saint Joseph Health Center	Saint Charles	100%	447
SSM Saint Joseph Hospital West	Lake Saint Louis	100%	236
University of Missouri Health Care	Columbia	100%	515
Barnes-Jewish Saint Peters Hospital	Saint Peters	99%	100
Barnes-Jewish West County Hospital	Creve Coeur	99%	282
Capital Region Medical Center	Jefferson City	99%	219
Christian Hospital Northeast - Northwest	Saint Louis	99%	377
Cox Medical Center	Springfield	99%	798
Lake Regional Health System	Osage Beach	99%	177
Lee's Summit Medical Center	Lees Summit	99%	143
Mercy Hospital Saint Louis	Saint Louis	99%	884
Mercy Hospital Springfield	Springfield	99%	756
Mercy Hospital Washington	Washington	99%	272
Missouri Baptist Medical Center	Town & Country	99%	637
Missouri Baptist Sullivan Hospital	Sullivan	99%	74
Moberly Regional Medical Center	Moberly	99%	103
North Kansas City Hospital	N Kansas City	99%	643
Research Medical Center	Kansas City	99%	533
Saint Anthony's Medical Center	Saint Louis	99%	688
SSM Saint Clare Health Center	Fenton	99%	422
SSM Saint Marys Health Center	Richmond Hghts	99%	493
Audrain Medical Center	Mexico	98%	182
Citizens Memorial Hospital	Bolivar	98%	151
Des Peres Hospital	Saint Louis	98%	422
Freeman Health System - Freeman West	Joplin	98%	584
Mercy Hospital Lebanon	Lebanon	98%	46
Poplar Bluff Regional Medical Center	Poplar Bluff	98%	314
Saint Francis Medical Center	Cape Girardeau	98%	676
Saint Joseph Medical Center	Kansas City	98%	320
Saint Luke's Hospital	Chesterfield	98%	930
Saint Luke's Hospital of Kansas City	Kansas City	98%	580
Saint Luke's Northland Hospital	Kansas City	98%	54
Southeast Missouri Hospital	Cape Girardeau	98%	557
Barnes-Jewish Hospital	Saint Louis	97%	773
Liberty Hospital	Liberty	97%	297
Ozarks Medical Center	West Plains	97%	184
Parkland Health Center	Farmington	97%	60
Saint Louis University Hospital	Saint Louis	97%	172
SSM Depaul Health Center	Bridgeton	97%	471
Hannibal Regional Hospital	Hannibal	95%	101
Phelps County Regional Medical Center	Rolla	95%	177
Truman Medical Center Hospital Hill	Kansas City	95%	149
Cox Medical Center Branson	Branson	94%	126
Mercy Hospital Joplin[3]	Joplin	94%	191
Nevada Regional Medical Center	Nevada	94%	31
Western Missouri Medical Center	Warrensburg	93%	54
Bothwell Regional Health Center	Sedalia	92%	159
Saint Francis Hospital & Health Services	Maryville	92%	39
Truman Medical Center Lakewood	Kansas City	92%	26
Mercy Mccune Brooks Hospital[3]	Carthage	83%	52
Saint Alexius Hospital	Saint Louis	79%	39

Urinary Catheter Removal

Hospital Name	City	Rate	Cases
Belton Regional Medical Center	Belton	100%	267
Capital Region Medical Center[2]	Jefferson City	100%	284
Fitzgibbon Hospital	Marshall	100%	45
Golden Valley Memorial Hospital	Clinton	100%	184
Heartland Regional Medical Center[2]	Saint Joseph	100%	663
Lee's Summit Medical Center	Lees Summit	100%	87
Lincoln County Medical Center	Troy	100%	28
Mercy Mccune Brooks Hospital[2,3]	Carthage	100%	38
Missouri Baptist Medical Center[2]	Town & Country	100%	419
Moberly Regional Medical Center	Moberly	100%	33
Northeast Regional Medical Center	Kirksville	100%	128
Perry County Memorial Hospital	Perryville	100%	63
Progress West Hospital[2]	O Fallon	100%	163
Saint Mary's Health Center[2]	Jefferson City	100%	355
Truman Medical Center Lakewood	Kansas City	100%	38
University of Missouri Health Care[2]	Columbia	100%	528
Barnes-Jewish West County Hospital[2]	Creve Coeur	99%	305
Cass Regional Medical Center	Harrisonville	99%	87
Centerpoint Medical Center[2]	Independence	99%	243
Christian Hospital Northeast - Northwest[2]	Saint Louis	99%	205
Columbia MO VA Medical Center[2]	Columbia	99%	195
Cox Medical Center Branson[2]	Branson	99%	205
Lake Regional Health System	Osage Beach	99%	239
Mercy Hospital Jefferson	Crystal City	99%	151
Mercy Hospital Lebanon[2]	Lebanon	99%	142
Mercy Hospital Saint Louis[2]	Saint Louis	99%	302
Mercy Hospital Springfield[2]	Springfield	99%	298
Missouri Delta Medical Center	Sikeston	99%	124
Research Medical Center[2]	Kansas City	99%	293
Saint Luke's Hospital of Kansas City[2]	Kansas City	99%	554
Saint Mary's Medical Center[2]	Blue Springs	99%	140
SSM Saint Clare Health Center[2]	Fenton	99%	287

NOTE: Hospital profiles are in alphabetical order by state, then city, then hospital within the city; Rankings exclude hospitals with less than 25 cases except for patient surveys which excludes hospitals with less than 100 cases; (a) 100-299 cases; (1) The number of cases/patients is too few to report; (2) Data submitted were based on a sample of cases/patients; (3) Results are based on a shorter time period than required; (4) Data suppressed by CMS for one or more quarters; (5) Results are not available for this reporting period; (6) Fewer than 100 patients completed the HCAHPS survey; (7) No cases met the criteria for this measure; (8) The lower limit of the confidence interval cannot be calculated if the number of observed infections equals zero; (9) No data are available from the state/territory for this reporting period; (10) The scores shown reflect fewer than 50 completed surveys; (11) There were discrepancies in the data collection process; (12) This measure does not apply to this hospital for this reporting period; (13) Results cannot be calculated for this reporting period; (14) The results for this state are combined with nearby states to protect confidentiality; Please refer to the User's Guide for a full explanation of data.

SSM Saint Joseph Health Center[2]	Saint Charles	99%	276
SSM Saint Joseph Hospital West[2]	Lake Saint Louis	99%	191
Western Missouri Medical Center	Warrensburg	99%	155
Barnes-Jewish Hospital[2]	Saint Louis	98%	396
Boone Hospital Center[2]	Columbia	98%	527
Citizens Memorial Hospital	Bolivar	98%	189
Mercy Hospital Washington[2]	Washington	98%	255
Mineral Area Regional Medical Center	Farmington	98%	89
North Kansas City Hospital[2]	N Kansas City	98%	428
St Louis-John Cochran VA Med Ctr[2]	Saint Louis	98%	234
Saint Louis University Hospital[2]	Saint Louis	98%	169
Twin Rivers Regional Medical Center	Kennett	98%	42
Barton County Memorial Hospital	Lamar	97%	36
Des Peres Hospital[2]	Saint Louis	97%	256
SSM Depaul Health Center[2]	Bridgeton	97%	146
SSM Saint Marys Health Center[2]	Richmond Hghts	97%	158
Kansas City VA Medical Center[2]	Kansas City	96%	134
Mercy Hospital Joplin[2,3]	Joplin	96%	166
Ozarks Community Hospital	Springfield	96%	50
Phelps County Regional Medical Center	Rolla	96%	296
Saint Francis Hospital & Health Services	Maryville	96%	54
Saint Luke's East Lee's Summit Hospital	Lees Summit	96%	142
Saint Luke's Hospital[2]	Chesterfield	96%	408
Barnes-Jewish Saint Peters Hospital[2]	Saint Peters	95%	235
Liberty Hospital	Liberty	95%	267
Parkland Health Center	Farmington	95%	55
Freeman Health System - Freeman West[2]	Joplin	93%	395
Poplar Bluff Regional Medical Center	Poplar Bluff	93%	259
Saint Anthony's Medical Center[2]	Saint Louis	93%	270
Saint Francis Medical Center	Cape Girardeau	93%	665
Southeast Missouri Hospital[2]	Cape Girardeau	93%	315
Truman Medical Center Hospital Hill[2]	Kansas City	92%	145
Cox Medical Center[2]	Springfield	91%	289
Ozarks Medical Center	West Plains	91%	105
Saint Luke's Northland Hospital	Kansas City	91%	149
Hannibal Regional Hospital	Hannibal	90%	135
Saint Joseph Medical Center[2]	Kansas City	90%	182
Bothwell Regional Health Center	Sedalia	86%	210
Cameron Regional Medical Center	Cameron	86%	86
Saint Alexius Hospital	Saint Louis	38%	39

Survey of Patients' Hospital Experiences

Area Around Room 'Always' Quiet at Night

Hospital Name	City	Rate	Cases
Wright Memorial Hospital	Trenton	76%	(a)
SSM Saint Clare Health Center[11]	Fenton	74%	300+
Barton County Memorial Hospital	Lamar	73%	(a)
Nevada Regional Medical Center	Nevada	73%	(a)
Cooper County Memorial Hospital	Boonville	72%	(a)
Christian Hospital Northeast - Northwest	Saint Louis	71%	300+
Cass Regional Medical Center	Harrisonville	70%	300+
Missouri Delta Medical Center	Sikeston	70%	300+
Saint Francis Hospital & Health Services	Maryville	70%	(a)
Western Missouri Medical Center	Warrensburg	70%	300+
Capital Region Medical Center	Jefferson City	68%	300+
Missouri Baptist Sullivan Hospital	Sullivan	68%	300+
University of Missouri Health Care	Columbia	68%	300+
Hedrick Medical Center	Chillicothe	67%	(a)
Saint Luke's Hospital of Kansas City	Kansas City	67%	300+
Community Hospital Association	Fairfax	66%	(a)
Freeman Neosho Hospital	Neosho	66%	(a)
Lee's Summit Medical Center	Lees Summit	66%	300+
Ozarks Community Hospital	Springfield	66%	(a)
Research Medical Center	Kansas City	66%	300+
Southeast Missouri Hospital	Cape Girardeau	66%	300+
Truman Medical Center Hospital Hill	Kansas City	66%	300+
Mercy Hospital Saint Louis[11]	Saint Louis	65%	300+
Northeast Regional Medical Center	Kirksville	65%	300+
Twin Rivers Regional Medical Center	Kennett	65%	(a)
Bothwell Regional Health Center	Sedalia	64%	300+
Centerpoint Medical Center	Independence	64%	300+
Golden Valley Memorial Hospital	Clinton	64%	300+
Saint Luke's Northland Hospital	Kansas City	64%	300+
Truman Medical Center Lakewood	Kansas City	64%	(a)
Boone Hospital Center	Columbia	63%	300+
Saint Francis Medical Center	Cape Girardeau	63%	300+
Belton Regional Medical Center	Belton	62%	300+
Mercy Hospital Joplin[11]	Joplin	62%	300+
North Kansas City Hospital	N Kansas City	62%	300+
Saint Luke's East Lee's Summit Hospital	Lees Summit	62%	300+
Saint Luke's Hospital	Chesterfield	62%	300+
SSM Depaul Health Center	Bridgeton	62%	300+
Cox Medical Center Branson	Branson	61%	300+
Heartland Regional Medical Center	Saint Joseph	61%	300+
Lincoln County Medical Center	Troy	61%	(a)
Texas County Memorial Hospital	Houston	61%	300+
Liberty Hospital	Liberty	60%	300+
Moberly Regional Medical Center	Moberly	60%	300+
Phelps County Regional Medical Center	Rolla	60%	300+
Saint Anthony's Medical Center	Saint Louis	60%	300+
Saint Joseph Medical Center	Kansas City	60%	300+
Sainte Genevieve County Memorial Hospital	Ste Genevieve	60%	(a)
Southeasthealth Center of Stoddard County	Dexter	60%	(a)
SSM Saint Marys Health Center	Richmond Hghts	60%	300+
Barnes-Jewish West County Hospital	Creve Coeur	59%	300+
Citizens Memorial Hospital	Bolivar	59%	300+
Mercy Hospital Springfield[11]	Springfield	59%	300+
Saint Alexius Hospital	Saint Louis	59%	300+
Saint Louis University Hospital	Saint Louis	59%	300+
Mercy Hospital Washington[11]	Washington	58%	300+
Mineral Area Regional Medical Center	Farmington	58%	300+
Des Peres Hospital	Saint Louis	57%	300+
Northwest Medical Center[3]	Albany	57%	(a)
Saint Mary's Medical Center	Blue Springs	57%	300+
SSM Saint Joseph Health Center	Saint Charles	57%	300+
Lafayette Regional Health Center	Lexington	56%	(a)
Saint Mary's Health Center	Jefferson City	56%	300+
Barnes-Jewish Hospital	Saint Louis	55%	300+
Fitzgibbon Hospital	Marshall	55%	300+
Hannibal Regional Hospital	Hannibal	55%	300+
Lake Regional Health System	Osage Beach	55%	300+
Parkland Health Center	Farmington	55%	300+
Poplar Bluff Regional Medical Center	Poplar Bluff	55%	300+
SSM Saint Joseph Hospital West	Lake Saint Louis	55%	300+
Barnes-Jewish Saint Peters Hospital	Saint Peters	54%	300+
Freeman Health System - Freeman West	Joplin	54%	300+
Mercy Hospital Jefferson	Crystal City	54%	300+
Progress West Hospital	O Fallon	54%	300+
Cox Medical Center	Springfield	53%	300+
Ozarks Medical Center	West Plains	53%	300+
Bates County Memorial Hospital	Butler	52%	(a)
Audrain Medical Center	Mexico	50%	300+
Mercy Hospital Lebanon[11]	Lebanon	50%	300+
Pemiscot County Memorial Hospital	Hayti	50%	(a)
Cameron Regional Medical Center	Cameron	49%	(a)
Missouri Baptist Medical Center	Town & Country	47%	300+

Doctors 'Always' Communicated Well

Hospital Name	City	Rate	Cases
Wright Memorial Hospital	Trenton	94%	(a)
Barton County Memorial Hospital	Lamar	90%	(a)
Parkland Health Center	Farmington	88%	300+
Texas County Memorial Hospital	Houston	88%	300+
Lafayette Regional Health Center	Lexington	87%	(a)
Missouri Delta Medical Center	Sikeston	87%	300+
Sainte Genevieve County Memorial Hospital	Ste Genevieve	87%	(a)
Barnes-Jewish West County Hospital	Creve Coeur	86%	300+
Community Hospital Association	Fairfax	86%	(a)
Mercy Hospital Joplin[11]	Joplin	86%	300+
Boone Hospital Center	Columbia	85%	300+
Capital Region Medical Center	Jefferson City	85%	300+
Des Peres Hospital	Saint Louis	85%	300+
Mercy Hospital Lebanon[11]	Lebanon	85%	300+
Ozarks Community Hospital	Springfield	85%	(a)
Ozarks Medical Center	West Plains	85%	300+
Cass Regional Medical Center	Harrisonville	84%	300+
Freeman Neosho Hospital	Neosho	84%	(a)
Missouri Baptist Sullivan Hospital	Sullivan	84%	300+
Pemiscot County Memorial Hospital	Hayti	84%	(a)
Phelps County Regional Medical Center	Rolla	84%	300+
Saint Francis Medical Center	Cape Girardeau	84%	300+
Saint Luke's Hospital	Chesterfield	84%	300+
Bothwell Regional Health Center	Sedalia	83%	300+
Citizens Memorial Hospital	Bolivar	83%	300+
Hannibal Regional Hospital	Hannibal	83%	300+
Hedrick Medical Center	Chillicothe	83%	(a)
Mercy Hospital Washington[11]	Washington	83%	300+
Progress West Hospital	O Fallon	83%	300+
SSM Depaul Health Center	Bridgeton	83%	300+
Barnes-Jewish Hospital	Saint Louis	82%	300+
Mercy Hospital Saint Louis[11]	Saint Louis	82%	300+
Mercy Hospital Springfield[11]	Springfield	82%	300+
Nevada Regional Medical Center	Nevada	82%	(a)
Northeast Regional Medical Center	Kirksville	82%	300+
Northwest Medical Center[3]	Albany	82%	(a)
Saint Joseph Medical Center	Kansas City	82%	300+
Saint Louis University Hospital	Saint Louis	82%	300+
Saint Luke's Hospital of Kansas City	Kansas City	82%	300+
Saint Mary's Health Center	Jefferson City	82%	300+
Twin Rivers Regional Medical Center	Kennett	82%	(a)
Western Missouri Medical Center	Warrensburg	82%	300+
Barnes-Jewish Saint Peters Hospital	Saint Peters	81%	300+
Cameron Regional Medical Center	Cameron	81%	(a)
Christian Hospital Northeast - Northwest	Saint Louis	81%	300+
Cooper County Memorial Hospital	Boonville	81%	(a)
Freeman Health System - Freeman West	Joplin	81%	300+
Heartland Regional Medical Center	Saint Joseph	81%	300+
Lee's Summit Medical Center	Lees Summit	81%	300+
Liberty Hospital	Liberty	81%	300+
Moberly Regional Medical Center	Moberly	81%	300+
North Kansas City Hospital	N Kansas City	81%	300+
Saint Alexius Hospital	Saint Louis	81%	300+
Saint Francis Hospital & Health Services	Maryville	81%	(a)
Saint Luke's Northland Hospital	Kansas City	81%	300+
Southeast Missouri Hospital	Cape Girardeau	81%	300+
Southeasthealth Center of Stoddard County	Dexter	81%	(a)
Cox Medical Center	Springfield	80%	300+
Golden Valley Memorial Hospital	Clinton	80%	300+
Missouri Baptist Medical Center	Town & Country	80%	300+
Saint Luke's East Lee's Summit Hospital	Lees Summit	80%	300+
SSM Saint Joseph Hospital West	Lake Saint Louis	80%	300+
SSM Saint Marys Health Center	Richmond Hghts	80%	300+
Truman Medical Center Lakewood	Kansas City	80%	(a)
Audrain Medical Center	Mexico	79%	300+
Belton Regional Medical Center	Belton	79%	300+
Cox Medical Center Branson	Branson	79%	300+
Fitzgibbon Hospital	Marshall	79%	300+
Lincoln County Medical Center	Troy	79%	(a)
Mineral Area Regional Medical Center	Farmington	79%	300+
Research Medical Center	Kansas City	79%	300+
Saint Mary's Medical Center	Blue Springs	79%	300+
SSM Saint Clare Health Center[11]	Fenton	79%	300+
SSM Saint Joseph Health Center	Saint Charles	79%	300+
Mercy Hospital Jefferson	Crystal City	78%	300+
University of Missouri Health Care	Columbia	78%	300+
Bates County Memorial Hospital	Butler	77%	(a)
Centerpoint Medical Center	Independence	77%	300+
Lake Regional Health System	Osage Beach	77%	300+
Saint Anthony's Medical Center	Saint Louis	77%	300+
Truman Medical Center Hospital Hill	Kansas City	77%	300+
Poplar Bluff Regional Medical Center	Poplar Bluff	76%	300+

Home Recovery Information Given

Hospital Name	City	Rate	Cases
Lafayette Regional Health Center	Lexington	92%	(a)
Barnes-Jewish Hospital	Saint Louis	91%	300+
Hedrick Medical Center	Chillicothe	91%	(a)
Moberly Regional Medical Center	Moberly	91%	300+
Progress West Hospital	O Fallon	91%	300+
Saint Luke's East Lee's Summit Hospital	Lees Summit	91%	300+
Sainte Genevieve County Memorial Hospital	Ste Genevieve	91%	(a)
Audrain Medical Center	Mexico	90%	300+
Boone Hospital Center	Columbia	90%	300+
Cass Regional Medical Center	Harrisonville	90%	300+
Des Peres Hospital	Saint Louis	90%	300+
Freeman Neosho Hospital	Neosho	90%	(a)
Mercy Hospital Joplin[11]	Joplin	90%	300+
Mercy Hospital Lebanon[11]	Lebanon	90%	300+
Missouri Baptist Sullivan Hospital	Sullivan	90%	300+
Northeast Regional Medical Center	Kirksville	90%	300+
Southeast Missouri Hospital	Cape Girardeau	90%	300+
SSM Saint Joseph Health Center	Saint Charles	90%	300+
Wright Memorial Hospital	Trenton	90%	(a)
Barnes-Jewish West County Hospital	Creve Coeur	89%	300+
Bates County Memorial Hospital	Butler	89%	(a)
Capital Region Medical Center	Jefferson City	89%	300+
Centerpoint Medical Center	Independence	89%	300+
Cox Medical Center	Springfield	89%	300+
Heartland Regional Medical Center	Saint Joseph	89%	300+
Lee's Summit Medical Center	Lees Summit	89%	300+
Liberty Hospital	Liberty	89%	300+
Mercy Hospital Washington[11]	Washington	89%	300+
Ozarks Community Hospital	Springfield	89%	(a)
Phelps County Regional Medical Center	Rolla	89%	300+
Saint Joseph Medical Center	Kansas City	89%	300+
SSM Depaul Health Center	Bridgeton	89%	300+
Texas County Memorial Hospital	Houston	89%	300+
Barnes-Jewish Saint Peters Hospital	Saint Peters	88%	300+
Citizens Memorial Hospital	Bolivar	88%	300+
Fitzgibbon Hospital	Marshall	88%	300+
Mercy Hospital Saint Louis[11]	Saint Louis	88%	300+
North Kansas City Hospital	N Kansas City	88%	300+
Parkland Health Center	Farmington	88%	300+
Saint Francis Hospital & Health Services	Maryville	88%	(a)
Saint Louis University Hospital	Saint Louis	88%	300+
Saint Mary's Medical Center	Blue Springs	88%	300+
Belton Regional Medical Center	Belton	87%	300+
Freeman Health System - Freeman West	Joplin	87%	300+
Golden Valley Memorial Hospital	Clinton	87%	300+
Hannibal Regional Hospital	Hannibal	87%	300+
Mercy Hospital Springfield[11]	Springfield	87%	300+
Saint Anthony's Medical Center	Saint Louis	87%	300+
Saint Luke's Hospital	Chesterfield	87%	300+
Saint Luke's Hospital of Kansas City	Kansas City	87%	300+
Saint Luke's Northland Hospital	Kansas City	87%	300+
SSM Saint Joseph Hospital West	Lake Saint Louis	87%	300+
Western Missouri Medical Center	Warrensburg	87%	300+
Barton County Memorial Hospital	Lamar	86%	(a)
Bothwell Regional Health Center	Sedalia	86%	300+
Cameron Regional Medical Center	Cameron	86%	(a)
Christian Hospital Northeast - Northwest	Saint Louis	86%	300+

NOTE: Hospital profiles are in alphabetical order by state, then city, then hospital within the city; Rankings exclude hospitals with less than 25 cases except for patient surveys which excludes hospitals with less than 100 cases; (a) 100-299 cases; (1) The number of cases/patients is too few to report; (2) Data submitted were based on a sample of cases/patients; (3) Results are based on a shorter time period than required; (4) Data suppressed by CMS for one or more quarters; (5) Results are not available for this reporting period; (6) Fewer than 100 patients completed the HCAHPS survey; (7) No cases met the criteria for this measure; (8) The lower limit of the confidence interval cannot be calculated if the number of observed infections equals zero; (9) No data are available from the state/territory for this reporting period; (10) The scores shown reflect fewer than 50 completed surveys; (11) There were discrepancies in the data collection process; (12) This measure does not apply to this hospital for this reporting period; (13) Results cannot be calculated for this reporting period; (14) The results for this state are combined with nearby states to protect confidentiality; Please refer to the User's Guide for a full explanation of data.

Hospital Name	City	Rate	Cases
Cox Medical Center Branson	Branson	86%	300+
Mercy Hospital Jefferson	Crystal City	86%	300+
Research Medical Center	Kansas City	86%	300+
Saint Francis Medical Center	Cape Girardeau	86%	300+
SSM Saint Marys Health Center	Richmond Hghts	86%	300+
Lincoln County Medical Center	Troy	85%	(a)
Missouri Baptist Medical Center	Town & Country	85%	300+
Saint Mary's Health Center	Jefferson City	85%	300+
Truman Medical Center Lakewood	Kansas City	85%	(a)
Twin Rivers Regional Medical Center	Kennett	85%	(a)
University of Missouri Health Care	Columbia	85%	300+
Cooper County Memorial Hospital	Boonville	84%	(a)
Missouri Delta Medical Center	Sikeston	84%	300+
SSM Saint Clare Health Center[11]	Fenton	84%	300+
Truman Medical Center Hospital Hill	Kansas City	84%	300+
Mineral Area Regional Medical Center	Farmington	83%	300+
Nevada Regional Medical Center	Nevada	83%	(a)
Ozarks Medical Center	West Plains	82%	300+
Lake Regional Health System	Osage Beach	81%	300+
Saint Alexius Hospital	Saint Louis	80%	300+
Southeasthealth Center of Stoddard County	Dexter	80%	(a)
Community Hospital Association	Fairfax	79%	(a)
Northwest Medical Center[3]	Albany	79%	(a)
Poplar Bluff Regional Medical Center	Poplar Bluff	73%	300+
Pemiscot County Memorial Hospital	Hayti	66%	(a)

Hospital Given 9 or 10 on 10 Point Scale

Hospital Name	City	Rate	Cases
Saint Luke's Hospital	Chesterfield	85%	300+
Wright Memorial Hospital	Trenton	85%	(a)
Boone Hospital Center	Columbia	83%	300+
Progress West Hospital	O Fallon	81%	300+
SSM Saint Clare Health Center[11]	Fenton	81%	300+
Mercy Hospital Joplin[11]	Joplin	80%	300+
Barton County Memorial Hospital	Lamar	79%	(a)
Capital Region Medical Center	Jefferson City	79%	300+
Parkland Health Center	Farmington	79%	300+
Saint Francis Medical Center	Cape Girardeau	79%	300+
Southeast Missouri Hospital	Cape Girardeau	79%	300+
Missouri Baptist Sullivan Hospital	Sullivan	78%	300+
Saint Luke's East Lee's Summit Hospital	Lees Summit	78%	300+
SSM Saint Joseph Hospital West	Lake Saint Louis	78%	300+
Barnes-Jewish Hospital	Saint Louis	77%	300+
Freeman Neosho Hospital	Neosho	77%	(a)
Mercy Hospital Saint Louis[11]	Saint Louis	77%	300+
Saint Luke's Hospital of Kansas City	Kansas City	77%	300+
SSM Depaul Health Center	Bridgeton	77%	300+
Cass Regional Medical Center	Harrisonville	76%	300+
Hannibal Regional Hospital	Hannibal	76%	300+
Hedrick Medical Center	Chillicothe	76%	(a)
North Kansas City Hospital	N Kansas City	76%	300+
Ozarks Community Hospital	Springfield	76%	(a)
University of Missouri Health Care	Columbia	76%	300+
Barnes-Jewish West County Hospital	Creve Coeur	75%	300+
Mercy Hospital Springfield[11]	Springfield	75%	300+
Saint Luke's Northland Hospital	Kansas City	75%	300+
Saint Mary's Medical Center	Blue Springs	75%	300+
Barnes-Jewish Saint Peters Hospital	Saint Peters	74%	300+
Des Peres Hospital	Saint Louis	74%	300+
Lafayette Regional Health Center	Lexington	74%	(a)
Lee's Summit Medical Center	Lees Summit	74%	300+
Northwest Medical Center[3]	Albany	74%	(a)
Saint Francis Hospital & Health Services	Maryville	74%	(a)
Sainte Genevieve County Memorial Hospital	Ste Genevieve	74%	(a)
SSM Saint Marys Health Center	Richmond Hghts	74%	300+
Bothwell Regional Health Center	Sedalia	73%	300+
Mercy Hospital Lebanon[11]	Lebanon	73%	300+
Citizens Memorial Hospital	Bolivar	72%	300+
Missouri Baptist Medical Center	Town & Country	72%	300+
Northeast Regional Medical Center	Kirksville	72%	300+
Saint Louis University Hospital	Saint Louis	72%	300+
Western Missouri Medical Center	Warrensburg	72%	300+
Golden Valley Memorial Hospital	Clinton	71%	300+
Mercy Hospital Washington[11]	Washington	71%	300+
Saint Mary's Health Center	Jefferson City	71%	300+
SSM Saint Joseph Health Center	Saint Charles	71%	300+
Community Hospital Association	Fairfax	70%	(a)
Liberty Hospital	Liberty	70%	300+
Missouri Delta Medical Center	Sikeston	70%	300+
Phelps County Regional Medical Center	Rolla	70%	300+
Saint Anthony's Medical Center	Saint Louis	70%	300+
Saint Joseph Medical Center	Kansas City	70%	300+
Truman Medical Center Lakewood	Kansas City	70%	(a)
Audrain Medical Center	Mexico	69%	300+
Heartland Regional Medical Center	Saint Joseph	69%	300+
Centerpoint Medical Center	Independence	68%	300+
Christian Hospital Northeast - Northwest	Saint Louis	68%	300+
Cox Medical Center	Springfield	68%	300+
Cox Medical Center Branson	Branson	68%	300+
Freeman Health System - Freeman West	Joplin	68%	300+
Southeasthealth Center of Stoddard County	Dexter	68%	(a)
Lake Regional Health System	Osage Beach	67%	300+
Moberly Regional Medical Center	Moberly	67%	300+
Cameron Regional Medical Center	Cameron	66%	(a)
Nevada Regional Medical Center	Nevada	66%	(a)
Research Medical Center	Kansas City	66%	300+
Truman Medical Center Hospital Hill	Kansas City	65%	300+
Bates County Memorial Hospital	Butler	64%	(a)
Belton Regional Medical Center	Belton	64%	300+
Ozarks Medical Center	West Plains	64%	300+
Texas County Memorial Hospital	Houston	64%	300+
Mercy Hospital Jefferson	Crystal City	63%	300+
Mineral Area Regional Medical Center	Farmington	63%	300+
Fitzgibbon Hospital	Marshall	61%	300+
Twin Rivers Regional Medical Center	Kennett	61%	(a)
Lincoln County Medical Center	Troy	60%	(a)
Saint Alexius Hospital	Saint Louis	60%	300+
Cooper County Memorial Hospital	Boonville	58%	(a)
Poplar Bluff Regional Medical Center	Poplar Bluff	48%	300+
Pemiscot County Memorial Hospital	Hayti	39%	(a)

Meds 'Always' Explained Before Given

Hospital Name	City	Rate	Cases
Wright Memorial Hospital	Trenton	75%	(a)
Lafayette Regional Health Center	Lexington	72%	(a)
Community Hospital Association	Fairfax	70%	(a)
Golden Valley Memorial Hospital	Clinton	70%	300+
Missouri Delta Medical Center	Sikeston	70%	300+
Barton County Memorial Hospital	Lamar	69%	(a)
Saint Francis Medical Center	Cape Girardeau	69%	300+
Southeast Missouri Hospital	Cape Girardeau	69%	300+
Cass Regional Medical Center	Harrisonville	68%	300+
Hedrick Medical Center	Chillicothe	68%	(a)
Mercy Hospital Lebanon[11]	Lebanon	68%	300+
Phelps County Regional Medical Center	Rolla	68%	300+
Capital Region Medical Center	Jefferson City	67%	300+
Missouri Baptist Sullivan Hospital	Sullivan	67%	300+
Parkland Health Center	Farmington	67%	300+
Progress West Hospital	O Fallon	67%	300+
Saint Luke's Hospital	Chesterfield	67%	300+
SSM Saint Joseph Hospital West	Lake Saint Louis	67%	300+
Texas County Memorial Hospital	Houston	67%	300+
Western Missouri Medical Center	Warrensburg	67%	300+
Barnes-Jewish Hospital	Saint Louis	66%	300+
Hannibal Regional Hospital	Hannibal	66%	300+
Mercy Hospital Joplin[11]	Joplin	66%	300+
Ozarks Community Hospital	Springfield	66%	(a)
Ozarks Medical Center	West Plains	66%	300+
Saint Mary's Health Center	Jefferson City	66%	300+
SSM Saint Marys Health Center	Richmond Hghts	66%	300+
Twin Rivers Regional Medical Center	Kennett	66%	(a)
Bothwell Regional Health Center	Sedalia	65%	300+
Des Peres Hospital	Saint Louis	65%	300+
Heartland Regional Medical Center	Saint Joseph	65%	300+
Northeast Regional Medical Center	Kirksville	65%	300+
Saint Louis University Hospital	Saint Louis	65%	300+
Sainte Genevieve County Memorial Hospital	Ste Genevieve	65%	(a)
Cameron Regional Medical Center	Cameron	64%	(a)
Christian Hospital Northeast - Northwest	Saint Louis	64%	300+
Freeman Neosho Hospital	Neosho	64%	(a)
Saint Luke's Hospital of Kansas City	Kansas City	64%	300+
Truman Medical Center Lakewood	Kansas City	64%	(a)
Audrain Medical Center	Mexico	63%	300+
Barnes-Jewish West County Hospital	Creve Coeur	63%	300+
Boone Hospital Center	Columbia	63%	300+
Centerpoint Medical Center	Independence	63%	300+
Lee's Summit Medical Center	Lees Summit	63%	300+
Liberty Hospital	Liberty	63%	300+
Mercy Hospital Washington[11]	Washington	63%	300+
Saint Francis Hospital & Health Services	Maryville	63%	(a)
Saint Luke's East Lee's Summit Hospital	Lees Summit	63%	300+
SSM Depaul Health Center	Bridgeton	63%	300+
SSM Saint Clare Health Center[11]	Fenton	63%	300+
University of Missouri Health Care	Columbia	63%	300+
Lake Regional Health System	Osage Beach	62%	300+
Mercy Hospital Saint Louis[11]	Saint Louis	62%	300+
Moberly Regional Medical Center	Moberly	62%	300+
Nevada Regional Medical Center	Nevada	62%	(a)
Saint Joseph Medical Center	Kansas City	62%	300+
Saint Luke's Northland Hospital	Kansas City	62%	300+
Saint Mary's Medical Center	Blue Springs	62%	300+
Belton Regional Medical Center	Belton	61%	300+
Fitzgibbon Hospital	Marshall	61%	300+
Freeman Health System - Freeman West	Joplin	61%	300+
Mercy Hospital Jefferson	Crystal City	61%	300+
Mercy Hospital Springfield[11]	Springfield	61%	300+
North Kansas City Hospital	N Kansas City	61%	300+
Research Medical Center	Kansas City	61%	300+
Saint Anthony's Medical Center	Saint Louis	61%	300+
Cooper County Memorial Hospital	Boonville	60%	(a)
Cox Medical Center	Springfield	60%	300+
Cox Medical Center Branson	Branson	60%	300+
Mineral Area Regional Medical Center	Farmington	60%	300+
SSM Saint Joseph Health Center	Saint Charles	60%	300+
Truman Medical Center Hospital Hill	Kansas City	60%	300+
Bates County Memorial Hospital	Butler	59%	(a)
Citizens Memorial Hospital	Bolivar	59%	300+
Missouri Baptist Medical Center	Town & Country	59%	300+
Lincoln County Medical Center	Troy	58%	(a)
Barnes-Jewish Saint Peters Hospital	Saint Peters	54%	300+
Northwest Medical Center[3]	Albany	54%	(a)
Poplar Bluff Regional Medical Center	Poplar Bluff	52%	300+
Saint Alexius Hospital	Saint Louis	51%	300+
Southeasthealth Center of Stoddard County	Dexter	51%	(a)
Pemiscot County Memorial Hospital	Hayti	46%	(a)

Nurses 'Always' Communicated Well

Hospital Name	City	Rate	Cases
Barton County Memorial Hospital	Lamar	88%	(a)
Wright Memorial Hospital	Trenton	88%	(a)
Missouri Delta Medical Center	Sikeston	86%	300+
SSM Depaul Health Center	Bridgeton	85%	300+
Audrain Medical Center	Mexico	84%	300+
Hannibal Regional Hospital	Hannibal	84%	300+
Parkland Health Center	Farmington	84%	300+
Bothwell Regional Health Center	Sedalia	83%	300+
Lafayette Regional Health Center	Lexington	83%	(a)
Missouri Baptist Sullivan Hospital	Sullivan	83%	300+
Ozarks Community Hospital	Springfield	83%	(a)
Saint Francis Medical Center	Cape Girardeau	83%	300+
Sainte Genevieve County Memorial Hospital	Ste Genevieve	83%	(a)
Southeast Missouri Hospital	Cape Girardeau	83%	300+
SSM Saint Joseph Hospital West	Lake Saint Louis	83%	300+
Capital Region Medical Center	Jefferson City	82%	300+
Cass Regional Medical Center	Harrisonville	82%	300+
Freeman Neosho Hospital	Neosho	82%	(a)
Golden Valley Memorial Hospital	Clinton	82%	300+
Heartland Regional Medical Center	Saint Joseph	82%	300+
Saint Francis Hospital & Health Services	Maryville	82%	(a)
Saint Luke's Hospital	Chesterfield	82%	300+
SSM Saint Marys Health Center	Richmond Hghts	82%	300+
Barnes-Jewish Saint Peters Hospital	Saint Peters	81%	300+
Community Hospital Association	Fairfax	81%	(a)
Mercy Hospital Joplin[11]	Joplin	81%	300+
Mercy Hospital Lebanon[11]	Lebanon	81%	300+
Ozarks Medical Center	West Plains	81%	300+
Phelps County Regional Medical Center	Rolla	81%	300+
Saint Luke's Hospital of Kansas City	Kansas City	81%	300+
Texas County Memorial Hospital	Houston	81%	300+
Western Missouri Medical Center	Warrensburg	81%	300+
Barnes-Jewish Hospital	Saint Louis	80%	300+
Boone Hospital Center	Columbia	80%	300+
Christian Hospital Northeast - Northwest	Saint Louis	80%	300+
Hedrick Medical Center	Chillicothe	80%	(a)
Northeast Regional Medical Center	Kirksville	80%	300+
Progress West Hospital	O Fallon	80%	300+
Saint Luke's East Lee's Summit Hospital	Lees Summit	80%	300+
Saint Mary's Health Center	Jefferson City	80%	300+
Saint Mary's Medical Center	Blue Springs	80%	300+
University of Missouri Health Care	Columbia	80%	300+
Barnes-Jewish West County Hospital	Creve Coeur	79%	300+
Citizens Memorial Hospital	Bolivar	79%	300+
Lincoln County Medical Center	Troy	79%	(a)
Mercy Hospital Saint Louis[11]	Saint Louis	79%	300+
Mercy Hospital Springfield[11]	Springfield	79%	300+
Northwest Medical Center[3]	Albany	79%	(a)
SSM Saint Clare Health Center[11]	Fenton	79%	300+
Truman Medical Center Hospital Hill	Kansas City	79%	300+
Lee's Summit Medical Center	Lees Summit	78%	300+
Mercy Hospital Washington[11]	Washington	78%	300+
Moberly Regional Medical Center	Moberly	78%	300+
Southeasthealth Center of Stoddard County	Dexter	78%	(a)
Cox Medical Center Branson	Branson	77%	300+
Des Peres Hospital	Saint Louis	77%	300+
Fitzgibbon Hospital	Marshall	77%	300+
Lake Regional Health System	Osage Beach	77%	300+
North Kansas City Hospital	N Kansas City	77%	300+
Saint Joseph Medical Center	Kansas City	77%	300+
Saint Louis University Hospital	Saint Louis	77%	300+
Saint Luke's Northland Hospital	Kansas City	77%	300+
SSM Saint Joseph Health Center	Saint Charles	77%	300+
Twin Rivers Regional Medical Center	Kennett	77%	(a)
Belton Regional Medical Center	Belton	76%	300+
Centerpoint Medical Center	Independence	76%	300+
Liberty Hospital	Liberty	76%	300+
Truman Medical Center Lakewood	Kansas City	76%	(a)
Cameron Regional Medical Center	Cameron	75%	(a)
Cooper County Memorial Hospital	Boonville	75%	(a)
Cox Medical Center	Springfield	75%	300+
Freeman Health System - Freeman West	Joplin	75%	300+
Missouri Baptist Medical Center	Town & Country	75%	300+
Nevada Regional Medical Center	Nevada	75%	(a)
Saint Anthony's Medical Center	Saint Louis	75%	300+

NOTE: Hospital profiles are in alphabetical order by state, then city, then hospital within the city; Rankings exclude hospitals with less than 25 cases except for patient surveys which excludes hospitals with less than 100 cases; (a) 100-299 cases; (1) The number of cases/patients is too few to report; (2) Data submitted were based on a sample of cases/patients; (3) Results are based on a shorter time period than required; (4) Data suppressed by CMS for one or more quarters; (5) Results are not available for this reporting period; (6) Fewer than 100 patients completed the HCAHPS survey; (7) No cases met the criteria for this measure; (8) The lower limit of the confidence interval cannot be calculated if the number of observed infections equals zero; (9) No data are available from the state/territory for this reporting period; (10) The scores shown reflect fewer than 50 completed surveys; (11) There were discrepancies in the data collection process; (12) This measure does not apply to this hospital for this reporting period; (13) Results cannot be calculated for this reporting period; (14) The results for this state are combined with nearby states to protect confidentiality; Please refer to the User's Guide for a full explanation of data.

Hospital Name	City	Rate	Cases
Mercy Hospital Jefferson	Crystal City	74%	300+
Mineral Area Regional Medical Center	Farmington	74%	300+
Research Medical Center	Kansas City	74%	300+
Bates County Memorial Hospital	Butler	73%	(a)
Saint Alexius Hospital	Saint Louis	72%	300+
Poplar Bluff Regional Medical Center	Poplar Bluff	69%	300+
Pemiscot County Memorial Hospital	Hayti	61%	(a)

Pain 'Always' Well Controlled

Hospital Name	City	Rate	Cases
Barton County Memorial Hospital	Lamar	82%	(a)
Missouri Delta Medical Center	Sikeston	81%	300+
Wright Memorial Hospital	Trenton	81%	(a)
Lafayette Regional Health Center	Lexington	76%	(a)
Saint Luke's Hospital of Kansas City	Kansas City	76%	300+
Southeast Missouri Hospital	Cape Girardeau	76%	300+
Freeman Neosho Hospital	Neosho	75%	(a)
Heartland Regional Medical Center	Saint Joseph	75%	300+
Hedrick Medical Center	Chillicothe	75%	(a)
Mercy Hospital Joplin[11]	Joplin	75%	300+
Sainte Genevieve County Memorial Hospital	Ste Genevieve	75%	(a)
Boone Hospital Center	Columbia	74%	300+
Bothwell Regional Health Center	Sedalia	74%	300+
Hannibal Regional Hospital	Hannibal	74%	300+
Parkland Health Center	Farmington	74%	300+
Saint Francis Hospital & Health Services	Maryville	74%	(a)
Saint Francis Medical Center	Cape Girardeau	74%	300+
Saint Luke's Hospital	Chesterfield	74%	300+
Saint Mary's Health Center	Jefferson City	74%	300+
SSM Saint Marys Health Center	Richmond Hghts	74%	300+
Texas County Memorial Hospital	Houston	74%	300+
Barnes-Jewish Hospital	Saint Louis	73%	300+
Barnes-Jewish Saint Peters Hospital	Saint Peters	73%	300+
Capital Region Medical Center	Jefferson City	73%	300+
Mercy Hospital Lebanon[11]	Lebanon	73%	300+
Moberly Regional Medical Center	Moberly	73%	300+
Saint Mary's Medical Center	Blue Springs	73%	300+
SSM Depaul Health Center	Bridgeton	73%	300+
SSM Saint Joseph Hospital West	Lake Saint Louis	73%	300+
Western Missouri Medical Center	Warrensburg	73%	300+
Barnes-Jewish West County Hospital	Creve Coeur	72%	300+
Belton Regional Medical Center	Belton	72%	300+
Christian Hospital Northeast - Northwest	Saint Louis	72%	300+
Des Peres Hospital	Saint Louis	72%	300+
Lee's Summit Medical Center	Lees Summit	72%	300+
Northeast Regional Medical Center	Kirksville	72%	300+
Ozarks Medical Center	West Plains	72%	300+
Progress West Hospital	O Fallon	72%	300+
Saint Louis University Hospital	Saint Louis	72%	300+
Saint Luke's East Lee's Summit Hospital	Lees Summit	72%	300+
SSM Saint Clare Health Center[11]	Fenton	72%	300+
Mercy Hospital Saint Louis[11]	Saint Louis	71%	300+
Missouri Baptist Sullivan Hospital	Sullivan	71%	300+
Ozarks Community Hospital	Springfield	71%	(a)
Audrain Medical Center	Mexico	70%	300+
Cass Regional Medical Center	Harrisonville	70%	300+
Golden Valley Memorial Hospital	Clinton	70%	300+
North Kansas City Hospital	N Kansas City	70%	300+
Saint Luke's Northland Hospital	Kansas City	70%	300+
Truman Medical Center Lakewood	Kansas City	70%	(a)
Twin Rivers Regional Medical Center	Kennett	70%	(a)
Citizens Memorial Hospital	Bolivar	69%	300+
Freeman Health System - Freeman West	Joplin	69%	300+
Liberty Hospital	Liberty	69%	300+
Mercy Hospital Springfield[11]	Springfield	69%	300+
Northwest Medical Center[3]	Albany	69%	(a)
Research Medical Center	Kansas City	69%	300+
SSM Saint Joseph Health Center	Saint Charles	69%	300+
Truman Medical Center Hospital Hill	Kansas City	69%	300+
Cameron Regional Medical Center	Cameron	68%	(a)
Centerpoint Medical Center	Independence	68%	300+
Community Hospital Association	Fairfax	68%	(a)
Mercy Hospital Washington[11]	Washington	68%	300+
Phelps County Regional Medical Center	Rolla	68%	300+
Saint Anthony's Medical Center	Saint Louis	68%	300+
Saint Joseph Medical Center	Kansas City	68%	300+
Cooper County Memorial Hospital	Boonville	67%	(a)
Fitzgibbon Hospital	Marshall	67%	300+
Mercy Hospital Jefferson	Crystal City	67%	300+
Mineral Area Regional Medical Center	Farmington	67%	300+
Missouri Baptist Medical Center	Town & Country	67%	300+
University of Missouri Health Care	Columbia	67%	300+
Cox Medical Center	Springfield	66%	300+
Lake Regional Health System	Osage Beach	66%	300+
Saint Alexius Hospital	Saint Louis	66%	300+
Cox Medical Center Branson	Branson	65%	300+
Nevada Regional Medical Center	Nevada	65%	(a)
Southeasthealth Center of Stoddard County	Dexter	65%	(a)
Bates County Memorial Hospital	Butler	64%	(a)
Lincoln County Medical Center	Troy	64%	(a)
Poplar Bluff Regional Medical Center	Poplar Bluff	59%	300+
Pemiscot County Memorial Hospital	Hayti	53%	(a)

Room and Bathroom 'Always' Clean

Hospital Name	City	Rate	Cases
Sainte Genevieve County Memorial Hospital	Ste Genevieve	88%	(a)
Community Hospital Association	Fairfax	87%	(a)
Missouri Delta Medical Center	Sikeston	86%	300+
Saint Francis Hospital & Health Services	Maryville	86%	(a)
Barton County Memorial Hospital	Lamar	85%	(a)
Ozarks Community Hospital	Springfield	85%	(a)
Northwest Medical Center[3]	Albany	81%	(a)
Southeast Missouri Hospital	Cape Girardeau	81%	300+
Western Missouri Medical Center	Warrensburg	81%	300+
Lincoln County Medical Center	Troy	80%	(a)
Missouri Baptist Sullivan Hospital	Sullivan	80%	300+
Texas County Memorial Hospital	Houston	80%	300+
Audrain Medical Center	Mexico	79%	300+
Capital Region Medical Center	Jefferson City	79%	300+
Cass Regional Medical Center	Harrisonville	79%	300+
Golden Valley Memorial Hospital	Clinton	79%	300+
Hedrick Medical Center	Chillicothe	79%	(a)
Bates County Memorial Hospital	Butler	78%	(a)
Ozarks Medical Center	West Plains	78%	300+
Wright Memorial Hospital	Trenton	78%	(a)
Hannibal Regional Hospital	Hannibal	77%	300+
Mercy Hospital Lebanon[11]	Lebanon	77%	300+
Southeasthealth Center of Stoddard County	Dexter	77%	(a)
University of Missouri Health Care	Columbia	77%	300+
Phelps County Regional Medical Center	Rolla	76%	300+
Saint Luke's East Lee's Summit Hospital	Lees Summit	76%	300+
Saint Luke's Hospital	Chesterfield	76%	300+
SSM Saint Joseph Hospital West	Lake Saint Louis	76%	300+
Citizens Memorial Hospital	Bolivar	75%	300+
Lake Regional Health System	Osage Beach	75%	300+
Saint Francis Medical Center	Cape Girardeau	75%	300+
Saint Mary's Medical Center	Blue Springs	75%	300+
Truman Medical Center Lakewood	Kansas City	75%	(a)
Heartland Regional Medical Center	Saint Joseph	74%	300+
Lee's Summit Medical Center	Lees Summit	74%	300+
Mercy Hospital Joplin[11]	Joplin	74%	300+
Northeast Regional Medical Center	Kirksville	74%	300+
Saint Mary's Health Center	Jefferson City	74%	300+
Cooper County Memorial Hospital	Boonville	73%	(a)
Lafayette Regional Health Center	Lexington	73%	(a)
Saint Luke's Northland Hospital	Kansas City	73%	300+
Bothwell Regional Health Center	Sedalia	72%	300+
Cox Medical Center Branson	Branson	72%	300+
Mercy Hospital Jefferson	Crystal City	72%	300+
Mercy Hospital Springfield[11]	Springfield	72%	300+
Mercy Hospital Washington[11]	Washington	72%	300+
Moberly Regional Medical Center	Moberly	72%	300+
Nevada Regional Medical Center	Nevada	72%	(a)
North Kansas City Hospital	N Kansas City	72%	300+
Saint Joseph Medical Center	Kansas City	72%	300+
SSM Saint Joseph Health Center	Saint Charles	72%	300+
Des Peres Hospital	Saint Louis	71%	300+
Parkland Health Center	Farmington	71%	300+
SSM Saint Clare Health Center[11]	Fenton	71%	300+
Freeman Neosho Hospital	Neosho	70%	(a)
Saint Luke's Hospital of Kansas City	Kansas City	70%	300+
Centerpoint Medical Center	Independence	69%	300+
Liberty Hospital	Liberty	69%	300+
SSM Depaul Health Center	Bridgeton	69%	300+
SSM Saint Marys Health Center	Richmond Hghts	69%	300+
Truman Medical Center Hospital Hill	Kansas City	69%	300+
Twin Rivers Regional Medical Center	Kennett	69%	(a)
Boone Hospital Center	Columbia	68%	300+
Mineral Area Regional Medical Center	Farmington	68%	300+
Research Medical Center	Kansas City	68%	300+
Saint Anthony's Medical Center	Saint Louis	68%	300+
Saint Louis University Hospital	Saint Louis	67%	300+
Barnes-Jewish Hospital	Saint Louis	66%	300+
Fitzgibbon Hospital	Marshall	66%	300+
Cameron Regional Medical Center	Cameron	65%	(a)
Cox Medical Center	Springfield	65%	300+
Freeman Health System - Freeman West	Joplin	65%	300+
Poplar Bluff Regional Medical Center	Poplar Bluff	65%	300+
Mercy Hospital Saint Louis[11]	Saint Louis	64%	300+
Missouri Baptist Medical Center	Town & Country	64%	300+
Progress West Hospital	O Fallon	64%	300+
Belton Regional Medical Center	Belton	63%	300+
Barnes-Jewish Saint Peters Hospital	Saint Peters	62%	300+
Barnes-Jewish West County Hospital	Creve Coeur	62%	300+
Christian Hospital Northeast - Northwest	Saint Louis	60%	300+
Pemiscot County Memorial Hospital	Hayti	58%	(a)
Saint Alexius Hospital	Saint Louis	58%	300+

Timely Help 'Always' Received

Hospital Name	City	Rate	Cases
Wright Memorial Hospital	Trenton	82%	(a)
Community Hospital Association	Fairfax	81%	(a)
Missouri Delta Medical Center	Sikeston	79%	300+
Saint Francis Hospital & Health Services	Maryville	79%	(a)
Barton County Memorial Hospital	Lamar	77%	(a)
Bothwell Regional Health Center	Sedalia	75%	300+
Missouri Baptist Sullivan Hospital	Sullivan	75%	300+
Freeman Neosho Hospital	Neosho	74%	(a)
Lafayette Regional Health Center	Lexington	74%	(a)
Ozarks Community Hospital	Springfield	73%	(a)
Audrain Medical Center	Mexico	72%	300+
Hannibal Regional Hospital	Hannibal	72%	300+
Sainte Genevieve County Memorial Hospital	Ste Genevieve	72%	(a)
Bates County Memorial Hospital	Butler	71%	(a)
Fitzgibbon Hospital	Marshall	71%	300+
Hedrick Medical Center	Chillicothe	71%	(a)
Lee's Summit Medical Center	Lees Summit	71%	300+
Mercy Hospital Joplin[11]	Joplin	71%	300+
Mercy Hospital Lebanon[11]	Lebanon	71%	300+
Northwest Medical Center[3]	Albany	71%	(a)
Ozarks Medical Center	West Plains	71%	300+
Saint Mary's Health Center	Jefferson City	71%	300+
Southeast Missouri Hospital	Cape Girardeau	71%	300+
University of Missouri Health Care	Columbia	71%	300+
Capital Region Medical Center	Jefferson City	70%	300+
Cooper County Memorial Hospital	Boonville	70%	(a)
Golden Valley Memorial Hospital	Clinton	70%	300+
Lake Regional Health System	Osage Beach	70%	300+
Boone Hospital Center	Columbia	69%	300+
Citizens Memorial Hospital	Bolivar	69%	300+
Nevada Regional Medical Center	Nevada	69%	(a)
Parkland Health Center	Farmington	69%	300+
Western Missouri Medical Center	Warrensburg	69%	300+
Cass Regional Medical Center	Harrisonville	68%	300+
Saint Mary's Medical Center	Blue Springs	68%	300+
Lincoln County Medical Center	Troy	67%	(a)
Northeast Regional Medical Center	Kirksville	67%	300+
Saint Francis Medical Center	Cape Girardeau	67%	300+
SSM Saint Joseph Hospital West	Lake Saint Louis	67%	300+
Texas County Memorial Hospital	Houston	67%	300+
Cox Medical Center Branson	Branson	66%	300+
Saint Luke's Hospital	Chesterfield	66%	300+
Southeasthealth Center of Stoddard County	Dexter	66%	(a)
SSM Saint Clare Health Center[11]	Fenton	66%	300+
SSM Saint Joseph Health Center	Saint Charles	66%	300+
Twin Rivers Regional Medical Center	Kennett	66%	(a)
Belton Regional Medical Center	Belton	65%	300+
Centerpoint Medical Center	Independence	65%	300+
Mercy Hospital Jefferson	Crystal City	65%	300+
Phelps County Regional Medical Center	Rolla	65%	300+
Saint Luke's Hospital of Kansas City	Kansas City	65%	300+
SSM Depaul Health Center	Bridgeton	65%	300+
SSM Saint Marys Health Center	Richmond Hghts	65%	300+
Truman Medical Center Lakewood	Kansas City	65%	(a)
Barnes-Jewish West County Hospital	Creve Coeur	64%	300+
Christian Hospital Northeast - Northwest	Saint Louis	64%	300+
Heartland Regional Medical Center	Saint Joseph	64%	300+
Liberty Hospital	Liberty	64%	300+
Mercy Hospital Saint Louis[11]	Saint Louis	64%	300+
Mercy Hospital Springfield[11]	Springfield	64%	300+
Mercy Hospital Washington[11]	Washington	64%	300+
Saint Louis University Hospital	Saint Louis	64%	300+
Barnes-Jewish Saint Peters Hospital	Saint Peters	63%	300+
Moberly Regional Medical Center	Moberly	63%	300+
Des Peres Hospital	Saint Louis	62%	300+
Saint Luke's East Lee's Summit Hospital	Lees Summit	62%	300+
Truman Medical Center Hospital Hill	Kansas City	62%	300+
Barnes-Jewish Hospital	Saint Louis	61%	300+
Cox Medical Center	Springfield	61%	300+
Mineral Area Regional Medical Center	Farmington	61%	300+
Missouri Baptist Medical Center	Town & Country	61%	300+
North Kansas City Hospital	N Kansas City	61%	300+
Progress West Hospital	O Fallon	61%	300+
Research Medical Center	Kansas City	61%	300+
Saint Anthony's Medical Center	Saint Louis	61%	300+
Saint Joseph Medical Center	Kansas City	61%	300+
Saint Luke's Northland Hospital	Kansas City	61%	300+
Freeman Health System - Freeman West	Joplin	58%	300+
Cameron Regional Medical Center	Cameron	56%	(a)
Poplar Bluff Regional Medical Center	Poplar Bluff	53%	300+
Pemiscot County Memorial Hospital	Hayti	49%	(a)
Saint Alexius Hospital	Saint Louis	46%	300+

Would Definitely Recommend Hospital

Hospital Name	City	Rate	Cases
Saint Luke's Hospital	Chesterfield	86%	300+
SSM Saint Clare Health Center[11]	Fenton	85%	300+
Boone Hospital Center	Columbia	84%	300+
Mercy Hospital Joplin[11]	Joplin	83%	300+
Saint Luke's East Lee's Summit Hospital	Lees Summit	83%	300+
Progress West Hospital	O Fallon	82%	300+
Saint Francis Medical Center	Cape Girardeau	82%	300+

NOTE: Hospital profiles are in alphabetical order by state, then city, then hospital within the city; Rankings exclude hospitals with less than 25 cases except for patient surveys which excludes hospitals with less than 100 cases; (a) 100-299 cases; (1) The number of cases/patients is too few to report; (2) Data submitted were based on a sample of cases/patients; (3) Results are based on a shorter time period than required; (4) Data suppressed by CMS for one or more quarters; (5) Results are not available for this reporting period; (6) Fewer than 100 patients completed the HCAHPS survey; (7) No cases met the criteria for this measure; (8) The lower limit of the confidence interval cannot be calculated if the number of observed infections equals zero; (9) No data are available from the state/territory for this reporting period; (10) The scores shown reflect fewer than 50 completed surveys; (11) There were discrepancies in the data collection process; (12) This measure does not apply to this hospital for this reporting period; (13) Results cannot be calculated for this reporting period; (14) The results for this state are combined with nearby states to protect confidentiality; Please refer to the User's Guide for a full explanation of data.

Saint Luke's Hospital of Kansas City	Kansas City	82%	300+
Mercy Hospital Saint Louis[11]	Saint Louis	81%	300+
Southeast Missouri Hospital	Cape Girardeau	81%	300+
Barnes-Jewish Saint Peters Hospital	Saint Peters	80%	300+
Barton County Memorial Hospital	Lamar	80%	(a)
Capital Region Medical Center	Jefferson City	80%	300+
Mercy Hospital Springfield[11]	Springfield	80%	300+
SSM Saint Joseph Hospital West	Lake Saint Louis	80%	300+
University of Missouri Health Care	Columbia	80%	300+
North Kansas City Hospital	N Kansas City	79%	300+
Barnes-Jewish Hospital	Saint Louis	78%	300+
Ozarks Community Hospital	Springfield	78%	(a)
Parkland Health Center	Farmington	78%	300+
Barnes-Jewish West County Hospital	Creve Coeur	77%	300+
Saint Louis University Hospital	Saint Louis	77%	300+
Saint Luke's Northland Hospital	Kansas City	77%	300+
Freeman Neosho Hospital	Neosho	76%	(a)
Missouri Baptist Medical Center	Town & Country	76%	300+
SSM Depaul Health Center	Bridgeton	76%	300+
Truman Medical Center Lakewood	Kansas City	76%	(a)
Cass Regional Medical Center	Harrisonville	75%	300+
Liberty Hospital	Liberty	75%	300+
SSM Saint Marys Health Center	Richmond Hghts	75%	300+
Community Hospital Association	Fairfax	74%	(a)
Saint Mary's Health Center	Jefferson City	74%	300+
Sainte Genevieve County Memorial Hospital	Ste Genevieve	74%	(a)
Cox Medical Center	Springfield	73%	300+
Des Peres Hospital	Saint Louis	73%	300+
Missouri Baptist Sullivan Hospital	Sullivan	73%	300+
Lee's Summit Medical Center	Lees Summit	72%	300+
Saint Joseph Medical Center	Kansas City	72%	300+
Saint Mary's Medical Center	Blue Springs	72%	300+
SSM Saint Joseph Health Center	Saint Charles	72%	300+
Freeman Health System - Freeman West	Joplin	71%	300+
Wright Memorial Hospital	Trenton	71%	(a)
Citizens Memorial Hospital	Bolivar	70%	300+
Hannibal Regional Hospital	Hannibal	70%	300+
Western Missouri Medical Center	Warrensburg	70%	300+
Cox Medical Center Branson	Branson	69%	300+
Lafayette Regional Health Center	Lexington	69%	(a)
Mercy Hospital Lebanon[11]	Lebanon	69%	300+
Mercy Hospital Washington[11]	Washington	69%	300+
Saint Anthony's Medical Center	Saint Louis	69%	300+
Saint Francis Hospital & Health Services	Maryville	69%	(a)
Heartland Regional Medical Center	Saint Joseph	68%	300+
Missouri Delta Medical Center	Sikeston	68%	300+
Phelps County Regional Medical Center	Rolla	68%	300+
Golden Valley Memorial Hospital	Clinton	67%	300+
Bates County Memorial Hospital	Butler	66%	(a)
Christian Hospital Northeast - Northwest	Saint Louis	66%	300+
Northwest Medical Center[3]	Albany	66%	(a)
Audrain Medical Center	Mexico	65%	300+
Centerpoint Medical Center	Independence	65%	300+
Hedrick Medical Center	Chillicothe	65%	(a)
Northeast Regional Medical Center	Kirksville	65%	300+
Ozarks Medical Center	West Plains	65%	300+
Belton Regional Medical Center	Belton	64%	300+
Lake Regional Health System	Osage Beach	64%	300+
Mineral Area Regional Medical Center	Farmington	64%	300+
Research Medical Center	Kansas City	64%	300+
Bothwell Regional Health Center	Sedalia	63%	300+
Cameron Regional Medical Center	Cameron	63%	(a)
Mercy Hospital Jefferson	Crystal City	63%	300+
Southeasthealth Center of Stoddard County	Dexter	63%	(a)
Nevada Regional Medical Center	Nevada	61%	(a)
Texas County Memorial Hospital	Houston	61%	300+
Moberly Regional Medical Center	Moberly	60%	300+
Truman Medical Center Hospital Hill	Kansas City	60%	300+
Lincoln County Medical Center	Troy	57%	(a)
Fitzgibbon Hospital	Marshall	56%	300+
Twin Rivers Regional Medical Center	Kennett	56%	(a)
Cooper County Memorial Hospital	Boonville	55%	(a)
Saint Alexius Hospital	Saint Louis	51%	300+
Poplar Bluff Regional Medical Center	Poplar Bluff	47%	300+
Pemiscot County Memorial Hospital	Hayti	38%	(a)

Use of Medical Imaging

Cardiac Imaging Stress Test before OP Surgery

Hospital Name	City	Rate	Cases
Missouri Baptist Sullivan Hospital	Sullivan	0.0%	140
Des Peres Hospital	Saint Louis	1.9%	107
Saint Luke's Northland Hospital	Kansas City	2.0%	202
Sainte Genevieve County Memorial Hospital	Ste Genevieve	2.5%	118
Audrain Medical Center	Mexico	3.2%	154
Hannibal Regional Hospital	Hannibal	3.2%	125
Missouri Delta Medical Center	Sikeston	3.2%	125
Western Missouri Medical Center	Warrensburg	3.3%	211
Barnes-Jewish West County Hospital	Creve Coeur	3.5%	115
Truman Medical Center Hospital Hill	Kansas City	3.6%	195
Lake Regional Health System	Osage Beach	3.7%	953
Phelps County Regional Medical Center	Rolla	3.7%	410
Citizens Memorial Hospital	Bolivar	3.8%	263
Belton Regional Medical Center	Belton	4.0%	124
Lee's Summit Medical Center	Lees Summit	4.0%	100
Saint Francis Medical Center	Cape Girardeau	4.0%	810
Ozarks Medical Center	West Plains	4.1%	493
SSM Saint Joseph Health Center	Saint Charles	4.2%	980
Golden Valley Memorial Hospital	Clinton	4.3%	231
Mercy Hospital Joplin	Joplin	4.4%	834
Research Medical Center	Kansas City	4.4%	274
Saint Joseph Medical Center	Kansas City	4.4%	780
Saint Luke's Hospital of Kansas City	Kansas City	4.4%	666
Cox Medical Center Branson	Branson	4.5%	684
Northeast Regional Medical Center	Kirksville	4.5%	243
Mercy Hospital Washington	Washington	4.6%	741
Christian Hospital Northeast - Northwest	Saint Louis	4.7%	275
Bothwell Regional Health Center	Sedalia	4.8%	416
Cameron Regional Medical Center	Cameron	4.8%	166
Freeman Health System - Freeman West	Joplin	4.8%	1429
Mercy Hospital Lebanon	Lebanon	4.8%	227
Mercy Hospital Saint Louis	Saint Louis	4.9%	1757
Barnes-Jewish Saint Peters Hospital	Saint Peters	5.0%	499
Cox Medical Center	Springfield	5.1%	1430
Saint Luke's Hospital	Chesterfield	5.1%	962
Twin Rivers Regional Medical Center	Kennett	5.1%	196
Saint Luke's East Lee's Summit Hospital	Lees Summit	5.2%	367
Saint Mary's Medical Center	Blue Springs	5.2%	250
Barnes-Jewish Hospital	Saint Louis	5.3%	1260
Missouri Baptist Medical Center	Town & Country	5.5%	1642
Mercy Hospital Springfield	Springfield	5.8%	569
North Kansas City Hospital	N Kansas City	5.8%	1338
Southeast Missouri Hospital	Cape Girardeau	5.8%	1191
Black River Community Medical Center	Poplar Bluff	5.9%	202
Heartland Regional Medical Center	Saint Joseph	5.9%	1074
Boone Hospital Center	Columbia	6.0%	1414
Saint Mary's Health Center	Jefferson City	6.0%	184
SSM Depaul Health Center	Bridgeton	6.0%	518
SSM Saint Joseph Hospital West	Lake Saint Louis	6.1%	540
SSM Saint Marys Health Center	Richmond Hghts	6.1%	593
University of Missouri Health Care	Columbia	6.1%	475
Ozarks Community Hospital	Springfield	6.2%	145
Saint Louis University Hospital	Saint Louis	6.3%	128
Moberly Regional Medical Center	Moberly	6.7%	224
Parkland Health Center	Farmington	6.9%	320
Centerpoint Medical Center	Independence	7.0%	316
Texas County Memorial Hospital	Houston	7.1%	70
Liberty Hospital	Liberty	7.9%	316
Saint Anthony's Medical Center	Saint Louis	8.3%	420
Progress West Hospital	O Fallon	8.6%	163
Fitzgibbon Hospital	Marshall	9.0%	122
Poplar Bluff Regional Medical Center	Poplar Bluff	9.3%	150
SSM Saint Clare Health Center	Fenton	9.6%	334
Mineral Area Regional Medical Center	Farmington	10.0%	100
Capital Region Medical Center	Jefferson City	10.5%	228

Combination Abdominal CT Scan

Hospital Name	City	Rate	Cases
Pemiscot County Memorial Hospital	Hayti	0.5%	213
Parkland Health Center	Farmington	1.3%	991
Sac-Osage Hospital	Osceola	1.6%	61
Saint Francis Hospital & Health Services	Maryville	1.7%	295
Heartland Regional Medical Center	Saint Joseph	1.8%	1578
Progress West Hospital	O Fallon	1.9%	207
Saint Luke's Hospital of Kansas City	Kansas City	1.9%	376
Lake Regional Health System	Osage Beach	2.0%	636
Missouri Baptist Sullivan Hospital	Sullivan	2.0%	301
Barnes-Jewish Saint Peters Hospital	Saint Peters	2.1%	846
Christian Hospital Northeast - Northwest	Saint Louis	2.2%	889
Saint Luke's East Lee's Summit Hospital	Lees Summit	2.2%	1044
Citizens Memorial Hospital	Bolivar	2.3%	598
Sainte Genevieve County Memorial Hospital	Ste Genevieve	2.5%	278
Mercy Hospital Springfield	Springfield	2.6%	2789
Southeast Health Center of Ripley County	Doniphan	2.6%	156
Saint Mary's Medical Center	Blue Springs	3.1%	489
Saint Luke's Hospital	Chesterfield	3.2%	1699
Nevada Regional Medical Center	Nevada	3.3%	213
Belton Regional Medical Center	Belton	3.5%	316
Mercy Hospital Lebanon	Lebanon	3.6%	604
Missouri Baptist Medical Center	Town & Country	3.7%	1914
Audrain Medical Center	Mexico	3.9%	309
Freeman Health System - Freeman West	Joplin	3.9%	1531
Boone Hospital Center	Columbia	4.0%	1113
SSM Saint Joseph Health Center	Saint Charles	4.0%	708
Fitzgibbon Hospital	Marshall	4.1%	320
Mercy Hospital Saint Louis	Saint Louis	4.3%	1910
Western Missouri Medical Center	Warrensburg	4.6%	461
Wright Memorial Hospital	Trenton	4.8%	145
SSM Saint Joseph Hospital West	Lake Saint Louis	5.0%	837
Barnes-Jewish Hospital	Saint Louis	5.5%	4956
SSM Depaul Health Center	Bridgeton	5.5%	1062
Barnes-Jewish West County Hospital	Creve Coeur	6.0%	1361
Golden Valley Memorial Hospital	Clinton	6.2%	530
Saint Luke's Northland Hospital	Kansas City	6.2%	433
Des Peres Hospital	Saint Louis	6.4%	220
Missouri Delta Medical Center	Sikeston	6.5%	371
Cox Medical Center	Springfield	6.7%	2279
Lafayette Regional Health Center	Lexington	6.7%	223
Mercy Hospital Joplin	Joplin	7.1%	756
Texas County Memorial Hospital	Houston	7.4%	231
Research Medical Center	Kansas City	7.6%	724
Centerpoint Medical Center	Independence	8.4%	874
Saint Mary's Health Center	Jefferson City	8.5%	399
Community Hospital Association	Fairfax	9.2%	120
Saint Alexius Hospital	Saint Louis	9.9%	111
Cooper County Memorial Hospital	Boonville	10.2%	98
Moberly Regional Medical Center	Moberly	10.7%	206
Cox Medical Center Branson	Branson	11.0%	816
Lee's Summit Medical Center	Lees Summit	11.3%	265
Cameron Regional Medical Center	Cameron	11.5%	304
Saint Louis University Hospital	Saint Louis	11.7%	677
Twin Rivers Regional Medical Center	Kennett	11.8%	502
North Kansas City Hospital	N Kansas City	12.1%	1435
Mineral Area Regional Medical Center	Farmington	12.2%	327
Truman Medical Center Hospital Hill	Kansas City	13.3%	248
Mercy Hospital Jefferson	Crystal City	13.6%	782
Truman Medical Center Lakewood	Kansas City	13.7%	161
Liberty Hospital	Liberty	14.2%	1167
Saint Joseph Medical Center	Kansas City	15.4%	869
Capital Region Medical Center	Jefferson City	15.9%	898
SSM Saint Clare Health Center	Fenton	16.4%	700
Saint Anthony's Medical Center	Saint Louis	16.8%	1618
SSM Saint Marys Health Center	Richmond Hghts	16.9%	663
Ozarks Community Hospital	Springfield	17.8%	135
Bates County Memorial Hospital	Butler	18.3%	262
University of Missouri Health Care	Columbia	20.5%	938
Hannibal Regional Hospital	Hannibal	20.7%	411
Southeasthealth Center of Stoddard County	Dexter	21.3%	244
Phelps County Regional Medical Center	Rolla	21.9%	699
Black River Community Medical Center	Poplar Bluff	22.4%	450
Mercy Hospital Washington	Washington	22.8%	839
Poplar Bluff Regional Medical Center	Poplar Bluff	23.7%	651
Northeast Regional Medical Center	Kirksville	30.1%	365
Saint Francis Medical Center	Cape Girardeau	30.4%	1810
Mercy Mccune Brooks Hospital	Carthage	35.2%	105
Callaway Community Hospital	Fulton	55.1%	127
Bothwell Regional Health Center	Sedalia	59.4%	907
Southeast Missouri Hospital	Cape Girardeau	61.0%	1108
Ozarks Medical Center	West Plains	61.3%	767

Combination Brain/Sinus CT Scan

Hospital Name	City	Rate	Cases
Des Peres Hospital	Saint Louis	0.0%	156
Cooper County Memorial Hospital	Boonville	1.1%	176
Citizens Memorial Hospital	Bolivar	1.4%	484
Mercy Hospital Joplin	Joplin	1.5%	666
SSM Saint Joseph Health Center	Saint Charles	1.5%	582
Mineral Area Regional Medical Center	Farmington	1.7%	363
Saint Mary's Health Center	Jefferson City	1.7%	460
Barnes-Jewish Hospital	Saint Louis	2.1%	1557
Cox Medical Center Branson	Branson	2.1%	665
Freeman Health System - Freeman West	Joplin	2.1%	998
Heartland Regional Medical Center	Saint Joseph	2.2%	1345
Mercy Hospital Lebanon	Lebanon	2.2%	597
Saint Joseph Medical Center	Kansas City	2.3%	954
Phelps County Regional Medical Center	Rolla	2.5%	842
SSM Depaul Health Center	Bridgeton	2.5%	1089
Poplar Bluff Regional Medical Center	Poplar Bluff	2.6%	729
Mercy Hospital Washington	Washington	2.7%	590
Missouri Baptist Medical Center	Town & Country	2.7%	1269
Saint Luke's Hospital	Chesterfield	2.7%	1111
Cox Medical Center	Springfield	2.8%	1802
Mercy Hospital Springfield	Springfield	2.8%	1817
Twin Rivers Regional Medical Center	Kennett	2.8%	703
Lake Regional Health System	Osage Beach	3.0%	700
Southeast Missouri Hospital	Cape Girardeau	3.0%	776
University of Missouri Health Care	Columbia	3.0%	725
SSM Saint Joseph Hospital West	Lake Saint Louis	3.1%	687
Boone Hospital Center	Columbia	3.4%	754
Saint Anthony's Medical Center	Saint Louis	3.4%	1288
Saint Luke's East Lee's Summit Hospital	Lees Summit	3.4%	865
SSM Saint Clare Health Center	Fenton	3.4%	730
Saint Luke's Hospital of Kansas City	Kansas City	3.6%	695
Ozarks Medical Center	West Plains	3.7%	778
Saint Francis Medical Center	Cape Girardeau	3.7%	1423
Liberty Hospital	Liberty	3.8%	852
North Kansas City Hospital	N Kansas City	3.9%	1321
Centerpoint Medical Center	Independence	4.0%	1015
SSM Saint Marys Health Center	Richmond Hghts	4.0%	695
Parkland Health Center	Farmington	4.1%	765
Christian Hospital Northeast - Northwest	Saint Louis	4.2%	975
Saint Louis University Hospital	Saint Louis	4.2%	500

NOTE: Hospital profiles are in alphabetical order by state, then city, then hospital within the city; Rankings exclude hospitals with less than 25 cases except for patient surveys which excludes hospitals with less than 100 cases; (a) 100-299 cases; (1) The number of cases/patients is too few to report; (2) Data submitted were based on a sample of cases/patients; (3) Results are based on a shorter time period than required; (4) Data suppressed by CMS for one or more quarters; (5) Results are not available for this reporting period; (6) Fewer than 100 patients completed the HCAHPS survey; (7) No cases met the criteria for this measure; (8) The lower limit of the confidence interval cannot be calculated if the number of observed infections equals zero; (9) No data are available from the state/territory for this reporting period; (10) The scores shown reflect fewer than 50 completed surveys; (11) There were discrepancies in the data collection process; (12) This measure does not apply to this hospital for this reporting period; (13) Results cannot be calculated for this reporting period; (14) The results for this state are combined with nearby states to protect confidentiality; Please refer to the User's Guide for a full explanation of data.

Hospital Name	City	Rate	Cases
Barnes-Jewish Saint Peters Hospital	Saint Peters	4.3%	464
Barnes-Jewish West County Hospital	Creve Coeur	4.4%	361
Bates County Memorial Hospital	Butler	4.4%	274
Hannibal Regional Hospital	Hannibal	4.6%	505
Pemiscot County Memorial Hospital	Hayti	4.8%	227
Research Medical Center	Kansas City	4.9%	749
Mercy Hospital Saint Louis	Saint Louis	5.3%	867
Bothwell Regional Health Center	Sedalia	5.9%	607
Southeast Health Center of Ripley County	Doniphan	7.2%	125
Texas County Memorial Hospital	Houston	8.1%	248
Ozarks Community Hospital	Springfield	8.8%	113

Combination Chest CT Scan

Hospital Name	City	Rate	Cases
Audrain Medical Center	Mexico	0.0%	316
Barnes-Jewish Saint Peters Hospital	Saint Peters	0.0%	906
Black River Community Medical Center	Poplar Bluff	0.0%	259
Citizens Memorial Hospital	Bolivar	0.0%	344
Cox Medical Center	Springfield	0.0%	1855
Des Peres Hospital	Saint Louis	0.0%	75
Lafayette Regional Health Center	Lexington	0.0%	171
Missouri Baptist Sullivan Hospital	Sullivan	0.0%	350
Nevada Regional Medical Center	Nevada	0.0%	91
Progress West Hospital	O Fallon	0.0%	190
Saint Luke's East Lee's Summit Hospital	Lees Summit	0.0%	643
Southeast Health Center of Ripley County	Doniphan	0.0%	91
Christian Hospital Northeast - Northwest	Saint Louis	0.1%	835
Mercy Hospital Springfield	Springfield	0.1%	1726
Saint Francis Medical Center	Cape Girardeau	0.1%	1190
Capital Region Medical Center	Jefferson City	0.2%	917
Phelps County Regional Medical Center	Rolla	0.2%	511
Freeman Health System - Freeman West	Joplin	0.3%	1240
Golden Valley Memorial Hospital	Clinton	0.3%	287
Missouri Baptist Medical Center	Town & Country	0.3%	1925
SSM Saint Marys Health Center	Richmond Hghts	0.3%	325
Mercy Hospital Saint Louis	Saint Louis	0.4%	1775
Truman Medical Center Hospital Hill	Kansas City	0.4%	255
Boone Hospital Center	Columbia	0.5%	934
Ozarks Medical Center	West Plains	0.5%	569
Saint Mary's Health Center	Jefferson City	0.5%	202
Belton Regional Medical Center	Belton	0.6%	169
Mercy Hospital Joplin	Joplin	0.6%	634
Mercy Hospital Washington	Washington	0.6%	679
Saint Anthony's Medical Center	Saint Louis	0.6%	853
Saint Luke's Hospital	Chesterfield	0.6%	1553
Barnes-Jewish West County Hospital	Creve Coeur	0.7%	1812
SSM Saint Joseph Hospital West	Lake Saint Louis	0.7%	535
Barnes-Jewish Hospital	Saint Louis	0.8%	6283
Missouri Delta Medical Center	Sikeston	0.8%	254
Southeast Missouri Hospital	Cape Girardeau	0.8%	926
Western Missouri Medical Center	Warrensburg	0.8%	254
Fitzgibbon Hospital	Marshall	1.0%	197
Parkland Health Center	Farmington	1.2%	513
Saint Francis Hospital & Health Services	Maryville	1.2%	257
SSM Depaul Health Center	Bridgeton	1.4%	490
Lake Regional Health System	Osage Beach	1.5%	341
SSM Saint Clare Health Center	Fenton	1.5%	469
SSM Saint Joseph Health Center	Saint Charles	1.5%	518
Centerpoint Medical Center	Independence	1.6%	369
University of Missouri Health Care	Columbia	1.6%	1167
Pemiscot County Memorial Hospital	Hayti	1.7%	59
Sainte Genevieve County Memorial Hospital	Ste Genevieve	1.7%	119
Saint Luke's Northland Hospital	Kansas City	1.8%	223
Research Medical Center	Kansas City	2.0%	564
Wright Memorial Hospital	Trenton	2.1%	144
Truman Medical Center Lakewood	Kansas City	2.2%	91
Heartland Regional Medical Center	Saint Joseph	2.4%	1407
North Kansas City Hospital	N Kansas City	2.5%	1220
Lee's Summit Medical Center	Lees Summit	2.6%	115
Saint Mary's Medical Center	Blue Springs	2.7%	185
Callaway Community Hospital	Fulton	2.9%	70
Community Hospital Association	Fairfax	3.4%	58
Cameron Regional Medical Center	Cameron	3.6%	138
Saint Louis University Hospital	Saint Louis	3.7%	657
Texas County Memorial Hospital	Houston	4.0%	124
Saint Joseph Medical Center	Kansas City	4.3%	397
Liberty Hospital	Liberty	4.5%	662
Mercy Hospital Jefferson	Crystal City	5.6%	647
Mercy Hospital Lebanon	Lebanon	5.6%	338
Cox Medical Center Branson	Branson	5.9%	545
Poplar Bluff Regional Medical Center	Poplar Bluff	6.4%	405
Mineral Area Regional Medical Center	Farmington	7.9%	126
Southeasthealth Center of Stoddard County	Dexter	8.5%	117
Hannibal Regional Hospital	Hannibal	9.2%	98
Moberly Regional Medical Center	Moberly	9.8%	92
Bates County Memorial Hospital	Butler	12.2%	164
Saint Luke's Hospital of Kansas City	Kansas City	13.9%	101
Bothwell Regional Health Center	Sedalia	15.2%	554
Twin Rivers Regional Medical Center	Kennett	21.5%	219
Northeast Regional Medical Center	Kirksville	24.1%	270

Follow-up Mammogram/Ultrasound

A follow-up rate near zero may indicate missed cancer; a rate higher than 14% may mean there is unnecessary follow up.

Hospital Name	City	Rate	Cases
Mercy Mccune Brooks Hospital	Carthage	2.7%	146
Pemiscot County Memorial Hospital	Hayti	3.1%	163
Sac-Osage Hospital	Osceola	3.4%	88
Southeast Missouri Hospital	Cape Girardeau	4.2%	1774
Boone Hospital Center	Columbia	4.3%	3870
Freeman Health System - Freeman West	Joplin	4.7%	3032
Nevada Regional Medical Center	Nevada	5.1%	431
Bothwell Regional Health Center	Sedalia	5.3%	1244
Golden Valley Memorial Hospital	Clinton	5.3%	848
Sainte Genevieve County Memorial Hospital	Ste Genevieve	5.5%	237
Research Medical Center	Kansas City	5.6%	1122
Saint Anthony's Medical Center	Saint Louis	5.6%	3400
Mercy Hospital Washington	Washington	5.7%	1690
Missouri Baptist Medical Center	Town & Country	5.7%	3320
Parkland Health Center	Farmington	5.8%	1392
Progress West Hospital	O Fallon	5.8%	257
Missouri Delta Medical Center	Sikeston	5.9%	666
Saint Luke's Hospital	Chesterfield	5.9%	5868
Mineral Area Regional Medical Center	Farmington	6.0%	546
Poplar Bluff Regional Medical Center	Poplar Bluff	6.1%	407
Belton Regional Medical Center	Belton	6.2%	545
Missouri Baptist Sullivan Hospital	Sullivan	6.4%	327
SSM Saint Joseph Hospital West	Lake Saint Louis	6.4%	1306
SSM Depaul Health Center	Bridgeton	6.5%	1181
Citizens Memorial Hospital	Bolivar	6.6%	817
Black River Community Medical Center	Poplar Bluff	6.7%	1072
Mercy Hospital Lebanon	Lebanon	6.8%	1021
Cameron Regional Medical Center	Cameron	6.9%	334
Saint Francis Hospital & Health Services	Maryville	6.9%	550
Mercy Hospital Saint Louis	Saint Louis	7.2%	5563
Fitzgibbon Hospital	Marshall	7.5%	589
Liberty Hospital	Liberty	7.6%	2047
Saint Mary's Medical Center	Blue Springs	7.7%	829
Heartland Regional Medical Center	Saint Joseph	8.1%	2992
Mercy Hospital Jefferson	Crystal City	8.3%	940
Texas County Memorial Hospital	Houston	8.3%	351
Saint Luke's East Lee's Summit Hospital	Lees Summit	8.4%	1037
Barnes-Jewish Hospital	Saint Louis	8.8%	5075
Barnes-Jewish West County Hospital	Creve Coeur	8.8%	786
Capital Region Medical Center	Jefferson City	8.8%	1417
Saint Luke's Northland Hospital	Kansas City	8.8%	762
Barnes-Jewish Saint Peters Hospital	Saint Peters	9.0%	1047
Des Peres Hospital	Saint Louis	9.0%	155
Ozarks Medical Center	West Plains	9.0%	879
Audrain Medical Center	Mexico	9.1%	1059
Saint Louis University Hospital	Saint Louis	9.1%	328
Southeasthealth Center of Stoddard County	Dexter	9.1%	384
Cox Medical Center	Springfield	9.4%	3875
Mercy Hospital Springfield	Springfield	10.1%	5510
SSM Saint Marys Health Center	Richmond Hghts	10.1%	1583
Lafayette Regional Health Center	Lexington	10.2%	275
SSM Saint Clare Health Center	Fenton	10.2%	1014
Saint Francis Medical Center	Cape Girardeau	10.3%	2066
Bates County Memorial Hospital	Butler	10.4%	260
Phelps County Regional Medical Center	Rolla	10.4%	1556
Saint Joseph Medical Center	Kansas City	10.4%	1405
Truman Medical Center Lakewood	Kansas City	10.5%	401
Centerpoint Medical Center	Independence	10.6%	1393
Lee's Summit Medical Center	Lees Summit	10.7%	450
Cox Medical Center Branson	Branson	10.8%	1441
Community Hospital Association	Fairfax	11.0%	172
SSM Saint Joseph Health Center	Saint Charles	11.0%	1294
Western Missouri Medical Center	Warrensburg	11.0%	599
Saint Mary's Health Center	Jefferson City	11.9%	846
Moberly Regional Medical Center	Moberly	12.1%	223
Twin Rivers Regional Medical Center	Kennett	12.1%	431
Hannibal Regional Hospital	Hannibal	12.2%	197
Saint Luke's Hospital of Kansas City	Kansas City	12.2%	998
Christian Hospital Northeast - Northwest	Saint Louis	12.8%	1410
Callaway Community Hospital	Fulton	14.5%	200
Northeast Regional Medical Center	Kirksville	15.3%	765
University of Missouri Health Care	Columbia	15.4%	3287
North Kansas City Hospital	N Kansas City	16.2%	1559
Truman Medical Center Hospital Hill	Kansas City	17.1%	613
Mercy Hospital Joplin	Joplin	17.2%	646
Saint Alexius Hospital	Saint Louis	22.1%	249
Wright Memorial Hospital	Trenton	65.5%	278

Lumbar Spine MRI for Low Back Pain

Hospital Name	City	Rate	Cases
Twin Rivers Regional Medical Center	Kennett	25.4%	142
SSM Saint Clare Health Center	Fenton	28.6%	185
Saint Francis Hospital & Health Services	Maryville	30.6%	62
Mineral Area Regional Medical Center	Farmington	30.9%	81
Missouri Delta Medical Center	Sikeston	31.0%	71
Black River Community Medical Center	Poplar Bluff	31.3%	224
Mercy Hospital Washington	Washington	32.1%	196
Barnes-Jewish Hospital	Saint Louis	32.3%	443
Barnes-Jewish Saint Peters Hospital	Saint Peters	32.9%	73
Saint Luke's Hospital	Chesterfield	32.9%	508
Christian Hospital Northeast - Northwest	Saint Louis	33.0%	94
Research Medical Center	Kansas City	33.0%	94
University of Missouri Health Care	Columbia	33.2%	235
Saint Anthony's Medical Center	Saint Louis	33.3%	165
SSM Depaul Health Center	Bridgeton	33.3%	153
Mercy Hospital Jefferson	Crystal City	34.4%	128
Barnes-Jewish West County Hospital	Creve Coeur	35.4%	113
Freeman Health System - Freeman West	Joplin	35.4%	407
SSM Saint Joseph Hospital West	Lake Saint Louis	35.5%	141
Saint Mary's Medical Center	Blue Springs	36.1%	83
Cox Medical Center Branson	Branson	36.8%	152
Southeast Missouri Hospital	Cape Girardeau	36.9%	203
Belton Regional Medical Center	Belton	37.0%	73
Cameron Regional Medical Center	Cameron	37.0%	46
Parkland Health Center	Farmington	37.5%	136
Missouri Baptist Medical Center	Town & Country	38.0%	279
Des Peres Hospital	Saint Louis	38.1%	126
Heartland Regional Medical Center	Saint Joseph	38.2%	275
Capital Region Medical Center	Jefferson City	38.7%	191
Saint Joseph Medical Center	Kansas City	38.8%	160
Golden Valley Memorial Hospital	Clinton	39.2%	130
Poplar Bluff Regional Medical Center	Poplar Bluff	39.2%	148
Liberty Hospital	Liberty	39.3%	173
SSM Saint Marys Health Center	Richmond Hghts	39.4%	94
Hannibal Regional Hospital	Hannibal	39.7%	73
SSM Saint Joseph Health Center	Saint Charles	39.7%	131
Western Missouri Medical Center	Warrensburg	42.1%	107
Centerpoint Medical Center	Independence	42.3%	111
North Kansas City Hospital	N Kansas City	42.5%	497
Cox Medical Center	Springfield	42.7%	581
Ozarks Medical Center	West Plains	42.7%	164
Mercy Hospital Springfield	Springfield	43.5%	543
Saint Francis Medical Center	Cape Girardeau	43.5%	271
Audrain Medical Center	Mexico	43.9%	82
Lee's Summit Medical Center	Lees Summit	43.9%	41
Mercy Hospital Joplin	Joplin	44.2%	129
Saint Luke's East Lee's Summit Hospital	Lees Summit	44.2%	120
Mercy Hospital Saint Louis	Saint Louis	44.4%	363
Saint Louis University Hospital	Saint Louis	44.7%	38
Truman Medical Center Hospital Hill	Kansas City	45.7%	35
Boone Hospital Center	Columbia	47.1%	223
Saint Luke's Northland Hospital	Kansas City	48.3%	89
Bothwell Regional Health Center	Sedalia	48.7%	113
Nevada Regional Medical Center	Nevada	49.1%	57
Saint Mary's Health Center	Jefferson City	50.8%	122
Citizens Memorial Hospital	Bolivar	51.3%	113
Truman Medical Center Lakewood	Kansas City	51.3%	39
Phelps County Regional Medical Center	Rolla	52.0%	175
Sainte Genevieve County Memorial Hospital	Ste Genevieve	53.1%	49
Missouri Baptist Sullivan Hospital	Sullivan	53.8%	52
Bates County Memorial Hospital	Butler	54.8%	73
Fitzgibbon Hospital	Marshall	60.0%	55
Mercy Hospital Lebanon	Lebanon	67.7%	133

NOTE: Hospital profiles are in alphabetical order by state, then city, then hospital within the city; Rankings exclude hospitals with less than 25 cases except for patient surveys which excludes hospitals with less than 100 cases; (a) 100-299 cases; (1) The number of cases/patients is too few to report; (2) Data submitted were based on a sample of cases/patients; (3) Results are based on a shorter time period than required; (4) Data suppressed by CMS for one or more quarters; (5) Results are not available for this reporting period; (6) Fewer than 100 patients completed the HCAHPS survey; (7) No cases met the criteria for this measure; (8) The lower limit of the confidence interval cannot be calculated if the number of observed infections equals zero; (9) No data are available from the state/territory for this reporting period; (10) The scores shown reflect fewer than 50 completed surveys; (11) There were discrepancies in the data collection process; (12) This measure does not apply to this hospital for this reporting period; (13) Results cannot be calculated for this reporting period; (14) The results for this state are combined with nearby states to protect confidentiality; Please refer to the User's Guide for a full explanation of data.

Northwest Medical Center

705 N College Street
Albany, MO 64402
Phone: 660-726-3941
Fax: 660-726-3647
URL: www.gcmh.org
Type: Critical Access Hospitals
Emergency Services: Yes
Ownership: Voluntary non-profit - Private
Beds: 45

Key Personnel:
CEO/President. . . . . Angelia Martin, MD
Chief of Medical Staff . . . . Angelia Martin

Measure	Cases	This Hosp.	State Avg.	U.S. Avg.
Blood Clot Prevention and Treatment				
Anticoagulation Overlap Therapy[5]	-	-	94%	93%
ICU Venous Thromboembolism Prophylaxis[5]	-	-	91%	92%
Incidence of Potentially Preventable VTE[5]	-	-	7%	10%
UFH with Dosages/Platelet Monitoring[5]	-	-	96%	97%
Venous Thromboembolism Prophylaxis[5]	-	-	85%	85%
Warfarin Therapy Discharge Instructions[5]	-	-	76%	75%
Chest Pain/Possible Heart Attack Care				
Aspirin Given Within 24 Hours of Arrival	-	-	95%	96%
Fibrinolytic Meds Within 30 Min. of Arrival	-	-	53%	58%
Average Time to ECG (minutes)	-	-	7	7
Average Time to Transfer (minutes)	-	-	53	60
Children's Asthma Care				
Received Home Management Plan of Care	-	-	-	88%
Received Reliever Medication	-	-	-	100%
Received Systemic Corticosteroids	-	-	-	100%
Emergency Department				
Admittance Decision Time (minutes)[5]	-	-	81	98
Head CT Results Within 45 Min. of Arrival	-	-	63%	57%
Patients Who Left ER Before Being Seen	-	-	3%	2%
Time from ER Arrival to Admit. (minutes)[5]	-	-	238	274
Time from ER Arrival to Discharge (minutes)	-	-	136	134
Time in ER Before Being Evaluated (minutes)	-	-	26	26
Time to Pain Meds for Fractures (minutes)	-	-	52	57
Heart Attack Care				
Aspirin Given at Discharge[1,3]	-	-	99%	99%
Fibrinolytic Meds Within 30 Min. of Arrival[3,7]	-	-	-	54%
PCI Within 90 Minutes of Arrival[3,7]	-	-	97%	96%
Statin Prescribed at Discharge[1,3]	-	-	98%	98%
Heart Failure Care				
ACE Inhibitor or ARB for LVSD[1,3]	-	-	96%	97%
Discharge Instructions Given[1,3]	-	-	94%	94%
Evaluation of LVS Function[3]	16	75%	98%	99%
Medicare Spending				
Medicare Spending per Patient (ratio)	-	-	0.95	0.98
Pneumonia Care				
Appropriate Initial Antibiotic Given[3]	12	92%	95%	95%
Blood Culture Timing[1,3]	-	-	98%	98%
Pregnancy and Delivery Care				
Newborn Deliveries Scheduled Early[5]	-	-	5%	6%
Preventive Care				
Immunization for Influenza[5]	-	-	92%	90%
Immunization for Pneumonia[5]	-	-	93%	92%
Stroke Care				
Anticoagulation Therapy for Atrial Fibrillation[5]	-	-	94%	95%
Antithrombotic Therapy Timing[5]	-	-	98%	98%
Assessed for Rehabilitation[5]	-	-	98%	97%
Discharged on Antithrombotic Therapy[5]	-	-	99%	99%
Discharged on Statin Medication[5]	-	-	95%	94%
Thrombolytic Therapy Timing[5]	-	-	67%	66%
Venous Thromboembolism Prophylaxis[5]	-	-	95%	94%
Written Stroke Educational Materials Given[5]	-	-	88%	88%
Surgical Care Improvement Project				
Appropriate Beta Blocker Usage[5]	-	-	98%	98%
Appropriate VTP Within 24 Hours[5]	-	-	98%	98%
Controlled Postoperative Blood Glucose[5]	-	-	97%	97%
Perioperative Temperature Management[5]	-	-	100%	100%
Prophylactic Antibiotic Selection[5]	-	-	99%	99%
Prophylactic Antibiotic Selection (Outpatient)	-	-	98%	98%
Prophylactic Antibiotic Stopped[5]	-	-	98%	98%
Prophylactic Antibiotic Timing[5]	-	-	99%	99%
Prophylactic Antibiotic Timing (Outpatient)	-	-	98%	98%
Urinary Catheter Removal[5]	-	-	97%	97%
Survey of Patients' Hospital Experiences				
Area Around Room 'Always' Quiet at Night[3]	(a)	57%	61%	61%
Doctors 'Always' Communicated Well[3]	(a)	82%	82%	82%
Home Recovery Information Given[3]	(a)	79%	87%	85%
Hospital Given 9 or 10 on 10 Point Scale[3]	(a)	74%	71%	71%
Meds 'Always' Explained Before Given[3]	(a)	54%	63%	64%
Nurses 'Always' Communicated Well[3]	(a)	79%	79%	79%
Pain 'Always' Well Controlled[3]	(a)	69%	71%	71%
Room and Bathroom 'Always' Clean[3]	(a)	81%	73%	73%
Timely Help 'Always' Received[3]	(a)	71%	68%	68%
Would Definitely Recommend Hospital[3]	(a)	66%	70%	71%
Use of Medical Imaging				
Cardiac Imaging Stress Test before Surgery	-	-	5.2%	5.3%
Combination Abdominal CT Scan	-	-	11.2%	10.5%
Combination Brain/Sinus CT Scan	-	-	3.2%	2.7%
Combination Chest CT Scan	-	-	1.9%	2.7%
Follow-up Mammogram/Ultrasound	-	-	8.6%	8.8%
Lumbar Spine MRI for Low Back Pain	-	-	39.6%	37.2%

Mercy Hospital Aurora

500 Porter Avenue
Aurora, MO 65605
Phone: 417-678-2122
Fax: 417-678-7877
E-mail: ach@achmo.com
URL: www.achmo.com
Type: Critical Access Hospitals
Emergency Services: Yes
Ownership: Voluntary non-profit - Church
Beds: 25

Key Personnel:
Chief of Medical Staff. . . . . Joseph Bizek
CEO/President. . . . . Lynn Britton
Cardiac Laboratory. . . . . Dave Dickson
Operating Room. . . . . Debbie Ehase
Quality Assurance . . . . Cathy Munden
Infection Control. . . . . Debbie Nelson
Emergency Room . . . . Kent Stringer

Measure	Cases	This Hosp.	State Avg.	U.S. Avg.
Blood Clot Prevention and Treatment				
Anticoagulation Overlap Therapy[5]	-	-	94%	93%
ICU Venous Thromboembolism Prophylaxis[5]	-	-	91%	92%
Incidence of Potentially Preventable VTE[5]	-	-	7%	10%
UFH with Dosages/Platelet Monitoring[5]	-	-	96%	97%
Venous Thromboembolism Prophylaxis[5]	-	-	85%	85%
Warfarin Therapy Discharge Instructions[5]	-	-	76%	75%
Chest Pain/Possible Heart Attack Care				
Aspirin Given Within 24 Hours of Arrival	-	-	95%	96%
Fibrinolytic Meds Within 30 Min. of Arrival	-	-	53%	58%
Average Time to ECG (minutes)	-	-	7	7
Average Time to Transfer (minutes)	-	-	53	60
Children's Asthma Care				
Received Home Management Plan of Care	-	-	-	88%
Received Reliever Medication	-	-	-	100%
Received Systemic Corticosteroids	-	-	-	100%
Emergency Department				
Admittance Decision Time (minutes)[2]	200	55	81	98
Head CT Results Within 45 Min. of Arrival	-	-	63%	57%
Patients Who Left ER Before Being Seen	-	-	3%	2%
Time from ER Arrival to Admit. (minutes)[2]	205	236	238	274
Time from ER Arrival to Discharge (minutes)	-	-	136	134
Time in ER Before Being Evaluated (minutes)	-	-	26	26
Time to Pain Meds for Fractures (minutes)	-	-	52	57
Heart Attack Care				
Aspirin Given at Discharge[5]	-	-	99%	99%
Fibrinolytic Meds Within 30 Min. of Arrival[5]	-	-	-	54%
PCI Within 90 Minutes of Arrival[5]	-	-	97%	96%
Statin Prescribed at Discharge[5]	-	-	98%	98%
Heart Failure Care				
ACE Inhibitor or ARB for LVSD[3,7]	-	-	96%	97%
Discharge Instructions Given[1,3]	-	-	94%	94%
Evaluation of LVS Function[1,3]	-	-	98%	99%
Medicare Spending				
Medicare Spending per Patient (ratio)	-	-	0.95	0.98
Pneumonia Care				
Appropriate Initial Antibiotic Given	25	88%	95%	95%
Blood Culture Timing	33	94%	98%	98%
Pregnancy and Delivery Care				
Newborn Deliveries Scheduled Early[5]	-	-	5%	6%
Preventive Care				
Immunization for Influenza[2]	310	82%	92%	90%
Immunization for Pneumonia[2]	259	97%	93%	92%
Stroke Care				
Anticoagulation Therapy for Atrial Fibrillation[5]	-	-	94%	95%
Antithrombotic Therapy Timing[5]	-	-	98%	98%
Assessed for Rehabilitation[5]	-	-	98%	97%
Discharged on Antithrombotic Therapy[5]	-	-	99%	99%
Discharged on Statin Medication[5]	-	-	95%	94%
Thrombolytic Therapy Timing[5]	-	-	67%	66%
Venous Thromboembolism Prophylaxis[5]	-	-	95%	94%
Written Stroke Educational Materials Given[5]	-	-	88%	88%
Surgical Care Improvement Project				
Appropriate Beta Blocker Usage[5]	-	-	98%	98%
Appropriate VTP Within 24 Hours[5]	-	-	98%	98%
Controlled Postoperative Blood Glucose[5]	-	-	97%	97%
Perioperative Temperature Management[5]	-	-	100%	100%
Prophylactic Antibiotic Selection[5]	-	-	99%	99%
Prophylactic Antibiotic Selection (Outpatient)	-	-	98%	98%
Prophylactic Antibiotic Stopped[5]	-	-	98%	98%
Prophylactic Antibiotic Timing[5]	-	-	99%	99%
Prophylactic Antibiotic Timing (Outpatient)	-	-	98%	98%
Urinary Catheter Removal[5]	-	-	97%	97%
Survey of Patients' Hospital Experiences				
Area Around Room 'Always' Quiet at Night[5]	-	-	61%	61%
Doctors 'Always' Communicated Well[5]	-	-	82%	82%
Home Recovery Information Given[5]	-	-	87%	85%
Hospital Given 9 or 10 on 10 Point Scale[5]	-	-	71%	71%
Meds 'Always' Explained Before Given[5]	-	-	63%	64%
Nurses 'Always' Communicated Well[5]	-	-	79%	79%
Pain 'Always' Well Controlled[5]	-	-	71%	71%
Room and Bathroom 'Always' Clean[5]	-	-	73%	73%
Timely Help 'Always' Received[5]	-	-	68%	68%
Would Definitely Recommend Hospital[5]	-	-	70%	71%
Use of Medical Imaging				
Cardiac Imaging Stress Test before Surgery	-	-	5.2%	5.3%
Combination Abdominal CT Scan	-	-	11.2%	10.5%
Combination Brain/Sinus CT Scan	-	-	3.2%	2.7%
Combination Chest CT Scan	-	-	1.9%	2.7%
Follow-up Mammogram/Ultrasound	-	-	8.6%	8.8%
Lumbar Spine MRI for Low Back Pain	-	-	39.6%	37.2%

Belton Regional Medical Center

17065 S 71 Highway
Belton, MO 64012
Phone: 816-348-1236
Fax: 816-348-1293
URL: www.beltonregionalmedicalcenter.com
Type: Acute Care Hospitals
Emergency Services: Yes
Ownership: Voluntary non-profit - Private
Beds: 75

Key Personnel:
Chief of Medical Staff . . . . Kirk Barnett
Emergency Room . . . . Carol Creek, RN
Operating Room. . . . . Carol Creek, RN
Infection Control. . . . . Cheryl Davis
Intensive Care Unit. . . . . Fran Florea, RN
Radiology. . . . . Barry A Gubin
CEO/President. . . . . Steve Newton

Measure	Cases	This Hosp.	State Avg.	U.S. Avg.
Blood Clot Prevention and Treatment				
Anticoagulation Overlap Therapy[2]	22	100%	94%	93%
ICU Venous Thromboembolism Prophylaxis[2]	43	100%	91%	92%
Incidence of Potentially Preventable VTE[1,2]	-	-	7%	10%
UFH with Dosages/Platelet Monitoring[1,2]	-	-	96%	97%
Venous Thromboembolism Prophylaxis[2]	184	100%	85%	85%
Warfarin Therapy Discharge Instructions[2]	12	100%	76%	75%
Chest Pain/Possible Heart Attack Care				
Aspirin Given Within 24 Hours of Arrival	38	100%	95%	96%
Fibrinolytic Meds Within 30 Min. of Arrival[7]	-	-	53%	58%
Average Time to ECG (minutes)	42	9	7	7
Average Time to Transfer (minutes)[1]	-	-	53	60
Children's Asthma Care				
Received Home Management Plan of Care	-	-	-	88%
Received Reliever Medication	-	-	-	100%
Received Systemic Corticosteroids	-	-	-	100%

NOTE: Hospital profiles are in alphabetical order by state, then city, then hospital within the city; Rankings exclude hospitals with less than 25 cases except for patient surveys which excludes hospitals with less than 100 cases; (a) 100-299 cases; (1) The number of cases/patients is too few to report; (2) Data submitted were based on a sample of cases/patients; (3) Results are based on a shorter time period than required; (4) Data suppressed by CMS for one or more quarters; (5) Results are not available for this reporting period; (6) Fewer than 100 patients completed the HCAHPS survey; (7) No cases met the criteria for this measure; (8) The lower limit of the confidence interval cannot be calculated if the number of observed infections equals zero; (9) No data are available from the state/territory for this reporting period; (10) The scores shown reflect fewer than 50 completed surveys; (11) There were discrepancies in the data collection process; (12) This measure does not apply to this hospital for this reporting period; (13) Results cannot be calculated for this reporting period; (14) The results for this state are combined with nearby states to protect confidentiality; Please refer to the User's Guide for a full explanation of data.

Measure	Cases	This Hosp.	State Avg.	U.S. Avg.
Emergency Department				
Admittance Decision Time (minutes)[2]	344	85	81	98
Head CT Results Within 45 Min. of Arrival[1]	-	-	63%	57%
Patients Who Left ER Before Being Seen	19,595	2%	3%	2%
Time from ER Arrival to Admit. (minutes)[2]	367	248	238	274
Time from ER Arrival to Discharge (minutes)	432	118	136	134
Time in ER Before Being Evaluated (minutes)	475	17	26	26
Time to Pain Meds for Fractures (minutes)	65	49	52	57
Heart Attack Care				
Aspirin Given at Discharge[1]	-	-	99%	99%
Fibrinolytic Meds Within 30 Min. of Arrival[7]	-	-	-	54%
PCI Within 90 Minutes of Arrival[7]	-	-	97%	96%
Statin Prescribed at Discharge[1]	-	-	98%	98%
Heart Failure Care				
ACE Inhibitor or ARB for LVSD	15	100%	96%	97%
Discharge Instructions Given	37	100%	94%	94%
Evaluation of LVS Function	50	100%	98%	99%
Medicare Spending				
Medicare Spending per Patient (ratio)	-	0.95	0.95	0.98
Pneumonia Care				
Appropriate Initial Antibiotic Given	36	100%	95%	95%
Blood Culture Timing	45	98%	98%	98%
Pregnancy and Delivery Care				
Newborn Deliveries Scheduled Early[2,7]	-	-	5%	6%
Preventive Care				
Immunization for Influenza[2]	307	100%	92%	90%
Immunization for Pneumonia[2]	463	100%	93%	92%
Stroke Care				
Anticoagulation Therapy for Atrial Fibrillation[1]	-	-	94%	95%
Antithrombotic Therapy Timing[1]	-	-	98%	98%
Assessed for Rehabilitation	11	100%	98%	97%
Discharged on Antithrombotic Therapy	11	100%	99%	99%
Discharged on Statin Medication[1]	-	-	95%	94%
Thrombolytic Therapy Timing[7]	-	-	67%	66%
Venous Thromboembolism Prophylaxis[1]	-	-	95%	94%
Written Stroke Educational Materials Given[1]	-	-	88%	88%
Surgical Care Improvement Project				
Appropriate Beta Blocker Usage	49	100%	98%	98%
Appropriate VTP Within 24 Hours	287	100%	98%	98%
Controlled Postoperative Blood Glucose[7]	-	-	97%	97%
Perioperative Temperature Management	303	100%	100%	100%
Prophylactic Antibiotic Selection	255	100%	99%	99%
Prophylactic Antibiotic Selection (Outpatient)	55	100%	98%	98%
Prophylactic Antibiotic Stopped	254	100%	98%	98%
Prophylactic Antibiotic Timing	255	100%	99%	99%
Prophylactic Antibiotic Timing (Outpatient)	55	100%	98%	98%
Urinary Catheter Removal	267	100%	97%	97%
Survey of Patients' Hospital Experiences				
Area Around Room 'Always' Quiet at Night	300+	62%	61%	61%
Doctors 'Always' Communicated Well	300+	79%	82%	82%
Home Recovery Information Given	300+	87%	87%	85%
Hospital Given 9 or 10 on 10 Point Scale	300+	64%	71%	71%
Meds 'Always' Explained Before Given	300+	61%	63%	64%
Nurses 'Always' Communicated Well	300+	76%	79%	79%
Pain 'Always' Well Controlled	300+	72%	71%	71%
Room and Bathroom 'Always' Clean	300+	63%	73%	73%
Timely Help 'Always' Received	300+	65%	68%	68%
Would Definitely Recommend Hospital	300+	64%	70%	71%
Use of Medical Imaging				
Cardiac Imaging Stress Test before Surgery	124	4.0%	5.2%	5.3%
Combination Abdominal CT Scan	316	3.5%	11.2%	10.5%
Combination Brain/Sinus CT Scan[1]	-	-	3.2%	2.7%
Combination Chest CT Scan	169	0.6%	1.9%	2.7%
Follow-up Mammogram/Ultrasound	545	6.2%	8.6%	8.8%
Lumbar Spine MRI for Low Back Pain	73	37.0%	39.6%	37.2%

Harrison County Community Hospital

2600 Miller Street
Bethany, MO 64424
Phone: 660-425-0284
Fax: 660-425-8535
URL: www.hcchospital.org
Type: Critical Access Hospitals
Emergency Services: Yes
Ownership: Govt - Hospital Dist/Auth
Beds: 17

Key Personnel:
Emergency Room . . . . Crystal Hicks
Chief of Medical Staff . . . . Natu Patel
Cardiac Laboratory. . . . . Kaeitie Smith

Measure	Cases	This Hosp.	State Avg.	U.S. Avg.
Blood Clot Prevention and Treatment				
Anticoagulation Overlap Therapy[5]	-	-	94%	93%
ICU Venous Thromboembolism Prophylaxis[5]	-	-	91%	92%
Incidence of Potentially Preventable VTE[5]	-	-	7%	10%
UFH with Dosages/Platelet Monitoring[5]	-	-	96%	97%
Venous Thromboembolism Prophylaxis[5]	-	-	85%	85%
Warfarin Therapy Discharge Instructions[5]	-	-	76%	75%
Chest Pain/Possible Heart Attack Care				
Aspirin Given Within 24 Hours of Arrival	-	-	95%	96%
Fibrinolytic Meds Within 30 Min. of Arrival	-	-	53%	58%
Average Time to ECG (minutes)	-	-	7	7
Average Time to Transfer (minutes)	-	-	53	60
Children's Asthma Care				
Received Home Management Plan of Care	-	-	-	88%
Received Reliever Medication	-	-	-	100%
Received Systemic Corticosteroids	-	-	-	100%
Emergency Department				
Admittance Decision Time (minutes)[5]	-	-	81	98
Head CT Results Within 45 Min. of Arrival	-	-	63%	57%
Patients Who Left ER Before Being Seen	-	-	3%	2%
Time from ER Arrival to Admit. (minutes)[5]	-	-	238	274
Time from ER Arrival to Discharge (minutes)	-	-	136	134
Time in ER Before Being Evaluated (minutes)	-	-	26	26
Time to Pain Meds for Fractures (minutes)	-	-	52	57
Heart Attack Care				
Aspirin Given at Discharge[1,3]	-	-	99%	99%
Fibrinolytic Meds Within 30 Min. of Arrival[3,7]	-	-	-	54%
PCI Within 90 Minutes of Arrival[3,7]	-	-	97%	96%
Statin Prescribed at Discharge[1,3]	-	-	98%	98%
Heart Failure Care				
ACE Inhibitor or ARB for LVSD[1]	-	-	96%	97%
Discharge Instructions Given[1]	-	-	94%	94%
Evaluation of LVS Function	15	47%	98%	99%
Medicare Spending				
Medicare Spending per Patient (ratio)	-	-	0.95	0.98
Pneumonia Care				
Appropriate Initial Antibiotic Given	23	96%	95%	95%
Blood Culture Timing	14	100%	98%	98%
Pregnancy and Delivery Care				
Newborn Deliveries Scheduled Early[5]	-	-	5%	6%
Preventive Care				
Immunization for Influenza[5]	-	-	92%	90%
Immunization for Pneumonia[5]	-	-	93%	92%
Stroke Care				
Anticoagulation Therapy for Atrial Fibrillation[5]	-	-	94%	95%
Antithrombotic Therapy Timing[5]	-	-	98%	98%
Assessed for Rehabilitation[5]	-	-	98%	97%
Discharged on Antithrombotic Therapy[5]	-	-	99%	99%
Discharged on Statin Medication[5]	-	-	95%	94%
Thrombolytic Therapy Timing[5]	-	-	67%	66%
Venous Thromboembolism Prophylaxis[5]	-	-	95%	94%
Written Stroke Educational Materials Given[5]	-	-	88%	88%
Surgical Care Improvement Project				
Appropriate Beta Blocker Usage[5]	-	-	98%	98%
Appropriate VTP Within 24 Hours[5]	-	-	98%	98%
Controlled Postoperative Blood Glucose[5]	-	-	97%	97%
Perioperative Temperature Management[5]	-	-	100%	100%
Prophylactic Antibiotic Selection[5]	-	-	99%	99%
Prophylactic Antibiotic Selection (Outpatient)	-	-	98%	98%
Prophylactic Antibiotic Stopped[5]	-	-	98%	98%
Prophylactic Antibiotic Timing[5]	-	-	99%	99%
Prophylactic Antibiotic Timing (Outpatient)	-	-	98%	98%
Urinary Catheter Removal[5]	-	-	97%	97%
Survey of Patients' Hospital Experiences				
Area Around Room 'Always' Quiet at Night[5]	-	-	61%	61%
Doctors 'Always' Communicated Well[5]	-	-	82%	82%
Home Recovery Information Given[5]	-	-	87%	85%
Hospital Given 9 or 10 on 10 Point Scale[5]	-	-	71%	71%
Meds 'Always' Explained Before Given[5]	-	-	63%	64%
Nurses 'Always' Communicated Well[5]	-	-	79%	79%
Pain 'Always' Well Controlled[5]	-	-	71%	71%
Room and Bathroom 'Always' Clean[5]	-	-	73%	73%
Timely Help 'Always' Received[5]	-	-	68%	68%
Would Definitely Recommend Hospital[5]	-	-	70%	71%
Use of Medical Imaging				
Cardiac Imaging Stress Test before Surgery	-	-	5.2%	5.3%
Combination Abdominal CT Scan	-	-	11.2%	10.5%
Combination Brain/Sinus CT Scan	-	-	3.2%	2.7%
Combination Chest CT Scan	-	-	1.9%	2.7%
Follow-up Mammogram/Ultrasound	-	-	8.6%	8.8%
Lumbar Spine MRI for Low Back Pain	-	-	39.6%	37.2%

Saint Mary's Medical Center

201 Nw R D Mize Rd
Blue Springs, MO 64014
Phone: 816-228-5900
Fax: 816-655-5649
URL: www.stmaryskc.com
Type: Acute Care Hospitals
Emergency Services: Yes
Ownership: Voluntary non-profit - Church
Beds: 143

Key Personnel:
Emergency Room . . . . Judy Avise
CEO/President. . . . . Gordon Docking
Cardiac Laboratory. . . . . Cynthia Peters
Chief of Medical Staff . . . . Steve Sanders

Measure	Cases	This Hosp.	State Avg.	U.S. Avg.
Blood Clot Prevention and Treatment				
Anticoagulation Overlap Therapy[2]	48	100%	94%	93%
ICU Venous Thromboembolism Prophylaxis[2]	62	100%	91%	92%
Incidence of Potentially Preventable VTE[1,2]	-	-	7%	10%
UFH with Dosages/Platelet Monitoring[2]	26	100%	96%	97%
Venous Thromboembolism Prophylaxis[2]	328	100%	85%	85%
Warfarin Therapy Discharge Instructions[2]	41	98%	76%	75%
Chest Pain/Possible Heart Attack Care				
Aspirin Given Within 24 Hours of Arrival[1,3]	-	-	95%	96%
Fibrinolytic Meds Within 30 Min. of Arrival[5]	-	-	53%	58%
Average Time to ECG (minutes)[1,3]	-	-	7	7
Average Time to Transfer (minutes)[5]	-	-	53	60
Children's Asthma Care				
Received Home Management Plan of Care	-	-	-	88%
Received Reliever Medication	-	-	-	100%
Received Systemic Corticosteroids	-	-	-	100%
Emergency Department				
Admittance Decision Time (minutes)[2]	630	110	81	98
Head CT Results Within 45 Min. of Arrival[1]	-	-	63%	57%
Patients Who Left ER Before Being Seen	29,376	2%	3%	2%
Time from ER Arrival to Admit. (minutes)[2]	639	258	238	274
Time from ER Arrival to Discharge (minutes)	358	114	136	134
Time in ER Before Being Evaluated (minutes)	383	17	26	26
Time to Pain Meds for Fractures (minutes)	106	44	52	57
Heart Attack Care				
Aspirin Given at Discharge	127	100%	99%	99%
Fibrinolytic Meds Within 30 Min. of Arrival[7]	-	-	-	54%
PCI Within 90 Minutes of Arrival	37	97%	97%	96%
Statin Prescribed at Discharge	124	98%	98%	98%
Heart Failure Care				
ACE Inhibitor or ARB for LVSD	26	88%	96%	97%
Discharge Instructions Given	81	74%	94%	94%
Evaluation of LVS Function	106	100%	98%	99%
Medicare Spending				
Medicare Spending per Patient (ratio)	-	1.02	0.95	0.98
Pneumonia Care				
Appropriate Initial Antibiotic Given	139	98%	95%	95%
Blood Culture Timing	190	98%	98%	98%
Pregnancy and Delivery Care				
Newborn Deliveries Scheduled Early[2]	17	0%	5%	6%
Preventive Care				
Immunization for Influenza[2]	474	95%	92%	90%
Immunization for Pneumonia[2]	582	96%	93%	92%
Stroke Care				
Anticoagulation Therapy for Atrial Fibrillation[1]	-	-	94%	95%
Antithrombotic Therapy Timing	34	100%	98%	98%
Assessed for Rehabilitation	37	97%	98%	97%
Discharged on Antithrombotic Therapy	34	100%	99%	99%

NOTE: Hospital profiles are in alphabetical order by state, then city, then hospital within the city; Rankings exclude hospitals with less than 25 cases except for patient surveys which excludes hospitals with less than 100 cases; (a) 100-299 cases; (1) The number of cases/patients is too few to report; (2) Data submitted were based on a sample of cases/patients; (3) Results are based on a shorter time period than required; (4) Data suppressed by CMS for one or more quarters; (5) Results are not available for this reporting period; (6) Fewer than 100 patients completed the HCAHPS survey; (7) No cases met the criteria for this measure; (8) The lower limit of the confidence interval cannot be calculated if the number of observed infections equals zero; (9) No data are available from the state/territory for this reporting period; (10) The scores shown reflect fewer than 50 completed surveys; (11) There were discrepancies in the data collection process; (12) This measure does not apply to this hospital for this reporting period; (13) Results cannot be calculated for this reporting period; (14) The results for this state are combined with nearby states to protect confidentiality; Please refer to the User's Guide for a full explanation of data.

Measure	Cases	This Hosp.	State Avg.	U.S. Avg.
Discharged on Statin Medication	25	100%	95%	94%
Thrombolytic Therapy Timing[1]	-	-	67%	66%
Venous Thromboembolism Prophylaxis	38	100%	95%	94%
Written Stroke Educational Materials Given	18	94%	88%	88%
Surgical Care Improvement Project				
Appropriate Beta Blocker Usage[2]	63	100%	98%	98%
Appropriate VTP Within 24 Hours[2]	234	99%	98%	98%
Controlled Postoperative Blood Glucose[2,7]	-	-	97%	97%
Perioperative Temperature Management[2]	265	100%	100%	100%
Prophylactic Antibiotic Selection[2]	175	97%	99%	99%
Prophylactic Antibiotic Selection (Outpatient)	24	96%	98%	98%
Prophylactic Antibiotic Stopped[2]	175	99%	98%	98%
Prophylactic Antibiotic Timing[2]	176	99%	99%	99%
Prophylactic Antibiotic Timing (Outpatient)	24	100%	98%	98%
Urinary Catheter Removal[2]	140	99%	97%	97%
Survey of Patients' Hospital Experiences				
Area Around Room 'Always' Quiet at Night	300+	57%	61%	61%
Doctors 'Always' Communicated Well	300+	79%	82%	82%
Home Recovery Information Given	300+	88%	87%	85%
Hospital Given 9 or 10 on 10 Point Scale	300+	75%	71%	71%
Meds 'Always' Explained Before Given	300+	62%	63%	64%
Nurses 'Always' Communicated Well	300+	80%	79%	79%
Pain 'Always' Well Controlled	300+	73%	71%	71%
Room and Bathroom 'Always' Clean	300+	75%	73%	73%
Timely Help 'Always' Received	300+	68%	68%	68%
Would Definitely Recommend Hospital	300+	72%	70%	71%
Use of Medical Imaging				
Cardiac Imaging Stress Test before Surgery	250	5.2%	5.2%	5.3%
Combination Abdominal CT Scan	489	3.1%	11.2%	10.5%
Combination Brain/Sinus CT Scan[1]	-	-	3.2%	2.7%
Combination Chest CT Scan	185	2.7%	1.9%	2.7%
Follow-up Mammogram/Ultrasound	829	7.7%	8.6%	8.8%
Lumbar Spine MRI for Low Back Pain	83	36.1%	39.6%	37.2%

Citizens Memorial Hospital

1500 N Oakland
Bolivar, MO 65613
Phone: 417-326-6000
Fax: 417-326-0338
URL: www.citizensmemorial.com
Type: Acute Care Hospitals
Emergency Services: Yes
Ownership: Govt - Hospital Dist/Auth
Beds: 74

Key Personnel:
CEO/President. . . . . Donald J Babb
Chief of Medical Staff. . . . . Dennis Boeke, DO
Radiology. . . . . John Gamble, III
Quality Assurance . . . . Karen Keeton
Infection Control. . . . . Helen Molchan, RN
Operating Room. . . . . Nancy Nickos

Measure	Cases	This Hosp.	State Avg.	U.S. Avg.
Blood Clot Prevention and Treatment				
Anticoagulation Overlap Therapy[2]	11	73%	94%	93%
ICU Venous Thromboembolism Prophylaxis[2]	63	78%	91%	92%
Incidence of Potentially Preventable VTE[1,2]	-	-	7%	10%
UFH with Dosages/Platelet Monitoring[1,2]	-	-	96%	97%
Venous Thromboembolism Prophylaxis[2]	129	84%	85%	85%
Warfarin Therapy Discharge Instructions[1,2]	-	-	76%	75%
Chest Pain/Possible Heart Attack Care				
Aspirin Given Within 24 Hours of Arrival	39	100%	95%	96%
Fibrinolytic Meds Within 30 Min. of Arrival[1]	-	-	53%	58%
Average Time to ECG (minutes)	39	6	7	7
Average Time to Transfer (minutes)[1]	-	-	53	60
Children's Asthma Care				
Received Home Management Plan of Care	-	-	-	88%
Received Reliever Medication	-	-	-	100%
Received Systemic Corticosteroids	-	-	-	100%
Emergency Department				
Admittance Decision Time (minutes)[2]	288	88	81	98
Head CT Results Within 45 Min. of Arrival	12	92%	63%	57%
Patients Who Left ER Before Being Seen	19,357	2%	3%	2%
Time from ER Arrival to Admit. (minutes)[2]	299	219	238	274
Time from ER Arrival to Discharge (minutes)	1,091	142	136	134
Time in ER Before Being Evaluated (minutes)	1,196	26	26	26
Time to Pain Meds for Fractures (minutes)	87	56	52	57
Heart Attack Care				
Aspirin Given at Discharge	52	98%	99%	99%
Fibrinolytic Meds Within 30 Min. of Arrival[7]	-	-	-	54%
PCI Within 90 Minutes of Arrival[1]	-	-	97%	96%
Statin Prescribed at Discharge	52	83%	98%	98%
Heart Failure Care				
ACE Inhibitor or ARB for LVSD	14	100%	96%	97%
Discharge Instructions Given	36	94%	94%	94%
Evaluation of LVS Function	43	100%	98%	99%
Medicare Spending				
Medicare Spending per Patient (ratio)	-	0.93	0.95	0.98
Pneumonia Care				
Appropriate Initial Antibiotic Given	70	93%	95%	95%
Blood Culture Timing	119	97%	98%	98%
Pregnancy and Delivery Care				
Newborn Deliveries Scheduled Early	49	4%	5%	6%
Preventive Care				
Immunization for Influenza[2]	292	86%	92%	90%
Immunization for Pneumonia[2]	365	90%	93%	92%
Stroke Care				
Anticoagulation Therapy for Atrial Fibrillation[1]	-	-	94%	95%
Antithrombotic Therapy Timing	21	100%	98%	98%
Assessed for Rehabilitation	26	88%	98%	97%
Discharged on Antithrombotic Therapy	24	100%	99%	99%
Discharged on Statin Medication	23	83%	95%	94%
Thrombolytic Therapy Timing[1]	-	-	67%	66%
Venous Thromboembolism Prophylaxis	22	86%	95%	94%
Written Stroke Educational Materials Given	15	40%	88%	88%
Surgical Care Improvement Project				
Appropriate Beta Blocker Usage	60	92%	98%	98%
Appropriate VTP Within 24 Hours	202	97%	98%	98%
Controlled Postoperative Blood Glucose[7]	-	-	97%	97%
Perioperative Temperature Management	218	100%	100%	100%
Prophylactic Antibiotic Selection	184	99%	99%	99%
Prophylactic Antibiotic Selection (Outpatient)	149	97%	98%	98%
Prophylactic Antibiotic Stopped	182	99%	98%	98%
Prophylactic Antibiotic Timing	184	98%	99%	99%
Prophylactic Antibiotic Timing (Outpatient)	151	98%	98%	98%
Urinary Catheter Removal	189	98%	97%	97%
Survey of Patients' Hospital Experiences				
Area Around Room 'Always' Quiet at Night	300+	59%	61%	61%
Doctors 'Always' Communicated Well	300+	83%	82%	82%
Home Recovery Information Given	300+	88%	87%	85%
Hospital Given 9 or 10 on 10 Point Scale	300+	72%	71%	71%
Meds 'Always' Explained Before Given	300+	59%	63%	64%
Nurses 'Always' Communicated Well	300+	79%	79%	79%
Pain 'Always' Well Controlled	300+	69%	71%	71%
Room and Bathroom 'Always' Clean	300+	75%	73%	73%
Timely Help 'Always' Received	300+	69%	68%	68%
Would Definitely Recommend Hospital	300+	70%	70%	71%
Use of Medical Imaging				
Cardiac Imaging Stress Test before Surgery	263	3.8%	5.2%	5.3%
Combination Abdominal CT Scan	598	2.3%	11.2%	10.5%
Combination Brain/Sinus CT Scan	484	1.4%	3.2%	2.7%
Combination Chest CT Scan	344	0.0%	1.9%	2.7%
Follow-up Mammogram/Ultrasound	817	6.6%	8.6%	8.8%
Lumbar Spine MRI for Low Back Pain	113	51.3%	39.6%	37.2%

Cooper County Memorial Hospital

17651 B Hwy
Boonville, MO 65233
Phone: 660-882-7461
Fax: 660-882-6093
Type: Acute Care Hospitals
Emergency Services: Yes
Ownership: Government - Local
Beds: 70

Key Personnel:
Cardiology . . . . William Fay, MD
CEO/President. . . . . Matt Waterman

Measure	Cases	This Hosp.	State Avg.	U.S. Avg.
Blood Clot Prevention and Treatment				
Anticoagulation Overlap Therapy[7]	-	-	94%	93%
ICU Venous Thromboembolism Prophylaxis[7]	-	-	91%	92%
Incidence of Potentially Preventable VTE[7]	-	-	7%	10%
UFH with Dosages/Platelet Monitoring[7]	-	-	96%	97%
Venous Thromboembolism Prophylaxis	93	81%	85%	85%
Warfarin Therapy Discharge Instructions[7]	-	-	76%	75%
Chest Pain/Possible Heart Attack Care				
Aspirin Given Within 24 Hours of Arrival	19	100%	95%	96%
Fibrinolytic Meds Within 30 Min. of Arrival[7]	-	-	53%	58%
Average Time to ECG (minutes)	24	11	7	7
Average Time to Transfer (minutes)[1]	-	-	53	60
Children's Asthma Care				
Received Home Management Plan of Care	-	-	-	88%
Received Reliever Medication	-	-	-	100%
Received Systemic Corticosteroids	-	-	-	100%
Emergency Department				
Admittance Decision Time (minutes)	143	30	81	98
Head CT Results Within 45 Min. of Arrival[1]	-	-	63%	57%
Patients Who Left ER Before Being Seen	7,272	1%	3%	2%
Time from ER Arrival to Admit. (minutes)	157	185	238	274
Time from ER Arrival to Discharge (minutes)	359	93	136	134
Time in ER Before Being Evaluated (minutes)	407	20	26	26
Time to Pain Meds for Fractures (minutes)	38	42	52	57
Heart Attack Care				
Aspirin Given at Discharge[1,3]	-	-	99%	99%
Fibrinolytic Meds Within 30 Min. of Arrival[3,7]	-	-	-	54%
PCI Within 90 Minutes of Arrival[3,7]	-	-	97%	96%
Statin Prescribed at Discharge[1,3]	-	-	98%	98%
Heart Failure Care				
ACE Inhibitor or ARB for LVSD[1]	-	-	96%	97%
Discharge Instructions Given	14	100%	94%	94%
Evaluation of LVS Function	22	100%	98%	99%
Medicare Spending				
Medicare Spending per Patient (ratio)	-	0.85	0.95	0.98
Pneumonia Care				
Appropriate Initial Antibiotic Given	12	100%	95%	95%
Blood Culture Timing	28	93%	98%	98%
Pregnancy and Delivery Care				
Newborn Deliveries Scheduled Early[7]	-	-	5%	6%
Preventive Care				
Immunization for Influenza	106	76%	92%	90%
Immunization for Pneumonia	164	90%	93%	92%
Stroke Care				
Anticoagulation Therapy for Atrial Fibrillation[5]	-	-	94%	95%
Antithrombotic Therapy Timing[5]	-	-	98%	98%
Assessed for Rehabilitation[5]	-	-	98%	97%
Discharged on Antithrombotic Therapy[5]	-	-	99%	99%
Discharged on Statin Medication[5]	-	-	95%	94%
Thrombolytic Therapy Timing[5]	-	-	67%	66%
Venous Thromboembolism Prophylaxis[5]	-	-	95%	94%
Written Stroke Educational Materials Given[5]	-	-	88%	88%
Surgical Care Improvement Project				
Appropriate Beta Blocker Usage[5]	-	-	98%	98%
Appropriate VTP Within 24 Hours[5]	-	-	98%	98%
Controlled Postoperative Blood Glucose[5]	-	-	97%	97%
Perioperative Temperature Management[5]	-	-	100%	100%
Prophylactic Antibiotic Selection[5]	-	-	99%	99%
Prophylactic Antibiotic Selection (Outpatient)[5]	-	-	98%	98%
Prophylactic Antibiotic Stopped[5]	-	-	98%	98%
Prophylactic Antibiotic Timing[5]	-	-	99%	99%
Prophylactic Antibiotic Timing (Outpatient)[5]	-	-	98%	98%
Urinary Catheter Removal[5]	-	-	97%	97%
Survey of Patients' Hospital Experiences				
Area Around Room 'Always' Quiet at Night	(a)	72%	61%	61%
Doctors 'Always' Communicated Well	(a)	81%	82%	82%
Home Recovery Information Given	(a)	84%	87%	85%
Hospital Given 9 or 10 on 10 Point Scale	(a)	58%	71%	71%
Meds 'Always' Explained Before Given	(a)	60%	63%	64%
Nurses 'Always' Communicated Well	(a)	75%	79%	79%
Pain 'Always' Well Controlled	(a)	67%	71%	71%
Room and Bathroom 'Always' Clean	(a)	73%	73%	73%
Timely Help 'Always' Received	(a)	70%	68%	68%
Would Definitely Recommend Hospital	(a)	55%	70%	71%
Use of Medical Imaging				
Cardiac Imaging Stress Test before Surgery[1]	-	-	5.2%	5.3%
Combination Abdominal CT Scan	98	10.2%	11.2%	10.5%
Combination Brain/Sinus CT Scan	176	1.1%	3.2%	2.7%
Combination Chest CT Scan[1]	-	-	1.9%	2.7%
Follow-up Mammogram/Ultrasound[7]	-	-	8.6%	8.8%

NOTE: Hospital profiles are in alphabetical order by state, then city, then hospital within the city; Rankings exclude hospitals with less than 25 cases except for patient surveys which excludes hospitals with less than 100 cases; (a) 100-299 cases; (1) The number of cases/patients is too few to report; (2) Data submitted were based on a sample of cases/patients; (3) Results are based on a shorter time period than required; (4) Data suppressed by CMS for one or more quarters; (5) Results are not available for this reporting period; (6) Fewer than 100 patients completed the HCAHPS survey; (7) No cases met the criteria for this measure; (8) The lower limit of the confidence interval cannot be calculated if the number of observed infections equals zero; (9) No data are available from the state/territory for this reporting period; (10) The scores shown reflect fewer than 50 completed surveys; (11) There were discrepancies in the data collection process; (12) This measure does not apply to this hospital for this reporting period; (13) Results cannot be calculated for this reporting period; (14) The results for this state are combined with nearby states to protect confidentiality; Please refer to the User's Guide for a full explanation of data.

Measure	Cases	This Hosp.	State Avg.	U.S. Avg.
Lumbar Spine MRI for Low Back Pain[1]	-	-	39.6%	37.2%

Cox Medical Center Branson

525 Branson Landing Blvd, PO Box 650
Branson, MO 65615
URL: www.skaggs.net
Type: Acute Care Hospitals
Ownership: Voluntary non-profit - Private
Phone: 417-335-7000
Fax: 417-334-1505
Emergency Services: Yes
Beds: 177

Key Personnel:
Infection Control. . . . . Ann Erving
Quality Assurance . . . . Cindy Gaddie
Cardiac Laboratory. . . . . Jon Jenkins
President . . . . William K. Mahoney, FACHE
Radiology. . . . . Richard S Makuch
Chief of Medical Staff. . . . . Peter Marcellus, MD
Intensive Care Unit. . . . . Angilee McPathe
Operating Room. . . . . Jackie Rozell

Measure	Cases	This Hosp.	State Avg.	U.S. Avg.
Blood Clot Prevention and Treatment				
Anticoagulation Overlap Therapy[2]	68	97%	94%	93%
ICU Venous Thromboembolism Prophylaxis[2]	113	89%	91%	92%
Incidence of Potentially Preventable VTE[1,2]	-	-	7%	10%
UFH with Dosages/Platelet Monitoring[2]	65	100%	96%	97%
Venous Thromboembolism Prophylaxis[2]	329	89%	85%	85%
Warfarin Therapy Discharge Instructions[2]	48	98%	76%	75%
Chest Pain/Possible Heart Attack Care				
Aspirin Given Within 24 Hours of Arrival[1]	-	-	95%	96%
Fibrinolytic Meds Within 30 Min. of Arrival[3,7]	-	-	53%	58%
Average Time to ECG (minutes)[1]	-	-	7	7
Average Time to Transfer (minutes)[3,7]	-	-	53	60
Children's Asthma Care				
Received Home Management Plan of Care	-	-	-	88%
Received Reliever Medication	-	-	-	100%
Received Systemic Corticosteroids	-	-	-	100%
Emergency Department				
Admittance Decision Time (minutes)[2]	695	133	81	98
Head CT Results Within 45 Min. of Arrival[1]	-	-	63%	57%
Patients Who Left ER Before Being Seen	35,423	1%	3%	2%
Time from ER Arrival to Admit. (minutes)[2]	696	267	238	274
Time from ER Arrival to Discharge (minutes)	448	89	136	134
Time in ER Before Being Evaluated (minutes)	490	29	26	26
Time to Pain Meds for Fractures (minutes)	82	66	52	57
Heart Attack Care				
Aspirin Given at Discharge	181	100%	99%	99%
Fibrinolytic Meds Within 30 Min. of Arrival[7]	-	-	-	54%
PCI Within 90 Minutes of Arrival	37	100%	97%	96%
Statin Prescribed at Discharge	172	98%	98%	98%
Heart Failure Care				
ACE Inhibitor or ARB for LVSD	58	97%	96%	97%
Discharge Instructions Given	182	97%	94%	94%
Evaluation of LVS Function	199	100%	98%	99%
Medicare Spending				
Medicare Spending per Patient (ratio)	-	0.95	0.95	0.98
Pneumonia Care				
Appropriate Initial Antibiotic Given[2]	105	98%	95%	95%
Blood Culture Timing[2]	166	99%	98%	98%
Pregnancy and Delivery Care				
Newborn Deliveries Scheduled Early[2]	77	0%	5%	6%
Preventive Care				
Immunization for Influenza[2]	516	95%	92%	90%
Immunization for Pneumonia[2]	743	98%	93%	92%
Stroke Care				
Anticoagulation Therapy for Atrial Fibrillation[1]	-	-	94%	95%
Antithrombotic Therapy Timing	59	100%	98%	98%
Assessed for Rehabilitation	58	100%	98%	97%
Discharged on Antithrombotic Therapy	57	100%	99%	99%
Discharged on Statin Medication	43	100%	95%	94%
Thrombolytic Therapy Timing[1]	-	-	67%	66%
Venous Thromboembolism Prophylaxis	61	98%	95%	94%
Written Stroke Educational Materials Given	36	100%	88%	88%
Surgical Care Improvement Project				
Appropriate Beta Blocker Usage[2]	80	98%	98%	98%
Appropriate VTP Within 24 Hours[2]	223	99%	98%	98%
Controlled Postoperative Blood Glucose[2,7]	-	-	97%	97%
Perioperative Temperature Management[2]	243	100%	100%	100%
Prophylactic Antibiotic Selection[2]	174	99%	99%	99%
Prophylactic Antibiotic Selection (Outpatient)	122	98%	98%	98%
Prophylactic Antibiotic Stopped[2]	167	99%	98%	98%
Prophylactic Antibiotic Timing[2]	174	100%	99%	99%
Prophylactic Antibiotic Timing (Outpatient)	126	94%	98%	98%
Urinary Catheter Removal[2]	205	99%	97%	97%
Survey of Patients' Hospital Experiences				
Area Around Room 'Always' Quiet at Night	300+	61%	61%	61%
Doctors 'Always' Communicated Well	300+	79%	82%	82%
Home Recovery Information Given	300+	86%	87%	85%
Hospital Given 9 or 10 on 10 Point Scale	300+	68%	71%	71%
Meds 'Always' Explained Before Given	300+	60%	63%	64%
Nurses 'Always' Communicated Well	300+	77%	79%	79%
Pain 'Always' Well Controlled	300+	65%	71%	71%
Room and Bathroom 'Always' Clean	300+	72%	73%	73%
Timely Help 'Always' Received	300+	66%	68%	68%
Would Definitely Recommend Hospital	300+	69%	70%	71%
Use of Medical Imaging				
Cardiac Imaging Stress Test before Surgery	684	4.5%	5.2%	5.3%
Combination Abdominal CT Scan	816	11.0%	11.2%	10.5%
Combination Brain/Sinus CT Scan	665	2.1%	3.2%	2.7%
Combination Chest CT Scan	545	5.9%	1.9%	2.7%
Follow-up Mammogram/Ultrasound	1,441	10.8%	8.6%	8.8%
Lumbar Spine MRI for Low Back Pain	152	36.8%	39.6%	37.2%

SSM Depaul Health Center

12303 Depaul Drive
Bridgeton, MO 63044
URL: www.ssmdepaul.com
Type: Acute Care Hospitals
Ownership: Voluntary non-profit - Private
Phone: 314-344-6000
Fax: 314-344-6840
Emergency Services: Yes
Beds: 476

Key Personnel:
Chief of Medical Staff. . . . . Jim E Bieser, MD
CEO/President. . . . . Pat Komoroski
Cardiac Laboratory. . . . . Mindy Manley
Quality Assurance . . . . PamAnn McDonald
Emergency Room . . . . Clare Mir

Measure	Cases	This Hosp.	State Avg.	U.S. Avg.
Blood Clot Prevention and Treatment				
Anticoagulation Overlap Therapy[2]	145	92%	94%	93%
ICU Venous Thromboembolism Prophylaxis[2]	48	100%	91%	92%
Incidence of Potentially Preventable VTE[2]	18	17%	7%	10%
UFH with Dosages/Platelet Monitoring[2]	80	88%	96%	97%
Venous Thromboembolism Prophylaxis[2]	296	85%	85%	85%
Warfarin Therapy Discharge Instructions[2]	115	35%	76%	75%
Chest Pain/Possible Heart Attack Care				
Aspirin Given Within 24 Hours of Arrival[1,3]	-	-	95%	96%
Fibrinolytic Meds Within 30 Min. of Arrival[3,7]	-	-	53%	58%
Average Time to ECG (minutes)[1,3]	-	-	7	7
Average Time to Transfer (minutes)[3,7]	-	-	53	60
Children's Asthma Care				
Received Home Management Plan of Care	-	-	-	88%
Received Reliever Medication	-	-	-	100%
Received Systemic Corticosteroids	-	-	-	100%
Emergency Department				
Admittance Decision Time (minutes)[2]	353	162	81	98
Head CT Results Within 45 Min. of Arrival[1]	-	-	63%	57%
Patients Who Left ER Before Being Seen	65,703	1%	3%	2%
Time from ER Arrival to Admit. (minutes)[2]	403	302	238	274
Time from ER Arrival to Discharge (minutes)	341	178	136	134
Time in ER Before Being Evaluated (minutes)	402	46	26	26
Time to Pain Meds for Fractures (minutes)	50	83	52	57
Heart Attack Care				
Aspirin Given at Discharge	273	100%	99%	99%
Fibrinolytic Meds Within 30 Min. of Arrival[7]	-	-	-	54%
PCI Within 90 Minutes of Arrival	56	100%	97%	96%
Statin Prescribed at Discharge	267	100%	98%	98%
Heart Failure Care				
ACE Inhibitor or ARB for LVSD[2]	79	100%	96%	97%
Discharge Instructions Given[2]	215	100%	94%	94%
Evaluation of LVS Function[2]	287	100%	98%	99%
Medicare Spending				
Medicare Spending per Patient (ratio)	-	1.00	0.95	0.98
Pneumonia Care				
Appropriate Initial Antibiotic Given[2]	61	100%	95%	95%
Blood Culture Timing[2]	117	98%	98%	98%
Pregnancy and Delivery Care				
Newborn Deliveries Scheduled Early[2]	31	13%	5%	6%
Preventive Care				
Immunization for Influenza[2]	567	99%	92%	90%
Immunization for Pneumonia[2]	757	98%	93%	92%
Stroke Care				
Anticoagulation Therapy for Atrial Fibrillation	38	92%	94%	95%
Antithrombotic Therapy Timing	217	99%	98%	98%
Assessed for Rehabilitation	338	99%	98%	97%
Discharged on Antithrombotic Therapy	295	100%	99%	99%
Discharged on Statin Medication	220	99%	95%	94%
Thrombolytic Therapy Timing	33	97%	67%	66%
Venous Thromboembolism Prophylaxis	321	100%	95%	94%
Written Stroke Educational Materials Given	165	98%	88%	88%
Surgical Care Improvement Project				
Appropriate Beta Blocker Usage[2]	260	99%	98%	98%
Appropriate VTP Within 24 Hours[2]	446	99%	98%	98%
Controlled Postoperative Blood Glucose[2]	148	99%	97%	97%
Perioperative Temperature Management[2]	527	100%	100%	100%
Prophylactic Antibiotic Selection[2]	472	99%	99%	99%
Prophylactic Antibiotic Selection (Outpatient)	461	99%	98%	98%
Prophylactic Antibiotic Stopped[2]	454	99%	98%	98%
Prophylactic Antibiotic Timing[2]	472	98%	99%	99%
Prophylactic Antibiotic Timing (Outpatient)	471	97%	98%	98%
Urinary Catheter Removal[2]	146	97%	97%	97%
Survey of Patients' Hospital Experiences				
Area Around Room 'Always' Quiet at Night	300+	62%	61%	61%
Doctors 'Always' Communicated Well	300+	83%	82%	82%
Home Recovery Information Given	300+	89%	87%	85%
Hospital Given 9 or 10 on 10 Point Scale	300+	77%	71%	71%
Meds 'Always' Explained Before Given	300+	63%	63%	64%
Nurses 'Always' Communicated Well	300+	85%	79%	79%
Pain 'Always' Well Controlled	300+	73%	71%	71%
Room and Bathroom 'Always' Clean	300+	69%	73%	73%
Timely Help 'Always' Received	300+	65%	68%	68%
Would Definitely Recommend Hospital	300+	76%	70%	71%
Use of Medical Imaging				
Cardiac Imaging Stress Test before Surgery	518	6.0%	5.2%	5.3%
Combination Abdominal CT Scan	1,062	5.5%	11.2%	10.5%
Combination Brain/Sinus CT Scan	1,089	2.5%	3.2%	2.7%
Combination Chest CT Scan	490	1.4%	1.9%	2.7%
Follow-up Mammogram/Ultrasound	1,181	6.5%	8.6%	8.8%
Lumbar Spine MRI for Low Back Pain	153	33.3%	39.6%	37.2%

Pershing Memorial Hospital

130 East Lockling
Brookfield, MO 64628
Type: Critical Access Hospitals
Ownership: Voluntary non-profit - Private
Phone: 660-258-2222
Fax: 660-258-5668
Emergency Services: Yes
Beds: 57

Key Personnel:
CEO/President. . . . . Phil Hamilton
Chief of Medical Staff. . . . . BD Howell, MD
Infection Control. . . . . Randy Kieffer
Emergency Room . . . . PC Rivera, MD
Quality Assurance . . . . Elaine Sutton
Ambulatory Care . . . . Betty Williams, CNE

Measure	Cases	This Hosp.	State Avg.	U.S. Avg.
Blood Clot Prevention and Treatment				
Anticoagulation Overlap Therapy[5]	-	-	94%	93%
ICU Venous Thromboembolism Prophylaxis[5]	-	-	91%	92%
Incidence of Potentially Preventable VTE[5]	-	-	7%	10%
UFH with Dosages/Platelet Monitoring[5]	-	-	96%	97%
Venous Thromboembolism Prophylaxis[5]	-	-	85%	85%
Warfarin Therapy Discharge Instructions[5]	-	-	76%	75%
Chest Pain/Possible Heart Attack Care				
Aspirin Given Within 24 Hours of Arrival	-	-	95%	96%
Fibrinolytic Meds Within 30 Min. of Arrival	-	-	53%	58%
Average Time to ECG (minutes)	-	-	7	7
Average Time to Transfer (minutes)	-	-	53	60

NOTE: Hospital profiles are in alphabetical order by state, then city, then hospital within the city; Rankings exclude hospitals with less than 25 cases except for patient surveys which excludes hospitals with less than 100 cases; (a) 100-299 cases; (1) The number of cases/patients is too few to report; (2) Data submitted were based on a sample of cases/patients; (3) Results are based on a shorter time period than required; (4) Data suppressed by CMS for one or more quarters; (5) Results are not available for this reporting period; (6) Fewer than 100 patients completed the HCAHPS survey; (7) No cases met the criteria for this measure; (8) The lower limit of the confidence interval cannot be calculated if the number of observed infections equals zero; (9) No data are available from the state/territory for this reporting period; (10) The scores shown reflect fewer than 50 completed surveys; (11) There were discrepancies in the data collection process; (12) This measure does not apply to this hospital for this reporting period; (13) Results cannot be calculated for this reporting period; (14) The results for this state are combined with nearby states to protect confidentiality; Please refer to the User's Guide for a full explanation of data.

Measure	Cases	This Hosp.	State Avg.	U.S. Avg.
Children's Asthma Care				
Received Home Management Plan of Care	-	-	-	88%
Received Reliever Medication	-	-	-	100%
Received Systemic Corticosteroids	-	-	-	100%
Emergency Department				
Admittance Decision Time (minutes)[5]	-	-	81	98
Head CT Results Within 45 Min. of Arrival	-	-	63%	57%
Patients Who Left ER Before Being Seen	-	-	3%	2%
Time from ER Arrival to Admit. (minutes)[5]	-	-	238	274
Time from ER Arrival to Discharge (minutes)	-	-	136	134
Time in ER Before Being Evaluated (minutes)	-	-	26	26
Time to Pain Meds for Fractures (minutes)	-	-	52	57
Heart Attack Care				
Aspirin Given at Discharge[3,7]	-	-	99%	99%
Fibrinolytic Meds Within 30 Min. of Arrival[3,7]	-	-	-	54%
PCI Within 90 Minutes of Arrival[3,7]	-	-	97%	96%
Statin Prescribed at Discharge[3,7]	-	-	98%	98%
Heart Failure Care				
ACE Inhibitor or ARB for LVSD[1,3]	-	-	96%	97%
Discharge Instructions Given[3]	21	90%	94%	94%
Evaluation of LVS Function[3]	37	19%	98%	99%
Medicare Spending				
Medicare Spending per Patient (ratio)	-	-	0.95	0.98
Pneumonia Care				
Appropriate Initial Antibiotic Given	25	44%	95%	95%
Blood Culture Timing	18	61%	98%	98%
Pregnancy and Delivery Care				
Newborn Deliveries Scheduled Early[5]	-	-	5%	6%
Preventive Care				
Immunization for Influenza[5]	-	-	92%	90%
Immunization for Pneumonia[5]	-	-	93%	92%
Stroke Care				
Anticoagulation Therapy for Atrial Fibrillation[5]	-	-	94%	95%
Antithrombotic Therapy Timing[5]	-	-	98%	98%
Assessed for Rehabilitation[5]	-	-	98%	97%
Discharged on Antithrombotic Therapy[5]	-	-	99%	99%
Discharged on Statin Medication[5]	-	-	95%	94%
Thrombolytic Therapy Timing[5]	-	-	67%	66%
Venous Thromboembolism Prophylaxis[5]	-	-	95%	94%
Written Stroke Educational Materials Given[5]	-	-	88%	88%
Surgical Care Improvement Project				
Appropriate Beta Blocker Usage[5]	-	-	98%	98%
Appropriate VTP Within 24 Hours[5]	-	-	98%	98%
Controlled Postoperative Blood Glucose[5]	-	-	97%	97%
Perioperative Temperature Management[5]	-	-	100%	100%
Prophylactic Antibiotic Selection[5]	-	-	99%	99%
Prophylactic Antibiotic Selection (Outpatient)	-	-	98%	98%
Prophylactic Antibiotic Stopped[5]	-	-	98%	98%
Prophylactic Antibiotic Timing[5]	-	-	99%	99%
Prophylactic Antibiotic Timing (Outpatient)	-	-	98%	98%
Urinary Catheter Removal[5]	-	-	97%	97%
Survey of Patients' Hospital Experiences				
Area Around Room 'Always' Quiet at Night[5]	-	-	61%	61%
Doctors 'Always' Communicated Well[5]	-	-	82%	82%
Home Recovery Information Given[5]	-	-	87%	85%
Hospital Given 9 or 10 on 10 Point Scale[5]	-	-	71%	71%
Meds 'Always' Explained Before Given[5]	-	-	63%	64%
Nurses 'Always' Communicated Well[5]	-	-	79%	79%
Pain 'Always' Well Controlled[5]	-	-	71%	71%
Room and Bathroom 'Always' Clean[5]	-	-	73%	73%
Timely Help 'Always' Received[5]	-	-	68%	68%
Would Definitely Recommend Hospital[5]	-	-	70%	71%
Use of Medical Imaging				
Cardiac Imaging Stress Test before Surgery	-	-	5.2%	5.3%
Combination Abdominal CT Scan	-	-	11.2%	10.5%
Combination Brain/Sinus CT Scan	-	-	3.2%	2.7%
Combination Chest CT Scan	-	-	1.9%	2.7%
Follow-up Mammogram/Ultrasound	-	-	8.6%	8.8%
Lumbar Spine MRI for Low Back Pain	-	-	39.6%	37.2%

Bates County Memorial Hospital

615 W Nursery St
Butler, MO 64730
URL: www.bcmhospital.com
Type: Acute Care Hospitals
Ownership: Government - Local

Phone: 660-200-7000
Fax: 660-200-7016
Emergency Services: Yes
Beds: 60

Key Personnel:
Chief of Medical Staff.......... Joseph Brewster, MD
CEO/President.............. Edward Hannon
Quality Assurance.......... Carol Lewis
Infection Control.......... Carmen Matter, RN
Operating Room.......... Kristie McKee, RN
Patient Relations.......... Cheryl Mohr
Radiology.......... Chris Pope
Intensive Care Unit.......... Donna Short, RN

Measure	Cases	This Hosp.	State Avg.	U.S. Avg.
Blood Clot Prevention and Treatment				
Anticoagulation Overlap Therapy[1,2]	-	-	94%	93%
ICU Venous Thromboembolism Prophylaxis[2]	35	94%	91%	92%
Incidence of Potentially Preventable VTE[2,7]	-	-	7%	10%
UFH with Dosages/Platelet Monitoring[2,7]	-	-	96%	97%
Venous Thromboembolism Prophylaxis[2]	183	95%	85%	85%
Warfarin Therapy Discharge Instructions[1,2]	-	-	76%	75%
Chest Pain/Possible Heart Attack Care				
Aspirin Given Within 24 Hours of Arrival	26	96%	95%	96%
Fibrinolytic Meds Within 30 Min. of Arrival[7]	-	-	53%	58%
Average Time to ECG (minutes)	28	8	7	7
Average Time to Transfer (minutes)[1]	-	-	53	60
Children's Asthma Care				
Received Home Management Plan of Care	-	-	-	88%
Received Reliever Medication	-	-	-	100%
Received Systemic Corticosteroids	-	-	-	100%
Emergency Department				
Admittance Decision Time (minutes)[2]	214	37	81	98
Head CT Results Within 45 Min. of Arrival[1]	-	-	63%	57%
Patients Who Left ER Before Being Seen	8,322	0%	3%	2%
Time from ER Arrival to Admit. (minutes)[2]	287	159	238	274
Time from ER Arrival to Discharge (minutes)	386	98	136	134
Time in ER Before Being Evaluated (minutes)	409	17	26	26
Time to Pain Meds for Fractures (minutes)	25	33	52	57
Heart Attack Care				
Aspirin Given at Discharge[1,3]	-	-	99%	99%
Fibrinolytic Meds Within 30 Min. of Arrival[3,7]	-	-	-	54%
PCI Within 90 Minutes of Arrival[3,7]	-	-	97%	96%
Statin Prescribed at Discharge[1,3]	-	-	98%	98%
Heart Failure Care				
ACE Inhibitor or ARB for LVSD[1]	-	-	96%	97%
Discharge Instructions Given	22	95%	94%	94%
Evaluation of LVS Function	40	98%	98%	99%
Medicare Spending				
Medicare Spending per Patient (ratio)	-	0.94	0.95	0.98
Pneumonia Care				
Appropriate Initial Antibiotic Given	59	92%	95%	95%
Blood Culture Timing	75	95%	98%	98%
Pregnancy and Delivery Care				
Newborn Deliveries Scheduled Early[7]	-	-	5%	6%
Preventive Care				
Immunization for Influenza[2]	321	99%	92%	90%
Immunization for Pneumonia[2]	498	98%	93%	92%
Stroke Care				
Anticoagulation Therapy for Atrial Fibrillation[3,7]	-	-	94%	95%
Antithrombotic Therapy Timing[1,3]	-	-	98%	98%
Assessed for Rehabilitation[1,3]	-	-	98%	97%
Discharged on Antithrombotic Therapy[1,3]	-	-	99%	99%
Discharged on Statin Medication[1,3]	-	-	95%	94%
Thrombolytic Therapy Timing[1,3]	-	-	67%	66%
Venous Thromboembolism Prophylaxis[1,3]	-	-	95%	94%
Written Stroke Educational Materials Given[1,3]	-	-	88%	88%
Surgical Care Improvement Project				
Appropriate Beta Blocker Usage[1]	-	-	98%	98%
Appropriate VTP Within 24 Hours	26	96%	98%	98%
Controlled Postoperative Blood Glucose[7]	-	-	97%	97%
Perioperative Temperature Management	28	96%	100%	100%
Prophylactic Antibiotic Selection	26	100%	99%	99%
Prophylactic Antibiotic Selection (Outpatient)[1]	-	-	98%	98%
Prophylactic Antibiotic Stopped	25	92%	98%	98%
Prophylactic Antibiotic Timing	26	96%	99%	99%
Prophylactic Antibiotic Timing (Outpatient)[1]	-	-	98%	98%
Urinary Catheter Removal	19	100%	97%	97%
Survey of Patients' Hospital Experiences				
Area Around Room 'Always' Quiet at Night	(a)	52%	61%	61%
Doctors 'Always' Communicated Well	(a)	77%	82%	82%
Home Recovery Information Given	(a)	89%	87%	85%
Hospital Given 9 or 10 on 10 Point Scale	(a)	64%	71%	71%
Meds 'Always' Explained Before Given	(a)	59%	63%	64%
Nurses 'Always' Communicated Well	(a)	73%	79%	79%
Pain 'Always' Well Controlled	(a)	64%	71%	71%
Room and Bathroom 'Always' Clean	(a)	78%	73%	73%
Timely Help 'Always' Received	(a)	71%	68%	68%
Would Definitely Recommend Hospital	(a)	66%	70%	71%
Use of Medical Imaging				
Cardiac Imaging Stress Test before Surgery[1]	-	-	5.2%	5.3%
Combination Abdominal CT Scan	262	18.3%	11.2%	10.5%
Combination Brain/Sinus CT Scan	274	4.4%	3.2%	2.7%
Combination Chest CT Scan	164	12.2%	1.9%	2.7%
Follow-up Mammogram/Ultrasound	260	10.4%	8.6%	8.8%
Lumbar Spine MRI for Low Back Pain	73	54.8%	39.6%	37.2%

Cameron Regional Medical Center

1600 E Evergreen
Cameron, MO 64429
URL: www.cameronregional.org
Type: Acute Care Hospitals
Ownership: Voluntary non-profit - Private

Phone: 816-632-2101
Fax: 816-649-3206
Emergency Services: Yes
Beds: 57

Key Personnel:
Quality Assurance.......... Joseph Abrutz, Jr
CEO/President.......... Joseph F Abrutz, Jr
Operating Room.......... Maria Cowell, RN
Infection Control.......... Ginger Graham, RN
Intensive Care Unit.......... Barbara Guernsey, RN
Chief of Medical Staff.......... Fred Kiehl, DO
Emergency Room.......... Fred Kiehl, DO
Anesthesiology.......... Steve Walker, CRNA

Measure	Cases	This Hosp.	State Avg.	U.S. Avg.
Blood Clot Prevention and Treatment				
Anticoagulation Overlap Therapy[2]	14	86%	94%	93%
ICU Venous Thromboembolism Prophylaxis[2]	55	67%	91%	92%
Incidence of Potentially Preventable VTE[1,2]	-	-	7%	10%
UFH with Dosages/Platelet Monitoring[2,7]	-	-	96%	97%
Venous Thromboembolism Prophylaxis[2]	200	47%	85%	85%
Warfarin Therapy Discharge Instructions[1,2]	-	-	76%	75%
Chest Pain/Possible Heart Attack Care				
Aspirin Given Within 24 Hours of Arrival	49	96%	95%	96%
Fibrinolytic Meds Within 30 Min. of Arrival[7]	-	-	53%	58%
Average Time to ECG (minutes)	49	8	7	7
Average Time to Transfer (minutes)	11	40	53	60
Children's Asthma Care				
Received Home Management Plan of Care	-	-	-	88%
Received Reliever Medication	-	-	-	100%
Received Systemic Corticosteroids	-	-	-	100%
Emergency Department				
Admittance Decision Time (minutes)[2]	401	50	81	98
Head CT Results Within 45 Min. of Arrival[1]	-	-	63%	57%
Patients Who Left ER Before Being Seen	9,256	0%	3%	2%
Time from ER Arrival to Admit. (minutes)[2]	474	140	238	274
Time from ER Arrival to Discharge (minutes)	452	70	136	134
Time in ER Before Being Evaluated (minutes)	512	10	26	26
Time to Pain Meds for Fractures (minutes)	32	28	52	57
Heart Attack Care				
Aspirin Given at Discharge[1]	-	-	99%	99%
Fibrinolytic Meds Within 30 Min. of Arrival[7]	-	-	-	54%
PCI Within 90 Minutes of Arrival[7]	-	-	97%	96%
Statin Prescribed at Discharge[1]	-	-	98%	98%
Heart Failure Care				
ACE Inhibitor or ARB for LVSD[1]	-	-	96%	97%
Discharge Instructions Given	24	88%	94%	94%
Evaluation of LVS Function	47	96%	98%	99%
Medicare Spending				

NOTE: Hospital profiles are in alphabetical order by state, then city, then hospital within the city; Rankings exclude hospitals with less than 25 cases except for patient surveys which excludes hospitals with less than 100 cases; (a) 100-299 cases; (1) The number of cases/patients is too few to report; (2) Data submitted were based on a sample of cases/patients; (3) Results are based on a shorter time period than required; (4) Data suppressed by CMS for one or more quarters; (5) Results are not available for this reporting period; (6) Fewer than 100 patients completed the HCAHPS survey; (7) No cases met the criteria for this measure; (8) The lower limit of the confidence interval cannot be calculated if the number of observed infections equals zero; (9) No data are available from the state/territory for this reporting period; (10) The scores shown reflect fewer than 50 completed surveys; (11) There were discrepancies in the data collection process; (12) This measure does not apply to this hospital for this reporting period; (13) Results cannot be calculated for this reporting period; (14) The results for this state are combined with nearby states to protect confidentiality; Please refer to the User's Guide for a full explanation of data.

Measure	Cases	This Hosp.	State Avg.	U.S. Avg.
Medicare Spending per Patient (ratio)	-	0.98	0.95	0.98
Pneumonia Care				
Appropriate Initial Antibiotic Given	50	86%	95%	95%
Blood Culture Timing	54	100%	98%	98%
Pregnancy and Delivery Care				
Newborn Deliveries Scheduled Early[2]	13	0%	5%	6%
Preventive Care				
Immunization for Influenza[2]	329	91%	92%	90%
Immunization for Pneumonia[2]	463	94%	93%	92%
Stroke Care				
Anticoagulation Therapy for Atrial Fibrillation[1]	-	-	94%	95%
Antithrombotic Therapy Timing[1]	-	-	98%	98%
Assessed for Rehabilitation[1]	-	-	98%	97%
Discharged on Antithrombotic Therapy[1]	-	-	99%	99%
Discharged on Statin Medication[1]	-	-	95%	94%
Thrombolytic Therapy Timing[7]	-	-	67%	66%
Venous Thromboembolism Prophylaxis[1]	-	-	95%	94%
Written Stroke Educational Materials Given[7]	-	-	88%	88%
Surgical Care Improvement Project				
Appropriate Beta Blocker Usage	33	94%	98%	98%
Appropriate VTP Within 24 Hours	101	92%	98%	98%
Controlled Postoperative Blood Glucose[7]	-	-	97%	97%
Perioperative Temperature Management	120	100%	100%	100%
Prophylactic Antibiotic Selection	85	86%	99%	99%
Prophylactic Antibiotic Selection (Outpatient)	20	90%	98%	98%
Prophylactic Antibiotic Stopped	82	93%	98%	98%
Prophylactic Antibiotic Timing	85	99%	99%	99%
Prophylactic Antibiotic Timing (Outpatient)[1]	-	-	98%	98%
Urinary Catheter Removal	86	86%	97%	97%
Survey of Patients' Hospital Experiences				
Area Around Room 'Always' Quiet at Night	(a)	49%	61%	61%
Doctors 'Always' Communicated Well	(a)	81%	82%	82%
Home Recovery Information Given	(a)	86%	87%	85%
Hospital Given 9 or 10 on 10 Point Scale	(a)	66%	71%	71%
Meds 'Always' Explained Before Given	(a)	64%	63%	64%
Nurses 'Always' Communicated Well	(a)	75%	79%	79%
Pain 'Always' Well Controlled	(a)	68%	71%	71%
Room and Bathroom 'Always' Clean	(a)	65%	73%	73%
Timely Help 'Always' Received	(a)	56%	68%	68%
Would Definitely Recommend Hospital	(a)	63%	70%	71%
Use of Medical Imaging				
Cardiac Imaging Stress Test before Surgery	166	4.8%	5.2%	5.3%
Combination Abdominal CT Scan	304	11.5%	11.2%	10.5%
Combination Brain/Sinus CT Scan[1]	-	-	3.2%	2.7%
Combination Chest CT Scan	138	3.6%	1.9%	2.7%
Follow-up Mammogram/Ultrasound	334	6.9%	8.6%	8.8%
Lumbar Spine MRI for Low Back Pain	46	37.0%	39.6%	37.2%

Saint Francis Medical Center

211 Saint Francis Dr
Cape Girardeau, MO 63703
Phone: 573-331-3000
Fax: 573-331-5009
E-mail: sfmc@sfmc.net
URL: www.sfmc.net
Type: Acute Care Hospitals
Emergency Services: Yes
Ownership: Voluntary non-profit - Church
Beds: 264

Key Personnel:

Emergency Room . . . . Marcia Abernathy
CEO/President. . . . . Stephen C. Bjelich, FACHE-D
Quality Assurance . . . . Rick Fehr
Chief of Medical Staff. . . . . Billy Hammond, MD
Pediatric Ambulatory Care . . . . . . John Russell, MD
Pediatric In-Patient Care . . . . John Russell, MD
Cardiac Laboratory. . . . . Savid Stagner
Radiology. . . . . WJ Stoecker, MD

Measure	Cases	This Hosp.	State Avg.	U.S. Avg.
Blood Clot Prevention and Treatment				
Anticoagulation Overlap Therapy[2]	45	98%	94%	93%
ICU Venous Thromboembolism Prophylaxis[2]	109	80%	91%	92%
Incidence of Potentially Preventable VTE[1,2]	-	-	7%	10%
UFH with Dosages/Platelet Monitoring[2]	23	100%	96%	97%
Venous Thromboembolism Prophylaxis[2]	322	79%	85%	85%
Warfarin Therapy Discharge Instructions[2]	38	79%	76%	75%
Chest Pain/Possible Heart Attack Care				
Aspirin Given Within 24 Hours of Arrival[5]	-	-	95%	96%
Fibrinolytic Meds Within 30 Min. of Arrival[5]	-	-	53%	58%
Average Time to ECG (minutes)[5]	-	-	7	7
Average Time to Transfer (minutes)[5]	-	-	53	60
Children's Asthma Care				
Received Home Management Plan of Care	-	-	-	88%
Received Reliever Medication	-	-	-	100%
Received Systemic Corticosteroids	-	-	-	100%
Emergency Department				
Admittance Decision Time (minutes)[2]	406	65	81	98
Head CT Results Within 45 Min. of Arrival[1,3]	-	-	63%	57%
Patients Who Left ER Before Being Seen	39,137	2%	3%	2%
Time from ER Arrival to Admit. (minutes)[2]	430	212	238	274
Time from ER Arrival to Discharge (minutes)	365	163	136	134
Time in ER Before Being Evaluated (minutes)	396	40	26	26
Time to Pain Meds for Fractures (minutes)	130	64	52	57
Heart Attack Care				
Aspirin Given at Discharge	185	100%	99%	99%
Fibrinolytic Meds Within 30 Min. of Arrival[7]	-	-	-	54%
PCI Within 90 Minutes of Arrival	36	97%	97%	96%
Statin Prescribed at Discharge	178	98%	98%	98%
Heart Failure Care				
ACE Inhibitor or ARB for LVSD	103	95%	96%	97%
Discharge Instructions Given	279	91%	94%	94%
Evaluation of LVS Function	338	99%	98%	99%
Medicare Spending				
Medicare Spending per Patient (ratio)	-	1.02	0.95	0.98
Pneumonia Care				
Appropriate Initial Antibiotic Given	220	91%	95%	95%
Blood Culture Timing	439	98%	98%	98%
Pregnancy and Delivery Care				
Newborn Deliveries Scheduled Early	101	9%	5%	6%
Preventive Care				
Immunization for Influenza[2]	570	87%	92%	90%
Immunization for Pneumonia[2]	762	93%	93%	92%
Stroke Care				
Anticoagulation Therapy for Atrial Fibrillation	22	100%	94%	95%
Antithrombotic Therapy Timing	156	99%	98%	98%
Assessed for Rehabilitation	182	100%	98%	97%
Discharged on Antithrombotic Therapy	157	99%	99%	99%
Discharged on Statin Medication	127	98%	95%	94%
Thrombolytic Therapy Timing[1]	-	-	67%	66%
Venous Thromboembolism Prophylaxis	187	96%	95%	94%
Written Stroke Educational Materials Given	77	94%	88%	88%
Surgical Care Improvement Project				
Appropriate Beta Blocker Usage	400	96%	98%	98%
Appropriate VTP Within 24 Hours	926	93%	98%	98%
Controlled Postoperative Blood Glucose	214	94%	97%	97%
Perioperative Temperature Management	1,090	100%	100%	100%
Prophylactic Antibiotic Selection	866	98%	99%	99%
Prophylactic Antibiotic Selection (Outpatient)	670	96%	98%	98%
Prophylactic Antibiotic Stopped	853	97%	98%	98%
Prophylactic Antibiotic Timing	867	98%	99%	99%
Prophylactic Antibiotic Timing (Outpatient)	676	98%	98%	98%
Urinary Catheter Removal	665	93%	97%	97%
Survey of Patients' Hospital Experiences				
Area Around Room 'Always' Quiet at Night	300+	63%	61%	61%
Doctors 'Always' Communicated Well	300+	84%	82%	82%
Home Recovery Information Given	300+	86%	87%	85%
Hospital Given 9 or 10 on 10 Point Scale	300+	79%	71%	71%
Meds 'Always' Explained Before Given	300+	69%	63%	64%
Nurses 'Always' Communicated Well	300+	83%	79%	79%
Pain 'Always' Well Controlled	300+	74%	71%	71%
Room and Bathroom 'Always' Clean	300+	75%	73%	73%
Timely Help 'Always' Received	300+	67%	68%	68%
Would Definitely Recommend Hospital	300+	82%	70%	71%
Use of Medical Imaging				
Cardiac Imaging Stress Test before Surgery	810	4.0%	5.2%	5.3%
Combination Abdominal CT Scan	1,810	30.4%	11.2%	10.5%
Combination Brain/Sinus CT Scan	1,423	3.7%	3.2%	2.7%
Combination Chest CT Scan	1,190	0.1%	1.9%	2.7%
Follow-up Mammogram/Ultrasound	2,066	10.3%	8.6%	8.8%
Lumbar Spine MRI for Low Back Pain	271	43.5%	39.6%	37.2%

Southeast Missouri Hospital

1701 Lacey St
Cape Girardeau, MO 63701
Phone: 573-334-4822
Fax: 573-651-5850
URL: www.southeastmissourihospital.com
Type: Acute Care Hospitals
Emergency Services: Yes
Ownership: Voluntary non-profit - Private
Beds: 269

Key Personnel:

Radiology. . . . . Jagan Ailinani
CEO/President. . . . . Wayne Smith
Chief of Medical Staff . . . . E Lee Taylor

Measure	Cases	This Hosp.	State Avg.	U.S. Avg.
Blood Clot Prevention and Treatment				
Anticoagulation Overlap Therapy[2]	53	83%	94%	93%
ICU Venous Thromboembolism Prophylaxis[2]	85	86%	91%	92%
Incidence of Potentially Preventable VTE[2]	12	8%	7%	10%
UFH with Dosages/Platelet Monitoring[2]	32	94%	96%	97%
Venous Thromboembolism Prophylaxis[2]	311	82%	85%	85%
Warfarin Therapy Discharge Instructions[2]	36	75%	76%	75%
Chest Pain/Possible Heart Attack Care				
Aspirin Given Within 24 Hours of Arrival[5]	-	-	95%	96%
Fibrinolytic Meds Within 30 Min. of Arrival[5]	-	-	53%	58%
Average Time to ECG (minutes)[5]	-	-	7	7
Average Time to Transfer (minutes)[5]	-	-	53	60
Children's Asthma Care				
Received Home Management Plan of Care	-	-	-	88%
Received Reliever Medication	-	-	-	100%
Received Systemic Corticosteroids	-	-	-	100%
Emergency Department				
Admittance Decision Time (minutes)[2]	478	58	81	98
Head CT Results Within 45 Min. of Arrival[1]	-	-	63%	57%
Patients Who Left ER Before Being Seen	40,379	4%	3%	2%
Time from ER Arrival to Admit. (minutes)[2]	481	240	238	274
Time from ER Arrival to Discharge (minutes)	558	205	136	134
Time in ER Before Being Evaluated (minutes)	551	81	26	26
Time to Pain Meds for Fractures (minutes)	80	92	52	57
Heart Attack Care				
Aspirin Given at Discharge	205	100%	99%	99%
Fibrinolytic Meds Within 30 Min. of Arrival[7]	-	-	-	54%
PCI Within 90 Minutes of Arrival	32	100%	97%	96%
Statin Prescribed at Discharge	202	99%	98%	98%
Heart Failure Care				
ACE Inhibitor or ARB for LVSD	75	100%	96%	97%
Discharge Instructions Given	176	79%	94%	94%
Evaluation of LVS Function	230	99%	98%	99%
Medicare Spending				
Medicare Spending per Patient (ratio)	-	0.95	0.95	0.98
Pneumonia Care				
Appropriate Initial Antibiotic Given	222	99%	95%	95%
Blood Culture Timing	371	99%	98%	98%
Pregnancy and Delivery Care				
Newborn Deliveries Scheduled Early	71	1%	5%	6%
Preventive Care				
Immunization for Influenza[2]	602	92%	92%	90%
Immunization for Pneumonia[2]	730	75%	93%	92%
Stroke Care				
Anticoagulation Therapy for Atrial Fibrillation	18	100%	94%	95%
Antithrombotic Therapy Timing	125	98%	98%	98%
Assessed for Rehabilitation	157	96%	98%	97%
Discharged on Antithrombotic Therapy	131	100%	99%	99%
Discharged on Statin Medication	115	96%	95%	94%
Thrombolytic Therapy Timing	12	42%	67%	66%
Venous Thromboembolism Prophylaxis	152	97%	95%	94%
Written Stroke Educational Materials Given	88	76%	88%	88%
Surgical Care Improvement Project				
Appropriate Beta Blocker Usage[2]	241	96%	98%	98%
Appropriate VTP Within 24 Hours[2]	374	95%	98%	98%
Controlled Postoperative Blood Glucose[2]	106	99%	97%	97%
Perioperative Temperature Management[2]	529	100%	100%	100%
Prophylactic Antibiotic Selection[2]	396	99%	99%	99%
Prophylactic Antibiotic Selection (Outpatient)	555	98%	98%	98%
Prophylactic Antibiotic Stopped[2]	386	97%	98%	98%
Prophylactic Antibiotic Timing[2]	402	97%	99%	99%
Prophylactic Antibiotic Timing (Outpatient)	557	98%	98%	98%

NOTE: Hospital profiles are in alphabetical order by state, then city, then hospital within the city; Rankings exclude hospitals with less than 25 cases except for patient surveys which excludes hospitals with less than 100 cases; (a) 100-299 cases; (1) The number of cases/patients is too few to report; (2) Data submitted were based on a sample of cases/patients; (3) Results are based on a shorter time period than required; (4) Data suppressed by CMS for one or more quarters; (5) Results are not available for this reporting period; (6) Fewer than 100 patients completed the HCAHPS survey; (7) No cases met the criteria for this measure; (8) The lower limit of the confidence interval cannot be calculated if the number of observed infections equals zero; (9) No data are available from the state/territory for this reporting period; (10) The scores shown reflect fewer than 50 completed surveys; (11) There were discrepancies in the data collection process; (12) This measure does not apply to this hospital for this reporting period; (13) Results cannot be calculated for this reporting period; (14) The results for this state are combined with nearby states to protect confidentiality; Please refer to the User's Guide for a full explanation of data.

Urinary Catheter Removal[2]	315	93%	97%	97%
Survey of Patients' Hospital Experiences				
Area Around Room 'Always' Quiet at Night	300+	66%	61%	61%
Doctors 'Always' Communicated Well	300+	81%	82%	82%
Home Recovery Information Given	300+	90%	87%	85%
Hospital Given 9 or 10 on 10 Point Scale	300+	79%	71%	71%
Meds 'Always' Explained Before Given	300+	69%	63%	64%
Nurses 'Always' Communicated Well	300+	83%	79%	79%
Pain 'Always' Well Controlled	300+	76%	71%	71%
Room and Bathroom 'Always' Clean	300+	81%	73%	73%
Timely Help 'Always' Received	300+	71%	68%	68%
Would Definitely Recommend Hospital	300+	81%	70%	71%
Use of Medical Imaging				
Cardiac Imaging Stress Test before Surgery	1,191	5.8%	5.2%	5.3%
Combination Abdominal CT Scan	1,108	61.0%	11.2%	10.5%
Combination Brain/Sinus CT Scan	776	3.0%	3.2%	2.7%
Combination Chest CT Scan	926	0.8%	1.9%	2.7%
Follow-up Mammogram/Ultrasound	1,774	4.2%	8.6%	8.8%
Lumbar Spine MRI for Low Back Pain	203	36.9%	39.6%	37.2%

Carroll County Memorial Hospital

1502 North Jefferson Phone: 660-542-1695
Carrollton, MO 64633 Fax: 660-542-0363
URL: www.carrollcountyhospital.org
Type: Critical Access Hospitals Emergency Services: Yes
Ownership: Voluntary non-profit - Private Beds: 25

Key Personnel:
Pediatric Ambulatory Care . . . . . . Dr Grace Dymek, MD
Infection Control. . . . . Vicki Lyon, RN
Quality Assurance . . . . Vicki Lyon, RN
Surgery . . . . Dr. Daniel Mrosak
Radiology. . . . . Jamie Ross
Chief of Medical Staff . . . . Marvin E Ross, DO
CEO/President. . . . . Jeff Tindle, M.H.A.

Measure	Cases	This Hosp.	State Avg.	U.S. Avg.
Blood Clot Prevention and Treatment				
Anticoagulation Overlap Therapy[3,7]	-	-	94%	93%
ICU Venous Thromboembolism Prophylaxis[3,7]	-	-	91%	92%
Incidence of Potentially Preventable VTE[3,7]	-	-	7%	10%
UFH with Dosages/Platelet Monitoring[3,7]	-	-	96%	97%
Venous Thromboembolism Prophylaxis[3]	11	82%	85%	85%
Warfarin Therapy Discharge Instructions[3,7]	-	-	76%	75%
Chest Pain/Possible Heart Attack Care				
Aspirin Given Within 24 Hours of Arrival	-	-	95%	96%
Fibrinolytic Meds Within 30 Min. of Arrival	-	-	53%	58%
Average Time to ECG (minutes)	-	-	7	7
Average Time to Transfer (minutes)	-	-	53	60
Children's Asthma Care				
Received Home Management Plan of Care	-	-	-	88%
Received Reliever Medication	-	-	-	100%
Received Systemic Corticosteroids	-	-	-	100%
Emergency Department				
Admittance Decision Time (minutes)	91	34	81	98
Head CT Results Within 45 Min. of Arrival	-	-	63%	57%
Patients Who Left ER Before Being Seen	-	-	3%	2%
Time from ER Arrival to Admit. (minutes)	95	125	238	274
Time from ER Arrival to Discharge (minutes)	-	-	136	134
Time in ER Before Being Evaluated (minutes)	-	-	26	26
Time to Pain Meds for Fractures (minutes)	-	-	52	57
Heart Attack Care				
Aspirin Given at Discharge[1,3]	-	-	99%	99%
Fibrinolytic Meds Within 30 Min. of Arrival[3,7]	-	-	-	54%
PCI Within 90 Minutes of Arrival[3,7]	-	-	97%	96%
Statin Prescribed at Discharge[1,3]	-	-	98%	98%
Heart Failure Care				
ACE Inhibitor or ARB for LVSD[1]	-	-	96%	97%
Discharge Instructions Given[1]	-	-	94%	94%
Evaluation of LVS Function	11	100%	98%	99%
Medicare Spending				
Medicare Spending per Patient (ratio)	-	-	0.95	0.98
Pneumonia Care				
Appropriate Initial Antibiotic Given	30	87%	95%	95%
Blood Culture Timing	13	100%	98%	98%
Pregnancy and Delivery Care				
Newborn Deliveries Scheduled Early[5]	-	-	5%	6%
Preventive Care				
Immunization for Influenza	140	64%	92%	90%
Immunization for Pneumonia	193	82%	93%	92%
Stroke Care				
Anticoagulation Therapy for Atrial Fibrillation[3,7]	-	-	94%	95%
Antithrombotic Therapy Timing[1,3]	-	-	98%	98%
Assessed for Rehabilitation[1,3]	-	-	98%	97%
Discharged on Antithrombotic Therapy[1,3]	-	-	99%	99%
Discharged on Statin Medication[1,3]	-	-	95%	94%
Thrombolytic Therapy Timing[1,3]	-	-	67%	66%
Venous Thromboembolism Prophylaxis[1,3]	-	-	95%	94%
Written Stroke Educational Materials Given[1,3]	-	-	88%	88%
Surgical Care Improvement Project				
Appropriate Beta Blocker Usage[5]	-	-	98%	98%
Appropriate VTP Within 24 Hours[5]	-	-	98%	98%
Controlled Postoperative Blood Glucose[5]	-	-	97%	97%
Perioperative Temperature Management[5]	-	-	100%	100%
Prophylactic Antibiotic Selection[5]	-	-	99%	99%
Prophylactic Antibiotic Selection (Outpatient)	-	-	98%	98%
Prophylactic Antibiotic Stopped[5]	-	-	98%	98%
Prophylactic Antibiotic Timing[5]	-	-	99%	99%
Prophylactic Antibiotic Timing (Outpatient)	-	-	98%	98%
Urinary Catheter Removal[5]	-	-	97%	97%
Survey of Patients' Hospital Experiences				
Area Around Room 'Always' Quiet at Night[5]	-	-	61%	61%
Doctors 'Always' Communicated Well[5]	-	-	82%	82%
Home Recovery Information Given[5]	-	-	87%	85%
Hospital Given 9 or 10 on 10 Point Scale[5]	-	-	71%	71%
Meds 'Always' Explained Before Given[5]	-	-	63%	64%
Nurses 'Always' Communicated Well[5]	-	-	79%	79%
Pain 'Always' Well Controlled[5]	-	-	71%	71%
Room and Bathroom 'Always' Clean[5]	-	-	73%	73%
Timely Help 'Always' Received[5]	-	-	68%	68%
Would Definitely Recommend Hospital[5]	-	-	70%	71%
Use of Medical Imaging				
Cardiac Imaging Stress Test before Surgery	-	-	5.2%	5.3%
Combination Abdominal CT Scan	-	-	11.2%	10.5%
Combination Brain/Sinus CT Scan	-	-	3.2%	2.7%
Combination Chest CT Scan	-	-	1.9%	2.7%
Follow-up Mammogram/Ultrasound	-	-	8.6%	8.8%
Lumbar Spine MRI for Low Back Pain	-	-	39.6%	37.2%

Mercy Mccune Brooks Hospital

3125 Dr Russell Smith Way Phone: 417-358-8121
Carthage, MO 64836
Type: Acute Care Hospitals Emergency Services: Yes
Ownership: Voluntary non-profit - Church

Measure	Cases	This Hosp.	State Avg.	U.S. Avg.
Blood Clot Prevention and Treatment				
Anticoagulation Overlap Therapy[1,2]	-	-	94%	93%
ICU Venous Thromboembolism Prophylaxis[1,2]	-	-	91%	92%
Incidence of Potentially Preventable VTE[1,2]	-	-	7%	10%
UFH with Dosages/Platelet Monitoring[1,2]	-	-	96%	97%
Venous Thromboembolism Prophylaxis[2,3]	29	90%	85%	85%
Warfarin Therapy Discharge Instructions[1,2]	-	-	76%	75%
Chest Pain/Possible Heart Attack Care				
Aspirin Given Within 24 Hours of Arrival[3]	33	100%	95%	96%
Fibrinolytic Meds Within 30 Min. of Arrival[3,7]	-	-	53%	58%
Average Time to ECG (minutes)[3]	33	5	7	7
Average Time to Transfer (minutes)[1,3]	-	-	53	60
Children's Asthma Care				
Received Home Management Plan of Care	-	-	-	88%
Received Reliever Medication	-	-	-	100%
Received Systemic Corticosteroids	-	-	-	100%
Emergency Department				
Admittance Decision Time (minutes)[2,3]	50	53	81	98
Head CT Results Within 45 Min. of Arrival[1,3]	-	-	63%	57%
Patients Who Left ER Before Being Seen	19,056	1%	3%	2%
Time from ER Arrival to Admit. (minutes)[2,3]	50	170	238	274
Time from ER Arrival to Discharge (minutes)[3]	264	97	136	134
Time in ER Before Being Evaluated (minutes)[3]	291	18	26	26
Time to Pain Meds for Fractures (minutes)[3]	36	58	52	57
Heart Attack Care				
Aspirin Given at Discharge[1,3]	-	-	99%	99%
Fibrinolytic Meds Within 30 Min. of Arrival[3,7]	-	-	-	54%
PCI Within 90 Minutes of Arrival[3,7]	-	-	97%	96%
Statin Prescribed at Discharge[1,3]	-	-	98%	98%
Heart Failure Care				
ACE Inhibitor or ARB for LVSD[1,3]	-	-	96%	97%
Discharge Instructions Given[3]	24	88%	94%	94%
Evaluation of LVS Function[3]	32	100%	98%	99%
Medicare Spending				
Medicare Spending per Patient (ratio)	-	-	0.95	0.98
Pneumonia Care				
Appropriate Initial Antibiotic Given[3]	36	94%	95%	95%
Blood Culture Timing[3]	65	97%	98%	98%
Pregnancy and Delivery Care				
Newborn Deliveries Scheduled Early[1,2]	-	-	5%	6%
Preventive Care				
Immunization for Influenza[5]	-	-	92%	90%
Immunization for Pneumonia[2,3]	68	88%	93%	92%
Stroke Care				
Anticoagulation Therapy for Atrial Fibrillation[1,3]	-	-	94%	95%
Antithrombotic Therapy Timing[1,3]	-	-	98%	98%
Assessed for Rehabilitation[1,3]	-	-	98%	97%
Discharged on Antithrombotic Therapy[1,3]	-	-	99%	99%
Discharged on Statin Medication[1,3]	-	-	95%	94%
Thrombolytic Therapy Timing[3,7]	-	-	67%	66%
Venous Thromboembolism Prophylaxis[1,3]	-	-	95%	94%
Written Stroke Educational Materials Given[1,3]	-	-	88%	88%
Surgical Care Improvement Project				
Appropriate Beta Blocker Usage[2,3]	47	98%	98%	98%
Appropriate VTP Within 24 Hours[2,3]	143	100%	98%	98%
Controlled Postoperative Blood Glucose[2,3]	-	-	97%	97%
Perioperative Temperature Management[2,3]	165	100%	100%	100%
Prophylactic Antibiotic Selection[2,3]	122	98%	99%	99%
Prophylactic Antibiotic Selection (Outpatient)[3]	51	88%	98%	98%
Prophylactic Antibiotic Stopped[2,3]	120	91%	98%	98%
Prophylactic Antibiotic Timing[2,3]	123	88%	99%	99%
Prophylactic Antibiotic Timing (Outpatient)[3]	52	83%	98%	98%
Urinary Catheter Removal[2,3]	38	100%	97%	97%
Survey of Patients' Hospital Experiences				
Area Around Room 'Always' Quiet at Night[5]	-	-	61%	61%
Doctors 'Always' Communicated Well[5]	-	-	82%	82%
Home Recovery Information Given[5]	-	-	87%	85%
Hospital Given 9 or 10 on 10 Point Scale[5]	-	-	71%	71%
Meds 'Always' Explained Before Given[5]	-	-	63%	64%
Nurses 'Always' Communicated Well[5]	-	-	79%	79%
Pain 'Always' Well Controlled[5]	-	-	71%	71%
Room and Bathroom 'Always' Clean[5]	-	-	73%	73%
Timely Help 'Always' Received[5]	-	-	68%	68%
Would Definitely Recommend Hospital[5]	-	-	70%	71%
Use of Medical Imaging				
Cardiac Imaging Stress Test before Surgery[1]	-	-	5.2%	5.3%
Combination Abdominal CT Scan	105	35.2%	11.2%	10.5%
Combination Brain/Sinus CT Scan[1]	-	-	3.2%	2.7%
Combination Chest CT Scan[1]	-	-	1.9%	2.7%
Follow-up Mammogram/Ultrasound	146	2.7%	8.6%	8.8%
Lumbar Spine MRI for Low Back Pain[1]	-	-	39.6%	37.2%

Mercy Hospital Cassville

94 Main Street Phone: 417-847-6065
Cassville, MO 65625 Fax: 417-847-6047
URL: www.southbarrycountyhospital.com
Type: Critical Access Hospitals Emergency Services: Yes
Ownership: Voluntary non-profit - Church Beds: 18

Key Personnel:
Chief of Medical Staff . . . . K Duane Cox, MD
CEO/President. . . . . Gary Jordan
Emergency Room . . . . Jerry Jumper
Infection Control. . . . . Joyce Noland, RN
Quality Assurance . . . . Joyce Noland

Measure	Cases	This Hosp.	State Avg.	U.S. Avg.
Blood Clot Prevention and Treatment				
Anticoagulation Overlap Therapy[5]	-	-	94%	93%

NOTE: Hospital profiles are in alphabetical order by state, then city, then hospital within the city; Rankings exclude hospitals with less than 25 cases except for patient surveys which excludes hospitals with less than 100 cases; (a) 100-299 cases; (1) The number of cases/patients is too few to report; (2) Data submitted were based on a sample of cases/patients; (3) Results are based on a shorter time period than required; (4) Data suppressed by CMS for one or more quarters; (5) Results are not available for this reporting period; (6) Fewer than 100 patients completed the HCAHPS survey; (7) No cases met the criteria for this measure; (8) The lower limit of the confidence interval cannot be calculated if the number of observed infections equals zero; (9) No data are available from the state/territory for this reporting period; (10) The scores shown reflect fewer than 50 completed surveys; (11) There were discrepancies in the data collection process; (12) This measure does not apply to this hospital for this reporting period; (13) Results cannot be calculated for this reporting period; (14) The results for this state are combined with nearby states to protect confidentiality; Please refer to the User's Guide for a full explanation of data.

Measure	Cases	This Hosp.	State Avg.	U.S. Avg.
ICU Venous Thromboembolism Prophylaxis[5]	-	-	91%	92%
Incidence of Potentially Preventable VTE[5]	-	-	7%	10%
UFH with Dosages/Platelet Monitoring[5]	-	-	96%	97%
Venous Thromboembolism Prophylaxis[5]	-	-	85%	85%
Warfarin Therapy Discharge Instructions[5]	-	-	76%	75%
Chest Pain/Possible Heart Attack Care				
Aspirin Given Within 24 Hours of Arrival	-	-	95%	96%
Fibrinolytic Meds Within 30 Min. of Arrival	-	-	53%	58%
Average Time to ECG (minutes)	-	-	7	7
Average Time to Transfer (minutes)	-	-	53	60
Children's Asthma Care				
Received Home Management Plan of Care	-	-	-	88%
Received Reliever Medication	-	-	-	100%
Received Systemic Corticosteroids	-	-	-	100%
Emergency Department				
Admittance Decision Time (minutes)	196	48	81	98
Head CT Results Within 45 Min. of Arrival	-	-	63%	57%
Patients Who Left ER Before Being Seen	-	-	3%	2%
Time from ER Arrival to Admit. (minutes)	202	246	238	274
Time from ER Arrival to Discharge (minutes)	-	-	136	134
Time in ER Before Being Evaluated (minutes)	-	-	26	26
Time to Pain Meds for Fractures (minutes)	-	-	52	57
Heart Attack Care				
Aspirin Given at Discharge[5]	-	-	99%	99%
Fibrinolytic Meds Within 30 Min. of Arrival[5]	-	-	-	54%
PCI Within 90 Minutes of Arrival[5]	-	-	97%	96%
Statin Prescribed at Discharge[5]	-	-	98%	98%
Heart Failure Care				
ACE Inhibitor or ARB for LVSD[1]	-	-	96%	97%
Discharge Instructions Given	12	58%	94%	94%
Evaluation of LVS Function	15	93%	98%	99%
Medicare Spending				
Medicare Spending per Patient (ratio)	-	-	0.95	0.98
Pneumonia Care				
Appropriate Initial Antibiotic Given	17	88%	95%	95%
Blood Culture Timing	20	95%	98%	98%
Pregnancy and Delivery Care				
Newborn Deliveries Scheduled Early[5]	-	-	5%	6%
Preventive Care				
Immunization for Influenza	130	97%	92%	90%
Immunization for Pneumonia	194	96%	93%	92%
Stroke Care				
Anticoagulation Therapy for Atrial Fibrillation[5]	-	-	94%	95%
Antithrombotic Therapy Timing[5]	-	-	98%	98%
Assessed for Rehabilitation[5]	-	-	98%	97%
Discharged on Antithrombotic Therapy[5]	-	-	99%	99%
Discharged on Statin Medication[5]	-	-	95%	94%
Thrombolytic Therapy Timing[5]	-	-	67%	66%
Venous Thromboembolism Prophylaxis[5]	-	-	95%	94%
Written Stroke Educational Materials Given[5]	-	-	88%	88%
Surgical Care Improvement Project				
Appropriate Beta Blocker Usage[5]	-	-	98%	98%
Appropriate VTP Within 24 Hours[5]	-	-	98%	98%
Controlled Postoperative Blood Glucose[5]	-	-	97%	97%
Perioperative Temperature Management[5]	-	-	100%	100%
Prophylactic Antibiotic Selection[5]	-	-	99%	99%
Prophylactic Antibiotic Selection (Outpatient)	-	-	98%	98%
Prophylactic Antibiotic Stopped[5]	-	-	98%	98%
Prophylactic Antibiotic Timing[5]	-	-	99%	99%
Prophylactic Antibiotic Timing (Outpatient)	-	-	98%	98%
Urinary Catheter Removal[5]	-	-	97%	97%
Survey of Patients' Hospital Experiences				
Area Around Room 'Always' Quiet at Night[5]	-	-	61%	61%
Doctors 'Always' Communicated Well[5]	-	-	82%	82%
Home Recovery Information Given[5]	-	-	87%	85%
Hospital Given 9 or 10 on 10 Point Scale[5]	-	-	71%	71%
Meds 'Always' Explained Before Given[5]	-	-	63%	64%
Nurses 'Always' Communicated Well[5]	-	-	79%	79%
Pain 'Always' Well Controlled[5]	-	-	71%	71%
Room and Bathroom 'Always' Clean[5]	-	-	73%	73%
Timely Help 'Always' Received[5]	-	-	68%	68%
Would Definitely Recommend Hospital[5]	-	-	70%	71%
Use of Medical Imaging				
Cardiac Imaging Stress Test before Surgery	-	-	5.2%	5.3%
Combination Abdominal CT Scan	-	-	11.2%	10.5%
Combination Brain/Sinus CT Scan	-	-	3.2%	2.7%
Combination Chest CT Scan	-	-	1.9%	2.7%
Follow-up Mammogram/Ultrasound	-	-	8.6%	8.8%
Lumbar Spine MRI for Low Back Pain	-	-	39.6%	37.2%

Saint Luke's Hospital

232 S Woods Mill Rd
Chesterfield, MO 63017
URL: www.goodhealthmatters.com
Type: Acute Care Hospitals
Ownership: Voluntary non-profit - Private
Phone: 314-434-1500
Fax: 314-205-6865
Emergency Services: Yes
Beds: 493

Key Personnel:

- Radiology . . . . Reggie Hicks
- Cardiac Laboratory. . . . . John Hilden
- Quality Assurance . . . . Linda Koste, RN
- Chief of Medical Staff . . . . Paul A Mennes, MD
- CEO/President. . . . . Gary Olson, MD
- Infection Control. . . . . Leon Robison, MD
- Pediatric Ambulatory Care . . . . . . Janet Ruzycler, MD
- Pediatric In-Patient Care . . . . Janet Ruzycler, MD

Measure	Cases	This Hosp.	State Avg.	U.S. Avg.
Blood Clot Prevention and Treatment				
Anticoagulation Overlap Therapy[2]	140	98%	94%	93%
ICU Venous Thromboembolism Prophylaxis[2]	65	95%	91%	92%
Incidence of Potentially Preventable VTE[2]	36	17%	7%	10%
UFH with Dosages/Platelet Monitoring[2]	81	99%	96%	97%
Venous Thromboembolism Prophylaxis[2]	348	80%	85%	85%
Warfarin Therapy Discharge Instructions[2]	88	84%	76%	75%
Chest Pain/Possible Heart Attack Care				
Aspirin Given Within 24 Hours of Arrival[3,7]	-	-	95%	96%
Fibrinolytic Meds Within 30 Min. of Arrival[5]	-	-	53%	58%
Average Time to ECG (minutes)[3,7]	-	-	7	7
Average Time to Transfer (minutes)[5]	-	-	53	60
Children's Asthma Care				
Received Home Management Plan of Care	-	-	-	88%
Received Reliever Medication	-	-	-	100%
Received Systemic Corticosteroids	-	-	-	100%
Emergency Department				
Admittance Decision Time (minutes)[2]	646	82	81	98
Head CT Results Within 45 Min. of Arrival[1]	-	-	63%	57%
Patients Who Left ER Before Being Seen	30,287	0%	3%	2%
Time from ER Arrival to Admit. (minutes)[2]	652	221	238	274
Time from ER Arrival to Discharge (minutes)	683	159	136	134
Time in ER Before Being Evaluated (minutes)	722	28	26	26
Time to Pain Meds for Fractures (minutes)	111	61	52	57
Heart Attack Care				
Aspirin Given at Discharge	285	100%	99%	99%
Fibrinolytic Meds Within 30 Min. of Arrival[7]	-	-	-	54%
PCI Within 90 Minutes of Arrival	45	100%	97%	96%
Statin Prescribed at Discharge	282	97%	98%	98%
Heart Failure Care				
ACE Inhibitor or ARB for LVSD[2]	78	100%	96%	97%
Discharge Instructions Given[2]	280	98%	94%	94%
Evaluation of LVS Function[2]	374	100%	98%	99%
Medicare Spending				
Medicare Spending per Patient (ratio)	-	0.95	0.95	0.98
Pneumonia Care				
Appropriate Initial Antibiotic Given[2]	102	96%	95%	95%
Blood Culture Timing[2]	129	100%	98%	98%
Pregnancy and Delivery Care				
Newborn Deliveries Scheduled Early[2]	73	0%	5%	6%
Preventive Care				
Immunization for Influenza[2]	564	94%	92%	90%
Immunization for Pneumonia[2]	749	95%	93%	92%
Stroke Care				
Anticoagulation Therapy for Atrial Fibrillation	32	97%	94%	95%
Antithrombotic Therapy Timing	122	100%	98%	98%
Assessed for Rehabilitation	164	99%	98%	97%
Discharged on Antithrombotic Therapy	148	100%	99%	99%
Discharged on Statin Medication	121	92%	95%	94%
Thrombolytic Therapy Timing	12	50%	67%	66%
Venous Thromboembolism Prophylaxis	152	89%	95%	94%
Written Stroke Educational Materials Given	95	87%	88%	88%
Surgical Care Improvement Project				
Appropriate Beta Blocker Usage[2]	308	99%	98%	98%
Appropriate VTP Within 24 Hours[2]	634	98%	98%	98%
Controlled Postoperative Blood Glucose[2]	202	97%	97%	97%
Perioperative Temperature Management[2]	842	98%	100%	100%
Prophylactic Antibiotic Selection[2]	703	100%	99%	99%
Prophylactic Antibiotic Selection (Outpatient)	924	99%	98%	98%
Prophylactic Antibiotic Stopped[2]	684	96%	98%	98%
Prophylactic Antibiotic Timing[2]	704	99%	99%	99%
Prophylactic Antibiotic Timing (Outpatient)	930	98%	98%	98%
Urinary Catheter Removal[2]	408	96%	97%	97%
Survey of Patients' Hospital Experiences				
Area Around Room 'Always' Quiet at Night	300+	62%	61%	61%
Doctors 'Always' Communicated Well	300+	84%	82%	82%
Home Recovery Information Given	300+	87%	87%	85%
Hospital Given 9 or 10 on 10 Point Scale	300+	85%	71%	71%
Meds 'Always' Explained Before Given	300+	67%	63%	64%
Nurses 'Always' Communicated Well	300+	82%	79%	79%
Pain 'Always' Well Controlled	300+	74%	71%	71%
Room and Bathroom 'Always' Clean	300+	76%	73%	73%
Timely Help 'Always' Received	300+	66%	68%	68%
Would Definitely Recommend Hospital	300+	86%	70%	71%
Use of Medical Imaging				
Cardiac Imaging Stress Test before Surgery	962	5.1%	5.2%	5.3%
Combination Abdominal CT Scan	1,699	3.2%	11.2%	10.5%
Combination Brain/Sinus CT Scan	1,111	2.7%	3.2%	2.7%
Combination Chest CT Scan	1,553	0.6%	1.9%	2.7%
Follow-up Mammogram/Ultrasound	5,868	5.9%	8.6%	8.8%
Lumbar Spine MRI for Low Back Pain	508	32.9%	39.6%	37.2%

Hedrick Medical Center

2799 North Washington Street
Chillicothe, MO 64601
URL: www.saintlukeshealthsystem.org
Type: Critical Access Hospitals
Ownership: Voluntary non-profit - Private
Phone: 660-646-1480
Fax: 660-646-6024
Emergency Services: Yes
Beds: 49

Key Personnel:

- Chief of Medical Staff . . . . Rick A Bonnette
- CEO/President. . . . . Brian Johnston
- CEO . . . . Matthew Wenzel

Measure	Cases	This Hosp.	State Avg.	U.S. Avg.
Blood Clot Prevention and Treatment				
Anticoagulation Overlap Therapy[1,2]	-	-	94%	93%
ICU Venous Thromboembolism Prophylaxis[1,2]	-	-	91%	92%
Incidence of Potentially Preventable VTE[2,3]	-	-	7%	10%
UFH with Dosages/Platelet Monitoring[2,3]	-	-	96%	97%
Venous Thromboembolism Prophylaxis[2,3]	45	60%	85%	85%
Warfarin Therapy Discharge Instructions[1,2]	-	-	76%	75%
Chest Pain/Possible Heart Attack Care				
Aspirin Given Within 24 Hours of Arrival	-	-	95%	96%
Fibrinolytic Meds Within 30 Min. of Arrival	-	-	53%	58%
Average Time to ECG (minutes)	-	-	7	7
Average Time to Transfer (minutes)	-	-	53	60
Children's Asthma Care				
Received Home Management Plan of Care	-	-	-	88%
Received Reliever Medication	-	-	-	100%
Received Systemic Corticosteroids	-	-	-	100%
Emergency Department				
Admittance Decision Time (minutes)[5]	-	-	81	98
Head CT Results Within 45 Min. of Arrival	-	-	63%	57%
Patients Who Left ER Before Being Seen	-	-	3%	2%
Time from ER Arrival to Admit. (minutes)[5]	-	-	238	274
Time from ER Arrival to Discharge (minutes)	-	-	136	134
Time in ER Before Being Evaluated (minutes)	-	-	26	26
Time to Pain Meds for Fractures (minutes)	-	-	52	57
Heart Attack Care				
Aspirin Given at Discharge[1,3]	-	-	99%	99%
Fibrinolytic Meds Within 30 Min. of Arrival[3,7]	-	-	-	54%
PCI Within 90 Minutes of Arrival[3,7]	-	-	97%	96%
Statin Prescribed at Discharge[1,3]	-	-	98%	98%
Heart Failure Care				

NOTE: Hospital profiles are in alphabetical order by state, then city, then hospital within the city; Rankings exclude hospitals with less than 25 cases except for patient surveys which excludes hospitals with less than 100 cases; (a) 100-299 cases; (1) The number of cases/patients is too few to report; (2) Data submitted were based on a sample of cases/patients; (3) Results are based on a shorter time period than required; (4) Data suppressed by CMS for one or more quarters; (5) Results are not available for this reporting period; (6) Fewer than 100 patients completed the HCAHPS survey; (7) No cases met the criteria for this measure; (8) The lower limit of the confidence interval cannot be calculated if the number of observed infections equals zero; (9) No data are available from the state/territory for this reporting period; (10) The scores shown reflect fewer than 50 completed surveys; (11) There were discrepancies in the data collection process; (12) This measure does not apply to this hospital for this reporting period; (13) Results cannot be calculated for this reporting period; (14) The results for this state are combined with nearby states to protect confidentiality; Please refer to the User's Guide for a full explanation of data.

Measure	Cases	This Hosp.	State Avg.	U.S. Avg.
ACE Inhibitor or ARB for LVSD[1]	-	-	96%	97%
Discharge Instructions Given	14	100%	94%	94%
Evaluation of LVS Function	24	100%	98%	99%
Medicare Spending				
Medicare Spending per Patient (ratio)	-	-	0.95	0.98
Pneumonia Care				
Appropriate Initial Antibiotic Given	29	93%	95%	95%
Blood Culture Timing	33	97%	98%	98%
Pregnancy and Delivery Care				
Newborn Deliveries Scheduled Early[5]	-	-	5%	6%
Preventive Care				
Immunization for Influenza[2,3]	144	100%	92%	90%
Immunization for Pneumonia[2,3]	89	100%	93%	92%
Stroke Care				
Anticoagulation Therapy for Atrial Fibrillation[5]	-	-	94%	95%
Antithrombotic Therapy Timing[5]	-	-	98%	98%
Assessed for Rehabilitation[5]	-	-	98%	97%
Discharged on Antithrombotic Therapy[5]	-	-	99%	99%
Discharged on Statin Medication[5]	-	-	95%	94%
Thrombolytic Therapy Timing[5]	-	-	67%	66%
Venous Thromboembolism Prophylaxis[5]	-	-	95%	94%
Written Stroke Educational Materials Given[5]	-	-	88%	88%
Surgical Care Improvement Project				
Appropriate Beta Blocker Usage[1]	-	-	98%	98%
Appropriate VTP Within 24 Hours	18	100%	98%	98%
Controlled Postoperative Blood Glucose[7]	-	-	97%	97%
Perioperative Temperature Management	21	100%	100%	100%
Prophylactic Antibiotic Selection	12	83%	99%	99%
Prophylactic Antibiotic Selection (Outpatient)	-	-	98%	98%
Prophylactic Antibiotic Stopped	12	100%	98%	98%
Prophylactic Antibiotic Timing	12	100%	99%	99%
Prophylactic Antibiotic Timing (Outpatient)	-	-	98%	98%
Urinary Catheter Removal[1]	-	-	97%	97%
Survey of Patients' Hospital Experiences				
Area Around Room 'Always' Quiet at Night	(a)	67%	61%	61%
Doctors 'Always' Communicated Well	(a)	83%	82%	82%
Home Recovery Information Given	(a)	91%	87%	85%
Hospital Given 9 or 10 on 10 Point Scale	(a)	76%	71%	71%
Meds 'Always' Explained Before Given	(a)	68%	63%	64%
Nurses 'Always' Communicated Well	(a)	80%	79%	79%
Pain 'Always' Well Controlled	(a)	75%	71%	71%
Room and Bathroom 'Always' Clean	(a)	79%	73%	73%
Timely Help 'Always' Received	(a)	71%	68%	68%
Would Definitely Recommend Hospital	(a)	65%	70%	71%
Use of Medical Imaging				
Cardiac Imaging Stress Test before Surgery	-	-	5.2%	5.3%
Combination Abdominal CT Scan	-	-	11.2%	10.5%
Combination Brain/Sinus CT Scan	-	-	3.2%	2.7%
Combination Chest CT Scan	-	-	1.9%	2.7%
Follow-up Mammogram/Ultrasound	-	-	8.6%	8.8%
Lumbar Spine MRI for Low Back Pain	-	-	39.6%	37.2%

Golden Valley Memorial Hospital

1600 N 2nd St
Clinton, MO 64735
Phone: 660-885-5511
Fax: 660-885-5012
URL: www.gvmh.org
Type: Acute Care Hospitals
Emergency Services: Yes
Ownership: Govt - Hospital Dist/Auth
Beds: 84

Key Personnel:

Emergency Room . . . . Richard F Beamon
Chief of Medical Staff . . . . Bruce Bellmay, MD
Infection Control . . . . Claudia Gibson
Radiology . . . . Douglas Walrath
CEO/President . . . . Randy S Wertz
Operating Room . . . . Gus S Wetzel II

Measure	Cases	This Hosp.	State Avg.	U.S. Avg.
Blood Clot Prevention and Treatment				
Anticoagulation Overlap Therapy[2]	11	91%	94%	93%
ICU Venous Thromboembolism Prophylaxis[2]	37	95%	91%	92%
Incidence of Potentially Preventable VTE[1,2]	-	-	7%	10%
UFH with Dosages/Platelet Monitoring[2,7]	-	-	96%	97%
Venous Thromboembolism Prophylaxis[2]	201	75%	85%	85%
Warfarin Therapy Discharge Instructions[1,2]	-	-	76%	75%
Chest Pain/Possible Heart Attack Care				
Aspirin Given Within 24 Hours of Arrival	109	96%	95%	96%
Fibrinolytic Meds Within 30 Min. of Arrival[1]	-	-	53%	58%
Average Time to ECG (minutes)	116	2	7	7
Average Time to Transfer (minutes)[7]	-	-	53	60
Children's Asthma Care				
Received Home Management Plan of Care	-	-	-	88%
Received Reliever Medication	-	-	-	100%
Received Systemic Corticosteroids	-	-	-	100%
Emergency Department				
Admittance Decision Time (minutes)[2]	280	59	81	98
Head CT Results Within 45 Min. of Arrival	12	83%	63%	57%
Patients Who Left ER Before Being Seen	14,965	2%	3%	2%
Time from ER Arrival to Admit. (minutes)[2]	289	198	238	274
Time from ER Arrival to Discharge (minutes)	385	117	136	134
Time in ER Before Being Evaluated (minutes)	443	15	26	26
Time to Pain Meds for Fractures (minutes)	51	50	52	57
Heart Attack Care				
Aspirin Given at Discharge[1]	-	-	99%	99%
Fibrinolytic Meds Within 30 Min. of Arrival[7]	-	-	-	54%
PCI Within 90 Minutes of Arrival[7]	-	-	97%	96%
Statin Prescribed at Discharge[1]	-	-	98%	98%
Heart Failure Care				
ACE Inhibitor or ARB for LVSD	31	90%	96%	97%
Discharge Instructions Given	56	95%	94%	94%
Evaluation of LVS Function	94	95%	98%	99%
Medicare Spending				
Medicare Spending per Patient (ratio)	-	0.94	0.95	0.98
Pneumonia Care				
Appropriate Initial Antibiotic Given	81	98%	95%	95%
Blood Culture Timing	101	94%	98%	98%
Pregnancy and Delivery Care				
Newborn Deliveries Scheduled Early	59	3%	5%	6%
Preventive Care				
Immunization for Influenza[2]	284	89%	92%	90%
Immunization for Pneumonia[2]	365	96%	93%	92%
Stroke Care				
Anticoagulation Therapy for Atrial Fibrillation[1,3]	-	-	94%	95%
Antithrombotic Therapy Timing[1,3]	-	-	98%	98%
Assessed for Rehabilitation[1,3]	-	-	98%	97%
Discharged on Antithrombotic Therapy[1,3]	-	-	99%	99%
Discharged on Statin Medication[1,3]	-	-	95%	94%
Thrombolytic Therapy Timing[1,3]	-	-	67%	66%
Venous Thromboembolism Prophylaxis[1,3]	-	-	95%	94%
Written Stroke Educational Materials Given[1,3]	-	-	88%	88%
Surgical Care Improvement Project				
Appropriate Beta Blocker Usage	72	99%	98%	98%
Appropriate VTP Within 24 Hours	258	98%	98%	98%
Controlled Postoperative Blood Glucose[7]	-	-	97%	97%
Perioperative Temperature Management	274	100%	100%	100%
Prophylactic Antibiotic Selection	210	99%	99%	99%
Prophylactic Antibiotic Selection (Outpatient)	12	100%	98%	98%
Prophylactic Antibiotic Stopped	207	98%	98%	98%
Prophylactic Antibiotic Timing	211	99%	99%	99%
Prophylactic Antibiotic Timing (Outpatient)	12	100%	98%	98%
Urinary Catheter Removal	184	100%	97%	97%
Survey of Patients' Hospital Experiences				
Area Around Room 'Always' Quiet at Night	300+	64%	61%	61%
Doctors 'Always' Communicated Well	300+	80%	82%	82%
Home Recovery Information Given	300+	87%	87%	85%
Hospital Given 9 or 10 on 10 Point Scale	300+	71%	71%	71%
Meds 'Always' Explained Before Given	300+	70%	63%	64%
Nurses 'Always' Communicated Well	300+	82%	79%	79%
Pain 'Always' Well Controlled	300+	70%	71%	71%
Room and Bathroom 'Always' Clean	300+	79%	73%	73%
Timely Help 'Always' Received	300+	70%	68%	68%
Would Definitely Recommend Hospital	300+	67%	70%	71%
Use of Medical Imaging				
Cardiac Imaging Stress Test before Surgery	231	4.3%	5.2%	5.3%
Combination Abdominal CT Scan	530	6.2%	11.2%	10.5%
Combination Brain/Sinus CT Scan[1]	-	-	3.2%	2.7%
Combination Chest CT Scan	287	0.3%	1.9%	2.7%
Follow-up Mammogram/Ultrasound	848	5.3%	8.6%	8.8%
Lumbar Spine MRI for Low Back Pain	130	39.2%	39.6%	37.2%

Boone Hospital Center

1600 E Broadway
Columbia, MO 65201
Phone: 573-815-8000
URL: www.boone.org
Type: Acute Care Hospitals
Emergency Services: Yes
Ownership: Voluntary non-profit - Other

Key Personnel:

Chief of Medical Staff . . . . Carol B Danuser
CEO/President . . . . Dan Rothery

Measure	Cases	This Hosp.	State Avg.	U.S. Avg.
Blood Clot Prevention and Treatment				
Anticoagulation Overlap Therapy[2]	95	97%	94%	93%
ICU Venous Thromboembolism Prophylaxis[2]	69	100%	91%	92%
Incidence of Potentially Preventable VTE[2]	45	7%	7%	10%
UFH with Dosages/Platelet Monitoring[2]	16	100%	96%	97%
Venous Thromboembolism Prophylaxis[2]	280	97%	85%	85%
Warfarin Therapy Discharge Instructions[2]	64	100%	76%	75%
Chest Pain/Possible Heart Attack Care				
Aspirin Given Within 24 Hours of Arrival[5]	-	-	95%	96%
Fibrinolytic Meds Within 30 Min. of Arrival[5]	-	-	53%	58%
Average Time to ECG (minutes)[5]	-	-	7	7
Average Time to Transfer (minutes)[5]	-	-	53	60
Children's Asthma Care				
Received Home Management Plan of Care	-	-	-	88%
Received Reliever Medication	-	-	-	100%
Received Systemic Corticosteroids	-	-	-	100%
Emergency Department				
Admittance Decision Time (minutes)[2]	217	59	81	98
Head CT Results Within 45 Min. of Arrival[1]	-	-	63%	57%
Patients Who Left ER Before Being Seen	31,987	2%	3%	2%
Time from ER Arrival to Admit. (minutes)[2]	300	194	238	274
Time from ER Arrival to Discharge (minutes)	613	150	136	134
Time in ER Before Being Evaluated (minutes)	301	59	26	26
Time to Pain Meds for Fractures (minutes)	116	66	52	57
Heart Attack Care				
Aspirin Given at Discharge	378	100%	99%	99%
Fibrinolytic Meds Within 30 Min. of Arrival[7]	-	-	-	54%
PCI Within 90 Minutes of Arrival	44	98%	97%	96%
Statin Prescribed at Discharge	369	100%	98%	98%
Heart Failure Care				
ACE Inhibitor or ARB for LVSD[2]	133	99%	96%	97%
Discharge Instructions Given[2]	346	99%	94%	94%
Evaluation of LVS Function[2]	406	100%	98%	99%
Medicare Spending				
Medicare Spending per Patient (ratio)	-	0.93	0.95	0.98
Pneumonia Care				
Appropriate Initial Antibiotic Given[2]	144	94%	95%	95%
Blood Culture Timing[2]	188	99%	98%	98%
Pregnancy and Delivery Care				
Newborn Deliveries Scheduled Early[2]	34	3%	5%	6%
Preventive Care				
Immunization for Influenza[2]	517	96%	92%	90%
Immunization for Pneumonia[2]	639	95%	93%	92%
Stroke Care				
Anticoagulation Therapy for Atrial Fibrillation[2]	29	97%	94%	95%
Antithrombotic Therapy Timing[2]	166	99%	98%	98%
Assessed for Rehabilitation[2]	228	98%	98%	97%
Discharged on Antithrombotic Therapy[2]	197	100%	99%	99%
Discharged on Statin Medication[2]	158	94%	95%	94%
Thrombolytic Therapy Timing[2]	18	100%	67%	66%
Venous Thromboembolism Prophylaxis[2]	223	98%	95%	94%
Written Stroke Educational Materials Given[2]	132	100%	88%	88%
Surgical Care Improvement Project				
Appropriate Beta Blocker Usage[2]	220	97%	98%	98%
Appropriate VTP Within 24 Hours[2]	427	100%	98%	98%
Controlled Postoperative Blood Glucose[2]	138	96%	97%	97%
Perioperative Temperature Management[2]	563	100%	100%	100%
Prophylactic Antibiotic Selection[2]	536	100%	99%	99%
Prophylactic Antibiotic Selection (Outpatient)	729	99%	98%	98%
Prophylactic Antibiotic Stopped[2]	534	98%	98%	98%
Prophylactic Antibiotic Timing[2]	536	99%	99%	99%

NOTE: Hospital profiles are in alphabetical order by state, then city, then hospital within the city; Rankings exclude hospitals with less than 25 cases except for patient surveys which excludes hospitals with less than 100 cases; (a) 100-299 cases; (1) The number of cases/patients is too few to report; (2) Data submitted were based on a sample of cases/patients; (3) Results are based on a shorter time period than required; (4) Data suppressed by CMS for one or more quarters; (5) Results are not available for this reporting period; (6) Fewer than 100 patients completed the HCAHPS survey; (7) No cases met the criteria for this measure; (8) The lower limit of the confidence interval cannot be calculated if the number of observed infections equals zero; (9) No data are available from the state/territory for this reporting period; (10) The scores shown reflect fewer than 50 completed surveys; (11) There were discrepancies in the data collection process; (12) This measure does not apply to this hospital for this reporting period; (13) Results cannot be calculated for this reporting period; (14) The results for this state are combined with nearby states to protect confidentiality; Please refer to the User's Guide for a full explanation of data.

Measure	Cases	This Hosp.	State Avg.	U.S. Avg.
Prophylactic Antibiotic Timing (Outpatient)	729	100%	98%	98%
Urinary Catheter Removal[2]	527	98%	97%	97%
Survey of Patients' Hospital Experiences				
Area Around Room 'Always' Quiet at Night	300+	63%	61%	61%
Doctors 'Always' Communicated Well	300+	85%	82%	82%
Home Recovery Information Given	300+	90%	87%	85%
Hospital Given 9 or 10 on 10 Point Scale	300+	83%	71%	71%
Meds 'Always' Explained Before Given	300+	63%	63%	64%
Nurses 'Always' Communicated Well	300+	80%	79%	79%
Pain 'Always' Well Controlled	300+	74%	71%	71%
Room and Bathroom 'Always' Clean	300+	68%	73%	73%
Timely Help 'Always' Received	300+	69%	68%	68%
Would Definitely Recommend Hospital	300+	84%	70%	71%
Use of Medical Imaging				
Cardiac Imaging Stress Test before Surgery	1,414	6.0%	5.2%	5.3%
Combination Abdominal CT Scan	1,113	4.0%	11.2%	10.5%
Combination Brain/Sinus CT Scan	754	3.4%	3.2%	2.7%
Combination Chest CT Scan	934	0.5%	1.9%	2.7%
Follow-up Mammogram/Ultrasound	3,870	4.3%	8.6%	8.8%
Lumbar Spine MRI for Low Back Pain	223	47.1%	39.6%	37.2%

Columbia MO VA Medical Center

800 Hospital Dr
Columbia, MO 65201
Phone: 573-814-6000
Fax: 573-814-6600
URL: www.columbiamo.va.gov
Type: Acute Care - VA
Emergency Services: No
Ownership: Government Federal
Beds: 123

Key Personnel:

Quality Assurance . . . . Crystal Aholt, RN
Patient Relations . . . . Debbie Canow, RN
Intensive Care Unit. . . . . Stephanie Carter, RN
Coronary Care . . . . Hunter Hofmann, MD
Emergency Room . . . . Lula Johnson, RN
CEO/President. . . . . Sallie Houser- Manfelder, FACHE
Anesthesiology. . . . . John Turchiano, MD
Cardiac Laboratory. . . . . Lana Zerrer, MD

Measure	Cases	This Hosp.	State Avg.	U.S. Avg.
Blood Clot Prevention and Treatment				
Anticoagulation Overlap Therapy	-	-	94%	93%
ICU Venous Thromboembolism Prophylaxis	-	-	91%	92%
Incidence of Potentially Preventable VTE	-	-	7%	10%
UFH with Dosages/Platelet Monitoring	-	-	96%	97%
Venous Thromboembolism Prophylaxis	-	-	85%	85%
Warfarin Therapy Discharge Instructions	-	-	76%	75%
Chest Pain/Possible Heart Attack Care				
Aspirin Given Within 24 Hours of Arrival	-	-	95%	96%
Fibrinolytic Meds Within 30 Min. of Arrival	-	-	53%	58%
Average Time to ECG (minutes)	-	-	7	7
Average Time to Transfer (minutes)	-	-	53	60
Children's Asthma Care				
Received Home Management Plan of Care	-	-	-	88%
Received Reliever Medication	-	-	-	100%
Received Systemic Corticosteroids	-	-	-	100%
Emergency Department				
Admittance Decision Time (minutes)	-	-	81	98
Head CT Results Within 45 Min. of Arrival	-	-	63%	57%
Patients Who Left ER Before Being Seen	-	-	3%	2%
Time from ER Arrival to Admit. (minutes)	-	-	238	274
Time from ER Arrival to Discharge (minutes)	-	-	136	134
Time in ER Before Being Evaluated (minutes)	-	-	26	26
Time to Pain Meds for Fractures (minutes)	-	-	52	57
Heart Attack Care				
Aspirin Given at Discharge	44	100%	99%	99%
Fibrinolytic Meds Within 30 Min. of Arrival[5]	-	-	-	54%
PCI Within 90 Minutes of Arrival[1]	-	-	97%	96%
Statin Prescribed at Discharge	44	98%	98%	98%
Heart Failure Care				
ACE Inhibitor or ARB for LVSD	50	98%	96%	97%
Discharge Instructions Given	118	90%	94%	94%
Evaluation of LVS Function	133	100%	98%	99%
Medicare Spending				
Medicare Spending per Patient (ratio)	-	-	0.95	0.98
Pneumonia Care				
Appropriate Initial Antibiotic Given	33	91%	95%	95%
Blood Culture Timing	62	100%	98%	98%
Pregnancy and Delivery Care				
Newborn Deliveries Scheduled Early	-	-	5%	6%
Preventive Care				
Immunization for Influenza[5]	-	-	92%	90%
Immunization for Pneumonia[5]	-	-	93%	92%
Stroke Care				
Anticoagulation Therapy for Atrial Fibrillation	-	-	94%	95%
Antithrombotic Therapy Timing	-	-	98%	98%
Assessed for Rehabilitation	-	-	98%	97%
Discharged on Antithrombotic Therapy	-	-	99%	99%
Discharged on Statin Medication	-	-	95%	94%
Thrombolytic Therapy Timing	-	-	67%	66%
Venous Thromboembolism Prophylaxis	-	-	95%	94%
Written Stroke Educational Materials Given	-	-	88%	88%
Surgical Care Improvement Project				
Appropriate Beta Blocker Usage[2]	180	97%	98%	98%
Appropriate VTP Within 24 Hours[2]	171	96%	98%	98%
Controlled Postoperative Blood Glucose[2]	153	97%	97%	97%
Perioperative Temperature Management[2]	202	100%	100%	100%
Prophylactic Antibiotic Selection	264	100%	99%	99%
Prophylactic Antibiotic Selection (Outpatient)	-	-	98%	98%
Prophylactic Antibiotic Stopped	264	99%	98%	98%
Prophylactic Antibiotic Timing	265	98%	99%	99%
Prophylactic Antibiotic Timing (Outpatient)	-	-	98%	98%
Urinary Catheter Removal[2]	195	99%	97%	97%
Survey of Patients' Hospital Experiences				
Area Around Room 'Always' Quiet at Night	-	-	61%	61%
Doctors 'Always' Communicated Well	-	-	82%	82%
Home Recovery Information Given	-	-	87%	85%
Hospital Given 9 or 10 on 10 Point Scale	-	-	71%	71%
Meds 'Always' Explained Before Given	-	-	63%	64%
Nurses 'Always' Communicated Well	-	-	79%	79%
Pain 'Always' Well Controlled	-	-	71%	71%
Room and Bathroom 'Always' Clean	-	-	73%	73%
Timely Help 'Always' Received	-	-	68%	68%
Would Definitely Recommend Hospital	-	-	70%	71%
Use of Medical Imaging				
Cardiac Imaging Stress Test before Surgery	-	-	5.2%	5.3%
Combination Abdominal CT Scan	-	-	11.2%	10.5%
Combination Brain/Sinus CT Scan	-	-	3.2%	2.7%
Combination Chest CT Scan	-	-	1.9%	2.7%
Follow-up Mammogram/Ultrasound	-	-	8.6%	8.8%
Lumbar Spine MRI for Low Back Pain	-	-	39.6%	37.2%

University of Missouri Health Care

One Hospital Drive, Room Ce121, Dc031,00
Phone: 573-882-4141
Columbia, MO 65212
Fax: 573-884-7470
URL: www.missouri.edu
Type: Acute Care Hospitals
Emergency Services: Yes
Ownership: Government - State
Beds: 495

Key Personnel:

Emergency Room . . . . Gwen Burley
Infection Control. . . . . E Dale Everett
CEO/President. . . . . Patsy J Hart
Radiology. . . . . Larry Kirschner
Anesthesiology. . . . . Noel Lawson, MD
Quality Assurance . . . . Myra McCoig
Operating Room. . . . . Amy Tinsley
Chief of Medical Staff. . . . . Karl Weber, MD

Measure	Cases	This Hosp.	State Avg.	U.S. Avg.
Blood Clot Prevention and Treatment				
Anticoagulation Overlap Therapy[2]	111	98%	94%	93%
ICU Venous Thromboembolism Prophylaxis[2]	140	98%	91%	92%
Incidence of Potentially Preventable VTE[2]	31	0%	7%	10%
UFH with Dosages/Platelet Monitoring[2]	82	100%	96%	97%
Venous Thromboembolism Prophylaxis[2]	277	90%	85%	85%
Warfarin Therapy Discharge Instructions[2]	81	77%	76%	75%
Chest Pain/Possible Heart Attack Care				
Aspirin Given Within 24 Hours of Arrival[1,3]	-	-	95%	96%
Fibrinolytic Meds Within 30 Min. of Arrival[3,7]	-	-	53%	58%
Average Time to ECG (minutes)[1,3]	-	-	7	7
Average Time to Transfer (minutes)[3,7]	-	-	53	60
Children's Asthma Care				
Received Home Management Plan of Care	-	-	-	88%
Received Reliever Medication	-	-	-	100%
Received Systemic Corticosteroids	-	-	-	100%
Emergency Department				
Admittance Decision Time (minutes)[2]	337	76	81	98
Head CT Results Within 45 Min. of Arrival[1]	-	-	63%	57%
Patients Who Left ER Before Being Seen	56,099	3%	3%	2%
Time from ER Arrival to Admit. (minutes)[2]	366	254	238	274
Time from ER Arrival to Discharge (minutes)	454	152	136	134
Time in ER Before Being Evaluated (minutes)	437	23	26	26
Time to Pain Meds for Fractures (minutes)	162	56	52	57
Heart Attack Care				
Aspirin Given at Discharge	284	100%	99%	99%
Fibrinolytic Meds Within 30 Min. of Arrival[7]	-	-	-	54%
PCI Within 90 Minutes of Arrival	39	100%	97%	96%
Statin Prescribed at Discharge	284	99%	98%	98%
Heart Failure Care				
ACE Inhibitor or ARB for LVSD	94	96%	96%	97%
Discharge Instructions Given	172	99%	94%	94%
Evaluation of LVS Function	231	100%	98%	99%
Medicare Spending				
Medicare Spending per Patient (ratio)	-	0.97	0.95	0.98
Pneumonia Care				
Appropriate Initial Antibiotic Given	68	87%	95%	95%
Blood Culture Timing	125	98%	98%	98%
Pregnancy and Delivery Care				
Newborn Deliveries Scheduled Early[2]	22	5%	5%	6%
Preventive Care				
Immunization for Influenza[2]	658	93%	92%	90%
Immunization for Pneumonia[2]	600	93%	93%	92%
Stroke Care				
Anticoagulation Therapy for Atrial Fibrillation	24	92%	94%	95%
Antithrombotic Therapy Timing	158	94%	98%	98%
Assessed for Rehabilitation	255	97%	98%	97%
Discharged on Antithrombotic Therapy	208	100%	99%	99%
Discharged on Statin Medication	156	96%	95%	94%
Thrombolytic Therapy Timing	16	100%	67%	66%
Venous Thromboembolism Prophylaxis	265	98%	95%	94%
Written Stroke Educational Materials Given	123	85%	88%	88%
Surgical Care Improvement Project				
Appropriate Beta Blocker Usage[2]	302	100%	98%	98%
Appropriate VTP Within 24 Hours[2]	606	100%	98%	98%
Controlled Postoperative Blood Glucose[2]	147	98%	97%	97%
Perioperative Temperature Management[2]	755	100%	100%	100%
Prophylactic Antibiotic Selection[2]	571	100%	99%	99%
Prophylactic Antibiotic Selection (Outpatient)	592	99%	98%	98%
Prophylactic Antibiotic Stopped[2]	547	99%	98%	98%
Prophylactic Antibiotic Timing[2]	572	99%	99%	99%
Prophylactic Antibiotic Timing (Outpatient)	515	100%	98%	98%
Urinary Catheter Removal[2]	528	100%	97%	97%
Survey of Patients' Hospital Experiences				
Area Around Room 'Always' Quiet at Night	300+	68%	61%	61%
Doctors 'Always' Communicated Well	300+	78%	82%	82%
Home Recovery Information Given	300+	85%	87%	85%
Hospital Given 9 or 10 on 10 Point Scale	300+	76%	71%	71%
Meds 'Always' Explained Before Given	300+	63%	63%	64%
Nurses 'Always' Communicated Well	300+	80%	79%	79%
Pain 'Always' Well Controlled	300+	67%	71%	71%
Room and Bathroom 'Always' Clean	300+	77%	73%	73%
Timely Help 'Always' Received	300+	71%	68%	68%
Would Definitely Recommend Hospital	300+	80%	70%	71%
Use of Medical Imaging				
Cardiac Imaging Stress Test before Surgery	475	6.1%	5.2%	5.3%
Combination Abdominal CT Scan	938	20.5%	11.2%	10.5%
Combination Brain/Sinus CT Scan	725	3.0%	3.2%	2.7%
Combination Chest CT Scan	1,167	1.6%	1.9%	2.7%
Follow-up Mammogram/Ultrasound	3,287	15.4%	8.6%	8.8%
Lumbar Spine MRI for Low Back Pain	235	33.2%	39.6%	37.2%

NOTE: Hospital profiles are in alphabetical order by state, then city, then hospital within the city; Rankings exclude hospitals with less than 25 cases except for patient surveys which excludes hospitals with less than 100 cases; (a) 100-299 cases; (1) The number of cases/patients is too few to report; (2) Data submitted were based on a sample of cases/patients; (3) Results are based on a shorter time period than required; (4) Data suppressed by CMS for one or more quarters; (5) Results are not available for this reporting period; (6) Fewer than 100 patients completed the HCAHPS survey; (7) No cases met the criteria for this measure; (8) The lower limit of the confidence interval cannot be calculated if the number of observed infections equals zero; (9) No data are available from the state/territory for this reporting period; (10) The scores shown reflect fewer than 50 completed surveys; (11) There were discrepancies in the data collection process; (12) This measure does not apply to this hospital for this reporting period; (13) Results cannot be calculated for this reporting period; (14) The results for this state are combined with nearby states to protect confidentiality; Please refer to the User's Guide for a full explanation of data.

Barnes-Jewish West County Hospital

12634 Olive Boulevard Phone: 314-996-8000
Creve Coeur, MO 63141 Fax: 314-286-0305
URL: www.barnesjewishwestcounty.org
Type: Acute Care Hospitals Emergency Services: Yes
Ownership: Voluntary non-profit - Private Beds: 113

Key Personnel:
Emergency Room . . . . Ren Kozikowski
Chief of Medical Staff. . . . . Alan Londe
Quality Assurance . . . . Mary Mantese
CEO/President. . . . . Pat Mohrman, RN, MSN

Measure	Cases	This Hosp.	State Avg.	U.S. Avg.
Blood Clot Prevention and Treatment				
Anticoagulation Overlap Therapy[1,2]	-	-	94%	93%
ICU Venous Thromboembolism Prophylaxis[2]	21	100%	91%	92%
Incidence of Potentially Preventable VTE[1,2]	-	-	7%	10%
UFH with Dosages/Platelet Monitoring[1,2]	-	-	96%	97%
Venous Thromboembolism Prophylaxis[2]	123	97%	85%	85%
Warfarin Therapy Discharge Instructions[1,2]	-	-	76%	75%
Chest Pain/Possible Heart Attack Care				
Aspirin Given Within 24 Hours of Arrival	42	95%	95%	96%
Fibrinolytic Meds Within 30 Min. of Arrival[7]	-	-	53%	58%
Average Time to ECG (minutes)	42	10	7	7
Average Time to Transfer (minutes)[1]	-	-	53	60
Children's Asthma Care				
Received Home Management Plan of Care	-	-	-	88%
Received Reliever Medication	-	-	-	100%
Received Systemic Corticosteroids	-	-	-	100%
Emergency Department				
Admittance Decision Time (minutes)[2]	104	50	81	98
Head CT Results Within 45 Min. of Arrival[1]	-	-	63%	57%
Patients Who Left ER Before Being Seen	12,021	2%	3%	2%
Time from ER Arrival to Admit. (minutes)[2]	106	226	238	274
Time from ER Arrival to Discharge (minutes)	633	142	136	134
Time in ER Before Being Evaluated (minutes)	546	48	26	26
Time to Pain Meds for Fractures (minutes)	26	73	52	57
Heart Attack Care				
Aspirin Given at Discharge[1,3]	-	-	99%	99%
Fibrinolytic Meds Within 30 Min. of Arrival[3,7]	-	-	-	54%
PCI Within 90 Minutes of Arrival[3,7]	-	-	97%	96%
Statin Prescribed at Discharge[1,3]	-	-	98%	98%
Heart Failure Care				
ACE Inhibitor or ARB for LVSD[1]	-	-	96%	97%
Discharge Instructions Given	37	100%	94%	94%
Evaluation of LVS Function	42	100%	98%	99%
Medicare Spending				
Medicare Spending per Patient (ratio)	-	0.88	0.95	0.98
Pneumonia Care				
Appropriate Initial Antibiotic Given[1]	-	-	95%	95%
Blood Culture Timing	23	100%	98%	98%
Pregnancy and Delivery Care				
Newborn Deliveries Scheduled Early[7]	-	-	5%	6%
Preventive Care				
Immunization for Influenza[2]	306	93%	92%	90%
Immunization for Pneumonia[2]	336	92%	93%	92%
Stroke Care				
Anticoagulation Therapy for Atrial Fibrillation[7]	-	-	94%	95%
Antithrombotic Therapy Timing[1]	-	-	98%	98%
Assessed for Rehabilitation[1]	-	-	98%	97%
Discharged on Antithrombotic Therapy[1]	-	-	99%	99%
Discharged on Statin Medication[1]	-	-	95%	94%
Thrombolytic Therapy Timing[7]	-	-	67%	66%
Venous Thromboembolism Prophylaxis[1]	-	-	95%	94%
Written Stroke Educational Materials Given[1]	-	-	88%	88%
Surgical Care Improvement Project				
Appropriate Beta Blocker Usage[2]	107	99%	98%	98%
Appropriate VTP Within 24 Hours[2]	457	100%	98%	98%
Controlled Postoperative Blood Glucose[2,7]	-	-	97%	97%
Perioperative Temperature Management[2]	640	100%	100%	100%
Prophylactic Antibiotic Selection[2]	437	100%	99%	99%
Prophylactic Antibiotic Selection (Outpatient)	282	99%	98%	98%
Prophylactic Antibiotic Stopped[2]	433	100%	98%	98%
Prophylactic Antibiotic Timing[2]	437	99%	99%	99%
Prophylactic Antibiotic Timing (Outpatient)	282	99%	98%	98%
Urinary Catheter Removal[2]	305	99%	97%	97%
Survey of Patients' Hospital Experiences				
Area Around Room 'Always' Quiet at Night	300+	59%	61%	61%
Doctors 'Always' Communicated Well	300+	86%	82%	82%
Home Recovery Information Given	300+	89%	87%	85%
Hospital Given 9 or 10 on 10 Point Scale	300+	75%	71%	71%
Meds 'Always' Explained Before Given	300+	63%	63%	64%
Nurses 'Always' Communicated Well	300+	79%	79%	79%
Pain 'Always' Well Controlled	300+	72%	71%	71%
Room and Bathroom 'Always' Clean	300+	62%	73%	73%
Timely Help 'Always' Received	300+	64%	68%	68%
Would Definitely Recommend Hospital	300+	77%	70%	71%
Use of Medical Imaging				
Cardiac Imaging Stress Test before Surgery	115	3.5%	5.2%	5.3%
Combination Abdominal CT Scan	1,361	6.0%	11.2%	10.5%
Combination Brain/Sinus CT Scan	361	4.4%	3.2%	2.7%
Combination Chest CT Scan	1,812	0.7%	1.9%	2.7%
Follow-up Mammogram/Ultrasound	786	8.8%	8.6%	8.8%
Lumbar Spine MRI for Low Back Pain	113	35.4%	39.6%	37.2%

Mercy Hospital Jefferson

1400 Highway 61 South Phone: 636-933-1000
Crystal City, MO 63019 Fax: 636-933-1119
E-mail: info@jeffersonmemorial.org
URL: www.jeffersonmemorial.org
Type: Acute Care Hospitals Emergency Services: Yes
Ownership: Voluntary non-profit - Private Beds: 240

Key Personnel:
Pediatric In-Patient Care . . . . Linda Blanc
CEO/President. . . . . Lindell Carter
Radiology. . . . . Jonathan Dehner, MD
Infection Control. . . . . Linda Ferrara
Operating Room. . . . . Lana Gladhill
Quality Assurance . . . . Sarah Johnson
Pediatric Ambulatory Care . . . . . . Sarah Moerschel, MD
Chief of Medical Staff . . . . Indu Patel

Measure	Cases	This Hosp.	State Avg.	U.S. Avg.
Blood Clot Prevention and Treatment				
Anticoagulation Overlap Therapy[2]	66	94%	94%	93%
ICU Venous Thromboembolism Prophylaxis[2]	72	89%	91%	92%
Incidence of Potentially Preventable VTE[2]	13	0%	7%	10%
UFH with Dosages/Platelet Monitoring[2]	27	100%	96%	97%
Venous Thromboembolism Prophylaxis[2]	347	89%	85%	85%
Warfarin Therapy Discharge Instructions[2]	41	98%	76%	75%
Chest Pain/Possible Heart Attack Care				
Aspirin Given Within 24 Hours of Arrival	12	100%	95%	96%
Fibrinolytic Meds Within 30 Min. of Arrival[3,7]	-	-	53%	58%
Average Time to ECG (minutes)	12	4	7	7
Average Time to Transfer (minutes)[3,7]	-	-	53	60
Children's Asthma Care				
Received Home Management Plan of Care	-	-	-	88%
Received Reliever Medication	-	-	-	100%
Received Systemic Corticosteroids	-	-	-	100%
Emergency Department				
Admittance Decision Time (minutes)[2]	748	78	81	98
Head CT Results Within 45 Min. of Arrival	20	85%	63%	57%
Patients Who Left ER Before Being Seen	32,695	1%	3%	2%
Time from ER Arrival to Admit. (minutes)[2]	753	270	238	274
Time from ER Arrival to Discharge (minutes)	382	162	136	134
Time in ER Before Being Evaluated (minutes)	398	61	26	26
Time to Pain Meds for Fractures (minutes)	123	57	52	57
Heart Attack Care				
Aspirin Given at Discharge[2]	289	97%	99%	99%
Fibrinolytic Meds Within 30 Min. of Arrival[2,7]	-	-	-	54%
PCI Within 90 Minutes of Arrival[2]	55	96%	97%	96%
Statin Prescribed at Discharge[2]	278	98%	98%	98%
Heart Failure Care				
ACE Inhibitor or ARB for LVSD[2]	72	96%	96%	97%
Discharge Instructions Given[2]	229	92%	94%	94%
Evaluation of LVS Function[2]	302	100%	98%	99%
Medicare Spending				
Medicare Spending per Patient (ratio)	-	1.00	0.95	0.98
Pneumonia Care				
Appropriate Initial Antibiotic Given[2]	116	97%	95%	95%
Blood Culture Timing[2]	161	99%	98%	98%
Pregnancy and Delivery Care				
Newborn Deliveries Scheduled Early	31	3%	5%	6%
Preventive Care				
Immunization for Influenza[2]	578	95%	92%	90%
Immunization for Pneumonia[2]	813	97%	93%	92%
Stroke Care				
Anticoagulation Therapy for Atrial Fibrillation	14	100%	94%	95%
Antithrombotic Therapy Timing	98	100%	98%	98%
Assessed for Rehabilitation	101	97%	98%	97%
Discharged on Antithrombotic Therapy	96	100%	99%	99%
Discharged on Statin Medication	89	98%	95%	94%
Thrombolytic Therapy Timing[1]	-	-	67%	66%
Venous Thromboembolism Prophylaxis	106	97%	95%	94%
Written Stroke Educational Materials Given	58	97%	88%	88%
Surgical Care Improvement Project				
Appropriate Beta Blocker Usage	194	96%	98%	98%
Appropriate VTP Within 24 Hours	400	99%	98%	98%
Controlled Postoperative Blood Glucose	52	87%	97%	97%
Perioperative Temperature Management	472	100%	100%	100%
Prophylactic Antibiotic Selection	333	99%	99%	99%
Prophylactic Antibiotic Selection (Outpatient)	128	99%	98%	98%
Prophylactic Antibiotic Stopped	313	96%	98%	98%
Prophylactic Antibiotic Timing	333	100%	99%	99%
Prophylactic Antibiotic Timing (Outpatient)	128	100%	98%	98%
Urinary Catheter Removal	151	99%	97%	97%
Survey of Patients' Hospital Experiences				
Area Around Room 'Always' Quiet at Night	300+	54%	61%	61%
Doctors 'Always' Communicated Well	300+	78%	82%	82%
Home Recovery Information Given	300+	86%	87%	85%
Hospital Given 9 or 10 on 10 Point Scale	300+	63%	71%	71%
Meds 'Always' Explained Before Given	300+	61%	63%	64%
Nurses 'Always' Communicated Well	300+	74%	79%	79%
Pain 'Always' Well Controlled	300+	67%	71%	71%
Room and Bathroom 'Always' Clean	300+	72%	73%	73%
Timely Help 'Always' Received	300+	65%	68%	68%
Would Definitely Recommend Hospital	300+	63%	70%	71%
Use of Medical Imaging				
Cardiac Imaging Stress Test before Surgery[1]	-	-	5.2%	5.3%
Combination Abdominal CT Scan	782	13.6%	11.2%	10.5%
Combination Brain/Sinus CT Scan[1]	-	-	3.2%	2.7%
Combination Chest CT Scan	647	5.6%	1.9%	2.7%
Follow-up Mammogram/Ultrasound	940	8.3%	8.6%	8.8%
Lumbar Spine MRI for Low Back Pain	128	34.4%	39.6%	37.2%

Southeasthealth Center of Stoddard County

1200 N One Mile Rd Phone: 573-624-5566
Dexter, MO 63841 Fax: 573-624-6265
Type: Acute Care Hospitals Emergency Services: Yes
Ownership: Proprietary Beds: 50

Key Personnel:
Intensive Care Unit. . . . . Christie DeArmen
Emergency Room . . . . Cathy Hawthorne
Chief of Medical Staff . . . . Reza Jalal, MD
Infection Control. . . . . Christine Neuber
Radiology. . . . . Christopher Newberry
Quality Assurance . . . . Judy Pedigo
Operating Room. . . . . Patti Shell
CEO/President. . . . . Wayne Smith

Measure	Cases	This Hosp.	State Avg.	U.S. Avg.
Blood Clot Prevention and Treatment				
Anticoagulation Overlap Therapy[2]	15	80%	94%	93%
ICU Venous Thromboembolism Prophylaxis[2]	36	67%	91%	92%
Incidence of Potentially Preventable VTE[1,2]	-	-	7%	10%
UFH with Dosages/Platelet Monitoring[1,2]	-	-	96%	97%
Venous Thromboembolism Prophylaxis[2]	417	73%	85%	85%
Warfarin Therapy Discharge Instructions[1,2]	-	-	76%	75%
Chest Pain/Possible Heart Attack Care				
Aspirin Given Within 24 Hours of Arrival	75	97%	95%	96%
Fibrinolytic Meds Within 30 Min. of Arrival[1]	-	-	53%	58%
Average Time to ECG (minutes)	79	9	7	7
Average Time to Transfer (minutes)[1]	-	-	53	60
Children's Asthma Care				

NOTE: *Hospital profiles are in alphabetical order by state, then city, then hospital within the city; Rankings exclude hospitals with less than 25 cases except for patient surveys which excludes hospitals with less than 100 cases; (a) 100-299 cases; (1) The number of cases/patients is too few to report; (2) Data submitted were based on a sample of cases/patients; (3) Results are based on a shorter time period than required; (4) Data suppressed by CMS for one or more quarters; (5) Results are not available for this reporting period; (6) Fewer than 100 patients completed the HCAHPS survey; (7) No cases met the criteria for this measure; (8) The lower limit of the confidence interval cannot be calculated if the number of observed infections equals zero; (9) No data are available from the state/territory for this reporting period; (10) The scores shown reflect fewer than 50 completed surveys; (11) There were discrepancies in the data collection process; (12) This measure does not apply to this hospital for this reporting period; (13) Results cannot be calculated for this reporting period; (14) The results for this state are combined with nearby states to protect confidentiality; Please refer to the User's Guide for a full explanation of data.*

Measure	Cases	This Hosp.	State Avg.	U.S. Avg.
Received Home Management Plan of Care	-	-	-	88%
Received Reliever Medication	-	-	-	100%
Received Systemic Corticosteroids	-	-	-	100%
Emergency Department				
Admittance Decision Time (minutes)	592	55	81	98
Head CT Results Within 45 Min. of Arrival[1]	-	-	63%	57%
Patients Who Left ER Before Being Seen	10,989	7%	3%	2%
Time from ER Arrival to Admit. (minutes)	630	191	238	274
Time from ER Arrival to Discharge (minutes)	404	99	136	134
Time in ER Before Being Evaluated (minutes)	369	46	26	26
Time to Pain Meds for Fractures (minutes)	57	53	52	57
Heart Attack Care				
Aspirin Given at Discharge[1,3]	-	-	99%	99%
Fibrinolytic Meds Within 30 Min. of Arrival[3,7]	-	-	-	54%
PCI Within 90 Minutes of Arrival[3,7]	-	-	97%	96%
Statin Prescribed at Discharge[1,3]	-	-	98%	98%
Heart Failure Care				
ACE Inhibitor or ARB for LVSD[1]	-	-	96%	97%
Discharge Instructions Given	29	45%	94%	94%
Evaluation of LVS Function	50	76%	98%	99%
Medicare Spending				
Medicare Spending per Patient (ratio)	-	0.99	0.95	0.98
Pneumonia Care				
Appropriate Initial Antibiotic Given	59	81%	95%	95%
Blood Culture Timing	57	96%	98%	98%
Pregnancy and Delivery Care				
Newborn Deliveries Scheduled Early[7]	-	-	5%	6%
Preventive Care				
Immunization for Influenza[2]	409	77%	92%	90%
Immunization for Pneumonia[2]	639	87%	93%	92%
Stroke Care				
Anticoagulation Therapy for Atrial Fibrillation[3,7]	-	-	94%	95%
Antithrombotic Therapy Timing[1,3]	-	-	98%	98%
Assessed for Rehabilitation[1,3]	-	-	98%	97%
Discharged on Antithrombotic Therapy[1,3]	-	-	99%	99%
Discharged on Statin Medication[1,3]	-	-	95%	94%
Thrombolytic Therapy Timing[3,7]	-	-	67%	66%
Venous Thromboembolism Prophylaxis[1,3]	-	-	95%	94%
Written Stroke Educational Materials Given[3,7]	-	-	88%	88%
Surgical Care Improvement Project				
Appropriate Beta Blocker Usage[1]	-	-	98%	98%
Appropriate VTP Within 24 Hours[1]	-	-	98%	98%
Controlled Postoperative Blood Glucose[7]	-	-	97%	97%
Perioperative Temperature Management[1]	-	-	100%	100%
Prophylactic Antibiotic Selection[1]	-	-	99%	99%
Prophylactic Antibiotic Selection (Outpatient)[1,3]	-	-	98%	98%
Prophylactic Antibiotic Stopped[1]	-	-	98%	98%
Prophylactic Antibiotic Timing[1]	-	-	99%	99%
Prophylactic Antibiotic Timing (Outpatient)[1,3]	-	-	98%	98%
Urinary Catheter Removal[1]	-	-	97%	97%
Survey of Patients' Hospital Experiences				
Area Around Room 'Always' Quiet at Night	(a)	60%	61%	61%
Doctors 'Always' Communicated Well	(a)	81%	82%	82%
Home Recovery Information Given	(a)	80%	87%	85%
Hospital Given 9 or 10 on 10 Point Scale	(a)	68%	71%	71%
Meds 'Always' Explained Before Given	(a)	51%	63%	64%
Nurses 'Always' Communicated Well	(a)	78%	79%	79%
Pain 'Always' Well Controlled	(a)	65%	71%	71%
Room and Bathroom 'Always' Clean	(a)	77%	73%	73%
Timely Help 'Always' Received	(a)	66%	68%	68%
Would Definitely Recommend Hospital	(a)	63%	70%	71%
Use of Medical Imaging				
Cardiac Imaging Stress Test before Surgery[1]	-	-	5.2%	5.3%
Combination Abdominal CT Scan	244	21.3%	11.2%	10.5%
Combination Brain/Sinus CT Scan[1]	-	-	3.2%	2.7%
Combination Chest CT Scan	117	8.5%	1.9%	2.7%
Follow-up Mammogram/Ultrasound	384	9.1%	8.6%	8.8%
Lumbar Spine MRI for Low Back Pain[1]	-	-	39.6%	37.2%

Southeast Health Center of Ripley County

109 Plum St
Doniphan, MO 63935
Phone: 573-996-2141
Fax: 573-996-3949
Type: Acute Care Hospitals
Emergency Services: Yes
Ownership: Government - Local
Beds: 30

Key Personnel:
Operating Room. . . . . Phyllis Featherston
CEO/President. . . . . Ray Freeman
Quality Assurance . . . . Jackie Johnson
Emergency Room . . . . Tamy Ryan
Chief of Medical Staff. . . . . Gary Ward

Measure	Cases	This Hosp.	State Avg.	U.S. Avg.
Blood Clot Prevention and Treatment				
Anticoagulation Overlap Therapy[1]	-	-	94%	93%
ICU Venous Thromboembolism Prophylaxis[7]	-	-	91%	92%
Incidence of Potentially Preventable VTE[7]	-	-	7%	10%
UFH with Dosages/Platelet Monitoring[7]	-	-	96%	97%
Venous Thromboembolism Prophylaxis	160	56%	85%	85%
Warfarin Therapy Discharge Instructions[7]	-	-	76%	75%
Chest Pain/Possible Heart Attack Care				
Aspirin Given Within 24 Hours of Arrival	32	91%	95%	96%
Fibrinolytic Meds Within 30 Min. of Arrival[7]	-	-	53%	58%
Average Time to ECG (minutes)	34	6	7	7
Average Time to Transfer (minutes)[1]	-	-	53	60
Children's Asthma Care				
Received Home Management Plan of Care	-	-	-	88%
Received Reliever Medication	-	-	-	100%
Received Systemic Corticosteroids	-	-	-	100%
Emergency Department				
Admittance Decision Time (minutes)[2]	163	85	81	98
Head CT Results Within 45 Min. of Arrival[1,3]	-	-	63%	57%
Patients Who Left ER Before Being Seen	6,202	2%	3%	2%
Time from ER Arrival to Admit. (minutes)[2]	197	222	238	274
Time from ER Arrival to Discharge (minutes)	452	107	136	134
Time in ER Before Being Evaluated (minutes)	709	16	26	26
Time to Pain Meds for Fractures (minutes)	30	52	52	57
Heart Attack Care				
Aspirin Given at Discharge[3,7]	-	-	99%	99%
Fibrinolytic Meds Within 30 Min. of Arrival[3,7]	-	-	-	54%
PCI Within 90 Minutes of Arrival[3,7]	-	-	97%	96%
Statin Prescribed at Discharge[3,7]	-	-	98%	98%
Heart Failure Care				
ACE Inhibitor or ARB for LVSD[1]	-	-	96%	97%
Discharge Instructions Given[1]	-	-	94%	94%
Evaluation of LVS Function[1]	-	-	98%	99%
Medicare Spending				
Medicare Spending per Patient (ratio)	-	1.01	0.95	0.98
Pneumonia Care				
Appropriate Initial Antibiotic Given	38	71%	95%	95%
Blood Culture Timing	49	94%	98%	98%
Pregnancy and Delivery Care				
Newborn Deliveries Scheduled Early[2,7]	-	-	5%	6%
Preventive Care				
Immunization for Influenza[2]	146	95%	92%	90%
Immunization for Pneumonia[2]	194	97%	93%	92%
Stroke Care				
Anticoagulation Therapy for Atrial Fibrillation[5]	-	-	94%	95%
Antithrombotic Therapy Timing[5]	-	-	98%	98%
Assessed for Rehabilitation[5]	-	-	98%	97%
Discharged on Antithrombotic Therapy[5]	-	-	99%	99%
Discharged on Statin Medication[5]	-	-	95%	94%
Thrombolytic Therapy Timing[5]	-	-	67%	66%
Venous Thromboembolism Prophylaxis[5]	-	-	95%	94%
Written Stroke Educational Materials Given[5]	-	-	88%	88%
Surgical Care Improvement Project				
Appropriate Beta Blocker Usage[5]	-	-	98%	98%
Appropriate VTP Within 24 Hours[5]	-	-	98%	98%
Controlled Postoperative Blood Glucose[5]	-	-	97%	97%
Perioperative Temperature Management[5]	-	-	100%	100%
Prophylactic Antibiotic Selection[5]	-	-	99%	99%
Prophylactic Antibiotic Selection (Outpatient)[5]	-	-	98%	98%
Prophylactic Antibiotic Stopped[5]	-	-	98%	98%
Prophylactic Antibiotic Timing[5]	-	-	99%	99%
Prophylactic Antibiotic Timing (Outpatient)[5]	-	-	98%	98%
Urinary Catheter Removal[5]	-	-	97%	97%
Survey of Patients' Hospital Experiences				
Area Around Room 'Always' Quiet at Night[6]	<100	69%	61%	61%
Doctors 'Always' Communicated Well[6]	<100	86%	82%	82%
Home Recovery Information Given[6]	<100	86%	87%	85%
Hospital Given 9 or 10 on 10 Point Scale[6]	<100	66%	71%	71%
Meds 'Always' Explained Before Given[6]	<100	52%	63%	64%
Nurses 'Always' Communicated Well[6]	<100	83%	79%	79%
Pain 'Always' Well Controlled[6]	<100	70%	71%	71%
Room and Bathroom 'Always' Clean[6]	<100	77%	73%	73%
Timely Help 'Always' Received[6]	<100	85%	68%	68%
Would Definitely Recommend Hospital[6]	<100	65%	70%	71%
Use of Medical Imaging				
Cardiac Imaging Stress Test before Surgery[7]	-	-	5.2%	5.3%
Combination Abdominal CT Scan	156	2.6%	11.2%	10.5%
Combination Brain/Sinus CT Scan	125	7.2%	3.2%	2.7%
Combination Chest CT Scan	91	0.0%	1.9%	2.7%
Follow-up Mammogram/Ultrasound[7]	-	-	8.6%	8.8%
Lumbar Spine MRI for Low Back Pain[7]	-	-	39.6%	37.2%

Southeast Health Center of Reynolds County

100 Hwy 21 N
Ellington, MO 63638
Phone: 573-334-4822
Type: Acute Care Hospitals
Emergency Services: Yes
Ownership: Voluntary non-profit - Private

Measure	Cases	This Hosp.	State Avg.	U.S. Avg.
Blood Clot Prevention and Treatment				
Anticoagulation Overlap Therapy[5]	-	-	94%	93%
ICU Venous Thromboembolism Prophylaxis[5]	-	-	91%	92%
Incidence of Potentially Preventable VTE[5]	-	-	7%	10%
UFH with Dosages/Platelet Monitoring[5]	-	-	96%	97%
Venous Thromboembolism Prophylaxis[5]	-	-	85%	85%
Warfarin Therapy Discharge Instructions[5]	-	-	76%	75%
Chest Pain/Possible Heart Attack Care				
Aspirin Given Within 24 Hours of Arrival[5]	-	-	95%	96%
Fibrinolytic Meds Within 30 Min. of Arrival[5]	-	-	53%	58%
Average Time to ECG (minutes)[5]	-	-	7	7
Average Time to Transfer (minutes)[5]	-	-	53	60
Children's Asthma Care				
Received Home Management Plan of Care	-	-	-	88%
Received Reliever Medication	-	-	-	100%
Received Systemic Corticosteroids	-	-	-	100%
Emergency Department				
Admittance Decision Time (minutes)[5]	-	-	81	98
Head CT Results Within 45 Min. of Arrival[5]	-	-	63%	57%
Patients Who Left ER Before Being Seen[5]	-	-	3%	2%
Time from ER Arrival to Admit. (minutes)[5]	-	-	238	274
Time from ER Arrival to Discharge (minutes)[5]	-	-	136	134
Time in ER Before Being Evaluated (minutes)[5]	-	-	26	26
Time to Pain Meds for Fractures (minutes)[5]	-	-	52	57
Heart Attack Care				
Aspirin Given at Discharge[5]	-	-	99%	99%
Fibrinolytic Meds Within 30 Min. of Arrival[5]	-	-	-	54%
PCI Within 90 Minutes of Arrival[5]	-	-	97%	96%
Statin Prescribed at Discharge[5]	-	-	98%	98%
Heart Failure Care				
ACE Inhibitor or ARB for LVSD[3,7]	-	-	96%	97%
Discharge Instructions Given[3,7]	-	-	94%	94%
Evaluation of LVS Function[1,3]	-	-	98%	99%
Medicare Spending				
Medicare Spending per Patient (ratio)	-	-	0.95	0.98
Pneumonia Care				
Appropriate Initial Antibiotic Given[3,7]	-	-	95%	95%
Blood Culture Timing[3,7]	-	-	98%	98%
Pregnancy and Delivery Care				
Newborn Deliveries Scheduled Early[5]	-	-	5%	6%
Preventive Care				
Immunization for Influenza[5]	-	-	92%	90%
Immunization for Pneumonia[5]	-	-	93%	92%
Stroke Care				
Anticoagulation Therapy for Atrial Fibrillation[5]	-	-	94%	95%

NOTE: Hospital profiles are in alphabetical order by state, then city, then hospital within the city; Rankings exclude hospitals with less than 25 cases except for patient surveys which excludes hospitals with less than 100 cases; (a) 100-299 cases; (1) The number of cases/patients is too few to report; (2) Data submitted were based on a sample of cases/patients; (3) Results are based on a shorter time period than required; (4) Data suppressed by CMS for one or more quarters; (5) Results are not available for this reporting period; (6) Fewer than 100 patients completed the HCAHPS survey; (7) No cases met the criteria for this measure; (8) The lower limit of the confidence interval cannot be calculated if the number of observed infections equals zero; (9) No data are available from the state/territory for this reporting period; (10) The scores shown reflect fewer than 50 completed surveys; (11) There were discrepancies in the data collection process; (12) This measure does not apply to this hospital for this reporting period; (13) Results cannot be calculated for this reporting period; (14) The results for this state are combined with nearby states to protect confidentiality; Please refer to the User's Guide for a full explanation of data.

Measure	Cases	This Hosp.	State Avg.	U.S. Avg.
Antithrombotic Therapy Timing[5]	-	-	98%	98%
Assessed for Rehabilitation[5]	-	-	98%	97%
Discharged on Antithrombotic Therapy[5]	-	-	99%	99%
Discharged on Statin Medication[5]	-	-	95%	94%
Thrombolytic Therapy Timing[5]	-	-	67%	66%
Venous Thromboembolism Prophylaxis[5]	-	-	95%	94%
Written Stroke Educational Materials Given[5]	-	-	88%	88%
Surgical Care Improvement Project				
Appropriate Beta Blocker Usage[5]	-	-	98%	98%
Appropriate VTP Within 24 Hours[5]	-	-	98%	98%
Controlled Postoperative Blood Glucose[5]	-	-	97%	97%
Perioperative Temperature Management[5]	-	-	100%	100%
Prophylactic Antibiotic Selection[5]	-	-	99%	99%
Prophylactic Antibiotic Selection (Outpatient)[5]	-	-	98%	98%
Prophylactic Antibiotic Stopped[5]	-	-	98%	98%
Prophylactic Antibiotic Timing[5]	-	-	99%	99%
Prophylactic Antibiotic Timing (Outpatient)[5]	-	-	98%	98%
Urinary Catheter Removal[5]	-	-	97%	97%
Survey of Patients' Hospital Experiences				
Area Around Room 'Always' Quiet at Night[5]	-	-	61%	61%
Doctors 'Always' Communicated Well[5]	-	-	82%	82%
Home Recovery Information Given[5]	-	-	87%	85%
Hospital Given 9 or 10 on 10 Point Scale[5]	-	-	71%	71%
Meds 'Always' Explained Before Given[5]	-	-	63%	64%
Nurses 'Always' Communicated Well[5]	-	-	79%	79%
Pain 'Always' Well Controlled[5]	-	-	71%	71%
Room and Bathroom 'Always' Clean[5]	-	-	73%	73%
Timely Help 'Always' Received[5]	-	-	68%	68%
Would Definitely Recommend Hospital[5]	-	-	70%	71%
Use of Medical Imaging				
Cardiac Imaging Stress Test before Surgery[7]	-	-	5.2%	5.3%
Combination Abdominal CT Scan[7]	-	-	11.2%	10.5%
Combination Brain/Sinus CT Scan[7]	-	-	3.2%	2.7%
Combination Chest CT Scan[7]	-	-	1.9%	2.7%
Follow-up Mammogram/Ultrasound[7]	-	-	8.6%	8.8%
Lumbar Spine MRI for Low Back Pain[7]	-	-	39.6%	37.2%

Community Hospital Association

26136 Us Highway 59, PO Box 107
Fairfax, MO 64446
Phone: 660-686-2111
Fax: 660-686-2618
Type: Critical Access Hospitals
Emergency Services: Yes
Ownership: Voluntary non-profit - Private
Beds: 25

Key Personnel:

- Radiology. . . . . Jack Bridges
- Anesthesiology. . . . . Mary Coleman, CRNA
- Ambulatory Care . . . . Betty Goins, RN
- Operating Room. . . . . Betty Goins, RN
- Chief of Medical Staff. . . . . James Humphrey, MD
- Emergency Room . . . . Teresa Oylear, FNP
- Infection Control. . . . . Linda Winkelman, RN

Measure	Cases	This Hosp.	State Avg.	U.S. Avg.
Blood Clot Prevention and Treatment				
Anticoagulation Overlap Therapy[5]	-	-	94%	93%
ICU Venous Thromboembolism Prophylaxis[5]	-	-	91%	92%
Incidence of Potentially Preventable VTE[5]	-	-	7%	10%
UFH with Dosages/Platelet Monitoring[5]	-	-	96%	97%
Venous Thromboembolism Prophylaxis[5]	-	-	85%	85%
Warfarin Therapy Discharge Instructions[5]	-	-	76%	75%
Chest Pain/Possible Heart Attack Care				
Aspirin Given Within 24 Hours of Arrival[5]	-	-	95%	96%
Fibrinolytic Meds Within 30 Min. of Arrival[5]	-	-	53%	58%
Average Time to ECG (minutes)[5]	-	-	7	7
Average Time to Transfer (minutes)[5]	-	-	53	60
Children's Asthma Care				
Received Home Management Plan of Care	-	-	-	88%
Received Reliever Medication	-	-	-	100%
Received Systemic Corticosteroids	-	-	-	100%
Emergency Department				
Admittance Decision Time (minutes)[5]	-	-	81	98
Head CT Results Within 45 Min. of Arrival[5]	-	-	63%	57%
Patients Who Left ER Before Being Seen[5]	-	-	3%	2%
Time from ER Arrival to Admit. (minutes)[5]	-	-	238	274
Time from ER Arrival to Discharge (minutes)[5]	-	-	136	134
Time in ER Before Being Evaluated (minutes)[5]	-	-	26	26
Time to Pain Meds for Fractures (minutes)[5]	-	-	52	57
Heart Attack Care				
Aspirin Given at Discharge[5]	-	-	99%	99%
Fibrinolytic Meds Within 30 Min. of Arrival[5]	-	-	-	54%
PCI Within 90 Minutes of Arrival[5]	-	-	97%	96%
Statin Prescribed at Discharge[5]	-	-	98%	98%
Heart Failure Care				
ACE Inhibitor or ARB for LVSD[1,3]	-	-	96%	97%
Discharge Instructions Given[1,3]	-	-	94%	94%
Evaluation of LVS Function[1,3]	-	-	98%	99%
Medicare Spending				
Medicare Spending per Patient (ratio)	-	-	0.95	0.98
Pneumonia Care				
Appropriate Initial Antibiotic Given	14	57%	95%	95%
Blood Culture Timing[7]	-	-	98%	98%
Pregnancy and Delivery Care				
Newborn Deliveries Scheduled Early[5]	-	-	5%	6%
Preventive Care				
Immunization for Influenza[5]	-	-	92%	90%
Immunization for Pneumonia[5]	-	-	93%	92%
Stroke Care				
Anticoagulation Therapy for Atrial Fibrillation[5]	-	-	94%	95%
Antithrombotic Therapy Timing[5]	-	-	98%	98%
Assessed for Rehabilitation[5]	-	-	98%	97%
Discharged on Antithrombotic Therapy[5]	-	-	99%	99%
Discharged on Statin Medication[5]	-	-	95%	94%
Thrombolytic Therapy Timing[5]	-	-	67%	66%
Venous Thromboembolism Prophylaxis[5]	-	-	95%	94%
Written Stroke Educational Materials Given[5]	-	-	88%	88%
Surgical Care Improvement Project				
Appropriate Beta Blocker Usage[5]	-	-	98%	98%
Appropriate VTP Within 24 Hours[5]	-	-	98%	98%
Controlled Postoperative Blood Glucose[5]	-	-	97%	97%
Perioperative Temperature Management[5]	-	-	100%	100%
Prophylactic Antibiotic Selection[5]	-	-	99%	99%
Prophylactic Antibiotic Selection (Outpatient)[5]	-	-	98%	98%
Prophylactic Antibiotic Stopped[5]	-	-	98%	98%
Prophylactic Antibiotic Timing[5]	-	-	99%	99%
Prophylactic Antibiotic Timing (Outpatient)[5]	-	-	98%	98%
Urinary Catheter Removal[5]	-	-	97%	97%
Survey of Patients' Hospital Experiences				
Area Around Room 'Always' Quiet at Night	(a)	66%	61%	61%
Doctors 'Always' Communicated Well	(a)	86%	82%	82%
Home Recovery Information Given	(a)	79%	87%	85%
Hospital Given 9 or 10 on 10 Point Scale	(a)	70%	71%	71%
Meds 'Always' Explained Before Given	(a)	70%	63%	64%
Nurses 'Always' Communicated Well	(a)	81%	79%	79%
Pain 'Always' Well Controlled	(a)	68%	71%	71%
Room and Bathroom 'Always' Clean	(a)	87%	73%	73%
Timely Help 'Always' Received	(a)	81%	68%	68%
Would Definitely Recommend Hospital	(a)	74%	70%	71%
Use of Medical Imaging				
Cardiac Imaging Stress Test before Surgery[1]	-	-	5.2%	5.3%
Combination Abdominal CT Scan	120	9.2%	11.2%	10.5%
Combination Brain/Sinus CT Scan[1]	-	-	3.2%	2.7%
Combination Chest CT Scan	58	3.4%	1.9%	2.7%
Follow-up Mammogram/Ultrasound	172	11.0%	8.6%	8.8%
Lumbar Spine MRI for Low Back Pain[1]	-	-	39.6%	37.2%

Mineral Area Regional Medical Center

1212 Weber Rd
Farmington, MO 63640
Phone: 573-756-4581
Fax: 573-756-5834
URL: www.marmc.org
Type: Acute Care Hospitals
Emergency Services: Yes
Ownership: Proprietary
Beds: 141

Key Personnel:

- CEO/President. . . . . Stephen L Crain
- Chair/CEO . . . . Gil Kennon
- Infection Control. . . . . Jack Marler
- CEO . . . . Lynn Mergen
- Emergency Room . . . . Beth Skaggs
- Quality Assurance . . . . LaDonna Smith
- Operating Room. . . . . John Spurgin
- Chief of Medical Staff. . . . . Henry Steele

Measure	Cases	This Hosp.	State Avg.	U.S. Avg.
Blood Clot Prevention and Treatment				
Anticoagulation Overlap Therapy[1,2]	-	-	94%	93%
ICU Venous Thromboembolism Prophylaxis[2]	43	91%	91%	92%
Incidence of Potentially Preventable VTE[1,2]	-	-	7%	10%
UFH with Dosages/Platelet Monitoring[1,2]	-	-	96%	97%
Venous Thromboembolism Prophylaxis[2]	154	92%	85%	85%
Warfarin Therapy Discharge Instructions[1,2]	-	-	76%	75%
Chest Pain/Possible Heart Attack Care				
Aspirin Given Within 24 Hours of Arrival	60	100%	95%	96%
Fibrinolytic Meds Within 30 Min. of Arrival[1]	-	-	53%	58%
Average Time to ECG (minutes)	61	5	7	7
Average Time to Transfer (minutes)	16	44	53	60
Children's Asthma Care				
Received Home Management Plan of Care	-	-	-	88%
Received Reliever Medication	-	-	-	100%
Received Systemic Corticosteroids	-	-	-	100%
Emergency Department				
Admittance Decision Time (minutes)[2]	380	101	81	98
Head CT Results Within 45 Min. of Arrival[1]	-	-	63%	57%
Patients Who Left ER Before Being Seen	18,793	0%	3%	2%
Time from ER Arrival to Admit. (minutes)[2]	380	253	238	274
Time from ER Arrival to Discharge (minutes)	385	108	136	134
Time in ER Before Being Evaluated (minutes)	433	18	26	26
Time to Pain Meds for Fractures (minutes)	52	49	52	57
Heart Attack Care				
Aspirin Given at Discharge[7]	-	-	99%	99%
Fibrinolytic Meds Within 30 Min. of Arrival[7]	-	-	-	54%
PCI Within 90 Minutes of Arrival[7]	-	-	97%	96%
Statin Prescribed at Discharge[7]	-	-	98%	98%
Heart Failure Care				
ACE Inhibitor or ARB for LVSD[1]	-	-	96%	97%
Discharge Instructions Given	29	86%	94%	94%
Evaluation of LVS Function	49	98%	98%	99%
Medicare Spending				
Medicare Spending per Patient (ratio)	-	0.91	0.95	0.98
Pneumonia Care				
Appropriate Initial Antibiotic Given	55	96%	95%	95%
Blood Culture Timing	104	99%	98%	98%
Pregnancy and Delivery Care				
Newborn Deliveries Scheduled Early[2]	28	7%	5%	6%
Preventive Care				
Immunization for Influenza[2]	452	97%	92%	90%
Immunization for Pneumonia[2]	351	98%	93%	92%
Stroke Care				
Anticoagulation Therapy for Atrial Fibrillation[1]	-	-	94%	95%
Antithrombotic Therapy Timing[1]	-	-	98%	98%
Assessed for Rehabilitation[1]	-	-	98%	97%
Discharged on Antithrombotic Therapy[1]	-	-	99%	99%
Discharged on Statin Medication[1]	-	-	95%	94%
Thrombolytic Therapy Timing[7]	-	-	67%	66%
Venous Thromboembolism Prophylaxis[1]	-	-	95%	94%
Written Stroke Educational Materials Given[1]	-	-	88%	88%
Surgical Care Improvement Project				
Appropriate Beta Blocker Usage	38	82%	98%	98%
Appropriate VTP Within 24 Hours	107	100%	98%	98%
Controlled Postoperative Blood Glucose[7]	-	-	97%	97%
Perioperative Temperature Management	119	100%	100%	100%
Prophylactic Antibiotic Selection	81	98%	99%	99%
Prophylactic Antibiotic Selection (Outpatient)	26	96%	98%	98%
Prophylactic Antibiotic Stopped	79	94%	98%	98%
Prophylactic Antibiotic Timing	81	99%	99%	99%
Prophylactic Antibiotic Timing (Outpatient)	26	100%	98%	98%
Urinary Catheter Removal	89	98%	97%	97%
Survey of Patients' Hospital Experiences				
Area Around Room 'Always' Quiet at Night	300+	58%	61%	61%
Doctors 'Always' Communicated Well	300+	79%	82%	82%
Home Recovery Information Given	300+	83%	87%	85%
Hospital Given 9 or 10 on 10 Point Scale	300+	63%	71%	71%
Meds 'Always' Explained Before Given	300+	60%	63%	64%
Nurses 'Always' Communicated Well	300+	74%	79%	79%
Pain 'Always' Well Controlled	300+	67%	71%	71%

NOTE: Hospital profiles are in alphabetical order by state, then city, then hospital within the city; Rankings exclude hospitals with less than 25 cases except for patient surveys which excludes hospitals with less than 100 cases; (a) 100-299 cases; (1) The number of cases/patients is too few to report; (2) Data submitted were based on a sample of cases/patients; (3) Results are based on a shorter time period than required; (4) Data suppressed by CMS for one or more quarters; (5) Results are not available for this reporting period; (6) Fewer than 100 patients completed the HCAHPS survey; (7) No cases met the criteria for this measure; (8) The lower limit of the confidence interval cannot be calculated if the number of observed infections equals zero; (9) No data are available from the state/territory for this reporting period; (10) The scores shown reflect fewer than 50 completed surveys; (11) There were discrepancies in the data collection process; (12) This measure does not apply to this hospital for this reporting period; (13) Results cannot be calculated for this reporting period; (14) The results for this state are combined with nearby states to protect confidentiality; Please refer to the User's Guide for a full explanation of data.

Measure	Cases	This Hosp.	State Avg.	U.S. Avg.
Room and Bathroom 'Always' Clean	300+	68%	73%	73%
Timely Help 'Always' Received	300+	61%	68%	68%
Would Definitely Recommend Hospital	300+	64%	70%	71%
Use of Medical Imaging				
Cardiac Imaging Stress Test before Surgery	100	10.0%	5.2%	5.3%
Combination Abdominal CT Scan	327	12.2%	11.2%	10.5%
Combination Brain/Sinus CT Scan	363	1.7%	3.2%	2.7%
Combination Chest CT Scan	126	7.9%	1.9%	2.7%
Follow-up Mammogram/Ultrasound	546	6.0%	8.6%	8.8%
Lumbar Spine MRI for Low Back Pain	81	30.9%	39.6%	37.2%

Parkland Health Center

1101 W Liberty
Farmington, MO 63640
E-mail: ssg.2352@bjc.org
URL: www.bjc.org
Phone: 573-431-6005
Fax: 573-760-8171
Type: Acute Care Hospitals
Emergency Services: Yes
Ownership: Voluntary non-profit - Private
Beds: 130

Key Personnel:

Intensive Care Unit. . . . . Patty Coleman
CEO/President. . . . . Richard Conklin
Quality Assurance . . . . Carol Coulter
Emergency Room . . . . Dana Day
Chief of Medical Staff. . . . . Gary Grix

Measure	Cases	This Hosp.	State Avg.	U.S. Avg.
Blood Clot Prevention and Treatment				
Anticoagulation Overlap Therapy[2]	14	93%	94%	93%
ICU Venous Thromboembolism Prophylaxis[2]	50	84%	91%	92%
Incidence of Potentially Preventable VTE[1,2]	-	-	7%	10%
UFH with Dosages/Platelet Monitoring[1,2]	-	-	96%	97%
Venous Thromboembolism Prophylaxis[2]	246	87%	85%	85%
Warfarin Therapy Discharge Instructions[1,2]	-	-	76%	75%
Chest Pain/Possible Heart Attack Care				
Aspirin Given Within 24 Hours of Arrival	219	97%	95%	96%
Fibrinolytic Meds Within 30 Min. of Arrival[7]	-	-	53%	58%
Average Time to ECG (minutes)	232	3	7	7
Average Time to Transfer (minutes)	16	43	53	60
Children's Asthma Care				
Received Home Management Plan of Care	-	-	-	88%
Received Reliever Medication	-	-	-	100%
Received Systemic Corticosteroids	-	-	-	100%
Emergency Department				
Admittance Decision Time (minutes)[2]	332	65	81	98
Head CT Results Within 45 Min. of Arrival	15	53%	63%	57%
Patients Who Left ER Before Being Seen	26,144	3%	3%	2%
Time from ER Arrival to Admit. (minutes)[2]	361	248	238	274
Time from ER Arrival to Discharge (minutes)	728	130	136	134
Time in ER Before Being Evaluated (minutes)	740	46	26	26
Time to Pain Meds for Fractures (minutes)	95	62	52	57
Heart Attack Care				
Aspirin Given at Discharge	11	100%	99%	99%
Fibrinolytic Meds Within 30 Min. of Arrival[7]	-	-	-	54%
PCI Within 90 Minutes of Arrival[7]	-	-	97%	96%
Statin Prescribed at Discharge[1]	-	-	98%	98%
Heart Failure Care				
ACE Inhibitor or ARB for LVSD	33	82%	96%	97%
Discharge Instructions Given	92	89%	94%	94%
Evaluation of LVS Function	134	100%	98%	99%
Medicare Spending				
Medicare Spending per Patient (ratio)	-	0.90	0.95	0.98
Pneumonia Care				
Appropriate Initial Antibiotic Given[2]	107	94%	95%	95%
Blood Culture Timing[2]	182	100%	98%	98%
Pregnancy and Delivery Care				
Newborn Deliveries Scheduled Early[2]	26	23%	5%	6%
Preventive Care				
Immunization for Influenza[2]	331	94%	92%	90%
Immunization for Pneumonia[2]	439	91%	93%	92%
Stroke Care				
Anticoagulation Therapy for Atrial Fibrillation[1]	-	-	94%	95%
Antithrombotic Therapy Timing[1]	-	-	98%	98%
Assessed for Rehabilitation	12	92%	98%	97%
Discharged on Antithrombotic Therapy	12	100%	99%	99%
Discharged on Statin Medication[1]	-	-	95%	94%
Thrombolytic Therapy Timing[1]	-	-	67%	66%
Venous Thromboembolism Prophylaxis	12	100%	95%	94%
Written Stroke Educational Materials Given[1]	-	-	88%	88%
Surgical Care Improvement Project				
Appropriate Beta Blocker Usage	20	85%	98%	98%
Appropriate VTP Within 24 Hours	66	100%	98%	98%
Controlled Postoperative Blood Glucose[7]	-	-	97%	97%
Perioperative Temperature Management	74	99%	100%	100%
Prophylactic Antibiotic Selection	65	98%	99%	99%
Prophylactic Antibiotic Selection (Outpatient)	60	97%	98%	98%
Prophylactic Antibiotic Stopped	61	93%	98%	98%
Prophylactic Antibiotic Timing	65	95%	99%	99%
Prophylactic Antibiotic Timing (Outpatient)	60	97%	98%	98%
Urinary Catheter Removal	55	95%	97%	97%
Survey of Patients' Hospital Experiences				
Area Around Room 'Always' Quiet at Night	300+	55%	61%	61%
Doctors 'Always' Communicated Well	300+	88%	82%	82%
Home Recovery Information Given	300+	88%	87%	85%
Hospital Given 9 or 10 on 10 Point Scale	300+	79%	71%	71%
Meds 'Always' Explained Before Given	300+	67%	63%	64%
Nurses 'Always' Communicated Well	300+	84%	79%	79%
Pain 'Always' Well Controlled	300+	74%	71%	71%
Room and Bathroom 'Always' Clean	300+	71%	73%	73%
Timely Help 'Always' Received	300+	69%	68%	68%
Would Definitely Recommend Hospital	300+	78%	70%	71%
Use of Medical Imaging				
Cardiac Imaging Stress Test before Surgery	320	6.9%	5.2%	5.3%
Combination Abdominal CT Scan	991	1.3%	11.2%	10.5%
Combination Brain/Sinus CT Scan	765	4.1%	3.2%	2.7%
Combination Chest CT Scan	513	1.2%	1.9%	2.7%
Follow-up Mammogram/Ultrasound	1,392	5.8%	8.6%	8.8%
Lumbar Spine MRI for Low Back Pain	136	37.5%	39.6%	37.2%

SSM Saint Clare Health Center

1015 Bowles
Fenton, MO 63026
URL: www.ssmstclare.com
Phone: 636-496-2000
Type: Acute Care Hospitals
Emergency Services: Yes
Ownership: Voluntary non-profit - Private
Beds: 180

Key Personnel:

Chair/CEO . . . . Christopher Howard

Measure	Cases	This Hosp.	State Avg.	U.S. Avg.
Blood Clot Prevention and Treatment				
Anticoagulation Overlap Therapy[2]	63	95%	94%	93%
ICU Venous Thromboembolism Prophylaxis[2]	78	94%	91%	92%
Incidence of Potentially Preventable VTE[1,2]	-	-	7%	10%
UFH with Dosages/Platelet Monitoring[2]	34	76%	96%	97%
Venous Thromboembolism Prophylaxis[2]	297	85%	85%	85%
Warfarin Therapy Discharge Instructions[2]	53	47%	76%	75%
Chest Pain/Possible Heart Attack Care				
Aspirin Given Within 24 Hours of Arrival[1,3]	-	-	95%	96%
Fibrinolytic Meds Within 30 Min. of Arrival[5]	-	-	53%	58%
Average Time to ECG (minutes)[1,3]	-	-	7	7
Average Time to Transfer (minutes)[5]	-	-	53	60
Children's Asthma Care				
Received Home Management Plan of Care	-	-	-	88%
Received Reliever Medication	-	-	-	100%
Received Systemic Corticosteroids	-	-	-	100%
Emergency Department				
Admittance Decision Time (minutes)[2]	486	166	81	98
Head CT Results Within 45 Min. of Arrival[1]	-	-	63%	57%
Patients Who Left ER Before Being Seen	43,462	1%	3%	2%
Time from ER Arrival to Admit. (minutes)[2]	530	276	238	274
Time from ER Arrival to Discharge (minutes)	365	187	136	134
Time in ER Before Being Evaluated (minutes)	407	45	26	26
Time to Pain Meds for Fractures (minutes)	70	39	52	57
Heart Attack Care				
Aspirin Given at Discharge	307	100%	99%	99%
Fibrinolytic Meds Within 30 Min. of Arrival[7]	-	-	-	54%
PCI Within 90 Minutes of Arrival	62	100%	97%	96%
Statin Prescribed at Discharge	299	100%	98%	98%
Heart Failure Care				
ACE Inhibitor or ARB for LVSD[2]	58	100%	96%	97%
Discharge Instructions Given[2]	199	99%	94%	94%
Evaluation of LVS Function[2]	240	100%	98%	99%
Medicare Spending				
Medicare Spending per Patient (ratio)	-	0.97	0.95	0.98
Pneumonia Care				
Appropriate Initial Antibiotic Given[2]	93	99%	95%	95%
Blood Culture Timing[2]	129	98%	98%	98%
Pregnancy and Delivery Care				
Newborn Deliveries Scheduled Early[2]	30	7%	5%	6%
Preventive Care				
Immunization for Influenza[2]	576	98%	92%	90%
Immunization for Pneumonia[2]	702	97%	93%	92%
Stroke Care				
Anticoagulation Therapy for Atrial Fibrillation	34	88%	94%	95%
Antithrombotic Therapy Timing	156	98%	98%	98%
Assessed for Rehabilitation	203	100%	98%	97%
Discharged on Antithrombotic Therapy	182	100%	99%	99%
Discharged on Statin Medication	128	96%	95%	94%
Thrombolytic Therapy Timing	23	96%	67%	66%
Venous Thromboembolism Prophylaxis	204	98%	95%	94%
Written Stroke Educational Materials Given	103	98%	88%	88%
Surgical Care Improvement Project				
Appropriate Beta Blocker Usage[2]	186	99%	98%	98%
Appropriate VTP Within 24 Hours[2]	366	98%	98%	98%
Controlled Postoperative Blood Glucose[2]	112	97%	97%	97%
Perioperative Temperature Management[2]	462	100%	100%	100%
Prophylactic Antibiotic Selection[2]	356	100%	99%	99%
Prophylactic Antibiotic Selection (Outpatient)	422	99%	98%	98%
Prophylactic Antibiotic Stopped[2]	344	99%	98%	98%
Prophylactic Antibiotic Timing[2]	358	99%	99%	99%
Prophylactic Antibiotic Timing (Outpatient)	422	99%	98%	98%
Urinary Catheter Removal[2]	287	99%	97%	97%
Survey of Patients' Hospital Experiences				
Area Around Room 'Always' Quiet at Night[11]	300+	74%	61%	61%
Doctors 'Always' Communicated Well[11]	300+	79%	82%	82%
Home Recovery Information Given[11]	300+	84%	87%	85%
Hospital Given 9 or 10 on 10 Point Scale[11]	300+	81%	71%	71%
Meds 'Always' Explained Before Given[11]	300+	63%	63%	64%
Nurses 'Always' Communicated Well[11]	300+	79%	79%	79%
Pain 'Always' Well Controlled[11]	300+	72%	71%	71%
Room and Bathroom 'Always' Clean[11]	300+	71%	73%	73%
Timely Help 'Always' Received[11]	300+	66%	68%	68%
Would Definitely Recommend Hospital[11]	300+	85%	70%	71%
Use of Medical Imaging				
Cardiac Imaging Stress Test before Surgery	334	9.6%	5.2%	5.3%
Combination Abdominal CT Scan	700	16.4%	11.2%	10.5%
Combination Brain/Sinus CT Scan	730	3.4%	3.2%	2.7%
Combination Chest CT Scan	469	1.5%	1.9%	2.7%
Follow-up Mammogram/Ultrasound	1,014	10.2%	8.6%	8.8%
Lumbar Spine MRI for Low Back Pain	185	28.6%	39.6%	37.2%

Callaway Community Hospital

10 South Hospital Drive
Fulton, MO 65251
URL: www.cchfulton.com
Phone: 573-642-3376
Fax: 573-592-6679
Type: Acute Care Hospitals
Emergency Services: Yes
Ownership: Proprietary
Beds: 53

Key Personnel:

Quality Assurance . . . . Simone Camp
CEO/President. . . . . John T Graves
Infection Control. . . . . Terri Herold
Radiology. . . . . Alan Hillard
Intensive Care Unit. . . . . Martin Parks, RN
Operating Room. . . . . Dilip Parulekar, RN
Emergency Room . . . . Riley Selby
Chief of Medical Staff. . . . . Michael Wilson, MD

Measure	Cases	This Hosp.	State Avg.	U.S. Avg.
Blood Clot Prevention and Treatment				
Anticoagulation Overlap Therapy[1,2]	-	-	94%	93%
ICU Venous Thromboembolism Prophylaxis[2,7]	-	-	91%	92%
Incidence of Potentially Preventable VTE[2,7]	-	-	7%	10%
UFH with Dosages/Platelet Monitoring[2,7]	-	-	96%	97%
Venous Thromboembolism Prophylaxis[2]	124	73%	85%	85%
Warfarin Therapy Discharge Instructions[1,2]	-	-	76%	75%

NOTE: Hospital profiles are in alphabetical order by state, then city, then hospital within the city; Rankings exclude hospitals with less than 25 cases except for patient surveys which excludes hospitals with less than 100 cases; (a) 100-299 cases; (1) The number of cases/patients is too few to report; (2) Data submitted were based on a sample of cases/patients; (3) Results are based on a shorter time period than required; (4) Data suppressed by CMS for one or more quarters; (5) Results are not available for this reporting period; (6) Fewer than 100 patients completed the HCAHPS survey; (7) No cases met the criteria for this measure; (8) The lower limit of the confidence interval cannot be calculated if the number of observed infections equals zero; (9) No data are available from the state/territory for this reporting period; (10) The scores shown reflect fewer than 50 completed surveys; (11) There were discrepancies in the data collection process; (12) This measure does not apply to this hospital for this reporting period; (13) Results cannot be calculated for this reporting period; (14) The results for this state are combined with nearby states to protect confidentiality; Please refer to the User's Guide for a full explanation of data.

Measure	Cases	This Hosp.	State Avg.	U.S. Avg.
Chest Pain/Possible Heart Attack Care				
Aspirin Given Within 24 Hours of Arrival	25	96%	95%	96%
Fibrinolytic Meds Within 30 Min. of Arrival[3,7]	-	-	53%	58%
Average Time to ECG (minutes)	26	10	7	7
Average Time to Transfer (minutes)[1,3]	-	-	53	60
Children's Asthma Care				
Received Home Management Plan of Care	-	-	-	88%
Received Reliever Medication	-	-	-	100%
Received Systemic Corticosteroids	-	-	-	100%
Emergency Department				
Admittance Decision Time (minutes)	215	60	81	98
Head CT Results Within 45 Min. of Arrival[1]	-	-	63%	57%
Patients Who Left ER Before Being Seen	10,380	1%	3%	2%
Time from ER Arrival to Admit. (minutes)	222	204	238	274
Time from ER Arrival to Discharge (minutes)	435	88	136	134
Time in ER Before Being Evaluated (minutes)	451	23	26	26
Time to Pain Meds for Fractures (minutes)	45	39	52	57
Heart Attack Care				
Aspirin Given at Discharge[1,3]	-	-	99%	99%
Fibrinolytic Meds Within 30 Min. of Arrival[3,7]	-	-	-	54%
PCI Within 90 Minutes of Arrival[3,7]	-	-	97%	96%
Statin Prescribed at Discharge[1,3]	-	-	98%	98%
Heart Failure Care				
ACE Inhibitor or ARB for LVSD[1]	-	-	96%	97%
Discharge Instructions Given[1]	-	-	94%	94%
Evaluation of LVS Function	12	83%	98%	99%
Medicare Spending				
Medicare Spending per Patient (ratio)	-	0.87	0.95	0.98
Pneumonia Care				
Appropriate Initial Antibiotic Given	19	84%	95%	95%
Blood Culture Timing	19	95%	98%	98%
Pregnancy and Delivery Care				
Newborn Deliveries Scheduled Early[7]	-	-	5%	6%
Preventive Care				
Immunization for Influenza	159	84%	92%	90%
Immunization for Pneumonia	236	78%	93%	92%
Stroke Care				
Anticoagulation Therapy for Atrial Fibrillation[5]	-	-	94%	95%
Antithrombotic Therapy Timing[5]	-	-	98%	98%
Assessed for Rehabilitation[5]	-	-	98%	97%
Discharged on Antithrombotic Therapy[5]	-	-	99%	99%
Discharged on Statin Medication[5]	-	-	95%	94%
Thrombolytic Therapy Timing[5]	-	-	67%	66%
Venous Thromboembolism Prophylaxis[5]	-	-	95%	94%
Written Stroke Educational Materials Given[5]	-	-	88%	88%
Surgical Care Improvement Project				
Appropriate Beta Blocker Usage[5]	-	-	98%	98%
Appropriate VTP Within 24 Hours[5]	-	-	98%	98%
Controlled Postoperative Blood Glucose[5]	-	-	97%	97%
Perioperative Temperature Management[5]	-	-	100%	100%
Prophylactic Antibiotic Selection[5]	-	-	99%	99%
Prophylactic Antibiotic Selection (Outpatient)[5]	-	-	98%	98%
Prophylactic Antibiotic Stopped[5]	-	-	98%	98%
Prophylactic Antibiotic Timing[5]	-	-	99%	99%
Prophylactic Antibiotic Timing (Outpatient)[5]	-	-	98%	98%
Urinary Catheter Removal[5]	-	-	97%	97%
Survey of Patients' Hospital Experiences				
Area Around Room 'Always' Quiet at Night[10]	<100	63%	61%	61%
Doctors 'Always' Communicated Well[10]	<100	78%	82%	82%
Home Recovery Information Given[10]	<100	83%	87%	85%
Hospital Given 9 or 10 on 10 Point Scale[10]	<100	53%	71%	71%
Meds 'Always' Explained Before Given[10]	<100	59%	63%	64%
Nurses 'Always' Communicated Well[10]	<100	74%	79%	79%
Pain 'Always' Well Controlled[10]	<100	74%	71%	71%
Room and Bathroom 'Always' Clean[10]	<100	53%	73%	73%
Timely Help 'Always' Received[10]	<100	82%	68%	68%
Would Definitely Recommend Hospital[10]	<100	43%	70%	71%
Use of Medical Imaging				
Cardiac Imaging Stress Test before Surgery[1]	-	-	5.2%	5.3%
Combination Abdominal CT Scan	127	55.1%	11.2%	10.5%
Combination Brain/Sinus CT Scan[1]	-	-	3.2%	2.7%
Combination Chest CT Scan	70	2.9%	1.9%	2.7%
Follow-up Mammogram/Ultrasound	200	14.5%	8.6%	8.8%
Lumbar Spine MRI for Low Back Pain[1]	-	-	39.6%	37.2%

Hannibal Regional Hospital

6000 Hospital Dr
Hannibal, MO 63401
Phone: 573-248-1300
Fax: 573-248-5264
E-mail: webmaster@hrhonline.org
URL: www.hrhonline.org
Type: Acute Care Hospitals
Emergency Services: Yes
Ownership: Voluntary non-profit - Private
Beds: 105

Key Personnel:

Chief of Medical Staff.......... Sebastian Baginski, MD
Operating Room.............. Michael Bukstei, RN
Radiology..................... Raman Danrad, MD
Infection Control.............. Leanna Darnold
CEO/President................ John C Grossmeier
Quality Assurance .... David Hevel
Pediatric Ambulatory Care ...... Patrick Hirner, MD
Coronary Care................ Laura Miller, RN

Measure	Cases	This Hosp.	State Avg.	U.S. Avg.
Blood Clot Prevention and Treatment				
Anticoagulation Overlap Therapy[2]	42	74%	94%	93%
ICU Venous Thromboembolism Prophylaxis[2]	88	72%	91%	92%
Incidence of Potentially Preventable VTE[2]	11	27%	7%	10%
UFH with Dosages/Platelet Monitoring[2]	17	100%	96%	97%
Venous Thromboembolism Prophylaxis[2]	326	67%	85%	85%
Warfarin Therapy Discharge Instructions[2]	29	62%	76%	75%
Chest Pain/Possible Heart Attack Care				
Aspirin Given Within 24 Hours of Arrival[1]	-	-	95%	96%
Fibrinolytic Meds Within 30 Min. of Arrival[3,7]	-	-	53%	58%
Average Time to ECG (minutes)[1]	-	-	7	7
Average Time to Transfer (minutes)[3,7]	-	-	53	60
Children's Asthma Care				
Received Home Management Plan of Care	-	-	-	88%
Received Reliever Medication	-	-	-	100%
Received Systemic Corticosteroids	-	-	-	100%
Emergency Department				
Admittance Decision Time (minutes)[2]	427	71	81	98
Head CT Results Within 45 Min. of Arrival	19	42%	63%	57%
Patients Who Left ER Before Being Seen	19,937	2%	3%	2%
Time from ER Arrival to Admit. (minutes)[2]	445	288	238	274
Time from ER Arrival to Discharge (minutes)	1,837	190	136	134
Time in ER Before Being Evaluated (minutes)	1,129	40	26	26
Time to Pain Meds for Fractures (minutes)	106	72	52	57
Heart Attack Care				
Aspirin Given at Discharge	80	99%	99%	99%
Fibrinolytic Meds Within 30 Min. of Arrival[7]	-	-	-	54%
PCI Within 90 Minutes of Arrival	30	87%	97%	96%
Statin Prescribed at Discharge	78	97%	98%	98%
Heart Failure Care				
ACE Inhibitor or ARB for LVSD	52	96%	96%	97%
Discharge Instructions Given	118	67%	94%	94%
Evaluation of LVS Function	167	96%	98%	99%
Medicare Spending				
Medicare Spending per Patient (ratio)	-	0.93	0.95	0.98
Pneumonia Care				
Appropriate Initial Antibiotic Given	115	90%	95%	95%
Blood Culture Timing	155	96%	98%	98%
Pregnancy and Delivery Care				
Newborn Deliveries Scheduled Early[2]	33	3%	5%	6%
Preventive Care				
Immunization for Influenza[2]	484	86%	92%	90%
Immunization for Pneumonia[2]	640	85%	93%	92%
Stroke Care				
Anticoagulation Therapy for Atrial Fibrillation[1]	-	-	94%	95%
Antithrombotic Therapy Timing	31	97%	98%	98%
Assessed for Rehabilitation	33	97%	98%	97%
Discharged on Antithrombotic Therapy	32	100%	99%	99%
Discharged on Statin Medication	27	81%	95%	94%
Thrombolytic Therapy Timing[1]	-	-	67%	66%
Venous Thromboembolism Prophylaxis	33	67%	95%	94%
Written Stroke Educational Materials Given	19	63%	88%	88%
Surgical Care Improvement Project				
Appropriate Beta Blocker Usage	222	93%	98%	98%
Appropriate VTP Within 24 Hours	443	93%	98%	98%
Controlled Postoperative Blood Glucose[7]	-	-	97%	97%
Perioperative Temperature Management	596	100%	100%	100%
Prophylactic Antibiotic Selection	470	99%	99%	99%
Prophylactic Antibiotic Selection (Outpatient)	98	98%	98%	98%
Prophylactic Antibiotic Stopped	461	97%	98%	98%
Prophylactic Antibiotic Timing	470	98%	99%	99%
Prophylactic Antibiotic Timing (Outpatient)	101	95%	98%	98%
Urinary Catheter Removal	135	90%	97%	97%
Survey of Patients' Hospital Experiences				
Area Around Room 'Always' Quiet at Night	300+	55%	61%	61%
Doctors 'Always' Communicated Well	300+	83%	82%	82%
Home Recovery Information Given	300+	87%	87%	85%
Hospital Given 9 or 10 on 10 Point Scale	300+	76%	71%	71%
Meds 'Always' Explained Before Given	300+	66%	63%	64%
Nurses 'Always' Communicated Well	300+	84%	79%	79%
Pain 'Always' Well Controlled	300+	74%	71%	71%
Room and Bathroom 'Always' Clean	300+	77%	73%	73%
Timely Help 'Always' Received	300+	72%	68%	68%
Would Definitely Recommend Hospital	300+	70%	70%	71%
Use of Medical Imaging				
Cardiac Imaging Stress Test before Surgery	125	3.2%	5.2%	5.3%
Combination Abdominal CT Scan	411	20.7%	11.2%	10.5%
Combination Brain/Sinus CT Scan	505	4.6%	3.2%	2.7%
Combination Chest CT Scan	98	9.2%	1.9%	2.7%
Follow-up Mammogram/Ultrasound	197	12.2%	8.6%	8.8%
Lumbar Spine MRI for Low Back Pain	73	39.7%	39.6%	37.2%

Cass Regional Medical Center

2800 E Rock Haven Road
Harrisonville, MO 64701
Phone: 816-380-5888
Fax: 816-380-4639
URL: www.cassregional.org
Type: Critical Access Hospitals
Emergency Services: Yes
Ownership: Government - Local
Beds: 49

Key Personnel:

Radiology.................. Ellen Clements, ARRT
Operating Room............. Linda Dawson, RN
Infection Control............ Melinda Flanner
CEO/President............... Chris Lang
Chief of Medical Staff......... Christopher D Maxwell
Quality Assurance .... Kendra McClellan, RN BSN
Intensive Care Unit........... Jill Slade, RN CCRN
Emergency Room .... Violet Warren

Measure	Cases	This Hosp.	State Avg.	U.S. Avg.
Blood Clot Prevention and Treatment				
Anticoagulation Overlap Therapy[5]	-	-	94%	93%
ICU Venous Thromboembolism Prophylaxis[5]	-	-	91%	92%
Incidence of Potentially Preventable VTE[5]	-	-	7%	10%
UFH with Dosages/Platelet Monitoring[5]	-	-	96%	97%
Venous Thromboembolism Prophylaxis[5]	-	-	85%	85%
Warfarin Therapy Discharge Instructions[5]	-	-	76%	75%
Chest Pain/Possible Heart Attack Care				
Aspirin Given Within 24 Hours of Arrival	-	-	95%	96%
Fibrinolytic Meds Within 30 Min. of Arrival	-	-	53%	58%
Average Time to ECG (minutes)	-	-	7	7
Average Time to Transfer (minutes)	-	-	53	60
Children's Asthma Care				
Received Home Management Plan of Care	-	-	-	88%
Received Reliever Medication	-	-	-	100%
Received Systemic Corticosteroids	-	-	-	100%
Emergency Department				
Admittance Decision Time (minutes)[5]	-	-	81	98
Head CT Results Within 45 Min. of Arrival	-	-	63%	57%
Patients Who Left ER Before Being Seen	-	-	3%	2%
Time from ER Arrival to Admit. (minutes)[5]	-	-	238	274
Time from ER Arrival to Discharge (minutes)	-	-	136	134
Time in ER Before Being Evaluated (minutes)	-	-	26	26
Time to Pain Meds for Fractures (minutes)	-	-	52	57
Heart Attack Care				
Aspirin Given at Discharge[5]	-	-	99%	99%
Fibrinolytic Meds Within 30 Min. of Arrival[5]	-	-	-	54%
PCI Within 90 Minutes of Arrival[5]	-	-	97%	96%
Statin Prescribed at Discharge[5]	-	-	98%	98%
Heart Failure Care				

NOTE: Hospital profiles are in alphabetical order by state, then city, then hospital within the city; Rankings exclude hospitals with less than 25 cases except for patient surveys which excludes hospitals with less than 100 cases; (a) 100-299 cases; (1) The number of cases/patients is too few to report; (2) Data submitted were based on a sample of cases/patients; (3) Results are based on a shorter time period than required; (4) Data suppressed by CMS for one or more quarters; (5) Results are not available for this reporting period; (6) Fewer than 100 patients completed the HCAHPS survey; (7) No cases met the criteria for this measure; (8) The lower limit of the confidence interval cannot be calculated if the number of observed infections equals zero; (9) No data are available from the state/territory for this reporting period; (10) The scores shown reflect fewer than 50 completed surveys; (11) There were discrepancies in the data collection process; (12) This measure does not apply to this hospital for this reporting period; (13) Results cannot be calculated for this reporting period; (14) The results for this state are combined with nearby states to protect confidentiality; Please refer to the User's Guide for a full explanation of data.

Measure	Cases	This Hosp.	State Avg.	U.S. Avg.
ACE Inhibitor or ARB for LVSD	12	92%	96%	97%
Discharge Instructions Given	43	98%	94%	94%
Evaluation of LVS Function	75	100%	98%	99%
Medicare Spending				
Medicare Spending per Patient (ratio)	-	-	0.95	0.98
Pneumonia Care				
Appropriate Initial Antibiotic Given	67	93%	95%	95%
Blood Culture Timing	91	98%	98%	98%
Pregnancy and Delivery Care				
Newborn Deliveries Scheduled Early[5]	-	-	5%	6%
Preventive Care				
Immunization for Influenza[5]	-	-	92%	90%
Immunization for Pneumonia[5]	-	-	93%	92%
Stroke Care				
Anticoagulation Therapy for Atrial Fibrillation[5]	-	-	94%	95%
Antithrombotic Therapy Timing[5]	-	-	98%	98%
Assessed for Rehabilitation[5]	-	-	98%	97%
Discharged on Antithrombotic Therapy[5]	-	-	99%	99%
Discharged on Statin Medication[5]	-	-	95%	94%
Thrombolytic Therapy Timing[5]	-	-	67%	66%
Venous Thromboembolism Prophylaxis[5]	-	-	95%	94%
Written Stroke Educational Materials Given[5]	-	-	88%	88%
Surgical Care Improvement Project				
Appropriate Beta Blocker Usage	29	100%	98%	98%
Appropriate VTP Within 24 Hours	88	99%	98%	98%
Controlled Postoperative Blood Glucose[7]	-	-	97%	97%
Perioperative Temperature Management	96	100%	100%	100%
Prophylactic Antibiotic Selection	79	100%	99%	99%
Prophylactic Antibiotic Selection (Outpatient)	-	-	98%	98%
Prophylactic Antibiotic Stopped	78	99%	98%	98%
Prophylactic Antibiotic Timing	79	100%	99%	99%
Prophylactic Antibiotic Timing (Outpatient)	-	-	98%	98%
Urinary Catheter Removal	87	99%	97%	97%
Survey of Patients' Hospital Experiences				
Area Around Room 'Always' Quiet at Night	300+	70%	61%	61%
Doctors 'Always' Communicated Well	300+	84%	82%	82%
Home Recovery Information Given	300+	90%	87%	85%
Hospital Given 9 or 10 on 10 Point Scale	300+	76%	71%	71%
Meds 'Always' Explained Before Given	300+	68%	63%	64%
Nurses 'Always' Communicated Well	300+	82%	79%	79%
Pain 'Always' Well Controlled	300+	70%	71%	71%
Room and Bathroom 'Always' Clean	300+	79%	73%	73%
Timely Help 'Always' Received	300+	68%	68%	68%
Would Definitely Recommend Hospital	300+	75%	70%	71%
Use of Medical Imaging				
Cardiac Imaging Stress Test before Surgery	-	-	5.2%	5.3%
Combination Abdominal CT Scan	-	-	11.2%	10.5%
Combination Brain/Sinus CT Scan	-	-	3.2%	2.7%
Combination Chest CT Scan	-	-	1.9%	2.7%
Follow-up Mammogram/Ultrasound	-	-	8.6%	8.8%
Lumbar Spine MRI for Low Back Pain	-	-	39.6%	37.2%

Pemiscot County Memorial Hospital

946 East Reed
Hayti, MO 63851
Phone: 573-359-1372
Fax: 573-359-3601
Type: Acute Care Hospitals
Emergency Services: Yes
Ownership: Govt - Hospital Dist/Auth
Beds: 245

Key Personnel:
Chief of Medical Staff.......... Jafer Gheraibeh, MD
Administrator................ Kerry Nobie
Quality Assurance............ Donna Sanders
Infection Control............. Micky Wilkerson, RN

Measure	Cases	This Hosp.	State Avg.	U.S. Avg.
Blood Clot Prevention and Treatment				
Anticoagulation Overlap Therapy[1,2]	-	-	94%	93%
ICU Venous Thromboembolism Prophylaxis[2]	48	40%	91%	92%
Incidence of Potentially Preventable VTE[2,7]	-	-	7%	10%
UFH with Dosages/Platelet Monitoring[1,2]	-	-	96%	97%
Venous Thromboembolism Prophylaxis[2]	104	8%	85%	85%
Warfarin Therapy Discharge Instructions[1,2]	-	-	76%	75%
Chest Pain/Possible Heart Attack Care				
Aspirin Given Within 24 Hours of Arrival	20	95%	95%	96%
Fibrinolytic Meds Within 30 Min. of Arrival[1]	-	-	53%	58%
Average Time to ECG (minutes)	18	16	7	7
Average Time to Transfer (minutes)[1]	-	-	53	60
Children's Asthma Care				
Received Home Management Plan of Care	-	-	-	88%
Received Reliever Medication	-	-	-	100%
Received Systemic Corticosteroids	-	-	-	100%
Emergency Department				
Admittance Decision Time (minutes)[2]	236	60	81	98
Head CT Results Within 45 Min. of Arrival[7]	-	-	63%	57%
Patients Who Left ER Before Being Seen	8,641	7%	3%	2%
Time from ER Arrival to Admit. (minutes)[2]	294	252	238	274
Time from ER Arrival to Discharge (minutes)	268	184	136	134
Time in ER Before Being Evaluated (minutes)	220	29	26	26
Time to Pain Meds for Fractures (minutes)	15	52	52	57
Heart Attack Care				
Aspirin Given at Discharge[1,3]	-	-	99%	99%
Fibrinolytic Meds Within 30 Min. of Arrival[3,7]	-	-	-	54%
PCI Within 90 Minutes of Arrival[3,7]	-	-	97%	96%
Statin Prescribed at Discharge[1,3]	-	-	98%	98%
Heart Failure Care				
ACE Inhibitor or ARB for LVSD[2]	18	67%	96%	97%
Discharge Instructions Given[2]	86	23%	94%	94%
Evaluation of LVS Function[2]	100	53%	98%	99%
Medicare Spending				
Medicare Spending per Patient (ratio)	-	0.87	0.95	0.98
Pneumonia Care				
Appropriate Initial Antibiotic Given[2]	20	40%	95%	95%
Blood Culture Timing[1,2]	-	-	98%	98%
Pregnancy and Delivery Care				
Newborn Deliveries Scheduled Early	15	0%	5%	6%
Preventive Care				
Immunization for Influenza[2]	291	16%	92%	90%
Immunization for Pneumonia[2]	567	14%	93%	92%
Stroke Care				
Anticoagulation Therapy for Atrial Fibrillation[1,2]	-	-	94%	95%
Antithrombotic Therapy Timing[1,2]	-	-	98%	98%
Assessed for Rehabilitation[1,2]	-	-	98%	97%
Discharged on Antithrombotic Therapy[1,2]	-	-	99%	99%
Discharged on Statin Medication[1,2]	-	-	95%	94%
Thrombolytic Therapy Timing[1,2]	-	-	67%	66%
Venous Thromboembolism Prophylaxis[1,2]	-	-	95%	94%
Written Stroke Educational Materials Given[1,2]	-	-	88%	88%
Surgical Care Improvement Project				
Appropriate Beta Blocker Usage[1,2]	-	-	98%	98%
Appropriate VTP Within 24 Hours[1,2]	-	-	98%	98%
Controlled Postoperative Blood Glucose[2,7]	-	-	97%	97%
Perioperative Temperature Management[1,2]	-	-	100%	100%
Prophylactic Antibiotic Selection[1,2]	-	-	99%	99%
Prophylactic Antibiotic Selection (Outpatient)[1,3]	-	-	98%	98%
Prophylactic Antibiotic Stopped[1,2]	-	-	98%	98%
Prophylactic Antibiotic Timing[1,2]	-	-	99%	99%
Prophylactic Antibiotic Timing (Outpatient)[1,3]	-	-	98%	98%
Urinary Catheter Removal[1,2]	-	-	97%	97%
Survey of Patients' Hospital Experiences				
Area Around Room 'Always' Quiet at Night	(a)	50%	61%	61%
Doctors 'Always' Communicated Well	(a)	84%	82%	82%
Home Recovery Information Given	(a)	66%	87%	85%
Hospital Given 9 or 10 on 10 Point Scale	(a)	39%	71%	71%
Meds 'Always' Explained Before Given	(a)	46%	63%	64%
Nurses 'Always' Communicated Well	(a)	61%	79%	79%
Pain 'Always' Well Controlled	(a)	53%	71%	71%
Room and Bathroom 'Always' Clean	(a)	58%	73%	73%
Timely Help 'Always' Received	(a)	49%	68%	68%
Would Definitely Recommend Hospital	(a)	38%	70%	71%
Use of Medical Imaging				
Cardiac Imaging Stress Test before Surgery[1]	-	-	5.2%	5.3%
Combination Abdominal CT Scan	213	0.5%	11.2%	10.5%
Combination Brain/Sinus CT Scan	227	4.8%	3.2%	2.7%
Combination Chest CT Scan	59	1.7%	1.9%	2.7%
Follow-up Mammogram/Ultrasound	163	3.1%	8.6%	8.8%
Lumbar Spine MRI for Low Back Pain[1]	-	-	39.6%	37.2%

Hermann Area District Hospital

509 W 18th St
Hermann, MO 65041
Phone: 573-486-2191
Fax: 573-486-3743
E-mail: hadh@ktif.net
URL: www.hadh.org
Type: Critical Access Hospitals
Emergency Services: Yes
Ownership: Govt - Hospital Dist/Auth
Beds: 44

Key Personnel:
Quality Assurance............ Holly Bloch, LPN
Anesthesiology............... Robert E Henson, D.O.
Chief of Medical Staff.......... Robert E Henson
Pediatric In-Patient Care .... Michael W Mahoney, DO
Emergency Room .... Jaya Parker, DO
Infection Control.............. James T Shaw, MD
Radiology.................... Matthew Siebert, MD
Operating Room.............. David Weston, MD

Measure	Cases	This Hosp.	State Avg.	U.S. Avg.
Blood Clot Prevention and Treatment				
Anticoagulation Overlap Therapy[5]	-	-	94%	93%
ICU Venous Thromboembolism Prophylaxis[5]	-	-	91%	92%
Incidence of Potentially Preventable VTE[5]	-	-	7%	10%
UFH with Dosages/Platelet Monitoring[5]	-	-	96%	97%
Venous Thromboembolism Prophylaxis[5]	-	-	85%	85%
Warfarin Therapy Discharge Instructions[5]	-	-	76%	75%
Chest Pain/Possible Heart Attack Care				
Aspirin Given Within 24 Hours of Arrival	-	-	95%	96%
Fibrinolytic Meds Within 30 Min. of Arrival	-	-	53%	58%
Average Time to ECG (minutes)	-	-	7	7
Average Time to Transfer (minutes)	-	-	53	60
Children's Asthma Care				
Received Home Management Plan of Care	-	-	-	88%
Received Reliever Medication	-	-	-	100%
Received Systemic Corticosteroids	-	-	-	100%
Emergency Department				
Admittance Decision Time (minutes)[5]	-	-	81	98
Head CT Results Within 45 Min. of Arrival	-	-	63%	57%
Patients Who Left ER Before Being Seen	-	-	3%	2%
Time from ER Arrival to Admit. (minutes)[5]	-	-	238	274
Time from ER Arrival to Discharge (minutes)	-	-	136	134
Time in ER Before Being Evaluated (minutes)	-	-	26	26
Time to Pain Meds for Fractures (minutes)	-	-	52	57
Heart Attack Care				
Aspirin Given at Discharge[5]	-	-	99%	99%
Fibrinolytic Meds Within 30 Min. of Arrival[5]	-	-	-	54%
PCI Within 90 Minutes of Arrival[5]	-	-	97%	96%
Statin Prescribed at Discharge[5]	-	-	98%	98%
Heart Failure Care				
ACE Inhibitor or ARB for LVSD[1]	-	-	96%	97%
Discharge Instructions Given[1]	-	-	94%	94%
Evaluation of LVS Function	13	54%	98%	99%
Medicare Spending				
Medicare Spending per Patient (ratio)	-	-	0.95	0.98
Pneumonia Care				
Appropriate Initial Antibiotic Given[1]	-	-	95%	95%
Blood Culture Timing	14	71%	98%	98%
Pregnancy and Delivery Care				
Newborn Deliveries Scheduled Early[5]	-	-	5%	6%
Preventive Care				
Immunization for Influenza[5]	-	-	92%	90%
Immunization for Pneumonia[5]	-	-	93%	92%
Stroke Care				
Anticoagulation Therapy for Atrial Fibrillation[5]	-	-	94%	95%
Antithrombotic Therapy Timing[5]	-	-	98%	98%
Assessed for Rehabilitation[5]	-	-	98%	97%
Discharged on Antithrombotic Therapy[5]	-	-	99%	99%
Discharged on Statin Medication[5]	-	-	95%	94%
Thrombolytic Therapy Timing[5]	-	-	67%	66%
Venous Thromboembolism Prophylaxis[5]	-	-	95%	94%
Written Stroke Educational Materials Given[5]	-	-	88%	88%
Surgical Care Improvement Project				
Appropriate Beta Blocker Usage[5]	-	-	98%	98%
Appropriate VTP Within 24 Hours[5]	-	-	98%	98%
Controlled Postoperative Blood Glucose[5]	-	-	97%	97%
Perioperative Temperature Management[5]	-	-	100%	100%

NOTE: Hospital profiles are in alphabetical order by state, then city, then hospital within the city; Rankings exclude hospitals with less than 25 cases except for patient surveys which excludes hospitals with less than 100 cases; (a) 100-299 cases; (1) The number of cases/patients is too few to report; (2) Data submitted were based on a sample of cases/patients; (3) Results are based on a shorter time period than required; (4) Data suppressed by CMS for one or more quarters; (5) Results are not available for this reporting period; (6) Fewer than 100 patients completed the HCAHPS survey; (7) No cases met the criteria for this measure; (8) The lower limit of the confidence interval cannot be calculated if the number of observed infections equals zero; (9) No data are available from the state/territory for this reporting period; (10) The scores shown reflect fewer than 50 completed surveys; (11) There were discrepancies in the data collection process; (12) This measure does not apply to this hospital for this reporting period; (13) Results cannot be calculated for this reporting period; (14) The results for this state are combined with nearby states to protect confidentiality; Please refer to the User's Guide for a full explanation of data.

Measure	Cases	This Hosp.	State Avg.	U.S. Avg.
Prophylactic Antibiotic Selection[5]	-	-	99%	99%
Prophylactic Antibiotic Selection (Outpatient)	-	-	98%	98%
Prophylactic Antibiotic Stopped[5]	-	-	98%	98%
Prophylactic Antibiotic Timing[5]	-	-	99%	99%
Prophylactic Antibiotic Timing (Outpatient)	-	-	98%	98%
Urinary Catheter Removal[5]	-	-	97%	97%
Survey of Patients' Hospital Experiences				
Area Around Room 'Always' Quiet at Night[5]	-	-	61%	61%
Doctors 'Always' Communicated Well[5]	-	-	82%	82%
Home Recovery Information Given[5]	-	-	87%	85%
Hospital Given 9 or 10 on 10 Point Scale[5]	-	-	71%	71%
Meds 'Always' Explained Before Given[5]	-	-	63%	64%
Nurses 'Always' Communicated Well[5]	-	-	79%	79%
Pain 'Always' Well Controlled[5]	-	-	71%	71%
Room and Bathroom 'Always' Clean[5]	-	-	73%	73%
Timely Help 'Always' Received[5]	-	-	68%	68%
Would Definitely Recommend Hospital[5]	-	-	70%	71%
Use of Medical Imaging				
Cardiac Imaging Stress Test before Surgery	-	-	5.2%	5.3%
Combination Abdominal CT Scan	-	-	11.2%	10.5%
Combination Brain/Sinus CT Scan	-	-	3.2%	2.7%
Combination Chest CT Scan	-	-	1.9%	2.7%
Follow-up Mammogram/Ultrasound	-	-	8.6%	8.8%
Lumbar Spine MRI for Low Back Pain	-	-	39.6%	37.2%

Texas County Memorial Hospital

1333 Sam Houston Boulevard
Houston, MO 65483
Phone: 417-967-3311
Fax: 417-967-1234
URL: www.tcmh.org
Type: Acute Care Hospitals
Emergency Services: Yes
Ownership: Voluntary non-profit - Other
Beds: 66

Key Personnel:
Emergency Room . . . . Mary Barnes
Infection Control. . . . . Tasaduq Fazili, MD
Chief of Medical Staff. . . . . Charles Mueller, MD
Operating Room. . . . . Charles Mueller, RN
CEO/President. . . . . Wes Murray

Measure	Cases	This Hosp.	State Avg.	U.S. Avg.
Blood Clot Prevention and Treatment				
Anticoagulation Overlap Therapy[2]	11	100%	94%	93%
ICU Venous Thromboembolism Prophylaxis[2]	31	94%	91%	92%
Incidence of Potentially Preventable VTE[2,7]	-	-	7%	10%
UFH with Dosages/Platelet Monitoring[2,7]	-	-	96%	97%
Venous Thromboembolism Prophylaxis[2]	125	82%	85%	85%
Warfarin Therapy Discharge Instructions[1,2]	-	-	76%	75%
Chest Pain/Possible Heart Attack Care				
Aspirin Given Within 24 Hours of Arrival	101	96%	95%	96%
Fibrinolytic Meds Within 30 Min. of Arrival[1]	-	-	53%	58%
Average Time to ECG (minutes)	103	10	7	7
Average Time to Transfer (minutes)[1]	-	-	53	60
Children's Asthma Care				
Received Home Management Plan of Care	-	-	-	88%
Received Reliever Medication	-	-	-	100%
Received Systemic Corticosteroids	-	-	-	100%
Emergency Department				
Admittance Decision Time (minutes)[2]	353	44	81	98
Head CT Results Within 45 Min. of Arrival[1]	-	-	63%	57%
Patients Who Left ER Before Being Seen	12,438	4%	3%	2%
Time from ER Arrival to Admit. (minutes)[2]	353	235	238	274
Time from ER Arrival to Discharge (minutes)	286	144	136	134
Time in ER Before Being Evaluated (minutes)	425	20	26	26
Time to Pain Meds for Fractures (minutes)	49	75	52	57
Heart Attack Care				
Aspirin Given at Discharge[5]	-	-	99%	99%
Fibrinolytic Meds Within 30 Min. of Arrival[5]	-	-	-	54%
PCI Within 90 Minutes of Arrival[5]	-	-	97%	96%
Statin Prescribed at Discharge[5]	-	-	98%	98%
Heart Failure Care				
ACE Inhibitor or ARB for LVSD	12	92%	96%	97%
Discharge Instructions Given	22	100%	94%	94%
Evaluation of LVS Function	36	97%	98%	99%
Medicare Spending				
Medicare Spending per Patient (ratio)	-	0.89	0.95	0.98
Pneumonia Care				
Appropriate Initial Antibiotic Given	82	99%	95%	95%
Blood Culture Timing	133	97%	98%	98%
Pregnancy and Delivery Care				
Newborn Deliveries Scheduled Early	50	6%	5%	6%
Preventive Care				
Immunization for Influenza[2]	243	86%	92%	90%
Immunization for Pneumonia[2]	293	90%	93%	92%
Stroke Care				
Anticoagulation Therapy for Atrial Fibrillation[1]	-	-	94%	95%
Antithrombotic Therapy Timing	13	100%	98%	98%
Assessed for Rehabilitation	13	100%	98%	97%
Discharged on Antithrombotic Therapy	13	100%	99%	99%
Discharged on Statin Medication[1]	-	-	95%	94%
Thrombolytic Therapy Timing[7]	-	-	67%	66%
Venous Thromboembolism Prophylaxis	16	88%	95%	94%
Written Stroke Educational Materials Given[1]	-	-	88%	88%
Surgical Care Improvement Project				
Appropriate Beta Blocker Usage[1,3]	-	-	98%	98%
Appropriate VTP Within 24 Hours[1,3]	-	-	98%	98%
Controlled Postoperative Blood Glucose[3,7]	-	-	97%	97%
Perioperative Temperature Management[1,3]	-	-	100%	100%
Prophylactic Antibiotic Selection[1,3]	-	-	99%	99%
Prophylactic Antibiotic Selection (Outpatient)[5]	-	-	98%	98%
Prophylactic Antibiotic Stopped[1,3]	-	-	98%	98%
Prophylactic Antibiotic Timing[1,3]	-	-	99%	99%
Prophylactic Antibiotic Timing (Outpatient)[5]	-	-	98%	98%
Urinary Catheter Removal[1,3]	-	-	97%	97%
Survey of Patients' Hospital Experiences				
Area Around Room 'Always' Quiet at Night	300+	61%	61%	61%
Doctors 'Always' Communicated Well	300+	88%	82%	82%
Home Recovery Information Given	300+	89%	87%	85%
Hospital Given 9 or 10 on 10 Point Scale	300+	64%	71%	71%
Meds 'Always' Explained Before Given	300+	67%	63%	64%
Nurses 'Always' Communicated Well	300+	81%	79%	79%
Pain 'Always' Well Controlled	300+	74%	71%	71%
Room and Bathroom 'Always' Clean	300+	80%	73%	73%
Timely Help 'Always' Received	300+	67%	68%	68%
Would Definitely Recommend Hospital	300+	61%	70%	71%
Use of Medical Imaging				
Cardiac Imaging Stress Test before Surgery	70	7.1%	5.2%	5.3%
Combination Abdominal CT Scan	231	7.4%	11.2%	10.5%
Combination Brain/Sinus CT Scan	248	8.1%	3.2%	2.7%
Combination Chest CT Scan	124	4.0%	1.9%	2.7%
Follow-up Mammogram/Ultrasound	351	8.3%	8.6%	8.8%
Lumbar Spine MRI for Low Back Pain[1]	-	-	39.6%	37.2%

Centerpoint Medical Center

19600 East 39th Street
Independence, MO 64057
Phone: 816-698-7000
URL: www.centerpointmedical.com
Type: Acute Care Hospitals
Emergency Services: Yes
Ownership: Voluntary non-profit - Private

Key Personnel:
CEO/President. . . . . Carolyn Caldwell
Radiology. . . . . Linda Dunaway
Operating Room. . . . . Pascal Spehar

Measure	Cases	This Hosp.	State Avg.	U.S. Avg.
Blood Clot Prevention and Treatment				
Anticoagulation Overlap Therapy[2]	104	100%	94%	93%
ICU Venous Thromboembolism Prophylaxis[2]	72	100%	91%	92%
Incidence of Potentially Preventable VTE[2]	16	6%	7%	10%
UFH with Dosages/Platelet Monitoring[2]	25	100%	96%	97%
Venous Thromboembolism Prophylaxis[2]	346	99%	85%	85%
Warfarin Therapy Discharge Instructions[2]	78	100%	76%	75%
Chest Pain/Possible Heart Attack Care				
Aspirin Given Within 24 Hours of Arrival[1,3]	-	-	95%	96%
Fibrinolytic Meds Within 30 Min. of Arrival[3,7]	-	-	53%	58%
Average Time to ECG (minutes)[1,3]	-	-	7	7
Average Time to Transfer (minutes)[3,7]	-	-	53	60
Children's Asthma Care				
Received Home Management Plan of Care	-	-	-	88%
Received Reliever Medication	-	-	-	100%
Received Systemic Corticosteroids	-	-	-	100%
Emergency Department				
Admittance Decision Time (minutes)[2]	825	84	81	98
Head CT Results Within 45 Min. of Arrival	12	83%	63%	57%
Patients Who Left ER Before Being Seen	62,216	1%	3%	2%
Time from ER Arrival to Admit. (minutes)[2]	825	253	238	274
Time from ER Arrival to Discharge (minutes)	493	135	136	134
Time in ER Before Being Evaluated (minutes)	521	17	26	26
Time to Pain Meds for Fractures (minutes)	148	64	52	57
Heart Attack Care				
Aspirin Given at Discharge	284	100%	99%	99%
Fibrinolytic Meds Within 30 Min. of Arrival[7]	-	-	-	54%
PCI Within 90 Minutes of Arrival	66	95%	97%	96%
Statin Prescribed at Discharge	281	100%	98%	98%
Heart Failure Care				
ACE Inhibitor or ARB for LVSD	109	100%	96%	97%
Discharge Instructions Given	269	100%	94%	94%
Evaluation of LVS Function	368	100%	98%	99%
Medicare Spending				
Medicare Spending per Patient (ratio)	-	1.01	0.95	0.98
Pneumonia Care				
Appropriate Initial Antibiotic Given	221	99%	95%	95%
Blood Culture Timing	416	100%	98%	98%
Pregnancy and Delivery Care				
Newborn Deliveries Scheduled Early[2]	22	5%	5%	6%
Preventive Care				
Immunization for Influenza[2]	634	100%	92%	90%
Immunization for Pneumonia[2]	817	100%	93%	92%
Stroke Care				
Anticoagulation Therapy for Atrial Fibrillation[1,2]	-	-	94%	95%
Antithrombotic Therapy Timing[2]	74	99%	98%	98%
Assessed for Rehabilitation[2]	106	100%	98%	97%
Discharged on Antithrombotic Therapy[2]	88	100%	99%	99%
Discharged on Statin Medication[2]	68	99%	95%	94%
Thrombolytic Therapy Timing[2]	16	100%	67%	66%
Venous Thromboembolism Prophylaxis[2]	107	99%	95%	94%
Written Stroke Educational Materials Given[2]	58	100%	88%	88%
Surgical Care Improvement Project				
Appropriate Beta Blocker Usage[2]	173	99%	98%	98%
Appropriate VTP Within 24 Hours[2]	423	99%	98%	98%
Controlled Postoperative Blood Glucose[2]	94	95%	97%	97%
Perioperative Temperature Management[2]	492	100%	100%	100%
Prophylactic Antibiotic Selection[2]	364	99%	99%	99%
Prophylactic Antibiotic Selection (Outpatient)	395	99%	98%	98%
Prophylactic Antibiotic Stopped[2]	349	99%	98%	98%
Prophylactic Antibiotic Timing[2]	364	100%	99%	99%
Prophylactic Antibiotic Timing (Outpatient)	395	100%	98%	98%
Urinary Catheter Removal[2]	243	99%	97%	97%
Survey of Patients' Hospital Experiences				
Area Around Room 'Always' Quiet at Night	300+	64%	61%	61%
Doctors 'Always' Communicated Well	300+	77%	82%	82%
Home Recovery Information Given	300+	89%	87%	85%
Hospital Given 9 or 10 on 10 Point Scale	300+	68%	71%	71%
Meds 'Always' Explained Before Given	300+	63%	63%	64%
Nurses 'Always' Communicated Well	300+	76%	79%	79%
Pain 'Always' Well Controlled	300+	68%	71%	71%
Room and Bathroom 'Always' Clean	300+	69%	73%	73%
Timely Help 'Always' Received	300+	65%	68%	68%
Would Definitely Recommend Hospital	300+	65%	70%	71%
Use of Medical Imaging				
Cardiac Imaging Stress Test before Surgery	316	7.0%	5.2%	5.3%
Combination Abdominal CT Scan	874	8.4%	11.2%	10.5%
Combination Brain/Sinus CT Scan	1,015	4.0%	3.2%	2.7%
Combination Chest CT Scan	369	1.6%	1.9%	2.7%
Follow-up Mammogram/Ultrasound	1,393	10.6%	8.6%	8.8%
Lumbar Spine MRI for Low Back Pain	111	42.3%	39.6%	37.2%

NOTE: Hospital profiles are in alphabetical order by state, then city, then hospital within the city; Rankings exclude hospitals with less than 25 cases except for patient surveys which excludes hospitals with less than 100 cases; (a) 100-299 cases; (1) The number of cases/patients is too few to report; (2) Data submitted were based on a sample of cases/patients; (3) Results are based on a shorter time period than required; (4) Data suppressed by CMS for one or more quarters; (5) Results are not available for this reporting period; (6) Fewer than 100 patients completed the HCAHPS survey; (7) No cases met the criteria for this measure; (8) The lower limit of the confidence interval cannot be calculated if the number of observed infections equals zero; (9) No data are available from the state/territory for this reporting period; (10) The scores shown reflect fewer than 50 completed surveys; (11) There were discrepancies in the data collection process; (12) This measure does not apply to this hospital for this reporting period; (13) Results cannot be calculated for this reporting period; (14) The results for this state are combined with nearby states to protect confidentiality; Please refer to the User's Guide for a full explanation of data.

Capital Region Medical Center

1125 Madison St
Jefferson City, MO 65102
E-mail: info@mail.crmc.org
URL: www.crmc.org
Type: Acute Care Hospitals
Ownership: Voluntary non-profit - Private
Phone: 573-632-5000
Fax: 573-632-5880
Emergency Services: Yes
Beds: 114

Key Personnel:
Patient Relations . . . . Joyce Corman
President . . . . Edward F. Farnsworth
Radiology. . . . . Mitchell Godbee
Operating Room. . . . . Chris Medlin
Chief of Medical Staff. . . . . Jake Tomblinson
Quality Assurance . . . . Janet Weckenborg

Measure	Cases	This Hosp.	State Avg.	U.S. Avg.
Blood Clot Prevention and Treatment				
Anticoagulation Overlap Therapy[2]	29	97%	94%	93%
ICU Venous Thromboembolism Prophylaxis[2]	70	97%	91%	92%
Incidence of Potentially Preventable VTE[1,2]	-	-	7%	10%
UFH with Dosages/Platelet Monitoring[2]	11	100%	96%	97%
Venous Thromboembolism Prophylaxis[2]	323	97%	85%	85%
Warfarin Therapy Discharge Instructions[2]	23	96%	76%	75%
Chest Pain/Possible Heart Attack Care				
Aspirin Given Within 24 Hours of Arrival[1,3]	-	-	95%	96%
Fibrinolytic Meds Within 30 Min. of Arrival[5]	-	-	53%	58%
Average Time to ECG (minutes)[1,3]	-	-	7	7
Average Time to Transfer (minutes)[5]	-	-	53	60
Children's Asthma Care				
Received Home Management Plan of Care	-	-	-	88%
Received Reliever Medication	-	-	-	100%
Received Systemic Corticosteroids	-	-	-	100%
Emergency Department				
Admittance Decision Time (minutes)[2]	515	87	81	98
Head CT Results Within 45 Min. of Arrival	25	88%	63%	57%
Patients Who Left ER Before Being Seen	32,866	1%	3%	2%
Time from ER Arrival to Admit. (minutes)[2]	540	227	238	274
Time from ER Arrival to Discharge (minutes)	384	130	136	134
Time in ER Before Being Evaluated (minutes)	402	17	26	26
Time to Pain Meds for Fractures (minutes)	131	55	52	57
Heart Attack Care				
Aspirin Given at Discharge	139	100%	99%	99%
Fibrinolytic Meds Within 30 Min. of Arrival[7]	-	-	-	54%
PCI Within 90 Minutes of Arrival	29	100%	97%	96%
Statin Prescribed at Discharge	140	100%	98%	98%
Heart Failure Care				
ACE Inhibitor or ARB for LVSD	51	100%	96%	97%
Discharge Instructions Given	139	96%	94%	94%
Evaluation of LVS Function	170	100%	98%	99%
Medicare Spending				
Medicare Spending per Patient (ratio)	-	0.94	0.95	0.98
Pneumonia Care				
Appropriate Initial Antibiotic Given	109	97%	95%	95%
Blood Culture Timing	179	98%	98%	98%
Pregnancy and Delivery Care				
Newborn Deliveries Scheduled Early	86	13%	5%	6%
Preventive Care				
Immunization for Influenza[2]	505	98%	92%	90%
Immunization for Pneumonia[2]	605	98%	93%	92%
Stroke Care				
Anticoagulation Therapy for Atrial Fibrillation[1]	-	-	94%	95%
Antithrombotic Therapy Timing	42	98%	98%	98%
Assessed for Rehabilitation	48	88%	98%	97%
Discharged on Antithrombotic Therapy	47	100%	99%	99%
Discharged on Statin Medication	39	87%	95%	94%
Thrombolytic Therapy Timing[1]	-	-	67%	66%
Venous Thromboembolism Prophylaxis	37	100%	95%	94%
Written Stroke Educational Materials Given	33	100%	88%	88%
Surgical Care Improvement Project				
Appropriate Beta Blocker Usage[2]	169	99%	98%	98%
Appropriate VTP Within 24 Hours[2]	316	99%	98%	98%
Controlled Postoperative Blood Glucose[2]	63	90%	97%	97%
Perioperative Temperature Management[2]	414	100%	100%	100%
Prophylactic Antibiotic Selection[2]	320	98%	99%	99%
Prophylactic Antibiotic Selection (Outpatient)	219	97%	98%	98%
Prophylactic Antibiotic Stopped[2]	307	97%	98%	98%
Prophylactic Antibiotic Timing[2]	320	100%	99%	99%
Prophylactic Antibiotic Timing (Outpatient)	219	99%	98%	98%
Urinary Catheter Removal[2]	284	100%	97%	97%
Survey of Patients' Hospital Experiences				
Area Around Room 'Always' Quiet at Night	300+	68%	61%	61%
Doctors 'Always' Communicated Well	300+	85%	82%	82%
Home Recovery Information Given	300+	89%	87%	85%
Hospital Given 9 or 10 on 10 Point Scale	300+	79%	71%	71%
Meds 'Always' Explained Before Given	300+	67%	63%	64%
Nurses 'Always' Communicated Well	300+	82%	79%	79%
Pain 'Always' Well Controlled	300+	73%	71%	71%
Room and Bathroom 'Always' Clean	300+	79%	73%	73%
Timely Help 'Always' Received	300+	70%	68%	68%
Would Definitely Recommend Hospital	300+	80%	70%	71%
Use of Medical Imaging				
Cardiac Imaging Stress Test before Surgery	228	10.5%	5.2%	5.3%
Combination Abdominal CT Scan	898	15.9%	11.2%	10.5%
Combination Brain/Sinus CT Scan[1]	-	-	3.2%	2.7%
Combination Chest CT Scan	917	0.2%	1.9%	2.7%
Follow-up Mammogram/Ultrasound	1,417	8.8%	8.6%	8.8%
Lumbar Spine MRI for Low Back Pain	191	38.7%	39.6%	37.2%

Saint Mary's Health Center

100 Saint Mary's Medical Plaza
Jefferson City, MO 65101
URL: www.stmarys-jeffcity.com
Type: Acute Care Hospitals
Ownership: Proprietary
Phone: 573-761-7000
Fax: 573-636-5733
Emergency Services: Yes
Beds: 167

Key Personnel:
CEO/President. . . . . Elizabeth Aderholdt
Pediatric In-Patient Care . . . . Chris Brandel
Radiology. . . . . Ralph Buettner
Coronary Care . . . . Gwen Douglas
Infection Control. . . . . Kathy Kormann
Chief of Medical Staff. . . . . John Lucia
Pediatric Ambulatory Care . . . . . . Barb Woods
Quality Assurance . . . . Jan Zimmerman

Measure	Cases	This Hosp.	State Avg.	U.S. Avg.
Blood Clot Prevention and Treatment				
Anticoagulation Overlap Therapy[2]	38	100%	94%	93%
ICU Venous Thromboembolism Prophylaxis[2]	70	100%	91%	92%
Incidence of Potentially Preventable VTE[1,2]	-	-	7%	10%
UFH with Dosages/Platelet Monitoring[2]	17	100%	96%	97%
Venous Thromboembolism Prophylaxis[2]	282	97%	85%	85%
Warfarin Therapy Discharge Instructions[2]	31	87%	76%	75%
Chest Pain/Possible Heart Attack Care				
Aspirin Given Within 24 Hours of Arrival[1,3]	-	-	95%	96%
Fibrinolytic Meds Within 30 Min. of Arrival[3,7]	-	-	53%	58%
Average Time to ECG (minutes)[1,3]	-	-	7	7
Average Time to Transfer (minutes)[3,7]	-	-	53	60
Children's Asthma Care				
Received Home Management Plan of Care	-	-	-	88%
Received Reliever Medication	-	-	-	100%
Received Systemic Corticosteroids	-	-	-	100%
Emergency Department				
Admittance Decision Time (minutes)[2]	516	72	81	98
Head CT Results Within 45 Min. of Arrival[1]	-	-	63%	57%
Patients Who Left ER Before Being Seen	34,388	2%	3%	2%
Time from ER Arrival to Admit. (minutes)[2]	525	258	238	274
Time from ER Arrival to Discharge (minutes)	371	150	136	134
Time in ER Before Being Evaluated (minutes)	206	23	26	26
Time to Pain Meds for Fractures (minutes)	112	39	52	57
Heart Attack Care				
Aspirin Given at Discharge	112	100%	99%	99%
Fibrinolytic Meds Within 30 Min. of Arrival[7]	-	-	-	54%
PCI Within 90 Minutes of Arrival	27	100%	97%	96%
Statin Prescribed at Discharge	105	100%	98%	98%
Heart Failure Care				
ACE Inhibitor or ARB for LVSD	92	100%	96%	97%
Discharge Instructions Given	210	100%	94%	94%
Evaluation of LVS Function	233	100%	98%	99%
Medicare Spending				
Medicare Spending per Patient (ratio)	-	0.92	0.95	0.98
Pneumonia Care				
Appropriate Initial Antibiotic Given	24	96%	95%	95%
Blood Culture Timing	151	99%	98%	98%
Pregnancy and Delivery Care				
Newborn Deliveries Scheduled Early[2]	39	3%	5%	6%
Preventive Care				
Immunization for Influenza[2]	545	100%	92%	90%
Immunization for Pneumonia[2]	617	100%	93%	92%
Stroke Care				
Anticoagulation Therapy for Atrial Fibrillation[1]	-	-	94%	95%
Antithrombotic Therapy Timing	45	93%	98%	98%
Assessed for Rehabilitation	42	100%	98%	97%
Discharged on Antithrombotic Therapy	41	100%	99%	99%
Discharged on Statin Medication	31	100%	95%	94%
Thrombolytic Therapy Timing[1]	-	-	67%	66%
Venous Thromboembolism Prophylaxis	51	90%	95%	94%
Written Stroke Educational Materials Given	27	56%	88%	88%
Surgical Care Improvement Project				
Appropriate Beta Blocker Usage[2]	149	100%	98%	98%
Appropriate VTP Within 24 Hours[2]	422	99%	98%	98%
Controlled Postoperative Blood Glucose[2]	40	98%	97%	97%
Perioperative Temperature Management[2]	455	100%	100%	100%
Prophylactic Antibiotic Selection[2]	354	100%	99%	99%
Prophylactic Antibiotic Selection (Outpatient)	285	99%	98%	98%
Prophylactic Antibiotic Stopped[2]	345	99%	98%	98%
Prophylactic Antibiotic Timing[2]	354	100%	99%	99%
Prophylactic Antibiotic Timing (Outpatient)	285	100%	98%	98%
Urinary Catheter Removal[2]	355	100%	97%	97%
Survey of Patients' Hospital Experiences				
Area Around Room 'Always' Quiet at Night	300+	56%	61%	61%
Doctors 'Always' Communicated Well	300+	82%	82%	82%
Home Recovery Information Given	300+	85%	87%	85%
Hospital Given 9 or 10 on 10 Point Scale	300+	71%	71%	71%
Meds 'Always' Explained Before Given	300+	66%	63%	64%
Nurses 'Always' Communicated Well	300+	80%	79%	79%
Pain 'Always' Well Controlled	300+	74%	71%	71%
Room and Bathroom 'Always' Clean	300+	74%	73%	73%
Timely Help 'Always' Received	300+	71%	68%	68%
Would Definitely Recommend Hospital	300+	74%	70%	71%
Use of Medical Imaging				
Cardiac Imaging Stress Test before Surgery	184	6.0%	5.2%	5.3%
Combination Abdominal CT Scan	399	8.5%	11.2%	10.5%
Combination Brain/Sinus CT Scan	460	1.7%	3.2%	2.7%
Combination Chest CT Scan	202	0.5%	1.9%	2.7%
Follow-up Mammogram/Ultrasound	846	11.9%	8.6%	8.8%
Lumbar Spine MRI for Low Back Pain	122	50.8%	39.6%	37.2%

Freeman Health System - Freeman West

1102 West 32nd Street
Joplin, MO 64804
URL: www.freemanhealth.com
Type: Acute Care Hospitals
Ownership: Voluntary non-profit - Other
Phone: 417-347-1111
Fax: 417-647-3716
Emergency Services: Yes
Beds: 203

Key Personnel:
Chief of Medical Staff. . . . . Christopher Andrew, MD
Operating Room. . . . . Patti Boman, RN
Infection Control. . . . . Madonna Briley
Radiology. . . . . Mark E Franham
Pediatric Ambulatory Care . . . . . . Denise Hamar, DO
Pediatric In-Patient Care . . . . Denise Hamar, DO
Quality Assurance . . . . Kathy Schurman

Measure	Cases	This Hosp.	State Avg.	U.S. Avg.
Blood Clot Prevention and Treatment				
Anticoagulation Overlap Therapy[2]	84	100%	94%	93%
ICU Venous Thromboembolism Prophylaxis[2]	93	96%	91%	92%
Incidence of Potentially Preventable VTE[2]	12	8%	7%	10%
UFH with Dosages/Platelet Monitoring[2]	100	100%	96%	97%
Venous Thromboembolism Prophylaxis[2]	267	89%	85%	85%
Warfarin Therapy Discharge Instructions[2]	41	61%	76%	75%
Chest Pain/Possible Heart Attack Care				
Aspirin Given Within 24 Hours of Arrival[1,3]	-	-	95%	96%
Fibrinolytic Meds Within 30 Min. of Arrival[5]	-	-	53%	58%
Average Time to ECG (minutes)[1,3]	-	-	7	7
Average Time to Transfer (minutes)[5]	-	-	53	60

NOTE: Hospital profiles are in alphabetical order by state, then city, then hospital within the city; Rankings exclude hospitals with less than 25 cases except for patient surveys which excludes hospitals with less than 100 cases; (a) 100-299 cases; (1) The number of cases/patients is too few to report; (2) Data submitted were based on a sample of cases/patients; (3) Results are based on a shorter time period than required; (4) Data suppressed by CMS for one or more quarters; (5) Results are not available for this reporting period; (6) Fewer than 100 patients completed the HCAHPS survey; (7) No cases met the criteria for this measure; (8) The lower limit of the confidence interval cannot be calculated if the number of observed infections equals zero; (9) No data are available from the state/territory for this reporting period; (10) The scores shown reflect fewer than 50 completed surveys; (11) There were discrepancies in the data collection process; (12) This measure does not apply to this hospital for this reporting period; (13) Results cannot be calculated for this reporting period; (14) The results for this state are combined with nearby states to protect confidentiality; Please refer to the User's Guide for a full explanation of data.

Measure	Cases	This Hosp.	State Avg.	U.S. Avg.
Children's Asthma Care				
Received Home Management Plan of Care	-	-	-	88%
Received Reliever Medication	-	-	-	100%
Received Systemic Corticosteroids	-	-	-	100%
Emergency Department				
Admittance Decision Time (minutes)[2]	351	188	81	98
Head CT Results Within 45 Min. of Arrival[1]	-	-	63%	57%
Patients Who Left ER Before Being Seen	50,971	8%	3%	2%
Time from ER Arrival to Admit. (minutes)[2]	365	343	238	274
Time from ER Arrival to Discharge (minutes)	342	208	136	134
Time in ER Before Being Evaluated (minutes)	375	39	26	26
Time to Pain Meds for Fractures (minutes)	221	76	52	57
Heart Attack Care				
Aspirin Given at Discharge	538	100%	99%	99%
Fibrinolytic Meds Within 30 Min. of Arrival[7]	-	-	-	54%
PCI Within 90 Minutes of Arrival	69	100%	97%	96%
Statin Prescribed at Discharge	489	100%	98%	98%
Heart Failure Care				
ACE Inhibitor or ARB for LVSD	90	98%	96%	97%
Discharge Instructions Given	227	89%	94%	94%
Evaluation of LVS Function	290	100%	98%	99%
Medicare Spending				
Medicare Spending per Patient (ratio)	-	0.94	0.95	0.98
Pneumonia Care				
Appropriate Initial Antibiotic Given[2]	57	95%	95%	95%
Blood Culture Timing[2]	117	97%	98%	98%
Pregnancy and Delivery Care				
Newborn Deliveries Scheduled Early[2]	47	2%	5%	6%
Preventive Care				
Immunization for Influenza[2]	525	94%	92%	90%
Immunization for Pneumonia[2]	602	91%	93%	92%
Stroke Care				
Anticoagulation Therapy for Atrial Fibrillation	33	97%	94%	95%
Antithrombotic Therapy Timing	172	98%	98%	98%
Assessed for Rehabilitation	201	94%	98%	97%
Discharged on Antithrombotic Therapy	182	100%	99%	99%
Discharged on Statin Medication	133	92%	95%	94%
Thrombolytic Therapy Timing[1]	-	-	67%	66%
Venous Thromboembolism Prophylaxis	217	89%	95%	94%
Written Stroke Educational Materials Given	110	43%	88%	88%
Surgical Care Improvement Project				
Appropriate Beta Blocker Usage[2]	314	98%	98%	98%
Appropriate VTP Within 24 Hours[2]	601	98%	98%	98%
Controlled Postoperative Blood Glucose[2]	186	97%	97%	97%
Perioperative Temperature Management[2]	733	100%	100%	100%
Prophylactic Antibiotic Selection[2]	656	100%	99%	99%
Prophylactic Antibiotic Selection (Outpatient)	581	99%	98%	98%
Prophylactic Antibiotic Stopped[2]	637	99%	98%	98%
Prophylactic Antibiotic Timing[2]	656	99%	99%	99%
Prophylactic Antibiotic Timing (Outpatient)	584	98%	98%	98%
Urinary Catheter Removal[2]	395	93%	97%	97%
Survey of Patients' Hospital Experiences				
Area Around Room 'Always' Quiet at Night	300+	54%	61%	61%
Doctors 'Always' Communicated Well	300+	81%	82%	82%
Home Recovery Information Given	300+	87%	87%	85%
Hospital Given 9 or 10 on 10 Point Scale	300+	68%	71%	71%
Meds 'Always' Explained Before Given	300+	61%	63%	64%
Nurses 'Always' Communicated Well	300+	75%	79%	79%
Pain 'Always' Well Controlled	300+	69%	71%	71%
Room and Bathroom 'Always' Clean	300+	65%	73%	73%
Timely Help 'Always' Received	300+	58%	68%	68%
Would Definitely Recommend Hospital	300+	71%	70%	71%
Use of Medical Imaging				
Cardiac Imaging Stress Test before Surgery	1,429	4.8%	5.2%	5.3%
Combination Abdominal CT Scan	1,531	3.9%	11.2%	10.5%
Combination Brain/Sinus CT Scan	998	2.1%	3.2%	2.7%
Combination Chest CT Scan	1,240	0.3%	1.9%	2.7%
Follow-up Mammogram/Ultrasound	3,032	4.7%	8.6%	8.8%
Lumbar Spine MRI for Low Back Pain	407	35.4%	39.6%	37.2%

Mercy Hospital Joplin

2817 Saint Johns Blvd
Joplin, MO 64804
URL: www.stj.com
Type: Acute Care Hospitals
Ownership: Voluntary non-profit - Church

Phone: 417-781-2727
Fax: 417-625-2910

Emergency Services: Yes
Beds: 367

Key Personnel:
Pediatric Ambulatory Care . . . . . . Barbara Chilton, DO
Pediatric In-Patient Care . . . . Barbara Chilton, DO
Radiology. . . . . Curtis Hammerman, MD
Operating Room. . . . . Christie Joyce
Quality Assurance . . . . Dennis Manley
Chief of Medical Staff . . . . J Marhnez, MD
CEO/President. . . . . Gary Rowe
Infection Control. . . . . Donna Stokes

Measure	Cases	This Hosp.	State Avg.	U.S. Avg.
Blood Clot Prevention and Treatment				
Anticoagulation Overlap Therapy[2]	52	92%	94%	93%
ICU Venous Thromboembolism Prophylaxis[2]	64	92%	91%	92%
Incidence of Potentially Preventable VTE[1,2]	-	-	7%	10%
UFH with Dosages/Platelet Monitoring[2]	44	100%	96%	97%
Venous Thromboembolism Prophylaxis[2]	248	85%	85%	85%
Warfarin Therapy Discharge Instructions[2]	43	65%	76%	75%
Chest Pain/Possible Heart Attack Care				
Aspirin Given Within 24 Hours of Arrival[1,3]	-	-	95%	96%
Fibrinolytic Meds Within 30 Min. of Arrival[5]	-	-	53%	58%
Average Time to ECG (minutes)[1,3]	-	-	7	7
Average Time to Transfer (minutes)[5]	-	-	53	60
Children's Asthma Care				
Received Home Management Plan of Care	-	-	-	88%
Received Reliever Medication	-	-	-	100%
Received Systemic Corticosteroids	-	-	-	100%
Emergency Department				
Admittance Decision Time (minutes)[2,3]	273	103	81	98
Head CT Results Within 45 Min. of Arrival[3,7]	-	-	63%	57%
Patients Who Left ER Before Being Seen	28,446	1%	3%	2%
Time from ER Arrival to Admit. (minutes)[2,3]	288	252	238	274
Time from ER Arrival to Discharge (minutes)[3]	281	149	136	134
Time in ER Before Being Evaluated (minutes)[3]	294	27	26	26
Time to Pain Meds for Fractures (minutes)[3]	38	66	52	57
Heart Attack Care				
Aspirin Given at Discharge[3]	126	98%	99%	99%
Fibrinolytic Meds Within 30 Min. of Arrival[3,7]	-	-	-	54%
PCI Within 90 Minutes of Arrival[3]	25	100%	97%	96%
Statin Prescribed at Discharge[3]	127	96%	98%	98%
Heart Failure Care				
ACE Inhibitor or ARB for LVSD[3]	52	92%	96%	97%
Discharge Instructions Given[3]	100	94%	94%	94%
Evaluation of LVS Function[3]	141	100%	98%	99%
Medicare Spending				
Medicare Spending per Patient (ratio)	-	0.93	0.95	0.98
Pneumonia Care				
Appropriate Initial Antibiotic Given[2,3]	40	98%	95%	95%
Blood Culture Timing[2,3]	83	99%	98%	98%
Pregnancy and Delivery Care				
Newborn Deliveries Scheduled Early[2]	27	4%	5%	6%
Preventive Care				
Immunization for Influenza[2,3]	279	94%	92%	90%
Immunization for Pneumonia[2,3]	517	94%	93%	92%
Stroke Care				
Anticoagulation Therapy for Atrial Fibrillation[2]	14	86%	94%	95%
Antithrombotic Therapy Timing[2]	62	97%	98%	98%
Assessed for Rehabilitation[2]	81	94%	98%	97%
Discharged on Antithrombotic Therapy[2]	76	93%	99%	99%
Discharged on Statin Medication[2]	56	86%	95%	94%
Thrombolytic Therapy Timing[2]	14	14%	67%	66%
Venous Thromboembolism Prophylaxis[2]	73	78%	95%	94%
Written Stroke Educational Materials Given[2]	51	43%	88%	88%
Surgical Care Improvement Project				
Appropriate Beta Blocker Usage[2,3]	109	99%	98%	98%
Appropriate VTP Within 24 Hours[2,3]	147	97%	98%	98%
Controlled Postoperative Blood Glucose[2,3]	81	91%	97%	97%
Perioperative Temperature Management[2,3]	211	99%	100%	100%
Prophylactic Antibiotic Selection[2,3]	181	98%	99%	99%
Prophylactic Antibiotic Selection (Outpatient)[3]	188	99%	98%	98%
Prophylactic Antibiotic Stopped[2,3]	171	98%	98%	98%
Prophylactic Antibiotic Timing[2,3]	183	94%	99%	99%
Prophylactic Antibiotic Timing (Outpatient)[3]	191	94%	98%	98%
Urinary Catheter Removal[2,3]	166	96%	97%	97%
Survey of Patients' Hospital Experiences				
Area Around Room 'Always' Quiet at Night[11]	300+	62%	61%	61%
Doctors 'Always' Communicated Well[11]	300+	86%	82%	82%
Home Recovery Information Given[11]	300+	90%	87%	85%
Hospital Given 9 or 10 on 10 Point Scale[11]	300+	80%	71%	71%
Meds 'Always' Explained Before Given[11]	300+	66%	63%	64%
Nurses 'Always' Communicated Well[11]	300+	81%	79%	79%
Pain 'Always' Well Controlled[11]	300+	75%	71%	71%
Room and Bathroom 'Always' Clean[11]	300+	74%	73%	73%
Timely Help 'Always' Received[11]	300+	71%	68%	68%
Would Definitely Recommend Hospital[11]	300+	83%	70%	71%
Use of Medical Imaging				
Cardiac Imaging Stress Test before Surgery	834	4.4%	5.2%	5.3%
Combination Abdominal CT Scan	756	7.1%	11.2%	10.5%
Combination Brain/Sinus CT Scan	666	1.5%	3.2%	2.7%
Combination Chest CT Scan	634	0.6%	1.9%	2.7%
Follow-up Mammogram/Ultrasound	646	17.2%	8.6%	8.8%
Lumbar Spine MRI for Low Back Pain	129	44.2%	39.6%	37.2%

Childrens Mercy Hospital

2401 Gillham Road
Kansas City, MO 64108
URL: www.childrens-mercy.org
Type: Childrens
Ownership: Voluntary non-profit - Private

Phone: 816-234-3000
Fax: 816-842-6107

Emergency Services: Yes
Beds: 241

Key Personnel:
Radiology. . . . . James C Brown, MD
Chief of Medical Staff . . . . V Fred Burry, MD
CEO/President. . . . . Randall L O'Donnell, PhD
Infection Control. . . . . Cindy Olson - Burgess, RN

Measure	Cases	This Hosp.	State Avg.	U.S. Avg.
Blood Clot Prevention and Treatment				
Anticoagulation Overlap Therapy[5]	-	-	94%	93%
ICU Venous Thromboembolism Prophylaxis[5]	-	-	91%	92%
Incidence of Potentially Preventable VTE[5]	-	-	7%	10%
UFH with Dosages/Platelet Monitoring[5]	-	-	96%	97%
Venous Thromboembolism Prophylaxis[5]	-	-	85%	85%
Warfarin Therapy Discharge Instructions[5]	-	-	76%	75%
Chest Pain/Possible Heart Attack Care				
Aspirin Given Within 24 Hours of Arrival	-	-	95%	96%
Fibrinolytic Meds Within 30 Min. of Arrival	-	-	53%	58%
Average Time to ECG (minutes)	-	-	7	7
Average Time to Transfer (minutes)	-	-	53	60
Children's Asthma Care				
Received Home Management Plan of Care[2]	323	90%	-	88%
Received Reliever Medication[2]	323	100%	-	100%
Received Systemic Corticosteroids[2]	318	99%	-	100%
Emergency Department				
Admittance Decision Time (minutes)[5]	-	-	81	98
Head CT Results Within 45 Min. of Arrival	-	-	63%	57%
Patients Who Left ER Before Being Seen	-	-	3%	2%
Time from ER Arrival to Admit. (minutes)[5]	-	-	238	274
Time from ER Arrival to Discharge (minutes)	-	-	136	134
Time in ER Before Being Evaluated (minutes)	-	-	26	26
Time to Pain Meds for Fractures (minutes)	-	-	52	57
Heart Attack Care				
Aspirin Given at Discharge[5]	-	-	99%	99%
Fibrinolytic Meds Within 30 Min. of Arrival[5]	-	-	-	54%
PCI Within 90 Minutes of Arrival[5]	-	-	97%	96%
Statin Prescribed at Discharge[5]	-	-	98%	98%
Heart Failure Care				
ACE Inhibitor or ARB for LVSD[5]	-	-	96%	97%
Discharge Instructions Given[5]	-	-	94%	94%
Evaluation of LVS Function[5]	-	-	98%	99%
Medicare Spending				
Medicare Spending per Patient (ratio)	-	-	0.95	0.98
Pneumonia Care				
Appropriate Initial Antibiotic Given[5]	-	-	95%	95%

NOTE: Hospital profiles are in alphabetical order by state, then city, then hospital within the city; Rankings exclude hospitals with less than 25 cases except for patient surveys which excludes hospitals with less than 100 cases; (a) 100-299 cases; (1) The number of cases/patients is too few to report; (2) Data submitted were based on a sample of cases/patients; (3) Results are based on a shorter time period than required; (4) Data suppressed by CMS for one or more quarters; (5) Results are not available for this reporting period; (6) Fewer than 100 patients completed the HCAHPS survey; (7) No cases met the criteria for this measure; (8) The lower limit of the confidence interval cannot be calculated if the number of observed infections equals zero; (9) No data are available from the state/territory for this reporting period; (10) The scores shown reflect fewer than 50 completed surveys; (11) There were discrepancies in the data collection process; (12) This measure does not apply to this hospital for this reporting period; (13) Results cannot be calculated for this reporting period; (14) The results for this state are combined with nearby states to protect confidentiality; Please refer to the User's Guide for a full explanation of data.

Measure	Cases	This Hosp.	State Avg.	U.S. Avg.
Blood Culture Timing[5]	-	-	98%	98%
Pregnancy and Delivery Care				
Newborn Deliveries Scheduled Early[5]	-	-	5%	6%
Preventive Care				
Immunization for Influenza[5]	-	-	92%	90%
Immunization for Pneumonia[5]	-	-	93%	92%
Stroke Care				
Anticoagulation Therapy for Atrial Fibrillation[5]	-	-	94%	95%
Antithrombotic Therapy Timing[5]	-	-	98%	98%
Assessed for Rehabilitation[5]	-	-	98%	97%
Discharged on Antithrombotic Therapy[5]	-	-	99%	99%
Discharged on Statin Medication[5]	-	-	95%	94%
Thrombolytic Therapy Timing[5]	-	-	67%	66%
Venous Thromboembolism Prophylaxis[5]	-	-	95%	94%
Written Stroke Educational Materials Given[5]	-	-	88%	88%
Surgical Care Improvement Project				
Appropriate Beta Blocker Usage[5]	-	-	98%	98%
Appropriate VTP Within 24 Hours[5]	-	-	98%	98%
Controlled Postoperative Blood Glucose[5]	-	-	97%	97%
Perioperative Temperature Management[5]	-	-	100%	100%
Prophylactic Antibiotic Selection[5]	-	-	99%	99%
Prophylactic Antibiotic Selection (Outpatient)	-	-	98%	98%
Prophylactic Antibiotic Stopped[5]	-	-	98%	98%
Prophylactic Antibiotic Timing[5]	-	-	99%	99%
Prophylactic Antibiotic Timing (Outpatient)	-	-	98%	98%
Urinary Catheter Removal[5]	-	-	97%	97%
Survey of Patients' Hospital Experiences				
Area Around Room 'Always' Quiet at Night[5]	-	-	61%	61%
Doctors 'Always' Communicated Well[5]	-	-	82%	82%
Home Recovery Information Given[5]	-	-	87%	85%
Hospital Given 9 or 10 on 10 Point Scale[5]	-	-	71%	71%
Meds 'Always' Explained Before Given[5]	-	-	63%	64%
Nurses 'Always' Communicated Well[5]	-	-	79%	79%
Pain 'Always' Well Controlled[5]	-	-	71%	71%
Room and Bathroom 'Always' Clean[5]	-	-	73%	73%
Timely Help 'Always' Received[5]	-	-	68%	68%
Would Definitely Recommend Hospital[5]	-	-	70%	71%
Use of Medical Imaging				
Cardiac Imaging Stress Test before Surgery	-	-	5.2%	5.3%
Combination Abdominal CT Scan	-	-	11.2%	10.5%
Combination Brain/Sinus CT Scan	-	-	3.2%	2.7%
Combination Chest CT Scan	-	-	1.9%	2.7%
Follow-up Mammogram/Ultrasound	-	-	8.6%	8.8%
Lumbar Spine MRI for Low Back Pain	-	-	39.6%	37.2%

Kansas City VA Medical Center

4801 Linwood Blvd.
Kansas City, MO 64128
Phone: 816-861-4700
Fax: 816-861-1110
Type: Acute Care - VA
Emergency Services: No
Ownership: Government Federal
Beds: 213

Key Personnel:

CEO/President. . . . . Hugh Doran
Chief of Medical Staff. . . . . James Kennedy, MD
Operating Room. . . . . Norman Probst, RN
Quality Assurance . . . . Barbara Shatto, RN
Emergency Room . . . . Robert Talley, MD

Measure	Cases	This Hosp.	State Avg.	U.S. Avg.
Blood Clot Prevention and Treatment				
Anticoagulation Overlap Therapy	-	-	94%	93%
ICU Venous Thromboembolism Prophylaxis	-	-	91%	92%
Incidence of Potentially Preventable VTE	-	-	7%	10%
UFH with Dosages/Platelet Monitoring	-	-	96%	97%
Venous Thromboembolism Prophylaxis	-	-	85%	85%
Warfarin Therapy Discharge Instructions	-	-	76%	75%
Chest Pain/Possible Heart Attack Care				
Aspirin Given Within 24 Hours of Arrival	-	-	95%	96%
Fibrinolytic Meds Within 30 Min. of Arrival	-	-	53%	58%
Average Time to ECG (minutes)	-	-	7	7
Average Time to Transfer (minutes)	-	-	53	60
Children's Asthma Care				
Received Home Management Plan of Care	-	-	-	88%
Received Reliever Medication	-	-	-	100%
Received Systemic Corticosteroids	-	-	-	100%
Emergency Department				
Admittance Decision Time (minutes)	-	-	81	98
Head CT Results Within 45 Min. of Arrival	-	-	63%	57%
Patients Who Left ER Before Being Seen	-	-	3%	2%
Time from ER Arrival to Admit. (minutes)	-	-	238	274
Time from ER Arrival to Discharge (minutes)	-	-	136	134
Time in ER Before Being Evaluated (minutes)	-	-	26	26
Time to Pain Meds for Fractures (minutes)	-	-	52	57
Heart Attack Care				
Aspirin Given at Discharge[1]	12	100%	99%	99%
Fibrinolytic Meds Within 30 Min. of Arrival[5]	-	-	-	54%
PCI Within 90 Minutes of Arrival[1]	-	-	97%	96%
Statin Prescribed at Discharge[1]	12	100%	98%	98%
Heart Failure Care				
ACE Inhibitor or ARB for LVSD	77	100%	96%	97%
Discharge Instructions Given	139	91%	94%	94%
Evaluation of LVS Function	167	100%	98%	99%
Medicare Spending				
Medicare Spending per Patient (ratio)	-	-	0.95	0.98
Pneumonia Care				
Appropriate Initial Antibiotic Given	73	92%	95%	95%
Blood Culture Timing	139	100%	98%	98%
Pregnancy and Delivery Care				
Newborn Deliveries Scheduled Early	-	-	5%	6%
Preventive Care				
Immunization for Influenza[5]	-	-	92%	90%
Immunization for Pneumonia[5]	-	-	93%	92%
Stroke Care				
Anticoagulation Therapy for Atrial Fibrillation	-	-	94%	95%
Antithrombotic Therapy Timing	-	-	98%	98%
Assessed for Rehabilitation	-	-	98%	97%
Discharged on Antithrombotic Therapy	-	-	99%	99%
Discharged on Statin Medication	-	-	95%	94%
Thrombolytic Therapy Timing	-	-	67%	66%
Venous Thromboembolism Prophylaxis	-	-	95%	94%
Written Stroke Educational Materials Given	-	-	88%	88%
Surgical Care Improvement Project				
Appropriate Beta Blocker Usage[2]	60	88%	98%	98%
Appropriate VTP Within 24 Hours[2]	192	96%	98%	98%
Controlled Postoperative Blood Glucose[5]	-	-	97%	97%
Perioperative Temperature Management[2]	215	99%	100%	100%
Prophylactic Antibiotic Selection	116	100%	99%	99%
Prophylactic Antibiotic Selection (Outpatient)	-	-	98%	98%
Prophylactic Antibiotic Stopped	114	96%	98%	98%
Prophylactic Antibiotic Timing	116	99%	99%	99%
Prophylactic Antibiotic Timing (Outpatient)	-	-	98%	98%
Urinary Catheter Removal[2]	134	96%	97%	97%
Survey of Patients' Hospital Experiences				
Area Around Room 'Always' Quiet at Night	-	-	61%	61%
Doctors 'Always' Communicated Well	-	-	82%	82%
Home Recovery Information Given	-	-	87%	85%
Hospital Given 9 or 10 on 10 Point Scale	-	-	71%	71%
Meds 'Always' Explained Before Given	-	-	63%	64%
Nurses 'Always' Communicated Well	-	-	79%	79%
Pain 'Always' Well Controlled	-	-	71%	71%
Room and Bathroom 'Always' Clean	-	-	73%	73%
Timely Help 'Always' Received	-	-	68%	68%
Would Definitely Recommend Hospital	-	-	70%	71%
Use of Medical Imaging				
Cardiac Imaging Stress Test before Surgery	-	-	5.2%	5.3%
Combination Abdominal CT Scan	-	-	11.2%	10.5%
Combination Brain/Sinus CT Scan	-	-	3.2%	2.7%
Combination Chest CT Scan	-	-	1.9%	2.7%
Follow-up Mammogram/Ultrasound	-	-	8.6%	8.8%
Lumbar Spine MRI for Low Back Pain	-	-	39.6%	37.2%

Research Medical Center

2316 E Meyer Blvd
Kansas City, MO 64132
Phone: 816-276-4000
URL: www.researchmedicalcenter.com
Type: Acute Care Hospitals
Emergency Services: Yes
Ownership: Proprietary
Beds: 511

Measure	Cases	This Hosp.	State Avg.	U.S. Avg.
Blood Clot Prevention and Treatment				
Anticoagulation Overlap Therapy[2]	105	97%	94%	93%
ICU Venous Thromboembolism Prophylaxis[2]	90	98%	91%	92%
Incidence of Potentially Preventable VTE[2]	28	0%	7%	10%
UFH with Dosages/Platelet Monitoring[2]	50	98%	96%	97%
Venous Thromboembolism Prophylaxis[2]	321	99%	85%	85%
Warfarin Therapy Discharge Instructions[2]	64	100%	76%	75%
Chest Pain/Possible Heart Attack Care				
Aspirin Given Within 24 Hours of Arrival[5]	-	-	95%	96%
Fibrinolytic Meds Within 30 Min. of Arrival[5]	-	-	53%	58%
Average Time to ECG (minutes)[5]	-	-	7	7
Average Time to Transfer (minutes)[5]	-	-	53	60
Children's Asthma Care				
Received Home Management Plan of Care	-	-	-	88%
Received Reliever Medication	-	-	-	100%
Received Systemic Corticosteroids	-	-	-	100%
Emergency Department				
Admittance Decision Time (minutes)[2]	556	98	81	98
Head CT Results Within 45 Min. of Arrival[7]	-	-	63%	57%
Patients Who Left ER Before Being Seen	65,857	4%	3%	2%
Time from ER Arrival to Admit. (minutes)[2]	556	234	238	274
Time from ER Arrival to Discharge (minutes)	465	94	136	134
Time in ER Before Being Evaluated (minutes)	503	15	26	26
Time to Pain Meds for Fractures (minutes)	72	54	52	57
Heart Attack Care				
Aspirin Given at Discharge	187	100%	99%	99%
Fibrinolytic Meds Within 30 Min. of Arrival[7]	-	-	-	54%
PCI Within 90 Minutes of Arrival	29	97%	97%	96%
Statin Prescribed at Discharge	182	100%	98%	98%
Heart Failure Care				
ACE Inhibitor or ARB for LVSD	112	100%	96%	97%
Discharge Instructions Given	278	100%	94%	94%
Evaluation of LVS Function	326	100%	98%	99%
Medicare Spending				
Medicare Spending per Patient (ratio)	-	1.02	0.95	0.98
Pneumonia Care				
Appropriate Initial Antibiotic Given	104	99%	95%	95%
Blood Culture Timing	238	100%	98%	98%
Pregnancy and Delivery Care				
Newborn Deliveries Scheduled Early[2]	30	3%	5%	6%
Preventive Care				
Immunization for Influenza[2]	630	100%	92%	90%
Immunization for Pneumonia[2]	798	100%	93%	92%
Stroke Care				
Anticoagulation Therapy for Atrial Fibrillation[1,2]	-	-	94%	95%
Antithrombotic Therapy Timing[2]	73	100%	98%	98%
Assessed for Rehabilitation[2]	106	100%	98%	97%
Discharged on Antithrombotic Therapy[2]	89	100%	99%	99%
Discharged on Statin Medication[2]	71	100%	95%	94%
Thrombolytic Therapy Timing[1,2]	-	-	67%	66%
Venous Thromboembolism Prophylaxis[2]	117	100%	95%	94%
Written Stroke Educational Materials Given[2]	46	91%	88%	88%
Surgical Care Improvement Project				
Appropriate Beta Blocker Usage[2]	215	100%	98%	98%
Appropriate VTP Within 24 Hours[2]	420	98%	98%	98%
Controlled Postoperative Blood Glucose[2]	114	98%	97%	97%
Perioperative Temperature Management[2]	534	100%	100%	100%
Prophylactic Antibiotic Selection[2]	432	100%	99%	99%
Prophylactic Antibiotic Selection (Outpatient)	539	99%	98%	98%
Prophylactic Antibiotic Stopped[2]	404	98%	98%	98%
Prophylactic Antibiotic Timing[2]	433	100%	99%	99%
Prophylactic Antibiotic Timing (Outpatient)	533	99%	98%	98%
Urinary Catheter Removal[2]	293	99%	97%	97%
Survey of Patients' Hospital Experiences				
Area Around Room 'Always' Quiet at Night	300+	66%	61%	61%

NOTE: Hospital profiles are in alphabetical order by state, then city, then hospital within the city; Rankings exclude hospitals with less than 25 cases except for patient surveys which excludes hospitals with less than 100 cases; (a) 100-299 cases; (1) The number of cases/patients is too few to report; (2) Data submitted were based on a sample of cases/patients; (3) Results are based on a shorter time period than required; (4) Data suppressed by CMS for one or more quarters; (5) Results are not available for this reporting period; (6) Fewer than 100 patients completed the HCAHPS survey; (7) No cases met the criteria for this measure; (8) The lower limit of the confidence interval cannot be calculated if the number of observed infections equals zero; (9) No data are available from the state/territory for this reporting period; (10) The scores shown reflect fewer than 50 completed surveys; (11) There were discrepancies in the data collection process; (12) This measure does not apply to this hospital for this reporting period; (13) Results cannot be calculated for this reporting period; (14) The results for this state are combined with nearby states to protect confidentiality; Please refer to the User's Guide for a full explanation of data.

Measure	Cases	This Hosp.	State Avg.	U.S. Avg.
Doctors 'Always' Communicated Well	300+	79%	82%	82%
Home Recovery Information Given	300+	86%	87%	85%
Hospital Given 9 or 10 on 10 Point Scale	300+	66%	71%	71%
Meds 'Always' Explained Before Given	300+	61%	63%	64%
Nurses 'Always' Communicated Well	300+	74%	79%	79%
Pain 'Always' Well Controlled	300+	69%	71%	71%
Room and Bathroom 'Always' Clean	300+	68%	73%	73%
Timely Help 'Always' Received	300+	61%	68%	68%
Would Definitely Recommend Hospital	300+	64%	70%	71%
Use of Medical Imaging				
Cardiac Imaging Stress Test before Surgery	274	4.4%	5.2%	5.3%
Combination Abdominal CT Scan	724	7.6%	11.2%	10.5%
Combination Brain/Sinus CT Scan	749	4.9%	3.2%	2.7%
Combination Chest CT Scan	564	2.0%	1.9%	2.7%
Follow-up Mammogram/Ultrasound	1,122	5.6%	8.6%	8.8%
Lumbar Spine MRI for Low Back Pain	94	33.0%	39.6%	37.2%

Saint Joseph Medical Center

1000 Carondelet Dr
Kansas City, MO 64114
Phone: 816-942-4000
Fax: 816-943-2840
URL: www.stjosehkc.com
Type: Acute Care Hospitals
Emergency Services: Yes
Ownership: Voluntary non-profit - Private
Beds: 300

Key Personnel:
Operating Room. . . . . Bev Camelia
CEO/President. . . . . Michael Dorsey
Radiology. . . . . Gord Hesse
Chief of Medical Staff. . . . . Stephen L. Stoops, MD
Quality Assurance . . . . Lisa Thacker
Emergency Room . . . . Kara Wineinger

Measure	Cases	This Hosp.	State Avg.	U.S. Avg.
Blood Clot Prevention and Treatment				
Anticoagulation Overlap Therapy[2]	89	98%	94%	93%
ICU Venous Thromboembolism Prophylaxis[2]	78	100%	91%	92%
Incidence of Potentially Preventable VTE[2]	25	4%	7%	10%
UFH with Dosages/Platelet Monitoring[2]	44	100%	96%	97%
Venous Thromboembolism Prophylaxis[2]	339	98%	85%	85%
Warfarin Therapy Discharge Instructions[2]	57	39%	76%	75%
Chest Pain/Possible Heart Attack Care				
Aspirin Given Within 24 Hours of Arrival[3,7]	-	-	95%	96%
Fibrinolytic Meds Within 30 Min. of Arrival[5]	-	-	53%	58%
Average Time to ECG (minutes)[3,7]	-	-	7	7
Average Time to Transfer (minutes)[5]	-	-	53	60
Children's Asthma Care				
Received Home Management Plan of Care	-	-	-	88%
Received Reliever Medication	-	-	-	100%
Received Systemic Corticosteroids	-	-	-	100%
Emergency Department				
Admittance Decision Time (minutes)[2]	605	106	81	98
Head CT Results Within 45 Min. of Arrival[1]	-	-	63%	57%
Patients Who Left ER Before Being Seen	34,064	2%	3%	2%
Time from ER Arrival to Admit. (minutes)[2]	608	255	238	274
Time from ER Arrival to Discharge (minutes)	353	145	136	134
Time in ER Before Being Evaluated (minutes)	384	13	26	26
Time to Pain Meds for Fractures (minutes)	113	42	52	57
Heart Attack Care				
Aspirin Given at Discharge	266	99%	99%	99%
Fibrinolytic Meds Within 30 Min. of Arrival[7]	-	-	-	54%
PCI Within 90 Minutes of Arrival	39	92%	97%	96%
Statin Prescribed at Discharge	263	99%	98%	98%
Heart Failure Care				
ACE Inhibitor or ARB for LVSD	106	98%	96%	97%
Discharge Instructions Given	229	77%	94%	94%
Evaluation of LVS Function	312	100%	98%	99%
Medicare Spending				
Medicare Spending per Patient (ratio)	-	1.06	0.95	0.98
Pneumonia Care				
Appropriate Initial Antibiotic Given	145	96%	95%	95%
Blood Culture Timing	256	97%	98%	98%
Pregnancy and Delivery Care				
Newborn Deliveries Scheduled Early[2]	25	8%	5%	6%
Preventive Care				
Immunization for Influenza[2]	526	92%	92%	90%
Immunization for Pneumonia[2]	715	93%	93%	92%
Stroke Care				
Anticoagulation Therapy for Atrial Fibrillation	19	100%	94%	95%
Antithrombotic Therapy Timing	73	100%	98%	98%
Assessed for Rehabilitation	101	100%	98%	97%
Discharged on Antithrombotic Therapy	88	100%	99%	99%
Discharged on Statin Medication	60	100%	95%	94%
Thrombolytic Therapy Timing	13	23%	67%	66%
Venous Thromboembolism Prophylaxis	103	98%	95%	94%
Written Stroke Educational Materials Given	42	100%	88%	88%
Surgical Care Improvement Project				
Appropriate Beta Blocker Usage[2]	153	96%	98%	98%
Appropriate VTP Within 24 Hours[2]	301	97%	98%	98%
Controlled Postoperative Blood Glucose[2]	98	93%	97%	97%
Perioperative Temperature Management[2]	354	100%	100%	100%
Prophylactic Antibiotic Selection[2]	318	98%	99%	99%
Prophylactic Antibiotic Selection (Outpatient)	320	96%	98%	98%
Prophylactic Antibiotic Stopped[2]	312	96%	98%	98%
Prophylactic Antibiotic Timing[2]	318	99%	99%	99%
Prophylactic Antibiotic Timing (Outpatient)	320	98%	98%	98%
Urinary Catheter Removal[2]	182	90%	97%	97%
Survey of Patients' Hospital Experiences				
Area Around Room 'Always' Quiet at Night	300+	60%	61%	61%
Doctors 'Always' Communicated Well	300+	82%	82%	82%
Home Recovery Information Given	300+	89%	87%	85%
Hospital Given 9 or 10 on 10 Point Scale	300+	70%	71%	71%
Meds 'Always' Explained Before Given	300+	62%	63%	64%
Nurses 'Always' Communicated Well	300+	77%	79%	79%
Pain 'Always' Well Controlled	300+	68%	71%	71%
Room and Bathroom 'Always' Clean	300+	72%	73%	73%
Timely Help 'Always' Received	300+	61%	68%	68%
Would Definitely Recommend Hospital	300+	72%	70%	71%
Use of Medical Imaging				
Cardiac Imaging Stress Test before Surgery	780	4.4%	5.2%	5.3%
Combination Abdominal CT Scan	869	15.4%	11.2%	10.5%
Combination Brain/Sinus CT Scan	954	2.3%	3.2%	2.7%
Combination Chest CT Scan	397	4.3%	1.9%	2.7%
Follow-up Mammogram/Ultrasound	1,405	10.4%	8.6%	8.8%
Lumbar Spine MRI for Low Back Pain	160	38.8%	39.6%	37.2%

Saint Luke's Hospital of Kansas City

4401 Wornall Road
Kansas City, MO 64111
Phone: 816-932-2000
Fax: 816-932-3599
URL: www.saintlukeshealthsystem.org
Type: Acute Care Hospitals
Emergency Services: Yes
Ownership: Govt - Hospital Dist/Auth
Beds: 629

Key Personnel:
CEO/President. . . . . Melinda L. Estes, MD
Emergency Room . . . . Denise Kintigh
CEO . . . . Julie Quirin

Measure	Cases	This Hosp.	State Avg.	U.S. Avg.
Blood Clot Prevention and Treatment				
Anticoagulation Overlap Therapy[2]	152	97%	94%	93%
ICU Venous Thromboembolism Prophylaxis[2]	118	92%	91%	92%
Incidence of Potentially Preventable VTE[2]	32	9%	7%	10%
UFH with Dosages/Platelet Monitoring[2]	128	98%	96%	97%
Venous Thromboembolism Prophylaxis[2]	328	70%	85%	85%
Warfarin Therapy Discharge Instructions[2]	108	55%	76%	75%
Chest Pain/Possible Heart Attack Care				
Aspirin Given Within 24 Hours of Arrival[1,3]	-	-	95%	96%
Fibrinolytic Meds Within 30 Min. of Arrival[5]	-	-	53%	58%
Average Time to ECG (minutes)[1,3]	-	-	7	7
Average Time to Transfer (minutes)[5]	-	-	53	60
Children's Asthma Care				
Received Home Management Plan of Care	-	-	-	88%
Received Reliever Medication	-	-	-	100%
Received Systemic Corticosteroids	-	-	-	100%
Emergency Department				
Admittance Decision Time (minutes)[2]	450	78	81	98
Head CT Results Within 45 Min. of Arrival[1]	-	-	63%	57%
Patients Who Left ER Before Being Seen	36,698	3%	3%	2%
Time from ER Arrival to Admit. (minutes)[2]	467	234	238	274
Time from ER Arrival to Discharge (minutes)	435	186	136	134
Time in ER Before Being Evaluated (minutes)	363	43	26	26
Time to Pain Meds for Fractures (minutes)	67	58	52	57
Heart Attack Care				
Aspirin Given at Discharge	348	100%	99%	99%
Fibrinolytic Meds Within 30 Min. of Arrival[7]	-	-	-	54%
PCI Within 90 Minutes of Arrival	21	100%	97%	96%
Statin Prescribed at Discharge	345	99%	98%	98%
Heart Failure Care				
ACE Inhibitor or ARB for LVSD	237	100%	96%	97%
Discharge Instructions Given	590	92%	94%	94%
Evaluation of LVS Function	692	100%	98%	99%
Medicare Spending				
Medicare Spending per Patient (ratio)	-	1.00	0.95	0.98
Pneumonia Care				
Appropriate Initial Antibiotic Given	104	94%	95%	95%
Blood Culture Timing	188	97%	98%	98%
Pregnancy and Delivery Care				
Newborn Deliveries Scheduled Early[2]	45	9%	5%	6%
Preventive Care				
Immunization for Influenza[2]	570	82%	92%	90%
Immunization for Pneumonia[2]	705	89%	93%	92%
Stroke Care				
Anticoagulation Therapy for Atrial Fibrillation	86	97%	94%	95%
Antithrombotic Therapy Timing	399	98%	98%	98%
Assessed for Rehabilitation	643	98%	98%	97%
Discharged on Antithrombotic Therapy	497	99%	99%	99%
Discharged on Statin Medication	367	96%	95%	94%
Thrombolytic Therapy Timing	48	88%	67%	66%
Venous Thromboembolism Prophylaxis	671	97%	95%	94%
Written Stroke Educational Materials Given	340	89%	88%	88%
Surgical Care Improvement Project				
Appropriate Beta Blocker Usage[2]	566	100%	98%	98%
Appropriate VTP Within 24 Hours[2]	551	98%	98%	98%
Controlled Postoperative Blood Glucose[2]	414	99%	97%	97%
Perioperative Temperature Management[2]	696	100%	100%	100%
Prophylactic Antibiotic Selection[2]	788	99%	99%	99%
Prophylactic Antibiotic Selection (Outpatient)	578	99%	98%	98%
Prophylactic Antibiotic Stopped[2]	770	98%	98%	98%
Prophylactic Antibiotic Timing[2]	788	100%	99%	99%
Prophylactic Antibiotic Timing (Outpatient)	580	98%	98%	98%
Urinary Catheter Removal[2]	554	99%	97%	97%
Survey of Patients' Hospital Experiences				
Area Around Room 'Always' Quiet at Night	300+	67%	61%	61%
Doctors 'Always' Communicated Well	300+	82%	82%	82%
Home Recovery Information Given	300+	87%	87%	85%
Hospital Given 9 or 10 on 10 Point Scale	300+	77%	71%	71%
Meds 'Always' Explained Before Given	300+	64%	63%	64%
Nurses 'Always' Communicated Well	300+	81%	79%	79%
Pain 'Always' Well Controlled	300+	76%	71%	71%
Room and Bathroom 'Always' Clean	300+	70%	73%	73%
Timely Help 'Always' Received	300+	65%	68%	68%
Would Definitely Recommend Hospital	300+	82%	70%	71%
Use of Medical Imaging				
Cardiac Imaging Stress Test before Surgery	666	4.4%	5.2%	5.3%
Combination Abdominal CT Scan	376	1.9%	11.2%	10.5%
Combination Brain/Sinus CT Scan	695	3.6%	3.2%	2.7%
Combination Chest CT Scan	101	13.9%	1.9%	2.7%
Follow-up Mammogram/Ultrasound	998	12.2%	8.6%	8.8%
Lumbar Spine MRI for Low Back Pain[1]	-	-	39.6%	37.2%

Saint Luke's Northland Hospital

5830 N W Barry Road
Kansas City, MO 64154
Phone: 816-891-6000
Fax: 816-880-6155
URL: www.saintlukeshealthsystem.org
Type: Acute Care Hospitals
Emergency Services: Yes
Ownership: Voluntary non-profit - Private
Beds: 84

Key Personnel:
Radiology. . . . . Julie F Harthung
CEO/President. . . . . Gary Wages
Chief of Medical Staff. . . . . Lance B Waldo

Measure	Cases	This Hosp.	State Avg.	U.S. Avg.
Blood Clot Prevention and Treatment				
Anticoagulation Overlap Therapy[2]	29	100%	94%	93%
ICU Venous Thromboembolism Prophylaxis[2]	66	79%	91%	92%

NOTE: Hospital profiles are in alphabetical order by state, then city, then hospital within the city; Rankings exclude hospitals with less than 25 cases except for patient surveys which excludes hospitals with less than 100 cases; (a) 100-299 cases; (1) The number of cases/patients is too few to report; (2) Data submitted were based on a sample of cases/patients; (3) Results are based on a shorter time period than required; (4) Data suppressed by CMS for one or more quarters; (5) Results are not available for this reporting period; (6) Fewer than 100 patients completed the HCAHPS survey; (7) No cases met the criteria for this measure; (8) The lower limit of the confidence interval cannot be calculated if the number of observed infections equals zero; (9) No data are available from the state/territory for this reporting period; (10) The scores shown reflect fewer than 50 completed surveys; (11) There were discrepancies in the data collection process; (12) This measure does not apply to this hospital for this reporting period; (13) Results cannot be calculated for this reporting period; (14) The results for this state are combined with nearby states to protect confidentiality; Please refer to the User's Guide for a full explanation of data.

Measure	Cases	This Hosp.	State Avg.	U.S. Avg.
Incidence of Potentially Preventable VTE[1,2]	-	-	7%	10%
UFH with Dosages/Platelet Monitoring[2]	19	100%	96%	97%
Venous Thromboembolism Prophylaxis[2]	351	78%	85%	85%
Warfarin Therapy Discharge Instructions[2]	22	64%	76%	75%
Chest Pain/Possible Heart Attack Care				
Aspirin Given Within 24 Hours of Arrival	16	75%	95%	96%
Fibrinolytic Meds Within 30 Min. of Arrival[1]	-	-	53%	58%
Average Time to ECG (minutes)	17	5	7	7
Average Time to Transfer (minutes)[1]	-	-	53	60
Children's Asthma Care				
Received Home Management Plan of Care	-	-	-	88%
Received Reliever Medication	-	-	-	100%
Received Systemic Corticosteroids	-	-	-	100%
Emergency Department				
Admittance Decision Time (minutes)[2]	505	94	81	98
Head CT Results Within 45 Min. of Arrival	24	62%	63%	57%
Patients Who Left ER Before Being Seen	33,308	2%	3%	2%
Time from ER Arrival to Admit. (minutes)[2]	506	248	238	274
Time from ER Arrival to Discharge (minutes)	380	132	136	134
Time in ER Before Being Evaluated (minutes)	296	33	26	26
Time to Pain Meds for Fractures (minutes)	88	51	52	57
Heart Attack Care				
Aspirin Given at Discharge	127	100%	99%	99%
Fibrinolytic Meds Within 30 Min. of Arrival[7]	-	-	-	54%
PCI Within 90 Minutes of Arrival	31	97%	97%	96%
Statin Prescribed at Discharge	122	99%	98%	98%
Heart Failure Care				
ACE Inhibitor or ARB for LVSD	38	100%	96%	97%
Discharge Instructions Given	120	90%	94%	94%
Evaluation of LVS Function	160	100%	98%	99%
Medicare Spending				
Medicare Spending per Patient (ratio)	-	0.98	0.95	0.98
Pneumonia Care				
Appropriate Initial Antibiotic Given	87	100%	95%	95%
Blood Culture Timing	106	99%	98%	98%
Pregnancy and Delivery Care				
Newborn Deliveries Scheduled Early[2]	40	5%	5%	6%
Preventive Care				
Immunization for Influenza[2]	483	92%	92%	90%
Immunization for Pneumonia[2]	524	93%	93%	92%
Stroke Care				
Anticoagulation Therapy for Atrial Fibrillation[1]	-	-	94%	95%
Antithrombotic Therapy Timing	53	98%	98%	98%
Assessed for Rehabilitation	61	98%	98%	97%
Discharged on Antithrombotic Therapy	59	100%	99%	99%
Discharged on Statin Medication	50	92%	95%	94%
Thrombolytic Therapy Timing[1]	-	-	67%	66%
Venous Thromboembolism Prophylaxis	52	92%	95%	94%
Written Stroke Educational Materials Given	40	55%	88%	88%
Surgical Care Improvement Project				
Appropriate Beta Blocker Usage	88	94%	98%	98%
Appropriate VTP Within 24 Hours	267	94%	98%	98%
Controlled Postoperative Blood Glucose[7]	-	-	97%	97%
Perioperative Temperature Management	298	94%	100%	100%
Prophylactic Antibiotic Selection	186	100%	99%	99%
Prophylactic Antibiotic Selection (Outpatient)	53	94%	98%	98%
Prophylactic Antibiotic Stopped	181	99%	98%	98%
Prophylactic Antibiotic Timing	186	98%	99%	99%
Prophylactic Antibiotic Timing (Outpatient)	54	98%	98%	98%
Urinary Catheter Removal	149	91%	97%	97%
Survey of Patients' Hospital Experiences				
Area Around Room 'Always' Quiet at Night	300+	64%	61%	61%
Doctors 'Always' Communicated Well	300+	81%	82%	82%
Home Recovery Information Given	300+	87%	87%	85%
Hospital Given 9 or 10 on 10 Point Scale	300+	75%	71%	71%
Meds 'Always' Explained Before Given	300+	62%	63%	64%
Nurses 'Always' Communicated Well	300+	77%	79%	79%
Pain 'Always' Well Controlled	300+	70%	71%	71%
Room and Bathroom 'Always' Clean	300+	73%	73%	73%
Timely Help 'Always' Received	300+	61%	68%	68%
Would Definitely Recommend Hospital	300+	77%	70%	71%
Use of Medical Imaging				
Cardiac Imaging Stress Test before Surgery	202	2.0%	5.2%	5.3%
Combination Abdominal CT Scan	433	6.2%	11.2%	10.5%
Combination Brain/Sinus CT Scan[1]	-	-	3.2%	2.7%
Combination Chest CT Scan	223	1.8%	1.9%	2.7%
Follow-up Mammogram/Ultrasound	762	8.8%	8.6%	8.8%
Lumbar Spine MRI for Low Back Pain	89	48.3%	39.6%	37.2%

Truman Medical Center Hospital Hill

2301 Holmes Street
Kansas City, MO 64108
URL: www.trumed.org
Type: Acute Care Hospitals
Ownership: Voluntary non-profit - Private
Phone: 816-404-1000
Fax: 816-404-3779
Emergency Services: Yes
Beds: 651

Key Personnel:

Operating Room. . . . . Todd Clayman
Infection Control. . . . . Jette Hogenmiller, PhD
Radiology. . . . . Lawrence Ricci, MD
Quality Assurance . . . . Shauna Roberts, MD
Pediatric In-Patient Care . . . . . . Michael Sheehan, MD
CEO/President. . . . . Charlie Shields
Coronary Care . . . . Sharon Snow
Chief of Medical Staff. . . . . Mark T. Steele, MD

Measure	Cases	This Hosp.	State Avg.	U.S. Avg.
Blood Clot Prevention and Treatment				
Anticoagulation Overlap Therapy[2]	58	100%	94%	93%
ICU Venous Thromboembolism Prophylaxis[2]	68	97%	91%	92%
Incidence of Potentially Preventable VTE[1,2]	-	-	7%	10%
UFH with Dosages/Platelet Monitoring[2]	46	100%	96%	97%
Venous Thromboembolism Prophylaxis[2]	314	95%	85%	85%
Warfarin Therapy Discharge Instructions[2]	56	96%	76%	75%
Chest Pain/Possible Heart Attack Care				
Aspirin Given Within 24 Hours of Arrival	119	97%	95%	96%
Fibrinolytic Meds Within 30 Min. of Arrival[7]	-	-	53%	58%
Average Time to ECG (minutes)	111	8	7	7
Average Time to Transfer (minutes)	22	86	53	60
Children's Asthma Care				
Received Home Management Plan of Care	-	-	-	88%
Received Reliever Medication	-	-	-	100%
Received Systemic Corticosteroids	-	-	-	100%
Emergency Department				
Admittance Decision Time (minutes)[2]	539	161	81	98
Head CT Results Within 45 Min. of Arrival[1]	-	-	63%	57%
Patients Who Left ER Before Being Seen	67,130	14%	3%	2%
Time from ER Arrival to Admit. (minutes)[2]	546	451	238	274
Time from ER Arrival to Discharge (minutes)	376	257	136	134
Time in ER Before Being Evaluated (minutes)	357	94	26	26
Time to Pain Meds for Fractures (minutes)	109	92	52	57
Heart Attack Care				
Aspirin Given at Discharge	167	100%	99%	99%
Fibrinolytic Meds Within 30 Min. of Arrival[7]	-	-	-	54%
PCI Within 90 Minutes of Arrival	17	94%	97%	96%
Statin Prescribed at Discharge	161	100%	98%	98%
Heart Failure Care				
ACE Inhibitor or ARB for LVSD	196	100%	96%	97%
Discharge Instructions Given	313	97%	94%	94%
Evaluation of LVS Function	338	100%	98%	99%
Medicare Spending				
Medicare Spending per Patient (ratio)	-	0.93	0.95	0.98
Pneumonia Care				
Appropriate Initial Antibiotic Given	111	99%	95%	95%
Blood Culture Timing	175	97%	98%	98%
Pregnancy and Delivery Care				
Newborn Deliveries Scheduled Early[2]	24	8%	5%	6%
Preventive Care				
Immunization for Influenza[2]	481	91%	92%	90%
Immunization for Pneumonia[2]	458	89%	93%	92%
Stroke Care				
Anticoagulation Therapy for Atrial Fibrillation[1]	-	-	94%	95%
Antithrombotic Therapy Timing	25	88%	98%	98%
Assessed for Rehabilitation	39	95%	98%	97%
Discharged on Antithrombotic Therapy	32	91%	99%	99%
Discharged on Statin Medication	33	91%	95%	94%
Thrombolytic Therapy Timing[1]	-	-	67%	66%
Venous Thromboembolism Prophylaxis	43	95%	95%	94%
Written Stroke Educational Materials Given	25	92%	88%	88%
Surgical Care Improvement Project				
Appropriate Beta Blocker Usage[2]	77	95%	98%	98%
Appropriate VTP Within 24 Hours[2]	287	97%	98%	98%
Controlled Postoperative Blood Glucose[1,2]	-	-	97%	97%
Perioperative Temperature Management[2]	350	100%	100%	100%
Prophylactic Antibiotic Selection[2]	238	100%	99%	99%
Prophylactic Antibiotic Selection (Outpatient)	187	97%	98%	98%
Prophylactic Antibiotic Stopped[2]	234	99%	98%	98%
Prophylactic Antibiotic Timing[2]	239	100%	99%	99%
Prophylactic Antibiotic Timing (Outpatient)	149	95%	98%	98%
Urinary Catheter Removal[2]	145	92%	97%	97%
Survey of Patients' Hospital Experiences				
Area Around Room 'Always' Quiet at Night	300+	66%	61%	61%
Doctors 'Always' Communicated Well	300+	77%	82%	82%
Home Recovery Information Given	300+	84%	87%	85%
Hospital Given 9 or 10 on 10 Point Scale	300+	65%	71%	71%
Meds 'Always' Explained Before Given	300+	60%	63%	64%
Nurses 'Always' Communicated Well	300+	79%	79%	79%
Pain 'Always' Well Controlled	300+	69%	71%	71%
Room and Bathroom 'Always' Clean	300+	69%	73%	73%
Timely Help 'Always' Received	300+	62%	68%	68%
Would Definitely Recommend Hospital	300+	60%	70%	71%
Use of Medical Imaging				
Cardiac Imaging Stress Test before Surgery	195	3.6%	5.2%	5.3%
Combination Abdominal CT Scan	248	13.3%	11.2%	10.5%
Combination Brain/Sinus CT Scan[1]	-	-	3.2%	2.7%
Combination Chest CT Scan	255	0.4%	1.9%	2.7%
Follow-up Mammogram/Ultrasound	613	17.1%	8.6%	8.8%
Lumbar Spine MRI for Low Back Pain	35	45.7%	39.6%	37.2%

Truman Medical Center Lakewood

7900 Lee's Summit Rd
Kansas City, MO 64139
URL: www.trumed.org
Type: Acute Care Hospitals
Ownership: Voluntary non-profit - Private
Phone: 816-404-7000
Fax: 816-404-8038
Emergency Services: Yes
Beds: 314

Key Personnel:

Infection Control. . . . . Jette Hogenmiller, PhD
Coronary Care . . . . Darinda Reberry, RN
Radiology. . . . . Lawrence Ricci, MD
Quality Assurance . . . . Shauna Roberts, MD
CEO/President. . . . . Charlie Shields
Chief of Medical Staff. . . . . Mark T. Steele, MD
Pediatric Ambulatory Care . . . . . Mark Woodring
Pediatric In-Patient Care . . . . . . Mark Woodring

Measure	Cases	This Hosp.	State Avg.	U.S. Avg.
Blood Clot Prevention and Treatment				
Anticoagulation Overlap Therapy[2]	13	100%	94%	93%
ICU Venous Thromboembolism Prophylaxis[2]	28	93%	91%	92%
Incidence of Potentially Preventable VTE[2,7]	-	-	7%	10%
UFH with Dosages/Platelet Monitoring[1,2]	-	-	96%	97%
Venous Thromboembolism Prophylaxis[2]	178	89%	85%	85%
Warfarin Therapy Discharge Instructions[2]	12	100%	76%	75%
Chest Pain/Possible Heart Attack Care				
Aspirin Given Within 24 Hours of Arrival	57	93%	95%	96%
Fibrinolytic Meds Within 30 Min. of Arrival[7]	-	-	53%	58%
Average Time to ECG (minutes)	54	2	7	7
Average Time to Transfer (minutes)	23	79	53	60
Children's Asthma Care				
Received Home Management Plan of Care	-	-	-	88%
Received Reliever Medication	-	-	-	100%
Received Systemic Corticosteroids	-	-	-	100%
Emergency Department				
Admittance Decision Time (minutes)[2]	263	94	81	98
Head CT Results Within 45 Min. of Arrival[3,7]	-	-	63%	57%
Patients Who Left ER Before Being Seen	33,486	6%	3%	2%
Time from ER Arrival to Admit. (minutes)[2]	284	272	238	274
Time from ER Arrival to Discharge (minutes)	379	169	136	134
Time in ER Before Being Evaluated (minutes)	41	90	26	26
Time to Pain Meds for Fractures (minutes)	28	88	52	57
Heart Attack Care				
Aspirin Given at Discharge[1]	-	-	99%	99%
Fibrinolytic Meds Within 30 Min. of Arrival[7]	-	-	-	54%

NOTE: Hospital profiles are in alphabetical order by state, then city, then hospital within the city; Rankings exclude hospitals with less than 25 cases except for patient surveys which excludes hospitals with less than 100 cases; (a) 100-299 cases; (1) The number of cases/patients is too few to report; (2) Data submitted were based on a sample of cases/patients; (3) Results are based on a shorter time period than required; (4) Data suppressed by CMS for one or more quarters; (5) Results are not available for this reporting period; (6) Fewer than 100 patients completed the HCAHPS survey; (7) No cases met the criteria for this measure; (8) The lower limit of the confidence interval cannot be calculated if the number of observed infections equals zero; (9) No data are available from the state/territory for this reporting period; (10) The scores shown reflect fewer than 50 completed surveys; (11) There were discrepancies in the data collection process; (12) This measure does not apply to this hospital for this reporting period; (13) Results cannot be calculated for this reporting period; (14) The results for this state are combined with nearby states to protect confidentiality; Please refer to the User's Guide for a full explanation of data.

Measure	Cases	This Hosp.	State Avg.	U.S. Avg.
PCI Within 90 Minutes of Arrival[7]	-	-	97%	96%
Statin Prescribed at Discharge[1]	-	-	98%	98%
Heart Failure Care				
ACE Inhibitor or ARB for LVSD	28	100%	96%	97%
Discharge Instructions Given	53	87%	94%	94%
Evaluation of LVS Function	63	98%	98%	99%
Medicare Spending				
Medicare Spending per Patient (ratio)	-	0.89	0.95	0.98
Pneumonia Care				
Appropriate Initial Antibiotic Given	71	97%	95%	95%
Blood Culture Timing	97	97%	98%	98%
Pregnancy and Delivery Care				
Newborn Deliveries Scheduled Early[2]	22	9%	5%	6%
Preventive Care				
Immunization for Influenza[2]	371	96%	92%	90%
Immunization for Pneumonia[2]	241	93%	93%	92%
Stroke Care				
Anticoagulation Therapy for Atrial Fibrillation[1]	-	-	94%	95%
Antithrombotic Therapy Timing	11	100%	98%	98%
Assessed for Rehabilitation	14	100%	98%	97%
Discharged on Antithrombotic Therapy	14	100%	99%	99%
Discharged on Statin Medication	11	82%	95%	94%
Thrombolytic Therapy Timing[7]	-	-	67%	66%
Venous Thromboembolism Prophylaxis	12	92%	95%	94%
Written Stroke Educational Materials Given	13	92%	88%	88%
Surgical Care Improvement Project				
Appropriate Beta Blocker Usage	49	100%	98%	98%
Appropriate VTP Within 24 Hours	154	97%	98%	98%
Controlled Postoperative Blood Glucose[7]	-	-	97%	97%
Perioperative Temperature Management	223	100%	100%	100%
Prophylactic Antibiotic Selection	169	99%	99%	99%
Prophylactic Antibiotic Selection (Outpatient)	24	96%	98%	98%
Prophylactic Antibiotic Stopped	169	100%	98%	98%
Prophylactic Antibiotic Timing	169	99%	99%	99%
Prophylactic Antibiotic Timing (Outpatient)	26	92%	98%	98%
Urinary Catheter Removal	38	100%	97%	97%
Survey of Patients' Hospital Experiences				
Area Around Room 'Always' Quiet at Night	(a)	64%	61%	61%
Doctors 'Always' Communicated Well	(a)	80%	82%	82%
Home Recovery Information Given	(a)	85%	87%	85%
Hospital Given 9 or 10 on 10 Point Scale	(a)	70%	71%	71%
Meds 'Always' Explained Before Given	(a)	64%	63%	64%
Nurses 'Always' Communicated Well	(a)	76%	79%	79%
Pain 'Always' Well Controlled	(a)	70%	71%	71%
Room and Bathroom 'Always' Clean	(a)	75%	73%	73%
Timely Help 'Always' Received	(a)	65%	68%	68%
Would Definitely Recommend Hospital	(a)	76%	70%	71%
Use of Medical Imaging				
Cardiac Imaging Stress Test before Surgery[1]	-	-	5.2%	5.3%
Combination Abdominal CT Scan	161	13.7%	11.2%	10.5%
Combination Brain/Sinus CT Scan[1]	-	-	3.2%	2.7%
Combination Chest CT Scan	91	2.2%	1.9%	2.7%
Follow-up Mammogram/Ultrasound	401	10.5%	8.6%	8.8%
Lumbar Spine MRI for Low Back Pain	39	51.3%	39.6%	37.2%

Twin Rivers Regional Medical Center

1301 First St
Kennett, MO 63857
Phone: 573-888-4522
Fax: 573-888-5525
URL: www.twinrivermedcenter.com
Type: Acute Care Hospitals
Ownership: Proprietary
Emergency Services: Yes
Beds: 116

Key Personnel:
Intensive Care Unit. . . . . Cathy Bradford, RN
Infection Control. . . . . Joanne Burton, RN
Operating Room. . . . . Joyce Danels, RN
Radiology. . . . . James G Hazel
Quality Assurance . . . . Geraldine Looney, RN
CEO/President. . . . . John McClellan
Emergency Room . . . . Bobby Sibbens, DO
Chief of Medical Staff. . . . . Maynard Sisler, MD

Measure	Cases	This Hosp.	State Avg.	U.S. Avg.
Blood Clot Prevention and Treatment				
Anticoagulation Overlap Therapy[1,2]	-	-	94%	93%
ICU Venous Thromboembolism Prophylaxis[2]	41	95%	91%	92%
Incidence of Potentially Preventable VTE[1,2]	-	-	7%	10%
UFH with Dosages/Platelet Monitoring[1,2]	-	-	96%	97%
Venous Thromboembolism Prophylaxis[2]	91	93%	85%	85%
Warfarin Therapy Discharge Instructions[1,2]	-	-	76%	75%
Chest Pain/Possible Heart Attack Care				
Aspirin Given Within 24 Hours of Arrival	105	97%	95%	96%
Fibrinolytic Meds Within 30 Min. of Arrival[1]	-	-	53%	58%
Average Time to ECG (minutes)	110	0	7	7
Average Time to Transfer (minutes)[7]	-	-	53	60
Children's Asthma Care				
Received Home Management Plan of Care	-	-	-	88%
Received Reliever Medication	-	-	-	100%
Received Systemic Corticosteroids	-	-	-	100%
Emergency Department				
Admittance Decision Time (minutes)[2]	253	62	81	98
Head CT Results Within 45 Min. of Arrival[1]	-	-	63%	57%
Patients Who Left ER Before Being Seen	23,434	2%	3%	2%
Time from ER Arrival to Admit. (minutes)[2]	253	208	238	274
Time from ER Arrival to Discharge (minutes)	329	114	136	134
Time in ER Before Being Evaluated (minutes)	385	16	26	26
Time to Pain Meds for Fractures (minutes)	31	44	52	57
Heart Attack Care				
Aspirin Given at Discharge[1]	-	-	99%	99%
Fibrinolytic Meds Within 30 Min. of Arrival[7]	-	-	-	54%
PCI Within 90 Minutes of Arrival[7]	-	-	97%	96%
Statin Prescribed at Discharge[1]	-	-	98%	98%
Heart Failure Care				
ACE Inhibitor or ARB for LVSD	17	100%	96%	97%
Discharge Instructions Given	43	88%	94%	94%
Evaluation of LVS Function	66	100%	98%	99%
Medicare Spending				
Medicare Spending per Patient (ratio)	-	0.95	0.95	0.98
Pneumonia Care				
Appropriate Initial Antibiotic Given	61	97%	95%	95%
Blood Culture Timing	131	100%	98%	98%
Pregnancy and Delivery Care				
Newborn Deliveries Scheduled Early	95	4%	5%	6%
Preventive Care				
Immunization for Influenza[2]	327	99%	92%	90%
Immunization for Pneumonia[2]	274	98%	93%	92%
Stroke Care				
Anticoagulation Therapy for Atrial Fibrillation[1]	-	-	94%	95%
Antithrombotic Therapy Timing[1]	-	-	98%	98%
Assessed for Rehabilitation[1]	-	-	98%	97%
Discharged on Antithrombotic Therapy[1]	-	-	99%	99%
Discharged on Statin Medication[1]	-	-	95%	94%
Thrombolytic Therapy Timing[7]	-	-	67%	66%
Venous Thromboembolism Prophylaxis[1]	-	-	95%	94%
Written Stroke Educational Materials Given[1]	-	-	88%	88%
Surgical Care Improvement Project				
Appropriate Beta Blocker Usage	23	100%	98%	98%
Appropriate VTP Within 24 Hours	80	100%	98%	98%
Controlled Postoperative Blood Glucose[7]	-	-	97%	97%
Perioperative Temperature Management	83	100%	100%	100%
Prophylactic Antibiotic Selection	55	100%	99%	99%
Prophylactic Antibiotic Selection (Outpatient)[1,3]	-	-	98%	98%
Prophylactic Antibiotic Stopped	53	98%	98%	98%
Prophylactic Antibiotic Timing	55	98%	99%	99%
Prophylactic Antibiotic Timing (Outpatient)[1,3]	-	-	98%	98%
Urinary Catheter Removal	42	98%	97%	97%
Survey of Patients' Hospital Experiences				
Area Around Room 'Always' Quiet at Night	(a)	65%	61%	61%
Doctors 'Always' Communicated Well	(a)	82%	82%	82%
Home Recovery Information Given	(a)	85%	87%	85%
Hospital Given 9 or 10 on 10 Point Scale	(a)	61%	71%	71%
Meds 'Always' Explained Before Given	(a)	66%	63%	64%
Nurses 'Always' Communicated Well	(a)	77%	79%	79%
Pain 'Always' Well Controlled	(a)	70%	71%	71%
Room and Bathroom 'Always' Clean	(a)	69%	73%	73%
Timely Help 'Always' Received	(a)	66%	68%	68%
Would Definitely Recommend Hospital	(a)	56%	70%	71%
Use of Medical Imaging				
Cardiac Imaging Stress Test before Surgery	196	5.1%	5.2%	5.3%
Combination Abdominal CT Scan	502	11.8%	11.2%	10.5%
Combination Brain/Sinus CT Scan	703	2.8%	3.2%	2.7%
Combination Chest CT Scan	219	21.5%	1.9%	2.7%
Follow-up Mammogram/Ultrasound	431	12.1%	8.6%	8.8%
Lumbar Spine MRI for Low Back Pain	142	25.4%	39.6%	37.2%

Northeast Regional Medical Center

315 S Osteopathy
Kirksville, MO 63501
Phone: 660-785-1000
Fax: 660-785-1110
URL: www.nermc.com
Type: Acute Care Hospitals
Ownership: Proprietary
Emergency Services: Yes
Beds: 109

Key Personnel:
Radiology. . . . . Thomas Bryce
Infection Control. . . . . Nita Coale, RN
Quality Assurance . . . . Cindy Dixon, RN
CEO/President. . . . . Robert Moore
Pediatric Ambulatory Care . . . . . . Paul Petry DO
Pediatric In-Patient Care . . . . Paul Petry DO
Chief of Medical Staff. . . . . Ronald Phillips, MD
Operating Room. . . . . Becky Taylor

Measure	Cases	This Hosp.	State Avg.	U.S. Avg.
Blood Clot Prevention and Treatment				
Anticoagulation Overlap Therapy[1,2]	-	-	94%	93%
ICU Venous Thromboembolism Prophylaxis[2]	100	100%	91%	92%
Incidence of Potentially Preventable VTE[2,7]	-	-	7%	10%
UFH with Dosages/Platelet Monitoring[1,2]	-	-	96%	97%
Venous Thromboembolism Prophylaxis[2]	150	100%	85%	85%
Warfarin Therapy Discharge Instructions[1,2]	-	-	76%	75%
Chest Pain/Possible Heart Attack Care				
Aspirin Given Within 24 Hours of Arrival	81	100%	95%	96%
Fibrinolytic Meds Within 30 Min. of Arrival[1]	-	-	53%	58%
Average Time to ECG (minutes)	82	3	7	7
Average Time to Transfer (minutes)[7]	-	-	53	60
Children's Asthma Care				
Received Home Management Plan of Care	-	-	-	88%
Received Reliever Medication	-	-	-	100%
Received Systemic Corticosteroids	-	-	-	100%
Emergency Department				
Admittance Decision Time (minutes)[2]	359	49	81	98
Head CT Results Within 45 Min. of Arrival[1]	-	-	63%	57%
Patients Who Left ER Before Being Seen	12,615	1%	3%	2%
Time from ER Arrival to Admit. (minutes)[2]	359	181	238	274
Time from ER Arrival to Discharge (minutes)	362	116	136	134
Time in ER Before Being Evaluated (minutes)	423	15	26	26
Time to Pain Meds for Fractures (minutes)	61	51	52	57
Heart Attack Care				
Aspirin Given at Discharge[1]	-	-	99%	99%
Fibrinolytic Meds Within 30 Min. of Arrival[7]	-	-	-	54%
PCI Within 90 Minutes of Arrival[1]	-	-	97%	96%
Statin Prescribed at Discharge[1]	-	-	98%	98%
Heart Failure Care				
ACE Inhibitor or ARB for LVSD	22	100%	96%	97%
Discharge Instructions Given	49	100%	94%	94%
Evaluation of LVS Function	71	100%	98%	99%
Medicare Spending				
Medicare Spending per Patient (ratio)	-	0.88	0.95	0.98
Pneumonia Care				
Appropriate Initial Antibiotic Given	33	100%	95%	95%
Blood Culture Timing	117	100%	98%	98%
Pregnancy and Delivery Care				
Newborn Deliveries Scheduled Early[2]	36	0%	5%	6%
Preventive Care				
Immunization for Influenza[2]	315	100%	92%	90%
Immunization for Pneumonia[2]	350	100%	93%	92%
Stroke Care				
Anticoagulation Therapy for Atrial Fibrillation[1]	-	-	94%	95%
Antithrombotic Therapy Timing[1]	-	-	98%	98%
Assessed for Rehabilitation[1]	-	-	98%	97%
Discharged on Antithrombotic Therapy[1]	-	-	99%	99%
Discharged on Statin Medication[1]	-	-	95%	94%
Thrombolytic Therapy Timing[7]	-	-	67%	66%
Venous Thromboembolism Prophylaxis[1]	-	-	95%	94%

NOTE: Hospital profiles are in alphabetical order by state, then city, then hospital within the city; Rankings exclude hospitals with less than 25 cases except for patient surveys which excludes hospitals with less than 100 cases; (a) 100-299 cases; (1) The number of cases/patients is too few to report; (2) Data submitted were based on a sample of cases/patients; (3) Results are based on a shorter time period than required; (4) Data suppressed by CMS for one or more quarters; (5) Results are not available for this reporting period; (6) Fewer than 100 patients completed the HCAHPS survey; (7) No cases met the criteria for this measure; (8) The lower limit of the confidence interval cannot be calculated if the number of observed infections equals zero; (9) No data are available from the state/territory for this reporting period; (10) The scores shown reflect fewer than 50 completed surveys; (11) There were discrepancies in the data collection process; (12) This measure does not apply to this hospital for this reporting period; (13) Results cannot be calculated for this reporting period; (14) The results for this state are combined with nearby states to protect confidentiality; Please refer to the User's Guide for a full explanation of data.

Measure	Cases	This Hosp.	State Avg.	U.S. Avg.
Written Stroke Educational Materials Given[1]	-	-	88%	88%
Surgical Care Improvement Project				
Appropriate Beta Blocker Usage	74	100%	98%	98%
Appropriate VTP Within 24 Hours	165	100%	98%	98%
Controlled Postoperative Blood Glucose[7]	-	-	97%	97%
Perioperative Temperature Management	194	100%	100%	100%
Prophylactic Antibiotic Selection	120	100%	99%	99%
Prophylactic Antibiotic Selection (Outpatient)	113	99%	98%	98%
Prophylactic Antibiotic Stopped	105	96%	98%	98%
Prophylactic Antibiotic Timing	120	100%	99%	99%
Prophylactic Antibiotic Timing (Outpatient)	97	100%	98%	98%
Urinary Catheter Removal	128	100%	97%	97%
Survey of Patients' Hospital Experiences				
Area Around Room 'Always' Quiet at Night	300+	65%	61%	61%
Doctors 'Always' Communicated Well	300+	82%	82%	82%
Home Recovery Information Given	300+	90%	87%	85%
Hospital Given 9 or 10 on 10 Point Scale	300+	72%	71%	71%
Meds 'Always' Explained Before Given	300+	65%	63%	64%
Nurses 'Always' Communicated Well	300+	80%	79%	79%
Pain 'Always' Well Controlled	300+	72%	71%	71%
Room and Bathroom 'Always' Clean	300+	74%	73%	73%
Timely Help 'Always' Received	300+	67%	68%	68%
Would Definitely Recommend Hospital	300+	65%	70%	71%
Use of Medical Imaging				
Cardiac Imaging Stress Test before Surgery	243	4.5%	5.2%	5.3%
Combination Abdominal CT Scan	365	30.1%	11.2%	10.5%
Combination Brain/Sinus CT Scan[1]	-	-	3.2%	2.7%
Combination Chest CT Scan	270	24.1%	1.9%	2.7%
Follow-up Mammogram/Ultrasound	765	15.3%	8.6%	8.8%
Lumbar Spine MRI for Low Back Pain[1]	-	-	39.6%	37.2%

SSM Saint Joseph Hospital West

100 Medical Plaza
Lake Saint Louis, MO 63367
Phone: 636-625-5200
Fax: 636-625-5314
Type: Acute Care Hospitals
Emergency Services: Yes
Ownership: Voluntary non-profit - Church
Beds: 100

Key Personnel:

Chief of Medical Staff.......... James Freeman, MD
CEO/President.............. Kevin Kast
Quality Assurance .... Pat Smith, RN
Emergency Room .... Tim Thompson, MD

Measure	Cases	This Hosp.	State Avg.	U.S. Avg.
Blood Clot Prevention and Treatment				
Anticoagulation Overlap Therapy[2]	57	91%	94%	93%
ICU Venous Thromboembolism Prophylaxis[2]	51	96%	91%	92%
Incidence of Potentially Preventable VTE[1,2]	-	-	7%	10%
UFH with Dosages/Platelet Monitoring[2]	23	74%	96%	97%
Venous Thromboembolism Prophylaxis[2]	321	95%	85%	85%
Warfarin Therapy Discharge Instructions[2]	49	65%	76%	75%
Chest Pain/Possible Heart Attack Care				
Aspirin Given Within 24 Hours of Arrival	34	94%	95%	96%
Fibrinolytic Meds Within 30 Min. of Arrival[3,7]	-	-	53%	58%
Average Time to ECG (minutes)	36	8	7	7
Average Time to Transfer (minutes)[3,7]	-	-	53	60
Children's Asthma Care				
Received Home Management Plan of Care	-	-	-	88%
Received Reliever Medication	-	-	-	100%
Received Systemic Corticosteroids	-	-	-	100%
Emergency Department				
Admittance Decision Time (minutes)[2]	429	103	81	98
Head CT Results Within 45 Min. of Arrival	19	95%	63%	57%
Patients Who Left ER Before Being Seen	41,416	0%	3%	2%
Time from ER Arrival to Admit. (minutes)[2]	502	220	238	274
Time from ER Arrival to Discharge (minutes)	377	155	136	134
Time in ER Before Being Evaluated (minutes)	406	28	26	26
Time to Pain Meds for Fractures (minutes)	92	34	52	57
Heart Attack Care				
Aspirin Given at Discharge	249	100%	99%	99%
Fibrinolytic Meds Within 30 Min. of Arrival[7]	-	-	-	54%
PCI Within 90 Minutes of Arrival	33	100%	97%	96%
Statin Prescribed at Discharge	247	100%	98%	98%
Heart Failure Care				
ACE Inhibitor or ARB for LVSD[2]	50	100%	96%	97%
Discharge Instructions Given[2]	198	99%	94%	94%
Evaluation of LVS Function[2]	265	100%	98%	99%
Medicare Spending				
Medicare Spending per Patient (ratio)	-	0.94	0.95	0.98
Pneumonia Care				
Appropriate Initial Antibiotic Given[2]	80	95%	95%	95%
Blood Culture Timing[2]	111	97%	98%	98%
Pregnancy and Delivery Care				
Newborn Deliveries Scheduled Early[2]	26	4%	5%	6%
Preventive Care				
Immunization for Influenza[2]	520	99%	92%	90%
Immunization for Pneumonia[2]	628	100%	93%	92%
Stroke Care				
Anticoagulation Therapy for Atrial Fibrillation[1]	-	-	94%	95%
Antithrombotic Therapy Timing	88	99%	98%	98%
Assessed for Rehabilitation	103	100%	98%	97%
Discharged on Antithrombotic Therapy	100	99%	99%	99%
Discharged on Statin Medication	77	99%	95%	94%
Thrombolytic Therapy Timing	14	100%	67%	66%
Venous Thromboembolism Prophylaxis	93	100%	95%	94%
Written Stroke Educational Materials Given	61	97%	88%	88%
Surgical Care Improvement Project				
Appropriate Beta Blocker Usage[2]	98	97%	98%	98%
Appropriate VTP Within 24 Hours[2]	307	100%	98%	98%
Controlled Postoperative Blood Glucose[2,7]	-	-	97%	97%
Perioperative Temperature Management[2]	334	100%	100%	100%
Prophylactic Antibiotic Selection[2]	191	100%	99%	99%
Prophylactic Antibiotic Selection (Outpatient)	236	99%	98%	98%
Prophylactic Antibiotic Stopped[2]	187	100%	98%	98%
Prophylactic Antibiotic Timing[2]	192	100%	99%	99%
Prophylactic Antibiotic Timing (Outpatient)	236	100%	98%	98%
Urinary Catheter Removal[2]	191	99%	97%	97%
Survey of Patients' Hospital Experiences				
Area Around Room 'Always' Quiet at Night	300+	55%	61%	61%
Doctors 'Always' Communicated Well	300+	80%	82%	82%
Home Recovery Information Given	300+	87%	87%	85%
Hospital Given 9 or 10 on 10 Point Scale	300+	78%	71%	71%
Meds 'Always' Explained Before Given	300+	67%	63%	64%
Nurses 'Always' Communicated Well	300+	83%	79%	79%
Pain 'Always' Well Controlled	300+	73%	71%	71%
Room and Bathroom 'Always' Clean	300+	76%	73%	73%
Timely Help 'Always' Received	300+	67%	68%	68%
Would Definitely Recommend Hospital	300+	80%	70%	71%
Use of Medical Imaging				
Cardiac Imaging Stress Test before Surgery	540	6.1%	5.2%	5.3%
Combination Abdominal CT Scan	837	5.0%	11.2%	10.5%
Combination Brain/Sinus CT Scan	687	3.1%	3.2%	2.7%
Combination Chest CT Scan	535	0.7%	1.9%	2.7%
Follow-up Mammogram/Ultrasound	1,306	6.4%	8.6%	8.8%
Lumbar Spine MRI for Low Back Pain	141	35.5%	39.6%	37.2%

Barton County Memorial Hospital

29 Nw 1st Lane
Lamar, MO 64759
Phone: 417-682-6081
Fax: 417-682-2138
URL: www.bcmh.net
Type: Critical Access Hospitals
Emergency Services: Yes
Ownership: Government - Local
Beds: 49

Key Personnel:

CEO .... Wendy Duvall
Quality Assurance .... Kathleen Jones
Emergency Room .... Kate Mallumian
CEO/President............. Rudy Snedigar
Chairman/CEO .... Karen O'S Wegener
Chief of Medical Staff.......... Joseph Wilson

Measure	Cases	This Hosp.	State Avg.	U.S. Avg.
Blood Clot Prevention and Treatment				
Anticoagulation Overlap Therapy[1,3]	-	-	94%	93%
ICU Venous Thromboembolism Prophylaxis[3,7]	-	-	91%	92%
Incidence of Potentially Preventable VTE[3,7]	-	-	7%	10%
UFH with Dosages/Platelet Monitoring[1,3]	-	-	96%	97%
Venous Thromboembolism Prophylaxis[3,7]	-	-	85%	85%
Warfarin Therapy Discharge Instructions[3,7]	-	-	76%	75%
Chest Pain/Possible Heart Attack Care				
Aspirin Given Within 24 Hours of Arrival	-	-	95%	96%
Fibrinolytic Meds Within 30 Min. of Arrival	-	-	53%	58%
Average Time to ECG (minutes)	-	-	7	7
Average Time to Transfer (minutes)	-	-	53	60
Children's Asthma Care				
Received Home Management Plan of Care	-	-	-	88%
Received Reliever Medication	-	-	-	100%
Received Systemic Corticosteroids	-	-	-	100%
Emergency Department				
Admittance Decision Time (minutes)[5]	-	-	81	98
Head CT Results Within 45 Min. of Arrival	-	-	63%	57%
Patients Who Left ER Before Being Seen	-	-	3%	2%
Time from ER Arrival to Admit. (minutes)[5]	-	-	238	274
Time from ER Arrival to Discharge (minutes)	-	-	136	134
Time in ER Before Being Evaluated (minutes)	-	-	26	26
Time to Pain Meds for Fractures (minutes)	-	-	52	57
Heart Attack Care				
Aspirin Given at Discharge[1,3]	-	-	99%	99%
Fibrinolytic Meds Within 30 Min. of Arrival[3,7]	-	-	-	54%
PCI Within 90 Minutes of Arrival[3,7]	-	-	97%	96%
Statin Prescribed at Discharge[1,3]	-	-	98%	98%
Heart Failure Care				
ACE Inhibitor or ARB for LVSD[1]	-	-	96%	97%
Discharge Instructions Given	24	67%	94%	94%
Evaluation of LVS Function	34	82%	98%	99%
Medicare Spending				
Medicare Spending per Patient (ratio)	-	-	0.95	0.98
Pneumonia Care				
Appropriate Initial Antibiotic Given	60	88%	95%	95%
Blood Culture Timing	43	93%	98%	98%
Pregnancy and Delivery Care				
Newborn Deliveries Scheduled Early[5]	-	-	5%	6%
Preventive Care				
Immunization for Influenza[5]	-	-	92%	90%
Immunization for Pneumonia[5]	-	-	93%	92%
Stroke Care				
Anticoagulation Therapy for Atrial Fibrillation[5]	-	-	94%	95%
Antithrombotic Therapy Timing[5]	-	-	98%	98%
Assessed for Rehabilitation[5]	-	-	98%	97%
Discharged on Antithrombotic Therapy[5]	-	-	99%	99%
Discharged on Statin Medication[5]	-	-	95%	94%
Thrombolytic Therapy Timing[5]	-	-	67%	66%
Venous Thromboembolism Prophylaxis[5]	-	-	95%	94%
Written Stroke Educational Materials Given[5]	-	-	88%	88%
Surgical Care Improvement Project				
Appropriate Beta Blocker Usage	12	83%	98%	98%
Appropriate VTP Within 24 Hours[3]	15	100%	98%	98%
Controlled Postoperative Blood Glucose[3,7]	-	-	97%	97%
Perioperative Temperature Management	46	100%	100%	100%
Prophylactic Antibiotic Selection[3]	14	100%	99%	99%
Prophylactic Antibiotic Selection (Outpatient)	-	-	98%	98%
Prophylactic Antibiotic Stopped[3]	14	100%	98%	98%
Prophylactic Antibiotic Timing[3]	14	86%	99%	99%
Prophylactic Antibiotic Timing (Outpatient)	-	-	98%	98%
Urinary Catheter Removal	36	97%	97%	97%
Survey of Patients' Hospital Experiences				
Area Around Room 'Always' Quiet at Night	(a)	73%	61%	61%
Doctors 'Always' Communicated Well	(a)	90%	82%	82%
Home Recovery Information Given	(a)	86%	87%	85%
Hospital Given 9 or 10 on 10 Point Scale	(a)	79%	71%	71%
Meds 'Always' Explained Before Given	(a)	69%	63%	64%
Nurses 'Always' Communicated Well	(a)	88%	79%	79%
Pain 'Always' Well Controlled	(a)	82%	71%	71%
Room and Bathroom 'Always' Clean	(a)	85%	73%	73%
Timely Help 'Always' Received	(a)	77%	68%	68%
Would Definitely Recommend Hospital	(a)	80%	70%	71%
Use of Medical Imaging				
Cardiac Imaging Stress Test before Surgery	-	-	5.2%	5.3%
Combination Abdominal CT Scan	-	-	11.2%	10.5%
Combination Brain/Sinus CT Scan	-	-	3.2%	2.7%
Combination Chest CT Scan	-	-	1.9%	2.7%
Follow-up Mammogram/Ultrasound	-	-	8.6%	8.8%
Lumbar Spine MRI for Low Back Pain	-	-	39.6%	37.2%

NOTE: Hospital profiles are in alphabetical order by state, then city, then hospital within the city; Rankings exclude hospitals with less than 25 cases except for patient surveys which excludes hospitals with less than 100 cases; (a) 100-299 cases; (1) The number of cases/patients is too few to report; (2) Data submitted were based on a sample of cases/patients; (3) Results are based on a shorter time period than required; (4) Data suppressed by CMS for one or more quarters; (5) Results are not available for this reporting period; (6) Fewer than 100 patients completed the HCAHPS survey; (7) No cases met the criteria for this measure; (8) The lower limit of the confidence interval cannot be calculated if the number of observed infections equals zero; (9) No data are available from the state/territory for this reporting period; (10) The scores shown reflect fewer than 50 completed surveys; (11) There were discrepancies in the data collection process; (12) This measure does not apply to this hospital for this reporting period; (13) Results cannot be calculated for this reporting period; (14) The results for this state are combined with nearby states to protect confidentiality; Please refer to the User's Guide for a full explanation of data.

Mercy Hospital Lebanon

100 Hospital Drive — Phone: 417-533-6100
Lebanon, MO 65536 — Fax: 417-533-6040
E-mail: rttinshaw@sprg.smhs.com
Type: Acute Care Hospitals — Emergency Services: Yes
Ownership: Voluntary non-profit - Church — Beds: 41

Key Personnel:
Radiology. . . . . Barbara Groves
Surgery . . . . Samira M. Hasan, DO
CEO/President. . . . . Gary Pulsipher
Patient Relations . . . . Sue Sturgill

Measure	Cases	This Hosp.	State Avg.	U.S. Avg.
Blood Clot Prevention and Treatment				
Anticoagulation Overlap Therapy[2]	19	79%	94%	93%
ICU Venous Thromboembolism Prophylaxis[2]	54	94%	91%	92%
Incidence of Potentially Preventable VTE[1,2]	-	-	7%	10%
UFH with Dosages/Platelet Monitoring[2]	16	100%	96%	97%
Venous Thromboembolism Prophylaxis[2]	165	95%	85%	85%
Warfarin Therapy Discharge Instructions[2]	12	58%	76%	75%
Chest Pain/Possible Heart Attack Care				
Aspirin Given Within 24 Hours of Arrival	138	98%	95%	96%
Fibrinolytic Meds Within 30 Min. of Arrival[1]	-	-	53%	58%
Average Time to ECG (minutes)	140	10	7	7
Average Time to Transfer (minutes)	11	53	53	60
Children's Asthma Care				
Received Home Management Plan of Care	-	-	-	88%
Received Reliever Medication	-	-	-	100%
Received Systemic Corticosteroids	-	-	-	100%
Emergency Department				
Admittance Decision Time (minutes)[2]	222	88	81	98
Head CT Results Within 45 Min. of Arrival	14	50%	63%	57%
Patients Who Left ER Before Being Seen	29,143	1%	3%	2%
Time from ER Arrival to Admit. (minutes)[2]	231	250	238	274
Time from ER Arrival to Discharge (minutes)	338	139	136	134
Time in ER Before Being Evaluated (minutes)	394	14	26	26
Time to Pain Meds for Fractures (minutes)	56	44	52	57
Heart Attack Care				
Aspirin Given at Discharge[1]	-	-	99%	99%
Fibrinolytic Meds Within 30 Min. of Arrival[7]	-	-	-	54%
PCI Within 90 Minutes of Arrival[7]	-	-	97%	96%
Statin Prescribed at Discharge[1]	-	-	98%	98%
Heart Failure Care				
ACE Inhibitor or ARB for LVSD	40	88%	96%	97%
Discharge Instructions Given	95	95%	94%	94%
Evaluation of LVS Function	118	100%	98%	99%
Medicare Spending				
Medicare Spending per Patient (ratio)	-	0.89	0.95	0.98
Pneumonia Care				
Appropriate Initial Antibiotic Given[2]	67	99%	95%	95%
Blood Culture Timing[2]	101	99%	98%	98%
Pregnancy and Delivery Care				
Newborn Deliveries Scheduled Early[2]	26	4%	5%	6%
Preventive Care				
Immunization for Influenza[2]	271	89%	92%	90%
Immunization for Pneumonia[2]	354	99%	93%	92%
Stroke Care				
Anticoagulation Therapy for Atrial Fibrillation[1]	-	-	94%	95%
Antithrombotic Therapy Timing	12	100%	98%	98%
Assessed for Rehabilitation	14	86%	98%	97%
Discharged on Antithrombotic Therapy	14	100%	99%	99%
Discharged on Statin Medication	11	91%	95%	94%
Thrombolytic Therapy Timing[7]	-	-	67%	66%
Venous Thromboembolism Prophylaxis	11	82%	95%	94%
Written Stroke Educational Materials Given	12	50%	88%	88%
Surgical Care Improvement Project				
Appropriate Beta Blocker Usage[2]	52	98%	98%	98%
Appropriate VTP Within 24 Hours[2]	153	98%	98%	98%
Controlled Postoperative Blood Glucose[2,7]	-	-	97%	97%
Perioperative Temperature Management[2]	168	98%	100%	100%
Prophylactic Antibiotic Selection[2]	134	100%	99%	99%
Prophylactic Antibiotic Selection (Outpatient)	45	98%	98%	98%
Prophylactic Antibiotic Stopped[2]	134	97%	98%	98%
Prophylactic Antibiotic Timing[2]	134	99%	99%	99%
Prophylactic Antibiotic Timing (Outpatient)	46	98%	98%	98%
Urinary Catheter Removal[2]	142	99%	97%	97%
Survey of Patients' Hospital Experiences				
Area Around Room 'Always' Quiet at Night[11]	300+	50%	61%	61%
Doctors 'Always' Communicated Well[11]	300+	85%	82%	82%
Home Recovery Information Given[11]	300+	90%	87%	85%
Hospital Given 9 or 10 on 10 Point Scale[11]	300+	73%	71%	71%
Meds 'Always' Explained Before Given[11]	300+	68%	63%	64%
Nurses 'Always' Communicated Well[11]	300+	81%	79%	79%
Pain 'Always' Well Controlled[11]	300+	73%	71%	71%
Room and Bathroom 'Always' Clean[11]	300+	77%	73%	73%
Timely Help 'Always' Received[11]	300+	71%	68%	68%
Would Definitely Recommend Hospital[11]	300+	69%	70%	71%
Use of Medical Imaging				
Cardiac Imaging Stress Test before Surgery	227	4.8%	5.2%	5.3%
Combination Abdominal CT Scan	604	3.6%	11.2%	10.5%
Combination Brain/Sinus CT Scan	597	2.2%	3.2%	2.7%
Combination Chest CT Scan	338	5.6%	1.9%	2.7%
Follow-up Mammogram/Ultrasound	1,021	6.8%	8.6%	8.8%
Lumbar Spine MRI for Low Back Pain	133	67.7%	39.6%	37.2%

Lee's Summit Medical Center

2100 Se Blue Parkway — Phone: 816-282-5000
Lees Summit, MO 64063 — Fax: 816-969-6523
URL: www.leessummithospital.com
Type: Acute Care Hospitals — Emergency Services: Yes
Ownership: Proprietary — Beds: 83

Key Personnel:
CEO/President. . . . . Carolyn W Caldwell
Chief of Medical Staff. . . . . Andrew S Pavlovich, MD

Measure	Cases	This Hosp.	State Avg.	U.S. Avg.
Blood Clot Prevention and Treatment				
Anticoagulation Overlap Therapy[2]	20	100%	94%	93%
ICU Venous Thromboembolism Prophylaxis[2]	93	100%	91%	92%
Incidence of Potentially Preventable VTE[1,2]	-	-	7%	10%
UFH with Dosages/Platelet Monitoring[1,2]	-	-	96%	97%
Venous Thromboembolism Prophylaxis[2]	271	100%	85%	85%
Warfarin Therapy Discharge Instructions[2]	12	92%	76%	75%
Chest Pain/Possible Heart Attack Care				
Aspirin Given Within 24 Hours of Arrival[5]	-	-	95%	96%
Fibrinolytic Meds Within 30 Min. of Arrival[5]	-	-	53%	58%
Average Time to ECG (minutes)[5]	-	-	7	7
Average Time to Transfer (minutes)[5]	-	-	53	60
Children's Asthma Care				
Received Home Management Plan of Care	-	-	-	88%
Received Reliever Medication	-	-	-	100%
Received Systemic Corticosteroids	-	-	-	100%
Emergency Department				
Admittance Decision Time (minutes)[2]	361	59	81	98
Head CT Results Within 45 Min. of Arrival[1]	-	-	63%	57%
Patients Who Left ER Before Being Seen	16,699	0%	3%	2%
Time from ER Arrival to Admit. (minutes)[2]	422	188	238	274
Time from ER Arrival to Discharge (minutes)	428	112	136	134
Time in ER Before Being Evaluated (minutes)	478	13	26	26
Time to Pain Meds for Fractures (minutes)	70	40	52	57
Heart Attack Care				
Aspirin Given at Discharge	93	100%	99%	99%
Fibrinolytic Meds Within 30 Min. of Arrival[7]	-	-	-	54%
PCI Within 90 Minutes of Arrival	13	92%	97%	96%
Statin Prescribed at Discharge	92	100%	98%	98%
Heart Failure Care				
ACE Inhibitor or ARB for LVSD	34	100%	96%	97%
Discharge Instructions Given	90	99%	94%	94%
Evaluation of LVS Function	127	100%	98%	99%
Medicare Spending				
Medicare Spending per Patient (ratio)	-	1.01	0.95	0.98
Pneumonia Care				
Appropriate Initial Antibiotic Given	41	100%	95%	95%
Blood Culture Timing	75	100%	98%	98%
Pregnancy and Delivery Care				
Newborn Deliveries Scheduled Early[2,7]	-	-	5%	6%
Preventive Care				
Immunization for Influenza[2]	425	100%	92%	90%
Immunization for Pneumonia[2]	632	99%	93%	92%
Stroke Care				
Anticoagulation Therapy for Atrial Fibrillation[1]	-	-	94%	95%
Antithrombotic Therapy Timing	38	100%	98%	98%
Assessed for Rehabilitation	43	100%	98%	97%
Discharged on Antithrombotic Therapy	43	100%	99%	99%
Discharged on Statin Medication	30	100%	95%	94%
Thrombolytic Therapy Timing[1]	-	-	67%	66%
Venous Thromboembolism Prophylaxis	36	100%	95%	94%
Written Stroke Educational Materials Given	17	100%	88%	88%
Surgical Care Improvement Project				
Appropriate Beta Blocker Usage	88	100%	98%	98%
Appropriate VTP Within 24 Hours	273	100%	98%	98%
Controlled Postoperative Blood Glucose[7]	-	-	97%	97%
Perioperative Temperature Management	316	100%	100%	100%
Prophylactic Antibiotic Selection	220	100%	99%	99%
Prophylactic Antibiotic Selection (Outpatient)	142	99%	98%	98%
Prophylactic Antibiotic Stopped	215	100%	98%	98%
Prophylactic Antibiotic Timing	220	100%	99%	99%
Prophylactic Antibiotic Timing (Outpatient)	143	99%	98%	98%
Urinary Catheter Removal	87	100%	97%	97%
Survey of Patients' Hospital Experiences				
Area Around Room 'Always' Quiet at Night	300+	66%	61%	61%
Doctors 'Always' Communicated Well	300+	81%	82%	82%
Home Recovery Information Given	300+	89%	87%	85%
Hospital Given 9 or 10 on 10 Point Scale	300+	74%	71%	71%
Meds 'Always' Explained Before Given	300+	63%	63%	64%
Nurses 'Always' Communicated Well	300+	78%	79%	79%
Pain 'Always' Well Controlled	300+	72%	71%	71%
Room and Bathroom 'Always' Clean	300+	74%	73%	73%
Timely Help 'Always' Received	300+	71%	68%	68%
Would Definitely Recommend Hospital	300+	72%	70%	71%
Use of Medical Imaging				
Cardiac Imaging Stress Test before Surgery	100	4.0%	5.2%	5.3%
Combination Abdominal CT Scan	265	11.3%	11.2%	10.5%
Combination Brain/Sinus CT Scan[1]	-	-	3.2%	2.7%
Combination Chest CT Scan	115	2.6%	1.9%	2.7%
Follow-up Mammogram/Ultrasound	450	10.7%	8.6%	8.8%
Lumbar Spine MRI for Low Back Pain	41	43.9%	39.6%	37.2%

Saint Luke's East Lee's Summit Hospital

100 N E Saint Luke's Boulevard — Phone: 816-347-5000
Lees Summit, MO 64086
Type: Acute Care Hospitals — Emergency Services: Yes
Ownership: Voluntary non-profit - Private — Beds: 57

Key Personnel:
CEO/President. . . . . Ron Baker, FACHE, CPME

Measure	Cases	This Hosp.	State Avg.	U.S. Avg.
Blood Clot Prevention and Treatment				
Anticoagulation Overlap Therapy[2]	59	100%	94%	93%
ICU Venous Thromboembolism Prophylaxis[2]	61	82%	91%	92%
Incidence of Potentially Preventable VTE[1,2]	-	-	7%	10%
UFH with Dosages/Platelet Monitoring[2]	70	99%	96%	97%
Venous Thromboembolism Prophylaxis[2]	316	72%	85%	85%
Warfarin Therapy Discharge Instructions[2]	38	63%	76%	75%
Chest Pain/Possible Heart Attack Care				
Aspirin Given Within 24 Hours of Arrival	15	93%	95%	96%
Fibrinolytic Meds Within 30 Min. of Arrival[3,7]	-	-	53%	58%
Average Time to ECG (minutes)	15	8	7	7
Average Time to Transfer (minutes)[3,7]	-	-	53	60
Children's Asthma Care				
Received Home Management Plan of Care	-	-	-	88%
Received Reliever Medication	-	-	-	100%
Received Systemic Corticosteroids	-	-	-	100%
Emergency Department				
Admittance Decision Time (minutes)[2]	490	134	81	98
Head CT Results Within 45 Min. of Arrival	21	90%	63%	57%
Patients Who Left ER Before Being Seen	38,727	2%	3%	2%
Time from ER Arrival to Admit. (minutes)[2]	491	266	238	274
Time from ER Arrival to Discharge (minutes)	353	144	136	134
Time in ER Before Being Evaluated (minutes)	317	30	26	26
Time to Pain Meds for Fractures (minutes)	123	56	52	57

NOTE: Hospital profiles are in alphabetical order by state, then city, then hospital within the city; Rankings exclude hospitals with less than 25 cases except for patient surveys which excludes hospitals with less than 100 cases; (a) 100-299 cases; (1) The number of cases/patients is too few to report; (2) Data submitted were based on a sample of cases/patients; (3) Results are based on a shorter time period than required; (4) Data suppressed by CMS for one or more quarters; (5) Results are not available for this reporting period; (6) Fewer than 100 patients completed the HCAHPS survey; (7) No cases met the criteria for this measure; (8) The lower limit of the confidence interval cannot be calculated if the number of observed infections equals zero; (9) No data are available from the state/territory for this reporting period; (10) The scores shown reflect fewer than 50 completed surveys; (11) There were discrepancies in the data collection process; (12) This measure does not apply to this hospital for this reporting period; (13) Results cannot be calculated for this reporting period; (14) The results for this state are combined with nearby states to protect confidentiality; Please refer to the User's Guide for a full explanation of data.

Measure	Cases	This Hosp.	State Avg.	U.S. Avg.
Heart Attack Care				
Aspirin Given at Discharge	164	100%	99%	99%
Fibrinolytic Meds Within 30 Min. of Arrival[7]	-	-	-	54%
PCI Within 90 Minutes of Arrival	36	97%	97%	96%
Statin Prescribed at Discharge	164	100%	98%	98%
Heart Failure Care				
ACE Inhibitor or ARB for LVSD	78	100%	96%	97%
Discharge Instructions Given	239	96%	94%	94%
Evaluation of LVS Function	305	100%	98%	99%
Medicare Spending				
Medicare Spending per Patient (ratio)	-	0.99	0.95	0.98
Pneumonia Care				
Appropriate Initial Antibiotic Given	169	98%	95%	95%
Blood Culture Timing	285	100%	98%	98%
Pregnancy and Delivery Care				
Newborn Deliveries Scheduled Early[2]	26	0%	5%	6%
Preventive Care				
Immunization for Influenza[2]	512	97%	92%	90%
Immunization for Pneumonia[2]	608	97%	93%	92%
Stroke Care				
Anticoagulation Therapy for Atrial Fibrillation	13	100%	94%	95%
Antithrombotic Therapy Timing	77	97%	98%	98%
Assessed for Rehabilitation	109	100%	98%	97%
Discharged on Antithrombotic Therapy	106	100%	99%	99%
Discharged on Statin Medication	76	99%	95%	94%
Thrombolytic Therapy Timing[1]	-	-	67%	66%
Venous Thromboembolism Prophylaxis	82	96%	95%	94%
Written Stroke Educational Materials Given	69	83%	88%	88%
Surgical Care Improvement Project				
Appropriate Beta Blocker Usage	158	99%	98%	98%
Appropriate VTP Within 24 Hours	503	100%	98%	98%
Controlled Postoperative Blood Glucose[7]	-	-	97%	97%
Perioperative Temperature Management	594	100%	100%	100%
Prophylactic Antibiotic Selection	344	99%	99%	99%
Prophylactic Antibiotic Selection (Outpatient)	299	99%	98%	98%
Prophylactic Antibiotic Stopped	335	100%	98%	98%
Prophylactic Antibiotic Timing	344	100%	99%	99%
Prophylactic Antibiotic Timing (Outpatient)	299	100%	98%	98%
Urinary Catheter Removal	142	96%	97%	97%
Survey of Patients' Hospital Experiences				
Area Around Room 'Always' Quiet at Night	300+	62%	61%	61%
Doctors 'Always' Communicated Well	300+	80%	82%	82%
Home Recovery Information Given	300+	91%	87%	85%
Hospital Given 9 or 10 on 10 Point Scale	300+	78%	71%	71%
Meds 'Always' Explained Before Given	300+	63%	63%	64%
Nurses 'Always' Communicated Well	300+	80%	79%	79%
Pain 'Always' Well Controlled	300+	72%	71%	71%
Room and Bathroom 'Always' Clean	300+	76%	73%	73%
Timely Help 'Always' Received	300+	62%	68%	68%
Would Definitely Recommend Hospital	300+	83%	70%	71%
Use of Medical Imaging				
Cardiac Imaging Stress Test before Surgery	367	5.2%	5.2%	5.3%
Combination Abdominal CT Scan	1,044	2.2%	11.2%	10.5%
Combination Brain/Sinus CT Scan	865	3.4%	3.2%	2.7%
Combination Chest CT Scan	643	0.0%	1.9%	2.7%
Follow-up Mammogram/Ultrasound	1,037	8.4%	8.6%	8.8%
Lumbar Spine MRI for Low Back Pain	120	44.2%	39.6%	37.2%

Lafayette Regional Health Center

1500 State Street
Lexington, MO 64067
URL: www.lafayetteregionalhealthcenter.com
Type: Critical Access Hospitals
Ownership: Proprietary
Phone: 660-259-2203
Fax: 660-259-6819
Emergency Services: Yes
Beds: 49

Key Personnel:
Infection Control. . . . . Jeannette Buckets, RN
Quality Assurance . . . . Debbie Green, RN
CEO/President. . . . . Bret Kolmant
Radiology. . . . . Teresa Mannick
Operating Room. . . . . Julie Osman, RN
Emergency Room . . . . Deb Peck, RN
Chief of Medical Staff. . . . . Clint Pickett, DO
Intensive Care Unit. . . . . Dena Stark, RN

Measure	Cases	This Hosp.	State Avg.	U.S. Avg.
Blood Clot Prevention and Treatment				
Anticoagulation Overlap Therapy[1,2]	-	-	94%	93%
ICU Venous Thromboembolism Prophylaxis[2]	22	100%	91%	92%
Incidence of Potentially Preventable VTE[1,2]	-	-	7%	10%
UFH with Dosages/Platelet Monitoring[2,7]	-	-	96%	97%
Venous Thromboembolism Prophylaxis[2]	122	100%	85%	85%
Warfarin Therapy Discharge Instructions[1,2]	-	-	76%	75%
Chest Pain/Possible Heart Attack Care				
Aspirin Given Within 24 Hours of Arrival	20	100%	95%	96%
Fibrinolytic Meds Within 30 Min. of Arrival[7]	-	-	53%	58%
Average Time to ECG (minutes)	21	5	7	7
Average Time to Transfer (minutes)[1]	-	-	53	60
Children's Asthma Care				
Received Home Management Plan of Care	-	-	-	88%
Received Reliever Medication	-	-	-	100%
Received Systemic Corticosteroids	-	-	-	100%
Emergency Department				
Admittance Decision Time (minutes)[2]	408	76	81	98
Head CT Results Within 45 Min. of Arrival[1]	-	-	63%	57%
Patients Who Left ER Before Being Seen	9,175	1%	3%	2%
Time from ER Arrival to Admit. (minutes)[2]	410	162	238	274
Time from ER Arrival to Discharge (minutes)	410	87	136	134
Time in ER Before Being Evaluated (minutes)	469	9	26	26
Time to Pain Meds for Fractures (minutes)	37	37	52	57
Heart Attack Care				
Aspirin Given at Discharge[1,3]	-	-	99%	99%
Fibrinolytic Meds Within 30 Min. of Arrival[3,7]	-	-	-	54%
PCI Within 90 Minutes of Arrival[3,7]	-	-	97%	96%
Statin Prescribed at Discharge[1,3]	-	-	98%	98%
Heart Failure Care				
ACE Inhibitor or ARB for LVSD[1]	-	-	96%	97%
Discharge Instructions Given	12	100%	94%	94%
Evaluation of LVS Function	16	100%	98%	99%
Medicare Spending				
Medicare Spending per Patient (ratio)	-	-	0.95	0.98
Pneumonia Care				
Appropriate Initial Antibiotic Given	23	100%	95%	95%
Blood Culture Timing	43	100%	98%	98%
Pregnancy and Delivery Care				
Newborn Deliveries Scheduled Early[2,7]	-	-	5%	6%
Preventive Care				
Immunization for Influenza[2]	301	100%	92%	90%
Immunization for Pneumonia[2]	435	100%	93%	92%
Stroke Care				
Anticoagulation Therapy for Atrial Fibrillation[7]	-	-	94%	95%
Antithrombotic Therapy Timing	13	100%	98%	98%
Assessed for Rehabilitation[1]	-	-	98%	97%
Discharged on Antithrombotic Therapy[1]	-	-	99%	99%
Discharged on Statin Medication[1]	-	-	95%	94%
Thrombolytic Therapy Timing[7]	-	-	67%	66%
Venous Thromboembolism Prophylaxis	12	100%	95%	94%
Written Stroke Educational Materials Given[1]	-	-	88%	88%
Surgical Care Improvement Project				
Appropriate Beta Blocker Usage[1]	-	-	98%	98%
Appropriate VTP Within 24 Hours	21	100%	98%	98%
Controlled Postoperative Blood Glucose[7]	-	-	97%	97%
Perioperative Temperature Management	22	100%	100%	100%
Prophylactic Antibiotic Selection	14	100%	99%	99%
Prophylactic Antibiotic Selection (Outpatient)	17	94%	98%	98%
Prophylactic Antibiotic Stopped	14	100%	98%	98%
Prophylactic Antibiotic Timing	15	100%	99%	99%
Prophylactic Antibiotic Timing (Outpatient)	17	100%	98%	98%
Urinary Catheter Removal[1]	-	-	97%	97%
Survey of Patients' Hospital Experiences				
Area Around Room 'Always' Quiet at Night	(a)	56%	61%	61%
Doctors 'Always' Communicated Well	(a)	87%	82%	82%
Home Recovery Information Given	(a)	92%	87%	85%
Hospital Given 9 or 10 on 10 Point Scale	(a)	74%	71%	71%
Meds 'Always' Explained Before Given	(a)	72%	63%	64%
Nurses 'Always' Communicated Well	(a)	83%	79%	79%
Pain 'Always' Well Controlled	(a)	76%	71%	71%
Room and Bathroom 'Always' Clean	(a)	73%	73%	73%
Timely Help 'Always' Received	(a)	74%	68%	68%
Would Definitely Recommend Hospital	(a)	69%	70%	71%
Use of Medical Imaging				
Cardiac Imaging Stress Test before Surgery[1]	-	-	5.2%	5.3%
Combination Abdominal CT Scan	223	6.7%	11.2%	10.5%
Combination Brain/Sinus CT Scan[1]	-	-	3.2%	2.7%
Combination Chest CT Scan	171	0.0%	1.9%	2.7%
Follow-up Mammogram/Ultrasound	275	10.2%	8.6%	8.8%
Lumbar Spine MRI for Low Back Pain[1]	-	-	39.6%	37.2%

Liberty Hospital

2525 Glenn Hendren Dr
Liberty, MO 64069
URL: www.libertyhospital.org
Type: Acute Care Hospitals
Ownership: Govt - Hospital Dist/Auth
Phone: 816-781-7200
Fax: 816-792-7117
Emergency Services: Yes
Beds: 202

Key Personnel:
Radiology. . . . . Joseph Caresio
President/CEO. . . . . David Feess
Infection Control. . . . . Maggie Hagan, MD
Operating Room. . . . . Shelly Moore
Quality Assurance . . . . Sharon Sirridge
Cardiac Laboratory. . . . . Georgia Solovic
Chief of Medical Staff . . . . Steve Starr, MD

Measure	Cases	This Hosp.	State Avg.	U.S. Avg.
Blood Clot Prevention and Treatment				
Anticoagulation Overlap Therapy[2]	80	89%	94%	93%
ICU Venous Thromboembolism Prophylaxis[2]	100	99%	91%	92%
Incidence of Potentially Preventable VTE[1,2]	-	-	7%	10%
UFH with Dosages/Platelet Monitoring[2]	45	100%	96%	97%
Venous Thromboembolism Prophylaxis[2]	494	94%	85%	85%
Warfarin Therapy Discharge Instructions[2]	62	87%	76%	75%
Chest Pain/Possible Heart Attack Care				
Aspirin Given Within 24 Hours of Arrival[1,3]	-	-	95%	96%
Fibrinolytic Meds Within 30 Min. of Arrival[5]	-	-	53%	58%
Average Time to ECG (minutes)[1,3]	-	-	7	7
Average Time to Transfer (minutes)[5]	-	-	53	60
Children's Asthma Care				
Received Home Management Plan of Care	-	-	-	88%
Received Reliever Medication	-	-	-	100%
Received Systemic Corticosteroids	-	-	-	100%
Emergency Department				
Admittance Decision Time (minutes)[2]	492	55	81	98
Head CT Results Within 45 Min. of Arrival[1]	-	-	63%	57%
Patients Who Left ER Before Being Seen	37,895	2%	3%	2%
Time from ER Arrival to Admit. (minutes)[2]	565	232	238	274
Time from ER Arrival to Discharge (minutes)	631	176	136	134
Time in ER Before Being Evaluated (minutes)	743	39	26	26
Time to Pain Meds for Fractures (minutes)	118	82	52	57
Heart Attack Care				
Aspirin Given at Discharge	168	99%	99%	99%
Fibrinolytic Meds Within 30 Min. of Arrival[7]	-	-	-	54%
PCI Within 90 Minutes of Arrival	34	91%	97%	96%
Statin Prescribed at Discharge	158	97%	98%	98%
Heart Failure Care				
ACE Inhibitor or ARB for LVSD	58	86%	96%	97%
Discharge Instructions Given	172	87%	94%	94%
Evaluation of LVS Function	214	100%	98%	99%
Medicare Spending				
Medicare Spending per Patient (ratio)	-	0.99	0.95	0.98
Pneumonia Care				
Appropriate Initial Antibiotic Given	209	96%	95%	95%
Blood Culture Timing	234	98%	98%	98%
Pregnancy and Delivery Care				
Newborn Deliveries Scheduled Early[2]	45	0%	5%	6%
Preventive Care				
Immunization for Influenza[2]	701	95%	92%	90%
Immunization for Pneumonia[2]	859	96%	93%	92%
Stroke Care				
Anticoagulation Therapy for Atrial Fibrillation[2]	12	92%	94%	95%
Antithrombotic Therapy Timing[2]	83	95%	98%	98%
Assessed for Rehabilitation[2]	89	91%	98%	97%
Discharged on Antithrombotic Therapy[2]	80	99%	99%	99%
Discharged on Statin Medication[2]	66	86%	95%	94%

NOTE: Hospital profiles are in alphabetical order by state, then city, then hospital within the city; Rankings exclude hospitals with less than 25 cases except for patient surveys which excludes hospitals with less than 100 cases; (a) 100-299 cases; (1) The number of cases/patients is too few to report; (2) Data submitted were based on a sample of cases/patients; (3) Results are based on a shorter time period than required; (4) Data suppressed by CMS for one or more quarters; (5) Results are not available for this reporting period; (6) Fewer than 100 patients completed the HCAHPS survey; (7) No cases met the criteria for this measure; (8) The lower limit of the confidence interval cannot be calculated if the number of observed infections equals zero; (9) No data are available from the state/territory for this reporting period; (10) The scores shown reflect fewer than 50 completed surveys; (11) There were discrepancies in the data collection process; (12) This measure does not apply to this hospital for this reporting period; (13) Results cannot be calculated for this reporting period; (14) The results for this state are combined with nearby states to protect confidentiality; Please refer to the User's Guide for a full explanation of data.

Measure	Cases	This Hosp.	State Avg.	U.S. Avg.
Thrombolytic Therapy Timing[1,2]	-	-	67%	66%
Venous Thromboembolism Prophylaxis[2]	86	90%	95%	94%
Written Stroke Educational Materials Given[2]	61	79%	88%	88%
Surgical Care Improvement Project				
Appropriate Beta Blocker Usage	249	97%	98%	98%
Appropriate VTP Within 24 Hours	635	99%	98%	98%
Controlled Postoperative Blood Glucose	83	99%	97%	97%
Perioperative Temperature Management	723	100%	100%	100%
Prophylactic Antibiotic Selection	501	100%	99%	99%
Prophylactic Antibiotic Selection (Outpatient)	295	98%	98%	98%
Prophylactic Antibiotic Stopped	489	98%	98%	98%
Prophylactic Antibiotic Timing	501	97%	99%	99%
Prophylactic Antibiotic Timing (Outpatient)	297	97%	98%	98%
Urinary Catheter Removal	267	95%	97%	97%
Survey of Patients' Hospital Experiences				
Area Around Room 'Always' Quiet at Night	300+	60%	61%	61%
Doctors 'Always' Communicated Well	300+	81%	82%	82%
Home Recovery Information Given	300+	89%	87%	85%
Hospital Given 9 or 10 on 10 Point Scale	300+	70%	71%	71%
Meds 'Always' Explained Before Given	300+	63%	63%	64%
Nurses 'Always' Communicated Well	300+	76%	79%	79%
Pain 'Always' Well Controlled	300+	69%	71%	71%
Room and Bathroom 'Always' Clean	300+	69%	73%	73%
Timely Help 'Always' Received	300+	64%	68%	68%
Would Definitely Recommend Hospital	300+	75%	70%	71%
Use of Medical Imaging				
Cardiac Imaging Stress Test before Surgery	316	7.9%	5.2%	5.3%
Combination Abdominal CT Scan	1,167	14.2%	11.2%	10.5%
Combination Brain/Sinus CT Scan	852	3.8%	3.2%	2.7%
Combination Chest CT Scan	662	4.5%	1.9%	2.7%
Follow-up Mammogram/Ultrasound	2,047	7.6%	8.6%	8.8%
Lumbar Spine MRI for Low Back Pain	173	39.3%	39.6%	37.2%

Pike County Memorial Hospital

2305 West Georgia Street
Louisiana, MO 63353
Phone: 573-754-5531
Fax: 573-754-5874
E-mail: djones@pcmhmo.org
URL: www.pcmh-mo.org
Type: Critical Access Hospitals
Emergency Services: Yes
Ownership: Government - Local
Beds: 25

Key Personnel:
Emergency Room . . . . Dolly Giles, RN
CEO/President. . . . . Lorraine Harness
Chief of Medical Staff. . . . . Casey Jennings, DO
Operating Room. . . . . Dianne Oliver
Infection Control . . . . Paulette Powelson, RN
Quality Assurance . . . . Paulette Powelson
Radiology. . . . . Rebekka Thornton

Measure	Cases	This Hosp.	State Avg.	U.S. Avg.
Blood Clot Prevention and Treatment				
Anticoagulation Overlap Therapy[5]	-	-	94%	93%
ICU Venous Thromboembolism Prophylaxis[5]	-	-	91%	92%
Incidence of Potentially Preventable VTE[5]	-	-	7%	10%
UFH with Dosages/Platelet Monitoring[5]	-	-	96%	97%
Venous Thromboembolism Prophylaxis[5]	-	-	85%	85%
Warfarin Therapy Discharge Instructions[5]	-	-	76%	75%
Chest Pain/Possible Heart Attack Care				
Aspirin Given Within 24 Hours of Arrival	-	-	95%	96%
Fibrinolytic Meds Within 30 Min. of Arrival	-	-	53%	58%
Average Time to ECG (minutes)	-	-	7	7
Average Time to Transfer (minutes)	-	-	53	60
Children's Asthma Care				
Received Home Management Plan of Care	-	-	-	88%
Received Reliever Medication	-	-	-	100%
Received Systemic Corticosteroids	-	-	-	100%
Emergency Department				
Admittance Decision Time (minutes)[5]	-	-	81	98
Head CT Results Within 45 Min. of Arrival	-	-	63%	57%
Patients Who Left ER Before Being Seen	-	-	3%	2%
Time from ER Arrival to Admit. (minutes)[5]	-	-	238	274
Time from ER Arrival to Discharge (minutes)	-	-	136	134
Time in ER Before Being Evaluated (minutes)	-	-	26	26
Time to Pain Meds for Fractures (minutes)	-	-	52	57
Heart Attack Care				
Aspirin Given at Discharge[3,7]	-	-	99%	99%
Fibrinolytic Meds Within 30 Min. of Arrival[3,7]	-	-	-	54%
PCI Within 90 Minutes of Arrival[3,7]	-	-	97%	96%
Statin Prescribed at Discharge[3,7]	-	-	98%	98%
Heart Failure Care				
ACE Inhibitor or ARB for LVSD[1,2]	-	-	96%	97%
Discharge Instructions Given[2]	38	100%	94%	94%
Evaluation of LVS Function[2]	50	100%	98%	99%
Medicare Spending				
Medicare Spending per Patient (ratio)	-	-	0.95	0.98
Pneumonia Care				
Appropriate Initial Antibiotic Given[2]	33	91%	95%	95%
Blood Culture Timing[2]	50	92%	98%	98%
Pregnancy and Delivery Care				
Newborn Deliveries Scheduled Early[5]	-	-	5%	6%
Preventive Care				
Immunization for Influenza[5]	-	-	92%	90%
Immunization for Pneumonia[5]	-	-	93%	92%
Stroke Care				
Anticoagulation Therapy for Atrial Fibrillation[5]	-	-	94%	95%
Antithrombotic Therapy Timing[5]	-	-	98%	98%
Assessed for Rehabilitation[5]	-	-	98%	97%
Discharged on Antithrombotic Therapy[5]	-	-	99%	99%
Discharged on Statin Medication[5]	-	-	95%	94%
Thrombolytic Therapy Timing[5]	-	-	67%	66%
Venous Thromboembolism Prophylaxis[5]	-	-	95%	94%
Written Stroke Educational Materials Given[5]	-	-	88%	88%
Surgical Care Improvement Project				
Appropriate Beta Blocker Usage[5]	-	-	98%	98%
Appropriate VTP Within 24 Hours[5]	-	-	98%	98%
Controlled Postoperative Blood Glucose[5]	-	-	97%	97%
Perioperative Temperature Management[5]	-	-	100%	100%
Prophylactic Antibiotic Selection[5]	-	-	99%	99%
Prophylactic Antibiotic Selection (Outpatient)	-	-	98%	98%
Prophylactic Antibiotic Stopped[5]	-	-	98%	98%
Prophylactic Antibiotic Timing[5]	-	-	99%	99%
Prophylactic Antibiotic Timing (Outpatient)	-	-	98%	98%
Urinary Catheter Removal[5]	-	-	97%	97%
Survey of Patients' Hospital Experiences				
Area Around Room 'Always' Quiet at Night[5]	-	-	61%	61%
Doctors 'Always' Communicated Well[5]	-	-	82%	82%
Home Recovery Information Given[5]	-	-	87%	85%
Hospital Given 9 or 10 on 10 Point Scale[5]	-	-	71%	71%
Meds 'Always' Explained Before Given[5]	-	-	63%	64%
Nurses 'Always' Communicated Well[5]	-	-	79%	79%
Pain 'Always' Well Controlled[5]	-	-	71%	71%
Room and Bathroom 'Always' Clean[5]	-	-	73%	73%
Timely Help 'Always' Received[5]	-	-	68%	68%
Would Definitely Recommend Hospital[5]	-	-	70%	71%
Use of Medical Imaging				
Cardiac Imaging Stress Test before Surgery	-	-	5.2%	5.3%
Combination Abdominal CT Scan	-	-	11.2%	10.5%
Combination Brain/Sinus CT Scan	-	-	3.2%	2.7%
Combination Chest CT Scan	-	-	1.9%	2.7%
Follow-up Mammogram/Ultrasound	-	-	8.6%	8.8%
Lumbar Spine MRI for Low Back Pain	-	-	39.6%	37.2%

Fitzgibbon Hospital

2305 S 65 Highway
Marshall, MO 65340
Phone: 660-886-7431
Fax: 660-886-9001
E-mail: snewman@murlin.com
URL: www.fitzgibbon.org
Type: Acute Care Hospitals
Emergency Services: Yes
Ownership: Voluntary non-profit - Private
Beds: 60

Key Personnel:
Quality Assurance . . . . R Bruce Blalock
Infection Control. . . . . Linda Cook, RN
Chief of Medical Staff . . . . Dr. Darin Haug
Operating Room. . . . . Millie Langan, RN
Radiology. . . . . H T Lee
CEO/President. . . . . Ronald A Ott
Pediatric Ambulatory Care . . . . . . C Alan Scott, MD
Pediatric In-Patient Care . . . . C Alan Scott, MD

Measure	Cases	This Hosp.	State Avg.	U.S. Avg.
Blood Clot Prevention and Treatment				
Anticoagulation Overlap Therapy[2]	13	100%	94%	93%
ICU Venous Thromboembolism Prophylaxis[1,2]	-	-	91%	92%
Incidence of Potentially Preventable VTE[1,2]	-	-	7%	10%
UFH with Dosages/Platelet Monitoring[1,2]	-	-	96%	97%
Venous Thromboembolism Prophylaxis[2]	168	78%	85%	85%
Warfarin Therapy Discharge Instructions[1,2]	-	-	76%	75%
Chest Pain/Possible Heart Attack Care				
Aspirin Given Within 24 Hours of Arrival	51	98%	95%	96%
Fibrinolytic Meds Within 30 Min. of Arrival[1,3]	-	-	53%	58%
Average Time to ECG (minutes)	54	24	7	7
Average Time to Transfer (minutes)[1,3]	-	-	53	60
Children's Asthma Care				
Received Home Management Plan of Care	-	-	-	88%
Received Reliever Medication	-	-	-	100%
Received Systemic Corticosteroids	-	-	-	100%
Emergency Department				
Admittance Decision Time (minutes)[2]	390	28	81	98
Head CT Results Within 45 Min. of Arrival[1,3]	-	-	63%	57%
Patients Who Left ER Before Being Seen	10,851	3%	3%	2%
Time from ER Arrival to Admit. (minutes)[2]	410	136	238	274
Time from ER Arrival to Discharge (minutes)	396	98	136	134
Time in ER Before Being Evaluated (minutes)	469	24	26	26
Time to Pain Meds for Fractures (minutes)	53	59	52	57
Heart Attack Care				
Aspirin Given at Discharge[1,3]	-	-	99%	99%
Fibrinolytic Meds Within 30 Min. of Arrival[3,7]	-	-	-	54%
PCI Within 90 Minutes of Arrival[3,7]	-	-	97%	96%
Statin Prescribed at Discharge[1,3]	-	-	98%	98%
Heart Failure Care				
ACE Inhibitor or ARB for LVSD	14	71%	96%	97%
Discharge Instructions Given	64	100%	94%	94%
Evaluation of LVS Function	95	98%	98%	99%
Medicare Spending				
Medicare Spending per Patient (ratio)	-	0.90	0.95	0.98
Pneumonia Care				
Appropriate Initial Antibiotic Given	45	98%	95%	95%
Blood Culture Timing	65	98%	98%	98%
Pregnancy and Delivery Care				
Newborn Deliveries Scheduled Early	40	8%	5%	6%
Preventive Care				
Immunization for Influenza[2]	280	90%	92%	90%
Immunization for Pneumonia[2]	395	96%	93%	92%
Stroke Care				
Anticoagulation Therapy for Atrial Fibrillation[3,7]	-	-	94%	95%
Antithrombotic Therapy Timing[1,3]	-	-	98%	98%
Assessed for Rehabilitation[1,3]	-	-	98%	97%
Discharged on Antithrombotic Therapy[1,3]	-	-	99%	99%
Discharged on Statin Medication[1,3]	-	-	95%	94%
Thrombolytic Therapy Timing[3,7]	-	-	67%	66%
Venous Thromboembolism Prophylaxis[1,3]	-	-	95%	94%
Written Stroke Educational Materials Given[1,3]	-	-	88%	88%
Surgical Care Improvement Project				
Appropriate Beta Blocker Usage	22	100%	98%	98%
Appropriate VTP Within 24 Hours	54	100%	98%	98%
Controlled Postoperative Blood Glucose[7]	-	-	97%	97%
Perioperative Temperature Management	57	100%	100%	100%
Prophylactic Antibiotic Selection	52	100%	99%	99%
Prophylactic Antibiotic Selection (Outpatient)[3]	19	95%	98%	98%
Prophylactic Antibiotic Stopped	49	96%	98%	98%
Prophylactic Antibiotic Timing	52	88%	99%	99%
Prophylactic Antibiotic Timing (Outpatient)[3]	20	95%	98%	98%
Urinary Catheter Removal	45	100%	97%	97%
Survey of Patients' Hospital Experiences				
Area Around Room 'Always' Quiet at Night	300+	55%	61%	61%
Doctors 'Always' Communicated Well	300+	79%	82%	82%
Home Recovery Information Given	300+	88%	87%	85%
Hospital Given 9 or 10 on 10 Point Scale	300+	61%	71%	71%
Meds 'Always' Explained Before Given	300+	61%	63%	64%
Nurses 'Always' Communicated Well	300+	77%	79%	79%
Pain 'Always' Well Controlled	300+	67%	71%	71%
Room and Bathroom 'Always' Clean	300+	66%	73%	73%

NOTE: Hospital profiles are in alphabetical order by state, then city, then hospital within the city; Rankings exclude hospitals with less than 25 cases except for patient surveys which excludes hospitals with less than 100 cases; (a) 100-299 cases; (1) The number of cases/patients is too few to report; (2) Data submitted were based on a sample of cases/patients; (3) Results are based on a shorter time period than required; (4) Data suppressed by CMS for one or more quarters; (5) Results are not available for this reporting period; (6) Fewer than 100 patients completed the HCAHPS survey; (7) No cases met the criteria for this measure; (8) The lower limit of the confidence interval cannot be calculated if the number of observed infections equals zero; (9) No data are available from the state/territory for this reporting period; (10) The scores shown reflect fewer than 50 completed surveys; (11) There were discrepancies in the data collection process; (12) This measure does not apply to this hospital for this reporting period; (13) Results cannot be calculated for this reporting period; (14) The results for this state are combined with nearby states to protect confidentiality; Please refer to the User's Guide for a full explanation of data.

Timely Help 'Always' Received	300+	71%	68%	68%
Would Definitely Recommend Hospital	300+	56%	70%	71%
Use of Medical Imaging				
Cardiac Imaging Stress Test before Surgery	122	9.0%	5.2%	5.3%
Combination Abdominal CT Scan	320	4.1%	11.2%	10.5%
Combination Brain/Sinus CT Scan[1]	-	-	3.2%	2.7%
Combination Chest CT Scan	197	1.0%	1.9%	2.7%
Follow-up Mammogram/Ultrasound	589	7.5%	8.6%	8.8%
Lumbar Spine MRI for Low Back Pain	55	60.0%	39.6%	37.2%

Saint Francis Hospital & Health Services

2016 South Main St
Maryville, MO 64468
Phone: 660-562-2600
Fax: 660-562-7911
URL: www.stfrancismaryville.com
Type: Acute Care Hospitals
Emergency Services: Yes
Ownership: Voluntary non-profit - Church
Beds: 81

Key Personnel:
Radiology. Edward Stevens
Chief of Medical Staff . . . . Michael Wurm
CEO/President. . . . . John Yancey, FSM

Measure	Cases	This Hosp.	State Avg.	U.S. Avg.
Blood Clot Prevention and Treatment				
Anticoagulation Overlap Therapy[1]	-	-	94%	93%
ICU Venous Thromboembolism Prophylaxis[7]	-	-	91%	92%
Incidence of Potentially Preventable VTE[7]	-	-	7%	10%
UFH with Dosages/Platelet Monitoring[1]	-	-	96%	97%
Venous Thromboembolism Prophylaxis	183	90%	85%	85%
Warfarin Therapy Discharge Instructions[1]	-	-	76%	75%
Chest Pain/Possible Heart Attack Care				
Aspirin Given Within 24 Hours of Arrival	29	100%	95%	96%
Fibrinolytic Meds Within 30 Min. of Arrival[1]	-	-	53%	58%
Average Time to ECG (minutes)	31	4	7	7
Average Time to Transfer (minutes)[1]	-	-	53	60
Children's Asthma Care				
Received Home Management Plan of Care	-	-	-	88%
Received Reliever Medication	-	-	-	100%
Received Systemic Corticosteroids	-	-	-	100%
Emergency Department				
Admittance Decision Time (minutes)	126	39	81	98
Head CT Results Within 45 Min. of Arrival[1]	-	-	63%	57%
Patients Who Left ER Before Being Seen	7,719	1%	3%	2%
Time from ER Arrival to Admit. (minutes)	129	197	238	274
Time from ER Arrival to Discharge (minutes)	338	100	136	134
Time in ER Before Being Evaluated (minutes)	404	19	26	26
Time to Pain Meds for Fractures (minutes)	43	52	52	57
Heart Attack Care				
Aspirin Given at Discharge[3,7]	-	-	99%	99%
Fibrinolytic Meds Within 30 Min. of Arrival[3,7]	-	-	-	54%
PCI Within 90 Minutes of Arrival[3,7]	-	-	97%	96%
Statin Prescribed at Discharge[3,7]	-	-	98%	98%
Heart Failure Care				
ACE Inhibitor or ARB for LVSD[1]	-	-	96%	97%
Discharge Instructions Given[1]	-	-	94%	94%
Evaluation of LVS Function[1]	-	-	98%	99%
Medicare Spending				
Medicare Spending per Patient (ratio)	-	0.97	0.95	0.98
Pneumonia Care				
Appropriate Initial Antibiotic Given	17	88%	95%	95%
Blood Culture Timing	12	92%	98%	98%
Pregnancy and Delivery Care				
Newborn Deliveries Scheduled Early	36	19%	5%	6%
Preventive Care				
Immunization for Influenza	389	94%	92%	90%
Immunization for Pneumonia	303	94%	93%	92%
Stroke Care				
Anticoagulation Therapy for Atrial Fibrillation[3,7]	-	-	94%	95%
Antithrombotic Therapy Timing[1,3]	-	-	98%	98%
Assessed for Rehabilitation[1,3]	-	-	98%	97%
Discharged on Antithrombotic Therapy[1,3]	-	-	99%	99%
Discharged on Statin Medication[1,3]	-	-	95%	94%
Thrombolytic Therapy Timing[3,7]	-	-	67%	66%
Venous Thromboembolism Prophylaxis[1,3]	-	-	95%	94%
Written Stroke Educational Materials Given[3,7]	-	-	88%	88%
Surgical Care Improvement Project				
Appropriate Beta Blocker Usage	24	100%	98%	98%
Appropriate VTP Within 24 Hours	77	100%	98%	98%
Controlled Postoperative Blood Glucose[7]	-	-	97%	97%
Perioperative Temperature Management	83	100%	100%	100%
Prophylactic Antibiotic Selection	66	100%	99%	99%
Prophylactic Antibiotic Selection (Outpatient)	38	95%	98%	98%
Prophylactic Antibiotic Stopped	65	95%	98%	98%
Prophylactic Antibiotic Timing	66	92%	99%	99%
Prophylactic Antibiotic Timing (Outpatient)	39	92%	98%	98%
Urinary Catheter Removal	54	96%	97%	97%
Survey of Patients' Hospital Experiences				
Area Around Room 'Always' Quiet at Night	(a)	70%	61%	61%
Doctors 'Always' Communicated Well	(a)	81%	82%	82%
Home Recovery Information Given	(a)	88%	87%	85%
Hospital Given 9 or 10 on 10 Point Scale	(a)	74%	71%	71%
Meds 'Always' Explained Before Given	(a)	63%	63%	64%
Nurses 'Always' Communicated Well	(a)	82%	79%	79%
Pain 'Always' Well Controlled	(a)	74%	71%	71%
Room and Bathroom 'Always' Clean	(a)	86%	73%	73%
Timely Help 'Always' Received	(a)	79%	68%	68%
Would Definitely Recommend Hospital	(a)	69%	70%	71%
Use of Medical Imaging				
Cardiac Imaging Stress Test before Surgery[7]	-	-	5.2%	5.3%
Combination Abdominal CT Scan	295	1.7%	11.2%	10.5%
Combination Brain/Sinus CT Scan[1]	-	-	3.2%	2.7%
Combination Chest CT Scan	257	1.2%	1.9%	2.7%
Follow-up Mammogram/Ultrasound	550	6.9%	8.6%	8.8%
Lumbar Spine MRI for Low Back Pain	62	30.6%	39.6%	37.2%

Scotland County Hospital

450 E Sigler Avenue
Memphis, MO 63555
Phone: 660-465-8511
Fax: 660-465-2513
E-mail: dialm@scotlandcountyhospital.com
Type: Critical Access Hospitals
Emergency Services: Yes
Ownership: Govt - Hospital Dist/Auth
Beds: 40

Key Personnel:
Anesthesiology. . . . . Michael Browning, CRNA
CEO/President. . . . . Marcia R Dial
Chairman/CEO . . . . Curtis Ebeling
Radiology. . . . . Angela Hawes, R.T. (R.)(C.T.)
Surgery . . . . Celeste Miller-Parish, DO
Emergency Room . . . . Thelma Norton, RN
Chief of Medical Staff . . . . Randy Tobler, MD, FACOG
Operating Room. . . . . Debbie Ward

Measure	Cases	This Hosp.	State Avg.	U.S. Avg.
Blood Clot Prevention and Treatment				
Anticoagulation Overlap Therapy[2,7]	-	-	94%	93%
ICU Venous Thromboembolism Prophylaxis[1,2]	-	-	91%	92%
Incidence of Potentially Preventable VTE[2,7]	-	-	7%	10%
UFH with Dosages/Platelet Monitoring[2,7]	-	-	96%	97%
Venous Thromboembolism Prophylaxis[2]	217	94%	85%	85%
Warfarin Therapy Discharge Instructions[2,7]	-	-	76%	75%
Chest Pain/Possible Heart Attack Care				
Aspirin Given Within 24 Hours of Arrival	-	-	95%	96%
Fibrinolytic Meds Within 30 Min. of Arrival	-	-	53%	58%
Average Time to ECG (minutes)	-	-	7	7
Average Time to Transfer (minutes)	-	-	53	60
Children's Asthma Care				
Received Home Management Plan of Care	-	-	-	88%
Received Reliever Medication	-	-	-	100%
Received Systemic Corticosteroids	-	-	-	100%
Emergency Department				
Admittance Decision Time (minutes)[2]	372	50	81	98
Head CT Results Within 45 Min. of Arrival	-	-	63%	57%
Patients Who Left ER Before Being Seen	-	-	3%	2%
Time from ER Arrival to Admit. (minutes)[2]	394	210	238	274
Time from ER Arrival to Discharge (minutes)	-	-	136	134
Time in ER Before Being Evaluated (minutes)	-	-	26	26
Time to Pain Meds for Fractures (minutes)	-	-	52	57
Heart Attack Care				
Aspirin Given at Discharge[1,3]	-	-	99%	99%
Fibrinolytic Meds Within 30 Min. of Arrival[3,7]	-	-	-	54%
PCI Within 90 Minutes of Arrival[3,7]	-	-	97%	96%
Statin Prescribed at Discharge[1,3]	-	-	98%	98%
Heart Failure Care				
ACE Inhibitor or ARB for LVSD[1]	-	-	96%	97%
Discharge Instructions Given	16	94%	94%	94%
Evaluation of LVS Function	20	95%	98%	99%
Medicare Spending				
Medicare Spending per Patient (ratio)	-	-	0.95	0.98
Pneumonia Care				
Appropriate Initial Antibiotic Given	17	71%	95%	95%
Blood Culture Timing	31	100%	98%	98%
Pregnancy and Delivery Care				
Newborn Deliveries Scheduled Early[5]	-	-	5%	6%
Preventive Care				
Immunization for Influenza[2]	260	82%	92%	90%
Immunization for Pneumonia[2]	376	82%	93%	92%
Stroke Care				
Anticoagulation Therapy for Atrial Fibrillation[1]	-	-	94%	95%
Antithrombotic Therapy Timing[1]	-	-	98%	98%
Assessed for Rehabilitation[1]	-	-	98%	97%
Discharged on Antithrombotic Therapy[1]	-	-	99%	99%
Discharged on Statin Medication[1]	-	-	95%	94%
Thrombolytic Therapy Timing[1]	-	-	67%	66%
Venous Thromboembolism Prophylaxis[1]	-	-	95%	94%
Written Stroke Educational Materials Given[7]	-	-	88%	88%
Surgical Care Improvement Project				
Appropriate Beta Blocker Usage[1]	-	-	98%	98%
Appropriate VTP Within 24 Hours	20	95%	98%	98%
Controlled Postoperative Blood Glucose[7]	-	-	97%	97%
Perioperative Temperature Management	29	100%	100%	100%
Prophylactic Antibiotic Selection[7]	-	-	99%	99%
Prophylactic Antibiotic Selection (Outpatient)	-	-	98%	98%
Prophylactic Antibiotic Stopped[7]	-	-	98%	98%
Prophylactic Antibiotic Timing[7]	-	-	99%	99%
Prophylactic Antibiotic Timing (Outpatient)	-	-	98%	98%
Urinary Catheter Removal	11	91%	97%	97%
Survey of Patients' Hospital Experiences				
Area Around Room 'Always' Quiet at Night[5]	-	-	61%	61%
Doctors 'Always' Communicated Well[5]	-	-	82%	82%
Home Recovery Information Given[5]	-	-	87%	85%
Hospital Given 9 or 10 on 10 Point Scale[5]	-	-	71%	71%
Meds 'Always' Explained Before Given[5]	-	-	63%	64%
Nurses 'Always' Communicated Well[5]	-	-	79%	79%
Pain 'Always' Well Controlled[5]	-	-	71%	71%
Room and Bathroom 'Always' Clean[5]	-	-	73%	73%
Timely Help 'Always' Received[5]	-	-	68%	68%
Would Definitely Recommend Hospital[5]	-	-	70%	71%
Use of Medical Imaging				
Cardiac Imaging Stress Test before Surgery	-	-	5.2%	5.3%
Combination Abdominal CT Scan	-	-	11.2%	10.5%
Combination Brain/Sinus CT Scan	-	-	3.2%	2.7%
Combination Chest CT Scan	-	-	1.9%	2.7%
Follow-up Mammogram/Ultrasound	-	-	8.6%	8.8%
Lumbar Spine MRI for Low Back Pain	-	-	39.6%	37.2%

Audrain Medical Center

620 E Monroe
Mexico, MO 65265
Phone: 573-582-5000
Fax: 573-582-3700
URL: www.audrainmedicalcenter.com
Type: Acute Care Hospitals
Emergency Services: Yes
Ownership: Voluntary non-profit - Private
Beds: 92

Key Personnel:
Radiology. George Kutty Cyriac
Chief of Medical Staff . . . . Justin Jones, MD
CEO/President. . . . . David A Neuendorf

Measure	Cases	This Hosp.	State Avg.	U.S. Avg.
Blood Clot Prevention and Treatment				
Anticoagulation Overlap Therapy[2]	24	88%	94%	93%
ICU Venous Thromboembolism Prophylaxis[2]	44	82%	91%	92%
Incidence of Potentially Preventable VTE[1,2]	-	-	7%	10%
UFH with Dosages/Platelet Monitoring[1,2]	-	-	96%	97%
Venous Thromboembolism Prophylaxis[2]	178	76%	85%	85%
Warfarin Therapy Discharge Instructions[2]	19	84%	76%	75%
Chest Pain/Possible Heart Attack Care				

NOTE: Hospital profiles are in alphabetical order by state, then city, then hospital within the city; Rankings exclude hospitals with less than 25 cases except for patient surveys which excludes hospitals with less than 100 cases; (a) 100-299 cases; (1) The number of cases/patients is too few to report; (2) Data submitted were based on a sample of cases/patients; (3) Results are based on a shorter time period than required; (4) Data suppressed by CMS for one or more quarters; (5) Results are not available for this reporting period; (6) Fewer than 100 patients completed the HCAHPS survey; (7) No cases met the criteria for this measure; (8) The lower limit of the confidence interval cannot be calculated if the number of observed infections equals zero; (9) No data are available from the state/territory for this reporting period; (10) The scores shown reflect fewer than 50 completed surveys; (11) There were discrepancies in the data collection process; (12) This measure does not apply to this hospital for this reporting period; (13) Results cannot be calculated for this reporting period; (14) The results for this state are combined with nearby states to protect confidentiality; Please refer to the User's Guide for a full explanation of data.

Measure	Cases	This Hosp.	State Avg.	U.S. Avg.
Aspirin Given Within 24 Hours of Arrival[1,3]	-	-	95%	96%
Fibrinolytic Meds Within 30 Min. of Arrival[3,7]	-	-	53%	58%
Average Time to ECG (minutes)[1,3]	-	-	7	7
Average Time to Transfer (minutes)[1,3]	-	-	53	60
Children's Asthma Care				
Received Home Management Plan of Care	-	-	-	88%
Received Reliever Medication	-	-	-	100%
Received Systemic Corticosteroids	-	-	-	100%
Emergency Department				
Admittance Decision Time (minutes)[2]	219	60	81	98
Head CT Results Within 45 Min. of Arrival[1]	-	-	63%	57%
Patients Who Left ER Before Being Seen	>100k	0%	3%	2%
Time from ER Arrival to Admit. (minutes)[2]	262	181	238	274
Time from ER Arrival to Discharge (minutes)	371	102	136	134
Time in ER Before Being Evaluated (minutes)	383	16	26	26
Time to Pain Meds for Fractures (minutes)	82	40	52	57
Heart Attack Care				
Aspirin Given at Discharge	56	100%	99%	99%
Fibrinolytic Meds Within 30 Min. of Arrival[7]	-	-	-	54%
PCI Within 90 Minutes of Arrival	25	88%	97%	96%
Statin Prescribed at Discharge	54	93%	98%	98%
Heart Failure Care				
ACE Inhibitor or ARB for LVSD	37	89%	96%	97%
Discharge Instructions Given	89	93%	94%	94%
Evaluation of LVS Function	128	99%	98%	99%
Medicare Spending				
Medicare Spending per Patient (ratio)	-	0.92	0.95	0.98
Pneumonia Care				
Appropriate Initial Antibiotic Given	74	99%	95%	95%
Blood Culture Timing	114	99%	98%	98%
Pregnancy and Delivery Care				
Newborn Deliveries Scheduled Early	21	0%	5%	6%
Preventive Care				
Immunization for Influenza[2]	261	94%	92%	90%
Immunization for Pneumonia[2]	387	97%	93%	92%
Stroke Care				
Anticoagulation Therapy for Atrial Fibrillation[1]	-	-	94%	95%
Antithrombotic Therapy Timing	12	58%	98%	98%
Assessed for Rehabilitation	11	100%	98%	97%
Discharged on Antithrombotic Therapy[1]	-	-	99%	99%
Discharged on Statin Medication[1]	-	-	95%	94%
Thrombolytic Therapy Timing[1]	-	-	67%	66%
Venous Thromboembolism Prophylaxis	12	75%	95%	94%
Written Stroke Educational Materials Given[1]	-	-	88%	88%
Surgical Care Improvement Project				
Appropriate Beta Blocker Usage	38	92%	98%	98%
Appropriate VTP Within 24 Hours	97	98%	98%	98%
Controlled Postoperative Blood Glucose[7]	-	-	97%	97%
Perioperative Temperature Management	131	95%	100%	100%
Prophylactic Antibiotic Selection	101	99%	99%	99%
Prophylactic Antibiotic Selection (Outpatient)	182	99%	98%	98%
Prophylactic Antibiotic Stopped	99	87%	98%	98%
Prophylactic Antibiotic Timing	101	98%	99%	99%
Prophylactic Antibiotic Timing (Outpatient)	182	98%	98%	98%
Urinary Catheter Removal	16	81%	97%	97%
Survey of Patients' Hospital Experiences				
Area Around Room 'Always' Quiet at Night	300+	50%	61%	61%
Doctors 'Always' Communicated Well	300+	79%	82%	82%
Home Recovery Information Given	300+	90%	87%	85%
Hospital Given 9 or 10 on 10 Point Scale	300+	69%	71%	71%
Meds 'Always' Explained Before Given	300+	63%	63%	64%
Nurses 'Always' Communicated Well	300+	84%	79%	79%
Pain 'Always' Well Controlled	300+	70%	71%	71%
Room and Bathroom 'Always' Clean	300+	79%	73%	73%
Timely Help 'Always' Received	300+	72%	68%	68%
Would Definitely Recommend Hospital	300+	65%	70%	71%
Use of Medical Imaging				
Cardiac Imaging Stress Test before Surgery	154	3.2%	5.2%	5.3%
Combination Abdominal CT Scan	309	3.9%	11.2%	10.5%
Combination Brain/Sinus CT Scan[1]	-	-	3.2%	2.7%
Combination Chest CT Scan	316	0.0%	1.9%	2.7%
Follow-up Mammogram/Ultrasound	1,059	9.1%	8.6%	8.8%
Lumbar Spine MRI for Low Back Pain	82	43.9%	39.6%	37.2%

Sullivan County Memorial Hospital

630 West Third Street
Milan, MO 63556
Phone: 660-265-4212
Fax: 660-265-3609
Type: Critical Access Hospitals
Emergency Services: Yes
Ownership: Government - Local
Beds: 39

Key Personnel:

Radiology.................... Mary Christians
CEO/President................ Martha Gragg
Chairman/CEO .... Keith Maggart
Infection Control............ Kim Ray, RN
Quality Assurance .... Kim Ray, RN
Emergency Room .... Thomas Williams, RN
Chief of Medical Staff....... Tom Williams

Measure	Cases	This Hosp.	State Avg.	U.S. Avg.
Blood Clot Prevention and Treatment				
Anticoagulation Overlap Therapy[5]	-	-	94%	93%
ICU Venous Thromboembolism Prophylaxis[5]	-	-	91%	92%
Incidence of Potentially Preventable VTE[5]	-	-	7%	10%
UFH with Dosages/Platelet Monitoring[5]	-	-	96%	97%
Venous Thromboembolism Prophylaxis[5]	-	-	85%	85%
Warfarin Therapy Discharge Instructions[5]	-	-	76%	75%
Chest Pain/Possible Heart Attack Care				
Aspirin Given Within 24 Hours of Arrival[5]	-	-	95%	96%
Fibrinolytic Meds Within 30 Min. of Arrival[5]	-	-	53%	58%
Average Time to ECG (minutes)[5]	-	-	7	7
Average Time to Transfer (minutes)[5]	-	-	53	60
Children's Asthma Care				
Received Home Management Plan of Care	-	-	-	88%
Received Reliever Medication	-	-	-	100%
Received Systemic Corticosteroids	-	-	-	100%
Emergency Department				
Admittance Decision Time (minutes)[5]	-	-	81	98
Head CT Results Within 45 Min. of Arrival[5]	-	-	63%	57%
Patients Who Left ER Before Being Seen[5]	-	-	3%	2%
Time from ER Arrival to Admit. (minutes)[5]	-	-	238	274
Time from ER Arrival to Discharge (minutes)[3]	78	60	136	134
Time in ER Before Being Evaluated (minutes)[3]	97	15	26	26
Time to Pain Meds for Fractures (minutes)[5]	-	-	52	57
Heart Attack Care				
Aspirin Given at Discharge[5]	-	-	99%	99%
Fibrinolytic Meds Within 30 Min. of Arrival[5]	-	-	-	54%
PCI Within 90 Minutes of Arrival[5]	-	-	97%	96%
Statin Prescribed at Discharge[5]	-	-	98%	98%
Heart Failure Care				
ACE Inhibitor or ARB for LVSD[1,3]	-	-	96%	97%
Discharge Instructions Given[1,3]	-	-	94%	94%
Evaluation of LVS Function[1,3]	-	-	98%	99%
Medicare Spending				
Medicare Spending per Patient (ratio)	-	-	0.95	0.98
Pneumonia Care				
Appropriate Initial Antibiotic Given[1,3]	-	-	95%	95%
Blood Culture Timing[1,3]	-	-	98%	98%
Pregnancy and Delivery Care				
Newborn Deliveries Scheduled Early[5]	-	-	5%	6%
Preventive Care				
Immunization for Influenza[5]	-	-	92%	90%
Immunization for Pneumonia[5]	-	-	93%	92%
Stroke Care				
Anticoagulation Therapy for Atrial Fibrillation[5]	-	-	94%	95%
Antithrombotic Therapy Timing[5]	-	-	98%	98%
Assessed for Rehabilitation[5]	-	-	98%	97%
Discharged on Antithrombotic Therapy[5]	-	-	99%	99%
Discharged on Statin Medication[5]	-	-	95%	94%
Thrombolytic Therapy Timing[5]	-	-	67%	66%
Venous Thromboembolism Prophylaxis[5]	-	-	95%	94%
Written Stroke Educational Materials Given[5]	-	-	88%	88%
Surgical Care Improvement Project				
Appropriate Beta Blocker Usage[5]	-	-	98%	98%
Appropriate VTP Within 24 Hours[5]	-	-	98%	98%
Controlled Postoperative Blood Glucose[5]	-	-	97%	97%
Perioperative Temperature Management[5]	-	-	100%	100%
Prophylactic Antibiotic Selection[5]	-	-	99%	99%
Prophylactic Antibiotic Selection (Outpatient)[5]	-	-	98%	98%
Prophylactic Antibiotic Stopped[5]	-	-	98%	98%
Prophylactic Antibiotic Timing[5]	-	-	99%	99%
Prophylactic Antibiotic Timing (Outpatient)[5]	-	-	98%	98%
Urinary Catheter Removal[5]	-	-	97%	97%
Survey of Patients' Hospital Experiences				
Area Around Room 'Always' Quiet at Night[5]	-	-	61%	61%
Doctors 'Always' Communicated Well[5]	-	-	82%	82%
Home Recovery Information Given[5]	-	-	87%	85%
Hospital Given 9 or 10 on 10 Point Scale[5]	-	-	71%	71%
Meds 'Always' Explained Before Given[5]	-	-	63%	64%
Nurses 'Always' Communicated Well[5]	-	-	79%	79%
Pain 'Always' Well Controlled[5]	-	-	71%	71%
Room and Bathroom 'Always' Clean[5]	-	-	73%	73%
Timely Help 'Always' Received[5]	-	-	68%	68%
Would Definitely Recommend Hospital[5]	-	-	70%	71%
Use of Medical Imaging				
Cardiac Imaging Stress Test before Surgery[7]	-	-	5.2%	5.3%
Combination Abdominal CT Scan[1]	-	-	11.2%	10.5%
Combination Brain/Sinus CT Scan[1]	-	-	3.2%	2.7%
Combination Chest CT Scan[1]	-	-	1.9%	2.7%
Follow-up Mammogram/Ultrasound[7]	-	-	8.6%	8.8%
Lumbar Spine MRI for Low Back Pain[1]	-	-	39.6%	37.2%

Moberly Regional Medical Center

1515 Union Ave
Moberly, MO 65270
Phone: 660-263-8400
Fax: 660-269-3091
URL: www.moberlyhospital.com
Type: Acute Care Hospitals
Emergency Services: Yes
Ownership: Proprietary
Beds: 114

Key Personnel:

Emergency Room .... Eric Bettis
Infection Control.......... Roanetta Bodgers
Intensive Care Unit........ Pat Fischer, RN
Cardiac Laboratory......... Ahmed Habib, MD
Chief of Medical Staff..... Ahmed Habib
CEO .... Chris Jones
Operating Room............. Sonja Nelson
Quality Assurance .... Roanetta Rodgers

Measure	Cases	This Hosp.	State Avg.	U.S. Avg.
Blood Clot Prevention and Treatment				
Anticoagulation Overlap Therapy[1,2]	-	-	94%	93%
ICU Venous Thromboembolism Prophylaxis[2]	71	100%	91%	92%
Incidence of Potentially Preventable VTE[2,7]	-	-	7%	10%
UFH with Dosages/Platelet Monitoring[1,2]	-	-	96%	97%
Venous Thromboembolism Prophylaxis[2]	200	100%	85%	85%
Warfarin Therapy Discharge Instructions[1,2]	-	-	76%	75%
Chest Pain/Possible Heart Attack Care				
Aspirin Given Within 24 Hours of Arrival	16	100%	95%	96%
Fibrinolytic Meds Within 30 Min. of Arrival[7]	-	-	53%	58%
Average Time to ECG (minutes)	16	5	7	7
Average Time to Transfer (minutes)[1]	-	-	53	60
Children's Asthma Care				
Received Home Management Plan of Care	-	-	-	88%
Received Reliever Medication	-	-	-	100%
Received Systemic Corticosteroids	-	-	-	100%
Emergency Department				
Admittance Decision Time (minutes)[2]	338	45	81	98
Head CT Results Within 45 Min. of Arrival[1]	-	-	63%	57%
Patients Who Left ER Before Being Seen	14,776	2%	3%	2%
Time from ER Arrival to Admit. (minutes)[2]	347	189	238	274
Time from ER Arrival to Discharge (minutes)	375	117	136	134
Time in ER Before Being Evaluated (minutes)	422	20	26	26
Time to Pain Meds for Fractures (minutes)	61	31	52	57
Heart Attack Care				
Aspirin Given at Discharge	45	100%	99%	99%
Fibrinolytic Meds Within 30 Min. of Arrival[7]	-	-	-	54%
PCI Within 90 Minutes of Arrival	12	100%	97%	96%
Statin Prescribed at Discharge	44	100%	98%	98%
Heart Failure Care				
ACE Inhibitor or ARB for LVSD	22	100%	96%	97%
Discharge Instructions Given	52	96%	94%	94%
Evaluation of LVS Function	85	100%	98%	99%
Medicare Spending				

NOTE: Hospital profiles are in alphabetical order by state, then city, then hospital within the city; Rankings exclude hospitals with less than 25 cases except for patient surveys which excludes hospitals with less than 100 cases; (a) 100-299 cases; (1) The number of cases/patients is too few to report; (2) Data submitted were based on a sample of cases/patients; (3) Results are based on a shorter time period than required; (4) Data suppressed by CMS for one or more quarters; (5) Results are not available for this reporting period; (6) Fewer than 100 patients completed the HCAHPS survey; (7) No cases met the criteria for this measure; (8) The lower limit of the confidence interval cannot be calculated if the number of observed infections equals zero; (9) No data are available from the state/territory for this reporting period; (10) The scores shown reflect fewer than 50 completed surveys; (11) There were discrepancies in the data collection process; (12) This measure does not apply to this hospital for this reporting period; (13) Results cannot be calculated for this reporting period; (14) The results for this state are combined with nearby states to protect confidentiality; Please refer to the User's Guide for a full explanation of data.

Measure	Cases	This Hosp.	State Avg.	U.S. Avg.
Medicare Spending per Patient (ratio)		-	0.93	0.95	0.98
Pneumonia Care				
Appropriate Initial Antibiotic Given	48	100%	95%	95%
Blood Culture Timing	95	100%	98%	98%
Pregnancy and Delivery Care				
Newborn Deliveries Scheduled Early[2]	15	0%	5%	6%
Preventive Care				
Immunization for Influenza[2]	297	100%	92%	90%
Immunization for Pneumonia[2]	398	100%	93%	92%
Stroke Care				
Anticoagulation Therapy for Atrial Fibrillation[1]	-	-	94%	95%
Antithrombotic Therapy Timing	11	100%	98%	98%
Assessed for Rehabilitation	11	100%	98%	97%
Discharged on Antithrombotic Therapy	11	100%	99%	99%
Discharged on Statin Medication[1]	-	-	95%	94%
Thrombolytic Therapy Timing[7]	-	-	67%	66%
Venous Thromboembolism Prophylaxis[1]	-	-	95%	94%
Written Stroke Educational Materials Given[1]	-	-	88%	88%
Surgical Care Improvement Project				
Appropriate Beta Blocker Usage	22	100%	98%	98%
Appropriate VTP Within 24 Hours	67	100%	98%	98%
Controlled Postoperative Blood Glucose[7]	-	-	97%	97%
Perioperative Temperature Management	73	100%	100%	100%
Prophylactic Antibiotic Selection	47	100%	99%	99%
Prophylactic Antibiotic Selection (Outpatient)	102	99%	98%	98%
Prophylactic Antibiotic Stopped	44	98%	98%	98%
Prophylactic Antibiotic Timing	47	100%	99%	99%
Prophylactic Antibiotic Timing (Outpatient)	103	99%	98%	98%
Urinary Catheter Removal	33	100%	97%	97%
Survey of Patients' Hospital Experiences				
Area Around Room 'Always' Quiet at Night	300+	60%	61%	61%
Doctors 'Always' Communicated Well	300+	81%	82%	82%
Home Recovery Information Given	300+	91%	87%	85%
Hospital Given 9 or 10 on 10 Point Scale	300+	67%	71%	71%
Meds 'Always' Explained Before Given	300+	62%	63%	64%
Nurses 'Always' Communicated Well	300+	78%	79%	79%
Pain 'Always' Well Controlled	300+	73%	71%	71%
Room and Bathroom 'Always' Clean	300+	72%	73%	73%
Timely Help 'Always' Received	300+	63%	68%	68%
Would Definitely Recommend Hospital	300+	60%	70%	71%
Use of Medical Imaging				
Cardiac Imaging Stress Test before Surgery	224	6.7%	5.2%	5.3%
Combination Abdominal CT Scan	206	10.7%	11.2%	10.5%
Combination Brain/Sinus CT Scan[1]	-	-	3.2%	2.7%
Combination Chest CT Scan	92	9.8%	1.9%	2.7%
Follow-up Mammogram/Ultrasound	223	12.1%	8.6%	8.8%
Lumbar Spine MRI for Low Back Pain[1]	-	-	39.6%	37.2%

Cox Monett Hospital

801 North Lincoln Avenue
Monett, MO 65708
Phone: 417-354-1400
Fax: 417-354-1412
Type: Critical Access Hospitals
Emergency Services: Yes
Ownership: Voluntary non-profit - Private
Beds: 25

Key Personnel:

Emergency Room . . . . Stephen Dennis, MD
Chief of Medical Staff. . . . . Amber Ecomomu, MD
President/CEO. . . . . Steven D. Edwards
Quality Assurance . . . . Jana Perall

Measure	Cases	This Hosp.	State Avg.	U.S. Avg.
Blood Clot Prevention and Treatment				
Anticoagulation Overlap Therapy[5]	-	-	94%	93%
ICU Venous Thromboembolism Prophylaxis[5]	-	-	91%	92%
Incidence of Potentially Preventable VTE[5]	-	-	7%	10%
UFH with Dosages/Platelet Monitoring[5]	-	-	96%	97%
Venous Thromboembolism Prophylaxis[5]	-	-	85%	85%
Warfarin Therapy Discharge Instructions[5]	-	-	76%	75%
Chest Pain/Possible Heart Attack Care				
Aspirin Given Within 24 Hours of Arrival	-	-	95%	96%
Fibrinolytic Meds Within 30 Min. of Arrival	-	-	53%	58%
Average Time to ECG (minutes)	-	-	7	7
Average Time to Transfer (minutes)	-	-	53	60
Children's Asthma Care				
Received Home Management Plan of Care	-	-	-	88%
Received Reliever Medication	-	-	-	100%
Received Systemic Corticosteroids	-	-	-	100%
Emergency Department				
Admittance Decision Time (minutes)[5]	-	-	81	98
Head CT Results Within 45 Min. of Arrival	-	-	63%	57%
Patients Who Left ER Before Being Seen	-	-	3%	2%
Time from ER Arrival to Admit. (minutes)[5]	-	-	238	274
Time from ER Arrival to Discharge (minutes)	-	-	136	134
Time in ER Before Being Evaluated (minutes)	-	-	26	26
Time to Pain Meds for Fractures (minutes)	-	-	52	57
Heart Attack Care				
Aspirin Given at Discharge[1,3]	-	-	99%	99%
Fibrinolytic Meds Within 30 Min. of Arrival[3,7]	-	-	-	54%
PCI Within 90 Minutes of Arrival[3,7]	-	-	97%	96%
Statin Prescribed at Discharge[1,3]	-	-	98%	98%
Heart Failure Care				
ACE Inhibitor or ARB for LVSD[1]	-	-	96%	97%
Discharge Instructions Given[1]	-	-	94%	94%
Evaluation of LVS Function	14	93%	98%	99%
Medicare Spending				
Medicare Spending per Patient (ratio)		-	0.95	0.98
Pneumonia Care				
Appropriate Initial Antibiotic Given	46	91%	95%	95%
Blood Culture Timing	69	94%	98%	98%
Pregnancy and Delivery Care				
Newborn Deliveries Scheduled Early[5]	-	-	5%	6%
Preventive Care				
Immunization for Influenza[5]	-	-	92%	90%
Immunization for Pneumonia[5]	-	-	93%	92%
Stroke Care				
Anticoagulation Therapy for Atrial Fibrillation[5]	-	-	94%	95%
Antithrombotic Therapy Timing[5]	-	-	98%	98%
Assessed for Rehabilitation[5]	-	-	98%	97%
Discharged on Antithrombotic Therapy[5]	-	-	99%	99%
Discharged on Statin Medication[5]	-	-	95%	94%
Thrombolytic Therapy Timing[5]	-	-	67%	66%
Venous Thromboembolism Prophylaxis[5]	-	-	95%	94%
Written Stroke Educational Materials Given[5]	-	-	88%	88%
Surgical Care Improvement Project				
Appropriate Beta Blocker Usage[1,3]	-	-	98%	98%
Appropriate VTP Within 24 Hours[1,3]	-	-	98%	98%
Controlled Postoperative Blood Glucose[3,7]	-	-	97%	97%
Perioperative Temperature Management[1,3]	-	-	100%	100%
Prophylactic Antibiotic Selection[1,3]	-	-	99%	99%
Prophylactic Antibiotic Selection (Outpatient)	-	-	98%	98%
Prophylactic Antibiotic Stopped[1,3]	-	-	98%	98%
Prophylactic Antibiotic Timing[1,3]	-	-	99%	99%
Prophylactic Antibiotic Timing (Outpatient)	-	-	98%	98%
Urinary Catheter Removal[1,3]	-	-	97%	97%
Survey of Patients' Hospital Experiences				
Area Around Room 'Always' Quiet at Night[6]	<100	71%	61%	61%
Doctors 'Always' Communicated Well[6]	<100	87%	82%	82%
Home Recovery Information Given[6]	<100	89%	87%	85%
Hospital Given 9 or 10 on 10 Point Scale[6]	<100	75%	71%	71%
Meds 'Always' Explained Before Given[6]	<100	70%	63%	64%
Nurses 'Always' Communicated Well[6]	<100	78%	79%	79%
Pain 'Always' Well Controlled[6]	<100	68%	71%	71%
Room and Bathroom 'Always' Clean[6]	<100	70%	73%	73%
Timely Help 'Always' Received[6]	<100	69%	68%	68%
Would Definitely Recommend Hospital[6]	<100	69%	70%	71%
Use of Medical Imaging				
Cardiac Imaging Stress Test before Surgery	-	-	5.2%	5.3%
Combination Abdominal CT Scan	-	-	11.2%	10.5%
Combination Brain/Sinus CT Scan	-	-	3.2%	2.7%
Combination Chest CT Scan	-	-	1.9%	2.7%
Follow-up Mammogram/Ultrasound	-	-	8.6%	8.8%
Lumbar Spine MRI for Low Back Pain	-	-	39.6%	37.2%

Mercy Saint Francis Hospital

100 West Highway 60, PO Box 82
Mountain View, MO 65548
Phone: 417-934-7000
Fax: 417-934-6024
Type: Critical Access Hospitals
Emergency Services: Yes
Ownership: Voluntary non-profit - Private
Beds: 42

Key Personnel:

CEO/President. . . . . Lynn Britton
Emergency Room . . . . Ernest L Carampatan, MD
Radiology. . . . . Brian Denton, RT
Operating Room. . . . . Janet Kile, RN
Infection Control. . . . . Jill Mundt, MT ASCP
Administrator . . . . Robert Rogers
Chief of Medical Staff. . . . . Mohammed Tabibi, DO
Anesthesiology. . . . . Cheryl Thurman, CRNA

Measure	Cases	This Hosp.	State Avg.	U.S. Avg.
Blood Clot Prevention and Treatment				
Anticoagulation Overlap Therapy[5]	-	-	94%	93%
ICU Venous Thromboembolism Prophylaxis[5]	-	-	91%	92%
Incidence of Potentially Preventable VTE[5]	-	-	7%	10%
UFH with Dosages/Platelet Monitoring[5]	-	-	96%	97%
Venous Thromboembolism Prophylaxis[5]	-	-	85%	85%
Warfarin Therapy Discharge Instructions[5]	-	-	76%	75%
Chest Pain/Possible Heart Attack Care				
Aspirin Given Within 24 Hours of Arrival	-	-	95%	96%
Fibrinolytic Meds Within 30 Min. of Arrival	-	-	53%	58%
Average Time to ECG (minutes)	-	-	7	7
Average Time to Transfer (minutes)	-	-	53	60
Children's Asthma Care				
Received Home Management Plan of Care	-	-	-	88%
Received Reliever Medication	-	-	-	100%
Received Systemic Corticosteroids	-	-	-	100%
Emergency Department				
Admittance Decision Time (minutes)	221	36	81	98
Head CT Results Within 45 Min. of Arrival	-	-	63%	57%
Patients Who Left ER Before Being Seen	-	-	3%	2%
Time from ER Arrival to Admit. (minutes)	229	184	238	274
Time from ER Arrival to Discharge (minutes)	-	-	136	134
Time in ER Before Being Evaluated (minutes)	-	-	26	26
Time to Pain Meds for Fractures (minutes)	-	-	52	57
Heart Attack Care				
Aspirin Given at Discharge[5]	-	-	99%	99%
Fibrinolytic Meds Within 30 Min. of Arrival[5]	-	-	-	54%
PCI Within 90 Minutes of Arrival[5]	-	-	97%	96%
Statin Prescribed at Discharge[5]	-	-	98%	98%
Heart Failure Care				
ACE Inhibitor or ARB for LVSD[1]	-	-	96%	97%
Discharge Instructions Given[1]	-	-	94%	94%
Evaluation of LVS Function	15	100%	98%	99%
Medicare Spending				
Medicare Spending per Patient (ratio)		-	0.95	0.98
Pneumonia Care				
Appropriate Initial Antibiotic Given	31	94%	95%	95%
Blood Culture Timing	25	100%	98%	98%
Pregnancy and Delivery Care				
Newborn Deliveries Scheduled Early[5]	-	-	5%	6%
Preventive Care				
Immunization for Influenza	171	82%	92%	90%
Immunization for Pneumonia	254	91%	93%	92%
Stroke Care				
Anticoagulation Therapy for Atrial Fibrillation[5]	-	-	94%	95%
Antithrombotic Therapy Timing[5]	-	-	98%	98%
Assessed for Rehabilitation[5]	-	-	98%	97%
Discharged on Antithrombotic Therapy[5]	-	-	99%	99%
Discharged on Statin Medication[5]	-	-	95%	94%
Thrombolytic Therapy Timing[5]	-	-	67%	66%
Venous Thromboembolism Prophylaxis[5]	-	-	95%	94%
Written Stroke Educational Materials Given[5]	-	-	88%	88%
Surgical Care Improvement Project				
Appropriate Beta Blocker Usage[5]	-	-	98%	98%
Appropriate VTP Within 24 Hours[5]	-	-	98%	98%
Controlled Postoperative Blood Glucose[5]	-	-	97%	97%
Perioperative Temperature Management[5]	-	-	100%	100%
Prophylactic Antibiotic Selection[5]	-	-	99%	99%
Prophylactic Antibiotic Selection (Outpatient)	-	-	98%	98%

NOTE: Hospital profiles are in alphabetical order by state, then city, then hospital within the city; Rankings exclude hospitals with less than 25 cases except for patient surveys which excludes hospitals with less than 100 cases; (a) 100-299 cases; (1) The number of cases/patients is too few to report; (2) Data submitted were based on a sample of cases/patients; (3) Results are based on a shorter time period than required; (4) Data suppressed by CMS for one or more quarters; (5) Results are not available for this reporting period; (6) Fewer than 100 patients completed the HCAHPS survey; (7) No cases met the criteria for this measure; (8) The lower limit of the confidence interval cannot be calculated if the number of observed infections equals zero; (9) No data are available from the state/territory for this reporting period; (10) The scores shown reflect fewer than 50 completed surveys; (11) There were discrepancies in the data collection process; (12) This measure does not apply to this hospital for this reporting period; (13) Results cannot be calculated for this reporting period; (14) The results for this state are combined with nearby states to protect confidentiality; Please refer to the User's Guide for a full explanation of data.

Measure	Cases	This Hosp.	State Avg.	U.S. Avg.
Prophylactic Antibiotic Stopped[5]	-	-	98%	98%
Prophylactic Antibiotic Timing[5]	-	-	99%	99%
Prophylactic Antibiotic Timing (Outpatient)	-	-	98%	98%
Urinary Catheter Removal[5]	-	-	97%	97%
Survey of Patients' Hospital Experiences				
Area Around Room 'Always' Quiet at Night[5]	-	-	61%	61%
Doctors 'Always' Communicated Well[5]	-	-	82%	82%
Home Recovery Information Given[5]	-	-	87%	85%
Hospital Given 9 or 10 on 10 Point Scale[5]	-	-	71%	71%
Meds 'Always' Explained Before Given[5]	-	-	63%	64%
Nurses 'Always' Communicated Well[5]	-	-	79%	79%
Pain 'Always' Well Controlled[5]	-	-	71%	71%
Room and Bathroom 'Always' Clean[5]	-	-	73%	73%
Timely Help 'Always' Received[5]	-	-	68%	68%
Would Definitely Recommend Hospital[5]	-	-	70%	71%
Use of Medical Imaging				
Cardiac Imaging Stress Test before Surgery	-	-	5.2%	5.3%
Combination Abdominal CT Scan	-	-	11.2%	10.5%
Combination Brain/Sinus CT Scan	-	-	3.2%	2.7%
Combination Chest CT Scan	-	-	1.9%	2.7%
Follow-up Mammogram/Ultrasound	-	-	8.6%	8.8%
Lumbar Spine MRI for Low Back Pain	-	-	39.6%	37.2%

Freeman Neosho Hospital

113 West Hickory Street
Neosho, MO 64850
Phone: 417-451-1234
Fax: 417-347-3716
URL: www.freemanhealth.com
Type: Critical Access Hospitals
Emergency Services: Yes
Ownership: Voluntary non-profit - Private
Beds: 67

Key Personnel:
CEO/President. . . . . Paula Baker
Radiology. . . . . Roger A Francis

Measure	Cases	This Hosp.	State Avg.	U.S. Avg.
Blood Clot Prevention and Treatment				
Anticoagulation Overlap Therapy[5]	-	-	94%	93%
ICU Venous Thromboembolism Prophylaxis[5]	-	-	91%	92%
Incidence of Potentially Preventable VTE[5]	-	-	7%	10%
UFH with Dosages/Platelet Monitoring[5]	-	-	96%	97%
Venous Thromboembolism Prophylaxis[5]	-	-	85%	85%
Warfarin Therapy Discharge Instructions[5]	-	-	76%	75%
Chest Pain/Possible Heart Attack Care				
Aspirin Given Within 24 Hours of Arrival	-	-	95%	96%
Fibrinolytic Meds Within 30 Min. of Arrival	-	-	53%	58%
Average Time to ECG (minutes)	-	-	7	7
Average Time to Transfer (minutes)	-	-	53	60
Children's Asthma Care				
Received Home Management Plan of Care	-	-	-	88%
Received Reliever Medication	-	-	-	100%
Received Systemic Corticosteroids	-	-	-	100%
Emergency Department				
Admittance Decision Time (minutes)[2,3]	319	65	81	98
Head CT Results Within 45 Min. of Arrival	-	-	63%	57%
Patients Who Left ER Before Being Seen	-	-	3%	2%
Time from ER Arrival to Admit. (minutes)[2,3]	341	208	238	274
Time from ER Arrival to Discharge (minutes)	-	-	136	134
Time in ER Before Being Evaluated (minutes)	-	-	26	26
Time to Pain Meds for Fractures (minutes)	-	-	52	57
Heart Attack Care				
Aspirin Given at Discharge[5]	-	-	99%	99%
Fibrinolytic Meds Within 30 Min. of Arrival[5]	-	-	-	54%
PCI Within 90 Minutes of Arrival[5]	-	-	97%	96%
Statin Prescribed at Discharge[5]	-	-	98%	98%
Heart Failure Care				
ACE Inhibitor or ARB for LVSD	20	100%	96%	97%
Discharge Instructions Given	28	89%	94%	94%
Evaluation of LVS Function	49	100%	98%	99%
Medicare Spending				
Medicare Spending per Patient (ratio)	-	-	0.95	0.98
Pneumonia Care				
Appropriate Initial Antibiotic Given	62	98%	95%	95%
Blood Culture Timing	109	99%	98%	98%
Pregnancy and Delivery Care				
Newborn Deliveries Scheduled Early[5]	-	-	5%	6%
Preventive Care				
Immunization for Influenza[5]	-	-	92%	90%
Immunization for Pneumonia[5]	-	-	93%	92%
Stroke Care				
Anticoagulation Therapy for Atrial Fibrillation[5]	-	-	94%	95%
Antithrombotic Therapy Timing[5]	-	-	98%	98%
Assessed for Rehabilitation[5]	-	-	98%	97%
Discharged on Antithrombotic Therapy[5]	-	-	99%	99%
Discharged on Statin Medication[5]	-	-	95%	94%
Thrombolytic Therapy Timing[5]	-	-	67%	66%
Venous Thromboembolism Prophylaxis[5]	-	-	95%	94%
Written Stroke Educational Materials Given[5]	-	-	88%	88%
Surgical Care Improvement Project				
Appropriate Beta Blocker Usage[1,3]	-	-	98%	98%
Appropriate VTP Within 24 Hours[1,3]	-	-	98%	98%
Controlled Postoperative Blood Glucose[3,7]	-	-	97%	97%
Perioperative Temperature Management[1,3]	-	-	100%	100%
Prophylactic Antibiotic Selection[1,3]	-	-	99%	99%
Prophylactic Antibiotic Selection (Outpatient)	-	-	98%	98%
Prophylactic Antibiotic Stopped[1,3]	-	-	98%	98%
Prophylactic Antibiotic Timing[1,3]	-	-	99%	99%
Prophylactic Antibiotic Timing (Outpatient)	-	-	98%	98%
Urinary Catheter Removal[1,3]	-	-	97%	97%
Survey of Patients' Hospital Experiences				
Area Around Room 'Always' Quiet at Night	(a)	66%	61%	61%
Doctors 'Always' Communicated Well	(a)	84%	82%	82%
Home Recovery Information Given	(a)	90%	87%	85%
Hospital Given 9 or 10 on 10 Point Scale	(a)	77%	71%	71%
Meds 'Always' Explained Before Given	(a)	64%	63%	64%
Nurses 'Always' Communicated Well	(a)	82%	79%	79%
Pain 'Always' Well Controlled	(a)	75%	71%	71%
Room and Bathroom 'Always' Clean	(a)	70%	73%	73%
Timely Help 'Always' Received	(a)	74%	68%	68%
Would Definitely Recommend Hospital	(a)	76%	70%	71%
Use of Medical Imaging				
Cardiac Imaging Stress Test before Surgery	-	-	5.2%	5.3%
Combination Abdominal CT Scan	-	-	11.2%	10.5%
Combination Brain/Sinus CT Scan	-	-	3.2%	2.7%
Combination Chest CT Scan	-	-	1.9%	2.7%
Follow-up Mammogram/Ultrasound	-	-	8.6%	8.8%
Lumbar Spine MRI for Low Back Pain	-	-	39.6%	37.2%

Nevada Regional Medical Center

800 S Ash St
Nevada, MO 64772
Phone: 417-667-3355
Fax: 417-448-3848
URL: www.nrmchealth.com
Type: Acute Care Hospitals
Emergency Services: Yes
Ownership: Government - Local
Beds: 53

Key Personnel:
Emergency Room . . . . Holly Busher, RN
Chief of Medical Staff. . . . . Michael Crim
Quality Assurance . . . . Janie Dickey
CEO/President. . . . . Judith Feuquay
Radiology. . . . . Roger Francis
CEO . . . . David Hample
Operating Room. . . . . Joy Jefferies
Chairman/CEO . . . . Glen Rogers, PhD

Measure	Cases	This Hosp.	State Avg.	U.S. Avg.
Blood Clot Prevention and Treatment				
Anticoagulation Overlap Therapy[1,2]	-	-	94%	93%
ICU Venous Thromboembolism Prophylaxis[2]	51	49%	91%	92%
Incidence of Potentially Preventable VTE[2,7]	-	-	7%	10%
UFH with Dosages/Platelet Monitoring[1,2]	-	-	96%	97%
Venous Thromboembolism Prophylaxis[2]	154	47%	85%	85%
Warfarin Therapy Discharge Instructions[1,2]	-	-	76%	75%
Chest Pain/Possible Heart Attack Care				
Aspirin Given Within 24 Hours of Arrival	31	100%	95%	96%
Fibrinolytic Meds Within 30 Min. of Arrival[1,3]	-	-	53%	58%
Average Time to ECG (minutes)	30	8	7	7
Average Time to Transfer (minutes)[1,3]	-	-	53	60
Children's Asthma Care				
Received Home Management Plan of Care	-	-	-	88%
Received Reliever Medication	-	-	-	100%
Received Systemic Corticosteroids	-	-	-	100%
Emergency Department				
Admittance Decision Time (minutes)[2]	176	60	81	98
Head CT Results Within 45 Min. of Arrival	14	43%	63%	57%
Patients Who Left ER Before Being Seen	9,893	2%	3%	2%
Time from ER Arrival to Admit. (minutes)[2]	201	171	238	274
Time from ER Arrival to Discharge (minutes)	448	75	136	134
Time in ER Before Being Evaluated (minutes)	497	19	26	26
Time to Pain Meds for Fractures (minutes)	42	38	52	57
Heart Attack Care				
Aspirin Given at Discharge[1,3]	-	-	99%	99%
Fibrinolytic Meds Within 30 Min. of Arrival[3,7]	-	-	-	54%
PCI Within 90 Minutes of Arrival[3,7]	-	-	97%	96%
Statin Prescribed at Discharge[1,3]	-	-	98%	98%
Heart Failure Care				
ACE Inhibitor or ARB for LVSD[1]	-	-	96%	97%
Discharge Instructions Given	26	65%	94%	94%
Evaluation of LVS Function	30	90%	98%	99%
Medicare Spending				
Medicare Spending per Patient (ratio)	-	0.87	0.95	0.98
Pneumonia Care				
Appropriate Initial Antibiotic Given	27	89%	95%	95%
Blood Culture Timing	36	97%	98%	98%
Pregnancy and Delivery Care				
Newborn Deliveries Scheduled Early[2]	20	0%	5%	6%
Preventive Care				
Immunization for Influenza[2]	329	92%	92%	90%
Immunization for Pneumonia[2]	317	83%	93%	92%
Stroke Care				
Anticoagulation Therapy for Atrial Fibrillation[3,7]	-	-	94%	95%
Antithrombotic Therapy Timing[1,3]	-	-	98%	98%
Assessed for Rehabilitation[1,3]	-	-	98%	97%
Discharged on Antithrombotic Therapy[1,3]	-	-	99%	99%
Discharged on Statin Medication[1,3]	-	-	95%	94%
Thrombolytic Therapy Timing[3,7]	-	-	67%	66%
Venous Thromboembolism Prophylaxis[1,3]	-	-	95%	94%
Written Stroke Educational Materials Given[1,3]	-	-	88%	88%
Surgical Care Improvement Project				
Appropriate Beta Blocker Usage[1]	-	-	98%	98%
Appropriate VTP Within 24 Hours	18	83%	98%	98%
Controlled Postoperative Blood Glucose[7]	-	-	97%	97%
Perioperative Temperature Management	18	100%	100%	100%
Prophylactic Antibiotic Selection[1]	-	-	99%	99%
Prophylactic Antibiotic Selection (Outpatient)	38	100%	98%	98%
Prophylactic Antibiotic Stopped[1]	-	-	98%	98%
Prophylactic Antibiotic Timing[1]	-	-	99%	99%
Prophylactic Antibiotic Timing (Outpatient)	31	94%	98%	98%
Urinary Catheter Removal	17	88%	97%	97%
Survey of Patients' Hospital Experiences				
Area Around Room 'Always' Quiet at Night	(a)	73%	61%	61%
Doctors 'Always' Communicated Well	(a)	82%	82%	82%
Home Recovery Information Given	(a)	83%	87%	85%
Hospital Given 9 or 10 on 10 Point Scale	(a)	66%	71%	71%
Meds 'Always' Explained Before Given	(a)	62%	63%	64%
Nurses 'Always' Communicated Well	(a)	75%	79%	79%
Pain 'Always' Well Controlled	(a)	65%	71%	71%
Room and Bathroom 'Always' Clean	(a)	72%	73%	73%
Timely Help 'Always' Received	(a)	69%	68%	68%
Would Definitely Recommend Hospital	(a)	61%	70%	71%
Use of Medical Imaging				
Cardiac Imaging Stress Test before Surgery[1]	-	-	5.2%	5.3%
Combination Abdominal CT Scan	213	3.3%	11.2%	10.5%
Combination Brain/Sinus CT Scan[1]	-	-	3.2%	2.7%
Combination Chest CT Scan	91	0.0%	1.9%	2.7%
Follow-up Mammogram/Ultrasound	431	5.1%	8.6%	8.8%
Lumbar Spine MRI for Low Back Pain	57	49.1%	39.6%	37.2%

North Kansas City Hospital

2800 Clay Edwards Drive
North Kansas City, MO 64116
Phone: 816-691-2000
Fax: 816-346-7020
URL: www.nkch.org
Type: Acute Care Hospitals
Emergency Services: Yes
Ownership: Government - Local
Beds: 451

Key Personnel:
CEO/President. . . . . David Carpenter

NOTE: Hospital profiles are in alphabetical order by state, then city, then hospital within the city; Rankings exclude hospitals with less than 25 cases except for patient surveys which excludes hospitals with less than 100 cases; (a) 100-299 cases; (1) The number of cases/patients is too few to report; (2) Data submitted were based on a sample of cases/patients; (3) Results are based on a shorter time period than required; (4) Data suppressed by CMS for one or more quarters; (5) Results are not available for this reporting period; (6) Fewer than 100 patients completed the HCAHPS survey; (7) No cases met the criteria for this measure; (8) The lower limit of the confidence interval cannot be calculated if the number of observed infections equals zero; (9) No data are available from the state/territory for this reporting period; (10) The scores shown reflect fewer than 50 completed surveys; (11) There were discrepancies in the data collection process; (12) This measure does not apply to this hospital for this reporting period; (13) Results cannot be calculated for this reporting period; (14) The results for this state are combined with nearby states to protect confidentiality; Please refer to the User's Guide for a full explanation of data.

Operating Room. . . . . Dewayne Gossett
Quality Assurance . . . . Connie Griffith
Infection Control. . . . . Tina Harvey
Cardiac Laboratory. . . . . Fran Marencik
Coronary Care . . . . April Patten
Radiology. . . . . Hanamel Rada
Chief of Medical Staff. . . . . Leslie Thomas, MD

Measure	Cases	This Hosp.	State Avg.	U.S. Avg.
Blood Clot Prevention and Treatment				
Anticoagulation Overlap Therapy[2]	160	94%	94%	93%
ICU Venous Thromboembolism Prophylaxis[2]	74	86%	91%	92%
Incidence of Potentially Preventable VTE[2]	20	15%	7%	10%
UFH with Dosages/Platelet Monitoring[2]	116	98%	96%	97%
Venous Thromboembolism Prophylaxis[2]	321	74%	85%	85%
Warfarin Therapy Discharge Instructions[2]	113	79%	76%	75%
Chest Pain/Possible Heart Attack Care				
Aspirin Given Within 24 Hours of Arrival[5]	-	-	95%	96%
Fibrinolytic Meds Within 30 Min. of Arrival[5]	-	-	53%	58%
Average Time to ECG (minutes)[5]	-	-	7	7
Average Time to Transfer (minutes)[5]	-	-	53	60
Children's Asthma Care				
Received Home Management Plan of Care	-	-	-	88%
Received Reliever Medication	-	-	-	100%
Received Systemic Corticosteroids	-	-	-	100%
Emergency Department				
Admittance Decision Time (minutes)[2]	458	104	81	98
Head CT Results Within 45 Min. of Arrival	14	57%	63%	57%
Patients Who Left ER Before Being Seen	63,178	1%	3%	2%
Time from ER Arrival to Admit. (minutes)[2]	479	212	238	274
Time from ER Arrival to Discharge (minutes)	1,312	128	136	134
Time in ER Before Being Evaluated (minutes)	1,483	20	26	26
Time to Pain Meds for Fractures (minutes)	156	50	52	57
Heart Attack Care				
Aspirin Given at Discharge[2]	296	100%	99%	99%
Fibrinolytic Meds Within 30 Min. of Arrival[2,7]	-	-	-	54%
PCI Within 90 Minutes of Arrival[2]	67	94%	97%	96%
Statin Prescribed at Discharge[2]	284	100%	98%	98%
Heart Failure Care				
ACE Inhibitor or ARB for LVSD[2]	137	98%	96%	97%
Discharge Instructions Given[2]	358	94%	94%	94%
Evaluation of LVS Function[2]	409	100%	98%	99%
Medicare Spending				
Medicare Spending per Patient (ratio)	-	0.95	0.95	0.98
Pneumonia Care				
Appropriate Initial Antibiotic Given[2]	152	97%	95%	95%
Blood Culture Timing[2]	162	99%	98%	98%
Pregnancy and Delivery Care				
Newborn Deliveries Scheduled Early	121	4%	5%	6%
Preventive Care				
Immunization for Influenza[2]	559	99%	92%	90%
Immunization for Pneumonia[2]	761	99%	93%	92%
Stroke Care				
Anticoagulation Therapy for Atrial Fibrillation	20	95%	94%	95%
Antithrombotic Therapy Timing	146	97%	98%	98%
Assessed for Rehabilitation	171	92%	98%	97%
Discharged on Antithrombotic Therapy	152	99%	99%	99%
Discharged on Statin Medication	122	90%	95%	94%
Thrombolytic Therapy Timing	16	12%	67%	66%
Venous Thromboembolism Prophylaxis	168	57%	95%	94%
Written Stroke Educational Materials Given	99	58%	88%	88%
Surgical Care Improvement Project				
Appropriate Beta Blocker Usage[2]	298	99%	98%	98%
Appropriate VTP Within 24 Hours[2]	514	97%	98%	98%
Controlled Postoperative Blood Glucose[2]	157	98%	97%	97%
Perioperative Temperature Management[2]	614	100%	100%	100%
Prophylactic Antibiotic Selection[2]	524	100%	99%	99%
Prophylactic Antibiotic Selection (Outpatient)	641	98%	98%	98%
Prophylactic Antibiotic Stopped[2]	500	98%	98%	98%
Prophylactic Antibiotic Timing[2]	525	100%	99%	99%
Prophylactic Antibiotic Timing (Outpatient)	643	99%	98%	98%
Urinary Catheter Removal[2]	428	98%	97%	97%
Survey of Patients' Hospital Experiences				
Area Around Room 'Always' Quiet at Night	300+	62%	61%	61%
Doctors 'Always' Communicated Well	300+	81%	82%	82%
Home Recovery Information Given	300+	88%	87%	85%
Hospital Given 9 or 10 on 10 Point Scale	300+	76%	71%	71%
Meds 'Always' Explained Before Given	300+	61%	63%	64%
Nurses 'Always' Communicated Well	300+	77%	79%	79%
Pain 'Always' Well Controlled	300+	70%	71%	71%
Room and Bathroom 'Always' Clean	300+	72%	73%	73%
Timely Help 'Always' Received	300+	61%	68%	68%
Would Definitely Recommend Hospital	300+	79%	70%	71%
Use of Medical Imaging				
Cardiac Imaging Stress Test before Surgery	1,338	5.8%	5.2%	5.3%
Combination Abdominal CT Scan	1,435	12.1%	11.2%	10.5%
Combination Brain/Sinus CT Scan	1,321	3.9%	3.2%	2.7%
Combination Chest CT Scan	1,220	2.5%	1.9%	2.7%
Follow-up Mammogram/Ultrasound	1,559	16.2%	8.6%	8.8%
Lumbar Spine MRI for Low Back Pain	497	42.5%	39.6%	37.2%

Progress West Hospital

2 Progress Point Pkwy
O Fallon, MO 63368
Phone: 636-344-1000
URL: www.progresswesthealthcare.org
Type: Acute Care Hospitals
Emergency Services: Yes
Ownership: Voluntary non-profit - Private
Key Personnel:
Cardiology . . . . Jeff Haile

Measure	Cases	This Hosp.	State Avg.	U.S. Avg.
Blood Clot Prevention and Treatment				
Anticoagulation Overlap Therapy[2]	15	93%	94%	93%
ICU Venous Thromboembolism Prophylaxis[2]	32	94%	91%	92%
Incidence of Potentially Preventable VTE[1,2]	-	-	7%	10%
UFH with Dosages/Platelet Monitoring[1,2]	-	-	96%	97%
Venous Thromboembolism Prophylaxis[2]	186	96%	85%	85%
Warfarin Therapy Discharge Instructions[2]	12	100%	76%	75%
Chest Pain/Possible Heart Attack Care				
Aspirin Given Within 24 Hours of Arrival[1,3]	-	-	95%	96%
Fibrinolytic Meds Within 30 Min. of Arrival[3,7]	-	-	53%	58%
Average Time to ECG (minutes)[1,3]	-	-	7	7
Average Time to Transfer (minutes)[3,7]	-	-	53	60
Children's Asthma Care				
Received Home Management Plan of Care	-	-	-	88%
Received Reliever Medication	-	-	-	100%
Received Systemic Corticosteroids	-	-	-	100%
Emergency Department				
Admittance Decision Time (minutes)[2]	305	52	81	98
Head CT Results Within 45 Min. of Arrival	15	80%	63%	57%
Patients Who Left ER Before Being Seen	24,586	2%	3%	2%
Time from ER Arrival to Admit. (minutes)[2]	335	209	238	274
Time from ER Arrival to Discharge (minutes)	793	138	136	134
Time in ER Before Being Evaluated (minutes)	763	50	26	26
Time to Pain Meds for Fractures (minutes)	198	36	52	57
Heart Attack Care				
Aspirin Given at Discharge	71	100%	99%	99%
Fibrinolytic Meds Within 30 Min. of Arrival[7]	-	-	-	54%
PCI Within 90 Minutes of Arrival	25	96%	97%	96%
Statin Prescribed at Discharge	70	97%	98%	98%
Heart Failure Care				
ACE Inhibitor or ARB for LVSD	15	100%	96%	97%
Discharge Instructions Given	47	98%	94%	94%
Evaluation of LVS Function	61	100%	98%	99%
Medicare Spending				
Medicare Spending per Patient (ratio)	-	0.93	0.95	0.98
Pneumonia Care				
Appropriate Initial Antibiotic Given	63	100%	95%	95%
Blood Culture Timing	86	99%	98%	98%
Pregnancy and Delivery Care				
Newborn Deliveries Scheduled Early[2]	21	0%	5%	6%
Preventive Care				
Immunization for Influenza[2]	297	91%	92%	90%
Immunization for Pneumonia[2]	313	96%	93%	92%
Stroke Care				
Anticoagulation Therapy for Atrial Fibrillation[1,2]	-	-	94%	95%
Antithrombotic Therapy Timing[2]	20	100%	98%	98%
Assessed for Rehabilitation[2]	23	91%	98%	97%
Discharged on Antithrombotic Therapy[2]	21	100%	99%	99%
Discharged on Statin Medication[2]	16	94%	95%	94%
Thrombolytic Therapy Timing[1,2]	-	-	67%	66%
Venous Thromboembolism Prophylaxis[2]	22	95%	95%	94%
Written Stroke Educational Materials Given[2]	11	100%	88%	88%
Surgical Care Improvement Project				
Appropriate Beta Blocker Usage[2]	80	100%	98%	98%
Appropriate VTP Within 24 Hours[2]	262	99%	98%	98%
Controlled Postoperative Blood Glucose[2,7]	-	-	97%	97%
Perioperative Temperature Management[2]	273	100%	100%	100%
Prophylactic Antibiotic Selection[2]	222	100%	99%	99%
Prophylactic Antibiotic Selection (Outpatient)	40	98%	98%	98%
Prophylactic Antibiotic Stopped[2]	215	97%	98%	98%
Prophylactic Antibiotic Timing[2]	222	100%	99%	99%
Prophylactic Antibiotic Timing (Outpatient)	40	100%	98%	98%
Urinary Catheter Removal[2]	163	100%	97%	97%
Survey of Patients' Hospital Experiences				
Area Around Room 'Always' Quiet at Night	300+	54%	61%	61%
Doctors 'Always' Communicated Well	300+	83%	82%	82%
Home Recovery Information Given	300+	91%	87%	85%
Hospital Given 9 or 10 on 10 Point Scale	300+	81%	71%	71%
Meds 'Always' Explained Before Given	300+	67%	63%	64%
Nurses 'Always' Communicated Well	300+	80%	79%	79%
Pain 'Always' Well Controlled	300+	72%	71%	71%
Room and Bathroom 'Always' Clean	300+	64%	73%	73%
Timely Help 'Always' Received	300+	61%	68%	68%
Would Definitely Recommend Hospital	300+	82%	70%	71%
Use of Medical Imaging				
Cardiac Imaging Stress Test before Surgery	163	8.6%	5.2%	5.3%
Combination Abdominal CT Scan	207	1.9%	11.2%	10.5%
Combination Brain/Sinus CT Scan[1]	-	-	3.2%	2.7%
Combination Chest CT Scan	190	0.0%	1.9%	2.7%
Follow-up Mammogram/Ultrasound	257	5.8%	8.6%	8.8%
Lumbar Spine MRI for Low Back Pain[1]	-	-	39.6%	37.2%

Lake Regional Health System

54 Hospital Drive
Osage Beach, MO 65065
Phone: 573-348-8000
Fax: 573-348-8268
E-mail: dwakeford@socket.net
URL: www.lakeregional.com
Type: Acute Care Hospitals
Emergency Services: Yes
Ownership: Voluntary non-profit - Other
Beds: 140
Key Personnel:
Chief of Medical Staff . . . . Grant Barnum, MD
Emergency Room . . . . Terry L Berry
Operating Room. . . . . Michael M Duff, RN
Quality Assurance . . . . Sue Fletcher
CEO . . . . Michael E Henze
Anesthesiology. . . . . Alan Meade, MD
Cardiac Laboratory. . . . . Tonnie Rugen
Intensive Care Unit. . . . . Cathlene Vybee

Measure	Cases	This Hosp.	State Avg.	U.S. Avg.
Blood Clot Prevention and Treatment				
Anticoagulation Overlap Therapy[2]	12	100%	94%	93%
ICU Venous Thromboembolism Prophylaxis[2]	122	97%	91%	92%
Incidence of Potentially Preventable VTE[1,2]	-	-	7%	10%
UFH with Dosages/Platelet Monitoring[1,2]	-	-	96%	97%
Venous Thromboembolism Prophylaxis[2]	481	93%	85%	85%
Warfarin Therapy Discharge Instructions[2]	12	100%	76%	75%
Chest Pain/Possible Heart Attack Care				
Aspirin Given Within 24 Hours of Arrival[1]	-	-	95%	96%
Fibrinolytic Meds Within 30 Min. of Arrival[3,7]	-	-	53%	58%
Average Time to ECG (minutes)[1]	-	-	7	7
Average Time to Transfer (minutes)[3,7]	-	-	53	60
Children's Asthma Care				
Received Home Management Plan of Care	-	-	-	88%
Received Reliever Medication	-	-	-	100%
Received Systemic Corticosteroids	-	-	-	100%
Emergency Department				
Admittance Decision Time (minutes)[2]	690	83	81	98
Head CT Results Within 45 Min. of Arrival	22	36%	63%	57%
Patients Who Left ER Before Being Seen	36,778	1%	3%	2%
Time from ER Arrival to Admit. (minutes)[2]	765	233	238	274
Time from ER Arrival to Discharge (minutes)	667	111	136	134

NOTE: Hospital profiles are in alphabetical order by state, then city, then hospital within the city; Rankings exclude hospitals with less than 25 cases except for patient surveys which excludes hospitals with less than 100 cases; (a) 100-299 cases; (1) The number of cases/patients is too few to report; (2) Data submitted were based on a sample of cases/patients; (3) Results are based on a shorter time period than required; (4) Data suppressed by CMS for one or more quarters; (5) Results are not available for this reporting period; (6) Fewer than 100 patients completed the HCAHPS survey; (7) No cases met the criteria for this measure; (8) The lower limit of the confidence interval cannot be calculated if the number of observed infections equals zero; (9) No data are available from the state/territory for this reporting period; (10) The scores shown reflect fewer than 50 completed surveys; (11) There were discrepancies in the data collection process; (12) This measure does not apply to this hospital for this reporting period; (13) Results cannot be calculated for this reporting period; (14) The results for this state are combined with nearby states to protect confidentiality; Please refer to the User's Guide for a full explanation of data.

Time in ER Before Being Evaluated (minutes)	743	9	26	26
Time to Pain Meds for Fractures (minutes)	203	54	52	57
Heart Attack Care				
Aspirin Given at Discharge	237	98%	99%	99%
Fibrinolytic Meds Within 30 Min. of Arrival[7]	-	-	-	54%
PCI Within 90 Minutes of Arrival	45	100%	97%	96%
Statin Prescribed at Discharge	220	98%	98%	98%
Heart Failure Care				
ACE Inhibitor or ARB for LVSD	64	97%	96%	97%
Discharge Instructions Given	148	93%	94%	94%
Evaluation of LVS Function	184	99%	98%	99%
Medicare Spending				
Medicare Spending per Patient (ratio)	-	0.92	0.95	0.98
Pneumonia Care				
Appropriate Initial Antibiotic Given	150	96%	95%	95%
Blood Culture Timing	225	99%	98%	98%
Pregnancy and Delivery Care				
Newborn Deliveries Scheduled Early[2]	67	3%	5%	6%
Preventive Care				
Immunization for Influenza[2]	600	94%	92%	90%
Immunization for Pneumonia[2]	770	91%	93%	92%
Stroke Care				
Anticoagulation Therapy for Atrial Fibrillation	11	91%	94%	95%
Antithrombotic Therapy Timing	66	97%	98%	98%
Assessed for Rehabilitation	74	96%	98%	97%
Discharged on Antithrombotic Therapy	73	99%	99%	99%
Discharged on Statin Medication	55	89%	95%	94%
Thrombolytic Therapy Timing[1]	-	-	67%	66%
Venous Thromboembolism Prophylaxis	75	95%	95%	94%
Written Stroke Educational Materials Given	48	81%	88%	88%
Surgical Care Improvement Project				
Appropriate Beta Blocker Usage	122	99%	98%	98%
Appropriate VTP Within 24 Hours	261	100%	98%	98%
Controlled Postoperative Blood Glucose	39	92%	97%	97%
Perioperative Temperature Management	303	100%	100%	100%
Prophylactic Antibiotic Selection	222	100%	99%	99%
Prophylactic Antibiotic Selection (Outpatient)	177	98%	98%	98%
Prophylactic Antibiotic Stopped	212	94%	98%	98%
Prophylactic Antibiotic Timing	222	99%	99%	99%
Prophylactic Antibiotic Timing (Outpatient)	177	99%	98%	98%
Urinary Catheter Removal	239	99%	97%	97%
Survey of Patients' Hospital Experiences				
Area Around Room 'Always' Quiet at Night	300+	55%	61%	61%
Doctors 'Always' Communicated Well	300+	77%	82%	82%
Home Recovery Information Given	300+	81%	87%	85%
Hospital Given 9 or 10 on 10 Point Scale	300+	67%	71%	71%
Meds 'Always' Explained Before Given	300+	62%	63%	64%
Nurses 'Always' Communicated Well	300+	77%	79%	79%
Pain 'Always' Well Controlled	300+	66%	71%	71%
Room and Bathroom 'Always' Clean	300+	75%	73%	73%
Timely Help 'Always' Received	300+	70%	68%	68%
Would Definitely Recommend Hospital	300+	64%	70%	71%
Use of Medical Imaging				
Cardiac Imaging Stress Test before Surgery	953	3.7%	5.2%	5.3%
Combination Abdominal CT Scan	636	2.0%	11.2%	10.5%
Combination Brain/Sinus CT Scan	700	3.0%	3.2%	2.7%
Combination Chest CT Scan	341	1.5%	1.9%	2.7%
Follow-up Mammogram/Ultrasound[7]	-	-	8.6%	8.8%
Lumbar Spine MRI for Low Back Pain[1]	-	-	39.6%	37.2%

Sac-Osage Hospital

700 Giesler Drive
Osceola, MO 64776
Phone: 417-646-8181
Fax: 417-646-8416
Type: Acute Care Hospitals
Emergency Services: No
Ownership: Govt - Hospital Dist/Auth
Beds: 47

Key Personnel:
CEO/President.............. Harrell Conelly
Operating Room.............. Mary Locke, RN
Chief of Medical Staff.......... Wayne L Morton, MD

Measure	Cases	This Hosp.	State Avg.	U.S. Avg.
Blood Clot Prevention and Treatment				
Anticoagulation Overlap Therapy[1,2]	-	-	94%	93%
ICU Venous Thromboembolism Prophylaxis[2,7]	-	-	91%	92%
Incidence of Potentially Preventable VTE[2,7]	-	-	7%	10%
UFH with Dosages/Platelet Monitoring[2,7]	-	-	96%	97%
Venous Thromboembolism Prophylaxis[2]	123	9%	85%	85%
Warfarin Therapy Discharge Instructions[1,2]	-	-	76%	75%
Chest Pain/Possible Heart Attack Care				
Aspirin Given Within 24 Hours of Arrival[3]	12	83%	95%	96%
Fibrinolytic Meds Within 30 Min. of Arrival[3,7]	-	-	53%	58%
Average Time to ECG (minutes)[3]	12	11	7	7
Average Time to Transfer (minutes)[3,7]	-	-	53	60
Children's Asthma Care				
Received Home Management Plan of Care	-	-	-	88%
Received Reliever Medication	-	-	-	100%
Received Systemic Corticosteroids	-	-	-	100%
Emergency Department				
Admittance Decision Time (minutes)[2]	170	45	81	98
Head CT Results Within 45 Min. of Arrival[3,7]	-	-	63%	57%
Patients Who Left ER Before Being Seen	2,014	1%	3%	2%
Time from ER Arrival to Admit. (minutes)[2]	176	174	238	274
Time from ER Arrival to Discharge (minutes)	210	115	136	134
Time in ER Before Being Evaluated (minutes)	244	22	26	26
Time to Pain Meds for Fractures (minutes)[1]	-	-	52	57
Heart Attack Care				
Aspirin Given at Discharge[1,2]	-	-	99%	99%
Fibrinolytic Meds Within 30 Min. of Arrival[2,3]	-	-	-	54%
PCI Within 90 Minutes of Arrival[2,3]	-	-	97%	96%
Statin Prescribed at Discharge[1,2]	-	-	98%	98%
Heart Failure Care				
ACE Inhibitor or ARB for LVSD[1,2]	-	-	96%	97%
Discharge Instructions Given[2]	15	73%	94%	94%
Evaluation of LVS Function[2]	20	0%	98%	99%
Medicare Spending				
Medicare Spending per Patient (ratio)	-	0.84	0.95	0.98
Pneumonia Care				
Appropriate Initial Antibiotic Given[2]	12	58%	95%	95%
Blood Culture Timing[1,2]	-	-	98%	98%
Pregnancy and Delivery Care				
Newborn Deliveries Scheduled Early[2,7]	-	-	5%	6%
Preventive Care				
Immunization for Influenza[2]	134	54%	92%	90%
Immunization for Pneumonia[2]	193	60%	93%	92%
Stroke Care				
Anticoagulation Therapy for Atrial Fibrillation[2,3]	-	-	94%	95%
Antithrombotic Therapy Timing[1,2]	-	-	98%	98%
Assessed for Rehabilitation[1,2]	-	-	98%	97%
Discharged on Antithrombotic Therapy[1,2]	-	-	99%	99%
Discharged on Statin Medication[1,2]	-	-	95%	94%
Thrombolytic Therapy Timing[2,3]	-	-	67%	66%
Venous Thromboembolism Prophylaxis[1,2]	-	-	95%	94%
Written Stroke Educational Materials Given[2,3]	-	-	88%	88%
Surgical Care Improvement Project				
Appropriate Beta Blocker Usage[5]	-	-	98%	98%
Appropriate VTP Within 24 Hours[5]	-	-	98%	98%
Controlled Postoperative Blood Glucose[5]	-	-	97%	97%
Perioperative Temperature Management[5]	-	-	100%	100%
Prophylactic Antibiotic Selection[5]	-	-	99%	99%
Prophylactic Antibiotic Selection (Outpatient)[5]	-	-	98%	98%
Prophylactic Antibiotic Stopped[5]	-	-	98%	98%
Prophylactic Antibiotic Timing[5]	-	-	99%	99%
Prophylactic Antibiotic Timing (Outpatient)[5]	-	-	98%	98%
Urinary Catheter Removal[5]	-	-	97%	97%
Survey of Patients' Hospital Experiences				
Area Around Room 'Always' Quiet at Night[6]	<100	68%	61%	61%
Doctors 'Always' Communicated Well[6]	<100	83%	82%	82%
Home Recovery Information Given[6]	<100	80%	87%	85%
Hospital Given 9 or 10 on 10 Point Scale[6]	<100	67%	71%	71%
Meds 'Always' Explained Before Given[6]	<100	69%	63%	64%
Nurses 'Always' Communicated Well[6]	<100	82%	79%	79%
Pain 'Always' Well Controlled[6]	<100	75%	71%	71%
Room and Bathroom 'Always' Clean[6]	<100	74%	73%	73%
Timely Help 'Always' Received[6]	<100	87%	68%	68%
Would Definitely Recommend Hospital[6]	<100	67%	70%	71%
Use of Medical Imaging				
Cardiac Imaging Stress Test before Surgery[7]	-	-	5.2%	5.3%
Combination Abdominal CT Scan	61	1.6%	11.2%	10.5%
Combination Brain/Sinus CT Scan[1]	-	-	3.2%	2.7%
Combination Chest CT Scan[1]	-	-	1.9%	2.7%
Follow-up Mammogram/Ultrasound	88	3.4%	8.6%	8.8%
Lumbar Spine MRI for Low Back Pain[1]	-	-	39.6%	37.2%

Perry County Memorial Hospital

434 North West Street
Perryville, MO 63775
Phone: 573-547-2530
Fax: 573-547-3776
URL: www.pchmo.org
Type: Critical Access Hospitals
Emergency Services: Yes
Ownership: Government - Local
Beds: 51

Key Personnel:
Quality Assurance.............. Linda Brown
CEO/President.............. Patrick Carron
Patient Relations.............. Barbara Ernst
Infection Control.............. Katie Godsey
Emergency Room.............. Melissa Hayden
Chief of Medical Staff.......... Mohammad Moaddabi
Operating Room.............. Lois Prost
Radiology.............. Christopher Wibbenme

Measure	Cases	This Hosp.	State Avg.	U.S. Avg.
Blood Clot Prevention and Treatment				
Anticoagulation Overlap Therapy[5]	-	-	94%	93%
ICU Venous Thromboembolism Prophylaxis[5]	-	-	91%	92%
Incidence of Potentially Preventable VTE[5]	-	-	7%	10%
UFH with Dosages/Platelet Monitoring[5]	-	-	96%	97%
Venous Thromboembolism Prophylaxis[5]	-	-	85%	85%
Warfarin Therapy Discharge Instructions[5]	-	-	76%	75%
Chest Pain/Possible Heart Attack Care				
Aspirin Given Within 24 Hours of Arrival	-	-	95%	96%
Fibrinolytic Meds Within 30 Min. of Arrival	-	-	53%	58%
Average Time to ECG (minutes)	-	-	7	7
Average Time to Transfer (minutes)	-	-	53	60
Children's Asthma Care				
Received Home Management Plan of Care	-	-	-	88%
Received Reliever Medication	-	-	-	100%
Received Systemic Corticosteroids	-	-	-	100%
Emergency Department				
Admittance Decision Time (minutes)[5]	-	-	81	98
Head CT Results Within 45 Min. of Arrival	-	-	63%	57%
Patients Who Left ER Before Being Seen	-	-	3%	2%
Time from ER Arrival to Admit. (minutes)[5]	-	-	238	274
Time from ER Arrival to Discharge (minutes)	-	-	136	134
Time in ER Before Being Evaluated (minutes)	-	-	26	26
Time to Pain Meds for Fractures (minutes)	-	-	52	57
Heart Attack Care				
Aspirin Given at Discharge[1,3]	-	-	99%	99%
Fibrinolytic Meds Within 30 Min. of Arrival[3,7]	-	-	-	54%
PCI Within 90 Minutes of Arrival[3,7]	-	-	97%	96%
Statin Prescribed at Discharge[1,3]	-	-	98%	98%
Heart Failure Care				
ACE Inhibitor or ARB for LVSD[1]	-	-	96%	97%
Discharge Instructions Given[1]	-	-	94%	94%
Evaluation of LVS Function	14	93%	98%	99%
Medicare Spending				
Medicare Spending per Patient (ratio)	-	-	0.95	0.98
Pneumonia Care				
Appropriate Initial Antibiotic Given[2]	11	100%	95%	95%
Blood Culture Timing[2]	61	100%	98%	98%
Pregnancy and Delivery Care				
Newborn Deliveries Scheduled Early[5]	-	-	5%	6%
Preventive Care				
Immunization for Influenza[5]	-	-	92%	90%
Immunization for Pneumonia[5]	-	-	93%	92%
Stroke Care				
Anticoagulation Therapy for Atrial Fibrillation[5]	-	-	94%	95%
Antithrombotic Therapy Timing[5]	-	-	98%	98%
Assessed for Rehabilitation[5]	-	-	98%	97%
Discharged on Antithrombotic Therapy[5]	-	-	99%	99%
Discharged on Statin Medication[5]	-	-	95%	94%
Thrombolytic Therapy Timing[5]	-	-	67%	66%
Venous Thromboembolism Prophylaxis[5]	-	-	95%	94%

NOTE: Hospital profiles are in alphabetical order by state, then city, then hospital within the city; Rankings exclude hospitals with less than 25 cases except for patient surveys which excludes hospitals with less than 100 cases; (a) 100-299 cases; (1) The number of cases/patients is too few to report; (2) Data submitted were based on a sample of cases/patients; (3) Results are based on a shorter time period than required; (4) Data suppressed by CMS for one or more quarters; (5) Results are not available for this reporting period; (6) Fewer than 100 patients completed the HCAHPS survey; (7) No cases met the criteria for this measure; (8) The lower limit of the confidence interval cannot be calculated if the number of observed infections equals zero; (9) No data are available from the state/territory for this reporting period; (10) The scores shown reflect fewer than 50 completed surveys; (11) There were discrepancies in the data collection process; (12) This measure does not apply to this hospital for this reporting period; (13) Results cannot be calculated for this reporting period; (14) The results for this state are combined with nearby states to protect confidentiality; Please refer to the User's Guide for a full explanation of data.

Measure	Cases	This Hosp.	State Avg.	U.S. Avg.
Written Stroke Educational Materials Given[5]	-	-	88%	88%
Surgical Care Improvement Project				
Appropriate Beta Blocker Usage	22	100%	98%	98%
Appropriate VTP Within 24 Hours	65	100%	98%	98%
Controlled Postoperative Blood Glucose[7]	-	-	97%	97%
Perioperative Temperature Management	73	100%	100%	100%
Prophylactic Antibiotic Selection	62	100%	99%	99%
Prophylactic Antibiotic Selection (Outpatient)	-	-	98%	98%
Prophylactic Antibiotic Stopped	61	100%	98%	98%
Prophylactic Antibiotic Timing	62	100%	99%	99%
Prophylactic Antibiotic Timing (Outpatient)	-	-	98%	98%
Urinary Catheter Removal	63	100%	97%	97%
Survey of Patients' Hospital Experiences				
Area Around Room 'Always' Quiet at Night[5]	-	-	61%	61%
Doctors 'Always' Communicated Well[5]	-	-	82%	82%
Home Recovery Information Given[5]	-	-	87%	85%
Hospital Given 9 or 10 on 10 Point Scale[5]	-	-	71%	71%
Meds 'Always' Explained Before Given[5]	-	-	63%	64%
Nurses 'Always' Communicated Well[5]	-	-	79%	79%
Pain 'Always' Well Controlled[5]	-	-	71%	71%
Room and Bathroom 'Always' Clean[5]	-	-	73%	73%
Timely Help 'Always' Received[5]	-	-	68%	68%
Would Definitely Recommend Hospital[5]	-	-	70%	71%
Use of Medical Imaging				
Cardiac Imaging Stress Test before Surgery	-	-	5.2%	5.3%
Combination Abdominal CT Scan	-	-	11.2%	10.5%
Combination Brain/Sinus CT Scan	-	-	3.2%	2.7%
Combination Chest CT Scan	-	-	1.9%	2.7%
Follow-up Mammogram/Ultrasound	-	-	8.6%	8.8%
Lumbar Spine MRI for Low Back Pain	-	-	39.6%	37.2%

Black River Community Medical Center

217 Physicians Park Drive
Poplar Bluff, MO 63901
Phone: 573-686-6001
Type: Acute Care Hospitals
Emergency Services: Yes
Ownership: Voluntary non-profit - Private

Measure	Cases	This Hosp.	State Avg.	U.S. Avg.
Blood Clot Prevention and Treatment				
Anticoagulation Overlap Therapy[1,2]	-	-	94%	93%
ICU Venous Thromboembolism Prophylaxis[2,7]	-	-	91%	92%
Incidence of Potentially Preventable VTE[2,7]	-	-	7%	10%
UFH with Dosages/Platelet Monitoring[1,2]	-	-	96%	97%
Venous Thromboembolism Prophylaxis[2]	144	42%	85%	85%
Warfarin Therapy Discharge Instructions[1,2]	-	-	76%	75%
Chest Pain/Possible Heart Attack Care				
Aspirin Given Within 24 Hours of Arrival[3]	33	94%	95%	96%
Fibrinolytic Meds Within 30 Min. of Arrival[3,7]	-	-	53%	58%
Average Time to ECG (minutes)[3]	33	7	7	7
Average Time to Transfer (minutes)[1,3]	-	-	53	60
Children's Asthma Care				
Received Home Management Plan of Care	-	-	-	88%
Received Reliever Medication	-	-	-	100%
Received Systemic Corticosteroids	-	-	-	100%
Emergency Department				
Admittance Decision Time (minutes)[2,3]	88	34	81	98
Head CT Results Within 45 Min. of Arrival[5]	-	-	63%	57%
Patients Who Left ER Before Being Seen	4,338	6%	3%	2%
Time from ER Arrival to Admit. (minutes)[2,3]	89	173	238	274
Time from ER Arrival to Discharge (minutes)[3]	291	103	136	134
Time in ER Before Being Evaluated (minutes)[3]	337	25	26	26
Time to Pain Meds for Fractures (minutes)[3]	25	76	52	57
Heart Attack Care				
Aspirin Given at Discharge[5]	-	-	99%	99%
Fibrinolytic Meds Within 30 Min. of Arrival[5]	-	-	-	54%
PCI Within 90 Minutes of Arrival[5]	-	-	97%	96%
Statin Prescribed at Discharge[5]	-	-	98%	98%
Heart Failure Care				
ACE Inhibitor or ARB for LVSD[1,3]	-	-	96%	97%
Discharge Instructions Given[1,3]	-	-	94%	94%
Evaluation of LVS Function[1,3]	-	-	98%	99%
Medicare Spending				
Medicare Spending per Patient (ratio)[1]	-	-	0.95	0.98
Pneumonia Care				
Appropriate Initial Antibiotic Given[2,3]	13	92%	95%	95%
Blood Culture Timing[1,2]	-	-	98%	98%
Pregnancy and Delivery Care				
Newborn Deliveries Scheduled Early[7]	-	-	5%	6%
Preventive Care				
Immunization for Influenza[2,3]	63	63%	92%	90%
Immunization for Pneumonia[2,3]	141	74%	93%	92%
Stroke Care				
Anticoagulation Therapy for Atrial Fibrillation[5]	-	-	94%	95%
Antithrombotic Therapy Timing[5]	-	-	98%	98%
Assessed for Rehabilitation[5]	-	-	98%	97%
Discharged on Antithrombotic Therapy[5]	-	-	99%	99%
Discharged on Statin Medication[5]	-	-	95%	94%
Thrombolytic Therapy Timing[5]	-	-	67%	66%
Venous Thromboembolism Prophylaxis[5]	-	-	95%	94%
Written Stroke Educational Materials Given[5]	-	-	88%	88%
Surgical Care Improvement Project				
Appropriate Beta Blocker Usage[5]	-	-	98%	98%
Appropriate VTP Within 24 Hours[5]	-	-	98%	98%
Controlled Postoperative Blood Glucose[5]	-	-	97%	97%
Perioperative Temperature Management[5]	-	-	100%	100%
Prophylactic Antibiotic Selection[5]	-	-	99%	99%
Prophylactic Antibiotic Selection (Outpatient)[5]	-	-	98%	98%
Prophylactic Antibiotic Stopped[5]	-	-	98%	98%
Prophylactic Antibiotic Timing[5]	-	-	99%	99%
Prophylactic Antibiotic Timing (Outpatient)[5]	-	-	98%	98%
Urinary Catheter Removal[5]	-	-	97%	97%
Survey of Patients' Hospital Experiences				
Area Around Room 'Always' Quiet at Night[5]	-	-	61%	61%
Doctors 'Always' Communicated Well[5]	-	-	82%	82%
Home Recovery Information Given[5]	-	-	87%	85%
Hospital Given 9 or 10 on 10 Point Scale[5]	-	-	71%	71%
Meds 'Always' Explained Before Given[5]	-	-	63%	64%
Nurses 'Always' Communicated Well[5]	-	-	79%	79%
Pain 'Always' Well Controlled[5]	-	-	71%	71%
Room and Bathroom 'Always' Clean[5]	-	-	73%	73%
Timely Help 'Always' Received[5]	-	-	68%	68%
Would Definitely Recommend Hospital[5]	-	-	70%	71%
Use of Medical Imaging				
Cardiac Imaging Stress Test before Surgery	202	5.9%	5.2%	5.3%
Combination Abdominal CT Scan	450	22.4%	11.2%	10.5%
Combination Brain/Sinus CT Scan[1]	-	-	3.2%	2.7%
Combination Chest CT Scan	259	0.0%	1.9%	2.7%
Follow-up Mammogram/Ultrasound	1,072	6.7%	8.6%	8.8%
Lumbar Spine MRI for Low Back Pain	224	31.3%	39.6%	37.2%

Poplar Bluff Regional Medical Center

3100 Oak Grove Road
Poplar Bluff, MO 63901
Phone: 573-785-7721
Fax: 573-686-5388
E-mail: info@pbrmc.hma-corp.com
URL: www.poplarbluffregional.com
Type: Acute Care Hospitals
Emergency Services: Yes
Ownership: Proprietary
Beds: 423
Key Personnel:
CEO/President. . . . . Kenneth James

Measure	Cases	This Hosp.	State Avg.	U.S. Avg.
Blood Clot Prevention and Treatment				
Anticoagulation Overlap Therapy[2]	85	98%	94%	93%
ICU Venous Thromboembolism Prophylaxis[2]	94	94%	91%	92%
Incidence of Potentially Preventable VTE[2]	16	12%	7%	10%
UFH with Dosages/Platelet Monitoring[2]	82	100%	96%	97%
Venous Thromboembolism Prophylaxis[2]	623	90%	85%	85%
Warfarin Therapy Discharge Instructions[2]	68	87%	76%	75%
Chest Pain/Possible Heart Attack Care				
Aspirin Given Within 24 Hours of Arrival	75	99%	95%	96%
Fibrinolytic Meds Within 30 Min. of Arrival[7]	-	-	53%	58%
Average Time to ECG (minutes)	78	10	7	7
Average Time to Transfer (minutes)[7]	-	-	53	60
Children's Asthma Care				
Received Home Management Plan of Care	-	-	-	88%
Received Reliever Medication	-	-	-	100%
Received Systemic Corticosteroids	-	-	-	100%
Emergency Department				
Admittance Decision Time (minutes)[2]	504	144	81	98
Head CT Results Within 45 Min. of Arrival[1]	-	-	63%	57%
Patients Who Left ER Before Being Seen	33,095	4%	3%	2%
Time from ER Arrival to Admit. (minutes)[2]	504	321	238	274
Time from ER Arrival to Discharge (minutes)	336	156	136	134
Time in ER Before Being Evaluated (minutes)	383	17	26	26
Time to Pain Meds for Fractures (minutes)	90	57	52	57
Heart Attack Care				
Aspirin Given at Discharge	171	100%	99%	99%
Fibrinolytic Meds Within 30 Min. of Arrival[7]	-	-	-	54%
PCI Within 90 Minutes of Arrival	35	97%	97%	96%
Statin Prescribed at Discharge	169	98%	98%	98%
Heart Failure Care				
ACE Inhibitor or ARB for LVSD	96	100%	96%	97%
Discharge Instructions Given	264	99%	94%	94%
Evaluation of LVS Function	316	100%	98%	99%
Medicare Spending				
Medicare Spending per Patient (ratio)	-	0.94	0.95	0.98
Pneumonia Care				
Appropriate Initial Antibiotic Given	186	98%	95%	95%
Blood Culture Timing	274	97%	98%	98%
Pregnancy and Delivery Care				
Newborn Deliveries Scheduled Early[2]	84	27%	5%	6%
Preventive Care				
Immunization for Influenza[2]	503	95%	92%	90%
Immunization for Pneumonia[2]	567	97%	93%	92%
Stroke Care				
Anticoagulation Therapy for Atrial Fibrillation	12	100%	94%	95%
Antithrombotic Therapy Timing	96	99%	98%	98%
Assessed for Rehabilitation	89	97%	98%	97%
Discharged on Antithrombotic Therapy	87	99%	99%	99%
Discharged on Statin Medication	62	81%	95%	94%
Thrombolytic Therapy Timing[1]	-	-	67%	66%
Venous Thromboembolism Prophylaxis	102	92%	95%	94%
Written Stroke Educational Materials Given	45	98%	88%	88%
Surgical Care Improvement Project				
Appropriate Beta Blocker Usage	167	98%	98%	98%
Appropriate VTP Within 24 Hours	303	97%	98%	98%
Controlled Postoperative Blood Glucose	80	98%	97%	97%
Perioperative Temperature Management	422	100%	100%	100%
Prophylactic Antibiotic Selection	316	100%	99%	99%
Prophylactic Antibiotic Selection (Outpatient)	312	96%	98%	98%
Prophylactic Antibiotic Stopped	286	98%	98%	98%
Prophylactic Antibiotic Timing	319	97%	99%	99%
Prophylactic Antibiotic Timing (Outpatient)	314	98%	98%	98%
Urinary Catheter Removal	259	93%	97%	97%
Survey of Patients' Hospital Experiences				
Area Around Room 'Always' Quiet at Night	300+	55%	61%	61%
Doctors 'Always' Communicated Well	300+	76%	82%	82%
Home Recovery Information Given	300+	73%	87%	85%
Hospital Given 9 or 10 on 10 Point Scale	300+	48%	71%	71%
Meds 'Always' Explained Before Given	300+	52%	63%	64%
Nurses 'Always' Communicated Well	300+	69%	79%	79%
Pain 'Always' Well Controlled	300+	59%	71%	71%
Room and Bathroom 'Always' Clean	300+	65%	73%	73%
Timely Help 'Always' Received	300+	53%	68%	68%
Would Definitely Recommend Hospital	300+	47%	70%	71%
Use of Medical Imaging				
Cardiac Imaging Stress Test before Surgery	150	9.3%	5.2%	5.3%
Combination Abdominal CT Scan	651	23.7%	11.2%	10.5%
Combination Brain/Sinus CT Scan	729	2.6%	3.2%	2.7%
Combination Chest CT Scan	405	6.4%	1.9%	2.7%
Follow-up Mammogram/Ultrasound	407	6.1%	8.6%	8.8%
Lumbar Spine MRI for Low Back Pain	148	39.2%	39.6%	37.2%

Poplar Bluff VA Medical Center

1500 N. Westwood Blvd.
Poplar Bluff, MO 63901
Phone: 573-686-4151
Fax: 573-778-4699
URL: www.poplarbluff.va.gov
Type: Acute Care - VA
Emergency Services: No
Ownership: Government Federal
Beds: 16
Key Personnel:
CEO/President. . . . . Nancy Arnold

NOTE: Hospital profiles are in alphabetical order by state, then city, then hospital within the city; Rankings exclude hospitals with less than 25 cases except for patient surveys which excludes hospitals with less than 100 cases; (a) 100-299 cases; (1) The number of cases/patients is too few to report; (2) Data submitted were based on a sample of cases/patients; (3) Results are based on a shorter time period than required; (4) Data suppressed by CMS for one or more quarters; (5) Results are not available for this reporting period; (6) Fewer than 100 patients completed the HCAHPS survey; (7) No cases met the criteria for this measure; (8) The lower limit of the confidence interval cannot be calculated if the number of observed infections equals zero; (9) No data are available from the state/territory for this reporting period; (10) The scores shown reflect fewer than 50 completed surveys; (11) There were discrepancies in the data collection process; (12) This measure does not apply to this hospital for this reporting period; (13) Results cannot be calculated for this reporting period; (14) The results for this state are combined with nearby states to protect confidentiality; Please refer to the User's Guide for a full explanation of data.

Chief of Medical Staff.......... Jose D. Riojas

Measure	Cases	This Hosp.	State Avg.	U.S. Avg.
Blood Clot Prevention and Treatment				
Anticoagulation Overlap Therapy	-	-	94%	93%
ICU Venous Thromboembolism Prophylaxis	-	-	91%	92%
Incidence of Potentially Preventable VTE	-	-	7%	10%
UFH with Dosages/Platelet Monitoring	-	-	96%	97%
Venous Thromboembolism Prophylaxis	-	-	85%	85%
Warfarin Therapy Discharge Instructions	-	-	76%	75%
Chest Pain/Possible Heart Attack Care				
Aspirin Given Within 24 Hours of Arrival	-	-	95%	96%
Fibrinolytic Meds Within 30 Min. of Arrival	-	-	53%	58%
Average Time to ECG (minutes)	-	-	7	7
Average Time to Transfer (minutes)	-	-	53	60
Children's Asthma Care				
Received Home Management Plan of Care	-	-	-	88%
Received Reliever Medication	-	-	-	100%
Received Systemic Corticosteroids	-	-	-	100%
Emergency Department				
Admittance Decision Time (minutes)	-	-	81	98
Head CT Results Within 45 Min. of Arrival	-	-	63%	57%
Patients Who Left ER Before Being Seen	-	-	3%	2%
Time from ER Arrival to Admit. (minutes)	-	-	238	274
Time from ER Arrival to Discharge (minutes)	-	-	136	134
Time in ER Before Being Evaluated (minutes)	-	-	26	26
Time to Pain Meds for Fractures (minutes)	-	-	52	57
Heart Attack Care				
Aspirin Given at Discharge[5]	-	-	99%	99%
Fibrinolytic Meds Within 30 Min. of Arrival[5]	-	-	-	54%
PCI Within 90 Minutes of Arrival[5]	-	-	97%	96%
Statin Prescribed at Discharge[5]	-	-	98%	98%
Heart Failure Care				
ACE Inhibitor or ARB for LVSD[1]	19	79%	96%	97%
Discharge Instructions Given	72	100%	94%	94%
Evaluation of LVS Function	75	100%	98%	99%
Medicare Spending				
Medicare Spending per Patient (ratio)	-	-	0.95	0.98
Pneumonia Care				
Appropriate Initial Antibiotic Given	52	98%	95%	95%
Blood Culture Timing[5]	-	-	98%	98%
Pregnancy and Delivery Care				
Newborn Deliveries Scheduled Early	-	-	5%	6%
Preventive Care				
Immunization for Influenza[2,3]	123	98%	92%	90%
Immunization for Pneumonia[2,3]	303	99%	93%	92%
Stroke Care				
Anticoagulation Therapy for Atrial Fibrillation	-	-	94%	95%
Antithrombotic Therapy Timing	-	-	98%	98%
Assessed for Rehabilitation	-	-	98%	97%
Discharged on Antithrombotic Therapy	-	-	99%	99%
Discharged on Statin Medication	-	-	95%	94%
Thrombolytic Therapy Timing	-	-	67%	66%
Venous Thromboembolism Prophylaxis	-	-	95%	94%
Written Stroke Educational Materials Given	-	-	88%	88%
Surgical Care Improvement Project				
Appropriate Beta Blocker Usage[5]	-	-	98%	98%
Appropriate VTP Within 24 Hours[5]	-	-	98%	98%
Controlled Postoperative Blood Glucose[5]	-	-	97%	97%
Perioperative Temperature Management[5]	-	-	100%	100%
Prophylactic Antibiotic Selection[5]	-	-	99%	99%
Prophylactic Antibiotic Selection (Outpatient)	-	-	98%	98%
Prophylactic Antibiotic Stopped[5]	-	-	98%	98%
Prophylactic Antibiotic Timing[5]	-	-	99%	99%
Prophylactic Antibiotic Timing (Outpatient)	-	-	98%	98%
Urinary Catheter Removal[5]	-	-	97%	97%
Survey of Patients' Hospital Experiences				
Area Around Room 'Always' Quiet at Night	-	-	61%	61%
Doctors 'Always' Communicated Well	-	-	82%	82%
Home Recovery Information Given	-	-	87%	85%
Hospital Given 9 or 10 on 10 Point Scale	-	-	71%	71%
Meds 'Always' Explained Before Given	-	-	63%	64%
Nurses 'Always' Communicated Well	-	-	79%	79%
Pain 'Always' Well Controlled	-	-	71%	71%
Room and Bathroom 'Always' Clean	-	-	73%	73%
Timely Help 'Always' Received	-	-	68%	68%
Would Definitely Recommend Hospital	-	-	70%	71%
Use of Medical Imaging				
Cardiac Imaging Stress Test before Surgery	-	-	5.2%	5.3%
Combination Abdominal CT Scan	-	-	11.2%	10.5%
Combination Brain/Sinus CT Scan	-	-	3.2%	2.7%
Combination Chest CT Scan	-	-	1.9%	2.7%
Follow-up Mammogram/Ultrasound	-	-	8.6%	8.8%
Lumbar Spine MRI for Low Back Pain	-	-	39.6%	37.2%

Washington County Memorial Hospital

300 Health Way
Potosi, MO 63664
E-mail: wcmhadm@mail.potosi.k12.mo.us
URL: www.wcmhosp.org
Type: Critical Access Hospitals
Ownership: Government - Local

Phone: 573-438-5451
Fax: 573-438-2399
Emergency Services: Yes
Beds: 42

Key Personnel:
Radiology.................... Aona DeClue
Cardiac Laboratory............ Bobin Delfield
CEO/President............... H Clark Duncan
Chief of Medical Staff.......... Frezerick Fyat, MD
Emergency Room .... A Minichuck

Measure	Cases	This Hosp.	State Avg.	U.S. Avg.
Blood Clot Prevention and Treatment				
Anticoagulation Overlap Therapy[5]	-	-	94%	93%
ICU Venous Thromboembolism Prophylaxis[5]	-	-	91%	92%
Incidence of Potentially Preventable VTE[5]	-	-	7%	10%
UFH with Dosages/Platelet Monitoring[5]	-	-	96%	97%
Venous Thromboembolism Prophylaxis[5]	-	-	85%	85%
Warfarin Therapy Discharge Instructions[5]	-	-	76%	75%
Chest Pain/Possible Heart Attack Care				
Aspirin Given Within 24 Hours of Arrival	-	-	95%	96%
Fibrinolytic Meds Within 30 Min. of Arrival	-	-	53%	58%
Average Time to ECG (minutes)	-	-	7	7
Average Time to Transfer (minutes)	-	-	53	60
Children's Asthma Care				
Received Home Management Plan of Care	-	-	-	88%
Received Reliever Medication	-	-	-	100%
Received Systemic Corticosteroids	-	-	-	100%
Emergency Department				
Admittance Decision Time (minutes)[5]	-	-	81	98
Head CT Results Within 45 Min. of Arrival	-	-	63%	57%
Patients Who Left ER Before Being Seen	-	-	3%	2%
Time from ER Arrival to Admit. (minutes)[5]	-	-	238	274
Time from ER Arrival to Discharge (minutes)	-	-	136	134
Time in ER Before Being Evaluated (minutes)	-	-	26	26
Time to Pain Meds for Fractures (minutes)	-	-	52	57
Heart Attack Care				
Aspirin Given at Discharge[1,3]	-	-	99%	99%
Fibrinolytic Meds Within 30 Min. of Arrival[3,7]	-	-	-	54%
PCI Within 90 Minutes of Arrival[3,7]	-	-	97%	96%
Statin Prescribed at Discharge[1,3]	-	-	98%	98%
Heart Failure Care				
ACE Inhibitor or ARB for LVSD[1]	-	-	96%	97%
Discharge Instructions Given	30	97%	94%	94%
Evaluation of LVS Function	43	86%	98%	99%
Medicare Spending				
Medicare Spending per Patient (ratio)	-	-	0.95	0.98
Pneumonia Care				
Appropriate Initial Antibiotic Given	60	88%	95%	95%
Blood Culture Timing	75	93%	98%	98%
Pregnancy and Delivery Care				
Newborn Deliveries Scheduled Early[5]	-	-	5%	6%
Preventive Care				
Immunization for Influenza[5]	-	-	92%	90%
Immunization for Pneumonia[5]	-	-	93%	92%
Stroke Care				
Anticoagulation Therapy for Atrial Fibrillation[5]	-	-	94%	95%
Antithrombotic Therapy Timing[5]	-	-	98%	98%
Assessed for Rehabilitation[5]	-	-	98%	97%
Discharged on Antithrombotic Therapy[5]	-	-	99%	99%
Discharged on Statin Medication[5]	-	-	95%	94%
Thrombolytic Therapy Timing[5]	-	-	67%	66%
Venous Thromboembolism Prophylaxis[5]	-	-	95%	94%
Written Stroke Educational Materials Given[5]	-	-	88%	88%
Surgical Care Improvement Project				
Appropriate Beta Blocker Usage[5]	-	-	98%	98%
Appropriate VTP Within 24 Hours[5]	-	-	98%	98%
Controlled Postoperative Blood Glucose[5]	-	-	97%	97%
Perioperative Temperature Management[5]	-	-	100%	100%
Prophylactic Antibiotic Selection[5]	-	-	99%	99%
Prophylactic Antibiotic Selection (Outpatient)	-	-	98%	98%
Prophylactic Antibiotic Stopped[5]	-	-	98%	98%
Prophylactic Antibiotic Timing[5]	-	-	99%	99%
Prophylactic Antibiotic Timing (Outpatient)	-	-	98%	98%
Urinary Catheter Removal[5]	-	-	97%	97%
Survey of Patients' Hospital Experiences				
Area Around Room 'Always' Quiet at Night[5]	-	-	61%	61%
Doctors 'Always' Communicated Well[5]	-	-	82%	82%
Home Recovery Information Given[5]	-	-	87%	85%
Hospital Given 9 or 10 on 10 Point Scale[5]	-	-	71%	71%
Meds 'Always' Explained Before Given[5]	-	-	63%	64%
Nurses 'Always' Communicated Well[5]	-	-	79%	79%
Pain 'Always' Well Controlled[5]	-	-	71%	71%
Room and Bathroom 'Always' Clean[5]	-	-	73%	73%
Timely Help 'Always' Received[5]	-	-	68%	68%
Would Definitely Recommend Hospital[5]	-	-	70%	71%
Use of Medical Imaging				
Cardiac Imaging Stress Test before Surgery	-	-	5.2%	5.3%
Combination Abdominal CT Scan	-	-	11.2%	10.5%
Combination Brain/Sinus CT Scan	-	-	3.2%	2.7%
Combination Chest CT Scan	-	-	1.9%	2.7%
Follow-up Mammogram/Ultrasound	-	-	8.6%	8.8%
Lumbar Spine MRI for Low Back Pain	-	-	39.6%	37.2%

Ray County Memorial Hospital

904 Wollard Boulevard
Richmond, MO 64085
Type: Critical Access Hospitals
Ownership: Government - Local

Phone: 816-470-5432
Fax: 816-470-8382
Emergency Services: Yes
Beds: 63

Key Personnel:
Infection Control............. Jackie Devaul, RN
Quality Assurance .... Donna Lamar
Operating Room.............. Cindy Rogers
Chief of Medical Staff.......... Daniel M Rosak, MD

Measure	Cases	This Hosp.	State Avg.	U.S. Avg.
Blood Clot Prevention and Treatment				
Anticoagulation Overlap Therapy[5]	-	-	94%	93%
ICU Venous Thromboembolism Prophylaxis[5]	-	-	91%	92%
Incidence of Potentially Preventable VTE[5]	-	-	7%	10%
UFH with Dosages/Platelet Monitoring[5]	-	-	96%	97%
Venous Thromboembolism Prophylaxis[5]	-	-	85%	85%
Warfarin Therapy Discharge Instructions[5]	-	-	76%	75%
Chest Pain/Possible Heart Attack Care				
Aspirin Given Within 24 Hours of Arrival	-	-	95%	96%
Fibrinolytic Meds Within 30 Min. of Arrival	-	-	53%	58%
Average Time to ECG (minutes)	-	-	7	7
Average Time to Transfer (minutes)	-	-	53	60
Children's Asthma Care				
Received Home Management Plan of Care	-	-	-	88%
Received Reliever Medication	-	-	-	100%
Received Systemic Corticosteroids	-	-	-	100%
Emergency Department				
Admittance Decision Time (minutes)[5]	-	-	81	98
Head CT Results Within 45 Min. of Arrival	-	-	63%	57%
Patients Who Left ER Before Being Seen	-	-	3%	2%
Time from ER Arrival to Admit. (minutes)[5]	-	-	238	274
Time from ER Arrival to Discharge (minutes)	-	-	136	134
Time in ER Before Being Evaluated (minutes)	-	-	26	26
Time to Pain Meds for Fractures (minutes)	-	-	52	57
Heart Attack Care				
Aspirin Given at Discharge[1,3]	-	-	99%	99%
Fibrinolytic Meds Within 30 Min. of Arrival[3,7]	-	-	-	54%

NOTE: Hospital profiles are in alphabetical order by state, then city, then hospital within the city; Rankings exclude hospitals with less than 25 cases except for patient surveys which excludes hospitals with less than 100 cases; (a) 100-299 cases; (1) The number of cases/patients is too few to report; (2) Data submitted were based on a sample of cases/patients; (3) Results are based on a shorter time period than required; (4) Data suppressed by CMS for one or more quarters; (5) Results are not available for this reporting period; (6) Fewer than 100 patients completed the HCAHPS survey; (7) No cases met the criteria for this measure; (8) The lower limit of the confidence interval cannot be calculated if the number of observed infections equals zero; (9) No data are available from the state/territory for this reporting period; (10) The scores shown reflect fewer than 50 completed surveys; (11) There were discrepancies in the data collection process; (12) This measure does not apply to this hospital for this reporting period; (13) Results cannot be calculated for this reporting period; (14) The results for this state are combined with nearby states to protect confidentiality; Please refer to the User's Guide for a full explanation of data.

Measure	Cases	This Hosp.	State Avg.	U.S. Avg.
PCI Within 90 Minutes of Arrival[3,7]	-	-	97%	96%
Statin Prescribed at Discharge[1,3]	-	-	98%	98%
Heart Failure Care				
ACE Inhibitor or ARB for LVSD[1,3]	-	-	96%	97%
Discharge Instructions Given[1,3]	-	-	94%	94%
Evaluation of LVS Function[3]	19	68%	98%	99%
Medicare Spending				
Medicare Spending per Patient (ratio)	-	-	0.95	0.98
Pneumonia Care				
Appropriate Initial Antibiotic Given[1,3]	-	-	95%	95%
Blood Culture Timing[1,3]	-	-	98%	98%
Pregnancy and Delivery Care				
Newborn Deliveries Scheduled Early[5]	-	-	5%	6%
Preventive Care				
Immunization for Influenza[5]	-	-	92%	90%
Immunization for Pneumonia[5]	-	-	93%	92%
Stroke Care				
Anticoagulation Therapy for Atrial Fibrillation[5]	-	-	94%	95%
Antithrombotic Therapy Timing[5]	-	-	98%	98%
Assessed for Rehabilitation[5]	-	-	98%	97%
Discharged on Antithrombotic Therapy[5]	-	-	99%	99%
Discharged on Statin Medication[5]	-	-	95%	94%
Thrombolytic Therapy Timing[5]	-	-	67%	66%
Venous Thromboembolism Prophylaxis[5]	-	-	95%	94%
Written Stroke Educational Materials Given[5]	-	-	88%	88%
Surgical Care Improvement Project				
Appropriate Beta Blocker Usage[5]	-	-	98%	98%
Appropriate VTP Within 24 Hours[5]	-	-	98%	98%
Controlled Postoperative Blood Glucose[5]	-	-	97%	97%
Perioperative Temperature Management[5]	-	-	100%	100%
Prophylactic Antibiotic Selection[5]	-	-	99%	99%
Prophylactic Antibiotic Selection (Outpatient)	-	-	98%	98%
Prophylactic Antibiotic Stopped[5]	-	-	98%	98%
Prophylactic Antibiotic Timing[5]	-	-	99%	99%
Prophylactic Antibiotic Timing (Outpatient)	-	-	98%	98%
Urinary Catheter Removal[5]	-	-	97%	97%
Survey of Patients' Hospital Experiences				
Area Around Room 'Always' Quiet at Night[5]	-	-	61%	61%
Doctors 'Always' Communicated Well[5]	-	-	82%	82%
Home Recovery Information Given[5]	-	-	87%	85%
Hospital Given 9 or 10 on 10 Point Scale[5]	-	-	71%	71%
Meds 'Always' Explained Before Given[5]	-	-	63%	64%
Nurses 'Always' Communicated Well[5]	-	-	79%	79%
Pain 'Always' Well Controlled[5]	-	-	71%	71%
Room and Bathroom 'Always' Clean[5]	-	-	73%	73%
Timely Help 'Always' Received[5]	-	-	68%	68%
Would Definitely Recommend Hospital[5]	-	-	70%	71%
Use of Medical Imaging				
Cardiac Imaging Stress Test before Surgery	-	-	5.2%	5.3%
Combination Abdominal CT Scan	-	-	11.2%	10.5%
Combination Brain/Sinus CT Scan	-	-	3.2%	2.7%
Combination Chest CT Scan	-	-	1.9%	2.7%
Follow-up Mammogram/Ultrasound	-	-	8.6%	8.8%
Lumbar Spine MRI for Low Back Pain	-	-	39.6%	37.2%

SSM Saint Marys Health Center

6420 Clayton Rd
Richmond Heights, MO 63117
URL: www.ssmhealth.com/stmarys
Type: Acute Care Hospitals
Ownership: Voluntary non-profit - Private

Phone: 314-768-8000
Fax: 314-768-7131
Emergency Services: Yes
Beds: 622

Key Personnel:
CEO/President. . . . . Kathleen Becker
Infection Control. . . . . Theresa Grattan
Chief of Medical Staff. . . . . Kevin Johnson, MD
Quality Assurance . . . . Shelly Pierce

Measure	Cases	This Hosp.	State Avg.	U.S. Avg.
Blood Clot Prevention and Treatment				
Anticoagulation Overlap Therapy[2]	97	93%	94%	93%
ICU Venous Thromboembolism Prophylaxis[2]	54	100%	91%	92%
Incidence of Potentially Preventable VTE[2]	14	0%	7%	10%
UFH with Dosages/Platelet Monitoring[2]	48	81%	96%	97%
Venous Thromboembolism Prophylaxis[2]	333	92%	85%	85%
Warfarin Therapy Discharge Instructions[2]	67	79%	76%	75%
Chest Pain/Possible Heart Attack Care				
Aspirin Given Within 24 Hours of Arrival[1]	-	-	95%	96%
Fibrinolytic Meds Within 30 Min. of Arrival[5]	-	-	53%	58%
Average Time to ECG (minutes)[1]	-	-	7	7
Average Time to Transfer (minutes)[5]	-	-	53	60
Children's Asthma Care				
Received Home Management Plan of Care[2]	240	98%	-	88%
Received Reliever Medication[2]	239	100%	-	100%
Received Systemic Corticosteroids[2]	240	100%	-	100%
Emergency Department				
Admittance Decision Time (minutes)[2]	421	124	81	98
Head CT Results Within 45 Min. of Arrival[1]	-	-	63%	57%
Patients Who Left ER Before Being Seen	54,056	1%	3%	2%
Time from ER Arrival to Admit. (minutes)[2]	457	267	238	274
Time from ER Arrival to Discharge (minutes)	372	124	136	134
Time in ER Before Being Evaluated (minutes)	402	32	26	26
Time to Pain Meds for Fractures (minutes)	133	27	52	57
Heart Attack Care				
Aspirin Given at Discharge	209	100%	99%	99%
Fibrinolytic Meds Within 30 Min. of Arrival[7]	-	-	-	54%
PCI Within 90 Minutes of Arrival	24	100%	97%	96%
Statin Prescribed at Discharge	208	100%	98%	98%
Heart Failure Care				
ACE Inhibitor or ARB for LVSD[2]	66	100%	96%	97%
Discharge Instructions Given[2]	261	100%	94%	94%
Evaluation of LVS Function[2]	297	100%	98%	99%
Medicare Spending				
Medicare Spending per Patient (ratio)	-	0.98	0.95	0.98
Pneumonia Care				
Appropriate Initial Antibiotic Given[2]	75	99%	95%	95%
Blood Culture Timing[2]	136	100%	98%	98%
Pregnancy and Delivery Care				
Newborn Deliveries Scheduled Early[2]	41	0%	5%	6%
Preventive Care				
Immunization for Influenza[2]	543	98%	92%	90%
Immunization for Pneumonia[2]	446	97%	93%	92%
Stroke Care				
Anticoagulation Therapy for Atrial Fibrillation	15	100%	94%	95%
Antithrombotic Therapy Timing	125	98%	98%	98%
Assessed for Rehabilitation	138	99%	98%	97%
Discharged on Antithrombotic Therapy	130	100%	99%	99%
Discharged on Statin Medication	98	99%	95%	94%
Thrombolytic Therapy Timing	12	75%	67%	66%
Venous Thromboembolism Prophylaxis	134	99%	95%	94%
Written Stroke Educational Materials Given	53	100%	88%	88%
Surgical Care Improvement Project				
Appropriate Beta Blocker Usage[2]	172	99%	98%	98%
Appropriate VTP Within 24 Hours[2]	386	99%	98%	98%
Controlled Postoperative Blood Glucose[2]	77	99%	97%	97%
Perioperative Temperature Management[2]	500	100%	100%	100%
Prophylactic Antibiotic Selection[2]	385	99%	99%	99%
Prophylactic Antibiotic Selection (Outpatient)	493	99%	98%	98%
Prophylactic Antibiotic Stopped[2]	369	98%	98%	98%
Prophylactic Antibiotic Timing[2]	385	100%	99%	99%
Prophylactic Antibiotic Timing (Outpatient)	493	99%	98%	98%
Urinary Catheter Removal[2]	158	97%	97%	97%
Survey of Patients' Hospital Experiences				
Area Around Room 'Always' Quiet at Night	300+	60%	61%	61%
Doctors 'Always' Communicated Well	300+	80%	82%	82%
Home Recovery Information Given	300+	86%	87%	85%
Hospital Given 9 or 10 on 10 Point Scale	300+	74%	71%	71%
Meds 'Always' Explained Before Given	300+	66%	63%	64%
Nurses 'Always' Communicated Well	300+	82%	79%	79%
Pain 'Always' Well Controlled	300+	74%	71%	71%
Room and Bathroom 'Always' Clean	300+	69%	73%	73%
Timely Help 'Always' Received	300+	65%	68%	68%
Would Definitely Recommend Hospital	300+	75%	70%	71%
Use of Medical Imaging				
Cardiac Imaging Stress Test before Surgery	593	6.1%	5.2%	5.3%
Combination Abdominal CT Scan	663	16.9%	11.2%	10.5%
Combination Brain/Sinus CT Scan	695	4.0%	3.2%	2.7%
Combination Chest CT Scan	325	0.3%	1.9%	2.7%
Follow-up Mammogram/Ultrasound	1,583	10.1%	8.6%	8.8%
Lumbar Spine MRI for Low Back Pain	94	39.4%	39.6%	37.2%

Phelps County Regional Medical Center

1000 W 10th St
Rolla, MO 65401
E-mail: bharvey@rollanet.org
URL: www.rollanet.org/~pcrmc
Type: Acute Care Hospitals
Ownership: Government - Local

Phone: 573-458-8899
Fax: 573-458-8413
Emergency Services: Yes
Beds: 232

Key Personnel:
Operating Room. . . . . Michael Beard
Pediatric Ambulatory Care . . . . . Katherine Cook, MD
Pediatric In-Patient Care . . . . Katherine Cook, MD
Radiology. . . . . Edward Downey, MD
Emergency Room . . . . Jeff Folhein
Chief of Medical Staff. . . . . Don James
CEO/President. . . . . David Ross
Quality Assurance . . . . Jean Waterman

Measure	Cases	This Hosp.	State Avg.	U.S. Avg.
Blood Clot Prevention and Treatment				
Anticoagulation Overlap Therapy[2]	17	59%	94%	93%
ICU Venous Thromboembolism Prophylaxis[2]	88	91%	91%	92%
Incidence of Potentially Preventable VTE[1,2]	-	-	7%	10%
UFH with Dosages/Platelet Monitoring[1,2]	-	-	96%	97%
Venous Thromboembolism Prophylaxis[2]	291	80%	85%	85%
Warfarin Therapy Discharge Instructions[2]	14	93%	76%	75%
Chest Pain/Possible Heart Attack Care				
Aspirin Given Within 24 Hours of Arrival	132	98%	95%	96%
Fibrinolytic Meds Within 30 Min. of Arrival[1]	-	-	53%	58%
Average Time to ECG (minutes)	139	8	7	7
Average Time to Transfer (minutes)[1]	-	-	53	60
Children's Asthma Care				
Received Home Management Plan of Care	-	-	-	88%
Received Reliever Medication	-	-	-	100%
Received Systemic Corticosteroids	-	-	-	100%
Emergency Department				
Admittance Decision Time (minutes)[2]	385	72	81	98
Head CT Results Within 45 Min. of Arrival[1]	-	-	63%	57%
Patients Who Left ER Before Being Seen	37,357	1%	3%	2%
Time from ER Arrival to Admit. (minutes)[2]	421	249	238	274
Time from ER Arrival to Discharge (minutes)	171	169	136	134
Time in ER Before Being Evaluated (minutes)	418	17	26	26
Time to Pain Meds for Fractures (minutes)	93	59	52	57
Heart Attack Care				
Aspirin Given at Discharge	49	94%	99%	99%
Fibrinolytic Meds Within 30 Min. of Arrival[7]	-	-	-	54%
PCI Within 90 Minutes of Arrival[7]	-	-	97%	96%
Statin Prescribed at Discharge	51	80%	98%	98%
Heart Failure Care				
ACE Inhibitor or ARB for LVSD	54	94%	96%	97%
Discharge Instructions Given	91	96%	94%	94%
Evaluation of LVS Function	127	99%	98%	99%
Medicare Spending				
Medicare Spending per Patient (ratio)	-	0.98	0.95	0.98
Pneumonia Care				
Appropriate Initial Antibiotic Given	116	96%	95%	95%
Blood Culture Timing	179	95%	98%	98%
Pregnancy and Delivery Care				
Newborn Deliveries Scheduled Early[2]	12	8%	5%	6%
Preventive Care				
Immunization for Influenza[2]	416	94%	92%	90%
Immunization for Pneumonia[2]	533	95%	93%	92%
Stroke Care				
Anticoagulation Therapy for Atrial Fibrillation[1]	-	-	94%	95%
Antithrombotic Therapy Timing	33	100%	98%	98%
Assessed for Rehabilitation	45	98%	98%	97%
Discharged on Antithrombotic Therapy	43	98%	99%	99%
Discharged on Statin Medication	35	89%	95%	94%
Thrombolytic Therapy Timing[1]	-	-	67%	66%
Venous Thromboembolism Prophylaxis	42	83%	95%	94%
Written Stroke Educational Materials Given	14	57%	88%	88%
Surgical Care Improvement Project				

NOTE: Hospital profiles are in alphabetical order by state, then city, then hospital within the city; Rankings exclude hospitals with less than 25 cases except for patient surveys which excludes hospitals with less than 100 cases; (a) 100-299 cases; (1) The number of cases/patients is too few to report; (2) Data submitted were based on a sample of cases/patients; (3) Results are based on a shorter time period than required; (4) Data suppressed by CMS for one or more quarters; (5) Results are not available for this reporting period; (6) Fewer than 100 patients completed the HCAHPS survey; (7) No cases met the criteria for this measure; (8) The lower limit of the confidence interval cannot be calculated if the number of observed infections equals zero; (9) No data are available from the state/territory for this reporting period; (10) The scores shown reflect fewer than 50 completed surveys; (11) There were discrepancies in the data collection process; (12) This measure does not apply to this hospital for this reporting period; (13) Results cannot be calculated for this reporting period; (14) The results for this state are combined with nearby states to protect confidentiality; Please refer to the User's Guide for a full explanation of data.

Measure	Cases	This Hosp.	State Avg.	U.S. Avg.
Appropriate Beta Blocker Usage	107	93%	98%	98%
Appropriate VTP Within 24 Hours	344	99%	98%	98%
Controlled Postoperative Blood Glucose[7]	-	-	97%	97%
Perioperative Temperature Management	385	100%	100%	100%
Prophylactic Antibiotic Selection	267	99%	99%	99%
Prophylactic Antibiotic Selection (Outpatient)	170	98%	98%	98%
Prophylactic Antibiotic Stopped	261	97%	98%	98%
Prophylactic Antibiotic Timing	267	99%	99%	99%
Prophylactic Antibiotic Timing (Outpatient)	177	95%	98%	98%
Urinary Catheter Removal	296	96%	97%	97%
Survey of Patients' Hospital Experiences				
Area Around Room 'Always' Quiet at Night	300+	60%	61%	61%
Doctors 'Always' Communicated Well	300+	84%	82%	82%
Home Recovery Information Given	300+	89%	87%	85%
Hospital Given 9 or 10 on 10 Point Scale	300+	70%	71%	71%
Meds 'Always' Explained Before Given	300+	68%	63%	64%
Nurses 'Always' Communicated Well	300+	81%	79%	79%
Pain 'Always' Well Controlled	300+	68%	71%	71%
Room and Bathroom 'Always' Clean	300+	76%	73%	73%
Timely Help 'Always' Received	300+	65%	68%	68%
Would Definitely Recommend Hospital	300+	68%	70%	71%
Use of Medical Imaging				
Cardiac Imaging Stress Test before Surgery	410	3.7%	5.2%	5.3%
Combination Abdominal CT Scan	699	21.9%	11.2%	10.5%
Combination Brain/Sinus CT Scan	842	2.5%	3.2%	2.7%
Combination Chest CT Scan	511	0.2%	1.9%	2.7%
Follow-up Mammogram/Ultrasound	1,556	10.4%	8.6%	8.8%
Lumbar Spine MRI for Low Back Pain	175	52.0%	39.6%	37.2%

SSM Saint Joseph Health Center

300 1st Capitol Dr
Saint Charles, MO 63301
Phone: 636-947-5000
Fax: 636-947-5609
E-mail: mblamy@ssmhc.com
Type: Acute Care Hospitals
Emergency Services: Yes
Ownership: Voluntary non-profit - Private
Beds: 433

Key Personnel:
Pediatric Ambulatory Care . . . . . . Nadira Adil
Pediatric In-Patient Care . . . . Nadira Adil
CEO/President. . . . . Lee Bernstein
Radiology. . . . . Lewis Halberson
Chief of Medical Staff . . . . Kevin Johnson, MD
Quality Assurance . . . . Lois Kohler
Operating Room. . . . . Joseph Seger
Cardiac Laboratory. . . . . Mark Taber

Measure	Cases	This Hosp.	State Avg.	U.S. Avg.
Blood Clot Prevention and Treatment				
Anticoagulation Overlap Therapy[2]	57	95%	94%	93%
ICU Venous Thromboembolism Prophylaxis[2]	56	95%	91%	92%
Incidence of Potentially Preventable VTE[1,2]	-	-	7%	10%
UFH with Dosages/Platelet Monitoring[2]	22	91%	96%	97%
Venous Thromboembolism Prophylaxis[2]	373	85%	85%	85%
Warfarin Therapy Discharge Instructions[2]	49	59%	76%	75%
Chest Pain/Possible Heart Attack Care				
Aspirin Given Within 24 Hours of Arrival[1]	-	-	95%	96%
Fibrinolytic Meds Within 30 Min. of Arrival[5]	-	-	53%	58%
Average Time to ECG (minutes)[1]	-	-	7	7
Average Time to Transfer (minutes)[5]	-	-	53	60
Children's Asthma Care				
Received Home Management Plan of Care	-	-	-	88%
Received Reliever Medication	-	-	-	100%
Received Systemic Corticosteroids	-	-	-	100%
Emergency Department				
Admittance Decision Time (minutes)[2]	503	139	81	98
Head CT Results Within 45 Min. of Arrival	13	92%	63%	57%
Patients Who Left ER Before Being Seen	40,645	1%	3%	2%
Time from ER Arrival to Admit. (minutes)[2]	552	224	238	274
Time from ER Arrival to Discharge (minutes)	346	136	136	134
Time in ER Before Being Evaluated (minutes)	404	22	26	26
Time to Pain Meds for Fractures (minutes)	45	33	52	57
Heart Attack Care				
Aspirin Given at Discharge	231	100%	99%	99%
Fibrinolytic Meds Within 30 Min. of Arrival[7]	-	-	-	54%
PCI Within 90 Minutes of Arrival	26	100%	97%	96%
Statin Prescribed at Discharge	231	100%	98%	98%
Heart Failure Care				
ACE Inhibitor or ARB for LVSD[2]	75	100%	96%	97%
Discharge Instructions Given[2]	219	98%	94%	94%
Evaluation of LVS Function[2]	253	100%	98%	99%
Medicare Spending				
Medicare Spending per Patient (ratio)	-	0.99	0.95	0.98
Pneumonia Care				
Appropriate Initial Antibiotic Given[2]	67	97%	95%	95%
Blood Culture Timing[2]	131	99%	98%	98%
Pregnancy and Delivery Care				
Newborn Deliveries Scheduled Early[2]	29	17%	5%	6%
Preventive Care				
Immunization for Influenza[2]	563	99%	92%	90%
Immunization for Pneumonia[2]	764	98%	93%	92%
Stroke Care				
Anticoagulation Therapy for Atrial Fibrillation	20	100%	94%	95%
Antithrombotic Therapy Timing	87	98%	98%	98%
Assessed for Rehabilitation	106	98%	98%	97%
Discharged on Antithrombotic Therapy	92	100%	99%	99%
Discharged on Statin Medication	71	97%	95%	94%
Thrombolytic Therapy Timing	11	82%	67%	66%
Venous Thromboembolism Prophylaxis	111	98%	95%	94%
Written Stroke Educational Materials Given	55	98%	88%	88%
Surgical Care Improvement Project				
Appropriate Beta Blocker Usage[2]	210	100%	98%	98%
Appropriate VTP Within 24 Hours[2]	350	99%	98%	98%
Controlled Postoperative Blood Glucose[2]	95	100%	97%	97%
Perioperative Temperature Management[2]	435	100%	100%	100%
Prophylactic Antibiotic Selection[2]	328	100%	99%	99%
Prophylactic Antibiotic Selection (Outpatient)	446	100%	98%	98%
Prophylactic Antibiotic Stopped[2]	312	99%	98%	98%
Prophylactic Antibiotic Timing[2]	328	99%	99%	99%
Prophylactic Antibiotic Timing (Outpatient)	447	100%	98%	98%
Urinary Catheter Removal[2]	276	99%	97%	97%
Survey of Patients' Hospital Experiences				
Area Around Room 'Always' Quiet at Night	300+	57%	61%	61%
Doctors 'Always' Communicated Well	300+	79%	82%	82%
Home Recovery Information Given	300+	90%	87%	85%
Hospital Given 9 or 10 on 10 Point Scale	300+	71%	71%	71%
Meds 'Always' Explained Before Given	300+	60%	63%	64%
Nurses 'Always' Communicated Well	300+	77%	79%	79%
Pain 'Always' Well Controlled	300+	69%	71%	71%
Room and Bathroom 'Always' Clean	300+	72%	73%	73%
Timely Help 'Always' Received	300+	66%	68%	68%
Would Definitely Recommend Hospital	300+	72%	70%	71%
Use of Medical Imaging				
Cardiac Imaging Stress Test before Surgery	980	4.2%	5.2%	5.3%
Combination Abdominal CT Scan	708	4.0%	11.2%	10.5%
Combination Brain/Sinus CT Scan	582	1.5%	3.2%	2.7%
Combination Chest CT Scan	518	1.5%	1.9%	2.7%
Follow-up Mammogram/Ultrasound	1,294	11.0%	8.6%	8.8%
Lumbar Spine MRI for Low Back Pain	131	39.7%	39.6%	37.2%

Heartland Regional Medical Center

5325 Faraon Street
Saint Joseph, MO 64506
Phone: 816-271-6000
Fax: 816-271-6656
URL: www.heartland-health.com
Type: Acute Care Hospitals
Emergency Services: Yes
Ownership: Voluntary non-profit - Private
Beds: 690

Key Personnel:
Radiology. . . . . Larry Kirschner
CEO/President. . . . . Lowell C Kruse
Chief of Medical Staff. . . . . Dr Robert Permut, MD
Quality Assurance . . . . Julie Ryder
Infection Control. . . . . Betty Shellenberder
Pediatric Ambulatory Care . . . . . . Robert B Sturdevant DO
Pediatric In-Patient Care . . . . Robert B Sturdevant DO

Measure	Cases	This Hosp.	State Avg.	U.S. Avg.
Blood Clot Prevention and Treatment				
Anticoagulation Overlap Therapy[2]	102	99%	94%	93%
ICU Venous Thromboembolism Prophylaxis[2]	56	96%	91%	92%
Incidence of Potentially Preventable VTE[2]	14	0%	7%	10%
UFH with Dosages/Platelet Monitoring[2]	61	100%	96%	97%
Venous Thromboembolism Prophylaxis[2]	296	96%	85%	85%
Warfarin Therapy Discharge Instructions[2]	81	100%	76%	75%
Chest Pain/Possible Heart Attack Care				
Aspirin Given Within 24 Hours of Arrival[1,3]	-	-	95%	96%
Fibrinolytic Meds Within 30 Min. of Arrival[5]	-	-	53%	58%
Average Time to ECG (minutes)[1,3]	-	-	7	7
Average Time to Transfer (minutes)[5]	-	-	53	60
Children's Asthma Care				
Received Home Management Plan of Care	-	-	-	88%
Received Reliever Medication	-	-	-	100%
Received Systemic Corticosteroids	-	-	-	100%
Emergency Department				
Admittance Decision Time (minutes)[2]	473	66	81	98
Head CT Results Within 45 Min. of Arrival[1]	-	-	63%	57%
Patients Who Left ER Before Being Seen	60,378	1%	3%	2%
Time from ER Arrival to Admit. (minutes)[2]	477	203	238	274
Time from ER Arrival to Discharge (minutes)	357	119	136	134
Time in ER Before Being Evaluated (minutes)	336	16	26	26
Time to Pain Meds for Fractures (minutes)	192	32	52	57
Heart Attack Care				
Aspirin Given at Discharge	321	100%	99%	99%
Fibrinolytic Meds Within 30 Min. of Arrival[7]	-	-	-	54%
PCI Within 90 Minutes of Arrival	49	98%	97%	96%
Statin Prescribed at Discharge	314	100%	98%	98%
Heart Failure Care				
ACE Inhibitor or ARB for LVSD	71	100%	96%	97%
Discharge Instructions Given	238	99%	94%	94%
Evaluation of LVS Function	332	100%	98%	99%
Medicare Spending				
Medicare Spending per Patient (ratio)	-	0.95	0.95	0.98
Pneumonia Care				
Appropriate Initial Antibiotic Given	338	99%	95%	95%
Blood Culture Timing	567	100%	98%	98%
Pregnancy and Delivery Care				
Newborn Deliveries Scheduled Early[2]	23	4%	5%	6%
Preventive Care				
Immunization for Influenza[2]	528	98%	92%	90%
Immunization for Pneumonia[2]	622	97%	93%	92%
Stroke Care				
Anticoagulation Therapy for Atrial Fibrillation[1]	-	-	94%	95%
Antithrombotic Therapy Timing	123	100%	98%	98%
Assessed for Rehabilitation	147	99%	98%	97%
Discharged on Antithrombotic Therapy	129	100%	99%	99%
Discharged on Statin Medication	109	100%	95%	94%
Thrombolytic Therapy Timing	11	100%	67%	66%
Venous Thromboembolism Prophylaxis	150	99%	95%	94%
Written Stroke Educational Materials Given	78	100%	88%	88%
Surgical Care Improvement Project				
Appropriate Beta Blocker Usage[2]	434	100%	98%	98%
Appropriate VTP Within 24 Hours[2]	704	100%	98%	98%
Controlled Postoperative Blood Glucose[2]	218	97%	97%	97%
Perioperative Temperature Management[2]	799	100%	100%	100%
Prophylactic Antibiotic Selection[2]	792	100%	99%	99%
Prophylactic Antibiotic Selection (Outpatient)	568	99%	98%	98%
Prophylactic Antibiotic Stopped[2]	749	100%	98%	98%
Prophylactic Antibiotic Timing[2]	795	100%	99%	99%
Prophylactic Antibiotic Timing (Outpatient)	569	100%	98%	98%
Urinary Catheter Removal[2]	663	100%	97%	97%
Survey of Patients' Hospital Experiences				
Area Around Room 'Always' Quiet at Night	300+	61%	61%	61%
Doctors 'Always' Communicated Well	300+	81%	82%	82%
Home Recovery Information Given	300+	89%	87%	85%
Hospital Given 9 or 10 on 10 Point Scale	300+	69%	71%	71%
Meds 'Always' Explained Before Given	300+	65%	63%	64%
Nurses 'Always' Communicated Well	300+	82%	79%	79%
Pain 'Always' Well Controlled	300+	75%	71%	71%
Room and Bathroom 'Always' Clean	300+	74%	73%	73%
Timely Help 'Always' Received	300+	64%	68%	68%
Would Definitely Recommend Hospital	300+	68%	70%	71%
Use of Medical Imaging				
Cardiac Imaging Stress Test before Surgery	1,074	5.9%	5.2%	5.3%
Combination Abdominal CT Scan	1,578	1.8%	11.2%	10.5%
Combination Brain/Sinus CT Scan	1,345	2.2%	3.2%	2.7%

NOTE: Hospital profiles are in alphabetical order by state, then city, then hospital within the city; Rankings exclude hospitals with less than 25 cases except for patient surveys which excludes hospitals with less than 100 cases; (a) 100-299 cases; (1) The number of cases/patients is too few to report; (2) Data submitted were based on a sample of cases/patients; (3) Results are based on a shorter time period than required; (4) Data suppressed by CMS for one or more quarters; (5) Results are not available for this reporting period; (6) Fewer than 100 patients completed the HCAHPS survey; (7) No cases met the criteria for this measure; (8) The lower limit of the confidence interval cannot be calculated if the number of observed infections equals zero; (9) No data are available from the state/territory for this reporting period; (10) The scores shown reflect fewer than 50 completed surveys; (11) There were discrepancies in the data collection process; (12) This measure does not apply to this hospital for this reporting period; (13) Results cannot be calculated for this reporting period; (14) The results for this state are combined with nearby states to protect confidentiality; Please refer to the User's Guide for a full explanation of data.

Combination Chest CT Scan	1,407	2.4%	1.9%	2.7%
Follow-up Mammogram/Ultrasound	2,992	8.1%	8.6%	8.8%
Lumbar Spine MRI for Low Back Pain	275	38.2%	39.6%	37.2%

Barnes-Jewish Hospital

One Barnes - Jewish Hospital Plaza
Saint Louis, MO 63110
Phone: 314-747-3000
Fax: 314-362-3421
URL: www.barnesjewish.org
Type: Acute Care Hospitals
Emergency Services: Yes
Ownership: Voluntary non-profit - Other
Beds: 1,252

Key Personnel:
Operating Room. . . . . David Jaques, MD
CEO/President. . . . . Richard Liekweg
Chief of Medical Staff . . . . John Lynch, MD
Quality Assurance . . . . Denise Murphy
Chair/CEO . . . . Craig D. Schnuck
Patient Relations . . . . Coreen Vlodarchyk

Measure	Cases	This Hosp.	State Avg.	U.S. Avg.
Blood Clot Prevention and Treatment				
Anticoagulation Overlap Therapy[2]	310	97%	94%	93%
ICU Venous Thromboembolism Prophylaxis[2]	65	98%	91%	92%
Incidence of Potentially Preventable VTE[2]	191	4%	7%	10%
UFH with Dosages/Platelet Monitoring[2]	410	100%	96%	97%
Venous Thromboembolism Prophylaxis[2]	300	94%	85%	85%
Warfarin Therapy Discharge Instructions[2]	208	95%	76%	75%
Chest Pain/Possible Heart Attack Care				
Aspirin Given Within 24 Hours of Arrival[1]	-	-	95%	96%
Fibrinolytic Meds Within 30 Min. of Arrival[3,7]	-	-	53%	58%
Average Time to ECG (minutes)[1]	-	-	7	7
Average Time to Transfer (minutes)[3,7]	-	-	53	60
Children's Asthma Care				
Received Home Management Plan of Care	-	-	-	88%
Received Reliever Medication	-	-	-	100%
Received Systemic Corticosteroids	-	-	-	100%
Emergency Department				
Admittance Decision Time (minutes)[2]	351	169	81	98
Head CT Results Within 45 Min. of Arrival[1]	-	-	63%	57%
Patients Who Left ER Before Being Seen	98,239	8%	3%	2%
Time from ER Arrival to Admit. (minutes)[2]	352	394	238	274
Time from ER Arrival to Discharge (minutes)	744	262	136	134
Time in ER Before Being Evaluated (minutes)	825	131	26	26
Time to Pain Meds for Fractures (minutes)	155	84	52	57
Heart Attack Care				
Aspirin Given at Discharge	545	100%	99%	99%
Fibrinolytic Meds Within 30 Min. of Arrival[7]	-	-	-	54%
PCI Within 90 Minutes of Arrival	27	100%	97%	96%
Statin Prescribed at Discharge	509	100%	98%	98%
Heart Failure Care				
ACE Inhibitor or ARB for LVSD[2]	276	99%	96%	97%
Discharge Instructions Given[2]	506	99%	94%	94%
Evaluation of LVS Function[2]	570	100%	98%	99%
Medicare Spending				
Medicare Spending per Patient (ratio)	-	0.98	0.95	0.98
Pneumonia Care				
Appropriate Initial Antibiotic Given[2]	80	98%	95%	95%
Blood Culture Timing[2]	112	99%	98%	98%
Pregnancy and Delivery Care				
Newborn Deliveries Scheduled Early[2]	30	0%	5%	6%
Preventive Care				
Immunization for Influenza[2]	553	89%	92%	90%
Immunization for Pneumonia[2]	652	88%	93%	92%
Stroke Care				
Anticoagulation Therapy for Atrial Fibrillation[2]	92	100%	94%	95%
Antithrombotic Therapy Timing[2]	412	99%	98%	98%
Assessed for Rehabilitation[2]	732	99%	98%	97%
Discharged on Antithrombotic Therapy[2]	545	100%	99%	99%
Discharged on Statin Medication[2]	371	99%	95%	94%
Thrombolytic Therapy Timing[2]	14	93%	67%	66%
Venous Thromboembolism Prophylaxis[2]	680	98%	95%	94%
Written Stroke Educational Materials Given[2]	332	99%	88%	88%
Surgical Care Improvement Project				
Appropriate Beta Blocker Usage[2]	236	99%	98%	98%
Appropriate VTP Within 24 Hours[2]	452	99%	98%	98%
Controlled Postoperative Blood Glucose[2]	125	90%	97%	97%
Perioperative Temperature Management[2]	650	100%	100%	100%
Prophylactic Antibiotic Selection[2]	416	99%	99%	99%
Prophylactic Antibiotic Selection (Outpatient)	766	99%	98%	98%
Prophylactic Antibiotic Stopped[2]	400	100%	98%	98%
Prophylactic Antibiotic Timing[2]	419	97%	99%	99%
Prophylactic Antibiotic Timing (Outpatient)	773	97%	98%	98%
Urinary Catheter Removal[2]	396	98%	97%	97%
Survey of Patients' Hospital Experiences				
Area Around Room 'Always' Quiet at Night	300+	55%	61%	61%
Doctors 'Always' Communicated Well	300+	82%	82%	82%
Home Recovery Information Given	300+	91%	87%	85%
Hospital Given 9 or 10 on 10 Point Scale	300+	77%	71%	71%
Meds 'Always' Explained Before Given	300+	66%	63%	64%
Nurses 'Always' Communicated Well	300+	80%	79%	79%
Pain 'Always' Well Controlled	300+	73%	71%	71%
Room and Bathroom 'Always' Clean	300+	66%	73%	73%
Timely Help 'Always' Received	300+	61%	68%	68%
Would Definitely Recommend Hospital	300+	78%	70%	71%
Use of Medical Imaging				
Cardiac Imaging Stress Test before Surgery	1,260	5.3%	5.2%	5.3%
Combination Abdominal CT Scan	4,956	5.5%	11.2%	10.5%
Combination Brain/Sinus CT Scan	1,557	2.1%	3.2%	2.7%
Combination Chest CT Scan	6,283	0.8%	1.9%	2.7%
Follow-up Mammogram/Ultrasound	5,075	8.8%	8.6%	8.8%
Lumbar Spine MRI for Low Back Pain	443	32.3%	39.6%	37.2%

Christian Hospital Northeast - Northwest

11133 Dunn Road
Saint Louis, MO 63136
Phone: 314-653-5000
Fax: 314-653-4130
URL: www.christianhospital.org
Type: Acute Care Hospitals
Emergency Services: Yes
Ownership: Voluntary non-profit - Private
Beds: 493

Key Personnel:
Anesthesiology. . . . . Stephen Feit, MD
CEO/President. . . . . Ronald B McMullen
Chief of Medical Staff . . . . Sebastian Rueckert, MD
Emergency Room . . . . Sebastian Rueckert, MD

Measure	Cases	This Hosp.	State Avg.	U.S. Avg.
Blood Clot Prevention and Treatment				
Anticoagulation Overlap Therapy[2]	150	95%	94%	93%
ICU Venous Thromboembolism Prophylaxis[2]	29	90%	91%	92%
Incidence of Potentially Preventable VTE[2]	24	0%	7%	10%
UFH with Dosages/Platelet Monitoring[2]	55	100%	96%	97%
Venous Thromboembolism Prophylaxis[2]	387	94%	85%	85%
Warfarin Therapy Discharge Instructions[2]	113	87%	76%	75%
Chest Pain/Possible Heart Attack Care				
Aspirin Given Within 24 Hours of Arrival	15	93%	95%	96%
Fibrinolytic Meds Within 30 Min. of Arrival[3,7]	-	-	53%	58%
Average Time to ECG (minutes)	15	7	7	7
Average Time to Transfer (minutes)[1,3]	-	-	53	60
Children's Asthma Care				
Received Home Management Plan of Care	-	-	-	88%
Received Reliever Medication	-	-	-	100%
Received Systemic Corticosteroids	-	-	-	100%
Emergency Department				
Admittance Decision Time (minutes)[2]	707	127	81	98
Head CT Results Within 45 Min. of Arrival	32	78%	63%	57%
Patients Who Left ER Before Being Seen	>100k	1%	3%	2%
Time from ER Arrival to Admit. (minutes)[2]	720	308	238	274
Time from ER Arrival to Discharge (minutes)	783	147	136	134
Time in ER Before Being Evaluated (minutes)	779	64	26	26
Time to Pain Meds for Fractures (minutes)	77	55	52	57
Heart Attack Care				
Aspirin Given at Discharge	330	99%	99%	99%
Fibrinolytic Meds Within 30 Min. of Arrival[7]	-	-	-	54%
PCI Within 90 Minutes of Arrival	31	94%	97%	96%
Statin Prescribed at Discharge	299	99%	98%	98%
Heart Failure Care				
ACE Inhibitor or ARB for LVSD[2]	159	97%	96%	97%
Discharge Instructions Given[2]	443	98%	94%	94%
Evaluation of LVS Function[2]	523	100%	98%	99%
Medicare Spending				
Medicare Spending per Patient (ratio)	-	1.00	0.95	0.98
Pneumonia Care				
Appropriate Initial Antibiotic Given[2]	115	98%	95%	95%
Blood Culture Timing[2]	253	98%	98%	98%
Pregnancy and Delivery Care				
Newborn Deliveries Scheduled Early[7]	-	-	5%	6%
Preventive Care				
Immunization for Influenza[2]	584	99%	92%	90%
Immunization for Pneumonia[2]	828	98%	93%	92%
Stroke Care				
Anticoagulation Therapy for Atrial Fibrillation[2]	14	100%	94%	95%
Antithrombotic Therapy Timing[2]	177	100%	98%	98%
Assessed for Rehabilitation[2]	179	99%	98%	97%
Discharged on Antithrombotic Therapy[2]	176	100%	99%	99%
Discharged on Statin Medication[2]	143	97%	95%	94%
Thrombolytic Therapy Timing[2]	20	75%	67%	66%
Venous Thromboembolism Prophylaxis[2]	189	99%	95%	94%
Written Stroke Educational Materials Given[2]	97	98%	88%	88%
Surgical Care Improvement Project				
Appropriate Beta Blocker Usage[2]	201	100%	98%	98%
Appropriate VTP Within 24 Hours[2]	308	97%	98%	98%
Controlled Postoperative Blood Glucose[2]	167	98%	97%	97%
Perioperative Temperature Management[2]	407	100%	100%	100%
Prophylactic Antibiotic Selection[2]	336	99%	99%	99%
Prophylactic Antibiotic Selection (Outpatient)	377	99%	98%	98%
Prophylactic Antibiotic Stopped[2]	303	98%	98%	98%
Prophylactic Antibiotic Timing[2]	336	99%	99%	99%
Prophylactic Antibiotic Timing (Outpatient)	377	99%	98%	98%
Urinary Catheter Removal[2]	205	99%	97%	97%
Survey of Patients' Hospital Experiences				
Area Around Room 'Always' Quiet at Night	300+	71%	61%	61%
Doctors 'Always' Communicated Well	300+	81%	82%	82%
Home Recovery Information Given	300+	86%	87%	85%
Hospital Given 9 or 10 on 10 Point Scale	300+	68%	71%	71%
Meds 'Always' Explained Before Given	300+	64%	63%	64%
Nurses 'Always' Communicated Well	300+	80%	79%	79%
Pain 'Always' Well Controlled	300+	72%	71%	71%
Room and Bathroom 'Always' Clean	300+	60%	73%	73%
Timely Help 'Always' Received	300+	64%	68%	68%
Would Definitely Recommend Hospital	300+	66%	70%	71%
Use of Medical Imaging				
Cardiac Imaging Stress Test before Surgery	275	4.7%	5.2%	5.3%
Combination Abdominal CT Scan	889	2.2%	11.2%	10.5%
Combination Brain/Sinus CT Scan	975	4.2%	3.2%	2.7%
Combination Chest CT Scan	835	0.1%	1.9%	2.7%
Follow-up Mammogram/Ultrasound	1,410	12.8%	8.6%	8.8%
Lumbar Spine MRI for Low Back Pain	94	33.0%	39.6%	37.2%

Des Peres Hospital

2345 Dougherty Ferry Road
Saint Louis, MO 63122
Phone: 314-966-9100
Fax: 314-966-9274
URL: www.desperesshospital.com
Type: Acute Care Hospitals
Emergency Services: Yes
Ownership: Proprietary
Beds: 167

Key Personnel:
Chief of Medical Staff . . . . Micheal Chablt
Quality Assurance . . . . Maryann Dundon
Emergency Room . . . . Thomas Hartmann
CEO/President. . . . . Michele Meyer
Radiology. . . . . James Schoen, MD

Measure	Cases	This Hosp.	State Avg.	U.S. Avg.
Blood Clot Prevention and Treatment				
Anticoagulation Overlap Therapy[2]	32	91%	94%	93%
ICU Venous Thromboembolism Prophylaxis[2]	76	99%	91%	92%
Incidence of Potentially Preventable VTE[1,2]	-	-	7%	10%
UFH with Dosages/Platelet Monitoring[2]	17	100%	96%	97%
Venous Thromboembolism Prophylaxis[2]	323	94%	85%	85%
Warfarin Therapy Discharge Instructions[2]	24	100%	76%	75%
Chest Pain/Possible Heart Attack Care				
Aspirin Given Within 24 Hours of Arrival[5]	-	-	95%	96%
Fibrinolytic Meds Within 30 Min. of Arrival[5]	-	-	53%	58%
Average Time to ECG (minutes)[5]	-	-	7	7
Average Time to Transfer (minutes)[5]	-	-	53	60
Children's Asthma Care				

NOTE: Hospital profiles are in alphabetical order by state, then city, then hospital within the city; Rankings exclude hospitals with less than 25 cases except for patient surveys which excludes hospitals with less than 100 cases; (a) 100-299 cases; (1) The number of cases/patients is too few to report; (2) Data submitted were based on a sample of cases/patients; (3) Results are based on a shorter time period than required; (4) Data suppressed by CMS for one or more quarters; (5) Results are not available for this reporting period; (6) Fewer than 100 patients completed the HCAHPS survey; (7) No cases met the criteria for this measure; (8) The lower limit of the confidence interval cannot be calculated if the number of observed infections equals zero; (9) No data are available from the state/territory for this reporting period; (10) The scores shown reflect fewer than 50 completed surveys; (11) There were discrepancies in the data collection process; (12) This measure does not apply to this hospital for this reporting period; (13) Results cannot be calculated for this reporting period; (14) The results for this state are combined with nearby states to protect confidentiality; Please refer to the User's Guide for a full explanation of data.

Received Home Management Plan of Care	-	-	-	88%
Received Reliever Medication	-	-	-	100%
Received Systemic Corticosteroids	-	-	-	100%
Emergency Department				
Admittance Decision Time (minutes)[2]	481	88	81	98
Head CT Results Within 45 Min. of Arrival[1]	-	-	63%	57%
Patients Who Left ER Before Being Seen	9,601	1%	3%	2%
Time from ER Arrival to Admit. (minutes)[2]	481	218	238	274
Time from ER Arrival to Discharge (minutes)	421	137	136	134
Time in ER Before Being Evaluated (minutes)	459	21	26	26
Time to Pain Meds for Fractures (minutes)	28	57	52	57
Heart Attack Care				
Aspirin Given at Discharge	103	100%	99%	99%
Fibrinolytic Meds Within 30 Min. of Arrival[7]	-	-	-	54%
PCI Within 90 Minutes of Arrival[1]	-	-	97%	96%
Statin Prescribed at Discharge	101	100%	98%	98%
Heart Failure Care				
ACE Inhibitor or ARB for LVSD	36	100%	96%	97%
Discharge Instructions Given	113	97%	94%	94%
Evaluation of LVS Function	149	99%	98%	99%
Medicare Spending				
Medicare Spending per Patient (ratio)	-	0.99	0.95	0.98
Pneumonia Care				
Appropriate Initial Antibiotic Given	59	97%	95%	95%
Blood Culture Timing	136	100%	98%	98%
Pregnancy and Delivery Care				
Newborn Deliveries Scheduled Early[7]	-	-	5%	6%
Preventive Care				
Immunization for Influenza[2]	600	99%	92%	90%
Immunization for Pneumonia[2]	857	99%	93%	92%
Stroke Care				
Anticoagulation Therapy for Atrial Fibrillation[1]	-	-	94%	95%
Antithrombotic Therapy Timing	16	100%	98%	98%
Assessed for Rehabilitation	18	100%	98%	97%
Discharged on Antithrombotic Therapy	18	100%	99%	99%
Discharged on Statin Medication	14	100%	95%	94%
Thrombolytic Therapy Timing[1]	-	-	67%	66%
Venous Thromboembolism Prophylaxis	18	94%	95%	94%
Written Stroke Educational Materials Given	15	87%	88%	88%
Surgical Care Improvement Project				
Appropriate Beta Blocker Usage[2]	144	94%	98%	98%
Appropriate VTP Within 24 Hours[2]	293	98%	98%	98%
Controlled Postoperative Blood Glucose[2]	53	92%	97%	97%
Perioperative Temperature Management[2]	333	100%	100%	100%
Prophylactic Antibiotic Selection[2]	231	100%	99%	99%
Prophylactic Antibiotic Selection (Outpatient)	422	99%	98%	98%
Prophylactic Antibiotic Stopped[2]	212	97%	98%	98%
Prophylactic Antibiotic Timing[2]	231	99%	99%	99%
Prophylactic Antibiotic Timing (Outpatient)	422	98%	98%	98%
Urinary Catheter Removal[2]	256	97%	97%	97%
Survey of Patients' Hospital Experiences				
Area Around Room 'Always' Quiet at Night	300+	57%	61%	61%
Doctors 'Always' Communicated Well	300+	85%	82%	82%
Home Recovery Information Given	300+	90%	87%	85%
Hospital Given 9 or 10 on 10 Point Scale	300+	74%	71%	71%
Meds 'Always' Explained Before Given	300+	65%	63%	64%
Nurses 'Always' Communicated Well	300+	77%	79%	79%
Pain 'Always' Well Controlled	300+	72%	71%	71%
Room and Bathroom 'Always' Clean	300+	71%	73%	73%
Timely Help 'Always' Received	300+	62%	68%	68%
Would Definitely Recommend Hospital	300+	73%	70%	71%
Use of Medical Imaging				
Cardiac Imaging Stress Test before Surgery	107	1.9%	5.2%	5.3%
Combination Abdominal CT Scan	220	6.4%	11.2%	10.5%
Combination Brain/Sinus CT Scan	156	0.0%	3.2%	2.7%
Combination Chest CT Scan	75	0.0%	1.9%	2.7%
Follow-up Mammogram/Ultrasound	155	9.0%	8.6%	8.8%
Lumbar Spine MRI for Low Back Pain	126	38.1%	39.6%	37.2%

Mercy Hospital Saint Louis

615 New Ballas Road
Saint Louis, MO 63141
URL: www.stjohnsmercy.org
Type: Acute Care Hospitals
Ownership: Voluntary non-profit - Private
Phone: 314-569-6000
Fax: 314-251-4719
Emergency Services: Yes
Beds: 787

Key Personnel:
Chief of Medical Staff . . . . Martin Bell
Cardiac Laboratory. . . . . John W Hubert, MD
CEO/President . . . . Jeff Johnston
Coronary Care . . . . James A Stokes, MD, FACC

Measure	Cases	This Hosp.	State Avg.	U.S. Avg.
Blood Clot Prevention and Treatment				
Anticoagulation Overlap Therapy[2]	171	98%	94%	93%
ICU Venous Thromboembolism Prophylaxis[2]	84	99%	91%	92%
Incidence of Potentially Preventable VTE[2]	41	10%	7%	10%
UFH with Dosages/Platelet Monitoring[2]	64	100%	96%	97%
Venous Thromboembolism Prophylaxis[2]	287	90%	85%	85%
Warfarin Therapy Discharge Instructions[2]	137	47%	76%	75%
Chest Pain/Possible Heart Attack Care				
Aspirin Given Within 24 Hours of Arrival[5]	-	-	95%	96%
Fibrinolytic Meds Within 30 Min. of Arrival[5]	-	-	53%	58%
Average Time to ECG (minutes)[5]	-	-	7	7
Average Time to Transfer (minutes)[5]	-	-	53	60
Children's Asthma Care				
Received Home Management Plan of Care	177	93%	-	88%
Received Reliever Medication	177	100%	-	100%
Received Systemic Corticosteroids	177	100%	-	100%
Emergency Department				
Admittance Decision Time (minutes)[2]	377	115	81	98
Head CT Results Within 45 Min. of Arrival[1]	-	-	63%	57%
Patients Who Left ER Before Being Seen	81,500	1%	3%	2%
Time from ER Arrival to Admit. (minutes)[2]	398	243	238	274
Time from ER Arrival to Discharge (minutes)	349	164	136	134
Time in ER Before Being Evaluated (minutes)	406	24	26	26
Time to Pain Meds for Fractures (minutes)	235	29	52	57
Heart Attack Care				
Aspirin Given at Discharge[2]	262	100%	99%	99%
Fibrinolytic Meds Within 30 Min. of Arrival[2,7]	-	-	-	54%
PCI Within 90 Minutes of Arrival[2]	37	95%	97%	96%
Statin Prescribed at Discharge[2]	264	98%	98%	98%
Heart Failure Care				
ACE Inhibitor or ARB for LVSD[2]	74	99%	96%	97%
Discharge Instructions Given[2]	244	95%	94%	94%
Evaluation of LVS Function[2]	300	100%	98%	99%
Medicare Spending				
Medicare Spending per Patient (ratio)	-	0.98	0.95	0.98
Pneumonia Care				
Appropriate Initial Antibiotic Given[2]	64	95%	95%	95%
Blood Culture Timing[2]	106	99%	98%	98%
Pregnancy and Delivery Care				
Newborn Deliveries Scheduled Early[2]	102	0%	5%	6%
Preventive Care				
Immunization for Influenza[2]	492	90%	92%	90%
Immunization for Pneumonia[2]	436	92%	93%	92%
Stroke Care				
Anticoagulation Therapy for Atrial Fibrillation	47	91%	94%	95%
Antithrombotic Therapy Timing	217	100%	98%	98%
Assessed for Rehabilitation	334	98%	98%	97%
Discharged on Antithrombotic Therapy	274	100%	99%	99%
Discharged on Statin Medication	199	99%	95%	94%
Thrombolytic Therapy Timing	24	100%	67%	66%
Venous Thromboembolism Prophylaxis	313	97%	95%	94%
Written Stroke Educational Materials Given	183	94%	88%	88%
Surgical Care Improvement Project				
Appropriate Beta Blocker Usage[2]	224	99%	98%	98%
Appropriate VTP Within 24 Hours[2]	364	100%	98%	98%
Controlled Postoperative Blood Glucose[2]	136	97%	97%	97%
Perioperative Temperature Management[2]	503	100%	100%	100%
Prophylactic Antibiotic Selection[2]	442	100%	99%	99%
Prophylactic Antibiotic Selection (Outpatient)	888	99%	98%	98%
Prophylactic Antibiotic Stopped[2]	431	98%	98%	98%
Prophylactic Antibiotic Timing[2]	443	99%	99%	99%
Prophylactic Antibiotic Timing (Outpatient)	884	99%	98%	98%
Urinary Catheter Removal[2]	302	99%	97%	97%
Survey of Patients' Hospital Experiences				
Area Around Room 'Always' Quiet at Night[11]	300+	65%	61%	61%
Doctors 'Always' Communicated Well[11]	300+	82%	82%	82%
Home Recovery Information Given[11]	300+	88%	87%	85%
Hospital Given 9 or 10 on 10 Point Scale[11]	300+	77%	71%	71%
Meds 'Always' Explained Before Given[11]	300+	62%	63%	64%
Nurses 'Always' Communicated Well[11]	300+	79%	79%	79%
Pain 'Always' Well Controlled[11]	300+	71%	71%	71%
Room and Bathroom 'Always' Clean[11]	300+	64%	73%	73%
Timely Help 'Always' Received[11]	300+	64%	68%	68%
Would Definitely Recommend Hospital[11]	300+	81%	70%	71%
Use of Medical Imaging				
Cardiac Imaging Stress Test before Surgery	1,757	4.9%	5.2%	5.3%
Combination Abdominal CT Scan	1,910	4.3%	11.2%	10.5%
Combination Brain/Sinus CT Scan	867	5.3%	3.2%	2.7%
Combination Chest CT Scan	1,775	0.4%	1.9%	2.7%
Follow-up Mammogram/Ultrasound	5,563	7.2%	8.6%	8.8%
Lumbar Spine MRI for Low Back Pain	363	44.4%	39.6%	37.2%

Saint Alexius Hospital

3933 S Broadway
Saint Louis, MO 63118
URL: www.stalexiushospital.com
Type: Acute Care Hospitals
Ownership: Proprietary
Phone: 314-865-7000
Fax: 314-865-7938
Emergency Services: Yes
Beds: 203

Key Personnel:
Anesthesiology. . . . . Brad Berstein, MD
Radiology. . . . . Patrick Cabrera, D.O.
Chief of Medical Staff . . . . Patrick Durbin, MD
Operating Room. . . . . Bonnie Henry, RN
Surgery . . . . Russell Kraeger, MD
Emergency Room . . . . Michael Kyzer, MD
President . . . . Mike Kyzer, MD
Quality Assurance . . . . Karen Salamone

Measure	Cases	This Hosp.	State Avg.	U.S. Avg.
Blood Clot Prevention and Treatment				
Anticoagulation Overlap Therapy[1,2]	-	-	94%	93%
ICU Venous Thromboembolism Prophylaxis[2]	53	85%	91%	92%
Incidence of Potentially Preventable VTE[1,2]	-	-	7%	10%
UFH with Dosages/Platelet Monitoring[1,2]	-	-	96%	97%
Venous Thromboembolism Prophylaxis[2]	148	78%	85%	85%
Warfarin Therapy Discharge Instructions[1,2]	-	-	76%	75%
Chest Pain/Possible Heart Attack Care				
Aspirin Given Within 24 Hours of Arrival[1,3]	-	-	95%	96%
Fibrinolytic Meds Within 30 Min. of Arrival[3,7]	-	-	53%	58%
Average Time to ECG (minutes)[1,3]	-	-	7	7
Average Time to Transfer (minutes)[1,3]	-	-	53	60
Children's Asthma Care				
Received Home Management Plan of Care	-	-	-	88%
Received Reliever Medication	-	-	-	100%
Received Systemic Corticosteroids	-	-	-	100%
Emergency Department				
Admittance Decision Time (minutes)[2]	225	86	81	98
Head CT Results Within 45 Min. of Arrival[1]	-	-	63%	57%
Patients Who Left ER Before Being Seen	19,217	14%	3%	2%
Time from ER Arrival to Admit. (minutes)[2]	240	377	238	274
Time from ER Arrival to Discharge (minutes)	286	206	136	134
Time in ER Before Being Evaluated (minutes)	314	81	26	26
Time to Pain Meds for Fractures (minutes)	32	91	52	57
Heart Attack Care				
Aspirin Given at Discharge[1]	-	-	99%	99%
Fibrinolytic Meds Within 30 Min. of Arrival[7]	-	-	-	54%
PCI Within 90 Minutes of Arrival[7]	-	-	97%	96%
Statin Prescribed at Discharge[1]	-	-	98%	98%
Heart Failure Care				
ACE Inhibitor or ARB for LVSD	24	88%	96%	97%
Discharge Instructions Given	52	40%	94%	94%
Evaluation of LVS Function	67	100%	98%	99%
Medicare Spending				
Medicare Spending per Patient (ratio)	-	1.04	0.95	0.98
Pneumonia Care				
Appropriate Initial Antibiotic Given	50	88%	95%	95%

NOTE: Hospital profiles are in alphabetical order by state, then city, then hospital within the city; Rankings exclude hospitals with less than 25 cases except for patient surveys which excludes hospitals with less than 100 cases; (a) 100-299 cases; (1) The number of cases/patients is too few to report; (2) Data submitted were based on a sample of cases/patients; (3) Results are based on a shorter time period than required; (4) Data suppressed by CMS for one or more quarters; (5) Results are not available for this reporting period; (6) Fewer than 100 patients completed the HCAHPS survey; (7) No cases met the criteria for this measure; (8) The lower limit of the confidence interval cannot be calculated if the number of observed infections equals zero; (9) No data are available from the state/territory for this reporting period; (10) The scores shown reflect fewer than 50 completed surveys; (11) There were discrepancies in the data collection process; (12) This measure does not apply to this hospital for this reporting period; (13) Results cannot be calculated for this reporting period; (14) The results for this state are combined with nearby states to protect confidentiality; Please refer to the User's Guide for a full explanation of data.

Measure	Cases	This Hosp.	State Avg.	U.S. Avg.
Blood Culture Timing	73	99%	98%	98%
Pregnancy and Delivery Care				
Newborn Deliveries Scheduled Early[7]	-	-	5%	6%
Preventive Care				
Immunization for Influenza[2]	439	49%	92%	90%
Immunization for Pneumonia[2]	487	57%	93%	92%
Stroke Care				
Anticoagulation Therapy for Atrial Fibrillation[7]	-	-	94%	95%
Antithrombotic Therapy Timing[1]	-	-	98%	98%
Assessed for Rehabilitation[1]	-	-	98%	97%
Discharged on Antithrombotic Therapy[1]	-	-	99%	99%
Discharged on Statin Medication[1]	-	-	95%	94%
Thrombolytic Therapy Timing[7]	-	-	67%	66%
Venous Thromboembolism Prophylaxis[1]	-	-	95%	94%
Written Stroke Educational Materials Given[1]	-	-	88%	88%
Surgical Care Improvement Project				
Appropriate Beta Blocker Usage	13	85%	98%	98%
Appropriate VTP Within 24 Hours	49	92%	98%	98%
Controlled Postoperative Blood Glucose[7]	-	-	97%	97%
Perioperative Temperature Management	62	100%	100%	100%
Prophylactic Antibiotic Selection	36	94%	99%	99%
Prophylactic Antibiotic Selection (Outpatient)	45	87%	98%	98%
Prophylactic Antibiotic Stopped	32	88%	98%	98%
Prophylactic Antibiotic Timing	36	94%	99%	99%
Prophylactic Antibiotic Timing (Outpatient)	39	79%	98%	98%
Urinary Catheter Removal	39	38%	97%	97%
Survey of Patients' Hospital Experiences				
Area Around Room 'Always' Quiet at Night	300+	59%	61%	61%
Doctors 'Always' Communicated Well	300+	81%	82%	82%
Home Recovery Information Given	300+	80%	87%	85%
Hospital Given 9 or 10 on 10 Point Scale	300+	60%	71%	71%
Meds 'Always' Explained Before Given	300+	51%	63%	64%
Nurses 'Always' Communicated Well	300+	72%	79%	79%
Pain 'Always' Well Controlled	300+	66%	71%	71%
Room and Bathroom 'Always' Clean	300+	58%	73%	73%
Timely Help 'Always' Received	300+	46%	68%	68%
Would Definitely Recommend Hospital	300+	51%	70%	71%
Use of Medical Imaging				
Cardiac Imaging Stress Test before Surgery[1]	-	-	5.2%	5.3%
Combination Abdominal CT Scan	111	9.9%	11.2%	10.5%
Combination Brain/Sinus CT Scan[1]	-	-	3.2%	2.7%
Combination Chest CT Scan[1]	-	-	1.9%	2.7%
Follow-up Mammogram/Ultrasound	249	22.1%	8.6%	8.8%
Lumbar Spine MRI for Low Back Pain[1]	-	-	39.6%	37.2%

Saint Anthony's Medical Center

10010 Kennerly Road
Saint Louis, MO 63128
Phone: 314-525-1000
Fax: 314-525-4040
E-mail: webmaster@samcstl.org
URL: www.samcstl.org
Type: Acute Care Hospitals
Emergency Services: Yes
Ownership: Voluntary non-profit - Private
Beds: 767

Key Personnel:

Chief of Medical Staff.......... Robert F Beckman, MD
Cardiac Laboratory............ David J Dobmeyer, MD
Hemotology Center .... R William Morris, MD
Radiology.................. Paul A Oberle, MD
Anesthesiology............... Armin Rahimi, DO
CEO/President............... Thomas H Rockers
Operating Room.............. David M Schuval, MD

Measure	Cases	This Hosp.	State Avg.	U.S. Avg.
Blood Clot Prevention and Treatment				
Anticoagulation Overlap Therapy[2]	150	92%	94%	93%
ICU Venous Thromboembolism Prophylaxis[2]	69	100%	91%	92%
Incidence of Potentially Preventable VTE[2]	37	8%	7%	10%
UFH with Dosages/Platelet Monitoring[2]	110	100%	96%	97%
Venous Thromboembolism Prophylaxis[2]	312	82%	85%	85%
Warfarin Therapy Discharge Instructions[2]	110	35%	76%	75%
Chest Pain/Possible Heart Attack Care				
Aspirin Given Within 24 Hours of Arrival[1]	-	-	95%	96%
Fibrinolytic Meds Within 30 Min. of Arrival[3,7]	-	-	53%	58%
Average Time to ECG (minutes)[1]	-	-	7	7
Average Time to Transfer (minutes)[3,7]	-	-	53	60
Children's Asthma Care				
Received Home Management Plan of Care	-	-	-	88%
Received Reliever Medication	-	-	-	100%
Received Systemic Corticosteroids	-	-	-	100%
Emergency Department				
Admittance Decision Time (minutes)[2]	728	143	81	98
Head CT Results Within 45 Min. of Arrival[1]	-	-	63%	57%
Patients Who Left ER Before Being Seen	72,325	3%	3%	2%
Time from ER Arrival to Admit. (minutes)[2]	747	254	238	274
Time from ER Arrival to Discharge (minutes)	382	182	136	134
Time in ER Before Being Evaluated (minutes)	236	35	26	26
Time to Pain Meds for Fractures (minutes)	258	46	52	57
Heart Attack Care				
Aspirin Given at Discharge[2]	304	99%	99%	99%
Fibrinolytic Meds Within 30 Min. of Arrival[2,7]	-	-	-	54%
PCI Within 90 Minutes of Arrival[2]	81	98%	97%	96%
Statin Prescribed at Discharge[2]	291	98%	98%	98%
Heart Failure Care				
ACE Inhibitor or ARB for LVSD[2]	82	96%	96%	97%
Discharge Instructions Given[2]	218	91%	94%	94%
Evaluation of LVS Function[2]	307	100%	98%	99%
Medicare Spending				
Medicare Spending per Patient (ratio)	-	0.98	0.95	0.98
Pneumonia Care				
Appropriate Initial Antibiotic Given[2]	90	98%	95%	95%
Blood Culture Timing[2]	179	98%	98%	98%
Pregnancy and Delivery Care				
Newborn Deliveries Scheduled Early	128	5%	5%	6%
Preventive Care				
Immunization for Influenza[2]	578	90%	92%	90%
Immunization for Pneumonia[2]	823	91%	93%	92%
Stroke Care				
Anticoagulation Therapy for Atrial Fibrillation	60	90%	94%	95%
Antithrombotic Therapy Timing	266	97%	98%	98%
Assessed for Rehabilitation	365	98%	98%	97%
Discharged on Antithrombotic Therapy	329	99%	99%	99%
Discharged on Statin Medication	260	93%	95%	94%
Thrombolytic Therapy Timing	21	67%	67%	66%
Venous Thromboembolism Prophylaxis	325	94%	95%	94%
Written Stroke Educational Materials Given	191	79%	88%	88%
Surgical Care Improvement Project				
Appropriate Beta Blocker Usage[2]	221	98%	98%	98%
Appropriate VTP Within 24 Hours[2]	443	98%	98%	98%
Controlled Postoperative Blood Glucose[2]	136	100%	97%	97%
Perioperative Temperature Management[2]	574	100%	100%	100%
Prophylactic Antibiotic Selection[2]	513	100%	99%	99%
Prophylactic Antibiotic Selection (Outpatient)	685	98%	98%	98%
Prophylactic Antibiotic Stopped[2]	505	99%	98%	98%
Prophylactic Antibiotic Timing[2]	515	99%	99%	99%
Prophylactic Antibiotic Timing (Outpatient)	688	99%	98%	98%
Urinary Catheter Removal[2]	270	93%	97%	97%
Survey of Patients' Hospital Experiences				
Area Around Room 'Always' Quiet at Night	300+	60%	61%	61%
Doctors 'Always' Communicated Well	300+	77%	82%	82%
Home Recovery Information Given	300+	87%	87%	85%
Hospital Given 9 or 10 on 10 Point Scale	300+	70%	71%	71%
Meds 'Always' Explained Before Given	300+	61%	63%	64%
Nurses 'Always' Communicated Well	300+	75%	79%	79%
Pain 'Always' Well Controlled	300+	68%	71%	71%
Room and Bathroom 'Always' Clean	300+	68%	73%	73%
Timely Help 'Always' Received	300+	61%	68%	68%
Would Definitely Recommend Hospital	300+	69%	70%	71%
Use of Medical Imaging				
Cardiac Imaging Stress Test before Surgery	420	8.3%	5.2%	5.3%
Combination Abdominal CT Scan	1,618	16.8%	11.2%	10.5%
Combination Brain/Sinus CT Scan	1,288	3.4%	3.2%	2.7%
Combination Chest CT Scan	853	0.6%	1.9%	2.7%
Follow-up Mammogram/Ultrasound	3,400	5.6%	8.6%	8.8%
Lumbar Spine MRI for Low Back Pain	165	33.3%	39.6%	37.2%

Saint Louis - John Cochran VA Medical Center

915 North Grand
Saint Louis, MO 63106
Phone: 314-652-4100
Fax: 314-894-6682
URL: www.stlouis.va.gov
Type: Acute Care - VA
Emergency Services: No
Ownership: Government Federal
Beds: 684

Key Personnel:

Chief of Medical Staff.......... Margarete Hageman, MD
Hemotology Center .... Scot Hichman
Anesthesiology............... Shigemasa Ikeda, MD
Emergency Room .... Laura Kroupa, MD
Quality Assurance .... Thomas Lewis

Measure	Cases	This Hosp.	State Avg.	U.S. Avg.
Blood Clot Prevention and Treatment				
Anticoagulation Overlap Therapy	-	-	94%	93%
ICU Venous Thromboembolism Prophylaxis	-	-	91%	92%
Incidence of Potentially Preventable VTE	-	-	7%	10%
UFH with Dosages/Platelet Monitoring	-	-	96%	97%
Venous Thromboembolism Prophylaxis	-	-	85%	85%
Warfarin Therapy Discharge Instructions	-	-	76%	75%
Chest Pain/Possible Heart Attack Care				
Aspirin Given Within 24 Hours of Arrival	-	-	95%	96%
Fibrinolytic Meds Within 30 Min. of Arrival	-	-	53%	58%
Average Time to ECG (minutes)	-	-	7	7
Average Time to Transfer (minutes)	-	-	53	60
Children's Asthma Care				
Received Home Management Plan of Care	-	-	-	88%
Received Reliever Medication	-	-	-	100%
Received Systemic Corticosteroids	-	-	-	100%
Emergency Department				
Admittance Decision Time (minutes)	-	-	81	98
Head CT Results Within 45 Min. of Arrival	-	-	63%	57%
Patients Who Left ER Before Being Seen	-	-	3%	2%
Time from ER Arrival to Admit. (minutes)	-	-	238	274
Time from ER Arrival to Discharge (minutes)	-	-	136	134
Time in ER Before Being Evaluated (minutes)	-	-	26	26
Time to Pain Meds for Fractures (minutes)	-	-	52	57
Heart Attack Care				
Aspirin Given at Discharge	81	100%	99%	99%
Fibrinolytic Meds Within 30 Min. of Arrival[5]	-	-	-	54%
PCI Within 90 Minutes of Arrival[1]	11	91%	97%	96%
Statin Prescribed at Discharge	78	100%	98%	98%
Heart Failure Care				
ACE Inhibitor or ARB for LVSD	154	99%	96%	97%
Discharge Instructions Given	349	88%	94%	94%
Evaluation of LVS Function	395	99%	98%	99%
Medicare Spending				
Medicare Spending per Patient (ratio)	-	-	0.95	0.98
Pneumonia Care				
Appropriate Initial Antibiotic Given	37	97%	95%	95%
Blood Culture Timing	62	94%	98%	98%
Pregnancy and Delivery Care				
Newborn Deliveries Scheduled Early	-	-	5%	6%
Preventive Care				
Immunization for Influenza[5]	-	-	92%	90%
Immunization for Pneumonia[5]	-	-	93%	92%
Stroke Care				
Anticoagulation Therapy for Atrial Fibrillation	-	-	94%	95%
Antithrombotic Therapy Timing	-	-	98%	98%
Assessed for Rehabilitation	-	-	98%	97%
Discharged on Antithrombotic Therapy	-	-	99%	99%
Discharged on Statin Medication	-	-	95%	94%
Thrombolytic Therapy Timing	-	-	67%	66%
Venous Thromboembolism Prophylaxis	-	-	95%	94%
Written Stroke Educational Materials Given	-	-	88%	88%
Surgical Care Improvement Project				
Appropriate Beta Blocker Usage[2]	93	99%	98%	98%
Appropriate VTP Within 24 Hours[2]	348	96%	98%	98%
Controlled Postoperative Blood Glucose[5]	-	-	97%	97%
Perioperative Temperature Management[2]	374	99%	100%	100%
Prophylactic Antibiotic Selection	249	99%	99%	99%
Prophylactic Antibiotic Selection (Outpatient)	-	-	98%	98%
Prophylactic Antibiotic Stopped	248	95%	98%	98%

NOTE: Hospital profiles are in alphabetical order by state, then city, then hospital within the city; Rankings exclude hospitals with less than 25 cases except for patient surveys which excludes hospitals with less than 100 cases; (a) 100-299 cases; (1) The number of cases/patients is too few to report; (2) Data submitted were based on a sample of cases/patients; (3) Results are based on a shorter time period than required; (4) Data suppressed by CMS for one or more quarters; (5) Results are not available for this reporting period; (6) Fewer than 100 patients completed the HCAHPS survey; (7) No cases met the criteria for this measure; (8) The lower limit of the confidence interval cannot be calculated if the number of observed infections equals zero; (9) No data are available from the state/territory for this reporting period; (10) The scores shown reflect fewer than 50 completed surveys; (11) There were discrepancies in the data collection process; (12) This measure does not apply to this hospital for this reporting period; (13) Results cannot be calculated for this reporting period; (14) The results for this state are combined with nearby states to protect confidentiality; Please refer to the User's Guide for a full explanation of data.

Prophylactic Antibiotic Timing	254	96%	99%	99%
Prophylactic Antibiotic Timing (Outpatient)	-	-	98%	98%
Urinary Catheter Removal[2]	234	98%	97%	97%
Survey of Patients' Hospital Experiences				
Area Around Room 'Always' Quiet at Night	-	-	61%	61%
Doctors 'Always' Communicated Well	-	-	82%	82%
Home Recovery Information Given	-	-	87%	85%
Hospital Given 9 or 10 on 10 Point Scale	-	-	71%	71%
Meds 'Always' Explained Before Given	-	-	63%	64%
Nurses 'Always' Communicated Well	-	-	79%	79%
Pain 'Always' Well Controlled	-	-	71%	71%
Room and Bathroom 'Always' Clean	-	-	73%	73%
Timely Help 'Always' Received	-	-	68%	68%
Would Definitely Recommend Hospital	-	-	70%	71%
Use of Medical Imaging				
Cardiac Imaging Stress Test before Surgery	-	-	5.2%	5.3%
Combination Abdominal CT Scan	-	-	11.2%	10.5%
Combination Brain/Sinus CT Scan	-	-	3.2%	2.7%
Combination Chest CT Scan	-	-	1.9%	2.7%
Follow-up Mammogram/Ultrasound	-	-	8.6%	8.8%
Lumbar Spine MRI for Low Back Pain	-	-	39.6%	37.2%

Saint Louis University Hospital

3635 Vista Ave
Saint Louis, MO 63110
E-mail: slucare@slu.edu
URL: www.slucare.edu/clinical
Phone: 314-577-8000
Fax: 314-577-8825
Type: Acute Care Hospitals
Ownership: Proprietary
Emergency Services: Yes
Beds: 356

Key Personnel:
Anesthesiology. . . . . Larry Baudendistel, MD
Chief of Medical Staff. . . . . Coy Fitch, MD
Radiology. . . . . Ben Frey
Infection Control. . . . . Donald J Kennedy, MD
Operating Room. . . . . Judy Mai Lombardo, RN
Pediatric Ambulatory Care . . . . . . George Ray, MD
Pediatric In-Patient Care . . . . George Ray, MD
CEO/President. . . . . Phillip E. Sowa

Measure	Cases	This Hosp.	State Avg.	U.S. Avg.
Blood Clot Prevention and Treatment				
Anticoagulation Overlap Therapy[2]	105	89%	94%	93%
ICU Venous Thromboembolism Prophylaxis[2]	155	97%	91%	92%
Incidence of Potentially Preventable VTE[2]	49	2%	7%	10%
UFH with Dosages/Platelet Monitoring[2]	61	97%	96%	97%
Venous Thromboembolism Prophylaxis[2]	284	89%	85%	85%
Warfarin Therapy Discharge Instructions[2]	74	99%	76%	75%
Chest Pain/Possible Heart Attack Care				
Aspirin Given Within 24 Hours of Arrival[1,3]	-	-	95%	96%
Fibrinolytic Meds Within 30 Min. of Arrival[5]	-	-	53%	58%
Average Time to ECG (minutes)[1,3]	-	-	7	7
Average Time to Transfer (minutes)[5]	-	-	53	60
Children's Asthma Care				
Received Home Management Plan of Care	-	-	-	88%
Received Reliever Medication	-	-	-	100%
Received Systemic Corticosteroids	-	-	-	100%
Emergency Department				
Admittance Decision Time (minutes)[2]	484	192	81	98
Head CT Results Within 45 Min. of Arrival[7]	-	-	63%	57%
Patients Who Left ER Before Being Seen	39,404	3%	3%	2%
Time from ER Arrival to Admit. (minutes)[2]	503	273	238	274
Time from ER Arrival to Discharge (minutes)	398	168	136	134
Time in ER Before Being Evaluated (minutes)	447	27	26	26
Time to Pain Meds for Fractures (minutes)	47	41	52	57
Heart Attack Care				
Aspirin Given at Discharge	168	100%	99%	99%
Fibrinolytic Meds Within 30 Min. of Arrival[1]	-	-	-	54%
PCI Within 90 Minutes of Arrival	40	98%	97%	96%
Statin Prescribed at Discharge	165	99%	98%	98%
Heart Failure Care				
ACE Inhibitor or ARB for LVSD	165	99%	96%	97%
Discharge Instructions Given	266	97%	94%	94%
Evaluation of LVS Function	298	100%	98%	99%
Medicare Spending				
Medicare Spending per Patient (ratio)	-	1.03	0.95	0.98
Pneumonia Care				
Appropriate Initial Antibiotic Given[2]	73	97%	95%	95%
Blood Culture Timing[2]	104	98%	98%	98%
Pregnancy and Delivery Care				
Newborn Deliveries Scheduled Early[7]	-	-	5%	6%
Preventive Care				
Immunization for Influenza[2]	630	98%	92%	90%
Immunization for Pneumonia[2]	737	97%	93%	92%
Stroke Care				
Anticoagulation Therapy for Atrial Fibrillation[2]	25	92%	94%	95%
Antithrombotic Therapy Timing[2]	129	98%	98%	98%
Assessed for Rehabilitation[2]	251	100%	98%	97%
Discharged on Antithrombotic Therapy[2]	173	100%	99%	99%
Discharged on Statin Medication[2]	131	99%	95%	94%
Thrombolytic Therapy Timing[2]	14	100%	67%	66%
Venous Thromboembolism Prophylaxis[2]	260	98%	95%	94%
Written Stroke Educational Materials Given[2]	130	98%	88%	88%
Surgical Care Improvement Project				
Appropriate Beta Blocker Usage[2]	139	99%	98%	98%
Appropriate VTP Within 24 Hours[2]	249	100%	98%	98%
Controlled Postoperative Blood Glucose[2]	62	90%	97%	97%
Perioperative Temperature Management[2]	301	99%	100%	100%
Prophylactic Antibiotic Selection[2]	129	99%	99%	99%
Prophylactic Antibiotic Selection (Outpatient)	170	99%	98%	98%
Prophylactic Antibiotic Stopped[2]	115	98%	98%	98%
Prophylactic Antibiotic Timing[2]	130	99%	99%	99%
Prophylactic Antibiotic Timing (Outpatient)	172	97%	98%	98%
Urinary Catheter Removal[2]	169	98%	97%	97%
Survey of Patients' Hospital Experiences				
Area Around Room 'Always' Quiet at Night	300+	59%	61%	61%
Doctors 'Always' Communicated Well	300+	82%	82%	82%
Home Recovery Information Given	300+	88%	87%	85%
Hospital Given 9 or 10 on 10 Point Scale	300+	72%	71%	71%
Meds 'Always' Explained Before Given	300+	65%	63%	64%
Nurses 'Always' Communicated Well	300+	77%	79%	79%
Pain 'Always' Well Controlled	300+	72%	71%	71%
Room and Bathroom 'Always' Clean	300+	67%	73%	73%
Timely Help 'Always' Received	300+	64%	68%	68%
Would Definitely Recommend Hospital	300+	77%	70%	71%
Use of Medical Imaging				
Cardiac Imaging Stress Test before Surgery	128	6.3%	5.2%	5.3%
Combination Abdominal CT Scan	677	11.7%	11.2%	10.5%
Combination Brain/Sinus CT Scan	500	4.2%	3.2%	2.7%
Combination Chest CT Scan	657	3.7%	1.9%	2.7%
Follow-up Mammogram/Ultrasound	328	9.1%	8.6%	8.8%
Lumbar Spine MRI for Low Back Pain	38	44.7%	39.6%	37.2%

Barnes-Jewish Saint Peters Hospital

10 Hospital Dr
Saint Peters, MO 63376
URL: www.bjsph.org
Phone: 636-916-9000
Fax: 636-916-9127
Type: Acute Care Hospitals
Ownership: Voluntary non-profit - Other
Emergency Services: Yes
Beds: 111

Key Personnel:
Chief of Medical Staff. . . . . Timothy Cooper, MD
Pediatric Ambulatory Care . . . . . . Michael Dauter
Pediatric In-Patient Care . . . . Michael Dauter
Quality Assurance . . . . Lois Koehler
Operating Room. . . . . Mindy Manly
Anesthesiology. . . . . John Menius, MD
CEO/President. . . . . David Ross
Infection Control. . . . . Janice Setzer

Measure	Cases	This Hosp.	State Avg.	U.S. Avg.
Blood Clot Prevention and Treatment				
Anticoagulation Overlap Therapy[2]	64	97%	94%	93%
ICU Venous Thromboembolism Prophylaxis[2]	50	98%	91%	92%
Incidence of Potentially Preventable VTE[2]	24	0%	7%	10%
UFH with Dosages/Platelet Monitoring[2]	19	100%	96%	97%
Venous Thromboembolism Prophylaxis[2]	334	93%	85%	85%
Warfarin Therapy Discharge Instructions[2]	51	86%	76%	75%
Chest Pain/Possible Heart Attack Care				
Aspirin Given Within 24 Hours of Arrival	12	83%	95%	96%
Fibrinolytic Meds Within 30 Min. of Arrival[3,7]	-	-	53%	58%
Average Time to ECG (minutes)	12	8	7	7
Average Time to Transfer (minutes)[3,7]	-	-	53	60
Children's Asthma Care				
Received Home Management Plan of Care	-	-	-	88%
Received Reliever Medication	-	-	-	100%
Received Systemic Corticosteroids	-	-	-	100%
Emergency Department				
Admittance Decision Time (minutes)[2]	711	66	81	98
Head CT Results Within 45 Min. of Arrival[1]	-	-	63%	57%
Patients Who Left ER Before Being Seen	29,998	1%	3%	2%
Time from ER Arrival to Admit. (minutes)[2]	729	234	238	274
Time from ER Arrival to Discharge (minutes)	791	142	136	134
Time in ER Before Being Evaluated (minutes)	798	50	26	26
Time to Pain Meds for Fractures (minutes)	171	38	52	57
Heart Attack Care				
Aspirin Given at Discharge	91	100%	99%	99%
Fibrinolytic Meds Within 30 Min. of Arrival[7]	-	-	-	54%
PCI Within 90 Minutes of Arrival	54	98%	97%	96%
Statin Prescribed at Discharge	91	100%	98%	98%
Heart Failure Care				
ACE Inhibitor or ARB for LVSD[2]	47	98%	96%	97%
Discharge Instructions Given[2]	159	97%	94%	94%
Evaluation of LVS Function[2]	190	100%	98%	99%
Medicare Spending				
Medicare Spending per Patient (ratio)	-	0.94	0.95	0.98
Pneumonia Care				
Appropriate Initial Antibiotic Given[2]	108	98%	95%	95%
Blood Culture Timing[2]	238	100%	98%	98%
Pregnancy and Delivery Care				
Newborn Deliveries Scheduled Early[2]	24	0%	5%	6%
Preventive Care				
Immunization for Influenza[2]	546	93%	92%	90%
Immunization for Pneumonia[2]	754	94%	93%	92%
Stroke Care				
Anticoagulation Therapy for Atrial Fibrillation[2]	11	100%	94%	95%
Antithrombotic Therapy Timing[2]	62	100%	98%	98%
Assessed for Rehabilitation[2]	83	95%	98%	97%
Discharged on Antithrombotic Therapy[2]	81	99%	99%	99%
Discharged on Statin Medication[2]	60	95%	95%	94%
Thrombolytic Therapy Timing[1,2]	-	-	67%	66%
Venous Thromboembolism Prophylaxis[2]	79	91%	95%	94%
Written Stroke Educational Materials Given[2]	54	98%	88%	88%
Surgical Care Improvement Project				
Appropriate Beta Blocker Usage[2]	103	99%	98%	98%
Appropriate VTP Within 24 Hours[2]	342	98%	98%	98%
Controlled Postoperative Blood Glucose[2,7]	-	-	97%	97%
Perioperative Temperature Management[2]	370	100%	100%	100%
Prophylactic Antibiotic Selection[2]	237	99%	99%	99%
Prophylactic Antibiotic Selection (Outpatient)	100	92%	98%	98%
Prophylactic Antibiotic Stopped[2]	232	99%	98%	98%
Prophylactic Antibiotic Timing[2]	238	97%	99%	99%
Prophylactic Antibiotic Timing (Outpatient)	100	99%	98%	98%
Urinary Catheter Removal[2]	235	95%	97%	97%
Survey of Patients' Hospital Experiences				
Area Around Room 'Always' Quiet at Night	300+	54%	61%	61%
Doctors 'Always' Communicated Well	300+	81%	82%	82%
Home Recovery Information Given	300+	88%	87%	85%
Hospital Given 9 or 10 on 10 Point Scale	300+	74%	71%	71%
Meds 'Always' Explained Before Given	300+	54%	63%	64%
Nurses 'Always' Communicated Well	300+	81%	79%	79%
Pain 'Always' Well Controlled	300+	73%	71%	71%
Room and Bathroom 'Always' Clean	300+	62%	73%	73%
Timely Help 'Always' Received	300+	63%	68%	68%
Would Definitely Recommend Hospital	300+	80%	70%	71%
Use of Medical Imaging				
Cardiac Imaging Stress Test before Surgery	499	5.0%	5.2%	5.3%
Combination Abdominal CT Scan	846	2.1%	11.2%	10.5%
Combination Brain/Sinus CT Scan	464	4.3%	3.2%	2.7%
Combination Chest CT Scan	906	0.0%	1.9%	2.7%
Follow-up Mammogram/Ultrasound	1,047	9.0%	8.6%	8.8%
Lumbar Spine MRI for Low Back Pain	73	32.9%	39.6%	37.2%

NOTE: Hospital profiles are in alphabetical order by state, then city, then hospital within the city; Rankings exclude hospitals with less than 25 cases except for patient surveys which excludes hospitals with less than 100 cases; (a) 100-299 cases; (1) The number of cases/patients is too few to report; (2) Data submitted were based on a sample of cases/patients; (3) Results are based on a shorter time period than required; (4) Data suppressed by CMS for one or more quarters; (5) Results are not available for this reporting period; (6) Fewer than 100 patients completed the HCAHPS survey; (7) No cases met the criteria for this measure; (8) The lower limit of the confidence interval cannot be calculated if the number of observed infections equals zero; (9) No data are available from the state/territory for this reporting period; (10) The scores shown reflect fewer than 50 completed surveys; (11) There were discrepancies in the data collection process; (12) This measure does not apply to this hospital for this reporting period; (13) Results cannot be calculated for this reporting period; (14) The results for this state are combined with nearby states to protect confidentiality; Please refer to the User's Guide for a full explanation of data.

Sainte Genevieve County Memorial Hospital

800 Ste Genevieve Drive, PO Box 468 Phone: 573-883-2751
Sainte Genevieve, MO 63670
Type: Critical Access Hospitals Emergency Services: Yes
Ownership: Govt - Hospital Dist/Auth
Key Personnel:
Radiology. . . . . Patrick Cabrera
CEO/President. . . . . Thomas Keim

Measure	Cases	This Hosp.	State Avg.	U.S. Avg.
Blood Clot Prevention and Treatment				
Anticoagulation Overlap Therapy[5]	-	-	94%	93%
ICU Venous Thromboembolism Prophylaxis[5]	-	-	91%	92%
Incidence of Potentially Preventable VTE[5]	-	-	7%	10%
UFH with Dosages/Platelet Monitoring[5]	-	-	96%	97%
Venous Thromboembolism Prophylaxis[5]	-	-	85%	85%
Warfarin Therapy Discharge Instructions[5]	-	-	76%	75%
Chest Pain/Possible Heart Attack Care				
Aspirin Given Within 24 Hours of Arrival[1,3]	-	-	95%	96%
Fibrinolytic Meds Within 30 Min. of Arrival[3,7]	-	-	53%	58%
Average Time to ECG (minutes)[1,3]	-	-	7	7
Average Time to Transfer (minutes)[1,3]	-	-	53	60
Children's Asthma Care				
Received Home Management Plan of Care	-	-	-	88%
Received Reliever Medication	-	-	-	100%
Received Systemic Corticosteroids	-	-	-	100%
Emergency Department				
Admittance Decision Time (minutes)[5]	-	-	81	98
Head CT Results Within 45 Min. of Arrival[5]	-	-	63%	57%
Patients Who Left ER Before Being Seen[5]	-	-	3%	2%
Time from ER Arrival to Admit. (minutes)[5]	-	-	238	274
Time from ER Arrival to Discharge (minutes)[5]	-	-	136	134
Time in ER Before Being Evaluated (minutes)[5]	-	-	26	26
Time to Pain Meds for Fractures (minutes)[5]	-	-	52	57
Heart Attack Care				
Aspirin Given at Discharge[5]	-	-	99%	99%
Fibrinolytic Meds Within 30 Min. of Arrival[5]	-	-	-	54%
PCI Within 90 Minutes of Arrival[5]	-	-	97%	96%
Statin Prescribed at Discharge[5]	-	-	98%	98%
Heart Failure Care				
ACE Inhibitor or ARB for LVSD[1]	-	-	96%	97%
Discharge Instructions Given	17	94%	94%	94%
Evaluation of LVS Function	36	100%	98%	99%
Medicare Spending				
Medicare Spending per Patient (ratio)	-	-	0.95	0.98
Pneumonia Care				
Appropriate Initial Antibiotic Given	26	85%	95%	95%
Blood Culture Timing	40	100%	98%	98%
Pregnancy and Delivery Care				
Newborn Deliveries Scheduled Early[5]	-	-	5%	6%
Preventive Care				
Immunization for Influenza[5]	-	-	92%	90%
Immunization for Pneumonia[5]	-	-	93%	92%
Stroke Care				
Anticoagulation Therapy for Atrial Fibrillation[5]	-	-	94%	95%
Antithrombotic Therapy Timing[5]	-	-	98%	98%
Assessed for Rehabilitation[5]	-	-	98%	97%
Discharged on Antithrombotic Therapy[5]	-	-	99%	99%
Discharged on Statin Medication[5]	-	-	95%	94%
Thrombolytic Therapy Timing[5]	-	-	67%	66%
Venous Thromboembolism Prophylaxis[5]	-	-	95%	94%
Written Stroke Educational Materials Given[5]	-	-	88%	88%
Surgical Care Improvement Project				
Appropriate Beta Blocker Usage[1]	-	-	98%	98%
Appropriate VTP Within 24 Hours[1,3]	-	-	98%	98%
Controlled Postoperative Blood Glucose[3,7]	-	-	97%	97%
Perioperative Temperature Management	42	100%	100%	100%
Prophylactic Antibiotic Selection	34	100%	99%	99%
Prophylactic Antibiotic Selection (Outpatient)[5]	-	-	98%	98%
Prophylactic Antibiotic Stopped	33	100%	98%	98%
Prophylactic Antibiotic Timing	34	100%	99%	99%
Prophylactic Antibiotic Timing (Outpatient)[5]	-	-	98%	98%
Urinary Catheter Removal	20	100%	97%	97%
Survey of Patients' Hospital Experiences				
Area Around Room 'Always' Quiet at Night	(a)	60%	61%	61%
Doctors 'Always' Communicated Well	(a)	87%	82%	82%
Home Recovery Information Given	(a)	91%	87%	85%
Hospital Given 9 or 10 on 10 Point Scale	(a)	74%	71%	71%
Meds 'Always' Explained Before Given	(a)	65%	63%	64%
Nurses 'Always' Communicated Well	(a)	83%	79%	79%
Pain 'Always' Well Controlled	(a)	75%	71%	71%
Room and Bathroom 'Always' Clean	(a)	88%	73%	73%
Timely Help 'Always' Received	(a)	72%	68%	68%
Would Definitely Recommend Hospital	(a)	74%	70%	71%
Use of Medical Imaging				
Cardiac Imaging Stress Test before Surgery	118	2.5%	5.2%	5.3%
Combination Abdominal CT Scan	278	2.5%	11.2%	10.5%
Combination Brain/Sinus CT Scan[1]	-	-	3.2%	2.7%
Combination Chest CT Scan	119	1.7%	1.9%	2.7%
Follow-up Mammogram/Ultrasound	237	5.5%	8.6%	8.8%
Lumbar Spine MRI for Low Back Pain	49	53.1%	39.6%	37.2%

Salem Memorial District Hospital

PO Box 774 Phone: 573-729-6626
Salem, MO 65560 Fax: 573-729-4511
Type: Critical Access Hospitals Emergency Services: Yes
Ownership: Govt - Hospital Dist/Auth Beds: 59
Key Personnel:
Chairman/CEO . . . . Joe Brand
Quality Assurance . . . . Arlene Cornell
Operating Room. . . . . Lowell Fisher
Infection Control. . . . . Cliff Free
Emergency Room . . . . Brenda Gott
Administrator . . . . Dennis P. Pryor

Measure	Cases	This Hosp.	State Avg.	U.S. Avg.
Blood Clot Prevention and Treatment				
Anticoagulation Overlap Therapy[5]	-	-	94%	93%
ICU Venous Thromboembolism Prophylaxis[5]	-	-	91%	92%
Incidence of Potentially Preventable VTE[5]	-	-	7%	10%
UFH with Dosages/Platelet Monitoring[5]	-	-	96%	97%
Venous Thromboembolism Prophylaxis[5]	-	-	85%	85%
Warfarin Therapy Discharge Instructions[5]	-	-	76%	75%
Chest Pain/Possible Heart Attack Care				
Aspirin Given Within 24 Hours of Arrival	-	-	95%	96%
Fibrinolytic Meds Within 30 Min. of Arrival	-	-	53%	58%
Average Time to ECG (minutes)	-	-	7	7
Average Time to Transfer (minutes)	-	-	53	60
Children's Asthma Care				
Received Home Management Plan of Care	-	-	-	88%
Received Reliever Medication	-	-	-	100%
Received Systemic Corticosteroids	-	-	-	100%
Emergency Department				
Admittance Decision Time (minutes)[5]	-	-	81	98
Head CT Results Within 45 Min. of Arrival	-	-	63%	57%
Patients Who Left ER Before Being Seen	-	-	3%	2%
Time from ER Arrival to Admit. (minutes)[5]	-	-	238	274
Time from ER Arrival to Discharge (minutes)	-	-	136	134
Time in ER Before Being Evaluated (minutes)	-	-	26	26
Time to Pain Meds for Fractures (minutes)	-	-	52	57
Heart Attack Care				
Aspirin Given at Discharge[5]	-	-	99%	99%
Fibrinolytic Meds Within 30 Min. of Arrival[5]	-	-	-	54%
PCI Within 90 Minutes of Arrival[5]	-	-	97%	96%
Statin Prescribed at Discharge[5]	-	-	98%	98%
Heart Failure Care				
ACE Inhibitor or ARB for LVSD	14	100%	96%	97%
Discharge Instructions Given	31	90%	94%	94%
Evaluation of LVS Function	35	66%	98%	99%
Medicare Spending				
Medicare Spending per Patient (ratio)	-	-	0.95	0.98
Pneumonia Care				
Appropriate Initial Antibiotic Given	42	79%	95%	95%
Blood Culture Timing	55	100%	98%	98%
Pregnancy and Delivery Care				
Newborn Deliveries Scheduled Early[5]	-	-	5%	6%
Preventive Care				
Immunization for Influenza[5]	-	-	92%	90%
Immunization for Pneumonia[5]	-	-	93%	92%
Stroke Care				
Anticoagulation Therapy for Atrial Fibrillation[5]	-	-	94%	95%
Antithrombotic Therapy Timing[5]	-	-	98%	98%
Assessed for Rehabilitation[5]	-	-	98%	97%
Discharged on Antithrombotic Therapy[5]	-	-	99%	99%
Discharged on Statin Medication[5]	-	-	95%	94%
Thrombolytic Therapy Timing[5]	-	-	67%	66%
Venous Thromboembolism Prophylaxis[5]	-	-	95%	94%
Written Stroke Educational Materials Given[5]	-	-	88%	88%
Surgical Care Improvement Project				
Appropriate Beta Blocker Usage[5]	-	-	98%	98%
Appropriate VTP Within 24 Hours[5]	-	-	98%	98%
Controlled Postoperative Blood Glucose[5]	-	-	97%	97%
Perioperative Temperature Management[5]	-	-	100%	100%
Prophylactic Antibiotic Selection[5]	-	-	99%	99%
Prophylactic Antibiotic Selection (Outpatient)	-	-	98%	98%
Prophylactic Antibiotic Stopped[5]	-	-	98%	98%
Prophylactic Antibiotic Timing[5]	-	-	99%	99%
Prophylactic Antibiotic Timing (Outpatient)	-	-	98%	98%
Urinary Catheter Removal[5]	-	-	97%	97%
Survey of Patients' Hospital Experiences				
Area Around Room 'Always' Quiet at Night[5]	-	-	61%	61%
Doctors 'Always' Communicated Well[5]	-	-	82%	82%
Home Recovery Information Given[5]	-	-	87%	85%
Hospital Given 9 or 10 on 10 Point Scale[5]	-	-	71%	71%
Meds 'Always' Explained Before Given[5]	-	-	63%	64%
Nurses 'Always' Communicated Well[5]	-	-	79%	79%
Pain 'Always' Well Controlled[5]	-	-	71%	71%
Room and Bathroom 'Always' Clean[5]	-	-	73%	73%
Timely Help 'Always' Received[5]	-	-	68%	68%
Would Definitely Recommend Hospital[5]	-	-	70%	71%
Use of Medical Imaging				
Cardiac Imaging Stress Test before Surgery	-	-	5.2%	5.3%
Combination Abdominal CT Scan	-	-	11.2%	10.5%
Combination Brain/Sinus CT Scan	-	-	3.2%	2.7%
Combination Chest CT Scan	-	-	1.9%	2.7%
Follow-up Mammogram/Ultrasound	-	-	8.6%	8.8%
Lumbar Spine MRI for Low Back Pain	-	-	39.6%	37.2%

Bothwell Regional Health Center

601 E 14th St Phone: 660-826-8833
Sedalia, MO 65302 Fax: 660-827-6784
URL: www.brhc.org
Type: Acute Care Hospitals Emergency Services: Yes
Ownership: Government - Local Beds: 170
Key Personnel:
Quality Assurance . . . . Connie Chappel
CEO/President. . . . . John Dawes
Chief of Medical Staff . . . . Phillip Horneospel
Operating Room. . . . . Bobbi McNims, RN
Radiology. . . . . David H Roehrs, MD
Chair/CEO. . . . . Rob Rollings
Emergency Room . . . . Karen Toy

Measure	Cases	This Hosp.	State Avg.	U.S. Avg.
Blood Clot Prevention and Treatment				
Anticoagulation Overlap Therapy[2]	19	74%	94%	93%
ICU Venous Thromboembolism Prophylaxis[2]	39	44%	91%	92%
Incidence of Potentially Preventable VTE[1,2]	-	-	7%	10%
UFH with Dosages/Platelet Monitoring[1,2]	-	-	96%	97%
Venous Thromboembolism Prophylaxis[2]	374	40%	85%	85%
Warfarin Therapy Discharge Instructions[2]	15	53%	76%	75%
Chest Pain/Possible Heart Attack Care				
Aspirin Given Within 24 Hours of Arrival	121	88%	95%	96%
Fibrinolytic Meds Within 30 Min. of Arrival[1]	-	-	53%	58%
Average Time to ECG (minutes)	123	9	7	7
Average Time to Transfer (minutes)	11	60	53	60
Children's Asthma Care				
Received Home Management Plan of Care	-	-	-	88%
Received Reliever Medication	-	-	-	100%
Received Systemic Corticosteroids	-	-	-	100%
Emergency Department				
Admittance Decision Time (minutes)[2]	540	60	81	98
Head CT Results Within 45 Min. of Arrival	20	50%	63%	57%
Patients Who Left ER Before Being Seen	24,868	1%	3%	2%

NOTE: Hospital profiles are in alphabetical order by state, then city, then hospital within the city; Rankings exclude hospitals with less than 25 cases except for patient surveys which excludes hospitals with less than 100 cases; (a) 100-299 cases; (1) The number of cases/patients is too few to report; (2) Data submitted were based on a sample of cases/patients; (3) Results are based on a shorter time period than required; (4) Data suppressed by CMS for one or more quarters; (5) Results are not available for this reporting period; (6) Fewer than 100 patients completed the HCAHPS survey; (7) No cases met the criteria for this measure; (8) The lower limit of the confidence interval cannot be calculated if the number of observed infections equals zero; (9) No data are available from the state/territory for this reporting period; (10) The scores shown reflect fewer than 50 completed surveys; (11) There were discrepancies in the data collection process; (12) This measure does not apply to this hospital for this reporting period; (13) Results cannot be calculated for this reporting period; (14) The results for this state are combined with nearby states to protect confidentiality; Please refer to the User's Guide for a full explanation of data.

Measure	Cases	This Hosp.	State Avg.	U.S. Avg.
Time from ER Arrival to Admit. (minutes)[2]	558	187	238	274
Time from ER Arrival to Discharge (minutes)	419	128	136	134
Time in ER Before Being Evaluated (minutes)	460	20	26	26
Time to Pain Meds for Fractures (minutes)	85	66	52	57
Heart Attack Care				
Aspirin Given at Discharge	26	88%	99%	99%
Fibrinolytic Meds Within 30 Min. of Arrival[1]	-	-	-	54%
PCI Within 90 Minutes of Arrival[7]	-	-	97%	96%
Statin Prescribed at Discharge	23	74%	98%	98%
Heart Failure Care				
ACE Inhibitor or ARB for LVSD	64	72%	96%	97%
Discharge Instructions Given	123	89%	94%	94%
Evaluation of LVS Function	159	99%	98%	99%
Medicare Spending				
Medicare Spending per Patient (ratio)	-	0.85	0.95	0.98
Pneumonia Care				
Appropriate Initial Antibiotic Given	100	91%	95%	95%
Blood Culture Timing	78	96%	98%	98%
Pregnancy and Delivery Care				
Newborn Deliveries Scheduled Early	34	0%	5%	6%
Preventive Care				
Immunization for Influenza[2]	502	88%	92%	90%
Immunization for Pneumonia[2]	666	98%	93%	92%
Stroke Care				
Anticoagulation Therapy for Atrial Fibrillation[1]	-	-	94%	95%
Antithrombotic Therapy Timing	46	96%	98%	98%
Assessed for Rehabilitation	46	80%	98%	97%
Discharged on Antithrombotic Therapy	46	96%	99%	99%
Discharged on Statin Medication	43	58%	95%	94%
Thrombolytic Therapy Timing[1]	-	-	67%	66%
Venous Thromboembolism Prophylaxis	48	58%	95%	94%
Written Stroke Educational Materials Given	24	25%	88%	88%
Surgical Care Improvement Project				
Appropriate Beta Blocker Usage	100	79%	98%	98%
Appropriate VTP Within 24 Hours	320	92%	98%	98%
Controlled Postoperative Blood Glucose[7]	-	-	97%	97%
Perioperative Temperature Management	368	99%	100%	100%
Prophylactic Antibiotic Selection	250	89%	99%	99%
Prophylactic Antibiotic Selection (Outpatient)	156	88%	98%	98%
Prophylactic Antibiotic Stopped	246	97%	98%	98%
Prophylactic Antibiotic Timing	250	100%	99%	99%
Prophylactic Antibiotic Timing (Outpatient)	159	92%	98%	98%
Urinary Catheter Removal	210	86%	97%	97%
Survey of Patients' Hospital Experiences				
Area Around Room 'Always' Quiet at Night	300+	64%	61%	61%
Doctors 'Always' Communicated Well	300+	83%	82%	82%
Home Recovery Information Given	300+	86%	87%	85%
Hospital Given 9 or 10 on 10 Point Scale	300+	73%	71%	71%
Meds 'Always' Explained Before Given	300+	65%	63%	64%
Nurses 'Always' Communicated Well	300+	83%	79%	79%
Pain 'Always' Well Controlled	300+	74%	71%	71%
Room and Bathroom 'Always' Clean	300+	72%	73%	73%
Timely Help 'Always' Received	300+	75%	68%	68%
Would Definitely Recommend Hospital	300+	63%	70%	71%
Use of Medical Imaging				
Cardiac Imaging Stress Test before Surgery	416	4.8%	5.2%	5.3%
Combination Abdominal CT Scan	907	59.4%	11.2%	10.5%
Combination Brain/Sinus CT Scan	607	5.9%	3.2%	2.7%
Combination Chest CT Scan	554	15.2%	1.9%	2.7%
Follow-up Mammogram/Ultrasound	1,244	5.3%	8.6%	8.8%
Lumbar Spine MRI for Low Back Pain	113	48.7%	39.6%	37.2%

Missouri Delta Medical Center

1008 North Main St
Sikeston, MO 63801
Phone: 573-471-1600
Fax: 573-472-7606
URL: www.missouridelta.com
Type: Acute Care Hospitals
Emergency Services: Yes
Ownership: Voluntary non-profit - Other
Beds: 188

Key Personnel:
Pediatric Ambulatory Care . . . . . . Joseph Blanton, MD
Pediatric In-Patient Care . . . . Joseph Blanton, MD
Infection Control. . . . . Joy Cauthorn
Quality Assurance . . . . Linda Culbertson
Operating Room. . . . . Libby Kliptel
Chief of Medical Staff . . . . Mowaffaq Said, MD
Cardiac Laboratory. . . . . Cindy Shands
Radiology. . . . . Mahmaud Ziaee

Measure	Cases	This Hosp.	State Avg.	U.S. Avg.
Blood Clot Prevention and Treatment				
Anticoagulation Overlap Therapy[2]	19	95%	94%	93%
ICU Venous Thromboembolism Prophylaxis[2]	91	97%	91%	92%
Incidence of Potentially Preventable VTE[1,2]	-	-	7%	10%
UFH with Dosages/Platelet Monitoring[2]	16	100%	96%	97%
Venous Thromboembolism Prophylaxis[2]	282	94%	85%	85%
Warfarin Therapy Discharge Instructions[2]	14	71%	76%	75%
Chest Pain/Possible Heart Attack Care				
Aspirin Given Within 24 Hours of Arrival	95	89%	95%	96%
Fibrinolytic Meds Within 30 Min. of Arrival[7]	-	-	53%	58%
Average Time to ECG (minutes)	97	10	7	7
Average Time to Transfer (minutes)	20	50	53	60
Children's Asthma Care				
Received Home Management Plan of Care	-	-	-	88%
Received Reliever Medication	-	-	-	100%
Received Systemic Corticosteroids	-	-	-	100%
Emergency Department				
Admittance Decision Time (minutes)[2]	337	60	81	98
Head CT Results Within 45 Min. of Arrival[1]	-	-	63%	57%
Patients Who Left ER Before Being Seen	17,251	9%	3%	2%
Time from ER Arrival to Admit. (minutes)[2]	372	274	238	274
Time from ER Arrival to Discharge (minutes)	381	166	136	134
Time in ER Before Being Evaluated (minutes)	444	51	26	26
Time to Pain Meds for Fractures (minutes)	69	84	52	57
Heart Attack Care				
Aspirin Given at Discharge[1]	-	-	99%	99%
Fibrinolytic Meds Within 30 Min. of Arrival[7]	-	-	-	54%
PCI Within 90 Minutes of Arrival[7]	-	-	97%	96%
Statin Prescribed at Discharge[1]	-	-	98%	98%
Heart Failure Care				
ACE Inhibitor or ARB for LVSD	69	100%	96%	97%
Discharge Instructions Given	126	100%	94%	94%
Evaluation of LVS Function	159	100%	98%	99%
Medicare Spending				
Medicare Spending per Patient (ratio)	-	1.00	0.95	0.98
Pneumonia Care				
Appropriate Initial Antibiotic Given	82	96%	95%	95%
Blood Culture Timing	107	99%	98%	98%
Pregnancy and Delivery Care				
Newborn Deliveries Scheduled Early[2]	48	6%	5%	6%
Preventive Care				
Immunization for Influenza[2]	381	93%	92%	90%
Immunization for Pneumonia[2]	456	90%	93%	92%
Stroke Care				
Anticoagulation Therapy for Atrial Fibrillation[7]	-	-	94%	95%
Antithrombotic Therapy Timing	12	92%	98%	98%
Assessed for Rehabilitation	11	82%	98%	97%
Discharged on Antithrombotic Therapy[1]	-	-	99%	99%
Discharged on Statin Medication	11	73%	95%	94%
Thrombolytic Therapy Timing[1]	-	-	67%	66%
Venous Thromboembolism Prophylaxis	16	94%	95%	94%
Written Stroke Educational Materials Given[1]	-	-	88%	88%
Surgical Care Improvement Project				
Appropriate Beta Blocker Usage	60	100%	98%	98%
Appropriate VTP Within 24 Hours	162	100%	98%	98%
Controlled Postoperative Blood Glucose[7]	-	-	97%	97%
Perioperative Temperature Management	185	100%	100%	100%
Prophylactic Antibiotic Selection	116	98%	99%	99%
Prophylactic Antibiotic Selection (Outpatient)	86	100%	98%	98%
Prophylactic Antibiotic Stopped	107	99%	98%	98%
Prophylactic Antibiotic Timing	116	100%	99%	99%
Prophylactic Antibiotic Timing (Outpatient)	86	100%	98%	98%
Urinary Catheter Removal	124	99%	97%	97%
Survey of Patients' Hospital Experiences				
Area Around Room 'Always' Quiet at Night	300+	70%	61%	61%
Doctors 'Always' Communicated Well	300+	87%	82%	82%
Home Recovery Information Given	300+	84%	87%	85%
Hospital Given 9 or 10 on 10 Point Scale	300+	70%	71%	71%
Meds 'Always' Explained Before Given	300+	70%	63%	64%
Nurses 'Always' Communicated Well	300+	86%	79%	79%
Pain 'Always' Well Controlled	300+	81%	71%	71%
Room and Bathroom 'Always' Clean	300+	86%	73%	73%
Timely Help 'Always' Received	300+	79%	68%	68%
Would Definitely Recommend Hospital	300+	68%	70%	71%
Use of Medical Imaging				
Cardiac Imaging Stress Test before Surgery	125	3.2%	5.2%	5.3%
Combination Abdominal CT Scan	371	6.5%	11.2%	10.5%
Combination Brain/Sinus CT Scan[1]	-	-	3.2%	2.7%
Combination Chest CT Scan	254	0.8%	1.9%	2.7%
Follow-up Mammogram/Ultrasound	666	5.9%	8.6%	8.8%
Lumbar Spine MRI for Low Back Pain	71	31.0%	39.6%	37.2%

Cox Medical Center

3801 South National Avenue
Springfield, MO 65807
Phone: 417-269-6000
URL: www.coxhealth.com
Type: Acute Care Hospitals
Emergency Services: Yes
Ownership: Voluntary non-profit - Private
Beds: 596

Key Personnel:
President/CEO. . . . . Steven D. Edwards
Chairman/CEO . . . . James W. Hutcheson
Chief of Medical Staff . . . . Frank Romero, MD

Measure	Cases	This Hosp.	State Avg.	U.S. Avg.
Blood Clot Prevention and Treatment				
Anticoagulation Overlap Therapy[2]	159	89%	94%	93%
ICU Venous Thromboembolism Prophylaxis[2]	85	89%	91%	92%
Incidence of Potentially Preventable VTE[2]	27	19%	7%	10%
UFH with Dosages/Platelet Monitoring[2]	82	28%	96%	97%
Venous Thromboembolism Prophylaxis[2]	288	85%	85%	85%
Warfarin Therapy Discharge Instructions[2]	121	74%	76%	75%
Chest Pain/Possible Heart Attack Care				
Aspirin Given Within 24 Hours of Arrival[1,3]	-	-	95%	96%
Fibrinolytic Meds Within 30 Min. of Arrival[5]	-	-	53%	58%
Average Time to ECG (minutes)[1,3]	-	-	7	7
Average Time to Transfer (minutes)[5]	-	-	53	60
Children's Asthma Care				
Received Home Management Plan of Care	-	-	-	88%
Received Reliever Medication	-	-	-	100%
Received Systemic Corticosteroids	-	-	-	100%
Emergency Department				
Admittance Decision Time (minutes)[2]	479	124	81	98
Head CT Results Within 45 Min. of Arrival[1]	-	-	63%	57%
Patients Who Left ER Before Being Seen	>100k	4%	3%	2%
Time from ER Arrival to Admit. (minutes)[2]	481	296	238	274
Time from ER Arrival to Discharge (minutes)	363	142	136	134
Time in ER Before Being Evaluated (minutes)	455	27	26	26
Time to Pain Meds for Fractures (minutes)	331	61	52	57
Heart Attack Care				
Aspirin Given at Discharge[2]	385	99%	99%	99%
Fibrinolytic Meds Within 30 Min. of Arrival[2,7]	-	-	-	54%
PCI Within 90 Minutes of Arrival[2]	70	93%	97%	96%
Statin Prescribed at Discharge[2]	374	94%	98%	98%
Heart Failure Care				
ACE Inhibitor or ARB for LVSD[2]	104	86%	96%	97%
Discharge Instructions Given[2]	334	100%	94%	94%
Evaluation of LVS Function[2]	401	100%	98%	99%
Medicare Spending				
Medicare Spending per Patient (ratio)	-	0.94	0.95	0.98
Pneumonia Care				
Appropriate Initial Antibiotic Given[2]	111	95%	95%	95%
Blood Culture Timing[2]	243	100%	98%	98%
Pregnancy and Delivery Care				
Newborn Deliveries Scheduled Early[2]	54	9%	5%	6%
Preventive Care				
Immunization for Influenza[2]	549	88%	92%	90%
Immunization for Pneumonia[2]	600	86%	93%	92%
Stroke Care				
Anticoagulation Therapy for Atrial Fibrillation[2]	13	77%	94%	95%
Antithrombotic Therapy Timing[2]	87	98%	98%	98%
Assessed for Rehabilitation[2]	123	98%	98%	97%
Discharged on Antithrombotic Therapy[2]	102	98%	99%	99%
Discharged on Statin Medication[2]	92	96%	95%	94%

NOTE: Hospital profiles are in alphabetical order by state, then city, then hospital within the city; Rankings exclude hospitals with less than 25 cases except for patient surveys which excludes hospitals with less than 100 cases; (a) 100-299 cases; (1) The number of cases/patients is too few to report; (2) Data submitted were based on a sample of cases/patients; (3) Results are based on a shorter time period than required; (4) Data suppressed by CMS for one or more quarters; (5) Results are not available for this reporting period; (6) Fewer than 100 patients completed the HCAHPS survey; (7) No cases met the criteria for this measure; (8) The lower limit of the confidence interval cannot be calculated if the number of observed infections equals zero; (9) No data are available from the state/territory for this reporting period; (10) The scores shown reflect fewer than 50 completed surveys; (11) There were discrepancies in the data collection process; (12) This measure does not apply to this hospital for this reporting period; (13) Results cannot be calculated for this reporting period; (14) The results for this state are combined with nearby states to protect confidentiality; Please refer to the User's Guide for a full explanation of data.

Measure	Cases	This Hosp.	State Avg.	U.S. Avg.
Thrombolytic Therapy Timing[1,2]	-	-	67%	66%
Venous Thromboembolism Prophylaxis[2]	116	97%	95%	94%
Written Stroke Educational Materials Given[2]	70	90%	88%	88%
Surgical Care Improvement Project				
Appropriate Beta Blocker Usage[2]	210	95%	98%	98%
Appropriate VTP Within 24 Hours[2]	379	97%	98%	98%
Controlled Postoperative Blood Glucose[2]	152	99%	97%	97%
Perioperative Temperature Management[2]	518	100%	100%	100%
Prophylactic Antibiotic Selection[2]	490	99%	99%	99%
Prophylactic Antibiotic Selection (Outpatient)	794	98%	98%	98%
Prophylactic Antibiotic Stopped[2]	485	97%	98%	98%
Prophylactic Antibiotic Timing[2]	492	98%	99%	99%
Prophylactic Antibiotic Timing (Outpatient)	798	99%	98%	98%
Urinary Catheter Removal[2]	289	91%	97%	97%
Survey of Patients' Hospital Experiences				
Area Around Room 'Always' Quiet at Night	300+	53%	61%	61%
Doctors 'Always' Communicated Well	300+	80%	82%	82%
Home Recovery Information Given	300+	89%	87%	85%
Hospital Given 9 or 10 on 10 Point Scale	300+	68%	71%	71%
Meds 'Always' Explained Before Given	300+	60%	63%	64%
Nurses 'Always' Communicated Well	300+	75%	79%	79%
Pain 'Always' Well Controlled	300+	66%	71%	71%
Room and Bathroom 'Always' Clean	300+	65%	73%	73%
Timely Help 'Always' Received	300+	61%	68%	68%
Would Definitely Recommend Hospital	300+	73%	70%	71%
Use of Medical Imaging				
Cardiac Imaging Stress Test before Surgery	1,430	5.1%	5.2%	5.3%
Combination Abdominal CT Scan	2,279	6.7%	11.2%	10.5%
Combination Brain/Sinus CT Scan	1,802	2.8%	3.2%	2.7%
Combination Chest CT Scan	1,855	0.0%	1.9%	2.7%
Follow-up Mammogram/Ultrasound	3,875	9.4%	8.6%	8.8%
Lumbar Spine MRI for Low Back Pain	581	42.7%	39.6%	37.2%

Mercy Hospital Springfield

1235 E Cherokee
Springfield, MO 65804
Phone: 417-820-2000
Fax: 417-820-6996
URL: www.stjohns.com
Type: Acute Care Hospitals
Emergency Services: Yes
Ownership: Voluntary non-profit - Church
Beds: 758

Key Personnel:

Radiology. . . . . Julie A Alford
CEO/President. . . . . David Barbe, MD
Quality Assurance . . . . Kathy Coleman
Chief of Medical Staff . . . . J Kent Dexter, MD
Pediatric Ambulatory Care . . . . . . Bernard Griesemer, MD
Pediatric In-Patient Care . . . . Bernard Griesemer, MD
Operating Room. . . . . Joe A Olivi
Infection Control. . . . . Patti Reynolds

Measure	Cases	This Hosp.	State Avg.	U.S. Avg.
Blood Clot Prevention and Treatment				
Anticoagulation Overlap Therapy[2]	242	94%	94%	93%
ICU Venous Thromboembolism Prophylaxis[2]	73	97%	91%	92%
Incidence of Potentially Preventable VTE[2]	51	10%	7%	10%
UFH with Dosages/Platelet Monitoring[2]	152	100%	96%	97%
Venous Thromboembolism Prophylaxis[2]	299	83%	85%	85%
Warfarin Therapy Discharge Instructions[2]	185	78%	76%	75%
Chest Pain/Possible Heart Attack Care				
Aspirin Given Within 24 Hours of Arrival[1]	-	-	95%	96%
Fibrinolytic Meds Within 30 Min. of Arrival[3,7]	-	-	53%	58%
Average Time to ECG (minutes)[1]	-	-	7	7
Average Time to Transfer (minutes)[1,3]	-	-	53	60
Children's Asthma Care				
Received Home Management Plan of Care	-	-	-	88%
Received Reliever Medication	-	-	-	100%
Received Systemic Corticosteroids	-	-	-	100%
Emergency Department				
Admittance Decision Time (minutes)[2]	402	86	81	98
Head CT Results Within 45 Min. of Arrival[1]	-	-	63%	57%
Patients Who Left ER Before Being Seen	96,706	5%	3%	2%
Time from ER Arrival to Admit. (minutes)[2]	445	235	238	274
Time from ER Arrival to Discharge (minutes)	351	189	136	134
Time in ER Before Being Evaluated (minutes)	391	14	26	26
Time to Pain Meds for Fractures (minutes)	128	48	52	57
Heart Attack Care				
Aspirin Given at Discharge[2]	281	100%	99%	99%
Fibrinolytic Meds Within 30 Min. of Arrival[2,7]	-	-	-	54%
PCI Within 90 Minutes of Arrival[2]	44	100%	97%	96%
Statin Prescribed at Discharge[2]	268	97%	98%	98%
Heart Failure Care				
ACE Inhibitor or ARB for LVSD[2]	90	97%	96%	97%
Discharge Instructions Given[2]	203	96%	94%	94%
Evaluation of LVS Function[2]	272	100%	98%	99%
Medicare Spending				
Medicare Spending per Patient (ratio)	-	0.95	0.95	0.98
Pneumonia Care				
Appropriate Initial Antibiotic Given[2]	75	93%	95%	95%
Blood Culture Timing[2]	164	99%	98%	98%
Pregnancy and Delivery Care				
Newborn Deliveries Scheduled Early[2]	47	0%	5%	6%
Preventive Care				
Immunization for Influenza[2]	535	90%	92%	90%
Immunization for Pneumonia[2]	660	91%	93%	92%
Stroke Care				
Anticoagulation Therapy for Atrial Fibrillation	76	89%	94%	95%
Antithrombotic Therapy Timing	394	97%	98%	98%
Assessed for Rehabilitation	571	98%	98%	97%
Discharged on Antithrombotic Therapy	463	99%	99%	99%
Discharged on Statin Medication	355	95%	95%	94%
Thrombolytic Therapy Timing	60	47%	67%	66%
Venous Thromboembolism Prophylaxis	580	96%	95%	94%
Written Stroke Educational Materials Given	329	96%	88%	88%
Surgical Care Improvement Project				
Appropriate Beta Blocker Usage[2]	247	98%	98%	98%
Appropriate VTP Within 24 Hours[2]	385	98%	98%	98%
Controlled Postoperative Blood Glucose[2]	147	96%	97%	97%
Perioperative Temperature Management[2]	540	99%	100%	100%
Prophylactic Antibiotic Selection[2]	478	100%	99%	99%
Prophylactic Antibiotic Selection (Outpatient)	756	99%	98%	98%
Prophylactic Antibiotic Stopped[2]	464	99%	98%	98%
Prophylactic Antibiotic Timing[2]	479	100%	99%	99%
Prophylactic Antibiotic Timing (Outpatient)	756	99%	98%	98%
Urinary Catheter Removal[2]	298	99%	97%	97%
Survey of Patients' Hospital Experiences				
Area Around Room 'Always' Quiet at Night[11]	300+	59%	61%	61%
Doctors 'Always' Communicated Well[11]	300+	82%	82%	82%
Home Recovery Information Given[11]	300+	87%	87%	85%
Hospital Given 9 or 10 on 10 Point Scale[11]	300+	75%	71%	71%
Meds 'Always' Explained Before Given[11]	300+	61%	63%	64%
Nurses 'Always' Communicated Well[11]	300+	79%	79%	79%
Pain 'Always' Well Controlled[11]	300+	69%	71%	71%
Room and Bathroom 'Always' Clean[11]	300+	72%	73%	73%
Timely Help 'Always' Received[11]	300+	64%	68%	68%
Would Definitely Recommend Hospital[11]	300+	80%	70%	71%
Use of Medical Imaging				
Cardiac Imaging Stress Test before Surgery	569	5.8%	5.2%	5.3%
Combination Abdominal CT Scan	2,789	2.6%	11.2%	10.5%
Combination Brain/Sinus CT Scan	1,817	2.8%	3.2%	2.7%
Combination Chest CT Scan	1,726	0.1%	1.9%	2.7%
Follow-up Mammogram/Ultrasound	5,510	10.1%	8.6%	8.8%
Lumbar Spine MRI for Low Back Pain	543	43.5%	39.6%	37.2%

Ozarks Community Hospital

2828 North National
Springfield, MO 65803
Phone: 417-837-4000
E-mail: info@ochonline.com
URL: www.ochonline.com
Type: Acute Care Hospitals
Emergency Services: Yes
Ownership: Proprietary
Beds: 45

Key Personnel:

CEO . . . . Paul Taylor

Measure	Cases	This Hosp.	State Avg.	U.S. Avg.
Blood Clot Prevention and Treatment				
Anticoagulation Overlap Therapy[1,2]	-	-	94%	93%
ICU Venous Thromboembolism Prophylaxis[2,7]	-	-	91%	92%
Incidence of Potentially Preventable VTE[2,7]	-	-	7%	10%
UFH with Dosages/Platelet Monitoring[1,2]	-	-	96%	97%
Venous Thromboembolism Prophylaxis[2]	103	22%	85%	85%
Warfarin Therapy Discharge Instructions[1,2]	-	-	76%	75%
Chest Pain/Possible Heart Attack Care				
Aspirin Given Within 24 Hours of Arrival	16	94%	95%	96%
Fibrinolytic Meds Within 30 Min. of Arrival[1]	-	-	53%	58%
Average Time to ECG (minutes)	16	20	7	7
Average Time to Transfer (minutes)[1]	-	-	53	60
Children's Asthma Care				
Received Home Management Plan of Care	-	-	-	88%
Received Reliever Medication	-	-	-	100%
Received Systemic Corticosteroids	-	-	-	100%
Emergency Department				
Admittance Decision Time (minutes)	346	58	81	98
Head CT Results Within 45 Min. of Arrival[3,7]	-	-	63%	57%
Patients Who Left ER Before Being Seen	19,052	3%	3%	2%
Time from ER Arrival to Admit. (minutes)	407	260	238	274
Time from ER Arrival to Discharge (minutes)	362	86	136	134
Time in ER Before Being Evaluated (minutes)	385	40	26	26
Time to Pain Meds for Fractures (minutes)	27	57	52	57
Heart Attack Care				
Aspirin Given at Discharge[1,3]	-	-	99%	99%
Fibrinolytic Meds Within 30 Min. of Arrival[3,7]	-	-	-	54%
PCI Within 90 Minutes of Arrival[3,7]	-	-	97%	96%
Statin Prescribed at Discharge[1,3]	-	-	98%	98%
Heart Failure Care				
ACE Inhibitor or ARB for LVSD[1]	-	-	96%	97%
Discharge Instructions Given[1]	-	-	94%	94%
Evaluation of LVS Function	12	92%	98%	99%
Medicare Spending				
Medicare Spending per Patient (ratio)	-	1.06	0.95	0.98
Pneumonia Care				
Appropriate Initial Antibiotic Given	33	91%	95%	95%
Blood Culture Timing	41	98%	98%	98%
Pregnancy and Delivery Care				
Newborn Deliveries Scheduled Early[7]	-	-	5%	6%
Preventive Care				
Immunization for Influenza	276	98%	92%	90%
Immunization for Pneumonia	440	95%	93%	92%
Stroke Care				
Anticoagulation Therapy for Atrial Fibrillation[7]	-	-	94%	95%
Antithrombotic Therapy Timing[1]	-	-	98%	98%
Assessed for Rehabilitation[1]	-	-	98%	97%
Discharged on Antithrombotic Therapy[1]	-	-	99%	99%
Discharged on Statin Medication[1]	-	-	95%	94%
Thrombolytic Therapy Timing[7]	-	-	67%	66%
Venous Thromboembolism Prophylaxis[1]	-	-	95%	94%
Written Stroke Educational Materials Given[1]	-	-	88%	88%
Surgical Care Improvement Project				
Appropriate Beta Blocker Usage	16	100%	98%	98%
Appropriate VTP Within 24 Hours	58	83%	98%	98%
Controlled Postoperative Blood Glucose[7]	-	-	97%	97%
Perioperative Temperature Management	64	100%	100%	100%
Prophylactic Antibiotic Selection	53	98%	99%	99%
Prophylactic Antibiotic Selection (Outpatient)	52	94%	98%	98%
Prophylactic Antibiotic Stopped	53	100%	98%	98%
Prophylactic Antibiotic Timing	53	91%	99%	99%
Prophylactic Antibiotic Timing (Outpatient)	52	100%	98%	98%
Urinary Catheter Removal	50	96%	97%	97%
Survey of Patients' Hospital Experiences				
Area Around Room 'Always' Quiet at Night	(a)	66%	61%	61%
Doctors 'Always' Communicated Well	(a)	85%	82%	82%
Home Recovery Information Given	(a)	89%	87%	85%
Hospital Given 9 or 10 on 10 Point Scale	(a)	76%	71%	71%
Meds 'Always' Explained Before Given	(a)	66%	63%	64%
Nurses 'Always' Communicated Well	(a)	83%	79%	79%
Pain 'Always' Well Controlled	(a)	71%	71%	71%
Room and Bathroom 'Always' Clean	(a)	85%	73%	73%
Timely Help 'Always' Received	(a)	73%	68%	68%
Would Definitely Recommend Hospital	(a)	78%	70%	71%
Use of Medical Imaging				
Cardiac Imaging Stress Test before Surgery	145	6.2%	5.2%	5.3%
Combination Abdominal CT Scan	135	17.8%	11.2%	10.5%
Combination Brain/Sinus CT Scan	113	8.8%	3.2%	2.7%

NOTE: Hospital profiles are in alphabetical order by state, then city, then hospital within the city; Rankings exclude hospitals with less than 25 cases except for patient surveys which excludes hospitals with less than 100 cases; (a) 100-299 cases; (1) The number of cases/patients is too few to report; (2) Data submitted were based on a sample of cases/patients; (3) Results are based on a shorter time period than required; (4) Data suppressed by CMS for one or more quarters; (5) Results are not available for this reporting period; (6) Fewer than 100 patients completed the HCAHPS survey; (7) No cases met the criteria for this measure; (8) The lower limit of the confidence interval cannot be calculated if the number of observed infections equals zero; (9) No data are available from the state/territory for this reporting period; (10) The scores shown reflect fewer than 50 completed surveys; (11) There were discrepancies in the data collection process; (12) This measure does not apply to this hospital for this reporting period; (13) Results cannot be calculated for this reporting period; (14) The results for this state are combined with nearby states to protect confidentiality; Please refer to the User's Guide for a full explanation of data.

Measure	Cases	This Hosp.	State Avg.	U.S. Avg.
Combination Chest CT Scan[1]	-	-	1.9%	2.7%
Follow-up Mammogram/Ultrasound[7]	-	-	8.6%	8.8%
Lumbar Spine MRI for Low Back Pain[1]	-	-	39.6%	37.2%

Missouri Baptist Sullivan Hospital

751 Sappington Bridge Rd
Sullivan, MO 63080
Phone: 573-468-4186
Type: Critical Access Hospitals
Emergency Services: Yes
Ownership: Voluntary non-profit - Private

Measure	Cases	This Hosp.	State Avg.	U.S. Avg.
Blood Clot Prevention and Treatment				
Anticoagulation Overlap Therapy[1,2]	-	-	94%	93%
ICU Venous Thromboembolism Prophylaxis[2]	15	93%	91%	92%
Incidence of Potentially Preventable VTE[1,2]	-	-	7%	10%
UFH with Dosages/Platelet Monitoring[2,7]	-	-	96%	97%
Venous Thromboembolism Prophylaxis[2]	112	96%	85%	85%
Warfarin Therapy Discharge Instructions[1,2]	-	-	76%	75%
Chest Pain/Possible Heart Attack Care				
Aspirin Given Within 24 Hours of Arrival	104	96%	95%	96%
Fibrinolytic Meds Within 30 Min. of Arrival[7]	-	-	53%	58%
Average Time to ECG (minutes)	108	6	7	7
Average Time to Transfer (minutes)[7]	-	-	53	60
Children's Asthma Care				
Received Home Management Plan of Care	-	-	-	88%
Received Reliever Medication	-	-	-	100%
Received Systemic Corticosteroids	-	-	-	100%
Emergency Department				
Admittance Decision Time (minutes)[2]	209	41	81	98
Head CT Results Within 45 Min. of Arrival[1]	-	-	63%	57%
Patients Who Left ER Before Being Seen	22,367	2%	3%	2%
Time from ER Arrival to Admit. (minutes)[2]	210	251	238	274
Time from ER Arrival to Discharge (minutes)	757	127	136	134
Time in ER Before Being Evaluated (minutes)	654	30	26	26
Time to Pain Meds for Fractures (minutes)	99	45	52	57
Heart Attack Care				
Aspirin Given at Discharge[3,7]	-	-	99%	99%
Fibrinolytic Meds Within 30 Min. of Arrival[3,7]	-	-	-	54%
PCI Within 90 Minutes of Arrival[3,7]	-	-	97%	96%
Statin Prescribed at Discharge[3,7]	-	-	98%	98%
Heart Failure Care				
ACE Inhibitor or ARB for LVSD[1]	-	-	96%	97%
Discharge Instructions Given	44	100%	94%	94%
Evaluation of LVS Function	72	100%	98%	99%
Medicare Spending				
Medicare Spending per Patient (ratio)	-	-	0.95	0.98
Pneumonia Care				
Appropriate Initial Antibiotic Given	40	95%	95%	95%
Blood Culture Timing	61	100%	98%	98%
Pregnancy and Delivery Care				
Newborn Deliveries Scheduled Early[2]	37	8%	5%	6%
Preventive Care				
Immunization for Influenza[2]	253	97%	92%	90%
Immunization for Pneumonia[2]	228	99%	93%	92%
Stroke Care				
Anticoagulation Therapy for Atrial Fibrillation[1]	-	-	94%	95%
Antithrombotic Therapy Timing[1]	-	-	98%	98%
Assessed for Rehabilitation	13	100%	98%	97%
Discharged on Antithrombotic Therapy	13	100%	99%	99%
Discharged on Statin Medication[1]	-	-	95%	94%
Thrombolytic Therapy Timing[1]	-	-	67%	66%
Venous Thromboembolism Prophylaxis[1]	-	-	95%	94%
Written Stroke Educational Materials Given[1]	-	-	88%	88%
Surgical Care Improvement Project				
Appropriate Beta Blocker Usage[1]	-	-	98%	98%
Appropriate VTP Within 24 Hours	19	100%	98%	98%
Controlled Postoperative Blood Glucose[7]	-	-	97%	97%
Perioperative Temperature Management	33	100%	100%	100%
Prophylactic Antibiotic Selection[1]	-	-	99%	99%
Prophylactic Antibiotic Selection (Outpatient)	80	99%	98%	98%
Prophylactic Antibiotic Stopped[1]	-	-	98%	98%
Prophylactic Antibiotic Timing[1]	-	-	99%	99%
Prophylactic Antibiotic Timing (Outpatient)	74	99%	98%	98%
Urinary Catheter Removal[1]	-	-	97%	97%
Survey of Patients' Hospital Experiences				
Area Around Room 'Always' Quiet at Night	300+	68%	61%	61%
Doctors 'Always' Communicated Well	300+	84%	82%	82%
Home Recovery Information Given	300+	90%	87%	85%
Hospital Given 9 or 10 on 10 Point Scale	300+	78%	71%	71%
Meds 'Always' Explained Before Given	300+	67%	63%	64%
Nurses 'Always' Communicated Well	300+	83%	79%	79%
Pain 'Always' Well Controlled	300+	71%	71%	71%
Room and Bathroom 'Always' Clean	300+	80%	73%	73%
Timely Help 'Always' Received	300+	75%	68%	68%
Would Definitely Recommend Hospital	300+	73%	70%	71%
Use of Medical Imaging				
Cardiac Imaging Stress Test before Surgery	140	0.0%	5.2%	5.3%
Combination Abdominal CT Scan	301	2.0%	11.2%	10.5%
Combination Brain/Sinus CT Scan[1]	-	-	3.2%	2.7%
Combination Chest CT Scan	350	0.0%	1.9%	2.7%
Follow-up Mammogram/Ultrasound	327	6.4%	8.6%	8.8%
Lumbar Spine MRI for Low Back Pain	52	53.8%	39.6%	37.2%

Missouri Baptist Medical Center

3015 N Ballas Rd
Town & Country, MO 63131
Phone: 314-996-5000
Fax: 314-432-1024
URL: www.missouribaptistmedicalcenter.org
Type: Acute Care Hospitals
Emergency Services: Yes
Ownership: Voluntary non-profit - Private
Beds: 489

Key Personnel:
CEO/President. . . . . John Antes
Chief of Medical Staff. . . . . Mitchell Botney, MD
Pediatric Ambulatory Care . . . . . . Renee Fishering
Operating Room. . . . . Nancy Hesselbach
Radiology. . . . . Vivian Prinster
Quality Assurance . . . . Carolyn Roth
Cardiac Laboratory. . . . . Douglas Sohn

Measure	Cases	This Hosp.	State Avg.	U.S. Avg.
Blood Clot Prevention and Treatment				
Anticoagulation Overlap Therapy[2]	47	94%	94%	93%
ICU Venous Thromboembolism Prophylaxis[2]	40	100%	91%	92%
Incidence of Potentially Preventable VTE[2]	26	4%	7%	10%
UFH with Dosages/Platelet Monitoring[2]	36	97%	96%	97%
Venous Thromboembolism Prophylaxis[2]	340	99%	85%	85%
Warfarin Therapy Discharge Instructions[2]	26	96%	76%	75%
Chest Pain/Possible Heart Attack Care				
Aspirin Given Within 24 Hours of Arrival[1,3]	-	-	95%	96%
Fibrinolytic Meds Within 30 Min. of Arrival[5]	-	-	53%	58%
Average Time to ECG (minutes)[1,3]	-	-	7	7
Average Time to Transfer (minutes)[5]	-	-	53	60
Children's Asthma Care				
Received Home Management Plan of Care	-	-	-	88%
Received Reliever Medication	-	-	-	100%
Received Systemic Corticosteroids	-	-	-	100%
Emergency Department				
Admittance Decision Time (minutes)[2]	460	69	81	98
Head CT Results Within 45 Min. of Arrival[1]	-	-	63%	57%
Patients Who Left ER Before Being Seen	42,542	1%	3%	2%
Time from ER Arrival to Admit. (minutes)[2]	463	278	238	274
Time from ER Arrival to Discharge (minutes)	800	192	136	134
Time in ER Before Being Evaluated (minutes)	812	27	26	26
Time to Pain Meds for Fractures (minutes)	237	34	52	57
Heart Attack Care				
Aspirin Given at Discharge	494	100%	99%	99%
Fibrinolytic Meds Within 30 Min. of Arrival[7]	-	-	-	54%
PCI Within 90 Minutes of Arrival	37	100%	97%	96%
Statin Prescribed at Discharge	477	100%	98%	98%
Heart Failure Care				
ACE Inhibitor or ARB for LVSD[2]	114	98%	96%	97%
Discharge Instructions Given[2]	412	100%	94%	94%
Evaluation of LVS Function[2]	510	100%	98%	99%
Medicare Spending				
Medicare Spending per Patient (ratio)	-	0.95	0.95	0.98
Pneumonia Care				
Appropriate Initial Antibiotic Given[2]	129	97%	95%	95%
Blood Culture Timing[2]	289	99%	98%	98%
Pregnancy and Delivery Care				
Newborn Deliveries Scheduled Early[2]	64	2%	5%	6%
Preventive Care				
Immunization for Influenza[2]	490	99%	92%	90%
Immunization for Pneumonia[2]	612	98%	93%	92%
Stroke Care				
Anticoagulation Therapy for Atrial Fibrillation	35	97%	94%	95%
Antithrombotic Therapy Timing	163	100%	98%	98%
Assessed for Rehabilitation	210	99%	98%	97%
Discharged on Antithrombotic Therapy	191	100%	99%	99%
Discharged on Statin Medication	149	99%	95%	94%
Thrombolytic Therapy Timing	13	100%	67%	66%
Venous Thromboembolism Prophylaxis	184	100%	95%	94%
Written Stroke Educational Materials Given	113	100%	88%	88%
Surgical Care Improvement Project				
Appropriate Beta Blocker Usage[2]	206	99%	98%	98%
Appropriate VTP Within 24 Hours[2]	437	100%	98%	98%
Controlled Postoperative Blood Glucose[2]	151	100%	97%	97%
Perioperative Temperature Management[2]	576	100%	100%	100%
Prophylactic Antibiotic Selection[2]	522	99%	99%	99%
Prophylactic Antibiotic Selection (Outpatient)	633	98%	98%	98%
Prophylactic Antibiotic Stopped[2]	506	100%	98%	98%
Prophylactic Antibiotic Timing[2]	522	98%	99%	99%
Prophylactic Antibiotic Timing (Outpatient)	637	99%	98%	98%
Urinary Catheter Removal[2]	419	100%	97%	97%
Survey of Patients' Hospital Experiences				
Area Around Room 'Always' Quiet at Night	300+	47%	61%	61%
Doctors 'Always' Communicated Well	300+	80%	82%	82%
Home Recovery Information Given	300+	85%	87%	85%
Hospital Given 9 or 10 on 10 Point Scale	300+	72%	71%	71%
Meds 'Always' Explained Before Given	300+	59%	63%	64%
Nurses 'Always' Communicated Well	300+	75%	79%	79%
Pain 'Always' Well Controlled	300+	67%	71%	71%
Room and Bathroom 'Always' Clean	300+	64%	73%	73%
Timely Help 'Always' Received	300+	61%	68%	68%
Would Definitely Recommend Hospital	300+	76%	70%	71%
Use of Medical Imaging				
Cardiac Imaging Stress Test before Surgery	1,642	5.5%	5.2%	5.3%
Combination Abdominal CT Scan	1,914	3.7%	11.2%	10.5%
Combination Brain/Sinus CT Scan	1,269	2.7%	3.2%	2.7%
Combination Chest CT Scan	1,925	0.3%	1.9%	2.7%
Follow-up Mammogram/Ultrasound	3,320	5.7%	8.6%	8.8%
Lumbar Spine MRI for Low Back Pain	279	38.0%	39.6%	37.2%

Wright Memorial Hospital

191 Iowa Boulevard
Trenton, MO 64683
Phone: 660-359-5621
URL: www.saintlukeshealthsystem.org
Type: Critical Access Hospitals
Emergency Services: Yes
Ownership: Voluntary non-profit - Private
Beds: 78

Key Personnel:
CEO/President. . . . . Karen Cole
Radiology. . . . . Pablo N Delgado
Pediatrics. . . . . Lori A Golon
Anesthesiology. . . . . Lisa D Health
Cardiology . . . . Kenneth C Huber
Anesthesiology. . . . . Patricia A Martin
Cardiology . . . . Barry D Rutherford

Measure	Cases	This Hosp.	State Avg.	U.S. Avg.
Blood Clot Prevention and Treatment				
Anticoagulation Overlap Therapy[1,2]	-	-	94%	93%
ICU Venous Thromboembolism Prophylaxis[2,3]	-	-	91%	92%
Incidence of Potentially Preventable VTE[2,3]	-	-	7%	10%
UFH with Dosages/Platelet Monitoring[1,2]	-	-	96%	97%
Venous Thromboembolism Prophylaxis[2,3]	141	89%	85%	85%
Warfarin Therapy Discharge Instructions[1,2]	-	-	76%	75%
Chest Pain/Possible Heart Attack Care				
Aspirin Given Within 24 Hours of Arrival	36	81%	95%	96%
Fibrinolytic Meds Within 30 Min. of Arrival[7]	-	-	53%	58%
Average Time to ECG (minutes)	40	10	7	7
Average Time to Transfer (minutes)[1]	-	-	53	60
Children's Asthma Care				
Received Home Management Plan of Care	-	-	-	88%
Received Reliever Medication	-	-	-	100%
Received Systemic Corticosteroids	-	-	-	100%

NOTE: Hospital profiles are in alphabetical order by state, then city, then hospital within the city; Rankings exclude hospitals with less than 25 cases except for patient surveys which excludes hospitals with less than 100 cases; (a) 100-299 cases; (1) The number of cases/patients is too few to report; (2) Data submitted were based on a sample of cases/patients; (3) Results are based on a shorter time period than required; (4) Data suppressed by CMS for one or more quarters; (5) Results are not available for this reporting period; (6) Fewer than 100 patients completed the HCAHPS survey; (7) No cases met the criteria for this measure; (8) The lower limit of the confidence interval cannot be calculated if the number of observed infections equals zero; (9) No data are available from the state/territory for this reporting period; (10) The scores shown reflect fewer than 50 completed surveys; (11) There were discrepancies in the data collection process; (12) This measure does not apply to this hospital for this reporting period; (13) Results cannot be calculated for this reporting period; (14) The results for this state are combined with nearby states to protect confidentiality; Please refer to the User's Guide for a full explanation of data.

Measure	Cases	This Hosp.	State Avg.	U.S. Avg.
Emergency Department				
Admittance Decision Time (minutes)[2]	229	37	81	98
Head CT Results Within 45 Min. of Arrival[1,3]	-	-	63%	57%
Patients Who Left ER Before Being Seen[5]	-	-	3%	2%
Time from ER Arrival to Admit. (minutes)[2]	301	181	238	274
Time from ER Arrival to Discharge (minutes)[5]	-	-	136	134
Time in ER Before Being Evaluated (minutes)[5]	-	-	26	26
Time to Pain Meds for Fractures (minutes)	51	47	52	57
Heart Attack Care				
Aspirin Given at Discharge[1,3]	-	-	99%	99%
Fibrinolytic Meds Within 30 Min. of Arrival[3,7]	-	-	-	54%
PCI Within 90 Minutes of Arrival[3,7]	-	-	97%	96%
Statin Prescribed at Discharge[1,3]	-	-	98%	98%
Heart Failure Care				
ACE Inhibitor or ARB for LVSD	12	75%	96%	97%
Discharge Instructions Given	38	95%	94%	94%
Evaluation of LVS Function	52	98%	98%	99%
Medicare Spending				
Medicare Spending per Patient (ratio)	-	-	0.95	0.98
Pneumonia Care				
Appropriate Initial Antibiotic Given	19	79%	95%	95%
Blood Culture Timing	34	100%	98%	98%
Pregnancy and Delivery Care				
Newborn Deliveries Scheduled Early[5]	-	-	5%	6%
Preventive Care				
Immunization for Influenza[2]	296	87%	92%	90%
Immunization for Pneumonia[2]	317	91%	93%	92%
Stroke Care				
Anticoagulation Therapy for Atrial Fibrillation[5]	-	-	94%	95%
Antithrombotic Therapy Timing[5]	-	-	98%	98%
Assessed for Rehabilitation[5]	-	-	98%	97%
Discharged on Antithrombotic Therapy[5]	-	-	99%	99%
Discharged on Statin Medication[5]	-	-	95%	94%
Thrombolytic Therapy Timing[5]	-	-	67%	66%
Venous Thromboembolism Prophylaxis[5]	-	-	95%	94%
Written Stroke Educational Materials Given[5]	-	-	88%	88%
Surgical Care Improvement Project				
Appropriate Beta Blocker Usage[5]	-	-	98%	98%
Appropriate VTP Within 24 Hours[5]	-	-	98%	98%
Controlled Postoperative Blood Glucose[5]	-	-	97%	97%
Perioperative Temperature Management[5]	-	-	100%	100%
Prophylactic Antibiotic Selection[5]	-	-	99%	99%
Prophylactic Antibiotic Selection (Outpatient)[5]	-	-	98%	98%
Prophylactic Antibiotic Stopped[5]	-	-	98%	98%
Prophylactic Antibiotic Timing[5]	-	-	99%	99%
Prophylactic Antibiotic Timing (Outpatient)[5]	-	-	98%	98%
Urinary Catheter Removal[5]	-	-	97%	97%
Survey of Patients' Hospital Experiences				
Area Around Room 'Always' Quiet at Night	(a)	76%	61%	61%
Doctors 'Always' Communicated Well	(a)	94%	82%	82%
Home Recovery Information Given	(a)	90%	87%	85%
Hospital Given 9 or 10 on 10 Point Scale	(a)	85%	71%	71%
Meds 'Always' Explained Before Given	(a)	75%	63%	64%
Nurses 'Always' Communicated Well	(a)	88%	79%	79%
Pain 'Always' Well Controlled	(a)	81%	71%	71%
Room and Bathroom 'Always' Clean	(a)	78%	73%	73%
Timely Help 'Always' Received	(a)	82%	68%	68%
Would Definitely Recommend Hospital	(a)	71%	70%	71%
Use of Medical Imaging				
Cardiac Imaging Stress Test before Surgery[7]	-	-	5.2%	5.3%
Combination Abdominal CT Scan	145	4.8%	11.2%	10.5%
Combination Brain/Sinus CT Scan[1]	-	-	3.2%	2.7%
Combination Chest CT Scan	144	2.1%	1.9%	2.7%
Follow-up Mammogram/Ultrasound	278	65.5%	8.6%	8.8%
Lumbar Spine MRI for Low Back Pain[1]	-	-	39.6%	37.2%

Lincoln County Medical Center

1000 East Cherry Street
Troy, MO 63379 Phone: 636-528-8551
Type: Critical Access Hospitals Emergency Services: Yes
Ownership: Government - Local

Key Personnel:

CEO . . . . Patrick Bira, FACHE, MHA, JD
Quality Assurance . . . . Marie Collinson
Emergency Room . . . . Mike Dach
Anesthesiology. . . . . Lisa Dugan
Radiology. . . . . Greg Heidbrier
Intensive Care Unit. . . . . Jamie Keiser
Infection Control. . . . . Becky O'Neal
Chief of Medical Staff . . . . Dale Reinker DO

Measure	Cases	This Hosp.	State Avg.	U.S. Avg.
Blood Clot Prevention and Treatment				
Anticoagulation Overlap Therapy[1]	-	-	94%	93%
ICU Venous Thromboembolism Prophylaxis	124	85%	91%	92%
Incidence of Potentially Preventable VTE[1]	-	-	7%	10%
UFH with Dosages/Platelet Monitoring[7]	-	-	96%	97%
Venous Thromboembolism Prophylaxis	293	77%	85%	85%
Warfarin Therapy Discharge Instructions[1]	-	-	76%	75%
Chest Pain/Possible Heart Attack Care				
Aspirin Given Within 24 Hours of Arrival	-	-	95%	96%
Fibrinolytic Meds Within 30 Min. of Arrival	-	-	53%	58%
Average Time to ECG (minutes)	-	-	7	7
Average Time to Transfer (minutes)	-	-	53	60
Children's Asthma Care				
Received Home Management Plan of Care	-	-	-	88%
Received Reliever Medication	-	-	-	100%
Received Systemic Corticosteroids	-	-	-	100%
Emergency Department				
Admittance Decision Time (minutes)[5]	-	-	81	98
Head CT Results Within 45 Min. of Arrival	-	-	63%	57%
Patients Who Left ER Before Being Seen	-	-	3%	2%
Time from ER Arrival to Admit. (minutes)[5]	-	-	238	274
Time from ER Arrival to Discharge (minutes)	-	-	136	134
Time in ER Before Being Evaluated (minutes)	-	-	26	26
Time to Pain Meds for Fractures (minutes)	-	-	52	57
Heart Attack Care				
Aspirin Given at Discharge[3,7]	-	-	99%	99%
Fibrinolytic Meds Within 30 Min. of Arrival[3,7]	-	-	-	54%
PCI Within 90 Minutes of Arrival[3,7]	-	-	97%	96%
Statin Prescribed at Discharge[3,7]	-	-	98%	98%
Heart Failure Care				
ACE Inhibitor or ARB for LVSD[1]	-	-	96%	97%
Discharge Instructions Given	15	73%	94%	94%
Evaluation of LVS Function	22	100%	98%	99%
Medicare Spending				
Medicare Spending per Patient (ratio)	-	-	0.95	0.98
Pneumonia Care				
Appropriate Initial Antibiotic Given	25	84%	95%	95%
Blood Culture Timing	73	96%	98%	98%
Pregnancy and Delivery Care				
Newborn Deliveries Scheduled Early[5]	-	-	5%	6%
Preventive Care				
Immunization for Influenza[5]	-	-	92%	90%
Immunization for Pneumonia[5]	-	-	93%	92%
Stroke Care				
Anticoagulation Therapy for Atrial Fibrillation[5]	-	-	94%	95%
Antithrombotic Therapy Timing[5]	-	-	98%	98%
Assessed for Rehabilitation[5]	-	-	98%	97%
Discharged on Antithrombotic Therapy[5]	-	-	99%	99%
Discharged on Statin Medication[5]	-	-	95%	94%
Thrombolytic Therapy Timing[5]	-	-	67%	66%
Venous Thromboembolism Prophylaxis[5]	-	-	95%	94%
Written Stroke Educational Materials Given[5]	-	-	88%	88%
Surgical Care Improvement Project				
Appropriate Beta Blocker Usage[1]	-	-	98%	98%
Appropriate VTP Within 24 Hours	29	97%	98%	98%
Controlled Postoperative Blood Glucose[7]	-	-	97%	97%
Perioperative Temperature Management	30	100%	100%	100%
Prophylactic Antibiotic Selection	24	100%	99%	99%
Prophylactic Antibiotic Selection (Outpatient)	-	-	98%	98%
Prophylactic Antibiotic Stopped	22	100%	98%	98%
Prophylactic Antibiotic Timing	24	100%	99%	99%
Prophylactic Antibiotic Timing (Outpatient)	-	-	98%	98%
Urinary Catheter Removal	28	100%	97%	97%
Survey of Patients' Hospital Experiences				
Area Around Room 'Always' Quiet at Night	(a)	61%	61%	61%
Doctors 'Always' Communicated Well	(a)	79%	82%	82%
Home Recovery Information Given	(a)	85%	87%	85%
Hospital Given 9 or 10 on 10 Point Scale	(a)	60%	71%	71%
Meds 'Always' Explained Before Given	(a)	58%	63%	64%
Nurses 'Always' Communicated Well	(a)	79%	79%	79%
Pain 'Always' Well Controlled	(a)	64%	71%	71%
Room and Bathroom 'Always' Clean	(a)	80%	73%	73%
Timely Help 'Always' Received	(a)	67%	68%	68%
Would Definitely Recommend Hospital	(a)	57%	70%	71%
Use of Medical Imaging				
Cardiac Imaging Stress Test before Surgery	-	-	5.2%	5.3%
Combination Abdominal CT Scan	-	-	11.2%	10.5%
Combination Brain/Sinus CT Scan	-	-	3.2%	2.7%
Combination Chest CT Scan	-	-	1.9%	2.7%
Follow-up Mammogram/Ultrasound	-	-	8.6%	8.8%
Lumbar Spine MRI for Low Back Pain	-	-	39.6%	37.2%

Putnam County Memorial Hospital

1926 Oak Street, PO Box 389 Phone: 660-947-2411
Unionville, MO 63565 Fax: 660-947-3825
E-mail: rmagers@istlaplata.net
Type: Critical Access Hospitals Emergency Services: Yes
Ownership: Voluntary non-profit - Other Beds: 40

Key Personnel:

Chief of Medical Staff . . . . W Stephen Casady
Quality Assurance . . . . Ediph Haffner
Chairman/CEO . . . . Howard Luscan
CEO/President. . . . . Ray Magers
Emergency Room . . . . James Pigg
Infection Control. . . . . Deb Smith, RN

Measure	Cases	This Hosp.	State Avg.	U.S. Avg.
Blood Clot Prevention and Treatment				
Anticoagulation Overlap Therapy[1,2]	-	-	94%	93%
ICU Venous Thromboembolism Prophylaxis[2,7]	-	-	91%	92%
Incidence of Potentially Preventable VTE[2,7]	-	-	7%	10%
UFH with Dosages/Platelet Monitoring[1,2]	-	-	96%	97%
Venous Thromboembolism Prophylaxis[1,2]	-	-	85%	85%
Warfarin Therapy Discharge Instructions[1,2]	-	-	76%	75%
Chest Pain/Possible Heart Attack Care				
Aspirin Given Within 24 Hours of Arrival	-	-	95%	96%
Fibrinolytic Meds Within 30 Min. of Arrival	-	-	53%	58%
Average Time to ECG (minutes)	-	-	7	7
Average Time to Transfer (minutes)	-	-	53	60
Children's Asthma Care				
Received Home Management Plan of Care	-	-	-	88%
Received Reliever Medication	-	-	-	100%
Received Systemic Corticosteroids	-	-	-	100%
Emergency Department				
Admittance Decision Time (minutes)[5]	-	-	81	98
Head CT Results Within 45 Min. of Arrival	-	-	63%	57%
Patients Who Left ER Before Being Seen	-	-	3%	2%
Time from ER Arrival to Admit. (minutes)[5]	-	-	238	274
Time from ER Arrival to Discharge (minutes)	-	-	136	134
Time in ER Before Being Evaluated (minutes)	-	-	26	26
Time to Pain Meds for Fractures (minutes)	-	-	52	57
Heart Attack Care				
Aspirin Given at Discharge[3,7]	-	-	99%	99%
Fibrinolytic Meds Within 30 Min. of Arrival[3,7]	-	-	-	54%
PCI Within 90 Minutes of Arrival[3,7]	-	-	97%	96%
Statin Prescribed at Discharge[1,3]	-	-	98%	98%
Heart Failure Care				
ACE Inhibitor or ARB for LVSD[1,2]	-	-	96%	97%
Discharge Instructions Given[1,2]	-	-	94%	94%
Evaluation of LVS Function[1,2]	-	-	98%	99%
Medicare Spending				
Medicare Spending per Patient (ratio)	-	-	0.95	0.98
Pneumonia Care				
Appropriate Initial Antibiotic Given[2,7]	-	-	95%	95%
Blood Culture Timing[2,7]	-	-	98%	98%
Pregnancy and Delivery Care				
Newborn Deliveries Scheduled Early[5]	-	-	5%	6%
Preventive Care				
Immunization for Influenza[5]	-	-	92%	90%
Immunization for Pneumonia[5]	-	-	93%	92%
Stroke Care				

NOTE: Hospital profiles are in alphabetical order by state, then city, then hospital within the city; Rankings exclude hospitals with less than 25 cases except for patient surveys which excludes hospitals with less than 100 cases; (a) 100-299 cases; (1) The number of cases/patients is too few to report; (2) Data submitted were based on a sample of cases/patients; (3) Results are based on a shorter time period than required; (4) Data suppressed by CMS for one or more quarters; (5) Results are not available for this reporting period; (6) Fewer than 100 patients completed the HCAHPS survey; (7) No cases met the criteria for this measure; (8) The lower limit of the confidence interval cannot be calculated if the number of observed infections equals zero; (9) No data are available from the state/territory for this reporting period; (10) The scores shown reflect fewer than 50 completed surveys; (11) There were discrepancies in the data collection process; (12) This measure does not apply to this hospital for this reporting period; (13) Results cannot be calculated for this reporting period; (14) The results for this state are combined with nearby states to protect confidentiality; Please refer to the User's Guide for a full explanation of data.

Measure	Cases	This Hosp.	State Avg.	U.S. Avg.
Anticoagulation Therapy for Atrial Fibrillation[5]	-	-	94%	95%
Antithrombotic Therapy Timing[5]	-	-	98%	98%
Assessed for Rehabilitation[5]	-	-	98%	97%
Discharged on Antithrombotic Therapy[5]	-	-	99%	99%
Discharged on Statin Medication[5]	-	-	95%	94%
Thrombolytic Therapy Timing[5]	-	-	67%	66%
Venous Thromboembolism Prophylaxis[5]	-	-	95%	94%
Written Stroke Educational Materials Given[5]	-	-	88%	88%
Surgical Care Improvement Project				
Appropriate Beta Blocker Usage[5]	-	-	98%	98%
Appropriate VTP Within 24 Hours[5]	-	-	98%	98%
Controlled Postoperative Blood Glucose[5]	-	-	97%	97%
Perioperative Temperature Management[5]	-	-	100%	100%
Prophylactic Antibiotic Selection[5]	-	-	99%	99%
Prophylactic Antibiotic Selection (Outpatient)	-	-	98%	98%
Prophylactic Antibiotic Stopped[5]	-	-	98%	98%
Prophylactic Antibiotic Timing[5]	-	-	99%	99%
Prophylactic Antibiotic Timing (Outpatient)	-	-	98%	98%
Urinary Catheter Removal[5]	-	-	97%	97%
Survey of Patients' Hospital Experiences				
Area Around Room 'Always' Quiet at Night[5]	-	-	61%	61%
Doctors 'Always' Communicated Well[5]	-	-	82%	82%
Home Recovery Information Given[5]	-	-	87%	85%
Hospital Given 9 or 10 on 10 Point Scale[5]	-	-	71%	71%
Meds 'Always' Explained Before Given[5]	-	-	63%	64%
Nurses 'Always' Communicated Well[5]	-	-	79%	79%
Pain 'Always' Well Controlled[5]	-	-	71%	71%
Room and Bathroom 'Always' Clean[5]	-	-	73%	73%
Timely Help 'Always' Received[5]	-	-	68%	68%
Would Definitely Recommend Hospital[5]	-	-	70%	71%
Use of Medical Imaging				
Cardiac Imaging Stress Test before Surgery	-	-	5.2%	5.3%
Combination Abdominal CT Scan	-	-	11.2%	10.5%
Combination Brain/Sinus CT Scan	-	-	3.2%	2.7%
Combination Chest CT Scan	-	-	1.9%	2.7%
Follow-up Mammogram/Ultrasound	-	-	8.6%	8.8%
Lumbar Spine MRI for Low Back Pain	-	-	39.6%	37.2%

Western Missouri Medical Center

403 Burkarth Road
Warrensburg, MO 64093
URL: www.wmmc.com
Phone: 660-747-2500
Fax: 660-747-8455
Type: Acute Care Hospitals
Ownership: Govt - Hospital Dist/Auth
Emergency Services: Yes
Beds: 92

Key Personnel:

Quality Assurance . . . . Deborah Haller
Infection Control. . . . . Carol Kientzy, RN
Operating Room. . . . . Linda Pai
Chief of Medical Staff. . . . . Linda Pal, MD
Emergency Room . . . . Laura Pinson, RN
CEO/President. . . . . Gregory B Vinardi
Radiology. . . . . John J Wadell
Intensive Care Unit. . . . . Rosemary Zelazek, RN

Measure	Cases	This Hosp.	State Avg.	U.S. Avg.
Blood Clot Prevention and Treatment				
Anticoagulation Overlap Therapy[2]	21	67%	94%	93%
ICU Venous Thromboembolism Prophylaxis[2]	55	82%	91%	92%
Incidence of Potentially Preventable VTE[1,2]	-	-	7%	10%
UFH with Dosages/Platelet Monitoring[1,2]	-	-	96%	97%
Venous Thromboembolism Prophylaxis[2]	234	61%	85%	85%
Warfarin Therapy Discharge Instructions[2]	18	72%	76%	75%
Chest Pain/Possible Heart Attack Care				
Aspirin Given Within 24 Hours of Arrival	83	99%	95%	96%
Fibrinolytic Meds Within 30 Min. of Arrival[7]	-	-	53%	58%
Average Time to ECG (minutes)	88	7	7	7
Average Time to Transfer (minutes)[1]	-	-	53	60
Children's Asthma Care				
Received Home Management Plan of Care	-	-	-	88%
Received Reliever Medication	-	-	-	100%
Received Systemic Corticosteroids	-	-	-	100%
Emergency Department				
Admittance Decision Time (minutes)[2]	215	75	81	98
Head CT Results Within 45 Min. of Arrival	13	23%	63%	57%
Patients Who Left ER Before Being Seen	20,098	2%	3%	2%
Time from ER Arrival to Admit. (minutes)[2]	247	238	238	274
Time from ER Arrival to Discharge (minutes)	388	152	136	134
Time in ER Before Being Evaluated (minutes)	392	37	26	26
Time to Pain Meds for Fractures (minutes)	72	72	52	57
Heart Attack Care				
Aspirin Given at Discharge[1]	-	-	99%	99%
Fibrinolytic Meds Within 30 Min. of Arrival[7]	-	-	-	54%
PCI Within 90 Minutes of Arrival[7]	-	-	97%	96%
Statin Prescribed at Discharge[1]	-	-	98%	98%
Heart Failure Care				
ACE Inhibitor or ARB for LVSD[1]	-	-	96%	97%
Discharge Instructions Given	31	77%	94%	94%
Evaluation of LVS Function	53	96%	98%	99%
Medicare Spending				
Medicare Spending per Patient (ratio)	-	0.92	0.95	0.98
Pneumonia Care				
Appropriate Initial Antibiotic Given	76	91%	95%	95%
Blood Culture Timing	94	99%	98%	98%
Pregnancy and Delivery Care				
Newborn Deliveries Scheduled Early[2]	26	4%	5%	6%
Preventive Care				
Immunization for Influenza[2]	320	85%	92%	90%
Immunization for Pneumonia[2]	327	90%	93%	92%
Stroke Care				
Anticoagulation Therapy for Atrial Fibrillation[7]	-	-	94%	95%
Antithrombotic Therapy Timing[1]	-	-	98%	98%
Assessed for Rehabilitation[1]	-	-	98%	97%
Discharged on Antithrombotic Therapy[1]	-	-	99%	99%
Discharged on Statin Medication[1]	-	-	95%	94%
Thrombolytic Therapy Timing[7]	-	-	67%	66%
Venous Thromboembolism Prophylaxis[1]	-	-	95%	94%
Written Stroke Educational Materials Given[1]	-	-	88%	88%
Surgical Care Improvement Project				
Appropriate Beta Blocker Usage	57	93%	98%	98%
Appropriate VTP Within 24 Hours	171	98%	98%	98%
Controlled Postoperative Blood Glucose[7]	-	-	97%	97%
Perioperative Temperature Management	199	100%	100%	100%
Prophylactic Antibiotic Selection	155	90%	99%	99%
Prophylactic Antibiotic Selection (Outpatient)	53	98%	98%	98%
Prophylactic Antibiotic Stopped	149	99%	98%	98%
Prophylactic Antibiotic Timing	157	96%	99%	99%
Prophylactic Antibiotic Timing (Outpatient)	54	93%	98%	98%
Urinary Catheter Removal	155	99%	97%	97%
Survey of Patients' Hospital Experiences				
Area Around Room 'Always' Quiet at Night	300+	70%	61%	61%
Doctors 'Always' Communicated Well	300+	82%	82%	82%
Home Recovery Information Given	300+	87%	87%	85%
Hospital Given 9 or 10 on 10 Point Scale	300+	72%	71%	71%
Meds 'Always' Explained Before Given	300+	67%	63%	64%
Nurses 'Always' Communicated Well	300+	81%	79%	79%
Pain 'Always' Well Controlled	300+	73%	71%	71%
Room and Bathroom 'Always' Clean	300+	81%	73%	73%
Timely Help 'Always' Received	300+	69%	68%	68%
Would Definitely Recommend Hospital	300+	70%	70%	71%
Use of Medical Imaging				
Cardiac Imaging Stress Test before Surgery	211	3.3%	5.2%	5.3%
Combination Abdominal CT Scan	461	4.6%	11.2%	10.5%
Combination Brain/Sinus CT Scan[1]	-	-	3.2%	2.7%
Combination Chest CT Scan	254	0.8%	1.9%	2.7%
Follow-up Mammogram/Ultrasound	599	11.0%	8.6%	8.8%
Lumbar Spine MRI for Low Back Pain	107	42.1%	39.6%	37.2%

Mercy Hospital Washington

901 East 5th Street
Washington, MO 63090
URL: www.stjohnsmercy.org
Phone: 636-239-8000
Fax: 314-569-6733
Type: Acute Care Hospitals
Ownership: Voluntary non-profit - Private
Emergency Services: Yes
Beds: 187

Key Personnel:

Infection Control. . . . . Phyllis Cassette, RN
Quality Assurance . . . . Phyllis Cassette, RN
Radiology. . . . . Marc F Clemente
Operating Room. . . . . Kathleen Gnavi, RN
Chief of Medical Staff. . . . . Thomas B Riechers, MD, FACS
CEO/President. . . . . Michael Zilm
Pediatric Ambulatory Care . . . . . . Andrew Zupan, MD
Pediatric In-Patient Care . . . . Andrew Zupan, MD

Measure	Cases	This Hosp.	State Avg.	U.S. Avg.
Blood Clot Prevention and Treatment				
Anticoagulation Overlap Therapy[2]	33	88%	94%	93%
ICU Venous Thromboembolism Prophylaxis[2]	69	93%	91%	92%
Incidence of Potentially Preventable VTE[2]	15	7%	7%	10%
UFH with Dosages/Platelet Monitoring[1,2]	-	-	96%	97%
Venous Thromboembolism Prophylaxis[2]	305	83%	85%	85%
Warfarin Therapy Discharge Instructions[2]	27	41%	76%	75%
Chest Pain/Possible Heart Attack Care				
Aspirin Given Within 24 Hours of Arrival[1,3]	-	-	95%	96%
Fibrinolytic Meds Within 30 Min. of Arrival[3,7]	-	-	53%	58%
Average Time to ECG (minutes)[1,3]	-	-	7	7
Average Time to Transfer (minutes)[3,7]	-	-	53	60
Children's Asthma Care				
Received Home Management Plan of Care	-	-	-	88%
Received Reliever Medication	-	-	-	100%
Received Systemic Corticosteroids	-	-	-	100%
Emergency Department				
Admittance Decision Time (minutes)[2]	477	99	81	98
Head CT Results Within 45 Min. of Arrival	11	36%	63%	57%
Patients Who Left ER Before Being Seen	35,005	0%	3%	2%
Time from ER Arrival to Admit. (minutes)[2]	512	242	238	274
Time from ER Arrival to Discharge (minutes)	368	116	136	134
Time in ER Before Being Evaluated (minutes)	393	13	26	26
Time to Pain Meds for Fractures (minutes)	76	42	52	57
Heart Attack Care				
Aspirin Given at Discharge	151	100%	99%	99%
Fibrinolytic Meds Within 30 Min. of Arrival[7]	-	-	-	54%
PCI Within 90 Minutes of Arrival	29	93%	97%	96%
Statin Prescribed at Discharge	145	98%	98%	98%
Heart Failure Care				
ACE Inhibitor or ARB for LVSD[2]	59	100%	96%	97%
Discharge Instructions Given[2]	180	93%	94%	94%
Evaluation of LVS Function[2]	224	100%	98%	99%
Medicare Spending				
Medicare Spending per Patient (ratio)	-	0.93	0.95	0.98
Pneumonia Care				
Appropriate Initial Antibiotic Given[2]	75	97%	95%	95%
Blood Culture Timing[2]	93	99%	98%	98%
Pregnancy and Delivery Care				
Newborn Deliveries Scheduled Early[2]	24	0%	5%	6%
Preventive Care				
Immunization for Influenza[2]	520	97%	92%	90%
Immunization for Pneumonia[2]	685	97%	93%	92%
Stroke Care				
Anticoagulation Therapy for Atrial Fibrillation	17	94%	94%	95%
Antithrombotic Therapy Timing	72	97%	98%	98%
Assessed for Rehabilitation	79	99%	98%	97%
Discharged on Antithrombotic Therapy	79	99%	99%	99%
Discharged on Statin Medication	65	91%	95%	94%
Thrombolytic Therapy Timing[1]	-	-	67%	66%
Venous Thromboembolism Prophylaxis	79	91%	95%	94%
Written Stroke Educational Materials Given	42	86%	88%	88%
Surgical Care Improvement Project				
Appropriate Beta Blocker Usage[2]	100	97%	98%	98%
Appropriate VTP Within 24 Hours[2]	299	98%	98%	98%
Controlled Postoperative Blood Glucose[2,7]	-	-	97%	97%
Perioperative Temperature Management[2]	349	100%	100%	100%
Prophylactic Antibiotic Selection[2]	203	100%	99%	99%
Prophylactic Antibiotic Selection (Outpatient)	271	100%	98%	98%
Prophylactic Antibiotic Stopped[2]	196	98%	98%	98%
Prophylactic Antibiotic Timing[2]	203	99%	99%	99%
Prophylactic Antibiotic Timing (Outpatient)	272	99%	98%	98%
Urinary Catheter Removal[2]	255	98%	97%	97%
Survey of Patients' Hospital Experiences				
Area Around Room 'Always' Quiet at Night[11]	300+	58%	61%	61%
Doctors 'Always' Communicated Well[11]	300+	83%	82%	82%
Home Recovery Information Given[11]	300+	89%	87%	85%
Hospital Given 9 or 10 on 10 Point Scale[11]	300+	71%	71%	71%
Meds 'Always' Explained Before Given[11]	300+	63%	63%	64%

NOTE: Hospital profiles are in alphabetical order by state, then city, then hospital within the city; Rankings exclude hospitals with less than 25 cases except for patient surveys which excludes hospitals with less than 100 cases; (a) 100-299 cases; (1) The number of cases/patients is too few to report; (2) Data submitted were based on a sample of cases/patients; (3) Results are based on a shorter time period than required; (4) Data suppressed by CMS for one or more quarters; (5) Results are not available for this reporting period; (6) Fewer than 100 patients completed the HCAHPS survey; (7) No cases met the criteria for this measure; (8) The lower limit of the confidence interval cannot be calculated if the number of observed infections equals zero; (9) No data are available from the state/territory for this reporting period; (10) The scores shown reflect fewer than 50 completed surveys; (11) There were discrepancies in the data collection process; (12) This measure does not apply to this hospital for this reporting period; (13) Results cannot be calculated for this reporting period; (14) The results for this state are combined with nearby states to protect confidentiality; Please refer to the User's Guide for a full explanation of data.

Nurses 'Always' Communicated Well[11]	300+	78%	79%	79%
Pain 'Always' Well Controlled[11]	300+	68%	71%	71%
Room and Bathroom 'Always' Clean[11]	300+	72%	73%	73%
Timely Help 'Always' Received[11]	300+	64%	68%	68%
Would Definitely Recommend Hospital[11]	300+	69%	70%	71%
Use of Medical Imaging				
Cardiac Imaging Stress Test before Surgery	741	4.6%	5.2%	5.3%
Combination Abdominal CT Scan	839	22.8%	11.2%	10.5%
Combination Brain/Sinus CT Scan	590	2.7%	3.2%	2.7%
Combination Chest CT Scan	679	0.6%	1.9%	2.7%
Follow-up Mammogram/Ultrasound	1,690	5.7%	8.6%	8.8%
Lumbar Spine MRI for Low Back Pain	196	32.1%	39.6%	37.2%

Ozarks Medical Center

1100 Kentucky Ave
West Plains, MO 65775
URL: www.ozarksmedicalcenter.com
Type: Acute Care Hospitals
Ownership: Voluntary non-profit - Other
Phone: 417-256-9111
Fax: 417-257-6770
Emergency Services: Yes
Beds: 114

Key Personnel:

Chief of Medical Staff.......... Edward Henegar, DO
Infection Control............ Torrance Hughes
President/CEO............ Thomas Keller, OMC
Hemotology Center........... Susan Kenolow, RN
Cardiac Laboratory............ Tim Kimball, RN
Emergency Room........... Dennise Lawson, RN
Quality Assurance........... Dona Paschall, RN
Operating Room............ Jill Tate, RN

Measure	Cases	This Hosp.	State Avg.	U.S. Avg.
Blood Clot Prevention and Treatment				
Anticoagulation Overlap Therapy[2]	35	80%	94%	93%
ICU Venous Thromboembolism Prophylaxis[2]	379	89%	91%	92%
Incidence of Potentially Preventable VTE[1,2]	-	-	7%	10%
UFH with Dosages/Platelet Monitoring[1,2]	-	-	96%	97%
Venous Thromboembolism Prophylaxis[2]	618	89%	85%	85%
Warfarin Therapy Discharge Instructions[2]	27	89%	76%	75%
Chest Pain/Possible Heart Attack Care				
Aspirin Given Within 24 Hours of Arrival[1]	-	-	95%	96%
Fibrinolytic Meds Within 30 Min. of Arrival[3,7]	-	-	53%	58%
Average Time to ECG (minutes)[1]	-	-	7	7
Average Time to Transfer (minutes)[3,7]	-	-	53	60
Children's Asthma Care				
Received Home Management Plan of Care	-	-	-	88%
Received Reliever Medication	-	-	-	100%
Received Systemic Corticosteroids	-	-	-	100%
Emergency Department				
Admittance Decision Time (minutes)[2]	1,182	113	81	98
Head CT Results Within 45 Min. of Arrival[1]	-	-	63%	57%
Patients Who Left ER Before Being Seen	26,498	1%	3%	2%
Time from ER Arrival to Admit. (minutes)[2]	1,270	289	238	274
Time from ER Arrival to Discharge (minutes)	676	166	136	134
Time in ER Before Being Evaluated (minutes)	618	29	26	26
Time to Pain Meds for Fractures (minutes)	125	61	52	57
Heart Attack Care				
Aspirin Given at Discharge	155	97%	99%	99%
Fibrinolytic Meds Within 30 Min. of Arrival[7]	-	-	-	54%
PCI Within 90 Minutes of Arrival	18	72%	97%	96%
Statin Prescribed at Discharge	148	89%	98%	98%
Heart Failure Care				
ACE Inhibitor or ARB for LVSD	37	97%	96%	97%
Discharge Instructions Given	73	89%	94%	94%
Evaluation of LVS Function	107	98%	98%	99%
Medicare Spending				
Medicare Spending per Patient (ratio)	-	0.90	0.95	0.98
Pneumonia Care				
Appropriate Initial Antibiotic Given	129	93%	95%	95%
Blood Culture Timing	234	98%	98%	98%
Pregnancy and Delivery Care				
Newborn Deliveries Scheduled Early	15	7%	5%	6%
Preventive Care				
Immunization for Influenza[2]	978	96%	92%	90%
Immunization for Pneumonia[2]	1,425	92%	93%	92%
Stroke Care				
Anticoagulation Therapy for Atrial Fibrillation[1]	-	-	94%	95%
Antithrombotic Therapy Timing	41	100%	98%	98%
Assessed for Rehabilitation	62	98%	98%	97%
Discharged on Antithrombotic Therapy	57	98%	99%	99%
Discharged on Statin Medication	43	86%	95%	94%
Thrombolytic Therapy Timing	20	70%	67%	66%
Venous Thromboembolism Prophylaxis	58	88%	95%	94%
Written Stroke Educational Materials Given	39	79%	88%	88%
Surgical Care Improvement Project				
Appropriate Beta Blocker Usage	63	98%	98%	98%
Appropriate VTP Within 24 Hours	129	94%	98%	98%
Controlled Postoperative Blood Glucose	14	100%	97%	97%
Perioperative Temperature Management	170	98%	100%	100%
Prophylactic Antibiotic Selection	122	98%	99%	99%
Prophylactic Antibiotic Selection (Outpatient)	183	89%	98%	98%
Prophylactic Antibiotic Stopped	117	94%	98%	98%
Prophylactic Antibiotic Timing	122	98%	99%	99%
Prophylactic Antibiotic Timing (Outpatient)	184	97%	98%	98%
Urinary Catheter Removal	105	91%	97%	97%
Survey of Patients' Hospital Experiences				
Area Around Room 'Always' Quiet at Night	300+	53%	61%	61%
Doctors 'Always' Communicated Well	300+	85%	82%	82%
Home Recovery Information Given	300+	82%	87%	85%
Hospital Given 9 or 10 on 10 Point Scale	300+	64%	71%	71%
Meds 'Always' Explained Before Given	300+	66%	63%	64%
Nurses 'Always' Communicated Well	300+	81%	79%	79%
Pain 'Always' Well Controlled	300+	72%	71%	71%
Room and Bathroom 'Always' Clean	300+	78%	73%	73%
Timely Help 'Always' Received	300+	71%	68%	68%
Would Definitely Recommend Hospital	300+	65%	70%	71%
Use of Medical Imaging				
Cardiac Imaging Stress Test before Surgery	493	4.1%	5.2%	5.3%
Combination Abdominal CT Scan	767	61.3%	11.2%	10.5%
Combination Brain/Sinus CT Scan	778	3.7%	3.2%	2.7%
Combination Chest CT Scan	569	0.5%	1.9%	2.7%
Follow-up Mammogram/Ultrasound	879	9.0%	8.6%	8.8%
Lumbar Spine MRI for Low Back Pain	164	42.7%	39.6%	37.2%

NOTE: Hospital profiles are in alphabetical order by state, then city, then hospital within the city; Rankings exclude hospitals with less than 25 cases except for patient surveys which excludes hospitals with less than 100 cases; (a) 100-299 cases; (1) The number of cases/patients is too few to report; (2) Data submitted were based on a sample of cases/patients; (3) Results are based on a shorter time period than required; (4) Data suppressed by CMS for one or more quarters; (5) Results are not available for this reporting period; (6) Fewer than 100 patients completed the HCAHPS survey; (7) No cases met the criteria for this measure; (8) The lower limit of the confidence interval cannot be calculated if the number of observed infections equals zero; (9) No data are available from the state/territory for this reporting period; (10) The scores shown reflect fewer than 50 completed surveys; (11) There were discrepancies in the data collection process; (12) This measure does not apply to this hospital for this reporting period; (13) Results cannot be calculated for this reporting period; (14) The results for this state are combined with nearby states to protect confidentiality; Please refer to the User's Guide for a full explanation of data.

Blood Clot Prevention and Treatment

Anticoagulation Overlap Therapy

Hospital Name	City	Rate	Cases
Fremont Area Medical Center[2]	Fremont	100%	31
Saint Elizabeth Regional Medical Center[2]	Lincoln	100%	61
Alegent Creighton-Lakeside Hosp[2]	Omaha	99%	86
Alegent Creighton-Bergan Mercy Med Ctr[2]	Omaha	98%	94
Alegent Creighton-Immanuel Med Ctr[2]	Omaha	98%	43
Bryan Medical Center[2]	Lincoln	98%	95
The Nebraska Methodist Hospital[2]	Omaha	95%	114
Good Samaritan Hospital[2]	Kearney	94%	50
Regional West Medical Center[2]	Scottsbluff	92%	48
Alegent Creighton-Creighton Univ Med[2]	Omaha	91%	47
Alegent Creighton-Midlands Hosp[2]	Papillion	89%	35
Faith Regional Health Services[2]	Norfolk	87%	39
The Nebraska Medical Center[2]	Omaha	86%	138
Great Plains Regional Medical Center[2]	North Platte	82%	49
Saint Francis Medical Center[2]	Grand Island	77%	39

ICU Venous Thromboembolism Prophylaxis

Hospital Name	City	Rate	Cases
Alegent Creighton-Lakeside Hosp[2]	Omaha	100%	67
Beatrice Comm Hosp & Health Ctr	Beatrice	100%	48
Alegent Creighton-Creighton Univ Med[2]	Omaha	99%	145
Alegent Creighton-Bergan Mercy Med Ctr[2]	Omaha	98%	56
Alegent Creighton-Immanuel Med Ctr[2]	Omaha	98%	54
Bryan Medical Center[2]	Lincoln	97%	70
Bellevue Medical Center[2]	Bellevue	96%	46
Faith Regional Health Services[2]	Norfolk	96%	71
Fremont Area Medical Center[2]	Fremont	96%	49
The Nebraska Medical Center[2]	Omaha	96%	80
The Nebraska Methodist Hospital[2]	Omaha	96%	57
Alegent Creighton-Midlands Hosp[2]	Papillion	93%	84
Good Samaritan Hospital[2]	Kearney	92%	37
Mary Lanning Healthcare[2]	Hastings	91%	33
Saint Elizabeth Regional Medical Center[2]	Lincoln	91%	33
Nebraska Heart Hospital	Lincoln	88%	504
Saint Francis Medical Center[2]	Grand Island	86%	57
Regional West Medical Center[2]	Scottsbluff	79%	76
Columbus Community Hospital[2]	Columbus	76%	131
Great Plains Regional Medical Center[2]	North Platte	70%	60

Incidence of Potentially Preventable VTE

Hospital Name	City	Rate	Cases
The Nebraska Medical Center[2]	Omaha	5%	56

UFH with Dosages/Platelet Count Monitoring

Hospital Name	City	Rate	Cases
Alegent Creighton-Midlands Hosp[2]	Papillion	100%	25
Good Samaritan Hospital[2]	Kearney	100%	49
The Nebraska Medical Center[2]	Omaha	100%	140
The Nebraska Methodist Hospital[2]	Omaha	100%	124
Saint Francis Medical Center[2]	Grand Island	100%	54
Alegent Creighton-Bergan Mercy Med Ctr[2]	Omaha	99%	95
Alegent Creighton-Lakeside Hosp[2]	Omaha	99%	69
Alegent Creighton-Immanuel Med Ctr[2]	Omaha	98%	49
Alegent Creighton-Creighton Univ Med[2]	Omaha	97%	29
Bryan Medical Center[2]	Lincoln	97%	36

Venous Thromboembolism Prophylaxis

Hospital Name	City	Rate	Cases
Beatrice Comm Hosp & Health Ctr	Beatrice	100%	149
Memorial Community Hospital[3]	Blair	99%	82
Nebraska Spine Hospital[2]	Omaha	99%	335
Alegent Creighton-Immanuel Med Ctr[2]	Omaha	98%	218
Alegent Creighton-Lakeside Hosp[2]	Omaha	98%	301
Alegent Creighton-Mem Hosp, Schuyl	Schuyler	97%	34
Midwest Surgical Hospital	Omaha	97%	267
Nebraska Orthopaedic Hospital[2]	Omaha	97%	29
Alegent Creighton-Creighton Univ Med[2]	Omaha	95%	335
Alegent Creighton-Plainview Hosp[3]	Plainview	94%	53
Alegent Creighton-Bergan Mercy Med Ctr[2]	Omaha	93%	252
Bryan Medical Center[2]	Lincoln	91%	288
Good Samaritan Hospital[2]	Kearney	90%	326
The Nebraska Medical Center[2]	Omaha	90%	313
Saint Elizabeth Regional Medical Center[2]	Lincoln	90%	331
Alegent Creighton-Midlands Hosp[2]	Papillion	89%	112
Bellevue Medical Center[2]	Bellevue	89%	194
Fremont Area Medical Center[2]	Fremont	89%	212
Faith Regional Health Services[2]	Norfolk	87%	285
Mary Lanning Healthcare[2]	Hastings	86%	212
Community Medical Center[3]	Falls City	84%	86
Regional West Medical Center[2]	Scottsbluff	84%	340
The Nebraska Methodist Hospital[2]	Omaha	83%	372
Columbus Community Hospital[2]	Columbus	80%	187
Nebraska Heart Hospital	Lincoln	79%	560
Saint Francis Medical Center[2]	Grand Island	75%	307
Great Plains Regional Medical Center[2]	North Platte	68%	330

Warfarin Therapy Discharge Instructions

Hospital Name	City	Rate	Cases
Great Plains Regional Medical Center[2]	North Platte	97%	34
Saint Francis Medical Center[2]	Grand Island	96%	26
The Nebraska Methodist Hospital[2]	Omaha	92%	87
Alegent Creighton-Bergan Mercy Med Ctr[2]	Omaha	89%	71
Alegent Creighton-Creighton Univ Med[2]	Omaha	89%	38
Saint Elizabeth Regional Medical Center[2]	Lincoln	85%	40
Alegent Creighton-Midlands Hosp[2]	Papillion	81%	26
Bryan Medical Center[2]	Lincoln	80%	70
The Nebraska Medical Center[2]	Omaha	80%	96
Alegent Creighton-Lakeside Hosp[2]	Omaha	73%	59
Good Samaritan Hospital[2]	Kearney	72%	43
Regional West Medical Center[2]	Scottsbluff	56%	34
Faith Regional Health Services[2]	Norfolk	20%	25

Chest Pain/Possible Heart Attack Care

Aspirin Given Within 24 Hours of Arrival

Hospital Name	City	Rate	Cases
Regional West Medical Center	Scottsbluff	100%	54
Beatrice Comm Hosp & Health Ctr	Beatrice	98%	44
Columbus Community Hospital	Columbus	98%	40
Nebraska Orthopaedic Hospital	Omaha	97%	34
Community Hospital	Mccook	94%	33
Pawnee County Memorial Hospital	Pawnee City	93%	27
Nemaha County Hospital	Auburn	90%	31

Average Time to ECG (minutes)

Hospital Name	City	Min.	Cases
Community Hospital	Mccook	5	35
Beatrice Comm Hosp & Health Ctr	Beatrice	6	45
Nebraska Orthopaedic Hospital	Omaha	6	33
Nemaha County Hospital	Auburn	7	35
Pawnee County Memorial Hospital	Pawnee City	7	27
Regional West Medical Center	Scottsbluff	7	56
Phelps Memorial Health Center	Holdrege	8	25
Columbus Community Hospital	Columbus	12	42

Children's Asthma Care

Received Home Management Plan of Care

Hospital Name	City	Rate	Cases
Children's Hospital & Medical Center	Omaha	93%	85

Received Reliever Medication

Hospital Name	City	Rate	Cases
Children's Hospital & Medical Center	Omaha	100%	85

Received Systemic Corticosteroids

Hospital Name	City	Rate	Cases
Children's Hospital & Medical Center	Omaha	100%	86

Emergency Department

Admittance Decision Time (minutes)

Hospital Name	City	Min.	Cases
Community Medical Center[2,3]	Falls City	30	47
Fremont Area Medical Center[2]	Fremont	30	257
Saint Francis Medical Center[2]	Grand Island	50	428
Box Butte General Hospital	Alliance	55	401
Mary Lanning Healthcare[2]	Hastings	55	217
Columbus Community Hospital[2]	Columbus	56	347
Faith Regional Health Services[2]	Norfolk	57	268
Good Samaritan Hospital[2]	Kearney	66	314
Bryan Medical Center[2]	Lincoln	69	342
Alegent Creighton-Bergan Mercy Med Ctr[2]	Omaha	76	289
The Nebraska Medical Center[2]	Omaha	76	307
The Nebraska Methodist Hospital[2]	Omaha	77	242
Bellevue Medical Center[2]	Bellevue	82	311
Alegent Creighton-Midlands Hosp[2]	Papillion	84	398
Great Plains Regional Medical Center[2]	North Platte	85	474
Regional West Medical Center[2]	Scottsbluff	85	482
Alegent Creighton-Lakeside Hosp[2]	Omaha	86	640
Alegent Creighton-Immanuel Med Ctr[2]	Omaha	107	397
Saint Elizabeth Regional Medical Center[2]	Lincoln	108	218
Alegent Creighton-Creighton Univ Med[2]	Omaha	171	508

Patients Who Left ER Before Being Seen

Hospital Name	City	Rate	Cases
Alegent Creighton-Lakeside Hosp	Omaha	0%	23159
Alegent Creighton-Midlands Hosp	Papillion	0%	13469
Bryan Medical Center	Lincoln	0%	71640
Columbus Community Hospital	Columbus	0%	11036
Fremont Area Medical Center	Fremont	0%	14590
Good Samaritan Hospital	Kearney	0%	15412
Great Plains Regional Medical Center	North Platte	0%	18217
Mary Lanning Healthcare	Hastings	0%	12547
Nebraska Orthopaedic Hospital	Omaha	0%	8850
Ogallala Community Hospital	Ogallala	0%	3303
Providence Medical Center	Wayne	0%	1749
Alegent Creighton-Bergan Mercy Med Ctr	Omaha	1%	26610
Alegent Creighton-Creighton Univ Med	Omaha	1%	35441
Bellevue Medical Center	Bellevue	1%	24996
Faith Regional Health Services	Norfolk	1%	11713
The Nebraska Methodist Hospital	Omaha	1%	29687
Regional West Medical Center	Scottsbluff	1%	16366
Saint Elizabeth Regional Medical Center	Lincoln	1%	32875
Saint Francis Medical Center	Grand Island	1%	24093
Alegent Creighton-Immanuel Med Ctr	Omaha	2%	33770
The Nebraska Medical Center	Omaha	2%	51834

Time from ER Arrival to Being Admitted (minutes)

Hospital Name	City	Min.	Cases
Community Medical Center[2,3]	Falls City	111	52
Mary Lanning Healthcare[2]	Hastings	156	218
Good Samaritan Hospital[2]	Kearney	168	334
Saint Francis Medical Center[2]	Grand Island	177	435
Columbus Community Hospital[2]	Columbus	179	390
Box Butte General Hospital	Alliance	188	401
Faith Regional Health Services[2]	Norfolk	188	288
Alegent Creighton-Bergan Mercy Med Ctr[2]	Omaha	192	299
Fremont Area Medical Center[2]	Fremont	194	264
Bryan Medical Center[2]	Lincoln	196	352
The Nebraska Methodist Hospital[2]	Omaha	198	244
Alegent Creighton-Lakeside Hosp[2]	Omaha	201	651
Alegent Creighton-Midlands Hosp[2]	Papillion	212	405
Bellevue Medical Center[2]	Bellevue	215	314
Great Plains Regional Medical Center[2]	North Platte	233	495
Regional West Medical Center[2]	Scottsbluff	238	495
Alegent Creighton-Immanuel Med Ctr[2]	Omaha	241	401
Saint Elizabeth Regional Medical Center[2]	Lincoln	242	398
Alegent Creighton-Creighton Univ Med[2]	Omaha	256	513
The Nebraska Medical Center[2]	Omaha	264	317

Time from ER Arrival to Discharge (minutes)

Hospital Name	City	Min.	Cases
Saint Mary's Community Hospital[3]	Nebraska City	76	80
Nebraska Orthopaedic Hospital	Omaha	78	378
Good Samaritan Hospital	Kearney	81	370
Fremont Area Medical Center	Fremont	85	348
Mary Lanning Healthcare	Hastings	89	516
Bryan Medical Center	Lincoln	94	342
Saint Francis Medical Center	Grand Island	102	346
Columbus Community Hospital	Columbus	107	414
Bellevue Medical Center	Bellevue	110	364
Alegent Creighton-Creighton Univ Med	Omaha	113	420
Alegent Creighton-Bergan Mercy Med Ctr	Omaha	114	389
Box Butte General Hospital	Alliance	115	373
Great Plains Regional Medical Center	North Platte	120	374
Faith Regional Health Services	Norfolk	125	409
Alegent Creighton-Lakeside Hosp	Omaha	126	382
Alegent Creighton-Midlands Hosp	Papillion	126	378
Alegent Creighton-Immanuel Med Ctr	Omaha	131	356
The Nebraska Medical Center	Omaha	147	359
Saint Elizabeth Regional Medical Center	Lincoln	149	576
Regional West Medical Center	Scottsbluff	154	402
The Nebraska Methodist Hospital	Omaha	211	543

Time in ER Before Being Evaluated (minutes)

Hospital Name	City	Min.	Cases
Fremont Area Medical Center	Fremont	0	325
Saint Mary's Community Hospital[3]	Nebraska City	6	94
Good Samaritan Hospital	Kearney	10	349
Bellevue Medical Center	Bellevue	15	280
Great Plains Regional Medical Center	North Platte	15	421
Mary Lanning Healthcare	Hastings	17	576
Alegent Creighton-Creighton Univ Med	Omaha	18	473
Nebraska Orthopaedic Hospital	Omaha	18	417
Saint Francis Medical Center	Grand Island	18	355
The Nebraska Methodist Hospital	Omaha	20	1108
Columbus Community Hospital	Columbus	21	454
Faith Regional Health Services	Norfolk	21	453
Regional West Medical Center	Scottsbluff	21	422
Alegent Creighton-Lakeside Hosp	Omaha	26	360
Saint Elizabeth Regional Medical Center	Lincoln	27	531
The Nebraska Medical Center	Omaha	30	369
Box Butte General Hospital	Alliance	31	407
Bryan Medical Center	Lincoln	36	329
Alegent Creighton-Bergan Mercy Med Ctr	Omaha	38	350
Alegent Creighton-Midlands Hosp	Papillion	39	352
Alegent Creighton-Immanuel Med Ctr	Omaha	45	383

NOTE: Hospital profiles are in alphabetical order by state, then city, then hospital within the city; Rankings exclude hospitals with less than 25 cases except for patient surveys which excludes hospitals with less than 100 cases; (a) 100-299 cases; (1) The number of cases/patients is too few to report; (2) Data submitted were based on a sample of cases/patients; (3) Results are based on a shorter time period than required; (4) Data suppressed by CMS for one or more quarters; (5) Results are not available for this reporting period; (6) Fewer than 100 patients completed the HCAHPS survey; (7) No cases met the criteria for this measure; (8) The lower limit of the confidence interval cannot be calculated if the number of observed infections equals zero; (9) No data are available from the state/territory for this reporting period; (10) The scores shown reflect fewer than 50 completed surveys; (11) There were discrepancies in the data collection process; (12) This measure does not apply to this hospital for this reporting period; (13) Results cannot be calculated for this reporting period; (14) The results for this state are combined with nearby states to protect confidentiality; Please refer to the User's Guide for a full explanation of data.

Time to Pain Meds for Bone Fractures (minutes)

Hospital Name	City	Min.	Cases
Fremont Area Medical Center	Fremont	22	74
Mary Lanning Healthcare	Hastings	29	63
Alegent Creighton-Creighton Univ Med	Omaha	30	106
Nebraska Orthopaedic Hospital	Omaha	30	45
Regional West Medical Center	Scottsbluff	32	44
Good Samaritan Hospital	Kearney	34	62
Great Plains Regional Medical Center	North Platte	36	61
Columbus Community Hospital	Columbus	37	51
Bryan Medical Center	Lincoln	41	216
Saint Francis Medical Center	Grand Island	44	124
Bellevue Medical Center	Bellevue	46	117
Faith Regional Health Services	Norfolk	46	80
Saint Elizabeth Regional Medical Center	Lincoln	48	141
Alegent Creighton-Lakeside Hosp	Omaha	49	143
Alegent Creighton-Midlands Hosp	Papillion	52	70
The Nebraska Medical Center	Omaha	55	116
Alegent Creighton-Immanuel Med Ctr	Omaha	56	61
Alegent Creighton-Bergan Mercy Med Ctr	Omaha	59	76
The Nebraska Methodist Hospital	Omaha	62	32

Heart Attack Care

Aspirin Given at Discharge

Hospital Name	City	Rate	Cases
Alegent Creighton-Bergan Mercy Med Ctr	Omaha	100%	210
Alegent Creighton-Creighton Univ Med	Omaha	100%	218
Alegent Creighton-Immanuel Med Ctr	Omaha	100%	111
Alegent Creighton-Lakeside Hosp	Omaha	100%	121
Alegent Creighton-Midlands Hosp	Papillion	100%	46
Bellevue Medical Center	Bellevue	100%	72
Bryan Medical Center	Lincoln	100%	447
Faith Regional Health Services	Norfolk	100%	108
Fremont Area Medical Center	Fremont	100%	39
The Nebraska Medical Center[2]	Omaha	100%	213
The Nebraska Methodist Hospital	Omaha	100%	193
Good Samaritan Hospital	Kearney	99%	198
Great Plains Regional Medical Center	North Platte	99%	82
Nebraska Heart Hospital	Lincoln	99%	279
Saint Elizabeth Regional Medical Center	Lincoln	99%	101
Saint Francis Medical Center	Grand Island	99%	76

PCI Within 90 Minutes of Arrival

Hospital Name	City	Rate	Cases
Alegent Creighton-Bergan Mercy Med Ctr	Omaha	100%	25
Saint Elizabeth Regional Medical Center	Lincoln	100%	35
Bryan Medical Center	Lincoln	98%	47
The Nebraska Methodist Hospital	Omaha	96%	28
Alegent Creighton-Lakeside Hosp	Omaha	93%	30

Statin Prescribed at Discharge

Hospital Name	City	Rate	Cases
Alegent Creighton-Bergan Mercy Med Ctr	Omaha	100%	204
Alegent Creighton-Creighton Univ Med	Omaha	100%	215
Alegent Creighton-Immanuel Med Ctr	Omaha	100%	109
Alegent Creighton-Midlands Hosp	Papillion	100%	46
Bellevue Medical Center	Bellevue	100%	70
Bryan Medical Center	Lincoln	100%	431
Great Plains Regional Medical Center	North Platte	100%	82
The Nebraska Medical Center[2]	Omaha	100%	209
Alegent Creighton-Lakeside Hosp	Omaha	99%	114
Faith Regional Health Services	Norfolk	99%	109
Nebraska Heart Hospital	Lincoln	99%	266
The Nebraska Methodist Hospital	Omaha	99%	191
Saint Elizabeth Regional Medical Center	Lincoln	98%	94
Fremont Area Medical Center	Fremont	97%	36
Good Samaritan Hospital	Kearney	97%	189
Saint Francis Medical Center	Grand Island	96%	76

Heart Failure Care

ACE Inhibitor or ARB for LVSD

Hospital Name	City	Rate	Cases
Alegent Creighton-Immanuel Med Ctr	Omaha	100%	31
Bryan Medical Center	Lincoln	100%	117
The Nebraska Medical Center[2]	Omaha	100%	89
The Nebraska Methodist Hospital	Omaha	100%	88
Alegent Creighton-Creighton Univ Med	Omaha	99%	99
Omaha VA Medical Center	Omaha	98%	54
Saint Elizabeth Regional Medical Center	Lincoln	98%	43
Mary Lanning Healthcare	Hastings	97%	33
Alegent Creighton-Bergan Mercy Med Ctr	Omaha	96%	56
Nebraska Heart Hospital	Lincoln	95%	130
Faith Regional Health Services	Norfolk	94%	34
Great Plains Regional Medical Center	North Platte	94%	34
Good Samaritan Hospital	Kearney	92%	37

Discharge Instructions Given

Hospital Name	City	Rate	Cases
Alegent Creighton-Immanuel Med Ctr	Omaha	100%	88
Alegent Creighton-Midlands Hosp	Papillion	100%	38
Bellevue Medical Center	Bellevue	100%	52
Community Hospital	Mccook	100%	25
Alegent Creighton-Bergan Mercy Med Ctr	Omaha	99%	199
Alegent Creighton-Lakeside Hosp	Omaha	99%	78
Columbus Community Hospital	Columbus	98%	43
Faith Regional Health Services	Norfolk	98%	63
The Nebraska Methodist Hospital	Omaha	97%	206
Great Plains Regional Medical Center	North Platte	96%	95
Fremont Area Medical Center	Fremont	95%	44
The Nebraska Medical Center[2]	Omaha	95%	241
Alegent Creighton-Creighton Univ Med	Omaha	94%	214
Bryan Medical Center	Lincoln	94%	299
Saint Elizabeth Regional Medical Center	Lincoln	94%	148
Good Samaritan Hospital	Kearney	93%	110
Mary Lanning Healthcare	Hastings	89%	56
Omaha VA Medical Center	Omaha	89%	137
Regional West Medical Center	Scottsbluff	88%	67
Nebraska Heart Hospital	Lincoln	85%	204
Saint Francis Medical Center	Grand Island	82%	88

Evaluation of LVS Function

Hospital Name	City	Rate	Cases
Alegent Creighton-Bergan Mercy Med Ctr	Omaha	100%	276
Alegent Creighton-Creighton Univ Med	Omaha	100%	261
Alegent Creighton-Immanuel Med Ctr	Omaha	100%	118
Alegent Creighton-Lakeside Hosp	Omaha	100%	116
Alegent Creighton-Midlands Hosp	Papillion	100%	56
Bellevue Medical Center	Bellevue	100%	71
Bryan Medical Center	Lincoln	100%	391
Columbus Community Hospital	Columbus	100%	61
Community Hospital	Mccook	100%	31
Good Samaritan Hospital	Kearney	100%	142
Great Plains Regional Medical Center	North Platte	100%	126
Nebraska Heart Hospital	Lincoln	100%	245
The Nebraska Medical Center[2]	Omaha	100%	281
The Nebraska Methodist Hospital	Omaha	100%	277
Omaha VA Medical Center	Omaha	100%	156
Regional West Medical Center	Scottsbluff	100%	90
Saint Elizabeth Regional Medical Center	Lincoln	100%	215
Saint Francis Medical Center	Grand Island	100%	129
Fremont Area Medical Center	Fremont	99%	77
Faith Regional Health Services	Norfolk	97%	113
Phelps Memorial Health Center	Holdrege	97%	29
Mary Lanning Healthcare	Hastings	96%	79

Medicare Spending

Medicare Spending per Patient (ratio)

Hospital Name	City	Ratio	Cases
Midwest Surgical Hospital	Omaha	0.88	-
Regional West Medical Center	Scottsbluff	0.90	-
Lincoln Surgical Hospital	Lincoln	0.91	-
Columbus Community Hospital	Columbus	0.93	-
Nebraska Orthopaedic Hospital	Omaha	0.93	-
Mary Lanning Healthcare	Hastings	0.95	-
Great Plains Regional Medical Center	North Platte	0.96	-
Good Samaritan Hospital	Kearney	0.98	-
Nebraska Heart Hospital	Lincoln	0.98	-
The Nebraska Medical Center	Omaha	0.98	-
Saint Francis Medical Center	Grand Island	0.98	-
Alegent Creighton-Bergan Mercy Med Ctr	Omaha	1.00	-
Saint Elizabeth Regional Medical Center	Lincoln	1.00	-
Alegent Creighton-Lakeside Hosp	Omaha	1.01	-
Alegent Creighton-Immanuel Med Ctr	Omaha	1.02	-
Bryan Medical Center	Lincoln	1.02	-
Fremont Area Medical Center	Fremont	1.02	-
The Nebraska Methodist Hospital	Omaha	1.02	-
Faith Regional Health Services	Norfolk	1.03	-
Nebraska Spine Hospital	Omaha	1.03	-
Alegent Creighton-Creighton Univ Med	Omaha	1.04	-
Bellevue Medical Center	Bellevue	1.05	-
Alegent Creighton-Midlands Hosp	Papillion	1.06	-

Pneumonia Care

Appropriate Initial Antibiotic Given

Hospital Name	City	Rate	Cases
Alegent Creighton-Creighton Univ Med	Omaha	100%	55
Alegent Creighton-Midlands Hosp	Papillion	100%	49
Bellevue Medical Center	Bellevue	100%	49
Boone County Health Center	Albion	100%	30
Faith Regional Health Services	Norfolk	100%	48
Phelps Memorial Health Center	Holdrege	100%	25
Valley County Health System	Ord	100%	28
Alegent Creighton-Bergan Mercy Med Ctr[2]	Omaha	99%	87
Alegent Creighton-Immanuel Med Ctr	Omaha	99%	86
Alegent Creighton-Lakeside Hosp	Omaha	99%	83
Regional West Medical Center	Scottsbluff	98%	59
Beatrice Comm Hosp & Health Ctr	Beatrice	97%	38
Bryan Medical Center[2]	Lincoln	97%	94
Great Plains Regional Medical Center[2]	North Platte	97%	97
Lexington Regional Health Center	Lexington	97%	30
The Nebraska Methodist Hospital	Omaha	97%	148
Saint Elizabeth Regional Medical Center[2]	Lincoln	97%	77
Good Samaritan Hospital	Kearney	96%	69
Omaha VA Medical Center	Omaha	96%	28
The Nebraska Medical Center[2]	Omaha	95%	37
Saint Francis Medical Center	Grand Island	95%	131
Mary Lanning Healthcare	Hastings	93%	58
Avera Saint Anthony's Hospital	O' Neill	92%	26
Fremont Area Medical Center	Fremont	92%	62
Jennie M Melham Memorial Medical Center	Broken Bow	91%	47
Box Butte General Hospital	Alliance	83%	48
Howard County Medical Center	Saint Paul	81%	27

Blood Culture Timing

Hospital Name	City	Rate	Cases
Alegent Creighton-Bergan Mercy Med Ctr[2]	Omaha	100%	116
Alegent Creighton-Creighton Univ Med	Omaha	100%	64
Alegent Creighton-Immanuel Med Ctr	Omaha	100%	122
Alegent Creighton-Midlands Hosp	Papillion	100%	86
Bellevue Medical Center	Bellevue	100%	115
Columbus Community Hospital	Columbus	100%	27
Community Hospital	Mccook	100%	34
Faith Regional Health Services	Norfolk	100%	113
York General Hospital	York	100%	26
Alegent Creighton-Lakeside Hosp	Omaha	99%	161
Beatrice Comm Hosp & Health Ctr	Beatrice	99%	75
Fremont Area Medical Center	Fremont	99%	96
Good Samaritan Hospital	Kearney	99%	114
Great Plains Regional Medical Center[2]	North Platte	99%	170
The Nebraska Methodist Hospital	Omaha	99%	232
Saint Francis Medical Center	Grand Island	99%	217
Bryan Medical Center[2]	Lincoln	98%	159
Mary Lanning Healthcare	Hastings	98%	64
The Nebraska Medical Center[2]	Omaha	98%	115
Omaha VA Medical Center	Omaha	98%	50
Saint Elizabeth Regional Medical Center[2]	Lincoln	98%	120
Regional West Medical Center	Scottsbluff	96%	112
Box Butte General Hospital	Alliance	85%	34

Pregnancy and Delivery Care

Newborns whose Deliveries were Scheduled Early

Hospital Name	City	Rate	Cases
Alegent Creighton-Immanuel Med Ctr[2]	Omaha	0%	54
Faith Regional Health Services[2]	Norfolk	0%	34
Fremont Area Medical Center	Fremont	0%	54
Alegent Creighton-Bergan Mercy Med Ctr[2]	Omaha	2%	54
Alegent Creighton-Creighton Univ Med[2]	Omaha	2%	41
Bryan Medical Center[2]	Lincoln	2%	50
The Nebraska Methodist Hospital[2]	Omaha	2%	89
Saint Francis Medical Center[2]	Grand Island	2%	58
Regional West Medical Center	Scottsbluff	3%	64
Bellevue Medical Center[2]	Bellevue	5%	42
Good Samaritan Hospital[2]	Kearney	7%	27
Alegent Creighton-Midlands Hosp	Papillion	8%	26
Columbus Community Hospital	Columbus	9%	65
Saint Elizabeth Regional Medical Center[2]	Lincoln	15%	26
Great Plains Regional Medical Center	North Platte	22%	58

Preventive Care

Immunization for Influenza

Hospital Name	City	Rate	Cases
Alegent Creighton-Midlands Hosp[2]	Papillion	100%	275
Alegent Creighton-Bergan Mercy Med Ctr[2]	Omaha	99%	498
Alegent Creighton-Creighton Univ Med[2]	Omaha	99%	567
Nebraska Spine Hospital[2]	Omaha	99%	311
Alegent Creighton-Lakeside Hosp[2]	Omaha	98%	542
Columbus Community Hospital[2]	Columbus	98%	311
Alegent Creighton-Immanuel Med Ctr[2]	Omaha	96%	576
Bryan Medical Center[2]	Lincoln	95%	534
Faith Regional Health Services[2]	Norfolk	95%	510
Nebraska Heart Hospital[2]	Lincoln	95%	320
Saint Elizabeth Regional Medical Center[2]	Lincoln	95%	536
Saint Francis Medical Center[2]	Grand Island	95%	507
Bellevue Medical Center[2]	Bellevue	94%	306
Fremont Area Medical Center[2]	Fremont	94%	305
Great Plains Regional Medical Center[2]	North Platte	94%	435
Nebraska Orthopaedic Hospital[2]	Omaha	94%	321
Community Medical Center	Falls City	93%	270
Lincoln Surgical Hospital[2]	Lincoln	93%	439
Good Samaritan Hospital[2]	Kearney	92%	532

NOTE: Hospital profiles are in alphabetical order by state, then city, then hospital within the city; Rankings exclude hospitals with less than 25 cases except for patient surveys which excludes hospitals with less than 100 cases; (a) 100-299 cases; (1) The number of cases/patients is too few to report; (2) Data submitted were based on a sample of cases/patients; (3) Results are based on a shorter time period than required; (4) Data suppressed by CMS for one or more quarters; (5) Results are not available for this reporting period; (6) Fewer than 100 patients completed the HCAHPS survey; (7) No cases met the criteria for this measure; (8) The lower limit of the confidence interval cannot be calculated if the number of observed infections equals zero; (9) No data are available from the state/territory for this reporting period; (10) The scores shown reflect fewer than 50 completed surveys; (11) There were discrepancies in the data collection process; (12) This measure does not apply to this hospital for this reporting period; (13) Results cannot be calculated for this reporting period; (14) The results for this state are combined with nearby states to protect confidentiality; Please refer to the User's Guide for a full explanation of data.

Hospital Name	City	Rate	Cases
The Nebraska Methodist Hospital[2]	Omaha	85%	560
The Nebraska Medical Center[2]	Omaha	83%	531
Midwest Surgical Hospital	Omaha	76%	443
Box Butte General Hospital	Alliance	72%	53
Mary Lanning Healthcare[2]	Hastings	65%	544
Regional West Medical Center[2]	Scottsbluff	44%	566

Immunization for Pneumonia

Hospital Name	City	Rate	Cases
Alegent Creighton-Creighton Univ Med[2]	Omaha	99%	605
Alegent Creighton-Midlands Hosp[2]	Papillion	99%	328
Columbus Community Hospital[2]	Columbus	99%	416
Alegent Creighton-Bergan Mercy Med Ctr[2]	Omaha	97%	467
Alegent Creighton-Immanuel Med Ctr[2]	Omaha	97%	473
Fremont Area Medical Center[2]	Fremont	97%	358
Saint Elizabeth Regional Medical Center[2]	Lincoln	97%	574
Saint Francis Medical Center[2]	Grand Island	96%	600
Bellevue Medical Center[2]	Bellevue	95%	353
Bryan Medical Center[2]	Lincoln	95%	529
Faith Regional Health Services[2]	Norfolk	94%	517
Alegent Creighton-Lakeside Hosp[2]	Omaha	93%	572
Good Samaritan Hospital[2]	Kearney	93%	637
Great Plains Regional Medical Center[2]	North Platte	93%	555
Nebraska Heart Hospital[2]	Lincoln	91%	538
Community Medical Center	Falls City	89%	319
Lincoln Surgical Hospital[2]	Lincoln	89%	525
Nebraska Orthopaedic Hospital[2]	Omaha	89%	403
Nebraska Spine Hospital[2]	Omaha	89%	337
The Nebraska Medical Center[2]	Omaha	87%	584
Mary Lanning Healthcare[2]	Hastings	86%	455
The Nebraska Methodist Hospital[2]	Omaha	76%	595
Midwest Surgical Hospital	Omaha	72%	272
Regional West Medical Center[2]	Scottsbluff	67%	656
Box Butte General Hospital	Alliance	60%	72

Stroke Care

Anticoagulation Therapy for Atrial Fibrillation

Hospital Name	City	Rate	Cases
Bryan Medical Center	Lincoln	100%	45

Antithrombotic Therapy Timing

Hospital Name	City	Rate	Cases
Alegent Creighton-Creighton Univ Med	Omaha	100%	65
Bellevue Medical Center	Bellevue	100%	52
Faith Regional Health Services	Norfolk	100%	29
Mary Lanning Healthcare	Hastings	100%	35
The Nebraska Medical Center[2]	Omaha	100%	40
Regional West Medical Center	Scottsbluff	100%	32
Saint Elizabeth Regional Medical Center	Lincoln	100%	91
Alegent Creighton-Bergan Mercy Med Ctr	Omaha	99%	71
Alegent Creighton-Immanuel Med Ctr	Omaha	99%	72
Alegent Creighton-Lakeside Hosp	Omaha	99%	85
Bryan Medical Center	Lincoln	99%	167
Good Samaritan Hospital	Kearney	99%	76
Great Plains Regional Medical Center	North Platte	98%	45
Saint Francis Medical Center	Grand Island	98%	53
The Nebraska Methodist Hospital	Omaha	97%	100

Assessed for Rehabilitation

Hospital Name	City	Rate	Cases
Alegent Creighton-Bergan Mercy Med Ctr	Omaha	100%	100
Alegent Creighton-Immanuel Med Ctr	Omaha	100%	89
Alegent Creighton-Lakeside Hosp	Omaha	100%	105
Bellevue Medical Center	Bellevue	100%	51
Bryan Medical Center	Lincoln	100%	221
Mary Lanning Healthcare	Hastings	100%	64
The Nebraska Medical Center[2]	Omaha	100%	95
Regional West Medical Center	Scottsbluff	100%	49
Saint Elizabeth Regional Medical Center	Lincoln	100%	113
Alegent Creighton-Creighton Univ Med	Omaha	97%	96
Faith Regional Health Services	Norfolk	97%	33
Good Samaritan Hospital	Kearney	97%	107
Great Plains Regional Medical Center	North Platte	96%	46
Saint Francis Medical Center	Grand Island	96%	57
The Nebraska Methodist Hospital	Omaha	95%	109

Discharged on Antithrombotic Therapy

Hospital Name	City	Rate	Cases
Alegent Creighton-Bergan Mercy Med Ctr	Omaha	100%	87
Alegent Creighton-Creighton Univ Med	Omaha	100%	76
Alegent Creighton-Immanuel Med Ctr	Omaha	100%	76
Bellevue Medical Center	Bellevue	100%	51
Bryan Medical Center	Lincoln	100%	194
Faith Regional Health Services	Norfolk	100%	31
Good Samaritan Hospital	Kearney	100%	82
Great Plains Regional Medical Center	North Platte	100%	45
Mary Lanning Healthcare	Hastings	100%	58
The Nebraska Medical Center[2]	Omaha	100%	61
Saint Elizabeth Regional Medical Center	Lincoln	100%	105
Saint Francis Medical Center	Grand Island	100%	54
Alegent Creighton-Lakeside Hosp	Omaha	99%	94
The Nebraska Methodist Hospital	Omaha	97%	92
Regional West Medical Center	Scottsbluff	97%	39

Discharged on Statin Medication

Hospital Name	City	Rate	Cases
Alegent Creighton-Bergan Mercy Med Ctr	Omaha	100%	61
Bellevue Medical Center	Bellevue	100%	36
Alegent Creighton-Immanuel Med Ctr	Omaha	98%	66
Mary Lanning Healthcare	Hastings	98%	42
Alegent Creighton-Lakeside Hosp	Omaha	97%	73
Bryan Medical Center	Lincoln	97%	142
Great Plains Regional Medical Center	North Platte	97%	39
Regional West Medical Center	Scottsbluff	97%	29
The Nebraska Medical Center[2]	Omaha	96%	45
Alegent Creighton-Creighton Univ Med	Omaha	94%	54
Saint Elizabeth Regional Medical Center	Lincoln	94%	77
Good Samaritan Hospital	Kearney	88%	68
Faith Regional Health Services	Norfolk	86%	29
Saint Francis Medical Center	Grand Island	81%	43
The Nebraska Methodist Hospital	Omaha	80%	75

Venous Thromboembolism (VTE) Prophylaxis

Hospital Name	City	Rate	Cases
Faith Regional Health Services	Norfolk	100%	32
The Nebraska Medical Center[2]	Omaha	100%	96
Alegent Creighton-Immanuel Med Ctr	Omaha	99%	90
Saint Elizabeth Regional Medical Center	Lincoln	99%	104
Alegent Creighton-Creighton Univ Med	Omaha	98%	97
Bellevue Medical Center	Bellevue	98%	56
Bryan Medical Center	Lincoln	98%	212
Mary Lanning Healthcare	Hastings	98%	48
Alegent Creighton-Bergan Mercy Med Ctr	Omaha	96%	84
Alegent Creighton-Lakeside Hosp	Omaha	96%	105
Good Samaritan Hospital	Kearney	93%	109
Regional West Medical Center	Scottsbluff	93%	46
Great Plains Regional Medical Center	North Platte	92%	48
Saint Francis Medical Center	Grand Island	81%	62
The Nebraska Methodist Hospital	Omaha	79%	135

Written Stroke Educational Materials Given

Hospital Name	City	Rate	Cases
Alegent Creighton-Immanuel Med Ctr	Omaha	100%	41
Bellevue Medical Center	Bellevue	100%	31
The Nebraska Medical Center[2]	Omaha	98%	43
Alegent Creighton-Bergan Mercy Med Ctr	Omaha	97%	59
Alegent Creighton-Creighton Univ Med	Omaha	96%	57
Mary Lanning Healthcare	Hastings	96%	26
Alegent Creighton-Lakeside Hosp	Omaha	94%	52
Saint Elizabeth Regional Medical Center	Lincoln	93%	60
Bryan Medical Center	Lincoln	91%	91
Good Samaritan Hospital	Kearney	62%	48
The Nebraska Methodist Hospital	Omaha	59%	46
Saint Francis Medical Center	Grand Island	39%	28

Surgical Care Improvement Project

Appropriate Beta Blocker Usage

Hospital Name	City	Rate	Cases
Alegent Creighton-Creighton Univ Med[2]	Omaha	100%	205
Bellevue Medical Center	Bellevue	100%	43
Faith Regional Health Services	Norfolk	100%	284
Lincoln Surgical Hospital[2]	Lincoln	100%	49
The Nebraska Medical Center[2]	Omaha	100%	231
Alegent Creighton-Bergan Mercy Med Ctr[2]	Omaha	99%	353
Alegent Creighton-Immanuel Med Ctr[2]	Omaha	99%	135
Alegent Creighton-Lakeside Hosp[2]	Omaha	99%	125
Bryan Medical Center[2]	Lincoln	99%	411
The Nebraska Methodist Hospital	Omaha	99%	378
Regional West Medical Center[2]	Scottsbluff	99%	122
Saint Francis Medical Center	Grand Island	99%	212
Columbus Community Hospital	Columbus	98%	63
Community Medical Center	Falls City	98%	40
Great Plains Regional Medical Center	North Platte	98%	112
Nebraska Heart Hospital[2]	Lincoln	98%	164
Nebraska Orthopaedic Hospital[2]	Omaha	98%	97
Saint Elizabeth Regional Medical Center[2]	Lincoln	98%	113
Midwest Surgical Hospital	Omaha	97%	74
Good Samaritan Hospital	Kearney	96%	443
Phelps Memorial Health Center	Holdrege	96%	25
Omaha VA Medical Center[2]	Omaha	95%	94
Mary Lanning Healthcare	Hastings	93%	159
Fremont Area Medical Center[2]	Fremont	89%	102

Appropriate VTP Within 24 Hours

Hospital Name	City	Rate	Cases
Alegent Creighton-Creighton Univ Med[2]	Omaha	100%	297
Alegent Creighton-Immanuel Med Ctr[2]	Omaha	100%	305
Butler County Health Care Center	David City	100%	32
Community Hospital	Mccook	100%	72
Faith Regional Health Services	Norfolk	100%	459
Lincoln Surgical Hospital[2]	Lincoln	100%	235
Midwest Surgical Hospital	Omaha	100%	194
Saint Francis Memorial Hospital	West Point	100%	36
Sidney Regional Medical Center	Sidney	100%	40
York General Hospital	York	100%	51
Alegent Creighton-Bergan Mercy Med Ctr[2]	Omaha	99%	423
Alegent Creighton-Lakeside Hosp[2]	Omaha	99%	362
Alegent Creighton-Midlands Hosp	Papillion	99%	79
Bellevue Medical Center	Bellevue	99%	136
Columbus Community Hospital	Columbus	99%	153
Fremont Area Medical Center[2]	Fremont	99%	318
Good Samaritan Hospital	Kearney	99%	1019
Great Plains Regional Medical Center	North Platte	99%	272
The Nebraska Medical Center[2]	Omaha	99%	308
Nebraska Orthopaedic Hospital[2]	Omaha	99%	261
Omaha VA Medical Center[2]	Omaha	99%	195
Phelps Memorial Health Center	Holdrege	99%	78
Saint Elizabeth Regional Medical Center[2]	Lincoln	99%	332
Saint Francis Medical Center	Grand Island	99%	490
Community Medical Center	Falls City	98%	104
The Nebraska Methodist Hospital	Omaha	98%	1873
Regional West Medical Center[2]	Scottsbluff	98%	397
Avera Saint Anthony's Hospital	O'Neill	97%	38
Bryan Medical Center[2]	Lincoln	97%	583
Mary Lanning Healthcare	Hastings	97%	421
Lexington Regional Health Center	Lexington	95%	39
Beatrice Comm Hosp & Health Ctr	Beatrice	94%	51

Controlled Postoperative Blood Glucose

Hospital Name	City	Rate	Cases
Alegent Creighton-Bergan Mercy Med Ctr[2]	Omaha	99%	184
Bryan Medical Center[2]	Lincoln	98%	251
The Nebraska Medical Center[2]	Omaha	98%	131
Faith Regional Health Services	Norfolk	97%	76
Good Samaritan Hospital	Kearney	95%	99
Alegent Creighton-Creighton Univ Med[2]	Omaha	94%	140
Nebraska Heart Hospital[2]	Lincoln	93%	176
The Nebraska Methodist Hospital	Omaha	92%	250

Perioperative Temperature Management

Hospital Name	City	Rate	Cases
Alegent Creighton-Bergan Mercy Med Ctr[2]	Omaha	100%	687
Alegent Creighton-Creighton Univ Med[2]	Omaha	100%	340
Alegent Creighton-Immanuel Med Ctr[2]	Omaha	100%	337
Alegent Creighton-Lakeside Hosp[2]	Omaha	100%	402
Alegent Creighton-Midlands Hosp	Papillion	100%	85
Avera Saint Anthony's Hospital	O'Neill	100%	40
Beatrice Comm Hosp & Health Ctr	Beatrice	100%	58
Bellevue Medical Center	Bellevue	100%	153
Bryan Medical Center[2]	Lincoln	100%	802
Butler County Health Care Center	David City	100%	32
Columbus Community Hospital	Columbus	100%	170
Community Hospital	Mccook	100%	79
Community Medical Center	Falls City	100%	108
Faith Regional Health Services	Norfolk	100%	531
Fremont Area Medical Center[2]	Fremont	100%	362
Good Samaritan Hospital	Kearney	100%	1184
Great Plains Regional Medical Center	North Platte	100%	299
Jefferson Community Health Center	Fairbury	100%	28
Lexington Regional Health Center	Lexington	100%	45
Mary Lanning Healthcare	Hastings	100%	469
Memorial Hospital	Aurora	100%	25
Midwest Surgical Hospital	Omaha	100%	259
Nebraska Heart Hospital[2]	Lincoln	100%	153
The Nebraska Medical Center[2]	Omaha	100%	426
The Nebraska Methodist Hospital	Omaha	100%	2288
Nebraska Orthopaedic Hospital[2]	Omaha	100%	277
Omaha VA Medical Center[2]	Omaha	100%	235
Saint Elizabeth Regional Medical Center[2]	Lincoln	100%	391
Saint Francis Medical Center	Grand Island	100%	647
Saint Francis Memorial Hospital	West Point	100%	36
York General Hospital	York	100%	58
Lincoln Surgical Hospital[2]	Lincoln	99%	240
Regional West Medical Center[2]	Scottsbluff	99%	538
Sidney Regional Medical Center	Sidney	98%	57
Phelps Memorial Health Center	Holdrege	94%	87

Prophylactic Antibiotic Selection

Hospital Name	City	Rate	Cases
Alegent Creighton-Creighton Univ Med[2]	Omaha	100%	321
Alegent Creighton-Immanuel Med Ctr[2]	Omaha	100%	190
Alegent Creighton-Lakeside Hosp[2]	Omaha	100%	251

NOTE: Hospital profiles are in alphabetical order by state, then city, then hospital within the city; Rankings exclude hospitals with less than 25 cases except for patient surveys which excludes hospitals with less than 100 cases; (a) 100-299 cases; (1) The number of cases/patients is too few to report; (2) Data submitted were based on a sample of cases/patients; (3) Results are based on a shorter time period than required; (4) Data suppressed by CMS for one or more quarters; (5) Results are not available for this reporting period; (6) Fewer than 100 patients completed the HCAHPS survey; (7) No cases met the criteria for this measure; (8) The lower limit of the confidence interval cannot be calculated if the number of observed infections equals zero; (9) No data are available from the state/territory for this reporting period; (10) The scores shown reflect fewer than 50 completed surveys; (11) There were discrepancies in the data collection process; (12) This measure does not apply to this hospital for this reporting period; (13) Results cannot be calculated for this reporting period; (14) The results for this state are combined with nearby states to protect confidentiality; Please refer to the User's Guide for a full explanation of data.

Hospital Name	City	Rate	Cases
Alegent Creighton-Midlands Hosp	Papillion	100%	44
Beatrice Comm Hosp & Health Ctr	Beatrice	100%	47
Bellevue Medical Center	Bellevue	100%	99
Community Hospital	Mccook	100%	62
Faith Regional Health Services	Norfolk	100%	460
Good Samaritan Hospital	Kearney	100%	862
Great Plains Regional Medical Center	North Platte	100%	207
Jefferson Community Health Center	Fairbury	100%	25
Lexington Regional Health Center	Lexington	100%	40
Lincoln Surgical Hospital[2]	Lincoln	100%	179
Midwest Surgical Hospital	Omaha	100%	224
The Nebraska Methodist Hospital	Omaha	100%	1449
Nebraska Orthopaedic Hospital[2]	Omaha	100%	192
Saint Francis Medical Center	Grand Island	100%	423
York General Hospital	York	100%	61
Alegent Creighton-Bergan Mercy Med Ctr[2]	Omaha	99%	582
Bryan Medical Center[2]	Lincoln	99%	643
Columbus Community Hospital	Columbus	99%	127
Mary Lanning Healthcare	Hastings	99%	345
The Nebraska Medical Center[2]	Omaha	99%	391
Omaha VA Medical Center	Omaha	99%	151
Phelps Memorial Health Center	Holdrege	99%	85
Saint Elizabeth Regional Medical Center[2]	Lincoln	99%	207
Fremont Area Medical Center[2]	Fremont	98%	254
Nebraska Heart Hospital[2]	Lincoln	98%	194
Regional West Medical Center[2]	Scottsbluff	98%	344
Avera Saint Anthony's Hospital	O'Neill	97%	37
Butler County Health Care Center	David City	97%	31
Community Medical Center	Falls City	97%	101
Sidney Regional Medical Center	Sidney	95%	61
Saint Francis Memorial Hospital	West Point	92%	37

Prophylactic Antibiotic Selection (Outpatient)

Hospital Name	City	Rate	Cases
Alegent Creighton-Immanuel Med Ctr	Omaha	100%	152
Alegent Creighton-Lakeside Hosp	Omaha	100%	259
Alegent Creighton-Midlands Hosp	Papillion	100%	110
Faith Regional Health Services	Norfolk	100%	233
Midwest Surgical Hospital	Omaha	100%	346
Nebraska Orthopaedic Hospital	Omaha	100%	77
Nebraska Spine Hospital	Omaha	100%	331
Alegent Creighton-Bergan Mercy Med Ctr	Omaha	99%	646
Alegent Creighton-Creighton Univ Med	Omaha	99%	224
Bryan Medical Center	Lincoln	99%	808
Columbus Community Hospital	Columbus	99%	68
Fremont Area Medical Center	Fremont	99%	84
Lincoln Surgical Hospital	Lincoln	99%	186
Nebraska Heart Hospital	Lincoln	99%	415
Regional West Medical Center	Scottsbluff	99%	134
Saint Elizabeth Regional Medical Center	Lincoln	99%	419
Saint Francis Medical Center	Grand Island	99%	114
Good Samaritan Hospital	Kearney	98%	364
Mary Lanning Healthcare	Hastings	98%	164
The Nebraska Medical Center	Omaha	98%	320
The Nebraska Methodist Hospital	Omaha	98%	1099
Beatrice Comm Hosp & Health Ctr	Beatrice	97%	34
Bellevue Medical Center	Bellevue	96%	51
Great Plains Regional Medical Center	North Platte	95%	164

Prophylactic Antibiotic Stopped

Hospital Name	City	Rate	Cases
Alegent Creighton-Creighton Univ Med[2]	Omaha	100%	312
Alegent Creighton-Lakeside Hosp[2]	Omaha	100%	247
Beatrice Comm Hosp & Health Ctr	Beatrice	100%	47
Bellevue Medical Center	Bellevue	100%	96
Butler County Health Care Center	David City	100%	30
Jefferson Community Health Center	Fairbury	100%	25
Lexington Regional Health Center	Lexington	100%	40
Lincoln Surgical Hospital[2]	Lincoln	100%	179
Midwest Surgical Hospital	Omaha	100%	224
The Nebraska Medical Center[2]	Omaha	100%	384
Sidney Regional Medical Center	Sidney	100%	61
York General Hospital	York	100%	61
Alegent Creighton-Bergan Mercy Med Ctr[2]	Omaha	99%	568
Alegent Creighton-Immanuel Med Ctr[2]	Omaha	99%	185
Columbus Community Hospital	Columbus	99%	123
Faith Regional Health Services	Norfolk	99%	446
Saint Elizabeth Regional Medical Center[2]	Lincoln	99%	206
Community Hospital	Mccook	98%	62
The Nebraska Methodist Hospital	Omaha	98%	1405
Nebraska Orthopaedic Hospital[2]	Omaha	98%	190
Saint Francis Medical Center	Grand Island	98%	410
Avera Saint Anthony's Hospital	O'Neill	97%	37
Bryan Medical Center[2]	Lincoln	97%	600
Good Samaritan Hospital	Kearney	97%	846
Omaha VA Medical Center	Omaha	97%	151
Saint Francis Memorial Hospital	West Point	97%	37
Great Plains Regional Medical Center	North Platte	96%	200
Mary Lanning Healthcare	Hastings	96%	333
Alegent Creighton-Midlands Hosp	Papillion	95%	44

Hospital Name	City	Rate	Cases
Community Medical Center	Falls City	95%	99
Regional West Medical Center[2]	Scottsbluff	95%	340
Fremont Area Medical Center[2]	Fremont	94%	251
Phelps Memorial Health Center	Holdrege	93%	85
Nebraska Heart Hospital[2]	Lincoln	90%	190

Prophylactic Antibiotic Timing

Hospital Name	City	Rate	Cases
Alegent Creighton-Midlands Hosp	Papillion	100%	44
Beatrice Comm Hosp & Health Ctr	Beatrice	100%	47
Bellevue Medical Center	Bellevue	100%	99
Columbus Community Hospital	Columbus	100%	127
Community Hospital	Mccook	100%	62
Faith Regional Health Services	Norfolk	100%	460
Good Samaritan Hospital	Kearney	100%	863
Great Plains Regional Medical Center	North Platte	100%	207
Lexington Regional Health Center	Lexington	100%	40
Nebraska Heart Hospital[2]	Lincoln	100%	195
Saint Elizabeth Regional Medical Center[2]	Lincoln	100%	207
Saint Francis Medical Center	Grand Island	100%	423
Alegent Creighton-Bergan Mercy Med Ctr[2]	Omaha	99%	583
Alegent Creighton-Creighton Univ Med[2]	Omaha	99%	323
Alegent Creighton-Immanuel Med Ctr[2]	Omaha	99%	190
Alegent Creighton-Lakeside Hosp[2]	Omaha	99%	251
Lincoln Surgical Hospital[2]	Lincoln	99%	179
Mary Lanning Healthcare	Hastings	99%	345
Nebraska Orthopaedic Hospital[2]	Omaha	99%	192
Regional West Medical Center[2]	Scottsbluff	99%	344
Bryan Medical Center[2]	Lincoln	98%	645
Fremont Area Medical Center[2]	Fremont	98%	254
Phelps Memorial Health Center	Holdrege	98%	85
York General Hospital	York	98%	61
Avera Saint Anthony's Hospital	O'Neill	97%	37
The Nebraska Methodist Hospital	Omaha	97%	1450
The Nebraska Medical Center[2]	Omaha	96%	394
Community Medical Center	Falls City	95%	101
Midwest Surgical Hospital	Omaha	93%	224
Jefferson Community Health Center	Fairbury	92%	25
Sidney Regional Medical Center	Sidney	92%	62
Butler County Health Care Center	David City	90%	31
Saint Francis Memorial Hospital	West Point	89%	37
Omaha VA Medical Center	Omaha	79%	154

Prophylactic Antibiotic Timing (Outpatient)

Hospital Name	City	Rate	Cases
Alegent Creighton-Creighton Univ Med	Omaha	100%	224
Alegent Creighton-Immanuel Med Ctr	Omaha	100%	151
Alegent Creighton-Lakeside Hosp	Omaha	100%	259
Faith Regional Health Services	Norfolk	100%	226
Nebraska Orthopaedic Hospital	Omaha	100%	77
Alegent Creighton-Bergan Mercy Med Ctr	Omaha	99%	649
Lincoln Surgical Hospital	Lincoln	99%	188
Nebraska Spine Hospital	Omaha	99%	331
Regional West Medical Center	Scottsbluff	99%	134
Saint Elizabeth Regional Medical Center	Lincoln	99%	420
Saint Francis Medical Center	Grand Island	99%	115
Alegent Creighton-Midlands Hosp	Papillion	98%	111
Bellevue Medical Center	Bellevue	98%	51
Bryan Medical Center	Lincoln	98%	813
The Nebraska Methodist Hospital	Omaha	98%	1112
Beatrice Comm Hosp & Health Ctr	Beatrice	97%	35
Great Plains Regional Medical Center	North Platte	97%	165
Columbus Community Hospital	Columbus	96%	70
Fremont Area Medical Center	Fremont	96%	84
Good Samaritan Hospital	Kearney	96%	364
Midwest Surgical Hospital	Omaha	96%	347
The Nebraska Medical Center	Omaha	92%	331
Mary Lanning Healthcare	Hastings	90%	173
Nebraska Heart Hospital	Lincoln	88%	420

Urinary Catheter Removal

Hospital Name	City	Rate	Cases
Alegent Creighton-Immanuel Med Ctr[2]	Omaha	100%	246
Alegent Creighton-Lakeside Hosp[2]	Omaha	100%	290
Alegent Creighton-Midlands Hosp	Papillion	100%	55
Avera Saint Anthony's Hospital	O'Neill	100%	37
Bellevue Medical Center	Bellevue	100%	76
Community Hospital	Mccook	100%	32
Faith Regional Health Services	Norfolk	100%	446
Great Plains Regional Medical Center	North Platte	100%	241
Lexington Regional Health Center	Lexington	100%	28
Midwest Surgical Hospital	Omaha	100%	175
Phelps Memorial Health Center	Holdrege	100%	49
York General Hospital	York	100%	46
Alegent Creighton-Bergan Mercy Med Ctr[2]	Omaha	99%	501
Lincoln Surgical Hospital[2]	Lincoln	99%	151
Mary Lanning Healthcare	Hastings	99%	276
The Nebraska Medical Center[2]	Omaha	99%	296
Nebraska Orthopaedic Hospital[2]	Omaha	99%	141
Omaha VA Medical Center[2]	Omaha	99%	158

Hospital Name	City	Rate	Cases
Saint Francis Medical Center	Grand Island	98%	425
Alegent Creighton-Creighton Univ Med[2]	Omaha	97%	199
Columbus Community Hospital	Columbus	97%	30
The Nebraska Methodist Hospital	Omaha	97%	1393
Fremont Area Medical Center[2]	Fremont	96%	80
Good Samaritan Hospital	Kearney	96%	521
Saint Elizabeth Regional Medical Center[2]	Lincoln	96%	217
Bryan Medical Center[2]	Lincoln	94%	456
Nebraska Heart Hospital[2]	Lincoln	93%	213
Regional West Medical Center[2]	Scottsbluff	93%	320

Survey of Patients' Hospital Experiences

Area Around Room 'Always' Quiet at Night

Hospital Name	City	Rate	Cases
Midwest Surgical Hospital	Omaha	91%	300+
Nebraska Orthopaedic Hospital	Omaha	85%	300+
Pender Community Hospital	Pender	79%	(a)
Brodstone Memorial Hospital	Superior	76%	(a)
Avera Saint Anthony's Hospital	O'Neill	75%	(a)
Community Medical Center	Falls City	74%	(a)
Lincoln Surgical Hospital	Lincoln	74%	300+
Chadron Comm Hosp & Health Services	Chadron	73%	(a)
Community Hospital	Mccook	71%	(a)
Nebraska Spine Hospital	Omaha	71%	300+
Bellevue Medical Center	Bellevue	69%	300+
Cherry County Hospital	Valentine	69%	(a)
Butler County Health Care Center	David City	68%	(a)
Ogallala Community Hospital[11]	Ogallala	68%	(a)
Faith Regional Health Services	Norfolk	67%	300+
Phelps Memorial Health Center	Holdrege	67%	(a)
Boone County Health Center	Albion	65%	(a)
Bryan Medical Center	Lincoln	65%	300+
Gothenburg Memorial Hospital	Gothenburg	65%	(a)
York General Hospital	York	65%	(a)
Saint Francis Medical Center	Grand Island	64%	300+
Alegent Creighton-Lakeside Hosp	Omaha	63%	300+
Alegent Creighton-Midlands Hosp	Papillion	63%	(a)
Beatrice Comm Hosp & Health Ctr	Beatrice	63%	(a)
Alegent Creighton-Bergan Mercy Med Ctr	Omaha	62%	300+
Saint Elizabeth Regional Medical Center	Lincoln	62%	300+
Alegent Creighton-Immanuel Med Ctr	Omaha	61%	300+
Good Samaritan Hospital	Kearney	61%	300+
Lexington Regional Health Center	Lexington	61%	(a)
Mary Lanning Healthcare	Hastings	61%	300+
The Nebraska Medical Center	Omaha	58%	300+
Columbus Community Hospital	Columbus	57%	300+
The Nebraska Methodist Hospital	Omaha	57%	300+
Regional West Medical Center	Scottsbluff	57%	300+
Tri Valley Health System	Cambridge	57%	(a)
Jennie M Melham Memorial Medical Center	Broken Bow	56%	(a)
Alegent Creighton-Creighton Univ Med	Omaha	54%	300+
Sidney Regional Medical Center	Sidney	54%	(a)
Nebraska Heart Hospital	Lincoln	53%	300+
Box Butte General Hospital	Alliance	51%	(a)
Great Plains Regional Medical Center	North Platte	51%	300+
Fremont Area Medical Center	Fremont	48%	300+

Doctors 'Always' Communicated Well

Hospital Name	City	Rate	Cases
Pender Community Hospital	Pender	95%	(a)
Boone County Health Center	Albion	93%	(a)
Ogallala Community Hospital[11]	Ogallala	92%	(a)
Beatrice Comm Hosp & Health Ctr	Beatrice	91%	(a)
Brodstone Memorial Hospital	Superior	91%	(a)
Butler County Health Care Center	David City	91%	(a)
Community Medical Center	Falls City	90%	(a)
Midwest Surgical Hospital	Omaha	90%	300+
Community Hospital	Mccook	89%	(a)
Avera Saint Anthony's Hospital	O'Neill	88%	(a)
Lincoln Surgical Hospital	Lincoln	88%	300+
Chadron Comm Hosp & Health Services	Chadron	87%	(a)
Gothenburg Memorial Hospital	Gothenburg	87%	(a)
Nebraska Orthopaedic Hospital	Omaha	87%	300+
Phelps Memorial Health Center	Holdrege	85%	(a)
Tri Valley Health System	Cambridge	85%	(a)
York General Hospital	York	85%	(a)
Alegent Creighton-Lakeside Hosp	Omaha	84%	300+
Box Butte General Hospital	Alliance	84%	(a)
Jennie M Melham Memorial Medical Center	Broken Bow	84%	(a)
Lexington Regional Health Center	Lexington	84%	(a)
Sidney Regional Medical Center	Sidney	84%	(a)
Alegent Creighton-Immanuel Med Ctr	Omaha	83%	300+
Cherry County Hospital	Valentine	83%	(a)
Mary Lanning Healthcare	Hastings	83%	300+
The Nebraska Methodist Hospital	Omaha	83%	300+
Alegent Creighton-Bergan Mercy Med Ctr	Omaha	82%	300+
Alegent Creighton-Midlands Hosp	Papillion	82%	(a)
Bellevue Medical Center	Bellevue	82%	300+
Nebraska Heart Hospital	Lincoln	82%	300+

NOTE: Hospital profiles are in alphabetical order by state, then city, then hospital within the city; Rankings exclude hospitals with less than 25 cases except for patient surveys which excludes hospitals with less than 100 cases; (a) 100-299 cases; (1) The number of cases/patients is too few to report; (2) Data submitted were based on a sample of cases/patients; (3) Results are based on a shorter time period than required; (4) Data suppressed by CMS for one or more quarters; (5) Results are not available for this reporting period; (6) Fewer than 100 patients completed the HCAHPS survey; (7) No cases met the criteria for this measure; (8) The lower limit of the confidence interval cannot be calculated if the number of observed infections equals zero; (9) No data are available from the state/territory for this reporting period; (10) The scores shown reflect fewer than 50 completed surveys; (11) There were discrepancies in the data collection process; (12) This measure does not apply to this hospital for this reporting period; (13) Results cannot be calculated for this reporting period; (14) The results for this state are combined with nearby states to protect confidentiality; Please refer to the User's Guide for a full explanation of data.

Hospital Name	City	Rate	Cases
Nebraska Spine Hospital	Omaha	82%	300+
Faith Regional Health Services	Norfolk	81%	300+
Good Samaritan Hospital	Kearney	81%	300+
Great Plains Regional Medical Center	North Platte	81%	300+
Saint Elizabeth Regional Medical Center	Lincoln	81%	300+
Saint Francis Medical Center	Grand Island	81%	300+
Bryan Medical Center	Lincoln	80%	300+
Columbus Community Hospital	Columbus	80%	300+
Fremont Area Medical Center	Fremont	80%	300+
Regional West Medical Center	Scottsbluff	79%	300+
Alegent Creighton-Creighton Univ Med	Omaha	78%	300+
The Nebraska Medical Center	Omaha	78%	300+

Home Recovery Information Given

Hospital Name	City	Rate	Cases
Lincoln Surgical Hospital	Lincoln	95%	300+
Nebraska Orthopaedic Hospital	Omaha	94%	300+
Ogallala Community Hospital[11]	Ogallala	94%	(a)
Avera Saint Anthony's Hospital	O' Neill	93%	(a)
Box Butte General Hospital	Alliance	93%	(a)
Nebraska Spine Hospital	Omaha	93%	300+
Alegent Creighton-Immanuel Med Ctr	Omaha	92%	300+
Beatrice Comm Hosp & Health Ctr	Beatrice	92%	(a)
Nebraska Heart Hospital	Lincoln	92%	300+
Pender Community Hospital	Pender	92%	(a)
Sidney Regional Medical Center	Sidney	92%	(a)
Brodstone Memorial Hospital	Superior	91%	(a)
Bryan Medical Center	Lincoln	91%	300+
Lexington Regional Health Center	Lexington	91%	(a)
Midwest Surgical Hospital	Omaha	91%	300+
Alegent Creighton-Lakeside Hosp	Omaha	90%	300+
Alegent Creighton-Midlands Hosp	Papillion	90%	(a)
Cherry County Hospital	Valentine	90%	(a)
Columbus Community Hospital	Columbus	90%	300+
Community Medical Center	Falls City	90%	(a)
Fremont Area Medical Center	Fremont	90%	300+
Great Plains Regional Medical Center	North Platte	90%	300+
The Nebraska Methodist Hospital	Omaha	90%	300+
Saint Elizabeth Regional Medical Center	Lincoln	90%	300+
Saint Francis Medical Center	Grand Island	90%	300+
Alegent Creighton-Bergan Mercy Med Ctr	Omaha	89%	300+
Boone County Health Center	Albion	89%	(a)
Butler County Health Care Center	David City	89%	(a)
Faith Regional Health Services	Norfolk	89%	300+
Mary Lanning Healthcare	Hastings	89%	300+
The Nebraska Medical Center	Omaha	89%	300+
Phelps Memorial Health Center	Holdrege	89%	(a)
Regional West Medical Center	Scottsbluff	89%	300+
Community Hospital	Mccook	88%	(a)
Good Samaritan Hospital	Kearney	88%	300+
Alegent Creighton-Creighton Univ Med	Omaha	85%	300+
Bellevue Medical Center	Bellevue	85%	300+
Jennie M Melham Memorial Medical Center	Broken Bow	85%	(a)
Tri Valley Health System	Cambridge	84%	(a)
York General Hospital	York	84%	(a)
Chadron Comm Hosp & Health Services	Chadron	82%	(a)
Gothenburg Memorial Hospital	Gothenburg	81%	(a)

Hospital Given 9 or 10 on 10 Point Scale

Hospital Name	City	Rate	Cases
Nebraska Orthopaedic Hospital	Omaha	92%	300+
Midwest Surgical Hospital	Omaha	91%	300+
Boone County Health Center	Albion	88%	(a)
Avera Saint Anthony's Hospital	O' Neill	87%	(a)
Butler County Health Care Center	David City	86%	(a)
Pender Community Hospital	Pender	86%	(a)
Lincoln Surgical Hospital	Lincoln	85%	300+
Ogallala Community Hospital[11]	Ogallala	83%	(a)
Phelps Memorial Health Center	Holdrege	83%	(a)
Community Medical Center	Falls City	82%	(a)
Nebraska Spine Hospital	Omaha	82%	300+
Brodstone Memorial Hospital	Superior	81%	(a)
Nebraska Heart Hospital	Lincoln	81%	300+
Alegent Creighton-Lakeside Hosp	Omaha	79%	300+
The Nebraska Methodist Hospital	Omaha	79%	300+
York General Hospital	York	79%	(a)
Alegent Creighton-Midlands Hosp	Papillion	78%	(a)
Community Hospital	Mccook	78%	(a)
Alegent Creighton-Immanuel Med Ctr	Omaha	77%	300+
Beatrice Comm Hosp & Health Ctr	Beatrice	77%	(a)
Bryan Medical Center	Lincoln	77%	300+
Saint Elizabeth Regional Medical Center	Lincoln	77%	300+
Saint Francis Medical Center	Grand Island	77%	300+
Alegent Creighton-Bergan Mercy Med Ctr	Omaha	76%	300+
Cherry County Hospital	Valentine	76%	(a)
Gothenburg Memorial Hospital	Gothenburg	76%	(a)
Bellevue Medical Center	Bellevue	75%	300+
Lexington Regional Health Center	Lexington	75%	(a)
Sidney Regional Medical Center	Sidney	75%	(a)
Columbus Community Hospital	Columbus	74%	300+

Hospital Name	City	Rate	Cases
Jennie M Melham Memorial Medical Center	Broken Bow	74%	(a)
Mary Lanning Healthcare	Hastings	74%	300+
The Nebraska Medical Center	Omaha	74%	300+
Good Samaritan Hospital	Kearney	73%	300+
Fremont Area Medical Center	Fremont	72%	300+
Faith Regional Health Services	Norfolk	70%	300+
Alegent Creighton-Creighton Univ Med	Omaha	67%	300+
Chadron Comm Hosp & Health Services	Chadron	67%	(a)
Tri Valley Health System	Cambridge	67%	(a)
Regional West Medical Center	Scottsbluff	66%	300+
Great Plains Regional Medical Center	North Platte	61%	300+
Box Butte General Hospital	Alliance	53%	(a)

Meds 'Always' Explained Before Given

Hospital Name	City	Rate	Cases
Chadron Comm Hosp & Health Services	Chadron	78%	(a)
Nebraska Orthopaedic Hospital	Omaha	77%	300+
Pender Community Hospital	Pender	77%	(a)
Lincoln Surgical Hospital	Lincoln	76%	300+
Boone County Health Center	Albion	74%	(a)
Brodstone Memorial Hospital	Superior	74%	(a)
Midwest Surgical Hospital	Omaha	74%	300+
Avera Saint Anthony's Hospital	O' Neill	73%	(a)
Beatrice Comm Hosp & Health Ctr	Beatrice	73%	(a)
Community Medical Center	Falls City	73%	(a)
Box Butte General Hospital	Alliance	72%	(a)
Cherry County Hospital	Valentine	72%	(a)
Nebraska Spine Hospital	Omaha	71%	300+
Community Hospital	Mccook	70%	(a)
Lexington Regional Health Center	Lexington	70%	(a)
Ogallala Community Hospital[11]	Ogallala	69%	(a)
Sidney Regional Medical Center	Sidney	69%	(a)
Phelps Memorial Health Center	Holdrege	68%	(a)
Alegent Creighton-Immanuel Med Ctr	Omaha	67%	300+
Fremont Area Medical Center	Fremont	67%	300+
Nebraska Heart Hospital	Lincoln	67%	300+
Alegent Creighton-Lakeside Hosp	Omaha	66%	300+
Saint Francis Medical Center	Grand Island	66%	300+
York General Hospital	York	66%	(a)
Bryan Medical Center	Lincoln	65%	300+
Gothenburg Memorial Hospital	Gothenburg	65%	(a)
Mary Lanning Healthcare	Hastings	65%	300+
Saint Elizabeth Regional Medical Center	Lincoln	65%	300+
Alegent Creighton-Bergan Mercy Med Ctr	Omaha	64%	300+
Alegent Creighton-Midlands Hosp	Papillion	64%	(a)
Good Samaritan Hospital	Kearney	64%	300+
Regional West Medical Center	Scottsbluff	64%	300+
Bellevue Medical Center	Bellevue	63%	300+
Jennie M Melham Memorial Medical Center	Broken Bow	63%	(a)
Tri Valley Health System	Cambridge	63%	(a)
Columbus Community Hospital	Columbus	62%	300+
The Nebraska Medical Center	Omaha	62%	300+
The Nebraska Methodist Hospital	Omaha	62%	300+
Alegent Creighton-Creighton Univ Med	Omaha	61%	300+
Great Plains Regional Medical Center	North Platte	61%	300+
Butler County Health Care Center	David City	58%	(a)
Faith Regional Health Services	Norfolk	57%	300+

Nurses 'Always' Communicated Well

Hospital Name	City	Rate	Cases
Nebraska Orthopaedic Hospital	Omaha	91%	300+
Pender Community Hospital	Pender	91%	(a)
Beatrice Comm Hosp & Health Ctr	Beatrice	90%	(a)
Community Medical Center	Falls City	90%	(a)
Midwest Surgical Hospital	Omaha	90%	300+
Avera Saint Anthony's Hospital	O' Neill	87%	(a)
Butler County Health Care Center	David City	86%	(a)
Lincoln Surgical Hospital	Lincoln	86%	300+
Boone County Health Center	Albion	85%	(a)
Brodstone Memorial Hospital	Superior	85%	(a)
Ogallala Community Hospital[11]	Ogallala	85%	(a)
Nebraska Spine Hospital	Omaha	84%	300+
Community Hospital	Mccook	83%	(a)
The Nebraska Methodist Hospital	Omaha	83%	300+
Alegent Creighton-Lakeside Hosp	Omaha	82%	300+
Alegent Creighton-Midlands Hosp	Papillion	82%	(a)
Gothenburg Memorial Hospital	Gothenburg	82%	(a)
Jennie M Melham Memorial Medical Center	Broken Bow	82%	(a)
Nebraska Heart Hospital	Lincoln	82%	300+
Bellevue Medical Center	Bellevue	81%	300+
Alegent Creighton-Immanuel Med Ctr	Omaha	80%	300+
Saint Francis Medical Center	Grand Island	80%	300+
Sidney Regional Medical Center	Sidney	80%	(a)
Alegent Creighton-Bergan Mercy Med Ctr	Omaha	79%	300+
Bryan Medical Center	Lincoln	79%	300+
Chadron Comm Hosp & Health Services	Chadron	79%	(a)
Cherry County Hospital	Valentine	79%	(a)
Faith Regional Health Services	Norfolk	79%	300+
Mary Lanning Healthcare	Hastings	79%	300+
Phelps Memorial Health Center	Holdrege	79%	(a)

Hospital Name	City	Rate	Cases
Saint Elizabeth Regional Medical Center	Lincoln	79%	300+
York General Hospital	York	79%	(a)
Columbus Community Hospital	Columbus	78%	300+
Fremont Area Medical Center	Fremont	78%	300+
Good Samaritan Hospital	Kearney	78%	300+
Lexington Regional Health Center	Lexington	78%	(a)
The Nebraska Medical Center	Omaha	78%	300+
Great Plains Regional Medical Center	North Platte	76%	300+
Regional West Medical Center	Scottsbluff	76%	300+
Box Butte General Hospital	Alliance	75%	(a)
Alegent Creighton-Creighton Univ Med	Omaha	74%	300+
Tri Valley Health System	Cambridge	71%	(a)

Pain 'Always' Well Controlled

Hospital Name	City	Rate	Cases
Ogallala Community Hospital[11]	Ogallala	82%	(a)
Midwest Surgical Hospital	Omaha	81%	300+
Avera Saint Anthony's Hospital	O' Neill	79%	(a)
Pender Community Hospital	Pender	79%	(a)
Nebraska Orthopaedic Hospital	Omaha	78%	300+
Butler County Health Care Center	David City	76%	(a)
Lincoln Surgical Hospital	Lincoln	76%	300+
Nebraska Heart Hospital	Lincoln	76%	300+
Alegent Creighton-Midlands Hosp	Papillion	75%	(a)
Community Medical Center	Falls City	75%	(a)
Lexington Regional Health Center	Lexington	75%	(a)
Alegent Creighton-Lakeside Hosp	Omaha	74%	300+
Beatrice Comm Hosp & Health Ctr	Beatrice	74%	(a)
Boone County Health Center	Albion	74%	(a)
Alegent Creighton-Immanuel Med Ctr	Omaha	73%	300+
Fremont Area Medical Center	Fremont	73%	300+
Alegent Creighton-Bergan Mercy Med Ctr	Omaha	72%	300+
Box Butte General Hospital	Alliance	72%	(a)
The Nebraska Methodist Hospital	Omaha	72%	300+
Phelps Memorial Health Center	Holdrege	72%	(a)
Saint Francis Medical Center	Grand Island	72%	300+
Sidney Regional Medical Center	Sidney	72%	(a)
Bryan Medical Center	Lincoln	71%	300+
Mary Lanning Healthcare	Hastings	71%	300+
Saint Elizabeth Regional Medical Center	Lincoln	71%	300+
Brodstone Memorial Hospital	Superior	70%	(a)
Columbus Community Hospital	Columbus	70%	300+
Community Hospital	Mccook	70%	(a)
Bellevue Medical Center	Bellevue	69%	300+
Chadron Comm Hosp & Health Services	Chadron	69%	(a)
Great Plains Regional Medical Center	North Platte	69%	300+
Jennie M Melham Memorial Medical Center	Broken Bow	69%	(a)
Regional West Medical Center	Scottsbluff	69%	300+
Faith Regional Health Services	Norfolk	68%	300+
Gothenburg Memorial Hospital	Gothenburg	68%	(a)
The Nebraska Medical Center	Omaha	68%	300+
Nebraska Spine Hospital	Omaha	68%	300+
Cherry County Hospital	Valentine	67%	(a)
Good Samaritan Hospital	Kearney	67%	300+
York General Hospital	York	66%	(a)
Alegent Creighton-Creighton Univ Med	Omaha	65%	300+
Tri Valley Health System	Cambridge	60%	(a)

Room and Bathroom 'Always' Clean

Hospital Name	City	Rate	Cases
York General Hospital	York	90%	(a)
Pender Community Hospital	Pender	89%	(a)
Butler County Health Care Center	David City	88%	(a)
Boone County Health Center	Albion	87%	(a)
Beatrice Comm Hosp & Health Ctr	Beatrice	86%	(a)
Box Butte General Hospital	Alliance	86%	(a)
Community Medical Center	Falls City	86%	(a)
Gothenburg Memorial Hospital	Gothenburg	86%	(a)
Lincoln Surgical Hospital	Lincoln	86%	300+
Midwest Surgical Hospital	Omaha	86%	300+
Ogallala Community Hospital[11]	Ogallala	86%	(a)
Phelps Memorial Health Center	Holdrege	85%	(a)
Cherry County Hospital	Valentine	84%	(a)
Community Hospital	Mccook	84%	(a)
Nebraska Orthopaedic Hospital	Omaha	84%	300+
Brodstone Memorial Hospital	Superior	83%	(a)
Tri Valley Health System	Cambridge	81%	(a)
Chadron Comm Hosp & Health Services	Chadron	79%	(a)
Alegent Creighton-Midlands Hosp	Papillion	78%	(a)
Nebraska Heart Hospital	Lincoln	78%	300+
Avera Saint Anthony's Hospital	O' Neill	77%	(a)
Jennie M Melham Memorial Medical Center	Broken Bow	77%	(a)
Alegent Creighton-Immanuel Med Ctr	Omaha	76%	300+
Sidney Regional Medical Center	Sidney	76%	(a)
Bellevue Medical Center	Bellevue	75%	300+
Faith Regional Health Services	Norfolk	75%	300+
Good Samaritan Hospital	Kearney	75%	300+
Nebraska Spine Hospital	Omaha	75%	300+
Mary Lanning Healthcare	Hastings	74%	300+
Alegent Creighton-Bergan Mercy Med Ctr	Omaha	73%	300+

NOTE: Hospital profiles are in alphabetical order by state, then city, then hospital within the city; Rankings exclude hospitals with less than 25 cases except for patient surveys which excludes hospitals with less than 100 cases; (a) 100-299 cases; (1) The number of cases/patients is too few to report; (2) Data submitted were based on a sample of cases/patients; (3) Results are based on a shorter time period than required; (4) Data suppressed by CMS for one or more quarters; (5) Results are not available for this reporting period; (6) Fewer than 100 patients completed the HCAHPS survey; (7) No cases met the criteria for this measure; (8) The lower limit of the confidence interval cannot be calculated if the number of observed infections equals zero; (9) No data are available from the state/territory for this reporting period; (10) The scores shown reflect fewer than 50 completed surveys; (11) There were discrepancies in the data collection process; (12) This measure does not apply to this hospital for this reporting period; (13) Results cannot be calculated for this reporting period; (14) The results for this state are combined with nearby states to protect confidentiality; Please refer to the User's Guide for a full explanation of data.

Hospital Name	City	Rate	Cases
Fremont Area Medical Center	Fremont	73%	300+
Lexington Regional Health Center	Lexington	73%	(a)
Saint Francis Medical Center	Grand Island	73%	300+
Columbus Community Hospital	Columbus	72%	300+
The Nebraska Medical Center	Omaha	72%	300+
Bryan Medical Center	Lincoln	71%	300+
Saint Elizabeth Regional Medical Center	Lincoln	70%	300+
The Nebraska Methodist Hospital	Omaha	69%	300+
Alegent Creighton-Creighton Univ Med	Omaha	66%	300+
Alegent Creighton-Lakeside Hosp	Omaha	66%	300+
Great Plains Regional Medical Center	North Platte	63%	300+
Regional West Medical Center	Scottsbluff	63%	300+

Timely Help 'Always' Received

Hospital Name	City	Rate	Cases
Midwest Surgical Hospital	Omaha	90%	300+
Nebraska Orthopaedic Hospital	Omaha	88%	300+
Brodstone Memorial Hospital	Superior	83%	(a)
Lincoln Surgical Hospital	Lincoln	81%	300+
Community Medical Center	Falls City	80%	(a)
Pender Community Hospital	Pender	80%	(a)
Boone County Health Center	Albion	79%	(a)
Butler County Health Care Center	David City	77%	(a)
Beatrice Comm Hosp & Health Ctr	Beatrice	76%	(a)
Cherry County Hospital	Valentine	76%	(a)
Nebraska Heart Hospital	Lincoln	76%	300+
Gothenburg Memorial Hospital	Gothenburg	75%	(a)
Ogallala Community Hospital[11]	Ogallala	74%	(a)
Avera Saint Anthony's Hospital	O' Neill	73%	(a)
Community Hospital	Mccook	73%	(a)
Phelps Memorial Health Center	Holdrege	73%	(a)
Nebraska Spine Hospital	Omaha	72%	300+
Lexington Regional Health Center	Lexington	71%	(a)
Fremont Area Medical Center	Fremont	70%	300+
York General Hospital	York	70%	(a)
Box Butte General Hospital	Alliance	69%	(a)
Chadron Comm Hosp & Health Services	Chadron	69%	(a)
Jennie M Melham Memorial Medical Center	Broken Bow	69%	(a)
The Nebraska Methodist Hospital	Omaha	69%	300+
Sidney Regional Medical Center	Sidney	69%	(a)
Bellevue Medical Center	Bellevue	68%	300+
Columbus Community Hospital	Columbus	68%	300+
Alegent Creighton-Midlands Hosp	Papillion	67%	(a)
Bryan Medical Center	Lincoln	67%	300+
Mary Lanning Healthcare	Hastings	66%	300+
Saint Francis Medical Center	Grand Island	66%	300+
Alegent Creighton-Bergan Mercy Med Ctr	Omaha	65%	300+
Alegent Creighton-Immanuel Med Ctr	Omaha	65%	300+
Great Plains Regional Medical Center	North Platte	65%	300+
Regional West Medical Center	Scottsbluff	65%	300+
Alegent Creighton-Lakeside Hosp	Omaha	63%	300+
The Nebraska Medical Center	Omaha	63%	300+
Tri Valley Health System	Cambridge	63%	(a)
Faith Regional Health Services	Norfolk	62%	300+
Good Samaritan Hospital	Kearney	62%	300+
Saint Elizabeth Regional Medical Center	Lincoln	59%	300+
Alegent Creighton-Creighton Univ Med	Omaha	56%	300+

Would Definitely Recommend Hospital

Hospital Name	City	Rate	Cases
Nebraska Orthopaedic Hospital	Omaha	94%	300+
Midwest Surgical Hospital	Omaha	91%	300+
Brodstone Memorial Hospital	Superior	89%	(a)
Pender Community Hospital	Pender	88%	(a)
Boone County Health Center	Albion	87%	(a)
Avera Saint Anthony's Hospital	O' Neill	86%	(a)
Lincoln Surgical Hospital	Lincoln	86%	300+
Nebraska Heart Hospital	Lincoln	85%	300+
Butler County Health Care Center	David City	83%	(a)
Ogallala Community Hospital[11]	Ogallala	83%	(a)
Phelps Memorial Health Center	Holdrege	83%	(a)
The Nebraska Methodist Hospital	Omaha	82%	300+
Nebraska Spine Hospital	Omaha	82%	300+
Community Medical Center	Falls City	81%	(a)
Alegent Creighton-Lakeside Hosp	Omaha	80%	300+
The Nebraska Medical Center	Omaha	79%	300+
Saint Elizabeth Regional Medical Center	Lincoln	79%	300+
Alegent Creighton-Immanuel Med Ctr	Omaha	78%	300+
Bellevue Medical Center	Bellevue	78%	300+
Bryan Medical Center	Lincoln	78%	300+
Beatrice Comm Hosp & Health Ctr	Beatrice	77%	(a)
Jennie M Melham Memorial Medical Center	Broken Bow	77%	(a)
Alegent Creighton-Bergan Mercy Med Ctr	Omaha	76%	300+
Alegent Creighton-Midlands Hosp	Papillion	76%	(a)
Community Hospital	Mccook	76%	(a)
Good Samaritan Hospital	Kearney	76%	300+
Gothenburg Memorial Hospital	Gothenburg	76%	(a)
Saint Francis Medical Center	Grand Island	76%	300+
Tri Valley Health System	Cambridge	74%	(a)
Mary Lanning Healthcare	Hastings	73%	300+

Hospital Name	City	Rate	Cases
York General Hospital	York	73%	(a)
Cherry County Hospital	Valentine	72%	(a)
Lexington Regional Health Center	Lexington	72%	(a)
Sidney Regional Medical Center	Sidney	70%	(a)
Alegent Creighton-Creighton Univ Med	Omaha	67%	300+
Faith Regional Health Services	Norfolk	67%	300+
Chadron Comm Hosp & Health Services	Chadron	66%	(a)
Great Plains Regional Medical Center	North Platte	66%	300+
Regional West Medical Center	Scottsbluff	66%	300+
Columbus Community Hospital	Columbus	64%	300+
Box Butte General Hospital	Alliance	61%	(a)
Fremont Area Medical Center	Fremont	61%	300+

Use of Medical Imaging

Cardiac Imaging Stress Test before OP Surgery

Hospital Name	City	Rate	Cases
Community Medical Center	Falls City	0.0%	49
Jennie M Melham Memorial Medical Center	Broken Bow	1.2%	84
Valley County Health System	Ord	1.2%	82
Thayer County Health Services	Hebron	1.5%	68
Memorial Community Hospital	Blair	1.9%	54
Chase County Community Hospital	Imperial	2.1%	48
Saint Mary's Community Hospital	Nebraska City	2.1%	95
Avera Creighton Hospital	Creighton	2.2%	45
Good Samaritan Hospital	Kearney	2.4%	210
Howard County Medical Center	Saint Paul	2.7%	73
Mary Lanning Healthcare	Hastings	3.1%	97
Tri Valley Health System	Cambridge	3.2%	62
Saunders Medical Center	Wahoo	3.6%	55
Perkins County Health Services	Grant	3.9%	51
Columbus Community Hospital	Columbus	4.1%	220
Alegent Creighton-Lakeside Hosp	Omaha	4.3%	140
Lexington Regional Health Center	Lexington	4.3%	46
Phelps Memorial Health Center	Holdrege	4.4%	114
Ogallala Community Hospital	Ogallala	4.5%	66
Saint Elizabeth Regional Medical Center	Lincoln	4.5%	287
Cherry County Hospital	Valentine	4.8%	62
Memorial Hospital	Aurora	4.8%	83
Nebraska Heart Hospital	Lincoln	4.8%	913
Bryan Medical Center	Lincoln	4.9%	1052
The Nebraska Methodist Hospital	Omaha	5.2%	1135
Beatrice Comm Hosp & Health Ctr	Beatrice	5.7%	141
Brodstone Memorial Hospital	Superior	5.8%	69
Faith Regional Health Services	Norfolk	5.9%	443
Alegent Creighton-Creighton Univ Med	Omaha	6.0%	299
Alegent Creighton-Bergan Mercy Med Ctr	Omaha	6.1%	808
Sidney Regional Medical Center	Sidney	6.1%	66
Fremont Area Medical Center	Fremont	6.2%	406
York General Hospital	York	6.4%	157
Community Hospital	Mccook	6.5%	169
Avera Saint Anthony's Hospital	O' Neill	6.6%	121
Antelope Memorial Hospital	Neligh	6.7%	60
Regional West Medical Center	Scottsbluff	6.8%	370
Alegent Creighton-Immanuel Med Ctr	Omaha	7.1%	182
The Nebraska Medical Center	Omaha	7.1%	675
Great Plains Regional Medical Center	North Platte	7.4%	393
Alegent Creighton-Midlands Hosp	Papillion	8.1%	271
Bellevue Medical Center	Bellevue	10.8%	111

Combination Abdominal CT Scan

Hospital Name	City	Rate	Cases
Gordon Memorial Hospital District	Gordon	0.0%	69
Cherry County Hospital	Valentine	1.3%	78
Saint Francis Medical Center	Grand Island	1.3%	299
Valley County Health System	Ord	1.4%	74
Box Butte General Hospital	Alliance	1.8%	111
The Nebraska Methodist Hospital	Omaha	2.0%	1470
Saint Francis Memorial Hospital	West Point	2.2%	90
Phelps Memorial Health Center	Holdrege	2.3%	177
Bellevue Medical Center	Bellevue	2.7%	409
Brodstone Memorial Hospital	Superior	2.9%	105
The Nebraska Medical Center	Omaha	3.0%	1490
Chadron Comm Hosp & Health Services	Chadron	3.2%	62
Harlan County Health System	Alma	3.2%	62
Alegent Creighton-Bergan Mercy Med Ctr	Omaha	3.4%	930
Boone County Health Center	Albion	3.6%	139
Chase County Community Hospital	Imperial	3.6%	56
Johnson County Hospital	Tecumseh	3.7%	54
Providence Medical Center	Wayne	3.7%	82
Mary Lanning Healthcare	Hastings	3.9%	490
Nemaha County Hospital	Auburn	3.9%	77
Saunders Medical Center	Wahoo	4.0%	125
Memorial Hospital	Aurora	4.4%	68
Tri Valley Health System	Cambridge	4.6%	65
Alegent Creighton-Immanuel Med Ctr	Omaha	4.7%	449
Gothenburg Memorial Hospital	Gothenburg	4.8%	63
Jennie M Melham Memorial Medical Center	Broken Bow	5.0%	120
Saint Elizabeth Regional Medical Center	Lincoln	5.1%	891
Columbus Community Hospital	Columbus	5.7%	435

Hospital Name	City	Rate	Cases
Sidney Regional Medical Center	Sidney	5.7%	106
Saint Mary's Community Hospital	Nebraska City	5.8%	103
Alegent Creighton-Creighton Univ Med	Omaha	5.9%	256
Good Samaritan Hospital	Kearney	6.0%	514
Perkins County Health Services	Grant	6.0%	67
Alegent Creighton-Lakeside Hosp	Omaha	6.2%	533
Memorial Community Hospital	Blair	6.6%	198
York General Hospital	York	7.0%	128
Bryan Medical Center	Lincoln	7.1%	1285
Butler County Health Care Center	David City	7.2%	69
Community Medical Center	Falls City	7.7%	117
Jefferson Community Health Center	Fairbury	8.0%	87
Lexington Regional Health Center	Lexington	8.1%	74
Beatrice Comm Hosp & Health Ctr	Beatrice	8.4%	296
Great Plains Regional Medical Center	North Platte	8.8%	706
Thayer County Health Services	Hebron	9.3%	75
Avera Saint Anthony's Hospital	O' Neill	9.5%	168
Litzenberg Memorial County Hospital	Central City	11.4%	79
Alegent Creighton-Midlands Hosp	Papillion	12.2%	312
Ogallala Community Hospital	Ogallala	12.3%	146
Regional West Medical Center	Scottsbluff	13.1%	647
Community Hospital	Mccook	16.2%	204
Howard County Medical Center	Saint Paul	17.7%	113
Fremont Area Medical Center	Fremont	32.7%	511
Osmond General Hospital	Osmond	54.1%	37
Faith Regional Health Services	Norfolk	65.0%	565
Antelope Memorial Hospital	Neligh	68.4%	79

Combination Brain/Sinus CT Scan

Hospital Name	City	Rate	Cases
Avera Creighton Hospital	Creighton	0.0%	54
Butler County Health Care Center	David City	0.0%	56
Chadron Comm Hosp & Health Services	Chadron	0.0%	50
Dundy County Hospital	Benkelman	0.0%	36
Fillmore County Hospital	Geneva	0.0%	58
Jefferson Community Health Center	Fairbury	0.0%	64
Oakland Mercy Hospital	Oakland	0.0%	44
Saint Francis Memorial Hospital	West Point	0.0%	78
Saint Francis Medical Center	Grand Island	0.6%	321
Fremont Area Medical Center	Fremont	0.8%	500
Columbus Community Hospital	Columbus	0.9%	348
York General Hospital	York	1.2%	163
The Nebraska Methodist Hospital	Omaha	1.3%	783
Bellevue Medical Center	Bellevue	1.6%	449
Faith Regional Health Services	Norfolk	1.7%	419
Saint Elizabeth Regional Medical Center	Lincoln	1.7%	688
Bryan Medical Center	Lincoln	3.4%	1428
The Nebraska Medical Center	Omaha	3.8%	871
Alegent Creighton-Lakeside Hosp	Omaha	4.4%	340
Cherry County Hospital	Valentine	5.8%	120
Regional West Medical Center	Scottsbluff	6.8%	457
Howard County Medical Center	Saint Paul	7.0%	114
Gothenburg Memorial Hospital	Gothenburg	10.6%	47

Combination Chest CT Scan

Hospital Name	City	Rate	Cases
Alegent Creighton-Bergan Mercy Med Ctr	Omaha	0.0%	789
Alegent Creighton-Immanuel Med Ctr	Omaha	0.0%	375
Alegent Creighton-Lakeside Hosp	Omaha	0.0%	341
Box Butte General Hospital	Alliance	0.0%	49
Chase County Community Hospital	Imperial	0.0%	53
Cherry County Hospital	Valentine	0.0%	50
Fremont Area Medical Center	Fremont	0.0%	455
Gothenburg Memorial Hospital	Gothenburg	0.0%	49
Jennie M Melham Memorial Medical Center	Broken Bow	0.0%	106
The Nebraska Methodist Hospital	Omaha	0.0%	1238
Ogallala Community Hospital	Ogallala	0.0%	71
Regional West Medical Center	Scottsbluff	0.0%	345
Saint Elizabeth Regional Medical Center	Lincoln	0.0%	505
Saunders Medical Center	Wahoo	0.0%	62
Valley County Health System	Ord	0.0%	55
York General Hospital	York	0.0%	127
The Nebraska Medical Center	Omaha	0.2%	1876
Columbus Community Hospital	Columbus	0.3%	315
Good Samaritan Hospital	Kearney	0.5%	440
Bellevue Medical Center	Bellevue	0.6%	165
Alegent Creighton-Creighton Univ Med	Omaha	0.9%	326
Great Plains Regional Medical Center	North Platte	1.0%	520
Antelope Memorial Hospital	Neligh	1.1%	91
Phelps Memorial Health Center	Holdrege	1.3%	152
Saint Francis Medical Center	Grand Island	1.5%	136
Faith Regional Health Services	Norfolk	1.6%	693
Mary Lanning Healthcare	Hastings	1.6%	443
Tri Valley Health System	Cambridge	1.7%	59
Brodstone Memorial Hospital	Superior	1.8%	114
Boone County Health Center	Albion	1.9%	108
Saint Mary's Community Hospital	Nebraska City	2.0%	98
Nemaha County Hospital	Auburn	2.1%	48
Beatrice Comm Hosp & Health Ctr	Beatrice	2.5%	199
Saint Francis Memorial Hospital	West Point	2.9%	69

NOTE: Hospital profiles are in alphabetical order by state, then city, then hospital within the city; Rankings exclude hospitals with less than 25 cases except for patient surveys which excludes hospitals with less than 100 cases; (a) 100-299 cases; (1) The number of cases/patients is too few to report; (2) Data submitted were based on a sample of cases/patients; (3) Results are based on a shorter time period than required; (4) Data suppressed by CMS for one or more quarters; (5) Results are not available for this reporting period; (6) Fewer than 100 patients completed the HCAHPS survey; (7) No cases met the criteria for this measure; (8) The lower limit of the confidence interval cannot be calculated if the number of observed infections equals zero; (9) No data are available from the state/territory for this reporting period; (10) The scores shown reflect fewer than 50 completed surveys; (11) There were discrepancies in the data collection process; (12) This measure does not apply to this hospital for this reporting period; (13) Results cannot be calculated for this reporting period; (14) The results for this state are combined with nearby states to protect confidentiality; Please refer to the User's Guide for a full explanation of data.

Hospital Name	City	Rate	Cases
Memorial Hospital	Aurora	3.0%	67
Lexington Regional Health Center	Lexington	3.3%	60
Jefferson Community Health Center	Fairbury	3.6%	56
Memorial Community Hospital	Blair	3.8%	130
Alegent Creighton-Midlands Hosp	Papillion	4.1%	220
Bryan Medical Center	Lincoln	4.1%	812
Community Medical Center	Falls City	4.9%	61
Avera Saint Anthony's Hospital	O' Neill	5.5%	110
Howard County Medical Center	Saint Paul	9.4%	85
Community Hospital	Mccook	9.7%	196

Follow-up Mammogram/Ultrasound

A follow-up rate near zero may indicate missed cancer; a rate higher than 14% may mean there is unnecessary follow up.

Hospital Name	City	Rate	Cases
Brown County Hospital	Ainsworth	1.3%	76
Alegent Creighton-Mem Hosp, Schuyl	Schuyler	1.6%	122
Columbus Community Hospital	Columbus	1.9%	899
Franklin County Memorial Hospital	Franklin	2.2%	46
Tri Valley Health System	Cambridge	2.7%	146
Boone County Health Center	Albion	3.0%	367
Fremont Area Medical Center	Fremont	3.2%	1376
Pender Community Hospital	Pender	3.6%	112
Good Samaritan Hospital	Kearney	3.7%	924
Phelps Memorial Health Center	Holdrege	3.7%	492
Callaway District Hospital	Callaway	4.0%	75
Alegent Creighton-Bergan Mercy Med Ctr	Omaha	4.3%	1353
Antelope Memorial Hospital	Neligh	4.4%	158
Alegent Creighton-Midlands Hosp	Papillion	4.7%	1173
Litzenberg Memorial County Hospital	Central City	5.0%	200
Chadron Comm Hosp & Health Services	Chadron	5.1%	255
Kearney County Health Services Hospital	Minden	5.3%	94
West Holt Memorial Hospital	Atkinson	5.4%	92
Butler County Health Care Center	David City	5.8%	171
Osmond General Hospital	Osmond	5.9%	68
Howard County Medical Center	Saint Paul	6.3%	174
Avera Creighton Hospital	Creighton	6.5%	139
Brodstone Memorial Hospital	Superior	6.6%	319
The Nebraska Medical Center	Omaha	7.3%	2022
Alegent Creighton-Lakeside Hosp	Omaha	7.4%	1756
Saint Francis Medical Center	Grand Island	7.4%	1826
Gothenburg Memorial Hospital	Gothenburg	7.6%	132
Sidney Regional Medical Center	Sidney	7.7%	209
Webster County Community Hospital	Red Cloud	7.7%	78
Saint Francis Memorial Hospital	West Point	7.8%	400
Annie Jeffrey Mem County Health Ctr	Osceola	7.9%	76
Bryan Medical Center	Lincoln	7.9%	2938
The Nebraska Methodist Hospital	Omaha	7.9%	1390
Regional West Medical Center	Scottsbluff	7.9%	1578
Thayer County Health Services	Hebron	7.9%	178
Box Butte General Hospital	Alliance	8.0%	175
Harlan County Health System	Alma	8.0%	112
Saunders Medical Center	Wahoo	8.0%	137
Alegent Creighton-Creighton Univ Med	Omaha	8.2%	388
Mary Lanning Healthcare	Hastings	8.2%	915
Avera Saint Anthony's Hospital	O' Neill	8.3%	254
Alegent Creighton-Immanuel Med Ctr	Omaha	8.4%	811
Henderson Health Care Services	Henderson	8.7%	69
Faith Regional Health Services	Norfolk	9.1%	804
Pawnee County Memorial Hospital	Pawnee City	9.2%	120
Valley County Health System	Ord	9.2%	130
Chase County Community Hospital	Imperial	9.4%	127
Providence Medical Center	Wayne	9.6%	187
Fillmore County Hospital	Geneva	10.2%	206
Saint Mary's Community Hospital	Nebraska City	10.4%	250
Community Medical Center	Falls City	10.5%	133
Nemaha County Hospital	Auburn	10.8%	194
Bellevue Medical Center	Bellevue	11.6%	398
Jennie M Melham Memorial Medical Center	Broken Bow	11.6%	181
Lexington Regional Health Center	Lexington	11.7%	239
Jefferson Community Health Center	Fairbury	11.8%	220
Great Plains Regional Medical Center	North Platte	12.2%	995
Beatrice Comm Hosp & Health Ctr	Beatrice	12.7%	629
Memorial Community Hospital	Blair	12.9%	341
Saint Elizabeth Regional Medical Center	Lincoln	13.1%	1905
Johnson County Hospital	Tecumseh	13.3%	181
Ogallala Community Hospital	Ogallala	13.4%	232
Perkins County Health Services	Grant	13.7%	161
Memorial Hospital	Aurora	14.6%	178
York General Hospital	York	15.1%	411
Community Hospital	Mccook	15.3%	131
Cherry County Hospital	Valentine	15.6%	122

Lumbar Spine MRI for Low Back Pain

Hospital Name	City	Rate	Cases
Columbus Community Hospital	Columbus	28.4%	67
Good Samaritan Hospital	Kearney	29.2%	130
Regional West Medical Center	Scottsbluff	29.6%	199
Fremont Area Medical Center	Fremont	30.8%	117
Faith Regional Health Services	Norfolk	31.0%	84
Bryan Medical Center	Lincoln	31.5%	108
Great Plains Regional Medical Center	North Platte	31.5%	200
Alegent Creighton-Midlands Hosp	Papillion	35.6%	73
Nebraska Orthopaedic Hospital	Omaha	36.2%	69
Mary Lanning Healthcare	Hastings	36.3%	113
Phelps Memorial Health Center	Holdrege	36.4%	55
Bellevue Medical Center	Bellevue	36.9%	65
Community Hospital	Mccook	37.2%	43
The Nebraska Medical Center	Omaha	38.6%	153
Saint Elizabeth Regional Medical Center	Lincoln	38.9%	72
Memorial Community Hospital	Blair	42.2%	45
Alegent Creighton-Lakeside Hosp	Omaha	42.6%	54
Alegent Creighton-Immanuel Med Ctr	Omaha	43.1%	123
The Nebraska Methodist Hospital	Omaha	44.6%	271
Beatrice Comm Hosp & Health Ctr	Beatrice	45.8%	59
Alegent Creighton-Bergan Mercy Med Ctr	Omaha	48.2%	199
Boone County Health Center	Albion	51.4%	35

NOTE: Hospital profiles are in alphabetical order by state, then city, then hospital within the city; Rankings exclude hospitals with less than 25 cases except for patient surveys which excludes hospitals with less than 100 cases; (a) 100-299 cases; (1) The number of cases/patients is too few to report; (2) Data submitted were based on a sample of cases/patients; (3) Results are based on a shorter time period than required; (4) Data suppressed by CMS for one or more quarters; (5) Results are not available for this reporting period; (6) Fewer than 100 patients completed the HCAHPS survey; (7) No cases met the criteria for this measure; (8) The lower limit of the confidence interval cannot be calculated if the number of observed infections equals zero; (9) No data are available from the state/territory for this reporting period; (10) The scores shown reflect fewer than 50 completed surveys; (11) There were discrepancies in the data collection process; (12) This measure does not apply to this hospital for this reporting period; (13) Results cannot be calculated for this reporting period; (14) The results for this state are combined with nearby states to protect confidentiality; Please refer to the User's Guide for a full explanation of data.

Brown County Hospital

945 East Zero St Phone: 402-387-2800
Ainsworth, NE 69210 Fax: 402-387-2804
URL: www.browncountyhospital.org
Type: Critical Access Hospitals Emergency Services: Yes
Ownership: Government - Local Beds: 25

Key Personnel:
Infection Control. . . . . Shelly Doyle
Quality Assurance . . . . Connie Gouchey
Radiology. . . . . Jennifer Krysi
Operating Room. . . . . Jayce Linse
Chief of Medical Staff . . . . Annette Miller, MD
CEO/President. . . . . Shannon Sorensen, CEO

Measure	Cases	This Hosp.	State Avg.	U.S. Avg.
Blood Clot Prevention and Treatment				
Anticoagulation Overlap Therapy[5]	-	-	93%	93%
ICU Venous Thromboembolism Prophylaxis[5]	-	-	91%	92%
Incidence of Potentially Preventable VTE[5]	-	-	11%	10%
UFH with Dosages/Platelet Monitoring[5]	-	-	98%	97%
Venous Thromboembolism Prophylaxis[5]	-	-	88%	85%
Warfarin Therapy Discharge Instructions[5]	-	-	81%	75%
Chest Pain/Possible Heart Attack Care				
Aspirin Given Within 24 Hours of Arrival[1]	-	-	96%	96%
Fibrinolytic Meds Within 30 Min. of Arrival[1,3]	-	-	53%	58%
Average Time to ECG (minutes)[1]	-	-	8	7
Average Time to Transfer (minutes)[3,7]	-	-	76	60
Children's Asthma Care				
Received Home Management Plan of Care	-	-	-	88%
Received Reliever Medication	-	-	-	100%
Received Systemic Corticosteroids	-	-	-	100%
Emergency Department				
Admittance Decision Time (minutes)[5]	-	-	75	98
Head CT Results Within 45 Min. of Arrival[5]	-	-	61%	57%
Patients Who Left ER Before Being Seen[5]	-	-	1%	2%
Time from ER Arrival to Admit. (minutes)[5]	-	-	207	274
Time from ER Arrival to Discharge (minutes)[5]	-	-	118	134
Time in ER Before Being Evaluated (minutes)[5]	-	-	21	26
Time to Pain Meds for Fractures (minutes)[5]	-	-	42	57
Heart Attack Care				
Aspirin Given at Discharge[3,7]	-	-	100%	99%
Fibrinolytic Meds Within 30 Min. of Arrival[3,7]	-	-	-	54%
PCI Within 90 Minutes of Arrival[3,7]	-	-	96%	96%
Statin Prescribed at Discharge[3,7]	-	-	99%	98%
Heart Failure Care				
ACE Inhibitor or ARB for LVSD[1,3]	-	-	96%	97%
Discharge Instructions Given[1,3]	-	-	93%	94%
Evaluation of LVS Function[1,3]	-	-	98%	99%
Medicare Spending				
Medicare Spending per Patient (ratio)	-	-	0.97	0.98
Pneumonia Care				
Appropriate Initial Antibiotic Given[1]	-	-	95%	95%
Blood Culture Timing[1]	-	-	99%	98%
Pregnancy and Delivery Care				
Newborn Deliveries Scheduled Early[5]	-	-	5%	6%
Preventive Care				
Immunization for Influenza[5]	-	-	89%	90%
Immunization for Pneumonia[5]	-	-	90%	92%
Stroke Care				
Anticoagulation Therapy for Atrial Fibrillation[5]	-	-	95%	95%
Antithrombotic Therapy Timing[5]	-	-	99%	98%
Assessed for Rehabilitation[5]	-	-	99%	97%
Discharged on Antithrombotic Therapy[5]	-	-	100%	99%
Discharged on Statin Medication[5]	-	-	93%	94%
Thrombolytic Therapy Timing[5]	-	-	75%	66%
Venous Thromboembolism Prophylaxis[5]	-	-	94%	94%
Written Stroke Educational Materials Given[5]	-	-	84%	88%
Surgical Care Improvement Project				
Appropriate Beta Blocker Usage[5]	-	-	98%	98%
Appropriate VTP Within 24 Hours[5]	-	-	99%	98%
Controlled Postoperative Blood Glucose[5]	-	-	96%	97%
Perioperative Temperature Management[5]	-	-	100%	100%
Prophylactic Antibiotic Selection[5]	-	-	99%	99%
Prophylactic Antibiotic Selection (Outpatient)[5]	-	-	99%	98%
Prophylactic Antibiotic Stopped[5]	-	-	98%	98%
Prophylactic Antibiotic Timing[5]	-	-	98%	99%
Prophylactic Antibiotic Timing (Outpatient)[5]	-	-	97%	98%
Urinary Catheter Removal[5]	-	-	98%	97%
Survey of Patients' Hospital Experiences				
Area Around Room 'Always' Quiet at Night[10]	<100	84%	67%	61%
Doctors 'Always' Communicated Well[10]	<100	84%	86%	82%
Home Recovery Information Given[10]	<100	89%	88%	85%
Hospital Given 9 or 10 on 10 Point Scale[10]	<100	89%	78%	71%
Meds 'Always' Explained Before Given[10]	<100	78%	68%	64%
Nurses 'Always' Communicated Well[10]	<100	86%	83%	79%
Pain 'Always' Well Controlled[10]	<100	93%	73%	71%
Room and Bathroom 'Always' Clean[10]	<100	75%	81%	73%
Timely Help 'Always' Received[10]	<100	79%	75%	68%
Would Definitely Recommend Hospital[10]	<100	82%	77%	71%
Use of Medical Imaging				
Cardiac Imaging Stress Test before Surgery[1]	-	-	5.4%	5.3%
Combination Abdominal CT Scan[1]	-	-	9.3%	10.5%
Combination Brain/Sinus CT Scan[1]	-	-	2.7%	2.7%
Combination Chest CT Scan[1]	-	-	1.7%	2.7%
Follow-up Mammogram/Ultrasound	76	1.3%	8%	8.8%
Lumbar Spine MRI for Low Back Pain[1]	-	-	36.5%	37.2%

Boone County Health Center

PO Box 151, 723 West Fairview St Phone: 402-395-2191
Albion, NE 68620 Fax: 402-395-5165
E-mail: bchc@boonecohealth.org
URL: www.boonecohealth.org
Type: Critical Access Hospitals Emergency Services: Yes
Ownership: Government - Local Beds: 30

Key Personnel:
Operating Room. . . . . Marna Ellenwood, RN
Chief of Medical Staff . . . . Dr. Lynette Kramer
CEO/President. . . . . Vic Lee, FACHE
Quality Assurance . . . . Jeanne Temme

Measure	Cases	This Hosp.	State Avg.	U.S. Avg.
Blood Clot Prevention and Treatment				
Anticoagulation Overlap Therapy[5]	-	-	93%	93%
ICU Venous Thromboembolism Prophylaxis[5]	-	-	91%	92%
Incidence of Potentially Preventable VTE[5]	-	-	11%	10%
UFH with Dosages/Platelet Monitoring[5]	-	-	98%	97%
Venous Thromboembolism Prophylaxis[5]	-	-	88%	85%
Warfarin Therapy Discharge Instructions[5]	-	-	81%	75%
Chest Pain/Possible Heart Attack Care				
Aspirin Given Within 24 Hours of Arrival[3]	11	100%	96%	96%
Fibrinolytic Meds Within 30 Min. of Arrival[1,3]	-	-	53%	58%
Average Time to ECG (minutes)[3]	12	15	8	7
Average Time to Transfer (minutes)[1,3]	-	-	76	60
Children's Asthma Care				
Received Home Management Plan of Care	-	-	-	88%
Received Reliever Medication	-	-	-	100%
Received Systemic Corticosteroids	-	-	-	100%
Emergency Department				
Admittance Decision Time (minutes)[5]	-	-	75	98
Head CT Results Within 45 Min. of Arrival[5]	-	-	61%	57%
Patients Who Left ER Before Being Seen[5]	-	-	1%	2%
Time from ER Arrival to Admit. (minutes)[5]	-	-	207	274
Time from ER Arrival to Discharge (minutes)[5]	-	-	118	134
Time in ER Before Being Evaluated (minutes)[5]	-	-	21	26
Time to Pain Meds for Fractures (minutes)[5]	-	-	42	57
Heart Attack Care				
Aspirin Given at Discharge[5]	-	-	100%	99%
Fibrinolytic Meds Within 30 Min. of Arrival[5]	-	-	-	54%
PCI Within 90 Minutes of Arrival[5]	-	-	96%	96%
Statin Prescribed at Discharge[5]	-	-	99%	98%
Heart Failure Care				
ACE Inhibitor or ARB for LVSD[1]	-	-	96%	97%
Discharge Instructions Given[1]	-	-	93%	94%
Evaluation of LVS Function	19	100%	98%	99%
Medicare Spending				
Medicare Spending per Patient (ratio)	-	-	0.97	0.98
Pneumonia Care				
Appropriate Initial Antibiotic Given	30	100%	95%	95%
Blood Culture Timing[1]	-	-	99%	98%
Pregnancy and Delivery Care				
Newborn Deliveries Scheduled Early[5]	-	-	5%	6%
Preventive Care				
Immunization for Influenza[5]	-	-	89%	90%
Immunization for Pneumonia[5]	-	-	90%	92%
Stroke Care				
Anticoagulation Therapy for Atrial Fibrillation[5]	-	-	95%	95%
Antithrombotic Therapy Timing[5]	-	-	99%	98%
Assessed for Rehabilitation[5]	-	-	99%	97%
Discharged on Antithrombotic Therapy[5]	-	-	100%	99%
Discharged on Statin Medication[5]	-	-	93%	94%
Thrombolytic Therapy Timing[5]	-	-	75%	66%
Venous Thromboembolism Prophylaxis[5]	-	-	94%	94%
Written Stroke Educational Materials Given[5]	-	-	84%	88%
Surgical Care Improvement Project				
Appropriate Beta Blocker Usage[1,3]	-	-	98%	98%
Appropriate VTP Within 24 Hours[3]	16	100%	99%	98%
Controlled Postoperative Blood Glucose[3,7]	-	-	96%	97%
Perioperative Temperature Management[3]	18	100%	100%	100%
Prophylactic Antibiotic Selection[3]	17	100%	99%	99%
Prophylactic Antibiotic Selection (Outpatient)	19	95%	99%	98%
Prophylactic Antibiotic Stopped[3]	17	100%	98%	98%
Prophylactic Antibiotic Timing[3]	17	100%	98%	99%
Prophylactic Antibiotic Timing (Outpatient)[1]	-	-	97%	98%
Urinary Catheter Removal[3,7]	-	-	98%	97%
Survey of Patients' Hospital Experiences				
Area Around Room 'Always' Quiet at Night	(a)	65%	67%	61%
Doctors 'Always' Communicated Well	(a)	93%	86%	82%
Home Recovery Information Given	(a)	89%	88%	85%
Hospital Given 9 or 10 on 10 Point Scale	(a)	88%	78%	71%
Meds 'Always' Explained Before Given	(a)	74%	68%	64%
Nurses 'Always' Communicated Well	(a)	85%	83%	79%
Pain 'Always' Well Controlled	(a)	74%	73%	71%
Room and Bathroom 'Always' Clean	(a)	87%	81%	73%
Timely Help 'Always' Received	(a)	79%	75%	68%
Would Definitely Recommend Hospital	(a)	87%	77%	71%
Use of Medical Imaging				
Cardiac Imaging Stress Test before Surgery[1]	-	-	5.4%	5.3%
Combination Abdominal CT Scan	139	3.6%	9.3%	10.5%
Combination Brain/Sinus CT Scan[1]	-	-	2.7%	2.7%
Combination Chest CT Scan	108	1.9%	1.7%	2.7%
Follow-up Mammogram/Ultrasound	367	3.0%	8%	8.8%
Lumbar Spine MRI for Low Back Pain	35	51.4%	36.5%	37.2%

Box Butte General Hospital

PO Box 810, 2101 Box Butte Ave Phone: 308-762-6660
Alliance, NE 69301 Fax: 308-762-1923
E-mail: boxbutte@btigate.com
URL: www.bbgh.org
Type: Critical Access Hospitals Emergency Services: Yes
Ownership: Government - Local Beds: 44

Key Personnel:
Operating Room. . . . . Glen Forney, RN
CEO/President. . . . . Dan Griess
Hemotology Center . . . . Sharon Groskopf, RN
Chief of Medical Staff . . . . David Luedke, MD
Infection Control. . . . . Mary Mockerman
Quality Assurance . . . . Mary Mockerman
Emergency Room . . . . Nancy Ross, RN
Intensive Care Unit. . . . . Dewitt Shannon, MD

Measure	Cases	This Hosp.	State Avg.	U.S. Avg.
Blood Clot Prevention and Treatment				
Anticoagulation Overlap Therapy[5]	-	-	93%	93%
ICU Venous Thromboembolism Prophylaxis[5]	-	-	91%	92%
Incidence of Potentially Preventable VTE[5]	-	-	11%	10%
UFH with Dosages/Platelet Monitoring[5]	-	-	98%	97%
Venous Thromboembolism Prophylaxis[5]	-	-	88%	85%
Warfarin Therapy Discharge Instructions[5]	-	-	81%	75%
Chest Pain/Possible Heart Attack Care				
Aspirin Given Within 24 Hours of Arrival	12	100%	96%	96%
Fibrinolytic Meds Within 30 Min. of Arrival[1]	-	-	53%	58%
Average Time to ECG (minutes)	12	7	8	7
Average Time to Transfer (minutes)[1]	-	-	76	60
Children's Asthma Care				
Received Home Management Plan of Care	-	-	-	88%

NOTE: *Hospital profiles are in alphabetical order by state, then city, then hospital within the city; Rankings exclude hospitals with less than 25 cases except for patient surveys which excludes hospitals with less than 100 cases; (a) 100-299 cases; (1) The number of cases/patients is too few to report; (2) Data submitted were based on a sample of cases/patients; (3) Results are based on a shorter time period than required; (4) Data suppressed by CMS for one or more quarters; (5) Results are not available for this reporting period; (6) Fewer than 100 patients completed the HCAHPS survey; (7) No cases met the criteria for this measure; (8) The lower limit of the confidence interval cannot be calculated if the number of observed infections equals zero; (9) No data are available from the state/territory for this reporting period; (10) The scores shown reflect fewer than 50 completed surveys; (11) There were discrepancies in the data collection process; (12) This measure does not apply to this hospital for this reporting period; (13) Results cannot be calculated for this reporting period; (14) The results for this state are combined with nearby states to protect confidentiality; Please refer to the User's Guide for a full explanation of data.*

Measure	Cases	This Hosp.	State Avg.	U.S. Avg.
Received Reliever Medication	-	-	-	100%
Received Systemic Corticosteroids	-	-	-	100%
Emergency Department				
Admittance Decision Time (minutes)	401	55	75	98
Head CT Results Within 45 Min. of Arrival[5]	-	-	61%	57%
Patients Who Left ER Before Being Seen[5]	-	-	1%	2%
Time from ER Arrival to Admit. (minutes)	401	188	207	274
Time from ER Arrival to Discharge (minutes)	373	115	118	134
Time in ER Before Being Evaluated (minutes)	407	31	21	26
Time to Pain Meds for Fractures (minutes)	18	28	42	57
Heart Attack Care				
Aspirin Given at Discharge[5]	-	-	100%	99%
Fibrinolytic Meds Within 30 Min. of Arrival[5]	-	-	-	54%
PCI Within 90 Minutes of Arrival[5]	-	-	96%	96%
Statin Prescribed at Discharge[5]	-	-	99%	98%
Heart Failure Care				
ACE Inhibitor or ARB for LVSD[1]	-	-	96%	97%
Discharge Instructions Given[1]	-	-	93%	94%
Evaluation of LVS Function	20	70%	98%	99%
Medicare Spending				
Medicare Spending per Patient (ratio)	-	-	0.97	0.98
Pneumonia Care				
Appropriate Initial Antibiotic Given	48	83%	95%	95%
Blood Culture Timing	34	85%	99%	98%
Pregnancy and Delivery Care				
Newborn Deliveries Scheduled Early[1]	-	-	5%	6%
Preventive Care				
Immunization for Influenza	53	72%	89%	90%
Immunization for Pneumonia	72	60%	90%	92%
Stroke Care				
Anticoagulation Therapy for Atrial Fibrillation[5]	-	-	95%	95%
Antithrombotic Therapy Timing[5]	-	-	99%	98%
Assessed for Rehabilitation[5]	-	-	99%	97%
Discharged on Antithrombotic Therapy[5]	-	-	100%	99%
Discharged on Statin Medication[5]	-	-	93%	94%
Thrombolytic Therapy Timing[5]	-	-	75%	66%
Venous Thromboembolism Prophylaxis[5]	-	-	94%	94%
Written Stroke Educational Materials Given[5]	-	-	84%	88%
Surgical Care Improvement Project				
Appropriate Beta Blocker Usage[1,3]	-	-	98%	98%
Appropriate VTP Within 24 Hours[3]	19	84%	99%	98%
Controlled Postoperative Blood Glucose[3,7]	-	-	96%	97%
Perioperative Temperature Management[3]	20	100%	100%	100%
Prophylactic Antibiotic Selection[3]	15	100%	99%	99%
Prophylactic Antibiotic Selection (Outpatient)[5]	-	-	99%	98%
Prophylactic Antibiotic Stopped[3]	15	87%	98%	98%
Prophylactic Antibiotic Timing[3]	15	60%	98%	99%
Prophylactic Antibiotic Timing (Outpatient)[5]	-	-	97%	98%
Urinary Catheter Removal[3]	19	100%	98%	97%
Survey of Patients' Hospital Experiences				
Area Around Room 'Always' Quiet at Night	(a)	51%	67%	61%
Doctors 'Always' Communicated Well	(a)	84%	86%	82%
Home Recovery Information Given	(a)	93%	88%	85%
Hospital Given 9 or 10 on 10 Point Scale	(a)	53%	78%	71%
Meds 'Always' Explained Before Given	(a)	72%	68%	64%
Nurses 'Always' Communicated Well	(a)	75%	83%	79%
Pain 'Always' Well Controlled	(a)	72%	73%	71%
Room and Bathroom 'Always' Clean	(a)	86%	81%	73%
Timely Help 'Always' Received	(a)	69%	75%	68%
Would Definitely Recommend Hospital	(a)	61%	77%	71%
Use of Medical Imaging				
Cardiac Imaging Stress Test before Surgery[1]	-	-	5.4%	5.3%
Combination Abdominal CT Scan	111	1.8%	9.3%	10.5%
Combination Brain/Sinus CT Scan[1]	-	-	2.7%	2.7%
Combination Chest CT Scan	49	0.0%	1.7%	2.7%
Follow-up Mammogram/Ultrasound	175	8.0%	8%	8.8%
Lumbar Spine MRI for Low Back Pain[1]	-	-	36.5%	37.2%

Harlan County Health System

PO Box 836, 717 North Brown St
Alma, NE 68920
Phone: 308-928-2151
Fax: 308-928-2774
Type: Critical Access Hospitals
Emergency Services: Yes
Ownership: Voluntary non-profit - Other
Beds: 25

Key Personnel:
Operating Room. . . . . Diane Fegter, RN
Infection Control. . . . . Sharee Ring, RN
Quality Assurance . . . . Sharee Ring, RN
CEO . . . . Manuela Wolf

Measure	Cases	This Hosp.	State Avg.	U.S. Avg.
Blood Clot Prevention and Treatment				
Anticoagulation Overlap Therapy[5]	-	-	93%	93%
ICU Venous Thromboembolism Prophylaxis[5]	-	-	91%	92%
Incidence of Potentially Preventable VTE[5]	-	-	11%	10%
UFH with Dosages/Platelet Monitoring[5]	-	-	98%	97%
Venous Thromboembolism Prophylaxis[5]	-	-	88%	85%
Warfarin Therapy Discharge Instructions[5]	-	-	81%	75%
Chest Pain/Possible Heart Attack Care				
Aspirin Given Within 24 Hours of Arrival	15	93%	96%	96%
Fibrinolytic Meds Within 30 Min. of Arrival[5]	-	-	53%	58%
Average Time to ECG (minutes)	14	10	8	7
Average Time to Transfer (minutes)[5]	-	-	76	60
Children's Asthma Care				
Received Home Management Plan of Care	-	-	-	88%
Received Reliever Medication	-	-	-	100%
Received Systemic Corticosteroids	-	-	-	100%
Emergency Department				
Admittance Decision Time (minutes)[5]	-	-	75	98
Head CT Results Within 45 Min. of Arrival[5]	-	-	61%	57%
Patients Who Left ER Before Being Seen[5]	-	-	1%	2%
Time from ER Arrival to Admit. (minutes)[5]	-	-	207	274
Time from ER Arrival to Discharge (minutes)[5]	-	-	118	134
Time in ER Before Being Evaluated (minutes)[5]	-	-	21	26
Time to Pain Meds for Fractures (minutes)[5]	-	-	42	57
Heart Attack Care				
Aspirin Given at Discharge[3,7]	-	-	100%	99%
Fibrinolytic Meds Within 30 Min. of Arrival[3,7]	-	-	-	54%
PCI Within 90 Minutes of Arrival[3,7]	-	-	96%	96%
Statin Prescribed at Discharge[3,7]	-	-	99%	98%
Heart Failure Care				
ACE Inhibitor or ARB for LVSD[1,3]	-	-	96%	97%
Discharge Instructions Given[3,7]	-	-	93%	94%
Evaluation of LVS Function[3,7]	-	-	98%	99%
Medicare Spending				
Medicare Spending per Patient (ratio)	-	-	0.97	0.98
Pneumonia Care				
Appropriate Initial Antibiotic Given[1]	-	-	95%	95%
Blood Culture Timing[1]	-	-	99%	98%
Pregnancy and Delivery Care				
Newborn Deliveries Scheduled Early[5]	-	-	5%	6%
Preventive Care				
Immunization for Influenza[5]	-	-	89%	90%
Immunization for Pneumonia[5]	-	-	90%	92%
Stroke Care				
Anticoagulation Therapy for Atrial Fibrillation[5]	-	-	95%	95%
Antithrombotic Therapy Timing[5]	-	-	99%	98%
Assessed for Rehabilitation[5]	-	-	99%	97%
Discharged on Antithrombotic Therapy[5]	-	-	100%	99%
Discharged on Statin Medication[5]	-	-	93%	94%
Thrombolytic Therapy Timing[5]	-	-	75%	66%
Venous Thromboembolism Prophylaxis[5]	-	-	94%	94%
Written Stroke Educational Materials Given[5]	-	-	84%	88%
Surgical Care Improvement Project				
Appropriate Beta Blocker Usage[5]	-	-	98%	98%
Appropriate VTP Within 24 Hours[5]	-	-	99%	98%
Controlled Postoperative Blood Glucose[5]	-	-	96%	97%
Perioperative Temperature Management[5]	-	-	100%	100%
Prophylactic Antibiotic Selection[5]	-	-	99%	99%
Prophylactic Antibiotic Selection (Outpatient)[5]	-	-	99%	98%
Prophylactic Antibiotic Stopped[5]	-	-	98%	98%
Prophylactic Antibiotic Timing[5]	-	-	98%	99%
Prophylactic Antibiotic Timing (Outpatient)[5]	-	-	97%	98%
Urinary Catheter Removal[5]	-	-	98%	97%
Survey of Patients' Hospital Experiences				
Area Around Room 'Always' Quiet at Night[10]	<100	77%	67%	61%
Doctors 'Always' Communicated Well[10]	<100	78%	86%	82%
Home Recovery Information Given[10]	<100	80%	88%	85%
Hospital Given 9 or 10 on 10 Point Scale[10]	<100	77%	78%	71%
Meds 'Always' Explained Before Given[10]	<100	58%	68%	64%
Nurses 'Always' Communicated Well[10]	<100	86%	83%	79%
Pain 'Always' Well Controlled[10]	<100	82%	73%	71%
Room and Bathroom 'Always' Clean[10]	<100	95%	81%	73%
Timely Help 'Always' Received[10]	<100	69%	75%	68%
Would Definitely Recommend Hospital[10]	<100	84%	77%	71%
Use of Medical Imaging				
Cardiac Imaging Stress Test before Surgery[1]	-	-	5.4%	5.3%
Combination Abdominal CT Scan	62	3.2%	9.3%	10.5%
Combination Brain/Sinus CT Scan[1]	-	-	2.7%	2.7%
Combination Chest CT Scan[1]	-	-	1.7%	2.7%
Follow-up Mammogram/Ultrasound	112	8.0%	8%	8.8%
Lumbar Spine MRI for Low Back Pain[1]	-	-	36.5%	37.2%

West Holt Memorial Hospital

406 W Neely St
Atkinson, NE 68713
Phone: 402-925-2811
Fax: 402-925-2810
URL: www.westholtmed.org
Type: Critical Access Hospitals
Emergency Services: Yes
Ownership: Voluntary non-profit - Private
Beds: 18

Key Personnel:
Emergency Room . . . . Jay Kennedy, M.D.
CEO/President. . . . . John Olson
Radiology. . . . . Mari Osborne, RT(R)
Patient Relations . . . . Sandra Schrunk
Chief of Medical Staff . . . . Talaha Shamim, MD
Operating Room. . . . . Peggy Tejral
Chief of Medical Staff. . . . . John Tubbs, M.D.

Measure	Cases	This Hosp.	State Avg.	U.S. Avg.
Blood Clot Prevention and Treatment				
Anticoagulation Overlap Therapy[5]	-	-	93%	93%
ICU Venous Thromboembolism Prophylaxis[5]	-	-	91%	92%
Incidence of Potentially Preventable VTE[5]	-	-	11%	10%
UFH with Dosages/Platelet Monitoring[5]	-	-	98%	97%
Venous Thromboembolism Prophylaxis[5]	-	-	88%	85%
Warfarin Therapy Discharge Instructions[5]	-	-	81%	75%
Chest Pain/Possible Heart Attack Care				
Aspirin Given Within 24 Hours of Arrival[1]	-	-	96%	96%
Fibrinolytic Meds Within 30 Min. of Arrival[1,3]	-	-	53%	58%
Average Time to ECG (minutes)[1]	-	-	8	7
Average Time to Transfer (minutes)[3,7]	-	-	76	60
Children's Asthma Care				
Received Home Management Plan of Care	-	-	-	88%
Received Reliever Medication	-	-	-	100%
Received Systemic Corticosteroids	-	-	-	100%
Emergency Department				
Admittance Decision Time (minutes)[5]	-	-	75	98
Head CT Results Within 45 Min. of Arrival[3,7]	-	-	61%	57%
Patients Who Left ER Before Being Seen[5]	-	-	1%	2%
Time from ER Arrival to Admit. (minutes)[5]	-	-	207	274
Time from ER Arrival to Discharge (minutes)[5]	-	-	118	134
Time in ER Before Being Evaluated (minutes)[5]	-	-	21	26
Time to Pain Meds for Fractures (minutes)[5]	-	-	42	57
Heart Attack Care				
Aspirin Given at Discharge[5]	-	-	100%	99%
Fibrinolytic Meds Within 30 Min. of Arrival[5]	-	-	-	54%
PCI Within 90 Minutes of Arrival[5]	-	-	96%	96%
Statin Prescribed at Discharge[5]	-	-	99%	98%
Heart Failure Care				
ACE Inhibitor or ARB for LVSD[1,3]	-	-	96%	97%
Discharge Instructions Given[1,3]	-	-	93%	94%
Evaluation of LVS Function[1,3]	-	-	98%	99%
Medicare Spending				
Medicare Spending per Patient (ratio)	-	-	0.97	0.98
Pneumonia Care				
Appropriate Initial Antibiotic Given[1]	-	-	95%	95%
Blood Culture Timing[7]	-	-	99%	98%
Pregnancy and Delivery Care				

NOTE: Hospital profiles are in alphabetical order by state, then city, then hospital within the city; Rankings exclude hospitals with less than 25 cases except for patient surveys which excludes hospitals with less than 100 cases; (a) 100-299 cases; (1) The number of cases/patients is too few to report; (2) Data submitted were based on a sample of cases/patients; (3) Results are based on a shorter time period than required; (4) Data suppressed by CMS for one or more quarters; (5) Results are not available for this reporting period; (6) Fewer than 100 patients completed the HCAHPS survey; (7) No cases met the criteria for this measure; (8) The lower limit of the confidence interval cannot be calculated if the number of observed infections equals zero; (9) No data are available from the state/territory for this reporting period; (10) The scores shown reflect fewer than 50 completed surveys; (11) There were discrepancies in the data collection process; (12) This measure does not apply to this hospital for this reporting period; (13) Results cannot be calculated for this reporting period; (14) The results for this state are combined with nearby states to protect confidentiality; Please refer to the User's Guide for a full explanation of data.

Measure	Cases	This Hosp.	State Avg.	U.S. Avg.
Newborn Deliveries Scheduled Early[5]	-	-	5%	6%
Preventive Care				
Immunization for Influenza[5]	-	-	89%	90%
Immunization for Pneumonia[5]	-	-	90%	92%
Stroke Care				
Anticoagulation Therapy for Atrial Fibrillation[5]	-	-	95%	95%
Antithrombotic Therapy Timing[5]	-	-	99%	98%
Assessed for Rehabilitation[5]	-	-	99%	97%
Discharged on Antithrombotic Therapy[5]	-	-	100%	99%
Discharged on Statin Medication[5]	-	-	93%	94%
Thrombolytic Therapy Timing[5]	-	-	75%	66%
Venous Thromboembolism Prophylaxis[5]	-	-	94%	94%
Written Stroke Educational Materials Given[5]	-	-	84%	88%
Surgical Care Improvement Project				
Appropriate Beta Blocker Usage[5]	-	-	98%	98%
Appropriate VTP Within 24 Hours[5]	-	-	99%	98%
Controlled Postoperative Blood Glucose[5]	-	-	96%	97%
Perioperative Temperature Management[5]	-	-	100%	100%
Prophylactic Antibiotic Selection[5]	-	-	99%	99%
Prophylactic Antibiotic Selection (Outpatient)[5]	-	-	99%	98%
Prophylactic Antibiotic Stopped[5]	-	-	98%	98%
Prophylactic Antibiotic Timing[5]	-	-	98%	99%
Prophylactic Antibiotic Timing (Outpatient)[5]	-	-	97%	98%
Urinary Catheter Removal[5]	-	-	98%	97%
Survey of Patients' Hospital Experiences				
Area Around Room 'Always' Quiet at Night[6]	<100	64%	67%	61%
Doctors 'Always' Communicated Well[6]	<100	83%	86%	82%
Home Recovery Information Given[6]	<100	83%	88%	85%
Hospital Given 9 or 10 on 10 Point Scale[6]	<100	83%	78%	71%
Meds 'Always' Explained Before Given[6]	<100	66%	68%	64%
Nurses 'Always' Communicated Well[6]	<100	82%	83%	79%
Pain 'Always' Well Controlled[6]	<100	72%	73%	71%
Room and Bathroom 'Always' Clean[6]	<100	91%	81%	73%
Timely Help 'Always' Received[6]	<100	83%	75%	68%
Would Definitely Recommend Hospital[6]	<100	81%	77%	71%
Use of Medical Imaging				
Cardiac Imaging Stress Test before Surgery[1]	-	-	5.4%	5.3%
Combination Abdominal CT Scan[1]	-	-	9.3%	10.5%
Combination Brain/Sinus CT Scan[1]	-	-	2.7%	2.7%
Combination Chest CT Scan[1]	-	-	1.7%	2.7%
Follow-up Mammogram/Ultrasound	92	5.4%	8%	8.8%
Lumbar Spine MRI for Low Back Pain[1]	-	-	36.5%	37.2%

Nemaha County Hospital

2022 13th St
Auburn, NE 68305
Phone: 402-274-4366
Fax: 402-274-4399
E-mail: info@nchnet.org
URL: www.nchnet.org
Type: Critical Access Hospitals
Emergency Services: Yes
Ownership: Government - Local
Beds: 20

Key Personnel:

Quality Assurance . . . . Marilyn Belding
CEO . . . . Marty Fattig
Infection Control. . . . . Pam John
Intensive Care Unit. . . . . Susan Joy
Operating Room. . . . . Jackie Obermeyer
Emergency Room . . . . Barb Ramer
Chief of Medical Staff. . . . . Mike Zaruba

Measure	Cases	This Hosp.	State Avg.	U.S. Avg.
Blood Clot Prevention and Treatment				
Anticoagulation Overlap Therapy[5]	-	-	93%	93%
ICU Venous Thromboembolism Prophylaxis[5]	-	-	91%	92%
Incidence of Potentially Preventable VTE[5]	-	-	11%	10%
UFH with Dosages/Platelet Monitoring[5]	-	-	98%	97%
Venous Thromboembolism Prophylaxis[5]	-	-	88%	85%
Warfarin Therapy Discharge Instructions[5]	-	-	81%	75%
Chest Pain/Possible Heart Attack Care				
Aspirin Given Within 24 Hours of Arrival	31	90%	96%	96%
Fibrinolytic Meds Within 30 Min. of Arrival[3,7]	-	-	53%	58%
Average Time to ECG (minutes)	35	7	8	7
Average Time to Transfer (minutes)[1,3]	-	-	76	60
Children's Asthma Care				
Received Home Management Plan of Care	-	-	-	88%
Received Reliever Medication	-	-	-	100%
Received Systemic Corticosteroids	-	-	-	100%
Emergency Department				
Admittance Decision Time (minutes)[5]	-	-	75	98
Head CT Results Within 45 Min. of Arrival[5]	-	-	61%	57%
Patients Who Left ER Before Being Seen[5]	-	-	1%	2%
Time from ER Arrival to Admit. (minutes)[5]	-	-	207	274
Time from ER Arrival to Discharge (minutes)[5]	-	-	118	134
Time in ER Before Being Evaluated (minutes)[5]	-	-	21	26
Time to Pain Meds for Fractures (minutes)[5]	-	-	42	57
Heart Attack Care				
Aspirin Given at Discharge[3,7]	-	-	100%	99%
Fibrinolytic Meds Within 30 Min. of Arrival[3,7]	-	-	-	54%
PCI Within 90 Minutes of Arrival[3,7]	-	-	96%	96%
Statin Prescribed at Discharge[3,7]	-	-	99%	98%
Heart Failure Care				
ACE Inhibitor or ARB for LVSD[1,3]	-	-	96%	97%
Discharge Instructions Given[3,7]	-	-	93%	94%
Evaluation of LVS Function[1,3]	-	-	98%	99%
Medicare Spending				
Medicare Spending per Patient (ratio)	-	-	0.97	0.98
Pneumonia Care				
Appropriate Initial Antibiotic Given[1]	-	-	95%	95%
Blood Culture Timing[1]	-	-	99%	98%
Pregnancy and Delivery Care				
Newborn Deliveries Scheduled Early[5]	-	-	5%	6%
Preventive Care				
Immunization for Influenza[5]	-	-	89%	90%
Immunization for Pneumonia[5]	-	-	90%	92%
Stroke Care				
Anticoagulation Therapy for Atrial Fibrillation[5]	-	-	95%	95%
Antithrombotic Therapy Timing[5]	-	-	99%	98%
Assessed for Rehabilitation[5]	-	-	99%	97%
Discharged on Antithrombotic Therapy[5]	-	-	100%	99%
Discharged on Statin Medication[5]	-	-	93%	94%
Thrombolytic Therapy Timing[5]	-	-	75%	66%
Venous Thromboembolism Prophylaxis[5]	-	-	94%	94%
Written Stroke Educational Materials Given[5]	-	-	84%	88%
Surgical Care Improvement Project				
Appropriate Beta Blocker Usage[3,7]	-	-	98%	98%
Appropriate VTP Within 24 Hours[1,3]	-	-	99%	98%
Controlled Postoperative Blood Glucose[3,7]	-	-	96%	97%
Perioperative Temperature Management[1,3]	-	-	100%	100%
Prophylactic Antibiotic Selection[3,7]	-	-	99%	99%
Prophylactic Antibiotic Selection (Outpatient)[5]	-	-	99%	98%
Prophylactic Antibiotic Stopped[3,7]	-	-	98%	98%
Prophylactic Antibiotic Timing[3,7]	-	-	98%	99%
Prophylactic Antibiotic Timing (Outpatient)[5]	-	-	97%	98%
Urinary Catheter Removal[3,7]	-	-	98%	97%
Survey of Patients' Hospital Experiences				
Area Around Room 'Always' Quiet at Night[10]	<100	56%	67%	61%
Doctors 'Always' Communicated Well[10]	<100	89%	86%	82%
Home Recovery Information Given[10]	<100	89%	88%	85%
Hospital Given 9 or 10 on 10 Point Scale[10]	<100	87%	78%	71%
Meds 'Always' Explained Before Given[10]	<100	78%	68%	64%
Nurses 'Always' Communicated Well[10]	<100	92%	83%	79%
Pain 'Always' Well Controlled[10]	<100	74%	73%	71%
Room and Bathroom 'Always' Clean[10]	<100	96%	81%	73%
Timely Help 'Always' Received[10]	<100	84%	75%	68%
Would Definitely Recommend Hospital[10]	<100	89%	77%	71%
Use of Medical Imaging				
Cardiac Imaging Stress Test before Surgery[1]	-	-	5.4%	5.3%
Combination Abdominal CT Scan	77	3.9%	9.3%	10.5%
Combination Brain/Sinus CT Scan[1]	-	-	2.7%	2.7%
Combination Chest CT Scan	48	2.1%	1.7%	2.7%
Follow-up Mammogram/Ultrasound	194	10.8%	8%	8.8%
Lumbar Spine MRI for Low Back Pain[1]	-	-	36.5%	37.2%

Memorial Hospital

1423 Seventh St
Aurora, NE 68818
Phone: 402-694-3171
Fax: 402-694-3177
URL: www.memorialcommunityhealth.net
Type: Critical Access Hospitals
Emergency Services: Yes
Ownership: Voluntary non-profit - Private
Beds: 75

Key Personnel:

Infection Control. . . . . Laurie Andrews
Anesthesiology. . . . . Timothy Arthur, CRNA
Emergency Room . . . . Chaeryl Ericson
CEO/President. . . . . Diane Keller
Operating Room. . . . . Teresa Wall, RN
Chief of Medical Staff. . . . . John Wilcox, MD

Measure	Cases	This Hosp.	State Avg.	U.S. Avg.
Blood Clot Prevention and Treatment				
Anticoagulation Overlap Therapy[5]	-	-	93%	93%
ICU Venous Thromboembolism Prophylaxis[5]	-	-	91%	92%
Incidence of Potentially Preventable VTE[5]	-	-	11%	10%
UFH with Dosages/Platelet Monitoring[5]	-	-	98%	97%
Venous Thromboembolism Prophylaxis[5]	-	-	88%	85%
Warfarin Therapy Discharge Instructions[5]	-	-	81%	75%
Chest Pain/Possible Heart Attack Care				
Aspirin Given Within 24 Hours of Arrival	15	100%	96%	96%
Fibrinolytic Meds Within 30 Min. of Arrival[1]	-	-	53%	58%
Average Time to ECG (minutes)	16	4	8	7
Average Time to Transfer (minutes)[7]	-	-	76	60
Children's Asthma Care				
Received Home Management Plan of Care	-	-	-	88%
Received Reliever Medication	-	-	-	100%
Received Systemic Corticosteroids	-	-	-	100%
Emergency Department				
Admittance Decision Time (minutes)[5]	-	-	75	98
Head CT Results Within 45 Min. of Arrival[5]	-	-	61%	57%
Patients Who Left ER Before Being Seen[5]	-	-	1%	2%
Time from ER Arrival to Admit. (minutes)[5]	-	-	207	274
Time from ER Arrival to Discharge (minutes)[5]	-	-	118	134
Time in ER Before Being Evaluated (minutes)[5]	-	-	21	26
Time to Pain Meds for Fractures (minutes)[5]	-	-	42	57
Heart Attack Care				
Aspirin Given at Discharge[1,3]	-	-	100%	99%
Fibrinolytic Meds Within 30 Min. of Arrival[3,7]	-	-	-	54%
PCI Within 90 Minutes of Arrival[3,7]	-	-	96%	96%
Statin Prescribed at Discharge[1,3]	-	-	99%	98%
Heart Failure Care				
ACE Inhibitor or ARB for LVSD[3,7]	-	-	96%	97%
Discharge Instructions Given[1,3]	-	-	93%	94%
Evaluation of LVS Function[1,3]	-	-	98%	99%
Medicare Spending				
Medicare Spending per Patient (ratio)	-	-	0.97	0.98
Pneumonia Care				
Appropriate Initial Antibiotic Given	15	100%	95%	95%
Blood Culture Timing[1]	-	-	99%	98%
Pregnancy and Delivery Care				
Newborn Deliveries Scheduled Early[5]	-	-	5%	6%
Preventive Care				
Immunization for Influenza[5]	-	-	89%	90%
Immunization for Pneumonia[5]	-	-	90%	92%
Stroke Care				
Anticoagulation Therapy for Atrial Fibrillation[5]	-	-	95%	95%
Antithrombotic Therapy Timing[5]	-	-	99%	98%
Assessed for Rehabilitation[5]	-	-	99%	97%
Discharged on Antithrombotic Therapy[5]	-	-	100%	99%
Discharged on Statin Medication[5]	-	-	93%	94%
Thrombolytic Therapy Timing[5]	-	-	75%	66%
Venous Thromboembolism Prophylaxis[5]	-	-	94%	94%
Written Stroke Educational Materials Given[5]	-	-	84%	88%
Surgical Care Improvement Project				
Appropriate Beta Blocker Usage[1]	-	-	98%	98%
Appropriate VTP Within 24 Hours	24	100%	99%	98%
Controlled Postoperative Blood Glucose[7]	-	-	96%	97%
Perioperative Temperature Management	25	100%	100%	100%
Prophylactic Antibiotic Selection	24	100%	99%	99%
Prophylactic Antibiotic Selection (Outpatient)	16	100%	99%	98%
Prophylactic Antibiotic Stopped	24	100%	98%	98%

NOTE: Hospital profiles are in alphabetical order by state, then city, then hospital within the city; Rankings exclude hospitals with less than 25 cases except for patient surveys which excludes hospitals with less than 100 cases; (a) 100-299 cases; (1) The number of cases/patients is too few to report; (2) Data submitted were based on a sample of cases/patients; (3) Results are based on a shorter time period than required; (4) Data suppressed by CMS for one or more quarters; (5) Results are not available for this reporting period; (6) Fewer than 100 patients completed the HCAHPS survey; (7) No cases met the criteria for this measure; (8) The lower limit of the confidence interval cannot be calculated if the number of observed infections equals zero; (9) No data are available from the state/territory for this reporting period; (10) The scores shown reflect fewer than 50 completed surveys; (11) There were discrepancies in the data collection process; (12) This measure does not apply to this hospital for this reporting period; (13) Results cannot be calculated for this reporting period; (14) The results for this state are combined with nearby states to protect confidentiality; Please refer to the User's Guide for a full explanation of data.

Measure	Cases	This Hosp.	State Avg.	U.S. Avg.
Prophylactic Antibiotic Timing	24	96%	98%	99%
Prophylactic Antibiotic Timing (Outpatient)	16	100%	97%	98%
Urinary Catheter Removal	24	100%	98%	97%
Survey of Patients' Hospital Experiences				
Area Around Room 'Always' Quiet at Night[6]	<100	72%	67%	61%
Doctors 'Always' Communicated Well[6]	<100	87%	86%	82%
Home Recovery Information Given[6]	<100	91%	88%	85%
Hospital Given 9 or 10 on 10 Point Scale[6]	<100	81%	78%	71%
Meds 'Always' Explained Before Given[6]	<100	71%	68%	64%
Nurses 'Always' Communicated Well[6]	<100	80%	83%	79%
Pain 'Always' Well Controlled[6]	<100	67%	73%	71%
Room and Bathroom 'Always' Clean[6]	<100	85%	81%	73%
Timely Help 'Always' Received[6]	<100	70%	75%	68%
Would Definitely Recommend Hospital[6]	<100	78%	77%	71%
Use of Medical Imaging				
Cardiac Imaging Stress Test before Surgery	83	4.8%	5.4%	5.3%
Combination Abdominal CT Scan	68	4.4%	9.3%	10.5%
Combination Brain/Sinus CT Scan[1]	-	-	2.7%	2.7%
Combination Chest CT Scan	67	3.0%	1.7%	2.7%
Follow-up Mammogram/Ultrasound	178	14.6%	8%	8.8%
Lumbar Spine MRI for Low Back Pain[1]	-	-	36.5%	37.2%

Rock County Hospital

102 East South Street
Bassett, NE 68714
Phone: 402-684-3366
Fax: 402-684-3677
E-mail: rch@huntel.net
URL: www.rockcountyhospital.com
Type: Critical Access Hospitals
Emergency Services: Yes
Ownership: Government - Local
Beds: 17

Key Personnel:
Chief of Medical Staff . . . . John Cherry, MD
Operating Room. . . . . Carolyn Doke, RN
Infection Control. . . . . Barb Kaup
Administrator . . . . Stacey Knox
Emergency Room . . . . Teresa Patrick, RN, MSN

Measure	Cases	This Hosp.	State Avg.	U.S. Avg.
Blood Clot Prevention and Treatment				
Anticoagulation Overlap Therapy[5]	-	-	93%	93%
ICU Venous Thromboembolism Prophylaxis[5]	-	-	91%	92%
Incidence of Potentially Preventable VTE[5]	-	-	11%	10%
UFH with Dosages/Platelet Monitoring[5]	-	-	98%	97%
Venous Thromboembolism Prophylaxis[5]	-	-	88%	85%
Warfarin Therapy Discharge Instructions[5]	-	-	81%	75%
Chest Pain/Possible Heart Attack Care				
Aspirin Given Within 24 Hours of Arrival[5]	-	-	96%	96%
Fibrinolytic Meds Within 30 Min. of Arrival[5]	-	-	53%	58%
Average Time to ECG (minutes)[5]	-	-	8	7
Average Time to Transfer (minutes)[5]	-	-	76	60
Children's Asthma Care				
Received Home Management Plan of Care	-	-	-	88%
Received Reliever Medication	-	-	-	100%
Received Systemic Corticosteroids	-	-	-	100%
Emergency Department				
Admittance Decision Time (minutes)[5]	-	-	75	98
Head CT Results Within 45 Min. of Arrival[5]	-	-	61%	57%
Patients Who Left ER Before Being Seen[5]	-	-	1%	2%
Time from ER Arrival to Admit. (minutes)[5]	-	-	207	274
Time from ER Arrival to Discharge (minutes)[5]	-	-	118	134
Time in ER Before Being Evaluated (minutes)[5]	-	-	21	26
Time to Pain Meds for Fractures (minutes)[5]	-	-	42	57
Heart Attack Care				
Aspirin Given at Discharge[5]	-	-	100%	99%
Fibrinolytic Meds Within 30 Min. of Arrival[5]	-	-	-	54%
PCI Within 90 Minutes of Arrival[5]	-	-	96%	96%
Statin Prescribed at Discharge[5]	-	-	99%	98%
Heart Failure Care				
ACE Inhibitor or ARB for LVSD[3,7]	-	-	96%	97%
Discharge Instructions Given[1,3]	-	-	93%	94%
Evaluation of LVS Function[1,3]	-	-	98%	99%
Medicare Spending				
Medicare Spending per Patient (ratio)	-	-	0.97	0.98
Pneumonia Care				
Appropriate Initial Antibiotic Given[1,3]	-	-	95%	95%
Blood Culture Timing[3,7]	-	-	99%	98%
Pregnancy and Delivery Care				
Newborn Deliveries Scheduled Early[5]	-	-	5%	6%
Preventive Care				
Immunization for Influenza[5]	-	-	89%	90%
Immunization for Pneumonia[5]	-	-	90%	92%
Stroke Care				
Anticoagulation Therapy for Atrial Fibrillation[5]	-	-	95%	95%
Antithrombotic Therapy Timing[5]	-	-	99%	98%
Assessed for Rehabilitation[5]	-	-	99%	97%
Discharged on Antithrombotic Therapy[5]	-	-	100%	99%
Discharged on Statin Medication[5]	-	-	93%	94%
Thrombolytic Therapy Timing[5]	-	-	75%	66%
Venous Thromboembolism Prophylaxis[5]	-	-	94%	94%
Written Stroke Educational Materials Given[5]	-	-	84%	88%
Surgical Care Improvement Project				
Appropriate Beta Blocker Usage[5]	-	-	98%	98%
Appropriate VTP Within 24 Hours[5]	-	-	99%	98%
Controlled Postoperative Blood Glucose[5]	-	-	96%	97%
Perioperative Temperature Management[5]	-	-	100%	100%
Prophylactic Antibiotic Selection[5]	-	-	99%	99%
Prophylactic Antibiotic Selection (Outpatient)[5]	-	-	99%	98%
Prophylactic Antibiotic Stopped[5]	-	-	98%	98%
Prophylactic Antibiotic Timing[5]	-	-	98%	99%
Prophylactic Antibiotic Timing (Outpatient)[5]	-	-	97%	98%
Urinary Catheter Removal[5]	-	-	98%	97%
Survey of Patients' Hospital Experiences				
Area Around Room 'Always' Quiet at Night[6]	<100	82%	67%	61%
Doctors 'Always' Communicated Well[6]	<100	92%	86%	82%
Home Recovery Information Given[6]	<100	83%	88%	85%
Hospital Given 9 or 10 on 10 Point Scale[6]	<100	71%	78%	71%
Meds 'Always' Explained Before Given[6]	<100	65%	68%	64%
Nurses 'Always' Communicated Well[6]	<100	91%	83%	79%
Pain 'Always' Well Controlled[6]	<100	79%	73%	71%
Room and Bathroom 'Always' Clean[6]	<100	95%	81%	73%
Timely Help 'Always' Received[6]	<100	82%	75%	68%
Would Definitely Recommend Hospital[6]	<100	88%	77%	71%
Use of Medical Imaging				
Cardiac Imaging Stress Test before Surgery[1]	-	-	5.4%	5.3%
Combination Abdominal CT Scan[1]	-	-	9.3%	10.5%
Combination Brain/Sinus CT Scan[1]	-	-	2.7%	2.7%
Combination Chest CT Scan[1]	-	-	1.7%	2.7%
Follow-up Mammogram/Ultrasound[1]	-	-	8%	8.8%
Lumbar Spine MRI for Low Back Pain[1]	-	-	36.5%	37.2%

Beatrice Community Hospital & Health Center

PO Box 278, 4800 Hospital Parkway
Beatrice, NE 68310
Phone: 402-228-3344
Fax: 402-223-7299
E-mail: info@bchhc.org
URL: www.beatricecommunityhospital.com
Type: Critical Access Hospitals
Emergency Services: Yes
Ownership: Voluntary non-profit - Private
Beds: 47

Key Personnel:
CEO/President. . . . . Larry Emerson
Chief of Medical Staff . . . . Darin Hoffman
Operating Room. . . . . Karen Johnson, RN
Coronary Care . . . . Sue Schouboe
Infection Control. . . . . Rose Wischmeir
Quality Assurance . . . . Dorothy Zimmerman

Measure	Cases	This Hosp.	State Avg.	U.S. Avg.
Blood Clot Prevention and Treatment				
Anticoagulation Overlap Therapy[1]	-	-	93%	93%
ICU Venous Thromboembolism Prophylaxis	48	100%	91%	92%
Incidence of Potentially Preventable VTE[1]	-	-	11%	10%
UFH with Dosages/Platelet Monitoring[1]	-	-	98%	97%
Venous Thromboembolism Prophylaxis	149	100%	88%	85%
Warfarin Therapy Discharge Instructions[1]	-	-	81%	75%
Chest Pain/Possible Heart Attack Care				
Aspirin Given Within 24 Hours of Arrival	44	98%	96%	96%
Fibrinolytic Meds Within 30 Min. of Arrival[1]	-	-	53%	58%
Average Time to ECG (minutes)	45	6	8	7
Average Time to Transfer (minutes)[1]	-	-	76	60
Children's Asthma Care				
Received Home Management Plan of Care	-	-	-	88%
Received Reliever Medication	-	-	-	100%
Received Systemic Corticosteroids	-	-	-	100%
Emergency Department				
Admittance Decision Time (minutes)[5]	-	-	75	98
Head CT Results Within 45 Min. of Arrival[5]	-	-	61%	57%
Patients Who Left ER Before Being Seen[5]	-	-	1%	2%
Time from ER Arrival to Admit. (minutes)[5]	-	-	207	274
Time from ER Arrival to Discharge (minutes)[5]	-	-	118	134
Time in ER Before Being Evaluated (minutes)[5]	-	-	21	26
Time to Pain Meds for Fractures (minutes)[5]	-	-	42	57
Heart Attack Care				
Aspirin Given at Discharge[5]	-	-	100%	99%
Fibrinolytic Meds Within 30 Min. of Arrival[5]	-	-	-	54%
PCI Within 90 Minutes of Arrival[5]	-	-	96%	96%
Statin Prescribed at Discharge[5]	-	-	99%	98%
Heart Failure Care				
ACE Inhibitor or ARB for LVSD[1]	-	-	96%	97%
Discharge Instructions Given	13	85%	93%	94%
Evaluation of LVS Function	24	100%	98%	99%
Medicare Spending				
Medicare Spending per Patient (ratio)	-	-	0.97	0.98
Pneumonia Care				
Appropriate Initial Antibiotic Given	38	97%	95%	95%
Blood Culture Timing	75	99%	99%	98%
Pregnancy and Delivery Care				
Newborn Deliveries Scheduled Early[5]	-	-	5%	6%
Preventive Care				
Immunization for Influenza[5]	-	-	89%	90%
Immunization for Pneumonia[5]	-	-	90%	92%
Stroke Care				
Anticoagulation Therapy for Atrial Fibrillation[5]	-	-	95%	95%
Antithrombotic Therapy Timing[5]	-	-	99%	98%
Assessed for Rehabilitation[5]	-	-	99%	97%
Discharged on Antithrombotic Therapy[5]	-	-	100%	99%
Discharged on Statin Medication[5]	-	-	93%	94%
Thrombolytic Therapy Timing[5]	-	-	75%	66%
Venous Thromboembolism Prophylaxis[5]	-	-	94%	94%
Written Stroke Educational Materials Given[5]	-	-	84%	88%
Surgical Care Improvement Project				
Appropriate Beta Blocker Usage	24	100%	98%	98%
Appropriate VTP Within 24 Hours	51	94%	99%	98%
Controlled Postoperative Blood Glucose[7]	-	-	96%	97%
Perioperative Temperature Management	58	100%	100%	100%
Prophylactic Antibiotic Selection	47	100%	99%	99%
Prophylactic Antibiotic Selection (Outpatient)	34	97%	99%	98%
Prophylactic Antibiotic Stopped	47	100%	98%	98%
Prophylactic Antibiotic Timing	47	100%	98%	99%
Prophylactic Antibiotic Timing (Outpatient)	35	97%	97%	98%
Urinary Catheter Removal	20	100%	98%	97%
Survey of Patients' Hospital Experiences				
Area Around Room 'Always' Quiet at Night	(a)	63%	67%	61%
Doctors 'Always' Communicated Well	(a)	91%	86%	82%
Home Recovery Information Given	(a)	92%	88%	85%
Hospital Given 9 or 10 on 10 Point Scale	(a)	77%	78%	71%
Meds 'Always' Explained Before Given	(a)	73%	68%	64%
Nurses 'Always' Communicated Well	(a)	90%	83%	79%
Pain 'Always' Well Controlled	(a)	74%	73%	71%
Room and Bathroom 'Always' Clean	(a)	86%	81%	73%
Timely Help 'Always' Received	(a)	76%	75%	68%
Would Definitely Recommend Hospital	(a)	77%	77%	71%
Use of Medical Imaging				
Cardiac Imaging Stress Test before Surgery	141	5.7%	5.4%	5.3%
Combination Abdominal CT Scan	296	8.4%	9.3%	10.5%
Combination Brain/Sinus CT Scan[1]	-	-	2.7%	2.7%
Combination Chest CT Scan	199	2.5%	1.7%	2.7%
Follow-up Mammogram/Ultrasound	629	12.7%	8%	8.8%
Lumbar Spine MRI for Low Back Pain	59	45.8%	36.5%	37.2%

NOTE: Hospital profiles are in alphabetical order by state, then city, then hospital within the city; Rankings exclude hospitals with less than 25 cases except for patient surveys which excludes hospitals with less than 100 cases; (a) 100-299 cases; (1) The number of cases/patients is too few to report; (2) Data submitted were based on a sample of cases/patients; (3) Results are based on a shorter time period than required; (4) Data suppressed by CMS for one or more quarters; (5) Results are not available for this reporting period; (6) Fewer than 100 patients completed the HCAHPS survey; (7) No cases met the criteria for this measure; (8) The lower limit of the confidence interval cannot be calculated if the number of observed infections equals zero; (9) No data are available from the state/territory for this reporting period; (10) The scores shown reflect fewer than 50 completed surveys; (11) There were discrepancies in the data collection process; (12) This measure does not apply to this hospital for this reporting period; (13) Results cannot be calculated for this reporting period; (14) The results for this state are combined with nearby states to protect confidentiality; Please refer to the User's Guide for a full explanation of data.

Bellevue Medical Center

2500 Bellevue Medical Center Dr Phone: 402-763-3600
Bellevue, NE 68123
URL: www.bellevuemed.com
Type: Acute Care Hospitals Emergency Services: Yes
Ownership: Proprietary

Measure	Cases	This Hosp.	State Avg.	U.S. Avg.
Blood Clot Prevention and Treatment				
Anticoagulation Overlap Therapy[2]	16	100%	93%	93%
ICU Venous Thromboembolism Prophylaxis[2]	46	96%	91%	92%
Incidence of Potentially Preventable VTE[1,2]	-	-	11%	10%
UFH with Dosages/Platelet Monitoring[2]	18	94%	98%	97%
Venous Thromboembolism Prophylaxis[2]	194	89%	88%	85%
Warfarin Therapy Discharge Instructions[1,2]	-	-	81%	75%
Chest Pain/Possible Heart Attack Care				
Aspirin Given Within 24 Hours of Arrival[1,3]	-	-	96%	96%
Fibrinolytic Meds Within 30 Min. of Arrival[3,7]	-	-	53%	58%
Average Time to ECG (minutes)[1,3]	-	-	8	7
Average Time to Transfer (minutes)[3,7]	-	-	76	60
Children's Asthma Care				
Received Home Management Plan of Care	-	-	-	88%
Received Reliever Medication	-	-	-	100%
Received Systemic Corticosteroids	-	-	-	100%
Emergency Department				
Admittance Decision Time (minutes)[2]	311	82	75	98
Head CT Results Within 45 Min. of Arrival[1]	-	-	61%	57%
Patients Who Left ER Before Being Seen	24,996	1%	1%	2%
Time from ER Arrival to Admit. (minutes)[2]	314	215	207	274
Time from ER Arrival to Discharge (minutes)	364	110	118	134
Time in ER Before Being Evaluated (minutes)	280	15	21	26
Time to Pain Meds for Fractures (minutes)	117	46	42	57
Heart Attack Care				
Aspirin Given at Discharge	72	100%	100%	99%
Fibrinolytic Meds Within 30 Min. of Arrival[7]	-	-	-	54%
PCI Within 90 Minutes of Arrival	19	95%	96%	96%
Statin Prescribed at Discharge	70	100%	99%	98%
Heart Failure Care				
ACE Inhibitor or ARB for LVSD	22	100%	96%	97%
Discharge Instructions Given	52	100%	93%	94%
Evaluation of LVS Function	71	100%	98%	99%
Medicare Spending				
Medicare Spending per Patient (ratio)	-	1.05	0.97	0.98
Pneumonia Care				
Appropriate Initial Antibiotic Given	49	100%	95%	95%
Blood Culture Timing	115	100%	99%	98%
Pregnancy and Delivery Care				
Newborn Deliveries Scheduled Early[2]	42	5%	5%	6%
Preventive Care				
Immunization for Influenza[2]	306	94%	89%	90%
Immunization for Pneumonia[2]	353	95%	90%	92%
Stroke Care				
Anticoagulation Therapy for Atrial Fibrillation[1]	-	-	95%	95%
Antithrombotic Therapy Timing	52	100%	99%	98%
Assessed for Rehabilitation	51	100%	99%	97%
Discharged on Antithrombotic Therapy	51	100%	100%	99%
Discharged on Statin Medication	36	100%	93%	94%
Thrombolytic Therapy Timing[1]	-	-	75%	66%
Venous Thromboembolism Prophylaxis	56	98%	94%	94%
Written Stroke Educational Materials Given	31	100%	84%	88%
Surgical Care Improvement Project				
Appropriate Beta Blocker Usage	43	100%	98%	98%
Appropriate VTP Within 24 Hours	136	99%	99%	98%
Controlled Postoperative Blood Glucose[7]	-	-	96%	97%
Perioperative Temperature Management	153	100%	100%	100%
Prophylactic Antibiotic Selection	99	100%	99%	99%
Prophylactic Antibiotic Selection (Outpatient)	51	96%	99%	98%
Prophylactic Antibiotic Stopped	96	100%	98%	98%
Prophylactic Antibiotic Timing	99	100%	98%	99%
Prophylactic Antibiotic Timing (Outpatient)	51	98%	97%	98%
Urinary Catheter Removal	76	100%	98%	97%
Survey of Patients' Hospital Experiences				
Area Around Room 'Always' Quiet at Night	300+	69%	67%	61%
Doctors 'Always' Communicated Well	300+	82%	86%	82%
Home Recovery Information Given	300+	85%	88%	85%
Hospital Given 9 or 10 on 10 Point Scale	300+	75%	78%	71%
Meds 'Always' Explained Before Given	300+	63%	68%	64%
Nurses 'Always' Communicated Well	300+	81%	83%	79%
Pain 'Always' Well Controlled	300+	69%	73%	71%
Room and Bathroom 'Always' Clean	300+	75%	81%	73%
Timely Help 'Always' Received	300+	68%	75%	68%
Would Definitely Recommend Hospital	300+	78%	77%	71%
Use of Medical Imaging				
Cardiac Imaging Stress Test before Surgery	111	10.8%	5.4%	5.3%
Combination Abdominal CT Scan	409	2.7%	9.3%	10.5%
Combination Brain/Sinus CT Scan	449	1.6%	2.7%	2.7%
Combination Chest CT Scan	165	0.6%	1.7%	2.7%
Follow-up Mammogram/Ultrasound	398	11.6%	8%	8.8%
Lumbar Spine MRI for Low Back Pain	65	36.9%	36.5%	37.2%

Dundy County Hospital

PO Box 626, 1313 North Cheyenne St Phone: 308-423-2204
Benkelman, NE 69021 Fax: 308-423-2298
URL: www.bwtelcom.net/dch
Type: Critical Access Hospitals Emergency Services: Yes
Ownership: Government - Local Beds: 14

Key Personnel:
Radiology. . . . . Kelly Custer, RT
Chief of Medical Staff . . . . Jose Garcia
Infection Control. . . . . Jennifer Hansen
Quality Assurance . . . . Jennifer Hansen
Emergency Room . . . . Kellie Minor, RN
Patient Relations . . . . Nola Pollman, RN
Hemotology Center . . . . Kathy Walgren, RN
Anesthesiology. . . . . Kim Zweygardt, CRNA

Measure	Cases	This Hosp.	State Avg.	U.S. Avg.
Blood Clot Prevention and Treatment				
Anticoagulation Overlap Therapy[5]	-	-	93%	93%
ICU Venous Thromboembolism Prophylaxis[5]	-	-	91%	92%
Incidence of Potentially Preventable VTE[5]	-	-	11%	10%
UFH with Dosages/Platelet Monitoring[5]	-	-	98%	97%
Venous Thromboembolism Prophylaxis[5]	-	-	88%	85%
Warfarin Therapy Discharge Instructions[5]	-	-	81%	75%
Chest Pain/Possible Heart Attack Care				
Aspirin Given Within 24 Hours of Arrival[1,3]	-	-	96%	96%
Fibrinolytic Meds Within 30 Min. of Arrival[1,3]	-	-	53%	58%
Average Time to ECG (minutes)[1,3]	-	-	8	7
Average Time to Transfer (minutes)[3,7]	-	-	76	60
Children's Asthma Care				
Received Home Management Plan of Care	-	-	-	88%
Received Reliever Medication	-	-	-	100%
Received Systemic Corticosteroids	-	-	-	100%
Emergency Department				
Admittance Decision Time (minutes)[5]	-	-	75	98
Head CT Results Within 45 Min. of Arrival[5]	-	-	61%	57%
Patients Who Left ER Before Being Seen[5]	-	-	1%	2%
Time from ER Arrival to Admit. (minutes)[5]	-	-	207	274
Time from ER Arrival to Discharge (minutes)[5]	-	-	118	134
Time in ER Before Being Evaluated (minutes)[5]	-	-	21	26
Time to Pain Meds for Fractures (minutes)[5]	-	-	42	57
Heart Attack Care				
Aspirin Given at Discharge[1,3]	-	-	100%	99%
Fibrinolytic Meds Within 30 Min. of Arrival[3,7]	-	-	-	54%
PCI Within 90 Minutes of Arrival[3,7]	-	-	96%	96%
Statin Prescribed at Discharge[1,3]	-	-	99%	98%
Heart Failure Care				
ACE Inhibitor or ARB for LVSD[3,7]	-	-	96%	97%
Discharge Instructions Given[1,3]	-	-	93%	94%
Evaluation of LVS Function[1,3]	-	-	98%	99%
Medicare Spending				
Medicare Spending per Patient (ratio)	-	-	0.97	0.98
Pneumonia Care				
Appropriate Initial Antibiotic Given[1,3]	-	-	95%	95%
Blood Culture Timing[1,3]	-	-	99%	98%
Pregnancy and Delivery Care				
Newborn Deliveries Scheduled Early[5]	-	-	5%	6%
Preventive Care				
Immunization for Influenza[5]	-	-	89%	90%
Immunization for Pneumonia[5]	-	-	90%	92%
Stroke Care				
Anticoagulation Therapy for Atrial Fibrillation[5]	-	-	95%	95%
Antithrombotic Therapy Timing[5]	-	-	99%	98%
Assessed for Rehabilitation[5]	-	-	99%	97%
Discharged on Antithrombotic Therapy[5]	-	-	100%	99%
Discharged on Statin Medication[5]	-	-	93%	94%
Thrombolytic Therapy Timing[5]	-	-	75%	66%
Venous Thromboembolism Prophylaxis[5]	-	-	94%	94%
Written Stroke Educational Materials Given[5]	-	-	84%	88%
Surgical Care Improvement Project				
Appropriate Beta Blocker Usage[1,3]	-	-	98%	98%
Appropriate VTP Within 24 Hours[1,3]	-	-	99%	98%
Controlled Postoperative Blood Glucose[3,7]	-	-	96%	97%
Perioperative Temperature Management[1,3]	-	-	100%	100%
Prophylactic Antibiotic Selection[1,3]	-	-	99%	99%
Prophylactic Antibiotic Selection (Outpatient)[5]	-	-	99%	98%
Prophylactic Antibiotic Stopped[1,3]	-	-	98%	98%
Prophylactic Antibiotic Timing[1,3]	-	-	98%	99%
Prophylactic Antibiotic Timing (Outpatient)[5]	-	-	97%	98%
Urinary Catheter Removal[3,7]	-	-	98%	97%
Survey of Patients' Hospital Experiences				
Area Around Room 'Always' Quiet at Night[10]	<100	73%	67%	61%
Doctors 'Always' Communicated Well[10]	<100	74%	86%	82%
Home Recovery Information Given[10]	<100	75%	88%	85%
Hospital Given 9 or 10 on 10 Point Scale[10]	<100	73%	78%	71%
Meds 'Always' Explained Before Given[10]	<100	63%	68%	64%
Nurses 'Always' Communicated Well[10]	<100	78%	83%	79%
Pain 'Always' Well Controlled[10]	<100	65%	73%	71%
Room and Bathroom 'Always' Clean[10]	<100	80%	81%	73%
Timely Help 'Always' Received[10]	<100	76%	75%	68%
Would Definitely Recommend Hospital[10]	<100	81%	77%	71%
Use of Medical Imaging				
Cardiac Imaging Stress Test before Surgery[1]	-	-	5.4%	5.3%
Combination Abdominal CT Scan[1]	-	-	9.3%	10.5%
Combination Brain/Sinus CT Scan	36	0.0%	2.7%	2.7%
Combination Chest CT Scan[1]	-	-	1.7%	2.7%
Follow-up Mammogram/Ultrasound[1]	-	-	8%	8.8%
Lumbar Spine MRI for Low Back Pain[1]	-	-	36.5%	37.2%

Memorial Community Hospital

810 North 22nd St Phone: 402-426-2182
Blair, NE 68008 Fax: 402-426-1439
E-mail: jtriplett@mchhs.org
URL: www.mchhs.org
Type: Critical Access Hospitals Emergency Services: Yes
Ownership: Voluntary non-profit - Private Beds: 29

Key Personnel:
Operating Room. . . . . Michael Bittles
CEO . . . . Robert Copple
Chief of Medical Staff . . . . Brad Sawtelle, MD
Infection Control. . . . . Annette Spooner

Measure	Cases	This Hosp.	State Avg.	U.S. Avg.
Blood Clot Prevention and Treatment				
Anticoagulation Overlap Therapy[3,7]	-	-	93%	93%
ICU Venous Thromboembolism Prophylaxis[1,3]	-	-	91%	92%
Incidence of Potentially Preventable VTE[3,7]	-	-	11%	10%
UFH with Dosages/Platelet Monitoring[3,7]	-	-	98%	97%
Venous Thromboembolism Prophylaxis[3]	82	99%	88%	85%
Warfarin Therapy Discharge Instructions[3,7]	-	-	81%	75%
Chest Pain/Possible Heart Attack Care				
Aspirin Given Within 24 Hours of Arrival	20	100%	96%	96%
Fibrinolytic Meds Within 30 Min. of Arrival[7]	-	-	53%	58%
Average Time to ECG (minutes)	20	6	8	7
Average Time to Transfer (minutes)[1]	-	-	76	60
Children's Asthma Care				
Received Home Management Plan of Care	-	-	-	88%
Received Reliever Medication	-	-	-	100%
Received Systemic Corticosteroids	-	-	-	100%
Emergency Department				
Admittance Decision Time (minutes)[5]	-	-	75	98
Head CT Results Within 45 Min. of Arrival[5]	-	-	61%	57%

NOTE: Hospital profiles are in alphabetical order by state, then city, then hospital within the city; Rankings exclude hospitals with less than 25 cases except for patient surveys which excludes hospitals with less than 100 cases; (a) 100-299 cases; (1) The number of cases/patients is too few to report; (2) Data submitted were based on a sample of cases/patients; (3) Results are based on a shorter time period than required; (4) Data suppressed by CMS for one or more quarters; (5) Results are not available for this reporting period; (6) Fewer than 100 patients completed the HCAHPS survey; (7) No cases met the criteria for this measure; (8) The lower limit of the confidence interval cannot be calculated if the number of observed infections equals zero; (9) No data are available from the state/territory for this reporting period; (10) The scores shown reflect fewer than 50 completed surveys; (11) There were discrepancies in the data collection process; (12) This measure does not apply to this hospital for this reporting period; (13) Results cannot be calculated for this reporting period; (14) The results for this state are combined with nearby states to protect confidentiality; Please refer to the User's Guide for a full explanation of data.

Measure	Cases	This Hosp.	State Avg.	U.S. Avg.
Patients Who Left ER Before Being Seen[5]	-	-	1%	2%
Time from ER Arrival to Admit. (minutes)[5]	-	-	207	274
Time from ER Arrival to Discharge (minutes)[5]	-	-	118	134
Time in ER Before Being Evaluated (minutes)[5]	-	-	21	26
Time to Pain Meds for Fractures (minutes)[5]	-	-	42	57
Heart Attack Care				
Aspirin Given at Discharge[3,7]	-	-	100%	99%
Fibrinolytic Meds Within 30 Min. of Arrival[3,7]	-	-	-	54%
PCI Within 90 Minutes of Arrival[3,7]	-	-	96%	96%
Statin Prescribed at Discharge[3,7]	-	-	99%	98%
Heart Failure Care				
ACE Inhibitor or ARB for LVSD[1]	-	-	96%	97%
Discharge Instructions Given[1]	-	-	93%	94%
Evaluation of LVS Function	11	91%	98%	99%
Medicare Spending				
Medicare Spending per Patient (ratio)	-	-	0.97	0.98
Pneumonia Care				
Appropriate Initial Antibiotic Given[2]	12	92%	95%	95%
Blood Culture Timing[2]	22	100%	99%	98%
Pregnancy and Delivery Care				
Newborn Deliveries Scheduled Early[5]	-	-	5%	6%
Preventive Care				
Immunization for Influenza[5]	-	-	89%	90%
Immunization for Pneumonia[5]	-	-	90%	92%
Stroke Care				
Anticoagulation Therapy for Atrial Fibrillation[5]	-	-	95%	95%
Antithrombotic Therapy Timing[5]	-	-	99%	98%
Assessed for Rehabilitation[5]	-	-	99%	97%
Discharged on Antithrombotic Therapy[5]	-	-	100%	99%
Discharged on Statin Medication[5]	-	-	93%	94%
Thrombolytic Therapy Timing[5]	-	-	75%	66%
Venous Thromboembolism Prophylaxis[5]	-	-	94%	94%
Written Stroke Educational Materials Given[5]	-	-	84%	88%
Surgical Care Improvement Project				
Appropriate Beta Blocker Usage[1,3]	-	-	98%	98%
Appropriate VTP Within 24 Hours[1,3]	-	-	99%	98%
Controlled Postoperative Blood Glucose[3,7]	-	-	96%	97%
Perioperative Temperature Management[1,3]	-	-	100%	100%
Prophylactic Antibiotic Selection[1,3]	-	-	99%	99%
Prophylactic Antibiotic Selection (Outpatient)[1,3]	-	-	99%	98%
Prophylactic Antibiotic Stopped[1,3]	-	-	98%	98%
Prophylactic Antibiotic Timing[1,3]	-	-	98%	99%
Prophylactic Antibiotic Timing (Outpatient)[1,3]	-	-	97%	98%
Urinary Catheter Removal[1,3]	-	-	98%	97%
Survey of Patients' Hospital Experiences				
Area Around Room 'Always' Quiet at Night[3,6,11]	<100	72%	67%	61%
Doctors 'Always' Communicated Well[3,6,11]	<100	90%	86%	82%
Home Recovery Information Given[3,6,11]	<100	98%	88%	85%
Hospital Given 9 or 10 on 10 Point Scale[3,6,11]	<100	87%	78%	71%
Meds 'Always' Explained Before Given[3,6,11]	<100	74%	68%	64%
Nurses 'Always' Communicated Well[3,6,11]	<100	86%	83%	79%
Pain 'Always' Well Controlled[3,6,11]	<100	82%	73%	71%
Room and Bathroom 'Always' Clean[3,6,11]	<100	83%	81%	73%
Timely Help 'Always' Received[3,6,11]	<100	80%	75%	68%
Would Definitely Recommend Hospital[3,6,11]	<100	85%	77%	71%
Use of Medical Imaging				
Cardiac Imaging Stress Test before Surgery	54	1.9%	5.4%	5.3%
Combination Abdominal CT Scan	198	6.6%	9.3%	10.5%
Combination Brain/Sinus CT Scan[1]	-	-	2.7%	2.7%
Combination Chest CT Scan	130	3.8%	1.7%	2.7%
Follow-up Mammogram/Ultrasound	341	12.9%	8%	8.8%
Lumbar Spine MRI for Low Back Pain	45	42.2%	36.5%	37.2%

Morrill County Community Hospital

PO Box 579, 1313 S Street — Phone: 308-262-1616
Bridgeport, NE 69336 — Fax: 308-262-0843
E-mail: morrow@hamilton.net
URL: www.morrillcountyhospital.org
Type: Critical Access Hospitals — Emergency Services: Yes
Ownership: Government - Local — Beds: 20

Key Personnel:
Quality Assurance . . . . Craig Krantz
CEO/President. . . . . Julie Morrow
Chief of Medical Staff . . . . Dr John Post

Measure	Cases	This Hosp.	State Avg.	U.S. Avg.
Blood Clot Prevention and Treatment				
Anticoagulation Overlap Therapy[5]	-	-	93%	93%
ICU Venous Thromboembolism Prophylaxis[5]	-	-	91%	92%
Incidence of Potentially Preventable VTE[5]	-	-	11%	10%
UFH with Dosages/Platelet Monitoring[5]	-	-	98%	97%
Venous Thromboembolism Prophylaxis[5]	-	-	88%	85%
Warfarin Therapy Discharge Instructions[5]	-	-	81%	75%
Chest Pain/Possible Heart Attack Care				
Aspirin Given Within 24 Hours of Arrival[1]	-	-	96%	96%
Fibrinolytic Meds Within 30 Min. of Arrival[1,3]	-	-	53%	58%
Average Time to ECG (minutes)[1]	-	-	8	7
Average Time to Transfer (minutes)[3,7]	-	-	76	60
Children's Asthma Care				
Received Home Management Plan of Care	-	-	-	88%
Received Reliever Medication	-	-	-	100%
Received Systemic Corticosteroids	-	-	-	100%
Emergency Department				
Admittance Decision Time (minutes)[5]	-	-	75	98
Head CT Results Within 45 Min. of Arrival[5]	-	-	61%	57%
Patients Who Left ER Before Being Seen[5]	-	-	1%	2%
Time from ER Arrival to Admit. (minutes)[5]	-	-	207	274
Time from ER Arrival to Discharge (minutes)[5]	-	-	118	134
Time in ER Before Being Evaluated (minutes)[5]	-	-	21	26
Time to Pain Meds for Fractures (minutes)[5]	-	-	42	57
Heart Attack Care				
Aspirin Given at Discharge[5]	-	-	100%	99%
Fibrinolytic Meds Within 30 Min. of Arrival[5]	-	-	-	54%
PCI Within 90 Minutes of Arrival[5]	-	-	96%	96%
Statin Prescribed at Discharge[5]	-	-	99%	98%
Heart Failure Care				
ACE Inhibitor or ARB for LVSD[2,3]	-	-	96%	97%
Discharge Instructions Given[1,2]	-	-	93%	94%
Evaluation of LVS Function[1,2]	-	-	98%	99%
Medicare Spending				
Medicare Spending per Patient (ratio)	-	-	0.97	0.98
Pneumonia Care				
Appropriate Initial Antibiotic Given[1,2]	-	-	95%	95%
Blood Culture Timing[1,2]	-	-	99%	98%
Pregnancy and Delivery Care				
Newborn Deliveries Scheduled Early[5]	-	-	5%	6%
Preventive Care				
Immunization for Influenza[5]	-	-	89%	90%
Immunization for Pneumonia[5]	-	-	90%	92%
Stroke Care				
Anticoagulation Therapy for Atrial Fibrillation[5]	-	-	95%	95%
Antithrombotic Therapy Timing[5]	-	-	99%	98%
Assessed for Rehabilitation[5]	-	-	99%	97%
Discharged on Antithrombotic Therapy[5]	-	-	100%	99%
Discharged on Statin Medication[5]	-	-	93%	94%
Thrombolytic Therapy Timing[5]	-	-	75%	66%
Venous Thromboembolism Prophylaxis[5]	-	-	94%	94%
Written Stroke Educational Materials Given[5]	-	-	84%	88%
Surgical Care Improvement Project				
Appropriate Beta Blocker Usage[5]	-	-	98%	98%
Appropriate VTP Within 24 Hours[5]	-	-	99%	98%
Controlled Postoperative Blood Glucose[5]	-	-	96%	97%
Perioperative Temperature Management[5]	-	-	100%	100%
Prophylactic Antibiotic Selection[5]	-	-	99%	99%
Prophylactic Antibiotic Selection (Outpatient)[1,3]	-	-	99%	98%
Prophylactic Antibiotic Stopped[5]	-	-	98%	98%
Prophylactic Antibiotic Timing[5]	-	-	98%	99%
Prophylactic Antibiotic Timing (Outpatient)[3,7]	-	-	97%	98%
Urinary Catheter Removal[5]	-	-	98%	97%
Survey of Patients' Hospital Experiences				
Area Around Room 'Always' Quiet at Night[5]	-	-	67%	61%
Doctors 'Always' Communicated Well[5]	-	-	86%	82%
Home Recovery Information Given[5]	-	-	88%	85%
Hospital Given 9 or 10 on 10 Point Scale[5]	-	-	78%	71%
Meds 'Always' Explained Before Given[5]	-	-	68%	64%
Nurses 'Always' Communicated Well[5]	-	-	83%	79%
Pain 'Always' Well Controlled[5]	-	-	73%	71%
Room and Bathroom 'Always' Clean[5]	-	-	81%	73%
Timely Help 'Always' Received[5]	-	-	75%	68%
Would Definitely Recommend Hospital[5]	-	-	77%	71%
Use of Medical Imaging				
Cardiac Imaging Stress Test before Surgery[1]	-	-	5.4%	5.3%
Combination Abdominal CT Scan[1]	-	-	9.3%	10.5%
Combination Brain/Sinus CT Scan[1]	-	-	2.7%	2.7%
Combination Chest CT Scan[1]	-	-	1.7%	2.7%
Follow-up Mammogram/Ultrasound[7]	-	-	8%	8.8%
Lumbar Spine MRI for Low Back Pain[1]	-	-	36.5%	37.2%

Jennie M Melham Memorial Medical Center

145 Memorial Drive — Phone: 308-872-4100
Broken Bow, NE 68822 — Fax: 308-872-6116
URL: www.brokenbow-ne.com/community/healthcare/melham.htm
Type: Critical Access Hospitals — Emergency Services: Yes
Ownership: Voluntary non-profit - Private — Beds: 39

Key Personnel:
Anesthesiology. . . . . Tim Johnson
Infection Control . . . . Steve Osborn
CEO/President . . . . Michael Steckler

Measure	Cases	This Hosp.	State Avg.	U.S. Avg.
Blood Clot Prevention and Treatment				
Anticoagulation Overlap Therapy[5]	-	-	93%	93%
ICU Venous Thromboembolism Prophylaxis[5]	-	-	91%	92%
Incidence of Potentially Preventable VTE[5]	-	-	11%	10%
UFH with Dosages/Platelet Monitoring[5]	-	-	98%	97%
Venous Thromboembolism Prophylaxis[5]	-	-	88%	85%
Warfarin Therapy Discharge Instructions[5]	-	-	81%	75%
Chest Pain/Possible Heart Attack Care				
Aspirin Given Within 24 Hours of Arrival[1]	-	-	96%	96%
Fibrinolytic Meds Within 30 Min. of Arrival[1,3]	-	-	53%	58%
Average Time to ECG (minutes)[1]	-	-	8	7
Average Time to Transfer (minutes)[1,3]	-	-	76	60
Children's Asthma Care				
Received Home Management Plan of Care	-	-	-	88%
Received Reliever Medication	-	-	-	100%
Received Systemic Corticosteroids	-	-	-	100%
Emergency Department				
Admittance Decision Time (minutes)[5]	-	-	75	98
Head CT Results Within 45 Min. of Arrival[5]	-	-	61%	57%
Patients Who Left ER Before Being Seen[5]	-	-	1%	2%
Time from ER Arrival to Admit. (minutes)[5]	-	-	207	274
Time from ER Arrival to Discharge (minutes)[5]	-	-	118	134
Time in ER Before Being Evaluated (minutes)[5]	-	-	21	26
Time to Pain Meds for Fractures (minutes)[5]	-	-	42	57
Heart Attack Care				
Aspirin Given at Discharge[5]	-	-	100%	99%
Fibrinolytic Meds Within 30 Min. of Arrival[5]	-	-	-	54%
PCI Within 90 Minutes of Arrival[5]	-	-	96%	96%
Statin Prescribed at Discharge[5]	-	-	99%	98%
Heart Failure Care				
ACE Inhibitor or ARB for LVSD[1]	-	-	96%	97%
Discharge Instructions Given[1]	-	-	93%	94%
Evaluation of LVS Function	15	93%	98%	99%
Medicare Spending				
Medicare Spending per Patient (ratio)	-	-	0.97	0.98
Pneumonia Care				
Appropriate Initial Antibiotic Given	47	91%	95%	95%
Blood Culture Timing	14	86%	99%	98%
Pregnancy and Delivery Care				
Newborn Deliveries Scheduled Early[5]	-	-	5%	6%
Preventive Care				
Immunization for Influenza[5]	-	-	89%	90%
Immunization for Pneumonia[5]	-	-	90%	92%
Stroke Care				
Anticoagulation Therapy for Atrial Fibrillation[5]	-	-	95%	95%
Antithrombotic Therapy Timing[5]	-	-	99%	98%
Assessed for Rehabilitation[5]	-	-	99%	97%
Discharged on Antithrombotic Therapy[5]	-	-	100%	99%
Discharged on Statin Medication[5]	-	-	93%	94%
Thrombolytic Therapy Timing[5]	-	-	75%	66%
Venous Thromboembolism Prophylaxis[5]	-	-	94%	94%

NOTE: Hospital profiles are in alphabetical order by state, then city, then hospital within the city; Rankings exclude hospitals with less than 25 cases except for patient surveys which excludes hospitals with less than 100 cases; (a) 100-299 cases; (1) The number of cases/patients is too few to report; (2) Data submitted were based on a sample of cases/patients; (3) Results are based on a shorter time period than required; (4) Data suppressed by CMS for one or more quarters; (5) Results are not available for this reporting period; (6) Fewer than 100 patients completed the HCAHPS survey; (7) No cases met the criteria for this measure; (8) The lower limit of the confidence interval cannot be calculated if the number of observed infections equals zero; (9) No data are available from the state/territory for this reporting period; (10) The scores shown reflect fewer than 50 completed surveys; (11) There were discrepancies in the data collection process; (12) This measure does not apply to this hospital for this reporting period; (13) Results cannot be calculated for this reporting period; (14) The results for this state are combined with nearby states to protect confidentiality; Please refer to the User's Guide for a full explanation of data.

Measure	Cases	This Hosp.	State Avg.	U.S. Avg.
Written Stroke Educational Materials Given[5]	-	-	84%	88%
Surgical Care Improvement Project				
Appropriate Beta Blocker Usage[3,7]	-	-	98%	98%
Appropriate VTP Within 24 Hours[3,7]	-	-	99%	98%
Controlled Postoperative Blood Glucose[3,7]	-	-	96%	97%
Perioperative Temperature Management[3,7]	-	-	100%	100%
Prophylactic Antibiotic Selection[3,7]	-	-	99%	99%
Prophylactic Antibiotic Selection (Outpatient)	12	75%	99%	98%
Prophylactic Antibiotic Stopped[3,7]	-	-	98%	98%
Prophylactic Antibiotic Timing[3,7]	-	-	98%	99%
Prophylactic Antibiotic Timing (Outpatient)	13	92%	97%	98%
Urinary Catheter Removal[3,7]	-	-	98%	97%
Survey of Patients' Hospital Experiences				
Area Around Room 'Always' Quiet at Night	(a)	56%	67%	61%
Doctors 'Always' Communicated Well	(a)	84%	86%	82%
Home Recovery Information Given	(a)	85%	88%	85%
Hospital Given 9 or 10 on 10 Point Scale	(a)	74%	78%	71%
Meds 'Always' Explained Before Given	(a)	63%	68%	64%
Nurses 'Always' Communicated Well	(a)	82%	83%	79%
Pain 'Always' Well Controlled	(a)	69%	73%	71%
Room and Bathroom 'Always' Clean	(a)	77%	81%	73%
Timely Help 'Always' Received	(a)	69%	75%	68%
Would Definitely Recommend Hospital	(a)	77%	77%	71%
Use of Medical Imaging				
Cardiac Imaging Stress Test before Surgery	84	1.2%	5.4%	5.3%
Combination Abdominal CT Scan	120	5.0%	9.3%	10.5%
Combination Brain/Sinus CT Scan[1]	-	-	2.7%	2.7%
Combination Chest CT Scan	106	0.0%	1.7%	2.7%
Follow-up Mammogram/Ultrasound	181	11.6%	8%	8.8%
Lumbar Spine MRI for Low Back Pain[1]	-	-	36.5%	37.2%

Callaway District Hospital

PO Box 100, 211 E Kimball St
Callaway, NE 68825
Phone: 308-836-2228
Fax: 308-836-2733
URL: www.callaway-ne.com/hospital
Type: Critical Access Hospitals
Emergency Services: Yes
Ownership: Govt - Hospital Dist/Auth
Beds: 12

Measure	Cases	This Hosp.	State Avg.	U.S. Avg.
Blood Clot Prevention and Treatment				
Anticoagulation Overlap Therapy[5]	-	-	93%	93%
ICU Venous Thromboembolism Prophylaxis[5]	-	-	91%	92%
Incidence of Potentially Preventable VTE[5]	-	-	11%	10%
UFH with Dosages/Platelet Monitoring[5]	-	-	98%	97%
Venous Thromboembolism Prophylaxis[5]	-	-	88%	85%
Warfarin Therapy Discharge Instructions[5]	-	-	81%	75%
Chest Pain/Possible Heart Attack Care				
Aspirin Given Within 24 Hours of Arrival[1,3]	-	-	96%	96%
Fibrinolytic Meds Within 30 Min. of Arrival[3,7]	-	-	53%	58%
Average Time to ECG (minutes)[1,3]	-	-	8	7
Average Time to Transfer (minutes)[3,7]	-	-	76	60
Children's Asthma Care				
Received Home Management Plan of Care	-	-	-	88%
Received Reliever Medication	-	-	-	100%
Received Systemic Corticosteroids	-	-	-	100%
Emergency Department				
Admittance Decision Time (minutes)[5]	-	-	75	98
Head CT Results Within 45 Min. of Arrival[5]	-	-	61%	57%
Patients Who Left ER Before Being Seen[5]	-	-	1%	2%
Time from ER Arrival to Admit. (minutes)[5]	-	-	207	274
Time from ER Arrival to Discharge (minutes)[5]	-	-	118	134
Time in ER Before Being Evaluated (minutes)[5]	-	-	21	26
Time to Pain Meds for Fractures (minutes)[5]	-	-	42	57
Heart Attack Care				
Aspirin Given at Discharge[1,3]	-	-	100%	99%
Fibrinolytic Meds Within 30 Min. of Arrival[3,7]	-	-	-	54%
PCI Within 90 Minutes of Arrival[3,7]	-	-	96%	96%
Statin Prescribed at Discharge[3,7]	-	-	99%	98%
Heart Failure Care				
ACE Inhibitor or ARB for LVSD[3,7]	-	-	96%	97%
Discharge Instructions Given[1,3]	-	-	93%	94%
Evaluation of LVS Function[1,3]	-	-	98%	99%
Medicare Spending				
Medicare Spending per Patient (ratio)	-	-	0.97	0.98
Pneumonia Care				
Appropriate Initial Antibiotic Given[7]	-	-	95%	95%
Blood Culture Timing[7]	-	-	99%	98%
Pregnancy and Delivery Care				
Newborn Deliveries Scheduled Early[5]	-	-	5%	6%
Preventive Care				
Immunization for Influenza[5]	-	-	89%	90%
Immunization for Pneumonia[5]	-	-	90%	92%
Stroke Care				
Anticoagulation Therapy for Atrial Fibrillation[5]	-	-	95%	95%
Antithrombotic Therapy Timing[5]	-	-	99%	98%
Assessed for Rehabilitation[5]	-	-	99%	97%
Discharged on Antithrombotic Therapy[5]	-	-	100%	99%
Discharged on Statin Medication[5]	-	-	93%	94%
Thrombolytic Therapy Timing[5]	-	-	75%	66%
Venous Thromboembolism Prophylaxis[5]	-	-	94%	94%
Written Stroke Educational Materials Given[5]	-	-	84%	88%
Surgical Care Improvement Project				
Appropriate Beta Blocker Usage[5]	-	-	98%	98%
Appropriate VTP Within 24 Hours[5]	-	-	99%	98%
Controlled Postoperative Blood Glucose[5]	-	-	96%	97%
Perioperative Temperature Management[5]	-	-	100%	100%
Prophylactic Antibiotic Selection[5]	-	-	99%	99%
Prophylactic Antibiotic Selection (Outpatient)[5]	-	-	99%	98%
Prophylactic Antibiotic Stopped[5]	-	-	98%	98%
Prophylactic Antibiotic Timing[5]	-	-	98%	99%
Prophylactic Antibiotic Timing (Outpatient)[5]	-	-	97%	98%
Urinary Catheter Removal[5]	-	-	98%	97%
Survey of Patients' Hospital Experiences				
Area Around Room 'Always' Quiet at Night[5]	-	-	67%	61%
Doctors 'Always' Communicated Well[5]	-	-	86%	82%
Home Recovery Information Given[5]	-	-	88%	85%
Hospital Given 9 or 10 on 10 Point Scale[5]	-	-	78%	71%
Meds 'Always' Explained Before Given[5]	-	-	68%	64%
Nurses 'Always' Communicated Well[5]	-	-	83%	79%
Pain 'Always' Well Controlled[5]	-	-	73%	71%
Room and Bathroom 'Always' Clean[5]	-	-	81%	73%
Timely Help 'Always' Received[5]	-	-	75%	68%
Would Definitely Recommend Hospital[5]	-	-	77%	71%
Use of Medical Imaging				
Cardiac Imaging Stress Test before Surgery[1]	-	-	5.4%	5.3%
Combination Abdominal CT Scan[1]	-	-	9.3%	10.5%
Combination Brain/Sinus CT Scan[1]	-	-	2.7%	2.7%
Combination Chest CT Scan[1]	-	-	1.7%	2.7%
Follow-up Mammogram/Ultrasound	75	4.0%	8%	8.8%
Lumbar Spine MRI for Low Back Pain[1]	-	-	36.5%	37.2%

Tri Valley Health System

1305 West Highway 6/34
Cambridge, NE 69022
Phone: 308-697-3329
Fax: 308-697-4918
URL: www.trivalleyhealth.com
Type: Critical Access Hospitals
Emergency Services: Yes
Ownership: Voluntary non-profit - Private
Beds: 25

Key Personnel:

Chief of Medical Staff.......... Lennis Deaver, MD
Anesthesiology.............. Rachelle Kaspor-Cope
CEO/President.............. Lynn Milnes
Infection Control.............. Shelly Shellabarger
Quality Assurance .... Shelly Shellabarger
Emergency Room .... Rhonda Sherman
Ambulatory Care .... Joyce Thompson, RN
Operating Room.............. Joyce Thompson, RN

Measure	Cases	This Hosp.	State Avg.	U.S. Avg.
Blood Clot Prevention and Treatment				
Anticoagulation Overlap Therapy[5]	-	-	93%	93%
ICU Venous Thromboembolism Prophylaxis[5]	-	-	91%	92%
Incidence of Potentially Preventable VTE[5]	-	-	11%	10%
UFH with Dosages/Platelet Monitoring[5]	-	-	98%	97%
Venous Thromboembolism Prophylaxis[5]	-	-	88%	85%
Warfarin Therapy Discharge Instructions[5]	-	-	81%	75%
Chest Pain/Possible Heart Attack Care				
Aspirin Given Within 24 Hours of Arrival	18	89%	96%	96%
Fibrinolytic Meds Within 30 Min. of Arrival[1,3]	-	-	53%	58%
Average Time to ECG (minutes)	19	6	8	7
Average Time to Transfer (minutes)[3,7]	-	-	76	60
Children's Asthma Care				
Received Home Management Plan of Care	-	-	-	88%
Received Reliever Medication	-	-	-	100%
Received Systemic Corticosteroids	-	-	-	100%
Emergency Department				
Admittance Decision Time (minutes)[5]	-	-	75	98
Head CT Results Within 45 Min. of Arrival[5]	-	-	61%	57%
Patients Who Left ER Before Being Seen[5]	-	-	1%	2%
Time from ER Arrival to Admit. (minutes)[5]	-	-	207	274
Time from ER Arrival to Discharge (minutes)[5]	-	-	118	134
Time in ER Before Being Evaluated (minutes)[5]	-	-	21	26
Time to Pain Meds for Fractures (minutes)[5]	-	-	42	57
Heart Attack Care				
Aspirin Given at Discharge[5]	-	-	100%	99%
Fibrinolytic Meds Within 30 Min. of Arrival[5]	-	-	-	54%
PCI Within 90 Minutes of Arrival[5]	-	-	96%	96%
Statin Prescribed at Discharge[5]	-	-	99%	98%
Heart Failure Care				
ACE Inhibitor or ARB for LVSD[1]	-	-	96%	97%
Discharge Instructions Given[1]	-	-	93%	94%
Evaluation of LVS Function	11	45%	98%	99%
Medicare Spending				
Medicare Spending per Patient (ratio)	-	-	0.97	0.98
Pneumonia Care				
Appropriate Initial Antibiotic Given[2]	11	82%	95%	95%
Blood Culture Timing[2,7]	-	-	99%	98%
Pregnancy and Delivery Care				
Newborn Deliveries Scheduled Early[5]	-	-	5%	6%
Preventive Care				
Immunization for Influenza[5]	-	-	89%	90%
Immunization for Pneumonia[5]	-	-	90%	92%
Stroke Care				
Anticoagulation Therapy for Atrial Fibrillation[5]	-	-	95%	95%
Antithrombotic Therapy Timing[5]	-	-	99%	98%
Assessed for Rehabilitation[5]	-	-	99%	97%
Discharged on Antithrombotic Therapy[5]	-	-	100%	99%
Discharged on Statin Medication[5]	-	-	93%	94%
Thrombolytic Therapy Timing[5]	-	-	75%	66%
Venous Thromboembolism Prophylaxis[5]	-	-	94%	94%
Written Stroke Educational Materials Given[5]	-	-	84%	88%
Surgical Care Improvement Project				
Appropriate Beta Blocker Usage[1,3]	-	-	98%	98%
Appropriate VTP Within 24 Hours[1,3]	-	-	99%	98%
Controlled Postoperative Blood Glucose[3,7]	-	-	96%	97%
Perioperative Temperature Management[1,3]	-	-	100%	100%
Prophylactic Antibiotic Selection[3,7]	-	-	99%	99%
Prophylactic Antibiotic Selection (Outpatient)[3]	11	73%	99%	98%
Prophylactic Antibiotic Stopped[3,7]	-	-	98%	98%
Prophylactic Antibiotic Timing[3,7]	-	-	98%	99%
Prophylactic Antibiotic Timing (Outpatient)[3]	14	71%	97%	98%
Urinary Catheter Removal[3,7]	-	-	98%	97%
Survey of Patients' Hospital Experiences				
Area Around Room 'Always' Quiet at Night	(a)	57%	67%	61%
Doctors 'Always' Communicated Well	(a)	85%	86%	82%
Home Recovery Information Given	(a)	84%	88%	85%
Hospital Given 9 or 10 on 10 Point Scale	(a)	67%	78%	71%
Meds 'Always' Explained Before Given	(a)	63%	68%	64%
Nurses 'Always' Communicated Well	(a)	71%	83%	79%
Pain 'Always' Well Controlled	(a)	60%	73%	71%
Room and Bathroom 'Always' Clean	(a)	81%	81%	73%
Timely Help 'Always' Received	(a)	63%	75%	68%
Would Definitely Recommend Hospital	(a)	74%	77%	71%
Use of Medical Imaging				
Cardiac Imaging Stress Test before Surgery	62	3.2%	5.4%	5.3%
Combination Abdominal CT Scan	65	4.6%	9.3%	10.5%
Combination Brain/Sinus CT Scan[1]	-	-	2.7%	2.7%
Combination Chest CT Scan	59	1.7%	1.7%	2.7%
Follow-up Mammogram/Ultrasound	146	2.7%	8%	8.8%
Lumbar Spine MRI for Low Back Pain[1]	-	-	36.5%	37.2%

NOTE: Hospital profiles are in alphabetical order by state, then city, then hospital within the city; Rankings exclude hospitals with less than 25 cases except for patient surveys which excludes hospitals with less than 100 cases; (a) 100-299 cases; (1) The number of cases/patients is too few to report; (2) Data submitted were based on a sample of cases/patients; (3) Results are based on a shorter time period than required; (4) Data suppressed by CMS for one or more quarters; (5) Results are not available for this reporting period; (6) Fewer than 100 patients completed the HCAHPS survey; (7) No cases met the criteria for this measure; (8) The lower limit of the confidence interval cannot be calculated if the number of observed infections equals zero; (9) No data are available from the state/territory for this reporting period; (10) The scores shown reflect fewer than 50 completed surveys; (11) There were discrepancies in the data collection process; (12) This measure does not apply to this hospital for this reporting period; (13) Results cannot be calculated for this reporting period; (14) The results for this state are combined with nearby states to protect confidentiality; Please refer to the User's Guide for a full explanation of data.

Litzenberg Memorial County Hospital

1715 26th St Phone: 308-946-3015
Central City, NE 68826 Fax: 308-946-2633
E-mail: mbowman@lmchealth.com
URL: www.lmchealth.com
Type: Critical Access Hospitals Emergency Services: Yes
Ownership: Government - Local Beds: 25

Key Personnel:
Radiology.................... John Allen
Chief of Medical Staff.......... Gerome Dackey
CEO.......................... Julie M. Murray
Emergency Room .... Diane Schoch
Infection Control.............. Lavonne Solomon, LPN
Quality Assurance .... Penny Wetovick

Measure	Cases	This Hosp.	State Avg.	U.S. Avg.
Blood Clot Prevention and Treatment				
Anticoagulation Overlap Therapy[5]	-	-	93%	93%
ICU Venous Thromboembolism Prophylaxis[5]	-	-	91%	92%
Incidence of Potentially Preventable VTE[5]	-	-	11%	10%
UFH with Dosages/Platelet Monitoring[5]	-	-	98%	97%
Venous Thromboembolism Prophylaxis[5]	-	-	88%	85%
Warfarin Therapy Discharge Instructions[5]	-	-	81%	75%
Chest Pain/Possible Heart Attack Care				
Aspirin Given Within 24 Hours of Arrival	11	91%	96%	96%
Fibrinolytic Meds Within 30 Min. of Arrival[3,7]	-	-	53%	58%
Average Time to ECG (minutes)	11	10	8	7
Average Time to Transfer (minutes)[3,7]	-	-	76	60
Children's Asthma Care				
Received Home Management Plan of Care	-	-	-	88%
Received Reliever Medication	-	-	-	100%
Received Systemic Corticosteroids	-	-	-	100%
Emergency Department				
Admittance Decision Time (minutes)[5]	-	-	75	98
Head CT Results Within 45 Min. of Arrival[5]	-	-	61%	57%
Patients Who Left ER Before Being Seen[5]	-	-	1%	2%
Time from ER Arrival to Admit. (minutes)[5]	-	-	207	274
Time from ER Arrival to Discharge (minutes)[5]	-	-	118	134
Time in ER Before Being Evaluated (minutes)[5]	-	-	21	26
Time to Pain Meds for Fractures (minutes)[5]	-	-	42	57
Heart Attack Care				
Aspirin Given at Discharge[5]	-	-	100%	99%
Fibrinolytic Meds Within 30 Min. of Arrival[5]	-	-	-	54%
PCI Within 90 Minutes of Arrival[5]	-	-	96%	96%
Statin Prescribed at Discharge[5]	-	-	99%	98%
Heart Failure Care				
ACE Inhibitor or ARB for LVSD[1]	-	-	96%	97%
Discharge Instructions Given[1]	-	-	93%	94%
Evaluation of LVS Function[1]	-	-	98%	99%
Medicare Spending				
Medicare Spending per Patient (ratio)	-	-	0.97	0.98
Pneumonia Care				
Appropriate Initial Antibiotic Given	20	100%	95%	95%
Blood Culture Timing[1]	-	-	99%	98%
Pregnancy and Delivery Care				
Newborn Deliveries Scheduled Early[5]	-	-	5%	6%
Preventive Care				
Immunization for Influenza[5]	-	-	89%	90%
Immunization for Pneumonia[5]	-	-	90%	92%
Stroke Care				
Anticoagulation Therapy for Atrial Fibrillation[5]	-	-	95%	95%
Antithrombotic Therapy Timing[5]	-	-	99%	98%
Assessed for Rehabilitation[5]	-	-	99%	97%
Discharged on Antithrombotic Therapy[5]	-	-	100%	99%
Discharged on Statin Medication[5]	-	-	93%	94%
Thrombolytic Therapy Timing[5]	-	-	75%	66%
Venous Thromboembolism Prophylaxis[5]	-	-	94%	94%
Written Stroke Educational Materials Given[5]	-	-	84%	88%
Surgical Care Improvement Project				
Appropriate Beta Blocker Usage[5]	-	-	98%	98%
Appropriate VTP Within 24 Hours[5]	-	-	99%	98%
Controlled Postoperative Blood Glucose[5]	-	-	96%	97%
Perioperative Temperature Management[5]	-	-	100%	100%
Prophylactic Antibiotic Selection[5]	-	-	99%	99%
Prophylactic Antibiotic Selection (Outpatient)[1,3]	-	-	99%	98%
Prophylactic Antibiotic Stopped[5]	-	-	98%	98%
Prophylactic Antibiotic Timing[5]	-	-	98%	99%
Prophylactic Antibiotic Timing (Outpatient)[1,3]	-	-	97%	98%
Urinary Catheter Removal[5]	-	-	98%	97%
Survey of Patients' Hospital Experiences				
Area Around Room 'Always' Quiet at Night[6]	<100	59%	67%	61%
Doctors 'Always' Communicated Well[6]	<100	73%	86%	82%
Home Recovery Information Given[6]	<100	71%	88%	85%
Hospital Given 9 or 10 on 10 Point Scale[6]	<100	43%	78%	71%
Meds 'Always' Explained Before Given[6]	<100	54%	68%	64%
Nurses 'Always' Communicated Well[6]	<100	64%	83%	79%
Pain 'Always' Well Controlled[6]	<100	61%	73%	71%
Room and Bathroom 'Always' Clean[6]	<100	69%	81%	73%
Timely Help 'Always' Received[6]	<100	64%	75%	68%
Would Definitely Recommend Hospital[6]	<100	46%	77%	71%
Use of Medical Imaging				
Cardiac Imaging Stress Test before Surgery[1]	-	-	5.4%	5.3%
Combination Abdominal CT Scan	79	11.4%	9.3%	10.5%
Combination Brain/Sinus CT Scan[1]	-	-	2.7%	2.7%
Combination Chest CT Scan[1]	-	-	1.7%	2.7%
Follow-up Mammogram/Ultrasound	200	5.0%	8%	8.8%
Lumbar Spine MRI for Low Back Pain[1]	-	-	36.5%	37.2%

Chadron Community Hospital & Health Services

825 Centennial Drive Phone: 308-432-5586
Chadron, NE 69337 Fax: 308-432-2737
E-mail: ceo@chadronhospital.com
URL: www.chadronhospital.com
Type: Critical Access Hospitals Emergency Services: Yes
Ownership: Voluntary non-profit - Private Beds: 25

Key Personnel:
Operating Room.............. Elinrey D Burgess
Infection Control.............. Cheryl Cassiday
Intensive Care Unit............ Cheryl Cassiday
Radiology..................... Jodi Dannar
Quality Assurance .... Amy Hindman
Emergency Room .... Sandra Ingwersen
CEO/President................ Harold Krueger, Jr
Chief of Medical Staff.......... Jeffrey Lias

Measure	Cases	This Hosp.	State Avg.	U.S. Avg.
Blood Clot Prevention and Treatment				
Anticoagulation Overlap Therapy[5]	-	-	93%	93%
ICU Venous Thromboembolism Prophylaxis[5]	-	-	91%	92%
Incidence of Potentially Preventable VTE[5]	-	-	11%	10%
UFH with Dosages/Platelet Monitoring[5]	-	-	98%	97%
Venous Thromboembolism Prophylaxis[5]	-	-	88%	85%
Warfarin Therapy Discharge Instructions[5]	-	-	81%	75%
Chest Pain/Possible Heart Attack Care				
Aspirin Given Within 24 Hours of Arrival[1]	-	-	96%	96%
Fibrinolytic Meds Within 30 Min. of Arrival[5]	-	-	53%	58%
Average Time to ECG (minutes)[1]	-	-	8	7
Average Time to Transfer (minutes)[5]	-	-	76	60
Children's Asthma Care				
Received Home Management Plan of Care	-	-	-	88%
Received Reliever Medication	-	-	-	100%
Received Systemic Corticosteroids	-	-	-	100%
Emergency Department				
Admittance Decision Time (minutes)[5]	-	-	75	98
Head CT Results Within 45 Min. of Arrival[5]	-	-	61%	57%
Patients Who Left ER Before Being Seen[5]	-	-	1%	2%
Time from ER Arrival to Admit. (minutes)[5]	-	-	207	274
Time from ER Arrival to Discharge (minutes)[5]	-	-	118	134
Time in ER Before Being Evaluated (minutes)[5]	-	-	21	26
Time to Pain Meds for Fractures (minutes)[5]	-	-	42	57
Heart Attack Care				
Aspirin Given at Discharge[5]	-	-	100%	99%
Fibrinolytic Meds Within 30 Min. of Arrival[3,7]	-	-	-	54%
PCI Within 90 Minutes of Arrival[5]	-	-	96%	96%
Statin Prescribed at Discharge[3,7]	-	-	99%	98%
Heart Failure Care				
ACE Inhibitor or ARB for LVSD[7]	-	-	96%	97%
Discharge Instructions Given[1]	-	-	93%	94%
Evaluation of LVS Function	11	64%	98%	99%
Medicare Spending				
Medicare Spending per Patient (ratio)	-	-	0.97	0.98
Pneumonia Care				
Appropriate Initial Antibiotic Given	11	100%	95%	95%
Blood Culture Timing[3,7]	-	-	99%	98%
Pregnancy and Delivery Care				
Newborn Deliveries Scheduled Early[5]	-	-	5%	6%
Preventive Care				
Immunization for Influenza[5]	-	-	89%	90%
Immunization for Pneumonia[5]	-	-	90%	92%
Stroke Care				
Anticoagulation Therapy for Atrial Fibrillation[5]	-	-	95%	95%
Antithrombotic Therapy Timing[5]	-	-	99%	98%
Assessed for Rehabilitation[5]	-	-	99%	97%
Discharged on Antithrombotic Therapy[5]	-	-	100%	99%
Discharged on Statin Medication[5]	-	-	93%	94%
Thrombolytic Therapy Timing[5]	-	-	75%	66%
Venous Thromboembolism Prophylaxis[5]	-	-	94%	94%
Written Stroke Educational Materials Given[5]	-	-	84%	88%
Surgical Care Improvement Project				
Appropriate Beta Blocker Usage[1,3]	-	-	98%	98%
Appropriate VTP Within 24 Hours[1,3]	-	-	99%	98%
Controlled Postoperative Blood Glucose[5]	-	-	96%	97%
Perioperative Temperature Management[1,3]	-	-	100%	100%
Prophylactic Antibiotic Selection[1,3]	-	-	99%	99%
Prophylactic Antibiotic Selection (Outpatient)[5]	-	-	99%	98%
Prophylactic Antibiotic Stopped[1,3]	-	-	98%	98%
Prophylactic Antibiotic Timing[1,3]	-	-	98%	99%
Prophylactic Antibiotic Timing (Outpatient)[5]	-	-	97%	98%
Urinary Catheter Removal[1,3]	-	-	98%	97%
Survey of Patients' Hospital Experiences				
Area Around Room 'Always' Quiet at Night	(a)	73%	67%	61%
Doctors 'Always' Communicated Well	(a)	87%	86%	82%
Home Recovery Information Given	(a)	82%	88%	85%
Hospital Given 9 or 10 on 10 Point Scale	(a)	67%	78%	71%
Meds 'Always' Explained Before Given	(a)	78%	68%	64%
Nurses 'Always' Communicated Well	(a)	79%	83%	79%
Pain 'Always' Well Controlled	(a)	69%	73%	71%
Room and Bathroom 'Always' Clean	(a)	79%	81%	73%
Timely Help 'Always' Received	(a)	69%	75%	68%
Would Definitely Recommend Hospital	(a)	66%	77%	71%
Use of Medical Imaging				
Cardiac Imaging Stress Test before Surgery[1]	-	-	5.4%	5.3%
Combination Abdominal CT Scan	62	3.2%	9.3%	10.5%
Combination Brain/Sinus CT Scan	50	0.0%	2.7%	2.7%
Combination Chest CT Scan[1]	-	-	1.7%	2.7%
Follow-up Mammogram/Ultrasound	255	5.1%	8%	8.8%
Lumbar Spine MRI for Low Back Pain[1]	-	-	36.5%	37.2%

Columbus Community Hospital

4600 38th St Phone: 402-564-7118
Columbus, NE 68601 Fax: 402-563-3267
E-mail: info@columbushosp.org
URL: www.columbushosp.org
Type: Acute Care Hospitals Emergency Services: Yes
Ownership: Voluntary non-profit - Other Beds: 81

Key Personnel:
Radiology..................... John P Beauvais
Operating Room.............. Marlene Engel
Emergency Room .... Cathy Hare
Infection Control.............. Cookie Walsh
Quality Assurance .... Cookie Walsh
CEO/President................ Donald Zornes

Measure	Cases	This Hosp.	State Avg.	U.S. Avg.
Blood Clot Prevention and Treatment				
Anticoagulation Overlap Therapy[1,2]	-	-	93%	93%
ICU Venous Thromboembolism Prophylaxis[2]	131	76%	91%	92%
Incidence of Potentially Preventable VTE[2,7]	-	-	11%	10%
UFH with Dosages/Platelet Monitoring[1,2]	-	-	98%	97%
Venous Thromboembolism Prophylaxis[2]	187	80%	88%	85%
Warfarin Therapy Discharge Instructions[1,2]	-	-	81%	75%
Chest Pain/Possible Heart Attack Care				
Aspirin Given Within 24 Hours of Arrival	40	98%	96%	96%
Fibrinolytic Meds Within 30 Min. of Arrival[1]	-	-	53%	58%
Average Time to ECG (minutes)	42	12	8	7

NOTE: Hospital profiles are in alphabetical order by state, then city, then hospital within the city; Rankings exclude hospitals with less than 25 cases except for patient surveys which excludes hospitals with less than 100 cases; (a) 100-299 cases; (1) The number of cases/patients is too few to report; (2) Data submitted were based on a sample of cases/patients; (3) Results are based on a shorter time period than required; (4) Data suppressed by CMS for one or more quarters; (5) Results are not available for this reporting period; (6) Fewer than 100 patients completed the HCAHPS survey; (7) No cases met the criteria for this measure; (8) The lower limit of the confidence interval cannot be calculated if the number of observed infections equals zero; (9) No data are available from the state/territory for this reporting period; (10) The scores shown reflect fewer than 50 completed surveys; (11) There were discrepancies in the data collection process; (12) This measure does not apply to this hospital for this reporting period; (13) Results cannot be calculated for this reporting period; (14) The results for this state are combined with nearby states to protect confidentiality; Please refer to the User's Guide for a full explanation of data.

Measure	Cases	This Hosp.	State Avg.	U.S. Avg.
Average Time to Transfer (minutes)[1]	-	-	76	60
Children's Asthma Care				
Received Home Management Plan of Care	-	-	-	88%
Received Reliever Medication	-	-	-	100%
Received Systemic Corticosteroids	-	-	-	100%
Emergency Department				
Admittance Decision Time (minutes)[2]	347	56	75	98
Head CT Results Within 45 Min. of Arrival[1]	-	-	61%	57%
Patients Who Left ER Before Being Seen	11,036	0%	1%	2%
Time from ER Arrival to Admit. (minutes)[2]	390	179	207	274
Time from ER Arrival to Discharge (minutes)	414	107	118	134
Time in ER Before Being Evaluated (minutes)	454	21	21	26
Time to Pain Meds for Fractures (minutes)	51	37	42	57
Heart Attack Care				
Aspirin Given at Discharge[1]	-	-	100%	99%
Fibrinolytic Meds Within 30 Min. of Arrival[7]	-	-	-	54%
PCI Within 90 Minutes of Arrival[7]	-	-	96%	96%
Statin Prescribed at Discharge[1]	-	-	99%	98%
Heart Failure Care				
ACE Inhibitor or ARB for LVSD	11	100%	96%	97%
Discharge Instructions Given	43	98%	93%	94%
Evaluation of LVS Function	61	100%	98%	99%
Medicare Spending				
Medicare Spending per Patient (ratio)	-	0.93	0.97	0.98
Pneumonia Care				
Appropriate Initial Antibiotic Given	15	100%	95%	95%
Blood Culture Timing	27	100%	99%	98%
Pregnancy and Delivery Care				
Newborn Deliveries Scheduled Early	65	9%	5%	6%
Preventive Care				
Immunization for Influenza[2]	311	98%	89%	90%
Immunization for Pneumonia[2]	416	99%	90%	92%
Stroke Care				
Anticoagulation Therapy for Atrial Fibrillation[1]	-	-	95%	95%
Antithrombotic Therapy Timing	11	91%	99%	98%
Assessed for Rehabilitation	12	100%	99%	97%
Discharged on Antithrombotic Therapy	12	100%	100%	99%
Discharged on Statin Medication[1]	-	-	93%	94%
Thrombolytic Therapy Timing[1]	-	-	75%	66%
Venous Thromboembolism Prophylaxis	12	75%	94%	94%
Written Stroke Educational Materials Given[1]	-	-	84%	88%
Surgical Care Improvement Project				
Appropriate Beta Blocker Usage	63	98%	98%	98%
Appropriate VTP Within 24 Hours	153	99%	99%	98%
Controlled Postoperative Blood Glucose[7]	-	-	96%	97%
Perioperative Temperature Management	170	100%	100%	100%
Prophylactic Antibiotic Selection	127	99%	99%	99%
Prophylactic Antibiotic Selection (Outpatient)	68	99%	99%	98%
Prophylactic Antibiotic Stopped	123	99%	98%	98%
Prophylactic Antibiotic Timing	127	100%	98%	99%
Prophylactic Antibiotic Timing (Outpatient)	70	96%	97%	98%
Urinary Catheter Removal	30	97%	98%	97%
Survey of Patients' Hospital Experiences				
Area Around Room 'Always' Quiet at Night	300+	57%	67%	61%
Doctors 'Always' Communicated Well	300+	80%	86%	82%
Home Recovery Information Given	300+	90%	88%	85%
Hospital Given 9 or 10 on 10 Point Scale	300+	74%	78%	71%
Meds 'Always' Explained Before Given	300+	62%	68%	64%
Nurses 'Always' Communicated Well	300+	78%	83%	79%
Pain 'Always' Well Controlled	300+	70%	73%	71%
Room and Bathroom 'Always' Clean	300+	72%	81%	73%
Timely Help 'Always' Received	300+	68%	75%	68%
Would Definitely Recommend Hospital	300+	64%	77%	71%
Use of Medical Imaging				
Cardiac Imaging Stress Test before Surgery	220	4.1%	5.4%	5.3%
Combination Abdominal CT Scan	435	5.7%	9.3%	10.5%
Combination Brain/Sinus CT Scan	348	0.9%	2.7%	2.7%
Combination Chest CT Scan	315	0.3%	1.7%	2.7%
Follow-up Mammogram/Ultrasound	899	1.9%	8%	8.8%
Lumbar Spine MRI for Low Back Pain	67	28.4%	36.5%	37.2%

Cozad Community Hospital

PO Box 108, 300 East 12th St
Cozad, NE 69130
Phone: 308-784-2261
Fax: 308-784-4691
E-mail: info@cozadcommunityhealth.com
URL: www.cozadhealthcare.com
Type: Critical Access Hospitals
Emergency Services: Yes
Ownership: Govt - Hospital Dist/Auth
Beds: 23

Key Personnel:

Operating Room. . . . . Cheryl Brooks
Infection Control. . . . . Jo Griffith
Emergency Room . . . . Tammy McMichael
Quality Assurance . . . . Shirley Urwiller

Measure	Cases	This Hosp.	State Avg.	U.S. Avg.
Blood Clot Prevention and Treatment				
Anticoagulation Overlap Therapy[5]	-	-	93%	93%
ICU Venous Thromboembolism Prophylaxis[5]	-	-	91%	92%
Incidence of Potentially Preventable VTE[5]	-	-	11%	10%
UFH with Dosages/Platelet Monitoring[5]	-	-	98%	97%
Venous Thromboembolism Prophylaxis[5]	-	-	88%	85%
Warfarin Therapy Discharge Instructions[5]	-	-	81%	75%
Chest Pain/Possible Heart Attack Care				
Aspirin Given Within 24 Hours of Arrival	-	-	96%	96%
Fibrinolytic Meds Within 30 Min. of Arrival	-	-	53%	58%
Average Time to ECG (minutes)	-	-	8	7
Average Time to Transfer (minutes)	-	-	76	60
Children's Asthma Care				
Received Home Management Plan of Care	-	-	-	88%
Received Reliever Medication	-	-	-	100%
Received Systemic Corticosteroids	-	-	-	100%
Emergency Department				
Admittance Decision Time (minutes)[5]	-	-	75	98
Head CT Results Within 45 Min. of Arrival	-	-	61%	57%
Patients Who Left ER Before Being Seen	-	-	1%	2%
Time from ER Arrival to Admit. (minutes)[5]	-	-	207	274
Time from ER Arrival to Discharge (minutes)	-	-	118	134
Time in ER Before Being Evaluated (minutes)	-	-	21	26
Time to Pain Meds for Fractures (minutes)	-	-	42	57
Heart Attack Care				
Aspirin Given at Discharge[5]	-	-	100%	99%
Fibrinolytic Meds Within 30 Min. of Arrival[5]	-	-	-	54%
PCI Within 90 Minutes of Arrival[5]	-	-	96%	96%
Statin Prescribed at Discharge[5]	-	-	99%	98%
Heart Failure Care				
ACE Inhibitor or ARB for LVSD[1,3]	-	-	96%	97%
Discharge Instructions Given[1,3]	-	-	93%	94%
Evaluation of LVS Function[1,3]	-	-	98%	99%
Medicare Spending				
Medicare Spending per Patient (ratio)	-	-	0.97	0.98
Pneumonia Care				
Appropriate Initial Antibiotic Given	16	81%	95%	95%
Blood Culture Timing[1]	-	-	99%	98%
Pregnancy and Delivery Care				
Newborn Deliveries Scheduled Early[5]	-	-	5%	6%
Preventive Care				
Immunization for Influenza[5]	-	-	89%	90%
Immunization for Pneumonia[5]	-	-	90%	92%
Stroke Care				
Anticoagulation Therapy for Atrial Fibrillation[5]	-	-	95%	95%
Antithrombotic Therapy Timing[5]	-	-	99%	98%
Assessed for Rehabilitation[5]	-	-	99%	97%
Discharged on Antithrombotic Therapy[5]	-	-	100%	99%
Discharged on Statin Medication[5]	-	-	93%	94%
Thrombolytic Therapy Timing[5]	-	-	75%	66%
Venous Thromboembolism Prophylaxis[5]	-	-	94%	94%
Written Stroke Educational Materials Given[5]	-	-	84%	88%
Surgical Care Improvement Project				
Appropriate Beta Blocker Usage[5]	-	-	98%	98%
Appropriate VTP Within 24 Hours[5]	-	-	99%	98%
Controlled Postoperative Blood Glucose[5]	-	-	96%	97%
Perioperative Temperature Management[5]	-	-	100%	100%
Prophylactic Antibiotic Selection[5]	-	-	99%	99%
Prophylactic Antibiotic Selection (Outpatient)	-	-	99%	98%
Prophylactic Antibiotic Stopped[5]	-	-	98%	98%
Prophylactic Antibiotic Timing[5]	-	-	98%	99%
Prophylactic Antibiotic Timing (Outpatient)	-	-	97%	98%
Urinary Catheter Removal[5]	-	-	98%	97%
Survey of Patients' Hospital Experiences				
Area Around Room 'Always' Quiet at Night[6]	<100	59%	67%	61%
Doctors 'Always' Communicated Well[6]	<100	85%	86%	82%
Home Recovery Information Given[6]	<100	77%	88%	85%
Hospital Given 9 or 10 on 10 Point Scale[6]	<100	69%	78%	71%
Meds 'Always' Explained Before Given[6]	<100	57%	68%	64%
Nurses 'Always' Communicated Well[6]	<100	85%	83%	79%
Pain 'Always' Well Controlled[6]	<100	65%	73%	71%
Room and Bathroom 'Always' Clean[6]	<100	78%	81%	73%
Timely Help 'Always' Received[6]	<100	80%	75%	68%
Would Definitely Recommend Hospital[6]	<100	60%	77%	71%
Use of Medical Imaging				
Cardiac Imaging Stress Test before Surgery	-	-	5.4%	5.3%
Combination Abdominal CT Scan	-	-	9.3%	10.5%
Combination Brain/Sinus CT Scan	-	-	2.7%	2.7%
Combination Chest CT Scan	-	-	1.7%	2.7%
Follow-up Mammogram/Ultrasound	-	-	8%	8.8%
Lumbar Spine MRI for Low Back Pain	-	-	36.5%	37.2%

Avera Creighton Hospital

PO Box 186, 1503 Main St
Creighton, NE 68729
Phone: 402-358-5700
Fax: 402-358-5769
E-mail: marketing@cahs-ne.org
Type: Critical Access Hospitals
Emergency Services: Yes
Ownership: Voluntary non-profit - Private
Beds: 69

Key Personnel:

Infection Control. . . . . Jean Henes
Chief of Medical Staff. . . . . Ron Morris
Operating Room. . . . . Barbara Nielsen
CEO . . . . Mark Schulte

Measure	Cases	This Hosp.	State Avg.	U.S. Avg.
Blood Clot Prevention and Treatment				
Anticoagulation Overlap Therapy[5]	-	-	93%	93%
ICU Venous Thromboembolism Prophylaxis[5]	-	-	91%	92%
Incidence of Potentially Preventable VTE[5]	-	-	11%	10%
UFH with Dosages/Platelet Monitoring[5]	-	-	98%	97%
Venous Thromboembolism Prophylaxis[5]	-	-	88%	85%
Warfarin Therapy Discharge Instructions[5]	-	-	81%	75%
Chest Pain/Possible Heart Attack Care				
Aspirin Given Within 24 Hours of Arrival[1]	-	-	96%	96%
Fibrinolytic Meds Within 30 Min. of Arrival[1,3]	-	-	53%	58%
Average Time to ECG (minutes)[1]	-	-	8	7
Average Time to Transfer (minutes)[1,3]	-	-	76	60
Children's Asthma Care				
Received Home Management Plan of Care	-	-	-	88%
Received Reliever Medication	-	-	-	100%
Received Systemic Corticosteroids	-	-	-	100%
Emergency Department				
Admittance Decision Time (minutes)[5]	-	-	75	98
Head CT Results Within 45 Min. of Arrival[3,7]	-	-	61%	57%
Patients Who Left ER Before Being Seen[5]	-	-	1%	2%
Time from ER Arrival to Admit. (minutes)[5]	-	-	207	274
Time from ER Arrival to Discharge (minutes)[5]	-	-	118	134
Time in ER Before Being Evaluated (minutes)[5]	-	-	21	26
Time to Pain Meds for Fractures (minutes)[5]	-	-	42	57
Heart Attack Care				
Aspirin Given at Discharge[3,7]	-	-	100%	99%
Fibrinolytic Meds Within 30 Min. of Arrival[3,7]	-	-	-	54%
PCI Within 90 Minutes of Arrival[3,7]	-	-	96%	96%
Statin Prescribed at Discharge[3,7]	-	-	99%	98%
Heart Failure Care				
ACE Inhibitor or ARB for LVSD[5]	-	-	96%	97%
Discharge Instructions Given[5]	-	-	93%	94%
Evaluation of LVS Function[5]	-	-	98%	99%
Medicare Spending				
Medicare Spending per Patient (ratio)	-	-	0.97	0.98
Pneumonia Care				
Appropriate Initial Antibiotic Given	23	100%	95%	95%
Blood Culture Timing[7]	-	-	99%	98%
Pregnancy and Delivery Care				

NOTE: Hospital profiles are in alphabetical order by state, then city, then hospital within the city; Rankings exclude hospitals with less than 25 cases except for patient surveys which excludes hospitals with less than 100 cases; (a) 100-299 cases; (1) The number of cases/patients is too few to report; (2) Data submitted were based on a sample of cases/patients; (3) Results are based on a shorter time period than required; (4) Data suppressed by CMS for one or more quarters; (5) Results are not available for this reporting period; (6) Fewer than 100 patients completed the HCAHPS survey; (7) No cases met the criteria for this measure; (8) The lower limit of the confidence interval cannot be calculated if the number of observed infections equals zero; (9) No data are available from the state/territory for this reporting period; (10) The scores shown reflect fewer than 50 completed surveys; (11) There were discrepancies in the data collection process; (12) This measure does not apply to this hospital for this reporting period; (13) Results cannot be calculated for this reporting period; (14) The results for this state are combined with nearby states to protect confidentiality; Please refer to the User's Guide for a full explanation of data.

Measure	Cases	This Hosp.	State Avg.	U.S. Avg.
Newborn Deliveries Scheduled Early[5]	-	-	5%	6%
Preventive Care				
Immunization for Influenza[5]	-	-	89%	90%
Immunization for Pneumonia[5]	-	-	90%	92%
Stroke Care				
Anticoagulation Therapy for Atrial Fibrillation[5]	-	-	95%	95%
Antithrombotic Therapy Timing[5]	-	-	99%	98%
Assessed for Rehabilitation[5]	-	-	99%	97%
Discharged on Antithrombotic Therapy[5]	-	-	100%	99%
Discharged on Statin Medication[5]	-	-	93%	94%
Thrombolytic Therapy Timing[5]	-	-	75%	66%
Venous Thromboembolism Prophylaxis[5]	-	-	94%	94%
Written Stroke Educational Materials Given[5]	-	-	84%	88%
Surgical Care Improvement Project				
Appropriate Beta Blocker Usage[5]	-	-	98%	98%
Appropriate VTP Within 24 Hours[5]	-	-	99%	98%
Controlled Postoperative Blood Glucose[5]	-	-	96%	97%
Perioperative Temperature Management[5]	-	-	100%	100%
Prophylactic Antibiotic Selection[5]	-	-	99%	99%
Prophylactic Antibiotic Selection (Outpatient)[1,3]	-	-	99%	98%
Prophylactic Antibiotic Stopped[5]	-	-	98%	98%
Prophylactic Antibiotic Timing[5]	-	-	98%	99%
Prophylactic Antibiotic Timing (Outpatient)[1,3]	-	-	97%	98%
Urinary Catheter Removal[5]	-	-	98%	97%
Survey of Patients' Hospital Experiences				
Area Around Room 'Always' Quiet at Night[10]	<100	55%	67%	61%
Doctors 'Always' Communicated Well[10]	<100	90%	86%	82%
Home Recovery Information Given[10]	<100	85%	88%	85%
Hospital Given 9 or 10 on 10 Point Scale[10]	<100	85%	78%	71%
Meds 'Always' Explained Before Given[10]	<100	79%	68%	64%
Nurses 'Always' Communicated Well[10]	<100	84%	83%	79%
Pain 'Always' Well Controlled[10]	<100	75%	73%	71%
Room and Bathroom 'Always' Clean[10]	<100	70%	81%	73%
Timely Help 'Always' Received[10]	<100	77%	75%	68%
Would Definitely Recommend Hospital[10]	<100	82%	77%	71%
Use of Medical Imaging				
Cardiac Imaging Stress Test before Surgery	45	2.2%	5.4%	5.3%
Combination Abdominal CT Scan[1]	-	-	9.3%	10.5%
Combination Brain/Sinus CT Scan	54	0.0%	2.7%	2.7%
Combination Chest CT Scan[1]	-	-	1.7%	2.7%
Follow-up Mammogram/Ultrasound	139	6.5%	8%	8.8%
Lumbar Spine MRI for Low Back Pain[1]	-	-	36.5%	37.2%

Crete Area Medical Center

PO Box 220, 2910 Betten Dr
Crete, NE 68333
Phone: 402-826-2102
Fax: 402-826-7950
URL: www.creteareamedicalcenter.com
Type: Critical Access Hospitals
Emergency Services: Yes
Ownership: Voluntary non-profit - Private
Beds: 57

Key Personnel:
Chairman/CEO . . . . Tad Eickman
Chief of Medical Staff . . . . Jasson Hasser, MD
CEO/President . . . . Tad Hunt

Measure	Cases	This Hosp.	State Avg.	U.S. Avg.
Blood Clot Prevention and Treatment				
Anticoagulation Overlap Therapy[5]	-	-	93%	93%
ICU Venous Thromboembolism Prophylaxis[5]	-	-	91%	92%
Incidence of Potentially Preventable VTE[5]	-	-	11%	10%
UFH with Dosages/Platelet Monitoring[5]	-	-	98%	97%
Venous Thromboembolism Prophylaxis[5]	-	-	88%	85%
Warfarin Therapy Discharge Instructions[5]	-	-	81%	75%
Chest Pain/Possible Heart Attack Care				
Aspirin Given Within 24 Hours of Arrival	-	-	96%	96%
Fibrinolytic Meds Within 30 Min. of Arrival	-	-	53%	58%
Average Time to ECG (minutes)	-	-	8	7
Average Time to Transfer (minutes)	-	-	76	60
Children's Asthma Care				
Received Home Management Plan of Care	-	-	-	88%
Received Reliever Medication	-	-	-	100%
Received Systemic Corticosteroids	-	-	-	100%
Emergency Department				
Admittance Decision Time (minutes)[5]	-	-	75	98
Head CT Results Within 45 Min. of Arrival	-	-	61%	57%
Patients Who Left ER Before Being Seen	-	-	1%	2%
Time from ER Arrival to Admit. (minutes)[5]	-	-	207	274
Time from ER Arrival to Discharge (minutes)	-	-	118	134
Time in ER Before Being Evaluated (minutes)	-	-	21	26
Time to Pain Meds for Fractures (minutes)	-	-	42	57
Heart Attack Care				
Aspirin Given at Discharge[5]	-	-	100%	99%
Fibrinolytic Meds Within 30 Min. of Arrival[5]	-	-	-	54%
PCI Within 90 Minutes of Arrival[5]	-	-	96%	96%
Statin Prescribed at Discharge[5]	-	-	99%	98%
Heart Failure Care				
ACE Inhibitor or ARB for LVSD[1,3]	-	-	96%	97%
Discharge Instructions Given[1,3]	-	-	93%	94%
Evaluation of LVS Function[1,3]	-	-	98%	99%
Medicare Spending				
Medicare Spending per Patient (ratio)	-	-	0.97	0.98
Pneumonia Care				
Appropriate Initial Antibiotic Given	12	92%	95%	95%
Blood Culture Timing[1]	-	-	99%	98%
Pregnancy and Delivery Care				
Newborn Deliveries Scheduled Early[5]	-	-	5%	6%
Preventive Care				
Immunization for Influenza[5]	-	-	89%	90%
Immunization for Pneumonia[5]	-	-	90%	92%
Stroke Care				
Anticoagulation Therapy for Atrial Fibrillation[5]	-	-	95%	95%
Antithrombotic Therapy Timing[5]	-	-	99%	98%
Assessed for Rehabilitation[5]	-	-	99%	97%
Discharged on Antithrombotic Therapy[5]	-	-	100%	99%
Discharged on Statin Medication[5]	-	-	93%	94%
Thrombolytic Therapy Timing[5]	-	-	75%	66%
Venous Thromboembolism Prophylaxis[5]	-	-	94%	94%
Written Stroke Educational Materials Given[5]	-	-	84%	88%
Surgical Care Improvement Project				
Appropriate Beta Blocker Usage[1]	-	-	98%	98%
Appropriate VTP Within 24 Hours	15	100%	99%	98%
Controlled Postoperative Blood Glucose[7]	-	-	96%	97%
Perioperative Temperature Management	20	100%	100%	100%
Prophylactic Antibiotic Selection	17	100%	99%	99%
Prophylactic Antibiotic Selection (Outpatient)	-	-	99%	98%
Prophylactic Antibiotic Stopped	17	100%	98%	98%
Prophylactic Antibiotic Timing	17	94%	98%	99%
Prophylactic Antibiotic Timing (Outpatient)	-	-	97%	98%
Urinary Catheter Removal[1]	-	-	98%	97%
Survey of Patients' Hospital Experiences				
Area Around Room 'Always' Quiet at Night[6]	<100	68%	67%	61%
Doctors 'Always' Communicated Well[6]	<100	87%	86%	82%
Home Recovery Information Given[6]	<100	88%	88%	85%
Hospital Given 9 or 10 on 10 Point Scale[6]	<100	75%	78%	71%
Meds 'Always' Explained Before Given[6]	<100	64%	68%	64%
Nurses 'Always' Communicated Well[6]	<100	80%	83%	79%
Pain 'Always' Well Controlled[6]	<100	72%	73%	71%
Room and Bathroom 'Always' Clean[6]	<100	69%	81%	73%
Timely Help 'Always' Received[6]	<100	69%	75%	68%
Would Definitely Recommend Hospital[6]	<100	75%	77%	71%
Use of Medical Imaging				
Cardiac Imaging Stress Test before Surgery	-	-	5.4%	5.3%
Combination Abdominal CT Scan	-	-	9.3%	10.5%
Combination Brain/Sinus CT Scan	-	-	2.7%	2.7%
Combination Chest CT Scan	-	-	1.7%	2.7%
Follow-up Mammogram/Ultrasound	-	-	8%	8.8%
Lumbar Spine MRI for Low Back Pain	-	-	36.5%	37.2%

Butler County Health Care Center

372 South 9th St
David City, NE 68632
Phone: 402-367-1200
Fax: 402-367-1350
URL: www.bchccnet.org
Type: Critical Access Hospitals
Emergency Services: Yes
Ownership: Government - Local
Beds: 20

Key Personnel:
Emergency Room . . . . Sue Birkel, RN
Infection Control . . . . Connie Janicek, RN
Operating Room . . . . Joyce Jelinek, RN
Anesthesiology . . . . Corey Kavan, CRNA
CEO/President . . . . Donald T Naiberk
Quality Assurance . . . . Lucy Roberts, RN
Radiology . . . . Allan Steinberg
Chief of Medical Staff . . . . Victor Thoendel, MD

Measure	Cases	This Hosp.	State Avg.	U.S. Avg.
Blood Clot Prevention and Treatment				
Anticoagulation Overlap Therapy[5]	-	-	93%	93%
ICU Venous Thromboembolism Prophylaxis[5]	-	-	91%	92%
Incidence of Potentially Preventable VTE[5]	-	-	11%	10%
UFH with Dosages/Platelet Monitoring[5]	-	-	98%	97%
Venous Thromboembolism Prophylaxis[5]	-	-	88%	85%
Warfarin Therapy Discharge Instructions[5]	-	-	81%	75%
Chest Pain/Possible Heart Attack Care				
Aspirin Given Within 24 Hours of Arrival[1]	-	-	96%	96%
Fibrinolytic Meds Within 30 Min. of Arrival[1,3]	-	-	53%	58%
Average Time to ECG (minutes)[1]	-	-	8	7
Average Time to Transfer (minutes)[3,7]	-	-	76	60
Children's Asthma Care				
Received Home Management Plan of Care	-	-	-	88%
Received Reliever Medication	-	-	-	100%
Received Systemic Corticosteroids	-	-	-	100%
Emergency Department				
Admittance Decision Time (minutes)[5]	-	-	75	98
Head CT Results Within 45 Min. of Arrival[5]	-	-	61%	57%
Patients Who Left ER Before Being Seen[5]	-	-	1%	2%
Time from ER Arrival to Admit. (minutes)[5]	-	-	207	274
Time from ER Arrival to Discharge (minutes)[5]	-	-	118	134
Time in ER Before Being Evaluated (minutes)[5]	-	-	21	26
Time to Pain Meds for Fractures (minutes)[5]	-	-	42	57
Heart Attack Care				
Aspirin Given at Discharge[1,3]	-	-	100%	99%
Fibrinolytic Meds Within 30 Min. of Arrival[3,7]	-	-	-	54%
PCI Within 90 Minutes of Arrival[3,7]	-	-	96%	96%
Statin Prescribed at Discharge[1,3]	-	-	99%	98%
Heart Failure Care				
ACE Inhibitor or ARB for LVSD[1]	-	-	96%	97%
Discharge Instructions Given[1]	-	-	93%	94%
Evaluation of LVS Function	16	75%	98%	99%
Medicare Spending				
Medicare Spending per Patient (ratio)	-	-	0.97	0.98
Pneumonia Care				
Appropriate Initial Antibiotic Given[1]	-	-	95%	95%
Blood Culture Timing[1]	-	-	99%	98%
Pregnancy and Delivery Care				
Newborn Deliveries Scheduled Early[5]	-	-	5%	6%
Preventive Care				
Immunization for Influenza[5]	-	-	89%	90%
Immunization for Pneumonia[5]	-	-	90%	92%
Stroke Care				
Anticoagulation Therapy for Atrial Fibrillation[5]	-	-	95%	95%
Antithrombotic Therapy Timing[5]	-	-	99%	98%
Assessed for Rehabilitation[5]	-	-	99%	97%
Discharged on Antithrombotic Therapy[5]	-	-	100%	99%
Discharged on Statin Medication[5]	-	-	93%	94%
Thrombolytic Therapy Timing[5]	-	-	75%	66%
Venous Thromboembolism Prophylaxis[5]	-	-	94%	94%
Written Stroke Educational Materials Given[5]	-	-	84%	88%
Surgical Care Improvement Project				
Appropriate Beta Blocker Usage[1]	-	-	98%	98%
Appropriate VTP Within 24 Hours	32	100%	99%	98%
Controlled Postoperative Blood Glucose[7]	-	-	96%	97%
Perioperative Temperature Management	32	100%	100%	100%
Prophylactic Antibiotic Selection	31	97%	99%	99%
Prophylactic Antibiotic Selection (Outpatient)[1,3]	-	-	99%	98%
Prophylactic Antibiotic Stopped	30	100%	98%	98%
Prophylactic Antibiotic Timing	31	90%	98%	99%
Prophylactic Antibiotic Timing (Outpatient)[3,7]	-	-	97%	98%
Urinary Catheter Removal	21	100%	98%	97%
Survey of Patients' Hospital Experiences				
Area Around Room 'Always' Quiet at Night	(a)	68%	67%	61%
Doctors 'Always' Communicated Well	(a)	91%	86%	82%
Home Recovery Information Given	(a)	89%	88%	85%
Hospital Given 9 or 10 on 10 Point Scale	(a)	86%	78%	71%

NOTE: Hospital profiles are in alphabetical order by state, then city, then hospital within the city; Rankings exclude hospitals with less than 25 cases except for patient surveys which excludes hospitals with less than 100 cases; (a) 100-299 cases; (1) The number of cases/patients is too few to report; (2) Data submitted were based on a sample of cases/patients; (3) Results are based on a shorter time period than required; (4) Data suppressed by CMS for one or more quarters; (5) Results are not available for this reporting period; (6) Fewer than 100 patients completed the HCAHPS survey; (7) No cases met the criteria for this measure; (8) The lower limit of the confidence interval cannot be calculated if the number of observed infections equals zero; (9) No data are available from the state/territory for this reporting period; (10) The scores shown reflect fewer than 50 completed surveys; (11) There were discrepancies in the data collection process; (12) This measure does not apply to this hospital for this reporting period; (13) Results cannot be calculated for this reporting period; (14) The results for this state are combined with nearby states to protect confidentiality; Please refer to the User's Guide for a full explanation of data.

Measure	Cases	This Hosp.	State Avg.	U.S. Avg.
Meds 'Always' Explained Before Given	(a)	58%	68%	64%
Nurses 'Always' Communicated Well	(a)	86%	83%	79%
Pain 'Always' Well Controlled	(a)	76%	73%	71%
Room and Bathroom 'Always' Clean	(a)	88%	81%	73%
Timely Help 'Always' Received	(a)	77%	75%	68%
Would Definitely Recommend Hospital	(a)	83%	77%	71%
Use of Medical Imaging				
Cardiac Imaging Stress Test before Surgery[1]	-	-	5.4%	5.3%
Combination Abdominal CT Scan	69	7.2%	9.3%	10.5%
Combination Brain/Sinus CT Scan	56	0.0%	2.7%	2.7%
Combination Chest CT Scan[1]	-	-	1.7%	2.7%
Follow-up Mammogram/Ultrasound	171	5.8%	8%	8.8%
Lumbar Spine MRI for Low Back Pain[1]	-	-	36.5%	37.2%

Jefferson Community Health Center

PO Box 277, 2200 H St
Fairbury, NE 68352
Phone: 402-729-3351
Fax: 402-729-2102
E-mail: lana.likens@jchc.us
URL: www.jchc.us
Type: Critical Access Hospitals
Emergency Services: Yes
Ownership: Voluntary non-profit - Private
Beds: 33

Key Personnel:
Radiology. . . . . Caryn Bales, RT
Infection Control. . . . . Mary Heidemann
Operating Room. . . . . Ermel Heuer, RN
Cardiac Laboratory. . . . . Elsiee Houser
Emergency Room . . . . Judy McGee, CNE
Chief of Medical Staff . . . . Craig Shumard, MD
Quality Assurance . . . . Sharon Vandegrift
CEO . . . . Shondra Williams

Measure	Cases	This Hosp.	State Avg.	U.S. Avg.
Blood Clot Prevention and Treatment				
Anticoagulation Overlap Therapy[5]	-	-	93%	93%
ICU Venous Thromboembolism Prophylaxis[5]	-	-	91%	92%
Incidence of Potentially Preventable VTE[5]	-	-	11%	10%
UFH with Dosages/Platelet Monitoring[5]	-	-	98%	97%
Venous Thromboembolism Prophylaxis[5]	-	-	88%	85%
Warfarin Therapy Discharge Instructions[5]	-	-	81%	75%
Chest Pain/Possible Heart Attack Care				
Aspirin Given Within 24 Hours of Arrival	20	100%	96%	96%
Fibrinolytic Meds Within 30 Min. of Arrival[1,3]	-	-	53%	58%
Average Time to ECG (minutes)	21	6	8	7
Average Time to Transfer (minutes)[3,7]	-	-	76	60
Children's Asthma Care				
Received Home Management Plan of Care	-	-	-	88%
Received Reliever Medication	-	-	-	100%
Received Systemic Corticosteroids	-	-	-	100%
Emergency Department				
Admittance Decision Time (minutes)[5]	-	-	75	98
Head CT Results Within 45 Min. of Arrival[5]	-	-	61%	57%
Patients Who Left ER Before Being Seen[5]	-	-	1%	2%
Time from ER Arrival to Admit. (minutes)[5]	-	-	207	274
Time from ER Arrival to Discharge (minutes)[5]	-	-	118	134
Time in ER Before Being Evaluated (minutes)[5]	-	-	21	26
Time to Pain Meds for Fractures (minutes)[5]	-	-	42	57
Heart Attack Care				
Aspirin Given at Discharge[1,3]	-	-	100%	99%
Fibrinolytic Meds Within 30 Min. of Arrival[3,7]	-	-	-	54%
PCI Within 90 Minutes of Arrival[3,7]	-	-	96%	96%
Statin Prescribed at Discharge[1,3]	-	-	99%	98%
Heart Failure Care				
ACE Inhibitor or ARB for LVSD[1]	-	-	96%	97%
Discharge Instructions Given[1]	-	-	93%	94%
Evaluation of LVS Function[1]	-	-	98%	99%
Medicare Spending				
Medicare Spending per Patient (ratio)	-	-	0.97	0.98
Pneumonia Care				
Appropriate Initial Antibiotic Given[1]	-	-	95%	95%
Blood Culture Timing[1]	-	-	99%	98%
Pregnancy and Delivery Care				
Newborn Deliveries Scheduled Early[5]	-	-	5%	6%
Preventive Care				
Immunization for Influenza[5]	-	-	89%	90%
Immunization for Pneumonia[5]	-	-	90%	92%
Stroke Care				
Anticoagulation Therapy for Atrial Fibrillation[5]	-	-	95%	95%
Antithrombotic Therapy Timing[5]	-	-	99%	98%
Assessed for Rehabilitation[5]	-	-	99%	97%
Discharged on Antithrombotic Therapy[5]	-	-	100%	99%
Discharged on Statin Medication[5]	-	-	93%	94%
Thrombolytic Therapy Timing[5]	-	-	75%	66%
Venous Thromboembolism Prophylaxis[5]	-	-	94%	94%
Written Stroke Educational Materials Given[5]	-	-	84%	88%
Surgical Care Improvement Project				
Appropriate Beta Blocker Usage[1]	-	-	98%	98%
Appropriate VTP Within 24 Hours	24	100%	99%	98%
Controlled Postoperative Blood Glucose[7]	-	-	96%	97%
Perioperative Temperature Management	28	100%	100%	100%
Prophylactic Antibiotic Selection	25	100%	99%	99%
Prophylactic Antibiotic Selection (Outpatient)[5]	-	-	99%	98%
Prophylactic Antibiotic Stopped	25	100%	98%	98%
Prophylactic Antibiotic Timing	25	92%	98%	99%
Prophylactic Antibiotic Timing (Outpatient)[5]	-	-	97%	98%
Urinary Catheter Removal	21	100%	98%	97%
Survey of Patients' Hospital Experiences				
Area Around Room 'Always' Quiet at Night[6]	<100	63%	67%	61%
Doctors 'Always' Communicated Well[6]	<100	87%	86%	82%
Home Recovery Information Given[6]	<100	84%	88%	85%
Hospital Given 9 or 10 on 10 Point Scale[6]	<100	73%	78%	71%
Meds 'Always' Explained Before Given[6]	<100	51%	68%	64%
Nurses 'Always' Communicated Well[6]	<100	84%	83%	79%
Pain 'Always' Well Controlled[6]	<100	68%	73%	71%
Room and Bathroom 'Always' Clean[6]	<100	90%	81%	73%
Timely Help 'Always' Received[6]	<100	72%	75%	68%
Would Definitely Recommend Hospital[6]	<100	72%	77%	71%
Use of Medical Imaging				
Cardiac Imaging Stress Test before Surgery[1]	-	-	5.4%	5.3%
Combination Abdominal CT Scan	87	8.0%	9.3%	10.5%
Combination Brain/Sinus CT Scan	64	0.0%	2.7%	2.7%
Combination Chest CT Scan	56	3.6%	1.7%	2.7%
Follow-up Mammogram/Ultrasound	220	11.8%	8%	8.8%
Lumbar Spine MRI for Low Back Pain[1]	-	-	36.5%	37.2%

Community Medical Center

PO Box 399, 3307 Barada St
Falls City, NE 68355
Phone: 402-245-2428
Fax: 402-245-4841
URL: www.hhs.state.ne.us/index.htm
Type: Critical Access Hospitals
Emergency Services: Yes
Ownership: Voluntary non-profit - Private
Beds: 35

Key Personnel:
Chief of Medical Staff. . . . . Joann Schaefer

Measure	Cases	This Hosp.	State Avg.	U.S. Avg.
Blood Clot Prevention and Treatment				
Anticoagulation Overlap Therapy[1,3]	-	-	93%	93%
ICU Venous Thromboembolism Prophylaxis[1,3]	-	-	91%	92%
Incidence of Potentially Preventable VTE[3,7]	-	-	11%	10%
UFH with Dosages/Platelet Monitoring[3,7]	-	-	98%	97%
Venous Thromboembolism Prophylaxis[3]	86	84%	88%	85%
Warfarin Therapy Discharge Instructions[1,3]	-	-	81%	75%
Chest Pain/Possible Heart Attack Care				
Aspirin Given Within 24 Hours of Arrival[1,3]	-	-	96%	96%
Fibrinolytic Meds Within 30 Min. of Arrival[3,7]	-	-	53%	58%
Average Time to ECG (minutes)[1,3]	-	-	8	7
Average Time to Transfer (minutes)[3,7]	-	-	76	60
Children's Asthma Care				
Received Home Management Plan of Care	-	-	-	88%
Received Reliever Medication	-	-	-	100%
Received Systemic Corticosteroids	-	-	-	100%
Emergency Department				
Admittance Decision Time (minutes)[2,3]	47	30	75	98
Head CT Results Within 45 Min. of Arrival[5]	-	-	61%	57%
Patients Who Left ER Before Being Seen[5]	-	-	1%	2%
Time from ER Arrival to Admit. (minutes)[2,3]	52	111	207	274
Time from ER Arrival to Discharge (minutes)[5]	-	-	118	134
Time in ER Before Being Evaluated (minutes)[5]	-	-	21	26
Time to Pain Meds for Fractures (minutes)[5]	-	-	42	57
Heart Attack Care				
Aspirin Given at Discharge[5]	-	-	100%	99%
Fibrinolytic Meds Within 30 Min. of Arrival[5]	-	-	-	54%
PCI Within 90 Minutes of Arrival[5]	-	-	96%	96%
Statin Prescribed at Discharge[5]	-	-	99%	98%
Heart Failure Care				
ACE Inhibitor or ARB for LVSD[1,2]	-	-	96%	97%
Discharge Instructions Given[2]	11	91%	93%	94%
Evaluation of LVS Function[2]	18	89%	98%	99%
Medicare Spending				
Medicare Spending per Patient (ratio)	-	-	0.97	0.98
Pneumonia Care				
Appropriate Initial Antibiotic Given[1,2]	-	-	95%	95%
Blood Culture Timing[1,2]	-	-	99%	98%
Pregnancy and Delivery Care				
Newborn Deliveries Scheduled Early[5]	-	-	5%	6%
Preventive Care				
Immunization for Influenza	270	93%	89%	90%
Immunization for Pneumonia	319	89%	90%	92%
Stroke Care				
Anticoagulation Therapy for Atrial Fibrillation[5]	-	-	95%	95%
Antithrombotic Therapy Timing[5]	-	-	99%	98%
Assessed for Rehabilitation[5]	-	-	99%	97%
Discharged on Antithrombotic Therapy[5]	-	-	100%	99%
Discharged on Statin Medication[5]	-	-	93%	94%
Thrombolytic Therapy Timing[5]	-	-	75%	66%
Venous Thromboembolism Prophylaxis[5]	-	-	94%	94%
Written Stroke Educational Materials Given[5]	-	-	84%	88%
Surgical Care Improvement Project				
Appropriate Beta Blocker Usage	40	98%	98%	98%
Appropriate VTP Within 24 Hours	104	98%	99%	98%
Controlled Postoperative Blood Glucose[7]	-	-	96%	97%
Perioperative Temperature Management	108	100%	100%	100%
Prophylactic Antibiotic Selection	101	97%	99%	99%
Prophylactic Antibiotic Selection (Outpatient)[5]	-	-	99%	98%
Prophylactic Antibiotic Stopped	99	95%	98%	98%
Prophylactic Antibiotic Timing	101	95%	98%	99%
Prophylactic Antibiotic Timing (Outpatient)[5]	-	-	97%	98%
Urinary Catheter Removal[1]	-	-	98%	97%
Survey of Patients' Hospital Experiences				
Area Around Room 'Always' Quiet at Night	(a)	74%	67%	61%
Doctors 'Always' Communicated Well	(a)	90%	86%	82%
Home Recovery Information Given	(a)	90%	88%	85%
Hospital Given 9 or 10 on 10 Point Scale	(a)	82%	78%	71%
Meds 'Always' Explained Before Given	(a)	73%	68%	64%
Nurses 'Always' Communicated Well	(a)	90%	83%	79%
Pain 'Always' Well Controlled	(a)	75%	73%	71%
Room and Bathroom 'Always' Clean	(a)	86%	81%	73%
Timely Help 'Always' Received	(a)	80%	75%	68%
Would Definitely Recommend Hospital	(a)	81%	77%	71%
Use of Medical Imaging				
Cardiac Imaging Stress Test before Surgery	49	0.0%	5.4%	5.3%
Combination Abdominal CT Scan	117	7.7%	9.3%	10.5%
Combination Brain/Sinus CT Scan[1]	-	-	2.7%	2.7%
Combination Chest CT Scan	61	4.9%	1.7%	2.7%
Follow-up Mammogram/Ultrasound	133	10.5%	8%	8.8%
Lumbar Spine MRI for Low Back Pain[1]	-	-	36.5%	37.2%

Franklin County Memorial Hospital

PO Box 315, 1406 Q St
Franklin, NE 68939
Phone: 308-425-6221
Fax: 308-425-3164
URL: www.franklincountymemorialhospital.org
Type: Critical Access Hospitals
Emergency Services: Yes
Ownership: Government - Local
Beds: 12

Key Personnel:
CEO/President. . . . . Jerrell F Gerdes, FACHE
Chief of Medical Staff . . . . Linda Mazour
Cardiac Laboratory. . . . . Gaylene Wentworth

Measure	Cases	This Hosp.	State Avg.	U.S. Avg.
Blood Clot Prevention and Treatment				
Anticoagulation Overlap Therapy[5]	-	-	93%	93%
ICU Venous Thromboembolism Prophylaxis[5]	-	-	91%	92%
Incidence of Potentially Preventable VTE[5]	-	-	11%	10%
UFH with Dosages/Platelet Monitoring[5]	-	-	98%	97%

NOTE: Hospital profiles are in alphabetical order by state, then city, then hospital within the city; Rankings exclude hospitals with less than 25 cases except for patient surveys which excludes hospitals with less than 100 cases; (a) 100-299 cases; (1) The number of cases/patients is too few to report; (2) Data submitted were based on a sample of cases/patients; (3) Results are based on a shorter time period than required; (4) Data suppressed by CMS for one or more quarters; (5) Results are not available for this reporting period; (6) Fewer than 100 patients completed the HCAHPS survey; (7) No cases met the criteria for this measure; (8) The lower limit of the confidence interval cannot be calculated if the number of observed infections equals zero; (9) No data are available from the state/territory for this reporting period; (10) The scores shown reflect fewer than 50 completed surveys; (11) There were discrepancies in the data collection process; (12) This measure does not apply to this hospital for this reporting period; (13) Results cannot be calculated for this reporting period; (14) The results for this state are combined with nearby states to protect confidentiality; Please refer to the User's Guide for a full explanation of data.

Venous Thromboembolism Prophylaxis[5]	-	-	88%	85%
Warfarin Therapy Discharge Instructions[5]	-	-	81%	75%
Chest Pain/Possible Heart Attack Care				
Aspirin Given Within 24 Hours of Arrival[5]	-	-	96%	96%
Fibrinolytic Meds Within 30 Min. of Arrival[5]	-	-	53%	58%
Average Time to ECG (minutes)[5]	-	-	8	7
Average Time to Transfer (minutes)[5]	-	-	76	60
Children's Asthma Care				
Received Home Management Plan of Care	-	-	-	88%
Received Reliever Medication	-	-	-	100%
Received Systemic Corticosteroids	-	-	-	100%
Emergency Department				
Admittance Decision Time (minutes)[5]	-	-	75	98
Head CT Results Within 45 Min. of Arrival[1,3]	-	-	61%	57%
Patients Who Left ER Before Being Seen[5]	-	-	1%	2%
Time from ER Arrival to Admit. (minutes)[5]	-	-	207	274
Time from ER Arrival to Discharge (minutes)[5]	-	-	118	134
Time in ER Before Being Evaluated (minutes)[5]	-	-	21	26
Time to Pain Meds for Fractures (minutes)[5]	-	-	42	57
Heart Attack Care				
Aspirin Given at Discharge[5]	-	-	100%	99%
Fibrinolytic Meds Within 30 Min. of Arrival[5]	-	-	-	54%
PCI Within 90 Minutes of Arrival[5]	-	-	96%	96%
Statin Prescribed at Discharge[5]	-	-	99%	98%
Heart Failure Care				
ACE Inhibitor or ARB for LVSD[1,3]	-	-	96%	97%
Discharge Instructions Given[1,3]	-	-	93%	94%
Evaluation of LVS Function[1,3]	-	-	98%	99%
Medicare Spending				
Medicare Spending per Patient (ratio)	-	-	0.97	0.98
Pneumonia Care				
Appropriate Initial Antibiotic Given[1]	-	-	95%	95%
Blood Culture Timing[7]	-	-	99%	98%
Pregnancy and Delivery Care				
Newborn Deliveries Scheduled Early[5]	-	-	5%	6%
Preventive Care				
Immunization for Influenza[5]	-	-	89%	90%
Immunization for Pneumonia[5]	-	-	90%	92%
Stroke Care				
Anticoagulation Therapy for Atrial Fibrillation[5]	-	-	95%	95%
Antithrombotic Therapy Timing[5]	-	-	99%	98%
Assessed for Rehabilitation[5]	-	-	99%	97%
Discharged on Antithrombotic Therapy[5]	-	-	100%	99%
Discharged on Statin Medication[5]	-	-	93%	94%
Thrombolytic Therapy Timing[5]	-	-	75%	66%
Venous Thromboembolism Prophylaxis[5]	-	-	94%	94%
Written Stroke Educational Materials Given[5]	-	-	84%	88%
Surgical Care Improvement Project				
Appropriate Beta Blocker Usage[5]	-	-	98%	98%
Appropriate VTP Within 24 Hours[5]	-	-	99%	98%
Controlled Postoperative Blood Glucose[5]	-	-	96%	97%
Perioperative Temperature Management[5]	-	-	100%	100%
Prophylactic Antibiotic Selection[5]	-	-	99%	99%
Prophylactic Antibiotic Selection (Outpatient)[5]	-	-	99%	98%
Prophylactic Antibiotic Stopped[5]	-	-	98%	98%
Prophylactic Antibiotic Timing[5]	-	-	98%	99%
Prophylactic Antibiotic Timing (Outpatient)[5]	-	-	97%	98%
Urinary Catheter Removal[5]	-	-	98%	97%
Survey of Patients' Hospital Experiences				
Area Around Room 'Always' Quiet at Night[5]	-	-	67%	61%
Doctors 'Always' Communicated Well[5]	-	-	86%	82%
Home Recovery Information Given[5]	-	-	88%	85%
Hospital Given 9 or 10 on 10 Point Scale[5]	-	-	78%	71%
Meds 'Always' Explained Before Given[5]	-	-	68%	64%
Nurses 'Always' Communicated Well[5]	-	-	83%	79%
Pain 'Always' Well Controlled[5]	-	-	73%	71%
Room and Bathroom 'Always' Clean[5]	-	-	81%	73%
Timely Help 'Always' Received[5]	-	-	75%	68%
Would Definitely Recommend Hospital[5]	-	-	77%	71%
Use of Medical Imaging				
Cardiac Imaging Stress Test before Surgery[1]	-	-	5.4%	5.3%
Combination Abdominal CT Scan[1]	-	-	9.3%	10.5%
Combination Brain/Sinus CT Scan[1]	-	-	2.7%	2.7%
Combination Chest CT Scan[1]	-	-	1.7%	2.7%
Follow-up Mammogram/Ultrasound	46	2.2%	8%	8.8%
Lumbar Spine MRI for Low Back Pain[1]	-	-	36.5%	37.2%

Fremont Area Medical Center

450 East 23rd St
Fremont, NE 68025
URL: www.famc.org
Type: Acute Care Hospitals
Ownership: Government - Local
Phone: 402-721-1610
Fax: 402-727-3433
Emergency Services: Yes
Beds: 262

Key Personnel:
CEO/President. . . . . Patrick Booth
Cardiac Laboratory. . . . . Brian Brodd
Emergency Room . . . . Brian K Elliott, MD
Anesthesiology. . . . . Jeffrey N Hawthorne, MD
Chairman/CEO . . . . Joel Jelkin
Radiology. . . . . Duane Krause, MD
Infection Control. . . . . Gerri Means
Operating Room. . . . . Don Tricarico

Measure	Cases	This Hosp.	State Avg.	U.S. Avg.
Blood Clot Prevention and Treatment				
Anticoagulation Overlap Therapy[2]	31	100%	93%	93%
ICU Venous Thromboembolism Prophylaxis[2]	49	96%	91%	92%
Incidence of Potentially Preventable VTE[2,7]	-	-	11%	10%
UFH with Dosages/Platelet Monitoring[2]	11	100%	98%	97%
Venous Thromboembolism Prophylaxis[2]	212	89%	88%	85%
Warfarin Therapy Discharge Instructions[2]	17	94%	81%	75%
Chest Pain/Possible Heart Attack Care				
Aspirin Given Within 24 Hours of Arrival	23	96%	96%	96%
Fibrinolytic Meds Within 30 Min. of Arrival[7]	-	-	53%	58%
Average Time to ECG (minutes)	23	8	8	7
Average Time to Transfer (minutes)[1]	-	-	76	60
Children's Asthma Care				
Received Home Management Plan of Care	-	-	-	88%
Received Reliever Medication	-	-	-	100%
Received Systemic Corticosteroids	-	-	-	100%
Emergency Department				
Admittance Decision Time (minutes)[2]	257	30	75	98
Head CT Results Within 45 Min. of Arrival	12	42%	61%	57%
Patients Who Left ER Before Being Seen	14,590	0%	1%	2%
Time from ER Arrival to Admit. (minutes)[2]	264	194	207	274
Time from ER Arrival to Discharge (minutes)	348	85	118	134
Time in ER Before Being Evaluated (minutes)	325	0	21	26
Time to Pain Meds for Fractures (minutes)	74	22	42	57
Heart Attack Care				
Aspirin Given at Discharge	39	100%	100%	99%
Fibrinolytic Meds Within 30 Min. of Arrival[7]	-	-	-	54%
PCI Within 90 Minutes of Arrival[1]	-	-	96%	96%
Statin Prescribed at Discharge	36	97%	99%	98%
Heart Failure Care				
ACE Inhibitor or ARB for LVSD	15	100%	96%	97%
Discharge Instructions Given	44	95%	93%	94%
Evaluation of LVS Function	77	99%	98%	99%
Medicare Spending				
Medicare Spending per Patient (ratio)	-	1.02	0.97	0.98
Pneumonia Care				
Appropriate Initial Antibiotic Given	62	92%	95%	95%
Blood Culture Timing	96	99%	99%	98%
Pregnancy and Delivery Care				
Newborn Deliveries Scheduled Early	54	0%	5%	6%
Preventive Care				
Immunization for Influenza[2]	305	94%	89%	90%
Immunization for Pneumonia[2]	358	97%	90%	92%
Stroke Care				
Anticoagulation Therapy for Atrial Fibrillation[1]	-	-	95%	95%
Antithrombotic Therapy Timing	21	100%	99%	98%
Assessed for Rehabilitation	21	95%	99%	97%
Discharged on Antithrombotic Therapy	20	100%	100%	99%
Discharged on Statin Medication	15	67%	93%	94%
Thrombolytic Therapy Timing[1]	-	-	75%	66%
Venous Thromboembolism Prophylaxis	22	95%	94%	94%
Written Stroke Educational Materials Given[1]	-	-	84%	88%
Surgical Care Improvement Project				
Appropriate Beta Blocker Usage[2]	102	89%	98%	98%
Appropriate VTP Within 24 Hours[2]	318	99%	99%	98%
Controlled Postoperative Blood Glucose[2,7]	-	-	96%	97%
Perioperative Temperature Management[2]	362	100%	100%	100%
Prophylactic Antibiotic Selection[2]	254	98%	99%	99%
Prophylactic Antibiotic Selection (Outpatient)	84	99%	99%	98%
Prophylactic Antibiotic Stopped[2]	251	94%	98%	98%
Prophylactic Antibiotic Timing[2]	254	98%	98%	99%
Prophylactic Antibiotic Timing (Outpatient)	84	96%	97%	98%
Urinary Catheter Removal[2]	80	96%	98%	97%
Survey of Patients' Hospital Experiences				
Area Around Room 'Always' Quiet at Night	300+	48%	67%	61%
Doctors 'Always' Communicated Well	300+	80%	86%	82%
Home Recovery Information Given	300+	90%	88%	85%
Hospital Given 9 or 10 on 10 Point Scale	300+	72%	78%	71%
Meds 'Always' Explained Before Given	300+	67%	68%	64%
Nurses 'Always' Communicated Well	300+	78%	83%	79%
Pain 'Always' Well Controlled	300+	73%	73%	71%
Room and Bathroom 'Always' Clean	300+	73%	81%	73%
Timely Help 'Always' Received	300+	70%	75%	68%
Would Definitely Recommend Hospital	300+	61%	77%	71%
Use of Medical Imaging				
Cardiac Imaging Stress Test before Surgery	406	6.2%	5.4%	5.3%
Combination Abdominal CT Scan	511	32.7%	9.3%	10.5%
Combination Brain/Sinus CT Scan	500	0.8%	2.7%	2.7%
Combination Chest CT Scan	455	0.0%	1.7%	2.7%
Follow-up Mammogram/Ultrasound	1,376	3.2%	8%	8.8%
Lumbar Spine MRI for Low Back Pain	117	30.8%	36.5%	37.2%

Warren Memorial Hospital

905 Second St
Friend, NE 68359
URL: www.warrenmemorialhospital.org
Type: Critical Access Hospitals
Ownership: Government - Local
Phone: 402-947-2541
Fax: 402-947-2881
Emergency Services: Yes
Beds: 15

Key Personnel:
CEO . . . . Chris Bjornberg
Quality Assurance . . . . Deb Gates
Chief of Medical Staff . . . . Dr Roger Meyer
Radiology. . . . . Tiphanie Potter

Measure	Cases	This Hosp.	State Avg.	U.S. Avg.
Blood Clot Prevention and Treatment				
Anticoagulation Overlap Therapy[5]	-	-	93%	93%
ICU Venous Thromboembolism Prophylaxis[5]	-	-	91%	92%
Incidence of Potentially Preventable VTE[5]	-	-	11%	10%
UFH with Dosages/Platelet Monitoring[5]	-	-	98%	97%
Venous Thromboembolism Prophylaxis[5]	-	-	88%	85%
Warfarin Therapy Discharge Instructions[5]	-	-	81%	75%
Chest Pain/Possible Heart Attack Care				
Aspirin Given Within 24 Hours of Arrival[5]	-	-	96%	96%
Fibrinolytic Meds Within 30 Min. of Arrival[5]	-	-	53%	58%
Average Time to ECG (minutes)[5]	-	-	8	7
Average Time to Transfer (minutes)[5]	-	-	76	60
Children's Asthma Care				
Received Home Management Plan of Care	-	-	-	88%
Received Reliever Medication	-	-	-	100%
Received Systemic Corticosteroids	-	-	-	100%
Emergency Department				
Admittance Decision Time (minutes)[5]	-	-	75	98
Head CT Results Within 45 Min. of Arrival[5]	-	-	61%	57%
Patients Who Left ER Before Being Seen[5]	-	-	1%	2%
Time from ER Arrival to Admit. (minutes)[5]	-	-	207	274
Time from ER Arrival to Discharge (minutes)[5]	-	-	118	134
Time in ER Before Being Evaluated (minutes)[5]	-	-	21	26
Time to Pain Meds for Fractures (minutes)[5]	-	-	42	57
Heart Attack Care				
Aspirin Given at Discharge[5]	-	-	100%	99%
Fibrinolytic Meds Within 30 Min. of Arrival[5]	-	-	-	54%
PCI Within 90 Minutes of Arrival[5]	-	-	96%	96%
Statin Prescribed at Discharge[5]	-	-	99%	98%
Heart Failure Care				
ACE Inhibitor or ARB for LVSD[5]	-	-	96%	97%
Discharge Instructions Given[5]	-	-	93%	94%

NOTE: Hospital profiles are in alphabetical order by state, then city, then hospital within the city; Rankings exclude hospitals with less than 25 cases except for patient surveys which excludes hospitals with less than 100 cases; (a) 100-299 cases; (1) The number of cases/patients is too few to report; (2) Data submitted were based on a sample of cases/patients; (3) Results are based on a shorter time period than required; (4) Data suppressed by CMS for one or more quarters; (5) Results are not available for this reporting period; (6) Fewer than 100 patients completed the HCAHPS survey; (7) No cases met the criteria for this measure; (8) The lower limit of the confidence interval cannot be calculated if the number of observed infections equals zero; (9) No data are available from the state/territory for this reporting period; (10) The scores shown reflect fewer than 50 completed surveys; (11) There were discrepancies in the data collection process; (12) This measure does not apply to this hospital for this reporting period; (13) Results cannot be calculated for this reporting period; (14) The results for this state are combined with nearby states to protect confidentiality; Please refer to the User's Guide for a full explanation of data.

Measure	Cases	This Hosp.	State Avg.	U.S. Avg.
Evaluation of LVS Function[5]	-	-	98%	99%
Medicare Spending				
Medicare Spending per Patient (ratio)	-	-	0.97	0.98
Pneumonia Care				
Appropriate Initial Antibiotic Given[5]	-	-	95%	95%
Blood Culture Timing[5]	-	-	99%	98%
Pregnancy and Delivery Care				
Newborn Deliveries Scheduled Early[5]	-	-	5%	6%
Preventive Care				
Immunization for Influenza[5]	-	-	89%	90%
Immunization for Pneumonia[5]	-	-	90%	92%
Stroke Care				
Anticoagulation Therapy for Atrial Fibrillation[5]	-	-	95%	95%
Antithrombotic Therapy Timing[5]	-	-	99%	98%
Assessed for Rehabilitation[5]	-	-	99%	97%
Discharged on Antithrombotic Therapy[5]	-	-	100%	99%
Discharged on Statin Medication[5]	-	-	93%	94%
Thrombolytic Therapy Timing[5]	-	-	75%	66%
Venous Thromboembolism Prophylaxis[5]	-	-	94%	94%
Written Stroke Educational Materials Given[5]	-	-	84%	88%
Surgical Care Improvement Project				
Appropriate Beta Blocker Usage[5]	-	-	98%	98%
Appropriate VTP Within 24 Hours[5]	-	-	99%	98%
Controlled Postoperative Blood Glucose[5]	-	-	96%	97%
Perioperative Temperature Management[5]	-	-	100%	100%
Prophylactic Antibiotic Selection[5]	-	-	99%	99%
Prophylactic Antibiotic Selection (Outpatient)[5]	-	-	99%	98%
Prophylactic Antibiotic Stopped[5]	-	-	98%	98%
Prophylactic Antibiotic Timing[5]	-	-	98%	99%
Prophylactic Antibiotic Timing (Outpatient)[5]	-	-	97%	98%
Urinary Catheter Removal[5]	-	-	98%	97%
Survey of Patients' Hospital Experiences				
Area Around Room 'Always' Quiet at Night[5]	-	-	67%	61%
Doctors 'Always' Communicated Well[5]	-	-	86%	82%
Home Recovery Information Given[5]	-	-	88%	85%
Hospital Given 9 or 10 on 10 Point Scale[5]	-	-	78%	71%
Meds 'Always' Explained Before Given[5]	-	-	68%	64%
Nurses 'Always' Communicated Well[5]	-	-	83%	79%
Pain 'Always' Well Controlled[5]	-	-	73%	71%
Room and Bathroom 'Always' Clean[5]	-	-	81%	73%
Timely Help 'Always' Received[5]	-	-	75%	68%
Would Definitely Recommend Hospital[5]	-	-	77%	71%
Use of Medical Imaging				
Cardiac Imaging Stress Test before Surgery[7]	-	-	5.4%	5.3%
Combination Abdominal CT Scan[1]	-	-	9.3%	10.5%
Combination Brain/Sinus CT Scan[1]	-	-	2.7%	2.7%
Combination Chest CT Scan[1]	-	-	1.7%	2.7%
Follow-up Mammogram/Ultrasound[1]	-	-	8%	8.8%
Lumbar Spine MRI for Low Back Pain[1]	-	-	36.5%	37.2%

Fillmore County Hospital

PO Box 193, 1900 F Street
Geneva, NE 68361
Phone: 402-759-3167
Fax: 402-759-3093
URL: www.fhsofgeneva.org
Type: Critical Access Hospitals
Ownership: Government - Local
Emergency Services: Yes
Beds: 25

Key Personnel:
Cardiac Laboratory. . . . . Ron Fleecs
President . . . . DeBorah Hoarty
CEO/President. . . . . Paul Utemark

Measure	Cases	This Hosp.	State Avg.	U.S. Avg.
Blood Clot Prevention and Treatment				
Anticoagulation Overlap Therapy[5]	-	-	93%	93%
ICU Venous Thromboembolism Prophylaxis[5]	-	-	91%	92%
Incidence of Potentially Preventable VTE[5]	-	-	11%	10%
UFH with Dosages/Platelet Monitoring[5]	-	-	98%	97%
Venous Thromboembolism Prophylaxis[5]	-	-	88%	85%
Warfarin Therapy Discharge Instructions[5]	-	-	81%	75%
Chest Pain/Possible Heart Attack Care				
Aspirin Given Within 24 Hours of Arrival[1]	-	-	96%	96%
Fibrinolytic Meds Within 30 Min. of Arrival[1,3]	-	-	53%	58%
Average Time to ECG (minutes)[1]	-	-	8	7
Average Time to Transfer (minutes)[3,7]	-	-	76	60
Children's Asthma Care				
Received Home Management Plan of Care	-	-	-	88%
Received Reliever Medication	-	-	-	100%
Received Systemic Corticosteroids	-	-	-	100%
Emergency Department				
Admittance Decision Time (minutes)[5]	-	-	75	98
Head CT Results Within 45 Min. of Arrival[5]	-	-	61%	57%
Patients Who Left ER Before Being Seen[5]	-	-	1%	2%
Time from ER Arrival to Admit. (minutes)[5]	-	-	207	274
Time from ER Arrival to Discharge (minutes)[5]	-	-	118	134
Time in ER Before Being Evaluated (minutes)[5]	-	-	21	26
Time to Pain Meds for Fractures (minutes)[5]	-	-	42	57
Heart Attack Care				
Aspirin Given at Discharge[5]	-	-	100%	99%
Fibrinolytic Meds Within 30 Min. of Arrival[5]	-	-	-	54%
PCI Within 90 Minutes of Arrival[5]	-	-	96%	96%
Statin Prescribed at Discharge[5]	-	-	99%	98%
Heart Failure Care				
ACE Inhibitor or ARB for LVSD[3,7]	-	-	96%	97%
Discharge Instructions Given[1,3]	-	-	93%	94%
Evaluation of LVS Function[1,3]	-	-	98%	99%
Medicare Spending				
Medicare Spending per Patient (ratio)	-	-	0.97	0.98
Pneumonia Care				
Appropriate Initial Antibiotic Given	12	92%	95%	95%
Blood Culture Timing[7]	-	-	99%	98%
Pregnancy and Delivery Care				
Newborn Deliveries Scheduled Early[5]	-	-	5%	6%
Preventive Care				
Immunization for Influenza[5]	-	-	89%	90%
Immunization for Pneumonia[5]	-	-	90%	92%
Stroke Care				
Anticoagulation Therapy for Atrial Fibrillation[5]	-	-	95%	95%
Antithrombotic Therapy Timing[5]	-	-	99%	98%
Assessed for Rehabilitation[5]	-	-	99%	97%
Discharged on Antithrombotic Therapy[5]	-	-	100%	99%
Discharged on Statin Medication[5]	-	-	93%	94%
Thrombolytic Therapy Timing[5]	-	-	75%	66%
Venous Thromboembolism Prophylaxis[5]	-	-	94%	94%
Written Stroke Educational Materials Given[5]	-	-	84%	88%
Surgical Care Improvement Project				
Appropriate Beta Blocker Usage[1,3]	-	-	98%	98%
Appropriate VTP Within 24 Hours[3]	14	100%	99%	98%
Controlled Postoperative Blood Glucose[3,7]	-	-	96%	97%
Perioperative Temperature Management[3]	16	100%	100%	100%
Prophylactic Antibiotic Selection[3]	16	100%	99%	99%
Prophylactic Antibiotic Selection (Outpatient)[1,3]	-	-	99%	98%
Prophylactic Antibiotic Stopped[3]	16	94%	98%	98%
Prophylactic Antibiotic Timing[3]	16	100%	98%	99%
Prophylactic Antibiotic Timing (Outpatient)[1,3]	-	-	97%	98%
Urinary Catheter Removal[3]	13	100%	98%	97%
Survey of Patients' Hospital Experiences				
Area Around Room 'Always' Quiet at Night[6]	<100	70%	67%	61%
Doctors 'Always' Communicated Well[6]	<100	85%	86%	82%
Home Recovery Information Given[6]	<100	78%	88%	85%
Hospital Given 9 or 10 on 10 Point Scale[6]	<100	71%	78%	71%
Meds 'Always' Explained Before Given[6]	<100	60%	68%	64%
Nurses 'Always' Communicated Well[6]	<100	70%	83%	79%
Pain 'Always' Well Controlled[6]	<100	67%	73%	71%
Room and Bathroom 'Always' Clean[6]	<100	85%	81%	73%
Timely Help 'Always' Received[6]	<100	66%	75%	68%
Would Definitely Recommend Hospital[6]	<100	71%	77%	71%
Use of Medical Imaging				
Cardiac Imaging Stress Test before Surgery[1]	-	-	5.4%	5.3%
Combination Abdominal CT Scan[1]	-	-	9.3%	10.5%
Combination Brain/Sinus CT Scan	58	0.0%	2.7%	2.7%
Combination Chest CT Scan[1]	-	-	1.7%	2.7%
Follow-up Mammogram/Ultrasound	206	10.2%	8%	8.8%
Lumbar Spine MRI for Low Back Pain[1]	-	-	36.5%	37.2%

Genoa Community Hospital

PO Box 310, 606/706 Ewing Ave
Genoa, NE 68640
Phone: 402-993-2283
Type: Critical Access Hospitals
Ownership: Government - Local
Emergency Services: Yes

Measure	Cases	This Hosp.	State Avg.	U.S. Avg.
Blood Clot Prevention and Treatment				
Anticoagulation Overlap Therapy[5]	-	-	93%	93%
ICU Venous Thromboembolism Prophylaxis[5]	-	-	91%	92%
Incidence of Potentially Preventable VTE[5]	-	-	11%	10%
UFH with Dosages/Platelet Monitoring[5]	-	-	98%	97%
Venous Thromboembolism Prophylaxis[5]	-	-	88%	85%
Warfarin Therapy Discharge Instructions[5]	-	-	81%	75%
Chest Pain/Possible Heart Attack Care				
Aspirin Given Within 24 Hours of Arrival[5]	-	-	96%	96%
Fibrinolytic Meds Within 30 Min. of Arrival[5]	-	-	53%	58%
Average Time to ECG (minutes)[5]	-	-	8	7
Average Time to Transfer (minutes)[5]	-	-	76	60
Children's Asthma Care				
Received Home Management Plan of Care	-	-	-	88%
Received Reliever Medication	-	-	-	100%
Received Systemic Corticosteroids	-	-	-	100%
Emergency Department				
Admittance Decision Time (minutes)[5]	-	-	75	98
Head CT Results Within 45 Min. of Arrival[5]	-	-	61%	57%
Patients Who Left ER Before Being Seen[5]	-	-	1%	2%
Time from ER Arrival to Admit. (minutes)[5]	-	-	207	274
Time from ER Arrival to Discharge (minutes)[5]	-	-	118	134
Time in ER Before Being Evaluated (minutes)[5]	-	-	21	26
Time to Pain Meds for Fractures (minutes)[5]	-	-	42	57
Heart Attack Care				
Aspirin Given at Discharge[5]	-	-	100%	99%
Fibrinolytic Meds Within 30 Min. of Arrival[5]	-	-	-	54%
PCI Within 90 Minutes of Arrival[5]	-	-	96%	96%
Statin Prescribed at Discharge[5]	-	-	99%	98%
Heart Failure Care				
ACE Inhibitor or ARB for LVSD[3,7]	-	-	96%	97%
Discharge Instructions Given[3,7]	-	-	93%	94%
Evaluation of LVS Function[1,3]	-	-	98%	99%
Medicare Spending				
Medicare Spending per Patient (ratio)	-	-	0.97	0.98
Pneumonia Care				
Appropriate Initial Antibiotic Given[1,3]	-	-	95%	95%
Blood Culture Timing[3,7]	-	-	99%	98%
Pregnancy and Delivery Care				
Newborn Deliveries Scheduled Early[5]	-	-	5%	6%
Preventive Care				
Immunization for Influenza[5]	-	-	89%	90%
Immunization for Pneumonia[5]	-	-	90%	92%
Stroke Care				
Anticoagulation Therapy for Atrial Fibrillation[5]	-	-	95%	95%
Antithrombotic Therapy Timing[5]	-	-	99%	98%
Assessed for Rehabilitation[5]	-	-	99%	97%
Discharged on Antithrombotic Therapy[5]	-	-	100%	99%
Discharged on Statin Medication[5]	-	-	93%	94%
Thrombolytic Therapy Timing[5]	-	-	75%	66%
Venous Thromboembolism Prophylaxis[5]	-	-	94%	94%
Written Stroke Educational Materials Given[5]	-	-	84%	88%
Surgical Care Improvement Project				
Appropriate Beta Blocker Usage[5]	-	-	98%	98%
Appropriate VTP Within 24 Hours[5]	-	-	99%	98%
Controlled Postoperative Blood Glucose[5]	-	-	96%	97%
Perioperative Temperature Management[5]	-	-	100%	100%
Prophylactic Antibiotic Selection[5]	-	-	99%	99%
Prophylactic Antibiotic Selection (Outpatient)[5]	-	-	99%	98%
Prophylactic Antibiotic Stopped[5]	-	-	98%	98%
Prophylactic Antibiotic Timing[5]	-	-	98%	99%
Prophylactic Antibiotic Timing (Outpatient)[5]	-	-	97%	98%
Urinary Catheter Removal[5]	-	-	98%	97%
Survey of Patients' Hospital Experiences				
Area Around Room 'Always' Quiet at Night[5]	-	-	67%	61%
Doctors 'Always' Communicated Well[5]	-	-	86%	82%

NOTE: Hospital profiles are in alphabetical order by state, then city, then hospital within the city; Rankings exclude hospitals with less than 25 cases except for patient surveys which excludes hospitals with less than 100 cases; (a) 100-299 cases; (1) The number of cases/patients is too few to report; (2) Data submitted were based on a sample of cases/patients; (3) Results are based on a shorter time period than required; (4) Data suppressed by CMS for one or more quarters; (5) Results are not available for this reporting period; (6) Fewer than 100 patients completed the HCAHPS survey; (7) No cases met the criteria for this measure; (8) The lower limit of the confidence interval cannot be calculated if the number of observed infections equals zero; (9) No data are available from the state/territory for this reporting period; (10) The scores shown reflect fewer than 50 completed surveys; (11) There were discrepancies in the data collection process; (12) This measure does not apply to this hospital for this reporting period; (13) Results cannot be calculated for this reporting period; (14) The results for this state are combined with nearby states to protect confidentiality; Please refer to the User's Guide for a full explanation of data.

Measure	Cases	This Hosp.	State Avg.	U.S. Avg.
Home Recovery Information Given[5]	-	-	88%	85%
Hospital Given 9 or 10 on 10 Point Scale[5]	-	-	78%	71%
Meds 'Always' Explained Before Given[5]	-	-	68%	64%
Nurses 'Always' Communicated Well[5]	-	-	83%	79%
Pain 'Always' Well Controlled[5]	-	-	73%	71%
Room and Bathroom 'Always' Clean[5]	-	-	81%	73%
Timely Help 'Always' Received[5]	-	-	75%	68%
Would Definitely Recommend Hospital[5]	-	-	77%	71%
Use of Medical Imaging				
Cardiac Imaging Stress Test before Surgery[1]	-	-	5.4%	5.3%
Combination Abdominal CT Scan[1]	-	-	9.3%	10.5%
Combination Brain/Sinus CT Scan[1]	-	-	2.7%	2.7%
Combination Chest CT Scan[1]	-	-	1.7%	2.7%
Follow-up Mammogram/Ultrasound[7]	-	-	8%	8.8%
Lumbar Spine MRI for Low Back Pain[1]	-	-	36.5%	37.2%

Gordon Memorial Hospital District

300 East 8th St
Gordon, NE 69343
Phone: 308-282-0401
Fax: 308-282-0431
URL: www.gordonhospital.org
Type: Critical Access Hospitals
Emergency Services: Yes
Ownership: Govt - Hospital Dist/Auth
Beds: 25

Key Personnel:
Infection Control. . . . . Kathie King, RN BSN
Quality Assurance . . . . Kathy King, RN BSN
Anesthesiology. . . . . Marty Lambert
Radiology. . . . . Corrinew Larson, RT, ARRT
CEO/President. . . . . Jim Lebrun
Operating Room. . . . . Andrea Parks, RN
Chief of Medical Staff . . . . Anthony Van Bang, MD

Measure	Cases	This Hosp.	State Avg.	U.S. Avg.
Blood Clot Prevention and Treatment				
Anticoagulation Overlap Therapy[5]	-	-	93%	93%
ICU Venous Thromboembolism Prophylaxis[5]	-	-	91%	92%
Incidence of Potentially Preventable VTE[5]	-	-	11%	10%
UFH with Dosages/Platelet Monitoring[5]	-	-	98%	97%
Venous Thromboembolism Prophylaxis[5]	-	-	88%	85%
Warfarin Therapy Discharge Instructions[5]	-	-	81%	75%
Chest Pain/Possible Heart Attack Care				
Aspirin Given Within 24 Hours of Arrival[1]	-	-	96%	96%
Fibrinolytic Meds Within 30 Min. of Arrival[3,7]	-	-	53%	58%
Average Time to ECG (minutes)[1]	-	-	8	7
Average Time to Transfer (minutes)[1,3]	-	-	76	60
Children's Asthma Care				
Received Home Management Plan of Care	-	-	-	88%
Received Reliever Medication	-	-	-	100%
Received Systemic Corticosteroids	-	-	-	100%
Emergency Department				
Admittance Decision Time (minutes)[5]	-	-	75	98
Head CT Results Within 45 Min. of Arrival[5]	-	-	61%	57%
Patients Who Left ER Before Being Seen[5]	-	-	1%	2%
Time from ER Arrival to Admit. (minutes)[5]	-	-	207	274
Time from ER Arrival to Discharge (minutes)[5]	-	-	118	134
Time in ER Before Being Evaluated (minutes)[5]	-	-	21	26
Time to Pain Meds for Fractures (minutes)[5]	-	-	42	57
Heart Attack Care				
Aspirin Given at Discharge[5]	-	-	100%	99%
Fibrinolytic Meds Within 30 Min. of Arrival[5]	-	-	-	54%
PCI Within 90 Minutes of Arrival[5]	-	-	96%	96%
Statin Prescribed at Discharge[5]	-	-	99%	98%
Heart Failure Care				
ACE Inhibitor or ARB for LVSD[7]	-	-	96%	97%
Discharge Instructions Given[1]	-	-	93%	94%
Evaluation of LVS Function[1]	-	-	98%	99%
Medicare Spending				
Medicare Spending per Patient (ratio)	-	-	0.97	0.98
Pneumonia Care				
Appropriate Initial Antibiotic Given	13	100%	95%	95%
Blood Culture Timing[1]	-	-	99%	98%
Pregnancy and Delivery Care				
Newborn Deliveries Scheduled Early[5]	-	-	5%	6%
Preventive Care				
Immunization for Influenza[5]	-	-	89%	90%
Immunization for Pneumonia[5]	-	-	90%	92%
Stroke Care				
Anticoagulation Therapy for Atrial Fibrillation[5]	-	-	95%	95%
Antithrombotic Therapy Timing[5]	-	-	99%	98%
Assessed for Rehabilitation[5]	-	-	99%	97%
Discharged on Antithrombotic Therapy[5]	-	-	100%	99%
Discharged on Statin Medication[5]	-	-	93%	94%
Thrombolytic Therapy Timing[5]	-	-	75%	66%
Venous Thromboembolism Prophylaxis[5]	-	-	94%	94%
Written Stroke Educational Materials Given[5]	-	-	84%	88%
Surgical Care Improvement Project				
Appropriate Beta Blocker Usage[5]	-	-	98%	98%
Appropriate VTP Within 24 Hours[5]	-	-	99%	98%
Controlled Postoperative Blood Glucose[5]	-	-	96%	97%
Perioperative Temperature Management[5]	-	-	100%	100%
Prophylactic Antibiotic Selection[5]	-	-	99%	99%
Prophylactic Antibiotic Selection (Outpatient)[5]	-	-	99%	98%
Prophylactic Antibiotic Stopped[5]	-	-	98%	98%
Prophylactic Antibiotic Timing[5]	-	-	98%	99%
Prophylactic Antibiotic Timing (Outpatient)[5]	-	-	97%	98%
Urinary Catheter Removal[5]	-	-	98%	97%
Survey of Patients' Hospital Experiences				
Area Around Room 'Always' Quiet at Night[6]	<100	51%	67%	61%
Doctors 'Always' Communicated Well[6]	<100	84%	86%	82%
Home Recovery Information Given[6]	<100	82%	88%	85%
Hospital Given 9 or 10 on 10 Point Scale[6]	<100	75%	78%	71%
Meds 'Always' Explained Before Given[6]	<100	74%	68%	64%
Nurses 'Always' Communicated Well[6]	<100	81%	83%	79%
Pain 'Always' Well Controlled[6]	<100	73%	73%	71%
Room and Bathroom 'Always' Clean[6]	<100	89%	81%	73%
Timely Help 'Always' Received[6]	<100	81%	75%	68%
Would Definitely Recommend Hospital[6]	<100	71%	77%	71%
Use of Medical Imaging				
Cardiac Imaging Stress Test before Surgery[7]	-	-	5.4%	5.3%
Combination Abdominal CT Scan	69	0.0%	9.3%	10.5%
Combination Brain/Sinus CT Scan[1]	-	-	2.7%	2.7%
Combination Chest CT Scan[1]	-	-	1.7%	2.7%
Follow-up Mammogram/Ultrasound[1]	-	-	8%	8.8%
Lumbar Spine MRI for Low Back Pain[1]	-	-	36.5%	37.2%

Gothenburg Memorial Hospital

910 20th St
Gothenburg, NE 69138
Phone: 308-537-3661
Fax: 308-537-3048
URL: www.ghospital.org
Type: Critical Access Hospitals
Emergency Services: Yes
Ownership: Govt - Hospital Dist/Auth
Beds: 25

Key Personnel:
CEO . . . . Mick Brant, Administrator
Operating Room. . . . . Carolyn Evenson
Cardiac Laboratory. . . . . Myra Gronewold
Quality Assurance . . . . Jeanine Kline
Radiology. . . . . Julie Koehler
Anesthesiology. . . . . Stanley Roethemeyer

Measure	Cases	This Hosp.	State Avg.	U.S. Avg.
Blood Clot Prevention and Treatment				
Anticoagulation Overlap Therapy[5]	-	-	93%	93%
ICU Venous Thromboembolism Prophylaxis[5]	-	-	91%	92%
Incidence of Potentially Preventable VTE[5]	-	-	11%	10%
UFH with Dosages/Platelet Monitoring[5]	-	-	98%	97%
Venous Thromboembolism Prophylaxis[5]	-	-	88%	85%
Warfarin Therapy Discharge Instructions[5]	-	-	81%	75%
Chest Pain/Possible Heart Attack Care				
Aspirin Given Within 24 Hours of Arrival	11	100%	96%	96%
Fibrinolytic Meds Within 30 Min. of Arrival[1,3]	-	-	53%	58%
Average Time to ECG (minutes)	11	7	8	7
Average Time to Transfer (minutes)[3,7]	-	-	76	60
Children's Asthma Care				
Received Home Management Plan of Care	-	-	-	88%
Received Reliever Medication	-	-	-	100%
Received Systemic Corticosteroids	-	-	-	100%
Emergency Department				
Admittance Decision Time (minutes)[5]	-	-	75	98
Head CT Results Within 45 Min. of Arrival[5]	-	-	61%	57%
Patients Who Left ER Before Being Seen[5]	-	-	1%	2%
Time from ER Arrival to Admit. (minutes)[5]	-	-	207	274
Time from ER Arrival to Discharge (minutes)[5]	-	-	118	134
Time in ER Before Being Evaluated (minutes)[5]	-	-	21	26
Time to Pain Meds for Fractures (minutes)[5]	-	-	42	57
Heart Attack Care				
Aspirin Given at Discharge[5]	-	-	100%	99%
Fibrinolytic Meds Within 30 Min. of Arrival[5]	-	-	-	54%
PCI Within 90 Minutes of Arrival[5]	-	-	96%	96%
Statin Prescribed at Discharge[5]	-	-	99%	98%
Heart Failure Care				
ACE Inhibitor or ARB for LVSD[1,3]	-	-	96%	97%
Discharge Instructions Given[1,3]	-	-	93%	94%
Evaluation of LVS Function[1,3]	-	-	98%	99%
Medicare Spending				
Medicare Spending per Patient (ratio)	-	-	0.97	0.98
Pneumonia Care				
Appropriate Initial Antibiotic Given[1]	-	-	95%	95%
Blood Culture Timing[1]	-	-	99%	98%
Pregnancy and Delivery Care				
Newborn Deliveries Scheduled Early[5]	-	-	5%	6%
Preventive Care				
Immunization for Influenza[5]	-	-	89%	90%
Immunization for Pneumonia[5]	-	-	90%	92%
Stroke Care				
Anticoagulation Therapy for Atrial Fibrillation[5]	-	-	95%	95%
Antithrombotic Therapy Timing[5]	-	-	99%	98%
Assessed for Rehabilitation[5]	-	-	99%	97%
Discharged on Antithrombotic Therapy[5]	-	-	100%	99%
Discharged on Statin Medication[5]	-	-	93%	94%
Thrombolytic Therapy Timing[5]	-	-	75%	66%
Venous Thromboembolism Prophylaxis[5]	-	-	94%	94%
Written Stroke Educational Materials Given[5]	-	-	84%	88%
Surgical Care Improvement Project				
Appropriate Beta Blocker Usage[5]	-	-	98%	98%
Appropriate VTP Within 24 Hours[5]	-	-	99%	98%
Controlled Postoperative Blood Glucose[5]	-	-	96%	97%
Perioperative Temperature Management[5]	-	-	100%	100%
Prophylactic Antibiotic Selection[5]	-	-	99%	99%
Prophylactic Antibiotic Selection (Outpatient)[1,3]	-	-	99%	98%
Prophylactic Antibiotic Stopped[5]	-	-	98%	98%
Prophylactic Antibiotic Timing[5]	-	-	98%	99%
Prophylactic Antibiotic Timing (Outpatient)[1,3]	-	-	97%	98%
Urinary Catheter Removal[5]	-	-	98%	97%
Survey of Patients' Hospital Experiences				
Area Around Room 'Always' Quiet at Night	(a)	65%	67%	61%
Doctors 'Always' Communicated Well	(a)	87%	86%	82%
Home Recovery Information Given	(a)	81%	88%	85%
Hospital Given 9 or 10 on 10 Point Scale	(a)	76%	78%	71%
Meds 'Always' Explained Before Given	(a)	65%	68%	64%
Nurses 'Always' Communicated Well	(a)	82%	83%	79%
Pain 'Always' Well Controlled	(a)	68%	73%	71%
Room and Bathroom 'Always' Clean	(a)	86%	81%	73%
Timely Help 'Always' Received	(a)	75%	75%	68%
Would Definitely Recommend Hospital	(a)	76%	77%	71%
Use of Medical Imaging				
Cardiac Imaging Stress Test before Surgery[1]	-	-	5.4%	5.3%
Combination Abdominal CT Scan	63	4.8%	9.3%	10.5%
Combination Brain/Sinus CT Scan	47	10.6%	2.7%	2.7%
Combination Chest CT Scan	49	0.0%	1.7%	2.7%
Follow-up Mammogram/Ultrasound	132	7.6%	8%	8.8%
Lumbar Spine MRI for Low Back Pain[1]	-	-	36.5%	37.2%

Saint Francis Medical Center

2620 West Faidley Ave
Grand Island, NE 68803
Phone: 308-384-4600
Fax: 308-398-5589
URL: www.saintfrancisgi.org
Type: Acute Care Hospitals
Emergency Services: Yes
Ownership: Voluntary non-profit - Church
Beds: 200

Key Personnel:
Operating Room. . . . . Dee Donaldson, RN
Chief of Medical Staff . . . . Michael Hein, MD
Radiology. . . . . Jackie Huldt
Patient Relations . . . . Joan Jensen
Quality Assurance . . . . Charlene L'Heureux
President . . . . Dan McElligott, FACHE
Hemotology Center . . . . Max Norvell

NOTE: Hospital profiles are in alphabetical order by state, then city, then hospital within the city; Rankings exclude hospitals with less than 25 cases except for patient surveys which excludes hospitals with less than 100 cases; (a) 100-299 cases; (1) The number of cases/patients is too few to report; (2) Data submitted were based on a sample of cases/patients; (3) Results are based on a shorter time period than required; (4) Data suppressed by CMS for one or more quarters; (5) Results are not available for this reporting period; (6) Fewer than 100 patients completed the HCAHPS survey; (7) No cases met the criteria for this measure; (8) The lower limit of the confidence interval cannot be calculated if the number of observed infections equals zero; (9) No data are available from the state/territory for this reporting period; (10) The scores shown reflect fewer than 50 completed surveys; (11) There were discrepancies in the data collection process; (12) This measure does not apply to this hospital for this reporting period; (13) Results cannot be calculated for this reporting period; (14) The results for this state are combined with nearby states to protect confidentiality; Please refer to the User's Guide for a full explanation of data.

Pediatric In-Patient Care . . . . Jan Spale

Measure	Cases	This Hosp.	State Avg.	U.S. Avg.
Blood Clot Prevention and Treatment				
Anticoagulation Overlap Therapy[2]	39	77%	93%	93%
ICU Venous Thromboembolism Prophylaxis[2]	57	86%	91%	92%
Incidence of Potentially Preventable VTE[1,2]	-	-	11%	10%
UFH with Dosages/Platelet Monitoring[2]	54	100%	98%	97%
Venous Thromboembolism Prophylaxis[2]	307	75%	88%	85%
Warfarin Therapy Discharge Instructions[2]	26	96%	81%	75%
Chest Pain/Possible Heart Attack Care				
Aspirin Given Within 24 Hours of Arrival	12	100%	96%	96%
Fibrinolytic Meds Within 30 Min. of Arrival[1]	-	-	53%	58%
Average Time to ECG (minutes)	14	8	8	7
Average Time to Transfer (minutes)[7]	-	-	76	60
Children's Asthma Care				
Received Home Management Plan of Care	-	-	-	88%
Received Reliever Medication	-	-	-	100%
Received Systemic Corticosteroids	-	-	-	100%
Emergency Department				
Admittance Decision Time (minutes)[2]	428	50	75	98
Head CT Results Within 45 Min. of Arrival[1]	-	-	61%	57%
Patients Who Left ER Before Being Seen	24,093	1%	1%	2%
Time from ER Arrival to Admit. (minutes)[2]	435	177	207	274
Time from ER Arrival to Discharge (minutes)	346	102	118	134
Time in ER Before Being Evaluated (minutes)	355	18	21	26
Time to Pain Meds for Fractures (minutes)	124	44	42	57
Heart Attack Care				
Aspirin Given at Discharge	76	99%	100%	99%
Fibrinolytic Meds Within 30 Min. of Arrival[7]	-	-	-	54%
PCI Within 90 Minutes of Arrival	12	100%	96%	96%
Statin Prescribed at Discharge	76	96%	99%	98%
Heart Failure Care				
ACE Inhibitor or ARB for LVSD	24	100%	96%	97%
Discharge Instructions Given	88	82%	93%	94%
Evaluation of LVS Function	129	100%	98%	99%
Medicare Spending				
Medicare Spending per Patient (ratio)	-	0.98	0.97	0.98
Pneumonia Care				
Appropriate Initial Antibiotic Given	131	95%	95%	95%
Blood Culture Timing	217	99%	99%	98%
Pregnancy and Delivery Care				
Newborn Deliveries Scheduled Early[2]	58	2%	5%	6%
Preventive Care				
Immunization for Influenza[2]	507	95%	89%	90%
Immunization for Pneumonia[2]	600	96%	90%	92%
Stroke Care				
Anticoagulation Therapy for Atrial Fibrillation	19	95%	95%	95%
Antithrombotic Therapy Timing	53	98%	99%	98%
Assessed for Rehabilitation	57	96%	99%	97%
Discharged on Antithrombotic Therapy	54	100%	100%	99%
Discharged on Statin Medication	43	81%	93%	94%
Thrombolytic Therapy Timing[1]	-	-	75%	66%
Venous Thromboembolism Prophylaxis	62	81%	94%	94%
Written Stroke Educational Materials Given	28	39%	84%	88%
Surgical Care Improvement Project				
Appropriate Beta Blocker Usage	212	99%	98%	98%
Appropriate VTP Within 24 Hours	490	99%	99%	98%
Controlled Postoperative Blood Glucose[7]	-	-	96%	97%
Perioperative Temperature Management	647	100%	100%	100%
Prophylactic Antibiotic Selection	423	100%	99%	99%
Prophylactic Antibiotic Selection (Outpatient)	114	99%	99%	98%
Prophylactic Antibiotic Stopped	410	98%	98%	98%
Prophylactic Antibiotic Timing	423	100%	98%	99%
Prophylactic Antibiotic Timing (Outpatient)	115	99%	97%	98%
Urinary Catheter Removal	425	98%	98%	97%
Survey of Patients' Hospital Experiences				
Area Around Room 'Always' Quiet at Night	300+	64%	67%	61%
Doctors 'Always' Communicated Well	300+	81%	86%	82%
Home Recovery Information Given	300+	90%	88%	85%
Hospital Given 9 or 10 on 10 Point Scale	300+	77%	78%	71%
Meds 'Always' Explained Before Given	300+	66%	68%	64%
Nurses 'Always' Communicated Well	300+	80%	83%	79%
Pain 'Always' Well Controlled	300+	72%	73%	71%
Room and Bathroom 'Always' Clean	300+	73%	81%	73%
Timely Help 'Always' Received	300+	66%	75%	68%
Would Definitely Recommend Hospital	300+	76%	77%	71%
Use of Medical Imaging				
Cardiac Imaging Stress Test before Surgery[1]	-	-	5.4%	5.3%
Combination Abdominal CT Scan	299	1.3%	9.3%	10.5%
Combination Brain/Sinus CT Scan	321	0.6%	2.7%	2.7%
Combination Chest CT Scan	136	1.5%	1.7%	2.7%
Follow-up Mammogram/Ultrasound	1,826	7.4%	8%	8.8%
Lumbar Spine MRI for Low Back Pain[1]	-	-	36.5%	37.2%

Perkins County Health Services

900 Lincoln Ave
Grant, NE 69140
Phone: 308-352-7200
Fax: 308-352-7291
URL: www.pchsgrant.com
Type: Critical Access Hospitals
Emergency Services: Yes
Ownership: Govt - Hospital Dist/Auth
Beds: 20

Key Personnel:
Cardiology . . . . Arshad Ali
Anesthesiology. . . . . Brian Bielicki, CRNA
Radiology. . . . . Clark Diffendaffer
CEO . . . . Jim LeBrun
Pulmonology . . . . Michael Shedd, MD

Measure	Cases	This Hosp.	State Avg.	U.S. Avg.
Blood Clot Prevention and Treatment				
Anticoagulation Overlap Therapy[5]	-	-	93%	93%
ICU Venous Thromboembolism Prophylaxis[5]	-	-	91%	92%
Incidence of Potentially Preventable VTE[5]	-	-	11%	10%
UFH with Dosages/Platelet Monitoring[5]	-	-	98%	97%
Venous Thromboembolism Prophylaxis[5]	-	-	88%	85%
Warfarin Therapy Discharge Instructions[5]	-	-	81%	75%
Chest Pain/Possible Heart Attack Care				
Aspirin Given Within 24 Hours of Arrival[1,3]	-	-	96%	96%
Fibrinolytic Meds Within 30 Min. of Arrival[3,7]	-	-	53%	58%
Average Time to ECG (minutes)[1,3]	-	-	8	7
Average Time to Transfer (minutes)[3,7]	-	-	76	60
Children's Asthma Care				
Received Home Management Plan of Care	-	-	-	88%
Received Reliever Medication	-	-	-	100%
Received Systemic Corticosteroids	-	-	-	100%
Emergency Department				
Admittance Decision Time (minutes)[5]	-	-	75	98
Head CT Results Within 45 Min. of Arrival[5]	-	-	61%	57%
Patients Who Left ER Before Being Seen[5]	-	-	1%	2%
Time from ER Arrival to Admit. (minutes)[5]	-	-	207	274
Time from ER Arrival to Discharge (minutes)[5]	-	-	118	134
Time in ER Before Being Evaluated (minutes)[5]	-	-	21	26
Time to Pain Meds for Fractures (minutes)[5]	-	-	42	57
Heart Attack Care				
Aspirin Given at Discharge[5]	-	-	100%	99%
Fibrinolytic Meds Within 30 Min. of Arrival[5]	-	-	-	54%
PCI Within 90 Minutes of Arrival[5]	-	-	96%	96%
Statin Prescribed at Discharge[5]	-	-	99%	98%
Heart Failure Care				
ACE Inhibitor or ARB for LVSD[5]	-	-	96%	97%
Discharge Instructions Given[5]	-	-	93%	94%
Evaluation of LVS Function[5]	-	-	98%	99%
Medicare Spending				
Medicare Spending per Patient (ratio)	-	-	0.97	0.98
Pneumonia Care				
Appropriate Initial Antibiotic Given	20	85%	95%	95%
Blood Culture Timing[1]	-	-	99%	98%
Pregnancy and Delivery Care				
Newborn Deliveries Scheduled Early[5]	-	-	5%	6%
Preventive Care				
Immunization for Influenza[5]	-	-	89%	90%
Immunization for Pneumonia[5]	-	-	90%	92%
Stroke Care				
Anticoagulation Therapy for Atrial Fibrillation[5]	-	-	95%	95%
Antithrombotic Therapy Timing[5]	-	-	99%	98%
Assessed for Rehabilitation[5]	-	-	99%	97%
Discharged on Antithrombotic Therapy[5]	-	-	100%	99%
Discharged on Statin Medication[5]	-	-	93%	94%
Thrombolytic Therapy Timing[5]	-	-	75%	66%
Venous Thromboembolism Prophylaxis[5]	-	-	94%	94%
Written Stroke Educational Materials Given[5]	-	-	84%	88%
Surgical Care Improvement Project				
Appropriate Beta Blocker Usage[5]	-	-	98%	98%
Appropriate VTP Within 24 Hours[5]	-	-	99%	98%
Controlled Postoperative Blood Glucose[5]	-	-	96%	97%
Perioperative Temperature Management[5]	-	-	100%	100%
Prophylactic Antibiotic Selection[5]	-	-	99%	99%
Prophylactic Antibiotic Selection (Outpatient)[3,7]	-	-	99%	98%
Prophylactic Antibiotic Stopped[5]	-	-	98%	98%
Prophylactic Antibiotic Timing[5]	-	-	98%	99%
Prophylactic Antibiotic Timing (Outpatient)[1,3]	-	-	97%	98%
Urinary Catheter Removal[5]	-	-	98%	97%
Survey of Patients' Hospital Experiences				
Area Around Room 'Always' Quiet at Night[6]	<100	53%	67%	61%
Doctors 'Always' Communicated Well[6]	<100	88%	86%	82%
Home Recovery Information Given[6]	<100	87%	88%	85%
Hospital Given 9 or 10 on 10 Point Scale[6]	<100	76%	78%	71%
Meds 'Always' Explained Before Given[6]	<100	63%	68%	64%
Nurses 'Always' Communicated Well[6]	<100	83%	83%	79%
Pain 'Always' Well Controlled[6]	<100	64%	73%	71%
Room and Bathroom 'Always' Clean[6]	<100	78%	81%	73%
Timely Help 'Always' Received[6]	<100	79%	75%	68%
Would Definitely Recommend Hospital[6]	<100	81%	77%	71%
Use of Medical Imaging				
Cardiac Imaging Stress Test before Surgery	51	3.9%	5.4%	5.3%
Combination Abdominal CT Scan	67	6.0%	9.3%	10.5%
Combination Brain/Sinus CT Scan[1]	-	-	2.7%	2.7%
Combination Chest CT Scan[1]	-	-	1.7%	2.7%
Follow-up Mammogram/Ultrasound	161	13.7%	8%	8.8%
Lumbar Spine MRI for Low Back Pain[1]	-	-	36.5%	37.2%

Mary Lanning Healthcare

715 N Saint Joseph Ave
Hastings, NE 68901
Phone: 402-463-4521
Fax: 402-461-5321
URL: www.marylanning.org
Type: Acute Care Hospitals
Emergency Services: Yes
Ownership: Voluntary non-profit - Other
Beds: 183

Key Personnel:
Anesthesiology. . . . . Mark S. Brosnihan, MD
Chief of Medical Staff . . . . Gary Caingren
Emergency Room . . . . Ronda Ehly
Radiology. . . . . Jonathan Hart, MD
Infection Control. . . . . Connie Hyde
CEO/President. . . . . W Michael Kearney
Cardiac Laboratory. . . . . Dave Patterson
Quality Assurance . . . . Leota Roll

Measure	Cases	This Hosp.	State Avg.	U.S. Avg.
Blood Clot Prevention and Treatment				
Anticoagulation Overlap Therapy[2]	22	86%	93%	93%
ICU Venous Thromboembolism Prophylaxis[2]	33	91%	91%	92%
Incidence of Potentially Preventable VTE[1,2]	-	-	11%	10%
UFH with Dosages/Platelet Monitoring[2]	21	100%	98%	97%
Venous Thromboembolism Prophylaxis[2]	212	86%	88%	85%
Warfarin Therapy Discharge Instructions[2]	13	85%	81%	75%
Chest Pain/Possible Heart Attack Care				
Aspirin Given Within 24 Hours of Arrival	21	95%	96%	96%
Fibrinolytic Meds Within 30 Min. of Arrival[1]	-	-	53%	58%
Average Time to ECG (minutes)	23	11	8	7
Average Time to Transfer (minutes)[1]	-	-	76	60
Children's Asthma Care				
Received Home Management Plan of Care	-	-	-	88%
Received Reliever Medication	-	-	-	100%
Received Systemic Corticosteroids	-	-	-	100%
Emergency Department				
Admittance Decision Time (minutes)[2]	217	55	75	98
Head CT Results Within 45 Min. of Arrival[1]	-	-	61%	57%
Patients Who Left ER Before Being Seen	12,547	0%	1%	2%
Time from ER Arrival to Admit. (minutes)[2]	218	156	207	274
Time from ER Arrival to Discharge (minutes)	516	89	118	134
Time in ER Before Being Evaluated (minutes)	576	17	21	26
Time to Pain Meds for Fractures (minutes)	63	29	42	57

NOTE: Hospital profiles are in alphabetical order by state, then city, then hospital within the city; Rankings exclude hospitals with less than 25 cases except for patient surveys which excludes hospitals with less than 100 cases; (a) 100-299 cases; (1) The number of cases/patients is too few to report; (2) Data submitted were based on a sample of cases/patients; (3) Results are based on a shorter time period than required; (4) Data suppressed by CMS for one or more quarters; (5) Results are not available for this reporting period; (6) Fewer than 100 patients completed the HCAHPS survey; (7) No cases met the criteria for this measure; (8) The lower limit of the confidence interval cannot be calculated if the number of observed infections equals zero; (9) No data are available from the state/territory for this reporting period; (10) The scores shown reflect fewer than 50 completed surveys; (11) There were discrepancies in the data collection process; (12) This measure does not apply to this hospital for this reporting period; (13) Results cannot be calculated for this reporting period; (14) The results for this state are combined with nearby states to protect confidentiality; Please refer to the User's Guide for a full explanation of data.

Heart Attack Care				
Aspirin Given at Discharge[1,3]	-	-	100%	99%
Fibrinolytic Meds Within 30 Min. of Arrival[3,7]	-	-	-	54%
PCI Within 90 Minutes of Arrival[1,3]	-	-	96%	96%
Statin Prescribed at Discharge[1,3]	-	-	99%	98%
Heart Failure Care				
ACE Inhibitor or ARB for LVSD	33	97%	96%	97%
Discharge Instructions Given	56	89%	93%	94%
Evaluation of LVS Function	79	96%	98%	99%
Medicare Spending				
Medicare Spending per Patient (ratio)	-	0.95	0.97	0.98
Pneumonia Care				
Appropriate Initial Antibiotic Given	58	93%	95%	95%
Blood Culture Timing	64	98%	99%	98%
Pregnancy and Delivery Care				
Newborn Deliveries Scheduled Early[2]	11	0%	5%	6%
Preventive Care				
Immunization for Influenza[2]	544	65%	89%	90%
Immunization for Pneumonia[2]	455	86%	90%	92%
Stroke Care				
Anticoagulation Therapy for Atrial Fibrillation	14	93%	95%	95%
Antithrombotic Therapy Timing	35	100%	99%	98%
Assessed for Rehabilitation	64	100%	99%	97%
Discharged on Antithrombotic Therapy	58	100%	100%	99%
Discharged on Statin Medication	42	98%	93%	94%
Thrombolytic Therapy Timing	11	100%	75%	66%
Venous Thromboembolism Prophylaxis	48	98%	94%	94%
Written Stroke Educational Materials Given	26	96%	84%	88%
Surgical Care Improvement Project				
Appropriate Beta Blocker Usage	159	93%	98%	98%
Appropriate VTP Within 24 Hours	421	97%	99%	98%
Controlled Postoperative Blood Glucose[7]	-	-	96%	97%
Perioperative Temperature Management	469	100%	100%	100%
Prophylactic Antibiotic Selection	345	99%	99%	99%
Prophylactic Antibiotic Selection (Outpatient)	164	98%	99%	98%
Prophylactic Antibiotic Stopped	333	96%	98%	98%
Prophylactic Antibiotic Timing	345	99%	98%	99%
Prophylactic Antibiotic Timing (Outpatient)	173	90%	97%	98%
Urinary Catheter Removal	276	99%	98%	97%
Survey of Patients' Hospital Experiences				
Area Around Room 'Always' Quiet at Night	300+	61%	67%	61%
Doctors 'Always' Communicated Well	300+	83%	86%	82%
Home Recovery Information Given	300+	89%	88%	85%
Hospital Given 9 or 10 on 10 Point Scale	300+	74%	78%	71%
Meds 'Always' Explained Before Given	300+	65%	68%	64%
Nurses 'Always' Communicated Well	300+	79%	83%	79%
Pain 'Always' Well Controlled	300+	71%	73%	71%
Room and Bathroom 'Always' Clean	300+	74%	81%	73%
Timely Help 'Always' Received	300+	66%	75%	68%
Would Definitely Recommend Hospital	300+	73%	77%	71%
Use of Medical Imaging				
Cardiac Imaging Stress Test before Surgery	97	3.1%	5.4%	5.3%
Combination Abdominal CT Scan	490	3.9%	9.3%	10.5%
Combination Brain/Sinus CT Scan[1]	-	-	2.7%	2.7%
Combination Chest CT Scan	443	1.6%	1.7%	2.7%
Follow-up Mammogram/Ultrasound	915	8.2%	8%	8.8%
Lumbar Spine MRI for Low Back Pain	113	36.3%	36.5%	37.2%

Thayer County Health Services

120 Park Ave
Hebron, NE 68370
Phone: 402-768-6041
Fax: 402-768-4669
E-mail: info@thayercountyhealth.com
URL: www.thayercountyhealth.com
Type: Critical Access Hospitals
Emergency Services: Yes
Ownership: Government - Local
Beds: 14

Key Personnel:

Chief of Medical Staff . . . . Marlin Bauhard, MD
CEO/President . . . . Joyce Beck
Intensive Care Unit . . . . Jolynn Hacker, RN
Infection Control . . . . Marla Heitmann, RN
Radiology . . . . Audra Hergott

Measure	Cases	This Hosp.	State Avg.	U.S. Avg.
Blood Clot Prevention and Treatment				
Anticoagulation Overlap Therapy[5]	-	-	93%	93%
ICU Venous Thromboembolism Prophylaxis[5]	-	-	91%	92%
Incidence of Potentially Preventable VTE[5]	-	-	11%	10%
UFH with Dosages/Platelet Monitoring[5]	-	-	98%	97%
Venous Thromboembolism Prophylaxis[5]	-	-	88%	85%
Warfarin Therapy Discharge Instructions[5]	-	-	81%	75%
Chest Pain/Possible Heart Attack Care				
Aspirin Given Within 24 Hours of Arrival	12	100%	96%	96%
Fibrinolytic Meds Within 30 Min. of Arrival[1,3]	-	-	53%	58%
Average Time to ECG (minutes)	12	8	8	7
Average Time to Transfer (minutes)[3,7]	-	-	76	60
Children's Asthma Care				
Received Home Management Plan of Care	-	-	-	88%
Received Reliever Medication	-	-	-	100%
Received Systemic Corticosteroids	-	-	-	100%
Emergency Department				
Admittance Decision Time (minutes)[5]	-	-	75	98
Head CT Results Within 45 Min. of Arrival[5]	-	-	61%	57%
Patients Who Left ER Before Being Seen[5]	-	-	1%	2%
Time from ER Arrival to Admit. (minutes)[5]	-	-	207	274
Time from ER Arrival to Discharge (minutes)[5]	-	-	118	134
Time in ER Before Being Evaluated (minutes)[5]	-	-	21	26
Time to Pain Meds for Fractures (minutes)[5]	-	-	42	57
Heart Attack Care				
Aspirin Given at Discharge[5]	-	-	100%	99%
Fibrinolytic Meds Within 30 Min. of Arrival[5]	-	-	-	54%
PCI Within 90 Minutes of Arrival[5]	-	-	96%	96%
Statin Prescribed at Discharge[5]	-	-	99%	98%
Heart Failure Care				
ACE Inhibitor or ARB for LVSD[1]	-	-	96%	97%
Discharge Instructions Given[1]	-	-	93%	94%
Evaluation of LVS Function[1]	-	-	98%	99%
Medicare Spending				
Medicare Spending per Patient (ratio)	-	-	0.97	0.98
Pneumonia Care				
Appropriate Initial Antibiotic Given[1]	-	-	95%	95%
Blood Culture Timing[1]	-	-	99%	98%
Pregnancy and Delivery Care				
Newborn Deliveries Scheduled Early[5]	-	-	5%	6%
Preventive Care				
Immunization for Influenza[5]	-	-	89%	90%
Immunization for Pneumonia[5]	-	-	90%	92%
Stroke Care				
Anticoagulation Therapy for Atrial Fibrillation[5]	-	-	95%	95%
Antithrombotic Therapy Timing[5]	-	-	99%	98%
Assessed for Rehabilitation[5]	-	-	99%	97%
Discharged on Antithrombotic Therapy[5]	-	-	100%	99%
Discharged on Statin Medication[5]	-	-	93%	94%
Thrombolytic Therapy Timing[5]	-	-	75%	66%
Venous Thromboembolism Prophylaxis[5]	-	-	94%	94%
Written Stroke Educational Materials Given[5]	-	-	84%	88%
Surgical Care Improvement Project				
Appropriate Beta Blocker Usage[7]	-	-	98%	98%
Appropriate VTP Within 24 Hours[1]	-	-	99%	98%
Controlled Postoperative Blood Glucose[7]	-	-	96%	97%
Perioperative Temperature Management[1]	-	-	100%	100%
Prophylactic Antibiotic Selection[1]	-	-	99%	99%
Prophylactic Antibiotic Selection (Outpatient)[1,3]	-	-	99%	98%
Prophylactic Antibiotic Stopped[1]	-	-	98%	98%
Prophylactic Antibiotic Timing[1]	-	-	98%	99%
Prophylactic Antibiotic Timing (Outpatient)[1,3]	-	-	97%	98%
Urinary Catheter Removal[1]	-	-	98%	97%
Survey of Patients' Hospital Experiences				
Area Around Room 'Always' Quiet at Night[10]	<100	73%	67%	61%
Doctors 'Always' Communicated Well[10]	<100	90%	86%	82%
Home Recovery Information Given[10]	<100	81%	88%	85%
Hospital Given 9 or 10 on 10 Point Scale[10]	<100	84%	78%	71%
Meds 'Always' Explained Before Given[10]	<100	72%	68%	64%
Nurses 'Always' Communicated Well[10]	<100	84%	83%	79%
Pain 'Always' Well Controlled[10]	<100	72%	73%	71%
Room and Bathroom 'Always' Clean[10]	<100	94%	81%	73%
Timely Help 'Always' Received[10]	<100	85%	75%	68%
Would Definitely Recommend Hospital[10]	<100	83%	77%	71%
Use of Medical Imaging				
Cardiac Imaging Stress Test before Surgery	68	1.5%	5.4%	5.3%
Combination Abdominal CT Scan	75	9.3%	9.3%	10.5%
Combination Brain/Sinus CT Scan[1]	-	-	2.7%	2.7%
Combination Chest CT Scan[1]	-	-	1.7%	2.7%
Follow-up Mammogram/Ultrasound	178	7.9%	8%	8.8%
Lumbar Spine MRI for Low Back Pain[1]	-	-	36.5%	37.2%

Henderson Health Care Services

1621 Front Street
Henderson, NE 68371
Phone: 402-723-4512
Fax: 402-723-4520
Type: Critical Access Hospitals
Emergency Services: Yes
Ownership: Voluntary non-profit - Private
Beds: 59

Key Personnel:

CEO . . . . Cheryl Brown
Quality Assurance . . . . Rita Kroeker
Operating Room. . . . . Lela Regier
Chief of Medical Staff . . . . Robet J Wochner, MD

Measure	Cases	This Hosp.	State Avg.	U.S. Avg.
Blood Clot Prevention and Treatment				
Anticoagulation Overlap Therapy[5]	-	-	93%	93%
ICU Venous Thromboembolism Prophylaxis[5]	-	-	91%	92%
Incidence of Potentially Preventable VTE[5]	-	-	11%	10%
UFH with Dosages/Platelet Monitoring[5]	-	-	98%	97%
Venous Thromboembolism Prophylaxis[5]	-	-	88%	85%
Warfarin Therapy Discharge Instructions[5]	-	-	81%	75%
Chest Pain/Possible Heart Attack Care				
Aspirin Given Within 24 Hours of Arrival[5]	-	-	96%	96%
Fibrinolytic Meds Within 30 Min. of Arrival[5]	-	-	53%	58%
Average Time to ECG (minutes)[5]	-	-	8	7
Average Time to Transfer (minutes)[5]	-	-	76	60
Children's Asthma Care				
Received Home Management Plan of Care	-	-	-	88%
Received Reliever Medication	-	-	-	100%
Received Systemic Corticosteroids	-	-	-	100%
Emergency Department				
Admittance Decision Time (minutes)[5]	-	-	75	98
Head CT Results Within 45 Min. of Arrival[5]	-	-	61%	57%
Patients Who Left ER Before Being Seen[5]	-	-	1%	2%
Time from ER Arrival to Admit. (minutes)[5]	-	-	207	274
Time from ER Arrival to Discharge (minutes)[5]	-	-	118	134
Time in ER Before Being Evaluated (minutes)[5]	-	-	21	26
Time to Pain Meds for Fractures (minutes)[5]	-	-	42	57
Heart Attack Care				
Aspirin Given at Discharge[5]	-	-	100%	99%
Fibrinolytic Meds Within 30 Min. of Arrival[5]	-	-	-	54%
PCI Within 90 Minutes of Arrival[5]	-	-	96%	96%
Statin Prescribed at Discharge[5]	-	-	99%	98%
Heart Failure Care				
ACE Inhibitor or ARB for LVSD[3,7]	-	-	96%	97%
Discharge Instructions Given[1,3]	-	-	93%	94%
Evaluation of LVS Function[1,3]	-	-	98%	99%
Medicare Spending				
Medicare Spending per Patient (ratio)	-	-	0.97	0.98
Pneumonia Care				
Appropriate Initial Antibiotic Given[1,3]	-	-	95%	95%
Blood Culture Timing[1,3]	-	-	99%	98%
Pregnancy and Delivery Care				
Newborn Deliveries Scheduled Early[5]	-	-	5%	6%
Preventive Care				
Immunization for Influenza[5]	-	-	89%	90%
Immunization for Pneumonia[5]	-	-	90%	92%
Stroke Care				
Anticoagulation Therapy for Atrial Fibrillation[5]	-	-	95%	95%
Antithrombotic Therapy Timing[5]	-	-	99%	98%
Assessed for Rehabilitation[5]	-	-	99%	97%
Discharged on Antithrombotic Therapy[5]	-	-	100%	99%
Discharged on Statin Medication[5]	-	-	93%	94%
Thrombolytic Therapy Timing[5]	-	-	75%	66%
Venous Thromboembolism Prophylaxis[5]	-	-	94%	94%
Written Stroke Educational Materials Given[5]	-	-	84%	88%
Surgical Care Improvement Project				
Appropriate Beta Blocker Usage[5]	-	-	98%	98%

NOTE: Hospital profiles are in alphabetical order by state, then city, then hospital within the city; Rankings exclude hospitals with less than 25 cases except for patient surveys which excludes hospitals with less than 100 cases; (a) 100-299 cases; (1) The number of cases/patients is too few to report; (2) Data submitted were based on a sample of cases/patients; (3) Results are based on a shorter time period than required; (4) Data suppressed by CMS for one or more quarters; (5) Results are not available for this reporting period; (6) Fewer than 100 patients completed the HCAHPS survey; (7) No cases met the criteria for this measure; (8) The lower limit of the confidence interval cannot be calculated if the number of observed infections equals zero; (9) No data are available from the state/territory for this reporting period; (10) The scores shown reflect fewer than 50 completed surveys; (11) There were discrepancies in the data collection process; (12) This measure does not apply to this hospital for this reporting period; (13) Results cannot be calculated for this reporting period; (14) The results for this state are combined with nearby states to protect confidentiality; Please refer to the User's Guide for a full explanation of data.

Measure	Cases	This Hosp.	State Avg.	U.S. Avg.
Appropriate VTP Within 24 Hours[5]	-	-	99%	98%
Controlled Postoperative Blood Glucose[5]	-	-	96%	97%
Perioperative Temperature Management[5]	-	-	100%	100%
Prophylactic Antibiotic Selection[5]	-	-	99%	99%
Prophylactic Antibiotic Selection (Outpatient)[5]	-	-	99%	98%
Prophylactic Antibiotic Stopped[5]	-	-	98%	98%
Prophylactic Antibiotic Timing[5]	-	-	98%	99%
Prophylactic Antibiotic Timing (Outpatient)[5]	-	-	97%	98%
Urinary Catheter Removal[5]	-	-	98%	97%
Survey of Patients' Hospital Experiences				
Area Around Room 'Always' Quiet at Night[6]	<100	96%	67%	61%
Doctors 'Always' Communicated Well[6]	<100	93%	86%	82%
Home Recovery Information Given[6]	<100	87%	88%	85%
Hospital Given 9 or 10 on 10 Point Scale[6]	<100	88%	78%	71%
Meds 'Always' Explained Before Given[6]	<100	74%	68%	64%
Nurses 'Always' Communicated Well[6]	<100	89%	83%	79%
Pain 'Always' Well Controlled[6]	<100	84%	73%	71%
Room and Bathroom 'Always' Clean[6]	<100	84%	81%	73%
Timely Help 'Always' Received[6]	<100	91%	75%	68%
Would Definitely Recommend Hospital[6]	<100	86%	77%	71%
Use of Medical Imaging				
Cardiac Imaging Stress Test before Surgery[1]	-	-	5.4%	5.3%
Combination Abdominal CT Scan[1]	-	-	9.3%	10.5%
Combination Brain/Sinus CT Scan[1]	-	-	2.7%	2.7%
Combination Chest CT Scan[1]	-	-	1.7%	2.7%
Follow-up Mammogram/Ultrasound	69	8.7%	8%	8.8%
Lumbar Spine MRI for Low Back Pain[1]	-	-	36.5%	37.2%

Phelps Memorial Health Center

1215 Tibbals St
Holdrege, NE 68949
Phone: 308-995-2211
Fax: 308-995-3333
URL: www.phelpsmemorial.com
Type: Critical Access Hospitals
Emergency Services: Yes
Ownership: Voluntary non-profit - Private
Beds: 49

Key Personnel:

CEO/President. . . . . Mark Harrel
Operating Room. . . . . Tammy Nelson, RN
Infection Control. . . . . Laurie Raboin
Quality Assurance . . . . Bill Redinger
Coronary Care. . . . . Susan Rieker
Emergency Room . . . . Susan Rieker
Intensive Care Unit. . . . . Susan Rieker
Chief of Medical Staff. . . . . Charlotte Wirges, MD

Measure	Cases	This Hosp.	State Avg.	U.S. Avg.
Blood Clot Prevention and Treatment				
Anticoagulation Overlap Therapy[5]	-	-	93%	93%
ICU Venous Thromboembolism Prophylaxis[5]	-	-	91%	92%
Incidence of Potentially Preventable VTE[5]	-	-	11%	10%
UFH with Dosages/Platelet Monitoring[5]	-	-	98%	97%
Venous Thromboembolism Prophylaxis[5]	-	-	88%	85%
Warfarin Therapy Discharge Instructions[5]	-	-	81%	75%
Chest Pain/Possible Heart Attack Care				
Aspirin Given Within 24 Hours of Arrival	24	100%	96%	96%
Fibrinolytic Meds Within 30 Min. of Arrival[1,3]	-	-	53%	58%
Average Time to ECG (minutes)	25	8	8	7
Average Time to Transfer (minutes)[1,3]	-	-	76	60
Children's Asthma Care				
Received Home Management Plan of Care	-	-	-	88%
Received Reliever Medication	-	-	-	100%
Received Systemic Corticosteroids	-	-	-	100%
Emergency Department				
Admittance Decision Time (minutes)[5]	-	-	75	98
Head CT Results Within 45 Min. of Arrival[5]	-	-	61%	57%
Patients Who Left ER Before Being Seen[5]	-	-	1%	2%
Time from ER Arrival to Admit. (minutes)[5]	-	-	207	274
Time from ER Arrival to Discharge (minutes)[5]	-	-	118	134
Time in ER Before Being Evaluated (minutes)[5]	-	-	21	26
Time to Pain Meds for Fractures (minutes)[5]	-	-	42	57
Heart Attack Care				
Aspirin Given at Discharge[1,3]	-	-	100%	99%
Fibrinolytic Meds Within 30 Min. of Arrival[1,3]	-	-	-	54%
PCI Within 90 Minutes of Arrival[3,7]	-	-	96%	96%
Statin Prescribed at Discharge[1,3]	-	-	99%	98%
Heart Failure Care				
ACE Inhibitor or ARB for LVSD[1]	-	-	96%	97%
Discharge Instructions Given	17	82%	93%	94%
Evaluation of LVS Function	29	97%	98%	99%
Medicare Spending				
Medicare Spending per Patient (ratio)	-	-	0.97	0.98
Pneumonia Care				
Appropriate Initial Antibiotic Given	25	100%	95%	95%
Blood Culture Timing[1]	-	-	99%	98%
Pregnancy and Delivery Care				
Newborn Deliveries Scheduled Early[5]	-	-	5%	6%
Preventive Care				
Immunization for Influenza[5]	-	-	89%	90%
Immunization for Pneumonia[5]	-	-	90%	92%
Stroke Care				
Anticoagulation Therapy for Atrial Fibrillation[5]	-	-	95%	95%
Antithrombotic Therapy Timing[5]	-	-	99%	98%
Assessed for Rehabilitation[5]	-	-	99%	97%
Discharged on Antithrombotic Therapy[5]	-	-	100%	99%
Discharged on Statin Medication[5]	-	-	93%	94%
Thrombolytic Therapy Timing[5]	-	-	75%	66%
Venous Thromboembolism Prophylaxis[5]	-	-	94%	94%
Written Stroke Educational Materials Given[5]	-	-	84%	88%
Surgical Care Improvement Project				
Appropriate Beta Blocker Usage	25	96%	98%	98%
Appropriate VTP Within 24 Hours	78	99%	99%	98%
Controlled Postoperative Blood Glucose[7]	-	-	96%	97%
Perioperative Temperature Management	87	94%	100%	100%
Prophylactic Antibiotic Selection	85	99%	99%	99%
Prophylactic Antibiotic Selection (Outpatient)	16	100%	99%	98%
Prophylactic Antibiotic Stopped	85	93%	98%	98%
Prophylactic Antibiotic Timing	85	98%	98%	99%
Prophylactic Antibiotic Timing (Outpatient)	18	89%	97%	98%
Urinary Catheter Removal	49	100%	98%	97%
Survey of Patients' Hospital Experiences				
Area Around Room 'Always' Quiet at Night	(a)	67%	67%	61%
Doctors 'Always' Communicated Well	(a)	85%	86%	82%
Home Recovery Information Given	(a)	89%	88%	85%
Hospital Given 9 or 10 on 10 Point Scale	(a)	83%	78%	71%
Meds 'Always' Explained Before Given	(a)	68%	68%	64%
Nurses 'Always' Communicated Well	(a)	79%	83%	79%
Pain 'Always' Well Controlled	(a)	72%	73%	71%
Room and Bathroom 'Always' Clean	(a)	85%	81%	73%
Timely Help 'Always' Received	(a)	73%	75%	68%
Would Definitely Recommend Hospital	(a)	83%	77%	71%
Use of Medical Imaging				
Cardiac Imaging Stress Test before Surgery	114	4.4%	5.4%	5.3%
Combination Abdominal CT Scan	177	2.3%	9.3%	10.5%
Combination Brain/Sinus CT Scan[1]	-	-	2.7%	2.7%
Combination Chest CT Scan	152	1.3%	1.7%	2.7%
Follow-up Mammogram/Ultrasound	492	3.7%	8%	8.8%
Lumbar Spine MRI for Low Back Pain	55	36.4%	36.5%	37.2%

Chase County Community Hospital

PO Box 819, 600 W 12th St
Imperial, NE 69033
Phone: 308-882-7111
Fax: 308-882-5950
E-mail: ccch@chasecountyhospital.com
URL: www.chasecountyhospital.com
Type: Critical Access Hospitals
Emergency Services: Yes
Ownership: Government - Local
Beds: 25

Key Personnel:

Radiology. . . . . Doug Douglas

Measure	Cases	This Hosp.	State Avg.	U.S. Avg.
Blood Clot Prevention and Treatment				
Anticoagulation Overlap Therapy[5]	-	-	93%	93%
ICU Venous Thromboembolism Prophylaxis[5]	-	-	91%	92%
Incidence of Potentially Preventable VTE[5]	-	-	11%	10%
UFH with Dosages/Platelet Monitoring[5]	-	-	98%	97%
Venous Thromboembolism Prophylaxis[5]	-	-	88%	85%
Warfarin Therapy Discharge Instructions[5]	-	-	81%	75%
Chest Pain/Possible Heart Attack Care				
Aspirin Given Within 24 Hours of Arrival[1,3]	-	-	96%	96%
Fibrinolytic Meds Within 30 Min. of Arrival[1,3]	-	-	53%	58%
Average Time to ECG (minutes)[1,3]	-	-	8	7
Average Time to Transfer (minutes)[1,3]	-	-	76	60
Children's Asthma Care				
Received Home Management Plan of Care	-	-	-	88%
Received Reliever Medication	-	-	-	100%
Received Systemic Corticosteroids	-	-	-	100%
Emergency Department				
Admittance Decision Time (minutes)[5]	-	-	75	98
Head CT Results Within 45 Min. of Arrival[5]	-	-	61%	57%
Patients Who Left ER Before Being Seen[5]	-	-	1%	2%
Time from ER Arrival to Admit. (minutes)[5]	-	-	207	274
Time from ER Arrival to Discharge (minutes)[5]	-	-	118	134
Time in ER Before Being Evaluated (minutes)[5]	-	-	21	26
Time to Pain Meds for Fractures (minutes)[5]	-	-	42	57
Heart Attack Care				
Aspirin Given at Discharge[5]	-	-	100%	99%
Fibrinolytic Meds Within 30 Min. of Arrival[5]	-	-	-	54%
PCI Within 90 Minutes of Arrival[5]	-	-	96%	96%
Statin Prescribed at Discharge[5]	-	-	99%	98%
Heart Failure Care				
ACE Inhibitor or ARB for LVSD[1,3]	-	-	96%	97%
Discharge Instructions Given[1,3]	-	-	93%	94%
Evaluation of LVS Function[1,3]	-	-	98%	99%
Medicare Spending				
Medicare Spending per Patient (ratio)	-	-	0.97	0.98
Pneumonia Care				
Appropriate Initial Antibiotic Given[1]	-	-	95%	95%
Blood Culture Timing[1]	-	-	99%	98%
Pregnancy and Delivery Care				
Newborn Deliveries Scheduled Early[5]	-	-	5%	6%
Preventive Care				
Immunization for Influenza[5]	-	-	89%	90%
Immunization for Pneumonia[5]	-	-	90%	92%
Stroke Care				
Anticoagulation Therapy for Atrial Fibrillation[5]	-	-	95%	95%
Antithrombotic Therapy Timing[5]	-	-	99%	98%
Assessed for Rehabilitation[5]	-	-	99%	97%
Discharged on Antithrombotic Therapy[5]	-	-	100%	99%
Discharged on Statin Medication[5]	-	-	93%	94%
Thrombolytic Therapy Timing[5]	-	-	75%	66%
Venous Thromboembolism Prophylaxis[5]	-	-	94%	94%
Written Stroke Educational Materials Given[5]	-	-	84%	88%
Surgical Care Improvement Project				
Appropriate Beta Blocker Usage[5]	-	-	98%	98%
Appropriate VTP Within 24 Hours[5]	-	-	99%	98%
Controlled Postoperative Blood Glucose[5]	-	-	96%	97%
Perioperative Temperature Management[5]	-	-	100%	100%
Prophylactic Antibiotic Selection[5]	-	-	99%	99%
Prophylactic Antibiotic Selection (Outpatient)[1,3]	-	-	99%	98%
Prophylactic Antibiotic Stopped[5]	-	-	98%	98%
Prophylactic Antibiotic Timing[5]	-	-	98%	99%
Prophylactic Antibiotic Timing (Outpatient)[1,3]	-	-	97%	98%
Urinary Catheter Removal[5]	-	-	98%	97%
Survey of Patients' Hospital Experiences				
Area Around Room 'Always' Quiet at Night[10]	<100	66%	67%	61%
Doctors 'Always' Communicated Well[10]	<100	81%	86%	82%
Home Recovery Information Given[10]	<100	81%	88%	85%
Hospital Given 9 or 10 on 10 Point Scale[10]	<100	59%	78%	71%
Meds 'Always' Explained Before Given[10]	<100	70%	68%	64%
Nurses 'Always' Communicated Well[10]	<100	81%	83%	79%
Pain 'Always' Well Controlled[10]	<100	77%	73%	71%
Room and Bathroom 'Always' Clean[10]	<100	80%	81%	73%
Timely Help 'Always' Received[10]	<100	84%	75%	68%
Would Definitely Recommend Hospital[10]	<100	46%	77%	71%
Use of Medical Imaging				
Cardiac Imaging Stress Test before Surgery	48	2.1%	5.4%	5.3%
Combination Abdominal CT Scan	56	3.6%	9.3%	10.5%
Combination Brain/Sinus CT Scan[1]	-	-	2.7%	2.7%
Combination Chest CT Scan	53	0.0%	1.7%	2.7%
Follow-up Mammogram/Ultrasound	127	9.4%	8%	8.8%
Lumbar Spine MRI for Low Back Pain[1]	-	-	36.5%	37.2%

NOTE: Hospital profiles are in alphabetical order by state, then city, then hospital within the city; Rankings exclude hospitals with less than 25 cases except for patient surveys which excludes hospitals with less than 100 cases; (a) 100-299 cases; (1) The number of cases/patients is too few to report; (2) Data submitted were based on a sample of cases/patients; (3) Results are based on a shorter time period than required; (4) Data suppressed by CMS for one or more quarters; (5) Results are not available for this reporting period; (6) Fewer than 100 patients completed the HCAHPS survey; (7) No cases met the criteria for this measure; (8) The lower limit of the confidence interval cannot be calculated if the number of observed infections equals zero; (9) No data are available from the state/territory for this reporting period; (10) The scores shown reflect fewer than 50 completed surveys; (11) There were discrepancies in the data collection process; (12) This measure does not apply to this hospital for this reporting period; (13) Results cannot be calculated for this reporting period; (14) The results for this state are combined with nearby states to protect confidentiality; Please refer to the User's Guide for a full explanation of data.

Good Samaritan Hospital

PO Box 1990, 10 East 31st St
Kearney, NE 68848
URL: www.gshs.org
Phone: 308-865-7100
Fax: 308-865-2924
Type: Acute Care Hospitals
Emergency Services: Yes
Ownership: Voluntary non-profit - Church
Beds: 287

Key Personnel:
CEO/President. . . . . John W Allen
Quality Assurance . . . . Judy Dady
Radiology. . . . . Chuck Day
Intensive Care Unit. . . . . Valerie Fredericksen
Operating Room. . . . . Ron Langford
Emergency Room . . . . Paul O'Connell
Pediatric In-Patient Care . . . . Coni Rinaker
Patient Relations . . . . Carol Wahl

Measure	Cases	This Hosp.	State Avg.	U.S. Avg.
Blood Clot Prevention and Treatment				
Anticoagulation Overlap Therapy[2]	50	94%	93%	93%
ICU Venous Thromboembolism Prophylaxis[2]	37	92%	91%	92%
Incidence of Potentially Preventable VTE[1,2]	-	-	11%	10%
UFH with Dosages/Platelet Monitoring[2]	49	100%	98%	97%
Venous Thromboembolism Prophylaxis[2]	326	90%	88%	85%
Warfarin Therapy Discharge Instructions[2]	43	72%	81%	75%
Chest Pain/Possible Heart Attack Care				
Aspirin Given Within 24 Hours of Arrival[5]	-	-	96%	96%
Fibrinolytic Meds Within 30 Min. of Arrival[5]	-	-	53%	58%
Average Time to ECG (minutes)[5]	-	-	8	7
Average Time to Transfer (minutes)[5]	-	-	76	60
Children's Asthma Care				
Received Home Management Plan of Care	-	-	-	88%
Received Reliever Medication	-	-	-	100%
Received Systemic Corticosteroids	-	-	-	100%
Emergency Department				
Admittance Decision Time (minutes)[2]	314	66	75	98
Head CT Results Within 45 Min. of Arrival[7]	-	-	61%	57%
Patients Who Left ER Before Being Seen	15,412	0%	1%	2%
Time from ER Arrival to Admit. (minutes)[2]	334	168	207	274
Time from ER Arrival to Discharge (minutes)	370	81	118	134
Time in ER Before Being Evaluated (minutes)	349	10	21	26
Time to Pain Meds for Fractures (minutes)	62	34	42	57
Heart Attack Care				
Aspirin Given at Discharge	198	99%	100%	99%
Fibrinolytic Meds Within 30 Min. of Arrival[7]	-	-	-	54%
PCI Within 90 Minutes of Arrival	12	83%	96%	96%
Statin Prescribed at Discharge	189	97%	99%	98%
Heart Failure Care				
ACE Inhibitor or ARB for LVSD	37	92%	96%	97%
Discharge Instructions Given	110	93%	93%	94%
Evaluation of LVS Function	142	100%	98%	99%
Medicare Spending				
Medicare Spending per Patient (ratio)	-	0.98	0.97	0.98
Pneumonia Care				
Appropriate Initial Antibiotic Given	69	96%	95%	95%
Blood Culture Timing	114	99%	99%	98%
Pregnancy and Delivery Care				
Newborn Deliveries Scheduled Early[2]	27	7%	5%	6%
Preventive Care				
Immunization for Influenza[2]	532	92%	89%	90%
Immunization for Pneumonia[2]	637	93%	90%	92%
Stroke Care				
Anticoagulation Therapy for Atrial Fibrillation	19	100%	95%	95%
Antithrombotic Therapy Timing	76	99%	99%	98%
Assessed for Rehabilitation	107	97%	99%	97%
Discharged on Antithrombotic Therapy	82	100%	100%	99%
Discharged on Statin Medication	68	88%	93%	94%
Thrombolytic Therapy Timing[1]	-	-	75%	66%
Venous Thromboembolism Prophylaxis	109	93%	94%	94%
Written Stroke Educational Materials Given	48	62%	84%	88%
Surgical Care Improvement Project				
Appropriate Beta Blocker Usage	443	96%	98%	98%
Appropriate VTP Within 24 Hours	1,019	99%	99%	98%
Controlled Postoperative Blood Glucose	99	95%	96%	97%
Perioperative Temperature Management	1,184	100%	100%	100%
Prophylactic Antibiotic Selection	862	100%	99%	99%
Prophylactic Antibiotic Selection (Outpatient)	364	98%	99%	98%
Prophylactic Antibiotic Stopped	846	97%	98%	98%
Prophylactic Antibiotic Timing	863	100%	98%	99%
Prophylactic Antibiotic Timing (Outpatient)	364	96%	97%	98%
Urinary Catheter Removal	521	96%	98%	97%
Survey of Patients' Hospital Experiences				
Area Around Room 'Always' Quiet at Night	300+	61%	67%	61%
Doctors 'Always' Communicated Well	300+	81%	86%	82%
Home Recovery Information Given	300+	88%	88%	85%
Hospital Given 9 or 10 on 10 Point Scale	300+	73%	78%	71%
Meds 'Always' Explained Before Given	300+	64%	68%	64%
Nurses 'Always' Communicated Well	300+	78%	83%	79%
Pain 'Always' Well Controlled	300+	67%	73%	71%
Room and Bathroom 'Always' Clean	300+	75%	81%	73%
Timely Help 'Always' Received	300+	62%	75%	68%
Would Definitely Recommend Hospital	300+	76%	77%	71%
Use of Medical Imaging				
Cardiac Imaging Stress Test before Surgery	210	2.4%	5.4%	5.3%
Combination Abdominal CT Scan	514	6.0%	9.3%	10.5%
Combination Brain/Sinus CT Scan[1]	-	-	2.7%	2.7%
Combination Chest CT Scan	440	0.5%	1.7%	2.7%
Follow-up Mammogram/Ultrasound	924	3.7%	8%	8.8%
Lumbar Spine MRI for Low Back Pain	130	29.2%	36.5%	37.2%

Kimball Health Services

505 South Burg St
Kimball, NE 69145
URL: www.kimballhealth.org
Phone: 308-235-1952
Type: Critical Access Hospitals
Emergency Services: Yes
Ownership: Government - Local
Beds: 20

Key Personnel:
CEO . . . . Kenneth H. Hunter, RN, BSN

Measure	Cases	This Hosp.	State Avg.	U.S. Avg.
Blood Clot Prevention and Treatment				
Anticoagulation Overlap Therapy[5]	-	-	93%	93%
ICU Venous Thromboembolism Prophylaxis[5]	-	-	91%	92%
Incidence of Potentially Preventable VTE[5]	-	-	11%	10%
UFH with Dosages/Platelet Monitoring[5]	-	-	98%	97%
Venous Thromboembolism Prophylaxis[5]	-	-	88%	85%
Warfarin Therapy Discharge Instructions[5]	-	-	81%	75%
Chest Pain/Possible Heart Attack Care				
Aspirin Given Within 24 Hours of Arrival[1,3]	-	-	96%	96%
Fibrinolytic Meds Within 30 Min. of Arrival[3,7]	-	-	53%	58%
Average Time to ECG (minutes)[1,3]	-	-	8	7
Average Time to Transfer (minutes)[1,3]	-	-	76	60
Children's Asthma Care				
Received Home Management Plan of Care	-	-	-	88%
Received Reliever Medication	-	-	-	100%
Received Systemic Corticosteroids	-	-	-	100%
Emergency Department				
Admittance Decision Time (minutes)[5]	-	-	75	98
Head CT Results Within 45 Min. of Arrival[5]	-	-	61%	57%
Patients Who Left ER Before Being Seen[5]	-	-	1%	2%
Time from ER Arrival to Admit. (minutes)[5]	-	-	207	274
Time from ER Arrival to Discharge (minutes)[5]	-	-	118	134
Time in ER Before Being Evaluated (minutes)[5]	-	-	21	26
Time to Pain Meds for Fractures (minutes)[5]	-	-	42	57
Heart Attack Care				
Aspirin Given at Discharge[5]	-	-	100%	99%
Fibrinolytic Meds Within 30 Min. of Arrival[5]	-	-	-	54%
PCI Within 90 Minutes of Arrival[5]	-	-	96%	96%
Statin Prescribed at Discharge[5]	-	-	99%	98%
Heart Failure Care				
ACE Inhibitor or ARB for LVSD[3,7]	-	-	96%	97%
Discharge Instructions Given[1,3]	-	-	93%	94%
Evaluation of LVS Function[1,3]	-	-	98%	99%
Medicare Spending				
Medicare Spending per Patient (ratio)	-	-	0.97	0.98
Pneumonia Care				
Appropriate Initial Antibiotic Given[1]	-	-	95%	95%
Blood Culture Timing[1]	-	-	99%	98%
Pregnancy and Delivery Care				
Newborn Deliveries Scheduled Early[5]	-	-	5%	6%
Preventive Care				
Immunization for Influenza[5]	-	-	89%	90%
Immunization for Pneumonia[3]	15	93%	90%	92%
Stroke Care				
Anticoagulation Therapy for Atrial Fibrillation[5]	-	-	95%	95%
Antithrombotic Therapy Timing[5]	-	-	99%	98%
Assessed for Rehabilitation[5]	-	-	99%	97%
Discharged on Antithrombotic Therapy[5]	-	-	100%	99%
Discharged on Statin Medication[5]	-	-	93%	94%
Thrombolytic Therapy Timing[5]	-	-	75%	66%
Venous Thromboembolism Prophylaxis[5]	-	-	94%	94%
Written Stroke Educational Materials Given[5]	-	-	84%	88%
Surgical Care Improvement Project				
Appropriate Beta Blocker Usage[5]	-	-	98%	98%
Appropriate VTP Within 24 Hours[5]	-	-	99%	98%
Controlled Postoperative Blood Glucose[5]	-	-	96%	97%
Perioperative Temperature Management[5]	-	-	100%	100%
Prophylactic Antibiotic Selection[5]	-	-	99%	99%
Prophylactic Antibiotic Selection (Outpatient)[5]	-	-	99%	98%
Prophylactic Antibiotic Stopped[5]	-	-	98%	98%
Prophylactic Antibiotic Timing[5]	-	-	98%	99%
Prophylactic Antibiotic Timing (Outpatient)[5]	-	-	97%	98%
Urinary Catheter Removal[5]	-	-	98%	97%
Survey of Patients' Hospital Experiences				
Area Around Room 'Always' Quiet at Night[3,10]	<100	72%	67%	61%
Doctors 'Always' Communicated Well[3,10]	<100	80%	86%	82%
Home Recovery Information Given[3,10]	<100	90%	88%	85%
Hospital Given 9 or 10 on 10 Point Scale[3,10]	<100	73%	78%	71%
Meds 'Always' Explained Before Given[3,10]	<100	52%	68%	64%
Nurses 'Always' Communicated Well[3,10]	<100	87%	83%	79%
Pain 'Always' Well Controlled[3,10]	<100	77%	73%	71%
Room and Bathroom 'Always' Clean[3,10]	<100	81%	81%	73%
Timely Help 'Always' Received[3,10]	<100	98%	75%	68%
Would Definitely Recommend Hospital[3,10]	<100	62%	77%	71%
Use of Medical Imaging				
Cardiac Imaging Stress Test before Surgery[1]	-	-	5.4%	5.3%
Combination Abdominal CT Scan[1]	-	-	9.3%	10.5%
Combination Brain/Sinus CT Scan[1]	-	-	2.7%	2.7%
Combination Chest CT Scan[1]	-	-	1.7%	2.7%
Follow-up Mammogram/Ultrasound[7]	-	-	8%	8.8%
Lumbar Spine MRI for Low Back Pain[1]	-	-	36.5%	37.2%

Lexington Regional Health Center

PO Box 980, 1201 North Erie St
Lexington, NE 68850
URL: www.tricountyhospital.com
Phone: 308-324-5651
Fax: 308-324-8359
Type: Critical Access Hospitals
Emergency Services: Yes
Ownership: Govt - Hospital Dist/Auth
Beds: 40

Key Personnel:
Chief of Medical Staff. . . . . Fran Acosta-Carlson, MD
President/CEO. . . . . Joel Beiswenger
Infection Control. . . . . Hawley Lister
Quality Assurance . . . . Sandy Nichelson
Cardiac Laboratory. . . . . Mary Kay Rhone
Radiology. . . . . Jo Swartz
Operating Room. . . . . Pam Teten

Measure	Cases	This Hosp.	State Avg.	U.S. Avg.
Blood Clot Prevention and Treatment				
Anticoagulation Overlap Therapy[5]	-	-	93%	93%
ICU Venous Thromboembolism Prophylaxis[5]	-	-	91%	92%
Incidence of Potentially Preventable VTE[5]	-	-	11%	10%
UFH with Dosages/Platelet Monitoring[5]	-	-	98%	97%
Venous Thromboembolism Prophylaxis[5]	-	-	88%	85%
Warfarin Therapy Discharge Instructions[5]	-	-	81%	75%
Chest Pain/Possible Heart Attack Care				
Aspirin Given Within 24 Hours of Arrival	17	100%	96%	96%
Fibrinolytic Meds Within 30 Min. of Arrival[7]	-	-	53%	58%
Average Time to ECG (minutes)	17	10	8	7
Average Time to Transfer (minutes)[1]	-	-	76	60
Children's Asthma Care				
Received Home Management Plan of Care	-	-	-	88%
Received Reliever Medication	-	-	-	100%
Received Systemic Corticosteroids	-	-	-	100%
Emergency Department				

NOTE: Hospital profiles are in alphabetical order by state, then city, then hospital within the city; Rankings exclude hospitals with less than 25 cases except for patient surveys which excludes hospitals with less than 100 cases; (a) 100-299 cases; (1) The number of cases/patients is too few to report; (2) Data submitted were based on a sample of cases/patients; (3) Results are based on a shorter time period than required; (4) Data suppressed by CMS for one or more quarters; (5) Results are not available for this reporting period; (6) Fewer than 100 patients completed the HCAHPS survey; (7) No cases met the criteria for this measure; (8) The lower limit of the confidence interval cannot be calculated if the number of observed infections equals zero; (9) No data are available from the state/territory for this reporting period; (10) The scores shown reflect fewer than 50 completed surveys; (11) There were discrepancies in the data collection process; (12) This measure does not apply to this hospital for this reporting period; (13) Results cannot be calculated for this reporting period; (14) The results for this state are combined with nearby states to protect confidentiality; Please refer to the User's Guide for a full explanation of data.

Measure	Cases	This Hosp.	State Avg.	U.S. Avg.
Admittance Decision Time (minutes)[5]	-	-	75	98
Head CT Results Within 45 Min. of Arrival[5]	-	-	61%	57%
Patients Who Left ER Before Being Seen[5]	-	-	1%	2%
Time from ER Arrival to Admit. (minutes)[5]	-	-	207	274
Time from ER Arrival to Discharge (minutes)[5]	-	-	118	134
Time in ER Before Being Evaluated (minutes)[5]	-	-	21	26
Time to Pain Meds for Fractures (minutes)[5]	-	-	42	57
Heart Attack Care				
Aspirin Given at Discharge[3,7]	-	-	100%	99%
Fibrinolytic Meds Within 30 Min. of Arrival[3,7]	-	-	-	54%
PCI Within 90 Minutes of Arrival[3,7]	-	-	96%	96%
Statin Prescribed at Discharge[3,7]	-	-	99%	98%
Heart Failure Care				
ACE Inhibitor or ARB for LVSD[1]	-	-	96%	97%
Discharge Instructions Given	13	100%	93%	94%
Evaluation of LVS Function	16	100%	98%	99%
Medicare Spending				
Medicare Spending per Patient (ratio)	-	-	0.97	0.98
Pneumonia Care				
Appropriate Initial Antibiotic Given	30	97%	95%	95%
Blood Culture Timing[1]	-	-	99%	98%
Pregnancy and Delivery Care				
Newborn Deliveries Scheduled Early[5]	-	-	5%	6%
Preventive Care				
Immunization for Influenza[5]	-	-	89%	90%
Immunization for Pneumonia[5]	-	-	90%	92%
Stroke Care				
Anticoagulation Therapy for Atrial Fibrillation[5]	-	-	95%	95%
Antithrombotic Therapy Timing[5]	-	-	99%	98%
Assessed for Rehabilitation[5]	-	-	99%	97%
Discharged on Antithrombotic Therapy[5]	-	-	100%	99%
Discharged on Statin Medication[5]	-	-	93%	94%
Thrombolytic Therapy Timing[5]	-	-	75%	66%
Venous Thromboembolism Prophylaxis[5]	-	-	94%	94%
Written Stroke Educational Materials Given[5]	-	-	84%	88%
Surgical Care Improvement Project				
Appropriate Beta Blocker Usage	19	100%	98%	98%
Appropriate VTP Within 24 Hours	39	95%	99%	98%
Controlled Postoperative Blood Glucose[7]	-	-	96%	97%
Perioperative Temperature Management	45	100%	100%	100%
Prophylactic Antibiotic Selection	40	100%	99%	99%
Prophylactic Antibiotic Selection (Outpatient)[1,3]	-	-	99%	98%
Prophylactic Antibiotic Stopped	40	100%	98%	98%
Prophylactic Antibiotic Timing	40	100%	98%	99%
Prophylactic Antibiotic Timing (Outpatient)[1,3]	-	-	97%	98%
Urinary Catheter Removal	28	100%	98%	97%
Survey of Patients' Hospital Experiences				
Area Around Room 'Always' Quiet at Night	(a)	61%	67%	61%
Doctors 'Always' Communicated Well	(a)	84%	86%	82%
Home Recovery Information Given	(a)	91%	88%	85%
Hospital Given 9 or 10 on 10 Point Scale	(a)	75%	78%	71%
Meds 'Always' Explained Before Given	(a)	70%	68%	64%
Nurses 'Always' Communicated Well	(a)	78%	83%	79%
Pain 'Always' Well Controlled	(a)	75%	73%	71%
Room and Bathroom 'Always' Clean	(a)	73%	81%	73%
Timely Help 'Always' Received	(a)	71%	75%	68%
Would Definitely Recommend Hospital	(a)	72%	77%	71%
Use of Medical Imaging				
Cardiac Imaging Stress Test before Surgery	46	4.3%	5.4%	5.3%
Combination Abdominal CT Scan	74	8.1%	9.3%	10.5%
Combination Brain/Sinus CT Scan[1]	-	-	2.7%	2.7%
Combination Chest CT Scan	60	3.3%	1.7%	2.7%
Follow-up Mammogram/Ultrasound	239	11.7%	8%	8.8%
Lumbar Spine MRI for Low Back Pain[1]	-	-	36.5%	37.2%

Bryan Medical Center

1600 South 48th St
Lincoln, NE 68506
Phone: 402-481-1111
Fax: 402-481-8306
URL: www.bryan.org
Type: Acute Care Hospitals
Emergency Services: Yes
Ownership: Voluntary non-profit - Private
Beds: 316

Key Personnel:
Quality Assurance .... Debbie Fisher
Radiology.................... Sharon Harms
Infection Control.................. Larry Krebsbach
Anesthesiology................ Elizabeth Lau, MD
Operating Room.............. Charles Meyer
Emergency Room .... Ed Mlinek, MD
Chief of Medical Staff........... Kevin Mota, MD
CEO/President............. John Woodrich

Measure	Cases	This Hosp.	State Avg.	U.S. Avg.
Blood Clot Prevention and Treatment				
Anticoagulation Overlap Therapy[2]	95	98%	93%	93%
ICU Venous Thromboembolism Prophylaxis[2]	70	97%	91%	92%
Incidence of Potentially Preventable VTE[2]	12	8%	11%	10%
UFH with Dosages/Platelet Monitoring[2]	36	97%	98%	97%
Venous Thromboembolism Prophylaxis[2]	288	91%	88%	85%
Warfarin Therapy Discharge Instructions[2]	70	80%	81%	75%
Chest Pain/Possible Heart Attack Care				
Aspirin Given Within 24 Hours of Arrival[3,7]	-	-	96%	96%
Fibrinolytic Meds Within 30 Min. of Arrival[5]	-	-	53%	58%
Average Time to ECG (minutes)[3,7]	-	-	8	7
Average Time to Transfer (minutes)[5]	-	-	76	60
Children's Asthma Care				
Received Home Management Plan of Care	-	-	-	88%
Received Reliever Medication	-	-	-	100%
Received Systemic Corticosteroids	-	-	-	100%
Emergency Department				
Admittance Decision Time (minutes)[2]	342	69	75	98
Head CT Results Within 45 Min. of Arrival[1]	-	-	61%	57%
Patients Who Left ER Before Being Seen	71,640	0%	1%	2%
Time from ER Arrival to Admit. (minutes)[2]	352	196	207	274
Time from ER Arrival to Discharge (minutes)	342	94	118	134
Time in ER Before Being Evaluated (minutes)	329	36	21	26
Time to Pain Meds for Fractures (minutes)	216	41	42	57
Heart Attack Care				
Aspirin Given at Discharge	447	100%	100%	99%
Fibrinolytic Meds Within 30 Min. of Arrival[7]	-	-	-	54%
PCI Within 90 Minutes of Arrival	47	98%	96%	96%
Statin Prescribed at Discharge	431	100%	99%	98%
Heart Failure Care				
ACE Inhibitor or ARB for LVSD	117	100%	96%	97%
Discharge Instructions Given	299	94%	93%	94%
Evaluation of LVS Function	391	100%	98%	99%
Medicare Spending				
Medicare Spending per Patient (ratio)	-	1.02	0.97	0.98
Pneumonia Care				
Appropriate Initial Antibiotic Given[2]	94	97%	95%	95%
Blood Culture Timing[2]	159	98%	99%	98%
Pregnancy and Delivery Care				
Newborn Deliveries Scheduled Early[2]	50	2%	5%	6%
Preventive Care				
Immunization for Influenza[2]	534	95%	89%	90%
Immunization for Pneumonia[2]	529	95%	90%	92%
Stroke Care				
Anticoagulation Therapy for Atrial Fibrillation	45	100%	95%	95%
Antithrombotic Therapy Timing	167	99%	99%	98%
Assessed for Rehabilitation	221	100%	99%	97%
Discharged on Antithrombotic Therapy	194	100%	100%	99%
Discharged on Statin Medication	142	97%	93%	94%
Thrombolytic Therapy Timing[1]	-	-	75%	66%
Venous Thromboembolism Prophylaxis	212	98%	94%	94%
Written Stroke Educational Materials Given	91	91%	84%	88%
Surgical Care Improvement Project				
Appropriate Beta Blocker Usage[2]	411	99%	98%	98%
Appropriate VTP Within 24 Hours[2]	583	97%	99%	98%
Controlled Postoperative Blood Glucose[2]	251	98%	96%	97%
Perioperative Temperature Management[2]	802	100%	100%	100%
Prophylactic Antibiotic Selection[2]	643	99%	99%	99%
Prophylactic Antibiotic Selection (Outpatient)	808	99%	99%	98%
Prophylactic Antibiotic Stopped[2]	600	97%	98%	98%
Prophylactic Antibiotic Timing[2]	645	98%	98%	99%
Prophylactic Antibiotic Timing (Outpatient)	813	98%	97%	98%
Urinary Catheter Removal[2]	456	94%	98%	97%
Survey of Patients' Hospital Experiences				
Area Around Room 'Always' Quiet at Night	300+	65%	67%	61%
Doctors 'Always' Communicated Well	300+	80%	86%	82%
Home Recovery Information Given	300+	91%	88%	85%
Hospital Given 9 or 10 on 10 Point Scale	300+	77%	78%	71%
Meds 'Always' Explained Before Given	300+	65%	68%	64%
Nurses 'Always' Communicated Well	300+	79%	83%	79%
Pain 'Always' Well Controlled	300+	71%	73%	71%
Room and Bathroom 'Always' Clean	300+	71%	81%	73%
Timely Help 'Always' Received	300+	67%	75%	68%
Would Definitely Recommend Hospital	300+	78%	77%	71%
Use of Medical Imaging				
Cardiac Imaging Stress Test before Surgery	1,052	4.9%	5.4%	5.3%
Combination Abdominal CT Scan	1,285	7.1%	9.3%	10.5%
Combination Brain/Sinus CT Scan	1,428	3.4%	2.7%	2.7%
Combination Chest CT Scan	812	4.1%	1.7%	2.7%
Follow-up Mammogram/Ultrasound	2,938	7.9%	8%	8.8%
Lumbar Spine MRI for Low Back Pain	108	31.5%	36.5%	37.2%

Lincoln Surgical Hospital

1710 South 70th St, Suite 200
Phone: 402-484-9090
Lincoln, NE 68506
URL: www.lincolnsurgery.com
Type: Acute Care Hospitals
Emergency Services: No
Ownership: Proprietary

Key Personnel:
Anesthesiology............... Stephanie L. Barry, M.D.
CEO .... Rob Linafelter

Measure	Cases	This Hosp.	State Avg.	U.S. Avg.
Blood Clot Prevention and Treatment				
Anticoagulation Overlap Therapy[2,7]	-	-	93%	93%
ICU Venous Thromboembolism Prophylaxis[2,7]	-	-	91%	92%
Incidence of Potentially Preventable VTE[2,7]	-	-	11%	10%
UFH with Dosages/Platelet Monitoring[2,7]	-	-	98%	97%
Venous Thromboembolism Prophylaxis[2]	17	100%	88%	85%
Warfarin Therapy Discharge Instructions[2,7]	-	-	81%	75%
Chest Pain/Possible Heart Attack Care				
Aspirin Given Within 24 Hours of Arrival[5]	-	-	96%	96%
Fibrinolytic Meds Within 30 Min. of Arrival[5]	-	-	53%	58%
Average Time to ECG (minutes)[5]	-	-	8	7
Average Time to Transfer (minutes)[5]	-	-	76	60
Children's Asthma Care				
Received Home Management Plan of Care	-	-	-	88%
Received Reliever Medication	-	-	-	100%
Received Systemic Corticosteroids	-	-	-	100%
Emergency Department				
Admittance Decision Time (minutes)[7]	-	-	75	98
Head CT Results Within 45 Min. of Arrival[5]	-	-	61%	57%
Patients Who Left ER Before Being Seen[5]	-	-	1%	2%
Time from ER Arrival to Admit. (minutes)[7]	-	-	207	274
Time from ER Arrival to Discharge (minutes)[5]	-	-	118	134
Time in ER Before Being Evaluated (minutes)[5]	-	-	21	26
Time to Pain Meds for Fractures (minutes)[5]	-	-	42	57
Heart Attack Care				
Aspirin Given at Discharge[5]	-	-	100%	99%
Fibrinolytic Meds Within 30 Min. of Arrival[5]	-	-	-	54%
PCI Within 90 Minutes of Arrival[5]	-	-	96%	96%
Statin Prescribed at Discharge[5]	-	-	99%	98%
Heart Failure Care				
ACE Inhibitor or ARB for LVSD[5]	-	-	96%	97%
Discharge Instructions Given[5]	-	-	93%	94%
Evaluation of LVS Function[5]	-	-	98%	99%
Medicare Spending				
Medicare Spending per Patient (ratio)	-	0.91	0.97	0.98
Pneumonia Care				
Appropriate Initial Antibiotic Given[5]	-	-	95%	95%
Blood Culture Timing[5]	-	-	99%	98%
Pregnancy and Delivery Care				
Newborn Deliveries Scheduled Early[7]	-	-	5%	6%
Preventive Care				
Immunization for Influenza[2]	439	93%	89%	90%
Immunization for Pneumonia[2]	525	89%	90%	92%
Stroke Care				
Anticoagulation Therapy for Atrial Fibrillation[5]	-	-	95%	95%
Antithrombotic Therapy Timing[5]	-	-	99%	98%
Assessed for Rehabilitation[5]	-	-	99%	97%

NOTE: Hospital profiles are in alphabetical order by state, then city, then hospital within the city; Rankings exclude hospitals with less than 25 cases except for patient surveys which excludes hospitals with less than 100 cases; (a) 100-299 cases; (1) The number of cases/patients is too few to report; (2) Data submitted were based on a sample of cases/patients; (3) Results are based on a shorter time period than required; (4) Data suppressed by CMS for one or more quarters; (5) Results are not available for this reporting period; (6) Fewer than 100 patients completed the HCAHPS survey; (7) No cases met the criteria for this measure; (8) The lower limit of the confidence interval cannot be calculated if the number of observed infections equals zero; (9) No data are available from the state/territory for this reporting period; (10) The scores shown reflect fewer than 50 completed surveys; (11) There were discrepancies in the data collection process; (12) This measure does not apply to this hospital for this reporting period; (13) Results cannot be calculated for this reporting period; (14) The results for this state are combined with nearby states to protect confidentiality; Please refer to the User's Guide for a full explanation of data.

Measure	Cases	This Hosp.	State Avg.	U.S. Avg.
Discharged on Antithrombotic Therapy[5]	-	-	100%	99%
Discharged on Statin Medication[5]	-	-	93%	94%
Thrombolytic Therapy Timing[5]	-	-	75%	66%
Venous Thromboembolism Prophylaxis[5]	-	-	94%	94%
Written Stroke Educational Materials Given[5]	-	-	84%	88%
Surgical Care Improvement Project				
Appropriate Beta Blocker Usage[2]	49	100%	98%	98%
Appropriate VTP Within 24 Hours[2]	235	100%	99%	98%
Controlled Postoperative Blood Glucose[2,7]	-	-	96%	97%
Perioperative Temperature Management[2]	240	99%	100%	100%
Prophylactic Antibiotic Selection[2]	179	100%	99%	99%
Prophylactic Antibiotic Selection (Outpatient)	186	99%	99%	98%
Prophylactic Antibiotic Stopped[2]	179	100%	98%	98%
Prophylactic Antibiotic Timing[2]	179	99%	98%	99%
Prophylactic Antibiotic Timing (Outpatient)	188	99%	97%	98%
Urinary Catheter Removal[2]	151	99%	98%	97%
Survey of Patients' Hospital Experiences				
Area Around Room 'Always' Quiet at Night	300+	74%	67%	61%
Doctors 'Always' Communicated Well	300+	88%	86%	82%
Home Recovery Information Given	300+	95%	88%	85%
Hospital Given 9 or 10 on 10 Point Scale	300+	85%	78%	71%
Meds 'Always' Explained Before Given	300+	76%	68%	64%
Nurses 'Always' Communicated Well	300+	86%	83%	79%
Pain 'Always' Well Controlled	300+	76%	73%	71%
Room and Bathroom 'Always' Clean	300+	86%	81%	73%
Timely Help 'Always' Received	300+	81%	75%	68%
Would Definitely Recommend Hospital	300+	86%	77%	71%
Use of Medical Imaging				
Cardiac Imaging Stress Test before Surgery[7]	-	-	5.4%	5.3%
Combination Abdominal CT Scan[7]	-	-	9.3%	10.5%
Combination Brain/Sinus CT Scan[7]	-	-	2.7%	2.7%
Combination Chest CT Scan[7]	-	-	1.7%	2.7%
Follow-up Mammogram/Ultrasound[7]	-	-	8%	8.8%
Lumbar Spine MRI for Low Back Pain[7]	-	-	36.5%	37.2%

Nebraska Heart Hospital

7500 South 91st St
Lincoln, NE 68526
Phone: 402-328-3000
Fax: 402-328-3010
URL: www.neheart.com
Type: Acute Care Hospitals
Ownership: Proprietary
Emergency Services: No
Beds: 54

Key Personnel:

Cardiology . . . . Stephen J. Ackerman, MD
Surgery . . . . Michael Bibler, MD
Anesthesiology. . . . . Erick J. Crimminns, MD
CEO/President. . . . . Sheryl D Dodds

Measure	Cases	This Hosp.	State Avg.	U.S. Avg.
Blood Clot Prevention and Treatment				
Anticoagulation Overlap Therapy[1]	-	-	93%	93%
ICU Venous Thromboembolism Prophylaxis	504	88%	91%	92%
Incidence of Potentially Preventable VTE[1]	-	-	11%	10%
UFH with Dosages/Platelet Monitoring[1]	-	-	98%	97%
Venous Thromboembolism Prophylaxis	560	79%	88%	85%
Warfarin Therapy Discharge Instructions[1]	-	-	81%	75%
Chest Pain/Possible Heart Attack Care				
Aspirin Given Within 24 Hours of Arrival[5]	-	-	96%	96%
Fibrinolytic Meds Within 30 Min. of Arrival[5]	-	-	53%	58%
Average Time to ECG (minutes)[5]	-	-	8	7
Average Time to Transfer (minutes)[5]	-	-	76	60
Children's Asthma Care				
Received Home Management Plan of Care	-	-	-	88%
Received Reliever Medication	-	-	-	100%
Received Systemic Corticosteroids	-	-	-	100%
Emergency Department				
Admittance Decision Time (minutes)[2,7]	-	-	75	98
Head CT Results Within 45 Min. of Arrival[5]	-	-	61%	57%
Patients Who Left ER Before Being Seen[5]	-	-	1%	2%
Time from ER Arrival to Admit. (minutes)[2,7]	-	-	207	274
Time from ER Arrival to Discharge (minutes)[5]	-	-	118	134
Time in ER Before Being Evaluated (minutes)[5]	-	-	21	26
Time to Pain Meds for Fractures (minutes)[5]	-	-	42	57
Heart Attack Care				
Aspirin Given at Discharge	279	99%	100%	99%
Fibrinolytic Meds Within 30 Min. of Arrival[7]	-	-	-	54%
PCI Within 90 Minutes of Arrival[1]	-	-	96%	96%
Statin Prescribed at Discharge	266	99%	99%	98%
Heart Failure Care				
ACE Inhibitor or ARB for LVSD	130	95%	96%	97%
Discharge Instructions Given	204	85%	93%	94%
Evaluation of LVS Function	245	100%	98%	99%
Medicare Spending				
Medicare Spending per Patient (ratio)	-	0.98	0.97	0.98
Pneumonia Care				
Appropriate Initial Antibiotic Given[5]	-	-	95%	95%
Blood Culture Timing[5]	-	-	99%	98%
Pregnancy and Delivery Care				
Newborn Deliveries Scheduled Early[2,7]	-	-	5%	6%
Preventive Care				
Immunization for Influenza[2]	320	95%	89%	90%
Immunization for Pneumonia[2]	538	91%	90%	92%
Stroke Care				
Anticoagulation Therapy for Atrial Fibrillation[1]	-	-	95%	95%
Antithrombotic Therapy Timing[1]	-	-	99%	98%
Assessed for Rehabilitation[1]	-	-	99%	97%
Discharged on Antithrombotic Therapy[1]	-	-	100%	99%
Discharged on Statin Medication[1]	-	-	93%	94%
Thrombolytic Therapy Timing[7]	-	-	75%	66%
Venous Thromboembolism Prophylaxis[1]	-	-	94%	94%
Written Stroke Educational Materials Given[7]	-	-	84%	88%
Surgical Care Improvement Project				
Appropriate Beta Blocker Usage[2]	164	98%	98%	98%
Appropriate VTP Within 24 Hours[2]	17	88%	99%	98%
Controlled Postoperative Blood Glucose[2]	176	93%	96%	97%
Perioperative Temperature Management[2]	153	100%	100%	100%
Prophylactic Antibiotic Selection[2]	194	98%	99%	99%
Prophylactic Antibiotic Selection (Outpatient)	415	99%	99%	98%
Prophylactic Antibiotic Stopped[2]	190	90%	98%	98%
Prophylactic Antibiotic Timing[2]	195	100%	98%	99%
Prophylactic Antibiotic Timing (Outpatient)	420	88%	97%	98%
Urinary Catheter Removal[2]	213	93%	98%	97%
Survey of Patients' Hospital Experiences				
Area Around Room 'Always' Quiet at Night	300+	53%	67%	61%
Doctors 'Always' Communicated Well	300+	82%	86%	82%
Home Recovery Information Given	300+	92%	88%	85%
Hospital Given 9 or 10 on 10 Point Scale	300+	81%	78%	71%
Meds 'Always' Explained Before Given	300+	67%	68%	64%
Nurses 'Always' Communicated Well	300+	82%	83%	79%
Pain 'Always' Well Controlled	300+	76%	73%	71%
Room and Bathroom 'Always' Clean	300+	78%	81%	73%
Timely Help 'Always' Received	300+	76%	75%	68%
Would Definitely Recommend Hospital	300+	85%	77%	71%
Use of Medical Imaging				
Cardiac Imaging Stress Test before Surgery	913	4.8%	5.4%	5.3%
Combination Abdominal CT Scan[1]	-	-	9.3%	10.5%
Combination Brain/Sinus CT Scan[1]	-	-	2.7%	2.7%
Combination Chest CT Scan[1]	-	-	1.7%	2.7%
Follow-up Mammogram/Ultrasound[7]	-	-	8%	8.8%
Lumbar Spine MRI for Low Back Pain[7]	-	-	36.5%	37.2%

Saint Elizabeth Regional Medical Center

555 South 70th St
Lincoln, NE 68510
Phone: 402-219-7700
Fax: 402-219-7673
URL: www.stelizabethonline.com
Type: Acute Care Hospitals
Ownership: Voluntary non-profit - Private
Emergency Services: Yes
Beds: 197

Key Personnel:

Quality Assurance . . . . Lori Burkett, RN
Pediatric In-Patient Care . . . . . . Kurstin Friesen, MD
Operating Room. . . . . Nancy Gondringer, RN
Chief of Medical Staff. . . . . Greg Heidrick, MD
CEO/President. . . . . Robert J Lanik

Measure	Cases	This Hosp.	State Avg.	U.S. Avg.
Blood Clot Prevention and Treatment				
Anticoagulation Overlap Therapy[2]	61	100%	93%	93%
ICU Venous Thromboembolism Prophylaxis[2]	33	91%	91%	92%
Incidence of Potentially Preventable VTE[1,2]	-	-	11%	10%
UFH with Dosages/Platelet Monitoring[2]	15	93%	98%	97%
Venous Thromboembolism Prophylaxis[2]	331	90%	88%	85%
Warfarin Therapy Discharge Instructions[2]	40	85%	81%	75%
Chest Pain/Possible Heart Attack Care				
Aspirin Given Within 24 Hours of Arrival	22	100%	96%	96%
Fibrinolytic Meds Within 30 Min. of Arrival[3,7]	-	-	53%	58%
Average Time to ECG (minutes)	23	1	8	7
Average Time to Transfer (minutes)[3,7]	-	-	76	60
Children's Asthma Care				
Received Home Management Plan of Care	-	-	-	88%
Received Reliever Medication	-	-	-	100%
Received Systemic Corticosteroids	-	-	-	100%
Emergency Department				
Admittance Decision Time (minutes)[2]	218	108	75	98
Head CT Results Within 45 Min. of Arrival[1]	-	-	61%	57%
Patients Who Left ER Before Being Seen	32,875	1%	1%	2%
Time from ER Arrival to Admit. (minutes)[2]	398	242	207	274
Time from ER Arrival to Discharge (minutes)	576	149	118	134
Time in ER Before Being Evaluated (minutes)	531	27	21	26
Time to Pain Meds for Fractures (minutes)	141	48	42	57
Heart Attack Care				
Aspirin Given at Discharge	101	99%	100%	99%
Fibrinolytic Meds Within 30 Min. of Arrival[7]	-	-	-	54%
PCI Within 90 Minutes of Arrival	35	100%	96%	96%
Statin Prescribed at Discharge	94	98%	99%	98%
Heart Failure Care				
ACE Inhibitor or ARB for LVSD	43	98%	96%	97%
Discharge Instructions Given	148	94%	93%	94%
Evaluation of LVS Function	215	100%	98%	99%
Medicare Spending				
Medicare Spending per Patient (ratio)	-	1.00	0.97	0.98
Pneumonia Care				
Appropriate Initial Antibiotic Given[2]	77	97%	95%	95%
Blood Culture Timing[2]	120	98%	99%	98%
Pregnancy and Delivery Care				
Newborn Deliveries Scheduled Early[2]	26	15%	5%	6%
Preventive Care				
Immunization for Influenza[2]	536	95%	89%	90%
Immunization for Pneumonia[2]	574	97%	90%	92%
Stroke Care				
Anticoagulation Therapy for Atrial Fibrillation	17	94%	95%	95%
Antithrombotic Therapy Timing	91	100%	99%	98%
Assessed for Rehabilitation	113	100%	99%	97%
Discharged on Antithrombotic Therapy	105	100%	100%	99%
Discharged on Statin Medication	77	94%	93%	94%
Thrombolytic Therapy Timing[1]	-	-	75%	66%
Venous Thromboembolism Prophylaxis	104	99%	94%	94%
Written Stroke Educational Materials Given	60	93%	84%	88%
Surgical Care Improvement Project				
Appropriate Beta Blocker Usage[2]	113	98%	98%	98%
Appropriate VTP Within 24 Hours[2]	332	99%	99%	98%
Controlled Postoperative Blood Glucose[2,7]	-	-	96%	97%
Perioperative Temperature Management[2]	391	100%	100%	100%
Prophylactic Antibiotic Selection[2]	207	99%	99%	99%
Prophylactic Antibiotic Selection (Outpatient)	419	99%	99%	98%
Prophylactic Antibiotic Stopped[2]	206	99%	98%	98%
Prophylactic Antibiotic Timing[2]	207	100%	98%	99%
Prophylactic Antibiotic Timing (Outpatient)	420	99%	97%	98%
Urinary Catheter Removal[2]	217	96%	98%	97%
Survey of Patients' Hospital Experiences				
Area Around Room 'Always' Quiet at Night	300+	62%	67%	61%
Doctors 'Always' Communicated Well	300+	81%	86%	82%
Home Recovery Information Given	300+	90%	88%	85%
Hospital Given 9 or 10 on 10 Point Scale	300+	77%	78%	71%
Meds 'Always' Explained Before Given	300+	65%	68%	64%
Nurses 'Always' Communicated Well	300+	79%	83%	79%
Pain 'Always' Well Controlled	300+	71%	73%	71%
Room and Bathroom 'Always' Clean	300+	70%	81%	73%
Timely Help 'Always' Received	300+	59%	75%	68%
Would Definitely Recommend Hospital	300+	79%	77%	71%
Use of Medical Imaging				
Cardiac Imaging Stress Test before Surgery	287	4.5%	5.4%	5.3%

NOTE: Hospital profiles are in alphabetical order by state, then city, then hospital within the city; Rankings exclude hospitals with less than 25 cases except for patient surveys which excludes hospitals with less than 100 cases; (a) 100-299 cases; (1) The number of cases/patients is too few to report; (2) Data submitted were based on a sample of cases/patients; (3) Results are based on a shorter time period than required; (4) Data suppressed by CMS for one or more quarters; (5) Results are not available for this reporting period; (6) Fewer than 100 patients completed the HCAHPS survey; (7) No cases met the criteria for this measure; (8) The lower limit of the confidence interval cannot be calculated if the number of observed infections equals zero; (9) No data are available from the state/territory for this reporting period; (10) The scores shown reflect fewer than 50 completed surveys; (11) There were discrepancies in the data collection process; (12) This measure does not apply to this hospital for this reporting period; (13) Results cannot be calculated for this reporting period; (14) The results for this state are combined with nearby states to protect confidentiality; Please refer to the User's Guide for a full explanation of data.

Combination Abdominal CT Scan	891	5.1%	9.3%	10.5%
Combination Brain/Sinus CT Scan	688	1.7%	2.7%	2.7%
Combination Chest CT Scan	505	0.0%	1.7%	2.7%
Follow-up Mammogram/Ultrasound	1,905	13.1%	8%	8.8%
Lumbar Spine MRI for Low Back Pain	72	38.9%	36.5%	37.2%

Niobrara Valley Hospital

PO Box 118, 401 South 5th Street
Lynch, NE 68746
Phone: 402-569-2451
Fax: 402-569-2474
Type: Critical Access Hospitals
Emergency Services: Yes
Ownership: Voluntary non-profit - Private
Beds: 20

Key Personnel:
Quality Assurance . . . . Karlene Classen
Infection Control. . . . . Barb Hart, RN
CEO/President. . . . . Kelly Kalkowski
Operating Room. . . . . April Micanek, RN
Cardiology . . . . Ekanka Mukhopadhyay

Measure	Cases	This Hosp.	State Avg.	U.S. Avg.
Blood Clot Prevention and Treatment				
Anticoagulation Overlap Therapy[5]	-	-	93%	93%
ICU Venous Thromboembolism Prophylaxis[5]	-	-	91%	92%
Incidence of Potentially Preventable VTE[5]	-	-	11%	10%
UFH with Dosages/Platelet Monitoring[5]	-	-	98%	97%
Venous Thromboembolism Prophylaxis[5]	-	-	88%	85%
Warfarin Therapy Discharge Instructions[5]	-	-	81%	75%
Chest Pain/Possible Heart Attack Care				
Aspirin Given Within 24 Hours of Arrival[1,3]	-	-	96%	96%
Fibrinolytic Meds Within 30 Min. of Arrival[3,7]	-	-	53%	58%
Average Time to ECG (minutes)[1,3]	-	-	8	7
Average Time to Transfer (minutes)[3,7]	-	-	76	60
Children's Asthma Care				
Received Home Management Plan of Care	-	-	-	88%
Received Reliever Medication	-	-	-	100%
Received Systemic Corticosteroids	-	-	-	100%
Emergency Department				
Admittance Decision Time (minutes)[5]	-	-	75	98
Head CT Results Within 45 Min. of Arrival[5]	-	-	61%	57%
Patients Who Left ER Before Being Seen[5]	-	-	1%	2%
Time from ER Arrival to Admit. (minutes)[5]	-	-	207	274
Time from ER Arrival to Discharge (minutes)[5]	-	-	118	134
Time in ER Before Being Evaluated (minutes)[5]	-	-	21	26
Time to Pain Meds for Fractures (minutes)[5]	-	-	42	57
Heart Attack Care				
Aspirin Given at Discharge[5]	-	-	100%	99%
Fibrinolytic Meds Within 30 Min. of Arrival[5]	-	-	-	54%
PCI Within 90 Minutes of Arrival[5]	-	-	96%	96%
Statin Prescribed at Discharge[5]	-	-	99%	98%
Heart Failure Care				
ACE Inhibitor or ARB for LVSD[5]	-	-	96%	97%
Discharge Instructions Given[5]	-	-	93%	94%
Evaluation of LVS Function[5]	-	-	98%	99%
Medicare Spending				
Medicare Spending per Patient (ratio)	-	-	0.97	0.98
Pneumonia Care				
Appropriate Initial Antibiotic Given[3,7]	-	-	95%	95%
Blood Culture Timing[3,7]	-	-	99%	98%
Pregnancy and Delivery Care				
Newborn Deliveries Scheduled Early[5]	-	-	5%	6%
Preventive Care				
Immunization for Influenza[5]	-	-	89%	90%
Immunization for Pneumonia[5]	-	-	90%	92%
Stroke Care				
Anticoagulation Therapy for Atrial Fibrillation[5]	-	-	95%	95%
Antithrombotic Therapy Timing[5]	-	-	99%	98%
Assessed for Rehabilitation[5]	-	-	99%	97%
Discharged on Antithrombotic Therapy[5]	-	-	100%	99%
Discharged on Statin Medication[5]	-	-	93%	94%
Thrombolytic Therapy Timing[5]	-	-	75%	66%
Venous Thromboembolism Prophylaxis[5]	-	-	94%	94%
Written Stroke Educational Materials Given[5]	-	-	84%	88%
Surgical Care Improvement Project				
Appropriate Beta Blocker Usage[5]	-	-	98%	98%
Appropriate VTP Within 24 Hours[5]	-	-	99%	98%
Controlled Postoperative Blood Glucose[5]	-	-	96%	97%
Perioperative Temperature Management[5]	-	-	100%	100%
Prophylactic Antibiotic Selection[5]	-	-	99%	99%
Prophylactic Antibiotic Selection (Outpatient)[5]	-	-	99%	98%
Prophylactic Antibiotic Stopped[5]	-	-	98%	98%
Prophylactic Antibiotic Timing[5]	-	-	98%	99%
Prophylactic Antibiotic Timing (Outpatient)[5]	-	-	97%	98%
Urinary Catheter Removal[5]	-	-	98%	97%
Survey of Patients' Hospital Experiences				
Area Around Room 'Always' Quiet at Night[3,10]	<100	98%	67%	61%
Doctors 'Always' Communicated Well[3,10]	<100	100%	86%	82%
Home Recovery Information Given[3,10]	<100	83%	88%	85%
Hospital Given 9 or 10 on 10 Point Scale[3,10]	<100	86%	78%	71%
Meds 'Always' Explained Before Given[3,10]	<100	-	68%	64%
Nurses 'Always' Communicated Well[3,10]	<100	89%	83%	79%
Pain 'Always' Well Controlled[3,10]	<100	61%	73%	71%
Room and Bathroom 'Always' Clean[3,10]	<100	100%	81%	73%
Timely Help 'Always' Received[3,10]	<100	100%	75%	68%
Would Definitely Recommend Hospital[3,10]	<100	75%	77%	71%
Use of Medical Imaging				
Cardiac Imaging Stress Test before Surgery[7]	-	-	5.4%	5.3%
Combination Abdominal CT Scan[1]	-	-	9.3%	10.5%
Combination Brain/Sinus CT Scan[1]	-	-	2.7%	2.7%
Combination Chest CT Scan[1]	-	-	1.7%	2.7%
Follow-up Mammogram/Ultrasound[1]	-	-	8%	8.8%
Lumbar Spine MRI for Low Back Pain[1]	-	-	36.5%	37.2%

Community Hospital

PO Box 1328, 1301 East H St
Mccook, NE 69001
Phone: 308-344-2650
Fax: 308-344-8358
E-mail: communityhospital@chmccook.org
URL: www.chmccook.orgerson.com
Type: Critical Access Hospitals
Emergency Services: Yes
Ownership: Voluntary non-profit - Other
Beds: 25

Key Personnel:
Operating Room. . . . . Joseph C Baer
Coronary Care . . . . Michael Ball
Intensive Care Unit. . . . . Evelyn Bertram
Radiology. . . . . Roger E Brockman
Infection Control. . . . . Linda Robinson
Pediatric In-Patient Care . . . . Wilfredo Souchet, MD
CEO/President. . . . . James P Ulrich, Jr
Quality Assurance . . . . Natalie Webb

Measure	Cases	This Hosp.	State Avg.	U.S. Avg.
Blood Clot Prevention and Treatment				
Anticoagulation Overlap Therapy[5]	-	-	93%	93%
ICU Venous Thromboembolism Prophylaxis[5]	-	-	91%	92%
Incidence of Potentially Preventable VTE[5]	-	-	11%	10%
UFH with Dosages/Platelet Monitoring[5]	-	-	98%	97%
Venous Thromboembolism Prophylaxis[5]	-	-	88%	85%
Warfarin Therapy Discharge Instructions[5]	-	-	81%	75%
Chest Pain/Possible Heart Attack Care				
Aspirin Given Within 24 Hours of Arrival	33	94%	96%	96%
Fibrinolytic Meds Within 30 Min. of Arrival[1,3]	-	-	53%	58%
Average Time to ECG (minutes)	35	5	8	7
Average Time to Transfer (minutes)[1,3]	-	-	76	60
Children's Asthma Care				
Received Home Management Plan of Care	-	-	-	88%
Received Reliever Medication	-	-	-	100%
Received Systemic Corticosteroids	-	-	-	100%
Emergency Department				
Admittance Decision Time (minutes)[5]	-	-	75	98
Head CT Results Within 45 Min. of Arrival[5]	-	-	61%	57%
Patients Who Left ER Before Being Seen[5]	-	-	1%	2%
Time from ER Arrival to Admit. (minutes)[5]	-	-	207	274
Time from ER Arrival to Discharge (minutes)[5]	-	-	118	134
Time in ER Before Being Evaluated (minutes)[5]	-	-	21	26
Time to Pain Meds for Fractures (minutes)[5]	-	-	42	57
Heart Attack Care				
Aspirin Given at Discharge[3,7]	-	-	100%	99%
Fibrinolytic Meds Within 30 Min. of Arrival[3,7]	-	-	-	54%
PCI Within 90 Minutes of Arrival[3,7]	-	-	96%	96%
Statin Prescribed at Discharge[3,7]	-	-	99%	98%
Heart Failure Care				
ACE Inhibitor or ARB for LVSD[1]	-	-	96%	97%
Discharge Instructions Given	25	100%	93%	94%
Evaluation of LVS Function	31	100%	98%	99%
Medicare Spending				
Medicare Spending per Patient (ratio)	-	-	0.97	0.98
Pneumonia Care				
Appropriate Initial Antibiotic Given	18	83%	95%	95%
Blood Culture Timing	34	100%	99%	98%
Pregnancy and Delivery Care				
Newborn Deliveries Scheduled Early[5]	-	-	5%	6%
Preventive Care				
Immunization for Influenza[5]	-	-	89%	90%
Immunization for Pneumonia[5]	-	-	90%	92%
Stroke Care				
Anticoagulation Therapy for Atrial Fibrillation[5]	-	-	95%	95%
Antithrombotic Therapy Timing[5]	-	-	99%	98%
Assessed for Rehabilitation[5]	-	-	99%	97%
Discharged on Antithrombotic Therapy[5]	-	-	100%	99%
Discharged on Statin Medication[5]	-	-	93%	94%
Thrombolytic Therapy Timing[5]	-	-	75%	66%
Venous Thromboembolism Prophylaxis[5]	-	-	94%	94%
Written Stroke Educational Materials Given[5]	-	-	84%	88%
Surgical Care Improvement Project				
Appropriate Beta Blocker Usage	23	100%	98%	98%
Appropriate VTP Within 24 Hours	72	100%	99%	98%
Controlled Postoperative Blood Glucose[3,7]	-	-	96%	97%
Perioperative Temperature Management	79	100%	100%	100%
Prophylactic Antibiotic Selection	62	100%	99%	99%
Prophylactic Antibiotic Selection (Outpatient)[1,3]	-	-	99%	98%
Prophylactic Antibiotic Stopped	62	98%	98%	98%
Prophylactic Antibiotic Timing	62	100%	98%	99%
Prophylactic Antibiotic Timing (Outpatient)[1,3]	-	-	97%	98%
Urinary Catheter Removal	32	100%	98%	97%
Survey of Patients' Hospital Experiences				
Area Around Room 'Always' Quiet at Night	(a)	71%	67%	61%
Doctors 'Always' Communicated Well	(a)	89%	86%	82%
Home Recovery Information Given	(a)	88%	88%	85%
Hospital Given 9 or 10 on 10 Point Scale	(a)	78%	78%	71%
Meds 'Always' Explained Before Given	(a)	70%	68%	64%
Nurses 'Always' Communicated Well	(a)	83%	83%	79%
Pain 'Always' Well Controlled	(a)	70%	73%	71%
Room and Bathroom 'Always' Clean	(a)	84%	81%	73%
Timely Help 'Always' Received	(a)	73%	75%	68%
Would Definitely Recommend Hospital	(a)	76%	77%	71%
Use of Medical Imaging				
Cardiac Imaging Stress Test before Surgery	169	6.5%	5.4%	5.3%
Combination Abdominal CT Scan	204	16.2%	9.3%	10.5%
Combination Brain/Sinus CT Scan[1]	-	-	2.7%	2.7%
Combination Chest CT Scan	196	9.7%	1.7%	2.7%
Follow-up Mammogram/Ultrasound	131	15.3%	8%	8.8%
Lumbar Spine MRI for Low Back Pain	43	37.2%	36.5%	37.2%

Kearney County Health Services Hospital

727 East 1st St
Minden, NE 68959
Phone: 308-832-3400
Fax: 308-832-3417
URL: www.kchs.org
Type: Critical Access Hospitals
Emergency Services: Yes
Ownership: Government - Local
Beds: 25

Key Personnel:
Emergency Room . . . . Mary Bunger
Radiology. . . . . Shelly Hawthorne
Quality Assurance . . . . Connie Jorgensen
CEO/President. . . . . Fred Meis
Chief of Medical Staff. . . . . Eddie Pierce, MD

Measure	Cases	This Hosp.	State Avg.	U.S. Avg.
Blood Clot Prevention and Treatment				
Anticoagulation Overlap Therapy[5]	-	-	93%	93%
ICU Venous Thromboembolism Prophylaxis[5]	-	-	91%	92%
Incidence of Potentially Preventable VTE[5]	-	-	11%	10%
UFH with Dosages/Platelet Monitoring[5]	-	-	98%	97%
Venous Thromboembolism Prophylaxis[5]	-	-	88%	85%
Warfarin Therapy Discharge Instructions[5]	-	-	81%	75%
Chest Pain/Possible Heart Attack Care				

NOTE: Hospital profiles are in alphabetical order by state, then city, then hospital within the city; Rankings exclude hospitals with less than 25 cases except for patient surveys which excludes hospitals with less than 100 cases; (a) 100-299 cases; (1) The number of cases/patients is too few to report; (2) Data submitted were based on a sample of cases/patients; (3) Results are based on a shorter time period than required; (4) Data suppressed by CMS for one or more quarters; (5) Results are not available for this reporting period; (6) Fewer than 100 patients completed the HCAHPS survey; (7) No cases met the criteria for this measure; (8) The lower limit of the confidence interval cannot be calculated if the number of observed infections equals zero; (9) No data are available from the state/territory for this reporting period; (10) The scores shown reflect fewer than 50 completed surveys; (11) There were discrepancies in the data collection process; (12) This measure does not apply to this hospital for this reporting period; (13) Results cannot be calculated for this reporting period; (14) The results for this state are combined with nearby states to protect confidentiality; Please refer to the User's Guide for a full explanation of data.

Measure	Cases	This Hosp.	State Avg.	U.S. Avg.
Aspirin Given Within 24 Hours of Arrival[5]	-	-	96%	96%
Fibrinolytic Meds Within 30 Min. of Arrival[5]	-	-	53%	58%
Average Time to ECG (minutes)[5]	-	-	8	7
Average Time to Transfer (minutes)[5]	-	-	76	60
Children's Asthma Care				
Received Home Management Plan of Care	-	-	-	88%
Received Reliever Medication	-	-	-	100%
Received Systemic Corticosteroids	-	-	-	100%
Emergency Department				
Admittance Decision Time (minutes)[5]	-	-	75	98
Head CT Results Within 45 Min. of Arrival[5]	-	-	61%	57%
Patients Who Left ER Before Being Seen[5]	-	-	1%	2%
Time from ER Arrival to Admit. (minutes)[5]	-	-	207	274
Time from ER Arrival to Discharge (minutes)[5]	-	-	118	134
Time in ER Before Being Evaluated (minutes)[5]	-	-	21	26
Time to Pain Meds for Fractures (minutes)[5]	-	-	42	57
Heart Attack Care				
Aspirin Given at Discharge[1,3]	-	-	100%	99%
Fibrinolytic Meds Within 30 Min. of Arrival[3,7]	-	-	-	54%
PCI Within 90 Minutes of Arrival[3,7]	-	-	96%	96%
Statin Prescribed at Discharge[3,7]	-	-	99%	98%
Heart Failure Care				
ACE Inhibitor or ARB for LVSD[1,3]	-	-	96%	97%
Discharge Instructions Given[1,3]	-	-	93%	94%
Evaluation of LVS Function[1,3]	-	-	98%	99%
Medicare Spending				
Medicare Spending per Patient (ratio)	-	-	0.97	0.98
Pneumonia Care				
Appropriate Initial Antibiotic Given[1]	-	-	95%	95%
Blood Culture Timing[1]	-	-	99%	98%
Pregnancy and Delivery Care				
Newborn Deliveries Scheduled Early[5]	-	-	5%	6%
Preventive Care				
Immunization for Influenza[5]	-	-	89%	90%
Immunization for Pneumonia[5]	-	-	90%	92%
Stroke Care				
Anticoagulation Therapy for Atrial Fibrillation[5]	-	-	95%	95%
Antithrombotic Therapy Timing[5]	-	-	99%	98%
Assessed for Rehabilitation[5]	-	-	99%	97%
Discharged on Antithrombotic Therapy[5]	-	-	100%	99%
Discharged on Statin Medication[5]	-	-	93%	94%
Thrombolytic Therapy Timing[5]	-	-	75%	66%
Venous Thromboembolism Prophylaxis[5]	-	-	94%	94%
Written Stroke Educational Materials Given[5]	-	-	84%	88%
Surgical Care Improvement Project				
Appropriate Beta Blocker Usage[5]	-	-	98%	98%
Appropriate VTP Within 24 Hours[5]	-	-	99%	98%
Controlled Postoperative Blood Glucose[5]	-	-	96%	97%
Perioperative Temperature Management[5]	-	-	100%	100%
Prophylactic Antibiotic Selection[5]	-	-	99%	99%
Prophylactic Antibiotic Selection (Outpatient)[5]	-	-	99%	98%
Prophylactic Antibiotic Stopped[5]	-	-	98%	98%
Prophylactic Antibiotic Timing[5]	-	-	98%	99%
Prophylactic Antibiotic Timing (Outpatient)[5]	-	-	97%	98%
Urinary Catheter Removal[5]	-	-	98%	97%
Survey of Patients' Hospital Experiences				
Area Around Room 'Always' Quiet at Night[10]	<100	83%	67%	61%
Doctors 'Always' Communicated Well[10]	<100	87%	86%	82%
Home Recovery Information Given[10]	<100	95%	88%	85%
Hospital Given 9 or 10 on 10 Point Scale[10]	<100	76%	78%	71%
Meds 'Always' Explained Before Given[10]	<100	59%	68%	64%
Nurses 'Always' Communicated Well[10]	<100	79%	83%	79%
Pain 'Always' Well Controlled[10]	<100	76%	73%	71%
Room and Bathroom 'Always' Clean[10]	<100	92%	81%	73%
Timely Help 'Always' Received[10]	<100	82%	75%	68%
Would Definitely Recommend Hospital[10]	<100	77%	77%	71%
Use of Medical Imaging				
Cardiac Imaging Stress Test before Surgery[1]	-	-	5.4%	5.3%
Combination Abdominal CT Scan[1]	-	-	9.3%	10.5%
Combination Brain/Sinus CT Scan[1]	-	-	2.7%	2.7%
Combination Chest CT Scan[1]	-	-	1.7%	2.7%
Follow-up Mammogram/Ultrasound	94	5.3%	8%	8.8%
Lumbar Spine MRI for Low Back Pain[7]	-	-	36.5%	37.2%

Saint Mary's Community Hospital

1314 3rd Ave
Nebraska City, NE 68410
Phone: 402-873-3321
Fax: 402-873-9033
URL: www.stmaryshospitalnecity.com
Type: Critical Access Hospitals
Emergency Services: Yes
Ownership: Voluntary non-profit - Church
Beds: 18

Key Personnel:
Radiology. . . . . Curtis R Burhoop
CEO . . . . Daniel Kelly
Operating Room. . . . . Tamela Osborn, RN
Infection Control . . . . Charisse Spitzer, RN
Quality Assurance . . . . Charisse Spitzer, RN
Chief of Medical Staff. . . . . Dr Jonathan Stelling

Measure	Cases	This Hosp.	State Avg.	U.S. Avg.
Blood Clot Prevention and Treatment				
Anticoagulation Overlap Therapy[5]	-	-	93%	93%
ICU Venous Thromboembolism Prophylaxis[5]	-	-	91%	92%
Incidence of Potentially Preventable VTE[5]	-	-	11%	10%
UFH with Dosages/Platelet Monitoring[5]	-	-	98%	97%
Venous Thromboembolism Prophylaxis[5]	-	-	88%	85%
Warfarin Therapy Discharge Instructions[5]	-	-	81%	75%
Chest Pain/Possible Heart Attack Care				
Aspirin Given Within 24 Hours of Arrival	12	100%	96%	96%
Fibrinolytic Meds Within 30 Min. of Arrival[1]	-	-	53%	58%
Average Time to ECG (minutes)	12	11	8	7
Average Time to Transfer (minutes)[7]	-	-	76	60
Children's Asthma Care				
Received Home Management Plan of Care	-	-	-	88%
Received Reliever Medication	-	-	-	100%
Received Systemic Corticosteroids	-	-	-	100%
Emergency Department				
Admittance Decision Time (minutes)[5]	-	-	75	98
Head CT Results Within 45 Min. of Arrival[1,3]	-	-	61%	57%
Patients Who Left ER Before Being Seen[5]	-	-	1%	2%
Time from ER Arrival to Admit. (minutes)[5]	-	-	207	274
Time from ER Arrival to Discharge (minutes)[3]	80	76	118	134
Time in ER Before Being Evaluated (minutes)[3]	94	6	21	26
Time to Pain Meds for Fractures (minutes)[5]	-	-	42	57
Heart Attack Care				
Aspirin Given at Discharge[1,3]	-	-	100%	99%
Fibrinolytic Meds Within 30 Min. of Arrival[3,7]	-	-	-	54%
PCI Within 90 Minutes of Arrival[3,7]	-	-	96%	96%
Statin Prescribed at Discharge[1,3]	-	-	99%	98%
Heart Failure Care				
ACE Inhibitor or ARB for LVSD[7]	-	-	96%	97%
Discharge Instructions Given[1]	-	-	93%	94%
Evaluation of LVS Function[1]	-	-	98%	99%
Medicare Spending				
Medicare Spending per Patient (ratio)	-	-	0.97	0.98
Pneumonia Care				
Appropriate Initial Antibiotic Given	14	100%	95%	95%
Blood Culture Timing[1]	-	-	99%	98%
Pregnancy and Delivery Care				
Newborn Deliveries Scheduled Early[5]	-	-	5%	6%
Preventive Care				
Immunization for Influenza[5]	-	-	89%	90%
Immunization for Pneumonia[5]	-	-	90%	92%
Stroke Care				
Anticoagulation Therapy for Atrial Fibrillation[5]	-	-	95%	95%
Antithrombotic Therapy Timing[5]	-	-	99%	98%
Assessed for Rehabilitation[5]	-	-	99%	97%
Discharged on Antithrombotic Therapy[5]	-	-	100%	99%
Discharged on Statin Medication[5]	-	-	93%	94%
Thrombolytic Therapy Timing[5]	-	-	75%	66%
Venous Thromboembolism Prophylaxis[5]	-	-	94%	94%
Written Stroke Educational Materials Given[5]	-	-	84%	88%
Surgical Care Improvement Project				
Appropriate Beta Blocker Usage[1]	-	-	98%	98%
Appropriate VTP Within 24 Hours	21	90%	99%	98%
Controlled Postoperative Blood Glucose[7]	-	-	96%	97%
Perioperative Temperature Management	21	100%	100%	100%
Prophylactic Antibiotic Selection	17	100%	99%	99%
Prophylactic Antibiotic Selection (Outpatient)[1,3]	-	-	99%	98%
Prophylactic Antibiotic Stopped	14	93%	98%	98%
Prophylactic Antibiotic Timing	17	94%	98%	99%
Prophylactic Antibiotic Timing (Outpatient)[1,3]	-	-	97%	98%
Urinary Catheter Removal	20	100%	98%	97%
Survey of Patients' Hospital Experiences				
Area Around Room 'Always' Quiet at Night[5]	-	-	67%	61%
Doctors 'Always' Communicated Well[5]	-	-	86%	82%
Home Recovery Information Given[5]	-	-	88%	85%
Hospital Given 9 or 10 on 10 Point Scale[5]	-	-	78%	71%
Meds 'Always' Explained Before Given[5]	-	-	68%	64%
Nurses 'Always' Communicated Well[5]	-	-	83%	79%
Pain 'Always' Well Controlled[5]	-	-	73%	71%
Room and Bathroom 'Always' Clean[5]	-	-	81%	73%
Timely Help 'Always' Received[5]	-	-	75%	68%
Would Definitely Recommend Hospital[5]	-	-	77%	71%
Use of Medical Imaging				
Cardiac Imaging Stress Test before Surgery	95	2.1%	5.4%	5.3%
Combination Abdominal CT Scan	103	5.8%	9.3%	10.5%
Combination Brain/Sinus CT Scan[1]	-	-	2.7%	2.7%
Combination Chest CT Scan	98	2.0%	1.7%	2.7%
Follow-up Mammogram/Ultrasound	250	10.4%	8%	8.8%
Lumbar Spine MRI for Low Back Pain[1]	-	-	36.5%	37.2%

Antelope Memorial Hospital

PO Box 229, 102 West 9th St
Neligh, NE 68756
Phone: 402-887-4151
Fax: 402-887-4092
URL: www.amhne.org
Type: Critical Access Hospitals
Emergency Services: Yes
Ownership: Voluntary non-profit - Private
Beds: 20

Key Personnel:
Pulmonology . . . . Francois Abi Fadel, MD
Anesthesiology. . . . . Jennifer Anson, CRNA
Radiology. . . . . Philip Eckstrom, MD
CEO/President. . . . . Jack Greene
Cardiology . . . . Maryanne Hartzell, MD

Measure	Cases	This Hosp.	State Avg.	U.S. Avg.
Blood Clot Prevention and Treatment				
Anticoagulation Overlap Therapy[5]	-	-	93%	93%
ICU Venous Thromboembolism Prophylaxis[5]	-	-	91%	92%
Incidence of Potentially Preventable VTE[5]	-	-	11%	10%
UFH with Dosages/Platelet Monitoring[5]	-	-	98%	97%
Venous Thromboembolism Prophylaxis[5]	-	-	88%	85%
Warfarin Therapy Discharge Instructions[5]	-	-	81%	75%
Chest Pain/Possible Heart Attack Care				
Aspirin Given Within 24 Hours of Arrival[1,3]	-	-	96%	96%
Fibrinolytic Meds Within 30 Min. of Arrival[1,3]	-	-	53%	58%
Average Time to ECG (minutes)[1,3]	-	-	8	7
Average Time to Transfer (minutes)[3,7]	-	-	76	60
Children's Asthma Care				
Received Home Management Plan of Care	-	-	-	88%
Received Reliever Medication	-	-	-	100%
Received Systemic Corticosteroids	-	-	-	100%
Emergency Department				
Admittance Decision Time (minutes)[5]	-	-	75	98
Head CT Results Within 45 Min. of Arrival[5]	-	-	61%	57%
Patients Who Left ER Before Being Seen[5]	-	-	1%	2%
Time from ER Arrival to Admit. (minutes)[5]	-	-	207	274
Time from ER Arrival to Discharge (minutes)[5]	-	-	118	134
Time in ER Before Being Evaluated (minutes)[5]	-	-	21	26
Time to Pain Meds for Fractures (minutes)[5]	-	-	42	57
Heart Attack Care				
Aspirin Given at Discharge[5]	-	-	100%	99%
Fibrinolytic Meds Within 30 Min. of Arrival[5]	-	-	-	54%
PCI Within 90 Minutes of Arrival[5]	-	-	96%	96%
Statin Prescribed at Discharge[5]	-	-	99%	98%
Heart Failure Care				
ACE Inhibitor or ARB for LVSD[1,3]	-	-	96%	97%
Discharge Instructions Given[1,3]	-	-	93%	94%
Evaluation of LVS Function[1,3]	-	-	98%	99%
Medicare Spending				
Medicare Spending per Patient (ratio)	-	-	0.97	0.98
Pneumonia Care				

NOTE: *Hospital profiles are in alphabetical order by state, then city, then hospital within the city; Rankings exclude hospitals with less than 25 cases except for patient surveys which excludes hospitals with less than 100 cases; (a) 100-299 cases; (1) The number of cases/patients is too few to report; (2) Data submitted were based on a sample of cases/patients; (3) Results are based on a shorter time period than required; (4) Data suppressed by CMS for one or more quarters; (5) Results are not available for this reporting period; (6) Fewer than 100 patients completed the HCAHPS survey; (7) No cases met the criteria for this measure; (8) The lower limit of the confidence interval cannot be calculated if the number of observed infections equals zero; (9) No data are available from the state/territory for this reporting period; (10) The scores shown reflect fewer than 50 completed surveys; (11) There were discrepancies in the data collection process; (12) This measure does not apply to this hospital for this reporting period; (13) Results cannot be calculated for this reporting period; (14) The results for this state are combined with nearby states to protect confidentiality; Please refer to the User's Guide for a full explanation of data.*

Measure	Cases	This Hosp.	State Avg.	U.S. Avg.
Appropriate Initial Antibiotic Given[1]	-	-	95%	95%
Blood Culture Timing[1]	-	-	99%	98%
Pregnancy and Delivery Care				
Newborn Deliveries Scheduled Early[5]	-	-	5%	6%
Preventive Care				
Immunization for Influenza[5]	-	-	89%	90%
Immunization for Pneumonia[5]	-	-	90%	92%
Stroke Care				
Anticoagulation Therapy for Atrial Fibrillation[5]	-	-	95%	95%
Antithrombotic Therapy Timing[5]	-	-	99%	98%
Assessed for Rehabilitation[5]	-	-	99%	97%
Discharged on Antithrombotic Therapy[5]	-	-	100%	99%
Discharged on Statin Medication[5]	-	-	93%	94%
Thrombolytic Therapy Timing[5]	-	-	75%	66%
Venous Thromboembolism Prophylaxis[5]	-	-	94%	94%
Written Stroke Educational Materials Given[5]	-	-	84%	88%
Surgical Care Improvement Project				
Appropriate Beta Blocker Usage[5]	-	-	98%	98%
Appropriate VTP Within 24 Hours[5]	-	-	99%	98%
Controlled Postoperative Blood Glucose[5]	-	-	96%	97%
Perioperative Temperature Management[5]	-	-	100%	100%
Prophylactic Antibiotic Selection[5]	-	-	99%	99%
Prophylactic Antibiotic Selection (Outpatient)[3,7]	-	-	99%	98%
Prophylactic Antibiotic Stopped[5]	-	-	98%	98%
Prophylactic Antibiotic Timing[5]	-	-	98%	99%
Prophylactic Antibiotic Timing (Outpatient)[1,3]	-	-	97%	98%
Urinary Catheter Removal[5]	-	-	98%	97%
Survey of Patients' Hospital Experiences				
Area Around Room 'Always' Quiet at Night[6]	<100	61%	67%	61%
Doctors 'Always' Communicated Well[6]	<100	83%	86%	82%
Home Recovery Information Given[6]	<100	92%	88%	85%
Hospital Given 9 or 10 on 10 Point Scale[6]	<100	80%	78%	71%
Meds 'Always' Explained Before Given[6]	<100	59%	68%	64%
Nurses 'Always' Communicated Well[6]	<100	88%	83%	79%
Pain 'Always' Well Controlled[6]	<100	73%	73%	71%
Room and Bathroom 'Always' Clean[6]	<100	79%	81%	73%
Timely Help 'Always' Received[6]	<100	78%	75%	68%
Would Definitely Recommend Hospital[6]	<100	78%	77%	71%
Use of Medical Imaging				
Cardiac Imaging Stress Test before Surgery	60	6.7%	5.4%	5.3%
Combination Abdominal CT Scan	79	68.4%	9.3%	10.5%
Combination Brain/Sinus CT Scan[1]	-	-	2.7%	2.7%
Combination Chest CT Scan	91	1.1%	1.7%	2.7%
Follow-up Mammogram/Ultrasound	158	4.4%	8%	8.8%
Lumbar Spine MRI for Low Back Pain[1]	-	-	36.5%	37.2%

Faith Regional Health Services

2700 West Norfolk Ave
Norfolk, NE 68701
Phone: 402-371-4880
Fax: 402-644-7324
URL: www.frhs.org
Type: Acute Care Hospitals
Emergency Services: Yes
Ownership: Voluntary non-profit - Private
Beds: 166

Key Personnel:
Chief of Medical Staff.......... Tim Davy
Intensive Care Unit............ Brenda Hokamp, RN
Infection Control............... Laura Hoogestradt
CEO/President................ Mark Klosterman
Quality Assurance .... Mary Meyer
Operating Room............... Mick Pick
Radiology....................... Brian Vonk
Hemotology Center .... Jan With

Measure	Cases	This Hosp.	State Avg.	U.S. Avg.
Blood Clot Prevention and Treatment				
Anticoagulation Overlap Therapy[2]	39	87%	93%	93%
ICU Venous Thromboembolism Prophylaxis[2]	71	96%	91%	92%
Incidence of Potentially Preventable VTE[1,2]	-	-	11%	10%
UFH with Dosages/Platelet Monitoring[2]	17	29%	98%	97%
Venous Thromboembolism Prophylaxis[2]	285	87%	88%	85%
Warfarin Therapy Discharge Instructions[2]	25	20%	81%	75%
Chest Pain/Possible Heart Attack Care				
Aspirin Given Within 24 Hours of Arrival[5]	-	-	96%	96%
Fibrinolytic Meds Within 30 Min. of Arrival[5]	-	-	53%	58%
Average Time to ECG (minutes)[5]	-	-	8	7
Average Time to Transfer (minutes)[5]	-	-	76	60
Children's Asthma Care				
Received Home Management Plan of Care	-	-	-	88%
Received Reliever Medication	-	-	-	100%
Received Systemic Corticosteroids	-	-	-	100%
Emergency Department				
Admittance Decision Time (minutes)[2]	268	57	75	98
Head CT Results Within 45 Min. of Arrival[1]	-	-	61%	57%
Patients Who Left ER Before Being Seen	11,713	1%	1%	2%
Time from ER Arrival to Admit. (minutes)[2]	288	188	207	274
Time from ER Arrival to Discharge (minutes)	409	125	118	134
Time in ER Before Being Evaluated (minutes)	453	21	21	26
Time to Pain Meds for Fractures (minutes)	80	46	42	57
Heart Attack Care				
Aspirin Given at Discharge	108	100%	100%	99%
Fibrinolytic Meds Within 30 Min. of Arrival[7]	-	-	-	54%
PCI Within 90 Minutes of Arrival	13	85%	96%	96%
Statin Prescribed at Discharge	109	99%	99%	98%
Heart Failure Care				
ACE Inhibitor or ARB for LVSD	34	94%	96%	97%
Discharge Instructions Given	63	98%	93%	94%
Evaluation of LVS Function	113	97%	98%	99%
Medicare Spending				
Medicare Spending per Patient (ratio)	-	1.03	0.97	0.98
Pneumonia Care				
Appropriate Initial Antibiotic Given	48	100%	95%	95%
Blood Culture Timing	113	100%	99%	98%
Pregnancy and Delivery Care				
Newborn Deliveries Scheduled Early[2]	34	0%	5%	6%
Preventive Care				
Immunization for Influenza[2]	510	95%	89%	90%
Immunization for Pneumonia[2]	517	94%	90%	92%
Stroke Care				
Anticoagulation Therapy for Atrial Fibrillation[1]	-	-	95%	95%
Antithrombotic Therapy Timing	29	100%	99%	98%
Assessed for Rehabilitation	33	97%	99%	97%
Discharged on Antithrombotic Therapy	31	100%	100%	99%
Discharged on Statin Medication	29	86%	93%	94%
Thrombolytic Therapy Timing[1]	-	-	75%	66%
Venous Thromboembolism Prophylaxis	32	100%	94%	94%
Written Stroke Educational Materials Given	13	69%	84%	88%
Surgical Care Improvement Project				
Appropriate Beta Blocker Usage	284	100%	98%	98%
Appropriate VTP Within 24 Hours	459	100%	99%	98%
Controlled Postoperative Blood Glucose	76	97%	96%	97%
Perioperative Temperature Management	531	100%	100%	100%
Prophylactic Antibiotic Selection	460	100%	99%	99%
Prophylactic Antibiotic Selection (Outpatient)	233	100%	99%	98%
Prophylactic Antibiotic Stopped	446	99%	98%	98%
Prophylactic Antibiotic Timing	460	100%	98%	99%
Prophylactic Antibiotic Timing (Outpatient)	226	100%	97%	98%
Urinary Catheter Removal	446	100%	98%	97%
Survey of Patients' Hospital Experiences				
Area Around Room 'Always' Quiet at Night	300+	67%	67%	61%
Doctors 'Always' Communicated Well	300+	81%	86%	82%
Home Recovery Information Given	300+	89%	88%	85%
Hospital Given 9 or 10 on 10 Point Scale	300+	70%	78%	71%
Meds 'Always' Explained Before Given	300+	57%	68%	64%
Nurses 'Always' Communicated Well	300+	79%	83%	79%
Pain 'Always' Well Controlled	300+	68%	73%	71%
Room and Bathroom 'Always' Clean	300+	75%	81%	73%
Timely Help 'Always' Received	300+	62%	75%	68%
Would Definitely Recommend Hospital	300+	67%	77%	71%
Use of Medical Imaging				
Cardiac Imaging Stress Test before Surgery	443	5.9%	5.4%	5.3%
Combination Abdominal CT Scan	565	65.0%	9.3%	10.5%
Combination Brain/Sinus CT Scan	419	1.7%	2.7%	2.7%
Combination Chest CT Scan	693	1.6%	1.7%	2.7%
Follow-up Mammogram/Ultrasound	804	9.1%	8%	8.8%
Lumbar Spine MRI for Low Back Pain	84	31.0%	36.5%	37.2%

Great Plains Regional Medical Center

601 West Leota St
North Platte, NE 69101
Phone: 308-696-8000
Fax: 308-535-3410
Type: Acute Care Hospitals
Emergency Services: Yes
Ownership: Voluntary non-profit - Private
Beds: 116

Key Personnel:
CEO/President.............. Lucinda A Bradley
Radiology.................... Douglas Child
Operating Room.............. Margaret Emme
Pediatric In-Patient Care .... Lisa Kosmarek
CEO .... Paul Kumpf
Infection Control............... Teresa Mowak
Chief of Medical Staff .... Clint Schafer, MD
Quality Assurance .... Pam Sweeney

Measure	Cases	This Hosp.	State Avg.	U.S. Avg.
Blood Clot Prevention and Treatment				
Anticoagulation Overlap Therapy[2]	49	82%	93%	93%
ICU Venous Thromboembolism Prophylaxis[2]	60	70%	91%	92%
Incidence of Potentially Preventable VTE[1,2]	-	-	11%	10%
UFH with Dosages/Platelet Monitoring[2]	19	100%	98%	97%
Venous Thromboembolism Prophylaxis[2]	330	68%	88%	85%
Warfarin Therapy Discharge Instructions[2]	34	97%	81%	75%
Chest Pain/Possible Heart Attack Care				
Aspirin Given Within 24 Hours of Arrival	15	93%	96%	96%
Fibrinolytic Meds Within 30 Min. of Arrival[7]	-	-	53%	58%
Average Time to ECG (minutes)	15	11	8	7
Average Time to Transfer (minutes)[7]	-	-	76	60
Children's Asthma Care				
Received Home Management Plan of Care	-	-	-	88%
Received Reliever Medication	-	-	-	100%
Received Systemic Corticosteroids	-	-	-	100%
Emergency Department				
Admittance Decision Time (minutes)[2]	474	85	75	98
Head CT Results Within 45 Min. of Arrival[1]	-	-	61%	57%
Patients Who Left ER Before Being Seen	18,217	0%	1%	2%
Time from ER Arrival to Admit. (minutes)[2]	495	233	207	274
Time from ER Arrival to Discharge (minutes)	374	120	118	134
Time in ER Before Being Evaluated (minutes)	421	15	21	26
Time to Pain Meds for Fractures (minutes)	61	36	42	57
Heart Attack Care				
Aspirin Given at Discharge	82	99%	100%	99%
Fibrinolytic Meds Within 30 Min. of Arrival[7]	-	-	-	54%
PCI Within 90 Minutes of Arrival	21	95%	96%	96%
Statin Prescribed at Discharge	82	100%	99%	98%
Heart Failure Care				
ACE Inhibitor or ARB for LVSD	34	94%	96%	97%
Discharge Instructions Given	95	96%	93%	94%
Evaluation of LVS Function	126	100%	98%	99%
Medicare Spending				
Medicare Spending per Patient (ratio)	-	0.96	0.97	0.98
Pneumonia Care				
Appropriate Initial Antibiotic Given[2]	97	97%	95%	95%
Blood Culture Timing[2]	170	99%	99%	98%
Pregnancy and Delivery Care				
Newborn Deliveries Scheduled Early	58	22%	5%	6%
Preventive Care				
Immunization for Influenza[2]	435	94%	89%	90%
Immunization for Pneumonia[2]	555	93%	90%	92%
Stroke Care				
Anticoagulation Therapy for Atrial Fibrillation[1]	-	-	95%	95%
Antithrombotic Therapy Timing	45	98%	99%	98%
Assessed for Rehabilitation	46	96%	99%	97%
Discharged on Antithrombotic Therapy	45	100%	100%	99%
Discharged on Statin Medication	39	97%	93%	94%
Thrombolytic Therapy Timing[1]	-	-	75%	66%
Venous Thromboembolism Prophylaxis	48	92%	94%	94%
Written Stroke Educational Materials Given	23	83%	84%	88%
Surgical Care Improvement Project				
Appropriate Beta Blocker Usage	112	98%	98%	98%
Appropriate VTP Within 24 Hours	272	99%	99%	98%
Controlled Postoperative Blood Glucose[7]	-	-	96%	97%
Perioperative Temperature Management	299	100%	100%	100%
Prophylactic Antibiotic Selection	207	100%	99%	99%
Prophylactic Antibiotic Selection (Outpatient)	164	95%	99%	98%

NOTE: Hospital profiles are in alphabetical order by state, then city, then hospital within the city; Rankings exclude hospitals with less than 25 cases except for patient surveys which excludes hospitals with less than 100 cases; (a) 100-299 cases; (1) The number of cases/patients is too few to report; (2) Data submitted were based on a sample of cases/patients; (3) Results are based on a shorter time period than required; (4) Data suppressed by CMS for one or more quarters; (5) Results are not available for this reporting period; (6) Fewer than 100 patients completed the HCAHPS survey; (7) No cases met the criteria for this measure; (8) The lower limit of the confidence interval cannot be calculated if the number of observed infections equals zero; (9) No data are available from the state/territory for this reporting period; (10) The scores shown reflect fewer than 50 completed surveys; (11) There were discrepancies in the data collection process; (12) This measure does not apply to this hospital for this reporting period; (13) Results cannot be calculated for this reporting period; (14) The results for this state are combined with nearby states to protect confidentiality; Please refer to the User's Guide for a full explanation of data.

Measure	Cases	This Hosp.	State Avg.	U.S. Avg.
Prophylactic Antibiotic Stopped	200	96%	98%	98%
Prophylactic Antibiotic Timing	207	100%	98%	99%
Prophylactic Antibiotic Timing (Outpatient)	165	97%	97%	98%
Urinary Catheter Removal	241	100%	98%	97%
Survey of Patients' Hospital Experiences				
Area Around Room 'Always' Quiet at Night	300+	51%	67%	61%
Doctors 'Always' Communicated Well	300+	81%	86%	82%
Home Recovery Information Given	300+	90%	88%	85%
Hospital Given 9 or 10 on 10 Point Scale	300+	61%	78%	71%
Meds 'Always' Explained Before Given	300+	61%	68%	64%
Nurses 'Always' Communicated Well	300+	76%	83%	79%
Pain 'Always' Well Controlled	300+	69%	73%	71%
Room and Bathroom 'Always' Clean	300+	63%	81%	73%
Timely Help 'Always' Received	300+	65%	75%	68%
Would Definitely Recommend Hospital	300+	66%	77%	71%
Use of Medical Imaging				
Cardiac Imaging Stress Test before Surgery	393	7.4%	5.4%	5.3%
Combination Abdominal CT Scan	706	8.8%	9.3%	10.5%
Combination Brain/Sinus CT Scan[1]	-	-	2.7%	2.7%
Combination Chest CT Scan	520	1.0%	1.7%	2.7%
Follow-up Mammogram/Ultrasound	995	12.2%	8%	8.8%
Lumbar Spine MRI for Low Back Pain	200	31.5%	36.5%	37.2%

Avera Saint Anthony's Hospital

300 North 2nd St
O' Neill, NE 68763
Phone: 402-336-2611
Fax: 402-336-5145
URL: www.avera-sta.org
Type: Critical Access Hospitals
Emergency Services: Yes
Ownership: Voluntary non-profit - Church
Beds: 25

Key Personnel:
CEO/President . . . . Ronald J Cork
Quality Assurance . . . . Maureen Haggerty, RN
Operating Room . . . . Vicky Harvey, RN
Radiology . . . . Lawrence Leon
Emergency Room . . . . Mark J Ptacek, MD
Chief of Medical Staff . . . . Robi Singh, MD
Ambulatory Care . . . . Wendell Spencer
Infection Control . . . . Val Wecker, RN

Measure	Cases	This Hosp.	State Avg.	U.S. Avg.
Blood Clot Prevention and Treatment				
Anticoagulation Overlap Therapy[5]	-	-	93%	93%
ICU Venous Thromboembolism Prophylaxis[5]	-	-	91%	92%
Incidence of Potentially Preventable VTE[5]	-	-	11%	10%
UFH with Dosages/Platelet Monitoring[5]	-	-	98%	97%
Venous Thromboembolism Prophylaxis[5]	-	-	88%	85%
Warfarin Therapy Discharge Instructions[5]	-	-	81%	75%
Chest Pain/Possible Heart Attack Care				
Aspirin Given Within 24 Hours of Arrival	15	80%	96%	96%
Fibrinolytic Meds Within 30 Min. of Arrival[3,7]	-	-	53%	58%
Average Time to ECG (minutes)	14	12	8	7
Average Time to Transfer (minutes)[1,3]	-	-	76	60
Children's Asthma Care				
Received Home Management Plan of Care	-	-	-	88%
Received Reliever Medication	-	-	-	100%
Received Systemic Corticosteroids	-	-	-	100%
Emergency Department				
Admittance Decision Time (minutes)[5]	-	-	75	98
Head CT Results Within 45 Min. of Arrival[5]	-	-	61%	57%
Patients Who Left ER Before Being Seen[5]	-	-	1%	2%
Time from ER Arrival to Admit. (minutes)[5]	-	-	207	274
Time from ER Arrival to Discharge (minutes)[5]	-	-	118	134
Time in ER Before Being Evaluated (minutes)[5]	-	-	21	26
Time to Pain Meds for Fractures (minutes)[5]	-	-	42	57
Heart Attack Care				
Aspirin Given at Discharge[1,3]	-	-	100%	99%
Fibrinolytic Meds Within 30 Min. of Arrival[3,7]	-	-	-	54%
PCI Within 90 Minutes of Arrival[3,7]	-	-	96%	96%
Statin Prescribed at Discharge[3,7]	-	-	99%	98%
Heart Failure Care				
ACE Inhibitor or ARB for LVSD[1]	-	-	96%	97%
Discharge Instructions Given[1]	-	-	93%	94%
Evaluation of LVS Function	17	65%	98%	99%
Medicare Spending				
Medicare Spending per Patient (ratio)	-	-	0.97	0.98
Pneumonia Care				
Appropriate Initial Antibiotic Given	26	92%	95%	95%
Blood Culture Timing[1]	-	-	99%	98%
Pregnancy and Delivery Care				
Newborn Deliveries Scheduled Early[5]	-	-	5%	6%
Preventive Care				
Immunization for Influenza[5]	-	-	89%	90%
Immunization for Pneumonia[5]	-	-	90%	92%
Stroke Care				
Anticoagulation Therapy for Atrial Fibrillation[5]	-	-	95%	95%
Antithrombotic Therapy Timing[5]	-	-	99%	98%
Assessed for Rehabilitation[5]	-	-	99%	97%
Discharged on Antithrombotic Therapy[5]	-	-	100%	99%
Discharged on Statin Medication[5]	-	-	93%	94%
Thrombolytic Therapy Timing[5]	-	-	75%	66%
Venous Thromboembolism Prophylaxis[5]	-	-	94%	94%
Written Stroke Educational Materials Given[5]	-	-	84%	88%
Surgical Care Improvement Project				
Appropriate Beta Blocker Usage[1]	-	-	98%	98%
Appropriate VTP Within 24 Hours	38	97%	99%	98%
Controlled Postoperative Blood Glucose[7]	-	-	96%	97%
Perioperative Temperature Management	40	100%	100%	100%
Prophylactic Antibiotic Selection	37	97%	99%	99%
Prophylactic Antibiotic Selection (Outpatient)[5]	-	-	99%	98%
Prophylactic Antibiotic Stopped	37	97%	98%	98%
Prophylactic Antibiotic Timing	37	97%	98%	99%
Prophylactic Antibiotic Timing (Outpatient)[5]	-	-	97%	98%
Urinary Catheter Removal	37	100%	98%	97%
Survey of Patients' Hospital Experiences				
Area Around Room 'Always' Quiet at Night	(a)	75%	67%	61%
Doctors 'Always' Communicated Well	(a)	88%	86%	82%
Home Recovery Information Given	(a)	93%	88%	85%
Hospital Given 9 or 10 on 10 Point Scale	(a)	87%	78%	71%
Meds 'Always' Explained Before Given	(a)	73%	68%	64%
Nurses 'Always' Communicated Well	(a)	87%	83%	79%
Pain 'Always' Well Controlled	(a)	79%	73%	71%
Room and Bathroom 'Always' Clean	(a)	77%	81%	73%
Timely Help 'Always' Received	(a)	73%	75%	68%
Would Definitely Recommend Hospital	(a)	86%	77%	71%
Use of Medical Imaging				
Cardiac Imaging Stress Test before Surgery	121	6.6%	5.4%	5.3%
Combination Abdominal CT Scan	168	9.5%	9.3%	10.5%
Combination Brain/Sinus CT Scan[1]	-	-	2.7%	2.7%
Combination Chest CT Scan	110	5.5%	1.7%	2.7%
Follow-up Mammogram/Ultrasound	254	8.3%	8%	8.8%
Lumbar Spine MRI for Low Back Pain[1]	-	-	36.5%	37.2%

Oakland Mercy Hospital

601 East Second St
Oakland, NE 68045
Phone: 402-685-5601
Fax: 402-685-6223
URL: www.oaklandhospital.org
Type: Critical Access Hospitals
Emergency Services: Yes
Ownership: Voluntary non-profit - Church
Beds: 17

Key Personnel:
Infection Control . . . . Mary Fran Bacon
Quality Assurance . . . . Roy Blomquist
CEO/President . . . . Tim Fischer
Chief of Medical Staff . . . . Tracy Martin
Emergency Room . . . . GE Petersons

Measure	Cases	This Hosp.	State Avg.	U.S. Avg.
Blood Clot Prevention and Treatment				
Anticoagulation Overlap Therapy[5]	-	-	93%	93%
ICU Venous Thromboembolism Prophylaxis[5]	-	-	91%	92%
Incidence of Potentially Preventable VTE[5]	-	-	11%	10%
UFH with Dosages/Platelet Monitoring[5]	-	-	98%	97%
Venous Thromboembolism Prophylaxis[5]	-	-	88%	85%
Warfarin Therapy Discharge Instructions[5]	-	-	81%	75%
Chest Pain/Possible Heart Attack Care				
Aspirin Given Within 24 Hours of Arrival[1]	-	-	96%	96%
Fibrinolytic Meds Within 30 Min. of Arrival[1,3]	-	-	53%	58%
Average Time to ECG (minutes)[1]	-	-	8	7
Average Time to Transfer (minutes)[3,7]	-	-	76	60
Children's Asthma Care				
Received Home Management Plan of Care	-	-	-	88%
Received Reliever Medication	-	-	-	100%
Received Systemic Corticosteroids	-	-	-	100%
Emergency Department				
Admittance Decision Time (minutes)[5]	-	-	75	98
Head CT Results Within 45 Min. of Arrival[5]	-	-	61%	57%
Patients Who Left ER Before Being Seen[5]	-	-	1%	2%
Time from ER Arrival to Admit. (minutes)[5]	-	-	207	274
Time from ER Arrival to Discharge (minutes)[5]	-	-	118	134
Time in ER Before Being Evaluated (minutes)[5]	-	-	21	26
Time to Pain Meds for Fractures (minutes)[5]	-	-	42	57
Heart Attack Care				
Aspirin Given at Discharge[5]	-	-	100%	99%
Fibrinolytic Meds Within 30 Min. of Arrival[5]	-	-	-	54%
PCI Within 90 Minutes of Arrival[5]	-	-	96%	96%
Statin Prescribed at Discharge[5]	-	-	99%	98%
Heart Failure Care				
ACE Inhibitor or ARB for LVSD[1,3]	-	-	96%	97%
Discharge Instructions Given[1,3]	-	-	93%	94%
Evaluation of LVS Function[1,3]	-	-	98%	99%
Medicare Spending				
Medicare Spending per Patient (ratio)	-	-	0.97	0.98
Pneumonia Care				
Appropriate Initial Antibiotic Given[1]	-	-	95%	95%
Blood Culture Timing[1]	-	-	99%	98%
Pregnancy and Delivery Care				
Newborn Deliveries Scheduled Early[5]	-	-	5%	6%
Preventive Care				
Immunization for Influenza[5]	-	-	89%	90%
Immunization for Pneumonia[5]	-	-	90%	92%
Stroke Care				
Anticoagulation Therapy for Atrial Fibrillation[5]	-	-	95%	95%
Antithrombotic Therapy Timing[5]	-	-	99%	98%
Assessed for Rehabilitation[5]	-	-	99%	97%
Discharged on Antithrombotic Therapy[5]	-	-	100%	99%
Discharged on Statin Medication[5]	-	-	93%	94%
Thrombolytic Therapy Timing[5]	-	-	75%	66%
Venous Thromboembolism Prophylaxis[5]	-	-	94%	94%
Written Stroke Educational Materials Given[5]	-	-	84%	88%
Surgical Care Improvement Project				
Appropriate Beta Blocker Usage[5]	-	-	98%	98%
Appropriate VTP Within 24 Hours[5]	-	-	99%	98%
Controlled Postoperative Blood Glucose[5]	-	-	96%	97%
Perioperative Temperature Management[5]	-	-	100%	100%
Prophylactic Antibiotic Selection[5]	-	-	99%	99%
Prophylactic Antibiotic Selection (Outpatient)[5]	-	-	99%	98%
Prophylactic Antibiotic Stopped[5]	-	-	98%	98%
Prophylactic Antibiotic Timing[5]	-	-	98%	99%
Prophylactic Antibiotic Timing (Outpatient)[5]	-	-	97%	98%
Urinary Catheter Removal[5]	-	-	98%	97%
Survey of Patients' Hospital Experiences				
Area Around Room 'Always' Quiet at Night[10]	<100	54%	67%	61%
Doctors 'Always' Communicated Well[10]	<100	73%	86%	82%
Home Recovery Information Given[10]	<100	67%	88%	85%
Hospital Given 9 or 10 on 10 Point Scale[10]	<100	57%	78%	71%
Meds 'Always' Explained Before Given[10]	<100	65%	68%	64%
Nurses 'Always' Communicated Well[10]	<100	72%	83%	79%
Pain 'Always' Well Controlled[10]	<100	61%	73%	71%
Room and Bathroom 'Always' Clean[10]	<100	63%	81%	73%
Timely Help 'Always' Received[10]	<100	69%	75%	68%
Would Definitely Recommend Hospital[10]	<100	75%	77%	71%
Use of Medical Imaging				
Cardiac Imaging Stress Test before Surgery[7]	-	-	5.4%	5.3%
Combination Abdominal CT Scan[1]	-	-	9.3%	10.5%
Combination Brain/Sinus CT Scan	44	0.0%	2.7%	2.7%
Combination Chest CT Scan[1]	-	-	1.7%	2.7%
Follow-up Mammogram/Ultrasound[1]	-	-	8%	8.8%
Lumbar Spine MRI for Low Back Pain[1]	-	-	36.5%	37.2%

NOTE: Hospital profiles are in alphabetical order by state, then city, then hospital within the city; Rankings exclude hospitals with less than 25 cases except for patient surveys which excludes hospitals with less than 100 cases; (a) 100-299 cases; (1) The number of cases/patients is too few to report; (2) Data submitted were based on a sample of cases/patients; (3) Results are based on a shorter time period than required; (4) Data suppressed by CMS for one or more quarters; (5) Results are not available for this reporting period; (6) Fewer than 100 patients completed the HCAHPS survey; (7) No cases met the criteria for this measure; (8) The lower limit of the confidence interval cannot be calculated if the number of observed infections equals zero; (9) No data are available from the state/territory for this reporting period; (10) The scores shown reflect fewer than 50 completed surveys; (11) There were discrepancies in the data collection process; (12) This measure does not apply to this hospital for this reporting period; (13) Results cannot be calculated for this reporting period; (14) The results for this state are combined with nearby states to protect confidentiality; Please refer to the User's Guide for a full explanation of data.

Ogallala Community Hospital

2601 North Spruce St
Ogallala, NE 69153
URL: www.bannerhealth.com
Type: Critical Access Hospitals
Ownership: Govt - Hospital Dist/Auth

Phone: 308-284-4011
Fax: 308-284-7262
Emergency Services: Yes
Beds: 18

Key Personnel:
Emergency Room . . . . Aric DeYoung
Quality Assurance . . . . Sue Hordessen
Anesthesiology. . . . . Michael Martinson
CEO/President. . . . . Margie Molitor
Infection Control. . . . . Stacy Olea
Operating Room. . . . . Kathy Vacura

Measure	Cases	This Hosp.	State Avg.	U.S. Avg.
Blood Clot Prevention and Treatment				
Anticoagulation Overlap Therapy[5]	-	-	93%	93%
ICU Venous Thromboembolism Prophylaxis[5]	-	-	91%	92%
Incidence of Potentially Preventable VTE[5]	-	-	11%	10%
UFH with Dosages/Platelet Monitoring[5]	-	-	98%	97%
Venous Thromboembolism Prophylaxis[5]	-	-	88%	85%
Warfarin Therapy Discharge Instructions[5]	-	-	81%	75%
Chest Pain/Possible Heart Attack Care				
Aspirin Given Within 24 Hours of Arrival	22	95%	96%	96%
Fibrinolytic Meds Within 30 Min. of Arrival[1]	-	-	53%	58%
Average Time to ECG (minutes)	23	6	8	7
Average Time to Transfer (minutes)[7]	-	-	76	60
Children's Asthma Care				
Received Home Management Plan of Care	-	-	-	88%
Received Reliever Medication	-	-	-	100%
Received Systemic Corticosteroids	-	-	-	100%
Emergency Department				
Admittance Decision Time (minutes)[5]	-	-	75	98
Head CT Results Within 45 Min. of Arrival[5]	-	-	61%	57%
Patients Who Left ER Before Being Seen	3,303	0%	1%	2%
Time from ER Arrival to Admit. (minutes)[5]	-	-	207	274
Time from ER Arrival to Discharge (minutes)[5]	-	-	118	134
Time in ER Before Being Evaluated (minutes)[5]	-	-	21	26
Time to Pain Meds for Fractures (minutes)[5]	-	-	42	57
Heart Attack Care				
Aspirin Given at Discharge[1]	-	-	100%	99%
Fibrinolytic Meds Within 30 Min. of Arrival[7]	-	-	-	54%
PCI Within 90 Minutes of Arrival[7]	-	-	96%	96%
Statin Prescribed at Discharge[1]	-	-	99%	98%
Heart Failure Care				
ACE Inhibitor or ARB for LVSD[1,2]	-	-	96%	97%
Discharge Instructions Given[2]	19	100%	93%	94%
Evaluation of LVS Function[2]	22	100%	98%	99%
Medicare Spending				
Medicare Spending per Patient (ratio)	-	-	0.97	0.98
Pneumonia Care				
Appropriate Initial Antibiotic Given	16	94%	95%	95%
Blood Culture Timing	15	93%	99%	98%
Pregnancy and Delivery Care				
Newborn Deliveries Scheduled Early[3,7]	-	-	5%	6%
Preventive Care				
Immunization for Influenza[5]	-	-	89%	90%
Immunization for Pneumonia[5]	-	-	90%	92%
Stroke Care				
Anticoagulation Therapy for Atrial Fibrillation[5]	-	-	95%	95%
Antithrombotic Therapy Timing[5]	-	-	99%	98%
Assessed for Rehabilitation[5]	-	-	99%	97%
Discharged on Antithrombotic Therapy[5]	-	-	100%	99%
Discharged on Statin Medication[5]	-	-	93%	94%
Thrombolytic Therapy Timing[5]	-	-	75%	66%
Venous Thromboembolism Prophylaxis[5]	-	-	94%	94%
Written Stroke Educational Materials Given[5]	-	-	84%	88%
Surgical Care Improvement Project				
Appropriate Beta Blocker Usage[1]	-	-	98%	98%
Appropriate VTP Within 24 Hours	15	100%	99%	98%
Controlled Postoperative Blood Glucose[7]	-	-	96%	97%
Perioperative Temperature Management	15	100%	100%	100%
Prophylactic Antibiotic Selection[1]	-	-	99%	99%
Prophylactic Antibiotic Selection (Outpatient)[1]	-	-	99%	98%
Prophylactic Antibiotic Stopped[1]	-	-	98%	98%
Prophylactic Antibiotic Timing[1]	-	-	98%	99%
Prophylactic Antibiotic Timing (Outpatient)[1]	-	-	97%	98%
Urinary Catheter Removal[1]	-	-	98%	97%
Survey of Patients' Hospital Experiences				
Area Around Room 'Always' Quiet at Night[11]	(a)	68%	67%	61%
Doctors 'Always' Communicated Well[11]	(a)	92%	86%	82%
Home Recovery Information Given[11]	(a)	94%	88%	85%
Hospital Given 9 or 10 on 10 Point Scale[11]	(a)	83%	78%	71%
Meds 'Always' Explained Before Given[11]	(a)	69%	68%	64%
Nurses 'Always' Communicated Well[11]	(a)	85%	83%	79%
Pain 'Always' Well Controlled[11]	(a)	82%	73%	71%
Room and Bathroom 'Always' Clean[11]	(a)	86%	81%	73%
Timely Help 'Always' Received[11]	(a)	74%	75%	68%
Would Definitely Recommend Hospital[11]	(a)	83%	77%	71%
Use of Medical Imaging				
Cardiac Imaging Stress Test before Surgery	66	4.5%	5.4%	5.3%
Combination Abdominal CT Scan	146	12.3%	9.3%	10.5%
Combination Brain/Sinus CT Scan[1]	-	-	2.7%	2.7%
Combination Chest CT Scan	71	0.0%	1.7%	2.7%
Follow-up Mammogram/Ultrasound	232	13.4%	8%	8.8%
Lumbar Spine MRI for Low Back Pain[1]	-	-	36.5%	37.2%

Alegent Creighton Health Bergan Mercy Medical Center

7500 Mercy Rd
Omaha, NE 68124
URL: www.alegent.com
Type: Acute Care Hospitals
Ownership: Voluntary non-profit - Private

Phone: 402-398-6060
Fax: 402-343-4316
Emergency Services: Yes
Beds: 400

Key Personnel:
Pediatric Ambulatory Care . . . . . . Shahab F Abdessalam, MD
Radiology. . . . . Kimberly A Apker, MD
CEO/President. . . . . Charles Brummund
Chief of Medical Staff. . . . . Joseph A Jarzobski
Operating Room. . . . . Joanne Kennebeck
Infection Control. . . . . Peggy Leubbert
Quality Assurance . . . . David Parks
Pediatric In-Patient Care . . . . Charles T Rush, MD

Measure	Cases	This Hosp.	State Avg.	U.S. Avg.
Blood Clot Prevention and Treatment				
Anticoagulation Overlap Therapy[2]	94	98%	93%	93%
ICU Venous Thromboembolism Prophylaxis[2]	56	98%	91%	92%
Incidence of Potentially Preventable VTE[2]	14	7%	11%	10%
UFH with Dosages/Platelet Monitoring[2]	95	99%	98%	97%
Venous Thromboembolism Prophylaxis[2]	252	93%	88%	85%
Warfarin Therapy Discharge Instructions[2]	71	89%	81%	75%
Chest Pain/Possible Heart Attack Care				
Aspirin Given Within 24 Hours of Arrival[5]	-	-	96%	96%
Fibrinolytic Meds Within 30 Min. of Arrival[5]	-	-	53%	58%
Average Time to ECG (minutes)[5]	-	-	8	7
Average Time to Transfer (minutes)[5]	-	-	76	60
Children's Asthma Care				
Received Home Management Plan of Care	-	-	-	88%
Received Reliever Medication	-	-	-	100%
Received Systemic Corticosteroids	-	-	-	100%
Emergency Department				
Admittance Decision Time (minutes)[2]	289	76	75	98
Head CT Results Within 45 Min. of Arrival[1,3]	-	-	61%	57%
Patients Who Left ER Before Being Seen	26,610	1%	1%	2%
Time from ER Arrival to Admit. (minutes)[2]	299	192	207	274
Time from ER Arrival to Discharge (minutes)	389	114	118	134
Time in ER Before Being Evaluated (minutes)	350	38	21	26
Time to Pain Meds for Fractures (minutes)	76	59	42	57
Heart Attack Care				
Aspirin Given at Discharge	210	100%	100%	99%
Fibrinolytic Meds Within 30 Min. of Arrival[7]	-	-	-	54%
PCI Within 90 Minutes of Arrival	25	100%	96%	96%
Statin Prescribed at Discharge	204	100%	99%	98%
Heart Failure Care				
ACE Inhibitor or ARB for LVSD	56	96%	96%	97%
Discharge Instructions Given	199	99%	93%	94%
Evaluation of LVS Function	276	100%	98%	99%
Medicare Spending				
Medicare Spending per Patient (ratio)	-	1.00	0.97	0.98
Pneumonia Care				
Appropriate Initial Antibiotic Given[2]	87	99%	95%	95%
Blood Culture Timing[2]	116	100%	99%	98%
Pregnancy and Delivery Care				
Newborn Deliveries Scheduled Early[2]	54	2%	5%	6%
Preventive Care				
Immunization for Influenza[2]	498	99%	89%	90%
Immunization for Pneumonia[2]	467	97%	90%	92%
Stroke Care				
Anticoagulation Therapy for Atrial Fibrillation	11	82%	95%	95%
Antithrombotic Therapy Timing	71	99%	99%	98%
Assessed for Rehabilitation	100	100%	99%	97%
Discharged on Antithrombotic Therapy	87	100%	100%	99%
Discharged on Statin Medication	61	100%	93%	94%
Thrombolytic Therapy Timing[1]	-	-	75%	66%
Venous Thromboembolism Prophylaxis	84	96%	94%	94%
Written Stroke Educational Materials Given	59	97%	84%	88%
Surgical Care Improvement Project				
Appropriate Beta Blocker Usage[2]	353	99%	98%	98%
Appropriate VTP Within 24 Hours[2]	423	99%	99%	98%
Controlled Postoperative Blood Glucose[2]	184	99%	96%	97%
Perioperative Temperature Management[2]	687	100%	100%	100%
Prophylactic Antibiotic Selection[2]	582	99%	99%	99%
Prophylactic Antibiotic Selection (Outpatient)	646	99%	99%	98%
Prophylactic Antibiotic Stopped[2]	568	99%	98%	98%
Prophylactic Antibiotic Timing[2]	583	99%	98%	99%
Prophylactic Antibiotic Timing (Outpatient)	649	99%	97%	98%
Urinary Catheter Removal[2]	501	99%	98%	97%
Survey of Patients' Hospital Experiences				
Area Around Room 'Always' Quiet at Night	300+	62%	67%	61%
Doctors 'Always' Communicated Well	300+	82%	86%	82%
Home Recovery Information Given	300+	89%	88%	85%
Hospital Given 9 or 10 on 10 Point Scale	300+	76%	78%	71%
Meds 'Always' Explained Before Given	300+	64%	68%	64%
Nurses 'Always' Communicated Well	300+	79%	83%	79%
Pain 'Always' Well Controlled	300+	72%	73%	71%
Room and Bathroom 'Always' Clean	300+	73%	81%	73%
Timely Help 'Always' Received	300+	65%	75%	68%
Would Definitely Recommend Hospital	300+	76%	77%	71%
Use of Medical Imaging				
Cardiac Imaging Stress Test before Surgery	808	6.1%	5.4%	5.3%
Combination Abdominal CT Scan	930	3.4%	9.3%	10.5%
Combination Brain/Sinus CT Scan[1]	-	-	2.7%	2.7%
Combination Chest CT Scan	789	0.0%	1.7%	2.7%
Follow-up Mammogram/Ultrasound	1,353	4.3%	8%	8.8%
Lumbar Spine MRI for Low Back Pain	199	48.2%	36.5%	37.2%

Alegent Creighton Health Creighton University Med

601 North 30th St
Omaha, NE 68131
URL: www.creightonhospital.com
Type: Acute Care Hospitals
Ownership: Voluntary non-profit - Other

Phone: 402-449-4000
Fax: 402-449-5020
Emergency Services: Yes
Beds: 404

Key Personnel:
Quality Assurance . . . . Dina Belfare
Pediatric Ambulatory Care . . . . . . Stephen A Chartrand, MD
Pediatric In-Patient Care . . . . Stephen A Chartrand, MD
Radiology. . . . . Charles Lemer, MD
Infection Control. . . . . Ann Lorenzen
CEO/President. . . . . Richard Rolston, MD, FAAP
Chief of Medical Staff. . . . . Cary Ward, MD
Operating Room. . . . . Gary Welch, RN

Measure	Cases	This Hosp.	State Avg.	U.S. Avg.
Blood Clot Prevention and Treatment				
Anticoagulation Overlap Therapy[2]	47	91%	93%	93%
ICU Venous Thromboembolism Prophylaxis[2]	145	99%	91%	92%
Incidence of Potentially Preventable VTE[1,2]	-	-	11%	10%
UFH with Dosages/Platelet Monitoring[2]	29	97%	98%	97%
Venous Thromboembolism Prophylaxis[2]	335	95%	88%	85%
Warfarin Therapy Discharge Instructions[2]	38	89%	81%	75%
Chest Pain/Possible Heart Attack Care				
Aspirin Given Within 24 Hours of Arrival[5]	-	-	96%	96%
Fibrinolytic Meds Within 30 Min. of Arrival[5]	-	-	53%	58%
Average Time to ECG (minutes)[5]	-	-	8	7

NOTE: Hospital profiles are in alphabetical order by state, then city, then hospital within the city; Rankings exclude hospitals with less than 25 cases except for patient surveys which excludes hospitals with less than 100 cases; (a) 100-299 cases; (1) The number of cases/patients is too few to report; (2) Data submitted were based on a sample of cases/patients; (3) Results are based on a shorter time period than required; (4) Data suppressed by CMS for one or more quarters; (5) Results are not available for this reporting period; (6) Fewer than 100 patients completed the HCAHPS survey; (7) No cases met the criteria for this measure; (8) The lower limit of the confidence interval cannot be calculated if the number of observed infections equals zero; (9) No data are available from the state/territory for this reporting period; (10) The scores shown reflect fewer than 50 completed surveys; (11) There were discrepancies in the data collection process; (12) This measure does not apply to this hospital for this reporting period; (13) Results cannot be calculated for this reporting period; (14) The results for this state are combined with nearby states to protect confidentiality; Please refer to the User's Guide for a full explanation of data.

Measure	Cases	This Hosp.	State Avg.	U.S. Avg.
Average Time to Transfer (minutes)[5]	-	-	76	60
Children's Asthma Care				
Received Home Management Plan of Care	-	-	-	88%
Received Reliever Medication	-	-	-	100%
Received Systemic Corticosteroids	-	-	-	100%
Emergency Department				
Admittance Decision Time (minutes)[2]	508	171	75	98
Head CT Results Within 45 Min. of Arrival[7]	-	-	61%	57%
Patients Who Left ER Before Being Seen	35,441	1%	1%	2%
Time from ER Arrival to Admit. (minutes)[2]	513	256	207	274
Time from ER Arrival to Discharge (minutes)	420	113	118	134
Time in ER Before Being Evaluated (minutes)	473	18	21	26
Time to Pain Meds for Fractures (minutes)	106	30	42	57
Heart Attack Care				
Aspirin Given at Discharge	218	100%	100%	99%
Fibrinolytic Meds Within 30 Min. of Arrival[7]	-	-	-	54%
PCI Within 90 Minutes of Arrival	24	96%	96%	96%
Statin Prescribed at Discharge	215	100%	99%	98%
Heart Failure Care				
ACE Inhibitor or ARB for LVSD	99	99%	96%	97%
Discharge Instructions Given	214	94%	93%	94%
Evaluation of LVS Function	261	100%	98%	99%
Medicare Spending				
Medicare Spending per Patient (ratio)	-	1.04	0.97	0.98
Pneumonia Care				
Appropriate Initial Antibiotic Given	55	100%	95%	95%
Blood Culture Timing	64	100%	99%	98%
Pregnancy and Delivery Care				
Newborn Deliveries Scheduled Early[2]	41	2%	5%	6%
Preventive Care				
Immunization for Influenza[2]	567	99%	89%	90%
Immunization for Pneumonia[2]	605	99%	90%	92%
Stroke Care				
Anticoagulation Therapy for Atrial Fibrillation[1]	-	-	95%	95%
Antithrombotic Therapy Timing	65	100%	99%	98%
Assessed for Rehabilitation	96	97%	99%	97%
Discharged on Antithrombotic Therapy	76	100%	100%	99%
Discharged on Statin Medication	54	94%	93%	94%
Thrombolytic Therapy Timing[1]	-	-	75%	66%
Venous Thromboembolism Prophylaxis	97	98%	94%	94%
Written Stroke Educational Materials Given	57	96%	84%	88%
Surgical Care Improvement Project				
Appropriate Beta Blocker Usage[2]	205	100%	98%	98%
Appropriate VTP Within 24 Hours[2]	297	100%	99%	98%
Controlled Postoperative Blood Glucose[2]	140	94%	96%	97%
Perioperative Temperature Management[2]	340	100%	100%	100%
Prophylactic Antibiotic Selection[2]	321	100%	99%	99%
Prophylactic Antibiotic Selection (Outpatient)	224	99%	99%	98%
Prophylactic Antibiotic Stopped[2]	312	100%	98%	98%
Prophylactic Antibiotic Timing[2]	323	99%	98%	99%
Prophylactic Antibiotic Timing (Outpatient)	224	100%	97%	98%
Urinary Catheter Removal[2]	199	97%	98%	97%
Survey of Patients' Hospital Experiences				
Area Around Room 'Always' Quiet at Night	300+	54%	67%	61%
Doctors 'Always' Communicated Well	300+	78%	86%	82%
Home Recovery Information Given	300+	85%	88%	85%
Hospital Given 9 or 10 on 10 Point Scale	300+	67%	78%	71%
Meds 'Always' Explained Before Given	300+	61%	68%	64%
Nurses 'Always' Communicated Well	300+	74%	83%	79%
Pain 'Always' Well Controlled	300+	65%	73%	71%
Room and Bathroom 'Always' Clean	300+	66%	81%	73%
Timely Help 'Always' Received	300+	56%	75%	68%
Would Definitely Recommend Hospital	300+	67%	77%	71%
Use of Medical Imaging				
Cardiac Imaging Stress Test before Surgery	299	6.0%	5.4%	5.3%
Combination Abdominal CT Scan	256	5.9%	9.3%	10.5%
Combination Brain/Sinus CT Scan[1]	-	-	2.7%	2.7%
Combination Chest CT Scan	326	0.9%	1.7%	2.7%
Follow-up Mammogram/Ultrasound	388	8.2%	8%	8.8%
Lumbar Spine MRI for Low Back Pain[1]	-	-	36.5%	37.2%

Alegent Creighton Health Immanuel Medical Center

6901 North 72nd St
Omaha, NE 68122
URL: www.alegent.com
Type: Acute Care Hospitals
Ownership: Voluntary non-profit - Private
Phone: 402-572-2121
Fax: 402-572-2268
Emergency Services: Yes
Beds: 601

Key Personnel:
Emergency Room . . . . Richard Alarid
Radiology. Kimberly Apker, MD
Quality Assurance . . . . David Parks
CEO/President. . . . . Richard Rolston, MD, F.A.A.P.
Chief of Medical Staff . . . . Cary Ward, MD

Measure	Cases	This Hosp.	State Avg.	U.S. Avg.
Blood Clot Prevention and Treatment				
Anticoagulation Overlap Therapy[2]	43	98%	93%	93%
ICU Venous Thromboembolism Prophylaxis[2]	54	98%	91%	92%
Incidence of Potentially Preventable VTE[1,2]	-	-	11%	10%
UFH with Dosages/Platelet Monitoring[2]	49	98%	98%	97%
Venous Thromboembolism Prophylaxis[2]	218	98%	88%	85%
Warfarin Therapy Discharge Instructions[2]	21	71%	81%	75%
Chest Pain/Possible Heart Attack Care				
Aspirin Given Within 24 Hours of Arrival[3,7]	-	-	96%	96%
Fibrinolytic Meds Within 30 Min. of Arrival[5]	-	-	53%	58%
Average Time to ECG (minutes)[3,7]	-	-	8	7
Average Time to Transfer (minutes)[5]	-	-	76	60
Children's Asthma Care				
Received Home Management Plan of Care	-	-	-	88%
Received Reliever Medication	-	-	-	100%
Received Systemic Corticosteroids	-	-	-	100%
Emergency Department				
Admittance Decision Time (minutes)[2]	397	107	75	98
Head CT Results Within 45 Min. of Arrival[1,3]	-	-	61%	57%
Patients Who Left ER Before Being Seen	33,770	2%	1%	2%
Time from ER Arrival to Admit. (minutes)[2]	401	241	207	274
Time from ER Arrival to Discharge (minutes)	356	131	118	134
Time in ER Before Being Evaluated (minutes)	383	45	21	26
Time to Pain Meds for Fractures (minutes)	61	56	42	57
Heart Attack Care				
Aspirin Given at Discharge	111	100%	100%	99%
Fibrinolytic Meds Within 30 Min. of Arrival[7]	-	-	-	54%
PCI Within 90 Minutes of Arrival	23	96%	96%	96%
Statin Prescribed at Discharge	109	100%	99%	98%
Heart Failure Care				
ACE Inhibitor or ARB for LVSD	31	100%	96%	97%
Discharge Instructions Given	88	100%	93%	94%
Evaluation of LVS Function	118	100%	98%	99%
Medicare Spending				
Medicare Spending per Patient (ratio)	-	1.02	0.97	0.98
Pneumonia Care				
Appropriate Initial Antibiotic Given	86	99%	95%	95%
Blood Culture Timing	122	100%	99%	98%
Pregnancy and Delivery Care				
Newborn Deliveries Scheduled Early[2]	54	0%	5%	6%
Preventive Care				
Immunization for Influenza[2]	576	96%	89%	90%
Immunization for Pneumonia[2]	473	97%	90%	92%
Stroke Care				
Anticoagulation Therapy for Atrial Fibrillation[1]	-	-	95%	95%
Antithrombotic Therapy Timing	72	99%	99%	98%
Assessed for Rehabilitation	89	100%	99%	97%
Discharged on Antithrombotic Therapy	76	100%	100%	99%
Discharged on Statin Medication	66	98%	93%	94%
Thrombolytic Therapy Timing[1]	-	-	75%	66%
Venous Thromboembolism Prophylaxis	90	99%	94%	94%
Written Stroke Educational Materials Given	41	100%	84%	88%
Surgical Care Improvement Project				
Appropriate Beta Blocker Usage[2]	135	99%	98%	98%
Appropriate VTP Within 24 Hours[2]	305	100%	99%	98%
Controlled Postoperative Blood Glucose[2,7]	-	-	96%	97%
Perioperative Temperature Management[2]	337	100%	100%	100%
Prophylactic Antibiotic Selection[2]	190	100%	99%	99%
Prophylactic Antibiotic Selection (Outpatient)	152	100%	99%	98%
Prophylactic Antibiotic Stopped[2]	185	99%	98%	98%
Prophylactic Antibiotic Timing[2]	190	99%	98%	99%
Prophylactic Antibiotic Timing (Outpatient)	151	100%	97%	98%
Urinary Catheter Removal[2]	246	100%	98%	97%
Survey of Patients' Hospital Experiences				
Area Around Room 'Always' Quiet at Night	300+	61%	67%	61%
Doctors 'Always' Communicated Well	300+	83%	86%	82%
Home Recovery Information Given	300+	92%	88%	85%
Hospital Given 9 or 10 on 10 Point Scale	300+	77%	78%	71%
Meds 'Always' Explained Before Given	300+	67%	68%	64%
Nurses 'Always' Communicated Well	300+	80%	83%	79%
Pain 'Always' Well Controlled	300+	73%	73%	71%
Room and Bathroom 'Always' Clean	300+	76%	81%	73%
Timely Help 'Always' Received	300+	65%	75%	68%
Would Definitely Recommend Hospital	300+	78%	77%	71%
Use of Medical Imaging				
Cardiac Imaging Stress Test before Surgery	182	7.1%	5.4%	5.3%
Combination Abdominal CT Scan	449	4.7%	9.3%	10.5%
Combination Brain/Sinus CT Scan[1]	-	-	2.7%	2.7%
Combination Chest CT Scan	375	0.0%	1.7%	2.7%
Follow-up Mammogram/Ultrasound	811	8.4%	8%	8.8%
Lumbar Spine MRI for Low Back Pain	123	43.1%	36.5%	37.2%

Alegent Creighton Health Lakeside Hospital

16901 Lakeside Hills Ct
Omaha, NE 68130
URL: www.alegent.com
Type: Acute Care Hospitals
Ownership: Voluntary non-profit - Church
Phone: 402-717-8000
Emergency Services: Yes
Beds: 77

Key Personnel:
CEO/President. . . . . Wayne Sensor

Measure	Cases	This Hosp.	State Avg.	U.S. Avg.
Blood Clot Prevention and Treatment				
Anticoagulation Overlap Therapy[2]	86	99%	93%	93%
ICU Venous Thromboembolism Prophylaxis[2]	67	100%	91%	92%
Incidence of Potentially Preventable VTE[2]	13	8%	11%	10%
UFH with Dosages/Platelet Monitoring[2]	69	99%	98%	97%
Venous Thromboembolism Prophylaxis[2]	301	98%	88%	85%
Warfarin Therapy Discharge Instructions[2]	59	73%	81%	75%
Chest Pain/Possible Heart Attack Care				
Aspirin Given Within 24 Hours of Arrival[1,3]	-	-	96%	96%
Fibrinolytic Meds Within 30 Min. of Arrival[3,7]	-	-	53%	58%
Average Time to ECG (minutes)[1,3]	-	-	8	7
Average Time to Transfer (minutes)[3,7]	-	-	76	60
Children's Asthma Care				
Received Home Management Plan of Care	-	-	-	88%
Received Reliever Medication	-	-	-	100%
Received Systemic Corticosteroids	-	-	-	100%
Emergency Department				
Admittance Decision Time (minutes)[2]	640	86	75	98
Head CT Results Within 45 Min. of Arrival[3,7]	-	-	61%	57%
Patients Who Left ER Before Being Seen	23,159	0%	1%	2%
Time from ER Arrival to Admit. (minutes)[2]	651	201	207	274
Time from ER Arrival to Discharge (minutes)	382	126	118	134
Time in ER Before Being Evaluated (minutes)	360	26	21	26
Time to Pain Meds for Fractures (minutes)	143	49	42	57
Heart Attack Care				
Aspirin Given at Discharge	121	100%	100%	99%
Fibrinolytic Meds Within 30 Min. of Arrival[7]	-	-	-	54%
PCI Within 90 Minutes of Arrival	30	93%	96%	96%
Statin Prescribed at Discharge	114	99%	99%	98%
Heart Failure Care				
ACE Inhibitor or ARB for LVSD	23	100%	96%	97%
Discharge Instructions Given	78	99%	93%	94%
Evaluation of LVS Function	116	100%	98%	99%
Medicare Spending				
Medicare Spending per Patient (ratio)	-	1.01	0.97	0.98
Pneumonia Care				
Appropriate Initial Antibiotic Given	83	99%	95%	95%
Blood Culture Timing	161	99%	99%	98%
Pregnancy and Delivery Care				
Newborn Deliveries Scheduled Early[2]	22	5%	5%	6%
Preventive Care				
Immunization for Influenza[2]	542	98%	89%	90%

NOTE: Hospital profiles are in alphabetical order by state, then city, then hospital within the city; Rankings exclude hospitals with less than 25 cases except for patient surveys which excludes hospitals with less than 100 cases; (a) 100-299 cases; (1) The number of cases/patients is too few to report; (2) Data submitted were based on a sample of cases/patients; (3) Results are based on a shorter time period than required; (4) Data suppressed by CMS for one or more quarters; (5) Results are not available for this reporting period; (6) Fewer than 100 patients completed the HCAHPS survey; (7) No cases met the criteria for this measure; (8) The lower limit of the confidence interval cannot be calculated if the number of observed infections equals zero; (9) No data are available from the state/territory for this reporting period; (10) The scores shown reflect fewer than 50 completed surveys; (11) There were discrepancies in the data collection process; (12) This measure does not apply to this hospital for this reporting period; (13) Results cannot be calculated for this reporting period; (14) The results for this state are combined with nearby states to protect confidentiality; Please refer to the User's Guide for a full explanation of data.

Measure	Cases	This Hosp.	State Avg.	U.S. Avg.
Immunization for Pneumonia[2]	572	93%	90%	92%
Stroke Care				
Anticoagulation Therapy for Atrial Fibrillation	15	93%	95%	95%
Antithrombotic Therapy Timing	85	99%	99%	98%
Assessed for Rehabilitation	105	100%	99%	97%
Discharged on Antithrombotic Therapy	94	99%	100%	99%
Discharged on Statin Medication	73	97%	93%	94%
Thrombolytic Therapy Timing[1]	-	-	75%	66%
Venous Thromboembolism Prophylaxis	105	96%	94%	94%
Written Stroke Educational Materials Given	52	94%	84%	88%
Surgical Care Improvement Project				
Appropriate Beta Blocker Usage[2]	125	99%	98%	98%
Appropriate VTP Within 24 Hours[2]	362	99%	99%	98%
Controlled Postoperative Blood Glucose[2,7]	-	-	96%	97%
Perioperative Temperature Management[2]	402	100%	100%	100%
Prophylactic Antibiotic Selection[2]	251	100%	99%	99%
Prophylactic Antibiotic Selection (Outpatient)	259	100%	99%	98%
Prophylactic Antibiotic Stopped[2]	247	100%	98%	98%
Prophylactic Antibiotic Timing[2]	251	99%	98%	99%
Prophylactic Antibiotic Timing (Outpatient)	259	100%	97%	98%
Urinary Catheter Removal[2]	290	100%	98%	97%
Survey of Patients' Hospital Experiences				
Area Around Room 'Always' Quiet at Night	300+	63%	67%	61%
Doctors 'Always' Communicated Well	300+	84%	86%	82%
Home Recovery Information Given	300+	90%	88%	85%
Hospital Given 9 or 10 on 10 Point Scale	300+	79%	78%	71%
Meds 'Always' Explained Before Given	300+	66%	68%	64%
Nurses 'Always' Communicated Well	300+	82%	83%	79%
Pain 'Always' Well Controlled	300+	74%	73%	71%
Room and Bathroom 'Always' Clean	300+	66%	81%	73%
Timely Help 'Always' Received	300+	63%	75%	68%
Would Definitely Recommend Hospital	300+	80%	77%	71%
Use of Medical Imaging				
Cardiac Imaging Stress Test before Surgery	140	4.3%	5.4%	5.3%
Combination Abdominal CT Scan	533	6.2%	9.3%	10.5%
Combination Brain/Sinus CT Scan	340	4.4%	2.7%	2.7%
Combination Chest CT Scan	341	0.0%	1.7%	2.7%
Follow-up Mammogram/Ultrasound	1,756	7.4%	8%	8.8%
Lumbar Spine MRI for Low Back Pain	54	42.6%	36.5%	37.2%

Children's Hospital & Medical Center

8200 Dodge St
Phone: 402-955-5400
Omaha, NE 68114
URL: www.childrensomaha.org
Type: Childrens
Emergency Services: Yes
Ownership: Voluntary non-profit - Private
Beds: 145
Key Personnel:
President/CEO. . . . . Gary A Perkins

Measure	Cases	This Hosp.	State Avg.	U.S. Avg.
Blood Clot Prevention and Treatment				
Anticoagulation Overlap Therapy[5]	-	-	93%	93%
ICU Venous Thromboembolism Prophylaxis[5]	-	-	91%	92%
Incidence of Potentially Preventable VTE[5]	-	-	11%	10%
UFH with Dosages/Platelet Monitoring[5]	-	-	98%	97%
Venous Thromboembolism Prophylaxis[5]	-	-	88%	85%
Warfarin Therapy Discharge Instructions[5]	-	-	81%	75%
Chest Pain/Possible Heart Attack Care				
Aspirin Given Within 24 Hours of Arrival	-	-	96%	96%
Fibrinolytic Meds Within 30 Min. of Arrival	-	-	53%	58%
Average Time to ECG (minutes)	-	-	8	7
Average Time to Transfer (minutes)	-	-	76	60
Children's Asthma Care				
Received Home Management Plan of Care	85	93%	-	88%
Received Reliever Medication	85	100%	-	100%
Received Systemic Corticosteroids	86	100%	-	100%
Emergency Department				
Admittance Decision Time (minutes)[5]	-	-	75	98
Head CT Results Within 45 Min. of Arrival	-	-	61%	57%
Patients Who Left ER Before Being Seen	-	-	1%	2%
Time from ER Arrival to Admit. (minutes)[5]	-	-	207	274
Time from ER Arrival to Discharge (minutes)	-	-	118	134
Time in ER Before Being Evaluated (minutes)	-	-	21	26
Time to Pain Meds for Fractures (minutes)	-	-	42	57
Heart Attack Care				
Aspirin Given at Discharge[5]	-	-	100%	99%
Fibrinolytic Meds Within 30 Min. of Arrival[5]		-	-	54%
PCI Within 90 Minutes of Arrival[5]	-	-	96%	96%
Statin Prescribed at Discharge[5]	-	-	99%	98%
Heart Failure Care				
ACE Inhibitor or ARB for LVSD[5]	-	-	96%	97%
Discharge Instructions Given[5]	-	-	93%	94%
Evaluation of LVS Function[5]	-	-	98%	99%
Medicare Spending				
Medicare Spending per Patient (ratio)	-	-	0.97	0.98
Pneumonia Care				
Appropriate Initial Antibiotic Given[5]	-	-	95%	95%
Blood Culture Timing[5]	-	-	99%	98%
Pregnancy and Delivery Care				
Newborn Deliveries Scheduled Early[5]	-	-	5%	6%
Preventive Care				
Immunization for Influenza[5]	-	-	89%	90%
Immunization for Pneumonia[5]	-	-	90%	92%
Stroke Care				
Anticoagulation Therapy for Atrial Fibrillation[5]	-	-	95%	95%
Antithrombotic Therapy Timing[5]	-	-	99%	98%
Assessed for Rehabilitation[5]	-	-	99%	97%
Discharged on Antithrombotic Therapy[5]	-	-	100%	99%
Discharged on Statin Medication[5]	-	-	93%	94%
Thrombolytic Therapy Timing[5]	-	-	75%	66%
Venous Thromboembolism Prophylaxis[5]	-	-	94%	94%
Written Stroke Educational Materials Given[5]	-	-	84%	88%
Surgical Care Improvement Project				
Appropriate Beta Blocker Usage[5]	-	-	98%	98%
Appropriate VTP Within 24 Hours[5]	-	-	99%	98%
Controlled Postoperative Blood Glucose[5]	-	-	96%	97%
Perioperative Temperature Management[5]	-	-	100%	100%
Prophylactic Antibiotic Selection[5]	-	-	99%	99%
Prophylactic Antibiotic Selection (Outpatient)	-	-	99%	98%
Prophylactic Antibiotic Stopped[5]	-	-	98%	98%
Prophylactic Antibiotic Timing[5]	-	-	98%	99%
Prophylactic Antibiotic Timing (Outpatient)	-	-	97%	98%
Urinary Catheter Removal[5]	-	-	98%	97%
Survey of Patients' Hospital Experiences				
Area Around Room 'Always' Quiet at Night[5]	-	-	67%	61%
Doctors 'Always' Communicated Well[5]	-	-	86%	82%
Home Recovery Information Given[5]	-	-	88%	85%
Hospital Given 9 or 10 on 10 Point Scale[5]	-	-	78%	71%
Meds 'Always' Explained Before Given[5]	-	-	68%	64%
Nurses 'Always' Communicated Well[5]	-	-	83%	79%
Pain 'Always' Well Controlled[5]	-	-	73%	71%
Room and Bathroom 'Always' Clean[5]	-	-	81%	73%
Timely Help 'Always' Received[5]	-	-	75%	68%
Would Definitely Recommend Hospital[5]	-	-	77%	71%
Use of Medical Imaging				
Cardiac Imaging Stress Test before Surgery	-	-	5.4%	5.3%
Combination Abdominal CT Scan	-	-	9.3%	10.5%
Combination Brain/Sinus CT Scan	-	-	2.7%	2.7%
Combination Chest CT Scan	-	-	1.7%	2.7%
Follow-up Mammogram/Ultrasound	-	-	8%	8.8%
Lumbar Spine MRI for Low Back Pain	-	-	36.5%	37.2%

Midwest Surgical Hospital

7915 Farnam Drive
Phone: 402-399-1900
Omaha, NE 68114
URL: www.mwsurgicalhospital.com
Type: Acute Care Hospitals
Emergency Services: No
Ownership: Physician
Key Personnel:
Administrator . . . . Charles Livingston

Measure	Cases	This Hosp.	State Avg.	U.S. Avg.
Blood Clot Prevention and Treatment				
Anticoagulation Overlap Therapy[7]	-	-	93%	93%
ICU Venous Thromboembolism Prophylaxis[7]	-	-	91%	92%
Incidence of Potentially Preventable VTE[7]	-	-	11%	10%
UFH with Dosages/Platelet Monitoring[7]	-	-	98%	97%
Venous Thromboembolism Prophylaxis	267	97%	88%	85%
Warfarin Therapy Discharge Instructions[7]	-	-	81%	75%
Chest Pain/Possible Heart Attack Care				
Aspirin Given Within 24 Hours of Arrival[5]	-	-	96%	96%
Fibrinolytic Meds Within 30 Min. of Arrival[5]	-	-	53%	58%
Average Time to ECG (minutes)[5]	-	-	8	7
Average Time to Transfer (minutes)[5]	-	-	76	60
Children's Asthma Care				
Received Home Management Plan of Care	-	-	-	88%
Received Reliever Medication	-	-	-	100%
Received Systemic Corticosteroids	-	-	-	100%
Emergency Department				
Admittance Decision Time (minutes)[7]	-	-	75	98
Head CT Results Within 45 Min. of Arrival[5]	-	-	61%	57%
Patients Who Left ER Before Being Seen[5]	-	-	1%	2%
Time from ER Arrival to Admit. (minutes)[7]	-	-	207	274
Time from ER Arrival to Discharge (minutes)[5]	-	-	118	134
Time in ER Before Being Evaluated (minutes)[5]	-	-	21	26
Time to Pain Meds for Fractures (minutes)[5]	-	-	42	57
Heart Attack Care				
Aspirin Given at Discharge[5]	-	-	100%	99%
Fibrinolytic Meds Within 30 Min. of Arrival[5]			-	54%
PCI Within 90 Minutes of Arrival[5]	-	-	96%	96%
Statin Prescribed at Discharge[5]	-	-	99%	98%
Heart Failure Care				
ACE Inhibitor or ARB for LVSD[5]	-	-	96%	97%
Discharge Instructions Given[5]	-	-	93%	94%
Evaluation of LVS Function[5]	-	-	98%	99%
Medicare Spending				
Medicare Spending per Patient (ratio)	-	0.88	0.97	0.98
Pneumonia Care				
Appropriate Initial Antibiotic Given[5]	-	-	95%	95%
Blood Culture Timing[5]	-	-	99%	98%
Pregnancy and Delivery Care				
Newborn Deliveries Scheduled Early[7]	-	-	5%	6%
Preventive Care				
Immunization for Influenza	443	76%	89%	90%
Immunization for Pneumonia	272	72%	90%	92%
Stroke Care				
Anticoagulation Therapy for Atrial Fibrillation[5]	-	-	95%	95%
Antithrombotic Therapy Timing[5]	-	-	99%	98%
Assessed for Rehabilitation[5]	-	-	99%	97%
Discharged on Antithrombotic Therapy[5]	-	-	100%	99%
Discharged on Statin Medication[5]	-	-	93%	94%
Thrombolytic Therapy Timing[5]	-	-	75%	66%
Venous Thromboembolism Prophylaxis[5]	-	-	94%	94%
Written Stroke Educational Materials Given[5]	-	-	84%	88%
Surgical Care Improvement Project				
Appropriate Beta Blocker Usage	74	97%	98%	98%
Appropriate VTP Within 24 Hours	194	100%	99%	98%
Controlled Postoperative Blood Glucose[7]	-	-	96%	97%
Perioperative Temperature Management	259	100%	100%	100%
Prophylactic Antibiotic Selection	224	100%	99%	99%
Prophylactic Antibiotic Selection (Outpatient)	346	100%	99%	98%
Prophylactic Antibiotic Stopped	224	100%	98%	98%
Prophylactic Antibiotic Timing	224	93%	98%	99%
Prophylactic Antibiotic Timing (Outpatient)	347	96%	97%	98%
Urinary Catheter Removal	175	100%	98%	97%
Survey of Patients' Hospital Experiences				
Area Around Room 'Always' Quiet at Night	300+	91%	67%	61%
Doctors 'Always' Communicated Well	300+	90%	86%	82%
Home Recovery Information Given	300+	91%	88%	85%
Hospital Given 9 or 10 on 10 Point Scale	300+	91%	78%	71%
Meds 'Always' Explained Before Given	300+	74%	68%	64%
Nurses 'Always' Communicated Well	300+	90%	83%	79%
Pain 'Always' Well Controlled	300+	81%	73%	71%
Room and Bathroom 'Always' Clean	300+	86%	81%	73%
Timely Help 'Always' Received	300+	90%	75%	68%
Would Definitely Recommend Hospital	300+	91%	77%	71%
Use of Medical Imaging				
Cardiac Imaging Stress Test before Surgery[7]	-	-	5.4%	5.3%
Combination Abdominal CT Scan[7]	-	-	9.3%	10.5%
Combination Brain/Sinus CT Scan[7]	-	-	2.7%	2.7%

NOTE: Hospital profiles are in alphabetical order by state, then city, then hospital within the city; Rankings exclude hospitals with less than 25 cases except for patient surveys which excludes hospitals with less than 100 cases; (a) 100-299 cases; (1) The number of cases/patients is too few to report; (2) Data submitted were based on a sample of cases/patients; (3) Results are based on a shorter time period than required; (4) Data suppressed by CMS for one or more quarters; (5) Results are not available for this reporting period; (6) Fewer than 100 patients completed the HCAHPS survey; (7) No cases met the criteria for this measure; (8) The lower limit of the confidence interval cannot be calculated if the number of observed infections equals zero; (9) No data are available from the state/territory for this reporting period; (10) The scores shown reflect fewer than 50 completed surveys; (11) There were discrepancies in the data collection process; (12) This measure does not apply to this hospital for this reporting period; (13) Results cannot be calculated for this reporting period; (14) The results for this state are combined with nearby states to protect confidentiality; Please refer to the User's Guide for a full explanation of data.

Measure	Cases	This Hosp.	State Avg.	U.S. Avg.
Combination Chest CT Scan[7]	-	-	1.7%	2.7%
Follow-up Mammogram/Ultrasound[7]	-	-	8%	8.8%
Lumbar Spine MRI for Low Back Pain[7]	-	-	36.5%	37.2%

The Nebraska Medical Center

987400 Nebraska Medical Center
Omaha, NE 68198
Phone: 402-552-2040
Fax: 402-595-1091
URL: www.nebraskamed.com
Type: Acute Care Hospitals
Emergency Services: Yes
Ownership: Voluntary non-profit - Private
Beds: 624

Key Personnel:

CEO/President. . . . . Jennifer Bartelt
Infection Control. . . . . Theresa Franco
Coronary Care. . . . . Maureen Kelpe
Quality Assurance . . . . Sue Korth
Pediatric In-Patient Care . . . . Jackie Parmenter, RN
Radiology. . . . . Terri Paulsen
Operating Room. . . . . Shelley Schwedhelm, RN
Chief of Medical Staff. . . . . Stephen Smith, MD

Measure	Cases	This Hosp.	State Avg.	U.S. Avg.
Blood Clot Prevention and Treatment				
Anticoagulation Overlap Therapy[2]	138	86%	93%	93%
ICU Venous Thromboembolism Prophylaxis[2]	80	96%	91%	92%
Incidence of Potentially Preventable VTE[2]	56	5%	11%	10%
UFH with Dosages/Platelet Monitoring[2]	140	100%	98%	97%
Venous Thromboembolism Prophylaxis[2]	313	90%	88%	85%
Warfarin Therapy Discharge Instructions[2]	96	80%	81%	75%
Chest Pain/Possible Heart Attack Care				
Aspirin Given Within 24 Hours of Arrival[5]	-	-	96%	96%
Fibrinolytic Meds Within 30 Min. of Arrival[5]	-	-	53%	58%
Average Time to ECG (minutes)[5]	-	-	8	7
Average Time to Transfer (minutes)[5]	-	-	76	60
Children's Asthma Care				
Received Home Management Plan of Care	-	-	-	88%
Received Reliever Medication	-	-	-	100%
Received Systemic Corticosteroids	-	-	-	100%
Emergency Department				
Admittance Decision Time (minutes)[2]	307	76	75	98
Head CT Results Within 45 Min. of Arrival[1,3]	-	-	61%	57%
Patients Who Left ER Before Being Seen	51,834	2%	1%	2%
Time from ER Arrival to Admit. (minutes)[2]	317	264	207	274
Time from ER Arrival to Discharge (minutes)	359	147	118	134
Time in ER Before Being Evaluated (minutes)	369	30	21	26
Time to Pain Meds for Fractures (minutes)	116	55	42	57
Heart Attack Care				
Aspirin Given at Discharge[2]	213	100%	100%	99%
Fibrinolytic Meds Within 30 Min. of Arrival[2,7]	-	-	-	54%
PCI Within 90 Minutes of Arrival[2]	14	93%	96%	96%
Statin Prescribed at Discharge[2]	209	100%	99%	98%
Heart Failure Care				
ACE Inhibitor or ARB for LVSD[2]	89	100%	96%	97%
Discharge Instructions Given[2]	241	95%	93%	94%
Evaluation of LVS Function[2]	281	100%	98%	99%
Medicare Spending				
Medicare Spending per Patient (ratio)	-	0.98	0.97	0.98
Pneumonia Care				
Appropriate Initial Antibiotic Given[2]	37	95%	95%	95%
Blood Culture Timing[2]	115	98%	99%	98%
Pregnancy and Delivery Care				
Newborn Deliveries Scheduled Early[2]	20	0%	5%	6%
Preventive Care				
Immunization for Influenza[2]	531	83%	89%	90%
Immunization for Pneumonia[2]	584	87%	90%	92%
Stroke Care				
Anticoagulation Therapy for Atrial Fibrillation[2]	16	100%	95%	95%
Antithrombotic Therapy Timing[2]	40	100%	99%	98%
Assessed for Rehabilitation[2]	95	100%	99%	97%
Discharged on Antithrombotic Therapy[2]	61	100%	100%	99%
Discharged on Statin Medication[2]	45	96%	93%	94%
Thrombolytic Therapy Timing[1,2]	-	-	75%	66%
Venous Thromboembolism Prophylaxis[2]	96	100%	94%	94%
Written Stroke Educational Materials Given[2]	43	98%	84%	88%
Surgical Care Improvement Project				
Appropriate Beta Blocker Usage[2]	231	100%	98%	98%
Appropriate VTP Within 24 Hours[2]	308	99%	99%	98%
Controlled Postoperative Blood Glucose[2]	131	98%	96%	97%
Perioperative Temperature Management[2]	426	100%	100%	100%
Prophylactic Antibiotic Selection[2]	391	99%	99%	99%
Prophylactic Antibiotic Selection (Outpatient)	320	98%	99%	98%
Prophylactic Antibiotic Stopped[2]	384	100%	98%	98%
Prophylactic Antibiotic Timing[2]	394	96%	98%	99%
Prophylactic Antibiotic Timing (Outpatient)	331	92%	97%	98%
Urinary Catheter Removal[2]	296	99%	98%	97%
Survey of Patients' Hospital Experiences				
Area Around Room 'Always' Quiet at Night	300+	58%	67%	61%
Doctors 'Always' Communicated Well	300+	78%	86%	82%
Home Recovery Information Given	300+	89%	88%	85%
Hospital Given 9 or 10 on 10 Point Scale	300+	74%	78%	71%
Meds 'Always' Explained Before Given	300+	62%	68%	64%
Nurses 'Always' Communicated Well	300+	78%	83%	79%
Pain 'Always' Well Controlled	300+	68%	73%	71%
Room and Bathroom 'Always' Clean	300+	72%	81%	73%
Timely Help 'Always' Received	300+	63%	75%	68%
Would Definitely Recommend Hospital	300+	79%	77%	71%
Use of Medical Imaging				
Cardiac Imaging Stress Test before Surgery	675	7.1%	5.4%	5.3%
Combination Abdominal CT Scan	1,490	3.0%	9.3%	10.5%
Combination Brain/Sinus CT Scan	871	3.8%	2.7%	2.7%
Combination Chest CT Scan	1,876	0.2%	1.7%	2.7%
Follow-up Mammogram/Ultrasound	2,022	7.3%	8%	8.8%
Lumbar Spine MRI for Low Back Pain	153	38.6%	36.5%	37.2%

The Nebraska Methodist Hospital

8303 Dodge St
Omaha, NE 68114
Phone: 402-354-4000
Fax: 402-354-8735
URL: www.bestcare.org
Type: Acute Care Hospitals
Emergency Services: Yes
Ownership: Voluntary non-profit - Private
Beds: 430

Key Personnel:

CEO/President. . . . . Stephen L Goeser
Radiology. . . . . Brad Hansen
Quality Assurance . . . . Sara Juster
Chief of Medical Staff. . . . . William Shiffermiller
Operating Room. . . . . Diana Whittle

Measure	Cases	This Hosp.	State Avg.	U.S. Avg.
Blood Clot Prevention and Treatment				
Anticoagulation Overlap Therapy[2]	114	95%	93%	93%
ICU Venous Thromboembolism Prophylaxis[2]	57	96%	91%	92%
Incidence of Potentially Preventable VTE[2]	20	10%	11%	10%
UFH with Dosages/Platelet Monitoring[2]	124	100%	98%	97%
Venous Thromboembolism Prophylaxis[2]	372	83%	88%	85%
Warfarin Therapy Discharge Instructions[2]	87	92%	81%	75%
Chest Pain/Possible Heart Attack Care				
Aspirin Given Within 24 Hours of Arrival	18	94%	96%	96%
Fibrinolytic Meds Within 30 Min. of Arrival[5]	-	-	53%	58%
Average Time to ECG (minutes)	19	1	8	7
Average Time to Transfer (minutes)[5]	-	-	76	60
Children's Asthma Care				
Received Home Management Plan of Care	-	-	-	88%
Received Reliever Medication	-	-	-	100%
Received Systemic Corticosteroids	-	-	-	100%
Emergency Department				
Admittance Decision Time (minutes)[2]	242	77	75	98
Head CT Results Within 45 Min. of Arrival[1]	-	-	61%	57%
Patients Who Left ER Before Being Seen	29,687	1%	1%	2%
Time from ER Arrival to Admit. (minutes)[2]	244	198	207	274
Time from ER Arrival to Discharge (minutes)	543	211	118	134
Time in ER Before Being Evaluated (minutes)	1,108	20	21	26
Time to Pain Meds for Fractures (minutes)	32	62	42	57
Heart Attack Care				
Aspirin Given at Discharge	193	100%	100%	99%
Fibrinolytic Meds Within 30 Min. of Arrival[7]	-	-	-	54%
PCI Within 90 Minutes of Arrival	28	96%	96%	96%
Statin Prescribed at Discharge	191	99%	99%	98%
Heart Failure Care				
ACE Inhibitor or ARB for LVSD	88	100%	96%	97%
Discharge Instructions Given	206	97%	93%	94%
Evaluation of LVS Function	277	100%	98%	99%
Medicare Spending				
Medicare Spending per Patient (ratio)	-	1.02	0.97	0.98
Pneumonia Care				
Appropriate Initial Antibiotic Given	148	97%	95%	95%
Blood Culture Timing	232	99%	99%	98%
Pregnancy and Delivery Care				
Newborn Deliveries Scheduled Early[2]	89	2%	5%	6%
Preventive Care				
Immunization for Influenza[2]	560	85%	89%	90%
Immunization for Pneumonia[2]	595	76%	90%	92%
Stroke Care				
Anticoagulation Therapy for Atrial Fibrillation	20	85%	95%	95%
Antithrombotic Therapy Timing	100	97%	99%	98%
Assessed for Rehabilitation	109	95%	99%	97%
Discharged on Antithrombotic Therapy	92	97%	100%	99%
Discharged on Statin Medication	75	80%	93%	94%
Thrombolytic Therapy Timing	14	29%	75%	66%
Venous Thromboembolism Prophylaxis	135	79%	94%	94%
Written Stroke Educational Materials Given	46	59%	84%	88%
Surgical Care Improvement Project				
Appropriate Beta Blocker Usage	378	99%	98%	98%
Appropriate VTP Within 24 Hours	1,873	98%	99%	98%
Controlled Postoperative Blood Glucose	250	92%	96%	97%
Perioperative Temperature Management	2,288	100%	100%	100%
Prophylactic Antibiotic Selection	1,449	100%	99%	99%
Prophylactic Antibiotic Selection (Outpatient)	1,099	98%	99%	98%
Prophylactic Antibiotic Stopped	1,405	98%	98%	98%
Prophylactic Antibiotic Timing	1,450	97%	98%	99%
Prophylactic Antibiotic Timing (Outpatient)	1,112	98%	97%	98%
Urinary Catheter Removal	1,393	97%	98%	97%
Survey of Patients' Hospital Experiences				
Area Around Room 'Always' Quiet at Night	300+	57%	67%	61%
Doctors 'Always' Communicated Well	300+	83%	86%	82%
Home Recovery Information Given	300+	90%	88%	85%
Hospital Given 9 or 10 on 10 Point Scale	300+	79%	78%	71%
Meds 'Always' Explained Before Given	300+	62%	68%	64%
Nurses 'Always' Communicated Well	300+	83%	83%	79%
Pain 'Always' Well Controlled	300+	72%	73%	71%
Room and Bathroom 'Always' Clean	300+	69%	81%	73%
Timely Help 'Always' Received	300+	69%	75%	68%
Would Definitely Recommend Hospital	300+	82%	77%	71%
Use of Medical Imaging				
Cardiac Imaging Stress Test before Surgery	1,135	5.2%	5.4%	5.3%
Combination Abdominal CT Scan	1,470	2.0%	9.3%	10.5%
Combination Brain/Sinus CT Scan	783	1.3%	2.7%	2.7%
Combination Chest CT Scan	1,238	0.0%	1.7%	2.7%
Follow-up Mammogram/Ultrasound	1,390	7.9%	8%	8.8%
Lumbar Spine MRI for Low Back Pain	271	44.6%	36.5%	37.2%

Nebraska Orthopaedic Hospital

2808 South 143rd Plz
Omaha, NE 68144
Phone: 402-609-1600
URL: www.neorthohospital.com
Type: Acute Care Hospitals
Emergency Services: Yes
Ownership: Physician

Measure	Cases	This Hosp.	State Avg.	U.S. Avg.
Blood Clot Prevention and Treatment				
Anticoagulation Overlap Therapy[2,7]	-	-	93%	93%
ICU Venous Thromboembolism Prophylaxis[2,7]	-	-	91%	92%
Incidence of Potentially Preventable VTE[2,7]	-	-	11%	10%
UFH with Dosages/Platelet Monitoring[2,7]	-	-	98%	97%
Venous Thromboembolism Prophylaxis[2]	29	97%	88%	85%
Warfarin Therapy Discharge Instructions[2,7]	-	-	81%	75%
Chest Pain/Possible Heart Attack Care				
Aspirin Given Within 24 Hours of Arrival	34	97%	96%	96%
Fibrinolytic Meds Within 30 Min. of Arrival[3,7]	-	-	53%	58%
Average Time to ECG (minutes)	33	6	8	7
Average Time to Transfer (minutes)[3,7]	-	-	76	60
Children's Asthma Care				
Received Home Management Plan of Care	-	-	-	88%
Received Reliever Medication	-	-	-	100%

NOTE: Hospital profiles are in alphabetical order by state, then city, then hospital within the city; Rankings exclude hospitals with less than 25 cases except for patient surveys which excludes hospitals with less than 100 cases; (a) 100-299 cases; (1) The number of cases/patients is too few to report; (2) Data submitted were based on a sample of cases/patients; (3) Results are based on a shorter time period than required; (4) Data suppressed by CMS for one or more quarters; (5) Results are not available for this reporting period; (6) Fewer than 100 patients completed the HCAHPS survey; (7) No cases met the criteria for this measure; (8) The lower limit of the confidence interval cannot be calculated if the number of observed infections equals zero; (9) No data are available from the state/territory for this reporting period; (10) The scores shown reflect fewer than 50 completed surveys; (11) There were discrepancies in the data collection process; (12) This measure does not apply to this hospital for this reporting period; (13) Results cannot be calculated for this reporting period; (14) The results for this state are combined with nearby states to protect confidentiality; Please refer to the User's Guide for a full explanation of data.

Measure	Cases	This Hosp.	State Avg.	U.S. Avg.
Received Systemic Corticosteroids	-	-	-	100%
Emergency Department				
Admittance Decision Time (minutes)[1,2]	-	-	75	98
Head CT Results Within 45 Min. of Arrival[1]	-	-	61%	57%
Patients Who Left ER Before Being Seen	8,850	0%	1%	2%
Time from ER Arrival to Admit. (minutes)[1,2]	-	-	207	274
Time from ER Arrival to Discharge (minutes)	378	78	118	134
Time in ER Before Being Evaluated (minutes)	417	18	21	26
Time to Pain Meds for Fractures (minutes)	45	30	42	57
Heart Attack Care				
Aspirin Given at Discharge[5]	-	-	100%	99%
Fibrinolytic Meds Within 30 Min. of Arrival[5]	-	-	-	54%
PCI Within 90 Minutes of Arrival[5]	-	-	96%	96%
Statin Prescribed at Discharge[5]	-	-	99%	98%
Heart Failure Care				
ACE Inhibitor or ARB for LVSD[5]	-	-	96%	97%
Discharge Instructions Given[5]	-	-	93%	94%
Evaluation of LVS Function[5]	-	-	98%	99%
Medicare Spending				
Medicare Spending per Patient (ratio)	-	0.93	0.97	0.98
Pneumonia Care				
Appropriate Initial Antibiotic Given[5]	-	-	95%	95%
Blood Culture Timing[5]	-	-	99%	98%
Pregnancy and Delivery Care				
Newborn Deliveries Scheduled Early[7]	-	-	5%	6%
Preventive Care				
Immunization for Influenza[2]	321	94%	89%	90%
Immunization for Pneumonia[2]	403	89%	90%	92%
Stroke Care				
Anticoagulation Therapy for Atrial Fibrillation[5]	-	-	95%	95%
Antithrombotic Therapy Timing[5]	-	-	99%	98%
Assessed for Rehabilitation[5]	-	-	99%	97%
Discharged on Antithrombotic Therapy[5]	-	-	100%	99%
Discharged on Statin Medication[5]	-	-	93%	94%
Thrombolytic Therapy Timing[5]	-	-	75%	66%
Venous Thromboembolism Prophylaxis[5]	-	-	94%	94%
Written Stroke Educational Materials Given[5]	-	-	84%	88%
Surgical Care Improvement Project				
Appropriate Beta Blocker Usage[2]	97	98%	98%	98%
Appropriate VTP Within 24 Hours[2]	261	99%	99%	98%
Controlled Postoperative Blood Glucose[2,7]	-	-	96%	97%
Perioperative Temperature Management[2]	277	100%	100%	100%
Prophylactic Antibiotic Selection[2]	192	100%	99%	99%
Prophylactic Antibiotic Selection (Outpatient)	77	100%	99%	98%
Prophylactic Antibiotic Stopped[2]	190	98%	98%	98%
Prophylactic Antibiotic Timing[2]	192	99%	98%	99%
Prophylactic Antibiotic Timing (Outpatient)	77	100%	97%	98%
Urinary Catheter Removal[2]	141	99%	98%	97%
Survey of Patients' Hospital Experiences				
Area Around Room 'Always' Quiet at Night	300+	85%	67%	61%
Doctors 'Always' Communicated Well	300+	87%	86%	82%
Home Recovery Information Given	300+	94%	88%	85%
Hospital Given 9 or 10 on 10 Point Scale	300+	92%	78%	71%
Meds 'Always' Explained Before Given	300+	77%	68%	64%
Nurses 'Always' Communicated Well	300+	91%	83%	79%
Pain 'Always' Well Controlled	300+	78%	73%	71%
Room and Bathroom 'Always' Clean	300+	84%	81%	73%
Timely Help 'Always' Received	300+	88%	75%	68%
Would Definitely Recommend Hospital	300+	94%	77%	71%
Use of Medical Imaging				
Cardiac Imaging Stress Test before Surgery[7]	-	-	5.4%	5.3%
Combination Abdominal CT Scan[1]	-	-	9.3%	10.5%
Combination Brain/Sinus CT Scan[1]	-	-	2.7%	2.7%
Combination Chest CT Scan[1]	-	-	1.7%	2.7%
Follow-up Mammogram/Ultrasound[7]	-	-	8%	8.8%
Lumbar Spine MRI for Low Back Pain	69	36.2%	36.5%	37.2%

Nebraska Spine Hospital

6901 North 72nd Street, Suite 20300
Omaha, NE 68122
Phone: 402-572-3000
Type: Acute Care Hospitals
Emergency Services: No
Ownership: Proprietary

Measure	Cases	This Hosp.	State Avg.	U.S. Avg.
Blood Clot Prevention and Treatment				
Anticoagulation Overlap Therapy[1,2]	-	-	93%	93%
ICU Venous Thromboembolism Prophylaxis[2,7]	-	-	91%	92%
Incidence of Potentially Preventable VTE[1,2]	-	-	11%	10%
UFH with Dosages/Platelet Monitoring[1,2]	-	-	98%	97%
Venous Thromboembolism Prophylaxis[2]	335	99%	88%	85%
Warfarin Therapy Discharge Instructions[1,2]	-	-	81%	75%
Chest Pain/Possible Heart Attack Care				
Aspirin Given Within 24 Hours of Arrival[5]	-	-	96%	96%
Fibrinolytic Meds Within 30 Min. of Arrival[5]	-	-	53%	58%
Average Time to ECG (minutes)[5]	-	-	8	7
Average Time to Transfer (minutes)[5]	-	-	76	60
Children's Asthma Care				
Received Home Management Plan of Care	-	-	-	88%
Received Reliever Medication	-	-	-	100%
Received Systemic Corticosteroids	-	-	-	100%
Emergency Department				
Admittance Decision Time (minutes)[2,7]	-	-	75	98
Head CT Results Within 45 Min. of Arrival[5]	-	-	61%	57%
Patients Who Left ER Before Being Seen[5]	-	-	1%	2%
Time from ER Arrival to Admit. (minutes)[2,7]	-	-	207	274
Time from ER Arrival to Discharge (minutes)[5]	-	-	118	134
Time in ER Before Being Evaluated (minutes)[5]	-	-	21	26
Time to Pain Meds for Fractures (minutes)[5]	-	-	42	57
Heart Attack Care				
Aspirin Given at Discharge[5]	-	-	100%	99%
Fibrinolytic Meds Within 30 Min. of Arrival[5]	-	-	-	54%
PCI Within 90 Minutes of Arrival[5]	-	-	96%	96%
Statin Prescribed at Discharge[5]	-	-	99%	98%
Heart Failure Care				
ACE Inhibitor or ARB for LVSD[5]	-	-	96%	97%
Discharge Instructions Given[5]	-	-	93%	94%
Evaluation of LVS Function[5]	-	-	98%	99%
Medicare Spending				
Medicare Spending per Patient (ratio)	-	1.03	0.97	0.98
Pneumonia Care				
Appropriate Initial Antibiotic Given[5]	-	-	95%	95%
Blood Culture Timing[5]	-	-	99%	98%
Pregnancy and Delivery Care				
Newborn Deliveries Scheduled Early[7]	-	-	5%	6%
Preventive Care				
Immunization for Influenza[2]	311	99%	89%	90%
Immunization for Pneumonia[2]	337	89%	90%	92%
Stroke Care				
Anticoagulation Therapy for Atrial Fibrillation[5]	-	-	95%	95%
Antithrombotic Therapy Timing[5]	-	-	99%	98%
Assessed for Rehabilitation[5]	-	-	99%	97%
Discharged on Antithrombotic Therapy[5]	-	-	100%	99%
Discharged on Statin Medication[5]	-	-	93%	94%
Thrombolytic Therapy Timing[5]	-	-	75%	66%
Venous Thromboembolism Prophylaxis[5]	-	-	94%	94%
Written Stroke Educational Materials Given[5]	-	-	84%	88%
Surgical Care Improvement Project				
Appropriate Beta Blocker Usage[5]	-	-	98%	98%
Appropriate VTP Within 24 Hours[5]	-	-	99%	98%
Controlled Postoperative Blood Glucose[5]	-	-	96%	97%
Perioperative Temperature Management[5]	-	-	100%	100%
Prophylactic Antibiotic Selection[5]	-	-	99%	99%
Prophylactic Antibiotic Selection (Outpatient)	331	100%	99%	98%
Prophylactic Antibiotic Stopped[5]	-	-	98%	98%
Prophylactic Antibiotic Timing[5]	-	-	98%	99%
Prophylactic Antibiotic Timing (Outpatient)	331	99%	97%	98%
Urinary Catheter Removal[5]	-	-	98%	97%
Survey of Patients' Hospital Experiences				
Area Around Room 'Always' Quiet at Night	300+	71%	67%	61%
Doctors 'Always' Communicated Well	300+	82%	86%	82%
Home Recovery Information Given	300+	93%	88%	85%
Hospital Given 9 or 10 on 10 Point Scale	300+	82%	78%	71%
Meds 'Always' Explained Before Given	300+	71%	68%	64%
Nurses 'Always' Communicated Well	300+	84%	83%	79%
Pain 'Always' Well Controlled	300+	68%	73%	71%
Room and Bathroom 'Always' Clean	300+	75%	81%	73%
Timely Help 'Always' Received	300+	72%	75%	68%
Would Definitely Recommend Hospital	300+	82%	77%	71%
Use of Medical Imaging				
Cardiac Imaging Stress Test before Surgery[7]	-	-	5.4%	5.3%
Combination Abdominal CT Scan[7]	-	-	9.3%	10.5%
Combination Brain/Sinus CT Scan[7]	-	-	2.7%	2.7%
Combination Chest CT Scan[7]	-	-	1.7%	2.7%
Follow-up Mammogram/Ultrasound[7]	-	-	8%	8.8%
Lumbar Spine MRI for Low Back Pain[7]	-	-	36.5%	37.2%

Omaha VA Medical Center

4101 Woolworth Avenue
Omaha, NE 68105
URL: www.va.gov
Phone: 402-346-8800
Fax: 402-449-0618
Type: Acute Care - VA
Emergency Services: No
Ownership: Government Federal
Beds: 100

Key Personnel:
CEO/President. . . . . John J Phillips
Quality Assurance . . . . Shirley A Simons
Chief of Medical Staff. . . . . Rowen K Zetterman, MD

Measure	Cases	This Hosp.	State Avg.	U.S. Avg.
Blood Clot Prevention and Treatment				
Anticoagulation Overlap Therapy	-	-	93%	93%
ICU Venous Thromboembolism Prophylaxis	-	-	91%	92%
Incidence of Potentially Preventable VTE	-	-	11%	10%
UFH with Dosages/Platelet Monitoring	-	-	98%	97%
Venous Thromboembolism Prophylaxis	-	-	88%	85%
Warfarin Therapy Discharge Instructions	-	-	81%	75%
Chest Pain/Possible Heart Attack Care				
Aspirin Given Within 24 Hours of Arrival	-	-	96%	96%
Fibrinolytic Meds Within 30 Min. of Arrival	-	-	53%	58%
Average Time to ECG (minutes)	-	-	8	7
Average Time to Transfer (minutes)	-	-	76	60
Children's Asthma Care				
Received Home Management Plan of Care	-	-	-	88%
Received Reliever Medication	-	-	-	100%
Received Systemic Corticosteroids	-	-	-	100%
Emergency Department				
Admittance Decision Time (minutes)	-	-	75	98
Head CT Results Within 45 Min. of Arrival	-	-	61%	57%
Patients Who Left ER Before Being Seen	-	-	1%	2%
Time from ER Arrival to Admit. (minutes)	-	-	207	274
Time from ER Arrival to Discharge (minutes)	-	-	118	134
Time in ER Before Being Evaluated (minutes)	-	-	21	26
Time to Pain Meds for Fractures (minutes)	-	-	42	57
Heart Attack Care				
Aspirin Given at Discharge[5]	-	-	100%	99%
Fibrinolytic Meds Within 30 Min. of Arrival[5]	-	-	-	54%
PCI Within 90 Minutes of Arrival[5]	-	-	96%	96%
Statin Prescribed at Discharge[5]	-	-	99%	98%
Heart Failure Care				
ACE Inhibitor or ARB for LVSD	54	98%	96%	97%
Discharge Instructions Given	137	89%	93%	94%
Evaluation of LVS Function	156	100%	98%	99%
Medicare Spending				
Medicare Spending per Patient (ratio)	-	-	0.97	0.98
Pneumonia Care				
Appropriate Initial Antibiotic Given	28	96%	95%	95%
Blood Culture Timing	50	98%	99%	98%
Pregnancy and Delivery Care				
Newborn Deliveries Scheduled Early	-	-	5%	6%
Preventive Care				
Immunization for Influenza[5]	-	-	89%	90%
Immunization for Pneumonia[5]	-	-	90%	92%
Stroke Care				
Anticoagulation Therapy for Atrial Fibrillation	-	-	95%	95%
Antithrombotic Therapy Timing	-	-	99%	98%

NOTE: Hospital profiles are in alphabetical order by state, then city, then hospital within the city; Rankings exclude hospitals with less than 25 cases except for patient surveys which excludes hospitals with less than 100 cases; (a) 100-299 cases; (1) The number of cases/patients is too few to report; (2) Data submitted were based on a sample of cases/patients; (3) Results are based on a shorter time period than required; (4) Data suppressed by CMS for one or more quarters; (5) Results are not available for this reporting period; (6) Fewer than 100 patients completed the HCAHPS survey; (7) No cases met the criteria for this measure; (8) The lower limit of the confidence interval cannot be calculated if the number of observed infections equals zero; (9) No data are available from the state/territory for this reporting period; (10) The scores shown reflect fewer than 50 completed surveys; (11) There were discrepancies in the data collection process; (12) This measure does not apply to this hospital for this reporting period; (13) Results cannot be calculated for this reporting period; (14) The results for this state are combined with nearby states to protect confidentiality; Please refer to the User's Guide for a full explanation of data.

Measure	Cases	This Hosp.	State Avg.	U.S. Avg.
Assessed for Rehabilitation	-	-	99%	97%
Discharged on Antithrombotic Therapy	-	-	100%	99%
Discharged on Statin Medication	-	-	93%	94%
Thrombolytic Therapy Timing	-	-	75%	66%
Venous Thromboembolism Prophylaxis	-	-	94%	94%
Written Stroke Educational Materials Given	-	-	84%	88%
Surgical Care Improvement Project				
Appropriate Beta Blocker Usage[2]	94	95%	98%	98%
Appropriate VTP Within 24 Hours[2]	195	99%	99%	98%
Controlled Postoperative Blood Glucose[5]	-	-	96%	97%
Perioperative Temperature Management[2]	235	100%	100%	100%
Prophylactic Antibiotic Selection	151	99%	99%	99%
Prophylactic Antibiotic Selection (Outpatient)	-	-	99%	98%
Prophylactic Antibiotic Stopped	151	97%	98%	98%
Prophylactic Antibiotic Timing	154	79%	98%	99%
Prophylactic Antibiotic Timing (Outpatient)	-	-	97%	98%
Urinary Catheter Removal[2]	158	99%	98%	97%
Survey of Patients' Hospital Experiences				
Area Around Room 'Always' Quiet at Night	-	-	67%	61%
Doctors 'Always' Communicated Well	-	-	86%	82%
Home Recovery Information Given	-	-	88%	85%
Hospital Given 9 or 10 on 10 Point Scale	-	-	78%	71%
Meds 'Always' Explained Before Given	-	-	68%	64%
Nurses 'Always' Communicated Well	-	-	83%	79%
Pain 'Always' Well Controlled	-	-	73%	71%
Room and Bathroom 'Always' Clean	-	-	81%	73%
Timely Help 'Always' Received	-	-	75%	68%
Would Definitely Recommend Hospital	-	-	77%	71%
Use of Medical Imaging				
Cardiac Imaging Stress Test before Surgery	-	-	5.4%	5.3%
Combination Abdominal CT Scan	-	-	9.3%	10.5%
Combination Brain/Sinus CT Scan	-	-	2.7%	2.7%
Combination Chest CT Scan	-	-	1.7%	2.7%
Follow-up Mammogram/Ultrasound	-	-	8%	8.8%
Lumbar Spine MRI for Low Back Pain	-	-	36.5%	37.2%

Valley County Health System

2707 L Street
Ord, NE 68862
Phone: 308-728-4200
Fax: 308-728-7809
URL: www.valleycountyhospital.org
Type: Critical Access Hospitals
Emergency Services: Yes
Ownership: Government - Local
Beds: 25

Key Personnel:
Chief of Medical Staff . . . . Jennifer Bengston
CEO/President. . . . . Dean Bither

Measure	Cases	This Hosp.	State Avg.	U.S. Avg.
Blood Clot Prevention and Treatment				
Anticoagulation Overlap Therapy[5]	-	-	93%	93%
ICU Venous Thromboembolism Prophylaxis[5]	-	-	91%	92%
Incidence of Potentially Preventable VTE[5]	-	-	11%	10%
UFH with Dosages/Platelet Monitoring[5]	-	-	98%	97%
Venous Thromboembolism Prophylaxis[5]	-	-	88%	85%
Warfarin Therapy Discharge Instructions[5]	-	-	81%	75%
Chest Pain/Possible Heart Attack Care				
Aspirin Given Within 24 Hours of Arrival	21	95%	96%	96%
Fibrinolytic Meds Within 30 Min. of Arrival[1]	-	-	53%	58%
Average Time to ECG (minutes)	21	9	8	7
Average Time to Transfer (minutes)[1]	-	-	76	60
Children's Asthma Care				
Received Home Management Plan of Care	-	-	-	88%
Received Reliever Medication	-	-	-	100%
Received Systemic Corticosteroids	-	-	-	100%
Emergency Department				
Admittance Decision Time (minutes)[5]	-	-	75	98
Head CT Results Within 45 Min. of Arrival[5]	-	-	61%	57%
Patients Who Left ER Before Being Seen[5]	-	-	1%	2%
Time from ER Arrival to Admit. (minutes)[5]	-	-	207	274
Time from ER Arrival to Discharge (minutes)[5]	-	-	118	134
Time in ER Before Being Evaluated (minutes)[5]	-	-	21	26
Time to Pain Meds for Fractures (minutes)[5]	-	-	42	57
Heart Attack Care				
Aspirin Given at Discharge[5]	-	-	100%	99%
Fibrinolytic Meds Within 30 Min. of Arrival[5]	-	-	-	54%
PCI Within 90 Minutes of Arrival[5]	-	-	96%	96%
Statin Prescribed at Discharge[5]	-	-	99%	98%
Heart Failure Care				
ACE Inhibitor or ARB for LVSD[1]	-	-	96%	97%
Discharge Instructions Given[1]	-	-	93%	94%
Evaluation of LVS Function[1]	-	-	98%	99%
Medicare Spending				
Medicare Spending per Patient (ratio)	-	-	0.97	0.98
Pneumonia Care				
Appropriate Initial Antibiotic Given	28	100%	95%	95%
Blood Culture Timing	21	100%	99%	98%
Pregnancy and Delivery Care				
Newborn Deliveries Scheduled Early[5]	-	-	5%	6%
Preventive Care				
Immunization for Influenza[5]	-	-	89%	90%
Immunization for Pneumonia[5]	-	-	90%	92%
Stroke Care				
Anticoagulation Therapy for Atrial Fibrillation[5]	-	-	95%	95%
Antithrombotic Therapy Timing[5]	-	-	99%	98%
Assessed for Rehabilitation[5]	-	-	99%	97%
Discharged on Antithrombotic Therapy[5]	-	-	100%	99%
Discharged on Statin Medication[5]	-	-	93%	94%
Thrombolytic Therapy Timing[5]	-	-	75%	66%
Venous Thromboembolism Prophylaxis[5]	-	-	94%	94%
Written Stroke Educational Materials Given[5]	-	-	84%	88%
Surgical Care Improvement Project				
Appropriate Beta Blocker Usage[5]	-	-	98%	98%
Appropriate VTP Within 24 Hours[5]	-	-	99%	98%
Controlled Postoperative Blood Glucose[5]	-	-	96%	97%
Perioperative Temperature Management[5]	-	-	100%	100%
Prophylactic Antibiotic Selection[5]	-	-	99%	99%
Prophylactic Antibiotic Selection (Outpatient)[5]	-	-	99%	98%
Prophylactic Antibiotic Stopped[5]	-	-	98%	98%
Prophylactic Antibiotic Timing[5]	-	-	98%	99%
Prophylactic Antibiotic Timing (Outpatient)[5]	-	-	97%	98%
Urinary Catheter Removal[5]	-	-	98%	97%
Survey of Patients' Hospital Experiences				
Area Around Room 'Always' Quiet at Night[10]	<100	55%	67%	61%
Doctors 'Always' Communicated Well[10]	<100	90%	86%	82%
Home Recovery Information Given[10]	<100	79%	88%	85%
Hospital Given 9 or 10 on 10 Point Scale[10]	<100	80%	78%	71%
Meds 'Always' Explained Before Given[10]	<100	81%	68%	64%
Nurses 'Always' Communicated Well[10]	<100	82%	83%	79%
Pain 'Always' Well Controlled[10]	<100	66%	73%	71%
Room and Bathroom 'Always' Clean[10]	<100	80%	81%	73%
Timely Help 'Always' Received[10]	<100	66%	75%	68%
Would Definitely Recommend Hospital[10]	<100	69%	77%	71%
Use of Medical Imaging				
Cardiac Imaging Stress Test before Surgery	82	1.2%	5.4%	5.3%
Combination Abdominal CT Scan	74	1.4%	9.3%	10.5%
Combination Brain/Sinus CT Scan[1]	-	-	2.7%	2.7%
Combination Chest CT Scan	55	0.0%	1.7%	2.7%
Follow-up Mammogram/Ultrasound	130	9.2%	8%	8.8%
Lumbar Spine MRI for Low Back Pain[1]	-	-	36.5%	37.2%

Annie Jeffrey Memorial County Health Center

PO Box 428, 531 Beebe St
Osceola, NE 68651
Phone: 402-747-2031
Fax: 402-747-1405
E-mail: smjohnston89@yahoo.com
URL: www.anniejeffreyhospital.org
Type: Critical Access Hospitals
Emergency Services: Yes
Ownership: Government - Local
Beds: 21

Key Personnel:
CEO/President. . . . . Kevin A Foote
Emergency Room . . . . Chris Gabel
Quality Assurance . . . . Chassidy McCreless
Anesthesiology. . . . . Tom McKenny
Operating Room. . . . . Stephen Nagengast

Measure	Cases	This Hosp.	State Avg.	U.S. Avg.
Blood Clot Prevention and Treatment				
Anticoagulation Overlap Therapy[5]	-	-	93%	93%
ICU Venous Thromboembolism Prophylaxis[5]	-	-	91%	92%
Incidence of Potentially Preventable VTE[5]	-	-	11%	10%
UFH with Dosages/Platelet Monitoring[5]	-	-	98%	97%
Venous Thromboembolism Prophylaxis[5]	-	-	88%	85%
Warfarin Therapy Discharge Instructions[5]	-	-	81%	75%
Chest Pain/Possible Heart Attack Care				
Aspirin Given Within 24 Hours of Arrival[1,3]	-	-	96%	96%
Fibrinolytic Meds Within 30 Min. of Arrival[5]	-	-	53%	58%
Average Time to ECG (minutes)[1,3]	-	-	8	7
Average Time to Transfer (minutes)[5]	-	-	76	60
Children's Asthma Care				
Received Home Management Plan of Care	-	-	-	88%
Received Reliever Medication	-	-	-	100%
Received Systemic Corticosteroids	-	-	-	100%
Emergency Department				
Admittance Decision Time (minutes)[5]	-	-	75	98
Head CT Results Within 45 Min. of Arrival[5]	-	-	61%	57%
Patients Who Left ER Before Being Seen[5]	-	-	1%	2%
Time from ER Arrival to Admit. (minutes)[5]	-	-	207	274
Time from ER Arrival to Discharge (minutes)[5]	-	-	118	134
Time in ER Before Being Evaluated (minutes)[5]	-	-	21	26
Time to Pain Meds for Fractures (minutes)[5]	-	-	42	57
Heart Attack Care				
Aspirin Given at Discharge[5]	-	-	100%	99%
Fibrinolytic Meds Within 30 Min. of Arrival[5]	-	-	-	54%
PCI Within 90 Minutes of Arrival[5]	-	-	96%	96%
Statin Prescribed at Discharge[5]	-	-	99%	98%
Heart Failure Care				
ACE Inhibitor or ARB for LVSD[1,3]	-	-	96%	97%
Discharge Instructions Given[1,3]	-	-	93%	94%
Evaluation of LVS Function[1,3]	-	-	98%	99%
Medicare Spending				
Medicare Spending per Patient (ratio)	-	-	0.97	0.98
Pneumonia Care				
Appropriate Initial Antibiotic Given[1]	-	-	95%	95%
Blood Culture Timing[1]	-	-	99%	98%
Pregnancy and Delivery Care				
Newborn Deliveries Scheduled Early[5]	-	-	5%	6%
Preventive Care				
Immunization for Influenza[5]	-	-	89%	90%
Immunization for Pneumonia[5]	-	-	90%	92%
Stroke Care				
Anticoagulation Therapy for Atrial Fibrillation[5]	-	-	95%	95%
Antithrombotic Therapy Timing[5]	-	-	99%	98%
Assessed for Rehabilitation[5]	-	-	99%	97%
Discharged on Antithrombotic Therapy[5]	-	-	100%	99%
Discharged on Statin Medication[5]	-	-	93%	94%
Thrombolytic Therapy Timing[5]	-	-	75%	66%
Venous Thromboembolism Prophylaxis[5]	-	-	94%	94%
Written Stroke Educational Materials Given[5]	-	-	84%	88%
Surgical Care Improvement Project				
Appropriate Beta Blocker Usage[5]	-	-	98%	98%
Appropriate VTP Within 24 Hours[5]	-	-	99%	98%
Controlled Postoperative Blood Glucose[5]	-	-	96%	97%
Perioperative Temperature Management[5]	-	-	100%	100%
Prophylactic Antibiotic Selection[5]	-	-	99%	99%
Prophylactic Antibiotic Selection (Outpatient)[5]	-	-	99%	98%
Prophylactic Antibiotic Stopped[5]	-	-	98%	98%
Prophylactic Antibiotic Timing[5]	-	-	98%	99%
Prophylactic Antibiotic Timing (Outpatient)[5]	-	-	97%	98%
Urinary Catheter Removal[5]	-	-	98%	97%
Survey of Patients' Hospital Experiences				
Area Around Room 'Always' Quiet at Night[10]	<100	63%	67%	61%
Doctors 'Always' Communicated Well[10]	<100	86%	86%	82%
Home Recovery Information Given[10]	<100	81%	88%	85%
Hospital Given 9 or 10 on 10 Point Scale[10]	<100	79%	78%	71%
Meds 'Always' Explained Before Given[10]	<100	72%	68%	64%
Nurses 'Always' Communicated Well[10]	<100	83%	83%	79%
Pain 'Always' Well Controlled[10]	<100	63%	73%	71%
Room and Bathroom 'Always' Clean[10]	<100	87%	81%	73%
Timely Help 'Always' Received[10]	<100	83%	75%	68%
Would Definitely Recommend Hospital[10]	<100	70%	77%	71%
Use of Medical Imaging				
Cardiac Imaging Stress Test before Surgery[1]	-	-	5.4%	5.3%
Combination Abdominal CT Scan[1]	-	-	9.3%	10.5%

NOTE: Hospital profiles are in alphabetical order by state, then city, then hospital within the city; Rankings exclude hospitals with less than 25 cases except for patient surveys which excludes hospitals with less than 100 cases; (a) 100-299 cases; (1) The number of cases/patients is too few to report; (2) Data submitted were based on a sample of cases/patients; (3) Results are based on a shorter time period than required; (4) Data suppressed by CMS for one or more quarters; (5) Results are not available for this reporting period; (6) Fewer than 100 patients completed the HCAHPS survey; (7) No cases met the criteria for this measure; (8) The lower limit of the confidence interval cannot be calculated if the number of observed infections equals zero; (9) No data are available from the state/territory for this reporting period; (10) The scores shown reflect fewer than 50 completed surveys; (11) There were discrepancies in the data collection process; (12) This measure does not apply to this hospital for this reporting period; (13) Results cannot be calculated for this reporting period; (14) The results for this state are combined with nearby states to protect confidentiality; Please refer to the User's Guide for a full explanation of data.

Measure	Cases	This Hosp.	State Avg.	U.S. Avg.
Combination Brain/Sinus CT Scan[1]	-	-	2.7%	2.7%
Combination Chest CT Scan[1]	-	-	1.7%	2.7%
Follow-up Mammogram/Ultrasound	76	7.9%	8%	8.8%
Lumbar Spine MRI for Low Back Pain[1]	-	-	36.5%	37.2%

Garden County Health Services

1100 West 2nd St
Oshkosh, NE 69154
E-mail: ceo@gchealth.org
URL: www.gchealth.org
Phone: 308-772-3283
Fax: 308-772-0143

Type: Critical Access Hospitals
Ownership: Government - Local
Emergency Services: Yes
Beds: 10

Key Personnel:
CEO . . . . Jimmie Hansel
Chief of Medical Staff . . . . Harold Keenan, MD
Radiology . . . . Nancy Loomis

Measure	Cases	This Hosp.	State Avg.	U.S. Avg.
Blood Clot Prevention and Treatment				
Anticoagulation Overlap Therapy[5]	-	-	93%	93%
ICU Venous Thromboembolism Prophylaxis[5]	-	-	91%	92%
Incidence of Potentially Preventable VTE[5]	-	-	11%	10%
UFH with Dosages/Platelet Monitoring[5]	-	-	98%	97%
Venous Thromboembolism Prophylaxis[5]	-	-	88%	85%
Warfarin Therapy Discharge Instructions[5]	-	-	81%	75%
Chest Pain/Possible Heart Attack Care				
Aspirin Given Within 24 Hours of Arrival[1,3]	-	-	96%	96%
Fibrinolytic Meds Within 30 Min. of Arrival[3,7]	-	-	53%	58%
Average Time to ECG (minutes)[1,3]	-	-	8	7
Average Time to Transfer (minutes)[3,7]	-	-	76	60
Children's Asthma Care				
Received Home Management Plan of Care	-	-	-	88%
Received Reliever Medication	-	-	-	100%
Received Systemic Corticosteroids	-	-	-	100%
Emergency Department				
Admittance Decision Time (minutes)[5]	-	-	75	98
Head CT Results Within 45 Min. of Arrival[5]	-	-	61%	57%
Patients Who Left ER Before Being Seen[5]	-	-	1%	2%
Time from ER Arrival to Admit. (minutes)[5]	-	-	207	274
Time from ER Arrival to Discharge (minutes)[5]	-	-	118	134
Time in ER Before Being Evaluated (minutes)[5]	-	-	21	26
Time to Pain Meds for Fractures (minutes)[5]	-	-	42	57
Heart Attack Care				
Aspirin Given at Discharge[5]	-	-	100%	99%
Fibrinolytic Meds Within 30 Min. of Arrival[5]	-	-	-	54%
PCI Within 90 Minutes of Arrival[5]	-	-	96%	96%
Statin Prescribed at Discharge[5]	-	-	99%	98%
Heart Failure Care				
ACE Inhibitor or ARB for LVSD[3,7]	-	-	96%	97%
Discharge Instructions Given[1,3]	-	-	93%	94%
Evaluation of LVS Function[1,3]	-	-	98%	99%
Medicare Spending				
Medicare Spending per Patient (ratio)	-	-	0.97	0.98
Pneumonia Care				
Appropriate Initial Antibiotic Given[1]	-	-	95%	95%
Blood Culture Timing[7]	-	-	99%	98%
Pregnancy and Delivery Care				
Newborn Deliveries Scheduled Early[5]	-	-	5%	6%
Preventive Care				
Immunization for Influenza[5]	-	-	89%	90%
Immunization for Pneumonia[5]	-	-	90%	92%
Stroke Care				
Anticoagulation Therapy for Atrial Fibrillation[5]	-	-	95%	95%
Antithrombotic Therapy Timing[5]	-	-	99%	98%
Assessed for Rehabilitation[5]	-	-	99%	97%
Discharged on Antithrombotic Therapy[5]	-	-	100%	99%
Discharged on Statin Medication[5]	-	-	93%	94%
Thrombolytic Therapy Timing[5]	-	-	75%	66%
Venous Thromboembolism Prophylaxis[5]	-	-	94%	94%
Written Stroke Educational Materials Given[5]	-	-	84%	88%
Surgical Care Improvement Project				
Appropriate Beta Blocker Usage[5]	-	-	98%	98%
Appropriate VTP Within 24 Hours[5]	-	-	99%	98%
Controlled Postoperative Blood Glucose[5]	-	-	96%	97%
Perioperative Temperature Management[5]	-	-	100%	100%
Prophylactic Antibiotic Selection[5]	-	-	99%	99%
Prophylactic Antibiotic Selection (Outpatient)[5]	-	-	99%	98%
Prophylactic Antibiotic Stopped[5]	-	-	98%	98%
Prophylactic Antibiotic Timing[5]	-	-	98%	99%
Prophylactic Antibiotic Timing (Outpatient)[5]	-	-	97%	98%
Urinary Catheter Removal[5]	-	-	98%	97%
Survey of Patients' Hospital Experiences				
Area Around Room 'Always' Quiet at Night[10]	<100	80%	67%	61%
Doctors 'Always' Communicated Well[10]	<100	100%	86%	82%
Home Recovery Information Given[10]	<100	86%	88%	85%
Hospital Given 9 or 10 on 10 Point Scale[10]	<100	98%	78%	71%
Meds 'Always' Explained Before Given[10]	<100	-	68%	64%
Nurses 'Always' Communicated Well[10]	<100	99%	83%	79%
Pain 'Always' Well Controlled[10]	<100	76%	73%	71%
Room and Bathroom 'Always' Clean[10]	<100	95%	81%	73%
Timely Help 'Always' Received[10]	<100	88%	75%	68%
Would Definitely Recommend Hospital[10]	<100	98%	77%	71%
Use of Medical Imaging				
Cardiac Imaging Stress Test before Surgery[1]	-	-	5.4%	5.3%
Combination Abdominal CT Scan[1]	-	-	9.3%	10.5%
Combination Brain/Sinus CT Scan[1]	-	-	2.7%	2.7%
Combination Chest CT Scan[1]	-	-	1.7%	2.7%
Follow-up Mammogram/Ultrasound[7]	-	-	8%	8.8%
Lumbar Spine MRI for Low Back Pain[1]	-	-	36.5%	37.2%

Osmond General Hospital

PO Box 429, 402 North Maple St
Osmond, NE 68765
URL: www.osmondhospital.com
Phone: 402-748-3393
Fax: 402-748-3349

Type: Critical Access Hospitals
Ownership: Voluntary non-profit - Private
Emergency Services: Yes
Beds: 21

Key Personnel:
CEO . . . . Celine M Mlady
Infection Control . . . . Lynn Riedmiller

Measure	Cases	This Hosp.	State Avg.	U.S. Avg.
Blood Clot Prevention and Treatment				
Anticoagulation Overlap Therapy[5]	-	-	93%	93%
ICU Venous Thromboembolism Prophylaxis[5]	-	-	91%	92%
Incidence of Potentially Preventable VTE[5]	-	-	11%	10%
UFH with Dosages/Platelet Monitoring[5]	-	-	98%	97%
Venous Thromboembolism Prophylaxis[5]	-	-	88%	85%
Warfarin Therapy Discharge Instructions[5]	-	-	81%	75%
Chest Pain/Possible Heart Attack Care				
Aspirin Given Within 24 Hours of Arrival[5]	-	-	96%	96%
Fibrinolytic Meds Within 30 Min. of Arrival[5]	-	-	53%	58%
Average Time to ECG (minutes)[5]	-	-	8	7
Average Time to Transfer (minutes)[5]	-	-	76	60
Children's Asthma Care				
Received Home Management Plan of Care	-	-	-	88%
Received Reliever Medication	-	-	-	100%
Received Systemic Corticosteroids	-	-	-	100%
Emergency Department				
Admittance Decision Time (minutes)[5]	-	-	75	98
Head CT Results Within 45 Min. of Arrival[5]	-	-	61%	57%
Patients Who Left ER Before Being Seen[5]	-	-	1%	2%
Time from ER Arrival to Admit. (minutes)[5]	-	-	207	274
Time from ER Arrival to Discharge (minutes)[5]	-	-	118	134
Time in ER Before Being Evaluated (minutes)[5]	-	-	21	26
Time to Pain Meds for Fractures (minutes)[5]	-	-	42	57
Heart Attack Care				
Aspirin Given at Discharge[1,3]	-	-	100%	99%
Fibrinolytic Meds Within 30 Min. of Arrival[3,7]	-	-	-	54%
PCI Within 90 Minutes of Arrival[3,7]	-	-	96%	96%
Statin Prescribed at Discharge[1,3]	-	-	99%	98%
Heart Failure Care				
ACE Inhibitor or ARB for LVSD[3,7]	-	-	96%	97%
Discharge Instructions Given[1,3]	-	-	93%	94%
Evaluation of LVS Function[1,3]	-	-	98%	99%
Medicare Spending				
Medicare Spending per Patient (ratio)	-	-	0.97	0.98
Pneumonia Care				
Appropriate Initial Antibiotic Given[1]	-	-	95%	95%
Blood Culture Timing[7]	-	-	99%	98%
Pregnancy and Delivery Care				
Newborn Deliveries Scheduled Early[5]	-	-	5%	6%
Preventive Care				
Immunization for Influenza[5]	-	-	89%	90%
Immunization for Pneumonia[5]	-	-	90%	92%
Stroke Care				
Anticoagulation Therapy for Atrial Fibrillation[5]	-	-	95%	95%
Antithrombotic Therapy Timing[5]	-	-	99%	98%
Assessed for Rehabilitation[5]	-	-	99%	97%
Discharged on Antithrombotic Therapy[5]	-	-	100%	99%
Discharged on Statin Medication[5]	-	-	93%	94%
Thrombolytic Therapy Timing[5]	-	-	75%	66%
Venous Thromboembolism Prophylaxis[5]	-	-	94%	94%
Written Stroke Educational Materials Given[5]	-	-	84%	88%
Surgical Care Improvement Project				
Appropriate Beta Blocker Usage[5]	-	-	98%	98%
Appropriate VTP Within 24 Hours[5]	-	-	99%	98%
Controlled Postoperative Blood Glucose[5]	-	-	96%	97%
Perioperative Temperature Management[5]	-	-	100%	100%
Prophylactic Antibiotic Selection[5]	-	-	99%	99%
Prophylactic Antibiotic Selection (Outpatient)[5]	-	-	99%	98%
Prophylactic Antibiotic Stopped[5]	-	-	98%	98%
Prophylactic Antibiotic Timing[5]	-	-	98%	99%
Prophylactic Antibiotic Timing (Outpatient)[5]	-	-	97%	98%
Urinary Catheter Removal[5]	-	-	98%	97%
Survey of Patients' Hospital Experiences				
Area Around Room 'Always' Quiet at Night[6]	<100	80%	67%	61%
Doctors 'Always' Communicated Well[6]	<100	83%	86%	82%
Home Recovery Information Given[6]	<100	81%	88%	85%
Hospital Given 9 or 10 on 10 Point Scale[6]	<100	79%	78%	71%
Meds 'Always' Explained Before Given[6]	<100	75%	68%	64%
Nurses 'Always' Communicated Well[6]	<100	81%	83%	79%
Pain 'Always' Well Controlled[6]	<100	81%	73%	71%
Room and Bathroom 'Always' Clean[6]	<100	82%	81%	73%
Timely Help 'Always' Received[6]	<100	79%	75%	68%
Would Definitely Recommend Hospital[6]	<100	80%	77%	71%
Use of Medical Imaging				
Cardiac Imaging Stress Test before Surgery[1]	-	-	5.4%	5.3%
Combination Abdominal CT Scan	37	54.1%	9.3%	10.5%
Combination Brain/Sinus CT Scan[1]	-	-	2.7%	2.7%
Combination Chest CT Scan[1]	-	-	1.7%	2.7%
Follow-up Mammogram/Ultrasound	68	5.9%	8%	8.8%
Lumbar Spine MRI for Low Back Pain[1]	-	-	36.5%	37.2%

Alegent Creighton Health Midlands Hospital

11111 South 84th St
Papillion, NE 68046
URL: www.alegent.com
Phone: 402-593-3000
Fax: 402-593-3117

Type: Acute Care Hospitals
Ownership: Voluntary non-profit - Church
Emergency Services: Yes
Beds: 208

Key Personnel:
Emergency Room . . . . Maurice Birdwell
Radiology . . . . Jon Bleicher
Cardiac Laboratory . . . . Georgia Blobaum
Operating Room . . . . Lisa Campbell
Intensive Care Unit . . . . Tami Field
President/CEO . . . . Cliff Robertson, MD, MBA

Measure	Cases	This Hosp.	State Avg.	U.S. Avg.
Blood Clot Prevention and Treatment				
Anticoagulation Overlap Therapy[2]	35	89%	93%	93%
ICU Venous Thromboembolism Prophylaxis[2]	84	93%	91%	92%
Incidence of Potentially Preventable VTE[1,2]	-	-	11%	10%
UFH with Dosages/Platelet Monitoring[2]	25	100%	98%	97%
Venous Thromboembolism Prophylaxis[2]	112	89%	88%	85%
Warfarin Therapy Discharge Instructions[2]	26	81%	81%	75%
Chest Pain/Possible Heart Attack Care				
Aspirin Given Within 24 Hours of Arrival[1,3]	-	-	96%	96%
Fibrinolytic Meds Within 30 Min. of Arrival[3,7]	-	-	53%	58%
Average Time to ECG (minutes)[1,3]	-	-	8	7
Average Time to Transfer (minutes)[3,7]	-	-	76	60
Children's Asthma Care				
Received Home Management Plan of Care	-	-	-	88%
Received Reliever Medication	-	-	-	100%

NOTE: Hospital profiles are in alphabetical order by state, then city, then hospital within the city; Rankings exclude hospitals with less than 25 cases except for patient surveys which excludes hospitals with less than 100 cases; (a) 100-299 cases; (1) The number of cases/patients is too few to report; (2) Data submitted were based on a sample of cases/patients; (3) Results are based on a shorter time period than required; (4) Data suppressed by CMS for one or more quarters; (5) Results are not available for this reporting period; (6) Fewer than 100 patients completed the HCAHPS survey; (7) No cases met the criteria for this measure; (8) The lower limit of the confidence interval cannot be calculated if the number of observed infections equals zero; (9) No data are available from the state/territory for this reporting period; (10) The scores shown reflect fewer than 50 completed surveys; (11) There were discrepancies in the data collection process; (12) This measure does not apply to this hospital for this reporting period; (13) Results cannot be calculated for this reporting period; (14) The results for this state are combined with nearby states to protect confidentiality; Please refer to the User's Guide for a full explanation of data.

Measure	Cases	This Hosp.	State Avg.	U.S. Avg.
Received Systemic Corticosteroids	-	-	-	100%
Emergency Department				
Admittance Decision Time (minutes)[2]	398	84	75	98
Head CT Results Within 45 Min. of Arrival	21	86%	61%	57%
Patients Who Left ER Before Being Seen	13,469	0%	1%	2%
Time from ER Arrival to Admit. (minutes)[2]	405	212	207	274
Time from ER Arrival to Discharge (minutes)	378	126	118	134
Time in ER Before Being Evaluated (minutes)	352	39	21	26
Time to Pain Meds for Fractures (minutes)	70	52	42	57
Heart Attack Care				
Aspirin Given at Discharge	46	100%	100%	99%
Fibrinolytic Meds Within 30 Min. of Arrival[7]	-	-	-	54%
PCI Within 90 Minutes of Arrival	17	100%	96%	96%
Statin Prescribed at Discharge	46	100%	99%	98%
Heart Failure Care				
ACE Inhibitor or ARB for LVSD	18	100%	96%	97%
Discharge Instructions Given	38	100%	93%	94%
Evaluation of LVS Function	56	100%	98%	99%
Medicare Spending				
Medicare Spending per Patient (ratio)	-	1.06	0.97	0.98
Pneumonia Care				
Appropriate Initial Antibiotic Given	49	100%	95%	95%
Blood Culture Timing	86	100%	99%	98%
Pregnancy and Delivery Care				
Newborn Deliveries Scheduled Early	26	8%	5%	6%
Preventive Care				
Immunization for Influenza[2]	275	100%	89%	90%
Immunization for Pneumonia[2]	328	99%	90%	92%
Stroke Care				
Anticoagulation Therapy for Atrial Fibrillation[1]	-	-	95%	95%
Antithrombotic Therapy Timing[1]	-	-	99%	98%
Assessed for Rehabilitation[1]	-	-	99%	97%
Discharged on Antithrombotic Therapy[1]	-	-	100%	99%
Discharged on Statin Medication[1]	-	-	93%	94%
Thrombolytic Therapy Timing[7]	-	-	75%	66%
Venous Thromboembolism Prophylaxis[1]	-	-	94%	94%
Written Stroke Educational Materials Given[1]	-	-	84%	88%
Surgical Care Improvement Project				
Appropriate Beta Blocker Usage	23	96%	98%	98%
Appropriate VTP Within 24 Hours	79	99%	99%	98%
Controlled Postoperative Blood Glucose[7]	-	-	96%	97%
Perioperative Temperature Management	85	100%	100%	100%
Prophylactic Antibiotic Selection	44	100%	99%	99%
Prophylactic Antibiotic Selection (Outpatient)	110	100%	99%	98%
Prophylactic Antibiotic Stopped	44	95%	98%	98%
Prophylactic Antibiotic Timing	44	100%	98%	99%
Prophylactic Antibiotic Timing (Outpatient)	111	98%	97%	98%
Urinary Catheter Removal	55	100%	98%	97%
Survey of Patients' Hospital Experiences				
Area Around Room 'Always' Quiet at Night	(a)	63%	67%	61%
Doctors 'Always' Communicated Well	(a)	82%	86%	82%
Home Recovery Information Given	(a)	90%	88%	85%
Hospital Given 9 or 10 on 10 Point Scale	(a)	78%	78%	71%
Meds 'Always' Explained Before Given	(a)	64%	68%	64%
Nurses 'Always' Communicated Well	(a)	82%	83%	79%
Pain 'Always' Well Controlled	(a)	75%	73%	71%
Room and Bathroom 'Always' Clean	(a)	78%	81%	73%
Timely Help 'Always' Received	(a)	67%	75%	68%
Would Definitely Recommend Hospital	(a)	76%	77%	71%
Use of Medical Imaging				
Cardiac Imaging Stress Test before Surgery	271	8.1%	5.4%	5.3%
Combination Abdominal CT Scan	312	12.2%	9.3%	10.5%
Combination Brain/Sinus CT Scan[1]	-	-	2.7%	2.7%
Combination Chest CT Scan	220	4.1%	1.7%	2.7%
Follow-up Mammogram/Ultrasound	1,173	4.7%	8%	8.8%
Lumbar Spine MRI for Low Back Pain	73	35.6%	36.5%	37.2%

Pawnee County Memorial Hospital

PO Box 433, 600 I St — Phone: 402-852-2231
Pawnee City, NE 68420 — Fax: 402-852-2098
Type: Critical Access Hospitals — Emergency Services: Yes
Ownership: Government - Local — Beds: 17
Key Personnel:
Chief of Medical Staff.......... Richard Jackson

Measure	Cases	This Hosp.	State Avg.	U.S. Avg.
Blood Clot Prevention and Treatment				
Anticoagulation Overlap Therapy[5]	-	-	93%	93%
ICU Venous Thromboembolism Prophylaxis[5]	-	-	91%	92%
Incidence of Potentially Preventable VTE[5]	-	-	11%	10%
UFH with Dosages/Platelet Monitoring[5]	-	-	98%	97%
Venous Thromboembolism Prophylaxis[5]	-	-	88%	85%
Warfarin Therapy Discharge Instructions[5]	-	-	81%	75%
Chest Pain/Possible Heart Attack Care				
Aspirin Given Within 24 Hours of Arrival	27	93%	96%	96%
Fibrinolytic Meds Within 30 Min. of Arrival[1]	-	-	53%	58%
Average Time to ECG (minutes)	27	7	8	7
Average Time to Transfer (minutes)[7]	-	-	76	60
Children's Asthma Care				
Received Home Management Plan of Care	-	-	-	88%
Received Reliever Medication	-	-	-	100%
Received Systemic Corticosteroids	-	-	-	100%
Emergency Department				
Admittance Decision Time (minutes)[5]	-	-	75	98
Head CT Results Within 45 Min. of Arrival[5]	-	-	61%	57%
Patients Who Left ER Before Being Seen[5]	-	-	1%	2%
Time from ER Arrival to Admit. (minutes)[5]	-	-	207	274
Time from ER Arrival to Discharge (minutes)[5]	-	-	118	134
Time in ER Before Being Evaluated (minutes)[5]	-	-	21	26
Time to Pain Meds for Fractures (minutes)[5]	-	-	42	57
Heart Attack Care				
Aspirin Given at Discharge[5]	-	-	100%	99%
Fibrinolytic Meds Within 30 Min. of Arrival[5]	-	-	-	54%
PCI Within 90 Minutes of Arrival[5]	-	-	96%	96%
Statin Prescribed at Discharge[5]	-	-	99%	98%
Heart Failure Care				
ACE Inhibitor or ARB for LVSD[1,3]	-	-	96%	97%
Discharge Instructions Given[1,3]	-	-	93%	94%
Evaluation of LVS Function[1,3]	-	-	98%	99%
Medicare Spending				
Medicare Spending per Patient (ratio)	-	-	0.97	0.98
Pneumonia Care				
Appropriate Initial Antibiotic Given[1,3]	-	-	95%	95%
Blood Culture Timing[1,3]	-	-	99%	98%
Pregnancy and Delivery Care				
Newborn Deliveries Scheduled Early[5]	-	-	5%	6%
Preventive Care				
Immunization for Influenza[5]	-	-	89%	90%
Immunization for Pneumonia[5]	-	-	90%	92%
Stroke Care				
Anticoagulation Therapy for Atrial Fibrillation[5]	-	-	95%	95%
Antithrombotic Therapy Timing[5]	-	-	99%	98%
Assessed for Rehabilitation[5]	-	-	99%	97%
Discharged on Antithrombotic Therapy[5]	-	-	100%	99%
Discharged on Statin Medication[5]	-	-	93%	94%
Thrombolytic Therapy Timing[5]	-	-	75%	66%
Venous Thromboembolism Prophylaxis[5]	-	-	94%	94%
Written Stroke Educational Materials Given[5]	-	-	84%	88%
Surgical Care Improvement Project				
Appropriate Beta Blocker Usage[5]	-	-	98%	98%
Appropriate VTP Within 24 Hours[5]	-	-	99%	98%
Controlled Postoperative Blood Glucose[5]	-	-	96%	97%
Perioperative Temperature Management[5]	-	-	100%	100%
Prophylactic Antibiotic Selection[5]	-	-	99%	99%
Prophylactic Antibiotic Selection (Outpatient)[5]	-	-	99%	98%
Prophylactic Antibiotic Stopped[5]	-	-	98%	98%
Prophylactic Antibiotic Timing[5]	-	-	98%	99%
Prophylactic Antibiotic Timing (Outpatient)[5]	-	-	97%	98%
Urinary Catheter Removal[5]	-	-	98%	97%
Survey of Patients' Hospital Experiences				
Area Around Room 'Always' Quiet at Night[5]	-	-	67%	61%
Doctors 'Always' Communicated Well[5]	-	-	86%	82%
Home Recovery Information Given[5]	-	-	88%	85%
Hospital Given 9 or 10 on 10 Point Scale[5]	-	-	78%	71%
Meds 'Always' Explained Before Given[5]	-	-	68%	64%
Nurses 'Always' Communicated Well[5]	-	-	83%	79%
Pain 'Always' Well Controlled[5]	-	-	73%	71%
Room and Bathroom 'Always' Clean[5]	-	-	81%	73%
Timely Help 'Always' Received[5]	-	-	75%	68%
Would Definitely Recommend Hospital[5]	-	-	77%	71%
Use of Medical Imaging				
Cardiac Imaging Stress Test before Surgery[1]	-	-	5.4%	5.3%
Combination Abdominal CT Scan[1]	-	-	9.3%	10.5%
Combination Brain/Sinus CT Scan[1]	-	-	2.7%	2.7%
Combination Chest CT Scan[1]	-	-	1.7%	2.7%
Follow-up Mammogram/Ultrasound	120	9.2%	8%	8.8%
Lumbar Spine MRI for Low Back Pain[1]	-	-	36.5%	37.2%

Pender Community Hospital

PO Box 100, 100 Hospital Drive — Phone: 402-385-3083
Pender, NE 68047 — Fax: 402-385-2155
URL: www.pendercommunityhospital.com
Type: Critical Access Hospitals — Emergency Services: Yes
Ownership: Govt - Hospital Dist/Auth — Beds: 47
Key Personnel:
Quality Assurance .... Gail Brondum
CEO/President.............. Michael Hansen, FACHE
Operating Room.............. Sue Hansen, RN
Chief of Medical Staff.......... David Hollting
Chairman/CEO .... Brian Kent
Radiology.................. Flora Lehmkuhl
Emergency Room .... Dee Moeller
Anesthesiology.............. Jerry VandeBrug

Measure	Cases	This Hosp.	State Avg.	U.S. Avg.
Blood Clot Prevention and Treatment				
Anticoagulation Overlap Therapy[5]	-	-	93%	93%
ICU Venous Thromboembolism Prophylaxis[5]	-	-	91%	92%
Incidence of Potentially Preventable VTE[5]	-	-	11%	10%
UFH with Dosages/Platelet Monitoring[5]	-	-	98%	97%
Venous Thromboembolism Prophylaxis[5]	-	-	88%	85%
Warfarin Therapy Discharge Instructions[5]	-	-	81%	75%
Chest Pain/Possible Heart Attack Care				
Aspirin Given Within 24 Hours of Arrival	11	91%	96%	96%
Fibrinolytic Meds Within 30 Min. of Arrival[1,3]	-	-	53%	58%
Average Time to ECG (minutes)	11	9	8	7
Average Time to Transfer (minutes)[1,3]	-	-	76	60
Children's Asthma Care				
Received Home Management Plan of Care	-	-	-	88%
Received Reliever Medication	-	-	-	100%
Received Systemic Corticosteroids	-	-	-	100%
Emergency Department				
Admittance Decision Time (minutes)[5]	-	-	75	98
Head CT Results Within 45 Min. of Arrival[5]	-	-	61%	57%
Patients Who Left ER Before Being Seen[5]	-	-	1%	2%
Time from ER Arrival to Admit. (minutes)[5]	-	-	207	274
Time from ER Arrival to Discharge (minutes)[5]	-	-	118	134
Time in ER Before Being Evaluated (minutes)[5]	-	-	21	26
Time to Pain Meds for Fractures (minutes)[5]	-	-	42	57
Heart Attack Care				
Aspirin Given at Discharge[1,3]	-	-	100%	99%
Fibrinolytic Meds Within 30 Min. of Arrival[3,7]	-	-	-	54%
PCI Within 90 Minutes of Arrival[3,7]	-	-	96%	96%
Statin Prescribed at Discharge[1,3]	-	-	99%	98%
Heart Failure Care				
ACE Inhibitor or ARB for LVSD[1,3]	-	-	96%	97%
Discharge Instructions Given[1,3]	-	-	93%	94%
Evaluation of LVS Function[3]	15	93%	98%	99%
Medicare Spending				
Medicare Spending per Patient (ratio)	-	-	0.97	0.98
Pneumonia Care				
Appropriate Initial Antibiotic Given	22	100%	95%	95%
Blood Culture Timing[1]	-	-	99%	98%
Pregnancy and Delivery Care				
Newborn Deliveries Scheduled Early[5]	-	-	5%	6%
Preventive Care				
Immunization for Influenza[5]	-	-	89%	90%
Immunization for Pneumonia[5]	-	-	90%	92%
Stroke Care				
Anticoagulation Therapy for Atrial Fibrillation[5]	-	-	95%	95%
Antithrombotic Therapy Timing[5]	-	-	99%	98%
Assessed for Rehabilitation[5]	-	-	99%	97%

NOTE: Hospital profiles are in alphabetical order by state, then city, then hospital within the city; Rankings exclude hospitals with less than 25 cases except for patient surveys which excludes hospitals with less than 100 cases; (a) 100-299 cases; (1) The number of cases/patients is too few to report; (2) Data submitted were based on a sample of cases/patients; (3) Results are based on a shorter time period than required; (4) Data suppressed by CMS for one or more quarters; (5) Results are not available for this reporting period; (6) Fewer than 100 patients completed the HCAHPS survey; (7) No cases met the criteria for this measure; (8) The lower limit of the confidence interval cannot be calculated if the number of observed infections equals zero; (9) No data are available from the state/territory for this reporting period; (10) The scores shown reflect fewer than 50 completed surveys; (11) There were discrepancies in the data collection process; (12) This measure does not apply to this hospital for this reporting period; (13) Results cannot be calculated for this reporting period; (14) The results for this state are combined with nearby states to protect confidentiality; Please refer to the User's Guide for a full explanation of data.

Measure	Cases	This Hosp.	State Avg.	U.S. Avg.
Discharged on Antithrombotic Therapy[5]	-	-	100%	99%
Discharged on Statin Medication[5]	-	-	93%	94%
Thrombolytic Therapy Timing[5]	-	-	75%	66%
Venous Thromboembolism Prophylaxis[5]	-	-	94%	94%
Written Stroke Educational Materials Given[5]	-	-	84%	88%
Surgical Care Improvement Project				
Appropriate Beta Blocker Usage[1]	-	-	98%	98%
Appropriate VTP Within 24 Hours[1]	-	-	99%	98%
Controlled Postoperative Blood Glucose[7]	-	-	96%	97%
Perioperative Temperature Management[1]	-	-	100%	100%
Prophylactic Antibiotic Selection[1]	-	-	99%	99%
Prophylactic Antibiotic Selection (Outpatient)[1]	-	-	99%	98%
Prophylactic Antibiotic Stopped[1]	-	-	98%	98%
Prophylactic Antibiotic Timing[1]	-	-	98%	99%
Prophylactic Antibiotic Timing (Outpatient)[1]	-	-	97%	98%
Urinary Catheter Removal[1]	-	-	98%	97%
Survey of Patients' Hospital Experiences				
Area Around Room 'Always' Quiet at Night	(a)	79%	67%	61%
Doctors 'Always' Communicated Well	(a)	95%	86%	82%
Home Recovery Information Given	(a)	92%	88%	85%
Hospital Given 9 or 10 on 10 Point Scale	(a)	86%	78%	71%
Meds 'Always' Explained Before Given	(a)	77%	68%	64%
Nurses 'Always' Communicated Well	(a)	91%	83%	79%
Pain 'Always' Well Controlled	(a)	79%	73%	71%
Room and Bathroom 'Always' Clean	(a)	89%	81%	73%
Timely Help 'Always' Received	(a)	80%	75%	68%
Would Definitely Recommend Hospital	(a)	88%	77%	71%
Use of Medical Imaging				
Cardiac Imaging Stress Test before Surgery[1]	-	-	5.4%	5.3%
Combination Abdominal CT Scan[1]	-	-	9.3%	10.5%
Combination Brain/Sinus CT Scan[1]	-	-	2.7%	2.7%
Combination Chest CT Scan[1]	-	-	1.7%	2.7%
Follow-up Mammogram/Ultrasound	112	3.6%	8%	8.8%
Lumbar Spine MRI for Low Back Pain[1]	-	-	36.5%	37.2%

Alegent Creighton Health Plainview Hospital

PO Box 489, 704 North Third St
Plainview, NE 68769
Type: Critical Access Hospitals
Ownership: Government - Local
Phone: 402-582-4245
Fax: 402-582-3940
Emergency Services: Yes
Beds: 20

Key Personnel:
Cardiac Laboratory............ Jill Anson, RN
Chief of Medical Staff.......... Edward Botha, MD
Operating Room............. Nancy Green, RD
CEO/President............... Bryan Roby
Emergency Room .... Deb Rutledge, RN

Measure	Cases	This Hosp.	State Avg.	U.S. Avg.
Blood Clot Prevention and Treatment				
Anticoagulation Overlap Therapy[3,7]	-	-	93%	93%
ICU Venous Thromboembolism Prophylaxis[3,7]	-	-	91%	92%
Incidence of Potentially Preventable VTE[3,7]	-	-	11%	10%
UFH with Dosages/Platelet Monitoring[3,7]	-	-	98%	97%
Venous Thromboembolism Prophylaxis[3]	53	94%	88%	85%
Warfarin Therapy Discharge Instructions[3,7]	-	-	81%	75%
Chest Pain/Possible Heart Attack Care				
Aspirin Given Within 24 Hours of Arrival[5]	-	-	96%	96%
Fibrinolytic Meds Within 30 Min. of Arrival[5]	-	-	53%	58%
Average Time to ECG (minutes)[5]	-	-	8	7
Average Time to Transfer (minutes)[5]	-	-	76	60
Children's Asthma Care				
Received Home Management Plan of Care	-	-	-	88%
Received Reliever Medication	-	-	-	100%
Received Systemic Corticosteroids	-	-	-	100%
Emergency Department				
Admittance Decision Time (minutes)[5]	-	-	75	98
Head CT Results Within 45 Min. of Arrival[5]	-	-	61%	57%
Patients Who Left ER Before Being Seen[5]	-	-	1%	2%
Time from ER Arrival to Admit. (minutes)[5]	-	-	207	274
Time from ER Arrival to Discharge (minutes)[5]	-	-	118	134
Time in ER Before Being Evaluated (minutes)[5]	-	-	21	26
Time to Pain Meds for Fractures (minutes)[5]	-	-	42	57
Heart Attack Care				
Aspirin Given at Discharge[1,3]	-	-	100%	99%
Fibrinolytic Meds Within 30 Min. of Arrival[3,7]	-	-	-	54%
PCI Within 90 Minutes of Arrival[3,7]	-	-	96%	96%
Statin Prescribed at Discharge[1,3]	-	-	99%	98%
Heart Failure Care				
ACE Inhibitor or ARB for LVSD[3,7]	-	-	96%	97%
Discharge Instructions Given[1,3]	-	-	93%	94%
Evaluation of LVS Function[1,3]	-	-	98%	99%
Medicare Spending				
Medicare Spending per Patient (ratio)	-	-	0.97	0.98
Pneumonia Care				
Appropriate Initial Antibiotic Given[1]	-	-	95%	95%
Blood Culture Timing[1]	-	-	99%	98%
Pregnancy and Delivery Care				
Newborn Deliveries Scheduled Early[5]	-	-	5%	6%
Preventive Care				
Immunization for Influenza[5]	-	-	89%	90%
Immunization for Pneumonia[5]	-	-	90%	92%
Stroke Care				
Anticoagulation Therapy for Atrial Fibrillation[5]	-	-	95%	95%
Antithrombotic Therapy Timing[5]	-	-	99%	98%
Assessed for Rehabilitation[5]	-	-	99%	97%
Discharged on Antithrombotic Therapy[5]	-	-	100%	99%
Discharged on Statin Medication[5]	-	-	93%	94%
Thrombolytic Therapy Timing[5]	-	-	75%	66%
Venous Thromboembolism Prophylaxis[5]	-	-	94%	94%
Written Stroke Educational Materials Given[5]	-	-	84%	88%
Surgical Care Improvement Project				
Appropriate Beta Blocker Usage[5]	-	-	98%	98%
Appropriate VTP Within 24 Hours[5]	-	-	99%	98%
Controlled Postoperative Blood Glucose[5]	-	-	96%	97%
Perioperative Temperature Management[5]	-	-	100%	100%
Prophylactic Antibiotic Selection[5]	-	-	99%	99%
Prophylactic Antibiotic Selection (Outpatient)[1,3]	-	-	99%	98%
Prophylactic Antibiotic Stopped[5]	-	-	98%	98%
Prophylactic Antibiotic Timing[5]	-	-	98%	99%
Prophylactic Antibiotic Timing (Outpatient)[3,7]	-	-	97%	98%
Urinary Catheter Removal[5]	-	-	98%	97%
Survey of Patients' Hospital Experiences				
Area Around Room 'Always' Quiet at Night[10]	<100	62%	67%	61%
Doctors 'Always' Communicated Well[10]	<100	88%	86%	82%
Home Recovery Information Given[10]	<100	96%	88%	85%
Hospital Given 9 or 10 on 10 Point Scale[10]	<100	90%	78%	71%
Meds 'Always' Explained Before Given[10]	<100	85%	68%	64%
Nurses 'Always' Communicated Well[10]	<100	85%	83%	79%
Pain 'Always' Well Controlled[10]	<100	84%	73%	71%
Room and Bathroom 'Always' Clean[10]	<100	85%	81%	73%
Timely Help 'Always' Received[10]	<100	83%	75%	68%
Would Definitely Recommend Hospital[10]	<100	82%	77%	71%
Use of Medical Imaging				
Cardiac Imaging Stress Test before Surgery[1]	-	-	5.4%	5.3%
Combination Abdominal CT Scan[1]	-	-	9.3%	10.5%
Combination Brain/Sinus CT Scan[1]	-	-	2.7%	2.7%
Combination Chest CT Scan[1]	-	-	1.7%	2.7%
Follow-up Mammogram/Ultrasound[1]	-	-	8%	8.8%
Lumbar Spine MRI for Low Back Pain[1]	-	-	36.5%	37.2%

Webster County Community Hospital

PO Box 465, 621 N Franklin St
Red Cloud, NE 68970
URL: www.websterhospital.org
Type: Critical Access Hospitals
Ownership: Government - Local
Phone: 402-746-5600
Fax: 402-746-2910
Emergency Services: Yes
Beds: 16

Key Personnel:
Chief of Medical Staff.......... Della Chan
Quality Assurance .... Terry Hoffart
Operating Room.............. Diane Hoffman
CEO/President................ Robert Sheckler

Measure	Cases	This Hosp.	State Avg.	U.S. Avg.
Blood Clot Prevention and Treatment				
Anticoagulation Overlap Therapy[5]	-	-	93%	93%
ICU Venous Thromboembolism Prophylaxis[5]	-	-	91%	92%
Incidence of Potentially Preventable VTE[5]	-	-	11%	10%
UFH with Dosages/Platelet Monitoring[5]	-	-	98%	97%
Venous Thromboembolism Prophylaxis[5]	-	-	88%	85%
Warfarin Therapy Discharge Instructions[5]	-	-	81%	75%
Chest Pain/Possible Heart Attack Care				
Aspirin Given Within 24 Hours of Arrival[1,3]	-	-	96%	96%
Fibrinolytic Meds Within 30 Min. of Arrival[3,7]	-	-	53%	58%
Average Time to ECG (minutes)[1,3]	-	-	8	7
Average Time to Transfer (minutes)[1,3]	-	-	76	60
Children's Asthma Care				
Received Home Management Plan of Care	-	-	-	88%
Received Reliever Medication	-	-	-	100%
Received Systemic Corticosteroids	-	-	-	100%
Emergency Department				
Admittance Decision Time (minutes)[5]	-	-	75	98
Head CT Results Within 45 Min. of Arrival[5]	-	-	61%	57%
Patients Who Left ER Before Being Seen[5]	-	-	1%	2%
Time from ER Arrival to Admit. (minutes)[5]	-	-	207	274
Time from ER Arrival to Discharge (minutes)[5]	-	-	118	134
Time in ER Before Being Evaluated (minutes)[5]	-	-	21	26
Time to Pain Meds for Fractures (minutes)[5]	-	-	42	57
Heart Attack Care				
Aspirin Given at Discharge[5]	-	-	100%	99%
Fibrinolytic Meds Within 30 Min. of Arrival[5]	-	-	-	54%
PCI Within 90 Minutes of Arrival[5]	-	-	96%	96%
Statin Prescribed at Discharge[5]	-	-	99%	98%
Heart Failure Care				
ACE Inhibitor or ARB for LVSD[3,7]	-	-	96%	97%
Discharge Instructions Given[3,7]	-	-	93%	94%
Evaluation of LVS Function[1,3]	-	-	98%	99%
Medicare Spending				
Medicare Spending per Patient (ratio)	-	-	0.97	0.98
Pneumonia Care				
Appropriate Initial Antibiotic Given[1]	-	-	95%	95%
Blood Culture Timing[7]	-	-	99%	98%
Pregnancy and Delivery Care				
Newborn Deliveries Scheduled Early[5]	-	-	5%	6%
Preventive Care				
Immunization for Influenza[5]	-	-	89%	90%
Immunization for Pneumonia[5]	-	-	90%	92%
Stroke Care				
Anticoagulation Therapy for Atrial Fibrillation[5]	-	-	95%	95%
Antithrombotic Therapy Timing[5]	-	-	99%	98%
Assessed for Rehabilitation[5]	-	-	99%	97%
Discharged on Antithrombotic Therapy[5]	-	-	100%	99%
Discharged on Statin Medication[5]	-	-	93%	94%
Thrombolytic Therapy Timing[5]	-	-	75%	66%
Venous Thromboembolism Prophylaxis[5]	-	-	94%	94%
Written Stroke Educational Materials Given[5]	-	-	84%	88%
Surgical Care Improvement Project				
Appropriate Beta Blocker Usage[5]	-	-	98%	98%
Appropriate VTP Within 24 Hours[5]	-	-	99%	98%
Controlled Postoperative Blood Glucose[5]	-	-	96%	97%
Perioperative Temperature Management[5]	-	-	100%	100%
Prophylactic Antibiotic Selection[5]	-	-	99%	99%
Prophylactic Antibiotic Selection (Outpatient)[5]	-	-	99%	98%
Prophylactic Antibiotic Stopped[5]	-	-	98%	98%
Prophylactic Antibiotic Timing[5]	-	-	98%	99%
Prophylactic Antibiotic Timing (Outpatient)[5]	-	-	97%	98%
Urinary Catheter Removal[5]	-	-	98%	97%
Survey of Patients' Hospital Experiences				
Area Around Room 'Always' Quiet at Night[10]	<100	72%	67%	61%
Doctors 'Always' Communicated Well[10]	<100	93%	86%	82%
Home Recovery Information Given[10]	<100	94%	88%	85%
Hospital Given 9 or 10 on 10 Point Scale[10]	<100	96%	78%	71%
Meds 'Always' Explained Before Given[10]	<100	72%	68%	64%
Nurses 'Always' Communicated Well[10]	<100	99%	83%	79%
Pain 'Always' Well Controlled[10]	<100	83%	73%	71%
Room and Bathroom 'Always' Clean[10]	<100	99%	81%	73%
Timely Help 'Always' Received[10]	<100	92%	75%	68%
Would Definitely Recommend Hospital[10]	<100	87%	77%	71%
Use of Medical Imaging				
Cardiac Imaging Stress Test before Surgery[1]	-	-	5.4%	5.3%
Combination Abdominal CT Scan[1]	-	-	9.3%	10.5%

NOTE: Hospital profiles are in alphabetical order by state, then city, then hospital within the city; Rankings exclude hospitals with less than 25 cases except for patient surveys which excludes hospitals with less than 100 cases; (a) 100-299 cases; (1) The number of cases/patients is too few to report; (2) Data submitted were based on a sample of cases/patients; (3) Results are based on a shorter time period than required; (4) Data suppressed by CMS for one or more quarters; (5) Results are not available for this reporting period; (6) Fewer than 100 patients completed the HCAHPS survey; (7) No cases met the criteria for this measure; (8) The lower limit of the confidence interval cannot be calculated if the number of observed infections equals zero; (9) No data are available from the state/territory for this reporting period; (10) The scores shown reflect fewer than 50 completed surveys; (11) There were discrepancies in the data collection process; (12) This measure does not apply to this hospital for this reporting period; (13) Results cannot be calculated for this reporting period; (14) The results for this state are combined with nearby states to protect confidentiality; Please refer to the User's Guide for a full explanation of data.

Combination Brain/Sinus CT Scan[1]	-	-	2.7%	2.7%
Combination Chest CT Scan[1]	-	-	1.7%	2.7%
Follow-up Mammogram/Ultrasound	78	7.7%	8%	8.8%
Lumbar Spine MRI for Low Back Pain[1]	-	-	36.5%	37.2%

Howard County Medical Center

PO Box 406, 1113 Sherman St
Saint Paul, NE 68873
Phone: 308-754-4421
Fax: 308-754-4429
Type: Critical Access Hospitals
Emergency Services: Yes
Ownership: Voluntary non-profit - Other
Beds: 25

Key Personnel:
CEO . . . . Arlan Johson

Measure	Cases	This Hosp.	State Avg.	U.S. Avg.
Blood Clot Prevention and Treatment				
Anticoagulation Overlap Therapy[5]	-	-	93%	93%
ICU Venous Thromboembolism Prophylaxis[5]	-	-	91%	92%
Incidence of Potentially Preventable VTE[5]	-	-	11%	10%
UFH with Dosages/Platelet Monitoring[5]	-	-	98%	97%
Venous Thromboembolism Prophylaxis[5]	-	-	88%	85%
Warfarin Therapy Discharge Instructions[5]	-	-	81%	75%
Chest Pain/Possible Heart Attack Care				
Aspirin Given Within 24 Hours of Arrival[1]	-	-	96%	96%
Fibrinolytic Meds Within 30 Min. of Arrival[1,3]	-	-	53%	58%
Average Time to ECG (minutes)[1]	-	-	8	7
Average Time to Transfer (minutes)[3,7]	-	-	76	60
Children's Asthma Care				
Received Home Management Plan of Care	-	-	-	88%
Received Reliever Medication	-	-	-	100%
Received Systemic Corticosteroids	-	-	-	100%
Emergency Department				
Admittance Decision Time (minutes)[5]	-	-	75	98
Head CT Results Within 45 Min. of Arrival[1]	-	-	61%	57%
Patients Who Left ER Before Being Seen[5]	-	-	1%	2%
Time from ER Arrival to Admit. (minutes)[5]	-	-	207	274
Time from ER Arrival to Discharge (minutes)[5]	-	-	118	134
Time in ER Before Being Evaluated (minutes)[5]	-	-	21	26
Time to Pain Meds for Fractures (minutes)[5]	-	-	42	57
Heart Attack Care				
Aspirin Given at Discharge[5]	-	-	100%	99%
Fibrinolytic Meds Within 30 Min. of Arrival[5]	-	-	-	54%
PCI Within 90 Minutes of Arrival[5]	-	-	96%	96%
Statin Prescribed at Discharge[5]	-	-	99%	98%
Heart Failure Care				
ACE Inhibitor or ARB for LVSD[7]	-	-	96%	97%
Discharge Instructions Given[1]	-	-	93%	94%
Evaluation of LVS Function[1]	-	-	98%	99%
Medicare Spending				
Medicare Spending per Patient (ratio)	-	-	0.97	0.98
Pneumonia Care				
Appropriate Initial Antibiotic Given	27	81%	95%	95%
Blood Culture Timing[1]	-	-	99%	98%
Pregnancy and Delivery Care				
Newborn Deliveries Scheduled Early[5]	-	-	5%	6%
Preventive Care				
Immunization for Influenza[5]	-	-	89%	90%
Immunization for Pneumonia[5]	-	-	90%	92%
Stroke Care				
Anticoagulation Therapy for Atrial Fibrillation[5]	-	-	95%	95%
Antithrombotic Therapy Timing[5]	-	-	99%	98%
Assessed for Rehabilitation[5]	-	-	99%	97%
Discharged on Antithrombotic Therapy[5]	-	-	100%	99%
Discharged on Statin Medication[5]	-	-	93%	94%
Thrombolytic Therapy Timing[5]	-	-	75%	66%
Venous Thromboembolism Prophylaxis[5]	-	-	94%	94%
Written Stroke Educational Materials Given[5]	-	-	84%	88%
Surgical Care Improvement Project				
Appropriate Beta Blocker Usage[5]	-	-	98%	98%
Appropriate VTP Within 24 Hours[5]	-	-	99%	98%
Controlled Postoperative Blood Glucose[5]	-	-	96%	97%
Perioperative Temperature Management[5]	-	-	100%	100%
Prophylactic Antibiotic Selection[5]	-	-	99%	99%
Prophylactic Antibiotic Selection (Outpatient)[5]	-	-	99%	98%
Prophylactic Antibiotic Stopped[5]	-	-	98%	98%
Prophylactic Antibiotic Timing[5]	-	-	98%	99%
Prophylactic Antibiotic Timing (Outpatient)[5]	-	-	97%	98%
Urinary Catheter Removal[5]	-	-	98%	97%
Survey of Patients' Hospital Experiences				
Area Around Room 'Always' Quiet at Night[6]	<100	57%	67%	61%
Doctors 'Always' Communicated Well[6]	<100	89%	86%	82%
Home Recovery Information Given[6]	<100	94%	88%	85%
Hospital Given 9 or 10 on 10 Point Scale[6]	<100	81%	78%	71%
Meds 'Always' Explained Before Given[6]	<100	64%	68%	64%
Nurses 'Always' Communicated Well[6]	<100	72%	83%	79%
Pain 'Always' Well Controlled[6]	<100	75%	73%	71%
Room and Bathroom 'Always' Clean[6]	<100	80%	81%	73%
Timely Help 'Always' Received[6]	<100	78%	75%	68%
Would Definitely Recommend Hospital[6]	<100	82%	77%	71%
Use of Medical Imaging				
Cardiac Imaging Stress Test before Surgery	73	2.7%	5.4%	5.3%
Combination Abdominal CT Scan	113	17.7%	9.3%	10.5%
Combination Brain/Sinus CT Scan	114	7.0%	2.7%	2.7%
Combination Chest CT Scan	85	9.4%	1.7%	2.7%
Follow-up Mammogram/Ultrasound	174	6.3%	8%	8.8%
Lumbar Spine MRI for Low Back Pain[1]	-	-	36.5%	37.2%

Alegent Creighton Health Memorial Hospital - Schuyl

104 West 17th St
Schuyler, NE 68661
Phone: 402-352-2441
Fax: 402-352-2643
URL: www.algent.com
Type: Critical Access Hospitals
Emergency Services: Yes
Ownership: Voluntary non-profit - Private
Beds: 49

Key Personnel:
Quality Assurance . . . . Al Klaasmeyer
Radiology. . . . . Elisa Morgan
Infection Control. . . . . Rose Neuhaus, RN
CEO/President. . . . . Richard Rolson, MD, FAAP
Chief of Medical Staff. . . . . Cary Ward, MD
Emergency Room . . . . Rita Zelda, RN

Measure	Cases	This Hosp.	State Avg.	U.S. Avg.
Blood Clot Prevention and Treatment				
Anticoagulation Overlap Therapy[7]	-	-	93%	93%
ICU Venous Thromboembolism Prophylaxis[7]	-	-	91%	92%
Incidence of Potentially Preventable VTE[7]	-	-	11%	10%
UFH with Dosages/Platelet Monitoring[7]	-	-	98%	97%
Venous Thromboembolism Prophylaxis	34	97%	88%	85%
Warfarin Therapy Discharge Instructions[7]	-	-	81%	75%
Chest Pain/Possible Heart Attack Care				
Aspirin Given Within 24 Hours of Arrival	11	100%	96%	96%
Fibrinolytic Meds Within 30 Min. of Arrival[1,3]	-	-	53%	58%
Average Time to ECG (minutes)	14	12	8	7
Average Time to Transfer (minutes)[3,7]	-	-	76	60
Children's Asthma Care				
Received Home Management Plan of Care	-	-	-	88%
Received Reliever Medication	-	-	-	100%
Received Systemic Corticosteroids	-	-	-	100%
Emergency Department				
Admittance Decision Time (minutes)[5]	-	-	75	98
Head CT Results Within 45 Min. of Arrival[5]	-	-	61%	57%
Patients Who Left ER Before Being Seen[5]	-	-	1%	2%
Time from ER Arrival to Admit. (minutes)[5]	-	-	207	274
Time from ER Arrival to Discharge (minutes)[5]	-	-	118	134
Time in ER Before Being Evaluated (minutes)[5]	-	-	21	26
Time to Pain Meds for Fractures (minutes)[5]	-	-	42	57
Heart Attack Care				
Aspirin Given at Discharge[3,7]	-	-	100%	99%
Fibrinolytic Meds Within 30 Min. of Arrival[3,7]	-	-	-	54%
PCI Within 90 Minutes of Arrival[3,7]	-	-	96%	96%
Statin Prescribed at Discharge[3,7]	-	-	99%	98%
Heart Failure Care				
ACE Inhibitor or ARB for LVSD[1]	-	-	96%	97%
Discharge Instructions Given[1]	-	-	93%	94%
Evaluation of LVS Function[1]	-	-	98%	99%
Medicare Spending				
Medicare Spending per Patient (ratio)	-	-	0.97	0.98
Pneumonia Care				
Appropriate Initial Antibiotic Given[7]	-	-	95%	95%
Blood Culture Timing[1]	-	-	99%	98%
Pregnancy and Delivery Care				
Newborn Deliveries Scheduled Early[5]	-	-	5%	6%
Preventive Care				
Immunization for Influenza[5]	-	-	89%	90%
Immunization for Pneumonia[5]	-	-	90%	92%
Stroke Care				
Anticoagulation Therapy for Atrial Fibrillation[5]	-	-	95%	95%
Antithrombotic Therapy Timing[5]	-	-	99%	98%
Assessed for Rehabilitation[5]	-	-	99%	97%
Discharged on Antithrombotic Therapy[5]	-	-	100%	99%
Discharged on Statin Medication[5]	-	-	93%	94%
Thrombolytic Therapy Timing[5]	-	-	75%	66%
Venous Thromboembolism Prophylaxis[5]	-	-	94%	94%
Written Stroke Educational Materials Given[5]	-	-	84%	88%
Surgical Care Improvement Project				
Appropriate Beta Blocker Usage[1,3]	-	-	98%	98%
Appropriate VTP Within 24 Hours[1,3]	-	-	99%	98%
Controlled Postoperative Blood Glucose[3,7]	-	-	96%	97%
Perioperative Temperature Management[1,3]	-	-	100%	100%
Prophylactic Antibiotic Selection[1,3]	-	-	99%	99%
Prophylactic Antibiotic Selection (Outpatient)[1,3]	-	-	99%	98%
Prophylactic Antibiotic Stopped[1,3]	-	-	98%	98%
Prophylactic Antibiotic Timing[1,3]	-	-	98%	99%
Prophylactic Antibiotic Timing (Outpatient)[1,3]	-	-	97%	98%
Urinary Catheter Removal[3,7]	-	-	98%	97%
Survey of Patients' Hospital Experiences				
Area Around Room 'Always' Quiet at Night[10]	<100	84%	67%	61%
Doctors 'Always' Communicated Well[10]	<100	91%	86%	82%
Home Recovery Information Given[10]	<100	87%	88%	85%
Hospital Given 9 or 10 on 10 Point Scale[10]	<100	76%	78%	71%
Meds 'Always' Explained Before Given[10]	<100	57%	68%	64%
Nurses 'Always' Communicated Well[10]	<100	91%	83%	79%
Pain 'Always' Well Controlled[10]	<100	93%	73%	71%
Room and Bathroom 'Always' Clean[10]	<100	87%	81%	73%
Timely Help 'Always' Received[10]	<100	73%	75%	68%
Would Definitely Recommend Hospital[10]	<100	79%	77%	71%
Use of Medical Imaging				
Cardiac Imaging Stress Test before Surgery[1]	-	-	5.4%	5.3%
Combination Abdominal CT Scan[1]	-	-	9.3%	10.5%
Combination Brain/Sinus CT Scan[1]	-	-	2.7%	2.7%
Combination Chest CT Scan[1]	-	-	1.7%	2.7%
Follow-up Mammogram/Ultrasound	122	1.6%	8%	8.8%
Lumbar Spine MRI for Low Back Pain[1]	-	-	36.5%	37.2%

Regional West Medical Center

4021 Ave B
Scottsbluff, NE 69361
Phone: 308-635-3711
Fax: 308-630-1815
URL: www.rwmc.net
Type: Acute Care Hospitals
Emergency Services: Yes
Ownership: Voluntary non-profit - Private
Beds: 203

Key Personnel:
Coronary Care . . . . Shirley Barlow
Pediatric In-Patient Care . . . . Robert Flynn
Radiology. . . . . Dan Gilbert
Operating Room. . . . . Linda Lund
Quality Assurance . . . . Barb Lundgner
Chief of Medical Staff . . . . James McHugh, MD
Infection Control. . . . . Marsha Meyer
President/CEO. . . . . Todd S Sorensen, MD

Measure	Cases	This Hosp.	State Avg.	U.S. Avg.
Blood Clot Prevention and Treatment				
Anticoagulation Overlap Therapy[2]	48	92%	93%	93%
ICU Venous Thromboembolism Prophylaxis[2]	76	79%	91%	92%
Incidence of Potentially Preventable VTE[2]	11	18%	11%	10%
UFH with Dosages/Platelet Monitoring[2]	20	100%	98%	97%
Venous Thromboembolism Prophylaxis[2]	340	84%	88%	85%
Warfarin Therapy Discharge Instructions[2]	34	56%	81%	75%
Chest Pain/Possible Heart Attack Care				
Aspirin Given Within 24 Hours of Arrival	54	100%	96%	96%
Fibrinolytic Meds Within 30 Min. of Arrival	18	78%	53%	58%
Average Time to ECG (minutes)	56	7	8	7
Average Time to Transfer (minutes)[1]	-	-	76	60
Children's Asthma Care				

NOTE: Hospital profiles are in alphabetical order by state, then city, then hospital within the city; Rankings exclude hospitals with less than 25 cases except for patient surveys which excludes hospitals with less than 100 cases; (a) 100-299 cases; (1) The number of cases/patients is too few to report; (2) Data submitted were based on a sample of cases/patients; (3) Results are based on a shorter time period than required; (4) Data suppressed by CMS for one or more quarters; (5) Results are not available for this reporting period; (6) Fewer than 100 patients completed the HCAHPS survey; (7) No cases met the criteria for this measure; (8) The lower limit of the confidence interval cannot be calculated if the number of observed infections equals zero; (9) No data are available from the state/territory for this reporting period; (10) The scores shown reflect fewer than 50 completed surveys; (11) There were discrepancies in the data collection process; (12) This measure does not apply to this hospital for this reporting period; (13) Results cannot be calculated for this reporting period; (14) The results for this state are combined with nearby states to protect confidentiality; Please refer to the User's Guide for a full explanation of data.

Measure	Cases	This Hosp.	State Avg.	U.S. Avg.
Received Home Management Plan of Care	-	-	-	88%
Received Reliever Medication	-	-	-	100%
Received Systemic Corticosteroids	-	-	-	100%
Emergency Department				
Admittance Decision Time (minutes)[2]	482	85	75	98
Head CT Results Within 45 Min. of Arrival[1]	-	-	61%	57%
Patients Who Left ER Before Being Seen	16,366	1%	1%	2%
Time from ER Arrival to Admit. (minutes)[2]	495	238	207	274
Time from ER Arrival to Discharge (minutes)	402	154	118	134
Time in ER Before Being Evaluated (minutes)	422	21	21	26
Time to Pain Meds for Fractures (minutes)	44	32	42	57
Heart Attack Care				
Aspirin Given at Discharge	21	100%	100%	99%
Fibrinolytic Meds Within 30 Min. of Arrival[7]	-	-	-	54%
PCI Within 90 Minutes of Arrival[7]	-	-	96%	96%
Statin Prescribed at Discharge	19	100%	99%	98%
Heart Failure Care				
ACE Inhibitor or ARB for LVSD	23	96%	96%	97%
Discharge Instructions Given	67	88%	93%	94%
Evaluation of LVS Function	90	100%	98%	99%
Medicare Spending				
Medicare Spending per Patient (ratio)	-	0.90	0.97	0.98
Pneumonia Care				
Appropriate Initial Antibiotic Given	59	98%	95%	95%
Blood Culture Timing	112	96%	99%	98%
Pregnancy and Delivery Care				
Newborn Deliveries Scheduled Early	64	3%	5%	6%
Preventive Care				
Immunization for Influenza[2]	566	44%	89%	90%
Immunization for Pneumonia[2]	656	67%	90%	92%
Stroke Care				
Anticoagulation Therapy for Atrial Fibrillation[1]	-	-	95%	95%
Antithrombotic Therapy Timing	32	100%	99%	98%
Assessed for Rehabilitation	49	100%	99%	97%
Discharged on Antithrombotic Therapy	39	97%	100%	99%
Discharged on Statin Medication	29	97%	93%	94%
Thrombolytic Therapy Timing[1]	-	-	75%	66%
Venous Thromboembolism Prophylaxis	46	93%	94%	94%
Written Stroke Educational Materials Given	23	4%	84%	88%
Surgical Care Improvement Project				
Appropriate Beta Blocker Usage[2]	122	99%	98%	98%
Appropriate VTP Within 24 Hours[2]	397	98%	99%	98%
Controlled Postoperative Blood Glucose[2,7]	-	-	96%	97%
Perioperative Temperature Management[2]	538	99%	100%	100%
Prophylactic Antibiotic Selection[2]	344	98%	99%	99%
Prophylactic Antibiotic Selection (Outpatient)	134	99%	99%	98%
Prophylactic Antibiotic Stopped[2]	340	95%	98%	98%
Prophylactic Antibiotic Timing[2]	344	99%	98%	99%
Prophylactic Antibiotic Timing (Outpatient)	134	99%	97%	98%
Urinary Catheter Removal[2]	320	93%	98%	97%
Survey of Patients' Hospital Experiences				
Area Around Room 'Always' Quiet at Night	300+	57%	67%	61%
Doctors 'Always' Communicated Well	300+	79%	86%	82%
Home Recovery Information Given	300+	89%	88%	85%
Hospital Given 9 or 10 on 10 Point Scale	300+	66%	78%	71%
Meds 'Always' Explained Before Given	300+	64%	68%	64%
Nurses 'Always' Communicated Well	300+	76%	83%	79%
Pain 'Always' Well Controlled	300+	69%	73%	71%
Room and Bathroom 'Always' Clean	300+	63%	81%	73%
Timely Help 'Always' Received	300+	65%	75%	68%
Would Definitely Recommend Hospital	300+	66%	77%	71%
Use of Medical Imaging				
Cardiac Imaging Stress Test before Surgery	370	6.8%	5.4%	5.3%
Combination Abdominal CT Scan	647	13.1%	9.3%	10.5%
Combination Brain/Sinus CT Scan	457	6.8%	2.7%	2.7%
Combination Chest CT Scan	345	0.0%	1.7%	2.7%
Follow-up Mammogram/Ultrasound	1,578	7.9%	8%	8.8%
Lumbar Spine MRI for Low Back Pain	199	29.6%	36.5%	37.2%

Memorial Health Care Systems

300 North Columbia Ave
Seward, NE 68434
URL: www.mhcs-seward.org
Type: Critical Access Hospitals
Ownership: Voluntary non-profit - Private
Phone: 402-643-2971
Fax: 402-646-4639
Emergency Services: Yes
Beds: 115

Key Personnel:
Cardiac Laboratory. . . . . Darcy Friedli, RN
Chief of Medical Staff . . . . Barbara E Froehner
Anesthesiology. . . . . Mike George, CRNA
Chairman/CEO . . . . Mike Hecker
Quality Assurance . . . . Kathi Kelly
Infection Control. . . . . Jan Lucas
Administrator . . . . Roger Reamer
Pediatric Ambulatory Care . . . . . . Judy Rehmer

Measure	Cases	This Hosp.	State Avg.	U.S. Avg.
Blood Clot Prevention and Treatment				
Anticoagulation Overlap Therapy[5]	-	-	93%	93%
ICU Venous Thromboembolism Prophylaxis[5]	-	-	91%	92%
Incidence of Potentially Preventable VTE[5]	-	-	11%	10%
UFH with Dosages/Platelet Monitoring[5]	-	-	98%	97%
Venous Thromboembolism Prophylaxis[5]	-	-	88%	85%
Warfarin Therapy Discharge Instructions[5]	-	-	81%	75%
Chest Pain/Possible Heart Attack Care				
Aspirin Given Within 24 Hours of Arrival	-	-	96%	96%
Fibrinolytic Meds Within 30 Min. of Arrival	-	-	53%	58%
Average Time to ECG (minutes)	-	-	8	7
Average Time to Transfer (minutes)	-	-	76	60
Children's Asthma Care				
Received Home Management Plan of Care	-	-	-	88%
Received Reliever Medication	-	-	-	100%
Received Systemic Corticosteroids	-	-	-	100%
Emergency Department				
Admittance Decision Time (minutes)[5]	-	-	75	98
Head CT Results Within 45 Min. of Arrival	-	-	61%	57%
Patients Who Left ER Before Being Seen	-	-	1%	2%
Time from ER Arrival to Admit. (minutes)[5]	-	-	207	274
Time from ER Arrival to Discharge (minutes)	-	-	118	134
Time in ER Before Being Evaluated (minutes)	-	-	21	26
Time to Pain Meds for Fractures (minutes)	-	-	42	57
Heart Attack Care				
Aspirin Given at Discharge[5]	-	-	100%	99%
Fibrinolytic Meds Within 30 Min. of Arrival[5]	-	-	-	54%
PCI Within 90 Minutes of Arrival[5]	-	-	96%	96%
Statin Prescribed at Discharge[5]	-	-	99%	98%
Heart Failure Care				
ACE Inhibitor or ARB for LVSD[1]	-	-	96%	97%
Discharge Instructions Given	12	42%	93%	94%
Evaluation of LVS Function	13	77%	98%	99%
Medicare Spending				
Medicare Spending per Patient (ratio)	-	-	0.97	0.98
Pneumonia Care				
Appropriate Initial Antibiotic Given	15	93%	95%	95%
Blood Culture Timing[1]	-	-	99%	98%
Pregnancy and Delivery Care				
Newborn Deliveries Scheduled Early[5]	-	-	5%	6%
Preventive Care				
Immunization for Influenza[5]	-	-	89%	90%
Immunization for Pneumonia[5]	-	-	90%	92%
Stroke Care				
Anticoagulation Therapy for Atrial Fibrillation[5]	-	-	95%	95%
Antithrombotic Therapy Timing[5]	-	-	99%	98%
Assessed for Rehabilitation[5]	-	-	99%	97%
Discharged on Antithrombotic Therapy[5]	-	-	100%	99%
Discharged on Statin Medication[5]	-	-	93%	94%
Thrombolytic Therapy Timing[5]	-	-	75%	66%
Venous Thromboembolism Prophylaxis[5]	-	-	94%	94%
Written Stroke Educational Materials Given[5]	-	-	84%	88%
Surgical Care Improvement Project				
Appropriate Beta Blocker Usage[5]	-	-	98%	98%
Appropriate VTP Within 24 Hours[5]	-	-	99%	98%
Controlled Postoperative Blood Glucose[5]	-	-	96%	97%
Perioperative Temperature Management[5]	-	-	100%	100%
Prophylactic Antibiotic Selection[5]	-	-	99%	99%
Prophylactic Antibiotic Selection (Outpatient)	-	-	99%	98%
Prophylactic Antibiotic Stopped[5]	-	-	98%	98%
Prophylactic Antibiotic Timing[5]	-	-	98%	99%
Prophylactic Antibiotic Timing (Outpatient)	-	-	97%	98%
Urinary Catheter Removal[5]	-	-	98%	97%
Survey of Patients' Hospital Experiences				
Area Around Room 'Always' Quiet at Night[6]	<100	69%	67%	61%
Doctors 'Always' Communicated Well[6]	<100	93%	86%	82%
Home Recovery Information Given[6]	<100	84%	88%	85%
Hospital Given 9 or 10 on 10 Point Scale[6]	<100	81%	78%	71%
Meds 'Always' Explained Before Given[6]	<100	69%	68%	64%
Nurses 'Always' Communicated Well[6]	<100	77%	83%	79%
Pain 'Always' Well Controlled[6]	<100	71%	73%	71%
Room and Bathroom 'Always' Clean[6]	<100	78%	81%	73%
Timely Help 'Always' Received[6]	<100	67%	75%	68%
Would Definitely Recommend Hospital[6]	<100	76%	77%	71%
Use of Medical Imaging				
Cardiac Imaging Stress Test before Surgery	-	-	5.4%	5.3%
Combination Abdominal CT Scan	-	-	9.3%	10.5%
Combination Brain/Sinus CT Scan	-	-	2.7%	2.7%
Combination Chest CT Scan	-	-	1.7%	2.7%
Follow-up Mammogram/Ultrasound	-	-	8%	8.8%
Lumbar Spine MRI for Low Back Pain	-	-	36.5%	37.2%

Sidney Regional Medical Center

645 Osage St
Sidney, NE 69162
E-mail: mhchk@wheatbelt.com
URL: www.memorialhealthcenter.org
Type: Critical Access Hospitals
Ownership: Voluntary non-profit - Private
Phone: 308-254-5825
Fax: 308-254-2300
Emergency Services: Yes
Beds: 25

Key Personnel:
Quality Assurance . . . . Greg Dyson, RN
CEO . . . . Jason Petik
Chief of Medical Staff . . . . Mandy Shaw, M.D.
Anesthesiology. . . . . Linda Shoemaker
Radiology. . . . . Randy Sonnie

Measure	Cases	This Hosp.	State Avg.	U.S. Avg.
Blood Clot Prevention and Treatment				
Anticoagulation Overlap Therapy[5]	-	-	93%	93%
ICU Venous Thromboembolism Prophylaxis[5]	-	-	91%	92%
Incidence of Potentially Preventable VTE[5]	-	-	11%	10%
UFH with Dosages/Platelet Monitoring[5]	-	-	98%	97%
Venous Thromboembolism Prophylaxis[5]	-	-	88%	85%
Warfarin Therapy Discharge Instructions[5]	-	-	81%	75%
Chest Pain/Possible Heart Attack Care				
Aspirin Given Within 24 Hours of Arrival[1,3]	-	-	96%	96%
Fibrinolytic Meds Within 30 Min. of Arrival[1,3]	-	-	53%	58%
Average Time to ECG (minutes)[1,3]	-	-	8	7
Average Time to Transfer (minutes)[3,7]	-	-	76	60
Children's Asthma Care				
Received Home Management Plan of Care	-	-	-	88%
Received Reliever Medication	-	-	-	100%
Received Systemic Corticosteroids	-	-	-	100%
Emergency Department				
Admittance Decision Time (minutes)[5]	-	-	75	98
Head CT Results Within 45 Min. of Arrival[5]	-	-	61%	57%
Patients Who Left ER Before Being Seen[5]	-	-	1%	2%
Time from ER Arrival to Admit. (minutes)[5]	-	-	207	274
Time from ER Arrival to Discharge (minutes)[5]	-	-	118	134
Time in ER Before Being Evaluated (minutes)[5]	-	-	21	26
Time to Pain Meds for Fractures (minutes)[5]	-	-	42	57
Heart Attack Care				
Aspirin Given at Discharge[3,7]	-	-	100%	99%
Fibrinolytic Meds Within 30 Min. of Arrival[3,7]	-	-	-	54%
PCI Within 90 Minutes of Arrival[3,7]	-	-	96%	96%
Statin Prescribed at Discharge[3,7]	-	-	99%	98%
Heart Failure Care				
ACE Inhibitor or ARB for LVSD[1,3]	-	-	96%	97%
Discharge Instructions Given[1,3]	-	-	93%	94%
Evaluation of LVS Function[3]	12	67%	98%	99%
Medicare Spending				
Medicare Spending per Patient (ratio)	-	-	0.97	0.98
Pneumonia Care				

NOTE: Hospital profiles are in alphabetical order by state, then city, then hospital within the city; Rankings exclude hospitals with less than 25 cases except for patient surveys which excludes hospitals with less than 100 cases; (a) 100-299 cases; (1) The number of cases/patients is too few to report; (2) Data submitted were based on a sample of cases/patients; (3) Results are based on a shorter time period than required; (4) Data suppressed by CMS for one or more quarters; (5) Results are not available for this reporting period; (6) Fewer than 100 patients completed the HCAHPS survey; (7) No cases met the criteria for this measure; (8) The lower limit of the confidence interval cannot be calculated if the number of observed infections equals zero; (9) No data are available from the state/territory for this reporting period; (10) The scores shown reflect fewer than 50 completed surveys; (11) There were discrepancies in the data collection process; (12) This measure does not apply to this hospital for this reporting period; (13) Results cannot be calculated for this reporting period; (14) The results for this state are combined with nearby states to protect confidentiality; Please refer to the User's Guide for a full explanation of data.

Appropriate Initial Antibiotic Given[2]	21	81%	95%	95%
Blood Culture Timing[2]	15	73%	99%	98%
Pregnancy and Delivery Care				
Newborn Deliveries Scheduled Early[5]	-	-	5%	6%
Preventive Care				
Immunization for Influenza[5]	-	-	89%	90%
Immunization for Pneumonia[5]	-	-	90%	92%
Stroke Care				
Anticoagulation Therapy for Atrial Fibrillation[5]	-	-	95%	95%
Antithrombotic Therapy Timing[5]	-	-	99%	98%
Assessed for Rehabilitation[5]	-	-	99%	97%
Discharged on Antithrombotic Therapy[5]	-	-	100%	99%
Discharged on Statin Medication[5]	-	-	93%	94%
Thrombolytic Therapy Timing[5]	-	-	75%	66%
Venous Thromboembolism Prophylaxis[5]	-	-	94%	94%
Written Stroke Educational Materials Given[5]	-	-	84%	88%
Surgical Care Improvement Project				
Appropriate Beta Blocker Usage[1]	-	-	98%	98%
Appropriate VTP Within 24 Hours	40	100%	99%	98%
Controlled Postoperative Blood Glucose[7]	-	-	96%	97%
Perioperative Temperature Management	57	98%	100%	100%
Prophylactic Antibiotic Selection	61	95%	99%	99%
Prophylactic Antibiotic Selection (Outpatient)[3]	23	100%	99%	98%
Prophylactic Antibiotic Stopped	61	100%	98%	98%
Prophylactic Antibiotic Timing	62	92%	98%	99%
Prophylactic Antibiotic Timing (Outpatient)[1,3]	-	-	97%	98%
Urinary Catheter Removal	13	85%	98%	97%
Survey of Patients' Hospital Experiences				
Area Around Room 'Always' Quiet at Night	(a)	54%	67%	61%
Doctors 'Always' Communicated Well	(a)	84%	86%	82%
Home Recovery Information Given	(a)	92%	88%	85%
Hospital Given 9 or 10 on 10 Point Scale	(a)	75%	78%	71%
Meds 'Always' Explained Before Given	(a)	69%	68%	64%
Nurses 'Always' Communicated Well	(a)	80%	83%	79%
Pain 'Always' Well Controlled	(a)	72%	73%	71%
Room and Bathroom 'Always' Clean	(a)	76%	81%	73%
Timely Help 'Always' Received	(a)	69%	75%	68%
Would Definitely Recommend Hospital	(a)	70%	77%	71%
Use of Medical Imaging				
Cardiac Imaging Stress Test before Surgery	66	6.1%	5.4%	5.3%
Combination Abdominal CT Scan	106	5.7%	9.3%	10.5%
Combination Brain/Sinus CT Scan[1]	-	-	2.7%	2.7%
Combination Chest CT Scan[1]	-	-	1.7%	2.7%
Follow-up Mammogram/Ultrasound	209	7.7%	8%	8.8%
Lumbar Spine MRI for Low Back Pain[1]	-	-	36.5%	37.2%

Brodstone Memorial Hospital

PO Box 187, 520 East 10th St
Superior, NE 68978
Phone: 402-879-3281
Fax: 402-879-3401
E-mail: jkeelan@brodstonehospital.org
URL: www.brodstonehospital.org
Type: Critical Access Hospitals
Emergency Services: Yes
Ownership: Voluntary non-profit - Private
Beds: 25

Key Personnel:
Infection Control. . . . . Pam Bower
Operating Room. . . . . Kathe Ely
CEO/President. . . . . John Keelan
Chief of Medical Staff . . . . Robert Leibel, MD

Measure	Cases	This Hosp.	State Avg.	U.S. Avg.
Blood Clot Prevention and Treatment				
Anticoagulation Overlap Therapy[5]	-	-	93%	93%
ICU Venous Thromboembolism Prophylaxis[5]	-	-	91%	92%
Incidence of Potentially Preventable VTE[5]	-	-	11%	10%
UFH with Dosages/Platelet Monitoring[5]	-	-	98%	97%
Venous Thromboembolism Prophylaxis[5]	-	-	88%	85%
Warfarin Therapy Discharge Instructions[5]	-	-	81%	75%
Chest Pain/Possible Heart Attack Care				
Aspirin Given Within 24 Hours of Arrival[1]	-	-	96%	96%
Fibrinolytic Meds Within 30 Min. of Arrival[1]	-	-	53%	58%
Average Time to ECG (minutes)[1]	-	-	8	7
Average Time to Transfer (minutes)[7]	-	-	76	60
Children's Asthma Care				
Received Home Management Plan of Care	-	-	-	88%
Received Reliever Medication	-	-	-	100%
Received Systemic Corticosteroids	-	-	-	100%
Emergency Department				
Admittance Decision Time (minutes)[5]	-	-	75	98
Head CT Results Within 45 Min. of Arrival[5]	-	-	61%	57%
Patients Who Left ER Before Being Seen[5]	-	-	1%	2%
Time from ER Arrival to Admit. (minutes)[5]	-	-	207	274
Time from ER Arrival to Discharge (minutes)[5]	-	-	118	134
Time in ER Before Being Evaluated (minutes)[5]	-	-	21	26
Time to Pain Meds for Fractures (minutes)[5]	-	-	42	57
Heart Attack Care				
Aspirin Given at Discharge[5]	-	-	100%	99%
Fibrinolytic Meds Within 30 Min. of Arrival[5]	-	-	-	54%
PCI Within 90 Minutes of Arrival[5]	-	-	96%	96%
Statin Prescribed at Discharge[5]	-	-	99%	98%
Heart Failure Care				
ACE Inhibitor or ARB for LVSD[1,2]	-	-	96%	97%
Discharge Instructions Given[2]	12	83%	93%	94%
Evaluation of LVS Function[2]	16	94%	98%	99%
Medicare Spending				
Medicare Spending per Patient (ratio)	-	-	0.97	0.98
Pneumonia Care				
Appropriate Initial Antibiotic Given	11	82%	95%	95%
Blood Culture Timing[1]	-	-	99%	98%
Pregnancy and Delivery Care				
Newborn Deliveries Scheduled Early[5]	-	-	5%	6%
Preventive Care				
Immunization for Influenza[5]	-	-	89%	90%
Immunization for Pneumonia[5]	-	-	90%	92%
Stroke Care				
Anticoagulation Therapy for Atrial Fibrillation[5]	-	-	95%	95%
Antithrombotic Therapy Timing[5]	-	-	99%	98%
Assessed for Rehabilitation[5]	-	-	99%	97%
Discharged on Antithrombotic Therapy[5]	-	-	100%	99%
Discharged on Statin Medication[5]	-	-	93%	94%
Thrombolytic Therapy Timing[5]	-	-	75%	66%
Venous Thromboembolism Prophylaxis[5]	-	-	94%	94%
Written Stroke Educational Materials Given[5]	-	-	84%	88%
Surgical Care Improvement Project				
Appropriate Beta Blocker Usage[5]	-	-	98%	98%
Appropriate VTP Within 24 Hours[5]	-	-	99%	98%
Controlled Postoperative Blood Glucose[5]	-	-	96%	97%
Perioperative Temperature Management[5]	-	-	100%	100%
Prophylactic Antibiotic Selection[5]	-	-	99%	99%
Prophylactic Antibiotic Selection (Outpatient)[5]	-	-	99%	98%
Prophylactic Antibiotic Stopped[5]	-	-	98%	98%
Prophylactic Antibiotic Timing[5]	-	-	98%	99%
Prophylactic Antibiotic Timing (Outpatient)[5]	-	-	97%	98%
Urinary Catheter Removal[5]	-	-	98%	97%
Survey of Patients' Hospital Experiences				
Area Around Room 'Always' Quiet at Night	(a)	76%	67%	61%
Doctors 'Always' Communicated Well	(a)	91%	86%	82%
Home Recovery Information Given	(a)	91%	88%	85%
Hospital Given 9 or 10 on 10 Point Scale	(a)	81%	78%	71%
Meds 'Always' Explained Before Given	(a)	74%	68%	64%
Nurses 'Always' Communicated Well	(a)	85%	83%	79%
Pain 'Always' Well Controlled	(a)	70%	73%	71%
Room and Bathroom 'Always' Clean	(a)	83%	81%	73%
Timely Help 'Always' Received	(a)	83%	75%	68%
Would Definitely Recommend Hospital	(a)	89%	77%	71%
Use of Medical Imaging				
Cardiac Imaging Stress Test before Surgery	69	5.8%	5.4%	5.3%
Combination Abdominal CT Scan	105	2.9%	9.3%	10.5%
Combination Brain/Sinus CT Scan[1]	-	-	2.7%	2.7%
Combination Chest CT Scan	114	1.8%	1.7%	2.7%
Follow-up Mammogram/Ultrasound	319	6.6%	8%	8.8%
Lumbar Spine MRI for Low Back Pain[1]	-	-	36.5%	37.2%

Community Memorial Hospital

PO Box N, 1579 Midland St
Syracuse, NE 68446
Phone: 402-269-2011
Fax: 402-269-2795
URL: www.syracusecmh.org
Type: Critical Access Hospitals
Emergency Services: Yes
Ownership: Govt - Hospital Dist/Auth
Beds: 18

Key Personnel:
CEO/President. . . . . Michael Harvey
Chief of Medical Staff . . . . Erin Haubschman, MD
Hemotology Center . . . . Jerel Katen
Ambulatory Care . . . . Bev Sporhase
Operating Room. . . . . Susan Wilson, RN
Anesthesiology. . . . . Suzanne Wilson

Measure	Cases	This Hosp.	State Avg.	U.S. Avg.
Blood Clot Prevention and Treatment				
Anticoagulation Overlap Therapy[5]	-	-	93%	93%
ICU Venous Thromboembolism Prophylaxis[5]	-	-	91%	92%
Incidence of Potentially Preventable VTE[5]	-	-	11%	10%
UFH with Dosages/Platelet Monitoring[5]	-	-	98%	97%
Venous Thromboembolism Prophylaxis[5]	-	-	88%	85%
Warfarin Therapy Discharge Instructions[5]	-	-	81%	75%
Chest Pain/Possible Heart Attack Care				
Aspirin Given Within 24 Hours of Arrival	-	-	96%	96%
Fibrinolytic Meds Within 30 Min. of Arrival	-	-	53%	58%
Average Time to ECG (minutes)	-	-	8	7
Average Time to Transfer (minutes)	-	-	76	60
Children's Asthma Care				
Received Home Management Plan of Care	-	-	-	88%
Received Reliever Medication	-	-	-	100%
Received Systemic Corticosteroids	-	-	-	100%
Emergency Department				
Admittance Decision Time (minutes)[5]	-	-	75	98
Head CT Results Within 45 Min. of Arrival	-	-	61%	57%
Patients Who Left ER Before Being Seen	-	-	1%	2%
Time from ER Arrival to Admit. (minutes)[5]	-	-	207	274
Time from ER Arrival to Discharge (minutes)	-	-	118	134
Time in ER Before Being Evaluated (minutes)	-	-	21	26
Time to Pain Meds for Fractures (minutes)	-	-	42	57
Heart Attack Care				
Aspirin Given at Discharge[5]	-	-	100%	99%
Fibrinolytic Meds Within 30 Min. of Arrival[5]	-	-	-	54%
PCI Within 90 Minutes of Arrival[5]	-	-	96%	96%
Statin Prescribed at Discharge[5]	-	-	99%	98%
Heart Failure Care				
ACE Inhibitor or ARB for LVSD[1,3]	-	-	96%	97%
Discharge Instructions Given[1,3]	-	-	93%	94%
Evaluation of LVS Function[1,3]	-	-	98%	99%
Medicare Spending				
Medicare Spending per Patient (ratio)	-	-	0.97	0.98
Pneumonia Care				
Appropriate Initial Antibiotic Given[1,3]	-	-	95%	95%
Blood Culture Timing[1,3]	-	-	99%	98%
Pregnancy and Delivery Care				
Newborn Deliveries Scheduled Early[5]	-	-	5%	6%
Preventive Care				
Immunization for Influenza[5]	-	-	89%	90%
Immunization for Pneumonia[5]	-	-	90%	92%
Stroke Care				
Anticoagulation Therapy for Atrial Fibrillation[5]	-	-	95%	95%
Antithrombotic Therapy Timing[5]	-	-	99%	98%
Assessed for Rehabilitation[5]	-	-	99%	97%
Discharged on Antithrombotic Therapy[5]	-	-	100%	99%
Discharged on Statin Medication[5]	-	-	93%	94%
Thrombolytic Therapy Timing[5]	-	-	75%	66%
Venous Thromboembolism Prophylaxis[5]	-	-	94%	94%
Written Stroke Educational Materials Given[5]	-	-	84%	88%
Surgical Care Improvement Project				
Appropriate Beta Blocker Usage[5]	-	-	98%	98%
Appropriate VTP Within 24 Hours[5]	-	-	99%	98%
Controlled Postoperative Blood Glucose[5]	-	-	96%	97%
Perioperative Temperature Management[5]	-	-	100%	100%
Prophylactic Antibiotic Selection[5]	-	-	99%	99%
Prophylactic Antibiotic Selection (Outpatient)	-	-	99%	98%
Prophylactic Antibiotic Stopped[5]	-	-	98%	98%

NOTE: Hospital profiles are in alphabetical order by state, then city, then hospital within the city; Rankings exclude hospitals with less than 25 cases except for patient surveys which excludes hospitals with less than 100 cases; (a) 100-299 cases; (1) The number of cases/patients is too few to report; (2) Data submitted were based on a sample of cases/patients; (3) Results are based on a shorter time period than required; (4) Data suppressed by CMS for one or more quarters; (5) Results are not available for this reporting period; (6) Fewer than 100 patients completed the HCAHPS survey; (7) No cases met the criteria for this measure; (8) The lower limit of the confidence interval cannot be calculated if the number of observed infections equals zero; (9) No data are available from the state/territory for this reporting period; (10) The scores shown reflect fewer than 50 completed surveys; (11) There were discrepancies in the data collection process; (12) This measure does not apply to this hospital for this reporting period; (13) Results cannot be calculated for this reporting period; (14) The results for this state are combined with nearby states to protect confidentiality; Please refer to the User's Guide for a full explanation of data.

Measure	Cases	This Hosp.	State Avg.	U.S. Avg.
Prophylactic Antibiotic Timing[5]	-	-	98%	99%
Prophylactic Antibiotic Timing (Outpatient)	-	-	97%	98%
Urinary Catheter Removal[5]	-	-	98%	97%
Survey of Patients' Hospital Experiences				
Area Around Room 'Always' Quiet at Night[6]	<100	62%	67%	61%
Doctors 'Always' Communicated Well[6]	<100	89%	86%	82%
Home Recovery Information Given[6]	<100	91%	88%	85%
Hospital Given 9 or 10 on 10 Point Scale[6]	<100	87%	78%	71%
Meds 'Always' Explained Before Given[6]	<100	86%	68%	64%
Nurses 'Always' Communicated Well[6]	<100	86%	83%	79%
Pain 'Always' Well Controlled[6]	<100	81%	73%	71%
Room and Bathroom 'Always' Clean[6]	<100	83%	81%	73%
Timely Help 'Always' Received[6]	<100	76%	75%	68%
Would Definitely Recommend Hospital[6]	<100	72%	77%	71%
Use of Medical Imaging				
Cardiac Imaging Stress Test before Surgery	-	-	5.4%	5.3%
Combination Abdominal CT Scan	-	-	9.3%	10.5%
Combination Brain/Sinus CT Scan	-	-	2.7%	2.7%
Combination Chest CT Scan	-	-	1.7%	2.7%
Follow-up Mammogram/Ultrasound	-	-	8%	8.8%
Lumbar Spine MRI for Low Back Pain	-	-	36.5%	37.2%

Johnson County Hospital

202 High St
Tecumseh, NE 68450
Phone: 402-335-3361
Fax: 402-335-6342
Type: Critical Access Hospitals
Emergency Services: Yes
Ownership: Government - Local
Beds: 18

Key Personnel:
Cardiac Laboratory. . . . . J Badertscher
Anesthesiology. . . . . James I DeFreece
Chief of Medical Staff . . . . Stacey Goodrich
Administrator . . . . Diane Newman
CEO/President. . . . . Dianne Newman
Operating Room. . . . . Jeanne Wolken

Measure	Cases	This Hosp.	State Avg.	U.S. Avg.
Blood Clot Prevention and Treatment				
Anticoagulation Overlap Therapy[5]	-	-	93%	93%
ICU Venous Thromboembolism Prophylaxis[5]	-	-	91%	92%
Incidence of Potentially Preventable VTE[5]	-	-	11%	10%
UFH with Dosages/Platelet Monitoring[5]	-	-	98%	97%
Venous Thromboembolism Prophylaxis[5]	-	-	88%	85%
Warfarin Therapy Discharge Instructions[5]	-	-	81%	75%
Chest Pain/Possible Heart Attack Care				
Aspirin Given Within 24 Hours of Arrival[1,3]	-	-	96%	96%
Fibrinolytic Meds Within 30 Min. of Arrival[1,3]	-	-	53%	58%
Average Time to ECG (minutes)[1,3]	-	-	8	7
Average Time to Transfer (minutes)[3,7]	-	-	76	60
Children's Asthma Care				
Received Home Management Plan of Care	-	-	-	88%
Received Reliever Medication	-	-	-	100%
Received Systemic Corticosteroids	-	-	-	100%
Emergency Department				
Admittance Decision Time (minutes)[5]	-	-	75	98
Head CT Results Within 45 Min. of Arrival[5]	-	-	61%	57%
Patients Who Left ER Before Being Seen[5]	-	-	1%	2%
Time from ER Arrival to Admit. (minutes)[5]	-	-	207	274
Time from ER Arrival to Discharge (minutes)[5]	-	-	118	134
Time in ER Before Being Evaluated (minutes)[5]	-	-	21	26
Time to Pain Meds for Fractures (minutes)[5]	-	-	42	57
Heart Attack Care				
Aspirin Given at Discharge[5]	-	-	100%	99%
Fibrinolytic Meds Within 30 Min. of Arrival[5]	-	-	-	54%
PCI Within 90 Minutes of Arrival[5]	-	-	96%	96%
Statin Prescribed at Discharge[5]	-	-	99%	98%
Heart Failure Care				
ACE Inhibitor or ARB for LVSD[1]	-	-	96%	97%
Discharge Instructions Given[1]	-	-	93%	94%
Evaluation of LVS Function[1]	-	-	98%	99%
Medicare Spending				
Medicare Spending per Patient (ratio)	-	-	0.97	0.98
Pneumonia Care				
Appropriate Initial Antibiotic Given	12	100%	95%	95%
Blood Culture Timing[1]	-	-	99%	98%
Pregnancy and Delivery Care				
Newborn Deliveries Scheduled Early[5]	-	-	5%	6%
Preventive Care				
Immunization for Influenza[5]	-	-	89%	90%
Immunization for Pneumonia[5]	-	-	90%	92%
Stroke Care				
Anticoagulation Therapy for Atrial Fibrillation[5]	-	-	95%	95%
Antithrombotic Therapy Timing[5]	-	-	99%	98%
Assessed for Rehabilitation[5]	-	-	99%	97%
Discharged on Antithrombotic Therapy[5]	-	-	100%	99%
Discharged on Statin Medication[5]	-	-	93%	94%
Thrombolytic Therapy Timing[5]	-	-	75%	66%
Venous Thromboembolism Prophylaxis[5]	-	-	94%	94%
Written Stroke Educational Materials Given[5]	-	-	84%	88%
Surgical Care Improvement Project				
Appropriate Beta Blocker Usage[3,7]	-	-	98%	98%
Appropriate VTP Within 24 Hours[1,3]	-	-	99%	98%
Controlled Postoperative Blood Glucose[3,7]	-	-	96%	97%
Perioperative Temperature Management[1,3]	-	-	100%	100%
Prophylactic Antibiotic Selection[1,3]	-	-	99%	99%
Prophylactic Antibiotic Selection (Outpatient)[5]	-	-	99%	98%
Prophylactic Antibiotic Stopped[1,3]	-	-	98%	98%
Prophylactic Antibiotic Timing[1,3]	-	-	98%	99%
Prophylactic Antibiotic Timing (Outpatient)[5]	-	-	97%	98%
Urinary Catheter Removal[3,7]	-	-	98%	97%
Survey of Patients' Hospital Experiences				
Area Around Room 'Always' Quiet at Night[6]	<100	63%	67%	61%
Doctors 'Always' Communicated Well[6]	<100	88%	86%	82%
Home Recovery Information Given[6]	<100	89%	88%	85%
Hospital Given 9 or 10 on 10 Point Scale[6]	<100	71%	78%	71%
Meds 'Always' Explained Before Given[6]	<100	62%	68%	64%
Nurses 'Always' Communicated Well[6]	<100	84%	83%	79%
Pain 'Always' Well Controlled[6]	<100	70%	73%	71%
Room and Bathroom 'Always' Clean[6]	<100	90%	81%	73%
Timely Help 'Always' Received[6]	<100	77%	75%	68%
Would Definitely Recommend Hospital[6]	<100	78%	77%	71%
Use of Medical Imaging				
Cardiac Imaging Stress Test before Surgery[1]	-	-	5.4%	5.3%
Combination Abdominal CT Scan	54	3.7%	9.3%	10.5%
Combination Brain/Sinus CT Scan[1]	-	-	2.7%	2.7%
Combination Chest CT Scan[1]	-	-	1.7%	2.7%
Follow-up Mammogram/Ultrasound	181	13.3%	8%	8.8%
Lumbar Spine MRI for Low Back Pain[1]	-	-	36.5%	37.2%

Tilden Community Hospital

PO Box 340, 308 West 2nd
Tilden, NE 68781
Phone: 402-368-5343
Fax: 402-368-7746
E-mail: info@tildenhospital.org
URL: www.tildenhospital.org
Type: Critical Access Hospitals
Emergency Services: Yes
Ownership: Government - Local
Beds: 20

Key Personnel:
Chief of Medical Staff . . . . Kelly Ellis
CEO/President. . . . . Lon Knievel
Ambulatory Care . . . . Anita Morrison
Anesthesiology. . . . . Anita Morrison
Emergency Room . . . . Anita Morrison
Intensive Care Unit. . . . . Anita Morrison
Quality Assurance . . . . Anita Morrison
Radiology. . . . . Judy Stout

Measure	Cases	This Hosp.	State Avg.	U.S. Avg.
Blood Clot Prevention and Treatment				
Anticoagulation Overlap Therapy[5]	-	-	93%	93%
ICU Venous Thromboembolism Prophylaxis[5]	-	-	91%	92%
Incidence of Potentially Preventable VTE[5]	-	-	11%	10%
UFH with Dosages/Platelet Monitoring[5]	-	-	98%	97%
Venous Thromboembolism Prophylaxis[5]	-	-	88%	85%
Warfarin Therapy Discharge Instructions[5]	-	-	81%	75%
Chest Pain/Possible Heart Attack Care				
Aspirin Given Within 24 Hours of Arrival[1,3]	-	-	96%	96%
Fibrinolytic Meds Within 30 Min. of Arrival[3,7]	-	-	53%	58%
Average Time to ECG (minutes)[1,3]	-	-	8	7
Average Time to Transfer (minutes)[1,3]	-	-	76	60
Children's Asthma Care				
Received Home Management Plan of Care	-	-	-	88%
Received Reliever Medication	-	-	-	100%
Received Systemic Corticosteroids	-	-	-	100%
Emergency Department				
Admittance Decision Time (minutes)[5]	-	-	75	98
Head CT Results Within 45 Min. of Arrival[5]	-	-	61%	57%
Patients Who Left ER Before Being Seen[5]	-	-	1%	2%
Time from ER Arrival to Admit. (minutes)[5]	-	-	207	274
Time from ER Arrival to Discharge (minutes)[5]	-	-	118	134
Time in ER Before Being Evaluated (minutes)[5]	-	-	21	26
Time to Pain Meds for Fractures (minutes)[5]	-	-	42	57
Heart Attack Care				
Aspirin Given at Discharge[5]	-	-	100%	99%
Fibrinolytic Meds Within 30 Min. of Arrival[5]	-	-	-	54%
PCI Within 90 Minutes of Arrival[5]	-	-	96%	96%
Statin Prescribed at Discharge[5]	-	-	99%	98%
Heart Failure Care				
ACE Inhibitor or ARB for LVSD[3,7]	-	-	96%	97%
Discharge Instructions Given[3,7]	-	-	93%	94%
Evaluation of LVS Function[3,7]	-	-	98%	99%
Medicare Spending				
Medicare Spending per Patient (ratio)	-	-	0.97	0.98
Pneumonia Care				
Appropriate Initial Antibiotic Given[1]	-	-	95%	95%
Blood Culture Timing[1]	-	-	99%	98%
Pregnancy and Delivery Care				
Newborn Deliveries Scheduled Early[5]	-	-	5%	6%
Preventive Care				
Immunization for Influenza[5]	-	-	89%	90%
Immunization for Pneumonia[5]	-	-	90%	92%
Stroke Care				
Anticoagulation Therapy for Atrial Fibrillation[5]	-	-	95%	95%
Antithrombotic Therapy Timing[5]	-	-	99%	98%
Assessed for Rehabilitation[5]	-	-	99%	97%
Discharged on Antithrombotic Therapy[5]	-	-	100%	99%
Discharged on Statin Medication[5]	-	-	93%	94%
Thrombolytic Therapy Timing[5]	-	-	75%	66%
Venous Thromboembolism Prophylaxis[5]	-	-	94%	94%
Written Stroke Educational Materials Given[5]	-	-	84%	88%
Surgical Care Improvement Project				
Appropriate Beta Blocker Usage[5]	-	-	98%	98%
Appropriate VTP Within 24 Hours[5]	-	-	99%	98%
Controlled Postoperative Blood Glucose[5]	-	-	96%	97%
Perioperative Temperature Management[5]	-	-	100%	100%
Prophylactic Antibiotic Selection[5]	-	-	99%	99%
Prophylactic Antibiotic Selection (Outpatient)[5]	-	-	99%	98%
Prophylactic Antibiotic Stopped[5]	-	-	98%	98%
Prophylactic Antibiotic Timing[5]	-	-	98%	99%
Prophylactic Antibiotic Timing (Outpatient)[5]	-	-	97%	98%
Urinary Catheter Removal[5]	-	-	98%	97%
Survey of Patients' Hospital Experiences				
Area Around Room 'Always' Quiet at Night[10]	<100	88%	67%	61%
Doctors 'Always' Communicated Well[10]	<100	96%	86%	82%
Home Recovery Information Given[10]	<100	95%	88%	85%
Hospital Given 9 or 10 on 10 Point Scale[10]	<100	81%	78%	71%
Meds 'Always' Explained Before Given[10]	<100	82%	68%	64%
Nurses 'Always' Communicated Well[10]	<100	99%	83%	79%
Pain 'Always' Well Controlled[10]	<100	100%	73%	71%
Room and Bathroom 'Always' Clean[10]	<100	97%	81%	73%
Timely Help 'Always' Received[10]	<100	100%	75%	68%
Would Definitely Recommend Hospital[10]	<100	90%	77%	71%
Use of Medical Imaging				
Cardiac Imaging Stress Test before Surgery[1]	-	-	5.4%	5.3%
Combination Abdominal CT Scan[1]	-	-	9.3%	10.5%
Combination Brain/Sinus CT Scan[1]	-	-	2.7%	2.7%
Combination Chest CT Scan[1]	-	-	1.7%	2.7%
Follow-up Mammogram/Ultrasound[1]	-	-	8%	8.8%
Lumbar Spine MRI for Low Back Pain[7]	-	-	36.5%	37.2%

NOTE: Hospital profiles are in alphabetical order by state, then city, then hospital within the city; Rankings exclude hospitals with less than 25 cases except for patient surveys which excludes hospitals with less than 100 cases; (a) 100-299 cases; (1) The number of cases/patients is too few to report; (2) Data submitted were based on a sample of cases/patients; (3) Results are based on a shorter time period than required; (4) Data suppressed by CMS for one or more quarters; (5) Results are not available for this reporting period; (6) Fewer than 100 patients completed the HCAHPS survey; (7) No cases met the criteria for this measure; (8) The lower limit of the confidence interval cannot be calculated if the number of observed infections equals zero; (9) No data are available from the state/territory for this reporting period; (10) The scores shown reflect fewer than 50 completed surveys; (11) There were discrepancies in the data collection process; (12) This measure does not apply to this hospital for this reporting period; (13) Results cannot be calculated for this reporting period; (14) The results for this state are combined with nearby states to protect confidentiality; Please refer to the User's Guide for a full explanation of data.

Cherry County Hospital

PO Box 410, 510 North Green St | Phone: 402-376-2525
Valentine, NE 69201 | Fax: 402-376-1627
URL: www.cchospital.net
Type: Critical Access Hospitals | Emergency Services: Yes
Ownership: Government - Local | Beds: 25

Key Personnel:
Surgery . . . . Morris C. Benson, MD
Cardiology . . . . Scott Coatsworth, MD
Pulmonology . . . . Lon W. Keim, MD
Emergency Room . . . . Shawn S. Lawrence, MD
Infection Control . . . . Darlene Myer
Operating Room . . . . Lyreva Nollette

Measure	Cases	This Hosp.	State Avg.	U.S. Avg.
Blood Clot Prevention and Treatment				
Anticoagulation Overlap Therapy[5]	-	-	93%	93%
ICU Venous Thromboembolism Prophylaxis[5]	-	-	91%	92%
Incidence of Potentially Preventable VTE[5]	-	-	11%	10%
UFH with Dosages/Platelet Monitoring[5]	-	-	98%	97%
Venous Thromboembolism Prophylaxis[5]	-	-	88%	85%
Warfarin Therapy Discharge Instructions[5]	-	-	81%	75%
Chest Pain/Possible Heart Attack Care				
Aspirin Given Within 24 Hours of Arrival[1]	-	-	96%	96%
Fibrinolytic Meds Within 30 Min. of Arrival[3,7]	-	-	53%	58%
Average Time to ECG (minutes)[1]	-	-	8	7
Average Time to Transfer (minutes)[3,7]	-	-	76	60
Children's Asthma Care				
Received Home Management Plan of Care	-	-	-	88%
Received Reliever Medication	-	-	-	100%
Received Systemic Corticosteroids	-	-	-	100%
Emergency Department				
Admittance Decision Time (minutes)[5]	-	-	75	98
Head CT Results Within 45 Min. of Arrival[5]	-	-	61%	57%
Patients Who Left ER Before Being Seen[5]	-	-	1%	2%
Time from ER Arrival to Admit. (minutes)[5]	-	-	207	274
Time from ER Arrival to Discharge (minutes)[5]	-	-	118	134
Time in ER Before Being Evaluated (minutes)[5]	-	-	21	26
Time to Pain Meds for Fractures (minutes)[5]	-	-	42	57
Heart Attack Care				
Aspirin Given at Discharge[5]	-	-	100%	99%
Fibrinolytic Meds Within 30 Min. of Arrival[5]	-	-	-	54%
PCI Within 90 Minutes of Arrival[5]	-	-	96%	96%
Statin Prescribed at Discharge[5]	-	-	99%	98%
Heart Failure Care				
ACE Inhibitor or ARB for LVSD[1,3]	-	-	96%	97%
Discharge Instructions Given[1,3]	-	-	93%	94%
Evaluation of LVS Function[1,3]	-	-	98%	99%
Medicare Spending				
Medicare Spending per Patient (ratio)	-	-	0.97	0.98
Pneumonia Care				
Appropriate Initial Antibiotic Given	11	100%	95%	95%
Blood Culture Timing[1]	-	-	99%	98%
Pregnancy and Delivery Care				
Newborn Deliveries Scheduled Early[5]	-	-	5%	6%
Preventive Care				
Immunization for Influenza[5]	-	-	89%	90%
Immunization for Pneumonia[5]	-	-	90%	92%
Stroke Care				
Anticoagulation Therapy for Atrial Fibrillation[5]	-	-	95%	95%
Antithrombotic Therapy Timing[5]	-	-	99%	98%
Assessed for Rehabilitation[5]	-	-	99%	97%
Discharged on Antithrombotic Therapy[5]	-	-	100%	99%
Discharged on Statin Medication[5]	-	-	93%	94%
Thrombolytic Therapy Timing[5]	-	-	75%	66%
Venous Thromboembolism Prophylaxis[5]	-	-	94%	94%
Written Stroke Educational Materials Given[5]	-	-	84%	88%
Surgical Care Improvement Project				
Appropriate Beta Blocker Usage[5]	-	-	98%	98%
Appropriate VTP Within 24 Hours[5]	-	-	99%	98%
Controlled Postoperative Blood Glucose[5]	-	-	96%	97%
Perioperative Temperature Management[5]	-	-	100%	100%
Prophylactic Antibiotic Selection[5]	-	-	99%	99%
Prophylactic Antibiotic Selection (Outpatient)[5]	-	-	99%	98%
Prophylactic Antibiotic Stopped[5]	-	-	98%	98%
Prophylactic Antibiotic Timing[5]	-	-	98%	99%
Prophylactic Antibiotic Timing (Outpatient)[5]	-	-	97%	98%
Urinary Catheter Removal[5]	-	-	98%	97%
Survey of Patients' Hospital Experiences				
Area Around Room 'Always' Quiet at Night	(a)	69%	67%	61%
Doctors 'Always' Communicated Well	(a)	83%	86%	82%
Home Recovery Information Given	(a)	90%	88%	85%
Hospital Given 9 or 10 on 10 Point Scale	(a)	76%	78%	71%
Meds 'Always' Explained Before Given	(a)	72%	68%	64%
Nurses 'Always' Communicated Well	(a)	79%	83%	79%
Pain 'Always' Well Controlled	(a)	67%	73%	71%
Room and Bathroom 'Always' Clean	(a)	84%	81%	73%
Timely Help 'Always' Received	(a)	76%	75%	68%
Would Definitely Recommend Hospital	(a)	72%	77%	71%
Use of Medical Imaging				
Cardiac Imaging Stress Test before Surgery	62	4.8%	5.4%	5.3%
Combination Abdominal CT Scan	78	1.3%	9.3%	10.5%
Combination Brain/Sinus CT Scan	120	5.8%	2.7%	2.7%
Combination Chest CT Scan	50	0.0%	1.7%	2.7%
Follow-up Mammogram/Ultrasound	122	15.6%	8%	8.8%
Lumbar Spine MRI for Low Back Pain[1]	-	-	36.5%	37.2%

Saunders Medical Center

1760 County Rd J | Phone: 402-443-4191
Wahoo, NE 68066 | Fax: 402-443-1401
E-mail: info@saunders-health.org
URL: www.saunders-health.org
Type: Critical Access Hospitals | Emergency Services: Yes
Ownership: Government - Local | Beds: 25

Key Personnel:
CEO . . . . Ken Archer
Infection Control . . . . Bev Janacek, RN
Chief of Medical Staff . . . . Leo Meduna, MD

Measure	Cases	This Hosp.	State Avg.	U.S. Avg.
Blood Clot Prevention and Treatment				
Anticoagulation Overlap Therapy[5]	-	-	93%	93%
ICU Venous Thromboembolism Prophylaxis[5]	-	-	91%	92%
Incidence of Potentially Preventable VTE[5]	-	-	11%	10%
UFH with Dosages/Platelet Monitoring[5]	-	-	98%	97%
Venous Thromboembolism Prophylaxis[5]	-	-	88%	85%
Warfarin Therapy Discharge Instructions[5]	-	-	81%	75%
Chest Pain/Possible Heart Attack Care				
Aspirin Given Within 24 Hours of Arrival	21	90%	96%	96%
Fibrinolytic Meds Within 30 Min. of Arrival[1]	-	-	53%	58%
Average Time to ECG (minutes)	23	11	8	7
Average Time to Transfer (minutes)[1]	-	-	76	60
Children's Asthma Care				
Received Home Management Plan of Care	-	-	-	88%
Received Reliever Medication	-	-	-	100%
Received Systemic Corticosteroids	-	-	-	100%
Emergency Department				
Admittance Decision Time (minutes)[5]	-	-	75	98
Head CT Results Within 45 Min. of Arrival[5]	-	-	61%	57%
Patients Who Left ER Before Being Seen[5]	-	-	1%	2%
Time from ER Arrival to Admit. (minutes)[5]	-	-	207	274
Time from ER Arrival to Discharge (minutes)[5]	-	-	118	134
Time in ER Before Being Evaluated (minutes)[5]	-	-	21	26
Time to Pain Meds for Fractures (minutes)[5]	-	-	42	57
Heart Attack Care				
Aspirin Given at Discharge[1,3]	-	-	100%	99%
Fibrinolytic Meds Within 30 Min. of Arrival[3,7]	-	-	-	54%
PCI Within 90 Minutes of Arrival[3,7]	-	-	96%	96%
Statin Prescribed at Discharge[1,3]	-	-	99%	98%
Heart Failure Care				
ACE Inhibitor or ARB for LVSD[1]	-	-	96%	97%
Discharge Instructions Given[1]	-	-	93%	94%
Evaluation of LVS Function	15	93%	98%	99%
Medicare Spending				
Medicare Spending per Patient (ratio)	-	-	0.97	0.98
Pneumonia Care				
Appropriate Initial Antibiotic Given	19	95%	95%	95%
Blood Culture Timing[1]	-	-	99%	98%
Pregnancy and Delivery Care				
Newborn Deliveries Scheduled Early[5]	-	-	5%	6%
Preventive Care				
Immunization for Influenza[5]	-	-	89%	90%
Immunization for Pneumonia[5]	-	-	90%	92%
Stroke Care				
Anticoagulation Therapy for Atrial Fibrillation[5]	-	-	95%	95%
Antithrombotic Therapy Timing[5]	-	-	99%	98%
Assessed for Rehabilitation[5]	-	-	99%	97%
Discharged on Antithrombotic Therapy[5]	-	-	100%	99%
Discharged on Statin Medication[5]	-	-	93%	94%
Thrombolytic Therapy Timing[5]	-	-	75%	66%
Venous Thromboembolism Prophylaxis[5]	-	-	94%	94%
Written Stroke Educational Materials Given[5]	-	-	84%	88%
Surgical Care Improvement Project				
Appropriate Beta Blocker Usage[5]	-	-	98%	98%
Appropriate VTP Within 24 Hours[5]	-	-	99%	98%
Controlled Postoperative Blood Glucose[5]	-	-	96%	97%
Perioperative Temperature Management[5]	-	-	100%	100%
Prophylactic Antibiotic Selection[5]	-	-	99%	99%
Prophylactic Antibiotic Selection (Outpatient)[5]	-	-	99%	98%
Prophylactic Antibiotic Stopped[5]	-	-	98%	98%
Prophylactic Antibiotic Timing[5]	-	-	98%	99%
Prophylactic Antibiotic Timing (Outpatient)[5]	-	-	97%	98%
Urinary Catheter Removal[5]	-	-	98%	97%
Survey of Patients' Hospital Experiences				
Area Around Room 'Always' Quiet at Night[6]	<100	76%	67%	61%
Doctors 'Always' Communicated Well[6]	<100	89%	86%	82%
Home Recovery Information Given[6]	<100	89%	88%	85%
Hospital Given 9 or 10 on 10 Point Scale[6]	<100	79%	78%	71%
Meds 'Always' Explained Before Given[6]	<100	69%	68%	64%
Nurses 'Always' Communicated Well[6]	<100	87%	83%	79%
Pain 'Always' Well Controlled[6]	<100	72%	73%	71%
Room and Bathroom 'Always' Clean[6]	<100	98%	81%	73%
Timely Help 'Always' Received[6]	<100	72%	75%	68%
Would Definitely Recommend Hospital[6]	<100	84%	77%	71%
Use of Medical Imaging				
Cardiac Imaging Stress Test before Surgery	55	3.6%	5.4%	5.3%
Combination Abdominal CT Scan	125	4.0%	9.3%	10.5%
Combination Brain/Sinus CT Scan[1]	-	-	2.7%	2.7%
Combination Chest CT Scan	62	0.0%	1.7%	2.7%
Follow-up Mammogram/Ultrasound	137	8.0%	8%	8.8%
Lumbar Spine MRI for Low Back Pain[1]	-	-	36.5%	37.2%

Providence Medical Center

1200 Providence Rd | Phone: 402-375-3800
Wayne, NE 68787 | Fax: 402-375-7989
URL: www.providencemedical.com
Type: Critical Access Hospitals | Emergency Services: Yes
Ownership: Voluntary non-profit - Private | Beds: 25

Key Personnel:
Radiology . . . . Jeffry Ailes
Operating Room . . . . Michael Bittles
Pulmonology . . . . Fawad Chaudry, MD
Chief of Medical Staff . . . . Matthew Felber
Cardiology . . . . Maryanne Hartzell, MD
Infection Control . . . . Kathy Hillier
Quality Assurance . . . . Dennis Spangler
Surgery . . . . Keith Vollstedt, MD

Measure	Cases	This Hosp.	State Avg.	U.S. Avg.
Blood Clot Prevention and Treatment				
Anticoagulation Overlap Therapy[5]	-	-	93%	93%
ICU Venous Thromboembolism Prophylaxis[5]	-	-	91%	92%
Incidence of Potentially Preventable VTE[5]	-	-	11%	10%
UFH with Dosages/Platelet Monitoring[5]	-	-	98%	97%
Venous Thromboembolism Prophylaxis[5]	-	-	88%	85%
Warfarin Therapy Discharge Instructions[5]	-	-	81%	75%
Chest Pain/Possible Heart Attack Care				
Aspirin Given Within 24 Hours of Arrival[1]	-	-	96%	96%
Fibrinolytic Meds Within 30 Min. of Arrival[3,7]	-	-	53%	58%
Average Time to ECG (minutes)[1]	-	-	8	7
Average Time to Transfer (minutes)[3,7]	-	-	76	60
Children's Asthma Care				
Received Home Management Plan of Care	-	-	-	88%
Received Reliever Medication	-	-	-	100%

NOTE: Hospital profiles are in alphabetical order by state, then city, then hospital within the city; Rankings exclude hospitals with less than 25 cases except for patient surveys which excludes hospitals with less than 100 cases; (a) 100-299 cases; (1) The number of cases/patients is too few to report; (2) Data submitted were based on a sample of cases/patients; (3) Results are based on a shorter time period than required; (4) Data suppressed by CMS for one or more quarters; (5) Results are not available for this reporting period; (6) Fewer than 100 patients completed the HCAHPS survey; (7) No cases met the criteria for this measure; (8) The lower limit of the confidence interval cannot be calculated if the number of observed infections equals zero; (9) No data are available from the state/territory for this reporting period; (10) The scores shown reflect fewer than 50 completed surveys; (11) There were discrepancies in the data collection process; (12) This measure does not apply to this hospital for this reporting period; (13) Results cannot be calculated for this reporting period; (14) The results for this state are combined with nearby states to protect confidentiality; Please refer to the User's Guide for a full explanation of data.

Measure	Cases	This Hosp.	State Avg.	U.S. Avg.
Received Systemic Corticosteroids	-	-	-	100%
Emergency Department				
Admittance Decision Time (minutes)[5]	-	-	75	98
Head CT Results Within 45 Min. of Arrival[5]	-	-	61%	57%
Patients Who Left ER Before Being Seen	1,749	0%	1%	2%
Time from ER Arrival to Admit. (minutes)[5]	-	-	207	274
Time from ER Arrival to Discharge (minutes)[5]	-	-	118	134
Time in ER Before Being Evaluated (minutes)[5]	-	-	21	26
Time to Pain Meds for Fractures (minutes)[5]	-	-	42	57
Heart Attack Care				
Aspirin Given at Discharge[1,3]	-	-	100%	99%
Fibrinolytic Meds Within 30 Min. of Arrival[3,7]	-	-	-	54%
PCI Within 90 Minutes of Arrival[3,7]	-	-	96%	96%
Statin Prescribed at Discharge[1,3]	-	-	99%	98%
Heart Failure Care				
ACE Inhibitor or ARB for LVSD[1]	-	-	96%	97%
Discharge Instructions Given[1]	-	-	93%	94%
Evaluation of LVS Function	13	92%	98%	99%
Medicare Spending				
Medicare Spending per Patient (ratio)	-	-	0.97	0.98
Pneumonia Care				
Appropriate Initial Antibiotic Given	13	100%	95%	95%
Blood Culture Timing[1]	-	-	99%	98%
Pregnancy and Delivery Care				
Newborn Deliveries Scheduled Early[5]	-	-	5%	6%
Preventive Care				
Immunization for Influenza[5]	-	-	89%	90%
Immunization for Pneumonia[5]	-	-	90%	92%
Stroke Care				
Anticoagulation Therapy for Atrial Fibrillation[5]	-	-	95%	95%
Antithrombotic Therapy Timing[5]	-	-	99%	98%
Assessed for Rehabilitation[5]	-	-	99%	97%
Discharged on Antithrombotic Therapy[5]	-	-	100%	99%
Discharged on Statin Medication[5]	-	-	93%	94%
Thrombolytic Therapy Timing[5]	-	-	75%	66%
Venous Thromboembolism Prophylaxis[5]	-	-	94%	94%
Written Stroke Educational Materials Given[5]	-	-	84%	88%
Surgical Care Improvement Project				
Appropriate Beta Blocker Usage[1]	-	-	98%	98%
Appropriate VTP Within 24 Hours	14	100%	99%	98%
Controlled Postoperative Blood Glucose[7]	-	-	96%	97%
Perioperative Temperature Management	17	94%	100%	100%
Prophylactic Antibiotic Selection	14	100%	99%	99%
Prophylactic Antibiotic Selection (Outpatient)[1,3]	-	-	99%	98%
Prophylactic Antibiotic Stopped	14	93%	98%	98%
Prophylactic Antibiotic Timing	14	86%	98%	99%
Prophylactic Antibiotic Timing (Outpatient)[1,3]	-	-	97%	98%
Urinary Catheter Removal[1]	-	-	98%	97%
Survey of Patients' Hospital Experiences				
Area Around Room 'Always' Quiet at Night[6]	<100	61%	67%	61%
Doctors 'Always' Communicated Well[6]	<100	92%	86%	82%
Home Recovery Information Given[6]	<100	88%	88%	85%
Hospital Given 9 or 10 on 10 Point Scale[6]	<100	82%	78%	71%
Meds 'Always' Explained Before Given[6]	<100	76%	68%	64%
Nurses 'Always' Communicated Well[6]	<100	86%	83%	79%
Pain 'Always' Well Controlled[6]	<100	69%	73%	71%
Room and Bathroom 'Always' Clean[6]	<100	86%	81%	73%
Timely Help 'Always' Received[6]	<100	82%	75%	68%
Would Definitely Recommend Hospital[6]	<100	74%	77%	71%
Use of Medical Imaging				
Cardiac Imaging Stress Test before Surgery[1]	-	-	5.4%	5.3%
Combination Abdominal CT Scan	82	3.7%	9.3%	10.5%
Combination Brain/Sinus CT Scan[1]	-	-	2.7%	2.7%
Combination Chest CT Scan[1]	-	-	1.7%	2.7%
Follow-up Mammogram/Ultrasound	187	9.6%	8%	8.8%
Lumbar Spine MRI for Low Back Pain[1]	-	-	36.5%	37.2%

Saint Francis Memorial Hospital

430 North Monitor St
West Point, NE 68788
E-mail: jmeiergerd@fcswp.org
URL: www.fcswp.org/sfmh
Phone: 402-372-2404
Fax: 402-372-2360
Type: Critical Access Hospitals
Emergency Services: Yes
Ownership: Voluntary non-profit - Private
Beds: 25

Key Personnel:
CEO/President. . . . . Ronald O Briggs
Chief of Medical Staff. . . . . Scott Green
Patient Relations . . . . Eileen Schlecht, RN
Infection Control. . . . . Karen Spenner, RN
Operating Room. . . . . Gloria Wellman, RN

Measure	Cases	This Hosp.	State Avg.	U.S. Avg.
Blood Clot Prevention and Treatment				
Anticoagulation Overlap Therapy[5]	-	-	93%	93%
ICU Venous Thromboembolism Prophylaxis[5]	-	-	91%	92%
Incidence of Potentially Preventable VTE[5]	-	-	11%	10%
UFH with Dosages/Platelet Monitoring[5]	-	-	98%	97%
Venous Thromboembolism Prophylaxis[5]	-	-	88%	85%
Warfarin Therapy Discharge Instructions[5]	-	-	81%	75%
Chest Pain/Possible Heart Attack Care				
Aspirin Given Within 24 Hours of Arrival	15	87%	96%	96%
Fibrinolytic Meds Within 30 Min. of Arrival[1]	-	-	53%	58%
Average Time to ECG (minutes)	15	6	8	7
Average Time to Transfer (minutes)[1]	-	-	76	60
Children's Asthma Care				
Received Home Management Plan of Care	-	-	-	88%
Received Reliever Medication	-	-	-	100%
Received Systemic Corticosteroids	-	-	-	100%
Emergency Department				
Admittance Decision Time (minutes)[5]	-	-	75	98
Head CT Results Within 45 Min. of Arrival[5]	-	-	61%	57%
Patients Who Left ER Before Being Seen[5]	-	-	1%	2%
Time from ER Arrival to Admit. (minutes)[5]	-	-	207	274
Time from ER Arrival to Discharge (minutes)[5]	-	-	118	134
Time in ER Before Being Evaluated (minutes)[5]	-	-	21	26
Time to Pain Meds for Fractures (minutes)[5]	-	-	42	57
Heart Attack Care				
Aspirin Given at Discharge[1,3]	-	-	100%	99%
Fibrinolytic Meds Within 30 Min. of Arrival[3,7]	-	-	-	54%
PCI Within 90 Minutes of Arrival[3,7]	-	-	96%	96%
Statin Prescribed at Discharge[1,3]	-	-	99%	98%
Heart Failure Care				
ACE Inhibitor or ARB for LVSD[1]	-	-	96%	97%
Discharge Instructions Given	11	91%	93%	94%
Evaluation of LVS Function	18	78%	98%	99%
Medicare Spending				
Medicare Spending per Patient (ratio)	-	-	0.97	0.98
Pneumonia Care				
Appropriate Initial Antibiotic Given	11	91%	95%	95%
Blood Culture Timing	11	100%	99%	98%
Pregnancy and Delivery Care				
Newborn Deliveries Scheduled Early[5]	-	-	5%	6%
Preventive Care				
Immunization for Influenza[5]	-	-	89%	90%
Immunization for Pneumonia[5]	-	-	90%	92%
Stroke Care				
Anticoagulation Therapy for Atrial Fibrillation[5]	-	-	95%	95%
Antithrombotic Therapy Timing[5]	-	-	99%	98%
Assessed for Rehabilitation[5]	-	-	99%	97%
Discharged on Antithrombotic Therapy[5]	-	-	100%	99%
Discharged on Statin Medication[5]	-	-	93%	94%
Thrombolytic Therapy Timing[5]	-	-	75%	66%
Venous Thromboembolism Prophylaxis[5]	-	-	94%	94%
Written Stroke Educational Materials Given[5]	-	-	84%	88%
Surgical Care Improvement Project				
Appropriate Beta Blocker Usage[1]	-	-	98%	98%
Appropriate VTP Within 24 Hours	36	100%	99%	98%
Controlled Postoperative Blood Glucose[7]	-	-	96%	97%
Perioperative Temperature Management	36	100%	100%	100%
Prophylactic Antibiotic Selection	37	92%	99%	99%
Prophylactic Antibiotic Selection (Outpatient)[1,3]	-	-	99%	98%
Prophylactic Antibiotic Stopped	37	97%	98%	98%
Prophylactic Antibiotic Timing	37	89%	98%	99%
Prophylactic Antibiotic Timing (Outpatient)[1,3]	-	-	97%	98%
Urinary Catheter Removal[1]	-	-	98%	97%
Survey of Patients' Hospital Experiences				
Area Around Room 'Always' Quiet at Night[6]	<100	72%	67%	61%
Doctors 'Always' Communicated Well[6]	<100	86%	86%	82%
Home Recovery Information Given[6]	<100	93%	88%	85%
Hospital Given 9 or 10 on 10 Point Scale[6]	<100	82%	78%	71%
Meds 'Always' Explained Before Given[6]	<100	73%	68%	64%
Nurses 'Always' Communicated Well[6]	<100	85%	83%	79%
Pain 'Always' Well Controlled[6]	<100	69%	73%	71%
Room and Bathroom 'Always' Clean[6]	<100	88%	81%	73%
Timely Help 'Always' Received[6]	<100	75%	75%	68%
Would Definitely Recommend Hospital[6]	<100	83%	77%	71%
Use of Medical Imaging				
Cardiac Imaging Stress Test before Surgery[1]	-	-	5.4%	5.3%
Combination Abdominal CT Scan	90	2.2%	9.3%	10.5%
Combination Brain/Sinus CT Scan	78	0.0%	2.7%	2.7%
Combination Chest CT Scan	69	2.9%	1.7%	2.7%
Follow-up Mammogram/Ultrasound	400	7.8%	8%	8.8%
Lumbar Spine MRI for Low Back Pain[1]	-	-	36.5%	37.2%

York General Hospital

2222 Lincoln Ave
York, NE 68467
E-mail: yorkgenhosp@navix.net
URL: www.yorkgeneral.org
Phone: 402-362-6671
Fax: 402-362-0499
Type: Critical Access Hospitals
Emergency Services: Yes
Ownership: Voluntary non-profit - Private
Beds: 25

Key Personnel:
Chief of Medical Staff. . . . . Todd Fago, MD
President. . . . . Charles Harris
Quality Assurance . . . . Linda Zieg

Measure	Cases	This Hosp.	State Avg.	U.S. Avg.
Blood Clot Prevention and Treatment				
Anticoagulation Overlap Therapy[5]	-	-	93%	93%
ICU Venous Thromboembolism Prophylaxis[5]	-	-	91%	92%
Incidence of Potentially Preventable VTE[5]	-	-	11%	10%
UFH with Dosages/Platelet Monitoring[5]	-	-	98%	97%
Venous Thromboembolism Prophylaxis[5]	-	-	88%	85%
Warfarin Therapy Discharge Instructions[5]	-	-	81%	75%
Chest Pain/Possible Heart Attack Care				
Aspirin Given Within 24 Hours of Arrival	13	100%	96%	96%
Fibrinolytic Meds Within 30 Min. of Arrival[1]	-	-	53%	58%
Average Time to ECG (minutes)	13	6	8	7
Average Time to Transfer (minutes)[1]	-	-	76	60
Children's Asthma Care				
Received Home Management Plan of Care	-	-	-	88%
Received Reliever Medication	-	-	-	100%
Received Systemic Corticosteroids	-	-	-	100%
Emergency Department				
Admittance Decision Time (minutes)[5]	-	-	75	98
Head CT Results Within 45 Min. of Arrival[5]	-	-	61%	57%
Patients Who Left ER Before Being Seen[5]	-	-	1%	2%
Time from ER Arrival to Admit. (minutes)[5]	-	-	207	274
Time from ER Arrival to Discharge (minutes)[5]	-	-	118	134
Time in ER Before Being Evaluated (minutes)[5]	-	-	21	26
Time to Pain Meds for Fractures (minutes)[5]	-	-	42	57
Heart Attack Care				
Aspirin Given at Discharge[5]	-	-	100%	99%
Fibrinolytic Meds Within 30 Min. of Arrival[5]	-	-	-	54%
PCI Within 90 Minutes of Arrival[5]	-	-	96%	96%
Statin Prescribed at Discharge[5]	-	-	99%	98%
Heart Failure Care				
ACE Inhibitor or ARB for LVSD[1]	-	-	96%	97%
Discharge Instructions Given[1]	-	-	93%	94%
Evaluation of LVS Function	18	100%	98%	99%
Medicare Spending				
Medicare Spending per Patient (ratio)	-	-	0.97	0.98
Pneumonia Care				
Appropriate Initial Antibiotic Given	21	100%	95%	95%
Blood Culture Timing	26	100%	99%	98%
Pregnancy and Delivery Care				

NOTE: Hospital profiles are in alphabetical order by state, then city, then hospital within the city; Rankings exclude hospitals with less than 25 cases except for patient surveys which excludes hospitals with less than 100 cases; (a) 100-299 cases; (1) The number of cases/patients is too few to report; (2) Data submitted were based on a sample of cases/patients; (3) Results are based on a shorter time period than required; (4) Data suppressed by CMS for one or more quarters; (5) Results are not available for this reporting period; (6) Fewer than 100 patients completed the HCAHPS survey; (7) No cases met the criteria for this measure; (8) The lower limit of the confidence interval cannot be calculated if the number of observed infections equals zero; (9) No data are available from the state/territory for this reporting period; (10) The scores shown reflect fewer than 50 completed surveys; (11) There were discrepancies in the data collection process; (12) This measure does not apply to this hospital for this reporting period; (13) Results cannot be calculated for this reporting period; (14) The results for this state are combined with nearby states to protect confidentiality; Please refer to the User's Guide for a full explanation of data.

Newborn Deliveries Scheduled Early[5]	-	-	5%	6%
Preventive Care				
Immunization for Influenza[5]	-	-	89%	90%
Immunization for Pneumonia[5]	-	-	90%	92%
Stroke Care				
Anticoagulation Therapy for Atrial Fibrillation[5]	-	-	95%	95%
Antithrombotic Therapy Timing[5]	-	-	99%	98%
Assessed for Rehabilitation[5]	-	-	99%	97%
Discharged on Antithrombotic Therapy[5]	-	-	100%	99%
Discharged on Statin Medication[5]	-	-	93%	94%
Thrombolytic Therapy Timing[5]	-	-	75%	66%
Venous Thromboembolism Prophylaxis[5]	-	-	94%	94%
Written Stroke Educational Materials Given[5]	-	-	84%	88%
Surgical Care Improvement Project				
Appropriate Beta Blocker Usage	16	100%	98%	98%
Appropriate VTP Within 24 Hours	51	100%	99%	98%
Controlled Postoperative Blood Glucose[7]	-	-	96%	97%
Perioperative Temperature Management	58	100%	100%	100%
Prophylactic Antibiotic Selection	61	100%	99%	99%
Prophylactic Antibiotic Selection (Outpatient)[1,3]	-	-	99%	98%
Prophylactic Antibiotic Stopped	61	100%	98%	98%
Prophylactic Antibiotic Timing	61	98%	98%	99%
Prophylactic Antibiotic Timing (Outpatient)[1,3]	-	-	97%	98%
Urinary Catheter Removal	46	100%	98%	97%
Survey of Patients' Hospital Experiences				
Area Around Room 'Always' Quiet at Night	(a)	65%	67%	61%
Doctors 'Always' Communicated Well	(a)	85%	86%	82%
Home Recovery Information Given	(a)	84%	88%	85%
Hospital Given 9 or 10 on 10 Point Scale	(a)	79%	78%	71%
Meds 'Always' Explained Before Given	(a)	66%	68%	64%
Nurses 'Always' Communicated Well	(a)	79%	83%	79%
Pain 'Always' Well Controlled	(a)	66%	73%	71%
Room and Bathroom 'Always' Clean	(a)	90%	81%	73%
Timely Help 'Always' Received	(a)	70%	75%	68%
Would Definitely Recommend Hospital	(a)	73%	77%	71%
Use of Medical Imaging				
Cardiac Imaging Stress Test before Surgery	157	6.4%	5.4%	5.3%
Combination Abdominal CT Scan	128	7.0%	9.3%	10.5%
Combination Brain/Sinus CT Scan	163	1.2%	2.7%	2.7%
Combination Chest CT Scan	127	0.0%	1.7%	2.7%
Follow-up Mammogram/Ultrasound	411	15.1%	8%	8.8%
Lumbar Spine MRI for Low Back Pain[1]	-	-	36.5%	37.2%

NOTE: Hospital profiles are in alphabetical order by state, then city, then hospital within the city; Rankings exclude hospitals with less than 25 cases except for patient surveys which excludes hospitals with less than 100 cases; (a) 100-299 cases; (1) The number of cases/patients is too few to report; (2) Data submitted were based on a sample of cases/patients; (3) Results are based on a shorter time period than required; (4) Data suppressed by CMS for one or more quarters; (5) Results are not available for this reporting period; (6) Fewer than 100 patients completed the HCAHPS survey; (7) No cases met the criteria for this measure; (8) The lower limit of the confidence interval cannot be calculated if the number of observed infections equals zero; (9) No data are available from the state/territory for this reporting period; (10) The scores shown reflect fewer than 50 completed surveys; (11) There were discrepancies in the data collection process; (12) This measure does not apply to this hospital for this reporting period; (13) Results cannot be calculated for this reporting period; (14) The results for this state are combined with nearby states to protect confidentiality; Please refer to the User's Guide for a full explanation of data.

Blood Clot Prevention and Treatment

Anticoagulation Overlap Therapy

Hospital Name	City	Rate	Cases
Essentia Health - Fargo[2]	Fargo	100%	48
Sanford Medical Center Fargo[2]	Fargo	100%	99
Trinity Hospitals[2]	Minot	97%	70
Altru Hospital[2]	Grand Forks	96%	70
Saint Alexius Medical Center[2]	Bismarck	95%	73
Sanford Medical Center Bismarck[2]	Bismarck	94%	79

ICU Venous Thromboembolism Prophylaxis

Hospital Name	City	Rate	Cases
Essentia Health - Fargo[2]	Fargo	96%	81
Saint Alexius Medical Center[2]	Bismarck	95%	40
Sanford Medical Center Fargo[2]	Fargo	94%	69
Sanford Medical Center Bismarck[2]	Bismarck	86%	37
Trinity Hospitals[2]	Minot	86%	133
Altru Hospital[2]	Grand Forks	77%	105

Incidence of Potentially Preventable VTE

Hospital Name	City	Rate	Cases
Sanford Medical Center Fargo[2]	Fargo	8%	25

UFH with Dosages/Platelet Count Monitoring

Hospital Name	City	Rate	Cases
Altru Hospital[2]	Grand Forks	100%	75
Essentia Health - Fargo[2]	Fargo	100%	36
Sanford Medical Center Bismarck[2]	Bismarck	100%	78
Sanford Medical Center Fargo[2]	Fargo	99%	78

Venous Thromboembolism Prophylaxis

Hospital Name	City	Rate	Cases
Mercy Medical Center[2]	Williston	94%	90
Essentia Health - Fargo[2]	Fargo	90%	300
Sanford Medical Center Fargo[2]	Fargo	90%	327
Saint Alexius Medical Center[2]	Bismarck	82%	391
Altru Hospital[2]	Grand Forks	79%	321
Sanford Medical Center Bismarck[2]	Bismarck	78%	329
Trinity Hospitals[2]	Minot	77%	328
PHS Indian Hosp at Belcourt-Quentin[2]	Belcourt	30%	142

Warfarin Therapy Discharge Instructions

Hospital Name	City	Rate	Cases
Essentia Health - Fargo[2]	Fargo	100%	40
Saint Alexius Medical Center[2]	Bismarck	96%	52
Sanford Medical Center Bismarck[2]	Bismarck	96%	67
Trinity Hospitals[2]	Minot	91%	55
Sanford Medical Center Fargo[2]	Fargo	42%	77
Altru Hospital[2]	Grand Forks	26%	53

Chest Pain/Possible Heart Attack Care

Aspirin Given Within 24 Hours of Arrival

Hospital Name	City	Rate	Cases
Saint Joseph's Hospital & Health Center	Dickinson	100%	56
Mercy Hospital of Valley City	Valley City	97%	29
Jamestown Regional Medical Center	Jamestown	95%	78
The Mercy Hospital of Devils Lake	Devils Lake	84%	37

Average Time to ECG (minutes)

Hospital Name	City	Min.	Cases
Mercy Hospital of Valley City	Valley City	3	29
Jamestown Regional Medical Center	Jamestown	8	78
The Mercy Hospital of Devils Lake	Devils Lake	9	37
Saint Joseph's Hospital & Health Center	Dickinson	11	57

Children's Asthma Care

No hospitals met the 25 case threshold.

Emergency Department

Admittance Decision Time (minutes)

Hospital Name	City	Min.	Cases
Mercy Hospital of Valley City[2,3]	Valley City	14	33
Lisbon Area Health Services[2,3]	Lisbon	15	41
PHS Indian Hosp at Belcourt-Quentin[2]	Belcourt	22	138
Mercy Medical Center[2]	Williston	44	168
Sanford Medical Center Bismarck[2]	Bismarck	45	65
Sanford Medical Center Fargo[2]	Fargo	63	205
Saint Alexius Medical Center[2]	Bismarck	69	269
Trinity Hospitals[2]	Minot	73	458
Essentia Health - Fargo[2]	Fargo	83	466
Altru Hospital[2]	Grand Forks	88	347

Patients Who Left ER Before Being Seen

Hospital Name	City	Rate	Cases
Ashley Medical Center	Ashley	0%	338
Carrington Health Center	Carrington	0%	1868
Community Memorial Hospital	Turtle Lake	0%	459
Cooperstown Medical Center	Cooperstown	0%	372
Essentia Health - Fargo	Fargo	0%	32699
First Care Health Center	Park River	0%	1218
Garrison Memorial Hospital	Garrison	0%	1411
Heart of America Medical Center	Rugby	0%	2549
Jamestown Regional Medical Center	Jamestown	0%	8246
Kenmare Community Hospital	Kenmare	0%	553
Linton Hospital	Linton	0%	957
Lisbon Area Health Services	Lisbon	0%	2226
McKenzie County Healthcare Systems	Watford City	0%	5298
The Mercy Hospital of Devils Lake	Devils Lake	0%	10797
Mercy Hospital of Valley City	Valley City	0%	3294
Nelson County Health System	Mcville	0%	402
Oakes Community Hospital	Oakes	0%	703
Pembina County Memorial Hospital	Cavalier	0%	1428
Saint Alexius Medical Center	Bismarck	0%	29082
Saint Aloisius Medical Center	Harvey	0%	1317
Saint Andrews Health Center	Bottineau	0%	1554
Saint Luke's Hospital	Crosby	0%	994
Sanford Hillsboro	Hillsboro	0%	943
Sanford Mayville	Mayville	0%	1082
Southwest Healthcare Services	Bowman	0%	863
Towner County Medical Center	Cando	0%	828
West River Regional Medical Center	Hettinger	0%	1697
Wishek Community Hospital	Wishek	0%	895
Altru Hospital	Grand Forks	1%	31244
Cavalier County Memorial Hospital	Langdon	1%	1095
Northwood Deaconess Health Center	Northwood	1%	505
Saint Joseph's Hospital & Health Center	Dickinson	1%	15501
Sakakawea Medical Center	Hazen	1%	2759
Sanford Medical Center Bismarck	Bismarck	1%	28866
Tioga Medical Center	Tioga	1%	2110
Unity Medical Center	Grafton	1%	2340
Presentation Medical Center	Rolla	2%	5923
Sanford Medical Center Fargo	Fargo	2%	55305
Trinity Hospitals	Minot	2%	35857
Mercy Medical Center	Williston	4%	17362

Time from ER Arrival to Being Admitted (minutes)

Hospital Name	City	Min.	Cases
Lisbon Area Health Services[2,3]	Lisbon	97	41
Mercy Hospital of Valley City[2,3]	Valley City	115	33
The Mercy Hospital of Devils Lake[2,3]	Devils Lake	140	106
PHS Indian Hosp at Belcourt-Quentin[2]	Belcourt	151	316
Sanford Medical Center Bismarck[2]	Bismarck	161	79
Saint Alexius Medical Center[2]	Bismarck	198	438
Sanford Medical Center Fargo[2]	Fargo	205	321
Mercy Medical Center[2]	Williston	208	209
Essentia Health - Fargo[2]	Fargo	214	469
Trinity Hospitals[2]	Minot	218	533
Altru Hospital[2]	Grand Forks	222	393

Time from ER Arrival to Discharge (minutes)

Hospital Name	City	Min.	Cases
The Mercy Hospital of Devils Lake	Devils Lake	59	375
Sanford Medical Center Bismarck	Bismarck	82	128
Lisbon Area Health Services[3]	Lisbon	83	50
Essentia Health - Fargo	Fargo	92	393
Jamestown Regional Medical Center	Jamestown	99	367
Mercy Medical Center	Williston	107	399
Saint Alexius Medical Center	Bismarck	113	381
Sanford Medical Center Fargo	Fargo	143	517
Altru Hospital	Grand Forks	153	416
Trinity Hospitals	Minot	167	341

Time in ER Before Being Evaluated (minutes)

Hospital Name	City	Min.	Cases
The Mercy Hospital of Devils Lake	Devils Lake	10	257
Saint Alexius Medical Center	Bismarck	13	322
Essentia Health - Fargo	Fargo	15	109
Sanford Medical Center Fargo	Fargo	15	492
Lisbon Area Health Services[3]	Lisbon	18	62
Jamestown Regional Medical Center	Jamestown	19	364
Sanford Medical Center Bismarck	Bismarck	22	152
Altru Hospital	Grand Forks	40	376
Mercy Medical Center	Williston	40	425
Trinity Hospitals	Minot	42	320

Time to Pain Meds for Bone Fractures (minutes)

Hospital Name	City	Min.	Cases
The Mercy Hospital of Devils Lake	Devils Lake	36	57
Sanford Medical Center Bismarck	Bismarck	37	139
Jamestown Regional Medical Center	Jamestown	39	43
Essentia Health - Fargo	Fargo	46	107
Saint Alexius Medical Center	Bismarck	46	86
Sanford Medical Center Fargo	Fargo	50	190
Mercy Medical Center	Williston	61	78
Trinity Hospitals	Minot	68	152
Altru Hospital	Grand Forks	70	132

Heart Attack Care

Aspirin Given at Discharge

Hospital Name	City	Rate	Cases
Altru Hospital	Grand Forks	100%	270
Saint Alexius Medical Center	Bismarck	100%	249
Sanford Medical Center Bismarck	Bismarck	100%	154
Trinity Hospitals	Minot	100%	249
Essentia Health - Fargo	Fargo	99%	217
Sanford Medical Center Fargo	Fargo	99%	581

PCI Within 90 Minutes of Arrival

Hospital Name	City	Rate	Cases
Saint Alexius Medical Center	Bismarck	94%	33
Sanford Medical Center Fargo	Fargo	94%	35
Altru Hospital	Grand Forks	89%	37

Statin Prescribed at Discharge

Hospital Name	City	Rate	Cases
Essentia Health - Fargo	Fargo	100%	211
Sanford Medical Center Bismarck	Bismarck	100%	140
Altru Hospital	Grand Forks	99%	265
Saint Alexius Medical Center	Bismarck	99%	244
Trinity Hospitals	Minot	98%	233
Sanford Medical Center Fargo	Fargo	97%	576

Heart Failure Care

ACE Inhibitor or ARB for LVSD

Hospital Name	City	Rate	Cases
Saint Alexius Medical Center	Bismarck	100%	49
Sanford Medical Center Bismarck	Bismarck	100%	58
Trinity Hospitals	Minot	100%	61
Altru Hospital	Grand Forks	98%	48
Sanford Medical Center Fargo	Fargo	94%	118
Essentia Health - Fargo	Fargo	93%	41

Discharge Instructions Given

Hospital Name	City	Rate	Cases
Sanford Medical Center Bismarck	Bismarck	100%	160
West River Regional Medical Center[2]	Hettinger	100%	43
Trinity Hospitals	Minot	99%	141
Altru Hospital	Grand Forks	98%	193
Essentia Health - Fargo	Fargo	96%	116
Saint Alexius Medical Center	Bismarck	96%	164
Saint Joseph's Hospital & Health Center	Dickinson	96%	57
Fargo VA Medical Center	Fargo	93%	57
Sanford Medical Center Fargo	Fargo	90%	382

Evaluation of LVS Function

Hospital Name	City	Rate	Cases
Altru Hospital	Grand Forks	100%	231
Fargo VA Medical Center	Fargo	100%	61
Saint Alexius Medical Center	Bismarck	100%	226
Saint Joseph's Hospital & Health Center	Dickinson	100%	72
Sanford Medical Center Bismarck	Bismarck	100%	195
Sanford Medical Center Fargo	Fargo	100%	487
Trinity Hospitals	Minot	100%	196
West River Regional Medical Center[2]	Hettinger	98%	55
Essentia Health - Fargo	Fargo	97%	152
Jamestown Regional Medical Center	Jamestown	95%	43
Oakes Community Hospital[2]	Oakes	88%	25

Medicare Spending

Medicare Spending per Patient (ratio)

Hospital Name	City	Ratio	Cases
PHS Indian Hosp at Belcourt-Quentin	Belcourt	0.67	-
Saint Alexius Medical Center	Bismarck	0.90	-
Sanford Medical Center Bismarck	Bismarck	0.92	-
Trinity Hospitals	Minot	0.94	-
Altru Hospital	Grand Forks	0.96	-
Sanford Medical Center Fargo	Fargo	0.97	-
Essentia Health - Fargo	Fargo	0.99	-

Pneumonia Care

Appropriate Initial Antibiotic Given

Hospital Name	City	Rate	Cases
Saint Joseph's Hospital & Health Center	Dickinson	100%	38

NOTE: Hospital profiles are in alphabetical order by state, then city, then hospital within the city; Rankings exclude hospitals with less than 25 cases except for patient surveys which excludes hospitals with less than 100 cases; (a) 100-299 cases; (1) The number of cases/patients is too few to report; (2) Data submitted were based on a sample of cases/patients; (3) Results are based on a shorter time period than required; (4) Data suppressed by CMS for one or more quarters; (5) Results are not available for this reporting period; (6) Fewer than 100 patients completed the HCAHPS survey; (7) No cases met the criteria for this measure; (8) The lower limit of the confidence interval cannot be calculated if the number of observed infections equals zero; (9) No data are available from the state/territory for this reporting period; (10) The scores shown reflect fewer than 50 completed surveys; (11) There were discrepancies in the data collection process; (12) This measure does not apply to this hospital for this reporting period; (13) Results cannot be calculated for this reporting period; (14) The results for this state are combined with nearby states to protect confidentiality; Please refer to the User's Guide for a full explanation of data.

Hospital Name	City	Rate	Cases
Sanford Medical Center Fargo	Fargo	100%	127
Trinity Hospitals	Minot	99%	142
Essentia Health - Fargo	Fargo	98%	49
Jamestown Regional Medical Center	Jamestown	98%	52
Sanford Medical Center Bismarck	Bismarck	98%	88
Saint Alexius Medical Center[2]	Bismarck	95%	129
West River Regional Medical Center[2]	Hettinger	95%	39
Altru Hospital	Grand Forks	94%	145
The Mercy Hospital of Devils Lake[2]	Devils Lake	94%	35
Mercy Medical Center	Williston	87%	45
Heart of America Medical Center[2]	Rugby	83%	30

Blood Culture Timing

Hospital Name	City	Rate	Cases
Altru Hospital	Grand Forks	100%	248
Essentia Health - Fargo	Fargo	100%	88
Sanford Medical Center Fargo	Fargo	99%	232
Saint Joseph's Hospital & Health Center	Dickinson	98%	63
Sanford Medical Center Bismarck	Bismarck	98%	184
Saint Alexius Medical Center[2]	Bismarck	97%	143
Trinity Hospitals	Minot	97%	289
Jamestown Regional Medical Center	Jamestown	96%	50
Mercy Medical Center	Williston	95%	58
The Mercy Hospital of Devils Lake[2]	Devils Lake	93%	45
Heart of America Medical Center[2]	Rugby	92%	26

Pregnancy and Delivery Care

Newborns whose Deliveries were Scheduled Early

Hospital Name	City	Rate	Cases
Sanford Medical Center Fargo[2]	Fargo	0%	43
Sanford Medical Center Bismarck	Bismarck	1%	127
Essentia Health - Fargo	Fargo	2%	128
Altru Hospital[2]	Grand Forks	6%	51
Trinity Hospitals[2]	Minot	6%	71
Saint Alexius Medical Center[2]	Bismarck	7%	28
Mercy Medical Center[3]	Williston	11%	28
PHS Indian Hosp at Belcourt-Quentin[2]	Belcourt	47%	32

Preventive Care

Immunization for Influenza

Hospital Name	City	Rate	Cases
Carrington Health Center[2]	Carrington	100%	144
Sanford Medical Center Bismarck[2]	Bismarck	95%	551
Essentia Health - Fargo[2]	Fargo	93%	521
Trinity Hospitals[2]	Minot	93%	515
Linton Hospital[3]	Linton	92%	38
The Mercy Hospital of Devils Lake[2,3]	Devils Lake	92%	113
Sanford Medical Center Fargo[2]	Fargo	89%	615
Saint Alexius Medical Center[2]	Bismarck	86%	535
Mercy Hospital of Valley City[2]	Valley City	79%	39
First Care Health Center[2]	Park River	73%	26
Mercy Medical Center[2]	Williston	73%	250
Altru Hospital[2]	Grand Forks	67%	520
PHS Indian Hosp at Belcourt-Quentin[2]	Belcourt	54%	288

Immunization for Pneumonia

Hospital Name	City	Rate	Cases
Carrington Health Center[2]	Carrington	100%	241
Essentia Health - Fargo[2]	Fargo	98%	570
The Mercy Hospital of Devils Lake[2,3]	Devils Lake	98%	144
Linton Hospital[2,3]	Linton	96%	49
Sanford Medical Center Bismarck[2]	Bismarck	96%	618
Saint Alexius Medical Center[2]	Bismarck	90%	563
Sanford Medical Center Fargo[2]	Fargo	90%	670
Mercy Hospital of Valley City[2,3]	Valley City	88%	50
Sanford Mayville	Mayville	88%	34
Trinity Hospitals[2]	Minot	88%	552
PHS Indian Hosp at Belcourt-Quentin[2]	Belcourt	79%	230
Altru Hospital[2]	Grand Forks	72%	605
Lisbon Area Health Services[2,3]	Lisbon	71%	38
Mercy Medical Center[2]	Williston	71%	180

Stroke Care

Antithrombotic Therapy Timing

Hospital Name	City	Rate	Cases
Altru Hospital	Grand Forks	100%	88
Saint Alexius Medical Center	Bismarck	100%	85
Essentia Health - Fargo	Fargo	99%	93
Sanford Medical Center Fargo[2]	Fargo	99%	93
Sanford Medical Center Bismarck	Bismarck	97%	69
Trinity Hospitals	Minot	97%	98

Assessed for Rehabilitation

Hospital Name	City	Rate	Cases
Altru Hospital	Grand Forks	100%	108
Sanford Medical Center Bismarck	Bismarck	100%	77
Saint Alexius Medical Center	Bismarck	99%	103
Trinity Hospitals	Minot	99%	111
Essentia Health - Fargo	Fargo	97%	137
Sanford Medical Center Fargo[2]	Fargo	92%	123

Discharged on Antithrombotic Therapy

Hospital Name	City	Rate	Cases
Altru Hospital	Grand Forks	100%	98
Essentia Health - Fargo	Fargo	100%	110
Saint Alexius Medical Center	Bismarck	100%	89
Trinity Hospitals	Minot	100%	102
Sanford Medical Center Bismarck	Bismarck	99%	68
Sanford Medical Center Fargo[2]	Fargo	99%	106

Discharged on Statin Medication

Hospital Name	City	Rate	Cases
Saint Alexius Medical Center	Bismarck	99%	69
Essentia Health - Fargo	Fargo	98%	83
Trinity Hospitals	Minot	97%	77
Sanford Medical Center Fargo[2]	Fargo	95%	84
Sanford Medical Center Bismarck	Bismarck	83%	54
Altru Hospital	Grand Forks	77%	83

Venous Thromboembolism (VTE) Prophylaxis

Hospital Name	City	Rate	Cases
Essentia Health - Fargo	Fargo	99%	139
Trinity Hospitals	Minot	96%	123
Altru Hospital	Grand Forks	95%	110
Saint Alexius Medical Center	Bismarck	95%	110
Sanford Medical Center Bismarck	Bismarck	95%	76
Sanford Medical Center Fargo[2]	Fargo	94%	122

Written Stroke Educational Materials Given

Hospital Name	City	Rate	Cases
Saint Alexius Medical Center	Bismarck	98%	46
Sanford Medical Center Bismarck	Bismarck	98%	46
Trinity Hospitals	Minot	97%	61
Essentia Health - Fargo	Fargo	96%	79
Sanford Medical Center Fargo[2]	Fargo	73%	64
Altru Hospital	Grand Forks	54%	54

Surgical Care Improvement Project

Appropriate Beta Blocker Usage

Hospital Name	City	Rate	Cases
Essentia Health - Fargo[2]	Fargo	100%	166
Fargo VA Medical Center[2]	Fargo	100%	56
Sanford Medical Center Bismarck[2]	Bismarck	100%	237
Trinity Hospitals	Minot	100%	217
Sanford Medical Center Fargo[2]	Fargo	99%	302
Jamestown Regional Medical Center	Jamestown	98%	42
Saint Alexius Medical Center[2]	Bismarck	98%	186
Altru Hospital[2]	Grand Forks	97%	240

Appropriate VTP Within 24 Hours

Hospital Name	City	Rate	Cases
Saint Joseph's Hospital & Health Center	Dickinson	100%	40
Sanford Medical Center Bismarck[2]	Bismarck	100%	503
Essentia Health - Fargo[2]	Fargo	99%	311
Fargo VA Medical Center[2]	Fargo	99%	143
Mercy Medical Center	Williston	98%	94
Sanford Medical Center Fargo[2]	Fargo	98%	524
Jamestown Regional Medical Center	Jamestown	97%	148
Trinity Hospitals	Minot	97%	508
Altru Hospital[2]	Grand Forks	96%	464
Saint Alexius Medical Center[2]	Bismarck	96%	368

Controlled Postoperative Blood Glucose

Hospital Name	City	Rate	Cases
Saint Alexius Medical Center[2]	Bismarck	99%	103
Sanford Medical Center Fargo[2]	Fargo	95%	195
Essentia Health - Fargo[2]	Fargo	94%	90
Sanford Medical Center Bismarck[2]	Bismarck	94%	125
Altru Hospital[2]	Grand Forks	93%	127
Trinity Hospitals	Minot	91%	58

Perioperative Temperature Management

Hospital Name	City	Rate	Cases
Essentia Health - Fargo[2]	Fargo	100%	401
Fargo VA Medical Center[2]	Fargo	100%	157
Jamestown Regional Medical Center	Jamestown	100%	166
Mercy Medical Center	Williston	100%	100
Saint Alexius Medical Center[2]	Bismarck	100%	477
Saint Joseph's Hospital & Health Center	Dickinson	100%	57
Sanford Medical Center Bismarck[2]	Bismarck	100%	610
Sanford Medical Center Fargo[2]	Fargo	100%	735
Trinity Hospitals	Minot	100%	594
Altru Hospital[2]	Grand Forks	99%	556

Prophylactic Antibiotic Selection

Hospital Name	City	Rate	Cases
Mercy Medical Center	Williston	100%	60
Saint Alexius Medical Center[2]	Bismarck	100%	427
Saint Joseph's Hospital & Health Center	Dickinson	100%	34
Trinity Hospitals	Minot	100%	428
Altru Hospital[2]	Grand Forks	99%	526
Essentia Health - Fargo[2]	Fargo	99%	353
Fargo VA Medical Center	Fargo	99%	121
Jamestown Regional Medical Center	Jamestown	99%	142
Sanford Medical Center Bismarck[2]	Bismarck	99%	565
Sanford Medical Center Fargo[2]	Fargo	99%	631

Prophylactic Antibiotic Selection (Outpatient)

Hospital Name	City	Rate	Cases
Mercy Medical Center	Williston	100%	49
Essentia Health - Fargo	Fargo	99%	333
Saint Alexius Medical Center	Bismarck	99%	475
Saint Joseph's Hospital & Health Center	Dickinson	98%	43
Sanford Medical Center Bismarck	Bismarck	98%	329
Altru Hospital	Grand Forks	97%	553
Sanford Medical Center Fargo	Fargo	96%	783
Trinity Hospitals	Minot	96%	395

Prophylactic Antibiotic Stopped

Hospital Name	City	Rate	Cases
Essentia Health - Fargo[2]	Fargo	100%	339
Saint Joseph's Hospital & Health Center	Dickinson	100%	33
Sanford Medical Center Fargo[2]	Fargo	100%	622
Fargo VA Medical Center	Fargo	99%	120
Jamestown Regional Medical Center	Jamestown	99%	141
Saint Alexius Medical Center[2]	Bismarck	99%	418
Sanford Medical Center Bismarck[2]	Bismarck	99%	555
Altru Hospital[2]	Grand Forks	98%	509
Trinity Hospitals	Minot	98%	407
Mercy Medical Center	Williston	97%	60

Prophylactic Antibiotic Timing

Hospital Name	City	Rate	Cases
Essentia Health - Fargo[2]	Fargo	100%	353
Trinity Hospitals	Minot	100%	430
Jamestown Regional Medical Center	Jamestown	99%	143
Saint Alexius Medical Center[2]	Bismarck	99%	427
Sanford Medical Center Bismarck[2]	Bismarck	99%	568
Sanford Medical Center Fargo[2]	Fargo	99%	632
Saint Joseph's Hospital & Health Center	Dickinson	97%	34
Altru Hospital[2]	Grand Forks	96%	527
Fargo VA Medical Center	Fargo	95%	121
Mercy Medical Center	Williston	90%	61

Prophylactic Antibiotic Timing (Outpatient)

Hospital Name	City	Rate	Cases
Essentia Health - Fargo	Fargo	100%	266
Saint Joseph's Hospital & Health Center	Dickinson	100%	43
Trinity Hospitals	Minot	100%	389
Saint Alexius Medical Center	Bismarck	97%	351
Sanford Medical Center Bismarck	Bismarck	97%	244
Sanford Medical Center Fargo	Fargo	96%	684
Mercy Medical Center	Williston	92%	49
Altru Hospital	Grand Forks	90%	439

Urinary Catheter Removal

Hospital Name	City	Rate	Cases
Saint Joseph's Hospital & Health Center	Dickinson	100%	26
Jamestown Regional Medical Center	Jamestown	99%	135
Saint Alexius Medical Center[2]	Bismarck	99%	254
Sanford Medical Center Fargo[2]	Fargo	99%	566
Essentia Health - Fargo[2]	Fargo	98%	219
Fargo VA Medical Center[2]	Fargo	98%	126
Mercy Medical Center	Williston	98%	44
Sanford Medical Center Bismarck[2]	Bismarck	98%	260
Trinity Hospitals	Minot	98%	491
Altru Hospital[2]	Grand Forks	93%	338

Survey of Patients' Hospital Experiences

Area Around Room 'Always' Quiet at Night

Hospital Name	City	Rate	Cases
Cavalier County Memorial Hospital	Langdon	78%	(a)
Mercy Medical Center	Williston	67%	300+
First Care Health Center	Park River	66%	(a)
Jamestown Regional Medical Center	Jamestown	66%	300+
Saint Alexius Medical Center	Bismarck	60%	300+
Saint Aloisius Medical Center	Harvey	60%	(a)

NOTE: Hospital profiles are in alphabetical order by state, then city, then hospital within the city; Rankings exclude hospitals with less than 25 cases except for patient surveys which excludes hospitals with less than 100 cases; (a) 100-299 cases; (1) The number of cases/patients is too few to report; (2) Data submitted were based on a sample of cases/patients; (3) Results are based on a shorter time period than required; (4) Data suppressed by CMS for one or more quarters; (5) Results are not available for this reporting period; (6) Fewer than 100 patients completed the HCAHPS survey; (7) No cases met the criteria for this measure; (8) The lower limit of the confidence interval cannot be calculated if the number of observed infections equals zero; (9) No data are available from the state/territory for this reporting period; (10) The scores shown reflect fewer than 50 completed surveys; (11) There were discrepancies in the data collection process; (12) This measure does not apply to this hospital for this reporting period; (13) Results cannot be calculated for this reporting period; (14) The results for this state are combined with nearby states to protect confidentiality; Please refer to the User's Guide for a full explanation of data.

Sanford Medical Center Bismarck	Bismarck	57%	300+
Essentia Health - Fargo	Fargo	56%	300+
Saint Joseph's Hospital & Health Center	Dickinson	56%	300+
West River Regional Medical Center	Hettinger	54%	300+
Sanford Medical Center Fargo	Fargo	53%	300+
Trinity Hospitals	Minot	49%	300+
Altru Hospital	Grand Forks	46%	300+

Doctors 'Always' Communicated Well

Hospital Name	City	Rate	Cases
First Care Health Center	Park River	91%	(a)
West River Regional Medical Center	Hettinger	88%	300+
Jamestown Regional Medical Center	Jamestown	85%	300+
Saint Aloisius Medical Center	Harvey	82%	(a)
Mercy Medical Center	Williston	81%	300+
Essentia Health - Fargo	Fargo	79%	300+
Sanford Medical Center Bismarck	Bismarck	79%	300+
Saint Alexius Medical Center	Bismarck	78%	300+
Sanford Medical Center Fargo	Fargo	77%	300+
Trinity Hospitals	Minot	77%	300+
Altru Hospital	Grand Forks	75%	300+
Saint Joseph's Hospital & Health Center	Dickinson	75%	300+
Cavalier County Memorial Hospital	Langdon	74%	(a)

Home Recovery Information Given

Hospital Name	City	Rate	Cases
Jamestown Regional Medical Center	Jamestown	91%	300+
Sanford Medical Center Bismarck	Bismarck	91%	300+
Mercy Medical Center	Williston	89%	300+
Essentia Health - Fargo	Fargo	88%	300+
Saint Joseph's Hospital & Health Center	Dickinson	87%	300+
Sanford Medical Center Fargo	Fargo	87%	300+
Saint Alexius Medical Center	Bismarck	86%	300+
West River Regional Medical Center	Hettinger	85%	300+
Altru Hospital	Grand Forks	84%	300+
Trinity Hospitals	Minot	82%	300+
First Care Health Center	Park River	80%	(a)
Saint Aloisius Medical Center	Harvey	79%	(a)
Cavalier County Memorial Hospital	Langdon	75%	(a)

Hospital Given 9 or 10 on 10 Point Scale

Hospital Name	City	Rate	Cases
First Care Health Center	Park River	86%	(a)
West River Regional Medical Center	Hettinger	80%	300+
Jamestown Regional Medical Center	Jamestown	76%	300+
Essentia Health - Fargo	Fargo	75%	300+
Sanford Medical Center Bismarck	Bismarck	74%	300+
Cavalier County Memorial Hospital	Langdon	73%	(a)
Saint Alexius Medical Center	Bismarck	73%	300+
Sanford Medical Center Fargo	Fargo	67%	300+
Altru Hospital	Grand Forks	62%	300+
Saint Joseph's Hospital & Health Center	Dickinson	61%	300+
Saint Aloisius Medical Center	Harvey	60%	(a)
Mercy Medical Center	Williston	55%	300+
Trinity Hospitals	Minot	49%	300+

Meds 'Always' Explained Before Given

Hospital Name	City	Rate	Cases
First Care Health Center	Park River	79%	(a)
West River Regional Medical Center	Hettinger	68%	300+
Mercy Medical Center	Williston	67%	300+
Jamestown Regional Medical Center	Jamestown	65%	300+
Sanford Medical Center Fargo	Fargo	64%	300+
Essentia Health - Fargo	Fargo	63%	300+
Sanford Medical Center Bismarck	Bismarck	63%	300+
Saint Alexius Medical Center	Bismarck	62%	300+
Saint Joseph's Hospital & Health Center	Dickinson	61%	300+
Cavalier County Memorial Hospital	Langdon	59%	(a)
Saint Aloisius Medical Center	Harvey	58%	(a)
Altru Hospital	Grand Forks	57%	300+
Trinity Hospitals	Minot	52%	300+

Nurses 'Always' Communicated Well

Hospital Name	City	Rate	Cases
West River Regional Medical Center	Hettinger	85%	300+
First Care Health Center	Park River	84%	(a)
Jamestown Regional Medical Center	Jamestown	82%	300+
Cavalier County Memorial Hospital	Langdon	80%	(a)
Sanford Medical Center Fargo	Fargo	80%	300+
Essentia Health - Fargo	Fargo	79%	300+
Sanford Medical Center Bismarck	Bismarck	79%	300+
Saint Alexius Medical Center	Bismarck	78%	300+
Altru Hospital	Grand Forks	76%	300+
Saint Joseph's Hospital & Health Center	Dickinson	76%	300+
Mercy Medical Center	Williston	73%	300+
Saint Aloisius Medical Center	Harvey	70%	(a)
Trinity Hospitals	Minot	68%	300+

Pain 'Always' Well Controlled

Hospital Name	City	Rate	Cases
West River Regional Medical Center	Hettinger	80%	300+
Jamestown Regional Medical Center	Jamestown	74%	300+
Cavalier County Memorial Hospital	Langdon	71%	(a)
Essentia Health - Fargo	Fargo	70%	300+
First Care Health Center	Park River	69%	(a)
Saint Alexius Medical Center	Bismarck	69%	300+
Saint Joseph's Hospital & Health Center	Dickinson	68%	300+
Sanford Medical Center Bismarck	Bismarck	68%	300+
Sanford Medical Center Fargo	Fargo	68%	300+
Altru Hospital	Grand Forks	66%	300+
Saint Aloisius Medical Center	Harvey	64%	(a)
Mercy Medical Center	Williston	63%	300+
Trinity Hospitals	Minot	62%	300+

Room and Bathroom 'Always' Clean

Hospital Name	City	Rate	Cases
First Care Health Center	Park River	92%	(a)
West River Regional Medical Center	Hettinger	88%	300+
Cavalier County Memorial Hospital	Langdon	83%	(a)
Jamestown Regional Medical Center	Jamestown	74%	300+
Saint Alexius Medical Center	Bismarck	72%	300+
Sanford Medical Center Bismarck	Bismarck	72%	300+
Sanford Medical Center Fargo	Fargo	71%	300+
Altru Hospital	Grand Forks	70%	300+
Saint Aloisius Medical Center	Harvey	68%	(a)
Trinity Hospitals	Minot	65%	300+
Essentia Health - Fargo	Fargo	64%	300+
Mercy Medical Center	Williston	62%	300+
Saint Joseph's Hospital & Health Center	Dickinson	59%	300+

Timely Help 'Always' Received

Hospital Name	City	Rate	Cases
Cavalier County Memorial Hospital	Langdon	79%	(a)
First Care Health Center	Park River	79%	(a)
West River Regional Medical Center	Hettinger	74%	300+
Jamestown Regional Medical Center	Jamestown	73%	300+
Saint Joseph's Hospital & Health Center	Dickinson	71%	300+
Saint Aloisius Medical Center	Harvey	70%	(a)
Sanford Medical Center Bismarck	Bismarck	68%	300+
Essentia Health - Fargo	Fargo	66%	300+
Saint Alexius Medical Center	Bismarck	66%	300+
Mercy Medical Center	Williston	65%	300+
Sanford Medical Center Fargo	Fargo	63%	300+
Altru Hospital	Grand Forks	59%	300+
Trinity Hospitals	Minot	58%	300+

Would Definitely Recommend Hospital

Hospital Name	City	Rate	Cases
First Care Health Center	Park River	91%	(a)
West River Regional Medical Center	Hettinger	80%	300+
Essentia Health - Fargo	Fargo	79%	300+
Sanford Medical Center Bismarck	Bismarck	79%	300+
Saint Alexius Medical Center	Bismarck	78%	300+
Jamestown Regional Medical Center	Jamestown	77%	300+
Sanford Medical Center Fargo	Fargo	73%	300+
Saint Aloisius Medical Center	Harvey	64%	(a)
Cavalier County Memorial Hospital	Langdon	61%	(a)
Altru Hospital	Grand Forks	59%	300+
Saint Joseph's Hospital & Health Center	Dickinson	59%	300+
Mercy Medical Center	Williston	58%	300+
Trinity Hospitals	Minot	49%	300+

Use of Medical Imaging

Cardiac Imaging Stress Test before OP Surgery

Hospital Name	City	Rate	Cases
Trinity Hospitals	Minot	2.2%	370
The Mercy Hospital of Devils Lake	Devils Lake	2.8%	108
Essentia Health - Fargo	Fargo	3.0%	301
Altru Hospital	Grand Forks	3.6%	858
Jamestown Regional Medical Center	Jamestown	3.8%	80
Saint Joseph's Hospital & Health Center	Dickinson	5.2%	192
Sanford Medical Center Fargo	Fargo	5.8%	639
Sanford Medical Center Bismarck	Bismarck	6.0%	685
West River Regional Medical Center	Hettinger	6.3%	95
Saint Alexius Medical Center	Bismarck	6.4%	581

Combination Abdominal CT Scan

Hospital Name	City	Rate	Cases
Saint Aloisius Medical Center	Harvey	0.0%	65
Pembina County Memorial Hospital	Cavalier	0.7%	141
Carrington Health Center	Carrington	3.1%	159
Heart of America Medical Center	Rugby	3.2%	93
Unity Medical Center	Grafton	4.2%	48
Cavalier County Memorial Hospital	Langdon	4.5%	66
The Mercy Hospital of Devils Lake	Devils Lake	4.9%	244
Sanford Medical Center Bismarck	Bismarck	5.2%	943
Altru Hospital	Grand Forks	5.5%	959
Jamestown Regional Medical Center	Jamestown	5.5%	256
West River Regional Medical Center	Hettinger	5.8%	139
Trinity Hospitals	Minot	6.2%	902
Mercy Hospital of Valley City	Valley City	7.0%	71
Essentia Health - Fargo	Fargo	7.2%	489
Saint Joseph's Hospital & Health Center	Dickinson	7.7%	390
Saint Andrews Health Center	Bottineau	8.9%	79
Mercy Medical Center	Williston	14.3%	245
Sanford Medical Center Fargo	Fargo	21.2%	1451
Sakakawea Medical Center	Hazen	22.2%	135
Garrison Memorial Hospital	Garrison	25.7%	70
Saint Alexius Medical Center	Bismarck	27.7%	480
Oakes Community Hospital	Oakes	51.4%	109

Combination Brain/Sinus CT Scan

Hospital Name	City	Rate	Cases
Carrington Health Center	Carrington	0.0%	114
Cavalier County Memorial Hospital	Langdon	0.0%	67
First Care Health Center	Park River	0.0%	55
Linton Hospital	Linton	0.0%	45
Oakes Community Hospital	Oakes	0.0%	73
Saint Andrews Health Center	Bottineau	0.0%	56
West River Regional Medical Center	Hettinger	0.0%	41
Sanford Medical Center Fargo	Fargo	1.2%	687
Saint Alexius Medical Center	Bismarck	1.4%	357
Essentia Health - Fargo	Fargo	1.5%	403
Trinity Hospitals	Minot	1.8%	603
Southwest Healthcare Services	Bowman	20.0%	30

Combination Chest CT Scan

Hospital Name	City	Rate	Cases
Carrington Health Center	Carrington	0.0%	79
Essentia Health - Fargo	Fargo	0.0%	213
Mercy Hospital of Valley City	Valley City	0.0%	71
Pembina County Memorial Hospital	Cavalier	0.0%	68
Sanford Medical Center Bismarck	Bismarck	0.0%	847
Trinity Hospitals	Minot	0.2%	612
Altru Hospital	Grand Forks	0.3%	1099
Saint Alexius Medical Center	Bismarck	0.7%	454
Oakes Community Hospital	Oakes	1.6%	63
West River Regional Medical Center	Hettinger	1.6%	64
Sanford Medical Center Fargo	Fargo	1.8%	1080
Jamestown Regional Medical Center	Jamestown	1.9%	158
Saint Andrews Health Center	Bottineau	3.0%	67
The Mercy Hospital of Devils Lake	Devils Lake	3.6%	111
Saint Joseph's Hospital & Health Center	Dickinson	3.6%	193
Mercy Medical Center	Williston	9.2%	131
Sakakawea Medical Center	Hazen	9.3%	86
Garrison Memorial Hospital	Garrison	16.3%	80

Follow-up Mammogram/Ultrasound

A follow-up rate near zero may indicate missed cancer; a rate higher than 14% may mean there is unnecessary follow up.

Hospital Name	City	Rate	Cases
First Care Health Center	Park River	2.8%	144
Wishek Community Hospital	Wishek	3.0%	100
Saint Andrews Health Center	Bottineau	3.2%	186
Saint Aloisius Medical Center	Harvey	3.3%	150
Trinity Hospitals	Minot	3.3%	2314
Saint Alexius Medical Center	Bismarck	3.8%	399
Cavalier County Memorial Hospital	Langdon	4.2%	215
Southwest Healthcare Services	Bowman	4.2%	95
Heart of America Medical Center	Rugby	4.7%	236
Pembina County Memorial Hospital	Cavalier	4.9%	144
Garrison Memorial Hospital	Garrison	5.4%	112
Sanford Medical Center Fargo	Fargo	5.6%	2576
Unity Medical Center	Grafton	5.6%	126
Linton Hospital	Linton	5.7%	105
Sakakawea Medical Center	Hazen	5.7%	244
Jamestown Regional Medical Center	Jamestown	6.3%	555
Carrington Health Center	Carrington	6.8%	294
Towner County Medical Center	Cando	7.1%	98
Saint Joseph's Hospital & Health Center	Dickinson	7.7%	117
West River Regional Medical Center	Hettinger	8.6%	303
Lisbon Area Health Services	Lisbon	10.2%	128
Mercy Medical Center	Williston	10.7%	318
Presentation Medical Center	Rolla	11.5%	87
Sanford Medical Center Bismarck	Bismarck	11.7%	1606
Altru Hospital	Grand Forks	16.2%	1900

Lumbar Spine MRI for Low Back Pain

Hospital Name	City	Rate	Cases
Essentia Health - Fargo	Fargo	27.1%	107
Saint Alexius Medical Center	Bismarck	27.4%	190
Sanford Medical Center Fargo	Fargo	27.8%	295
Saint Joseph's Hospital & Health Center	Dickinson	29.2%	106
Sanford Medical Center Bismarck	Bismarck	32.4%	136
Altru Hospital	Grand Forks	32.9%	155
Trinity Hospitals	Minot	38.3%	154

NOTE: Hospital profiles are in alphabetical order by state, then city, then hospital within the city; Rankings exclude hospitals with less than 25 cases except for patient surveys which excludes hospitals with less than 100 cases; (a) 100-299 cases; (1) The number of cases/patients is too few to report; (2) Data submitted were based on a sample of cases/patients; (3) Results are based on a shorter time period than required; (4) Data suppressed by CMS for one or more quarters; (5) Results are not available for this reporting period; (6) Fewer than 100 patients completed the HCAHPS survey; (7) No cases met the criteria for this measure; (8) The lower limit of the confidence interval cannot be calculated if the number of observed infections equals zero; (9) No data are available from the state/territory for this reporting period; (10) The scores shown reflect fewer than 50 completed surveys; (11) There were discrepancies in the data collection process; (12) This measure does not apply to this hospital for this reporting period; (13) Results cannot be calculated for this reporting period; (14) The results for this state are combined with nearby states to protect confidentiality; Please refer to the User's Guide for a full explanation of data.

Ashley Medical Center

612 Center Avenue N
Ashley, ND 58413
Phone: 701-288-3433
Type: Critical Access Hospitals
Emergency Services: Yes
Ownership: Voluntary non-profit - Private

Measure	Cases	This Hosp.	State Avg.	U.S. Avg.
Blood Clot Prevention and Treatment				
Anticoagulation Overlap Therapy[5]	-	-	97%	93%
ICU Venous Thromboembolism Prophylaxis[5]	-	-	88%	92%
Incidence of Potentially Preventable VTE[5]	-	-	16%	10%
UFH with Dosages/Platelet Monitoring[5]	-	-	100%	97%
Venous Thromboembolism Prophylaxis[5]	-	-	80%	85%
Warfarin Therapy Discharge Instructions[5]	-	-	72%	75%
Chest Pain/Possible Heart Attack Care				
Aspirin Given Within 24 Hours of Arrival[1,3]	-	-	95%	96%
Fibrinolytic Meds Within 30 Min. of Arrival[1,3]	-	-	51%	58%
Average Time to ECG (minutes)[1,3]	-	-	11	7
Average Time to Transfer (minutes)[1,3]	-	-	114	60
Children's Asthma Care				
Received Home Management Plan of Care	-	-	-	88%
Received Reliever Medication	-	-	-	100%
Received Systemic Corticosteroids	-	-	-	100%
Emergency Department				
Admittance Decision Time (minutes)[5]	-	-	66	98
Head CT Results Within 45 Min. of Arrival[5]	-	-	25%	57%
Patients Who Left ER Before Being Seen	338	0%	1%	2%
Time from ER Arrival to Admit. (minutes)[5]	-	-	201	274
Time from ER Arrival to Discharge (minutes)[5]	-	-	112	134
Time in ER Before Being Evaluated (minutes)[5]	-	-	22	26
Time to Pain Meds for Fractures (minutes)[5]	-	-	52	57
Heart Attack Care				
Aspirin Given at Discharge[1,2]	-	-	99%	99%
Fibrinolytic Meds Within 30 Min. of Arrival[2,3]	-	-	17%	54%
PCI Within 90 Minutes of Arrival[2,3]	-	-	93%	96%
Statin Prescribed at Discharge[1,2]	-	-	98%	98%
Heart Failure Care				
ACE Inhibitor or ARB for LVSD[1,3]	-	-	96%	97%
Discharge Instructions Given[3,7]	-	-	94%	94%
Evaluation of LVS Function[1,3]	-	-	96%	99%
Medicare Spending				
Medicare Spending per Patient (ratio)		-	0.9	0.98
Pneumonia Care				
Appropriate Initial Antibiotic Given[1,3]	-	-	94%	95%
Blood Culture Timing[3,7]	-	-	97%	98%
Pregnancy and Delivery Care				
Newborn Deliveries Scheduled Early[5]	-	-	6%	6%
Preventive Care				
Immunization for Influenza[5]	-	-	84%	90%
Immunization for Pneumonia[5]	-	-	88%	92%
Stroke Care				
Anticoagulation Therapy for Atrial Fibrillation[5]	-	-	96%	95%
Antithrombotic Therapy Timing[5]	-	-	98%	98%
Assessed for Rehabilitation[5]	-	-	97%	97%
Discharged on Antithrombotic Therapy[5]	-	-	100%	99%
Discharged on Statin Medication[5]	-	-	91%	94%
Thrombolytic Therapy Timing[5]	-	-	96%	66%
Venous Thromboembolism Prophylaxis[5]	-	-	96%	94%
Written Stroke Educational Materials Given[5]	-	-	86%	88%
Surgical Care Improvement Project				
Appropriate Beta Blocker Usage[5]	-	-	99%	98%
Appropriate VTP Within 24 Hours[5]	-	-	98%	98%
Controlled Postoperative Blood Glucose[5]	-	-	95%	97%
Perioperative Temperature Management[5]	-	-	100%	100%
Prophylactic Antibiotic Selection[5]	-	-	99%	99%
Prophylactic Antibiotic Selection (Outpatient)[5]	-	-	97%	98%
Prophylactic Antibiotic Stopped[5]	-	-	99%	98%
Prophylactic Antibiotic Timing[5]	-	-	98%	99%
Prophylactic Antibiotic Timing (Outpatient)[5]	-	-	96%	98%
Urinary Catheter Removal[5]	-	-	97%	97%
Survey of Patients' Hospital Experiences				
Area Around Room 'Always' Quiet at Night[10]	<100	82%	66%	61%
Doctors 'Always' Communicated Well[10]	<100	91%	84%	82%
Home Recovery Information Given[10]	<100	84%	82%	85%
Hospital Given 9 or 10 on 10 Point Scale[10]	<100	91%	70%	71%
Meds 'Always' Explained Before Given[10]	<100	95%	67%	64%
Nurses 'Always' Communicated Well[10]	<100	86%	80%	79%
Pain 'Always' Well Controlled[10]	<100	80%	69%	71%
Room and Bathroom 'Always' Clean[10]	<100	99%	78%	73%
Timely Help 'Always' Received[10]	<100	95%	74%	68%
Would Definitely Recommend Hospital[10]	<100	95%	73%	71%
Use of Medical Imaging				
Cardiac Imaging Stress Test before Surgery[7]	-	-	4.6%	5.3%
Combination Abdominal CT Scan[1]	-	-	11.8%	10.5%
Combination Brain/Sinus CT Scan[1]	-	-	2.2%	2.7%
Combination Chest CT Scan[1]	-	-	2%	2.7%
Follow-up Mammogram/Ultrasound[1]	-	-	7.8%	8.8%
Lumbar Spine MRI for Low Back Pain[1]	-	-	32.9%	37.2%

P H S Indian Hospital at Belcourt - Quentin N Burdick

PO Box 160
Belcourt, ND 58316
Phone: 701-477-6111
Fax: 701-477-8410
Type: Acute Care Hospitals
Emergency Services: Yes
Ownership: Government - Federal
Beds: 29

Key Personnel:
Quality Assurance . . . . Dale Buckles
Operating Room. . . . . Yvonne Graber
Emergency Room . . . . Cheryl LaVallie
Intensive Care Unit. . . . . Cheryl LaVallie
CEO/President. . . . . Levern Parker
Infection Control. . . . . Virginia Thomas
Chief of Medical Staff. . . . . Penny Wilkie, MD

Measure	Cases	This Hosp.	State Avg.	U.S. Avg.
Blood Clot Prevention and Treatment				
Anticoagulation Overlap Therapy[1,2]	-	-	97%	93%
ICU Venous Thromboembolism Prophylaxis[2,7]	-	-	88%	92%
Incidence of Potentially Preventable VTE[1,2]	-	-	16%	10%
UFH with Dosages/Platelet Monitoring[2,7]	-	-	100%	97%
Venous Thromboembolism Prophylaxis[2]	142	30%	80%	85%
Warfarin Therapy Discharge Instructions[1,2]	-	-	72%	75%
Chest Pain/Possible Heart Attack Care				
Aspirin Given Within 24 Hours of Arrival	-	-	95%	96%
Fibrinolytic Meds Within 30 Min. of Arrival	-	-	51%	58%
Average Time to ECG (minutes)	-	-	11	7
Average Time to Transfer (minutes)	-	-	114	60
Children's Asthma Care				
Received Home Management Plan of Care	-	-	-	88%
Received Reliever Medication	-	-	-	100%
Received Systemic Corticosteroids	-	-	-	100%
Emergency Department				
Admittance Decision Time (minutes)[2]	138	22	66	98
Head CT Results Within 45 Min. of Arrival	-	-	25%	57%
Patients Who Left ER Before Being Seen	-	-	1%	2%
Time from ER Arrival to Admit. (minutes)[2]	316	151	201	274
Time from ER Arrival to Discharge (minutes)	-	-	112	134
Time in ER Before Being Evaluated (minutes)	-	-	22	26
Time to Pain Meds for Fractures (minutes)	-	-	52	57
Heart Attack Care				
Aspirin Given at Discharge[1,2]	-	-	99%	99%
Fibrinolytic Meds Within 30 Min. of Arrival[2,3]	-	-	17%	54%
PCI Within 90 Minutes of Arrival[2,3]	-	-	93%	96%
Statin Prescribed at Discharge[1,2]	-	-	98%	98%
Heart Failure Care				
ACE Inhibitor or ARB for LVSD[1,2]	-	-	96%	97%
Discharge Instructions Given[1,2]	-	-	94%	94%
Evaluation of LVS Function[1,2]	-	-	96%	99%
Medicare Spending				
Medicare Spending per Patient (ratio)		0.67	0.9	0.98
Pneumonia Care				
Appropriate Initial Antibiotic Given[2]	17	76%	94%	95%
Blood Culture Timing[2]	17	65%	97%	98%
Pregnancy and Delivery Care				
Newborn Deliveries Scheduled Early[2]	32	47%	6%	6%
Preventive Care				
Immunization for Influenza[2]	288	54%	84%	90%
Immunization for Pneumonia[2]	230	79%	88%	92%
Stroke Care				
Anticoagulation Therapy for Atrial Fibrillation[2,3]	-	-	96%	95%
Antithrombotic Therapy Timing[1,2]	-	-	98%	98%
Assessed for Rehabilitation[1,2]	-	-	97%	97%
Discharged on Antithrombotic Therapy[1,2]	-	-	100%	99%
Discharged on Statin Medication[1,2]	-	-	91%	94%
Thrombolytic Therapy Timing[2,3]	-	-	96%	66%
Venous Thromboembolism Prophylaxis[1,2]	-	-	96%	94%
Written Stroke Educational Materials Given[2,3]	-	-	86%	88%
Surgical Care Improvement Project				
Appropriate Beta Blocker Usage[1,2]	-	-	99%	98%
Appropriate VTP Within 24 Hours[1,2]	-	-	98%	98%
Controlled Postoperative Blood Glucose[2,7]	-	-	95%	97%
Perioperative Temperature Management[1,2]	-	-	100%	100%
Prophylactic Antibiotic Selection[1,2]	-	-	99%	99%
Prophylactic Antibiotic Selection (Outpatient)	-	-	97%	98%
Prophylactic Antibiotic Stopped[1,2]	-	-	99%	98%
Prophylactic Antibiotic Timing[1,2]	-	-	98%	99%
Prophylactic Antibiotic Timing (Outpatient)	-	-	96%	98%
Urinary Catheter Removal[2,7]	-	-	97%	97%
Survey of Patients' Hospital Experiences				
Area Around Room 'Always' Quiet at Night[6]	<100	70%	66%	61%
Doctors 'Always' Communicated Well[6]	<100	71%	84%	82%
Home Recovery Information Given[6]	<100	81%	82%	85%
Hospital Given 9 or 10 on 10 Point Scale[6]	<100	39%	70%	71%
Meds 'Always' Explained Before Given[6]	<100	58%	67%	64%
Nurses 'Always' Communicated Well[6]	<100	61%	80%	79%
Pain 'Always' Well Controlled[6]	<100	65%	69%	71%
Room and Bathroom 'Always' Clean[6]	<100	74%	78%	73%
Timely Help 'Always' Received[6]	<100	64%	74%	68%
Would Definitely Recommend Hospital[6]	<100	45%	73%	71%
Use of Medical Imaging				
Cardiac Imaging Stress Test before Surgery	-	-	4.6%	5.3%
Combination Abdominal CT Scan	-	-	11.8%	10.5%
Combination Brain/Sinus CT Scan	-	-	2.2%	2.7%
Combination Chest CT Scan	-	-	2%	2.7%
Follow-up Mammogram/Ultrasound	-	-	7.8%	8.8%
Lumbar Spine MRI for Low Back Pain	-	-	32.9%	37.2%

Saint Alexius Medical Center

900 E Broadway
Bismarck, ND 58501
Phone: 701-530-7000
Fax: 701-530-7161
URL: www.st.alexius.org
Type: Acute Care Hospitals
Emergency Services: Yes
Ownership: Voluntary non-profit - Church
Beds: 307

Key Personnel:
Operating Room. . . . . Sue Ebertowski, RN
Pediatric Ambulatory Care . . . . . . Atef Gayed
Pediatric In-Patient Care . . . . Atef Gayed
Quality Assurance . . . . Pam Heinrich
CEO/President. . . . . Gary P. Miller
Radiology. . . . . Doug Peterson
Emergency Room . . . . Kathy Seidel

Measure	Cases	This Hosp.	State Avg.	U.S. Avg.
Blood Clot Prevention and Treatment				
Anticoagulation Overlap Therapy[2]	73	95%	97%	93%
ICU Venous Thromboembolism Prophylaxis[2]	40	95%	88%	92%
Incidence of Potentially Preventable VTE[2]	11	9%	16%	10%
UFH with Dosages/Platelet Monitoring[2]	23	100%	100%	97%
Venous Thromboembolism Prophylaxis[2]	391	82%	80%	85%
Warfarin Therapy Discharge Instructions[2]	52	96%	72%	75%
Chest Pain/Possible Heart Attack Care				
Aspirin Given Within 24 Hours of Arrival[3,7]	-	-	95%	96%
Fibrinolytic Meds Within 30 Min. of Arrival[5]	-	-	51%	58%
Average Time to ECG (minutes)[3,7]	-	-	11	7
Average Time to Transfer (minutes)[5]	-	-	114	60
Children's Asthma Care				
Received Home Management Plan of Care	-	-	-	88%
Received Reliever Medication	-	-	-	100%
Received Systemic Corticosteroids	-	-	-	100%
Emergency Department				
Admittance Decision Time (minutes)[2]	269	69	66	98
Head CT Results Within 45 Min. of Arrival[7]	-	-	25%	57%
Patients Who Left ER Before Being Seen	29,082	0%	1%	2%

NOTE: Hospital profiles are in alphabetical order by state, then city, then hospital within the city; Rankings exclude hospitals with less than 25 cases except for patient surveys which excludes hospitals with less than 100 cases; (a) 100-299 cases; (1) The number of cases/patients is too few to report; (2) Data submitted were based on a sample of cases/patients; (3) Results are based on a shorter time period than required; (4) Data suppressed by CMS for one or more quarters; (5) Results are not available for this reporting period; (6) Fewer than 100 patients completed the HCAHPS survey; (7) No cases met the criteria for this measure; (8) The lower limit of the confidence interval cannot be calculated if the number of observed infections equals zero; (9) No data are available from the state/territory for this reporting period; (10) The scores shown reflect fewer than 50 completed surveys; (11) There were discrepancies in the data collection process; (12) This measure does not apply to this hospital for this reporting period; (13) Results cannot be calculated for this reporting period; (14) The results for this state are combined with nearby states to protect confidentiality; Please refer to the User's Guide for a full explanation of data.

Measure	Cases	This Hosp.	State Avg.	U.S. Avg.
Time from ER Arrival to Admit. (minutes)[2]	438	198	201	274
Time from ER Arrival to Discharge (minutes)	381	113	112	134
Time in ER Before Being Evaluated (minutes)	322	13	22	26
Time to Pain Meds for Fractures (minutes)	86	46	52	57
Heart Attack Care				
Aspirin Given at Discharge	249	100%	99%	99%
Fibrinolytic Meds Within 30 Min. of Arrival[7]	-	-	17%	54%
PCI Within 90 Minutes of Arrival	33	94%	93%	96%
Statin Prescribed at Discharge	244	99%	98%	98%
Heart Failure Care				
ACE Inhibitor or ARB for LVSD	49	100%	96%	97%
Discharge Instructions Given	164	96%	94%	94%
Evaluation of LVS Function	226	100%	96%	99%
Medicare Spending				
Medicare Spending per Patient (ratio)	-	0.90	0.9	0.98
Pneumonia Care				
Appropriate Initial Antibiotic Given[2]	129	95%	94%	95%
Blood Culture Timing[2]	143	97%	97%	98%
Pregnancy and Delivery Care				
Newborn Deliveries Scheduled Early[2]	28	7%	6%	6%
Preventive Care				
Immunization for Influenza[2]	535	86%	84%	90%
Immunization for Pneumonia[2]	563	90%	88%	92%
Stroke Care				
Anticoagulation Therapy for Atrial Fibrillation	19	100%	96%	95%
Antithrombotic Therapy Timing	85	100%	98%	98%
Assessed for Rehabilitation	103	99%	97%	97%
Discharged on Antithrombotic Therapy	89	100%	100%	99%
Discharged on Statin Medication	69	99%	91%	94%
Thrombolytic Therapy Timing[1]	-	-	96%	66%
Venous Thromboembolism Prophylaxis	110	95%	96%	94%
Written Stroke Educational Materials Given	46	98%	86%	88%
Surgical Care Improvement Project				
Appropriate Beta Blocker Usage[2]	186	98%	99%	98%
Appropriate VTP Within 24 Hours[2]	368	96%	98%	98%
Controlled Postoperative Blood Glucose[2]	103	99%	95%	97%
Perioperative Temperature Management[2]	477	100%	100%	100%
Prophylactic Antibiotic Selection[2]	427	100%	99%	99%
Prophylactic Antibiotic Selection (Outpatient)	475	99%	97%	98%
Prophylactic Antibiotic Stopped[2]	418	99%	99%	98%
Prophylactic Antibiotic Timing[2]	427	99%	98%	99%
Prophylactic Antibiotic Timing (Outpatient)	351	97%	96%	98%
Urinary Catheter Removal[2]	254	99%	97%	97%
Survey of Patients' Hospital Experiences				
Area Around Room 'Always' Quiet at Night	300+	60%	66%	61%
Doctors 'Always' Communicated Well	300+	78%	84%	82%
Home Recovery Information Given	300+	86%	82%	85%
Hospital Given 9 or 10 on 10 Point Scale	300+	73%	70%	71%
Meds 'Always' Explained Before Given	300+	62%	67%	64%
Nurses 'Always' Communicated Well	300+	78%	80%	79%
Pain 'Always' Well Controlled	300+	69%	69%	71%
Room and Bathroom 'Always' Clean	300+	72%	78%	73%
Timely Help 'Always' Received	300+	66%	74%	68%
Would Definitely Recommend Hospital	300+	78%	73%	71%
Use of Medical Imaging				
Cardiac Imaging Stress Test before Surgery	581	6.4%	4.6%	5.3%
Combination Abdominal CT Scan	480	27.7%	11.8%	10.5%
Combination Brain/Sinus CT Scan	357	1.4%	2.2%	2.7%
Combination Chest CT Scan	454	0.7%	2%	2.7%
Follow-up Mammogram/Ultrasound	399	3.8%	7.8%	8.8%
Lumbar Spine MRI for Low Back Pain	190	27.4%	32.9%	37.2%

Sanford Medical Center Bismarck

300 N 7th St
Bismarck, ND 58506
URL: www.medcenterone.com
Type: Acute Care Hospitals
Ownership: Voluntary non-profit - Private
Phone: 701-323-6000
Fax: 701-323-5221
Emergency Services: Yes
Beds: 196

Key Personnel:
Infection Control. . . . . Jodi Barnum
Operating Room. . . . . Douglas Berglund
Radiology. . . . . William Cain
CEO/President. . . . . James C Cooper
Pediatric Ambulatory Care . . . . . . Rafael Ocejo, MD
Quality Assurance . . . . Evy Olson
Chief of Medical Staff. . . . . Les Rainwater, MD
Pediatric In-Patient Care . . . . Randi Schaeffer

Measure	Cases	This Hosp.	State Avg.	U.S. Avg.
Blood Clot Prevention and Treatment				
Anticoagulation Overlap Therapy[2]	79	94%	97%	93%
ICU Venous Thromboembolism Prophylaxis[2]	37	86%	88%	92%
Incidence of Potentially Preventable VTE[1,2]	-	-	16%	10%
UFH with Dosages/Platelet Monitoring[2]	78	100%	100%	97%
Venous Thromboembolism Prophylaxis[2]	329	78%	80%	85%
Warfarin Therapy Discharge Instructions[2]	67	96%	72%	75%
Chest Pain/Possible Heart Attack Care				
Aspirin Given Within 24 Hours of Arrival[3,7]	-	-	95%	96%
Fibrinolytic Meds Within 30 Min. of Arrival[5]	-	-	51%	58%
Average Time to ECG (minutes)[3,7]	-	-	11	7
Average Time to Transfer (minutes)[5]	-	-	114	60
Children's Asthma Care				
Received Home Management Plan of Care	-	-	-	88%
Received Reliever Medication	-	-	-	100%
Received Systemic Corticosteroids	-	-	-	100%
Emergency Department				
Admittance Decision Time (minutes)[2]	65	45	66	98
Head CT Results Within 45 Min. of Arrival[1,3]	-	-	25%	57%
Patients Who Left ER Before Being Seen	28,866	1%	1%	2%
Time from ER Arrival to Admit. (minutes)[2]	79	161	201	274
Time from ER Arrival to Discharge (minutes)	128	82	112	134
Time in ER Before Being Evaluated (minutes)	152	22	22	26
Time to Pain Meds for Fractures (minutes)	139	37	52	57
Heart Attack Care				
Aspirin Given at Discharge	154	100%	99%	99%
Fibrinolytic Meds Within 30 Min. of Arrival[7]	-	-	17%	54%
PCI Within 90 Minutes of Arrival	16	100%	93%	96%
Statin Prescribed at Discharge	140	100%	98%	98%
Heart Failure Care				
ACE Inhibitor or ARB for LVSD	58	100%	96%	97%
Discharge Instructions Given	160	100%	94%	94%
Evaluation of LVS Function	195	100%	96%	99%
Medicare Spending				
Medicare Spending per Patient (ratio)	-	0.92	0.9	0.98
Pneumonia Care				
Appropriate Initial Antibiotic Given	88	98%	94%	95%
Blood Culture Timing	184	98%	97%	98%
Pregnancy and Delivery Care				
Newborn Deliveries Scheduled Early	127	1%	6%	6%
Preventive Care				
Immunization for Influenza[2]	551	95%	84%	90%
Immunization for Pneumonia[2]	618	96%	88%	92%
Stroke Care				
Anticoagulation Therapy for Atrial Fibrillation	14	79%	96%	95%
Antithrombotic Therapy Timing	69	97%	98%	98%
Assessed for Rehabilitation	77	100%	97%	97%
Discharged on Antithrombotic Therapy	68	99%	100%	99%
Discharged on Statin Medication	54	83%	91%	94%
Thrombolytic Therapy Timing[7]	-	-	96%	66%
Venous Thromboembolism Prophylaxis	76	95%	96%	94%
Written Stroke Educational Materials Given	46	98%	86%	88%
Surgical Care Improvement Project				
Appropriate Beta Blocker Usage[2]	237	100%	99%	98%
Appropriate VTP Within 24 Hours[2]	503	100%	98%	98%
Controlled Postoperative Blood Glucose[2]	125	94%	95%	97%
Perioperative Temperature Management[2]	610	100%	100%	100%
Prophylactic Antibiotic Selection[2]	565	99%	99%	99%
Prophylactic Antibiotic Selection (Outpatient)	329	98%	97%	98%
Prophylactic Antibiotic Stopped[2]	555	99%	99%	98%
Prophylactic Antibiotic Timing[2]	568	99%	98%	99%
Prophylactic Antibiotic Timing (Outpatient)	244	97%	96%	98%
Urinary Catheter Removal[2]	260	98%	97%	97%
Survey of Patients' Hospital Experiences				
Area Around Room 'Always' Quiet at Night	300+	57%	66%	61%
Doctors 'Always' Communicated Well	300+	79%	84%	82%
Home Recovery Information Given	300+	91%	82%	85%
Hospital Given 9 or 10 on 10 Point Scale	300+	74%	70%	71%
Meds 'Always' Explained Before Given	300+	63%	67%	64%
Nurses 'Always' Communicated Well	300+	79%	80%	79%
Pain 'Always' Well Controlled	300+	68%	69%	71%
Room and Bathroom 'Always' Clean	300+	72%	78%	73%
Timely Help 'Always' Received	300+	68%	74%	68%
Would Definitely Recommend Hospital	300+	79%	73%	71%
Use of Medical Imaging				
Cardiac Imaging Stress Test before Surgery	685	6.0%	4.6%	5.3%
Combination Abdominal CT Scan	943	5.2%	11.8%	10.5%
Combination Brain/Sinus CT Scan[1]	-	-	2.2%	2.7%
Combination Chest CT Scan	847	0.0%	2%	2.7%
Follow-up Mammogram/Ultrasound	1,606	11.7%	7.8%	8.8%
Lumbar Spine MRI for Low Back Pain	136	32.4%	32.9%	37.2%

Saint Andrews Health Center

316 Ohmer Street
Bottineau, ND 58318
E-mail: sahc@utma.com
URL: www.standrewshealth.us
Type: Critical Access Hospitals
Ownership: Voluntary non-profit - Church
Phone: 701-228-9300
Fax: 701-228-9384
Emergency Services: Yes
Beds: 25

Key Personnel:
Radiology. . . . . Brenda Aberle
Chief of Medical Staff. . . . . Dinesh Agnihotri, MD
CEO/President. . . . . Jodi Atkinson
Infection Control. . . . . Debra Kleven
Quality Assurance . . . . Jeanne McGuire
Emergency Room . . . . Gwen Wall

Measure	Cases	This Hosp.	State Avg.	U.S. Avg.
Blood Clot Prevention and Treatment				
Anticoagulation Overlap Therapy[5]	-	-	97%	93%
ICU Venous Thromboembolism Prophylaxis[5]	-	-	88%	92%
Incidence of Potentially Preventable VTE[5]	-	-	16%	10%
UFH with Dosages/Platelet Monitoring[5]	-	-	100%	97%
Venous Thromboembolism Prophylaxis[5]	-	-	80%	85%
Warfarin Therapy Discharge Instructions[5]	-	-	72%	75%
Chest Pain/Possible Heart Attack Care				
Aspirin Given Within 24 Hours of Arrival[1]	-	-	95%	96%
Fibrinolytic Meds Within 30 Min. of Arrival[3,7]	-	-	51%	58%
Average Time to ECG (minutes)[1]	-	-	11	7
Average Time to Transfer (minutes)[3,7]	-	-	114	60
Children's Asthma Care				
Received Home Management Plan of Care	-	-	-	88%
Received Reliever Medication	-	-	-	100%
Received Systemic Corticosteroids	-	-	-	100%
Emergency Department				
Admittance Decision Time (minutes)[5]	-	-	66	98
Head CT Results Within 45 Min. of Arrival[5]	-	-	25%	57%
Patients Who Left ER Before Being Seen	1,554	0%	1%	2%
Time from ER Arrival to Admit. (minutes)[5]	-	-	201	274
Time from ER Arrival to Discharge (minutes)[5]	-	-	112	134
Time in ER Before Being Evaluated (minutes)[5]	-	-	22	26
Time to Pain Meds for Fractures (minutes)[5]	-	-	52	57
Heart Attack Care				
Aspirin Given at Discharge[1,3]	-	-	99%	99%
Fibrinolytic Meds Within 30 Min. of Arrival[3,7]	-	-	17%	54%
PCI Within 90 Minutes of Arrival[3,7]	-	-	93%	96%
Statin Prescribed at Discharge[1,3]	-	-	98%	98%
Heart Failure Care				
ACE Inhibitor or ARB for LVSD[3,7]	-	-	96%	97%
Discharge Instructions Given[1,3]	-	-	94%	94%
Evaluation of LVS Function[1,3]	-	-	96%	99%
Medicare Spending				
Medicare Spending per Patient (ratio)	-	-	0.9	0.98
Pneumonia Care				
Appropriate Initial Antibiotic Given[1]	-	-	94%	95%
Blood Culture Timing[1]	-	-	97%	98%
Pregnancy and Delivery Care				
Newborn Deliveries Scheduled Early[5]	-	-	6%	6%
Preventive Care				
Immunization for Influenza[5]	-	-	84%	90%
Immunization for Pneumonia[5]	-	-	88%	92%
Stroke Care				
Anticoagulation Therapy for Atrial Fibrillation[5]	-	-	96%	95%
Antithrombotic Therapy Timing[5]	-	-	98%	98%

NOTE: Hospital profiles are in alphabetical order by state, then city, then hospital within the city; Rankings exclude hospitals with less than 25 cases except for patient surveys which excludes hospitals with less than 100 cases; (a) 100-299 cases; (1) The number of cases/patients is too few to report; (2) Data submitted were based on a sample of cases/patients; (3) Results are based on a shorter time period than required; (4) Data suppressed by CMS for one or more quarters; (5) Results are not available for this reporting period; (6) Fewer than 100 patients completed the HCAHPS survey; (7) No cases met the criteria for this measure; (8) The lower limit of the confidence interval cannot be calculated if the number of observed infections equals zero; (9) No data are available from the state/territory for this reporting period; (10) The scores shown reflect fewer than 50 completed surveys; (11) There were discrepancies in the data collection process; (12) This measure does not apply to this hospital for this reporting period; (13) Results cannot be calculated for this reporting period; (14) The results for this state are combined with nearby states to protect confidentiality; Please refer to the User's Guide for a full explanation of data.

Measure	Cases	This Hosp.	State Avg.	U.S. Avg.
Assessed for Rehabilitation[5]	-	-	97%	97%
Discharged on Antithrombotic Therapy[5]	-	-	100%	99%
Discharged on Statin Medication[5]	-	-	91%	94%
Thrombolytic Therapy Timing[5]	-	-	96%	66%
Venous Thromboembolism Prophylaxis[5]	-	-	96%	94%
Written Stroke Educational Materials Given[5]	-	-	86%	88%
Surgical Care Improvement Project				
Appropriate Beta Blocker Usage[5]	-	-	99%	98%
Appropriate VTP Within 24 Hours[5]	-	-	98%	98%
Controlled Postoperative Blood Glucose[5]	-	-	95%	97%
Perioperative Temperature Management[5]	-	-	100%	100%
Prophylactic Antibiotic Selection[5]	-	-	99%	99%
Prophylactic Antibiotic Selection (Outpatient)[5]	-	-	97%	98%
Prophylactic Antibiotic Stopped[5]	-	-	99%	98%
Prophylactic Antibiotic Timing[5]	-	-	98%	99%
Prophylactic Antibiotic Timing (Outpatient)[5]	-	-	96%	98%
Urinary Catheter Removal[5]	-	-	97%	97%
Survey of Patients' Hospital Experiences				
Area Around Room 'Always' Quiet at Night[10]	<100	90%	66%	61%
Doctors 'Always' Communicated Well[10]	<100	93%	84%	82%
Home Recovery Information Given[10]	<100	84%	82%	85%
Hospital Given 9 or 10 on 10 Point Scale[10]	<100	91%	70%	71%
Meds 'Always' Explained Before Given[10]	<100	78%	67%	64%
Nurses 'Always' Communicated Well[10]	<100	93%	80%	79%
Pain 'Always' Well Controlled[10]	<100	79%	69%	71%
Room and Bathroom 'Always' Clean[10]	<100	84%	78%	73%
Timely Help 'Always' Received[10]	<100	77%	74%	68%
Would Definitely Recommend Hospital[10]	<100	86%	73%	71%
Use of Medical Imaging				
Cardiac Imaging Stress Test before Surgery[1]	-	-	4.6%	5.3%
Combination Abdominal CT Scan	79	8.9%	11.8%	10.5%
Combination Brain/Sinus CT Scan	56	0.0%	2.2%	2.7%
Combination Chest CT Scan	67	3.0%	2%	2.7%
Follow-up Mammogram/Ultrasound	186	3.2%	7.8%	8.8%
Lumbar Spine MRI for Low Back Pain[1]	-	-	32.9%	37.2%

Southwest Healthcare Services

14 6th Ave Sw
Phone: 701-523-5265
Bowman, ND 58623
Type: Critical Access Hospitals
Emergency Services: Yes
Ownership: Voluntary non-profit - Private

Measure	Cases	This Hosp.	State Avg.	U.S. Avg.
Blood Clot Prevention and Treatment				
Anticoagulation Overlap Therapy[5]	-	-	97%	93%
ICU Venous Thromboembolism Prophylaxis[5]	-	-	88%	92%
Incidence of Potentially Preventable VTE[5]	-	-	16%	10%
UFH with Dosages/Platelet Monitoring[5]	-	-	100%	97%
Venous Thromboembolism Prophylaxis[5]	-	-	80%	85%
Warfarin Therapy Discharge Instructions[5]	-	-	72%	75%
Chest Pain/Possible Heart Attack Care				
Aspirin Given Within 24 Hours of Arrival[5]	-	-	95%	96%
Fibrinolytic Meds Within 30 Min. of Arrival[5]	-	-	51%	58%
Average Time to ECG (minutes)[5]	-	-	11	7
Average Time to Transfer (minutes)[5]	-	-	114	60
Children's Asthma Care				
Received Home Management Plan of Care	-	-	-	88%
Received Reliever Medication	-	-	-	100%
Received Systemic Corticosteroids	-	-	-	100%
Emergency Department				
Admittance Decision Time (minutes)[5]	-	-	66	98
Head CT Results Within 45 Min. of Arrival[5]	-	-	25%	57%
Patients Who Left ER Before Being Seen	863	0%	1%	2%
Time from ER Arrival to Admit. (minutes)[5]	-	-	201	274
Time from ER Arrival to Discharge (minutes)[5]	-	-	112	134
Time in ER Before Being Evaluated (minutes)[5]	-	-	22	26
Time to Pain Meds for Fractures (minutes)[5]	-	-	52	57
Heart Attack Care				
Aspirin Given at Discharge[1,3]	-	-	99%	99%
Fibrinolytic Meds Within 30 Min. of Arrival[3,7]	-	-	17%	54%
PCI Within 90 Minutes of Arrival[3,7]	-	-	93%	96%
Statin Prescribed at Discharge[3,7]	-	-	98%	98%
Heart Failure Care				
ACE Inhibitor or ARB for LVSD[1,3]	-	-	96%	97%
Discharge Instructions Given[1,3]	-	-	94%	94%
Evaluation of LVS Function[1,3]	-	-	96%	99%
Medicare Spending				
Medicare Spending per Patient (ratio)	-	-	0.9	0.98
Pneumonia Care				
Appropriate Initial Antibiotic Given[3,7]	-	-	94%	95%
Blood Culture Timing[3,7]	-	-	97%	98%
Pregnancy and Delivery Care				
Newborn Deliveries Scheduled Early[5]	-	-	6%	6%
Preventive Care				
Immunization for Influenza[5]	-	-	84%	90%
Immunization for Pneumonia[5]	-	-	88%	92%
Stroke Care				
Anticoagulation Therapy for Atrial Fibrillation[5]	-	-	96%	95%
Antithrombotic Therapy Timing[5]	-	-	98%	98%
Assessed for Rehabilitation[5]	-	-	97%	97%
Discharged on Antithrombotic Therapy[5]	-	-	100%	99%
Discharged on Statin Medication[5]	-	-	91%	94%
Thrombolytic Therapy Timing[5]	-	-	96%	66%
Venous Thromboembolism Prophylaxis[5]	-	-	96%	94%
Written Stroke Educational Materials Given[5]	-	-	86%	88%
Surgical Care Improvement Project				
Appropriate Beta Blocker Usage[5]	-	-	99%	98%
Appropriate VTP Within 24 Hours[5]	-	-	98%	98%
Controlled Postoperative Blood Glucose[5]	-	-	95%	97%
Perioperative Temperature Management[5]	-	-	100%	100%
Prophylactic Antibiotic Selection[5]	-	-	99%	99%
Prophylactic Antibiotic Selection (Outpatient)[5]	-	-	97%	98%
Prophylactic Antibiotic Stopped[5]	-	-	99%	98%
Prophylactic Antibiotic Timing[5]	-	-	98%	99%
Prophylactic Antibiotic Timing (Outpatient)[5]	-	-	96%	98%
Urinary Catheter Removal[5]	-	-	97%	97%
Survey of Patients' Hospital Experiences				
Area Around Room 'Always' Quiet at Night[10]	<100	66%	66%	61%
Doctors 'Always' Communicated Well[10]	<100	77%	84%	82%
Home Recovery Information Given[10]	<100	83%	82%	85%
Hospital Given 9 or 10 on 10 Point Scale[10]	<100	62%	70%	71%
Meds 'Always' Explained Before Given[10]	<100	76%	67%	64%
Nurses 'Always' Communicated Well[10]	<100	78%	80%	79%
Pain 'Always' Well Controlled[10]	<100	66%	69%	71%
Room and Bathroom 'Always' Clean[10]	<100	81%	78%	73%
Timely Help 'Always' Received[10]	<100	78%	74%	68%
Would Definitely Recommend Hospital[10]	<100	87%	73%	71%
Use of Medical Imaging				
Cardiac Imaging Stress Test before Surgery[7]	-	-	4.6%	5.3%
Combination Abdominal CT Scan[1]	-	-	11.8%	10.5%
Combination Brain/Sinus CT Scan	30	20.0%	2.2%	2.7%
Combination Chest CT Scan[1]	-	-	2%	2.7%
Follow-up Mammogram/Ultrasound	95	4.2%	7.8%	8.8%
Lumbar Spine MRI for Low Back Pain[1]	-	-	32.9%	37.2%

Towner County Medical Center

Hwy 281 N
Phone: 701-968-4411
Cando, ND 58324
Type: Critical Access Hospitals
Emergency Services: Yes
Ownership: Voluntary non-profit - Private

Measure	Cases	This Hosp.	State Avg.	U.S. Avg.
Blood Clot Prevention and Treatment				
Anticoagulation Overlap Therapy[5]	-	-	97%	93%
ICU Venous Thromboembolism Prophylaxis[5]	-	-	88%	92%
Incidence of Potentially Preventable VTE[5]	-	-	16%	10%
UFH with Dosages/Platelet Monitoring[5]	-	-	100%	97%
Venous Thromboembolism Prophylaxis[5]	-	-	80%	85%
Warfarin Therapy Discharge Instructions[5]	-	-	72%	75%
Chest Pain/Possible Heart Attack Care				
Aspirin Given Within 24 Hours of Arrival[1,3]	-	-	95%	96%
Fibrinolytic Meds Within 30 Min. of Arrival[5]	-	-	51%	58%
Average Time to ECG (minutes)[1,3]	-	-	11	7
Average Time to Transfer (minutes)[5]	-	-	114	60
Children's Asthma Care				
Received Home Management Plan of Care	-	-	-	88%
Received Reliever Medication	-	-	-	100%
Received Systemic Corticosteroids	-	-	-	100%
Emergency Department				
Admittance Decision Time (minutes)[5]	-	-	66	98
Head CT Results Within 45 Min. of Arrival[5]	-	-	25%	57%
Patients Who Left ER Before Being Seen	828	0%	1%	2%
Time from ER Arrival to Admit. (minutes)[5]	-	-	201	274
Time from ER Arrival to Discharge (minutes)[5]	-	-	112	134
Time in ER Before Being Evaluated (minutes)[5]	-	-	22	26
Time to Pain Meds for Fractures (minutes)[5]	-	-	52	57
Heart Attack Care				
Aspirin Given at Discharge[1,3]	-	-	99%	99%
Fibrinolytic Meds Within 30 Min. of Arrival[3,7]	-	-	17%	54%
PCI Within 90 Minutes of Arrival[3,7]	-	-	93%	96%
Statin Prescribed at Discharge[1,3]	-	-	98%	98%
Heart Failure Care				
ACE Inhibitor or ARB for LVSD[7]	-	-	96%	97%
Discharge Instructions Given[1]	-	-	94%	94%
Evaluation of LVS Function[1]	-	-	96%	99%
Medicare Spending				
Medicare Spending per Patient (ratio)	-	-	0.9	0.98
Pneumonia Care				
Appropriate Initial Antibiotic Given	17	88%	94%	95%
Blood Culture Timing[1]	-	-	97%	98%
Pregnancy and Delivery Care				
Newborn Deliveries Scheduled Early[5]	-	-	6%	6%
Preventive Care				
Immunization for Influenza[5]	-	-	84%	90%
Immunization for Pneumonia[5]	-	-	88%	92%
Stroke Care				
Anticoagulation Therapy for Atrial Fibrillation[5]	-	-	96%	95%
Antithrombotic Therapy Timing[5]	-	-	98%	98%
Assessed for Rehabilitation[5]	-	-	97%	97%
Discharged on Antithrombotic Therapy[5]	-	-	100%	99%
Discharged on Statin Medication[5]	-	-	91%	94%
Thrombolytic Therapy Timing[5]	-	-	96%	66%
Venous Thromboembolism Prophylaxis[5]	-	-	96%	94%
Written Stroke Educational Materials Given[5]	-	-	86%	88%
Surgical Care Improvement Project				
Appropriate Beta Blocker Usage[5]	-	-	99%	98%
Appropriate VTP Within 24 Hours[5]	-	-	98%	98%
Controlled Postoperative Blood Glucose[5]	-	-	95%	97%
Perioperative Temperature Management[5]	-	-	100%	100%
Prophylactic Antibiotic Selection[5]	-	-	99%	99%
Prophylactic Antibiotic Selection (Outpatient)[5]	-	-	97%	98%
Prophylactic Antibiotic Stopped[5]	-	-	99%	98%
Prophylactic Antibiotic Timing[5]	-	-	98%	99%
Prophylactic Antibiotic Timing (Outpatient)[5]	-	-	96%	98%
Urinary Catheter Removal[5]	-	-	97%	97%
Survey of Patients' Hospital Experiences				
Area Around Room 'Always' Quiet at Night[3,10]	<100	78%	66%	61%
Doctors 'Always' Communicated Well[3,10]	<100	88%	84%	82%
Home Recovery Information Given[3,10]	<100	74%	82%	85%
Hospital Given 9 or 10 on 10 Point Scale[3,10]	<100	85%	70%	71%
Meds 'Always' Explained Before Given[3,10]	<100	67%	67%	64%
Nurses 'Always' Communicated Well[3,10]	<100	86%	80%	79%
Pain 'Always' Well Controlled[3,10]	<100	69%	69%	71%
Room and Bathroom 'Always' Clean[3,10]	<100	88%	78%	73%
Timely Help 'Always' Received[3,10]	<100	72%	74%	68%
Would Definitely Recommend Hospital[3,10]	<100	69%	73%	71%
Use of Medical Imaging				
Cardiac Imaging Stress Test before Surgery[1]	-	-	4.6%	5.3%
Combination Abdominal CT Scan[1]	-	-	11.8%	10.5%
Combination Brain/Sinus CT Scan[1]	-	-	2.2%	2.7%
Combination Chest CT Scan[1]	-	-	2%	2.7%
Follow-up Mammogram/Ultrasound	98	7.1%	7.8%	8.8%
Lumbar Spine MRI for Low Back Pain[1]	-	-	32.9%	37.2%

NOTE: Hospital profiles are in alphabetical order by state, then city, then hospital within the city; Rankings exclude hospitals with less than 25 cases except for patient surveys which excludes hospitals with less than 100 cases; (a) 100-299 cases; (1) The number of cases/patients is too few to report; (2) Data submitted were based on a sample of cases/patients; (3) Results are based on a shorter time period than required; (4) Data suppressed by CMS for one or more quarters; (5) Results are not available for this reporting period; (6) Fewer than 100 patients completed the HCAHPS survey; (7) No cases met the criteria for this measure; (8) The lower limit of the confidence interval cannot be calculated if the number of observed infections equals zero; (9) No data are available from the state/territory for this reporting period; (10) The scores shown reflect fewer than 50 completed surveys; (11) There were discrepancies in the data collection process; (12) This measure does not apply to this hospital for this reporting period; (13) Results cannot be calculated for this reporting period; (14) The results for this state are combined with nearby states to protect confidentiality; Please refer to the User's Guide for a full explanation of data.

Carrington Health Center

PO Box 461
Carrington, ND 58421
URL: www.carringtonhealthcenter.net
Phone: 701-652-3141
Fax: 701-652-2884

Type: Critical Access Hospitals
Emergency Services: Yes
Ownership: Voluntary non-profit - Private
Beds: 25

Key Personnel:
Operating Room. . . . . Bernadin Anderson
Infection Control. . . . . Bernardine Anderson
Quality Assurance . . . . Mariann Doeling
CEO/President. . . . . Johnson Smith

Measure	Cases	This Hosp.	State Avg.	U.S. Avg.
Blood Clot Prevention and Treatment				
Anticoagulation Overlap Therapy[5]	-	-	97%	93%
ICU Venous Thromboembolism Prophylaxis[5]	-	-	88%	92%
Incidence of Potentially Preventable VTE[5]	-	-	16%	10%
UFH with Dosages/Platelet Monitoring[5]	-	-	100%	97%
Venous Thromboembolism Prophylaxis[5]	-	-	80%	85%
Warfarin Therapy Discharge Instructions[5]	-	-	72%	75%
Chest Pain/Possible Heart Attack Care				
Aspirin Given Within 24 Hours of Arrival	11	100%	95%	96%
Fibrinolytic Meds Within 30 Min. of Arrival[3,7]	-	-	51%	58%
Average Time to ECG (minutes)	11	16	11	7
Average Time to Transfer (minutes)[3,7]	-	-	114	60
Children's Asthma Care				
Received Home Management Plan of Care	-	-	-	88%
Received Reliever Medication	-	-	-	100%
Received Systemic Corticosteroids	-	-	-	100%
Emergency Department				
Admittance Decision Time (minutes)[2,3]	16	12	66	98
Head CT Results Within 45 Min. of Arrival[5]	-	-	25%	57%
Patients Who Left ER Before Being Seen	1,868	0%	1%	2%
Time from ER Arrival to Admit. (minutes)[2,3]	19	85	201	274
Time from ER Arrival to Discharge (minutes)[5]	-	-	112	134
Time in ER Before Being Evaluated (minutes)[5]	-	-	22	26
Time to Pain Meds for Fractures (minutes)[5]	-	-	52	57
Heart Attack Care				
Aspirin Given at Discharge[1,2]	-	-	99%	99%
Fibrinolytic Meds Within 30 Min. of Arrival[2,3]	-	-	17%	54%
PCI Within 90 Minutes of Arrival[2,3]	-	-	93%	96%
Statin Prescribed at Discharge[1,2]	-	-	98%	98%
Heart Failure Care				
ACE Inhibitor or ARB for LVSD[1,2]	-	-	96%	97%
Discharge Instructions Given[1,2]	-	-	94%	94%
Evaluation of LVS Function[2]	19	100%	96%	99%
Medicare Spending				
Medicare Spending per Patient (ratio)	-	-	0.9	0.98
Pneumonia Care				
Appropriate Initial Antibiotic Given[2]	16	88%	94%	95%
Blood Culture Timing[1,2]	-	-	97%	98%
Pregnancy and Delivery Care				
Newborn Deliveries Scheduled Early[5]	-	-	6%	6%
Preventive Care				
Immunization for Influenza[2]	144	100%	84%	90%
Immunization for Pneumonia[2]	241	100%	88%	92%
Stroke Care				
Anticoagulation Therapy for Atrial Fibrillation[5]	-	-	96%	95%
Antithrombotic Therapy Timing[5]	-	-	98%	98%
Assessed for Rehabilitation[5]	-	-	97%	97%
Discharged on Antithrombotic Therapy[5]	-	-	100%	99%
Discharged on Statin Medication[5]	-	-	91%	94%
Thrombolytic Therapy Timing[5]	-	-	96%	66%
Venous Thromboembolism Prophylaxis[5]	-	-	96%	94%
Written Stroke Educational Materials Given[5]	-	-	86%	88%
Surgical Care Improvement Project				
Appropriate Beta Blocker Usage[5]	-	-	99%	98%
Appropriate VTP Within 24 Hours[5]	-	-	98%	98%
Controlled Postoperative Blood Glucose[5]	-	-	95%	97%
Perioperative Temperature Management[5]	-	-	100%	100%
Prophylactic Antibiotic Selection[5]	-	-	99%	99%
Prophylactic Antibiotic Selection (Outpatient)[5]	-	-	97%	98%
Prophylactic Antibiotic Stopped[5]	-	-	99%	98%
Prophylactic Antibiotic Timing[5]	-	-	98%	99%
Prophylactic Antibiotic Timing (Outpatient)[5]	-	-	96%	98%
Urinary Catheter Removal[5]	-	-	97%	97%
Survey of Patients' Hospital Experiences				
Area Around Room 'Always' Quiet at Night[6]	<100	78%	66%	61%
Doctors 'Always' Communicated Well[6]	<100	89%	84%	82%
Home Recovery Information Given[6]	<100	89%	82%	85%
Hospital Given 9 or 10 on 10 Point Scale[6]	<100	82%	70%	71%
Meds 'Always' Explained Before Given[6]	<100	72%	67%	64%
Nurses 'Always' Communicated Well[6]	<100	79%	80%	79%
Pain 'Always' Well Controlled[6]	<100	77%	69%	71%
Room and Bathroom 'Always' Clean[6]	<100	81%	78%	73%
Timely Help 'Always' Received[6]	<100	80%	74%	68%
Would Definitely Recommend Hospital[6]	<100	84%	73%	71%
Use of Medical Imaging				
Cardiac Imaging Stress Test before Surgery[1]	-	-	4.6%	5.3%
Combination Abdominal CT Scan	159	3.1%	11.8%	10.5%
Combination Brain/Sinus CT Scan	114	0.0%	2.2%	2.7%
Combination Chest CT Scan	79	0.0%	2%	2.7%
Follow-up Mammogram/Ultrasound	294	6.8%	7.8%	8.8%
Lumbar Spine MRI for Low Back Pain[1]	-	-	32.9%	37.2%

Pembina County Memorial Hospital

Box 380
Cavalier, ND 58220
URL: www.cavalierhospital.com
Phone: 701-265-8461
Fax: 701-265-8752

Type: Critical Access Hospitals
Emergency Services: Yes
Ownership: Voluntary non-profit - Private
Beds: 29

Key Personnel:
Chief of Medical Staff. . . . . Hassan Abul-Khoudoud
CEO/President. . . . . Everett Butler
Emergency Room . . . . Kathelen Duff
Patient Relations . . . . Kathy Duff
Surgery . . . . Inder Khokha, MD
Quality Assurance . . . . Jodi Thoreson

Measure	Cases	This Hosp.	State Avg.	U.S. Avg.
Blood Clot Prevention and Treatment				
Anticoagulation Overlap Therapy[5]	-	-	97%	93%
ICU Venous Thromboembolism Prophylaxis[5]	-	-	88%	92%
Incidence of Potentially Preventable VTE[5]	-	-	16%	10%
UFH with Dosages/Platelet Monitoring[5]	-	-	100%	97%
Venous Thromboembolism Prophylaxis[5]	-	-	80%	85%
Warfarin Therapy Discharge Instructions[5]	-	-	72%	75%
Chest Pain/Possible Heart Attack Care				
Aspirin Given Within 24 Hours of Arrival[1,3]	-	-	95%	96%
Fibrinolytic Meds Within 30 Min. of Arrival[5]	-	-	51%	58%
Average Time to ECG (minutes)[1,3]	-	-	11	7
Average Time to Transfer (minutes)[5]	-	-	114	60
Children's Asthma Care				
Received Home Management Plan of Care	-	-	-	88%
Received Reliever Medication	-	-	-	100%
Received Systemic Corticosteroids	-	-	-	100%
Emergency Department				
Admittance Decision Time (minutes)[5]	-	-	66	98
Head CT Results Within 45 Min. of Arrival[1,3]	-	-	25%	57%
Patients Who Left ER Before Being Seen	1,428	0%	1%	2%
Time from ER Arrival to Admit. (minutes)[5]	-	-	201	274
Time from ER Arrival to Discharge (minutes)[5]	-	-	112	134
Time in ER Before Being Evaluated (minutes)[5]	-	-	22	26
Time to Pain Meds for Fractures (minutes)[5]	-	-	52	57
Heart Attack Care				
Aspirin Given at Discharge[5]	-	-	99%	99%
Fibrinolytic Meds Within 30 Min. of Arrival[5]	-	-	17%	54%
PCI Within 90 Minutes of Arrival[5]	-	-	93%	96%
Statin Prescribed at Discharge[5]	-	-	98%	98%
Heart Failure Care				
ACE Inhibitor or ARB for LVSD[1,2]	-	-	96%	97%
Discharge Instructions Given[1,2]	-	-	94%	94%
Evaluation of LVS Function[1,2]	-	-	96%	99%
Medicare Spending				
Medicare Spending per Patient (ratio)	-	-	0.9	0.98
Pneumonia Care				
Appropriate Initial Antibiotic Given[1,2]	-	-	94%	95%
Blood Culture Timing[2,7]	-	-	97%	98%
Pregnancy and Delivery Care				
Newborn Deliveries Scheduled Early[5]	-	-	6%	6%
Preventive Care				
Immunization for Influenza[5]	-	-	84%	90%
Immunization for Pneumonia[5]	-	-	88%	92%
Stroke Care				
Anticoagulation Therapy for Atrial Fibrillation[5]	-	-	96%	95%
Antithrombotic Therapy Timing[5]	-	-	98%	98%
Assessed for Rehabilitation[5]	-	-	97%	97%
Discharged on Antithrombotic Therapy[5]	-	-	100%	99%
Discharged on Statin Medication[5]	-	-	91%	94%
Thrombolytic Therapy Timing[5]	-	-	96%	66%
Venous Thromboembolism Prophylaxis[5]	-	-	96%	94%
Written Stroke Educational Materials Given[5]	-	-	86%	88%
Surgical Care Improvement Project				
Appropriate Beta Blocker Usage[5]	-	-	99%	98%
Appropriate VTP Within 24 Hours[5]	-	-	98%	98%
Controlled Postoperative Blood Glucose[5]	-	-	95%	97%
Perioperative Temperature Management[5]	-	-	100%	100%
Prophylactic Antibiotic Selection[5]	-	-	99%	99%
Prophylactic Antibiotic Selection (Outpatient)[5]	-	-	97%	98%
Prophylactic Antibiotic Stopped[5]	-	-	99%	98%
Prophylactic Antibiotic Timing[5]	-	-	98%	99%
Prophylactic Antibiotic Timing (Outpatient)[5]	-	-	96%	98%
Urinary Catheter Removal[5]	-	-	97%	97%
Survey of Patients' Hospital Experiences				
Area Around Room 'Always' Quiet at Night[6]	<100	61%	66%	61%
Doctors 'Always' Communicated Well[6]	<100	86%	84%	82%
Home Recovery Information Given[6]	<100	66%	82%	85%
Hospital Given 9 or 10 on 10 Point Scale[6]	<100	69%	70%	71%
Meds 'Always' Explained Before Given[6]	<100	75%	67%	64%
Nurses 'Always' Communicated Well[6]	<100	80%	80%	79%
Pain 'Always' Well Controlled[6]	<100	73%	69%	71%
Room and Bathroom 'Always' Clean[6]	<100	91%	78%	73%
Timely Help 'Always' Received[6]	<100	79%	74%	68%
Would Definitely Recommend Hospital[6]	<100	72%	73%	71%
Use of Medical Imaging				
Cardiac Imaging Stress Test before Surgery[7]	-	-	4.6%	5.3%
Combination Abdominal CT Scan	141	0.7%	11.8%	10.5%
Combination Brain/Sinus CT Scan[1]	-	-	2.2%	2.7%
Combination Chest CT Scan	68	0.0%	2%	2.7%
Follow-up Mammogram/Ultrasound	144	4.9%	7.8%	8.8%
Lumbar Spine MRI for Low Back Pain[1]	-	-	32.9%	37.2%

Cooperstown Medical Center

1200 Roberts Ave Ne
Cooperstown, ND 58425
Phone: 701-797-2221

Type: Critical Access Hospitals
Emergency Services: Yes
Ownership: Voluntary non-profit - Private

Measure	Cases	This Hosp.	State Avg.	U.S. Avg.
Blood Clot Prevention and Treatment				
Anticoagulation Overlap Therapy[5]	-	-	97%	93%
ICU Venous Thromboembolism Prophylaxis[5]	-	-	88%	92%
Incidence of Potentially Preventable VTE[5]	-	-	16%	10%
UFH with Dosages/Platelet Monitoring[5]	-	-	100%	97%
Venous Thromboembolism Prophylaxis[5]	-	-	80%	85%
Warfarin Therapy Discharge Instructions[5]	-	-	72%	75%
Chest Pain/Possible Heart Attack Care				
Aspirin Given Within 24 Hours of Arrival[1,3]	-	-	95%	96%
Fibrinolytic Meds Within 30 Min. of Arrival[3,7]	-	-	51%	58%
Average Time to ECG (minutes)[1,3]	-	-	11	7
Average Time to Transfer (minutes)[1,3]	-	-	114	60
Children's Asthma Care				
Received Home Management Plan of Care	-	-	-	88%
Received Reliever Medication	-	-	-	100%
Received Systemic Corticosteroids	-	-	-	100%
Emergency Department				
Admittance Decision Time (minutes)[5]	-	-	66	98
Head CT Results Within 45 Min. of Arrival[5]	-	-	25%	57%
Patients Who Left ER Before Being Seen	372	0%	1%	2%
Time from ER Arrival to Admit. (minutes)[5]	-	-	201	274
Time from ER Arrival to Discharge (minutes)[5]	-	-	112	134
Time in ER Before Being Evaluated (minutes)[5]	-	-	22	26

NOTE: Hospital profiles are in alphabetical order by state, then city, then hospital within the city; Rankings exclude hospitals with less than 25 cases except for patient surveys which excludes hospitals with less than 100 cases; (a) 100-299 cases; (1) The number of cases/patients is too few to report; (2) Data submitted were based on a sample of cases/patients; (3) Results are based on a shorter time period than required; (4) Data suppressed by CMS for one or more quarters; (5) Results are not available for this reporting period; (6) Fewer than 100 patients completed the HCAHPS survey; (7) No cases met the criteria for this measure; (8) The lower limit of the confidence interval cannot be calculated if the number of observed infections equals zero; (9) No data are available from the state/territory for this reporting period; (10) The scores shown reflect fewer than 50 completed surveys; (11) There were discrepancies in the data collection process; (12) This measure does not apply to this hospital for this reporting period; (13) Results cannot be calculated for this reporting period; (14) The results for this state are combined with nearby states to protect confidentiality; Please refer to the User's Guide for a full explanation of data.

Measure	Cases	This Hosp.	State Avg.	U.S. Avg.
Time to Pain Meds for Fractures (minutes)[5]	-	-	52	57
Heart Attack Care				
Aspirin Given at Discharge[5]	-	-	99%	99%
Fibrinolytic Meds Within 30 Min. of Arrival[5]	-	-	17%	54%
PCI Within 90 Minutes of Arrival[5]	-	-	93%	96%
Statin Prescribed at Discharge[5]	-	-	98%	98%
Heart Failure Care				
ACE Inhibitor or ARB for LVSD[3,7]	-	-	96%	97%
Discharge Instructions Given[1,3]	-	-	94%	94%
Evaluation of LVS Function[1,3]	-	-	96%	99%
Medicare Spending				
Medicare Spending per Patient (ratio)	-	-	0.9	0.98
Pneumonia Care				
Appropriate Initial Antibiotic Given[1]	-	-	94%	95%
Blood Culture Timing[1]	-	-	97%	98%
Pregnancy and Delivery Care				
Newborn Deliveries Scheduled Early[5]	-	-	6%	6%
Preventive Care				
Immunization for Influenza[5]	-	-	84%	90%
Immunization for Pneumonia[5]	-	-	88%	92%
Stroke Care				
Anticoagulation Therapy for Atrial Fibrillation[5]	-	-	96%	95%
Antithrombotic Therapy Timing[5]	-	-	98%	98%
Assessed for Rehabilitation[5]	-	-	97%	97%
Discharged on Antithrombotic Therapy[5]	-	-	100%	99%
Discharged on Statin Medication[5]	-	-	91%	94%
Thrombolytic Therapy Timing[5]	-	-	96%	66%
Venous Thromboembolism Prophylaxis[5]	-	-	96%	94%
Written Stroke Educational Materials Given[5]	-	-	86%	88%
Surgical Care Improvement Project				
Appropriate Beta Blocker Usage[5]	-	-	99%	98%
Appropriate VTP Within 24 Hours[5]	-	-	98%	98%
Controlled Postoperative Blood Glucose[5]	-	-	95%	97%
Perioperative Temperature Management[5]	-	-	100%	100%
Prophylactic Antibiotic Selection[5]	-	-	99%	99%
Prophylactic Antibiotic Selection (Outpatient)[5]	-	-	97%	98%
Prophylactic Antibiotic Stopped[5]	-	-	99%	98%
Prophylactic Antibiotic Timing[5]	-	-	98%	99%
Prophylactic Antibiotic Timing (Outpatient)[5]	-	-	96%	98%
Urinary Catheter Removal[5]	-	-	97%	97%
Survey of Patients' Hospital Experiences				
Area Around Room 'Always' Quiet at Night[10]	<100	90%	66%	61%
Doctors 'Always' Communicated Well[10]	<100	99%	84%	82%
Home Recovery Information Given[10]	<100	94%	82%	85%
Hospital Given 9 or 10 on 10 Point Scale[10]	<100	84%	70%	71%
Meds 'Always' Explained Before Given[10]	<100	83%	67%	64%
Nurses 'Always' Communicated Well[10]	<100	97%	80%	79%
Pain 'Always' Well Controlled[10]	<100	76%	69%	71%
Room and Bathroom 'Always' Clean[10]	<100	96%	78%	73%
Timely Help 'Always' Received[10]	<100	85%	74%	68%
Would Definitely Recommend Hospital[10]	<100	93%	73%	71%
Use of Medical Imaging				
Cardiac Imaging Stress Test before Surgery[7]	-	-	4.6%	5.3%
Combination Abdominal CT Scan[1]	-	-	11.8%	10.5%
Combination Brain/Sinus CT Scan[7]	-	-	2.2%	2.7%
Combination Chest CT Scan[1]	-	-	2%	2.7%
Follow-up Mammogram/Ultrasound[1]	-	-	7.8%	8.8%
Lumbar Spine MRI for Low Back Pain[7]	-	-	32.9%	37.2%

Saint Luke's Hospital

702 1st Saint Sw
Crosby, ND 58730
Phone: 701-965-6384
Type: Critical Access Hospitals
Emergency Services: Yes
Ownership: Voluntary non-profit - Private

Measure	Cases	This Hosp.	State Avg.	U.S. Avg.
Blood Clot Prevention and Treatment				
Anticoagulation Overlap Therapy[5]	-	-	97%	93%
ICU Venous Thromboembolism Prophylaxis[5]	-	-	88%	92%
Incidence of Potentially Preventable VTE[5]	-	-	16%	10%
UFH with Dosages/Platelet Monitoring[5]	-	-	100%	97%
Venous Thromboembolism Prophylaxis[5]	-	-	80%	85%
Warfarin Therapy Discharge Instructions[5]	-	-	72%	75%
Chest Pain/Possible Heart Attack Care				
Aspirin Given Within 24 Hours of Arrival[1,3]	-	-	95%	96%
Fibrinolytic Meds Within 30 Min. of Arrival[3,7]	-	-	51%	58%
Average Time to ECG (minutes)[1,3]	-	-	11	7
Average Time to Transfer (minutes)[3,7]	-	-	114	60
Children's Asthma Care				
Received Home Management Plan of Care	-	-	-	88%
Received Reliever Medication	-	-	-	100%
Received Systemic Corticosteroids	-	-	-	100%
Emergency Department				
Admittance Decision Time (minutes)[5]	-	-	66	98
Head CT Results Within 45 Min. of Arrival[3,7]	-	-	25%	57%
Patients Who Left ER Before Being Seen	994	0%	1%	2%
Time from ER Arrival to Admit. (minutes)[5]	-	-	201	274
Time from ER Arrival to Discharge (minutes)[5]	-	-	112	134
Time in ER Before Being Evaluated (minutes)[5]	-	-	22	26
Time to Pain Meds for Fractures (minutes)[5]	-	-	52	57
Heart Attack Care				
Aspirin Given at Discharge[1,3]	-	-	99%	99%
Fibrinolytic Meds Within 30 Min. of Arrival[3,7]	-	-	17%	54%
PCI Within 90 Minutes of Arrival[3,7]	-	-	93%	96%
Statin Prescribed at Discharge[1,3]	-	-	98%	98%
Heart Failure Care				
ACE Inhibitor or ARB for LVSD[3,7]	-	-	96%	97%
Discharge Instructions Given[1,3]	-	-	94%	94%
Evaluation of LVS Function[1,3]	-	-	96%	99%
Medicare Spending				
Medicare Spending per Patient (ratio)	-	-	0.9	0.98
Pneumonia Care				
Appropriate Initial Antibiotic Given[1,3]	-	-	94%	95%
Blood Culture Timing[1,3]	-	-	97%	98%
Pregnancy and Delivery Care				
Newborn Deliveries Scheduled Early[5]	-	-	6%	6%
Preventive Care				
Immunization for Influenza	12	33%	84%	90%
Immunization for Pneumonia[3]	15	40%	88%	92%
Stroke Care				
Anticoagulation Therapy for Atrial Fibrillation[5]	-	-	96%	95%
Antithrombotic Therapy Timing[5]	-	-	98%	98%
Assessed for Rehabilitation[5]	-	-	97%	97%
Discharged on Antithrombotic Therapy[5]	-	-	100%	99%
Discharged on Statin Medication[5]	-	-	91%	94%
Thrombolytic Therapy Timing[5]	-	-	96%	66%
Venous Thromboembolism Prophylaxis[5]	-	-	96%	94%
Written Stroke Educational Materials Given[5]	-	-	86%	88%
Surgical Care Improvement Project				
Appropriate Beta Blocker Usage[5]	-	-	99%	98%
Appropriate VTP Within 24 Hours[5]	-	-	98%	98%
Controlled Postoperative Blood Glucose[5]	-	-	95%	97%
Perioperative Temperature Management[5]	-	-	100%	100%
Prophylactic Antibiotic Selection[5]	-	-	99%	99%
Prophylactic Antibiotic Selection (Outpatient)[5]	-	-	97%	98%
Prophylactic Antibiotic Stopped[5]	-	-	99%	98%
Prophylactic Antibiotic Timing[5]	-	-	98%	99%
Prophylactic Antibiotic Timing (Outpatient)[5]	-	-	96%	98%
Urinary Catheter Removal[5]	-	-	97%	97%
Survey of Patients' Hospital Experiences				
Area Around Room 'Always' Quiet at Night[3,10]	<100	72%	66%	61%
Doctors 'Always' Communicated Well[3,10]	<100	82%	84%	82%
Home Recovery Information Given[3,10]	<100	69%	82%	85%
Hospital Given 9 or 10 on 10 Point Scale[3,10]	<100	69%	70%	71%
Meds 'Always' Explained Before Given[3,10]	<100	76%	67%	64%
Nurses 'Always' Communicated Well[3,10]	<100	85%	80%	79%
Pain 'Always' Well Controlled[3,10]	<100	72%	69%	71%
Room and Bathroom 'Always' Clean[3,10]	<100	84%	78%	73%
Timely Help 'Always' Received[3,10]	<100	82%	74%	68%
Would Definitely Recommend Hospital[3,10]	<100	64%	73%	71%
Use of Medical Imaging				
Cardiac Imaging Stress Test before Surgery[7]	-	-	4.6%	5.3%
Combination Abdominal CT Scan[1]	-	-	11.8%	10.5%
Combination Brain/Sinus CT Scan[1]	-	-	2.2%	2.7%
Combination Chest CT Scan[1]	-	-	2%	2.7%
Follow-up Mammogram/Ultrasound[7]	-	-	7.8%	8.8%
Lumbar Spine MRI for Low Back Pain[7]	-	-	32.9%	37.2%

The Mercy Hospital of Devils Lake

1031 7th Saint Ne
Phone: 701-662-2131
Devils Lake, ND 58301
Type: Critical Access Hospitals
Emergency Services: Yes
Ownership: Voluntary non-profit - Private

Measure	Cases	This Hosp.	State Avg.	U.S. Avg.
Blood Clot Prevention and Treatment				
Anticoagulation Overlap Therapy[5]	-	-	97%	93%
ICU Venous Thromboembolism Prophylaxis[5]	-	-	88%	92%
Incidence of Potentially Preventable VTE[5]	-	-	16%	10%
UFH with Dosages/Platelet Monitoring[5]	-	-	100%	97%
Venous Thromboembolism Prophylaxis[5]	-	-	80%	85%
Warfarin Therapy Discharge Instructions[5]	-	-	72%	75%
Chest Pain/Possible Heart Attack Care				
Aspirin Given Within 24 Hours of Arrival	37	84%	95%	96%
Fibrinolytic Meds Within 30 Min. of Arrival[1,3]	-	-	51%	58%
Average Time to ECG (minutes)	37	9	11	7
Average Time to Transfer (minutes)[1,3]	-	-	114	60
Children's Asthma Care				
Received Home Management Plan of Care	-	-	-	88%
Received Reliever Medication	-	-	-	100%
Received Systemic Corticosteroids	-	-	-	100%
Emergency Department				
Admittance Decision Time (minutes)[1,2]	-	-	66	98
Head CT Results Within 45 Min. of Arrival	11	18%	25%	57%
Patients Who Left ER Before Being Seen	10,797	0%	1%	2%
Time from ER Arrival to Admit. (minutes)[2,3]	106	140	201	274
Time from ER Arrival to Discharge (minutes)	375	59	112	134
Time in ER Before Being Evaluated (minutes)	257	10	22	26
Time to Pain Meds for Fractures (minutes)	57	36	52	57
Heart Attack Care				
Aspirin Given at Discharge[1,2]	-	-	99%	99%
Fibrinolytic Meds Within 30 Min. of Arrival[2,3]	-	-	17%	54%
PCI Within 90 Minutes of Arrival[2,3]	-	-	93%	96%
Statin Prescribed at Discharge[1,2]	-	-	98%	98%
Heart Failure Care				
ACE Inhibitor or ARB for LVSD[1,2]	-	-	96%	97%
Discharge Instructions Given[2]	11	100%	94%	94%
Evaluation of LVS Function[2]	23	100%	96%	99%
Medicare Spending				
Medicare Spending per Patient (ratio)	-	-	0.9	0.98
Pneumonia Care				
Appropriate Initial Antibiotic Given[2]	35	94%	94%	95%
Blood Culture Timing[2]	45	93%	97%	98%
Pregnancy and Delivery Care				
Newborn Deliveries Scheduled Early[5]	-	-	6%	6%
Preventive Care				
Immunization for Influenza[2,3]	113	92%	84%	90%
Immunization for Pneumonia[2,3]	144	98%	88%	92%
Stroke Care				
Anticoagulation Therapy for Atrial Fibrillation[5]	-	-	96%	95%
Antithrombotic Therapy Timing[5]	-	-	98%	98%
Assessed for Rehabilitation[5]	-	-	97%	97%
Discharged on Antithrombotic Therapy[5]	-	-	100%	99%
Discharged on Statin Medication[5]	-	-	91%	94%
Thrombolytic Therapy Timing[5]	-	-	96%	66%
Venous Thromboembolism Prophylaxis[5]	-	-	96%	94%
Written Stroke Educational Materials Given[5]	-	-	86%	88%
Surgical Care Improvement Project				
Appropriate Beta Blocker Usage[3,7]	-	-	99%	98%
Appropriate VTP Within 24 Hours[1,3]	-	-	98%	98%
Controlled Postoperative Blood Glucose[3,7]	-	-	95%	97%
Perioperative Temperature Management[1,3]	-	-	100%	100%
Prophylactic Antibiotic Selection[3,7]	-	-	99%	99%
Prophylactic Antibiotic Selection (Outpatient)[5]	-	-	97%	98%
Prophylactic Antibiotic Stopped[3,7]	-	-	99%	98%
Prophylactic Antibiotic Timing[3,7]	-	-	98%	99%
Prophylactic Antibiotic Timing (Outpatient)[5]	-	-	96%	98%
Urinary Catheter Removal[3,7]	-	-	97%	97%

NOTE: Hospital profiles are in alphabetical order by state, then city, then hospital within the city; Rankings exclude hospitals with less than 25 cases except for patient surveys which excludes hospitals with less than 100 cases; (a) 100-299 cases; (1) The number of cases/patients is too few to report; (2) Data submitted were based on a sample of cases/patients; (3) Results are based on a shorter time period than required; (4) Data suppressed by CMS for one or more quarters; (5) Results are not available for this reporting period; (6) Fewer than 100 patients completed the HCAHPS survey; (7) No cases met the criteria for this measure; (8) The lower limit of the confidence interval cannot be calculated if the number of observed infections equals zero; (9) No data are available from the state/territory for this reporting period; (10) The scores shown reflect fewer than 50 completed surveys; (11) There were discrepancies in the data collection process; (12) This measure does not apply to this hospital for this reporting period; (13) Results cannot be calculated for this reporting period; (14) The results for this state are combined with nearby states to protect confidentiality; Please refer to the User's Guide for a full explanation of data.

Measure	Cases	This Hosp.	State Avg.	U.S. Avg.
Survey of Patients' Hospital Experiences				
Area Around Room 'Always' Quiet at Night[5]	-	-	66%	61%
Doctors 'Always' Communicated Well[5]	-	-	84%	82%
Home Recovery Information Given[5]	-	-	82%	85%
Hospital Given 9 or 10 on 10 Point Scale[5]	-	-	70%	71%
Meds 'Always' Explained Before Given[5]	-	-	67%	64%
Nurses 'Always' Communicated Well[5]	-	-	80%	79%
Pain 'Always' Well Controlled[5]	-	-	69%	71%
Room and Bathroom 'Always' Clean[5]	-	-	78%	73%
Timely Help 'Always' Received[5]	-	-	74%	68%
Would Definitely Recommend Hospital[5]	-	-	73%	71%
Use of Medical Imaging				
Cardiac Imaging Stress Test before Surgery	108	2.8%	4.6%	5.3%
Combination Abdominal CT Scan	244	4.9%	11.8%	10.5%
Combination Brain/Sinus CT Scan[1]	-	-	2.2%	2.7%
Combination Chest CT Scan	111	3.6%	2%	2.7%
Follow-up Mammogram/Ultrasound[7]	-	-	7.8%	8.8%
Lumbar Spine MRI for Low Back Pain[1]	-	-	32.9%	37.2%

Saint Joseph's Hospital & Health Center

30 West 7th St
Dickinson, ND 58601
Phone: 701-456-4000
Fax: 701-456-4829
E-mail: stjoesinfo@catholichealth.net
URL: www.stjoeshospital.org
Type: Critical Access Hospitals
Emergency Services: Yes
Ownership: Voluntary non-profit - Church
Beds: 106

Key Personnel:
Radiology. . . . . Garry Dunn
Operating Room. . . . . Janis Gartner
Intensive Care Unit. . . . . Denette Lothspeich
Chief of Medical Staff . . . . Amy Okasa, MD
Hemotology Center . . . . Curtis Prevost
President/CEO. . . . . Reed E. Reyman
Infection Control. . . . . Tavia Voll
Quality Assurance . . . . Tavia Voll

Measure	Cases	This Hosp.	State Avg.	U.S. Avg.
Blood Clot Prevention and Treatment				
Anticoagulation Overlap Therapy[5]	-	-	97%	93%
ICU Venous Thromboembolism Prophylaxis[5]	-	-	88%	92%
Incidence of Potentially Preventable VTE[5]	-	-	16%	10%
UFH with Dosages/Platelet Monitoring[5]	-	-	100%	97%
Venous Thromboembolism Prophylaxis[5]	-	-	80%	85%
Warfarin Therapy Discharge Instructions[5]	-	-	72%	75%
Chest Pain/Possible Heart Attack Care				
Aspirin Given Within 24 Hours of Arrival	56	100%	95%	96%
Fibrinolytic Meds Within 30 Min. of Arrival[1]	-	-	51%	58%
Average Time to ECG (minutes)	57	11	11	7
Average Time to Transfer (minutes)[7]	-	-	114	60
Children's Asthma Care				
Received Home Management Plan of Care	-	-	-	88%
Received Reliever Medication	-	-	-	100%
Received Systemic Corticosteroids	-	-	-	100%
Emergency Department				
Admittance Decision Time (minutes)[5]	-	-	66	98
Head CT Results Within 45 Min. of Arrival[5]	-	-	25%	57%
Patients Who Left ER Before Being Seen	15,501	1%	1%	2%
Time from ER Arrival to Admit. (minutes)[5]	-	-	201	274
Time from ER Arrival to Discharge (minutes)[5]	-	-	112	134
Time in ER Before Being Evaluated (minutes)[5]	-	-	22	26
Time to Pain Meds for Fractures (minutes)[5]	-	-	52	57
Heart Attack Care				
Aspirin Given at Discharge[1,3]	-	-	99%	99%
Fibrinolytic Meds Within 30 Min. of Arrival[3,7]	-	-	17%	54%
PCI Within 90 Minutes of Arrival[3,7]	-	-	93%	96%
Statin Prescribed at Discharge[1,3]	-	-	98%	98%
Heart Failure Care				
ACE Inhibitor or ARB for LVSD	13	92%	96%	97%
Discharge Instructions Given	57	96%	94%	94%
Evaluation of LVS Function	72	100%	96%	99%
Medicare Spending				
Medicare Spending per Patient (ratio)	-	-	0.9	0.98
Pneumonia Care				
Appropriate Initial Antibiotic Given	38	100%	94%	95%
Blood Culture Timing	63	98%	97%	98%
Pregnancy and Delivery Care				
Newborn Deliveries Scheduled Early[2,3]	19	0%	6%	6%
Preventive Care				
Immunization for Influenza[5]	-	-	84%	90%
Immunization for Pneumonia[5]	-	-	88%	92%
Stroke Care				
Anticoagulation Therapy for Atrial Fibrillation[5]	-	-	96%	95%
Antithrombotic Therapy Timing[5]	-	-	98%	98%
Assessed for Rehabilitation[5]	-	-	97%	97%
Discharged on Antithrombotic Therapy[5]	-	-	100%	99%
Discharged on Statin Medication[5]	-	-	91%	94%
Thrombolytic Therapy Timing[5]	-	-	96%	66%
Venous Thromboembolism Prophylaxis[5]	-	-	96%	94%
Written Stroke Educational Materials Given[5]	-	-	86%	88%
Surgical Care Improvement Project				
Appropriate Beta Blocker Usage	12	100%	99%	98%
Appropriate VTP Within 24 Hours	40	100%	98%	98%
Controlled Postoperative Blood Glucose[7]	-	-	95%	97%
Perioperative Temperature Management	57	100%	100%	100%
Prophylactic Antibiotic Selection	34	100%	99%	99%
Prophylactic Antibiotic Selection (Outpatient)	43	98%	97%	98%
Prophylactic Antibiotic Stopped	33	100%	99%	98%
Prophylactic Antibiotic Timing	34	97%	98%	99%
Prophylactic Antibiotic Timing (Outpatient)	43	100%	96%	98%
Urinary Catheter Removal	26	100%	97%	97%
Survey of Patients' Hospital Experiences				
Area Around Room 'Always' Quiet at Night	300+	56%	66%	61%
Doctors 'Always' Communicated Well	300+	75%	84%	82%
Home Recovery Information Given	300+	87%	82%	85%
Hospital Given 9 or 10 on 10 Point Scale	300+	61%	70%	71%
Meds 'Always' Explained Before Given	300+	61%	67%	64%
Nurses 'Always' Communicated Well	300+	76%	80%	79%
Pain 'Always' Well Controlled	300+	68%	69%	71%
Room and Bathroom 'Always' Clean	300+	59%	78%	73%
Timely Help 'Always' Received	300+	71%	74%	68%
Would Definitely Recommend Hospital	300+	59%	73%	71%
Use of Medical Imaging				
Cardiac Imaging Stress Test before Surgery	192	5.2%	4.6%	5.3%
Combination Abdominal CT Scan	390	7.7%	11.8%	10.5%
Combination Brain/Sinus CT Scan[1]	-	-	2.2%	2.7%
Combination Chest CT Scan	193	3.6%	2%	2.7%
Follow-up Mammogram/Ultrasound	117	7.7%	7.8%	8.8%
Lumbar Spine MRI for Low Back Pain	106	29.2%	32.9%	37.2%

Jacobson Memorial Hospital Care Center

601 East Saint N
Elgin, ND 58533
Phone: 701-584-2792
Fax: 701-584-3348
Type: Critical Access Hospitals
Emergency Services: Yes
Ownership: Voluntary non-profit - Private
Beds: 50

Key Personnel:
Emergency Room . . . . Marcy Dawson, RN
Chief of Medical Staff. . . . . Dr. Deepak Manmohan Goyal, MD
Operating Room. . . . . Thomas Matheson, MD
Chairman/CEO . . . . Leslie Niederman
CEO . . . . Theo Stoller
Infection Control. . . . . Nadia Tymkowych
CEO/President. . . . . Douglas W Wamack
Quality Assurance . . . . Marian Will

Measure	Cases	This Hosp.	State Avg.	U.S. Avg.
Blood Clot Prevention and Treatment				
Anticoagulation Overlap Therapy[5]	-	-	97%	93%
ICU Venous Thromboembolism Prophylaxis[5]	-	-	88%	92%
Incidence of Potentially Preventable VTE[5]	-	-	16%	10%
UFH with Dosages/Platelet Monitoring[5]	-	-	100%	97%
Venous Thromboembolism Prophylaxis[5]	-	-	80%	85%
Warfarin Therapy Discharge Instructions[5]	-	-	72%	75%
Chest Pain/Possible Heart Attack Care				
Aspirin Given Within 24 Hours of Arrival[3]	11	100%	95%	96%
Fibrinolytic Meds Within 30 Min. of Arrival[3,7]	-	-	51%	58%
Average Time to ECG (minutes)[3]	11	16	11	7
Average Time to Transfer (minutes)[3,7]	-	-	114	60
Children's Asthma Care				
Received Home Management Plan of Care	-	-	-	88%
Received Reliever Medication	-	-	-	100%
Received Systemic Corticosteroids	-	-	-	100%
Emergency Department				
Admittance Decision Time (minutes)[5]	-	-	66	98
Head CT Results Within 45 Min. of Arrival[5]	-	-	25%	57%
Patients Who Left ER Before Being Seen[1]	-	-	1%	2%
Time from ER Arrival to Admit. (minutes)[5]	-	-	201	274
Time from ER Arrival to Discharge (minutes)[5]	-	-	112	134
Time in ER Before Being Evaluated (minutes)[5]	-	-	22	26
Time to Pain Meds for Fractures (minutes)[5]	-	-	52	57
Heart Attack Care				
Aspirin Given at Discharge[1,3]	-	-	99%	99%
Fibrinolytic Meds Within 30 Min. of Arrival[3,7]	-	-	17%	54%
PCI Within 90 Minutes of Arrival[3,7]	-	-	93%	96%
Statin Prescribed at Discharge[3,7]	-	-	98%	98%
Heart Failure Care				
ACE Inhibitor or ARB for LVSD[3,7]	-	-	96%	97%
Discharge Instructions Given[1,3]	-	-	94%	94%
Evaluation of LVS Function[1,3]	-	-	96%	99%
Medicare Spending				
Medicare Spending per Patient (ratio)	-	-	0.9	0.98
Pneumonia Care				
Appropriate Initial Antibiotic Given[1]	-	-	94%	95%
Blood Culture Timing[1]	-	-	97%	98%
Pregnancy and Delivery Care				
Newborn Deliveries Scheduled Early[5]	-	-	6%	6%
Preventive Care				
Immunization for Influenza[5]	-	-	84%	90%
Immunization for Pneumonia[5]	-	-	88%	92%
Stroke Care				
Anticoagulation Therapy for Atrial Fibrillation[5]	-	-	96%	95%
Antithrombotic Therapy Timing[5]	-	-	98%	98%
Assessed for Rehabilitation[5]	-	-	97%	97%
Discharged on Antithrombotic Therapy[5]	-	-	100%	99%
Discharged on Statin Medication[5]	-	-	91%	94%
Thrombolytic Therapy Timing[5]	-	-	96%	66%
Venous Thromboembolism Prophylaxis[5]	-	-	96%	94%
Written Stroke Educational Materials Given[5]	-	-	86%	88%
Surgical Care Improvement Project				
Appropriate Beta Blocker Usage[5]	-	-	99%	98%
Appropriate VTP Within 24 Hours[5]	-	-	98%	98%
Controlled Postoperative Blood Glucose[5]	-	-	95%	97%
Perioperative Temperature Management[5]	-	-	100%	100%
Prophylactic Antibiotic Selection[5]	-	-	99%	99%
Prophylactic Antibiotic Selection (Outpatient)[5]	-	-	97%	98%
Prophylactic Antibiotic Stopped[5]	-	-	99%	98%
Prophylactic Antibiotic Timing[5]	-	-	98%	99%
Prophylactic Antibiotic Timing (Outpatient)[5]	-	-	96%	98%
Urinary Catheter Removal[5]	-	-	97%	97%
Survey of Patients' Hospital Experiences				
Area Around Room 'Always' Quiet at Night[10]	<100	57%	66%	61%
Doctors 'Always' Communicated Well[10]	<100	90%	84%	82%
Home Recovery Information Given[10]	<100	84%	82%	85%
Hospital Given 9 or 10 on 10 Point Scale[10]	<100	68%	70%	71%
Meds 'Always' Explained Before Given[10]	<100	78%	67%	64%
Nurses 'Always' Communicated Well[10]	<100	88%	80%	79%
Pain 'Always' Well Controlled[10]	<100	94%	69%	71%
Room and Bathroom 'Always' Clean[10]	<100	86%	78%	73%
Timely Help 'Always' Received[10]	<100	83%	74%	68%
Would Definitely Recommend Hospital[10]	<100	68%	73%	71%
Use of Medical Imaging				
Cardiac Imaging Stress Test before Surgery[7]	-	-	4.6%	5.3%
Combination Abdominal CT Scan[1]	-	-	11.8%	10.5%
Combination Brain/Sinus CT Scan[1]	-	-	2.2%	2.7%
Combination Chest CT Scan[1]	-	-	2%	2.7%
Follow-up Mammogram/Ultrasound[1]	-	-	7.8%	8.8%
Lumbar Spine MRI for Low Back Pain[1]	-	-	32.9%	37.2%

NOTE: Hospital profiles are in alphabetical order by state, then city, then hospital within the city; Rankings exclude hospitals with less than 25 cases except for patient surveys which excludes hospitals with less than 100 cases; (a) 100-299 cases; (1) The number of cases/patients is too few to report; (2) Data submitted were based on a sample of cases/patients; (3) Results are based on a shorter time period than required; (4) Data suppressed by CMS for one or more quarters; (5) Results are not available for this reporting period; (6) Fewer than 100 patients completed the HCAHPS survey; (7) No cases met the criteria for this measure; (8) The lower limit of the confidence interval cannot be calculated if the number of observed infections equals zero; (9) No data are available from the state/territory for this reporting period; (10) The scores shown reflect fewer than 50 completed surveys; (11) There were discrepancies in the data collection process; (12) This measure does not apply to this hospital for this reporting period; (13) Results cannot be calculated for this reporting period; (14) The results for this state are combined with nearby states to protect confidentiality; Please refer to the User's Guide for a full explanation of data.

Essentia Health - Fargo

3000 32nd Ave South
Fargo, ND 58104
Phone: 701-364-8000
Fax: 701-364-8078
URL: www.dakotaclinic.com
Type: Acute Care Hospitals
Emergency Services: Yes
Ownership: Voluntary non-profit - Private
Beds: 74

Key Personnel:
Emergency Room . . . . John R Baugh
Chief of Medical Staff . . . . Michael Priggs
CEO/President . . . . Paul Wilson

Measure	Cases	This Hosp.	State Avg.	U.S. Avg.
Blood Clot Prevention and Treatment				
Anticoagulation Overlap Therapy[2]	48	100%	97%	93%
ICU Venous Thromboembolism Prophylaxis[2]	81	96%	88%	92%
Incidence of Potentially Preventable VTE[1,2]	-	-	16%	10%
UFH with Dosages/Platelet Monitoring[2]	36	100%	100%	97%
Venous Thromboembolism Prophylaxis[2]	300	90%	80%	85%
Warfarin Therapy Discharge Instructions[2]	40	100%	72%	75%
Chest Pain/Possible Heart Attack Care				
Aspirin Given Within 24 Hours of Arrival[5]	-	-	95%	96%
Fibrinolytic Meds Within 30 Min. of Arrival[5]	-	-	51%	58%
Average Time to ECG (minutes)[5]	-	-	11	7
Average Time to Transfer (minutes)[5]	-	-	114	60
Children's Asthma Care				
Received Home Management Plan of Care	-	-	-	88%
Received Reliever Medication	-	-	-	100%
Received Systemic Corticosteroids	-	-	-	100%
Emergency Department				
Admittance Decision Time (minutes)[2]	466	83	66	98
Head CT Results Within 45 Min. of Arrival[1,3]	-	-	25%	57%
Patients Who Left ER Before Being Seen	32,699	0%	1%	2%
Time from ER Arrival to Admit. (minutes)[2]	469	214	201	274
Time from ER Arrival to Discharge (minutes)	393	92	112	134
Time in ER Before Being Evaluated (minutes)	109	15	22	26
Time to Pain Meds for Fractures (minutes)	107	46	52	57
Heart Attack Care				
Aspirin Given at Discharge	217	99%	99%	99%
Fibrinolytic Meds Within 30 Min. of Arrival[7]	-	-	17%	54%
PCI Within 90 Minutes of Arrival	24	100%	93%	96%
Statin Prescribed at Discharge	211	100%	98%	98%
Heart Failure Care				
ACE Inhibitor or ARB for LVSD	41	93%	96%	97%
Discharge Instructions Given	116	96%	94%	94%
Evaluation of LVS Function	152	97%	96%	99%
Medicare Spending				
Medicare Spending per Patient (ratio)	-	0.99	0.9	0.98
Pneumonia Care				
Appropriate Initial Antibiotic Given	49	98%	94%	95%
Blood Culture Timing	88	100%	97%	98%
Pregnancy and Delivery Care				
Newborn Deliveries Scheduled Early	128	2%	6%	6%
Preventive Care				
Immunization for Influenza[2]	521	93%	84%	90%
Immunization for Pneumonia[2]	570	98%	88%	92%
Stroke Care				
Anticoagulation Therapy for Atrial Fibrillation	19	100%	96%	95%
Antithrombotic Therapy Timing	93	99%	98%	98%
Assessed for Rehabilitation	137	97%	97%	97%
Discharged on Antithrombotic Therapy	110	100%	100%	99%
Discharged on Statin Medication	83	98%	91%	94%
Thrombolytic Therapy Timing[1]	-	-	96%	66%
Venous Thromboembolism Prophylaxis	139	99%	96%	94%
Written Stroke Educational Materials Given	79	96%	86%	88%
Surgical Care Improvement Project				
Appropriate Beta Blocker Usage[2]	166	100%	99%	98%
Appropriate VTP Within 24 Hours[2]	311	99%	98%	98%
Controlled Postoperative Blood Glucose[2]	90	94%	95%	97%
Perioperative Temperature Management[2]	401	100%	100%	100%
Prophylactic Antibiotic Selection[2]	353	99%	99%	99%
Prophylactic Antibiotic Selection (Outpatient)	333	99%	97%	98%
Prophylactic Antibiotic Stopped[2]	339	100%	99%	98%
Prophylactic Antibiotic Timing[2]	353	100%	98%	99%
Prophylactic Antibiotic Timing (Outpatient)	266	100%	96%	98%
Urinary Catheter Removal[2]	219	98%	97%	97%
Survey of Patients' Hospital Experiences				
Area Around Room 'Always' Quiet at Night	300+	56%	66%	61%
Doctors 'Always' Communicated Well	300+	79%	84%	82%
Home Recovery Information Given	300+	88%	82%	85%
Hospital Given 9 or 10 on 10 Point Scale	300+	75%	70%	71%
Meds 'Always' Explained Before Given	300+	63%	67%	64%
Nurses 'Always' Communicated Well	300+	79%	80%	79%
Pain 'Always' Well Controlled	300+	70%	69%	71%
Room and Bathroom 'Always' Clean	300+	64%	78%	73%
Timely Help 'Always' Received	300+	66%	74%	68%
Would Definitely Recommend Hospital	300+	79%	73%	71%
Use of Medical Imaging				
Cardiac Imaging Stress Test before Surgery	301	3.0%	4.6%	5.3%
Combination Abdominal CT Scan	489	7.2%	11.8%	10.5%
Combination Brain/Sinus CT Scan	403	1.5%	2.2%	2.7%
Combination Chest CT Scan	213	0.0%	2%	2.7%
Follow-up Mammogram/Ultrasound[1]	-	-	7.8%	8.8%
Lumbar Spine MRI for Low Back Pain	107	27.1%	32.9%	37.2%

Fargo VA Medical Center

2101 Elm Street
Fargo, ND 58102
Phone: 701-232-3241
Fax: 701-239-3705
URL: www.fargo.va.gov
Type: Acute Care - VA
Emergency Services: No
Ownership: Government Federal
Beds: 109

Key Personnel:
Quality Assurance . . . . Julie Bruhn, RN
Operating Room. . . . . Barbara Franke, RN
Intensive Care Unit. . . . . Kye Grundyson, RN
Infection Control. . . . . Jan Holmes, RN
Emergency Room . . . . Ronald Johnson, MD
Chief of Medical Staff . . . . Steven Julius, MD
CEO/President. . . . . Douglas M Kenyon
Patient Relations . . . . Victor Martinez

Measure	Cases	This Hosp.	State Avg.	U.S. Avg.
Blood Clot Prevention and Treatment				
Anticoagulation Overlap Therapy	-	-	97%	93%
ICU Venous Thromboembolism Prophylaxis	-	-	88%	92%
Incidence of Potentially Preventable VTE	-	-	16%	10%
UFH with Dosages/Platelet Monitoring	-	-	100%	97%
Venous Thromboembolism Prophylaxis	-	-	80%	85%
Warfarin Therapy Discharge Instructions	-	-	72%	75%
Chest Pain/Possible Heart Attack Care				
Aspirin Given Within 24 Hours of Arrival	-	-	95%	96%
Fibrinolytic Meds Within 30 Min. of Arrival	-	-	51%	58%
Average Time to ECG (minutes)	-	-	11	7
Average Time to Transfer (minutes)	-	-	114	60
Children's Asthma Care				
Received Home Management Plan of Care	-	-	-	88%
Received Reliever Medication	-	-	-	100%
Received Systemic Corticosteroids	-	-	-	100%
Emergency Department				
Admittance Decision Time (minutes)	-	-	66	98
Head CT Results Within 45 Min. of Arrival	-	-	25%	57%
Patients Who Left ER Before Being Seen	-	-	1%	2%
Time from ER Arrival to Admit. (minutes)	-	-	201	274
Time from ER Arrival to Discharge (minutes)	-	-	112	134
Time in ER Before Being Evaluated (minutes)	-	-	22	26
Time to Pain Meds for Fractures (minutes)	-	-	52	57
Heart Attack Care				
Aspirin Given at Discharge[5]	-	-	99%	99%
Fibrinolytic Meds Within 30 Min. of Arrival[5]	-	-	17%	54%
PCI Within 90 Minutes of Arrival[5]	-	-	93%	96%
Statin Prescribed at Discharge[5]	-	-	98%	98%
Heart Failure Care				
ACE Inhibitor or ARB for LVSD[1]	21	100%	96%	97%
Discharge Instructions Given	57	93%	94%	94%
Evaluation of LVS Function	61	100%	96%	99%
Medicare Spending				
Medicare Spending per Patient (ratio)	-	-	0.9	0.98
Pneumonia Care				
Appropriate Initial Antibiotic Given[1]	21	100%	94%	95%
Blood Culture Timing[1]	24	96%	97%	98%
Pregnancy and Delivery Care				
Newborn Deliveries Scheduled Early	-	-	6%	6%
Preventive Care				
Immunization for Influenza[5]	-	-	84%	90%
Immunization for Pneumonia[5]	-	-	88%	92%
Stroke Care				
Anticoagulation Therapy for Atrial Fibrillation	-	-	96%	95%
Antithrombotic Therapy Timing	-	-	98%	98%
Assessed for Rehabilitation	-	-	97%	97%
Discharged on Antithrombotic Therapy	-	-	100%	99%
Discharged on Statin Medication	-	-	91%	94%
Thrombolytic Therapy Timing	-	-	96%	66%
Venous Thromboembolism Prophylaxis	-	-	96%	94%
Written Stroke Educational Materials Given	-	-	86%	88%
Surgical Care Improvement Project				
Appropriate Beta Blocker Usage[2]	56	100%	99%	98%
Appropriate VTP Within 24 Hours[2]	143	99%	98%	98%
Controlled Postoperative Blood Glucose[5]	-	-	95%	97%
Perioperative Temperature Management[2]	157	100%	100%	100%
Prophylactic Antibiotic Selection	121	99%	99%	99%
Prophylactic Antibiotic Selection (Outpatient)	-	-	97%	98%
Prophylactic Antibiotic Stopped	120	99%	99%	98%
Prophylactic Antibiotic Timing	121	95%	98%	99%
Prophylactic Antibiotic Timing (Outpatient)	-	-	96%	98%
Urinary Catheter Removal[2]	126	98%	97%	97%
Survey of Patients' Hospital Experiences				
Area Around Room 'Always' Quiet at Night	-	-	66%	61%
Doctors 'Always' Communicated Well	-	-	84%	82%
Home Recovery Information Given	-	-	82%	85%
Hospital Given 9 or 10 on 10 Point Scale	-	-	70%	71%
Meds 'Always' Explained Before Given	-	-	67%	64%
Nurses 'Always' Communicated Well	-	-	80%	79%
Pain 'Always' Well Controlled	-	-	69%	71%
Room and Bathroom 'Always' Clean	-	-	78%	73%
Timely Help 'Always' Received	-	-	74%	68%
Would Definitely Recommend Hospital	-	-	73%	71%
Use of Medical Imaging				
Cardiac Imaging Stress Test before Surgery	-	-	4.6%	5.3%
Combination Abdominal CT Scan	-	-	11.8%	10.5%
Combination Brain/Sinus CT Scan	-	-	2.2%	2.7%
Combination Chest CT Scan	-	-	2%	2.7%
Follow-up Mammogram/Ultrasound	-	-	7.8%	8.8%
Lumbar Spine MRI for Low Back Pain	-	-	32.9%	37.2%

Sanford Medical Center Fargo

801 Broadway North
Fargo, ND 58122
Phone: 701-234-2000
Fax: 701-234-6979
E-mail: feedback@meritcare.com
URL: www.meritcare.com
Type: Acute Care Hospitals
Emergency Services: Yes
Ownership: Voluntary non-profit - Private
Beds: 583

Key Personnel:
Operating Room. . . . . Vicki Beaton
Infection Control. . . . . Joan Cook
Quality Assurance . . . . Rhonda Ketterling, MD
CEO/President. . . . . Kelby K. Krabbenhoft, MD
Radiology. . . . . Daniel Mickelso, MD
Pediatric Ambulatory Care . . . . . Ron Miller, MD
Pediatric In-Patient Care . . . . . . Ron Miller, MD
Chief of Medical Staff. . . . . Gregory Post, MD

Measure	Cases	This Hosp.	State Avg.	U.S. Avg.
Blood Clot Prevention and Treatment				
Anticoagulation Overlap Therapy[2]	99	100%	97%	93%
ICU Venous Thromboembolism Prophylaxis[2]	69	94%	88%	92%
Incidence of Potentially Preventable VTE[2]	25	8%	16%	10%
UFH with Dosages/Platelet Monitoring[2]	78	99%	100%	97%
Venous Thromboembolism Prophylaxis[2]	327	90%	80%	85%
Warfarin Therapy Discharge Instructions[2]	77	42%	72%	75%
Chest Pain/Possible Heart Attack Care				
Aspirin Given Within 24 Hours of Arrival[5]	-	-	95%	96%
Fibrinolytic Meds Within 30 Min. of Arrival[5]	-	-	51%	58%
Average Time to ECG (minutes)[5]	-	-	11	7
Average Time to Transfer (minutes)[5]	-	-	114	60
Children's Asthma Care				

NOTE: Hospital profiles are in alphabetical order by state, then city, then hospital within the city; Rankings exclude hospitals with less than 25 cases except for patient surveys which excludes hospitals with less than 100 cases; (a) 100-299 cases; (1) The number of cases/patients is too few to report; (2) Data submitted were based on a sample of cases/patients; (3) Results are based on a shorter time period than required; (4) Data suppressed by CMS for one or more quarters; (5) Results are not available for this reporting period; (6) Fewer than 100 patients completed the HCAHPS survey; (7) No cases met the criteria for this measure; (8) The lower limit of the confidence interval cannot be calculated if the number of observed infections equals zero; (9) No data are available from the state/territory for this reporting period; (10) The scores shown reflect fewer than 50 completed surveys; (11) There were discrepancies in the data collection process; (12) This measure does not apply to this hospital for this reporting period; (13) Results cannot be calculated for this reporting period; (14) The results for this state are combined with nearby states to protect confidentiality; Please refer to the User's Guide for a full explanation of data.

Measure	Cases	This Hosp.	State Avg.	U.S. Avg.
Received Home Management Plan of Care	-	-	-	88%
Received Reliever Medication	-	-	-	100%
Received Systemic Corticosteroids	-	-	-	100%
Emergency Department				
Admittance Decision Time (minutes)[2]	205	63	66	98
Head CT Results Within 45 Min. of Arrival[1]	-	-	25%	57%
Patients Who Left ER Before Being Seen	55,305	2%	1%	2%
Time from ER Arrival to Admit. (minutes)[2]	321	205	201	274
Time from ER Arrival to Discharge (minutes)	517	143	112	134
Time in ER Before Being Evaluated (minutes)	492	15	22	26
Time to Pain Meds for Fractures (minutes)	190	50	52	57
Heart Attack Care				
Aspirin Given at Discharge	581	99%	99%	99%
Fibrinolytic Meds Within 30 Min. of Arrival[7]	-	-	17%	54%
PCI Within 90 Minutes of Arrival	35	94%	93%	96%
Statin Prescribed at Discharge	576	97%	98%	98%
Heart Failure Care				
ACE Inhibitor or ARB for LVSD	118	94%	96%	97%
Discharge Instructions Given	382	90%	94%	94%
Evaluation of LVS Function	487	100%	96%	99%
Medicare Spending				
Medicare Spending per Patient (ratio)	-	0.97	0.9	0.98
Pneumonia Care				
Appropriate Initial Antibiotic Given	127	100%	94%	95%
Blood Culture Timing	232	99%	97%	98%
Pregnancy and Delivery Care				
Newborn Deliveries Scheduled Early[2]	43	0%	6%	6%
Preventive Care				
Immunization for Influenza[2]	615	89%	84%	90%
Immunization for Pneumonia[2]	670	90%	88%	92%
Stroke Care				
Anticoagulation Therapy for Atrial Fibrillation[2]	15	93%	96%	95%
Antithrombotic Therapy Timing[2]	93	99%	98%	98%
Assessed for Rehabilitation[2]	123	92%	97%	97%
Discharged on Antithrombotic Therapy[2]	106	99%	100%	99%
Discharged on Statin Medication[2]	84	95%	91%	94%
Thrombolytic Therapy Timing[1,2]	-	-	96%	66%
Venous Thromboembolism Prophylaxis[2]	122	94%	96%	94%
Written Stroke Educational Materials Given[2]	64	73%	86%	88%
Surgical Care Improvement Project				
Appropriate Beta Blocker Usage[2]	302	99%	99%	98%
Appropriate VTP Within 24 Hours[2]	524	98%	98%	98%
Controlled Postoperative Blood Glucose[2]	195	95%	95%	97%
Perioperative Temperature Management[2]	735	100%	100%	100%
Prophylactic Antibiotic Selection[2]	631	99%	99%	99%
Prophylactic Antibiotic Selection (Outpatient)	783	96%	97%	98%
Prophylactic Antibiotic Stopped[2]	622	100%	99%	98%
Prophylactic Antibiotic Timing[2]	632	99%	98%	99%
Prophylactic Antibiotic Timing (Outpatient)	684	96%	96%	98%
Urinary Catheter Removal[2]	566	99%	97%	97%
Survey of Patients' Hospital Experiences				
Area Around Room 'Always' Quiet at Night	300+	53%	66%	61%
Doctors 'Always' Communicated Well	300+	77%	84%	82%
Home Recovery Information Given	300+	87%	82%	85%
Hospital Given 9 or 10 on 10 Point Scale	300+	67%	70%	71%
Meds 'Always' Explained Before Given	300+	64%	67%	64%
Nurses 'Always' Communicated Well	300+	80%	80%	79%
Pain 'Always' Well Controlled	300+	68%	69%	71%
Room and Bathroom 'Always' Clean	300+	71%	78%	73%
Timely Help 'Always' Received	300+	63%	74%	68%
Would Definitely Recommend Hospital	300+	73%	73%	71%
Use of Medical Imaging				
Cardiac Imaging Stress Test before Surgery	639	5.8%	4.6%	5.3%
Combination Abdominal CT Scan	1,451	21.2%	11.8%	10.5%
Combination Brain/Sinus CT Scan	687	1.2%	2.2%	2.7%
Combination Chest CT Scan	1,080	1.8%	2%	2.7%
Follow-up Mammogram/Ultrasound	2,576	5.6%	7.8%	8.8%
Lumbar Spine MRI for Low Back Pain	295	27.8%	32.9%	37.2%

Standing Rock Indian Health Service Hospital

10 North River Road
Fort Yates, ND 58538
Type: Acute Care Hospitals
Ownership: Government - Federal
Phone: 701-854-3831
Fax: 701-854-7399
Emergency Services: Yes
Beds: 12

Key Personnel:
CEO/President. . . . . Lisa Guardipee

Measure	Cases	This Hosp.	State Avg.	U.S. Avg.
Blood Clot Prevention and Treatment				
Anticoagulation Overlap Therapy[3,7]	-	-	97%	93%
ICU Venous Thromboembolism Prophylaxis[3,7]	-	-	88%	92%
Incidence of Potentially Preventable VTE[3,7]	-	-	16%	10%
UFH with Dosages/Platelet Monitoring[3,7]	-	-	100%	97%
Venous Thromboembolism Prophylaxis[1,3]	-	-	80%	85%
Warfarin Therapy Discharge Instructions[3,7]	-	-	72%	75%
Chest Pain/Possible Heart Attack Care				
Aspirin Given Within 24 Hours of Arrival	-	-	95%	96%
Fibrinolytic Meds Within 30 Min. of Arrival	-	-	51%	58%
Average Time to ECG (minutes)	-	-	11	7
Average Time to Transfer (minutes)	-	-	114	60
Children's Asthma Care				
Received Home Management Plan of Care	-	-	-	88%
Received Reliever Medication	-	-	-	100%
Received Systemic Corticosteroids	-	-	-	100%
Emergency Department				
Admittance Decision Time (minutes)[1,3]	-	-	66	98
Head CT Results Within 45 Min. of Arrival	-	-	25%	57%
Patients Who Left ER Before Being Seen	-	-	1%	2%
Time from ER Arrival to Admit. (minutes)[1,3]	-	-	201	274
Time from ER Arrival to Discharge (minutes)	-	-	112	134
Time in ER Before Being Evaluated (minutes)	-	-	22	26
Time to Pain Meds for Fractures (minutes)	-	-	52	57
Heart Attack Care				
Aspirin Given at Discharge[5]	-	-	99%	99%
Fibrinolytic Meds Within 30 Min. of Arrival[5]	-	-	17%	54%
PCI Within 90 Minutes of Arrival[5]	-	-	93%	96%
Statin Prescribed at Discharge[5]	-	-	98%	98%
Heart Failure Care				
ACE Inhibitor or ARB for LVSD[5]	-	-	96%	97%
Discharge Instructions Given[5]	-	-	94%	94%
Evaluation of LVS Function[5]	-	-	96%	99%
Medicare Spending				
Medicare Spending per Patient (ratio)	-	-	0.9	0.98
Pneumonia Care				
Appropriate Initial Antibiotic Given[3,7]	-	-	94%	95%
Blood Culture Timing[3,7]	-	-	97%	98%
Pregnancy and Delivery Care				
Newborn Deliveries Scheduled Early[2,7]	-	-	6%	6%
Preventive Care				
Immunization for Influenza[1,3]	-	-	84%	90%
Immunization for Pneumonia[3,7]	-	-	88%	92%
Stroke Care				
Anticoagulation Therapy for Atrial Fibrillation[5]	-	-	96%	95%
Antithrombotic Therapy Timing[5]	-	-	98%	98%
Assessed for Rehabilitation[5]	-	-	97%	97%
Discharged on Antithrombotic Therapy[5]	-	-	100%	99%
Discharged on Statin Medication[5]	-	-	91%	94%
Thrombolytic Therapy Timing[5]	-	-	96%	66%
Venous Thromboembolism Prophylaxis[5]	-	-	96%	94%
Written Stroke Educational Materials Given[5]	-	-	86%	88%
Surgical Care Improvement Project				
Appropriate Beta Blocker Usage[5]	-	-	99%	98%
Appropriate VTP Within 24 Hours[5]	-	-	98%	98%
Controlled Postoperative Blood Glucose[5]	-	-	95%	97%
Perioperative Temperature Management[5]	-	-	100%	100%
Prophylactic Antibiotic Selection[5]	-	-	99%	99%
Prophylactic Antibiotic Selection (Outpatient)	-	-	97%	98%
Prophylactic Antibiotic Stopped[5]	-	-	99%	98%
Prophylactic Antibiotic Timing[5]	-	-	98%	99%
Prophylactic Antibiotic Timing (Outpatient)	-	-	96%	98%
Urinary Catheter Removal[5]	-	-	97%	97%
Survey of Patients' Hospital Experiences				
Area Around Room 'Always' Quiet at Night[1]	-	-	66%	61%
Doctors 'Always' Communicated Well[1]	-	-	84%	82%
Home Recovery Information Given[1]	-	-	82%	85%
Hospital Given 9 or 10 on 10 Point Scale[1]	-	-	70%	71%
Meds 'Always' Explained Before Given[1]	-	-	67%	64%
Nurses 'Always' Communicated Well[1]	-	-	80%	79%
Pain 'Always' Well Controlled[1]	-	-	69%	71%
Room and Bathroom 'Always' Clean[1]	-	-	78%	73%
Timely Help 'Always' Received[1]	-	-	74%	68%
Would Definitely Recommend Hospital[1]	-	-	73%	71%
Use of Medical Imaging				
Cardiac Imaging Stress Test before Surgery	-	-	4.6%	5.3%
Combination Abdominal CT Scan	-	-	11.8%	10.5%
Combination Brain/Sinus CT Scan	-	-	2.2%	2.7%
Combination Chest CT Scan	-	-	2%	2.7%
Follow-up Mammogram/Ultrasound	-	-	7.8%	8.8%
Lumbar Spine MRI for Low Back Pain	-	-	32.9%	37.2%

Garrison Memorial Hospital

407 3rd Ave Se
Garrison, ND 58540
Type: Critical Access Hospitals
Ownership: Voluntary non-profit - Church
Phone: 701-463-2275
Emergency Services: Yes

Measure	Cases	This Hosp.	State Avg.	U.S. Avg.
Blood Clot Prevention and Treatment				
Anticoagulation Overlap Therapy[5]	-	-	97%	93%
ICU Venous Thromboembolism Prophylaxis[5]	-	-	88%	92%
Incidence of Potentially Preventable VTE[5]	-	-	16%	10%
UFH with Dosages/Platelet Monitoring[5]	-	-	100%	97%
Venous Thromboembolism Prophylaxis[5]	-	-	80%	85%
Warfarin Therapy Discharge Instructions[5]	-	-	72%	75%
Chest Pain/Possible Heart Attack Care				
Aspirin Given Within 24 Hours of Arrival[1,3]	-	-	95%	96%
Fibrinolytic Meds Within 30 Min. of Arrival[5]	-	-	51%	58%
Average Time to ECG (minutes)[1,3]	-	-	11	7
Average Time to Transfer (minutes)[5]	-	-	114	60
Children's Asthma Care				
Received Home Management Plan of Care	-	-	-	88%
Received Reliever Medication	-	-	-	100%
Received Systemic Corticosteroids	-	-	-	100%
Emergency Department				
Admittance Decision Time (minutes)[5]	-	-	66	98
Head CT Results Within 45 Min. of Arrival[5]	-	-	25%	57%
Patients Who Left ER Before Being Seen	1,411	0%	1%	2%
Time from ER Arrival to Admit. (minutes)[5]	-	-	201	274
Time from ER Arrival to Discharge (minutes)[5]	-	-	112	134
Time in ER Before Being Evaluated (minutes)[5]	-	-	22	26
Time to Pain Meds for Fractures (minutes)[5]	-	-	52	57
Heart Attack Care				
Aspirin Given at Discharge[5]	-	-	99%	99%
Fibrinolytic Meds Within 30 Min. of Arrival[5]	-	-	17%	54%
PCI Within 90 Minutes of Arrival[5]	-	-	93%	96%
Statin Prescribed at Discharge[5]	-	-	98%	98%
Heart Failure Care				
ACE Inhibitor or ARB for LVSD[5]	-	-	96%	97%
Discharge Instructions Given[5]	-	-	94%	94%
Evaluation of LVS Function[5]	-	-	96%	99%
Medicare Spending				
Medicare Spending per Patient (ratio)	-	-	0.9	0.98
Pneumonia Care				
Appropriate Initial Antibiotic Given[2,7]	-	-	94%	95%
Blood Culture Timing[1,2]	-	-	97%	98%
Pregnancy and Delivery Care				
Newborn Deliveries Scheduled Early[5]	-	-	6%	6%
Preventive Care				
Immunization for Influenza[5]	-	-	84%	90%
Immunization for Pneumonia[5]	-	-	88%	92%
Stroke Care				
Anticoagulation Therapy for Atrial Fibrillation[5]	-	-	96%	95%
Antithrombotic Therapy Timing[5]	-	-	98%	98%
Assessed for Rehabilitation[5]	-	-	97%	97%
Discharged on Antithrombotic Therapy[5]	-	-	100%	99%

NOTE: Hospital profiles are in alphabetical order by state, then city, then hospital within the city; Rankings exclude hospitals with less than 25 cases except for patient surveys which excludes hospitals with less than 100 cases; (a) 100-299 cases; (1) The number of cases/patients is too few to report; (2) Data submitted were based on a sample of cases/patients; (3) Results are based on a shorter time period than required; (4) Data suppressed by CMS for one or more quarters; (5) Results are not available for this reporting period; (6) Fewer than 100 patients completed the HCAHPS survey; (7) No cases met the criteria for this measure; (8) The lower limit of the confidence interval cannot be calculated if the number of observed infections equals zero; (9) No data are available from the state/territory for this reporting period; (10) The scores shown reflect fewer than 50 completed surveys; (11) There were discrepancies in the data collection process; (12) This measure does not apply to this hospital for this reporting period; (13) Results cannot be calculated for this reporting period; (14) The results for this state are combined with nearby states to protect confidentiality; Please refer to the User's Guide for a full explanation of data.

Measure	Cases	This Hosp.	State Avg.	U.S. Avg.
Discharged on Statin Medication[5]	-	-	91%	94%
Thrombolytic Therapy Timing[5]	-	-	96%	66%
Venous Thromboembolism Prophylaxis[5]	-	-	96%	94%
Written Stroke Educational Materials Given[5]	-	-	86%	88%
Surgical Care Improvement Project				
Appropriate Beta Blocker Usage[5]	-	-	99%	98%
Appropriate VTP Within 24 Hours[5]	-	-	98%	98%
Controlled Postoperative Blood Glucose[5]	-	-	95%	97%
Perioperative Temperature Management[5]	-	-	100%	100%
Prophylactic Antibiotic Selection[5]	-	-	99%	99%
Prophylactic Antibiotic Selection (Outpatient)[5]	-	-	97%	98%
Prophylactic Antibiotic Stopped[5]	-	-	99%	98%
Prophylactic Antibiotic Timing[5]	-	-	98%	99%
Prophylactic Antibiotic Timing (Outpatient)[5]	-	-	96%	98%
Urinary Catheter Removal[5]	-	-	97%	97%
Survey of Patients' Hospital Experiences				
Area Around Room 'Always' Quiet at Night[5]	-	-	66%	61%
Doctors 'Always' Communicated Well[5]	-	-	84%	82%
Home Recovery Information Given[5]	-	-	82%	85%
Hospital Given 9 or 10 on 10 Point Scale[5]	-	-	70%	71%
Meds 'Always' Explained Before Given[5]	-	-	67%	64%
Nurses 'Always' Communicated Well[5]	-	-	80%	79%
Pain 'Always' Well Controlled[5]	-	-	69%	71%
Room and Bathroom 'Always' Clean[5]	-	-	78%	73%
Timely Help 'Always' Received[5]	-	-	74%	68%
Would Definitely Recommend Hospital[5]	-	-	73%	71%
Use of Medical Imaging				
Cardiac Imaging Stress Test before Surgery[7]	-	-	4.6%	5.3%
Combination Abdominal CT Scan	70	25.7%	11.8%	10.5%
Combination Brain/Sinus CT Scan[1]	-	-	2.2%	2.7%
Combination Chest CT Scan	80	16.3%	2%	2.7%
Follow-up Mammogram/Ultrasound	112	5.4%	7.8%	8.8%
Lumbar Spine MRI for Low Back Pain[1]	-	-	32.9%	37.2%

Unity Medical Center

164 W 13th Street
Grafton, ND 58237
Phone: 701-352-1620
Fax: 701-352-1671
URL: www.unitymedcenter.com
Type: Critical Access Hospitals
Emergency Services: Yes
Ownership: Voluntary non-profit - Other
Beds: 50

Key Personnel:
CEO/President. . . . . Evett A Butler
Infection Control. . . . . Marlene Quanrud
Operating Room. . . . . Delaine Russum
President . . . . Keith Zikmund

Measure	Cases	This Hosp.	State Avg.	U.S. Avg.
Blood Clot Prevention and Treatment				
Anticoagulation Overlap Therapy[5]	-	-	97%	93%
ICU Venous Thromboembolism Prophylaxis[5]	-	-	88%	92%
Incidence of Potentially Preventable VTE[5]	-	-	16%	10%
UFH with Dosages/Platelet Monitoring[5]	-	-	100%	97%
Venous Thromboembolism Prophylaxis[5]	-	-	80%	85%
Warfarin Therapy Discharge Instructions[5]	-	-	72%	75%
Chest Pain/Possible Heart Attack Care				
Aspirin Given Within 24 Hours of Arrival[1,3]	-	-	95%	96%
Fibrinolytic Meds Within 30 Min. of Arrival[3,7]	-	-	51%	58%
Average Time to ECG (minutes)[1,3]	-	-	11	7
Average Time to Transfer (minutes)[3,7]	-	-	114	60
Children's Asthma Care				
Received Home Management Plan of Care	-	-	-	88%
Received Reliever Medication	-	-	-	100%
Received Systemic Corticosteroids	-	-	-	100%
Emergency Department				
Admittance Decision Time (minutes)[5]	-	-	66	98
Head CT Results Within 45 Min. of Arrival[5]	-	-	25%	57%
Patients Who Left ER Before Being Seen	2,340	1%	1%	2%
Time from ER Arrival to Admit. (minutes)[5]	-	-	201	274
Time from ER Arrival to Discharge (minutes)[5]	-	-	112	134
Time in ER Before Being Evaluated (minutes)[5]	-	-	22	26
Time to Pain Meds for Fractures (minutes)[5]	-	-	52	57
Heart Attack Care				
Aspirin Given at Discharge[5]	-	-	99%	99%
Fibrinolytic Meds Within 30 Min. of Arrival[5]	-	-	17%	54%
PCI Within 90 Minutes of Arrival[5]	-	-	93%	96%
Statin Prescribed at Discharge[5]	-	-	98%	98%
Heart Failure Care				
ACE Inhibitor or ARB for LVSD[5]	-	-	96%	97%
Discharge Instructions Given[5]	-	-	94%	94%
Evaluation of LVS Function[5]	-	-	96%	99%
Medicare Spending				
Medicare Spending per Patient (ratio)	-	-	0.9	0.98
Pneumonia Care				
Appropriate Initial Antibiotic Given	13	92%	94%	95%
Blood Culture Timing[1]	-	-	97%	98%
Pregnancy and Delivery Care				
Newborn Deliveries Scheduled Early[5]	-	-	6%	6%
Preventive Care				
Immunization for Influenza	17	71%	84%	90%
Immunization for Pneumonia	21	81%	88%	92%
Stroke Care				
Anticoagulation Therapy for Atrial Fibrillation[5]	-	-	96%	95%
Antithrombotic Therapy Timing[5]	-	-	98%	98%
Assessed for Rehabilitation[5]	-	-	97%	97%
Discharged on Antithrombotic Therapy[5]	-	-	100%	99%
Discharged on Statin Medication[5]	-	-	91%	94%
Thrombolytic Therapy Timing[5]	-	-	96%	66%
Venous Thromboembolism Prophylaxis[5]	-	-	96%	94%
Written Stroke Educational Materials Given[5]	-	-	86%	88%
Surgical Care Improvement Project				
Appropriate Beta Blocker Usage[5]	-	-	99%	98%
Appropriate VTP Within 24 Hours[5]	-	-	98%	98%
Controlled Postoperative Blood Glucose[5]	-	-	95%	97%
Perioperative Temperature Management[5]	-	-	100%	100%
Prophylactic Antibiotic Selection[5]	-	-	99%	99%
Prophylactic Antibiotic Selection (Outpatient)[5]	-	-	97%	98%
Prophylactic Antibiotic Stopped[5]	-	-	99%	98%
Prophylactic Antibiotic Timing[5]	-	-	98%	99%
Prophylactic Antibiotic Timing (Outpatient)[5]	-	-	96%	98%
Urinary Catheter Removal[5]	-	-	97%	97%
Survey of Patients' Hospital Experiences				
Area Around Room 'Always' Quiet at Night[10]	<100	49%	66%	61%
Doctors 'Always' Communicated Well[10]	<100	86%	84%	82%
Home Recovery Information Given[10]	<100	72%	82%	85%
Hospital Given 9 or 10 on 10 Point Scale[10]	<100	56%	70%	71%
Meds 'Always' Explained Before Given[10]	<100	70%	67%	64%
Nurses 'Always' Communicated Well[10]	<100	74%	80%	79%
Pain 'Always' Well Controlled[10]	<100	32%	69%	71%
Room and Bathroom 'Always' Clean[10]	<100	63%	78%	73%
Timely Help 'Always' Received[10]	<100	53%	74%	68%
Would Definitely Recommend Hospital[10]	<100	51%	73%	71%
Use of Medical Imaging				
Cardiac Imaging Stress Test before Surgery[7]	-	-	4.6%	5.3%
Combination Abdominal CT Scan	48	4.2%	11.8%	10.5%
Combination Brain/Sinus CT Scan[1]	-	-	2.2%	2.7%
Combination Chest CT Scan[1]	-	-	2%	2.7%
Follow-up Mammogram/Ultrasound	126	5.6%	7.8%	8.8%
Lumbar Spine MRI for Low Back Pain[1]	-	-	32.9%	37.2%

Altru Hospital

1200 S Columbia Rd
Grand Forks, ND 58201
Phone: 701-780-5000
Fax: 701-780-1093
E-mail: contactus@altru.org
URL: www.altru.org
Type: Acute Care Hospitals
Emergency Services: Yes
Ownership: Government - Local
Beds: 352

Key Personnel:
Emergency Room . . . . Tom Alinder
Operating Room. . . . . Mary Herbeck
Chief of Medical Staff. . . . . Eric Lunn, MD
Radiology. . . . . Steve Metcaff
Quality Assurance . . . . Ben Ronstrom
Intensive Care Unit. . . . . Wanda Rosenquist
CEO/President. . . . . Casey Ryan, MD
Patient Relations . . . . Marilyn Troftgrubeen

Measure	Cases	This Hosp.	State Avg.	U.S. Avg.
Blood Clot Prevention and Treatment				
Anticoagulation Overlap Therapy[2]	70	96%	97%	93%
ICU Venous Thromboembolism Prophylaxis[2]	105	77%	88%	92%
Incidence of Potentially Preventable VTE[2]	16	19%	16%	10%
UFH with Dosages/Platelet Monitoring[2]	75	100%	100%	97%
Venous Thromboembolism Prophylaxis[2]	321	79%	80%	85%
Warfarin Therapy Discharge Instructions[2]	53	26%	72%	75%
Chest Pain/Possible Heart Attack Care				
Aspirin Given Within 24 Hours of Arrival[5]	-	-	95%	96%
Fibrinolytic Meds Within 30 Min. of Arrival[5]	-	-	51%	58%
Average Time to ECG (minutes)[5]	-	-	11	7
Average Time to Transfer (minutes)[5]	-	-	114	60
Children's Asthma Care				
Received Home Management Plan of Care	-	-	-	88%
Received Reliever Medication	-	-	-	100%
Received Systemic Corticosteroids	-	-	-	100%
Emergency Department				
Admittance Decision Time (minutes)[2]	347	88	66	98
Head CT Results Within 45 Min. of Arrival[1]	-	-	25%	57%
Patients Who Left ER Before Being Seen	31,244	1%	1%	2%
Time from ER Arrival to Admit. (minutes)[2]	393	222	201	274
Time from ER Arrival to Discharge (minutes)	416	153	112	134
Time in ER Before Being Evaluated (minutes)	376	40	22	26
Time to Pain Meds for Fractures (minutes)	132	70	52	57
Heart Attack Care				
Aspirin Given at Discharge	270	100%	99%	99%
Fibrinolytic Meds Within 30 Min. of Arrival[7]	-	-	17%	54%
PCI Within 90 Minutes of Arrival	37	89%	93%	96%
Statin Prescribed at Discharge	265	99%	98%	98%
Heart Failure Care				
ACE Inhibitor or ARB for LVSD	48	98%	96%	97%
Discharge Instructions Given	193	98%	94%	94%
Evaluation of LVS Function	231	100%	96%	99%
Medicare Spending				
Medicare Spending per Patient (ratio)	-	0.96	0.9	0.98
Pneumonia Care				
Appropriate Initial Antibiotic Given	145	94%	94%	95%
Blood Culture Timing	248	100%	97%	98%
Pregnancy and Delivery Care				
Newborn Deliveries Scheduled Early[2]	51	6%	6%	6%
Preventive Care				
Immunization for Influenza[2]	520	67%	84%	90%
Immunization for Pneumonia[2]	605	72%	88%	92%
Stroke Care				
Anticoagulation Therapy for Atrial Fibrillation	16	100%	96%	95%
Antithrombotic Therapy Timing	88	100%	98%	98%
Assessed for Rehabilitation	108	100%	97%	97%
Discharged on Antithrombotic Therapy	98	100%	100%	99%
Discharged on Statin Medication	83	77%	91%	94%
Thrombolytic Therapy Timing[1]	-	-	96%	66%
Venous Thromboembolism Prophylaxis	110	95%	96%	94%
Written Stroke Educational Materials Given	54	54%	86%	88%
Surgical Care Improvement Project				
Appropriate Beta Blocker Usage[2]	240	97%	99%	98%
Appropriate VTP Within 24 Hours[2]	464	96%	98%	98%
Controlled Postoperative Blood Glucose[2]	127	93%	95%	97%
Perioperative Temperature Management[2]	556	99%	100%	100%
Prophylactic Antibiotic Selection[2]	526	99%	99%	99%
Prophylactic Antibiotic Selection (Outpatient)	553	97%	97%	98%
Prophylactic Antibiotic Stopped[2]	509	98%	99%	98%
Prophylactic Antibiotic Timing[2]	527	96%	98%	99%
Prophylactic Antibiotic Timing (Outpatient)	439	90%	96%	98%
Urinary Catheter Removal[2]	338	93%	97%	97%
Survey of Patients' Hospital Experiences				
Area Around Room 'Always' Quiet at Night	300+	46%	66%	61%
Doctors 'Always' Communicated Well	300+	75%	84%	82%
Home Recovery Information Given	300+	84%	82%	85%
Hospital Given 9 or 10 on 10 Point Scale	300+	62%	70%	71%
Meds 'Always' Explained Before Given	300+	57%	67%	64%
Nurses 'Always' Communicated Well	300+	76%	80%	79%
Pain 'Always' Well Controlled	300+	66%	69%	71%
Room and Bathroom 'Always' Clean	300+	70%	78%	73%
Timely Help 'Always' Received	300+	59%	74%	68%
Would Definitely Recommend Hospital	300+	59%	73%	71%

NOTE: Hospital profiles are in alphabetical order by state, then city, then hospital within the city; Rankings exclude hospitals with less than 25 cases except for patient surveys which excludes hospitals with less than 100 cases; (a) 100-299 cases; (1) The number of cases/patients is too few to report; (2) Data submitted were based on a sample of cases/patients; (3) Results are based on a shorter time period than required; (4) Data suppressed by CMS for one or more quarters; (5) Results are not available for this reporting period; (6) Fewer than 100 patients completed the HCAHPS survey; (7) No cases met the criteria for this measure; (8) The lower limit of the confidence interval cannot be calculated if the number of observed infections equals zero; (9) No data are available from the state/territory for this reporting period; (10) The scores shown reflect fewer than 50 completed surveys; (11) There were discrepancies in the data collection process; (12) This measure does not apply to this hospital for this reporting period; (13) Results cannot be calculated for this reporting period; (14) The results for this state are combined with nearby states to protect confidentiality; Please refer to the User's Guide for a full explanation of data.

Use of Medical Imaging				
Cardiac Imaging Stress Test before Surgery	858	3.6%	4.6%	5.3%
Combination Abdominal CT Scan	959	5.5%	11.8%	10.5%
Combination Brain/Sinus CT Scan[1]	-	-	2.2%	2.7%
Combination Chest CT Scan	1,099	0.3%	2%	2.7%
Follow-up Mammogram/Ultrasound	1,900	16.2%	7.8%	8.8%
Lumbar Spine MRI for Low Back Pain	155	32.9%	32.9%	37.2%

Saint Aloisius Medical Center

325 E Brewster St
Harvey, ND 58341
URL: www.staloisius.com
Type: Critical Access Hospitals
Ownership: Voluntary non-profit - Private

Phone: 701-324-4651
Fax: 701-324-4651
Emergency Services: Yes
Beds: 131

Key Personnel:
Operating Room. . . . . Susanne Levene, RN
Chief of Medical Staff. . . . . Charles Nyhus, MD
Hemotology Center . . . . Candice Thompson
Cardiac Laboratory. . . . . Wayne Zahy

Measure	Cases	This Hosp.	State Avg.	U.S. Avg.
Blood Clot Prevention and Treatment				
Anticoagulation Overlap Therapy[5]	-	-	97%	93%
ICU Venous Thromboembolism Prophylaxis[5]	-	-	88%	92%
Incidence of Potentially Preventable VTE[5]	-	-	16%	10%
UFH with Dosages/Platelet Monitoring[5]	-	-	100%	97%
Venous Thromboembolism Prophylaxis[5]	-	-	80%	85%
Warfarin Therapy Discharge Instructions[5]	-	-	72%	75%
Chest Pain/Possible Heart Attack Care				
Aspirin Given Within 24 Hours of Arrival[1]	-	-	95%	96%
Fibrinolytic Meds Within 30 Min. of Arrival[1,3]	-	-	51%	58%
Average Time to ECG (minutes)[1]	-	-	11	7
Average Time to Transfer (minutes)[1,3]	-	-	114	60
Children's Asthma Care				
Received Home Management Plan of Care	-	-	-	88%
Received Reliever Medication	-	-	-	100%
Received Systemic Corticosteroids	-	-	-	100%
Emergency Department				
Admittance Decision Time (minutes)[5]	-	-	66	98
Head CT Results Within 45 Min. of Arrival[5]	-	-	25%	57%
Patients Who Left ER Before Being Seen	1,317	0%	1%	2%
Time from ER Arrival to Admit. (minutes)[5]	-	-	201	274
Time from ER Arrival to Discharge (minutes)[5]	-	-	112	134
Time in ER Before Being Evaluated (minutes)[5]	-	-	22	26
Time to Pain Meds for Fractures (minutes)[5]	-	-	52	57
Heart Attack Care				
Aspirin Given at Discharge[5]	-	-	99%	99%
Fibrinolytic Meds Within 30 Min. of Arrival[5]	-	-	17%	54%
PCI Within 90 Minutes of Arrival[5]	-	-	93%	96%
Statin Prescribed at Discharge[5]	-	-	98%	98%
Heart Failure Care				
ACE Inhibitor or ARB for LVSD[7]	-	-	96%	97%
Discharge Instructions Given[1]	-	-	94%	94%
Evaluation of LVS Function	15	7%	96%	99%
Medicare Spending				
Medicare Spending per Patient (ratio)	-	-	0.9	0.98
Pneumonia Care				
Appropriate Initial Antibiotic Given	11	55%	94%	95%
Blood Culture Timing[1]	-	-	97%	98%
Pregnancy and Delivery Care				
Newborn Deliveries Scheduled Early[5]	-	-	6%	6%
Preventive Care				
Immunization for Influenza[5]	-	-	84%	90%
Immunization for Pneumonia[5]	-	-	88%	92%
Stroke Care				
Anticoagulation Therapy for Atrial Fibrillation[5]	-	-	96%	95%
Antithrombotic Therapy Timing[5]	-	-	98%	98%
Assessed for Rehabilitation[5]	-	-	97%	97%
Discharged on Antithrombotic Therapy[5]	-	-	100%	99%
Discharged on Statin Medication[5]	-	-	91%	94%
Thrombolytic Therapy Timing[5]	-	-	96%	66%
Venous Thromboembolism Prophylaxis[5]	-	-	96%	94%
Written Stroke Educational Materials Given[5]	-	-	86%	88%
Surgical Care Improvement Project				
Appropriate Beta Blocker Usage[5]	-	-	99%	98%
Appropriate VTP Within 24 Hours[5]	-	-	98%	98%
Controlled Postoperative Blood Glucose[5]	-	-	95%	97%
Perioperative Temperature Management[5]	-	-	100%	100%
Prophylactic Antibiotic Selection[5]	-	-	99%	99%
Prophylactic Antibiotic Selection (Outpatient)[5]	-	-	97%	98%
Prophylactic Antibiotic Stopped[5]	-	-	99%	98%
Prophylactic Antibiotic Timing[5]	-	-	98%	99%
Prophylactic Antibiotic Timing (Outpatient)[5]	-	-	96%	98%
Urinary Catheter Removal[5]	-	-	97%	97%
Survey of Patients' Hospital Experiences				
Area Around Room 'Always' Quiet at Night	(a)	60%	66%	61%
Doctors 'Always' Communicated Well	(a)	82%	84%	82%
Home Recovery Information Given	(a)	79%	82%	85%
Hospital Given 9 or 10 on 10 Point Scale	(a)	60%	70%	71%
Meds 'Always' Explained Before Given	(a)	58%	67%	64%
Nurses 'Always' Communicated Well	(a)	70%	80%	79%
Pain 'Always' Well Controlled	(a)	64%	69%	71%
Room and Bathroom 'Always' Clean	(a)	68%	78%	73%
Timely Help 'Always' Received	(a)	70%	74%	68%
Would Definitely Recommend Hospital	(a)	64%	73%	71%
Use of Medical Imaging				
Cardiac Imaging Stress Test before Surgery[1]	-	-	4.6%	5.3%
Combination Abdominal CT Scan	65	0.0%	11.8%	10.5%
Combination Brain/Sinus CT Scan[1]	-	-	2.2%	2.7%
Combination Chest CT Scan[1]	-	-	2%	2.7%
Follow-up Mammogram/Ultrasound	150	3.3%	7.8%	8.8%
Lumbar Spine MRI for Low Back Pain[1]	-	-	32.9%	37.2%

Sakakawea Medical Center

510 8th Avenue Ne
Hazen, ND 58545
Type: Critical Access Hospitals
Ownership: Voluntary non-profit - Private

Phone: 701-748-2225
Emergency Services: Yes

Measure	Cases	This Hosp.	State Avg.	U.S. Avg.
Blood Clot Prevention and Treatment				
Anticoagulation Overlap Therapy[5]	-	-	97%	93%
ICU Venous Thromboembolism Prophylaxis[5]	-	-	88%	92%
Incidence of Potentially Preventable VTE[5]	-	-	16%	10%
UFH with Dosages/Platelet Monitoring[5]	-	-	100%	97%
Venous Thromboembolism Prophylaxis[5]	-	-	80%	85%
Warfarin Therapy Discharge Instructions[5]	-	-	72%	75%
Chest Pain/Possible Heart Attack Care				
Aspirin Given Within 24 Hours of Arrival[1,3]	-	-	95%	96%
Fibrinolytic Meds Within 30 Min. of Arrival[5]	-	-	51%	58%
Average Time to ECG (minutes)[3]	12	17	11	7
Average Time to Transfer (minutes)[5]	-	-	114	60
Children's Asthma Care				
Received Home Management Plan of Care	-	-	-	88%
Received Reliever Medication	-	-	-	100%
Received Systemic Corticosteroids	-	-	-	100%
Emergency Department				
Admittance Decision Time (minutes)[5]	-	-	66	98
Head CT Results Within 45 Min. of Arrival[3,7]	-	-	25%	57%
Patients Who Left ER Before Being Seen	2,759	1%	1%	2%
Time from ER Arrival to Admit. (minutes)[5]	-	-	201	274
Time from ER Arrival to Discharge (minutes)[5]	-	-	112	134
Time in ER Before Being Evaluated (minutes)[5]	-	-	22	26
Time to Pain Meds for Fractures (minutes)[5]	-	-	52	57
Heart Attack Care				
Aspirin Given at Discharge[5]	-	-	99%	99%
Fibrinolytic Meds Within 30 Min. of Arrival[5]	-	-	17%	54%
PCI Within 90 Minutes of Arrival[5]	-	-	93%	96%
Statin Prescribed at Discharge[5]	-	-	98%	98%
Heart Failure Care				
ACE Inhibitor or ARB for LVSD[1,2]	-	-	96%	97%
Discharge Instructions Given[1,2]	-	-	94%	94%
Evaluation of LVS Function[1,2]	-	-	96%	99%
Medicare Spending				
Medicare Spending per Patient (ratio)	-	-	0.9	0.98
Pneumonia Care				
Appropriate Initial Antibiotic Given[1,2]	-	-	94%	95%
Blood Culture Timing[1,2]	-	-	97%	98%
Pregnancy and Delivery Care				
Newborn Deliveries Scheduled Early[5]	-	-	6%	6%
Preventive Care				
Immunization for Influenza[5]	-	-	84%	90%
Immunization for Pneumonia[5]	-	-	88%	92%
Stroke Care				
Anticoagulation Therapy for Atrial Fibrillation[5]	-	-	96%	95%
Antithrombotic Therapy Timing[5]	-	-	98%	98%
Assessed for Rehabilitation[5]	-	-	97%	97%
Discharged on Antithrombotic Therapy[5]	-	-	100%	99%
Discharged on Statin Medication[5]	-	-	91%	94%
Thrombolytic Therapy Timing[5]	-	-	96%	66%
Venous Thromboembolism Prophylaxis[5]	-	-	96%	94%
Written Stroke Educational Materials Given[5]	-	-	86%	88%
Surgical Care Improvement Project				
Appropriate Beta Blocker Usage[5]	-	-	99%	98%
Appropriate VTP Within 24 Hours[5]	-	-	98%	98%
Controlled Postoperative Blood Glucose[5]	-	-	95%	97%
Perioperative Temperature Management[5]	-	-	100%	100%
Prophylactic Antibiotic Selection[5]	-	-	99%	99%
Prophylactic Antibiotic Selection (Outpatient)[5]	-	-	97%	98%
Prophylactic Antibiotic Stopped[5]	-	-	99%	98%
Prophylactic Antibiotic Timing[5]	-	-	98%	99%
Prophylactic Antibiotic Timing (Outpatient)[5]	-	-	96%	98%
Urinary Catheter Removal[5]	-	-	97%	97%
Survey of Patients' Hospital Experiences				
Area Around Room 'Always' Quiet at Night[6]	<100	66%	66%	61%
Doctors 'Always' Communicated Well[6]	<100	93%	84%	82%
Home Recovery Information Given[6]	<100	84%	82%	85%
Hospital Given 9 or 10 on 10 Point Scale[6]	<100	71%	70%	71%
Meds 'Always' Explained Before Given[6]	<100	62%	67%	64%
Nurses 'Always' Communicated Well[6]	<100	80%	80%	79%
Pain 'Always' Well Controlled[6]	<100	72%	69%	71%
Room and Bathroom 'Always' Clean[6]	<100	84%	78%	73%
Timely Help 'Always' Received[6]	<100	71%	74%	68%
Would Definitely Recommend Hospital[6]	<100	69%	73%	71%
Use of Medical Imaging				
Cardiac Imaging Stress Test before Surgery[1]	-	-	4.6%	5.3%
Combination Abdominal CT Scan	135	22.2%	11.8%	10.5%
Combination Brain/Sinus CT Scan[1]	-	-	2.2%	2.7%
Combination Chest CT Scan	86	9.3%	2%	2.7%
Follow-up Mammogram/Ultrasound	244	5.7%	7.8%	8.8%
Lumbar Spine MRI for Low Back Pain[1]	-	-	32.9%	37.2%

West River Regional Medical Center

1000 Highway 12
Hettinger, ND 58639
E-mail: jiml@wrhs.com
URL: www.wrhs.com
Type: Critical Access Hospitals
Ownership: Voluntary non-profit - Private

Phone: 701-567-4561
Fax: 701-567-6364
Emergency Services: Yes
Beds: 25

Key Personnel:
Quality Assurance . . . . Dana And
Operating Room. . . . . Leah Gunther
CEO/President. . . . . James K Long

Measure	Cases	This Hosp.	State Avg.	U.S. Avg.
Blood Clot Prevention and Treatment				
Anticoagulation Overlap Therapy[5]	-	-	97%	93%
ICU Venous Thromboembolism Prophylaxis[5]	-	-	88%	92%
Incidence of Potentially Preventable VTE[5]	-	-	16%	10%
UFH with Dosages/Platelet Monitoring[5]	-	-	100%	97%
Venous Thromboembolism Prophylaxis[5]	-	-	80%	85%
Warfarin Therapy Discharge Instructions[5]	-	-	72%	75%
Chest Pain/Possible Heart Attack Care				
Aspirin Given Within 24 Hours of Arrival[1,3]	-	-	95%	96%
Fibrinolytic Meds Within 30 Min. of Arrival[3,7]	-	-	51%	58%
Average Time to ECG (minutes)[1,3]	-	-	11	7
Average Time to Transfer (minutes)[3,7]	-	-	114	60
Children's Asthma Care				
Received Home Management Plan of Care	-	-	-	88%
Received Reliever Medication	-	-	-	100%
Received Systemic Corticosteroids	-	-	-	100%

NOTE: Hospital profiles are in alphabetical order by state, then city, then hospital within the city; Rankings exclude hospitals with less than 25 cases except for patient surveys which excludes hospitals with less than 100 cases; (a) 100-299 cases; (1) The number of cases/patients is too few to report; (2) Data submitted were based on a sample of cases/patients; (3) Results are based on a shorter time period than required; (4) Data suppressed by CMS for one or more quarters; (5) Results are not available for this reporting period; (6) Fewer than 100 patients completed the HCAHPS survey; (7) No cases met the criteria for this measure; (8) The lower limit of the confidence interval cannot be calculated if the number of observed infections equals zero; (9) No data are available from the state/territory for this reporting period; (10) The scores shown reflect fewer than 50 completed surveys; (11) There were discrepancies in the data collection process; (12) This measure does not apply to this hospital for this reporting period; (13) Results cannot be calculated for this reporting period; (14) The results for this state are combined with nearby states to protect confidentiality; Please refer to the User's Guide for a full explanation of data.

Measure	Cases	This Hosp.	State Avg.	U.S. Avg.
Emergency Department				
Admittance Decision Time (minutes)[5]	-	-	66	98
Head CT Results Within 45 Min. of Arrival[5]	-	-	25%	57%
Patients Who Left ER Before Being Seen	1,697	0%	1%	2%
Time from ER Arrival to Admit. (minutes)[5]	-	-	201	274
Time from ER Arrival to Discharge (minutes)[5]	-	-	112	134
Time in ER Before Being Evaluated (minutes)[5]	-	-	22	26
Time to Pain Meds for Fractures (minutes)[5]	-	-	52	57
Heart Attack Care				
Aspirin Given at Discharge[1,2]	-	-	99%	99%
Fibrinolytic Meds Within 30 Min. of Arrival[1,2]	-	-	17%	54%
PCI Within 90 Minutes of Arrival[2,7]	-	-	93%	96%
Statin Prescribed at Discharge[1,2]	-	-	98%	98%
Heart Failure Care				
ACE Inhibitor or ARB for LVSD[1,2]	-	-	96%	97%
Discharge Instructions Given[2]	43	100%	94%	94%
Evaluation of LVS Function[2]	55	98%	96%	99%
Medicare Spending				
Medicare Spending per Patient (ratio)	-	-	0.9	0.98
Pneumonia Care				
Appropriate Initial Antibiotic Given[2]	39	95%	94%	95%
Blood Culture Timing[2]	12	100%	97%	98%
Pregnancy and Delivery Care				
Newborn Deliveries Scheduled Early[5]	-	-	6%	6%
Preventive Care				
Immunization for Influenza[5]	-	-	84%	90%
Immunization for Pneumonia[5]	-	-	88%	92%
Stroke Care				
Anticoagulation Therapy for Atrial Fibrillation[5]	-	-	96%	95%
Antithrombotic Therapy Timing[5]	-	-	98%	98%
Assessed for Rehabilitation[5]	-	-	97%	97%
Discharged on Antithrombotic Therapy[5]	-	-	100%	99%
Discharged on Statin Medication[5]	-	-	91%	94%
Thrombolytic Therapy Timing[5]	-	-	96%	66%
Venous Thromboembolism Prophylaxis[5]	-	-	96%	94%
Written Stroke Educational Materials Given[5]	-	-	86%	88%
Surgical Care Improvement Project				
Appropriate Beta Blocker Usage[3,7]	-	-	99%	98%
Appropriate VTP Within 24 Hours[1,3]	-	-	98%	98%
Controlled Postoperative Blood Glucose[3,7]	-	-	95%	97%
Perioperative Temperature Management[1,3]	-	-	100%	100%
Prophylactic Antibiotic Selection[1,3]	-	-	99%	99%
Prophylactic Antibiotic Selection (Outpatient)[5]	-	-	97%	98%
Prophylactic Antibiotic Stopped[1,3]	-	-	99%	98%
Prophylactic Antibiotic Timing[1,3]	-	-	98%	99%
Prophylactic Antibiotic Timing (Outpatient)[5]	-	-	96%	98%
Urinary Catheter Removal[1,3]	-	-	97%	97%
Survey of Patients' Hospital Experiences				
Area Around Room 'Always' Quiet at Night	300+	54%	66%	61%
Doctors 'Always' Communicated Well	300+	88%	84%	82%
Home Recovery Information Given	300+	85%	82%	85%
Hospital Given 9 or 10 on 10 Point Scale	300+	80%	70%	71%
Meds 'Always' Explained Before Given	300+	68%	67%	64%
Nurses 'Always' Communicated Well	300+	85%	80%	79%
Pain 'Always' Well Controlled	300+	80%	69%	71%
Room and Bathroom 'Always' Clean	300+	88%	78%	73%
Timely Help 'Always' Received	300+	74%	74%	68%
Would Definitely Recommend Hospital	300+	80%	73%	71%
Use of Medical Imaging				
Cardiac Imaging Stress Test before Surgery	95	6.3%	4.6%	5.3%
Combination Abdominal CT Scan	139	5.8%	11.8%	10.5%
Combination Brain/Sinus CT Scan	41	0.0%	2.2%	2.7%
Combination Chest CT Scan	64	1.6%	2%	2.7%
Follow-up Mammogram/Ultrasound	303	8.6%	7.8%	8.8%
Lumbar Spine MRI for Low Back Pain[1]	-	-	32.9%	37.2%

Sanford Hillsboro

12 Third Street South East
Hillsboro, ND 58045
E-mail: darleneswanson@meritcare.com
Type: Critical Access Hospitals
Ownership: Voluntary non-profit - Private
Phone: 701-636-3200
Fax: 701-636-3206
Emergency Services: Yes
Beds: 20

Key Personnel:
Chief of Medical Staff . . . . Charles Breen
Quality Assurance . . . . Jennifer Jacobson
Infection Control. . . . . Julieeen Rosenberg

Measure	Cases	This Hosp.	State Avg.	U.S. Avg.
Blood Clot Prevention and Treatment				
Anticoagulation Overlap Therapy[5]	-	-	97%	93%
ICU Venous Thromboembolism Prophylaxis[5]	-	-	88%	92%
Incidence of Potentially Preventable VTE[5]	-	-	16%	10%
UFH with Dosages/Platelet Monitoring[5]	-	-	100%	97%
Venous Thromboembolism Prophylaxis[5]	-	-	80%	85%
Warfarin Therapy Discharge Instructions[5]	-	-	72%	75%
Chest Pain/Possible Heart Attack Care				
Aspirin Given Within 24 Hours of Arrival[1,3]	-	-	95%	96%
Fibrinolytic Meds Within 30 Min. of Arrival[3,7]	-	-	51%	58%
Average Time to ECG (minutes)[1,3]	-	-	11	7
Average Time to Transfer (minutes)[3,7]	-	-	114	60
Children's Asthma Care				
Received Home Management Plan of Care	-	-	-	88%
Received Reliever Medication	-	-	-	100%
Received Systemic Corticosteroids	-	-	-	100%
Emergency Department				
Admittance Decision Time (minutes)[5]	-	-	66	98
Head CT Results Within 45 Min. of Arrival[5]	-	-	25%	57%
Patients Who Left ER Before Being Seen	943	0%	1%	2%
Time from ER Arrival to Admit. (minutes)[5]	-	-	201	274
Time from ER Arrival to Discharge (minutes)[5]	-	-	112	134
Time in ER Before Being Evaluated (minutes)[5]	-	-	22	26
Time to Pain Meds for Fractures (minutes)[5]	-	-	52	57
Heart Attack Care				
Aspirin Given at Discharge[1,2]	-	-	99%	99%
Fibrinolytic Meds Within 30 Min. of Arrival[1,2]	-	-	17%	54%
PCI Within 90 Minutes of Arrival[2,3]	-	-	93%	96%
Statin Prescribed at Discharge[1,2]	-	-	98%	98%
Heart Failure Care				
ACE Inhibitor or ARB for LVSD[1,2]	-	-	96%	97%
Discharge Instructions Given[1,2]	-	-	94%	94%
Evaluation of LVS Function[1,2]	-	-	96%	99%
Medicare Spending				
Medicare Spending per Patient (ratio)	-	-	0.9	0.98
Pneumonia Care				
Appropriate Initial Antibiotic Given[1,2]	-	-	94%	95%
Blood Culture Timing[2,7]	-	-	97%	98%
Pregnancy and Delivery Care				
Newborn Deliveries Scheduled Early[5]	-	-	6%	6%
Preventive Care				
Immunization for Influenza[5]	-	-	84%	90%
Immunization for Pneumonia[5]	-	-	88%	92%
Stroke Care				
Anticoagulation Therapy for Atrial Fibrillation[5]	-	-	96%	95%
Antithrombotic Therapy Timing[5]	-	-	98%	98%
Assessed for Rehabilitation[5]	-	-	97%	97%
Discharged on Antithrombotic Therapy[5]	-	-	100%	99%
Discharged on Statin Medication[5]	-	-	91%	94%
Thrombolytic Therapy Timing[5]	-	-	96%	66%
Venous Thromboembolism Prophylaxis[5]	-	-	96%	94%
Written Stroke Educational Materials Given[5]	-	-	86%	88%
Surgical Care Improvement Project				
Appropriate Beta Blocker Usage[5]	-	-	99%	98%
Appropriate VTP Within 24 Hours[5]	-	-	98%	98%
Controlled Postoperative Blood Glucose[5]	-	-	95%	97%
Perioperative Temperature Management[5]	-	-	100%	100%
Prophylactic Antibiotic Selection[5]	-	-	99%	99%
Prophylactic Antibiotic Selection (Outpatient)[5]	-	-	97%	98%
Prophylactic Antibiotic Stopped[5]	-	-	99%	98%
Prophylactic Antibiotic Timing[5]	-	-	98%	99%
Prophylactic Antibiotic Timing (Outpatient)[5]	-	-	96%	98%
Urinary Catheter Removal[5]	-	-	97%	97%
Survey of Patients' Hospital Experiences				
Area Around Room 'Always' Quiet at Night[5]	-	-	66%	61%
Doctors 'Always' Communicated Well[5]	-	-	84%	82%
Home Recovery Information Given[5]	-	-	82%	85%
Hospital Given 9 or 10 on 10 Point Scale[5]	-	-	70%	71%
Meds 'Always' Explained Before Given[5]	-	-	67%	64%
Nurses 'Always' Communicated Well[5]	-	-	80%	79%
Pain 'Always' Well Controlled[5]	-	-	69%	71%
Room and Bathroom 'Always' Clean[5]	-	-	78%	73%
Timely Help 'Always' Received[5]	-	-	74%	68%
Would Definitely Recommend Hospital[5]	-	-	73%	71%
Use of Medical Imaging				
Cardiac Imaging Stress Test before Surgery[7]	-	-	4.6%	5.3%
Combination Abdominal CT Scan[1]	-	-	11.8%	10.5%
Combination Brain/Sinus CT Scan[7]	-	-	2.2%	2.7%
Combination Chest CT Scan[1]	-	-	2%	2.7%
Follow-up Mammogram/Ultrasound[7]	-	-	7.8%	8.8%
Lumbar Spine MRI for Low Back Pain[1]	-	-	32.9%	37.2%

Jamestown Regional Medical Center

2422 20th Saint Sw
Jamestown, ND 58401
URL: www.jamestownhospital.com
Type: Critical Access Hospitals
Ownership: Voluntary non-profit - Other
Phone: 701-252-1050
Fax: 701-952-3270
Emergency Services: Yes
Beds: 85

Key Personnel:
Radiology. . . . . Alfonso C Findley
Emergency Room . . . . Scott Goecke
Ambulatory Care . . . . Sheila Krapp
Pediatrics. . . . . Myra QUANRUD
Radiology. . . . . Madhu Reddy
CEO/President. . . . . Martin I Richman
Radiology. . . . . Gary Wade, RN
Surgery . . . . Patrick Walter, MD

Measure	Cases	This Hosp.	State Avg.	U.S. Avg.
Blood Clot Prevention and Treatment				
Anticoagulation Overlap Therapy[5]	-	-	97%	93%
ICU Venous Thromboembolism Prophylaxis[5]	-	-	88%	92%
Incidence of Potentially Preventable VTE[5]	-	-	16%	10%
UFH with Dosages/Platelet Monitoring[5]	-	-	100%	97%
Venous Thromboembolism Prophylaxis[5]	-	-	80%	85%
Warfarin Therapy Discharge Instructions[5]	-	-	72%	75%
Chest Pain/Possible Heart Attack Care				
Aspirin Given Within 24 Hours of Arrival	78	95%	95%	96%
Fibrinolytic Meds Within 30 Min. of Arrival[1]	-	-	51%	58%
Average Time to ECG (minutes)	78	8	11	7
Average Time to Transfer (minutes)[7]	-	-	114	60
Children's Asthma Care				
Received Home Management Plan of Care	-	-	-	88%
Received Reliever Medication	-	-	-	100%
Received Systemic Corticosteroids	-	-	-	100%
Emergency Department				
Admittance Decision Time (minutes)[5]	-	-	66	98
Head CT Results Within 45 Min. of Arrival[1]	-	-	25%	57%
Patients Who Left ER Before Being Seen	8,246	0%	1%	2%
Time from ER Arrival to Admit. (minutes)[5]	-	-	201	274
Time from ER Arrival to Discharge (minutes)	367	99	112	134
Time in ER Before Being Evaluated (minutes)	364	19	22	26
Time to Pain Meds for Fractures (minutes)	43	39	52	57
Heart Attack Care				
Aspirin Given at Discharge[1]	-	-	99%	99%
Fibrinolytic Meds Within 30 Min. of Arrival[7]	-	-	17%	54%
PCI Within 90 Minutes of Arrival[7]	-	-	93%	96%
Statin Prescribed at Discharge[1]	-	-	98%	98%
Heart Failure Care				
ACE Inhibitor or ARB for LVSD[1]	-	-	96%	97%
Discharge Instructions Given	20	100%	94%	94%
Evaluation of LVS Function	43	95%	96%	99%
Medicare Spending				
Medicare Spending per Patient (ratio)	-	-	0.9	0.98
Pneumonia Care				
Appropriate Initial Antibiotic Given	52	98%	94%	95%
Blood Culture Timing	50	96%	97%	98%
Pregnancy and Delivery Care				
Newborn Deliveries Scheduled Early[5]	-	-	6%	6%
Preventive Care				
Immunization for Influenza[5]	-	-	84%	90%
Immunization for Pneumonia[5]	-	-	88%	92%
Stroke Care				
Anticoagulation Therapy for Atrial Fibrillation[5]	-	-	96%	95%

NOTE: Hospital profiles are in alphabetical order by state, then city, then hospital within the city; Rankings exclude hospitals with less than 25 cases except for patient surveys which excludes hospitals with less than 100 cases; (a) 100-299 cases; (1) The number of cases/patients is too few to report; (2) Data submitted were based on a sample of cases/patients; (3) Results are based on a shorter time period than required; (4) Data suppressed by CMS for one or more quarters; (5) Results are not available for this reporting period; (6) Fewer than 100 patients completed the HCAHPS survey; (7) No cases met the criteria for this measure; (8) The lower limit of the confidence interval cannot be calculated if the number of observed infections equals zero; (9) No data are available from the state/territory for this reporting period; (10) The scores shown reflect fewer than 50 completed surveys; (11) There were discrepancies in the data collection process; (12) This measure does not apply to this hospital for this reporting period; (13) Results cannot be calculated for this reporting period; (14) The results for this state are combined with nearby states to protect confidentiality; Please refer to the User's Guide for a full explanation of data.

Measure	Cases	This Hosp.	State Avg.	U.S. Avg.
Antithrombotic Therapy Timing[5]	-	-	98%	98%
Assessed for Rehabilitation[5]	-	-	97%	97%
Discharged on Antithrombotic Therapy[5]	-	-	100%	99%
Discharged on Statin Medication[5]	-	-	91%	94%
Thrombolytic Therapy Timing[5]	-	-	96%	66%
Venous Thromboembolism Prophylaxis[5]	-	-	96%	94%
Written Stroke Educational Materials Given[5]	-	-	86%	88%
Surgical Care Improvement Project				
Appropriate Beta Blocker Usage	42	98%	99%	98%
Appropriate VTP Within 24 Hours	148	97%	98%	98%
Controlled Postoperative Blood Glucose[7]	-	-	95%	97%
Perioperative Temperature Management	166	100%	100%	100%
Prophylactic Antibiotic Selection	142	99%	99%	99%
Prophylactic Antibiotic Selection (Outpatient)[1]	-	-	97%	98%
Prophylactic Antibiotic Stopped	141	99%	99%	98%
Prophylactic Antibiotic Timing	143	99%	98%	99%
Prophylactic Antibiotic Timing (Outpatient)[1]	-	-	96%	98%
Urinary Catheter Removal	135	99%	97%	97%
Survey of Patients' Hospital Experiences				
Area Around Room 'Always' Quiet at Night	300+	66%	66%	61%
Doctors 'Always' Communicated Well	300+	85%	84%	82%
Home Recovery Information Given	300+	91%	82%	85%
Hospital Given 9 or 10 on 10 Point Scale	300+	76%	70%	71%
Meds 'Always' Explained Before Given	300+	65%	67%	64%
Nurses 'Always' Communicated Well	300+	82%	80%	79%
Pain 'Always' Well Controlled	300+	74%	69%	71%
Room and Bathroom 'Always' Clean	300+	74%	78%	73%
Timely Help 'Always' Received	300+	73%	74%	68%
Would Definitely Recommend Hospital	300+	77%	73%	71%
Use of Medical Imaging				
Cardiac Imaging Stress Test before Surgery	80	3.8%	4.6%	5.3%
Combination Abdominal CT Scan	256	5.5%	11.8%	10.5%
Combination Brain/Sinus CT Scan[1]	-	-	2.2%	2.7%
Combination Chest CT Scan	158	1.9%	2%	2.7%
Follow-up Mammogram/Ultrasound	555	6.3%	7.8%	8.8%
Lumbar Spine MRI for Low Back Pain[1]	-	-	32.9%	37.2%

Kenmare Community Hospital

PO Box 697
Kenmare, ND 58746
Phone: 701-385-4296
Type: Critical Access Hospitals
Emergency Services: Yes
Ownership: Voluntary non-profit - Private

Measure	Cases	This Hosp.	State Avg.	U.S. Avg.
Blood Clot Prevention and Treatment				
Anticoagulation Overlap Therapy[5]	-	-	97%	93%
ICU Venous Thromboembolism Prophylaxis[5]	-	-	88%	92%
Incidence of Potentially Preventable VTE[5]	-	-	16%	10%
UFH with Dosages/Platelet Monitoring[5]	-	-	100%	97%
Venous Thromboembolism Prophylaxis[5]	-	-	80%	85%
Warfarin Therapy Discharge Instructions[5]	-	-	72%	75%
Chest Pain/Possible Heart Attack Care				
Aspirin Given Within 24 Hours of Arrival[1,3]	-	-	95%	96%
Fibrinolytic Meds Within 30 Min. of Arrival[3,7]	-	-	51%	58%
Average Time to ECG (minutes)[1,3]	-	-	11	7
Average Time to Transfer (minutes)[3,7]	-	-	114	60
Children's Asthma Care				
Received Home Management Plan of Care	-	-	-	88%
Received Reliever Medication	-	-	-	100%
Received Systemic Corticosteroids	-	-	-	100%
Emergency Department				
Admittance Decision Time (minutes)[5]	-	-	66	98
Head CT Results Within 45 Min. of Arrival[5]	-	-	25%	57%
Patients Who Left ER Before Being Seen	553	0%	1%	2%
Time from ER Arrival to Admit. (minutes)[5]	-	-	201	274
Time from ER Arrival to Discharge (minutes)[5]	-	-	112	134
Time in ER Before Being Evaluated (minutes)[5]	-	-	22	26
Time to Pain Meds for Fractures (minutes)[5]	-	-	52	57
Heart Attack Care				
Aspirin Given at Discharge[5]	-	-	99%	99%
Fibrinolytic Meds Within 30 Min. of Arrival[5]	-	-	17%	54%
PCI Within 90 Minutes of Arrival[5]	-	-	93%	96%
Statin Prescribed at Discharge[5]	-	-	98%	98%
Heart Failure Care				
ACE Inhibitor or ARB for LVSD[5]	-	-	96%	97%
Discharge Instructions Given[5]	-	-	94%	94%
Evaluation of LVS Function[5]	-	-	96%	99%
Medicare Spending				
Medicare Spending per Patient (ratio)	-	-	0.9	0.98
Pneumonia Care				
Appropriate Initial Antibiotic Given[5]	-	-	94%	95%
Blood Culture Timing[5]	-	-	97%	98%
Pregnancy and Delivery Care				
Newborn Deliveries Scheduled Early[5]	-	-	6%	6%
Preventive Care				
Immunization for Influenza[5]	-	-	84%	90%
Immunization for Pneumonia[5]	-	-	88%	92%
Stroke Care				
Anticoagulation Therapy for Atrial Fibrillation[5]	-	-	96%	95%
Antithrombotic Therapy Timing[5]	-	-	98%	98%
Assessed for Rehabilitation[5]	-	-	97%	97%
Discharged on Antithrombotic Therapy[5]	-	-	100%	99%
Discharged on Statin Medication[5]	-	-	91%	94%
Thrombolytic Therapy Timing[5]	-	-	96%	66%
Venous Thromboembolism Prophylaxis[5]	-	-	96%	94%
Written Stroke Educational Materials Given[5]	-	-	86%	88%
Surgical Care Improvement Project				
Appropriate Beta Blocker Usage[5]	-	-	99%	98%
Appropriate VTP Within 24 Hours[5]	-	-	98%	98%
Controlled Postoperative Blood Glucose[5]	-	-	95%	97%
Perioperative Temperature Management[5]	-	-	100%	100%
Prophylactic Antibiotic Selection[5]	-	-	99%	99%
Prophylactic Antibiotic Selection (Outpatient)[5]	-	-	97%	98%
Prophylactic Antibiotic Stopped[5]	-	-	99%	98%
Prophylactic Antibiotic Timing[5]	-	-	98%	99%
Prophylactic Antibiotic Timing (Outpatient)[5]	-	-	96%	98%
Urinary Catheter Removal[5]	-	-	97%	97%
Survey of Patients' Hospital Experiences				
Area Around Room 'Always' Quiet at Night[5]	-	-	66%	61%
Doctors 'Always' Communicated Well[5]	-	-	84%	82%
Home Recovery Information Given[5]	-	-	82%	85%
Hospital Given 9 or 10 on 10 Point Scale[5]	-	-	70%	71%
Meds 'Always' Explained Before Given[5]	-	-	67%	64%
Nurses 'Always' Communicated Well[5]	-	-	80%	79%
Pain 'Always' Well Controlled[5]	-	-	69%	71%
Room and Bathroom 'Always' Clean[5]	-	-	78%	73%
Timely Help 'Always' Received[5]	-	-	74%	68%
Would Definitely Recommend Hospital[5]	-	-	73%	71%
Use of Medical Imaging				
Cardiac Imaging Stress Test before Surgery[7]	-	-	4.6%	5.3%
Combination Abdominal CT Scan[1]	-	-	11.8%	10.5%
Combination Brain/Sinus CT Scan[1]	-	-	2.2%	2.7%
Combination Chest CT Scan[1]	-	-	2%	2.7%
Follow-up Mammogram/Ultrasound[7]	-	-	7.8%	8.8%
Lumbar Spine MRI for Low Back Pain[7]	-	-	32.9%	37.2%

Cavalier County Memorial Hospital

909 2nd St
Langdon, ND 58249
Phone: 701-256-6100
Type: Critical Access Hospitals
Emergency Services: Yes
Ownership: Voluntary non-profit - Other

Measure	Cases	This Hosp.	State Avg.	U.S. Avg.
Blood Clot Prevention and Treatment				
Anticoagulation Overlap Therapy[5]	-	-	97%	93%
ICU Venous Thromboembolism Prophylaxis[5]	-	-	88%	92%
Incidence of Potentially Preventable VTE[5]	-	-	16%	10%
UFH with Dosages/Platelet Monitoring[5]	-	-	100%	97%
Venous Thromboembolism Prophylaxis[5]	-	-	80%	85%
Warfarin Therapy Discharge Instructions[5]	-	-	72%	75%
Chest Pain/Possible Heart Attack Care				
Aspirin Given Within 24 Hours of Arrival[1,3]	-	-	95%	96%
Fibrinolytic Meds Within 30 Min. of Arrival[1,3]	-	-	51%	58%
Average Time to ECG (minutes)[1,3]	-	-	11	7
Average Time to Transfer (minutes)[3,7]	-	-	114	60
Children's Asthma Care				
Received Home Management Plan of Care	-	-	-	88%
Received Reliever Medication	-	-	-	100%
Received Systemic Corticosteroids	-	-	-	100%
Emergency Department				
Admittance Decision Time (minutes)[5]	-	-	66	98
Head CT Results Within 45 Min. of Arrival[5]	-	-	25%	57%
Patients Who Left ER Before Being Seen	1,095	1%	1%	2%
Time from ER Arrival to Admit. (minutes)[5]	-	-	201	274
Time from ER Arrival to Discharge (minutes)[5]	-	-	112	134
Time in ER Before Being Evaluated (minutes)[5]	-	-	22	26
Time to Pain Meds for Fractures (minutes)[5]	-	-	52	57
Heart Attack Care				
Aspirin Given at Discharge[5]	-	-	99%	99%
Fibrinolytic Meds Within 30 Min. of Arrival[5]	-	-	17%	54%
PCI Within 90 Minutes of Arrival[5]	-	-	93%	96%
Statin Prescribed at Discharge[5]	-	-	98%	98%
Heart Failure Care				
ACE Inhibitor or ARB for LVSD[1,3]	-	-	96%	97%
Discharge Instructions Given[1,3]	-	-	94%	94%
Evaluation of LVS Function[1,3]	-	-	96%	99%
Medicare Spending				
Medicare Spending per Patient (ratio)	-	-	0.9	0.98
Pneumonia Care				
Appropriate Initial Antibiotic Given	15	60%	94%	95%
Blood Culture Timing[1]	-	-	97%	98%
Pregnancy and Delivery Care				
Newborn Deliveries Scheduled Early[5]	-	-	6%	6%
Preventive Care				
Immunization for Influenza[5]	-	-	84%	90%
Immunization for Pneumonia[5]	-	-	88%	92%
Stroke Care				
Anticoagulation Therapy for Atrial Fibrillation[5]	-	-	96%	95%
Antithrombotic Therapy Timing[5]	-	-	98%	98%
Assessed for Rehabilitation[5]	-	-	97%	97%
Discharged on Antithrombotic Therapy[5]	-	-	100%	99%
Discharged on Statin Medication[5]	-	-	91%	94%
Thrombolytic Therapy Timing[5]	-	-	96%	66%
Venous Thromboembolism Prophylaxis[5]	-	-	96%	94%
Written Stroke Educational Materials Given[5]	-	-	86%	88%
Surgical Care Improvement Project				
Appropriate Beta Blocker Usage[5]	-	-	99%	98%
Appropriate VTP Within 24 Hours[5]	-	-	98%	98%
Controlled Postoperative Blood Glucose[5]	-	-	95%	97%
Perioperative Temperature Management[5]	-	-	100%	100%
Prophylactic Antibiotic Selection[5]	-	-	99%	99%
Prophylactic Antibiotic Selection (Outpatient)[5]	-	-	97%	98%
Prophylactic Antibiotic Stopped[5]	-	-	99%	98%
Prophylactic Antibiotic Timing[5]	-	-	98%	99%
Prophylactic Antibiotic Timing (Outpatient)[5]	-	-	96%	98%
Urinary Catheter Removal[5]	-	-	97%	97%
Survey of Patients' Hospital Experiences				
Area Around Room 'Always' Quiet at Night	(a)	78%	66%	61%
Doctors 'Always' Communicated Well	(a)	74%	84%	82%
Home Recovery Information Given	(a)	75%	82%	85%
Hospital Given 9 or 10 on 10 Point Scale	(a)	73%	70%	71%
Meds 'Always' Explained Before Given	(a)	59%	67%	64%
Nurses 'Always' Communicated Well	(a)	80%	80%	79%
Pain 'Always' Well Controlled	(a)	71%	69%	71%
Room and Bathroom 'Always' Clean	(a)	83%	78%	73%
Timely Help 'Always' Received	(a)	79%	74%	68%
Would Definitely Recommend Hospital	(a)	61%	73%	71%
Use of Medical Imaging				
Cardiac Imaging Stress Test before Surgery[1]	-	-	4.6%	5.3%
Combination Abdominal CT Scan	66	4.5%	11.8%	10.5%
Combination Brain/Sinus CT Scan	67	0.0%	2.2%	2.7%
Combination Chest CT Scan[1]	-	-	2%	2.7%
Follow-up Mammogram/Ultrasound	215	4.2%	7.8%	8.8%
Lumbar Spine MRI for Low Back Pain[1]	-	-	32.9%	37.2%

NOTE: Hospital profiles are in alphabetical order by state, then city, then hospital within the city; Rankings exclude hospitals with less than 25 cases except for patient surveys which excludes hospitals with less than 100 cases; (a) 100-299 cases; (1) The number of cases/patients is too few to report; (2) Data submitted were based on a sample of cases/patients; (3) Results are based on a shorter time period than required; (4) Data suppressed by CMS for one or more quarters; (5) Results are not available for this reporting period; (6) Fewer than 100 patients completed the HCAHPS survey; (7) No cases met the criteria for this measure; (8) The lower limit of the confidence interval cannot be calculated if the number of observed infections equals zero; (9) No data are available from the state/territory for this reporting period; (10) The scores shown reflect fewer than 50 completed surveys; (11) There were discrepancies in the data collection process; (12) This measure does not apply to this hospital for this reporting period; (13) Results cannot be calculated for this reporting period; (14) The results for this state are combined with nearby states to protect confidentiality; Please refer to the User's Guide for a full explanation of data.

Linton Hospital

518 North Broadway
Linton, ND 58552
Phone: 701-254-4511
Fax: 701-254-4578
E-mail: info@lintonhospital.com
URL: www.lintonhospital.com
Type: Critical Access Hospitals
Emergency Services: Yes
Ownership: Government - Local
Beds: 25

Key Personnel:
Chief of Medical Staff.......... Donald Grinz
Quality Assurance .... Nadine Held, LPN
Infection Control............. Melanie Jangula, RN
Radiology.................. Dennis Kress
Emergency Room .... Roger Martin
CEO/President............... Roger Unger
Operating Room.............. Joan Wittmeier, RN

Measure	Cases	This Hosp.	State Avg.	U.S. Avg.
Blood Clot Prevention and Treatment				
Anticoagulation Overlap Therapy[5]	-	-	97%	93%
ICU Venous Thromboembolism Prophylaxis[5]	-	-	88%	92%
Incidence of Potentially Preventable VTE[5]	-	-	16%	10%
UFH with Dosages/Platelet Monitoring[5]	-	-	100%	97%
Venous Thromboembolism Prophylaxis[5]	-	-	80%	85%
Warfarin Therapy Discharge Instructions[5]	-	-	72%	75%
Chest Pain/Possible Heart Attack Care				
Aspirin Given Within 24 Hours of Arrival[1]	-	-	95%	96%
Fibrinolytic Meds Within 30 Min. of Arrival[7]	-	-	51%	58%
Average Time to ECG (minutes)[1]	-	-	11	7
Average Time to Transfer (minutes)[1]	-	-	114	60
Children's Asthma Care				
Received Home Management Plan of Care	-	-	-	88%
Received Reliever Medication	-	-	-	100%
Received Systemic Corticosteroids	-	-	-	100%
Emergency Department				
Admittance Decision Time (minutes)[5]	-	-	66	98
Head CT Results Within 45 Min. of Arrival[5]	-	-	25%	57%
Patients Who Left ER Before Being Seen	957	0%	1%	2%
Time from ER Arrival to Admit. (minutes)[5]	-	-	201	274
Time from ER Arrival to Discharge (minutes)[5]	-	-	112	134
Time in ER Before Being Evaluated (minutes)[5]	-	-	22	26
Time to Pain Meds for Fractures (minutes)[5]	-	-	52	57
Heart Attack Care				
Aspirin Given at Discharge[1,3]	-	-	99%	99%
Fibrinolytic Meds Within 30 Min. of Arrival[3,7]	-	-	17%	54%
PCI Within 90 Minutes of Arrival[3,7]	-	-	93%	96%
Statin Prescribed at Discharge[1,3]	-	-	98%	98%
Heart Failure Care				
ACE Inhibitor or ARB for LVSD[3,7]	-	-	96%	97%
Discharge Instructions Given[1,3]	-	-	94%	94%
Evaluation of LVS Function[3]	11	64%	96%	99%
Medicare Spending				
Medicare Spending per Patient (ratio)	-	-	0.9	0.98
Pneumonia Care				
Appropriate Initial Antibiotic Given[1]	-	-	94%	95%
Blood Culture Timing[1]	-	-	97%	98%
Pregnancy and Delivery Care				
Newborn Deliveries Scheduled Early[5]	-	-	6%	6%
Preventive Care				
Immunization for Influenza[3]	38	92%	84%	90%
Immunization for Pneumonia[2,3]	49	96%	88%	92%
Stroke Care				
Anticoagulation Therapy for Atrial Fibrillation[5]	-	-	96%	95%
Antithrombotic Therapy Timing[5]	-	-	98%	98%
Assessed for Rehabilitation[5]	-	-	97%	97%
Discharged on Antithrombotic Therapy[5]	-	-	100%	99%
Discharged on Statin Medication[5]	-	-	91%	94%
Thrombolytic Therapy Timing[5]	-	-	96%	66%
Venous Thromboembolism Prophylaxis[5]	-	-	96%	94%
Written Stroke Educational Materials Given[5]	-	-	86%	88%
Surgical Care Improvement Project				
Appropriate Beta Blocker Usage[5]	-	-	99%	98%
Appropriate VTP Within 24 Hours[5]	-	-	98%	98%
Controlled Postoperative Blood Glucose[5]	-	-	95%	97%
Perioperative Temperature Management[5]	-	-	100%	100%
Prophylactic Antibiotic Selection[5]	-	-	99%	99%
Prophylactic Antibiotic Selection (Outpatient)[5]	-	-	97%	98%
Prophylactic Antibiotic Stopped[5]	-	-	99%	98%
Prophylactic Antibiotic Timing[5]	-	-	98%	99%
Prophylactic Antibiotic Timing (Outpatient)[5]	-	-	96%	98%
Urinary Catheter Removal[5]	-	-	97%	97%
Survey of Patients' Hospital Experiences				
Area Around Room 'Always' Quiet at Night[6]	<100	81%	66%	61%
Doctors 'Always' Communicated Well[6]	<100	75%	84%	82%
Home Recovery Information Given[6]	<100	75%	82%	85%
Hospital Given 9 or 10 on 10 Point Scale[6]	<100	78%	70%	71%
Meds 'Always' Explained Before Given[6]	<100	58%	67%	64%
Nurses 'Always' Communicated Well[6]	<100	83%	80%	79%
Pain 'Always' Well Controlled[6]	<100	95%	69%	71%
Room and Bathroom 'Always' Clean[6]	<100	88%	78%	73%
Timely Help 'Always' Received[6]	<100	88%	74%	68%
Would Definitely Recommend Hospital[6]	<100	74%	73%	71%
Use of Medical Imaging				
Cardiac Imaging Stress Test before Surgery[7]	-	-	4.6%	5.3%
Combination Abdominal CT Scan[1]	-	-	11.8%	10.5%
Combination Brain/Sinus CT Scan	45	0.0%	2.2%	2.7%
Combination Chest CT Scan[1]	-	-	2%	2.7%
Follow-up Mammogram/Ultrasound	105	5.7%	7.8%	8.8%
Lumbar Spine MRI for Low Back Pain[1]	-	-	32.9%	37.2%

Lisbon Area Health Services

905 Main St
Lisbon, ND 58054
Phone: 701-683-5241
Type: Critical Access Hospitals
Emergency Services: Yes
Ownership: Voluntary non-profit - Private

Measure	Cases	This Hosp.	State Avg.	U.S. Avg.
Blood Clot Prevention and Treatment				
Anticoagulation Overlap Therapy[5]	-	-	97%	93%
ICU Venous Thromboembolism Prophylaxis[5]	-	-	88%	92%
Incidence of Potentially Preventable VTE[5]	-	-	16%	10%
UFH with Dosages/Platelet Monitoring[5]	-	-	100%	97%
Venous Thromboembolism Prophylaxis[5]	-	-	80%	85%
Warfarin Therapy Discharge Instructions[5]	-	-	72%	75%
Chest Pain/Possible Heart Attack Care				
Aspirin Given Within 24 Hours of Arrival[3]	21	100%	95%	96%
Fibrinolytic Meds Within 30 Min. of Arrival[3,7]	-	-	51%	58%
Average Time to ECG (minutes)[3]	22	22	11	7
Average Time to Transfer (minutes)[1,3]	-	-	114	60
Children's Asthma Care				
Received Home Management Plan of Care	-	-	-	88%
Received Reliever Medication	-	-	-	100%
Received Systemic Corticosteroids	-	-	-	100%
Emergency Department				
Admittance Decision Time (minutes)[2,3]	41	15	66	98
Head CT Results Within 45 Min. of Arrival[1,3]	-	-	25%	57%
Patients Who Left ER Before Being Seen	2,226	0%	1%	2%
Time from ER Arrival to Admit. (minutes)[2,3]	41	97	201	274
Time from ER Arrival to Discharge (minutes)[3]	50	83	112	134
Time in ER Before Being Evaluated (minutes)[3]	62	18	22	26
Time to Pain Meds for Fractures (minutes)[1,3]	-	-	52	57
Heart Attack Care				
Aspirin Given at Discharge[1,2]	-	-	99%	99%
Fibrinolytic Meds Within 30 Min. of Arrival[2,7]	-	-	17%	54%
PCI Within 90 Minutes of Arrival[2,7]	-	-	93%	96%
Statin Prescribed at Discharge[1,2]	-	-	98%	98%
Heart Failure Care				
ACE Inhibitor or ARB for LVSD[1,2]	-	-	96%	97%
Discharge Instructions Given[2]	11	100%	94%	94%
Evaluation of LVS Function[2]	23	91%	96%	99%
Medicare Spending				
Medicare Spending per Patient (ratio)	-	-	0.9	0.98
Pneumonia Care				
Appropriate Initial Antibiotic Given[1,2]	-	-	94%	95%
Blood Culture Timing[1,2]	-	-	97%	98%
Pregnancy and Delivery Care				
Newborn Deliveries Scheduled Early[5]	-	-	6%	6%
Preventive Care				
Immunization for Influenza[5]	-	-	84%	90%
Immunization for Pneumonia[2,3]	38	71%	88%	92%
Stroke Care				
Anticoagulation Therapy for Atrial Fibrillation[5]	-	-	96%	95%
Antithrombotic Therapy Timing[5]	-	-	98%	98%
Assessed for Rehabilitation[5]	-	-	97%	97%
Discharged on Antithrombotic Therapy[5]	-	-	100%	99%
Discharged on Statin Medication[5]	-	-	91%	94%
Thrombolytic Therapy Timing[5]	-	-	96%	66%
Venous Thromboembolism Prophylaxis[5]	-	-	96%	94%
Written Stroke Educational Materials Given[5]	-	-	86%	88%
Surgical Care Improvement Project				
Appropriate Beta Blocker Usage[5]	-	-	99%	98%
Appropriate VTP Within 24 Hours[5]	-	-	98%	98%
Controlled Postoperative Blood Glucose[5]	-	-	95%	97%
Perioperative Temperature Management[5]	-	-	100%	100%
Prophylactic Antibiotic Selection[5]	-	-	99%	99%
Prophylactic Antibiotic Selection (Outpatient)[5]	-	-	97%	98%
Prophylactic Antibiotic Stopped[5]	-	-	99%	98%
Prophylactic Antibiotic Timing[5]	-	-	98%	99%
Prophylactic Antibiotic Timing (Outpatient)[5]	-	-	96%	98%
Urinary Catheter Removal[5]	-	-	97%	97%
Survey of Patients' Hospital Experiences				
Area Around Room 'Always' Quiet at Night[5]	-	-	66%	61%
Doctors 'Always' Communicated Well[5]	-	-	84%	82%
Home Recovery Information Given[5]	-	-	82%	85%
Hospital Given 9 or 10 on 10 Point Scale[5]	-	-	70%	71%
Meds 'Always' Explained Before Given[5]	-	-	67%	64%
Nurses 'Always' Communicated Well[5]	-	-	80%	79%
Pain 'Always' Well Controlled[5]	-	-	69%	71%
Room and Bathroom 'Always' Clean[5]	-	-	78%	73%
Timely Help 'Always' Received[5]	-	-	74%	68%
Would Definitely Recommend Hospital[5]	-	-	73%	71%
Use of Medical Imaging				
Cardiac Imaging Stress Test before Surgery[1]	-	-	4.6%	5.3%
Combination Abdominal CT Scan[1]	-	-	11.8%	10.5%
Combination Brain/Sinus CT Scan[1]	-	-	2.2%	2.7%
Combination Chest CT Scan[1]	-	-	2%	2.7%
Follow-up Mammogram/Ultrasound	128	10.2%	7.8%	8.8%
Lumbar Spine MRI for Low Back Pain[1]	-	-	32.9%	37.2%

Sanford Mayville

42 6th Avenue Se
Mayville, ND 58257
Phone: 701-786-3800
Fax: 701-788-2145
Type: Critical Access Hospitals
Emergency Services: Yes
Ownership: Voluntary non-profit - Private
Beds: 25

Key Personnel:
Radiology.................. Lorell Carlson
CEO/President............... Kelby K. Krabbenhoft
Chief of Medical Staff.......... Janus McHus
Operating Room.............. Cindy Petersen
Quality Assurance .... Cynthia Thompson
Emergency Room .... Doris Vigen, RN

Measure	Cases	This Hosp.	State Avg.	U.S. Avg.
Blood Clot Prevention and Treatment				
Anticoagulation Overlap Therapy[5]	-	-	97%	93%
ICU Venous Thromboembolism Prophylaxis[5]	-	-	88%	92%
Incidence of Potentially Preventable VTE[5]	-	-	16%	10%
UFH with Dosages/Platelet Monitoring[5]	-	-	100%	97%
Venous Thromboembolism Prophylaxis[5]	-	-	80%	85%
Warfarin Therapy Discharge Instructions[5]	-	-	72%	75%
Chest Pain/Possible Heart Attack Care				
Aspirin Given Within 24 Hours of Arrival[1,3]	-	-	95%	96%
Fibrinolytic Meds Within 30 Min. of Arrival[3,7]	-	-	51%	58%
Average Time to ECG (minutes)[1,3]	-	-	11	7
Average Time to Transfer (minutes)[1,3]	-	-	114	60
Children's Asthma Care				
Received Home Management Plan of Care	-	-	-	88%
Received Reliever Medication	-	-	-	100%
Received Systemic Corticosteroids	-	-	-	100%
Emergency Department				
Admittance Decision Time (minutes)[5]	-	-	66	98
Head CT Results Within 45 Min. of Arrival[5]	-	-	25%	57%
Patients Who Left ER Before Being Seen	1,082	0%	1%	2%

NOTE: Hospital profiles are in alphabetical order by state, then city, then hospital within the city; Rankings exclude hospitals with less than 25 cases except for patient surveys which excludes hospitals with less than 100 cases; (a) 100-299 cases; (1) The number of cases/patients is too few to report; (2) Data submitted were based on a sample of cases/patients; (3) Results are based on a shorter time period than required; (4) Data suppressed by CMS for one or more quarters; (5) Results are not available for this reporting period; (6) Fewer than 100 patients completed the HCAHPS survey; (7) No cases met the criteria for this measure; (8) The lower limit of the confidence interval cannot be calculated if the number of observed infections equals zero; (9) No data are available from the state/territory for this reporting period; (10) The scores shown reflect fewer than 50 completed surveys; (11) There were discrepancies in the data collection process; (12) This measure does not apply to this hospital for this reporting period; (13) Results cannot be calculated for this reporting period; (14) The results for this state are combined with nearby states to protect confidentiality; Please refer to the User's Guide for a full explanation of data.

Measure	Cases	This Hosp.	State Avg.	U.S. Avg.
Time from ER Arrival to Admit. (minutes)[5]	-	-	201	274
Time from ER Arrival to Discharge (minutes)[5]	-	-	112	134
Time in ER Before Being Evaluated (minutes)[5]	-	-	22	26
Time to Pain Meds for Fractures (minutes)[5]	-	-	52	57
Heart Attack Care				
Aspirin Given at Discharge[1,3]	-	-	99%	99%
Fibrinolytic Meds Within 30 Min. of Arrival[3,7]	-	-	17%	54%
PCI Within 90 Minutes of Arrival[3,7]	-	-	93%	96%
Statin Prescribed at Discharge[1,3]	-	-	98%	98%
Heart Failure Care				
ACE Inhibitor or ARB for LVSD[1,3]	-	-	96%	97%
Discharge Instructions Given[1,3]	-	-	94%	94%
Evaluation of LVS Function[3]	11	100%	96%	99%
Medicare Spending				
Medicare Spending per Patient (ratio)	-	-	0.9	0.98
Pneumonia Care				
Appropriate Initial Antibiotic Given[1,2]	-	-	94%	95%
Blood Culture Timing[1,2]	-	-	97%	98%
Pregnancy and Delivery Care				
Newborn Deliveries Scheduled Early[5]	-	-	6%	6%
Preventive Care				
Immunization for Influenza	17	94%	84%	90%
Immunization for Pneumonia	34	88%	88%	92%
Stroke Care				
Anticoagulation Therapy for Atrial Fibrillation[5]	-	-	96%	95%
Antithrombotic Therapy Timing[5]	-	-	98%	98%
Assessed for Rehabilitation[5]	-	-	97%	97%
Discharged on Antithrombotic Therapy[5]	-	-	100%	99%
Discharged on Statin Medication[5]	-	-	91%	94%
Thrombolytic Therapy Timing[5]	-	-	96%	66%
Venous Thromboembolism Prophylaxis[5]	-	-	96%	94%
Written Stroke Educational Materials Given[5]	-	-	86%	88%
Surgical Care Improvement Project				
Appropriate Beta Blocker Usage[5]	-	-	99%	98%
Appropriate VTP Within 24 Hours[5]	-	-	98%	98%
Controlled Postoperative Blood Glucose[5]	-	-	95%	97%
Perioperative Temperature Management[5]	-	-	100%	100%
Prophylactic Antibiotic Selection[5]	-	-	99%	99%
Prophylactic Antibiotic Selection (Outpatient)[5]	-	-	97%	98%
Prophylactic Antibiotic Stopped[5]	-	-	99%	98%
Prophylactic Antibiotic Timing[5]	-	-	98%	99%
Prophylactic Antibiotic Timing (Outpatient)[5]	-	-	96%	98%
Urinary Catheter Removal[5]	-	-	97%	97%
Survey of Patients' Hospital Experiences				
Area Around Room 'Always' Quiet at Night[5]	-	-	66%	61%
Doctors 'Always' Communicated Well[5]	-	-	84%	82%
Home Recovery Information Given[5]	-	-	82%	85%
Hospital Given 9 or 10 on 10 Point Scale[5]	-	-	70%	71%
Meds 'Always' Explained Before Given[5]	-	-	67%	64%
Nurses 'Always' Communicated Well[5]	-	-	80%	79%
Pain 'Always' Well Controlled[5]	-	-	69%	71%
Room and Bathroom 'Always' Clean[5]	-	-	78%	73%
Timely Help 'Always' Received[5]	-	-	74%	68%
Would Definitely Recommend Hospital[5]	-	-	73%	71%
Use of Medical Imaging				
Cardiac Imaging Stress Test before Surgery[1]	-	-	4.6%	5.3%
Combination Abdominal CT Scan[1]	-	-	11.8%	10.5%
Combination Brain/Sinus CT Scan[1]	-	-	2.2%	2.7%
Combination Chest CT Scan[1]	-	-	2%	2.7%
Follow-up Mammogram/Ultrasound[7]	-	-	7.8%	8.8%
Lumbar Spine MRI for Low Back Pain[1]	-	-	32.9%	37.2%

Nelson County Health System

200 N Main St
Mcville, ND 58254
Phone: 701-322-4328
Type: Critical Access Hospitals
Emergency Services: Yes
Ownership: Voluntary non-profit - Private

Measure	Cases	This Hosp.	State Avg.	U.S. Avg.
Blood Clot Prevention and Treatment				
Anticoagulation Overlap Therapy[5]	-	-	97%	93%
ICU Venous Thromboembolism Prophylaxis[5]	-	-	88%	92%
Incidence of Potentially Preventable VTE[5]	-	-	16%	10%
UFH with Dosages/Platelet Monitoring[5]	-	-	100%	97%
Venous Thromboembolism Prophylaxis[5]	-	-	80%	85%
Warfarin Therapy Discharge Instructions[5]	-	-	72%	75%
Chest Pain/Possible Heart Attack Care				
Aspirin Given Within 24 Hours of Arrival[1,3]	-	-	95%	96%
Fibrinolytic Meds Within 30 Min. of Arrival[1,3]	-	-	51%	58%
Average Time to ECG (minutes)[1,3]	-	-	11	7
Average Time to Transfer (minutes)[3,7]	-	-	114	60
Children's Asthma Care				
Received Home Management Plan of Care	-	-	-	88%
Received Reliever Medication	-	-	-	100%
Received Systemic Corticosteroids	-	-	-	100%
Emergency Department				
Admittance Decision Time (minutes)[5]	-	-	66	98
Head CT Results Within 45 Min. of Arrival[5]	-	-	25%	57%
Patients Who Left ER Before Being Seen	402	0%	1%	2%
Time from ER Arrival to Admit. (minutes)[5]	-	-	201	274
Time from ER Arrival to Discharge (minutes)[5]	-	-	112	134
Time in ER Before Being Evaluated (minutes)[5]	-	-	22	26
Time to Pain Meds for Fractures (minutes)[5]	-	-	52	57
Heart Attack Care				
Aspirin Given at Discharge[5]	-	-	99%	99%
Fibrinolytic Meds Within 30 Min. of Arrival[5]	-	-	17%	54%
PCI Within 90 Minutes of Arrival[5]	-	-	93%	96%
Statin Prescribed at Discharge[5]	-	-	98%	98%
Heart Failure Care				
ACE Inhibitor or ARB for LVSD[5]	-	-	96%	97%
Discharge Instructions Given[5]	-	-	94%	94%
Evaluation of LVS Function[5]	-	-	96%	99%
Medicare Spending				
Medicare Spending per Patient (ratio)	-	-	0.9	0.98
Pneumonia Care				
Appropriate Initial Antibiotic Given[1,3]	-	-	94%	95%
Blood Culture Timing[3,7]	-	-	97%	98%
Pregnancy and Delivery Care				
Newborn Deliveries Scheduled Early[5]	-	-	6%	6%
Preventive Care				
Immunization for Influenza[5]	-	-	84%	90%
Immunization for Pneumonia[5]	-	-	88%	92%
Stroke Care				
Anticoagulation Therapy for Atrial Fibrillation[3,7]	-	-	96%	95%
Antithrombotic Therapy Timing[3,7]	-	-	98%	98%
Assessed for Rehabilitation[3,7]	-	-	97%	97%
Discharged on Antithrombotic Therapy[3,7]	-	-	100%	99%
Discharged on Statin Medication[3,7]	-	-	91%	94%
Thrombolytic Therapy Timing[3,7]	-	-	96%	66%
Venous Thromboembolism Prophylaxis[3,7]	-	-	96%	94%
Written Stroke Educational Materials Given[3,7]	-	-	86%	88%
Surgical Care Improvement Project				
Appropriate Beta Blocker Usage[5]	-	-	99%	98%
Appropriate VTP Within 24 Hours[5]	-	-	98%	98%
Controlled Postoperative Blood Glucose[5]	-	-	95%	97%
Perioperative Temperature Management[5]	-	-	100%	100%
Prophylactic Antibiotic Selection[5]	-	-	99%	99%
Prophylactic Antibiotic Selection (Outpatient)[5]	-	-	97%	98%
Prophylactic Antibiotic Stopped[5]	-	-	99%	98%
Prophylactic Antibiotic Timing[5]	-	-	98%	99%
Prophylactic Antibiotic Timing (Outpatient)[5]	-	-	96%	98%
Urinary Catheter Removal[5]	-	-	97%	97%
Survey of Patients' Hospital Experiences				
Area Around Room 'Always' Quiet at Night[10]	<100	65%	66%	61%
Doctors 'Always' Communicated Well[10]	<100	89%	84%	82%
Home Recovery Information Given[10]	<100	81%	82%	85%
Hospital Given 9 or 10 on 10 Point Scale[10]	<100	100%	70%	71%
Meds 'Always' Explained Before Given[10]	<100	92%	67%	64%
Nurses 'Always' Communicated Well[10]	<100	92%	80%	79%
Pain 'Always' Well Controlled[10]	<100	68%	69%	71%
Room and Bathroom 'Always' Clean[10]	<100	87%	78%	73%
Timely Help 'Always' Received[10]	<100	100%	74%	68%
Would Definitely Recommend Hospital[10]	<100	96%	73%	71%
Use of Medical Imaging				
Cardiac Imaging Stress Test before Surgery[7]	-	-	4.6%	5.3%
Combination Abdominal CT Scan[1]	-	-	11.8%	10.5%
Combination Brain/Sinus CT Scan[1]	-	-	2.2%	2.7%
Combination Chest CT Scan[1]	-	-	2%	2.7%
Follow-up Mammogram/Ultrasound[1]	-	-	7.8%	8.8%
Lumbar Spine MRI for Low Back Pain[7]	-	-	32.9%	37.2%

Trinity Hospitals

407 3rd Saint Se
Minot, ND 58701
Phone: 701-857-5000
Fax: 701-857-5408
E-mail: info@trinityhealth.org
URL: www.trinityhealth.org
Type: Acute Care Hospitals
Emergency Services: Yes
Ownership: Voluntary non-profit - Private
Beds: 441

Key Personnel:

Radiology. . . . . James Call
Chief of Medical Staff . . . . Kevin Collins
Intensive Care Unit. . . . . Donna Hegle
Chairman/CEO . . . . Patrick Holien
Operating Room. . . . . Nancy Holmes
CEO/President. . . . . John M. Kutch
Infection Control. . . . . Brenda Lokken
Quality Assurance . . . . Julie Waldera, RN

Measure	Cases	This Hosp.	State Avg.	U.S. Avg.
Blood Clot Prevention and Treatment				
Anticoagulation Overlap Therapy[2]	70	97%	97%	93%
ICU Venous Thromboembolism Prophylaxis[2]	133	86%	88%	92%
Incidence of Potentially Preventable VTE[1,2]	-	-	16%	10%
UFH with Dosages/Platelet Monitoring[1,2]	-	-	100%	97%
Venous Thromboembolism Prophylaxis[2]	328	77%	80%	85%
Warfarin Therapy Discharge Instructions[2]	55	91%	72%	75%
Chest Pain/Possible Heart Attack Care				
Aspirin Given Within 24 Hours of Arrival[3,7]	-	-	95%	96%
Fibrinolytic Meds Within 30 Min. of Arrival[5]	-	-	51%	58%
Average Time to ECG (minutes)[1,3]	-	-	11	7
Average Time to Transfer (minutes)[5]	-	-	114	60
Children's Asthma Care				
Received Home Management Plan of Care	-	-	-	88%
Received Reliever Medication	-	-	-	100%
Received Systemic Corticosteroids	-	-	-	100%
Emergency Department				
Admittance Decision Time (minutes)[2]	458	73	66	98
Head CT Results Within 45 Min. of Arrival[1]	-	-	25%	57%
Patients Who Left ER Before Being Seen	35,857	2%	1%	2%
Time from ER Arrival to Admit. (minutes)[2]	533	218	201	274
Time from ER Arrival to Discharge (minutes)	341	167	112	134
Time in ER Before Being Evaluated (minutes)	320	42	22	26
Time to Pain Meds for Fractures (minutes)	152	68	52	57
Heart Attack Care				
Aspirin Given at Discharge	249	100%	99%	99%
Fibrinolytic Meds Within 30 Min. of Arrival[7]	-	-	17%	54%
PCI Within 90 Minutes of Arrival	24	83%	93%	96%
Statin Prescribed at Discharge	233	98%	98%	98%
Heart Failure Care				
ACE Inhibitor or ARB for LVSD	61	100%	96%	97%
Discharge Instructions Given	141	99%	94%	94%
Evaluation of LVS Function	196	100%	96%	99%
Medicare Spending				
Medicare Spending per Patient (ratio)	-	0.94	0.9	0.98
Pneumonia Care				
Appropriate Initial Antibiotic Given	142	99%	94%	95%
Blood Culture Timing	289	97%	97%	98%
Pregnancy and Delivery Care				
Newborn Deliveries Scheduled Early[2]	71	6%	6%	6%
Preventive Care				
Immunization for Influenza[2]	515	93%	84%	90%
Immunization for Pneumonia[2]	552	88%	88%	92%
Stroke Care				
Anticoagulation Therapy for Atrial Fibrillation	11	100%	96%	95%
Antithrombotic Therapy Timing	98	97%	98%	98%
Assessed for Rehabilitation	111	99%	97%	97%
Discharged on Antithrombotic Therapy	102	100%	100%	99%
Discharged on Statin Medication	77	97%	91%	94%
Thrombolytic Therapy Timing[1]	-	-	96%	66%
Venous Thromboembolism Prophylaxis	123	96%	96%	94%

NOTE: Hospital profiles are in alphabetical order by state, then city, then hospital within the city; Rankings exclude hospitals with less than 25 cases except for patient surveys which excludes hospitals with less than 100 cases; (a) 100-299 cases; (1) The number of cases/patients is too few to report; (2) Data submitted were based on a sample of cases/patients; (3) Results are based on a shorter time period than required; (4) Data suppressed by CMS for one or more quarters; (5) Results are not available for this reporting period; (6) Fewer than 100 patients completed the HCAHPS survey; (7) No cases met the criteria for this measure; (8) The lower limit of the confidence interval cannot be calculated if the number of observed infections equals zero; (9) No data are available from the state/territory for this reporting period; (10) The scores shown reflect fewer than 50 completed surveys; (11) There were discrepancies in the data collection process; (12) This measure does not apply to this hospital for this reporting period; (13) Results cannot be calculated for this reporting period; (14) The results for this state are combined with nearby states to protect confidentiality; Please refer to the User's Guide for a full explanation of data.

Measure	Cases	This Hosp.	State Avg.	U.S. Avg.
Written Stroke Educational Materials Given	61	97%	86%	88%
Surgical Care Improvement Project				
Appropriate Beta Blocker Usage	217	100%	99%	98%
Appropriate VTP Within 24 Hours	508	97%	98%	98%
Controlled Postoperative Blood Glucose	58	91%	95%	97%
Perioperative Temperature Management	594	100%	100%	100%
Prophylactic Antibiotic Selection	428	100%	99%	99%
Prophylactic Antibiotic Selection (Outpatient)	395	96%	97%	98%
Prophylactic Antibiotic Stopped	407	98%	99%	98%
Prophylactic Antibiotic Timing	430	100%	98%	99%
Prophylactic Antibiotic Timing (Outpatient)	389	100%	96%	98%
Urinary Catheter Removal	491	98%	97%	97%
Survey of Patients' Hospital Experiences				
Area Around Room 'Always' Quiet at Night	300+	49%	66%	61%
Doctors 'Always' Communicated Well	300+	77%	84%	82%
Home Recovery Information Given	300+	82%	82%	85%
Hospital Given 9 or 10 on 10 Point Scale	300+	49%	70%	71%
Meds 'Always' Explained Before Given	300+	52%	67%	64%
Nurses 'Always' Communicated Well	300+	68%	80%	79%
Pain 'Always' Well Controlled	300+	62%	69%	71%
Room and Bathroom 'Always' Clean	300+	65%	78%	73%
Timely Help 'Always' Received	300+	58%	74%	68%
Would Definitely Recommend Hospital	300+	49%	73%	71%
Use of Medical Imaging				
Cardiac Imaging Stress Test before Surgery	370	2.2%	4.6%	5.3%
Combination Abdominal CT Scan	902	6.2%	11.8%	10.5%
Combination Brain/Sinus CT Scan	603	1.8%	2.2%	2.7%
Combination Chest CT Scan	612	0.2%	2%	2.7%
Follow-up Mammogram/Ultrasound	2,314	3.3%	7.8%	8.8%
Lumbar Spine MRI for Low Back Pain	154	38.3%	32.9%	37.2%

Northwood Deaconess Health Center

PO Box 190
Northwood, ND 58267
URL: www.ndhc.net
Type: Critical Access Hospitals
Ownership: Voluntary non-profit - Church
Phone: 701-587-6060
Fax: 701-587-6479
Emergency Services: Yes
Beds: 89

Key Personnel:
CEO/President. . . . . Pete Antonson
Chief of Medical Staff . . . . Dr Jon Berg
Quality Assurance . . . . Colleen Bomber

Measure	Cases	This Hosp.	State Avg.	U.S. Avg.
Blood Clot Prevention and Treatment				
Anticoagulation Overlap Therapy[5]	-	-	97%	93%
ICU Venous Thromboembolism Prophylaxis[5]	-	-	88%	92%
Incidence of Potentially Preventable VTE[5]	-	-	16%	10%
UFH with Dosages/Platelet Monitoring[5]	-	-	100%	97%
Venous Thromboembolism Prophylaxis[5]	-	-	80%	85%
Warfarin Therapy Discharge Instructions[5]	-	-	72%	75%
Chest Pain/Possible Heart Attack Care				
Aspirin Given Within 24 Hours of Arrival[1,3]	-	-	95%	96%
Fibrinolytic Meds Within 30 Min. of Arrival[1,3]	-	-	51%	58%
Average Time to ECG (minutes)[1,3]	-	-	11	7
Average Time to Transfer (minutes)[3,7]	-	-	114	60
Children's Asthma Care				
Received Home Management Plan of Care	-	-	-	88%
Received Reliever Medication	-	-	-	100%
Received Systemic Corticosteroids	-	-	-	100%
Emergency Department				
Admittance Decision Time (minutes)[5]	-	-	66	98
Head CT Results Within 45 Min. of Arrival[5]	-	-	25%	57%
Patients Who Left ER Before Being Seen	505	1%	1%	2%
Time from ER Arrival to Admit. (minutes)[5]	-	-	201	274
Time from ER Arrival to Discharge (minutes)[5]	-	-	112	134
Time in ER Before Being Evaluated (minutes)[5]	-	-	22	26
Time to Pain Meds for Fractures (minutes)[5]	-	-	52	57
Heart Attack Care				
Aspirin Given at Discharge[5]	-	-	99%	99%
Fibrinolytic Meds Within 30 Min. of Arrival[5]	-	-	17%	54%
PCI Within 90 Minutes of Arrival[5]	-	-	93%	96%
Statin Prescribed at Discharge[5]	-	-	98%	98%
Heart Failure Care				
ACE Inhibitor or ARB for LVSD[1,2]	-	-	96%	97%
Discharge Instructions Given[1,2]	-	-	94%	94%
Evaluation of LVS Function[1,2]	-	-	96%	99%
Medicare Spending				
Medicare Spending per Patient (ratio)	-	-	0.9	0.98
Pneumonia Care				
Appropriate Initial Antibiotic Given[1,2]	-	-	94%	95%
Blood Culture Timing[1,2]	-	-	97%	98%
Pregnancy and Delivery Care				
Newborn Deliveries Scheduled Early[5]	-	-	6%	6%
Preventive Care				
Immunization for Influenza[1]	-	-	84%	90%
Immunization for Pneumonia	14	86%	88%	92%
Stroke Care				
Anticoagulation Therapy for Atrial Fibrillation[5]	-	-	96%	95%
Antithrombotic Therapy Timing[5]	-	-	98%	98%
Assessed for Rehabilitation[5]	-	-	97%	97%
Discharged on Antithrombotic Therapy[5]	-	-	100%	99%
Discharged on Statin Medication[5]	-	-	91%	94%
Thrombolytic Therapy Timing[5]	-	-	96%	66%
Venous Thromboembolism Prophylaxis[5]	-	-	96%	94%
Written Stroke Educational Materials Given[5]	-	-	86%	88%
Surgical Care Improvement Project				
Appropriate Beta Blocker Usage[5]	-	-	99%	98%
Appropriate VTP Within 24 Hours[5]	-	-	98%	98%
Controlled Postoperative Blood Glucose[5]	-	-	95%	97%
Perioperative Temperature Management[5]	-	-	100%	100%
Prophylactic Antibiotic Selection[5]	-	-	99%	99%
Prophylactic Antibiotic Selection (Outpatient)[5]	-	-	97%	98%
Prophylactic Antibiotic Stopped[5]	-	-	99%	98%
Prophylactic Antibiotic Timing[5]	-	-	98%	99%
Prophylactic Antibiotic Timing (Outpatient)[5]	-	-	96%	98%
Urinary Catheter Removal[5]	-	-	97%	97%
Survey of Patients' Hospital Experiences				
Area Around Room 'Always' Quiet at Night[3,10]	<100	100%	66%	61%
Doctors 'Always' Communicated Well[3,10]	<100	100%	84%	82%
Home Recovery Information Given[3,10]	<100	83%	82%	85%
Hospital Given 9 or 10 on 10 Point Scale[3,10]	<100	81%	70%	71%
Meds 'Always' Explained Before Given[3,10]	<100	-	67%	64%
Nurses 'Always' Communicated Well[3,10]	<100	100%	80%	79%
Pain 'Always' Well Controlled[3,10]	<100	64%	69%	71%
Room and Bathroom 'Always' Clean[3,10]	<100	77%	78%	73%
Timely Help 'Always' Received[3,10]	<100	73%	74%	68%
Would Definitely Recommend Hospital[3,10]	<100	100%	73%	71%
Use of Medical Imaging				
Cardiac Imaging Stress Test before Surgery[7]	-	-	4.6%	5.3%
Combination Abdominal CT Scan[1]	-	-	11.8%	10.5%
Combination Brain/Sinus CT Scan[1]	-	-	2.2%	2.7%
Combination Chest CT Scan[1]	-	-	2%	2.7%
Follow-up Mammogram/Ultrasound[1]	-	-	7.8%	8.8%
Lumbar Spine MRI for Low Back Pain[1]	-	-	32.9%	37.2%

Oakes Community Hospital

1200 N 7th St
Oakes, ND 58474
Type: Critical Access Hospitals
Ownership: Voluntary non-profit - Private
Phone: 701-742-3291
Emergency Services: Yes

Measure	Cases	This Hosp.	State Avg.	U.S. Avg.
Blood Clot Prevention and Treatment				
Anticoagulation Overlap Therapy[5]	-	-	97%	93%
ICU Venous Thromboembolism Prophylaxis[5]	-	-	88%	92%
Incidence of Potentially Preventable VTE[5]	-	-	16%	10%
UFH with Dosages/Platelet Monitoring[5]	-	-	100%	97%
Venous Thromboembolism Prophylaxis[5]	-	-	80%	85%
Warfarin Therapy Discharge Instructions[5]	-	-	72%	75%
Chest Pain/Possible Heart Attack Care				
Aspirin Given Within 24 Hours of Arrival[3,7]	-	-	95%	96%
Fibrinolytic Meds Within 30 Min. of Arrival[3,7]	-	-	51%	58%
Average Time to ECG (minutes)[1,3]	-	-	11	7
Average Time to Transfer (minutes)[3,7]	-	-	114	60
Children's Asthma Care				
Received Home Management Plan of Care	-	-	-	88%
Received Reliever Medication	-	-	-	100%
Received Systemic Corticosteroids	-	-	-	100%
Emergency Department				
Admittance Decision Time (minutes)[5]	-	-	66	98
Head CT Results Within 45 Min. of Arrival[5]	-	-	25%	57%
Patients Who Left ER Before Being Seen	703	0%	1%	2%
Time from ER Arrival to Admit. (minutes)[5]	-	-	201	274
Time from ER Arrival to Discharge (minutes)[5]	-	-	112	134
Time in ER Before Being Evaluated (minutes)[5]	-	-	22	26
Time to Pain Meds for Fractures (minutes)[5]	-	-	52	57
Heart Attack Care				
Aspirin Given at Discharge[1,2]	-	-	99%	99%
Fibrinolytic Meds Within 30 Min. of Arrival[2,7]	-	-	17%	54%
PCI Within 90 Minutes of Arrival[2,7]	-	-	93%	96%
Statin Prescribed at Discharge[1,2]	-	-	98%	98%
Heart Failure Care				
ACE Inhibitor or ARB for LVSD[1,2]	-	-	96%	97%
Discharge Instructions Given[1,2]	-	-	94%	94%
Evaluation of LVS Function[2]	25	88%	96%	99%
Medicare Spending				
Medicare Spending per Patient (ratio)	-	-	0.9	0.98
Pneumonia Care				
Appropriate Initial Antibiotic Given[2]	11	100%	94%	95%
Blood Culture Timing[2]	13	100%	97%	98%
Pregnancy and Delivery Care				
Newborn Deliveries Scheduled Early[5]	-	-	6%	6%
Preventive Care				
Immunization for Influenza[5]	-	-	84%	90%
Immunization for Pneumonia[5]	-	-	88%	92%
Stroke Care				
Anticoagulation Therapy for Atrial Fibrillation[5]	-	-	96%	95%
Antithrombotic Therapy Timing[5]	-	-	98%	98%
Assessed for Rehabilitation[5]	-	-	97%	97%
Discharged on Antithrombotic Therapy[5]	-	-	100%	99%
Discharged on Statin Medication[5]	-	-	91%	94%
Thrombolytic Therapy Timing[5]	-	-	96%	66%
Venous Thromboembolism Prophylaxis[5]	-	-	96%	94%
Written Stroke Educational Materials Given[5]	-	-	86%	88%
Surgical Care Improvement Project				
Appropriate Beta Blocker Usage[2,3]	-	-	99%	98%
Appropriate VTP Within 24 Hours[1,2]	-	-	98%	98%
Controlled Postoperative Blood Glucose[2,3]	-	-	95%	97%
Perioperative Temperature Management[1,2]	-	-	100%	100%
Prophylactic Antibiotic Selection[1,2]	-	-	99%	99%
Prophylactic Antibiotic Selection (Outpatient)[5]	-	-	97%	98%
Prophylactic Antibiotic Stopped[1,2]	-	-	99%	98%
Prophylactic Antibiotic Timing[1,2]	-	-	98%	99%
Prophylactic Antibiotic Timing (Outpatient)[5]	-	-	96%	98%
Urinary Catheter Removal[2,3]	-	-	97%	97%
Survey of Patients' Hospital Experiences				
Area Around Room 'Always' Quiet at Night[5]	-	-	66%	61%
Doctors 'Always' Communicated Well[5]	-	-	84%	82%
Home Recovery Information Given[5]	-	-	82%	85%
Hospital Given 9 or 10 on 10 Point Scale[5]	-	-	70%	71%
Meds 'Always' Explained Before Given[5]	-	-	67%	64%
Nurses 'Always' Communicated Well[5]	-	-	80%	79%
Pain 'Always' Well Controlled[5]	-	-	69%	71%
Room and Bathroom 'Always' Clean[5]	-	-	78%	73%
Timely Help 'Always' Received[5]	-	-	74%	68%
Would Definitely Recommend Hospital[5]	-	-	73%	71%
Use of Medical Imaging				
Cardiac Imaging Stress Test before Surgery[1]	-	-	4.6%	5.3%
Combination Abdominal CT Scan	109	51.4%	11.8%	10.5%
Combination Brain/Sinus CT Scan	73	0.0%	2.2%	2.7%
Combination Chest CT Scan	63	1.6%	2%	2.7%
Follow-up Mammogram/Ultrasound[1]	-	-	7.8%	8.8%
Lumbar Spine MRI for Low Back Pain[1]	-	-	32.9%	37.2%

NOTE: Hospital profiles are in alphabetical order by state, then city, then hospital within the city; Rankings exclude hospitals with less than 25 cases except for patient surveys which excludes hospitals with less than 100 cases; (a) 100-299 cases; (1) The number of cases/patients is too few to report; (2) Data submitted were based on a sample of cases/patients; (3) Results are based on a shorter time period than required; (4) Data suppressed by CMS for one or more quarters; (5) Results are not available for this reporting period; (6) Fewer than 100 patients completed the HCAHPS survey; (7) No cases met the criteria for this measure; (8) The lower limit of the confidence interval cannot be calculated if the number of observed infections equals zero; (9) No data are available from the state/territory for this reporting period; (10) The scores shown reflect fewer than 50 completed surveys; (11) There were discrepancies in the data collection process; (12) This measure does not apply to this hospital for this reporting period; (13) Results cannot be calculated for this reporting period; (14) The results for this state are combined with nearby states to protect confidentiality; Please refer to the User's Guide for a full explanation of data.

First Care Health Center

115 Vivian St | Phone: 701-284-7500
Park River, ND 58270
URL: www.firstcarehc.com
Type: Critical Access Hospitals | Emergency Services: Yes
Ownership: Voluntary non-profit - Private

Measure	Cases	This Hosp.	State Avg.	U.S. Avg.
Blood Clot Prevention and Treatment				
Anticoagulation Overlap Therapy[5]	-	-	97%	93%
ICU Venous Thromboembolism Prophylaxis[5]	-	-	88%	92%
Incidence of Potentially Preventable VTE[5]	-	-	16%	10%
UFH with Dosages/Platelet Monitoring[5]	-	-	100%	97%
Venous Thromboembolism Prophylaxis[5]	-	-	80%	85%
Warfarin Therapy Discharge Instructions[5]	-	-	72%	75%
Chest Pain/Possible Heart Attack Care				
Aspirin Given Within 24 Hours of Arrival[1,3]	-	-	95%	96%
Fibrinolytic Meds Within 30 Min. of Arrival[1,3]	-	-	51%	58%
Average Time to ECG (minutes)[1,3]	-	-	11	7
Average Time to Transfer (minutes)[3,7]	-	-	114	60
Children's Asthma Care				
Received Home Management Plan of Care	-	-	-	88%
Received Reliever Medication	-	-	-	100%
Received Systemic Corticosteroids	-	-	-	100%
Emergency Department				
Admittance Decision Time (minutes)[5]	-	-	66	98
Head CT Results Within 45 Min. of Arrival[5]	-	-	25%	57%
Patients Who Left ER Before Being Seen	1,218	0%	1%	2%
Time from ER Arrival to Admit. (minutes)[5]	-	-	201	274
Time from ER Arrival to Discharge (minutes)[5]	-	-	112	134
Time in ER Before Being Evaluated (minutes)[5]	-	-	22	26
Time to Pain Meds for Fractures (minutes)[5]	-	-	52	57
Heart Attack Care				
Aspirin Given at Discharge[5]	-	-	99%	99%
Fibrinolytic Meds Within 30 Min. of Arrival[5]	-	-	17%	54%
PCI Within 90 Minutes of Arrival[5]	-	-	93%	96%
Statin Prescribed at Discharge[5]	-	-	98%	98%
Heart Failure Care				
ACE Inhibitor or ARB for LVSD[1]	-	-	96%	97%
Discharge Instructions Given[1]	-	-	94%	94%
Evaluation of LVS Function	12	83%	96%	99%
Medicare Spending				
Medicare Spending per Patient (ratio)	-	-	0.9	0.98
Pneumonia Care				
Appropriate Initial Antibiotic Given	14	100%	94%	95%
Blood Culture Timing[1]	-	-	97%	98%
Pregnancy and Delivery Care				
Newborn Deliveries Scheduled Early[5]	-	-	6%	6%
Preventive Care				
Immunization for Influenza[2]	26	73%	84%	90%
Immunization for Pneumonia[2,3]	22	77%	88%	92%
Stroke Care				
Anticoagulation Therapy for Atrial Fibrillation[5]	-	-	96%	95%
Antithrombotic Therapy Timing[5]	-	-	98%	98%
Assessed for Rehabilitation[5]	-	-	97%	97%
Discharged on Antithrombotic Therapy[5]	-	-	100%	99%
Discharged on Statin Medication[5]	-	-	91%	94%
Thrombolytic Therapy Timing[5]	-	-	96%	66%
Venous Thromboembolism Prophylaxis[5]	-	-	96%	94%
Written Stroke Educational Materials Given[5]	-	-	86%	88%
Surgical Care Improvement Project				
Appropriate Beta Blocker Usage[5]	-	-	99%	98%
Appropriate VTP Within 24 Hours[5]	-	-	98%	98%
Controlled Postoperative Blood Glucose[5]	-	-	95%	97%
Perioperative Temperature Management[5]	-	-	100%	100%
Prophylactic Antibiotic Selection[5]	-	-	99%	99%
Prophylactic Antibiotic Selection (Outpatient)[5]	-	-	97%	98%
Prophylactic Antibiotic Stopped[5]	-	-	99%	98%
Prophylactic Antibiotic Timing[5]	-	-	98%	99%
Prophylactic Antibiotic Timing (Outpatient)[5]	-	-	96%	98%
Urinary Catheter Removal[5]	-	-	97%	97%
Survey of Patients' Hospital Experiences				
Area Around Room 'Always' Quiet at Night	(a)	66%	66%	61%
Doctors 'Always' Communicated Well	(a)	91%	84%	82%
Home Recovery Information Given	(a)	80%	82%	85%
Hospital Given 9 or 10 on 10 Point Scale	(a)	86%	70%	71%
Meds 'Always' Explained Before Given	(a)	79%	67%	64%
Nurses 'Always' Communicated Well	(a)	84%	80%	79%
Pain 'Always' Well Controlled	(a)	69%	69%	71%
Room and Bathroom 'Always' Clean	(a)	92%	78%	73%
Timely Help 'Always' Received	(a)	79%	74%	68%
Would Definitely Recommend Hospital	(a)	91%	73%	71%
Use of Medical Imaging				
Cardiac Imaging Stress Test before Surgery[7]	-	-	4.6%	5.3%
Combination Abdominal CT Scan[1]	-	-	11.8%	10.5%
Combination Brain/Sinus CT Scan	55	0.0%	2.2%	2.7%
Combination Chest CT Scan[1]	-	-	2%	2.7%
Follow-up Mammogram/Ultrasound	144	2.8%	7.8%	8.8%
Lumbar Spine MRI for Low Back Pain[1]	-	-	32.9%	37.2%

Presentation Medical Center

213 Second Ave Ne | Phone: 701-477-3161
Rolla, ND 58367 | Fax: 701-477-5564
URL: www.pmc-rolla.com
Type: Critical Access Hospitals | Emergency Services: Yes
Ownership: Voluntary non-profit - Private | Beds: 54

Key Personnel:
Operating Room. . . . . Peggy Hendrickson, RN
Radiology. . . . . Kim Kakela
CEO/President. . . . . Mark Kerr, CHE
Emergency Room . . . . Bonnie McDougall
Infection Control. . . . . Bonnie McDougall, RN
Intensive Care Unit. . . . . Peggy McPougall

Measure	Cases	This Hosp.	State Avg.	U.S. Avg.
Blood Clot Prevention and Treatment				
Anticoagulation Overlap Therapy[5]	-	-	97%	93%
ICU Venous Thromboembolism Prophylaxis[5]	-	-	88%	92%
Incidence of Potentially Preventable VTE[5]	-	-	16%	10%
UFH with Dosages/Platelet Monitoring[5]	-	-	100%	97%
Venous Thromboembolism Prophylaxis[5]	-	-	80%	85%
Warfarin Therapy Discharge Instructions[5]	-	-	72%	75%
Chest Pain/Possible Heart Attack Care				
Aspirin Given Within 24 Hours of Arrival[1]	-	-	95%	96%
Fibrinolytic Meds Within 30 Min. of Arrival[1,3]	-	-	51%	58%
Average Time to ECG (minutes)[1]	-	-	11	7
Average Time to Transfer (minutes)[3,7]	-	-	114	60
Children's Asthma Care				
Received Home Management Plan of Care	-	-	-	88%
Received Reliever Medication	-	-	-	100%
Received Systemic Corticosteroids	-	-	-	100%
Emergency Department				
Admittance Decision Time (minutes)[5]	-	-	66	98
Head CT Results Within 45 Min. of Arrival[5]	-	-	25%	57%
Patients Who Left ER Before Being Seen	5,923	2%	1%	2%
Time from ER Arrival to Admit. (minutes)[5]	-	-	201	274
Time from ER Arrival to Discharge (minutes)[5]	-	-	112	134
Time in ER Before Being Evaluated (minutes)[5]	-	-	22	26
Time to Pain Meds for Fractures (minutes)[5]	-	-	52	57
Heart Attack Care				
Aspirin Given at Discharge[5]	-	-	99%	99%
Fibrinolytic Meds Within 30 Min. of Arrival[5]	-	-	17%	54%
PCI Within 90 Minutes of Arrival[5]	-	-	93%	96%
Statin Prescribed at Discharge[5]	-	-	98%	98%
Heart Failure Care				
ACE Inhibitor or ARB for LVSD[7]	-	-	96%	97%
Discharge Instructions Given[1]	-	-	94%	94%
Evaluation of LVS Function[1]	-	-	96%	99%
Medicare Spending				
Medicare Spending per Patient (ratio)	-	-	0.9	0.98
Pneumonia Care				
Appropriate Initial Antibiotic Given	14	100%	94%	95%
Blood Culture Timing[1]	-	-	97%	98%
Pregnancy and Delivery Care				
Newborn Deliveries Scheduled Early[5]	-	-	6%	6%
Preventive Care				
Immunization for Influenza[5]	-	-	84%	90%
Immunization for Pneumonia[5]	-	-	88%	92%
Stroke Care				
Anticoagulation Therapy for Atrial Fibrillation[5]	-	-	96%	95%
Antithrombotic Therapy Timing[5]	-	-	98%	98%
Assessed for Rehabilitation[5]	-	-	97%	97%
Discharged on Antithrombotic Therapy[5]	-	-	100%	99%
Discharged on Statin Medication[5]	-	-	91%	94%
Thrombolytic Therapy Timing[5]	-	-	96%	66%
Venous Thromboembolism Prophylaxis[5]	-	-	96%	94%
Written Stroke Educational Materials Given[5]	-	-	86%	88%
Surgical Care Improvement Project				
Appropriate Beta Blocker Usage[5]	-	-	99%	98%
Appropriate VTP Within 24 Hours[5]	-	-	98%	98%
Controlled Postoperative Blood Glucose[5]	-	-	95%	97%
Perioperative Temperature Management[5]	-	-	100%	100%
Prophylactic Antibiotic Selection[5]	-	-	99%	99%
Prophylactic Antibiotic Selection (Outpatient)[5]	-	-	97%	98%
Prophylactic Antibiotic Stopped[5]	-	-	99%	98%
Prophylactic Antibiotic Timing[5]	-	-	98%	99%
Prophylactic Antibiotic Timing (Outpatient)[5]	-	-	96%	98%
Urinary Catheter Removal[5]	-	-	97%	97%
Survey of Patients' Hospital Experiences				
Area Around Room 'Always' Quiet at Night[5]	-	-	66%	61%
Doctors 'Always' Communicated Well[5]	-	-	84%	82%
Home Recovery Information Given[5]	-	-	82%	85%
Hospital Given 9 or 10 on 10 Point Scale[5]	-	-	70%	71%
Meds 'Always' Explained Before Given[5]	-	-	67%	64%
Nurses 'Always' Communicated Well[5]	-	-	80%	79%
Pain 'Always' Well Controlled[5]	-	-	69%	71%
Room and Bathroom 'Always' Clean[5]	-	-	78%	73%
Timely Help 'Always' Received[5]	-	-	74%	68%
Would Definitely Recommend Hospital[5]	-	-	73%	71%
Use of Medical Imaging				
Cardiac Imaging Stress Test before Surgery[7]	-	-	4.6%	5.3%
Combination Abdominal CT Scan[1]	-	-	11.8%	10.5%
Combination Brain/Sinus CT Scan[1]	-	-	2.2%	2.7%
Combination Chest CT Scan[1]	-	-	2%	2.7%
Follow-up Mammogram/Ultrasound	87	11.5%	7.8%	8.8%
Lumbar Spine MRI for Low Back Pain[1]	-	-	32.9%	37.2%

Heart of America Medical Center

800 S Main Ave | Phone: 701-776-5261
Rugby, ND 58368 | Fax: 701-776-5448
E-mail: admin@hamc.com
URL: www.hamc.com
Type: Critical Access Hospitals | Emergency Services: Yes
Ownership: Voluntary non-profit - Other | Beds: 118

Key Personnel:
Infection Control. . . . . Mary Haugen
CEO/President. . . . . Jerry E Jurena
CEO . . . . Jeff Lingerfelt
Chairman/CEO . . . . Jon Nelson
Chief of Medical Staff. . . . . Ron Skipper
Cardiac Laboratory. . . . . Keri Weick

Measure	Cases	This Hosp.	State Avg.	U.S. Avg.
Blood Clot Prevention and Treatment				
Anticoagulation Overlap Therapy[5]	-	-	97%	93%
ICU Venous Thromboembolism Prophylaxis[5]	-	-	88%	92%
Incidence of Potentially Preventable VTE[5]	-	-	16%	10%
UFH with Dosages/Platelet Monitoring[5]	-	-	100%	97%
Venous Thromboembolism Prophylaxis[5]	-	-	80%	85%
Warfarin Therapy Discharge Instructions[5]	-	-	72%	75%
Chest Pain/Possible Heart Attack Care				
Aspirin Given Within 24 Hours of Arrival[1]	-	-	95%	96%
Fibrinolytic Meds Within 30 Min. of Arrival[3,7]	-	-	51%	58%
Average Time to ECG (minutes)[1]	-	-	11	7
Average Time to Transfer (minutes)[1,3]	-	-	114	60
Children's Asthma Care				
Received Home Management Plan of Care	-	-	-	88%
Received Reliever Medication	-	-	-	100%
Received Systemic Corticosteroids	-	-	-	100%
Emergency Department				
Admittance Decision Time (minutes)[5]	-	-	66	98
Head CT Results Within 45 Min. of Arrival[5]	-	-	25%	57%
Patients Who Left ER Before Being Seen	2,549	0%	1%	2%

NOTE: Hospital profiles are in alphabetical order by state, then city, then hospital within the city; Rankings exclude hospitals with less than 25 cases except for patient surveys which excludes hospitals with less than 100 cases; (a) 100-299 cases; (1) The number of cases/patients is too few to report; (2) Data submitted were based on a sample of cases/patients; (3) Results are based on a shorter time period than required; (4) Data suppressed by CMS for one or more quarters; (5) Results are not available for this reporting period; (6) Fewer than 100 patients completed the HCAHPS survey; (7) No cases met the criteria for this measure; (8) The lower limit of the confidence interval cannot be calculated if the number of observed infections equals zero; (9) No data are available from the state/territory for this reporting period; (10) The scores shown reflect fewer than 50 completed surveys; (11) There were discrepancies in the data collection process; (12) This measure does not apply to this hospital for this reporting period; (13) Results cannot be calculated for this reporting period; (14) The results for this state are combined with nearby states to protect confidentiality; Please refer to the User's Guide for a full explanation of data.

Measure	Cases	This Hosp.	State Avg.	U.S. Avg.
Time from ER Arrival to Admit. (minutes)[5]	-	-	201	274
Time from ER Arrival to Discharge (minutes)[5]	-	-	112	134
Time in ER Before Being Evaluated (minutes)[5]	-	-	22	26
Time to Pain Meds for Fractures (minutes)[5]	-	-	52	57
Heart Attack Care				
Aspirin Given at Discharge[1,2]	-	-	99%	99%
Fibrinolytic Meds Within 30 Min. of Arrival[2,3]	-	-	17%	54%
PCI Within 90 Minutes of Arrival[2,3]	-	-	93%	96%
Statin Prescribed at Discharge[1,2]	-	-	98%	98%
Heart Failure Care				
ACE Inhibitor or ARB for LVSD[2,7]	-	-	96%	97%
Discharge Instructions Given[1,2]	-	-	94%	94%
Evaluation of LVS Function[2]	17	88%	96%	99%
Medicare Spending				
Medicare Spending per Patient (ratio)	-	-	0.9	0.98
Pneumonia Care				
Appropriate Initial Antibiotic Given[2]	30	83%	94%	95%
Blood Culture Timing[2]	26	92%	97%	98%
Pregnancy and Delivery Care				
Newborn Deliveries Scheduled Early[5]	-	-	6%	6%
Preventive Care				
Immunization for Influenza[5]	-	-	84%	90%
Immunization for Pneumonia[5]	-	-	88%	92%
Stroke Care				
Anticoagulation Therapy for Atrial Fibrillation[5]	-	-	96%	95%
Antithrombotic Therapy Timing[5]	-	-	98%	98%
Assessed for Rehabilitation[5]	-	-	97%	97%
Discharged on Antithrombotic Therapy[5]	-	-	100%	99%
Discharged on Statin Medication[5]	-	-	91%	94%
Thrombolytic Therapy Timing[5]	-	-	96%	66%
Venous Thromboembolism Prophylaxis[5]	-	-	96%	94%
Written Stroke Educational Materials Given[5]	-	-	86%	88%
Surgical Care Improvement Project				
Appropriate Beta Blocker Usage[1,3]	-	-	99%	98%
Appropriate VTP Within 24 Hours[1,3]	-	-	98%	98%
Controlled Postoperative Blood Glucose[3,7]	-	-	95%	97%
Perioperative Temperature Management[1,3]	-	-	100%	100%
Prophylactic Antibiotic Selection[1,3]	-	-	99%	99%
Prophylactic Antibiotic Selection (Outpatient)[1]	-	-	97%	98%
Prophylactic Antibiotic Stopped[1,3]	-	-	99%	98%
Prophylactic Antibiotic Timing[1,3]	-	-	98%	99%
Prophylactic Antibiotic Timing (Outpatient)[1]	-	-	96%	98%
Urinary Catheter Removal[1,3]	-	-	97%	97%
Survey of Patients' Hospital Experiences				
Area Around Room 'Always' Quiet at Night[6]	<100	61%	66%	61%
Doctors 'Always' Communicated Well[6]	<100	82%	84%	82%
Home Recovery Information Given[6]	<100	83%	82%	85%
Hospital Given 9 or 10 on 10 Point Scale[6]	<100	66%	70%	71%
Meds 'Always' Explained Before Given[6]	<100	62%	67%	64%
Nurses 'Always' Communicated Well[6]	<100	82%	80%	79%
Pain 'Always' Well Controlled[6]	<100	70%	69%	71%
Room and Bathroom 'Always' Clean[6]	<100	75%	78%	73%
Timely Help 'Always' Received[6]	<100	67%	74%	68%
Would Definitely Recommend Hospital[6]	<100	65%	73%	71%
Use of Medical Imaging				
Cardiac Imaging Stress Test before Surgery[1]	-	-	4.6%	5.3%
Combination Abdominal CT Scan	93	3.2%	11.8%	10.5%
Combination Brain/Sinus CT Scan[1]	-	-	2.2%	2.7%
Combination Chest CT Scan[1]	-	-	2%	2.7%
Follow-up Mammogram/Ultrasound	236	4.7%	7.8%	8.8%
Lumbar Spine MRI for Low Back Pain[1]	-	-	32.9%	37.2%

Mountrail County Medical Center

615 6th Saint Se
Stanley, ND 58784
Phone: 701-628-2424
Fax: 701-628-3274
URL: www.stanleyhealth.org
Type: Critical Access Hospitals
Emergency Services: Yes
Ownership: Voluntary non-profit - Other
Beds: 25

Key Personnel:

Cardiac Laboratory. . . . . Judy Hove
Chief of Medical Staff. . . . . Tyrone Langer, MD
Quality Assurance . . . . Ann Nelson

Measure	Cases	This Hosp.	State Avg.	U.S. Avg.
Blood Clot Prevention and Treatment				
Anticoagulation Overlap Therapy[5]	-	-	97%	93%
ICU Venous Thromboembolism Prophylaxis[5]	-	-	88%	92%
Incidence of Potentially Preventable VTE[5]	-	-	16%	10%
UFH with Dosages/Platelet Monitoring[5]	-	-	100%	97%
Venous Thromboembolism Prophylaxis[5]	-	-	80%	85%
Warfarin Therapy Discharge Instructions[5]	-	-	72%	75%
Chest Pain/Possible Heart Attack Care				
Aspirin Given Within 24 Hours of Arrival[5]	-	-	95%	96%
Fibrinolytic Meds Within 30 Min. of Arrival[5]	-	-	51%	58%
Average Time to ECG (minutes)[5]	-	-	11	7
Average Time to Transfer (minutes)[5]	-	-	114	60
Children's Asthma Care				
Received Home Management Plan of Care	-	-	-	88%
Received Reliever Medication	-	-	-	100%
Received Systemic Corticosteroids	-	-	-	100%
Emergency Department				
Admittance Decision Time (minutes)[5]	-	-	66	98
Head CT Results Within 45 Min. of Arrival[5]	-	-	25%	57%
Patients Who Left ER Before Being Seen[1]	-	-	1%	2%
Time from ER Arrival to Admit. (minutes)[5]	-	-	201	274
Time from ER Arrival to Discharge (minutes)[5]	-	-	112	134
Time in ER Before Being Evaluated (minutes)[5]	-	-	22	26
Time to Pain Meds for Fractures (minutes)[5]	-	-	52	57
Heart Attack Care				
Aspirin Given at Discharge[5]	-	-	99%	99%
Fibrinolytic Meds Within 30 Min. of Arrival[5]	-	-	17%	54%
PCI Within 90 Minutes of Arrival[5]	-	-	93%	96%
Statin Prescribed at Discharge[5]	-	-	98%	98%
Heart Failure Care				
ACE Inhibitor or ARB for LVSD[3,7]	-	-	96%	97%
Discharge Instructions Given[3,7]	-	-	94%	94%
Evaluation of LVS Function[1,3]	-	-	96%	99%
Medicare Spending				
Medicare Spending per Patient (ratio)	-	-	0.9	0.98
Pneumonia Care				
Appropriate Initial Antibiotic Given[1]	-	-	94%	95%
Blood Culture Timing[1]	-	-	97%	98%
Pregnancy and Delivery Care				
Newborn Deliveries Scheduled Early[5]	-	-	6%	6%
Preventive Care				
Immunization for Influenza[5]	-	-	84%	90%
Immunization for Pneumonia[5]	-	-	88%	92%
Stroke Care				
Anticoagulation Therapy for Atrial Fibrillation[5]	-	-	96%	95%
Antithrombotic Therapy Timing[5]	-	-	98%	98%
Assessed for Rehabilitation[5]	-	-	97%	97%
Discharged on Antithrombotic Therapy[5]	-	-	100%	99%
Discharged on Statin Medication[5]	-	-	91%	94%
Thrombolytic Therapy Timing[5]	-	-	96%	66%
Venous Thromboembolism Prophylaxis[5]	-	-	96%	94%
Written Stroke Educational Materials Given[5]	-	-	86%	88%
Surgical Care Improvement Project				
Appropriate Beta Blocker Usage[5]	-	-	99%	98%
Appropriate VTP Within 24 Hours[5]	-	-	98%	98%
Controlled Postoperative Blood Glucose[5]	-	-	95%	97%
Perioperative Temperature Management[5]	-	-	100%	100%
Prophylactic Antibiotic Selection[5]	-	-	99%	99%
Prophylactic Antibiotic Selection (Outpatient)[5]	-	-	97%	98%
Prophylactic Antibiotic Stopped[5]	-	-	99%	98%
Prophylactic Antibiotic Timing[5]	-	-	98%	99%
Prophylactic Antibiotic Timing (Outpatient)[5]	-	-	96%	98%
Urinary Catheter Removal[5]	-	-	97%	97%
Survey of Patients' Hospital Experiences				
Area Around Room 'Always' Quiet at Night[5]	-	-	66%	61%
Doctors 'Always' Communicated Well[5]	-	-	84%	82%
Home Recovery Information Given[5]	-	-	82%	85%
Hospital Given 9 or 10 on 10 Point Scale[5]	-	-	70%	71%
Meds 'Always' Explained Before Given[5]	-	-	67%	64%
Nurses 'Always' Communicated Well[5]	-	-	80%	79%
Pain 'Always' Well Controlled[5]	-	-	69%	71%
Room and Bathroom 'Always' Clean[5]	-	-	78%	73%
Timely Help 'Always' Received[5]	-	-	74%	68%
Would Definitely Recommend Hospital[5]	-	-	73%	71%
Use of Medical Imaging				
Cardiac Imaging Stress Test before Surgery[7]	-	-	4.6%	5.3%
Combination Abdominal CT Scan[1]	-	-	11.8%	10.5%
Combination Brain/Sinus CT Scan[1]	-	-	2.2%	2.7%
Combination Chest CT Scan[1]	-	-	2%	2.7%
Follow-up Mammogram/Ultrasound[7]	-	-	7.8%	8.8%
Lumbar Spine MRI for Low Back Pain[1]	-	-	32.9%	37.2%

Tioga Medical Center

810 N Welo St
Tioga, ND 58852
Phone: 701-664-3305
Fax: 701-664-3644
URL: www.tiogahealth.org
Type: Critical Access Hospitals
Emergency Services: Yes
Ownership: Voluntary non-profit - Private
Beds: 29

Key Personnel:

Operating Room. . . . . Ardith Bingeman, RN
Infection Control. . . . . Shelley Eide, RN
Quality Assurance . . . . Roger Endres
CEO/President. . . . . Randy Paderson
Chief of Medical Staff . . . . MV Patel, MD

Measure	Cases	This Hosp.	State Avg.	U.S. Avg.
Blood Clot Prevention and Treatment				
Anticoagulation Overlap Therapy[5]	-	-	97%	93%
ICU Venous Thromboembolism Prophylaxis[5]	-	-	88%	92%
Incidence of Potentially Preventable VTE[5]	-	-	16%	10%
UFH with Dosages/Platelet Monitoring[5]	-	-	100%	97%
Venous Thromboembolism Prophylaxis[5]	-	-	80%	85%
Warfarin Therapy Discharge Instructions[5]	-	-	72%	75%
Chest Pain/Possible Heart Attack Care				
Aspirin Given Within 24 Hours of Arrival[1]	-	-	95%	96%
Fibrinolytic Meds Within 30 Min. of Arrival[1]	-	-	51%	58%
Average Time to ECG (minutes)[1]	-	-	11	7
Average Time to Transfer (minutes)[1]	-	-	114	60
Children's Asthma Care				
Received Home Management Plan of Care	-	-	-	88%
Received Reliever Medication	-	-	-	100%
Received Systemic Corticosteroids	-	-	-	100%
Emergency Department				
Admittance Decision Time (minutes)[5]	-	-	66	98
Head CT Results Within 45 Min. of Arrival[5]	-	-	25%	57%
Patients Who Left ER Before Being Seen	2,110	1%	1%	2%
Time from ER Arrival to Admit. (minutes)[5]	-	-	201	274
Time from ER Arrival to Discharge (minutes)[5]	-	-	112	134
Time in ER Before Being Evaluated (minutes)[5]	-	-	22	26
Time to Pain Meds for Fractures (minutes)[5]	-	-	52	57
Heart Attack Care				
Aspirin Given at Discharge[1,3]	-	-	99%	99%
Fibrinolytic Meds Within 30 Min. of Arrival[3,7]	-	-	17%	54%
PCI Within 90 Minutes of Arrival[3,7]	-	-	93%	96%
Statin Prescribed at Discharge[1,3]	-	-	98%	98%
Heart Failure Care				
ACE Inhibitor or ARB for LVSD[1,3]	-	-	96%	97%
Discharge Instructions Given[1,3]	-	-	94%	94%
Evaluation of LVS Function[1,3]	-	-	96%	99%
Medicare Spending				
Medicare Spending per Patient (ratio)	-	-	0.9	0.98
Pneumonia Care				
Appropriate Initial Antibiotic Given[1]	-	-	94%	95%
Blood Culture Timing[1]	-	-	97%	98%
Pregnancy and Delivery Care				
Newborn Deliveries Scheduled Early[5]	-	-	6%	6%
Preventive Care				
Immunization for Influenza[5]	-	-	84%	90%
Immunization for Pneumonia[5]	-	-	88%	92%
Stroke Care				
Anticoagulation Therapy for Atrial Fibrillation[5]	-	-	96%	95%
Antithrombotic Therapy Timing[5]	-	-	98%	98%
Assessed for Rehabilitation[5]	-	-	97%	97%
Discharged on Antithrombotic Therapy[5]	-	-	100%	99%
Discharged on Statin Medication[5]	-	-	91%	94%
Thrombolytic Therapy Timing[5]	-	-	96%	66%
Venous Thromboembolism Prophylaxis[5]	-	-	96%	94%

NOTE: Hospital profiles are in alphabetical order by state, then city, then hospital within the city; Rankings exclude hospitals with less than 25 cases except for patient surveys which excludes hospitals with less than 100 cases; (a) 100-299 cases; (1) The number of cases/patients is too few to report; (2) Data submitted were based on a sample of cases/patients; (3) Results are based on a shorter time period than required; (4) Data suppressed by CMS for one or more quarters; (5) Results are not available for this reporting period; (6) Fewer than 100 patients completed the HCAHPS survey; (7) No cases met the criteria for this measure; (8) The lower limit of the confidence interval cannot be calculated if the number of observed infections equals zero; (9) No data are available from the state/territory for this reporting period; (10) The scores shown reflect fewer than 50 completed surveys; (11) There were discrepancies in the data collection process; (12) This measure does not apply to this hospital for this reporting period; (13) Results cannot be calculated for this reporting period; (14) The results for this state are combined with nearby states to protect confidentiality; Please refer to the User's Guide for a full explanation of data.

Measure	Cases	This Hosp.	State Avg.	U.S. Avg.
Written Stroke Educational Materials Given[5]	-	-	86%	88%
Surgical Care Improvement Project				
Appropriate Beta Blocker Usage[5]	-	-	99%	98%
Appropriate VTP Within 24 Hours[5]	-	-	98%	98%
Controlled Postoperative Blood Glucose[5]	-	-	95%	97%
Perioperative Temperature Management[5]	-	-	100%	100%
Prophylactic Antibiotic Selection[5]	-	-	99%	99%
Prophylactic Antibiotic Selection (Outpatient)[5]	-	-	97%	98%
Prophylactic Antibiotic Stopped[5]	-	-	99%	98%
Prophylactic Antibiotic Timing[5]	-	-	98%	99%
Prophylactic Antibiotic Timing (Outpatient)[5]	-	-	96%	98%
Urinary Catheter Removal[5]	-	-	97%	97%
Survey of Patients' Hospital Experiences				
Area Around Room 'Always' Quiet at Night[10]	<100	67%	66%	61%
Doctors 'Always' Communicated Well[10]	<100	87%	84%	82%
Home Recovery Information Given[10]	<100	89%	82%	85%
Hospital Given 9 or 10 on 10 Point Scale[10]	<100	64%	70%	71%
Meds 'Always' Explained Before Given[10]	<100	76%	67%	64%
Nurses 'Always' Communicated Well[10]	<100	72%	80%	79%
Pain 'Always' Well Controlled[10]	<100	81%	69%	71%
Room and Bathroom 'Always' Clean[10]	<100	74%	78%	73%
Timely Help 'Always' Received[10]	<100	88%	74%	68%
Would Definitely Recommend Hospital[10]	<100	85%	73%	71%
Use of Medical Imaging				
Cardiac Imaging Stress Test before Surgery[7]	-	-	4.6%	5.3%
Combination Abdominal CT Scan[1]	-	-	11.8%	10.5%
Combination Brain/Sinus CT Scan[1]	-	-	2.2%	2.7%
Combination Chest CT Scan[1]	-	-	2%	2.7%
Follow-up Mammogram/Ultrasound[7]	-	-	7.8%	8.8%
Lumbar Spine MRI for Low Back Pain[1]	-	-	32.9%	37.2%

Community Memorial Hospital

220 5th Ave W
Turtle Lake, ND 58575
Phone: 701-448-2331
Type: Critical Access Hospitals
Emergency Services: Yes
Ownership: Voluntary non-profit - Church

Measure	Cases	This Hosp.	State Avg.	U.S. Avg.
Blood Clot Prevention and Treatment				
Anticoagulation Overlap Therapy[5]	-	-	97%	93%
ICU Venous Thromboembolism Prophylaxis[5]	-	-	88%	92%
Incidence of Potentially Preventable VTE[5]	-	-	16%	10%
UFH with Dosages/Platelet Monitoring[5]	-	-	100%	97%
Venous Thromboembolism Prophylaxis[5]	-	-	80%	85%
Warfarin Therapy Discharge Instructions[5]	-	-	72%	75%
Chest Pain/Possible Heart Attack Care				
Aspirin Given Within 24 Hours of Arrival[5]	-	-	95%	96%
Fibrinolytic Meds Within 30 Min. of Arrival[5]	-	-	51%	58%
Average Time to ECG (minutes)[5]	-	-	11	7
Average Time to Transfer (minutes)[5]	-	-	114	60
Children's Asthma Care				
Received Home Management Plan of Care	-	-	-	88%
Received Reliever Medication	-	-	-	100%
Received Systemic Corticosteroids	-	-	-	100%
Emergency Department				
Admittance Decision Time (minutes)[5]	-	-	66	98
Head CT Results Within 45 Min. of Arrival[5]	-	-	25%	57%
Patients Who Left ER Before Being Seen	459	0%	1%	2%
Time from ER Arrival to Admit. (minutes)[5]	-	-	201	274
Time from ER Arrival to Discharge (minutes)[5]	-	-	112	134
Time in ER Before Being Evaluated (minutes)[5]	-	-	22	26
Time to Pain Meds for Fractures (minutes)[5]	-	-	52	57
Heart Attack Care				
Aspirin Given at Discharge[5]	-	-	99%	99%
Fibrinolytic Meds Within 30 Min. of Arrival[5]	-	-	17%	54%
PCI Within 90 Minutes of Arrival[5]	-	-	93%	96%
Statin Prescribed at Discharge[5]	-	-	98%	98%
Heart Failure Care				
ACE Inhibitor or ARB for LVSD[5]	-	-	96%	97%
Discharge Instructions Given[5]	-	-	94%	94%
Evaluation of LVS Function[5]	-	-	96%	99%
Medicare Spending				
Medicare Spending per Patient (ratio)	-	-	0.9	0.98
Pneumonia Care				
Appropriate Initial Antibiotic Given[1,2]	-	-	94%	95%
Blood Culture Timing[1,2]	-	-	97%	98%
Pregnancy and Delivery Care				
Newborn Deliveries Scheduled Early[5]	-	-	6%	6%
Preventive Care				
Immunization for Influenza[5]	-	-	84%	90%
Immunization for Pneumonia[5]	-	-	88%	92%
Stroke Care				
Anticoagulation Therapy for Atrial Fibrillation[5]	-	-	96%	95%
Antithrombotic Therapy Timing[5]	-	-	98%	98%
Assessed for Rehabilitation[5]	-	-	97%	97%
Discharged on Antithrombotic Therapy[5]	-	-	100%	99%
Discharged on Statin Medication[5]	-	-	91%	94%
Thrombolytic Therapy Timing[5]	-	-	96%	66%
Venous Thromboembolism Prophylaxis[5]	-	-	96%	94%
Written Stroke Educational Materials Given[5]	-	-	86%	88%
Surgical Care Improvement Project				
Appropriate Beta Blocker Usage[5]	-	-	99%	98%
Appropriate VTP Within 24 Hours[5]	-	-	98%	98%
Controlled Postoperative Blood Glucose[5]	-	-	95%	97%
Perioperative Temperature Management[5]	-	-	100%	100%
Prophylactic Antibiotic Selection[5]	-	-	99%	99%
Prophylactic Antibiotic Selection (Outpatient)[5]	-	-	97%	98%
Prophylactic Antibiotic Stopped[5]	-	-	99%	98%
Prophylactic Antibiotic Timing[5]	-	-	98%	99%
Prophylactic Antibiotic Timing (Outpatient)[5]	-	-	96%	98%
Urinary Catheter Removal[5]	-	-	97%	97%
Survey of Patients' Hospital Experiences				
Area Around Room 'Always' Quiet at Night[5]	-	-	66%	61%
Doctors 'Always' Communicated Well[5]	-	-	84%	82%
Home Recovery Information Given[5]	-	-	82%	85%
Hospital Given 9 or 10 on 10 Point Scale[5]	-	-	70%	71%
Meds 'Always' Explained Before Given[5]	-	-	67%	64%
Nurses 'Always' Communicated Well[5]	-	-	80%	79%
Pain 'Always' Well Controlled[5]	-	-	69%	71%
Room and Bathroom 'Always' Clean[5]	-	-	78%	73%
Timely Help 'Always' Received[5]	-	-	74%	68%
Would Definitely Recommend Hospital[5]	-	-	73%	71%
Use of Medical Imaging				
Cardiac Imaging Stress Test before Surgery[7]	-	-	4.6%	5.3%
Combination Abdominal CT Scan[1]	-	-	11.8%	10.5%
Combination Brain/Sinus CT Scan[1]	-	-	2.2%	2.7%
Combination Chest CT Scan[1]	-	-	2%	2.7%
Follow-up Mammogram/Ultrasound[7]	-	-	7.8%	8.8%
Lumbar Spine MRI for Low Back Pain[7]	-	-	32.9%	37.2%

Mercy Hospital of Valley City

570 Chautauqua Blvd
Valley City, ND 58072
Phone: 701-845-6400
Type: Critical Access Hospitals
Emergency Services: Yes
Ownership: Voluntary non-profit - Church

Measure	Cases	This Hosp.	State Avg.	U.S. Avg.
Blood Clot Prevention and Treatment				
Anticoagulation Overlap Therapy[5]	-	-	97%	93%
ICU Venous Thromboembolism Prophylaxis[5]	-	-	88%	92%
Incidence of Potentially Preventable VTE[5]	-	-	16%	10%
UFH with Dosages/Platelet Monitoring[5]	-	-	100%	97%
Venous Thromboembolism Prophylaxis[5]	-	-	80%	85%
Warfarin Therapy Discharge Instructions[5]	-	-	72%	75%
Chest Pain/Possible Heart Attack Care				
Aspirin Given Within 24 Hours of Arrival	29	97%	95%	96%
Fibrinolytic Meds Within 30 Min. of Arrival[7]	-	-	51%	58%
Average Time to ECG (minutes)	29	3	11	7
Average Time to Transfer (minutes)[7]	-	-	114	60
Children's Asthma Care				
Received Home Management Plan of Care	-	-	-	88%
Received Reliever Medication	-	-	-	100%
Received Systemic Corticosteroids	-	-	-	100%
Emergency Department				
Admittance Decision Time (minutes)[2,3]	33	14	66	98
Head CT Results Within 45 Min. of Arrival[5]	-	-	25%	57%
Patients Who Left ER Before Being Seen	3,294	0%	1%	2%
Time from ER Arrival to Admit. (minutes)[2,3]	33	115	201	274
Time from ER Arrival to Discharge (minutes)[5]	-	-	112	134
Time in ER Before Being Evaluated (minutes)[5]	-	-	22	26
Time to Pain Meds for Fractures (minutes)[5]	-	-	52	57
Heart Attack Care				
Aspirin Given at Discharge[1]	-	-	99%	99%
Fibrinolytic Meds Within 30 Min. of Arrival[7]	-	-	17%	54%
PCI Within 90 Minutes of Arrival[7]	-	-	93%	96%
Statin Prescribed at Discharge[1]	-	-	98%	98%
Heart Failure Care				
ACE Inhibitor or ARB for LVSD[1]	-	-	96%	97%
Discharge Instructions Given[1]	-	-	94%	94%
Evaluation of LVS Function	17	100%	96%	99%
Medicare Spending				
Medicare Spending per Patient (ratio)	-	-	0.9	0.98
Pneumonia Care				
Appropriate Initial Antibiotic Given	18	100%	94%	95%
Blood Culture Timing	21	95%	97%	98%
Pregnancy and Delivery Care				
Newborn Deliveries Scheduled Early[5]	-	-	6%	6%
Preventive Care				
Immunization for Influenza[2]	39	79%	84%	90%
Immunization for Pneumonia[2,3]	50	88%	88%	92%
Stroke Care				
Anticoagulation Therapy for Atrial Fibrillation[5]	-	-	96%	95%
Antithrombotic Therapy Timing[5]	-	-	98%	98%
Assessed for Rehabilitation[5]	-	-	97%	97%
Discharged on Antithrombotic Therapy[5]	-	-	100%	99%
Discharged on Statin Medication[5]	-	-	91%	94%
Thrombolytic Therapy Timing[5]	-	-	96%	66%
Venous Thromboembolism Prophylaxis[5]	-	-	96%	94%
Written Stroke Educational Materials Given[5]	-	-	86%	88%
Surgical Care Improvement Project				
Appropriate Beta Blocker Usage[5]	-	-	99%	98%
Appropriate VTP Within 24 Hours[5]	-	-	98%	98%
Controlled Postoperative Blood Glucose[5]	-	-	95%	97%
Perioperative Temperature Management[5]	-	-	100%	100%
Prophylactic Antibiotic Selection[5]	-	-	99%	99%
Prophylactic Antibiotic Selection (Outpatient)[5]	-	-	97%	98%
Prophylactic Antibiotic Stopped[5]	-	-	99%	98%
Prophylactic Antibiotic Timing[5]	-	-	98%	99%
Prophylactic Antibiotic Timing (Outpatient)[5]	-	-	96%	98%
Urinary Catheter Removal[5]	-	-	97%	97%
Survey of Patients' Hospital Experiences				
Area Around Room 'Always' Quiet at Night[6]	<100	70%	66%	61%
Doctors 'Always' Communicated Well[6]	<100	83%	84%	82%
Home Recovery Information Given[6]	<100	85%	82%	85%
Hospital Given 9 or 10 on 10 Point Scale[6]	<100	65%	70%	71%
Meds 'Always' Explained Before Given[6]	<100	66%	67%	64%
Nurses 'Always' Communicated Well[6]	<100	82%	80%	79%
Pain 'Always' Well Controlled[6]	<100	74%	69%	71%
Room and Bathroom 'Always' Clean[6]	<100	75%	78%	73%
Timely Help 'Always' Received[6]	<100	74%	74%	68%
Would Definitely Recommend Hospital[6]	<100	64%	73%	71%
Use of Medical Imaging				
Cardiac Imaging Stress Test before Surgery[1]	-	-	4.6%	5.3%
Combination Abdominal CT Scan	71	7.0%	11.8%	10.5%
Combination Brain/Sinus CT Scan[1]	-	-	2.2%	2.7%
Combination Chest CT Scan	71	0.0%	2%	2.7%
Follow-up Mammogram/Ultrasound[1]	-	-	7.8%	8.8%
Lumbar Spine MRI for Low Back Pain[1]	-	-	32.9%	37.2%

McKenzie County Healthcare Systems

516 North Main St
Watford City, ND 58854
Phone: 701-842-3000
Fax: 701-842-6248
Type: Critical Access Hospitals
Emergency Services: Yes
Ownership: Voluntary non-profit - Private
Beds: 24

Key Personnel:

CEO . . . . Daniel Kelly
Cardiology . . . . Robert Oatfield
Chief of Medical Staff. . . . . Gary Ramage, MD

Measure	Cases	This Hosp.	State Avg.	U.S. Avg.

NOTE: Hospital profiles are in alphabetical order by state, then city, then hospital within the city; Rankings exclude hospitals with less than 25 cases except for patient surveys which excludes hospitals with less than 100 cases; (a) 100-299 cases; (1) The number of cases/patients is too few to report; (2) Data submitted were based on a sample of cases/patients; (3) Results are based on a shorter time period than required; (4) Data suppressed by CMS for one or more quarters; (5) Results are not available for this reporting period; (6) Fewer than 100 patients completed the HCAHPS survey; (7) No cases met the criteria for this measure; (8) The lower limit of the confidence interval cannot be calculated if the number of observed infections equals zero; (9) No data are available from the state/territory for this reporting period; (10) The scores shown reflect fewer than 50 completed surveys; (11) There were discrepancies in the data collection process; (12) This measure does not apply to this hospital for this reporting period; (13) Results cannot be calculated for this reporting period; (14) The results for this state are combined with nearby states to protect confidentiality; Please refer to the User's Guide for a full explanation of data.

Measure	Cases	This Hosp.	State Avg.	U.S. Avg.
Blood Clot Prevention and Treatment				
Anticoagulation Overlap Therapy[5]	-	-	97%	93%
ICU Venous Thromboembolism Prophylaxis[5]	-	-	88%	92%
Incidence of Potentially Preventable VTE[5]	-	-	16%	10%
UFH with Dosages/Platelet Monitoring[5]	-	-	100%	97%
Venous Thromboembolism Prophylaxis[5]	-	-	80%	85%
Warfarin Therapy Discharge Instructions[5]	-	-	72%	75%
Chest Pain/Possible Heart Attack Care				
Aspirin Given Within 24 Hours of Arrival	13	77%	95%	96%
Fibrinolytic Meds Within 30 Min. of Arrival[1,3]	-	-	51%	58%
Average Time to ECG (minutes)	13	5	11	7
Average Time to Transfer (minutes)[1,3]	-	-	114	60
Children's Asthma Care				
Received Home Management Plan of Care	-	-	-	88%
Received Reliever Medication	-	-	-	100%
Received Systemic Corticosteroids	-	-	-	100%
Emergency Department				
Admittance Decision Time (minutes)[5]	-	-	66	98
Head CT Results Within 45 Min. of Arrival[5]	-	-	25%	57%
Patients Who Left ER Before Being Seen	5,298	0%	1%	2%
Time from ER Arrival to Admit. (minutes)[5]	-	-	201	274
Time from ER Arrival to Discharge (minutes)[5]	-	-	112	134
Time in ER Before Being Evaluated (minutes)[5]	-	-	22	26
Time to Pain Meds for Fractures (minutes)[5]	-	-	52	57
Heart Attack Care				
Aspirin Given at Discharge[5]	-	-	99%	99%
Fibrinolytic Meds Within 30 Min. of Arrival[5]	-	-	17%	54%
PCI Within 90 Minutes of Arrival[5]	-	-	93%	96%
Statin Prescribed at Discharge[5]	-	-	98%	98%
Heart Failure Care				
ACE Inhibitor or ARB for LVSD[1,2]	-	-	96%	97%
Discharge Instructions Given[1,2]	-	-	94%	94%
Evaluation of LVS Function[1,2]	-	-	96%	99%
Medicare Spending				
Medicare Spending per Patient (ratio)	-	-	0.9	0.98
Pneumonia Care				
Appropriate Initial Antibiotic Given[2]	22	86%	94%	95%
Blood Culture Timing[1,2]	-	-	97%	98%
Pregnancy and Delivery Care				
Newborn Deliveries Scheduled Early[5]	-	-	6%	6%
Preventive Care				
Immunization for Influenza[5]	-	-	84%	90%
Immunization for Pneumonia[5]	-	-	88%	92%
Stroke Care				
Anticoagulation Therapy for Atrial Fibrillation[5]	-	-	96%	95%
Antithrombotic Therapy Timing[5]	-	-	98%	98%
Assessed for Rehabilitation[5]	-	-	97%	97%
Discharged on Antithrombotic Therapy[5]	-	-	100%	99%
Discharged on Statin Medication[5]	-	-	91%	94%
Thrombolytic Therapy Timing[5]	-	-	96%	66%
Venous Thromboembolism Prophylaxis[5]	-	-	96%	94%
Written Stroke Educational Materials Given[5]	-	-	86%	88%
Surgical Care Improvement Project				
Appropriate Beta Blocker Usage[5]	-	-	99%	98%
Appropriate VTP Within 24 Hours[5]	-	-	98%	98%
Controlled Postoperative Blood Glucose[5]	-	-	95%	97%
Perioperative Temperature Management[5]	-	-	100%	100%
Prophylactic Antibiotic Selection[5]	-	-	99%	99%
Prophylactic Antibiotic Selection (Outpatient)[5]	-	-	97%	98%
Prophylactic Antibiotic Stopped[5]	-	-	99%	98%
Prophylactic Antibiotic Timing[5]	-	-	98%	99%
Prophylactic Antibiotic Timing (Outpatient)[5]	-	-	96%	98%
Urinary Catheter Removal[5]	-	-	97%	97%
Survey of Patients' Hospital Experiences				
Area Around Room 'Always' Quiet at Night[10]	<100	67%	66%	61%
Doctors 'Always' Communicated Well[10]	<100	75%	84%	82%
Home Recovery Information Given[10]	<100	76%	82%	85%
Hospital Given 9 or 10 on 10 Point Scale[10]	<100	35%	70%	71%
Meds 'Always' Explained Before Given[10]	<100	47%	67%	64%
Nurses 'Always' Communicated Well[10]	<100	69%	80%	79%
Pain 'Always' Well Controlled[10]	<100	38%	69%	71%
Room and Bathroom 'Always' Clean[10]	<100	85%	78%	73%
Timely Help 'Always' Received[10]	<100	74%	74%	68%
Would Definitely Recommend Hospital[10]	<100	45%	73%	71%
Use of Medical Imaging				
Cardiac Imaging Stress Test before Surgery[7]	-	-	4.6%	5.3%
Combination Abdominal CT Scan[1]	-	-	11.8%	10.5%
Combination Brain/Sinus CT Scan[1]	-	-	2.2%	2.7%
Combination Chest CT Scan[1]	-	-	2%	2.7%
Follow-up Mammogram/Ultrasound[1]	-	-	7.8%	8.8%
Lumbar Spine MRI for Low Back Pain[7]	-	-	32.9%	37.2%

Mercy Medical Center

1301 15th Ave W
Williston, ND 58801
URL: www.mercy-williston.org
Type: Critical Access Hospitals
Ownership: Voluntary non-profit - Church
Phone: 701-774-7400
Fax: 701-774-7479
Emergency Services: Yes
Beds: 25

Key Personnel:
Intensive Care Unit. . . . . Lorrie Antos
Radiology. . . . . Barb Cook
Cardiac Laboratory. . . . . Gloria Fenster
Quality Assurance . . . . Lori Hahn
Operating Room. . . . . Rod Kerzmann
Infection Control. . . . . James Moe
Patient Relations . . . . Tami Solberg
Chief of Medical Staff. . . . . B K Vibeto, MD

Measure	Cases	This Hosp.	State Avg.	U.S. Avg.
Blood Clot Prevention and Treatment				
Anticoagulation Overlap Therapy[1,2]	-	-	97%	93%
ICU Venous Thromboembolism Prophylaxis[1,2]	-	-	88%	92%
Incidence of Potentially Preventable VTE[2,7]	-	-	16%	10%
UFH with Dosages/Platelet Monitoring[1,2]	-	-	100%	97%
Venous Thromboembolism Prophylaxis[2]	90	94%	80%	85%
Warfarin Therapy Discharge Instructions[1,2]	-	-	72%	75%
Chest Pain/Possible Heart Attack Care				
Aspirin Given Within 24 Hours of Arrival	14	100%	95%	96%
Fibrinolytic Meds Within 30 Min. of Arrival[1]	-	-	51%	58%
Average Time to ECG (minutes)	14	16	11	7
Average Time to Transfer (minutes)[1]	-	-	114	60
Children's Asthma Care				
Received Home Management Plan of Care	-	-	-	88%
Received Reliever Medication	-	-	-	100%
Received Systemic Corticosteroids	-	-	-	100%
Emergency Department				
Admittance Decision Time (minutes)[2]	168	44	66	98
Head CT Results Within 45 Min. of Arrival	20	25%	25%	57%
Patients Who Left ER Before Being Seen	17,362	4%	1%	2%
Time from ER Arrival to Admit. (minutes)[2]	209	208	201	274
Time from ER Arrival to Discharge (minutes)	399	107	112	134
Time in ER Before Being Evaluated (minutes)	425	40	22	26
Time to Pain Meds for Fractures (minutes)	78	61	52	57
Heart Attack Care				
Aspirin Given at Discharge[3,7]	-	-	99%	99%
Fibrinolytic Meds Within 30 Min. of Arrival[3,7]	-	-	17%	54%
PCI Within 90 Minutes of Arrival[3,7]	-	-	93%	96%
Statin Prescribed at Discharge[3,7]	-	-	98%	98%
Heart Failure Care				
ACE Inhibitor or ARB for LVSD[1]	-	-	96%	97%
Discharge Instructions Given	21	90%	94%	94%
Evaluation of LVS Function	23	91%	96%	99%
Medicare Spending				
Medicare Spending per Patient (ratio)	-	-	0.9	0.98
Pneumonia Care				
Appropriate Initial Antibiotic Given	45	87%	94%	95%
Blood Culture Timing	58	95%	97%	98%
Pregnancy and Delivery Care				
Newborn Deliveries Scheduled Early[3]	28	11%	6%	6%
Preventive Care				
Immunization for Influenza[2]	250	73%	84%	90%
Immunization for Pneumonia[2]	180	71%	88%	92%
Stroke Care				
Anticoagulation Therapy for Atrial Fibrillation[1,3]	-	-	96%	95%
Antithrombotic Therapy Timing[1,3]	-	-	98%	98%
Assessed for Rehabilitation[1,3]	-	-	97%	97%
Discharged on Antithrombotic Therapy[1,3]	-	-	100%	99%
Discharged on Statin Medication[1,3]	-	-	91%	94%
Thrombolytic Therapy Timing[1,3]	-	-	96%	66%
Venous Thromboembolism Prophylaxis[1,3]	-	-	96%	94%
Written Stroke Educational Materials Given[3,7]	-	-	86%	88%
Surgical Care Improvement Project				
Appropriate Beta Blocker Usage	21	95%	99%	98%
Appropriate VTP Within 24 Hours	94	98%	98%	98%
Controlled Postoperative Blood Glucose[7]	-	-	95%	97%
Perioperative Temperature Management	100	100%	100%	100%
Prophylactic Antibiotic Selection	60	100%	99%	99%
Prophylactic Antibiotic Selection (Outpatient)	49	100%	97%	98%
Prophylactic Antibiotic Stopped	60	97%	99%	98%
Prophylactic Antibiotic Timing	61	90%	98%	99%
Prophylactic Antibiotic Timing (Outpatient)	49	92%	96%	98%
Urinary Catheter Removal	44	98%	97%	97%
Survey of Patients' Hospital Experiences				
Area Around Room 'Always' Quiet at Night	300+	67%	66%	61%
Doctors 'Always' Communicated Well	300+	81%	84%	82%
Home Recovery Information Given	300+	89%	82%	85%
Hospital Given 9 or 10 on 10 Point Scale	300+	55%	70%	71%
Meds 'Always' Explained Before Given	300+	67%	67%	64%
Nurses 'Always' Communicated Well	300+	73%	80%	79%
Pain 'Always' Well Controlled	300+	63%	69%	71%
Room and Bathroom 'Always' Clean	300+	62%	78%	73%
Timely Help 'Always' Received	300+	65%	74%	68%
Would Definitely Recommend Hospital	300+	58%	73%	71%
Use of Medical Imaging				
Cardiac Imaging Stress Test before Surgery[1]	-	-	4.6%	5.3%
Combination Abdominal CT Scan	245	14.3%	11.8%	10.5%
Combination Brain/Sinus CT Scan[1]	-	-	2.2%	2.7%
Combination Chest CT Scan	131	9.2%	2%	2.7%
Follow-up Mammogram/Ultrasound	318	10.7%	7.8%	8.8%
Lumbar Spine MRI for Low Back Pain[1]	-	-	32.9%	37.2%

Wishek Community Hospital

1007 4th Ave S
Wishek, ND 58495
E-mail: wchcbek@bektel.com
URL: www.wishekhospital.com
Type: Critical Access Hospitals
Ownership: Voluntary non-profit - Private
Phone: 701-452-2326
Fax: 701-452-2392
Emergency Services: Yes
Beds: 24

Key Personnel:
Quality Assurance . . . . Shelly Glaseman
Emergency Room . . . . Calli Klusmann
Operating Room. . . . . Calli Klusmann
Patient Relations . . . . Katie Lu Bvee
CEO . . . . Mark Rinehardt
Chief of Medical Staff. . . . . Amy Smittle, D.O.
Radiology. . . . . Jo Vilhauer
Infection Control. . . . . Stacy Wiest

Measure	Cases	This Hosp.	State Avg.	U.S. Avg.
Blood Clot Prevention and Treatment				
Anticoagulation Overlap Therapy[5]	-	-	97%	93%
ICU Venous Thromboembolism Prophylaxis[5]	-	-	88%	92%
Incidence of Potentially Preventable VTE[5]	-	-	16%	10%
UFH with Dosages/Platelet Monitoring[5]	-	-	100%	97%
Venous Thromboembolism Prophylaxis[5]	-	-	80%	85%
Warfarin Therapy Discharge Instructions[5]	-	-	72%	75%
Chest Pain/Possible Heart Attack Care				
Aspirin Given Within 24 Hours of Arrival[1,3]	-	-	95%	96%
Fibrinolytic Meds Within 30 Min. of Arrival[3,7]	-	-	51%	58%
Average Time to ECG (minutes)[1,3]	-	-	11	7
Average Time to Transfer (minutes)[1,3]	-	-	114	60
Children's Asthma Care				
Received Home Management Plan of Care	-	-	-	88%
Received Reliever Medication	-	-	-	100%
Received Systemic Corticosteroids	-	-	-	100%
Emergency Department				
Admittance Decision Time (minutes)[5]	-	-	66	98
Head CT Results Within 45 Min. of Arrival[5]	-	-	25%	57%
Patients Who Left ER Before Being Seen	895	0%	1%	2%
Time from ER Arrival to Admit. (minutes)[5]	-	-	201	274
Time from ER Arrival to Discharge (minutes)[5]	-	-	112	134
Time in ER Before Being Evaluated (minutes)[5]	-	-	22	26

NOTE: Hospital profiles are in alphabetical order by state, then city, then hospital within the city; Rankings exclude hospitals with less than 25 cases except for patient surveys which excludes hospitals with less than 100 cases; (a) 100-299 cases; (1) The number of cases/patients is too few to report; (2) Data submitted were based on a sample of cases/patients; (3) Results are based on a shorter time period than required; (4) Data suppressed by CMS for one or more quarters; (5) Results are not available for this reporting period; (6) Fewer than 100 patients completed the HCAHPS survey; (7) No cases met the criteria for this measure; (8) The lower limit of the confidence interval cannot be calculated if the number of observed infections equals zero; (9) No data are available from the state/territory for this reporting period; (10) The scores shown reflect fewer than 50 completed surveys; (11) There were discrepancies in the data collection process; (12) This measure does not apply to this hospital for this reporting period; (13) Results cannot be calculated for this reporting period; (14) The results for this state are combined with nearby states to protect confidentiality; Please refer to the User's Guide for a full explanation of data.

Time to Pain Meds for Fractures (minutes)[5]	-	-	52	57
Heart Attack Care				
Aspirin Given at Discharge[1,3]	-	-	99%	99%
Fibrinolytic Meds Within 30 Min. of Arrival[3,7]	-	-	17%	54%
PCI Within 90 Minutes of Arrival[3,7]	-	-	93%	96%
Statin Prescribed at Discharge[1,3]	-	-	98%	98%
Heart Failure Care				
ACE Inhibitor or ARB for LVSD[1]	-	-	96%	97%
Discharge Instructions Given[1]	-	-	94%	94%
Evaluation of LVS Function[1]	-	-	96%	99%
Medicare Spending				
Medicare Spending per Patient (ratio)	-	-	0.9	0.98
Pneumonia Care				
Appropriate Initial Antibiotic Given	17	82%	94%	95%
Blood Culture Timing[1]	-	-	97%	98%
Pregnancy and Delivery Care				
Newborn Deliveries Scheduled Early[5]	-	-	6%	6%
Preventive Care				
Immunization for Influenza[5]	-	-	84%	90%
Immunization for Pneumonia[5]	-	-	88%	92%
Stroke Care				
Anticoagulation Therapy for Atrial Fibrillation[5]	-	-	96%	95%
Antithrombotic Therapy Timing[5]	-	-	98%	98%
Assessed for Rehabilitation[5]	-	-	97%	97%
Discharged on Antithrombotic Therapy[5]	-	-	100%	99%
Discharged on Statin Medication[5]	-	-	91%	94%
Thrombolytic Therapy Timing[5]	-	-	96%	66%
Venous Thromboembolism Prophylaxis[5]	-	-	96%	94%
Written Stroke Educational Materials Given[5]	-	-	86%	88%
Surgical Care Improvement Project				
Appropriate Beta Blocker Usage[5]	-	-	99%	98%
Appropriate VTP Within 24 Hours[5]	-	-	98%	98%
Controlled Postoperative Blood Glucose[5]	-	-	95%	97%
Perioperative Temperature Management[5]	-	-	100%	100%
Prophylactic Antibiotic Selection[5]	-	-	99%	99%
Prophylactic Antibiotic Selection (Outpatient)[5]	-	-	97%	98%
Prophylactic Antibiotic Stopped[5]	-	-	99%	98%
Prophylactic Antibiotic Timing[5]	-	-	98%	99%
Prophylactic Antibiotic Timing (Outpatient)[5]	-	-	96%	98%
Urinary Catheter Removal[5]	-	-	97%	97%
Survey of Patients' Hospital Experiences				
Area Around Room 'Always' Quiet at Night[6]	<100	54%	66%	61%
Doctors 'Always' Communicated Well[6]	<100	86%	84%	82%
Home Recovery Information Given[6]	<100	76%	82%	85%
Hospital Given 9 or 10 on 10 Point Scale[6]	<100	50%	70%	71%
Meds 'Always' Explained Before Given[6]	<100	44%	67%	64%
Nurses 'Always' Communicated Well[6]	<100	72%	80%	79%
Pain 'Always' Well Controlled[6]	<100	54%	69%	71%
Room and Bathroom 'Always' Clean[6]	<100	75%	78%	73%
Timely Help 'Always' Received[6]	<100	74%	74%	68%
Would Definitely Recommend Hospital[6]	<100	75%	73%	71%
Use of Medical Imaging				
Cardiac Imaging Stress Test before Surgery[1]	-	-	4.6%	5.3%
Combination Abdominal CT Scan[1]	-	-	11.8%	10.5%
Combination Brain/Sinus CT Scan[1]	-	-	2.2%	2.7%
Combination Chest CT Scan[1]	-	-	2%	2.7%
Follow-up Mammogram/Ultrasound	100	3.0%	7.8%	8.8%
Lumbar Spine MRI for Low Back Pain[1]	-	-	32.9%	37.2%

NOTE: Hospital profiles are in alphabetical order by state, then city, then hospital within the city; Rankings exclude hospitals with less than 25 cases except for patient surveys which excludes hospitals with less than 100 cases; (a) 100-299 cases; (1) The number of cases/patients is too few to report; (2) Data submitted were based on a sample of cases/patients; (3) Results are based on a shorter time period than required; (4) Data suppressed by CMS for one or more quarters; (5) Results are not available for this reporting period; (6) Fewer than 100 patients completed the HCAHPS survey; (7) No cases met the criteria for this measure; (8) The lower limit of the confidence interval cannot be calculated if the number of observed infections equals zero; (9) No data are available from the state/territory for this reporting period; (10) The scores shown reflect fewer than 50 completed surveys; (11) There were discrepancies in the data collection process; (12) This measure does not apply to this hospital for this reporting period; (13) Results cannot be calculated for this reporting period; (14) The results for this state are combined with nearby states to protect confidentiality; Please refer to the User's Guide for a full explanation of data.

Blood Clot Prevention and Treatment

Anticoagulation Overlap Therapy

Hospital Name	City	Rate	Cases
Hillcrest Hospital South[2]	Tulsa	100%	28
Mercy Hospital Ada[2]	Ada	100%	27
Hillcrest Medical Center[2]	Tulsa	98%	98
O U Medical Center[2]	Oklahoma City	98%	124
Duncan Regional Hospital[2]	Duncan	97%	30
Comanche County Memorial Hospital[2]	Lawton	94%	36
Eastar Health System[2]	Muskogee	93%	59
Midwest Regional Medical Center[2]	Midwest City	93%	45
Saint Anthony Hospital[2]	Oklahoma City	93%	117
Mercy Memorial Health Center[2]	Ardmore	92%	38
Norman Regional Health System[2]	Norman	92%	128
Oklahoma Heart Hospital[2]	Oklahoma City	92%	40
Saint Anthony Shawnee Hospital[2]	Shawnee	92%	25
Saint John Medical Center[2]	Tulsa	92%	142
Oklahoma State University Medical Center[2]	Tulsa	90%	42
Integris Baptist Medical Center[2]	Oklahoma City	89%	134
Integris Southwest Medical Center[2]	Oklahoma City	85%	67
Deaconess Hospital[2]	Oklahoma City	84%	43
Mercy Hospital Oklahoma City[2]	Oklahoma City	84%	93
Saint Francis Hospital[2]	Tulsa	82%	155

ICU Venous Thromboembolism Prophylaxis

Hospital Name	City	Rate	Cases
Hillcrest Medical Center[2]	Tulsa	100%	101
Mercy Hospital Oklahoma City[2]	Oklahoma City	100%	74
Oklahoma Heart Hospital[2]	Oklahoma City	100%	100
Oklahoma Heart Hospital South[2]	Oklahoma City	100%	84
Woodward Regional Hospital[2]	Woodward	100%	88
Jane Phillips Medical Center[2]	Bartlesville	98%	63
Saint Anthony Shawnee Hospital[2]	Shawnee	98%	94
O U Medical Center[2]	Oklahoma City	97%	114
W W Hastings Indian Hospital[2]	Tahlequah	96%	57
Claremore Indian Hospital[2]	Claremore	95%	44
Saint Anthony Hospital[2]	Oklahoma City	95%	103
Saint Francis Hospital[2]	Tulsa	95%	116
Hillcrest Hospital South[2]	Tulsa	94%	84
Integris Baptist Regional Health Center[2]	Miami	94%	33
Medical Center of Southeastern Oklahoma[2]	Durant	94%	53
Saint Francis Hospital South[2]	Tulsa	94%	62
Saint John Medical Center[2]	Tulsa	94%	90
Integris Southwest Medical Center[2]	Oklahoma City	93%	81
Ponca City Medical Center[2]	Ponca City	93%	42
Eastar Health System[2]	Muskogee	91%	131
Duncan Regional Hospital[2]	Duncan	90%	78
Southwestern Medical Center[2]	Lawton	90%	63
Saint Mary's Regional Medical Center[2]	Enid	89%	62
Southwestern Regional Medical Center[2]	Tulsa	89%	28
Mercy Memorial Health Center[2]	Ardmore	88%	51
Deaconess Hospital[2]	Oklahoma City	87%	54
Stillwater Medical Center[2]	Stillwater	87%	55
Norman Regional Health System[2]	Norman	86%	69
Comanche County Memorial Hospital[2]	Lawton	84%	86
Integris Baptist Medical Center[2]	Oklahoma City	84%	105
Great Plains Regional Medical Center[2]	Elk City	83%	48
Hillcrest Hospital Claremore[2]	Claremore	82%	55
Tahlequah City Hospital[2]	Tahlequah	82%	87
Integris Health Edmond[2]	Edmond	80%	25
Eastern Oklahoma Medical Center[2]	Poteau	78%	184
Oklahoma State University Medical Center[2]	Tulsa	78%	166
Integris Canadian Valley Hospital[2]	Yukon	77%	44
McAlester Regional Health Center[2]	Mcalester	77%	98
Mercy Hospital Ada[2]	Ada	76%	49
Midwest Regional Medical Center[2]	Midwest City	74%	87
Integris Grove Hospital[2]	Grove	71%	35
Chickasaw Nation Medical Center[2]	Ada	70%	37
Grady Memorial Hospital[2]	Chickasha	70%	27
Jackson County Memorial Hospital[2]	Altus	63%	51
Integris Bass Baptist Health Center[2]	Enid	61%	44
McCurtain Memorial Hospital[2]	Idabel	55%	53

Incidence of Potentially Preventable VTE

Hospital Name	City	Rate	Cases
O U Medical Center[2]	Oklahoma City	1%	122
Saint John Medical Center[2]	Tulsa	2%	51
Saint Francis Hospital[2]	Tulsa	6%	64
Integris Baptist Medical Center[2]	Oklahoma City	9%	34

UFH with Dosages/Platelet Count Monitoring

Hospital Name	City	Rate	Cases
Hillcrest Medical Center[2]	Tulsa	100%	51
O U Medical Center[2]	Oklahoma City	100%	80
Saint John Medical Center[2]	Tulsa	100%	61
Integris Baptist Medical Center[2]	Oklahoma City	98%	41
Saint Francis Hospital[2]	Tulsa	83%	60

Venous Thromboembolism Prophylaxis

Hospital Name	City	Rate	Cases
Bailey Medical Center[2]	Owasso	100%	86
Orthopedic Hospital[2]	Oklahoma City	100%	34
Surgical Hospital of Oklahoma	Oklahoma City	100%	37
Woodward Regional Hospital[2]	Woodward	100%	143
Hillcrest Hospital Cushing[2]	Cushing	99%	121
Oklahoma Heart Hospital[2]	Oklahoma City	99%	323
Oklahoma Heart Hospital South[2]	Oklahoma City	99%	272
Oklahoma Spine Hospital[2]	Oklahoma City	99%	155
Oklahoma Surgical Hospital[2]	Tulsa	99%	135
Tulsa Spine & Specialty Hospital[2]	Tulsa	99%	210
Jane Phillips Medical Center[2]	Bartlesville	98%	295
Ponca City Medical Center[2]	Ponca City	98%	203
Community Hospital[2]	Oklahoma City	97%	157
Northwest Surgical Hospital	Oklahoma City	97%	96
Saint Anthony Shawnee Hospital[2]	Shawnee	97%	270
Integris Mayes County Medical Center[2]	Pryor	95%	117
Claremore Indian Hospital[2]	Claremore	94%	54
Hillcrest Hospital South[2]	Tulsa	94%	327
Medical Center of Southeastern Oklahoma[2]	Durant	94%	340
Hillcrest Medical Center[2]	Tulsa	93%	320
O U Medical Center[2]	Oklahoma City	93%	414
Saint Francis Hospital[2]	Tulsa	93%	320
Saint John Broken Arrow[2]	Broken Arrow	93%	116
Saint John Owasso[2]	Owasso	93%	112
Saint Anthony Hospital[2]	Oklahoma City	92%	314
Saint Francis Hospital South[2]	Tulsa	92%	255
Integris Marshall County Medical Center[2]	Madill	91%	110
Saint John Medical Center[2]	Tulsa	91%	292
Summit Medical Center	Edmond	90%	60
Hillcrest Hospital Henryetta[2]	Henryetta	89%	75
Integris Baptist Regional Health Center[2]	Miami	89%	141
Eastar Health System[2]	Muskogee	88%	295
Integris Clinton Regional Hospital[2]	Clinton	88%	100
McBride Clinic Orthopedic Hospital[2]	Oklahoma City	88%	160
Stillwater Medical Center[2]	Stillwater	87%	229
W W Hastings Indian Hospital[2]	Tahlequah	86%	111
Mercy Hospital Oklahoma City[2]	Oklahoma City	85%	321
Saint Mary's Regional Medical Center[2]	Enid	85%	343
Mercy Hospital Ada[2]	Ada	82%	179
Mercy Memorial Health Center[2]	Ardmore	81%	317
Great Plains Regional Medical Center[2]	Elk City	79%	85
Oklahoma State University Medical Center[2]	Tulsa	79%	283
Southwestern Regional Medical Center[2]	Tulsa	79%	85
Comanche County Memorial Hospital[2]	Lawton	78%	370
McAlester Regional Health Center[2]	Mcalester	76%	261
Norman Regional Health System[2]	Norman	76%	320
Deaconess Hospital[2]	Oklahoma City	75%	336
Memorial Hospital of Stilwell[2]	Stilwell	75%	175
Duncan Regional Hospital[2]	Duncan	74%	264
Southwestern Medical Center[2]	Lawton	74%	235
Chickasaw Nation Medical Center[2]	Ada	73%	150
Integris Canadian Valley Hospital[2]	Yukon	73%	132
Integris Southwest Medical Center[2]	Oklahoma City	73%	343
Hillcrest Hospital Claremore[2]	Claremore	71%	194
Integris Grove Hospital[2]	Grove	71%	155
Tahlequah City Hospital[2]	Tahlequah	68%	171
Jackson County Memorial Hospital[2]	Altus	67%	235
Integris Seminole Medical Center[2]	Seminole	63%	149
Midwest Regional Medical Center[2]	Midwest City	62%	372
Integris Baptist Medical Center[2]	Oklahoma City	58%	285
Integris Blackwell Regional Hospital[2]	Blackwell	58%	161
Integris Health Edmond[2]	Edmond	58%	88
Mercy Hospital El Reno[2]	El Reno	56%	111
Integris Bass Baptist Health Center[2]	Enid	55%	251
Share Memorial Hospital	Alva	55%	87
Grady Memorial Hospital[2]	Chickasha	54%	155
Eastern Oklahoma Medical Center[2]	Poteau	53%	579
Memorial Hospital of Texas County[2]	Guymon	50%	121
USPHS Lawton Indian Hospital[2]	Lawton	45%	127
Elkview General Hospital[2]	Hobart	44%	107
Perry Memorial Hospital	Perry	44%	174
Purcell Municipal Hospital[2]	Purcell	43%	115
Newman Memorial Hospital	Shattuck	41%	81
McCurtain Memorial Hospital[2]	Idabel	38%	146
Sequoyah Co-Sallisaw Hosp Auth[2]	Sallisaw	36%	260
Pauls Valley General Hospital[2]	Pauls Valley	24%	120
Bristow Medical Center[2]	Bristow	23%	141
Wagoner Community Hospital[2]	Wagoner	22%	286
Choctaw Nation Healthcare[2]	Talihina	20%	111
Craig General Hospital[2]	Vinita	20%	152
Epic Medical Center	Eufaula	16%	77
Muscogee (Creek) Nation Medical Center[2]	Okmulgee	15%	157
Memorial Hospital & Physician Group[2]	Frederick	14%	112
Sayre Memorial Hospital[2]	Sayre	11%	155
Pushmataha Co-Antlers Town Hosp Auth[2]	Antlers	3%	110
Choctaw Memorial Hospital[2]	Hugo	2%	211
Harmon Memorial Hospital[2]	Hollis	0%	115
Latimer County General Hospital	Wilburton	0%	108

Warfarin Therapy Discharge Instructions

Hospital Name	City	Rate	Cases
Midwest Regional Medical Center[2]	Midwest City	100%	34
Oklahoma Heart Hospital[2]	Oklahoma City	100%	31
Norman Regional Health System[2]	Norman	99%	96
O U Medical Center[2]	Oklahoma City	99%	93
Deaconess Hospital[2]	Oklahoma City	97%	29
Hillcrest Medical Center[2]	Tulsa	96%	70
Eastar Health System[2]	Muskogee	90%	39
Saint Anthony Hospital[2]	Oklahoma City	83%	83
Comanche County Memorial Hospital[2]	Lawton	81%	26
Saint Francis Hospital[2]	Tulsa	74%	114
Integris Southwest Medical Center[2]	Oklahoma City	64%	53
Mercy Hospital Oklahoma City[2]	Oklahoma City	52%	66
Mercy Memorial Health Center[2]	Ardmore	42%	31
Integris Baptist Medical Center[2]	Oklahoma City	37%	101
Saint John Medical Center[2]	Tulsa	27%	101
Oklahoma State University Medical Center[2]	Tulsa	21%	28

Chest Pain/Possible Heart Attack Care

Aspirin Given Within 24 Hours of Arrival

Hospital Name	City	Rate	Cases
Bailey Medical Center	Owasso	100%	29
Great Plains Regional Medical Center	Elk City	100%	28
Integris Blackwell Regional Hospital	Blackwell	100%	26
Mercy Hospital Ada	Ada	100%	52
Mercy Hospital Oklahoma City	Oklahoma City	100%	61
Mercy Memorial Health Center	Ardmore	100%	27
O U Medical Center	Oklahoma City	100%	29
Ponca City Medical Center	Ponca City	100%	51
Saint Anthony Shawnee Hospital	Shawnee	100%	92
Saint Francis Hospital South	Tulsa	100%	32
Saint John Broken Arrow	Broken Arrow	100%	79
Woodward Regional Hospital	Woodward	100%	39
Grady Memorial Hospital	Chickasha	98%	59
Hillcrest Hospital Cushing	Cushing	98%	116
Integris Baptist Regional Health Center	Miami	98%	81
Integris Canadian Valley Hospital	Yukon	98%	59
Jackson County Memorial Hospital	Altus	98%	51
Saint John Sapulpa	Sapulpa	98%	44
Stillwater Medical Center	Stillwater	98%	48
Atoka County Medical Center	Atoka	97%	29
Cleveland Area Hospital	Cleveland	97%	29
Duncan Regional Hospital	Duncan	97%	106
Integris Grove Hospital	Grove	97%	36
Memorial Hospital of Texas County	Guymon	97%	31
Saint John Owasso	Owasso	97%	69
Hillcrest Hospital Henryetta	Henryetta	96%	46
Integris Seminole Medical Center	Seminole	96%	67
Medical Center of Southeastern Oklahoma	Durant	96%	47
Muscogee (Creek) Nation Medical Center	Okmulgee	96%	56
Bristow Medical Center	Bristow	95%	75
Integris Mayes County Medical Center	Pryor	95%	80
Midwest Regional Medical Center	Midwest City	95%	170
Arbuckle Memorial Hospital	Sulphur	94%	33
Craig General Hospital	Vinita	94%	67
Eastar Health System	Muskogee	94%	79
Pauls Valley General Hospital	Pauls Valley	93%	46
Hillcrest Hospital Claremore	Claremore	92%	38
Integris Clinton Regional Hospital	Clinton	92%	36
Weatherford Regional Hospital	Weatherford	92%	37
McAlester Regional Health Center	Mcalester	91%	57
Holdenville Hospital Authority	Holdenville	90%	51
Integris Marshall County Medical Center	Madill	90%	29
Eastern Oklahoma Medical Center	Poteau	87%	47
McCurtain Memorial Hospital	Idabel	85%	41
Sequoyah Co-Sallisaw Hosp Auth	Sallisaw	85%	46

Average Time to ECG (minutes)

Hospital Name	City	Min.	Cases
Jackson County Memorial Hospital	Altus	0	51
Saint Anthony Shawnee Hospital	Shawnee	1	95
Craig General Hospital	Vinita	3	65
Duncan Regional Hospital	Duncan	3	106
McAlester Regional Health Center	Mcalester	4	57
O U Medical Center	Oklahoma City	4	30
Woodward Regional Hospital	Woodward	4	39
Atoka County Medical Center	Atoka	5	35
Hillcrest Hospital Claremore	Claremore	5	39
Integris Baptist Regional Health Center	Miami	5	83
Integris Blackwell Regional Hospital	Blackwell	5	26
Mercy Memorial Health Center	Ardmore	5	28
Ponca City Medical Center	Ponca City	5	52
Bailey Medical Center	Owasso	6	30
Integris Canadian Valley Hospital	Yukon	6	62
Midwest Regional Medical Center	Midwest City	6	196
Saint John Owasso	Owasso	6	72
Stillwater Medical Center	Stillwater	6	50

NOTE: Hospital profiles are in alphabetical order by state, then city, then hospital within the city; Rankings exclude hospitals with less than 25 cases except for patient surveys which excludes hospitals with less than 100 cases; (a) 100-299 cases; (1) The number of cases/patients is too few to report; (2) Data submitted were based on a sample of cases/patients; (3) Results are based on a shorter time period than required; (4) Data suppressed by CMS for one or more quarters; (5) Results are not available for this reporting period; (6) Fewer than 100 patients completed the HCAHPS survey; (7) No cases met the criteria for this measure; (8) The lower limit of the confidence interval cannot be calculated if the number of observed infections equals zero; (9) No data are available from the state/territory for this reporting period; (10) The scores shown reflect fewer than 50 completed surveys; (11) There were discrepancies in the data collection process; (12) This measure does not apply to this hospital for this reporting period; (13) Results cannot be calculated for this reporting period; (14) The results for this state are combined with nearby states to protect confidentiality; Please refer to the User's Guide for a full explanation of data.

Hospital Name	City	Value	Cases
Eastern Oklahoma Medical Center	Poteau	7	44
Hillcrest Hospital Henryetta	Henryetta	7	45
Integris Clinton Regional Hospital	Clinton	7	37
Memorial Hospital of Texas County	Guymon	7	34
Saint Francis Hospital South	Tulsa	7	34
Saint John Sapulpa	Sapulpa	7	44
Eastar Health System	Muskogee	8	81
Hillcrest Hospital Cushing	Cushing	8	122
Holdenville Hospital Authority	Holdenville	8	52
Integris Seminole Medical Center	Seminole	8	72
Mercy Hospital Ada	Ada	8	54
Saint John Broken Arrow	Broken Arrow	8	81
Great Plains Regional Medical Center	Elk City	9	31
Mercy Hospital Oklahoma City	Oklahoma City	9	63
Sequoyah Co-Sallisaw Hosp Auth	Sallisaw	9	47
Arbuckle Memorial Hospital	Sulphur	10	31
Medical Center of Southeastern Oklahoma	Durant	10	52
McCurtain Memorial Hospital	Idabel	11	43
Muscogee (Creek) Nation Medical Center	Okmulgee	12	54
Cleveland Area Hospital	Cleveland	14	30
Integris Mayes County Medical Center	Pryor	14	84
Bristow Medical Center	Bristow	15	76
Grady Memorial Hospital	Chickasha	15	61
Integris Grove Hospital	Grove	15	36
Pauls Valley General Hospital	Pauls Valley	18	54
Integris Marshall County Medical Center	Madill	22	32
Weatherford Regional Hospital	Weatherford	22	39

Children's Asthma Care

Received Home Management Plan of Care

Hospital Name	City	Rate	Cases
O U Medical Center	Oklahoma City	94%	454

Received Reliever Medication

Hospital Name	City	Rate	Cases
O U Medical Center	Oklahoma City	100%	456

Received Systemic Corticosteroids

Hospital Name	City	Rate	Cases
O U Medical Center	Oklahoma City	100%	456

Emergency Department

Admittance Decision Time (minutes)

Hospital Name	City	Min.	Cases
Memorial Hospital & Physician Group[2]	Frederick	0	282
Elkview General Hospital[2]	Hobart	10	32
Harmon Memorial Hospital	Hollis	10	210
Share Memorial Hospital	Alva	15	111
Sayre Memorial Hospital[2]	Sayre	17	155
Latimer County General Hospital	Wilburton	20	266
Mary Hurley Hospital[3]	Coalgate	20	36
Memorial Hospital of Stilwell[2]	Stilwell	21	222
Drumright Regional Hospital	Drumright	27	231
Perry Memorial Hospital[2]	Perry	30	172
Woodward Regional Hospital[2]	Woodward	33	339
Mercy Hospital Ada[2]	Ada	34	268
Choctaw Nation Healthcare[2]	Talihina	35	346
USPHS Lawton Indian Hospital[2]	Lawton	37	278
Epic Medical Center[2]	Eufaula	40	53
Integris Marshall County Medical Center[2]	Madill	41	200
Holdenville Hospital Authority	Holdenville	44	43
Bailey Medical Center[2]	Owasso	47	119
Oklahoma Heart Hospital[2]	Oklahoma City	47	203
Sequoyah Co-Sallisaw Hosp Auth[2]	Sallisaw	47	297
Chickasaw Nation Medical Center[2]	Ada	48	240
Mercy Hospital Logan County[2]	Guthrie	48	342
Purcell Municipal Hospital[2]	Purcell	48	359
Bristow Medical Center	Bristow	49	147
Community Hospital[2]	Oklahoma City	50	189
Craig General Hospital[2]	Vinita	50	449
McBride Clinic Orthopedic Hospital[2]	Oklahoma City	50	69
Muscogee (Creek) Nation Medical Center[2]	Okmulgee	50	460
Newman Memorial Hospital	Shattuck	50	107
Saint Mary's Regional Medical Center[2]	Enid	50	418
Integris Baptist Regional Health Center[2]	Miami	51	282
Duncan Regional Hospital[2]	Duncan	52	499
Integris Blackwell Regional Hospital[2]	Blackwell	52	511
Hillcrest Hospital Cushing[2]	Cushing	53	310
Claremore Indian Hospital[2]	Claremore	54	204
Great Plains Regional Medical Center[2]	Elk City	54	215
Jackson County Memorial Hospital[2]	Altus	54	319
Integris Health Edmond[2]	Edmond	55	270
Integris Seminole Medical Center[2]	Seminole	55	470
Stillwater Medical Center[2]	Stillwater	55	408
Tahlequah City Hospital[2]	Tahlequah	55	271
Hillcrest Hospital Henryetta[2]	Henryetta	57	258
Choctaw Memorial Hospital[2]	Hugo	60	106
Integris Grove Hospital[2]	Grove	60	240
McAlester Regional Health Center[2]	Mcalester	60	472
Saint Anthony Shawnee Hospital[2]	Shawnee	60	502
Saint John Sapulpa[2,3]	Sapulpa	60	57
Hillcrest Hospital Claremore[2]	Claremore	61	457
Integris Bass Baptist Health Center[2]	Enid	61	350
Integris Canadian Valley Hospital[2]	Yukon	61	231
Integris Clinton Regional Hospital[2]	Clinton	61	316
Integris Mayes County Medical Center[2]	Pryor	61	394
Integris Southwest Medical Center[2]	Oklahoma City	61	599
Mercy Hospital Kingfisher	Kingfisher	62	26
Saint John Owasso[2]	Owasso	62	207
Grady Memorial Hospital[2]	Chickasha	63	198
McCurtain Memorial Hospital[2]	Idabel	64	422
Pauls Valley General Hospital[2]	Pauls Valley	65	209
Ponca City Medical Center[2]	Ponca City	65	429
Saint Francis Hospital South[2]	Tulsa	65	411
Weatherford Regional Hospital	Weatherford	66	112
Saint John Broken Arrow[2]	Broken Arrow	68	167
Pushmataha Co-Antlers Town Hosp Auth[2]	Antlers	70	429
Wagoner Community Hospital[2]	Wagoner	72	209
Eastern Oklahoma Medical Center[2]	Poteau	75	156
Jane Phillips Medical Center[2]	Bartlesville	75	294
Mercy Hospital Oklahoma City[2]	Oklahoma City	75	367
Southwestern Medical Center[2]	Lawton	75	273
Medical Center of Southeastern Oklahoma[2]	Durant	80	492
Deaconess Hospital[2]	Oklahoma City	82	574
Mercy Hospital El Reno	El Reno	82	236
Saint Francis Hospital[2]	Tulsa	84	627
Eastar Health System[2]	Muskogee	86	494
Hillcrest Hospital South[2]	Tulsa	86	490
W W Hastings Indian Hospital[2]	Tahlequah	86	169
Mercy Memorial Health Center[2]	Ardmore	88	594
Saint John Medical Center[2]	Tulsa	88	548
Memorial Hospital of Texas County[2]	Guymon	90	125
Integris Baptist Medical Center[2]	Oklahoma City	94	451
Saint Anthony Hospital[2]	Oklahoma City	95	437
Oklahoma State University Medical Center[2]	Tulsa	99	418
O U Medical Center[2]	Oklahoma City	102	602
Hillcrest Medical Center[2]	Tulsa	104	431
Midwest Regional Medical Center[2]	Midwest City	105	913
Comanche County Memorial Hospital[2]	Lawton	109	308
Oklahoma Heart Hospital South[2]	Oklahoma City	116	298
Norman Regional Health System[2]	Norman	126	410

Head CT Results Within 45 Minutes of Arrival

Hospital Name	City	Rate	Cases
McAlester Regional Health Center	Mcalester	53%	38

Patients Who Left ER Before Being Seen

Hospital Name	City	Rate	Cases
Duncan Regional Hospital	Duncan	0%	33465
Integris Health Edmond	Edmond	0%	11280
Lakeside Women's Hospital	Oklahoma City	0%	50
McBride Clinic Orthopedic Hospital	Oklahoma City	0%	3234
Norman Regional Health System	Norman	0%	109631
Oklahoma Heart Hospital	Oklahoma City	0%	11871
Oklahoma State University Medical Center	Tulsa	0%	48197
Sayre Memorial Hospital	Sayre	0%	4046
Share Memorial Hospital	Alva	0%	5026
Summit Medical Center	Edmond	0%	115
Tulsa Spine & Specialty Hospital	Tulsa	0%	79
Comanche County Memorial Hospital	Lawton	1%	52559
Community Hospital	Oklahoma City	1%	7046
Craig General Hospital	Vinita	1%	10871
Elkview General Hospital	Hobart	1%	4262
Great Plains Regional Medical Center	Elk City	1%	12698
Harmon Memorial Hospital	Hollis	1%	1970
Hillcrest Hospital Claremore	Claremore	1%	19070
Hillcrest Hospital South	Tulsa	1%	23071
Holdenville Hospital Authority	Holdenville	1%	7625
Integris Blackwell Regional Hospital	Blackwell	1%	6260
Integris Canadian Valley Hospital	Yukon	1%	28881
Integris Clinton Regional Hospital	Clinton	1%	9358
Integris Marshall County Medical Center	Madill	1%	8623
Integris Seminole Medical Center	Seminole	1%	11089
Jane Phillips Medical Center	Bartlesville	1%	34827
Latimer County General Hospital	Wilburton	1%	3440
Medical Center of Southeastern Oklahoma	Durant	1%	24032
Mercy Hospital El Reno	El Reno	1%	9639
Mercy Hospital Oklahoma City	Oklahoma City	1%	54395
Oklahoma Heart Hospital South	Oklahoma City	1%	11886
Oklahoma Surgical Hospital	Tulsa	1%	145
Perry Memorial Hospital	Perry	1%	2912
Saint Francis Hospital South	Tulsa	1%	24598
Saint John Owasso	Owasso	1%	21597
Woodward Regional Hospital	Woodward	1%	12846
Bailey Medical Center	Owasso	2%	12273
Bristow Medical Center	Bristow	2%	5646
Cleveland Area Hospital	Cleveland	2%	5300
Epic Medical Center	Eufaula	2%	5870
Grady Memorial Hospital	Chickasha	2%	18649
Integris Grove Hospital	Grove	2%	17129
Memorial Hospital & Physician Group	Frederick	2%	3188
Memorial Hospital of Stilwell	Stilwell	2%	8205
Memorial Hospital of Texas County	Guymon	2%	5016
Mercy Hospital Ada	Ada	2%	21539
Muscogee (Creek) Nation Medical Center	Okmulgee	2%	13598
Ponca City Medical Center	Ponca City	2%	26376
Saint Anthony Shawnee Hospital	Shawnee	2%	37769
Saint Francis Hospital	Tulsa	2%	97379
Saint John Broken Arrow	Broken Arrow	2%	23633
Saint Mary's Regional Medical Center	Enid	2%	18861
Southwestern Medical Center	Lawton	2%	18915
Tahlequah City Hospital	Tahlequah	2%	24422
Deaconess Hospital	Oklahoma City	3%	40348
Eastern Oklahoma Medical Center	Poteau	3%	15372
Integris Baptist Regional Health Center	Miami	3%	20147
Integris Bass Baptist Health Center	Enid	3%	22166
Integris Southwest Medical Center	Oklahoma City	3%	83666
O U Medical Center	Oklahoma City	3%	115525
Pauls Valley General Hospital	Pauls Valley	3%	8702
Purcell Municipal Hospital	Purcell	3%	12636
Pushmataha Co-Antlers Town Hosp Auth	Antlers	3%	5438
Hillcrest Hospital Henryetta	Henryetta	4%	7720
Integris Mayes County Medical Center	Pryor	4%	15903
Jackson County Memorial Hospital	Altus	4%	21097
Midwest Regional Medical Center	Midwest City	4%	40859
Saint John Medical Center	Tulsa	4%	61858
Sequoyah Co-Sallisaw Hosp Auth	Sallisaw	4%	15591
Stillwater Medical Center	Stillwater	4%	27936
Eastar Health System	Muskogee	5%	33065
Hillcrest Hospital Cushing	Cushing	5%	10465
Hillcrest Medical Center	Tulsa	5%	47642
McAlester Regional Health Center	Mcalester	5%	20956
McCurtain Memorial Hospital	Idabel	5%	13406
Mercy Memorial Health Center	Ardmore	5%	39518
Newman Memorial Hospital	Shattuck	5%	3125
Wagoner Community Hospital	Wagoner	5%	8052
Choctaw Memorial Hospital	Hugo	6%	6531
Saint Anthony Hospital	Oklahoma City	6%	59728
Integris Baptist Medical Center	Oklahoma City	7%	57548

Time from ER Arrival to Being Admitted (minutes)

Hospital Name	City	Min.	Cases
Mary Hurley Hospital[3]	Coalgate	83	36
Latimer County General Hospital	Wilburton	110	289
Memorial Hospital & Physician Group[2]	Frederick	110	282
Elkview General Hospital[2]	Hobart	114	406
Harmon Memorial Hospital	Hollis	115	228
Drumright Regional Hospital	Drumright	124	236
Memorial Hospital of Stilwell[2]	Stilwell	134	282
Sayre Memorial Hospital[2]	Sayre	141	159
McBride Clinic Orthopedic Hospital[2]	Oklahoma City	150	69
Oklahoma Heart Hospital[2]	Oklahoma City	153	211
Sequoyah Co-Sallisaw Hosp Auth[2]	Sallisaw	153	312
Perry Memorial Hospital[2]	Perry	154	176
Woodward Regional Hospital[2]	Woodward	154	342
Epic Medical Center[2]	Eufaula	159	75
Share Memorial Hospital	Alva	162	115
Holdenville Hospital Authority	Holdenville	163	86
Integris Blackwell Regional Hospital[2]	Blackwell	166	513
Pushmataha Co-Antlers Town Hosp Auth[2]	Antlers	170	444
Integris Marshall County Medical Center[2]	Madill	172	371
Bristow Medical Center	Bristow	173	147
Craig General Hospital[2]	Vinita	175	497
Jackson County Memorial Hospital[2]	Altus	181	337
Integris Health Edmond[2]	Edmond	184	274
Stillwater Medical Center[2]	Stillwater	184	411
Mercy Hospital Logan County[2]	Guthrie	188	365
Mercy Memorial Health Center[2]	Ardmore	188	605
Community Hospital[2]	Oklahoma City	189	201
Muscogee (Creek) Nation Medical Center[2]	Okmulgee	189	483
Saint Anthony Shawnee Hospital[2]	Shawnee	190	511
Saint John Owasso[2]	Owasso	190	228
Integris Baptist Regional Health Center[2]	Miami	191	324
Ponca City Medical Center[2]	Ponca City	192	432
Integris Southwest Medical Center[2]	Oklahoma City	193	671
Saint Mary's Regional Medical Center[2]	Enid	194	473
Purcell Municipal Hospital[2]	Purcell	195	369
Integris Seminole Medical Center[2]	Seminole	196	499
Integris Clinton Regional Hospital[2]	Clinton	197	322
Bailey Medical Center[2]	Owasso	199	133
Jane Phillips Medical Center[2]	Bartlesville	200	359
Choctaw Nation Healthcare[2]	Talihina	202	412
Duncan Regional Hospital[2]	Duncan	202	526
Integris Grove Hospital[2]	Grove	204	332
Mercy Hospital Oklahoma City[2]	Oklahoma City	204	378
Oklahoma State University Medical Center[2]	Tulsa	204	476
Choctaw Memorial Hospital[2]	Hugo	206	117
Mercy Hospital Kingfisher	Kingfisher	206	34

NOTE: Hospital profiles are in alphabetical order by state, then city, then hospital within the city; Rankings exclude hospitals with less than 25 cases except for patient surveys which excludes hospitals with less than 100 cases; (a) 100-299 cases; (1) The number of cases/patients is too few to report; (2) Data submitted were based on a sample of cases/patients; (3) Results are based on a shorter time period than required; (4) Data suppressed by CMS for one or more quarters; (5) Results are not available for this reporting period; (6) Fewer than 100 patients completed the HCAHPS survey; (7) No cases met the criteria for this measure; (8) The lower limit of the confidence interval cannot be calculated if the number of observed infections equals zero; (9) No data are available from the state/territory for this reporting period; (10) The scores shown reflect fewer than 50 completed surveys; (11) There were discrepancies in the data collection process; (12) This measure does not apply to this hospital for this reporting period; (13) Results cannot be calculated for this reporting period; (14) The results for this state are combined with nearby states to protect confidentiality; Please refer to the User's Guide for a full explanation of data.

Hospital Name	City	Min.	Cases
Grady Memorial Hospital[2]	Chickasha	209	290
McAlester Regional Health Center[2]	Mcalester	212	499
Tahlequah City Hospital[2]	Tahlequah	212	277
Great Plains Regional Medical Center[2]	Elk City	213	242
Saint John Sapulpa[2,3]	Sapulpa	215	57
Integris Canadian Valley Hospital[2]	Yukon	216	252
Oklahoma Heart Hospital South[2]	Oklahoma City	218	302
Saint Francis Hospital[2]	Tulsa	218	627
Eastern Oklahoma Medical Center[2]	Poteau	222	175
Integris Bass Baptist Health Center[2]	Enid	222	363
Mercy Hospital Ada[2]	Ada	222	268
Mercy Hospital El Reno	El Reno	224	249
Integris Mayes County Medical Center[2]	Pryor	225	398
Saint John Broken Arrow[2]	Broken Arrow	225	189
Hillcrest Hospital Henryetta[2]	Henryetta	226	262
Medical Center of Southeastern Oklahoma[2]	Durant	232	493
Pauls Valley General Hospital[2]	Pauls Valley	233	224
Southwestern Medical Center[2]	Lawton	233	281
Newman Memorial Hospital	Shattuck	234	109
Memorial Hospital of Texas County[2]	Guymon	235	197
Chickasaw Nation Medical Center[2]	Ada	236	239
Hillcrest Hospital Cushing[2]	Cushing	236	316
Hillcrest Hospital South[2]	Tulsa	236	501
Deaconess Hospital[2]	Oklahoma City	237	577
Hillcrest Hospital Claremore[2]	Claremore	239	461
Saint Francis Hospital South[2]	Tulsa	249	413
USPHS Lawton Indian Hospital[2]	Lawton	253	278
Norman Regional Health System[2]	Norman	256	455
Weatherford Regional Hospital	Weatherford	262	115
Comanche County Memorial Hospital[2]	Lawton	267	319
Wagoner Community Hospital[2]	Wagoner	267	409
McCurtain Memorial Hospital[2]	Idabel	270	428
Saint John Medical Center[2]	Tulsa	271	578
Midwest Regional Medical Center[2]	Midwest City	272	913
Saint Anthony Hospital[2]	Oklahoma City	279	443
Eastar Health System[2]	Muskogee	283	500
O U Medical Center[2]	Oklahoma City	288	601
Integris Baptist Medical Center[2]	Oklahoma City	290	495
Hillcrest Medical Center[2]	Tulsa	298	460
W W Hastings Indian Hospital[2]	Tahlequah	312	264
Claremore Indian Hospital[2]	Claremore	343	205

Time from ER Arrival to Discharge (minutes)

Hospital Name	City	Min.	Cases
Oklahoma State University Medical Center	Tulsa	64	364
Drumright Regional Hospital	Drumright	67	239
Integris Marshall County Medical Center	Madill	69	584
Elkview General Hospital	Hobart	75	366
Integris Blackwell Regional Hospital	Blackwell	75	473
Latimer County General Hospital	Wilburton	75	175
Woodward Regional Hospital	Woodward	75	409
Sequoyah Co-Sallisaw Hosp Auth	Sallisaw	77	329
Mary Hurley Hospital	Coalgate	79	245
Holdenville Hospital Authority	Holdenville	80	49
Pushmataha Co-Antlers Town Hosp Auth	Antlers	80	368
Integris Southwest Medical Center	Oklahoma City	82	364
Ponca City Medical Center	Ponca City	82	376
Craig General Hospital	Vinita	84	445
McBride Clinic Orthopedic Hospital	Oklahoma City	84	291
Epic Medical Center	Eufaula	85	219
Norman Regional Health System	Norman	85	397
Community Hospital	Oklahoma City	87	1313
Perry Memorial Hospital	Perry	87	236
Share Memorial Hospital	Alva	87	350
Integris Seminole Medical Center	Seminole	88	340
Okeene Municipal Hospital[3]	Okeene	90	49
Integris Baptist Regional Health Center	Miami	92	386
Oklahoma Heart Hospital South	Oklahoma City	92	372
Bristow Medical Center	Bristow	93	238
Muscogee (Creek) Nation Medical Center	Okmulgee	93	247
Purcell Municipal Hospital	Purcell	94	351
Choctaw Memorial Hospital	Hugo	100	328
Newman Memorial Hospital	Shattuck	100	274
Saint Anthony Hospital	Oklahoma City	101	408
Saint John Owasso	Owasso	102	358
Sayre Memorial Hospital	Sayre	102	276
Integris Health Edmond	Edmond	104	356
Saint Anthony Shawnee Hospital	Shawnee	104	413
Harmon Memorial Hospital	Hollis	106	226
Integris Bass Baptist Health Center	Enid	106	368
Memorial Hospital of Stilwell	Stilwell	106	350
Comanche County Memorial Hospital	Lawton	109	475
Bailey Medical Center	Owasso	110	398
Grady Memorial Hospital	Chickasha	110	337
Integris Clinton Regional Hospital	Clinton	111	785
Jane Phillips Medical Center	Bartlesville	111	1218
Mercy Hospital El Reno	El Reno	111	357
Mercy Memorial Health Center	Ardmore	112	383
Integris Canadian Valley Hospital	Yukon	113	359
Integris Mayes County Medical Center	Pryor	114	343
Tulsa Spine & Specialty Hospital	Tulsa	114	57
Duncan Regional Hospital	Duncan	116	483
Great Plains Regional Medical Center	Elk City	116	381
Tahlequah City Hospital	Tahlequah	116	372
Medical Center of Southeastern Oklahoma	Durant	118	849
Deaconess Hospital	Oklahoma City	119	382
Memorial Hospital & Physician Group	Frederick	119	241
Oklahoma Heart Hospital	Oklahoma City	119	351
Eastern Oklahoma Medical Center	Poteau	120	1035
Mercy Hospital Oklahoma City	Oklahoma City	120	382
Hillcrest Hospital Henryetta	Henryetta	121	355
Jackson County Memorial Hospital	Altus	121	421
Memorial Hospital of Texas County	Guymon	121	283
Wagoner Community Hospital	Wagoner	122	318
Integris Grove Hospital	Grove	125	1011
Lakeside Women's Hospital[3]	Oklahoma City	127	45
Saint John Broken Arrow	Broken Arrow	128	368
Saint Mary's Regional Medical Center	Enid	128	411
McAlester Regional Health Center	Mcalester	129	355
Southwestern Medical Center	Lawton	130	431
Pauls Valley General Hospital	Pauls Valley	132	284
Stillwater Medical Center	Stillwater	132	402
O U Medical Center	Oklahoma City	134	482
Saint Francis Hospital South	Tulsa	138	383
Mercy Hospital Ada	Ada	141	353
Hillcrest Hospital Cushing	Cushing	143	323
Hillcrest Hospital South	Tulsa	146	588
Hillcrest Hospital Claremore	Claremore	150	498
Hillcrest Medical Center	Tulsa	150	381
Midwest Regional Medical Center	Midwest City	153	451
McCurtain Memorial Hospital	Idabel	156	384
Mercy Hospital Kingfisher	Kingfisher	158	37
Saint Francis Hospital	Tulsa	162	392
Claremore Indian Hospital[3]	Claremore	164	83
Oklahoma Surgical Hospital	Tulsa	180	92
Eastar Health System	Muskogee	201	397
Integris Baptist Medical Center	Oklahoma City	212	347
Saint John Medical Center	Tulsa	223	369
Summit Medical Center	Edmond	283	68

Time in ER Before Being Evaluated (minutes)

Hospital Name	City	Min.	Cases
Latimer County General Hospital	Wilburton	0	263
Okeene Municipal Hospital[3]	Okeene	10	60
Oklahoma Heart Hospital	Oklahoma City	10	408
Tulsa Spine & Specialty Hospital	Tulsa	11	58
Community Hospital	Oklahoma City	12	1365
Memorial Hospital of Texas County	Guymon	12	346
Mercy Hospital Oklahoma City	Oklahoma City	12	394
Oklahoma Heart Hospital South	Oklahoma City	12	419
Integris Health Edmond	Edmond	13	287
Wagoner Community Hospital	Wagoner	13	345
Woodward Regional Hospital	Woodward	13	441
Integris Blackwell Regional Hospital	Blackwell	14	480
Oklahoma State University Medical Center	Tulsa	14	411
Integris Seminole Medical Center	Seminole	15	352
Share Memorial Hospital	Alva	15	162
Holdenville Hospital Authority	Holdenville	16	114
Integris Mayes County Medical Center	Pryor	16	390
Medical Center of Southeastern Oklahoma	Durant	16	922
Norman Regional Health System	Norman	16	303
Integris Marshall County Medical Center	Madill	17	620
Mercy Memorial Health Center	Ardmore	17	403
Bristow Medical Center	Bristow	18	389
McBride Clinic Orthopedic Hospital	Oklahoma City	18	295
Pauls Valley General Hospital	Pauls Valley	18	388
Perry Memorial Hospital	Perry	18	248
Duncan Regional Hospital	Duncan	19	520
Mercy Hospital El Reno	El Reno	19	379
Mary Hurley Hospital	Coalgate	20	239
Mercy Hospital Kingfisher	Kingfisher	20	47
Ponca City Medical Center	Ponca City	20	421
Pushmataha Co-Antlers Town Hosp Auth	Antlers	20	387
Saint John Owasso	Owasso	20	361
Sequoyah Co-Sallisaw Hosp Auth	Sallisaw	20	453
Bailey Medical Center	Owasso	22	393
Craig General Hospital	Vinita	22	508
Deaconess Hospital	Oklahoma City	22	417
Muscogee (Creek) Nation Medical Center	Okmulgee	23	362
Saint Anthony Shawnee Hospital	Shawnee	23	463
Oklahoma Surgical Hospital	Tulsa	24	84
Epic Medical Center	Eufaula	25	246
Harmon Memorial Hospital	Hollis	25	240
Integris Baptist Regional Health Center	Miami	25	401
Purcell Municipal Hospital	Purcell	25	386
Saint Francis Hospital	Tulsa	25	421
Sayre Memorial Hospital	Sayre	25	319
Integris Clinton Regional Hospital	Clinton	26	874
Integris Southwest Medical Center	Oklahoma City	27	114
Tahlequah City Hospital	Tahlequah	27	315
Great Plains Regional Medical Center	Elk City	28	407
Hillcrest Hospital Cushing	Cushing	28	378
Drumright Regional Hospital	Drumright	29	246
Comanche County Memorial Hospital	Lawton	30	254
Grady Memorial Hospital	Chickasha	30	404
Saint John Broken Arrow	Broken Arrow	30	387
Hillcrest Hospital Henryetta	Henryetta	31	395
O U Medical Center	Oklahoma City	31	520
Stillwater Medical Center	Stillwater	31	423
Jane Phillips Medical Center	Bartlesville	32	1189
Saint Anthony Hospital	Oklahoma City	32	428
Saint Mary's Regional Medical Center	Enid	33	426
Hillcrest Hospital South	Tulsa	34	650
Jackson County Memorial Hospital	Altus	34	449
Southwestern Medical Center	Lawton	34	442
Choctaw Memorial Hospital	Hugo	36	294
Mercy Hospital Ada	Ada	36	384
Saint Francis Hospital South	Tulsa	39	411
Hillcrest Hospital Claremore	Claremore	40	561
Integris Grove Hospital	Grove	40	863
Memorial Hospital & Physician Group	Frederick	40	117
Eastern Oklahoma Medical Center	Poteau	42	1098
Integris Canadian Valley Hospital	Yukon	42	36
Newman Memorial Hospital	Shattuck	42	215
Midwest Regional Medical Center	Midwest City	43	499
Eastar Health System	Muskogee	46	462
Integris Bass Baptist Health Center	Enid	46	145
McAlester Regional Health Center	Mcalester	47	375
Hillcrest Medical Center	Tulsa	50	400
McCurtain Memorial Hospital	Idabel	52	216
Claremore Indian Hospital[3]	Claremore	61	94
Integris Baptist Medical Center	Oklahoma City	64	103
Memorial Hospital of Stilwell	Stilwell	66	388
Lakeside Women's Hospital[3]	Oklahoma City	77	27
Saint John Medical Center	Tulsa	102	373
Summit Medical Center	Edmond	122	40

Time to Pain Meds for Bone Fractures (minutes)

Hospital Name	City	Min.	Cases
Share Memorial Hospital	Alva	24	41
Mercy Hospital El Reno	El Reno	26	32
Hillcrest Hospital Henryetta	Henryetta	30	38
Ponca City Medical Center	Ponca City	35	107
Integris Blackwell Regional Hospital	Blackwell	36	29
Pushmataha Co-Antlers Town Hosp Auth[3]	Antlers	36	30
Holdenville Hospital Authority	Holdenville	37	31
Woodward Regional Hospital	Woodward	37	68
Integris Southwest Medical Center	Oklahoma City	38	163
Integris Health Edmond	Edmond	39	68
Tahlequah City Hospital	Tahlequah	40	82
Norman Regional Health System	Norman	41	265
Integris Canadian Valley Hospital	Yukon	42	135
Saint Mary's Regional Medical Center	Enid	42	82
Bailey Medical Center	Owasso	43	46
Mercy Hospital Oklahoma City	Oklahoma City	43	120
Mercy Memorial Health Center	Ardmore	43	125
Saint Francis Hospital	Tulsa	43	289
Integris Clinton Regional Hospital	Clinton	45	43
Saint John Owasso	Owasso	46	96
Saint John Broken Arrow	Broken Arrow	48	85
Duncan Regional Hospital	Duncan	49	151
Integris Marshall County Medical Center	Madill	49	31
Integris Baptist Regional Health Center	Miami	50	37
Integris Mayes County Medical Center	Pryor	50	82
Jane Phillips Medical Center	Bartlesville	50	156
Integris Bass Baptist Health Center	Enid	51	71
McBride Clinic Orthopedic Hospital	Oklahoma City	51	69
Saint Anthony Shawnee Hospital	Shawnee	51	165
Integris Seminole Medical Center	Seminole	52	48
Pauls Valley General Hospital	Pauls Valley	52	37
Hillcrest Medical Center	Tulsa	54	104
Muscogee (Creek) Nation Medical Center	Okmulgee	54	70
Great Plains Regional Medical Center	Elk City	55	60
Midwest Regional Medical Center	Midwest City	57	93
Comanche County Memorial Hospital	Lawton	58	95
Craig General Hospital	Vinita	58	45
Saint Anthony Hospital	Oklahoma City	60	277
Memorial Hospital of Texas County	Guymon	61	39
Stillwater Medical Center	Stillwater	61	107
Weatherford Regional Hospital	Weatherford	62	62
McAlester Regional Health Center	Mcalester	63	95
Hillcrest Hospital Cushing	Cushing	64	59
Integris Grove Hospital	Grove	64	110
Integris Baptist Medical Center	Oklahoma City	66	116
Saint Francis Hospital South	Tulsa	67	131
Deaconess Hospital	Oklahoma City	68	97
Hillcrest Hospital Claremore	Claremore	68	75
Oklahoma State University Medical Center	Tulsa	68	80
Purcell Municipal Hospital	Purcell	70	36
Choctaw Memorial Hospital	Hugo	71	25
Grady Memorial Hospital	Chickasha	73	76
Jackson County Memorial Hospital	Altus	74	90
O U Medical Center	Oklahoma City	74	291

NOTE: Hospital profiles are in alphabetical order by state, then city, then hospital within the city; Rankings exclude hospitals with less than 25 cases except for patient surveys which excludes hospitals with less than 100 cases; (a) 100-299 cases; (1) The number of cases/patients is too few to report; (2) Data submitted were based on a sample of cases/patients; (3) Results are based on a shorter time period than required; (4) Data suppressed by CMS for one or more quarters; (5) Results are not available for this reporting period; (6) Fewer than 100 patients completed the HCAHPS survey; (7) No cases met the criteria for this measure; (8) The lower limit of the confidence interval cannot be calculated if the number of observed infections equals zero; (9) No data are available from the state/territory for this reporting period; (10) The scores shown reflect fewer than 50 completed surveys; (11) There were discrepancies in the data collection process; (12) This measure does not apply to this hospital for this reporting period; (13) Results cannot be calculated for this reporting period; (14) The results for this state are combined with nearby states to protect confidentiality; Please refer to the User's Guide for a full explanation of data.

Hospital Name	City	Rate	Cases
Mercy Hospital Ada	Ada	78	81
Hillcrest Hospital South	Tulsa	80	78
Southwestern Medical Center	Lawton	81	61
Medical Center of Southeastern Oklahoma	Durant	82	93
Memorial Hospital of Stilwell	Stilwell	83	32
Eastar Health System	Muskogee	88	90
Eastern Oklahoma Medical Center	Poteau	91	80
McCurtain Memorial Hospital	Idabel	97	75
Saint John Medical Center	Tulsa	105	259

Heart Attack Care

Aspirin Given at Discharge

Hospital Name	City	Rate	Cases
Deaconess Hospital	Oklahoma City	100%	76
Eastar Health System	Muskogee	100%	50
Hillcrest Medical Center	Tulsa	100%	556
Integris Baptist Medical Center	Oklahoma City	100%	561
Mercy Memorial Health Center	Ardmore	100%	98
Norman Regional Health System[2]	Norman	100%	264
O U Medical Center	Oklahoma City	100%	132
Oklahoma Heart Hospital[2]	Oklahoma City	100%	327
Oklahoma Heart Hospital South[2]	Oklahoma City	100%	313
Saint Anthony Hospital	Oklahoma City	100%	285
Saint Anthony Shawnee Hospital	Shawnee	100%	53
Saint Francis Hospital	Tulsa	100%	674
Saint Francis Hospital South	Tulsa	100%	67
Stillwater Medical Center	Stillwater	100%	56
Tahlequah City Hospital	Tahlequah	100%	58
Comanche County Memorial Hospital[2]	Lawton	99%	307
Hillcrest Hospital South	Tulsa	99%	154
Jane Phillips Medical Center	Bartlesville	99%	147
Saint John Medical Center	Tulsa	99%	617
Integris Bass Baptist Health Center	Enid	98%	52
Integris Grove Hospital	Grove	98%	40
Integris Southwest Medical Center[2]	Oklahoma City	98%	214
Oklahoma State University Medical Center	Tulsa	98%	143
Saint Mary's Regional Medical Center	Enid	98%	48
Midwest Regional Medical Center	Midwest City	97%	173
Oklahoma City VA Medical Center	Oklahoma City	97%	104
Medical Center of Southeastern Oklahoma	Durant	92%	63
McAlester Regional Health Center	Mcalester	75%	36

PCI Within 90 Minutes of Arrival

Hospital Name	City	Rate	Cases
Norman Regional Health System[2]	Norman	100%	44
Oklahoma Heart Hospital[2]	Oklahoma City	100%	27
Hillcrest Medical Center	Tulsa	98%	48
Oklahoma Heart Hospital South[2]	Oklahoma City	97%	34
Comanche County Memorial Hospital[2]	Lawton	95%	42
Integris Southwest Medical Center[2]	Oklahoma City	95%	41
Saint John Medical Center	Tulsa	95%	94
Integris Baptist Medical Center	Oklahoma City	94%	50
Saint Francis Hospital	Tulsa	94%	80
Jane Phillips Medical Center	Bartlesville	91%	32
Hillcrest Hospital South	Tulsa	85%	27

Statin Prescribed at Discharge

Hospital Name	City	Rate	Cases
Deaconess Hospital	Oklahoma City	100%	77
Hillcrest Medical Center	Tulsa	100%	538
Integris Baptist Medical Center	Oklahoma City	100%	555
O U Medical Center	Oklahoma City	100%	127
Oklahoma Heart Hospital[2]	Oklahoma City	100%	316
Saint Anthony Hospital	Oklahoma City	100%	282
Saint Anthony Shawnee Hospital	Shawnee	100%	47
Saint Mary's Regional Medical Center	Enid	100%	39
Stillwater Medical Center	Stillwater	100%	60
Jane Phillips Medical Center	Bartlesville	99%	146
Oklahoma Heart Hospital South[2]	Oklahoma City	99%	305
Oklahoma State University Medical Center	Tulsa	99%	141
Saint Francis Hospital South	Tulsa	99%	67
Saint John Medical Center	Tulsa	99%	598
Eastar Health System	Muskogee	98%	46
Hillcrest Hospital South	Tulsa	98%	149
Norman Regional Health System[2]	Norman	98%	254
Oklahoma City VA Medical Center	Oklahoma City	98%	100
Saint Francis Hospital	Tulsa	98%	669
Comanche County Memorial Hospital[2]	Lawton	97%	301
Medical Center of Southeastern Oklahoma	Durant	97%	59
Mercy Memorial Health Center	Ardmore	97%	98
Integris Bass Baptist Health Center	Enid	96%	53
Integris Southwest Medical Center[2]	Oklahoma City	96%	212
Midwest Regional Medical Center	Midwest City	96%	156
Integris Grove Hospital	Grove	91%	43
Tahlequah City Hospital	Tahlequah	84%	57
McAlester Regional Health Center	Mcalester	82%	34

Heart Failure Care

ACE Inhibitor or ARB for LVSD

Hospital Name	City	Rate	Cases
Deaconess Hospital	Oklahoma City	100%	37
Duncan Regional Hospital	Duncan	100%	33
Hillcrest Hospital South	Tulsa	100%	38
Integris Bass Baptist Health Center	Enid	100%	40
Medical Center of Southeastern Oklahoma	Durant	100%	62
O U Medical Center	Oklahoma City	100%	114
Ponca City Medical Center	Ponca City	100%	41
Saint Anthony Hospital	Oklahoma City	100%	138
Saint Anthony Shawnee Hospital	Shawnee	100%	65
Saint Francis Hospital	Tulsa	100%	290
Saint Francis Hospital South	Tulsa	100%	48
Saint Mary's Regional Medical Center	Enid	100%	25
Hillcrest Medical Center	Tulsa	98%	165
Oklahoma Heart Hospital[2]	Oklahoma City	98%	114
Oklahoma State University Medical Center	Tulsa	98%	95
Saint John Medical Center	Tulsa	98%	234
Eastar Health System	Muskogee	97%	63
Jane Phillips Medical Center	Bartlesville	97%	38
Muskogee VA Medical Center	Muskogee	97%	61
Oklahoma Heart Hospital South[2]	Oklahoma City	97%	104
Integris Baptist Medical Center	Oklahoma City	96%	187
Norman Regional Health System[2]	Norman	96%	101
Comanche County Memorial Hospital[2]	Lawton	94%	98
Integris Southwest Medical Center[2]	Oklahoma City	94%	123
Jackson County Memorial Hospital	Altus	94%	34
Oklahoma City VA Medical Center	Oklahoma City	94%	83
Tahlequah City Hospital	Tahlequah	93%	42
Mercy Memorial Health Center	Ardmore	92%	72
Midwest Regional Medical Center	Midwest City	92%	100
Stillwater Medical Center	Stillwater	88%	34
McAlester Regional Health Center	Mcalester	70%	37

Discharge Instructions Given

Hospital Name	City	Rate	Cases
Chickasaw Nation Medical Center	Ada	100%	37
Craig General Hospital[2]	Vinita	100%	37
Duncan Regional Hospital	Duncan	100%	77
Elkview General Hospital[2]	Hobart	100%	25
Hillcrest Hospital Claremore	Claremore	100%	58
Hillcrest Hospital Cushing	Cushing	100%	59
Hillcrest Medical Center	Tulsa	100%	550
Integris Bass Baptist Health Center	Enid	100%	71
Integris Grove Hospital	Grove	100%	42
Jane Phillips Medical Center	Bartlesville	100%	84
Midwest Regional Medical Center	Midwest City	100%	240
Oklahoma Heart Hospital[2]	Oklahoma City	100%	283
Oklahoma Heart Hospital South[2]	Oklahoma City	100%	260
Saint Anthony Hospital	Oklahoma City	100%	330
Saint John Broken Arrow	Broken Arrow	100%	30
Stillwater Medical Center	Stillwater	100%	75
Saint Anthony Shawnee Hospital	Shawnee	99%	151
Hillcrest Hospital South	Tulsa	98%	123
Saint John Medical Center	Tulsa	98%	581
Mary Hurley Hospital	Coalgate	97%	34
Norman Regional Health System[2]	Norman	97%	246
Ponca City Medical Center	Ponca City	97%	104
Integris Baptist Medical Center	Oklahoma City	96%	360
Integris Baptist Regional Health Center	Miami	95%	44
Mercy Memorial Health Center	Ardmore	94%	136
O U Medical Center	Oklahoma City	94%	247
Saint Francis Hospital	Tulsa	94%	729
Saint John Owasso	Owasso	94%	33
Medical Center of Southeastern Oklahoma	Durant	93%	148
Southwestern Medical Center	Lawton	92%	36
Oklahoma City VA Medical Center	Oklahoma City	89%	178
Saint Francis Hospital South	Tulsa	89%	131
McAlester Regional Health Center	Mcalester	88%	68
Muskogee VA Medical Center	Muskogee	88%	93
Memorial Hospital of Stilwell[2]	Stilwell	87%	31
Mercy Hospital Ada	Ada	86%	35
Saint Mary's Regional Medical Center	Enid	86%	81
Eastern Oklahoma Medical Center	Poteau	85%	60
Deaconess Hospital	Oklahoma City	84%	67
Comanche County Memorial Hospital[2]	Lawton	83%	201
Eastar Health System	Muskogee	83%	167
Integris Canadian Valley Hospital	Yukon	81%	26
Mercy Hospital Oklahoma City	Oklahoma City	81%	47
Choctaw Memorial Hospital[2]	Hugo	80%	65
Integris Blackwell Regional Hospital	Blackwell	79%	47
Integris Southwest Medical Center[2]	Oklahoma City	79%	227
Oklahoma State University Medical Center	Tulsa	79%	169
Integris Clinton Regional Hospital	Clinton	77%	26
Integris Health Edmond	Edmond	77%	31
Jackson County Memorial Hospital	Altus	70%	77
Tahlequah City Hospital	Tahlequah	70%	88
Wagoner Community Hospital[2]	Wagoner	70%	27
Purcell Municipal Hospital	Purcell	67%	30
Muscogee (Creek) Nation Medical Center[2]	Okmulgee	66%	38
McCurtain Memorial Hospital[2]	Idabel	55%	60
Integris Seminole Medical Center	Seminole	53%	34

Evaluation of LVS Function

Hospital Name	City	Rate	Cases
Deaconess Hospital	Oklahoma City	100%	92
Duncan Regional Hospital	Duncan	100%	108
Eastar Health System	Muskogee	100%	223
Hillcrest Hospital Cushing	Cushing	100%	63
Hillcrest Medical Center	Tulsa	100%	593
Integris Baptist Medical Center	Oklahoma City	100%	423
Integris Baptist Regional Health Center	Miami	100%	57
Integris Bass Baptist Health Center	Enid	100%	106
Integris Clinton Regional Hospital	Clinton	100%	40
Jane Phillips Medical Center	Bartlesville	100%	110
Medical Center of Southeastern Oklahoma	Durant	100%	193
Mercy Hospital Ada	Ada	100%	43
Mercy Hospital Logan County	Guthrie	100%	25
Mercy Hospital Oklahoma City	Oklahoma City	100%	77
Mercy Memorial Health Center	Ardmore	100%	187
Muskogee VA Medical Center	Muskogee	100%	111
Norman Regional Health System[2]	Norman	100%	306
O U Medical Center	Oklahoma City	100%	279
Oklahoma City VA Medical Center	Oklahoma City	100%	201
Oklahoma Heart Hospital[2]	Oklahoma City	100%	311
Oklahoma Heart Hospital South[2]	Oklahoma City	100%	287
Ponca City Medical Center	Ponca City	100%	124
Saint Anthony Hospital	Oklahoma City	100%	376
Saint Anthony Shawnee Hospital	Shawnee	100%	188
Saint Francis Hospital	Tulsa	100%	893
Saint Francis Hospital South	Tulsa	100%	154
Saint John Broken Arrow	Broken Arrow	100%	37
Saint John Medical Center	Tulsa	100%	710
Saint John Owasso	Owasso	100%	38
Saint Mary's Regional Medical Center	Enid	100%	123
Southwestern Medical Center	Lawton	100%	55
Tahlequah City Hospital	Tahlequah	100%	107
Woodward Regional Hospital	Woodward	100%	32
Eastern Oklahoma Medical Center	Poteau	99%	90
Hillcrest Hospital South	Tulsa	99%	143
Integris Blackwell Regional Hospital	Blackwell	99%	72
Oklahoma State University Medical Center	Tulsa	99%	180
Stillwater Medical Center	Stillwater	99%	100
Comanche County Memorial Hospital[2]	Lawton	98%	250
Integris Grove Hospital	Grove	98%	54
Chickasaw Nation Medical Center	Ada	97%	38
Elkview General Hospital[2]	Hobart	97%	34
Great Plains Regional Medical Center	Elk City	97%	37
Hillcrest Hospital Claremore	Claremore	97%	71
Integris Southwest Medical Center[2]	Oklahoma City	97%	272
Midwest Regional Medical Center	Midwest City	97%	295
Grady Memorial Hospital	Chickasha	95%	44
McAlester Regional Health Center	Mcalester	95%	96
Integris Health Edmond	Edmond	94%	32
Jackson County Memorial Hospital	Altus	93%	114
Memorial Hospital of Stilwell[2]	Stilwell	93%	41
Craig General Hospital[2]	Vinita	92%	48
Integris Canadian Valley Hospital	Yukon	90%	31
Muscogee (Creek) Nation Medical Center[2]	Okmulgee	85%	59
Integris Seminole Medical Center	Seminole	84%	37
Mary Hurley Hospital	Coalgate	81%	67
Pauls Valley General Hospital[2]	Pauls Valley	79%	33
McCurtain Memorial Hospital[2]	Idabel	77%	64
Wagoner Community Hospital[2]	Wagoner	76%	29
Purcell Municipal Hospital	Purcell	74%	39
Choctaw Memorial Hospital[2]	Hugo	72%	101
Pushmataha Co-Antlers Town Hosp Auth	Antlers	67%	27
Sequoyah Co-Sallisaw Hosp Auth[2]	Sallisaw	62%	26
Memorial Hospital & Physician Group[2]	Frederick	52%	25

Medicare Spending

Medicare Spending per Patient (ratio)

Hospital Name	City	Ratio	Cases
USPHS Lawton Indian Hospital	Lawton	0.54	-
Harmon Memorial Hospital	Hollis	0.62	-
Newman Memorial Hospital	Shattuck	0.70	-
Epic Medical Center	Eufaula	0.73	-
Memorial Hospital of Texas County	Guymon	0.74	-
Share Memorial Hospital	Alva	0.76	-
Memorial Hospital & Physician Group	Frederick	0.78	-
Integris Blackwell Regional Hospital	Blackwell	0.79	-
Chickasaw Nation Medical Center	Ada	0.80	-
Choctaw Nation Healthcare	Talihina	0.81	-
Memorial Hospital of Stilwell	Stilwell	0.81	-
Sayre Memorial Hospital	Sayre	0.82	-
Elkview General Hospital	Hobart	0.83	-
Saint John Owasso	Owasso	0.83	-

NOTE: Hospital profiles are in alphabetical order by state, then city, then hospital within the city; Rankings exclude hospitals with less than 25 cases except for patient surveys which excludes hospitals with less than 100 cases; (a) 100-299 cases; (1) The number of cases/patients is too few to report; (2) Data submitted were based on a sample of cases/patients; (3) Results are based on a shorter time period than required; (4) Data suppressed by CMS for one or more quarters; (5) Results are not available for this reporting period; (6) Fewer than 100 patients completed the HCAHPS survey; (7) No cases met the criteria for this measure; (8) The lower limit of the confidence interval cannot be calculated if the number of observed infections equals zero; (9) No data are available from the state/territory for this reporting period; (10) The scores shown reflect fewer than 50 completed surveys; (11) There were discrepancies in the data collection process; (12) This measure does not apply to this hospital for this reporting period; (13) Results cannot be calculated for this reporting period; (14) The results for this state are combined with nearby states to protect confidentiality; Please refer to the User's Guide for a full explanation of data.

Claremore Indian Hospital	Claremore	0.84	-
Wagoner Community Hospital	Wagoner	0.84	-
Hillcrest Hospital Henryetta	Henryetta	0.85	-
Woodward Regional Hospital	Woodward	0.85	-
Bristow Medical Center	Bristow	0.86	-
Integris Baptist Regional Health Center	Miami	0.86	-
Oklahoma Surgical Hospital	Tulsa	0.86	-
Pauls Valley General Hospital	Pauls Valley	0.86	-
Hillcrest Hospital Cushing	Cushing	0.87	-
Saint John Broken Arrow	Broken Arrow	0.87	-
Integris Clinton Regional Hospital	Clinton	0.88	-
Craig General Hospital	Vinita	0.89	-
Oklahoma Spine Hospital	Oklahoma City	0.89	-
Ponca City Medical Center	Ponca City	0.89	-
Great Plains Regional Medical Center	Elk City	0.90	-
Hillcrest Hospital Claremore	Claremore	0.90	-
Integris Mayes County Medical Center	Pryor	0.90	-
Oklahoma Heart Hospital South	Oklahoma City	0.90	-
Perry Memorial Hospital	Perry	0.90	-
Sequoyah Co-Sallisaw Hosp Auth	Sallisaw	0.90	-
McBride Clinic Orthopedic Hospital	Oklahoma City	0.92	-
Oklahoma Heart Hospital	Oklahoma City	0.92	-
Tulsa Spine & Specialty Hospital	Tulsa	0.92	-
W W Hastings Indian Hospital	Tahlequah	0.92	-
Bailey Medical Center	Owasso	0.93	-
Comanche County Memorial Hospital	Lawton	0.93	-
Jackson County Memorial Hospital	Altus	0.93	-
Duncan Regional Hospital	Duncan	0.94	-
Grady Memorial Hospital	Chickasha	0.94	-
McCurtain Memorial Hospital	Idabel	0.94	-
Medical Center of Southeastern Oklahoma	Durant	0.94	-
Tahlequah City Hospital	Tahlequah	0.94	-
Saint Anthony Hospital	Oklahoma City	0.95	-
Saint Mary's Regional Medical Center	Enid	0.95	-
Southwestern Medical Center	Lawton	0.95	-
Jane Phillips Medical Center	Bartlesville	0.96	-
Latimer County General Hospital	Wilburton	0.96	-
Mercy Memorial Health Center	Ardmore	0.96	-
Purcell Municipal Hospital	Purcell	0.96	-
Hillcrest Medical Center	Tulsa	0.97	-
Oklahoma State University Medical Center	Tulsa	0.97	-
Saint Francis Hospital South	Tulsa	0.97	-
Saint John Medical Center	Tulsa	0.98	-
Integris Baptist Medical Center	Oklahoma City	0.99	-
Integris Grove Hospital	Grove	0.99	-
Saint Francis Hospital	Tulsa	0.99	-
Community Hospital	Oklahoma City	1.00	-
Eastern Oklahoma Medical Center	Poteau	1.00	-
Midwest Regional Medical Center	Midwest City	1.00	-
Norman Regional Health System	Norman	1.00	-
Oklahoma Ctr for Ortho & Multi-Spec	Oklahoma City	1.00	-
Pushmataha Co-Antlers Town Hosp Auth	Antlers	1.00	-
Saint Anthony Shawnee Hospital	Shawnee	1.00	-
Mercy Hospital Ada	Ada	1.01	-
Mercy Hospital Oklahoma City	Oklahoma City	1.01	-
Choctaw Memorial Hospital	Hugo	1.02	-
Integris Bass Baptist Health Center	Enid	1.02	-
Integris Southwest Medical Center	Oklahoma City	1.02	-
Muscogee (Creek) Nation Medical Center	Okmulgee	1.02	-
O U Medical Center	Oklahoma City	1.02	-
Stillwater Medical Center	Stillwater	1.02	-
McAlester Regional Health Center	Mcalester	1.03	-
Mercy Hospital El Reno	El Reno	1.03	-
Eastar Health System	Muskogee	1.04	-
Hillcrest Hospital South	Tulsa	1.04	-
Integris Health Edmond	Edmond	1.04	-
Deaconess Hospital	Oklahoma City	1.05	-
Integris Canadian Valley Hospital	Yukon	1.06	-
Integris Seminole Medical Center	Seminole	1.07	-
Orthopedic Hospital	Oklahoma City	1.08	-
Summit Medical Center	Edmond	1.11	-
Southwestern Regional Medical Center	Tulsa	1.40	-

Pneumonia Care

Appropriate Initial Antibiotic Given

Hospital Name	City	Rate	Cases
Duncan Regional Hospital	Duncan	100%	118
Integris Blackwell Regional Hospital	Blackwell	100%	43
Oklahoma Heart Hospital South	Oklahoma City	100%	30
Oklahoma State University Medical Center	Tulsa	100%	87
Saint Anthony Shawnee Hospital	Shawnee	100%	101
Woodward Regional Hospital	Woodward	100%	38
Deaconess Hospital	Oklahoma City	99%	96
Hillcrest Hospital Cushing	Cushing	99%	68
Hillcrest Hospital South	Tulsa	99%	100
Norman Regional Health System[2]	Norman	99%	95
Saint Anthony Hospital	Oklahoma City	99%	200
Arbuckle Memorial Hospital	Sulphur	98%	43
Hillcrest Hospital Claremore	Claremore	98%	87
Integris Southwest Medical Center[2]	Oklahoma City	98%	124
Mercy Hospital Oklahoma City[2]	Oklahoma City	98%	48
Saint Francis Hospital South	Tulsa	98%	107
Saint John Broken Arrow	Broken Arrow	98%	55
Hillcrest Medical Center	Tulsa	97%	137
Integris Baptist Regional Health Center	Miami	97%	96
Integris Bass Baptist Health Center	Enid	97%	59
Integris Mayes County Medical Center	Pryor	97%	35
Jackson County Memorial Hospital[2]	Altus	97%	67
Jane Phillips Medical Center	Bartlesville	97%	103
Muskogee VA Medical Center	Muskogee	97%	73
Ponca City Medical Center	Ponca City	97%	67
Saint John Sapulpa	Sapulpa	97%	32
Saint Mary's Regional Medical Center[2]	Enid	97%	79
Southwestern Medical Center	Lawton	97%	35
Integris Grove Hospital	Grove	96%	55
Medical Center of Southeastern Oklahoma	Durant	96%	141
Mercy Hospital Ada	Ada	96%	77
Midwest Regional Medical Center	Midwest City	96%	152
Oklahoma Heart Hospital[2]	Oklahoma City	96%	49
Hillcrest Hospital Henryetta	Henryetta	95%	41
Integris Baptist Medical Center[2]	Oklahoma City	95%	120
Integris Clinton Regional Hospital	Clinton	95%	59
Memorial Hospital of Stilwell[2]	Stilwell	95%	38
O U Medical Center	Oklahoma City	95%	126
Stillwater Medical Center	Stillwater	95%	110
Claremore Indian Hospital	Claremore	94%	31
Integris Marshall County Medical Center	Madill	94%	48
Mercy Hospital El Reno	El Reno	94%	34
Mercy Memorial Health Center[2]	Ardmore	94%	69
Saint John Owasso	Owasso	94%	51
McCurtain Memorial Hospital[2]	Idabel	93%	69
Oklahoma City VA Medical Center	Oklahoma City	93%	69
Saint John Medical Center[2]	Tulsa	93%	227
Integris Health Edmond	Edmond	92%	50
Saint Francis Hospital	Tulsa	92%	476
Tahlequah City Hospital[2]	Tahlequah	92%	77
Eastar Health System	Muskogee	91%	131
Comanche County Memorial Hospital[2]	Lawton	90%	78
Grady Memorial Hospital	Chickasha	90%	69
Integris Canadian Valley Hospital	Yukon	90%	80
Bristow Medical Center	Bristow	89%	28
Elkview General Hospital	Hobart	89%	27
Craig General Hospital[2]	Vinita	88%	80
Wagoner Community Hospital[2]	Wagoner	88%	40
Chickasaw Nation Medical Center	Ada	87%	47
W W Hastings Indian Hospital	Tahlequah	87%	52
Holdenville Hospital Authority	Holdenville	86%	42
McAlester Regional Health Center[2]	Mcalester	85%	107
Pushmataha Co-Antlers Town Hosp Auth	Antlers	85%	47
Weatherford Regional Hospital	Weatherford	85%	41
Memorial Hospital of Texas County[2]	Guymon	84%	25
Pauls Valley General Hospital[2]	Pauls Valley	84%	44
Purcell Municipal Hospital	Purcell	83%	63
Integris Seminole Medical Center	Seminole	82%	28
Choctaw Memorial Hospital	Hugo	79%	72
Sequoyah Co-Sallisaw Hosp Auth	Sallisaw	78%	55
Great Plains Regional Medical Center	Elk City	75%	40
Muscogee (Creek) Nation Medical Center[2]	Okmulgee	74%	61
Eastern Oklahoma Medical Center	Poteau	73%	62
Mercy Hospital Kingfisher[2]	Kingfisher	73%	41
Mercy Health Love County	Marietta	28%	25
Memorial Hospital & Physician Group[2]	Frederick	23%	30

Blood Culture Timing

Hospital Name	City	Rate	Cases
Bailey Medical Center	Owasso	100%	31
Claremore Indian Hospital	Claremore	100%	33
Integris Mayes County Medical Center	Pryor	100%	45
Mercy Hospital Logan County	Guthrie	100%	37
Mercy Hospital Oklahoma City[2]	Oklahoma City	100%	115
Oklahoma State University Medical Center	Tulsa	100%	108
Ponca City Medical Center	Ponca City	100%	80
Saint Anthony Hospital	Oklahoma City	100%	460
Saint Anthony Shawnee Hospital	Shawnee	100%	252
Saint John Sapulpa	Sapulpa	100%	55
Woodward Regional Hospital	Woodward	100%	57
Duncan Regional Hospital	Duncan	99%	218
Hillcrest Hospital Cushing	Cushing	99%	79
Integris Baptist Medical Center[2]	Oklahoma City	99%	270
Integris Baptist Regional Health Center	Miami	99%	105
Integris Bass Baptist Health Center	Enid	99%	116
Integris Clinton Regional Hospital	Clinton	99%	81
McCurtain Memorial Hospital[2]	Idabel	99%	81
Midwest Regional Medical Center	Midwest City	99%	173
Norman Regional Health System[2]	Norman	99%	160
O U Medical Center	Oklahoma City	99%	276
Saint Francis Hospital South	Tulsa	99%	140
Saint John Owasso	Owasso	99%	96
Saint Mary's Regional Medical Center[2]	Enid	99%	124
Stillwater Medical Center	Stillwater	99%	160
Arbuckle Memorial Hospital	Sulphur	98%	45
Deaconess Hospital	Oklahoma City	98%	173
Eastar Health System	Muskogee	98%	246
Grady Memorial Hospital	Chickasha	98%	116
Hillcrest Hospital South	Tulsa	98%	125
Integris Blackwell Regional Hospital	Blackwell	98%	46
Integris Southwest Medical Center[2]	Oklahoma City	98%	169
Tahlequah City Hospital[2]	Tahlequah	98%	175
Hillcrest Hospital Claremore	Claremore	97%	145
Hillcrest Medical Center	Tulsa	97%	264
Integris Health Edmond	Edmond	97%	62
Jackson County Memorial Hospital[2]	Altus	97%	97
Medical Center of Southeastern Oklahoma	Durant	97%	217
Mercy Hospital Ada	Ada	97%	157
Mercy Hospital El Reno	El Reno	97%	31
Mercy Memorial Health Center[2]	Ardmore	97%	77
Saint Francis Hospital	Tulsa	97%	642
Southwestern Medical Center	Lawton	97%	29
Weatherford Regional Hospital	Weatherford	97%	38
Elkview General Hospital	Hobart	96%	26
Integris Canadian Valley Hospital	Yukon	96%	108
Oklahoma City VA Medical Center	Oklahoma City	96%	164
Pauls Valley General Hospital[2]	Pauls Valley	96%	54
Saint John Broken Arrow	Broken Arrow	96%	79
Integris Grove Hospital	Grove	95%	108
Muskogee VA Medical Center	Muskogee	95%	131
Purcell Municipal Hospital	Purcell	95%	40
Jane Phillips Medical Center	Bartlesville	94%	158
McAlester Regional Health Center[2]	Mcalester	94%	159
Muscogee (Creek) Nation Medical Center[2]	Okmulgee	94%	36
Sequoyah Co-Sallisaw Hosp Auth	Sallisaw	94%	50
Saint John Medical Center[2]	Tulsa	93%	383
Chickasaw Nation Medical Center	Ada	92%	52
Comanche County Memorial Hospital[2]	Lawton	92%	123
Eastern Oklahoma Medical Center	Poteau	92%	74
Hillcrest Hospital Henryetta	Henryetta	92%	48
Holdenville Hospital Authority	Holdenville	92%	36
Pushmataha Co-Antlers Town Hosp Auth	Antlers	92%	25
Great Plains Regional Medical Center	Elk City	91%	101
Integris Seminole Medical Center	Seminole	90%	41
Integris Marshall County Medical Center	Madill	89%	36
Choctaw Nation Healthcare	Talihina	88%	25
W W Hastings Indian Hospital	Tahlequah	87%	61
Mercy Hospital Kingfisher[2]	Kingfisher	85%	27

Pregnancy and Delivery Care

Newborns whose Deliveries were Scheduled Early

Hospital Name	City	Rate	Cases
Deaconess Hospital[2]	Oklahoma City	0%	32
Duncan Regional Hospital	Duncan	0%	137
Integris Baptist Regional Health Center	Miami	0%	38
Jackson County Memorial Hospital[2]	Altus	0%	29
Mercy Hospital Ada[2]	Ada	0%	38
Southwestern Medical Center[2]	Lawton	0%	27
Stillwater Medical Center[2]	Stillwater	0%	115
Tahlequah City Hospital[2]	Tahlequah	0%	34
W W Hastings Indian Hospital	Tahlequah	0%	136
McCurtain Memorial Hospital[2]	Idabel	1%	88
Saint Anthony Shawnee Hospital	Shawnee	1%	97
Hillcrest Hospital Claremore	Claremore	2%	86
Integris Bass Baptist Health Center[2]	Enid	2%	127
Integris Clinton Regional Hospital	Clinton	2%	41
Jane Phillips Medical Center	Bartlesville	2%	44
O U Medical Center[2]	Oklahoma City	2%	60
Saint John Owasso	Owasso	2%	49
Woodward Regional Hospital[2]	Woodward	2%	62
Integris Baptist Medical Center	Oklahoma City	3%	369
Integris Canadian Valley Hospital	Yukon	3%	126
Comanche County Memorial Hospital[2]	Lawton	5%	42
Grady Memorial Hospital[2]	Chickasha	5%	96
McAlester Regional Health Center[2]	Mcalester	5%	44
Oklahoma State University Medical Center	Tulsa	5%	43
Ponca City Medical Center[2]	Ponca City	6%	34
Integris Grove Hospital	Grove	7%	28
Mercy Memorial Health Center[2]	Ardmore	7%	28
Midwest Regional Medical Center[2]	Midwest City	7%	68
Saint Anthony Hospital[2]	Oklahoma City	7%	82
Saint John Medical Center	Tulsa	9%	167
Hillcrest Hospital South	Tulsa	10%	143
Hillcrest Medical Center	Tulsa	10%	273
Integris Southwest Medical Center	Oklahoma City	10%	124
Saint Francis Hospital South	Tulsa	10%	134
Eastern Oklahoma Medical Center	Poteau	11%	27
Mercy Hospital Oklahoma City[2]	Oklahoma City	11%	56
Saint Mary's Regional Medical Center[2]	Enid	11%	27
Norman Regional Health System	Norman	12%	331
Integris Health Edmond	Edmond	13%	31
Choctaw Nation Healthcare[2]	Talihina	14%	121
Saint Francis Hospital	Tulsa	14%	437

NOTE: Hospital profiles are in alphabetical order by state, then city, then hospital within the city; Rankings exclude hospitals with less than 25 cases except for patient surveys which excludes hospitals with less than 100 cases; (a) 100-299 cases; (1) The number of cases/patients is too few to report; (2) Data submitted were based on a sample of cases/patients; (3) Results are based on a shorter time period than required; (4) Data suppressed by CMS for one or more quarters; (5) Results are not available for this reporting period; (6) Fewer than 100 patients completed the HCAHPS survey; (7) No cases met the criteria for this measure; (8) The lower limit of the confidence interval cannot be calculated if the number of observed infections equals zero; (9) No data are available from the state/territory for this reporting period; (10) The scores shown reflect fewer than 50 completed surveys; (11) There were discrepancies in the data collection process; (12) This measure does not apply to this hospital for this reporting period; (13) Results cannot be calculated for this reporting period; (14) The results for this state are combined with nearby states to protect confidentiality; Please refer to the User's Guide for a full explanation of data.

Hospital Name	City	Rate	Cases
Eastar Health System[2]	Muskogee	15%	34
Great Plains Regional Medical Center[2]	Elk City	15%	34
Lakeside Women's Hospital[2]	Oklahoma City	16%	93
Memorial Hospital of Texas County	Guymon	20%	86
Chickasaw Nation Medical Center[2]	Ada	32%	28
Medical Center of Southeastern Oklahoma	Durant	35%	120

Preventive Care

Immunization for Influenza

Hospital Name	City	Rate	Cases
Bailey Medical Center[2]	Owasso	100%	285
Integris Mayes County Medical Center[2]	Pryor	100%	276
Medical Center of Southeastern Oklahoma[2]	Durant	100%	498
Oklahoma Heart Hospital South[2]	Oklahoma City	100%	506
Oklahoma Surgical Hospital[2]	Tulsa	100%	365
Ponca City Medical Center[2]	Ponca City	100%	363
Woodward Regional Hospital[2]	Woodward	100%	289
Community Hospital[2]	Oklahoma City	99%	736
Hillcrest Hospital Cushing[2]	Cushing	99%	259
Hillcrest Hospital South[2]	Tulsa	99%	717
Integris Clinton Regional Hospital[2]	Clinton	99%	305
O U Medical Center[2]	Oklahoma City	99%	643
Oklahoma Heart Hospital[2]	Oklahoma City	99%	616
Saint John Broken Arrow[2]	Broken Arrow	99%	299
Deaconess Hospital[2]	Oklahoma City	98%	589
Integris Blackwell Regional Hospital[2]	Blackwell	98%	318
Integris Seminole Medical Center[2]	Seminole	98%	251
Midwest Regional Medical Center[2]	Midwest City	98%	621
Norman Regional Health System[2]	Norman	98%	517
Saint Anthony Hospital[2]	Oklahoma City	98%	567
Saint Francis Hospital South[2]	Tulsa	98%	395
Hillcrest Medical Center[2]	Tulsa	97%	639
Memorial Hospital of Stilwell[2]	Stilwell	97%	319
Orthopedic Hospital	Oklahoma City	97%	58
Saint Anthony Shawnee Hospital[2]	Shawnee	97%	451
Saint John Sapulpa[2]	Sapulpa	97%	60
Stillwater Medical Center[2]	Stillwater	97%	434
Hillcrest Hospital Claremore[2]	Claremore	96%	394
Hillcrest Hospital Henryetta[2]	Henryetta	96%	288
Integris Baptist Regional Health Center[2]	Miami	96%	250
Jane Phillips Medical Center[2]	Bartlesville	96%	419
Eastar Health System[2]	Muskogee	95%	532
Integris Bass Baptist Health Center[2]	Enid	95%	440
McBride Clinic Orthopedic Hospital[2]	Oklahoma City	95%	494
Mercy Hospital Logan County[2]	Guthrie	95%	319
Mercy Hospital Oklahoma City[2]	Oklahoma City	95%	502
Oklahoma Ctr for Ortho & Multi-Spec[2]	Oklahoma City	95%	228
Saint John Owasso[2]	Owasso	95%	233
Elkview General Hospital[2]	Hobart	94%	287
Integris Southwest Medical Center[2]	Oklahoma City	94%	522
Mercy Hospital Kingfisher[2]	Kingfisher	94%	31
Saint Francis Hospital[2]	Tulsa	94%	570
Saint John Medical Center[2]	Tulsa	94%	537
Southwestern Regional Medical Center[2]	Tulsa	94%	280
Weatherford Regional Hospital	Weatherford	94%	63
Integris Health Edmond[2]	Edmond	93%	237
Integris Marshall County Medical Center[2]	Madill	93%	251
Comanche County Memorial Hospital[2]	Lawton	92%	575
Mercy Hospital Ada[2]	Ada	92%	279
Tahlequah City Hospital[2]	Tahlequah	92%	348
McAlester Regional Health Center[2]	Mcalester	90%	490
Mercy Memorial Health Center[2]	Ardmore	90%	534
Share Memorial Hospital	Alva	90%	98
Integris Canadian Valley Hospital[2]	Yukon	89%	276
Duncan Regional Hospital[2]	Duncan	88%	490
Integris Baptist Medical Center[2]	Oklahoma City	88%	499
Jackson County Memorial Hospital[2]	Altus	88%	345
Memorial Hospital & Physician Group[2]	Frederick	88%	235
Mercy Hospital El Reno	El Reno	88%	251
Oklahoma State University Medical Center[2]	Tulsa	88%	555
Saint Mary's Regional Medical Center[2]	Enid	88%	469
Craig General Hospital[2]	Vinita	87%	287
Harmon Memorial Hospital	Hollis	87%	206
Muscogee (Creek) Nation Medical Center[2]	Okmulgee	86%	290
Claremore Indian Hospital[2]	Claremore	85%	259
Grady Memorial Hospital[2]	Chickasha	85%	295
Chickasaw Nation Medical Center[2]	Ada	84%	315
Great Plains Regional Medical Center[2]	Elk City	84%	236
Perry Memorial Hospital[2]	Perry	84%	159
Memorial Hospital of Texas County[2]	Guymon	83%	289
Northwest Surgical Hospital	Oklahoma City	81%	155
Holdenville Hospital Authority	Holdenville	80%	51
Southwestern Medical Center[2]	Lawton	80%	319
Sayre Memorial Hospital[2]	Sayre	78%	165
Oklahoma Spine Hospital[2]	Oklahoma City	77%	364
McCurtain Memorial Hospital[2]	Idabel	75%	264
Pushmataha Co-Antlers Town Hosp Auth[2]	Antlers	75%	283
Eastern Oklahoma Medical Center[2]	Poteau	73%	232
Integris Grove Hospital[2]	Grove	73%	270
Lakeside Women's Hospital[2]	Oklahoma City	73%	313
Latimer County General Hospital[2]	Wilburton	73%	255
Sequoyah Co-Sallisaw Hosp Auth	Sallisaw	73%	262
Tulsa Spine & Specialty Hospital[2]	Tulsa	73%	314
Surgical Hospital of Oklahoma	Oklahoma City	70%	143
Epic Medical Center	Eufaula	68%	50
USPHS Lawton Indian Hospital	Lawton	68%	202
Choctaw Memorial Hospital[2]	Hugo	67%	275
Purcell Municipal Hospital[2]	Purcell	64%	292
Bristow Medical Center[2]	Bristow	61%	148
Newman Memorial Hospital	Shattuck	58%	159
W W Hastings Indian Hospital[2]	Tahlequah	58%	289
Pauls Valley General Hospital[2]	Pauls Valley	56%	273
Drumright Regional Hospital	Drumright	53%	96
Wagoner Community Hospital[2]	Wagoner	50%	301
Choctaw Nation Healthcare[2]	Talihina	48%	363
Summit Medical Center	Edmond	19%	128

Immunization for Pneumonia

Hospital Name	City	Rate	Cases
Bailey Medical Center[2]	Owasso	100%	246
Harper County Community Hospital	Buffalo	100%	31
Hillcrest Hospital Cushing[2]	Cushing	100%	309
Integris Mayes County Medical Center[2]	Pryor	100%	461
Medical Center of Southeastern Oklahoma[2]	Durant	100%	607
Okeene Municipal Hospital	Okeene	100%	27
Oklahoma Heart Hospital South[2]	Oklahoma City	100%	782
Oklahoma Surgical Hospital[2]	Tulsa	100%	314
Ponca City Medical Center[2]	Ponca City	100%	383
Woodward Regional Hospital[2]	Woodward	100%	287
Midwest Regional Medical Center[2]	Midwest City	99%	775
Norman Regional Health System[2]	Norman	99%	584
Oklahoma Heart Hospital[2]	Oklahoma City	99%	1028
Hillcrest Hospital South[2]	Tulsa	98%	708
Integris Bass Baptist Health Center[2]	Enid	98%	405
Integris Blackwell Regional Hospital[2]	Blackwell	98%	463
Memorial Hospital of Stilwell[2]	Stilwell	98%	341
Saint John Broken Arrow[2]	Broken Arrow	98%	395
Stillwater Medical Center[2]	Stillwater	98%	402
Deaconess Hospital[2]	Oklahoma City	97%	648
Hillcrest Hospital Henryetta[2]	Henryetta	97%	296
Integris Clinton Regional Hospital[2]	Clinton	97%	276
Mercy Hospital Logan County[2]	Guthrie	97%	471
Mercy Hospital Oklahoma City[2]	Oklahoma City	97%	578
O U Medical Center[2]	Oklahoma City	97%	479
Saint Anthony Hospital[2]	Oklahoma City	97%	691
Saint Anthony Shawnee Hospital[2]	Shawnee	97%	556
Saint John Owasso[2]	Owasso	97%	239
Duncan Regional Hospital[2]	Duncan	96%	606
Integris Seminole Medical Center[2]	Seminole	96%	460
McBride Clinic Orthopedic Hospital[2]	Oklahoma City	96%	558
Orthopedic Hospital	Oklahoma City	96%	28
Southwestern Regional Medical Center[2]	Tulsa	96%	196
Hillcrest Medical Center[2]	Tulsa	95%	689
Integris Canadian Valley Hospital[2]	Yukon	95%	251
Integris Health Edmond[2]	Edmond	95%	256
Integris Southwest Medical Center[2]	Oklahoma City	95%	664
Weatherford Regional Hospital	Weatherford	95%	114
Integris Baptist Regional Health Center[2]	Miami	94%	320
Eastar Health System[2]	Muskogee	93%	614
McAlester Regional Health Center[2]	Mcalester	93%	578
Memorial Hospital of Texas County[2]	Guymon	93%	223
Mercy Hospital Kingfisher[2,3]	Kingfisher	93%	27
Saint John Sapulpa[2]	Sapulpa	93%	84
Tahlequah City Hospital[2]	Tahlequah	93%	414
Integris Baptist Medical Center[2]	Oklahoma City	92%	568
Jackson County Memorial Hospital[2]	Altus	92%	429
Jane Phillips Medical Center[2]	Bartlesville	92%	497
Mercy Hospital Ada[2]	Ada	92%	299
Mercy Memorial Health Center[2]	Ardmore	92%	693
Choctaw Nation Healthcare[2]	Talihina	91%	286
Mercy Hospital El Reno	El Reno	91%	379
Saint Francis Hospital South[2]	Tulsa	91%	449
Hillcrest Hospital Claremore[2]	Claremore	90%	407
Muscogee (Creek) Nation Medical Center[2]	Okmulgee	90%	406
Saint Francis Hospital[2]	Tulsa	90%	578
Community Hospital[2]	Oklahoma City	89%	809
Cordell Memorial Hospital	Cordell	89%	37
Great Plains Regional Medical Center[2]	Elk City	89%	235
Share Memorial Hospital	Alva	89%	138
Surgical Hospital of Oklahoma	Oklahoma City	89%	158
Craig General Hospital[2]	Vinita	88%	483
Integris Marshall County Medical Center[2]	Madill	88%	388
Oklahoma State University Medical Center[2]	Tulsa	88%	681
Saint Mary's Regional Medical Center[2]	Enid	88%	626
Comanche County Memorial Hospital[2]	Lawton	87%	718
Eastern Oklahoma Medical Center[2]	Poteau	87%	301
Grady Memorial Hospital[2]	Chickasha	87%	331
Saint John Medical Center[2]	Tulsa	87%	677
Elkview General Hospital[2]	Hobart	86%	409
Harmon Memorial Hospital	Hollis	86%	244
Holdenville Hospital Authority	Holdenville	85%	81
USPHS Lawton Indian Hospital[2]	Lawton	85%	142
Chickasaw Nation Medical Center[2]	Ada	84%	272
Tulsa Spine & Specialty Hospital[2]	Tulsa	83%	279
McCurtain Memorial Hospital[2]	Idabel	82%	385
Pushmataha Co-Antlers Town Hosp Auth[2]	Antlers	82%	415
Newman Memorial Hospital	Shattuck	81%	139
Northwest Surgical Hospital[2]	Oklahoma City	81%	99
Perry Memorial Hospital[2]	Perry	81%	229
Purcell Municipal Hospital[2]	Purcell	81%	466
Claremore Indian Hospital[2]	Claremore	80%	142
Sequoyah Co-Sallisaw Hosp Auth[2]	Sallisaw	80%	357
Integris Grove Hospital[2]	Grove	78%	369
Latimer County General Hospital[2]	Wilburton	77%	268
Memorial Hospital & Physician Group[2]	Frederick	77%	287
Choctaw Memorial Hospital[2]	Hugo	76%	454
Oklahoma Ctr for Ortho & Multi-Spec[2]	Oklahoma City	75%	316
Pauls Valley General Hospital[2]	Pauls Valley	72%	351
W W Hastings Indian Hospital[2]	Tahlequah	72%	270
Epic Medical Center	Eufaula	70%	76
Sayre Memorial Hospital[2]	Sayre	70%	185
Southwestern Medical Center[2]	Lawton	68%	279
Drumright Regional Hospital	Drumright	67%	121
Wagoner Community Hospital[2]	Wagoner	65%	225
Bristow Medical Center[2]	Bristow	61%	214
Oklahoma Spine Hospital[2]	Oklahoma City	53%	253
Summit Medical Center	Edmond	23%	52

Stroke Care

Anticoagulation Therapy for Atrial Fibrillation

Hospital Name	City	Rate	Cases
Saint John Medical Center	Tulsa	100%	91
Mercy Hospital Oklahoma City	Oklahoma City	94%	34
Saint Francis Hospital	Tulsa	87%	61
Norman Regional Health System	Norman	82%	39

Antithrombotic Therapy Timing

Hospital Name	City	Rate	Cases
Eastar Health System[2]	Muskogee	100%	57
Integris Bass Baptist Health Center	Enid	100%	35
Jane Phillips Medical Center	Bartlesville	100%	46
Medical Center of Southeastern Oklahoma	Durant	100%	53
Mercy Hospital Ada	Ada	100%	32
Mercy Hospital Oklahoma City	Oklahoma City	100%	220
Saint Francis Hospital South	Tulsa	100%	30
Saint Mary's Regional Medical Center	Enid	100%	45
Southwestern Medical Center	Lawton	100%	44
Hillcrest Medical Center	Tulsa	99%	171
Norman Regional Health System	Norman	99%	196
O U Medical Center[2]	Oklahoma City	99%	76
Comanche County Memorial Hospital[2]	Lawton	98%	86
Integris Southwest Medical Center[2]	Oklahoma City	98%	87
Midwest Regional Medical Center	Midwest City	98%	60
Integris Baptist Medical Center[2]	Oklahoma City	97%	91
Mercy Memorial Health Center[2]	Ardmore	97%	71
Ponca City Medical Center	Ponca City	97%	35
Saint Francis Hospital	Tulsa	97%	387
Saint Anthony Hospital	Oklahoma City	96%	185
Oklahoma State University Medical Center	Tulsa	94%	36
Stillwater Medical Center	Stillwater	93%	28
Saint John Medical Center	Tulsa	92%	459
Tahlequah City Hospital	Tahlequah	92%	26
McAlester Regional Health Center	Mcalester	91%	34
Saint Anthony Shawnee Hospital	Shawnee	91%	33
Deaconess Hospital	Oklahoma City	81%	36

Assessed for Rehabilitation

Hospital Name	City	Rate	Cases
Duncan Regional Hospital	Duncan	100%	42
Integris Baptist Medical Center[2]	Oklahoma City	100%	124
Integris Southwest Medical Center[2]	Oklahoma City	100%	135
Mercy Hospital Ada	Ada	100%	33
Mercy Hospital Oklahoma City	Oklahoma City	100%	388
Saint Francis Hospital South	Tulsa	100%	30
Saint Mary's Regional Medical Center	Enid	100%	55
Norman Regional Health System	Norman	99%	216
O U Medical Center[2]	Oklahoma City	99%	176
Saint John Medical Center	Tulsa	99%	623
Deaconess Hospital	Oklahoma City	98%	40
Eastar Health System[2]	Muskogee	98%	57
Hillcrest Medical Center	Tulsa	98%	192
Medical Center of Southeastern Oklahoma	Durant	98%	53
Ponca City Medical Center	Ponca City	98%	45
Saint Anthony Hospital	Oklahoma City	98%	228
Saint Anthony Shawnee Hospital	Shawnee	97%	31
Stillwater Medical Center	Stillwater	96%	26
Southwestern Medical Center	Lawton	95%	44
Saint Francis Hospital	Tulsa	94%	503

NOTE: Hospital profiles are in alphabetical order by state, then city, then hospital within the city; Rankings exclude hospitals with less than 25 cases except for patient surveys which excludes hospitals with less than 100 cases; (a) 100-299 cases; (1) The number of cases/patients is too few to report; (2) Data submitted were based on a sample of cases/patients; (3) Results are based on a shorter time period than required; (4) Data suppressed by CMS for one or more quarters; (5) Results are not available for this reporting period; (6) Fewer than 100 patients completed the HCAHPS survey; (7) No cases met the criteria for this measure; (8) The lower limit of the confidence interval cannot be calculated if the number of observed infections equals zero; (9) No data are available from the state/territory for this reporting period; (10) The scores shown reflect fewer than 50 completed surveys; (11) There were discrepancies in the data collection process; (12) This measure does not apply to this hospital for this reporting period; (13) Results cannot be calculated for this reporting period; (14) The results for this state are combined with nearby states to protect confidentiality; Please refer to the User's Guide for a full explanation of data.

Hospital Name	City	Rate	Cases
Tahlequah City Hospital	Tahlequah	93%	29
McAlester Regional Health Center	Mcalester	91%	34
Integris Bass Baptist Health Center	Enid	90%	42
Jane Phillips Medical Center	Bartlesville	90%	51
Comanche County Memorial Hospital[2]	Lawton	89%	91
Oklahoma State University Medical Center	Tulsa	88%	33
Midwest Regional Medical Center	Midwest City	86%	56
Mercy Memorial Health Center[2]	Ardmore	82%	72

Discharged on Antithrombotic Therapy

Hospital Name	City	Rate	Cases
Hillcrest Medical Center	Tulsa	100%	166
Integris Southwest Medical Center[2]	Oklahoma City	100%	127
Jane Phillips Medical Center	Bartlesville	100%	49
Medical Center of Southeastern Oklahoma	Durant	100%	53
Mercy Hospital Oklahoma City	Oklahoma City	100%	323
Norman Regional Health System	Norman	100%	206
O U Medical Center[2]	Oklahoma City	100%	107
Ponca City Medical Center	Ponca City	100%	42
Saint Anthony Shawnee Hospital	Shawnee	100%	31
Saint Francis Hospital South	Tulsa	100%	29
Saint Mary's Regional Medical Center	Enid	100%	49
Saint Anthony Hospital	Oklahoma City	99%	199
Saint Francis Hospital	Tulsa	99%	406
Saint John Medical Center	Tulsa	99%	532
Eastar Health System[2]	Muskogee	98%	54
Integris Baptist Medical Center[2]	Oklahoma City	98%	110
Southwestern Medical Center	Lawton	98%	42
Deaconess Hospital	Oklahoma City	97%	37
Mercy Hospital Ada	Ada	97%	33
Midwest Regional Medical Center	Midwest City	96%	54
Tahlequah City Hospital	Tahlequah	96%	26
Integris Bass Baptist Health Center	Enid	95%	37
Comanche County Memorial Hospital[2]	Lawton	94%	80
Oklahoma State University Medical Center	Tulsa	94%	32
Mercy Memorial Health Center[2]	Ardmore	93%	71
Duncan Regional Hospital	Duncan	92%	38
Stillwater Medical Center	Stillwater	92%	25
McAlester Regional Health Center	Mcalester	91%	34

Discharged on Statin Medication

Hospital Name	City	Rate	Cases
O U Medical Center[2]	Oklahoma City	100%	79
Hillcrest Medical Center	Tulsa	99%	134
Integris Southwest Medical Center[2]	Oklahoma City	98%	99
Mercy Hospital Oklahoma City	Oklahoma City	98%	223
Integris Baptist Medical Center[2]	Oklahoma City	97%	69
Jane Phillips Medical Center	Bartlesville	97%	38
Saint Mary's Regional Medical Center	Enid	97%	34
Ponca City Medical Center	Ponca City	95%	37
Norman Regional Health System	Norman	94%	156
Saint John Medical Center	Tulsa	94%	419
Deaconess Hospital	Oklahoma City	93%	28
Medical Center of Southeastern Oklahoma	Durant	93%	42
Saint Anthony Hospital	Oklahoma City	93%	149
Southwestern Medical Center	Lawton	89%	27
Saint Anthony Shawnee Hospital	Shawnee	88%	26
Comanche County Memorial Hospital[2]	Lawton	84%	62
Eastar Health System[2]	Muskogee	84%	45
Saint Francis Hospital	Tulsa	84%	341
Integris Bass Baptist Health Center	Enid	82%	33
Mercy Memorial Health Center[2]	Ardmore	80%	61
McAlester Regional Health Center	Mcalester	74%	27
Mercy Hospital Ada	Ada	68%	25
Midwest Regional Medical Center	Midwest City	68%	47

Thrombolytic Therapy Timing

Hospital Name	City	Rate	Cases
Saint John Medical Center	Tulsa	96%	69
Mercy Hospital Oklahoma City	Oklahoma City	94%	33

Venous Thromboembolism (VTE) Prophylaxis

Hospital Name	City	Rate	Cases
Ponca City Medical Center	Ponca City	100%	36
Saint Francis Hospital South	Tulsa	100%	30
O U Medical Center[2]	Oklahoma City	99%	192
Duncan Regional Hospital	Duncan	98%	44
Saint John Medical Center	Tulsa	98%	680
Hillcrest Medical Center	Tulsa	97%	192
Mercy Hospital Oklahoma City	Oklahoma City	97%	336
Integris Southwest Medical Center[2]	Oklahoma City	96%	135
Jane Phillips Medical Center	Bartlesville	96%	57
Medical Center of Southeastern Oklahoma	Durant	96%	56
Norman Regional Health System	Norman	96%	221
Saint Anthony Hospital	Oklahoma City	96%	247
Saint Francis Hospital	Tulsa	96%	512
Eastar Health System[2]	Muskogee	95%	61
Integris Baptist Medical Center[2]	Oklahoma City	94%	121
Saint Anthony Shawnee Hospital	Shawnee	94%	31
Southwestern Medical Center	Lawton	94%	47
Deaconess Hospital	Oklahoma City	92%	39
Mercy Memorial Health Center[2]	Ardmore	92%	72
Saint Mary's Regional Medical Center	Enid	92%	60
Oklahoma State University Medical Center	Tulsa	89%	38
Comanche County Memorial Hospital[2]	Lawton	88%	96
Stillwater Medical Center	Stillwater	82%	28
Mercy Hospital Ada	Ada	78%	37
Tahlequah City Hospital	Tahlequah	76%	25
Jackson County Memorial Hospital	Altus	73%	26
McAlester Regional Health Center	Mcalester	71%	34
Integris Bass Baptist Health Center	Enid	67%	43
Midwest Regional Medical Center	Midwest City	59%	59

Written Stroke Educational Materials Given

Hospital Name	City	Rate	Cases
Eastar Health System[2]	Muskogee	100%	31
Mercy Hospital Oklahoma City	Oklahoma City	100%	197
Integris Baptist Medical Center[2]	Oklahoma City	99%	76
Integris Southwest Medical Center[2]	Oklahoma City	99%	72
Saint Anthony Hospital	Oklahoma City	99%	140
Hillcrest Medical Center	Tulsa	98%	126
O U Medical Center[2]	Oklahoma City	97%	95
Saint John Medical Center	Tulsa	93%	336
Norman Regional Health System	Norman	84%	128
Medical Center of Southeastern Oklahoma	Durant	83%	36
Saint Francis Hospital	Tulsa	83%	274
Comanche County Memorial Hospital[2]	Lawton	69%	51
Mercy Memorial Health Center[2]	Ardmore	69%	39
Midwest Regional Medical Center	Midwest City	52%	33
Oklahoma State University Medical Center	Tulsa	20%	25

Surgical Care Improvement Project

Appropriate Beta Blocker Usage

Hospital Name	City	Rate	Cases
Community Hospital[2]	Oklahoma City	100%	54
Duncan Regional Hospital	Duncan	100%	108
Hillcrest Hospital Claremore	Claremore	100%	32
McBride Clinic Orthopedic Hospital[2]	Oklahoma City	100%	106
Muskogee VA Medical Center[2]	Muskogee	100%	39
Oklahoma Heart Hospital South	Oklahoma City	100%	241
Oklahoma Surgical Hospital[2]	Tulsa	100%	64
Saint Anthony Hospital[2]	Oklahoma City	100%	535
Saint Anthony Shawnee Hospital	Shawnee	100%	29
Integris Southwest Medical Center[2]	Oklahoma City	99%	149
Mercy Hospital Oklahoma City[2]	Oklahoma City	99%	102
Midwest Regional Medical Center[2]	Midwest City	99%	129
O U Medical Center[2]	Oklahoma City	99%	174
Oklahoma City VA Medical Center[2]	Oklahoma City	99%	159
Oklahoma Heart Hospital	Oklahoma City	99%	569
Saint John Medical Center[2]	Tulsa	99%	408
Saint Mary's Regional Medical Center[2]	Enid	99%	93
Hillcrest Medical Center[2]	Tulsa	98%	297
Integris Baptist Medical Center[2]	Oklahoma City	98%	266
Integris Canadian Valley Hospital[2]	Yukon	98%	50
Saint John Broken Arrow	Broken Arrow	98%	329
Stillwater Medical Center	Stillwater	98%	129
Tahlequah City Hospital	Tahlequah	98%	122
Comanche County Memorial Hospital[2]	Lawton	97%	230
Integris Health Edmond[2]	Edmond	97%	36
Northwest Surgical Hospital[2]	Oklahoma City	97%	37
Mercy Memorial Health Center[2]	Ardmore	96%	96
Norman Regional Health System[2]	Norman	96%	183
Ponca City Medical Center	Ponca City	96%	51
Surgical Hospital of Oklahoma	Oklahoma City	96%	48
Deaconess Hospital	Oklahoma City	95%	92
Jackson County Memorial Hospital[2]	Altus	95%	105
Jane Phillips Medical Center[2]	Bartlesville	95%	111
Oklahoma State University Medical Center[2]	Tulsa	95%	106
Saint Francis Hospital[2]	Tulsa	95%	644
Integris Baptist Regional Health Center	Miami	94%	32
McAlester Regional Health Center[2]	Mcalester	94%	83
Oklahoma Ctr for Ortho & Multi-Spec	Oklahoma City	94%	80
Saint John Owasso	Owasso	94%	32
Southwestern Medical Center	Lawton	93%	46
Eastar Health System	Muskogee	92%	152
Hillcrest Hospital South	Tulsa	92%	77
Saint Francis Hospital South	Tulsa	92%	80
Integris Bass Baptist Health Center	Enid	91%	78
Integris Grove Hospital	Grove	90%	30
Southwestern Regional Medical Center	Tulsa	88%	25
Mercy Hospital Ada	Ada	80%	61

Appropriate VTP Within 24 Hours

Hospital Name	City	Rate	Cases
Bailey Medical Center	Owasso	100%	81
Duncan Regional Hospital	Duncan	100%	323
Hillcrest Hospital Cushing	Cushing	100%	32
Integris Baptist Regional Health Center	Miami	100%	89
Integris Mayes County Medical Center	Pryor	100%	36
McCurtain Memorial Hospital	Idabel	100%	27
Muskogee VA Medical Center[2]	Muskogee	100%	91
Oklahoma Heart Hospital	Oklahoma City	100%	53
Oklahoma Surgical Hospital[2]	Tulsa	100%	279
Saint Anthony Hospital[2]	Oklahoma City	100%	1482
Saint John Broken Arrow	Broken Arrow	100%	983
Woodward Regional Hospital	Woodward	100%	45
Mercy Hospital Oklahoma City[2]	Oklahoma City	99%	350
Mercy Memorial Health Center[2]	Ardmore	99%	295
Norman Regional Health System[2]	Norman	99%	448
Northwest Surgical Hospital[2]	Oklahoma City	99%	173
O U Medical Center[2]	Oklahoma City	99%	494
Oklahoma City VA Medical Center[2]	Oklahoma City	99%	266
Ponca City Medical Center	Ponca City	99%	175
Saint Mary's Regional Medical Center[2]	Enid	99%	335
Stillwater Medical Center	Stillwater	99%	364
Elkview General Hospital	Hobart	98%	61
Hillcrest Hospital Claremore	Claremore	98%	129
Integris Baptist Medical Center[2]	Oklahoma City	98%	308
Oklahoma Ctr for Ortho & Multi-Spec	Oklahoma City	98%	373
Saint Anthony Shawnee Hospital	Shawnee	98%	164
Saint Francis Hospital South	Tulsa	98%	259
Comanche County Memorial Hospital[2]	Lawton	97%	386
Great Plains Regional Medical Center[2]	Elk City	97%	117
Hillcrest Hospital South	Tulsa	97%	293
Hillcrest Medical Center[2]	Tulsa	97%	475
Integris Canadian Valley Hospital[2]	Yukon	97%	225
Integris Grove Hospital	Grove	97%	97
Jane Phillips Medical Center[2]	Bartlesville	97%	383
McAlester Regional Health Center[2]	Mcalester	97%	307
McBride Clinic Orthopedic Hospital[2]	Oklahoma City	97%	340
Mercy Hospital Logan County	Guthrie	97%	38
Saint John Medical Center[2]	Tulsa	97%	616
Deaconess Hospital	Oklahoma City	96%	342
Integris Southwest Medical Center[2]	Oklahoma City	96%	246
Jackson County Memorial Hospital[2]	Altus	96%	271
Oklahoma State University Medical Center[2]	Tulsa	96%	170
Saint John Owasso	Owasso	96%	119
Southwestern Medical Center	Lawton	96%	200
Tulsa Spine & Specialty Hospital[2]	Tulsa	96%	55
W W Hastings Indian Hospital[2]	Tahlequah	96%	75
Community Hospital[2]	Oklahoma City	95%	191
Medical Center of Southeastern Oklahoma	Durant	95%	183
Midwest Regional Medical Center[2]	Midwest City	95%	356
Saint Francis Hospital[2]	Tulsa	95%	1288
Tahlequah City Hospital	Tahlequah	95%	257
Eastar Health System	Muskogee	94%	491
Mercy Hospital Ada	Ada	94%	156
Grady Memorial Hospital	Chickasha	93%	42
Integris Bass Baptist Health Center	Enid	93%	188
Southwestern Regional Medical Center	Tulsa	93%	158
Summit Medical Center	Edmond	93%	41
Chickasaw Nation Medical Center	Ada	92%	51
Integris Health Edmond[2]	Edmond	90%	130
Drumright Regional Hospital	Drumright	87%	39
Surgical Hospital of Oklahoma	Oklahoma City	77%	163
Lakeside Women's Hospital[2]	Oklahoma City	18%	33

Controlled Postoperative Blood Glucose

Hospital Name	City	Rate	Cases
Saint John Medical Center[2]	Tulsa	100%	321
Oklahoma Heart Hospital South	Oklahoma City	99%	338
Oklahoma State University Medical Center[2]	Tulsa	99%	78
Integris Bass Baptist Health Center	Enid	98%	49
Oklahoma Heart Hospital	Oklahoma City	98%	759
Norman Regional Health System[2]	Norman	97%	73
Integris Baptist Medical Center[2]	Oklahoma City	96%	161
Saint Anthony Hospital[2]	Oklahoma City	96%	140
Saint Francis Hospital[2]	Tulsa	96%	289
Hillcrest Medical Center[2]	Tulsa	95%	196
O U Medical Center[2]	Oklahoma City	95%	80
Oklahoma City VA Medical Center[2]	Oklahoma City	95%	41
Comanche County Memorial Hospital[2]	Lawton	92%	151
Integris Southwest Medical Center[2]	Oklahoma City	92%	76
Tahlequah City Hospital	Tahlequah	90%	50

Perioperative Temperature Management

Hospital Name	City	Rate	Cases
Bailey Medical Center	Owasso	100%	89
Chickasaw Nation Medical Center	Ada	100%	53
Choctaw Nation Healthcare	Talihina	100%	43
Claremore Indian Hospital	Claremore	100%	51
Community Hospital[2]	Oklahoma City	100%	203
Craig General Hospital[2]	Vinita	100%	32
Deaconess Hospital	Oklahoma City	100%	419
Drumright Regional Hospital	Drumright	100%	39
Duncan Regional Hospital	Duncan	100%	362
Eastar Health System	Muskogee	100%	548

NOTE: Hospital profiles are in alphabetical order by state, then city, then hospital within the city; Rankings exclude hospitals with less than 25 cases except for patient surveys which excludes hospitals with less than 100 cases; (a) 100-299 cases; (1) The number of cases/patients is too few to report; (2) Data submitted were based on a sample of cases/patients; (3) Results are based on a shorter time period than required; (4) Data suppressed by CMS for one or more quarters; (5) Results are not available for this reporting period; (6) Fewer than 100 patients completed the HCAHPS survey; (7) No cases met the criteria for this measure; (8) The lower limit of the confidence interval cannot be calculated if the number of observed infections equals zero; (9) No data are available from the state/territory for this reporting period; (10) The scores shown reflect fewer than 50 completed surveys; (11) There were discrepancies in the data collection process; (12) This measure does not apply to this hospital for this reporting period; (13) Results cannot be calculated for this reporting period; (14) The results for this state are combined with nearby states to protect confidentiality; Please refer to the User's Guide for a full explanation of data.

Hospital Name	City	Rate	Cases
Eastern Oklahoma Medical Center	Poteau	100%	40
Elkview General Hospital	Hobart	100%	67
Hillcrest Hospital Claremore	Claremore	100%	148
Hillcrest Hospital Cushing	Cushing	100%	38
Hillcrest Hospital South	Tulsa	100%	333
Hillcrest Medical Center[2]	Tulsa	100%	590
Integris Baptist Medical Center[2]	Oklahoma City	100%	443
Integris Bass Baptist Health Center	Enid	100%	254
Integris Blackwell Regional Hospital	Blackwell	100%	26
Integris Canadian Valley Hospital[2]	Yukon	100%	239
Integris Grove Hospital	Grove	100%	105
Integris Health Edmond[2]	Edmond	100%	141
Integris Mayes County Medical Center	Pryor	100%	39
Integris Southwest Medical Center[2]	Oklahoma City	100%	332
Jackson County Memorial Hospital[2]	Altus	100%	295
Jane Phillips Medical Center[2]	Bartlesville	100%	437
Lakeside Women's Hospital[2]	Oklahoma City	100%	33
McAlester Regional Health Center[2]	Mcalester	100%	324
McBride Clinic Orthopedic Hospital[2]	Oklahoma City	100%	355
McCurtain Memorial Hospital	Idabel	100%	29
Medical Center of Southeastern Oklahoma	Durant	100%	209
Mercy Hospital Ada	Ada	100%	173
Mercy Hospital Logan County	Guthrie	100%	40
Mercy Hospital Oklahoma City[2]	Oklahoma City	100%	413
Mercy Memorial Health Center[2]	Ardmore	100%	347
Midwest Regional Medical Center[2]	Midwest City	100%	416
Muskogee VA Medical Center[2]	Muskogee	100%	98
Norman Regional Health System[2]	Norman	100%	504
Northwest Surgical Hospital[2]	Oklahoma City	100%	178
O U Medical Center[2]	Oklahoma City	100%	635
Oklahoma City VA Medical Center[2]	Oklahoma City	100%	328
Oklahoma Heart Hospital	Oklahoma City	100%	393
Oklahoma Heart Hospital South	Oklahoma City	100%	131
Oklahoma State University Medical Center[2]	Tulsa	100%	244
Oklahoma Surgical Hospital[2]	Tulsa	100%	320
Ponca City Medical Center	Ponca City	100%	194
Saint Anthony Hospital[2]	Oklahoma City	100%	1664
Saint Anthony Shawnee Hospital	Shawnee	100%	197
Saint Francis Hospital[2]	Tulsa	100%	1494
Saint Francis Hospital South	Tulsa	100%	296
Saint John Broken Arrow	Broken Arrow	100%	1095
Saint John Medical Center[2]	Tulsa	100%	794
Saint John Owasso	Owasso	100%	141
Saint Mary's Regional Medical Center[2]	Enid	100%	382
Southwestern Medical Center	Lawton	100%	227
Southwestern Regional Medical Center	Tulsa	100%	169
Summit Medical Center	Edmond	100%	52
Tahlequah City Hospital	Tahlequah	100%	320
Tulsa Spine & Specialty Hospital[2]	Tulsa	100%	99
Woodward Regional Hospital	Woodward	100%	74
Comanche County Memorial Hospital[2]	Lawton	99%	473
Great Plains Regional Medical Center[2]	Elk City	99%	122
Integris Baptist Regional Health Center	Miami	99%	105
Stillwater Medical Center	Stillwater	99%	391
Surgical Hospital of Oklahoma	Oklahoma City	99%	174
Oklahoma Ctr for Ortho & Multi-Spec	Oklahoma City	97%	373
W W Hastings Indian Hospital[2]	Tahlequah	97%	92
Grady Memorial Hospital	Chickasha	94%	53

Prophylactic Antibiotic Selection

Hospital Name	City	Rate	Cases
Chickasaw Nation Medical Center	Ada	100%	36
Comanche County Memorial Hospital[2]	Lawton	100%	377
Community Hospital[2]	Oklahoma City	100%	172
Craig General Hospital[2]	Vinita	100%	29
Deaconess Hospital	Oklahoma City	100%	215
Duncan Regional Hospital	Duncan	100%	261
Elkview General Hospital	Hobart	100%	45
Hillcrest Hospital South	Tulsa	100%	217
Hillcrest Medical Center[2]	Tulsa	100%	595
Integris Canadian Valley Hospital[2]	Yukon	100%	158
Integris Mayes County Medical Center	Pryor	100%	33
McBride Clinic Orthopedic Hospital[2]	Oklahoma City	100%	274
Mercy Hospital Ada	Ada	100%	92
Mercy Hospital Logan County	Guthrie	100%	34
Mercy Hospital Oklahoma City[2]	Oklahoma City	100%	264
Oklahoma Ctr for Ortho & Multi-Spec	Oklahoma City	100%	345
Oklahoma Heart Hospital	Oklahoma City	100%	826
Oklahoma Heart Hospital South	Oklahoma City	100%	333
Oklahoma Surgical Hospital[2]	Tulsa	100%	225
Saint Anthony Hospital[2]	Oklahoma City	100%	1518
Saint Anthony Shawnee Hospital	Shawnee	100%	128
Saint John Broken Arrow	Broken Arrow	100%	984
Stillwater Medical Center	Stillwater	100%	302
Summit Medical Center	Edmond	100%	36
Woodward Regional Hospital	Woodward	100%	26
Hillcrest Hospital Claremore	Claremore	99%	113
Integris Baptist Medical Center[2]	Oklahoma City	99%	448
Integris Baptist Regional Health Center	Miami	99%	79
Integris Southwest Medical Center[2]	Oklahoma City	99%	265
Jackson County Memorial Hospital[2]	Altus	99%	194
Norman Regional Health System[2]	Norman	99%	383
Northwest Surgical Hospital[2]	Oklahoma City	99%	166
O U Medical Center[2]	Oklahoma City	99%	429
Oklahoma City VA Medical Center	Oklahoma City	99%	257
Saint John Medical Center[2]	Tulsa	99%	835
Saint John Owasso	Owasso	99%	112
Tahlequah City Hospital	Tahlequah	99%	303
Bailey Medical Center	Owasso	98%	66
Eastar Health System	Muskogee	98%	384
Integris Bass Baptist Health Center	Enid	98%	180
Integris Health Edmond[2]	Edmond	98%	101
Medical Center of Southeastern Oklahoma	Durant	98%	147
Mercy Memorial Health Center[2]	Ardmore	98%	196
Midwest Regional Medical Center[2]	Midwest City	98%	306
Ponca City Medical Center	Ponca City	98%	131
Saint Francis Hospital[2]	Tulsa	98%	1321
Saint Mary's Regional Medical Center[2]	Enid	98%	248
Surgical Hospital of Oklahoma	Oklahoma City	98%	126
Tulsa Spine & Specialty Hospital[2]	Tulsa	98%	65
W W Hastings Indian Hospital[2]	Tahlequah	98%	61
Claremore Indian Hospital	Claremore	97%	37
Drumright Regional Hospital	Drumright	97%	34
Hillcrest Hospital Cushing	Cushing	97%	32
Jane Phillips Medical Center[2]	Bartlesville	97%	316
Saint Francis Hospital South	Tulsa	97%	237
Southwestern Regional Medical Center	Tulsa	97%	32
Integris Grove Hospital	Grove	96%	79
McAlester Regional Health Center[2]	Mcalester	96%	250
Muskogee VA Medical Center	Muskogee	96%	27
Oklahoma State University Medical Center[2]	Tulsa	96%	192
Southwestern Medical Center	Lawton	96%	144
Grady Memorial Hospital	Chickasha	93%	42
Great Plains Regional Medical Center[2]	Elk City	93%	94
Lakeside Women's Hospital[2]	Oklahoma City	93%	29
Choctaw Nation Healthcare	Talihina	75%	40
Eastern Oklahoma Medical Center	Poteau	73%	37

Prophylactic Antibiotic Selection (Outpatient)

Hospital Name	City	Rate	Cases
Bailey Medical Center	Owasso	100%	47
Hillcrest Hospital South	Tulsa	100%	164
Hillcrest Medical Center	Tulsa	100%	629
Integris Baptist Regional Health Center	Miami	100%	37
McBride Clinic Orthopedic Hospital	Oklahoma City	100%	60
Oklahoma Heart Hospital	Oklahoma City	100%	518
Oklahoma Heart Hospital South	Oklahoma City	100%	188
Oklahoma Spine Hospital	Oklahoma City	100%	179
Oklahoma Surgical Hospital	Tulsa	100%	483
Ponca City Medical Center	Ponca City	100%	67
Saint John Broken Arrow	Broken Arrow	100%	31
Community Hospital	Oklahoma City	99%	159
Deaconess Hospital	Oklahoma City	99%	458
Integris Baptist Medical Center	Oklahoma City	99%	525
Integris Southwest Medical Center	Oklahoma City	99%	171
Mercy Hospital Ada	Ada	99%	221
Norman Regional Health System	Norman	99%	584
O U Medical Center	Oklahoma City	99%	709
Saint Anthony Hospital	Oklahoma City	99%	303
Summit Medical Center	Edmond	99%	171
Tulsa Spine & Specialty Hospital	Tulsa	99%	464
Duncan Regional Hospital	Duncan	98%	57
Eastar Health System	Muskogee	98%	113
Hillcrest Hospital Claremore	Claremore	98%	59
Integris Canadian Valley Hospital	Yukon	98%	124
Integris Grove Hospital	Grove	98%	41
Jane Phillips Medical Center	Bartlesville	98%	129
Medical Center of Southeastern Oklahoma	Durant	98%	228
Oklahoma Ctr for Ortho & Multi-Spec	Oklahoma City	98%	87
Saint Anthony Shawnee Hospital	Shawnee	98%	65
Saint Francis Hospital South	Tulsa	98%	60
Saint John Medical Center	Tulsa	98%	834
Tahlequah City Hospital	Tahlequah	98%	58
Woodward Regional Hospital	Woodward	98%	46
Comanche County Memorial Hospital	Lawton	97%	447
Hillcrest Hospital Cushing	Cushing	97%	29
Integris Bass Baptist Health Center	Enid	97%	69
Mercy Hospital Oklahoma City	Oklahoma City	97%	425
Midwest Regional Medical Center	Midwest City	97%	165
Oklahoma State University Medical Center	Tulsa	97%	86
Saint Francis Hospital	Tulsa	97%	716
Saint Mary's Regional Medical Center	Enid	97%	235
Southwestern Regional Medical Center	Tulsa	97%	66
Stillwater Medical Center	Stillwater	97%	117
Integris Health Edmond	Edmond	95%	38
Surgical Hospital of Oklahoma	Oklahoma City	94%	106
Mercy Memorial Health Center	Ardmore	93%	319
Southwestern Medical Center	Lawton	92%	158
McAlester Regional Health Center	Mcalester	91%	35
Lakeside Women's Hospital	Oklahoma City	90%	166
Northwest Surgical Hospital[3]	Oklahoma City	88%	25

Prophylactic Antibiotic Stopped

Hospital Name	City	Rate	Cases
Choctaw Nation Healthcare	Talihina	100%	40
Eastern Oklahoma Medical Center	Poteau	100%	37
Great Plains Regional Medical Center[2]	Elk City	100%	83
Integris Mayes County Medical Center	Pryor	100%	32
Lakeside Women's Hospital[2]	Oklahoma City	100%	29
McBride Clinic Orthopedic Hospital[2]	Oklahoma City	100%	274
Mercy Hospital Ada	Ada	100%	91
Oklahoma Heart Hospital South	Oklahoma City	100%	310
Oklahoma Surgical Hospital[2]	Tulsa	100%	224
Saint Anthony Hospital[2]	Oklahoma City	100%	1478
Saint Anthony Shawnee Hospital	Shawnee	100%	128
Saint John Broken Arrow	Broken Arrow	100%	982
Saint John Owasso	Owasso	100%	111
Saint Mary's Regional Medical Center[2]	Enid	100%	242
Summit Medical Center	Edmond	100%	36
Hillcrest Hospital South	Tulsa	99%	213
Integris Bass Baptist Health Center	Enid	99%	180
Integris Canadian Valley Hospital[2]	Yukon	99%	155
Integris Grove Hospital	Grove	99%	78
Medical Center of Southeastern Oklahoma	Durant	99%	142
Mercy Hospital Oklahoma City[2]	Oklahoma City	99%	250
Mercy Memorial Health Center[2]	Ardmore	99%	183
O U Medical Center[2]	Oklahoma City	99%	389
Oklahoma Ctr for Ortho & Multi-Spec	Oklahoma City	99%	345
Oklahoma Heart Hospital	Oklahoma City	99%	760
Ponca City Medical Center	Ponca City	99%	127
Saint Francis Hospital South	Tulsa	99%	235
Stillwater Medical Center	Stillwater	99%	299
Bailey Medical Center	Owasso	98%	65
Comanche County Memorial Hospital[2]	Lawton	98%	368
Community Hospital[2]	Oklahoma City	98%	172
Deaconess Hospital	Oklahoma City	98%	213
Duncan Regional Hospital	Duncan	98%	257
Eastar Health System	Muskogee	98%	373
Hillcrest Medical Center[2]	Tulsa	98%	575
Integris Baptist Medical Center[2]	Oklahoma City	98%	440
Jackson County Memorial Hospital[2]	Altus	98%	185
Jane Phillips Medical Center[2]	Bartlesville	98%	310
Norman Regional Health System[2]	Norman	98%	354
Northwest Surgical Hospital[2]	Oklahoma City	98%	166
Saint Francis Hospital[2]	Tulsa	98%	1291
Saint John Medical Center[2]	Tulsa	98%	815
Chickasaw Nation Medical Center	Ada	97%	36
Craig General Hospital[2]	Vinita	97%	29
Integris Health Edmond[2]	Edmond	97%	100
Integris Southwest Medical Center[2]	Oklahoma City	97%	240
Mercy Hospital Logan County	Guthrie	97%	32
Midwest Regional Medical Center[2]	Midwest City	97%	300
Oklahoma City VA Medical Center	Oklahoma City	97%	256
Southwestern Medical Center	Lawton	97%	141
Tahlequah City Hospital	Tahlequah	97%	298
Hillcrest Hospital Claremore	Claremore	96%	107
McAlester Regional Health Center[2]	Mcalester	96%	250
Integris Baptist Regional Health Center	Miami	95%	75
Tulsa Spine & Specialty Hospital[2]	Tulsa	95%	65
Claremore Indian Hospital	Claremore	94%	36
Hillcrest Hospital Cushing	Cushing	94%	32
Elkview General Hospital	Hobart	93%	45
W W Hastings Indian Hospital[2]	Tahlequah	93%	60
Muskogee VA Medical Center	Muskogee	92%	26
Oklahoma State University Medical Center[2]	Tulsa	89%	187
Southwestern Regional Medical Center	Tulsa	89%	28
Grady Memorial Hospital	Chickasha	88%	42
Drumright Regional Hospital	Drumright	50%	34
Surgical Hospital of Oklahoma	Oklahoma City	37%	126

Prophylactic Antibiotic Timing

Hospital Name	City	Rate	Cases
Chickasaw Nation Medical Center	Ada	100%	36
Deaconess Hospital	Oklahoma City	100%	215
Duncan Regional Hospital	Duncan	100%	261
Hillcrest Hospital Cushing	Cushing	100%	32
Hillcrest Hospital South	Tulsa	100%	217
Hillcrest Medical Center[2]	Tulsa	100%	596
Integris Baptist Medical Center[2]	Oklahoma City	100%	448
Integris Mayes County Medical Center	Pryor	100%	33
Integris Southwest Medical Center[2]	Oklahoma City	100%	266
McBride Clinic Orthopedic Hospital[2]	Oklahoma City	100%	274
Mercy Hospital Oklahoma City[2]	Oklahoma City	100%	264
Muskogee VA Medical Center	Muskogee	100%	27
O U Medical Center[2]	Oklahoma City	100%	430
Oklahoma Heart Hospital	Oklahoma City	100%	829
Oklahoma Surgical Hospital[2]	Tulsa	100%	225
Ponca City Medical Center	Ponca City	100%	131
Saint Anthony Hospital[2]	Oklahoma City	100%	1519
Saint John Broken Arrow	Broken Arrow	100%	984
Saint John Medical Center[2]	Tulsa	100%	836
Saint John Owasso	Owasso	100%	112

NOTE: Hospital profiles are in alphabetical order by state, then city, then hospital within the city; Rankings exclude hospitals with less than 25 cases except for patient surveys which excludes hospitals with less than 100 cases; (a) 100-299 cases; (1) The number of cases/patients is too few to report; (2) Data submitted were based on a sample of cases/patients; (3) Results are based on a shorter time period than required; (4) Data suppressed by CMS for one or more quarters; (5) Results are not available for this reporting period; (6) Fewer than 100 patients completed the HCAHPS survey; (7) No cases met the criteria for this measure; (8) The lower limit of the confidence interval cannot be calculated if the number of observed infections equals zero; (9) No data are available from the state/territory for this reporting period; (10) The scores shown reflect fewer than 50 completed surveys; (11) There were discrepancies in the data collection process; (12) This measure does not apply to this hospital for this reporting period; (13) Results cannot be calculated for this reporting period; (14) The results for this state are combined with nearby states to protect confidentiality; Please refer to the User's Guide for a full explanation of data.

Hospital Name	City	Rate	Cases
Summit Medical Center	Edmond	100%	36
Woodward Regional Hospital	Woodward	100%	26
Community Hospital[2]	Oklahoma City	99%	172
Hillcrest Hospital Claremore	Claremore	99%	113
Integris Health Edmond[2]	Edmond	99%	101
Jane Phillips Medical Center[2]	Bartlesville	99%	316
Medical Center of Southeastern Oklahoma	Durant	99%	148
Mercy Hospital Ada	Ada	99%	92
Midwest Regional Medical Center[2]	Midwest City	99%	307
Oklahoma State University Medical Center[2]	Tulsa	99%	194
Saint Anthony Shawnee Hospital	Shawnee	99%	128
Saint Francis Hospital South	Tulsa	99%	237
Southwestern Medical Center	Lawton	99%	144
Bailey Medical Center	Owasso	98%	66
Comanche County Memorial Hospital[2]	Lawton	98%	378
Eastar Health System	Muskogee	98%	384
Great Plains Regional Medical Center[2]	Elk City	98%	94
Integris Canadian Valley Hospital[2]	Yukon	98%	158
Integris Grove Hospital	Grove	98%	80
Norman Regional Health System[2]	Norman	98%	385
Northwest Surgical Hospital[2]	Oklahoma City	98%	166
Oklahoma City VA Medical Center	Oklahoma City	98%	257
Oklahoma Heart Hospital South	Oklahoma City	98%	336
Saint Mary's Regional Medical Center[2]	Enid	98%	248
Stillwater Medical Center	Stillwater	98%	302
Tulsa Spine & Specialty Hospital[2]	Tulsa	98%	65
Claremore Indian Hospital	Claremore	97%	38
Jackson County Memorial Hospital[2]	Altus	97%	195
Lakeside Women's Hospital[2]	Oklahoma City	97%	30
McAlester Regional Health Center[2]	Mcalester	97%	250
Saint Francis Hospital[2]	Tulsa	97%	1322
Southwestern Regional Medical Center	Tulsa	97%	32
Tahlequah City Hospital	Tahlequah	97%	303
Integris Baptist Regional Health Center	Miami	96%	79
Mercy Memorial Health Center[2]	Ardmore	95%	196
Drumright Regional Hospital	Drumright	94%	34
Integris Bass Baptist Health Center	Enid	94%	181
Mercy Hospital Logan County	Guthrie	94%	34
Craig General Hospital[2]	Vinita	93%	29
W W Hastings Indian Hospital[2]	Tahlequah	93%	61
Oklahoma Ctr for Ortho & Multi-Spec	Oklahoma City	92%	345
Surgical Hospital of Oklahoma	Oklahoma City	91%	127
Choctaw Nation Healthcare	Talihina	88%	43
Grady Memorial Hospital	Chickasha	88%	42
Elkview General Hospital	Hobart	87%	46
Eastern Oklahoma Medical Center	Poteau	61%	38

Prophylactic Antibiotic Timing (Outpatient)

Hospital Name	City	Rate	Cases
Bailey Medical Center	Owasso	100%	47
Community Hospital	Oklahoma City	100%	159
Hillcrest Hospital Claremore	Claremore	100%	59
Hillcrest Hospital Cushing	Cushing	100%	29
Hillcrest Hospital South	Tulsa	100%	164
McBride Clinic Orthopedic Hospital	Oklahoma City	100%	60
Oklahoma Heart Hospital	Oklahoma City	100%	518
Oklahoma Surgical Hospital	Tulsa	100%	483
Ponca City Medical Center	Ponca City	100%	67
Saint Francis Hospital South	Tulsa	100%	60
Saint John Broken Arrow	Broken Arrow	100%	31
Woodward Regional Hospital	Woodward	100%	46
Deaconess Hospital	Oklahoma City	99%	425
Hillcrest Medical Center	Tulsa	99%	579
Medical Center of Southeastern Oklahoma	Durant	99%	228
Midwest Regional Medical Center	Midwest City	99%	167
Norman Regional Health System	Norman	99%	585
O U Medical Center	Oklahoma City	99%	678
Oklahoma Heart Hospital South	Oklahoma City	99%	188
Oklahoma Spine Hospital	Oklahoma City	99%	179
Saint Mary's Regional Medical Center	Enid	99%	233
Southwestern Medical Center	Lawton	99%	159
Summit Medical Center	Edmond	99%	173
Tulsa Spine & Specialty Hospital	Tulsa	99%	465
Integris Baptist Medical Center	Oklahoma City	98%	522
Integris Canadian Valley Hospital	Yukon	98%	124
Integris Southwest Medical Center	Oklahoma City	98%	172
Mercy Hospital Oklahoma City	Oklahoma City	98%	420
Saint Anthony Hospital	Oklahoma City	98%	306
Saint Francis Hospital	Tulsa	98%	723
Saint John Medical Center	Tulsa	98%	841
Tahlequah City Hospital	Tahlequah	98%	59
Comanche County Memorial Hospital	Lawton	97%	453
Duncan Regional Hospital	Duncan	97%	58
Eastar Health System	Muskogee	97%	115
Mercy Hospital Ada	Ada	97%	226
Saint Anthony Shawnee Hospital	Shawnee	97%	67
Stillwater Medical Center	Stillwater	97%	118
Integris Bass Baptist Health Center	Enid	96%	71
Northwest Surgical Hospital[3]	Oklahoma City	96%	25
Integris Baptist Regional Health Center	Miami	95%	38
Lakeside Women's Hospital	Oklahoma City	95%	167

Hospital Name	City	Rate	Cases
Mercy Memorial Health Center	Ardmore	95%	321
Surgical Hospital of Oklahoma	Oklahoma City	95%	106
Oklahoma State University Medical Center	Tulsa	94%	86
Oklahoma Ctr for Ortho & Multi-Spec	Oklahoma City	92%	91
Southwestern Regional Medical Center	Tulsa	92%	66
Integris Grove Hospital	Grove	91%	44
McAlester Regional Health Center	Mcalester	89%	36
Jane Phillips Medical Center	Bartlesville	87%	148

Urinary Catheter Removal

Hospital Name	City	Rate	Cases
Bailey Medical Center	Owasso	100%	51
Integris Mayes County Medical Center	Pryor	100%	26
Muskogee VA Medical Center[2]	Muskogee	100%	61
Oklahoma Ctr for Ortho & Multi-Spec	Oklahoma City	100%	369
Oklahoma Heart Hospital	Oklahoma City	100%	860
Oklahoma Heart Hospital South	Oklahoma City	100%	248
Oklahoma Surgical Hospital[2]	Tulsa	100%	81
Ponca City Medical Center	Ponca City	100%	120
Saint Anthony Shawnee Hospital	Shawnee	100%	90
Hillcrest Medical Center[2]	Tulsa	99%	408
Stillwater Medical Center	Stillwater	99%	272
Community Hospital[2]	Oklahoma City	98%	62
Hillcrest Hospital Claremore	Claremore	98%	63
Integris Grove Hospital	Grove	98%	81
Saint Anthony Hospital[2]	Oklahoma City	98%	391
Saint John Broken Arrow	Broken Arrow	98%	58
Saint John Medical Center[2]	Tulsa	98%	548
Duncan Regional Hospital	Duncan	97%	77
Integris Baptist Regional Health Center	Miami	97%	68
Integris Canadian Valley Hospital[2]	Yukon	97%	144
Medical Center of Southeastern Oklahoma	Durant	97%	128
O U Medical Center[2]	Oklahoma City	97%	189
Oklahoma City VA Medical Center[2]	Oklahoma City	97%	39
Saint Mary's Regional Medical Center[2]	Enid	97%	87
Surgical Hospital of Oklahoma	Oklahoma City	97%	71
Tahlequah City Hospital	Tahlequah	97%	287
Integris Bass Baptist Health Center	Enid	96%	134
Integris Southwest Medical Center[2]	Oklahoma City	96%	294
Jackson County Memorial Hospital[2]	Altus	96%	168
Norman Regional Health System[2]	Norman	96%	292
Comanche County Memorial Hospital[2]	Lawton	95%	381
Deaconess Hospital	Oklahoma City	95%	117
Integris Baptist Medical Center[2]	Oklahoma City	95%	348
Integris Health Edmond[2]	Edmond	95%	40
Jane Phillips Medical Center[2]	Bartlesville	95%	196
Saint Francis Hospital South	Tulsa	95%	159
McAlester Regional Health Center[2]	Mcalester	94%	198
Mercy Hospital Oklahoma City[2]	Oklahoma City	94%	111
Eastar Health System	Muskogee	93%	274
Saint Francis Hospital[2]	Tulsa	93%	791
Hillcrest Hospital South	Tulsa	92%	205
Mercy Memorial Health Center[2]	Ardmore	92%	88
Oklahoma State University Medical Center[2]	Tulsa	92%	159
Great Plains Regional Medical Center[2]	Elk City	89%	27
Southwestern Medical Center	Lawton	89%	83
Mercy Hospital Ada	Ada	86%	78
Southwestern Regional Medical Center	Tulsa	85%	41
Midwest Regional Medical Center[2]	Midwest City	84%	113
Elkview General Hospital	Hobart	60%	57

Survey of Patients' Hospital Experiences

Area Around Room 'Always' Quiet at Night

Hospital Name	City	Rate	Cases
Tulsa Spine & Specialty Hospital	Tulsa	89%	300+
Oklahoma Spine Hospital	Oklahoma City	86%	300+
Integris Health Edmond	Edmond	85%	300+
Oklahoma Surgical Hospital	Tulsa	84%	300+
Northwest Surgical Hospital	Oklahoma City	83%	(a)
McBride Clinic Orthopedic Hospital	Oklahoma City	80%	300+
Oklahoma Ctr for Ortho & Multi-Spec	Oklahoma City	80%	(a)
Surgical Hospital of Oklahoma	Oklahoma City	80%	(a)
Bailey Medical Center	Owasso	78%	300+
Community Hospital	Oklahoma City	78%	300+
Oklahoma Heart Hospital South	Oklahoma City	78%	300+
Integris Marshall County Medical Center	Madill	77%	(a)
Muscogee (Creek) Nation Medical Center	Okmulgee	77%	(a)
Chickasaw Nation Medical Center	Ada	76%	300+
Choctaw Nation Healthcare	Talihina	75%	300+
Saint John Broken Arrow	Broken Arrow	75%	300+
Integris Blackwell Regional Hospital	Blackwell	73%	(a)
Integris Canadian Valley Hospital	Yukon	73%	300+
Oklahoma Heart Hospital	Oklahoma City	72%	300+
Hillcrest Hospital Henryetta	Henryetta	71%	(a)
Integris Mayes County Medical Center	Pryor	70%	(a)
Integris Seminole Medical Center	Seminole	69%	(a)
Jane Phillips Medical Center	Bartlesville	69%	300+
Pauls Valley General Hospital	Pauls Valley	69%	(a)
Great Plains Regional Medical Center	Elk City	68%	300+

Hospital Name	City	Rate	Cases
Saint John Sapulpa	Sapulpa	68%	(a)
Southwestern Regional Medical Center	Tulsa	68%	(a)
Integris Grove Hospital	Grove	67%	300+
Purcell Municipal Hospital	Purcell	67%	(a)
Saint Anthony Shawnee Hospital	Shawnee	67%	300+
Saint John Owasso	Owasso	67%	300+
Integris Baptist Medical Center	Oklahoma City	66%	300+
Memorial Hospital of Texas County	Guymon	66%	(a)
Stillwater Medical Center	Stillwater	66%	300+
Claremore Indian Hospital	Claremore	65%	(a)
Duncan Regional Hospital	Duncan	65%	300+
McCurtain Memorial Hospital	Idabel	65%	(a)
Memorial Hospital of Stilwell	Stilwell	64%	(a)
Southwestern Medical Center	Lawton	64%	300+
Wagoner Community Hospital	Wagoner	64%	(a)
Comanche County Memorial Hospital	Lawton	63%	300+
Deaconess Hospital	Oklahoma City	63%	300+
Integris Clinton Regional Hospital	Clinton	63%	(a)
Mercy Hospital Ada[11]	Ada	63%	300+
Norman Regional Health System	Norman	63%	300+
Saint Anthony Hospital	Oklahoma City	63%	300+
Woodward Regional Hospital	Woodward	63%	300+
Integris Southwest Medical Center	Oklahoma City	62%	300+
Lakeside Women's Hospital	Oklahoma City	62%	(a)
Mercy Hospital Oklahoma City[11]	Oklahoma City	62%	300+
Saint Mary's Regional Medical Center	Enid	62%	300+
Craig General Hospital	Vinita	61%	(a)
Hillcrest Hospital Cushing	Cushing	61%	300+
Hillcrest Hospital South	Tulsa	61%	300+
Mercy Memorial Health Center[11]	Ardmore	61%	300+
Ponca City Medical Center	Ponca City	61%	300+
Eastern Oklahoma Medical Center	Poteau	60%	300+
Grady Memorial Hospital	Chickasha	60%	300+
Hillcrest Medical Center	Tulsa	60%	300+
Jackson County Memorial Hospital	Altus	60%	300+
W W Hastings Indian Hospital	Tahlequah	60%	300+
Saint Francis Hospital	Tulsa	59%	300+
Integris Baptist Regional Health Center	Miami	58%	300+
Integris Bass Baptist Health Center	Enid	57%	300+
Medical Center of Southeastern Oklahoma	Durant	57%	300+
Saint John Medical Center	Tulsa	57%	300+
Choctaw Memorial Hospital	Hugo	56%	(a)
Elkview General Hospital	Hobart	56%	(a)
Midwest Regional Medical Center	Midwest City	56%	300+
Hillcrest Hospital Claremore	Claremore	55%	300+
Eastar Health System	Muskogee	54%	300+
McAlester Regional Health Center	Mcalester	54%	300+
O U Medical Center	Oklahoma City	54%	300+
Oklahoma State University Medical Center	Tulsa	54%	300+
Saint Francis Hospital South	Tulsa	54%	300+
Tahlequah City Hospital	Tahlequah	52%	300+

Doctors 'Always' Communicated Well

Hospital Name	City	Rate	Cases
Purcell Municipal Hospital	Purcell	94%	(a)
Integris Marshall County Medical Center	Madill	91%	(a)
Northwest Surgical Hospital	Oklahoma City	90%	(a)
Oklahoma Heart Hospital	Oklahoma City	90%	300+
Oklahoma Spine Hospital	Oklahoma City	90%	300+
Craig General Hospital	Vinita	89%	(a)
Elkview General Hospital	Hobart	89%	(a)
Integris Blackwell Regional Hospital	Blackwell	89%	(a)
Southwestern Regional Medical Center	Tulsa	89%	(a)
Eastern Oklahoma Medical Center	Poteau	88%	300+
Hillcrest Hospital Henryetta	Henryetta	88%	(a)
Integris Health Edmond	Edmond	88%	300+
Bailey Medical Center	Owasso	87%	300+
Integris Clinton Regional Hospital	Clinton	87%	(a)
McBride Clinic Orthopedic Hospital	Oklahoma City	87%	300+
Memorial Hospital of Stilwell	Stilwell	87%	(a)
Oklahoma Ctr for Ortho & Multi-Spec	Oklahoma City	87%	(a)
Oklahoma Heart Hospital South	Oklahoma City	87%	300+
Oklahoma Surgical Hospital	Tulsa	87%	300+
Woodward Regional Hospital	Woodward	87%	300+
Duncan Regional Hospital	Duncan	86%	300+
Integris Mayes County Medical Center	Pryor	86%	(a)
Saint John Owasso	Owasso	86%	300+
Saint John Sapulpa	Sapulpa	86%	(a)
Chickasaw Nation Medical Center	Ada	85%	300+
Choctaw Nation Healthcare	Talihina	85%	300+
Jackson County Memorial Hospital	Altus	85%	300+
Jane Phillips Medical Center	Bartlesville	85%	300+
Muscogee (Creek) Nation Medical Center	Okmulgee	85%	(a)
Saint Anthony Shawnee Hospital	Shawnee	85%	300+
Saint Mary's Regional Medical Center	Enid	85%	300+
Tulsa Spine & Specialty Hospital	Tulsa	85%	300+
Choctaw Memorial Hospital	Hugo	84%	(a)
Community Hospital	Oklahoma City	84%	300+
Integris Baptist Medical Center	Oklahoma City	84%	300+
Integris Baptist Regional Health Center	Miami	84%	300+
Integris Canadian Valley Hospital	Yukon	84%	300+

NOTE: Hospital profiles are in alphabetical order by state, then city, then hospital within the city; Rankings exclude hospitals with less than 25 cases except for patient surveys which excludes hospitals with less than 100 cases; (a) 100-299 cases; (1) The number of cases/patients is too few to report; (2) Data submitted were based on a sample of cases/patients; (3) Results are based on a shorter time period than required; (4) Data suppressed by CMS for one or more quarters; (5) Results are not available for this reporting period; (6) Fewer than 100 patients completed the HCAHPS survey; (7) No cases met the criteria for this measure; (8) The lower limit of the confidence interval cannot be calculated if the number of observed infections equals zero; (9) No data are available from the state/territory for this reporting period; (10) The scores shown reflect fewer than 50 completed surveys; (11) There were discrepancies in the data collection process; (12) This measure does not apply to this hospital for this reporting period; (13) Results cannot be calculated for this reporting period; (14) The results for this state are combined with nearby states to protect confidentiality; Please refer to the User's Guide for a full explanation of data.

Hospital Name	City	Rate	Cases
Integris Seminole Medical Center	Seminole	84%	(a)
Mercy Hospital Oklahoma City[11]	Oklahoma City	84%	300+
Ponca City Medical Center	Ponca City	84%	300+
Saint Anthony Hospital	Oklahoma City	84%	300+
Saint John Broken Arrow	Broken Arrow	84%	300+
Hillcrest Hospital Claremore	Claremore	83%	300+
Hillcrest Hospital Cushing	Cushing	83%	300+
Lakeside Women's Hospital	Oklahoma City	83%	(a)
Mercy Memorial Health Center[11]	Ardmore	83%	300+
Stillwater Medical Center	Stillwater	83%	300+
Claremore Indian Hospital	Claremore	82%	(a)
Comanche County Memorial Hospital	Lawton	82%	300+
Grady Memorial Hospital	Chickasha	82%	300+
Great Plains Regional Medical Center	Elk City	82%	300+
Integris Bass Baptist Health Center	Enid	82%	300+
Integris Grove Hospital	Grove	82%	300+
Memorial Hospital of Texas County	Guymon	82%	(a)
Saint Francis Hospital South	Tulsa	82%	300+
Southwestern Medical Center	Lawton	82%	300+
Wagoner Community Hospital	Wagoner	82%	(a)
Deaconess Hospital	Oklahoma City	81%	300+
Surgical Hospital of Oklahoma	Oklahoma City	81%	(a)
W W Hastings Indian Hospital	Tahlequah	81%	300+
Mercy Hospital Ada[11]	Ada	80%	300+
Pauls Valley General Hospital	Pauls Valley	80%	(a)
Medical Center of Southeastern Oklahoma	Durant	79%	300+
Norman Regional Health System	Norman	79%	300+
Saint John Medical Center	Tulsa	79%	300+
Eastar Health System	Muskogee	78%	300+
Hillcrest Hospital South	Tulsa	78%	300+
McCurtain Memorial Hospital	Idabel	78%	(a)
Oklahoma State University Medical Center	Tulsa	78%	300+
Saint Francis Hospital	Tulsa	77%	300+
Integris Southwest Medical Center	Oklahoma City	76%	300+
McAlester Regional Health Center	Mcalester	76%	300+
O U Medical Center	Oklahoma City	76%	300+
Tahlequah City Hospital	Tahlequah	76%	300+
Hillcrest Medical Center	Tulsa	75%	300+
Midwest Regional Medical Center	Midwest City	74%	300+

Home Recovery Information Given

Hospital Name	City	Rate	Cases
Bailey Medical Center	Owasso	91%	300+
McBride Clinic Orthopedic Hospital	Oklahoma City	91%	300+
Oklahoma Ctr for Ortho & Multi-Spec	Oklahoma City	91%	(a)
Eastern Oklahoma Medical Center	Poteau	90%	300+
Elkview General Hospital	Hobart	90%	(a)
Stillwater Medical Center	Stillwater	90%	300+
Integris Mayes County Medical Center	Pryor	89%	(a)
Oklahoma Heart Hospital South	Oklahoma City	89%	300+
Saint John Broken Arrow	Broken Arrow	89%	300+
Saint Mary's Regional Medical Center	Enid	89%	300+
Southwestern Regional Medical Center	Tulsa	89%	(a)
Integris Health Edmond	Edmond	88%	300+
Mercy Hospital Ada[11]	Ada	88%	300+
Norman Regional Health System	Norman	88%	300+
Northwest Surgical Hospital	Oklahoma City	88%	(a)
Oklahoma Heart Hospital	Oklahoma City	88%	300+
Oklahoma Spine Hospital	Oklahoma City	88%	300+
Tulsa Spine & Specialty Hospital	Tulsa	88%	300+
Woodward Regional Hospital	Woodward	88%	300+
Chickasaw Nation Medical Center	Ada	87%	300+
Community Hospital	Oklahoma City	87%	300+
Deaconess Hospital	Oklahoma City	87%	300+
Duncan Regional Hospital	Duncan	87%	300+
Grady Memorial Hospital	Chickasha	87%	300+
Jackson County Memorial Hospital	Altus	87%	300+
Mercy Hospital Oklahoma City[11]	Oklahoma City	87%	300+
Muscogee (Creek) Nation Medical Center	Okmulgee	87%	(a)
Oklahoma Surgical Hospital	Tulsa	87%	300+
Ponca City Medical Center	Ponca City	87%	300+
Saint Anthony Hospital	Oklahoma City	87%	300+
Choctaw Nation Healthcare	Talihina	86%	300+
Hillcrest Hospital Claremore	Claremore	86%	300+
Integris Baptist Regional Health Center	Miami	86%	300+
Lakeside Women's Hospital	Oklahoma City	86%	(a)
Hillcrest Hospital Cushing	Cushing	85%	300+
Hillcrest Hospital South	Tulsa	85%	300+
Integris Clinton Regional Hospital	Clinton	85%	(a)
Integris Southwest Medical Center	Oklahoma City	85%	300+
Memorial Hospital of Texas County	Guymon	85%	(a)
Saint Anthony Shawnee Hospital	Shawnee	85%	300+
Surgical Hospital of Oklahoma	Oklahoma City	85%	(a)
Claremore Indian Hospital	Claremore	84%	(a)
Hillcrest Hospital Henryetta	Henryetta	84%	(a)
Integris Baptist Medical Center	Oklahoma City	84%	300+
Integris Canadian Valley Hospital	Yukon	84%	300+
Integris Grove Hospital	Grove	84%	300+
Integris Marshall County Medical Center	Madill	84%	(a)
Mercy Memorial Health Center[11]	Ardmore	84%	300+
O U Medical Center	Oklahoma City	84%	300+
Southwestern Medical Center	Lawton	84%	300+
Comanche County Memorial Hospital	Lawton	83%	300+
Craig General Hospital	Vinita	83%	(a)
Great Plains Regional Medical Center	Elk City	83%	300+
Integris Blackwell Regional Hospital	Blackwell	83%	(a)
Integris Seminole Medical Center	Seminole	83%	(a)
Jane Phillips Medical Center	Bartlesville	83%	300+
Saint John Owasso	Owasso	83%	300+
Eastar Health System	Muskogee	82%	300+
Integris Bass Baptist Health Center	Enid	82%	300+
Memorial Hospital of Stilwell	Stilwell	82%	(a)
Saint Francis Hospital South	Tulsa	82%	300+
Tahlequah City Hospital	Tahlequah	82%	300+
Hillcrest Medical Center	Tulsa	81%	300+
Saint Francis Hospital	Tulsa	81%	300+
W W Hastings Indian Hospital	Tahlequah	81%	300+
Wagoner Community Hospital	Wagoner	81%	(a)
McCurtain Memorial Hospital	Idabel	79%	(a)
Oklahoma State University Medical Center	Tulsa	79%	300+
Saint John Medical Center	Tulsa	79%	300+
McAlester Regional Health Center	Mcalester	78%	300+
Midwest Regional Medical Center	Midwest City	78%	300+
Pauls Valley General Hospital	Pauls Valley	78%	(a)
Purcell Municipal Hospital	Purcell	78%	(a)
Medical Center of Southeastern Oklahoma	Durant	74%	300+
Saint John Sapulpa	Sapulpa	74%	(a)
Choctaw Memorial Hospital	Hugo	72%	(a)

Hospital Given 9 or 10 on 10 Point Scale

Hospital Name	City	Rate	Cases
Oklahoma Heart Hospital	Oklahoma City	94%	300+
Oklahoma Heart Hospital South	Oklahoma City	93%	300+
Southwestern Regional Medical Center	Tulsa	92%	(a)
Oklahoma Spine Hospital	Oklahoma City	89%	300+
Integris Health Edmond	Edmond	88%	300+
Tulsa Spine & Specialty Hospital	Tulsa	88%	300+
McBride Clinic Orthopedic Hospital	Oklahoma City	86%	300+
Bailey Medical Center	Owasso	85%	300+
Northwest Surgical Hospital	Oklahoma City	85%	(a)
Oklahoma Surgical Hospital	Tulsa	85%	300+
Chickasaw Nation Medical Center	Ada	84%	300+
Choctaw Nation Healthcare	Talihina	83%	300+
Oklahoma Ctr for Ortho & Multi-Spec	Oklahoma City	83%	(a)
Saint John Broken Arrow	Broken Arrow	82%	300+
Community Hospital	Oklahoma City	80%	300+
Integris Baptist Medical Center	Oklahoma City	80%	300+
Saint Anthony Hospital	Oklahoma City	80%	300+
Saint John Owasso	Owasso	79%	300+
Stillwater Medical Center	Stillwater	78%	300+
Surgical Hospital of Oklahoma	Oklahoma City	77%	(a)
Saint Francis Hospital South	Tulsa	76%	300+
Saint Mary's Regional Medical Center	Enid	76%	300+
Lakeside Women's Hospital	Oklahoma City	75%	(a)
Norman Regional Health System	Norman	74%	300+
Hillcrest Hospital Henryetta	Henryetta	73%	(a)
Integris Canadian Valley Hospital	Yukon	73%	300+
Saint Anthony Shawnee Hospital	Shawnee	73%	300+
Saint John Sapulpa	Sapulpa	73%	(a)
Comanche County Memorial Hospital	Lawton	72%	300+
Mercy Hospital Oklahoma City[11]	Oklahoma City	72%	300+
Purcell Municipal Hospital	Purcell	72%	(a)
Elkview General Hospital	Hobart	71%	(a)
Mercy Memorial Health Center[11]	Ardmore	71%	300+
Muscogee (Creek) Nation Medical Center	Okmulgee	71%	(a)
Hillcrest Hospital Cushing	Cushing	70%	300+
Jane Phillips Medical Center	Bartlesville	70%	300+
Saint John Medical Center	Tulsa	70%	300+
Duncan Regional Hospital	Duncan	69%	300+
Integris Grove Hospital	Grove	69%	300+
Integris Marshall County Medical Center	Madill	69%	(a)
Integris Seminole Medical Center	Seminole	69%	(a)
Memorial Hospital of Texas County	Guymon	69%	(a)
Ponca City Medical Center	Ponca City	69%	300+
Integris Baptist Regional Health Center	Miami	68%	300+
Integris Bass Baptist Health Center	Enid	68%	300+
Integris Blackwell Regional Hospital	Blackwell	68%	(a)
Integris Southwest Medical Center	Oklahoma City	68%	300+
Saint Francis Hospital	Tulsa	68%	300+
Craig General Hospital	Vinita	67%	(a)
Deaconess Hospital	Oklahoma City	67%	300+
Eastern Oklahoma Medical Center	Poteau	67%	300+
Jackson County Memorial Hospital	Altus	67%	300+
Mercy Hospital Ada[11]	Ada	67%	300+
Oklahoma State University Medical Center	Tulsa	67%	300+
Southwestern Medical Center	Lawton	67%	300+
Claremore Indian Hospital	Claremore	66%	(a)
Hillcrest Hospital South	Tulsa	66%	300+
W W Hastings Indian Hospital	Tahlequah	66%	300+
Woodward Regional Hospital	Woodward	66%	300+
Great Plains Regional Medical Center	Elk City	65%	300+
O U Medical Center	Oklahoma City	65%	300+
Grady Memorial Hospital	Chickasha	64%	300+
Hillcrest Hospital Claremore	Claremore	64%	300+
Integris Mayes County Medical Center	Pryor	63%	(a)
Tahlequah City Hospital	Tahlequah	63%	300+
Hillcrest Medical Center	Tulsa	61%	300+
Integris Clinton Regional Hospital	Clinton	59%	(a)
Medical Center of Southeastern Oklahoma	Durant	59%	300+
Memorial Hospital of Stilwell	Stilwell	59%	(a)
Pauls Valley General Hospital	Pauls Valley	58%	(a)
Wagoner Community Hospital	Wagoner	58%	(a)
McAlester Regional Health Center	Mcalester	55%	300+
Choctaw Memorial Hospital	Hugo	52%	(a)
Eastar Health System	Muskogee	51%	300+
McCurtain Memorial Hospital	Idabel	51%	(a)
Midwest Regional Medical Center	Midwest City	50%	300+

Meds 'Always' Explained Before Given

Hospital Name	City	Rate	Cases
Northwest Surgical Hospital	Oklahoma City	84%	(a)
Integris Marshall County Medical Center	Madill	80%	(a)
Choctaw Nation Healthcare	Talihina	76%	300+
Oklahoma Spine Hospital	Oklahoma City	75%	300+
Chickasaw Nation Medical Center	Ada	73%	300+
Hillcrest Hospital Henryetta	Henryetta	73%	(a)
Oklahoma Heart Hospital	Oklahoma City	73%	300+
Oklahoma Heart Hospital South	Oklahoma City	73%	300+
Pauls Valley General Hospital	Pauls Valley	73%	(a)
Surgical Hospital of Oklahoma	Oklahoma City	73%	(a)
Oklahoma Ctr for Ortho & Multi-Spec	Oklahoma City	72%	(a)
Southwestern Regional Medical Center	Tulsa	72%	(a)
Tulsa Spine & Specialty Hospital	Tulsa	72%	300+
Integris Baptist Regional Health Center	Miami	71%	300+
McBride Clinic Orthopedic Hospital	Oklahoma City	71%	300+
Woodward Regional Hospital	Woodward	71%	300+
Jackson County Memorial Hospital	Altus	70%	300+
Bailey Medical Center	Owasso	69%	300+
Claremore Indian Hospital	Claremore	69%	(a)
Oklahoma Surgical Hospital	Tulsa	69%	300+
Saint Anthony Shawnee Hospital	Shawnee	69%	300+
Community Hospital	Oklahoma City	68%	300+
Integris Health Edmond	Edmond	68%	300+
W W Hastings Indian Hospital	Tahlequah	68%	300+
Duncan Regional Hospital	Duncan	67%	300+
Integris Clinton Regional Hospital	Clinton	67%	(a)
Muscogee (Creek) Nation Medical Center	Okmulgee	67%	(a)
Ponca City Medical Center	Ponca City	67%	300+
Saint John Broken Arrow	Broken Arrow	67%	300+
Eastern Oklahoma Medical Center	Poteau	66%	300+
Lakeside Women's Hospital	Oklahoma City	65%	(a)
Mercy Hospital Ada[11]	Ada	65%	300+
Mercy Hospital Oklahoma City[11]	Oklahoma City	65%	300+
Saint John Owasso	Owasso	65%	300+
Stillwater Medical Center	Stillwater	65%	300+
Integris Blackwell Regional Hospital	Blackwell	64%	(a)
Integris Canadian Valley Hospital	Yukon	64%	300+
Integris Mayes County Medical Center	Pryor	64%	(a)
Memorial Hospital of Texas County	Guymon	64%	(a)
Saint Mary's Regional Medical Center	Enid	64%	300+
Comanche County Memorial Hospital	Lawton	63%	300+
Elkview General Hospital	Hobart	63%	(a)
Hillcrest Hospital Cushing	Cushing	63%	300+
Integris Baptist Medical Center	Oklahoma City	63%	300+
Memorial Hospital of Stilwell	Stilwell	63%	(a)
Purcell Municipal Hospital	Purcell	63%	(a)
Craig General Hospital	Vinita	62%	(a)
Deaconess Hospital	Oklahoma City	62%	300+
Integris Bass Baptist Health Center	Enid	62%	300+
Integris Grove Hospital	Grove	62%	300+
Southwestern Medical Center	Lawton	62%	300+
Hillcrest Hospital Claremore	Claremore	61%	300+
Jane Phillips Medical Center	Bartlesville	61%	300+
Mercy Memorial Health Center[11]	Ardmore	61%	300+
Saint Anthony Hospital	Oklahoma City	61%	300+
Saint Francis Hospital	Tulsa	61%	300+
Wagoner Community Hospital	Wagoner	61%	(a)
Norman Regional Health System	Norman	60%	300+
Saint John Sapulpa	Sapulpa	60%	(a)
Grady Memorial Hospital	Chickasha	59%	300+
Integris Seminole Medical Center	Seminole	59%	(a)
Integris Southwest Medical Center	Oklahoma City	59%	300+
Tahlequah City Hospital	Tahlequah	59%	300+
Choctaw Memorial Hospital	Hugo	58%	(a)
O U Medical Center	Oklahoma City	58%	300+
Hillcrest Medical Center	Tulsa	57%	300+
McAlester Regional Health Center	Mcalester	57%	300+
McCurtain Memorial Hospital	Idabel	57%	(a)
Oklahoma State University Medical Center	Tulsa	57%	300+
Saint Francis Hospital South	Tulsa	57%	300+
Hillcrest Hospital South	Tulsa	56%	300+
Medical Center of Southeastern Oklahoma	Durant	56%	300+
Saint John Medical Center	Tulsa	55%	300+

NOTE: Hospital profiles are in alphabetical order by state, then city, then hospital within the city; Rankings exclude hospitals with less than 25 cases except for patient surveys which excludes hospitals with less than 100 cases; (a) 100-299 cases; (1) The number of cases/patients is too few to report; (2) Data submitted were based on a sample of cases/patients; (3) Results are based on a shorter time period than required; (4) Data suppressed by CMS for one or more quarters; (5) Results are not available for this reporting period; (6) Fewer than 100 patients completed the HCAHPS survey; (7) No cases met the criteria for this measure; (8) The lower limit of the confidence interval cannot be calculated if the number of observed infections equals zero; (9) No data are available from the state/territory for this reporting period; (10) The scores shown reflect fewer than 50 completed surveys; (11) There were discrepancies in the data collection process; (12) This measure does not apply to this hospital for this reporting period; (13) Results cannot be calculated for this reporting period; (14) The results for this state are combined with nearby states to protect confidentiality; Please refer to the User's Guide for a full explanation of data.

Hospital Name	City	Rate	Cases
Eastar Health System	Muskogee	53%	300+
Great Plains Regional Medical Center	Elk City	53%	300+
Midwest Regional Medical Center	Midwest City	51%	300+

Nurses 'Always' Communicated Well

Hospital Name	City	Rate	Cases
Oklahoma Heart Hospital	Oklahoma City	90%	300+
Northwest Surgical Hospital	Oklahoma City	89%	(a)
Oklahoma Heart Hospital South	Oklahoma City	89%	300+
Southwestern Regional Medical Center	Tulsa	88%	(a)
Purcell Municipal Hospital	Purcell	87%	(a)
Choctaw Nation Healthcare	Talihina	86%	300+
Hillcrest Hospital Henryetta	Henryetta	86%	(a)
Integris Marshall County Medical Center	Madill	86%	(a)
Tulsa Spine & Specialty Hospital	Tulsa	86%	300+
Oklahoma Ctr for Ortho & Multi-Spec	Oklahoma City	85%	(a)
Oklahoma Spine Hospital	Oklahoma City	85%	300+
Surgical Hospital of Oklahoma	Oklahoma City	85%	(a)
Bailey Medical Center	Owasso	84%	300+
Chickasaw Nation Medical Center	Ada	84%	300+
Integris Health Edmond	Edmond	84%	300+
McBride Clinic Orthopedic Hospital	Oklahoma City	84%	300+
Oklahoma Surgical Hospital	Tulsa	84%	300+
Claremore Indian Hospital	Claremore	83%	(a)
Integris Baptist Regional Health Center	Miami	83%	300+
Jackson County Memorial Hospital	Altus	83%	300+
Community Hospital	Oklahoma City	82%	300+
Integris Mayes County Medical Center	Pryor	82%	(a)
Saint Anthony Shawnee Hospital	Shawnee	82%	300+
Saint John Owasso	Owasso	82%	300+
Stillwater Medical Center	Stillwater	82%	300+
Craig General Hospital	Vinita	81%	(a)
Elkview General Hospital	Hobart	81%	(a)
Integris Blackwell Regional Hospital	Blackwell	81%	(a)
Jane Phillips Medical Center	Bartlesville	81%	300+
Muscogee (Creek) Nation Medical Center	Okmulgee	81%	(a)
Saint Anthony Hospital	Oklahoma City	81%	300+
Saint John Broken Arrow	Broken Arrow	81%	300+
Integris Canadian Valley Hospital	Yukon	80%	300+
Mercy Memorial Health Center[11]	Ardmore	80%	300+
Pauls Valley General Hospital	Pauls Valley	80%	(a)
Comanche County Memorial Hospital	Lawton	79%	300+
Duncan Regional Hospital	Duncan	79%	300+
Hillcrest Hospital Cushing	Cushing	79%	300+
Integris Grove Hospital	Grove	79%	300+
Saint Mary's Regional Medical Center	Enid	79%	300+
W W Hastings Indian Hospital	Tahlequah	79%	300+
Woodward Regional Hospital	Woodward	79%	300+
Great Plains Regional Medical Center	Elk City	78%	300+
Integris Baptist Medical Center	Oklahoma City	78%	300+
Eastern Oklahoma Medical Center	Poteau	77%	300+
Integris Seminole Medical Center	Seminole	77%	(a)
Integris Southwest Medical Center	Oklahoma City	77%	300+
Lakeside Women's Hospital	Oklahoma City	77%	(a)
McCurtain Memorial Hospital	Idabel	77%	(a)
Memorial Hospital of Texas County	Guymon	77%	(a)
Ponca City Medical Center	Ponca City	77%	300+
Integris Bass Baptist Health Center	Enid	76%	300+
Mercy Hospital Ada[11]	Ada	76%	300+
Saint Francis Hospital South	Tulsa	76%	300+
Deaconess Hospital	Oklahoma City	75%	300+
Grady Memorial Hospital	Chickasha	75%	300+
Integris Clinton Regional Hospital	Clinton	75%	(a)
Norman Regional Health System	Norman	75%	300+
Saint John Medical Center	Tulsa	75%	300+
Wagoner Community Hospital	Wagoner	75%	(a)
Hillcrest Hospital Claremore	Claremore	74%	300+
Memorial Hospital of Stilwell	Stilwell	74%	(a)
Mercy Hospital Oklahoma City[11]	Oklahoma City	74%	300+
Choctaw Memorial Hospital	Hugo	73%	(a)
Saint Francis Hospital	Tulsa	73%	300+
Saint John Sapulpa	Sapulpa	73%	(a)
Southwestern Medical Center	Lawton	73%	300+
Hillcrest Hospital South	Tulsa	72%	300+
McAlester Regional Health Center	Mcalester	72%	300+
O U Medical Center	Oklahoma City	72%	300+
Oklahoma State University Medical Center	Tulsa	72%	300+
Tahlequah City Hospital	Tahlequah	72%	300+
Hillcrest Medical Center	Tulsa	71%	300+
Medical Center of Southeastern Oklahoma	Durant	69%	300+
Eastar Health System	Muskogee	64%	300+
Midwest Regional Medical Center	Midwest City	64%	300+

Pain 'Always' Well Controlled

Hospital Name	City	Rate	Cases
Hillcrest Hospital Henryetta	Henryetta	87%	(a)
Oklahoma Heart Hospital	Oklahoma City	82%	300+
Northwest Surgical Hospital	Oklahoma City	81%	(a)
Oklahoma Heart Hospital South	Oklahoma City	81%	300+
Chickasaw Nation Medical Center	Ada	80%	300+
Oklahoma Ctr for Ortho & Multi-Spec	Oklahoma City	79%	(a)
Oklahoma Spine Hospital	Oklahoma City	78%	300+
Integris Blackwell Regional Hospital	Blackwell	77%	(a)
Integris Health Edmond	Edmond	77%	300+
McBride Clinic Orthopedic Hospital	Oklahoma City	77%	300+
Tulsa Spine & Specialty Hospital	Tulsa	77%	300+
Integris Baptist Regional Health Center	Miami	76%	300+
Oklahoma Surgical Hospital	Tulsa	76%	300+
Surgical Hospital of Oklahoma	Oklahoma City	76%	(a)
Bailey Medical Center	Owasso	75%	300+
Choctaw Nation Healthcare	Talihina	75%	300+
Integris Marshall County Medical Center	Madill	75%	(a)
Purcell Municipal Hospital	Purcell	75%	(a)
Saint John Broken Arrow	Broken Arrow	75%	300+
Craig General Hospital	Vinita	74%	(a)
Duncan Regional Hospital	Duncan	74%	300+
Memorial Hospital of Texas County	Guymon	74%	(a)
Saint Anthony Shawnee Hospital	Shawnee	74%	300+
Saint John Owasso	Owasso	74%	300+
Saint John Sapulpa	Sapulpa	74%	(a)
Southwestern Regional Medical Center	Tulsa	74%	(a)
Stillwater Medical Center	Stillwater	74%	300+
Comanche County Memorial Hospital	Lawton	73%	300+
Integris Baptist Medical Center	Oklahoma City	73%	300+
Integris Clinton Regional Hospital	Clinton	73%	(a)
Jackson County Memorial Hospital	Altus	73%	300+
Lakeside Women's Hospital	Oklahoma City	73%	(a)
Muscogee (Creek) Nation Medical Center	Okmulgee	73%	(a)
Saint Anthony Hospital	Oklahoma City	73%	300+
Woodward Regional Hospital	Woodward	73%	300+
Claremore Indian Hospital	Claremore	72%	(a)
Integris Grove Hospital	Grove	72%	300+
Community Hospital	Oklahoma City	71%	300+
Deaconess Hospital	Oklahoma City	71%	300+
Integris Canadian Valley Hospital	Yukon	71%	300+
Integris Seminole Medical Center	Seminole	71%	(a)
Norman Regional Health System	Norman	71%	300+
Saint Francis Hospital	Tulsa	71%	300+
Saint Mary's Regional Medical Center	Enid	71%	300+
Eastern Oklahoma Medical Center	Poteau	70%	300+
Elkview General Hospital	Hobart	70%	(a)
Grady Memorial Hospital	Chickasha	70%	300+
Great Plains Regional Medical Center	Elk City	70%	300+
Hillcrest Hospital Cushing	Cushing	70%	300+
Integris Bass Baptist Health Center	Enid	70%	300+
Jane Phillips Medical Center	Bartlesville	70%	300+
Mercy Hospital Ada[11]	Ada	70%	300+
Mercy Memorial Health Center[11]	Ardmore	70%	300+
Ponca City Medical Center	Ponca City	70%	300+
Hillcrest Hospital Claremore	Claremore	69%	300+
McCurtain Memorial Hospital	Idabel	69%	(a)
Memorial Hospital of Stilwell	Stilwell	69%	(a)
Pauls Valley General Hospital	Pauls Valley	69%	(a)
W W Hastings Indian Hospital	Tahlequah	69%	300+
Integris Southwest Medical Center	Oklahoma City	68%	300+
Mercy Hospital Oklahoma City[11]	Oklahoma City	68%	300+
Saint Francis Hospital South	Tulsa	68%	300+
Integris Mayes County Medical Center	Pryor	67%	(a)
McAlester Regional Health Center	Mcalester	67%	300+
Saint John Medical Center	Tulsa	67%	300+
Hillcrest Hospital South	Tulsa	66%	300+
Southwestern Medical Center	Lawton	66%	300+
Hillcrest Medical Center	Tulsa	65%	300+
Medical Center of Southeastern Oklahoma	Durant	65%	300+
O U Medical Center	Oklahoma City	65%	300+
Wagoner Community Hospital	Wagoner	65%	(a)
Choctaw Memorial Hospital	Hugo	64%	(a)
Oklahoma State University Medical Center	Tulsa	63%	300+
Eastar Health System	Muskogee	62%	300+
Midwest Regional Medical Center	Midwest City	60%	300+
Tahlequah City Hospital	Tahlequah	59%	300+

Room and Bathroom 'Always' Clean

Hospital Name	City	Rate	Cases
Southwestern Regional Medical Center	Tulsa	87%	(a)
Oklahoma Ctr for Ortho & Multi-Spec	Oklahoma City	86%	(a)
Oklahoma Heart Hospital South	Oklahoma City	86%	300+
Tulsa Spine & Specialty Hospital	Tulsa	86%	300+
Integris Seminole Medical Center	Seminole	85%	(a)
Oklahoma Spine Hospital	Oklahoma City	85%	300+
Jane Phillips Medical Center	Bartlesville	84%	300+
Oklahoma Surgical Hospital	Tulsa	84%	300+
Oklahoma Heart Hospital	Oklahoma City	83%	300+
Chickasaw Nation Medical Center	Ada	82%	300+
Integris Canadian Valley Hospital	Yukon	81%	300+
Saint Anthony Shawnee Hospital	Shawnee	81%	300+
Community Hospital	Oklahoma City	80%	300+
McBride Clinic Orthopedic Hospital	Oklahoma City	80%	300+
Northwest Surgical Hospital	Oklahoma City	80%	(a)
Bailey Medical Center	Owasso	79%	300+
Choctaw Nation Healthcare	Talihina	79%	300+
Integris Health Edmond	Edmond	79%	300+
Integris Mayes County Medical Center	Pryor	79%	(a)
Saint John Broken Arrow	Broken Arrow	79%	300+
Memorial Hospital of Texas County	Guymon	77%	(a)
Hillcrest Hospital Henryetta	Henryetta	76%	(a)
Purcell Municipal Hospital	Purcell	76%	(a)
Saint John Sapulpa	Sapulpa	76%	(a)
Stillwater Medical Center	Stillwater	76%	300+
Woodward Regional Hospital	Woodward	76%	300+
Craig General Hospital	Vinita	75%	(a)
Integris Marshall County Medical Center	Madill	75%	(a)
Saint John Owasso	Owasso	75%	300+
Duncan Regional Hospital	Duncan	74%	300+
Integris Baptist Medical Center	Oklahoma City	74%	300+
Integris Baptist Regional Health Center	Miami	74%	300+
Integris Blackwell Regional Hospital	Blackwell	74%	(a)
Jackson County Memorial Hospital	Altus	74%	300+
Mercy Hospital Ada[11]	Ada	74%	300+
Pauls Valley General Hospital	Pauls Valley	74%	(a)
W W Hastings Indian Hospital	Tahlequah	74%	300+
Choctaw Memorial Hospital	Hugo	73%	(a)
Memorial Hospital of Stilwell	Stilwell	73%	(a)
Great Plains Regional Medical Center	Elk City	72%	300+
Lakeside Women's Hospital	Oklahoma City	72%	(a)
Saint Anthony Hospital	Oklahoma City	72%	300+
Saint Francis Hospital South	Tulsa	72%	300+
Comanche County Memorial Hospital	Lawton	70%	300+
McAlester Regional Health Center	Mcalester	70%	300+
Eastern Oklahoma Medical Center	Poteau	69%	300+
Hillcrest Hospital Claremore	Claremore	69%	300+
Muscogee (Creek) Nation Medical Center	Okmulgee	69%	(a)
Norman Regional Health System	Norman	69%	300+
Oklahoma State University Medical Center	Tulsa	69%	300+
Saint Mary's Regional Medical Center	Enid	69%	300+
Surgical Hospital of Oklahoma	Oklahoma City	69%	(a)
Saint Francis Hospital	Tulsa	68%	300+
Saint John Medical Center	Tulsa	68%	300+
Deaconess Hospital	Oklahoma City	67%	300+
Hillcrest Hospital South	Tulsa	67%	300+
Integris Bass Baptist Health Center	Enid	67%	300+
Southwestern Medical Center	Lawton	67%	300+
Grady Memorial Hospital	Chickasha	66%	300+
Integris Southwest Medical Center	Oklahoma City	66%	300+
Mercy Hospital Oklahoma City[11]	Oklahoma City	66%	300+
Mercy Memorial Health Center[11]	Ardmore	66%	300+
Hillcrest Hospital Cushing	Cushing	65%	300+
McCurtain Memorial Hospital	Idabel	65%	(a)
Ponca City Medical Center	Ponca City	65%	300+
Claremore Indian Hospital	Claremore	64%	(a)
Integris Grove Hospital	Grove	64%	300+
O U Medical Center	Oklahoma City	63%	300+
Wagoner Community Hospital	Wagoner	62%	(a)
Eastar Health System	Muskogee	60%	300+
Medical Center of Southeastern Oklahoma	Durant	60%	300+
Integris Clinton Regional Hospital	Clinton	59%	(a)
Tahlequah City Hospital	Tahlequah	58%	300+
Hillcrest Medical Center	Tulsa	57%	300+
Elkview General Hospital	Hobart	56%	(a)
Midwest Regional Medical Center	Midwest City	55%	300+

Timely Help 'Always' Received

Hospital Name	City	Rate	Cases
Oklahoma Heart Hospital	Oklahoma City	91%	300+
Northwest Surgical Hospital	Oklahoma City	88%	(a)
Oklahoma Heart Hospital South	Oklahoma City	88%	300+
Oklahoma Spine Hospital	Oklahoma City	83%	300+
Choctaw Nation Healthcare	Talihina	82%	300+
Oklahoma Ctr for Ortho & Multi-Spec	Oklahoma City	80%	(a)
Surgical Hospital of Oklahoma	Oklahoma City	80%	(a)
Integris Marshall County Medical Center	Madill	78%	(a)
Tulsa Spine & Specialty Hospital	Tulsa	78%	300+
Community Hospital	Oklahoma City	77%	300+
Chickasaw Nation Medical Center	Ada	76%	300+
Integris Baptist Regional Health Center	Miami	76%	300+
Muscogee (Creek) Nation Medical Center	Okmulgee	76%	(a)
Bailey Medical Center	Owasso	75%	300+
Elkview General Hospital	Hobart	75%	(a)
Integris Mayes County Medical Center	Pryor	75%	(a)
McBride Clinic Orthopedic Hospital	Oklahoma City	75%	300+
Purcell Municipal Hospital	Purcell	75%	(a)
Southwestern Regional Medical Center	Tulsa	75%	(a)
Integris Health Edmond	Edmond	74%	300+
Memorial Hospital of Texas County	Guymon	74%	(a)
Woodward Regional Hospital	Woodward	74%	300+
Claremore Indian Hospital	Claremore	73%	(a)
Comanche County Memorial Hospital	Lawton	73%	300+
Oklahoma Surgical Hospital	Tulsa	73%	300+
Duncan Regional Hospital	Duncan	72%	300+
Hillcrest Hospital Henryetta	Henryetta	72%	(a)
Jackson County Memorial Hospital	Altus	72%	300+
Saint Anthony Shawnee Hospital	Shawnee	72%	300+

NOTE: Hospital profiles are in alphabetical order by state, then city, then hospital within the city; Rankings exclude hospitals with less than 25 cases except for patient surveys which excludes hospitals with less than 100 cases; (a) 100-299 cases; (1) The number of cases/patients is too few to report; (2) Data submitted were based on a sample of cases/patients; (3) Results are based on a shorter time period than required; (4) Data suppressed by CMS for one or more quarters; (5) Results are not available for this reporting period; (6) Fewer than 100 patients completed the HCAHPS survey; (7) No cases met the criteria for this measure; (8) The lower limit of the confidence interval cannot be calculated if the number of observed infections equals zero; (9) No data are available from the state/territory for this reporting period; (10) The scores shown reflect fewer than 50 completed surveys; (11) There were discrepancies in the data collection process; (12) This measure does not apply to this hospital for this reporting period; (13) Results cannot be calculated for this reporting period; (14) The results for this state are combined with nearby states to protect confidentiality; Please refer to the User's Guide for a full explanation of data.

Hospital Name	City	Rate	Cases
Craig General Hospital	Vinita	71%	(a)
Great Plains Regional Medical Center	Elk City	71%	300+
Integris Clinton Regional Hospital	Clinton	71%	(a)
Jane Phillips Medical Center	Bartlesville	70%	300+
Pauls Valley General Hospital	Pauls Valley	70%	(a)
Saint John Broken Arrow	Broken Arrow	70%	300+
Saint John Owasso	Owasso	70%	300+
Stillwater Medical Center	Stillwater	70%	300+
W W Hastings Indian Hospital	Tahlequah	70%	300+
Eastern Oklahoma Medical Center	Poteau	69%	300+
Integris Bass Baptist Health Center	Enid	69%	300+
Mercy Hospital Ada[11]	Ada	69%	300+
Mercy Memorial Health Center[11]	Ardmore	68%	300+
Ponca City Medical Center	Ponca City	68%	300+
Hillcrest Hospital Cushing	Cushing	67%	300+
Integris Baptist Medical Center	Oklahoma City	67%	300+
McCurtain Memorial Hospital	Idabel	66%	(a)
Memorial Hospital of Stilwell	Stilwell	66%	(a)
Saint Anthony Hospital	Oklahoma City	66%	300+
Saint Mary's Regional Medical Center	Enid	66%	300+
Integris Grove Hospital	Grove	65%	300+
Integris Seminole Medical Center	Seminole	65%	(a)
Hillcrest Hospital Claremore	Claremore	64%	300+
Integris Canadian Valley Hospital	Yukon	64%	300+
Integris Southwest Medical Center	Oklahoma City	64%	300+
Saint John Sapulpa	Sapulpa	64%	(a)
Integris Blackwell Regional Hospital	Blackwell	63%	(a)
Southwestern Medical Center	Lawton	63%	300+
Grady Memorial Hospital	Chickasha	62%	300+
Wagoner Community Hospital	Wagoner	62%	(a)
Saint Francis Hospital South	Tulsa	61%	300+
Saint John Medical Center	Tulsa	61%	300+
Choctaw Memorial Hospital	Hugo	60%	(a)
Hillcrest Hospital South	Tulsa	60%	300+
Tahlequah City Hospital	Tahlequah	60%	300+
Deaconess Hospital	Oklahoma City	59%	300+
Lakeside Women's Hospital	Oklahoma City	59%	(a)
Mercy Hospital Oklahoma City[11]	Oklahoma City	59%	300+
Saint Francis Hospital	Tulsa	59%	300+
Norman Regional Health System	Norman	58%	300+
Oklahoma State University Medical Center	Tulsa	58%	300+
McAlester Regional Health Center	Mcalester	57%	300+
Medical Center of Southeastern Oklahoma	Durant	55%	300+
Hillcrest Medical Center	Tulsa	54%	300+
O U Medical Center	Oklahoma City	54%	300+
Eastar Health System	Muskogee	51%	300+
Midwest Regional Medical Center	Midwest City	45%	300+

Would Definitely Recommend Hospital

Hospital Name	City	Rate	Cases
Southwestern Regional Medical Center	Tulsa	97%	(a)
Oklahoma Heart Hospital	Oklahoma City	96%	300+
Oklahoma Heart Hospital South	Oklahoma City	95%	300+
Oklahoma Spine Hospital	Oklahoma City	90%	300+
Tulsa Spine & Specialty Hospital	Tulsa	90%	300+
McBride Clinic Orthopedic Hospital	Oklahoma City	89%	300+
Chickasaw Nation Medical Center	Ada	88%	300+
Integris Health Edmond	Edmond	88%	300+
Northwest Surgical Hospital	Oklahoma City	87%	(a)
Oklahoma Surgical Hospital	Tulsa	87%	300+
Oklahoma Ctr for Ortho & Multi-Spec	Oklahoma City	86%	(a)
Saint John Broken Arrow	Broken Arrow	86%	300+
Bailey Medical Center	Owasso	85%	300+
Saint John Owasso	Owasso	85%	300+
Choctaw Nation Healthcare	Talihina	84%	300+
Community Hospital	Oklahoma City	82%	300+
Integris Baptist Medical Center	Oklahoma City	81%	300+
Lakeside Women's Hospital	Oklahoma City	80%	(a)
Saint Anthony Hospital	Oklahoma City	80%	300+
Stillwater Medical Center	Stillwater	78%	300+
Mercy Hospital Oklahoma City[11]	Oklahoma City	77%	300+
Purcell Municipal Hospital	Purcell	77%	(a)
Saint Francis Hospital South	Tulsa	77%	300+
Surgical Hospital of Oklahoma	Oklahoma City	77%	(a)
Saint Francis Hospital	Tulsa	76%	300+
Saint Mary's Regional Medical Center	Enid	76%	300+
Elkview General Hospital	Hobart	75%	(a)
Integris Canadian Valley Hospital	Yukon	75%	300+
Comanche County Memorial Hospital	Lawton	73%	300+
Hillcrest Hospital Henryetta	Henryetta	73%	(a)
Norman Regional Health System	Norman	73%	300+
Integris Bass Baptist Health Center	Enid	72%	300+
Saint John Medical Center	Tulsa	72%	300+
Saint Anthony Shawnee Hospital	Shawnee	71%	300+
Hillcrest Hospital South	Tulsa	70%	300+
Southwestern Medical Center	Lawton	70%	300+
Deaconess Hospital	Oklahoma City	69%	300+
Jane Phillips Medical Center	Bartlesville	69%	300+
Integris Grove Hospital	Grove	68%	300+
Integris Southwest Medical Center	Oklahoma City	68%	300+
Oklahoma State University Medical Center	Tulsa	68%	300+
Jackson County Memorial Hospital	Altus	67%	300+
Claremore Indian Hospital	Claremore	66%	(a)
Duncan Regional Hospital	Duncan	66%	300+
Great Plains Regional Medical Center	Elk City	66%	300+
Hillcrest Hospital Cushing	Cushing	66%	300+
Muscogee (Creek) Nation Medical Center	Okmulgee	66%	(a)
O U Medical Center	Oklahoma City	66%	300+
Eastern Oklahoma Medical Center	Poteau	65%	300+
Integris Baptist Regional Health Center	Miami	65%	300+
Integris Marshall County Medical Center	Madill	65%	(a)
Integris Seminole Medical Center	Seminole	65%	(a)
Mercy Hospital Ada[11]	Ada	65%	300+
Saint John Sapulpa	Sapulpa	65%	(a)
Tahlequah City Hospital	Tahlequah	65%	300+
W W Hastings Indian Hospital	Tahlequah	65%	300+
Hillcrest Medical Center	Tulsa	64%	300+
Mercy Memorial Health Center[11]	Ardmore	64%	300+
Woodward Regional Hospital	Woodward	63%	300+
Craig General Hospital	Vinita	62%	(a)
Hillcrest Hospital Claremore	Claremore	62%	300+
Integris Blackwell Regional Hospital	Blackwell	62%	(a)
Integris Clinton Regional Hospital	Clinton	60%	(a)
Memorial Hospital of Texas County	Guymon	59%	(a)
Ponca City Medical Center	Ponca City	59%	300+
Wagoner Community Hospital	Wagoner	59%	(a)
Grady Memorial Hospital	Chickasha	58%	300+
Integris Mayes County Medical Center	Pryor	58%	(a)
Memorial Hospital of Stilwell	Stilwell	57%	(a)
Medical Center of Southeastern Oklahoma	Durant	55%	300+
Choctaw Memorial Hospital	Hugo	54%	(a)
Eastar Health System	Muskogee	52%	300+
McAlester Regional Health Center	Mcalester	51%	300+
Pauls Valley General Hospital	Pauls Valley	51%	(a)
McCurtain Memorial Hospital	Idabel	49%	(a)
Midwest Regional Medical Center	Midwest City	47%	300+

Use of Medical Imaging

Cardiac Imaging Stress Test before OP Surgery

Hospital Name	City	Rate	Cases
Grady Memorial Hospital	Chickasha	0.6%	154
Craig General Hospital	Vinita	1.7%	117
Weatherford Regional Hospital	Weatherford	1.9%	208
Stillwater Medical Center	Stillwater	2.2%	557
Hillcrest Hospital Cushing	Cushing	2.4%	84
Norman Regional Health System	Norman	2.4%	253
Tahlequah City Hospital	Tahlequah	2.4%	1011
Oklahoma State University Medical Center	Tulsa	2.6%	77
Elkview General Hospital	Hobart	2.9%	136
Integris Baptist Regional Health Center	Miami	2.9%	139
Purcell Municipal Hospital	Purcell	2.9%	68
Oklahoma Heart Hospital South	Oklahoma City	3.1%	196
Integris Mayes County Medical Center	Pryor	3.2%	216
Saint Anthony Hospital	Oklahoma City	3.6%	364
Jackson County Memorial Hospital	Altus	3.8%	105
Mercy Memorial Health Center	Ardmore	3.8%	425
O U Medical Center	Oklahoma City	3.8%	183
Saint Mary's Regional Medical Center	Enid	3.8%	185
Integris Bass Baptist Health Center	Enid	4.0%	403
Saint John Broken Arrow	Broken Arrow	4.0%	149
Saint Francis Hospital South	Tulsa	4.1%	390
Muscogee (Creek) Nation Medical Center	Okmulgee	4.3%	70
Hillcrest Medical Center	Tulsa	4.4%	1626
Integris Southwest Medical Center	Oklahoma City	4.4%	90
Wagoner Community Hospital	Wagoner	4.4%	45
Oklahoma Heart Hospital	Oklahoma City	4.5%	4303
Ponca City Medical Center	Ponca City	4.5%	89
Jane Phillips Medical Center	Bartlesville	4.6%	921
Hillcrest Hospital Claremore	Claremore	4.8%	310
Saint Francis Hospital	Tulsa	5.0%	1827
Comanche County Memorial Hospital	Lawton	5.2%	1211
Saint John Medical Center	Tulsa	5.2%	1098
Integris Baptist Medical Center	Oklahoma City	5.4%	821
Hillcrest Hospital South	Tulsa	5.6%	234
Integris Grove Hospital	Grove	5.7%	87
McAlester Regional Health Center	Mcalester	5.8%	294
Memorial Hospital of Texas County	Guymon	6.3%	80
Great Plains Regional Medical Center	Elk City	6.7%	119
Duncan Regional Hospital	Duncan	7.7%	168
Midwest Regional Medical Center	Midwest City	7.8%	77
Mercy Hospital Ada	Ada	7.9%	114
Southwestern Medical Center	Lawton	9.0%	89
Bailey Medical Center	Owasso	9.5%	148
Eastar Health System	Muskogee	10.7%	150

Combination Abdominal CT Scan

Hospital Name	City	Rate	Cases
Haskell County Community Hospital	Stigler	0.0%	106
Memorial Hospital of Stilwell	Stilwell	0.0%	88
Hillcrest Hospital Claremore	Claremore	1.5%	335
Saint John Owasso	Owasso	2.0%	406
Saint John Sapulpa	Sapulpa	2.2%	267
Integris Health Edmond	Edmond	2.5%	160
Stroud Regional Medical Center	Stroud	2.5%	80
Saint John Broken Arrow	Broken Arrow	2.8%	327
Mary Hurley Hospital	Coalgate	3.7%	81
Saint John Medical Center	Tulsa	3.7%	1066
Integris Marshall County Medical Center	Madill	3.8%	132
Integris Grove Hospital	Grove	4.1%	394
Jane Phillips Medical Center	Bartlesville	4.4%	1160
Mercy Hospital Kingfisher	Kingfisher	4.4%	160
Comanche County Memorial Hospital	Lawton	6.0%	1048
Ponca City Medical Center	Ponca City	6.0%	420
Sequoyah Co-Sallisaw Hosp Auth	Sallisaw	6.6%	241
Craig General Hospital	Vinita	7.2%	263
Integris Canadian Valley Hospital	Yukon	8.1%	322
Bailey Medical Center	Owasso	8.3%	264
Muscogee (Creek) Nation Medical Center	Okmulgee	8.8%	204
Integris Mayes County Medical Center	Pryor	9.1%	287
Grady Memorial Hospital	Chickasha	9.8%	275
Oklahoma State University Medical Center	Tulsa	10.3%	310
Deaconess Hospital	Oklahoma City	11.5%	486
Integris Bass Baptist Health Center	Enid	11.9%	477
Mercy Hospital El Reno	El Reno	11.9%	109
Mercy Hospital Logan County	Guthrie	12.5%	224
Creek Nation Community Hospital	Okemah	12.7%	102
Holdenville Hospital Authority	Holdenville	12.9%	163
Cleveland Area Hospital	Cleveland	13.2%	106
Arbuckle Memorial Hospital	Sulphur	13.3%	173
Integris Baptist Medical Center	Oklahoma City	14.0%	1063
Integris Blackwell Regional Hospital	Blackwell	14.0%	100
Share Memorial Hospital	Alva	14.5%	83
Mercy Memorial Health Center	Ardmore	15.6%	928
Medical Center of Southeastern Oklahoma	Durant	15.8%	444
Sayre Memorial Hospital	Sayre	16.0%	75
Norman Regional Health System	Norman	16.2%	1518
Bristow Medical Center	Bristow	16.7%	102
Southwestern Medical Center	Lawton	17.4%	219
Mercy Hospital Oklahoma City	Oklahoma City	17.8%	2438
Pushmataha Co-Antlers Town Hosp Auth	Antlers	18.3%	82
Tahlequah City Hospital	Tahlequah	18.4%	631
Atoka County Medical Center	Atoka	18.9%	122
Eastern Oklahoma Medical Center	Poteau	18.9%	227
Perry Memorial Hospital	Perry	19.4%	103
Saint Anthony Hospital	Oklahoma City	19.4%	969
Purcell Municipal Hospital	Purcell	19.5%	164
Integris Baptist Regional Health Center	Miami	20.1%	249
Saint Anthony Shawnee Hospital	Shawnee	20.1%	622
Integris Southwest Medical Center	Oklahoma City	21.0%	926
Midwest Regional Medical Center	Midwest City	21.0%	738
Saint Mary's Regional Medical Center	Enid	22.2%	662
Woodward Regional Hospital	Woodward	22.4%	183
Great Plains Regional Medical Center	Elk City	22.7%	255
Hillcrest Hospital Henryetta	Henryetta	22.9%	166
Eastar Health System	Muskogee	24.4%	823
Hillcrest Hospital South	Tulsa	24.4%	401
Memorial Hospital of Texas County	Guymon	25.3%	79
Stillwater Medical Center	Stillwater	25.5%	646
Duncan Regional Hospital	Duncan	26.1%	651
Pauls Valley General Hospital	Pauls Valley	28.6%	189
Hillcrest Medical Center	Tulsa	28.9%	588
Mercy Hospital Ada	Ada	28.9%	592
Southwestern Regional Medical Center	Tulsa	28.9%	443
Community Hospital	Oklahoma City	29.2%	106
Integris Seminole Medical Center	Seminole	29.6%	233
Hillcrest Hospital Cushing	Cushing	30.2%	199
McAlester Regional Health Center	Mcalester	39.3%	667
Mercy Hospital Tishomingo	Tishomingo	40.0%	50
Physicians' Hospital in Anadarko	Anadarko	41.7%	115
McCurtain Memorial Hospital	Idabel	42.2%	223
Saint Francis Hospital	Tulsa	43.2%	1714
Northwest Surgical Hospital	Oklahoma City	44.6%	56
Weatherford Regional Hospital	Weatherford	46.4%	194
Saint Francis Hospital South	Tulsa	47.1%	461
Fairview Regional Medical Center	Fairview	48.8%	41
Integris Clinton Regional Hospital	Clinton	49.3%	215
Oklahoma Heart Hospital South	Oklahoma City	51.0%	147
Drumright Regional Hospital	Drumright	51.1%	45
Choctaw Memorial Hospital	Hugo	53.8%	119
Elkview General Hospital	Hobart	55.7%	106
Wagoner Community Hospital	Wagoner	64.7%	85
Oklahoma Heart Hospital	Oklahoma City	64.8%	395
O U Medical Center	Oklahoma City	65.5%	1782
Newman Memorial Hospital	Shattuck	68.3%	63
Jackson County Memorial Hospital	Altus	73.1%	490

Combination Brain/Sinus CT Scan

Hospital Name	City	Rate	Cases
Bristow Medical Center	Bristow	0.0%	101
Carnegie Tri-County Municipal Hospital	Carnegie	0.0%	35
Community Hospital	Oklahoma City	0.0%	71

NOTE: Hospital profiles are in alphabetical order by state, then city, then hospital within the city; Rankings exclude hospitals with less than 25 cases except for patient surveys which excludes hospitals with less than 100 cases; (a) 100-299 cases; (1) The number of cases/patients is too few to report; (2) Data submitted were based on a sample of cases/patients; (3) Results are based on a shorter time period than required; (4) Data suppressed by CMS for one or more quarters; (5) Results are not available for this reporting period; (6) Fewer than 100 patients completed the HCAHPS survey; (7) No cases met the criteria for this measure; (8) The lower limit of the confidence interval cannot be calculated if the number of observed infections equals zero; (9) No data are available from the state/territory for this reporting period; (10) The scores shown reflect fewer than 50 completed surveys; (11) There were discrepancies in the data collection process; (12) This measure does not apply to this hospital for this reporting period; (13) Results cannot be calculated for this reporting period; (14) The results for this state are combined with nearby states to protect confidentiality; Please refer to the User's Guide for a full explanation of data.

Cordell Memorial Hospital	Cordell	0.0%	31
Fairfax Community Hospital	Fairfax	0.0%	59
Harmon Memorial Hospital	Hollis	0.0%	65
Integris Blackwell Regional Hospital	Blackwell	0.0%	96
Jefferson County Hospital	Waurika	0.0%	30
Latimer County General Hospital	Wilburton	0.0%	63
Mary Hurley Hospital	Coalgate	0.0%	101
Memorial Hospital of Texas County	Guymon	0.0%	80
Mercy Health Love County	Marietta	0.0%	45
Mercy Hospital Healdton	Healdton	0.0%	38
Mercy Hospital Tishomingo	Tishomingo	0.0%	63
Mercy Hospital Watonga	Watonga	0.0%	101
Prague Community Hospital	Prague	0.0%	35
Seiling Community Hospital	Seiling	0.0%	37
Oklahoma Heart Hospital South	Oklahoma City	0.3%	321
Saint John Sapulpa	Sapulpa	0.3%	325
Atoka County Medical Center	Atoka	0.5%	215
Oklahoma Heart Hospital	Oklahoma City	0.5%	382
Integris Southwest Medical Center	Oklahoma City	0.6%	633
Integris Mayes County Medical Center	Pryor	0.7%	294
Stillwater Medical Center	Stillwater	0.7%	545
Eastern Oklahoma Medical Center	Poteau	0.8%	240
Integris Canadian Valley Hospital	Yukon	0.8%	383
Saint Francis Hospital South	Tulsa	0.8%	353
Integris Seminole Medical Center	Seminole	0.9%	225
Muscogee (Creek) Nation Medical Center	Okmulgee	0.9%	339
Hillcrest Hospital Cushing	Cushing	1.0%	197
Hillcrest Medical Center	Tulsa	1.0%	511
Saint Francis Hospital	Tulsa	1.0%	1342
Tahlequah City Hospital	Tahlequah	1.2%	577
Integris Baptist Medical Center	Oklahoma City	1.3%	989
Saint Anthony Shawnee Hospital	Shawnee	1.4%	832
Duncan Regional Hospital	Duncan	1.5%	680
Grady Memorial Hospital	Chickasha	1.5%	338
Mercy Hospital Ada	Ada	1.5%	620
Jane Phillips Medical Center	Bartlesville	1.8%	1085
Saint John Medical Center	Tulsa	1.8%	1336
Comanche County Memorial Hospital	Lawton	1.9%	635
Saint Anthony Hospital	Oklahoma City	2.0%	855
Mercy Hospital Oklahoma City	Oklahoma City	2.3%	1757
Eastar Health System	Muskogee	2.9%	899
Norman Regional Health System	Norman	2.9%	1248
Deaconess Hospital	Oklahoma City	3.7%	712
O U Medical Center	Oklahoma City	3.9%	685
Ponca City Medical Center	Ponca City	4.2%	430
Medical Center of Southeastern Oklahoma	Durant	4.5%	508
McAlester Regional Health Center	Mcalester	4.6%	587
Midwest Regional Medical Center	Midwest City	4.6%	725
McCurtain Memorial Hospital	Idabel	4.8%	336
Purcell Municipal Hospital	Purcell	5.2%	230
Mercy Hospital Kingfisher	Kingfisher	5.8%	155
Elkview General Hospital	Hobart	8.9%	79

Combination Chest CT Scan

Hospital Name	City	Rate	Cases
Duncan Regional Hospital	Duncan	0.0%	518
Integris Health Edmond	Edmond	0.0%	75
Integris Marshall County Medical Center	Madill	0.0%	59
Integris Southwest Medical Center	Oklahoma City	0.0%	841
Saint Francis Hospital South	Tulsa	0.0%	373
Saint John Broken Arrow	Broken Arrow	0.0%	193
Saint John Sapulpa	Sapulpa	0.0%	158
Southwestern Regional Medical Center	Tulsa	0.0%	439
Saint Francis Hospital	Tulsa	0.2%	1460
Saint John Medical Center	Tulsa	0.2%	855
Comanche County Memorial Hospital	Lawton	0.3%	739
Integris Baptist Medical Center	Oklahoma City	0.3%	937
O U Medical Center	Oklahoma City	0.3%	1450
Integris Canadian Valley Hospital	Yukon	0.4%	235
Integris Grove Hospital	Grove	0.4%	250
Jackson County Memorial Hospital	Altus	0.4%	234
Ponca City Medical Center	Ponca City	0.4%	246
Medical Center of Southeastern Oklahoma	Durant	0.5%	190
Mercy Hospital Ada	Ada	0.9%	232
Norman Regional Health System	Norman	1.3%	1285
Saint John Owasso	Owasso	1.3%	238
Hillcrest Hospital Claremore	Claremore	1.4%	144
Integris Bass Baptist Health Center	Enid	1.4%	509
Mercy Hospital Kingfisher	Kingfisher	1.5%	133
Saint Anthony Shawnee Hospital	Shawnee	1.5%	199
Bristow Medical Center	Bristow	1.7%	58
Muscogee (Creek) Nation Medical Center	Okmulgee	1.8%	114
Saint Mary's Regional Medical Center	Enid	1.8%	440
Craig General Hospital	Vinita	2.1%	94
Oklahoma State University Medical Center	Tulsa	2.1%	143
Community Hospital	Oklahoma City	2.2%	45
Jane Phillips Medical Center	Bartlesville	2.6%	664
Arbuckle Memorial Hospital	Sulphur	2.8%	108
Saint Anthony Hospital	Oklahoma City	3.1%	387
Integris Blackwell Regional Hospital	Blackwell	3.4%	58
Deaconess Hospital	Oklahoma City	3.5%	346
Oklahoma Heart Hospital	Oklahoma City	3.5%	395
Mercy Hospital El Reno	El Reno	4.1%	49
Mercy Memorial Health Center	Ardmore	4.6%	479
Eastar Health System	Muskogee	5.2%	363
Integris Mayes County Medical Center	Pryor	5.2%	135
Mercy Hospital Logan County	Guthrie	5.5%	128
Grady Memorial Hospital	Chickasha	5.7%	140
Integris Seminole Medical Center	Seminole	6.7%	90
McAlester Regional Health Center	Mcalester	6.7%	580
Purcell Municipal Hospital	Purcell	7.5%	107
Mercy Hospital Oklahoma City	Oklahoma City	8.5%	1673
Stillwater Medical Center	Stillwater	8.6%	244
Oklahoma Heart Hospital South	Oklahoma City	8.8%	194
Bailey Medical Center	Owasso	10.1%	79
Hillcrest Hospital Cushing	Cushing	10.8%	120
Pauls Valley General Hospital	Pauls Valley	12.5%	72
Creek Nation Community Hospital	Okemah	12.8%	78
Woodward Regional Hospital	Woodward	13.7%	117
Southwestern Medical Center	Lawton	15.0%	120
Hillcrest Hospital South	Tulsa	15.3%	340
Integris Clinton Regional Hospital	Clinton	15.7%	89
Sequoyah Co-Sallisaw Hosp Auth	Sallisaw	16.7%	108
Hillcrest Medical Center	Tulsa	17.0%	548
Integris Baptist Regional Health Center	Miami	17.6%	148
Hillcrest Hospital Henryetta	Henryetta	19.3%	83
Great Plains Regional Medical Center	Elk City	19.6%	138
Midwest Regional Medical Center	Midwest City	19.9%	272
Tahlequah City Hospital	Tahlequah	23.4%	209
McCurtain Memorial Hospital	Idabel	23.8%	84
Weatherford Regional Hospital	Weatherford	24.3%	74
Eastern Oklahoma Medical Center	Poteau	28.6%	70
Elkview General Hospital	Hobart	33.3%	63
Physicians' Hospital in Anadarko	Anadarko	44.0%	75
Choctaw Memorial Hospital	Hugo	46.2%	78
Oklahoma Ctr for Ortho & Multi-Spec	Oklahoma City	52.9%	34

Follow-up Mammogram/Ultrasound

A follow-up rate near zero may indicate missed cancer; a rate higher than 14% may mean there is unnecessary follow up.

Hospital Name	City	Rate	Cases
Perry Memorial Hospital	Perry	0.8%	247
Integris Blackwell Regional Hospital	Blackwell	2.0%	101
Wagoner Community Hospital	Wagoner	2.7%	183
Midwest Regional Medical Center	Midwest City	3.7%	1736
Saint Francis Hospital South	Tulsa	3.8%	1018
Jane Phillips Medical Center	Bartlesville	4.0%	2396
Stillwater Medical Center	Stillwater	4.0%	955
Lakeside Women's Hospital	Oklahoma City	4.1%	716
Mercy Memorial Health Center	Ardmore	4.4%	1223
Pauls Valley General Hospital	Pauls Valley	4.6%	194
Deaconess Hospital	Oklahoma City	4.8%	903
Craig General Hospital	Vinita	4.9%	427
Hillcrest Hospital South	Tulsa	5.4%	741
Integris Grove Hospital	Grove	5.4%	716
Saint Francis Hospital	Tulsa	5.5%	4102
McCurtain Memorial Hospital	Idabel	5.6%	249
Integris Seminole Medical Center	Seminole	5.8%	326
Integris Mayes County Medical Center	Pryor	5.9%	427
Duncan Regional Hospital	Duncan	6.5%	847
Weatherford Regional Hospital	Weatherford	6.5%	201
Saint John Owasso	Owasso	6.8%	513
Share Memorial Hospital	Alva	7.0%	142
Woodward Regional Hospital	Woodward	7.0%	385
Tahlequah City Hospital	Tahlequah	7.1%	538
Grady Memorial Hospital	Chickasha	7.3%	593
Oklahoma State University Medical Center	Tulsa	7.3%	151
Saint Anthony Shawnee Hospital	Shawnee	7.3%	354
Eastern Oklahoma Medical Center	Poteau	7.5%	241
Mercy Hospital Ada	Ada	7.8%	663
Norman Regional Health System	Norman	7.8%	3017
Comanche County Memorial Hospital	Lawton	8.0%	1295
Hillcrest Hospital Claremore	Claremore	8.1%	531
Hillcrest Medical Center	Tulsa	8.3%	1595
Bailey Medical Center	Owasso	8.5%	270
Memorial Hospital of Texas County	Guymon	8.6%	139
Great Plains Regional Medical Center	Elk City	8.7%	275
Integris Clinton Regional Hospital	Clinton	8.7%	161
Choctaw Memorial Hospital	Hugo	8.8%	148
Saint Mary's Regional Medical Center	Enid	8.8%	1575
Newman Memorial Hospital	Shattuck	8.9%	112
Integris Baptist Regional Health Center	Miami	9.0%	578
Integris Bass Baptist Health Center	Enid	9.1%	722
Integris Southwest Medical Center	Oklahoma City	9.2%	1932
Mercy Hospital Kingfisher	Kingfisher	9.4%	170
McAlester Regional Health Center	Mcalester	9.7%	472
Ponca City Medical Center	Ponca City	10.0%	911
Eastar Health System	Muskogee	10.1%	1899
Sequoyah Co-Sallisaw Hosp Auth	Sallisaw	10.2%	177
Jackson County Memorial Hospital	Altus	10.3%	686
Integris Baptist Medical Center	Oklahoma City	10.5%	2024
Muscogee (Creek) Nation Medical Center	Okmulgee	10.8%	372
Purcell Municipal Hospital	Purcell	10.9%	174
Elkview General Hospital	Hobart	11.0%	181
Hillcrest Hospital Henryetta	Henryetta	11.1%	144
Integris Canadian Valley Hospital	Yukon	11.1%	416
Hillcrest Hospital Cushing	Cushing	11.2%	170
Mercy Hospital Oklahoma City	Oklahoma City	11.2%	2785
Medical Center of Southeastern Oklahoma	Durant	11.3%	690
Integris Health Edmond	Edmond	11.4%	88
Saint John Medical Center	Tulsa	12.0%	3119
Creek Nation Community Hospital	Okemah	13.7%	131
Haskell County Community Hospital	Stigler	14.1%	71
Saint Anthony Hospital	Oklahoma City	14.5%	1370
Mercy Hospital Logan County	Guthrie	17.3%	168
Saint John Sapulpa	Sapulpa	18.6%	307
Saint John Broken Arrow	Broken Arrow	22.9%	271

Lumbar Spine MRI for Low Back Pain

Hospital Name	City	Rate	Cases
Integris Baptist Regional Health Center	Miami	25.9%	58
Summit Medical Center	Edmond	30.6%	85
Hillcrest Medical Center	Tulsa	31.4%	121
Hillcrest Hospital Cushing	Cushing	32.7%	49
Medical Center of Southeastern Oklahoma	Durant	33.8%	80
McBride Clinic Orthopedic Hospital	Oklahoma City	34.5%	388
Stillwater Medical Center	Stillwater	34.6%	52
Saint Anthony Shawnee Hospital	Shawnee	34.8%	46
Deaconess Hospital	Oklahoma City	35.2%	105
Saint John Broken Arrow	Broken Arrow	36.7%	49
O U Medical Center	Oklahoma City	36.9%	122
Integris Grove Hospital	Grove	37.0%	100
Integris Southwest Medical Center	Oklahoma City	37.0%	173
McAlester Regional Health Center	Mcalester	37.7%	154
Midwest Regional Medical Center	Midwest City	37.7%	228
Tahlequah City Hospital	Tahlequah	37.8%	148
Mercy Hospital Oklahoma City	Oklahoma City	37.9%	441
Comanche County Memorial Hospital	Lawton	38.6%	202
Northwest Surgical Hospital	Oklahoma City	38.7%	119
Saint Anthony Hospital	Oklahoma City	38.7%	124
Saint John Medical Center	Tulsa	39.0%	195
Oklahoma Ctr for Ortho & Multi-Spec	Oklahoma City	39.2%	421
Oklahoma Surgical Hospital	Tulsa	39.4%	226
Tulsa Spine & Specialty Hospital	Tulsa	39.6%	225
Saint Francis Hospital South	Tulsa	40.3%	186
Bristow Medical Center	Bristow	40.5%	232
Mercy Memorial Health Center	Ardmore	40.5%	158
Saint Mary's Regional Medical Center	Enid	41.1%	168
Eastar Health System	Muskogee	42.1%	140
Great Plains Regional Medical Center	Elk City	42.1%	76
Saint Francis Hospital	Tulsa	42.6%	282
Duncan Regional Hospital	Duncan	43.2%	125
Mercy Hospital Ada	Ada	43.2%	95
Community Hospital	Oklahoma City	43.3%	178
Southwestern Medical Center	Lawton	44.2%	206
Jane Phillips Medical Center	Bartlesville	45.1%	286
Integris Bass Baptist Health Center	Enid	45.3%	95
Norman Regional Health System	Norman	45.3%	172
Grady Memorial Hospital	Chickasha	45.5%	55
Integris Canadian Valley Hospital	Yukon	47.8%	67
Ponca City Medical Center	Ponca City	48.3%	60
Jackson County Memorial Hospital	Altus	49.2%	63
Hillcrest Hospital South	Tulsa	51.2%	43
Hillcrest Hospital Henryetta	Henryetta	51.5%	33
Sequoyah Co-Sallisaw Hosp Auth	Sallisaw	52.4%	42
Bailey Medical Center	Owasso	55.0%	60
Hillcrest Hospital Claremore	Claremore	56.7%	60
Saint John Owasso	Owasso	57.6%	59
Choctaw Memorial Hospital	Hugo	60.8%	51

NOTE: Hospital profiles are in alphabetical order by state, then city, then hospital within the city; Rankings exclude hospitals with less than 25 cases except for patient surveys which excludes hospitals with less than 100 cases; (a) 100-299 cases; (1) The number of cases/patients is too few to report; (2) Data submitted were based on a sample of cases/patients; (3) Results are based on a shorter time period than required; (4) Data suppressed by CMS for one or more quarters; (5) Results are not available for this reporting period; (6) Fewer than 100 patients completed the HCAHPS survey; (7) No cases met the criteria for this measure; (8) The lower limit of the confidence interval cannot be calculated if the number of observed infections equals zero; (9) No data are available from the state/territory for this reporting period; (10) The scores shown reflect fewer than 50 completed surveys; (11) There were discrepancies in the data collection process; (12) This measure does not apply to this hospital for this reporting period; (13) Results cannot be calculated for this reporting period; (14) The results for this state are combined with nearby states to protect confidentiality; Please refer to the User's Guide for a full explanation of data.

Chickasaw Nation Medical Center

1921 Stonecipher Blvd Phone: 580-436-3980
Ada, OK 74820
URL: www.chickasaw.net
Type: Acute Care Hospitals Emergency Services: Yes
Ownership: Government - Local

Measure	Cases	This Hosp.	State Avg.	U.S. Avg.
Blood Clot Prevention and Treatment				
Anticoagulation Overlap Therapy[2]	11	100%	89%	93%
ICU Venous Thromboembolism Prophylaxis[2]	37	70%	87%	92%
Incidence of Potentially Preventable VTE[2,7]	-	-	8%	10%
UFH with Dosages/Platelet Monitoring[1,2]	-	-	97%	97%
Venous Thromboembolism Prophylaxis[2]	150	73%	72%	85%
Warfarin Therapy Discharge Instructions[1,2]	-	-	73%	75%
Chest Pain/Possible Heart Attack Care				
Aspirin Given Within 24 Hours of Arrival	-	-	95%	96%
Fibrinolytic Meds Within 30 Min. of Arrival	-	-	54%	58%
Average Time to ECG (minutes)	-	-	8	7
Average Time to Transfer (minutes)	-	-	77	60
Children's Asthma Care				
Received Home Management Plan of Care	-	-	-	88%
Received Reliever Medication	-	-	-	100%
Received Systemic Corticosteroids	-	-	-	100%
Emergency Department				
Admittance Decision Time (minutes)[2]	240	48	63	98
Head CT Results Within 45 Min. of Arrival	-	-	49%	57%
Patients Who Left ER Before Being Seen	-	-	2%	2%
Time from ER Arrival to Admit. (minutes)[2]	239	236	210	274
Time from ER Arrival to Discharge (minutes)	-	-	110	134
Time in ER Before Being Evaluated (minutes)	-	-	24	26
Time to Pain Meds for Fractures (minutes)	-	-	55	57
Heart Attack Care				
Aspirin Given at Discharge[3,7]	-	-	99%	99%
Fibrinolytic Meds Within 30 Min. of Arrival[3,7]	-	-	25%	54%
PCI Within 90 Minutes of Arrival[3,7]	-	-	95%	96%
Statin Prescribed at Discharge[3,7]	-	-	98%	98%
Heart Failure Care				
ACE Inhibitor or ARB for LVSD[1]	-	-	95%	97%
Discharge Instructions Given	37	100%	92%	94%
Evaluation of LVS Function	38	97%	96%	99%
Medicare Spending				
Medicare Spending per Patient (ratio)	-	0.80	0.93	0.98
Pneumonia Care				
Appropriate Initial Antibiotic Given	47	87%	92%	95%
Blood Culture Timing	52	92%	97%	98%
Pregnancy and Delivery Care				
Newborn Deliveries Scheduled Early[2]	28	32%	8%	6%
Preventive Care				
Immunization for Influenza[2]	315	84%	89%	90%
Immunization for Pneumonia[2]	272	84%	91%	92%
Stroke Care				
Anticoagulation Therapy for Atrial Fibrillation[7]	-	-	91%	95%
Antithrombotic Therapy Timing	11	100%	95%	98%
Assessed for Rehabilitation	12	75%	96%	97%
Discharged on Antithrombotic Therapy	11	82%	98%	99%
Discharged on Statin Medication	11	91%	88%	94%
Thrombolytic Therapy Timing[7]	-	-	61%	66%
Venous Thromboembolism Prophylaxis	11	73%	92%	94%
Written Stroke Educational Materials Given[1]	-	-	86%	88%
Surgical Care Improvement Project				
Appropriate Beta Blocker Usage	12	100%	97%	98%
Appropriate VTP Within 24 Hours	51	92%	97%	98%
Controlled Postoperative Blood Glucose[7]	-	-	97%	97%
Perioperative Temperature Management	53	100%	100%	100%
Prophylactic Antibiotic Selection	36	100%	99%	99%
Prophylactic Antibiotic Selection (Outpatient)	-	-	98%	98%
Prophylactic Antibiotic Stopped	36	97%	98%	98%
Prophylactic Antibiotic Timing	36	100%	98%	99%
Prophylactic Antibiotic Timing (Outpatient)	-	-	98%	98%
Urinary Catheter Removal	13	100%	96%	97%
Survey of Patients' Hospital Experiences				
Area Around Room 'Always' Quiet at Night	300+	76%	68%	61%
Doctors 'Always' Communicated Well	300+	85%	84%	82%
Home Recovery Information Given	300+	87%	84%	85%
Hospital Given 9 or 10 on 10 Point Scale	300+	84%	72%	71%
Meds 'Always' Explained Before Given	300+	73%	66%	64%
Nurses 'Always' Communicated Well	300+	84%	80%	79%
Pain 'Always' Well Controlled	300+	80%	72%	71%
Room and Bathroom 'Always' Clean	300+	82%	73%	73%
Timely Help 'Always' Received	300+	76%	71%	68%
Would Definitely Recommend Hospital	300+	88%	71%	71%
Use of Medical Imaging				
Cardiac Imaging Stress Test before Surgery	-	-	4.5%	5.3%
Combination Abdominal CT Scan	-	-	23%	10.5%
Combination Brain/Sinus CT Scan	-	-	2.2%	2.7%
Combination Chest CT Scan	-	-	5.1%	2.7%
Follow-up Mammogram/Ultrasound	-	-	8.1%	8.8%
Lumbar Spine MRI for Low Back Pain	-	-	39.9%	37.2%

Mercy Hospital Ada

430 North Monta Vista Phone: 580-332-2323
Ada, OK 74820 Fax: 580-421-1386
URL: www.valleyviewregional.org
Type: Acute Care Hospitals Emergency Services: Yes
Ownership: Voluntary non-profit - Private Beds: 180

Key Personnel:
Radiology. . . . . John Alcini
CEO/President. . . . . Lynn Britton
Chief of Medical Staff . . . . James R Powers, MD
Patient Relations . . . . Jackye Ward, MS, RN

Measure	Cases	This Hosp.	State Avg.	U.S. Avg.
Blood Clot Prevention and Treatment				
Anticoagulation Overlap Therapy[2]	27	100%	89%	93%
ICU Venous Thromboembolism Prophylaxis[2]	49	76%	87%	92%
Incidence of Potentially Preventable VTE[1,2]	-	-	8%	10%
UFH with Dosages/Platelet Monitoring[1,2]	-	-	97%	97%
Venous Thromboembolism Prophylaxis[2]	179	82%	72%	85%
Warfarin Therapy Discharge Instructions[2]	21	95%	73%	75%
Chest Pain/Possible Heart Attack Care				
Aspirin Given Within 24 Hours of Arrival	52	100%	95%	96%
Fibrinolytic Meds Within 30 Min. of Arrival[1]	-	-	54%	58%
Average Time to ECG (minutes)	54	8	8	7
Average Time to Transfer (minutes)[7]	-	-	77	60
Children's Asthma Care				
Received Home Management Plan of Care	-	-	-	88%
Received Reliever Medication	-	-	-	100%
Received Systemic Corticosteroids	-	-	-	100%
Emergency Department				
Admittance Decision Time (minutes)[2]	268	34	63	98
Head CT Results Within 45 Min. of Arrival[1]	-	-	49%	57%
Patients Who Left ER Before Being Seen	21,539	2%	2%	2%
Time from ER Arrival to Admit. (minutes)[2]	268	222	210	274
Time from ER Arrival to Discharge (minutes)	353	141	110	134
Time in ER Before Being Evaluated (minutes)	384	36	24	26
Time to Pain Meds for Fractures (minutes)	81	78	55	57
Heart Attack Care				
Aspirin Given at Discharge[1]	-	-	99%	99%
Fibrinolytic Meds Within 30 Min. of Arrival[7]	-	-	25%	54%
PCI Within 90 Minutes of Arrival[7]	-	-	95%	96%
Statin Prescribed at Discharge[1]	-	-	98%	98%
Heart Failure Care				
ACE Inhibitor or ARB for LVSD[1]	-	-	95%	97%
Discharge Instructions Given	35	86%	92%	94%
Evaluation of LVS Function	43	100%	96%	99%
Medicare Spending				
Medicare Spending per Patient (ratio)	-	1.01	0.93	0.98
Pneumonia Care				
Appropriate Initial Antibiotic Given	77	96%	92%	95%
Blood Culture Timing	157	97%	97%	98%
Pregnancy and Delivery Care				
Newborn Deliveries Scheduled Early[2]	38	0%	8%	6%
Preventive Care				
Immunization for Influenza[2]	279	92%	89%	90%
Immunization for Pneumonia[2]	299	92%	91%	92%
Stroke Care				
Anticoagulation Therapy for Atrial Fibrillation[1]	-	-	91%	95%
Antithrombotic Therapy Timing	32	100%	95%	98%
Assessed for Rehabilitation	33	100%	96%	97%
Discharged on Antithrombotic Therapy	33	97%	98%	99%
Discharged on Statin Medication	25	68%	88%	94%
Thrombolytic Therapy Timing[1]	-	-	61%	66%
Venous Thromboembolism Prophylaxis	37	78%	92%	94%
Written Stroke Educational Materials Given	13	15%	86%	88%
Surgical Care Improvement Project				
Appropriate Beta Blocker Usage	61	80%	97%	98%
Appropriate VTP Within 24 Hours	156	94%	97%	98%
Controlled Postoperative Blood Glucose[7]	-	-	97%	97%
Perioperative Temperature Management	173	100%	100%	100%
Prophylactic Antibiotic Selection	92	100%	99%	99%
Prophylactic Antibiotic Selection (Outpatient)	221	99%	98%	98%
Prophylactic Antibiotic Stopped	91	100%	98%	98%
Prophylactic Antibiotic Timing	92	99%	98%	99%
Prophylactic Antibiotic Timing (Outpatient)	226	97%	98%	98%
Urinary Catheter Removal	78	86%	96%	97%
Survey of Patients' Hospital Experiences				
Area Around Room 'Always' Quiet at Night[11]	300+	63%	68%	61%
Doctors 'Always' Communicated Well[11]	300+	80%	84%	82%
Home Recovery Information Given[11]	300+	88%	84%	85%
Hospital Given 9 or 10 on 10 Point Scale[11]	300+	67%	72%	71%
Meds 'Always' Explained Before Given[11]	300+	65%	66%	64%
Nurses 'Always' Communicated Well[11]	300+	76%	80%	79%
Pain 'Always' Well Controlled[11]	300+	70%	72%	71%
Room and Bathroom 'Always' Clean[11]	300+	74%	73%	73%
Timely Help 'Always' Received[11]	300+	69%	71%	68%
Would Definitely Recommend Hospital[11]	300+	65%	71%	71%
Use of Medical Imaging				
Cardiac Imaging Stress Test before Surgery	114	7.9%	4.5%	5.3%
Combination Abdominal CT Scan	592	28.9%	23%	10.5%
Combination Brain/Sinus CT Scan	620	1.5%	2.2%	2.7%
Combination Chest CT Scan	232	0.9%	5.1%	2.7%
Follow-up Mammogram/Ultrasound	663	7.8%	8.1%	8.8%
Lumbar Spine MRI for Low Back Pain	95	43.2%	39.9%	37.2%

Jackson County Memorial Hospital

1200 East Pecan St Phone: 580-379-5000
Altus, OK 73523 Fax: 580-379-5509
URL: www.jcmh.com
Type: Acute Care Hospitals Emergency Services: Yes
Ownership: Govt - Hospital Dist/Auth Beds: 156

Key Personnel:
Intensive Care Unit. . . . . Becky Braddock
Infection Control. . . . . Dorothy Butler
CEO/President. . . . . Steve Hartgraves
Chief of Medical Staff . . . . Richard Katseros, MD
Quality Assurance . . . . Jim King
Patient Relations . . . . Bonnie McAskill
Emergency Room . . . . Cheryl Simco
Operating Room. . . . . Mary Stuard

Measure	Cases	This Hosp.	State Avg.	U.S. Avg.
Blood Clot Prevention and Treatment				
Anticoagulation Overlap Therapy[2]	20	95%	89%	93%
ICU Venous Thromboembolism Prophylaxis[2]	51	63%	87%	92%
Incidence of Potentially Preventable VTE[1,2]	-	-	8%	10%
UFH with Dosages/Platelet Monitoring[1,2]	-	-	97%	97%
Venous Thromboembolism Prophylaxis[2]	235	67%	72%	85%
Warfarin Therapy Discharge Instructions[2]	13	46%	73%	75%
Chest Pain/Possible Heart Attack Care				
Aspirin Given Within 24 Hours of Arrival	51	98%	95%	96%
Fibrinolytic Meds Within 30 Min. of Arrival[1]	-	-	54%	58%
Average Time to ECG (minutes)	51	0	8	7
Average Time to Transfer (minutes)[1]	-	-	77	60
Children's Asthma Care				
Received Home Management Plan of Care	-	-	-	88%
Received Reliever Medication	-	-	-	100%
Received Systemic Corticosteroids	-	-	-	100%
Emergency Department				
Admittance Decision Time (minutes)[2]	319	54	63	98
Head CT Results Within 45 Min. of Arrival[1]	-	-	49%	57%
Patients Who Left ER Before Being Seen	21,097	4%	2%	2%

NOTE: Hospital profiles are in alphabetical order by state, then city, then hospital within the city; Rankings exclude hospitals with less than 25 cases except for patient surveys which excludes hospitals with less than 100 cases; (a) 100-299 cases; (1) The number of cases/patients is too few to report; (2) Data submitted were based on a sample of cases/patients; (3) Results are based on a shorter time period than required; (4) Data suppressed by CMS for one or more quarters; (5) Results are not available for this reporting period; (6) Fewer than 100 patients completed the HCAHPS survey; (7) No cases met the criteria for this measure; (8) The lower limit of the confidence interval cannot be calculated if the number of observed infections equals zero; (9) No data are available from the state/territory for this reporting period; (10) The scores shown reflect fewer than 50 completed surveys; (11) There were discrepancies in the data collection process; (12) This measure does not apply to this hospital for this reporting period; (13) Results cannot be calculated for this reporting period; (14) The results for this state are combined with nearby states to protect confidentiality; Please refer to the User's Guide for a full explanation of data.

Measure	Cases	This Hosp.	State Avg.	U.S. Avg.
Time from ER Arrival to Admit. (minutes)[2]	337	181	210	274
Time from ER Arrival to Discharge (minutes)	421	121	110	134
Time in ER Before Being Evaluated (minutes)	449	34	24	26
Time to Pain Meds for Fractures (minutes)	90	74	55	57
Heart Attack Care				
Aspirin Given at Discharge[1]	-	-	99%	99%
Fibrinolytic Meds Within 30 Min. of Arrival[7]	-	-	25%	54%
PCI Within 90 Minutes of Arrival[7]	-	-	95%	96%
Statin Prescribed at Discharge[1]	-	-	98%	98%
Heart Failure Care				
ACE Inhibitor or ARB for LVSD	34	94%	95%	97%
Discharge Instructions Given	77	70%	92%	94%
Evaluation of LVS Function	114	93%	96%	99%
Medicare Spending				
Medicare Spending per Patient (ratio)	-	0.93	0.93	0.98
Pneumonia Care				
Appropriate Initial Antibiotic Given[2]	67	97%	92%	95%
Blood Culture Timing[2]	97	97%	97%	98%
Pregnancy and Delivery Care				
Newborn Deliveries Scheduled Early[2]	29	0%	8%	6%
Preventive Care				
Immunization for Influenza[2]	345	88%	89%	90%
Immunization for Pneumonia[2]	429	92%	91%	92%
Stroke Care				
Anticoagulation Therapy for Atrial Fibrillation[1]	-	-	91%	95%
Antithrombotic Therapy Timing	21	100%	95%	98%
Assessed for Rehabilitation	24	96%	96%	97%
Discharged on Antithrombotic Therapy	22	95%	98%	99%
Discharged on Statin Medication	22	45%	88%	94%
Thrombolytic Therapy Timing[1]	-	-	61%	66%
Venous Thromboembolism Prophylaxis	26	73%	92%	94%
Written Stroke Educational Materials Given	12	17%	86%	88%
Surgical Care Improvement Project				
Appropriate Beta Blocker Usage[2]	105	95%	97%	98%
Appropriate VTP Within 24 Hours[2]	271	96%	97%	98%
Controlled Postoperative Blood Glucose[2,7]	-	-	97%	97%
Perioperative Temperature Management[2]	295	100%	100%	100%
Prophylactic Antibiotic Selection[2]	194	99%	99%	99%
Prophylactic Antibiotic Selection (Outpatient)	13	100%	98%	98%
Prophylactic Antibiotic Stopped[2]	185	98%	98%	98%
Prophylactic Antibiotic Timing[2]	195	97%	98%	99%
Prophylactic Antibiotic Timing (Outpatient)	13	100%	98%	98%
Urinary Catheter Removal[2]	168	96%	96%	97%
Survey of Patients' Hospital Experiences				
Area Around Room 'Always' Quiet at Night	300+	60%	68%	61%
Doctors 'Always' Communicated Well	300+	85%	84%	82%
Home Recovery Information Given	300+	87%	84%	85%
Hospital Given 9 or 10 on 10 Point Scale	300+	67%	72%	71%
Meds 'Always' Explained Before Given	300+	70%	66%	64%
Nurses 'Always' Communicated Well	300+	83%	80%	79%
Pain 'Always' Well Controlled	300+	73%	72%	71%
Room and Bathroom 'Always' Clean	300+	74%	73%	73%
Timely Help 'Always' Received	300+	72%	71%	68%
Would Definitely Recommend Hospital	300+	67%	71%	71%
Use of Medical Imaging				
Cardiac Imaging Stress Test before Surgery	105	3.8%	4.5%	5.3%
Combination Abdominal CT Scan	490	73.1%	23%	10.5%
Combination Brain/Sinus CT Scan[1]	-	-	2.2%	2.7%
Combination Chest CT Scan	234	0.4%	5.1%	2.7%
Follow-up Mammogram/Ultrasound	686	10.3%	8.1%	8.8%
Lumbar Spine MRI for Low Back Pain	63	49.2%	39.9%	37.2%

Share Memorial Hospital

800 Share Drive
Alva, OK 73717
Phone: 580-327-2800
Fax: 580-430-3332
URL: www.smcok.com
Type: Acute Care Hospitals
Ownership: Government - Local
Emergency Services: Yes
Beds: 37

Key Personnel:
Chief of Medical Staff. . . . . Kirtt Bierig, DO
Infection Control. . . . . Cheryl Ellis, RN
Quality Assurance . . . . Dottie Gatz
Operating Room. . . . . Kelly Hellar, RN, BSN
Emergency Room . . . . Barbara Louthan, RN
CEO/President. . . . . Barbara Oestmann

Measure	Cases	This Hosp.	State Avg.	U.S. Avg.
Blood Clot Prevention and Treatment				
Anticoagulation Overlap Therapy[1]	-	-	89%	93%
ICU Venous Thromboembolism Prophylaxis[7]	-	-	87%	92%
Incidence of Potentially Preventable VTE[7]	-	-	8%	10%
UFH with Dosages/Platelet Monitoring[7]	-	-	97%	97%
Venous Thromboembolism Prophylaxis	87	55%	72%	85%
Warfarin Therapy Discharge Instructions[1]	-	-	73%	75%
Chest Pain/Possible Heart Attack Care				
Aspirin Given Within 24 Hours of Arrival	19	84%	95%	96%
Fibrinolytic Meds Within 30 Min. of Arrival[1]	-	-	54%	58%
Average Time to ECG (minutes)	19	7	8	7
Average Time to Transfer (minutes)[1]	-	-	77	60
Children's Asthma Care				
Received Home Management Plan of Care	-	-	-	88%
Received Reliever Medication	-	-	-	100%
Received Systemic Corticosteroids	-	-	-	100%
Emergency Department				
Admittance Decision Time (minutes)	111	15	63	98
Head CT Results Within 45 Min. of Arrival[1]	-	-	49%	57%
Patients Who Left ER Before Being Seen	5,026	0%	2%	2%
Time from ER Arrival to Admit. (minutes)	115	162	210	274
Time from ER Arrival to Discharge (minutes)	350	87	110	134
Time in ER Before Being Evaluated (minutes)	162	15	24	26
Time to Pain Meds for Fractures (minutes)	41	24	55	57
Heart Attack Care				
Aspirin Given at Discharge[3,7]	-	-	99%	99%
Fibrinolytic Meds Within 30 Min. of Arrival[3,7]	-	-	25%	54%
PCI Within 90 Minutes of Arrival[3,7]	-	-	95%	96%
Statin Prescribed at Discharge[3,7]	-	-	98%	98%
Heart Failure Care				
ACE Inhibitor or ARB for LVSD[3,7]	-	-	95%	97%
Discharge Instructions Given[3,7]	-	-	92%	94%
Evaluation of LVS Function[1,3]	-	-	96%	99%
Medicare Spending				
Medicare Spending per Patient (ratio)	-	0.76	0.93	0.98
Pneumonia Care				
Appropriate Initial Antibiotic Given	21	81%	92%	95%
Blood Culture Timing	20	100%	97%	98%
Pregnancy and Delivery Care				
Newborn Deliveries Scheduled Early[7]	-	-	8%	6%
Preventive Care				
Immunization for Influenza	98	90%	89%	90%
Immunization for Pneumonia	138	89%	91%	92%
Stroke Care				
Anticoagulation Therapy for Atrial Fibrillation[1,3]	-	-	91%	95%
Antithrombotic Therapy Timing[1,3]	-	-	95%	98%
Assessed for Rehabilitation[1,3]	-	-	96%	97%
Discharged on Antithrombotic Therapy[1,3]	-	-	98%	99%
Discharged on Statin Medication[1,3]	-	-	88%	94%
Thrombolytic Therapy Timing[1,3]	-	-	61%	66%
Venous Thromboembolism Prophylaxis[1,3]	-	-	92%	94%
Written Stroke Educational Materials Given[1,3]	-	-	86%	88%
Surgical Care Improvement Project				
Appropriate Beta Blocker Usage[1,3]	-	-	97%	98%
Appropriate VTP Within 24 Hours[1,3]	-	-	97%	98%
Controlled Postoperative Blood Glucose[3,7]	-	-	97%	97%
Perioperative Temperature Management[1,3]	-	-	100%	100%
Prophylactic Antibiotic Selection[1,3]	-	-	99%	99%
Prophylactic Antibiotic Selection (Outpatient)[5]	-	-	98%	98%
Prophylactic Antibiotic Stopped[1,3]	-	-	98%	98%
Prophylactic Antibiotic Timing[1,3]	-	-	98%	99%
Prophylactic Antibiotic Timing (Outpatient)[5]	-	-	98%	98%
Urinary Catheter Removal[3,7]	-	-	96%	97%
Survey of Patients' Hospital Experiences				
Area Around Room 'Always' Quiet at Night[10]	<100	76%	68%	61%
Doctors 'Always' Communicated Well[10]	<100	84%	84%	82%
Home Recovery Information Given[10]	<100	82%	84%	85%
Hospital Given 9 or 10 on 10 Point Scale[10]	<100	68%	72%	71%
Meds 'Always' Explained Before Given[10]	<100	63%	66%	64%
Nurses 'Always' Communicated Well[10]	<100	78%	80%	79%
Pain 'Always' Well Controlled[10]	<100	67%	72%	71%
Room and Bathroom 'Always' Clean[10]	<100	63%	73%	73%
Timely Help 'Always' Received[10]	<100	75%	71%	68%
Would Definitely Recommend Hospital[10]	<100	57%	71%	71%
Use of Medical Imaging				
Cardiac Imaging Stress Test before Surgery[7]	-	-	4.5%	5.3%
Combination Abdominal CT Scan	83	14.5%	23%	10.5%
Combination Brain/Sinus CT Scan[1]	-	-	2.2%	2.7%
Combination Chest CT Scan[1]	-	-	5.1%	2.7%
Follow-up Mammogram/Ultrasound	142	7.0%	8.1%	8.8%
Lumbar Spine MRI for Low Back Pain[1]	-	-	39.9%	37.2%

Physicians' Hospital in Anadarko

1002 East Central Boulevard
Anadarko, OK 73005
Phone: 405-247-2551
Fax: 405-247-9407
Type: Critical Access Hospitals
Ownership: Proprietary
Emergency Services: Yes
Beds: 25

Key Personnel:
Surgery . . . . Roy Bankhead
Emergency Room . . . . Richard Carter
CEO . . . . Bart Daugherty
Radiology. . . . . Craig L Lastine
Chief of Medical Staff . . . . Roberta Martin

Measure	Cases	This Hosp.	State Avg.	U.S. Avg.
Blood Clot Prevention and Treatment				
Anticoagulation Overlap Therapy[5]	-	-	89%	93%
ICU Venous Thromboembolism Prophylaxis[5]	-	-	87%	92%
Incidence of Potentially Preventable VTE[5]	-	-	8%	10%
UFH with Dosages/Platelet Monitoring[5]	-	-	97%	97%
Venous Thromboembolism Prophylaxis[5]	-	-	72%	85%
Warfarin Therapy Discharge Instructions[5]	-	-	73%	75%
Chest Pain/Possible Heart Attack Care				
Aspirin Given Within 24 Hours of Arrival[1,3]	-	-	95%	96%
Fibrinolytic Meds Within 30 Min. of Arrival[1,3]	-	-	54%	58%
Average Time to ECG (minutes)[1,3]	-	-	8	7
Average Time to Transfer (minutes)[3,7]	-	-	77	60
Children's Asthma Care				
Received Home Management Plan of Care	-	-	-	88%
Received Reliever Medication	-	-	-	100%
Received Systemic Corticosteroids	-	-	-	100%
Emergency Department				
Admittance Decision Time (minutes)[5]	-	-	63	98
Head CT Results Within 45 Min. of Arrival[5]	-	-	49%	57%
Patients Who Left ER Before Being Seen[5]	-	-	2%	2%
Time from ER Arrival to Admit. (minutes)[5]	-	-	210	274
Time from ER Arrival to Discharge (minutes)[5]	-	-	110	134
Time in ER Before Being Evaluated (minutes)[5]	-	-	24	26
Time to Pain Meds for Fractures (minutes)[5]	-	-	55	57
Heart Attack Care				
Aspirin Given at Discharge[5]	-	-	99%	99%
Fibrinolytic Meds Within 30 Min. of Arrival[5]	-	-	25%	54%
PCI Within 90 Minutes of Arrival[5]	-	-	95%	96%
Statin Prescribed at Discharge[5]	-	-	98%	98%
Heart Failure Care				
ACE Inhibitor or ARB for LVSD[3,7]	-	-	95%	97%
Discharge Instructions Given[1,3]	-	-	92%	94%
Evaluation of LVS Function[3]	11	27%	96%	99%
Medicare Spending				
Medicare Spending per Patient (ratio)	-	-	0.93	0.98
Pneumonia Care				
Appropriate Initial Antibiotic Given	12	67%	92%	95%
Blood Culture Timing[1]	-	-	97%	98%
Pregnancy and Delivery Care				
Newborn Deliveries Scheduled Early[5]	-	-	8%	6%
Preventive Care				
Immunization for Influenza[5]	-	-	89%	90%
Immunization for Pneumonia[5]	-	-	91%	92%
Stroke Care				
Anticoagulation Therapy for Atrial Fibrillation[5]	-	-	91%	95%
Antithrombotic Therapy Timing[5]	-	-	95%	98%
Assessed for Rehabilitation[5]	-	-	96%	97%
Discharged on Antithrombotic Therapy[5]	-	-	98%	99%
Discharged on Statin Medication[5]	-	-	88%	94%
Thrombolytic Therapy Timing[5]	-	-	61%	66%

NOTE: Hospital profiles are in alphabetical order by state, then city, then hospital within the city; Rankings exclude hospitals with less than 25 cases except for patient surveys which excludes hospitals with less than 100 cases; (a) 100-299 cases; (1) The number of cases/patients is too few to report; (2) Data submitted were based on a sample of cases/patients; (3) Results are based on a shorter time period than required; (4) Data suppressed by CMS for one or more quarters; (5) Results are not available for this reporting period; (6) Fewer than 100 patients completed the HCAHPS survey; (7) No cases met the criteria for this measure; (8) The lower limit of the confidence interval cannot be calculated if the number of observed infections equals zero; (9) No data are available from the state/territory for this reporting period; (10) The scores shown reflect fewer than 50 completed surveys; (11) There were discrepancies in the data collection process; (12) This measure does not apply to this hospital for this reporting period; (13) Results cannot be calculated for this reporting period; (14) The results for this state are combined with nearby states to protect confidentiality; Please refer to the User's Guide for a full explanation of data.

Measure	Cases	This Hosp.	State Avg.	U.S. Avg.
Venous Thromboembolism Prophylaxis[5]	-	-	92%	94%
Written Stroke Educational Materials Given[5]	-	-	86%	88%
Surgical Care Improvement Project				
Appropriate Beta Blocker Usage[5]	-	-	97%	98%
Appropriate VTP Within 24 Hours[5]	-	-	97%	98%
Controlled Postoperative Blood Glucose[5]	-	-	97%	97%
Perioperative Temperature Management[5]	-	-	100%	100%
Prophylactic Antibiotic Selection[5]	-	-	99%	99%
Prophylactic Antibiotic Selection (Outpatient)[5]	-	-	98%	98%
Prophylactic Antibiotic Stopped[5]	-	-	98%	98%
Prophylactic Antibiotic Timing[5]	-	-	98%	99%
Prophylactic Antibiotic Timing (Outpatient)[5]	-	-	98%	98%
Urinary Catheter Removal[5]	-	-	96%	97%
Survey of Patients' Hospital Experiences				
Area Around Room 'Always' Quiet at Night[5]	-	-	68%	61%
Doctors 'Always' Communicated Well[5]	-	-	84%	82%
Home Recovery Information Given[5]	-	-	84%	85%
Hospital Given 9 or 10 on 10 Point Scale[5]	-	-	72%	71%
Meds 'Always' Explained Before Given[5]	-	-	66%	64%
Nurses 'Always' Communicated Well[5]	-	-	80%	79%
Pain 'Always' Well Controlled[5]	-	-	72%	71%
Room and Bathroom 'Always' Clean[5]	-	-	73%	73%
Timely Help 'Always' Received[5]	-	-	71%	68%
Would Definitely Recommend Hospital[5]	-	-	71%	71%
Use of Medical Imaging				
Cardiac Imaging Stress Test before Surgery[7]	-	-	4.5%	5.3%
Combination Abdominal CT Scan	115	41.7%	23%	10.5%
Combination Brain/Sinus CT Scan[1]	-	-	2.2%	2.7%
Combination Chest CT Scan	75	44.0%	5.1%	2.7%
Follow-up Mammogram/Ultrasound[7]	-	-	8.1%	8.8%
Lumbar Spine MRI for Low Back Pain[1]	-	-	39.9%	37.2%

Pushmataha County - Town of Antlers Hospital Authority

510 East Main Street
Antlers, OK 74523
Phone: 580-298-3341
Fax: 580-298-4713
E-mail: comments@pushhospital.com
URL: www.pushhospital.com
Type: Acute Care Hospitals
Emergency Services: Yes
Ownership: Govt - Hospital Dist/Auth
Beds: 48

Key Personnel:
Infection Control............Jane Bates
Emergency Room............Nadine David
CEO/President.............Denis Frank
Chief of Medical Staff..........Herbert Rowland

Measure	Cases	This Hosp.	State Avg.	U.S. Avg.
Blood Clot Prevention and Treatment				
Anticoagulation Overlap Therapy[1,2]	-	-	89%	93%
ICU Venous Thromboembolism Prophylaxis[2,7]	-	-	87%	92%
Incidence of Potentially Preventable VTE[1,2]	-	-	8%	10%
UFH with Dosages/Platelet Monitoring[2,7]	-	-	97%	97%
Venous Thromboembolism Prophylaxis[2]	110	3%	72%	85%
Warfarin Therapy Discharge Instructions[1,2]	-	-	73%	75%
Chest Pain/Possible Heart Attack Care				
Aspirin Given Within 24 Hours of Arrival[3]	11	73%	95%	96%
Fibrinolytic Meds Within 30 Min. of Arrival[1,3]	-	-	54%	58%
Average Time to ECG (minutes)[3]	11	15	8	7
Average Time to Transfer (minutes)[1,3]	-	-	77	60
Children's Asthma Care				
Received Home Management Plan of Care	-	-	-	88%
Received Reliever Medication	-	-	-	100%
Received Systemic Corticosteroids	-	-	-	100%
Emergency Department				
Admittance Decision Time (minutes)[2]	429	70	63	98
Head CT Results Within 45 Min. of Arrival[1,3]	-	-	49%	57%
Patients Who Left ER Before Being Seen	5,438	3%	2%	2%
Time from ER Arrival to Admit. (minutes)[2]	444	170	210	274
Time from ER Arrival to Discharge (minutes)	368	80	110	134
Time in ER Before Being Evaluated (minutes)	387	20	24	26
Time to Pain Meds for Fractures (minutes)[3]	30	36	55	57
Heart Attack Care				
Aspirin Given at Discharge[5]	-	-	99%	99%
Fibrinolytic Meds Within 30 Min. of Arrival[5]	-	-	25%	54%
PCI Within 90 Minutes of Arrival[5]	-	-	95%	96%
Statin Prescribed at Discharge[5]	-	-	98%	98%
Heart Failure Care				
ACE Inhibitor or ARB for LVSD[1]	-	-	95%	97%
Discharge Instructions Given	14	43%	92%	94%
Evaluation of LVS Function	27	67%	96%	99%
Medicare Spending				
Medicare Spending per Patient (ratio)	-	1.00	0.93	0.98
Pneumonia Care				
Appropriate Initial Antibiotic Given	47	85%	92%	95%
Blood Culture Timing	25	92%	97%	98%
Pregnancy and Delivery Care				
Newborn Deliveries Scheduled Early[7]	-	-	8%	6%
Preventive Care				
Immunization for Influenza[2]	283	75%	89%	90%
Immunization for Pneumonia[2]	415	82%	91%	92%
Stroke Care				
Anticoagulation Therapy for Atrial Fibrillation[3,7]	-	-	91%	95%
Antithrombotic Therapy Timing[1,3]	-	-	95%	98%
Assessed for Rehabilitation[1,3]	-	-	96%	97%
Discharged on Antithrombotic Therapy[1,3]	-	-	98%	99%
Discharged on Statin Medication[1,3]	-	-	88%	94%
Thrombolytic Therapy Timing[1,3]	-	-	61%	66%
Venous Thromboembolism Prophylaxis[1,3]	-	-	92%	94%
Written Stroke Educational Materials Given[1,3]	-	-	86%	88%
Surgical Care Improvement Project				
Appropriate Beta Blocker Usage[5]	-	-	97%	98%
Appropriate VTP Within 24 Hours[5]	-	-	97%	98%
Controlled Postoperative Blood Glucose[5]	-	-	97%	97%
Perioperative Temperature Management[5]	-	-	100%	100%
Prophylactic Antibiotic Selection[5]	-	-	99%	99%
Prophylactic Antibiotic Selection (Outpatient)[5]	-	-	98%	98%
Prophylactic Antibiotic Stopped[5]	-	-	98%	98%
Prophylactic Antibiotic Timing[5]	-	-	98%	99%
Prophylactic Antibiotic Timing (Outpatient)[5]	-	-	98%	98%
Urinary Catheter Removal[5]	-	-	96%	97%
Survey of Patients' Hospital Experiences				
Area Around Room 'Always' Quiet at Night[3,6]	<100	76%	68%	61%
Doctors 'Always' Communicated Well[3,6]	<100	80%	84%	82%
Home Recovery Information Given[3,6]	<100	76%	84%	85%
Hospital Given 9 or 10 on 10 Point Scale[3,6]	<100	59%	72%	71%
Meds 'Always' Explained Before Given[3,6]	<100	55%	66%	64%
Nurses 'Always' Communicated Well[3,6]	<100	74%	80%	79%
Pain 'Always' Well Controlled[3,6]	<100	67%	72%	71%
Room and Bathroom 'Always' Clean[3,6]	<100	83%	73%	73%
Timely Help 'Always' Received[3,6]	<100	68%	71%	68%
Would Definitely Recommend Hospital[3,6]	<100	52%	71%	71%
Use of Medical Imaging				
Cardiac Imaging Stress Test before Surgery[7]	-	-	4.5%	5.3%
Combination Abdominal CT Scan	82	18.3%	23%	10.5%
Combination Brain/Sinus CT Scan[1]	-	-	2.2%	2.7%
Combination Chest CT Scan[1]	-	-	5.1%	2.7%
Follow-up Mammogram/Ultrasound[7]	-	-	8.1%	8.8%
Lumbar Spine MRI for Low Back Pain[7]	-	-	39.9%	37.2%

Mercy Memorial Health Center

1011 Fourteenth Avenue, Northwest
Ardmore, OK 73401
Phone: 405-223-5400
Fax: 580-220-6580
URL: www.mercyok.com/mmhc
Type: Acute Care Hospitals
Emergency Services: Yes
Ownership: Voluntary non-profit - Private
Beds: 176

Key Personnel:
CEO/President..............Bobby G Thompson

Measure	Cases	This Hosp.	State Avg.	U.S. Avg.
Blood Clot Prevention and Treatment				
Anticoagulation Overlap Therapy[2]	38	92%	89%	93%
ICU Venous Thromboembolism Prophylaxis[2]	51	88%	87%	92%
Incidence of Potentially Preventable VTE[1,2]	-	-	8%	10%
UFH with Dosages/Platelet Monitoring[1,2]	-	-	97%	97%
Venous Thromboembolism Prophylaxis[2]	317	81%	72%	85%
Warfarin Therapy Discharge Instructions[2]	31	42%	73%	75%
Chest Pain/Possible Heart Attack Care				
Aspirin Given Within 24 Hours of Arrival	27	100%	95%	96%
Fibrinolytic Meds Within 30 Min. of Arrival[1,3]	-	-	54%	58%
Average Time to ECG (minutes)	28	5	8	7
Average Time to Transfer (minutes)[1,3]	-	-	77	60
Children's Asthma Care				
Received Home Management Plan of Care	-	-	-	88%
Received Reliever Medication	-	-	-	100%
Received Systemic Corticosteroids	-	-	-	100%
Emergency Department				
Admittance Decision Time (minutes)[2]	594	88	63	98
Head CT Results Within 45 Min. of Arrival	19	53%	49%	57%
Patients Who Left ER Before Being Seen	39,518	5%	2%	2%
Time from ER Arrival to Admit. (minutes)[2]	605	188	210	274
Time from ER Arrival to Discharge (minutes)	383	112	110	134
Time in ER Before Being Evaluated (minutes)	403	17	24	26
Time to Pain Meds for Fractures (minutes)	125	43	55	57
Heart Attack Care				
Aspirin Given at Discharge	98	100%	99%	99%
Fibrinolytic Meds Within 30 Min. of Arrival[7]	-	-	25%	54%
PCI Within 90 Minutes of Arrival	20	90%	95%	96%
Statin Prescribed at Discharge	98	97%	98%	98%
Heart Failure Care				
ACE Inhibitor or ARB for LVSD	72	92%	95%	97%
Discharge Instructions Given	136	94%	92%	94%
Evaluation of LVS Function	187	100%	96%	99%
Medicare Spending				
Medicare Spending per Patient (ratio)	-	0.96	0.93	0.98
Pneumonia Care				
Appropriate Initial Antibiotic Given[2]	69	94%	92%	95%
Blood Culture Timing[2]	77	97%	97%	98%
Pregnancy and Delivery Care				
Newborn Deliveries Scheduled Early[2]	28	7%	8%	6%
Preventive Care				
Immunization for Influenza[2]	534	90%	89%	90%
Immunization for Pneumonia[2]	693	92%	91%	92%
Stroke Care				
Anticoagulation Therapy for Atrial Fibrillation[1,2]	-	-	91%	95%
Antithrombotic Therapy Timing[2]	71	97%	95%	98%
Assessed for Rehabilitation[2]	72	82%	96%	97%
Discharged on Antithrombotic Therapy[2]	71	93%	98%	99%
Discharged on Statin Medication[2]	61	80%	88%	94%
Thrombolytic Therapy Timing[1,2]	-	-	61%	66%
Venous Thromboembolism Prophylaxis[2]	72	92%	92%	94%
Written Stroke Educational Materials Given[2]	39	69%	86%	88%
Surgical Care Improvement Project				
Appropriate Beta Blocker Usage[2]	96	96%	97%	98%
Appropriate VTP Within 24 Hours[2]	295	99%	97%	98%
Controlled Postoperative Blood Glucose[2,7]	-	-	97%	97%
Perioperative Temperature Management[2]	347	100%	100%	100%
Prophylactic Antibiotic Selection[2]	196	98%	99%	99%
Prophylactic Antibiotic Selection (Outpatient)	319	93%	98%	98%
Prophylactic Antibiotic Stopped[2]	183	99%	98%	98%
Prophylactic Antibiotic Timing[2]	196	95%	98%	99%
Prophylactic Antibiotic Timing (Outpatient)	321	95%	98%	98%
Urinary Catheter Removal[2]	88	92%	96%	97%
Survey of Patients' Hospital Experiences				
Area Around Room 'Always' Quiet at Night[11]	300+	61%	68%	61%
Doctors 'Always' Communicated Well[11]	300+	83%	84%	82%
Home Recovery Information Given[11]	300+	84%	84%	85%
Hospital Given 9 or 10 on 10 Point Scale[11]	300+	71%	72%	71%
Meds 'Always' Explained Before Given[11]	300+	61%	66%	64%
Nurses 'Always' Communicated Well[11]	300+	80%	80%	79%
Pain 'Always' Well Controlled[11]	300+	70%	72%	71%
Room and Bathroom 'Always' Clean[11]	300+	66%	73%	73%
Timely Help 'Always' Received[11]	300+	68%	71%	68%
Would Definitely Recommend Hospital[11]	300+	64%	71%	71%
Use of Medical Imaging				
Cardiac Imaging Stress Test before Surgery	425	3.8%	4.5%	5.3%
Combination Abdominal CT Scan	928	15.6%	23%	10.5%
Combination Brain/Sinus CT Scan[1]	-	-	2.2%	2.7%
Combination Chest CT Scan	479	4.6%	5.1%	2.7%
Follow-up Mammogram/Ultrasound	1,223	4.4%	8.1%	8.8%
Lumbar Spine MRI for Low Back Pain	158	40.5%	39.9%	37.2%

NOTE: Hospital profiles are in alphabetical order by state, then city, then hospital within the city; Rankings exclude hospitals with less than 25 cases except for patient surveys which excludes hospitals with less than 100 cases; (a) 100-299 cases; (1) The number of cases/patients is too few to report; (2) Data submitted were based on a sample of cases/patients; (3) Results are based on a shorter time period than required; (4) Data suppressed by CMS for one or more quarters; (5) Results are not available for this reporting period; (6) Fewer than 100 patients completed the HCAHPS survey; (7) No cases met the criteria for this measure; (8) The lower limit of the confidence interval cannot be calculated if the number of observed infections equals zero; (9) No data are available from the state/territory for this reporting period; (10) The scores shown reflect fewer than 50 completed surveys; (11) There were discrepancies in the data collection process; (12) This measure does not apply to this hospital for this reporting period; (13) Results cannot be calculated for this reporting period; (14) The results for this state are combined with nearby states to protect confidentiality; Please refer to the User's Guide for a full explanation of data.

Atoka County Medical Center

1200 West Liberty Road Phone: 580-889-3333
Atoka, OK 74525 Fax: 580-889-1948
URL: www.atoka-hosp.otnnet.net
Type: Critical Access Hospitals Emergency Services: Yes
Ownership: Govt - Hospital Dist/Auth Beds: 25
Key Personnel:
CEO/President. . . . . Charles Young

Measure	Cases	This Hosp.	State Avg.	U.S. Avg.
Blood Clot Prevention and Treatment				
Anticoagulation Overlap Therapy[5]	-	-	89%	93%
ICU Venous Thromboembolism Prophylaxis[5]	-	-	87%	92%
Incidence of Potentially Preventable VTE[5]	-	-	8%	10%
UFH with Dosages/Platelet Monitoring[5]	-	-	97%	97%
Venous Thromboembolism Prophylaxis[5]	-	-	72%	85%
Warfarin Therapy Discharge Instructions[5]	-	-	73%	75%
Chest Pain/Possible Heart Attack Care				
Aspirin Given Within 24 Hours of Arrival	29	97%	95%	96%
Fibrinolytic Meds Within 30 Min. of Arrival	14	14%	54%	58%
Average Time to ECG (minutes)	35	5	8	7
Average Time to Transfer (minutes)[7]	-	-	77	60
Children's Asthma Care				
Received Home Management Plan of Care	-	-	-	88%
Received Reliever Medication	-	-	-	100%
Received Systemic Corticosteroids	-	-	-	100%
Emergency Department				
Admittance Decision Time (minutes)[5]	-	-	63	98
Head CT Results Within 45 Min. of Arrival[5]	-	-	49%	57%
Patients Who Left ER Before Being Seen[5]	-	-	2%	2%
Time from ER Arrival to Admit. (minutes)[5]	-	-	210	274
Time from ER Arrival to Discharge (minutes)[5]	-	-	110	134
Time in ER Before Being Evaluated (minutes)[5]	-	-	24	26
Time to Pain Meds for Fractures (minutes)[5]	-	-	55	57
Heart Attack Care				
Aspirin Given at Discharge[1,3]	-	-	99%	99%
Fibrinolytic Meds Within 30 Min. of Arrival[3,7]	-	-	25%	54%
PCI Within 90 Minutes of Arrival[3,7]	-	-	95%	96%
Statin Prescribed at Discharge[1,3]	-	-	98%	98%
Heart Failure Care				
ACE Inhibitor or ARB for LVSD[1]	-	-	95%	97%
Discharge Instructions Given[1]	-	-	92%	94%
Evaluation of LVS Function	23	9%	96%	99%
Medicare Spending				
Medicare Spending per Patient (ratio)	-	-	0.93	0.98
Pneumonia Care				
Appropriate Initial Antibiotic Given[1]	-	-	92%	95%
Blood Culture Timing[1]	-	-	97%	98%
Pregnancy and Delivery Care				
Newborn Deliveries Scheduled Early[5]	-	-	8%	6%
Preventive Care				
Immunization for Influenza[5]	-	-	89%	90%
Immunization for Pneumonia[5]	-	-	91%	92%
Stroke Care				
Anticoagulation Therapy for Atrial Fibrillation[5]	-	-	91%	95%
Antithrombotic Therapy Timing[5]	-	-	95%	98%
Assessed for Rehabilitation[5]	-	-	96%	97%
Discharged on Antithrombotic Therapy[5]	-	-	98%	99%
Discharged on Statin Medication[5]	-	-	88%	94%
Thrombolytic Therapy Timing[5]	-	-	61%	66%
Venous Thromboembolism Prophylaxis[5]	-	-	92%	94%
Written Stroke Educational Materials Given[5]	-	-	86%	88%
Surgical Care Improvement Project				
Appropriate Beta Blocker Usage[5]	-	-	97%	98%
Appropriate VTP Within 24 Hours[5]	-	-	97%	98%
Controlled Postoperative Blood Glucose[5]	-	-	97%	97%
Perioperative Temperature Management[5]	-	-	100%	100%
Prophylactic Antibiotic Selection[5]	-	-	99%	99%
Prophylactic Antibiotic Selection (Outpatient)[5]	-	-	98%	98%
Prophylactic Antibiotic Stopped[5]	-	-	98%	98%
Prophylactic Antibiotic Timing[5]	-	-	98%	99%
Prophylactic Antibiotic Timing (Outpatient)[5]	-	-	98%	98%
Urinary Catheter Removal[5]	-	-	96%	97%
Survey of Patients' Hospital Experiences				
Area Around Room 'Always' Quiet at Night[6]	<100	49%	68%	61%
Doctors 'Always' Communicated Well[6]	<100	79%	84%	82%
Home Recovery Information Given[6]	<100	67%	84%	85%
Hospital Given 9 or 10 on 10 Point Scale[6]	<100	45%	72%	71%
Meds 'Always' Explained Before Given[6]	<100	49%	66%	64%
Nurses 'Always' Communicated Well[6]	<100	62%	80%	79%
Pain 'Always' Well Controlled[6]	<100	54%	72%	71%
Room and Bathroom 'Always' Clean[6]	<100	63%	73%	73%
Timely Help 'Always' Received[6]	<100	75%	71%	68%
Would Definitely Recommend Hospital[6]	<100	52%	71%	71%
Use of Medical Imaging				
Cardiac Imaging Stress Test before Surgery[7]	-	-	4.5%	5.3%
Combination Abdominal CT Scan	122	18.9%	23%	10.5%
Combination Brain/Sinus CT Scan	215	0.5%	2.2%	2.7%
Combination Chest CT Scan[1]	-	-	5.1%	2.7%
Follow-up Mammogram/Ultrasound[7]	-	-	8.1%	8.8%
Lumbar Spine MRI for Low Back Pain[7]	-	-	39.9%	37.2%

Jane Phillips Medical Center

3500 East Frank Phillips Boulevard Phone: 918-333-7200
Bartlesville, OK 74006 Fax: 918-331-1612
URL: www.jpmc.org
Type: Acute Care Hospitals Emergency Services: Yes
Ownership: Voluntary non-profit - Private Beds: 144
Key Personnel:
Quality Assurance . . . . Diane Garrett, RN
Chairman/CEO . . . . John B. Kane
Chief of Medical Staff. . . . . Paul W. McQuillen, MD
CEO/President. . . . . David R Stire

Measure	Cases	This Hosp.	State Avg.	U.S. Avg.
Blood Clot Prevention and Treatment				
Anticoagulation Overlap Therapy[2]	17	82%	89%	93%
ICU Venous Thromboembolism Prophylaxis[2]	63	98%	87%	92%
Incidence of Potentially Preventable VTE[1,2]	-	-	8%	10%
UFH with Dosages/Platelet Monitoring[1,2]	-	-	97%	97%
Venous Thromboembolism Prophylaxis[2]	295	98%	72%	85%
Warfarin Therapy Discharge Instructions[2]	14	100%	73%	75%
Chest Pain/Possible Heart Attack Care				
Aspirin Given Within 24 Hours of Arrival	11	91%	95%	96%
Fibrinolytic Meds Within 30 Min. of Arrival[5]	-	-	54%	58%
Average Time to ECG (minutes)	12	8	8	7
Average Time to Transfer (minutes)[5]	-	-	77	60
Children's Asthma Care				
Received Home Management Plan of Care	-	-	-	88%
Received Reliever Medication	-	-	-	100%
Received Systemic Corticosteroids	-	-	-	100%
Emergency Department				
Admittance Decision Time (minutes)[2]	294	75	63	98
Head CT Results Within 45 Min. of Arrival	23	52%	49%	57%
Patients Who Left ER Before Being Seen	34,827	1%	2%	2%
Time from ER Arrival to Admit. (minutes)[2]	359	200	210	274
Time from ER Arrival to Discharge (minutes)	1,218	111	110	134
Time in ER Before Being Evaluated (minutes)	1,189	32	24	26
Time to Pain Meds for Fractures (minutes)	156	50	55	57
Heart Attack Care				
Aspirin Given at Discharge	147	99%	99%	99%
Fibrinolytic Meds Within 30 Min. of Arrival[7]	-	-	25%	54%
PCI Within 90 Minutes of Arrival	32	91%	95%	96%
Statin Prescribed at Discharge	146	99%	98%	98%
Heart Failure Care				
ACE Inhibitor or ARB for LVSD	38	97%	95%	97%
Discharge Instructions Given	84	100%	92%	94%
Evaluation of LVS Function	110	100%	96%	99%
Medicare Spending				
Medicare Spending per Patient (ratio)	-	0.96	0.93	0.98
Pneumonia Care				
Appropriate Initial Antibiotic Given	103	97%	92%	95%
Blood Culture Timing	158	94%	97%	98%
Pregnancy and Delivery Care				
Newborn Deliveries Scheduled Early	44	2%	8%	6%
Preventive Care				
Immunization for Influenza[2]	419	96%	89%	90%
Immunization for Pneumonia[2]	497	92%	91%	92%
Stroke Care				
Anticoagulation Therapy for Atrial Fibrillation[1]	-	-	91%	95%
Antithrombotic Therapy Timing	46	100%	95%	98%
Assessed for Rehabilitation	51	90%	96%	97%
Discharged on Antithrombotic Therapy	49	100%	98%	99%
Discharged on Statin Medication	38	97%	88%	94%
Thrombolytic Therapy Timing	13	46%	61%	66%
Venous Thromboembolism Prophylaxis	57	96%	92%	94%
Written Stroke Educational Materials Given	20	95%	86%	88%
Surgical Care Improvement Project				
Appropriate Beta Blocker Usage[2]	111	95%	97%	98%
Appropriate VTP Within 24 Hours[2]	383	97%	97%	98%
Controlled Postoperative Blood Glucose[2,7]	-	-	97%	97%
Perioperative Temperature Management[2]	437	100%	100%	100%
Prophylactic Antibiotic Selection[2]	316	97%	99%	99%
Prophylactic Antibiotic Selection (Outpatient)	129	98%	98%	98%
Prophylactic Antibiotic Stopped[2]	310	98%	98%	98%
Prophylactic Antibiotic Timing[2]	316	99%	98%	99%
Prophylactic Antibiotic Timing (Outpatient)	148	87%	98%	98%
Urinary Catheter Removal[2]	196	95%	96%	97%
Survey of Patients' Hospital Experiences				
Area Around Room 'Always' Quiet at Night	300+	69%	68%	61%
Doctors 'Always' Communicated Well	300+	85%	84%	82%
Home Recovery Information Given	300+	83%	84%	85%
Hospital Given 9 or 10 on 10 Point Scale	300+	70%	72%	71%
Meds 'Always' Explained Before Given	300+	61%	66%	64%
Nurses 'Always' Communicated Well	300+	81%	80%	79%
Pain 'Always' Well Controlled	300+	70%	72%	71%
Room and Bathroom 'Always' Clean	300+	84%	73%	73%
Timely Help 'Always' Received	300+	70%	71%	68%
Would Definitely Recommend Hospital	300+	69%	71%	71%
Use of Medical Imaging				
Cardiac Imaging Stress Test before Surgery	921	4.6%	4.5%	5.3%
Combination Abdominal CT Scan	1,160	4.4%	23%	10.5%
Combination Brain/Sinus CT Scan	1,085	1.8%	2.2%	2.7%
Combination Chest CT Scan	664	2.6%	5.1%	2.7%
Follow-up Mammogram/Ultrasound	2,396	4.0%	8.1%	8.8%
Lumbar Spine MRI for Low Back Pain	286	45.1%	39.9%	37.2%

Beaver County Memorial Hospital

212 East 8th Street Phone: 580-625-4551
Beaver, OK 73932 Fax: 580-625-4212
Type: Critical Access Hospitals Emergency Services: Yes
Ownership: Govt - Hospital Dist/Auth Beds: 24
Key Personnel:
Emergency Room . . . . Deanna Brown

Measure	Cases	This Hosp.	State Avg.	U.S. Avg.
Blood Clot Prevention and Treatment				
Anticoagulation Overlap Therapy[5]	-	-	89%	93%
ICU Venous Thromboembolism Prophylaxis[5]	-	-	87%	92%
Incidence of Potentially Preventable VTE[5]	-	-	8%	10%
UFH with Dosages/Platelet Monitoring[5]	-	-	97%	97%
Venous Thromboembolism Prophylaxis[5]	-	-	72%	85%
Warfarin Therapy Discharge Instructions[5]	-	-	73%	75%
Chest Pain/Possible Heart Attack Care				
Aspirin Given Within 24 Hours of Arrival[5]	-	-	95%	96%
Fibrinolytic Meds Within 30 Min. of Arrival[5]	-	-	54%	58%
Average Time to ECG (minutes)[5]	-	-	8	7
Average Time to Transfer (minutes)[5]	-	-	77	60
Children's Asthma Care				
Received Home Management Plan of Care	-	-	-	88%
Received Reliever Medication	-	-	-	100%
Received Systemic Corticosteroids	-	-	-	100%
Emergency Department				
Admittance Decision Time (minutes)[5]	-	-	63	98
Head CT Results Within 45 Min. of Arrival[5]	-	-	49%	57%
Patients Who Left ER Before Being Seen[5]	-	-	2%	2%
Time from ER Arrival to Admit. (minutes)[5]	-	-	210	274
Time from ER Arrival to Discharge (minutes)[5]	-	-	110	134
Time in ER Before Being Evaluated (minutes)[5]	-	-	24	26
Time to Pain Meds for Fractures (minutes)[5]	-	-	55	57
Heart Attack Care				

NOTE: Hospital profiles are in alphabetical order by state, then city, then hospital within the city; Rankings exclude hospitals with less than 25 cases except for patient surveys which excludes hospitals with less than 100 cases; (a) 100-299 cases; (1) The number of cases/patients is too few to report; (2) Data submitted were based on a sample of cases/patients; (3) Results are based on a shorter time period than required; (4) Data suppressed by CMS for one or more quarters; (5) Results are not available for this reporting period; (6) Fewer than 100 patients completed the HCAHPS survey; (7) No cases met the criteria for this measure; (8) The lower limit of the confidence interval cannot be calculated if the number of observed infections equals zero; (9) No data are available from the state/territory for this reporting period; (10) The scores shown reflect fewer than 50 completed surveys; (11) There were discrepancies in the data collection process; (12) This measure does not apply to this hospital for this reporting period; (13) Results cannot be calculated for this reporting period; (14) The results for this state are combined with nearby states to protect confidentiality; Please refer to the User's Guide for a full explanation of data.

Measure	Cases	This Hosp.	State Avg.	U.S. Avg.
Aspirin Given at Discharge[5]	-	-	99%	99%
Fibrinolytic Meds Within 30 Min. of Arrival[5]	-	-	25%	54%
PCI Within 90 Minutes of Arrival[5]	-	-	95%	96%
Statin Prescribed at Discharge[5]	-	-	98%	98%
Heart Failure Care				
ACE Inhibitor or ARB for LVSD[3,7]	-	-	95%	97%
Discharge Instructions Given[1,3]	-	-	92%	94%
Evaluation of LVS Function[1,3]	-	-	96%	99%
Medicare Spending				
Medicare Spending per Patient (ratio)	-	-	0.93	0.98
Pneumonia Care				
Appropriate Initial Antibiotic Given[1]	-	-	92%	95%
Blood Culture Timing[7]	-	-	97%	98%
Pregnancy and Delivery Care				
Newborn Deliveries Scheduled Early[5]	-	-	8%	6%
Preventive Care				
Immunization for Influenza[5]	-	-	89%	90%
Immunization for Pneumonia[5]	-	-	91%	92%
Stroke Care				
Anticoagulation Therapy for Atrial Fibrillation[5]	-	-	91%	95%
Antithrombotic Therapy Timing[5]	-	-	95%	98%
Assessed for Rehabilitation[5]	-	-	96%	97%
Discharged on Antithrombotic Therapy[5]	-	-	98%	99%
Discharged on Statin Medication[5]	-	-	88%	94%
Thrombolytic Therapy Timing[5]	-	-	61%	66%
Venous Thromboembolism Prophylaxis[5]	-	-	92%	94%
Written Stroke Educational Materials Given[5]	-	-	86%	88%
Surgical Care Improvement Project				
Appropriate Beta Blocker Usage[5]	-	-	97%	98%
Appropriate VTP Within 24 Hours[5]	-	-	97%	98%
Controlled Postoperative Blood Glucose[5]	-	-	97%	97%
Perioperative Temperature Management[5]	-	-	100%	100%
Prophylactic Antibiotic Selection[5]	-	-	99%	99%
Prophylactic Antibiotic Selection (Outpatient)[5]	-	-	98%	98%
Prophylactic Antibiotic Stopped[5]	-	-	98%	98%
Prophylactic Antibiotic Timing[5]	-	-	98%	99%
Prophylactic Antibiotic Timing (Outpatient)[5]	-	-	98%	98%
Urinary Catheter Removal[5]	-	-	96%	97%
Survey of Patients' Hospital Experiences				
Area Around Room 'Always' Quiet at Night[5]	-	-	68%	61%
Doctors 'Always' Communicated Well[5]	-	-	84%	82%
Home Recovery Information Given[5]	-	-	84%	85%
Hospital Given 9 or 10 on 10 Point Scale[5]	-	-	72%	71%
Meds 'Always' Explained Before Given[5]	-	-	66%	64%
Nurses 'Always' Communicated Well[5]	-	-	80%	79%
Pain 'Always' Well Controlled[5]	-	-	72%	71%
Room and Bathroom 'Always' Clean[5]	-	-	73%	73%
Timely Help 'Always' Received[5]	-	-	71%	68%
Would Definitely Recommend Hospital[5]	-	-	71%	71%
Use of Medical Imaging				
Cardiac Imaging Stress Test before Surgery[7]	-	-	4.5%	5.3%
Combination Abdominal CT Scan[1]	-	-	23%	10.5%
Combination Brain/Sinus CT Scan[1]	-	-	2.2%	2.7%
Combination Chest CT Scan[7]	-	-	5.1%	2.7%
Follow-up Mammogram/Ultrasound[7]	-	-	8.1%	8.8%
Lumbar Spine MRI for Low Back Pain[7]	-	-	39.9%	37.2%

Integris Blackwell Regional Hospital

710 South 13th Street
Blackwell, OK 74631
URL: www.integrisblackwell.com
Phone: 580-363-2311
Fax: 580-363-2339
Type: Acute Care Hospitals
Emergency Services: Yes
Ownership: Voluntary non-profit - Private
Beds: 53

Key Personnel:
Chief of Medical Staff.......... Paul Briggs, MD
Chairman/CEO .... Bruce Dale
Patient Relations .... Cassie Leatherman
Infection Control........... Pam Lewellyn
CEO/President.............. James Moore
Quality Assurance .... Janet Reser, RN

Measure	Cases	This Hosp.	State Avg.	U.S. Avg.
Blood Clot Prevention and Treatment				
Anticoagulation Overlap Therapy[1,2]	-	-	89%	93%
ICU Venous Thromboembolism Prophylaxis[2,7]	-	-	87%	92%
Incidence of Potentially Preventable VTE[2,7]	-	-	8%	10%
UFH with Dosages/Platelet Monitoring[2,7]	-	-	97%	97%
Venous Thromboembolism Prophylaxis[2]	161	58%	72%	85%
Warfarin Therapy Discharge Instructions[1,2]	-	-	73%	75%
Chest Pain/Possible Heart Attack Care				
Aspirin Given Within 24 Hours of Arrival	26	100%	95%	96%
Fibrinolytic Meds Within 30 Min. of Arrival[1]	-	-	54%	58%
Average Time to ECG (minutes)	26	5	8	7
Average Time to Transfer (minutes)[1]	-	-	77	60
Children's Asthma Care				
Received Home Management Plan of Care	-	-	-	88%
Received Reliever Medication	-	-	-	100%
Received Systemic Corticosteroids	-	-	-	100%
Emergency Department				
Admittance Decision Time (minutes)[2]	511	52	63	98
Head CT Results Within 45 Min. of Arrival[1]	-	-	49%	57%
Patients Who Left ER Before Being Seen	6,260	1%	2%	2%
Time from ER Arrival to Admit. (minutes)[2]	513	166	210	274
Time from ER Arrival to Discharge (minutes)	473	75	110	134
Time in ER Before Being Evaluated (minutes)	480	14	24	26
Time to Pain Meds for Fractures (minutes)	29	36	55	57
Heart Attack Care				
Aspirin Given at Discharge[7]	-	-	99%	99%
Fibrinolytic Meds Within 30 Min. of Arrival[7]	-	-	25%	54%
PCI Within 90 Minutes of Arrival[7]	-	-	95%	96%
Statin Prescribed at Discharge[7]	-	-	98%	98%
Heart Failure Care				
ACE Inhibitor or ARB for LVSD	24	88%	95%	97%
Discharge Instructions Given	47	79%	92%	94%
Evaluation of LVS Function	72	99%	96%	99%
Medicare Spending				
Medicare Spending per Patient (ratio)	-	0.79	0.93	0.98
Pneumonia Care				
Appropriate Initial Antibiotic Given	43	100%	92%	95%
Blood Culture Timing	46	98%	97%	98%
Pregnancy and Delivery Care				
Newborn Deliveries Scheduled Early[2,7]	-	-	8%	6%
Preventive Care				
Immunization for Influenza[2]	318	98%	89%	90%
Immunization for Pneumonia[2]	463	98%	91%	92%
Stroke Care				
Anticoagulation Therapy for Atrial Fibrillation[1]	-	-	91%	95%
Antithrombotic Therapy Timing[1]	-	-	95%	98%
Assessed for Rehabilitation[1]	-	-	96%	97%
Discharged on Antithrombotic Therapy[1]	-	-	98%	99%
Discharged on Statin Medication[1]	-	-	88%	94%
Thrombolytic Therapy Timing[7]	-	-	61%	66%
Venous Thromboembolism Prophylaxis[1]	-	-	92%	94%
Written Stroke Educational Materials Given[1]	-	-	86%	88%
Surgical Care Improvement Project				
Appropriate Beta Blocker Usage[1]	-	-	97%	98%
Appropriate VTP Within 24 Hours	24	100%	97%	98%
Controlled Postoperative Blood Glucose[7]	-	-	97%	97%
Perioperative Temperature Management	26	100%	100%	100%
Prophylactic Antibiotic Selection	17	100%	99%	99%
Prophylactic Antibiotic Selection (Outpatient)[3,7]	-	-	98%	98%
Prophylactic Antibiotic Stopped	16	94%	98%	98%
Prophylactic Antibiotic Timing	17	100%	98%	99%
Prophylactic Antibiotic Timing (Outpatient)[3,7]	-	-	98%	98%
Urinary Catheter Removal	11	100%	96%	97%
Survey of Patients' Hospital Experiences				
Area Around Room 'Always' Quiet at Night	(a)	73%	68%	61%
Doctors 'Always' Communicated Well	(a)	89%	84%	82%
Home Recovery Information Given	(a)	83%	84%	85%
Hospital Given 9 or 10 on 10 Point Scale	(a)	68%	72%	71%
Meds 'Always' Explained Before Given	(a)	64%	66%	64%
Nurses 'Always' Communicated Well	(a)	81%	80%	79%
Pain 'Always' Well Controlled	(a)	77%	72%	71%
Room and Bathroom 'Always' Clean	(a)	74%	73%	73%
Timely Help 'Always' Received	(a)	63%	71%	68%
Would Definitely Recommend Hospital	(a)	62%	71%	71%
Use of Medical Imaging				
Cardiac Imaging Stress Test before Surgery[1]	-	-	4.5%	5.3%
Combination Abdominal CT Scan	100	14.0%	23%	10.5%
Combination Brain/Sinus CT Scan	96	0.0%	2.2%	2.7%
Combination Chest CT Scan	58	3.4%	5.1%	2.7%
Follow-up Mammogram/Ultrasound	101	2.0%	8.1%	8.8%
Lumbar Spine MRI for Low Back Pain[1]	-	-	39.9%	37.2%

Cimarron Memorial Hospital

100 South Ellis
Boise City, OK 73933
Phone: 580-544-2501
Fax: 580-544-2517
Type: Critical Access Hospitals
Emergency Services: Yes
Ownership: Govt - Hospital Dist/Auth
Beds: 64

Key Personnel:
CEO .... Tim Beard
Operating Room.............. Lois Burkhalter
Chairman/CEO .... Paul Toon
Quality Assurance .... Mary Van Leer
Chief of Medical Staff.......... JL Wheeler, MD

Measure	Cases	This Hosp.	State Avg.	U.S. Avg.
Blood Clot Prevention and Treatment				
Anticoagulation Overlap Therapy[5]	-	-	89%	93%
ICU Venous Thromboembolism Prophylaxis[5]	-	-	87%	92%
Incidence of Potentially Preventable VTE[5]	-	-	8%	10%
UFH with Dosages/Platelet Monitoring[5]	-	-	97%	97%
Venous Thromboembolism Prophylaxis[5]	-	-	72%	85%
Warfarin Therapy Discharge Instructions[5]	-	-	73%	75%
Chest Pain/Possible Heart Attack Care				
Aspirin Given Within 24 Hours of Arrival[1,3]	-	-	95%	96%
Fibrinolytic Meds Within 30 Min. of Arrival[3,7]	-	-	54%	58%
Average Time to ECG (minutes)[1,3]	-	-	8	7
Average Time to Transfer (minutes)[1,3]	-	-	77	60
Children's Asthma Care				
Received Home Management Plan of Care	-	-	-	88%
Received Reliever Medication	-	-	-	100%
Received Systemic Corticosteroids	-	-	-	100%
Emergency Department				
Admittance Decision Time (minutes)[5]	-	-	63	98
Head CT Results Within 45 Min. of Arrival[5]	-	-	49%	57%
Patients Who Left ER Before Being Seen[5]	-	-	2%	2%
Time from ER Arrival to Admit. (minutes)[5]	-	-	210	274
Time from ER Arrival to Discharge (minutes)[5]	-	-	110	134
Time in ER Before Being Evaluated (minutes)[5]	-	-	24	26
Time to Pain Meds for Fractures (minutes)[5]	-	-	55	57
Heart Attack Care				
Aspirin Given at Discharge[3,7]	-	-	99%	99%
Fibrinolytic Meds Within 30 Min. of Arrival[3,7]	-	-	25%	54%
PCI Within 90 Minutes of Arrival[3,7]	-	-	95%	96%
Statin Prescribed at Discharge[3,7]	-	-	98%	98%
Heart Failure Care				
ACE Inhibitor or ARB for LVSD[3,7]	-	-	95%	97%
Discharge Instructions Given[1,3]	-	-	92%	94%
Evaluation of LVS Function[1,3]	-	-	96%	99%
Medicare Spending				
Medicare Spending per Patient (ratio)	-	-	0.93	0.98
Pneumonia Care				
Appropriate Initial Antibiotic Given[1]	-	-	92%	95%
Blood Culture Timing[7]	-	-	97%	98%
Pregnancy and Delivery Care				
Newborn Deliveries Scheduled Early[5]	-	-	8%	6%
Preventive Care				
Immunization for Influenza[5]	-	-	89%	90%
Immunization for Pneumonia[5]	-	-	91%	92%
Stroke Care				
Anticoagulation Therapy for Atrial Fibrillation[5]	-	-	91%	95%
Antithrombotic Therapy Timing[5]	-	-	95%	98%
Assessed for Rehabilitation[5]	-	-	96%	97%
Discharged on Antithrombotic Therapy[5]	-	-	98%	99%
Discharged on Statin Medication[5]	-	-	88%	94%
Thrombolytic Therapy Timing[5]	-	-	61%	66%
Venous Thromboembolism Prophylaxis[5]	-	-	92%	94%
Written Stroke Educational Materials Given[5]	-	-	86%	88%
Surgical Care Improvement Project				
Appropriate Beta Blocker Usage[5]	-	-	97%	98%

NOTE: Hospital profiles are in alphabetical order by state, then city, then hospital within the city; Rankings exclude hospitals with less than 25 cases except for patient surveys which excludes hospitals with less than 100 cases; (a) 100-299 cases; (1) The number of cases/patients is too few to report; (2) Data submitted were based on a sample of cases/patients; (3) Results are based on a shorter time period than required; (4) Data suppressed by CMS for one or more quarters; (5) Results are not available for this reporting period; (6) Fewer than 100 patients completed the HCAHPS survey; (7) No cases met the criteria for this measure; (8) The lower limit of the confidence interval cannot be calculated if the number of observed infections equals zero; (9) No data are available from the state/territory for this reporting period; (10) The scores shown reflect fewer than 50 completed surveys; (11) There were discrepancies in the data collection process; (12) This measure does not apply to this hospital for this reporting period; (13) Results cannot be calculated for this reporting period; (14) The results for this state are combined with nearby states to protect confidentiality; Please refer to the User's Guide for a full explanation of data.

Measure	Cases	This Hosp.	State Avg.	U.S. Avg.
Appropriate VTP Within 24 Hours[5]	-	-	97%	98%
Controlled Postoperative Blood Glucose[5]	-	-	97%	97%
Perioperative Temperature Management[5]	-	-	100%	100%
Prophylactic Antibiotic Selection[5]	-	-	99%	99%
Prophylactic Antibiotic Selection (Outpatient)[5]	-	-	98%	98%
Prophylactic Antibiotic Stopped[5]	-	-	98%	98%
Prophylactic Antibiotic Timing[5]	-	-	98%	99%
Prophylactic Antibiotic Timing (Outpatient)[5]	-	-	98%	98%
Urinary Catheter Removal[5]	-	-	96%	97%
Survey of Patients' Hospital Experiences				
Area Around Room 'Always' Quiet at Night[10]	<100	76%	68%	61%
Doctors 'Always' Communicated Well[10]	<100	91%	84%	82%
Home Recovery Information Given[10]	<100	79%	84%	85%
Hospital Given 9 or 10 on 10 Point Scale[10]	<100	90%	72%	71%
Meds 'Always' Explained Before Given[10]	<100	84%	66%	64%
Nurses 'Always' Communicated Well[10]	<100	96%	80%	79%
Pain 'Always' Well Controlled[10]	<100	78%	72%	71%
Room and Bathroom 'Always' Clean[10]	<100	79%	73%	73%
Timely Help 'Always' Received[10]	<100	98%	71%	68%
Would Definitely Recommend Hospital[10]	<100	91%	71%	71%
Use of Medical Imaging				
Cardiac Imaging Stress Test before Surgery[7]	-	-	4.5%	5.3%
Combination Abdominal CT Scan[1]	-	-	23%	10.5%
Combination Brain/Sinus CT Scan[1]	-	-	2.2%	2.7%
Combination Chest CT Scan[1]	-	-	5.1%	2.7%
Follow-up Mammogram/Ultrasound[7]	-	-	8.1%	8.8%
Lumbar Spine MRI for Low Back Pain[7]	-	-	39.9%	37.2%

Bristow Medical Center

700 W. 7th Street
Bristow, OK 74010
Phone: 918-367-2215
Fax: 918-367-9190
Type: Acute Care Hospitals
Emergency Services: Yes
Ownership: Govt - Hospital Dist/Auth
Beds: 30

Key Personnel:
Quality Assurance . . . . Della Allison
Chief of Medical Staff . . . . Dennise Blackstad
Radiology . . . . Vivian J Mcdaniel
Infection Control . . . . Tina Ordway, RN
CEO . . . . Jan Winter Clark, RN, MHA

Measure	Cases	This Hosp.	State Avg.	U.S. Avg.
Blood Clot Prevention and Treatment				
Anticoagulation Overlap Therapy[1,2]	-	-	89%	93%
ICU Venous Thromboembolism Prophylaxis[2,7]	-	-	87%	92%
Incidence of Potentially Preventable VTE[2,7]	-	-	8%	10%
UFH with Dosages/Platelet Monitoring[2,7]	-	-	97%	97%
Venous Thromboembolism Prophylaxis[2]	141	23%	72%	85%
Warfarin Therapy Discharge Instructions[1,2]	-	-	73%	75%
Chest Pain/Possible Heart Attack Care				
Aspirin Given Within 24 Hours of Arrival	75	95%	95%	96%
Fibrinolytic Meds Within 30 Min. of Arrival[1]	-	-	54%	58%
Average Time to ECG (minutes)	76	15	8	7
Average Time to Transfer (minutes)[1]	-	-	77	60
Children's Asthma Care				
Received Home Management Plan of Care	-	-	-	88%
Received Reliever Medication	-	-	-	100%
Received Systemic Corticosteroids	-	-	-	100%
Emergency Department				
Admittance Decision Time (minutes)	147	49	63	98
Head CT Results Within 45 Min. of Arrival[3,7]	-	-	49%	57%
Patients Who Left ER Before Being Seen	5,646	2%	2%	2%
Time from ER Arrival to Admit. (minutes)	147	173	210	274
Time from ER Arrival to Discharge (minutes)	238	93	110	134
Time in ER Before Being Evaluated (minutes)	389	18	24	26
Time to Pain Meds for Fractures (minutes)	23	53	55	57
Heart Attack Care				
Aspirin Given at Discharge[1,3]	-	-	99%	99%
Fibrinolytic Meds Within 30 Min. of Arrival[3,7]	-	-	25%	54%
PCI Within 90 Minutes of Arrival[3,7]	-	-	95%	96%
Statin Prescribed at Discharge[1,3]	-	-	98%	98%
Heart Failure Care				
ACE Inhibitor or ARB for LVSD[1]	-	-	95%	97%
Discharge Instructions Given[1]	-	-	92%	94%
Evaluation of LVS Function[1]	-	-	96%	99%
Medicare Spending				
Medicare Spending per Patient (ratio)	-	0.86	0.93	0.98
Pneumonia Care				
Appropriate Initial Antibiotic Given	28	89%	92%	95%
Blood Culture Timing	20	85%	97%	98%
Pregnancy and Delivery Care				
Newborn Deliveries Scheduled Early[7]	-	-	8%	6%
Preventive Care				
Immunization for Influenza[2]	148	61%	89%	90%
Immunization for Pneumonia[2]	214	61%	91%	92%
Stroke Care				
Anticoagulation Therapy for Atrial Fibrillation[7]	-	-	91%	95%
Antithrombotic Therapy Timing[7]	-	-	95%	98%
Assessed for Rehabilitation[7]	-	-	96%	97%
Discharged on Antithrombotic Therapy[7]	-	-	98%	99%
Discharged on Statin Medication[7]	-	-	88%	94%
Thrombolytic Therapy Timing[7]	-	-	61%	66%
Venous Thromboembolism Prophylaxis[7]	-	-	92%	94%
Written Stroke Educational Materials Given[7]	-	-	86%	88%
Surgical Care Improvement Project				
Appropriate Beta Blocker Usage[5]	-	-	97%	98%
Appropriate VTP Within 24 Hours[5]	-	-	97%	98%
Controlled Postoperative Blood Glucose[5]	-	-	97%	97%
Perioperative Temperature Management[5]	-	-	100%	100%
Prophylactic Antibiotic Selection[5]	-	-	99%	99%
Prophylactic Antibiotic Selection (Outpatient)[5]	-	-	98%	98%
Prophylactic Antibiotic Stopped[5]	-	-	98%	98%
Prophylactic Antibiotic Timing[5]	-	-	98%	99%
Prophylactic Antibiotic Timing (Outpatient)[5]	-	-	98%	98%
Urinary Catheter Removal[5]	-	-	96%	97%
Survey of Patients' Hospital Experiences				
Area Around Room 'Always' Quiet at Night[6]	<100	69%	68%	61%
Doctors 'Always' Communicated Well[6]	<100	90%	84%	82%
Home Recovery Information Given[6]	<100	82%	84%	85%
Hospital Given 9 or 10 on 10 Point Scale[6]	<100	60%	72%	71%
Meds 'Always' Explained Before Given[6]	<100	66%	66%	64%
Nurses 'Always' Communicated Well[6]	<100	86%	80%	79%
Pain 'Always' Well Controlled[6]	<100	81%	72%	71%
Room and Bathroom 'Always' Clean[6]	<100	73%	73%	73%
Timely Help 'Always' Received[6]	<100	74%	71%	68%
Would Definitely Recommend Hospital[6]	<100	71%	71%	71%
Use of Medical Imaging				
Cardiac Imaging Stress Test before Surgery[7]	-	-	4.5%	5.3%
Combination Abdominal CT Scan	102	16.7%	23%	10.5%
Combination Brain/Sinus CT Scan	101	0.0%	2.2%	2.7%
Combination Chest CT Scan	58	1.7%	5.1%	2.7%
Follow-up Mammogram/Ultrasound[7]	-	-	8.1%	8.8%
Lumbar Spine MRI for Low Back Pain	232	40.5%	39.9%	37.2%

Saint John Broken Arrow

1000 West Boise Circle
Broken Arrow, OK 74012
Phone: 918-994-8199
Type: Acute Care Hospitals
Emergency Services: Yes
Ownership: Voluntary non-profit - Church

Measure	Cases	This Hosp.	State Avg.	U.S. Avg.
Blood Clot Prevention and Treatment				
Anticoagulation Overlap Therapy[1,2]	-	-	89%	93%
ICU Venous Thromboembolism Prophylaxis[2,7]	-	-	87%	92%
Incidence of Potentially Preventable VTE[2,7]	-	-	8%	10%
UFH with Dosages/Platelet Monitoring[1,2]	-	-	97%	97%
Venous Thromboembolism Prophylaxis[2]	116	93%	72%	85%
Warfarin Therapy Discharge Instructions[1,2]	-	-	73%	75%
Chest Pain/Possible Heart Attack Care				
Aspirin Given Within 24 Hours of Arrival	79	100%	95%	96%
Fibrinolytic Meds Within 30 Min. of Arrival[7]	-	-	54%	58%
Average Time to ECG (minutes)	81	8	8	7
Average Time to Transfer (minutes)[1]	-	-	77	60
Children's Asthma Care				
Received Home Management Plan of Care	-	-	-	88%
Received Reliever Medication	-	-	-	100%
Received Systemic Corticosteroids	-	-	-	100%
Emergency Department				
Admittance Decision Time (minutes)[2]	167	68	63	98
Head CT Results Within 45 Min. of Arrival[1]	-	-	49%	57%
Patients Who Left ER Before Being Seen	23,633	2%	2%	2%
Time from ER Arrival to Admit. (minutes)[2]	189	225	210	274
Time from ER Arrival to Discharge (minutes)	368	128	110	134
Time in ER Before Being Evaluated (minutes)	387	30	24	26
Time to Pain Meds for Fractures (minutes)	85	48	55	57
Heart Attack Care				
Aspirin Given at Discharge[5]	-	-	99%	99%
Fibrinolytic Meds Within 30 Min. of Arrival[5]	-	-	25%	54%
PCI Within 90 Minutes of Arrival[5]	-	-	95%	96%
Statin Prescribed at Discharge[5]	-	-	98%	98%
Heart Failure Care				
ACE Inhibitor or ARB for LVSD[1]	-	-	95%	97%
Discharge Instructions Given	30	100%	92%	94%
Evaluation of LVS Function	37	100%	96%	99%
Medicare Spending				
Medicare Spending per Patient (ratio)	-	0.87	0.93	0.98
Pneumonia Care				
Appropriate Initial Antibiotic Given	55	98%	92%	95%
Blood Culture Timing	79	96%	97%	98%
Pregnancy and Delivery Care				
Newborn Deliveries Scheduled Early[7]	-	-	8%	6%
Preventive Care				
Immunization for Influenza[2]	299	99%	89%	90%
Immunization for Pneumonia[2]	395	98%	91%	92%
Stroke Care				
Anticoagulation Therapy for Atrial Fibrillation[5]	-	-	91%	95%
Antithrombotic Therapy Timing[5]	-	-	95%	98%
Assessed for Rehabilitation[5]	-	-	96%	97%
Discharged on Antithrombotic Therapy[5]	-	-	98%	99%
Discharged on Statin Medication[5]	-	-	88%	94%
Thrombolytic Therapy Timing[5]	-	-	61%	66%
Venous Thromboembolism Prophylaxis[5]	-	-	92%	94%
Written Stroke Educational Materials Given[5]	-	-	86%	88%
Surgical Care Improvement Project				
Appropriate Beta Blocker Usage	329	98%	97%	98%
Appropriate VTP Within 24 Hours	983	100%	97%	98%
Controlled Postoperative Blood Glucose[7]	-	-	97%	97%
Perioperative Temperature Management	1,095	100%	100%	100%
Prophylactic Antibiotic Selection	984	100%	99%	99%
Prophylactic Antibiotic Selection (Outpatient)	31	100%	98%	98%
Prophylactic Antibiotic Stopped	982	100%	98%	98%
Prophylactic Antibiotic Timing	984	100%	98%	99%
Prophylactic Antibiotic Timing (Outpatient)	31	100%	98%	98%
Urinary Catheter Removal	58	98%	96%	97%
Survey of Patients' Hospital Experiences				
Area Around Room 'Always' Quiet at Night	300+	75%	68%	61%
Doctors 'Always' Communicated Well	300+	84%	84%	82%
Home Recovery Information Given	300+	89%	84%	85%
Hospital Given 9 or 10 on 10 Point Scale	300+	82%	72%	71%
Meds 'Always' Explained Before Given	300+	67%	66%	64%
Nurses 'Always' Communicated Well	300+	81%	80%	79%
Pain 'Always' Well Controlled	300+	75%	72%	71%
Room and Bathroom 'Always' Clean	300+	79%	73%	73%
Timely Help 'Always' Received	300+	70%	71%	68%
Would Definitely Recommend Hospital	300+	86%	71%	71%
Use of Medical Imaging				
Cardiac Imaging Stress Test before Surgery	149	4.0%	4.5%	5.3%
Combination Abdominal CT Scan	327	2.8%	23%	10.5%
Combination Brain/Sinus CT Scan[1]	-	-	2.2%	2.7%
Combination Chest CT Scan	193	0.0%	5.1%	2.7%
Follow-up Mammogram/Ultrasound	271	22.9%	8.1%	8.8%
Lumbar Spine MRI for Low Back Pain	49	36.7%	39.9%	37.2%

Harper County Community Hospital

1003 Us Highway 64 North
Buffalo, OK 73834
Phone: 580-735-2555
Fax: 580-735-2342
URL: www.hcchospital.com
Type: Critical Access Hospitals
Emergency Services: Yes
Ownership: Voluntary non-profit - Other
Beds: 25

Key Personnel:
Radiology . . . . Carl Fieser
Quality Assurance . . . . Kim Hudson

NOTE: Hospital profiles are in alphabetical order by state, then city, then hospital within the city; Rankings exclude hospitals with less than 25 cases except for patient surveys which excludes hospitals with less than 100 cases; (a) 100-299 cases; (1) The number of cases/patients is too few to report; (2) Data submitted were based on a sample of cases/patients; (3) Results are based on a shorter time period than required; (4) Data suppressed by CMS for one or more quarters; (5) Results are not available for this reporting period; (6) Fewer than 100 patients completed the HCAHPS survey; (7) No cases met the criteria for this measure; (8) The lower limit of the confidence interval cannot be calculated if the number of observed infections equals zero; (9) No data are available from the state/territory for this reporting period; (10) The scores shown reflect fewer than 50 completed surveys; (11) There were discrepancies in the data collection process; (12) This measure does not apply to this hospital for this reporting period; (13) Results cannot be calculated for this reporting period; (14) The results for this state are combined with nearby states to protect confidentiality; Please refer to the User's Guide for a full explanation of data.

Emergency Room . . . . Paula Lauer, RN
Operating Room. . . . . Paula Lauer, RN
Patient Relations . . . . Ronna McCubbin
Chief of Medical Staff. . . . . N Suthers

Measure	Cases	This Hosp.	State Avg.	U.S. Avg.
Blood Clot Prevention and Treatment				
Anticoagulation Overlap Therapy[1]	-	-	89%	93%
ICU Venous Thromboembolism Prophylaxis[7]	-	-	87%	92%
Incidence of Potentially Preventable VTE[7]	-	-	8%	10%
UFH with Dosages/Platelet Monitoring[7]	-	-	97%	97%
Venous Thromboembolism Prophylaxis[1]	-	-	72%	85%
Warfarin Therapy Discharge Instructions[1]	-	-	73%	75%
Chest Pain/Possible Heart Attack Care				
Aspirin Given Within 24 Hours of Arrival[1,3]	-	-	95%	96%
Fibrinolytic Meds Within 30 Min. of Arrival[3,7]	-	-	54%	58%
Average Time to ECG (minutes)[1,3]	-	-	8	7
Average Time to Transfer (minutes)[3,7]	-	-	77	60
Children's Asthma Care				
Received Home Management Plan of Care	-	-	-	88%
Received Reliever Medication	-	-	-	100%
Received Systemic Corticosteroids	-	-	-	100%
Emergency Department				
Admittance Decision Time (minutes)	22	0	63	98
Head CT Results Within 45 Min. of Arrival[5]	-	-	49%	57%
Patients Who Left ER Before Being Seen[5]	-	-	2%	2%
Time from ER Arrival to Admit. (minutes)	22	100	210	274
Time from ER Arrival to Discharge (minutes)[5]	-	-	110	134
Time in ER Before Being Evaluated (minutes)[5]	-	-	24	26
Time to Pain Meds for Fractures (minutes)[1,3]	-	-	55	57
Heart Attack Care				
Aspirin Given at Discharge[1,3]	-	-	99%	99%
Fibrinolytic Meds Within 30 Min. of Arrival[3,7]	-	-	25%	54%
PCI Within 90 Minutes of Arrival[3,7]	-	-	95%	96%
Statin Prescribed at Discharge[1,3]	-	-	98%	98%
Heart Failure Care				
ACE Inhibitor or ARB for LVSD[1]	-	-	95%	97%
Discharge Instructions Given[1]	-	-	92%	94%
Evaluation of LVS Function[1]	-	-	96%	99%
Medicare Spending				
Medicare Spending per Patient (ratio)	-	-	0.93	0.98
Pneumonia Care				
Appropriate Initial Antibiotic Given[1]	-	-	92%	95%
Blood Culture Timing[1]	-	-	97%	98%
Pregnancy and Delivery Care				
Newborn Deliveries Scheduled Early[5]	-	-	8%	6%
Preventive Care				
Immunization for Influenza	21	100%	89%	90%
Immunization for Pneumonia	31	100%	91%	92%
Stroke Care				
Anticoagulation Therapy for Atrial Fibrillation[3,7]	-	-	91%	95%
Antithrombotic Therapy Timing[3,7]	-	-	95%	98%
Assessed for Rehabilitation[3,7]	-	-	96%	97%
Discharged on Antithrombotic Therapy[3,7]	-	-	98%	99%
Discharged on Statin Medication[3,7]	-	-	88%	94%
Thrombolytic Therapy Timing[3,7]	-	-	61%	66%
Venous Thromboembolism Prophylaxis[3,7]	-	-	92%	94%
Written Stroke Educational Materials Given[3,7]	-	-	86%	88%
Surgical Care Improvement Project				
Appropriate Beta Blocker Usage[5]	-	-	97%	98%
Appropriate VTP Within 24 Hours[5]	-	-	97%	98%
Controlled Postoperative Blood Glucose[5]	-	-	97%	97%
Perioperative Temperature Management[5]	-	-	100%	100%
Prophylactic Antibiotic Selection[5]	-	-	99%	99%
Prophylactic Antibiotic Selection (Outpatient)[5]	-	-	98%	98%
Prophylactic Antibiotic Stopped[5]	-	-	98%	98%
Prophylactic Antibiotic Timing[5]	-	-	98%	99%
Prophylactic Antibiotic Timing (Outpatient)[5]	-	-	98%	98%
Urinary Catheter Removal[5]	-	-	96%	97%
Survey of Patients' Hospital Experiences				
Area Around Room 'Always' Quiet at Night[10]	<100	62%	68%	61%
Doctors 'Always' Communicated Well[10]	<100	87%	84%	82%
Home Recovery Information Given[10]	<100	81%	84%	85%
Hospital Given 9 or 10 on 10 Point Scale[10]	<100	79%	72%	71%
Meds 'Always' Explained Before Given[10]	<100	67%	66%	64%
Nurses 'Always' Communicated Well[10]	<100	85%	80%	79%
Pain 'Always' Well Controlled[10]	<100	84%	72%	71%
Room and Bathroom 'Always' Clean[10]	<100	84%	73%	73%
Timely Help 'Always' Received[10]	<100	77%	71%	68%
Would Definitely Recommend Hospital[10]	<100	76%	71%	71%
Use of Medical Imaging				
Cardiac Imaging Stress Test before Surgery[7]	-	-	4.5%	5.3%
Combination Abdominal CT Scan[1]	-	-	23%	10.5%
Combination Brain/Sinus CT Scan[1]	-	-	2.2%	2.7%
Combination Chest CT Scan[1]	-	-	5.1%	2.7%
Follow-up Mammogram/Ultrasound[7]	-	-	8.1%	8.8%
Lumbar Spine MRI for Low Back Pain[7]	-	-	39.9%	37.2%

Carnegie Tri-County Municipal Hospital

102 North Broadway
Carnegie, OK 73015
Phone: 580-654-1050
Fax: 580-654-2111
Type: Critical Access Hospitals
Emergency Services: Yes
Ownership: Govt - Hospital Dist/Auth
Beds: 28

Key Personnel:
Chief of Medical Staff. . . . . Ronald Hill, MD
CEO/President. . . . . Barbara Orrell

Measure	Cases	This Hosp.	State Avg.	U.S. Avg.
Blood Clot Prevention and Treatment				
Anticoagulation Overlap Therapy[5]	-	-	89%	93%
ICU Venous Thromboembolism Prophylaxis[5]	-	-	87%	92%
Incidence of Potentially Preventable VTE[5]	-	-	8%	10%
UFH with Dosages/Platelet Monitoring[5]	-	-	97%	97%
Venous Thromboembolism Prophylaxis[5]	-	-	72%	85%
Warfarin Therapy Discharge Instructions[5]	-	-	73%	75%
Chest Pain/Possible Heart Attack Care				
Aspirin Given Within 24 Hours of Arrival[1,3]	-	-	95%	96%
Fibrinolytic Meds Within 30 Min. of Arrival[3,7]	-	-	54%	58%
Average Time to ECG (minutes)[1,3]	-	-	8	7
Average Time to Transfer (minutes)[1,3]	-	-	77	60
Children's Asthma Care				
Received Home Management Plan of Care	-	-	-	88%
Received Reliever Medication	-	-	-	100%
Received Systemic Corticosteroids	-	-	-	100%
Emergency Department				
Admittance Decision Time (minutes)[5]	-	-	63	98
Head CT Results Within 45 Min. of Arrival[1,3]	-	-	49%	57%
Patients Who Left ER Before Being Seen[5]	-	-	2%	2%
Time from ER Arrival to Admit. (minutes)[5]	-	-	210	274
Time from ER Arrival to Discharge (minutes)[5]	-	-	110	134
Time in ER Before Being Evaluated (minutes)[5]	-	-	24	26
Time to Pain Meds for Fractures (minutes)[1,3]	-	-	55	57
Heart Attack Care				
Aspirin Given at Discharge[3,7]	-	-	99%	99%
Fibrinolytic Meds Within 30 Min. of Arrival[3,7]	-	-	25%	54%
PCI Within 90 Minutes of Arrival[3,7]	-	-	95%	96%
Statin Prescribed at Discharge[3,7]	-	-	98%	98%
Heart Failure Care				
ACE Inhibitor or ARB for LVSD[1]	-	-	95%	97%
Discharge Instructions Given[1]	-	-	92%	94%
Evaluation of LVS Function	13	31%	96%	99%
Medicare Spending				
Medicare Spending per Patient (ratio)	-	-	0.93	0.98
Pneumonia Care				
Appropriate Initial Antibiotic Given	17	71%	92%	95%
Blood Culture Timing[7]	-	-	97%	98%
Pregnancy and Delivery Care				
Newborn Deliveries Scheduled Early[5]	-	-	8%	6%
Preventive Care				
Immunization for Influenza[5]	-	-	89%	90%
Immunization for Pneumonia[5]	-	-	91%	92%
Stroke Care				
Anticoagulation Therapy for Atrial Fibrillation[3,7]	-	-	91%	95%
Antithrombotic Therapy Timing[3,7]	-	-	95%	98%
Assessed for Rehabilitation[3,7]	-	-	96%	97%
Discharged on Antithrombotic Therapy[3,7]	-	-	98%	99%
Discharged on Statin Medication[3,7]	-	-	88%	94%
Thrombolytic Therapy Timing[1,3]	-	-	61%	66%
Venous Thromboembolism Prophylaxis[1,3]	-	-	92%	94%
Written Stroke Educational Materials Given[3,7]	-	-	86%	88%
Surgical Care Improvement Project				
Appropriate Beta Blocker Usage[5]	-	-	97%	98%
Appropriate VTP Within 24 Hours[5]	-	-	97%	98%
Controlled Postoperative Blood Glucose[5]	-	-	97%	97%
Perioperative Temperature Management[5]	-	-	100%	100%
Prophylactic Antibiotic Selection[5]	-	-	99%	99%
Prophylactic Antibiotic Selection (Outpatient)[5]	-	-	98%	98%
Prophylactic Antibiotic Stopped[5]	-	-	98%	98%
Prophylactic Antibiotic Timing[5]	-	-	98%	99%
Prophylactic Antibiotic Timing (Outpatient)[5]	-	-	98%	98%
Urinary Catheter Removal[5]	-	-	96%	97%
Survey of Patients' Hospital Experiences				
Area Around Room 'Always' Quiet at Night[5]	-	-	68%	61%
Doctors 'Always' Communicated Well[5]	-	-	84%	82%
Home Recovery Information Given[5]	-	-	84%	85%
Hospital Given 9 or 10 on 10 Point Scale[5]	-	-	72%	71%
Meds 'Always' Explained Before Given[5]	-	-	66%	64%
Nurses 'Always' Communicated Well[5]	-	-	80%	79%
Pain 'Always' Well Controlled[5]	-	-	72%	71%
Room and Bathroom 'Always' Clean[5]	-	-	73%	73%
Timely Help 'Always' Received[5]	-	-	71%	68%
Would Definitely Recommend Hospital[5]	-	-	71%	71%
Use of Medical Imaging				
Cardiac Imaging Stress Test before Surgery[7]	-	-	4.5%	5.3%
Combination Abdominal CT Scan[1]	-	-	23%	10.5%
Combination Brain/Sinus CT Scan	35	0.0%	2.2%	2.7%
Combination Chest CT Scan[1]	-	-	5.1%	2.7%
Follow-up Mammogram/Ultrasound[7]	-	-	8.1%	8.8%
Lumbar Spine MRI for Low Back Pain[7]	-	-	39.9%	37.2%

Roger Mills Memorial Hospital

501 South L L Males Avenue
Cheyenne, OK 73628
Phone: 580-497-3336
Type: Critical Access Hospitals
Emergency Services: Yes
Ownership: Govt - Hospital Dist/Auth

Measure	Cases	This Hosp.	State Avg.	U.S. Avg.
Blood Clot Prevention and Treatment				
Anticoagulation Overlap Therapy[5]	-	-	89%	93%
ICU Venous Thromboembolism Prophylaxis[5]	-	-	87%	92%
Incidence of Potentially Preventable VTE[5]	-	-	8%	10%
UFH with Dosages/Platelet Monitoring[5]	-	-	97%	97%
Venous Thromboembolism Prophylaxis[5]	-	-	72%	85%
Warfarin Therapy Discharge Instructions[5]	-	-	73%	75%
Chest Pain/Possible Heart Attack Care				
Aspirin Given Within 24 Hours of Arrival[5]	-	-	95%	96%
Fibrinolytic Meds Within 30 Min. of Arrival[5]	-	-	54%	58%
Average Time to ECG (minutes)[5]	-	-	8	7
Average Time to Transfer (minutes)[5]	-	-	77	60
Children's Asthma Care				
Received Home Management Plan of Care	-	-	-	88%
Received Reliever Medication	-	-	-	100%
Received Systemic Corticosteroids	-	-	-	100%
Emergency Department				
Admittance Decision Time (minutes)[5]	-	-	63	98
Head CT Results Within 45 Min. of Arrival[5]	-	-	49%	57%
Patients Who Left ER Before Being Seen[5]	-	-	2%	2%
Time from ER Arrival to Admit. (minutes)[5]	-	-	210	274
Time from ER Arrival to Discharge (minutes)[5]	-	-	110	134
Time in ER Before Being Evaluated (minutes)[5]	-	-	24	26
Time to Pain Meds for Fractures (minutes)[5]	-	-	55	57
Heart Attack Care				
Aspirin Given at Discharge[5]	-	-	99%	99%
Fibrinolytic Meds Within 30 Min. of Arrival[5]	-	-	25%	54%
PCI Within 90 Minutes of Arrival[5]	-	-	95%	96%
Statin Prescribed at Discharge[5]	-	-	98%	98%
Heart Failure Care				
ACE Inhibitor or ARB for LVSD[5]	-	-	95%	97%
Discharge Instructions Given[5]	-	-	92%	94%
Evaluation of LVS Function[5]	-	-	96%	99%

NOTE: Hospital profiles are in alphabetical order by state, then city, then hospital within the city; Rankings exclude hospitals with less than 25 cases except for patient surveys which excludes hospitals with less than 100 cases; (a) 100-299 cases; (1) The number of cases/patients is too few to report; (2) Data submitted were based on a sample of cases/patients; (3) Results are based on a shorter time period than required; (4) Data suppressed by CMS for one or more quarters; (5) Results are not available for this reporting period; (6) Fewer than 100 patients completed the HCAHPS survey; (7) No cases met the criteria for this measure; (8) The lower limit of the confidence interval cannot be calculated if the number of observed infections equals zero; (9) No data are available from the state/territory for this reporting period; (10) The scores shown reflect fewer than 50 completed surveys; (11) There were discrepancies in the data collection process; (12) This measure does not apply to this hospital for this reporting period; (13) Results cannot be calculated for this reporting period; (14) The results for this state are combined with nearby states to protect confidentiality; Please refer to the User's Guide for a full explanation of data.

Measure	Cases	This Hosp.	State Avg.	U.S. Avg.
Medicare Spending				
Medicare Spending per Patient (ratio)	-	-	0.93	0.98
Pneumonia Care				
Appropriate Initial Antibiotic Given[5]	-	-	92%	95%
Blood Culture Timing[5]	-	-	97%	98%
Pregnancy and Delivery Care				
Newborn Deliveries Scheduled Early[5]	-	-	8%	6%
Preventive Care				
Immunization for Influenza[5]	-	-	89%	90%
Immunization for Pneumonia[5]	-	-	91%	92%
Stroke Care				
Anticoagulation Therapy for Atrial Fibrillation[5]	-	-	91%	95%
Antithrombotic Therapy Timing[5]	-	-	95%	98%
Assessed for Rehabilitation[5]	-	-	96%	97%
Discharged on Antithrombotic Therapy[5]	-	-	98%	99%
Discharged on Statin Medication[5]	-	-	88%	94%
Thrombolytic Therapy Timing[5]	-	-	61%	66%
Venous Thromboembolism Prophylaxis[5]	-	-	92%	94%
Written Stroke Educational Materials Given[5]	-	-	86%	88%
Surgical Care Improvement Project				
Appropriate Beta Blocker Usage[5]	-	-	97%	98%
Appropriate VTP Within 24 Hours[5]	-	-	97%	98%
Controlled Postoperative Blood Glucose[5]	-	-	97%	97%
Perioperative Temperature Management[5]	-	-	100%	100%
Prophylactic Antibiotic Selection[5]	-	-	99%	99%
Prophylactic Antibiotic Selection (Outpatient)[5]	-	-	98%	98%
Prophylactic Antibiotic Stopped[5]	-	-	98%	98%
Prophylactic Antibiotic Timing[5]	-	-	98%	99%
Prophylactic Antibiotic Timing (Outpatient)[5]	-	-	98%	98%
Urinary Catheter Removal[5]	-	-	96%	97%
Survey of Patients' Hospital Experiences				
Area Around Room 'Always' Quiet at Night[10]	<100	53%	68%	61%
Doctors 'Always' Communicated Well[10]	<100	100%	84%	82%
Home Recovery Information Given[10]	<100	100%	84%	85%
Hospital Given 9 or 10 on 10 Point Scale[10]	<100	100%	72%	71%
Meds 'Always' Explained Before Given[10]	<100	-	66%	64%
Nurses 'Always' Communicated Well[10]	<100	100%	80%	79%
Pain 'Always' Well Controlled[10]	<100	-	72%	71%
Room and Bathroom 'Always' Clean[10]	<100	100%	73%	73%
Timely Help 'Always' Received[10]	<100	100%	71%	68%
Would Definitely Recommend Hospital[10]	<100	100%	71%	71%
Use of Medical Imaging				
Cardiac Imaging Stress Test before Surgery[7]	-	-	4.5%	5.3%
Combination Abdominal CT Scan[1]	-	-	23%	10.5%
Combination Brain/Sinus CT Scan[1]	-	-	2.2%	2.7%
Combination Chest CT Scan[1]	-	-	5.1%	2.7%
Follow-up Mammogram/Ultrasound[7]	-	-	8.1%	8.8%
Lumbar Spine MRI for Low Back Pain[7]	-	-	39.9%	37.2%

Grady Memorial Hospital

2220 Iowa Street
Chickasha, OK 73018
Phone: 405-224-2300
Fax: 405-779-2413
E-mail: jcrump@gradymem.org
URL: www.gradymem.org
Type: Acute Care Hospitals
Emergency Services: Yes
Ownership: Govt - Hospital Dist/Auth
Beds: 99

Key Personnel:
Infection Control. . . . . Cathy Hamit, RN
Chief of Medical Staff . . . . Don R Hess, MD
Radiology. . . . . James E Milton
CEO/President. . . . . E Michael Nunamaker
Operating Room. . . . . Rick Warden, RN
Quality Assurance . . . . Tawina Wouldridge

Measure	Cases	This Hosp.	State Avg.	U.S. Avg.
Blood Clot Prevention and Treatment				
Anticoagulation Overlap Therapy[1,2]	-	-	89%	93%
ICU Venous Thromboembolism Prophylaxis[2]	27	70%	87%	92%
Incidence of Potentially Preventable VTE[1,2]	-	-	8%	10%
UFH with Dosages/Platelet Monitoring[2,7]	-	-	97%	97%
Venous Thromboembolism Prophylaxis[2]	155	54%	72%	85%
Warfarin Therapy Discharge Instructions[1,2]	-	-	73%	75%
Chest Pain/Possible Heart Attack Care				
Aspirin Given Within 24 Hours of Arrival	59	98%	95%	96%
Fibrinolytic Meds Within 30 Min. of Arrival	14	64%	54%	58%
Average Time to ECG (minutes)	61	15	8	7
Average Time to Transfer (minutes)[1]	-	-	77	60
Children's Asthma Care				
Received Home Management Plan of Care	-	-	-	88%
Received Reliever Medication	-	-	-	100%
Received Systemic Corticosteroids	-	-	-	100%
Emergency Department				
Admittance Decision Time (minutes)[2]	198	63	63	98
Head CT Results Within 45 Min. of Arrival	20	30%	49%	57%
Patients Who Left ER Before Being Seen	18,649	2%	2%	2%
Time from ER Arrival to Admit. (minutes)[2]	290	209	210	274
Time from ER Arrival to Discharge (minutes)	337	110	110	134
Time in ER Before Being Evaluated (minutes)	404	30	24	26
Time to Pain Meds for Fractures (minutes)	76	73	55	57
Heart Attack Care				
Aspirin Given at Discharge[1,3]	-	-	99%	99%
Fibrinolytic Meds Within 30 Min. of Arrival[3,7]	-	-	25%	54%
PCI Within 90 Minutes of Arrival[3,7]	-	-	95%	96%
Statin Prescribed at Discharge[3,7]	-	-	98%	98%
Heart Failure Care				
ACE Inhibitor or ARB for LVSD[1]	-	-	95%	97%
Discharge Instructions Given	23	96%	92%	94%
Evaluation of LVS Function	44	95%	96%	99%
Medicare Spending				
Medicare Spending per Patient (ratio)	-	0.94	0.93	0.98
Pneumonia Care				
Appropriate Initial Antibiotic Given	69	90%	92%	95%
Blood Culture Timing	116	98%	97%	98%
Pregnancy and Delivery Care				
Newborn Deliveries Scheduled Early[2]	96	5%	8%	6%
Preventive Care				
Immunization for Influenza[2]	295	85%	89%	90%
Immunization for Pneumonia[2]	331	87%	91%	92%
Stroke Care				
Anticoagulation Therapy for Atrial Fibrillation[1]	-	-	91%	95%
Antithrombotic Therapy Timing[1]	-	-	95%	98%
Assessed for Rehabilitation[1]	-	-	96%	97%
Discharged on Antithrombotic Therapy[1]	-	-	98%	99%
Discharged on Statin Medication[1]	-	-	88%	94%
Thrombolytic Therapy Timing[1]	-	-	61%	66%
Venous Thromboembolism Prophylaxis[1]	-	-	92%	94%
Written Stroke Educational Materials Given[1]	-	-	86%	88%
Surgical Care Improvement Project				
Appropriate Beta Blocker Usage[1]	-	-	97%	98%
Appropriate VTP Within 24 Hours	42	93%	97%	98%
Controlled Postoperative Blood Glucose[7]	-	-	97%	97%
Perioperative Temperature Management	53	94%	100%	100%
Prophylactic Antibiotic Selection	42	93%	99%	99%
Prophylactic Antibiotic Selection (Outpatient)	18	100%	98%	98%
Prophylactic Antibiotic Stopped	42	88%	98%	98%
Prophylactic Antibiotic Timing	42	88%	98%	99%
Prophylactic Antibiotic Timing (Outpatient)	19	95%	98%	98%
Urinary Catheter Removal	14	79%	96%	97%
Survey of Patients' Hospital Experiences				
Area Around Room 'Always' Quiet at Night	300+	60%	68%	61%
Doctors 'Always' Communicated Well	300+	82%	84%	82%
Home Recovery Information Given	300+	87%	84%	85%
Hospital Given 9 or 10 on 10 Point Scale	300+	64%	72%	71%
Meds 'Always' Explained Before Given	300+	59%	66%	64%
Nurses 'Always' Communicated Well	300+	75%	80%	79%
Pain 'Always' Well Controlled	300+	70%	72%	71%
Room and Bathroom 'Always' Clean	300+	66%	73%	73%
Timely Help 'Always' Received	300+	62%	71%	68%
Would Definitely Recommend Hospital	300+	58%	71%	71%
Use of Medical Imaging				
Cardiac Imaging Stress Test before Surgery	154	0.6%	4.5%	5.3%
Combination Abdominal CT Scan	275	9.8%	23%	10.5%
Combination Brain/Sinus CT Scan	338	1.5%	2.2%	2.7%
Combination Chest CT Scan	140	5.7%	5.1%	2.7%
Follow-up Mammogram/Ultrasound	593	7.3%	8.1%	8.8%
Lumbar Spine MRI for Low Back Pain	55	45.5%	39.9%	37.2%

Claremore Indian Hospital

101 South Moore Ave
Claremore, OK 74017
Phone: 918-341-8430
Fax: 918-342-6436
Type: Acute Care Hospitals
Emergency Services: Yes
Ownership: Government - Federal
Beds: 50

Key Personnel:
Anesthesiology. . . . . Jeff Belinski, MD
Emergency Room . . . . Donald Bobek
CEO/President. . . . . James Cussen
Quality Assurance . . . . Donna Francisco
Chief of Medical Staff . . . . Paul Mobley, DO
Infection Control. . . . . Patti V White

Measure	Cases	This Hosp.	State Avg.	U.S. Avg.
Blood Clot Prevention and Treatment				
Anticoagulation Overlap Therapy[2,7]	-	-	89%	93%
ICU Venous Thromboembolism Prophylaxis[2]	44	95%	87%	92%
Incidence of Potentially Preventable VTE[2,7]	-	-	8%	10%
UFH with Dosages/Platelet Monitoring[2,7]	-	-	97%	97%
Venous Thromboembolism Prophylaxis[2]	54	94%	72%	85%
Warfarin Therapy Discharge Instructions[2,7]	-	-	73%	75%
Chest Pain/Possible Heart Attack Care				
Aspirin Given Within 24 Hours of Arrival[3]	20	95%	95%	96%
Fibrinolytic Meds Within 30 Min. of Arrival[3,7]	-	-	54%	58%
Average Time to ECG (minutes)[3]	20	14	8	7
Average Time to Transfer (minutes)[3,7]	-	-	77	60
Children's Asthma Care				
Received Home Management Plan of Care	-	-	-	88%
Received Reliever Medication	-	-	-	100%
Received Systemic Corticosteroids	-	-	-	100%
Emergency Department				
Admittance Decision Time (minutes)[2]	204	54	63	98
Head CT Results Within 45 Min. of Arrival[1,3]	-	-	49%	57%
Patients Who Left ER Before Being Seen[5]	-	-	2%	2%
Time from ER Arrival to Admit. (minutes)[2]	205	343	210	274
Time from ER Arrival to Discharge (minutes)[3]	83	164	110	134
Time in ER Before Being Evaluated (minutes)[3]	94	61	24	26
Time to Pain Meds for Fractures (minutes)[1,3]	-	-	55	57
Heart Attack Care				
Aspirin Given at Discharge[5]	-	-	99%	99%
Fibrinolytic Meds Within 30 Min. of Arrival[5]	-	-	25%	54%
PCI Within 90 Minutes of Arrival[5]	-	-	95%	96%
Statin Prescribed at Discharge[5]	-	-	98%	98%
Heart Failure Care				
ACE Inhibitor or ARB for LVSD[1,3]	-	-	95%	97%
Discharge Instructions Given[1,3]	-	-	92%	94%
Evaluation of LVS Function[1,3]	-	-	96%	99%
Medicare Spending				
Medicare Spending per Patient (ratio)	-	0.84	0.93	0.98
Pneumonia Care				
Appropriate Initial Antibiotic Given	31	94%	92%	95%
Blood Culture Timing	33	100%	97%	98%
Pregnancy and Delivery Care				
Newborn Deliveries Scheduled Early[1]	-	-	8%	6%
Preventive Care				
Immunization for Influenza[2]	259	85%	89%	90%
Immunization for Pneumonia[2]	142	80%	91%	92%
Stroke Care				
Anticoagulation Therapy for Atrial Fibrillation[3,7]	-	-	91%	95%
Antithrombotic Therapy Timing[3,7]	-	-	95%	98%
Assessed for Rehabilitation[3,7]	-	-	96%	97%
Discharged on Antithrombotic Therapy[3,7]	-	-	98%	99%
Discharged on Statin Medication[3,7]	-	-	88%	94%
Thrombolytic Therapy Timing[3,7]	-	-	61%	66%
Venous Thromboembolism Prophylaxis[1,3]	-	-	92%	94%
Written Stroke Educational Materials Given[3,7]	-	-	86%	88%
Surgical Care Improvement Project				
Appropriate Beta Blocker Usage[1]	-	-	97%	98%
Appropriate VTP Within 24 Hours	20	100%	97%	98%
Controlled Postoperative Blood Glucose[7]	-	-	97%	97%
Perioperative Temperature Management	51	100%	100%	100%
Prophylactic Antibiotic Selection	37	97%	99%	99%
Prophylactic Antibiotic Selection (Outpatient)[5]	-	-	98%	98%
Prophylactic Antibiotic Stopped	36	94%	98%	98%

NOTE: Hospital profiles are in alphabetical order by state, then city, then hospital within the city; Rankings exclude hospitals with less than 25 cases except for patient surveys which excludes hospitals with less than 100 cases; (a) 100-299 cases; (1) The number of cases/patients is too few to report; (2) Data submitted were based on a sample of cases/patients; (3) Results are based on a shorter time period than required; (4) Data suppressed by CMS for one or more quarters; (5) Results are not available for this reporting period; (6) Fewer than 100 patients completed the HCAHPS survey; (7) No cases met the criteria for this measure; (8) The lower limit of the confidence interval cannot be calculated if the number of observed infections equals zero; (9) No data are available from the state/territory for this reporting period; (10) The scores shown reflect fewer than 50 completed surveys; (11) There were discrepancies in the data collection process; (12) This measure does not apply to this hospital for this reporting period; (13) Results cannot be calculated for this reporting period; (14) The results for this state are combined with nearby states to protect confidentiality; Please refer to the User's Guide for a full explanation of data.

Measure	Cases	This Hosp.	State Avg.	U.S. Avg.
Prophylactic Antibiotic Timing	38	97%	98%	99%
Prophylactic Antibiotic Timing (Outpatient)[5]	-	-	98%	98%
Urinary Catheter Removal	13	100%	96%	97%
Survey of Patients' Hospital Experiences				
Area Around Room 'Always' Quiet at Night	(a)	65%	68%	61%
Doctors 'Always' Communicated Well	(a)	82%	84%	82%
Home Recovery Information Given	(a)	84%	84%	85%
Hospital Given 9 or 10 on 10 Point Scale	(a)	66%	72%	71%
Meds 'Always' Explained Before Given	(a)	69%	66%	64%
Nurses 'Always' Communicated Well	(a)	83%	80%	79%
Pain 'Always' Well Controlled	(a)	72%	72%	71%
Room and Bathroom 'Always' Clean	(a)	64%	73%	73%
Timely Help 'Always' Received	(a)	73%	71%	68%
Would Definitely Recommend Hospital	(a)	66%	71%	71%
Use of Medical Imaging				
Cardiac Imaging Stress Test before Surgery[7]	-	-	4.5%	5.3%
Combination Abdominal CT Scan[7]	-	-	23%	10.5%
Combination Brain/Sinus CT Scan[7]	-	-	2.2%	2.7%
Combination Chest CT Scan[7]	-	-	5.1%	2.7%
Follow-up Mammogram/Ultrasound[7]	-	-	8.1%	8.8%
Lumbar Spine MRI for Low Back Pain[7]	-	-	39.9%	37.2%

Hillcrest Hospital Claremore

1202 N Muskogee Place
Claremore, OK 74017
Phone: 918-342-6777
Fax: 918-342-3330
URL: www.claremorereghospital.com
Type: Acute Care Hospitals
Emergency Services: Yes
Ownership: Proprietary
Beds: 73

Key Personnel:

Emergency Room .... Jimmy Bible
CEO/President............... David Chausard
Chief of Medical Staff.......... Karen Harris
Cardiac Laboratory............ Lilia Turner

Measure	Cases	This Hosp.	State Avg.	U.S. Avg.
Blood Clot Prevention and Treatment				
Anticoagulation Overlap Therapy[1,2]	-	-	89%	93%
ICU Venous Thromboembolism Prophylaxis[2]	55	82%	87%	92%
Incidence of Potentially Preventable VTE[1,2]	-	-	8%	10%
UFH with Dosages/Platelet Monitoring[1,2]	-	-	97%	97%
Venous Thromboembolism Prophylaxis[2]	194	71%	72%	85%
Warfarin Therapy Discharge Instructions[1,2]	-	-	73%	75%
Chest Pain/Possible Heart Attack Care				
Aspirin Given Within 24 Hours of Arrival	38	92%	95%	96%
Fibrinolytic Meds Within 30 Min. of Arrival[7]	-	-	54%	58%
Average Time to ECG (minutes)	39	5	8	7
Average Time to Transfer (minutes)	13	57	77	60
Children's Asthma Care				
Received Home Management Plan of Care	-	-	-	88%
Received Reliever Medication	-	-	-	100%
Received Systemic Corticosteroids	-	-	-	100%
Emergency Department				
Admittance Decision Time (minutes)[2]	457	61	63	98
Head CT Results Within 45 Min. of Arrival[1]	-	-	49%	57%
Patients Who Left ER Before Being Seen	19,070	1%	2%	2%
Time from ER Arrival to Admit. (minutes)[2]	461	239	210	274
Time from ER Arrival to Discharge (minutes)	498	150	110	134
Time in ER Before Being Evaluated (minutes)	561	40	24	26
Time to Pain Meds for Fractures (minutes)	75	68	55	57
Heart Attack Care				
Aspirin Given at Discharge	20	95%	99%	99%
Fibrinolytic Meds Within 30 Min. of Arrival[7]	-	-	25%	54%
PCI Within 90 Minutes of Arrival[1]	-	-	95%	96%
Statin Prescribed at Discharge	17	82%	98%	98%
Heart Failure Care				
ACE Inhibitor or ARB for LVSD	16	100%	95%	97%
Discharge Instructions Given	58	100%	92%	94%
Evaluation of LVS Function	71	97%	96%	99%
Medicare Spending				
Medicare Spending per Patient (ratio)	-	0.90	0.93	0.98
Pneumonia Care				
Appropriate Initial Antibiotic Given	87	98%	92%	95%
Blood Culture Timing	145	97%	97%	98%
Pregnancy and Delivery Care				
Newborn Deliveries Scheduled Early	86	2%	8%	6%
Preventive Care				
Immunization for Influenza[2]	394	96%	89%	90%
Immunization for Pneumonia[2]	407	90%	91%	92%
Stroke Care				
Anticoagulation Therapy for Atrial Fibrillation[7]	-	-	91%	95%
Antithrombotic Therapy Timing	12	92%	95%	98%
Assessed for Rehabilitation[1]	-	-	96%	97%
Discharged on Antithrombotic Therapy[1]	-	-	98%	99%
Discharged on Statin Medication[1]	-	-	88%	94%
Thrombolytic Therapy Timing[1]	-	-	61%	66%
Venous Thromboembolism Prophylaxis	13	69%	92%	94%
Written Stroke Educational Materials Given[1]	-	-	86%	88%
Surgical Care Improvement Project				
Appropriate Beta Blocker Usage	32	100%	97%	98%
Appropriate VTP Within 24 Hours	129	98%	97%	98%
Controlled Postoperative Blood Glucose[7]	-	-	97%	97%
Perioperative Temperature Management	148	100%	100%	100%
Prophylactic Antibiotic Selection	113	99%	99%	99%
Prophylactic Antibiotic Selection (Outpatient)	59	98%	98%	98%
Prophylactic Antibiotic Stopped	107	96%	98%	98%
Prophylactic Antibiotic Timing	113	99%	98%	99%
Prophylactic Antibiotic Timing (Outpatient)	59	100%	98%	98%
Urinary Catheter Removal	63	98%	96%	97%
Survey of Patients' Hospital Experiences				
Area Around Room 'Always' Quiet at Night	300+	55%	68%	61%
Doctors 'Always' Communicated Well	300+	83%	84%	82%
Home Recovery Information Given	300+	86%	84%	85%
Hospital Given 9 or 10 on 10 Point Scale	300+	64%	72%	71%
Meds 'Always' Explained Before Given	300+	61%	66%	64%
Nurses 'Always' Communicated Well	300+	74%	80%	79%
Pain 'Always' Well Controlled	300+	69%	72%	71%
Room and Bathroom 'Always' Clean	300+	69%	73%	73%
Timely Help 'Always' Received	300+	64%	71%	68%
Would Definitely Recommend Hospital	300+	62%	71%	71%
Use of Medical Imaging				
Cardiac Imaging Stress Test before Surgery	310	4.8%	4.5%	5.3%
Combination Abdominal CT Scan	335	1.5%	23%	10.5%
Combination Brain/Sinus CT Scan[1]	-	-	2.2%	2.7%
Combination Chest CT Scan	144	1.4%	5.1%	2.7%
Follow-up Mammogram/Ultrasound	531	8.1%	8.1%	8.8%
Lumbar Spine MRI for Low Back Pain	60	56.7%	39.9%	37.2%

Cleveland Area Hospital

1401 West Pawnee
Cleveland, OK 74020
Phone: 918-358-2501
Type: Critical Access Hospitals
Emergency Services: Yes
Ownership: Govt - Hospital Dist/Auth

Measure	Cases	This Hosp.	State Avg.	U.S. Avg.
Blood Clot Prevention and Treatment				
Anticoagulation Overlap Therapy[3,7]	-	-	89%	93%
ICU Venous Thromboembolism Prophylaxis[3,7]	-	-	87%	92%
Incidence of Potentially Preventable VTE[3,7]	-	-	8%	10%
UFH with Dosages/Platelet Monitoring[3,7]	-	-	97%	97%
Venous Thromboembolism Prophylaxis[1,3]	-	-	72%	85%
Warfarin Therapy Discharge Instructions[3,7]	-	-	73%	75%
Chest Pain/Possible Heart Attack Care				
Aspirin Given Within 24 Hours of Arrival	29	97%	95%	96%
Fibrinolytic Meds Within 30 Min. of Arrival[1]	-	-	54%	58%
Average Time to ECG (minutes)	30	14	8	7
Average Time to Transfer (minutes)[7]	-	-	77	60
Children's Asthma Care				
Received Home Management Plan of Care	-	-	-	88%
Received Reliever Medication	-	-	-	100%
Received Systemic Corticosteroids	-	-	-	100%
Emergency Department				
Admittance Decision Time (minutes)[5]	-	-	63	98
Head CT Results Within 45 Min. of Arrival[1,3]	-	-	49%	57%
Patients Who Left ER Before Being Seen	5,300	2%	2%	2%
Time from ER Arrival to Admit. (minutes)[5]	-	-	210	274
Time from ER Arrival to Discharge (minutes)[1]	-	-	110	134
Time in ER Before Being Evaluated (minutes)	16	28	24	26
Time to Pain Meds for Fractures (minutes)[3]	13	77	55	57
Heart Attack Care				
Aspirin Given at Discharge[3,7]	-	-	99%	99%
Fibrinolytic Meds Within 30 Min. of Arrival[3,7]	-	-	25%	54%
PCI Within 90 Minutes of Arrival[3,7]	-	-	95%	96%
Statin Prescribed at Discharge[3,7]	-	-	98%	98%
Heart Failure Care				
ACE Inhibitor or ARB for LVSD[3,7]	-	-	95%	97%
Discharge Instructions Given[1,3]	-	-	92%	94%
Evaluation of LVS Function[1,3]	-	-	96%	99%
Medicare Spending				
Medicare Spending per Patient (ratio)	-	-	0.93	0.98
Pneumonia Care				
Appropriate Initial Antibiotic Given	12	92%	92%	95%
Blood Culture Timing	12	92%	97%	98%
Pregnancy and Delivery Care				
Newborn Deliveries Scheduled Early[5]	-	-	8%	6%
Preventive Care				
Immunization for Influenza[5]	-	-	89%	90%
Immunization for Pneumonia[5]	-	-	91%	92%
Stroke Care				
Anticoagulation Therapy for Atrial Fibrillation[5]	-	-	91%	95%
Antithrombotic Therapy Timing[5]	-	-	95%	98%
Assessed for Rehabilitation[5]	-	-	96%	97%
Discharged on Antithrombotic Therapy[5]	-	-	98%	99%
Discharged on Statin Medication[5]	-	-	88%	94%
Thrombolytic Therapy Timing[5]	-	-	61%	66%
Venous Thromboembolism Prophylaxis[5]	-	-	92%	94%
Written Stroke Educational Materials Given[5]	-	-	86%	88%
Surgical Care Improvement Project				
Appropriate Beta Blocker Usage[5]	-	-	97%	98%
Appropriate VTP Within 24 Hours[5]	-	-	97%	98%
Controlled Postoperative Blood Glucose[5]	-	-	97%	97%
Perioperative Temperature Management[5]	-	-	100%	100%
Prophylactic Antibiotic Selection[5]	-	-	99%	99%
Prophylactic Antibiotic Selection (Outpatient)[5]	-	-	98%	98%
Prophylactic Antibiotic Stopped[5]	-	-	98%	98%
Prophylactic Antibiotic Timing[5]	-	-	98%	99%
Prophylactic Antibiotic Timing (Outpatient)[5]	-	-	98%	98%
Urinary Catheter Removal[5]	-	-	96%	97%
Survey of Patients' Hospital Experiences				
Area Around Room 'Always' Quiet at Night[5]	-	-	68%	61%
Doctors 'Always' Communicated Well[5]	-	-	84%	82%
Home Recovery Information Given[5]	-	-	84%	85%
Hospital Given 9 or 10 on 10 Point Scale[5]	-	-	72%	71%
Meds 'Always' Explained Before Given[5]	-	-	66%	64%
Nurses 'Always' Communicated Well[5]	-	-	80%	79%
Pain 'Always' Well Controlled[5]	-	-	72%	71%
Room and Bathroom 'Always' Clean[5]	-	-	73%	73%
Timely Help 'Always' Received[5]	-	-	71%	68%
Would Definitely Recommend Hospital[5]	-	-	71%	71%
Use of Medical Imaging				
Cardiac Imaging Stress Test before Surgery[1]	-	-	4.5%	5.3%
Combination Abdominal CT Scan	106	13.2%	23%	10.5%
Combination Brain/Sinus CT Scan[1]	-	-	2.2%	2.7%
Combination Chest CT Scan[1]	-	-	5.1%	2.7%
Follow-up Mammogram/Ultrasound[1]	-	-	8.1%	8.8%
Lumbar Spine MRI for Low Back Pain[1]	-	-	39.9%	37.2%

Integris Clinton Regional Hospital

100 North 30th Street
Clinton, OK 73601
Phone: 580-323-2363
Fax: 580-331-1463
URL: www.integris-health.com
Type: Acute Care Hospitals
Emergency Services: Yes
Ownership: Government - Local
Beds: 56

Key Personnel:

Operating Room.............. Tom Cashero, RN
Chief of Medical Staff.......... Stacy Clothier
Infection Control............. Karol Dillard, RN
CEO/President............... Stanley F Hupfeld
Quality Assurance .... Bill Kelton
Intensive Care Unit........... Carol Kish, RN
Emergency Room .... Tammy Martin, RN

Measure	Cases	This Hosp.	State Avg.	U.S. Avg.

NOTE: Hospital profiles are in alphabetical order by state, then city, then hospital within the city; Rankings exclude hospitals with less than 25 cases except for patient surveys which excludes hospitals with less than 100 cases; (a) 100-299 cases; (1) The number of cases/patients is too few to report; (2) Data submitted were based on a sample of cases/patients; (3) Results are based on a shorter time period than required; (4) Data suppressed by CMS for one or more quarters; (5) Results are not available for this reporting period; (6) Fewer than 100 patients completed the HCAHPS survey; (7) No cases met the criteria for this measure; (8) The lower limit of the confidence interval cannot be calculated if the number of observed infections equals zero; (9) No data are available from the state/territory for this reporting period; (10) The scores shown reflect fewer than 50 completed surveys; (11) There were discrepancies in the data collection process; (12) This measure does not apply to this hospital for this reporting period; (13) Results cannot be calculated for this reporting period; (14) The results for this state are combined with nearby states to protect confidentiality; Please refer to the User's Guide for a full explanation of data.

Measure	Cases	This Hosp.	State Avg.	U.S. Avg.
Blood Clot Prevention and Treatment				
Anticoagulation Overlap Therapy[1,2]	-	-	89%	93%
ICU Venous Thromboembolism Prophylaxis[2]	12	92%	87%	92%
Incidence of Potentially Preventable VTE[1,2]	-	-	8%	10%
UFH with Dosages/Platelet Monitoring[1,2]	-	-	97%	97%
Venous Thromboembolism Prophylaxis[2]	100	88%	72%	85%
Warfarin Therapy Discharge Instructions[1,2]	-	-	73%	75%
Chest Pain/Possible Heart Attack Care				
Aspirin Given Within 24 Hours of Arrival	36	92%	95%	96%
Fibrinolytic Meds Within 30 Min. of Arrival[1]	-	-	54%	58%
Average Time to ECG (minutes)	37	7	8	7
Average Time to Transfer (minutes)[1]	-	-	77	60
Children's Asthma Care				
Received Home Management Plan of Care	-	-	-	88%
Received Reliever Medication	-	-	-	100%
Received Systemic Corticosteroids	-	-	-	100%
Emergency Department				
Admittance Decision Time (minutes)[2]	316	61	63	98
Head CT Results Within 45 Min. of Arrival[1]	-	-	49%	57%
Patients Who Left ER Before Being Seen	9,358	1%	2%	2%
Time from ER Arrival to Admit. (minutes)[2]	322	197	210	274
Time from ER Arrival to Discharge (minutes)	785	111	110	134
Time in ER Before Being Evaluated (minutes)	874	26	24	26
Time to Pain Meds for Fractures (minutes)	43	45	55	57
Heart Attack Care				
Aspirin Given at Discharge[1]	-	-	99%	99%
Fibrinolytic Meds Within 30 Min. of Arrival[7]	-	-	25%	54%
PCI Within 90 Minutes of Arrival[7]	-	-	95%	96%
Statin Prescribed at Discharge[1]	-	-	98%	98%
Heart Failure Care				
ACE Inhibitor or ARB for LVSD[1]	-	-	95%	97%
Discharge Instructions Given	26	77%	92%	94%
Evaluation of LVS Function	40	100%	96%	99%
Medicare Spending				
Medicare Spending per Patient (ratio)	-	0.88	0.93	0.98
Pneumonia Care				
Appropriate Initial Antibiotic Given	59	95%	92%	95%
Blood Culture Timing	81	99%	97%	98%
Pregnancy and Delivery Care				
Newborn Deliveries Scheduled Early	41	2%	8%	6%
Preventive Care				
Immunization for Influenza[2]	305	99%	89%	90%
Immunization for Pneumonia[2]	276	97%	91%	92%
Stroke Care				
Anticoagulation Therapy for Atrial Fibrillation[7]	-	-	91%	95%
Antithrombotic Therapy Timing	13	100%	95%	98%
Assessed for Rehabilitation	11	100%	96%	97%
Discharged on Antithrombotic Therapy	11	100%	98%	99%
Discharged on Statin Medication[1]	-	-	88%	94%
Thrombolytic Therapy Timing[7]	-	-	61%	66%
Venous Thromboembolism Prophylaxis	13	92%	92%	94%
Written Stroke Educational Materials Given[1]	-	-	86%	88%
Surgical Care Improvement Project				
Appropriate Beta Blocker Usage[1,3]	-	-	97%	98%
Appropriate VTP Within 24 Hours[1,3]	-	-	97%	98%
Controlled Postoperative Blood Glucose[3,7]	-	-	97%	97%
Perioperative Temperature Management[3]	12	100%	100%	100%
Prophylactic Antibiotic Selection[1,3]	-	-	99%	99%
Prophylactic Antibiotic Selection (Outpatient)[1,3]	-	-	98%	98%
Prophylactic Antibiotic Stopped[1,3]	-	-	98%	98%
Prophylactic Antibiotic Timing[1,3]	-	-	98%	99%
Prophylactic Antibiotic Timing (Outpatient)[1,3]	-	-	98%	98%
Urinary Catheter Removal[1,3]	-	-	96%	97%
Survey of Patients' Hospital Experiences				
Area Around Room 'Always' Quiet at Night	(a)	63%	68%	61%
Doctors 'Always' Communicated Well	(a)	87%	84%	82%
Home Recovery Information Given	(a)	85%	84%	85%
Hospital Given 9 or 10 on 10 Point Scale	(a)	59%	72%	71%
Meds 'Always' Explained Before Given	(a)	67%	66%	64%
Nurses 'Always' Communicated Well	(a)	75%	80%	79%
Pain 'Always' Well Controlled	(a)	73%	72%	71%
Room and Bathroom 'Always' Clean	(a)	59%	73%	73%
Timely Help 'Always' Received	(a)	71%	71%	68%
Would Definitely Recommend Hospital	(a)	60%	71%	71%
Use of Medical Imaging				
Cardiac Imaging Stress Test before Surgery[7]	-	-	4.5%	5.3%
Combination Abdominal CT Scan	215	49.3%	23%	10.5%
Combination Brain/Sinus CT Scan[1]	-	-	2.2%	2.7%
Combination Chest CT Scan	89	15.7%	5.1%	2.7%
Follow-up Mammogram/Ultrasound	161	8.7%	8.1%	8.8%
Lumbar Spine MRI for Low Back Pain[1]	-	-	39.9%	37.2%

Mary Hurley Hospital

6 North Covington
Coalgate, OK 74538
Type: Critical Access Hospitals
Ownership: Voluntary non-profit - Private
Phone: 580-927-2327
Fax: 580-927-2432
Emergency Services: Yes
Beds: 20

Key Personnel:
Chief of Medical Staff .... R J Alton
CEO/President .... Dean Clements
Emergency Room .... Tommie Stanberry

Measure	Cases	This Hosp.	State Avg.	U.S. Avg.
Blood Clot Prevention and Treatment				
Anticoagulation Overlap Therapy[5]	-	-	89%	93%
ICU Venous Thromboembolism Prophylaxis[5]	-	-	87%	92%
Incidence of Potentially Preventable VTE[5]	-	-	8%	10%
UFH with Dosages/Platelet Monitoring[5]	-	-	97%	97%
Venous Thromboembolism Prophylaxis[5]	-	-	72%	85%
Warfarin Therapy Discharge Instructions[5]	-	-	73%	75%
Chest Pain/Possible Heart Attack Care				
Aspirin Given Within 24 Hours of Arrival[1,3]	-	-	95%	96%
Fibrinolytic Meds Within 30 Min. of Arrival[3,7]	-	-	54%	58%
Average Time to ECG (minutes)[1,3]	-	-	8	7
Average Time to Transfer (minutes)[1,3]	-	-	77	60
Children's Asthma Care				
Received Home Management Plan of Care	-	-	-	88%
Received Reliever Medication	-	-	-	100%
Received Systemic Corticosteroids	-	-	-	100%
Emergency Department				
Admittance Decision Time (minutes)[3]	36	20	63	98
Head CT Results Within 45 Min. of Arrival[1,3]	-	-	49%	57%
Patients Who Left ER Before Being Seen[5]	-	-	2%	2%
Time from ER Arrival to Admit. (minutes)[3]	36	83	210	274
Time from ER Arrival to Discharge (minutes)	245	79	110	134
Time in ER Before Being Evaluated (minutes)	239	20	24	26
Time to Pain Meds for Fractures (minutes)[1,3]	-	-	55	57
Heart Attack Care				
Aspirin Given at Discharge[3,7]	-	-	99%	99%
Fibrinolytic Meds Within 30 Min. of Arrival[3,7]	-	-	25%	54%
PCI Within 90 Minutes of Arrival[3,7]	-	-	95%	96%
Statin Prescribed at Discharge[3,7]	-	-	98%	98%
Heart Failure Care				
ACE Inhibitor or ARB for LVSD	17	100%	95%	97%
Discharge Instructions Given	34	97%	92%	94%
Evaluation of LVS Function	67	81%	96%	99%
Medicare Spending				
Medicare Spending per Patient (ratio)	-	-	0.93	0.98
Pneumonia Care				
Appropriate Initial Antibiotic Given	14	21%	92%	95%
Blood Culture Timing[1]	-	-	97%	98%
Pregnancy and Delivery Care				
Newborn Deliveries Scheduled Early[5]	-	-	8%	6%
Preventive Care				
Immunization for Influenza[5]	-	-	89%	90%
Immunization for Pneumonia[5]	-	-	91%	92%
Stroke Care				
Anticoagulation Therapy for Atrial Fibrillation[5]	-	-	91%	95%
Antithrombotic Therapy Timing[5]	-	-	95%	98%
Assessed for Rehabilitation[5]	-	-	96%	97%
Discharged on Antithrombotic Therapy[5]	-	-	98%	99%
Discharged on Statin Medication[5]	-	-	88%	94%
Thrombolytic Therapy Timing[5]	-	-	61%	66%
Venous Thromboembolism Prophylaxis[5]	-	-	92%	94%
Written Stroke Educational Materials Given[5]	-	-	86%	88%
Surgical Care Improvement Project				
Appropriate Beta Blocker Usage[5]	-	-	97%	98%
Appropriate VTP Within 24 Hours[5]	-	-	97%	98%
Controlled Postoperative Blood Glucose[5]	-	-	97%	97%
Perioperative Temperature Management[5]	-	-	100%	100%
Prophylactic Antibiotic Selection[5]	-	-	99%	99%
Prophylactic Antibiotic Selection (Outpatient)[5]	-	-	98%	98%
Prophylactic Antibiotic Stopped[5]	-	-	98%	98%
Prophylactic Antibiotic Timing[5]	-	-	98%	99%
Prophylactic Antibiotic Timing (Outpatient)[5]	-	-	98%	98%
Urinary Catheter Removal[5]	-	-	96%	97%
Survey of Patients' Hospital Experiences				
Area Around Room 'Always' Quiet at Night[5]	-	-	68%	61%
Doctors 'Always' Communicated Well[5]	-	-	84%	82%
Home Recovery Information Given[5]	-	-	84%	85%
Hospital Given 9 or 10 on 10 Point Scale[5]	-	-	72%	71%
Meds 'Always' Explained Before Given[5]	-	-	66%	64%
Nurses 'Always' Communicated Well[5]	-	-	80%	79%
Pain 'Always' Well Controlled[5]	-	-	72%	71%
Room and Bathroom 'Always' Clean[5]	-	-	73%	73%
Timely Help 'Always' Received[5]	-	-	71%	68%
Would Definitely Recommend Hospital[5]	-	-	71%	71%
Use of Medical Imaging				
Cardiac Imaging Stress Test before Surgery[7]	-	-	4.5%	5.3%
Combination Abdominal CT Scan	81	3.7%	23%	10.5%
Combination Brain/Sinus CT Scan	101	0.0%	2.2%	2.7%
Combination Chest CT Scan[1]	-	-	5.1%	2.7%
Follow-up Mammogram/Ultrasound[7]	-	-	8.1%	8.8%
Lumbar Spine MRI for Low Back Pain[7]	-	-	39.9%	37.2%

Cordell Memorial Hospital

1220 North Glenn English Street
Cordell, OK 73632
Type: Critical Access Hospitals
Ownership: Govt - Hospital Dist/Auth
Phone: 580-832-3339
Fax: 580-832-5076
Emergency Services: Yes
Beds: 25

Measure	Cases	This Hosp.	State Avg.	U.S. Avg.
Blood Clot Prevention and Treatment				
Anticoagulation Overlap Therapy[5]	-	-	89%	93%
ICU Venous Thromboembolism Prophylaxis[5]	-	-	87%	92%
Incidence of Potentially Preventable VTE[5]	-	-	8%	10%
UFH with Dosages/Platelet Monitoring[5]	-	-	97%	97%
Venous Thromboembolism Prophylaxis[5]	-	-	72%	85%
Warfarin Therapy Discharge Instructions[5]	-	-	73%	75%
Chest Pain/Possible Heart Attack Care				
Aspirin Given Within 24 Hours of Arrival[1,3]	-	-	95%	96%
Fibrinolytic Meds Within 30 Min. of Arrival[1,3]	-	-	54%	58%
Average Time to ECG (minutes)[1,3]	-	-	8	7
Average Time to Transfer (minutes)[3,7]	-	-	77	60
Children's Asthma Care				
Received Home Management Plan of Care	-	-	-	88%
Received Reliever Medication	-	-	-	100%
Received Systemic Corticosteroids	-	-	-	100%
Emergency Department				
Admittance Decision Time (minutes)[3]	23	0	63	98
Head CT Results Within 45 Min. of Arrival[3,7]	-	-	49%	57%
Patients Who Left ER Before Being Seen[5]	-	-	2%	2%
Time from ER Arrival to Admit. (minutes)[3]	23	85	210	274
Time from ER Arrival to Discharge (minutes)[1,3]	-	-	110	134
Time in ER Before Being Evaluated (minutes)[3,7]	-	-	24	26
Time to Pain Meds for Fractures (minutes)[1,3]	-	-	55	57
Heart Attack Care				
Aspirin Given at Discharge[1,3]	-	-	99%	99%
Fibrinolytic Meds Within 30 Min. of Arrival[3,7]	-	-	25%	54%
PCI Within 90 Minutes of Arrival[3,7]	-	-	95%	96%
Statin Prescribed at Discharge[1,3]	-	-	98%	98%
Heart Failure Care				
ACE Inhibitor or ARB for LVSD[1]	-	-	95%	97%
Discharge Instructions Given[1]	-	-	92%	94%
Evaluation of LVS Function	15	87%	96%	99%
Medicare Spending				
Medicare Spending per Patient (ratio)	-	-	0.93	0.98
Pneumonia Care				

NOTE: Hospital profiles are in alphabetical order by state, then city, then hospital within the city; Rankings exclude hospitals with less than 25 cases except for patient surveys which excludes hospitals with less than 100 cases; (a) 100-299 cases; (1) The number of cases/patients is too few to report; (2) Data submitted were based on a sample of cases/patients; (3) Results are based on a shorter time period than required; (4) Data suppressed by CMS for one or more quarters; (5) Results are not available for this reporting period; (6) Fewer than 100 patients completed the HCAHPS survey; (7) No cases met the criteria for this measure; (8) The lower limit of the confidence interval cannot be calculated if the number of observed infections equals zero; (9) No data are available from the state/territory for this reporting period; (10) The scores shown reflect fewer than 50 completed surveys; (11) There were discrepancies in the data collection process; (12) This measure does not apply to this hospital for this reporting period; (13) Results cannot be calculated for this reporting period; (14) The results for this state are combined with nearby states to protect confidentiality; Please refer to the User's Guide for a full explanation of data.

Measure	Cases	This Hosp.	State Avg.	U.S. Avg.
Appropriate Initial Antibiotic Given[1]	-	-	92%	95%
Blood Culture Timing[1]	-	-	97%	98%
Pregnancy and Delivery Care				
Newborn Deliveries Scheduled Early[5]	-	-	8%	6%
Preventive Care				
Immunization for Influenza	24	79%	89%	90%
Immunization for Pneumonia	37	89%	91%	92%
Stroke Care				
Anticoagulation Therapy for Atrial Fibrillation[3,7]	-	-	91%	95%
Antithrombotic Therapy Timing[1,3]	-	-	95%	98%
Assessed for Rehabilitation[1,3]	-	-	96%	97%
Discharged on Antithrombotic Therapy[1,3]	-	-	98%	99%
Discharged on Statin Medication[1,3]	-	-	88%	94%
Thrombolytic Therapy Timing[3,7]	-	-	61%	66%
Venous Thromboembolism Prophylaxis[1,3]	-	-	92%	94%
Written Stroke Educational Materials Given[1,3]	-	-	86%	88%
Surgical Care Improvement Project				
Appropriate Beta Blocker Usage[5]	-	-	97%	98%
Appropriate VTP Within 24 Hours[5]	-	-	97%	98%
Controlled Postoperative Blood Glucose[5]	-	-	97%	97%
Perioperative Temperature Management[5]	-	-	100%	100%
Prophylactic Antibiotic Selection[5]	-	-	99%	99%
Prophylactic Antibiotic Selection (Outpatient)[5]	-	-	98%	98%
Prophylactic Antibiotic Stopped[5]	-	-	98%	98%
Prophylactic Antibiotic Timing[5]	-	-	98%	99%
Prophylactic Antibiotic Timing (Outpatient)[5]	-	-	98%	98%
Urinary Catheter Removal[5]	-	-	96%	97%
Survey of Patients' Hospital Experiences				
Area Around Room 'Always' Quiet at Night[10]	<100	57%	68%	61%
Doctors 'Always' Communicated Well[10]	<100	89%	84%	82%
Home Recovery Information Given[10]	<100	86%	84%	85%
Hospital Given 9 or 10 on 10 Point Scale[10]	<100	95%	72%	71%
Meds 'Always' Explained Before Given[10]	<100	63%	66%	64%
Nurses 'Always' Communicated Well[10]	<100	90%	80%	79%
Pain 'Always' Well Controlled[10]	<100	79%	72%	71%
Room and Bathroom 'Always' Clean[10]	<100	93%	73%	73%
Timely Help 'Always' Received[10]	<100	92%	71%	68%
Would Definitely Recommend Hospital[10]	<100	89%	71%	71%
Use of Medical Imaging				
Cardiac Imaging Stress Test before Surgery[7]	-	-	4.5%	5.3%
Combination Abdominal CT Scan[1]	-	-	23%	10.5%
Combination Brain/Sinus CT Scan	31	0.0%	2.2%	2.7%
Combination Chest CT Scan[1]	-	-	5.1%	2.7%
Follow-up Mammogram/Ultrasound[7]	-	-	8.1%	8.8%
Lumbar Spine MRI for Low Back Pain[7]	-	-	39.9%	37.2%

Hillcrest Hospital Cushing

1027 East Cherry Street　　Phone: 918-225-2915
Cushing, OK 74023　　Fax: 918-225-8202
URL: www.hillcrest.com/cushing
Type: Acute Care Hospitals　　Emergency Services: Yes
Ownership: Proprietary　　Beds: 99

Key Personnel:
Infection Control. . . . . Bernadine Allen, RN
Quality Assurance . . . . Bernadine Allen, RN
CEO/President. . . . . Ron Cackler
Operating Room. . . . . Fred J Crapse
Emergency Room . . . . Tom Dotson, MD
Chief of Medical Staff. . . . . Marylin Peck
Anesthesiology. . . . . Ray Shofner
Intensive Care Unit. . . . . Jane Stephens

Measure	Cases	This Hosp.	State Avg.	U.S. Avg.
Blood Clot Prevention and Treatment				
Anticoagulation Overlap Therapy[1,2]	-	-	89%	93%
ICU Venous Thromboembolism Prophylaxis[1,2]	-	-	87%	92%
Incidence of Potentially Preventable VTE[2,7]	-	-	8%	10%
UFH with Dosages/Platelet Monitoring[2,7]	-	-	97%	97%
Venous Thromboembolism Prophylaxis[2]	121	99%	72%	85%
Warfarin Therapy Discharge Instructions[1,2]	-	-	73%	75%
Chest Pain/Possible Heart Attack Care				
Aspirin Given Within 24 Hours of Arrival	116	98%	95%	96%
Fibrinolytic Meds Within 30 Min. of Arrival[7]	-	-	54%	58%
Average Time to ECG (minutes)	122	8	8	7
Average Time to Transfer (minutes)[1]	-	-	77	60
Children's Asthma Care				
Received Home Management Plan of Care	-	-	-	88%
Received Reliever Medication	-	-	-	100%
Received Systemic Corticosteroids	-	-	-	100%
Emergency Department				
Admittance Decision Time (minutes)[2]	310	53	63	98
Head CT Results Within 45 Min. of Arrival	12	8%	49%	57%
Patients Who Left ER Before Being Seen	10,465	5%	2%	2%
Time from ER Arrival to Admit. (minutes)[2]	316	236	210	274
Time from ER Arrival to Discharge (minutes)	323	143	110	134
Time in ER Before Being Evaluated (minutes)	378	28	24	26
Time to Pain Meds for Fractures (minutes)	59	64	55	57
Heart Attack Care				
Aspirin Given at Discharge[1,3]	-	-	99%	99%
Fibrinolytic Meds Within 30 Min. of Arrival[3,7]	-	-	25%	54%
PCI Within 90 Minutes of Arrival[3,7]	-	-	95%	96%
Statin Prescribed at Discharge[1,3]	-	-	98%	98%
Heart Failure Care				
ACE Inhibitor or ARB for LVSD	15	93%	95%	97%
Discharge Instructions Given	59	100%	92%	94%
Evaluation of LVS Function	63	100%	96%	99%
Medicare Spending				
Medicare Spending per Patient (ratio)	-	0.87	0.93	0.98
Pneumonia Care				
Appropriate Initial Antibiotic Given	68	99%	92%	95%
Blood Culture Timing	79	99%	97%	98%
Pregnancy and Delivery Care				
Newborn Deliveries Scheduled Early	12	0%	8%	6%
Preventive Care				
Immunization for Influenza[2]	259	99%	89%	90%
Immunization for Pneumonia[2]	309	100%	91%	92%
Stroke Care				
Anticoagulation Therapy for Atrial Fibrillation[7]	-	-	91%	95%
Antithrombotic Therapy Timing[1]	-	-	95%	98%
Assessed for Rehabilitation[1]	-	-	96%	97%
Discharged on Antithrombotic Therapy[1]	-	-	98%	99%
Discharged on Statin Medication[1]	-	-	88%	94%
Thrombolytic Therapy Timing[1]	-	-	61%	66%
Venous Thromboembolism Prophylaxis	11	55%	92%	94%
Written Stroke Educational Materials Given[1]	-	-	86%	88%
Surgical Care Improvement Project				
Appropriate Beta Blocker Usage	13	85%	97%	98%
Appropriate VTP Within 24 Hours	32	100%	97%	98%
Controlled Postoperative Blood Glucose[7]	-	-	97%	97%
Perioperative Temperature Management	38	100%	100%	100%
Prophylactic Antibiotic Selection	32	97%	99%	99%
Prophylactic Antibiotic Selection (Outpatient)	29	97%	98%	98%
Prophylactic Antibiotic Stopped	32	94%	98%	98%
Prophylactic Antibiotic Timing	32	100%	98%	99%
Prophylactic Antibiotic Timing (Outpatient)	29	100%	98%	98%
Urinary Catheter Removal	21	90%	96%	97%
Survey of Patients' Hospital Experiences				
Area Around Room 'Always' Quiet at Night	300+	61%	68%	61%
Doctors 'Always' Communicated Well	300+	83%	84%	82%
Home Recovery Information Given	300+	85%	84%	85%
Hospital Given 9 or 10 on 10 Point Scale	300+	70%	72%	71%
Meds 'Always' Explained Before Given	300+	63%	66%	64%
Nurses 'Always' Communicated Well	300+	79%	80%	79%
Pain 'Always' Well Controlled	300+	70%	72%	71%
Room and Bathroom 'Always' Clean	300+	65%	73%	73%
Timely Help 'Always' Received	300+	67%	71%	68%
Would Definitely Recommend Hospital	300+	66%	71%	71%
Use of Medical Imaging				
Cardiac Imaging Stress Test before Surgery	84	2.4%	4.5%	5.3%
Combination Abdominal CT Scan	199	30.2%	23%	10.5%
Combination Brain/Sinus CT Scan	197	1.0%	2.2%	2.7%
Combination Chest CT Scan	120	10.8%	5.1%	2.7%
Follow-up Mammogram/Ultrasound	170	11.2%	8.1%	8.8%
Lumbar Spine MRI for Low Back Pain	49	32.7%	39.9%	37.2%

Drumright Regional Hospital

610 West Bypass　　Phone: 918-382-2300
Drumright, OK 74030
Type: Critical Access Hospitals　　Emergency Services: Yes
Ownership: Proprietary

Measure	Cases	This Hosp.	State Avg.	U.S. Avg.
Blood Clot Prevention and Treatment				
Anticoagulation Overlap Therapy[5]	-	-	89%	93%
ICU Venous Thromboembolism Prophylaxis[5]	-	-	87%	92%
Incidence of Potentially Preventable VTE[5]	-	-	8%	10%
UFH with Dosages/Platelet Monitoring[5]	-	-	97%	97%
Venous Thromboembolism Prophylaxis[5]	-	-	72%	85%
Warfarin Therapy Discharge Instructions[5]	-	-	73%	75%
Chest Pain/Possible Heart Attack Care				
Aspirin Given Within 24 Hours of Arrival[1,3]	-	-	95%	96%
Fibrinolytic Meds Within 30 Min. of Arrival[3,7]	-	-	54%	58%
Average Time to ECG (minutes)[1,3]	-	-	8	7
Average Time to Transfer (minutes)[1,3]	-	-	77	60
Children's Asthma Care				
Received Home Management Plan of Care	-	-	-	88%
Received Reliever Medication	-	-	-	100%
Received Systemic Corticosteroids	-	-	-	100%
Emergency Department				
Admittance Decision Time (minutes)	231	27	63	98
Head CT Results Within 45 Min. of Arrival[3,7]	-	-	49%	57%
Patients Who Left ER Before Being Seen[5]	-	-	2%	2%
Time from ER Arrival to Admit. (minutes)	236	124	210	274
Time from ER Arrival to Discharge (minutes)	239	67	110	134
Time in ER Before Being Evaluated (minutes)	246	29	24	26
Time to Pain Meds for Fractures (minutes)[1,3]	-	-	55	57
Heart Attack Care				
Aspirin Given at Discharge[5]	-	-	99%	99%
Fibrinolytic Meds Within 30 Min. of Arrival[5]	-	-	25%	54%
PCI Within 90 Minutes of Arrival[5]	-	-	95%	96%
Statin Prescribed at Discharge[5]	-	-	98%	98%
Heart Failure Care				
ACE Inhibitor or ARB for LVSD[7]	-	-	95%	97%
Discharge Instructions Given	11	64%	92%	94%
Evaluation of LVS Function	16	62%	96%	99%
Medicare Spending				
Medicare Spending per Patient (ratio)	-	-	0.93	0.98
Pneumonia Care				
Appropriate Initial Antibiotic Given	19	89%	92%	95%
Blood Culture Timing[1]	-	-	97%	98%
Pregnancy and Delivery Care				
Newborn Deliveries Scheduled Early[5]	-	-	8%	6%
Preventive Care				
Immunization for Influenza	96	53%	89%	90%
Immunization for Pneumonia	121	67%	91%	92%
Stroke Care				
Anticoagulation Therapy for Atrial Fibrillation[5]	-	-	91%	95%
Antithrombotic Therapy Timing[5]	-	-	95%	98%
Assessed for Rehabilitation[5]	-	-	96%	97%
Discharged on Antithrombotic Therapy[5]	-	-	98%	99%
Discharged on Statin Medication[5]	-	-	88%	94%
Thrombolytic Therapy Timing[5]	-	-	61%	66%
Venous Thromboembolism Prophylaxis[5]	-	-	92%	94%
Written Stroke Educational Materials Given[5]	-	-	86%	88%
Surgical Care Improvement Project				
Appropriate Beta Blocker Usage[1]	-	-	97%	98%
Appropriate VTP Within 24 Hours	39	87%	97%	98%
Controlled Postoperative Blood Glucose[7]	-	-	97%	97%
Perioperative Temperature Management	39	100%	100%	100%
Prophylactic Antibiotic Selection	34	97%	99%	99%
Prophylactic Antibiotic Selection (Outpatient)[5]	-	-	98%	98%
Prophylactic Antibiotic Stopped	34	50%	98%	98%
Prophylactic Antibiotic Timing	34	94%	98%	99%
Prophylactic Antibiotic Timing (Outpatient)[5]	-	-	98%	98%
Urinary Catheter Removal[1]	-	-	96%	97%
Survey of Patients' Hospital Experiences				
Area Around Room 'Always' Quiet at Night[5]	-	-	68%	61%
Doctors 'Always' Communicated Well[5]	-	-	84%	82%

NOTE: Hospital profiles are in alphabetical order by state, then city, then hospital within the city; Rankings exclude hospitals with less than 25 cases except for patient surveys which excludes hospitals with less than 100 cases; (a) 100-299 cases; (1) The number of cases/patients is too few to report; (2) Data submitted were based on a sample of cases/patients; (3) Results are based on a shorter time period than required; (4) Data suppressed by CMS for one or more quarters; (5) Results are not available for this reporting period; (6) Fewer than 100 patients completed the HCAHPS survey; (7) No cases met the criteria for this measure; (8) The lower limit of the confidence interval cannot be calculated if the number of observed infections equals zero; (9) No data are available from the state/territory for this reporting period; (10) The scores shown reflect fewer than 50 completed surveys; (11) There were discrepancies in the data collection process; (12) This measure does not apply to this hospital for this reporting period; (13) Results cannot be calculated for this reporting period; (14) The results for this state are combined with nearby states to protect confidentiality; Please refer to the User's Guide for a full explanation of data.

Home Recovery Information Given[5]	-	-	84%	85%
Hospital Given 9 or 10 on 10 Point Scale[5]	-	-	72%	71%
Meds 'Always' Explained Before Given[5]	-	-	66%	64%
Nurses 'Always' Communicated Well[5]	-	-	80%	79%
Pain 'Always' Well Controlled[5]	-	-	72%	71%
Room and Bathroom 'Always' Clean[5]	-	-	73%	73%
Timely Help 'Always' Received[5]	-	-	71%	68%
Would Definitely Recommend Hospital[5]	-	-	71%	71%
Use of Medical Imaging				
Cardiac Imaging Stress Test before Surgery[1]	-	-	4.5%	5.3%
Combination Abdominal CT Scan	45	51.1%	23%	10.5%
Combination Brain/Sinus CT Scan[1]	-	-	2.2%	2.7%
Combination Chest CT Scan[1]	-	-	5.1%	2.7%
Follow-up Mammogram/Ultrasound[7]	-	-	8.1%	8.8%
Lumbar Spine MRI for Low Back Pain[1]	-	-	39.9%	37.2%

Duncan Regional Hospital

1407 Whisenant Drive
Duncan, OK 73533
Phone: 580-252-5300
Fax: 580-251-8559
URL: www.duncanregional.com
Type: Acute Care Hospitals
Emergency Services: Yes
Ownership: Proprietary
Beds: 152

Key Personnel:

Radiology. . . . . Curtis Holmes
CEO/President. . . . . Jay R. Johnson
Chief of Medical Staff. . . . . Jim McGooran, MD
Quality Assurance . . . . Deborah G. Rodgers
Surgery. Kristen Webb

Measure	Cases	This Hosp.	State Avg.	U.S. Avg.
Blood Clot Prevention and Treatment				
Anticoagulation Overlap Therapy[2]	30	97%	89%	93%
ICU Venous Thromboembolism Prophylaxis[2]	78	90%	87%	92%
Incidence of Potentially Preventable VTE[1,2]	-	-	8%	10%
UFH with Dosages/Platelet Monitoring[1,2]	-	-	97%	97%
Venous Thromboembolism Prophylaxis[2]	264	74%	72%	85%
Warfarin Therapy Discharge Instructions[2]	20	90%	73%	75%
Chest Pain/Possible Heart Attack Care				
Aspirin Given Within 24 Hours of Arrival	106	97%	95%	96%
Fibrinolytic Meds Within 30 Min. of Arrival[1]	-	-	54%	58%
Average Time to ECG (minutes)	106	3	8	7
Average Time to Transfer (minutes)[1]	-	-	77	60
Children's Asthma Care				
Received Home Management Plan of Care	-	-	-	88%
Received Reliever Medication	-	-	-	100%
Received Systemic Corticosteroids	-	-	-	100%
Emergency Department				
Admittance Decision Time (minutes)[2]	499	52	63	98
Head CT Results Within 45 Min. of Arrival	22	77%	49%	57%
Patients Who Left ER Before Being Seen	33,465	0%	2%	2%
Time from ER Arrival to Admit. (minutes)[2]	526	202	210	274
Time from ER Arrival to Discharge (minutes)	483	116	110	134
Time in ER Before Being Evaluated (minutes)	520	19	24	26
Time to Pain Meds for Fractures (minutes)	151	49	55	57
Heart Attack Care				
Aspirin Given at Discharge[1]	-	-	99%	99%
Fibrinolytic Meds Within 30 Min. of Arrival[7]	-	-	25%	54%
PCI Within 90 Minutes of Arrival[7]	-	-	95%	96%
Statin Prescribed at Discharge[1]	-	-	98%	98%
Heart Failure Care				
ACE Inhibitor or ARB for LVSD	33	100%	95%	97%
Discharge Instructions Given	77	100%	92%	94%
Evaluation of LVS Function	108	100%	96%	99%
Medicare Spending				
Medicare Spending per Patient (ratio)	-	0.94	0.93	0.98
Pneumonia Care				
Appropriate Initial Antibiotic Given	118	100%	92%	95%
Blood Culture Timing	218	99%	97%	98%
Pregnancy and Delivery Care				
Newborn Deliveries Scheduled Early	137	0%	8%	6%
Preventive Care				
Immunization for Influenza[2]	490	88%	89%	90%
Immunization for Pneumonia[2]	606	96%	91%	92%
Stroke Care				
Anticoagulation Therapy for Atrial Fibrillation[1]	-	-	91%	95%
Antithrombotic Therapy Timing	23	87%	95%	98%
Assessed for Rehabilitation	42	100%	96%	97%
Discharged on Antithrombotic Therapy	38	92%	98%	99%
Discharged on Statin Medication	24	92%	88%	94%
Thrombolytic Therapy Timing[7]	-	-	61%	66%
Venous Thromboembolism Prophylaxis	44	98%	92%	94%
Written Stroke Educational Materials Given	24	100%	86%	88%
Surgical Care Improvement Project				
Appropriate Beta Blocker Usage	108	100%	97%	98%
Appropriate VTP Within 24 Hours	323	100%	97%	98%
Controlled Postoperative Blood Glucose[7]	-	-	97%	97%
Perioperative Temperature Management	362	100%	100%	100%
Prophylactic Antibiotic Selection	261	100%	99%	99%
Prophylactic Antibiotic Selection (Outpatient)	57	98%	98%	98%
Prophylactic Antibiotic Stopped	257	98%	98%	98%
Prophylactic Antibiotic Timing	261	100%	98%	99%
Prophylactic Antibiotic Timing (Outpatient)	58	97%	98%	98%
Urinary Catheter Removal	77	97%	96%	97%
Survey of Patients' Hospital Experiences				
Area Around Room 'Always' Quiet at Night	300+	65%	68%	61%
Doctors 'Always' Communicated Well	300+	86%	84%	82%
Home Recovery Information Given	300+	87%	84%	85%
Hospital Given 9 or 10 on 10 Point Scale	300+	69%	72%	71%
Meds 'Always' Explained Before Given	300+	67%	66%	64%
Nurses 'Always' Communicated Well	300+	79%	80%	79%
Pain 'Always' Well Controlled	300+	74%	72%	71%
Room and Bathroom 'Always' Clean	300+	74%	73%	73%
Timely Help 'Always' Received	300+	72%	71%	68%
Would Definitely Recommend Hospital	300+	66%	71%	71%
Use of Medical Imaging				
Cardiac Imaging Stress Test before Surgery	168	7.7%	4.5%	5.3%
Combination Abdominal CT Scan	651	26.1%	23%	10.5%
Combination Brain/Sinus CT Scan	680	1.5%	2.2%	2.7%
Combination Chest CT Scan	518	0.0%	5.1%	2.7%
Follow-up Mammogram/Ultrasound	847	6.5%	8.1%	8.8%
Lumbar Spine MRI for Low Back Pain	125	43.2%	39.9%	37.2%

Medical Center of Southeastern Oklahoma

1800 University Boulevard
Durant, OK 74702
Phone: 405-924-3080
Fax: 580-924-0422
E-mail: info@mcsohealth.com
URL: www.mcsohealth.com
Type: Acute Care Hospitals
Emergency Services: Yes
Ownership: Proprietary
Beds: 103

Key Personnel:

Quality Assurance . . . . Belinda Butlan, RN
CEO . . . . Patricia Dorris
Operating Room. . . . . Pat Ferreri, RN
Infection Control. . . . . Vicki Fridle, MT ASCP
Chief of Medical Staff. . . . . Peter Hedberg, MD

Measure	Cases	This Hosp.	State Avg.	U.S. Avg.
Blood Clot Prevention and Treatment				
Anticoagulation Overlap Therapy[2]	21	100%	89%	93%
ICU Venous Thromboembolism Prophylaxis[2]	53	94%	87%	92%
Incidence of Potentially Preventable VTE[1,2]	-	-	8%	10%
UFH with Dosages/Platelet Monitoring[2,7]	-	-	97%	97%
Venous Thromboembolism Prophylaxis[2]	340	94%	72%	85%
Warfarin Therapy Discharge Instructions[2]	14	100%	73%	75%
Chest Pain/Possible Heart Attack Care				
Aspirin Given Within 24 Hours of Arrival	47	96%	95%	96%
Fibrinolytic Meds Within 30 Min. of Arrival[1]	-	-	54%	58%
Average Time to ECG (minutes)	52	10	8	7
Average Time to Transfer (minutes)[1]	-	-	77	60
Children's Asthma Care				
Received Home Management Plan of Care	-	-	-	88%
Received Reliever Medication	-	-	-	100%
Received Systemic Corticosteroids	-	-	-	100%
Emergency Department				
Admittance Decision Time (minutes)[2]	492	80	63	98
Head CT Results Within 45 Min. of Arrival	11	91%	49%	57%
Patients Who Left ER Before Being Seen	24,032	1%	2%	2%
Time from ER Arrival to Admit. (minutes)[2]	493	232	210	274
Time from ER Arrival to Discharge (minutes)	849	118	110	134
Time in ER Before Being Evaluated (minutes)	922	16	24	26
Time to Pain Meds for Fractures (minutes)	93	82	55	57
Heart Attack Care				
Aspirin Given at Discharge	63	92%	99%	99%
Fibrinolytic Meds Within 30 Min. of Arrival[1]	-	-	25%	54%
PCI Within 90 Minutes of Arrival[1]	-	-	95%	96%
Statin Prescribed at Discharge	59	97%	98%	98%
Heart Failure Care				
ACE Inhibitor or ARB for LVSD	62	100%	95%	97%
Discharge Instructions Given	148	93%	92%	94%
Evaluation of LVS Function	193	100%	96%	99%
Medicare Spending				
Medicare Spending per Patient (ratio)	-	0.94	0.93	0.98
Pneumonia Care				
Appropriate Initial Antibiotic Given	141	96%	92%	95%
Blood Culture Timing	217	97%	97%	98%
Pregnancy and Delivery Care				
Newborn Deliveries Scheduled Early	120	35%	8%	6%
Preventive Care				
Immunization for Influenza[2]	498	100%	89%	90%
Immunization for Pneumonia[2]	607	100%	91%	92%
Stroke Care				
Anticoagulation Therapy for Atrial Fibrillation[1]	-	-	91%	95%
Antithrombotic Therapy Timing	53	100%	95%	98%
Assessed for Rehabilitation	53	98%	96%	97%
Discharged on Antithrombotic Therapy	53	100%	98%	99%
Discharged on Statin Medication	42	93%	88%	94%
Thrombolytic Therapy Timing[7]	-	-	61%	66%
Venous Thromboembolism Prophylaxis	56	96%	92%	94%
Written Stroke Educational Materials Given	36	83%	86%	88%
Surgical Care Improvement Project				
Appropriate Beta Blocker Usage	23	91%	97%	98%
Appropriate VTP Within 24 Hours	183	95%	97%	98%
Controlled Postoperative Blood Glucose[7]	-	-	97%	97%
Perioperative Temperature Management	209	100%	100%	100%
Prophylactic Antibiotic Selection	147	98%	99%	99%
Prophylactic Antibiotic Selection (Outpatient)	228	98%	98%	98%
Prophylactic Antibiotic Stopped	142	99%	98%	98%
Prophylactic Antibiotic Timing	148	99%	98%	99%
Prophylactic Antibiotic Timing (Outpatient)	228	99%	98%	98%
Urinary Catheter Removal	128	97%	96%	97%
Survey of Patients' Hospital Experiences				
Area Around Room 'Always' Quiet at Night	300+	57%	68%	61%
Doctors 'Always' Communicated Well	300+	79%	84%	82%
Home Recovery Information Given	300+	74%	84%	85%
Hospital Given 9 or 10 on 10 Point Scale	300+	59%	72%	71%
Meds 'Always' Explained Before Given	300+	56%	66%	64%
Nurses 'Always' Communicated Well	300+	69%	80%	79%
Pain 'Always' Well Controlled	300+	65%	72%	71%
Room and Bathroom 'Always' Clean	300+	60%	73%	73%
Timely Help 'Always' Received	300+	55%	71%	68%
Would Definitely Recommend Hospital	300+	55%	71%	71%
Use of Medical Imaging				
Cardiac Imaging Stress Test before Surgery[1]	-	-	4.5%	5.3%
Combination Abdominal CT Scan	444	15.8%	23%	10.5%
Combination Brain/Sinus CT Scan	508	4.5%	2.2%	2.7%
Combination Chest CT Scan	190	0.5%	5.1%	2.7%
Follow-up Mammogram/Ultrasound	690	11.3%	8.1%	8.8%
Lumbar Spine MRI for Low Back Pain	80	33.8%	39.9%	37.2%

Integris Health Edmond

4801 Integris Parkway
Edmond, OK 73034
Phone: 405-657-3000
URL: www.integrisok.com/integris-health-edmond-ok
Type: Acute Care Hospitals
Emergency Services: Yes
Ownership: Voluntary non-profit - Private

Measure	Cases	This Hosp.	State Avg.	U.S. Avg.
Blood Clot Prevention and Treatment				
Anticoagulation Overlap Therapy[2]	16	81%	89%	93%
ICU Venous Thromboembolism Prophylaxis[2]	25	80%	87%	92%
Incidence of Potentially Preventable VTE[1,2]	-	-	8%	10%
UFH with Dosages/Platelet Monitoring[2,7]	-	-	97%	97%
Venous Thromboembolism Prophylaxis[2]	88	58%	72%	85%

NOTE: Hospital profiles are in alphabetical order by state, then city, then hospital within the city; Rankings exclude hospitals with less than 25 cases except for patient surveys which excludes hospitals with less than 100 cases; (a) 100-299 cases; (1) The number of cases/patients is too few to report; (2) Data submitted were based on a sample of cases/patients; (3) Results are based on a shorter time period than required; (4) Data suppressed by CMS for one or more quarters; (5) Results are not available for this reporting period; (6) Fewer than 100 patients completed the HCAHPS survey; (7) No cases met the criteria for this measure; (8) The lower limit of the confidence interval cannot be calculated if the number of observed infections equals zero; (9) No data are available from the state/territory for this reporting period; (10) The scores shown reflect fewer than 50 completed surveys; (11) There were discrepancies in the data collection process; (12) This measure does not apply to this hospital for this reporting period; (13) Results cannot be calculated for this reporting period; (14) The results for this state are combined with nearby states to protect confidentiality; Please refer to the User's Guide for a full explanation of data.

Measure	Cases	This Hosp.	State Avg.	U.S. Avg.
Warfarin Therapy Discharge Instructions[2]	12	100%	73%	75%
Chest Pain/Possible Heart Attack Care				
Aspirin Given Within 24 Hours of Arrival	16	100%	95%	96%
Fibrinolytic Meds Within 30 Min. of Arrival[3,7]	-	-	54%	58%
Average Time to ECG (minutes)	17	5	8	7
Average Time to Transfer (minutes)[1,3]	-	-	77	60
Children's Asthma Care				
Received Home Management Plan of Care	-	-	-	88%
Received Reliever Medication	-	-	-	100%
Received Systemic Corticosteroids	-	-	-	100%
Emergency Department				
Admittance Decision Time (minutes)[2]	270	55	63	98
Head CT Results Within 45 Min. of Arrival[1]	-	-	49%	57%
Patients Who Left ER Before Being Seen	11,280	0%	2%	2%
Time from ER Arrival to Admit. (minutes)[2]	274	184	210	274
Time from ER Arrival to Discharge (minutes)	356	104	110	134
Time in ER Before Being Evaluated (minutes)	287	13	24	26
Time to Pain Meds for Fractures (minutes)	68	39	55	57
Heart Attack Care				
Aspirin Given at Discharge[1]	-	-	99%	99%
Fibrinolytic Meds Within 30 Min. of Arrival[7]	-	-	25%	54%
PCI Within 90 Minutes of Arrival[7]	-	-	95%	96%
Statin Prescribed at Discharge[1]	-	-	98%	98%
Heart Failure Care				
ACE Inhibitor or ARB for LVSD	12	92%	95%	97%
Discharge Instructions Given	31	77%	92%	94%
Evaluation of LVS Function	32	94%	96%	99%
Medicare Spending				
Medicare Spending per Patient (ratio)	-	1.04	0.93	0.98
Pneumonia Care				
Appropriate Initial Antibiotic Given	50	92%	92%	95%
Blood Culture Timing	62	97%	97%	98%
Pregnancy and Delivery Care				
Newborn Deliveries Scheduled Early	31	13%	8%	6%
Preventive Care				
Immunization for Influenza[2]	237	93%	89%	90%
Immunization for Pneumonia[2]	256	95%	91%	92%
Stroke Care				
Anticoagulation Therapy for Atrial Fibrillation[7]	-	-	91%	95%
Antithrombotic Therapy Timing	13	92%	95%	98%
Assessed for Rehabilitation	13	100%	96%	97%
Discharged on Antithrombotic Therapy	13	100%	98%	99%
Discharged on Statin Medication[1]	-	-	88%	94%
Thrombolytic Therapy Timing[1]	-	-	61%	66%
Venous Thromboembolism Prophylaxis	12	58%	92%	94%
Written Stroke Educational Materials Given[1]	-	-	86%	88%
Surgical Care Improvement Project				
Appropriate Beta Blocker Usage[2]	36	97%	97%	98%
Appropriate VTP Within 24 Hours[2]	130	90%	97%	98%
Controlled Postoperative Blood Glucose[2,7]	-	-	97%	97%
Perioperative Temperature Management[2]	141	100%	100%	100%
Prophylactic Antibiotic Selection[2]	101	98%	99%	99%
Prophylactic Antibiotic Selection (Outpatient)	38	95%	98%	98%
Prophylactic Antibiotic Stopped[2]	100	97%	98%	98%
Prophylactic Antibiotic Timing[2]	101	99%	98%	99%
Prophylactic Antibiotic Timing (Outpatient)	23	91%	98%	98%
Urinary Catheter Removal[2]	40	95%	96%	97%
Survey of Patients' Hospital Experiences				
Area Around Room 'Always' Quiet at Night	300+	85%	68%	61%
Doctors 'Always' Communicated Well	300+	88%	84%	82%
Home Recovery Information Given	300+	88%	84%	85%
Hospital Given 9 or 10 on 10 Point Scale	300+	88%	72%	71%
Meds 'Always' Explained Before Given	300+	68%	66%	64%
Nurses 'Always' Communicated Well	300+	84%	80%	79%
Pain 'Always' Well Controlled	300+	77%	72%	71%
Room and Bathroom 'Always' Clean	300+	79%	73%	73%
Timely Help 'Always' Received	300+	74%	71%	68%
Would Definitely Recommend Hospital	300+	88%	71%	71%
Use of Medical Imaging				
Cardiac Imaging Stress Test before Surgery[1]	-	-	4.5%	5.3%
Combination Abdominal CT Scan	160	2.5%	23%	10.5%
Combination Brain/Sinus CT Scan[1]	-	-	2.2%	2.7%
Combination Chest CT Scan	75	0.0%	5.1%	2.7%
Follow-up Mammogram/Ultrasound	88	11.4%	8.1%	8.8%
Lumbar Spine MRI for Low Back Pain[1]	-	-	39.9%	37.2%

Summit Medical Center

1800 South Renaissance Boulevard Phone: 405-359-2400
Edmond, OK 73013
URL: www.weightwise.com
Type: Acute Care Hospitals Emergency Services: Yes
Ownership: Physician

Measure	Cases	This Hosp.	State Avg.	U.S. Avg.
Blood Clot Prevention and Treatment				
Anticoagulation Overlap Therapy[7]	-	-	89%	93%
ICU Venous Thromboembolism Prophylaxis[7]	-	-	87%	92%
Incidence of Potentially Preventable VTE[7]	-	-	8%	10%
UFH with Dosages/Platelet Monitoring[7]	-	-	97%	97%
Venous Thromboembolism Prophylaxis	60	90%	72%	85%
Warfarin Therapy Discharge Instructions[7]	-	-	73%	75%
Chest Pain/Possible Heart Attack Care				
Aspirin Given Within 24 Hours of Arrival[5]	-	-	95%	96%
Fibrinolytic Meds Within 30 Min. of Arrival[5]	-	-	54%	58%
Average Time to ECG (minutes)[5]	-	-	8	7
Average Time to Transfer (minutes)[5]	-	-	77	60
Children's Asthma Care				
Received Home Management Plan of Care	-	-	-	88%
Received Reliever Medication	-	-	-	100%
Received Systemic Corticosteroids	-	-	-	100%
Emergency Department				
Admittance Decision Time (minutes)[1]	-	-	63	98
Head CT Results Within 45 Min. of Arrival[5]	-	-	49%	57%
Patients Who Left ER Before Being Seen	115	0%	2%	2%
Time from ER Arrival to Admit. (minutes)[1]	-	-	210	274
Time from ER Arrival to Discharge (minutes)	68	283	110	134
Time in ER Before Being Evaluated (minutes)	40	122	24	26
Time to Pain Meds for Fractures (minutes)[5]	-	-	55	57
Heart Attack Care				
Aspirin Given at Discharge[5]	-	-	99%	99%
Fibrinolytic Meds Within 30 Min. of Arrival[5]	-	-	25%	54%
PCI Within 90 Minutes of Arrival[5]	-	-	95%	96%
Statin Prescribed at Discharge[5]	-	-	98%	98%
Heart Failure Care				
ACE Inhibitor or ARB for LVSD[5]	-	-	95%	97%
Discharge Instructions Given[5]	-	-	92%	94%
Evaluation of LVS Function[5]	-	-	96%	99%
Medicare Spending				
Medicare Spending per Patient (ratio)	-	1.11	0.93	0.98
Pneumonia Care				
Appropriate Initial Antibiotic Given[5]	-	-	92%	95%
Blood Culture Timing[5]	-	-	97%	98%
Pregnancy and Delivery Care				
Newborn Deliveries Scheduled Early[7]	-	-	8%	6%
Preventive Care				
Immunization for Influenza	128	19%	89%	90%
Immunization for Pneumonia	52	23%	91%	92%
Stroke Care				
Anticoagulation Therapy for Atrial Fibrillation[5]	-	-	91%	95%
Antithrombotic Therapy Timing[5]	-	-	95%	98%
Assessed for Rehabilitation[5]	-	-	96%	97%
Discharged on Antithrombotic Therapy[5]	-	-	98%	99%
Discharged on Statin Medication[5]	-	-	88%	94%
Thrombolytic Therapy Timing[5]	-	-	61%	66%
Venous Thromboembolism Prophylaxis[5]	-	-	92%	94%
Written Stroke Educational Materials Given[5]	-	-	86%	88%
Surgical Care Improvement Project				
Appropriate Beta Blocker Usage[1]	-	-	97%	98%
Appropriate VTP Within 24 Hours	41	93%	97%	98%
Controlled Postoperative Blood Glucose[7]	-	-	97%	97%
Perioperative Temperature Management	52	100%	100%	100%
Prophylactic Antibiotic Selection	36	100%	99%	99%
Prophylactic Antibiotic Selection (Outpatient)	171	99%	98%	98%
Prophylactic Antibiotic Stopped	36	100%	98%	98%
Prophylactic Antibiotic Timing	36	100%	98%	99%
Prophylactic Antibiotic Timing (Outpatient)	173	99%	98%	98%
Urinary Catheter Removal[1]	-	-	96%	97%
Survey of Patients' Hospital Experiences				
Area Around Room 'Always' Quiet at Night[6]	<100	79%	68%	61%
Doctors 'Always' Communicated Well[6]	<100	88%	84%	82%
Home Recovery Information Given[6]	<100	85%	84%	85%
Hospital Given 9 or 10 on 10 Point Scale[6]	<100	79%	72%	71%
Meds 'Always' Explained Before Given[6]	<100	66%	66%	64%
Nurses 'Always' Communicated Well[6]	<100	75%	80%	79%
Pain 'Always' Well Controlled[6]	<100	76%	72%	71%
Room and Bathroom 'Always' Clean[6]	<100	70%	73%	73%
Timely Help 'Always' Received[6]	<100	79%	71%	68%
Would Definitely Recommend Hospital[6]	<100	74%	71%	71%
Use of Medical Imaging				
Cardiac Imaging Stress Test before Surgery[7]	-	-	4.5%	5.3%
Combination Abdominal CT Scan[1]	-	-	23%	10.5%
Combination Brain/Sinus CT Scan[1]	-	-	2.2%	2.7%
Combination Chest CT Scan[1]	-	-	5.1%	2.7%
Follow-up Mammogram/Ultrasound[7]	-	-	8.1%	8.8%
Lumbar Spine MRI for Low Back Pain	85	30.6%	39.9%	37.2%

Mercy Hospital El Reno

2115 Park View Drive Phone: 405-262-2640
El Reno, OK 73036 Fax: 405-422-2521
URL: www.parkview-hospital.com
Type: Acute Care Hospitals Emergency Services: Yes
Ownership: Voluntary non-profit - Church Beds: 54

Key Personnel:
Radiology. . . . . Jane Bates, RT(R)
CEO/President. . . . . Lynn Britton
Infection Control. . . . . Claudi Eaton, RN
Quality Assurance . . . . Claudia Eaton
Chief of Medical Staff. . . . . Dr Michael Sullivan

Measure	Cases	This Hosp.	State Avg.	U.S. Avg.
Blood Clot Prevention and Treatment				
Anticoagulation Overlap Therapy[1,2]	-	-	89%	93%
ICU Venous Thromboembolism Prophylaxis[2,7]	-	-	87%	92%
Incidence of Potentially Preventable VTE[2,7]	-	-	8%	10%
UFH with Dosages/Platelet Monitoring[2,7]	-	-	97%	97%
Venous Thromboembolism Prophylaxis[2]	111	56%	72%	85%
Warfarin Therapy Discharge Instructions[2,7]	-	-	73%	75%
Chest Pain/Possible Heart Attack Care				
Aspirin Given Within 24 Hours of Arrival	13	92%	95%	96%
Fibrinolytic Meds Within 30 Min. of Arrival[1]	-	-	54%	58%
Average Time to ECG (minutes)	14	6	8	7
Average Time to Transfer (minutes)[1]	-	-	77	60
Children's Asthma Care				
Received Home Management Plan of Care	-	-	-	88%
Received Reliever Medication	-	-	-	100%
Received Systemic Corticosteroids	-	-	-	100%
Emergency Department				
Admittance Decision Time (minutes)	236	82	63	98
Head CT Results Within 45 Min. of Arrival[1]	-	-	49%	57%
Patients Who Left ER Before Being Seen	9,639	1%	2%	2%
Time from ER Arrival to Admit. (minutes)	249	224	210	274
Time from ER Arrival to Discharge (minutes)	357	111	110	134
Time in ER Before Being Evaluated (minutes)	379	19	24	26
Time to Pain Meds for Fractures (minutes)	32	26	55	57
Heart Attack Care				
Aspirin Given at Discharge[5]	-	-	99%	99%
Fibrinolytic Meds Within 30 Min. of Arrival[5]	-	-	25%	54%
PCI Within 90 Minutes of Arrival[5]	-	-	95%	96%
Statin Prescribed at Discharge[5]	-	-	98%	98%
Heart Failure Care				
ACE Inhibitor or ARB for LVSD[1]	-	-	95%	97%
Discharge Instructions Given[1]	-	-	92%	94%
Evaluation of LVS Function	12	92%	96%	99%
Medicare Spending				
Medicare Spending per Patient (ratio)	-	1.03	0.93	0.98
Pneumonia Care				
Appropriate Initial Antibiotic Given	34	94%	92%	95%
Blood Culture Timing	31	97%	97%	98%
Pregnancy and Delivery Care				
Newborn Deliveries Scheduled Early[2,7]	-	-	8%	6%

NOTE: Hospital profiles are in alphabetical order by state, then city, then hospital within the city; Rankings exclude hospitals with less than 25 cases except for patient surveys which excludes hospitals with less than 100 cases; (a) 100-299 cases; (1) The number of cases/patients is too few to report; (2) Data submitted were based on a sample of cases/patients; (3) Results are based on a shorter time period than required; (4) Data suppressed by CMS for one or more quarters; (5) Results are not available for this reporting period; (6) Fewer than 100 patients completed the HCAHPS survey; (7) No cases met the criteria for this measure; (8) The lower limit of the confidence interval cannot be calculated if the number of observed infections equals zero; (9) No data are available from the state/territory for this reporting period; (10) The scores shown reflect fewer than 50 completed surveys; (11) There were discrepancies in the data collection process; (12) This measure does not apply to this hospital for this reporting period; (13) Results cannot be calculated for this reporting period; (14) The results for this state are combined with nearby states to protect confidentiality; Please refer to the User's Guide for a full explanation of data.

Preventive Care				
Immunization for Influenza	251	88%	89%	90%
Immunization for Pneumonia	379	91%	91%	92%
Stroke Care				
Anticoagulation Therapy for Atrial Fibrillation[7]	-	-	91%	95%
Antithrombotic Therapy Timing[1]	-	-	95%	98%
Assessed for Rehabilitation[1]	-	-	96%	97%
Discharged on Antithrombotic Therapy[1]	-	-	98%	99%
Discharged on Statin Medication[1]	-	-	88%	94%
Thrombolytic Therapy Timing[7]	-	-	61%	66%
Venous Thromboembolism Prophylaxis[1]	-	-	92%	94%
Written Stroke Educational Materials Given[1]	-	-	86%	88%
Surgical Care Improvement Project				
Appropriate Beta Blocker Usage[7]	-	-	97%	98%
Appropriate VTP Within 24 Hours[1]	-	-	97%	98%
Controlled Postoperative Blood Glucose[7]	-	-	97%	97%
Perioperative Temperature Management[1]	-	-	100%	100%
Prophylactic Antibiotic Selection[7]	-	-	99%	99%
Prophylactic Antibiotic Selection (Outpatient)[1,3]	-	-	98%	98%
Prophylactic Antibiotic Stopped[7]	-	-	98%	98%
Prophylactic Antibiotic Timing[1]	-	-	98%	99%
Prophylactic Antibiotic Timing (Outpatient)[1,3]	-	-	98%	98%
Urinary Catheter Removal[1]	-	-	96%	97%
Survey of Patients' Hospital Experiences				
Area Around Room 'Always' Quiet at Night[6,11]	<100	73%	68%	61%
Doctors 'Always' Communicated Well[6,11]	<100	87%	84%	82%
Home Recovery Information Given[6,11]	<100	85%	84%	85%
Hospital Given 9 or 10 on 10 Point Scale[6,11]	<100	64%	72%	71%
Meds 'Always' Explained Before Given[6,11]	<100	72%	66%	64%
Nurses 'Always' Communicated Well[6,11]	<100	76%	80%	79%
Pain 'Always' Well Controlled[6,11]	<100	72%	72%	71%
Room and Bathroom 'Always' Clean[6,11]	<100	63%	73%	73%
Timely Help 'Always' Received[6,11]	<100	65%	71%	68%
Would Definitely Recommend Hospital[6,11]	<100	61%	71%	71%
Use of Medical Imaging				
Cardiac Imaging Stress Test before Surgery[7]	-	-	4.5%	5.3%
Combination Abdominal CT Scan	109	11.9%	23%	10.5%
Combination Brain/Sinus CT Scan[1]	-	-	2.2%	2.7%
Combination Chest CT Scan	49	4.1%	5.1%	2.7%
Follow-up Mammogram/Ultrasound[7]	-	-	8.1%	8.8%
Lumbar Spine MRI for Low Back Pain[1]	-	-	39.9%	37.2%

Great Plains Regional Medical Center

1801 West 3rd Street
Elk City, OK 73644
Phone: 580-225-2511
Fax: 580-225-9143
URL: www.gprmc-ok.com
Type: Acute Care Hospitals
Emergency Services: Yes
Ownership: Voluntary non-profit - Private
Beds: 62

Key Personnel:
Chief of Medical Staff. . . . . Francis Abraham
Quality Assurance . . . . Kimmy Davis
Operating Room. . . . . Gwen Fuchs
Emergency Room . . . . Jacob Krajicek, DO
Chairman/CEO . . . . Paul Kumpf
CEO/President. . . . . Corey Lively
Radiology. . . . . Duane Mills
Intensive Care Unit. . . . . Debra Morris

Measure	Cases	This Hosp.	State Avg.	U.S. Avg.
Blood Clot Prevention and Treatment				
Anticoagulation Overlap Therapy[2]	11	82%	89%	93%
ICU Venous Thromboembolism Prophylaxis[2]	48	83%	87%	92%
Incidence of Potentially Preventable VTE[2,7]	-	-	8%	10%
UFH with Dosages/Platelet Monitoring[2,7]	-	-	97%	97%
Venous Thromboembolism Prophylaxis[2]	85	79%	72%	85%
Warfarin Therapy Discharge Instructions[1,2]	-	-	73%	75%
Chest Pain/Possible Heart Attack Care				
Aspirin Given Within 24 Hours of Arrival	28	100%	95%	96%
Fibrinolytic Meds Within 30 Min. of Arrival[1]	-	-	54%	58%
Average Time to ECG (minutes)	31	9	8	7
Average Time to Transfer (minutes)[1]	-	-	77	60
Children's Asthma Care				
Received Home Management Plan of Care	-	-	-	88%
Received Reliever Medication	-	-	-	100%
Received Systemic Corticosteroids	-	-	-	100%
Emergency Department				
Admittance Decision Time (minutes)[2]	215	54	63	98
Head CT Results Within 45 Min. of Arrival[1]	-	-	49%	57%
Patients Who Left ER Before Being Seen	12,698	1%	2%	2%
Time from ER Arrival to Admit. (minutes)[2]	242	213	210	274
Time from ER Arrival to Discharge (minutes)	381	116	110	134
Time in ER Before Being Evaluated (minutes)	407	28	24	26
Time to Pain Meds for Fractures (minutes)	60	55	55	57
Heart Attack Care				
Aspirin Given at Discharge[1,3]	-	-	99%	99%
Fibrinolytic Meds Within 30 Min. of Arrival[3,7]	-	-	25%	54%
PCI Within 90 Minutes of Arrival[3,7]	-	-	95%	96%
Statin Prescribed at Discharge[1,3]	-	-	98%	98%
Heart Failure Care				
ACE Inhibitor or ARB for LVSD	13	100%	95%	97%
Discharge Instructions Given	24	92%	92%	94%
Evaluation of LVS Function	37	97%	96%	99%
Medicare Spending				
Medicare Spending per Patient (ratio)	-	0.90	0.93	0.98
Pneumonia Care				
Appropriate Initial Antibiotic Given	40	75%	92%	95%
Blood Culture Timing	101	91%	97%	98%
Pregnancy and Delivery Care				
Newborn Deliveries Scheduled Early[2]	34	15%	8%	6%
Preventive Care				
Immunization for Influenza[2]	236	84%	89%	90%
Immunization for Pneumonia[2]	235	89%	91%	92%
Stroke Care				
Anticoagulation Therapy for Atrial Fibrillation[1]	-	-	91%	95%
Antithrombotic Therapy Timing	11	100%	95%	98%
Assessed for Rehabilitation	14	86%	96%	97%
Discharged on Antithrombotic Therapy	13	100%	98%	99%
Discharged on Statin Medication	12	75%	88%	94%
Thrombolytic Therapy Timing[1]	-	-	61%	66%
Venous Thromboembolism Prophylaxis	12	75%	92%	94%
Written Stroke Educational Materials Given[1]	-	-	86%	88%
Surgical Care Improvement Project				
Appropriate Beta Blocker Usage[2]	19	100%	97%	98%
Appropriate VTP Within 24 Hours[2]	117	97%	97%	98%
Controlled Postoperative Blood Glucose[2,7]	-	-	97%	97%
Perioperative Temperature Management[2]	122	99%	100%	100%
Prophylactic Antibiotic Selection[2]	94	93%	99%	99%
Prophylactic Antibiotic Selection (Outpatient)	18	100%	98%	98%
Prophylactic Antibiotic Stopped[2]	83	100%	98%	98%
Prophylactic Antibiotic Timing[2]	94	98%	98%	99%
Prophylactic Antibiotic Timing (Outpatient)	18	100%	98%	98%
Urinary Catheter Removal[2]	27	89%	96%	97%
Survey of Patients' Hospital Experiences				
Area Around Room 'Always' Quiet at Night	300+	68%	68%	61%
Doctors 'Always' Communicated Well	300+	82%	84%	82%
Home Recovery Information Given	300+	83%	84%	85%
Hospital Given 9 or 10 on 10 Point Scale	300+	65%	72%	71%
Meds 'Always' Explained Before Given	300+	53%	66%	64%
Nurses 'Always' Communicated Well	300+	78%	80%	79%
Pain 'Always' Well Controlled	300+	70%	72%	71%
Room and Bathroom 'Always' Clean	300+	72%	73%	73%
Timely Help 'Always' Received	300+	71%	71%	68%
Would Definitely Recommend Hospital	300+	66%	71%	71%
Use of Medical Imaging				
Cardiac Imaging Stress Test before Surgery	119	6.7%	4.5%	5.3%
Combination Abdominal CT Scan	255	22.7%	23%	10.5%
Combination Brain/Sinus CT Scan[1]	-	-	2.2%	2.7%
Combination Chest CT Scan	138	19.6%	5.1%	2.7%
Follow-up Mammogram/Ultrasound	275	8.7%	8.1%	8.8%
Lumbar Spine MRI for Low Back Pain	76	42.1%	39.9%	37.2%

Integris Bass Baptist Health Center

600 South Monroe
Enid, OK 73701
Phone: 580-233-2300
Fax: 580-233-8922
URL: www.integris-health.com/facilities
Type: Acute Care Hospitals
Emergency Services: Yes
Ownership: Voluntary non-profit - Private
Beds: 253

Measure	Cases	This Hosp.	State Avg.	U.S. Avg.
Blood Clot Prevention and Treatment				
Anticoagulation Overlap Therapy[2]	15	93%	89%	93%
ICU Venous Thromboembolism Prophylaxis[2]	44	61%	87%	92%
Incidence of Potentially Preventable VTE[1,2]	-	-	8%	10%
UFH with Dosages/Platelet Monitoring[1,2]	-	-	97%	97%
Venous Thromboembolism Prophylaxis[2]	251	55%	72%	85%
Warfarin Therapy Discharge Instructions[1,2]	-	-	73%	75%
Chest Pain/Possible Heart Attack Care				
Aspirin Given Within 24 Hours of Arrival[1,3]	-	-	95%	96%
Fibrinolytic Meds Within 30 Min. of Arrival[5]	-	-	54%	58%
Average Time to ECG (minutes)[1,3]	-	-	8	7
Average Time to Transfer (minutes)[5]	-	-	77	60
Children's Asthma Care				
Received Home Management Plan of Care	-	-	-	88%
Received Reliever Medication	-	-	-	100%
Received Systemic Corticosteroids	-	-	-	100%
Emergency Department				
Admittance Decision Time (minutes)[2]	350	61	63	98
Head CT Results Within 45 Min. of Arrival[1]	-	-	49%	57%
Patients Who Left ER Before Being Seen	22,166	3%	2%	2%
Time from ER Arrival to Admit. (minutes)[2]	363	222	210	274
Time from ER Arrival to Discharge (minutes)	368	106	110	134
Time in ER Before Being Evaluated (minutes)	145	46	24	26
Time to Pain Meds for Fractures (minutes)	71	51	55	57
Heart Attack Care				
Aspirin Given at Discharge	52	98%	99%	99%
Fibrinolytic Meds Within 30 Min. of Arrival[7]	-	-	25%	54%
PCI Within 90 Minutes of Arrival[1]	-	-	95%	96%
Statin Prescribed at Discharge	53	96%	98%	98%
Heart Failure Care				
ACE Inhibitor or ARB for LVSD	40	100%	95%	97%
Discharge Instructions Given	71	100%	92%	94%
Evaluation of LVS Function	106	100%	96%	99%
Medicare Spending				
Medicare Spending per Patient (ratio)	-	1.02	0.93	0.98
Pneumonia Care				
Appropriate Initial Antibiotic Given	59	97%	92%	95%
Blood Culture Timing	116	99%	97%	98%
Pregnancy and Delivery Care				
Newborn Deliveries Scheduled Early[2]	127	2%	8%	6%
Preventive Care				
Immunization for Influenza[2]	440	95%	89%	90%
Immunization for Pneumonia[2]	405	98%	91%	92%
Stroke Care				
Anticoagulation Therapy for Atrial Fibrillation[1]	-	-	91%	95%
Antithrombotic Therapy Timing	35	100%	95%	98%
Assessed for Rehabilitation	42	90%	96%	97%
Discharged on Antithrombotic Therapy	37	95%	98%	99%
Discharged on Statin Medication	33	82%	88%	94%
Thrombolytic Therapy Timing[1]	-	-	61%	66%
Venous Thromboembolism Prophylaxis	43	67%	92%	94%
Written Stroke Educational Materials Given	22	82%	86%	88%
Surgical Care Improvement Project				
Appropriate Beta Blocker Usage	78	91%	97%	98%
Appropriate VTP Within 24 Hours	188	93%	97%	98%
Controlled Postoperative Blood Glucose	49	98%	97%	97%
Perioperative Temperature Management	254	100%	100%	100%
Prophylactic Antibiotic Selection	180	98%	99%	99%
Prophylactic Antibiotic Selection (Outpatient)	69	97%	98%	98%
Prophylactic Antibiotic Stopped	180	99%	98%	98%
Prophylactic Antibiotic Timing	181	94%	98%	99%
Prophylactic Antibiotic Timing (Outpatient)	71	96%	98%	98%
Urinary Catheter Removal	134	96%	96%	97%
Survey of Patients' Hospital Experiences				
Area Around Room 'Always' Quiet at Night	300+	57%	68%	61%

NOTE: Hospital profiles are in alphabetical order by state, then city, then hospital within the city; Rankings exclude hospitals with less than 25 cases except for patient surveys which excludes hospitals with less than 100 cases; (a) 100-299 cases; (1) The number of cases/patients is too few to report; (2) Data submitted were based on a sample of cases/patients; (3) Results are based on a shorter time period than required; (4) Data suppressed by CMS for one or more quarters; (5) Results are not available for this reporting period; (6) Fewer than 100 patients completed the HCAHPS survey; (7) No cases met the criteria for this measure; (8) The lower limit of the confidence interval cannot be calculated if the number of observed infections equals zero; (9) No data are available from the state/territory for this reporting period; (10) The scores shown reflect fewer than 50 completed surveys; (11) There were discrepancies in the data collection process; (12) This measure does not apply to this hospital for this reporting period; (13) Results cannot be calculated for this reporting period; (14) The results for this state are combined with nearby states to protect confidentiality; Please refer to the User's Guide for a full explanation of data.

Measure	Cases	This Hosp.	State Avg.	U.S. Avg.
Doctors 'Always' Communicated Well	300+	82%	84%	82%
Home Recovery Information Given	300+	82%	84%	85%
Hospital Given 9 or 10 on 10 Point Scale	300+	68%	72%	71%
Meds 'Always' Explained Before Given	300+	62%	66%	64%
Nurses 'Always' Communicated Well	300+	76%	80%	79%
Pain 'Always' Well Controlled	300+	70%	72%	71%
Room and Bathroom 'Always' Clean	300+	67%	73%	73%
Timely Help 'Always' Received	300+	69%	71%	68%
Would Definitely Recommend Hospital	300+	72%	71%	71%
Use of Medical Imaging				
Cardiac Imaging Stress Test before Surgery	403	4.0%	4.5%	5.3%
Combination Abdominal CT Scan	477	11.9%	23%	10.5%
Combination Brain/Sinus CT Scan[1]	-	-	2.2%	2.7%
Combination Chest CT Scan	509	1.4%	5.1%	2.7%
Follow-up Mammogram/Ultrasound	722	9.1%	8.1%	8.8%
Lumbar Spine MRI for Low Back Pain	95	45.3%	39.9%	37.2%

Saint Mary's Regional Medical Center

305 South 5th Street
Enid, OK 73701
Phone: 580-233-6100
Fax: 580-249-3982
URL: www.stmarysregional.com
Type: Acute Care Hospitals
Emergency Services: Yes
Ownership: Proprietary
Beds: 245

Key Personnel:
Patient Relations . . . . Verla Holguin
Coronary Care . . . . Virginia McCall
Intensive Care Unit. . . . . Virginia McCall
Pediatric In-Patient Care . . . . . . Kathy Niswander
Operating Room. . . . . Robert Ritter
Quality Assurance . . . . Ann Thain
CEO/President. . . . . Rick Wallace
Infection Control. . . . . Janie Word

Measure	Cases	This Hosp.	State Avg.	U.S. Avg.
Blood Clot Prevention and Treatment				
Anticoagulation Overlap Therapy[2]	23	96%	89%	93%
ICU Venous Thromboembolism Prophylaxis[2]	62	89%	87%	92%
Incidence of Potentially Preventable VTE[1,2]	-	-	8%	10%
UFH with Dosages/Platelet Monitoring[1,2]	-	-	97%	97%
Venous Thromboembolism Prophylaxis[2]	343	85%	72%	85%
Warfarin Therapy Discharge Instructions[2]	13	85%	73%	75%
Chest Pain/Possible Heart Attack Care				
Aspirin Given Within 24 Hours of Arrival[1,3]	-	-	95%	96%
Fibrinolytic Meds Within 30 Min. of Arrival[3,7]	-	-	54%	58%
Average Time to ECG (minutes)[1,3]	-	-	8	7
Average Time to Transfer (minutes)[3,7]	-	-	77	60
Children's Asthma Care				
Received Home Management Plan of Care	-	-	-	88%
Received Reliever Medication	-	-	-	100%
Received Systemic Corticosteroids	-	-	-	100%
Emergency Department				
Admittance Decision Time (minutes)[2]	418	50	63	98
Head CT Results Within 45 Min. of Arrival[3,7]	-	-	49%	57%
Patients Who Left ER Before Being Seen	18,861	2%	2%	2%
Time from ER Arrival to Admit. (minutes)[2]	473	194	210	274
Time from ER Arrival to Discharge (minutes)	411	128	110	134
Time in ER Before Being Evaluated (minutes)	426	33	24	26
Time to Pain Meds for Fractures (minutes)	82	42	55	57
Heart Attack Care				
Aspirin Given at Discharge	48	98%	99%	99%
Fibrinolytic Meds Within 30 Min. of Arrival[7]	-	-	25%	54%
PCI Within 90 Minutes of Arrival[1]	-	-	95%	96%
Statin Prescribed at Discharge	39	100%	98%	98%
Heart Failure Care				
ACE Inhibitor or ARB for LVSD	25	100%	95%	97%
Discharge Instructions Given	81	86%	92%	94%
Evaluation of LVS Function	123	100%	96%	99%
Medicare Spending				
Medicare Spending per Patient (ratio)	-	0.95	0.93	0.98
Pneumonia Care				
Appropriate Initial Antibiotic Given[2]	79	97%	92%	95%
Blood Culture Timing[2]	124	99%	97%	98%
Pregnancy and Delivery Care				
Newborn Deliveries Scheduled Early[2]	27	11%	8%	6%
Preventive Care				
Immunization for Influenza[2]	469	88%	89%	90%
Immunization for Pneumonia[2]	626	88%	91%	92%
Stroke Care				
Anticoagulation Therapy for Atrial Fibrillation[1]	-	-	91%	95%
Antithrombotic Therapy Timing	45	100%	95%	98%
Assessed for Rehabilitation	55	100%	96%	97%
Discharged on Antithrombotic Therapy	49	100%	98%	99%
Discharged on Statin Medication	34	97%	88%	94%
Thrombolytic Therapy Timing[1]	-	-	61%	66%
Venous Thromboembolism Prophylaxis	60	92%	92%	94%
Written Stroke Educational Materials Given	20	90%	86%	88%
Surgical Care Improvement Project				
Appropriate Beta Blocker Usage[2]	93	99%	97%	98%
Appropriate VTP Within 24 Hours[2]	335	99%	97%	98%
Controlled Postoperative Blood Glucose[2,7]	-	-	97%	97%
Perioperative Temperature Management[2]	382	100%	100%	100%
Prophylactic Antibiotic Selection[2]	248	98%	99%	99%
Prophylactic Antibiotic Selection (Outpatient)	235	97%	98%	98%
Prophylactic Antibiotic Stopped[2]	242	100%	98%	98%
Prophylactic Antibiotic Timing[2]	248	98%	98%	99%
Prophylactic Antibiotic Timing (Outpatient)	233	99%	98%	98%
Urinary Catheter Removal[2]	87	97%	96%	97%
Survey of Patients' Hospital Experiences				
Area Around Room 'Always' Quiet at Night	300+	62%	68%	61%
Doctors 'Always' Communicated Well	300+	85%	84%	82%
Home Recovery Information Given	300+	89%	84%	85%
Hospital Given 9 or 10 on 10 Point Scale	300+	76%	72%	71%
Meds 'Always' Explained Before Given	300+	64%	66%	64%
Nurses 'Always' Communicated Well	300+	79%	80%	79%
Pain 'Always' Well Controlled	300+	71%	72%	71%
Room and Bathroom 'Always' Clean	300+	69%	73%	73%
Timely Help 'Always' Received	300+	66%	71%	68%
Would Definitely Recommend Hospital	300+	76%	71%	71%
Use of Medical Imaging				
Cardiac Imaging Stress Test before Surgery	185	3.8%	4.5%	5.3%
Combination Abdominal CT Scan	662	22.2%	23%	10.5%
Combination Brain/Sinus CT Scan[1]	-	-	2.2%	2.7%
Combination Chest CT Scan	440	1.8%	5.1%	2.7%
Follow-up Mammogram/Ultrasound	1,575	8.8%	8.1%	8.8%
Lumbar Spine MRI for Low Back Pain	168	41.1%	39.9%	37.2%

Epic Medical Center

1 Hospital Drive
Eufaula, OK 74432
Phone: 918-689-2535
Fax: 918-689-7285
Type: Acute Care Hospitals
Emergency Services: Yes
Ownership: Proprietary
Beds: 33

Key Personnel:
Quality Assurance . . . . Jerry Manning
Emergency Room . . . . Dorothy Merrick
Infection Control. . . . . Dorothy Merrick
CEO/President. . . . . Daniel Schaecvle
Operating Room. . . . . Vanessa Williams, RN

Measure	Cases	This Hosp.	State Avg.	U.S. Avg.
Blood Clot Prevention and Treatment				
Anticoagulation Overlap Therapy[7]	-	-	89%	93%
ICU Venous Thromboembolism Prophylaxis[7]	-	-	87%	92%
Incidence of Potentially Preventable VTE[7]	-	-	8%	10%
UFH with Dosages/Platelet Monitoring[7]	-	-	97%	97%
Venous Thromboembolism Prophylaxis	77	16%	72%	85%
Warfarin Therapy Discharge Instructions[7]	-	-	73%	75%
Chest Pain/Possible Heart Attack Care				
Aspirin Given Within 24 Hours of Arrival[3]	11	100%	95%	96%
Fibrinolytic Meds Within 30 Min. of Arrival[1,3]	-	-	54%	58%
Average Time to ECG (minutes)[3]	13	5	8	7
Average Time to Transfer (minutes)[1,3]	-	-	77	60
Children's Asthma Care				
Received Home Management Plan of Care	-	-	-	88%
Received Reliever Medication	-	-	-	100%
Received Systemic Corticosteroids	-	-	-	100%
Emergency Department				
Admittance Decision Time (minutes)[2]	53	40	63	98
Head CT Results Within 45 Min. of Arrival[7]	-	-	49%	57%
Patients Who Left ER Before Being Seen	5,870	2%	2%	2%
Time from ER Arrival to Admit. (minutes)[2]	75	159	210	274
Time from ER Arrival to Discharge (minutes)	219	85	110	134
Time in ER Before Being Evaluated (minutes)	246	25	24	26
Time to Pain Meds for Fractures (minutes)	13	70	55	57
Heart Attack Care				
Aspirin Given at Discharge[5]	-	-	99%	99%
Fibrinolytic Meds Within 30 Min. of Arrival[5]	-	-	25%	54%
PCI Within 90 Minutes of Arrival[5]	-	-	95%	96%
Statin Prescribed at Discharge[5]	-	-	98%	98%
Heart Failure Care				
ACE Inhibitor or ARB for LVSD[7]	-	-	95%	97%
Discharge Instructions Given[1]	-	-	92%	94%
Evaluation of LVS Function[1]	-	-	96%	99%
Medicare Spending				
Medicare Spending per Patient (ratio)	-	0.73	0.93	0.98
Pneumonia Care				
Appropriate Initial Antibiotic Given[1]	-	-	92%	95%
Blood Culture Timing[1]	-	-	97%	98%
Pregnancy and Delivery Care				
Newborn Deliveries Scheduled Early[7]	-	-	8%	6%
Preventive Care				
Immunization for Influenza	50	68%	89%	90%
Immunization for Pneumonia	76	70%	91%	92%
Stroke Care				
Anticoagulation Therapy for Atrial Fibrillation[5]	-	-	91%	95%
Antithrombotic Therapy Timing[5]	-	-	95%	98%
Assessed for Rehabilitation[5]	-	-	96%	97%
Discharged on Antithrombotic Therapy[5]	-	-	98%	99%
Discharged on Statin Medication[5]	-	-	88%	94%
Thrombolytic Therapy Timing[5]	-	-	61%	66%
Venous Thromboembolism Prophylaxis[5]	-	-	92%	94%
Written Stroke Educational Materials Given[5]	-	-	86%	88%
Surgical Care Improvement Project				
Appropriate Beta Blocker Usage[5]	-	-	97%	98%
Appropriate VTP Within 24 Hours[5]	-	-	97%	98%
Controlled Postoperative Blood Glucose[5]	-	-	97%	97%
Perioperative Temperature Management[5]	-	-	100%	100%
Prophylactic Antibiotic Selection[5]	-	-	99%	99%
Prophylactic Antibiotic Selection (Outpatient)[7]	-	-	98%	98%
Prophylactic Antibiotic Stopped[5]	-	-	98%	98%
Prophylactic Antibiotic Timing[5]	-	-	98%	99%
Prophylactic Antibiotic Timing (Outpatient)[1]	-	-	98%	98%
Urinary Catheter Removal[5]	-	-	96%	97%
Survey of Patients' Hospital Experiences				
Area Around Room 'Always' Quiet at Night[10]	<100	75%	68%	61%
Doctors 'Always' Communicated Well[10]	<100	85%	84%	82%
Home Recovery Information Given[10]	<100	90%	84%	85%
Hospital Given 9 or 10 on 10 Point Scale[10]	<100	60%	72%	71%
Meds 'Always' Explained Before Given[10]	<100	98%	66%	64%
Nurses 'Always' Communicated Well[10]	<100	85%	80%	79%
Pain 'Always' Well Controlled[10]	<100	81%	72%	71%
Room and Bathroom 'Always' Clean[10]	<100	56%	73%	73%
Timely Help 'Always' Received[10]	<100	92%	71%	68%
Would Definitely Recommend Hospital[10]	<100	64%	71%	71%
Use of Medical Imaging				
Cardiac Imaging Stress Test before Surgery[7]	-	-	4.5%	5.3%
Combination Abdominal CT Scan[7]	-	-	23%	10.5%
Combination Brain/Sinus CT Scan[7]	-	-	2.2%	2.7%
Combination Chest CT Scan[7]	-	-	5.1%	2.7%
Follow-up Mammogram/Ultrasound[7]	-	-	8.1%	8.8%
Lumbar Spine MRI for Low Back Pain[7]	-	-	39.9%	37.2%

Fairfax Community Hospital

40 Hospital Road
Fairfax, OK 74637
Phone: 918-642-3291
Fax: 918-642-5161
Type: Critical Access Hospitals
Emergency Services: Yes
Ownership: Proprietary
Beds: 21

Key Personnel:
Quality Assurance . . . . Tammy Gibson
Chief of Medical Staff . . . . James Graham
CEO . . . . Tina Steele

Measure	Cases	This Hosp.	State Avg.	U.S. Avg.
Blood Clot Prevention and Treatment				

NOTE: Hospital profiles are in alphabetical order by state, then city, then hospital within the city; Rankings exclude hospitals with less than 25 cases except for patient surveys which excludes hospitals with less than 100 cases; (a) 100-299 cases; (1) The number of cases/patients is too few to report; (2) Data submitted were based on a sample of cases/patients; (3) Results are based on a shorter time period than required; (4) Data suppressed by CMS for one or more quarters; (5) Results are not available for this reporting period; (6) Fewer than 100 patients completed the HCAHPS survey; (7) No cases met the criteria for this measure; (8) The lower limit of the confidence interval cannot be calculated if the number of observed infections equals zero; (9) No data are available from the state/territory for this reporting period; (10) The scores shown reflect fewer than 50 completed surveys; (11) There were discrepancies in the data collection process; (12) This measure does not apply to this hospital for this reporting period; (13) Results cannot be calculated for this reporting period; (14) The results for this state are combined with nearby states to protect confidentiality; Please refer to the User's Guide for a full explanation of data.

Measure	Cases	This Hosp.	State Avg.	U.S. Avg.
Anticoagulation Overlap Therapy[5]	-	-	89%	93%
ICU Venous Thromboembolism Prophylaxis[5]	-	-	87%	92%
Incidence of Potentially Preventable VTE[5]	-	-	8%	10%
UFH with Dosages/Platelet Monitoring[5]	-	-	97%	97%
Venous Thromboembolism Prophylaxis[5]	-	-	72%	85%
Warfarin Therapy Discharge Instructions[5]	-	-	73%	75%
Chest Pain/Possible Heart Attack Care				
Aspirin Given Within 24 Hours of Arrival[1,3]	-	-	95%	96%
Fibrinolytic Meds Within 30 Min. of Arrival[3,7]	-	-	54%	58%
Average Time to ECG (minutes)[1,3]	-	-	8	7
Average Time to Transfer (minutes)[1,3]	-	-	77	60
Children's Asthma Care				
Received Home Management Plan of Care	-	-	-	88%
Received Reliever Medication	-	-	-	100%
Received Systemic Corticosteroids	-	-	-	100%
Emergency Department				
Admittance Decision Time (minutes)[5]	-	-	63	98
Head CT Results Within 45 Min. of Arrival[3,7]	-	-	49%	57%
Patients Who Left ER Before Being Seen[5]	-	-	2%	2%
Time from ER Arrival to Admit. (minutes)[5]	-	-	210	274
Time from ER Arrival to Discharge (minutes)[5]	-	-	110	134
Time in ER Before Being Evaluated (minutes)[5]	-	-	24	26
Time to Pain Meds for Fractures (minutes)[1,3]	-	-	55	57
Heart Attack Care				
Aspirin Given at Discharge[5]	-	-	99%	99%
Fibrinolytic Meds Within 30 Min. of Arrival[5]	-	-	25%	54%
PCI Within 90 Minutes of Arrival[5]	-	-	95%	96%
Statin Prescribed at Discharge[5]	-	-	98%	98%
Heart Failure Care				
ACE Inhibitor or ARB for LVSD[3,7]	-	-	95%	97%
Discharge Instructions Given[1,3]	-	-	92%	94%
Evaluation of LVS Function[1,3]	-	-	96%	99%
Medicare Spending				
Medicare Spending per Patient (ratio)	-	-	0.93	0.98
Pneumonia Care				
Appropriate Initial Antibiotic Given[1]	-	-	92%	95%
Blood Culture Timing	11	100%	97%	98%
Pregnancy and Delivery Care				
Newborn Deliveries Scheduled Early[5]	-	-	8%	6%
Preventive Care				
Immunization for Influenza[1,3]	-	-	89%	90%
Immunization for Pneumonia[1,3]	-	-	91%	92%
Stroke Care				
Anticoagulation Therapy for Atrial Fibrillation[5]	-	-	91%	95%
Antithrombotic Therapy Timing[5]	-	-	95%	98%
Assessed for Rehabilitation[5]	-	-	96%	97%
Discharged on Antithrombotic Therapy[5]	-	-	98%	99%
Discharged on Statin Medication[5]	-	-	88%	94%
Thrombolytic Therapy Timing[5]	-	-	61%	66%
Venous Thromboembolism Prophylaxis[5]	-	-	92%	94%
Written Stroke Educational Materials Given[5]	-	-	86%	88%
Surgical Care Improvement Project				
Appropriate Beta Blocker Usage[5]	-	-	97%	98%
Appropriate VTP Within 24 Hours[5]	-	-	97%	98%
Controlled Postoperative Blood Glucose[5]	-	-	97%	97%
Perioperative Temperature Management[5]	-	-	100%	100%
Prophylactic Antibiotic Selection[5]	-	-	99%	99%
Prophylactic Antibiotic Selection (Outpatient)[5]	-	-	98%	98%
Prophylactic Antibiotic Stopped[5]	-	-	98%	98%
Prophylactic Antibiotic Timing[5]	-	-	98%	99%
Prophylactic Antibiotic Timing (Outpatient)[5]	-	-	98%	98%
Urinary Catheter Removal[5]	-	-	96%	97%
Survey of Patients' Hospital Experiences				
Area Around Room 'Always' Quiet at Night[5]	-	-	68%	61%
Doctors 'Always' Communicated Well[5]	-	-	84%	82%
Home Recovery Information Given[5]	-	-	84%	85%
Hospital Given 9 or 10 on 10 Point Scale[5]	-	-	72%	71%
Meds 'Always' Explained Before Given[5]	-	-	66%	64%
Nurses 'Always' Communicated Well[5]	-	-	80%	79%
Pain 'Always' Well Controlled[5]	-	-	72%	71%
Room and Bathroom 'Always' Clean[5]	-	-	73%	73%
Timely Help 'Always' Received[5]	-	-	71%	68%
Would Definitely Recommend Hospital[5]	-	-	71%	71%
Use of Medical Imaging				
Cardiac Imaging Stress Test before Surgery[1]	-	-	4.5%	5.3%
Combination Abdominal CT Scan[1]	-	-	23%	10.5%
Combination Brain/Sinus CT Scan	59	0.0%	2.2%	2.7%
Combination Chest CT Scan[1]	-	-	5.1%	2.7%
Follow-up Mammogram/Ultrasound[7]	-	-	8.1%	8.8%
Lumbar Spine MRI for Low Back Pain[1]	-	-	39.9%	37.2%

Fairview Regional Medical Center

523 East State Road
Fairview, OK 73737
URL: www.fairviewhospital.net
Phone: 580-227-3721
Fax: 580-227-2882
Type: Critical Access Hospitals
Ownership: Govt - Hospital Dist/Auth
Emergency Services: Yes
Beds: 25

Key Personnel:
Chief of Medical Staff. . . . . Kathy Cain
CEO . . . . Roger Knak

Measure	Cases	This Hosp.	State Avg.	U.S. Avg.
Blood Clot Prevention and Treatment				
Anticoagulation Overlap Therapy[5]	-	-	89%	93%
ICU Venous Thromboembolism Prophylaxis[5]	-	-	87%	92%
Incidence of Potentially Preventable VTE[5]	-	-	8%	10%
UFH with Dosages/Platelet Monitoring[5]	-	-	97%	97%
Venous Thromboembolism Prophylaxis[5]	-	-	72%	85%
Warfarin Therapy Discharge Instructions[5]	-	-	73%	75%
Chest Pain/Possible Heart Attack Care				
Aspirin Given Within 24 Hours of Arrival[5]	-	-	95%	96%
Fibrinolytic Meds Within 30 Min. of Arrival[5]	-	-	54%	58%
Average Time to ECG (minutes)[5]	-	-	8	7
Average Time to Transfer (minutes)[5]	-	-	77	60
Children's Asthma Care				
Received Home Management Plan of Care	-	-	-	88%
Received Reliever Medication	-	-	-	100%
Received Systemic Corticosteroids	-	-	-	100%
Emergency Department				
Admittance Decision Time (minutes)[5]	-	-	63	98
Head CT Results Within 45 Min. of Arrival[3,7]	-	-	49%	57%
Patients Who Left ER Before Being Seen[5]	-	-	2%	2%
Time from ER Arrival to Admit. (minutes)[5]	-	-	210	274
Time from ER Arrival to Discharge (minutes)[5]	-	-	110	134
Time in ER Before Being Evaluated (minutes)[5]	-	-	24	26
Time to Pain Meds for Fractures (minutes)[1,3]	-	-	55	57
Heart Attack Care				
Aspirin Given at Discharge[1,3]	-	-	99%	99%
Fibrinolytic Meds Within 30 Min. of Arrival[3,7]	-	-	25%	54%
PCI Within 90 Minutes of Arrival[3,7]	-	-	95%	96%
Statin Prescribed at Discharge[1,3]	-	-	98%	98%
Heart Failure Care				
ACE Inhibitor or ARB for LVSD[3,7]	-	-	95%	97%
Discharge Instructions Given[1,3]	-	-	92%	94%
Evaluation of LVS Function[1,3]	-	-	96%	99%
Medicare Spending				
Medicare Spending per Patient (ratio)	-	-	0.93	0.98
Pneumonia Care				
Appropriate Initial Antibiotic Given[3]	15	73%	92%	95%
Blood Culture Timing[1,3]	-	-	97%	98%
Pregnancy and Delivery Care				
Newborn Deliveries Scheduled Early[5]	-	-	8%	6%
Preventive Care				
Immunization for Influenza[5]	-	-	89%	90%
Immunization for Pneumonia[5]	-	-	91%	92%
Stroke Care				
Anticoagulation Therapy for Atrial Fibrillation[5]	-	-	91%	95%
Antithrombotic Therapy Timing[5]	-	-	95%	98%
Assessed for Rehabilitation[5]	-	-	96%	97%
Discharged on Antithrombotic Therapy[5]	-	-	98%	99%
Discharged on Statin Medication[5]	-	-	88%	94%
Thrombolytic Therapy Timing[5]	-	-	61%	66%
Venous Thromboembolism Prophylaxis[5]	-	-	92%	94%
Written Stroke Educational Materials Given[5]	-	-	86%	88%
Surgical Care Improvement Project				
Appropriate Beta Blocker Usage[5]	-	-	97%	98%
Appropriate VTP Within 24 Hours[5]	-	-	97%	98%
Controlled Postoperative Blood Glucose[5]	-	-	97%	97%
Perioperative Temperature Management[5]	-	-	100%	100%
Prophylactic Antibiotic Selection[5]	-	-	99%	99%
Prophylactic Antibiotic Selection (Outpatient)[5]	-	-	98%	98%
Prophylactic Antibiotic Stopped[5]	-	-	98%	98%
Prophylactic Antibiotic Timing[5]	-	-	98%	99%
Prophylactic Antibiotic Timing (Outpatient)[5]	-	-	98%	98%
Urinary Catheter Removal[5]	-	-	96%	97%
Survey of Patients' Hospital Experiences				
Area Around Room 'Always' Quiet at Night[5]	-	-	68%	61%
Doctors 'Always' Communicated Well[5]	-	-	84%	82%
Home Recovery Information Given[5]	-	-	84%	85%
Hospital Given 9 or 10 on 10 Point Scale[5]	-	-	72%	71%
Meds 'Always' Explained Before Given[5]	-	-	66%	64%
Nurses 'Always' Communicated Well[5]	-	-	80%	79%
Pain 'Always' Well Controlled[5]	-	-	72%	71%
Room and Bathroom 'Always' Clean[5]	-	-	73%	73%
Timely Help 'Always' Received[5]	-	-	71%	68%
Would Definitely Recommend Hospital[5]	-	-	71%	71%
Use of Medical Imaging				
Cardiac Imaging Stress Test before Surgery[7]	-	-	4.5%	5.3%
Combination Abdominal CT Scan	41	48.8%	23%	10.5%
Combination Brain/Sinus CT Scan[1]	-	-	2.2%	2.7%
Combination Chest CT Scan[1]	-	-	5.1%	2.7%
Follow-up Mammogram/Ultrasound[7]	-	-	8.1%	8.8%
Lumbar Spine MRI for Low Back Pain[1]	-	-	39.9%	37.2%

Memorial Hospital & Physician Group

319 East Josephine
Frederick, OK 73542
Phone: 580-335-7565
Fax: 580-335-7329
Type: Acute Care Hospitals
Ownership: Voluntary non-profit - Other
Emergency Services: Yes
Beds: 48

Key Personnel:
CEO/President. . . . . Al Allee
Chief of Medical Staff . . . . Maha Sultan, MD

Measure	Cases	This Hosp.	State Avg.	U.S. Avg.
Blood Clot Prevention and Treatment				
Anticoagulation Overlap Therapy[2,7]	-	-	89%	93%
ICU Venous Thromboembolism Prophylaxis[2,7]	-	-	87%	92%
Incidence of Potentially Preventable VTE[2,7]	-	-	8%	10%
UFH with Dosages/Platelet Monitoring[2,7]	-	-	97%	97%
Venous Thromboembolism Prophylaxis[2]	112	14%	72%	85%
Warfarin Therapy Discharge Instructions[2,7]	-	-	73%	75%
Chest Pain/Possible Heart Attack Care				
Aspirin Given Within 24 Hours of Arrival[1,3]	-	-	95%	96%
Fibrinolytic Meds Within 30 Min. of Arrival[3,7]	-	-	54%	58%
Average Time to ECG (minutes)[1,3]	-	-	8	7
Average Time to Transfer (minutes)[1,3]	-	-	77	60
Children's Asthma Care				
Received Home Management Plan of Care	-	-	-	88%
Received Reliever Medication	-	-	-	100%
Received Systemic Corticosteroids	-	-	-	100%
Emergency Department				
Admittance Decision Time (minutes)[2]	282	0	63	98
Head CT Results Within 45 Min. of Arrival[5]	-	-	49%	57%
Patients Who Left ER Before Being Seen	3,188	2%	2%	2%
Time from ER Arrival to Admit. (minutes)[2]	282	110	210	274
Time from ER Arrival to Discharge (minutes)	241	119	110	134
Time in ER Before Being Evaluated (minutes)	117	40	24	26
Time to Pain Meds for Fractures (minutes)[5]	-	-	55	57
Heart Attack Care				
Aspirin Given at Discharge[2,3]	-	-	99%	99%
Fibrinolytic Meds Within 30 Min. of Arrival[2,3]	-	-	25%	54%
PCI Within 90 Minutes of Arrival[2,3]	-	-	95%	96%
Statin Prescribed at Discharge[2,3]	-	-	98%	98%
Heart Failure Care				
ACE Inhibitor or ARB for LVSD[2,7]	-	-	95%	97%
Discharge Instructions Given[2]	16	94%	92%	94%
Evaluation of LVS Function[2]	25	52%	96%	99%
Medicare Spending				
Medicare Spending per Patient (ratio)	-	0.78	0.93	0.98
Pneumonia Care				

NOTE: Hospital profiles are in alphabetical order by state, then city, then hospital within the city; Rankings exclude hospitals with less than 25 cases except for patient surveys which excludes hospitals with less than 100 cases; (a) 100-299 cases; (1) The number of cases/patients is too few to report; (2) Data submitted were based on a sample of cases/patients; (3) Results are based on a shorter time period than required; (4) Data suppressed by CMS for one or more quarters; (5) Results are not available for this reporting period; (6) Fewer than 100 patients completed the HCAHPS survey; (7) No cases met the criteria for this measure; (8) The lower limit of the confidence interval cannot be calculated if the number of observed infections equals zero; (9) No data are available from the state/territory for this reporting period; (10) The scores shown reflect fewer than 50 completed surveys; (11) There were discrepancies in the data collection process; (12) This measure does not apply to this hospital for this reporting period; (13) Results cannot be calculated for this reporting period; (14) The results for this state are combined with nearby states to protect confidentiality; Please refer to the User's Guide for a full explanation of data.

Measure	Cases	This Hosp.	State Avg.	U.S. Avg.
Appropriate Initial Antibiotic Given[2]	30	23%	92%	95%
Blood Culture Timing[1,2]	-	-	97%	98%
Pregnancy and Delivery Care				
Newborn Deliveries Scheduled Early[2,7]	-	-	8%	6%
Preventive Care				
Immunization for Influenza[2]	235	88%	89%	90%
Immunization for Pneumonia[2]	287	77%	91%	92%
Stroke Care				
Anticoagulation Therapy for Atrial Fibrillation[5]	-	-	91%	95%
Antithrombotic Therapy Timing[5]	-	-	95%	98%
Assessed for Rehabilitation[5]	-	-	96%	97%
Discharged on Antithrombotic Therapy[5]	-	-	98%	99%
Discharged on Statin Medication[5]	-	-	88%	94%
Thrombolytic Therapy Timing[5]	-	-	61%	66%
Venous Thromboembolism Prophylaxis[5]	-	-	92%	94%
Written Stroke Educational Materials Given[5]	-	-	86%	88%
Surgical Care Improvement Project				
Appropriate Beta Blocker Usage[5]	-	-	97%	98%
Appropriate VTP Within 24 Hours[5]	-	-	97%	98%
Controlled Postoperative Blood Glucose[5]	-	-	97%	97%
Perioperative Temperature Management[5]	-	-	100%	100%
Prophylactic Antibiotic Selection[5]	-	-	99%	99%
Prophylactic Antibiotic Selection (Outpatient)[5]	-	-	98%	98%
Prophylactic Antibiotic Stopped[5]	-	-	98%	98%
Prophylactic Antibiotic Timing[5]	-	-	98%	99%
Prophylactic Antibiotic Timing (Outpatient)[5]	-	-	98%	98%
Urinary Catheter Removal[5]	-	-	96%	97%
Survey of Patients' Hospital Experiences				
Area Around Room 'Always' Quiet at Night[6]	<100	75%	68%	61%
Doctors 'Always' Communicated Well[6]	<100	92%	84%	82%
Home Recovery Information Given[6]	<100	84%	84%	85%
Hospital Given 9 or 10 on 10 Point Scale[6]	<100	66%	72%	71%
Meds 'Always' Explained Before Given[6]	<100	60%	66%	64%
Nurses 'Always' Communicated Well[6]	<100	74%	80%	79%
Pain 'Always' Well Controlled[6]	<100	81%	72%	71%
Room and Bathroom 'Always' Clean[6]	<100	82%	73%	73%
Timely Help 'Always' Received[6]	<100	70%	71%	68%
Would Definitely Recommend Hospital[6]	<100	58%	71%	71%
Use of Medical Imaging				
Cardiac Imaging Stress Test before Surgery[7]	-	-	4.5%	5.3%
Combination Abdominal CT Scan[1]	-	-	23%	10.5%
Combination Brain/Sinus CT Scan[1]	-	-	2.2%	2.7%
Combination Chest CT Scan[1]	-	-	5.1%	2.7%
Follow-up Mammogram/Ultrasound[7]	-	-	8.1%	8.8%
Lumbar Spine MRI for Low Back Pain[7]	-	-	39.9%	37.2%

Integris Grove Hospital

1001 East 18th Street Phone: 918-786-2243
Grove, OK 74344 Fax: 918-787-3403
E-mail: cathy.trewyn@integrisok.com
URL: www.integris-health.com
Type: Acute Care Hospitals Emergency Services: Yes
Ownership: Voluntary non-profit - Other Beds: 58
Key Personnel:
Operating Room. . . . . Debbie Berry, RN
Quality Assurance . . . . Dana Chouteau
Radiology. . . . . Michael Foster
Infection Control. . . . . Debbie Lawson
CEO/President. . . . . Greg Martin
Chief of Medical Staff. . . . . Richard Tidewell, MD
Emergency Room . . . . Diane Wilkie

Measure	Cases	This Hosp.	State Avg.	U.S. Avg.
Blood Clot Prevention and Treatment				
Anticoagulation Overlap Therapy[1,2]	-	-	89%	93%
ICU Venous Thromboembolism Prophylaxis[2]	35	71%	87%	92%
Incidence of Potentially Preventable VTE[2,7]	-	-	8%	10%
UFH with Dosages/Platelet Monitoring[1,2]	-	-	97%	97%
Venous Thromboembolism Prophylaxis[2]	155	71%	72%	85%
Warfarin Therapy Discharge Instructions[1,2]	-	-	73%	75%
Chest Pain/Possible Heart Attack Care				
Aspirin Given Within 24 Hours of Arrival	36	97%	95%	96%
Fibrinolytic Meds Within 30 Min. of Arrival[1]	-	-	54%	58%
Average Time to ECG (minutes)	36	15	8	7
Average Time to Transfer (minutes)[1]	-	-	77	60
Children's Asthma Care				
Received Home Management Plan of Care	-	-	-	88%
Received Reliever Medication	-	-	-	100%
Received Systemic Corticosteroids	-	-	-	100%
Emergency Department				
Admittance Decision Time (minutes)[2]	240	60	63	98
Head CT Results Within 45 Min. of Arrival	21	48%	49%	57%
Patients Who Left ER Before Being Seen	17,129	2%	2%	2%
Time from ER Arrival to Admit. (minutes)[2]	332	204	210	274
Time from ER Arrival to Discharge (minutes)	1,011	125	110	134
Time in ER Before Being Evaluated (minutes)	863	40	24	26
Time to Pain Meds for Fractures (minutes)	110	64	55	57
Heart Attack Care				
Aspirin Given at Discharge	40	98%	99%	99%
Fibrinolytic Meds Within 30 Min. of Arrival[7]	-	-	25%	54%
PCI Within 90 Minutes of Arrival[1]	-	-	95%	96%
Statin Prescribed at Discharge	43	91%	98%	98%
Heart Failure Care				
ACE Inhibitor or ARB for LVSD	19	89%	95%	97%
Discharge Instructions Given	42	100%	92%	94%
Evaluation of LVS Function	54	98%	96%	99%
Medicare Spending				
Medicare Spending per Patient (ratio)	-	0.99	0.93	0.98
Pneumonia Care				
Appropriate Initial Antibiotic Given	55	96%	92%	95%
Blood Culture Timing	108	95%	97%	98%
Pregnancy and Delivery Care				
Newborn Deliveries Scheduled Early	28	7%	8%	6%
Preventive Care				
Immunization for Influenza[2]	270	73%	89%	90%
Immunization for Pneumonia[2]	369	78%	91%	92%
Stroke Care				
Anticoagulation Therapy for Atrial Fibrillation[1]	-	-	91%	95%
Antithrombotic Therapy Timing	21	86%	95%	98%
Assessed for Rehabilitation	20	95%	96%	97%
Discharged on Antithrombotic Therapy	19	84%	98%	99%
Discharged on Statin Medication	20	85%	88%	94%
Thrombolytic Therapy Timing	12	0%	61%	66%
Venous Thromboembolism Prophylaxis	20	65%	92%	94%
Written Stroke Educational Materials Given	12	42%	86%	88%
Surgical Care Improvement Project				
Appropriate Beta Blocker Usage	30	90%	97%	98%
Appropriate VTP Within 24 Hours	97	97%	97%	98%
Controlled Postoperative Blood Glucose[7]	-	-	97%	97%
Perioperative Temperature Management	105	100%	100%	100%
Prophylactic Antibiotic Selection	79	96%	99%	99%
Prophylactic Antibiotic Selection (Outpatient)	41	98%	98%	98%
Prophylactic Antibiotic Stopped	78	99%	98%	98%
Prophylactic Antibiotic Timing	80	98%	98%	99%
Prophylactic Antibiotic Timing (Outpatient)	44	91%	98%	98%
Urinary Catheter Removal	81	98%	96%	97%
Survey of Patients' Hospital Experiences				
Area Around Room 'Always' Quiet at Night	300+	67%	68%	61%
Doctors 'Always' Communicated Well	300+	82%	84%	82%
Home Recovery Information Given	300+	84%	84%	85%
Hospital Given 9 or 10 on 10 Point Scale	300+	69%	72%	71%
Meds 'Always' Explained Before Given	300+	62%	66%	64%
Nurses 'Always' Communicated Well	300+	79%	80%	79%
Pain 'Always' Well Controlled	300+	72%	72%	71%
Room and Bathroom 'Always' Clean	300+	64%	73%	73%
Timely Help 'Always' Received	300+	65%	71%	68%
Would Definitely Recommend Hospital	300+	68%	71%	71%
Use of Medical Imaging				
Cardiac Imaging Stress Test before Surgery	87	5.7%	4.5%	5.3%
Combination Abdominal CT Scan	394	4.1%	23%	10.5%
Combination Brain/Sinus CT Scan[1]	-	-	2.2%	2.7%
Combination Chest CT Scan	250	0.4%	5.1%	2.7%
Follow-up Mammogram/Ultrasound	716	5.4%	8.1%	8.8%
Lumbar Spine MRI for Low Back Pain	100	37.0%	39.9%	37.2%

Mercy Hospital Logan County

200 South Academy Road Phone: 405-282-6700
Guthrie, OK 73044 Fax: 405-282-6790
URL: www.loganhosp.com
Type: Critical Access Hospitals Emergency Services: Yes
Ownership: Govt - Hospital Dist/Auth Beds: 25
Key Personnel:
Emergency Room . . . . Ann Campbell, MD
Infection Control. . . . . Kaye Freudenberger
Chief of Medical Staff. . . . . Todd Krehbiel, MD
CEO/President. . . . . Steve Rowley
Radiology. . . . . Abe Sims
Administrator . . . . Josh Tucker
Quality Assurance . . . . Anita Valentine, RN

Measure	Cases	This Hosp.	State Avg.	U.S. Avg.
Blood Clot Prevention and Treatment				
Anticoagulation Overlap Therapy[5]	-	-	89%	93%
ICU Venous Thromboembolism Prophylaxis[5]	-	-	87%	92%
Incidence of Potentially Preventable VTE[5]	-	-	8%	10%
UFH with Dosages/Platelet Monitoring[5]	-	-	97%	97%
Venous Thromboembolism Prophylaxis[5]	-	-	72%	85%
Warfarin Therapy Discharge Instructions[5]	-	-	73%	75%
Chest Pain/Possible Heart Attack Care				
Aspirin Given Within 24 Hours of Arrival[3]	18	100%	95%	96%
Fibrinolytic Meds Within 30 Min. of Arrival[3,7]	-	-	54%	58%
Average Time to ECG (minutes)[3]	18	6	8	7
Average Time to Transfer (minutes)[1,3]	-	-	77	60
Children's Asthma Care				
Received Home Management Plan of Care	-	-	-	88%
Received Reliever Medication	-	-	-	100%
Received Systemic Corticosteroids	-	-	-	100%
Emergency Department				
Admittance Decision Time (minutes)[2]	342	48	63	98
Head CT Results Within 45 Min. of Arrival[5]	-	-	49%	57%
Patients Who Left ER Before Being Seen[5]	-	-	2%	2%
Time from ER Arrival to Admit. (minutes)[2]	365	188	210	274
Time from ER Arrival to Discharge (minutes)[5]	-	-	110	134
Time in ER Before Being Evaluated (minutes)[5]	-	-	24	26
Time to Pain Meds for Fractures (minutes)[5]	-	-	55	57
Heart Attack Care				
Aspirin Given at Discharge[3,7]	-	-	99%	99%
Fibrinolytic Meds Within 30 Min. of Arrival[3,7]	-	-	25%	54%
PCI Within 90 Minutes of Arrival[3,7]	-	-	95%	96%
Statin Prescribed at Discharge[3,7]	-	-	98%	98%
Heart Failure Care				
ACE Inhibitor or ARB for LVSD[1]	-	-	95%	97%
Discharge Instructions Given	16	69%	92%	94%
Evaluation of LVS Function	25	100%	96%	99%
Medicare Spending				
Medicare Spending per Patient (ratio)	-	-	0.93	0.98
Pneumonia Care				
Appropriate Initial Antibiotic Given	23	100%	92%	95%
Blood Culture Timing	37	100%	97%	98%
Pregnancy and Delivery Care				
Newborn Deliveries Scheduled Early[5]	-	-	8%	6%
Preventive Care				
Immunization for Influenza[2]	319	95%	89%	90%
Immunization for Pneumonia[2]	471	97%	91%	92%
Stroke Care				
Anticoagulation Therapy for Atrial Fibrillation[5]	-	-	91%	95%
Antithrombotic Therapy Timing[5]	-	-	95%	98%
Assessed for Rehabilitation[5]	-	-	96%	97%
Discharged on Antithrombotic Therapy[5]	-	-	98%	99%
Discharged on Statin Medication[5]	-	-	88%	94%
Thrombolytic Therapy Timing[5]	-	-	61%	66%
Venous Thromboembolism Prophylaxis[5]	-	-	92%	94%
Written Stroke Educational Materials Given[5]	-	-	86%	88%
Surgical Care Improvement Project				
Appropriate Beta Blocker Usage[1]	-	-	97%	98%
Appropriate VTP Within 24 Hours	38	97%	97%	98%
Controlled Postoperative Blood Glucose[7]	-	-	97%	97%
Perioperative Temperature Management	40	100%	100%	100%
Prophylactic Antibiotic Selection	34	100%	99%	99%
Prophylactic Antibiotic Selection (Outpatient)[1,3]	-	-	98%	98%

NOTE: Hospital profiles are in alphabetical order by state, then city, then hospital within the city; Rankings exclude hospitals with less than 25 cases except for patient surveys which excludes hospitals with less than 100 cases; (a) 100-299 cases; (1) The number of cases/patients is too few to report; (2) Data submitted were based on a sample of cases/patients; (3) Results are based on a shorter time period than required; (4) Data suppressed by CMS for one or more quarters; (5) Results are not available for this reporting period; (6) Fewer than 100 patients completed the HCAHPS survey; (7) No cases met the criteria for this measure; (8) The lower limit of the confidence interval cannot be calculated if the number of observed infections equals zero; (9) No data are available from the state/territory for this reporting period; (10) The scores shown reflect fewer than 50 completed surveys; (11) There were discrepancies in the data collection process; (12) This measure does not apply to this hospital for this reporting period; (13) Results cannot be calculated for this reporting period; (14) The results for this state are combined with nearby states to protect confidentiality; Please refer to the User's Guide for a full explanation of data.

Measure	Cases	This Hosp.	State Avg.	U.S. Avg.
Prophylactic Antibiotic Stopped	32	97%	98%	98%
Prophylactic Antibiotic Timing	34	94%	98%	99%
Prophylactic Antibiotic Timing (Outpatient)[1,3]	-	-	98%	98%
Urinary Catheter Removal	24	100%	96%	97%
Survey of Patients' Hospital Experiences				
Area Around Room 'Always' Quiet at Night[5]	-	-	68%	61%
Doctors 'Always' Communicated Well[5]	-	-	84%	82%
Home Recovery Information Given[5]	-	-	84%	85%
Hospital Given 9 or 10 on 10 Point Scale[5]	-	-	72%	71%
Meds 'Always' Explained Before Given[5]	-	-	66%	64%
Nurses 'Always' Communicated Well[5]	-	-	80%	79%
Pain 'Always' Well Controlled[5]	-	-	72%	71%
Room and Bathroom 'Always' Clean[5]	-	-	73%	73%
Timely Help 'Always' Received[5]	-	-	71%	68%
Would Definitely Recommend Hospital[5]	-	-	71%	71%
Use of Medical Imaging				
Cardiac Imaging Stress Test before Surgery[7]	-	-	4.5%	5.3%
Combination Abdominal CT Scan	224	12.5%	23%	10.5%
Combination Brain/Sinus CT Scan[1]	-	-	2.2%	2.7%
Combination Chest CT Scan	128	5.5%	5.1%	2.7%
Follow-up Mammogram/Ultrasound	168	17.3%	8.1%	8.8%
Lumbar Spine MRI for Low Back Pain[1]	-	-	39.9%	37.2%

Memorial Hospital of Texas County

520 Medical Drive
Guymon, OK 73942
Phone: 580-338-6515
Fax: 580-338-5722
E-mail: mhtchr@iptsi.net
URL: www.mhtcguymon.org
Type: Acute Care Hospitals
Emergency Services: Yes
Ownership: Government - Local
Beds: 42

Key Personnel:

Intensive Care Unit. . . . . Jane Brown
Operating Room. . . . . Wayne Caniwell
Chief of Medical Staff. . . . . Kelly McNurry
CEO/President. . . . . Tim Starkey
Infection Control. . . . . Julie West
Quality Assurance . . . . Julie West

Measure	Cases	This Hosp.	State Avg.	U.S. Avg.
Blood Clot Prevention and Treatment				
Anticoagulation Overlap Therapy[1,2]	-	-	89%	93%
ICU Venous Thromboembolism Prophylaxis[2,7]	-	-	87%	92%
Incidence of Potentially Preventable VTE[1,2]	-	-	8%	10%
UFH with Dosages/Platelet Monitoring[2,7]	-	-	97%	97%
Venous Thromboembolism Prophylaxis[2]	121	50%	72%	85%
Warfarin Therapy Discharge Instructions[1,2]	-	-	73%	75%
Chest Pain/Possible Heart Attack Care				
Aspirin Given Within 24 Hours of Arrival	31	97%	95%	96%
Fibrinolytic Meds Within 30 Min. of Arrival[1]	-	-	54%	58%
Average Time to ECG (minutes)	34	7	8	7
Average Time to Transfer (minutes)[1]	-	-	77	60
Children's Asthma Care				
Received Home Management Plan of Care	-	-	-	88%
Received Reliever Medication	-	-	-	100%
Received Systemic Corticosteroids	-	-	-	100%
Emergency Department				
Admittance Decision Time (minutes)[2]	125	90	63	98
Head CT Results Within 45 Min. of Arrival[1]	-	-	49%	57%
Patients Who Left ER Before Being Seen	5,016	2%	2%	2%
Time from ER Arrival to Admit. (minutes)[2]	197	235	210	274
Time from ER Arrival to Discharge (minutes)	283	121	110	134
Time in ER Before Being Evaluated (minutes)	346	12	24	26
Time to Pain Meds for Fractures (minutes)	39	61	55	57
Heart Attack Care				
Aspirin Given at Discharge[5]	-	-	99%	99%
Fibrinolytic Meds Within 30 Min. of Arrival[5]	-	-	25%	54%
PCI Within 90 Minutes of Arrival[5]	-	-	95%	96%
Statin Prescribed at Discharge[5]	-	-	98%	98%
Heart Failure Care				
ACE Inhibitor or ARB for LVSD[1]	-	-	95%	97%
Discharge Instructions Given[1]	-	-	92%	94%
Evaluation of LVS Function	11	91%	96%	99%
Medicare Spending				
Medicare Spending per Patient (ratio)	-	0.74	0.93	0.98
Pneumonia Care				
Appropriate Initial Antibiotic Given[2]	25	84%	92%	95%
Blood Culture Timing[2]	13	92%	97%	98%
Pregnancy and Delivery Care				
Newborn Deliveries Scheduled Early	86	20%	8%	6%
Preventive Care				
Immunization for Influenza[2]	289	83%	89%	90%
Immunization for Pneumonia[2]	223	93%	91%	92%
Stroke Care				
Anticoagulation Therapy for Atrial Fibrillation[3,7]	-	-	91%	95%
Antithrombotic Therapy Timing[1,3]	-	-	95%	98%
Assessed for Rehabilitation[1,3]	-	-	96%	97%
Discharged on Antithrombotic Therapy[1,3]	-	-	98%	99%
Discharged on Statin Medication[1,3]	-	-	88%	94%
Thrombolytic Therapy Timing[3,7]	-	-	61%	66%
Venous Thromboembolism Prophylaxis[1,3]	-	-	92%	94%
Written Stroke Educational Materials Given[1,3]	-	-	86%	88%
Surgical Care Improvement Project				
Appropriate Beta Blocker Usage[1,2]	-	-	97%	98%
Appropriate VTP Within 24 Hours[2]	14	71%	97%	98%
Controlled Postoperative Blood Glucose[2,7]	-	-	97%	97%
Perioperative Temperature Management[2]	19	100%	100%	100%
Prophylactic Antibiotic Selection[1,2]	-	-	99%	99%
Prophylactic Antibiotic Selection (Outpatient)[1,3]	-	-	98%	98%
Prophylactic Antibiotic Stopped[1,2]	-	-	98%	98%
Prophylactic Antibiotic Timing[1,2]	-	-	98%	99%
Prophylactic Antibiotic Timing (Outpatient)[1,3]	-	-	98%	98%
Urinary Catheter Removal[1,2]	-	-	96%	97%
Survey of Patients' Hospital Experiences				
Area Around Room 'Always' Quiet at Night	(a)	66%	68%	61%
Doctors 'Always' Communicated Well	(a)	82%	84%	82%
Home Recovery Information Given	(a)	85%	84%	85%
Hospital Given 9 or 10 on 10 Point Scale	(a)	69%	72%	71%
Meds 'Always' Explained Before Given	(a)	64%	66%	64%
Nurses 'Always' Communicated Well	(a)	77%	80%	79%
Pain 'Always' Well Controlled	(a)	74%	72%	71%
Room and Bathroom 'Always' Clean	(a)	77%	73%	73%
Timely Help 'Always' Received	(a)	74%	71%	68%
Would Definitely Recommend Hospital	(a)	59%	71%	71%
Use of Medical Imaging				
Cardiac Imaging Stress Test before Surgery	80	6.3%	4.5%	5.3%
Combination Abdominal CT Scan	79	25.3%	23%	10.5%
Combination Brain/Sinus CT Scan	80	0.0%	2.2%	2.7%
Combination Chest CT Scan[1]	-	-	5.1%	2.7%
Follow-up Mammogram/Ultrasound	139	8.6%	8.1%	8.8%
Lumbar Spine MRI for Low Back Pain[1]	-	-	39.9%	37.2%

Mercy Hospital Healdton

3462 Hospital Rd
Healdton, OK 73438
Phone: 580-229-0701
Fax: 580-229-0691
Type: Critical Access Hospitals
Emergency Services: Yes
Ownership: Voluntary non-profit - Private
Beds: 25

Key Personnel:

Administrator . . . . Jeremy Jones
Infection Control. . . . . Larry Lovelace
CEO/President. . . . . Bob Thompson
Radiology. . . . . Johnny Walker

Measure	Cases	This Hosp.	State Avg.	U.S. Avg.
Blood Clot Prevention and Treatment				
Anticoagulation Overlap Therapy[5]	-	-	89%	93%
ICU Venous Thromboembolism Prophylaxis[5]	-	-	87%	92%
Incidence of Potentially Preventable VTE[5]	-	-	8%	10%
UFH with Dosages/Platelet Monitoring[5]	-	-	97%	97%
Venous Thromboembolism Prophylaxis[5]	-	-	72%	85%
Warfarin Therapy Discharge Instructions[5]	-	-	73%	75%
Chest Pain/Possible Heart Attack Care				
Aspirin Given Within 24 Hours of Arrival[1,3]	-	-	95%	96%
Fibrinolytic Meds Within 30 Min. of Arrival[3,7]	-	-	54%	58%
Average Time to ECG (minutes)[1,3]	-	-	8	7
Average Time to Transfer (minutes)[1,3]	-	-	77	60
Children's Asthma Care				
Received Home Management Plan of Care	-	-	-	88%
Received Reliever Medication	-	-	-	100%
Received Systemic Corticosteroids	-	-	-	100%
Emergency Department				
Admittance Decision Time (minutes)[5]	-	-	63	98
Head CT Results Within 45 Min. of Arrival[5]	-	-	49%	57%
Patients Who Left ER Before Being Seen[5]	-	-	2%	2%
Time from ER Arrival to Admit. (minutes)[5]	-	-	210	274
Time from ER Arrival to Discharge (minutes)[5]	-	-	110	134
Time in ER Before Being Evaluated (minutes)[5]	-	-	24	26
Time to Pain Meds for Fractures (minutes)[5]	-	-	55	57
Heart Attack Care				
Aspirin Given at Discharge[5]	-	-	99%	99%
Fibrinolytic Meds Within 30 Min. of Arrival[5]	-	-	25%	54%
PCI Within 90 Minutes of Arrival[5]	-	-	95%	96%
Statin Prescribed at Discharge[5]	-	-	98%	98%
Heart Failure Care				
ACE Inhibitor or ARB for LVSD[1,3]	-	-	95%	97%
Discharge Instructions Given[1,3]	-	-	92%	94%
Evaluation of LVS Function[1,3]	-	-	96%	99%
Medicare Spending				
Medicare Spending per Patient (ratio)	-	-	0.93	0.98
Pneumonia Care				
Appropriate Initial Antibiotic Given[3]	11	82%	92%	95%
Blood Culture Timing[3,7]	-	-	97%	98%
Pregnancy and Delivery Care				
Newborn Deliveries Scheduled Early[5]	-	-	8%	6%
Preventive Care				
Immunization for Influenza[5]	-	-	89%	90%
Immunization for Pneumonia[5]	-	-	91%	92%
Stroke Care				
Anticoagulation Therapy for Atrial Fibrillation[5]	-	-	91%	95%
Antithrombotic Therapy Timing[5]	-	-	95%	98%
Assessed for Rehabilitation[5]	-	-	96%	97%
Discharged on Antithrombotic Therapy[5]	-	-	98%	99%
Discharged on Statin Medication[5]	-	-	88%	94%
Thrombolytic Therapy Timing[5]	-	-	61%	66%
Venous Thromboembolism Prophylaxis[5]	-	-	92%	94%
Written Stroke Educational Materials Given[5]	-	-	86%	88%
Surgical Care Improvement Project				
Appropriate Beta Blocker Usage[5]	-	-	97%	98%
Appropriate VTP Within 24 Hours[5]	-	-	97%	98%
Controlled Postoperative Blood Glucose[5]	-	-	97%	97%
Perioperative Temperature Management[5]	-	-	100%	100%
Prophylactic Antibiotic Selection[5]	-	-	99%	99%
Prophylactic Antibiotic Selection (Outpatient)[5]	-	-	98%	98%
Prophylactic Antibiotic Stopped[5]	-	-	98%	98%
Prophylactic Antibiotic Timing[5]	-	-	98%	99%
Prophylactic Antibiotic Timing (Outpatient)[5]	-	-	98%	98%
Urinary Catheter Removal[5]	-	-	96%	97%
Survey of Patients' Hospital Experiences				
Area Around Room 'Always' Quiet at Night[5]	-	-	68%	61%
Doctors 'Always' Communicated Well[5]	-	-	84%	82%
Home Recovery Information Given[5]	-	-	84%	85%
Hospital Given 9 or 10 on 10 Point Scale[5]	-	-	72%	71%
Meds 'Always' Explained Before Given[5]	-	-	66%	64%
Nurses 'Always' Communicated Well[5]	-	-	80%	79%
Pain 'Always' Well Controlled[5]	-	-	72%	71%
Room and Bathroom 'Always' Clean[5]	-	-	73%	73%
Timely Help 'Always' Received[5]	-	-	71%	68%
Would Definitely Recommend Hospital[5]	-	-	71%	71%
Use of Medical Imaging				
Cardiac Imaging Stress Test before Surgery[7]	-	-	4.5%	5.3%
Combination Abdominal CT Scan[1]	-	-	23%	10.5%
Combination Brain/Sinus CT Scan	38	0.0%	2.2%	2.7%
Combination Chest CT Scan[1]	-	-	5.1%	2.7%
Follow-up Mammogram/Ultrasound[7]	-	-	8.1%	8.8%
Lumbar Spine MRI for Low Back Pain[7]	-	-	39.9%	37.2%

Hillcrest Hospital Henryetta

Dewey Bartlett Saint & Main St
Henryetta, OK 74437
Phone: 918-615-1100
Fax: 918-652-3675
URL: www.hillcrest.com/henryetta
Type: Acute Care Hospitals
Emergency Services: Yes
Ownership: Proprietary
Beds: 41

Key Personnel:

Quality Assurance . . . . Benita Casselman

NOTE: Hospital profiles are in alphabetical order by state, then city, then hospital within the city; Rankings exclude hospitals with less than 25 cases except for patient surveys which excludes hospitals with less than 100 cases; (a) 100-299 cases; (1) The number of cases/patients is too few to report; (2) Data submitted were based on a sample of cases/patients; (3) Results are based on a shorter time period than required; (4) Data suppressed by CMS for one or more quarters; (5) Results are not available for this reporting period; (6) Fewer than 100 patients completed the HCAHPS survey; (7) No cases met the criteria for this measure; (8) The lower limit of the confidence interval cannot be calculated if the number of observed infections equals zero; (9) No data are available from the state/territory for this reporting period; (10) The scores shown reflect fewer than 50 completed surveys; (11) There were discrepancies in the data collection process; (12) This measure does not apply to this hospital for this reporting period; (13) Results cannot be calculated for this reporting period; (14) The results for this state are combined with nearby states to protect confidentiality; Please refer to the User's Guide for a full explanation of data.

Chief of Medical Staff.......... Brent Davis, DO
Emergency Room............ Brent Davis, DO
Operating Room.............. James McGee, RN
Infection Control.............. Mike Patterson
Hemotology Center........... George Pikler, MD
CEO/President................ Dee Renshaw
Anesthesiology................ Tom Thompson, CRNA

Measure	Cases	This Hosp.	State Avg.	U.S. Avg.
Blood Clot Prevention and Treatment				
Anticoagulation Overlap Therapy[2,7]	-	-	89%	93%
ICU Venous Thromboembolism Prophylaxis[2,7]	-	-	87%	92%
Incidence of Potentially Preventable VTE[2,7]	-	-	8%	10%
UFH with Dosages/Platelet Monitoring[2,7]	-	-	97%	97%
Venous Thromboembolism Prophylaxis[2]	75	89%	72%	85%
Warfarin Therapy Discharge Instructions[2,7]	-	-	73%	75%
Chest Pain/Possible Heart Attack Care				
Aspirin Given Within 24 Hours of Arrival	46	96%	95%	96%
Fibrinolytic Meds Within 30 Min. of Arrival[3,7]	-	-	54%	58%
Average Time to ECG (minutes)	45	7	8	7
Average Time to Transfer (minutes)[1,3]	-	-	77	60
Children's Asthma Care				
Received Home Management Plan of Care	-	-	-	88%
Received Reliever Medication	-	-	-	100%
Received Systemic Corticosteroids	-	-	-	100%
Emergency Department				
Admittance Decision Time (minutes)[2]	258	57	63	98
Head CT Results Within 45 Min. of Arrival[1]	-	-	49%	57%
Patients Who Left ER Before Being Seen	7,720	4%	2%	2%
Time from ER Arrival to Admit. (minutes)[2]	262	226	210	274
Time from ER Arrival to Discharge (minutes)	355	121	110	134
Time in ER Before Being Evaluated (minutes)	395	31	24	26
Time to Pain Meds for Fractures (minutes)	38	30	55	57
Heart Attack Care				
Aspirin Given at Discharge[1,3]	-	-	99%	99%
Fibrinolytic Meds Within 30 Min. of Arrival[3,7]	-	-	25%	54%
PCI Within 90 Minutes of Arrival[3,7]	-	-	95%	96%
Statin Prescribed at Discharge[1,3]	-	-	98%	98%
Heart Failure Care				
ACE Inhibitor or ARB for LVSD[7]	-	-	95%	97%
Discharge Instructions Given	22	100%	92%	94%
Evaluation of LVS Function	21	100%	96%	99%
Medicare Spending				
Medicare Spending per Patient (ratio)	-	0.85	0.93	0.98
Pneumonia Care				
Appropriate Initial Antibiotic Given	41	95%	92%	95%
Blood Culture Timing	48	92%	97%	98%
Pregnancy and Delivery Care				
Newborn Deliveries Scheduled Early[7]	-	-	8%	6%
Preventive Care				
Immunization for Influenza[2]	288	96%	89%	90%
Immunization for Pneumonia[2]	296	97%	91%	92%
Stroke Care				
Anticoagulation Therapy for Atrial Fibrillation[3,7]	-	-	91%	95%
Antithrombotic Therapy Timing[1,3]	-	-	95%	98%
Assessed for Rehabilitation[3,7]	-	-	96%	97%
Discharged on Antithrombotic Therapy[3,7]	-	-	98%	99%
Discharged on Statin Medication[3,7]	-	-	88%	94%
Thrombolytic Therapy Timing[3,7]	-	-	61%	66%
Venous Thromboembolism Prophylaxis[1,3]	-	-	92%	94%
Written Stroke Educational Materials Given[3,7]	-	-	86%	88%
Surgical Care Improvement Project				
Appropriate Beta Blocker Usage[1,3]	-	-	97%	98%
Appropriate VTP Within 24 Hours[1,3]	-	-	97%	98%
Controlled Postoperative Blood Glucose[3,7]	-	-	97%	97%
Perioperative Temperature Management[1,3]	-	-	100%	100%
Prophylactic Antibiotic Selection[1,3]	-	-	99%	99%
Prophylactic Antibiotic Selection (Outpatient)[1]	-	-	98%	98%
Prophylactic Antibiotic Stopped[1,3]	-	-	98%	98%
Prophylactic Antibiotic Timing[1,3]	-	-	98%	99%
Prophylactic Antibiotic Timing (Outpatient)[1]	-	-	98%	98%
Urinary Catheter Removal[1,3]	-	-	96%	97%
Survey of Patients' Hospital Experiences				
Area Around Room 'Always' Quiet at Night	(a)	71%	68%	61%
Doctors 'Always' Communicated Well	(a)	88%	84%	82%
Home Recovery Information Given	(a)	84%	84%	85%
Hospital Given 9 or 10 on 10 Point Scale	(a)	73%	72%	71%
Meds 'Always' Explained Before Given	(a)	73%	66%	64%
Nurses 'Always' Communicated Well	(a)	86%	80%	79%
Pain 'Always' Well Controlled	(a)	87%	72%	71%
Room and Bathroom 'Always' Clean	(a)	76%	73%	73%
Timely Help 'Always' Received	(a)	72%	71%	68%
Would Definitely Recommend Hospital	(a)	73%	71%	71%
Use of Medical Imaging				
Cardiac Imaging Stress Test before Surgery[1]	-	-	4.5%	5.3%
Combination Abdominal CT Scan	166	22.9%	23%	10.5%
Combination Brain/Sinus CT Scan[1]	-	-	2.2%	2.7%
Combination Chest CT Scan	83	19.3%	5.1%	2.7%
Follow-up Mammogram/Ultrasound	144	11.1%	8.1%	8.8%
Lumbar Spine MRI for Low Back Pain	33	51.5%	39.9%	37.2%

Elkview General Hospital

429 West Elm Street
Hobart, OK 73651
URL: www.hobartok.com
Phone: 580-726-3324
Fax: 580-726-6041
Type: Acute Care Hospitals
Ownership: Govt - Hospital Dist/Auth
Emergency Services: Yes
Beds: 50

Measure	Cases	This Hosp.	State Avg.	U.S. Avg.
Blood Clot Prevention and Treatment				
Anticoagulation Overlap Therapy[1,2]	-	-	89%	93%
ICU Venous Thromboembolism Prophylaxis[2,7]	-	-	87%	92%
Incidence of Potentially Preventable VTE[2,7]	-	-	8%	10%
UFH with Dosages/Platelet Monitoring[1,2]	-	-	97%	97%
Venous Thromboembolism Prophylaxis[2]	107	44%	72%	85%
Warfarin Therapy Discharge Instructions[1,2]	-	-	73%	75%
Chest Pain/Possible Heart Attack Care				
Aspirin Given Within 24 Hours of Arrival[1]	-	-	95%	96%
Fibrinolytic Meds Within 30 Min. of Arrival[1]	-	-	54%	58%
Average Time to ECG (minutes)[1]	-	-	8	7
Average Time to Transfer (minutes)[1]	-	-	77	60
Children's Asthma Care				
Received Home Management Plan of Care	-	-	-	88%
Received Reliever Medication	-	-	-	100%
Received Systemic Corticosteroids	-	-	-	100%
Emergency Department				
Admittance Decision Time (minutes)[2]	32	10	63	98
Head CT Results Within 45 Min. of Arrival[1,3]	-	-	49%	57%
Patients Who Left ER Before Being Seen	4,262	1%	2%	2%
Time from ER Arrival to Admit. (minutes)[2]	406	114	210	274
Time from ER Arrival to Discharge (minutes)	366	75	110	134
Time in ER Before Being Evaluated (minutes)[7]	-	-	24	26
Time to Pain Meds for Fractures (minutes)[1]	-	-	55	57
Heart Attack Care				
Aspirin Given at Discharge[1]	-	-	99%	99%
Fibrinolytic Meds Within 30 Min. of Arrival[7]	-	-	25%	54%
PCI Within 90 Minutes of Arrival[7]	-	-	95%	96%
Statin Prescribed at Discharge[1]	-	-	98%	98%
Heart Failure Care				
ACE Inhibitor or ARB for LVSD[1,2]	-	-	95%	97%
Discharge Instructions Given[2]	25	100%	92%	94%
Evaluation of LVS Function[2]	34	97%	96%	99%
Medicare Spending				
Medicare Spending per Patient (ratio)	-	0.83	0.93	0.98
Pneumonia Care				
Appropriate Initial Antibiotic Given	27	89%	92%	95%
Blood Culture Timing	26	96%	97%	98%
Pregnancy and Delivery Care				
Newborn Deliveries Scheduled Early[7]	-	-	8%	6%
Preventive Care				
Immunization for Influenza[2]	287	94%	89%	90%
Immunization for Pneumonia[2]	409	86%	91%	92%
Stroke Care				
Anticoagulation Therapy for Atrial Fibrillation[1]	-	-	91%	95%
Antithrombotic Therapy Timing	11	82%	95%	98%
Assessed for Rehabilitation	11	100%	96%	97%
Discharged on Antithrombotic Therapy	11	91%	98%	99%
Discharged on Statin Medication[1]	-	-	88%	94%
Thrombolytic Therapy Timing[1]	-	-	61%	66%
Venous Thromboembolism Prophylaxis	13	46%	92%	94%
Written Stroke Educational Materials Given[1]	-	-	86%	88%
Surgical Care Improvement Project				
Appropriate Beta Blocker Usage[1]	-	-	97%	98%
Appropriate VTP Within 24 Hours	61	98%	97%	98%
Controlled Postoperative Blood Glucose[7]	-	-	97%	97%
Perioperative Temperature Management	67	100%	100%	100%
Prophylactic Antibiotic Selection	45	100%	99%	99%
Prophylactic Antibiotic Selection (Outpatient)[5]	-	-	98%	98%
Prophylactic Antibiotic Stopped	45	93%	98%	98%
Prophylactic Antibiotic Timing	46	87%	98%	99%
Prophylactic Antibiotic Timing (Outpatient)[5]	-	-	98%	98%
Urinary Catheter Removal	57	60%	96%	97%
Survey of Patients' Hospital Experiences				
Area Around Room 'Always' Quiet at Night	(a)	56%	68%	61%
Doctors 'Always' Communicated Well	(a)	89%	84%	82%
Home Recovery Information Given	(a)	90%	84%	85%
Hospital Given 9 or 10 on 10 Point Scale	(a)	71%	72%	71%
Meds 'Always' Explained Before Given	(a)	63%	66%	64%
Nurses 'Always' Communicated Well	(a)	81%	80%	79%
Pain 'Always' Well Controlled	(a)	70%	72%	71%
Room and Bathroom 'Always' Clean	(a)	56%	73%	73%
Timely Help 'Always' Received	(a)	75%	71%	68%
Would Definitely Recommend Hospital	(a)	75%	71%	71%
Use of Medical Imaging				
Cardiac Imaging Stress Test before Surgery	136	2.9%	4.5%	5.3%
Combination Abdominal CT Scan	106	55.7%	23%	10.5%
Combination Brain/Sinus CT Scan	79	8.9%	2.2%	2.7%
Combination Chest CT Scan	63	33.3%	5.1%	2.7%
Follow-up Mammogram/Ultrasound	181	11.0%	8.1%	8.8%
Lumbar Spine MRI for Low Back Pain[1]	-	-	39.9%	37.2%

Holdenville Hospital Authority

100 Mcdougal Drive
Holdenville, OK 74848
Phone: 405-379-4200
Type: Critical Access Hospitals
Ownership: Govt - Hospital Dist/Auth
Emergency Services: Yes
Beds: 25

Key Personnel:

Anesthesiology................ Bill Brasher
CEO/President................ Bridget Cosby, CEO
Emergency Room............ Evin Marshall
Chief of Medical Staff.......... Tom Osborn, DO
Operating Room.............. Jackie Smith

Measure	Cases	This Hosp.	State Avg.	U.S. Avg.
Blood Clot Prevention and Treatment				
Anticoagulation Overlap Therapy[5]	-	-	89%	93%
ICU Venous Thromboembolism Prophylaxis[5]	-	-	87%	92%
Incidence of Potentially Preventable VTE[5]	-	-	8%	10%
UFH with Dosages/Platelet Monitoring[5]	-	-	97%	97%
Venous Thromboembolism Prophylaxis[5]	-	-	72%	85%
Warfarin Therapy Discharge Instructions[5]	-	-	73%	75%
Chest Pain/Possible Heart Attack Care				
Aspirin Given Within 24 Hours of Arrival	51	90%	95%	96%
Fibrinolytic Meds Within 30 Min. of Arrival[1,3]	-	-	54%	58%
Average Time to ECG (minutes)	52	8	8	7
Average Time to Transfer (minutes)[3,7]	-	-	77	60
Children's Asthma Care				
Received Home Management Plan of Care	-	-	-	88%
Received Reliever Medication	-	-	-	100%
Received Systemic Corticosteroids	-	-	-	100%
Emergency Department				
Admittance Decision Time (minutes)	43	44	63	98
Head CT Results Within 45 Min. of Arrival[1]	-	-	49%	57%
Patients Who Left ER Before Being Seen	7,625	1%	2%	2%
Time from ER Arrival to Admit. (minutes)	86	163	210	274
Time from ER Arrival to Discharge (minutes)	49	80	110	134
Time in ER Before Being Evaluated (minutes)	114	16	24	26
Time to Pain Meds for Fractures (minutes)	31	37	55	57
Heart Attack Care				
Aspirin Given at Discharge[3,7]	-	-	99%	99%
Fibrinolytic Meds Within 30 Min. of Arrival[3,7]	-	-	25%	54%

NOTE: Hospital profiles are in alphabetical order by state, then city, then hospital within the city; Rankings exclude hospitals with less than 25 cases except for patient surveys which excludes hospitals with less than 100 cases; (a) 100-299 cases; (1) The number of cases/patients is too few to report; (2) Data submitted were based on a sample of cases/patients; (3) Results are based on a shorter time period than required; (4) Data suppressed by CMS for one or more quarters; (5) Results are not available for this reporting period; (6) Fewer than 100 patients completed the HCAHPS survey; (7) No cases met the criteria for this measure; (8) The lower limit of the confidence interval cannot be calculated if the number of observed infections equals zero; (9) No data are available from the state/territory for this reporting period; (10) The scores shown reflect fewer than 50 completed surveys; (11) There were discrepancies in the data collection process; (12) This measure does not apply to this hospital for this reporting period; (13) Results cannot be calculated for this reporting period; (14) The results for this state are combined with nearby states to protect confidentiality; Please refer to the User's Guide for a full explanation of data.

Measure	Cases	This Hosp.	State Avg.	U.S. Avg.
PCI Within 90 Minutes of Arrival[3,7]	-	-	95%	96%
Statin Prescribed at Discharge[3,7]	-	-	98%	98%
Heart Failure Care				
ACE Inhibitor or ARB for LVSD[1]	-	-	95%	97%
Discharge Instructions Given	13	62%	92%	94%
Evaluation of LVS Function	19	68%	96%	99%
Medicare Spending				
Medicare Spending per Patient (ratio)	-	-	0.93	0.98
Pneumonia Care				
Appropriate Initial Antibiotic Given	42	86%	92%	95%
Blood Culture Timing	36	92%	97%	98%
Pregnancy and Delivery Care				
Newborn Deliveries Scheduled Early[5]	-	-	8%	6%
Preventive Care				
Immunization for Influenza	51	80%	89%	90%
Immunization for Pneumonia	81	85%	91%	92%
Stroke Care				
Anticoagulation Therapy for Atrial Fibrillation[5]	-	-	91%	95%
Antithrombotic Therapy Timing[5]	-	-	95%	98%
Assessed for Rehabilitation[5]	-	-	96%	97%
Discharged on Antithrombotic Therapy[5]	-	-	98%	99%
Discharged on Statin Medication[5]	-	-	88%	94%
Thrombolytic Therapy Timing[5]	-	-	61%	66%
Venous Thromboembolism Prophylaxis[5]	-	-	92%	94%
Written Stroke Educational Materials Given[5]	-	-	86%	88%
Surgical Care Improvement Project				
Appropriate Beta Blocker Usage[5]	-	-	97%	98%
Appropriate VTP Within 24 Hours[5]	-	-	97%	98%
Controlled Postoperative Blood Glucose[5]	-	-	97%	97%
Perioperative Temperature Management[5]	-	-	100%	100%
Prophylactic Antibiotic Selection[5]	-	-	99%	99%
Prophylactic Antibiotic Selection (Outpatient)[5]	-	-	98%	98%
Prophylactic Antibiotic Stopped[5]	-	-	98%	98%
Prophylactic Antibiotic Timing[5]	-	-	98%	99%
Prophylactic Antibiotic Timing (Outpatient)[5]	-	-	98%	98%
Urinary Catheter Removal[5]	-	-	96%	97%
Survey of Patients' Hospital Experiences				
Area Around Room 'Always' Quiet at Night[5]	-	-	68%	61%
Doctors 'Always' Communicated Well[5]	-	-	84%	82%
Home Recovery Information Given[5]	-	-	84%	85%
Hospital Given 9 or 10 on 10 Point Scale[5]	-	-	72%	71%
Meds 'Always' Explained Before Given[5]	-	-	66%	64%
Nurses 'Always' Communicated Well[5]	-	-	80%	79%
Pain 'Always' Well Controlled[5]	-	-	72%	71%
Room and Bathroom 'Always' Clean[5]	-	-	73%	73%
Timely Help 'Always' Received[5]	-	-	71%	68%
Would Definitely Recommend Hospital[5]	-	-	71%	71%
Use of Medical Imaging				
Cardiac Imaging Stress Test before Surgery[7]	-	-	4.5%	5.3%
Combination Abdominal CT Scan	163	12.9%	23%	10.5%
Combination Brain/Sinus CT Scan[1]	-	-	2.2%	2.7%
Combination Chest CT Scan[1]	-	-	5.1%	2.7%
Follow-up Mammogram/Ultrasound[7]	-	-	8.1%	8.8%
Lumbar Spine MRI for Low Back Pain[1]	-	-	39.9%	37.2%

Harmon Memorial Hospital

400 East Chestnut Street
Hollis, OK 73550
Phone: 580-688-3363
Fax: 580-688-2246
Type: Acute Care Hospitals
Emergency Services: Yes
Ownership: Govt - Hospital Dist/Auth
Beds: 22

Measure	Cases	This Hosp.	State Avg.	U.S. Avg.
Blood Clot Prevention and Treatment				
Anticoagulation Overlap Therapy[1,2]	-	-	89%	93%
ICU Venous Thromboembolism Prophylaxis[2,7]	-	-	87%	92%
Incidence of Potentially Preventable VTE[2,7]	-	-	8%	10%
UFH with Dosages/Platelet Monitoring[2,7]	-	-	97%	97%
Venous Thromboembolism Prophylaxis[2]	115	0%	72%	85%
Warfarin Therapy Discharge Instructions[2,7]	-	-	73%	75%
Chest Pain/Possible Heart Attack Care				
Aspirin Given Within 24 Hours of Arrival[1,3]	-	-	95%	96%
Fibrinolytic Meds Within 30 Min. of Arrival[3,7]	-	-	54%	58%
Average Time to ECG (minutes)[1,3]	-	-	8	7
Average Time to Transfer (minutes)[3,7]	-	-	77	60
Children's Asthma Care				
Received Home Management Plan of Care	-	-	-	88%
Received Reliever Medication	-	-	-	100%
Received Systemic Corticosteroids	-	-	-	100%
Emergency Department				
Admittance Decision Time (minutes)	210	10	63	98
Head CT Results Within 45 Min. of Arrival[1,3]	-	-	49%	57%
Patients Who Left ER Before Being Seen	1,970	1%	2%	2%
Time from ER Arrival to Admit. (minutes)	228	115	210	274
Time from ER Arrival to Discharge (minutes)	226	106	110	134
Time in ER Before Being Evaluated (minutes)	240	25	24	26
Time to Pain Meds for Fractures (minutes)[5]	-	-	55	57
Heart Attack Care				
Aspirin Given at Discharge[1,3]	-	-	99%	99%
Fibrinolytic Meds Within 30 Min. of Arrival[3,7]	-	-	25%	54%
PCI Within 90 Minutes of Arrival[3,7]	-	-	95%	96%
Statin Prescribed at Discharge[1,3]	-	-	98%	98%
Heart Failure Care				
ACE Inhibitor or ARB for LVSD[1]	-	-	95%	97%
Discharge Instructions Given	19	79%	92%	94%
Evaluation of LVS Function	22	14%	96%	99%
Medicare Spending				
Medicare Spending per Patient (ratio)	-	0.62	0.93	0.98
Pneumonia Care				
Appropriate Initial Antibiotic Given	12	75%	92%	95%
Blood Culture Timing[1]	-	-	97%	98%
Pregnancy and Delivery Care				
Newborn Deliveries Scheduled Early[7]	-	-	8%	6%
Preventive Care				
Immunization for Influenza	206	87%	89%	90%
Immunization for Pneumonia	244	86%	91%	92%
Stroke Care				
Anticoagulation Therapy for Atrial Fibrillation[3,7]	-	-	91%	95%
Antithrombotic Therapy Timing[1,3]	-	-	95%	98%
Assessed for Rehabilitation[1,3]	-	-	96%	97%
Discharged on Antithrombotic Therapy[1,3]	-	-	98%	99%
Discharged on Statin Medication[1,3]	-	-	88%	94%
Thrombolytic Therapy Timing[1,3]	-	-	61%	66%
Venous Thromboembolism Prophylaxis[1,3]	-	-	92%	94%
Written Stroke Educational Materials Given[1,3]	-	-	86%	88%
Surgical Care Improvement Project				
Appropriate Beta Blocker Usage[5]	-	-	97%	98%
Appropriate VTP Within 24 Hours[5]	-	-	97%	98%
Controlled Postoperative Blood Glucose[5]	-	-	97%	97%
Perioperative Temperature Management[5]	-	-	100%	100%
Prophylactic Antibiotic Selection[5]	-	-	99%	99%
Prophylactic Antibiotic Selection (Outpatient)[5]	-	-	98%	98%
Prophylactic Antibiotic Stopped[5]	-	-	98%	98%
Prophylactic Antibiotic Timing[5]	-	-	98%	99%
Prophylactic Antibiotic Timing (Outpatient)[5]	-	-	98%	98%
Urinary Catheter Removal[5]	-	-	96%	97%
Survey of Patients' Hospital Experiences				
Area Around Room 'Always' Quiet at Night[10]	<100	61%	68%	61%
Doctors 'Always' Communicated Well[10]	<100	71%	84%	82%
Home Recovery Information Given[10]	<100	82%	84%	85%
Hospital Given 9 or 10 on 10 Point Scale[10]	<100	62%	72%	71%
Meds 'Always' Explained Before Given[10]	<100	80%	66%	64%
Nurses 'Always' Communicated Well[10]	<100	71%	80%	79%
Pain 'Always' Well Controlled[10]	<100	58%	72%	71%
Room and Bathroom 'Always' Clean[10]	<100	83%	73%	73%
Timely Help 'Always' Received[10]	<100	80%	71%	68%
Would Definitely Recommend Hospital[10]	<100	64%	71%	71%
Use of Medical Imaging				
Cardiac Imaging Stress Test before Surgery[7]	-	-	4.5%	5.3%
Combination Abdominal CT Scan[1]	-	-	23%	10.5%
Combination Brain/Sinus CT Scan	65	0.0%	2.2%	2.7%
Combination Chest CT Scan[1]	-	-	5.1%	2.7%
Follow-up Mammogram/Ultrasound[7]	-	-	8.1%	8.8%
Lumbar Spine MRI for Low Back Pain[7]	-	-	39.9%	37.2%

Choctaw Memorial Hospital

1405 East Kirk Road
Hugo, OK 74743
Phone: 580-317-9500
Fax: 580-326-3541
Type: Acute Care Hospitals
Emergency Services: Yes
Ownership: Govt - Hospital Dist/Auth
Beds: 34

Key Personnel:

Chief of Medical Staff. . . . . Ted Rowland, MD
CEO/President. . . . . Emmett Sthuster

Measure	Cases	This Hosp.	State Avg.	U.S. Avg.
Blood Clot Prevention and Treatment				
Anticoagulation Overlap Therapy[1,2]	-	-	89%	93%
ICU Venous Thromboembolism Prophylaxis[2,7]	-	-	87%	92%
Incidence of Potentially Preventable VTE[1,2]	-	-	8%	10%
UFH with Dosages/Platelet Monitoring[2,7]	-	-	97%	97%
Venous Thromboembolism Prophylaxis[2]	211	2%	72%	85%
Warfarin Therapy Discharge Instructions[1,2]	-	-	73%	75%
Chest Pain/Possible Heart Attack Care				
Aspirin Given Within 24 Hours of Arrival	18	72%	95%	96%
Fibrinolytic Meds Within 30 Min. of Arrival[1]	-	-	54%	58%
Average Time to ECG (minutes)	19	24	8	7
Average Time to Transfer (minutes)[1]	-	-	77	60
Children's Asthma Care				
Received Home Management Plan of Care	-	-	-	88%
Received Reliever Medication	-	-	-	100%
Received Systemic Corticosteroids	-	-	-	100%
Emergency Department				
Admittance Decision Time (minutes)[2]	106	60	63	98
Head CT Results Within 45 Min. of Arrival[1,3]	-	-	49%	57%
Patients Who Left ER Before Being Seen	6,531	6%	2%	2%
Time from ER Arrival to Admit. (minutes)[2]	117	206	210	274
Time from ER Arrival to Discharge (minutes)	328	100	110	134
Time in ER Before Being Evaluated (minutes)	294	36	24	26
Time to Pain Meds for Fractures (minutes)	25	71	55	57
Heart Attack Care				
Aspirin Given at Discharge[1,3]	-	-	99%	99%
Fibrinolytic Meds Within 30 Min. of Arrival[3,7]	-	-	25%	54%
PCI Within 90 Minutes of Arrival[3,7]	-	-	95%	96%
Statin Prescribed at Discharge[1,3]	-	-	98%	98%
Heart Failure Care				
ACE Inhibitor or ARB for LVSD[1,2]	-	-	95%	97%
Discharge Instructions Given[2]	65	80%	92%	94%
Evaluation of LVS Function[2]	101	72%	96%	99%
Medicare Spending				
Medicare Spending per Patient (ratio)	-	1.02	0.93	0.98
Pneumonia Care				
Appropriate Initial Antibiotic Given	72	79%	92%	95%
Blood Culture Timing	12	50%	97%	98%
Pregnancy and Delivery Care				
Newborn Deliveries Scheduled Early[7]	-	-	8%	6%
Preventive Care				
Immunization for Influenza[2]	275	67%	89%	90%
Immunization for Pneumonia[2]	454	76%	91%	92%
Stroke Care				
Anticoagulation Therapy for Atrial Fibrillation[1]	-	-	91%	95%
Antithrombotic Therapy Timing[1]	-	-	95%	98%
Assessed for Rehabilitation[1]	-	-	96%	97%
Discharged on Antithrombotic Therapy[1]	-	-	98%	99%
Discharged on Statin Medication[1]	-	-	88%	94%
Thrombolytic Therapy Timing[1]	-	-	61%	66%
Venous Thromboembolism Prophylaxis[1]	-	-	92%	94%
Written Stroke Educational Materials Given[1]	-	-	86%	88%
Surgical Care Improvement Project				
Appropriate Beta Blocker Usage[3,7]	-	-	97%	98%
Appropriate VTP Within 24 Hours[1,3]	-	-	97%	98%
Controlled Postoperative Blood Glucose[3,7]	-	-	97%	97%
Perioperative Temperature Management[1,3]	-	-	100%	100%
Prophylactic Antibiotic Selection[1,3]	-	-	99%	99%
Prophylactic Antibiotic Selection (Outpatient)[5]	-	-	98%	98%
Prophylactic Antibiotic Stopped[1,3]	-	-	98%	98%
Prophylactic Antibiotic Timing[1,3]	-	-	98%	99%
Prophylactic Antibiotic Timing (Outpatient)[5]	-	-	98%	98%
Urinary Catheter Removal[1,3]	-	-	96%	97%
Survey of Patients' Hospital Experiences				

NOTE: Hospital profiles are in alphabetical order by state, then city, then hospital within the city; Rankings exclude hospitals with less than 25 cases except for patient surveys which excludes hospitals with less than 100 cases; (a) 100-299 cases; (1) The number of cases/patients is too few to report; (2) Data submitted were based on a sample of cases/patients; (3) Results are based on a shorter time period than required; (4) Data suppressed by CMS for one or more quarters; (5) Results are not available for this reporting period; (6) Fewer than 100 patients completed the HCAHPS survey; (7) No cases met the criteria for this measure; (8) The lower limit of the confidence interval cannot be calculated if the number of observed infections equals zero; (9) No data are available from the state/territory for this reporting period; (10) The scores shown reflect fewer than 50 completed surveys; (11) There were discrepancies in the data collection process; (12) This measure does not apply to this hospital for this reporting period; (13) Results cannot be calculated for this reporting period; (14) The results for this state are combined with nearby states to protect confidentiality; Please refer to the User's Guide for a full explanation of data.

Measure	Cases	This Hosp.	State Avg.	U.S. Avg.
Area Around Room 'Always' Quiet at Night	(a)	56%	68%	61%
Doctors 'Always' Communicated Well	(a)	84%	84%	82%
Home Recovery Information Given	(a)	72%	84%	85%
Hospital Given 9 or 10 on 10 Point Scale	(a)	52%	72%	71%
Meds 'Always' Explained Before Given	(a)	58%	66%	64%
Nurses 'Always' Communicated Well	(a)	73%	80%	79%
Pain 'Always' Well Controlled	(a)	64%	72%	71%
Room and Bathroom 'Always' Clean	(a)	73%	73%	73%
Timely Help 'Always' Received	(a)	60%	71%	68%
Would Definitely Recommend Hospital	(a)	54%	71%	71%
Use of Medical Imaging				
Cardiac Imaging Stress Test before Surgery[7]	-	-	4.5%	5.3%
Combination Abdominal CT Scan	119	53.8%	23%	10.5%
Combination Brain/Sinus CT Scan[1]	-	-	2.2%	2.7%
Combination Chest CT Scan	78	46.2%	5.1%	2.7%
Follow-up Mammogram/Ultrasound	148	8.8%	8.1%	8.8%
Lumbar Spine MRI for Low Back Pain	51	60.8%	39.9%	37.2%

McCurtain Memorial Hospital

1301 Lincoln Road
Idabel, OK 74745
Phone: 580-286-7623
Fax: 580-208-3199
Type: Acute Care Hospitals
Emergency Services: Yes
Ownership: Voluntary non-profit - Private
Beds: 111

Key Personnel:

Intensive Care Unit. . . . . Debbie Adams, RN
Emergency Room . . . . Faye Gurley
Chief of Medical Staff . . . . Jon Maxwell, DO
Operating Room. . . . . Anne May
CEO/President. . . . . Brit Messer
Quality Assurance . . . . Carla Mitchell, RN
Radiology. . . . . R Pritchard, MD
Infection Control. . . . . Ella Ward, RN

Measure	Cases	This Hosp.	State Avg.	U.S. Avg.
Blood Clot Prevention and Treatment				
Anticoagulation Overlap Therapy[1,2]	-	-	89%	93%
ICU Venous Thromboembolism Prophylaxis[2]	53	55%	87%	92%
Incidence of Potentially Preventable VTE[2,7]	-	-	8%	10%
UFH with Dosages/Platelet Monitoring[2,7]	-	-	97%	97%
Venous Thromboembolism Prophylaxis[2]	146	38%	72%	85%
Warfarin Therapy Discharge Instructions[1,2]	-	-	73%	75%
Chest Pain/Possible Heart Attack Care				
Aspirin Given Within 24 Hours of Arrival	41	85%	95%	96%
Fibrinolytic Meds Within 30 Min. of Arrival[1]	-	-	54%	58%
Average Time to ECG (minutes)	43	11	8	7
Average Time to Transfer (minutes)[1]	-	-	77	60
Children's Asthma Care				
Received Home Management Plan of Care	-	-	-	88%
Received Reliever Medication	-	-	-	100%
Received Systemic Corticosteroids	-	-	-	100%
Emergency Department				
Admittance Decision Time (minutes)[2]	422	64	63	98
Head CT Results Within 45 Min. of Arrival	11	73%	49%	57%
Patients Who Left ER Before Being Seen	13,406	5%	2%	2%
Time from ER Arrival to Admit. (minutes)[2]	428	270	210	274
Time from ER Arrival to Discharge (minutes)	384	156	110	134
Time in ER Before Being Evaluated (minutes)	216	52	24	26
Time to Pain Meds for Fractures (minutes)	75	97	55	57
Heart Attack Care				
Aspirin Given at Discharge[3,7]	-	-	99%	99%
Fibrinolytic Meds Within 30 Minutes of Arrival[3,7]	-	-	25%	54%
PCI Within 90 Minutes of Arrival[3,7]	-	-	95%	96%
Statin Prescribed at Discharge[3,7]	-	-	98%	98%
Heart Failure Care				
ACE Inhibitor or ARB for LVSD[2]	11	100%	95%	97%
Discharge Instructions Given[2]	60	55%	92%	94%
Evaluation of LVS Function[2]	64	77%	96%	99%
Medicare Spending				
Medicare Spending per Patient (ratio)	-	0.94	0.93	0.98
Pneumonia Care				
Appropriate Initial Antibiotic Given[2]	69	93%	92%	95%
Blood Culture Timing[2]	81	99%	97%	98%
Pregnancy and Delivery Care				
Newborn Deliveries Scheduled Early	88	1%	8%	6%
Preventive Care				
Immunization for Influenza[2]	264	75%	89%	90%
Immunization for Pneumonia[2]	385	82%	91%	92%
Stroke Care				
Anticoagulation Therapy for Atrial Fibrillation[1]	-	-	91%	95%
Antithrombotic Therapy Timing[1]	-	-	95%	98%
Assessed for Rehabilitation[1]	-	-	96%	97%
Discharged on Antithrombotic Therapy[1]	-	-	98%	99%
Discharged on Statin Medication[1]	-	-	88%	94%
Thrombolytic Therapy Timing[1]	-	-	61%	66%
Venous Thromboembolism Prophylaxis[1]	-	-	92%	94%
Written Stroke Educational Materials Given[1]	-	-	86%	88%
Surgical Care Improvement Project				
Appropriate Beta Blocker Usage[1]	-	-	97%	98%
Appropriate VTP Within 24 Hours	27	100%	97%	98%
Controlled Postoperative Blood Glucose[7]	-	-	97%	97%
Perioperative Temperature Management	29	100%	100%	100%
Prophylactic Antibiotic Selection	17	88%	99%	99%
Prophylactic Antibiotic Selection (Outpatient)[1,3]	-	-	98%	98%
Prophylactic Antibiotic Stopped	17	76%	98%	98%
Prophylactic Antibiotic Timing	17	100%	98%	99%
Prophylactic Antibiotic Timing (Outpatient)[1,3]	-	-	98%	98%
Urinary Catheter Removal[1]	-	-	96%	97%
Survey of Patients' Hospital Experiences				
Area Around Room 'Always' Quiet at Night	(a)	65%	68%	61%
Doctors 'Always' Communicated Well	(a)	78%	84%	82%
Home Recovery Information Given	(a)	79%	84%	85%
Hospital Given 9 or 10 on 10 Point Scale	(a)	51%	72%	71%
Meds 'Always' Explained Before Given	(a)	57%	66%	64%
Nurses 'Always' Communicated Well	(a)	77%	80%	79%
Pain 'Always' Well Controlled	(a)	69%	72%	71%
Room and Bathroom 'Always' Clean	(a)	65%	73%	73%
Timely Help 'Always' Received	(a)	66%	71%	68%
Would Definitely Recommend Hospital	(a)	49%	71%	71%
Use of Medical Imaging				
Cardiac Imaging Stress Test before Surgery[7]	-	-	4.5%	5.3%
Combination Abdominal CT Scan	223	42.2%	23%	10.5%
Combination Brain/Sinus CT Scan	336	4.8%	2.2%	2.7%
Combination Chest CT Scan	84	23.8%	5.1%	2.7%
Follow-up Mammogram/Ultrasound	249	5.6%	8.1%	8.8%
Lumbar Spine MRI for Low Back Pain[1]	-	-	39.9%	37.2%

Mercy Hospital Kingfisher

1000 Kingfisher Hospital Drive
Kingfisher, OK 73750
Phone: 405-375-3141
Fax: 405-375-6983
E-mail: dbenson@krhhospital.com
URL: www.kingfisherhospital.com
Type: Critical Access Hospitals
Emergency Services: Yes
Ownership: Voluntary non-profit - Private
Beds: 25

Key Personnel:

Emergency Room . . . . Steve Arthurs
Administrator . . . . Brian Denton
CEO/President. . . . . Steve Jacobson
Chief of Medical Staff . . . . Jb Krablin
Infection Control. . . . . Amanda Mathews
Radiology. . . . . Ted Payne

Measure	Cases	This Hosp.	State Avg.	U.S. Avg.
Blood Clot Prevention and Treatment				
Anticoagulation Overlap Therapy[2,3]	-	-	89%	93%
ICU Venous Thromboembolism Prophylaxis[2,3]	-	-	87%	92%
Incidence of Potentially Preventable VTE[2,3]	-	-	8%	10%
UFH with Dosages/Platelet Monitoring[2,3]	-	-	97%	97%
Venous Thromboembolism Prophylaxis[2,3]	17	82%	72%	85%
Warfarin Therapy Discharge Instructions[2,3]	-	-	73%	75%
Chest Pain/Possible Heart Attack Care				
Aspirin Given Within 24 Hours of Arrival[1]	-	-	95%	96%
Fibrinolytic Meds Within 30 Min. of Arrival[1,3]	-	-	54%	58%
Average Time to ECG (minutes)[1]	-	-	8	7
Average Time to Transfer (minutes)[1,3]	-	-	77	60
Children's Asthma Care				
Received Home Management Plan of Care	-	-	-	88%
Received Reliever Medication	-	-	-	100%
Received Systemic Corticosteroids	-	-	-	100%
Emergency Department				
Admittance Decision Time (minutes)	26	62	63	98
Head CT Results Within 45 Min. of Arrival[3,7]	-	-	49%	57%
Patients Who Left ER Before Being Seen[5]	-	-	2%	2%
Time from ER Arrival to Admit. (minutes)	34	206	210	274
Time from ER Arrival to Discharge (minutes)	37	158	110	134
Time in ER Before Being Evaluated (minutes)	47	20	24	26
Time to Pain Meds for Fractures (minutes)[1,3]	-	-	55	57
Heart Attack Care				
Aspirin Given at Discharge[5]	-	-	99%	99%
Fibrinolytic Meds Within 30 Min. of Arrival[5]	-	-	25%	54%
PCI Within 90 Minutes of Arrival[5]	-	-	95%	96%
Statin Prescribed at Discharge[5]	-	-	98%	98%
Heart Failure Care				
ACE Inhibitor or ARB for LVSD[1]	-	-	95%	97%
Discharge Instructions Given[1]	-	-	92%	94%
Evaluation of LVS Function	23	74%	96%	99%
Medicare Spending				
Medicare Spending per Patient (ratio)	-	-	0.93	0.98
Pneumonia Care				
Appropriate Initial Antibiotic Given[2]	41	73%	92%	95%
Blood Culture Timing[2]	27	85%	97%	98%
Pregnancy and Delivery Care				
Newborn Deliveries Scheduled Early[5]	-	-	8%	6%
Preventive Care				
Immunization for Influenza[2]	31	94%	89%	90%
Immunization for Pneumonia[2,3]	27	93%	91%	92%
Stroke Care				
Anticoagulation Therapy for Atrial Fibrillation[3,7]	-	-	91%	95%
Antithrombotic Therapy Timing[1,3]	-	-	95%	98%
Assessed for Rehabilitation[1,3]	-	-	96%	97%
Discharged on Antithrombotic Therapy[1,3]	-	-	98%	99%
Discharged on Statin Medication[1,3]	-	-	88%	94%
Thrombolytic Therapy Timing[3,7]	-	-	61%	66%
Venous Thromboembolism Prophylaxis[1,3]	-	-	92%	94%
Written Stroke Educational Materials Given[3,7]	-	-	86%	88%
Surgical Care Improvement Project				
Appropriate Beta Blocker Usage[5]	-	-	97%	98%
Appropriate VTP Within 24 Hours[5]	-	-	97%	98%
Controlled Postoperative Blood Glucose[5]	-	-	97%	97%
Perioperative Temperature Management[5]	-	-	100%	100%
Prophylactic Antibiotic Selection[5]	-	-	99%	99%
Prophylactic Antibiotic Selection (Outpatient)[5]	-	-	98%	98%
Prophylactic Antibiotic Stopped[5]	-	-	98%	98%
Prophylactic Antibiotic Timing[5]	-	-	98%	99%
Prophylactic Antibiotic Timing (Outpatient)[5]	-	-	98%	98%
Urinary Catheter Removal[5]	-	-	96%	97%
Survey of Patients' Hospital Experiences				
Area Around Room 'Always' Quiet at Night[6]	<100	66%	68%	61%
Doctors 'Always' Communicated Well[6]	<100	88%	84%	82%
Home Recovery Information Given[6]	<100	85%	84%	85%
Hospital Given 9 or 10 on 10 Point Scale[6]	<100	76%	72%	71%
Meds 'Always' Explained Before Given[6]	<100	67%	66%	64%
Nurses 'Always' Communicated Well[6]	<100	79%	80%	79%
Pain 'Always' Well Controlled[6]	<100	70%	72%	71%
Room and Bathroom 'Always' Clean[6]	<100	81%	73%	73%
Timely Help 'Always' Received[6]	<100	82%	71%	68%
Would Definitely Recommend Hospital[6]	<100	72%	71%	71%
Use of Medical Imaging				
Cardiac Imaging Stress Test before Surgery[7]	-	-	4.5%	5.3%
Combination Abdominal CT Scan	160	4.4%	23%	10.5%
Combination Brain/Sinus CT Scan	155	5.8%	2.2%	2.7%
Combination Chest CT Scan	133	1.5%	5.1%	2.7%
Follow-up Mammogram/Ultrasound	170	9.4%	8.1%	8.8%
Lumbar Spine MRI for Low Back Pain[1]	-	-	39.9%	37.2%

Comanche County Memorial Hospital

3401 West Gore Boulvard
Lawton, OK 73505
Phone: 580-355-8620
Fax: 580-250-5868
URL: www.memorialhealthsource.org
Type: Acute Care Hospitals
Emergency Services: Yes
Ownership: Govt - Hospital Dist/Auth
Beds: 250

Key Personnel:

Chief of Medical Staff . . . . Rick Brittingham
Emergency Room . . . . Barbara Clyde, RN
Radiology. . . . . Mittie Dragodjvich, MD

NOTE: Hospital profiles are in alphabetical order by state, then city, then hospital within the city; Rankings exclude hospitals with less than 25 cases except for patient surveys which excludes hospitals with less than 100 cases; (a) 100-299 cases; (1) The number of cases/patients is too few to report; (2) Data submitted were based on a sample of cases/patients; (3) Results are based on a shorter time period than required; (4) Data suppressed by CMS for one or more quarters; (5) Results are not available for this reporting period; (6) Fewer than 100 patients completed the HCAHPS survey; (7) No cases met the criteria for this measure; (8) The lower limit of the confidence interval cannot be calculated if the number of observed infections equals zero; (9) No data are available from the state/territory for this reporting period; (10) The scores shown reflect fewer than 50 completed surveys; (11) There were discrepancies in the data collection process; (12) This measure does not apply to this hospital for this reporting period; (13) Results cannot be calculated for this reporting period; (14) The results for this state are combined with nearby states to protect confidentiality; Please refer to the User's Guide for a full explanation of data.

Quality Assurance . . . . Joanne Knecht
Operating Room. . . . . Marilyn Magid, RN
Pediatric Ambulatory Care . . . . . . Joseph Rarick, MD
Pediatric In-Patient Care . . . . Joseph Rarick, MD
CEO . . . . Randy Segler

Measure	Cases	This Hosp.	State Avg.	U.S. Avg.
Blood Clot Prevention and Treatment				
Anticoagulation Overlap Therapy[2]	36	94%	89%	93%
ICU Venous Thromboembolism Prophylaxis[2]	86	84%	87%	92%
Incidence of Potentially Preventable VTE[2]	11	0%	8%	10%
UFH with Dosages/Platelet Monitoring[1,2]	-	-	97%	97%
Venous Thromboembolism Prophylaxis[2]	370	78%	72%	85%
Warfarin Therapy Discharge Instructions[2]	26	81%	73%	75%
Chest Pain/Possible Heart Attack Care				
Aspirin Given Within 24 Hours of Arrival[1,3]	-	-	95%	96%
Fibrinolytic Meds Within 30 Min. of Arrival[5]	-	-	54%	58%
Average Time to ECG (minutes)[1,3]	-	-	8	7
Average Time to Transfer (minutes)[5]	-	-	77	60
Children's Asthma Care				
Received Home Management Plan of Care	-	-	-	88%
Received Reliever Medication	-	-	-	100%
Received Systemic Corticosteroids	-	-	-	100%
Emergency Department				
Admittance Decision Time (minutes)[2]	308	109	63	98
Head CT Results Within 45 Min. of Arrival	11	73%	49%	57%
Patients Who Left ER Before Being Seen	52,559	1%	2%	2%
Time from ER Arrival to Admit. (minutes)[2]	319	267	210	274
Time from ER Arrival to Discharge (minutes)	475	109	110	134
Time in ER Before Being Evaluated (minutes)	254	30	24	26
Time to Pain Meds for Fractures (minutes)	95	58	55	57
Heart Attack Care				
Aspirin Given at Discharge[2]	307	99%	99%	99%
Fibrinolytic Meds Within 30 Min. of Arrival[2,7]	-	-	25%	54%
PCI Within 90 Minutes of Arrival[2]	42	95%	95%	96%
Statin Prescribed at Discharge[2]	301	97%	98%	98%
Heart Failure Care				
ACE Inhibitor or ARB for LVSD[2]	98	94%	95%	97%
Discharge Instructions Given[2]	201	83%	92%	94%
Evaluation of LVS Function[2]	250	98%	96%	99%
Medicare Spending				
Medicare Spending per Patient (ratio)	-	0.93	0.93	0.98
Pneumonia Care				
Appropriate Initial Antibiotic Given[2]	78	90%	92%	95%
Blood Culture Timing[2]	123	92%	97%	98%
Pregnancy and Delivery Care				
Newborn Deliveries Scheduled Early[2]	42	5%	8%	6%
Preventive Care				
Immunization for Influenza[2]	575	92%	89%	90%
Immunization for Pneumonia[2]	718	87%	91%	92%
Stroke Care				
Anticoagulation Therapy for Atrial Fibrillation[2]	13	100%	91%	95%
Antithrombotic Therapy Timing[2]	86	98%	95%	98%
Assessed for Rehabilitation[2]	91	89%	96%	97%
Discharged on Antithrombotic Therapy[2]	80	94%	98%	99%
Discharged on Statin Medication[2]	62	84%	88%	94%
Thrombolytic Therapy Timing[1,2]	-	-	61%	66%
Venous Thromboembolism Prophylaxis[2]	96	88%	92%	94%
Written Stroke Educational Materials Given[2]	51	69%	86%	88%
Surgical Care Improvement Project				
Appropriate Beta Blocker Usage[2]	230	97%	97%	98%
Appropriate VTP Within 24 Hours[2]	386	97%	97%	98%
Controlled Postoperative Blood Glucose[2]	151	92%	97%	97%
Perioperative Temperature Management[2]	473	99%	100%	100%
Prophylactic Antibiotic Selection[2]	377	100%	99%	99%
Prophylactic Antibiotic Selection (Outpatient)	447	97%	98%	98%
Prophylactic Antibiotic Stopped[2]	368	98%	98%	98%
Prophylactic Antibiotic Timing[2]	378	98%	98%	99%
Prophylactic Antibiotic Timing (Outpatient)	453	97%	98%	98%
Urinary Catheter Removal[2]	381	95%	96%	97%
Survey of Patients' Hospital Experiences				
Area Around Room 'Always' Quiet at Night	300+	63%	68%	61%
Doctors 'Always' Communicated Well	300+	82%	84%	82%
Home Recovery Information Given	300+	83%	84%	85%
Hospital Given 9 or 10 on 10 Point Scale	300+	72%	72%	71%
Meds 'Always' Explained Before Given	300+	63%	66%	64%
Nurses 'Always' Communicated Well	300+	79%	80%	79%
Pain 'Always' Well Controlled	300+	73%	72%	71%
Room and Bathroom 'Always' Clean	300+	70%	73%	73%
Timely Help 'Always' Received	300+	73%	71%	68%
Would Definitely Recommend Hospital	300+	73%	71%	71%
Use of Medical Imaging				
Cardiac Imaging Stress Test before Surgery	1,211	5.2%	4.5%	5.3%
Combination Abdominal CT Scan	1,048	6.0%	23%	10.5%
Combination Brain/Sinus CT Scan	635	1.9%	2.2%	2.7%
Combination Chest CT Scan	739	0.3%	5.1%	2.7%
Follow-up Mammogram/Ultrasound	1,295	8.0%	8.1%	8.8%
Lumbar Spine MRI for Low Back Pain	202	38.6%	39.9%	37.2%

Southwestern Medical Center

5602 Southwest Lee Boulevard
Lawton, OK 73505
Phone: 580-531-4700
Fax: 580-531-4702
URL: www.swmconline.com
Type: Acute Care Hospitals
Emergency Services: Yes
Ownership: Proprietary
Beds: 162
Key Personnel:
Emergency Room . . . . David W Behm
Radiology. . . . . Randall D Behrmann
Administrator . . . . Lanya Doyle
CEO . . . . Steve Hyde
Quality Assurance . . . . Dinah Lazarte
President . . . . Daniel K. Podolsky, MD
CEO/President. . . . . Thomas L Rine
Chief of Medical Staff . . . . Shane Ross

Measure	Cases	This Hosp.	State Avg.	U.S. Avg.
Blood Clot Prevention and Treatment				
Anticoagulation Overlap Therapy[2]	12	50%	89%	93%
ICU Venous Thromboembolism Prophylaxis[2]	63	90%	87%	92%
Incidence of Potentially Preventable VTE[1,2]	-	-	8%	10%
UFH with Dosages/Platelet Monitoring[1,2]	-	-	97%	97%
Venous Thromboembolism Prophylaxis[2]	235	74%	72%	85%
Warfarin Therapy Discharge Instructions[1,2]	-	-	73%	75%
Chest Pain/Possible Heart Attack Care				
Aspirin Given Within 24 Hours of Arrival	11	100%	95%	96%
Fibrinolytic Meds Within 30 Min. of Arrival[7]	-	-	54%	58%
Average Time to ECG (minutes)	12	6	8	7
Average Time to Transfer (minutes)[1]	-	-	77	60
Children's Asthma Care				
Received Home Management Plan of Care	-	-	-	88%
Received Reliever Medication	-	-	-	100%
Received Systemic Corticosteroids	-	-	-	100%
Emergency Department				
Admittance Decision Time (minutes)[2]	273	75	63	98
Head CT Results Within 45 Min. of Arrival[3,7]	-	-	49%	57%
Patients Who Left ER Before Being Seen	18,915	2%	2%	2%
Time from ER Arrival to Admit. (minutes)[2]	281	233	210	274
Time from ER Arrival to Discharge (minutes)	431	130	110	134
Time in ER Before Being Evaluated (minutes)	442	34	24	26
Time to Pain Meds for Fractures (minutes)	61	81	55	57
Heart Attack Care				
Aspirin Given at Discharge[1,3]	-	-	99%	99%
Fibrinolytic Meds Within 30 Min. of Arrival[3,7]	-	-	25%	54%
PCI Within 90 Minutes of Arrival[3,7]	-	-	95%	96%
Statin Prescribed at Discharge[1,3]	-	-	98%	98%
Heart Failure Care				
ACE Inhibitor or ARB for LVSD	11	100%	95%	97%
Discharge Instructions Given	36	92%	92%	94%
Evaluation of LVS Function	55	100%	96%	99%
Medicare Spending				
Medicare Spending per Patient (ratio)	-	0.95	0.93	0.98
Pneumonia Care				
Appropriate Initial Antibiotic Given	35	97%	92%	95%
Blood Culture Timing	29	97%	97%	98%
Pregnancy and Delivery Care				
Newborn Deliveries Scheduled Early[2]	27	0%	8%	6%
Preventive Care				
Immunization for Influenza[2]	319	80%	89%	90%
Immunization for Pneumonia[2]	279	68%	91%	92%
Stroke Care				
Anticoagulation Therapy for Atrial Fibrillation[1]	-	-	91%	95%
Antithrombotic Therapy Timing	44	100%	95%	98%
Assessed for Rehabilitation	44	95%	96%	97%
Discharged on Antithrombotic Therapy	42	98%	98%	99%
Discharged on Statin Medication	27	89%	88%	94%
Thrombolytic Therapy Timing[7]	-	-	61%	66%
Venous Thromboembolism Prophylaxis	47	94%	92%	94%
Written Stroke Educational Materials Given	23	87%	86%	88%
Surgical Care Improvement Project				
Appropriate Beta Blocker Usage	46	93%	97%	98%
Appropriate VTP Within 24 Hours	200	96%	97%	98%
Controlled Postoperative Blood Glucose[7]	-	-	97%	97%
Perioperative Temperature Management	227	100%	100%	100%
Prophylactic Antibiotic Selection	144	96%	99%	99%
Prophylactic Antibiotic Selection (Outpatient)	158	92%	98%	98%
Prophylactic Antibiotic Stopped	141	97%	98%	98%
Prophylactic Antibiotic Timing	144	99%	98%	99%
Prophylactic Antibiotic Timing (Outpatient)	159	99%	98%	98%
Urinary Catheter Removal	83	89%	96%	97%
Survey of Patients' Hospital Experiences				
Area Around Room 'Always' Quiet at Night	300+	64%	68%	61%
Doctors 'Always' Communicated Well	300+	82%	84%	82%
Home Recovery Information Given	300+	84%	84%	85%
Hospital Given 9 or 10 on 10 Point Scale	300+	67%	72%	71%
Meds 'Always' Explained Before Given	300+	62%	66%	64%
Nurses 'Always' Communicated Well	300+	73%	80%	79%
Pain 'Always' Well Controlled	300+	66%	72%	71%
Room and Bathroom 'Always' Clean	300+	67%	73%	73%
Timely Help 'Always' Received	300+	63%	71%	68%
Would Definitely Recommend Hospital	300+	70%	71%	71%
Use of Medical Imaging				
Cardiac Imaging Stress Test before Surgery	89	9.0%	4.5%	5.3%
Combination Abdominal CT Scan	219	17.4%	23%	10.5%
Combination Brain/Sinus CT Scan[1]	-	-	2.2%	2.7%
Combination Chest CT Scan	120	15.0%	5.1%	2.7%
Follow-up Mammogram/Ultrasound[7]	-	-	8.1%	8.8%
Lumbar Spine MRI for Low Back Pain	206	44.2%	39.9%	37.2%

USPHS Lawton Indian Hospital

1515 Lawrie Tatum Road
Lawton, OK 73507
Phone: 580-354-5000
Fax: 580-353-2914
Type: Acute Care Hospitals
Emergency Services: Yes
Ownership: Government - Federal
Beds: 48
Key Personnel:
Infection Control. . . . . Sue Burgess
Operating Room. . . . . Dr Pilar
Pediatric Ambulatory Care . . . . . Bryce Poolaw, MD
Pediatric In-Patient Care . . . . . . Bryce Poolaw, MD
Chief of Medical Staff . . . . Dr Boyce Poolaw, MD
CEO/President. . . . . Hickory Starr, Jr
Quality Assurance . . . . Kevin Whitehead

Measure	Cases	This Hosp.	State Avg.	U.S. Avg.
Blood Clot Prevention and Treatment				
Anticoagulation Overlap Therapy[2,7]	-	-	89%	93%
ICU Venous Thromboembolism Prophylaxis[1,2]	-	-	87%	92%
Incidence of Potentially Preventable VTE[2,7]	-	-	8%	10%
UFH with Dosages/Platelet Monitoring[2,7]	-	-	97%	97%
Venous Thromboembolism Prophylaxis[2]	127	45%	72%	85%
Warfarin Therapy Discharge Instructions[2,7]	-	-	73%	75%
Chest Pain/Possible Heart Attack Care				
Aspirin Given Within 24 Hours of Arrival	-	-	95%	96%
Fibrinolytic Meds Within 30 Min. of Arrival	-	-	54%	58%
Average Time to ECG (minutes)	-	-	8	7
Average Time to Transfer (minutes)	-	-	77	60
Children's Asthma Care				
Received Home Management Plan of Care	-	-	-	88%
Received Reliever Medication	-	-	-	100%
Received Systemic Corticosteroids	-	-	-	100%
Emergency Department				
Admittance Decision Time (minutes)[2]	278	37	63	98
Head CT Results Within 45 Min. of Arrival	-	-	49%	57%
Patients Who Left ER Before Being Seen	-	-	2%	2%

NOTE: Hospital profiles are in alphabetical order by state, then city, then hospital within the city; Rankings exclude hospitals with less than 25 cases except for patient surveys which excludes hospitals with less than 100 cases; (a) 100-299 cases; (1) The number of cases/patients is too few to report; (2) Data submitted were based on a sample of cases/patients; (3) Results are based on a shorter time period than required; (4) Data suppressed by CMS for one or more quarters; (5) Results are not available for this reporting period; (6) Fewer than 100 patients completed the HCAHPS survey; (7) No cases met the criteria for this measure; (8) The lower limit of the confidence interval cannot be calculated if the number of observed infections equals zero; (9) No data are available from the state/territory for this reporting period; (10) The scores shown reflect fewer than 50 completed surveys; (11) There were discrepancies in the data collection process; (12) This measure does not apply to this hospital for this reporting period; (13) Results cannot be calculated for this reporting period; (14) The results for this state are combined with nearby states to protect confidentiality; Please refer to the User's Guide for a full explanation of data.

Time from ER Arrival to Admit. (minutes)[2]	278	253	210	274
Time from ER Arrival to Discharge (minutes)	-	-	110	134
Time in ER Before Being Evaluated (minutes)	-	-	24	26
Time to Pain Meds for Fractures (minutes)	-	-	55	57
Heart Attack Care				
Aspirin Given at Discharge[5]	-	-	99%	99%
Fibrinolytic Meds Within 30 Min. of Arrival[5]	-	-	25%	54%
PCI Within 90 Minutes of Arrival[5]	-	-	95%	96%
Statin Prescribed at Discharge[5]	-	-	98%	98%
Heart Failure Care				
ACE Inhibitor or ARB for LVSD[5]	-	-	95%	97%
Discharge Instructions Given[5]	-	-	92%	94%
Evaluation of LVS Function[5]	-	-	96%	99%
Medicare Spending				
Medicare Spending per Patient (ratio)	-	0.54	0.93	0.98
Pneumonia Care				
Appropriate Initial Antibiotic Given[3,7]	-	-	92%	95%
Blood Culture Timing[3,7]	-	-	97%	98%
Pregnancy and Delivery Care				
Newborn Deliveries Scheduled Early[7]	-	-	8%	6%
Preventive Care				
Immunization for Influenza	202	68%	89%	90%
Immunization for Pneumonia[2]	142	85%	91%	92%
Stroke Care				
Anticoagulation Therapy for Atrial Fibrillation[5]	-	-	91%	95%
Antithrombotic Therapy Timing[5]	-	-	95%	98%
Assessed for Rehabilitation[5]	-	-	96%	97%
Discharged on Antithrombotic Therapy[5]	-	-	98%	99%
Discharged on Statin Medication[5]	-	-	88%	94%
Thrombolytic Therapy Timing[5]	-	-	61%	66%
Venous Thromboembolism Prophylaxis[5]	-	-	92%	94%
Written Stroke Educational Materials Given[5]	-	-	86%	88%
Surgical Care Improvement Project				
Appropriate Beta Blocker Usage[5]	-	-	97%	98%
Appropriate VTP Within 24 Hours[5]	-	-	97%	98%
Controlled Postoperative Blood Glucose[5]	-	-	97%	97%
Perioperative Temperature Management[5]	-	-	100%	100%
Prophylactic Antibiotic Selection[5]	-	-	99%	99%
Prophylactic Antibiotic Selection (Outpatient)	-	-	98%	98%
Prophylactic Antibiotic Stopped[5]	-	-	98%	98%
Prophylactic Antibiotic Timing[5]	-	-	98%	99%
Prophylactic Antibiotic Timing (Outpatient)	-	-	98%	98%
Urinary Catheter Removal[5]	-	-	96%	97%
Survey of Patients' Hospital Experiences				
Area Around Room 'Always' Quiet at Night[10]	<100	78%	68%	61%
Doctors 'Always' Communicated Well[10]	<100	76%	84%	82%
Home Recovery Information Given[10]	<100	73%	84%	85%
Hospital Given 9 or 10 on 10 Point Scale[10]	<100	63%	72%	71%
Meds 'Always' Explained Before Given[10]	<100	62%	66%	64%
Nurses 'Always' Communicated Well[10]	<100	79%	80%	79%
Pain 'Always' Well Controlled[10]	<100	69%	72%	71%
Room and Bathroom 'Always' Clean[10]	<100	90%	73%	73%
Timely Help 'Always' Received[10]	<100	79%	71%	68%
Would Definitely Recommend Hospital[10]	<100	49%	71%	71%
Use of Medical Imaging				
Cardiac Imaging Stress Test before Surgery	-	-	4.5%	5.3%
Combination Abdominal CT Scan	-	-	23%	10.5%
Combination Brain/Sinus CT Scan	-	-	2.2%	2.7%
Combination Chest CT Scan	-	-	5.1%	2.7%
Follow-up Mammogram/Ultrasound	-	-	8.1%	8.8%
Lumbar Spine MRI for Low Back Pain	-	-	39.9%	37.2%

Lindsay Municipal Hospital

Highway 19 West
Lindsay, OK 73052
Phone: 405-756-1404
Fax: 405-756-1476
Type: Acute Care Hospitals
Ownership: Govt - Hospital Dist/Auth
Emergency Services: Yes
Beds: 25

Key Personnel:
Cardiac Laboratory. . . . . Lisa Davis
CEO/President. . . . . Norma Howard

Measure	Cases	This Hosp.	State Avg.	U.S. Avg.
Blood Clot Prevention and Treatment				
Anticoagulation Overlap Therapy[5]	-	-	89%	93%
ICU Venous Thromboembolism Prophylaxis[5]	-	-	87%	92%
Incidence of Potentially Preventable VTE[5]	-	-	8%	10%
UFH with Dosages/Platelet Monitoring[5]	-	-	97%	97%
Venous Thromboembolism Prophylaxis[5]	-	-	72%	85%
Warfarin Therapy Discharge Instructions[5]	-	-	73%	75%
Chest Pain/Possible Heart Attack Care				
Aspirin Given Within 24 Hours of Arrival	-	-	95%	96%
Fibrinolytic Meds Within 30 Min. of Arrival	-	-	54%	58%
Average Time to ECG (minutes)	-	-	8	7
Average Time to Transfer (minutes)	-	-	77	60
Children's Asthma Care				
Received Home Management Plan of Care	-	-	-	88%
Received Reliever Medication	-	-	-	100%
Received Systemic Corticosteroids	-	-	-	100%
Emergency Department				
Admittance Decision Time (minutes)[5]	-	-	63	98
Head CT Results Within 45 Min. of Arrival	-	-	49%	57%
Patients Who Left ER Before Being Seen	-	-	2%	2%
Time from ER Arrival to Admit. (minutes)[5]	-	-	210	274
Time from ER Arrival to Discharge (minutes)	-	-	110	134
Time in ER Before Being Evaluated (minutes)	-	-	24	26
Time to Pain Meds for Fractures (minutes)	-	-	55	57
Heart Attack Care				
Aspirin Given at Discharge[5]	-	-	99%	99%
Fibrinolytic Meds Within 30 Min. of Arrival[5]	-	-	25%	54%
PCI Within 90 Minutes of Arrival[5]	-	-	95%	96%
Statin Prescribed at Discharge[5]	-	-	98%	98%
Heart Failure Care				
ACE Inhibitor or ARB for LVSD[5]	-	-	95%	97%
Discharge Instructions Given[5]	-	-	92%	94%
Evaluation of LVS Function[5]	-	-	96%	99%
Medicare Spending				
Medicare Spending per Patient (ratio)[1]	-	-	0.93	0.98
Pneumonia Care				
Appropriate Initial Antibiotic Given[5]	-	-	92%	95%
Blood Culture Timing[5]	-	-	97%	98%
Pregnancy and Delivery Care				
Newborn Deliveries Scheduled Early[5]	-	-	8%	6%
Preventive Care				
Immunization for Influenza[5]	-	-	89%	90%
Immunization for Pneumonia[5]	-	-	91%	92%
Stroke Care				
Anticoagulation Therapy for Atrial Fibrillation[5]	-	-	91%	95%
Antithrombotic Therapy Timing[5]	-	-	95%	98%
Assessed for Rehabilitation[5]	-	-	96%	97%
Discharged on Antithrombotic Therapy[5]	-	-	98%	99%
Discharged on Statin Medication[5]	-	-	88%	94%
Thrombolytic Therapy Timing[5]	-	-	61%	66%
Venous Thromboembolism Prophylaxis[5]	-	-	92%	94%
Written Stroke Educational Materials Given[5]	-	-	86%	88%
Surgical Care Improvement Project				
Appropriate Beta Blocker Usage[5]	-	-	97%	98%
Appropriate VTP Within 24 Hours[5]	-	-	97%	98%
Controlled Postoperative Blood Glucose[5]	-	-	97%	97%
Perioperative Temperature Management[5]	-	-	100%	100%
Prophylactic Antibiotic Selection[5]	-	-	99%	99%
Prophylactic Antibiotic Selection (Outpatient)	-	-	98%	98%
Prophylactic Antibiotic Stopped[5]	-	-	98%	98%
Prophylactic Antibiotic Timing[5]	-	-	98%	99%
Prophylactic Antibiotic Timing (Outpatient)	-	-	98%	98%
Urinary Catheter Removal[5]	-	-	96%	97%
Survey of Patients' Hospital Experiences				
Area Around Room 'Always' Quiet at Night[5]	-	-	68%	61%
Doctors 'Always' Communicated Well[5]	-	-	84%	82%
Home Recovery Information Given[5]	-	-	84%	85%
Hospital Given 9 or 10 on 10 Point Scale[5]	-	-	72%	71%
Meds 'Always' Explained Before Given[5]	-	-	66%	64%
Nurses 'Always' Communicated Well[5]	-	-	80%	79%
Pain 'Always' Well Controlled[5]	-	-	72%	71%
Room and Bathroom 'Always' Clean[5]	-	-	73%	73%
Timely Help 'Always' Received[5]	-	-	71%	68%
Would Definitely Recommend Hospital[5]	-	-	71%	71%
Use of Medical Imaging				
Cardiac Imaging Stress Test before Surgery	-	-	4.5%	5.3%
Combination Abdominal CT Scan	-	-	23%	10.5%
Combination Brain/Sinus CT Scan	-	-	2.2%	2.7%
Combination Chest CT Scan	-	-	5.1%	2.7%
Follow-up Mammogram/Ultrasound	-	-	8.1%	8.8%
Lumbar Spine MRI for Low Back Pain	-	-	39.9%	37.2%

Integris Marshall County Medical Center

901 S 5th Ave
Madill, OK 73446
Phone: 580-795-3384
Fax: 580-795-7080
URL: www.integris-health.com/integris
Type: Critical Access Hospitals
Ownership: Proprietary
Emergency Services: Yes
Beds: 25

Key Personnel:
Infection Control. . . . . Lois Erwin
Emergency Room . . . . Carol Gay
Operating Room. . . . . Joy Henry, RN
Administrator . . . . Greg Holder
CEO . . . . Matt Lyden
CEO/President. . . . . Karen Reynolds
Chief of Medical Staff . . . . Bruck Zimmerman

Measure	Cases	This Hosp.	State Avg.	U.S. Avg.
Blood Clot Prevention and Treatment				
Anticoagulation Overlap Therapy[1,2]	-	-	89%	93%
ICU Venous Thromboembolism Prophylaxis[2,7]	-	-	87%	92%
Incidence of Potentially Preventable VTE[2,7]	-	-	8%	10%
UFH with Dosages/Platelet Monitoring[2,7]	-	-	97%	97%
Venous Thromboembolism Prophylaxis[2]	110	91%	72%	85%
Warfarin Therapy Discharge Instructions[1,2]	-	-	73%	75%
Chest Pain/Possible Heart Attack Care				
Aspirin Given Within 24 Hours of Arrival	29	90%	95%	96%
Fibrinolytic Meds Within 30 Min. of Arrival[1]	-	-	54%	58%
Average Time to ECG (minutes)	32	22	8	7
Average Time to Transfer (minutes)[1]	-	-	77	60
Children's Asthma Care				
Received Home Management Plan of Care	-	-	-	88%
Received Reliever Medication	-	-	-	100%
Received Systemic Corticosteroids	-	-	-	100%
Emergency Department				
Admittance Decision Time (minutes)[2]	200	41	63	98
Head CT Results Within 45 Min. of Arrival[1]	-	-	49%	57%
Patients Who Left ER Before Being Seen	8,623	1%	2%	2%
Time from ER Arrival to Admit. (minutes)[2]	371	172	210	274
Time from ER Arrival to Discharge (minutes)	584	69	110	134
Time in ER Before Being Evaluated (minutes)	620	17	24	26
Time to Pain Meds for Fractures (minutes)	31	49	55	57
Heart Attack Care				
Aspirin Given at Discharge[3,7]	-	-	99%	99%
Fibrinolytic Meds Within 30 Min. of Arrival[3,7]	-	-	25%	54%
PCI Within 90 Minutes of Arrival[3,7]	-	-	95%	96%
Statin Prescribed at Discharge[1,3]	-	-	98%	98%
Heart Failure Care				
ACE Inhibitor or ARB for LVSD[1]	-	-	95%	97%
Discharge Instructions Given	18	72%	92%	94%
Evaluation of LVS Function	23	61%	96%	99%
Medicare Spending				
Medicare Spending per Patient (ratio)	-	-	0.93	0.98
Pneumonia Care				
Appropriate Initial Antibiotic Given	48	94%	92%	95%
Blood Culture Timing	36	89%	97%	98%
Pregnancy and Delivery Care				
Newborn Deliveries Scheduled Early[5]	-	-	8%	6%
Preventive Care				
Immunization for Influenza[2]	251	93%	89%	90%
Immunization for Pneumonia[2]	388	88%	91%	92%
Stroke Care				
Anticoagulation Therapy for Atrial Fibrillation[3,7]	-	-	91%	95%
Antithrombotic Therapy Timing[1,3]	-	-	95%	98%
Assessed for Rehabilitation[1,3]	-	-	96%	97%
Discharged on Antithrombotic Therapy[1,3]	-	-	98%	99%
Discharged on Statin Medication[1,3]	-	-	88%	94%
Thrombolytic Therapy Timing[1,3]	-	-	61%	66%
Venous Thromboembolism Prophylaxis[1,3]	-	-	92%	94%

NOTE: Hospital profiles are in alphabetical order by state, then city, then hospital within the city; Rankings exclude hospitals with less than 25 cases except for patient surveys which excludes hospitals with less than 100 cases; (a) 100-299 cases; (1) The number of cases/patients is too few to report; (2) Data submitted were based on a sample of cases/patients; (3) Results are based on a shorter time period than required; (4) Data suppressed by CMS for one or more quarters; (5) Results are not available for this reporting period; (6) Fewer than 100 patients completed the HCAHPS survey; (7) No cases met the criteria for this measure; (8) The lower limit of the confidence interval cannot be calculated if the number of observed infections equals zero; (9) No data are available from the state/territory for this reporting period; (10) The scores shown reflect fewer than 50 completed surveys; (11) There were discrepancies in the data collection process; (12) This measure does not apply to this hospital for this reporting period; (13) Results cannot be calculated for this reporting period; (14) The results for this state are combined with nearby states to protect confidentiality; Please refer to the User's Guide for a full explanation of data.

Measure	Cases	This Hosp.	State Avg.	U.S. Avg.
Written Stroke Educational Materials Given[1,3]	-	-	86%	88%
Surgical Care Improvement Project				
Appropriate Beta Blocker Usage[1,3]	-	-	97%	98%
Appropriate VTP Within 24 Hours[1,3]	-	-	97%	98%
Controlled Postoperative Blood Glucose[3,7]	-	-	97%	97%
Perioperative Temperature Management[3,7]	-	-	100%	100%
Prophylactic Antibiotic Selection[3,7]	-	-	99%	99%
Prophylactic Antibiotic Selection (Outpatient)[3,7]	-	-	98%	98%
Prophylactic Antibiotic Stopped[3,7]	-	-	98%	98%
Prophylactic Antibiotic Timing[3,7]	-	-	98%	99%
Prophylactic Antibiotic Timing (Outpatient)[3,7]	-	-	98%	98%
Urinary Catheter Removal[3,7]	-	-	96%	97%
Survey of Patients' Hospital Experiences				
Area Around Room 'Always' Quiet at Night	(a)	77%	68%	61%
Doctors 'Always' Communicated Well	(a)	91%	84%	82%
Home Recovery Information Given	(a)	84%	84%	85%
Hospital Given 9 or 10 on 10 Point Scale	(a)	69%	72%	71%
Meds 'Always' Explained Before Given	(a)	80%	66%	64%
Nurses 'Always' Communicated Well	(a)	86%	80%	79%
Pain 'Always' Well Controlled	(a)	75%	72%	71%
Room and Bathroom 'Always' Clean	(a)	75%	73%	73%
Timely Help 'Always' Received	(a)	78%	71%	68%
Would Definitely Recommend Hospital	(a)	65%	71%	71%
Use of Medical Imaging				
Cardiac Imaging Stress Test before Surgery[7]	-	-	4.5%	5.3%
Combination Abdominal CT Scan	132	3.8%	23%	10.5%
Combination Brain/Sinus CT Scan[1]	-	-	2.2%	2.7%
Combination Chest CT Scan	59	0.0%	5.1%	2.7%
Follow-up Mammogram/Ultrasound[7]	-	-	8.1%	8.8%
Lumbar Spine MRI for Low Back Pain[1]	-	-	39.9%	37.2%

Quartz Mountain Medical Center

One Wickersham Drive
Mangum, OK 73554
Phone: 580-782-3353
Fax: 580-782-5944
URL: www.mangumhealth.com
Type: Critical Access Hospitals
Emergency Services: Yes
Ownership: Proprietary
Beds: 25
Key Personnel:
CEO/President. . . . . Jim Ivey

Measure	Cases	This Hosp.	State Avg.	U.S. Avg.
Blood Clot Prevention and Treatment				
Anticoagulation Overlap Therapy[1,3]	-	-	89%	93%
ICU Venous Thromboembolism Prophylaxis[3,7]	-	-	87%	92%
Incidence of Potentially Preventable VTE[3,7]	-	-	8%	10%
UFH with Dosages/Platelet Monitoring[3,7]	-	-	97%	97%
Venous Thromboembolism Prophylaxis[3,7]	-	-	72%	85%
Warfarin Therapy Discharge Instructions[1,3]	-	-	73%	75%
Chest Pain/Possible Heart Attack Care				
Aspirin Given Within 24 Hours of Arrival[1,3]	-	-	95%	96%
Fibrinolytic Meds Within 30 Min. of Arrival[3,7]	-	-	54%	58%
Average Time to ECG (minutes)[1,3]	-	-	8	7
Average Time to Transfer (minutes)[3,7]	-	-	77	60
Children's Asthma Care				
Received Home Management Plan of Care	-	-	-	88%
Received Reliever Medication	-	-	-	100%
Received Systemic Corticosteroids	-	-	-	100%
Emergency Department				
Admittance Decision Time (minutes)[3,7]	-	-	63	98
Head CT Results Within 45 Min. of Arrival[5]	-	-	49%	57%
Patients Who Left ER Before Being Seen[5]	-	-	2%	2%
Time from ER Arrival to Admit. (minutes)[3,7]	-	-	210	274
Time from ER Arrival to Discharge (minutes)[5]	-	-	110	134
Time in ER Before Being Evaluated (minutes)[5]	-	-	24	26
Time to Pain Meds for Fractures (minutes)[5]	-	-	55	57
Heart Attack Care				
Aspirin Given at Discharge[1,3]	-	-	99%	99%
Fibrinolytic Meds Within 30 Min. of Arrival[3,7]	-	-	25%	54%
PCI Within 90 Minutes of Arrival[3,7]	-	-	95%	96%
Statin Prescribed at Discharge[1,3]	-	-	98%	98%
Heart Failure Care				
ACE Inhibitor or ARB for LVSD[1,3]	-	-	95%	97%
Discharge Instructions Given[1,3]	-	-	92%	94%
Evaluation of LVS Function[1,3]	-	-	96%	99%
Medicare Spending				
Medicare Spending per Patient (ratio)	-	-	0.93	0.98
Pneumonia Care				
Appropriate Initial Antibiotic Given[3,7]	-	-	92%	95%
Blood Culture Timing[3,7]	-	-	97%	98%
Pregnancy and Delivery Care				
Newborn Deliveries Scheduled Early[5]	-	-	8%	6%
Preventive Care				
Immunization for Influenza[5]	-	-	89%	90%
Immunization for Pneumonia[5]	-	-	91%	92%
Stroke Care				
Anticoagulation Therapy for Atrial Fibrillation[5]	-	-	91%	95%
Antithrombotic Therapy Timing[5]	-	-	95%	98%
Assessed for Rehabilitation[5]	-	-	96%	97%
Discharged on Antithrombotic Therapy[5]	-	-	98%	99%
Discharged on Statin Medication[5]	-	-	88%	94%
Thrombolytic Therapy Timing[5]	-	-	61%	66%
Venous Thromboembolism Prophylaxis[5]	-	-	92%	94%
Written Stroke Educational Materials Given[5]	-	-	86%	88%
Surgical Care Improvement Project				
Appropriate Beta Blocker Usage[3,7]	-	-	97%	98%
Appropriate VTP Within 24 Hours[1,3]	-	-	97%	98%
Controlled Postoperative Blood Glucose[3,7]	-	-	97%	97%
Perioperative Temperature Management[3]	11	100%	100%	100%
Prophylactic Antibiotic Selection[1,3]	-	-	99%	99%
Prophylactic Antibiotic Selection (Outpatient)[5]	-	-	98%	98%
Prophylactic Antibiotic Stopped[1,3]	-	-	98%	98%
Prophylactic Antibiotic Timing[1,3]	-	-	98%	99%
Prophylactic Antibiotic Timing (Outpatient)[5]	-	-	98%	98%
Urinary Catheter Removal[3]	11	73%	96%	97%
Survey of Patients' Hospital Experiences				
Area Around Room 'Always' Quiet at Night[5]	-	-	68%	61%
Doctors 'Always' Communicated Well[5]	-	-	84%	82%
Home Recovery Information Given[5]	-	-	84%	85%
Hospital Given 9 or 10 on 10 Point Scale[5]	-	-	72%	71%
Meds 'Always' Explained Before Given[5]	-	-	66%	64%
Nurses 'Always' Communicated Well[5]	-	-	80%	79%
Pain 'Always' Well Controlled[5]	-	-	72%	71%
Room and Bathroom 'Always' Clean[5]	-	-	73%	73%
Timely Help 'Always' Received[5]	-	-	71%	68%
Would Definitely Recommend Hospital[5]	-	-	71%	71%
Use of Medical Imaging				
Cardiac Imaging Stress Test before Surgery[7]	-	-	4.5%	5.3%
Combination Abdominal CT Scan[1]	-	-	23%	10.5%
Combination Brain/Sinus CT Scan[1]	-	-	2.2%	2.7%
Combination Chest CT Scan[1]	-	-	5.1%	2.7%
Follow-up Mammogram/Ultrasound[7]	-	-	8.1%	8.8%
Lumbar Spine MRI for Low Back Pain[1]	-	-	39.9%	37.2%

Mercy Health Love County

300 Wanda Street
Marietta, OK 73448
Phone: 580-276-3347
Fax: 580-276-2182
URL: www.mercyok.net
Type: Critical Access Hospitals
Emergency Services: Yes
Ownership: Government - Local
Beds: 30
Key Personnel:
CEO/President. . . . . Lynn Britton

Measure	Cases	This Hosp.	State Avg.	U.S. Avg.
Blood Clot Prevention and Treatment				
Anticoagulation Overlap Therapy[5]	-	-	89%	93%
ICU Venous Thromboembolism Prophylaxis[5]	-	-	87%	92%
Incidence of Potentially Preventable VTE[5]	-	-	8%	10%
UFH with Dosages/Platelet Monitoring[5]	-	-	97%	97%
Venous Thromboembolism Prophylaxis[5]	-	-	72%	85%
Warfarin Therapy Discharge Instructions[5]	-	-	73%	75%
Chest Pain/Possible Heart Attack Care				
Aspirin Given Within 24 Hours of Arrival[1,3]	-	-	95%	96%
Fibrinolytic Meds Within 30 Min. of Arrival[1,3]	-	-	54%	58%
Average Time to ECG (minutes)[1,3]	-	-	8	7
Average Time to Transfer (minutes)[1,3]	-	-	77	60
Children's Asthma Care				
Received Home Management Plan of Care	-	-	-	88%
Received Reliever Medication	-	-	-	100%
Received Systemic Corticosteroids	-	-	-	100%
Emergency Department				
Admittance Decision Time (minutes)[5]	-	-	63	98
Head CT Results Within 45 Min. of Arrival[5]	-	-	49%	57%
Patients Who Left ER Before Being Seen[5]	-	-	2%	2%
Time from ER Arrival to Admit. (minutes)[5]	-	-	210	274
Time from ER Arrival to Discharge (minutes)[5]	-	-	110	134
Time in ER Before Being Evaluated (minutes)[5]	-	-	24	26
Time to Pain Meds for Fractures (minutes)[5]	-	-	55	57
Heart Attack Care				
Aspirin Given at Discharge[3,7]	-	-	99%	99%
Fibrinolytic Meds Within 30 Min. of Arrival[3,7]	-	-	25%	54%
PCI Within 90 Minutes of Arrival[3,7]	-	-	95%	96%
Statin Prescribed at Discharge[1,3]	-	-	98%	98%
Heart Failure Care				
ACE Inhibitor or ARB for LVSD[7]	-	-	95%	97%
Discharge Instructions Given[1]	-	-	92%	94%
Evaluation of LVS Function[1]	-	-	96%	99%
Medicare Spending				
Medicare Spending per Patient (ratio)	-	-	0.93	0.98
Pneumonia Care				
Appropriate Initial Antibiotic Given	25	28%	92%	95%
Blood Culture Timing[1]	-	-	97%	98%
Pregnancy and Delivery Care				
Newborn Deliveries Scheduled Early[5]	-	-	8%	6%
Preventive Care				
Immunization for Influenza[5]	-	-	89%	90%
Immunization for Pneumonia[5]	-	-	91%	92%
Stroke Care				
Anticoagulation Therapy for Atrial Fibrillation[5]	-	-	91%	95%
Antithrombotic Therapy Timing[5]	-	-	95%	98%
Assessed for Rehabilitation[5]	-	-	96%	97%
Discharged on Antithrombotic Therapy[5]	-	-	98%	99%
Discharged on Statin Medication[5]	-	-	88%	94%
Thrombolytic Therapy Timing[5]	-	-	61%	66%
Venous Thromboembolism Prophylaxis[5]	-	-	92%	94%
Written Stroke Educational Materials Given[5]	-	-	86%	88%
Surgical Care Improvement Project				
Appropriate Beta Blocker Usage[5]	-	-	97%	98%
Appropriate VTP Within 24 Hours[5]	-	-	97%	98%
Controlled Postoperative Blood Glucose[5]	-	-	97%	97%
Perioperative Temperature Management[5]	-	-	100%	100%
Prophylactic Antibiotic Selection[5]	-	-	99%	99%
Prophylactic Antibiotic Selection (Outpatient)[5]	-	-	98%	98%
Prophylactic Antibiotic Stopped[5]	-	-	98%	98%
Prophylactic Antibiotic Timing[5]	-	-	98%	99%
Prophylactic Antibiotic Timing (Outpatient)[5]	-	-	98%	98%
Urinary Catheter Removal[5]	-	-	96%	97%
Survey of Patients' Hospital Experiences				
Area Around Room 'Always' Quiet at Night[5]	-	-	68%	61%
Doctors 'Always' Communicated Well[5]	-	-	84%	82%
Home Recovery Information Given[5]	-	-	84%	85%
Hospital Given 9 or 10 on 10 Point Scale[5]	-	-	72%	71%
Meds 'Always' Explained Before Given[5]	-	-	66%	64%
Nurses 'Always' Communicated Well[5]	-	-	80%	79%
Pain 'Always' Well Controlled[5]	-	-	72%	71%
Room and Bathroom 'Always' Clean[5]	-	-	73%	73%
Timely Help 'Always' Received[5]	-	-	71%	68%
Would Definitely Recommend Hospital[5]	-	-	71%	71%
Use of Medical Imaging				
Cardiac Imaging Stress Test before Surgery[7]	-	-	4.5%	5.3%
Combination Abdominal CT Scan[1]	-	-	23%	10.5%
Combination Brain/Sinus CT Scan	45	0.0%	2.2%	2.7%
Combination Chest CT Scan[1]	-	-	5.1%	2.7%
Follow-up Mammogram/Ultrasound[7]	-	-	8.1%	8.8%
Lumbar Spine MRI for Low Back Pain[7]	-	-	39.9%	37.2%

NOTE: Hospital profiles are in alphabetical order by state, then city, then hospital within the city; Rankings exclude hospitals with less than 25 cases except for patient surveys which excludes hospitals with less than 100 cases; (a) 100-299 cases; (1) The number of cases/patients is too few to report; (2) Data submitted were based on a sample of cases/patients; (3) Results are based on a shorter time period than required; (4) Data suppressed by CMS for one or more quarters; (5) Results are not available for this reporting period; (6) Fewer than 100 patients completed the HCAHPS survey; (7) No cases met the criteria for this measure; (8) The lower limit of the confidence interval cannot be calculated if the number of observed infections equals zero; (9) No data are available from the state/territory for this reporting period; (10) The scores shown reflect fewer than 50 completed surveys; (11) There were discrepancies in the data collection process; (12) This measure does not apply to this hospital for this reporting period; (13) Results cannot be calculated for this reporting period; (14) The results for this state are combined with nearby states to protect confidentiality; Please refer to the User's Guide for a full explanation of data.

McAlester Regional Health Center

One Clark Bass Boulevard
Mcalester, OK 74501
E-mail: nbrinlee@mrhcok.com
URL: www.mrhcok.com
Type: Acute Care Hospitals
Ownership: Voluntary non-profit - Other
Phone: 918-426-1800
Fax: 918-421-8633
Emergency Services: Yes
Beds: 197

Key Personnel:
CEO/President. . . . . Sean Beggs
Operating Room. . . . . Lem Hodges, RN
Chief of Medical Staff. . . . . Milton James
Radiology. . . . . Bruce O'Brien, MD
Quality Assurance . . . . Kathy Rollins
Emergency Room . . . . Dennis Staggs

Measure	Cases	This Hosp.	State Avg.	U.S. Avg.
Blood Clot Prevention and Treatment				
Anticoagulation Overlap Therapy[2]	19	95%	89%	93%
ICU Venous Thromboembolism Prophylaxis[2]	98	77%	87%	92%
Incidence of Potentially Preventable VTE[2,7]	-	-	8%	10%
UFH with Dosages/Platelet Monitoring[1,2]	-	-	97%	97%
Venous Thromboembolism Prophylaxis[2]	261	76%	72%	85%
Warfarin Therapy Discharge Instructions[1,2]	-	-	73%	75%
Chest Pain/Possible Heart Attack Care				
Aspirin Given Within 24 Hours of Arrival	57	91%	95%	96%
Fibrinolytic Meds Within 30 Min. of Arrival[1]	-	-	54%	58%
Average Time to ECG (minutes)	57	4	8	7
Average Time to Transfer (minutes)[1]	-	-	77	60
Children's Asthma Care				
Received Home Management Plan of Care	-	-	-	88%
Received Reliever Medication	-	-	-	100%
Received Systemic Corticosteroids	-	-	-	100%
Emergency Department				
Admittance Decision Time (minutes)[2]	472	60	63	98
Head CT Results Within 45 Min. of Arrival	38	53%	49%	57%
Patients Who Left ER Before Being Seen	20,956	5%	2%	2%
Time from ER Arrival to Admit. (minutes)[2]	499	212	210	274
Time from ER Arrival to Discharge (minutes)	355	129	110	134
Time in ER Before Being Evaluated (minutes)	375	47	24	26
Time to Pain Meds for Fractures (minutes)	95	63	55	57
Heart Attack Care				
Aspirin Given at Discharge	36	75%	99%	99%
Fibrinolytic Meds Within 30 Min. of Arrival[7]	-	-	25%	54%
PCI Within 90 Minutes of Arrival[1]	-	-	95%	96%
Statin Prescribed at Discharge	34	82%	98%	98%
Heart Failure Care				
ACE Inhibitor or ARB for LVSD	37	70%	95%	97%
Discharge Instructions Given	68	88%	92%	94%
Evaluation of LVS Function	96	95%	96%	99%
Medicare Spending				
Medicare Spending per Patient (ratio)	-	1.03	0.93	0.98
Pneumonia Care				
Appropriate Initial Antibiotic Given[2]	107	85%	92%	95%
Blood Culture Timing[2]	159	94%	97%	98%
Pregnancy and Delivery Care				
Newborn Deliveries Scheduled Early[2]	44	5%	8%	6%
Preventive Care				
Immunization for Influenza[2]	490	90%	89%	90%
Immunization for Pneumonia[2]	578	93%	91%	92%
Stroke Care				
Anticoagulation Therapy for Atrial Fibrillation[1]	-	-	91%	95%
Antithrombotic Therapy Timing	34	91%	95%	98%
Assessed for Rehabilitation	34	91%	96%	97%
Discharged on Antithrombotic Therapy	34	91%	98%	99%
Discharged on Statin Medication	27	74%	88%	94%
Thrombolytic Therapy Timing[1]	-	-	61%	66%
Venous Thromboembolism Prophylaxis	34	71%	92%	94%
Written Stroke Educational Materials Given	11	36%	86%	88%
Surgical Care Improvement Project				
Appropriate Beta Blocker Usage[2]	83	94%	97%	98%
Appropriate VTP Within 24 Hours[2]	307	97%	97%	98%
Controlled Postoperative Blood Glucose[2,7]	-	-	97%	97%
Perioperative Temperature Management[2]	324	100%	100%	100%
Prophylactic Antibiotic Selection[2]	250	96%	99%	99%
Prophylactic Antibiotic Selection (Outpatient)	35	91%	98%	98%
Prophylactic Antibiotic Stopped[2]	250	96%	98%	98%
Prophylactic Antibiotic Timing[2]	250	97%	98%	99%
Prophylactic Antibiotic Timing (Outpatient)	36	89%	98%	98%
Urinary Catheter Removal[2]	198	94%	96%	97%
Survey of Patients' Hospital Experiences				
Area Around Room 'Always' Quiet at Night	300+	54%	68%	61%
Doctors 'Always' Communicated Well	300+	76%	84%	82%
Home Recovery Information Given	300+	78%	84%	85%
Hospital Given 9 or 10 on 10 Point Scale	300+	55%	72%	71%
Meds 'Always' Explained Before Given	300+	57%	66%	64%
Nurses 'Always' Communicated Well	300+	72%	80%	79%
Pain 'Always' Well Controlled	300+	67%	72%	71%
Room and Bathroom 'Always' Clean	300+	70%	73%	73%
Timely Help 'Always' Received	300+	57%	71%	68%
Would Definitely Recommend Hospital	300+	51%	71%	71%
Use of Medical Imaging				
Cardiac Imaging Stress Test before Surgery	294	5.8%	4.5%	5.3%
Combination Abdominal CT Scan	667	39.3%	23%	10.5%
Combination Brain/Sinus CT Scan	587	4.6%	2.2%	2.7%
Combination Chest CT Scan	580	6.7%	5.1%	2.7%
Follow-up Mammogram/Ultrasound	472	9.7%	8.1%	8.8%
Lumbar Spine MRI for Low Back Pain	154	37.7%	39.9%	37.2%

Integris Baptist Regional Health Center

200 Second Avenue Southwest, Box 1207
Miami, OK 74355
URL: www.integris-health.com
Type: Acute Care Hospitals
Ownership: Voluntary non-profit - Other
Phone: 918-542-6611
Fax: 918-540-7605
Emergency Services: Yes
Beds: 124

Key Personnel:
CEO/President. . . . . Bruce Lawrence
Chief of Medical Staff. . . . . James White, MD

Measure	Cases	This Hosp.	State Avg.	U.S. Avg.
Blood Clot Prevention and Treatment				
Anticoagulation Overlap Therapy[2]	14	79%	89%	93%
ICU Venous Thromboembolism Prophylaxis[2]	33	94%	87%	92%
Incidence of Potentially Preventable VTE[1,2]	-	-	8%	10%
UFH with Dosages/Platelet Monitoring[1,2]	-	-	97%	97%
Venous Thromboembolism Prophylaxis[2]	141	89%	72%	85%
Warfarin Therapy Discharge Instructions[1,2]	-	-	73%	75%
Chest Pain/Possible Heart Attack Care				
Aspirin Given Within 24 Hours of Arrival	81	98%	95%	96%
Fibrinolytic Meds Within 30 Min. of Arrival[1]	-	-	54%	58%
Average Time to ECG (minutes)	83	5	8	7
Average Time to Transfer (minutes)[1]	-	-	77	60
Children's Asthma Care				
Received Home Management Plan of Care	-	-	-	88%
Received Reliever Medication	-	-	-	100%
Received Systemic Corticosteroids	-	-	-	100%
Emergency Department				
Admittance Decision Time (minutes)[2]	282	51	63	98
Head CT Results Within 45 Min. of Arrival[1]	-	-	49%	57%
Patients Who Left ER Before Being Seen	20,147	3%	2%	2%
Time from ER Arrival to Admit. (minutes)[2]	324	191	210	274
Time from ER Arrival to Discharge (minutes)	386	92	110	134
Time in ER Before Being Evaluated (minutes)	401	25	24	26
Time to Pain Meds for Fractures (minutes)	37	50	55	57
Heart Attack Care				
Aspirin Given at Discharge[1,3]	-	-	99%	99%
Fibrinolytic Meds Within 30 Min. of Arrival[3,7]	-	-	25%	54%
PCI Within 90 Minutes of Arrival[3,7]	-	-	95%	96%
Statin Prescribed at Discharge[1,3]	-	-	98%	98%
Heart Failure Care				
ACE Inhibitor or ARB for LVSD	19	74%	95%	97%
Discharge Instructions Given	44	95%	92%	94%
Evaluation of LVS Function	57	100%	96%	99%
Medicare Spending				
Medicare Spending per Patient (ratio)	-	0.86	0.93	0.98
Pneumonia Care				
Appropriate Initial Antibiotic Given	96	97%	92%	95%
Blood Culture Timing	105	99%	97%	98%
Pregnancy and Delivery Care				
Newborn Deliveries Scheduled Early	38	0%	8%	6%
Preventive Care				
Immunization for Influenza[2]	250	96%	89%	90%
Immunization for Pneumonia[2]	320	94%	91%	92%
Stroke Care				
Anticoagulation Therapy for Atrial Fibrillation[7]	-	-	91%	95%
Antithrombotic Therapy Timing	13	92%	95%	98%
Assessed for Rehabilitation	19	89%	96%	97%
Discharged on Antithrombotic Therapy	16	100%	98%	99%
Discharged on Statin Medication	15	53%	88%	94%
Thrombolytic Therapy Timing[7]	-	-	61%	66%
Venous Thromboembolism Prophylaxis	12	92%	92%	94%
Written Stroke Educational Materials Given	11	45%	86%	88%
Surgical Care Improvement Project				
Appropriate Beta Blocker Usage	32	94%	97%	98%
Appropriate VTP Within 24 Hours	89	100%	97%	98%
Controlled Postoperative Blood Glucose[7]	-	-	97%	97%
Perioperative Temperature Management	105	99%	100%	100%
Prophylactic Antibiotic Selection	79	99%	99%	99%
Prophylactic Antibiotic Selection (Outpatient)	37	100%	98%	98%
Prophylactic Antibiotic Stopped	75	95%	98%	98%
Prophylactic Antibiotic Timing	79	96%	98%	99%
Prophylactic Antibiotic Timing (Outpatient)	38	95%	98%	98%
Urinary Catheter Removal	68	97%	96%	97%
Survey of Patients' Hospital Experiences				
Area Around Room 'Always' Quiet at Night	300+	58%	68%	61%
Doctors 'Always' Communicated Well	300+	84%	84%	82%
Home Recovery Information Given	300+	86%	84%	85%
Hospital Given 9 or 10 on 10 Point Scale	300+	68%	72%	71%
Meds 'Always' Explained Before Given	300+	71%	66%	64%
Nurses 'Always' Communicated Well	300+	83%	80%	79%
Pain 'Always' Well Controlled	300+	76%	72%	71%
Room and Bathroom 'Always' Clean	300+	74%	73%	73%
Timely Help 'Always' Received	300+	76%	71%	68%
Would Definitely Recommend Hospital	300+	65%	71%	71%
Use of Medical Imaging				
Cardiac Imaging Stress Test before Surgery	139	2.9%	4.5%	5.3%
Combination Abdominal CT Scan	249	20.1%	23%	10.5%
Combination Brain/Sinus CT Scan[1]	-	-	2.2%	2.7%
Combination Chest CT Scan	148	17.6%	5.1%	2.7%
Follow-up Mammogram/Ultrasound	578	9.0%	8.1%	8.8%
Lumbar Spine MRI for Low Back Pain	58	25.9%	39.9%	37.2%

Midwest Regional Medical Center

2825 Parklawn Drive
Midwest City, OK 73110
URL: www.midwestregional.com
Type: Acute Care Hospitals
Ownership: Proprietary
Phone: 405-610-8530
Fax: 405-610-1483
Emergency Services: Yes
Beds: 255

Key Personnel:
Chief of Medical Staff. . . . . M Terry Anderson
CEO . . . . Damon Brown
Radiology. . . . . Chris Degner
Emergency Room . . . . Joel III, MD

Measure	Cases	This Hosp.	State Avg.	U.S. Avg.
Blood Clot Prevention and Treatment				
Anticoagulation Overlap Therapy[2]	45	93%	89%	93%
ICU Venous Thromboembolism Prophylaxis[2]	87	74%	87%	92%
Incidence of Potentially Preventable VTE[1,2]	-	-	8%	10%
UFH with Dosages/Platelet Monitoring[1,2]	-	-	97%	97%
Venous Thromboembolism Prophylaxis[2]	372	62%	72%	85%
Warfarin Therapy Discharge Instructions[2]	34	100%	73%	75%
Chest Pain/Possible Heart Attack Care				
Aspirin Given Within 24 Hours of Arrival	170	95%	95%	96%
Fibrinolytic Meds Within 30 Min. of Arrival[3,7]	-	-	54%	58%
Average Time to ECG (minutes)	196	6	8	7
Average Time to Transfer (minutes)[3,7]	-	-	77	60
Children's Asthma Care				
Received Home Management Plan of Care	-	-	-	88%
Received Reliever Medication	-	-	-	100%
Received Systemic Corticosteroids	-	-	-	100%
Emergency Department				
Admittance Decision Time (minutes)[2]	913	105	63	98
Head CT Results Within 45 Min. of Arrival	13	62%	49%	57%

NOTE: Hospital profiles are in alphabetical order by state, then city, then hospital within the city; Rankings exclude hospitals with less than 25 cases except for patient surveys which excludes hospitals with less than 100 cases; (a) 100-299 cases; (1) The number of cases/patients is too few to report; (2) Data submitted were based on a sample of cases/patients; (3) Results are based on a shorter time period than required; (4) Data suppressed by CMS for one or more quarters; (5) Results are not available for this reporting period; (6) Fewer than 100 patients completed the HCAHPS survey; (7) No cases met the criteria for this measure; (8) The lower limit of the confidence interval cannot be calculated if the number of observed infections equals zero; (9) No data are available from the state/territory for this reporting period; (10) The scores shown reflect fewer than 50 completed surveys; (11) There were discrepancies in the data collection process; (12) This measure does not apply to this hospital for this reporting period; (13) Results cannot be calculated for this reporting period; (14) The results for this state are combined with nearby states to protect confidentiality; Please refer to the User's Guide for a full explanation of data.

Measure	Cases	This Hosp.	State Avg.	U.S. Avg.
Patients Who Left ER Before Being Seen	40,859	4%	2%	2%
Time from ER Arrival to Admit. (minutes)[2]	913	272	210	274
Time from ER Arrival to Discharge (minutes)	451	153	110	134
Time in ER Before Being Evaluated (minutes)	499	43	24	26
Time to Pain Meds for Fractures (minutes)	93	57	55	57
Heart Attack Care				
Aspirin Given at Discharge	173	97%	99%	99%
Fibrinolytic Meds Within 30 Min. of Arrival[7]	-	-	25%	54%
PCI Within 90 Minutes of Arrival	22	100%	95%	96%
Statin Prescribed at Discharge	156	96%	98%	98%
Heart Failure Care				
ACE Inhibitor or ARB for LVSD	100	92%	95%	97%
Discharge Instructions Given	240	100%	92%	94%
Evaluation of LVS Function	295	97%	96%	99%
Medicare Spending				
Medicare Spending per Patient (ratio)	-	1.00	0.93	0.98
Pneumonia Care				
Appropriate Initial Antibiotic Given	152	96%	92%	95%
Blood Culture Timing	173	99%	97%	98%
Pregnancy and Delivery Care				
Newborn Deliveries Scheduled Early[2]	68	7%	8%	6%
Preventive Care				
Immunization for Influenza[2]	621	98%	89%	90%
Immunization for Pneumonia[2]	775	99%	91%	92%
Stroke Care				
Anticoagulation Therapy for Atrial Fibrillation[1]	-	-	91%	95%
Antithrombotic Therapy Timing	60	98%	95%	98%
Assessed for Rehabilitation	56	86%	96%	97%
Discharged on Antithrombotic Therapy	54	96%	98%	99%
Discharged on Statin Medication	47	68%	88%	94%
Thrombolytic Therapy Timing[1]	-	-	61%	66%
Venous Thromboembolism Prophylaxis	59	59%	92%	94%
Written Stroke Educational Materials Given	33	52%	86%	88%
Surgical Care Improvement Project				
Appropriate Beta Blocker Usage[2]	129	99%	97%	98%
Appropriate VTP Within 24 Hours[2]	356	95%	97%	98%
Controlled Postoperative Blood Glucose[2]	11	91%	97%	97%
Perioperative Temperature Management[2]	416	100%	100%	100%
Prophylactic Antibiotic Selection[2]	306	98%	99%	99%
Prophylactic Antibiotic Selection (Outpatient)	165	97%	98%	98%
Prophylactic Antibiotic Stopped[2]	300	97%	98%	98%
Prophylactic Antibiotic Timing[2]	307	99%	98%	99%
Prophylactic Antibiotic Timing (Outpatient)	167	99%	98%	98%
Urinary Catheter Removal[2]	113	84%	96%	97%
Survey of Patients' Hospital Experiences				
Area Around Room 'Always' Quiet at Night	300+	56%	68%	61%
Doctors 'Always' Communicated Well	300+	74%	84%	82%
Home Recovery Information Given	300+	78%	84%	85%
Hospital Given 9 or 10 on 10 Point Scale	300+	50%	72%	71%
Meds 'Always' Explained Before Given	300+	51%	66%	64%
Nurses 'Always' Communicated Well	300+	64%	80%	79%
Pain 'Always' Well Controlled	300+	60%	72%	71%
Room and Bathroom 'Always' Clean	300+	55%	73%	73%
Timely Help 'Always' Received	300+	45%	71%	68%
Would Definitely Recommend Hospital	300+	47%	71%	71%
Use of Medical Imaging				
Cardiac Imaging Stress Test before Surgery	77	7.8%	4.5%	5.3%
Combination Abdominal CT Scan	738	21.0%	23%	10.5%
Combination Brain/Sinus CT Scan	725	4.6%	2.2%	2.7%
Combination Chest CT Scan	272	19.9%	5.1%	2.7%
Follow-up Mammogram/Ultrasound	1,736	3.7%	8.1%	8.8%
Lumbar Spine MRI for Low Back Pain	228	37.7%	39.9%	37.2%

Eastar Health System

300 Rockefeller Drive
Muskogee, OK 74401
Phone: 918-682-5501
Fax: 918-684-2552
URL: www.muskogeehealth.com
Type: Acute Care Hospitals
Emergency Services: Yes
Ownership: Proprietary
Beds: 366

Key Personnel:
Infection Control . . . . Becky Elliott
Chief of Medical Staff. . . . . Jay Gregory, MD
Chair/CEO . . . . Kathy Hewitt
Operating Room. . . . . Susan Julian
Surgery . . . . Dennis Rivero, MD
Radiology. . . . . Linda Stubbs
Quality Assurance . . . . Ched Wetz
CEO/President. . . . . Tony Young

Measure	Cases	This Hosp.	State Avg.	U.S. Avg.
Blood Clot Prevention and Treatment				
Anticoagulation Overlap Therapy[2]	59	93%	89%	93%
ICU Venous Thromboembolism Prophylaxis[2]	131	91%	87%	92%
Incidence of Potentially Preventable VTE[2]	11	9%	8%	10%
UFH with Dosages/Platelet Monitoring[2]	12	100%	97%	97%
Venous Thromboembolism Prophylaxis[2]	295	88%	72%	85%
Warfarin Therapy Discharge Instructions[2]	39	90%	73%	75%
Chest Pain/Possible Heart Attack Care				
Aspirin Given Within 24 Hours of Arrival	79	94%	95%	96%
Fibrinolytic Meds Within 30 Min. of Arrival	24	58%	54%	58%
Average Time to ECG (minutes)	81	8	8	7
Average Time to Transfer (minutes)	14	43	77	60
Children's Asthma Care				
Received Home Management Plan of Care	-	-	-	88%
Received Reliever Medication	-	-	-	100%
Received Systemic Corticosteroids	-	-	-	100%
Emergency Department				
Admittance Decision Time (minutes)[2]	494	86	63	98
Head CT Results Within 45 Min. of Arrival	23	87%	49%	57%
Patients Who Left ER Before Being Seen	33,065	5%	2%	2%
Time from ER Arrival to Admit. (minutes)[2]	500	283	210	274
Time from ER Arrival to Discharge (minutes)	397	201	110	134
Time in ER Before Being Evaluated (minutes)	462	46	24	26
Time to Pain Meds for Fractures (minutes)	90	88	55	57
Heart Attack Care				
Aspirin Given at Discharge	50	100%	99%	99%
Fibrinolytic Meds Within 30 Min. of Arrival[7]	-	-	25%	54%
PCI Within 90 Minutes of Arrival[7]	-	-	95%	96%
Statin Prescribed at Discharge	46	98%	98%	98%
Heart Failure Care				
ACE Inhibitor or ARB for LVSD	63	97%	95%	97%
Discharge Instructions Given	167	83%	92%	94%
Evaluation of LVS Function	223	100%	96%	99%
Medicare Spending				
Medicare Spending per Patient (ratio)	-	1.04	0.93	0.98
Pneumonia Care				
Appropriate Initial Antibiotic Given	131	91%	92%	95%
Blood Culture Timing	246	98%	97%	98%
Pregnancy and Delivery Care				
Newborn Deliveries Scheduled Early[2]	34	15%	8%	6%
Preventive Care				
Immunization for Influenza[2]	532	95%	89%	90%
Immunization for Pneumonia[2]	614	93%	91%	92%
Stroke Care				
Anticoagulation Therapy for Atrial Fibrillation[2]	11	100%	91%	95%
Antithrombotic Therapy Timing[2]	57	100%	95%	98%
Assessed for Rehabilitation[2]	57	98%	96%	97%
Discharged on Antithrombotic Therapy[2]	54	98%	98%	99%
Discharged on Statin Medication[2]	45	84%	88%	94%
Thrombolytic Therapy Timing[1,2]	-	-	61%	66%
Venous Thromboembolism Prophylaxis[2]	61	95%	92%	94%
Written Stroke Educational Materials Given[2]	31	100%	86%	88%
Surgical Care Improvement Project				
Appropriate Beta Blocker Usage	152	92%	97%	98%
Appropriate VTP Within 24 Hours	491	94%	97%	98%
Controlled Postoperative Blood Glucose[7]	-	-	97%	97%
Perioperative Temperature Management	548	100%	100%	100%
Prophylactic Antibiotic Selection	384	98%	99%	99%
Prophylactic Antibiotic Selection (Outpatient)	113	98%	98%	98%
Prophylactic Antibiotic Stopped	373	98%	98%	98%
Prophylactic Antibiotic Timing	384	98%	98%	99%
Prophylactic Antibiotic Timing (Outpatient)	115	97%	98%	98%
Urinary Catheter Removal	274	93%	96%	97%
Survey of Patients' Hospital Experiences				
Area Around Room 'Always' Quiet at Night	300+	54%	68%	61%
Doctors 'Always' Communicated Well	300+	78%	84%	82%
Home Recovery Information Given	300+	82%	84%	85%
Hospital Given 9 or 10 on 10 Point Scale	300+	51%	72%	71%
Meds 'Always' Explained Before Given	300+	53%	66%	64%
Nurses 'Always' Communicated Well	300+	64%	80%	79%
Pain 'Always' Well Controlled	300+	62%	72%	71%
Room and Bathroom 'Always' Clean	300+	60%	73%	73%
Timely Help 'Always' Received	300+	51%	71%	68%
Would Definitely Recommend Hospital	300+	52%	71%	71%
Use of Medical Imaging				
Cardiac Imaging Stress Test before Surgery	150	10.7%	4.5%	5.3%
Combination Abdominal CT Scan	823	24.4%	23%	10.5%
Combination Brain/Sinus CT Scan	899	2.9%	2.2%	2.7%
Combination Chest CT Scan	363	5.2%	5.1%	2.7%
Follow-up Mammogram/Ultrasound	1,899	10.1%	8.1%	8.8%
Lumbar Spine MRI for Low Back Pain	140	42.1%	39.9%	37.2%

Muskogee VA Medical Center

1011 Honor Heights Drive
Muskogee, OK 74401
Phone: 918-577-3000
Fax: 918-577-3648
URL: www.visn16.med.va.gov/muskogee.asp
Type: Acute Care - VA
Emergency Services: No
Ownership: Government Federal
Beds: 187

Key Personnel:
Patient Relations . . . . Margie Carlton
Quality Assurance . . . . Linda Fredrick, RN
Chief of Medical Staff . . . . Karen H Gribbin, MD
Operating Room. . . . . Susan McKinney

Measure	Cases	This Hosp.	State Avg.	U.S. Avg.
Blood Clot Prevention and Treatment				
Anticoagulation Overlap Therapy	-	-	89%	93%
ICU Venous Thromboembolism Prophylaxis	-	-	87%	92%
Incidence of Potentially Preventable VTE	-	-	8%	10%
UFH with Dosages/Platelet Monitoring	-	-	97%	97%
Venous Thromboembolism Prophylaxis	-	-	72%	85%
Warfarin Therapy Discharge Instructions	-	-	73%	75%
Chest Pain/Possible Heart Attack Care				
Aspirin Given Within 24 Hours of Arrival	-	-	95%	96%
Fibrinolytic Meds Within 30 Min. of Arrival	-	-	54%	58%
Average Time to ECG (minutes)	-	-	8	7
Average Time to Transfer (minutes)	-	-	77	60
Children's Asthma Care				
Received Home Management Plan of Care	-	-	-	88%
Received Reliever Medication	-	-	-	100%
Received Systemic Corticosteroids	-	-	-	100%
Emergency Department				
Admittance Decision Time (minutes)	-	-	63	98
Head CT Results Within 45 Min. of Arrival	-	-	49%	57%
Patients Who Left ER Before Being Seen	-	-	2%	2%
Time from ER Arrival to Admit. (minutes)	-	-	210	274
Time from ER Arrival to Discharge (minutes)	-	-	110	134
Time in ER Before Being Evaluated (minutes)	-	-	24	26
Time to Pain Meds for Fractures (minutes)	-	-	55	57
Heart Attack Care				
Aspirin Given at Discharge[5]	-	-	99%	99%
Fibrinolytic Meds Within 30 Min. of Arrival[5]	-	-	25%	54%
PCI Within 90 Minutes of Arrival[5]	-	-	95%	96%
Statin Prescribed at Discharge[5]	-	-	98%	98%
Heart Failure Care				
ACE Inhibitor or ARB for LVSD	61	97%	95%	97%
Discharge Instructions Given	93	88%	92%	94%
Evaluation of LVS Function	111	100%	96%	99%
Medicare Spending				
Medicare Spending per Patient (ratio)	-	-	0.93	0.98
Pneumonia Care				
Appropriate Initial Antibiotic Given	73	97%	92%	95%
Blood Culture Timing	131	95%	97%	98%
Pregnancy and Delivery Care				
Newborn Deliveries Scheduled Early	-	-	8%	6%
Preventive Care				
Immunization for Influenza[5]	-	-	89%	90%
Immunization for Pneumonia[5]	-	-	91%	92%
Stroke Care				
Anticoagulation Therapy for Atrial Fibrillation	-	-	91%	95%
Antithrombotic Therapy Timing	-	-	95%	98%
Assessed for Rehabilitation	-	-	96%	97%

NOTE: Hospital profiles are in alphabetical order by state, then city, then hospital within the city; Rankings exclude hospitals with less than 25 cases except for patient surveys which excludes hospitals with less than 100 cases; (a) 100-299 cases; (1) The number of cases/patients is too few to report; (2) Data submitted were based on a sample of cases/patients; (3) Results are based on a shorter time period than required; (4) Data suppressed by CMS for one or more quarters; (5) Results are not available for this reporting period; (6) Fewer than 100 patients completed the HCAHPS survey; (7) No cases met the criteria for this measure; (8) The lower limit of the confidence interval cannot be calculated if the number of observed infections equals zero; (9) No data are available from the state/territory for this reporting period; (10) The scores shown reflect fewer than 50 completed surveys; (11) There were discrepancies in the data collection process; (12) This measure does not apply to this hospital for this reporting period; (13) Results cannot be calculated for this reporting period; (14) The results for this state are combined with nearby states to protect confidentiality; Please refer to the User's Guide for a full explanation of data.

Measure	Cases	This Hosp.	State Avg.	U.S. Avg.
Discharged on Antithrombotic Therapy	-	-	98%	99%
Discharged on Statin Medication	-	-	88%	94%
Thrombolytic Therapy Timing	-	-	61%	66%
Venous Thromboembolism Prophylaxis	-	-	92%	94%
Written Stroke Educational Materials Given	-	-	86%	88%
Surgical Care Improvement Project				
Appropriate Beta Blocker Usage[2]	39	100%	97%	98%
Appropriate VTP Within 24 Hours[2]	91	100%	97%	98%
Controlled Postoperative Blood Glucose[5]	-	-	97%	97%
Perioperative Temperature Management[2]	98	100%	100%	100%
Prophylactic Antibiotic Selection	27	96%	99%	99%
Prophylactic Antibiotic Selection (Outpatient)	-	-	98%	98%
Prophylactic Antibiotic Stopped	26	92%	98%	98%
Prophylactic Antibiotic Timing	27	100%	98%	99%
Prophylactic Antibiotic Timing (Outpatient)	-	-	98%	98%
Urinary Catheter Removal[2]	61	100%	96%	97%
Survey of Patients' Hospital Experiences				
Area Around Room 'Always' Quiet at Night	-	-	68%	61%
Doctors 'Always' Communicated Well	-	-	84%	82%
Home Recovery Information Given	-	-	84%	85%
Hospital Given 9 or 10 on 10 Point Scale	-	-	72%	71%
Meds 'Always' Explained Before Given	-	-	66%	64%
Nurses 'Always' Communicated Well	-	-	80%	79%
Pain 'Always' Well Controlled	-	-	72%	71%
Room and Bathroom 'Always' Clean	-	-	73%	73%
Timely Help 'Always' Received	-	-	71%	68%
Would Definitely Recommend Hospital	-	-	71%	71%
Use of Medical Imaging				
Cardiac Imaging Stress Test before Surgery	-	-	4.5%	5.3%
Combination Abdominal CT Scan	-	-	23%	10.5%
Combination Brain/Sinus CT Scan	-	-	2.2%	2.7%
Combination Chest CT Scan	-	-	5.1%	2.7%
Follow-up Mammogram/Ultrasound	-	-	8.1%	8.8%
Lumbar Spine MRI for Low Back Pain	-	-	39.9%	37.2%

Norman Regional Health System

901 North Porter
Norman, OK 73070
Phone: 405-321-1700
Fax: 405-307-1548
URL: www.normanregional.com
Type: Acute Care Hospitals
Emergency Services: Yes
Ownership: Government - Local
Beds: 382
Key Personnel:
CEO/President. . . . . David D Whitaker, FACHE
Chair/CEO. . . . . Robin Wiens

Measure	Cases	This Hosp.	State Avg.	U.S. Avg.
Blood Clot Prevention and Treatment				
Anticoagulation Overlap Therapy[2]	128	92%	89%	93%
ICU Venous Thromboembolism Prophylaxis[2]	69	86%	87%	92%
Incidence of Potentially Preventable VTE[2]	15	20%	8%	10%
UFH with Dosages/Platelet Monitoring[2]	17	100%	97%	97%
Venous Thromboembolism Prophylaxis[2]	320	76%	72%	85%
Warfarin Therapy Discharge Instructions[2]	96	99%	73%	75%
Chest Pain/Possible Heart Attack Care				
Aspirin Given Within 24 Hours of Arrival[3,7]	-	-	95%	96%
Fibrinolytic Meds Within 30 Min. of Arrival[5]	-	-	54%	58%
Average Time to ECG (minutes)[3,7]	-	-	8	7
Average Time to Transfer (minutes)[5]	-	-	77	60
Children's Asthma Care				
Received Home Management Plan of Care	-	-	-	88%
Received Reliever Medication	-	-	-	100%
Received Systemic Corticosteroids	-	-	-	100%
Emergency Department				
Admittance Decision Time (minutes)[2]	410	126	63	98
Head CT Results Within 45 Min. of Arrival	12	67%	49%	57%
Patients Who Left ER Before Being Seen	>100k	0%	2%	2%
Time from ER Arrival to Admit. (minutes)[2]	455	256	210	274
Time from ER Arrival to Discharge (minutes)	397	85	110	134
Time in ER Before Being Evaluated (minutes)	303	16	24	26
Time to Pain Meds for Fractures (minutes)	265	41	55	57
Heart Attack Care				
Aspirin Given at Discharge[2]	264	100%	99%	99%
Fibrinolytic Meds Within 30 Min. of Arrival[2,7]	-	-	25%	54%
PCI Within 90 Minutes of Arrival[2]	44	100%	95%	96%
Statin Prescribed at Discharge[2]	254	98%	98%	98%
Heart Failure Care				
ACE Inhibitor or ARB for LVSD[2]	101	96%	95%	97%
Discharge Instructions Given[2]	246	97%	92%	94%
Evaluation of LVS Function[2]	306	100%	96%	99%
Medicare Spending				
Medicare Spending per Patient (ratio)	-	1.00	0.93	0.98
Pneumonia Care				
Appropriate Initial Antibiotic Given[2]	95	99%	92%	95%
Blood Culture Timing[2]	160	99%	97%	98%
Pregnancy and Delivery Care				
Newborn Deliveries Scheduled Early	331	12%	8%	6%
Preventive Care				
Immunization for Influenza[2]	517	98%	89%	90%
Immunization for Pneumonia[2]	584	99%	91%	92%
Stroke Care				
Anticoagulation Therapy for Atrial Fibrillation	39	82%	91%	95%
Antithrombotic Therapy Timing	196	99%	95%	98%
Assessed for Rehabilitation	216	99%	96%	97%
Discharged on Antithrombotic Therapy	206	100%	98%	99%
Discharged on Statin Medication	156	94%	88%	94%
Thrombolytic Therapy Timing	15	93%	61%	66%
Venous Thromboembolism Prophylaxis	221	96%	92%	94%
Written Stroke Educational Materials Given	128	84%	86%	88%
Surgical Care Improvement Project				
Appropriate Beta Blocker Usage[2]	183	96%	97%	98%
Appropriate VTP Within 24 Hours[2]	448	99%	97%	98%
Controlled Postoperative Blood Glucose[2]	73	97%	97%	97%
Perioperative Temperature Management[2]	504	100%	100%	100%
Prophylactic Antibiotic Selection[2]	383	99%	99%	99%
Prophylactic Antibiotic Selection (Outpatient)	584	99%	98%	98%
Prophylactic Antibiotic Stopped[2]	354	98%	98%	98%
Prophylactic Antibiotic Timing[2]	385	98%	98%	99%
Prophylactic Antibiotic Timing (Outpatient)	585	99%	98%	98%
Urinary Catheter Removal[2]	292	96%	96%	97%
Survey of Patients' Hospital Experiences				
Area Around Room 'Always' Quiet at Night	300+	63%	68%	61%
Doctors 'Always' Communicated Well	300+	79%	84%	82%
Home Recovery Information Given	300+	88%	84%	85%
Hospital Given 9 or 10 on 10 Point Scale	300+	74%	72%	71%
Meds 'Always' Explained Before Given	300+	60%	66%	64%
Nurses 'Always' Communicated Well	300+	75%	80%	79%
Pain 'Always' Well Controlled	300+	71%	72%	71%
Room and Bathroom 'Always' Clean	300+	69%	73%	73%
Timely Help 'Always' Received	300+	58%	71%	68%
Would Definitely Recommend Hospital	300+	73%	71%	71%
Use of Medical Imaging				
Cardiac Imaging Stress Test before Surgery	253	2.4%	4.5%	5.3%
Combination Abdominal CT Scan	1,518	16.2%	23%	10.5%
Combination Brain/Sinus CT Scan	1,248	2.9%	2.2%	2.7%
Combination Chest CT Scan	1,285	1.3%	5.1%	2.7%
Follow-up Mammogram/Ultrasound	3,017	7.8%	8.1%	8.8%
Lumbar Spine MRI for Low Back Pain	172	45.3%	39.9%	37.2%

Jane Phillips Nowata Health Center

237 South Locust Street
Nowata, OK 74048
Phone: 918-273-3102
Type: Critical Access Hospitals
Emergency Services: Yes
Ownership: Voluntary non-profit - Private

Measure	Cases	This Hosp.	State Avg.	U.S. Avg.
Blood Clot Prevention and Treatment				
Anticoagulation Overlap Therapy[5]	-	-	89%	93%
ICU Venous Thromboembolism Prophylaxis[5]	-	-	87%	92%
Incidence of Potentially Preventable VTE[5]	-	-	8%	10%
UFH with Dosages/Platelet Monitoring[5]	-	-	97%	97%
Venous Thromboembolism Prophylaxis[5]	-	-	72%	85%
Warfarin Therapy Discharge Instructions[5]	-	-	73%	75%
Chest Pain/Possible Heart Attack Care				
Aspirin Given Within 24 Hours of Arrival[1,3]	-	-	95%	96%
Fibrinolytic Meds Within 30 Min. of Arrival[3,7]	-	-	54%	58%
Average Time to ECG (minutes)[1,3]	-	-	8	7
Average Time to Transfer (minutes)[3,7]	-	-	77	60
Children's Asthma Care				
Received Home Management Plan of Care	-	-	-	88%
Received Reliever Medication	-	-	-	100%
Received Systemic Corticosteroids	-	-	-	100%
Emergency Department				
Admittance Decision Time (minutes)[5]	-	-	63	98
Head CT Results Within 45 Min. of Arrival[5]	-	-	49%	57%
Patients Who Left ER Before Being Seen[5]	-	-	2%	2%
Time from ER Arrival to Admit. (minutes)[5]	-	-	210	274
Time from ER Arrival to Discharge (minutes)[5]	-	-	110	134
Time in ER Before Being Evaluated (minutes)[5]	-	-	24	26
Time to Pain Meds for Fractures (minutes)[1,3]	-	-	55	57
Heart Attack Care				
Aspirin Given at Discharge[5]	-	-	99%	99%
Fibrinolytic Meds Within 30 Min. of Arrival[5]	-	-	25%	54%
PCI Within 90 Minutes of Arrival[5]	-	-	95%	96%
Statin Prescribed at Discharge[5]	-	-	98%	98%
Heart Failure Care				
ACE Inhibitor or ARB for LVSD[3,7]	-	-	95%	97%
Discharge Instructions Given[1,3]	-	-	92%	94%
Evaluation of LVS Function[1,3]	-	-	96%	99%
Medicare Spending				
Medicare Spending per Patient (ratio)	-	-	0.93	0.98
Pneumonia Care				
Appropriate Initial Antibiotic Given[1]	-	-	92%	95%
Blood Culture Timing[1]	-	-	97%	98%
Pregnancy and Delivery Care				
Newborn Deliveries Scheduled Early[5]	-	-	8%	6%
Preventive Care				
Immunization for Influenza[5]	-	-	89%	90%
Immunization for Pneumonia[5]	-	-	91%	92%
Stroke Care				
Anticoagulation Therapy for Atrial Fibrillation[5]	-	-	91%	95%
Antithrombotic Therapy Timing[5]	-	-	95%	98%
Assessed for Rehabilitation[5]	-	-	96%	97%
Discharged on Antithrombotic Therapy[5]	-	-	98%	99%
Discharged on Statin Medication[5]	-	-	88%	94%
Thrombolytic Therapy Timing[5]	-	-	61%	66%
Venous Thromboembolism Prophylaxis[5]	-	-	92%	94%
Written Stroke Educational Materials Given[5]	-	-	86%	88%
Surgical Care Improvement Project				
Appropriate Beta Blocker Usage[5]	-	-	97%	98%
Appropriate VTP Within 24 Hours[5]	-	-	97%	98%
Controlled Postoperative Blood Glucose[5]	-	-	97%	97%
Perioperative Temperature Management[5]	-	-	100%	100%
Prophylactic Antibiotic Selection[5]	-	-	99%	99%
Prophylactic Antibiotic Selection (Outpatient)[5]	-	-	98%	98%
Prophylactic Antibiotic Stopped[5]	-	-	98%	98%
Prophylactic Antibiotic Timing[5]	-	-	98%	99%
Prophylactic Antibiotic Timing (Outpatient)[5]	-	-	98%	98%
Urinary Catheter Removal[5]	-	-	96%	97%
Survey of Patients' Hospital Experiences				
Area Around Room 'Always' Quiet at Night[5]	-	-	68%	61%
Doctors 'Always' Communicated Well[5]	-	-	84%	82%
Home Recovery Information Given[5]	-	-	84%	85%
Hospital Given 9 or 10 on 10 Point Scale[5]	-	-	72%	71%
Meds 'Always' Explained Before Given[5]	-	-	66%	64%
Nurses 'Always' Communicated Well[5]	-	-	80%	79%
Pain 'Always' Well Controlled[5]	-	-	72%	71%
Room and Bathroom 'Always' Clean[5]	-	-	73%	73%
Timely Help 'Always' Received[5]	-	-	71%	68%
Would Definitely Recommend Hospital[5]	-	-	71%	71%
Use of Medical Imaging				
Cardiac Imaging Stress Test before Surgery[7]	-	-	4.5%	5.3%
Combination Abdominal CT Scan[7]	-	-	23%	10.5%
Combination Brain/Sinus CT Scan[7]	-	-	2.2%	2.7%
Combination Chest CT Scan[7]	-	-	5.1%	2.7%
Follow-up Mammogram/Ultrasound[7]	-	-	8.1%	8.8%
Lumbar Spine MRI for Low Back Pain[7]	-	-	39.9%	37.2%

NOTE: Hospital profiles are in alphabetical order by state, then city, then hospital within the city; Rankings exclude hospitals with less than 25 cases except for patient surveys which excludes hospitals with less than 100 cases; (a) 100-299 cases; (1) The number of cases/patients is too few to report; (2) Data submitted were based on a sample of cases/patients; (3) Results are based on a shorter time period than required; (4) Data suppressed by CMS for one or more quarters; (5) Results are not available for this reporting period; (6) Fewer than 100 patients completed the HCAHPS survey; (7) No cases met the criteria for this measure; (8) The lower limit of the confidence interval cannot be calculated if the number of observed infections equals zero; (9) No data are available from the state/territory for this reporting period; (10) The scores shown reflect fewer than 50 completed surveys; (11) There were discrepancies in the data collection process; (12) This measure does not apply to this hospital for this reporting period; (13) Results cannot be calculated for this reporting period; (14) The results for this state are combined with nearby states to protect confidentiality; Please refer to the User's Guide for a full explanation of data.

Okeene Municipal Hospital

207 East F Street
Okeene, OK 73763
Phone: 580-822-4417
Fax: 580-822-3018
E-mail: sdunham@okeenehospital.com
URL: www.okeenehospital.com
Type: Critical Access Hospitals
Emergency Services: Yes
Ownership: Govt - Hospital Dist/Auth
Beds: 17

Key Personnel:
Emergency Room . . . . A Atendido, MD
Cardiac Laboratory. . . . . Tammy Fisher
CEO/President. . . . . Sandra Lamie
Infection Control. . . . . Pat Lorenz, RN
Operating Room. . . . . Pat Lorenz
Quality Assurance . . . . Pat Lorenz
Anesthesiology. . . . . Ken Parrott, MD
Chief of Medical Staff . . . . Ken Parrott, MD

Measure	Cases	This Hosp.	State Avg.	U.S. Avg.
Blood Clot Prevention and Treatment				
Anticoagulation Overlap Therapy[5]	-	-	89%	93%
ICU Venous Thromboembolism Prophylaxis[5]	-	-	87%	92%
Incidence of Potentially Preventable VTE[5]	-	-	8%	10%
UFH with Dosages/Platelet Monitoring[5]	-	-	97%	97%
Venous Thromboembolism Prophylaxis[5]	-	-	72%	85%
Warfarin Therapy Discharge Instructions[5]	-	-	73%	75%
Chest Pain/Possible Heart Attack Care				
Aspirin Given Within 24 Hours of Arrival[1,3]	-	-	95%	96%
Fibrinolytic Meds Within 30 Min. of Arrival[3,7]	-	-	54%	58%
Average Time to ECG (minutes)[1,3]	-	-	8	7
Average Time to Transfer (minutes)[3,7]	-	-	77	60
Children's Asthma Care				
Received Home Management Plan of Care	-	-	-	88%
Received Reliever Medication	-	-	-	100%
Received Systemic Corticosteroids	-	-	-	100%
Emergency Department				
Admittance Decision Time (minutes)	21	0	63	98
Head CT Results Within 45 Min. of Arrival[1,3]	-	-	49%	57%
Patients Who Left ER Before Being Seen[5]	-	-	2%	2%
Time from ER Arrival to Admit. (minutes)	21	125	210	274
Time from ER Arrival to Discharge (minutes)[3]	49	90	110	134
Time in ER Before Being Evaluated (minutes)[3]	60	10	24	26
Time to Pain Meds for Fractures (minutes)	13	30	55	57
Heart Attack Care				
Aspirin Given at Discharge[5]	-	-	99%	99%
Fibrinolytic Meds Within 30 Min. of Arrival[5]	-	-	25%	54%
PCI Within 90 Minutes of Arrival[5]	-	-	95%	96%
Statin Prescribed at Discharge[5]	-	-	98%	98%
Heart Failure Care				
ACE Inhibitor or ARB for LVSD[1,3]	-	-	95%	97%
Discharge Instructions Given[1,3]	-	-	92%	94%
Evaluation of LVS Function[1,3]	-	-	96%	99%
Medicare Spending				
Medicare Spending per Patient (ratio)	-	-	0.93	0.98
Pneumonia Care				
Appropriate Initial Antibiotic Given	11	82%	92%	95%
Blood Culture Timing[1]	-	-	97%	98%
Pregnancy and Delivery Care				
Newborn Deliveries Scheduled Early[5]	-	-	8%	6%
Preventive Care				
Immunization for Influenza	19	84%	89%	90%
Immunization for Pneumonia	27	100%	91%	92%
Stroke Care				
Anticoagulation Therapy for Atrial Fibrillation[5]	-	-	91%	95%
Antithrombotic Therapy Timing[5]	-	-	95%	98%
Assessed for Rehabilitation[5]	-	-	96%	97%
Discharged on Antithrombotic Therapy[5]	-	-	98%	99%
Discharged on Statin Medication[5]	-	-	88%	94%
Thrombolytic Therapy Timing[5]	-	-	61%	66%
Venous Thromboembolism Prophylaxis[5]	-	-	92%	94%
Written Stroke Educational Materials Given[5]	-	-	86%	88%
Surgical Care Improvement Project				
Appropriate Beta Blocker Usage[5]	-	-	97%	98%
Appropriate VTP Within 24 Hours[5]	-	-	97%	98%
Controlled Postoperative Blood Glucose[5]	-	-	97%	97%
Perioperative Temperature Management[5]	-	-	100%	100%
Prophylactic Antibiotic Selection[5]	-	-	99%	99%
Prophylactic Antibiotic Selection (Outpatient)[5]	-	-	98%	98%
Prophylactic Antibiotic Stopped[5]	-	-	98%	98%
Prophylactic Antibiotic Timing[5]	-	-	98%	99%
Prophylactic Antibiotic Timing (Outpatient)[5]	-	-	98%	98%
Urinary Catheter Removal[5]	-	-	96%	97%
Survey of Patients' Hospital Experiences				
Area Around Room 'Always' Quiet at Night[10]	<100	90%	68%	61%
Doctors 'Always' Communicated Well[10]	<100	92%	84%	82%
Home Recovery Information Given[10]	<100	99%	84%	85%
Hospital Given 9 or 10 on 10 Point Scale[10]	<100	94%	72%	71%
Meds 'Always' Explained Before Given[10]	<100	76%	66%	64%
Nurses 'Always' Communicated Well[10]	<100	91%	80%	79%
Pain 'Always' Well Controlled[10]	<100	82%	72%	71%
Room and Bathroom 'Always' Clean[10]	<100	86%	73%	73%
Timely Help 'Always' Received[10]	<100	82%	71%	68%
Would Definitely Recommend Hospital[10]	<100	97%	71%	71%
Use of Medical Imaging				
Cardiac Imaging Stress Test before Surgery[7]	-	-	4.5%	5.3%
Combination Abdominal CT Scan[1]	-	-	23%	10.5%
Combination Brain/Sinus CT Scan[1]	-	-	2.2%	2.7%
Combination Chest CT Scan[1]	-	-	5.1%	2.7%
Follow-up Mammogram/Ultrasound[7]	-	-	8.1%	8.8%
Lumbar Spine MRI for Low Back Pain[1]	-	-	39.9%	37.2%

Creek Nation Community Hospital

309 North 14th
Okemah, OK 74859
Phone: 918-623-1424
Fax: 918-623-9016
URL: www.muscogeenation-nsn.gov
Type: Critical Access Hospitals
Emergency Services: Yes
Ownership: Tribal
Beds: 39

Key Personnel:
CEO/President. . . . . Judy Aaron
Infection Control. . . . . Betty Brown
Chief of Medical Staff . . . . Dr. Charles Colbert
Operating Room. . . . . Cindy Franks
Quality Assurance . . . . Rick Mathews
Emergency Room . . . . Mark Sullivan, MD

Measure	Cases	This Hosp.	State Avg.	U.S. Avg.
Blood Clot Prevention and Treatment				
Anticoagulation Overlap Therapy[5]	-	-	89%	93%
ICU Venous Thromboembolism Prophylaxis[5]	-	-	87%	92%
Incidence of Potentially Preventable VTE[5]	-	-	8%	10%
UFH with Dosages/Platelet Monitoring[5]	-	-	97%	97%
Venous Thromboembolism Prophylaxis[5]	-	-	72%	85%
Warfarin Therapy Discharge Instructions[5]	-	-	73%	75%
Chest Pain/Possible Heart Attack Care				
Aspirin Given Within 24 Hours of Arrival	12	92%	95%	96%
Fibrinolytic Meds Within 30 Min. of Arrival[3,7]	-	-	54%	58%
Average Time to ECG (minutes)	15	17	8	7
Average Time to Transfer (minutes)[1,3]	-	-	77	60
Children's Asthma Care				
Received Home Management Plan of Care	-	-	-	88%
Received Reliever Medication	-	-	-	100%
Received Systemic Corticosteroids	-	-	-	100%
Emergency Department				
Admittance Decision Time (minutes)[5]	-	-	63	98
Head CT Results Within 45 Min. of Arrival[1]	-	-	49%	57%
Patients Who Left ER Before Being Seen[5]	-	-	2%	2%
Time from ER Arrival to Admit. (minutes)[5]	-	-	210	274
Time from ER Arrival to Discharge (minutes)[5]	-	-	110	134
Time in ER Before Being Evaluated (minutes)[5]	-	-	24	26
Time to Pain Meds for Fractures (minutes)[1]	-	-	55	57
Heart Attack Care				
Aspirin Given at Discharge[3,7]	-	-	99%	99%
Fibrinolytic Meds Within 30 Min. of Arrival[3,7]	-	-	25%	54%
PCI Within 90 Minutes of Arrival[3,7]	-	-	95%	96%
Statin Prescribed at Discharge[3,7]	-	-	98%	98%
Heart Failure Care				
ACE Inhibitor or ARB for LVSD[1]	-	-	95%	97%
Discharge Instructions Given[1]	-	-	92%	94%
Evaluation of LVS Function[1]	-	-	96%	99%
Medicare Spending				
Medicare Spending per Patient (ratio)	-	-	0.93	0.98
Pneumonia Care				
Appropriate Initial Antibiotic Given	17	94%	92%	95%
Blood Culture Timing	11	82%	97%	98%
Pregnancy and Delivery Care				
Newborn Deliveries Scheduled Early[5]	-	-	8%	6%
Preventive Care				
Immunization for Influenza[5]	-	-	89%	90%
Immunization for Pneumonia[5]	-	-	91%	92%
Stroke Care				
Anticoagulation Therapy for Atrial Fibrillation[5]	-	-	91%	95%
Antithrombotic Therapy Timing[5]	-	-	95%	98%
Assessed for Rehabilitation[5]	-	-	96%	97%
Discharged on Antithrombotic Therapy[5]	-	-	98%	99%
Discharged on Statin Medication[5]	-	-	88%	94%
Thrombolytic Therapy Timing[5]	-	-	61%	66%
Venous Thromboembolism Prophylaxis[5]	-	-	92%	94%
Written Stroke Educational Materials Given[5]	-	-	86%	88%
Surgical Care Improvement Project				
Appropriate Beta Blocker Usage[5]	-	-	97%	98%
Appropriate VTP Within 24 Hours[5]	-	-	97%	98%
Controlled Postoperative Blood Glucose[5]	-	-	97%	97%
Perioperative Temperature Management[5]	-	-	100%	100%
Prophylactic Antibiotic Selection[5]	-	-	99%	99%
Prophylactic Antibiotic Selection (Outpatient)[5]	-	-	98%	98%
Prophylactic Antibiotic Stopped[5]	-	-	98%	98%
Prophylactic Antibiotic Timing[5]	-	-	98%	99%
Prophylactic Antibiotic Timing (Outpatient)[5]	-	-	98%	98%
Urinary Catheter Removal[5]	-	-	96%	97%
Survey of Patients' Hospital Experiences				
Area Around Room 'Always' Quiet at Night[5]	-	-	68%	61%
Doctors 'Always' Communicated Well[5]	-	-	84%	82%
Home Recovery Information Given[5]	-	-	84%	85%
Hospital Given 9 or 10 on 10 Point Scale[5]	-	-	72%	71%
Meds 'Always' Explained Before Given[5]	-	-	66%	64%
Nurses 'Always' Communicated Well[5]	-	-	80%	79%
Pain 'Always' Well Controlled[5]	-	-	72%	71%
Room and Bathroom 'Always' Clean[5]	-	-	73%	73%
Timely Help 'Always' Received[5]	-	-	71%	68%
Would Definitely Recommend Hospital[5]	-	-	71%	71%
Use of Medical Imaging				
Cardiac Imaging Stress Test before Surgery[1]	-	-	4.5%	5.3%
Combination Abdominal CT Scan	102	12.7%	23%	10.5%
Combination Brain/Sinus CT Scan[1]	-	-	2.2%	2.7%
Combination Chest CT Scan	78	12.8%	5.1%	2.7%
Follow-up Mammogram/Ultrasound	131	13.7%	8.1%	8.8%
Lumbar Spine MRI for Low Back Pain[7]	-	-	39.9%	37.2%

Community Hospital

3100 Southwest 89th Street
Oklahoma City, OK 73159
Phone: 405-602-8100
Type: Acute Care Hospitals
Emergency Services: Yes
Ownership: Physician

Measure	Cases	This Hosp.	State Avg.	U.S. Avg.
Blood Clot Prevention and Treatment				
Anticoagulation Overlap Therapy[1,2]	-	-	89%	93%
ICU Venous Thromboembolism Prophylaxis[1,2]	-	-	87%	92%
Incidence of Potentially Preventable VTE[2,7]	-	-	8%	10%
UFH with Dosages/Platelet Monitoring[2,7]	-	-	97%	97%
Venous Thromboembolism Prophylaxis[2]	157	97%	72%	85%
Warfarin Therapy Discharge Instructions[1,2]	-	-	73%	75%
Chest Pain/Possible Heart Attack Care				
Aspirin Given Within 24 Hours of Arrival[5]	-	-	95%	96%
Fibrinolytic Meds Within 30 Min. of Arrival[5]	-	-	54%	58%
Average Time to ECG (minutes)[5]	-	-	8	7
Average Time to Transfer (minutes)[5]	-	-	77	60
Children's Asthma Care				
Received Home Management Plan of Care	-	-	-	88%
Received Reliever Medication	-	-	-	100%
Received Systemic Corticosteroids	-	-	-	100%
Emergency Department				
Admittance Decision Time (minutes)[2]	189	50	63	98
Head CT Results Within 45 Min. of Arrival[1,3]	-	-	49%	57%

NOTE: Hospital profiles are in alphabetical order by state, then city, then hospital within the city; Rankings exclude hospitals with less than 25 cases except for patient surveys which excludes hospitals with less than 100 cases; (a) 100-299 cases; (1) The number of cases/patients is too few to report; (2) Data submitted were based on a sample of cases/patients; (3) Results are based on a shorter time period than required; (4) Data suppressed by CMS for one or more quarters; (5) Results are not available for this reporting period; (6) Fewer than 100 patients completed the HCAHPS survey; (7) No cases met the criteria for this measure; (8) The lower limit of the confidence interval cannot be calculated if the number of observed infections equals zero; (9) No data are available from the state/territory for this reporting period; (10) The scores shown reflect fewer than 50 completed surveys; (11) There were discrepancies in the data collection process; (12) This measure does not apply to this hospital for this reporting period; (13) Results cannot be calculated for this reporting period; (14) The results for this state are combined with nearby states to protect confidentiality; Please refer to the User's Guide for a full explanation of data.

Patients Who Left ER Before Being Seen	7,046	1%	2%	2%
Time from ER Arrival to Admit. (minutes)[2]	201	189	210	274
Time from ER Arrival to Discharge (minutes)	1,313	87	110	134
Time in ER Before Being Evaluated (minutes)	1,365	12	24	26
Time to Pain Meds for Fractures (minutes)	16	44	55	57
Heart Attack Care				
Aspirin Given at Discharge[5]	-	-	99%	99%
Fibrinolytic Meds Within 30 Min. of Arrival[5]	-	-	25%	54%
PCI Within 90 Minutes of Arrival[5]	-	-	95%	96%
Statin Prescribed at Discharge[5]	-	-	98%	98%
Heart Failure Care				
ACE Inhibitor or ARB for LVSD[3,7]	-	-	95%	97%
Discharge Instructions Given[1,3]	-	-	92%	94%
Evaluation of LVS Function[1,3]	-	-	96%	99%
Medicare Spending				
Medicare Spending per Patient (ratio)	-	1.00	0.93	0.98
Pneumonia Care				
Appropriate Initial Antibiotic Given[1]	-	-	92%	95%
Blood Culture Timing[1]	-	-	97%	98%
Pregnancy and Delivery Care				
Newborn Deliveries Scheduled Early[7]	-	-	8%	6%
Preventive Care				
Immunization for Influenza[2]	736	99%	89%	90%
Immunization for Pneumonia[2]	809	89%	91%	92%
Stroke Care				
Anticoagulation Therapy for Atrial Fibrillation[3,7]	-	-	91%	95%
Antithrombotic Therapy Timing[3,7]	-	-	95%	98%
Assessed for Rehabilitation[3,7]	-	-	96%	97%
Discharged on Antithrombotic Therapy[3,7]	-	-	98%	99%
Discharged on Statin Medication[3,7]	-	-	88%	94%
Thrombolytic Therapy Timing[3,7]	-	-	61%	66%
Venous Thromboembolism Prophylaxis[3,7]	-	-	92%	94%
Written Stroke Educational Materials Given[3,7]	-	-	86%	88%
Surgical Care Improvement Project				
Appropriate Beta Blocker Usage[2]	54	100%	97%	98%
Appropriate VTP Within 24 Hours[2]	191	95%	97%	98%
Controlled Postoperative Blood Glucose[2,7]	-	-	97%	97%
Perioperative Temperature Management[2]	203	100%	100%	100%
Prophylactic Antibiotic Selection[2]	172	100%	99%	99%
Prophylactic Antibiotic Selection (Outpatient)	159	99%	98%	98%
Prophylactic Antibiotic Stopped[2]	172	98%	98%	98%
Prophylactic Antibiotic Timing[2]	172	99%	98%	99%
Prophylactic Antibiotic Timing (Outpatient)	159	100%	98%	98%
Urinary Catheter Removal[2]	62	98%	96%	97%
Survey of Patients' Hospital Experiences				
Area Around Room 'Always' Quiet at Night	300+	78%	68%	61%
Doctors 'Always' Communicated Well	300+	84%	84%	82%
Home Recovery Information Given	300+	87%	84%	85%
Hospital Given 9 or 10 on 10 Point Scale	300+	80%	72%	71%
Meds 'Always' Explained Before Given	300+	68%	66%	64%
Nurses 'Always' Communicated Well	300+	82%	80%	79%
Pain 'Always' Well Controlled	300+	71%	72%	71%
Room and Bathroom 'Always' Clean	300+	80%	73%	73%
Timely Help 'Always' Received	300+	77%	71%	68%
Would Definitely Recommend Hospital	300+	82%	71%	71%
Use of Medical Imaging				
Cardiac Imaging Stress Test before Surgery[7]	-	-	4.5%	5.3%
Combination Abdominal CT Scan	106	29.2%	23%	10.5%
Combination Brain/Sinus CT Scan	71	0.0%	2.2%	2.7%
Combination Chest CT Scan	45	2.2%	5.1%	2.7%
Follow-up Mammogram/Ultrasound[7]	-	-	8.1%	8.8%
Lumbar Spine MRI for Low Back Pain	178	43.3%	39.9%	37.2%

Deaconess Hospital

5501 North Portland Avenue
Oklahoma City, OK 73112
URL: www.deaconessokc.com
Type: Acute Care Hospitals
Ownership: Proprietary
Phone: 405-604-6109
Fax: 405-604-4297
Emergency Services: Yes
Beds: 313

Key Personnel:
Anesthesiology. . . . . Robin Bayless, MD
CEO/President. . . . . Paul Dougherty
Intensive Care Unit. . . . . Michelle Engress, RN
Radiology. . . . . Kerri Kirchoff, MD
Emergency Room . . . . Judi Merning, RN
Quality Assurance . . . . Mary Quisenberg
Infection Control. . . . . Carol Shenold, ICP
Chief of Medical Staff . . . . Ken Whittington, MD

Measure	Cases	This Hosp.	State Avg.	U.S. Avg.
Blood Clot Prevention and Treatment				
Anticoagulation Overlap Therapy[2]	43	84%	89%	93%
ICU Venous Thromboembolism Prophylaxis[2]	54	87%	87%	92%
Incidence of Potentially Preventable VTE[1,2]	-	-	8%	10%
UFH with Dosages/Platelet Monitoring[1,2]	-	-	97%	97%
Venous Thromboembolism Prophylaxis[2]	336	75%	72%	85%
Warfarin Therapy Discharge Instructions[2]	29	97%	73%	75%
Chest Pain/Possible Heart Attack Care				
Aspirin Given Within 24 Hours of Arrival[3,7]	-	-	95%	96%
Fibrinolytic Meds Within 30 Min. of Arrival[5]	-	-	54%	58%
Average Time to ECG (minutes)[3,7]	-	-	8	7
Average Time to Transfer (minutes)[5]	-	-	77	60
Children's Asthma Care				
Received Home Management Plan of Care	-	-	-	88%
Received Reliever Medication	-	-	-	100%
Received Systemic Corticosteroids	-	-	-	100%
Emergency Department				
Admittance Decision Time (minutes)[2]	574	82	63	98
Head CT Results Within 45 Min. of Arrival[3,7]	-	-	49%	57%
Patients Who Left ER Before Being Seen	40,348	3%	2%	2%
Time from ER Arrival to Admit. (minutes)[2]	577	237	210	274
Time from ER Arrival to Discharge (minutes)	382	119	110	134
Time in ER Before Being Evaluated (minutes)	417	22	24	26
Time to Pain Meds for Fractures (minutes)	97	68	55	57
Heart Attack Care				
Aspirin Given at Discharge	76	100%	99%	99%
Fibrinolytic Meds Within 30 Min. of Arrival[7]	-	-	25%	54%
PCI Within 90 Minutes of Arrival	14	100%	95%	96%
Statin Prescribed at Discharge	77	100%	98%	98%
Heart Failure Care				
ACE Inhibitor or ARB for LVSD	37	100%	95%	97%
Discharge Instructions Given	67	84%	92%	94%
Evaluation of LVS Function	92	100%	96%	99%
Medicare Spending				
Medicare Spending per Patient (ratio)	-	1.05	0.93	0.98
Pneumonia Care				
Appropriate Initial Antibiotic Given	96	99%	92%	95%
Blood Culture Timing	173	98%	97%	98%
Pregnancy and Delivery Care				
Newborn Deliveries Scheduled Early[2]	32	0%	8%	6%
Preventive Care				
Immunization for Influenza[2]	589	98%	89%	90%
Immunization for Pneumonia[2]	648	97%	91%	92%
Stroke Care				
Anticoagulation Therapy for Atrial Fibrillation[1]	-	-	91%	95%
Antithrombotic Therapy Timing	36	81%	95%	98%
Assessed for Rehabilitation	40	98%	96%	97%
Discharged on Antithrombotic Therapy	37	97%	98%	99%
Discharged on Statin Medication	28	93%	88%	94%
Thrombolytic Therapy Timing[1]	-	-	61%	66%
Venous Thromboembolism Prophylaxis	39	92%	92%	94%
Written Stroke Educational Materials Given	21	95%	86%	88%
Surgical Care Improvement Project				
Appropriate Beta Blocker Usage	92	95%	97%	98%
Appropriate VTP Within 24 Hours	342	96%	97%	98%
Controlled Postoperative Blood Glucose	15	100%	97%	97%
Perioperative Temperature Management	419	100%	100%	100%
Prophylactic Antibiotic Selection	215	100%	99%	99%
Prophylactic Antibiotic Selection (Outpatient)	458	99%	98%	98%
Prophylactic Antibiotic Stopped	213	98%	98%	98%
Prophylactic Antibiotic Timing	215	100%	98%	99%
Prophylactic Antibiotic Timing (Outpatient)	425	99%	98%	98%
Urinary Catheter Removal	117	95%	96%	97%
Survey of Patients' Hospital Experiences				
Area Around Room 'Always' Quiet at Night	300+	63%	68%	61%
Doctors 'Always' Communicated Well	300+	81%	84%	82%
Home Recovery Information Given	300+	87%	84%	85%
Hospital Given 9 or 10 on 10 Point Scale	300+	67%	72%	71%
Meds 'Always' Explained Before Given	300+	62%	66%	64%
Nurses 'Always' Communicated Well	300+	75%	80%	79%
Pain 'Always' Well Controlled	300+	71%	72%	71%
Room and Bathroom 'Always' Clean	300+	67%	73%	73%
Timely Help 'Always' Received	300+	59%	71%	68%
Would Definitely Recommend Hospital	300+	69%	71%	71%
Use of Medical Imaging				
Cardiac Imaging Stress Test before Surgery[1]	-	-	4.5%	5.3%
Combination Abdominal CT Scan	486	11.5%	23%	10.5%
Combination Brain/Sinus CT Scan	712	3.7%	2.2%	2.7%
Combination Chest CT Scan	346	3.5%	5.1%	2.7%
Follow-up Mammogram/Ultrasound	903	4.8%	8.1%	8.8%
Lumbar Spine MRI for Low Back Pain	105	35.2%	39.9%	37.2%

Integris Baptist Medical Center

3300 Northwest Expressway
Oklahoma City, OK 73112
URL: www.integris-health.com
Type: Acute Care Hospitals
Ownership: Voluntary non-profit - Private
Phone: 405-951-8110
Fax: 405-945-4997
Emergency Services: Yes
Beds: 577

Key Personnel:
Operating Room. . . . . Connie Harper
CEO/President. . . . . Tim Johnsen
Pediatric Ambulatory Care . . . . . . Kevin Moore, MD
Pediatric In-Patient Care . . . . Kevin Moore, MD
Infection Control. . . . . V Ramgopal, MD
Radiology. . . . . Georgianne Snowden, MD
Quality Assurance . . . . Bill Wandel
Chief of Medical Staff . . . . James White, MD

Measure	Cases	This Hosp.	State Avg.	U.S. Avg.
Blood Clot Prevention and Treatment				
Anticoagulation Overlap Therapy[2]	134	89%	89%	93%
ICU Venous Thromboembolism Prophylaxis[2]	105	84%	87%	92%
Incidence of Potentially Preventable VTE[2]	34	9%	8%	10%
UFH with Dosages/Platelet Monitoring[2]	41	98%	97%	97%
Venous Thromboembolism Prophylaxis[2]	285	58%	72%	85%
Warfarin Therapy Discharge Instructions[2]	101	37%	73%	75%
Chest Pain/Possible Heart Attack Care				
Aspirin Given Within 24 Hours of Arrival[1,3]	-	-	95%	96%
Fibrinolytic Meds Within 30 Min. of Arrival[5]	-	-	54%	58%
Average Time to ECG (minutes)[1,3]	-	-	8	7
Average Time to Transfer (minutes)[5]	-	-	77	60
Children's Asthma Care				
Received Home Management Plan of Care	-	-	-	88%
Received Reliever Medication	-	-	-	100%
Received Systemic Corticosteroids	-	-	-	100%
Emergency Department				
Admittance Decision Time (minutes)[2]	451	94	63	98
Head CT Results Within 45 Min. of Arrival[1]	-	-	49%	57%
Patients Who Left ER Before Being Seen	57,548	7%	2%	2%
Time from ER Arrival to Admit. (minutes)[2]	495	290	210	274
Time from ER Arrival to Discharge (minutes)	347	212	110	134
Time in ER Before Being Evaluated (minutes)	103	64	24	26
Time to Pain Meds for Fractures (minutes)	116	66	55	57
Heart Attack Care				
Aspirin Given at Discharge	561	100%	99%	99%
Fibrinolytic Meds Within 30 Min. of Arrival[7]	-	-	25%	54%
PCI Within 90 Minutes of Arrival	50	94%	95%	96%
Statin Prescribed at Discharge	555	100%	98%	98%
Heart Failure Care				
ACE Inhibitor or ARB for LVSD	187	96%	95%	97%
Discharge Instructions Given	360	96%	92%	94%
Evaluation of LVS Function	423	100%	96%	99%
Medicare Spending				
Medicare Spending per Patient (ratio)	-	0.99	0.93	0.98
Pneumonia Care				
Appropriate Initial Antibiotic Given[2]	120	95%	92%	95%
Blood Culture Timing[2]	270	99%	97%	98%
Pregnancy and Delivery Care				
Newborn Deliveries Scheduled Early	369	3%	8%	6%
Preventive Care				
Immunization for Influenza[2]	499	88%	89%	90%
Immunization for Pneumonia[2]	568	92%	91%	92%
Stroke Care				

NOTE: Hospital profiles are in alphabetical order by state, then city, then hospital within the city; Rankings exclude hospitals with less than 25 cases except for patient surveys which excludes hospitals with less than 100 cases; (a) 100-299 cases; (1) The number of cases/patients is too few to report; (2) Data submitted were based on a sample of cases/patients; (3) Results are based on a shorter time period than required; (4) Data suppressed by CMS for one or more quarters; (5) Results are not available for this reporting period; (6) Fewer than 100 patients completed the HCAHPS survey; (7) No cases met the criteria for this measure; (8) The lower limit of the confidence interval cannot be calculated if the number of observed infections equals zero; (9) No data are available from the state/territory for this reporting period; (10) The scores shown reflect fewer than 50 completed surveys; (11) There were discrepancies in the data collection process; (12) This measure does not apply to this hospital for this reporting period; (13) Results cannot be calculated for this reporting period; (14) The results for this state are combined with nearby states to protect confidentiality; Please refer to the User's Guide for a full explanation of data.

Measure	Cases	This Hosp.	State Avg.	U.S. Avg.
Anticoagulation Therapy for Atrial Fibrillation[2]	22	100%	91%	95%
Antithrombotic Therapy Timing[2]	91	97%	95%	98%
Assessed for Rehabilitation[2]	124	100%	96%	97%
Discharged on Antithrombotic Therapy[2]	110	98%	98%	99%
Discharged on Statin Medication[2]	69	97%	88%	94%
Thrombolytic Therapy Timing[1,2]	-	-	61%	66%
Venous Thromboembolism Prophylaxis[2]	121	94%	92%	94%
Written Stroke Educational Materials Given[2]	76	99%	86%	88%
Surgical Care Improvement Project				
Appropriate Beta Blocker Usage[2]	266	98%	97%	98%
Appropriate VTP Within 24 Hours[2]	308	98%	97%	98%
Controlled Postoperative Blood Glucose[2]	161	96%	97%	97%
Perioperative Temperature Management[2]	443	100%	100%	100%
Prophylactic Antibiotic Selection[2]	448	99%	99%	99%
Prophylactic Antibiotic Selection (Outpatient)	525	99%	98%	98%
Prophylactic Antibiotic Stopped[2]	440	98%	98%	98%
Prophylactic Antibiotic Timing[2]	448	100%	98%	99%
Prophylactic Antibiotic Timing (Outpatient)	522	98%	98%	98%
Urinary Catheter Removal[2]	348	95%	96%	97%
Survey of Patients' Hospital Experiences				
Area Around Room 'Always' Quiet at Night	300+	66%	68%	61%
Doctors 'Always' Communicated Well	300+	84%	84%	82%
Home Recovery Information Given	300+	84%	84%	85%
Hospital Given 9 or 10 on 10 Point Scale	300+	80%	72%	71%
Meds 'Always' Explained Before Given	300+	63%	66%	64%
Nurses 'Always' Communicated Well	300+	78%	80%	79%
Pain 'Always' Well Controlled	300+	73%	72%	71%
Room and Bathroom 'Always' Clean	300+	74%	73%	73%
Timely Help 'Always' Received	300+	67%	71%	68%
Would Definitely Recommend Hospital	300+	81%	71%	71%
Use of Medical Imaging				
Cardiac Imaging Stress Test before Surgery	821	5.4%	4.5%	5.3%
Combination Abdominal CT Scan	1,063	14.0%	23%	10.5%
Combination Brain/Sinus CT Scan	989	1.3%	2.2%	2.7%
Combination Chest CT Scan	937	0.3%	5.1%	2.7%
Follow-up Mammogram/Ultrasound	2,024	10.5%	8.1%	8.8%
Lumbar Spine MRI for Low Back Pain[1]	-	-	39.9%	37.2%

Integris Southwest Medical Center

4401 South Western Avenue — Phone: 405-636-7000
Oklahoma City, OK 73109 — Fax: 405-636-7064
URL: www.integris-health.com
Type: Acute Care Hospitals — Emergency Services: No
Ownership: Proprietary — Beds: 369

Key Personnel:
Intensive Care Unit. . . . . Darlene Burton
Hemotology Center . . . . Hallie Ennis
Operating Room. . . . . Jim Lynch
CEO/President. . . . . James Moore
Infection Control. . . . . Jennifer Perry
Quality Assurance . . . . Joan Pierce, RN
Radiology. . . . . Dee Tucker
Chief of Medical Staff. . . . . James White, MD

Measure	Cases	This Hosp.	State Avg.	U.S. Avg.
Blood Clot Prevention and Treatment				
Anticoagulation Overlap Therapy[2]	67	85%	89%	93%
ICU Venous Thromboembolism Prophylaxis[2]	81	93%	87%	92%
Incidence of Potentially Preventable VTE[2]	18	6%	8%	10%
UFH with Dosages/Platelet Monitoring[1,2]	-	-	97%	97%
Venous Thromboembolism Prophylaxis[2]	343	73%	72%	85%
Warfarin Therapy Discharge Instructions[2]	53	64%	73%	75%
Chest Pain/Possible Heart Attack Care				
Aspirin Given Within 24 Hours of Arrival	20	95%	95%	96%
Fibrinolytic Meds Within 30 Min. of Arrival[3,7]	-	-	54%	58%
Average Time to ECG (minutes)	19	9	8	7
Average Time to Transfer (minutes)[3,7]	-	-	77	60
Children's Asthma Care				
Received Home Management Plan of Care	-	-	-	88%
Received Reliever Medication	-	-	-	100%
Received Systemic Corticosteroids	-	-	-	100%
Emergency Department				
Admittance Decision Time (minutes)[2]	599	61	63	98
Head CT Results Within 45 Min. of Arrival[1]	-	-	49%	57%
Patients Who Left ER Before Being Seen	83,666	3%	2%	2%
Time from ER Arrival to Admit. (minutes)[2]	671	193	210	274
Time from ER Arrival to Discharge (minutes)	364	82	110	134
Time in ER Before Being Evaluated (minutes)	114	27	24	26
Time to Pain Meds for Fractures (minutes)	163	38	55	57
Heart Attack Care				
Aspirin Given at Discharge[2]	214	98%	99%	99%
Fibrinolytic Meds Within 30 Min. of Arrival[2,7]	-	-	25%	54%
PCI Within 90 Minutes of Arrival[2]	41	95%	95%	96%
Statin Prescribed at Discharge[2]	212	96%	98%	98%
Heart Failure Care				
ACE Inhibitor or ARB for LVSD[2]	123	94%	95%	97%
Discharge Instructions Given[2]	227	79%	92%	94%
Evaluation of LVS Function[2]	272	97%	96%	99%
Medicare Spending				
Medicare Spending per Patient (ratio)	-	1.02	0.93	0.98
Pneumonia Care				
Appropriate Initial Antibiotic Given[2]	124	98%	92%	95%
Blood Culture Timing[2]	169	98%	97%	98%
Pregnancy and Delivery Care				
Newborn Deliveries Scheduled Early	124	10%	8%	6%
Preventive Care				
Immunization for Influenza[2]	522	94%	89%	90%
Immunization for Pneumonia[2]	664	95%	91%	92%
Stroke Care				
Anticoagulation Therapy for Atrial Fibrillation[2]	22	95%	91%	95%
Antithrombotic Therapy Timing[2]	87	98%	95%	98%
Assessed for Rehabilitation[2]	135	100%	96%	97%
Discharged on Antithrombotic Therapy[2]	127	100%	98%	99%
Discharged on Statin Medication[2]	99	98%	88%	94%
Thrombolytic Therapy Timing[2]	14	100%	61%	66%
Venous Thromboembolism Prophylaxis[2]	135	96%	92%	94%
Written Stroke Educational Materials Given[2]	72	99%	86%	88%
Surgical Care Improvement Project				
Appropriate Beta Blocker Usage[2]	149	99%	97%	98%
Appropriate VTP Within 24 Hours[2]	246	96%	97%	98%
Controlled Postoperative Blood Glucose[2]	76	92%	97%	97%
Perioperative Temperature Management[2]	332	100%	100%	100%
Prophylactic Antibiotic Selection[2]	265	99%	99%	99%
Prophylactic Antibiotic Selection (Outpatient)	171	99%	98%	98%
Prophylactic Antibiotic Stopped[2]	240	97%	98%	98%
Prophylactic Antibiotic Timing[2]	266	100%	98%	99%
Prophylactic Antibiotic Timing (Outpatient)	172	98%	98%	98%
Urinary Catheter Removal[2]	294	96%	96%	97%
Survey of Patients' Hospital Experiences				
Area Around Room 'Always' Quiet at Night	300+	62%	68%	61%
Doctors 'Always' Communicated Well	300+	76%	84%	82%
Home Recovery Information Given	300+	85%	84%	85%
Hospital Given 9 or 10 on 10 Point Scale	300+	68%	72%	71%
Meds 'Always' Explained Before Given	300+	59%	66%	64%
Nurses 'Always' Communicated Well	300+	77%	80%	79%
Pain 'Always' Well Controlled	300+	68%	72%	71%
Room and Bathroom 'Always' Clean	300+	66%	73%	73%
Timely Help 'Always' Received	300+	64%	71%	68%
Would Definitely Recommend Hospital	300+	68%	71%	71%
Use of Medical Imaging				
Cardiac Imaging Stress Test before Surgery	90	4.4%	4.5%	5.3%
Combination Abdominal CT Scan	926	21.0%	23%	10.5%
Combination Brain/Sinus CT Scan	633	0.6%	2.2%	2.7%
Combination Chest CT Scan	841	0.0%	5.1%	2.7%
Follow-up Mammogram/Ultrasound	1,932	9.2%	8.1%	8.8%
Lumbar Spine MRI for Low Back Pain	173	37.0%	39.9%	37.2%

Lakeside Women's Hospital

11200 North Portland Avenue — Phone: 405-936-1500
Oklahoma City, OK 73120
Type: Acute Care Hospitals — Emergency Services: Yes
Ownership: Proprietary

Key Personnel:
CEO/President. . . . . Kelley Brewer
Emergency Room . . . . Melinda Oldham

Measure	Cases	This Hosp.	State Avg.	U.S. Avg.
Blood Clot Prevention and Treatment				
Anticoagulation Overlap Therapy[2,7]	-	-	89%	93%
ICU Venous Thromboembolism Prophylaxis[2,7]	-	-	87%	92%
Incidence of Potentially Preventable VTE[2,7]	-	-	8%	10%
UFH with Dosages/Platelet Monitoring[2,7]	-	-	97%	97%
Venous Thromboembolism Prophylaxis[2,7]	-	-	72%	85%
Warfarin Therapy Discharge Instructions[2,7]	-	-	73%	75%
Chest Pain/Possible Heart Attack Care				
Aspirin Given Within 24 Hours of Arrival[5]	-	-	95%	96%
Fibrinolytic Meds Within 30 Min. of Arrival[5]	-	-	54%	58%
Average Time to ECG (minutes)[5]	-	-	8	7
Average Time to Transfer (minutes)[5]	-	-	77	60
Children's Asthma Care				
Received Home Management Plan of Care	-	-	-	88%
Received Reliever Medication	-	-	-	100%
Received Systemic Corticosteroids	-	-	-	100%
Emergency Department				
Admittance Decision Time (minutes)[2,7]	-	-	63	98
Head CT Results Within 45 Min. of Arrival[5]	-	-	49%	57%
Patients Who Left ER Before Being Seen	50	0%	2%	2%
Time from ER Arrival to Admit. (minutes)[2,7]	-	-	210	274
Time from ER Arrival to Discharge (minutes)[3]	45	127	110	134
Time in ER Before Being Evaluated (minutes)[3]	27	77	24	26
Time to Pain Meds for Fractures (minutes)[5]	-	-	55	57
Heart Attack Care				
Aspirin Given at Discharge[5]	-	-	99%	99%
Fibrinolytic Meds Within 30 Min. of Arrival[5]	-	-	25%	54%
PCI Within 90 Minutes of Arrival[5]	-	-	95%	96%
Statin Prescribed at Discharge[5]	-	-	98%	98%
Heart Failure Care				
ACE Inhibitor or ARB for LVSD[5]	-	-	95%	97%
Discharge Instructions Given[5]	-	-	92%	94%
Evaluation of LVS Function[5]	-	-	96%	99%
Medicare Spending				
Medicare Spending per Patient (ratio)[1]	-	-	0.93	0.98
Pneumonia Care				
Appropriate Initial Antibiotic Given[5]	-	-	92%	95%
Blood Culture Timing[5]	-	-	97%	98%
Pregnancy and Delivery Care				
Newborn Deliveries Scheduled Early[2]	93	16%	8%	6%
Preventive Care				
Immunization for Influenza[2]	313	73%	89%	90%
Immunization for Pneumonia[2]	13	15%	91%	92%
Stroke Care				
Anticoagulation Therapy for Atrial Fibrillation[5]	-	-	91%	95%
Antithrombotic Therapy Timing[5]	-	-	95%	98%
Assessed for Rehabilitation[5]	-	-	96%	97%
Discharged on Antithrombotic Therapy[5]	-	-	98%	99%
Discharged on Statin Medication[5]	-	-	88%	94%
Thrombolytic Therapy Timing[5]	-	-	61%	66%
Venous Thromboembolism Prophylaxis[5]	-	-	92%	94%
Written Stroke Educational Materials Given[5]	-	-	86%	88%
Surgical Care Improvement Project				
Appropriate Beta Blocker Usage[1,2]	-	-	97%	98%
Appropriate VTP Within 24 Hours[2]	33	18%	97%	98%
Controlled Postoperative Blood Glucose[2,7]	-	-	97%	97%
Perioperative Temperature Management[2]	33	100%	100%	100%
Prophylactic Antibiotic Selection[2]	29	93%	99%	99%
Prophylactic Antibiotic Selection (Outpatient)	166	90%	98%	98%
Prophylactic Antibiotic Stopped[2]	29	100%	98%	98%
Prophylactic Antibiotic Timing[2]	30	97%	98%	99%
Prophylactic Antibiotic Timing (Outpatient)	167	95%	98%	98%
Urinary Catheter Removal[2,7]	-	-	96%	97%
Survey of Patients' Hospital Experiences				
Area Around Room 'Always' Quiet at Night	(a)	62%	68%	61%
Doctors 'Always' Communicated Well	(a)	83%	84%	82%
Home Recovery Information Given	(a)	86%	84%	85%
Hospital Given 9 or 10 on 10 Point Scale	(a)	75%	72%	71%
Meds 'Always' Explained Before Given	(a)	65%	66%	64%
Nurses 'Always' Communicated Well	(a)	77%	80%	79%
Pain 'Always' Well Controlled	(a)	73%	72%	71%
Room and Bathroom 'Always' Clean	(a)	72%	73%	73%
Timely Help 'Always' Received	(a)	59%	71%	68%
Would Definitely Recommend Hospital	(a)	80%	71%	71%

NOTE: Hospital profiles are in alphabetical order by state, then city, then hospital within the city; Rankings exclude hospitals with less than 25 cases except for patient surveys which excludes hospitals with less than 100 cases; (a) 100-299 cases; (1) The number of cases/patients is too few to report; (2) Data submitted were based on a sample of cases/patients; (3) Results are based on a shorter time period than required; (4) Data suppressed by CMS for one or more quarters; (5) Results are not available for this reporting period; (6) Fewer than 100 patients completed the HCAHPS survey; (7) No cases met the criteria for this measure; (8) The lower limit of the confidence interval cannot be calculated if the number of observed infections equals zero; (9) No data are available from the state/territory for this reporting period; (10) The scores shown reflect fewer than 50 completed surveys; (11) There were discrepancies in the data collection process; (12) This measure does not apply to this hospital for this reporting period; (13) Results cannot be calculated for this reporting period; (14) The results for this state are combined with nearby states to protect confidentiality; Please refer to the User's Guide for a full explanation of data.

Measure	Cases	This Hosp.	State Avg.	U.S. Avg.
Use of Medical Imaging				
Cardiac Imaging Stress Test before Surgery[7]	-	-	4.5%	5.3%
Combination Abdominal CT Scan[7]	-	-	23%	10.5%
Combination Brain/Sinus CT Scan[7]	-	-	2.2%	2.7%
Combination Chest CT Scan[7]	-	-	5.1%	2.7%
Follow-up Mammogram/Ultrasound	716	4.1%	8.1%	8.8%
Lumbar Spine MRI for Low Back Pain[7]	-	-	39.9%	37.2%

McBride Clinic Orthopedic Hospital

9600 North Broadway Extension
Oklahoma City, OK 73114
URL: www.mcbrideclinic.com
Type: Acute Care Hospitals
Ownership: Proprietary
Phone: 405-478-1717
Fax: 405-486-2144
Emergency Services: Yes

Measure	Cases	This Hosp.	State Avg.	U.S. Avg.
Blood Clot Prevention and Treatment				
Anticoagulation Overlap Therapy[1,2]	-	-	89%	93%
ICU Venous Thromboembolism Prophylaxis[2,7]	-	-	87%	92%
Incidence of Potentially Preventable VTE[1,2]	-	-	8%	10%
UFH with Dosages/Platelet Monitoring[2,7]	-	-	97%	97%
Venous Thromboembolism Prophylaxis[2]	160	88%	72%	85%
Warfarin Therapy Discharge Instructions[1,2]	-	-	73%	75%
Chest Pain/Possible Heart Attack Care				
Aspirin Given Within 24 Hours of Arrival[1,3]	-	-	95%	96%
Fibrinolytic Meds Within 30 Min. of Arrival[5]	-	-	54%	58%
Average Time to ECG (minutes)[1,3]	-	-	8	7
Average Time to Transfer (minutes)[5]	-	-	77	60
Children's Asthma Care				
Received Home Management Plan of Care	-	-	-	88%
Received Reliever Medication	-	-	-	100%
Received Systemic Corticosteroids	-	-	-	100%
Emergency Department				
Admittance Decision Time (minutes)[2]	69	50	63	98
Head CT Results Within 45 Min. of Arrival[5]	-	-	49%	57%
Patients Who Left ER Before Being Seen	3,234	0%	2%	2%
Time from ER Arrival to Admit. (minutes)[2]	69	150	210	274
Time from ER Arrival to Discharge (minutes)	291	84	110	134
Time in ER Before Being Evaluated (minutes)	295	18	24	26
Time to Pain Meds for Fractures (minutes)	69	51	55	57
Heart Attack Care				
Aspirin Given at Discharge[5]	-	-	99%	99%
Fibrinolytic Meds Within 30 Min. of Arrival[5]	-	-	25%	54%
PCI Within 90 Minutes of Arrival[5]	-	-	95%	96%
Statin Prescribed at Discharge[5]	-	-	98%	98%
Heart Failure Care				
ACE Inhibitor or ARB for LVSD[5]	-	-	95%	97%
Discharge Instructions Given[5]	-	-	92%	94%
Evaluation of LVS Function[5]	-	-	96%	99%
Medicare Spending				
Medicare Spending per Patient (ratio)	-	0.92	0.93	0.98
Pneumonia Care				
Appropriate Initial Antibiotic Given[5]	-	-	92%	95%
Blood Culture Timing[5]	-	-	97%	98%
Pregnancy and Delivery Care				
Newborn Deliveries Scheduled Early[7]	-	-	8%	6%
Preventive Care				
Immunization for Influenza[2]	494	95%	89%	90%
Immunization for Pneumonia[2]	558	96%	91%	92%
Stroke Care				
Anticoagulation Therapy for Atrial Fibrillation[5]	-	-	91%	95%
Antithrombotic Therapy Timing[5]	-	-	95%	98%
Assessed for Rehabilitation[5]	-	-	96%	97%
Discharged on Antithrombotic Therapy[5]	-	-	98%	99%
Discharged on Statin Medication[5]	-	-	88%	94%
Thrombolytic Therapy Timing[5]	-	-	61%	66%
Venous Thromboembolism Prophylaxis[5]	-	-	92%	94%
Written Stroke Educational Materials Given[5]	-	-	86%	88%
Surgical Care Improvement Project				
Appropriate Beta Blocker Usage[2]	106	100%	97%	98%
Appropriate VTP Within 24 Hours[2]	340	97%	97%	98%
Controlled Postoperative Blood Glucose[2,7]	-	-	97%	97%
Perioperative Temperature Management[2]	355	100%	100%	100%
Prophylactic Antibiotic Selection[2]	274	100%	99%	99%
Prophylactic Antibiotic Selection (Outpatient)	60	100%	98%	98%
Prophylactic Antibiotic Stopped[2]	274	100%	98%	98%
Prophylactic Antibiotic Timing[2]	274	100%	98%	99%
Prophylactic Antibiotic Timing (Outpatient)	60	100%	98%	98%
Urinary Catheter Removal[1,2]	-	-	96%	97%
Survey of Patients' Hospital Experiences				
Area Around Room 'Always' Quiet at Night	300+	80%	68%	61%
Doctors 'Always' Communicated Well	300+	87%	84%	82%
Home Recovery Information Given	300+	91%	84%	85%
Hospital Given 9 or 10 on 10 Point Scale	300+	86%	72%	71%
Meds 'Always' Explained Before Given	300+	71%	66%	64%
Nurses 'Always' Communicated Well	300+	84%	80%	79%
Pain 'Always' Well Controlled	300+	77%	72%	71%
Room and Bathroom 'Always' Clean	300+	80%	73%	73%
Timely Help 'Always' Received	300+	75%	71%	68%
Would Definitely Recommend Hospital	300+	89%	71%	71%
Use of Medical Imaging				
Cardiac Imaging Stress Test before Surgery[7]	-	-	4.5%	5.3%
Combination Abdominal CT Scan[1]	-	-	23%	10.5%
Combination Brain/Sinus CT Scan[1]	-	-	2.2%	2.7%
Combination Chest CT Scan[1]	-	-	5.1%	2.7%
Follow-up Mammogram/Ultrasound[7]	-	-	8.1%	8.8%
Lumbar Spine MRI for Low Back Pain	388	34.5%	39.9%	37.2%

Mercy Hospital Oklahoma City

4300 West Memorial Road
Oklahoma City, OK 73120
URL: www.mercyok.net/mhc
Type: Acute Care Hospitals
Ownership: Voluntary non-profit - Church
Phone: 405-752-3754
Fax: 405-752-3811
Emergency Services: Yes
Beds: 351

Key Personnel:
Quality Assurance . . . . Cozy Armstrong
CEO/President. . . . . Bruce F Buchanan
Radiology. . . . . Richard Cooke, MD
Anesthesiology. . . . . Bennett Fuller
Chief of Medical Staff. . . . . William Hughes, MD
Emergency Room . . . . Paul Orchutt, MD
Pediatric In-Patient Care . . . . Merl Simmons, MD

Measure	Cases	This Hosp.	State Avg.	U.S. Avg.
Blood Clot Prevention and Treatment				
Anticoagulation Overlap Therapy[2]	93	84%	89%	93%
ICU Venous Thromboembolism Prophylaxis[2]	74	100%	87%	92%
Incidence of Potentially Preventable VTE[2]	19	16%	8%	10%
UFH with Dosages/Platelet Monitoring[2]	20	100%	97%	97%
Venous Thromboembolism Prophylaxis[2]	321	85%	72%	85%
Warfarin Therapy Discharge Instructions[2]	66	52%	73%	75%
Chest Pain/Possible Heart Attack Care				
Aspirin Given Within 24 Hours of Arrival	61	100%	95%	96%
Fibrinolytic Meds Within 30 Min. of Arrival[7]	-	-	54%	58%
Average Time to ECG (minutes)	63	9	8	7
Average Time to Transfer (minutes)[1]	-	-	77	60
Children's Asthma Care				
Received Home Management Plan of Care	-	-	-	88%
Received Reliever Medication	-	-	-	100%
Received Systemic Corticosteroids	-	-	-	100%
Emergency Department				
Admittance Decision Time (minutes)[2]	367	75	63	98
Head CT Results Within 45 Min. of Arrival[1]	-	-	49%	57%
Patients Who Left ER Before Being Seen	54,395	1%	2%	2%
Time from ER Arrival to Admit. (minutes)[2]	378	204	210	274
Time from ER Arrival to Discharge (minutes)	382	120	110	134
Time in ER Before Being Evaluated (minutes)	394	12	24	26
Time to Pain Meds for Fractures (minutes)	120	43	55	57
Heart Attack Care				
Aspirin Given at Discharge[1]	-	-	99%	99%
Fibrinolytic Meds Within 30 Min. of Arrival[7]	-	-	25%	54%
PCI Within 90 Minutes of Arrival[7]	-	-	95%	96%
Statin Prescribed at Discharge	11	91%	98%	98%
Heart Failure Care				
ACE Inhibitor or ARB for LVSD	17	94%	95%	97%
Discharge Instructions Given	47	81%	92%	94%
Evaluation of LVS Function	77	100%	96%	99%
Medicare Spending				
Medicare Spending per Patient (ratio)	-	1.01	0.93	0.98
Pneumonia Care				
Appropriate Initial Antibiotic Given[2]	48	98%	92%	95%
Blood Culture Timing[2]	115	100%	97%	98%
Pregnancy and Delivery Care				
Newborn Deliveries Scheduled Early[2]	56	11%	8%	6%
Preventive Care				
Immunization for Influenza[2]	502	95%	89%	90%
Immunization for Pneumonia[2]	578	97%	91%	92%
Stroke Care				
Anticoagulation Therapy for Atrial Fibrillation	34	94%	91%	95%
Antithrombotic Therapy Timing	220	100%	95%	98%
Assessed for Rehabilitation	388	100%	96%	97%
Discharged on Antithrombotic Therapy	323	100%	98%	99%
Discharged on Statin Medication	223	98%	88%	94%
Thrombolytic Therapy Timing	33	94%	61%	66%
Venous Thromboembolism Prophylaxis	336	97%	92%	94%
Written Stroke Educational Materials Given	197	100%	86%	88%
Surgical Care Improvement Project				
Appropriate Beta Blocker Usage[2]	102	99%	97%	98%
Appropriate VTP Within 24 Hours[2]	350	99%	97%	98%
Controlled Postoperative Blood Glucose[2,7]	-	-	97%	97%
Perioperative Temperature Management[2]	413	100%	100%	100%
Prophylactic Antibiotic Selection[2]	264	100%	99%	99%
Prophylactic Antibiotic Selection (Outpatient)	425	97%	98%	98%
Prophylactic Antibiotic Stopped[2]	250	99%	98%	98%
Prophylactic Antibiotic Timing[2]	264	100%	98%	99%
Prophylactic Antibiotic Timing (Outpatient)	420	98%	98%	98%
Urinary Catheter Removal[2]	111	94%	96%	97%
Survey of Patients' Hospital Experiences				
Area Around Room 'Always' Quiet at Night[11]	300+	62%	68%	61%
Doctors 'Always' Communicated Well[11]	300+	84%	84%	82%
Home Recovery Information Given[11]	300+	87%	84%	85%
Hospital Given 9 or 10 on 10 Point Scale[11]	300+	72%	72%	71%
Meds 'Always' Explained Before Given[11]	300+	65%	66%	64%
Nurses 'Always' Communicated Well[11]	300+	74%	80%	79%
Pain 'Always' Well Controlled[11]	300+	68%	72%	71%
Room and Bathroom 'Always' Clean[11]	300+	66%	73%	73%
Timely Help 'Always' Received[11]	300+	59%	71%	68%
Would Definitely Recommend Hospital[11]	300+	77%	71%	71%
Use of Medical Imaging				
Cardiac Imaging Stress Test before Surgery[7]	-	-	4.5%	5.3%
Combination Abdominal CT Scan	2,438	17.8%	23%	10.5%
Combination Brain/Sinus CT Scan	1,757	2.3%	2.2%	2.7%
Combination Chest CT Scan	1,673	8.5%	5.1%	2.7%
Follow-up Mammogram/Ultrasound	2,785	11.2%	8.1%	8.8%
Lumbar Spine MRI for Low Back Pain	441	37.9%	39.9%	37.2%

Northwest Surgical Hospital

9204 North May Avenue
Oklahoma City, OK 73120
URL: www.nwsurgicalokc.com
Type: Acute Care Hospitals
Ownership: Physician
Phone: 404-848-1918
Emergency Services: Yes
Beds: 9

Key Personnel:
Radiology. . . . . Byron Christie, M.D.
Anesthesiology. . . . . Phillip G. Doerner, Jr, M.D.
CEO/President. . . . . Debbie Foster

Measure	Cases	This Hosp.	State Avg.	U.S. Avg.
Blood Clot Prevention and Treatment				
Anticoagulation Overlap Therapy[7]	-	-	89%	93%
ICU Venous Thromboembolism Prophylaxis[7]	-	-	87%	92%
Incidence of Potentially Preventable VTE[7]	-	-	8%	10%
UFH with Dosages/Platelet Monitoring[7]	-	-	97%	97%
Venous Thromboembolism Prophylaxis	96	97%	72%	85%
Warfarin Therapy Discharge Instructions[7]	-	-	73%	75%
Chest Pain/Possible Heart Attack Care				
Aspirin Given Within 24 Hours of Arrival[5]	-	-	95%	96%
Fibrinolytic Meds Within 30 Min. of Arrival[5]	-	-	54%	58%
Average Time to ECG (minutes)[5]	-	-	8	7
Average Time to Transfer (minutes)[5]	-	-	77	60
Children's Asthma Care				
Received Home Management Plan of Care	-	-	-	88%

NOTE: Hospital profiles are in alphabetical order by state, then city, then hospital within the city; Rankings exclude hospitals with less than 25 cases except for patient surveys which excludes hospitals with less than 100 cases; (a) 100-299 cases; (1) The number of cases/patients is too few to report; (2) Data submitted were based on a sample of cases/patients; (3) Results are based on a shorter time period than required; (4) Data suppressed by CMS for one or more quarters; (5) Results are not available for this reporting period; (6) Fewer than 100 patients completed the HCAHPS survey; (7) No cases met the criteria for this measure; (8) The lower limit of the confidence interval cannot be calculated if the number of observed infections equals zero; (9) No data are available from the state/territory for this reporting period; (10) The scores shown reflect fewer than 50 completed surveys; (11) There were discrepancies in the data collection process; (12) This measure does not apply to this hospital for this reporting period; (13) Results cannot be calculated for this reporting period; (14) The results for this state are combined with nearby states to protect confidentiality; Please refer to the User's Guide for a full explanation of data.

Measure	Cases	This Hosp.	State Avg.	U.S. Avg.
Received Reliever Medication	-	-	-	100%
Received Systemic Corticosteroids	-	-	-	100%
Emergency Department				
Admittance Decision Time (minutes)[7]	-	-	63	98
Head CT Results Within 45 Min. of Arrival[5]	-	-	49%	57%
Patients Who Left ER Before Being Seen[5]	-	-	2%	2%
Time from ER Arrival to Admit. (minutes)[7]	-	-	210	274
Time from ER Arrival to Discharge (minutes)[5]	-	-	110	134
Time in ER Before Being Evaluated (minutes)[5]	-	-	24	26
Time to Pain Meds for Fractures (minutes)[5]	-	-	55	57
Heart Attack Care				
Aspirin Given at Discharge[5]	-	-	99%	99%
Fibrinolytic Meds Within 30 Min. of Arrival[5]	-	-	25%	54%
PCI Within 90 Minutes of Arrival[5]	-	-	95%	96%
Statin Prescribed at Discharge[5]	-	-	98%	98%
Heart Failure Care				
ACE Inhibitor or ARB for LVSD[5]	-	-	95%	97%
Discharge Instructions Given[5]	-	-	92%	94%
Evaluation of LVS Function[5]	-	-	96%	99%
Medicare Spending				
Medicare Spending per Patient (ratio)[1]	-	-	0.93	0.98
Pneumonia Care				
Appropriate Initial Antibiotic Given[5]	-	-	92%	95%
Blood Culture Timing[5]	-	-	97%	98%
Pregnancy and Delivery Care				
Newborn Deliveries Scheduled Early[2,7]	-	-	8%	6%
Preventive Care				
Immunization for Influenza	155	81%	89%	90%
Immunization for Pneumonia[2]	99	81%	91%	92%
Stroke Care				
Anticoagulation Therapy for Atrial Fibrillation[5]	-	-	91%	95%
Antithrombotic Therapy Timing[5]	-	-	95%	98%
Assessed for Rehabilitation[5]	-	-	96%	97%
Discharged on Antithrombotic Therapy[5]	-	-	98%	99%
Discharged on Statin Medication[5]	-	-	88%	94%
Thrombolytic Therapy Timing[5]	-	-	61%	66%
Venous Thromboembolism Prophylaxis[5]	-	-	92%	94%
Written Stroke Educational Materials Given[5]	-	-	86%	88%
Surgical Care Improvement Project				
Appropriate Beta Blocker Usage[2]	37	97%	97%	98%
Appropriate VTP Within 24 Hours[2]	173	99%	97%	98%
Controlled Postoperative Blood Glucose[2,7]	-	-	97%	97%
Perioperative Temperature Management[2]	178	100%	100%	100%
Prophylactic Antibiotic Selection[2]	166	99%	99%	99%
Prophylactic Antibiotic Selection (Outpatient)[3]	25	88%	98%	98%
Prophylactic Antibiotic Stopped[2]	166	98%	98%	98%
Prophylactic Antibiotic Timing[2]	166	98%	98%	99%
Prophylactic Antibiotic Timing (Outpatient)[3]	25	96%	98%	98%
Urinary Catheter Removal[1,2]	-	-	96%	97%
Survey of Patients' Hospital Experiences				
Area Around Room 'Always' Quiet at Night	(a)	83%	68%	61%
Doctors 'Always' Communicated Well	(a)	90%	84%	82%
Home Recovery Information Given	(a)	88%	84%	85%
Hospital Given 9 or 10 on 10 Point Scale	(a)	85%	72%	71%
Meds 'Always' Explained Before Given	(a)	84%	66%	64%
Nurses 'Always' Communicated Well	(a)	89%	80%	79%
Pain 'Always' Well Controlled	(a)	81%	72%	71%
Room and Bathroom 'Always' Clean	(a)	80%	73%	73%
Timely Help 'Always' Received	(a)	88%	71%	68%
Would Definitely Recommend Hospital	(a)	87%	71%	71%
Use of Medical Imaging				
Cardiac Imaging Stress Test before Surgery[7]	-	-	4.5%	5.3%
Combination Abdominal CT Scan	56	44.6%	23%	10.5%
Combination Brain/Sinus CT Scan[1]	-	-	2.2%	2.7%
Combination Chest CT Scan[1]	-	-	5.1%	2.7%
Follow-up Mammogram/Ultrasound[7]	-	-	8.1%	8.8%
Lumbar Spine MRI for Low Back Pain	119	38.7%	39.9%	37.2%

O U Medical Center

1200 Everett Drive
Oklahoma City, OK 73104
URL: www.oumedcenter.com
Type: Acute Care Hospitals
Ownership: Proprietary
Phone: 405-271-5911
Fax: 405-271-7344
Emergency Services: Yes
Beds: 394

Key Personnel:
Chief of Medical Staff. . . . . Timothy Coussons, MD
Quality Assurance . . . . John Douvillier
Radiology. . . . . Bob Eaton, MD
Operating Room. . . . . Susan Hollingsworth, RN
CEO/President. . . . . Charles L. Spicer, Jr., FACHE
Infection Control. . . . . Margaret Tannehill, RN
Pediatric Ambulatory Care . . . . . . Paul Toubas, MD
Pediatric In-Patient Care . . . . Paul Toubas, MD

Measure	Cases	This Hosp.	State Avg.	U.S. Avg.
Blood Clot Prevention and Treatment				
Anticoagulation Overlap Therapy[2]	124	98%	89%	93%
ICU Venous Thromboembolism Prophylaxis[2]	114	97%	87%	92%
Incidence of Potentially Preventable VTE[2]	122	1%	8%	10%
UFH with Dosages/Platelet Monitoring[2]	80	100%	97%	97%
Venous Thromboembolism Prophylaxis[2]	414	93%	72%	85%
Warfarin Therapy Discharge Instructions[2]	93	99%	73%	75%
Chest Pain/Possible Heart Attack Care				
Aspirin Given Within 24 Hours of Arrival	29	100%	95%	96%
Fibrinolytic Meds Within 30 Min. of Arrival[7]	-	-	54%	58%
Average Time to ECG (minutes)	30	4	8	7
Average Time to Transfer (minutes)[1]	-	-	77	60
Children's Asthma Care				
Received Home Management Plan of Care	454	94%	-	88%
Received Reliever Medication	456	100%	-	100%
Received Systemic Corticosteroids	456	100%	-	100%
Emergency Department				
Admittance Decision Time (minutes)[2]	602	102	63	98
Head CT Results Within 45 Min. of Arrival[1]	-	-	49%	57%
Patients Who Left ER Before Being Seen	>100k	3%	2%	2%
Time from ER Arrival to Admit. (minutes)[2]	601	288	210	274
Time from ER Arrival to Discharge (minutes)	482	134	110	134
Time in ER Before Being Evaluated (minutes)	520	31	24	26
Time to Pain Meds for Fractures (minutes)	291	74	55	57
Heart Attack Care				
Aspirin Given at Discharge	132	100%	99%	99%
Fibrinolytic Meds Within 30 Min. of Arrival[7]	-	-	25%	54%
PCI Within 90 Minutes of Arrival	21	100%	95%	96%
Statin Prescribed at Discharge	127	100%	98%	98%
Heart Failure Care				
ACE Inhibitor or ARB for LVSD	114	100%	95%	97%
Discharge Instructions Given	247	94%	92%	94%
Evaluation of LVS Function	279	100%	96%	99%
Medicare Spending				
Medicare Spending per Patient (ratio)	-	1.02	0.93	0.98
Pneumonia Care				
Appropriate Initial Antibiotic Given	126	95%	92%	95%
Blood Culture Timing	276	99%	97%	98%
Pregnancy and Delivery Care				
Newborn Deliveries Scheduled Early[2]	60	2%	8%	6%
Preventive Care				
Immunization for Influenza[2]	643	99%	89%	90%
Immunization for Pneumonia[2]	479	97%	91%	92%
Stroke Care				
Anticoagulation Therapy for Atrial Fibrillation[2]	19	100%	91%	95%
Antithrombotic Therapy Timing[2]	76	99%	95%	98%
Assessed for Rehabilitation[2]	176	99%	96%	97%
Discharged on Antithrombotic Therapy[2]	107	100%	98%	99%
Discharged on Statin Medication[2]	79	100%	88%	94%
Thrombolytic Therapy Timing[2]	18	94%	61%	66%
Venous Thromboembolism Prophylaxis[2]	192	99%	92%	94%
Written Stroke Educational Materials Given[2]	95	97%	86%	88%
Surgical Care Improvement Project				
Appropriate Beta Blocker Usage[2]	174	99%	97%	98%
Appropriate VTP Within 24 Hours[2]	494	99%	97%	98%
Controlled Postoperative Blood Glucose[2]	80	95%	97%	97%
Perioperative Temperature Management[2]	635	100%	100%	100%
Prophylactic Antibiotic Selection[2]	429	99%	99%	99%
Prophylactic Antibiotic Selection (Outpatient)	709	99%	98%	98%
Prophylactic Antibiotic Stopped[2]	389	99%	98%	98%
Prophylactic Antibiotic Timing[2]	430	100%	98%	99%
Prophylactic Antibiotic Timing (Outpatient)	678	99%	98%	98%
Urinary Catheter Removal[2]	189	97%	96%	97%
Survey of Patients' Hospital Experiences				
Area Around Room 'Always' Quiet at Night	300+	54%	68%	61%
Doctors 'Always' Communicated Well	300+	76%	84%	82%
Home Recovery Information Given	300+	84%	84%	85%
Hospital Given 9 or 10 on 10 Point Scale	300+	65%	72%	71%
Meds 'Always' Explained Before Given	300+	58%	66%	64%
Nurses 'Always' Communicated Well	300+	72%	80%	79%
Pain 'Always' Well Controlled	300+	65%	72%	71%
Room and Bathroom 'Always' Clean	300+	63%	73%	73%
Timely Help 'Always' Received	300+	54%	71%	68%
Would Definitely Recommend Hospital	300+	66%	71%	71%
Use of Medical Imaging				
Cardiac Imaging Stress Test before Surgery	183	3.8%	4.5%	5.3%
Combination Abdominal CT Scan	1,782	65.5%	23%	10.5%
Combination Brain/Sinus CT Scan	685	3.9%	2.2%	2.7%
Combination Chest CT Scan	1,450	0.3%	5.1%	2.7%
Follow-up Mammogram/Ultrasound[1]	-	-	8.1%	8.8%
Lumbar Spine MRI for Low Back Pain	122	36.9%	39.9%	37.2%

Oklahoma Center for Orthopaedic & Multi-Spec

330 Southwest 80th Street
Oklahoma City, OK 73139
URL: www.ocomhospital.com
Type: Acute Care Hospitals
Ownership: Proprietary
Phone: 405-602-6500
Emergency Services: No

Measure	Cases	This Hosp.	State Avg.	U.S. Avg.
Blood Clot Prevention and Treatment				
Anticoagulation Overlap Therapy[2,7]	-	-	89%	93%
ICU Venous Thromboembolism Prophylaxis[2,7]	-	-	87%	92%
Incidence of Potentially Preventable VTE[2,7]	-	-	8%	10%
UFH with Dosages/Platelet Monitoring[2,7]	-	-	97%	97%
Venous Thromboembolism Prophylaxis[2]	19	100%	72%	85%
Warfarin Therapy Discharge Instructions[2,7]	-	-	73%	75%
Chest Pain/Possible Heart Attack Care				
Aspirin Given Within 24 Hours of Arrival[5]	-	-	95%	96%
Fibrinolytic Meds Within 30 Min. of Arrival[5]	-	-	54%	58%
Average Time to ECG (minutes)[5]	-	-	8	7
Average Time to Transfer (minutes)[5]	-	-	77	60
Children's Asthma Care				
Received Home Management Plan of Care	-	-	-	88%
Received Reliever Medication	-	-	-	100%
Received Systemic Corticosteroids	-	-	-	100%
Emergency Department				
Admittance Decision Time (minutes)[2,7]	-	-	63	98
Head CT Results Within 45 Min. of Arrival[5]	-	-	49%	57%
Patients Who Left ER Before Being Seen	12	0%	2%	2%
Time from ER Arrival to Admit. (minutes)[2,7]	-	-	210	274
Time from ER Arrival to Discharge (minutes)	13	94	110	134
Time in ER Before Being Evaluated (minutes)	12	6	24	26
Time to Pain Meds for Fractures (minutes)[1,3]	-	-	55	57
Heart Attack Care				
Aspirin Given at Discharge[5]	-	-	99%	99%
Fibrinolytic Meds Within 30 Min. of Arrival[5]	-	-	25%	54%
PCI Within 90 Minutes of Arrival[5]	-	-	95%	96%
Statin Prescribed at Discharge[5]	-	-	98%	98%
Heart Failure Care				
ACE Inhibitor or ARB for LVSD[5]	-	-	95%	97%
Discharge Instructions Given[5]	-	-	92%	94%
Evaluation of LVS Function[5]	-	-	96%	99%
Medicare Spending				
Medicare Spending per Patient (ratio)	-	1.00	0.93	0.98
Pneumonia Care				
Appropriate Initial Antibiotic Given[5]	-	-	92%	95%
Blood Culture Timing[5]	-	-	97%	98%
Pregnancy and Delivery Care				
Newborn Deliveries Scheduled Early[7]	-	-	8%	6%
Preventive Care				

NOTE: Hospital profiles are in alphabetical order by state, then city, then hospital within the city; Rankings exclude hospitals with less than 25 cases except for patient surveys which excludes hospitals with less than 100 cases; (a) 100-299 cases; (1) The number of cases/patients is too few to report; (2) Data submitted were based on a sample of cases/patients; (3) Results are based on a shorter time period than required; (4) Data suppressed by CMS for one or more quarters; (5) Results are not available for this reporting period; (6) Fewer than 100 patients completed the HCAHPS survey; (7) No cases met the criteria for this measure; (8) The lower limit of the confidence interval cannot be calculated if the number of observed infections equals zero; (9) No data are available from the state/territory for this reporting period; (10) The scores shown reflect fewer than 50 completed surveys; (11) There were discrepancies in the data collection process; (12) This measure does not apply to this hospital for this reporting period; (13) Results cannot be calculated for this reporting period; (14) The results for this state are combined with nearby states to protect confidentiality; Please refer to the User's Guide for a full explanation of data.

Measure	Cases	This Hosp.	State Avg.	U.S. Avg.
Immunization for Influenza[2]	228	95%	89%	90%
Immunization for Pneumonia[2]	316	75%	91%	92%
Stroke Care				
Anticoagulation Therapy for Atrial Fibrillation[5]	-	-	91%	95%
Antithrombotic Therapy Timing[5]	-	-	95%	98%
Assessed for Rehabilitation[5]	-	-	96%	97%
Discharged on Antithrombotic Therapy[5]	-	-	98%	99%
Discharged on Statin Medication[5]	-	-	88%	94%
Thrombolytic Therapy Timing[5]	-	-	61%	66%
Venous Thromboembolism Prophylaxis[5]	-	-	92%	94%
Written Stroke Educational Materials Given[5]	-	-	86%	88%
Surgical Care Improvement Project				
Appropriate Beta Blocker Usage	80	94%	97%	98%
Appropriate VTP Within 24 Hours	373	98%	97%	98%
Controlled Postoperative Blood Glucose[7]	-	-	97%	97%
Perioperative Temperature Management	373	97%	100%	100%
Prophylactic Antibiotic Selection	345	100%	99%	99%
Prophylactic Antibiotic Selection (Outpatient)	87	98%	98%	98%
Prophylactic Antibiotic Stopped	345	99%	98%	98%
Prophylactic Antibiotic Timing	345	92%	98%	99%
Prophylactic Antibiotic Timing (Outpatient)	91	92%	98%	98%
Urinary Catheter Removal	369	100%	96%	97%
Survey of Patients' Hospital Experiences				
Area Around Room 'Always' Quiet at Night	(a)	80%	68%	61%
Doctors 'Always' Communicated Well	(a)	87%	84%	82%
Home Recovery Information Given	(a)	91%	84%	85%
Hospital Given 9 or 10 on 10 Point Scale	(a)	83%	72%	71%
Meds 'Always' Explained Before Given	(a)	72%	66%	64%
Nurses 'Always' Communicated Well	(a)	85%	80%	79%
Pain 'Always' Well Controlled	(a)	79%	72%	71%
Room and Bathroom 'Always' Clean	(a)	86%	73%	73%
Timely Help 'Always' Received	(a)	80%	71%	68%
Would Definitely Recommend Hospital	(a)	86%	71%	71%
Use of Medical Imaging				
Cardiac Imaging Stress Test before Surgery[7]	-	-	4.5%	5.3%
Combination Abdominal CT Scan[1]	-	-	23%	10.5%
Combination Brain/Sinus CT Scan[1]	-	-	2.2%	2.7%
Combination Chest CT Scan	34	52.9%	5.1%	2.7%
Follow-up Mammogram/Ultrasound[7]	-	-	8.1%	8.8%
Lumbar Spine MRI for Low Back Pain	421	39.2%	39.9%	37.2%

Oklahoma City VA Medical Center

921 Ne 13th Street
Oklahoma City, OK 73104
Phone: 405-270-0501
Fax: 405-270-1560
URL: www.va.gov
Type: Acute Care - VA
Ownership: Government Federal
Emergency Services: No
Beds: 245

Key Personnel:
Infection Control. . . . . Linda Adkins, RN
Anesthesiology. . . . . Raghuvender Gauta, MD
Operating Room. . . . . Deborah Hovarter
Quality Assurance . . . . Jennifer Kubiak
Chief of Medical Staff. . . . . D Robert McCaffree, MD
Ambulatory Care . . . . M Boyd Shook, MD
Emergency Room . . . . M Boyd Shook, MD
Radiology. . . . . Max Walters, MD

Measure	Cases	This Hosp.	State Avg.	U.S. Avg.
Blood Clot Prevention and Treatment				
Anticoagulation Overlap Therapy	-	-	89%	93%
ICU Venous Thromboembolism Prophylaxis	-	-	87%	92%
Incidence of Potentially Preventable VTE	-	-	8%	10%
UFH with Dosages/Platelet Monitoring	-	-	97%	97%
Venous Thromboembolism Prophylaxis	-	-	72%	85%
Warfarin Therapy Discharge Instructions	-	-	73%	75%
Chest Pain/Possible Heart Attack Care				
Aspirin Given Within 24 Hours of Arrival	-	-	95%	96%
Fibrinolytic Meds Within 30 Min. of Arrival	-	-	54%	58%
Average Time to ECG (minutes)	-	-	8	7
Average Time to Transfer (minutes)	-	-	77	60
Children's Asthma Care				
Received Home Management Plan of Care	-	-	-	88%
Received Reliever Medication	-	-	-	100%
Received Systemic Corticosteroids	-	-	-	100%
Emergency Department				
Admittance Decision Time (minutes)	-	-	63	98
Head CT Results Within 45 Min. of Arrival	-	-	49%	57%
Patients Who Left ER Before Being Seen	-	-	2%	2%
Time from ER Arrival to Admit. (minutes)	-	-	210	274
Time from ER Arrival to Discharge (minutes)	-	-	110	134
Time in ER Before Being Evaluated (minutes)	-	-	24	26
Time to Pain Meds for Fractures (minutes)	-	-	55	57
Heart Attack Care				
Aspirin Given at Discharge	104	97%	99%	99%
Fibrinolytic Meds Within 30 Min. of Arrival[5]	-	-	25%	54%
PCI Within 90 Minutes of Arrival[1]	-	-	95%	96%
Statin Prescribed at Discharge	100	98%	98%	98%
Heart Failure Care				
ACE Inhibitor or ARB for LVSD	83	94%	95%	97%
Discharge Instructions Given	178	89%	92%	94%
Evaluation of LVS Function	201	100%	96%	99%
Medicare Spending				
Medicare Spending per Patient (ratio)	-	-	0.93	0.98
Pneumonia Care				
Appropriate Initial Antibiotic Given	69	93%	92%	95%
Blood Culture Timing	164	96%	97%	98%
Pregnancy and Delivery Care				
Newborn Deliveries Scheduled Early	-	-	8%	6%
Preventive Care				
Immunization for Influenza[5]	-	-	89%	90%
Immunization for Pneumonia[5]	-	-	91%	92%
Stroke Care				
Anticoagulation Therapy for Atrial Fibrillation	-	-	91%	95%
Antithrombotic Therapy Timing	-	-	95%	98%
Assessed for Rehabilitation	-	-	96%	97%
Discharged on Antithrombotic Therapy	-	-	98%	99%
Discharged on Statin Medication	-	-	88%	94%
Thrombolytic Therapy Timing	-	-	61%	66%
Venous Thromboembolism Prophylaxis	-	-	92%	94%
Written Stroke Educational Materials Given	-	-	86%	88%
Surgical Care Improvement Project				
Appropriate Beta Blocker Usage[2]	159	99%	97%	98%
Appropriate VTP Within 24 Hours[2]	266	99%	97%	98%
Controlled Postoperative Blood Glucose[2]	41	95%	97%	97%
Perioperative Temperature Management[2]	328	100%	100%	100%
Prophylactic Antibiotic Selection	257	99%	99%	99%
Prophylactic Antibiotic Selection (Outpatient)	-	-	98%	98%
Prophylactic Antibiotic Stopped	256	97%	98%	98%
Prophylactic Antibiotic Timing	257	98%	98%	99%
Prophylactic Antibiotic Timing (Outpatient)	-	-	98%	98%
Urinary Catheter Removal[2]	39	97%	96%	97%
Survey of Patients' Hospital Experiences				
Area Around Room 'Always' Quiet at Night	-	-	68%	61%
Doctors 'Always' Communicated Well	-	-	84%	82%
Home Recovery Information Given	-	-	84%	85%
Hospital Given 9 or 10 on 10 Point Scale	-	-	72%	71%
Meds 'Always' Explained Before Given	-	-	66%	64%
Nurses 'Always' Communicated Well	-	-	80%	79%
Pain 'Always' Well Controlled	-	-	72%	71%
Room and Bathroom 'Always' Clean	-	-	73%	73%
Timely Help 'Always' Received	-	-	71%	68%
Would Definitely Recommend Hospital	-	-	71%	71%
Use of Medical Imaging				
Cardiac Imaging Stress Test before Surgery	-	-	4.5%	5.3%
Combination Abdominal CT Scan	-	-	23%	10.5%
Combination Brain/Sinus CT Scan	-	-	2.2%	2.7%
Combination Chest CT Scan	-	-	5.1%	2.7%
Follow-up Mammogram/Ultrasound	-	-	8.1%	8.8%
Lumbar Spine MRI for Low Back Pain	-	-	39.9%	37.2%

Oklahoma Heart Hospital

4050 West Memorial Road
Oklahoma City, OK 73120
Phone: 405-608-3200
Fax: 405-608-3396
URL: www.okheart.com
Type: Acute Care Hospitals
Ownership: Physician
Emergency Services: Yes
Beds: 78

Key Personnel:
CEO/President. . . . . John Harvey
Chief of Medical Staff. . . . . John Harvey, MD
Radiology. . . . . Vance E McCollom

Measure	Cases	This Hosp.	State Avg.	U.S. Avg.
Blood Clot Prevention and Treatment				
Anticoagulation Overlap Therapy[2]	40	92%	89%	93%
ICU Venous Thromboembolism Prophylaxis[2]	100	100%	87%	92%
Incidence of Potentially Preventable VTE[1,2]	-	-	8%	10%
UFH with Dosages/Platelet Monitoring[1,2]	-	-	97%	97%
Venous Thromboembolism Prophylaxis[2]	323	99%	72%	85%
Warfarin Therapy Discharge Instructions[2]	31	100%	73%	75%
Chest Pain/Possible Heart Attack Care				
Aspirin Given Within 24 Hours of Arrival[1,3]	-	-	95%	96%
Fibrinolytic Meds Within 30 Min. of Arrival[3,7]	-	-	54%	58%
Average Time to ECG (minutes)[1,3]	-	-	8	7
Average Time to Transfer (minutes)[3,7]	-	-	77	60
Children's Asthma Care				
Received Home Management Plan of Care	-	-	-	88%
Received Reliever Medication	-	-	-	100%
Received Systemic Corticosteroids	-	-	-	100%
Emergency Department				
Admittance Decision Time (minutes)[2]	203	47	63	98
Head CT Results Within 45 Min. of Arrival[1]	-	-	49%	57%
Patients Who Left ER Before Being Seen	11,871	0%	2%	2%
Time from ER Arrival to Admit. (minutes)[2]	211	153	210	274
Time from ER Arrival to Discharge (minutes)	351	119	110	134
Time in ER Before Being Evaluated (minutes)	408	10	24	26
Time to Pain Meds for Fractures (minutes)[1]	-	-	55	57
Heart Attack Care				
Aspirin Given at Discharge[2]	327	100%	99%	99%
Fibrinolytic Meds Within 30 Min. of Arrival[2,7]	-	-	25%	54%
PCI Within 90 Minutes of Arrival[2]	27	100%	95%	96%
Statin Prescribed at Discharge[2]	316	100%	98%	98%
Heart Failure Care				
ACE Inhibitor or ARB for LVSD[2]	114	98%	95%	97%
Discharge Instructions Given[2]	283	100%	92%	94%
Evaluation of LVS Function[2]	311	100%	96%	99%
Medicare Spending				
Medicare Spending per Patient (ratio)	-	0.92	0.93	0.98
Pneumonia Care				
Appropriate Initial Antibiotic Given[2]	49	96%	92%	95%
Blood Culture Timing[1,2]	-	-	97%	98%
Pregnancy and Delivery Care				
Newborn Deliveries Scheduled Early[7]	-	-	8%	6%
Preventive Care				
Immunization for Influenza[2]	616	99%	89%	90%
Immunization for Pneumonia[2]	1,028	99%	91%	92%
Stroke Care				
Anticoagulation Therapy for Atrial Fibrillation[2,7]	-	-	91%	95%
Antithrombotic Therapy Timing[1,2]	-	-	95%	98%
Assessed for Rehabilitation[2]	11	91%	96%	97%
Discharged on Antithrombotic Therapy[2]	11	100%	98%	99%
Discharged on Statin Medication[1,2]	-	-	88%	94%
Thrombolytic Therapy Timing[2,7]	-	-	61%	66%
Venous Thromboembolism Prophylaxis[1,2]	-	-	92%	94%
Written Stroke Educational Materials Given[1,2]	-	-	86%	88%
Surgical Care Improvement Project				
Appropriate Beta Blocker Usage	569	99%	97%	98%
Appropriate VTP Within 24 Hours	53	100%	97%	98%
Controlled Postoperative Blood Glucose	759	98%	97%	97%
Perioperative Temperature Management	393	100%	100%	100%
Prophylactic Antibiotic Selection	826	100%	99%	99%
Prophylactic Antibiotic Selection (Outpatient)	518	100%	98%	98%
Prophylactic Antibiotic Stopped	760	99%	98%	98%
Prophylactic Antibiotic Timing	829	100%	98%	99%
Prophylactic Antibiotic Timing (Outpatient)	518	100%	98%	98%
Urinary Catheter Removal	860	100%	96%	97%
Survey of Patients' Hospital Experiences				
Area Around Room 'Always' Quiet at Night	300+	72%	68%	61%
Doctors 'Always' Communicated Well	300+	90%	84%	82%
Home Recovery Information Given	300+	88%	84%	85%
Hospital Given 9 or 10 on 10 Point Scale	300+	94%	72%	71%
Meds 'Always' Explained Before Given	300+	73%	66%	64%

NOTE: Hospital profiles are in alphabetical order by state, then city, then hospital within the city; Rankings exclude hospitals with less than 25 cases except for patient surveys which excludes hospitals with less than 100 cases; (a) 100-299 cases; (1) The number of cases/patients is too few to report; (2) Data submitted were based on a sample of cases/patients; (3) Results are based on a shorter time period than required; (4) Data suppressed by CMS for one or more quarters; (5) Results are not available for this reporting period; (6) Fewer than 100 patients completed the HCAHPS survey; (7) No cases met the criteria for this measure; (8) The lower limit of the confidence interval cannot be calculated if the number of observed infections equals zero; (9) No data are available from the state/territory for this reporting period; (10) The scores shown reflect fewer than 50 completed surveys; (11) There were discrepancies in the data collection process; (12) This measure does not apply to this hospital for this reporting period; (13) Results cannot be calculated for this reporting period; (14) The results for this state are combined with nearby states to protect confidentiality; Please refer to the User's Guide for a full explanation of data.

Nurses 'Always' Communicated Well	300+	90%	80%	79%
Pain 'Always' Well Controlled	300+	82%	72%	71%
Room and Bathroom 'Always' Clean	300+	83%	73%	73%
Timely Help 'Always' Received	300+	91%	71%	68%
Would Definitely Recommend Hospital	300+	96%	71%	71%
Use of Medical Imaging				
Cardiac Imaging Stress Test before Surgery	4,303	4.5%	4.5%	5.3%
Combination Abdominal CT Scan	395	64.8%	23%	10.5%
Combination Brain/Sinus CT Scan	382	0.5%	2.2%	2.7%
Combination Chest CT Scan	395	3.5%	5.1%	2.7%
Follow-up Mammogram/Ultrasound[7]	-	-	8.1%	8.8%
Lumbar Spine MRI for Low Back Pain[1]	-	-	39.9%	37.2%

Oklahoma Heart Hospital South

5200 East I-240 Service Road
Oklahoma City, OK 73135
Phone: 405-628-6000
URL: www.okheart.com/south-campus
Type: Acute Care Hospitals
Emergency Services: Yes
Ownership: Physician
Key Personnel:
CEO . . . . John Harvey

Measure	Cases	This Hosp.	State Avg.	U.S. Avg.
Blood Clot Prevention and Treatment				
Anticoagulation Overlap Therapy[2]	24	100%	89%	93%
ICU Venous Thromboembolism Prophylaxis[2]	84	100%	87%	92%
Incidence of Potentially Preventable VTE[1,2]	-	-	8%	10%
UFH with Dosages/Platelet Monitoring[1,2]	-	-	97%	97%
Venous Thromboembolism Prophylaxis[2]	272	99%	72%	85%
Warfarin Therapy Discharge Instructions[2]	20	100%	73%	75%
Chest Pain/Possible Heart Attack Care				
Aspirin Given Within 24 Hours of Arrival[1]	-	-	95%	96%
Fibrinolytic Meds Within 30 Min. of Arrival[5]	-	-	54%	58%
Average Time to ECG (minutes)[1]	-	-	8	7
Average Time to Transfer (minutes)[5]	-	-	77	60
Children's Asthma Care				
Received Home Management Plan of Care	-	-	-	88%
Received Reliever Medication	-	-	-	100%
Received Systemic Corticosteroids	-	-	-	100%
Emergency Department				
Admittance Decision Time (minutes)[2]	298	116	63	98
Head CT Results Within 45 Min. of Arrival	11	36%	49%	57%
Patients Who Left ER Before Being Seen	11,886	1%	2%	2%
Time from ER Arrival to Admit. (minutes)[2]	302	218	210	274
Time from ER Arrival to Discharge (minutes)	372	92	110	134
Time in ER Before Being Evaluated (minutes)	419	12	24	26
Time to Pain Meds for Fractures (minutes)[1]	-	-	55	57
Heart Attack Care				
Aspirin Given at Discharge[2]	313	100%	99%	99%
Fibrinolytic Meds Within 30 Min. of Arrival[2,7]	-	-	25%	54%
PCI Within 90 Minutes of Arrival[2]	34	97%	95%	96%
Statin Prescribed at Discharge[2]	305	99%	98%	98%
Heart Failure Care				
ACE Inhibitor or ARB for LVSD[2]	104	97%	95%	97%
Discharge Instructions Given[2]	260	100%	92%	94%
Evaluation of LVS Function[2]	287	100%	96%	99%
Medicare Spending				
Medicare Spending per Patient (ratio)	-	0.90	0.93	0.98
Pneumonia Care				
Appropriate Initial Antibiotic Given	30	100%	92%	95%
Blood Culture Timing[1]	-	-	97%	98%
Pregnancy and Delivery Care				
Newborn Deliveries Scheduled Early[7]	-	-	8%	6%
Preventive Care				
Immunization for Influenza[2]	506	100%	89%	90%
Immunization for Pneumonia[2]	782	100%	91%	92%
Stroke Care				
Anticoagulation Therapy for Atrial Fibrillation[2,7]	-	-	91%	95%
Antithrombotic Therapy Timing[2]	12	100%	95%	98%
Assessed for Rehabilitation[2]	16	94%	96%	97%
Discharged on Antithrombotic Therapy[2]	15	100%	98%	99%
Discharged on Statin Medication[2]	12	100%	88%	94%
Thrombolytic Therapy Timing[2,7]	-	-	61%	66%
Venous Thromboembolism Prophylaxis[2]	12	100%	92%	94%
Written Stroke Educational Materials Given[1,2]	-	-	86%	88%
Surgical Care Improvement Project				
Appropriate Beta Blocker Usage	241	100%	97%	98%
Appropriate VTP Within 24 Hours	16	75%	97%	98%
Controlled Postoperative Blood Glucose	338	99%	97%	97%
Perioperative Temperature Management	131	100%	100%	100%
Prophylactic Antibiotic Selection	333	100%	99%	99%
Prophylactic Antibiotic Selection (Outpatient)	188	100%	98%	98%
Prophylactic Antibiotic Stopped	310	100%	98%	98%
Prophylactic Antibiotic Timing	336	98%	98%	99%
Prophylactic Antibiotic Timing (Outpatient)	188	99%	98%	98%
Urinary Catheter Removal	248	100%	96%	97%
Survey of Patients' Hospital Experiences				
Area Around Room 'Always' Quiet at Night	300+	78%	68%	61%
Doctors 'Always' Communicated Well	300+	87%	84%	82%
Home Recovery Information Given	300+	89%	84%	85%
Hospital Given 9 or 10 on 10 Point Scale	300+	93%	72%	71%
Meds 'Always' Explained Before Given	300+	73%	66%	64%
Nurses 'Always' Communicated Well	300+	89%	80%	79%
Pain 'Always' Well Controlled	300+	81%	72%	71%
Room and Bathroom 'Always' Clean	300+	86%	73%	73%
Timely Help 'Always' Received	300+	88%	71%	68%
Would Definitely Recommend Hospital	300+	95%	71%	71%
Use of Medical Imaging				
Cardiac Imaging Stress Test before Surgery	196	3.1%	4.5%	5.3%
Combination Abdominal CT Scan	147	51.0%	23%	10.5%
Combination Brain/Sinus CT Scan	321	0.3%	2.2%	2.7%
Combination Chest CT Scan	194	8.8%	5.1%	2.7%
Follow-up Mammogram/Ultrasound[7]	-	-	8.1%	8.8%
Lumbar Spine MRI for Low Back Pain[1]	-	-	39.9%	37.2%

Oklahoma Spine Hospital

14101 Parkway Commons Drive
Oklahoma City, OK 73134
Phone: 405-749-2700
Fax: 405-749-2783
URL: www.oklahomaspine.com
Type: Acute Care Hospitals
Emergency Services: Yes
Ownership: Physician
Beds: 18

Measure	Cases	This Hosp.	State Avg.	U.S. Avg.
Blood Clot Prevention and Treatment				
Anticoagulation Overlap Therapy[2,7]	-	-	89%	93%
ICU Venous Thromboembolism Prophylaxis[2,7]	-	-	87%	92%
Incidence of Potentially Preventable VTE[2,7]	-	-	8%	10%
UFH with Dosages/Platelet Monitoring[2,7]	-	-	97%	97%
Venous Thromboembolism Prophylaxis[2]	155	99%	72%	85%
Warfarin Therapy Discharge Instructions[2,7]	-	-	73%	75%
Chest Pain/Possible Heart Attack Care				
Aspirin Given Within 24 Hours of Arrival[5]	-	-	95%	96%
Fibrinolytic Meds Within 30 Min. of Arrival[5]	-	-	54%	58%
Average Time to ECG (minutes)[5]	-	-	8	7
Average Time to Transfer (minutes)[5]	-	-	77	60
Children's Asthma Care				
Received Home Management Plan of Care	-	-	-	88%
Received Reliever Medication	-	-	-	100%
Received Systemic Corticosteroids	-	-	-	100%
Emergency Department				
Admittance Decision Time (minutes)[1,2]	-	-	63	98
Head CT Results Within 45 Min. of Arrival[5]	-	-	49%	57%
Patients Who Left ER Before Being Seen	21	5%	2%	2%
Time from ER Arrival to Admit. (minutes)[1,2]	-	-	210	274
Time from ER Arrival to Discharge (minutes)[1]	-	-	110	134
Time in ER Before Being Evaluated (minutes)[1]	-	-	24	26
Time to Pain Meds for Fractures (minutes)[5]	-	-	55	57
Heart Attack Care				
Aspirin Given at Discharge[5]	-	-	99%	99%
Fibrinolytic Meds Within 30 Min. of Arrival[5]	-	-	25%	54%
PCI Within 90 Minutes of Arrival[5]	-	-	95%	96%
Statin Prescribed at Discharge[5]	-	-	98%	98%
Heart Failure Care				
ACE Inhibitor or ARB for LVSD[5]	-	-	95%	97%
Discharge Instructions Given[5]	-	-	92%	94%
Evaluation of LVS Function[5]	-	-	96%	99%
Medicare Spending				
Medicare Spending per Patient (ratio)	-	-	0.89	0.93	0.98
Pneumonia Care				
Appropriate Initial Antibiotic Given[5]	-	-	92%	95%
Blood Culture Timing[5]	-	-	97%	98%
Pregnancy and Delivery Care				
Newborn Deliveries Scheduled Early[7]	-	-	8%	6%
Preventive Care				
Immunization for Influenza[2]	364	77%	89%	90%
Immunization for Pneumonia[2]	253	53%	91%	92%
Stroke Care				
Anticoagulation Therapy for Atrial Fibrillation[5]	-	-	91%	95%
Antithrombotic Therapy Timing[5]	-	-	95%	98%
Assessed for Rehabilitation[5]	-	-	96%	97%
Discharged on Antithrombotic Therapy[5]	-	-	98%	99%
Discharged on Statin Medication[5]	-	-	88%	94%
Thrombolytic Therapy Timing[5]	-	-	61%	66%
Venous Thromboembolism Prophylaxis[5]	-	-	92%	94%
Written Stroke Educational Materials Given[5]	-	-	86%	88%
Surgical Care Improvement Project				
Appropriate Beta Blocker Usage[3,7]	-	-	97%	98%
Appropriate VTP Within 24 Hours[3,7]	-	-	97%	98%
Controlled Postoperative Blood Glucose[3,7]	-	-	97%	97%
Perioperative Temperature Management[3,7]	-	-	100%	100%
Prophylactic Antibiotic Selection[3,7]	-	-	99%	99%
Prophylactic Antibiotic Selection (Outpatient)	179	100%	98%	98%
Prophylactic Antibiotic Stopped[3,7]	-	-	98%	98%
Prophylactic Antibiotic Timing[3,7]	-	-	98%	99%
Prophylactic Antibiotic Timing (Outpatient)	179	99%	98%	98%
Urinary Catheter Removal[3,7]	-	-	96%	97%
Survey of Patients' Hospital Experiences				
Area Around Room 'Always' Quiet at Night	300+	86%	68%	61%
Doctors 'Always' Communicated Well	300+	90%	84%	82%
Home Recovery Information Given	300+	88%	84%	85%
Hospital Given 9 or 10 on 10 Point Scale	300+	89%	72%	71%
Meds 'Always' Explained Before Given	300+	75%	66%	64%
Nurses 'Always' Communicated Well	300+	85%	80%	79%
Pain 'Always' Well Controlled	300+	78%	72%	71%
Room and Bathroom 'Always' Clean	300+	85%	73%	73%
Timely Help 'Always' Received	300+	83%	71%	68%
Would Definitely Recommend Hospital	300+	90%	71%	71%
Use of Medical Imaging				
Cardiac Imaging Stress Test before Surgery[7]	-	-	4.5%	5.3%
Combination Abdominal CT Scan[1]	-	-	23%	10.5%
Combination Brain/Sinus CT Scan[1]	-	-	2.2%	2.7%
Combination Chest CT Scan[1]	-	-	5.1%	2.7%
Follow-up Mammogram/Ultrasound[7]	-	-	8.1%	8.8%
Lumbar Spine MRI for Low Back Pain[1]	-	-	39.9%	37.2%

Orthopedic Hospital

1044 Sw 44th, Suite 350
Oklahoma City, OK 73109
Phone: 405-631-3085
Fax: 405-616-2670
URL: www.ortho-ok.com/orthopedichospital
Type: Acute Care Hospitals
Emergency Services: Yes
Ownership: Physician
Key Personnel:
Patient Relations . . . . Pam Cannon
CEO/President. . . . . Joel Frazier, MD

Measure	Cases	This Hosp.	State Avg.	U.S. Avg.
Blood Clot Prevention and Treatment				
Anticoagulation Overlap Therapy[2,7]	-	-	89%	93%
ICU Venous Thromboembolism Prophylaxis[2,7]	-	-	87%	92%
Incidence of Potentially Preventable VTE[2,7]	-	-	8%	10%
UFH with Dosages/Platelet Monitoring[2,7]	-	-	97%	97%
Venous Thromboembolism Prophylaxis[2]	34	100%	72%	85%
Warfarin Therapy Discharge Instructions[2,7]	-	-	73%	75%
Chest Pain/Possible Heart Attack Care				
Aspirin Given Within 24 Hours of Arrival[5]	-	-	95%	96%
Fibrinolytic Meds Within 30 Min. of Arrival[5]	-	-	54%	58%
Average Time to ECG (minutes)[5]	-	-	8	7
Average Time to Transfer (minutes)[5]	-	-	77	60
Children's Asthma Care				
Received Home Management Plan of Care	-	-	-	88%
Received Reliever Medication	-	-	-	100%

NOTE: Hospital profiles are in alphabetical order by state, then city, then hospital within the city; Rankings exclude hospitals with less than 25 cases except for patient surveys which excludes hospitals with less than 100 cases; (a) 100-299 cases; (1) The number of cases/patients is too few to report; (2) Data submitted were based on a sample of cases/patients; (3) Results are based on a shorter time period than required; (4) Data suppressed by CMS for one or more quarters; (5) Results are not available for this reporting period; (6) Fewer than 100 patients completed the HCAHPS survey; (7) No cases met the criteria for this measure; (8) The lower limit of the confidence interval cannot be calculated if the number of observed infections equals zero; (9) No data are available from the state/territory for this reporting period; (10) The scores shown reflect fewer than 50 completed surveys; (11) There were discrepancies in the data collection process; (12) This measure does not apply to this hospital for this reporting period; (13) Results cannot be calculated for this reporting period; (14) The results for this state are combined with nearby states to protect confidentiality; Please refer to the User's Guide for a full explanation of data.

Measure	Cases	This Hosp.	State Avg.	U.S. Avg.
Received Systemic Corticosteroids	-	-	-	100%
Emergency Department				
Admittance Decision Time (minutes)[7]	-	-	63	98
Head CT Results Within 45 Min. of Arrival[5]	-	-	49%	57%
Patients Who Left ER Before Being Seen	16	12%	2%	2%
Time from ER Arrival to Admit. (minutes)[7]	-	-	210	274
Time from ER Arrival to Discharge (minutes)[1,3]	-	-	110	134
Time in ER Before Being Evaluated (minutes)[3,7]	-	-	24	26
Time to Pain Meds for Fractures (minutes)[5]	-	-	55	57
Heart Attack Care				
Aspirin Given at Discharge[5]	-	-	99%	99%
Fibrinolytic Meds Within 30 Min. of Arrival[5]	-	-	25%	54%
PCI Within 90 Minutes of Arrival[5]	-	-	95%	96%
Statin Prescribed at Discharge[5]	-	-	98%	98%
Heart Failure Care				
ACE Inhibitor or ARB for LVSD[5]	-	-	95%	97%
Discharge Instructions Given[5]	-	-	92%	94%
Evaluation of LVS Function[5]	-	-	96%	99%
Medicare Spending				
Medicare Spending per Patient (ratio)	-	1.08	0.93	0.98
Pneumonia Care				
Appropriate Initial Antibiotic Given[5]	-	-	92%	95%
Blood Culture Timing[5]	-	-	97%	98%
Pregnancy and Delivery Care				
Newborn Deliveries Scheduled Early[7]	-	-	8%	6%
Preventive Care				
Immunization for Influenza	58	97%	89%	90%
Immunization for Pneumonia	28	96%	91%	92%
Stroke Care				
Anticoagulation Therapy for Atrial Fibrillation[5]	-	-	91%	95%
Antithrombotic Therapy Timing[5]	-	-	95%	98%
Assessed for Rehabilitation[5]	-	-	96%	97%
Discharged on Antithrombotic Therapy[5]	-	-	98%	99%
Discharged on Statin Medication[5]	-	-	88%	94%
Thrombolytic Therapy Timing[5]	-	-	61%	66%
Venous Thromboembolism Prophylaxis[5]	-	-	92%	94%
Written Stroke Educational Materials Given[5]	-	-	86%	88%
Surgical Care Improvement Project				
Appropriate Beta Blocker Usage[5]	-	-	97%	98%
Appropriate VTP Within 24 Hours[5]	-	-	97%	98%
Controlled Postoperative Blood Glucose[5]	-	-	97%	97%
Perioperative Temperature Management[5]	-	-	100%	100%
Prophylactic Antibiotic Selection[5]	-	-	99%	99%
Prophylactic Antibiotic Selection (Outpatient)[1,3]	-	-	98%	98%
Prophylactic Antibiotic Stopped[5]	-	-	98%	98%
Prophylactic Antibiotic Timing[5]	-	-	98%	99%
Prophylactic Antibiotic Timing (Outpatient)[1,3]	-	-	98%	98%
Urinary Catheter Removal[5]	-	-	96%	97%
Survey of Patients' Hospital Experiences				
Area Around Room 'Always' Quiet at Night[10]	<100	99%	68%	61%
Doctors 'Always' Communicated Well[10]	<100	94%	84%	82%
Home Recovery Information Given[10]	<100	95%	84%	85%
Hospital Given 9 or 10 on 10 Point Scale[10]	<100	89%	72%	71%
Meds 'Always' Explained Before Given[10]	<100	98%	66%	64%
Nurses 'Always' Communicated Well[10]	<100	100%	80%	79%
Pain 'Always' Well Controlled[10]	<100	93%	72%	71%
Room and Bathroom 'Always' Clean[10]	<100	98%	73%	73%
Timely Help 'Always' Received[10]	<100	94%	71%	68%
Would Definitely Recommend Hospital[10]	<100	77%	71%	71%
Use of Medical Imaging				
Cardiac Imaging Stress Test before Surgery[7]	-	-	4.5%	5.3%
Combination Abdominal CT Scan[7]	-	-	23%	10.5%
Combination Brain/Sinus CT Scan[7]	-	-	2.2%	2.7%
Combination Chest CT Scan[7]	-	-	5.1%	2.7%
Follow-up Mammogram/Ultrasound[7]	-	-	8.1%	8.8%
Lumbar Spine MRI for Low Back Pain[7]	-	-	39.9%	37.2%

Saint Anthony Hospital

1000 North Lee Avenue
Oklahoma City, OK 73101
URL: www.saintsok.com
Type: Acute Care Hospitals
Ownership: Voluntary non-profit - Private
Phone: 405-272-7000
Fax: 405-272-6592
Emergency Services: Yes
Beds: 659

Key Personnel:
Emergency Room . . . . Jack Bair, MD
Infection Control . . . . Barbara Baker
Anesthesiology. . . . . Tin Chen
Chief of Medical Staff . . . . Susan Edwards, MD
Quality Assurance . . . . Wanda Fairless
CEO/President. . . . . Valinda Rutledge

Measure	Cases	This Hosp.	State Avg.	U.S. Avg.
Blood Clot Prevention and Treatment				
Anticoagulation Overlap Therapy[2]	117	93%	89%	93%
ICU Venous Thromboembolism Prophylaxis[2]	103	95%	87%	92%
Incidence of Potentially Preventable VTE[2]	19	16%	8%	10%
UFH with Dosages/Platelet Monitoring[2]	18	100%	97%	97%
Venous Thromboembolism Prophylaxis[2]	314	92%	72%	85%
Warfarin Therapy Discharge Instructions[2]	83	83%	73%	75%
Chest Pain/Possible Heart Attack Care				
Aspirin Given Within 24 Hours of Arrival[1,3]	-	-	95%	96%
Fibrinolytic Meds Within 30 Min. of Arrival[5]	-	-	54%	58%
Average Time to ECG (minutes)[1,3]	-	-	8	7
Average Time to Transfer (minutes)[5]	-	-	77	60
Children's Asthma Care				
Received Home Management Plan of Care	-	-	-	88%
Received Reliever Medication	-	-	-	100%
Received Systemic Corticosteroids	-	-	-	100%
Emergency Department				
Admittance Decision Time (minutes)[2]	437	95	63	98
Head CT Results Within 45 Min. of Arrival[1]	-	-	49%	57%
Patients Who Left ER Before Being Seen	59,728	6%	2%	2%
Time from ER Arrival to Admit. (minutes)[2]	443	279	210	274
Time from ER Arrival to Discharge (minutes)	408	101	110	134
Time in ER Before Being Evaluated (minutes)	428	32	24	26
Time to Pain Meds for Fractures (minutes)	277	60	55	57
Heart Attack Care				
Aspirin Given at Discharge	285	100%	99%	99%
Fibrinolytic Meds Within 30 Min. of Arrival[7]	-	-	25%	54%
PCI Within 90 Minutes of Arrival	23	100%	95%	96%
Statin Prescribed at Discharge	282	100%	98%	98%
Heart Failure Care				
ACE Inhibitor or ARB for LVSD	138	100%	95%	97%
Discharge Instructions Given	330	100%	92%	94%
Evaluation of LVS Function	376	100%	96%	99%
Medicare Spending				
Medicare Spending per Patient (ratio)	-	0.95	0.93	0.98
Pneumonia Care				
Appropriate Initial Antibiotic Given	200	99%	92%	95%
Blood Culture Timing	460	100%	97%	98%
Pregnancy and Delivery Care				
Newborn Deliveries Scheduled Early[2]	82	7%	8%	6%
Preventive Care				
Immunization for Influenza[2]	567	98%	89%	90%
Immunization for Pneumonia[2]	691	97%	91%	92%
Stroke Care				
Anticoagulation Therapy for Atrial Fibrillation	24	92%	91%	95%
Antithrombotic Therapy Timing	185	96%	95%	98%
Assessed for Rehabilitation	228	98%	96%	97%
Discharged on Antithrombotic Therapy	199	99%	98%	99%
Discharged on Statin Medication	149	93%	88%	94%
Thrombolytic Therapy Timing	11	73%	61%	66%
Venous Thromboembolism Prophylaxis	247	96%	92%	94%
Written Stroke Educational Materials Given	140	99%	86%	88%
Surgical Care Improvement Project				
Appropriate Beta Blocker Usage[2]	535	100%	97%	98%
Appropriate VTP Within 24 Hours[2]	1,482	100%	97%	98%
Controlled Postoperative Blood Glucose[2]	140	96%	97%	97%
Perioperative Temperature Management[2]	1,664	100%	100%	100%
Prophylactic Antibiotic Selection[2]	1,518	100%	99%	99%
Prophylactic Antibiotic Selection (Outpatient)	303	99%	98%	98%
Prophylactic Antibiotic Stopped[2]	1,478	100%	98%	98%
Prophylactic Antibiotic Timing[2]	1,519	100%	98%	99%
Prophylactic Antibiotic Timing (Outpatient)	306	98%	98%	98%
Urinary Catheter Removal[2]	391	98%	96%	97%
Survey of Patients' Hospital Experiences				
Area Around Room 'Always' Quiet at Night	300+	63%	68%	61%
Doctors 'Always' Communicated Well	300+	84%	84%	82%
Home Recovery Information Given	300+	87%	84%	85%
Hospital Given 9 or 10 on 10 Point Scale	300+	80%	72%	71%
Meds 'Always' Explained Before Given	300+	61%	66%	64%
Nurses 'Always' Communicated Well	300+	81%	80%	79%
Pain 'Always' Well Controlled	300+	73%	72%	71%
Room and Bathroom 'Always' Clean	300+	72%	73%	73%
Timely Help 'Always' Received	300+	66%	71%	68%
Would Definitely Recommend Hospital	300+	80%	71%	71%
Use of Medical Imaging				
Cardiac Imaging Stress Test before Surgery	364	3.6%	4.5%	5.3%
Combination Abdominal CT Scan	969	19.4%	23%	10.5%
Combination Brain/Sinus CT Scan	855	2.0%	2.2%	2.7%
Combination Chest CT Scan	387	3.1%	5.1%	2.7%
Follow-up Mammogram/Ultrasound	1,370	14.5%	8.1%	8.8%
Lumbar Spine MRI for Low Back Pain	124	38.7%	39.9%	37.2%

Surgical Hospital of Oklahoma

100 Southeast 59th Street
Oklahoma City, OK 73129
Type: Acute Care Hospitals
Ownership: Proprietary
Phone: 405-634-9300
Emergency Services: Yes
Beds: 12

Key Personnel:
Administrator . . . . Phil Ross
CEO/President. . . . . Phil Ross

Measure	Cases	This Hosp.	State Avg.	U.S. Avg.
Blood Clot Prevention and Treatment				
Anticoagulation Overlap Therapy[7]	-	-	89%	93%
ICU Venous Thromboembolism Prophylaxis[7]	-	-	87%	92%
Incidence of Potentially Preventable VTE[7]	-	-	8%	10%
UFH with Dosages/Platelet Monitoring[7]	-	-	97%	97%
Venous Thromboembolism Prophylaxis	37	100%	72%	85%
Warfarin Therapy Discharge Instructions[7]	-	-	73%	75%
Chest Pain/Possible Heart Attack Care				
Aspirin Given Within 24 Hours of Arrival[5]	-	-	95%	96%
Fibrinolytic Meds Within 30 Min. of Arrival[5]	-	-	54%	58%
Average Time to ECG (minutes)[5]	-	-	8	7
Average Time to Transfer (minutes)[5]	-	-	77	60
Children's Asthma Care				
Received Home Management Plan of Care	-	-	-	88%
Received Reliever Medication	-	-	-	100%
Received Systemic Corticosteroids	-	-	-	100%
Emergency Department				
Admittance Decision Time (minutes)[7]	-	-	63	98
Head CT Results Within 45 Min. of Arrival[5]	-	-	49%	57%
Patients Who Left ER Before Being Seen	15	0%	2%	2%
Time from ER Arrival to Admit. (minutes)[7]	-	-	210	274
Time from ER Arrival to Discharge (minutes)[1,3]	-	-	110	134
Time in ER Before Being Evaluated (minutes)[1,3]	-	-	24	26
Time to Pain Meds for Fractures (minutes)[5]	-	-	55	57
Heart Attack Care				
Aspirin Given at Discharge[5]	-	-	99%	99%
Fibrinolytic Meds Within 30 Min. of Arrival[5]	-	-	25%	54%
PCI Within 90 Minutes of Arrival[5]	-	-	95%	96%
Statin Prescribed at Discharge[5]	-	-	98%	98%
Heart Failure Care				
ACE Inhibitor or ARB for LVSD[5]	-	-	95%	97%
Discharge Instructions Given[5]	-	-	92%	94%
Evaluation of LVS Function[5]	-	-	96%	99%
Medicare Spending				
Medicare Spending per Patient (ratio)[1]	-	-	0.93	0.98
Pneumonia Care				
Appropriate Initial Antibiotic Given[5]	-	-	92%	95%
Blood Culture Timing[5]	-	-	97%	98%
Pregnancy and Delivery Care				
Newborn Deliveries Scheduled Early[7]	-	-	8%	6%
Preventive Care				

NOTE: Hospital profiles are in alphabetical order by state, then city, then hospital within the city; Rankings exclude hospitals with less than 25 cases except for patient surveys which excludes hospitals with less than 100 cases; (a) 100-299 cases; (1) The number of cases/patients is too few to report; (2) Data submitted were based on a sample of cases/patients; (3) Results are based on a shorter time period than required; (4) Data suppressed by CMS for one or more quarters; (5) Results are not available for this reporting period; (6) Fewer than 100 patients completed the HCAHPS survey; (7) No cases met the criteria for this measure; (8) The lower limit of the confidence interval cannot be calculated if the number of observed infections equals zero; (9) No data are available from the state/territory for this reporting period; (10) The scores shown reflect fewer than 50 completed surveys; (11) There were discrepancies in the data collection process; (12) This measure does not apply to this hospital for this reporting period; (13) Results cannot be calculated for this reporting period; (14) The results for this state are combined with nearby states to protect confidentiality; Please refer to the User's Guide for a full explanation of data.

Measure	Cases	This Hosp.	State Avg.	U.S. Avg.
Immunization for Influenza	143	70%	89%	90%
Immunization for Pneumonia	158	89%	91%	92%
Stroke Care				
Anticoagulation Therapy for Atrial Fibrillation[5]	-	-	91%	95%
Antithrombotic Therapy Timing[5]	-	-	95%	98%
Assessed for Rehabilitation[5]	-	-	96%	97%
Discharged on Antithrombotic Therapy[5]	-	-	98%	99%
Discharged on Statin Medication[5]	-	-	88%	94%
Thrombolytic Therapy Timing[5]	-	-	61%	66%
Venous Thromboembolism Prophylaxis[5]	-	-	92%	94%
Written Stroke Educational Materials Given[5]	-	-	86%	88%
Surgical Care Improvement Project				
Appropriate Beta Blocker Usage	48	96%	97%	98%
Appropriate VTP Within 24 Hours	163	77%	97%	98%
Controlled Postoperative Blood Glucose[7]	-	-	97%	97%
Perioperative Temperature Management	174	99%	100%	100%
Prophylactic Antibiotic Selection	126	98%	99%	99%
Prophylactic Antibiotic Selection (Outpatient)	106	94%	98%	98%
Prophylactic Antibiotic Stopped	126	37%	98%	98%
Prophylactic Antibiotic Timing	127	91%	98%	99%
Prophylactic Antibiotic Timing (Outpatient)	106	95%	98%	98%
Urinary Catheter Removal	71	97%	96%	97%
Survey of Patients' Hospital Experiences				
Area Around Room 'Always' Quiet at Night	(a)	80%	68%	61%
Doctors 'Always' Communicated Well	(a)	81%	84%	82%
Home Recovery Information Given	(a)	85%	84%	85%
Hospital Given 9 or 10 on 10 Point Scale	(a)	77%	72%	71%
Meds 'Always' Explained Before Given	(a)	73%	66%	64%
Nurses 'Always' Communicated Well	(a)	85%	80%	79%
Pain 'Always' Well Controlled	(a)	76%	72%	71%
Room and Bathroom 'Always' Clean	(a)	69%	73%	73%
Timely Help 'Always' Received	(a)	80%	71%	68%
Would Definitely Recommend Hospital	(a)	77%	71%	71%
Use of Medical Imaging				
Cardiac Imaging Stress Test before Surgery[7]	-	-	4.5%	5.3%
Combination Abdominal CT Scan[7]	-	-	23%	10.5%
Combination Brain/Sinus CT Scan[7]	-	-	2.2%	2.7%
Combination Chest CT Scan[7]	-	-	5.1%	2.7%
Follow-up Mammogram/Ultrasound[7]	-	-	8.1%	8.8%
Lumbar Spine MRI for Low Back Pain[7]	-	-	39.9%	37.2%

Muscogee (Creek) Nation Medical Center

1401 Morris Drive — Phone: 918-756-4233
Okmulgee, OK 74447 — Fax: 918-756-5968
URL: www.okmulgeehospital.com
Type: Acute Care Hospitals — Emergency Services: Yes
Ownership: Voluntary non-profit - Private — Beds: 66

Key Personnel:
Operating Room. . . . . Sara Davis, RN
Radiology. . . . . Dean Fullingim, DO
Emergency Room . . . . Kim Gage, MD
CEO/President. . . . . Rex Jones
Infection Control. . . . . Kahty Machetta, RN
Quality Assurance . . . . Anita Raley
Chief of Medical Staff. . . . . Tim Sanford, DO

Measure	Cases	This Hosp.	State Avg.	U.S. Avg.
Blood Clot Prevention and Treatment				
Anticoagulation Overlap Therapy[1,2]	-	-	89%	93%
ICU Venous Thromboembolism Prophylaxis[1,2]	-	-	87%	92%
Incidence of Potentially Preventable VTE[2,7]	-	-	8%	10%
UFH with Dosages/Platelet Monitoring[1,2]	-	-	97%	97%
Venous Thromboembolism Prophylaxis[2]	157	15%	72%	85%
Warfarin Therapy Discharge Instructions[1,2]	-	-	73%	75%
Chest Pain/Possible Heart Attack Care				
Aspirin Given Within 24 Hours of Arrival	56	96%	95%	96%
Fibrinolytic Meds Within 30 Min. of Arrival[1]	-	-	54%	58%
Average Time to ECG (minutes)	54	12	8	7
Average Time to Transfer (minutes)	15	185	77	60
Children's Asthma Care				
Received Home Management Plan of Care	-	-	-	88%
Received Reliever Medication	-	-	-	100%
Received Systemic Corticosteroids	-	-	-	100%
Emergency Department				
Admittance Decision Time (minutes)[2]	460	50	63	98
Head CT Results Within 45 Min. of Arrival	20	0%	49%	57%
Patients Who Left ER Before Being Seen	13,598	2%	2%	2%
Time from ER Arrival to Admit. (minutes)[2]	483	189	210	274
Time from ER Arrival to Discharge (minutes)	247	93	110	134
Time in ER Before Being Evaluated (minutes)	362	23	24	26
Time to Pain Meds for Fractures (minutes)	70	54	55	57
Heart Attack Care				
Aspirin Given at Discharge[1,2]	-	-	99%	99%
Fibrinolytic Meds Within 30 Min. of Arrival[2,3]	-	-	25%	54%
PCI Within 90 Minutes of Arrival[2,3]	-	-	95%	96%
Statin Prescribed at Discharge[1,2]	-	-	98%	98%
Heart Failure Care				
ACE Inhibitor or ARB for LVSD[2]	18	94%	95%	97%
Discharge Instructions Given[2]	38	66%	92%	94%
Evaluation of LVS Function[2]	59	85%	96%	99%
Medicare Spending				
Medicare Spending per Patient (ratio)	-	1.02	0.93	0.98
Pneumonia Care				
Appropriate Initial Antibiotic Given[2]	61	74%	92%	95%
Blood Culture Timing[2]	36	94%	97%	98%
Pregnancy and Delivery Care				
Newborn Deliveries Scheduled Early[2,7]	-	-	8%	6%
Preventive Care				
Immunization for Influenza[2]	290	86%	89%	90%
Immunization for Pneumonia[2]	406	90%	91%	92%
Stroke Care				
Anticoagulation Therapy for Atrial Fibrillation[3,7]	-	-	91%	95%
Antithrombotic Therapy Timing[1,3]	-	-	95%	98%
Assessed for Rehabilitation[1,3]	-	-	96%	97%
Discharged on Antithrombotic Therapy[1,3]	-	-	98%	99%
Discharged on Statin Medication[1,3]	-	-	88%	94%
Thrombolytic Therapy Timing[3,7]	-	-	61%	66%
Venous Thromboembolism Prophylaxis[1,3]	-	-	92%	94%
Written Stroke Educational Materials Given[1,3]	-	-	86%	88%
Surgical Care Improvement Project				
Appropriate Beta Blocker Usage[1,3]	-	-	97%	98%
Appropriate VTP Within 24 Hours[1,3]	-	-	97%	98%
Controlled Postoperative Blood Glucose[3,7]	-	-	97%	97%
Perioperative Temperature Management[1,3]	-	-	100%	100%
Prophylactic Antibiotic Selection[3,7]	-	-	99%	99%
Prophylactic Antibiotic Selection (Outpatient)[5]	-	-	98%	98%
Prophylactic Antibiotic Stopped[3,7]	-	-	98%	98%
Prophylactic Antibiotic Timing[3,7]	-	-	98%	99%
Prophylactic Antibiotic Timing (Outpatient)[5]	-	-	98%	98%
Urinary Catheter Removal[1,3]	-	-	96%	97%
Survey of Patients' Hospital Experiences				
Area Around Room 'Always' Quiet at Night	(a)	77%	68%	61%
Doctors 'Always' Communicated Well	(a)	85%	84%	82%
Home Recovery Information Given	(a)	87%	84%	85%
Hospital Given 9 or 10 on 10 Point Scale	(a)	71%	72%	71%
Meds 'Always' Explained Before Given	(a)	67%	66%	64%
Nurses 'Always' Communicated Well	(a)	81%	80%	79%
Pain 'Always' Well Controlled	(a)	73%	72%	71%
Room and Bathroom 'Always' Clean	(a)	69%	73%	73%
Timely Help 'Always' Received	(a)	76%	71%	68%
Would Definitely Recommend Hospital	(a)	66%	71%	71%
Use of Medical Imaging				
Cardiac Imaging Stress Test before Surgery	70	4.3%	4.5%	5.3%
Combination Abdominal CT Scan	204	8.8%	23%	10.5%
Combination Brain/Sinus CT Scan	339	0.9%	2.2%	2.7%
Combination Chest CT Scan	114	1.8%	5.1%	2.7%
Follow-up Mammogram/Ultrasound	372	10.8%	8.1%	8.8%
Lumbar Spine MRI for Low Back Pain[1]	-	-	39.9%	37.2%

Bailey Medical Center

10502 North 110th East Avenue — Phone: 918-376-8000
Owasso, OK 74055
URL: www.baileymedicalcenter.com
Type: Acute Care Hospitals — Emergency Services: Yes
Ownership: Proprietary — Beds: 73

Key Personnel:
Cardiology . . . . Eric G Auerbach, MD
Pediatrics. . . . . Lauri S Blesch, MD
Pulmonary Disease . . . . Mark P Britt, MD

Measure	Cases	This Hosp.	State Avg.	U.S. Avg.
Blood Clot Prevention and Treatment				
Anticoagulation Overlap Therapy[1,2]	-	-	89%	93%
ICU Venous Thromboembolism Prophylaxis[1,2]	-	-	87%	92%
Incidence of Potentially Preventable VTE[2,7]	-	-	8%	10%
UFH with Dosages/Platelet Monitoring[1,2]	-	-	97%	97%
Venous Thromboembolism Prophylaxis[2]	86	100%	72%	85%
Warfarin Therapy Discharge Instructions[1,2]	-	-	73%	75%
Chest Pain/Possible Heart Attack Care				
Aspirin Given Within 24 Hours of Arrival	29	100%	95%	96%
Fibrinolytic Meds Within 30 Min. of Arrival[7]	-	-	54%	58%
Average Time to ECG (minutes)	30	6	8	7
Average Time to Transfer (minutes)[1]	-	-	77	60
Children's Asthma Care				
Received Home Management Plan of Care	-	-	-	88%
Received Reliever Medication	-	-	-	100%
Received Systemic Corticosteroids	-	-	-	100%
Emergency Department				
Admittance Decision Time (minutes)[2]	119	47	63	98
Head CT Results Within 45 Min. of Arrival[1]	-	-	49%	57%
Patients Who Left ER Before Being Seen	12,273	2%	2%	2%
Time from ER Arrival to Admit. (minutes)[2]	133	199	210	274
Time from ER Arrival to Discharge (minutes)	398	110	110	134
Time in ER Before Being Evaluated (minutes)	393	22	24	26
Time to Pain Meds for Fractures (minutes)	46	43	55	57
Heart Attack Care				
Aspirin Given at Discharge[1,3]	-	-	99%	99%
Fibrinolytic Meds Within 30 Min. of Arrival[3,7]	-	-	25%	54%
PCI Within 90 Minutes of Arrival[3,7]	-	-	95%	96%
Statin Prescribed at Discharge[1,3]	-	-	98%	98%
Heart Failure Care				
ACE Inhibitor or ARB for LVSD[1]	-	-	95%	97%
Discharge Instructions Given	11	100%	92%	94%
Evaluation of LVS Function	14	100%	96%	99%
Medicare Spending				
Medicare Spending per Patient (ratio)	-	0.93	0.93	0.98
Pneumonia Care				
Appropriate Initial Antibiotic Given	22	100%	92%	95%
Blood Culture Timing	31	100%	97%	98%
Pregnancy and Delivery Care				
Newborn Deliveries Scheduled Early	17	6%	8%	6%
Preventive Care				
Immunization for Influenza[2]	285	100%	89%	90%
Immunization for Pneumonia[2]	246	100%	91%	92%
Stroke Care				
Anticoagulation Therapy for Atrial Fibrillation[3,7]	-	-	91%	95%
Antithrombotic Therapy Timing[1,3]	-	-	95%	98%
Assessed for Rehabilitation[1,3]	-	-	96%	97%
Discharged on Antithrombotic Therapy[1,3]	-	-	98%	99%
Discharged on Statin Medication[1,3]	-	-	88%	94%
Thrombolytic Therapy Timing[3,7]	-	-	61%	66%
Venous Thromboembolism Prophylaxis[1,3]	-	-	92%	94%
Written Stroke Educational Materials Given[1,3]	-	-	86%	88%
Surgical Care Improvement Project				
Appropriate Beta Blocker Usage	24	100%	97%	98%
Appropriate VTP Within 24 Hours	81	100%	97%	98%
Controlled Postoperative Blood Glucose[7]	-	-	97%	97%
Perioperative Temperature Management	89	100%	100%	100%
Prophylactic Antibiotic Selection	66	98%	99%	99%
Prophylactic Antibiotic Selection (Outpatient)	47	100%	98%	98%
Prophylactic Antibiotic Stopped	65	98%	98%	98%
Prophylactic Antibiotic Timing	66	98%	98%	99%
Prophylactic Antibiotic Timing (Outpatient)	47	100%	98%	98%
Urinary Catheter Removal	51	100%	96%	97%
Survey of Patients' Hospital Experiences				
Area Around Room 'Always' Quiet at Night	300+	78%	68%	61%
Doctors 'Always' Communicated Well	300+	87%	84%	82%
Home Recovery Information Given	300+	91%	84%	85%
Hospital Given 9 or 10 on 10 Point Scale	300+	85%	72%	71%
Meds 'Always' Explained Before Given	300+	69%	66%	64%
Nurses 'Always' Communicated Well	300+	84%	80%	79%
Pain 'Always' Well Controlled	300+	75%	72%	71%

NOTE: Hospital profiles are in alphabetical order by state, then city, then hospital within the city; Rankings exclude hospitals with less than 25 cases except for patient surveys which excludes hospitals with less than 100 cases; (a) 100-299 cases; (1) The number of cases/patients is too few to report; (2) Data submitted were based on a sample of cases/patients; (3) Results are based on a shorter time period than required; (4) Data suppressed by CMS for one or more quarters; (5) Results are not available for this reporting period; (6) Fewer than 100 patients completed the HCAHPS survey; (7) No cases met the criteria for this measure; (8) The lower limit of the confidence interval cannot be calculated if the number of observed infections equals zero; (9) No data are available from the state/territory for this reporting period; (10) The scores shown reflect fewer than 50 completed surveys; (11) There were discrepancies in the data collection process; (12) This measure does not apply to this hospital for this reporting period; (13) Results cannot be calculated for this reporting period; (14) The results for this state are combined with nearby states to protect confidentiality; Please refer to the User's Guide for a full explanation of data.

Room and Bathroom 'Always' Clean	300+	79%	73%	73%
Timely Help 'Always' Received	300+	75%	71%	68%
Would Definitely Recommend Hospital	300+	85%	71%	71%
Use of Medical Imaging				
Cardiac Imaging Stress Test before Surgery	148	9.5%	4.5%	5.3%
Combination Abdominal CT Scan	264	8.3%	23%	10.5%
Combination Brain/Sinus CT Scan[1]	-	-	2.2%	2.7%
Combination Chest CT Scan	79	10.1%	5.1%	2.7%
Follow-up Mammogram/Ultrasound	270	8.5%	8.1%	8.8%
Lumbar Spine MRI for Low Back Pain	60	55.0%	39.9%	37.2%

Saint John Owasso

12451 East 100th Street North
Owasso, OK 74055
Phone: 918-274-5100
URL: www.stjohnowasso.com
Type: Acute Care Hospitals
Emergency Services: Yes
Ownership: Voluntary non-profit - Church
Key Personnel:
President/CEO. . . . . M Therese Gottschalk

Measure	Cases	This Hosp.	State Avg.	U.S. Avg.
Blood Clot Prevention and Treatment				
Anticoagulation Overlap Therapy[1,2]	-	-	89%	93%
ICU Venous Thromboembolism Prophylaxis[2,7]	-	-	87%	92%
Incidence of Potentially Preventable VTE[2,7]	-	-	8%	10%
UFH with Dosages/Platelet Monitoring[2,7]	-	-	97%	97%
Venous Thromboembolism Prophylaxis[2]	112	93%	72%	85%
Warfarin Therapy Discharge Instructions[1,2]	-	-	73%	75%
Chest Pain/Possible Heart Attack Care				
Aspirin Given Within 24 Hours of Arrival	69	97%	95%	96%
Fibrinolytic Meds Within 30 Min. of Arrival[7]	-	-	54%	58%
Average Time to ECG (minutes)	72	6	8	7
Average Time to Transfer (minutes)	12	67	77	60
Children's Asthma Care				
Received Home Management Plan of Care	-	-	-	88%
Received Reliever Medication	-	-	-	100%
Received Systemic Corticosteroids	-	-	-	100%
Emergency Department				
Admittance Decision Time (minutes)[2]	207	62	63	98
Head CT Results Within 45 Min. of Arrival	15	87%	49%	57%
Patients Who Left ER Before Being Seen	21,597	1%	2%	2%
Time from ER Arrival to Admit. (minutes)[2]	228	190	210	274
Time from ER Arrival to Discharge (minutes)	358	102	110	134
Time in ER Before Being Evaluated (minutes)	361	20	24	26
Time to Pain Meds for Fractures (minutes)	96	46	55	57
Heart Attack Care				
Aspirin Given at Discharge[5]	-	-	99%	99%
Fibrinolytic Meds Within 30 Min. of Arrival[5]	-	-	25%	54%
PCI Within 90 Minutes of Arrival[5]	-	-	95%	96%
Statin Prescribed at Discharge[5]	-	-	98%	98%
Heart Failure Care				
ACE Inhibitor or ARB for LVSD	16	88%	95%	97%
Discharge Instructions Given	33	94%	92%	94%
Evaluation of LVS Function	38	100%	96%	99%
Medicare Spending				
Medicare Spending per Patient (ratio)	-	0.83	0.93	0.98
Pneumonia Care				
Appropriate Initial Antibiotic Given	51	94%	92%	95%
Blood Culture Timing	96	99%	97%	98%
Pregnancy and Delivery Care				
Newborn Deliveries Scheduled Early	49	2%	8%	6%
Preventive Care				
Immunization for Influenza[2]	233	95%	89%	90%
Immunization for Pneumonia[2]	239	97%	91%	92%
Stroke Care				
Anticoagulation Therapy for Atrial Fibrillation[5]	-	-	91%	95%
Antithrombotic Therapy Timing[5]	-	-	95%	98%
Assessed for Rehabilitation[5]	-	-	96%	97%
Discharged on Antithrombotic Therapy[5]	-	-	98%	99%
Discharged on Statin Medication[5]	-	-	88%	94%
Thrombolytic Therapy Timing[5]	-	-	61%	66%
Venous Thromboembolism Prophylaxis[5]	-	-	92%	94%
Written Stroke Educational Materials Given[5]	-	-	86%	88%
Surgical Care Improvement Project				
Appropriate Beta Blocker Usage	32	94%	97%	98%
Appropriate VTP Within 24 Hours	119	96%	97%	98%
Controlled Postoperative Blood Glucose[7]	-	-	97%	97%
Perioperative Temperature Management	141	100%	100%	100%
Prophylactic Antibiotic Selection	112	99%	99%	99%
Prophylactic Antibiotic Selection (Outpatient)[1]	-	-	98%	98%
Prophylactic Antibiotic Stopped	111	100%	98%	98%
Prophylactic Antibiotic Timing	112	100%	98%	99%
Prophylactic Antibiotic Timing (Outpatient)[1]	-	-	98%	98%
Urinary Catheter Removal[1]	-	-	96%	97%
Survey of Patients' Hospital Experiences				
Area Around Room 'Always' Quiet at Night	300+	67%	68%	61%
Doctors 'Always' Communicated Well	300+	86%	84%	82%
Home Recovery Information Given	300+	83%	84%	85%
Hospital Given 9 or 10 on 10 Point Scale	300+	79%	72%	71%
Meds 'Always' Explained Before Given	300+	65%	66%	64%
Nurses 'Always' Communicated Well	300+	82%	80%	79%
Pain 'Always' Well Controlled	300+	74%	72%	71%
Room and Bathroom 'Always' Clean	300+	75%	73%	73%
Timely Help 'Always' Received	300+	70%	71%	68%
Would Definitely Recommend Hospital	300+	85%	71%	71%
Use of Medical Imaging				
Cardiac Imaging Stress Test before Surgery[1]	-	-	4.5%	5.3%
Combination Abdominal CT Scan	406	2.0%	23%	10.5%
Combination Brain/Sinus CT Scan[1]	-	-	2.2%	2.7%
Combination Chest CT Scan	238	1.3%	5.1%	2.7%
Follow-up Mammogram/Ultrasound	513	6.8%	8.1%	8.8%
Lumbar Spine MRI for Low Back Pain	59	57.6%	39.9%	37.2%

Pauls Valley General Hospital

100 Valley Drive
Pauls Valley, OK 73075
Phone: 405-238-5501
Fax: 405-238-5926
URL: www.pvgh.net
Type: Acute Care Hospitals
Emergency Services: Yes
Ownership: Govt - Hospital Dist/Auth
Beds: 72
Key Personnel:
Operating Room. . . . . Marty Bashaw, CRNA
CEO/President. . . . . Bridget Copsy
Chief of Medical Staff. . . . . Charles H Mitchell, MD
Radiology. . . . . Mike Welborn

Measure	Cases	This Hosp.	State Avg.	U.S. Avg.
Blood Clot Prevention and Treatment				
Anticoagulation Overlap Therapy[1,2]	-	-	89%	93%
ICU Venous Thromboembolism Prophylaxis[2,7]	-	-	87%	92%
Incidence of Potentially Preventable VTE[1,2]	-	-	8%	10%
UFH with Dosages/Platelet Monitoring[2,7]	-	-	97%	97%
Venous Thromboembolism Prophylaxis[2]	120	24%	72%	85%
Warfarin Therapy Discharge Instructions[1,2]	-	-	73%	75%
Chest Pain/Possible Heart Attack Care				
Aspirin Given Within 24 Hours of Arrival	46	93%	95%	96%
Fibrinolytic Meds Within 30 Min. of Arrival[1]	-	-	54%	58%
Average Time to ECG (minutes)	54	18	8	7
Average Time to Transfer (minutes)[1]	-	-	77	60
Children's Asthma Care				
Received Home Management Plan of Care	-	-	-	88%
Received Reliever Medication	-	-	-	100%
Received Systemic Corticosteroids	-	-	-	100%
Emergency Department				
Admittance Decision Time (minutes)[2]	209	65	63	98
Head CT Results Within 45 Min. of Arrival	15	13%	49%	57%
Patients Who Left ER Before Being Seen	8,702	3%	2%	2%
Time from ER Arrival to Admit. (minutes)[2]	224	233	210	274
Time from ER Arrival to Discharge (minutes)	284	132	110	134
Time in ER Before Being Evaluated (minutes)	388	18	24	26
Time to Pain Meds for Fractures (minutes)	37	52	55	57
Heart Attack Care				
Aspirin Given at Discharge[2,3]	-	-	99%	99%
Fibrinolytic Meds Within 30 Min. of Arrival[2,3]	-	-	25%	54%
PCI Within 90 Minutes of Arrival[2,3]	-	-	95%	96%
Statin Prescribed at Discharge[2,3]	-	-	98%	98%
Heart Failure Care				
ACE Inhibitor or ARB for LVSD[1,2]	-	-	95%	97%
Discharge Instructions Given[2]	24	92%	92%	94%
Evaluation of LVS Function[2]	33	79%	96%	99%
Medicare Spending				
Medicare Spending per Patient (ratio)	-	0.86	0.93	0.98
Pneumonia Care				
Appropriate Initial Antibiotic Given[2]	44	84%	92%	95%
Blood Culture Timing[2]	54	96%	97%	98%
Pregnancy and Delivery Care				
Newborn Deliveries Scheduled Early[1,2]	-	-	8%	6%
Preventive Care				
Immunization for Influenza[2]	273	56%	89%	90%
Immunization for Pneumonia[2]	351	72%	91%	92%
Stroke Care				
Anticoagulation Therapy for Atrial Fibrillation[1,2]	-	-	91%	95%
Antithrombotic Therapy Timing[1,2]	-	-	95%	98%
Assessed for Rehabilitation[1,2]	-	-	96%	97%
Discharged on Antithrombotic Therapy[1,2]	-	-	98%	99%
Discharged on Statin Medication[1,2]	-	-	88%	94%
Thrombolytic Therapy Timing[1,2]	-	-	61%	66%
Venous Thromboembolism Prophylaxis[1,2]	-	-	92%	94%
Written Stroke Educational Materials Given[1,2]	-	-	86%	88%
Surgical Care Improvement Project				
Appropriate Beta Blocker Usage[2,3]	-	-	97%	98%
Appropriate VTP Within 24 Hours[1,2]	-	-	97%	98%
Controlled Postoperative Blood Glucose[2,3]	-	-	97%	97%
Perioperative Temperature Management[1,2]	-	-	100%	100%
Prophylactic Antibiotic Selection[2,3]	-	-	99%	99%
Prophylactic Antibiotic Selection (Outpatient)[5]	-	-	98%	98%
Prophylactic Antibiotic Stopped[2,3]	-	-	98%	98%
Prophylactic Antibiotic Timing[2,3]	-	-	98%	99%
Prophylactic Antibiotic Timing (Outpatient)[5]	-	-	98%	98%
Urinary Catheter Removal[2,3]	-	-	96%	97%
Survey of Patients' Hospital Experiences				
Area Around Room 'Always' Quiet at Night	(a)	69%	68%	61%
Doctors 'Always' Communicated Well	(a)	80%	84%	82%
Home Recovery Information Given	(a)	78%	84%	85%
Hospital Given 9 or 10 on 10 Point Scale	(a)	58%	72%	71%
Meds 'Always' Explained Before Given	(a)	73%	66%	64%
Nurses 'Always' Communicated Well	(a)	80%	80%	79%
Pain 'Always' Well Controlled	(a)	69%	72%	71%
Room and Bathroom 'Always' Clean	(a)	74%	73%	73%
Timely Help 'Always' Received	(a)	70%	71%	68%
Would Definitely Recommend Hospital	(a)	51%	71%	71%
Use of Medical Imaging				
Cardiac Imaging Stress Test before Surgery[7]	-	-	4.5%	5.3%
Combination Abdominal CT Scan	189	28.6%	23%	10.5%
Combination Brain/Sinus CT Scan[1]	-	-	2.2%	2.7%
Combination Chest CT Scan	72	12.5%	5.1%	2.7%
Follow-up Mammogram/Ultrasound	194	4.6%	8.1%	8.8%
Lumbar Spine MRI for Low Back Pain[1]	-	-	39.9%	37.2%

Pawhuska Hospital

1101 East 15th Street
Pawhuska, OK 74056
Phone: 918-287-3232
Fax: 918-287-5145
Type: Critical Access Hospitals
Emergency Services: Yes
Ownership: Government - Local
Beds: 15
Key Personnel:
Quality Assurance . . . . Karin Arrow Smith
Emergency Room . . . . Kelly Eaton, RN
Infection Control. . . . . Gertrude Greghoff
Chief of Medical Staff . . . . Mike Priest, DO

Measure	Cases	This Hosp.	State Avg.	U.S. Avg.
Blood Clot Prevention and Treatment				
Anticoagulation Overlap Therapy[5]	-	-	89%	93%
ICU Venous Thromboembolism Prophylaxis[5]	-	-	87%	92%
Incidence of Potentially Preventable VTE[5]	-	-	8%	10%
UFH with Dosages/Platelet Monitoring[5]	-	-	97%	97%
Venous Thromboembolism Prophylaxis[5]	-	-	72%	85%
Warfarin Therapy Discharge Instructions[5]	-	-	73%	75%
Chest Pain/Possible Heart Attack Care				
Aspirin Given Within 24 Hours of Arrival[1,3]	-	-	95%	96%
Fibrinolytic Meds Within 30 Min. of Arrival[5]	-	-	54%	58%
Average Time to ECG (minutes)[1,3]	-	-	8	7
Average Time to Transfer (minutes)[5]	-	-	77	60

NOTE: Hospital profiles are in alphabetical order by state, then city, then hospital within the city; Rankings exclude hospitals with less than 25 cases except for patient surveys which excludes hospitals with less than 100 cases; (a) 100-299 cases; (1) The number of cases/patients is too few to report; (2) Data submitted were based on a sample of cases/patients; (3) Results are based on a shorter time period than required; (4) Data suppressed by CMS for one or more quarters; (5) Results are not available for this reporting period; (6) Fewer than 100 patients completed the HCAHPS survey; (7) No cases met the criteria for this measure; (8) The lower limit of the confidence interval cannot be calculated if the number of observed infections equals zero; (9) No data are available from the state/territory for this reporting period; (10) The scores shown reflect fewer than 50 completed surveys; (11) There were discrepancies in the data collection process; (12) This measure does not apply to this hospital for this reporting period; (13) Results cannot be calculated for this reporting period; (14) The results for this state are combined with nearby states to protect confidentiality; Please refer to the User's Guide for a full explanation of data.

Measure	Cases	This Hosp.	State Avg.	U.S. Avg.
Children's Asthma Care				
Received Home Management Plan of Care	-	-	-	88%
Received Reliever Medication	-	-	-	100%
Received Systemic Corticosteroids	-	-	-	100%
Emergency Department				
Admittance Decision Time (minutes)[5]	-	-	63	98
Head CT Results Within 45 Min. of Arrival[5]	-	-	49%	57%
Patients Who Left ER Before Being Seen[5]	-	-	2%	2%
Time from ER Arrival to Admit. (minutes)[5]	-	-	210	274
Time from ER Arrival to Discharge (minutes)[5]	-	-	110	134
Time in ER Before Being Evaluated (minutes)[5]	-	-	24	26
Time to Pain Meds for Fractures (minutes)[5]	-	-	55	57
Heart Attack Care				
Aspirin Given at Discharge[5]	-	-	99%	99%
Fibrinolytic Meds Within 30 Min. of Arrival[5]	-	-	25%	54%
PCI Within 90 Minutes of Arrival[5]	-	-	95%	96%
Statin Prescribed at Discharge[5]	-	-	98%	98%
Heart Failure Care				
ACE Inhibitor or ARB for LVSD[3,7]	-	-	95%	97%
Discharge Instructions Given[1,3]	-	-	92%	94%
Evaluation of LVS Function[1,3]	-	-	96%	99%
Medicare Spending				
Medicare Spending per Patient (ratio)	-	-	0.93	0.98
Pneumonia Care				
Appropriate Initial Antibiotic Given[3,7]	-	-	92%	95%
Blood Culture Timing[3,7]	-	-	97%	98%
Pregnancy and Delivery Care				
Newborn Deliveries Scheduled Early[5]	-	-	8%	6%
Preventive Care				
Immunization for Influenza[5]	-	-	89%	90%
Immunization for Pneumonia[5]	-	-	91%	92%
Stroke Care				
Anticoagulation Therapy for Atrial Fibrillation[5]	-	-	91%	95%
Antithrombotic Therapy Timing[5]	-	-	95%	98%
Assessed for Rehabilitation[5]	-	-	96%	97%
Discharged on Antithrombotic Therapy[5]	-	-	98%	99%
Discharged on Statin Medication[5]	-	-	88%	94%
Thrombolytic Therapy Timing[5]	-	-	61%	66%
Venous Thromboembolism Prophylaxis[5]	-	-	92%	94%
Written Stroke Educational Materials Given[5]	-	-	86%	88%
Surgical Care Improvement Project				
Appropriate Beta Blocker Usage[5]	-	-	97%	98%
Appropriate VTP Within 24 Hours[5]	-	-	97%	98%
Controlled Postoperative Blood Glucose[5]	-	-	97%	97%
Perioperative Temperature Management[5]	-	-	100%	100%
Prophylactic Antibiotic Selection[5]	-	-	99%	99%
Prophylactic Antibiotic Selection (Outpatient)[5]	-	-	98%	98%
Prophylactic Antibiotic Stopped[5]	-	-	98%	98%
Prophylactic Antibiotic Timing[5]	-	-	98%	99%
Prophylactic Antibiotic Timing (Outpatient)[5]	-	-	98%	98%
Urinary Catheter Removal[5]	-	-	96%	97%
Survey of Patients' Hospital Experiences				
Area Around Room 'Always' Quiet at Night[5]	-	-	68%	61%
Doctors 'Always' Communicated Well[5]	-	-	84%	82%
Home Recovery Information Given[5]	-	-	84%	85%
Hospital Given 9 or 10 on 10 Point Scale[5]	-	-	72%	71%
Meds 'Always' Explained Before Given[5]	-	-	66%	64%
Nurses 'Always' Communicated Well[5]	-	-	80%	79%
Pain 'Always' Well Controlled[5]	-	-	72%	71%
Room and Bathroom 'Always' Clean[5]	-	-	73%	73%
Timely Help 'Always' Received[5]	-	-	71%	68%
Would Definitely Recommend Hospital[5]	-	-	71%	71%
Use of Medical Imaging				
Cardiac Imaging Stress Test before Surgery[7]	-	-	4.5%	5.3%
Combination Abdominal CT Scan[1]	-	-	23%	10.5%
Combination Brain/Sinus CT Scan[1]	-	-	2.2%	2.7%
Combination Chest CT Scan[1]	-	-	5.1%	2.7%
Follow-up Mammogram/Ultrasound[7]	-	-	8.1%	8.8%
Lumbar Spine MRI for Low Back Pain[7]	-	-	39.9%	37.2%

Perry Memorial Hospital

501 Fourteenth Street
Perry, OK 73077
URL: www.pmh-ok.org
Type: Acute Care Hospitals
Ownership: Govt - Hospital Dist/Auth

Phone: 580-336-3541
Fax: 580-336-7209

Emergency Services: Yes
Beds: 28

Key Personnel:
Radiology . . . . James Bullen
CEO . . . . Dean Turner

Measure	Cases	This Hosp.	State Avg.	U.S. Avg.
Blood Clot Prevention and Treatment				
Anticoagulation Overlap Therapy[1]	-	-	89%	93%
ICU Venous Thromboembolism Prophylaxis[7]	-	-	87%	92%
Incidence of Potentially Preventable VTE[7]	-	-	8%	10%
UFH with Dosages/Platelet Monitoring[7]	-	-	97%	97%
Venous Thromboembolism Prophylaxis	174	44%	72%	85%
Warfarin Therapy Discharge Instructions[7]	-	-	73%	75%
Chest Pain/Possible Heart Attack Care				
Aspirin Given Within 24 Hours of Arrival[1]	-	-	95%	96%
Fibrinolytic Meds Within 30 Min. of Arrival[3,7]	-	-	54%	58%
Average Time to ECG (minutes)[1]	-	-	8	7
Average Time to Transfer (minutes)[3,7]	-	-	77	60
Children's Asthma Care				
Received Home Management Plan of Care	-	-	-	88%
Received Reliever Medication	-	-	-	100%
Received Systemic Corticosteroids	-	-	-	100%
Emergency Department				
Admittance Decision Time (minutes)[2]	172	30	63	98
Head CT Results Within 45 Min. of Arrival[3,7]	-	-	49%	57%
Patients Who Left ER Before Being Seen	2,912	1%	2%	2%
Time from ER Arrival to Admit. (minutes)[2]	176	154	210	274
Time from ER Arrival to Discharge (minutes)	236	87	110	134
Time in ER Before Being Evaluated (minutes)	248	18	24	26
Time to Pain Meds for Fractures (minutes)[1]	-	-	55	57
Heart Attack Care				
Aspirin Given at Discharge[1,3]	-	-	99%	99%
Fibrinolytic Meds Within 30 Min. of Arrival[3,7]	-	-	25%	54%
PCI Within 90 Minutes of Arrival[3,7]	-	-	95%	96%
Statin Prescribed at Discharge[1,3]	-	-	98%	98%
Heart Failure Care				
ACE Inhibitor or ARB for LVSD[1,2]	-	-	95%	97%
Discharge Instructions Given[1,2]	-	-	92%	94%
Evaluation of LVS Function[2,3]	16	75%	96%	99%
Medicare Spending				
Medicare Spending per Patient (ratio)	-	0.90	0.93	0.98
Pneumonia Care				
Appropriate Initial Antibiotic Given[2]	18	78%	92%	95%
Blood Culture Timing[2]	12	83%	97%	98%
Pregnancy and Delivery Care				
Newborn Deliveries Scheduled Early[7]	-	-	8%	6%
Preventive Care				
Immunization for Influenza[2]	159	84%	89%	90%
Immunization for Pneumonia[2]	229	81%	91%	92%
Stroke Care				
Anticoagulation Therapy for Atrial Fibrillation[1,3]	-	-	91%	95%
Antithrombotic Therapy Timing[1,3]	-	-	95%	98%
Assessed for Rehabilitation[1,3]	-	-	96%	97%
Discharged on Antithrombotic Therapy[3,7]	-	-	98%	99%
Discharged on Statin Medication[1,3]	-	-	88%	94%
Thrombolytic Therapy Timing[1,3]	-	-	61%	66%
Venous Thromboembolism Prophylaxis[1,3]	-	-	92%	94%
Written Stroke Educational Materials Given[3,7]	-	-	86%	88%
Surgical Care Improvement Project				
Appropriate Beta Blocker Usage[5]	-	-	97%	98%
Appropriate VTP Within 24 Hours[5]	-	-	97%	98%
Controlled Postoperative Blood Glucose[5]	-	-	97%	97%
Perioperative Temperature Management[5]	-	-	100%	100%
Prophylactic Antibiotic Selection[5]	-	-	99%	99%
Prophylactic Antibiotic Selection (Outpatient)[5]	-	-	98%	98%
Prophylactic Antibiotic Stopped[5]	-	-	98%	98%
Prophylactic Antibiotic Timing[5]	-	-	98%	99%
Prophylactic Antibiotic Timing (Outpatient)[5]	-	-	98%	98%
Urinary Catheter Removal[5]	-	-	96%	97%
Survey of Patients' Hospital Experiences				
Area Around Room 'Always' Quiet at Night[6]	<100	69%	68%	61%
Doctors 'Always' Communicated Well[6]	<100	93%	84%	82%
Home Recovery Information Given[6]	<100	93%	84%	85%
Hospital Given 9 or 10 on 10 Point Scale[6]	<100	82%	72%	71%
Meds 'Always' Explained Before Given[6]	<100	64%	66%	64%
Nurses 'Always' Communicated Well[6]	<100	86%	80%	79%
Pain 'Always' Well Controlled[6]	<100	86%	72%	71%
Room and Bathroom 'Always' Clean[6]	<100	74%	73%	73%
Timely Help 'Always' Received[6]	<100	84%	71%	68%
Would Definitely Recommend Hospital[6]	<100	76%	71%	71%
Use of Medical Imaging				
Cardiac Imaging Stress Test before Surgery[7]	-	-	4.5%	5.3%
Combination Abdominal CT Scan	103	19.4%	23%	10.5%
Combination Brain/Sinus CT Scan[1]	-	-	2.2%	2.7%
Combination Chest CT Scan[1]	-	-	5.1%	2.7%
Follow-up Mammogram/Ultrasound	247	0.8%	8.1%	8.8%
Lumbar Spine MRI for Low Back Pain[1]	-	-	39.9%	37.2%

Ponca City Medical Center

1900 North 14th Street
Ponca City, OK 74601
URL: www.poncamedcenter.com
Type: Acute Care Hospitals
Ownership: Proprietary

Phone: 580-765-3321
Fax: 580-765-0341

Emergency Services: Yes
Beds: 140

Key Personnel:
CEO/President . . . . Dennis Barts
Emergency Room . . . . Danny Cassidy, MD
Infection Control . . . . Cheryle Hiebert
Radiology . . . . John Hoy
Quality Assurance . . . . Nancy Nebe
Coronary Care . . . . Jeanne Stara
Intensive Care Unit . . . . Jeanne Stara
Chief of Medical Staff . . . . Krishna Vaidya

Measure	Cases	This Hosp.	State Avg.	U.S. Avg.
Blood Clot Prevention and Treatment				
Anticoagulation Overlap Therapy[2]	15	100%	89%	93%
ICU Venous Thromboembolism Prophylaxis[2]	42	93%	87%	92%
Incidence of Potentially Preventable VTE[2,7]	-	-	8%	10%
UFH with Dosages/Platelet Monitoring[1,2]	-	-	97%	97%
Venous Thromboembolism Prophylaxis[2]	203	98%	72%	85%
Warfarin Therapy Discharge Instructions[2]	14	100%	73%	75%
Chest Pain/Possible Heart Attack Care				
Aspirin Given Within 24 Hours of Arrival	51	100%	95%	96%
Fibrinolytic Meds Within 30 Min. of Arrival[1]	-	-	54%	58%
Average Time to ECG (minutes)	52	5	8	7
Average Time to Transfer (minutes)[7]	-	-	77	60
Children's Asthma Care				
Received Home Management Plan of Care	-	-	-	88%
Received Reliever Medication	-	-	-	100%
Received Systemic Corticosteroids	-	-	-	100%
Emergency Department				
Admittance Decision Time (minutes)[2]	429	65	63	98
Head CT Results Within 45 Min. of Arrival[1]	-	-	49%	57%
Patients Who Left ER Before Being Seen	26,376	2%	2%	2%
Time from ER Arrival to Admit. (minutes)[2]	432	192	210	274
Time from ER Arrival to Discharge (minutes)	376	82	110	134
Time in ER Before Being Evaluated (minutes)	421	20	24	26
Time to Pain Meds for Fractures (minutes)	107	35	55	57
Heart Attack Care				
Aspirin Given at Discharge[1]	-	-	99%	99%
Fibrinolytic Meds Within 30 Min. of Arrival[7]	-	-	25%	54%
PCI Within 90 Minutes of Arrival[7]	-	-	95%	96%
Statin Prescribed at Discharge[1]	-	-	98%	98%
Heart Failure Care				
ACE Inhibitor or ARB for LVSD	41	100%	95%	97%
Discharge Instructions Given	104	97%	92%	94%
Evaluation of LVS Function	124	100%	96%	99%
Medicare Spending				
Medicare Spending per Patient (ratio)	-	0.89	0.93	0.98
Pneumonia Care				
Appropriate Initial Antibiotic Given	67	97%	92%	95%
Blood Culture Timing	80	100%	97%	98%
Pregnancy and Delivery Care				

NOTE: Hospital profiles are in alphabetical order by state, then city, then hospital within the city; Rankings exclude hospitals with less than 25 cases except for patient surveys which excludes hospitals with less than 100 cases; (a) 100-299 cases; (1) The number of cases/patients is too few to report; (2) Data submitted were based on a sample of cases/patients; (3) Results are based on a shorter time period than required; (4) Data suppressed by CMS for one or more quarters; (5) Results are not available for this reporting period; (6) Fewer than 100 patients completed the HCAHPS survey; (7) No cases met the criteria for this measure; (8) The lower limit of the confidence interval cannot be calculated if the number of observed infections equals zero; (9) No data are available from the state/territory for this reporting period; (10) The scores shown reflect fewer than 50 completed surveys; (11) There were discrepancies in the data collection process; (12) This measure does not apply to this hospital for this reporting period; (13) Results cannot be calculated for this reporting period; (14) The results for this state are combined with nearby states to protect confidentiality; Please refer to the User's Guide for a full explanation of data.

Newborn Deliveries Scheduled Early[2]	34	6%	8%	6%
Preventive Care				
Immunization for Influenza[2]	363	100%	89%	90%
Immunization for Pneumonia[2]	383	100%	91%	92%
Stroke Care				
Anticoagulation Therapy for Atrial Fibrillation[1]	-	-	91%	95%
Antithrombotic Therapy Timing	35	97%	95%	98%
Assessed for Rehabilitation	45	98%	96%	97%
Discharged on Antithrombotic Therapy	42	100%	98%	99%
Discharged on Statin Medication	37	95%	88%	94%
Thrombolytic Therapy Timing[1]	-	-	61%	66%
Venous Thromboembolism Prophylaxis	36	100%	92%	94%
Written Stroke Educational Materials Given	24	100%	86%	88%
Surgical Care Improvement Project				
Appropriate Beta Blocker Usage	51	96%	97%	98%
Appropriate VTP Within 24 Hours	175	99%	97%	98%
Controlled Postoperative Blood Glucose[7]	-	-	97%	97%
Perioperative Temperature Management	194	100%	100%	100%
Prophylactic Antibiotic Selection	131	98%	99%	99%
Prophylactic Antibiotic Selection (Outpatient)	67	100%	98%	98%
Prophylactic Antibiotic Stopped	127	99%	98%	98%
Prophylactic Antibiotic Timing	131	100%	98%	99%
Prophylactic Antibiotic Timing (Outpatient)	67	100%	98%	98%
Urinary Catheter Removal	120	100%	96%	97%
Survey of Patients' Hospital Experiences				
Area Around Room 'Always' Quiet at Night	300+	61%	68%	61%
Doctors 'Always' Communicated Well	300+	84%	84%	82%
Home Recovery Information Given	300+	87%	84%	85%
Hospital Given 9 or 10 on 10 Point Scale	300+	69%	72%	71%
Meds 'Always' Explained Before Given	300+	67%	66%	64%
Nurses 'Always' Communicated Well	300+	77%	80%	79%
Pain 'Always' Well Controlled	300+	70%	72%	71%
Room and Bathroom 'Always' Clean	300+	65%	73%	73%
Timely Help 'Always' Received	300+	68%	71%	68%
Would Definitely Recommend Hospital	300+	59%	71%	71%
Use of Medical Imaging				
Cardiac Imaging Stress Test before Surgery	89	4.5%	4.5%	5.3%
Combination Abdominal CT Scan	420	6.0%	23%	10.5%
Combination Brain/Sinus CT Scan	430	4.2%	2.2%	2.7%
Combination Chest CT Scan	246	0.4%	5.1%	2.7%
Follow-up Mammogram/Ultrasound	911	10.0%	8.1%	8.8%
Lumbar Spine MRI for Low Back Pain	60	48.3%	39.9%	37.2%

Eastern Oklahoma Medical Center

105 Wall Street
Poteau, OK 74953
Phone: 918-647-8161
Fax: 918-635-3358
URL: www.eomchospital.com
Type: Acute Care Hospitals
Emergency Services: Yes
Ownership: Voluntary non-profit - Other
Beds: 84

Key Personnel:
CEO/President. . . . . Terry Buckner
Emergency Room . . . . Jonathan Clark, MD
Intensive Care Unit. . . . . Sue Hall
Operating Room. . . . . Ron Huddleston, RN
Infection Control. . . . . Connie Moody
Quality Assurance . . . . Connie Moody
Anesthesiology. . . . . Vickie Smalley

Measure	Cases	This Hosp.	State Avg.	U.S. Avg.
Blood Clot Prevention and Treatment				
Anticoagulation Overlap Therapy[1,2]	-	-	89%	93%
ICU Venous Thromboembolism Prophylaxis[2]	184	78%	87%	92%
Incidence of Potentially Preventable VTE[2,7]	-	-	8%	10%
UFH with Dosages/Platelet Monitoring[1,2]	-	-	97%	97%
Venous Thromboembolism Prophylaxis[2]	579	53%	72%	85%
Warfarin Therapy Discharge Instructions[1,2]	-	-	73%	75%
Chest Pain/Possible Heart Attack Care				
Aspirin Given Within 24 Hours of Arrival	47	87%	95%	96%
Fibrinolytic Meds Within 30 Min. of Arrival[3,7]	-	-	54%	58%
Average Time to ECG (minutes)	44	7	8	7
Average Time to Transfer (minutes)[1,3]	-	-	77	60
Children's Asthma Care				
Received Home Management Plan of Care	-	-	-	88%
Received Reliever Medication	-	-	-	100%
Received Systemic Corticosteroids	-	-	-	100%
Emergency Department				
Admittance Decision Time (minutes)[2]	156	75	63	98
Head CT Results Within 45 Min. of Arrival[1]	-	-	49%	57%
Patients Who Left ER Before Being Seen	15,372	3%	2%	2%
Time from ER Arrival to Admit. (minutes)[2]	175	222	210	274
Time from ER Arrival to Discharge (minutes)	1,035	120	110	134
Time in ER Before Being Evaluated (minutes)	1,098	42	24	26
Time to Pain Meds for Fractures (minutes)	80	91	55	57
Heart Attack Care				
Aspirin Given at Discharge[1,3]	-	-	99%	99%
Fibrinolytic Meds Within 30 Min. of Arrival[3,7]	-	-	25%	54%
PCI Within 90 Minutes of Arrival[3,7]	-	-	95%	96%
Statin Prescribed at Discharge[1,3]	-	-	98%	98%
Heart Failure Care				
ACE Inhibitor or ARB for LVSD	24	71%	95%	97%
Discharge Instructions Given	60	85%	92%	94%
Evaluation of LVS Function	90	99%	96%	99%
Medicare Spending				
Medicare Spending per Patient (ratio)	-	1.00	0.93	0.98
Pneumonia Care				
Appropriate Initial Antibiotic Given	62	73%	92%	95%
Blood Culture Timing	74	92%	97%	98%
Pregnancy and Delivery Care				
Newborn Deliveries Scheduled Early	27	11%	8%	6%
Preventive Care				
Immunization for Influenza[2]	232	73%	89%	90%
Immunization for Pneumonia[2]	301	87%	91%	92%
Stroke Care				
Anticoagulation Therapy for Atrial Fibrillation[7]	-	-	91%	95%
Antithrombotic Therapy Timing[1]	-	-	95%	98%
Assessed for Rehabilitation[1]	-	-	96%	97%
Discharged on Antithrombotic Therapy[1]	-	-	98%	99%
Discharged on Statin Medication[1]	-	-	88%	94%
Thrombolytic Therapy Timing[1]	-	-	61%	66%
Venous Thromboembolism Prophylaxis[1]	-	-	92%	94%
Written Stroke Educational Materials Given[1]	-	-	86%	88%
Surgical Care Improvement Project				
Appropriate Beta Blocker Usage[1]	-	-	97%	98%
Appropriate VTP Within 24 Hours	18	28%	97%	98%
Controlled Postoperative Blood Glucose[7]	-	-	97%	97%
Perioperative Temperature Management	40	100%	100%	100%
Prophylactic Antibiotic Selection	37	73%	99%	99%
Prophylactic Antibiotic Selection (Outpatient)[1,3]	-	-	98%	98%
Prophylactic Antibiotic Stopped	37	100%	98%	98%
Prophylactic Antibiotic Timing	38	61%	98%	99%
Prophylactic Antibiotic Timing (Outpatient)[1,3]	-	-	98%	98%
Urinary Catheter Removal[1]	-	-	96%	97%
Survey of Patients' Hospital Experiences				
Area Around Room 'Always' Quiet at Night	300+	60%	68%	61%
Doctors 'Always' Communicated Well	300+	88%	84%	82%
Home Recovery Information Given	300+	90%	84%	85%
Hospital Given 9 or 10 on 10 Point Scale	300+	67%	72%	71%
Meds 'Always' Explained Before Given	300+	66%	66%	64%
Nurses 'Always' Communicated Well	300+	77%	80%	79%
Pain 'Always' Well Controlled	300+	70%	72%	71%
Room and Bathroom 'Always' Clean	300+	69%	73%	73%
Timely Help 'Always' Received	300+	69%	71%	68%
Would Definitely Recommend Hospital	300+	65%	71%	71%
Use of Medical Imaging				
Cardiac Imaging Stress Test before Surgery[7]	-	-	4.5%	5.3%
Combination Abdominal CT Scan	227	18.9%	23%	10.5%
Combination Brain/Sinus CT Scan	240	0.8%	2.2%	2.7%
Combination Chest CT Scan	70	28.6%	5.1%	2.7%
Follow-up Mammogram/Ultrasound	241	7.5%	8.1%	8.8%
Lumbar Spine MRI for Low Back Pain[1]	-	-	39.9%	37.2%

Prague Community Hospital

1322 Klabsuba Avenue
Prague, OK 74864
Phone: 405-567-4922
Fax: 405-567-4290
URL: www.praguehospital.com
Type: Critical Access Hospitals
Emergency Services: Yes
Ownership: Proprietary
Beds: 25

Key Personnel:
Chief of Medical Staff. . . . . Scott Fowler
Emergency Room . . . . Alexander Frank, MD
CEO/President. . . . . Joan Walters
Quality Assurance . . . . Joan Walters

Measure	Cases	This Hosp.	State Avg.	U.S. Avg.
Blood Clot Prevention and Treatment				
Anticoagulation Overlap Therapy[5]	-	-	89%	93%
ICU Venous Thromboembolism Prophylaxis[5]	-	-	87%	92%
Incidence of Potentially Preventable VTE[5]	-	-	8%	10%
UFH with Dosages/Platelet Monitoring[5]	-	-	97%	97%
Venous Thromboembolism Prophylaxis[5]	-	-	72%	85%
Warfarin Therapy Discharge Instructions[5]	-	-	73%	75%
Chest Pain/Possible Heart Attack Care				
Aspirin Given Within 24 Hours of Arrival[1,3]	-	-	95%	96%
Fibrinolytic Meds Within 30 Min. of Arrival[3,7]	-	-	54%	58%
Average Time to ECG (minutes)[1,3]	-	-	8	7
Average Time to Transfer (minutes)[3,7]	-	-	77	60
Children's Asthma Care				
Received Home Management Plan of Care	-	-	-	88%
Received Reliever Medication	-	-	-	100%
Received Systemic Corticosteroids	-	-	-	100%
Emergency Department				
Admittance Decision Time (minutes)[5]	-	-	63	98
Head CT Results Within 45 Min. of Arrival[3,7]	-	-	49%	57%
Patients Who Left ER Before Being Seen[5]	-	-	2%	2%
Time from ER Arrival to Admit. (minutes)[5]	-	-	210	274
Time from ER Arrival to Discharge (minutes)[5]	-	-	110	134
Time in ER Before Being Evaluated (minutes)[5]	-	-	24	26
Time to Pain Meds for Fractures (minutes)[1,3]	-	-	55	57
Heart Attack Care				
Aspirin Given at Discharge[5]	-	-	99%	99%
Fibrinolytic Meds Within 30 Min. of Arrival[5]	-	-	25%	54%
PCI Within 90 Minutes of Arrival[5]	-	-	95%	96%
Statin Prescribed at Discharge[5]	-	-	98%	98%
Heart Failure Care				
ACE Inhibitor or ARB for LVSD[3,7]	-	-	95%	97%
Discharge Instructions Given[1,3]	-	-	92%	94%
Evaluation of LVS Function[1,3]	-	-	96%	99%
Medicare Spending				
Medicare Spending per Patient (ratio)	-	-	0.93	0.98
Pneumonia Care				
Appropriate Initial Antibiotic Given[1,3]	-	-	92%	95%
Blood Culture Timing[1,3]	-	-	97%	98%
Pregnancy and Delivery Care				
Newborn Deliveries Scheduled Early[5]	-	-	8%	6%
Preventive Care				
Immunization for Influenza[5]	-	-	89%	90%
Immunization for Pneumonia[5]	-	-	91%	92%
Stroke Care				
Anticoagulation Therapy for Atrial Fibrillation[5]	-	-	91%	95%
Antithrombotic Therapy Timing[5]	-	-	95%	98%
Assessed for Rehabilitation[5]	-	-	96%	97%
Discharged on Antithrombotic Therapy[5]	-	-	98%	99%
Discharged on Statin Medication[5]	-	-	88%	94%
Thrombolytic Therapy Timing[5]	-	-	61%	66%
Venous Thromboembolism Prophylaxis[5]	-	-	92%	94%
Written Stroke Educational Materials Given[5]	-	-	86%	88%
Surgical Care Improvement Project				
Appropriate Beta Blocker Usage[5]	-	-	97%	98%
Appropriate VTP Within 24 Hours[5]	-	-	97%	98%
Controlled Postoperative Blood Glucose[5]	-	-	97%	97%
Perioperative Temperature Management[5]	-	-	100%	100%
Prophylactic Antibiotic Selection[5]	-	-	99%	99%
Prophylactic Antibiotic Selection (Outpatient)[5]	-	-	98%	98%
Prophylactic Antibiotic Stopped[5]	-	-	98%	98%
Prophylactic Antibiotic Timing[5]	-	-	98%	99%
Prophylactic Antibiotic Timing (Outpatient)[5]	-	-	98%	98%
Urinary Catheter Removal[5]	-	-	96%	97%
Survey of Patients' Hospital Experiences				
Area Around Room 'Always' Quiet at Night[5]	-	-	68%	61%
Doctors 'Always' Communicated Well[5]	-	-	84%	82%
Home Recovery Information Given[5]	-	-	84%	85%
Hospital Given 9 or 10 on 10 Point Scale[5]	-	-	72%	71%

NOTE: Hospital profiles are in alphabetical order by state, then city, then hospital within the city; Rankings exclude hospitals with less than 25 cases except for patient surveys which excludes hospitals with less than 100 cases; (a) 100-299 cases; (1) The number of cases/patients is too few to report; (2) Data submitted were based on a sample of cases/patients; (3) Results are based on a shorter time period than required; (4) Data suppressed by CMS for one or more quarters; (5) Results are not available for this reporting period; (6) Fewer than 100 patients completed the HCAHPS survey; (7) No cases met the criteria for this measure; (8) The lower limit of the confidence interval cannot be calculated if the number of observed infections equals zero; (9) No data are available from the state/territory for this reporting period; (10) The scores shown reflect fewer than 50 completed surveys; (11) There were discrepancies in the data collection process; (12) This measure does not apply to this hospital for this reporting period; (13) Results cannot be calculated for this reporting period; (14) The results for this state are combined with nearby states to protect confidentiality; Please refer to the User's Guide for a full explanation of data.

Measure	Cases	This Hosp.	State Avg.	U.S. Avg.
Meds 'Always' Explained Before Given[5]	-	-	66%	64%
Nurses 'Always' Communicated Well[5]	-	-	80%	79%
Pain 'Always' Well Controlled[5]	-	-	72%	71%
Room and Bathroom 'Always' Clean[5]	-	-	73%	73%
Timely Help 'Always' Received[5]	-	-	71%	68%
Would Definitely Recommend Hospital[5]	-	-	71%	71%
Use of Medical Imaging				
Cardiac Imaging Stress Test before Surgery[1]	-	-	4.5%	5.3%
Combination Abdominal CT Scan[1]	-	-	23%	10.5%
Combination Brain/Sinus CT Scan	35	0.0%	2.2%	2.7%
Combination Chest CT Scan[1]	-	-	5.1%	2.7%
Follow-up Mammogram/Ultrasound[7]	-	-	8.1%	8.8%
Lumbar Spine MRI for Low Back Pain[1]	-	-	39.9%	37.2%

Integris Mayes County Medical Center

111 North Bailey Street
Pryor, OK 74361
Phone: 918-825-1600
Fax: 918-825-7668
E-mail: white@integris-health.com
URL: www.integris-health.com
Type: Acute Care Hospitals
Emergency Services: No
Ownership: Voluntary non-profit - Other
Beds: 73

Key Personnel:
Emergency Room . . . . Chris DeLong, DO
President . . . . Eddie Herrman
President/CEO. . . . . Bruce Lawrence
Chief of Medical Staff . . . . James White, MD

Measure	Cases	This Hosp.	State Avg.	U.S. Avg.
Blood Clot Prevention and Treatment				
Anticoagulation Overlap Therapy[1,2]	-	-	89%	93%
ICU Venous Thromboembolism Prophylaxis[2,7]	-	-	87%	92%
Incidence of Potentially Preventable VTE[2,7]	-	-	8%	10%
UFH with Dosages/Platelet Monitoring[1,2]	-	-	97%	97%
Venous Thromboembolism Prophylaxis[2]	117	95%	72%	85%
Warfarin Therapy Discharge Instructions[1,2]	-	-	73%	75%
Chest Pain/Possible Heart Attack Care				
Aspirin Given Within 24 Hours of Arrival	80	95%	95%	96%
Fibrinolytic Meds Within 30 Min. of Arrival[1]	-	-	54%	58%
Average Time to ECG (minutes)	84	14	8	7
Average Time to Transfer (minutes)	14	67	77	60
Children's Asthma Care				
Received Home Management Plan of Care	-	-	-	88%
Received Reliever Medication	-	-	-	100%
Received Systemic Corticosteroids	-	-	-	100%
Emergency Department				
Admittance Decision Time (minutes)[2]	394	61	63	98
Head CT Results Within 45 Min. of Arrival[1]	-	-	49%	57%
Patients Who Left ER Before Being Seen	15,903	4%	2%	2%
Time from ER Arrival to Admit. (minutes)[2]	398	225	210	274
Time from ER Arrival to Discharge (minutes)	343	114	110	134
Time in ER Before Being Evaluated (minutes)	390	16	24	26
Time to Pain Meds for Fractures (minutes)	82	50	55	57
Heart Attack Care				
Aspirin Given at Discharge[3,7]	-	-	99%	99%
Fibrinolytic Meds Within 30 Min. of Arrival[3,7]	-	-	25%	54%
PCI Within 90 Minutes of Arrival[3,7]	-	-	95%	96%
Statin Prescribed at Discharge[3,7]	-	-	98%	98%
Heart Failure Care				
ACE Inhibitor or ARB for LVSD[1]	-	-	95%	97%
Discharge Instructions Given	13	92%	92%	94%
Evaluation of LVS Function	17	94%	96%	99%
Medicare Spending				
Medicare Spending per Patient (ratio)	-	0.90	0.93	0.98
Pneumonia Care				
Appropriate Initial Antibiotic Given	35	97%	92%	95%
Blood Culture Timing	45	100%	97%	98%
Pregnancy and Delivery Care				
Newborn Deliveries Scheduled Early[7]	-	-	8%	6%
Preventive Care				
Immunization for Influenza[2]	276	100%	89%	90%
Immunization for Pneumonia[2]	461	100%	91%	92%
Stroke Care				
Anticoagulation Therapy for Atrial Fibrillation[3,7]	-	-	91%	95%
Antithrombotic Therapy Timing[1,3]	-	-	95%	98%
Assessed for Rehabilitation[1,3]	-	-	96%	97%
Discharged on Antithrombotic Therapy[1,3]	-	-	98%	99%
Discharged on Statin Medication[1,3]	-	-	88%	94%
Thrombolytic Therapy Timing[3,7]	-	-	61%	66%
Venous Thromboembolism Prophylaxis[1,3]	-	-	92%	94%
Written Stroke Educational Materials Given[3,7]	-	-	86%	88%
Surgical Care Improvement Project				
Appropriate Beta Blocker Usage	11	100%	97%	98%
Appropriate VTP Within 24 Hours	36	100%	97%	98%
Controlled Postoperative Blood Glucose[7]	-	-	97%	97%
Perioperative Temperature Management	39	100%	100%	100%
Prophylactic Antibiotic Selection	33	100%	99%	99%
Prophylactic Antibiotic Selection (Outpatient)[3,7]	-	-	98%	98%
Prophylactic Antibiotic Stopped	32	100%	98%	98%
Prophylactic Antibiotic Timing	33	100%	98%	99%
Prophylactic Antibiotic Timing (Outpatient)[3,7]	-	-	98%	98%
Urinary Catheter Removal	26	100%	96%	97%
Survey of Patients' Hospital Experiences				
Area Around Room 'Always' Quiet at Night	(a)	70%	68%	61%
Doctors 'Always' Communicated Well	(a)	86%	84%	82%
Home Recovery Information Given	(a)	89%	84%	85%
Hospital Given 9 or 10 on 10 Point Scale	(a)	63%	72%	71%
Meds 'Always' Explained Before Given	(a)	64%	66%	64%
Nurses 'Always' Communicated Well	(a)	82%	80%	79%
Pain 'Always' Well Controlled	(a)	67%	72%	71%
Room and Bathroom 'Always' Clean	(a)	79%	73%	73%
Timely Help 'Always' Received	(a)	75%	71%	68%
Would Definitely Recommend Hospital	(a)	58%	71%	71%
Use of Medical Imaging				
Cardiac Imaging Stress Test before Surgery	216	3.2%	4.5%	5.3%
Combination Abdominal CT Scan	287	9.1%	23%	10.5%
Combination Brain/Sinus CT Scan	294	0.7%	2.2%	2.7%
Combination Chest CT Scan	135	5.2%	5.1%	2.7%
Follow-up Mammogram/Ultrasound	427	5.9%	8.1%	8.8%
Lumbar Spine MRI for Low Back Pain[1]	-	-	39.9%	37.2%

Purcell Municipal Hospital

1500 North Green Avenue
Purcell, OK 73080
Phone: 405-527-6524
Fax: 405-527-6963
Type: Acute Care Hospitals
Emergency Services: Yes
Ownership: Govt - Hospital Dist/Auth
Beds: 39

Key Personnel:
Emergency Room . . . . Donn A Avila, RN
Operating Room. . . . . Angela Garrett, RN
Infection Control. . . . . Pam Kaiser, RN
Quality Assurance . . . . Pam Kaiser, RN
Chair/CEO . . . . Gracie Montgomery
Chief of Medical Staff . . . . Sean A. Orlino, MD
CEO/President. . . . . Kem Scully

Measure	Cases	This Hosp.	State Avg.	U.S. Avg.
Blood Clot Prevention and Treatment				
Anticoagulation Overlap Therapy[2]	11	64%	89%	93%
ICU Venous Thromboembolism Prophylaxis[2,7]	-	-	87%	92%
Incidence of Potentially Preventable VTE[1,2]	-	-	8%	10%
UFH with Dosages/Platelet Monitoring[2,7]	-	-	97%	97%
Venous Thromboembolism Prophylaxis[2]	115	43%	72%	85%
Warfarin Therapy Discharge Instructions[1,2]	-	-	73%	75%
Chest Pain/Possible Heart Attack Care				
Aspirin Given Within 24 Hours of Arrival	17	82%	95%	96%
Fibrinolytic Meds Within 30 Min. of Arrival[7]	-	-	54%	58%
Average Time to ECG (minutes)	17	1	8	7
Average Time to Transfer (minutes)[7]	-	-	77	60
Children's Asthma Care				
Received Home Management Plan of Care	-	-	-	88%
Received Reliever Medication	-	-	-	100%
Received Systemic Corticosteroids	-	-	-	100%
Emergency Department				
Admittance Decision Time (minutes)[2]	359	48	63	98
Head CT Results Within 45 Min. of Arrival[1]	-	-	49%	57%
Patients Who Left ER Before Being Seen	12,636	3%	2%	2%
Time from ER Arrival to Admit. (minutes)[2]	369	195	210	274
Time from ER Arrival to Discharge (minutes)	351	94	110	134
Time in ER Before Being Evaluated (minutes)	386	25	24	26
Time to Pain Meds for Fractures (minutes)	36	70	55	57
Heart Attack Care				
Aspirin Given at Discharge[1]	-	-	99%	99%
Fibrinolytic Meds Within 30 Min. of Arrival[7]	-	-	25%	54%
PCI Within 90 Minutes of Arrival[7]	-	-	95%	96%
Statin Prescribed at Discharge[1]	-	-	98%	98%
Heart Failure Care				
ACE Inhibitor or ARB for LVSD[1]	-	-	95%	97%
Discharge Instructions Given	30	67%	92%	94%
Evaluation of LVS Function	39	74%	96%	99%
Medicare Spending				
Medicare Spending per Patient (ratio)	-	0.96	0.93	0.98
Pneumonia Care				
Appropriate Initial Antibiotic Given	63	83%	92%	95%
Blood Culture Timing	40	95%	97%	98%
Pregnancy and Delivery Care				
Newborn Deliveries Scheduled Early[1]	-	-	8%	6%
Preventive Care				
Immunization for Influenza[2]	292	64%	89%	90%
Immunization for Pneumonia[2]	466	81%	91%	92%
Stroke Care				
Anticoagulation Therapy for Atrial Fibrillation[3,7]	-	-	91%	95%
Antithrombotic Therapy Timing[1,3]	-	-	95%	98%
Assessed for Rehabilitation[1,3]	-	-	96%	97%
Discharged on Antithrombotic Therapy[1,3]	-	-	98%	99%
Discharged on Statin Medication[1,3]	-	-	88%	94%
Thrombolytic Therapy Timing[3,7]	-	-	61%	66%
Venous Thromboembolism Prophylaxis[1,3]	-	-	92%	94%
Written Stroke Educational Materials Given[3,7]	-	-	86%	88%
Surgical Care Improvement Project				
Appropriate Beta Blocker Usage[3,7]	-	-	97%	98%
Appropriate VTP Within 24 Hours[1,3]	-	-	97%	98%
Controlled Postoperative Blood Glucose[3,7]	-	-	97%	97%
Perioperative Temperature Management[1,3]	-	-	100%	100%
Prophylactic Antibiotic Selection[3,7]	-	-	99%	99%
Prophylactic Antibiotic Selection (Outpatient)[1,3]	-	-	98%	98%
Prophylactic Antibiotic Stopped[3,7]	-	-	98%	98%
Prophylactic Antibiotic Timing[3,7]	-	-	98%	99%
Prophylactic Antibiotic Timing (Outpatient)[1,3]	-	-	98%	98%
Urinary Catheter Removal[3,7]	-	-	96%	97%
Survey of Patients' Hospital Experiences				
Area Around Room 'Always' Quiet at Night	(a)	67%	68%	61%
Doctors 'Always' Communicated Well	(a)	94%	84%	82%
Home Recovery Information Given	(a)	78%	84%	85%
Hospital Given 9 or 10 on 10 Point Scale	(a)	72%	72%	71%
Meds 'Always' Explained Before Given	(a)	63%	66%	64%
Nurses 'Always' Communicated Well	(a)	87%	80%	79%
Pain 'Always' Well Controlled	(a)	75%	72%	71%
Room and Bathroom 'Always' Clean	(a)	76%	73%	73%
Timely Help 'Always' Received	(a)	75%	71%	68%
Would Definitely Recommend Hospital	(a)	77%	71%	71%
Use of Medical Imaging				
Cardiac Imaging Stress Test before Surgery	68	2.9%	4.5%	5.3%
Combination Abdominal CT Scan	164	19.5%	23%	10.5%
Combination Brain/Sinus CT Scan	230	5.2%	2.2%	2.7%
Combination Chest CT Scan	107	7.5%	5.1%	2.7%
Follow-up Mammogram/Ultrasound	174	10.9%	8.1%	8.8%
Lumbar Spine MRI for Low Back Pain[7]	-	-	39.9%	37.2%

Sequoyah County City of Sallisaw Hospital Authority

213 East Redwood
Sallisaw, OK 74955
Phone: 918-774-1100
Fax: 918-774-1142
URL: www.smhok.com
Type: Acute Care Hospitals
Emergency Services: Yes
Ownership: Govt - Hospital Dist/Auth
Beds: 41

Key Personnel:
CEO/President. . . . . Chuck Wade
Chief of Medical Staff . . . . William E Wood

Measure	Cases	This Hosp.	State Avg.	U.S. Avg.
Blood Clot Prevention and Treatment				
Anticoagulation Overlap Therapy[1,2]	-	-	89%	93%
ICU Venous Thromboembolism Prophylaxis[2,7]	-	-	87%	92%
Incidence of Potentially Preventable VTE[2,7]	-	-	8%	10%
UFH with Dosages/Platelet Monitoring[2,7]	-	-	97%	97%

NOTE: Hospital profiles are in alphabetical order by state, then city, then hospital within the city; Rankings exclude hospitals with less than 25 cases except for patient surveys which excludes hospitals with less than 100 cases; (a) 100-299 cases; (1) The number of cases/patients is too few to report; (2) Data submitted were based on a sample of cases/patients; (3) Results are based on a shorter time period than required; (4) Data suppressed by CMS for one or more quarters; (5) Results are not available for this reporting period; (6) Fewer than 100 patients completed the HCAHPS survey; (7) No cases met the criteria for this measure; (8) The lower limit of the confidence interval cannot be calculated if the number of observed infections equals zero; (9) No data are available from the state/territory for this reporting period; (10) The scores shown reflect fewer than 50 completed surveys; (11) There were discrepancies in the data collection process; (12) This measure does not apply to this hospital for this reporting period; (13) Results cannot be calculated for this reporting period; (14) The results for this state are combined with nearby states to protect confidentiality; Please refer to the User's Guide for a full explanation of data.

Measure	Cases	This Hosp.	State Avg.	U.S. Avg.
Venous Thromboembolism Prophylaxis[2]	260	36%	72%	85%
Warfarin Therapy Discharge Instructions[1,2]	-	-	73%	75%
Chest Pain/Possible Heart Attack Care				
Aspirin Given Within 24 Hours of Arrival	46	85%	95%	96%
Fibrinolytic Meds Within 30 Min. of Arrival[1]	-	-	54%	58%
Average Time to ECG (minutes)	47	9	8	7
Average Time to Transfer (minutes)[1]	-	-	77	60
Children's Asthma Care				
Received Home Management Plan of Care	-	-	-	88%
Received Reliever Medication	-	-	-	100%
Received Systemic Corticosteroids	-	-	-	100%
Emergency Department				
Admittance Decision Time (minutes)[2]	297	47	63	98
Head CT Results Within 45 Min. of Arrival[1]	-	-	49%	57%
Patients Who Left ER Before Being Seen	15,591	4%	2%	2%
Time from ER Arrival to Admit. (minutes)[2]	312	153	210	274
Time from ER Arrival to Discharge (minutes)	329	77	110	134
Time in ER Before Being Evaluated (minutes)	453	20	24	26
Time to Pain Meds for Fractures (minutes)	24	46	55	57
Heart Attack Care				
Aspirin Given at Discharge[1]	-	-	99%	99%
Fibrinolytic Meds Within 30 Min. of Arrival[7]	-	-	25%	54%
PCI Within 90 Minutes of Arrival[7]	-	-	95%	96%
Statin Prescribed at Discharge[1]	-	-	98%	98%
Heart Failure Care				
ACE Inhibitor or ARB for LVSD[1,2]	-	-	95%	97%
Discharge Instructions Given[2]	16	31%	92%	94%
Evaluation of LVS Function[2]	26	62%	96%	99%
Medicare Spending				
Medicare Spending per Patient (ratio)	-	0.90	0.93	0.98
Pneumonia Care				
Appropriate Initial Antibiotic Given	55	78%	92%	95%
Blood Culture Timing	50	94%	97%	98%
Pregnancy and Delivery Care				
Newborn Deliveries Scheduled Early[7]	-	-	8%	6%
Preventive Care				
Immunization for Influenza	262	73%	89%	90%
Immunization for Pneumonia[2]	357	80%	91%	92%
Stroke Care				
Anticoagulation Therapy for Atrial Fibrillation[3,7]	-	-	91%	95%
Antithrombotic Therapy Timing[1,3]	-	-	95%	98%
Assessed for Rehabilitation[1,3]	-	-	96%	97%
Discharged on Antithrombotic Therapy[1,3]	-	-	98%	99%
Discharged on Statin Medication[1,3]	-	-	88%	94%
Thrombolytic Therapy Timing[3,7]	-	-	61%	66%
Venous Thromboembolism Prophylaxis[1,3]	-	-	92%	94%
Written Stroke Educational Materials Given[3,7]	-	-	86%	88%
Surgical Care Improvement Project				
Appropriate Beta Blocker Usage[3,7]	-	-	97%	98%
Appropriate VTP Within 24 Hours[1,3]	-	-	97%	98%
Controlled Postoperative Blood Glucose[3,7]	-	-	97%	97%
Perioperative Temperature Management[1,3]	-	-	100%	100%
Prophylactic Antibiotic Selection[1,3]	-	-	99%	99%
Prophylactic Antibiotic Selection (Outpatient)[1,3]	-	-	98%	98%
Prophylactic Antibiotic Stopped[1,3]	-	-	98%	98%
Prophylactic Antibiotic Timing[1,3]	-	-	98%	99%
Prophylactic Antibiotic Timing (Outpatient)[1,3]	-	-	98%	98%
Urinary Catheter Removal[1,3]	-	-	96%	97%
Survey of Patients' Hospital Experiences				
Area Around Room 'Always' Quiet at Night[6]	<100	71%	68%	61%
Doctors 'Always' Communicated Well[6]	<100	88%	84%	82%
Home Recovery Information Given[6]	<100	91%	84%	85%
Hospital Given 9 or 10 on 10 Point Scale[6]	<100	63%	72%	71%
Meds 'Always' Explained Before Given[6]	<100	66%	66%	64%
Nurses 'Always' Communicated Well[6]	<100	79%	80%	79%
Pain 'Always' Well Controlled[6]	<100	64%	72%	71%
Room and Bathroom 'Always' Clean[6]	<100	77%	73%	73%
Timely Help 'Always' Received[6]	<100	69%	71%	68%
Would Definitely Recommend Hospital[6]	<100	64%	71%	71%
Use of Medical Imaging				
Cardiac Imaging Stress Test before Surgery[7]	-	-	4.5%	5.3%
Combination Abdominal CT Scan	241	6.6%	23%	10.5%
Combination Brain/Sinus CT Scan[1]	-	-	2.2%	2.7%
Combination Chest CT Scan	108	16.7%	5.1%	2.7%
Follow-up Mammogram/Ultrasound	177	10.2%	8.1%	8.8%
Lumbar Spine MRI for Low Back Pain	42	52.4%	39.9%	37.2%

Saint John Sapulpa

1004 East Bryan
Sapulpa, OK 74066
Type: Critical Access Hospitals
Ownership: Voluntary non-profit - Private
Phone: 918-224-4280
Fax: 918-224-4395
Emergency Services: Yes
Beds: 113

Key Personnel:

Infection Control . . . . Peggy Ault
Operating Room. . . . . Kurt Lane
Emergency Room . . . . Beatrice Lewis, RN
Quality Assurance . . . . Faye Massey
CEO/President. . . . . Raymond Replogle
Chief of Medical Staff . . . . Roger Wilson

Measure	Cases	This Hosp.	State Avg.	U.S. Avg.
Blood Clot Prevention and Treatment				
Anticoagulation Overlap Therapy[5]	-	-	89%	93%
ICU Venous Thromboembolism Prophylaxis[5]	-	-	87%	92%
Incidence of Potentially Preventable VTE[5]	-	-	8%	10%
UFH with Dosages/Platelet Monitoring[5]	-	-	97%	97%
Venous Thromboembolism Prophylaxis[5]	-	-	72%	85%
Warfarin Therapy Discharge Instructions[5]	-	-	73%	75%
Chest Pain/Possible Heart Attack Care				
Aspirin Given Within 24 Hours of Arrival	44	98%	95%	96%
Fibrinolytic Meds Within 30 Min. of Arrival[7]	-	-	54%	58%
Average Time to ECG (minutes)	44	7	8	7
Average Time to Transfer (minutes)[1]	-	-	77	60
Children's Asthma Care				
Received Home Management Plan of Care	-	-	-	88%
Received Reliever Medication	-	-	-	100%
Received Systemic Corticosteroids	-	-	-	100%
Emergency Department				
Admittance Decision Time (minutes)[2,3]	57	60	63	98
Head CT Results Within 45 Min. of Arrival[5]	-	-	49%	57%
Patients Who Left ER Before Being Seen[5]	-	-	2%	2%
Time from ER Arrival to Admit. (minutes)[2,3]	57	215	210	274
Time from ER Arrival to Discharge (minutes)[5]	-	-	110	134
Time in ER Before Being Evaluated (minutes)[5]	-	-	24	26
Time to Pain Meds for Fractures (minutes)[5]	-	-	55	57
Heart Attack Care				
Aspirin Given at Discharge[5]	-	-	99%	99%
Fibrinolytic Meds Within 30 Min. of Arrival[5]	-	-	25%	54%
PCI Within 90 Minutes of Arrival[5]	-	-	95%	96%
Statin Prescribed at Discharge[5]	-	-	98%	98%
Heart Failure Care				
ACE Inhibitor or ARB for LVSD[1]	-	-	95%	97%
Discharge Instructions Given	16	100%	92%	94%
Evaluation of LVS Function	19	74%	96%	99%
Medicare Spending				
Medicare Spending per Patient (ratio)	-	-	0.93	0.98
Pneumonia Care				
Appropriate Initial Antibiotic Given	32	97%	92%	95%
Blood Culture Timing	55	100%	97%	98%
Pregnancy and Delivery Care				
Newborn Deliveries Scheduled Early[5]	-	-	8%	6%
Preventive Care				
Immunization for Influenza[2]	60	97%	89%	90%
Immunization for Pneumonia[2]	84	93%	91%	92%
Stroke Care				
Anticoagulation Therapy for Atrial Fibrillation[5]	-	-	91%	95%
Antithrombotic Therapy Timing[5]	-	-	95%	98%
Assessed for Rehabilitation[5]	-	-	96%	97%
Discharged on Antithrombotic Therapy[5]	-	-	98%	99%
Discharged on Statin Medication[5]	-	-	88%	94%
Thrombolytic Therapy Timing[5]	-	-	61%	66%
Venous Thromboembolism Prophylaxis[5]	-	-	92%	94%
Written Stroke Educational Materials Given[5]	-	-	86%	88%
Surgical Care Improvement Project				
Appropriate Beta Blocker Usage[5]	-	-	97%	98%
Appropriate VTP Within 24 Hours[5]	-	-	97%	98%
Controlled Postoperative Blood Glucose[5]	-	-	97%	97%
Perioperative Temperature Management[5]	-	-	100%	100%
Prophylactic Antibiotic Selection[5]	-	-	99%	99%
Prophylactic Antibiotic Selection (Outpatient)[5]	-	-	98%	98%
Prophylactic Antibiotic Stopped[5]	-	-	98%	98%
Prophylactic Antibiotic Timing[5]	-	-	98%	99%
Prophylactic Antibiotic Timing (Outpatient)[5]	-	-	98%	98%
Urinary Catheter Removal[5]	-	-	96%	97%
Survey of Patients' Hospital Experiences				
Area Around Room 'Always' Quiet at Night	(a)	68%	68%	61%
Doctors 'Always' Communicated Well	(a)	86%	84%	82%
Home Recovery Information Given	(a)	74%	84%	85%
Hospital Given 9 or 10 on 10 Point Scale	(a)	73%	72%	71%
Meds 'Always' Explained Before Given	(a)	60%	66%	64%
Nurses 'Always' Communicated Well	(a)	73%	80%	79%
Pain 'Always' Well Controlled	(a)	74%	72%	71%
Room and Bathroom 'Always' Clean	(a)	76%	73%	73%
Timely Help 'Always' Received	(a)	64%	71%	68%
Would Definitely Recommend Hospital	(a)	65%	71%	71%
Use of Medical Imaging				
Cardiac Imaging Stress Test before Surgery[7]	-	-	4.5%	5.3%
Combination Abdominal CT Scan	267	2.2%	23%	10.5%
Combination Brain/Sinus CT Scan	325	0.3%	2.2%	2.7%
Combination Chest CT Scan	158	0.0%	5.1%	2.7%
Follow-up Mammogram/Ultrasound	307	18.6%	8.1%	8.8%
Lumbar Spine MRI for Low Back Pain[1]	-	-	39.9%	37.2%

Sayre Memorial Hospital

911 Hospital Drive
Sayre, OK 73662
Type: Acute Care Hospitals
Ownership: Voluntary non-profit - Private
Phone: 580-928-5541
Fax: 580-928-3523
Emergency Services: Yes
Beds: 46

Key Personnel:

Chairman/CEO . . . . Mike Blevins
CEO . . . . Brian Denton
Chief of Medical Staff . . . . Dr. Treva Graham, MD
Emergency Room . . . . Kenneth Whinery, MD

Measure	Cases	This Hosp.	State Avg.	U.S. Avg.
Blood Clot Prevention and Treatment				
Anticoagulation Overlap Therapy[2,7]	-	-	89%	93%
ICU Venous Thromboembolism Prophylaxis[2,7]	-	-	87%	92%
Incidence of Potentially Preventable VTE[2,7]	-	-	8%	10%
UFH with Dosages/Platelet Monitoring[2,7]	-	-	97%	97%
Venous Thromboembolism Prophylaxis[2]	155	11%	72%	85%
Warfarin Therapy Discharge Instructions[2,7]	-	-	73%	75%
Chest Pain/Possible Heart Attack Care				
Aspirin Given Within 24 Hours of Arrival	12	100%	95%	96%
Fibrinolytic Meds Within 30 Min. of Arrival[3,7]	-	-	54%	58%
Average Time to ECG (minutes)	12	23	8	7
Average Time to Transfer (minutes)[1,3]	-	-	77	60
Children's Asthma Care				
Received Home Management Plan of Care	-	-	-	88%
Received Reliever Medication	-	-	-	100%
Received Systemic Corticosteroids	-	-	-	100%
Emergency Department				
Admittance Decision Time (minutes)[2]	155	17	63	98
Head CT Results Within 45 Min. of Arrival[1]	-	-	49%	57%
Patients Who Left ER Before Being Seen	4,046	0%	2%	2%
Time from ER Arrival to Admit. (minutes)[2]	159	141	210	274
Time from ER Arrival to Discharge (minutes)	276	102	110	134
Time in ER Before Being Evaluated (minutes)	319	25	24	26
Time to Pain Meds for Fractures (minutes)[1,3]	-	-	55	57
Heart Attack Care				
Aspirin Given at Discharge[1,2]	-	-	99%	99%
Fibrinolytic Meds Within 30 Min. of Arrival[2,3]	-	-	25%	54%
PCI Within 90 Minutes of Arrival[2,3]	-	-	95%	96%
Statin Prescribed at Discharge[1,2]	-	-	98%	98%
Heart Failure Care				
ACE Inhibitor or ARB for LVSD[1,2]	-	-	95%	97%
Discharge Instructions Given[2]	11	91%	92%	94%
Evaluation of LVS Function[2]	18	67%	96%	99%
Medicare Spending				
Medicare Spending per Patient (ratio)	-	0.82	0.93	0.98
Pneumonia Care				

NOTE: Hospital profiles are in alphabetical order by state, then city, then hospital within the city; Rankings exclude hospitals with less than 25 cases except for patient surveys which excludes hospitals with less than 100 cases; (a) 100-299 cases; (1) The number of cases/patients is too few to report; (2) Data submitted were based on a sample of cases/patients; (3) Results are based on a shorter time period than required; (4) Data suppressed by CMS for one or more quarters; (5) Results are not available for this reporting period; (6) Fewer than 100 patients completed the HCAHPS survey; (7) No cases met the criteria for this measure; (8) The lower limit of the confidence interval cannot be calculated if the number of observed infections equals zero; (9) No data are available from the state/territory for this reporting period; (10) The scores shown reflect fewer than 50 completed surveys; (11) There were discrepancies in the data collection process; (12) This measure does not apply to this hospital for this reporting period; (13) Results cannot be calculated for this reporting period; (14) The results for this state are combined with nearby states to protect confidentiality; Please refer to the User's Guide for a full explanation of data.

Measure	Cases	This Hosp.	State Avg.	U.S. Avg.
Appropriate Initial Antibiotic Given[2]	14	50%	92%	95%
Blood Culture Timing[2]	11	36%	97%	98%
Pregnancy and Delivery Care				
Newborn Deliveries Scheduled Early[7]	-	-	8%	6%
Preventive Care				
Immunization for Influenza[2]	165	78%	89%	90%
Immunization for Pneumonia[2]	185	70%	91%	92%
Stroke Care				
Anticoagulation Therapy for Atrial Fibrillation[2,7]	-	-	91%	95%
Antithrombotic Therapy Timing[1,2]	-	-	95%	98%
Assessed for Rehabilitation[1,2]	-	-	96%	97%
Discharged on Antithrombotic Therapy[1,2]	-	-	98%	99%
Discharged on Statin Medication[1,2]	-	-	88%	94%
Thrombolytic Therapy Timing[1,2]	-	-	61%	66%
Venous Thromboembolism Prophylaxis[1,2]	-	-	92%	94%
Written Stroke Educational Materials Given[1,2]	-	-	86%	88%
Surgical Care Improvement Project				
Appropriate Beta Blocker Usage[5]	-	-	97%	98%
Appropriate VTP Within 24 Hours[5]	-	-	97%	98%
Controlled Postoperative Blood Glucose[5]	-	-	97%	97%
Perioperative Temperature Management[5]	-	-	100%	100%
Prophylactic Antibiotic Selection[5]	-	-	99%	99%
Prophylactic Antibiotic Selection (Outpatient)[5]	-	-	98%	98%
Prophylactic Antibiotic Stopped[5]	-	-	98%	98%
Prophylactic Antibiotic Timing[5]	-	-	98%	99%
Prophylactic Antibiotic Timing (Outpatient)[5]	-	-	98%	98%
Urinary Catheter Removal[5]	-	-	96%	97%
Survey of Patients' Hospital Experiences				
Area Around Room 'Always' Quiet at Night[10]	<100	78%	68%	61%
Doctors 'Always' Communicated Well[10]	<100	92%	84%	82%
Home Recovery Information Given[10]	<100	72%	84%	85%
Hospital Given 9 or 10 on 10 Point Scale[10]	<100	65%	72%	71%
Meds 'Always' Explained Before Given[10]	<100	63%	66%	64%
Nurses 'Always' Communicated Well[10]	<100	74%	80%	79%
Pain 'Always' Well Controlled[10]	<100	49%	72%	71%
Room and Bathroom 'Always' Clean[10]	<100	45%	73%	73%
Timely Help 'Always' Received[10]	<100	65%	71%	68%
Would Definitely Recommend Hospital[10]	<100	53%	71%	71%
Use of Medical Imaging				
Cardiac Imaging Stress Test before Surgery[7]	-	-	4.5%	5.3%
Combination Abdominal CT Scan	75	16.0%	23%	10.5%
Combination Brain/Sinus CT Scan[1]	-	-	2.2%	2.7%
Combination Chest CT Scan[1]	-	-	5.1%	2.7%
Follow-up Mammogram/Ultrasound[7]	-	-	8.1%	8.8%
Lumbar Spine MRI for Low Back Pain[1]	-	-	39.9%	37.2%

Seiling Community Hospital

Highway 60 & 281
Seiling, OK 73663
Type: Critical Access Hospitals
Ownership: Proprietary
Phone: 580-922-7361
Fax: 580-922-7718
Emergency Services: Yes
Beds: 18

Key Personnel:
CEO/President. . . . . Donald Buchanan

Measure	Cases	This Hosp.	State Avg.	U.S. Avg.
Blood Clot Prevention and Treatment				
Anticoagulation Overlap Therapy[3,7]	-	-	89%	93%
ICU Venous Thromboembolism Prophylaxis[3,7]	-	-	87%	92%
Incidence of Potentially Preventable VTE[3,7]	-	-	8%	10%
UFH with Dosages/Platelet Monitoring[3,7]	-	-	97%	97%
Venous Thromboembolism Prophylaxis[3,7]	-	-	72%	85%
Warfarin Therapy Discharge Instructions[3,7]	-	-	73%	75%
Chest Pain/Possible Heart Attack Care				
Aspirin Given Within 24 Hours of Arrival[5]	-	-	95%	96%
Fibrinolytic Meds Within 30 Min. of Arrival[5]	-	-	54%	58%
Average Time to ECG (minutes)[5]	-	-	8	7
Average Time to Transfer (minutes)[5]	-	-	77	60
Children's Asthma Care				
Received Home Management Plan of Care	-	-	-	88%
Received Reliever Medication	-	-	-	100%
Received Systemic Corticosteroids	-	-	-	100%
Emergency Department				
Admittance Decision Time (minutes)[5]	-	-	63	98
Head CT Results Within 45 Min. of Arrival[5]	-	-	49%	57%
Patients Who Left ER Before Being Seen[5]	-	-	2%	2%
Time from ER Arrival to Admit. (minutes)[5]	-	-	210	274
Time from ER Arrival to Discharge (minutes)[5]	-	-	110	134
Time in ER Before Being Evaluated (minutes)[5]	-	-	24	26
Time to Pain Meds for Fractures (minutes)[1,3]	-	-	55	57
Heart Attack Care				
Aspirin Given at Discharge[1,3]	-	-	99%	99%
Fibrinolytic Meds Within 30 Min. of Arrival[3,7]	-	-	25%	54%
PCI Within 90 Minutes of Arrival[3,7]	-	-	95%	96%
Statin Prescribed at Discharge[1,3]	-	-	98%	98%
Heart Failure Care				
ACE Inhibitor or ARB for LVSD[3,7]	-	-	95%	97%
Discharge Instructions Given[3,7]	-	-	92%	94%
Evaluation of LVS Function[1,3]	-	-	96%	99%
Medicare Spending				
Medicare Spending per Patient (ratio)	-	-	0.93	0.98
Pneumonia Care				
Appropriate Initial Antibiotic Given[1,3]	-	-	92%	95%
Blood Culture Timing[1,3]	-	-	97%	98%
Pregnancy and Delivery Care				
Newborn Deliveries Scheduled Early[5]	-	-	8%	6%
Preventive Care				
Immunization for Influenza[1,3]	-	-	89%	90%
Immunization for Pneumonia[1,3]	-	-	91%	92%
Stroke Care				
Anticoagulation Therapy for Atrial Fibrillation[2,3]	-	-	91%	95%
Antithrombotic Therapy Timing[1,2]	-	-	95%	98%
Assessed for Rehabilitation[1,2]	-	-	96%	97%
Discharged on Antithrombotic Therapy[1,2]	-	-	98%	99%
Discharged on Statin Medication[1,2]	-	-	88%	94%
Thrombolytic Therapy Timing[2,3]	-	-	61%	66%
Venous Thromboembolism Prophylaxis[1,2]	-	-	92%	94%
Written Stroke Educational Materials Given[2,3]	-	-	86%	88%
Surgical Care Improvement Project				
Appropriate Beta Blocker Usage[5]	-	-	97%	98%
Appropriate VTP Within 24 Hours[5]	-	-	97%	98%
Controlled Postoperative Blood Glucose[5]	-	-	97%	97%
Perioperative Temperature Management[5]	-	-	100%	100%
Prophylactic Antibiotic Selection[5]	-	-	99%	99%
Prophylactic Antibiotic Selection (Outpatient)[5]	-	-	98%	98%
Prophylactic Antibiotic Stopped[5]	-	-	98%	98%
Prophylactic Antibiotic Timing[5]	-	-	98%	99%
Prophylactic Antibiotic Timing (Outpatient)[5]	-	-	98%	98%
Urinary Catheter Removal[5]	-	-	96%	97%
Survey of Patients' Hospital Experiences				
Area Around Room 'Always' Quiet at Night[5]	-	-	68%	61%
Doctors 'Always' Communicated Well[5]	-	-	84%	82%
Home Recovery Information Given[5]	-	-	84%	85%
Hospital Given 9 or 10 on 10 Point Scale[5]	-	-	72%	71%
Meds 'Always' Explained Before Given[5]	-	-	66%	64%
Nurses 'Always' Communicated Well[5]	-	-	80%	79%
Pain 'Always' Well Controlled[5]	-	-	72%	71%
Room and Bathroom 'Always' Clean[5]	-	-	73%	73%
Timely Help 'Always' Received[5]	-	-	71%	68%
Would Definitely Recommend Hospital[5]	-	-	71%	71%
Use of Medical Imaging				
Cardiac Imaging Stress Test before Surgery[7]	-	-	4.5%	5.3%
Combination Abdominal CT Scan[1]	-	-	23%	10.5%
Combination Brain/Sinus CT Scan	37	0.0%	2.2%	2.7%
Combination Chest CT Scan[1]	-	-	5.1%	2.7%
Follow-up Mammogram/Ultrasound[7]	-	-	8.1%	8.8%
Lumbar Spine MRI for Low Back Pain[1]	-	-	39.9%	37.2%

Integris Seminole Medical Center

2401 Wrangler Boulevard
Seminole, OK 74868
URL: www.seminolemedicalcenter.com
Type: Acute Care Hospitals
Ownership: Proprietary
Phone: 405-303-4000
Fax: 405-303-4150
Emergency Services: Yes
Beds: 32

Key Personnel:
Patient Relations . . . . Darlene Cornelious
Emergency Room . . . . Mark Macklin, RN
Chief of Medical Staff. . . . . Rodney McCrory
Infection Control. . . . . Troy Sainder, RN
CEO . . . . Jimmy D. Stuart
Quality Assurance . . . . Brenda Swanson
Operating Room. . . . . Dana Taylor, RNFA

Measure	Cases	This Hosp.	State Avg.	U.S. Avg.
Blood Clot Prevention and Treatment				
Anticoagulation Overlap Therapy[1,2]	-	-	89%	93%
ICU Venous Thromboembolism Prophylaxis[2,7]	-	-	87%	92%
Incidence of Potentially Preventable VTE[2,7]	-	-	8%	10%
UFH with Dosages/Platelet Monitoring[1,2]	-	-	97%	97%
Venous Thromboembolism Prophylaxis[2]	149	63%	72%	85%
Warfarin Therapy Discharge Instructions[1,2]	-	-	73%	75%
Chest Pain/Possible Heart Attack Care				
Aspirin Given Within 24 Hours of Arrival	67	96%	95%	96%
Fibrinolytic Meds Within 30 Min. of Arrival[1]	-	-	54%	58%
Average Time to ECG (minutes)	72	8	8	7
Average Time to Transfer (minutes)[1]	-	-	77	60
Children's Asthma Care				
Received Home Management Plan of Care	-	-	-	88%
Received Reliever Medication	-	-	-	100%
Received Systemic Corticosteroids	-	-	-	100%
Emergency Department				
Admittance Decision Time (minutes)[2]	470	55	63	98
Head CT Results Within 45 Min. of Arrival[1]	-	-	49%	57%
Patients Who Left ER Before Being Seen	11,089	1%	2%	2%
Time from ER Arrival to Admit. (minutes)[2]	499	196	210	274
Time from ER Arrival to Discharge (minutes)	340	88	110	134
Time in ER Before Being Evaluated (minutes)	352	15	24	26
Time to Pain Meds for Fractures (minutes)	48	52	55	57
Heart Attack Care				
Aspirin Given at Discharge[1,3]	-	-	99%	99%
Fibrinolytic Meds Within 30 Min. of Arrival[3,7]	-	-	25%	54%
PCI Within 90 Minutes of Arrival[3,7]	-	-	95%	96%
Statin Prescribed at Discharge[1,3]	-	-	98%	98%
Heart Failure Care				
ACE Inhibitor or ARB for LVSD[1]	-	-	95%	97%
Discharge Instructions Given	34	53%	92%	94%
Evaluation of LVS Function	37	84%	96%	99%
Medicare Spending				
Medicare Spending per Patient (ratio)	-	1.07	0.93	0.98
Pneumonia Care				
Appropriate Initial Antibiotic Given	28	82%	92%	95%
Blood Culture Timing	41	90%	97%	98%
Pregnancy and Delivery Care				
Newborn Deliveries Scheduled Early[7]	-	-	8%	6%
Preventive Care				
Immunization for Influenza[2]	251	98%	89%	90%
Immunization for Pneumonia[2]	460	96%	91%	92%
Stroke Care				
Anticoagulation Therapy for Atrial Fibrillation[1]	-	-	91%	95%
Antithrombotic Therapy Timing[1]	-	-	95%	98%
Assessed for Rehabilitation[1]	-	-	96%	97%
Discharged on Antithrombotic Therapy[1]	-	-	98%	99%
Discharged on Statin Medication[1]	-	-	88%	94%
Thrombolytic Therapy Timing[1]	-	-	61%	66%
Venous Thromboembolism Prophylaxis[1]	-	-	92%	94%
Written Stroke Educational Materials Given[7]	-	-	86%	88%
Surgical Care Improvement Project				
Appropriate Beta Blocker Usage[1,3]	-	-	97%	98%
Appropriate VTP Within 24 Hours[1,3]	-	-	97%	98%
Controlled Postoperative Blood Glucose[3,7]	-	-	97%	97%
Perioperative Temperature Management[1,3]	-	-	100%	100%
Prophylactic Antibiotic Selection[1,3]	-	-	99%	99%
Prophylactic Antibiotic Selection (Outpatient)[1,3]	-	-	98%	98%
Prophylactic Antibiotic Stopped[1,3]	-	-	98%	98%
Prophylactic Antibiotic Timing[1,3]	-	-	98%	99%
Prophylactic Antibiotic Timing (Outpatient)[1,3]	-	-	98%	98%
Urinary Catheter Removal[1,3]	-	-	96%	97%
Survey of Patients' Hospital Experiences				
Area Around Room 'Always' Quiet at Night	(a)	69%	68%	61%
Doctors 'Always' Communicated Well	(a)	84%	84%	82%
Home Recovery Information Given	(a)	83%	84%	85%

NOTE: Hospital profiles are in alphabetical order by state, then city, then hospital within the city; Rankings exclude hospitals with less than 25 cases except for patient surveys which excludes hospitals with less than 100 cases; (a) 100-299 cases; (1) The number of cases/patients is too few to report; (2) Data submitted were based on a sample of cases/patients; (3) Results are based on a shorter time period than required; (4) Data suppressed by CMS for one or more quarters; (5) Results are not available for this reporting period; (6) Fewer than 100 patients completed the HCAHPS survey; (7) No cases met the criteria for this measure; (8) The lower limit of the confidence interval cannot be calculated if the number of observed infections equals zero; (9) No data are available from the state/territory for this reporting period; (10) The scores shown reflect fewer than 50 completed surveys; (11) There were discrepancies in the data collection process; (12) This measure does not apply to this hospital for this reporting period; (13) Results cannot be calculated for this reporting period; (14) The results for this state are combined with nearby states to protect confidentiality; Please refer to the User's Guide for a full explanation of data.

Measure	Cases	This Hosp.	State Avg.	U.S. Avg.
Hospital Given 9 or 10 on 10 Point Scale	(a)	69%	72%	71%
Meds 'Always' Explained Before Given	(a)	59%	66%	64%
Nurses 'Always' Communicated Well	(a)	77%	80%	79%
Pain 'Always' Well Controlled	(a)	71%	72%	71%
Room and Bathroom 'Always' Clean	(a)	85%	73%	73%
Timely Help 'Always' Received	(a)	65%	71%	68%
Would Definitely Recommend Hospital	(a)	65%	71%	71%
Use of Medical Imaging				
Cardiac Imaging Stress Test before Surgery[1]	-	-	4.5%	5.3%
Combination Abdominal CT Scan	233	29.6%	23%	10.5%
Combination Brain/Sinus CT Scan	225	0.9%	2.2%	2.7%
Combination Chest CT Scan	90	6.7%	5.1%	2.7%
Follow-up Mammogram/Ultrasound	326	5.8%	8.1%	8.8%
Lumbar Spine MRI for Low Back Pain[1]	-	-	39.9%	37.2%

Newman Memorial Hospital

905 South Main Street
Shattuck, OK 73858
Phone: 580-938-2551
Fax: 580-938-2309
Type: Acute Care Hospitals
Emergency Services: Yes
Ownership: Govt - Hospital Dist/Auth
Beds: 27

Key Personnel:
Surgery .... Brad Bunch, RRT, RN, RNFA
Anesthesiology.............. Greg Farrar, CRNA
Operating Room.............. Brenda Huenergardt
Radiology................... Nikki Ray, RT(R)
CEO .... Jeffery D. Shelton
Infection Control........... Gwen Stafford, RN

Measure	Cases	This Hosp.	State Avg.	U.S. Avg.
Blood Clot Prevention and Treatment				
Anticoagulation Overlap Therapy[7]	-	-	89%	93%
ICU Venous Thromboembolism Prophylaxis[7]	-	-	87%	92%
Incidence of Potentially Preventable VTE[7]	-	-	8%	10%
UFH with Dosages/Platelet Monitoring[7]	-	-	97%	97%
Venous Thromboembolism Prophylaxis	81	41%	72%	85%
Warfarin Therapy Discharge Instructions[7]	-	-	73%	75%
Chest Pain/Possible Heart Attack Care				
Aspirin Given Within 24 Hours of Arrival[1]	-	-	95%	96%
Fibrinolytic Meds Within 30 Min. of Arrival[3,7]	-	-	54%	58%
Average Time to ECG (minutes)[1]	-	-	8	7
Average Time to Transfer (minutes)[1,3]	-	-	77	60
Children's Asthma Care				
Received Home Management Plan of Care	-	-	-	88%
Received Reliever Medication	-	-	-	100%
Received Systemic Corticosteroids	-	-	-	100%
Emergency Department				
Admittance Decision Time (minutes)	107	50	63	98
Head CT Results Within 45 Min. of Arrival[1,3]	-	-	49%	57%
Patients Who Left ER Before Being Seen	3,125	5%	2%	2%
Time from ER Arrival to Admit. (minutes)	109	234	210	274
Time from ER Arrival to Discharge (minutes)	274	100	110	134
Time in ER Before Being Evaluated (minutes)	215	42	24	26
Time to Pain Meds for Fractures (minutes)	12	37	55	57
Heart Attack Care				
Aspirin Given at Discharge[3,7]	-	-	99%	99%
Fibrinolytic Meds Within 30 Min. of Arrival[3,7]	-	-	25%	54%
PCI Within 90 Minutes of Arrival[3,7]	-	-	95%	96%
Statin Prescribed at Discharge[3,7]	-	-	98%	98%
Heart Failure Care				
ACE Inhibitor or ARB for LVSD[1]	-	-	95%	97%
Discharge Instructions Given[1]	-	-	92%	94%
Evaluation of LVS Function[1]	-	-	96%	99%
Medicare Spending				
Medicare Spending per Patient (ratio)	-	0.70	0.93	0.98
Pneumonia Care				
Appropriate Initial Antibiotic Given	11	82%	92%	95%
Blood Culture Timing[1]	-	-	97%	98%
Pregnancy and Delivery Care				
Newborn Deliveries Scheduled Early	13	31%	8%	6%
Preventive Care				
Immunization for Influenza	159	58%	89%	90%
Immunization for Pneumonia	139	81%	91%	92%
Stroke Care				
Anticoagulation Therapy for Atrial Fibrillation[3,7]	-	-	91%	95%
Antithrombotic Therapy Timing[3,7]	-	-	95%	98%
Assessed for Rehabilitation[3,7]	-	-	96%	97%
Discharged on Antithrombotic Therapy[3,7]	-	-	98%	99%
Discharged on Statin Medication[3,7]	-	-	88%	94%
Thrombolytic Therapy Timing[1,3]	-	-	61%	66%
Venous Thromboembolism Prophylaxis[3,7]	-	-	92%	94%
Written Stroke Educational Materials Given[3,7]	-	-	86%	88%
Surgical Care Improvement Project				
Appropriate Beta Blocker Usage[1,3]	-	-	97%	98%
Appropriate VTP Within 24 Hours[1,3]	-	-	97%	98%
Controlled Postoperative Blood Glucose[3,7]	-	-	97%	97%
Perioperative Temperature Management[1,3]	-	-	100%	100%
Prophylactic Antibiotic Selection[1,3]	-	-	99%	99%
Prophylactic Antibiotic Selection (Outpatient)[5]	-	-	98%	98%
Prophylactic Antibiotic Stopped[1,3]	-	-	98%	98%
Prophylactic Antibiotic Timing[1,3]	-	-	98%	99%
Prophylactic Antibiotic Timing (Outpatient)[5]	-	-	98%	98%
Urinary Catheter Removal[1,3]	-	-	96%	97%
Survey of Patients' Hospital Experiences				
Area Around Room 'Always' Quiet at Night[6]	<100	75%	68%	61%
Doctors 'Always' Communicated Well[6]	<100	86%	84%	82%
Home Recovery Information Given[6]	<100	82%	84%	85%
Hospital Given 9 or 10 on 10 Point Scale[6]	<100	76%	72%	71%
Meds 'Always' Explained Before Given[6]	<100	74%	66%	64%
Nurses 'Always' Communicated Well[6]	<100	82%	80%	79%
Pain 'Always' Well Controlled[6]	<100	71%	72%	71%
Room and Bathroom 'Always' Clean[6]	<100	77%	73%	73%
Timely Help 'Always' Received[6]	<100	70%	71%	68%
Would Definitely Recommend Hospital[6]	<100	77%	71%	71%
Use of Medical Imaging				
Cardiac Imaging Stress Test before Surgery[7]	-	-	4.5%	5.3%
Combination Abdominal CT Scan	63	68.3%	23%	10.5%
Combination Brain/Sinus CT Scan[1]	-	-	2.2%	2.7%
Combination Chest CT Scan[1]	-	-	5.1%	2.7%
Follow-up Mammogram/Ultrasound	112	8.9%	8.1%	8.8%
Lumbar Spine MRI for Low Back Pain[1]	-	-	39.9%	37.2%

Saint Anthony Shawnee Hospital

1102 W Macarthur
Shawnee, OK 74804
Phone: 405-273-2270
E-mail: info@uhcenter.com
URL: www.unityhealthcenter.com
Type: Acute Care Hospitals
Emergency Services: Yes
Ownership: Voluntary non-profit - Private

Key Personnel:
Chief of Medical Staff.......... Linda E Brown
CEO/President................... Charles E Skillings

Measure	Cases	This Hosp.	State Avg.	U.S. Avg.
Blood Clot Prevention and Treatment				
Anticoagulation Overlap Therapy[2]	25	92%	89%	93%
ICU Venous Thromboembolism Prophylaxis[2]	94	98%	87%	92%
Incidence of Potentially Preventable VTE[1,2]	-	-	8%	10%
UFH with Dosages/Platelet Monitoring[1,2]	-	-	97%	97%
Venous Thromboembolism Prophylaxis[2]	270	97%	72%	85%
Warfarin Therapy Discharge Instructions[2]	21	95%	73%	75%
Chest Pain/Possible Heart Attack Care				
Aspirin Given Within 24 Hours of Arrival	92	100%	95%	96%
Fibrinolytic Meds Within 30 Min. of Arrival	23	87%	54%	58%
Average Time to ECG (minutes)	95	1	8	7
Average Time to Transfer (minutes)[1]	-	-	77	60
Children's Asthma Care				
Received Home Management Plan of Care	-	-	-	88%
Received Reliever Medication	-	-	-	100%
Received Systemic Corticosteroids	-	-	-	100%
Emergency Department				
Admittance Decision Time (minutes)[2]	502	60	63	98
Head CT Results Within 45 Min. of Arrival	15	60%	49%	57%
Patients Who Left ER Before Being Seen	37,769	2%	2%	2%
Time from ER Arrival to Admit. (minutes)[2]	511	190	210	274
Time from ER Arrival to Discharge (minutes)	413	104	110	134
Time in ER Before Being Evaluated (minutes)	463	23	24	26
Time to Pain Meds for Fractures (minutes)	165	51	55	57
Heart Attack Care				
Aspirin Given at Discharge	53	100%	99%	99%
Fibrinolytic Meds Within 30 Min. of Arrival[7]	-	-	25%	54%
PCI Within 90 Minutes of Arrival[7]	-	-	95%	96%
Statin Prescribed at Discharge	47	100%	98%	98%
Heart Failure Care				
ACE Inhibitor or ARB for LVSD	65	100%	95%	97%
Discharge Instructions Given	151	99%	92%	94%
Evaluation of LVS Function	188	100%	96%	99%
Medicare Spending				
Medicare Spending per Patient (ratio)	-	1.00	0.93	0.98
Pneumonia Care				
Appropriate Initial Antibiotic Given	101	100%	92%	95%
Blood Culture Timing	252	100%	97%	98%
Pregnancy and Delivery Care				
Newborn Deliveries Scheduled Early	97	1%	8%	6%
Preventive Care				
Immunization for Influenza[2]	451	97%	89%	90%
Immunization for Pneumonia[2]	556	97%	91%	92%
Stroke Care				
Anticoagulation Therapy for Atrial Fibrillation[1]	-	-	91%	95%
Antithrombotic Therapy Timing	33	91%	95%	98%
Assessed for Rehabilitation	31	97%	96%	97%
Discharged on Antithrombotic Therapy	31	100%	98%	99%
Discharged on Statin Medication	26	88%	88%	94%
Thrombolytic Therapy Timing[1]	-	-	61%	66%
Venous Thromboembolism Prophylaxis	31	94%	92%	94%
Written Stroke Educational Materials Given	16	100%	86%	88%
Surgical Care Improvement Project				
Appropriate Beta Blocker Usage	29	100%	97%	98%
Appropriate VTP Within 24 Hours	164	98%	97%	98%
Controlled Postoperative Blood Glucose[7]	-	-	97%	97%
Perioperative Temperature Management	197	100%	100%	100%
Prophylactic Antibiotic Selection	128	100%	99%	99%
Prophylactic Antibiotic Selection (Outpatient)	65	98%	98%	98%
Prophylactic Antibiotic Stopped	128	100%	98%	98%
Prophylactic Antibiotic Timing	128	99%	98%	99%
Prophylactic Antibiotic Timing (Outpatient)	67	97%	98%	98%
Urinary Catheter Removal	90	100%	96%	97%
Survey of Patients' Hospital Experiences				
Area Around Room 'Always' Quiet at Night	300+	67%	68%	61%
Doctors 'Always' Communicated Well	300+	85%	84%	82%
Home Recovery Information Given	300+	85%	84%	85%
Hospital Given 9 or 10 on 10 Point Scale	300+	73%	72%	71%
Meds 'Always' Explained Before Given	300+	69%	66%	64%
Nurses 'Always' Communicated Well	300+	82%	80%	79%
Pain 'Always' Well Controlled	300+	74%	72%	71%
Room and Bathroom 'Always' Clean	300+	81%	73%	73%
Timely Help 'Always' Received	300+	72%	71%	68%
Would Definitely Recommend Hospital	300+	71%	71%	71%
Use of Medical Imaging				
Cardiac Imaging Stress Test before Surgery[7]	-	-	4.5%	5.3%
Combination Abdominal CT Scan	622	20.1%	23%	10.5%
Combination Brain/Sinus CT Scan	832	1.4%	2.2%	2.7%
Combination Chest CT Scan	199	1.5%	5.1%	2.7%
Follow-up Mammogram/Ultrasound	354	7.3%	8.1%	8.8%
Lumbar Spine MRI for Low Back Pain	46	34.8%	39.9%	37.2%

Haskell County Community Hospital

401 Northwest H Street
Stigler, OK 74462
Phone: 918-967-4682
Type: Critical Access Hospitals
Emergency Services: Yes
Ownership: Govt - Hospital Dist/Auth

Measure	Cases	This Hosp.	State Avg.	U.S. Avg.
Blood Clot Prevention and Treatment				
Anticoagulation Overlap Therapy[5]	-	-	89%	93%
ICU Venous Thromboembolism Prophylaxis[5]	-	-	87%	92%
Incidence of Potentially Preventable VTE[5]	-	-	8%	10%
UFH with Dosages/Platelet Monitoring[5]	-	-	97%	97%
Venous Thromboembolism Prophylaxis[5]	-	-	72%	85%
Warfarin Therapy Discharge Instructions[5]	-	-	73%	75%
Chest Pain/Possible Heart Attack Care				
Aspirin Given Within 24 Hours of Arrival[3]	19	89%	95%	96%
Fibrinolytic Meds Within 30 Min. of Arrival[3,7]	-	-	54%	58%

NOTE: Hospital profiles are in alphabetical order by state, then city, then hospital within the city; Rankings exclude hospitals with less than 25 cases except for patient surveys which excludes hospitals with less than 100 cases; (a) 100-299 cases; (1) The number of cases/patients is too few to report; (2) Data submitted were based on a sample of cases/patients; (3) Results are based on a shorter time period than required; (4) Data suppressed by CMS for one or more quarters; (5) Results are not available for this reporting period; (6) Fewer than 100 patients completed the HCAHPS survey; (7) No cases met the criteria for this measure; (8) The lower limit of the confidence interval cannot be calculated if the number of observed infections equals zero; (9) No data are available from the state/territory for this reporting period; (10) The scores shown reflect fewer than 50 completed surveys; (11) There were discrepancies in the data collection process; (12) This measure does not apply to this hospital for this reporting period; (13) Results cannot be calculated for this reporting period; (14) The results for this state are combined with nearby states to protect confidentiality; Please refer to the User's Guide for a full explanation of data.

Measure	Cases	This Hosp.	State Avg.	U.S. Avg.
Average Time to ECG (minutes)[3]	18	30	8	7
Average Time to Transfer (minutes)[1,3]	-	-	77	60
Children's Asthma Care				
Received Home Management Plan of Care	-	-	-	88%
Received Reliever Medication	-	-	-	100%
Received Systemic Corticosteroids	-	-	-	100%
Emergency Department				
Admittance Decision Time (minutes)[5]	-	-	63	98
Head CT Results Within 45 Min. of Arrival[1,3]	-	-	49%	57%
Patients Who Left ER Before Being Seen[5]	-	-	2%	2%
Time from ER Arrival to Admit. (minutes)[5]	-	-	210	274
Time from ER Arrival to Discharge (minutes)[5]	-	-	110	134
Time in ER Before Being Evaluated (minutes)[5]	-	-	24	26
Time to Pain Meds for Fractures (minutes)[1,3]	-	-	55	57
Heart Attack Care				
Aspirin Given at Discharge[5]	-	-	99%	99%
Fibrinolytic Meds Within 30 Min. of Arrival[5]	-	-	25%	54%
PCI Within 90 Minutes of Arrival[5]	-	-	95%	96%
Statin Prescribed at Discharge[5]	-	-	98%	98%
Heart Failure Care				
ACE Inhibitor or ARB for LVSD[3,7]	-	-	95%	97%
Discharge Instructions Given[3,7]	-	-	92%	94%
Evaluation of LVS Function[3,7]	-	-	96%	99%
Medicare Spending				
Medicare Spending per Patient (ratio)		-	0.93	0.98
Pneumonia Care				
Appropriate Initial Antibiotic Given[3,7]	-	-	92%	95%
Blood Culture Timing[3,7]	-	-	97%	98%
Pregnancy and Delivery Care				
Newborn Deliveries Scheduled Early[5]	-	-	8%	6%
Preventive Care				
Immunization for Influenza[5]	-	-	89%	90%
Immunization for Pneumonia[5]	-	-	91%	92%
Stroke Care				
Anticoagulation Therapy for Atrial Fibrillation[5]	-	-	91%	95%
Antithrombotic Therapy Timing[5]	-	-	95%	98%
Assessed for Rehabilitation[5]	-	-	96%	97%
Discharged on Antithrombotic Therapy[5]	-	-	98%	99%
Discharged on Statin Medication[5]	-	-	88%	94%
Thrombolytic Therapy Timing[5]	-	-	61%	66%
Venous Thromboembolism Prophylaxis[5]	-	-	92%	94%
Written Stroke Educational Materials Given[5]	-	-	86%	88%
Surgical Care Improvement Project				
Appropriate Beta Blocker Usage[5]	-	-	97%	98%
Appropriate VTP Within 24 Hours[5]	-	-	97%	98%
Controlled Postoperative Blood Glucose[5]	-	-	97%	97%
Perioperative Temperature Management[5]	-	-	100%	100%
Prophylactic Antibiotic Selection[5]	-	-	99%	99%
Prophylactic Antibiotic Selection (Outpatient)[5]	-	-	98%	98%
Prophylactic Antibiotic Stopped[5]	-	-	98%	98%
Prophylactic Antibiotic Timing[5]	-	-	98%	99%
Prophylactic Antibiotic Timing (Outpatient)[5]	-	-	98%	98%
Urinary Catheter Removal[5]	-	-	96%	97%
Survey of Patients' Hospital Experiences				
Area Around Room 'Always' Quiet at Night[5]	-	-	68%	61%
Doctors 'Always' Communicated Well[5]	-	-	84%	82%
Home Recovery Information Given[5]	-	-	84%	85%
Hospital Given 9 or 10 on 10 Point Scale[5]	-	-	72%	71%
Meds 'Always' Explained Before Given[5]	-	-	66%	64%
Nurses 'Always' Communicated Well[5]	-	-	80%	79%
Pain 'Always' Well Controlled[5]	-	-	72%	71%
Room and Bathroom 'Always' Clean[5]	-	-	73%	73%
Timely Help 'Always' Received[5]	-	-	71%	68%
Would Definitely Recommend Hospital[5]	-	-	71%	71%
Use of Medical Imaging				
Cardiac Imaging Stress Test before Surgery[7]	-	-	4.5%	5.3%
Combination Abdominal CT Scan	106	0.0%	23%	10.5%
Combination Brain/Sinus CT Scan[1]	-	-	2.2%	2.7%
Combination Chest CT Scan[1]	-	-	5.1%	2.7%
Follow-up Mammogram/Ultrasound	71	14.1%	8.1%	8.8%
Lumbar Spine MRI for Low Back Pain[1]	-	-	39.9%	37.2%

Stillwater Medical Center

1323 West 6th Street
Stillwater, OK 74076
Phone: 405-372-1480
Fax: 405-372-9552
E-mail: info@stillwater-medical.org
URL: www.stillwater-medical.org
Type: Acute Care Hospitals
Emergency Services: Yes
Ownership: Govt - Hospital Dist/Auth
Beds: 128

Key Personnel:

Chairman/CEO .... Lowell Barto
Radiology.................. J Bullen
Chief of Medical Staff.......... Karen Hendren
CEO/President.............. Jerry Moeller
Patient Relations .... Bonnie Peterson
Quality Assurance .... Cheryl Wilkinson

Measure	Cases	This Hosp.	State Avg.	U.S. Avg.
Blood Clot Prevention and Treatment				
Anticoagulation Overlap Therapy[2]	16	100%	89%	93%
ICU Venous Thromboembolism Prophylaxis[2]	55	87%	87%	92%
Incidence of Potentially Preventable VTE[1,2]	-	-	8%	10%
UFH with Dosages/Platelet Monitoring[2,7]	-	-	97%	97%
Venous Thromboembolism Prophylaxis[2]	229	87%	72%	85%
Warfarin Therapy Discharge Instructions[2]	15	80%	73%	75%
Chest Pain/Possible Heart Attack Care				
Aspirin Given Within 24 Hours of Arrival	48	98%	95%	96%
Fibrinolytic Meds Within 30 Min. of Arrival[1]	-	-	54%	58%
Average Time to ECG (minutes)	50	6	8	7
Average Time to Transfer (minutes)[1]	-	-	77	60
Children's Asthma Care				
Received Home Management Plan of Care	-	-	-	88%
Received Reliever Medication	-	-	-	100%
Received Systemic Corticosteroids	-	-	-	100%
Emergency Department				
Admittance Decision Time (minutes)[2]	408	55	63	98
Head CT Results Within 45 Min. of Arrival	18	78%	49%	57%
Patients Who Left ER Before Being Seen	27,936	4%	2%	2%
Time from ER Arrival to Admit. (minutes)[2]	411	184	210	274
Time from ER Arrival to Discharge (minutes)	402	132	110	134
Time in ER Before Being Evaluated (minutes)	423	31	24	26
Time to Pain Meds for Fractures (minutes)	107	61	55	57
Heart Attack Care				
Aspirin Given at Discharge	56	100%	99%	99%
Fibrinolytic Meds Within 30 Min. of Arrival[7]	-	-	25%	54%
PCI Within 90 Minutes of Arrival	17	100%	95%	96%
Statin Prescribed at Discharge	60	100%	98%	98%
Heart Failure Care				
ACE Inhibitor or ARB for LVSD	34	88%	95%	97%
Discharge Instructions Given	75	100%	92%	94%
Evaluation of LVS Function	100	99%	96%	99%
Medicare Spending				
Medicare Spending per Patient (ratio)		1.02	0.93	0.98
Pneumonia Care				
Appropriate Initial Antibiotic Given	110	95%	92%	95%
Blood Culture Timing	160	99%	97%	98%
Pregnancy and Delivery Care				
Newborn Deliveries Scheduled Early[2]	115	0%	8%	6%
Preventive Care				
Immunization for Influenza[2]	434	97%	89%	90%
Immunization for Pneumonia[2]	402	98%	91%	92%
Stroke Care				
Anticoagulation Therapy for Atrial Fibrillation[1]	-	-	91%	95%
Antithrombotic Therapy Timing	28	93%	95%	98%
Assessed for Rehabilitation	26	96%	96%	97%
Discharged on Antithrombotic Therapy	25	92%	98%	99%
Discharged on Statin Medication	24	92%	88%	94%
Thrombolytic Therapy Timing[7]	-	-	61%	66%
Venous Thromboembolism Prophylaxis	28	82%	92%	94%
Written Stroke Educational Materials Given[1]	-	-	86%	88%
Surgical Care Improvement Project				
Appropriate Beta Blocker Usage	129	98%	97%	98%
Appropriate VTP Within 24 Hours	364	99%	97%	98%
Controlled Postoperative Blood Glucose[7]	-	-	97%	97%
Perioperative Temperature Management	391	99%	100%	100%
Prophylactic Antibiotic Selection	302	100%	99%	99%
Prophylactic Antibiotic Selection (Outpatient)	117	97%	98%	98%
Prophylactic Antibiotic Stopped	299	99%	98%	98%
Prophylactic Antibiotic Timing	302	98%	98%	99%
Prophylactic Antibiotic Timing (Outpatient)	118	97%	98%	98%
Urinary Catheter Removal	272	99%	96%	97%
Survey of Patients' Hospital Experiences				
Area Around Room 'Always' Quiet at Night	300+	66%	68%	61%
Doctors 'Always' Communicated Well	300+	83%	84%	82%
Home Recovery Information Given	300+	90%	84%	85%
Hospital Given 9 or 10 on 10 Point Scale	300+	78%	72%	71%
Meds 'Always' Explained Before Given	300+	65%	66%	64%
Nurses 'Always' Communicated Well	300+	82%	80%	79%
Pain 'Always' Well Controlled	300+	74%	72%	71%
Room and Bathroom 'Always' Clean	300+	76%	73%	73%
Timely Help 'Always' Received	300+	70%	71%	68%
Would Definitely Recommend Hospital	300+	78%	71%	71%
Use of Medical Imaging				
Cardiac Imaging Stress Test before Surgery	557	2.2%	4.5%	5.3%
Combination Abdominal CT Scan	646	25.5%	23%	10.5%
Combination Brain/Sinus CT Scan	545	0.7%	2.2%	2.7%
Combination Chest CT Scan	244	8.6%	5.1%	2.7%
Follow-up Mammogram/Ultrasound	955	4.0%	8.1%	8.8%
Lumbar Spine MRI for Low Back Pain	52	34.6%	39.9%	37.2%

Memorial Hospital of Stilwell

1401 West Locust
Stilwell, OK 74960
Phone: 918-696-3101
Fax: 918-696-3388
URL: www.stilwellmemorialhospital.com
Type: Acute Care Hospitals
Emergency Services: Yes
Ownership: Voluntary non-profit - Private
Beds: 50

Key Personnel:

CEO/President............... Alan L Adams

Measure	Cases	This Hosp.	State Avg.	U.S. Avg.
Blood Clot Prevention and Treatment				
Anticoagulation Overlap Therapy[1,2]	-	-	89%	93%
ICU Venous Thromboembolism Prophylaxis[2,7]	-	-	87%	92%
Incidence of Potentially Preventable VTE[1,2]	-	-	8%	10%
UFH with Dosages/Platelet Monitoring[2,7]	-	-	97%	97%
Venous Thromboembolism Prophylaxis[2]	175	75%	72%	85%
Warfarin Therapy Discharge Instructions[1,2]	-	-	73%	75%
Chest Pain/Possible Heart Attack Care				
Aspirin Given Within 24 Hours of Arrival	17	71%	95%	96%
Fibrinolytic Meds Within 30 Min. of Arrival[1]	-	-	54%	58%
Average Time to ECG (minutes)	19	15	8	7
Average Time to Transfer (minutes)[1]	-	-	77	60
Children's Asthma Care				
Received Home Management Plan of Care	-	-	-	88%
Received Reliever Medication	-	-	-	100%
Received Systemic Corticosteroids	-	-	-	100%
Emergency Department				
Admittance Decision Time (minutes)[2]	222	21	63	98
Head CT Results Within 45 Min. of Arrival[1]	-	-	49%	57%
Patients Who Left ER Before Being Seen	8,205	2%	2%	2%
Time from ER Arrival to Admit. (minutes)[2]	282	134	210	274
Time from ER Arrival to Discharge (minutes)	350	106	110	134
Time in ER Before Being Evaluated (minutes)	388	66	24	26
Time to Pain Meds for Fractures (minutes)	32	83	55	57
Heart Attack Care				
Aspirin Given at Discharge[1,2]	-	-	99%	99%
Fibrinolytic Meds Within 30 Min. of Arrival[2,3]	-	-	25%	54%
PCI Within 90 Minutes of Arrival[2,3]	-	-	95%	96%
Statin Prescribed at Discharge[1,2]	-	-	98%	98%
Heart Failure Care				
ACE Inhibitor or ARB for LVSD[2]	15	93%	95%	97%
Discharge Instructions Given[2]	31	87%	92%	94%
Evaluation of LVS Function[2]	41	93%	96%	99%
Medicare Spending				
Medicare Spending per Patient (ratio)	-	0.81	0.93	0.98
Pneumonia Care				
Appropriate Initial Antibiotic Given[2]	38	95%	92%	95%
Blood Culture Timing[2]	17	100%	97%	98%
Pregnancy and Delivery Care				
Newborn Deliveries Scheduled Early[2]	13	0%	8%	6%
Preventive Care				

NOTE: Hospital profiles are in alphabetical order by state, then city, then hospital within the city; Rankings exclude hospitals with less than 25 cases except for patient surveys which excludes hospitals with less than 100 cases; (a) 100-299 cases; (1) The number of cases/patients is too few to report; (2) Data submitted were based on a sample of cases/patients; (3) Results are based on a shorter time period than required; (4) Data suppressed by CMS for one or more quarters; (5) Results are not available for this reporting period; (6) Fewer than 100 patients completed the HCAHPS survey; (7) No cases met the criteria for this measure; (8) The lower limit of the confidence interval cannot be calculated if the number of observed infections equals zero; (9) No data are available from the state/territory for this reporting period; (10) The scores shown reflect fewer than 50 completed surveys; (11) There were discrepancies in the data collection process; (12) This measure does not apply to this hospital for this reporting period; (13) Results cannot be calculated for this reporting period; (14) The results for this state are combined with nearby states to protect confidentiality; Please refer to the User's Guide for a full explanation of data.

Measure	Cases	This Hosp.	State Avg.	U.S. Avg.
Immunization for Influenza[2]	319	97%	89%	90%
Immunization for Pneumonia[2]	341	98%	91%	92%
Stroke Care				
Anticoagulation Therapy for Atrial Fibrillation[1,2]	-	-	91%	95%
Antithrombotic Therapy Timing[1,2]	-	-	95%	98%
Assessed for Rehabilitation[1,2]	-	-	96%	97%
Discharged on Antithrombotic Therapy[1,2]	-	-	98%	99%
Discharged on Statin Medication[1,2]	-	-	88%	94%
Thrombolytic Therapy Timing[1,2]	-	-	61%	66%
Venous Thromboembolism Prophylaxis[1,2]	-	-	92%	94%
Written Stroke Educational Materials Given[1,2]	-	-	86%	88%
Surgical Care Improvement Project				
Appropriate Beta Blocker Usage[1,2]	-	-	97%	98%
Appropriate VTP Within 24 Hours[2,3]	13	100%	97%	98%
Controlled Postoperative Blood Glucose[2,3]	-	-	97%	97%
Perioperative Temperature Management[2,3]	15	100%	100%	100%
Prophylactic Antibiotic Selection[2,3]	15	100%	99%	99%
Prophylactic Antibiotic Selection (Outpatient)[1,3]	-	-	98%	98%
Prophylactic Antibiotic Stopped[2,3]	15	100%	98%	98%
Prophylactic Antibiotic Timing[2,3]	15	100%	98%	99%
Prophylactic Antibiotic Timing (Outpatient)[1,3]	-	-	98%	98%
Urinary Catheter Removal[1,2]	-	-	96%	97%
Survey of Patients' Hospital Experiences				
Area Around Room 'Always' Quiet at Night	(a)	64%	68%	61%
Doctors 'Always' Communicated Well	(a)	87%	84%	82%
Home Recovery Information Given	(a)	82%	84%	85%
Hospital Given 9 or 10 on 10 Point Scale	(a)	59%	72%	71%
Meds 'Always' Explained Before Given	(a)	63%	66%	64%
Nurses 'Always' Communicated Well	(a)	74%	80%	79%
Pain 'Always' Well Controlled	(a)	69%	72%	71%
Room and Bathroom 'Always' Clean	(a)	73%	73%	73%
Timely Help 'Always' Received	(a)	66%	71%	68%
Would Definitely Recommend Hospital	(a)	57%	71%	71%
Use of Medical Imaging				
Cardiac Imaging Stress Test before Surgery[7]	-	-	4.5%	5.3%
Combination Abdominal CT Scan	88	0.0%	23%	10.5%
Combination Brain/Sinus CT Scan[1]	-	-	2.2%	2.7%
Combination Chest CT Scan[1]	-	-	5.1%	2.7%
Follow-up Mammogram/Ultrasound[7]	-	-	8.1%	8.8%
Lumbar Spine MRI for Low Back Pain[1]	-	-	39.9%	37.2%

Stroud Regional Medical Center

2308 Highway 66 West
Stroud, OK 74079
Phone: 918-968-3571
Fax: 918-968-4814
Type: Critical Access Hospitals
Emergency Services: Yes
Ownership: Voluntary non-profit - Private
Beds: 25

Key Personnel:

Intensive Care Unit. . . . . Donna Buchanan
Quality Assurance . . . . Donna Buchanan
Chief of Medical Staff . . . . Ken Darvin, MD
Emergency Room . . . . Tammy McElroy
Radiology. . . . . Brenda McGinnis
Anesthesiology. . . . . Monica McKinney
CEO/President. . . . . Regina Peters
Infection Control. . . . . Linda Wolff

Measure	Cases	This Hosp.	State Avg.	U.S. Avg.
Blood Clot Prevention and Treatment				
Anticoagulation Overlap Therapy[5]	-	-	89%	93%
ICU Venous Thromboembolism Prophylaxis[5]	-	-	87%	92%
Incidence of Potentially Preventable VTE[5]	-	-	8%	10%
UFH with Dosages/Platelet Monitoring[5]	-	-	97%	97%
Venous Thromboembolism Prophylaxis[5]	-	-	72%	85%
Warfarin Therapy Discharge Instructions[5]	-	-	73%	75%
Chest Pain/Possible Heart Attack Care				
Aspirin Given Within 24 Hours of Arrival[1,3]	-	-	95%	96%
Fibrinolytic Meds Within 30 Min. of Arrival[3,7]	-	-	54%	58%
Average Time to ECG (minutes)[1,3]	-	-	8	7
Average Time to Transfer (minutes)[3,7]	-	-	77	60
Children's Asthma Care				
Received Home Management Plan of Care	-	-	-	88%
Received Reliever Medication	-	-	-	100%
Received Systemic Corticosteroids	-	-	-	100%
Emergency Department				
Admittance Decision Time (minutes)[5]	-	-	63	98
Head CT Results Within 45 Min. of Arrival[5]	-	-	49%	57%
Patients Who Left ER Before Being Seen[5]	-	-	2%	2%
Time from ER Arrival to Admit. (minutes)[5]	-	-	210	274
Time from ER Arrival to Discharge (minutes)[5]	-	-	110	134
Time in ER Before Being Evaluated (minutes)[5]	-	-	24	26
Time to Pain Meds for Fractures (minutes)[5]	-	-	55	57
Heart Attack Care				
Aspirin Given at Discharge[5]	-	-	99%	99%
Fibrinolytic Meds Within 30 Min. of Arrival[5]	-	-	25%	54%
PCI Within 90 Minutes of Arrival[5]	-	-	95%	96%
Statin Prescribed at Discharge[5]	-	-	98%	98%
Heart Failure Care				
ACE Inhibitor or ARB for LVSD[1,3]	-	-	95%	97%
Discharge Instructions Given[1,3]	-	-	92%	94%
Evaluation of LVS Function[1,3]	-	-	96%	99%
Medicare Spending				
Medicare Spending per Patient (ratio)	-	-	0.93	0.98
Pneumonia Care				
Appropriate Initial Antibiotic Given[1,2]	-	-	92%	95%
Blood Culture Timing[1,2]	-	-	97%	98%
Pregnancy and Delivery Care				
Newborn Deliveries Scheduled Early[5]	-	-	8%	6%
Preventive Care				
Immunization for Influenza[5]	-	-	89%	90%
Immunization for Pneumonia[5]	-	-	91%	92%
Stroke Care				
Anticoagulation Therapy for Atrial Fibrillation[5]	-	-	91%	95%
Antithrombotic Therapy Timing[5]	-	-	95%	98%
Assessed for Rehabilitation[5]	-	-	96%	97%
Discharged on Antithrombotic Therapy[5]	-	-	98%	99%
Discharged on Statin Medication[5]	-	-	88%	94%
Thrombolytic Therapy Timing[5]	-	-	61%	66%
Venous Thromboembolism Prophylaxis[5]	-	-	92%	94%
Written Stroke Educational Materials Given[5]	-	-	86%	88%
Surgical Care Improvement Project				
Appropriate Beta Blocker Usage[5]	-	-	97%	98%
Appropriate VTP Within 24 Hours[5]	-	-	97%	98%
Controlled Postoperative Blood Glucose[5]	-	-	97%	97%
Perioperative Temperature Management[5]	-	-	100%	100%
Prophylactic Antibiotic Selection[5]	-	-	99%	99%
Prophylactic Antibiotic Selection (Outpatient)[5]	-	-	98%	98%
Prophylactic Antibiotic Stopped[5]	-	-	98%	98%
Prophylactic Antibiotic Timing[5]	-	-	98%	99%
Prophylactic Antibiotic Timing (Outpatient)[5]	-	-	98%	98%
Urinary Catheter Removal[5]	-	-	96%	97%
Survey of Patients' Hospital Experiences				
Area Around Room 'Always' Quiet at Night[5]	-	-	68%	61%
Doctors 'Always' Communicated Well[5]	-	-	84%	82%
Home Recovery Information Given[5]	-	-	84%	85%
Hospital Given 9 or 10 on 10 Point Scale[5]	-	-	72%	71%
Meds 'Always' Explained Before Given[5]	-	-	66%	64%
Nurses 'Always' Communicated Well[5]	-	-	80%	79%
Pain 'Always' Well Controlled[5]	-	-	72%	71%
Room and Bathroom 'Always' Clean[5]	-	-	73%	73%
Timely Help 'Always' Received[5]	-	-	71%	68%
Would Definitely Recommend Hospital[5]	-	-	71%	71%
Use of Medical Imaging				
Cardiac Imaging Stress Test before Surgery[7]	-	-	4.5%	5.3%
Combination Abdominal CT Scan	80	2.5%	23%	10.5%
Combination Brain/Sinus CT Scan[1]	-	-	2.2%	2.7%
Combination Chest CT Scan[1]	-	-	5.1%	2.7%
Follow-up Mammogram/Ultrasound[7]	-	-	8.1%	8.8%
Lumbar Spine MRI for Low Back Pain[7]	-	-	39.9%	37.2%

Arbuckle Memorial Hospital

2011 West Broadway
Sulphur, OK 73086
Phone: 580-622-2161
Fax: 580-622-2763
E-mail: webmaster@arbucklehospital.com
URL: www.arbucklehospital.com
Type: Critical Access Hospitals
Emergency Services: Yes
Ownership: Voluntary non-profit - Other
Beds: 25

Key Personnel:

Chief of Medical Staff . . . . Atonio Lee, MD

Measure	Cases	This Hosp.	State Avg.	U.S. Avg.
Blood Clot Prevention and Treatment				
Anticoagulation Overlap Therapy[5]	-	-	89%	93%
ICU Venous Thromboembolism Prophylaxis[5]	-	-	87%	92%
Incidence of Potentially Preventable VTE[5]	-	-	8%	10%
UFH with Dosages/Platelet Monitoring[5]	-	-	97%	97%
Venous Thromboembolism Prophylaxis[5]	-	-	72%	85%
Warfarin Therapy Discharge Instructions[5]	-	-	73%	75%
Chest Pain/Possible Heart Attack Care				
Aspirin Given Within 24 Hours of Arrival	33	94%	95%	96%
Fibrinolytic Meds Within 30 Min. of Arrival[3,7]	-	-	54%	58%
Average Time to ECG (minutes)	31	10	8	7
Average Time to Transfer (minutes)[3,7]	-	-	77	60
Children's Asthma Care				
Received Home Management Plan of Care	-	-	-	88%
Received Reliever Medication	-	-	-	100%
Received Systemic Corticosteroids	-	-	-	100%
Emergency Department				
Admittance Decision Time (minutes)[5]	-	-	63	98
Head CT Results Within 45 Min. of Arrival[1]	-	-	49%	57%
Patients Who Left ER Before Being Seen[5]	-	-	2%	2%
Time from ER Arrival to Admit. (minutes)[5]	-	-	210	274
Time from ER Arrival to Discharge (minutes)[5]	-	-	110	134
Time in ER Before Being Evaluated (minutes)[5]	-	-	24	26
Time to Pain Meds for Fractures (minutes)[5]	-	-	55	57
Heart Attack Care				
Aspirin Given at Discharge[3,7]	-	-	99%	99%
Fibrinolytic Meds Within 30 Min. of Arrival[3,7]	-	-	25%	54%
PCI Within 90 Minutes of Arrival[3,7]	-	-	95%	96%
Statin Prescribed at Discharge[1,3]	-	-	98%	98%
Heart Failure Care				
ACE Inhibitor or ARB for LVSD[1]	-	-	95%	97%
Discharge Instructions Given[1]	-	-	92%	94%
Evaluation of LVS Function[1]	-	-	96%	99%
Medicare Spending				
Medicare Spending per Patient (ratio)	-	-	0.93	0.98
Pneumonia Care				
Appropriate Initial Antibiotic Given	43	98%	92%	95%
Blood Culture Timing	45	98%	97%	98%
Pregnancy and Delivery Care				
Newborn Deliveries Scheduled Early[5]	-	-	8%	6%
Preventive Care				
Immunization for Influenza[5]	-	-	89%	90%
Immunization for Pneumonia[5]	-	-	91%	92%
Stroke Care				
Anticoagulation Therapy for Atrial Fibrillation[5]	-	-	91%	95%
Antithrombotic Therapy Timing[5]	-	-	95%	98%
Assessed for Rehabilitation[5]	-	-	96%	97%
Discharged on Antithrombotic Therapy[5]	-	-	98%	99%
Discharged on Statin Medication[5]	-	-	88%	94%
Thrombolytic Therapy Timing[5]	-	-	61%	66%
Venous Thromboembolism Prophylaxis[5]	-	-	92%	94%
Written Stroke Educational Materials Given[5]	-	-	86%	88%
Surgical Care Improvement Project				
Appropriate Beta Blocker Usage[5]	-	-	97%	98%
Appropriate VTP Within 24 Hours[5]	-	-	97%	98%
Controlled Postoperative Blood Glucose[5]	-	-	97%	97%
Perioperative Temperature Management[5]	-	-	100%	100%
Prophylactic Antibiotic Selection[5]	-	-	99%	99%
Prophylactic Antibiotic Selection (Outpatient)[5]	-	-	98%	98%
Prophylactic Antibiotic Stopped[5]	-	-	98%	98%
Prophylactic Antibiotic Timing[5]	-	-	98%	99%
Prophylactic Antibiotic Timing (Outpatient)[5]	-	-	98%	98%
Urinary Catheter Removal[5]	-	-	96%	97%
Survey of Patients' Hospital Experiences				
Area Around Room 'Always' Quiet at Night[5]	-	-	68%	61%
Doctors 'Always' Communicated Well[5]	-	-	84%	82%
Home Recovery Information Given[5]	-	-	84%	85%
Hospital Given 9 or 10 on 10 Point Scale[5]	-	-	72%	71%
Meds 'Always' Explained Before Given[5]	-	-	66%	64%
Nurses 'Always' Communicated Well[5]	-	-	80%	79%
Pain 'Always' Well Controlled[5]	-	-	72%	71%

NOTE: Hospital profiles are in alphabetical order by state, then city, then hospital within the city; Rankings exclude hospitals with less than 25 cases except for patient surveys which excludes hospitals with less than 100 cases; (a) 100-299 cases; (1) The number of cases/patients is too few to report; (2) Data submitted were based on a sample of cases/patients; (3) Results are based on a shorter time period than required; (4) Data suppressed by CMS for one or more quarters; (5) Results are not available for this reporting period; (6) Fewer than 100 patients completed the HCAHPS survey; (7) No cases met the criteria for this measure; (8) The lower limit of the confidence interval cannot be calculated if the number of observed infections equals zero; (9) No data are available from the state/territory for this reporting period; (10) The scores shown reflect fewer than 50 completed surveys; (11) There were discrepancies in the data collection process; (12) This measure does not apply to this hospital for this reporting period; (13) Results cannot be calculated for this reporting period; (14) The results for this state are combined with nearby states to protect confidentiality; Please refer to the User's Guide for a full explanation of data.

Measure	Cases	This Hosp.	State Avg.	U.S. Avg.
Room and Bathroom 'Always' Clean[5]	-	-	73%	73%
Timely Help 'Always' Received[5]	-	-	71%	68%
Would Definitely Recommend Hospital[5]	-	-	71%	71%
Use of Medical Imaging				
Cardiac Imaging Stress Test before Surgery[7]	-	-	4.5%	5.3%
Combination Abdominal CT Scan	173	13.3%	23%	10.5%
Combination Brain/Sinus CT Scan[1]	-	-	2.2%	2.7%
Combination Chest CT Scan	108	2.8%	5.1%	2.7%
Follow-up Mammogram/Ultrasound[7]	-	-	8.1%	8.8%
Lumbar Spine MRI for Low Back Pain[7]	-	-	39.9%	37.2%

Tahlequah City Hospital

1400 East Downing Street
Tahlequah, OK 74465
Phone: 918-456-0641
Fax: 918-456-8886
Type: Acute Care Hospitals
Emergency Services: Yes
Ownership: Govt - Hospital Dist/Auth
Beds: 82

Key Personnel:
Emergency Room .... John Galdamez, DO
Quality Assurance .... Gloria Hoover
CEO/President............... Gary L Jepson
Anesthesiology.............. M Adele King, DO
Chief of Medical Staff.......... Herbert Littleton, DO
Infection Control............... Cheri Olgesbee, RN
Radiology.................... Mark Whitley, MD

Measure	Cases	This Hosp.	State Avg.	U.S. Avg.
Blood Clot Prevention and Treatment				
Anticoagulation Overlap Therapy[2]	22	100%	89%	93%
ICU Venous Thromboembolism Prophylaxis[2]	87	82%	87%	92%
Incidence of Potentially Preventable VTE[1,2]	-	-	8%	10%
UFH with Dosages/Platelet Monitoring[2]	11	100%	97%	97%
Venous Thromboembolism Prophylaxis[2]	171	68%	72%	85%
Warfarin Therapy Discharge Instructions[2]	16	31%	73%	75%
Chest Pain/Possible Heart Attack Care				
Aspirin Given Within 24 Hours of Arrival	20	95%	95%	96%
Fibrinolytic Meds Within 30 Min. of Arrival[3,7]	-	-	54%	58%
Average Time to ECG (minutes)	20	5	8	7
Average Time to Transfer (minutes)[1,3]	-	-	77	60
Children's Asthma Care				
Received Home Management Plan of Care	-	-	-	88%
Received Reliever Medication	-	-	-	100%
Received Systemic Corticosteroids	-	-	-	100%
Emergency Department				
Admittance Decision Time (minutes)[2]	271	55	63	98
Head CT Results Within 45 Min. of Arrival[1]	-	-	49%	57%
Patients Who Left ER Before Being Seen	24,422	2%	2%	2%
Time from ER Arrival to Admit. (minutes)[2]	277	212	210	274
Time from ER Arrival to Discharge (minutes)	372	116	110	134
Time in ER Before Being Evaluated (minutes)	315	27	24	26
Time to Pain Meds for Fractures (minutes)	82	40	55	57
Heart Attack Care				
Aspirin Given at Discharge	58	100%	99%	99%
Fibrinolytic Meds Within 30 Min. of Arrival[1]	-	-	25%	54%
PCI Within 90 Minutes of Arrival[1]	-	-	95%	96%
Statin Prescribed at Discharge	57	84%	98%	98%
Heart Failure Care				
ACE Inhibitor or ARB for LVSD	42	93%	95%	97%
Discharge Instructions Given	88	70%	92%	94%
Evaluation of LVS Function	107	100%	96%	99%
Medicare Spending				
Medicare Spending per Patient (ratio)	-	0.94	0.93	0.98
Pneumonia Care				
Appropriate Initial Antibiotic Given[2]	77	92%	92%	95%
Blood Culture Timing[2]	175	98%	97%	98%
Pregnancy and Delivery Care				
Newborn Deliveries Scheduled Early[2]	34	0%	8%	6%
Preventive Care				
Immunization for Influenza[2]	348	92%	89%	90%
Immunization for Pneumonia[2]	414	93%	91%	92%
Stroke Care				
Anticoagulation Therapy for Atrial Fibrillation[1]	-	-	91%	95%
Antithrombotic Therapy Timing	26	92%	95%	98%
Assessed for Rehabilitation	29	93%	96%	97%
Discharged on Antithrombotic Therapy	26	96%	98%	99%
Discharged on Statin Medication	23	78%	88%	94%
Thrombolytic Therapy Timing[7]	-	-	61%	66%
Venous Thromboembolism Prophylaxis	25	76%	92%	94%
Written Stroke Educational Materials Given	16	19%	86%	88%
Surgical Care Improvement Project				
Appropriate Beta Blocker Usage	122	98%	97%	98%
Appropriate VTP Within 24 Hours	257	95%	97%	98%
Controlled Postoperative Blood Glucose	50	90%	97%	97%
Perioperative Temperature Management	320	100%	100%	100%
Prophylactic Antibiotic Selection	303	99%	99%	99%
Prophylactic Antibiotic Selection (Outpatient)	58	98%	98%	98%
Prophylactic Antibiotic Stopped	298	97%	98%	98%
Prophylactic Antibiotic Timing	303	97%	98%	99%
Prophylactic Antibiotic Timing (Outpatient)	59	98%	98%	98%
Urinary Catheter Removal	287	97%	96%	97%
Survey of Patients' Hospital Experiences				
Area Around Room 'Always' Quiet at Night	300+	52%	68%	61%
Doctors 'Always' Communicated Well	300+	76%	84%	82%
Home Recovery Information Given	300+	82%	84%	85%
Hospital Given 9 or 10 on 10 Point Scale	300+	63%	72%	71%
Meds 'Always' Explained Before Given	300+	59%	66%	64%
Nurses 'Always' Communicated Well	300+	72%	80%	79%
Pain 'Always' Well Controlled	300+	59%	72%	71%
Room and Bathroom 'Always' Clean	300+	58%	73%	73%
Timely Help 'Always' Received	300+	60%	71%	68%
Would Definitely Recommend Hospital	300+	65%	71%	71%
Use of Medical Imaging				
Cardiac Imaging Stress Test before Surgery	1,011	2.4%	4.5%	5.3%
Combination Abdominal CT Scan	631	18.4%	23%	10.5%
Combination Brain/Sinus CT Scan	577	1.2%	2.2%	2.7%
Combination Chest CT Scan	209	23.4%	5.1%	2.7%
Follow-up Mammogram/Ultrasound	538	7.1%	8.1%	8.8%
Lumbar Spine MRI for Low Back Pain	148	37.8%	39.9%	37.2%

W W Hastings Indian Hospital

100 S Bliss Avenue
Tahlequah, OK 74464
Phone: 918-458-3100
Fax: 918-458-3262
URL: www.ihs.gov
Type: Acute Care Hospitals
Emergency Services: Yes
Ownership: Voluntary non-profit - Other
Beds: 58

Key Personnel:
Quality Assurance .... James Clevenger
CEO/President............... Edwin McLemore

Measure	Cases	This Hosp.	State Avg.	U.S. Avg.
Blood Clot Prevention and Treatment				
Anticoagulation Overlap Therapy[1,2]	-	-	89%	93%
ICU Venous Thromboembolism Prophylaxis[2]	57	96%	87%	92%
Incidence of Potentially Preventable VTE[1,2]	-	-	8%	10%
UFH with Dosages/Platelet Monitoring[2,7]	-	-	97%	97%
Venous Thromboembolism Prophylaxis[2]	111	86%	72%	85%
Warfarin Therapy Discharge Instructions[1,2]	-	-	73%	75%
Chest Pain/Possible Heart Attack Care				
Aspirin Given Within 24 Hours of Arrival	-	-	95%	96%
Fibrinolytic Meds Within 30 Min. of Arrival	-	-	54%	58%
Average Time to ECG (minutes)	-	-	8	7
Average Time to Transfer (minutes)	-	-	77	60
Children's Asthma Care				
Received Home Management Plan of Care	-	-	-	88%
Received Reliever Medication	-	-	-	100%
Received Systemic Corticosteroids	-	-	-	100%
Emergency Department				
Admittance Decision Time (minutes)[2]	169	86	63	98
Head CT Results Within 45 Min. of Arrival	-	-	49%	57%
Patients Who Left ER Before Being Seen	-	-	2%	2%
Time from ER Arrival to Admit. (minutes)[2]	264	312	210	274
Time from ER Arrival to Discharge (minutes)	-	-	110	134
Time in ER Before Being Evaluated (minutes)	-	-	24	26
Time to Pain Meds for Fractures (minutes)	-	-	55	57
Heart Attack Care				
Aspirin Given at Discharge[1,3]	-	-	99%	99%
Fibrinolytic Meds Within 30 Min. of Arrival[3,7]	-	-	25%	54%
PCI Within 90 Minutes of Arrival[3,7]	-	-	95%	96%
Statin Prescribed at Discharge[1,3]	-	-	98%	98%
Heart Failure Care				
ACE Inhibitor or ARB for LVSD[1]	-	-	95%	97%
Discharge Instructions Given	13	100%	92%	94%
Evaluation of LVS Function	14	86%	96%	99%
Medicare Spending				
Medicare Spending per Patient (ratio)	-	0.92	0.93	0.98
Pneumonia Care				
Appropriate Initial Antibiotic Given	52	87%	92%	95%
Blood Culture Timing	61	87%	97%	98%
Pregnancy and Delivery Care				
Newborn Deliveries Scheduled Early	136	0%	8%	6%
Preventive Care				
Immunization for Influenza[2]	289	58%	89%	90%
Immunization for Pneumonia[2]	270	72%	91%	92%
Stroke Care				
Anticoagulation Therapy for Atrial Fibrillation[5]	-	-	91%	95%
Antithrombotic Therapy Timing[5]	-	-	95%	98%
Assessed for Rehabilitation[5]	-	-	96%	97%
Discharged on Antithrombotic Therapy[5]	-	-	98%	99%
Discharged on Statin Medication[5]	-	-	88%	94%
Thrombolytic Therapy Timing[5]	-	-	61%	66%
Venous Thromboembolism Prophylaxis[5]	-	-	92%	94%
Written Stroke Educational Materials Given[5]	-	-	86%	88%
Surgical Care Improvement Project				
Appropriate Beta Blocker Usage[2]	13	77%	97%	98%
Appropriate VTP Within 24 Hours[2]	75	96%	97%	98%
Controlled Postoperative Blood Glucose[2,7]	-	-	97%	97%
Perioperative Temperature Management[2]	92	97%	100%	100%
Prophylactic Antibiotic Selection[2]	61	98%	99%	99%
Prophylactic Antibiotic Selection (Outpatient)	-	-	98%	98%
Prophylactic Antibiotic Stopped[2]	60	93%	98%	98%
Prophylactic Antibiotic Timing[2]	61	93%	98%	99%
Prophylactic Antibiotic Timing (Outpatient)	-	-	98%	98%
Urinary Catheter Removal[2]	22	50%	96%	97%
Survey of Patients' Hospital Experiences				
Area Around Room 'Always' Quiet at Night	300+	60%	68%	61%
Doctors 'Always' Communicated Well	300+	81%	84%	82%
Home Recovery Information Given	300+	81%	84%	85%
Hospital Given 9 or 10 on 10 Point Scale	300+	66%	72%	71%
Meds 'Always' Explained Before Given	300+	68%	66%	64%
Nurses 'Always' Communicated Well	300+	79%	80%	79%
Pain 'Always' Well Controlled	300+	69%	72%	71%
Room and Bathroom 'Always' Clean	300+	74%	73%	73%
Timely Help 'Always' Received	300+	70%	71%	68%
Would Definitely Recommend Hospital	300+	65%	71%	71%
Use of Medical Imaging				
Cardiac Imaging Stress Test before Surgery	-	-	4.5%	5.3%
Combination Abdominal CT Scan	-	-	23%	10.5%
Combination Brain/Sinus CT Scan	-	-	2.2%	2.7%
Combination Chest CT Scan	-	-	5.1%	2.7%
Follow-up Mammogram/Ultrasound	-	-	8.1%	8.8%
Lumbar Spine MRI for Low Back Pain	-	-	39.9%	37.2%

Choctaw Nation Healthcare

1 Choctaw Way
Talihina, OK 74571
Phone: 918-567-7000
Fax: 918-567-7026
URL: www.choctawnationhealth.com
Type: Acute Care Hospitals
Emergency Services: Yes
Ownership: Government - Federal
Beds: 37

Key Personnel:
Chief of Medical Staff.......... Dr Thomas Bonien
Patient Relations .... Maggie Hayes
Surgery .... Antoine Jumelle, MD
Pediatric Ambulatory Care ...... Valerie Taylor, LPN
Quality Assurance .... David Wharton

Measure	Cases	This Hosp.	State Avg.	U.S. Avg.
Blood Clot Prevention and Treatment				
Anticoagulation Overlap Therapy[1,2]	-	-	89%	93%
ICU Venous Thromboembolism Prophylaxis[1,2]	-	-	87%	92%
Incidence of Potentially Preventable VTE[2,7]	-	-	8%	10%
UFH with Dosages/Platelet Monitoring[2,7]	-	-	97%	97%
Venous Thromboembolism Prophylaxis[2]	111	20%	72%	85%
Warfarin Therapy Discharge Instructions[1,2]	-	-	73%	75%
Chest Pain/Possible Heart Attack Care				

NOTE: Hospital profiles are in alphabetical order by state, then city, then hospital within the city; Rankings exclude hospitals with less than 25 cases except for patient surveys which excludes hospitals with less than 100 cases; (a) 100-299 cases; (1) The number of cases/patients is too few to report; (2) Data submitted were based on a sample of cases/patients; (3) Results are based on a shorter time period than required; (4) Data suppressed by CMS for one or more quarters; (5) Results are not available for this reporting period; (6) Fewer than 100 patients completed the HCAHPS survey; (7) No cases met the criteria for this measure; (8) The lower limit of the confidence interval cannot be calculated if the number of observed infections equals zero; (9) No data are available from the state/territory for this reporting period; (10) The scores shown reflect fewer than 50 completed surveys; (11) There were discrepancies in the data collection process; (12) This measure does not apply to this hospital for this reporting period; (13) Results cannot be calculated for this reporting period; (14) The results for this state are combined with nearby states to protect confidentiality; Please refer to the User's Guide for a full explanation of data.

Measure	Cases	This Hosp.	State Avg.	U.S. Avg.
Aspirin Given Within 24 Hours of Arrival	-	-	95%	96%
Fibrinolytic Meds Within 30 Min. of Arrival	-	-	54%	58%
Average Time to ECG (minutes)	-	-	8	7
Average Time to Transfer (minutes)	-	-	77	60
Children's Asthma Care				
Received Home Management Plan of Care	-	-	-	88%
Received Reliever Medication	-	-	-	100%
Received Systemic Corticosteroids	-	-	-	100%
Emergency Department				
Admittance Decision Time (minutes)[2]	346	35	63	98
Head CT Results Within 45 Min. of Arrival	-	-	49%	57%
Patients Who Left ER Before Being Seen	-	-	2%	2%
Time from ER Arrival to Admit. (minutes)[2]	412	202	210	274
Time from ER Arrival to Discharge (minutes)	-	-	110	134
Time in ER Before Being Evaluated (minutes)	-	-	24	26
Time to Pain Meds for Fractures (minutes)	-	-	55	57
Heart Attack Care				
Aspirin Given at Discharge[1,3]	-	-	99%	99%
Fibrinolytic Meds Within 30 Min. of Arrival[3,7]	-	-	25%	54%
PCI Within 90 Minutes of Arrival[3,7]	-	-	95%	96%
Statin Prescribed at Discharge[1,3]	-	-	98%	98%
Heart Failure Care				
ACE Inhibitor or ARB for LVSD[1]	-	-	95%	97%
Discharge Instructions Given[1]	-	-	92%	94%
Evaluation of LVS Function	11	100%	96%	99%
Medicare Spending				
Medicare Spending per Patient (ratio)	-	0.81	0.93	0.98
Pneumonia Care				
Appropriate Initial Antibiotic Given	21	95%	92%	95%
Blood Culture Timing	25	88%	97%	98%
Pregnancy and Delivery Care				
Newborn Deliveries Scheduled Early[2]	121	14%	8%	6%
Preventive Care				
Immunization for Influenza[2]	363	48%	89%	90%
Immunization for Pneumonia[2]	286	91%	91%	92%
Stroke Care				
Anticoagulation Therapy for Atrial Fibrillation[3,7]	-	-	91%	95%
Antithrombotic Therapy Timing[1,3]	-	-	95%	98%
Assessed for Rehabilitation[1,3]	-	-	96%	97%
Discharged on Antithrombotic Therapy[1,3]	-	-	98%	99%
Discharged on Statin Medication[1,3]	-	-	88%	94%
Thrombolytic Therapy Timing[3,7]	-	-	61%	66%
Venous Thromboembolism Prophylaxis[1,3]	-	-	92%	94%
Written Stroke Educational Materials Given[1,3]	-	-	86%	88%
Surgical Care Improvement Project				
Appropriate Beta Blocker Usage[1]	-	-	97%	98%
Appropriate VTP Within 24 Hours	13	100%	97%	98%
Controlled Postoperative Blood Glucose[7]	-	-	97%	97%
Perioperative Temperature Management	43	100%	100%	100%
Prophylactic Antibiotic Selection	40	75%	99%	99%
Prophylactic Antibiotic Selection (Outpatient)	-	-	98%	98%
Prophylactic Antibiotic Stopped	40	100%	98%	98%
Prophylactic Antibiotic Timing	43	88%	98%	99%
Prophylactic Antibiotic Timing (Outpatient)	-	-	98%	98%
Urinary Catheter Removal[1]	-	-	96%	97%
Survey of Patients' Hospital Experiences				
Area Around Room 'Always' Quiet at Night	300+	75%	68%	61%
Doctors 'Always' Communicated Well	300+	85%	84%	82%
Home Recovery Information Given	300+	86%	84%	85%
Hospital Given 9 or 10 on 10 Point Scale	300+	83%	72%	71%
Meds 'Always' Explained Before Given	300+	76%	66%	64%
Nurses 'Always' Communicated Well	300+	86%	80%	79%
Pain 'Always' Well Controlled	300+	75%	72%	71%
Room and Bathroom 'Always' Clean	300+	79%	73%	73%
Timely Help 'Always' Received	300+	82%	71%	68%
Would Definitely Recommend Hospital	300+	84%	71%	71%
Use of Medical Imaging				
Cardiac Imaging Stress Test before Surgery	-	-	4.5%	5.3%
Combination Abdominal CT Scan	-	-	23%	10.5%
Combination Brain/Sinus CT Scan	-	-	2.2%	2.7%
Combination Chest CT Scan	-	-	5.1%	2.7%
Follow-up Mammogram/Ultrasound	-	-	8.1%	8.8%
Lumbar Spine MRI for Low Back Pain	-	-	39.9%	37.2%

Mercy Hospital Tishomingo

1000 South Byrd
Tishomingo, OK 73460
Phone: 580-371-2327
Fax: 580-371-2127
Type: Critical Access Hospitals
Emergency Services: Yes
Ownership: Voluntary non-profit - Church
Beds: 25

Key Personnel:
Operating Room. . . . . Carol Hewitt, RN
Infection Control. . . . . Carolyn Pearson, RN
Chief of Medical Staff. . . . . Richard H Tidwell, MD

Measure	Cases	This Hosp.	State Avg.	U.S. Avg.
Blood Clot Prevention and Treatment				
Anticoagulation Overlap Therapy[5]	-	-	89%	93%
ICU Venous Thromboembolism Prophylaxis[5]	-	-	87%	92%
Incidence of Potentially Preventable VTE[5]	-	-	8%	10%
UFH with Dosages/Platelet Monitoring[5]	-	-	97%	97%
Venous Thromboembolism Prophylaxis[5]	-	-	72%	85%
Warfarin Therapy Discharge Instructions[5]	-	-	73%	75%
Chest Pain/Possible Heart Attack Care				
Aspirin Given Within 24 Hours of Arrival[1,3]	-	-	95%	96%
Fibrinolytic Meds Within 30 Min. of Arrival[1,3]	-	-	54%	58%
Average Time to ECG (minutes)[1,3]	-	-	8	7
Average Time to Transfer (minutes)[3,7]	-	-	77	60
Children's Asthma Care				
Received Home Management Plan of Care	-	-	-	88%
Received Reliever Medication	-	-	-	100%
Received Systemic Corticosteroids	-	-	-	100%
Emergency Department				
Admittance Decision Time (minutes)[5]	-	-	63	98
Head CT Results Within 45 Min. of Arrival[5]	-	-	49%	57%
Patients Who Left ER Before Being Seen[5]	-	-	2%	2%
Time from ER Arrival to Admit. (minutes)[5]	-	-	210	274
Time from ER Arrival to Discharge (minutes)[5]	-	-	110	134
Time in ER Before Being Evaluated (minutes)[5]	-	-	24	26
Time to Pain Meds for Fractures (minutes)[5]	-	-	55	57
Heart Attack Care				
Aspirin Given at Discharge[5]	-	-	99%	99%
Fibrinolytic Meds Within 30 Min. of Arrival[5]	-	-	25%	54%
PCI Within 90 Minutes of Arrival[5]	-	-	95%	96%
Statin Prescribed at Discharge[5]	-	-	98%	98%
Heart Failure Care				
ACE Inhibitor or ARB for LVSD[1,3]	-	-	95%	97%
Discharge Instructions Given[1,3]	-	-	92%	94%
Evaluation of LVS Function[3]	14	71%	96%	99%
Medicare Spending				
Medicare Spending per Patient (ratio)	-	-	0.93	0.98
Pneumonia Care				
Appropriate Initial Antibiotic Given[1,3]	-	-	92%	95%
Blood Culture Timing[1,3]	-	-	97%	98%
Pregnancy and Delivery Care				
Newborn Deliveries Scheduled Early[5]	-	-	8%	6%
Preventive Care				
Immunization for Influenza[5]	-	-	89%	90%
Immunization for Pneumonia[5]	-	-	91%	92%
Stroke Care				
Anticoagulation Therapy for Atrial Fibrillation[5]	-	-	91%	95%
Antithrombotic Therapy Timing[5]	-	-	95%	98%
Assessed for Rehabilitation[5]	-	-	96%	97%
Discharged on Antithrombotic Therapy[5]	-	-	98%	99%
Discharged on Statin Medication[5]	-	-	88%	94%
Thrombolytic Therapy Timing[5]	-	-	61%	66%
Venous Thromboembolism Prophylaxis[5]	-	-	92%	94%
Written Stroke Educational Materials Given[5]	-	-	86%	88%
Surgical Care Improvement Project				
Appropriate Beta Blocker Usage[5]	-	-	97%	98%
Appropriate VTP Within 24 Hours[5]	-	-	97%	98%
Controlled Postoperative Blood Glucose[5]	-	-	97%	97%
Perioperative Temperature Management[5]	-	-	100%	100%
Prophylactic Antibiotic Selection[5]	-	-	99%	99%
Prophylactic Antibiotic Selection (Outpatient)[5]	-	-	98%	98%
Prophylactic Antibiotic Stopped[5]	-	-	98%	98%
Prophylactic Antibiotic Timing[5]	-	-	98%	99%
Prophylactic Antibiotic Timing (Outpatient)[5]	-	-	98%	98%
Urinary Catheter Removal[5]	-	-	96%	97%
Survey of Patients' Hospital Experiences				
Area Around Room 'Always' Quiet at Night[5]	-	-	68%	61%
Doctors 'Always' Communicated Well[5]	-	-	84%	82%
Home Recovery Information Given[5]	-	-	84%	85%
Hospital Given 9 or 10 on 10 Point Scale[5]	-	-	72%	71%
Meds 'Always' Explained Before Given[5]	-	-	66%	64%
Nurses 'Always' Communicated Well[5]	-	-	80%	79%
Pain 'Always' Well Controlled[5]	-	-	72%	71%
Room and Bathroom 'Always' Clean[5]	-	-	73%	73%
Timely Help 'Always' Received[5]	-	-	71%	68%
Would Definitely Recommend Hospital[5]	-	-	71%	71%
Use of Medical Imaging				
Cardiac Imaging Stress Test before Surgery[7]	-	-	4.5%	5.3%
Combination Abdominal CT Scan	50	40.0%	23%	10.5%
Combination Brain/Sinus CT Scan	63	0.0%	2.2%	2.7%
Combination Chest CT Scan[1]	-	-	5.1%	2.7%
Follow-up Mammogram/Ultrasound[7]	-	-	8.1%	8.8%
Lumbar Spine MRI for Low Back Pain[7]	-	-	39.9%	37.2%

Hillcrest Hospital South

8801 South 101st East Avenue
Tulsa, OK 74133
Phone: 918-294-4000
Fax: 918-294-4809
URL: www.southcresthospital.com
Type: Acute Care Hospitals
Emergency Services: No
Ownership: Proprietary
Beds: 180

Key Personnel:
Quality Assurance . . . . Judy Dodson
Radiology. . . . . M Nguyen
Cardiac Laboratory. . . . . Ernest Pickpring
CEO/President. . . . . Anthony R Young

Measure	Cases	This Hosp.	State Avg.	U.S. Avg.
Blood Clot Prevention and Treatment				
Anticoagulation Overlap Therapy[2]	28	100%	89%	93%
ICU Venous Thromboembolism Prophylaxis[2]	84	94%	87%	92%
Incidence of Potentially Preventable VTE[1,2]	-	-	8%	10%
UFH with Dosages/Platelet Monitoring[2]	15	100%	97%	97%
Venous Thromboembolism Prophylaxis[2]	327	94%	72%	85%
Warfarin Therapy Discharge Instructions[2]	15	100%	73%	75%
Chest Pain/Possible Heart Attack Care				
Aspirin Given Within 24 Hours of Arrival[1,3]	-	-	95%	96%
Fibrinolytic Meds Within 30 Min. of Arrival[5]	-	-	54%	58%
Average Time to ECG (minutes)[1,3]	-	-	8	7
Average Time to Transfer (minutes)[5]	-	-	77	60
Children's Asthma Care				
Received Home Management Plan of Care	-	-	-	88%
Received Reliever Medication	-	-	-	100%
Received Systemic Corticosteroids	-	-	-	100%
Emergency Department				
Admittance Decision Time (minutes)[2]	490	86	63	98
Head CT Results Within 45 Min. of Arrival[1]	-	-	49%	57%
Patients Who Left ER Before Being Seen	23,071	1%	2%	2%
Time from ER Arrival to Admit. (minutes)[2]	501	236	210	274
Time from ER Arrival to Discharge (minutes)	588	146	110	134
Time in ER Before Being Evaluated (minutes)	650	34	24	26
Time to Pain Meds for Fractures (minutes)	78	80	55	57
Heart Attack Care				
Aspirin Given at Discharge	154	99%	99%	99%
Fibrinolytic Meds Within 30 Min. of Arrival[7]	-	-	25%	54%
PCI Within 90 Minutes of Arrival	27	85%	95%	96%
Statin Prescribed at Discharge	149	98%	98%	98%
Heart Failure Care				
ACE Inhibitor or ARB for LVSD	38	100%	95%	97%
Discharge Instructions Given	123	98%	92%	94%
Evaluation of LVS Function	143	99%	96%	99%
Medicare Spending				
Medicare Spending per Patient (ratio)	-	1.04	0.93	0.98
Pneumonia Care				
Appropriate Initial Antibiotic Given	100	99%	92%	95%
Blood Culture Timing	125	98%	97%	98%
Pregnancy and Delivery Care				
Newborn Deliveries Scheduled Early	143	10%	8%	6%

NOTE: Hospital profiles are in alphabetical order by state, then city, then hospital within the city; Rankings exclude hospitals with less than 25 cases except for patient surveys which excludes hospitals with less than 100 cases; (a) 100-299 cases; (1) The number of cases/patients is too few to report; (2) Data submitted were based on a sample of cases/patients; (3) Results are based on a shorter time period than required; (4) Data suppressed by CMS for one or more quarters; (5) Results are not available for this reporting period; (6) Fewer than 100 patients completed the HCAHPS survey; (7) No cases met the criteria for this measure; (8) The lower limit of the confidence interval cannot be calculated if the number of observed infections equals zero; (9) No data are available from the state/territory for this reporting period; (10) The scores shown reflect fewer than 50 completed surveys; (11) There were discrepancies in the data collection process; (12) This measure does not apply to this hospital for this reporting period; (13) Results cannot be calculated for this reporting period; (14) The results for this state are combined with nearby states to protect confidentiality; Please refer to the User's Guide for a full explanation of data.

Preventive Care				
Immunization for Influenza[2]	717	99%	89%	90%
Immunization for Pneumonia[2]	708	98%	91%	92%
Stroke Care				
Anticoagulation Therapy for Atrial Fibrillation[1]	-	-	91%	95%
Antithrombotic Therapy Timing[1]	-	-	95%	98%
Assessed for Rehabilitation[1]	-	-	96%	97%
Discharged on Antithrombotic Therapy[1]	-	-	98%	99%
Discharged on Statin Medication[1]	-	-	88%	94%
Thrombolytic Therapy Timing[7]	-	-	61%	66%
Venous Thromboembolism Prophylaxis[1]	-	-	92%	94%
Written Stroke Educational Materials Given[1]	-	-	86%	88%
Surgical Care Improvement Project				
Appropriate Beta Blocker Usage	77	92%	97%	98%
Appropriate VTP Within 24 Hours	293	97%	97%	98%
Controlled Postoperative Blood Glucose[7]	-	-	97%	97%
Perioperative Temperature Management	333	100%	100%	100%
Prophylactic Antibiotic Selection	217	100%	99%	99%
Prophylactic Antibiotic Selection (Outpatient)	164	100%	98%	98%
Prophylactic Antibiotic Stopped	213	99%	98%	98%
Prophylactic Antibiotic Timing	217	100%	98%	99%
Prophylactic Antibiotic Timing (Outpatient)	164	100%	98%	98%
Urinary Catheter Removal	205	92%	96%	97%
Survey of Patients' Hospital Experiences				
Area Around Room 'Always' Quiet at Night	300+	61%	68%	61%
Doctors 'Always' Communicated Well	300+	78%	84%	82%
Home Recovery Information Given	300+	85%	84%	85%
Hospital Given 9 or 10 on 10 Point Scale	300+	66%	72%	71%
Meds 'Always' Explained Before Given	300+	56%	66%	64%
Nurses 'Always' Communicated Well	300+	72%	80%	79%
Pain 'Always' Well Controlled	300+	66%	72%	71%
Room and Bathroom 'Always' Clean	300+	67%	73%	73%
Timely Help 'Always' Received	300+	60%	71%	68%
Would Definitely Recommend Hospital	300+	70%	71%	71%
Use of Medical Imaging				
Cardiac Imaging Stress Test before Surgery	234	5.6%	4.5%	5.3%
Combination Abdominal CT Scan	401	24.4%	23%	10.5%
Combination Brain/Sinus CT Scan[1]	-	-	2.2%	2.7%
Combination Chest CT Scan	340	15.3%	5.1%	2.7%
Follow-up Mammogram/Ultrasound	741	5.4%	8.1%	8.8%
Lumbar Spine MRI for Low Back Pain	43	51.2%	39.9%	37.2%

Hillcrest Medical Center

1120 South Utica Avenue
Tulsa, OK 74104
Phone: 918-579-1000
Fax: 918-584-6636
URL: www.hillcrest.com
Type: Acute Care Hospitals
Ownership: Proprietary
Emergency Services: Yes
Beds: 607

Key Personnel:
Operating Room. . . . . Robert L Archer
Chief of Medical Staff . . . . D Decker, MD
CEO/President. . . . . Steve Dobbs
Emergency Room . . . . Susan Messon
Quality Assurance . . . . Liz Ross

Measure	Cases	This Hosp.	State Avg.	U.S. Avg.
Blood Clot Prevention and Treatment				
Anticoagulation Overlap Therapy[2]	98	98%	89%	93%
ICU Venous Thromboembolism Prophylaxis[2]	101	100%	87%	92%
Incidence of Potentially Preventable VTE[2]	18	0%	8%	10%
UFH with Dosages/Platelet Monitoring[2]	51	100%	97%	97%
Venous Thromboembolism Prophylaxis[2]	320	93%	72%	85%
Warfarin Therapy Discharge Instructions[2]	70	96%	73%	75%
Chest Pain/Possible Heart Attack Care				
Aspirin Given Within 24 Hours of Arrival[1,3]	-	-	95%	96%
Fibrinolytic Meds Within 30 Min. of Arrival[5]	-	-	54%	58%
Average Time to ECG (minutes)[1,3]	-	-	8	7
Average Time to Transfer (minutes)[5]	-	-	77	60
Children's Asthma Care				
Received Home Management Plan of Care	-	-	-	88%
Received Reliever Medication	-	-	-	100%
Received Systemic Corticosteroids	-	-	-	100%
Emergency Department				
Admittance Decision Time (minutes)[2]	431	104	63	98
Head CT Results Within 45 Min. of Arrival[1]	-	-	49%	57%
Patients Who Left ER Before Being Seen	47,642	5%	2%	2%
Time from ER Arrival to Admit. (minutes)[2]	460	298	210	274
Time from ER Arrival to Discharge (minutes)	381	150	110	134
Time in ER Before Being Evaluated (minutes)	400	50	24	26
Time to Pain Meds for Fractures (minutes)	104	54	55	57
Heart Attack Care				
Aspirin Given at Discharge	556	100%	99%	99%
Fibrinolytic Meds Within 30 Min. of Arrival[1]	-	-	25%	54%
PCI Within 90 Minutes of Arrival	48	98%	95%	96%
Statin Prescribed at Discharge	538	100%	98%	98%
Heart Failure Care				
ACE Inhibitor or ARB for LVSD	165	98%	95%	97%
Discharge Instructions Given	550	100%	92%	94%
Evaluation of LVS Function	593	100%	96%	99%
Medicare Spending				
Medicare Spending per Patient (ratio)	-	0.97	0.93	0.98
Pneumonia Care				
Appropriate Initial Antibiotic Given	137	97%	92%	95%
Blood Culture Timing	264	97%	97%	98%
Pregnancy and Delivery Care				
Newborn Deliveries Scheduled Early	273	10%	8%	6%
Preventive Care				
Immunization for Influenza[2]	639	97%	89%	90%
Immunization for Pneumonia[2]	689	95%	91%	92%
Stroke Care				
Anticoagulation Therapy for Atrial Fibrillation	13	100%	91%	95%
Antithrombotic Therapy Timing	171	99%	95%	98%
Assessed for Rehabilitation	192	98%	96%	97%
Discharged on Antithrombotic Therapy	166	100%	98%	99%
Discharged on Statin Medication	134	99%	88%	94%
Thrombolytic Therapy Timing[1]	-	-	61%	66%
Venous Thromboembolism Prophylaxis	192	97%	92%	94%
Written Stroke Educational Materials Given	126	98%	86%	88%
Surgical Care Improvement Project				
Appropriate Beta Blocker Usage[2]	297	98%	97%	98%
Appropriate VTP Within 24 Hours[2]	475	97%	97%	98%
Controlled Postoperative Blood Glucose[2]	196	95%	97%	97%
Perioperative Temperature Management[2]	590	100%	100%	100%
Prophylactic Antibiotic Selection[2]	595	100%	99%	99%
Prophylactic Antibiotic Selection (Outpatient)	629	100%	98%	98%
Prophylactic Antibiotic Stopped[2]	575	98%	98%	98%
Prophylactic Antibiotic Timing[2]	596	100%	98%	99%
Prophylactic Antibiotic Timing (Outpatient)	579	99%	98%	98%
Urinary Catheter Removal[2]	408	99%	96%	97%
Survey of Patients' Hospital Experiences				
Area Around Room 'Always' Quiet at Night	300+	60%	68%	61%
Doctors 'Always' Communicated Well	300+	75%	84%	82%
Home Recovery Information Given	300+	81%	84%	85%
Hospital Given 9 or 10 on 10 Point Scale	300+	61%	72%	71%
Meds 'Always' Explained Before Given	300+	57%	66%	64%
Nurses 'Always' Communicated Well	300+	71%	80%	79%
Pain 'Always' Well Controlled	300+	65%	72%	71%
Room and Bathroom 'Always' Clean	300+	57%	73%	73%
Timely Help 'Always' Received	300+	54%	71%	68%
Would Definitely Recommend Hospital	300+	64%	71%	71%
Use of Medical Imaging				
Cardiac Imaging Stress Test before Surgery	1,626	4.4%	4.5%	5.3%
Combination Abdominal CT Scan	588	28.9%	23%	10.5%
Combination Brain/Sinus CT Scan	511	1.0%	2.2%	2.7%
Combination Chest CT Scan	548	17.0%	5.1%	2.7%
Follow-up Mammogram/Ultrasound	1,595	8.3%	8.1%	8.8%
Lumbar Spine MRI for Low Back Pain	121	31.4%	39.9%	37.2%

Oklahoma State University Medical Center

744 West 9th Street
Tulsa, OK 74127
Phone: 918-587-2561
Fax: 918-599-1750
URL: www.tulsaregional.com
Type: Acute Care Hospitals
Ownership: Government - Local
Emergency Services: Yes
Beds: 415

Key Personnel:
Chief of Medical Staff . . . . Jenny Alexopulos, DO
Infection Control. . . . . Janet Bacon
Intensive Care Unit. . . . . Eric Burch
Anesthesiology. . . . . Kimberly Dullge
Emergency Room . . . . Jan Emmons
Radiology. . . . . Maureen Miller
Operating Room. . . . . Nellie Rhea
CEO/President. . . . . Jan Slater

Measure	Cases	This Hosp.	State Avg.	U.S. Avg.
Blood Clot Prevention and Treatment				
Anticoagulation Overlap Therapy[2]	42	90%	89%	93%
ICU Venous Thromboembolism Prophylaxis[2]	166	78%	87%	92%
Incidence of Potentially Preventable VTE[1,2]	-	-	8%	10%
UFH with Dosages/Platelet Monitoring[2]	14	86%	97%	97%
Venous Thromboembolism Prophylaxis[2]	283	79%	72%	85%
Warfarin Therapy Discharge Instructions[2]	28	21%	73%	75%
Chest Pain/Possible Heart Attack Care				
Aspirin Given Within 24 Hours of Arrival[3,7]	-	-	95%	96%
Fibrinolytic Meds Within 30 Min. of Arrival[5]	-	-	54%	58%
Average Time to ECG (minutes)[3,7]	-	-	8	7
Average Time to Transfer (minutes)[5]	-	-	77	60
Children's Asthma Care				
Received Home Management Plan of Care	-	-	-	88%
Received Reliever Medication	-	-	-	100%
Received Systemic Corticosteroids	-	-	-	100%
Emergency Department				
Admittance Decision Time (minutes)[2]	418	99	63	98
Head CT Results Within 45 Min. of Arrival[1]	-	-	49%	57%
Patients Who Left ER Before Being Seen	48,197	0%	2%	2%
Time from ER Arrival to Admit. (minutes)[2]	476	204	210	274
Time from ER Arrival to Discharge (minutes)	364	64	110	134
Time in ER Before Being Evaluated (minutes)	411	14	24	26
Time to Pain Meds for Fractures (minutes)	80	68	55	57
Heart Attack Care				
Aspirin Given at Discharge	143	98%	99%	99%
Fibrinolytic Meds Within 30 Min. of Arrival[7]	-	-	25%	54%
PCI Within 90 Minutes of Arrival[1]	-	-	95%	96%
Statin Prescribed at Discharge	141	99%	98%	98%
Heart Failure Care				
ACE Inhibitor or ARB for LVSD	95	98%	95%	97%
Discharge Instructions Given	169	79%	92%	94%
Evaluation of LVS Function	180	99%	96%	99%
Medicare Spending				
Medicare Spending per Patient (ratio)	-	0.97	0.93	0.98
Pneumonia Care				
Appropriate Initial Antibiotic Given	87	100%	92%	95%
Blood Culture Timing	108	100%	97%	98%
Pregnancy and Delivery Care				
Newborn Deliveries Scheduled Early	43	5%	8%	6%
Preventive Care				
Immunization for Influenza[2]	555	88%	89%	90%
Immunization for Pneumonia[2]	681	88%	91%	92%
Stroke Care				
Anticoagulation Therapy for Atrial Fibrillation[1]	-	-	91%	95%
Antithrombotic Therapy Timing	36	94%	95%	98%
Assessed for Rehabilitation	33	88%	96%	97%
Discharged on Antithrombotic Therapy	32	94%	98%	99%
Discharged on Statin Medication	23	91%	88%	94%
Thrombolytic Therapy Timing[1]	-	-	61%	66%
Venous Thromboembolism Prophylaxis	38	89%	92%	94%
Written Stroke Educational Materials Given	25	20%	86%	88%
Surgical Care Improvement Project				
Appropriate Beta Blocker Usage[2]	106	95%	97%	98%
Appropriate VTP Within 24 Hours[2]	170	96%	97%	98%
Controlled Postoperative Blood Glucose[2]	78	99%	97%	97%
Perioperative Temperature Management[2]	244	100%	100%	100%
Prophylactic Antibiotic Selection[2]	192	96%	99%	99%
Prophylactic Antibiotic Selection (Outpatient)	86	97%	98%	98%
Prophylactic Antibiotic Stopped[2]	187	89%	98%	98%
Prophylactic Antibiotic Timing[2]	194	99%	98%	99%
Prophylactic Antibiotic Timing (Outpatient)	86	94%	98%	98%
Urinary Catheter Removal[2]	159	92%	96%	97%
Survey of Patients' Hospital Experiences				
Area Around Room 'Always' Quiet at Night	300+	54%	68%	61%
Doctors 'Always' Communicated Well	300+	78%	84%	82%

NOTE: Hospital profiles are in alphabetical order by state, then city, then hospital within the city; Rankings exclude hospitals with less than 25 cases except for patient surveys which excludes hospitals with less than 100 cases; (a) 100-299 cases; (1) The number of cases/patients is too few to report; (2) Data submitted were based on a sample of cases/patients; (3) Results are based on a shorter time period than required; (4) Data suppressed by CMS for one or more quarters; (5) Results are not available for this reporting period; (6) Fewer than 100 patients completed the HCAHPS survey; (7) No cases met the criteria for this measure; (8) The lower limit of the confidence interval cannot be calculated if the number of observed infections equals zero; (9) No data are available from the state/territory for this reporting period; (10) The scores shown reflect fewer than 50 completed surveys; (11) There were discrepancies in the data collection process; (12) This measure does not apply to this hospital for this reporting period; (13) Results cannot be calculated for this reporting period; (14) The results for this state are combined with nearby states to protect confidentiality; Please refer to the User's Guide for a full explanation of data.

Measure	Cases	This Hosp.	State Avg.	U.S. Avg.
Home Recovery Information Given	300+	79%	84%	85%
Hospital Given 9 or 10 on 10 Point Scale	300+	67%	72%	71%
Meds 'Always' Explained Before Given	300+	57%	66%	64%
Nurses 'Always' Communicated Well	300+	72%	80%	79%
Pain 'Always' Well Controlled	300+	63%	72%	71%
Room and Bathroom 'Always' Clean	300+	69%	73%	73%
Timely Help 'Always' Received	300+	58%	71%	68%
Would Definitely Recommend Hospital	300+	68%	71%	71%
Use of Medical Imaging				
Cardiac Imaging Stress Test before Surgery	77	2.6%	4.5%	5.3%
Combination Abdominal CT Scan	310	10.3%	23%	10.5%
Combination Brain/Sinus CT Scan[1]	-	-	2.2%	2.7%
Combination Chest CT Scan	143	2.1%	5.1%	2.7%
Follow-up Mammogram/Ultrasound	151	7.3%	8.1%	8.8%
Lumbar Spine MRI for Low Back Pain[1]	-	-	39.9%	37.2%

Oklahoma Surgical Hospital

2408 East 81st Street, Suite 300 Phone: 918-477-5000
Tulsa, OK 74137
URL: www.oklahomasurgicalhospital.com
Type: Acute Care Hospitals Emergency Services: Yes
Ownership: Physician
Key Personnel:
President/CEO. . . . . Rick Ferguson

Measure	Cases	This Hosp.	State Avg.	U.S. Avg.
Blood Clot Prevention and Treatment				
Anticoagulation Overlap Therapy[1,2]	-	-	89%	93%
ICU Venous Thromboembolism Prophylaxis[2,7]	-	-	87%	92%
Incidence of Potentially Preventable VTE[1,2]	-	-	8%	10%
UFH with Dosages/Platelet Monitoring[2,7]	-	-	97%	97%
Venous Thromboembolism Prophylaxis[2]	135	99%	72%	85%
Warfarin Therapy Discharge Instructions[1,2]	-	-	73%	75%
Chest Pain/Possible Heart Attack Care				
Aspirin Given Within 24 Hours of Arrival[5]	-	-	95%	96%
Fibrinolytic Meds Within 30 Min. of Arrival[5]	-	-	54%	58%
Average Time to ECG (minutes)[5]	-	-	8	7
Average Time to Transfer (minutes)[5]	-	-	77	60
Children's Asthma Care				
Received Home Management Plan of Care	-	-	-	88%
Received Reliever Medication	-	-	-	100%
Received Systemic Corticosteroids	-	-	-	100%
Emergency Department				
Admittance Decision Time (minutes)[2,7]	-	-	63	98
Head CT Results Within 45 Min. of Arrival[5]	-	-	49%	57%
Patients Who Left ER Before Being Seen	145	1%	2%	2%
Time from ER Arrival to Admit. (minutes)[2,7]	-	-	210	274
Time from ER Arrival to Discharge (minutes)	92	180	110	134
Time in ER Before Being Evaluated (minutes)	84	24	24	26
Time to Pain Meds for Fractures (minutes)[5]	-	-	55	57
Heart Attack Care				
Aspirin Given at Discharge[5]	-	-	99%	99%
Fibrinolytic Meds Within 30 Min. of Arrival[5]	-	-	25%	54%
PCI Within 90 Minutes of Arrival[5]	-	-	95%	96%
Statin Prescribed at Discharge[5]	-	-	98%	98%
Heart Failure Care				
ACE Inhibitor or ARB for LVSD[5]	-	-	95%	97%
Discharge Instructions Given[5]	-	-	92%	94%
Evaluation of LVS Function[5]	-	-	96%	99%
Medicare Spending				
Medicare Spending per Patient (ratio)	-	0.86	0.93	0.98
Pneumonia Care				
Appropriate Initial Antibiotic Given[2,3]	-	-	92%	95%
Blood Culture Timing[2,3]	-	-	97%	98%
Pregnancy and Delivery Care				
Newborn Deliveries Scheduled Early[2,7]	-	-	8%	6%
Preventive Care				
Immunization for Influenza[2]	365	100%	89%	90%
Immunization for Pneumonia[2]	314	100%	91%	92%
Stroke Care				
Anticoagulation Therapy for Atrial Fibrillation[5]	-	-	91%	95%
Antithrombotic Therapy Timing[5]	-	-	95%	98%
Assessed for Rehabilitation[5]	-	-	96%	97%
Discharged on Antithrombotic Therapy[5]	-	-	98%	99%
Discharged on Statin Medication[5]	-	-	88%	94%
Thrombolytic Therapy Timing[5]	-	-	61%	66%
Venous Thromboembolism Prophylaxis[5]	-	-	92%	94%
Written Stroke Educational Materials Given[5]	-	-	86%	88%
Surgical Care Improvement Project				
Appropriate Beta Blocker Usage[2]	64	100%	97%	98%
Appropriate VTP Within 24 Hours[2]	279	100%	97%	98%
Controlled Postoperative Blood Glucose[2,7]	-	-	97%	97%
Perioperative Temperature Management[2]	320	100%	100%	100%
Prophylactic Antibiotic Selection[2]	225	100%	99%	99%
Prophylactic Antibiotic Selection (Outpatient)	483	100%	98%	98%
Prophylactic Antibiotic Stopped[2]	224	100%	98%	98%
Prophylactic Antibiotic Timing[2]	225	100%	98%	99%
Prophylactic Antibiotic Timing (Outpatient)	483	100%	98%	98%
Urinary Catheter Removal[2]	81	100%	96%	97%
Survey of Patients' Hospital Experiences				
Area Around Room 'Always' Quiet at Night	300+	84%	68%	61%
Doctors 'Always' Communicated Well	300+	87%	84%	82%
Home Recovery Information Given	300+	87%	84%	85%
Hospital Given 9 or 10 on 10 Point Scale	300+	85%	72%	71%
Meds 'Always' Explained Before Given	300+	69%	66%	64%
Nurses 'Always' Communicated Well	300+	84%	80%	79%
Pain 'Always' Well Controlled	300+	76%	72%	71%
Room and Bathroom 'Always' Clean	300+	84%	73%	73%
Timely Help 'Always' Received	300+	73%	71%	68%
Would Definitely Recommend Hospital	300+	87%	71%	71%
Use of Medical Imaging				
Cardiac Imaging Stress Test before Surgery[7]	-	-	4.5%	5.3%
Combination Abdominal CT Scan[1]	-	-	23%	10.5%
Combination Brain/Sinus CT Scan[1]	-	-	2.2%	2.7%
Combination Chest CT Scan[1]	-	-	5.1%	2.7%
Follow-up Mammogram/Ultrasound[7]	-	-	8.1%	8.8%
Lumbar Spine MRI for Low Back Pain	226	39.4%	39.9%	37.2%

Pinnacle Specialty Hospital

2408 East 81st Street, Suite 600 Phone: 918-392-2780
Tulsa, OK 74137
URL: www.pinnaclespecialtyhospital.com
Type: Acute Care Hospitals Emergency Services: Yes
Ownership: Proprietary

Measure	Cases	This Hosp.	State Avg.	U.S. Avg.
Blood Clot Prevention and Treatment				
Anticoagulation Overlap Therapy[7]	-	-	89%	93%
ICU Venous Thromboembolism Prophylaxis[7]	-	-	87%	92%
Incidence of Potentially Preventable VTE[7]	-	-	8%	10%
UFH with Dosages/Platelet Monitoring[7]	-	-	97%	97%
Venous Thromboembolism Prophylaxis[1]	-	-	72%	85%
Warfarin Therapy Discharge Instructions[7]	-	-	73%	75%
Chest Pain/Possible Heart Attack Care				
Aspirin Given Within 24 Hours of Arrival[5]	-	-	95%	96%
Fibrinolytic Meds Within 30 Min. of Arrival[5]	-	-	54%	58%
Average Time to ECG (minutes)[5]	-	-	8	7
Average Time to Transfer (minutes)[5]	-	-	77	60
Children's Asthma Care				
Received Home Management Plan of Care	-	-	-	88%
Received Reliever Medication	-	-	-	100%
Received Systemic Corticosteroids	-	-	-	100%
Emergency Department				
Admittance Decision Time (minutes)[7]	-	-	63	98
Head CT Results Within 45 Min. of Arrival[5]	-	-	49%	57%
Patients Who Left ER Before Being Seen[5]	-	-	2%	2%
Time from ER Arrival to Admit. (minutes)[7]	-	-	210	274
Time from ER Arrival to Discharge (minutes)[5]	-	-	110	134
Time in ER Before Being Evaluated (minutes)[5]	-	-	24	26
Time to Pain Meds for Fractures (minutes)[5]	-	-	55	57
Heart Attack Care				
Aspirin Given at Discharge[5]	-	-	99%	99%
Fibrinolytic Meds Within 30 Min. of Arrival[5]	-	-	25%	54%
PCI Within 90 Minutes of Arrival[5]	-	-	95%	96%
Statin Prescribed at Discharge[5]	-	-	98%	98%
Heart Failure Care				
ACE Inhibitor or ARB for LVSD[5]	-	-	95%	97%
Discharge Instructions Given[5]	-	-	92%	94%
Evaluation of LVS Function[5]	-	-	96%	99%
Medicare Spending				
Medicare Spending per Patient (ratio)	-	-	0.93	0.98
Pneumonia Care				
Appropriate Initial Antibiotic Given[5]	-	-	92%	95%
Blood Culture Timing[5]	-	-	97%	98%
Pregnancy and Delivery Care				
Newborn Deliveries Scheduled Early[7]	-	-	8%	6%
Preventive Care				
Immunization for Influenza	24	21%	89%	90%
Immunization for Pneumonia	11	55%	91%	92%
Stroke Care				
Anticoagulation Therapy for Atrial Fibrillation[5]	-	-	91%	95%
Antithrombotic Therapy Timing[5]	-	-	95%	98%
Assessed for Rehabilitation[5]	-	-	96%	97%
Discharged on Antithrombotic Therapy[5]	-	-	98%	99%
Discharged on Statin Medication[5]	-	-	88%	94%
Thrombolytic Therapy Timing[5]	-	-	61%	66%
Venous Thromboembolism Prophylaxis[5]	-	-	92%	94%
Written Stroke Educational Materials Given[5]	-	-	86%	88%
Surgical Care Improvement Project				
Appropriate Beta Blocker Usage[5]	-	-	97%	98%
Appropriate VTP Within 24 Hours[5]	-	-	97%	98%
Controlled Postoperative Blood Glucose[5]	-	-	97%	97%
Perioperative Temperature Management[5]	-	-	100%	100%
Prophylactic Antibiotic Selection[5]	-	-	99%	99%
Prophylactic Antibiotic Selection (Outpatient)[5]	-	-	98%	98%
Prophylactic Antibiotic Stopped[5]	-	-	98%	98%
Prophylactic Antibiotic Timing[5]	-	-	98%	99%
Prophylactic Antibiotic Timing (Outpatient)[5]	-	-	98%	98%
Urinary Catheter Removal[5]	-	-	96%	97%
Survey of Patients' Hospital Experiences				
Area Around Room 'Always' Quiet at Night[1]	-	-	68%	61%
Doctors 'Always' Communicated Well[1]	-	-	84%	82%
Home Recovery Information Given[1]	-	-	84%	85%
Hospital Given 9 or 10 on 10 Point Scale[1]	-	-	72%	71%
Meds 'Always' Explained Before Given[1]	-	-	66%	64%
Nurses 'Always' Communicated Well[1]	-	-	80%	79%
Pain 'Always' Well Controlled[1]	-	-	72%	71%
Room and Bathroom 'Always' Clean[1]	-	-	73%	73%
Timely Help 'Always' Received[1]	-	-	71%	68%
Would Definitely Recommend Hospital[1]	-	-	71%	71%
Use of Medical Imaging				
Cardiac Imaging Stress Test before Surgery[7]	-	-	4.5%	5.3%
Combination Abdominal CT Scan[7]	-	-	23%	10.5%
Combination Brain/Sinus CT Scan[7]	-	-	2.2%	2.7%
Combination Chest CT Scan[7]	-	-	5.1%	2.7%
Follow-up Mammogram/Ultrasound[7]	-	-	8.1%	8.8%
Lumbar Spine MRI for Low Back Pain[7]	-	-	39.9%	37.2%

Saint Francis Hospital

6161 South Yale Phone: 918-494-2200
Tulsa, OK 74136 Fax: 918-494-4501
E-mail: webadministrator@saintfrancis.com
URL: www.saintfrancis.com
Type: Acute Care Hospitals Emergency Services: Yes
Ownership: Voluntary non-profit - Private Beds: 918
Key Personnel:
Infection Control. . . . . Dee Copeland, RN
CEO/President. . . . . Jake Henry, Jr
Chairman/CEO . . . . John Kelly C Warren
Radiology. . . . . R Krieger, MD
Anesthesiology. . . . . Mel Mercer Jr, MD
Emergency Room . . . . Frank Mitchell, MD
Quality Assurance . . . . Jane Sharpe, RN
Administrator . . . . Lynn Sund

Measure	Cases	This Hosp.	State Avg.	U.S. Avg.
Blood Clot Prevention and Treatment				
Anticoagulation Overlap Therapy[2]	155	82%	89%	93%
ICU Venous Thromboembolism Prophylaxis[2]	116	95%	87%	92%
Incidence of Potentially Preventable VTE[2]	64	6%	8%	10%
UFH with Dosages/Platelet Monitoring[2]	60	83%	97%	97%
Venous Thromboembolism Prophylaxis[2]	320	93%	72%	85%

NOTE: Hospital profiles are in alphabetical order by state, then city, then hospital within the city; Rankings exclude hospitals with less than 25 cases except for patient surveys which excludes hospitals with less than 100 cases; (a) 100-299 cases; (1) The number of cases/patients is too few to report; (2) Data submitted were based on a sample of cases/patients; (3) Results are based on a shorter time period than required; (4) Data suppressed by CMS for one or more quarters; (5) Results are not available for this reporting period; (6) Fewer than 100 patients completed the HCAHPS survey; (7) No cases met the criteria for this measure; (8) The lower limit of the confidence interval cannot be calculated if the number of observed infections equals zero; (9) No data are available from the state/territory for this reporting period; (10) The scores shown reflect fewer than 50 completed surveys; (11) There were discrepancies in the data collection process; (12) This measure does not apply to this hospital for this reporting period; (13) Results cannot be calculated for this reporting period; (14) The results for this state are combined with nearby states to protect confidentiality; Please refer to the User's Guide for a full explanation of data.

Measure	Cases	This Hosp.	State Avg.	U.S. Avg.
Warfarin Therapy Discharge Instructions[2]	114	74%	73%	75%
Chest Pain/Possible Heart Attack Care				
Aspirin Given Within 24 Hours of Arrival[1,3]	-	-	95%	96%
Fibrinolytic Meds Within 30 Min. of Arrival[5]	-	-	54%	58%
Average Time to ECG (minutes)[1,3]	-	-	8	7
Average Time to Transfer (minutes)[5]	-	-	77	60
Children's Asthma Care				
Received Home Management Plan of Care	-	-	-	88%
Received Reliever Medication	-	-	-	100%
Received Systemic Corticosteroids	-	-	-	100%
Emergency Department				
Admittance Decision Time (minutes)[2]	627	84	63	98
Head CT Results Within 45 Min. of Arrival[1]	-	-	49%	57%
Patients Who Left ER Before Being Seen	97,379	2%	2%	2%
Time from ER Arrival to Admit. (minutes)[2]	627	218	210	274
Time from ER Arrival to Discharge (minutes)	392	162	110	134
Time in ER Before Being Evaluated (minutes)	421	25	24	26
Time to Pain Meds for Fractures (minutes)	289	43	55	57
Heart Attack Care				
Aspirin Given at Discharge	674	100%	99%	99%
Fibrinolytic Meds Within 30 Min. of Arrival[7]	-	-	25%	54%
PCI Within 90 Minutes of Arrival	80	94%	95%	96%
Statin Prescribed at Discharge	669	98%	98%	98%
Heart Failure Care				
ACE Inhibitor or ARB for LVSD	290	100%	95%	97%
Discharge Instructions Given	729	94%	92%	94%
Evaluation of LVS Function	893	100%	96%	99%
Medicare Spending				
Medicare Spending per Patient (ratio)	-	0.99	0.93	0.98
Pneumonia Care				
Appropriate Initial Antibiotic Given	476	92%	92%	95%
Blood Culture Timing	642	97%	97%	98%
Pregnancy and Delivery Care				
Newborn Deliveries Scheduled Early	437	14%	8%	6%
Preventive Care				
Immunization for Influenza[2]	570	94%	89%	90%
Immunization for Pneumonia[2]	578	90%	91%	92%
Stroke Care				
Anticoagulation Therapy for Atrial Fibrillation	61	87%	91%	95%
Antithrombotic Therapy Timing	387	97%	95%	98%
Assessed for Rehabilitation	503	94%	96%	97%
Discharged on Antithrombotic Therapy	406	99%	98%	99%
Discharged on Statin Medication	341	84%	88%	94%
Thrombolytic Therapy Timing	14	36%	61%	66%
Venous Thromboembolism Prophylaxis	512	96%	92%	94%
Written Stroke Educational Materials Given	274	83%	86%	88%
Surgical Care Improvement Project				
Appropriate Beta Blocker Usage[2]	644	95%	97%	98%
Appropriate VTP Within 24 Hours[2]	1,288	95%	97%	98%
Controlled Postoperative Blood Glucose[2]	289	96%	97%	97%
Perioperative Temperature Management[2]	1,494	100%	100%	100%
Prophylactic Antibiotic Selection[2]	1,321	98%	99%	99%
Prophylactic Antibiotic Selection (Outpatient)	716	97%	98%	98%
Prophylactic Antibiotic Stopped[2]	1,291	98%	98%	98%
Prophylactic Antibiotic Timing[2]	1,322	97%	98%	99%
Prophylactic Antibiotic Timing (Outpatient)	723	98%	98%	98%
Urinary Catheter Removal[2]	791	93%	96%	97%
Survey of Patients' Hospital Experiences				
Area Around Room 'Always' Quiet at Night	300+	59%	68%	61%
Doctors 'Always' Communicated Well	300+	77%	84%	82%
Home Recovery Information Given	300+	81%	84%	85%
Hospital Given 9 or 10 on 10 Point Scale	300+	68%	72%	71%
Meds 'Always' Explained Before Given	300+	61%	66%	64%
Nurses 'Always' Communicated Well	300+	73%	80%	79%
Pain 'Always' Well Controlled	300+	71%	72%	71%
Room and Bathroom 'Always' Clean	300+	68%	73%	73%
Timely Help 'Always' Received	300+	59%	71%	68%
Would Definitely Recommend Hospital	300+	76%	71%	71%
Use of Medical Imaging				
Cardiac Imaging Stress Test before Surgery	1,827	5.0%	4.5%	5.3%
Combination Abdominal CT Scan	1,714	43.2%	23%	10.5%
Combination Brain/Sinus CT Scan	1,342	1.0%	2.2%	2.7%
Combination Chest CT Scan	1,460	0.2%	5.1%	2.7%
Follow-up Mammogram/Ultrasound	4,102	5.5%	8.1%	8.8%
Lumbar Spine MRI for Low Back Pain	282	42.6%	39.9%	37.2%

Saint Francis Hospital South

10501 East 91st Street South | Phone: 918-307-6000
Tulsa, OK 74133
E-mail: webadministrator@saintfrancis.com
URL: www.saintfrancis.com
Type: Acute Care Hospitals | Emergency Services: Yes
Ownership: Voluntary non-profit - Private | Beds: 76

Key Personnel:
CEO/President . . . . Jake Henry, Jr
Administrator . . . . William Schloss
Chief of Medical Staff . . . . David Thomas

Measure	Cases	This Hosp.	State Avg.	U.S. Avg.
Blood Clot Prevention and Treatment				
Anticoagulation Overlap Therapy[2]	23	96%	89%	93%
ICU Venous Thromboembolism Prophylaxis[2]	62	94%	87%	92%
Incidence of Potentially Preventable VTE[1,2]	-	-	8%	10%
UFH with Dosages/Platelet Monitoring[1,2]	-	-	97%	97%
Venous Thromboembolism Prophylaxis[2]	255	92%	72%	85%
Warfarin Therapy Discharge Instructions[2]	18	78%	73%	75%
Chest Pain/Possible Heart Attack Care				
Aspirin Given Within 24 Hours of Arrival	32	100%	95%	96%
Fibrinolytic Meds Within 30 Min. of Arrival[7]	-	-	54%	58%
Average Time to ECG (minutes)	34	7	8	7
Average Time to Transfer (minutes)	11	55	77	60
Children's Asthma Care				
Received Home Management Plan of Care	-	-	-	88%
Received Reliever Medication	-	-	-	100%
Received Systemic Corticosteroids	-	-	-	100%
Emergency Department				
Admittance Decision Time (minutes)[2]	411	65	63	98
Head CT Results Within 45 Min. of Arrival[1]	-	-	49%	57%
Patients Who Left ER Before Being Seen	24,598	1%	2%	2%
Time from ER Arrival to Admit. (minutes)[2]	413	249	210	274
Time from ER Arrival to Discharge (minutes)	383	138	110	134
Time in ER Before Being Evaluated (minutes)	411	39	24	26
Time to Pain Meds for Fractures (minutes)	131	67	55	57
Heart Attack Care				
Aspirin Given at Discharge	67	100%	99%	99%
Fibrinolytic Meds Within 30 Min. of Arrival[7]	-	-	25%	54%
PCI Within 90 Minutes of Arrival[1]	-	-	95%	96%
Statin Prescribed at Discharge	67	99%	98%	98%
Heart Failure Care				
ACE Inhibitor or ARB for LVSD	48	100%	95%	97%
Discharge Instructions Given	131	89%	92%	94%
Evaluation of LVS Function	154	100%	96%	99%
Medicare Spending				
Medicare Spending per Patient (ratio)	-	0.97	0.93	0.98
Pneumonia Care				
Appropriate Initial Antibiotic Given	107	98%	92%	95%
Blood Culture Timing	140	99%	97%	98%
Pregnancy and Delivery Care				
Newborn Deliveries Scheduled Early	134	10%	8%	6%
Preventive Care				
Immunization for Influenza[2]	395	98%	89%	90%
Immunization for Pneumonia[2]	449	91%	91%	92%
Stroke Care				
Anticoagulation Therapy for Atrial Fibrillation[1]	-	-	91%	95%
Antithrombotic Therapy Timing	30	100%	95%	98%
Assessed for Rehabilitation	30	100%	96%	97%
Discharged on Antithrombotic Therapy	29	100%	98%	99%
Discharged on Statin Medication	20	95%	88%	94%
Thrombolytic Therapy Timing[1]	-	-	61%	66%
Venous Thromboembolism Prophylaxis	30	100%	92%	94%
Written Stroke Educational Materials Given	20	75%	86%	88%
Surgical Care Improvement Project				
Appropriate Beta Blocker Usage	80	92%	97%	98%
Appropriate VTP Within 24 Hours	259	98%	97%	98%
Controlled Postoperative Blood Glucose[7]	-	-	97%	97%
Perioperative Temperature Management	296	100%	100%	100%
Prophylactic Antibiotic Selection	237	97%	99%	99%
Prophylactic Antibiotic Selection (Outpatient)	60	98%	98%	98%
Prophylactic Antibiotic Stopped	235	99%	98%	98%
Prophylactic Antibiotic Timing	237	99%	98%	99%
Prophylactic Antibiotic Timing (Outpatient)	60	100%	98%	98%
Urinary Catheter Removal	159	95%	96%	97%
Survey of Patients' Hospital Experiences				
Area Around Room 'Always' Quiet at Night	300+	54%	68%	61%
Doctors 'Always' Communicated Well	300+	82%	84%	82%
Home Recovery Information Given	300+	82%	84%	85%
Hospital Given 9 or 10 on 10 Point Scale	300+	76%	72%	71%
Meds 'Always' Explained Before Given	300+	57%	66%	64%
Nurses 'Always' Communicated Well	300+	76%	80%	79%
Pain 'Always' Well Controlled	300+	68%	72%	71%
Room and Bathroom 'Always' Clean	300+	72%	73%	73%
Timely Help 'Always' Received	300+	61%	71%	68%
Would Definitely Recommend Hospital	300+	77%	71%	71%
Use of Medical Imaging				
Cardiac Imaging Stress Test before Surgery	390	4.1%	4.5%	5.3%
Combination Abdominal CT Scan	461	47.1%	23%	10.5%
Combination Brain/Sinus CT Scan	353	0.8%	2.2%	2.7%
Combination Chest CT Scan	373	0.0%	5.1%	2.7%
Follow-up Mammogram/Ultrasound	1,018	3.8%	8.1%	8.8%
Lumbar Spine MRI for Low Back Pain	186	40.3%	39.9%	37.2%

Saint John Medical Center

1923 South Utica Avenue | Phone: 918-744-3606
Tulsa, OK 74104
URL: www.sjmc.org
Type: Acute Care Hospitals | Emergency Services: Yes
Ownership: Voluntary non-profit - Church

Key Personnel:
CEO . . . . Charles Anderson

Measure	Cases	This Hosp.	State Avg.	U.S. Avg.
Blood Clot Prevention and Treatment				
Anticoagulation Overlap Therapy[2]	142	92%	89%	93%
ICU Venous Thromboembolism Prophylaxis[2]	90	94%	87%	92%
Incidence of Potentially Preventable VTE[2]	51	2%	8%	10%
UFH with Dosages/Platelet Monitoring[2]	61	100%	97%	97%
Venous Thromboembolism Prophylaxis[2]	292	91%	72%	85%
Warfarin Therapy Discharge Instructions[2]	101	27%	73%	75%
Chest Pain/Possible Heart Attack Care				
Aspirin Given Within 24 Hours of Arrival[1,3]	-	-	95%	96%
Fibrinolytic Meds Within 30 Min. of Arrival[5]	-	-	54%	58%
Average Time to ECG (minutes)[1,3]	-	-	8	7
Average Time to Transfer (minutes)[5]	-	-	77	60
Children's Asthma Care				
Received Home Management Plan of Care	-	-	-	88%
Received Reliever Medication	-	-	-	100%
Received Systemic Corticosteroids	-	-	-	100%
Emergency Department				
Admittance Decision Time (minutes)[2]	548	88	63	98
Head CT Results Within 45 Min. of Arrival[1]	-	-	49%	57%
Patients Who Left ER Before Being Seen	61,858	4%	2%	2%
Time from ER Arrival to Admit. (minutes)[2]	578	271	210	274
Time from ER Arrival to Discharge (minutes)	369	223	110	134
Time in ER Before Being Evaluated (minutes)	373	102	24	26
Time to Pain Meds for Fractures (minutes)	259	105	55	57
Heart Attack Care				
Aspirin Given at Discharge	617	99%	99%	99%
Fibrinolytic Meds Within 30 Min. of Arrival[7]	-	-	25%	54%
PCI Within 90 Minutes of Arrival	94	95%	95%	96%
Statin Prescribed at Discharge	598	99%	98%	98%
Heart Failure Care				
ACE Inhibitor or ARB for LVSD	234	98%	95%	97%
Discharge Instructions Given	581	98%	92%	94%
Evaluation of LVS Function	710	100%	96%	99%
Medicare Spending				
Medicare Spending per Patient (ratio)	-	0.98	0.93	0.98
Pneumonia Care				
Appropriate Initial Antibiotic Given[2]	227	93%	92%	95%
Blood Culture Timing[2]	383	93%	97%	98%
Pregnancy and Delivery Care				

NOTE: Hospital profiles are in alphabetical order by state, then city, then hospital within the city; Rankings exclude hospitals with less than 25 cases except for patient surveys which excludes hospitals with less than 100 cases; (a) 100-299 cases; (1) The number of cases/patients is too few to report; (2) Data submitted were based on a sample of cases/patients; (3) Results are based on a shorter time period than required; (4) Data suppressed by CMS for one or more quarters; (5) Results are not available for this reporting period; (6) Fewer than 100 patients completed the HCAHPS survey; (7) No cases met the criteria for this measure; (8) The lower limit of the confidence interval cannot be calculated if the number of observed infections equals zero; (9) No data are available from the state/territory for this reporting period; (10) The scores shown reflect fewer than 50 completed surveys; (11) There were discrepancies in the data collection process; (12) This measure does not apply to this hospital for this reporting period; (13) Results cannot be calculated for this reporting period; (14) The results for this state are combined with nearby states to protect confidentiality; Please refer to the User's Guide for a full explanation of data.

Measure	Cases	This Hosp.	State Avg.	U.S. Avg.
Newborn Deliveries Scheduled Early	167	9%	8%	6%
Preventive Care				
Immunization for Influenza[2]	537	94%	89%	90%
Immunization for Pneumonia[2]	677	87%	91%	92%
Stroke Care				
Anticoagulation Therapy for Atrial Fibrillation	91	100%	91%	95%
Antithrombotic Therapy Timing	459	92%	95%	98%
Assessed for Rehabilitation	623	99%	96%	97%
Discharged on Antithrombotic Therapy	532	99%	98%	99%
Discharged on Statin Medication	419	94%	88%	94%
Thrombolytic Therapy Timing	69	96%	61%	66%
Venous Thromboembolism Prophylaxis	680	98%	92%	94%
Written Stroke Educational Materials Given	336	93%	86%	88%
Surgical Care Improvement Project				
Appropriate Beta Blocker Usage[2]	408	99%	97%	98%
Appropriate VTP Within 24 Hours[2]	616	97%	97%	98%
Controlled Postoperative Blood Glucose[2]	321	100%	97%	97%
Perioperative Temperature Management[2]	794	100%	100%	100%
Prophylactic Antibiotic Selection[2]	835	99%	99%	99%
Prophylactic Antibiotic Selection (Outpatient)	834	98%	98%	98%
Prophylactic Antibiotic Stopped[2]	815	98%	98%	98%
Prophylactic Antibiotic Timing[2]	836	100%	98%	99%
Prophylactic Antibiotic Timing (Outpatient)	841	98%	98%	98%
Urinary Catheter Removal[2]	548	98%	96%	97%
Survey of Patients' Hospital Experiences				
Area Around Room 'Always' Quiet at Night	300+	57%	68%	61%
Doctors 'Always' Communicated Well	300+	79%	84%	82%
Home Recovery Information Given	300+	79%	84%	85%
Hospital Given 9 or 10 on 10 Point Scale	300+	70%	72%	71%
Meds 'Always' Explained Before Given	300+	55%	66%	64%
Nurses 'Always' Communicated Well	300+	75%	80%	79%
Pain 'Always' Well Controlled	300+	67%	72%	71%
Room and Bathroom 'Always' Clean	300+	68%	73%	73%
Timely Help 'Always' Received	300+	61%	71%	68%
Would Definitely Recommend Hospital	300+	72%	71%	71%
Use of Medical Imaging				
Cardiac Imaging Stress Test before Surgery	1,098	5.2%	4.5%	5.3%
Combination Abdominal CT Scan	1,066	3.7%	23%	10.5%
Combination Brain/Sinus CT Scan	1,336	1.8%	2.2%	2.7%
Combination Chest CT Scan	855	0.2%	5.1%	2.7%
Follow-up Mammogram/Ultrasound	3,119	12.0%	8.1%	8.8%
Lumbar Spine MRI for Low Back Pain	195	39.0%	39.9%	37.2%

Southwestern Regional Medical Center

10109 East 79th Street South
Tulsa, OK 74133
Phone: 918-496-5000
URL: www.cancercenter.com/southwestern
Type: Acute Care Hospitals
Emergency Services: Yes
Ownership: Proprietary
Beds: 42
Key Personnel:
CEO/President. . . . . Jim Brewer
Radiology. . . . . Ed McKay

Measure	Cases	This Hosp.	State Avg.	U.S. Avg.
Blood Clot Prevention and Treatment				
Anticoagulation Overlap Therapy[1,2]	-	-	89%	93%
ICU Venous Thromboembolism Prophylaxis[2]	28	89%	87%	92%
Incidence of Potentially Preventable VTE[1,2]	-	-	8%	10%
UFH with Dosages/Platelet Monitoring[1,2]	-	-	97%	97%
Venous Thromboembolism Prophylaxis[2]	85	79%	72%	85%
Warfarin Therapy Discharge Instructions[1,2]	-	-	73%	75%
Chest Pain/Possible Heart Attack Care				
Aspirin Given Within 24 Hours of Arrival[5]	-	-	95%	96%
Fibrinolytic Meds Within 30 Min. of Arrival[5]	-	-	54%	58%
Average Time to ECG (minutes)[5]	-	-	8	7
Average Time to Transfer (minutes)[5]	-	-	77	60
Children's Asthma Care				
Received Home Management Plan of Care	-	-	-	88%
Received Reliever Medication	-	-	-	100%
Received Systemic Corticosteroids	-	-	-	100%
Emergency Department				
Admittance Decision Time (minutes)[2,7]	-	-	63	98
Head CT Results Within 45 Min. of Arrival[5]	-	-	49%	57%
Patients Who Left ER Before Being Seen[5]	-	-	2%	2%
Time from ER Arrival to Admit. (minutes)[2,7]	-	-	210	274
Time from ER Arrival to Discharge (minutes)[5]	-	-	110	134
Time in ER Before Being Evaluated (minutes)[5]	-	-	24	26
Time to Pain Meds for Fractures (minutes)[5]	-	-	55	57
Heart Attack Care				
Aspirin Given at Discharge[3,7]	-	-	99%	99%
Fibrinolytic Meds Within 30 Min. of Arrival[3,7]	-	-	25%	54%
PCI Within 90 Minutes of Arrival[3,7]	-	-	95%	96%
Statin Prescribed at Discharge[3,7]	-	-	98%	98%
Heart Failure Care				
ACE Inhibitor or ARB for LVSD[1,3]	-	-	95%	97%
Discharge Instructions Given[1,3]	-	-	92%	94%
Evaluation of LVS Function[1,3]	-	-	96%	99%
Medicare Spending				
Medicare Spending per Patient (ratio)	-	1.40	0.93	0.98
Pneumonia Care				
Appropriate Initial Antibiotic Given[7]	-	-	92%	95%
Blood Culture Timing[7]	-	-	97%	98%
Pregnancy and Delivery Care				
Newborn Deliveries Scheduled Early[7]	-	-	8%	6%
Preventive Care				
Immunization for Influenza[2]	280	94%	89%	90%
Immunization for Pneumonia[2]	196	96%	91%	92%
Stroke Care				
Anticoagulation Therapy for Atrial Fibrillation[3,7]	-	-	91%	95%
Antithrombotic Therapy Timing[1,3]	-	-	95%	98%
Assessed for Rehabilitation[1,3]	-	-	96%	97%
Discharged on Antithrombotic Therapy[1,3]	-	-	98%	99%
Discharged on Statin Medication[1,3]	-	-	88%	94%
Thrombolytic Therapy Timing[3,7]	-	-	61%	66%
Venous Thromboembolism Prophylaxis[1,3]	-	-	92%	94%
Written Stroke Educational Materials Given[1,3]	-	-	86%	88%
Surgical Care Improvement Project				
Appropriate Beta Blocker Usage	25	88%	97%	98%
Appropriate VTP Within 24 Hours	158	93%	97%	98%
Controlled Postoperative Blood Glucose[7]	-	-	97%	97%
Perioperative Temperature Management	169	100%	100%	100%
Prophylactic Antibiotic Selection	32	97%	99%	99%
Prophylactic Antibiotic Selection (Outpatient)	66	97%	98%	98%
Prophylactic Antibiotic Stopped	28	89%	98%	98%
Prophylactic Antibiotic Timing	32	97%	98%	99%
Prophylactic Antibiotic Timing (Outpatient)	66	92%	98%	98%
Urinary Catheter Removal	41	85%	96%	97%
Survey of Patients' Hospital Experiences				
Area Around Room 'Always' Quiet at Night	(a)	68%	68%	61%
Doctors 'Always' Communicated Well	(a)	89%	84%	82%
Home Recovery Information Given	(a)	89%	84%	85%
Hospital Given 9 or 10 on 10 Point Scale	(a)	92%	72%	71%
Meds 'Always' Explained Before Given	(a)	72%	66%	64%
Nurses 'Always' Communicated Well	(a)	88%	80%	79%
Pain 'Always' Well Controlled	(a)	74%	72%	71%
Room and Bathroom 'Always' Clean	(a)	87%	73%	73%
Timely Help 'Always' Received	(a)	75%	71%	68%
Would Definitely Recommend Hospital	(a)	97%	71%	71%
Use of Medical Imaging				
Cardiac Imaging Stress Test before Surgery[1]	-	-	4.5%	5.3%
Combination Abdominal CT Scan	443	28.9%	23%	10.5%
Combination Brain/Sinus CT Scan[1]	-	-	2.2%	2.7%
Combination Chest CT Scan	439	0.0%	5.1%	2.7%
Follow-up Mammogram/Ultrasound[1]	-	-	8.1%	8.8%
Lumbar Spine MRI for Low Back Pain[7]	-	-	39.9%	37.2%

Tulsa Spine & Specialty Hospital

6901 South Olympia Avenue
Tulsa, OK 74132
Phone: 918-388-5701
URL: www.tulsaspinehospital.com
Type: Acute Care Hospitals
Emergency Services: Yes
Ownership: Physician

Measure	Cases	This Hosp.	State Avg.	U.S. Avg.
Blood Clot Prevention and Treatment				
Anticoagulation Overlap Therapy[2,7]	-	-	89%	93%
ICU Venous Thromboembolism Prophylaxis[2,7]	-	-	87%	92%
Incidence of Potentially Preventable VTE[2,7]	-	-	8%	10%
UFH with Dosages/Platelet Monitoring[2,7]	-	-	97%	97%
Venous Thromboembolism Prophylaxis[2]	210	99%	72%	85%
Warfarin Therapy Discharge Instructions[2,7]	-	-	73%	75%
Chest Pain/Possible Heart Attack Care				
Aspirin Given Within 24 Hours of Arrival[5]	-	-	95%	96%
Fibrinolytic Meds Within 30 Min. of Arrival[5]	-	-	54%	58%
Average Time to ECG (minutes)[5]	-	-	8	7
Average Time to Transfer (minutes)[5]	-	-	77	60
Children's Asthma Care				
Received Home Management Plan of Care	-	-	-	88%
Received Reliever Medication	-	-	-	100%
Received Systemic Corticosteroids	-	-	-	100%
Emergency Department				
Admittance Decision Time (minutes)[1,2]	-	-	63	98
Head CT Results Within 45 Min. of Arrival[5]	-	-	49%	57%
Patients Who Left ER Before Being Seen	79	0%	2%	2%
Time from ER Arrival to Admit. (minutes)[1,2]	-	-	210	274
Time from ER Arrival to Discharge (minutes)	57	114	110	134
Time in ER Before Being Evaluated (minutes)	58	11	24	26
Time to Pain Meds for Fractures (minutes)[5]	-	-	55	57
Heart Attack Care				
Aspirin Given at Discharge[5]	-	-	99%	99%
Fibrinolytic Meds Within 30 Min. of Arrival[5]	-	-	25%	54%
PCI Within 90 Minutes of Arrival[5]	-	-	95%	96%
Statin Prescribed at Discharge[5]	-	-	98%	98%
Heart Failure Care				
ACE Inhibitor or ARB for LVSD[5]	-	-	95%	97%
Discharge Instructions Given[5]	-	-	92%	94%
Evaluation of LVS Function[5]	-	-	96%	99%
Medicare Spending				
Medicare Spending per Patient (ratio)	-	0.92	0.93	0.98
Pneumonia Care				
Appropriate Initial Antibiotic Given[5]	-	-	92%	95%
Blood Culture Timing[5]	-	-	97%	98%
Pregnancy and Delivery Care				
Newborn Deliveries Scheduled Early[7]	-	-	8%	6%
Preventive Care				
Immunization for Influenza[2]	314	73%	89%	90%
Immunization for Pneumonia[2]	279	83%	91%	92%
Stroke Care				
Anticoagulation Therapy for Atrial Fibrillation[5]	-	-	91%	95%
Antithrombotic Therapy Timing[5]	-	-	95%	98%
Assessed for Rehabilitation[5]	-	-	96%	97%
Discharged on Antithrombotic Therapy[5]	-	-	98%	99%
Discharged on Statin Medication[5]	-	-	88%	94%
Thrombolytic Therapy Timing[5]	-	-	61%	66%
Venous Thromboembolism Prophylaxis[5]	-	-	92%	94%
Written Stroke Educational Materials Given[5]	-	-	86%	88%
Surgical Care Improvement Project				
Appropriate Beta Blocker Usage[2]	14	93%	97%	98%
Appropriate VTP Within 24 Hours[2]	55	96%	97%	98%
Controlled Postoperative Blood Glucose[2,7]	-	-	97%	97%
Perioperative Temperature Management[2]	99	100%	100%	100%
Prophylactic Antibiotic Selection[2]	65	98%	99%	99%
Prophylactic Antibiotic Selection (Outpatient)	464	99%	98%	98%
Prophylactic Antibiotic Stopped[2]	65	95%	98%	98%
Prophylactic Antibiotic Timing[2]	65	98%	98%	99%
Prophylactic Antibiotic Timing (Outpatient)	465	99%	98%	98%
Urinary Catheter Removal[1,2]	-	-	96%	97%
Survey of Patients' Hospital Experiences				
Area Around Room 'Always' Quiet at Night	300+	89%	68%	61%
Doctors 'Always' Communicated Well	300+	85%	84%	82%
Home Recovery Information Given	300+	88%	84%	85%
Hospital Given 9 or 10 on 10 Point Scale	300+	88%	72%	71%
Meds 'Always' Explained Before Given	300+	72%	66%	64%
Nurses 'Always' Communicated Well	300+	86%	80%	79%
Pain 'Always' Well Controlled	300+	77%	72%	71%
Room and Bathroom 'Always' Clean	300+	86%	73%	73%
Timely Help 'Always' Received	300+	78%	71%	68%
Would Definitely Recommend Hospital	300+	90%	71%	71%
Use of Medical Imaging				

NOTE: Hospital profiles are in alphabetical order by state, then city, then hospital within the city; Rankings exclude hospitals with less than 25 cases except for patient surveys which excludes hospitals with less than 100 cases; (a) 100-299 cases; (1) The number of cases/patients is too few to report; (2) Data submitted were based on a sample of cases/patients; (3) Results are based on a shorter time period than required; (4) Data suppressed by CMS for one or more quarters; (5) Results are not available for this reporting period; (6) Fewer than 100 patients completed the HCAHPS survey; (7) No cases met the criteria for this measure; (8) The lower limit of the confidence interval cannot be calculated if the number of observed infections equals zero; (9) No data are available from the state/territory for this reporting period; (10) The scores shown reflect fewer than 50 completed surveys; (11) There were discrepancies in the data collection process; (12) This measure does not apply to this hospital for this reporting period; (13) Results cannot be calculated for this reporting period; (14) The results for this state are combined with nearby states to protect confidentiality; Please refer to the User's Guide for a full explanation of data.

Measure	Cases	This Hosp.	State Avg.	U.S. Avg.
Cardiac Imaging Stress Test before Surgery[7]	-	-	4.5%	5.3%
Combination Abdominal CT Scan[1]	-	-	23%	10.5%
Combination Brain/Sinus CT Scan[1]	-	-	2.2%	2.7%
Combination Chest CT Scan[1]	-	-	5.1%	2.7%
Follow-up Mammogram/Ultrasound[7]	-	-	8.1%	8.8%
Lumbar Spine MRI for Low Back Pain	225	39.6%	39.9%	37.2%

Craig General Hospital

735 North Foreman
Vinita, OK 74301
Phone: 918-256-7551
Fax: 918-256-3703
URL: www.craiggeneralhospital.com
Type: Acute Care Hospitals
Emergency Services: Yes
Ownership: Voluntary non-profit - Other
Beds: 62

Key Personnel:
Radiology. Laura Arrowsmith
Infection Control. . . . . Gwen Barbaree
CEO/President. . . . . Steven Chase
Administrator . . . . Sandi Davis
Quality Assurance . . . . Bill Dennis
Chairman/CEO . . . . Cecil Egnor
Emergency Room . . . . Barbara Hodges
Chief of Medical Staff . . . . Robert F Villareal, MD

Measure	Cases	This Hosp.	State Avg.	U.S. Avg.
Blood Clot Prevention and Treatment				
Anticoagulation Overlap Therapy[1,2]	-	-	89%	93%
ICU Venous Thromboembolism Prophylaxis[2,7]	-	-	87%	92%
Incidence of Potentially Preventable VTE[2,7]	-	-	8%	10%
UFH with Dosages/Platelet Monitoring[2,7]	-	-	97%	97%
Venous Thromboembolism Prophylaxis[2]	152	20%	72%	85%
Warfarin Therapy Discharge Instructions[1,2]	-	-	73%	75%
Chest Pain/Possible Heart Attack Care				
Aspirin Given Within 24 Hours of Arrival	67	94%	95%	96%
Fibrinolytic Meds Within 30 Min. of Arrival[7]	-	-	54%	58%
Average Time to ECG (minutes)	65	3	8	7
Average Time to Transfer (minutes)[1]	-	-	77	60
Children's Asthma Care				
Received Home Management Plan of Care	-	-	-	88%
Received Reliever Medication	-	-	-	100%
Received Systemic Corticosteroids	-	-	-	100%
Emergency Department				
Admittance Decision Time (minutes)[2]	449	50	63	98
Head CT Results Within 45 Min. of Arrival[1]	-	-	49%	57%
Patients Who Left ER Before Being Seen	10,871	1%	2%	2%
Time from ER Arrival to Admit. (minutes)[2]	497	175	210	274
Time from ER Arrival to Discharge (minutes)	445	84	110	134
Time in ER Before Being Evaluated (minutes)	508	22	24	26
Time to Pain Meds for Fractures (minutes)	45	58	55	57
Heart Attack Care				
Aspirin Given at Discharge[1]	-	-	99%	99%
Fibrinolytic Meds Within 30 Min. of Arrival[7]	-	-	25%	54%
PCI Within 90 Minutes of Arrival[7]	-	-	95%	96%
Statin Prescribed at Discharge[1]	-	-	98%	98%
Heart Failure Care				
ACE Inhibitor or ARB for LVSD[2]	16	75%	95%	97%
Discharge Instructions Given[2]	37	100%	92%	94%
Evaluation of LVS Function[2]	48	92%	96%	99%
Medicare Spending				
Medicare Spending per Patient (ratio)	-	0.89	0.93	0.98
Pneumonia Care				
Appropriate Initial Antibiotic Given[2]	80	88%	92%	95%
Blood Culture Timing[2]	18	83%	97%	98%
Pregnancy and Delivery Care				
Newborn Deliveries Scheduled Early[1,2]	-	-	8%	6%
Preventive Care				
Immunization for Influenza[2]	287	87%	89%	90%
Immunization for Pneumonia[2]	483	88%	91%	92%
Stroke Care				
Anticoagulation Therapy for Atrial Fibrillation[7]	-	-	91%	95%
Antithrombotic Therapy Timing[1]	-	-	95%	98%
Assessed for Rehabilitation[1]	-	-	96%	97%
Discharged on Antithrombotic Therapy[1]	-	-	98%	99%
Discharged on Statin Medication[1]	-	-	88%	94%
Thrombolytic Therapy Timing[7]	-	-	61%	66%
Venous Thromboembolism Prophylaxis[1]	-	-	92%	94%
Written Stroke Educational Materials Given[1]	-	-	86%	88%
Surgical Care Improvement Project				
Appropriate Beta Blocker Usage[1,2]	-	-	97%	98%
Appropriate VTP Within 24 Hours[1,2]	-	-	97%	98%
Controlled Postoperative Blood Glucose[2,7]	-	-	97%	97%
Perioperative Temperature Management[2]	32	100%	100%	100%
Prophylactic Antibiotic Selection[2]	29	100%	99%	99%
Prophylactic Antibiotic Selection (Outpatient)[1,3]	-	-	98%	98%
Prophylactic Antibiotic Stopped[2]	29	97%	98%	98%
Prophylactic Antibiotic Timing[2]	29	93%	98%	99%
Prophylactic Antibiotic Timing (Outpatient)[3]	11	82%	98%	98%
Urinary Catheter Removal[2,7]	-	-	96%	97%
Survey of Patients' Hospital Experiences				
Area Around Room 'Always' Quiet at Night	(a)	61%	68%	61%
Doctors 'Always' Communicated Well	(a)	89%	84%	82%
Home Recovery Information Given	(a)	83%	84%	85%
Hospital Given 9 or 10 on 10 Point Scale	(a)	67%	72%	71%
Meds 'Always' Explained Before Given	(a)	62%	66%	64%
Nurses 'Always' Communicated Well	(a)	81%	80%	79%
Pain 'Always' Well Controlled	(a)	74%	72%	71%
Room and Bathroom 'Always' Clean	(a)	75%	73%	73%
Timely Help 'Always' Received	(a)	71%	71%	68%
Would Definitely Recommend Hospital	(a)	62%	71%	71%
Use of Medical Imaging				
Cardiac Imaging Stress Test before Surgery	117	1.7%	4.5%	5.3%
Combination Abdominal CT Scan	263	7.2%	23%	10.5%
Combination Brain/Sinus CT Scan[1]	-	-	2.2%	2.7%
Combination Chest CT Scan	94	2.1%	5.1%	2.7%
Follow-up Mammogram/Ultrasound	427	4.9%	8.1%	8.8%
Lumbar Spine MRI for Low Back Pain[1]	-	-	39.9%	37.2%

Wagoner Community Hospital

1200 West Cherokee Street
Wagoner, OK 74467
Phone: 918-485-5514
Fax: 918-485-9701
Type: Acute Care Hospitals
Emergency Services: Yes
Ownership: Govt - Hospital Dist/Auth
Beds: 100

Key Personnel:
CEO/President. . . . . John Crawford
Intensive Care Unit. . . . . Louie Easter
Chief of Medical Staff. . . . . Chris Roberts

Measure	Cases	This Hosp.	State Avg.	U.S. Avg.
Blood Clot Prevention and Treatment				
Anticoagulation Overlap Therapy[1,2]	-	-	89%	93%
ICU Venous Thromboembolism Prophylaxis[2]	13	23%	87%	92%
Incidence of Potentially Preventable VTE[2,7]	-	-	8%	10%
UFH with Dosages/Platelet Monitoring[2,7]	-	-	97%	97%
Venous Thromboembolism Prophylaxis[2]	286	22%	72%	85%
Warfarin Therapy Discharge Instructions[1,2]	-	-	73%	75%
Chest Pain/Possible Heart Attack Care				
Aspirin Given Within 24 Hours of Arrival[3]	19	95%	95%	96%
Fibrinolytic Meds Within 30 Min. of Arrival[1,3]	-	-	54%	58%
Average Time to ECG (minutes)[3]	20	8	8	7
Average Time to Transfer (minutes)[1,3]	-	-	77	60
Children's Asthma Care				
Received Home Management Plan of Care	-	-	-	88%
Received Reliever Medication	-	-	-	100%
Received Systemic Corticosteroids	-	-	-	100%
Emergency Department				
Admittance Decision Time (minutes)[2]	209	72	63	98
Head CT Results Within 45 Min. of Arrival[3,7]	-	-	49%	57%
Patients Who Left ER Before Being Seen	8,052	5%	2%	2%
Time from ER Arrival to Admit. (minutes)[2]	409	267	210	274
Time from ER Arrival to Discharge (minutes)	318	122	110	134
Time in ER Before Being Evaluated (minutes)	345	13	24	26
Time to Pain Meds for Fractures (minutes)[3]	24	58	55	57
Heart Attack Care				
Aspirin Given at Discharge[2,7]	-	-	99%	99%
Fibrinolytic Meds Within 30 Min. of Arrival[2,7]	-	-	25%	54%
PCI Within 90 Minutes of Arrival[2,7]	-	-	95%	96%
Statin Prescribed at Discharge[2,7]	-	-	98%	98%
Heart Failure Care				
ACE Inhibitor or ARB for LVSD[1,2]	-	-	95%	97%
Discharge Instructions Given[2]	27	70%	92%	94%
Evaluation of LVS Function[2]	29	76%	96%	99%
Medicare Spending				
Medicare Spending per Patient (ratio)	-	0.84	0.93	0.98
Pneumonia Care				
Appropriate Initial Antibiotic Given[2]	40	88%	92%	95%
Blood Culture Timing[2]	22	91%	97%	98%
Pregnancy and Delivery Care				
Newborn Deliveries Scheduled Early[7]	-	-	8%	6%
Preventive Care				
Immunization for Influenza[2]	301	50%	89%	90%
Immunization for Pneumonia[2]	225	65%	91%	92%
Stroke Care				
Anticoagulation Therapy for Atrial Fibrillation[2,3]	-	-	91%	95%
Antithrombotic Therapy Timing[1,2]	-	-	95%	98%
Assessed for Rehabilitation[1,2]	-	-	96%	97%
Discharged on Antithrombotic Therapy[1,2]	-	-	98%	99%
Discharged on Statin Medication[1,2]	-	-	88%	94%
Thrombolytic Therapy Timing[1,2]	-	-	61%	66%
Venous Thromboembolism Prophylaxis[1,2]	-	-	92%	94%
Written Stroke Educational Materials Given[1,2]	-	-	86%	88%
Surgical Care Improvement Project				
Appropriate Beta Blocker Usage[1,2]	-	-	97%	98%
Appropriate VTP Within 24 Hours[2]	13	100%	97%	98%
Controlled Postoperative Blood Glucose[2,7]	-	-	97%	97%
Perioperative Temperature Management[2]	18	100%	100%	100%
Prophylactic Antibiotic Selection[2]	15	93%	99%	99%
Prophylactic Antibiotic Selection (Outpatient)[5]	-	-	98%	98%
Prophylactic Antibiotic Stopped[2]	15	100%	98%	98%
Prophylactic Antibiotic Timing[2]	15	100%	98%	99%
Prophylactic Antibiotic Timing (Outpatient)[5]	-	-	98%	98%
Urinary Catheter Removal[2]	12	92%	96%	97%
Survey of Patients' Hospital Experiences				
Area Around Room 'Always' Quiet at Night	(a)	64%	68%	61%
Doctors 'Always' Communicated Well	(a)	82%	84%	82%
Home Recovery Information Given	(a)	81%	84%	85%
Hospital Given 9 or 10 on 10 Point Scale	(a)	58%	72%	71%
Meds 'Always' Explained Before Given	(a)	61%	66%	64%
Nurses 'Always' Communicated Well	(a)	75%	80%	79%
Pain 'Always' Well Controlled	(a)	65%	72%	71%
Room and Bathroom 'Always' Clean	(a)	62%	73%	73%
Timely Help 'Always' Received	(a)	62%	71%	68%
Would Definitely Recommend Hospital	(a)	59%	71%	71%
Use of Medical Imaging				
Cardiac Imaging Stress Test before Surgery	45	4.4%	4.5%	5.3%
Combination Abdominal CT Scan	85	64.7%	23%	10.5%
Combination Brain/Sinus CT Scan[1]	-	-	2.2%	2.7%
Combination Chest CT Scan[1]	-	-	5.1%	2.7%
Follow-up Mammogram/Ultrasound	183	2.7%	8.1%	8.8%
Lumbar Spine MRI for Low Back Pain[1]	-	-	39.9%	37.2%

Mercy Hospital Watonga

500 North Clarence Nash Boulevard
Watonga, OK 73772
Phone: 580-623-7211
Fax: 580-623-7206
E-mail: wmhosp@pldi.net
URL: www.watongahospital.com
Type: Critical Access Hospitals
Emergency Services: Yes
Ownership: Govt - Hospital Dist/Auth
Beds: 25

Key Personnel:
CEO/President. . . . . Brenda Doyel
Administrator . . . . Bobby Stitt
Quality Assurance . . . . Kathy Vermillion

Measure	Cases	This Hosp.	State Avg.	U.S. Avg.
Blood Clot Prevention and Treatment				
Anticoagulation Overlap Therapy[5]	-	-	89%	93%
ICU Venous Thromboembolism Prophylaxis[5]	-	-	87%	92%
Incidence of Potentially Preventable VTE[5]	-	-	8%	10%
UFH with Dosages/Platelet Monitoring[5]	-	-	97%	97%
Venous Thromboembolism Prophylaxis[5]	-	-	72%	85%
Warfarin Therapy Discharge Instructions[5]	-	-	73%	75%
Chest Pain/Possible Heart Attack Care				
Aspirin Given Within 24 Hours of Arrival[1,3]	-	-	95%	96%
Fibrinolytic Meds Within 30 Min. of Arrival[3,7]	-	-	54%	58%
Average Time to ECG (minutes)[1,3]	-	-	8	7

NOTE: Hospital profiles are in alphabetical order by state, then city, then hospital within the city; Rankings exclude hospitals with less than 25 cases except for patient surveys which excludes hospitals with less than 100 cases; (a) 100-299 cases; (1) The number of cases/patients is too few to report; (2) Data submitted were based on a sample of cases/patients; (3) Results are based on a shorter time period than required; (4) Data suppressed by CMS for one or more quarters; (5) Results are not available for this reporting period; (6) Fewer than 100 patients completed the HCAHPS survey; (7) No cases met the criteria for this measure; (8) The lower limit of the confidence interval cannot be calculated if the number of observed infections equals zero; (9) No data are available from the state/territory for this reporting period; (10) The scores shown reflect fewer than 50 completed surveys; (11) There were discrepancies in the data collection process; (12) This measure does not apply to this hospital for this reporting period; (13) Results cannot be calculated for this reporting period; (14) The results for this state are combined with nearby states to protect confidentiality; Please refer to the User's Guide for a full explanation of data.

Measure	Cases	This Hosp.	State Avg.	U.S. Avg.
Average Time to Transfer (minutes)[3,7]	-	-	77	60
Children's Asthma Care				
Received Home Management Plan of Care	-	-	-	88%
Received Reliever Medication	-	-	-	100%
Received Systemic Corticosteroids	-	-	-	100%
Emergency Department				
Admittance Decision Time (minutes)[5]	-	-	63	98
Head CT Results Within 45 Min. of Arrival[5]	-	-	49%	57%
Patients Who Left ER Before Being Seen[5]	-	-	2%	2%
Time from ER Arrival to Admit. (minutes)[5]	-	-	210	274
Time from ER Arrival to Discharge (minutes)[5]	-	-	110	134
Time in ER Before Being Evaluated (minutes)[5]	-	-	24	26
Time to Pain Meds for Fractures (minutes)[5]	-	-	55	57
Heart Attack Care				
Aspirin Given at Discharge[5]	-	-	99%	99%
Fibrinolytic Meds Within 30 Min. of Arrival[5]	-	-	25%	54%
PCI Within 90 Minutes of Arrival[5]	-	-	95%	96%
Statin Prescribed at Discharge[5]	-	-	98%	98%
Heart Failure Care				
ACE Inhibitor or ARB for LVSD[1,3]	-	-	95%	97%
Discharge Instructions Given[1,3]	-	-	92%	94%
Evaluation of LVS Function[1,3]	-	-	96%	99%
Medicare Spending				
Medicare Spending per Patient (ratio)	-	-	0.93	0.98
Pneumonia Care				
Appropriate Initial Antibiotic Given[1,3]	-	-	92%	95%
Blood Culture Timing[1,3]	-	-	97%	98%
Pregnancy and Delivery Care				
Newborn Deliveries Scheduled Early[5]	-	-	8%	6%
Preventive Care				
Immunization for Influenza[5]	-	-	89%	90%
Immunization for Pneumonia[5]	-	-	91%	92%
Stroke Care				
Anticoagulation Therapy for Atrial Fibrillation[5]	-	-	91%	95%
Antithrombotic Therapy Timing[5]	-	-	95%	98%
Assessed for Rehabilitation[5]	-	-	96%	97%
Discharged on Antithrombotic Therapy[5]	-	-	98%	99%
Discharged on Statin Medication[5]	-	-	88%	94%
Thrombolytic Therapy Timing[5]	-	-	61%	66%
Venous Thromboembolism Prophylaxis[5]	-	-	92%	94%
Written Stroke Educational Materials Given[5]	-	-	86%	88%
Surgical Care Improvement Project				
Appropriate Beta Blocker Usage[5]	-	-	97%	98%
Appropriate VTP Within 24 Hours[5]	-	-	97%	98%
Controlled Postoperative Blood Glucose[5]	-	-	97%	97%
Perioperative Temperature Management[5]	-	-	100%	100%
Prophylactic Antibiotic Selection[5]	-	-	99%	99%
Prophylactic Antibiotic Selection (Outpatient)[5]	-	-	98%	98%
Prophylactic Antibiotic Stopped[5]	-	-	98%	98%
Prophylactic Antibiotic Timing[5]	-	-	98%	99%
Prophylactic Antibiotic Timing (Outpatient)[5]	-	-	98%	98%
Urinary Catheter Removal[5]	-	-	96%	97%
Survey of Patients' Hospital Experiences				
Area Around Room 'Always' Quiet at Night[5]	-	-	68%	61%
Doctors 'Always' Communicated Well[5]	-	-	84%	82%
Home Recovery Information Given[5]	-	-	84%	85%
Hospital Given 9 or 10 on 10 Point Scale[5]	-	-	72%	71%
Meds 'Always' Explained Before Given[5]	-	-	66%	64%
Nurses 'Always' Communicated Well[5]	-	-	80%	79%
Pain 'Always' Well Controlled[5]	-	-	72%	71%
Room and Bathroom 'Always' Clean[5]	-	-	73%	73%
Timely Help 'Always' Received[5]	-	-	71%	68%
Would Definitely Recommend Hospital[5]	-	-	71%	71%
Use of Medical Imaging				
Cardiac Imaging Stress Test before Surgery[7]	-	-	4.5%	5.3%
Combination Abdominal CT Scan[1]	-	-	23%	10.5%
Combination Brain/Sinus CT Scan	101	0.0%	2.2%	2.7%
Combination Chest CT Scan[1]	-	-	5.1%	2.7%
Follow-up Mammogram/Ultrasound[7]	-	-	8.1%	8.8%
Lumbar Spine MRI for Low Back Pain[1]	-	-	39.9%	37.2%

Jefferson County Hospital

Intersection Hyws 81 & 70
Waurika, OK 73573
Phone: 580-228-2344
Fax: 580-228-3410
Type: Critical Access Hospitals
Emergency Services: Yes
Ownership: Govt - Hospital Dist/Auth
Beds: 25

Key Personnel:
Emergency Room . . . . Steven Hwshay, DO
Infection Control . . . . Pam Jackson, RN
Quality Assurance . . . . Buck McKinley, Jr
CEO/President. . . . . Buck McKinney Jr
Chief of Medical Staff . . . . Harold Start, MD
Chairman/CEO . . . . Carter Waid

Measure	Cases	This Hosp.	State Avg.	U.S. Avg.
Blood Clot Prevention and Treatment				
Anticoagulation Overlap Therapy[5]	-	-	89%	93%
ICU Venous Thromboembolism Prophylaxis[5]	-	-	87%	92%
Incidence of Potentially Preventable VTE[5]	-	-	8%	10%
UFH with Dosages/Platelet Monitoring[5]	-	-	97%	97%
Venous Thromboembolism Prophylaxis[5]	-	-	72%	85%
Warfarin Therapy Discharge Instructions[5]	-	-	73%	75%
Chest Pain/Possible Heart Attack Care				
Aspirin Given Within 24 Hours of Arrival[5]	-	-	95%	96%
Fibrinolytic Meds Within 30 Min. of Arrival[5]	-	-	54%	58%
Average Time to ECG (minutes)[5]	-	-	8	7
Average Time to Transfer (minutes)[5]	-	-	77	60
Children's Asthma Care				
Received Home Management Plan of Care	-	-	-	88%
Received Reliever Medication	-	-	-	100%
Received Systemic Corticosteroids	-	-	-	100%
Emergency Department				
Admittance Decision Time (minutes)[5]	-	-	63	98
Head CT Results Within 45 Min. of Arrival[5]	-	-	49%	57%
Patients Who Left ER Before Being Seen[5]	-	-	2%	2%
Time from ER Arrival to Admit. (minutes)[5]	-	-	210	274
Time from ER Arrival to Discharge (minutes)[5]	-	-	110	134
Time in ER Before Being Evaluated (minutes)[5]	-	-	24	26
Time to Pain Meds for Fractures (minutes)[5]	-	-	55	57
Heart Attack Care				
Aspirin Given at Discharge[5]	-	-	99%	99%
Fibrinolytic Meds Within 30 Min. of Arrival[5]	-	-	25%	54%
PCI Within 90 Minutes of Arrival[5]	-	-	95%	96%
Statin Prescribed at Discharge[5]	-	-	98%	98%
Heart Failure Care				
ACE Inhibitor or ARB for LVSD[5]	-	-	95%	97%
Discharge Instructions Given[5]	-	-	92%	94%
Evaluation of LVS Function[5]	-	-	96%	99%
Medicare Spending				
Medicare Spending per Patient (ratio)	-	-	0.93	0.98
Pneumonia Care				
Appropriate Initial Antibiotic Given[5]	-	-	92%	95%
Blood Culture Timing[5]	-	-	97%	98%
Pregnancy and Delivery Care				
Newborn Deliveries Scheduled Early[5]	-	-	8%	6%
Preventive Care				
Immunization for Influenza[5]	-	-	89%	90%
Immunization for Pneumonia[5]	-	-	91%	92%
Stroke Care				
Anticoagulation Therapy for Atrial Fibrillation[5]	-	-	91%	95%
Antithrombotic Therapy Timing[5]	-	-	95%	98%
Assessed for Rehabilitation[5]	-	-	96%	97%
Discharged on Antithrombotic Therapy[5]	-	-	98%	99%
Discharged on Statin Medication[5]	-	-	88%	94%
Thrombolytic Therapy Timing[5]	-	-	61%	66%
Venous Thromboembolism Prophylaxis[5]	-	-	92%	94%
Written Stroke Educational Materials Given[5]	-	-	86%	88%
Surgical Care Improvement Project				
Appropriate Beta Blocker Usage[5]	-	-	97%	98%
Appropriate VTP Within 24 Hours[5]	-	-	97%	98%
Controlled Postoperative Blood Glucose[5]	-	-	97%	97%
Perioperative Temperature Management[5]	-	-	100%	100%
Prophylactic Antibiotic Selection[5]	-	-	99%	99%
Prophylactic Antibiotic Selection (Outpatient)[5]	-	-	98%	98%
Prophylactic Antibiotic Stopped[5]	-	-	98%	98%
Prophylactic Antibiotic Timing[5]	-	-	98%	99%
Prophylactic Antibiotic Timing (Outpatient)[5]	-	-	98%	98%
Urinary Catheter Removal[5]	-	-	96%	97%
Survey of Patients' Hospital Experiences				
Area Around Room 'Always' Quiet at Night[5]	-	-	68%	61%
Doctors 'Always' Communicated Well[5]	-	-	84%	82%
Home Recovery Information Given[5]	-	-	84%	85%
Hospital Given 9 or 10 on 10 Point Scale[5]	-	-	72%	71%
Meds 'Always' Explained Before Given[5]	-	-	66%	64%
Nurses 'Always' Communicated Well[5]	-	-	80%	79%
Pain 'Always' Well Controlled[5]	-	-	72%	71%
Room and Bathroom 'Always' Clean[5]	-	-	73%	73%
Timely Help 'Always' Received[5]	-	-	71%	68%
Would Definitely Recommend Hospital[5]	-	-	71%	71%
Use of Medical Imaging				
Cardiac Imaging Stress Test before Surgery[7]	-	-	4.5%	5.3%
Combination Abdominal CT Scan[1]	-	-	23%	10.5%
Combination Brain/Sinus CT Scan	30	0.0%	2.2%	2.7%
Combination Chest CT Scan[1]	-	-	5.1%	2.7%
Follow-up Mammogram/Ultrasound[7]	-	-	8.1%	8.8%
Lumbar Spine MRI for Low Back Pain[7]	-	-	39.9%	37.2%

Weatherford Regional Hospital

3701 E Main
Weatherford, OK 73096
Phone: 580-772-5551
Fax: 580-774-4764
URL: www.weatherfordhospital.com
Type: Critical Access Hospitals
Emergency Services: Yes
Ownership: Govt - Hospital Dist/Auth
Beds: 49

Key Personnel:
Operating Room. . . . . Ollie Brooks
Emergency Room . . . . Sergio DeMier
Radiology. . . . . John Hamlin
CEO/President. . . . . Debbie Howe

Measure	Cases	This Hosp.	State Avg.	U.S. Avg.
Blood Clot Prevention and Treatment				
Anticoagulation Overlap Therapy[5]	-	-	89%	93%
ICU Venous Thromboembolism Prophylaxis[5]	-	-	87%	92%
Incidence of Potentially Preventable VTE[5]	-	-	8%	10%
UFH with Dosages/Platelet Monitoring[5]	-	-	97%	97%
Venous Thromboembolism Prophylaxis[5]	-	-	72%	85%
Warfarin Therapy Discharge Instructions[5]	-	-	73%	75%
Chest Pain/Possible Heart Attack Care				
Aspirin Given Within 24 Hours of Arrival	37	92%	95%	96%
Fibrinolytic Meds Within 30 Min. of Arrival[1]	-	-	54%	58%
Average Time to ECG (minutes)	39	22	8	7
Average Time to Transfer (minutes)[7]	-	-	77	60
Children's Asthma Care				
Received Home Management Plan of Care	-	-	-	88%
Received Reliever Medication	-	-	-	100%
Received Systemic Corticosteroids	-	-	-	100%
Emergency Department				
Admittance Decision Time (minutes)	112	66	63	98
Head CT Results Within 45 Min. of Arrival[1]	-	-	49%	57%
Patients Who Left ER Before Being Seen[5]	-	-	2%	2%
Time from ER Arrival to Admit. (minutes)	115	262	210	274
Time from ER Arrival to Discharge (minutes)[5]	-	-	110	134
Time in ER Before Being Evaluated (minutes)[5]	-	-	24	26
Time to Pain Meds for Fractures (minutes)	62	62	55	57
Heart Attack Care				
Aspirin Given at Discharge[1,3]	-	-	99%	99%
Fibrinolytic Meds Within 30 Min. of Arrival[3,7]	-	-	25%	54%
PCI Within 90 Minutes of Arrival[3,7]	-	-	95%	96%
Statin Prescribed at Discharge[1,3]	-	-	98%	98%
Heart Failure Care				
ACE Inhibitor or ARB for LVSD[1]	-	-	95%	97%
Discharge Instructions Given[1]	-	-	92%	94%
Evaluation of LVS Function	14	43%	96%	99%
Medicare Spending				
Medicare Spending per Patient (ratio)	-	-	0.93	0.98
Pneumonia Care				
Appropriate Initial Antibiotic Given	41	85%	92%	95%
Blood Culture Timing	38	97%	97%	98%
Pregnancy and Delivery Care				

NOTE: Hospital profiles are in alphabetical order by state, then city, then hospital within the city; Rankings exclude hospitals with less than 25 cases except for patient surveys which excludes hospitals with less than 100 cases; (a) 100-299 cases; (1) The number of cases/patients is too few to report; (2) Data submitted were based on a sample of cases/patients; (3) Results are based on a shorter time period than required; (4) Data suppressed by CMS for one or more quarters; (5) Results are not available for this reporting period; (6) Fewer than 100 patients completed the HCAHPS survey; (7) No cases met the criteria for this measure; (8) The lower limit of the confidence interval cannot be calculated if the number of observed infections equals zero; (9) No data are available from the state/territory for this reporting period; (10) The scores shown reflect fewer than 50 completed surveys; (11) There were discrepancies in the data collection process; (12) This measure does not apply to this hospital for this reporting period; (13) Results cannot be calculated for this reporting period; (14) The results for this state are combined with nearby states to protect confidentiality; Please refer to the User's Guide for a full explanation of data.

Measure	Cases	This Hosp.	State Avg.	U.S. Avg.
Newborn Deliveries Scheduled Early[5]	-	-	8%	6%
Preventive Care				
Immunization for Influenza	63	94%	89%	90%
Immunization for Pneumonia	114	95%	91%	92%
Stroke Care				
Anticoagulation Therapy for Atrial Fibrillation[3,7]	-	-	91%	95%
Antithrombotic Therapy Timing[1,3]	-	-	95%	98%
Assessed for Rehabilitation[1,3]	-	-	96%	97%
Discharged on Antithrombotic Therapy[1,3]	-	-	98%	99%
Discharged on Statin Medication[1,3]	-	-	88%	94%
Thrombolytic Therapy Timing[1,3]	-	-	61%	66%
Venous Thromboembolism Prophylaxis[1,3]	-	-	92%	94%
Written Stroke Educational Materials Given[3,7]	-	-	86%	88%
Surgical Care Improvement Project				
Appropriate Beta Blocker Usage[5]	-	-	97%	98%
Appropriate VTP Within 24 Hours[5]	-	-	97%	98%
Controlled Postoperative Blood Glucose[5]	-	-	97%	97%
Perioperative Temperature Management[5]	-	-	100%	100%
Prophylactic Antibiotic Selection[5]	-	-	99%	99%
Prophylactic Antibiotic Selection (Outpatient)[5]	-	-	98%	98%
Prophylactic Antibiotic Stopped[5]	-	-	98%	98%
Prophylactic Antibiotic Timing[5]	-	-	98%	99%
Prophylactic Antibiotic Timing (Outpatient)[5]	-	-	98%	98%
Urinary Catheter Removal[5]	-	-	96%	97%
Survey of Patients' Hospital Experiences				
Area Around Room 'Always' Quiet at Night[5]	-	-	68%	61%
Doctors 'Always' Communicated Well[5]	-	-	84%	82%
Home Recovery Information Given[5]	-	-	84%	85%
Hospital Given 9 or 10 on 10 Point Scale[5]	-	-	72%	71%
Meds 'Always' Explained Before Given[5]	-	-	66%	64%
Nurses 'Always' Communicated Well[5]	-	-	80%	79%
Pain 'Always' Well Controlled[5]	-	-	72%	71%
Room and Bathroom 'Always' Clean[5]	-	-	73%	73%
Timely Help 'Always' Received[5]	-	-	71%	68%
Would Definitely Recommend Hospital[5]	-	-	71%	71%
Use of Medical Imaging				
Cardiac Imaging Stress Test before Surgery	208	1.9%	4.5%	5.3%
Combination Abdominal CT Scan	194	46.4%	23%	10.5%
Combination Brain/Sinus CT Scan[1]	-	-	2.2%	2.7%
Combination Chest CT Scan	74	24.3%	5.1%	2.7%
Follow-up Mammogram/Ultrasound	201	6.5%	8.1%	8.8%
Lumbar Spine MRI for Low Back Pain[1]	-	-	39.9%	37.2%

Latimer County General Hospital

806 State Highway 2 North
Wilburton, OK 74578
Phone: 918-465-2391
Fax: 918-465-5169
Type: Acute Care Hospitals
Emergency Services: Yes
Ownership: Govt - Hospital Dist/Auth
Beds: 33

Key Personnel:
CEO/President. . . . . Sue Mings
Chief of Medical Staff. . . . . Ricardo Valbuena
Emergency Room . . . . Lynda Willmoen

Measure	Cases	This Hosp.	State Avg.	U.S. Avg.
Blood Clot Prevention and Treatment				
Anticoagulation Overlap Therapy[7]	-	-	89%	93%
ICU Venous Thromboembolism Prophylaxis[7]	-	-	87%	92%
Incidence of Potentially Preventable VTE[7]	-	-	8%	10%
UFH with Dosages/Platelet Monitoring[7]	-	-	97%	97%
Venous Thromboembolism Prophylaxis	108	0%	72%	85%
Warfarin Therapy Discharge Instructions[7]	-	-	73%	75%
Chest Pain/Possible Heart Attack Care				
Aspirin Given Within 24 Hours of Arrival[1,3]	-	-	95%	96%
Fibrinolytic Meds Within 30 Min. of Arrival[1,3]	-	-	54%	58%
Average Time to ECG (minutes)[1,3]	-	-	8	7
Average Time to Transfer (minutes)[1,3]	-	-	77	60
Children's Asthma Care				
Received Home Management Plan of Care	-	-	-	88%
Received Reliever Medication	-	-	-	100%
Received Systemic Corticosteroids	-	-	-	100%
Emergency Department				
Admittance Decision Time (minutes)	266	20	63	98
Head CT Results Within 45 Min. of Arrival[1]	-	-	49%	57%
Patients Who Left ER Before Being Seen	3,440	1%	2%	2%
Time from ER Arrival to Admit. (minutes)	289	110	210	274
Time from ER Arrival to Discharge (minutes)	175	75	110	134
Time in ER Before Being Evaluated (minutes)	263	0	24	26
Time to Pain Meds for Fractures (minutes)	11	45	55	57
Heart Attack Care				
Aspirin Given at Discharge[3,7]	-	-	99%	99%
Fibrinolytic Meds Within 30 Min. of Arrival[1,3]	-	-	25%	54%
PCI Within 90 Minutes of Arrival[3,7]	-	-	95%	96%
Statin Prescribed at Discharge[3,7]	-	-	98%	98%
Heart Failure Care				
ACE Inhibitor or ARB for LVSD[1,3]	-	-	95%	97%
Discharge Instructions Given[1,3]	-	-	92%	94%
Evaluation of LVS Function[1,3]	-	-	96%	99%
Medicare Spending				
Medicare Spending per Patient (ratio)	-	0.96	0.93	0.98
Pneumonia Care				
Appropriate Initial Antibiotic Given	15	53%	92%	95%
Blood Culture Timing[1]	-	-	97%	98%
Pregnancy and Delivery Care				
Newborn Deliveries Scheduled Early[7]	-	-	8%	6%
Preventive Care				
Immunization for Influenza[2]	255	73%	89%	90%
Immunization for Pneumonia[2]	268	77%	91%	92%
Stroke Care				
Anticoagulation Therapy for Atrial Fibrillation[5]	-	-	91%	95%
Antithrombotic Therapy Timing[5]	-	-	95%	98%
Assessed for Rehabilitation[5]	-	-	96%	97%
Discharged on Antithrombotic Therapy[5]	-	-	98%	99%
Discharged on Statin Medication[5]	-	-	88%	94%
Thrombolytic Therapy Timing[5]	-	-	61%	66%
Venous Thromboembolism Prophylaxis[5]	-	-	92%	94%
Written Stroke Educational Materials Given[5]	-	-	86%	88%
Surgical Care Improvement Project				
Appropriate Beta Blocker Usage[5]	-	-	97%	98%
Appropriate VTP Within 24 Hours[5]	-	-	97%	98%
Controlled Postoperative Blood Glucose[5]	-	-	97%	97%
Perioperative Temperature Management[5]	-	-	100%	100%
Prophylactic Antibiotic Selection[5]	-	-	99%	99%
Prophylactic Antibiotic Selection (Outpatient)[5]	-	-	98%	98%
Prophylactic Antibiotic Stopped[5]	-	-	98%	98%
Prophylactic Antibiotic Timing[5]	-	-	98%	99%
Prophylactic Antibiotic Timing (Outpatient)[5]	-	-	98%	98%
Urinary Catheter Removal[5]	-	-	96%	97%
Survey of Patients' Hospital Experiences				
Area Around Room 'Always' Quiet at Night[6]	<100	83%	68%	61%
Doctors 'Always' Communicated Well[6]	<100	85%	84%	82%
Home Recovery Information Given[6]	<100	78%	84%	85%
Hospital Given 9 or 10 on 10 Point Scale[6]	<100	66%	72%	71%
Meds 'Always' Explained Before Given[6]	<100	71%	66%	64%
Nurses 'Always' Communicated Well[6]	<100	87%	80%	79%
Pain 'Always' Well Controlled[6]	<100	83%	72%	71%
Room and Bathroom 'Always' Clean[6]	<100	78%	73%	73%
Timely Help 'Always' Received[6]	<100	82%	71%	68%
Would Definitely Recommend Hospital[6]	<100	62%	71%	71%
Use of Medical Imaging				
Cardiac Imaging Stress Test before Surgery[7]	-	-	4.5%	5.3%
Combination Abdominal CT Scan[1]	-	-	23%	10.5%
Combination Brain/Sinus CT Scan	63	0.0%	2.2%	2.7%
Combination Chest CT Scan[1]	-	-	5.1%	2.7%
Follow-up Mammogram/Ultrasound[7]	-	-	8.1%	8.8%
Lumbar Spine MRI for Low Back Pain[7]	-	-	39.9%	37.2%

Woodward Regional Hospital

900 17th Street
Woodward, OK 73801
Phone: 580-254-8492
Fax: 580-254-8431
E-mail: bhubbard@woodwardhospital.com
URL: www.woodwardhospital.com
Type: Acute Care Hospitals
Emergency Services: Yes
Ownership: Proprietary
Beds: 87

Key Personnel:
Radiology. . . . . Stephen Back
Emergency Room . . . . Jason Benn
Pediatrics. . . . . Janice Chleborad, MD
Emergency Room . . . . Kevin Hoos, DO
Emergency Room . . . . Liz Sizelove, RN
Quality Assurance . . . . Martha Syms, RN, BSN
CEO/President. . . . . Troy Taubenheim, CPA

Measure	Cases	This Hosp.	State Avg.	U.S. Avg.
Blood Clot Prevention and Treatment				
Anticoagulation Overlap Therapy[1,2]	-	-	89%	93%
ICU Venous Thromboembolism Prophylaxis[2]	88	100%	87%	92%
Incidence of Potentially Preventable VTE[2,7]	-	-	8%	10%
UFH with Dosages/Platelet Monitoring[2,7]	-	-	97%	97%
Venous Thromboembolism Prophylaxis[2]	143	100%	72%	85%
Warfarin Therapy Discharge Instructions[1,2]	-	-	73%	75%
Chest Pain/Possible Heart Attack Care				
Aspirin Given Within 24 Hours of Arrival	39	100%	95%	96%
Fibrinolytic Meds Within 30 Min. of Arrival[1]	-	-	54%	58%
Average Time to ECG (minutes)	39	4	8	7
Average Time to Transfer (minutes)[1]	-	-	77	60
Children's Asthma Care				
Received Home Management Plan of Care	-	-	-	88%
Received Reliever Medication	-	-	-	100%
Received Systemic Corticosteroids	-	-	-	100%
Emergency Department				
Admittance Decision Time (minutes)[2]	339	33	63	98
Head CT Results Within 45 Min. of Arrival[1]	-	-	49%	57%
Patients Who Left ER Before Being Seen	12,846	1%	2%	2%
Time from ER Arrival to Admit. (minutes)[2]	342	154	210	274
Time from ER Arrival to Discharge (minutes)	409	75	110	134
Time in ER Before Being Evaluated (minutes)	441	13	24	26
Time to Pain Meds for Fractures (minutes)	68	37	55	57
Heart Attack Care				
Aspirin Given at Discharge[1,3]	-	-	99%	99%
Fibrinolytic Meds Within 30 Min. of Arrival[3,7]	-	-	25%	54%
PCI Within 90 Minutes of Arrival[3,7]	-	-	95%	96%
Statin Prescribed at Discharge[1,3]	-	-	98%	98%
Heart Failure Care				
ACE Inhibitor or ARB for LVSD	17	100%	95%	97%
Discharge Instructions Given	23	100%	92%	94%
Evaluation of LVS Function	32	100%	96%	99%
Medicare Spending				
Medicare Spending per Patient (ratio)	-	0.85	0.93	0.98
Pneumonia Care				
Appropriate Initial Antibiotic Given	38	100%	92%	95%
Blood Culture Timing	57	100%	97%	98%
Pregnancy and Delivery Care				
Newborn Deliveries Scheduled Early[2]	62	2%	8%	6%
Preventive Care				
Immunization for Influenza[2]	289	100%	89%	90%
Immunization for Pneumonia[2]	287	100%	91%	92%
Stroke Care				
Anticoagulation Therapy for Atrial Fibrillation[1]	-	-	91%	95%
Antithrombotic Therapy Timing[1]	-	-	95%	98%
Assessed for Rehabilitation[1]	-	-	96%	97%
Discharged on Antithrombotic Therapy[1]	-	-	98%	99%
Discharged on Statin Medication[1]	-	-	88%	94%
Thrombolytic Therapy Timing[7]	-	-	61%	66%
Venous Thromboembolism Prophylaxis[1]	-	-	92%	94%
Written Stroke Educational Materials Given[1]	-	-	86%	88%
Surgical Care Improvement Project				
Appropriate Beta Blocker Usage	24	100%	97%	98%
Appropriate VTP Within 24 Hours	45	100%	97%	98%
Controlled Postoperative Blood Glucose[7]	-	-	97%	97%
Perioperative Temperature Management	74	100%	100%	100%
Prophylactic Antibiotic Selection	26	100%	99%	99%
Prophylactic Antibiotic Selection (Outpatient)	46	98%	98%	98%
Prophylactic Antibiotic Stopped	24	100%	98%	98%
Prophylactic Antibiotic Timing	26	100%	98%	99%
Prophylactic Antibiotic Timing (Outpatient)	46	100%	98%	98%
Urinary Catheter Removal	21	100%	96%	97%
Survey of Patients' Hospital Experiences				
Area Around Room 'Always' Quiet at Night	300+	63%	68%	61%
Doctors 'Always' Communicated Well	300+	87%	84%	82%
Home Recovery Information Given	300+	88%	84%	85%
Hospital Given 9 or 10 on 10 Point Scale	300+	66%	72%	71%
Meds 'Always' Explained Before Given	300+	71%	66%	64%

NOTE: Hospital profiles are in alphabetical order by state, then city, then hospital within the city; Rankings exclude hospitals with less than 25 cases except for patient surveys which excludes hospitals with less than 100 cases; (a) 100-299 cases; (1) The number of cases/patients is too few to report; (2) Data submitted were based on a sample of cases/patients; (3) Results are based on a shorter time period than required; (4) Data suppressed by CMS for one or more quarters; (5) Results are not available for this reporting period; (6) Fewer than 100 patients completed the HCAHPS survey; (7) No cases met the criteria for this measure; (8) The lower limit of the confidence interval cannot be calculated if the number of observed infections equals zero; (9) No data are available from the state/territory for this reporting period; (10) The scores shown reflect fewer than 50 completed surveys; (11) There were discrepancies in the data collection process; (12) This measure does not apply to this hospital for this reporting period; (13) Results cannot be calculated for this reporting period; (14) The results for this state are combined with nearby states to protect confidentiality; Please refer to the User's Guide for a full explanation of data.

Nurses 'Always' Communicated Well	300+	79%	80%	79%
Pain 'Always' Well Controlled	300+	73%	72%	71%
Room and Bathroom 'Always' Clean	300+	76%	73%	73%
Timely Help 'Always' Received	300+	74%	71%	68%
Would Definitely Recommend Hospital	300+	63%	71%	71%
Use of Medical Imaging				
Cardiac Imaging Stress Test before Surgery[1]	-	-	4.5%	5.3%
Combination Abdominal CT Scan	183	22.4%	23%	10.5%
Combination Brain/Sinus CT Scan[1]	-	-	2.2%	2.7%
Combination Chest CT Scan	117	13.7%	5.1%	2.7%
Follow-up Mammogram/Ultrasound	385	7.0%	8.1%	8.8%
Lumbar Spine MRI for Low Back Pain[1]	-	-	39.9%	37.2%

Integris Canadian Valley Hospital

1201 Health Center Parkway
Yukon, OK 73099
Phone: 405-717-6800
Type: Acute Care Hospitals
Emergency Services: No
Ownership: Voluntary non-profit - Other

Measure	Cases	This Hosp.	State Avg.	U.S. Avg.
Blood Clot Prevention and Treatment				
Anticoagulation Overlap Therapy[2]	24	67%	89%	93%
ICU Venous Thromboembolism Prophylaxis[2]	44	77%	87%	92%
Incidence of Potentially Preventable VTE[1,2]	-	-	8%	10%
UFH with Dosages/Platelet Monitoring[2,7]	-	-	97%	97%
Venous Thromboembolism Prophylaxis[2]	132	73%	72%	85%
Warfarin Therapy Discharge Instructions[2]	21	86%	73%	75%
Chest Pain/Possible Heart Attack Care				
Aspirin Given Within 24 Hours of Arrival	59	98%	95%	96%
Fibrinolytic Meds Within 30 Min. of Arrival[1]	-	-	54%	58%
Average Time to ECG (minutes)	62	6	8	7
Average Time to Transfer (minutes)	12	58	77	60
Children's Asthma Care				
Received Home Management Plan of Care	-	-	-	88%
Received Reliever Medication	-	-	-	100%
Received Systemic Corticosteroids	-	-	-	100%
Emergency Department				
Admittance Decision Time (minutes)[2]	231	61	63	98
Head CT Results Within 45 Min. of Arrival	16	69%	49%	57%
Patients Who Left ER Before Being Seen	28,881	1%	2%	2%
Time from ER Arrival to Admit. (minutes)[2]	252	216	210	274
Time from ER Arrival to Discharge (minutes)	359	113	110	134
Time in ER Before Being Evaluated (minutes)	36	42	24	26
Time to Pain Meds for Fractures (minutes)	135	42	55	57
Heart Attack Care				
Aspirin Given at Discharge[1,3]	-	-	99%	99%
Fibrinolytic Meds Within 30 Min. of Arrival[3,7]	-	-	25%	54%
PCI Within 90 Minutes of Arrival[3,7]	-	-	95%	96%
Statin Prescribed at Discharge[3,7]	-	-	98%	98%
Heart Failure Care				
ACE Inhibitor or ARB for LVSD	15	93%	95%	97%
Discharge Instructions Given	26	81%	92%	94%
Evaluation of LVS Function	31	90%	96%	99%
Medicare Spending				
Medicare Spending per Patient (ratio)	-	1.06	0.93	0.98
Pneumonia Care				
Appropriate Initial Antibiotic Given	80	90%	92%	95%
Blood Culture Timing	108	96%	97%	98%
Pregnancy and Delivery Care				
Newborn Deliveries Scheduled Early	126	3%	8%	6%
Preventive Care				
Immunization for Influenza[2]	276	89%	89%	90%
Immunization for Pneumonia[2]	251	95%	91%	92%
Stroke Care				
Anticoagulation Therapy for Atrial Fibrillation[1]	-	-	91%	95%
Antithrombotic Therapy Timing[1]	-	-	95%	98%
Assessed for Rehabilitation	11	82%	96%	97%
Discharged on Antithrombotic Therapy	11	100%	98%	99%
Discharged on Statin Medication[1]	-	-	88%	94%
Thrombolytic Therapy Timing[1]	-	-	61%	66%
Venous Thromboembolism Prophylaxis[1]	-	-	92%	94%
Written Stroke Educational Materials Given[1]	-	-	86%	88%
Surgical Care Improvement Project				
Appropriate Beta Blocker Usage[2]	50	98%	97%	98%
Appropriate VTP Within 24 Hours[2]	225	97%	97%	98%
Controlled Postoperative Blood Glucose[2,7]	-	-	97%	97%
Perioperative Temperature Management[2]	239	100%	100%	100%
Prophylactic Antibiotic Selection[2]	158	100%	99%	99%
Prophylactic Antibiotic Selection (Outpatient)	124	98%	98%	98%
Prophylactic Antibiotic Stopped[2]	155	99%	98%	98%
Prophylactic Antibiotic Timing[2]	158	98%	98%	99%
Prophylactic Antibiotic Timing (Outpatient)	124	98%	98%	98%
Urinary Catheter Removal[2]	144	97%	96%	97%
Survey of Patients' Hospital Experiences				
Area Around Room 'Always' Quiet at Night	300+	73%	68%	61%
Doctors 'Always' Communicated Well	300+	84%	84%	82%
Home Recovery Information Given	300+	84%	84%	85%
Hospital Given 9 or 10 on 10 Point Scale	300+	73%	72%	71%
Meds 'Always' Explained Before Given	300+	64%	66%	64%
Nurses 'Always' Communicated Well	300+	80%	80%	79%
Pain 'Always' Well Controlled	300+	71%	72%	71%
Room and Bathroom 'Always' Clean	300+	81%	73%	73%
Timely Help 'Always' Received	300+	64%	71%	68%
Would Definitely Recommend Hospital	300+	75%	71%	71%
Use of Medical Imaging				
Cardiac Imaging Stress Test before Surgery[1]	-	-	4.5%	5.3%
Combination Abdominal CT Scan	322	8.1%	23%	10.5%
Combination Brain/Sinus CT Scan	383	0.8%	2.2%	2.7%
Combination Chest CT Scan	235	0.4%	5.1%	2.7%
Follow-up Mammogram/Ultrasound	416	11.1%	8.1%	8.8%
Lumbar Spine MRI for Low Back Pain	67	47.8%	39.9%	37.2%

NOTE: Hospital profiles are in alphabetical order by state, then city, then hospital within the city; Rankings exclude hospitals with less than 25 cases except for patient surveys which excludes hospitals with less than 100 cases; (a) 100-299 cases; (1) The number of cases/patients is too few to report; (2) Data submitted were based on a sample of cases/patients; (3) Results are based on a shorter time period than required; (4) Data suppressed by CMS for one or more quarters; (5) Results are not available for this reporting period; (6) Fewer than 100 patients completed the HCAHPS survey; (7) No cases met the criteria for this measure; (8) The lower limit of the confidence interval cannot be calculated if the number of observed infections equals zero; (9) No data are available from the state/territory for this reporting period; (10) The scores shown reflect fewer than 50 completed surveys; (11) There were discrepancies in the data collection process; (12) This measure does not apply to this hospital for this reporting period; (13) Results cannot be calculated for this reporting period; (14) The results for this state are combined with nearby states to protect confidentiality; Please refer to the User's Guide for a full explanation of data.

Blood Clot Prevention and Treatment

Anticoagulation Overlap Therapy

Hospital Name	City	Rate	Cases
Avera Queen of Peace[2]	Mitchell	100%	26
Avera Mckennan Hosp & Univ Health Ctr[2]	Sioux Falls	99%	134
Avera Saint Lukes[2]	Aberdeen	96%	27
Sanford Usd Medical Center[2]	Sioux Falls	96%	158
Avera Sacred Heart Hospital[2]	Yankton	95%	39
Rapid City Regional Hospital[2]	Rapid City	95%	131
Prairie Lakes Hospital[2]	Watertown	90%	42
Avera Heart Hospital of South Dakota[2]	Sioux Falls	79%	42

ICU Venous Thromboembolism Prophylaxis

Hospital Name	City	Rate	Cases
Avera Queen of Peace[2]	Mitchell	100%	50
Rapid City Regional Hospital[2]	Rapid City	98%	89
Avera Sacred Heart Hospital[2]	Yankton	97%	62
Avera Saint Lukes[2]	Aberdeen	97%	68
Sanford Usd Medical Center[2]	Sioux Falls	97%	65
Avera Mckennan Hosp & Univ Health Ctr[2]	Sioux Falls	95%	63
Prairie Lakes Hospital[2]	Watertown	57%	74

Incidence of Potentially Preventable VTE

Hospital Name	City	Rate	Cases
Rapid City Regional Hospital[2]	Rapid City	9%	33
Sanford Usd Medical Center[2]	Sioux Falls	9%	33

UFH with Dosages/Platelet Count Monitoring

Hospital Name	City	Rate	Cases
Avera Heart Hospital of South Dakota[2]	Sioux Falls	100%	49
Avera Mckennan Hosp & Univ Health Ctr[2]	Sioux Falls	100%	69
Avera Queen of Peace[2]	Mitchell	100%	26
Avera Saint Lukes[2]	Aberdeen	100%	34
Prairie Lakes Hospital[2]	Watertown	100%	28
Rapid City Regional Hospital[2]	Rapid City	100%	62
Sanford Usd Medical Center[2]	Sioux Falls	100%	117

Venous Thromboembolism Prophylaxis

Hospital Name	City	Rate	Cases
Black Hills Surgical Hospital[2]	Rapid City	100%	105
Dakota Plains Surgical Center[2]	Aberdeen	100%	35
Sioux Falls Specialty Hospital[2]	Sioux Falls	100%	100
Siouxland Surgery Center	Dakota Dunes	100%	275
Avera Queen of Peace[2]	Mitchell	96%	163
Avera Sacred Heart Hospital[2]	Yankton	96%	199
Avera Heart Hospital of South Dakota[2]	Sioux Falls	95%	260
Avera Mckennan Hosp & Univ Health Ctr[2]	Sioux Falls	92%	254
Rapid City Regional Hospital[2]	Rapid City	90%	357
Spearfish Regional Hospital[2]	Spearfish	90%	240
Avera Saint Lukes[2]	Aberdeen	88%	187
Sanford Aberdeen Medical Center[2,3]	Aberdeen	84%	76
Sanford Usd Medical Center[2]	Sioux Falls	81%	286
Avera Saint Mary's Hospital[2]	Pierre	79%	72
Brookings Hospital[2]	Brookings	79%	124
Lewis & Clark Specialty Hospital	Yankton	72%	78
Custer Regional Hospital	Custer	71%	102
Sturgis Regional Hospital	Sturgis	60%	169
Prairie Lakes Hospital[2]	Watertown	59%	292
PHS Indian Hospital at Eagle Butte[2]	Eagle Butte	40%	82
PHS Indian Hospital at Rosebud[2]	Rosebud	4%	69
PHS Indian Hospital at Pine Ridge[2]	Pine Ridge	0%	145

Warfarin Therapy Discharge Instructions

Hospital Name	City	Rate	Cases
Avera Mckennan Hosp & Univ Health Ctr[2]	Sioux Falls	92%	96
Sanford Usd Medical Center[2]	Sioux Falls	90%	119
Avera Sacred Heart Hospital[2]	Yankton	88%	33
Avera Heart Hospital of South Dakota[2]	Sioux Falls	85%	34
Prairie Lakes Hospital[2]	Watertown	24%	34
Rapid City Regional Hospital[2]	Rapid City	9%	85

Chest Pain/Possible Heart Attack Care

Aspirin Given Within 24 Hours of Arrival

Hospital Name	City	Rate	Cases
Avera Queen of Peace	Mitchell	100%	29
Avera Sacred Heart Hospital	Yankton	100%	36
Brookings Hospital	Brookings	100%	27
Sturgis Regional Hospital	Sturgis	100%	25
Spearfish Regional Hospital	Spearfish	97%	37

Average Time to ECG (minutes)

Hospital Name	City	Min.	Cases
Avera Queen of Peace	Mitchell	5	29
Avera Sacred Heart Hospital	Yankton	5	37
Brookings Hospital	Brookings	5	28
Spearfish Regional Hospital	Spearfish	6	42
Sturgis Regional Hospital	Sturgis	7	25

Children's Asthma Care

Received Home Management Plan of Care

Hospital Name	City	Rate	Cases
Sanford Usd Medical Center	Sioux Falls	98%	50

Received Reliever Medication

Hospital Name	City	Rate	Cases
Sanford Usd Medical Center	Sioux Falls	100%	50

Received Systemic Corticosteroids

Hospital Name	City	Rate	Cases
Sanford Usd Medical Center	Sioux Falls	100%	50

Emergency Department

Admittance Decision Time (minutes)

Hospital Name	City	Min.	Cases
Custer Regional Hospital	Custer	15	95
Sturgis Regional Hospital	Sturgis	17	243
Avera Queen of Peace	Mitchell	28	833
Avera Heart Hospital of South Dakota[2]	Sioux Falls	31	29
Avera Saint Lukes	Aberdeen	36	1685
PHS Indian Hospital at Eagle Butte[2]	Eagle Butte	40	167
Prairie Lakes Hospital[2]	Watertown	40	374
Sanford Aberdeen Medical Center[2,3]	Aberdeen	40	138
Avera Sacred Heart Hospital	Yankton	46	1219
Brookings Hospital[2]	Brookings	52	222
PHS Indian Hospital at Pine Ridge[2]	Pine Ridge	53	175
Spearfish Regional Hospital[2]	Spearfish	53	114
Sanford Usd Medical Center[2]	Sioux Falls	56	305
Avera Saint Mary's Hospital[2]	Pierre	61	96
Avera Mckennan Hosp & Univ Health Ctr[2]	Sioux Falls	62	83
PHS Indian Hospital at Rosebud[2]	Rosebud	64	76
Rapid City Regional Hospital[2]	Rapid City	84	513

Patients Who Left ER Before Being Seen

Hospital Name	City	Rate	Cases
Avera Heart Hospital of South Dakota	Sioux Falls	0%	2821
Avera Queen of Peace	Mitchell	0%	7573
Avera Sacred Heart Hospital	Yankton	0%	10295
Avera Saint Benedict Health Center	Parkston	0%	883
Avera Saint Mary's Hospital	Pierre	0%	6783
Brookings Hospital	Brookings	0%	8035
Custer Regional Hospital	Custer	0%	2709
Platte Health Center	Platte	0%	614
Sanford Aberdeen Medical Center	Aberdeen	0%	1979
Spearfish Regional Surgery Center	Spearfish	0%	2302
Avera Mckennan Hosp & Univ Health Ctr	Sioux Falls	1%	26912
Avera Saint Lukes	Aberdeen	1%	13678
Prairie Lakes Hospital	Watertown	1%	12512
Rapid City Regional Hospital	Rapid City	1%	51454
Sanford Usd Medical Center	Sioux Falls	1%	41378
Spearfish Regional Hospital	Spearfish	1%	9199

Time from ER Arrival to Being Admitted (minutes)

Hospital Name	City	Min.	Cases
Avera Heart Hospital of South Dakota[2]	Sioux Falls	102	48
Sturgis Regional Hospital	Sturgis	126	247
Prairie Lakes Hospital[2]	Watertown	142	423
Avera Saint Mary's Hospital[2]	Pierre	150	164
Custer Regional Hospital	Custer	150	148
Brookings Hospital[2]	Brookings	152	224
Sanford Aberdeen Medical Center[2,3]	Aberdeen	160	140
Avera Mckennan Hosp & Univ Health Ctr[2]	Sioux Falls	162	83
Avera Saint Lukes	Aberdeen	166	1729
Avera Queen of Peace	Mitchell	167	833
Spearfish Regional Hospital[2]	Spearfish	169	189
Avera Sacred Heart Hospital	Yankton	171	1223
Sanford Usd Medical Center[2]	Sioux Falls	195	311
Rapid City Regional Hospital[2]	Rapid City	224	536
PHS Indian Hospital at Eagle Butte[2]	Eagle Butte	236	167
PHS Indian Hospital at Pine Ridge[2]	Pine Ridge	267	268
PHS Indian Hospital at Rosebud[2]	Rosebud	268	358

Time from ER Arrival to Discharge (minutes)

Hospital Name	City	Min.	Cases
Brookings Hospital	Brookings	70	456
Wagner Community Memorial Hospital[3]	Wagner	75	99
Avera Saint Mary's Hospital	Pierre	78	488
Prairie Lakes Hospital	Watertown	82	336
Lead - Deadwood Regional Hospital[3]	Deadwood	83	59
Spearfish Regional Hospital	Spearfish	87	512
Sturgis Regional Hospital	Sturgis	91	369
Custer Regional Hospital	Custer	95	285
Sanford Aberdeen Medical Center[3]	Aberdeen	104	211
Avera Heart Hospital of South Dakota	Sioux Falls	109	241
Avera Sacred Heart Hospital	Yankton	109	6874
Rapid City Regional Hospital	Rapid City	112	385
Avera Mckennan Hosp & Univ Health Ctr	Sioux Falls	116	13670
Avera Queen of Peace	Mitchell	116	5390
Avera Saint Lukes	Aberdeen	122	5921
Sanford Usd Medical Center	Sioux Falls	145	396

Time in ER Before Being Evaluated (minutes)

Hospital Name	City	Min.	Cases
Lead - Deadwood Regional Hospital[3]	Deadwood	0	61
Sanford Aberdeen Medical Center[3]	Aberdeen	3	227
Avera Heart Hospital of South Dakota	Sioux Falls	7	277
Sanford Usd Medical Center	Sioux Falls	14	345
Spearfish Regional Hospital	Spearfish	14	376
Prairie Lakes Hospital	Watertown	15	377
Sturgis Regional Hospital	Sturgis	16	376
Avera Sacred Heart Hospital	Yankton	17	6917
Avera Saint Lukes	Aberdeen	17	5320
Brookings Hospital	Brookings	17	505
Avera Mckennan Hosp & Univ Health Ctr	Sioux Falls	19	13359
Avera Saint Mary's Hospital	Pierre	19	457
Custer Regional Hospital	Custer	20	285
Wagner Community Memorial Hospital[3]	Wagner	20	133
Avera Queen of Peace	Mitchell	21	6166
Rapid City Regional Hospital	Rapid City	27	404

Time to Pain Meds for Bone Fractures (minutes)

Hospital Name	City	Min.	Cases
Custer Regional Hospital	Custer	26	28
Avera Sacred Heart Hospital	Yankton	28	69
Spearfish Regional Hospital	Spearfish	38	70
Brookings Hospital	Brookings	39	54
Avera Saint Mary's Hospital	Pierre	41	33
Prairie Lakes Hospital	Watertown	42	67
Avera Saint Lukes	Aberdeen	43	79
Avera Mckennan Hosp & Univ Health Ctr	Sioux Falls	48	121
Sanford Usd Medical Center	Sioux Falls	54	170
Avera Queen of Peace	Mitchell	56	43
Rapid City Regional Hospital	Rapid City	62	170

Heart Attack Care

Aspirin Given at Discharge

Hospital Name	City	Rate	Cases
Avera Heart Hospital of South Dakota	Sioux Falls	100%	444
Avera Mckennan Hosp & Univ Health Ctr	Sioux Falls	100%	50
Avera Saint Lukes	Aberdeen	100%	68
Prairie Lakes Hospital	Watertown	100%	55
Rapid City Regional Hospital	Rapid City	100%	398
Sanford Usd Medical Center	Sioux Falls	100%	494

PCI Within 90 Minutes of Arrival

Hospital Name	City	Rate	Cases
Sanford Usd Medical Center	Sioux Falls	100%	37
Rapid City Regional Hospital	Rapid City	89%	45

Statin Prescribed at Discharge

Hospital Name	City	Rate	Cases
Avera Heart Hospital of South Dakota	Sioux Falls	99%	419
Rapid City Regional Hospital	Rapid City	99%	399
Avera Mckennan Hosp & Univ Health Ctr	Sioux Falls	98%	45
Avera Saint Lukes	Aberdeen	98%	66
Prairie Lakes Hospital	Watertown	98%	46
Sanford Usd Medical Center	Sioux Falls	98%	465

Heart Failure Care

ACE Inhibitor or ARB for LVSD

Hospital Name	City	Rate	Cases
Sanford Usd Medical Center	Sioux Falls	100%	99
Sioux Falls VA Medical Center	Sioux Falls	100%	27
Avera Heart Hospital of South Dakota	Sioux Falls	98%	62
Rapid City Regional Hospital	Rapid City	98%	102
Avera Mckennan Hosp & Univ Health Ctr	Sioux Falls	89%	55
VA Black Hills Hlthcare Sys-Fort Meade	Fort Meade	88%	25

Discharge Instructions Given

Hospital Name	City	Rate	Cases
Avera Heart Hospital of South Dakota	Sioux Falls	100%	130
Avera Queen of Peace	Mitchell	100%	37
Avera Sacred Heart Hospital	Yankton	100%	48
Avera Saint Lukes	Aberdeen	100%	49
Sanford Usd Medical Center	Sioux Falls	98%	269
Brookings Hospital	Brookings	97%	30

NOTE: Hospital profiles are in alphabetical order by state, then city, then hospital within the city; Rankings exclude hospitals with less than 25 cases except for patient surveys which excludes hospitals with less than 100 cases; (a) 100-299 cases; (1) The number of cases/patients is too few to report; (2) Data submitted were based on a sample of cases/patients; (3) Results are based on a shorter time period than required; (4) Data suppressed by CMS for one or more quarters; (5) Results are not available for this reporting period; (6) Fewer than 100 patients completed the HCAHPS survey; (7) No cases met the criteria for this measure; (8) The lower limit of the confidence interval cannot be calculated if the number of observed infections equals zero; (9) No data are available from the state/territory for this reporting period; (10) The scores shown reflect fewer than 50 completed surveys; (11) There were discrepancies in the data collection process; (12) This measure does not apply to this hospital for this reporting period; (13) Results cannot be calculated for this reporting period; (14) The results for this state are combined with nearby states to protect confidentiality; Please refer to the User's Guide for a full explanation of data.

Sioux Falls VA Medical Center	Sioux Falls	97%	73
VA Black Hills Hlthcare Sys-Fort Meade	Fort Meade	95%	44
Avera Mckennan Hosp & Univ Health Ctr	Sioux Falls	91%	164
Prairie Lakes Hospital[2]	Watertown	90%	73
Rapid City Regional Hospital	Rapid City	80%	313

Evaluation of LVS Function

Hospital Name	City	Rate	Cases
Avera Heart Hospital of South Dakota	Sioux Falls	100%	156
Avera Mckennan Hosp & Univ Health Ctr	Sioux Falls	100%	218
Avera Queen of Peace	Mitchell	100%	65
Avera Sacred Heart Hospital	Yankton	100%	68
Avera Saint Lukes	Aberdeen	100%	101
Avera Saint Mary's Hospital	Pierre	100%	28
Sanford Usd Medical Center	Sioux Falls	100%	343
Sioux Falls VA Medical Center	Sioux Falls	100%	86
VA Black Hills Hlthcare Sys-Fort Meade	Fort Meade	100%	60
Rapid City Regional Hospital	Rapid City	99%	372
Brookings Hospital	Brookings	95%	40
Prairie Lakes Hospital[2]	Watertown	95%	97

Medicare Spending

Medicare Spending per Patient (ratio)

Hospital Name	City	Ratio	Cases
PHS Indian Hospital at Pine Ridge	Pine Ridge	0.69	-
PHS Indian Hospital at Rosebud	Rosebud	0.71	-
Avera Saint Mary's Hospital	Pierre	0.84	-
Brookings Hospital	Brookings	0.84	-
Sioux Falls Specialty Hospital	Sioux Falls	0.86	-
Avera Queen of Peace	Mitchell	0.87	-
Siouxland Surgery Center	Dakota Dunes	0.88	-
Black Hills Surgical Hospital	Rapid City	0.89	-
Prairie Lakes Hospital	Watertown	0.90	-
Spearfish Regional Hospital	Spearfish	0.91	-
Avera Mckennan Hosp & Univ Health Ctr	Sioux Falls	0.93	-
Sanford Aberdeen Medical Center	Aberdeen	0.94	-
Dakota Plains Surgical Center	Aberdeen	0.96	-
Sanford Usd Medical Center	Sioux Falls	0.96	-
Avera Sacred Heart Hospital	Yankton	0.97	-
Lewis & Clark Specialty Hospital	Yankton	0.97	-
Avera Heart Hospital of South Dakota	Sioux Falls	0.98	-
Rapid City Regional Hospital	Rapid City	0.98	-
Avera Saint Lukes	Aberdeen	0.99	-

Pneumonia Care

Appropriate Initial Antibiotic Given

Hospital Name	City	Rate	Cases
Brookings Hospital	Brookings	100%	39
Avera Queen of Peace	Mitchell	98%	90
Avera Saint Mary's Hospital	Pierre	97%	38
Sanford Usd Medical Center	Sioux Falls	97%	136
Sioux Falls VA Medical Center	Sioux Falls	97%	30
Avera Sacred Heart Hospital	Yankton	96%	85
Prairie Lakes Hospital[2]	Watertown	96%	75
Rapid City Regional Hospital	Rapid City	96%	187
Avera Mckennan Hosp & Univ Health Ctr	Sioux Falls	95%	87
Avera Saint Lukes	Aberdeen	95%	60
Sturgis Regional Hospital	Sturgis	93%	28
VA Black Hills Hlthcare Sys-Fort Meade	Fort Meade	91%	35
Spearfish Regional Hospital[2]	Spearfish	88%	25
Huron Regional Medical Center	Huron	75%	59
PHS Indian Hospital at Rosebud[2]	Rosebud	54%	26

Blood Culture Timing

Hospital Name	City	Rate	Cases
Avera Sacred Heart Hospital	Yankton	100%	86
Avera Saint Mary's Hospital	Pierre	100%	52
Brookings Hospital	Brookings	100%	40
Sanford Aberdeen Medical Center[3]	Aberdeen	100%	26
Sioux Falls VA Medical Center	Sioux Falls	100%	50
VA Black Hills Hlthcare Sys-Fort Meade	Fort Meade	100%	35
Avera Queen of Peace	Mitchell	99%	101
Prairie Lakes Hospital[2]	Watertown	99%	81
Avera Mckennan Hosp & Univ Health Ctr	Sioux Falls	97%	97
Avera Saint Lukes	Aberdeen	97%	116
Sanford Usd Medical Center	Sioux Falls	97%	199
Rapid City Regional Hospital	Rapid City	96%	290
Spearfish Regional Hospital[2]	Spearfish	96%	25
Huron Regional Medical Center	Huron	95%	61

Pregnancy and Delivery Care

Newborns whose Deliveries were Scheduled Early

Hospital Name	City	Rate	Cases
Sanford Usd Medical Center[2]	Sioux Falls	2%	51
Spearfish Regional Hospital	Spearfish	2%	48
Avera Saint Mary's Hospital[2]	Pierre	3%	29
Rapid City Regional Hospital[2]	Rapid City	3%	59
Avera Mckennan Hosp & Univ Health Ctr	Sioux Falls	4%	120
Prairie Lakes Hospital[2]	Watertown	4%	81
Avera Queen of Peace	Mitchell	12%	33
Avera Sacred Heart Hospital	Yankton	15%	67
PHS Indian Hospital at Pine Ridge	Pine Ridge	17%	84

Preventive Care

Immunization for Influenza

Hospital Name	City	Rate	Cases
Avera Heart Hospital of South Dakota[2]	Sioux Falls	100%	314
Dakota Plains Surgical Center[2]	Aberdeen	100%	179
Black Hills Surgical Hospital[2]	Rapid City	98%	406
Avera Queen of Peace	Mitchell	97%	1016
Avera Saint Benedict Health Center	Parkston	96%	28
Brookings Hospital[2]	Brookings	95%	254
Sanford Usd Medical Center[2]	Sioux Falls	94%	549
Sioux Falls Specialty Hospital[2]	Sioux Falls	94%	327
Avera Mckennan Hosp & Univ Health Ctr[2]	Sioux Falls	92%	582
Avera Sacred Heart Hospital	Yankton	92%	1594
Spearfish Regional Hospital[2]	Spearfish	92%	255
Avera Saint Lukes	Aberdeen	91%	1822
Avera Saint Mary's Hospital[2]	Pierre	90%	237
Siouxland Surgery Center	Dakota Dunes	90%	599
Sturgis Regional Hospital	Sturgis	89%	149
Rapid City Regional Hospital[2]	Rapid City	88%	546
PHS Indian Hospital at Rapid City[2]	Rapid City	86%	29
Same Day Surgery Center[2]	Rapid City	84%	55
Custer Regional Hospital	Custer	81%	88
Prairie Lakes Hospital[2]	Watertown	79%	513
Spearfish Regional Surgery Center	Spearfish	74%	34
PHS Indian Hospital at Pine Ridge[2]	Pine Ridge	53%	245
Lewis & Clark Specialty Hospital	Yankton	47%	89
PHS Indian Hospital at Rosebud[2]	Rosebud	46%	285
PHS Indian Hospital at Eagle Butte[2]	Eagle Butte	38%	74

Immunization for Pneumonia

Hospital Name	City	Rate	Cases
Avera Heart Hospital of South Dakota[2]	Sioux Falls	100%	485
Avera Saint Benedict Health Center[2,3]	Parkston	100%	33
Brookings Hospital[2]	Brookings	99%	284
Avera Saint Mary's Hospital[2]	Pierre	98%	229
Black Hills Surgical Hospital[2]	Rapid City	98%	408
Dakota Plains Surgical Center[2]	Aberdeen	95%	206
Sioux Falls Specialty Hospital[2]	Sioux Falls	95%	321
Avera Queen of Peace	Mitchell	94%	1193
Avera Sacred Heart Hospital	Yankton	94%	1805
Custer Regional Hospital	Custer	94%	127
Spearfish Regional Hospital[2]	Spearfish	94%	243
Sturgis Regional Hospital	Sturgis	91%	222
Siouxland Surgery Center	Dakota Dunes	89%	580
PHS Indian Hospital at Eagle Butte[2]	Eagle Butte	88%	86
Rapid City Regional Hospital[2]	Rapid City	88%	589
Sanford Aberdeen Medical Center[2,3]	Aberdeen	87%	179
Sanford Usd Medical Center[2]	Sioux Falls	86%	534
Avera Mckennan Hosp & Univ Health Ctr[2]	Sioux Falls	85%	533
PHS Indian Hospital at Pine Ridge[2]	Pine Ridge	84%	159
Avera Saint Lukes	Aberdeen	82%	2033
PHS Indian Hospital at Rosebud[2]	Rosebud	80%	153
Prairie Lakes Hospital[2]	Watertown	75%	821
Lewis & Clark Specialty Hospital	Yankton	69%	118
Spearfish Regional Surgery Center	Spearfish	65%	26
Same Day Surgery Center[2]	Rapid City	50%	32

Stroke Care

Anticoagulation Therapy for Atrial Fibrillation

Hospital Name	City	Rate	Cases
Sanford Usd Medical Center	Sioux Falls	100%	31
Avera Mckennan Hosp & Univ Health Ctr	Sioux Falls	93%	30

Antithrombotic Therapy Timing

Hospital Name	City	Rate	Cases
Rapid City Regional Hospital	Rapid City	100%	129
Avera Mckennan Hosp & Univ Health Ctr	Sioux Falls	99%	138
Sanford Usd Medical Center	Sioux Falls	99%	147
Prairie Lakes Hospital	Watertown	94%	35
Avera Saint Lukes	Aberdeen	93%	30

Assessed for Rehabilitation

Hospital Name	City	Rate	Cases
Sanford Usd Medical Center	Sioux Falls	100%	222
Rapid City Regional Hospital	Rapid City	99%	147
Avera Mckennan Hosp & Univ Health Ctr	Sioux Falls	98%	172
Avera Saint Lukes	Aberdeen	97%	37
Prairie Lakes Hospital	Watertown	93%	30

Discharged on Antithrombotic Therapy

Hospital Name	City	Rate	Cases
Avera Mckennan Hosp & Univ Health Ctr	Sioux Falls	100%	155
Avera Saint Lukes	Aberdeen	100%	35
Prairie Lakes Hospital	Watertown	100%	30
Rapid City Regional Hospital	Rapid City	100%	133
Sanford Usd Medical Center	Sioux Falls	100%	189

Discharged on Statin Medication

Hospital Name	City	Rate	Cases
Sanford Usd Medical Center	Sioux Falls	100%	129
Avera Mckennan Hosp & Univ Health Ctr	Sioux Falls	98%	121
Avera Saint Lukes	Aberdeen	96%	27
Rapid City Regional Hospital	Rapid City	96%	101
Prairie Lakes Hospital	Watertown	63%	27

Venous Thromboembolism (VTE) Prophylaxis

Hospital Name	City	Rate	Cases
Sanford Usd Medical Center	Sioux Falls	100%	200
Avera Mckennan Hosp & Univ Health Ctr	Sioux Falls	99%	170
Rapid City Regional Hospital	Rapid City	98%	160
Avera Saint Lukes	Aberdeen	94%	34
Prairie Lakes Hospital	Watertown	60%	35

Written Stroke Educational Materials Given

Hospital Name	City	Rate	Cases
Sanford Usd Medical Center	Sioux Falls	98%	121
Rapid City Regional Hospital	Rapid City	87%	84
Avera Mckennan Hosp & Univ Health Ctr	Sioux Falls	86%	92

Surgical Care Improvement Project

Appropriate Beta Blocker Usage

Hospital Name	City	Rate	Cases
Avera Sacred Heart Hospital	Yankton	100%	109
Avera Saint Mary's Hospital	Pierre	100%	47
Sioux Falls Specialty Hospital[2]	Sioux Falls	100%	76
Avera Heart Hospital of South Dakota[2]	Sioux Falls	99%	324
Avera Queen of Peace	Mitchell	99%	78
Dakota Plains Surgical Center[2]	Aberdeen	99%	71
Rapid City Regional Hospital[2]	Rapid City	99%	227
Avera Mckennan Hosp & Univ Health Ctr[2]	Sioux Falls	98%	124
Avera Saint Lukes	Aberdeen	98%	141
Black Hills Surgical Hospital[2]	Rapid City	98%	56
Sanford Usd Medical Center[2]	Sioux Falls	98%	416
Sioux Falls VA Medical Center[2]	Sioux Falls	97%	73
Spearfish Regional Hospital[2]	Spearfish	97%	79
Prairie Lakes Hospital[2]	Watertown	95%	125
Siouxland Surgery Center	Dakota Dunes	95%	194

Appropriate VTP Within 24 Hours

Hospital Name	City	Rate	Cases
Avera Queen of Peace	Mitchell	100%	204
Avera Sacred Heart Hospital	Yankton	100%	311
Dakota Plains Surgical Center[2]	Aberdeen	100%	287
Sioux Falls VA Medical Center[2]	Sioux Falls	100%	148
Siouxland Surgery Center	Dakota Dunes	100%	689
Spearfish Regional Surgery Center	Spearfish	100%	50
Avera Mckennan Hosp & Univ Health Ctr[2]	Sioux Falls	99%	336
Avera Saint Lukes	Aberdeen	99%	276
Black Hills Surgical Hospital[2]	Rapid City	99%	236
Sioux Falls Specialty Hospital[2]	Sioux Falls	99%	434
Prairie Lakes Hospital[2]	Watertown	98%	340
Sanford Aberdeen Medical Center[3]	Aberdeen	98%	41
Sanford Usd Medical Center[2]	Sioux Falls	98%	642
Avera Heart Hospital of South Dakota[2]	Sioux Falls	97%	39
Brookings Hospital	Brookings	97%	35
Lewis & Clark Specialty Hospital	Yankton	97%	79
Spearfish Regional Hospital[2]	Spearfish	97%	254
Avera Saint Mary's Hospital	Pierre	96%	137
Rapid City Regional Hospital[2]	Rapid City	96%	296
Huron Regional Medical Center	Huron	92%	40

Controlled Postoperative Blood Glucose

Hospital Name	City	Rate	Cases
Avera Heart Hospital of South Dakota[2]	Sioux Falls	98%	322
Sanford Usd Medical Center[2]	Sioux Falls	98%	198
Rapid City Regional Hospital[2]	Rapid City	97%	118

Perioperative Temperature Management

Hospital Name	City	Rate	Cases
Avera Mckennan Hosp & Univ Health Ctr[2]	Sioux Falls	100%	425
Avera Queen of Peace	Mitchell	100%	225
Avera Sacred Heart Hospital	Yankton	100%	377
Avera Saint Lukes	Aberdeen	100%	341
Avera Saint Mary's Hospital	Pierre	100%	149
Black Hills Surgical Hospital[2]	Rapid City	100%	261

NOTE: Hospital profiles are in alphabetical order by state, then city, then hospital within the city; Rankings exclude hospitals with less than 25 cases except for patient surveys which excludes hospitals with less than 100 cases; (a) 100-299 cases; (1) The number of cases/patients is too few to report; (2) Data submitted were based on a sample of cases/patients; (3) Results are based on a shorter time period than required; (4) Data suppressed by CMS for one or more quarters; (5) Results are not available for this reporting period; (6) Fewer than 100 patients completed the HCAHPS survey; (7) No cases met the criteria for this measure; (8) The lower limit of the confidence interval cannot be calculated if the number of observed infections equals zero; (9) No data are available from the state/territory for this reporting period; (10) The scores shown reflect fewer than 50 completed surveys; (11) There were discrepancies in the data collection process; (12) This measure does not apply to this hospital for this reporting period; (13) Results cannot be calculated for this reporting period; (14) The results for this state are combined with nearby states to protect confidentiality; Please refer to the User's Guide for a full explanation of data.

Brookings Hospital	Brookings	100%	47
Dakota Plains Surgical Center[2]	Aberdeen	100%	292
Huron Regional Medical Center	Huron	100%	42
Prairie Lakes Hospital[2]	Watertown	100%	410
Same Day Surgery Center[2]	Rapid City	100%	32
Sanford Aberdeen Medical Center[3]	Aberdeen	100%	51
Sanford Usd Medical Center[2]	Sioux Falls	100%	1054
Sioux Falls Specialty Hospital[2]	Sioux Falls	100%	475
Sioux Falls VA Medical Center[2]	Sioux Falls	100%	168
Spearfish Regional Hospital[2]	Spearfish	100%	311
Spearfish Regional Surgery Center	Spearfish	100%	57
Avera Heart Hospital of South Dakota[2]	Sioux Falls	99%	68
Siouxland Surgery Center	Dakota Dunes	99%	712
Rapid City Regional Hospital[2]	Rapid City	98%	400
Lewis & Clark Specialty Hospital	Yankton	90%	81

Prophylactic Antibiotic Selection

Hospital Name	City	Rate	Cases
Avera Heart Hospital of South Dakota[2]	Sioux Falls	100%	345
Avera Queen of Peace	Mitchell	100%	175
Avera Sacred Heart Hospital	Yankton	100%	259
Black Hills Surgical Hospital[2]	Rapid City	100%	214
Brookings Hospital	Brookings	100%	42
Dakota Plains Surgical Center[2]	Aberdeen	100%	283
Lewis & Clark Specialty Hospital	Yankton	100%	71
Prairie Lakes Hospital[2]	Watertown	100%	327
Sioux Falls Specialty Hospital[2]	Sioux Falls	100%	413
Sioux Falls VA Medical Center	Sioux Falls	100%	138
Siouxland Surgery Center	Dakota Dunes	100%	625
Spearfish Regional Hospital[2]	Spearfish	100%	263
Spearfish Regional Surgery Center	Spearfish	100%	55
Avera Mckennan Hosp & Univ Health Ctr[2]	Sioux Falls	99%	276
Avera Saint Mary's Hospital	Pierre	99%	120
Rapid City Regional Hospital[2]	Rapid City	99%	316
Sanford Usd Medical Center[2]	Sioux Falls	99%	920
Avera Saint Lukes	Aberdeen	98%	208
Sanford Aberdeen Medical Center[3]	Aberdeen	97%	34
Huron Regional Medical Center	Huron	93%	28
Same Day Surgery Center[2]	Rapid City	93%	30

Prophylactic Antibiotic Selection (Outpatient)

Hospital Name	City	Rate	Cases
Avera Queen of Peace	Mitchell	100%	66
Avera Sacred Heart Hospital	Yankton	100%	77
Black Hills Surgical Hospital	Rapid City	100%	512
Dakota Plains Surgical Center	Aberdeen	100%	34
Avera Heart Hospital of South Dakota	Sioux Falls	99%	309
Avera Mckennan Hosp & Univ Health Ctr	Sioux Falls	99%	322
Prairie Lakes Hospital	Watertown	99%	128
Rapid City Regional Hospital	Rapid City	99%	288
Sanford Usd Medical Center	Sioux Falls	99%	587
Sioux Falls Specialty Hospital	Sioux Falls	98%	254
Siouxland Surgery Center	Dakota Dunes	98%	302
Spearfish Regional Hospital	Spearfish	98%	66
Same Day Surgery Center	Rapid City	97%	176
Lewis & Clark Specialty Hospital	Yankton	96%	26
Avera Saint Lukes	Aberdeen	92%	148

Prophylactic Antibiotic Stopped

Hospital Name	City	Rate	Cases
Avera Heart Hospital of South Dakota[2]	Sioux Falls	100%	344
Avera Mckennan Hosp & Univ Health Ctr[2]	Sioux Falls	100%	272
Avera Queen of Peace	Mitchell	100%	164
Avera Saint Lukes	Aberdeen	100%	201
Black Hills Surgical Hospital[2]	Rapid City	100%	213
Huron Regional Medical Center	Huron	100%	27
Spearfish Regional Hospital[2]	Spearfish	100%	255
Spearfish Regional Surgery Center	Spearfish	100%	55
Avera Sacred Heart Hospital	Yankton	99%	255
Avera Saint Mary's Hospital	Pierre	99%	116
Lewis & Clark Specialty Hospital	Yankton	99%	71
Sioux Falls Specialty Hospital[2]	Sioux Falls	99%	413
Siouxland Surgery Center	Dakota Dunes	99%	616
Brookings Hospital	Brookings	98%	42
Prairie Lakes Hospital[2]	Watertown	98%	316
Sanford Usd Medical Center[2]	Sioux Falls	98%	895
Same Day Surgery Center[2]	Rapid City	97%	30
Rapid City Regional Hospital[2]	Rapid City	96%	300
Sioux Falls VA Medical Center	Sioux Falls	96%	138
Dakota Plains Surgical Center[2]	Aberdeen	95%	279
Sanford Aberdeen Medical Center[3]	Aberdeen	91%	32

Prophylactic Antibiotic Timing

Hospital Name	City	Rate	Cases
Avera Heart Hospital of South Dakota[2]	Sioux Falls	100%	345
Avera Mckennan Hosp & Univ Health Ctr[2]	Sioux Falls	100%	276
Avera Queen of Peace	Mitchell	100%	175
Avera Sacred Heart Hospital	Yankton	100%	259
Avera Saint Mary's Hospital	Pierre	100%	121
Black Hills Surgical Hospital[2]	Rapid City	100%	214
Brookings Hospital	Brookings	100%	42
Huron Regional Medical Center	Huron	100%	28
Spearfish Regional Surgery Center	Spearfish	100%	55
Avera Saint Lukes	Aberdeen	99%	209
Dakota Plains Surgical Center[2]	Aberdeen	99%	283
Rapid City Regional Hospital[2]	Rapid City	99%	316
Sioux Falls Specialty Hospital[2]	Sioux Falls	99%	413
Sioux Falls VA Medical Center	Sioux Falls	99%	138
Siouxland Surgery Center	Dakota Dunes	99%	626
Prairie Lakes Hospital[2]	Watertown	98%	327
Sanford Usd Medical Center[2]	Sioux Falls	98%	922
Lewis & Clark Specialty Hospital	Yankton	97%	71
Sanford Aberdeen Medical Center[3]	Aberdeen	97%	34
Spearfish Regional Hospital[2]	Spearfish	97%	263
Same Day Surgery Center[2]	Rapid City	93%	30

Prophylactic Antibiotic Timing (Outpatient)

Hospital Name	City	Rate	Cases
Avera Queen of Peace	Mitchell	100%	66
Avera Sacred Heart Hospital	Yankton	100%	77
Black Hills Surgical Hospital	Rapid City	100%	512
Dakota Plains Surgical Center	Aberdeen	100%	34
Avera Mckennan Hosp & Univ Health Ctr	Sioux Falls	99%	321
Siouxland Surgery Center	Dakota Dunes	99%	304
Same Day Surgery Center	Rapid City	98%	178
Sanford Usd Medical Center	Sioux Falls	98%	597
Sioux Falls Specialty Hospital	Sioux Falls	98%	255
Spearfish Regional Hospital	Spearfish	97%	66
Avera Heart Hospital of South Dakota	Sioux Falls	96%	311
Rapid City Regional Hospital	Rapid City	95%	291
Avera Saint Lukes	Aberdeen	94%	143
Prairie Lakes Hospital	Watertown	93%	83

Urinary Catheter Removal

Hospital Name	City	Rate	Cases
Avera Queen of Peace	Mitchell	100%	34
Black Hills Surgical Hospital[2]	Rapid City	100%	218
Brookings Hospital	Brookings	100%	33
Dakota Plains Surgical Center[2]	Aberdeen	100%	290
Sioux Falls Specialty Hospital[2]	Sioux Falls	100%	262
Spearfish Regional Surgery Center	Spearfish	100%	48
Avera Saint Lukes	Aberdeen	99%	216
Spearfish Regional Hospital[2]	Spearfish	99%	246
Sanford Aberdeen Medical Center[3]	Aberdeen	98%	40
Sioux Falls VA Medical Center[2]	Sioux Falls	98%	140
Prairie Lakes Hospital[2]	Watertown	97%	318
Avera Heart Hospital of South Dakota[2]	Sioux Falls	96%	277
Sanford Usd Medical Center[2]	Sioux Falls	96%	433
Avera Mckennan Hosp & Univ Health Ctr[2]	Sioux Falls	94%	179
Rapid City Regional Hospital[2]	Rapid City	89%	246

Survey of Patients' Hospital Experiences

Area Around Room 'Always' Quiet at Night

Hospital Name	City	Rate	Cases
Black Hills Surgical Hospital	Rapid City	90%	300+
Dakota Plains Surgical Center	Aberdeen	89%	(a)
Sioux Falls Specialty Hospital	Sioux Falls	88%	300+
Siouxland Surgery Center	Dakota Dunes	88%	300+
Brookings Hospital	Brookings	72%	300+
Winner Regional Healthcare Center	Winner	69%	(a)
Avera Heart Hospital of South Dakota	Sioux Falls	67%	300+
Sturgis Regional Hospital	Sturgis	65%	(a)
Avera Queen of Peace	Mitchell	64%	300+
Avera Sacred Heart Hospital	Yankton	63%	300+
Spearfish Regional Hospital	Spearfish	62%	300+
Avera Mckennan Hosp & Univ Health Ctr	Sioux Falls	60%	300+
Avera Saint Lukes	Aberdeen	60%	300+
Avera Saint Mary's Hospital	Pierre	59%	300+
Sanford Usd Medical Center	Sioux Falls	59%	300+
Prairie Lakes Hospital	Watertown	58%	300+
Rapid City Regional Hospital	Rapid City	54%	300+

Doctors 'Always' Communicated Well

Hospital Name	City	Rate	Cases
Dakota Plains Surgical Center	Aberdeen	91%	(a)
Black Hills Surgical Hospital	Rapid City	88%	300+
Sturgis Regional Hospital	Sturgis	88%	(a)
Winner Regional Healthcare Center	Winner	88%	(a)
Avera Heart Hospital of South Dakota	Sioux Falls	86%	300+
Avera Queen of Peace	Mitchell	85%	300+
Siouxland Surgery Center	Dakota Dunes	85%	300+
Brookings Hospital	Brookings	84%	300+
Sioux Falls Specialty Hospital	Sioux Falls	84%	300+
Avera Sacred Heart Hospital	Yankton	83%	300+
Avera Mckennan Hosp & Univ Health Ctr	Sioux Falls	81%	300+
Avera Saint Lukes	Aberdeen	81%	300+
Avera Saint Mary's Hospital	Pierre	81%	300+
Prairie Lakes Hospital	Watertown	81%	300+
Rapid City Regional Hospital	Rapid City	79%	300+
Sanford Usd Medical Center	Sioux Falls	78%	300+
Spearfish Regional Hospital	Spearfish	77%	300+

Home Recovery Information Given

Hospital Name	City	Rate	Cases
Black Hills Surgical Hospital	Rapid City	93%	300+
Avera Queen of Peace	Mitchell	92%	300+
Avera Saint Lukes	Aberdeen	92%	300+
Dakota Plains Surgical Center	Aberdeen	92%	(a)
Avera Heart Hospital of South Dakota	Sioux Falls	91%	300+
Avera Sacred Heart Hospital	Yankton	91%	300+
Sioux Falls Specialty Hospital	Sioux Falls	91%	300+
Siouxland Surgery Center	Dakota Dunes	91%	300+
Sturgis Regional Hospital	Sturgis	91%	(a)
Avera Mckennan Hosp & Univ Health Ctr	Sioux Falls	90%	300+
Prairie Lakes Hospital	Watertown	90%	300+
Sanford Usd Medical Center	Sioux Falls	89%	300+
Rapid City Regional Hospital	Rapid City	88%	300+
Spearfish Regional Hospital	Spearfish	88%	300+
Avera Saint Mary's Hospital	Pierre	86%	300+
Brookings Hospital	Brookings	86%	300+
Winner Regional Healthcare Center	Winner	82%	(a)

Hospital Given 9 or 10 on 10 Point Scale

Hospital Name	City	Rate	Cases
Dakota Plains Surgical Center	Aberdeen	93%	(a)
Avera Heart Hospital of South Dakota	Sioux Falls	91%	300+
Black Hills Surgical Hospital	Rapid City	91%	300+
Sioux Falls Specialty Hospital	Sioux Falls	90%	300+
Siouxland Surgery Center	Dakota Dunes	89%	300+
Avera Queen of Peace	Mitchell	77%	300+
Brookings Hospital	Brookings	77%	300+
Sturgis Regional Hospital	Sturgis	77%	(a)
Sanford Usd Medical Center	Sioux Falls	74%	300+
Avera Mckennan Hosp & Univ Health Ctr	Sioux Falls	73%	300+
Winner Regional Healthcare Center	Winner	73%	(a)
Prairie Lakes Hospital	Watertown	72%	300+
Spearfish Regional Hospital	Spearfish	72%	300+
Avera Sacred Heart Hospital	Yankton	71%	300+
Avera Saint Lukes	Aberdeen	71%	300+
Rapid City Regional Hospital	Rapid City	68%	300+
Avera Saint Mary's Hospital	Pierre	66%	300+

Meds 'Always' Explained Before Given

Hospital Name	City	Rate	Cases
Black Hills Surgical Hospital	Rapid City	76%	300+
Dakota Plains Surgical Center	Aberdeen	76%	(a)
Sioux Falls Specialty Hospital	Sioux Falls	76%	300+
Avera Heart Hospital of South Dakota	Sioux Falls	74%	300+
Winner Regional Healthcare Center	Winner	74%	(a)
Avera Queen of Peace	Mitchell	72%	300+
Siouxland Surgery Center	Dakota Dunes	72%	300+
Sturgis Regional Hospital	Sturgis	72%	(a)
Brookings Hospital	Brookings	67%	300+
Avera Mckennan Hosp & Univ Health Ctr	Sioux Falls	64%	300+
Rapid City Regional Hospital	Rapid City	64%	300+
Avera Saint Mary's Hospital	Pierre	63%	300+
Prairie Lakes Hospital	Watertown	63%	300+
Spearfish Regional Hospital	Spearfish	63%	300+
Avera Saint Lukes	Aberdeen	62%	300+
Sanford Usd Medical Center	Sioux Falls	62%	300+
Avera Sacred Heart Hospital	Yankton	61%	300+

Nurses 'Always' Communicated Well

Hospital Name	City	Rate	Cases
Dakota Plains Surgical Center	Aberdeen	93%	(a)
Sioux Falls Specialty Hospital	Sioux Falls	90%	300+
Avera Heart Hospital of South Dakota	Sioux Falls	89%	300+
Black Hills Surgical Hospital	Rapid City	88%	300+
Siouxland Surgery Center	Dakota Dunes	88%	300+
Sturgis Regional Hospital	Sturgis	88%	(a)
Brookings Hospital	Brookings	84%	300+
Avera Queen of Peace	Mitchell	82%	300+
Spearfish Regional Hospital	Spearfish	81%	300+
Winner Regional Healthcare Center	Winner	81%	(a)
Avera Sacred Heart Hospital	Yankton	79%	300+
Avera Saint Lukes	Aberdeen	78%	300+
Rapid City Regional Hospital	Rapid City	78%	300+
Sanford Usd Medical Center	Sioux Falls	78%	300+
Avera Mckennan Hosp & Univ Health Ctr	Sioux Falls	77%	300+
Prairie Lakes Hospital	Watertown	77%	300+
Avera Saint Mary's Hospital	Pierre	76%	300+

Pain 'Always' Well Controlled

Hospital Name	City	Rate	Cases
Sturgis Regional Hospital	Sturgis	85%	(a)
Dakota Plains Surgical Center	Aberdeen	82%	(a)

NOTE: Hospital profiles are in alphabetical order by state, then city, then hospital within the city; Rankings exclude hospitals with less than 25 cases except for patient surveys which excludes hospitals with less than 100 cases; (a) 100-299 cases; (1) The number of cases/patients is too few to report; (2) Data submitted were based on a sample of cases/patients; (3) Results are based on a shorter time period than required; (4) Data suppressed by CMS for one or more quarters; (5) Results are not available for this reporting period; (6) Fewer than 100 patients completed the HCAHPS survey; (7) No cases met the criteria for this measure; (8) The lower limit of the confidence interval cannot be calculated if the number of observed infections equals zero; (9) No data are available from the state/territory for this reporting period; (10) The scores shown reflect fewer than 50 completed surveys; (11) There were discrepancies in the data collection process; (12) This measure does not apply to this hospital for this reporting period; (13) Results cannot be calculated for this reporting period; (14) The results for this state are combined with nearby states to protect confidentiality; Please refer to the User's Guide for a full explanation of data.

Hospital Name	City	Rate	Cases
Avera Heart Hospital of South Dakota	Sioux Falls	80%	300+
Sioux Falls Specialty Hospital	Sioux Falls	80%	300+
Black Hills Surgical Hospital	Rapid City	78%	300+
Siouxland Surgery Center	Dakota Dunes	76%	300+
Avera Queen of Peace	Mitchell	75%	300+
Brookings Hospital	Brookings	75%	300+
Avera Sacred Heart Hospital	Yankton	71%	300+
Prairie Lakes Hospital	Watertown	71%	300+
Winner Regional Healthcare Center	Winner	71%	(a)
Rapid City Regional Hospital	Rapid City	70%	300+
Spearfish Regional Hospital	Spearfish	70%	300+
Sanford Usd Medical Center	Sioux Falls	69%	300+
Avera Mckennan Hosp & Univ Health Ctr	Sioux Falls	68%	300+
Avera Saint Mary's Hospital	Pierre	65%	300+
Avera Saint Lukes	Aberdeen	64%	300+

Room and Bathroom 'Always' Clean

Hospital Name	City	Rate	Cases
Dakota Plains Surgical Center	Aberdeen	88%	(a)
Siouxland Surgery Center	Dakota Dunes	87%	300+
Black Hills Surgical Hospital	Rapid City	86%	300+
Avera Heart Hospital of South Dakota	Sioux Falls	85%	300+
Sioux Falls Specialty Hospital	Sioux Falls	84%	300+
Brookings Hospital	Brookings	82%	300+
Sturgis Regional Hospital	Sturgis	82%	(a)
Winner Regional Healthcare Center	Winner	80%	(a)
Spearfish Regional Hospital	Spearfish	75%	300+
Avera Queen of Peace	Mitchell	73%	300+
Avera Sacred Heart Hospital	Yankton	73%	300+
Avera Saint Lukes	Aberdeen	73%	300+
Avera Mckennan Hosp & Univ Health Ctr	Sioux Falls	71%	300+
Prairie Lakes Hospital	Watertown	70%	300+
Rapid City Regional Hospital	Rapid City	70%	300+
Sanford Usd Medical Center	Sioux Falls	67%	300+
Avera Saint Mary's Hospital	Pierre	66%	300+

Timely Help 'Always' Received

Hospital Name	City	Rate	Cases
Dakota Plains Surgical Center	Aberdeen	93%	(a)
Black Hills Surgical Hospital	Rapid City	91%	300+
Siouxland Surgery Center	Dakota Dunes	90%	300+
Sioux Falls Specialty Hospital	Sioux Falls	88%	300+
Sturgis Regional Hospital	Sturgis	84%	(a)
Avera Heart Hospital of South Dakota	Sioux Falls	81%	300+
Spearfish Regional Hospital	Spearfish	78%	300+
Winner Regional Healthcare Center	Winner	76%	(a)
Brookings Hospital	Brookings	73%	300+
Avera Queen of Peace	Mitchell	71%	300+
Rapid City Regional Hospital	Rapid City	71%	300+
Avera Sacred Heart Hospital	Yankton	69%	300+
Avera Saint Mary's Hospital	Pierre	69%	300+
Prairie Lakes Hospital	Watertown	67%	300+
Sanford Usd Medical Center	Sioux Falls	67%	300+
Avera Mckennan Hosp & Univ Health Ctr	Sioux Falls	66%	300+
Avera Saint Lukes	Aberdeen	64%	300+

Would Definitely Recommend Hospital

Hospital Name	City	Rate	Cases
Dakota Plains Surgical Center	Aberdeen	94%	(a)
Avera Heart Hospital of South Dakota	Sioux Falls	92%	300+
Black Hills Surgical Hospital	Rapid City	92%	300+
Sioux Falls Specialty Hospital	Sioux Falls	92%	300+
Siouxland Surgery Center	Dakota Dunes	89%	300+
Avera Mckennan Hosp & Univ Health Ctr	Sioux Falls	77%	300+
Sanford Usd Medical Center	Sioux Falls	77%	300+
Avera Queen of Peace	Mitchell	75%	300+
Brookings Hospital	Brookings	75%	300+
Avera Saint Lukes	Aberdeen	73%	300+
Sturgis Regional Hospital	Sturgis	73%	(a)
Winner Regional Healthcare Center	Winner	73%	(a)
Avera Sacred Heart Hospital	Yankton	71%	300+
Prairie Lakes Hospital	Watertown	70%	300+
Spearfish Regional Hospital	Spearfish	70%	300+
Rapid City Regional Hospital	Rapid City	69%	300+
Avera Saint Mary's Hospital	Pierre	63%	300+

Use of Medical Imaging

Cardiac Imaging Stress Test before OP Surgery

Hospital Name	City	Rate	Cases
Avera Mckennan Hosp & Univ Health Ctr	Sioux Falls	1.5%	137
Avera Saint Lukes	Aberdeen	2.1%	289
Prairie Lakes Hospital	Watertown	2.6%	309
Rapid City Regional Hospital	Rapid City	3.8%	1278
Avera Heart Hospital of South Dakota	Sioux Falls	4.3%	765
Sanford Aberdeen Medical Center	Aberdeen	5.2%	97
Sanford Usd Medical Center	Sioux Falls	5.3%	1154
Avera Saint Mary's Hospital	Pierre	5.6%	107
Avera Sacred Heart Hospital	Yankton	6.3%	190

Combination Abdominal CT Scan

Hospital Name	City	Rate	Cases
Fall River Hospital	Hot Springs	0.0%	86
Custer Regional Hospital	Custer	0.9%	107
Lead - Deadwood Regional Hospital	Deadwood	1.7%	58
Avera Heart Hospital of South Dakota	Sioux Falls	1.9%	107
Sanford Usd Medical Center	Sioux Falls	1.9%	1252
Spearfish Regional Hospital	Spearfish	2.7%	262
Avera Saint Lukes	Aberdeen	4.3%	678
Avera Sacred Heart Hospital	Yankton	5.0%	140
Rapid City Regional Hospital	Rapid City	5.1%	939
Sturgis Regional Hospital	Sturgis	6.5%	93
Brookings Hospital	Brookings	6.9%	174
Avera Mckennan Hosp & Univ Health Ctr	Sioux Falls	10.6%	1101
Sanford Aberdeen Medical Center	Aberdeen	14.8%	128
Avera Queen of Peace	Mitchell	19.6%	286
Black Hills Surgical Hospital	Rapid City	50.0%	34
Prairie Lakes Hospital	Watertown	58.3%	254
Avera Saint Mary's Hospital	Pierre	65.9%	220

Combination Brain/Sinus CT Scan

Hospital Name	City	Rate	Cases
Avera Heart Hospital of South Dakota	Sioux Falls	0.0%	87
Avera Saint Benedict Health Center	Parkston	0.0%	53
Brookings Hospital	Brookings	0.0%	117
Sanford Aberdeen Medical Center	Aberdeen	0.0%	122
Avera Queen of Peace	Mitchell	1.1%	281
Rapid City Regional Hospital	Rapid City	2.9%	619
Sanford Usd Medical Center	Sioux Falls	2.9%	717

Combination Chest CT Scan

Hospital Name	City	Rate	Cases
Brookings Hospital	Brookings	0.0%	80
Fall River Hospital	Hot Springs	0.0%	47
Rapid City Regional Hospital	Rapid City	0.0%	627
Sanford Usd Medical Center	Sioux Falls	0.0%	1141
Avera Saint Lukes	Aberdeen	0.3%	613
Spearfish Regional Hospital	Spearfish	1.2%	169
Avera Saint Mary's Hospital	Pierre	1.7%	174
Avera Sacred Heart Hospital	Yankton	2.1%	47
Avera Mckennan Hosp & Univ Health Ctr	Sioux Falls	4.3%	967
Sanford Aberdeen Medical Center	Aberdeen	11.4%	70
Avera Queen of Peace	Mitchell	13.1%	175
Prairie Lakes Hospital	Watertown	64.3%	140

Follow-up Mammogram/Ultrasound

A follow-up rate near zero may indicate missed cancer; a rate higher than 14% may mean there is unnecessary follow up.

Hospital Name	City	Rate	Cases
Fall River Hospital	Hot Springs	1.5%	66
Spearfish Regional Hospital	Spearfish	5.5%	328
Avera Saint Mary's Hospital	Pierre	7.0%	700
Platte Health Center	Platte	7.5%	120
Avera Mckennan Hosp & Univ Health Ctr	Sioux Falls	8.4%	2053
Rapid City Regional Hospital	Rapid City	8.4%	370
Avera Saint Benedict Health Center	Parkston	8.5%	211
Lead - Deadwood Regional Hospital	Deadwood	8.6%	185
Sanford Aberdeen Medical Center	Aberdeen	9.4%	149
Avera Queen of Peace	Mitchell	10.1%	1005
Sturgis Regional Hospital	Sturgis	10.8%	166
Avera Sacred Heart Hospital	Yankton	11.2%	260
Avera Saint Lukes	Aberdeen	12.2%	1396
Wagner Community Memorial Hospital	Wagner	15.3%	72

Lumbar Spine MRI for Low Back Pain

Hospital Name	City	Rate	Cases
Dakota Plains Surgical Center	Aberdeen	16.2%	68
Sioux Falls Specialty Hospital	Sioux Falls	26.6%	128
Prairie Lakes Hospital	Watertown	29.2%	72
Rapid City Regional Hospital	Rapid City	30.7%	114
Sanford Usd Medical Center	Sioux Falls	31.7%	300
Avera Mckennan Hosp & Univ Health Ctr	Sioux Falls	33.1%	166
Avera Saint Lukes	Aberdeen	33.8%	77
Avera Queen of Peace	Mitchell	34.7%	124
Black Hills Surgical Hospital	Rapid City	36.5%	384
Spearfish Regional Hospital	Spearfish	48.2%	85

NOTE: Hospital profiles are in alphabetical order by state, then city, then hospital within the city; Rankings exclude hospitals with less than 25 cases except for patient surveys which excludes hospitals with less than 100 cases; (a) 100-299 cases; (1) The number of cases/patients is too few to report; (2) Data submitted were based on a sample of cases/patients; (3) Results are based on a shorter time period than required; (4) Data suppressed by CMS for one or more quarters; (5) Results are not available for this reporting period; (6) Fewer than 100 patients completed the HCAHPS survey; (7) No cases met the criteria for this measure; (8) The lower limit of the confidence interval cannot be calculated if the number of observed infections equals zero; (9) No data are available from the state/territory for this reporting period; (10) The scores shown reflect fewer than 50 completed surveys; (11) There were discrepancies in the data collection process; (12) This measure does not apply to this hospital for this reporting period; (13) Results cannot be calculated for this reporting period; (14) The results for this state are combined with nearby states to protect confidentiality; Please refer to the User's Guide for a full explanation of data.

Avera Saint Lukes

305 S State Saint Post Office Box 4450
Aberdeen, SD 57401
Phone: 605-622-5000
Fax: 605-622-5041
URL: www.averastlukes.org
Type: Acute Care Hospitals
Emergency Services: Yes
Ownership: Voluntary non-profit - Church
Beds: 137

Key Personnel:
Radiology. . . . . Melchor Aguilar, MD
Quality Assurance . . . . Pat Cavanaugh
CEO/President. . . . . Todd Forkel
Chief of Medical Staff. . . . . John Fritz
Operating Room. . . . . Kathy Nipp
Infection Control. . . . . Jolynn Zeller

Measure	Cases	This Hosp.	State Avg.	U.S. Avg.
Blood Clot Prevention and Treatment				
Anticoagulation Overlap Therapy[2]	27	96%	95%	93%
ICU Venous Thromboembolism Prophylaxis[2]	68	97%	91%	92%
Incidence of Potentially Preventable VTE[1,2]	-	-	5%	10%
UFH with Dosages/Platelet Monitoring[2]	34	100%	100%	97%
Venous Thromboembolism Prophylaxis[2]	187	88%	80%	85%
Warfarin Therapy Discharge Instructions[2]	20	90%	70%	75%
Chest Pain/Possible Heart Attack Care				
Aspirin Given Within 24 Hours of Arrival[1,3]	-	-	99%	96%
Fibrinolytic Meds Within 30 Min. of Arrival[3,7]	-	-	69%	58%
Average Time to ECG (minutes)[1,3]	-	-	5	7
Average Time to Transfer (minutes)[3,7]	-	-	66	60
Children's Asthma Care				
Received Home Management Plan of Care	-	-	-	88%
Received Reliever Medication	-	-	-	100%
Received Systemic Corticosteroids	-	-	-	100%
Emergency Department				
Admittance Decision Time (minutes)	1,685	36	41	98
Head CT Results Within 45 Min. of Arrival[7]	-	-	44%	57%
Patients Who Left ER Before Being Seen	13,678	1%	1%	2%
Time from ER Arrival to Admit. (minutes)	1,729	166	174	274
Time from ER Arrival to Discharge (minutes)	5,921	122	113	134
Time in ER Before Being Evaluated (minutes)	5,320	17	18	26
Time to Pain Meds for Fractures (minutes)	79	43	44	57
Heart Attack Care				
Aspirin Given at Discharge	68	100%	100%	99%
Fibrinolytic Meds Within 30 Min. of Arrival[1]	-	-	100%	54%
PCI Within 90 Minutes of Arrival	11	100%	94%	96%
Statin Prescribed at Discharge	66	98%	98%	98%
Heart Failure Care				
ACE Inhibitor or ARB for LVSD	20	95%	93%	97%
Discharge Instructions Given	49	100%	90%	94%
Evaluation of LVS Function	101	100%	97%	99%
Medicare Spending				
Medicare Spending per Patient (ratio)	-	0.99	0.9	0.98
Pneumonia Care				
Appropriate Initial Antibiotic Given	60	95%	90%	95%
Blood Culture Timing	116	97%	95%	98%
Pregnancy and Delivery Care				
Newborn Deliveries Scheduled Early[2]	18	0%	7%	6%
Preventive Care				
Immunization for Influenza	1,822	91%	89%	90%
Immunization for Pneumonia	2,033	82%	89%	92%
Stroke Care				
Anticoagulation Therapy for Atrial Fibrillation[1]	-	-	97%	95%
Antithrombotic Therapy Timing	30	93%	98%	98%
Assessed for Rehabilitation	37	97%	98%	97%
Discharged on Antithrombotic Therapy	35	100%	100%	99%
Discharged on Statin Medication	27	96%	93%	94%
Thrombolytic Therapy Timing[1]	-	-	51%	66%
Venous Thromboembolism Prophylaxis	34	94%	96%	94%
Written Stroke Educational Materials Given	18	100%	85%	88%
Surgical Care Improvement Project				
Appropriate Beta Blocker Usage	141	98%	98%	98%
Appropriate VTP Within 24 Hours	276	99%	98%	98%
Controlled Postoperative Blood Glucose[7]	-	-	98%	97%
Perioperative Temperature Management	341	100%	99%	100%
Prophylactic Antibiotic Selection	208	98%	99%	99%
Prophylactic Antibiotic Selection (Outpatient)	148	92%	99%	98%
Prophylactic Antibiotic Stopped	201	100%	98%	98%
Prophylactic Antibiotic Timing	209	99%	99%	99%
Prophylactic Antibiotic Timing (Outpatient)	143	94%	98%	98%
Urinary Catheter Removal	216	99%	97%	97%
Survey of Patients' Hospital Experiences				
Area Around Room 'Always' Quiet at Night	300+	60%	72%	61%
Doctors 'Always' Communicated Well	300+	81%	85%	82%
Home Recovery Information Given	300+	92%	87%	85%
Hospital Given 9 or 10 on 10 Point Scale	300+	71%	78%	71%
Meds 'Always' Explained Before Given	300+	62%	69%	64%
Nurses 'Always' Communicated Well	300+	78%	83%	79%
Pain 'Always' Well Controlled	300+	64%	72%	71%
Room and Bathroom 'Always' Clean	300+	73%	79%	73%
Timely Help 'Always' Received	300+	64%	77%	68%
Would Definitely Recommend Hospital	300+	73%	76%	71%
Use of Medical Imaging				
Cardiac Imaging Stress Test before Surgery	289	2.1%	4.4%	5.3%
Combination Abdominal CT Scan	678	4.3%	12.5%	10.5%
Combination Brain/Sinus CT Scan[1]	-	-	2%	2.7%
Combination Chest CT Scan	613	0.3%	4.5%	2.7%
Follow-up Mammogram/Ultrasound	1,396	12.2%	8.7%	8.8%
Lumbar Spine MRI for Low Back Pain	77	33.8%	33%	37.2%

Dakota Plains Surgical Center

701 8th Avenue Nw Suite C
Aberdeen, SD 57401
Phone: 605-225-3300
URL: www.orthopediccenterofthedakotas.com
Type: Acute Care Hospitals
Emergency Services: No
Ownership: Physician

Measure	Cases	This Hosp.	State Avg.	U.S. Avg.
Blood Clot Prevention and Treatment				
Anticoagulation Overlap Therapy[2,7]	-	-	95%	93%
ICU Venous Thromboembolism Prophylaxis[2,7]	-	-	91%	92%
Incidence of Potentially Preventable VTE[2,7]	-	-	5%	10%
UFH with Dosages/Platelet Monitoring[2,7]	-	-	100%	97%
Venous Thromboembolism Prophylaxis[2]	35	100%	80%	85%
Warfarin Therapy Discharge Instructions[2,7]	-	-	70%	75%
Chest Pain/Possible Heart Attack Care				
Aspirin Given Within 24 Hours of Arrival[5]	-	-	99%	96%
Fibrinolytic Meds Within 30 Min. of Arrival[5]	-	-	69%	58%
Average Time to ECG (minutes)[5]	-	-	5	7
Average Time to Transfer (minutes)[5]	-	-	66	60
Children's Asthma Care				
Received Home Management Plan of Care	-	-	-	88%
Received Reliever Medication	-	-	-	100%
Received Systemic Corticosteroids	-	-	-	100%
Emergency Department				
Admittance Decision Time (minutes)[2,7]	-	-	41	98
Head CT Results Within 45 Min. of Arrival[5]	-	-	44%	57%
Patients Who Left ER Before Being Seen[5]	-	-	1%	2%
Time from ER Arrival to Admit. (minutes)[2,7]	-	-	174	274
Time from ER Arrival to Discharge (minutes)[5]	-	-	113	134
Time in ER Before Being Evaluated (minutes)[5]	-	-	18	26
Time to Pain Meds for Fractures (minutes)[5]	-	-	44	57
Heart Attack Care				
Aspirin Given at Discharge[5]	-	-	100%	99%
Fibrinolytic Meds Within 30 Min. of Arrival[5]	-	-	100%	54%
PCI Within 90 Minutes of Arrival[5]	-	-	94%	96%
Statin Prescribed at Discharge[5]	-	-	98%	98%
Heart Failure Care				
ACE Inhibitor or ARB for LVSD[5]	-	-	93%	97%
Discharge Instructions Given[5]	-	-	90%	94%
Evaluation of LVS Function[5]	-	-	97%	99%
Medicare Spending				
Medicare Spending per Patient (ratio)	-	0.96	0.9	0.98
Pneumonia Care				
Appropriate Initial Antibiotic Given[5]	-	-	90%	95%
Blood Culture Timing[5]	-	-	95%	98%
Pregnancy and Delivery Care				
Newborn Deliveries Scheduled Early[7]	-	-	7%	6%
Preventive Care				
Immunization for Influenza[2]	179	100%	89%	90%
Immunization for Pneumonia[2]	206	95%	89%	92%
Stroke Care				
Anticoagulation Therapy for Atrial Fibrillation[5]	-	-	97%	95%
Antithrombotic Therapy Timing[5]	-	-	98%	98%
Assessed for Rehabilitation[5]	-	-	98%	97%
Discharged on Antithrombotic Therapy[5]	-	-	100%	99%
Discharged on Statin Medication[5]	-	-	93%	94%
Thrombolytic Therapy Timing[5]	-	-	51%	66%
Venous Thromboembolism Prophylaxis[5]	-	-	96%	94%
Written Stroke Educational Materials Given[5]	-	-	85%	88%
Surgical Care Improvement Project				
Appropriate Beta Blocker Usage[2]	71	99%	98%	98%
Appropriate VTP Within 24 Hours[2]	287	100%	98%	98%
Controlled Postoperative Blood Glucose[2,7]	-	-	98%	97%
Perioperative Temperature Management[2]	292	100%	99%	100%
Prophylactic Antibiotic Selection[2]	283	100%	99%	99%
Prophylactic Antibiotic Selection (Outpatient)	34	100%	99%	98%
Prophylactic Antibiotic Stopped[2]	279	95%	98%	98%
Prophylactic Antibiotic Timing[2]	283	99%	99%	99%
Prophylactic Antibiotic Timing (Outpatient)	34	100%	98%	98%
Urinary Catheter Removal[2]	290	100%	97%	97%
Survey of Patients' Hospital Experiences				
Area Around Room 'Always' Quiet at Night	(a)	89%	72%	61%
Doctors 'Always' Communicated Well	(a)	91%	85%	82%
Home Recovery Information Given	(a)	92%	87%	85%
Hospital Given 9 or 10 on 10 Point Scale	(a)	93%	78%	71%
Meds 'Always' Explained Before Given	(a)	76%	69%	64%
Nurses 'Always' Communicated Well	(a)	93%	83%	79%
Pain 'Always' Well Controlled	(a)	82%	72%	71%
Room and Bathroom 'Always' Clean	(a)	88%	79%	73%
Timely Help 'Always' Received	(a)	93%	77%	68%
Would Definitely Recommend Hospital	(a)	94%	76%	71%
Use of Medical Imaging				
Cardiac Imaging Stress Test before Surgery[7]	-	-	4.4%	5.3%
Combination Abdominal CT Scan[7]	-	-	12.5%	10.5%
Combination Brain/Sinus CT Scan[7]	-	-	2%	2.7%
Combination Chest CT Scan[7]	-	-	4.5%	2.7%
Follow-up Mammogram/Ultrasound[7]	-	-	8.7%	8.8%
Lumbar Spine MRI for Low Back Pain	68	16.2%	33%	37.2%

Sanford Aberdeen Medical Center

2905 3rd Ave Se Post Office Box 1770
Aberdeen, SD 57402
Phone: 605-626-4200
Type: Acute Care Hospitals
Emergency Services: Yes
Ownership: Voluntary non-profit - Private

Measure	Cases	This Hosp.	State Avg.	U.S. Avg.
Blood Clot Prevention and Treatment				
Anticoagulation Overlap Therapy[2,3]	11	91%	95%	93%
ICU Venous Thromboembolism Prophylaxis[1,2]	-	-	91%	92%
Incidence of Potentially Preventable VTE[1,2]	-	-	5%	10%
UFH with Dosages/Platelet Monitoring[1,2]	-	-	100%	97%
Venous Thromboembolism Prophylaxis[2,3]	76	84%	80%	85%
Warfarin Therapy Discharge Instructions[1,2]	-	-	70%	75%
Chest Pain/Possible Heart Attack Care				
Aspirin Given Within 24 Hours of Arrival[5]	-	-	99%	96%
Fibrinolytic Meds Within 30 Min. of Arrival[5]	-	-	69%	58%
Average Time to ECG (minutes)[5]	-	-	5	7
Average Time to Transfer (minutes)[5]	-	-	66	60
Children's Asthma Care				
Received Home Management Plan of Care	-	-	-	88%
Received Reliever Medication	-	-	-	100%
Received Systemic Corticosteroids	-	-	-	100%
Emergency Department				
Admittance Decision Time (minutes)[2,3]	138	40	41	98
Head CT Results Within 45 Min. of Arrival[3,7]	-	-	44%	57%
Patients Who Left ER Before Being Seen	1,979	0%	1%	2%
Time from ER Arrival to Admit. (minutes)[2,3]	140	160	174	274
Time from ER Arrival to Discharge (minutes)[3]	211	104	113	134
Time in ER Before Being Evaluated (minutes)[3]	227	3	18	26
Time to Pain Meds for Fractures (minutes)[3]	14	23	44	57
Heart Attack Care				
Aspirin Given at Discharge[3]	11	100%	100%	99%
Fibrinolytic Meds Within 30 Min. of Arrival[3,7]	-	-	100%	54%

NOTE: Hospital profiles are in alphabetical order by state, then city, then hospital within the city; Rankings exclude hospitals with less than 25 cases except for patient surveys which excludes hospitals with less than 100 cases; (a) 100-299 cases; (1) The number of cases/patients is too few to report; (2) Data submitted were based on a sample of cases/patients; (3) Results are based on a shorter time period than required; (4) Data suppressed by CMS for one or more quarters; (5) Results are not available for this reporting period; (6) Fewer than 100 patients completed the HCAHPS survey; (7) No cases met the criteria for this measure; (8) The lower limit of the confidence interval cannot be calculated if the number of observed infections equals zero; (9) No data are available from the state/territory for this reporting period; (10) The scores shown reflect fewer than 50 completed surveys; (11) There were discrepancies in the data collection process; (12) This measure does not apply to this hospital for this reporting period; (13) Results cannot be calculated for this reporting period; (14) The results for this state are combined with nearby states to protect confidentiality; Please refer to the User's Guide for a full explanation of data.

Measure	Cases	This Hosp.	State Avg.	U.S. Avg.
PCI Within 90 Minutes of Arrival[1,3]	-	-	94%	96%
Statin Prescribed at Discharge[3]	13	92%	98%	98%
Heart Failure Care				
ACE Inhibitor or ARB for LVSD[1,3]	-	-	93%	97%
Discharge Instructions Given[3]	17	100%	90%	94%
Evaluation of LVS Function[3]	24	100%	97%	99%
Medicare Spending				
Medicare Spending per Patient (ratio)	-	0.94	0.9	0.98
Pneumonia Care				
Appropriate Initial Antibiotic Given[3]	11	91%	90%	95%
Blood Culture Timing[3]	26	100%	95%	98%
Pregnancy and Delivery Care				
Newborn Deliveries Scheduled Early[3]	14	0%	7%	6%
Preventive Care				
Immunization for Influenza[5]	-	-	89%	90%
Immunization for Pneumonia[2,3]	179	87%	89%	92%
Stroke Care				
Anticoagulation Therapy for Atrial Fibrillation[1,3]	-	-	97%	95%
Antithrombotic Therapy Timing[1,3]	-	-	98%	98%
Assessed for Rehabilitation[1,3]	-	-	98%	97%
Discharged on Antithrombotic Therapy[1,3]	-	-	100%	99%
Discharged on Statin Medication[1,3]	-	-	93%	94%
Thrombolytic Therapy Timing[1,3]	-	-	51%	66%
Venous Thromboembolism Prophylaxis[1,3]	-	-	96%	94%
Written Stroke Educational Materials Given[1,3]	-	-	85%	88%
Surgical Care Improvement Project				
Appropriate Beta Blocker Usage[3]	18	89%	98%	98%
Appropriate VTP Within 24 Hours[3]	41	98%	98%	98%
Controlled Postoperative Blood Glucose[3,7]	-	-	98%	97%
Perioperative Temperature Management[3]	51	100%	99%	100%
Prophylactic Antibiotic Selection[3]	34	97%	99%	99%
Prophylactic Antibiotic Selection (Outpatient)[1,3]	-	-	99%	98%
Prophylactic Antibiotic Stopped[3]	32	91%	98%	98%
Prophylactic Antibiotic Timing[3]	34	97%	99%	99%
Prophylactic Antibiotic Timing (Outpatient)[1,3]	-	-	98%	98%
Urinary Catheter Removal[3]	40	98%	97%	97%
Survey of Patients' Hospital Experiences				
Area Around Room 'Always' Quiet at Night[5]	-	-	72%	61%
Doctors 'Always' Communicated Well[5]	-	-	85%	82%
Home Recovery Information Given[5]	-	-	87%	85%
Hospital Given 9 or 10 on 10 Point Scale[5]	-	-	78%	71%
Meds 'Always' Explained Before Given[5]	-	-	69%	64%
Nurses 'Always' Communicated Well[5]	-	-	83%	79%
Pain 'Always' Well Controlled[5]	-	-	72%	71%
Room and Bathroom 'Always' Clean[5]	-	-	79%	73%
Timely Help 'Always' Received[5]	-	-	77%	68%
Would Definitely Recommend Hospital[5]	-	-	76%	71%
Use of Medical Imaging				
Cardiac Imaging Stress Test before Surgery	97	5.2%	4.4%	5.3%
Combination Abdominal CT Scan	128	14.8%	12.5%	10.5%
Combination Brain/Sinus CT Scan	122	0.0%	2%	2.7%
Combination Chest CT Scan	70	11.4%	4.5%	2.7%
Follow-up Mammogram/Ultrasound	149	9.4%	8.7%	8.8%
Lumbar Spine MRI for Low Back Pain[1]	-	-	33%	37.2%

Bowdle Hospital

8001 W 5th PO Box 556
Bowdle, SD 57428
Phone: 605-285-6146
Fax: 605-285-6410
E-mail: kkarst@midca.net
URL: www.bowdlehealthcarecenter.com
Type: Critical Access Hospitals
Emergency Services: Yes
Ownership: Government - Local
Beds: 50

Key Personnel:
Quality Assurance . . . . Karen Karst
CEO/President. . . . . Mike Piper

Measure	Cases	This Hosp.	State Avg.	U.S. Avg.
Blood Clot Prevention and Treatment				
Anticoagulation Overlap Therapy	-	-	95%	93%
ICU Venous Thromboembolism Prophylaxis	-	-	91%	92%
Incidence of Potentially Preventable VTE	-	-	5%	10%
UFH with Dosages/Platelet Monitoring	-	-	100%	97%
Venous Thromboembolism Prophylaxis	-	-	80%	85%
Warfarin Therapy Discharge Instructions	-	-	70%	75%
Chest Pain/Possible Heart Attack Care				
Aspirin Given Within 24 Hours of Arrival[5]	-	-	99%	96%
Fibrinolytic Meds Within 30 Min. of Arrival[5]	-	-	69%	58%
Average Time to ECG (minutes)[5]	-	-	5	7
Average Time to Transfer (minutes)[5]	-	-	66	60
Children's Asthma Care				
Received Home Management Plan of Care	-	-	-	88%
Received Reliever Medication	-	-	-	100%
Received Systemic Corticosteroids	-	-	-	100%
Emergency Department				
Admittance Decision Time (minutes)	-	-	41	98
Head CT Results Within 45 Min. of Arrival[5]	-	-	44%	57%
Patients Who Left ER Before Being Seen[5]	-	-	1%	2%
Time from ER Arrival to Admit. (minutes)	-	-	174	274
Time from ER Arrival to Discharge (minutes)[5]	-	-	113	134
Time in ER Before Being Evaluated (minutes)[5]	-	-	18	26
Time to Pain Meds for Fractures (minutes)[5]	-	-	44	57
Heart Attack Care				
Aspirin Given at Discharge	-	-	100%	99%
Fibrinolytic Meds Within 30 Min. of Arrival	-	-	100%	54%
PCI Within 90 Minutes of Arrival	-	-	94%	96%
Statin Prescribed at Discharge	-	-	98%	98%
Heart Failure Care				
ACE Inhibitor or ARB for LVSD	-	-	93%	97%
Discharge Instructions Given	-	-	90%	94%
Evaluation of LVS Function	-	-	97%	99%
Medicare Spending				
Medicare Spending per Patient (ratio)	-	-	0.9	0.98
Pneumonia Care				
Appropriate Initial Antibiotic Given	-	-	90%	95%
Blood Culture Timing	-	-	95%	98%
Pregnancy and Delivery Care				
Newborn Deliveries Scheduled Early	-	-	7%	6%
Preventive Care				
Immunization for Influenza	-	-	89%	90%
Immunization for Pneumonia	-	-	89%	92%
Stroke Care				
Anticoagulation Therapy for Atrial Fibrillation	-	-	97%	95%
Antithrombotic Therapy Timing	-	-	98%	98%
Assessed for Rehabilitation	-	-	98%	97%
Discharged on Antithrombotic Therapy	-	-	100%	99%
Discharged on Statin Medication	-	-	93%	94%
Thrombolytic Therapy Timing	-	-	51%	66%
Venous Thromboembolism Prophylaxis	-	-	96%	94%
Written Stroke Educational Materials Given	-	-	85%	88%
Surgical Care Improvement Project				
Appropriate Beta Blocker Usage	-	-	98%	98%
Appropriate VTP Within 24 Hours	-	-	98%	98%
Controlled Postoperative Blood Glucose	-	-	98%	97%
Perioperative Temperature Management	-	-	99%	100%
Prophylactic Antibiotic Selection	-	-	99%	99%
Prophylactic Antibiotic Selection (Outpatient)[5]	-	-	99%	98%
Prophylactic Antibiotic Stopped	-	-	98%	98%
Prophylactic Antibiotic Timing	-	-	99%	99%
Prophylactic Antibiotic Timing (Outpatient)[5]	-	-	98%	98%
Urinary Catheter Removal	-	-	97%	97%
Survey of Patients' Hospital Experiences				
Area Around Room 'Always' Quiet at Night	-	-	72%	61%
Doctors 'Always' Communicated Well	-	-	85%	82%
Home Recovery Information Given	-	-	87%	85%
Hospital Given 9 or 10 on 10 Point Scale	-	-	78%	71%
Meds 'Always' Explained Before Given	-	-	69%	64%
Nurses 'Always' Communicated Well	-	-	83%	79%
Pain 'Always' Well Controlled	-	-	72%	71%
Room and Bathroom 'Always' Clean	-	-	79%	73%
Timely Help 'Always' Received	-	-	77%	68%
Would Definitely Recommend Hospital	-	-	76%	71%
Use of Medical Imaging				
Cardiac Imaging Stress Test before Surgery[7]	-	-	4.4%	5.3%
Combination Abdominal CT Scan[1]	-	-	12.5%	10.5%
Combination Brain/Sinus CT Scan[1]	-	-	2%	2.7%
Combination Chest CT Scan[1]	-	-	4.5%	2.7%
Follow-up Mammogram/Ultrasound[1]	-	-	8.7%	8.8%
Lumbar Spine MRI for Low Back Pain[1]	-	-	33%	37.2%

Marshall County Healthcare Center

413 9th Street
Britton, SD 57430
Phone: 605-448-2253
Type: Critical Access Hospitals
Emergency Services: Yes
Ownership: Voluntary non-profit - Private

Measure	Cases	This Hosp.	State Avg.	U.S. Avg.
Blood Clot Prevention and Treatment				
Anticoagulation Overlap Therapy[5]	-	-	95%	93%
ICU Venous Thromboembolism Prophylaxis[5]	-	-	91%	92%
Incidence of Potentially Preventable VTE[5]	-	-	5%	10%
UFH with Dosages/Platelet Monitoring[5]	-	-	100%	97%
Venous Thromboembolism Prophylaxis[5]	-	-	80%	85%
Warfarin Therapy Discharge Instructions[5]	-	-	70%	75%
Chest Pain/Possible Heart Attack Care				
Aspirin Given Within 24 Hours of Arrival	-	-	99%	96%
Fibrinolytic Meds Within 30 Min. of Arrival	-	-	69%	58%
Average Time to ECG (minutes)	-	-	5	7
Average Time to Transfer (minutes)	-	-	66	60
Children's Asthma Care				
Received Home Management Plan of Care	-	-	-	88%
Received Reliever Medication	-	-	-	100%
Received Systemic Corticosteroids	-	-	-	100%
Emergency Department				
Admittance Decision Time (minutes)[5]	-	-	41	98
Head CT Results Within 45 Min. of Arrival	-	-	44%	57%
Patients Who Left ER Before Being Seen	-	-	1%	2%
Time from ER Arrival to Admit. (minutes)[5]	-	-	174	274
Time from ER Arrival to Discharge (minutes)	-	-	113	134
Time in ER Before Being Evaluated (minutes)	-	-	18	26
Time to Pain Meds for Fractures (minutes)	-	-	44	57
Heart Attack Care				
Aspirin Given at Discharge[5]	-	-	100%	99%
Fibrinolytic Meds Within 30 Min. of Arrival[5]	-	-	100%	54%
PCI Within 90 Minutes of Arrival[5]	-	-	94%	96%
Statin Prescribed at Discharge[5]	-	-	98%	98%
Heart Failure Care				
ACE Inhibitor or ARB for LVSD[1,3]	-	-	93%	97%
Discharge Instructions Given[1,3]	-	-	90%	94%
Evaluation of LVS Function[1,3]	-	-	97%	99%
Medicare Spending				
Medicare Spending per Patient (ratio)	-	-	0.9	0.98
Pneumonia Care				
Appropriate Initial Antibiotic Given[1,3]	-	-	90%	95%
Blood Culture Timing[1,3]	-	-	95%	98%
Pregnancy and Delivery Care				
Newborn Deliveries Scheduled Early[5]	-	-	7%	6%
Preventive Care				
Immunization for Influenza[5]	-	-	89%	90%
Immunization for Pneumonia[5]	-	-	89%	92%
Stroke Care				
Anticoagulation Therapy for Atrial Fibrillation[5]	-	-	97%	95%
Antithrombotic Therapy Timing[5]	-	-	98%	98%
Assessed for Rehabilitation[5]	-	-	98%	97%
Discharged on Antithrombotic Therapy[5]	-	-	100%	99%
Discharged on Statin Medication[5]	-	-	93%	94%
Thrombolytic Therapy Timing[5]	-	-	51%	66%
Venous Thromboembolism Prophylaxis[5]	-	-	96%	94%
Written Stroke Educational Materials Given[5]	-	-	85%	88%
Surgical Care Improvement Project				
Appropriate Beta Blocker Usage[5]	-	-	98%	98%
Appropriate VTP Within 24 Hours[5]	-	-	98%	98%
Controlled Postoperative Blood Glucose[5]	-	-	98%	97%
Perioperative Temperature Management[5]	-	-	99%	100%
Prophylactic Antibiotic Selection[5]	-	-	99%	99%
Prophylactic Antibiotic Selection (Outpatient)	-	-	99%	98%
Prophylactic Antibiotic Stopped[5]	-	-	98%	98%
Prophylactic Antibiotic Timing[5]	-	-	99%	99%
Prophylactic Antibiotic Timing (Outpatient)	-	-	98%	98%
Urinary Catheter Removal[5]	-	-	97%	97%

NOTE: Hospital profiles are in alphabetical order by state, then city, then hospital within the city; Rankings exclude hospitals with less than 25 cases except for patient surveys which excludes hospitals with less than 100 cases; (a) 100-299 cases; (1) The number of cases/patients is too few to report; (2) Data submitted were based on a sample of cases/patients; (3) Results are based on a shorter time period than required; (4) Data suppressed by CMS for one or more quarters; (5) Results are not available for this reporting period; (6) Fewer than 100 patients completed the HCAHPS survey; (7) No cases met the criteria for this measure; (8) The lower limit of the confidence interval cannot be calculated if the number of observed infections equals zero; (9) No data are available from the state/territory for this reporting period; (10) The scores shown reflect fewer than 50 completed surveys; (11) There were discrepancies in the data collection process; (12) This measure does not apply to this hospital for this reporting period; (13) Results cannot be calculated for this reporting period; (14) The results for this state are combined with nearby states to protect confidentiality; Please refer to the User's Guide for a full explanation of data.

Survey of Patients' Hospital Experiences				
Area Around Room 'Always' Quiet at Night[10]	<100	81%	72%	61%
Doctors 'Always' Communicated Well[10]	<100	93%	85%	82%
Home Recovery Information Given[10]	<100	85%	87%	85%
Hospital Given 9 or 10 on 10 Point Scale[10]	<100	87%	78%	71%
Meds 'Always' Explained Before Given[10]	<100	86%	69%	64%
Nurses 'Always' Communicated Well[10]	<100	95%	83%	79%
Pain 'Always' Well Controlled[10]	<100	67%	72%	71%
Room and Bathroom 'Always' Clean[10]	<100	85%	79%	73%
Timely Help 'Always' Received[10]	<100	72%	77%	68%
Would Definitely Recommend Hospital[10]	<100	89%	76%	71%
Use of Medical Imaging				
Cardiac Imaging Stress Test before Surgery	-	-	4.4%	5.3%
Combination Abdominal CT Scan	-	-	12.5%	10.5%
Combination Brain/Sinus CT Scan	-	-	2%	2.7%
Combination Chest CT Scan	-	-	4.5%	2.7%
Follow-up Mammogram/Ultrasound	-	-	8.7%	8.8%
Lumbar Spine MRI for Low Back Pain	-	-	33%	37.2%

Brookings Hospital

300 22nd Ave
Brookings, SD 57006
Phone: 605-696-7701
Fax: 605-696-7770
URL: www.brookingshospital.org
Type: Acute Care Hospitals
Emergency Services: Yes
Ownership: Government - Local
Beds: 128

Key Personnel:
Chairman/CEO . . . . Al Baker
CEO/President. . . . . Kevin Coffey
Quality Assurance . . . . Dianna Eberf
Radiology. . . . . Randi Hart
Chief of Medical Staff. . . . . Richard S Hieb

Measure	Cases	This Hosp.	State Avg.	U.S. Avg.
Blood Clot Prevention and Treatment				
Anticoagulation Overlap Therapy[2]	13	85%	95%	93%
ICU Venous Thromboembolism Prophylaxis[1,2]	-	-	91%	92%
Incidence of Potentially Preventable VTE[1,2]	-	-	5%	10%
UFH with Dosages/Platelet Monitoring[1,2]	-	-	100%	97%
Venous Thromboembolism Prophylaxis[2]	124	79%	80%	85%
Warfarin Therapy Discharge Instructions[1,2]	-	-	70%	75%
Chest Pain/Possible Heart Attack Care				
Aspirin Given Within 24 Hours of Arrival	27	100%	99%	96%
Fibrinolytic Meds Within 30 Min. of Arrival[1]	-	-	69%	58%
Average Time to ECG (minutes)	28	5	5	7
Average Time to Transfer (minutes)[1]	-	-	66	60
Children's Asthma Care				
Received Home Management Plan of Care	-	-	-	88%
Received Reliever Medication	-	-	-	100%
Received Systemic Corticosteroids	-	-	-	100%
Emergency Department				
Admittance Decision Time (minutes)[2]	222	52	41	98
Head CT Results Within 45 Min. of Arrival[1]	-	-	44%	57%
Patients Who Left ER Before Being Seen	8,035	0%	1%	2%
Time from ER Arrival to Admit. (minutes)[2]	224	152	174	274
Time from ER Arrival to Discharge (minutes)	456	70	113	134
Time in ER Before Being Evaluated (minutes)	505	17	18	26
Time to Pain Meds for Fractures (minutes)	54	39	44	57
Heart Attack Care				
Aspirin Given at Discharge[1]	-	-	100%	99%
Fibrinolytic Meds Within 30 Min. of Arrival[7]	-	-	100%	54%
PCI Within 90 Minutes of Arrival[7]	-	-	94%	96%
Statin Prescribed at Discharge[1]	-	-	98%	98%
Heart Failure Care				
ACE Inhibitor or ARB for LVSD[1]	-	-	93%	97%
Discharge Instructions Given	30	97%	90%	94%
Evaluation of LVS Function	40	95%	97%	99%
Medicare Spending				
Medicare Spending per Patient (ratio)	-	0.84	0.9	0.98
Pneumonia Care				
Appropriate Initial Antibiotic Given	39	100%	90%	95%
Blood Culture Timing	40	100%	95%	98%
Pregnancy and Delivery Care				
Newborn Deliveries Scheduled Early	24	4%	7%	6%
Preventive Care				
Immunization for Influenza[2]	254	95%	89%	90%
Immunization for Pneumonia[2]	284	99%	89%	92%
Stroke Care				
Anticoagulation Therapy for Atrial Fibrillation[1]	-	-	97%	95%
Antithrombotic Therapy Timing[1]	-	-	98%	98%
Assessed for Rehabilitation[1]	-	-	98%	97%
Discharged on Antithrombotic Therapy[1]	-	-	100%	99%
Discharged on Statin Medication[1]	-	-	93%	94%
Thrombolytic Therapy Timing[1]	-	-	51%	66%
Venous Thromboembolism Prophylaxis[1]	-	-	96%	94%
Written Stroke Educational Materials Given[1]	-	-	85%	88%
Surgical Care Improvement Project				
Appropriate Beta Blocker Usage	13	100%	98%	98%
Appropriate VTP Within 24 Hours	35	97%	98%	98%
Controlled Postoperative Blood Glucose[7]	-	-	98%	97%
Perioperative Temperature Management	47	100%	99%	100%
Prophylactic Antibiotic Selection	42	100%	99%	99%
Prophylactic Antibiotic Selection (Outpatient)	24	100%	99%	98%
Prophylactic Antibiotic Stopped	42	98%	98%	98%
Prophylactic Antibiotic Timing	42	100%	99%	99%
Prophylactic Antibiotic Timing (Outpatient)	24	96%	98%	98%
Urinary Catheter Removal	33	100%	97%	97%
Survey of Patients' Hospital Experiences				
Area Around Room 'Always' Quiet at Night	300+	72%	72%	61%
Doctors 'Always' Communicated Well	300+	84%	85%	82%
Home Recovery Information Given	300+	86%	87%	85%
Hospital Given 9 or 10 on 10 Point Scale	300+	77%	78%	71%
Meds 'Always' Explained Before Given	300+	67%	69%	64%
Nurses 'Always' Communicated Well	300+	84%	83%	79%
Pain 'Always' Well Controlled	300+	75%	72%	71%
Room and Bathroom 'Always' Clean	300+	82%	79%	73%
Timely Help 'Always' Received	300+	73%	77%	68%
Would Definitely Recommend Hospital	300+	75%	76%	71%
Use of Medical Imaging				
Cardiac Imaging Stress Test before Surgery[1]	-	-	4.4%	5.3%
Combination Abdominal CT Scan	174	6.9%	12.5%	10.5%
Combination Brain/Sinus CT Scan	117	0.0%	2%	2.7%
Combination Chest CT Scan	80	0.0%	4.5%	2.7%
Follow-up Mammogram/Ultrasound[7]	-	-	8.7%	8.8%
Lumbar Spine MRI for Low Back Pain[1]	-	-	33%	37.2%

Community Memorial Hospital

809 Jackson PO Box 319
Burke, SD 57523
Phone: 605-775-2621
Type: Critical Access Hospitals
Emergency Services: Yes
Ownership: Voluntary non-profit - Private

Measure	Cases	This Hosp.	State Avg.	U.S. Avg.
Blood Clot Prevention and Treatment				
Anticoagulation Overlap Therapy[5]	-	-	95%	93%
ICU Venous Thromboembolism Prophylaxis[5]	-	-	91%	92%
Incidence of Potentially Preventable VTE[5]	-	-	5%	10%
UFH with Dosages/Platelet Monitoring[5]	-	-	100%	97%
Venous Thromboembolism Prophylaxis[5]	-	-	80%	85%
Warfarin Therapy Discharge Instructions[5]	-	-	70%	75%
Chest Pain/Possible Heart Attack Care				
Aspirin Given Within 24 Hours of Arrival	-	-	99%	96%
Fibrinolytic Meds Within 30 Min. of Arrival	-	-	69%	58%
Average Time to ECG (minutes)	-	-	5	7
Average Time to Transfer (minutes)	-	-	66	60
Children's Asthma Care				
Received Home Management Plan of Care	-	-	-	88%
Received Reliever Medication	-	-	-	100%
Received Systemic Corticosteroids	-	-	-	100%
Emergency Department				
Admittance Decision Time (minutes)[5]	-	-	41	98
Head CT Results Within 45 Min. of Arrival	-	-	44%	57%
Patients Who Left ER Before Being Seen	-	-	1%	2%
Time from ER Arrival to Admit. (minutes)[5]	-	-	174	274
Time from ER Arrival to Discharge (minutes)	-	-	113	134
Time in ER Before Being Evaluated (minutes)	-	-	18	26
Time to Pain Meds for Fractures (minutes)	-	-	44	57
Heart Attack Care				
Aspirin Given at Discharge[5]	-	-	100%	99%
Fibrinolytic Meds Within 30 Min. of Arrival[5]	-	-	100%	54%
PCI Within 90 Minutes of Arrival[5]	-	-	94%	96%
Statin Prescribed at Discharge[5]	-	-	98%	98%
Heart Failure Care				
ACE Inhibitor or ARB for LVSD[1,2]	-	-	93%	97%
Discharge Instructions Given[1,2]	-	-	90%	94%
Evaluation of LVS Function[1,2]	-	-	97%	99%
Medicare Spending				
Medicare Spending per Patient (ratio)	-	-	0.9	0.98
Pneumonia Care				
Appropriate Initial Antibiotic Given[2]	17	76%	90%	95%
Blood Culture Timing[1,2]	-	-	95%	98%
Pregnancy and Delivery Care				
Newborn Deliveries Scheduled Early[5]	-	-	7%	6%
Preventive Care				
Immunization for Influenza[5]	-	-	89%	90%
Immunization for Pneumonia[5]	-	-	89%	92%
Stroke Care				
Anticoagulation Therapy for Atrial Fibrillation[5]	-	-	97%	95%
Antithrombotic Therapy Timing[5]	-	-	98%	98%
Assessed for Rehabilitation[5]	-	-	98%	97%
Discharged on Antithrombotic Therapy[5]	-	-	100%	99%
Discharged on Statin Medication[5]	-	-	93%	94%
Thrombolytic Therapy Timing[5]	-	-	51%	66%
Venous Thromboembolism Prophylaxis[5]	-	-	96%	94%
Written Stroke Educational Materials Given[5]	-	-	85%	88%
Surgical Care Improvement Project				
Appropriate Beta Blocker Usage[5]	-	-	98%	98%
Appropriate VTP Within 24 Hours[5]	-	-	98%	98%
Controlled Postoperative Blood Glucose[5]	-	-	98%	97%
Perioperative Temperature Management[5]	-	-	99%	100%
Prophylactic Antibiotic Selection[5]	-	-	99%	99%
Prophylactic Antibiotic Selection (Outpatient)	-	-	99%	98%
Prophylactic Antibiotic Stopped[5]	-	-	98%	98%
Prophylactic Antibiotic Timing[5]	-	-	99%	99%
Prophylactic Antibiotic Timing (Outpatient)	-	-	98%	98%
Urinary Catheter Removal[5]	-	-	97%	97%
Survey of Patients' Hospital Experiences				
Area Around Room 'Always' Quiet at Night[5]	-	-	72%	61%
Doctors 'Always' Communicated Well[5]	-	-	85%	82%
Home Recovery Information Given[5]	-	-	87%	85%
Hospital Given 9 or 10 on 10 Point Scale[5]	-	-	78%	71%
Meds 'Always' Explained Before Given[5]	-	-	69%	64%
Nurses 'Always' Communicated Well[5]	-	-	83%	79%
Pain 'Always' Well Controlled[5]	-	-	72%	71%
Room and Bathroom 'Always' Clean[5]	-	-	79%	73%
Timely Help 'Always' Received[5]	-	-	77%	68%
Would Definitely Recommend Hospital[5]	-	-	76%	71%
Use of Medical Imaging				
Cardiac Imaging Stress Test before Surgery	-	-	4.4%	5.3%
Combination Abdominal CT Scan	-	-	12.5%	10.5%
Combination Brain/Sinus CT Scan	-	-	2%	2.7%
Combination Chest CT Scan	-	-	4.5%	2.7%
Follow-up Mammogram/Ultrasound	-	-	8.7%	8.8%
Lumbar Spine MRI for Low Back Pain	-	-	33%	37.2%

Sanford Canton - Inwood Medical Center

440 North Hiawatha Drive
Canton, SD 57013
Phone: 605-764-1400
Type: Critical Access Hospitals
Emergency Services: Yes
Ownership: Voluntary non-profit - Private

Measure	Cases	This Hosp.	State Avg.	U.S. Avg.
Blood Clot Prevention and Treatment				
Anticoagulation Overlap Therapy[5]	-	-	95%	93%
ICU Venous Thromboembolism Prophylaxis[5]	-	-	91%	92%
Incidence of Potentially Preventable VTE[5]	-	-	5%	10%
UFH with Dosages/Platelet Monitoring[5]	-	-	100%	97%
Venous Thromboembolism Prophylaxis[5]	-	-	80%	85%
Warfarin Therapy Discharge Instructions[5]	-	-	70%	75%
Chest Pain/Possible Heart Attack Care				
Aspirin Given Within 24 Hours of Arrival	-	-	99%	96%
Fibrinolytic Meds Within 30 Min. of Arrival	-	-	69%	58%

NOTE: Hospital profiles are in alphabetical order by state, then city, then hospital within the city; Rankings exclude hospitals with less than 25 cases except for patient surveys which excludes hospitals with less than 100 cases; (a) 100-299 cases; (1) The number of cases/patients is too few to report; (2) Data submitted were based on a sample of cases/patients; (3) Results are based on a shorter time period than required; (4) Data suppressed by CMS for one or more quarters; (5) Results are not available for this reporting period; (6) Fewer than 100 patients completed the HCAHPS survey; (7) No cases met the criteria for this measure; (8) The lower limit of the confidence interval cannot be calculated if the number of observed infections equals zero; (9) No data are available from the state/territory for this reporting period; (10) The scores shown reflect fewer than 50 completed surveys; (11) There were discrepancies in the data collection process; (12) This measure does not apply to this hospital for this reporting period; (13) Results cannot be calculated for this reporting period; (14) The results for this state are combined with nearby states to protect confidentiality; Please refer to the User's Guide for a full explanation of data.

Measure	Cases	This Hosp.	State Avg.	U.S. Avg.
Average Time to ECG (minutes)	-	-	5	7
Average Time to Transfer (minutes)	-	-	66	60
Children's Asthma Care				
Received Home Management Plan of Care	-	-	-	88%
Received Reliever Medication	-	-	-	100%
Received Systemic Corticosteroids	-	-	-	100%
Emergency Department				
Admittance Decision Time (minutes)[5]	-	-	41	98
Head CT Results Within 45 Min. of Arrival	-	-	44%	57%
Patients Who Left ER Before Being Seen	-	-	1%	2%
Time from ER Arrival to Admit. (minutes)[5]	-	-	174	274
Time from ER Arrival to Discharge (minutes)	-	-	113	134
Time in ER Before Being Evaluated (minutes)	-	-	18	26
Time to Pain Meds for Fractures (minutes)	-	-	44	57
Heart Attack Care				
Aspirin Given at Discharge[5]	-	-	100%	99%
Fibrinolytic Meds Within 30 Min. of Arrival[5]	-	-	100%	54%
PCI Within 90 Minutes of Arrival[5]	-	-	94%	96%
Statin Prescribed at Discharge[5]	-	-	98%	98%
Heart Failure Care				
ACE Inhibitor or ARB for LVSD[3,7]	-	-	93%	97%
Discharge Instructions Given[1,3]	-	-	90%	94%
Evaluation of LVS Function[1,3]	-	-	97%	99%
Medicare Spending				
Medicare Spending per Patient (ratio)	-	-	0.9	0.98
Pneumonia Care				
Appropriate Initial Antibiotic Given	12	100%	90%	95%
Blood Culture Timing[1]	-	-	95%	98%
Pregnancy and Delivery Care				
Newborn Deliveries Scheduled Early[5]	-	-	7%	6%
Preventive Care				
Immunization for Influenza[5]	-	-	89%	90%
Immunization for Pneumonia[5]	-	-	89%	92%
Stroke Care				
Anticoagulation Therapy for Atrial Fibrillation[5]	-	-	97%	95%
Antithrombotic Therapy Timing[5]	-	-	98%	98%
Assessed for Rehabilitation[5]	-	-	98%	97%
Discharged on Antithrombotic Therapy[5]	-	-	100%	99%
Discharged on Statin Medication[5]	-	-	93%	94%
Thrombolytic Therapy Timing[5]	-	-	51%	66%
Venous Thromboembolism Prophylaxis[5]	-	-	96%	94%
Written Stroke Educational Materials Given[5]	-	-	85%	88%
Surgical Care Improvement Project				
Appropriate Beta Blocker Usage[5]	-	-	98%	98%
Appropriate VTP Within 24 Hours[5]	-	-	98%	98%
Controlled Postoperative Blood Glucose[5]	-	-	98%	97%
Perioperative Temperature Management[5]	-	-	99%	100%
Prophylactic Antibiotic Selection[5]	-	-	99%	99%
Prophylactic Antibiotic Selection (Outpatient)	-	-	99%	98%
Prophylactic Antibiotic Stopped[5]	-	-	98%	98%
Prophylactic Antibiotic Timing[5]	-	-	99%	99%
Prophylactic Antibiotic Timing (Outpatient)	-	-	98%	98%
Urinary Catheter Removal[5]	-	-	97%	97%
Survey of Patients' Hospital Experiences				
Area Around Room 'Always' Quiet at Night[10]	<100	77%	72%	61%
Doctors 'Always' Communicated Well[10]	<100	88%	85%	82%
Home Recovery Information Given[10]	<100	85%	87%	85%
Hospital Given 9 or 10 on 10 Point Scale[10]	<100	90%	78%	71%
Meds 'Always' Explained Before Given[10]	<100	83%	69%	64%
Nurses 'Always' Communicated Well[10]	<100	93%	83%	79%
Pain 'Always' Well Controlled[10]	<100	82%	72%	71%
Room and Bathroom 'Always' Clean[10]	<100	90%	79%	73%
Timely Help 'Always' Received[10]	<100	89%	77%	68%
Would Definitely Recommend Hospital[10]	<100	80%	76%	71%
Use of Medical Imaging				
Cardiac Imaging Stress Test before Surgery	-	-	4.4%	5.3%
Combination Abdominal CT Scan	-	-	12.5%	10.5%
Combination Brain/Sinus CT Scan	-	-	2%	2.7%
Combination Chest CT Scan	-	-	4.5%	2.7%
Follow-up Mammogram/Ultrasound	-	-	8.7%	8.8%
Lumbar Spine MRI for Low Back Pain	-	-	33%	37.2%

Sanford Chamberlain Medical Center

300 S Byron   Phone: 605-234-5511
Chamberlain, SD 57325   Fax: 605-234-7118
URL: www.sanfordmiddakota.org
Type: Critical Access Hospitals   Emergency Services: Yes
Ownership: Voluntary non-profit - Private   Beds: 25

Key Personnel:
Infection Control. . . . . Diane Blasius
CEO/President. . . . . Maureen Cadwell, FHFMA
Radiology. . . . . Tom Davis
Emergency Room . . . . Stephanie Feltman, RN
Operating Room. . . . . Donna Greensfeild, RN
Chief of Medical Staff. . . . . John Jones, MD
Quality Assurance . . . . Nancy McDonald, RN
Intensive Care Unit. . . . . Jayson Pullman, RN

Measure	Cases	This Hosp.	State Avg.	U.S. Avg.
Blood Clot Prevention and Treatment				
Anticoagulation Overlap Therapy[5]	-	-	95%	93%
ICU Venous Thromboembolism Prophylaxis[5]	-	-	91%	92%
Incidence of Potentially Preventable VTE[5]	-	-	5%	10%
UFH with Dosages/Platelet Monitoring[5]	-	-	100%	97%
Venous Thromboembolism Prophylaxis[5]	-	-	80%	85%
Warfarin Therapy Discharge Instructions[5]	-	-	70%	75%
Chest Pain/Possible Heart Attack Care				
Aspirin Given Within 24 Hours of Arrival	-	-	99%	96%
Fibrinolytic Meds Within 30 Min. of Arrival	-	-	69%	58%
Average Time to ECG (minutes)	-	-	5	7
Average Time to Transfer (minutes)	-	-	66	60
Children's Asthma Care				
Received Home Management Plan of Care	-	-	-	88%
Received Reliever Medication	-	-	-	100%
Received Systemic Corticosteroids	-	-	-	100%
Emergency Department				
Admittance Decision Time (minutes)[5]	-	-	41	98
Head CT Results Within 45 Min. of Arrival	-	-	44%	57%
Patients Who Left ER Before Being Seen	-	-	1%	2%
Time from ER Arrival to Admit. (minutes)[5]	-	-	174	274
Time from ER Arrival to Discharge (minutes)	-	-	113	134
Time in ER Before Being Evaluated (minutes)	-	-	18	26
Time to Pain Meds for Fractures (minutes)	-	-	44	57
Heart Attack Care				
Aspirin Given at Discharge[3,7]	-	-	100%	99%
Fibrinolytic Meds Within 30 Min. of Arrival[3,7]	-	-	100%	54%
PCI Within 90 Minutes of Arrival[3,7]	-	-	94%	96%
Statin Prescribed at Discharge[3,7]	-	-	98%	98%
Heart Failure Care				
ACE Inhibitor or ARB for LVSD[1,3]	-	-	93%	97%
Discharge Instructions Given[1,3]	-	-	90%	94%
Evaluation of LVS Function[1,3]	-	-	97%	99%
Medicare Spending				
Medicare Spending per Patient (ratio)	-	-	0.9	0.98
Pneumonia Care				
Appropriate Initial Antibiotic Given[7]	-	-	90%	95%
Blood Culture Timing[7]	-	-	95%	98%
Pregnancy and Delivery Care				
Newborn Deliveries Scheduled Early[5]	-	-	7%	6%
Preventive Care				
Immunization for Influenza[5]	-	-	89%	90%
Immunization for Pneumonia[5]	-	-	89%	92%
Stroke Care				
Anticoagulation Therapy for Atrial Fibrillation[3,7]	-	-	97%	95%
Antithrombotic Therapy Timing[3,7]	-	-	98%	98%
Assessed for Rehabilitation[1,3]	-	-	98%	97%
Discharged on Antithrombotic Therapy[3,7]	-	-	100%	99%
Discharged on Statin Medication[1,3]	-	-	93%	94%
Thrombolytic Therapy Timing[3,7]	-	-	51%	66%
Venous Thromboembolism Prophylaxis[1,3]	-	-	96%	94%
Written Stroke Educational Materials Given[1,3]	-	-	85%	88%
Surgical Care Improvement Project				
Appropriate Beta Blocker Usage[3,7]	-	-	98%	98%
Appropriate VTP Within 24 Hours[1,3]	-	-	98%	98%
Controlled Postoperative Blood Glucose[3,7]	-	-	98%	97%
Perioperative Temperature Management[1,3]	-	-	99%	100%
Prophylactic Antibiotic Selection[1,3]	-	-	99%	99%
Prophylactic Antibiotic Selection (Outpatient)	-	-	99%	98%
Prophylactic Antibiotic Stopped[1,3]	-	-	98%	98%
Prophylactic Antibiotic Timing[1,3]	-	-	99%	99%
Prophylactic Antibiotic Timing (Outpatient)	-	-	98%	98%
Urinary Catheter Removal[1,3]	-	-	97%	97%
Survey of Patients' Hospital Experiences				
Area Around Room 'Always' Quiet at Night[10]	<100	72%	72%	61%
Doctors 'Always' Communicated Well[10]	<100	84%	85%	82%
Home Recovery Information Given[10]	<100	81%	87%	85%
Hospital Given 9 or 10 on 10 Point Scale[10]	<100	53%	78%	71%
Meds 'Always' Explained Before Given[10]	<100	53%	69%	64%
Nurses 'Always' Communicated Well[10]	<100	72%	83%	79%
Pain 'Always' Well Controlled[10]	<100	60%	72%	71%
Room and Bathroom 'Always' Clean[10]	<100	49%	79%	73%
Timely Help 'Always' Received[10]	<100	60%	77%	68%
Would Definitely Recommend Hospital[10]	<100	51%	76%	71%
Use of Medical Imaging				
Cardiac Imaging Stress Test before Surgery	-	-	4.4%	5.3%
Combination Abdominal CT Scan	-	-	12.5%	10.5%
Combination Brain/Sinus CT Scan	-	-	2%	2.7%
Combination Chest CT Scan	-	-	4.5%	2.7%
Follow-up Mammogram/Ultrasound	-	-	8.7%	8.8%
Lumbar Spine MRI for Low Back Pain	-	-	33%	37.2%

Sanford Clear Lake Medical Center

701 Third Avenue South   Phone: 605-874-2141
Clear Lake, SD 57226
Type: Critical Access Hospitals   Emergency Services: Yes
Ownership: Voluntary non-profit - Private

Measure	Cases	This Hosp.	State Avg.	U.S. Avg.
Blood Clot Prevention and Treatment				
Anticoagulation Overlap Therapy[5]	-	-	95%	93%
ICU Venous Thromboembolism Prophylaxis[5]	-	-	91%	92%
Incidence of Potentially Preventable VTE[5]	-	-	5%	10%
UFH with Dosages/Platelet Monitoring[5]	-	-	100%	97%
Venous Thromboembolism Prophylaxis[5]	-	-	80%	85%
Warfarin Therapy Discharge Instructions[5]	-	-	70%	75%
Chest Pain/Possible Heart Attack Care				
Aspirin Given Within 24 Hours of Arrival	-	-	99%	96%
Fibrinolytic Meds Within 30 Min. of Arrival	-	-	69%	58%
Average Time to ECG (minutes)	-	-	5	7
Average Time to Transfer (minutes)	-	-	66	60
Children's Asthma Care				
Received Home Management Plan of Care	-	-	-	88%
Received Reliever Medication	-	-	-	100%
Received Systemic Corticosteroids	-	-	-	100%
Emergency Department				
Admittance Decision Time (minutes)[5]	-	-	41	98
Head CT Results Within 45 Min. of Arrival	-	-	44%	57%
Patients Who Left ER Before Being Seen	-	-	1%	2%
Time from ER Arrival to Admit. (minutes)[5]	-	-	174	274
Time from ER Arrival to Discharge (minutes)	-	-	113	134
Time in ER Before Being Evaluated (minutes)	-	-	18	26
Time to Pain Meds for Fractures (minutes)	-	-	44	57
Heart Attack Care				
Aspirin Given at Discharge[5]	-	-	100%	99%
Fibrinolytic Meds Within 30 Min. of Arrival[5]	-	-	100%	54%
PCI Within 90 Minutes of Arrival[5]	-	-	94%	96%
Statin Prescribed at Discharge[5]	-	-	98%	98%
Heart Failure Care				
ACE Inhibitor or ARB for LVSD[1,3]	-	-	93%	97%
Discharge Instructions Given[1,3]	-	-	90%	94%
Evaluation of LVS Function[1,3]	-	-	97%	99%
Medicare Spending				
Medicare Spending per Patient (ratio)	-	-	0.9	0.98
Pneumonia Care				
Appropriate Initial Antibiotic Given[1,3]	-	-	90%	95%
Blood Culture Timing[3,7]	-	-	95%	98%
Pregnancy and Delivery Care				
Newborn Deliveries Scheduled Early[5]	-	-	7%	6%
Preventive Care				
Immunization for Influenza[5]	-	-	89%	90%

NOTE: Hospital profiles are in alphabetical order by state, then city, then hospital within the city; Rankings exclude hospitals with less than 25 cases except for patient surveys which excludes hospitals with less than 100 cases; (a) 100-299 cases; (1) The number of cases/patients is too few to report; (2) Data submitted were based on a sample of cases/patients; (3) Results are based on a shorter time period than required; (4) Data suppressed by CMS for one or more quarters; (5) Results are not available for this reporting period; (6) Fewer than 100 patients completed the HCAHPS survey; (7) No cases met the criteria for this measure; (8) The lower limit of the confidence interval cannot be calculated if the number of observed infections equals zero; (9) No data are available from the state/territory for this reporting period; (10) The scores shown reflect fewer than 50 completed surveys; (11) There were discrepancies in the data collection process; (12) This measure does not apply to this hospital for this reporting period; (13) Results cannot be calculated for this reporting period; (14) The results for this state are combined with nearby states to protect confidentiality; Please refer to the User's Guide for a full explanation of data.

Measure	Cases	This Hosp.	State Avg.	U.S. Avg.
Immunization for Pneumonia[5]	-	-	89%	92%
Stroke Care				
Anticoagulation Therapy for Atrial Fibrillation[3,7]	-	-	97%	95%
Antithrombotic Therapy Timing[3,7]	-	-	98%	98%
Assessed for Rehabilitation[1,3]	-	-	98%	97%
Discharged on Antithrombotic Therapy[1,3]	-	-	100%	99%
Discharged on Statin Medication[1,3]	-	-	93%	94%
Thrombolytic Therapy Timing[3,7]	-	-	51%	66%
Venous Thromboembolism Prophylaxis[1,3]	-	-	96%	94%
Written Stroke Educational Materials Given[3,7]	-	-	85%	88%
Surgical Care Improvement Project				
Appropriate Beta Blocker Usage[5]	-	-	98%	98%
Appropriate VTP Within 24 Hours[5]	-	-	98%	98%
Controlled Postoperative Blood Glucose[5]	-	-	98%	97%
Perioperative Temperature Management[5]	-	-	99%	100%
Prophylactic Antibiotic Selection[5]	-	-	99%	99%
Prophylactic Antibiotic Selection (Outpatient)	-	-	99%	98%
Prophylactic Antibiotic Stopped[5]	-	-	98%	98%
Prophylactic Antibiotic Timing[5]	-	-	99%	99%
Prophylactic Antibiotic Timing (Outpatient)	-	-	98%	98%
Urinary Catheter Removal[5]	-	-	97%	97%
Survey of Patients' Hospital Experiences				
Area Around Room 'Always' Quiet at Night[10]	<100	82%	72%	61%
Doctors 'Always' Communicated Well[10]	<100	80%	85%	82%
Home Recovery Information Given[10]	<100	80%	87%	85%
Hospital Given 9 or 10 on 10 Point Scale[10]	<100	84%	78%	71%
Meds 'Always' Explained Before Given[10]	<100	85%	69%	64%
Nurses 'Always' Communicated Well[10]	<100	90%	83%	79%
Pain 'Always' Well Controlled[10]	<100	63%	72%	71%
Room and Bathroom 'Always' Clean[10]	<100	92%	79%	73%
Timely Help 'Always' Received[10]	<100	84%	77%	68%
Would Definitely Recommend Hospital[10]	<100	87%	76%	71%
Use of Medical Imaging				
Cardiac Imaging Stress Test before Surgery	-	-	4.4%	5.3%
Combination Abdominal CT Scan	-	-	12.5%	10.5%
Combination Brain/Sinus CT Scan	-	-	2%	2.7%
Combination Chest CT Scan	-	-	4.5%	2.7%
Follow-up Mammogram/Ultrasound	-	-	8.7%	8.8%
Lumbar Spine MRI for Low Back Pain	-	-	33%	37.2%

Custer Regional Hospital

1039 Montgomery Street
Custer, SD 57730
Phone: 605-673-2229
Fax: 605-673-3586
URL: www.rcrh.org/facilities
Type: Critical Access Hospitals
Emergency Services: Yes
Ownership: Voluntary non-profit - Private
Beds: 16

Key Personnel:
Radiology. . . . . Brian R Baxter
Quality Assurance . . . . Nancy Hargens
Infection Control. . . . . Wendy Honomichl
Chief of Medical Staff. . . . . Sarah Schryvers

Measure	Cases	This Hosp.	State Avg.	U.S. Avg.
Blood Clot Prevention and Treatment				
Anticoagulation Overlap Therapy[1]	-	-	95%	93%
ICU Venous Thromboembolism Prophylaxis[7]	-	-	91%	92%
Incidence of Potentially Preventable VTE[7]	-	-	5%	10%
UFH with Dosages/Platelet Monitoring[7]	-	-	100%	97%
Venous Thromboembolism Prophylaxis	102	71%	80%	85%
Warfarin Therapy Discharge Instructions[1]	-	-	70%	75%
Chest Pain/Possible Heart Attack Care				
Aspirin Given Within 24 Hours of Arrival	20	100%	99%	96%
Fibrinolytic Meds Within 30 Min. of Arrival[1,3]	-	-	69%	58%
Average Time to ECG (minutes)	21	3	5	7
Average Time to Transfer (minutes)[3,7]	-	-	66	60
Children's Asthma Care				
Received Home Management Plan of Care	-	-	-	88%
Received Reliever Medication	-	-	-	100%
Received Systemic Corticosteroids	-	-	-	100%
Emergency Department				
Admittance Decision Time (minutes)	95	15	41	98
Head CT Results Within 45 Min. of Arrival[1,3]	-	-	44%	57%
Patients Who Left ER Before Being Seen	2,709	0%	1%	2%
Time from ER Arrival to Admit. (minutes)	148	150	174	274
Time from ER Arrival to Discharge (minutes)	285	95	113	134
Time in ER Before Being Evaluated (minutes)	285	20	18	26
Time to Pain Meds for Fractures (minutes)	28	26	44	57
Heart Attack Care				
Aspirin Given at Discharge[3,7]	-	-	100%	99%
Fibrinolytic Meds Within 30 Min. of Arrival[3,7]	-	-	100%	54%
PCI Within 90 Minutes of Arrival[3,7]	-	-	94%	96%
Statin Prescribed at Discharge[3,7]	-	-	98%	98%
Heart Failure Care				
ACE Inhibitor or ARB for LVSD[3,7]	-	-	93%	97%
Discharge Instructions Given[1,3]	-	-	90%	94%
Evaluation of LVS Function[1,3]	-	-	97%	99%
Medicare Spending				
Medicare Spending per Patient (ratio)	-	-	0.9	0.98
Pneumonia Care				
Appropriate Initial Antibiotic Given[3,7]	-	-	90%	95%
Blood Culture Timing[1,3]	-	-	95%	98%
Pregnancy and Delivery Care				
Newborn Deliveries Scheduled Early[3,7]	-	-	7%	6%
Preventive Care				
Immunization for Influenza	88	81%	89%	90%
Immunization for Pneumonia	127	94%	89%	92%
Stroke Care				
Anticoagulation Therapy for Atrial Fibrillation[3,7]	-	-	97%	95%
Antithrombotic Therapy Timing[1,3]	-	-	98%	98%
Assessed for Rehabilitation[1,3]	-	-	98%	97%
Discharged on Antithrombotic Therapy[1,3]	-	-	100%	99%
Discharged on Statin Medication[1,3]	-	-	93%	94%
Thrombolytic Therapy Timing[3,7]	-	-	51%	66%
Venous Thromboembolism Prophylaxis[1,3]	-	-	96%	94%
Written Stroke Educational Materials Given[3,7]	-	-	85%	88%
Surgical Care Improvement Project				
Appropriate Beta Blocker Usage[5]	-	-	98%	98%
Appropriate VTP Within 24 Hours[5]	-	-	98%	98%
Controlled Postoperative Blood Glucose[5]	-	-	98%	97%
Perioperative Temperature Management[5]	-	-	99%	100%
Prophylactic Antibiotic Selection[5]	-	-	99%	99%
Prophylactic Antibiotic Selection (Outpatient)[5]	-	-	99%	98%
Prophylactic Antibiotic Stopped[5]	-	-	98%	98%
Prophylactic Antibiotic Timing[5]	-	-	99%	99%
Prophylactic Antibiotic Timing (Outpatient)[5]	-	-	98%	98%
Urinary Catheter Removal[5]	-	-	97%	97%
Survey of Patients' Hospital Experiences				
Area Around Room 'Always' Quiet at Night[6]	<100	76%	72%	61%
Doctors 'Always' Communicated Well[6]	<100	87%	85%	82%
Home Recovery Information Given[6]	<100	87%	87%	85%
Hospital Given 9 or 10 on 10 Point Scale[6]	<100	83%	78%	71%
Meds 'Always' Explained Before Given[6]	<100	81%	69%	64%
Nurses 'Always' Communicated Well[6]	<100	81%	83%	79%
Pain 'Always' Well Controlled[6]	<100	69%	72%	71%
Room and Bathroom 'Always' Clean[6]	<100	73%	79%	73%
Timely Help 'Always' Received[6]	<100	74%	77%	68%
Would Definitely Recommend Hospital[6]	<100	80%	76%	71%
Use of Medical Imaging				
Cardiac Imaging Stress Test before Surgery[7]	-	-	4.4%	5.3%
Combination Abdominal CT Scan	107	0.9%	12.5%	10.5%
Combination Brain/Sinus CT Scan[1]	-	-	2%	2.7%
Combination Chest CT Scan[1]	-	-	4.5%	2.7%
Follow-up Mammogram/Ultrasound[7]	-	-	8.7%	8.8%
Lumbar Spine MRI for Low Back Pain[1]	-	-	33%	37.2%

Siouxland Surgery Center

600 Sioux Point Road
Dakota Dunes, SD 57049
Phone: 605-232-3332
URL: www.siouxlandsurg.com
Type: Acute Care Hospitals
Emergency Services: No
Ownership: Proprietary
Beds: 10

Key Personnel:
Cardiology . . . . Ramin Artang
Infection Control. . . . . Bertha Ayi
Pulmonology . . . . Ross N. Bacon
Radiology. . . . . James C. Beeler
Anesthesiology. . . . . John E. Cook
CEO/President. . . . . Greg Miner

Measure	Cases	This Hosp.	State Avg.	U.S. Avg.
Blood Clot Prevention and Treatment				
Anticoagulation Overlap Therapy[7]	-	-	95%	93%
ICU Venous Thromboembolism Prophylaxis[7]	-	-	91%	92%
Incidence of Potentially Preventable VTE[7]	-	-	5%	10%
UFH with Dosages/Platelet Monitoring[7]	-	-	100%	97%
Venous Thromboembolism Prophylaxis	275	100%	80%	85%
Warfarin Therapy Discharge Instructions[7]	-	-	70%	75%
Chest Pain/Possible Heart Attack Care				
Aspirin Given Within 24 Hours of Arrival[5]	-	-	99%	96%
Fibrinolytic Meds Within 30 Min. of Arrival[5]	-	-	69%	58%
Average Time to ECG (minutes)[5]	-	-	5	7
Average Time to Transfer (minutes)[5]	-	-	66	60
Children's Asthma Care				
Received Home Management Plan of Care	-	-	-	88%
Received Reliever Medication	-	-	-	100%
Received Systemic Corticosteroids	-	-	-	100%
Emergency Department				
Admittance Decision Time (minutes)[7]	-	-	41	98
Head CT Results Within 45 Min. of Arrival[5]	-	-	44%	57%
Patients Who Left ER Before Being Seen[5]	-	-	1%	2%
Time from ER Arrival to Admit. (minutes)[7]	-	-	174	274
Time from ER Arrival to Discharge (minutes)[5]	-	-	113	134
Time in ER Before Being Evaluated (minutes)[5]	-	-	18	26
Time to Pain Meds for Fractures (minutes)[5]	-	-	44	57
Heart Attack Care				
Aspirin Given at Discharge[5]	-	-	100%	99%
Fibrinolytic Meds Within 30 Min. of Arrival[5]	-	-	100%	54%
PCI Within 90 Minutes of Arrival[5]	-	-	94%	96%
Statin Prescribed at Discharge[5]	-	-	98%	98%
Heart Failure Care				
ACE Inhibitor or ARB for LVSD[5]	-	-	93%	97%
Discharge Instructions Given[5]	-	-	90%	94%
Evaluation of LVS Function[5]	-	-	97%	99%
Medicare Spending				
Medicare Spending per Patient (ratio)	-	0.88	0.9	0.98
Pneumonia Care				
Appropriate Initial Antibiotic Given[5]	-	-	90%	95%
Blood Culture Timing[5]	-	-	95%	98%
Pregnancy and Delivery Care				
Newborn Deliveries Scheduled Early[7]	-	-	7%	6%
Preventive Care				
Immunization for Influenza	599	90%	89%	90%
Immunization for Pneumonia	580	89%	89%	92%
Stroke Care				
Anticoagulation Therapy for Atrial Fibrillation[5]	-	-	97%	95%
Antithrombotic Therapy Timing[5]	-	-	98%	98%
Assessed for Rehabilitation[5]	-	-	98%	97%
Discharged on Antithrombotic Therapy[5]	-	-	100%	99%
Discharged on Statin Medication[5]	-	-	93%	94%
Thrombolytic Therapy Timing[5]	-	-	51%	66%
Venous Thromboembolism Prophylaxis[5]	-	-	96%	94%
Written Stroke Educational Materials Given[5]	-	-	85%	88%
Surgical Care Improvement Project				
Appropriate Beta Blocker Usage	194	95%	98%	98%
Appropriate VTP Within 24 Hours	689	100%	98%	98%
Controlled Postoperative Blood Glucose[7]	-	-	98%	97%
Perioperative Temperature Management	712	99%	99%	100%
Prophylactic Antibiotic Selection	625	100%	99%	99%
Prophylactic Antibiotic Selection (Outpatient)	302	98%	99%	98%
Prophylactic Antibiotic Stopped	616	99%	98%	98%
Prophylactic Antibiotic Timing	626	99%	99%	99%
Prophylactic Antibiotic Timing (Outpatient)	304	99%	98%	98%
Urinary Catheter Removal	18	94%	97%	97%
Survey of Patients' Hospital Experiences				
Area Around Room 'Always' Quiet at Night	300+	88%	72%	61%
Doctors 'Always' Communicated Well	300+	85%	85%	82%
Home Recovery Information Given	300+	91%	87%	85%
Hospital Given 9 or 10 on 10 Point Scale	300+	89%	78%	71%
Meds 'Always' Explained Before Given	300+	72%	69%	64%
Nurses 'Always' Communicated Well	300+	88%	83%	79%
Pain 'Always' Well Controlled	300+	76%	72%	71%

NOTE: Hospital profiles are in alphabetical order by state, then city, then hospital within the city; Rankings exclude hospitals with less than 25 cases except for patient surveys which excludes hospitals with less than 100 cases; (a) 100-299 cases; (1) The number of cases/patients is too few to report; (2) Data submitted were based on a sample of cases/patients; (3) Results are based on a shorter time period than required; (4) Data suppressed by CMS for one or more quarters; (5) Results are not available for this reporting period; (6) Fewer than 100 patients completed the HCAHPS survey; (7) No cases met the criteria for this measure; (8) The lower limit of the confidence interval cannot be calculated if the number of observed infections equals zero; (9) No data are available from the state/territory for this reporting period; (10) The scores shown reflect fewer than 50 completed surveys; (11) There were discrepancies in the data collection process; (12) This measure does not apply to this hospital for this reporting period; (13) Results cannot be calculated for this reporting period; (14) The results for this state are combined with nearby states to protect confidentiality; Please refer to the User's Guide for a full explanation of data.

Measure	Cases	This Hosp.	State Avg.	U.S. Avg.
Room and Bathroom 'Always' Clean	300+	87%	79%	73%
Timely Help 'Always' Received	300+	90%	77%	68%
Would Definitely Recommend Hospital	300+	89%	76%	71%
Use of Medical Imaging				
Cardiac Imaging Stress Test before Surgery[7]	-	-	4.4%	5.3%
Combination Abdominal CT Scan[1]	-	-	12.5%	10.5%
Combination Brain/Sinus CT Scan[1]	-	-	2%	2.7%
Combination Chest CT Scan[1]	-	-	4.5%	2.7%
Follow-up Mammogram/Ultrasound[7]	-	-	8.7%	8.8%
Lumbar Spine MRI for Low Back Pain[1]	-	-	33%	37.2%

Avera Desmet Memorial Hospital

306 Prairie Avenue Sw, PO Box 160
De Smet, SD 57231
Phone: 605-854-3329
Fax: 605-854-3161
E-mail: info@desmetmemorial.org
URL: www.desmetmemorial.org
Type: Critical Access Hospitals
Emergency Services: Yes
Ownership: Voluntary non-profit - Private
Beds: 17
Key Personnel:
Chief of Medical Staff. . . . . John A Berg

Measure	Cases	This Hosp.	State Avg.	U.S. Avg.
Blood Clot Prevention and Treatment				
Anticoagulation Overlap Therapy[5]	-	-	95%	93%
ICU Venous Thromboembolism Prophylaxis[5]	-	-	91%	92%
Incidence of Potentially Preventable VTE[5]	-	-	5%	10%
UFH with Dosages/Platelet Monitoring[5]	-	-	100%	97%
Venous Thromboembolism Prophylaxis[5]	-	-	80%	85%
Warfarin Therapy Discharge Instructions[5]	-	-	70%	75%
Chest Pain/Possible Heart Attack Care				
Aspirin Given Within 24 Hours of Arrival	-	-	99%	96%
Fibrinolytic Meds Within 30 Min. of Arrival	-	-	69%	58%
Average Time to ECG (minutes)	-	-	5	7
Average Time to Transfer (minutes)	-	-	66	60
Children's Asthma Care				
Received Home Management Plan of Care	-	-	-	88%
Received Reliever Medication	-	-	-	100%
Received Systemic Corticosteroids	-	-	-	100%
Emergency Department				
Admittance Decision Time (minutes)[5]	-	-	41	98
Head CT Results Within 45 Min. of Arrival	-	-	44%	57%
Patients Who Left ER Before Being Seen	-	-	1%	2%
Time from ER Arrival to Admit. (minutes)[5]	-	-	174	274
Time from ER Arrival to Discharge (minutes)	-	-	113	134
Time in ER Before Being Evaluated (minutes)	-	-	18	26
Time to Pain Meds for Fractures (minutes)	-	-	44	57
Heart Attack Care				
Aspirin Given at Discharge[5]	-	-	100%	99%
Fibrinolytic Meds Within 30 Min. of Arrival[5]	-	-	100%	54%
PCI Within 90 Minutes of Arrival[5]	-	-	94%	96%
Statin Prescribed at Discharge[5]	-	-	98%	98%
Heart Failure Care				
ACE Inhibitor or ARB for LVSD[1,3]	-	-	93%	97%
Discharge Instructions Given[1,3]	-	-	90%	94%
Evaluation of LVS Function[1,3]	-	-	97%	99%
Medicare Spending				
Medicare Spending per Patient (ratio)	-	-	0.9	0.98
Pneumonia Care				
Appropriate Initial Antibiotic Given[1,3]	-	-	90%	95%
Blood Culture Timing[3,7]	-	-	95%	98%
Pregnancy and Delivery Care				
Newborn Deliveries Scheduled Early[5]	-	-	7%	6%
Preventive Care				
Immunization for Influenza[5]	-	-	89%	90%
Immunization for Pneumonia[5]	-	-	89%	92%
Stroke Care				
Anticoagulation Therapy for Atrial Fibrillation[5]	-	-	97%	95%
Antithrombotic Therapy Timing[5]	-	-	98%	98%
Assessed for Rehabilitation[5]	-	-	98%	97%
Discharged on Antithrombotic Therapy[5]	-	-	100%	99%
Discharged on Statin Medication[5]	-	-	93%	94%
Thrombolytic Therapy Timing[5]	-	-	51%	66%
Venous Thromboembolism Prophylaxis[5]	-	-	96%	94%
Written Stroke Educational Materials Given[5]	-	-	85%	88%
Surgical Care Improvement Project				
Appropriate Beta Blocker Usage[5]	-	-	98%	98%
Appropriate VTP Within 24 Hours[5]	-	-	98%	98%
Controlled Postoperative Blood Glucose[5]	-	-	98%	97%
Perioperative Temperature Management[5]	-	-	99%	100%
Prophylactic Antibiotic Selection[5]	-	-	99%	99%
Prophylactic Antibiotic Selection (Outpatient)	-	-	99%	98%
Prophylactic Antibiotic Stopped[5]	-	-	98%	98%
Prophylactic Antibiotic Timing[5]	-	-	99%	99%
Prophylactic Antibiotic Timing (Outpatient)	-	-	98%	98%
Urinary Catheter Removal[5]	-	-	97%	97%
Survey of Patients' Hospital Experiences				
Area Around Room 'Always' Quiet at Night[10]	<100	77%	72%	61%
Doctors 'Always' Communicated Well[10]	<100	81%	85%	82%
Home Recovery Information Given[10]	<100	83%	87%	85%
Hospital Given 9 or 10 on 10 Point Scale[10]	<100	67%	78%	71%
Meds 'Always' Explained Before Given[10]	<100	67%	69%	64%
Nurses 'Always' Communicated Well[10]	<100	74%	83%	79%
Pain 'Always' Well Controlled[10]	<100	56%	72%	71%
Room and Bathroom 'Always' Clean[10]	<100	76%	79%	73%
Timely Help 'Always' Received[10]	<100	65%	77%	68%
Would Definitely Recommend Hospital[10]	<100	76%	76%	71%
Use of Medical Imaging				
Cardiac Imaging Stress Test before Surgery	-	-	4.4%	5.3%
Combination Abdominal CT Scan	-	-	12.5%	10.5%
Combination Brain/Sinus CT Scan	-	-	2%	2.7%
Combination Chest CT Scan	-	-	4.5%	2.7%
Follow-up Mammogram/Ultrasound	-	-	8.7%	8.8%
Lumbar Spine MRI for Low Back Pain	-	-	33%	37.2%

Lead - Deadwood Regional Hospital

61 Charles Street
Deadwood, SD 57732
Phone: 605-722-6101
Fax: 605-719-6163
Type: Critical Access Hospitals
Emergency Services: Yes
Ownership: Voluntary non-profit - Private
Beds: 18
Key Personnel:
Infection Control. . . . . Joanne Baer, RN
Quality Assurance . . . . Joanne Baer, RN
CEO/President. . . . . Charles E. Hart, M.D., M.S.
Chief of Medical Staff. . . . . James J Holloway, MD
Operating Room. . . . . Karen Schleenaut, MD

Measure	Cases	This Hosp.	State Avg.	U.S. Avg.
Blood Clot Prevention and Treatment				
Anticoagulation Overlap Therapy[5]	-	-	95%	93%
ICU Venous Thromboembolism Prophylaxis[5]	-	-	91%	92%
Incidence of Potentially Preventable VTE[5]	-	-	5%	10%
UFH with Dosages/Platelet Monitoring[5]	-	-	100%	97%
Venous Thromboembolism Prophylaxis[5]	-	-	80%	85%
Warfarin Therapy Discharge Instructions[5]	-	-	70%	75%
Chest Pain/Possible Heart Attack Care				
Aspirin Given Within 24 Hours of Arrival[1,3]	-	-	99%	96%
Fibrinolytic Meds Within 30 Min. of Arrival[3,7]	-	-	69%	58%
Average Time to ECG (minutes)[1,3]	-	-	5	7
Average Time to Transfer (minutes)[3,7]	-	-	66	60
Children's Asthma Care				
Received Home Management Plan of Care	-	-	-	88%
Received Reliever Medication	-	-	-	100%
Received Systemic Corticosteroids	-	-	-	100%
Emergency Department				
Admittance Decision Time (minutes)[1,3]	-	-	41	98
Head CT Results Within 45 Min. of Arrival[3,7]	-	-	44%	57%
Patients Who Left ER Before Being Seen[5]	-	-	1%	2%
Time from ER Arrival to Admit. (minutes)[1,3]	-	-	174	274
Time from ER Arrival to Discharge (minutes)[3]	59	83	113	134
Time in ER Before Being Evaluated (minutes)[3]	61	0	18	26
Time to Pain Meds for Fractures (minutes)[3]	23	19	44	57
Heart Attack Care				
Aspirin Given at Discharge[5]	-	-	100%	99%
Fibrinolytic Meds Within 30 Min. of Arrival[5]	-	-	100%	54%
PCI Within 90 Minutes of Arrival[5]	-	-	94%	96%
Statin Prescribed at Discharge[5]	-	-	98%	98%
Heart Failure Care				
ACE Inhibitor or ARB for LVSD[3,7]	-	-	93%	97%
Discharge Instructions Given[1,3]	-	-	90%	94%
Evaluation of LVS Function[1,3]	-	-	97%	99%
Medicare Spending				
Medicare Spending per Patient (ratio)	-	-	0.9	0.98
Pneumonia Care				
Appropriate Initial Antibiotic Given[1,3]	-	-	90%	95%
Blood Culture Timing[1,3]	-	-	95%	98%
Pregnancy and Delivery Care				
Newborn Deliveries Scheduled Early[5]	-	-	7%	6%
Preventive Care				
Immunization for Influenza[5]	-	-	89%	90%
Immunization for Pneumonia[3,7]	-	-	89%	92%
Stroke Care				
Anticoagulation Therapy for Atrial Fibrillation[5]	-	-	97%	95%
Antithrombotic Therapy Timing[5]	-	-	98%	98%
Assessed for Rehabilitation[5]	-	-	98%	97%
Discharged on Antithrombotic Therapy[5]	-	-	100%	99%
Discharged on Statin Medication[5]	-	-	93%	94%
Thrombolytic Therapy Timing[5]	-	-	51%	66%
Venous Thromboembolism Prophylaxis[5]	-	-	96%	94%
Written Stroke Educational Materials Given[5]	-	-	85%	88%
Surgical Care Improvement Project				
Appropriate Beta Blocker Usage[5]	-	-	98%	98%
Appropriate VTP Within 24 Hours[5]	-	-	98%	98%
Controlled Postoperative Blood Glucose[5]	-	-	98%	97%
Perioperative Temperature Management[5]	-	-	99%	100%
Prophylactic Antibiotic Selection[5]	-	-	99%	99%
Prophylactic Antibiotic Selection (Outpatient)[5]	-	-	99%	98%
Prophylactic Antibiotic Stopped[5]	-	-	98%	98%
Prophylactic Antibiotic Timing[5]	-	-	99%	99%
Prophylactic Antibiotic Timing (Outpatient)[5]	-	-	98%	98%
Urinary Catheter Removal[5]	-	-	97%	97%
Survey of Patients' Hospital Experiences				
Area Around Room 'Always' Quiet at Night[6]	<100	70%	72%	61%
Doctors 'Always' Communicated Well[6]	<100	91%	85%	82%
Home Recovery Information Given[6]	<100	87%	87%	85%
Hospital Given 9 or 10 on 10 Point Scale[6]	<100	77%	78%	71%
Meds 'Always' Explained Before Given[6]	<100	71%	69%	64%
Nurses 'Always' Communicated Well[6]	<100	79%	83%	79%
Pain 'Always' Well Controlled[6]	<100	61%	72%	71%
Room and Bathroom 'Always' Clean[6]	<100	91%	79%	73%
Timely Help 'Always' Received[6]	<100	78%	77%	68%
Would Definitely Recommend Hospital[6]	<100	79%	76%	71%
Use of Medical Imaging				
Cardiac Imaging Stress Test before Surgery[1]	-	-	4.4%	5.3%
Combination Abdominal CT Scan	58	1.7%	12.5%	10.5%
Combination Brain/Sinus CT Scan[1]	-	-	2%	2.7%
Combination Chest CT Scan[1]	-	-	4.5%	2.7%
Follow-up Mammogram/Ultrasound	185	8.6%	8.7%	8.8%
Lumbar Spine MRI for Low Back Pain[1]	-	-	33%	37.2%

Avera Dells Area Hospital

909 N Iowa Ave
Dell Rapids, SD 57022
Phone: 605-428-5431
Fax: 605-428-3906
URL: www.avera.org/avera/facilities
Type: Critical Access Hospitals
Emergency Services: Yes
Ownership: Voluntary non-profit - Private
Beds: 21
Key Personnel:
Chief of Medical Staff. . . . . Shawn Culey, MD
CEO/President. . . . . James A Faulwell
Radiology. . . . . Daryl C Rife

Measure	Cases	This Hosp.	State Avg.	U.S. Avg.
Blood Clot Prevention and Treatment				
Anticoagulation Overlap Therapy[5]	-	-	95%	93%
ICU Venous Thromboembolism Prophylaxis[5]	-	-	91%	92%
Incidence of Potentially Preventable VTE[5]	-	-	5%	10%
UFH with Dosages/Platelet Monitoring[5]	-	-	100%	97%
Venous Thromboembolism Prophylaxis[5]	-	-	80%	85%
Warfarin Therapy Discharge Instructions[5]	-	-	70%	75%
Chest Pain/Possible Heart Attack Care				
Aspirin Given Within 24 Hours of Arrival	-	-	99%	96%
Fibrinolytic Meds Within 30 Min. of Arrival	-	-	69%	58%
Average Time to ECG (minutes)	-	-	5	7

NOTE: Hospital profiles are in alphabetical order by state, then city, then hospital within the city; Rankings exclude hospitals with less than 25 cases except for patient surveys which excludes hospitals with less than 100 cases; (a) 100-299 cases; (1) The number of cases/patients is too few to report; (2) Data submitted were based on a sample of cases/patients; (3) Results are based on a shorter time period than required; (4) Data suppressed by CMS for one or more quarters; (5) Results are not available for this reporting period; (6) Fewer than 100 patients completed the HCAHPS survey; (7) No cases met the criteria for this measure; (8) The lower limit of the confidence interval cannot be calculated if the number of observed infections equals zero; (9) No data are available from the state/territory for this reporting period; (10) The scores shown reflect fewer than 50 completed surveys; (11) There were discrepancies in the data collection process; (12) This measure does not apply to this hospital for this reporting period; (13) Results cannot be calculated for this reporting period; (14) The results for this state are combined with nearby states to protect confidentiality; Please refer to the User's Guide for a full explanation of data.

Measure	Cases	This Hosp.	State Avg.	U.S. Avg.
Average Time to Transfer (minutes)	-	-	66	60
Children's Asthma Care				
Received Home Management Plan of Care	-	-	-	88%
Received Reliever Medication	-	-	-	100%
Received Systemic Corticosteroids	-	-	-	100%
Emergency Department				
Admittance Decision Time (minutes)[5]	-	-	41	98
Head CT Results Within 45 Min. of Arrival	-	-	44%	57%
Patients Who Left ER Before Being Seen	-	-	1%	2%
Time from ER Arrival to Admit. (minutes)[5]	-	-	174	274
Time from ER Arrival to Discharge (minutes)	-	-	113	134
Time in ER Before Being Evaluated (minutes)	-	-	18	26
Time to Pain Meds for Fractures (minutes)	-	-	44	57
Heart Attack Care				
Aspirin Given at Discharge[3,7]	-	-	100%	99%
Fibrinolytic Meds Within 30 Min. of Arrival[3,7]	-	-	100%	54%
PCI Within 90 Minutes of Arrival[3,7]	-	-	94%	96%
Statin Prescribed at Discharge[3,7]	-	-	98%	98%
Heart Failure Care				
ACE Inhibitor or ARB for LVSD[1]	-	-	93%	97%
Discharge Instructions Given[1]	-	-	90%	94%
Evaluation of LVS Function[1]	-	-	97%	99%
Medicare Spending				
Medicare Spending per Patient (ratio)	-	-	0.9	0.98
Pneumonia Care				
Appropriate Initial Antibiotic Given[1]	-	-	90%	95%
Blood Culture Timing[7]	-	-	95%	98%
Pregnancy and Delivery Care				
Newborn Deliveries Scheduled Early[5]	-	-	7%	6%
Preventive Care				
Immunization for Influenza[5]	-	-	89%	90%
Immunization for Pneumonia[5]	-	-	89%	92%
Stroke Care				
Anticoagulation Therapy for Atrial Fibrillation[5]	-	-	97%	95%
Antithrombotic Therapy Timing[5]	-	-	98%	98%
Assessed for Rehabilitation[5]	-	-	98%	97%
Discharged on Antithrombotic Therapy[5]	-	-	100%	99%
Discharged on Statin Medication[5]	-	-	93%	94%
Thrombolytic Therapy Timing[5]	-	-	51%	66%
Venous Thromboembolism Prophylaxis[5]	-	-	96%	94%
Written Stroke Educational Materials Given[5]	-	-	85%	88%
Surgical Care Improvement Project				
Appropriate Beta Blocker Usage[5]	-	-	98%	98%
Appropriate VTP Within 24 Hours[5]	-	-	98%	98%
Controlled Postoperative Blood Glucose[5]	-	-	98%	97%
Perioperative Temperature Management[5]	-	-	99%	100%
Prophylactic Antibiotic Selection[5]	-	-	99%	99%
Prophylactic Antibiotic Selection (Outpatient)	-	-	99%	98%
Prophylactic Antibiotic Stopped[5]	-	-	98%	98%
Prophylactic Antibiotic Timing[5]	-	-	99%	99%
Prophylactic Antibiotic Timing (Outpatient)	-	-	98%	98%
Urinary Catheter Removal[5]	-	-	97%	97%
Survey of Patients' Hospital Experiences				
Area Around Room 'Always' Quiet at Night[10]	<100	54%	72%	61%
Doctors 'Always' Communicated Well[10]	<100	81%	85%	82%
Home Recovery Information Given[10]	<100	85%	87%	85%
Hospital Given 9 or 10 on 10 Point Scale[10]	<100	79%	78%	71%
Meds 'Always' Explained Before Given[10]	<100	62%	69%	64%
Nurses 'Always' Communicated Well[10]	<100	78%	83%	79%
Pain 'Always' Well Controlled[10]	<100	60%	72%	71%
Room and Bathroom 'Always' Clean[10]	<100	90%	79%	73%
Timely Help 'Always' Received[10]	<100	75%	77%	68%
Would Definitely Recommend Hospital[10]	<100	86%	76%	71%
Use of Medical Imaging				
Cardiac Imaging Stress Test before Surgery	-	-	4.4%	5.3%
Combination Abdominal CT Scan	-	-	12.5%	10.5%
Combination Brain/Sinus CT Scan	-	-	2%	2.7%
Combination Chest CT Scan	-	-	4.5%	2.7%
Follow-up Mammogram/Ultrasound	-	-	8.7%	8.8%
Lumbar Spine MRI for Low Back Pain	-	-	33%	37.2%

PHS Indian Hospital at Eagle Butte

317 Main Street
Eagle Butte, SD 57625
URL: www.ihs.gov
Type: Acute Care Hospitals
Ownership: Government - Federal
Phone: 605-964-3005
Fax: 605-964-1169
Emergency Services: Yes
Beds: 27

Key Personnel:
Quality Assurance . . . . Cyndi Halfred
Chief of Medical Staff . . . . Margaret Upell
Infection Control . . . . Margaret Zephier, RN

Measure	Cases	This Hosp.	State Avg.	U.S. Avg.
Blood Clot Prevention and Treatment				
Anticoagulation Overlap Therapy[2,7]	-	-	95%	93%
ICU Venous Thromboembolism Prophylaxis[2,7]	-	-	91%	92%
Incidence of Potentially Preventable VTE[2,7]	-	-	5%	10%
UFH with Dosages/Platelet Monitoring[2,7]	-	-	100%	97%
Venous Thromboembolism Prophylaxis[2]	82	40%	80%	85%
Warfarin Therapy Discharge Instructions[2,7]	-	-	70%	75%
Chest Pain/Possible Heart Attack Care				
Aspirin Given Within 24 Hours of Arrival	-	-	99%	96%
Fibrinolytic Meds Within 30 Min. of Arrival	-	-	69%	58%
Average Time to ECG (minutes)	-	-	5	7
Average Time to Transfer (minutes)	-	-	66	60
Children's Asthma Care				
Received Home Management Plan of Care	-	-	-	88%
Received Reliever Medication	-	-	-	100%
Received Systemic Corticosteroids	-	-	-	100%
Emergency Department				
Admittance Decision Time (minutes)[2]	167	40	41	98
Head CT Results Within 45 Min. of Arrival	-	-	44%	57%
Patients Who Left ER Before Being Seen	-	-	1%	2%
Time from ER Arrival to Admit. (minutes)[2]	167	236	174	274
Time from ER Arrival to Discharge (minutes)	-	-	113	134
Time in ER Before Being Evaluated (minutes)	-	-	18	26
Time to Pain Meds for Fractures (minutes)	-	-	44	57
Heart Attack Care				
Aspirin Given at Discharge[5]	-	-	100%	99%
Fibrinolytic Meds Within 30 Min. of Arrival[5]	-	-	100%	54%
PCI Within 90 Minutes of Arrival[5]	-	-	94%	96%
Statin Prescribed at Discharge[5]	-	-	98%	98%
Heart Failure Care				
ACE Inhibitor or ARB for LVSD[5]	-	-	93%	97%
Discharge Instructions Given[5]	-	-	90%	94%
Evaluation of LVS Function[5]	-	-	97%	99%
Medicare Spending				
Medicare Spending per Patient (ratio)[1]	-	-	0.9	0.98
Pneumonia Care				
Appropriate Initial Antibiotic Given[1,2]	-	-	90%	95%
Blood Culture Timing[1,2]	-	-	95%	98%
Pregnancy and Delivery Care				
Newborn Deliveries Scheduled Early[2,7]	-	-	7%	6%
Preventive Care				
Immunization for Influenza[2]	74	38%	89%	90%
Immunization for Pneumonia[2]	86	88%	89%	92%
Stroke Care				
Anticoagulation Therapy for Atrial Fibrillation[5]	-	-	97%	95%
Antithrombotic Therapy Timing[5]	-	-	98%	98%
Assessed for Rehabilitation[5]	-	-	98%	97%
Discharged on Antithrombotic Therapy[5]	-	-	100%	99%
Discharged on Statin Medication[5]	-	-	93%	94%
Thrombolytic Therapy Timing[5]	-	-	51%	66%
Venous Thromboembolism Prophylaxis[5]	-	-	96%	94%
Written Stroke Educational Materials Given[5]	-	-	85%	88%
Surgical Care Improvement Project				
Appropriate Beta Blocker Usage[5]	-	-	98%	98%
Appropriate VTP Within 24 Hours[5]	-	-	98%	98%
Controlled Postoperative Blood Glucose[5]	-	-	98%	97%
Perioperative Temperature Management[5]	-	-	99%	100%
Prophylactic Antibiotic Selection[5]	-	-	99%	99%
Prophylactic Antibiotic Selection (Outpatient)	-	-	99%	98%
Prophylactic Antibiotic Stopped[5]	-	-	98%	98%
Prophylactic Antibiotic Timing[5]	-	-	99%	99%
Prophylactic Antibiotic Timing (Outpatient)	-	-	98%	98%
Urinary Catheter Removal[5]	-	-	97%	97%
Survey of Patients' Hospital Experiences				
Area Around Room 'Always' Quiet at Night[10,11]	<100	76%	72%	61%
Doctors 'Always' Communicated Well[10,11]	<100	78%	85%	82%
Home Recovery Information Given[10,11]	<100	81%	87%	85%
Hospital Given 9 or 10 on 10 Point Scale[10,11]	<100	62%	78%	71%
Meds 'Always' Explained Before Given[10,11]	<100	55%	69%	64%
Nurses 'Always' Communicated Well[10,11]	<100	81%	83%	79%
Pain 'Always' Well Controlled[10,11]	<100	68%	72%	71%
Room and Bathroom 'Always' Clean[10,11]	<100	77%	79%	73%
Timely Help 'Always' Received[10,11]	<100	91%	77%	68%
Would Definitely Recommend Hospital[10,11]	<100	33%	76%	71%
Use of Medical Imaging				
Cardiac Imaging Stress Test before Surgery	-	-	4.4%	5.3%
Combination Abdominal CT Scan	-	-	12.5%	10.5%
Combination Brain/Sinus CT Scan	-	-	2%	2.7%
Combination Chest CT Scan	-	-	4.5%	2.7%
Follow-up Mammogram/Ultrasound	-	-	8.7%	8.8%
Lumbar Spine MRI for Low Back Pain	-	-	33%	37.2%

Eureka Community Health Services

410 9th Saint PO Box 517
Eureka, SD 57437
Type: Critical Access Hospitals
Ownership: Government - Local
Phone: 605-284-2661
Emergency Services: Yes

Measure	Cases	This Hosp.	State Avg.	U.S. Avg.
Blood Clot Prevention and Treatment				
Anticoagulation Overlap Therapy[5]	-	-	95%	93%
ICU Venous Thromboembolism Prophylaxis[5]	-	-	91%	92%
Incidence of Potentially Preventable VTE[5]	-	-	5%	10%
UFH with Dosages/Platelet Monitoring[5]	-	-	100%	97%
Venous Thromboembolism Prophylaxis[5]	-	-	80%	85%
Warfarin Therapy Discharge Instructions[5]	-	-	70%	75%
Chest Pain/Possible Heart Attack Care				
Aspirin Given Within 24 Hours of Arrival	-	-	99%	96%
Fibrinolytic Meds Within 30 Min. of Arrival	-	-	69%	58%
Average Time to ECG (minutes)	-	-	5	7
Average Time to Transfer (minutes)	-	-	66	60
Children's Asthma Care				
Received Home Management Plan of Care	-	-	-	88%
Received Reliever Medication	-	-	-	100%
Received Systemic Corticosteroids	-	-	-	100%
Emergency Department				
Admittance Decision Time (minutes)[5]	-	-	41	98
Head CT Results Within 45 Min. of Arrival	-	-	44%	57%
Patients Who Left ER Before Being Seen	-	-	1%	2%
Time from ER Arrival to Admit. (minutes)[5]	-	-	174	274
Time from ER Arrival to Discharge (minutes)	-	-	113	134
Time in ER Before Being Evaluated (minutes)	-	-	18	26
Time to Pain Meds for Fractures (minutes)	-	-	44	57
Heart Attack Care				
Aspirin Given at Discharge[5]	-	-	100%	99%
Fibrinolytic Meds Within 30 Min. of Arrival[5]	-	-	100%	54%
PCI Within 90 Minutes of Arrival[5]	-	-	94%	96%
Statin Prescribed at Discharge[5]	-	-	98%	98%
Heart Failure Care				
ACE Inhibitor or ARB for LVSD[5]	-	-	93%	97%
Discharge Instructions Given[5]	-	-	90%	94%
Evaluation of LVS Function[5]	-	-	97%	99%
Medicare Spending				
Medicare Spending per Patient (ratio)	-	-	0.9	0.98
Pneumonia Care				
Appropriate Initial Antibiotic Given[5]	-	-	90%	95%
Blood Culture Timing[5]	-	-	95%	98%
Pregnancy and Delivery Care				
Newborn Deliveries Scheduled Early[5]	-	-	7%	6%
Preventive Care				
Immunization for Influenza[5]	-	-	89%	90%
Immunization for Pneumonia[5]	-	-	89%	92%
Stroke Care				
Anticoagulation Therapy for Atrial Fibrillation[5]	-	-	97%	95%
Antithrombotic Therapy Timing[5]	-	-	98%	98%

NOTE: Hospital profiles are in alphabetical order by state, then city, then hospital within the city; Rankings exclude hospitals with less than 25 cases except for patient surveys which excludes hospitals with less than 100 cases; (a) 100-299 cases; (1) The number of cases/patients is too few to report; (2) Data submitted were based on a sample of cases/patients; (3) Results are based on a shorter time period than required; (4) Data suppressed by CMS for one or more quarters; (5) Results are not available for this reporting period; (6) Fewer than 100 patients completed the HCAHPS survey; (7) No cases met the criteria for this measure; (8) The lower limit of the confidence interval cannot be calculated if the number of observed infections equals zero; (9) No data are available from the state/territory for this reporting period; (10) The scores shown reflect fewer than 50 completed surveys; (11) There were discrepancies in the data collection process; (12) This measure does not apply to this hospital for this reporting period; (13) Results cannot be calculated for this reporting period; (14) The results for this state are combined with nearby states to protect confidentiality; Please refer to the User's Guide for a full explanation of data.

Measure	Cases	This Hosp.	State Avg.	U.S. Avg.
Assessed for Rehabilitation[5]	-	-	98%	97%
Discharged on Antithrombotic Therapy[5]	-	-	100%	99%
Discharged on Statin Medication[5]	-	-	93%	94%
Thrombolytic Therapy Timing[5]	-	-	51%	66%
Venous Thromboembolism Prophylaxis[5]	-	-	96%	94%
Written Stroke Educational Materials Given[5]	-	-	85%	88%
Surgical Care Improvement Project				
Appropriate Beta Blocker Usage[5]	-	-	98%	98%
Appropriate VTP Within 24 Hours[5]	-	-	98%	98%
Controlled Postoperative Blood Glucose[5]	-	-	98%	97%
Perioperative Temperature Management[5]	-	-	99%	100%
Prophylactic Antibiotic Selection[5]	-	-	99%	99%
Prophylactic Antibiotic Selection (Outpatient)	-	-	99%	98%
Prophylactic Antibiotic Stopped[5]	-	-	98%	98%
Prophylactic Antibiotic Timing[5]	-	-	99%	99%
Prophylactic Antibiotic Timing (Outpatient)	-	-	98%	98%
Urinary Catheter Removal[5]	-	-	97%	97%
Survey of Patients' Hospital Experiences				
Area Around Room 'Always' Quiet at Night[10]	<100	69%	72%	61%
Doctors 'Always' Communicated Well[10]	<100	93%	85%	82%
Home Recovery Information Given[10]	<100	90%	87%	85%
Hospital Given 9 or 10 on 10 Point Scale[10]	<100	64%	78%	71%
Meds 'Always' Explained Before Given[10]	<100	50%	69%	64%
Nurses 'Always' Communicated Well[10]	<100	78%	83%	79%
Pain 'Always' Well Controlled[10]	<100	59%	72%	71%
Room and Bathroom 'Always' Clean[10]	<100	82%	79%	73%
Timely Help 'Always' Received[10]	<100	73%	77%	68%
Would Definitely Recommend Hospital[10]	<100	83%	76%	71%
Use of Medical Imaging				
Cardiac Imaging Stress Test before Surgery	-	-	4.4%	5.3%
Combination Abdominal CT Scan	-	-	12.5%	10.5%
Combination Brain/Sinus CT Scan	-	-	2%	2.7%
Combination Chest CT Scan	-	-	4.5%	2.7%
Follow-up Mammogram/Ultrasound	-	-	8.7%	8.8%
Lumbar Spine MRI for Low Back Pain	-	-	33%	37.2%

Avera Flandreau Hospital

214 North Prairie Avenue
Flandreau, SD 57028
URL: www.flandreaumedical.org
Phone: 605-997-2433
Fax: 605-997-3611
Type: Critical Access Hospitals
Ownership: Voluntary non-profit - Private
Emergency Services: Yes
Beds: 18

Key Personnel:
Chief of Medical Staff.......... Gary Bruning, DO
CEO .... Amanda Goostree
Patient Relations .... Marie Myers, RN

Measure	Cases	This Hosp.	State Avg.	U.S. Avg.
Blood Clot Prevention and Treatment				
Anticoagulation Overlap Therapy[5]	-	-	95%	93%
ICU Venous Thromboembolism Prophylaxis[5]	-	-	91%	92%
Incidence of Potentially Preventable VTE[5]	-	-	5%	10%
UFH with Dosages/Platelet Monitoring[5]	-	-	100%	97%
Venous Thromboembolism Prophylaxis[5]	-	-	80%	85%
Warfarin Therapy Discharge Instructions[5]	-	-	70%	75%
Chest Pain/Possible Heart Attack Care				
Aspirin Given Within 24 Hours of Arrival	-	-	99%	96%
Fibrinolytic Meds Within 30 Min. of Arrival	-	-	69%	58%
Average Time to ECG (minutes)	-	-	5	7
Average Time to Transfer (minutes)	-	-	66	60
Children's Asthma Care				
Received Home Management Plan of Care	-	-	-	88%
Received Reliever Medication	-	-	-	100%
Received Systemic Corticosteroids	-	-	-	100%
Emergency Department				
Admittance Decision Time (minutes)[5]	-	-	41	98
Head CT Results Within 45 Min. of Arrival	-	-	44%	57%
Patients Who Left ER Before Being Seen	-	-	1%	2%
Time from ER Arrival to Admit. (minutes)[5]	-	-	174	274
Time from ER Arrival to Discharge (minutes)	-	-	113	134
Time in ER Before Being Evaluated (minutes)	-	-	18	26
Time to Pain Meds for Fractures (minutes)	-	-	44	57
Heart Attack Care				
Aspirin Given at Discharge[5]	-	-	100%	99%
Fibrinolytic Meds Within 30 Min. of Arrival[5]	-	-	100%	54%
PCI Within 90 Minutes of Arrival[5]	-	-	94%	96%
Statin Prescribed at Discharge[5]	-	-	98%	98%
Heart Failure Care				
ACE Inhibitor or ARB for LVSD[1,3]	-	-	93%	97%
Discharge Instructions Given[1,3]	-	-	90%	94%
Evaluation of LVS Function[1,3]	-	-	97%	99%
Medicare Spending				
Medicare Spending per Patient (ratio)	-	-	0.9	0.98
Pneumonia Care				
Appropriate Initial Antibiotic Given[1,3]	-	-	90%	95%
Blood Culture Timing[3,7]	-	-	95%	98%
Pregnancy and Delivery Care				
Newborn Deliveries Scheduled Early[5]	-	-	7%	6%
Preventive Care				
Immunization for Influenza[5]	-	-	89%	90%
Immunization for Pneumonia[5]	-	-	89%	92%
Stroke Care				
Anticoagulation Therapy for Atrial Fibrillation[5]	-	-	97%	95%
Antithrombotic Therapy Timing[5]	-	-	98%	98%
Assessed for Rehabilitation[5]	-	-	98%	97%
Discharged on Antithrombotic Therapy[5]	-	-	100%	99%
Discharged on Statin Medication[5]	-	-	93%	94%
Thrombolytic Therapy Timing[5]	-	-	51%	66%
Venous Thromboembolism Prophylaxis[5]	-	-	96%	94%
Written Stroke Educational Materials Given[5]	-	-	85%	88%
Surgical Care Improvement Project				
Appropriate Beta Blocker Usage[5]	-	-	98%	98%
Appropriate VTP Within 24 Hours[5]	-	-	98%	98%
Controlled Postoperative Blood Glucose[5]	-	-	98%	97%
Perioperative Temperature Management[5]	-	-	99%	100%
Prophylactic Antibiotic Selection[5]	-	-	99%	99%
Prophylactic Antibiotic Selection (Outpatient)	-	-	99%	98%
Prophylactic Antibiotic Stopped[5]	-	-	98%	98%
Prophylactic Antibiotic Timing[5]	-	-	99%	99%
Prophylactic Antibiotic Timing (Outpatient)	-	-	98%	98%
Urinary Catheter Removal[5]	-	-	97%	97%
Survey of Patients' Hospital Experiences				
Area Around Room 'Always' Quiet at Night[10]	<100	70%	72%	61%
Doctors 'Always' Communicated Well[10]	<100	88%	85%	82%
Home Recovery Information Given[10]	<100	92%	87%	85%
Hospital Given 9 or 10 on 10 Point Scale[10]	<100	76%	78%	71%
Meds 'Always' Explained Before Given[10]	<100	81%	69%	64%
Nurses 'Always' Communicated Well[10]	<100	79%	83%	79%
Pain 'Always' Well Controlled[10]	<100	76%	72%	71%
Room and Bathroom 'Always' Clean[10]	<100	73%	79%	73%
Timely Help 'Always' Received[10]	<100	74%	77%	68%
Would Definitely Recommend Hospital[10]	<100	77%	76%	71%
Use of Medical Imaging				
Cardiac Imaging Stress Test before Surgery	-	-	4.4%	5.3%
Combination Abdominal CT Scan	-	-	12.5%	10.5%
Combination Brain/Sinus CT Scan	-	-	2%	2.7%
Combination Chest CT Scan	-	-	4.5%	2.7%
Follow-up Mammogram/Ultrasound	-	-	8.7%	8.8%
Lumbar Spine MRI for Low Back Pain	-	-	33%	37.2%

VA Black Hills Healthcare System - Fort Meade

113 Comanche Road
Fort Meade, SD 57741
URL: www.va.gov
Phone: 605-347-2511
Fax: 605-720-7171
Type: Acute Care - VA
Ownership: Government Federal
Emergency Services: No
Beds: 318

Key Personnel:
Chief of Medical Staff.......... Andrea R. Conti
Anesthesiology............... Rodney Hines
Radiology.................. Nathan Pulcher
Quality Assurance .... Sandra Simensen, RN
Intensive Care Unit........... Robert Vosler
Emergency Room .... Moriah Walker
Patient Relations .... Clyde Walton

Measure	Cases	This Hosp.	State Avg.	U.S. Avg.
Blood Clot Prevention and Treatment				
Anticoagulation Overlap Therapy	-	-	95%	93%
ICU Venous Thromboembolism Prophylaxis	-	-	91%	92%
Incidence of Potentially Preventable VTE	-	-	5%	10%
UFH with Dosages/Platelet Monitoring	-	-	100%	97%
Venous Thromboembolism Prophylaxis	-	-	80%	85%
Warfarin Therapy Discharge Instructions	-	-	70%	75%
Chest Pain/Possible Heart Attack Care				
Aspirin Given Within 24 Hours of Arrival	-	-	99%	96%
Fibrinolytic Meds Within 30 Min. of Arrival	-	-	69%	58%
Average Time to ECG (minutes)	-	-	5	7
Average Time to Transfer (minutes)	-	-	66	60
Children's Asthma Care				
Received Home Management Plan of Care	-	-	-	88%
Received Reliever Medication	-	-	-	100%
Received Systemic Corticosteroids	-	-	-	100%
Emergency Department				
Admittance Decision Time (minutes)	-	-	41	98
Head CT Results Within 45 Min. of Arrival	-	-	44%	57%
Patients Who Left ER Before Being Seen	-	-	1%	2%
Time from ER Arrival to Admit. (minutes)	-	-	174	274
Time from ER Arrival to Discharge (minutes)	-	-	113	134
Time in ER Before Being Evaluated (minutes)	-	-	18	26
Time to Pain Meds for Fractures (minutes)	-	-	44	57
Heart Attack Care				
Aspirin Given at Discharge[5]	-	-	100%	99%
Fibrinolytic Meds Within 30 Min. of Arrival[5]	-	-	100%	54%
PCI Within 90 Minutes of Arrival[5]	-	-	94%	96%
Statin Prescribed at Discharge[5]	-	-	98%	98%
Heart Failure Care				
ACE Inhibitor or ARB for LVSD	25	88%	93%	97%
Discharge Instructions Given	44	95%	90%	94%
Evaluation of LVS Function	60	100%	97%	99%
Medicare Spending				
Medicare Spending per Patient (ratio)	-	-	0.9	0.98
Pneumonia Care				
Appropriate Initial Antibiotic Given	35	91%	90%	95%
Blood Culture Timing	35	100%	95%	98%
Pregnancy and Delivery Care				
Newborn Deliveries Scheduled Early	-	-	7%	6%
Preventive Care				
Immunization for Influenza[5]	-	-	89%	90%
Immunization for Pneumonia[5]	-	-	89%	92%
Stroke Care				
Anticoagulation Therapy for Atrial Fibrillation	-	-	97%	95%
Antithrombotic Therapy Timing	-	-	98%	98%
Assessed for Rehabilitation	-	-	98%	97%
Discharged on Antithrombotic Therapy	-	-	100%	99%
Discharged on Statin Medication	-	-	93%	94%
Thrombolytic Therapy Timing	-	-	51%	66%
Venous Thromboembolism Prophylaxis	-	-	96%	94%
Written Stroke Educational Materials Given	-	-	85%	88%
Surgical Care Improvement Project				
Appropriate Beta Blocker Usage[5]	-	-	98%	98%
Appropriate VTP Within 24 Hours[5]	-	-	98%	98%
Controlled Postoperative Blood Glucose[5]	-	-	98%	97%
Perioperative Temperature Management[5]	-	-	99%	100%
Prophylactic Antibiotic Selection[5]	-	-	99%	99%
Prophylactic Antibiotic Selection (Outpatient)	-	-	99%	98%
Prophylactic Antibiotic Stopped[5]	-	-	98%	98%
Prophylactic Antibiotic Timing[5]	-	-	99%	99%
Prophylactic Antibiotic Timing (Outpatient)	-	-	98%	98%
Urinary Catheter Removal[5]	-	-	97%	97%
Survey of Patients' Hospital Experiences				
Area Around Room 'Always' Quiet at Night	-	-	72%	61%
Doctors 'Always' Communicated Well	-	-	85%	82%
Home Recovery Information Given	-	-	87%	85%
Hospital Given 9 or 10 on 10 Point Scale	-	-	78%	71%
Meds 'Always' Explained Before Given	-	-	69%	64%
Nurses 'Always' Communicated Well	-	-	83%	79%
Pain 'Always' Well Controlled	-	-	72%	71%
Room and Bathroom 'Always' Clean	-	-	79%	73%
Timely Help 'Always' Received	-	-	77%	68%
Would Definitely Recommend Hospital	-	-	76%	71%
Use of Medical Imaging				

NOTE: Hospital profiles are in alphabetical order by state, then city, then hospital within the city; Rankings exclude hospitals with less than 25 cases except for patient surveys which excludes hospitals with less than 100 cases; (a) 100-299 cases; (1) The number of cases/patients is too few to report; (2) Data submitted were based on a sample of cases/patients; (3) Results are based on a shorter time period than required; (4) Data suppressed by CMS for one or more quarters; (5) Results are not available for this reporting period; (6) Fewer than 100 patients completed the HCAHPS survey; (7) No cases met the criteria for this measure; (8) The lower limit of the confidence interval cannot be calculated if the number of observed infections equals zero; (9) No data are available from the state/territory for this reporting period; (10) The scores shown reflect fewer than 50 completed surveys; (11) There were discrepancies in the data collection process; (12) This measure does not apply to this hospital for this reporting period; (13) Results cannot be calculated for this reporting period; (14) The results for this state are combined with nearby states to protect confidentiality; Please refer to the User's Guide for a full explanation of data.

Measure	Cases	This Hosp.	State Avg.	U.S. Avg.
Cardiac Imaging Stress Test before Surgery	-	-	4.4%	5.3%
Combination Abdominal CT Scan	-	-	12.5%	10.5%
Combination Brain/Sinus CT Scan	-	-	2%	2.7%
Combination Chest CT Scan	-	-	4.5%	2.7%
Follow-up Mammogram/Ultrasound	-	-	8.7%	8.8%
Lumbar Spine MRI for Low Back Pain	-	-	33%	37.2%

Avera Gregory Hospital

400 Park Street PO Box 408 Phone: 605-835-8394
Gregory, SD 57533 Fax: 605-835-9422
URL: www.gregoryhealthcare.org
Type: Critical Access Hospitals Emergency Services: Yes
Ownership: Voluntary non-profit - Church Beds: 81
Key Personnel:
Chief of Medical Staff. . . . . R Nemer, MD
CEO/President. . . . . Carol Varland

Measure	Cases	This Hosp.	State Avg.	U.S. Avg.
Blood Clot Prevention and Treatment				
Anticoagulation Overlap Therapy[5]	-	-	95%	93%
ICU Venous Thromboembolism Prophylaxis[5]	-	-	91%	92%
Incidence of Potentially Preventable VTE[5]	-	-	5%	10%
UFH with Dosages/Platelet Monitoring[5]	-	-	100%	97%
Venous Thromboembolism Prophylaxis[5]	-	-	80%	85%
Warfarin Therapy Discharge Instructions[5]	-	-	70%	75%
Chest Pain/Possible Heart Attack Care				
Aspirin Given Within 24 Hours of Arrival	-	-	99%	96%
Fibrinolytic Meds Within 30 Min. of Arrival	-	-	69%	58%
Average Time to ECG (minutes)	-	-	5	7
Average Time to Transfer (minutes)	-	-	66	60
Children's Asthma Care				
Received Home Management Plan of Care	-	-	-	88%
Received Reliever Medication	-	-	-	100%
Received Systemic Corticosteroids	-	-	-	100%
Emergency Department				
Admittance Decision Time (minutes)[5]	-	-	41	98
Head CT Results Within 45 Min. of Arrival	-	-	44%	57%
Patients Who Left ER Before Being Seen	-	-	1%	2%
Time from ER Arrival to Admit. (minutes)[5]	-	-	174	274
Time from ER Arrival to Discharge (minutes)	-	-	113	134
Time in ER Before Being Evaluated (minutes)	-	-	18	26
Time to Pain Meds for Fractures (minutes)	-	-	44	57
Heart Attack Care				
Aspirin Given at Discharge[5]	-	-	100%	99%
Fibrinolytic Meds Within 30 Min. of Arrival[5]	-	-	100%	54%
PCI Within 90 Minutes of Arrival[5]	-	-	94%	96%
Statin Prescribed at Discharge[5]	-	-	98%	98%
Heart Failure Care				
ACE Inhibitor or ARB for LVSD[5]	-	-	93%	97%
Discharge Instructions Given[5]	-	-	90%	94%
Evaluation of LVS Function[5]	-	-	97%	99%
Medicare Spending				
Medicare Spending per Patient (ratio)	-	-	0.9	0.98
Pneumonia Care				
Appropriate Initial Antibiotic Given[5]	-	-	90%	95%
Blood Culture Timing[5]	-	-	95%	98%
Pregnancy and Delivery Care				
Newborn Deliveries Scheduled Early[5]	-	-	7%	6%
Preventive Care				
Immunization for Influenza[5]	-	-	89%	90%
Immunization for Pneumonia[5]	-	-	89%	92%
Stroke Care				
Anticoagulation Therapy for Atrial Fibrillation[5]	-	-	97%	95%
Antithrombotic Therapy Timing[5]	-	-	98%	98%
Assessed for Rehabilitation[5]	-	-	98%	97%
Discharged on Antithrombotic Therapy[5]	-	-	100%	99%
Discharged on Statin Medication[5]	-	-	93%	94%
Thrombolytic Therapy Timing[5]	-	-	51%	66%
Venous Thromboembolism Prophylaxis[5]	-	-	96%	94%
Written Stroke Educational Materials Given[5]	-	-	85%	88%
Surgical Care Improvement Project				
Appropriate Beta Blocker Usage[5]	-	-	98%	98%
Appropriate VTP Within 24 Hours[5]	-	-	98%	98%
Controlled Postoperative Blood Glucose[5]	-	-	98%	97%
Perioperative Temperature Management[5]	-	-	99%	100%
Prophylactic Antibiotic Selection[5]	-	-	99%	99%
Prophylactic Antibiotic Selection (Outpatient)	-	-	99%	98%
Prophylactic Antibiotic Stopped[5]	-	-	98%	98%
Prophylactic Antibiotic Timing[5]	-	-	99%	99%
Prophylactic Antibiotic Timing (Outpatient)	-	-	98%	98%
Urinary Catheter Removal[5]	-	-	97%	97%
Survey of Patients' Hospital Experiences				
Area Around Room 'Always' Quiet at Night[6]	<100	64%	72%	61%
Doctors 'Always' Communicated Well[6]	<100	83%	85%	82%
Home Recovery Information Given[6]	<100	88%	87%	85%
Hospital Given 9 or 10 on 10 Point Scale[6]	<100	79%	78%	71%
Meds 'Always' Explained Before Given[6]	<100	63%	69%	64%
Nurses 'Always' Communicated Well[6]	<100	80%	83%	79%
Pain 'Always' Well Controlled[6]	<100	69%	72%	71%
Room and Bathroom 'Always' Clean[6]	<100	84%	79%	73%
Timely Help 'Always' Received[6]	<100	71%	77%	68%
Would Definitely Recommend Hospital[6]	<100	72%	76%	71%
Use of Medical Imaging				
Cardiac Imaging Stress Test before Surgery	-	-	4.4%	5.3%
Combination Abdominal CT Scan	-	-	12.5%	10.5%
Combination Brain/Sinus CT Scan	-	-	2%	2.7%
Combination Chest CT Scan	-	-	4.5%	2.7%
Follow-up Mammogram/Ultrasound	-	-	8.7%	8.8%
Lumbar Spine MRI for Low Back Pain	-	-	33%	37.2%

Fall River Hospital

1201 Highway 71 South Phone: 605-745-8910
Hot Springs, SD 57747
URL: www.fallriverhealthservices.com/hospital.php
Type: Critical Access Hospitals Emergency Services: Yes
Ownership: Voluntary non-profit - Private Beds: 11

Measure	Cases	This Hosp.	State Avg.	U.S. Avg.
Blood Clot Prevention and Treatment				
Anticoagulation Overlap Therapy[5]	-	-	95%	93%
ICU Venous Thromboembolism Prophylaxis[5]	-	-	91%	92%
Incidence of Potentially Preventable VTE[5]	-	-	5%	10%
UFH with Dosages/Platelet Monitoring[5]	-	-	100%	97%
Venous Thromboembolism Prophylaxis[5]	-	-	80%	85%
Warfarin Therapy Discharge Instructions[5]	-	-	70%	75%
Chest Pain/Possible Heart Attack Care				
Aspirin Given Within 24 Hours of Arrival[5]	-	-	99%	96%
Fibrinolytic Meds Within 30 Min. of Arrival[5]	-	-	69%	58%
Average Time to ECG (minutes)[5]	-	-	5	7
Average Time to Transfer (minutes)[5]	-	-	66	60
Children's Asthma Care				
Received Home Management Plan of Care	-	-	-	88%
Received Reliever Medication	-	-	-	100%
Received Systemic Corticosteroids	-	-	-	100%
Emergency Department				
Admittance Decision Time (minutes)[5]	-	-	41	98
Head CT Results Within 45 Min. of Arrival[5]	-	-	44%	57%
Patients Who Left ER Before Being Seen[5]	-	-	1%	2%
Time from ER Arrival to Admit. (minutes)[5]	-	-	174	274
Time from ER Arrival to Discharge (minutes)[5]	-	-	113	134
Time in ER Before Being Evaluated (minutes)[5]	-	-	18	26
Time to Pain Meds for Fractures (minutes)[5]	-	-	44	57
Heart Attack Care				
Aspirin Given at Discharge[5]	-	-	100%	99%
Fibrinolytic Meds Within 30 Min. of Arrival[5]	-	-	100%	54%
PCI Within 90 Minutes of Arrival[5]	-	-	94%	96%
Statin Prescribed at Discharge[5]	-	-	98%	98%
Heart Failure Care				
ACE Inhibitor or ARB for LVSD[5]	-	-	93%	97%
Discharge Instructions Given[5]	-	-	90%	94%
Evaluation of LVS Function[5]	-	-	97%	99%
Medicare Spending				
Medicare Spending per Patient (ratio)	-	-	0.9	0.98
Pneumonia Care				
Appropriate Initial Antibiotic Given[5]	-	-	90%	95%
Blood Culture Timing[5]	-	-	95%	98%
Pregnancy and Delivery Care				
Newborn Deliveries Scheduled Early[5]	-	-	7%	6%
Preventive Care				
Immunization for Influenza[5]	-	-	89%	90%
Immunization for Pneumonia[5]	-	-	89%	92%
Stroke Care				
Anticoagulation Therapy for Atrial Fibrillation[5]	-	-	97%	95%
Antithrombotic Therapy Timing[5]	-	-	98%	98%
Assessed for Rehabilitation[5]	-	-	98%	97%
Discharged on Antithrombotic Therapy[5]	-	-	100%	99%
Discharged on Statin Medication[5]	-	-	93%	94%
Thrombolytic Therapy Timing[5]	-	-	51%	66%
Venous Thromboembolism Prophylaxis[5]	-	-	96%	94%
Written Stroke Educational Materials Given[5]	-	-	85%	88%
Surgical Care Improvement Project				
Appropriate Beta Blocker Usage[5]	-	-	98%	98%
Appropriate VTP Within 24 Hours[5]	-	-	98%	98%
Controlled Postoperative Blood Glucose[5]	-	-	98%	97%
Perioperative Temperature Management[5]	-	-	99%	100%
Prophylactic Antibiotic Selection[5]	-	-	99%	99%
Prophylactic Antibiotic Selection (Outpatient)[5]	-	-	99%	98%
Prophylactic Antibiotic Stopped[5]	-	-	98%	98%
Prophylactic Antibiotic Timing[5]	-	-	99%	99%
Prophylactic Antibiotic Timing (Outpatient)[5]	-	-	98%	98%
Urinary Catheter Removal[5]	-	-	97%	97%
Survey of Patients' Hospital Experiences				
Area Around Room 'Always' Quiet at Night[5]	-	-	72%	61%
Doctors 'Always' Communicated Well[5]	-	-	85%	82%
Home Recovery Information Given[5]	-	-	87%	85%
Hospital Given 9 or 10 on 10 Point Scale[5]	-	-	78%	71%
Meds 'Always' Explained Before Given[5]	-	-	69%	64%
Nurses 'Always' Communicated Well[5]	-	-	83%	79%
Pain 'Always' Well Controlled[5]	-	-	72%	71%
Room and Bathroom 'Always' Clean[5]	-	-	79%	73%
Timely Help 'Always' Received[5]	-	-	77%	68%
Would Definitely Recommend Hospital[5]	-	-	76%	71%
Use of Medical Imaging				
Cardiac Imaging Stress Test before Surgery[7]	-	-	4.4%	5.3%
Combination Abdominal CT Scan	86	0.0%	12.5%	10.5%
Combination Brain/Sinus CT Scan[1]	-	-	2%	2.7%
Combination Chest CT Scan	47	0.0%	4.5%	2.7%
Follow-up Mammogram/Ultrasound	66	1.5%	8.7%	8.8%
Lumbar Spine MRI for Low Back Pain[1]	-	-	33%	37.2%

Huron Regional Medical Center

172 Fourth Street Se Phone: 605-353-6200
Huron, SD 57350 Fax: 605-353-6300
URL: www.huronregional.org
Type: Critical Access Hospitals Emergency Services: Yes
Ownership: Voluntary non-profit - Private Beds: 25
Key Personnel:
Operating Room. . . . . Kris Brandt
Infection Control. . . . . Janice Farrar, RN
Quality Assurance . . . . Janice Farrar
Chief of Medical Staff. . . . . Cy Hartvedt
Radiology. . . . . Rick Janes
CEO/President. . . . . John Single
Emergency Room . . . . Pat Woulridge

Measure	Cases	This Hosp.	State Avg.	U.S. Avg.
Blood Clot Prevention and Treatment				
Anticoagulation Overlap Therapy[5]	-	-	95%	93%
ICU Venous Thromboembolism Prophylaxis[5]	-	-	91%	92%
Incidence of Potentially Preventable VTE[5]	-	-	5%	10%
UFH with Dosages/Platelet Monitoring[5]	-	-	100%	97%
Venous Thromboembolism Prophylaxis[5]	-	-	80%	85%
Warfarin Therapy Discharge Instructions[5]	-	-	70%	75%
Chest Pain/Possible Heart Attack Care				
Aspirin Given Within 24 Hours of Arrival	-	-	99%	96%
Fibrinolytic Meds Within 30 Min. of Arrival	-	-	69%	58%
Average Time to ECG (minutes)	-	-	5	7
Average Time to Transfer (minutes)	-	-	66	60
Children's Asthma Care				
Received Home Management Plan of Care	-	-	-	88%
Received Reliever Medication	-	-	-	100%
Received Systemic Corticosteroids	-	-	-	100%

NOTE: Hospital profiles are in alphabetical order by state, then city, then hospital within the city; Rankings exclude hospitals with less than 25 cases except for patient surveys which excludes hospitals with less than 100 cases; (a) 100-299 cases; (1) The number of cases/patients is too few to report; (2) Data submitted were based on a sample of cases/patients; (3) Results are based on a shorter time period than required; (4) Data suppressed by CMS for one or more quarters; (5) Results are not available for this reporting period; (6) Fewer than 100 patients completed the HCAHPS survey; (7) No cases met the criteria for this measure; (8) The lower limit of the confidence interval cannot be calculated if the number of observed infections equals zero; (9) No data are available from the state/territory for this reporting period; (10) The scores shown reflect fewer than 50 completed surveys; (11) There were discrepancies in the data collection process; (12) This measure does not apply to this hospital for this reporting period; (13) Results cannot be calculated for this reporting period; (14) The results for this state are combined with nearby states to protect confidentiality; Please refer to the User's Guide for a full explanation of data.

Measure	Cases	This Hosp.	State Avg.	U.S. Avg.
Emergency Department				
Admittance Decision Time (minutes)[5]	-	-	41	98
Head CT Results Within 45 Min. of Arrival	-	-	44%	57%
Patients Who Left ER Before Being Seen	-	-	1%	2%
Time from ER Arrival to Admit. (minutes)[5]	-	-	174	274
Time from ER Arrival to Discharge (minutes)	-	-	113	134
Time in ER Before Being Evaluated (minutes)	-	-	18	26
Time to Pain Meds for Fractures (minutes)	-	-	44	57
Heart Attack Care				
Aspirin Given at Discharge[5]	-	-	100%	99%
Fibrinolytic Meds Within 30 Min. of Arrival[5]	-	-	100%	54%
PCI Within 90 Minutes of Arrival[5]	-	-	94%	96%
Statin Prescribed at Discharge[5]	-	-	98%	98%
Heart Failure Care				
ACE Inhibitor or ARB for LVSD[1]	-	-	93%	97%
Discharge Instructions Given	14	93%	90%	94%
Evaluation of LVS Function	23	74%	97%	99%
Medicare Spending				
Medicare Spending per Patient (ratio)	-	-	0.9	0.98
Pneumonia Care				
Appropriate Initial Antibiotic Given	59	75%	90%	95%
Blood Culture Timing	61	95%	95%	98%
Pregnancy and Delivery Care				
Newborn Deliveries Scheduled Early[5]	-	-	7%	6%
Preventive Care				
Immunization for Influenza[5]	-	-	89%	90%
Immunization for Pneumonia[5]	-	-	89%	92%
Stroke Care				
Anticoagulation Therapy for Atrial Fibrillation[5]	-	-	97%	95%
Antithrombotic Therapy Timing[5]	-	-	98%	98%
Assessed for Rehabilitation[5]	-	-	98%	97%
Discharged on Antithrombotic Therapy[5]	-	-	100%	99%
Discharged on Statin Medication[5]	-	-	93%	94%
Thrombolytic Therapy Timing[5]	-	-	51%	66%
Venous Thromboembolism Prophylaxis[5]	-	-	96%	94%
Written Stroke Educational Materials Given[5]	-	-	85%	88%
Surgical Care Improvement Project				
Appropriate Beta Blocker Usage[5]	-	-	98%	98%
Appropriate VTP Within 24 Hours	40	92%	98%	98%
Controlled Postoperative Blood Glucose[5]	-	-	98%	97%
Perioperative Temperature Management	42	100%	99%	100%
Prophylactic Antibiotic Selection	28	93%	99%	99%
Prophylactic Antibiotic Selection (Outpatient)	-	-	99%	98%
Prophylactic Antibiotic Stopped	27	100%	98%	98%
Prophylactic Antibiotic Timing	28	100%	99%	99%
Prophylactic Antibiotic Timing (Outpatient)	-	-	98%	98%
Urinary Catheter Removal[1]	-	-	97%	97%
Survey of Patients' Hospital Experiences				
Area Around Room 'Always' Quiet at Night[5]	-	-	72%	61%
Doctors 'Always' Communicated Well[5]	-	-	85%	82%
Home Recovery Information Given[5]	-	-	87%	85%
Hospital Given 9 or 10 on 10 Point Scale[5]	-	-	78%	71%
Meds 'Always' Explained Before Given[5]	-	-	69%	64%
Nurses 'Always' Communicated Well[5]	-	-	83%	79%
Pain 'Always' Well Controlled[5]	-	-	72%	71%
Room and Bathroom 'Always' Clean[5]	-	-	79%	73%
Timely Help 'Always' Received[5]	-	-	77%	68%
Would Definitely Recommend Hospital[5]	-	-	76%	71%
Use of Medical Imaging				
Cardiac Imaging Stress Test before Surgery	-	-	4.4%	5.3%
Combination Abdominal CT Scan	-	-	12.5%	10.5%
Combination Brain/Sinus CT Scan	-	-	2%	2.7%
Combination Chest CT Scan	-	-	4.5%	2.7%
Follow-up Mammogram/Ultrasound	-	-	8.7%	8.8%
Lumbar Spine MRI for Low Back Pain	-	-	33%	37.2%

Madison Community Hospital

917 N Washington Ave
Madison, SD 57042
Phone: 605-256-6551
Fax: 605-256-6469
E-mail: info@madisonhospital.com
URL: www.madisonhospital.com
Type: Critical Access Hospitals
Emergency Services: Yes
Ownership: Voluntary non-profit - Private
Beds: 25

Key Personnel:
CEO . . . . Tamara Miller
Quality Assurance . . . . Jennifer Eimers
Infection Control. . . . . Kathy Hansen
Emergency Room . . . . Donna Quade
Chief of Medical Staff. . . . . RG Sample, MD

Measure	Cases	This Hosp.	State Avg.	U.S. Avg.
Blood Clot Prevention and Treatment				
Anticoagulation Overlap Therapy[5]	-	-	95%	93%
ICU Venous Thromboembolism Prophylaxis[5]	-	-	91%	92%
Incidence of Potentially Preventable VTE[5]	-	-	5%	10%
UFH with Dosages/Platelet Monitoring[5]	-	-	100%	97%
Venous Thromboembolism Prophylaxis[5]	-	-	80%	85%
Warfarin Therapy Discharge Instructions[5]	-	-	70%	75%
Chest Pain/Possible Heart Attack Care				
Aspirin Given Within 24 Hours of Arrival	-	-	99%	96%
Fibrinolytic Meds Within 30 Min. of Arrival	-	-	69%	58%
Average Time to ECG (minutes)	-	-	5	7
Average Time to Transfer (minutes)	-	-	66	60
Children's Asthma Care				
Received Home Management Plan of Care	-	-	-	88%
Received Reliever Medication	-	-	-	100%
Received Systemic Corticosteroids	-	-	-	100%
Emergency Department				
Admittance Decision Time (minutes)[5]	-	-	41	98
Head CT Results Within 45 Min. of Arrival	-	-	44%	57%
Patients Who Left ER Before Being Seen	-	-	1%	2%
Time from ER Arrival to Admit. (minutes)[5]	-	-	174	274
Time from ER Arrival to Discharge (minutes)	-	-	113	134
Time in ER Before Being Evaluated (minutes)	-	-	18	26
Time to Pain Meds for Fractures (minutes)	-	-	44	57
Heart Attack Care				
Aspirin Given at Discharge[3,7]	-	-	100%	99%
Fibrinolytic Meds Within 30 Min. of Arrival[3,7]	-	-	100%	54%
PCI Within 90 Minutes of Arrival[3,7]	-	-	94%	96%
Statin Prescribed at Discharge[3,7]	-	-	98%	98%
Heart Failure Care				
ACE Inhibitor or ARB for LVSD[1,3]	-	-	93%	97%
Discharge Instructions Given[1,3]	-	-	90%	94%
Evaluation of LVS Function[1,3]	-	-	97%	99%
Medicare Spending				
Medicare Spending per Patient (ratio)	-	-	0.9	0.98
Pneumonia Care				
Appropriate Initial Antibiotic Given[1]	-	-	90%	95%
Blood Culture Timing[1]	-	-	95%	98%
Pregnancy and Delivery Care				
Newborn Deliveries Scheduled Early[5]	-	-	7%	6%
Preventive Care				
Immunization for Influenza[5]	-	-	89%	90%
Immunization for Pneumonia[5]	-	-	89%	92%
Stroke Care				
Anticoagulation Therapy for Atrial Fibrillation[5]	-	-	97%	95%
Antithrombotic Therapy Timing[5]	-	-	98%	98%
Assessed for Rehabilitation[5]	-	-	98%	97%
Discharged on Antithrombotic Therapy[5]	-	-	100%	99%
Discharged on Statin Medication[5]	-	-	93%	94%
Thrombolytic Therapy Timing[5]	-	-	51%	66%
Venous Thromboembolism Prophylaxis[5]	-	-	96%	94%
Written Stroke Educational Materials Given[5]	-	-	85%	88%
Surgical Care Improvement Project				
Appropriate Beta Blocker Usage[1,3]	-	-	98%	98%
Appropriate VTP Within 24 Hours[1,3]	-	-	98%	98%
Controlled Postoperative Blood Glucose[3,7]	-	-	98%	97%
Perioperative Temperature Management[1,3]	-	-	99%	100%
Prophylactic Antibiotic Selection[1,3]	-	-	99%	99%
Prophylactic Antibiotic Selection (Outpatient)	-	-	99%	98%
Prophylactic Antibiotic Stopped[1,3]	-	-	98%	98%
Prophylactic Antibiotic Timing[1,3]	-	-	99%	99%
Prophylactic Antibiotic Timing (Outpatient)	-	-	98%	98%
Urinary Catheter Removal[1,3]	-	-	97%	97%
Survey of Patients' Hospital Experiences				
Area Around Room 'Always' Quiet at Night[6]	<100	76%	72%	61%
Doctors 'Always' Communicated Well[6]	<100	95%	85%	82%
Home Recovery Information Given[6]	<100	96%	87%	85%
Hospital Given 9 or 10 on 10 Point Scale[6]	<100	80%	78%	71%
Meds 'Always' Explained Before Given[6]	<100	86%	69%	64%
Nurses 'Always' Communicated Well[6]	<100	85%	83%	79%
Pain 'Always' Well Controlled[6]	<100	75%	72%	71%
Room and Bathroom 'Always' Clean[6]	<100	83%	79%	73%
Timely Help 'Always' Received[6]	<100	82%	77%	68%
Would Definitely Recommend Hospital[6]	<100	75%	76%	71%
Use of Medical Imaging				
Cardiac Imaging Stress Test before Surgery	-	-	4.4%	5.3%
Combination Abdominal CT Scan	-	-	12.5%	10.5%
Combination Brain/Sinus CT Scan	-	-	2%	2.7%
Combination Chest CT Scan	-	-	4.5%	2.7%
Follow-up Mammogram/Ultrasound	-	-	8.7%	8.8%
Lumbar Spine MRI for Low Back Pain	-	-	33%	37.2%

Milbank Area Hospital/Avera Health

901 E Virgil Ave
Milbank, SD 57252
Phone: 605-432-4538
URL: www1.averahealth.org
Type: Critical Access Hospitals
Emergency Services: Yes
Ownership: Voluntary non-profit - Private

Key Personnel:
Administrator . . . . Natalie Gauer
Radiology. . . . . Amanda Sommers

Measure	Cases	This Hosp.	State Avg.	U.S. Avg.
Blood Clot Prevention and Treatment				
Anticoagulation Overlap Therapy[5]	-	-	95%	93%
ICU Venous Thromboembolism Prophylaxis[5]	-	-	91%	92%
Incidence of Potentially Preventable VTE[5]	-	-	5%	10%
UFH with Dosages/Platelet Monitoring[5]	-	-	100%	97%
Venous Thromboembolism Prophylaxis[5]	-	-	80%	85%
Warfarin Therapy Discharge Instructions[5]	-	-	70%	75%
Chest Pain/Possible Heart Attack Care				
Aspirin Given Within 24 Hours of Arrival	-	-	99%	96%
Fibrinolytic Meds Within 30 Min. of Arrival	-	-	69%	58%
Average Time to ECG (minutes)	-	-	5	7
Average Time to Transfer (minutes)	-	-	66	60
Children's Asthma Care				
Received Home Management Plan of Care	-	-	-	88%
Received Reliever Medication	-	-	-	100%
Received Systemic Corticosteroids	-	-	-	100%
Emergency Department				
Admittance Decision Time (minutes)[5]	-	-	41	98
Head CT Results Within 45 Min. of Arrival	-	-	44%	57%
Patients Who Left ER Before Being Seen	-	-	1%	2%
Time from ER Arrival to Admit. (minutes)[5]	-	-	174	274
Time from ER Arrival to Discharge (minutes)	-	-	113	134
Time in ER Before Being Evaluated (minutes)	-	-	18	26
Time to Pain Meds for Fractures (minutes)	-	-	44	57
Heart Attack Care				
Aspirin Given at Discharge[1,3]	-	-	100%	99%
Fibrinolytic Meds Within 30 Min. of Arrival[3,7]	-	-	100%	54%
PCI Within 90 Minutes of Arrival[3,7]	-	-	94%	96%
Statin Prescribed at Discharge[1,3]	-	-	98%	98%
Heart Failure Care				
ACE Inhibitor or ARB for LVSD[3,7]	-	-	93%	97%
Discharge Instructions Given[1,3]	-	-	90%	94%
Evaluation of LVS Function[1,3]	-	-	97%	99%
Medicare Spending				
Medicare Spending per Patient (ratio)	-	-	0.9	0.98
Pneumonia Care				
Appropriate Initial Antibiotic Given	13	92%	90%	95%
Blood Culture Timing[1]	-	-	95%	98%
Pregnancy and Delivery Care				
Newborn Deliveries Scheduled Early[5]	-	-	7%	6%
Preventive Care				

NOTE: Hospital profiles are in alphabetical order by state, then city, then hospital within the city; Rankings exclude hospitals with less than 25 cases except for patient surveys which excludes hospitals with less than 100 cases; (a) 100-299 cases; (1) The number of cases/patients is too few to report; (2) Data submitted were based on a sample of cases/patients; (3) Results are based on a shorter time period than required; (4) Data suppressed by CMS for one or more quarters; (5) Results are not available for this reporting period; (6) Fewer than 100 patients completed the HCAHPS survey; (7) No cases met the criteria for this measure; (8) The lower limit of the confidence interval cannot be calculated if the number of observed infections equals zero; (9) No data are available from the state/territory for this reporting period; (10) The scores shown reflect fewer than 50 completed surveys; (11) There were discrepancies in the data collection process; (12) This measure does not apply to this hospital for this reporting period; (13) Results cannot be calculated for this reporting period; (14) The results for this state are combined with nearby states to protect confidentiality; Please refer to the User's Guide for a full explanation of data.

Measure	Cases	This Hosp.	State Avg.	U.S. Avg.
Immunization for Influenza[5]	-	-	89%	90%
Immunization for Pneumonia[5]	-	-	89%	92%
Stroke Care				
Anticoagulation Therapy for Atrial Fibrillation[5]	-	-	97%	95%
Antithrombotic Therapy Timing[5]	-	-	98%	98%
Assessed for Rehabilitation[5]	-	-	98%	97%
Discharged on Antithrombotic Therapy[5]	-	-	100%	99%
Discharged on Statin Medication[5]	-	-	93%	94%
Thrombolytic Therapy Timing[5]	-	-	51%	66%
Venous Thromboembolism Prophylaxis[5]	-	-	96%	94%
Written Stroke Educational Materials Given[5]	-	-	85%	88%
Surgical Care Improvement Project				
Appropriate Beta Blocker Usage[5]	-	-	98%	98%
Appropriate VTP Within 24 Hours[5]	-	-	98%	98%
Controlled Postoperative Blood Glucose[5]	-	-	98%	97%
Perioperative Temperature Management[5]	-	-	99%	100%
Prophylactic Antibiotic Selection[5]	-	-	99%	99%
Prophylactic Antibiotic Selection (Outpatient)	-	-	99%	98%
Prophylactic Antibiotic Stopped[5]	-	-	98%	98%
Prophylactic Antibiotic Timing[5]	-	-	99%	99%
Prophylactic Antibiotic Timing (Outpatient)	-	-	98%	98%
Urinary Catheter Removal[5]	-	-	97%	97%
Survey of Patients' Hospital Experiences				
Area Around Room 'Always' Quiet at Night[6]	<100	73%	72%	61%
Doctors 'Always' Communicated Well[6]	<100	87%	85%	82%
Home Recovery Information Given[6]	<100	89%	87%	85%
Hospital Given 9 or 10 on 10 Point Scale[6]	<100	69%	78%	71%
Meds 'Always' Explained Before Given[6]	<100	62%	69%	64%
Nurses 'Always' Communicated Well[6]	<100	84%	83%	79%
Pain 'Always' Well Controlled[6]	<100	70%	72%	71%
Room and Bathroom 'Always' Clean[6]	<100	77%	79%	73%
Timely Help 'Always' Received[6]	<100	70%	77%	68%
Would Definitely Recommend Hospital[6]	<100	67%	76%	71%
Use of Medical Imaging				
Cardiac Imaging Stress Test before Surgery	-	-	4.4%	5.3%
Combination Abdominal CT Scan	-	-	12.5%	10.5%
Combination Brain/Sinus CT Scan	-	-	2%	2.7%
Combination Chest CT Scan	-	-	4.5%	2.7%
Follow-up Mammogram/Ultrasound	-	-	8.7%	8.8%
Lumbar Spine MRI for Low Back Pain	-	-	33%	37.2%

Avera Hand County Memorial Hospital & Clinic

300 W 5th St
Miller, SD 57362
Phone: 605-853-2421
Fax: 605-853-0333
URL: www.avera.org
Type: Critical Access Hospitals
Emergency Services: No
Ownership: Voluntary non-profit - Private
Beds: 25

Key Personnel:
Chief of Medical Staff.......... Joel Huber
Radiology.................. Daryl C Rife

Measure	Cases	This Hosp.	State Avg.	U.S. Avg.
Blood Clot Prevention and Treatment				
Anticoagulation Overlap Therapy[5]	-	-	95%	93%
ICU Venous Thromboembolism Prophylaxis[5]	-	-	91%	92%
Incidence of Potentially Preventable VTE[5]	-	-	5%	10%
UFH with Dosages/Platelet Monitoring[5]	-	-	100%	97%
Venous Thromboembolism Prophylaxis[5]	-	-	80%	85%
Warfarin Therapy Discharge Instructions[5]	-	-	70%	75%
Chest Pain/Possible Heart Attack Care				
Aspirin Given Within 24 Hours of Arrival	-	-	99%	96%
Fibrinolytic Meds Within 30 Min. of Arrival	-	-	69%	58%
Average Time to ECG (minutes)	-	-	5	7
Average Time to Transfer (minutes)	-	-	66	60
Children's Asthma Care				
Received Home Management Plan of Care	-	-	-	88%
Received Reliever Medication	-	-	-	100%
Received Systemic Corticosteroids	-	-	-	100%
Emergency Department				
Admittance Decision Time (minutes)[5]	-	-	41	98
Head CT Results Within 45 Min. of Arrival	-	-	44%	57%
Patients Who Left ER Before Being Seen	-	-	1%	2%
Time from ER Arrival to Admit. (minutes)[5]	-	-	174	274
Time from ER Arrival to Discharge (minutes)	-	-	113	134
Time in ER Before Being Evaluated (minutes)	-	-	18	26
Time to Pain Meds for Fractures (minutes)	-	-	44	57
Heart Attack Care				
Aspirin Given at Discharge[5]	-	-	100%	99%
Fibrinolytic Meds Within 30 Min. of Arrival[5]	-	-	100%	54%
PCI Within 90 Minutes of Arrival[5]	-	-	94%	96%
Statin Prescribed at Discharge[5]	-	-	98%	98%
Heart Failure Care				
ACE Inhibitor or ARB for LVSD[1]	-	-	93%	97%
Discharge Instructions Given[1]	-	-	90%	94%
Evaluation of LVS Function	15	67%	97%	99%
Medicare Spending				
Medicare Spending per Patient (ratio)	-	-	0.9	0.98
Pneumonia Care				
Appropriate Initial Antibiotic Given	11	91%	90%	95%
Blood Culture Timing[1]	-	-	95%	98%
Pregnancy and Delivery Care				
Newborn Deliveries Scheduled Early[5]	-	-	7%	6%
Preventive Care				
Immunization for Influenza[5]	-	-	89%	90%
Immunization for Pneumonia[5]	-	-	89%	92%
Stroke Care				
Anticoagulation Therapy for Atrial Fibrillation[5]	-	-	97%	95%
Antithrombotic Therapy Timing[5]	-	-	98%	98%
Assessed for Rehabilitation[5]	-	-	98%	97%
Discharged on Antithrombotic Therapy[5]	-	-	100%	99%
Discharged on Statin Medication[5]	-	-	93%	94%
Thrombolytic Therapy Timing[5]	-	-	51%	66%
Venous Thromboembolism Prophylaxis[5]	-	-	96%	94%
Written Stroke Educational Materials Given[5]	-	-	85%	88%
Surgical Care Improvement Project				
Appropriate Beta Blocker Usage[5]	-	-	98%	98%
Appropriate VTP Within 24 Hours[5]	-	-	98%	98%
Controlled Postoperative Blood Glucose[5]	-	-	98%	97%
Perioperative Temperature Management[5]	-	-	99%	100%
Prophylactic Antibiotic Selection[5]	-	-	99%	99%
Prophylactic Antibiotic Selection (Outpatient)	-	-	99%	98%
Prophylactic Antibiotic Stopped[5]	-	-	98%	98%
Prophylactic Antibiotic Timing[5]	-	-	99%	99%
Prophylactic Antibiotic Timing (Outpatient)	-	-	98%	98%
Urinary Catheter Removal[5]	-	-	97%	97%
Survey of Patients' Hospital Experiences				
Area Around Room 'Always' Quiet at Night[6]	<100	70%	72%	61%
Doctors 'Always' Communicated Well[6]	<100	84%	85%	82%
Home Recovery Information Given[6]	<100	92%	87%	85%
Hospital Given 9 or 10 on 10 Point Scale[6]	<100	80%	78%	71%
Meds 'Always' Explained Before Given[6]	<100	58%	69%	64%
Nurses 'Always' Communicated Well[6]	<100	87%	83%	79%
Pain 'Always' Well Controlled[6]	<100	70%	72%	71%
Room and Bathroom 'Always' Clean[6]	<100	83%	79%	73%
Timely Help 'Always' Received[6]	<100	74%	77%	68%
Would Definitely Recommend Hospital[6]	<100	81%	76%	71%
Use of Medical Imaging				
Cardiac Imaging Stress Test before Surgery	-	-	4.4%	5.3%
Combination Abdominal CT Scan	-	-	12.5%	10.5%
Combination Brain/Sinus CT Scan	-	-	2%	2.7%
Combination Chest CT Scan	-	-	4.5%	2.7%
Follow-up Mammogram/Ultrasound	-	-	8.7%	8.8%
Lumbar Spine MRI for Low Back Pain	-	-	33%	37.2%

Avera Queen of Peace

525 N Foster
Mitchell, SD 57301
Phone: 605-995-2000
Fax: 605-995-2441
URL: www.averaqueenofpeace.org
Type: Acute Care Hospitals
Emergency Services: Yes
Ownership: Voluntary non-profit - Church
Beds: 120

Key Personnel:
Radiology.................. Calvin F Andersen
Emergency Room .... Kathy Herttinger, RN
Chief of Medical Staff........ Jerome Howe
Quality Assurance .... Brenda Olson
CEO/President.............. Thomas P Rasmusson

Measure	Cases	This Hosp.	State Avg.	U.S. Avg.
Blood Clot Prevention and Treatment				
Anticoagulation Overlap Therapy[2]	26	100%	95%	93%
ICU Venous Thromboembolism Prophylaxis[2]	50	100%	91%	92%
Incidence of Potentially Preventable VTE[1,2]	-	-	5%	10%
UFH with Dosages/Platelet Monitoring[2]	26	100%	100%	97%
Venous Thromboembolism Prophylaxis[2]	163	96%	80%	85%
Warfarin Therapy Discharge Instructions[2]	16	100%	70%	75%
Chest Pain/Possible Heart Attack Care				
Aspirin Given Within 24 Hours of Arrival	29	100%	99%	96%
Fibrinolytic Meds Within 30 Min. of Arrival[1]	-	-	69%	58%
Average Time to ECG (minutes)	29	5	5	7
Average Time to Transfer (minutes)[7]	-	-	66	60
Children's Asthma Care				
Received Home Management Plan of Care	-	-	-	88%
Received Reliever Medication	-	-	-	100%
Received Systemic Corticosteroids	-	-	-	100%
Emergency Department				
Admittance Decision Time (minutes)	833	28	41	98
Head CT Results Within 45 Min. of Arrival[1]	-	-	44%	57%
Patients Who Left ER Before Being Seen	7,573	0%	1%	2%
Time from ER Arrival to Admit. (minutes)	833	167	174	274
Time from ER Arrival to Discharge (minutes)	5,390	116	113	134
Time in ER Before Being Evaluated (minutes)	6,166	21	18	26
Time to Pain Meds for Fractures (minutes)	43	56	44	57
Heart Attack Care				
Aspirin Given at Discharge	12	100%	100%	99%
Fibrinolytic Meds Within 30 Min. of Arrival[7]	-	-	100%	54%
PCI Within 90 Minutes of Arrival[7]	-	-	94%	96%
Statin Prescribed at Discharge[1]	-	-	98%	98%
Heart Failure Care				
ACE Inhibitor or ARB for LVSD[1]	-	-	93%	97%
Discharge Instructions Given	37	100%	90%	94%
Evaluation of LVS Function	65	100%	97%	99%
Medicare Spending				
Medicare Spending per Patient (ratio)	-	0.87	0.9	0.98
Pneumonia Care				
Appropriate Initial Antibiotic Given	90	98%	90%	95%
Blood Culture Timing	101	99%	95%	98%
Pregnancy and Delivery Care				
Newborn Deliveries Scheduled Early	33	12%	7%	6%
Preventive Care				
Immunization for Influenza	1,016	97%	89%	90%
Immunization for Pneumonia	1,193	94%	89%	92%
Stroke Care				
Anticoagulation Therapy for Atrial Fibrillation[1]	-	-	97%	95%
Antithrombotic Therapy Timing	11	100%	98%	98%
Assessed for Rehabilitation	13	100%	98%	97%
Discharged on Antithrombotic Therapy[1]	-	-	100%	99%
Discharged on Statin Medication[1]	-	-	93%	94%
Thrombolytic Therapy Timing[7]	-	-	51%	66%
Venous Thromboembolism Prophylaxis	13	92%	96%	94%
Written Stroke Educational Materials Given[1]	-	-	85%	88%
Surgical Care Improvement Project				
Appropriate Beta Blocker Usage	78	99%	98%	98%
Appropriate VTP Within 24 Hours	204	100%	98%	98%
Controlled Postoperative Blood Glucose[7]	-	-	98%	97%
Perioperative Temperature Management	225	100%	99%	100%
Prophylactic Antibiotic Selection	175	100%	99%	99%
Prophylactic Antibiotic Selection (Outpatient)	66	100%	99%	98%
Prophylactic Antibiotic Stopped	164	100%	98%	98%
Prophylactic Antibiotic Timing	175	100%	99%	99%
Prophylactic Antibiotic Timing (Outpatient)	66	100%	98%	98%
Urinary Catheter Removal	34	100%	97%	97%
Survey of Patients' Hospital Experiences				
Area Around Room 'Always' Quiet at Night	300+	64%	72%	61%
Doctors 'Always' Communicated Well	300+	85%	85%	82%
Home Recovery Information Given	300+	92%	87%	85%
Hospital Given 9 or 10 on 10 Point Scale	300+	77%	78%	71%
Meds 'Always' Explained Before Given	300+	72%	69%	64%
Nurses 'Always' Communicated Well	300+	82%	83%	79%
Pain 'Always' Well Controlled	300+	75%	72%	71%
Room and Bathroom 'Always' Clean	300+	73%	79%	73%
Timely Help 'Always' Received	300+	71%	77%	68%

NOTE: Hospital profiles are in alphabetical order by state, then city, then hospital within the city; Rankings exclude hospitals with less than 25 cases except for patient surveys which excludes hospitals with less than 100 cases; (a) 100-299 cases; (1) The number of cases/patients is too few to report; (2) Data submitted were based on a sample of cases/patients; (3) Results are based on a shorter time period than required; (4) Data suppressed by CMS for one or more quarters; (5) Results are not available for this reporting period; (6) Fewer than 100 patients completed the HCAHPS survey; (7) No cases met the criteria for this measure; (8) The lower limit of the confidence interval cannot be calculated if the number of observed infections equals zero; (9) No data are available from the state/territory for this reporting period; (10) The scores shown reflect fewer than 50 completed surveys; (11) There were discrepancies in the data collection process; (12) This measure does not apply to this hospital for this reporting period; (13) Results cannot be calculated for this reporting period; (14) The results for this state are combined with nearby states to protect confidentiality; Please refer to the User's Guide for a full explanation of data.

Would Definitely Recommend Hospital	300+	75%	76%	71%
Use of Medical Imaging				
Cardiac Imaging Stress Test before Surgery[1]	-	-	4.4%	5.3%
Combination Abdominal CT Scan	286	19.6%	12.5%	10.5%
Combination Brain/Sinus CT Scan	281	1.1%	2%	2.7%
Combination Chest CT Scan	175	13.1%	4.5%	2.7%
Follow-up Mammogram/Ultrasound	1,005	10.1%	8.7%	8.8%
Lumbar Spine MRI for Low Back Pain	124	34.7%	33%	37.2%

Mobridge Regional Hospital

1401 10th Ave West
Mobridge, SD 57601
Phone: 605-845-3692
Fax: 605-845-8252
URL: www.mobridgehospital.org
Type: Critical Access Hospitals
Emergency Services: Yes
Ownership: Voluntary non-profit - Private
Beds: 25

Key Personnel:
Surgery . . . . Bela Csaki
Quality Assurance . . . . Diane Blom
Cardiac Laboratory. . . . . Deb Brekke
Radiology. . . . . Charles Peacock
CEO . . . . Angelia Svihovec
Infection Control. . . . . June Volk

Measure	Cases	This Hosp.	State Avg.	U.S. Avg.
Blood Clot Prevention and Treatment				
Anticoagulation Overlap Therapy[5]	-	-	95%	93%
ICU Venous Thromboembolism Prophylaxis[5]	-	-	91%	92%
Incidence of Potentially Preventable VTE[5]	-	-	5%	10%
UFH with Dosages/Platelet Monitoring[5]	-	-	100%	97%
Venous Thromboembolism Prophylaxis[5]	-	-	80%	85%
Warfarin Therapy Discharge Instructions[5]	-	-	70%	75%
Chest Pain/Possible Heart Attack Care				
Aspirin Given Within 24 Hours of Arrival	-	-	99%	96%
Fibrinolytic Meds Within 30 Min. of Arrival	-	-	69%	58%
Average Time to ECG (minutes)	-	-	5	7
Average Time to Transfer (minutes)	-	-	66	60
Children's Asthma Care				
Received Home Management Plan of Care	-	-	-	88%
Received Reliever Medication	-	-	-	100%
Received Systemic Corticosteroids	-	-	-	100%
Emergency Department				
Admittance Decision Time (minutes)[5]	-	-	41	98
Head CT Results Within 45 Min. of Arrival	-	-	44%	57%
Patients Who Left ER Before Being Seen	-	-	1%	2%
Time from ER Arrival to Admit. (minutes)[5]	-	-	174	274
Time from ER Arrival to Discharge (minutes)	-	-	113	134
Time in ER Before Being Evaluated (minutes)	-	-	18	26
Time to Pain Meds for Fractures (minutes)	-	-	44	57
Heart Attack Care				
Aspirin Given at Discharge[5]	-	-	100%	99%
Fibrinolytic Meds Within 30 Min. of Arrival[5]	-	-	100%	54%
PCI Within 90 Minutes of Arrival[5]	-	-	94%	96%
Statin Prescribed at Discharge[5]	-	-	98%	98%
Heart Failure Care				
ACE Inhibitor or ARB for LVSD[5]	-	-	93%	97%
Discharge Instructions Given[5]	-	-	90%	94%
Evaluation of LVS Function[5]	-	-	97%	99%
Medicare Spending				
Medicare Spending per Patient (ratio)	-	-	0.9	0.98
Pneumonia Care				
Appropriate Initial Antibiotic Given[5]	-	-	90%	95%
Blood Culture Timing[5]	-	-	95%	98%
Pregnancy and Delivery Care				
Newborn Deliveries Scheduled Early[5]	-	-	7%	6%
Preventive Care				
Immunization for Influenza[5]	-	-	89%	90%
Immunization for Pneumonia[5]	-	-	89%	92%
Stroke Care				
Anticoagulation Therapy for Atrial Fibrillation[5]	-	-	97%	95%
Antithrombotic Therapy Timing[5]	-	-	98%	98%
Assessed for Rehabilitation[5]	-	-	98%	97%
Discharged on Antithrombotic Therapy[5]	-	-	100%	99%
Discharged on Statin Medication[5]	-	-	93%	94%
Thrombolytic Therapy Timing[5]	-	-	51%	66%
Venous Thromboembolism Prophylaxis[5]	-	-	96%	94%
Written Stroke Educational Materials Given[5]	-	-	85%	88%
Surgical Care Improvement Project				
Appropriate Beta Blocker Usage[5]	-	-	98%	98%
Appropriate VTP Within 24 Hours[5]	-	-	98%	98%
Controlled Postoperative Blood Glucose[5]	-	-	98%	97%
Perioperative Temperature Management[5]	-	-	99%	100%
Prophylactic Antibiotic Selection[5]	-	-	99%	99%
Prophylactic Antibiotic Selection (Outpatient)	-	-	99%	98%
Prophylactic Antibiotic Stopped[5]	-	-	98%	98%
Prophylactic Antibiotic Timing[5]	-	-	99%	99%
Prophylactic Antibiotic Timing (Outpatient)	-	-	98%	98%
Urinary Catheter Removal[5]	-	-	97%	97%
Survey of Patients' Hospital Experiences				
Area Around Room 'Always' Quiet at Night[6]	<100	60%	72%	61%
Doctors 'Always' Communicated Well[6]	<100	87%	85%	82%
Home Recovery Information Given[6]	<100	84%	87%	85%
Hospital Given 9 or 10 on 10 Point Scale[6]	<100	64%	78%	71%
Meds 'Always' Explained Before Given[6]	<100	71%	69%	64%
Nurses 'Always' Communicated Well[6]	<100	81%	83%	79%
Pain 'Always' Well Controlled[6]	<100	76%	72%	71%
Room and Bathroom 'Always' Clean[6]	<100	77%	79%	73%
Timely Help 'Always' Received[6]	<100	77%	77%	68%
Would Definitely Recommend Hospital[6]	<100	68%	76%	71%
Use of Medical Imaging				
Cardiac Imaging Stress Test before Surgery	-	-	4.4%	5.3%
Combination Abdominal CT Scan	-	-	12.5%	10.5%
Combination Brain/Sinus CT Scan	-	-	2%	2.7%
Combination Chest CT Scan	-	-	4.5%	2.7%
Follow-up Mammogram/Ultrasound	-	-	8.7%	8.8%
Lumbar Spine MRI for Low Back Pain	-	-	33%	37.2%

Avera Saint Benedict Health Center

401 West Glynn Drive
Parkston, SD 57366
Phone: 605-928-3311
Fax: 605-928-7368
URL: www.averastbenedict.org
Type: Critical Access Hospitals
Emergency Services: Yes
Ownership: Voluntary non-profit - Private
Beds: 25

Key Personnel:
Emergency Room . . . . Phillip D Barker, DO
Radiology. . . . . Carey Buhler
Intensive Care Unit. . . . . Denise Muntefering
Infection Control. . . . . Brenda Stoebner
Quality Assurance . . . . Brenda Stoebner
Operating Room. . . . . Kynan Trail, RN
Anesthesiology. . . . . Ken Travnick
Chief of Medical Staff. . . . . Toni Vanderpol

Measure	Cases	This Hosp.	State Avg.	U.S. Avg.
Blood Clot Prevention and Treatment				
Anticoagulation Overlap Therapy[5]	-	-	95%	93%
ICU Venous Thromboembolism Prophylaxis[5]	-	-	91%	92%
Incidence of Potentially Preventable VTE[5]	-	-	5%	10%
UFH with Dosages/Platelet Monitoring[5]	-	-	100%	97%
Venous Thromboembolism Prophylaxis[5]	-	-	80%	85%
Warfarin Therapy Discharge Instructions[5]	-	-	70%	75%
Chest Pain/Possible Heart Attack Care				
Aspirin Given Within 24 Hours of Arrival[1,3]	-	-	99%	96%
Fibrinolytic Meds Within 30 Min. of Arrival[3,7]	-	-	69%	58%
Average Time to ECG (minutes)[1,3]	-	-	5	7
Average Time to Transfer (minutes)[3,7]	-	-	66	60
Children's Asthma Care				
Received Home Management Plan of Care	-	-	-	88%
Received Reliever Medication	-	-	-	100%
Received Systemic Corticosteroids	-	-	-	100%
Emergency Department				
Admittance Decision Time (minutes)[1,2]	-	-	41	98
Head CT Results Within 45 Min. of Arrival[3,7]	-	-	44%	57%
Patients Who Left ER Before Being Seen	883	0%	1%	2%
Time from ER Arrival to Admit. (minutes)[1,2]	-	-	174	274
Time from ER Arrival to Discharge (minutes)[3,7]	-	-	113	134
Time in ER Before Being Evaluated (minutes)[1,3]	-	-	18	26
Time to Pain Meds for Fractures (minutes)[3,7]	-	-	44	57
Heart Attack Care				
Aspirin Given at Discharge[1,3]	-	-	100%	99%
Fibrinolytic Meds Within 30 Min. of Arrival[3,7]	-	-	100%	54%
PCI Within 90 Minutes of Arrival[3,7]	-	-	94%	96%
Statin Prescribed at Discharge[1,3]	-	-	98%	98%
Heart Failure Care				
ACE Inhibitor or ARB for LVSD[1,3]	-	-	93%	97%
Discharge Instructions Given[1,3]	-	-	90%	94%
Evaluation of LVS Function[1,3]	-	-	97%	99%
Medicare Spending				
Medicare Spending per Patient (ratio)	-	-	0.9	0.98
Pneumonia Care				
Appropriate Initial Antibiotic Given[1,3]	-	-	90%	95%
Blood Culture Timing[1,3]	-	-	95%	98%
Pregnancy and Delivery Care				
Newborn Deliveries Scheduled Early[1,2]	-	-	7%	6%
Preventive Care				
Immunization for Influenza	28	96%	89%	90%
Immunization for Pneumonia[2,3]	33	100%	89%	92%
Stroke Care				
Anticoagulation Therapy for Atrial Fibrillation[5]	-	-	97%	95%
Antithrombotic Therapy Timing[5]	-	-	98%	98%
Assessed for Rehabilitation[5]	-	-	98%	97%
Discharged on Antithrombotic Therapy[5]	-	-	100%	99%
Discharged on Statin Medication[5]	-	-	93%	94%
Thrombolytic Therapy Timing[5]	-	-	51%	66%
Venous Thromboembolism Prophylaxis[5]	-	-	96%	94%
Written Stroke Educational Materials Given[5]	-	-	85%	88%
Surgical Care Improvement Project				
Appropriate Beta Blocker Usage[5]	-	-	98%	98%
Appropriate VTP Within 24 Hours[5]	-	-	98%	98%
Controlled Postoperative Blood Glucose[5]	-	-	98%	97%
Perioperative Temperature Management[5]	-	-	99%	100%
Prophylactic Antibiotic Selection[5]	-	-	99%	99%
Prophylactic Antibiotic Selection (Outpatient)[5]	-	-	99%	98%
Prophylactic Antibiotic Stopped[5]	-	-	98%	98%
Prophylactic Antibiotic Timing[5]	-	-	99%	99%
Prophylactic Antibiotic Timing (Outpatient)[5]	-	-	98%	98%
Urinary Catheter Removal[5]	-	-	97%	97%
Survey of Patients' Hospital Experiences				
Area Around Room 'Always' Quiet at Night[6]	<100	71%	72%	61%
Doctors 'Always' Communicated Well[6]	<100	82%	85%	82%
Home Recovery Information Given[6]	<100	91%	87%	85%
Hospital Given 9 or 10 on 10 Point Scale[6]	<100	80%	78%	71%
Meds 'Always' Explained Before Given[6]	<100	63%	69%	64%
Nurses 'Always' Communicated Well[6]	<100	77%	83%	79%
Pain 'Always' Well Controlled[6]	<100	59%	72%	71%
Room and Bathroom 'Always' Clean[6]	<100	84%	79%	73%
Timely Help 'Always' Received[6]	<100	68%	77%	68%
Would Definitely Recommend Hospital[6]	<100	87%	76%	71%
Use of Medical Imaging				
Cardiac Imaging Stress Test before Surgery[1]	-	-	4.4%	5.3%
Combination Abdominal CT Scan[1]	-	-	12.5%	10.5%
Combination Brain/Sinus CT Scan	53	0.0%	2%	2.7%
Combination Chest CT Scan[1]	-	-	4.5%	2.7%
Follow-up Mammogram/Ultrasound	211	8.5%	8.7%	8.8%
Lumbar Spine MRI for Low Back Pain[1]	-	-	33%	37.2%

Avera Saint Mary's Hospital

801 E Sioux
Pierre, SD 57501
Phone: 605-224-3100
Fax: 605-224-3429
URL: www.st-marys.com
Type: Acute Care Hospitals
Emergency Services: Yes
Ownership: Voluntary non-profit - Church
Beds: 83

Key Personnel:
Quality Assurance . . . . Anita Baker
Patient Relations . . . . Nick Brandner
CEO/President. . . . . Chad Cooper
Emergency Room . . . . Robin Gadd
Operating Room. . . . . Jackie Neilan
Radiology. . . . . Ben Shoup
Infection Control. . . . . Jeanne Vogel

Measure	Cases	This Hosp.	State Avg.	U.S. Avg.
Blood Clot Prevention and Treatment				
Anticoagulation Overlap Therapy[1,2]	-	-	95%	93%
ICU Venous Thromboembolism Prophylaxis[2]	23	83%	91%	92%

NOTE: Hospital profiles are in alphabetical order by state, then city, then hospital within the city; Rankings exclude hospitals with less than 25 cases except for patient surveys which excludes hospitals with less than 100 cases; (a) 100-299 cases; (1) The number of cases/patients is too few to report; (2) Data submitted were based on a sample of cases/patients; (3) Results are based on a shorter time period than required; (4) Data suppressed by CMS for one or more quarters; (5) Results are not available for this reporting period; (6) Fewer than 100 patients completed the HCAHPS survey; (7) No cases met the criteria for this measure; (8) The lower limit of the confidence interval cannot be calculated if the number of observed infections equals zero; (9) No data are available from the state/territory for this reporting period; (10) The scores shown reflect fewer than 50 completed surveys; (11) There were discrepancies in the data collection process; (12) This measure does not apply to this hospital for this reporting period; (13) Results cannot be calculated for this reporting period; (14) The results for this state are combined with nearby states to protect confidentiality; Please refer to the User's Guide for a full explanation of data.

Measure	Cases	This Hosp.	State Avg.	U.S. Avg.
Incidence of Potentially Preventable VTE[1,2]	-	-	5%	10%
UFH with Dosages/Platelet Monitoring[1,2]	-	-	100%	97%
Venous Thromboembolism Prophylaxis[2]	72	79%	80%	85%
Warfarin Therapy Discharge Instructions[1,2]	-	-	70%	75%
Chest Pain/Possible Heart Attack Care				
Aspirin Given Within 24 Hours of Arrival[3]	23	96%	99%	96%
Fibrinolytic Meds Within 30 Min. of Arrival[1,3]	-	-	69%	58%
Average Time to ECG (minutes)[3]	23	4	5	7
Average Time to Transfer (minutes)[3,7]	-	-	66	60
Children's Asthma Care				
Received Home Management Plan of Care	-	-	-	88%
Received Reliever Medication	-	-	-	100%
Received Systemic Corticosteroids	-	-	-	100%
Emergency Department				
Admittance Decision Time (minutes)[2]	96	61	41	98
Head CT Results Within 45 Min. of Arrival[1]	-	-	44%	57%
Patients Who Left ER Before Being Seen	6,783	0%	1%	2%
Time from ER Arrival to Admit. (minutes)[2]	164	150	174	274
Time from ER Arrival to Discharge (minutes)	488	78	113	134
Time in ER Before Being Evaluated (minutes)	457	19	18	26
Time to Pain Meds for Fractures (minutes)	33	41	44	57
Heart Attack Care				
Aspirin Given at Discharge[1]	-	-	100%	99%
Fibrinolytic Meds Within 30 Min. of Arrival[7]	-	-	100%	54%
PCI Within 90 Minutes of Arrival[7]	-	-	94%	96%
Statin Prescribed at Discharge[1]	-	-	98%	98%
Heart Failure Care				
ACE Inhibitor or ARB for LVSD[1]	-	-	93%	97%
Discharge Instructions Given	20	90%	90%	94%
Evaluation of LVS Function	28	100%	97%	99%
Medicare Spending				
Medicare Spending per Patient (ratio)	-	0.84	0.9	0.98
Pneumonia Care				
Appropriate Initial Antibiotic Given	38	97%	90%	95%
Blood Culture Timing	52	100%	95%	98%
Pregnancy and Delivery Care				
Newborn Deliveries Scheduled Early[2]	29	3%	7%	6%
Preventive Care				
Immunization for Influenza[2]	237	90%	89%	90%
Immunization for Pneumonia[2]	229	98%	89%	92%
Stroke Care				
Anticoagulation Therapy for Atrial Fibrillation[1]	-	-	97%	95%
Antithrombotic Therapy Timing	14	100%	98%	98%
Assessed for Rehabilitation	11	100%	98%	97%
Discharged on Antithrombotic Therapy[1]	-	-	100%	99%
Discharged on Statin Medication[1]	-	-	93%	94%
Thrombolytic Therapy Timing[1]	-	-	51%	66%
Venous Thromboembolism Prophylaxis	15	100%	96%	94%
Written Stroke Educational Materials Given[1]	-	-	85%	88%
Surgical Care Improvement Project				
Appropriate Beta Blocker Usage	47	100%	98%	98%
Appropriate VTP Within 24 Hours	137	96%	98%	98%
Controlled Postoperative Blood Glucose[7]	-	-	98%	97%
Perioperative Temperature Management	149	100%	99%	100%
Prophylactic Antibiotic Selection	120	99%	99%	99%
Prophylactic Antibiotic Selection (Outpatient)[3]	20	100%	99%	98%
Prophylactic Antibiotic Stopped	116	99%	98%	98%
Prophylactic Antibiotic Timing	121	100%	99%	99%
Prophylactic Antibiotic Timing (Outpatient)[3]	11	100%	98%	98%
Urinary Catheter Removal	21	100%	97%	97%
Survey of Patients' Hospital Experiences				
Area Around Room 'Always' Quiet at Night	300+	59%	72%	61%
Doctors 'Always' Communicated Well	300+	81%	85%	82%
Home Recovery Information Given	300+	86%	87%	85%
Hospital Given 9 or 10 on 10 Point Scale	300+	66%	78%	71%
Meds 'Always' Explained Before Given	300+	63%	69%	64%
Nurses 'Always' Communicated Well	300+	76%	83%	79%
Pain 'Always' Well Controlled	300+	65%	72%	71%
Room and Bathroom 'Always' Clean	300+	66%	79%	73%
Timely Help 'Always' Received	300+	69%	77%	68%
Would Definitely Recommend Hospital	300+	63%	76%	71%
Use of Medical Imaging				
Cardiac Imaging Stress Test before Surgery	107	5.6%	4.4%	5.3%
Combination Abdominal CT Scan	220	65.9%	12.5%	10.5%
Combination Brain/Sinus CT Scan[1]	-	-	2%	2.7%
Combination Chest CT Scan	174	1.7%	4.5%	2.7%
Follow-up Mammogram/Ultrasound	700	7.0%	8.7%	8.8%
Lumbar Spine MRI for Low Back Pain[1]	-	-	33%	37.2%

PHS Indian Hospital at Pine Ridge

East Highway 18
Pine Ridge, SD 57770
URL: www.ihs.gov
Type: Acute Care Hospitals
Ownership: Government - Federal
Phone: 605-867-5131
Fax: 605-867-3271
Emergency Services: Yes
Beds: 45

Key Personnel:
Quality Assurance . . . . Kathey Wilson Ecoffey
Chief of Medical Staff . . . . Andy Hurst, MD
Infection Control . . . . Alice Sierra

Measure	Cases	This Hosp.	State Avg.	U.S. Avg.
Blood Clot Prevention and Treatment				
Anticoagulation Overlap Therapy[2,7]	-	-	95%	93%
ICU Venous Thromboembolism Prophylaxis[2,7]	-	-	91%	92%
Incidence of Potentially Preventable VTE[2,7]	-	-	5%	10%
UFH with Dosages/Platelet Monitoring[2,7]	-	-	100%	97%
Venous Thromboembolism Prophylaxis[2]	145	0%	80%	85%
Warfarin Therapy Discharge Instructions[1,2]	-	-	70%	75%
Chest Pain/Possible Heart Attack Care				
Aspirin Given Within 24 Hours of Arrival	-	-	99%	96%
Fibrinolytic Meds Within 30 Min. of Arrival	-	-	69%	58%
Average Time to ECG (minutes)	-	-	5	7
Average Time to Transfer (minutes)	-	-	66	60
Children's Asthma Care				
Received Home Management Plan of Care	-	-	-	88%
Received Reliever Medication	-	-	-	100%
Received Systemic Corticosteroids	-	-	-	100%
Emergency Department				
Admittance Decision Time (minutes)[2]	175	53	41	98
Head CT Results Within 45 Min. of Arrival	-	-	44%	57%
Patients Who Left ER Before Being Seen	-	-	1%	2%
Time from ER Arrival to Admit. (minutes)[2]	268	267	174	274
Time from ER Arrival to Discharge (minutes)	-	-	113	134
Time in ER Before Being Evaluated (minutes)	-	-	18	26
Time to Pain Meds for Fractures (minutes)	-	-	44	57
Heart Attack Care				
Aspirin Given at Discharge[3,7]	-	-	100%	99%
Fibrinolytic Meds Within 30 Min. of Arrival[3,7]	-	-	100%	54%
PCI Within 90 Minutes of Arrival[3,7]	-	-	94%	96%
Statin Prescribed at Discharge[3,7]	-	-	98%	98%
Heart Failure Care				
ACE Inhibitor or ARB for LVSD[1,2]	-	-	93%	97%
Discharge Instructions Given[1,2]	-	-	90%	94%
Evaluation of LVS Function[1,2]	-	-	97%	99%
Medicare Spending				
Medicare Spending per Patient (ratio)	-	0.69	0.9	0.98
Pneumonia Care				
Appropriate Initial Antibiotic Given[1,2]	-	-	90%	95%
Blood Culture Timing[2]	21	81%	95%	98%
Pregnancy and Delivery Care				
Newborn Deliveries Scheduled Early	84	17%	7%	6%
Preventive Care				
Immunization for Influenza[2]	245	53%	89%	90%
Immunization for Pneumonia[2]	159	84%	89%	92%
Stroke Care				
Anticoagulation Therapy for Atrial Fibrillation[3,7]	-	-	97%	95%
Antithrombotic Therapy Timing[3,7]	-	-	98%	98%
Assessed for Rehabilitation[1,3]	-	-	98%	97%
Discharged on Antithrombotic Therapy[1,3]	-	-	100%	99%
Discharged on Statin Medication[1,3]	-	-	93%	94%
Thrombolytic Therapy Timing[3,7]	-	-	51%	66%
Venous Thromboembolism Prophylaxis[3,7]	-	-	96%	94%
Written Stroke Educational Materials Given[1,3]	-	-	85%	88%
Surgical Care Improvement Project				
Appropriate Beta Blocker Usage[1,2]	-	-	98%	98%
Appropriate VTP Within 24 Hours[1,2]	-	-	98%	98%
Controlled Postoperative Blood Glucose[2,7]	-	-	98%	97%
Perioperative Temperature Management[1,2]	-	-	99%	100%
Prophylactic Antibiotic Selection[1,2]	-	-	99%	99%
Prophylactic Antibiotic Selection (Outpatient)	-	-	99%	98%
Prophylactic Antibiotic Stopped[1,2]	-	-	98%	98%
Prophylactic Antibiotic Timing[1,2]	-	-	99%	99%
Prophylactic Antibiotic Timing (Outpatient)	-	-	98%	98%
Urinary Catheter Removal[1,2]	-	-	97%	97%
Survey of Patients' Hospital Experiences				
Area Around Room 'Always' Quiet at Night[6,11]	<100	66%	72%	61%
Doctors 'Always' Communicated Well[6,11]	<100	77%	85%	82%
Home Recovery Information Given[6,11]	<100	78%	87%	85%
Hospital Given 9 or 10 on 10 Point Scale[6,11]	<100	50%	78%	71%
Meds 'Always' Explained Before Given[6,11]	<100	62%	69%	64%
Nurses 'Always' Communicated Well[6,11]	<100	67%	83%	79%
Pain 'Always' Well Controlled[6,11]	<100	68%	72%	71%
Room and Bathroom 'Always' Clean[6,11]	<100	65%	79%	73%
Timely Help 'Always' Received[6,11]	<100	65%	77%	68%
Would Definitely Recommend Hospital[6,11]	<100	21%	76%	71%
Use of Medical Imaging				
Cardiac Imaging Stress Test before Surgery	-	-	4.4%	5.3%
Combination Abdominal CT Scan	-	-	12.5%	10.5%
Combination Brain/Sinus CT Scan	-	-	2%	2.7%
Combination Chest CT Scan	-	-	4.5%	2.7%
Follow-up Mammogram/Ultrasound	-	-	8.7%	8.8%
Lumbar Spine MRI for Low Back Pain	-	-	33%	37.2%

Platte Health Center

601 E 7th St
Platte, SD 57369
Type: Critical Access Hospitals
Ownership: Government - Local
Phone: 605-337-3364
Fax: 605-337-2670
Emergency Services: Yes
Beds: 15

Key Personnel:
Radiology. . . . . Calvin Andersen
Chief of Medical Staff . . . . John Bentv
Emergency Room . . . . Jerome Bentz, MD
CEO/President. . . . . Mark Burkett
Operating Room. . . . . Linda Fito
Quality Assurance . . . . Nancy Nachtigal
Infection Control. . . . . Jan Stahnke
Cardiology . . . . Galen N. Vonk

Measure	Cases	This Hosp.	State Avg.	U.S. Avg.
Blood Clot Prevention and Treatment				
Anticoagulation Overlap Therapy[5]	-	-	95%	93%
ICU Venous Thromboembolism Prophylaxis[5]	-	-	91%	92%
Incidence of Potentially Preventable VTE[5]	-	-	5%	10%
UFH with Dosages/Platelet Monitoring[5]	-	-	100%	97%
Venous Thromboembolism Prophylaxis[5]	-	-	80%	85%
Warfarin Therapy Discharge Instructions[5]	-	-	70%	75%
Chest Pain/Possible Heart Attack Care				
Aspirin Given Within 24 Hours of Arrival[5]	-	-	99%	96%
Fibrinolytic Meds Within 30 Min. of Arrival[5]	-	-	69%	58%
Average Time to ECG (minutes)[5]	-	-	5	7
Average Time to Transfer (minutes)[5]	-	-	66	60
Children's Asthma Care				
Received Home Management Plan of Care	-	-	-	88%
Received Reliever Medication	-	-	-	100%
Received Systemic Corticosteroids	-	-	-	100%
Emergency Department				
Admittance Decision Time (minutes)[5]	-	-	41	98
Head CT Results Within 45 Min. of Arrival[5]	-	-	44%	57%
Patients Who Left ER Before Being Seen	614	0%	1%	2%
Time from ER Arrival to Admit. (minutes)[5]	-	-	174	274
Time from ER Arrival to Discharge (minutes)[5]	-	-	113	134
Time in ER Before Being Evaluated (minutes)[5]	-	-	18	26
Time to Pain Meds for Fractures (minutes)[5]	-	-	44	57
Heart Attack Care				
Aspirin Given at Discharge[1,3]	-	-	100%	99%
Fibrinolytic Meds Within 30 Min. of Arrival[3,7]	-	-	100%	54%
PCI Within 90 Minutes of Arrival[3,7]	-	-	94%	96%
Statin Prescribed at Discharge[1,3]	-	-	98%	98%
Heart Failure Care				
ACE Inhibitor or ARB for LVSD[3,7]	-	-	93%	97%
Discharge Instructions Given[1,3]	-	-	90%	94%

NOTE: Hospital profiles are in alphabetical order by state, then city, then hospital within the city; Rankings exclude hospitals with less than 25 cases except for patient surveys which excludes hospitals with less than 100 cases; (a) 100-299 cases; (1) The number of cases/patients is too few to report; (2) Data submitted were based on a sample of cases/patients; (3) Results are based on a shorter time period than required; (4) Data suppressed by CMS for one or more quarters; (5) Results are not available for this reporting period; (6) Fewer than 100 patients completed the HCAHPS survey; (7) No cases met the criteria for this measure; (8) The lower limit of the confidence interval cannot be calculated if the number of observed infections equals zero; (9) No data are available from the state/territory for this reporting period; (10) The scores shown reflect fewer than 50 completed surveys; (11) There were discrepancies in the data collection process; (12) This measure does not apply to this hospital for this reporting period; (13) Results cannot be calculated for this reporting period; (14) The results for this state are combined with nearby states to protect confidentiality; Please refer to the User's Guide for a full explanation of data.

Measure	Cases	This Hosp.	State Avg.	U.S. Avg.
Evaluation of LVS Function[1,3]	-	-	97%	99%
Medicare Spending				
Medicare Spending per Patient (ratio)	-	-	0.9	0.98
Pneumonia Care				
Appropriate Initial Antibiotic Given[1]	-	-	90%	95%
Blood Culture Timing[1]	-	-	95%	98%
Pregnancy and Delivery Care				
Newborn Deliveries Scheduled Early[5]	-	-	7%	6%
Preventive Care				
Immunization for Influenza[5]	-	-	89%	90%
Immunization for Pneumonia[5]	-	-	89%	92%
Stroke Care				
Anticoagulation Therapy for Atrial Fibrillation[5]	-	-	97%	95%
Antithrombotic Therapy Timing[5]	-	-	98%	98%
Assessed for Rehabilitation[5]	-	-	98%	97%
Discharged on Antithrombotic Therapy[5]	-	-	100%	99%
Discharged on Statin Medication[5]	-	-	93%	94%
Thrombolytic Therapy Timing[5]	-	-	51%	66%
Venous Thromboembolism Prophylaxis[5]	-	-	96%	94%
Written Stroke Educational Materials Given[5]	-	-	85%	88%
Surgical Care Improvement Project				
Appropriate Beta Blocker Usage[5]	-	-	98%	98%
Appropriate VTP Within 24 Hours[5]	-	-	98%	98%
Controlled Postoperative Blood Glucose[5]	-	-	98%	97%
Perioperative Temperature Management[5]	-	-	99%	100%
Prophylactic Antibiotic Selection[5]	-	-	99%	99%
Prophylactic Antibiotic Selection (Outpatient)[5]	-	-	99%	98%
Prophylactic Antibiotic Stopped[5]	-	-	98%	98%
Prophylactic Antibiotic Timing[5]	-	-	99%	99%
Prophylactic Antibiotic Timing (Outpatient)[5]	-	-	98%	98%
Urinary Catheter Removal[5]	-	-	97%	97%
Survey of Patients' Hospital Experiences				
Area Around Room 'Always' Quiet at Night[10]	<100	71%	72%	61%
Doctors 'Always' Communicated Well[10]	<100	80%	85%	82%
Home Recovery Information Given[10]	<100	96%	87%	85%
Hospital Given 9 or 10 on 10 Point Scale[10]	<100	88%	78%	71%
Meds 'Always' Explained Before Given[10]	<100	60%	69%	64%
Nurses 'Always' Communicated Well[10]	<100	77%	83%	79%
Pain 'Always' Well Controlled[10]	<100	66%	72%	71%
Room and Bathroom 'Always' Clean[10]	<100	81%	79%	73%
Timely Help 'Always' Received[10]	<100	70%	77%	68%
Would Definitely Recommend Hospital[10]	<100	82%	76%	71%
Use of Medical Imaging				
Cardiac Imaging Stress Test before Surgery[1]	-	-	4.4%	5.3%
Combination Abdominal CT Scan[1]	-	-	12.5%	10.5%
Combination Brain/Sinus CT Scan[1]	-	-	2%	2.7%
Combination Chest CT Scan[1]	-	-	4.5%	2.7%
Follow-up Mammogram/Ultrasound	120	7.5%	8.7%	8.8%
Lumbar Spine MRI for Low Back Pain[1]	-	-	33%	37.2%

Black Hills Surgical Hospital

216 Anamaria Dr
Rapid City, SD 57703
Phone: 605-721-4700
URL: www.bhsh.com
Type: Acute Care Hospitals
Emergency Services: No
Ownership: Proprietary

Key Personnel:

Chief of Medical Staff.......... Dave Johnson, MD
CEO/President.............. William May
Patient Relations .... Debbie Mertes
Radiology.................. Nicholas Wilson

Measure	Cases	This Hosp.	State Avg.	U.S. Avg.
Blood Clot Prevention and Treatment				
Anticoagulation Overlap Therapy[1,2]	-	-	95%	93%
ICU Venous Thromboembolism Prophylaxis[2,7]	-	-	91%	92%
Incidence of Potentially Preventable VTE[1,2]	-	-	5%	10%
UFH with Dosages/Platelet Monitoring[1,2]	-	-	100%	97%
Venous Thromboembolism Prophylaxis[2]	105	100%	80%	85%
Warfarin Therapy Discharge Instructions[1,2]	-	-	70%	75%
Chest Pain/Possible Heart Attack Care				
Aspirin Given Within 24 Hours of Arrival[5]	-	-	99%	96%
Fibrinolytic Meds Within 30 Min. of Arrival[5]	-	-	69%	58%
Average Time to ECG (minutes)[5]	-	-	5	7
Average Time to Transfer (minutes)[5]	-	-	66	60
Children's Asthma Care				
Received Home Management Plan of Care	-	-	-	88%
Received Reliever Medication	-	-	-	100%
Received Systemic Corticosteroids	-	-	-	100%
Emergency Department				
Admittance Decision Time (minutes)[2,7]	-	-	41	98
Head CT Results Within 45 Min. of Arrival[5]	-	-	44%	57%
Patients Who Left ER Before Being Seen[5]	-	-	1%	2%
Time from ER Arrival to Admit. (minutes)[2,7]	-	-	174	274
Time from ER Arrival to Discharge (minutes)[5]	-	-	113	134
Time in ER Before Being Evaluated (minutes)[5]	-	-	18	26
Time to Pain Meds for Fractures (minutes)[5]	-	-	44	57
Heart Attack Care				
Aspirin Given at Discharge[5]	-	-	100%	99%
Fibrinolytic Meds Within 30 Min. of Arrival[5]	-	-	100%	54%
PCI Within 90 Minutes of Arrival[5]	-	-	94%	96%
Statin Prescribed at Discharge[5]	-	-	98%	98%
Heart Failure Care				
ACE Inhibitor or ARB for LVSD[5]	-	-	93%	97%
Discharge Instructions Given[5]	-	-	90%	94%
Evaluation of LVS Function[5]	-	-	97%	99%
Medicare Spending				
Medicare Spending per Patient (ratio)	-	0.89	0.9	0.98
Pneumonia Care				
Appropriate Initial Antibiotic Given[5]	-	-	90%	95%
Blood Culture Timing[5]	-	-	95%	98%
Pregnancy and Delivery Care				
Newborn Deliveries Scheduled Early[7]	-	-	7%	6%
Preventive Care				
Immunization for Influenza[2]	406	98%	89%	90%
Immunization for Pneumonia[2]	408	98%	89%	92%
Stroke Care				
Anticoagulation Therapy for Atrial Fibrillation[5]	-	-	97%	95%
Antithrombotic Therapy Timing[5]	-	-	98%	98%
Assessed for Rehabilitation[5]	-	-	98%	97%
Discharged on Antithrombotic Therapy[5]	-	-	100%	99%
Discharged on Statin Medication[5]	-	-	93%	94%
Thrombolytic Therapy Timing[5]	-	-	51%	66%
Venous Thromboembolism Prophylaxis[5]	-	-	96%	94%
Written Stroke Educational Materials Given[5]	-	-	85%	88%
Surgical Care Improvement Project				
Appropriate Beta Blocker Usage[2]	56	98%	98%	98%
Appropriate VTP Within 24 Hours[2]	236	99%	98%	98%
Controlled Postoperative Blood Glucose[2,7]	-	-	98%	97%
Perioperative Temperature Management[2]	261	100%	99%	100%
Prophylactic Antibiotic Selection[2]	214	100%	99%	99%
Prophylactic Antibiotic Selection (Outpatient)	512	100%	99%	98%
Prophylactic Antibiotic Stopped[2]	213	100%	98%	98%
Prophylactic Antibiotic Timing[2]	214	100%	99%	99%
Prophylactic Antibiotic Timing (Outpatient)	512	100%	98%	98%
Urinary Catheter Removal[2]	218	100%	97%	97%
Survey of Patients' Hospital Experiences				
Area Around Room 'Always' Quiet at Night	300+	90%	72%	61%
Doctors 'Always' Communicated Well	300+	88%	85%	82%
Home Recovery Information Given	300+	93%	87%	85%
Hospital Given 9 or 10 on 10 Point Scale	300+	91%	78%	71%
Meds 'Always' Explained Before Given	300+	76%	69%	64%
Nurses 'Always' Communicated Well	300+	88%	83%	79%
Pain 'Always' Well Controlled	300+	78%	72%	71%
Room and Bathroom 'Always' Clean	300+	86%	79%	73%
Timely Help 'Always' Received	300+	91%	77%	68%
Would Definitely Recommend Hospital	300+	92%	76%	71%
Use of Medical Imaging				
Cardiac Imaging Stress Test before Surgery[7]	-	-	4.4%	5.3%
Combination Abdominal CT Scan	34	50.0%	12.5%	10.5%
Combination Brain/Sinus CT Scan[1]	-	-	2%	2.7%
Combination Chest CT Scan[1]	-	-	4.5%	2.7%
Follow-up Mammogram/Ultrasound[7]	-	-	8.7%	8.8%
Lumbar Spine MRI for Low Back Pain	384	36.5%	33%	37.2%

PHS Indian Hospital at Rapid City

3200 Canyon Lake Dr
Rapid City, SD 57702
Phone: 605-355-2500
Fax: 605-355-2504
URL: www.ihs.gov
Type: Acute Care Hospitals
Emergency Services: Yes
Ownership: Government - Federal
Beds: 32

Measure	Cases	This Hosp.	State Avg.	U.S. Avg.
Blood Clot Prevention and Treatment				
Anticoagulation Overlap Therapy[2,7]	-	-	95%	93%
ICU Venous Thromboembolism Prophylaxis[2,7]	-	-	91%	92%
Incidence of Potentially Preventable VTE[2,7]	-	-	5%	10%
UFH with Dosages/Platelet Monitoring[2,7]	-	-	100%	97%
Venous Thromboembolism Prophylaxis[2]	24	0%	80%	85%
Warfarin Therapy Discharge Instructions[2,7]	-	-	70%	75%
Chest Pain/Possible Heart Attack Care				
Aspirin Given Within 24 Hours of Arrival	-	-	99%	96%
Fibrinolytic Meds Within 30 Min. of Arrival	-	-	69%	58%
Average Time to ECG (minutes)	-	-	5	7
Average Time to Transfer (minutes)	-	-	66	60
Children's Asthma Care				
Received Home Management Plan of Care	-	-	-	88%
Received Reliever Medication	-	-	-	100%
Received Systemic Corticosteroids	-	-	-	100%
Emergency Department				
Admittance Decision Time (minutes)[2]	15	38	41	98
Head CT Results Within 45 Min. of Arrival	-	-	44%	57%
Patients Who Left ER Before Being Seen	-	-	1%	2%
Time from ER Arrival to Admit. (minutes)[2]	19	193	174	274
Time from ER Arrival to Discharge (minutes)	-	-	113	134
Time in ER Before Being Evaluated (minutes)	-	-	18	26
Time to Pain Meds for Fractures (minutes)	-	-	44	57
Heart Attack Care				
Aspirin Given at Discharge[5]	-	-	100%	99%
Fibrinolytic Meds Within 30 Min. of Arrival[5]	-	-	100%	54%
PCI Within 90 Minutes of Arrival[5]	-	-	94%	96%
Statin Prescribed at Discharge[5]	-	-	98%	98%
Heart Failure Care				
ACE Inhibitor or ARB for LVSD[5]	-	-	93%	97%
Discharge Instructions Given[5]	-	-	90%	94%
Evaluation of LVS Function[5]	-	-	97%	99%
Medicare Spending				
Medicare Spending per Patient (ratio)	-	-	0.9	0.98
Pneumonia Care				
Appropriate Initial Antibiotic Given[2,3]	-	-	90%	95%
Blood Culture Timing[2,3]	-	-	95%	98%
Pregnancy and Delivery Care				
Newborn Deliveries Scheduled Early[2,7]	-	-	7%	6%
Preventive Care				
Immunization for Influenza[2]	29	86%	89%	90%
Immunization for Pneumonia[2]	20	100%	89%	92%
Stroke Care				
Anticoagulation Therapy for Atrial Fibrillation[5]	-	-	97%	95%
Antithrombotic Therapy Timing[5]	-	-	98%	98%
Assessed for Rehabilitation[5]	-	-	98%	97%
Discharged on Antithrombotic Therapy[5]	-	-	100%	99%
Discharged on Statin Medication[5]	-	-	93%	94%
Thrombolytic Therapy Timing[5]	-	-	51%	66%
Venous Thromboembolism Prophylaxis[5]	-	-	96%	94%
Written Stroke Educational Materials Given[5]	-	-	85%	88%
Surgical Care Improvement Project				
Appropriate Beta Blocker Usage[5]	-	-	98%	98%
Appropriate VTP Within 24 Hours[5]	-	-	98%	98%
Controlled Postoperative Blood Glucose[5]	-	-	98%	97%
Perioperative Temperature Management[5]	-	-	99%	100%
Prophylactic Antibiotic Selection[5]	-	-	99%	99%
Prophylactic Antibiotic Selection (Outpatient)	-	-	99%	98%
Prophylactic Antibiotic Stopped[5]	-	-	98%	98%
Prophylactic Antibiotic Timing[5]	-	-	99%	99%
Prophylactic Antibiotic Timing (Outpatient)	-	-	98%	98%
Urinary Catheter Removal[5]	-	-	97%	97%
Survey of Patients' Hospital Experiences				
Area Around Room 'Always' Quiet at Night[10]	<100	100%	72%	61%

NOTE: Hospital profiles are in alphabetical order by state, then city, then hospital within the city; Rankings exclude hospitals with less than 25 cases except for patient surveys which excludes hospitals with less than 100 cases; (a) 100-299 cases; (1) The number of cases/patients is too few to report; (2) Data submitted were based on a sample of cases/patients; (3) Results are based on a shorter time period than required; (4) Data suppressed by CMS for one or more quarters; (5) Results are not available for this reporting period; (6) Fewer than 100 patients completed the HCAHPS survey; (7) No cases met the criteria for this measure; (8) The lower limit of the confidence interval cannot be calculated if the number of observed infections equals zero; (9) No data are available from the state/territory for this reporting period; (10) The scores shown reflect fewer than 50 completed surveys; (11) There were discrepancies in the data collection process; (12) This measure does not apply to this hospital for this reporting period; (13) Results cannot be calculated for this reporting period; (14) The results for this state are combined with nearby states to protect confidentiality; Please refer to the User's Guide for a full explanation of data.

Measure	Cases	This Hosp.	State Avg.	U.S. Avg.
Doctors 'Always' Communicated Well[10]	<100	100%	85%	82%
Home Recovery Information Given[10]	<100	-	87%	85%
Hospital Given 9 or 10 on 10 Point Scale[10]	<100	100%	78%	71%
Meds 'Always' Explained Before Given[10]	<100	100%	69%	64%
Nurses 'Always' Communicated Well[10]	<100	100%	83%	79%
Pain 'Always' Well Controlled[10]	<100	88%	72%	71%
Room and Bathroom 'Always' Clean[10]	<100	100%	79%	73%
Timely Help 'Always' Received[10]	<100	91%	77%	68%
Would Definitely Recommend Hospital[10]	<100	100%	76%	71%
Use of Medical Imaging				
Cardiac Imaging Stress Test before Surgery	-	-	4.4%	5.3%
Combination Abdominal CT Scan	-	-	12.5%	10.5%
Combination Brain/Sinus CT Scan	-	-	2%	2.7%
Combination Chest CT Scan	-	-	4.5%	2.7%
Follow-up Mammogram/Ultrasound	-	-	8.7%	8.8%
Lumbar Spine MRI for Low Back Pain	-	-	33%	37.2%

Rapid City Regional Hospital

353 Fairmont Blvd Post Office Box 6000
Rapid City, SD 57701
Phone: 605-719-1000
Fax: 605-719-8053
E-mail: humanresources@rcrh.org
URL: www.rcrh.org
Type: Acute Care Hospitals
Emergency Services: Yes
Ownership: Voluntary non-profit - Private
Beds: 310

Key Personnel:

Chief of Medical Staff.......... David Klocke, MD
Quality Assurance .... Mary Masten
Cardiac Laboratory............ Alex Schabauer
Intensive Care Unit............ Sherry Smith
CEO/President................ Timothy Sughrue
Operating Room............... Marcia Taylor

Measure	Cases	This Hosp.	State Avg.	U.S. Avg.
Blood Clot Prevention and Treatment				
Anticoagulation Overlap Therapy[2]	131	95%	95%	93%
ICU Venous Thromboembolism Prophylaxis[2]	89	98%	91%	92%
Incidence of Potentially Preventable VTE[2]	33	9%	5%	10%
UFH with Dosages/Platelet Monitoring[2]	62	100%	100%	97%
Venous Thromboembolism Prophylaxis[2]	357	90%	80%	85%
Warfarin Therapy Discharge Instructions[2]	85	9%	70%	75%
Chest Pain/Possible Heart Attack Care				
Aspirin Given Within 24 Hours of Arrival[5]	-	-	99%	96%
Fibrinolytic Meds Within 30 Min. of Arrival[5]	-	-	69%	58%
Average Time to ECG (minutes)[5]	-	-	5	7
Average Time to Transfer (minutes)[5]	-	-	66	60
Children's Asthma Care				
Received Home Management Plan of Care	-	-	-	88%
Received Reliever Medication	-	-	-	100%
Received Systemic Corticosteroids	-	-	-	100%
Emergency Department				
Admittance Decision Time (minutes)[2]	513	84	41	98
Head CT Results Within 45 Min. of Arrival[1]	-	-	44%	57%
Patients Who Left ER Before Being Seen	51,454	1%	1%	2%
Time from ER Arrival to Admit. (minutes)[2]	536	224	174	274
Time from ER Arrival to Discharge (minutes)	385	112	113	134
Time in ER Before Being Evaluated (minutes)	404	27	18	26
Time to Pain Meds for Fractures (minutes)	170	62	44	57
Heart Attack Care				
Aspirin Given at Discharge	398	100%	100%	99%
Fibrinolytic Meds Within 30 Min. of Arrival[7]	-	-	100%	54%
PCI Within 90 Minutes of Arrival	45	89%	94%	96%
Statin Prescribed at Discharge	399	99%	98%	98%
Heart Failure Care				
ACE Inhibitor or ARB for LVSD	102	98%	93%	97%
Discharge Instructions Given	313	80%	90%	94%
Evaluation of LVS Function	372	99%	97%	99%
Medicare Spending				
Medicare Spending per Patient (ratio)	-	0.98	0.9	0.98
Pneumonia Care				
Appropriate Initial Antibiotic Given	187	96%	90%	95%
Blood Culture Timing	290	96%	95%	98%
Pregnancy and Delivery Care				
Newborn Deliveries Scheduled Early[2]	59	3%	7%	6%
Preventive Care				
Immunization for Influenza[2]	546	88%	89%	90%
Immunization for Pneumonia[2]	589	88%	89%	92%
Stroke Care				
Anticoagulation Therapy for Atrial Fibrillation	22	100%	97%	95%
Antithrombotic Therapy Timing	129	100%	98%	98%
Assessed for Rehabilitation	147	99%	98%	97%
Discharged on Antithrombotic Therapy	133	100%	100%	99%
Discharged on Statin Medication	101	96%	93%	94%
Thrombolytic Therapy Timing[1]	-	-	51%	66%
Venous Thromboembolism Prophylaxis	160	98%	96%	94%
Written Stroke Educational Materials Given	84	87%	85%	88%
Surgical Care Improvement Project				
Appropriate Beta Blocker Usage[2]	227	99%	98%	98%
Appropriate VTP Within 24 Hours[2]	296	96%	98%	98%
Controlled Postoperative Blood Glucose[2]	118	97%	98%	97%
Perioperative Temperature Management[2]	400	98%	99%	100%
Prophylactic Antibiotic Selection[2]	316	99%	99%	99%
Prophylactic Antibiotic Selection (Outpatient)	288	99%	99%	98%
Prophylactic Antibiotic Stopped[2]	300	96%	98%	98%
Prophylactic Antibiotic Timing[2]	316	99%	99%	99%
Prophylactic Antibiotic Timing (Outpatient)	291	95%	98%	98%
Urinary Catheter Removal[2]	246	89%	97%	97%
Survey of Patients' Hospital Experiences				
Area Around Room 'Always' Quiet at Night	300+	54%	72%	61%
Doctors 'Always' Communicated Well	300+	79%	85%	82%
Home Recovery Information Given	300+	88%	87%	85%
Hospital Given 9 or 10 on 10 Point Scale	300+	68%	78%	71%
Meds 'Always' Explained Before Given	300+	64%	69%	64%
Nurses 'Always' Communicated Well	300+	78%	83%	79%
Pain 'Always' Well Controlled	300+	70%	72%	71%
Room and Bathroom 'Always' Clean	300+	70%	79%	73%
Timely Help 'Always' Received	300+	71%	77%	68%
Would Definitely Recommend Hospital	300+	69%	76%	71%
Use of Medical Imaging				
Cardiac Imaging Stress Test before Surgery	1,278	3.8%	4.4%	5.3%
Combination Abdominal CT Scan	939	5.1%	12.5%	10.5%
Combination Brain/Sinus CT Scan	619	2.9%	2%	2.7%
Combination Chest CT Scan	627	0.0%	4.5%	2.7%
Follow-up Mammogram/Ultrasound	370	8.4%	8.7%	8.8%
Lumbar Spine MRI for Low Back Pain	114	30.7%	33%	37.2%

Same Day Surgery Center

651 Cathedral Drive
Rapid City, SD 57701
Phone: 605-755-9900
Fax: 605-719-5055
URL: www.samedaysurgerycenter.org
Type: Acute Care Hospitals
Emergency Services: No
Ownership: Proprietary
Beds: 8

Key Personnel:

CEO/President................ Doris Fritts

Measure	Cases	This Hosp.	State Avg.	U.S. Avg.
Blood Clot Prevention and Treatment				
Anticoagulation Overlap Therapy[2,7]	-	-	95%	93%
ICU Venous Thromboembolism Prophylaxis[1,2]	-	-	91%	92%
Incidence of Potentially Preventable VTE[2,7]	-	-	5%	10%
UFH with Dosages/Platelet Monitoring[2,7]	-	-	100%	97%
Venous Thromboembolism Prophylaxis[2]	16	94%	80%	85%
Warfarin Therapy Discharge Instructions[2,7]	-	-	70%	75%
Chest Pain/Possible Heart Attack Care				
Aspirin Given Within 24 Hours of Arrival[5]	-	-	99%	96%
Fibrinolytic Meds Within 30 Min. of Arrival[5]	-	-	69%	58%
Average Time to ECG (minutes)[5]	-	-	5	7
Average Time to Transfer (minutes)[5]	-	-	66	60
Children's Asthma Care				
Received Home Management Plan of Care	-	-	-	88%
Received Reliever Medication	-	-	-	100%
Received Systemic Corticosteroids	-	-	-	100%
Emergency Department				
Admittance Decision Time (minutes)[2,7]	-	-	41	98
Head CT Results Within 45 Min. of Arrival[5]	-	-	44%	57%
Patients Who Left ER Before Being Seen[5]	-	-	1%	2%
Time from ER Arrival to Admit. (minutes)[2,7]	-	-	174	274
Time from ER Arrival to Discharge (minutes)[5]	-	-	113	134
Time in ER Before Being Evaluated (minutes)[5]	-	-	18	26
Time to Pain Meds for Fractures (minutes)[5]	-	-	44	57
Heart Attack Care				
Aspirin Given at Discharge[5]	-	-	100%	99%
Fibrinolytic Meds Within 30 Min. of Arrival[5]	-	-	100%	54%
PCI Within 90 Minutes of Arrival[5]	-	-	94%	96%
Statin Prescribed at Discharge[5]	-	-	98%	98%
Heart Failure Care				
ACE Inhibitor or ARB for LVSD[5]	-	-	93%	97%
Discharge Instructions Given[5]	-	-	90%	94%
Evaluation of LVS Function[5]	-	-	97%	99%
Medicare Spending				
Medicare Spending per Patient (ratio)[1]	-	-	0.9	0.98
Pneumonia Care				
Appropriate Initial Antibiotic Given[5]	-	-	90%	95%
Blood Culture Timing[5]	-	-	95%	98%
Pregnancy and Delivery Care				
Newborn Deliveries Scheduled Early[7]	-	-	7%	6%
Preventive Care				
Immunization for Influenza[2]	55	84%	89%	90%
Immunization for Pneumonia[2]	32	50%	89%	92%
Stroke Care				
Anticoagulation Therapy for Atrial Fibrillation[5]	-	-	97%	95%
Antithrombotic Therapy Timing[5]	-	-	98%	98%
Assessed for Rehabilitation[5]	-	-	98%	97%
Discharged on Antithrombotic Therapy[5]	-	-	100%	99%
Discharged on Statin Medication[5]	-	-	93%	94%
Thrombolytic Therapy Timing[5]	-	-	51%	66%
Venous Thromboembolism Prophylaxis[5]	-	-	96%	94%
Written Stroke Educational Materials Given[5]	-	-	85%	88%
Surgical Care Improvement Project				
Appropriate Beta Blocker Usage[1,2]	-	-	98%	98%
Appropriate VTP Within 24 Hours[2]	17	100%	98%	98%
Controlled Postoperative Blood Glucose[2,7]	-	-	98%	97%
Perioperative Temperature Management[2]	32	100%	99%	100%
Prophylactic Antibiotic Selection[2]	30	93%	99%	99%
Prophylactic Antibiotic Selection (Outpatient)	176	97%	99%	98%
Prophylactic Antibiotic Stopped[2]	30	97%	98%	98%
Prophylactic Antibiotic Timing[2]	30	93%	99%	99%
Prophylactic Antibiotic Timing (Outpatient)	178	98%	98%	98%
Urinary Catheter Removal[2,7]	-	-	97%	97%
Survey of Patients' Hospital Experiences				
Area Around Room 'Always' Quiet at Night[6]	<100	89%	72%	61%
Doctors 'Always' Communicated Well[6]	<100	93%	85%	82%
Home Recovery Information Given[6]	<100	87%	87%	85%
Hospital Given 9 or 10 on 10 Point Scale[6]	<100	94%	78%	71%
Meds 'Always' Explained Before Given[6]	<100	85%	69%	64%
Nurses 'Always' Communicated Well[6]	<100	93%	83%	79%
Pain 'Always' Well Controlled[6]	<100	84%	72%	71%
Room and Bathroom 'Always' Clean[6]	<100	87%	79%	73%
Timely Help 'Always' Received[6]	<100	98%	77%	68%
Would Definitely Recommend Hospital[6]	<100	94%	76%	71%
Use of Medical Imaging				
Cardiac Imaging Stress Test before Surgery[7]	-	-	4.4%	5.3%
Combination Abdominal CT Scan[7]	-	-	12.5%	10.5%
Combination Brain/Sinus CT Scan[7]	-	-	2%	2.7%
Combination Chest CT Scan[7]	-	-	4.5%	2.7%
Follow-up Mammogram/Ultrasound[7]	-	-	8.7%	8.8%
Lumbar Spine MRI for Low Back Pain[7]	-	-	33%	37.2%

Community Memorial Hospital

111 W 10th Ave Post Office Box 420
Redfield, SD 57469
Phone: 605-472-1110
Fax: 605-472-0331
URL: www.redfield-sd.com/hospital
Type: Critical Access Hospitals
Emergency Services: Yes
Ownership: Government - Local
Beds: 25

Key Personnel:

CEO/President................ William E Bestor

Measure	Cases	This Hosp.	State Avg.	U.S. Avg.
Blood Clot Prevention and Treatment				
Anticoagulation Overlap Therapy[5]	-	-	95%	93%
ICU Venous Thromboembolism Prophylaxis[5]	-	-	91%	92%
Incidence of Potentially Preventable VTE[5]	-	-	5%	10%
UFH with Dosages/Platelet Monitoring[5]	-	-	100%	97%
Venous Thromboembolism Prophylaxis[5]	-	-	80%	85%

NOTE: Hospital profiles are in alphabetical order by state, then city, then hospital within the city; Rankings exclude hospitals with less than 25 cases except for patient surveys which excludes hospitals with less than 100 cases; (a) 100-299 cases; (1) The number of cases/patients is too few to report; (2) Data submitted were based on a sample of cases/patients; (3) Results are based on a shorter time period than required; (4) Data suppressed by CMS for one or more quarters; (5) Results are not available for this reporting period; (6) Fewer than 100 patients completed the HCAHPS survey; (7) No cases met the criteria for this measure; (8) The lower limit of the confidence interval cannot be calculated if the number of observed infections equals zero; (9) No data are available from the state/territory for this reporting period; (10) The scores shown reflect fewer than 50 completed surveys; (11) There were discrepancies in the data collection process; (12) This measure does not apply to this hospital for this reporting period; (13) Results cannot be calculated for this reporting period; (14) The results for this state are combined with nearby states to protect confidentiality; Please refer to the User's Guide for a full explanation of data.

Warfarin Therapy Discharge Instructions[5]	-	-	70%	75%
Chest Pain/Possible Heart Attack Care				
Aspirin Given Within 24 Hours of Arrival	-	-	99%	96%
Fibrinolytic Meds Within 30 Min. of Arrival	-	-	69%	58%
Average Time to ECG (minutes)	-	-	5	7
Average Time to Transfer (minutes)	-	-	66	60
Children's Asthma Care				
Received Home Management Plan of Care	-	-	-	88%
Received Reliever Medication	-	-	-	100%
Received Systemic Corticosteroids	-	-	-	100%
Emergency Department				
Admittance Decision Time (minutes)[5]	-	-	41	98
Head CT Results Within 45 Min. of Arrival	-	-	44%	57%
Patients Who Left ER Before Being Seen	-	-	1%	2%
Time from ER Arrival to Admit. (minutes)[5]	-	-	174	274
Time from ER Arrival to Discharge (minutes)	-	-	113	134
Time in ER Before Being Evaluated (minutes)	-	-	18	26
Time to Pain Meds for Fractures (minutes)	-	-	44	57
Heart Attack Care				
Aspirin Given at Discharge[5]	-	-	100%	99%
Fibrinolytic Meds Within 30 Min. of Arrival[5]	-	-	100%	54%
PCI Within 90 Minutes of Arrival[5]	-	-	94%	96%
Statin Prescribed at Discharge[5]	-	-	98%	98%
Heart Failure Care				
ACE Inhibitor or ARB for LVSD[5]	-	-	93%	97%
Discharge Instructions Given[5]	-	-	90%	94%
Evaluation of LVS Function[5]	-	-	97%	99%
Medicare Spending				
Medicare Spending per Patient (ratio)	-	-	0.9	0.98
Pneumonia Care				
Appropriate Initial Antibiotic Given[5]	-	-	90%	95%
Blood Culture Timing[5]	-	-	95%	98%
Pregnancy and Delivery Care				
Newborn Deliveries Scheduled Early[5]	-	-	7%	6%
Preventive Care				
Immunization for Influenza[5]	-	-	89%	90%
Immunization for Pneumonia[5]	-	-	89%	92%
Stroke Care				
Anticoagulation Therapy for Atrial Fibrillation[5]	-	-	97%	95%
Antithrombotic Therapy Timing[5]	-	-	98%	98%
Assessed for Rehabilitation[5]	-	-	98%	97%
Discharged on Antithrombotic Therapy[5]	-	-	100%	99%
Discharged on Statin Medication[5]	-	-	93%	94%
Thrombolytic Therapy Timing[5]	-	-	51%	66%
Venous Thromboembolism Prophylaxis[5]	-	-	96%	94%
Written Stroke Educational Materials Given[5]	-	-	85%	88%
Surgical Care Improvement Project				
Appropriate Beta Blocker Usage[5]	-	-	98%	98%
Appropriate VTP Within 24 Hours[5]	-	-	98%	98%
Controlled Postoperative Blood Glucose[5]	-	-	98%	97%
Perioperative Temperature Management[5]	-	-	99%	100%
Prophylactic Antibiotic Selection[5]	-	-	99%	99%
Prophylactic Antibiotic Selection (Outpatient)	-	-	99%	98%
Prophylactic Antibiotic Stopped[5]	-	-	98%	98%
Prophylactic Antibiotic Timing[5]	-	-	99%	99%
Prophylactic Antibiotic Timing (Outpatient)	-	-	98%	98%
Urinary Catheter Removal[5]	-	-	97%	97%
Survey of Patients' Hospital Experiences				
Area Around Room 'Always' Quiet at Night[5]	-	-	72%	61%
Doctors 'Always' Communicated Well[5]	-	-	85%	82%
Home Recovery Information Given[5]	-	-	87%	85%
Hospital Given 9 or 10 on 10 Point Scale[5]	-	-	78%	71%
Meds 'Always' Explained Before Given[5]	-	-	69%	64%
Nurses 'Always' Communicated Well[5]	-	-	83%	79%
Pain 'Always' Well Controlled[5]	-	-	72%	71%
Room and Bathroom 'Always' Clean[5]	-	-	79%	73%
Timely Help 'Always' Received[5]	-	-	77%	68%
Would Definitely Recommend Hospital[5]	-	-	76%	71%
Use of Medical Imaging				
Cardiac Imaging Stress Test before Surgery	-	-	4.4%	5.3%
Combination Abdominal CT Scan	-	-	12.5%	10.5%
Combination Brain/Sinus CT Scan	-	-	2%	2.7%
Combination Chest CT Scan	-	-	4.5%	2.7%
Follow-up Mammogram/Ultrasound	-	-	8.7%	8.8%
Lumbar Spine MRI for Low Back Pain	-	-	33%	37.2%

PHS Indian Hospital at Rosebud

400 Soldier Creek Road
Rosebud, SD 57570
URL: www.ihs.gov
Type: Acute Care Hospitals
Ownership: Government - Federal
Phone: 605-747-2231
Fax: 605-747-2216
Emergency Services: Yes
Beds: 35

Key Personnel:
Emergency Room . . . . Pam Pourier
Chief of Medical Staff . . . . Timothy Ryscon, MD

Measure	Cases	This Hosp.	State Avg.	U.S. Avg.
Blood Clot Prevention and Treatment				
Anticoagulation Overlap Therapy[2,7]	-	-	95%	93%
ICU Venous Thromboembolism Prophylaxis[2,7]	-	-	91%	92%
Incidence of Potentially Preventable VTE[2,7]	-	-	5%	10%
UFH with Dosages/Platelet Monitoring[2,7]	-	-	100%	97%
Venous Thromboembolism Prophylaxis[2]	69	4%	80%	85%
Warfarin Therapy Discharge Instructions[2,7]	-	-	70%	75%
Chest Pain/Possible Heart Attack Care				
Aspirin Given Within 24 Hours of Arrival[5]	-	-	99%	96%
Fibrinolytic Meds Within 30 Min. of Arrival[5]	-	-	69%	58%
Average Time to ECG (minutes)[5]	-	-	5	7
Average Time to Transfer (minutes)[5]	-	-	66	60
Children's Asthma Care				
Received Home Management Plan of Care	-	-	-	88%
Received Reliever Medication	-	-	-	100%
Received Systemic Corticosteroids	-	-	-	100%
Emergency Department				
Admittance Decision Time (minutes)[2]	76	64	41	98
Head CT Results Within 45 Min. of Arrival[5]	-	-	44%	57%
Patients Who Left ER Before Being Seen[5]	-	-	1%	2%
Time from ER Arrival to Admit. (minutes)[2]	358	268	174	274
Time from ER Arrival to Discharge (minutes)[5]	-	-	113	134
Time in ER Before Being Evaluated (minutes)[5]	-	-	18	26
Time to Pain Meds for Fractures (minutes)[5]	-	-	44	57
Heart Attack Care				
Aspirin Given at Discharge[2,3]	-	-	100%	99%
Fibrinolytic Meds Within 30 Min. of Arrival[2,3]	-	-	100%	54%
PCI Within 90 Minutes of Arrival[2,3]	-	-	94%	96%
Statin Prescribed at Discharge[2,3]	-	-	98%	98%
Heart Failure Care				
ACE Inhibitor or ARB for LVSD[2,7]	-	-	93%	97%
Discharge Instructions Given[1,2]	-	-	90%	94%
Evaluation of LVS Function[1,2]	-	-	97%	99%
Medicare Spending				
Medicare Spending per Patient (ratio)	-	0.71	0.9	0.98
Pneumonia Care				
Appropriate Initial Antibiotic Given[2]	26	54%	90%	95%
Blood Culture Timing[2]	24	8%	95%	98%
Pregnancy and Delivery Care				
Newborn Deliveries Scheduled Early[2]	21	10%	7%	6%
Preventive Care				
Immunization for Influenza[2]	285	46%	89%	90%
Immunization for Pneumonia[2]	153	80%	89%	92%
Stroke Care				
Anticoagulation Therapy for Atrial Fibrillation[5]	-	-	97%	95%
Antithrombotic Therapy Timing[5]	-	-	98%	98%
Assessed for Rehabilitation[5]	-	-	98%	97%
Discharged on Antithrombotic Therapy[5]	-	-	100%	99%
Discharged on Statin Medication[5]	-	-	93%	94%
Thrombolytic Therapy Timing[5]	-	-	51%	66%
Venous Thromboembolism Prophylaxis[5]	-	-	96%	94%
Written Stroke Educational Materials Given[5]	-	-	85%	88%
Surgical Care Improvement Project				
Appropriate Beta Blocker Usage[2,3]	-	-	98%	98%
Appropriate VTP Within 24 Hours[2,3]	-	-	98%	98%
Controlled Postoperative Blood Glucose[2,3]	-	-	98%	97%
Perioperative Temperature Management[1,2]	-	-	99%	100%
Prophylactic Antibiotic Selection[2,3]	-	-	99%	99%
Prophylactic Antibiotic Selection (Outpatient)[5]	-	-	99%	98%
Prophylactic Antibiotic Stopped[2,3]	-	-	98%	98%
Prophylactic Antibiotic Timing[2,3]	-	-	99%	99%
Prophylactic Antibiotic Timing (Outpatient)[5]	-	-	98%	98%
Urinary Catheter Removal[2,3]	-	-	97%	97%
Survey of Patients' Hospital Experiences				
Area Around Room 'Always' Quiet at Night[6,11]	<100	52%	72%	61%
Doctors 'Always' Communicated Well[6,11]	<100	69%	85%	82%
Home Recovery Information Given[6,11]	<100	74%	87%	85%
Hospital Given 9 or 10 on 10 Point Scale[6,11]	<100	49%	78%	71%
Meds 'Always' Explained Before Given[6,11]	<100	50%	69%	64%
Nurses 'Always' Communicated Well[6,11]	<100	71%	83%	79%
Pain 'Always' Well Controlled[6,11]	<100	76%	72%	71%
Room and Bathroom 'Always' Clean[6,11]	<100	75%	79%	73%
Timely Help 'Always' Received[6,11]	<100	69%	77%	68%
Would Definitely Recommend Hospital[6,11]	<100	23%	76%	71%
Use of Medical Imaging				
Cardiac Imaging Stress Test before Surgery[7]	-	-	4.4%	5.3%
Combination Abdominal CT Scan[7]	-	-	12.5%	10.5%
Combination Brain/Sinus CT Scan[7]	-	-	2%	2.7%
Combination Chest CT Scan[7]	-	-	4.5%	2.7%
Follow-up Mammogram/Ultrasound[7]	-	-	8.7%	8.8%
Lumbar Spine MRI for Low Back Pain[7]	-	-	33%	37.2%

Landmann - Jungman Memorial Hospital

600 Billars St
Scotland, SD 57059
E-mail: jay.plucker@mckennan.org
URL: www.ljmh.org
Type: Critical Access Hospitals
Ownership: Government - Local
Phone: 605-583-2226
Fax: 605-583-4557
Emergency Services: Yes
Beds: 25

Key Personnel:
Operating Room. . . . . Sherry Fisher, RN
Chief of Medical Staff . . . . Manuel Ramos, MD

Measure	Cases	This Hosp.	State Avg.	U.S. Avg.
Blood Clot Prevention and Treatment				
Anticoagulation Overlap Therapy[5]	-	-	95%	93%
ICU Venous Thromboembolism Prophylaxis[5]	-	-	91%	92%
Incidence of Potentially Preventable VTE[5]	-	-	5%	10%
UFH with Dosages/Platelet Monitoring[5]	-	-	100%	97%
Venous Thromboembolism Prophylaxis[5]	-	-	80%	85%
Warfarin Therapy Discharge Instructions[5]	-	-	70%	75%
Chest Pain/Possible Heart Attack Care				
Aspirin Given Within 24 Hours of Arrival	-	-	99%	96%
Fibrinolytic Meds Within 30 Min. of Arrival	-	-	69%	58%
Average Time to ECG (minutes)	-	-	5	7
Average Time to Transfer (minutes)	-	-	66	60
Children's Asthma Care				
Received Home Management Plan of Care	-	-	-	88%
Received Reliever Medication	-	-	-	100%
Received Systemic Corticosteroids	-	-	-	100%
Emergency Department				
Admittance Decision Time (minutes)[5]	-	-	41	98
Head CT Results Within 45 Min. of Arrival	-	-	44%	57%
Patients Who Left ER Before Being Seen	-	-	1%	2%
Time from ER Arrival to Admit. (minutes)[5]	-	-	174	274
Time from ER Arrival to Discharge (minutes)	-	-	113	134
Time in ER Before Being Evaluated (minutes)	-	-	18	26
Time to Pain Meds for Fractures (minutes)	-	-	44	57
Heart Attack Care				
Aspirin Given at Discharge[5]	-	-	100%	99%
Fibrinolytic Meds Within 30 Min. of Arrival[5]	-	-	100%	54%
PCI Within 90 Minutes of Arrival[5]	-	-	94%	96%
Statin Prescribed at Discharge[5]	-	-	98%	98%
Heart Failure Care				
ACE Inhibitor or ARB for LVSD[3,7]	-	-	93%	97%
Discharge Instructions Given[1,3]	-	-	90%	94%
Evaluation of LVS Function[1,3]	-	-	97%	99%
Medicare Spending				
Medicare Spending per Patient (ratio)	-	-	0.9	0.98
Pneumonia Care				
Appropriate Initial Antibiotic Given[1]	-	-	90%	95%
Blood Culture Timing[3,7]	-	-	95%	98%
Pregnancy and Delivery Care				

NOTE: Hospital profiles are in alphabetical order by state, then city, then hospital within the city; Rankings exclude hospitals with less than 25 cases except for patient surveys which excludes hospitals with less than 100 cases; (a) 100-299 cases; (1) The number of cases/patients is too few to report; (2) Data submitted were based on a sample of cases/patients; (3) Results are based on a shorter time period than required; (4) Data suppressed by CMS for one or more quarters; (5) Results are not available for this reporting period; (6) Fewer than 100 patients completed the HCAHPS survey; (7) No cases met the criteria for this measure; (8) The lower limit of the confidence interval cannot be calculated if the number of observed infections equals zero; (9) No data are available from the state/territory for this reporting period; (10) The scores shown reflect fewer than 50 completed surveys; (11) There were discrepancies in the data collection process; (12) This measure does not apply to this hospital for this reporting period; (13) Results cannot be calculated for this reporting period; (14) The results for this state are combined with nearby states to protect confidentiality; Please refer to the User's Guide for a full explanation of data.

Measure	Cases	This Hosp.	State Avg.	U.S. Avg.
Newborn Deliveries Scheduled Early[5]	-	-	7%	6%
Preventive Care				
Immunization for Influenza[5]	-	-	89%	90%
Immunization for Pneumonia[5]	-	-	89%	92%
Stroke Care				
Anticoagulation Therapy for Atrial Fibrillation[5]	-	-	97%	95%
Antithrombotic Therapy Timing[5]	-	-	98%	98%
Assessed for Rehabilitation[5]	-	-	98%	97%
Discharged on Antithrombotic Therapy[5]	-	-	100%	99%
Discharged on Statin Medication[5]	-	-	93%	94%
Thrombolytic Therapy Timing[5]	-	-	51%	66%
Venous Thromboembolism Prophylaxis[5]	-	-	96%	94%
Written Stroke Educational Materials Given[5]	-	-	85%	88%
Surgical Care Improvement Project				
Appropriate Beta Blocker Usage[5]	-	-	98%	98%
Appropriate VTP Within 24 Hours[5]	-	-	98%	98%
Controlled Postoperative Blood Glucose[5]	-	-	98%	97%
Perioperative Temperature Management[5]	-	-	99%	100%
Prophylactic Antibiotic Selection[5]	-	-	99%	99%
Prophylactic Antibiotic Selection (Outpatient)	-	-	99%	98%
Prophylactic Antibiotic Stopped[5]	-	-	98%	98%
Prophylactic Antibiotic Timing[5]	-	-	99%	99%
Prophylactic Antibiotic Timing (Outpatient)	-	-	98%	98%
Urinary Catheter Removal[5]	-	-	97%	97%
Survey of Patients' Hospital Experiences				
Area Around Room 'Always' Quiet at Night[5]	-	-	72%	61%
Doctors 'Always' Communicated Well[5]	-	-	85%	82%
Home Recovery Information Given[5]	-	-	87%	85%
Hospital Given 9 or 10 on 10 Point Scale[5]	-	-	78%	71%
Meds 'Always' Explained Before Given[5]	-	-	69%	64%
Nurses 'Always' Communicated Well[5]	-	-	83%	79%
Pain 'Always' Well Controlled[5]	-	-	72%	71%
Room and Bathroom 'Always' Clean[5]	-	-	79%	73%
Timely Help 'Always' Received[5]	-	-	77%	68%
Would Definitely Recommend Hospital[5]	-	-	76%	71%
Use of Medical Imaging				
Cardiac Imaging Stress Test before Surgery	-	-	4.4%	5.3%
Combination Abdominal CT Scan	-	-	12.5%	10.5%
Combination Brain/Sinus CT Scan	-	-	2%	2.7%
Combination Chest CT Scan	-	-	4.5%	2.7%
Follow-up Mammogram/Ultrasound	-	-	8.7%	8.8%
Lumbar Spine MRI for Low Back Pain	-	-	33%	37.2%

Avera Heart Hospital of South Dakota

4500 W 69th St
Sioux Falls, SD 57108
Phone: 605-977-7000
URL: www.avera.org/heart-hospital
Type: Acute Care Hospitals
Emergency Services: Yes
Ownership: Proprietary
Key Personnel:
CEO/President. . . . . John Soderholm
Anesthesiology. . . . . Ty White

Measure	Cases	This Hosp.	State Avg.	U.S. Avg.
Blood Clot Prevention and Treatment				
Anticoagulation Overlap Therapy[2]	42	79%	95%	93%
ICU Venous Thromboembolism Prophylaxis[2,7]	-	-	91%	92%
Incidence of Potentially Preventable VTE[2,7]	-	-	5%	10%
UFH with Dosages/Platelet Monitoring[2]	49	100%	100%	97%
Venous Thromboembolism Prophylaxis[2]	260	95%	80%	85%
Warfarin Therapy Discharge Instructions[2]	34	85%	70%	75%
Chest Pain/Possible Heart Attack Care				
Aspirin Given Within 24 Hours of Arrival[1]	-	-	99%	96%
Fibrinolytic Meds Within 30 Min. of Arrival[5]	-	-	69%	58%
Average Time to ECG (minutes)[1]	-	-	5	7
Average Time to Transfer (minutes)[5]	-	-	66	60
Children's Asthma Care				
Received Home Management Plan of Care	-	-	-	88%
Received Reliever Medication	-	-	-	100%
Received Systemic Corticosteroids	-	-	-	100%
Emergency Department				
Admittance Decision Time (minutes)[2]	29	31	41	98
Head CT Results Within 45 Min. of Arrival[3,7]	-	-	44%	57%
Patients Who Left ER Before Being Seen	2,821	0%	1%	2%
Time from ER Arrival to Admit. (minutes)[2]	48	102	174	274
Time from ER Arrival to Discharge (minutes)	241	109	113	134
Time in ER Before Being Evaluated (minutes)	277	7	18	26
Time to Pain Meds for Fractures (minutes)[5]	-	-	44	57
Heart Attack Care				
Aspirin Given at Discharge	444	100%	100%	99%
Fibrinolytic Meds Within 30 Min. of Arrival[7]	-	-	100%	54%
PCI Within 90 Minutes of Arrival	16	100%	94%	96%
Statin Prescribed at Discharge	419	99%	98%	98%
Heart Failure Care				
ACE Inhibitor or ARB for LVSD	62	98%	93%	97%
Discharge Instructions Given	130	100%	90%	94%
Evaluation of LVS Function	156	100%	97%	99%
Medicare Spending				
Medicare Spending per Patient (ratio)	-	0.98	0.9	0.98
Pneumonia Care				
Appropriate Initial Antibiotic Given[1]	-	-	90%	95%
Blood Culture Timing[1]	-	-	95%	98%
Pregnancy and Delivery Care				
Newborn Deliveries Scheduled Early[7]	-	-	7%	6%
Preventive Care				
Immunization for Influenza[2]	314	100%	89%	90%
Immunization for Pneumonia[2]	485	100%	89%	92%
Stroke Care				
Anticoagulation Therapy for Atrial Fibrillation[1]	-	-	97%	95%
Antithrombotic Therapy Timing	13	100%	98%	98%
Assessed for Rehabilitation	13	62%	98%	97%
Discharged on Antithrombotic Therapy	13	100%	100%	99%
Discharged on Statin Medication	12	75%	93%	94%
Thrombolytic Therapy Timing[7]	-	-	51%	66%
Venous Thromboembolism Prophylaxis	13	85%	96%	94%
Written Stroke Educational Materials Given[1]	-	-	85%	88%
Surgical Care Improvement Project				
Appropriate Beta Blocker Usage[2]	324	99%	98%	98%
Appropriate VTP Within 24 Hours[2]	39	97%	98%	98%
Controlled Postoperative Blood Glucose[2]	322	98%	98%	97%
Perioperative Temperature Management[2]	68	99%	99%	100%
Prophylactic Antibiotic Selection[2]	345	100%	99%	99%
Prophylactic Antibiotic Selection (Outpatient)	309	99%	99%	98%
Prophylactic Antibiotic Stopped[2]	344	100%	98%	98%
Prophylactic Antibiotic Timing[2]	345	100%	99%	99%
Prophylactic Antibiotic Timing (Outpatient)	311	96%	98%	98%
Urinary Catheter Removal[2]	277	96%	97%	97%
Survey of Patients' Hospital Experiences				
Area Around Room 'Always' Quiet at Night	300+	67%	72%	61%
Doctors 'Always' Communicated Well	300+	86%	85%	82%
Home Recovery Information Given	300+	91%	87%	85%
Hospital Given 9 or 10 on 10 Point Scale	300+	91%	78%	71%
Meds 'Always' Explained Before Given	300+	74%	69%	64%
Nurses 'Always' Communicated Well	300+	89%	83%	79%
Pain 'Always' Well Controlled	300+	80%	72%	71%
Room and Bathroom 'Always' Clean	300+	85%	79%	73%
Timely Help 'Always' Received	300+	81%	77%	68%
Would Definitely Recommend Hospital	300+	92%	76%	71%
Use of Medical Imaging				
Cardiac Imaging Stress Test before Surgery	765	4.3%	4.4%	5.3%
Combination Abdominal CT Scan	107	1.9%	12.5%	10.5%
Combination Brain/Sinus CT Scan	87	0.0%	2%	2.7%
Combination Chest CT Scan[1]	-	-	4.5%	2.7%
Follow-up Mammogram/Ultrasound[7]	-	-	8.7%	8.8%
Lumbar Spine MRI for Low Back Pain[7]	-	-	33%	37.2%

Avera Mckennan Hospital & University Health Center

1325 S Cliff Ave Post Office Box 5045
Sioux Falls, SD 57117
Phone: 605-322-8000
Fax: 605-322-7822
E-mail: info@mckennan.org
URL: www.mckennan.org
Type: Acute Care Hospitals
Emergency Services: Yes
Ownership: Voluntary non-profit - Private
Beds: 490
Key Personnel:
Emergency Room . . . . Howard Burns
Chief of Medical Staff. . . . . Michael Elliott, MD
CEO/President. . . . . Dr. David Kapaska
Infection Control. . . . . Don Tomac

Measure	Cases	This Hosp.	State Avg.	U.S. Avg.
Blood Clot Prevention and Treatment				
Anticoagulation Overlap Therapy[2]	134	99%	95%	93%
ICU Venous Thromboembolism Prophylaxis[2]	63	95%	91%	92%
Incidence of Potentially Preventable VTE[2]	24	0%	5%	10%
UFH with Dosages/Platelet Monitoring[2]	69	100%	100%	97%
Venous Thromboembolism Prophylaxis[2]	254	92%	80%	85%
Warfarin Therapy Discharge Instructions[2]	96	92%	70%	75%
Chest Pain/Possible Heart Attack Care				
Aspirin Given Within 24 Hours of Arrival[5]	-	-	99%	96%
Fibrinolytic Meds Within 30 Min. of Arrival[5]	-	-	69%	58%
Average Time to ECG (minutes)[5]	-	-	5	7
Average Time to Transfer (minutes)[5]	-	-	66	60
Children's Asthma Care				
Received Home Management Plan of Care	-	-	-	88%
Received Reliever Medication	-	-	-	100%
Received Systemic Corticosteroids	-	-	-	100%
Emergency Department				
Admittance Decision Time (minutes)[2]	83	62	41	98
Head CT Results Within 45 Min. of Arrival[3,7]	-	-	44%	57%
Patients Who Left ER Before Being Seen	26,912	1%	1%	2%
Time from ER Arrival to Admit. (minutes)[2]	83	162	174	274
Time from ER Arrival to Discharge (minutes)	13,670	116	113	134
Time in ER Before Being Evaluated (minutes)	13,359	19	18	26
Time to Pain Meds for Fractures (minutes)	121	48	44	57
Heart Attack Care				
Aspirin Given at Discharge	50	100%	100%	99%
Fibrinolytic Meds Within 30 Min. of Arrival[7]	-	-	100%	54%
PCI Within 90 Minutes of Arrival	16	100%	94%	96%
Statin Prescribed at Discharge	45	98%	98%	98%
Heart Failure Care				
ACE Inhibitor or ARB for LVSD	55	89%	93%	97%
Discharge Instructions Given	164	91%	90%	94%
Evaluation of LVS Function	218	100%	97%	99%
Medicare Spending				
Medicare Spending per Patient (ratio)	-	0.93	0.9	0.98
Pneumonia Care				
Appropriate Initial Antibiotic Given	87	95%	90%	95%
Blood Culture Timing	97	97%	95%	98%
Pregnancy and Delivery Care				
Newborn Deliveries Scheduled Early	120	4%	7%	6%
Preventive Care				
Immunization for Influenza[2]	582	92%	89%	90%
Immunization for Pneumonia[2]	533	85%	89%	92%
Stroke Care				
Anticoagulation Therapy for Atrial Fibrillation	30	93%	97%	95%
Antithrombotic Therapy Timing	138	99%	98%	98%
Assessed for Rehabilitation	172	98%	98%	97%
Discharged on Antithrombotic Therapy	155	100%	100%	99%
Discharged on Statin Medication	121	98%	93%	94%
Thrombolytic Therapy Timing[1]	-	-	51%	66%
Venous Thromboembolism Prophylaxis	170	99%	96%	94%
Written Stroke Educational Materials Given	92	86%	85%	88%
Surgical Care Improvement Project				
Appropriate Beta Blocker Usage[2]	124	98%	98%	98%
Appropriate VTP Within 24 Hours[2]	336	99%	98%	98%
Controlled Postoperative Blood Glucose[2,7]	-	-	98%	97%
Perioperative Temperature Management[2]	425	100%	99%	100%
Prophylactic Antibiotic Selection[2]	276	99%	99%	99%
Prophylactic Antibiotic Selection (Outpatient)	322	99%	99%	98%
Prophylactic Antibiotic Stopped[2]	272	100%	98%	98%
Prophylactic Antibiotic Timing[2]	276	100%	99%	99%
Prophylactic Antibiotic Timing (Outpatient)	321	99%	98%	98%
Urinary Catheter Removal[2]	179	94%	97%	97%
Survey of Patients' Hospital Experiences				
Area Around Room 'Always' Quiet at Night	300+	60%	72%	61%
Doctors 'Always' Communicated Well	300+	81%	85%	82%
Home Recovery Information Given	300+	90%	87%	85%
Hospital Given 9 or 10 on 10 Point Scale	300+	73%	78%	71%
Meds 'Always' Explained Before Given	300+	64%	69%	64%
Nurses 'Always' Communicated Well	300+	77%	83%	79%
Pain 'Always' Well Controlled	300+	68%	72%	71%

NOTE: Hospital profiles are in alphabetical order by state, then city, then hospital within the city; Rankings exclude hospitals with less than 25 cases except for patient surveys which excludes hospitals with less than 100 cases; (a) 100-299 cases; (1) The number of cases/patients is too few to report; (2) Data submitted were based on a sample of cases/patients; (3) Results are based on a shorter time period than required; (4) Data suppressed by CMS for one or more quarters; (5) Results are not available for this reporting period; (6) Fewer than 100 patients completed the HCAHPS survey; (7) No cases met the criteria for this measure; (8) The lower limit of the confidence interval cannot be calculated if the number of observed infections equals zero; (9) No data are available from the state/territory for this reporting period; (10) The scores shown reflect fewer than 50 completed surveys; (11) There were discrepancies in the data collection process; (12) This measure does not apply to this hospital for this reporting period; (13) Results cannot be calculated for this reporting period; (14) The results for this state are combined with nearby states to protect confidentiality; Please refer to the User's Guide for a full explanation of data.

Room and Bathroom 'Always' Clean	300+	71%	79%	73%
Timely Help 'Always' Received	300+	66%	77%	68%
Would Definitely Recommend Hospital	300+	77%	76%	71%
Use of Medical Imaging				
Cardiac Imaging Stress Test before Surgery	137	1.5%	4.4%	5.3%
Combination Abdominal CT Scan	1,101	10.6%	12.5%	10.5%
Combination Brain/Sinus CT Scan[1]	-	-	2%	2.7%
Combination Chest CT Scan	967	4.3%	4.5%	2.7%
Follow-up Mammogram/Ultrasound	2,053	8.4%	8.7%	8.8%
Lumbar Spine MRI for Low Back Pain	166	33.1%	33%	37.2%

Sanford Usd Medical Center

1305 W 18th Saint Post Office Box 5039
Sioux Falls, SD 57117
Phone: 605-333-1000
Fax: 605-328-1577
E-mail: info@sanfordhealth.org
URL: www.sanfordhealth.org
Type: Acute Care Hospitals
Emergency Services: Yes
Ownership: Voluntary non-profit - Other
Beds: 477

Key Personnel:

Infection Control. . . . . Lisa Docken, RN
Chief of Medical Staff. . . . . Barbara Hall, MD
CEO/President. . . . . Kelby K Krabbenhoft
Pediatric Ambulatory Care . . . . . . Dave Munson, MD
Pediatric In-Patient Care . . . . Dave Munson, MD
Emergency Room . . . . Becky Nelson, MD
Quality Assurance . . . . Jeannine Schwarting
Radiology. . . . . Daryl Wierda, MD

Measure	Cases	This Hosp.	State Avg.	U.S. Avg.
Blood Clot Prevention and Treatment				
Anticoagulation Overlap Therapy[2]	158	96%	95%	93%
ICU Venous Thromboembolism Prophylaxis[2]	65	97%	91%	92%
Incidence of Potentially Preventable VTE[2]	33	9%	5%	10%
UFH with Dosages/Platelet Monitoring[2]	117	100%	100%	97%
Venous Thromboembolism Prophylaxis[2]	286	81%	80%	85%
Warfarin Therapy Discharge Instructions[2]	119	90%	70%	75%
Chest Pain/Possible Heart Attack Care				
Aspirin Given Within 24 Hours of Arrival[5]	-	-	99%	96%
Fibrinolytic Meds Within 30 Min. of Arrival[5]	-	-	69%	58%
Average Time to ECG (minutes)[5]	-	-	5	7
Average Time to Transfer (minutes)[5]	-	-	66	60
Children's Asthma Care				
Received Home Management Plan of Care	50	98%	-	88%
Received Reliever Medication	50	100%	-	100%
Received Systemic Corticosteroids	50	100%	-	100%
Emergency Department				
Admittance Decision Time (minutes)[2]	305	56	41	98
Head CT Results Within 45 Min. of Arrival[1,3]	-	-	44%	57%
Patients Who Left ER Before Being Seen	41,378	1%	1%	2%
Time from ER Arrival to Admit. (minutes)[2]	311	195	174	274
Time from ER Arrival to Discharge (minutes)	396	145	113	134
Time in ER Before Being Evaluated (minutes)	345	14	18	26
Time to Pain Meds for Fractures (minutes)	170	54	44	57
Heart Attack Care				
Aspirin Given at Discharge	494	100%	100%	99%
Fibrinolytic Meds Within 30 Min. of Arrival[7]	-	-	100%	54%
PCI Within 90 Minutes of Arrival	37	100%	94%	96%
Statin Prescribed at Discharge	465	98%	98%	98%
Heart Failure Care				
ACE Inhibitor or ARB for LVSD	99	100%	93%	97%
Discharge Instructions Given	269	98%	90%	94%
Evaluation of LVS Function	343	100%	97%	99%
Medicare Spending				
Medicare Spending per Patient (ratio)	-	0.96	0.9	0.98
Pneumonia Care				
Appropriate Initial Antibiotic Given	136	97%	90%	95%
Blood Culture Timing	199	97%	95%	98%
Pregnancy and Delivery Care				
Newborn Deliveries Scheduled Early[2]	51	2%	7%	6%
Preventive Care				
Immunization for Influenza[2]	549	94%	89%	90%
Immunization for Pneumonia[2]	534	86%	89%	92%
Stroke Care				
Anticoagulation Therapy for Atrial Fibrillation	31	100%	97%	95%
Antithrombotic Therapy Timing	147	99%	98%	98%
Assessed for Rehabilitation	222	100%	98%	97%
Discharged on Antithrombotic Therapy	189	100%	100%	99%
Discharged on Statin Medication	129	100%	93%	94%
Thrombolytic Therapy Timing[1]	-	-	51%	66%
Venous Thromboembolism Prophylaxis	200	100%	96%	94%
Written Stroke Educational Materials Given	121	98%	85%	88%
Surgical Care Improvement Project				
Appropriate Beta Blocker Usage[2]	416	98%	98%	98%
Appropriate VTP Within 24 Hours[2]	642	98%	98%	98%
Controlled Postoperative Blood Glucose[2]	198	98%	98%	97%
Perioperative Temperature Management[2]	1,054	100%	99%	100%
Prophylactic Antibiotic Selection[2]	920	99%	99%	99%
Prophylactic Antibiotic Selection (Outpatient)	587	99%	99%	98%
Prophylactic Antibiotic Stopped[2]	895	98%	98%	98%
Prophylactic Antibiotic Timing[2]	922	98%	99%	99%
Prophylactic Antibiotic Timing (Outpatient)	597	98%	98%	98%
Urinary Catheter Removal[2]	433	96%	97%	97%
Survey of Patients' Hospital Experiences				
Area Around Room 'Always' Quiet at Night	300+	59%	72%	61%
Doctors 'Always' Communicated Well	300+	78%	85%	82%
Home Recovery Information Given	300+	89%	87%	85%
Hospital Given 9 or 10 on 10 Point Scale	300+	74%	78%	71%
Meds 'Always' Explained Before Given	300+	62%	69%	64%
Nurses 'Always' Communicated Well	300+	78%	83%	79%
Pain 'Always' Well Controlled	300+	69%	72%	71%
Room and Bathroom 'Always' Clean	300+	67%	79%	73%
Timely Help 'Always' Received	300+	67%	77%	68%
Would Definitely Recommend Hospital	300+	77%	76%	71%
Use of Medical Imaging				
Cardiac Imaging Stress Test before Surgery	1,154	5.3%	4.4%	5.3%
Combination Abdominal CT Scan	1,252	1.9%	12.5%	10.5%
Combination Brain/Sinus CT Scan	717	2.9%	2%	2.7%
Combination Chest CT Scan	1,141	0.0%	4.5%	2.7%
Follow-up Mammogram/Ultrasound[7]	-	-	8.7%	8.8%
Lumbar Spine MRI for Low Back Pain	300	31.7%	33%	37.2%

Sioux Falls Specialty Hospital

910 East 20th Street
Sioux Falls, SD 57105
Phone: 605-334-6730
Fax: 605-334-8096
URL: www.sfsurgical.com
Type: Acute Care Hospitals
Emergency Services: No
Ownership: Proprietary
Beds: 13

Key Personnel:

Cardiology . . . . Raymond Allen, MD
Anesthesiology. . . . . James Brunz, MD
Pulmonology . . . . Rizan Hajal, MD
CEO/President. . . . . Douglas V Johnson

Measure	Cases	This Hosp.	State Avg.	U.S. Avg.
Blood Clot Prevention and Treatment				
Anticoagulation Overlap Therapy[2,7]	-	-	95%	93%
ICU Venous Thromboembolism Prophylaxis[2,7]	-	-	91%	92%
Incidence of Potentially Preventable VTE[2,7]	-	-	5%	10%
UFH with Dosages/Platelet Monitoring[2,7]	-	-	100%	97%
Venous Thromboembolism Prophylaxis[2]	100	100%	80%	85%
Warfarin Therapy Discharge Instructions[2,7]	-	-	70%	75%
Chest Pain/Possible Heart Attack Care				
Aspirin Given Within 24 Hours of Arrival[5]	-	-	99%	96%
Fibrinolytic Meds Within 30 Min. of Arrival[5]	-	-	69%	58%
Average Time to ECG (minutes)[5]	-	-	5	7
Average Time to Transfer (minutes)[5]	-	-	66	60
Children's Asthma Care				
Received Home Management Plan of Care	-	-	-	88%
Received Reliever Medication	-	-	-	100%
Received Systemic Corticosteroids	-	-	-	100%
Emergency Department				
Admittance Decision Time (minutes)[2,7]	-	-	41	98
Head CT Results Within 45 Min. of Arrival[5]	-	-	44%	57%
Patients Who Left ER Before Being Seen	21	0%	1%	2%
Time from ER Arrival to Admit. (minutes)[2,7]	-	-	174	274
Time from ER Arrival to Discharge (minutes)[5]	-	-	113	134
Time in ER Before Being Evaluated (minutes)[5]	-	-	18	26
Time to Pain Meds for Fractures (minutes)[5]	-	-	44	57
Heart Attack Care				
Aspirin Given at Discharge[5]	-	-	100%	99%
Fibrinolytic Meds Within 30 Min. of Arrival[5]	-	-	100%	54%
PCI Within 90 Minutes of Arrival[5]	-	-	94%	96%
Statin Prescribed at Discharge[5]	-	-	98%	98%
Heart Failure Care				
ACE Inhibitor or ARB for LVSD[5]	-	-	93%	97%
Discharge Instructions Given[5]	-	-	90%	94%
Evaluation of LVS Function[5]	-	-	97%	99%
Medicare Spending				
Medicare Spending per Patient (ratio)	-	0.86	0.9	0.98
Pneumonia Care				
Appropriate Initial Antibiotic Given[5]	-	-	90%	95%
Blood Culture Timing[5]	-	-	95%	98%
Pregnancy and Delivery Care				
Newborn Deliveries Scheduled Early[7]	-	-	7%	6%
Preventive Care				
Immunization for Influenza[2]	327	94%	89%	90%
Immunization for Pneumonia[2]	321	95%	89%	92%
Stroke Care				
Anticoagulation Therapy for Atrial Fibrillation[5]	-	-	97%	95%
Antithrombotic Therapy Timing[5]	-	-	98%	98%
Assessed for Rehabilitation[5]	-	-	98%	97%
Discharged on Antithrombotic Therapy[5]	-	-	100%	99%
Discharged on Statin Medication[5]	-	-	93%	94%
Thrombolytic Therapy Timing[5]	-	-	51%	66%
Venous Thromboembolism Prophylaxis[5]	-	-	96%	94%
Written Stroke Educational Materials Given[5]	-	-	85%	88%
Surgical Care Improvement Project				
Appropriate Beta Blocker Usage[2]	76	100%	98%	98%
Appropriate VTP Within 24 Hours[2]	434	99%	98%	98%
Controlled Postoperative Blood Glucose[2,7]	-	-	98%	97%
Perioperative Temperature Management[2]	475	100%	99%	100%
Prophylactic Antibiotic Selection[2]	413	100%	99%	99%
Prophylactic Antibiotic Selection (Outpatient)	254	98%	99%	98%
Prophylactic Antibiotic Stopped[2]	413	99%	98%	98%
Prophylactic Antibiotic Timing[2]	413	99%	99%	99%
Prophylactic Antibiotic Timing (Outpatient)	255	98%	98%	98%
Urinary Catheter Removal[2]	262	100%	97%	97%
Survey of Patients' Hospital Experiences				
Area Around Room 'Always' Quiet at Night	300+	88%	72%	61%
Doctors 'Always' Communicated Well	300+	84%	85%	82%
Home Recovery Information Given	300+	91%	87%	85%
Hospital Given 9 or 10 on 10 Point Scale	300+	90%	78%	71%
Meds 'Always' Explained Before Given	300+	76%	69%	64%
Nurses 'Always' Communicated Well	300+	90%	83%	79%
Pain 'Always' Well Controlled	300+	80%	72%	71%
Room and Bathroom 'Always' Clean	300+	84%	79%	73%
Timely Help 'Always' Received	300+	88%	77%	68%
Would Definitely Recommend Hospital	300+	92%	76%	71%
Use of Medical Imaging				
Cardiac Imaging Stress Test before Surgery[7]	-	-	4.4%	5.3%
Combination Abdominal CT Scan[7]	-	-	12.5%	10.5%
Combination Brain/Sinus CT Scan[7]	-	-	2%	2.7%
Combination Chest CT Scan[7]	-	-	4.5%	2.7%
Follow-up Mammogram/Ultrasound[7]	-	-	8.7%	8.8%
Lumbar Spine MRI for Low Back Pain	128	26.6%	33%	37.2%

Sioux Falls VA Medical Center

2501 West 22nd Street
Sioux Falls, SD 57117
Phone: 605-336-3230
Fax: 605-333-6878
URL: www.va.gov
Type: Acute Care - VA
Emergency Services: No
Ownership: Government Federal
Beds: 259

Key Personnel:

Chief of Medical Staff. . . . . Vikrant Choudhry
CEO/President. . . . . Vincent Crawford
Intensive Care Unit. . . . . Elizabeth Flinn, RN
Quality Assurance . . . . Sandra Frazer
Patient Relations . . . . Rita Loving, RN
Hemotology Center . . . . Michael Robinson, MD
Infection Control. . . . . Jeanld Tjaden, RN
Operating Room. . . . . Sandra Vander Woude

Measure	Cases	This Hosp.	State Avg.	U.S. Avg.
Blood Clot Prevention and Treatment				

NOTE: Hospital profiles are in alphabetical order by state, then city, then hospital within the city; Rankings exclude hospitals with less than 25 cases except for patient surveys which excludes hospitals with less than 100 cases; (a) 100-299 cases; (1) The number of cases/patients is too few to report; (2) Data submitted were based on a sample of cases/patients; (3) Results are based on a shorter time period than required; (4) Data suppressed by CMS for one or more quarters; (5) Results are not available for this reporting period; (6) Fewer than 100 patients completed the HCAHPS survey; (7) No cases met the criteria for this measure; (8) The lower limit of the confidence interval cannot be calculated if the number of observed infections equals zero; (9) No data are available from the state/territory for this reporting period; (10) The scores shown reflect fewer than 50 completed surveys; (11) There were discrepancies in the data collection process; (12) This measure does not apply to this hospital for this reporting period; (13) Results cannot be calculated for this reporting period; (14) The results for this state are combined with nearby states to protect confidentiality; Please refer to the User's Guide for a full explanation of data.

Measure	Cases	This Hosp.	State Avg.	U.S. Avg.
Anticoagulation Overlap Therapy	-	-	95%	93%
ICU Venous Thromboembolism Prophylaxis	-	-	91%	92%
Incidence of Potentially Preventable VTE	-	-	5%	10%
UFH with Dosages/Platelet Monitoring	-	-	100%	97%
Venous Thromboembolism Prophylaxis	-	-	80%	85%
Warfarin Therapy Discharge Instructions	-	-	70%	75%
Chest Pain/Possible Heart Attack Care				
Aspirin Given Within 24 Hours of Arrival	-	-	99%	96%
Fibrinolytic Meds Within 30 Min. of Arrival	-	-	69%	58%
Average Time to ECG (minutes)	-	-	5	7
Average Time to Transfer (minutes)	-	-	66	60
Children's Asthma Care				
Received Home Management Plan of Care	-	-	-	88%
Received Reliever Medication	-	-	-	100%
Received Systemic Corticosteroids	-	-	-	100%
Emergency Department				
Admittance Decision Time (minutes)	-	-	41	98
Head CT Results Within 45 Min. of Arrival	-	-	44%	57%
Patients Who Left ER Before Being Seen	-	-	1%	2%
Time from ER Arrival to Admit. (minutes)	-	-	174	274
Time from ER Arrival to Discharge (minutes)	-	-	113	134
Time in ER Before Being Evaluated (minutes)	-	-	18	26
Time to Pain Meds for Fractures (minutes)	-	-	44	57
Heart Attack Care				
Aspirin Given at Discharge[5]	-	-	100%	99%
Fibrinolytic Meds Within 30 Min. of Arrival[5]	-	-	100%	54%
PCI Within 90 Minutes of Arrival[5]	-	-	94%	96%
Statin Prescribed at Discharge[5]	-	-	98%	98%
Heart Failure Care				
ACE Inhibitor or ARB for LVSD	27	100%	93%	97%
Discharge Instructions Given	73	97%	90%	94%
Evaluation of LVS Function	86	100%	97%	99%
Medicare Spending				
Medicare Spending per Patient (ratio)	-	-	0.9	0.98
Pneumonia Care				
Appropriate Initial Antibiotic Given	30	97%	90%	95%
Blood Culture Timing	50	100%	95%	98%
Pregnancy and Delivery Care				
Newborn Deliveries Scheduled Early	-	-	7%	6%
Preventive Care				
Immunization for Influenza[5]	-	-	89%	90%
Immunization for Pneumonia[5]	-	-	89%	92%
Stroke Care				
Anticoagulation Therapy for Atrial Fibrillation	-	-	97%	95%
Antithrombotic Therapy Timing	-	-	98%	98%
Assessed for Rehabilitation	-	-	98%	97%
Discharged on Antithrombotic Therapy	-	-	100%	99%
Discharged on Statin Medication	-	-	93%	94%
Thrombolytic Therapy Timing	-	-	51%	66%
Venous Thromboembolism Prophylaxis	-	-	96%	94%
Written Stroke Educational Materials Given	-	-	85%	88%
Surgical Care Improvement Project				
Appropriate Beta Blocker Usage[2]	73	97%	98%	98%
Appropriate VTP Within 24 Hours[2]	148	100%	98%	98%
Controlled Postoperative Blood Glucose[5]	-	-	98%	97%
Perioperative Temperature Management[2]	168	100%	99%	100%
Prophylactic Antibiotic Selection	138	100%	99%	99%
Prophylactic Antibiotic Selection (Outpatient)	-	-	99%	98%
Prophylactic Antibiotic Stopped	138	96%	98%	98%
Prophylactic Antibiotic Timing	138	99%	99%	99%
Prophylactic Antibiotic Timing (Outpatient)	-	-	98%	98%
Urinary Catheter Removal[2]	140	98%	97%	97%
Survey of Patients' Hospital Experiences				
Area Around Room 'Always' Quiet at Night	-	-	72%	61%
Doctors 'Always' Communicated Well	-	-	85%	82%
Home Recovery Information Given	-	-	87%	85%
Hospital Given 9 or 10 on 10 Point Scale	-	-	78%	71%
Meds 'Always' Explained Before Given	-	-	69%	64%
Nurses 'Always' Communicated Well	-	-	83%	79%
Pain 'Always' Well Controlled	-	-	72%	71%
Room and Bathroom 'Always' Clean	-	-	79%	73%
Timely Help 'Always' Received	-	-	77%	68%
Would Definitely Recommend Hospital	-	-	76%	71%
Use of Medical Imaging				
Cardiac Imaging Stress Test before Surgery	-	-	4.4%	5.3%
Combination Abdominal CT Scan	-	-	12.5%	10.5%
Combination Brain/Sinus CT Scan	-	-	2%	2.7%
Combination Chest CT Scan	-	-	4.5%	2.7%
Follow-up Mammogram/Ultrasound	-	-	8.7%	8.8%
Lumbar Spine MRI for Low Back Pain	-	-	33%	37.2%

Spearfish Regional Hospital

1440 N Main St
Spearfish, SD 57783
URL: www.rcrh.org
Phone: 605-644-4000
Fax: 605-644-4011
Type: Acute Care Hospitals
Emergency Services: Yes
Ownership: Voluntary non-profit - Private
Beds: 40

Key Personnel:

Anesthesiology. . . . . Chuck Austin
Emergency Room . . . . Kathy Culver
Radiology. . . . . Garry K. Dunn, MD
Surgery . . . . Steven A. Giuseffi, MD
CEO/President. . . . . Charles E. Hart, MD, MS
Infection Control. . . . . Jennifer Jones
Cardiac Laboratory. . . . . Dawn Koehler

Measure	Cases	This Hosp.	State Avg.	U.S. Avg.
Blood Clot Prevention and Treatment				
Anticoagulation Overlap Therapy[1,2]	-	-	95%	93%
ICU Venous Thromboembolism Prophylaxis[2]	22	100%	91%	92%
Incidence of Potentially Preventable VTE[2,7]	-	-	5%	10%
UFH with Dosages/Platelet Monitoring[2,7]	-	-	100%	97%
Venous Thromboembolism Prophylaxis[2]	240	90%	80%	85%
Warfarin Therapy Discharge Instructions[1,2]	-	-	70%	75%
Chest Pain/Possible Heart Attack Care				
Aspirin Given Within 24 Hours of Arrival	37	97%	99%	96%
Fibrinolytic Meds Within 30 Min. of Arrival	13	77%	69%	58%
Average Time to ECG (minutes)	42	6	5	7
Average Time to Transfer (minutes)[7]	-	-	66	60
Children's Asthma Care				
Received Home Management Plan of Care	-	-	-	88%
Received Reliever Medication	-	-	-	100%
Received Systemic Corticosteroids	-	-	-	100%
Emergency Department				
Admittance Decision Time (minutes)[2]	114	53	41	98
Head CT Results Within 45 Min. of Arrival[1]	-	-	44%	57%
Patients Who Left ER Before Being Seen	9,199	1%	1%	2%
Time from ER Arrival to Admit. (minutes)[2]	189	169	174	274
Time from ER Arrival to Discharge (minutes)	512	87	113	134
Time in ER Before Being Evaluated (minutes)	376	14	18	26
Time to Pain Meds for Fractures (minutes)	70	38	44	57
Heart Attack Care				
Aspirin Given at Discharge[1,2]	-	-	100%	99%
Fibrinolytic Meds Within 30 Min. of Arrival[2,7]	-	-	100%	54%
PCI Within 90 Minutes of Arrival[2,7]	-	-	94%	96%
Statin Prescribed at Discharge[1,2]	-	-	98%	98%
Heart Failure Care				
ACE Inhibitor or ARB for LVSD[1]	-	-	93%	97%
Discharge Instructions Given[1]	-	-	90%	94%
Evaluation of LVS Function	20	95%	97%	99%
Medicare Spending				
Medicare Spending per Patient (ratio)	-	0.91	0.9	0.98
Pneumonia Care				
Appropriate Initial Antibiotic Given[2]	25	88%	90%	95%
Blood Culture Timing[2]	25	96%	95%	98%
Pregnancy and Delivery Care				
Newborn Deliveries Scheduled Early	48	2%	7%	6%
Preventive Care				
Immunization for Influenza[2]	255	92%	89%	90%
Immunization for Pneumonia[2]	243	94%	89%	92%
Stroke Care				
Anticoagulation Therapy for Atrial Fibrillation[1]	-	-	97%	95%
Antithrombotic Therapy Timing[1]	-	-	98%	98%
Assessed for Rehabilitation[1]	-	-	98%	97%
Discharged on Antithrombotic Therapy[1]	-	-	100%	99%
Discharged on Statin Medication[1]	-	-	93%	94%
Thrombolytic Therapy Timing[7]	-	-	51%	66%
Venous Thromboembolism Prophylaxis[1]	-	-	96%	94%
Written Stroke Educational Materials Given[1]	-	-	85%	88%
Surgical Care Improvement Project				
Appropriate Beta Blocker Usage[2]	79	97%	98%	98%
Appropriate VTP Within 24 Hours[2]	254	97%	98%	98%
Controlled Postoperative Blood Glucose[2,7]	-	-	98%	97%
Perioperative Temperature Management[2]	311	100%	99%	100%
Prophylactic Antibiotic Selection[2]	263	100%	99%	99%
Prophylactic Antibiotic Selection (Outpatient)	66	98%	99%	98%
Prophylactic Antibiotic Stopped[2]	255	100%	98%	98%
Prophylactic Antibiotic Timing[2]	263	97%	99%	99%
Prophylactic Antibiotic Timing (Outpatient)	66	97%	98%	98%
Urinary Catheter Removal[2]	246	99%	97%	97%
Survey of Patients' Hospital Experiences				
Area Around Room 'Always' Quiet at Night	300+	62%	72%	61%
Doctors 'Always' Communicated Well	300+	77%	85%	82%
Home Recovery Information Given	300+	88%	87%	85%
Hospital Given 9 or 10 on 10 Point Scale	300+	72%	78%	71%
Meds 'Always' Explained Before Given	300+	63%	69%	64%
Nurses 'Always' Communicated Well	300+	81%	83%	79%
Pain 'Always' Well Controlled	300+	70%	72%	71%
Room and Bathroom 'Always' Clean	300+	75%	79%	73%
Timely Help 'Always' Received	300+	78%	77%	68%
Would Definitely Recommend Hospital	300+	70%	76%	71%
Use of Medical Imaging				
Cardiac Imaging Stress Test before Surgery[7]	-	-	4.4%	5.3%
Combination Abdominal CT Scan	262	2.7%	12.5%	10.5%
Combination Brain/Sinus CT Scan[1]	-	-	2%	2.7%
Combination Chest CT Scan	169	1.2%	4.5%	2.7%
Follow-up Mammogram/Ultrasound	328	5.5%	8.7%	8.8%
Lumbar Spine MRI for Low Back Pain	85	48.2%	33%	37.2%

Spearfish Regional Surgery Center

1316 10th St
Spearfish, SD 57783
Phone: 605-642-3113
Type: Acute Care Hospitals
Emergency Services: No
Ownership: Voluntary non-profit - Other
Beds: 6

Key Personnel:

CEO/President. . . . . Mike Delano
Radiology. . . . . Garry K. Dunn, MD

Measure	Cases	This Hosp.	State Avg.	U.S. Avg.
Blood Clot Prevention and Treatment				
Anticoagulation Overlap Therapy[1]	-	-	95%	93%
ICU Venous Thromboembolism Prophylaxis[7]	-	-	91%	92%
Incidence of Potentially Preventable VTE[1]	-	-	5%	10%
UFH with Dosages/Platelet Monitoring[7]	-	-	100%	97%
Venous Thromboembolism Prophylaxis[1]	-	-	80%	85%
Warfarin Therapy Discharge Instructions[7]	-	-	70%	75%
Chest Pain/Possible Heart Attack Care				
Aspirin Given Within 24 Hours of Arrival[5]	-	-	99%	96%
Fibrinolytic Meds Within 30 Min. of Arrival[5]	-	-	69%	58%
Average Time to ECG (minutes)[5]	-	-	5	7
Average Time to Transfer (minutes)[5]	-	-	66	60
Children's Asthma Care				
Received Home Management Plan of Care	-	-	-	88%
Received Reliever Medication	-	-	-	100%
Received Systemic Corticosteroids	-	-	-	100%
Emergency Department				
Admittance Decision Time (minutes)[7]	-	-	41	98
Head CT Results Within 45 Min. of Arrival[5]	-	-	44%	57%
Patients Who Left ER Before Being Seen	2,302	0%	1%	2%
Time from ER Arrival to Admit. (minutes)[7]	-	-	174	274
Time from ER Arrival to Discharge (minutes)[5]	-	-	113	134
Time in ER Before Being Evaluated (minutes)[5]	-	-	18	26
Time to Pain Meds for Fractures (minutes)[5]	-	-	44	57
Heart Attack Care				
Aspirin Given at Discharge[5]	-	-	100%	99%
Fibrinolytic Meds Within 30 Min. of Arrival[5]	-	-	100%	54%
PCI Within 90 Minutes of Arrival[5]	-	-	94%	96%
Statin Prescribed at Discharge[5]	-	-	98%	98%
Heart Failure Care				
ACE Inhibitor or ARB for LVSD[5]	-	-	93%	97%
Discharge Instructions Given[5]	-	-	90%	94%

NOTE: Hospital profiles are in alphabetical order by state, then city, then hospital within the city; Rankings exclude hospitals with less than 25 cases except for patient surveys which excludes hospitals with less than 100 cases; (a) 100-299 cases; (1) The number of cases/patients is too few to report; (2) Data submitted were based on a sample of cases/patients; (3) Results are based on a shorter time period than required; (4) Data suppressed by CMS for one or more quarters; (5) Results are not available for this reporting period; (6) Fewer than 100 patients completed the HCAHPS survey; (7) No cases met the criteria for this measure; (8) The lower limit of the confidence interval cannot be calculated if the number of observed infections equals zero; (9) No data are available from the state/territory for this reporting period; (10) The scores shown reflect fewer than 50 completed surveys; (11) There were discrepancies in the data collection process; (12) This measure does not apply to this hospital for this reporting period; (13) Results cannot be calculated for this reporting period; (14) The results for this state are combined with nearby states to protect confidentiality; Please refer to the User's Guide for a full explanation of data.

Measure	Cases	This Hosp.	State Avg.	U.S. Avg.
Evaluation of LVS Function[5]	-	-	97%	99%
Medicare Spending				
Medicare Spending per Patient (ratio)[1]	-	-	0.9	0.98
Pneumonia Care				
Appropriate Initial Antibiotic Given[5]	-	-	90%	95%
Blood Culture Timing[5]	-	-	95%	98%
Pregnancy and Delivery Care				
Newborn Deliveries Scheduled Early[7]	-	-	7%	6%
Preventive Care				
Immunization for Influenza	34	74%	89%	90%
Immunization for Pneumonia	26	65%	89%	92%
Stroke Care				
Anticoagulation Therapy for Atrial Fibrillation[5]	-	-	97%	95%
Antithrombotic Therapy Timing[5]	-	-	98%	98%
Assessed for Rehabilitation[5]	-	-	98%	97%
Discharged on Antithrombotic Therapy[5]	-	-	100%	99%
Discharged on Statin Medication[5]	-	-	93%	94%
Thrombolytic Therapy Timing[5]	-	-	51%	66%
Venous Thromboembolism Prophylaxis[5]	-	-	96%	94%
Written Stroke Educational Materials Given[5]	-	-	85%	88%
Surgical Care Improvement Project				
Appropriate Beta Blocker Usage[1]	-	-	98%	98%
Appropriate VTP Within 24 Hours	50	100%	98%	98%
Controlled Postoperative Blood Glucose[7]	-	-	98%	97%
Perioperative Temperature Management	57	100%	99%	100%
Prophylactic Antibiotic Selection	55	100%	99%	99%
Prophylactic Antibiotic Selection (Outpatient)[5]	-	-	99%	98%
Prophylactic Antibiotic Stopped	55	100%	98%	98%
Prophylactic Antibiotic Timing	55	100%	99%	99%
Prophylactic Antibiotic Timing (Outpatient)[5]	-	-	98%	98%
Urinary Catheter Removal	48	100%	97%	97%
Survey of Patients' Hospital Experiences				
Area Around Room 'Always' Quiet at Night[10]	<100	91%	72%	61%
Doctors 'Always' Communicated Well[10]	<100	97%	85%	82%
Home Recovery Information Given[10]	<100	92%	87%	85%
Hospital Given 9 or 10 on 10 Point Scale[10]	<100	87%	78%	71%
Meds 'Always' Explained Before Given[10]	<100	69%	69%	64%
Nurses 'Always' Communicated Well[10]	<100	88%	83%	79%
Pain 'Always' Well Controlled[10]	<100	79%	72%	71%
Room and Bathroom 'Always' Clean[10]	<100	77%	79%	73%
Timely Help 'Always' Received[10]	<100	81%	77%	68%
Would Definitely Recommend Hospital[10]	<100	86%	76%	71%
Use of Medical Imaging				
Cardiac Imaging Stress Test before Surgery[7]	-	-	4.4%	5.3%
Combination Abdominal CT Scan[7]	-	-	12.5%	10.5%
Combination Brain/Sinus CT Scan[7]	-	-	2%	2.7%
Combination Chest CT Scan[7]	-	-	4.5%	2.7%
Follow-up Mammogram/Ultrasound[7]	-	-	8.7%	8.8%
Lumbar Spine MRI for Low Back Pain[7]	-	-	33%	37.2%

Sturgis Regional Hospital

949 Harmon Street
Sturgis, SD 57785
Phone: 605-720-2400
Fax: 605-720-0338
URL: www.rcrh.org
Type: Critical Access Hospitals
Emergency Services: Yes
Ownership: Voluntary non-profit - Private
Beds: 25

Key Personnel:
Infection Control. . . . . Glea Beck
CEO/President. . . . . Charles E. Hart, MD, MS
Quality Assurance . . . . Marilyn Johnson
Operating Room. . . . . Ron Owen
Emergency Room . . . . Lynn Simons
Chief of Medical Staff. . . . . George Tenter

Measure	Cases	This Hosp.	State Avg.	U.S. Avg.
Blood Clot Prevention and Treatment				
Anticoagulation Overlap Therapy[1]	-	-	95%	93%
ICU Venous Thromboembolism Prophylaxis[1]	-	-	91%	92%
Incidence of Potentially Preventable VTE[1]	-	-	5%	10%
UFH with Dosages/Platelet Monitoring[7]	-	-	100%	97%
Venous Thromboembolism Prophylaxis	169	60%	80%	85%
Warfarin Therapy Discharge Instructions[1]	-	-	70%	75%
Chest Pain/Possible Heart Attack Care				
Aspirin Given Within 24 Hours of Arrival	25	100%	99%	96%
Fibrinolytic Meds Within 30 Min. of Arrival[3,7]	-	-	69%	58%
Average Time to ECG (minutes)	25	7	5	7
Average Time to Transfer (minutes)[1,3]	-	-	66	60
Children's Asthma Care				
Received Home Management Plan of Care	-	-	-	88%
Received Reliever Medication	-	-	-	100%
Received Systemic Corticosteroids	-	-	-	100%
Emergency Department				
Admittance Decision Time (minutes)	243	17	41	98
Head CT Results Within 45 Min. of Arrival[3,7]	-	-	44%	57%
Patients Who Left ER Before Being Seen[5]	-	-	1%	2%
Time from ER Arrival to Admit. (minutes)	247	126	174	274
Time from ER Arrival to Discharge (minutes)	369	91	113	134
Time in ER Before Being Evaluated (minutes)	376	16	18	26
Time to Pain Meds for Fractures (minutes)[1,3]	-	-	44	57
Heart Attack Care				
Aspirin Given at Discharge[5]	-	-	100%	99%
Fibrinolytic Meds Within 30 Min. of Arrival[5]	-	-	100%	54%
PCI Within 90 Minutes of Arrival[5]	-	-	94%	96%
Statin Prescribed at Discharge[5]	-	-	98%	98%
Heart Failure Care				
ACE Inhibitor or ARB for LVSD[7]	-	-	93%	97%
Discharge Instructions Given[1]	-	-	90%	94%
Evaluation of LVS Function[1]	-	-	97%	99%
Medicare Spending				
Medicare Spending per Patient (ratio)	-	-	0.9	0.98
Pneumonia Care				
Appropriate Initial Antibiotic Given	28	93%	90%	95%
Blood Culture Timing[1]	-	-	95%	98%
Pregnancy and Delivery Care				
Newborn Deliveries Scheduled Early[5]	-	-	7%	6%
Preventive Care				
Immunization for Influenza	149	89%	89%	90%
Immunization for Pneumonia	222	91%	89%	92%
Stroke Care				
Anticoagulation Therapy for Atrial Fibrillation[3,7]	-	-	97%	95%
Antithrombotic Therapy Timing[3,7]	-	-	98%	98%
Assessed for Rehabilitation[1,3]	-	-	98%	97%
Discharged on Antithrombotic Therapy[3,7]	-	-	100%	99%
Discharged on Statin Medication[1,3]	-	-	93%	94%
Thrombolytic Therapy Timing[3,7]	-	-	51%	66%
Venous Thromboembolism Prophylaxis[1,3]	-	-	96%	94%
Written Stroke Educational Materials Given[3,7]	-	-	85%	88%
Surgical Care Improvement Project				
Appropriate Beta Blocker Usage[5]	-	-	98%	98%
Appropriate VTP Within 24 Hours[5]	-	-	98%	98%
Controlled Postoperative Blood Glucose[5]	-	-	98%	97%
Perioperative Temperature Management[5]	-	-	99%	100%
Prophylactic Antibiotic Selection[5]	-	-	99%	99%
Prophylactic Antibiotic Selection (Outpatient)[5]	-	-	99%	98%
Prophylactic Antibiotic Stopped[5]	-	-	98%	98%
Prophylactic Antibiotic Timing[5]	-	-	99%	99%
Prophylactic Antibiotic Timing (Outpatient)[5]	-	-	98%	98%
Urinary Catheter Removal[5]	-	-	97%	97%
Survey of Patients' Hospital Experiences				
Area Around Room 'Always' Quiet at Night	(a)	65%	72%	61%
Doctors 'Always' Communicated Well	(a)	88%	85%	82%
Home Recovery Information Given	(a)	91%	87%	85%
Hospital Given 9 or 10 on 10 Point Scale	(a)	77%	78%	71%
Meds 'Always' Explained Before Given	(a)	72%	69%	64%
Nurses 'Always' Communicated Well	(a)	88%	83%	79%
Pain 'Always' Well Controlled	(a)	85%	72%	71%
Room and Bathroom 'Always' Clean	(a)	82%	79%	73%
Timely Help 'Always' Received	(a)	84%	77%	68%
Would Definitely Recommend Hospital	(a)	73%	76%	71%
Use of Medical Imaging				
Cardiac Imaging Stress Test before Surgery[7]	-	-	4.4%	5.3%
Combination Abdominal CT Scan	93	6.5%	12.5%	10.5%
Combination Brain/Sinus CT Scan[1]	-	-	2%	2.7%
Combination Chest CT Scan[1]	-	-	4.5%	2.7%
Follow-up Mammogram/Ultrasound	166	10.8%	8.7%	8.8%
Lumbar Spine MRI for Low Back Pain[1]	-	-	33%	37.2%

Saint Michael's Hospital

410 W 16th Ave
Phone: 605-589-3341
Tyndall, SD 57066
Type: Critical Access Hospitals
Emergency Services: Yes
Ownership: Government - Local

Measure	Cases	This Hosp.	State Avg.	U.S. Avg.
Blood Clot Prevention and Treatment				
Anticoagulation Overlap Therapy[5]	-	-	95%	93%
ICU Venous Thromboembolism Prophylaxis[5]	-	-	91%	92%
Incidence of Potentially Preventable VTE[5]	-	-	5%	10%
UFH with Dosages/Platelet Monitoring[5]	-	-	100%	97%
Venous Thromboembolism Prophylaxis[5]	-	-	80%	85%
Warfarin Therapy Discharge Instructions[5]	-	-	70%	75%
Chest Pain/Possible Heart Attack Care				
Aspirin Given Within 24 Hours of Arrival	-	-	99%	96%
Fibrinolytic Meds Within 30 Min. of Arrival	-	-	69%	58%
Average Time to ECG (minutes)	-	-	5	7
Average Time to Transfer (minutes)	-	-	66	60
Children's Asthma Care				
Received Home Management Plan of Care	-	-	-	88%
Received Reliever Medication	-	-	-	100%
Received Systemic Corticosteroids	-	-	-	100%
Emergency Department				
Admittance Decision Time (minutes)[5]	-	-	41	98
Head CT Results Within 45 Min. of Arrival	-	-	44%	57%
Patients Who Left ER Before Being Seen	-	-	1%	2%
Time from ER Arrival to Admit. (minutes)[5]	-	-	174	274
Time from ER Arrival to Discharge (minutes)	-	-	113	134
Time in ER Before Being Evaluated (minutes)	-	-	18	26
Time to Pain Meds for Fractures (minutes)	-	-	44	57
Heart Attack Care				
Aspirin Given at Discharge[3,7]	-	-	100%	99%
Fibrinolytic Meds Within 30 Min. of Arrival[3,7]	-	-	100%	54%
PCI Within 90 Minutes of Arrival[3,7]	-	-	94%	96%
Statin Prescribed at Discharge[3,7]	-	-	98%	98%
Heart Failure Care				
ACE Inhibitor or ARB for LVSD[1,3]	-	-	93%	97%
Discharge Instructions Given[1,3]	-	-	90%	94%
Evaluation of LVS Function[3]	12	92%	97%	99%
Medicare Spending				
Medicare Spending per Patient (ratio)	-	-	0.9	0.98
Pneumonia Care				
Appropriate Initial Antibiotic Given[1,3]	-	-	90%	95%
Blood Culture Timing[1,3]	-	-	95%	98%
Pregnancy and Delivery Care				
Newborn Deliveries Scheduled Early[5]	-	-	7%	6%
Preventive Care				
Immunization for Influenza[5]	-	-	89%	90%
Immunization for Pneumonia[5]	-	-	89%	92%
Stroke Care				
Anticoagulation Therapy for Atrial Fibrillation[5]	-	-	97%	95%
Antithrombotic Therapy Timing[5]	-	-	98%	98%
Assessed for Rehabilitation[5]	-	-	98%	97%
Discharged on Antithrombotic Therapy[5]	-	-	100%	99%
Discharged on Statin Medication[5]	-	-	93%	94%
Thrombolytic Therapy Timing[5]	-	-	51%	66%
Venous Thromboembolism Prophylaxis[5]	-	-	96%	94%
Written Stroke Educational Materials Given[5]	-	-	85%	88%
Surgical Care Improvement Project				
Appropriate Beta Blocker Usage[5]	-	-	98%	98%
Appropriate VTP Within 24 Hours[5]	-	-	98%	98%
Controlled Postoperative Blood Glucose[5]	-	-	98%	97%
Perioperative Temperature Management[5]	-	-	99%	100%
Prophylactic Antibiotic Selection[5]	-	-	99%	99%
Prophylactic Antibiotic Selection (Outpatient)	-	-	99%	98%
Prophylactic Antibiotic Stopped[5]	-	-	98%	98%
Prophylactic Antibiotic Timing[5]	-	-	99%	99%
Prophylactic Antibiotic Timing (Outpatient)	-	-	98%	98%
Urinary Catheter Removal[5]	-	-	97%	97%
Survey of Patients' Hospital Experiences				
Area Around Room 'Always' Quiet at Night[10]	<100	70%	72%	61%
Doctors 'Always' Communicated Well[10]	<100	90%	85%	82%

NOTE: Hospital profiles are in alphabetical order by state, then city, then hospital within the city; Rankings exclude hospitals with less than 25 cases except for patient surveys which excludes hospitals with less than 100 cases; (a) 100-299 cases; (1) The number of cases/patients is too few to report; (2) Data submitted were based on a sample of cases/patients; (3) Results are based on a shorter time period than required; (4) Data suppressed by CMS for one or more quarters; (5) Results are not available for this reporting period; (6) Fewer than 100 patients completed the HCAHPS survey; (7) No cases met the criteria for this measure; (8) The lower limit of the confidence interval cannot be calculated if the number of observed infections equals zero; (9) No data are available from the state/territory for this reporting period; (10) The scores shown reflect fewer than 50 completed surveys; (11) There were discrepancies in the data collection process; (12) This measure does not apply to this hospital for this reporting period; (13) Results cannot be calculated for this reporting period; (14) The results for this state are combined with nearby states to protect confidentiality; Please refer to the User's Guide for a full explanation of data.

Home Recovery Information Given[10]	<100	87%	87%	85%
Hospital Given 9 or 10 on 10 Point Scale[10]	<100	87%	78%	71%
Meds 'Always' Explained Before Given[10]	<100	47%	69%	64%
Nurses 'Always' Communicated Well[10]	<100	83%	83%	79%
Pain 'Always' Well Controlled[10]	<100	78%	72%	71%
Room and Bathroom 'Always' Clean[10]	<100	69%	79%	73%
Timely Help 'Always' Received[10]	<100	71%	77%	68%
Would Definitely Recommend Hospital[10]	<100	77%	76%	71%
Use of Medical Imaging				
Cardiac Imaging Stress Test before Surgery	-	-	4.4%	5.3%
Combination Abdominal CT Scan	-	-	12.5%	10.5%
Combination Brain/Sinus CT Scan	-	-	2%	2.7%
Combination Chest CT Scan	-	-	4.5%	2.7%
Follow-up Mammogram/Ultrasound	-	-	8.7%	8.8%
Lumbar Spine MRI for Low Back Pain	-	-	33%	37.2%

Sanford Vermillion Hospital

20 South Plum Street
Vermillion, SD 57069
Phone: 605-624-2611
Fax: 605-624-4001
E-mail: info@sanfordvermillion.org
URL: www.sanfordvermillion.org
Type: Critical Access Hospitals
Emergency Services: Yes
Ownership: Voluntary non-profit - Private
Beds: 25

Key Personnel:
Chief of Medical Staff.......... W Dendinger, MD
Operating Room.............. John Jorgensen
CEO/President............... John Paulsa
Infection Control.............. Tammy Spiers
Anesthesiology............... Jim Sundit

Measure	Cases	This Hosp.	State Avg.	U.S. Avg.
Blood Clot Prevention and Treatment				
Anticoagulation Overlap Therapy[5]	-	-	95%	93%
ICU Venous Thromboembolism Prophylaxis[5]	-	-	91%	92%
Incidence of Potentially Preventable VTE[5]	-	-	5%	10%
UFH with Dosages/Platelet Monitoring[5]	-	-	100%	97%
Venous Thromboembolism Prophylaxis[5]	-	-	80%	85%
Warfarin Therapy Discharge Instructions[5]	-	-	70%	75%
Chest Pain/Possible Heart Attack Care				
Aspirin Given Within 24 Hours of Arrival	-	-	99%	96%
Fibrinolytic Meds Within 30 Min. of Arrival	-	-	69%	58%
Average Time to ECG (minutes)	-	-	5	7
Average Time to Transfer (minutes)	-	-	66	60
Children's Asthma Care				
Received Home Management Plan of Care	-	-	-	88%
Received Reliever Medication	-	-	-	100%
Received Systemic Corticosteroids	-	-	-	100%
Emergency Department				
Admittance Decision Time (minutes)[5]	-	-	41	98
Head CT Results Within 45 Min. of Arrival	-	-	44%	57%
Patients Who Left ER Before Being Seen	-	-	1%	2%
Time from ER Arrival to Admit. (minutes)[5]	-	-	174	274
Time from ER Arrival to Discharge (minutes)	-	-	113	134
Time in ER Before Being Evaluated (minutes)	-	-	18	26
Time to Pain Meds for Fractures (minutes)	-	-	44	57
Heart Attack Care				
Aspirin Given at Discharge[3,7]	-	-	100%	99%
Fibrinolytic Meds Within 30 Min. of Arrival[3,7]	-	-	100%	54%
PCI Within 90 Minutes of Arrival[3,7]	-	-	94%	96%
Statin Prescribed at Discharge[3,7]	-	-	98%	98%
Heart Failure Care				
ACE Inhibitor or ARB for LVSD[1]	-	-	93%	97%
Discharge Instructions Given[1]	-	-	90%	94%
Evaluation of LVS Function	12	83%	97%	99%
Medicare Spending				
Medicare Spending per Patient (ratio)	-	-	0.9	0.98
Pneumonia Care				
Appropriate Initial Antibiotic Given	14	100%	90%	95%
Blood Culture Timing[1]	-	-	95%	98%
Pregnancy and Delivery Care				
Newborn Deliveries Scheduled Early[5]	-	-	7%	6%
Preventive Care				
Immunization for Influenza[5]	-	-	89%	90%
Immunization for Pneumonia[5]	-	-	89%	92%
Stroke Care				
Anticoagulation Therapy for Atrial Fibrillation[5]	-	-	97%	95%
Antithrombotic Therapy Timing[5]	-	-	98%	98%
Assessed for Rehabilitation[5]	-	-	98%	97%
Discharged on Antithrombotic Therapy[5]	-	-	100%	99%
Discharged on Statin Medication[5]	-	-	93%	94%
Thrombolytic Therapy Timing[5]	-	-	51%	66%
Venous Thromboembolism Prophylaxis[5]	-	-	96%	94%
Written Stroke Educational Materials Given[5]	-	-	85%	88%
Surgical Care Improvement Project				
Appropriate Beta Blocker Usage[5]	-	-	98%	98%
Appropriate VTP Within 24 Hours[5]	-	-	98%	98%
Controlled Postoperative Blood Glucose[5]	-	-	98%	97%
Perioperative Temperature Management[5]	-	-	99%	100%
Prophylactic Antibiotic Selection[5]	-	-	99%	99%
Prophylactic Antibiotic Selection (Outpatient)	-	-	99%	98%
Prophylactic Antibiotic Stopped[5]	-	-	98%	98%
Prophylactic Antibiotic Timing[5]	-	-	99%	99%
Prophylactic Antibiotic Timing (Outpatient)	-	-	98%	98%
Urinary Catheter Removal[5]	-	-	97%	97%
Survey of Patients' Hospital Experiences				
Area Around Room 'Always' Quiet at Night[6]	<100	76%	72%	61%
Doctors 'Always' Communicated Well[6]	<100	92%	85%	82%
Home Recovery Information Given[6]	<100	88%	87%	85%
Hospital Given 9 or 10 on 10 Point Scale[6]	<100	77%	78%	71%
Meds 'Always' Explained Before Given[6]	<100	67%	69%	64%
Nurses 'Always' Communicated Well[6]	<100	80%	83%	79%
Pain 'Always' Well Controlled[6]	<100	71%	72%	71%
Room and Bathroom 'Always' Clean[6]	<100	74%	79%	73%
Timely Help 'Always' Received[6]	<100	70%	77%	68%
Would Definitely Recommend Hospital[6]	<100	74%	76%	71%
Use of Medical Imaging				
Cardiac Imaging Stress Test before Surgery	-	-	4.4%	5.3%
Combination Abdominal CT Scan	-	-	12.5%	10.5%
Combination Brain/Sinus CT Scan	-	-	2%	2.7%
Combination Chest CT Scan	-	-	4.5%	2.7%
Follow-up Mammogram/Ultrasound	-	-	8.7%	8.8%
Lumbar Spine MRI for Low Back Pain	-	-	33%	37.2%

Wagner Community Memorial Hospital

513 3rd Saint Sw, Post Office Box 280
Wagner, SD 57380
Phone: 605-384-3611
Fax: 605-384-3232
URL: www.avera.org
Type: Critical Access Hospitals
Emergency Services: Yes
Ownership: Voluntary non-profit - Other
Beds: 20

Key Personnel:
Chief of Medical Staff.......... GA Bubak, MD
Emergency Room .... Judith Neilsen
Infection Control............. Marcia Podzimek

Measure	Cases	This Hosp.	State Avg.	U.S. Avg.
Blood Clot Prevention and Treatment				
Anticoagulation Overlap Therapy[5]	-	-	95%	93%
ICU Venous Thromboembolism Prophylaxis[5]	-	-	91%	92%
Incidence of Potentially Preventable VTE[5]	-	-	5%	10%
UFH with Dosages/Platelet Monitoring[5]	-	-	100%	97%
Venous Thromboembolism Prophylaxis[5]	-	-	80%	85%
Warfarin Therapy Discharge Instructions[5]	-	-	70%	75%
Chest Pain/Possible Heart Attack Care				
Aspirin Given Within 24 Hours of Arrival[5]	-	-	99%	96%
Fibrinolytic Meds Within 30 Min. of Arrival[5]	-	-	69%	58%
Average Time to ECG (minutes)[5]	-	-	5	7
Average Time to Transfer (minutes)[5]	-	-	66	60
Children's Asthma Care				
Received Home Management Plan of Care	-	-	-	88%
Received Reliever Medication	-	-	-	100%
Received Systemic Corticosteroids	-	-	-	100%
Emergency Department				
Admittance Decision Time (minutes)[5]	-	-	41	98
Head CT Results Within 45 Min. of Arrival[5]	-	-	44%	57%
Patients Who Left ER Before Being Seen[5]	-	-	1%	2%
Time from ER Arrival to Admit. (minutes)[5]	-	-	174	274
Time from ER Arrival to Discharge (minutes)[3]	99	75	113	134
Time in ER Before Being Evaluated (minutes)[3]	133	20	18	26
Time to Pain Meds for Fractures (minutes)[1,3]	-	-	44	57
Heart Attack Care				
Aspirin Given at Discharge[5]	-	-	100%	99%
Fibrinolytic Meds Within 30 Min. of Arrival[5]	-	-	100%	54%
PCI Within 90 Minutes of Arrival[5]	-	-	94%	96%
Statin Prescribed at Discharge[5]	-	-	98%	98%
Heart Failure Care				
ACE Inhibitor or ARB for LVSD[3,7]	-	-	93%	97%
Discharge Instructions Given[1,3]	-	-	90%	94%
Evaluation of LVS Function[1,3]	-	-	97%	99%
Medicare Spending				
Medicare Spending per Patient (ratio)	-	-	0.9	0.98
Pneumonia Care				
Appropriate Initial Antibiotic Given[1,3]	-	-	90%	95%
Blood Culture Timing[1,3]	-	-	95%	98%
Pregnancy and Delivery Care				
Newborn Deliveries Scheduled Early[5]	-	-	7%	6%
Preventive Care				
Immunization for Influenza[5]	-	-	89%	90%
Immunization for Pneumonia[5]	-	-	89%	92%
Stroke Care				
Anticoagulation Therapy for Atrial Fibrillation[5]	-	-	97%	95%
Antithrombotic Therapy Timing[5]	-	-	98%	98%
Assessed for Rehabilitation[5]	-	-	98%	97%
Discharged on Antithrombotic Therapy[5]	-	-	100%	99%
Discharged on Statin Medication[5]	-	-	93%	94%
Thrombolytic Therapy Timing[5]	-	-	51%	66%
Venous Thromboembolism Prophylaxis[5]	-	-	96%	94%
Written Stroke Educational Materials Given[5]	-	-	85%	88%
Surgical Care Improvement Project				
Appropriate Beta Blocker Usage[5]	-	-	98%	98%
Appropriate VTP Within 24 Hours[5]	-	-	98%	98%
Controlled Postoperative Blood Glucose[5]	-	-	98%	97%
Perioperative Temperature Management[5]	-	-	99%	100%
Prophylactic Antibiotic Selection[5]	-	-	99%	99%
Prophylactic Antibiotic Selection (Outpatient)[5]	-	-	99%	98%
Prophylactic Antibiotic Stopped[5]	-	-	98%	98%
Prophylactic Antibiotic Timing[5]	-	-	99%	99%
Prophylactic Antibiotic Timing (Outpatient)[5]	-	-	98%	98%
Urinary Catheter Removal[5]	-	-	97%	97%
Survey of Patients' Hospital Experiences				
Area Around Room 'Always' Quiet at Night[10]	<100	74%	72%	61%
Doctors 'Always' Communicated Well[10]	<100	89%	85%	82%
Home Recovery Information Given[10]	<100	88%	87%	85%
Hospital Given 9 or 10 on 10 Point Scale[10]	<100	65%	78%	71%
Meds 'Always' Explained Before Given[10]	<100	55%	69%	64%
Nurses 'Always' Communicated Well[10]	<100	86%	83%	79%
Pain 'Always' Well Controlled[10]	<100	79%	72%	71%
Room and Bathroom 'Always' Clean[10]	<100	68%	79%	73%
Timely Help 'Always' Received[10]	<100	74%	77%	68%
Would Definitely Recommend Hospital[10]	<100	72%	76%	71%
Use of Medical Imaging				
Cardiac Imaging Stress Test before Surgery[1]	-	-	4.4%	5.3%
Combination Abdominal CT Scan[1]	-	-	12.5%	10.5%
Combination Brain/Sinus CT Scan[1]	-	-	2%	2.7%
Combination Chest CT Scan[1]	-	-	4.5%	2.7%
Follow-up Mammogram/Ultrasound	72	15.3%	8.7%	8.8%
Lumbar Spine MRI for Low Back Pain[1]	-	-	33%	37.2%

Prairie Lakes Hospital

401 9th Avenue Nw Post Office Box 1210
Watertown, SD 57201
Phone: 605-882-7000
Fax: 605-882-7726
E-mail: info@prairielakes.com
URL: www.prairielakes.com
Type: Acute Care Hospitals
Emergency Services: Yes
Ownership: Voluntary non-profit - Private
Beds: 81

Key Personnel:
Anesthesiology.............. Jeffrey Bergsbaken, MD
Radiology.................. Jeffrey Brindle
Surgery.................... Alan Christensen
Radiology.................. Craig Crismon
Emergency Room .... Elliott Filler
Patient Relations .... Jill Fuller
CEO/President.............. Paul Hanson
Intensive Care Unit........... Debra Pederson

NOTE: Hospital profiles are in alphabetical order by state, then city, then hospital within the city; Rankings exclude hospitals with less than 25 cases except for patient surveys which excludes hospitals with less than 100 cases; (a) 100-299 cases; (1) The number of cases/patients is too few to report; (2) Data submitted were based on a sample of cases/patients; (3) Results are based on a shorter time period than required; (4) Data suppressed by CMS for one or more quarters; (5) Results are not available for this reporting period; (6) Fewer than 100 patients completed the HCAHPS survey; (7) No cases met the criteria for this measure; (8) The lower limit of the confidence interval cannot be calculated if the number of observed infections equals zero; (9) No data are available from the state/territory for this reporting period; (10) The scores shown reflect fewer than 50 completed surveys; (11) There were discrepancies in the data collection process; (12) This measure does not apply to this hospital for this reporting period; (13) Results cannot be calculated for this reporting period; (14) The results for this state are combined with nearby states to protect confidentiality; Please refer to the User's Guide for a full explanation of data.

Measure	Cases	This Hosp.	State Avg.	U.S. Avg.
Blood Clot Prevention and Treatment				
Anticoagulation Overlap Therapy[2]	42	90%	95%	93%
ICU Venous Thromboembolism Prophylaxis[2]	74	57%	91%	92%
Incidence of Potentially Preventable VTE[1,2]	-	-	5%	10%
UFH with Dosages/Platelet Monitoring[2]	28	100%	100%	97%
Venous Thromboembolism Prophylaxis[2]	292	59%	80%	85%
Warfarin Therapy Discharge Instructions[2]	34	24%	70%	75%
Chest Pain/Possible Heart Attack Care				
Aspirin Given Within 24 Hours of Arrival	15	100%	99%	96%
Fibrinolytic Meds Within 30 Min. of Arrival[3,7]	-	-	69%	58%
Average Time to ECG (minutes)	15	8	5	7
Average Time to Transfer (minutes)[3,7]	-	-	66	60
Children's Asthma Care				
Received Home Management Plan of Care	-	-	-	88%
Received Reliever Medication	-	-	-	100%
Received Systemic Corticosteroids	-	-	-	100%
Emergency Department				
Admittance Decision Time (minutes)[2]	374	40	41	98
Head CT Results Within 45 Min. of Arrival	12	50%	44%	57%
Patients Who Left ER Before Being Seen	12,512	1%	1%	2%
Time from ER Arrival to Admit. (minutes)[2]	423	142	174	274
Time from ER Arrival to Discharge (minutes)	336	82	113	134
Time in ER Before Being Evaluated (minutes)	377	15	18	26
Time to Pain Meds for Fractures (minutes)	67	42	44	57
Heart Attack Care				
Aspirin Given at Discharge	55	100%	100%	99%
Fibrinolytic Meds Within 30 Min. of Arrival[7]	-	-	100%	54%
PCI Within 90 Minutes of Arrival	14	86%	94%	96%
Statin Prescribed at Discharge	46	98%	98%	98%
Heart Failure Care				
ACE Inhibitor or ARB for LVSD[2]	24	71%	93%	97%
Discharge Instructions Given[2]	73	90%	90%	94%
Evaluation of LVS Function[2]	97	95%	97%	99%
Medicare Spending				
Medicare Spending per Patient (ratio)	-	0.90	0.9	0.98
Pneumonia Care				
Appropriate Initial Antibiotic Given[2]	75	96%	90%	95%
Blood Culture Timing[2]	81	99%	95%	98%
Pregnancy and Delivery Care				
Newborn Deliveries Scheduled Early	81	4%	7%	6%
Preventive Care				
Immunization for Influenza[2]	513	79%	89%	90%
Immunization for Pneumonia[2]	821	75%	89%	92%
Stroke Care				
Anticoagulation Therapy for Atrial Fibrillation[1]	-	-	97%	95%
Antithrombotic Therapy Timing	35	94%	98%	98%
Assessed for Rehabilitation	30	93%	98%	97%
Discharged on Antithrombotic Therapy	30	100%	100%	99%
Discharged on Statin Medication	27	63%	93%	94%
Thrombolytic Therapy Timing[1]	-	-	51%	66%
Venous Thromboembolism Prophylaxis	35	60%	96%	94%
Written Stroke Educational Materials Given	17	0%	85%	88%
Surgical Care Improvement Project				
Appropriate Beta Blocker Usage[2]	125	95%	98%	98%
Appropriate VTP Within 24 Hours[2]	340	98%	98%	98%
Controlled Postoperative Blood Glucose[2,7]	-	-	98%	97%
Perioperative Temperature Management[2]	410	100%	99%	100%
Prophylactic Antibiotic Selection[2]	327	100%	99%	99%
Prophylactic Antibiotic Selection (Outpatient)	128	99%	99%	98%
Prophylactic Antibiotic Stopped[2]	316	98%	98%	98%
Prophylactic Antibiotic Timing[2]	327	98%	99%	99%
Prophylactic Antibiotic Timing (Outpatient)	83	93%	98%	98%
Urinary Catheter Removal[2]	318	97%	97%	97%
Survey of Patients' Hospital Experiences				
Area Around Room 'Always' Quiet at Night	300+	58%	72%	61%
Doctors 'Always' Communicated Well	300+	81%	85%	82%
Home Recovery Information Given	300+	90%	87%	85%
Hospital Given 9 or 10 on 10 Point Scale	300+	72%	78%	71%
Meds 'Always' Explained Before Given	300+	63%	69%	64%
Nurses 'Always' Communicated Well	300+	77%	83%	79%
Pain 'Always' Well Controlled	300+	71%	72%	71%
Room and Bathroom 'Always' Clean	300+	70%	79%	73%
Timely Help 'Always' Received	300+	67%	77%	68%
Would Definitely Recommend Hospital	300+	70%	76%	71%
Use of Medical Imaging				
Cardiac Imaging Stress Test before Surgery	309	2.6%	4.4%	5.3%
Combination Abdominal CT Scan	254	58.3%	12.5%	10.5%
Combination Brain/Sinus CT Scan[1]	-	-	2%	2.7%
Combination Chest CT Scan	140	64.3%	4.5%	2.7%
Follow-up Mammogram/Ultrasound[7]	-	-	8.7%	8.8%
Lumbar Spine MRI for Low Back Pain	72	29.2%	33%	37.2%

Sanford Hospital Webster

1401 W First Saint Post Office Box 489 Phone: 605-345-3336
Webster, SD 57274
Type: Critical Access Hospitals Emergency Services: Yes
Ownership: Voluntary non-profit - Private

Measure	Cases	This Hosp.	State Avg.	U.S. Avg.
Blood Clot Prevention and Treatment				
Anticoagulation Overlap Therapy[5]	-	-	95%	93%
ICU Venous Thromboembolism Prophylaxis[5]	-	-	91%	92%
Incidence of Potentially Preventable VTE[5]	-	-	5%	10%
UFH with Dosages/Platelet Monitoring[5]	-	-	100%	97%
Venous Thromboembolism Prophylaxis[5]	-	-	80%	85%
Warfarin Therapy Discharge Instructions[5]	-	-	70%	75%
Chest Pain/Possible Heart Attack Care				
Aspirin Given Within 24 Hours of Arrival	-	-	99%	96%
Fibrinolytic Meds Within 30 Min. of Arrival	-	-	69%	58%
Average Time to ECG (minutes)	-	-	5	7
Average Time to Transfer (minutes)	-	-	66	60
Children's Asthma Care				
Received Home Management Plan of Care	-	-	-	88%
Received Reliever Medication	-	-	-	100%
Received Systemic Corticosteroids	-	-	-	100%
Emergency Department				
Admittance Decision Time (minutes)[5]	-	-	41	98
Head CT Results Within 45 Min. of Arrival	-	-	44%	57%
Patients Who Left ER Before Being Seen	-	-	1%	2%
Time from ER Arrival to Admit. (minutes)[5]	-	-	174	274
Time from ER Arrival to Discharge (minutes)	-	-	113	134
Time in ER Before Being Evaluated (minutes)	-	-	18	26
Time to Pain Meds for Fractures (minutes)	-	-	44	57
Heart Attack Care				
Aspirin Given at Discharge[1,3]	-	-	100%	99%
Fibrinolytic Meds Within 30 Min. of Arrival[3,7]	-	-	100%	54%
PCI Within 90 Minutes of Arrival[3,7]	-	-	94%	96%
Statin Prescribed at Discharge[1,3]	-	-	98%	98%
Heart Failure Care				
ACE Inhibitor or ARB for LVSD[1]	-	-	93%	97%
Discharge Instructions Given[1]	-	-	90%	94%
Evaluation of LVS Function[1]	-	-	97%	99%
Medicare Spending				
Medicare Spending per Patient (ratio)	-	-	0.9	0.98
Pneumonia Care				
Appropriate Initial Antibiotic Given[1]	-	-	90%	95%
Blood Culture Timing[1]	-	-	95%	98%
Pregnancy and Delivery Care				
Newborn Deliveries Scheduled Early[5]	-	-	7%	6%
Preventive Care				
Immunization for Influenza[1,3]	-	-	89%	90%
Immunization for Pneumonia[3]	18	72%	89%	92%
Stroke Care				
Anticoagulation Therapy for Atrial Fibrillation[1,3]	-	-	97%	95%
Antithrombotic Therapy Timing[3,7]	-	-	98%	98%
Assessed for Rehabilitation[1,3]	-	-	98%	97%
Discharged on Antithrombotic Therapy[1,3]	-	-	100%	99%
Discharged on Statin Medication[1,3]	-	-	93%	94%
Thrombolytic Therapy Timing[3,7]	-	-	51%	66%
Venous Thromboembolism Prophylaxis[1,3]	-	-	96%	94%
Written Stroke Educational Materials Given[3,7]	-	-	85%	88%
Surgical Care Improvement Project				
Appropriate Beta Blocker Usage[5]	-	-	98%	98%
Appropriate VTP Within 24 Hours[5]	-	-	98%	98%
Controlled Postoperative Blood Glucose[5]	-	-	98%	97%
Perioperative Temperature Management[5]	-	-	99%	100%
Prophylactic Antibiotic Selection[5]	-	-	99%	99%
Prophylactic Antibiotic Selection (Outpatient)	-	-	99%	98%
Prophylactic Antibiotic Stopped[5]	-	-	98%	98%
Prophylactic Antibiotic Timing[5]	-	-	99%	99%
Prophylactic Antibiotic Timing (Outpatient)	-	-	98%	98%
Urinary Catheter Removal[5]	-	-	97%	97%
Survey of Patients' Hospital Experiences				
Area Around Room 'Always' Quiet at Night[10]	<100	70%	72%	61%
Doctors 'Always' Communicated Well[10]	<100	84%	85%	82%
Home Recovery Information Given[10]	<100	88%	87%	85%
Hospital Given 9 or 10 on 10 Point Scale[10]	<100	80%	78%	71%
Meds 'Always' Explained Before Given[10]	<100	81%	69%	64%
Nurses 'Always' Communicated Well[10]	<100	85%	83%	79%
Pain 'Always' Well Controlled[10]	<100	74%	72%	71%
Room and Bathroom 'Always' Clean[10]	<100	81%	79%	73%
Timely Help 'Always' Received[10]	<100	90%	77%	68%
Would Definitely Recommend Hospital[10]	<100	78%	76%	71%
Use of Medical Imaging				
Cardiac Imaging Stress Test before Surgery	-	-	4.4%	5.3%
Combination Abdominal CT Scan	-	-	12.5%	10.5%
Combination Brain/Sinus CT Scan	-	-	2%	2.7%
Combination Chest CT Scan	-	-	4.5%	2.7%
Follow-up Mammogram/Ultrasound	-	-	8.7%	8.8%
Lumbar Spine MRI for Low Back Pain	-	-	33%	37.2%

Avera Weskota Memorial Medical Center

604 1st Saint Ne Phone: 605-539-1201
Wessington Springs, SD 57382 Fax: 605-995-2441
URL: www.averaweskota.org
Type: Critical Access Hospitals Emergency Services: Yes
Ownership: Voluntary non-profit - Church Beds: 28
Key Personnel:
Chief of Medical Staff . . . . Tom Dehan
Emergency Room . . . . Grace Edwyetr

Measure	Cases	This Hosp.	State Avg.	U.S. Avg.
Blood Clot Prevention and Treatment				
Anticoagulation Overlap Therapy[5]	-	-	95%	93%
ICU Venous Thromboembolism Prophylaxis[5]	-	-	91%	92%
Incidence of Potentially Preventable VTE[5]	-	-	5%	10%
UFH with Dosages/Platelet Monitoring[5]	-	-	100%	97%
Venous Thromboembolism Prophylaxis[5]	-	-	80%	85%
Warfarin Therapy Discharge Instructions[5]	-	-	70%	75%
Chest Pain/Possible Heart Attack Care				
Aspirin Given Within 24 Hours of Arrival	-	-	99%	96%
Fibrinolytic Meds Within 30 Min. of Arrival	-	-	69%	58%
Average Time to ECG (minutes)	-	-	5	7
Average Time to Transfer (minutes)	-	-	66	60
Children's Asthma Care				
Received Home Management Plan of Care	-	-	-	88%
Received Reliever Medication	-	-	-	100%
Received Systemic Corticosteroids	-	-	-	100%
Emergency Department				
Admittance Decision Time (minutes)[5]	-	-	41	98
Head CT Results Within 45 Min. of Arrival	-	-	44%	57%
Patients Who Left ER Before Being Seen	-	-	1%	2%
Time from ER Arrival to Admit. (minutes)[5]	-	-	174	274
Time from ER Arrival to Discharge (minutes)	-	-	113	134
Time in ER Before Being Evaluated (minutes)	-	-	18	26
Time to Pain Meds for Fractures (minutes)	-	-	44	57
Heart Attack Care				
Aspirin Given at Discharge[3,7]	-	-	100%	99%
Fibrinolytic Meds Within 30 Min. of Arrival[3,7]	-	-	100%	54%
PCI Within 90 Minutes of Arrival[3,7]	-	-	94%	96%
Statin Prescribed at Discharge[3,7]	-	-	98%	98%
Heart Failure Care				
ACE Inhibitor or ARB for LVSD[3,7]	-	-	93%	97%
Discharge Instructions Given[1,3]	-	-	90%	94%
Evaluation of LVS Function[1,3]	-	-	97%	99%
Medicare Spending				
Medicare Spending per Patient (ratio)	-	-	0.9	0.98
Pneumonia Care				

NOTE: Hospital profiles are in alphabetical order by state, then city, then hospital within the city; Rankings exclude hospitals with less than 25 cases except for patient surveys which excludes hospitals with less than 100 cases; (a) 100-299 cases; (1) The number of cases/patients is too few to report; (2) Data submitted were based on a sample of cases/patients; (3) Results are based on a shorter time period than required; (4) Data suppressed by CMS for one or more quarters; (5) Results are not available for this reporting period; (6) Fewer than 100 patients completed the HCAHPS survey; (7) No cases met the criteria for this measure; (8) The lower limit of the confidence interval cannot be calculated if the number of observed infections equals zero; (9) No data are available from the state/territory for this reporting period; (10) The scores shown reflect fewer than 50 completed surveys; (11) There were discrepancies in the data collection process; (12) This measure does not apply to this hospital for this reporting period; (13) Results cannot be calculated for this reporting period; (14) The results for this state are combined with nearby states to protect confidentiality; Please refer to the User's Guide for a full explanation of data.

Measure	Cases	This Hosp.	State Avg.	U.S. Avg.
Appropriate Initial Antibiotic Given[1]	-	-	90%	95%
Blood Culture Timing[1]	-	-	95%	98%
Pregnancy and Delivery Care				
Newborn Deliveries Scheduled Early[5]	-	-	7%	6%
Preventive Care				
Immunization for Influenza[5]	-	-	89%	90%
Immunization for Pneumonia[5]	-	-	89%	92%
Stroke Care				
Anticoagulation Therapy for Atrial Fibrillation[5]	-	-	97%	95%
Antithrombotic Therapy Timing[5]	-	-	98%	98%
Assessed for Rehabilitation[5]	-	-	98%	97%
Discharged on Antithrombotic Therapy[5]	-	-	100%	99%
Discharged on Statin Medication[5]	-	-	93%	94%
Thrombolytic Therapy Timing[5]	-	-	51%	66%
Venous Thromboembolism Prophylaxis[5]	-	-	96%	94%
Written Stroke Educational Materials Given[5]	-	-	85%	88%
Surgical Care Improvement Project				
Appropriate Beta Blocker Usage[5]	-	-	98%	98%
Appropriate VTP Within 24 Hours[5]	-	-	98%	98%
Controlled Postoperative Blood Glucose[5]	-	-	98%	97%
Perioperative Temperature Management[5]	-	-	99%	100%
Prophylactic Antibiotic Selection[5]	-	-	99%	99%
Prophylactic Antibiotic Selection (Outpatient)	-	-	99%	98%
Prophylactic Antibiotic Stopped[5]	-	-	98%	98%
Prophylactic Antibiotic Timing[5]	-	-	99%	99%
Prophylactic Antibiotic Timing (Outpatient)	-	-	98%	98%
Urinary Catheter Removal[5]	-	-	97%	97%
Survey of Patients' Hospital Experiences				
Area Around Room 'Always' Quiet at Night[10]	<100	51%	72%	61%
Doctors 'Always' Communicated Well[10]	<100	68%	85%	82%
Home Recovery Information Given[10]	<100	64%	87%	85%
Hospital Given 9 or 10 on 10 Point Scale[10]	<100	91%	78%	71%
Meds 'Always' Explained Before Given[10]	<100	71%	69%	64%
Nurses 'Always' Communicated Well[10]	<100	79%	83%	79%
Pain 'Always' Well Controlled[10]	<100	43%	72%	71%
Room and Bathroom 'Always' Clean[10]	<100	80%	79%	73%
Timely Help 'Always' Received[10]	<100	76%	77%	68%
Would Definitely Recommend Hospital[10]	<100	72%	76%	71%
Use of Medical Imaging				
Cardiac Imaging Stress Test before Surgery	-	-	4.4%	5.3%
Combination Abdominal CT Scan	-	-	12.5%	10.5%
Combination Brain/Sinus CT Scan	-	-	2%	2.7%
Combination Chest CT Scan	-	-	4.5%	2.7%
Follow-up Mammogram/Ultrasound	-	-	8.7%	8.8%
Lumbar Spine MRI for Low Back Pain	-	-	33%	37.2%

Winner Regional Healthcare Center

745 East 8th Street
Winner, SD 57580
Phone: 605-842-7100
Fax: 605-842-7198
E-mail: info@winnerregional.org
URL: www.winnerregional.org
Type: Critical Access Hospitals
Emergency Services: Yes
Ownership: Voluntary non-profit - Private
Beds: 97

Key Personnel:

Chief of Medical Staff.......... Tony Berg
CEO/President.............. Michael Hall
Quality Assurance .... Wendy Heath, PRO
Operating Room............ Thomas Kosina
Anesthesiology............ Nancy Rehr
Infection Control............ Ellen Storms
Emergency Room .... Gregg Tobin, MD

Measure	Cases	This Hosp.	State Avg.	U.S. Avg.
Blood Clot Prevention and Treatment				
Anticoagulation Overlap Therapy[5]	-	-	95%	93%
ICU Venous Thromboembolism Prophylaxis[5]	-	-	91%	92%
Incidence of Potentially Preventable VTE[5]	-	-	5%	10%
UFH with Dosages/Platelet Monitoring[5]	-	-	100%	97%
Venous Thromboembolism Prophylaxis[5]	-	-	80%	85%
Warfarin Therapy Discharge Instructions[5]	-	-	70%	75%
Chest Pain/Possible Heart Attack Care				
Aspirin Given Within 24 Hours of Arrival	-	-	99%	96%
Fibrinolytic Meds Within 30 Min. of Arrival	-	-	69%	58%
Average Time to ECG (minutes)	-	-	5	7
Average Time to Transfer (minutes)	-	-	66	60
Children's Asthma Care				
Received Home Management Plan of Care	-	-	-	88%
Received Reliever Medication	-	-	-	100%
Received Systemic Corticosteroids	-	-	-	100%
Emergency Department				
Admittance Decision Time (minutes)[5]	-	-	41	98
Head CT Results Within 45 Min. of Arrival	-	-	44%	57%
Patients Who Left ER Before Being Seen	-	-	1%	2%
Time from ER Arrival to Admit. (minutes)[5]	-	-	174	274
Time from ER Arrival to Discharge (minutes)	-	-	113	134
Time in ER Before Being Evaluated (minutes)	-	-	18	26
Time to Pain Meds for Fractures (minutes)	-	-	44	57
Heart Attack Care				
Aspirin Given at Discharge[1,3]	-	-	100%	99%
Fibrinolytic Meds Within 30 Min. of Arrival[3,7]	-	-	100%	54%
PCI Within 90 Minutes of Arrival[3,7]	-	-	94%	96%
Statin Prescribed at Discharge[1,3]	-	-	98%	98%
Heart Failure Care				
ACE Inhibitor or ARB for LVSD[1]	-	-	93%	97%
Discharge Instructions Given[1]	-	-	90%	94%
Evaluation of LVS Function	12	92%	97%	99%
Medicare Spending				
Medicare Spending per Patient (ratio)	-	-	0.9	0.98
Pneumonia Care				
Appropriate Initial Antibiotic Given[2]	23	57%	90%	95%
Blood Culture Timing[2]	11	45%	95%	98%
Pregnancy and Delivery Care				
Newborn Deliveries Scheduled Early[5]	-	-	7%	6%
Preventive Care				
Immunization for Influenza[5]	-	-	89%	90%
Immunization for Pneumonia[5]	-	-	89%	92%
Stroke Care				
Anticoagulation Therapy for Atrial Fibrillation[5]	-	-	97%	95%
Antithrombotic Therapy Timing[5]	-	-	98%	98%
Assessed for Rehabilitation[5]	-	-	98%	97%
Discharged on Antithrombotic Therapy[5]	-	-	100%	99%
Discharged on Statin Medication[5]	-	-	93%	94%
Thrombolytic Therapy Timing[5]	-	-	51%	66%
Venous Thromboembolism Prophylaxis[5]	-	-	96%	94%
Written Stroke Educational Materials Given[5]	-	-	85%	88%
Surgical Care Improvement Project				
Appropriate Beta Blocker Usage[1]	-	-	98%	98%
Appropriate VTP Within 24 Hours	17	53%	98%	98%
Controlled Postoperative Blood Glucose[7]	-	-	98%	97%
Perioperative Temperature Management	19	100%	99%	100%
Prophylactic Antibiotic Selection	16	88%	99%	99%
Prophylactic Antibiotic Selection (Outpatient)	-	-	99%	98%
Prophylactic Antibiotic Stopped	16	94%	98%	98%
Prophylactic Antibiotic Timing	16	88%	99%	99%
Prophylactic Antibiotic Timing (Outpatient)	-	-	98%	98%
Urinary Catheter Removal[1]	-	-	97%	97%
Survey of Patients' Hospital Experiences				
Area Around Room 'Always' Quiet at Night	(a)	69%	72%	61%
Doctors 'Always' Communicated Well	(a)	88%	85%	82%
Home Recovery Information Given	(a)	82%	87%	85%
Hospital Given 9 or 10 on 10 Point Scale	(a)	73%	78%	71%
Meds 'Always' Explained Before Given	(a)	74%	69%	64%
Nurses 'Always' Communicated Well	(a)	81%	83%	79%
Pain 'Always' Well Controlled	(a)	71%	72%	71%
Room and Bathroom 'Always' Clean	(a)	80%	79%	73%
Timely Help 'Always' Received	(a)	76%	77%	68%
Would Definitely Recommend Hospital	(a)	73%	76%	71%
Use of Medical Imaging				
Cardiac Imaging Stress Test before Surgery	-	-	4.4%	5.3%
Combination Abdominal CT Scan	-	-	12.5%	10.5%
Combination Brain/Sinus CT Scan	-	-	2%	2.7%
Combination Chest CT Scan	-	-	4.5%	2.7%
Follow-up Mammogram/Ultrasound	-	-	8.7%	8.8%
Lumbar Spine MRI for Low Back Pain	-	-	33%	37.2%

Avera Sacred Heart Hospital

501 Summit
Yankton, SD 57078
Phone: 605-668-8000
Fax: 605-665-0170
URL: www.avera.org/sacred-heart
Type: Acute Care Hospitals
Emergency Services: Yes
Ownership: Voluntary non-profit - Private
Beds: 144

Key Personnel:

Chief of Medical Staff.......... David Barnes
Pediatric In-Patient Care .... Mark Brown, MD
Quality Assurance .... Jean Hunhoff
Infection Control............ Jan Johnson
Operating Room............ Cindy Miller
Radiology................ Thomas Posch
CEO/President.............. Pamela Rezac, PhD
Pediatric Ambulatory Care ...... David Withrow, MD

Measure	Cases	This Hosp.	State Avg.	U.S. Avg.
Blood Clot Prevention and Treatment				
Anticoagulation Overlap Therapy[2]	39	95%	95%	93%
ICU Venous Thromboembolism Prophylaxis[2]	62	97%	91%	92%
Incidence of Potentially Preventable VTE[1,2]	-	-	5%	10%
UFH with Dosages/Platelet Monitoring[2]	17	100%	100%	97%
Venous Thromboembolism Prophylaxis[2]	199	96%	80%	85%
Warfarin Therapy Discharge Instructions[2]	33	88%	70%	75%
Chest Pain/Possible Heart Attack Care				
Aspirin Given Within 24 Hours of Arrival	36	100%	99%	96%
Fibrinolytic Meds Within 30 Min. of Arrival[1]	-	-	69%	58%
Average Time to ECG (minutes)	37	5	5	7
Average Time to Transfer (minutes)[1]	-	-	66	60
Children's Asthma Care				
Received Home Management Plan of Care	-	-	-	88%
Received Reliever Medication	-	-	-	100%
Received Systemic Corticosteroids	-	-	-	100%
Emergency Department				
Admittance Decision Time (minutes)	1,219	46	41	98
Head CT Results Within 45 Min. of Arrival[1,3]	-	-	44%	57%
Patients Who Left ER Before Being Seen	10,295	0%	1%	2%
Time from ER Arrival to Admit. (minutes)	1,223	171	174	274
Time from ER Arrival to Discharge (minutes)	6,874	109	113	134
Time in ER Before Being Evaluated (minutes)	6,917	17	18	26
Time to Pain Meds for Fractures (minutes)	69	28	44	57
Heart Attack Care				
Aspirin Given at Discharge	13	100%	100%	99%
Fibrinolytic Meds Within 30 Min. of Arrival[7]	-	-	100%	54%
PCI Within 90 Minutes of Arrival[7]	-	-	94%	96%
Statin Prescribed at Discharge	12	100%	98%	98%
Heart Failure Care				
ACE Inhibitor or ARB for LVSD	17	100%	93%	97%
Discharge Instructions Given	48	100%	90%	94%
Evaluation of LVS Function	68	100%	97%	99%
Medicare Spending				
Medicare Spending per Patient (ratio)	-	0.97	0.9	0.98
Pneumonia Care				
Appropriate Initial Antibiotic Given	85	96%	90%	95%
Blood Culture Timing	86	100%	95%	98%
Pregnancy and Delivery Care				
Newborn Deliveries Scheduled Early	67	15%	7%	6%
Preventive Care				
Immunization for Influenza	1,594	92%	89%	90%
Immunization for Pneumonia	1,805	94%	89%	92%
Stroke Care				
Anticoagulation Therapy for Atrial Fibrillation[1]	-	-	97%	95%
Antithrombotic Therapy Timing	16	94%	98%	98%
Assessed for Rehabilitation	17	100%	98%	97%
Discharged on Antithrombotic Therapy	16	100%	100%	99%
Discharged on Statin Medication	11	91%	93%	94%
Thrombolytic Therapy Timing[1]	-	-	51%	66%
Venous Thromboembolism Prophylaxis	16	88%	96%	94%
Written Stroke Educational Materials Given[1]	-	-	85%	88%
Surgical Care Improvement Project				
Appropriate Beta Blocker Usage	109	100%	98%	98%
Appropriate VTP Within 24 Hours	311	100%	98%	98%
Controlled Postoperative Blood Glucose[7]	-	-	98%	97%
Perioperative Temperature Management	377	100%	99%	100%
Prophylactic Antibiotic Selection	259	100%	99%	99%

NOTE: Hospital profiles are in alphabetical order by state, then city, then hospital within the city; Rankings exclude hospitals with less than 25 cases except for patient surveys which excludes hospitals with less than 100 cases; (a) 100-299 cases; (1) The number of cases/patients is too few to report; (2) Data submitted were based on a sample of cases/patients; (3) Results are based on a shorter time period than required; (4) Data suppressed by CMS for one or more quarters; (5) Results are not available for this reporting period; (6) Fewer than 100 patients completed the HCAHPS survey; (7) No cases met the criteria for this measure; (8) The lower limit of the confidence interval cannot be calculated if the number of observed infections equals zero; (9) No data are available from the state/territory for this reporting period; (10) The scores shown reflect fewer than 50 completed surveys; (11) There were discrepancies in the data collection process; (12) This measure does not apply to this hospital for this reporting period; (13) Results cannot be calculated for this reporting period; (14) The results for this state are combined with nearby states to protect confidentiality; Please refer to the User's Guide for a full explanation of data.

Measure	Cases	This Hosp.	State Avg.	U.S. Avg.
Prophylactic Antibiotic Selection (Outpatient)	77	100%	99%	98%
Prophylactic Antibiotic Stopped	255	99%	98%	98%
Prophylactic Antibiotic Timing	259	100%	99%	99%
Prophylactic Antibiotic Timing (Outpatient)	77	100%	98%	98%
Urinary Catheter Removal	23	100%	97%	97%
Survey of Patients' Hospital Experiences				
Area Around Room 'Always' Quiet at Night	300+	63%	72%	61%
Doctors 'Always' Communicated Well	300+	83%	85%	82%
Home Recovery Information Given	300+	91%	87%	85%
Hospital Given 9 or 10 on 10 Point Scale	300+	71%	78%	71%
Meds 'Always' Explained Before Given	300+	61%	69%	64%
Nurses 'Always' Communicated Well	300+	79%	83%	79%
Pain 'Always' Well Controlled	300+	71%	72%	71%
Room and Bathroom 'Always' Clean	300+	73%	79%	73%
Timely Help 'Always' Received	300+	69%	77%	68%
Would Definitely Recommend Hospital	300+	71%	76%	71%
Use of Medical Imaging				
Cardiac Imaging Stress Test before Surgery	190	6.3%	4.4%	5.3%
Combination Abdominal CT Scan	140	5.0%	12.5%	10.5%
Combination Brain/Sinus CT Scan[1]	-	-	2%	2.7%
Combination Chest CT Scan	47	2.1%	4.5%	2.7%
Follow-up Mammogram/Ultrasound	260	11.2%	8.7%	8.8%
Lumbar Spine MRI for Low Back Pain[1]	-	-	33%	37.2%

Lewis & Clark Specialty Hospital

2601 Fox Run Parkway
Yankton, SD 57078
Phone: 605-665-5100
Type: Acute Care Hospitals
Emergency Services: No
Ownership: Physician
Key Personnel:
CEO .... Doug Doorn, MBA

Measure	Cases	This Hosp.	State Avg.	U.S. Avg.
Blood Clot Prevention and Treatment				
Anticoagulation Overlap Therapy[7]	-	-	95%	93%
ICU Venous Thromboembolism Prophylaxis[7]	-	-	91%	92%
Incidence of Potentially Preventable VTE[7]	-	-	5%	10%
UFH with Dosages/Platelet Monitoring[7]	-	-	100%	97%
Venous Thromboembolism Prophylaxis	78	72%	80%	85%
Warfarin Therapy Discharge Instructions[7]	-	-	70%	75%
Chest Pain/Possible Heart Attack Care				
Aspirin Given Within 24 Hours of Arrival[5]	-	-	99%	96%
Fibrinolytic Meds Within 30 Min. of Arrival[5]	-	-	69%	58%
Average Time to ECG (minutes)[5]	-	-	5	7
Average Time to Transfer (minutes)[5]	-	-	66	60
Children's Asthma Care				
Received Home Management Plan of Care	-	-	-	88%
Received Reliever Medication	-	-	-	100%
Received Systemic Corticosteroids	-	-	-	100%
Emergency Department				
Admittance Decision Time (minutes)[7]	-	-	41	98
Head CT Results Within 45 Min. of Arrival[5]	-	-	44%	57%
Patients Who Left ER Before Being Seen[5]	-	-	1%	2%
Time from ER Arrival to Admit. (minutes)[7]	-	-	174	274
Time from ER Arrival to Discharge (minutes)[5]	-	-	113	134
Time in ER Before Being Evaluated (minutes)[5]	-	-	18	26
Time to Pain Meds for Fractures (minutes)[5]	-	-	44	57
Heart Attack Care				
Aspirin Given at Discharge[5]	-	-	100%	99%
Fibrinolytic Meds Within 30 Min. of Arrival[5]	-	-	100%	54%
PCI Within 90 Minutes of Arrival[5]	-	-	94%	96%
Statin Prescribed at Discharge[5]	-	-	98%	98%
Heart Failure Care				
ACE Inhibitor or ARB for LVSD[5]	-	-	93%	97%
Discharge Instructions Given[5]	-	-	90%	94%
Evaluation of LVS Function[5]	-	-	97%	99%
Medicare Spending				
Medicare Spending per Patient (ratio)	-	0.97	0.9	0.98
Pneumonia Care				
Appropriate Initial Antibiotic Given[3,7]	-	-	90%	95%
Blood Culture Timing[3,7]	-	-	95%	98%
Pregnancy and Delivery Care				
Newborn Deliveries Scheduled Early[7]	-	-	7%	6%
Preventive Care				
Immunization for Influenza	89	47%	89%	90%
Immunization for Pneumonia	118	69%	89%	92%
Stroke Care				
Anticoagulation Therapy for Atrial Fibrillation[5]	-	-	97%	95%
Antithrombotic Therapy Timing[5]	-	-	98%	98%
Assessed for Rehabilitation[5]	-	-	98%	97%
Discharged on Antithrombotic Therapy[5]	-	-	100%	99%
Discharged on Statin Medication[5]	-	-	93%	94%
Thrombolytic Therapy Timing[5]	-	-	51%	66%
Venous Thromboembolism Prophylaxis[5]	-	-	96%	94%
Written Stroke Educational Materials Given[5]	-	-	85%	88%
Surgical Care Improvement Project				
Appropriate Beta Blocker Usage	17	88%	98%	98%
Appropriate VTP Within 24 Hours	79	97%	98%	98%
Controlled Postoperative Blood Glucose[7]	-	-	98%	97%
Perioperative Temperature Management	81	90%	99%	100%
Prophylactic Antibiotic Selection	71	100%	99%	99%
Prophylactic Antibiotic Selection (Outpatient)	26	96%	99%	98%
Prophylactic Antibiotic Stopped	71	99%	98%	98%
Prophylactic Antibiotic Timing	71	97%	99%	99%
Prophylactic Antibiotic Timing (Outpatient)	18	94%	98%	98%
Urinary Catheter Removal[1]	-	-	97%	97%
Survey of Patients' Hospital Experiences				
Area Around Room 'Always' Quiet at Night[6]	<100	86%	72%	61%
Doctors 'Always' Communicated Well[6]	<100	90%	85%	82%
Home Recovery Information Given[6]	<100	87%	87%	85%
Hospital Given 9 or 10 on 10 Point Scale[6]	<100	88%	78%	71%
Meds 'Always' Explained Before Given[6]	<100	77%	69%	64%
Nurses 'Always' Communicated Well[6]	<100	89%	83%	79%
Pain 'Always' Well Controlled[6]	<100	82%	72%	71%
Room and Bathroom 'Always' Clean[6]	<100	84%	79%	73%
Timely Help 'Always' Received[6]	<100	85%	77%	68%
Would Definitely Recommend Hospital[6]	<100	84%	76%	71%
Use of Medical Imaging				
Cardiac Imaging Stress Test before Surgery[7]	-	-	4.4%	5.3%
Combination Abdominal CT Scan[1]	-	-	12.5%	10.5%
Combination Brain/Sinus CT Scan[1]	-	-	2%	2.7%
Combination Chest CT Scan[1]	-	-	4.5%	2.7%
Follow-up Mammogram/Ultrasound[7]	-	-	8.7%	8.8%
Lumbar Spine MRI for Low Back Pain[1]	-	-	33%	37.2%

NOTE: Hospital profiles are in alphabetical order by state, then city, then hospital within the city; Rankings exclude hospitals with less than 25 cases except for patient surveys which excludes hospitals with less than 100 cases; (a) 100-299 cases; (1) The number of cases/patients is too few to report; (2) Data submitted were based on a sample of cases/patients; (3) Results are based on a shorter time period than required; (4) Data suppressed by CMS for one or more quarters; (5) Results are not available for this reporting period; (6) Fewer than 100 patients completed the HCAHPS survey; (7) No cases met the criteria for this measure; (8) The lower limit of the confidence interval cannot be calculated if the number of observed infections equals zero; (9) No data are available from the state/territory for this reporting period; (10) The scores shown reflect fewer than 50 completed surveys; (11) There were discrepancies in the data collection process; (12) This measure does not apply to this hospital for this reporting period; (13) Results cannot be calculated for this reporting period; (14) The results for this state are combined with nearby states to protect confidentiality; Please refer to the User's Guide for a full explanation of data.

Blood Clot Prevention and Treatment

Anticoagulation Overlap Therapy

Hospital Name	City	Rate	Cases
Aurora Medical Center[2]	Summit	100%	26
Aurora Medical Center Oshkosh[2]	Oshkosh	100%	33
Aurora Medical Center Washington County[2]	Hartford	100%	32
Aurora Memorial Hospital Burlington[2]	Burlington	100%	31
Aurora Sheboygan Memorial Medical Center[2]	Sheboygan	100%	38
Bay Area Medical Center[2]	Marinette	100%	39
Beloit Memorial Hospital[2]	Beloit	100%	43
Gundersen Lutheran Medical Center[2]	La Crosse	100%	70
Lakeview Medical Center[2]	Rice Lake	100%	33
Meriter Hospital[2]	Madison	100%	96
Ministry Saint Josephs Hospital[2]	Marshfield	100%	154
Ministry Saint Marys Hospital[2]	Rhinelander	100%	33
Ministry St Michaels Hosp-Stevens Pt[2]	Stevens Point	100%	36
Saint Agnes Hospital[2]	Fond Du Lac	100%	63
Saint Clares Hospital of Weston[2]	Weston	100%	45
Columbia Saint Marys Hospital Milwaukee[2]	Milwaukee	99%	96
Froedtert Memorial Lutheran Hospital[2]	Milwaukee	99%	176
Mercy Health System Corp[2]	Janesville	99%	77
Saint Marys Hospital[2]	Madison	99%	157
Univ of WI Hosps & Clinics Authority[2]	Madison	99%	161
Waukesha Memorial Hospital[2]	Waukesha	99%	124
Mayo Clinic Hlth Sys Franciscan Med Ctr[2]	La Crosse	98%	42
Aspirus Wausau Hospital[2]	Wausau	97%	92
Aurora Baycare Medical Center[2]	Green Bay	97%	65
Aurora Lakeland Medical Center[2]	Elkhorn	97%	33
Bellin Memorial Hospital[2]	Green Bay	97%	69
Saint Marys Hospital Medical Center[2]	Green Bay	97%	37
Columbia Saint Marys Hospital Ozaukee[2]	Mequon	96%	56
Fort Memorial Hospital[2]	Fort Atkinson	96%	26
Mayo Clinic Hlth Sys-Eau Claire Hosp[2]	Eau Claire	96%	91
Saint Elizabeth Hospital[2]	Appleton	95%	59
Mercy Medical Center of Oshkosh[2]	Oshkosh	94%	31
St Joseph's Comm Hosp of West Bend[2]	West Bend	93%	57
Theda Clark Medical Center[2]	Neenah	92%	51
Wheaton Franciscan Healthcare All Saints[2]	Racine	92%	133
Wheaton Franciscan Healthcare Franklin[2]	Franklin	92%	48
Aurora Medical Center[2]	Grafton	91%	55
Aurora Saint Lukes Medical Center[2]	Milwaukee	91%	369
Aurora West Allis Medical Center[2]	West Allis	91%	91
Appleton Medical Center[2]	Appleton	90%	92
Aurora Medical Center Kenosha[2]	Kenosha	90%	48
Saint Vincent Hospital[2]	Green Bay	89%	80
United Hospital System[2]	Kenosha	89%	72
Community Memorial Hospital[2]	Menomonee Fls	87%	46
Sacred Heart Hospital[2]	Eau Claire	86%	81
Wheaton Franciscan Hlthcare St Francis[2]	Milwaukee	86%	79
Wheaton Franciscan Saint Joseph[2]	Milwaukee	84%	130
The Monroe Clinic[2]	Monroe	77%	31

ICU Venous Thromboembolism Prophylaxis

Hospital Name	City	Rate	Cases
Aurora Lakeland Medical Center[2]	Elkhorn	100%	84
Aurora Memorial Hospital Burlington[2]	Burlington	100%	87
Beaver Dam Com Hospital[2]	Beaver Dam	100%	26
Lakeview Medical Center[2]	Rice Lake	100%	29
Saint Clare Hospital Health Services[2]	Baraboo	100%	40
Saint Clares Hospital of Weston[2]	Weston	100%	64
Mayo Clinic Hlth Sys Franciscan Med Ctr[2]	La Crosse	98%	52
Ministry Saint Josephs Hospital[2]	Marshfield	98%	112
Oconomowoc Memorial Hospital[2]	Oconomowoc	98%	56
Aurora Medical Center[2]	Grafton	97%	79
Aurora Medical Center[2]	Summit	97%	68
Aurora Medical Center Washington County[2]	Hartford	97%	33
Aurora West Allis Medical Center[2]	West Allis	97%	71
Ministry St Michaels Hosp-Stevens Pt[2]	Stevens Point	97%	33
Saint Elizabeth Hospital[2]	Appleton	97%	70
Aurora Baycare Medical Center[2]	Green Bay	96%	102
Fort Memorial Hospital[2]	Fort Atkinson	96%	46
Froedtert Memorial Lutheran Hospital[2]	Milwaukee	96%	105
Riverview Hospital Assoc[2]	Wisc. Rapids	96%	47
Saint Marys Hospital[2]	Madison	96%	25
United Hospital System[2]	Kenosha	96%	77
Beloit Memorial Hospital[2]	Beloit	95%	56
Mayo Clinic Hlth Sys-Eau Claire Hosp[2]	Eau Claire	95%	93
Meriter Hospital[2]	Madison	95%	63
Theda Clark Medical Center[2]	Neenah	95%	59
Columbia Saint Marys Hospital Milwaukee[2]	Milwaukee	94%	139
Gundersen Lutheran Medical Center[2]	La Crosse	94%	112
Waukesha Memorial Hospital[2]	Waukesha	94%	89
Aurora Medical Center Oshkosh[2]	Oshkosh	93%	73
Aurora Saint Lukes Medical Center[2]	Milwaukee	93%	245
Aurora Sheboygan Memorial Medical Center[2]	Sheboygan	93%	30
Mercy Health System Corp[2]	Janesville	93%	57
Mercy Medical Center of Oshkosh[2]	Oshkosh	93%	61
St Joseph's Comm Hosp of West Bend[2]	West Bend	93%	72
Univ of WI Hosps & Clinics Authority[2]	Madison	93%	60
Aurora Medical Center Kenosha[2]	Kenosha	92%	51
Aurora Medical Center Manitowoc County[2]	Two Rivers	92%	25
Bay Area Medical Center[2]	Marinette	91%	55
Divine Savior Healthcare	Portage	91%	44
Saint Agnes Hospital[2]	Fond Du Lac	90%	62
Appleton Medical Center[2]	Appleton	88%	77
Sauk Prairie Hospital	Prairie Du Sac	88%	48
The Monroe Clinic[2]	Monroe	87%	149
Wheaton Franciscan Hlthcare St Francis[2]	Milwaukee	86%	71
Bellin Memorial Hospital[2]	Green Bay	85%	131
Saint Vincent Hospital[2]	Green Bay	85%	46
Wheaton Franciscan Healthcare All Saints[2]	Racine	84%	44
Columbia Saint Marys Hospital Ozaukee[2]	Mequon	83%	65
Community Memorial Hospital	Oconto Falls	81%	27
Aspirus Wausau Hospital[2]	Wausau	76%	82
Wheaton Franciscan Saint Joseph[2]	Milwaukee	74%	73
Holy Family Memorial[2]	Manitowoc	72%	60
Saint Nicholas Hospital[2]	Sheboygan	67%	43
Sacred Heart Hospital[2]	Eau Claire	58%	84

Incidence of Potentially Preventable VTE

Hospital Name	City	Rate	Cases
Ministry Saint Josephs Hospital[2]	Marshfield	0%	45
Froedtert Memorial Lutheran Hospital[2]	Milwaukee	2%	56
Univ of WI Hosps & Clinics Authority[2]	Madison	3%	61
Aurora Saint Lukes Medical Center[2]	Milwaukee	9%	74
Wheaton Franciscan Healthcare All Saints[2]	Racine	24%	25
Mayo Clinic Hlth Sys-Eau Claire Hosp[2]	Eau Claire	39%	28

UFH with Dosages/Platelet Count Monitoring

Hospital Name	City	Rate	Cases
Appleton Medical Center[2]	Appleton	100%	28
Aurora Saint Lukes Medical Center[2]	Milwaukee	100%	292
Aurora West Allis Medical Center[2]	West Allis	100%	39
Bellin Memorial Hospital[2]	Green Bay	100%	33
Columbia Saint Marys Hospital Milwaukee[2]	Milwaukee	100%	38
Froedtert Memorial Lutheran Hospital[2]	Milwaukee	100%	167
Mayo Clinic Hlth Sys Franciscan Med Ctr[2]	La Crosse	100%	34
Mayo Clinic Hlth Sys-Eau Claire Hosp[2]	Eau Claire	100%	83
Mercy Health System Corp[2]	Janesville	100%	42
Meriter Hospital[2]	Madison	100%	35
Ministry Saint Josephs Hospital[2]	Marshfield	100%	150
Sacred Heart Hospital[2]	Eau Claire	100%	51
Saint Clares Hospital of Weston[2]	Weston	100%	36
Saint Marys Hospital[2]	Madison	100%	102
Waukesha Memorial Hospital[2]	Waukesha	100%	38
Wheaton Franciscan Hlthcare St Francis[2]	Milwaukee	100%	56
Wheaton Franciscan Saint Joseph[2]	Milwaukee	99%	69
Aurora Medical Center[2]	Grafton	97%	30
Aspirus Wausau Hospital[2]	Wausau	93%	58
Wheaton Franciscan Healthcare All Saints[2]	Racine	93%	55
Gundersen Lutheran Medical Center[2]	La Crosse	88%	34
Saint Vincent Hospital[2]	Green Bay	78%	27
Univ of WI Hosps & Clinics Authority[2]	Madison	62%	121

Venous Thromboembolism Prophylaxis

Hospital Name	City	Rate	Cases
Good Samaritan Health Center[2]	Merrill	100%	91
Midwest Orthopedic Specialty Hospital[2]	Franklin	100%	48
Ministry Eagle River Memorial Hospital	Eagle River	100%	167
Orthopaedic Hospital of Wisconsin[2]	Glendale	100%	35
Saint Clares Hospital of Weston[2]	Weston	100%	367
Tomah Memorial Hospital	Tomah	100%	310
Howard Young Medical Center[2]	Woodruff	99%	221
Mercy Walworth Hospital & Medical Center[2]	Lake Geneva	99%	90
Aurora Lakeland Medical Center[2]	Elkhorn	98%	148
Lakeview Medical Center[2]	Rice Lake	98%	114
Ministry Sacred Heart Hospital[2]	Tomahawk	98%	131
Ministry St Michaels Hosp-Stevens Pt[2]	Stevens Point	98%	554
Saint Clare Hospital Health Services[2]	Baraboo	98%	132
Stoughton Hospital[2]	Stoughton	98%	92
United Hospital System[2]	Kenosha	98%	359
Fort Memorial Hospital[2]	Fort Atkinson	97%	130
Gundersen Lutheran Medical Center[2]	La Crosse	97%	281
Saint Elizabeth Hospital[2]	Appleton	97%	256
Mayo Clinic Hlth Sys-Eau Claire Hosp[2]	Eau Claire	96%	291
Mercy Medical Center of Oshkosh[2]	Oshkosh	95%	246
Aurora Memorial Hospital Burlington[2]	Burlington	94%	193
Ministry Saint Josephs Hospital[2]	Marshfield	94%	493
Riverview Hospital Assoc[2]	Wisc. Rapids	94%	146
Aurora Medical Center[2]	Summit	93%	151
Aurora Sheboygan Memorial Medical Center[2]	Sheboygan	93%	202
Mayo Clinic Hlth Sys Franciscan Med Ctr[2]	La Crosse	93%	235
River Falls Area Hospital[2]	River Falls	93%	133
UW Hlth Partners Watertown Reg Med Ctr[2]	Watertown	93%	113
Aurora Medical Center Washington County[2]	Hartford	92%	140
Beaver Dam Com Hospital[2]	Beaver Dam	92%	118
Froedtert Memorial Lutheran Hospital[2]	Milwaukee	92%	301
Mayo Clinic Hlth Sys Franciscan[2]	Sparta	92%	103
Oconomowoc Memorial Hospital[2]	Oconomowoc	92%	191
Theda Clark Medical Center[2]	Neenah	92%	284
Aurora Medical Center Kenosha[2]	Kenosha	91%	317
The Monroe Clinic[2]	Monroe	91%	722
Aurora Baycare Medical Center[2]	Green Bay	90%	241
Memorial Medical Center	Neillsville	90%	87
Mercy Health System Corp[2]	Janesville	90%	263
Aurora Medical Center Oshkosh[2]	Oshkosh	89%	151
Saint Agnes Hospital[2]	Fond Du Lac	89%	406
Aurora Medical Center Manitowoc County[2]	Two Rivers	88%	128
Meriter Hospital[2]	Madison	88%	431
Aurora Medical Center[2]	Grafton	87%	247
Bellin Memorial Hospital[2]	Green Bay	87%	232
Beloit Memorial Hospital[2]	Beloit	87%	297
Ministry Saint Marys Hospital[2]	Rhinelander	87%	194
Saint Joseph's Hospital[2]	Chippewa Falls	87%	134
Saint Marys Hospital[2]	Madison	87%	346
Sauk Prairie Hospital	Prairie Du Sac	87%	234
Univ of WI Hosps & Clinics Authority[2]	Madison	87%	311
Aurora West Allis Medical Center[2]	West Allis	86%	305
Memorial Hospital Lafayette Cty	Darlington	84%	160
St Joseph's Comm Hosp of West Bend[2]	West Bend	84%	227
Columbia Saint Marys Hospital Milwaukee[2]	Milwaukee	83%	234
Bay Area Medical Center[2]	Marinette	82%	305
Holy Family Memorial[2]	Manitowoc	82%	188
Columbia Saint Marys Hospital Ozaukee[2]	Mequon	80%	325
Community Memorial Hospital[2]	Menomonee Fls	80%	357
Waukesha Memorial Hospital[2]	Waukesha	80%	304
Wheaton Franciscan Healthcare Franklin[2]	Franklin	79%	193
Appleton Medical Center[2]	Appleton	78%	339
Saint Marys Hospital Superior[2]	Superior	78%	103
Saint Marys Janesville Hospital[2]	Janesville	78%	228
Wheaton Franciscan Saint Joseph[2]	Milwaukee	78%	334
Aspirus Wausau Hospital[2]	Wausau	77%	279
Aurora Saint Lukes Medical Center[2]	Milwaukee	77%	827
Mile Bluff Medical Center	Mauston	75%	523
Saint Marys Hospital Medical Center[2]	Green Bay	75%	292
Sacred Heart Hospital[2]	Eau Claire	73%	298
Saint Nicholas Hospital[2]	Sheboygan	73%	208
Saint Vincent Hospital[2]	Green Bay	73%	306
Wheaton Franciscan Healthcare All Saints[2]	Racine	73%	289
Vernon Memorial Hospital	Viroqua	64%	329
Divine Savior Healthcare	Portage	57%	626
Wheaton Franciscan Hlthcare St Francis[2]	Milwaukee	55%	300
Moundview Memorial Hospital & Clinics	Friendship	51%	71
Hayward Area Memorial Hospital[2]	Hayward	38%	114

Warfarin Therapy Discharge Instructions

Hospital Name	City	Rate	Cases
Aurora Lakeland Medical Center[2]	Elkhorn	100%	30
Aurora Medical Center Oshkosh[2]	Oshkosh	100%	30
Aurora Memorial Hospital Burlington[2]	Burlington	100%	30
Bellin Memorial Hospital[2]	Green Bay	100%	53
Lakeview Medical Center[2]	Rice Lake	100%	27
Mercy Medical Center of Oshkosh[2]	Oshkosh	100%	25
Saint Clares Hospital of Weston[2]	Weston	100%	35
United Hospital System[2]	Kenosha	98%	53
Ministry Saint Josephs Hospital[2]	Marshfield	97%	112
Aurora Sheboygan Memorial Medical Center[2]	Sheboygan	96%	28
Saint Elizabeth Hospital[2]	Appleton	96%	53
Bay Area Medical Center[2]	Marinette	93%	27
Meriter Hospital[2]	Madison	92%	74
Ministry St Michaels Hosp-Stevens Pt[2]	Stevens Point	91%	33
Saint Marys Hospital[2]	Madison	90%	125
Columbia Saint Marys Hospital Ozaukee[2]	Mequon	89%	45
Saint Agnes Hospital[2]	Fond Du Lac	89%	54
The Monroe Clinic[2]	Monroe	88%	25
Columbia Saint Marys Hospital Milwaukee[2]	Milwaukee	82%	84
Saint Marys Hospital Medical Center[2]	Green Bay	81%	31
Beloit Memorial Hospital[2]	Beloit	79%	39
Mercy Health System Corp[2]	Janesville	79%	63
Community Memorial Hospital[2]	Menomonee Fls	73%	30
Wheaton Franciscan Healthcare All Saints[2]	Racine	73%	106
Univ of WI Hosps & Clinics Authority[2]	Madison	70%	128
Froedtert Memorial Lutheran Hospital[2]	Milwaukee	69%	133
Aurora West Allis Medical Center[2]	West Allis	68%	72
Saint Vincent Hospital[2]	Green Bay	68%	68
Aurora Saint Lukes Medical Center[2]	Milwaukee	67%	270
Gundersen Lutheran Medical Center[2]	La Crosse	67%	52
Mayo Clinic Hlth Sys-Eau Claire Hosp[2]	Eau Claire	64%	77
Aurora Medical Center[2]	Grafton	61%	44
Aurora Medical Center Kenosha[2]	Kenosha	56%	36
Waukesha Memorial Hospital[2]	Waukesha	50%	100
Aurora Baycare Medical Center[2]	Green Bay	49%	55
St Joseph's Comm Hosp of West Bend[2]	West Bend	40%	43
Wheaton Franciscan Saint Joseph[2]	Milwaukee	40%	90
Mayo Clinic Hlth Sys Franciscan Med Ctr[2]	La Crosse	38%	34
Sacred Heart Hospital[2]	Eau Claire	37%	65
Wheaton Franciscan Hlthcare St Francis[2]	Milwaukee	34%	47
Aspirus Wausau Hospital[2]	Wausau	27%	77
Wheaton Franciscan Healthcare Franklin[2]	Franklin	18%	40
Appleton Medical Center[2]	Appleton	0%	75

NOTE: Hospital profiles are in alphabetical order by state, then city, then hospital within the city; Rankings exclude hospitals with less than 25 cases except for patient surveys which excludes hospitals with less than 100 cases; (a) 100-299 cases; (1) The number of cases/patients is too few to report; (2) Data submitted were based on a sample of cases/patients; (3) Results are based on a shorter time period than required; (4) Data suppressed by CMS for one or more quarters; (5) Results are not available for this reporting period; (6) Fewer than 100 patients completed the HCAHPS survey; (7) No cases met the criteria for this measure; (8) The lower limit of the confidence interval cannot be calculated if the number of observed infections equals zero; (9) No data are available from the state/territory for this reporting period; (10) The scores shown reflect fewer than 50 completed surveys; (11) There were discrepancies in the data collection process; (12) This measure does not apply to this hospital for this reporting period; (13) Results cannot be calculated for this reporting period; (14) The results for this state are combined with nearby states to protect confidentiality; Please refer to the User's Guide for a full explanation of data.

Hospital Name	City	Rate	Cases
Theda Clark Medical Center[2]	Neenah	0%	40

Chest Pain/Possible Heart Attack Care

Aspirin Given Within 24 Hours of Arrival

Hospital Name	City	Rate	Cases
Aurora Medical Center Washington County	Hartford	100%	47
Aurora Memorial Hospital Burlington	Burlington	100%	34
Aurora Sheboygan Memorial Medical Center	Sheboygan	100%	54
Aurora West Allis Medical Center	West Allis	100%	64
Berlin Memorial Hospital	Berlin	100%	40
Howard Young Medical Center	Woodruff	100%	100
Hudson Hospital	Hudson	100%	59
Lakeview Medical Center	Rice Lake	100%	96
Memorial Health Center	Medford	100%	37
Ministry Door County Medical Center[3]	Sturgeon Bay	100%	27
Ministry Eagle River Memorial Hospital	Eagle River	100%	45
Ministry Sacred Heart Hospital	Tomahawk	100%	30
Ministry Saint Marys Hospital	Rhinelander	100%	144
Reedsburg Area Medical Center	Reedsburg	100%	71
Saint Clare Hospital Health Services	Baraboo	100%	59
Saint Joseph's Hospital	Chippewa Falls	100%	50
Saint Marys Hospital Superior	Superior	100%	27
Vernon Memorial Hospital	Viroqua	100%	54
Wheaton Franciscan Healthcare Franklin	Franklin	100%	44
Bay Area Medical Center	Marinette	99%	83
Beaver Dam Com Hospital	Beaver Dam	99%	137
Ministry St Michaels Hosp-Stevens Pt	Stevens Point	99%	183
Riverview Hospital Assoc	Wisc. Rapids	99%	124
St Joseph's Comm Hosp of West Bend	West Bend	99%	95
Aurora Medical Center Manitowoc County	Two Rivers	98%	46
Divine Savior Healthcare	Portage	98%	45
Fort Memorial Hospital	Fort Atkinson	98%	91
Good Samaritan Health Center	Merrill	98%	46
Memorial Medical Center	Neillsville	98%	48
Mercy Walworth Hospital & Medical Center	Lake Geneva	98%	57
Prairie Du Chien Memorial Hospital	Prairie Du Chien	98%	43
Sauk Prairie Hospital	Prairie Du Sac	98%	43
UW Hlth Partners Watertown Reg Med Ctr	Watertown	98%	63
Aurora Lakeland Medical Center	Elkhorn	96%	51
Black River Memorial Hospital	Black River Falls	96%	53
Langlade Hospital	Antigo	96%	28
River Falls Area Hospital	River Falls	96%	46
Tomah Memorial Hospital	Tomah	96%	54
Mile Bluff Medical Center	Mauston	95%	65
Saint Marys Janesville Hospital	Janesville	95%	77
Moundview Memorial Hospital & Clinics	Friendship	94%	34
Hayward Area Memorial Hospital	Hayward	93%	43
Aurora Medical Center Kenosha	Kenosha	91%	33
Saint Nicholas Hospital	Sheboygan	91%	46
Spooner Health System	Spooner	88%	43

Average Time to ECG (minutes)

Hospital Name	City	Min.	Cases
Lakeview Medical Center	Rice Lake	1	96
Fort Memorial Hospital	Fort Atkinson	2	91
Aurora Lakeland Medical Center	Elkhorn	3	54
Ministry Sacred Heart Hospital	Tomahawk	3	33
Bay Area Medical Center	Marinette	4	84
Beaver Dam Com Hospital	Beaver Dam	4	138
Berlin Memorial Hospital	Berlin	4	41
Memorial Health Center	Medford	4	38
Reedsburg Area Medical Center	Reedsburg	4	72
Howard Young Medical Center	Woodruff	5	99
Memorial Medical Center	Neillsville	5	50
Prairie Du Chien Memorial Hospital	Prairie Du Chien	5	43
River Falls Area Hospital	River Falls	5	48
Spooner Health System	Spooner	5	46
Aurora Memorial Hospital Burlington	Burlington	6	36
Ministry Saint Marys Hospital	Rhinelander	6	154
Southwest Health Center	Platteville	6	25
UW Hlth Partners Watertown Reg Med Ctr	Watertown	6	64
Aurora Medical Center Kenosha	Kenosha	7	33
Aurora Sheboygan Memorial Medical Center	Sheboygan	7	55
Divine Savior Healthcare	Portage	7	52
Good Samaritan Health Center	Merrill	7	49
Hudson Hospital	Hudson	7	60
Mercy Walworth Hospital & Medical Center	Lake Geneva	7	63
Ministry St Michaels Hosp-Stevens Pt	Stevens Point	7	205
Tomah Memorial Hospital	Tomah	7	49
Wheaton Franciscan Healthcare Franklin	Franklin	7	45
Black River Memorial Hospital	Black River Falls	8	53
Boscobel Area Health Care	Boscobel	8	26
Langlade Hospital	Antigo	8	26
Mile Bluff Medical Center	Mauston	8	67
Moundview Memorial Hospital & Clinics	Friendship	8	34
Saint Marys Janesville Hospital	Janesville	8	78
Saint Clare Hospital Health Services	Baraboo	9	62
St Joseph's Comm Hosp of West Bend	West Bend	9	100
Vernon Memorial Hospital	Viroqua	9	55
Aurora Medical Center Manitowoc County	Two Rivers	10	47
Aurora Medical Center Washington County	Hartford	10	48
Ministry Door County Medical Center[3]	Sturgeon Bay	10	26
Ministry Eagle River Memorial Hospital	Eagle River	10	47
Riverview Hospital Assoc	Wisc. Rapids	10	126
Saint Nicholas Hospital	Sheboygan	10	48
Sauk Prairie Hospital	Prairie Du Sac	10	43
Saint Marys Hospital Superior	Superior	12	28
Saint Joseph's Hospital	Chippewa Falls	13	51
Aurora West Allis Medical Center	West Allis	15	65
Hayward Area Memorial Hospital	Hayward	18	44

Average Time to Transfer (minutes)

Hospital Name	City	Min.	Cases
St Joseph's Comm Hosp of West Bend	West Bend	50	26

Children's Asthma Care

No hospitals met the 25 case threshold.

Emergency Department

Admittance Decision Time (minutes)

Hospital Name	City	Min.	Cases
Saint Joseph's Health Services	Hillsboro	8	122
Good Samaritan Health Center[2]	Merrill	14	443
Memorial Hospital Lafayette Cty	Darlington	15	175
Bellin Health Oconto Hospital[3]	Oconto	19	53
Moundview Memorial Hospital & Clinics	Friendship	20	81
Cumberland Memorial Hospital[3]	Cumberland	28	99
Hayward Area Memorial Hospital[2]	Hayward	30	323
Appleton Medical Center[2]	Appleton	34	328
Spooner Health System	Spooner	35	242
Saint Marys Hospital Superior[2]	Superior	36	197
Ministry Sacred Heart Hospital[2]	Tomahawk	38	186
Mercy Walworth Hospital & Medical Center	Lake Geneva	40	626
Ministry Eagle River Memorial Hospital	Eagle River	40	299
Our Lady of Victory Hospital[2]	Stanley	40	278
Mercy Health System Corp[2]	Janesville	41	580
Flambeau Hospital	Park Falls	44	459
Froedtert Memorial Lutheran Hospital[2]	Milwaukee	44	494
Sauk Prairie Hospital[2]	Prairie Du Sac	45	147
Richland Hospital	Richland Center	46	560
Stoughton Hospital[2]	Stoughton	46	335
Saint Marys Janesville Hospital[2]	Janesville	48	264
Bellin Memorial Hospital[2]	Green Bay	49	389
Holy Family Memorial[2]	Manitowoc	49	286
Riverview Hospital Assoc[2]	Wisc. Rapids	49	288
Theda Clark Medical Center[2]	Neenah	50	340
Aurora Medical Center Washington County[2]	Hartford	52	395
Beaver Dam Com Hospital[2]	Beaver Dam	53	298
Lakeview Medical Center[2]	Rice Lake	53	195
Vernon Memorial Hospital[2]	Viroqua	53	344
Aspirus Wausau Hospital[2]	Wausau	54	393
Aurora Medical Center Manitowoc County[2]	Two Rivers	54	213
Boscobel Area Health Care	Boscobel	55	143
Prairie Du Chien Memorial Hospital	Prairie Du Chien	55	612
Beloit Memorial Hospital[2]	Beloit	56	439
Divine Savior Healthcare	Portage	56	1067
The Monroe Clinic[2]	Monroe	56	1226
Ministry St Michaels Hosp-Stevens Pt[2]	Stevens Point	58	504
Saint Clare Hospital Health Services[2]	Baraboo	59	181
Aurora Sheboygan Memorial Medical Center[2]	Sheboygan	60	265
Community Memorial Hospital[2]	Menomonee Fls	60	589
Community Memorial Hospital	Oconto Falls	60	103
Meriter Hospital[2]	Madison	62	482
Saint Elizabeth Hospital[2]	Appleton	63	454
Fort Memorial Hospital[2]	Fort Atkinson	64	282
Saint Agnes Hospital[2]	Fond Du Lac	64	536
St Joseph's Comm Hosp of West Bend[2]	West Bend	64	420
Memorial Medical Center	Neillsville	65	144
Ministry Saint Josephs Hospital[2]	Marshfield	65	758
Howard Young Medical Center[2]	Woodruff	66	278
UW Hlth Partners Watertown Reg Med Ctr[2]	Watertown	66	122
Saint Clares Hospital of Weston[2]	Weston	67	388
Saint Marys Hospital[2]	Madison	67	357
Aurora Medical Center Kenosha[2]	Kenosha	68	452
Gundersen Lutheran Medical Center[2]	La Crosse	68	377
Aurora Medical Center[2]	Grafton	69	464
Aurora Medical Center[2]	Summit	70	277
Bay Area Medical Center[2]	Marinette	70	522
Aurora Medical Center Oshkosh[2]	Oshkosh	71	183
Mercy Medical Center of Oshkosh[2]	Oshkosh	72	418
Sacred Heart Hospital[2]	Eau Claire	74	364
Univ of WI Hosps & Clinics Authority[2]	Madison	74	356
Aurora Baycare Medical Center[2]	Green Bay	75	211
River Falls Area Hospital[2]	River Falls	75	191
Saint Joseph's Hospital[2]	Chippewa Falls	76	192
Aurora Memorial Hospital Burlington[2]	Burlington	78	320
Columbia Saint Marys Hospital Ozaukee[2]	Mequon	78	648
Waukesha Memorial Hospital[2]	Waukesha	79	622
Tomah Memorial Hospital	Tomah	80	490
Wheaton Franciscan Healthcare Franklin[2]	Franklin	80	647
Oconomowoc Memorial Hospital[2]	Oconomowoc	82	358
Reedsburg Area Medical Center	Reedsburg	82	556
United Hospital System[2]	Kenosha	82	665
Aurora Lakeland Medical Center[2]	Elkhorn	83	295
Saint Nicholas Hospital[2]	Sheboygan	86	261
Wheaton Franciscan Saint Joseph[2]	Milwaukee	86	650
Ministry Saint Marys Hospital[2]	Rhinelander	90	171
Aurora West Allis Medical Center[2]	West Allis	91	458
Wheaton Franciscan Healthcare All Saints[2]	Racine	94	536
Columbia Saint Marys Hospital Milwaukee[2]	Milwaukee	96	490
Wheaton Franciscan Hlthcare St Francis[2]	Milwaukee	97	689
Mayo Clinic Hlth Sys Franciscan Med Ctr[2]	La Crosse	99	425
Aurora Saint Lukes Medical Center[2]	Milwaukee	100	1696
Mayo Clinic Hlth Sys-Eau Claire Hosp[2]	Eau Claire	102	445
Mile Bluff Medical Center	Mauston	106	533
Saint Vincent Hospital[2]	Green Bay	109	364
Saint Marys Hospital Medical Center[2]	Green Bay	129	421

Head CT Results Within 45 Minutes of Arrival

Hospital Name	City	Rate	Cases
Wheaton Franciscan Saint Joseph	Milwaukee	84%	32
United Hospital System	Kenosha	75%	32

Patients Who Left ER Before Being Seen

Hospital Name	City	Rate	Cases
Appleton Medical Center	Appleton	0%	21541
Aspirus Wausau Hospital	Wausau	0%	29086
Aurora Baycare Medical Center	Green Bay	0%	26292
Aurora Medical Center	Grafton	0%	11788
Aurora Medical Center	Summit	0%	11841
Aurora Medical Center Manitowoc County	Two Rivers	0%	12270
Aurora Medical Center Washington County	Hartford	0%	8564
Beaver Dam Com Hospital	Beaver Dam	0%	29940
Columbia Saint Marys Hospital Ozaukee	Mequon	0%	17354
Community Memorial Hospital	Menomonee Fls	0%	20263
Divine Savior Healthcare	Portage	0%	13144
Fort Memorial Hospital	Fort Atkinson	0%	16458
Good Samaritan Health Center	Merrill	0%	6063
Grant Regional Health Center	Lancaster	0%	5986
Holy Family Memorial	Manitowoc	0%	12884
Hudson Hospital	Hudson	0%	9919
Lakeview Medical Center	Rice Lake	0%	11471
Mayo Clinic Hlth Sys Franciscan Med Ctr	La Crosse	0%	33534
Mayo Clinic Hlth Sys-Eau Claire Hosp	Eau Claire	0%	30116
Memorial Health Center	Medford	0%	7213
Meriter Hospital	Madison	0%	44764
Mile Bluff Medical Center	Mauston	0%	7523
Ministry Sacred Heart Hospital	Tomahawk	0%	4194
Ministry Saint Josephs Hospital	Marshfield	0%	22095
Ministry Saint Marys Hospital	Rhinelander	0%	19395
Ministry St Michaels Hosp-Stevens Pt	Stevens Point	0%	19631
The Monroe Clinic	Monroe	0%	20480
New London Family Medical Center	New London	0%	8792
Oconomowoc Memorial Hospital	Oconomowoc	0%	13387
River Falls Area Hospital	River Falls	0%	5720
Riverside Medical Center	Waupaca	0%	12507
Saint Agnes Hospital	Fond Du Lac	0%	28614
Saint Clare Hospital Health Services	Baraboo	0%	19894
Saint Clares Hospital of Weston	Weston	0%	14731
Saint Elizabeth Hospital	Appleton	0%	31110
Saint Joseph's Hospital	Chippewa Falls	0%	16829
Saint Marys Hospital	Madison	0%	49988
Saint Marys Hospital Medical Center	Green Bay	0%	32670
Saint Marys Janesville Hospital	Janesville	0%	12343
Saint Nicholas Hospital	Sheboygan	0%	14293
Saint Vincent Hospital	Green Bay	0%	37289
Shawano Medical Center	Shawano	0%	19401
Theda Clark Medical Center	Neenah	0%	16381
United Hospital System	Kenosha	0%	70560
Univ of WI Hosps & Clinics Authority	Madison	0%	46937
UW Hlth Partners Watertown Reg Med Ctr	Watertown	0%	20343
Wheaton Franciscan Healthcare Franklin	Franklin	0%	22355
Aurora Lakeland Medical Center	Elkhorn	1%	16126
Aurora Medical Center Kenosha	Kenosha	1%	25070
Aurora Medical Center Oshkosh	Oshkosh	1%	12778
Aurora Memorial Hospital Burlington	Burlington	1%	14171
Aurora Sheboygan Memorial Medical Center	Sheboygan	1%	18591
Bay Area Medical Center	Marinette	1%	21795
Bellin Memorial Hospital	Green Bay	1%	31685
Gundersen Lutheran Medical Center	La Crosse	1%	29703
Howard Young Medical Center	Woodruff	1%	7686
Langlade Hospital	Antigo	1%	11319
Mercy Health System Corp	Janesville	1%	29768
Mercy Medical Center of Oshkosh	Oshkosh	1%	18436
Ministry Door County Medical Center	Sturgeon Bay	1%	9752
Ministry Eagle River Memorial Hospital	Eagle River	1%	5067
Riverview Hospital Assoc	Wisc. Rapids	1%	24911
Sacred Heart Hospital	Eau Claire	1%	19992

NOTE: Hospital profiles are in alphabetical order by state, then city, then hospital within the city; Rankings exclude hospitals with less than 25 cases except for patient surveys which excludes hospitals with less than 100 cases; (a) 100-299 cases; (1) The number of cases/patients is too few to report; (2) Data submitted were based on a sample of cases/patients; (3) Results are based on a shorter time period than required; (4) Data suppressed by CMS for one or more quarters; (5) Results are not available for this reporting period; (6) Fewer than 100 patients completed the HCAHPS survey; (7) No cases met the criteria for this measure; (8) The lower limit of the confidence interval cannot be calculated if the number of observed infections equals zero; (9) No data are available from the state/territory for this reporting period; (10) The scores shown reflect fewer than 50 completed surveys; (11) There were discrepancies in the data collection process; (12) This measure does not apply to this hospital for this reporting period; (13) Results cannot be calculated for this reporting period; (14) The results for this state are combined with nearby states to protect confidentiality; Please refer to the User's Guide for a full explanation of data.

St Joseph's Comm Hosp of West Bend	West Bend	1%	16689
Saint Marys Hospital Superior	Superior	1%	15211
Sauk Prairie Hospital	Prairie Du Sac	1%	6940
Waukesha Memorial Hospital	Waukesha	1%	39517
Wheaton Franciscan Healthcare All Saints	Racine	1%	59574
Wheaton Franciscan Hlthcare St Francis	Milwaukee	1%	48611
Aurora Saint Lukes Medical Center	Milwaukee	2%	136667
Aurora West Allis Medical Center	West Allis	2%	34374
Beloit Memorial Hospital	Beloit	2%	39846
Columbia Saint Marys Hospital Milwaukee	Milwaukee	2%	57146
Wheaton Franciscan Saint Joseph	Milwaukee	2%	131911
Froedtert Memorial Lutheran Hospital	Milwaukee	3%	64923

Time from ER Arrival to Being Admitted (minutes)

Hospital Name	City	Min.	Cases
Cumberland Memorial Hospital[3]	Cumberland	100	100
Saint Joseph's Health Services	Hillsboro	130	129
River Falls Area Hospital[2]	River Falls	141	199
Ministry Sacred Heart Hospital[2]	Tomahawk	148	216
Memorial Hospital Lafayette Cty	Darlington	152	175
Bellin Health Oconto Hospital[3]	Oconto	153	57
Flambeau Hospital	Park Falls	155	459
Holy Family Memorial[2]	Manitowoc	157	329
Moundview Memorial Hospital & Clinics	Friendship	159	96
Community Memorial Hospital	Oconto Falls	160	116
Mercy Health System Corp[2]	Janesville	163	583
Theda Clark Medical Center[2]	Neenah	169	350
Aspirus Wausau Hospital[2]	Wausau	172	402
Richland Hospital	Richland Center	173	560
Saint Clare Hospital Health Services[2]	Baraboo	180	182
Saint Vincent Hospital[2]	Green Bay	180	374
Appleton Medical Center[2]	Appleton	181	334
Gundersen Lutheran Medical Center[2]	La Crosse	181	391
Prairie Du Chien Memorial Hospital	Prairie Du Chien	181	614
Ministry Saint Josephs Hospital[2]	Marshfield	182	841
Saint Marys Hospital Medical Center[2]	Green Bay	182	430
Aurora Medical Center[2]	Summit	183	287
Stoughton Hospital[2]	Stoughton	183	335
Boscobel Area Health Care	Boscobel	184	154
Saint Marys Hospital Superior[2]	Superior	186	206
Vernon Memorial Hospital[2]	Viroqua	187	346
Aurora Medical Center[2]	Grafton	188	471
Ministry St Michaels Hosp-Stevens Pt[2]	Stevens Point	188	504
Saint Nicholas Hospital[2]	Sheboygan	188	264
Mercy Walworth Hospital & Medical Center	Lake Geneva	189	627
Meriter Hospital[2]	Madison	190	482
Our Lady of Victory Hospital[2]	Stanley	190	280
Riverview Hospital Assoc[2]	Wisc. Rapids	190	312
Saint Marys Hospital[2]	Madison	190	361
Spooner Health System	Spooner	191	286
Aurora Baycare Medical Center[2]	Green Bay	192	258
Aurora Sheboygan Memorial Medical Center[2]	Sheboygan	192	299
Hayward Area Memorial Hospital[2]	Hayward	192	323
Saint Marys Janesville Hospital[2]	Janesville	194	268
Sauk Prairie Hospital[2]	Prairie Du Sac	194	151
Saint Clares Hospital of Weston[2]	Weston	195	391
Bay Area Medical Center[2]	Marinette	196	522
Mercy Medical Center of Oshkosh[2]	Oshkosh	197	420
Berlin Memorial Hospital	Berlin	198	134
Saint Agnes Hospital[2]	Fond Du Lac	199	668
Aurora Medical Center Washington County[2]	Hartford	202	404
Memorial Medical Center	Neillsville	203	165
Mile Bluff Medical Center	Mauston	203	586
Saint Elizabeth Hospital[2]	Appleton	203	454
Bellin Memorial Hospital[2]	Green Bay	204	389
Lakeview Medical Center[2]	Rice Lake	204	213
Ministry Eagle River Memorial Hospital	Eagle River	206	300
Sacred Heart Hospital[2]	Eau Claire	207	365
Columbia Saint Marys Hospital Ozaukee[2]	Mequon	208	657
Aurora Medical Center Oshkosh[2]	Oshkosh	210	262
St Joseph's Comm Hosp of West Bend[2]	West Bend	212	420
Community Memorial Hospital[2]	Menomonee Fls	213	592
Edgerton Hospital & Health Services[3]	Edgerton	213	27
Good Samaritan Health Center[2]	Merrill	213	453
The Monroe Clinic[2]	Monroe	214	1256
Saint Joseph's Hospital[2]	Chippewa Falls	214	195
UW Hlth Partners Watertown Reg Med Ctr[2]	Watertown	215	171
Oconomowoc Memorial Hospital[2]	Oconomowoc	216	361
Aurora Medical Center Manitowoc County[2]	Two Rivers	217	255
Aurora Lakeland Medical Center[2]	Elkhorn	218	296
Beaver Dam Com Hospital[2]	Beaver Dam	220	299
Howard Young Medical Center[2]	Woodruff	220	279
Divine Savior Healthcare	Portage	221	1068
Mayo Clinic Hlth Sys Franciscan Med Ctr[2]	La Crosse	222	432
Aurora Medical Center Kenosha[2]	Kenosha	223	528
Reedsburg Area Medical Center	Reedsburg	223	624
Tomah Memorial Hospital	Tomah	224	490
Fort Memorial Hospital[2]	Fort Atkinson	225	295
Beloit Memorial Hospital[2]	Beloit	226	439
United Hospital System[2]	Kenosha	226	666
Waukesha Memorial Hospital[2]	Waukesha	233	625

Froedtert Memorial Lutheran Hospital[2]	Milwaukee	238	495
Wheaton Franciscan Healthcare Franklin[2]	Franklin	240	647
Wheaton Franciscan Saint Joseph[2]	Milwaukee	243	653
Aurora Memorial Hospital Burlington[2]	Burlington	246	356
Columbia Saint Marys Hospital Milwaukee[2]	Milwaukee	246	498
Mayo Clinic Hlth Sys-Eau Claire Hosp[2]	Eau Claire	247	474
Ministry Saint Marys Hospital[2]	Rhinelander	250	318
Aurora Saint Lukes Medical Center[2]	Milwaukee	252	1722
Aurora West Allis Medical Center[2]	West Allis	252	458
Wheaton Franciscan Hlthcare St Francis[2]	Milwaukee	264	689
Univ of WI Hosps & Clinics Authority[2]	Madison	267	366
Wheaton Franciscan Healthcare All Saints[2]	Racine	270	540

Time from ER Arrival to Discharge (minutes)

Hospital Name	City	Min.	Cases
Bellin Health Oconto Hospital[3]	Oconto	79	131
Moundview Memorial Hospital & Clinics	Friendship	83	550
Chippewa Valley Hospital	Durand	87	494
Ministry Sacred Heart Hospital	Tomahawk	88	661
Flambeau Hospital	Park Falls	90	383
River Falls Area Hospital	River Falls	92	353
Holy Family Memorial	Manitowoc	95	376
Aurora Medical Center Oshkosh	Oshkosh	96	358
Amery Regional Medical Center[3]	Amery	98	318
Memorial Hospital Lafayette Cty	Darlington	98	202
Memorial Medical Center	Neillsville	98	199
Saint Joseph's Health Services	Hillsboro	98	780
Saint Elizabeth Hospital	Appleton	100	349
Aurora Medical Center	Summit	101	356
Saint Marys Hospital Superior	Superior	102	394
Mercy Health System Corp	Janesville	103	440
Saint Clare Hospital Health Services	Baraboo	104	358
Saint Marys Janesville Hospital	Janesville	104	374
Mercy Medical Center of Oshkosh	Oshkosh	105	365
Meriter Hospital	Madison	105	1087
Bay Area Medical Center	Marinette	106	363
Prairie Du Chien Memorial Hospital	Prairie Du Chien	106	418
Hudson Hospital	Hudson	107	367
Lakeview Medical Center	Rice Lake	108	437
Saint Marys Hospital	Madison	108	376
Aurora Sheboygan Memorial Medical Center	Sheboygan	109	349
Aurora Baycare Medical Center	Green Bay	110	348
Aspirus Wausau Hospital	Wausau	112	363
Wheaton Franciscan Saint Joseph	Milwaukee	112	387
Divine Savior Healthcare	Portage	113	10990
Hayward Area Memorial Hospital	Hayward	113	399
Mercy Walworth Hospital & Medical Center	Lake Geneva	113	437
Saint Agnes Hospital	Fond Du Lac	113	562
Theda Clark Medical Center	Neenah	113	400
United Hospital System	Kenosha	113	351
Vernon Memorial Hospital	Viroqua	113	313
Ministry Eagle River Memorial Hospital	Eagle River	114	488
Tomah Memorial Hospital[3]	Tomah	114	290
UW Hlth Partners Watertown Reg Med Ctr	Watertown	114	408
Ministry Saint Josephs Hospital	Marshfield	115	669
Saint Marys Hospital Medical Center	Green Bay	115	391
Sauk Prairie Hospital	Prairie Du Sac	116	396
Riverview Hospital Assoc	Wisc. Rapids	117	360
Saint Clares Hospital of Weston	Weston	118	1022
Mile Bluff Medical Center	Mauston	119	390
Aurora Lakeland Medical Center	Elkhorn	120	332
Berlin Memorial Hospital	Berlin	120	337
Saint Vincent Hospital	Green Bay	120	385
Oconomowoc Memorial Hospital	Oconomowoc	122	382
Mayo Clinic Hlth Sys Franciscan Med Ctr	La Crosse	124	344
Aurora Medical Center	Grafton	125	347
Reedsburg Area Medical Center	Reedsburg	125	343
Aurora Medical Center Washington County	Hartford	126	351
Good Samaritan Health Center	Merrill	126	354
Langlade Hospital[3]	Antigo	126	208
Saint Nicholas Hospital	Sheboygan	126	380
Beloit Memorial Hospital	Beloit	127	397
Ministry Saint Marys Hospital	Rhinelander	127	749
Aurora Medical Center Manitowoc County	Two Rivers	128	344
Bellin Memorial Hospital	Green Bay	128	367
Ministry St Michaels Hosp-Stevens Pt	Stevens Point	128	1431
Gundersen Lutheran Medical Center	La Crosse	129	1406
Stoughton Hospital	Stoughton	129	338
Fort Memorial Hospital	Fort Atkinson	130	360
Appleton Medical Center	Appleton	134	401
Howard Young Medical Center	Woodruff	134	345
The Monroe Clinic	Monroe	134	10422
Sacred Heart Hospital	Eau Claire	134	370
St Joseph's Comm Hosp of West Bend	West Bend	134	373
Our Lady of Victory Hospital[3]	Stanley	136	33
Saint Joseph's Hospital	Chippewa Falls	137	443
Beaver Dam Com Hospital	Beaver Dam	138	368
Columbia Saint Marys Hospital Ozaukee	Mequon	138	368
Wheaton Franciscan Healthcare All Saints	Racine	140	379
Columbia Saint Marys Hospital Milwaukee	Milwaukee	144	367
Aurora Medical Center Kenosha	Kenosha	146	352

Mayo Clinic Hlth Sys-Eau Claire Hosp	Eau Claire	147	383
Aurora Memorial Hospital Burlington	Burlington	148	346
Aurora West Allis Medical Center	West Allis	152	339
Community Memorial Hospital	Menomonee Fls	154	371
Aurora Saint Lukes Medical Center	Milwaukee	155	1055
Waukesha Memorial Hospital	Waukesha	155	372
Wheaton Franciscan Healthcare Franklin	Franklin	156	375
Wheaton Franciscan Hlthcare St Francis	Milwaukee	164	364
Froedtert Memorial Lutheran Hospital	Milwaukee	184	371
Univ of WI Hosps & Clinics Authority	Madison	196	340

Time in ER Before Being Evaluated (minutes)

Hospital Name	City	Min.	Cases
Mile Bluff Medical Center	Mauston	4	423
River Falls Area Hospital	River Falls	7	425
Mercy Health System Corp	Janesville	8	472
Saint Marys Hospital	Madison	8	407
Stoughton Hospital	Stoughton	9	386
Aurora Medical Center	Grafton	10	369
Meriter Hospital	Madison	10	1149
Saint Clare Hospital Health Services	Baraboo	10	406
Aurora Medical Center	Summit	11	384
Our Lady of Victory Hospital[3]	Stanley	11	38
Saint Marys Janesville Hospital	Janesville	11	407
Aspirus Wausau Hospital	Wausau	12	246
Ministry St Michaels Hosp-Stevens Pt	Stevens Point	12	1597
Mayo Clinic Hlth Sys Franciscan Med Ctr	La Crosse	13	415
Prairie Du Chien Memorial Hospital	Prairie Du Chien	13	525
Berlin Memorial Hospital	Berlin	14	404
Mercy Walworth Hospital & Medical Center	Lake Geneva	14	537
Saint Joseph's Health Services	Hillsboro	14	868
Aurora Medical Center Washington County	Hartford	15	381
Flambeau Hospital	Park Falls	15	443
Gundersen Lutheran Medical Center	La Crosse	15	1566
Mayo Clinic Hlth Sys-Eau Claire Hosp	Eau Claire	15	414
Ministry Saint Marys Hospital	Rhinelander	15	611
Oconomowoc Memorial Hospital	Oconomowoc	15	263
Saint Elizabeth Hospital	Appleton	15	392
Chippewa Valley Hospital	Durand	16	569
Community Memorial Hospital	Menomonee Fls	16	421
Mercy Medical Center of Oshkosh	Oshkosh	16	392
Ministry Sacred Heart Hospital	Tomahawk	16	638
Tomah Memorial Hospital[3]	Tomah	16	93
Columbia Saint Marys Hospital Ozaukee	Mequon	17	406
Froedtert Memorial Lutheran Hospital	Milwaukee	17	407
Good Samaritan Health Center	Merrill	17	365
Hudson Hospital	Hudson	17	384
Saint Agnes Hospital	Fond Du Lac	17	617
UW Hlth Partners Watertown Reg Med Ctr	Watertown	17	450
Memorial Hospital Lafayette Cty	Darlington	18	258
The Monroe Clinic	Monroe	18	11678
Reedsburg Area Medical Center	Reedsburg	18	453
Riverview Hospital Assoc	Wisc. Rapids	18	380
Saint Joseph's Hospital	Chippewa Falls	18	501
Saint Marys Hospital Medical Center	Green Bay	18	374
Theda Clark Medical Center	Neenah	18	420
Wheaton Franciscan Healthcare Franklin	Franklin	18	396
Langlade Hospital[3]	Antigo	19	235
St Joseph's Comm Hosp of West Bend	West Bend	19	422
Saint Vincent Hospital	Green Bay	19	370
Appleton Medical Center	Appleton	20	424
Aurora Baycare Medical Center	Green Bay	20	360
Aurora Lakeland Medical Center	Elkhorn	20	373
Aurora Medical Center Oshkosh	Oshkosh	20	296
Bellin Health Oconto Hospital[3]	Oconto	20	30
Lakeview Medical Center	Rice Lake	20	334
Memorial Medical Center	Neillsville	20	230
Wheaton Franciscan Saint Joseph	Milwaukee	20	388
Aurora Medical Center Kenosha	Kenosha	21	295
Aurora Sheboygan Memorial Medical Center	Sheboygan	21	368
Bay Area Medical Center	Marinette	21	398
Saint Marys Hospital Superior	Superior	21	153
Univ of WI Hosps & Clinics Authority	Madison	21	380
Moundview Memorial Hospital & Clinics	Friendship	22	496
Sacred Heart Hospital	Eau Claire	22	397
Saint Nicholas Hospital	Sheboygan	22	370
Beaver Dam Com Hospital	Beaver Dam	23	412
Holy Family Memorial	Manitowoc	23	367
Vernon Memorial Hospital	Viroqua	23	377
Waukesha Memorial Hospital	Waukesha	23	339
Amery Regional Medical Center[3]	Amery	24	325
Aurora Memorial Hospital Burlington	Burlington	24	332
Divine Savior Healthcare	Portage	24	11929
Fort Memorial Hospital	Fort Atkinson	24	306
Sauk Prairie Hospital	Prairie Du Sac	24	443
Aurora Saint Lukes Medical Center	Milwaukee	25	978
Aurora West Allis Medical Center	West Allis	25	362
Columbia Saint Marys Hospital Milwaukee	Milwaukee	26	405
Ministry Saint Josephs Hospital	Marshfield	26	514
Saint Clares Hospital of Weston	Weston	26	1115
United Hospital System	Kenosha	26	381

NOTE: Hospital profiles are in alphabetical order by state, then city, then hospital within the city; Rankings exclude hospitals with less than 25 cases except for patient surveys which excludes hospitals with less than 100 cases; (a) 100-299 cases; (1) The number of cases/patients is too few to report; (2) Data submitted were based on a sample of cases/patients; (3) Results are based on a shorter time period than required; (4) Data suppressed by CMS for one or more quarters; (5) Results are not available for this reporting period; (6) Fewer than 100 patients completed the HCAHPS survey; (7) No cases met the criteria for this measure; (8) The lower limit of the confidence interval cannot be calculated if the number of observed infections equals zero; (9) No data are available from the state/territory for this reporting period; (10) The scores shown reflect fewer than 50 completed surveys; (11) There were discrepancies in the data collection process; (12) This measure does not apply to this hospital for this reporting period; (13) Results cannot be calculated for this reporting period; (14) The results for this state are combined with nearby states to protect confidentiality; Please refer to the User's Guide for a full explanation of data.

Aurora Medical Center Manitowoc County	Two Rivers	27	357
Howard Young Medical Center	Woodruff	27	384
Ministry Eagle River Memorial Hospital	Eagle River	27	556
Wheaton Franciscan Hlthcare St Francis	Milwaukee	27	397
Hayward Area Memorial Hospital	Hayward	31	444
Bellin Memorial Hospital	Green Bay	34	259
Wheaton Franciscan Healthcare All Saints	Racine	34	380
Beloit Memorial Hospital	Beloit	39	245

Time to Pain Meds for Bone Fractures (minutes)

Hospital Name	City	Min.	Cases
Prairie Du Chien Memorial Hospital	Prairie Du Chien	25	33
Saint Clare Hospital Health Services	Baraboo	26	66
Good Samaritan Health Center	Merrill	28	31
Ministry St Michaels Hosp-Stevens Pt	Stevens Point	30	59
Saint Marys Hospital	Madison	30	152
Meriter Hospital	Madison	31	89
Aspirus Wausau Hospital	Wausau	32	126
Aurora Medical Center	Summit	32	75
Bay Area Medical Center	Marinette	32	76
Wheaton Franciscan Healthcare Franklin	Franklin	32	53
Sauk Prairie Hospital	Prairie Du Sac	33	69
Hudson Hospital	Hudson	34	74
Mercy Medical Center of Oshkosh	Oshkosh	34	69
Oconomowoc Memorial Hospital	Oconomowoc	34	74
Saint Elizabeth Hospital	Appleton	34	125
Aurora Medical Center Washington County	Hartford	35	43
Reedsburg Area Medical Center	Reedsburg	35	59
Saint Marys Hospital Superior	Superior	35	38
Wheaton Franciscan Saint Joseph	Milwaukee	35	152
Mercy Health System Corp	Janesville	36	96
Saint Agnes Hospital	Fond Du Lac	36	94
Aurora Sheboygan Memorial Medical Center	Sheboygan	37	80
Mercy Walworth Hospital & Medical Center	Lake Geneva	37	88
Ministry Saint Marys Hospital	Rhinelander	37	47
Saint Clares Hospital of Weston	Weston	37	54
UW Hlth Partners Watertown Reg Med Ctr	Watertown	37	53
Divine Savior Healthcare	Portage	38	97
Aurora Medical Center	Grafton	39	91
Aurora Lakeland Medical Center	Elkhorn	40	105
Aurora Medical Center Oshkosh	Oshkosh	40	56
Mile Bluff Medical Center	Mauston	40	30
Saint Nicholas Hospital	Sheboygan	40	44
Wheaton Franciscan Hlthcare St Francis	Milwaukee	40	47
Aurora Memorial Hospital Burlington	Burlington	41	62
Beaver Dam Com Hospital	Beaver Dam	41	57
Mayo Clinic Hlth Sys Franciscan Med Ctr	La Crosse	41	50
Riverview Hospital Assoc	Wisc. Rapids	41	66
Saint Marys Janesville Hospital	Janesville	41	43
Aurora Medical Center Kenosha	Kenosha	42	79
Froedtert Memorial Lutheran Hospital	Milwaukee	42	148
Ministry Eagle River Memorial Hospital	Eagle River	42	26
Theda Clark Medical Center	Neenah	42	107
Howard Young Medical Center	Woodruff	43	59
Holy Family Memorial	Manitowoc	44	38
Mayo Clinic Hlth Sys-Eau Claire Hosp	Eau Claire	44	55
Ministry Saint Josephs Hospital	Marshfield	44	93
Community Memorial Hospital	Menomonee Fls	45	103
Lakeview Medical Center	Rice Lake	45	45
Saint Vincent Hospital	Green Bay	45	81
Aurora Baycare Medical Center	Green Bay	46	102
St Joseph's Comm Hosp of West Bend	West Bend	46	91
Waukesha Memorial Hospital	Waukesha	46	191
Appleton Medical Center	Appleton	47	191
Saint Joseph's Hospital	Chippewa Falls	48	37
The Monroe Clinic	Monroe	50	78
Hayward Area Memorial Hospital	Hayward	52	60
Sacred Heart Hospital	Eau Claire	52	89
Wheaton Franciscan Healthcare All Saints	Racine	52	178
Aurora Medical Center Manitowoc County	Two Rivers	53	46
Aurora Saint Lukes Medical Center	Milwaukee	53	173
Fort Memorial Hospital	Fort Atkinson	53	41
Gundersen Lutheran Medical Center	La Crosse	53	51
Univ of WI Hosps & Clinics Authority	Madison	53	108
Saint Marys Hospital Medical Center	Green Bay	54	71
Bellin Memorial Hospital	Green Bay	56	94
Columbia Saint Marys Hospital Ozaukee	Mequon	56	78
Aurora West Allis Medical Center	West Allis	58	63
United Hospital System	Kenosha	58	152
Columbia Saint Marys Hospital Milwaukee	Milwaukee	60	93
Beloit Memorial Hospital	Beloit	72	102

Heart Attack Care

Aspirin Given at Discharge

Hospital Name	City	Rate	Cases
Appleton Medical Center	Appleton	100%	273
Aurora Baycare Medical Center	Green Bay	100%	152
Aurora Medical Center	Summit	100%	43
Aurora Medical Center Oshkosh	Oshkosh	100%	58
Aurora Memorial Hospital Burlington	Burlington	100%	26
Aurora Saint Lukes Medical Center	Milwaukee	100%	916
Columbia Saint Marys Hospital Milwaukee	Milwaukee	100%	136
Community Memorial Hospital	Menomonee Fls	100%	117
Froedtert Memorial Lutheran Hospital	Milwaukee	100%	216
Holy Family Memorial	Manitowoc	100%	66
Madison VA Medical Center	Madison	100%	58
Mayo Clinic Hlth Sys-Eau Claire Hosp	Eau Claire	100%	218
Mercy Medical Center of Oshkosh	Oshkosh	100%	81
Meriter Hospital	Madison	100%	325
Ministry Saint Josephs Hospital	Marshfield	100%	352
The Monroe Clinic	Monroe	100%	31
Oconomowoc Memorial Hospital	Oconomowoc	100%	52
Sacred Heart Hospital[2]	Eau Claire	100%	285
Saint Clares Hospital of Weston	Weston	100%	260
Saint Elizabeth Hospital	Appleton	100%	125
Saint Marys Hospital	Madison	100%	488
Theda Clark Medical Center	Neenah	100%	50
United Hospital System	Kenosha	100%	120
Univ of WI Hosps & Clinics Authority[2]	Madison	100%	280
Waukesha Memorial Hospital[2]	Waukesha	100%	242
Wheaton Franciscan Healthcare All Saints	Racine	100%	178
Wheaton Franciscan Saint Joseph	Milwaukee	100%	299
Aspirus Wausau Hospital[2]	Wausau	99%	258
Aurora Medical Center	Grafton	99%	180
Bellin Memorial Hospital[2]	Green Bay	99%	378
Gundersen Lutheran Medical Center	La Crosse	99%	325
Mayo Clinic Hlth Sys Franciscan Med Ctr	La Crosse	99%	111
Mercy Health System Corp	Janesville	99%	166
Saint Agnes Hospital	Fond Du Lac	99%	229
Saint Marys Hospital Medical Center	Green Bay	99%	119
Bay Area Medical Center	Marinette	98%	83
Columbia Saint Marys Hospital Ozaukee	Mequon	98%	127
Milwaukee VA Medical Center	Milwaukee	98%	65
Wheaton Franciscan Hlthcare St Francis	Milwaukee	98%	118
Aurora Sheboygan Memorial Medical Center	Sheboygan	97%	36
Saint Vincent Hospital	Green Bay	97%	188
Beloit Memorial Hospital	Beloit	96%	90
Aurora West Allis Medical Center	West Allis	92%	26

PCI Within 90 Minutes of Arrival

Hospital Name	City	Rate	Cases
Aspirus Wausau Hospital[2]	Wausau	100%	46
Mercy Health System Corp	Janesville	100%	37
Ministry Saint Josephs Hospital	Marshfield	100%	31
Saint Agnes Hospital	Fond Du Lac	100%	37
Waukesha Memorial Hospital[2]	Waukesha	100%	60
Wheaton Franciscan Healthcare All Saints	Racine	100%	42
Aurora Saint Lukes Medical Center	Milwaukee	98%	111
Columbia Saint Marys Hospital Milwaukee	Milwaukee	97%	38
Mayo Clinic Hlth Sys-Eau Claire Hosp	Eau Claire	97%	29
Saint Marys Hospital	Madison	97%	39
Appleton Medical Center	Appleton	95%	39
Bellin Memorial Hospital[2]	Green Bay	95%	37
Froedtert Memorial Lutheran Hospital	Milwaukee	95%	40
Aurora Medical Center	Grafton	94%	32
Meriter Hospital	Madison	94%	50
Wheaton Franciscan Saint Joseph	Milwaukee	90%	77
United Hospital System	Kenosha	89%	28

Statin Prescribed at Discharge

Hospital Name	City	Rate	Cases
Appleton Medical Center	Appleton	100%	275
Aurora Baycare Medical Center	Green Bay	100%	148
Aurora Medical Center	Summit	100%	39
Aurora Medical Center Oshkosh	Oshkosh	100%	55
Aurora Saint Lukes Medical Center	Milwaukee	100%	884
Bellin Memorial Hospital[2]	Green Bay	100%	360
Community Memorial Hospital	Menomonee Fls	100%	106
Froedtert Memorial Lutheran Hospital	Milwaukee	100%	212
Gundersen Lutheran Medical Center	La Crosse	100%	321
Madison VA Medical Center	Madison	100%	57
Mayo Clinic Hlth Sys-Eau Claire Hosp	Eau Claire	100%	217
Mercy Medical Center of Oshkosh	Oshkosh	100%	77
Milwaukee VA Medical Center	Milwaukee	100%	62
Ministry Saint Josephs Hospital	Marshfield	100%	332
Saint Agnes Hospital	Fond Du Lac	100%	219
Saint Clares Hospital of Weston	Weston	100%	246
Saint Elizabeth Hospital	Appleton	100%	122
Saint Marys Hospital	Madison	100%	487
Saint Marys Hospital Medical Center	Green Bay	100%	114
Theda Clark Medical Center	Neenah	100%	50
Aspirus Wausau Hospital[2]	Wausau	99%	253
Aurora Medical Center	Grafton	99%	176
Columbia Saint Marys Hospital Milwaukee	Milwaukee	99%	138
Mayo Clinic Hlth Sys Franciscan Med Ctr	La Crosse	99%	109
United Hospital System	Kenosha	99%	109
Univ of WI Hosps & Clinics Authority[2]	Madison	99%	271
Wheaton Franciscan Healthcare All Saints	Racine	99%	171
Wheaton Franciscan Saint Joseph	Milwaukee	99%	303
Holy Family Memorial	Manitowoc	98%	62
Sacred Heart Hospital[2]	Eau Claire	98%	266
Waukesha Memorial Hospital[2]	Waukesha	98%	233
Aurora Sheboygan Memorial Medical Center	Sheboygan	97%	32
Columbia Saint Marys Hospital Ozaukee	Mequon	97%	119
Mercy Health System Corp	Janesville	97%	155
Meriter Hospital	Madison	97%	315
The Monroe Clinic	Monroe	97%	30
Wheaton Franciscan Hlthcare St Francis	Milwaukee	97%	124
Oconomowoc Memorial Hospital	Oconomowoc	96%	50
Saint Vincent Hospital	Green Bay	96%	184
Bay Area Medical Center	Marinette	95%	85
Beloit Memorial Hospital	Beloit	93%	91
Aurora West Allis Medical Center	West Allis	89%	27

Heart Failure Care

ACE Inhibitor or ARB for LVSD

Hospital Name	City	Rate	Cases
Aurora Medical Center	Grafton	100%	26
Aurora Medical Center Kenosha	Kenosha	100%	33
Aurora Saint Lukes Medical Center	Milwaukee	100%	457
Aurora Sheboygan Memorial Medical Center	Sheboygan	100%	29
Community Memorial Hospital	Menomonee Fls	100%	53
Froedtert Memorial Lutheran Hospital[2]	Milwaukee	100%	112
Mayo Clinic Hlth Sys Franciscan Med Ctr	La Crosse	100%	39
Mayo Clinic Hlth Sys-Eau Claire Hosp	Eau Claire	100%	50
Mercy Health System Corp	Janesville	100%	34
Mercy Medical Center of Oshkosh	Oshkosh	100%	31
Ministry Saint Josephs Hospital	Marshfield	100%	71
Ministry St Michaels Hosp-Stevens Pt	Stevens Point	100%	26
Saint Agnes Hospital	Fond Du Lac	100%	43
Wheaton Franciscan Healthcare All Saints	Racine	100%	72
Wheaton Franciscan Hlthcare St Francis	Milwaukee	100%	64
Columbia Saint Marys Hospital Milwaukee	Milwaukee	99%	100
Meriter Hospital	Madison	99%	71
United Hospital System	Kenosha	99%	106
Wheaton Franciscan Saint Joseph[2]	Milwaukee	99%	135
Bellin Memorial Hospital	Green Bay	98%	47
Columbia Saint Marys Hospital Ozaukee	Mequon	98%	55
Madison VA Medical Center	Madison	98%	50
Gundersen Lutheran Medical Center	La Crosse	97%	70
Milwaukee VA Medical Center	Milwaukee	97%	101
Aspirus Wausau Hospital[2]	Wausau	96%	56
Univ of WI Hosps & Clinics Authority[2]	Madison	96%	98
Appleton Medical Center	Appleton	95%	55
Saint Marys Hospital	Madison	95%	113
Waukesha Memorial Hospital[2]	Waukesha	94%	66
Saint Marys Hospital Medical Center	Green Bay	90%	31
Beloit Memorial Hospital	Beloit	89%	37
Saint Vincent Hospital	Green Bay	87%	30
Sacred Heart Hospital	Eau Claire	82%	44
Bay Area Medical Center	Marinette	81%	36

Discharge Instructions Given

Hospital Name	City	Rate	Cases
Aurora Medical Center Oshkosh	Oshkosh	100%	30
Aurora Sheboygan Memorial Medical Center	Sheboygan	100%	90
Flambeau Hospital	Park Falls	100%	28
Gundersen Lutheran Medical Center	La Crosse	100%	198
Howard Young Medical Center	Woodruff	100%	69
Lakeview Medical Center	Rice Lake	100%	34
Milwaukee VA Medical Center	Milwaukee	100%	257
Ministry Saint Marys Hospital	Rhinelander	100%	63
Saint Clare Hospital Health Services	Baraboo	100%	38
Saint Clares Hospital of Weston	Weston	100%	134
Saint Elizabeth Hospital	Appleton	100%	122
Tomah Memorial Hospital	Tomah	100%	29
Aurora Memorial Hospital Burlington	Burlington	99%	75
Community Memorial Hospital	Menomonee Fls	99%	170
Froedtert Memorial Lutheran Hospital[2]	Milwaukee	99%	274
Holy Family Memorial	Manitowoc	99%	81
Meriter Hospital	Madison	99%	251
Ministry Saint Josephs Hospital	Marshfield	99%	327
The Monroe Clinic	Monroe	99%	68
Saint Marys Hospital Medical Center	Green Bay	99%	77
Univ of WI Hosps & Clinics Authority[2]	Madison	99%	231
Wheaton Franciscan Saint Joseph[2]	Milwaukee	99%	358
Aspirus Wausau Hospital[2]	Wausau	98%	211
Aurora Baycare Medical Center	Green Bay	98%	50
Aurora Medical Center Washington County	Hartford	98%	59
Aurora Saint Lukes Medical Center	Milwaukee	98%	1166
Aurora West Allis Medical Center	West Allis	98%	95
Mayo Clinic Hlth Sys-Eau Claire Hosp	Eau Claire	98%	224
Mercy Health System Corp	Janesville	98%	129
Ministry St Michaels Hosp-Stevens Pt	Stevens Point	98%	101
Wheaton Franciscan Hlthcare St Francis	Milwaukee	98%	167
Appleton Medical Center	Appleton	97%	174
Aurora Medical Center	Grafton	97%	66
Columbia Saint Marys Hospital Milwaukee	Milwaukee	97%	242

NOTE: Hospital profiles are in alphabetical order by state, then city, then hospital within the city; Rankings exclude hospitals with less than 25 cases except for patient surveys which excludes hospitals with less than 100 cases; (a) 100-299 cases; (1) The number of cases/patients is too few to report; (2) Data submitted were based on a sample of cases/patients; (3) Results are based on a shorter time period than required; (4) Data suppressed by CMS for one or more quarters; (5) Results are not available for this reporting period; (6) Fewer than 100 patients completed the HCAHPS survey; (7) No cases met the criteria for this measure; (8) The lower limit of the confidence interval cannot be calculated if the number of observed infections equals zero; (9) No data are available from the state/territory for this reporting period; (10) The scores shown reflect fewer than 50 completed surveys; (11) There were discrepancies in the data collection process; (12) This measure does not apply to this hospital for this reporting period; (13) Results cannot be calculated for this reporting period; (14) The results for this state are combined with nearby states to protect confidentiality; Please refer to the User's Guide for a full explanation of data.

Columbia Saint Marys Hospital Ozaukee	Mequon	97%	125
Madison VA Medical Center	Madison	97%	159
Mercy Medical Center of Oshkosh	Oshkosh	97%	95
Oconomowoc Memorial Hospital	Oconomowoc	97%	61
Sacred Heart Hospital	Eau Claire	97%	119
Saint Croix Regional Medical Center	Saint Croix Falls	97%	35
Shawano Medical Center	Shawano	97%	35
Waukesha Memorial Hospital[2]	Waukesha	97%	221
Wheaton Franciscan Healthcare Franklin	Franklin	97%	36
Bellin Memorial Hospital	Green Bay	96%	157
Berlin Memorial Hospital	Berlin	96%	26
Mayo Clinic Health System - Red Cedar	Menomonie	96%	27
Saint Marys Hospital	Madison	96%	425
Southwest Health Center	Platteville	96%	25
Ministry Door County Medical Center	Sturgeon Bay	95%	59
Saint Vincent Hospital	Green Bay	95%	103
Langlade Hospital	Antigo	94%	34
Wheaton Franciscan Healthcare All Saints	Racine	94%	231
Aurora Lakeland Medical Center	Elkhorn	93%	30
Aurora Medical Center	Summit	93%	57
Bay Area Medical Center	Marinette	93%	134
Columbus Community Hospital	Columbus	93%	29
Aurora Medical Center Manitowoc County	Two Rivers	92%	39
Mayo Clinic Hlth Sys Franciscan Med Ctr	La Crosse	92%	98
Saint Agnes Hospital	Fond Du Lac	92%	158
Saint Nicholas Hospital	Sheboygan	92%	38
United Hospital System	Kenosha	92%	241
Beloit Memorial Hospital	Beloit	91%	115
St Joseph's Comm Hosp of West Bend	West Bend	91%	66
Saint Joseph's Hospital	Chippewa Falls	91%	32
Theda Clark Medical Center	Neenah	91%	75
Saint Marys Janesville Hospital	Janesville	90%	49
Beaver Dam Com Hospital	Beaver Dam	89%	46
Fort Memorial Hospital	Fort Atkinson	89%	54
Aurora Medical Center Kenosha	Kenosha	88%	81
Baldwin Area Medical Center	Baldwin	88%	25
Divine Savior Healthcare	Portage	88%	26
Mile Bluff Medical Center	Mauston	88%	26
Riverside Medical Center	Waupaca	82%	28
Memorial Medical Center	Ashland	81%	31
Reedsburg Area Medical Center	Reedsburg	75%	28
Riverview Hospital Assoc[2]	Wisc. Rapids	74%	54

Evaluation of LVS Function

Hospital Name	City	Rate	Cases
Aspirus Wausau Hospital[2]	Wausau	100%	261
Aurora Baycare Medical Center	Green Bay	100%	55
Aurora Lakeland Medical Center	Elkhorn	100%	44
Aurora Medical Center	Grafton	100%	103
Aurora Medical Center	Summit	100%	66
Aurora Medical Center Kenosha	Kenosha	100%	105
Aurora Medical Center Manitowoc County	Two Rivers	100%	51
Aurora Medical Center Oshkosh	Oshkosh	100%	39
Aurora Medical Center Washington County	Hartford	100%	83
Aurora Memorial Hospital Burlington	Burlington	100%	92
Aurora Saint Lukes Medical Center	Milwaukee	100%	1387
Aurora Sheboygan Memorial Medical Center	Sheboygan	100%	114
Aurora West Allis Medical Center	West Allis	100%	135
Bay Area Medical Center	Marinette	100%	174
Bellin Memorial Hospital	Green Bay	100%	195
Beloit Memorial Hospital	Beloit	100%	147
Columbia Saint Marys Hospital Milwaukee	Milwaukee	100%	299
Columbia Saint Marys Hospital Ozaukee	Mequon	100%	173
Columbus Community Hospital	Columbus	100%	36
Community Memorial Hospital	Menomonee Fls	100%	226
Fort Memorial Hospital	Fort Atkinson	100%	72
Froedtert Memorial Lutheran Hospital[2]	Milwaukee	100%	313
Gundersen Lutheran Medical Center	La Crosse	100%	240
Holy Family Memorial	Manitowoc	100%	104
Howard Young Medical Center	Woodruff	100%	90
Hudson Hospital	Hudson	100%	28
Lakeview Medical Center	Rice Lake	100%	52
Langlade Hospital	Antigo	100%	44
Madison VA Medical Center	Madison	100%	182
Mayo Clinic Hlth Sys Franciscan Med Ctr	La Crosse	100%	137
Mayo Clinic Hlth Sys-Eau Claire Hosp	Eau Claire	100%	317
Mayo Clinic Health System - Red Cedar	Menomonie	100%	39
Mercy Medical Center of Oshkosh	Oshkosh	100%	116
Meriter Hospital	Madison	100%	307
Milwaukee VA Medical Center	Milwaukee	100%	279
Ministry Saint Josephs Hospital	Marshfield	100%	410
Ministry Saint Marys Hospital	Rhinelander	100%	79
Ministry St Michaels Hosp-Stevens Pt	Stevens Point	100%	145
The Monroe Clinic	Monroe	100%	93
Oconomowoc Memorial Hospital	Oconomowoc	100%	95
Reedsburg Area Medical Center	Reedsburg	100%	38
Richland Hospital	Richland Center	100%	35
Saint Agnes Hospital	Fond Du Lac	100%	219
Saint Clare Hospital Health Services	Baraboo	100%	58
Saint Clares Hospital of Weston	Weston	100%	163
Saint Croix Regional Medical Center	Saint Croix Falls	100%	42
Saint Elizabeth Hospital	Appleton	100%	154
St Joseph's Comm Hosp of West Bend	West Bend	100%	85
Saint Joseph's Hospital	Chippewa Falls	100%	53
Saint Marys Hospital	Madison	100%	514
Saint Marys Hospital Medical Center	Green Bay	100%	94
Saint Marys Janesville Hospital	Janesville	100%	77
Tomah Memorial Hospital	Tomah	100%	33
United Hospital System	Kenosha	100%	313
Univ of WI Hosps & Clinics Authority[2]	Madison	100%	269
UW Hlth Partners Watertown Reg Med Ctr	Watertown	100%	29
Waukesha Memorial Hospital[2]	Waukesha	100%	291
Wheaton Franciscan Healthcare All Saints	Racine	100%	291
Wheaton Franciscan Healthcare Franklin	Franklin	100%	56
Wheaton Franciscan Saint Joseph[2]	Milwaukee	100%	410
Appleton Medical Center	Appleton	99%	206
Sacred Heart Hospital	Eau Claire	99%	178
Theda Clark Medical Center	Neenah	99%	99
Beaver Dam Com Hospital	Beaver Dam	98%	52
Saint Vincent Hospital	Green Bay	98%	124
Wheaton Franciscan Hlthcare St Francis	Milwaukee	98%	213
Black River Memorial Hospital	Black River Falls	97%	33
Mercy Health System Corp	Janesville	97%	155
Ministry Door County Medical Center	Sturgeon Bay	97%	66
Community Memorial Hospital	Oconto Falls	96%	25
Riverview Hospital Assoc[2]	Wisc. Rapids	96%	93
Shawano Medical Center	Shawano	96%	51
Hayward Area Memorial Hospital	Hayward	94%	33
Divine Savior Healthcare	Portage	92%	36
Southwest Health Center	Platteville	92%	39
Berlin Memorial Hospital	Berlin	90%	39
Riverside Medical Center	Waupaca	90%	42
Mile Bluff Medical Center	Mauston	89%	35
Memorial Medical Center	Ashland	88%	40
Saint Nicholas Hospital	Sheboygan	88%	64
Flambeau Hospital	Park Falls	87%	38
Prairie Du Chien Memorial Hospital	Prairie Du Chien	87%	31
New London Family Medical Center	New London	86%	36
Baldwin Area Medical Center	Baldwin	84%	37

Medicare Spending

Medicare Spending per Patient (ratio)

Hospital Name	City	Ratio	Cases
Riverview Hospital Assoc	Wisc. Rapids	0.82	-
Mile Bluff Medical Center	Mauston	0.84	-
Sauk Prairie Hospital	Prairie Du Sac	0.84	-
Howard Young Medical Center	Woodruff	0.85	-
Ministry St Michaels Hosp-Stevens Pt	Stevens Point	0.85	-
Saint Joseph's Hospital	Chippewa Falls	0.85	-
Lakeview Medical Center	Rice Lake	0.86	-
Orthopaedic Hospital of Wisconsin	Glendale	0.86	-
Fort Memorial Hospital	Fort Atkinson	0.87	-
Ministry Saint Marys Hospital	Rhinelander	0.87	-
Oak Leaf Surgical Hospital	Eau Claire	0.88	-
Gundersen Lutheran Medical Center	La Crosse	0.89	-
Saint Marys Hospital Medical Center	Green Bay	0.89	-
Aurora Sheboygan Memorial Medical Center	Sheboygan	0.90	-
Divine Savior Healthcare	Portage	0.90	-
Mayo Clinic Hlth Sys Franciscan Med Ctr	La Crosse	0.90	-
Mercy Medical Center of Oshkosh	Oshkosh	0.90	-
Saint Clares Hospital of Weston	Weston	0.90	-
Beaver Dam Com Hospital	Beaver Dam	0.91	-
Mercy Health System Corp	Janesville	0.91	-
Saint Vincent Hospital	Green Bay	0.92	-
Aspirus Wausau Hospital	Wausau	0.93	-
Aurora Memorial Hospital Burlington	Burlington	0.93	-
Meriter Hospital	Madison	0.93	-
Midwest Orthopedic Specialty Hospital	Franklin	0.93	-
Saint Elizabeth Hospital	Appleton	0.93	-
Bay Area Medical Center	Marinette	0.94	-
Holy Family Memorial	Manitowoc	0.94	-
Ministry Saint Josephs Hospital	Marshfield	0.94	-
Saint Agnes Hospital	Fond Du Lac	0.94	-
Theda Clark Medical Center	Neenah	0.94	-
Wheaton Franciscan Saint Joseph	Milwaukee	0.94	-
Appleton Medical Center	Appleton	0.95	-
Aurora Medical Center	Grafton	0.95	-
Columbia Saint Marys Hospital Milwaukee	Milwaukee	0.95	-
Froedtert Memorial Lutheran Hospital	Milwaukee	0.95	-
The Monroe Clinic	Monroe	0.95	-
Oconomowoc Memorial Hospital	Oconomowoc	0.95	-
Saint Marys Hospital	Madison	0.95	-
Saint Nicholas Hospital	Sheboygan	0.95	-
Univ of WI Hosps & Clinics Authority	Madison	0.95	-
Aurora Baycare Medical Center	Green Bay	0.96	-
Bellin Memorial Hospital	Green Bay	0.96	-
Sacred Heart Hospital	Eau Claire	0.96	-
St Joseph's Comm Hosp of West Bend	West Bend	0.96	-
UW Hlth Partners Watertown Reg Med Ctr	Watertown	0.96	-
Wheaton Franciscan Healthcare All Saints	Racine	0.96	-
Wheaton Franciscan Hlthcare St Francis	Milwaukee	0.96	-
Aurora Medical Center	Summit	0.97	-
Aurora Medical Center Oshkosh	Oshkosh	0.97	-
Saint Clare Hospital Health Services	Baraboo	0.97	-
Waukesha Memorial Hospital	Waukesha	0.97	-
Aurora Medical Center Manitowoc County	Two Rivers	0.98	-
Aurora Medical Center Washington County	Hartford	0.98	-
Columbia Saint Marys Hospital Ozaukee	Mequon	0.98	-
Mayo Clinic Hlth Sys-Eau Claire Hosp	Eau Claire	0.98	-
Aurora Saint Lukes Medical Center	Milwaukee	0.99	-
Beloit Memorial Hospital	Beloit	0.99	-
Aurora Lakeland Medical Center	Elkhorn	1.00	-
Aurora West Allis Medical Center	West Allis	1.00	-
Community Memorial Hospital	Menomonee Fls	1.00	-
Wheaton Franciscan Healthcare Franklin	Franklin	1.00	-
Saint Marys Janesville Hospital	Janesville	1.01	-
Aurora Medical Center Kenosha	Kenosha	1.03	-
United Hospital System	Kenosha	1.03	-

Pneumonia Care

Appropriate Initial Antibiotic Given

Hospital Name	City	Rate	Cases
Aurora Baycare Medical Center	Green Bay	100%	53
Aurora Medical Center Washington County	Hartford	100%	38
Aurora West Allis Medical Center	West Allis	100%	185
Black River Memorial Hospital	Black River Falls	100%	45
Holy Family Memorial	Manitowoc	100%	46
Hudson Hospital	Hudson	100%	26
Lakeview Medical Center	Rice Lake	100%	32
Mayo Clinic Hlth Sys Franciscan Med Ctr	La Crosse	100%	91
Mayo Clinic Health System - Northland	Barron	100%	25
Mayo Clinic Health System - Red Cedar	Menomonie	100%	32
Memorial Medical Center	Ashland	100%	54
Mercy Walworth Hospital & Medical Center	Lake Geneva	100%	30
Ministry Sacred Heart Hospital	Tomahawk	100%	27
Ministry Saint Marys Hospital	Rhinelander	100%	62
Ministry St Michaels Hosp-Stevens Pt	Stevens Point	100%	48
Saint Clare Hospital Health Services	Baraboo	100%	64
Saint Clares Hospital of Weston	Weston	100%	36
Saint Joseph's Hospital	Chippewa Falls	100%	30
United Hospital System	Kenosha	100%	154
Waupun Memorial Hospital	Waupun	100%	44
Wheaton Franciscan Healthcare All Saints[2]	Racine	100%	64
Aurora Lakeland Medical Center	Elkhorn	99%	80
Aurora Memorial Hospital Burlington	Burlington	99%	80
Mercy Health System Corp	Janesville	99%	82
Saint Elizabeth Hospital	Appleton	99%	90
St Joseph's Comm Hosp of West Bend	West Bend	99%	101
Saint Marys Hospital	Madison	99%	139
Shawano Medical Center	Shawano	99%	82
Aspirus Wausau Hospital[2]	Wausau	98%	64
Aurora Medical Center	Grafton	98%	61
Aurora Medical Center Kenosha	Kenosha	98%	123
Aurora Saint Lukes Medical Center	Milwaukee	98%	540
Aurora Sheboygan Memorial Medical Center	Sheboygan	98%	63
Columbia Saint Marys Hospital Milwaukee	Milwaukee	98%	183
Langlade Hospital	Antigo	98%	51
New London Family Medical Center	New London	98%	50
Reedsburg Area Medical Center	Reedsburg	98%	54
Theda Clark Medical Center	Neenah	98%	47
UW Hlth Partners Watertown Reg Med Ctr	Watertown	98%	52
Wheaton Franciscan Hlthcare St Francis[2]	Milwaukee	98%	103
Wheaton Franciscan Saint Joseph[2]	Milwaukee	98%	129
Aurora Medical Center Oshkosh	Oshkosh	97%	39
Community Memorial Hospital	Menomonee Fls	97%	114
Hayward Area Memorial Hospital	Hayward	97%	34
Mayo Clinic Hlth Sys-Eau Claire Hosp	Eau Claire	97%	119
Mercy Medical Center of Oshkosh	Oshkosh	97%	70
Oconomowoc Memorial Hospital	Oconomowoc	97%	69
Saint Nicholas Hospital	Sheboygan	97%	64
Univ of WI Hosps & Clinics Authority[2]	Madison	97%	37
Wheaton Franciscan Healthcare Franklin	Franklin	97%	68
Froedtert Memorial Lutheran Hospital[2]	Milwaukee	96%	72
Sacred Heart Hospital[2]	Eau Claire	96%	115
Southwest Health Center	Platteville	96%	26
Waukesha Memorial Hospital[2]	Waukesha	96%	99
Aurora Medical Center	Summit	95%	37
Divine Savior Healthcare	Portage	95%	58
Gundersen Lutheran Medical Center	La Crosse	95%	106
Howard Young Medical Center	Woodruff	95%	77
Meriter Hospital	Madison	95%	136
Ministry Saint Josephs Hospital	Marshfield	95%	82
Saint Agnes Hospital	Fond Du Lac	95%	127
Saint Marys Hospital Medical Center	Green Bay	95%	77
Saint Marys Janesville Hospital	Janesville	95%	56
Vernon Memorial Hospital	Viroqua	95%	65
Aurora Medical Center Manitowoc County	Two Rivers	94%	54
Beloit Memorial Hospital	Beloit	94%	35
Columbia Saint Marys Hospital Ozaukee	Mequon	94%	110

NOTE: Hospital profiles are in alphabetical order by state, then city, then hospital within the city; Rankings exclude hospitals with less than 25 cases except for patient surveys which excludes hospitals with less than 100 cases; (a) 100-299 cases; (1) The number of cases/patients is too few to report; (2) Data submitted were based on a sample of cases/patients; (3) Results are based on a shorter time period than required; (4) Data suppressed by CMS for one or more quarters; (5) Results are not available for this reporting period; (6) Fewer than 100 patients completed the HCAHPS survey; (7) No cases met the criteria for this measure; (8) The lower limit of the confidence interval cannot be calculated if the number of observed infections equals zero; (9) No data are available from the state/territory for this reporting period; (10) The scores shown reflect fewer than 50 completed surveys; (11) There were discrepancies in the data collection process; (12) This measure does not apply to this hospital for this reporting period; (13) Results cannot be calculated for this reporting period; (14) The results for this state are combined with nearby states to protect confidentiality; Please refer to the User's Guide for a full explanation of data.

The Monroe Clinic	Monroe	94%	87
Saint Vincent Hospital[2]	Green Bay	94%	80
Appleton Medical Center	Appleton	93%	127
Fort Memorial Hospital	Fort Atkinson	93%	55
Good Samaritan Health Center	Merrill	93%	30
Milwaukee VA Medical Center	Milwaukee	93%	43
Ministry Door County Medical Center	Sturgeon Bay	93%	43
Riverview Hospital Assoc[2]	Wisc. Rapids	93%	72
Tomah Memorial Hospital	Tomah	92%	50
Bay Area Medical Center	Marinette	91%	68
Beaver Dam Com Hospital	Beaver Dam	91%	53
Berlin Memorial Hospital	Berlin	88%	26
Spooner Health System	Spooner	88%	33
Wild Rose Com Memorial Hospital	Wild Rose	88%	25
Columbus Community Hospital	Columbus	87%	30
Bellin Memorial Hospital	Green Bay	85%	48
Riverside Medical Center	Waupaca	85%	34
Cumberland Memorial Hospital	Cumberland	84%	25

Blood Culture Timing

Hospital Name	City	Rate	Cases
Aurora Baycare Medical Center	Green Bay	100%	72
Aurora Lakeland Medical Center	Elkhorn	100%	124
Aurora Medical Center	Grafton	100%	103
Aurora Medical Center	Summit	100%	43
Aurora Medical Center Kenosha	Kenosha	100%	168
Aurora Medical Center Manitowoc County	Two Rivers	100%	53
Aurora Medical Center Oshkosh	Oshkosh	100%	71
Aurora Sheboygan Memorial Medical Center	Sheboygan	100%	82
Aurora West Allis Medical Center	West Allis	100%	207
Beloit Memorial Hospital	Beloit	100%	67
Berlin Memorial Hospital	Berlin	100%	54
Community Memorial Hospital	Menomonee Fls	100%	202
Holy Family Memorial	Manitowoc	100%	85
Lakeview Medical Center	Rice Lake	100%	61
Langlade Hospital	Antigo	100%	73
Mayo Clinic Health System - Northland	Barron	100%	40
Memorial Health Center	Medford	100%	31
Mercy Medical Center of Oshkosh	Oshkosh	100%	100
Ministry Door County Medical Center	Sturgeon Bay	100%	53
Ministry Sacred Heart Hospital	Tomahawk	100%	28
Ministry Saint Josephs Hospital	Marshfield	100%	87
Ministry Saint Marys Hospital	Rhinelander	100%	97
Ministry St Michaels Hosp-Stevens Pt	Stevens Point	100%	149
Oconomowoc Memorial Hospital	Oconomowoc	100%	97
Saint Clare Hospital Health Services	Baraboo	100%	96
Saint Clares Hospital of Weston	Weston	100%	67
Saint Croix Regional Medical Center	Saint Croix Falls	100%	31
Southwest Health Center	Platteville	100%	31
Stoughton Hospital	Stoughton	100%	28
Univ of WI Hosps & Clinics Authority[2]	Madison	100%	72
Waukesha Memorial Hospital[2]	Waukesha	100%	156
Waupun Memorial Hospital	Waupun	100%	53
Wild Rose Com Memorial Hospital	Wild Rose	100%	26
Appleton Medical Center	Appleton	99%	147
Aurora Memorial Hospital Burlington	Burlington	99%	170
Aurora Saint Lukes Medical Center	Milwaukee	99%	1046
Froedtert Memorial Lutheran Hospital[2]	Milwaukee	99%	170
Gundersen Lutheran Medical Center	La Crosse	99%	191
Madison VA Medical Center	Madison	99%	67
Mayo Clinic Hlth Sys-Eau Claire Hosp	Eau Claire	99%	178
Meriter Hospital	Madison	99%	174
Saint Elizabeth Hospital	Appleton	99%	118
Saint Joseph's Hospital	Chippewa Falls	99%	70
Saint Marys Hospital Medical Center	Green Bay	99%	118
Saint Nicholas Hospital	Sheboygan	99%	85
Shawano Medical Center	Shawano	99%	96
UW Hlth Partners Watertown Reg Med Ctr	Watertown	99%	91
Vernon Memorial Hospital	Viroqua	99%	70
Wheaton Franciscan Healthcare All Saints[2]	Racine	99%	187
Wheaton Franciscan Healthcare Franklin	Franklin	99%	136
Wheaton Franciscan Hlthcare St Francis[2]	Milwaukee	99%	205
Wheaton Franciscan Saint Joseph[2]	Milwaukee	99%	227
Bellin Memorial Hospital	Green Bay	98%	88
Columbia Saint Marys Hospital Milwaukee	Milwaukee	98%	267
Columbia Saint Marys Hospital Ozaukee	Mequon	98%	139
Divine Savior Healthcare	Portage	98%	58
Fort Memorial Hospital	Fort Atkinson	98%	88
Good Samaritan Health Center	Merrill	98%	47
Mercy Health System Corp	Janesville	98%	147
Mercy Walworth Hospital & Medical Center	Lake Geneva	98%	43
Reedsburg Area Medical Center	Reedsburg	98%	60
Saint Agnes Hospital	Fond Du Lac	98%	251
St Joseph's Comm Hosp of West Bend	West Bend	98%	169
Saint Vincent Hospital[2]	Green Bay	98%	130
Tomah Memorial Hospital	Tomah	98%	50
Aurora Medical Center Washington County	Hartford	97%	60
Milwaukee VA Medical Center	Milwaukee	97%	70
Prairie Du Chien Memorial Hospital	Prairie Du Chien	97%	39
Riverview Hospital Assoc[2]	Wisc. Rapids	97%	91
Sacred Heart Hospital[2]	Eau Claire	97%	144

Saint Marys Janesville Hospital	Janesville	97%	74
Spooner Health System	Spooner	97%	31
Bay Area Medical Center	Marinette	96%	101
Howard Young Medical Center	Woodruff	96%	99
Mayo Clinic Hlth Sys Franciscan Med Ctr	La Crosse	96%	136
The Monroe Clinic	Monroe	96%	158
Ripon Medical Center	Ripon	96%	26
Saint Marys Hospital	Madison	96%	269
United Hospital System	Kenosha	96%	308
Aspirus Wausau Hospital[2]	Wausau	95%	125
Beaver Dam Com Hospital	Beaver Dam	95%	77
Columbus Community Hospital	Columbus	95%	39
Mayo Clinic Health System - Red Cedar	Menomonie	95%	39
New London Family Medical Center	New London	95%	37
Riverside Medical Center	Waupaca	94%	53
Tri County Memorial Hospital	Whitehall	94%	32
Westfields Hospital	New Richmond	93%	28
Black River Memorial Hospital	Black River Falls	92%	38
Memorial Medical Center	Ashland	92%	66
Theda Clark Medical Center	Neenah	92%	49
Hayward Area Memorial Hospital	Hayward	84%	45

Pregnancy and Delivery Care

Newborns whose Deliveries were Scheduled Early

Hospital Name	City	Rate	Cases
Aurora Medical Center	Summit	0%	32
Aurora Medical Center Manitowoc County[2]	Two Rivers	0%	35
Aurora Medical Center Oshkosh	Oshkosh	0%	45
Bay Area Medical Center	Marinette	0%	28
Fort Memorial Hospital[2]	Fort Atkinson	0%	53
Gundersen Lutheran Medical Center	La Crosse	0%	99
Mayo Clinic Hlth Sys Franciscan Med Ctr	La Crosse	0%	36
Mayo Clinic Hlth Sys-Eau Claire Hosp[2]	Eau Claire	0%	28
Mercy Health System Corp	Janesville	0%	107
Mercy Walworth Hospital & Medical Center	Lake Geneva	0%	26
Meriter Hospital[2]	Madison	0%	52
Oconomowoc Memorial Hospital[2]	Oconomowoc	0%	44
Saint Nicholas Hospital[2]	Sheboygan	0%	25
Saint Vincent Hospital[2]	Green Bay	0%	30
United Hospital System[2]	Kenosha	0%	36
Waukesha Memorial Hospital[2]	Waukesha	0%	204
Aurora Baycare Medical Center	Green Bay	1%	156
Columbia Saint Marys Hospital Milwaukee	Milwaukee	1%	254
Aurora Saint Lukes Medical Center	Milwaukee	2%	181
Aurora West Allis Medical Center	West Allis	2%	294
Beloit Memorial Hospital	Beloit	2%	80
Ministry Saint Marys Hospital	Rhinelander	2%	48
Wheaton Franciscan Hlthcare St Francis[2]	Milwaukee	2%	92
Wheaton Franciscan Saint Joseph	Milwaukee	2%	334
The Monroe Clinic	Monroe	3%	38
Saint Marys Hospital Medical Center[2]	Green Bay	3%	31
Wheaton Franciscan Healthcare All Saints	Racine	3%	157
Aurora Medical Center	Grafton	4%	116
Lakeview Medical Center	Rice Lake	4%	55
Riverview Hospital Assoc	Wisc. Rapids	4%	47
Sacred Heart Hospital[2]	Eau Claire	4%	26
Saint Marys Hospital[2]	Madison	4%	53
Appleton Medical Center	Appleton	5%	111
Froedtert Memorial Lutheran Hospital	Milwaukee	5%	108
Saint Agnes Hospital	Fond Du Lac	5%	101
UW Hlth Partners Watertown Reg Med Ctr[2]	Watertown	5%	40
Aurora Medical Center Kenosha	Kenosha	6%	101
Aurora Sheboygan Memorial Medical Center	Sheboygan	6%	79
Community Memorial Hospital	Menomonee Fls	6%	108
Ministry Saint Josephs Hospital	Marshfield	6%	77
Bellin Memorial Hospital[2]	Green Bay	8%	108
Saint Elizabeth Hospital	Appleton	8%	97
Saint Clares Hospital of Weston[2]	Weston	9%	81
Theda Clark Medical Center	Neenah	9%	108
Aspirus Wausau Hospital	Wausau	10%	122
Aurora Lakeland Medical Center	Elkhorn	10%	50
Ministry St Michaels Hosp-Stevens Pt	Stevens Point	12%	41
Saint Marys Janesville Hospital	Janesville	12%	50
Grant Regional Health Center	Lancaster	17%	30
Mercy Medical Center of Oshkosh	Oshkosh	17%	77
St Joseph's Comm Hosp of West Bend[2]	West Bend	17%	29
Mile Bluff Medical Center	Mauston	43%	49

Preventive Care

Immunization for Influenza

Hospital Name	City	Rate	Cases
Ministry Eagle River Memorial Hospital	Eagle River	100%	189
Tomah Memorial Hospital[3]	Tomah	100%	221
Flambeau Hospital	Park Falls	99%	262
Ministry Sacred Heart Hospital[2]	Tomahawk	99%	151
Sauk Prairie Hospital[2]	Prairie Du Sac	99%	276
Stoughton Hospital[2]	Stoughton	99%	273
United Hospital System[2]	Kenosha	99%	578
Aurora Lakeland Medical Center[2]	Elkhorn	98%	291
Aurora Medical Center Manitowoc County[2]	Two Rivers	98%	248
Midwest Orthopedic Specialty Hospital[2]	Franklin	98%	320
Ministry Door County Medical Center[2]	Sturgeon Bay	98%	266
Sacred Heart Hospital[2]	Eau Claire	98%	545
Saint Clare Hospital Health Services[2]	Baraboo	98%	263
Saint Marys Hospital[2]	Madison	98%	522
Aurora Sheboygan Memorial Medical Center[2]	Sheboygan	97%	498
Aurora West Allis Medical Center[2]	West Allis	97%	416
Community Memorial Hospital	Oconto Falls	97%	72
Howard Young Medical Center[2]	Woodruff	97%	292
Mercy Health System Corp[2]	Janesville	97%	620
Mercy Walworth Hospital & Medical Center	Lake Geneva	97%	564
Ministry Saint Josephs Hospital[2]	Marshfield	97%	1091
Ministry Saint Marys Hospital[2]	Rhinelander	97%	278
Ministry St Michaels Hosp-Stevens Pt[2]	Stevens Point	97%	468
Our Lady of Victory Hospital	Stanley	97%	122
Saint Elizabeth Hospital[2]	Appleton	97%	557
Saint Marys Janesville Hospital[2]	Janesville	97%	304
Univ of WI Hosps & Clinics Authority[2]	Madison	97%	583
Aurora Medical Center[2]	Grafton	96%	545
Aurora Memorial Hospital Burlington[2]	Burlington	96%	271
Beloit Memorial Hospital[2]	Beloit	96%	366
Grant Regional Health Center	Lancaster	96%	289
Mercy Medical Center of Oshkosh[2]	Oshkosh	96%	532
Oak Leaf Surgical Hospital	Eau Claire	96%	259
Saint Agnes Hospital[2]	Fond Du Lac	96%	677
Vernon Memorial Hospital[2]	Viroqua	96%	507
Hayward Area Memorial Hospital[2]	Hayward	95%	242
Mayo Clinic Hlth Sys Franciscan Med Ctr[2]	La Crosse	95%	550
Mile Bluff Medical Center	Mauston	95%	609
Oconomowoc Memorial Hospital[2]	Oconomowoc	95%	295
River Falls Area Hospital[2]	River Falls	95%	251
Saint Clares Hospital of Weston[2]	Weston	95%	515
Tomah VA Medical Center[2,3]	Tomah	95%	147
Wheaton Franciscan Healthcare Franklin[2]	Franklin	95%	310
Appleton Medical Center[2]	Appleton	94%	555
Aurora Medical Center Washington County[2]	Hartford	94%	293
Fort Memorial Hospital[2]	Fort Atkinson	94%	256
Holy Family Memorial[2]	Manitowoc	94%	296
Columbia Saint Marys Hospital Ozaukee[2]	Mequon	93%	429
Saint Marys Hospital Superior[2]	Superior	93%	137
Lakeview Medical Center[2]	Rice Lake	92%	253
Wheaton Franciscan Hlthcare St Francis[2]	Milwaukee	92%	613
Aurora Baycare Medical Center[2]	Green Bay	91%	495
Bellin Memorial Hospital[2]	Green Bay	91%	584
UW Hlth Partners Watertown Reg Med Ctr[2]	Watertown	91%	255
Wheaton Franciscan Saint Joseph[2]	Milwaukee	91%	610
Saint Marys Hospital Medical Center[2]	Green Bay	90%	524
Aurora Saint Lukes Medical Center[2]	Milwaukee	89%	1581
Beaver Dam Com Hospital[2]	Beaver Dam	89%	271
Mayo Clinic Hlth Sys-Eau Claire Hosp[2]	Eau Claire	89%	555
Memorial Health Center	Medford	89%	232
Memorial Hospital Lafayette Cty	Darlington	89%	168
Reedsburg Area Medical Center	Reedsburg	89%	681
Riverview Hospital Assoc[2]	Wisc. Rapids	88%	292
St Joseph's Comm Hosp of West Bend[2]	West Bend	88%	360
Saint Vincent Hospital[2]	Green Bay	88%	549
Waukesha Memorial Hospital[2]	Waukesha	88%	544
Aurora Medical Center[2]	Summit	87%	306
Froedtert Memorial Lutheran Hospital[2]	Milwaukee	87%	572
Theda Clark Medical Center[2]	Neenah	87%	520
Aurora Medical Center Oshkosh[2]	Oshkosh	86%	286
Bay Area Medical Center[2]	Marinette	85%	378
Berlin Memorial Hospital	Berlin	85%	153
Community Memorial Hospital[2]	Menomonee Fls	85%	559
Good Samaritan Health Center[2]	Merrill	85%	275
Prairie Du Chien Memorial Hospital	Prairie Du Chien	85%	418
Wheaton Franciscan Healthcare All Saints[2]	Racine	85%	518
Saint Nicholas Hospital[2]	Sheboygan	84%	303
Divine Savior Healthcare	Portage	83%	874
Meriter Hospital[2]	Madison	83%	637
Aurora Medical Center Kenosha[2]	Kenosha	82%	473
Memorial Medical Center	Neillsville	82%	112
Columbia Saint Marys Hospital Milwaukee[2]	Milwaukee	81%	552
Saint Joseph's Hospital[2]	Chippewa Falls	79%	320
Moundview Memorial Hospital & Clinics	Friendship	77%	60
The Monroe Clinic[2]	Monroe	74%	1363
Aspirus Wausau Hospital[2]	Wausau	71%	538
Saint Joseph's Health Services	Hillsboro	70%	113
Gundersen Lutheran Medical Center[2]	La Crosse	55%	580
Orthopaedic Hospital of Wisconsin[2]	Glendale	39%	318

Immunization for Pneumonia

Hospital Name	City	Rate	Cases
Flambeau Hospital	Park Falls	100%	442
Howard Young Medical Center[2]	Woodruff	100%	392
Saint Marys Hospital Superior[2]	Superior	100%	207
Tomah Memorial Hospital[3]	Tomah	100%	321
United Hospital System[2]	Kenosha	100%	721
Aurora Lakeland Medical Center[2]	Elkhorn	99%	338

NOTE: Hospital profiles are in alphabetical order by state, then city, then hospital within the city; Rankings exclude hospitals with less than 25 cases except for patient surveys which excludes hospitals with less than 100 cases; (a) 100-299 cases; (1) The number of cases/patients is too few to report; (2) Data submitted were based on a sample of cases/patients; (3) Results are based on a shorter time period than required; (4) Data suppressed by CMS for one or more quarters; (5) Results are not available for this reporting period; (6) Fewer than 100 patients completed the HCAHPS survey; (7) No cases met the criteria for this measure; (8) The lower limit of the confidence interval cannot be calculated if the number of observed infections equals zero; (9) No data are available from the state/territory for this reporting period; (10) The scores shown reflect fewer than 50 completed surveys; (11) There were discrepancies in the data collection process; (12) This measure does not apply to this hospital for this reporting period; (13) Results cannot be calculated for this reporting period; (14) The results for this state are combined with nearby states to protect confidentiality; Please refer to the User's Guide for a full explanation of data.

Aurora Memorial Hospital Burlington[2]	Burlington	99%	387
Ministry Eagle River Memorial Hospital	Eagle River	99%	305
Ministry Sacred Heart Hospital[2]	Tomahawk	99%	267
Saint Clare Hospital Health Services[2]	Baraboo	99%	323
Stoughton Hospital[2]	Stoughton	99%	424
Aurora Medical Center Manitowoc County[2]	Two Rivers	98%	296
Mercy Medical Center of Oshkosh[2]	Oshkosh	98%	554
Saint Elizabeth Hospital[2]	Appleton	98%	518
Tomah VA Medical Center[2,3]	Tomah	98%	250
Aurora Medical Center Washington County[2]	Hartford	97%	433
Aurora West Allis Medical Center[2]	West Allis	97%	455
Beloit Memorial Hospital[2]	Beloit	97%	458
Mercy Health System Corp[2]	Janesville	97%	695
Ministry Door County Medical Center[2]	Sturgeon Bay	97%	381
Ministry Saint Josephs Hospital[2]	Marshfield	97%	1333
Ministry St Michaels Hosp-Stevens Pt[2]	Stevens Point	97%	542
Oak Leaf Surgical Hospital[2]	Eau Claire	97%	255
Our Lady of Victory Hospital[2]	Stanley	97%	216
River Falls Area Hospital[2]	River Falls	97%	292
Saint Marys Hospital[2]	Madison	97%	615
Saint Marys Janesville Hospital[2]	Janesville	97%	395
Univ of WI Hosps & Clinics Authority[2]	Madison	97%	588
Aurora Medical Center[2]	Grafton	96%	699
Aurora Sheboygan Memorial Medical Center[2]	Sheboygan	96%	487
Mayo Clinic Hlth Sys Franciscan Med Ctr[2]	La Crosse	96%	567
Memorial Hospital Lafayette Cty	Darlington	96%	237
Mercy Walworth Hospital & Medical Center	Lake Geneva	96%	661
Ministry Saint Marys Hospital[2]	Rhinelander	96%	405
Sauk Prairie Hospital[2]	Prairie Du Sac	96%	334
Bellin Memorial Hospital[2]	Green Bay	95%	722
Community Memorial Hospital	Oconto Falls	95%	114
Grant Regional Health Center	Lancaster	95%	330
Holy Family Memorial[2]	Manitowoc	95%	397
Oconomowoc Memorial Hospital[2]	Oconomowoc	95%	360
Prairie Du Chien Memorial Hospital	Prairie Du Chien	95%	572
Saint Clares Hospital of Weston[2]	Weston	95%	626
UW Hlth Partners Watertown Reg Med Ctr[2]	Watertown	95%	335
Vernon Memorial Hospital[2]	Viroqua	95%	718
Aurora Saint Lukes Medical Center[2]	Milwaukee	94%	2029
Community Memorial Hospital[2]	Menomonee Fls	94%	760
Saint Agnes Hospital[2]	Fond Du Lac	94%	758
Aurora Medical Center Kenosha[2]	Kenosha	93%	556
Beaver Dam Com Hospital[2]	Beaver Dam	93%	325
Columbia Saint Marys Hospital Ozaukee[2]	Mequon	93%	680
Fort Memorial Hospital[2]	Fort Atkinson	93%	310
Saint Marys Hospital Medical Center[2]	Green Bay	93%	600
Aurora Medical Center Oshkosh[2]	Oshkosh	92%	349
Froedtert Memorial Lutheran Hospital[2]	Milwaukee	92%	624
Lakeview Medical Center[2]	Rice Lake	92%	319
Mayo Clinic Hlth Sys-Eau Claire Hosp[2]	Eau Claire	92%	702
Memorial Health Center	Medford	92%	335
Meriter Hospital[2]	Madison	92%	583
Mile Bluff Medical Center	Mauston	92%	712
Riverview Hospital Assoc[2]	Wisc. Rapids	92%	329
Sacred Heart Hospital[2]	Eau Claire	92%	667
Waukesha Memorial Hospital[2]	Waukesha	92%	685
Appleton Medical Center[2]	Appleton	91%	663
Aurora Medical Center[2]	Summit	91%	338
Reedsburg Area Medical Center	Reedsburg	91%	797
St Joseph's Comm Hosp of West Bend[2]	West Bend	91%	430
Wheaton Franciscan Hlthcare St Francis[2]	Milwaukee	91%	794
Aurora Baycare Medical Center[2]	Green Bay	90%	459
Bay Area Medical Center[2]	Marinette	90%	519
Bellin Health Oconto Hospital[3]	Oconto	90%	63
Hayward Area Memorial Hospital[2]	Hayward	90%	318
Wheaton Franciscan Saint Joseph[2]	Milwaukee	90%	720
Wheaton Franciscan Healthcare Franklin[2]	Franklin	89%	512
Berlin Memorial Hospital	Berlin	88%	232
Saint Vincent Hospital[2]	Green Bay	88%	633
Columbia Saint Marys Hospital Milwaukee[2]	Milwaukee	87%	539
Divine Savior Healthcare	Portage	87%	989
Good Samaritan Health Center[2]	Merrill	87%	443
Memorial Medical Center	Neillsville	87%	146
Wheaton Franciscan Healthcare All Saints[2]	Racine	86%	633
Aspirus Wausau Hospital[2]	Wausau	85%	693
Midwest Orthopedic Specialty Hospital[2]	Franklin	84%	395
Saint Nicholas Hospital[2]	Sheboygan	84%	397
The Monroe Clinic[2]	Monroe	83%	1481
Saint Joseph's Health Services	Hillsboro	83%	183
Theda Clark Medical Center[2]	Neenah	83%	526
Gundersen Lutheran Medical Center[2]	La Crosse	81%	642
Moundview Memorial Hospital & Clinics	Friendship	72%	92
Cumberland Memorial Hospital[3]	Cumberland	71%	75
Orthopaedic Hospital of Wisconsin[2]	Glendale	69%	429
Saint Joseph's Hospital[2]	Chippewa Falls	68%	265

Stroke Care

Anticoagulation Therapy for Atrial Fibrillation

Hospital Name	City	Rate	Cases
Ministry Saint Josephs Hospital	Marshfield	100%	42
Waukesha Memorial Hospital	Waukesha	100%	25
Aurora Saint Lukes Medical Center	Milwaukee	98%	42
Gundersen Lutheran Medical Center	La Crosse	92%	26
Saint Marys Hospital	Madison	86%	35

Antithrombotic Therapy Timing

Hospital Name	City	Rate	Cases
Appleton Medical Center	Appleton	100%	41
Aurora Baycare Medical Center	Green Bay	100%	52
Aurora Medical Center	Grafton	100%	78
Aurora Medical Center Kenosha	Kenosha	100%	36
Aurora Saint Lukes Medical Center	Milwaukee	100%	326
Aurora Sheboygan Memorial Medical Center	Sheboygan	100%	36
Aurora West Allis Medical Center	West Allis	100%	78
Bay Area Medical Center	Marinette	100%	30
Columbia Saint Marys Hospital Milwaukee	Milwaukee	100%	104
Community Memorial Hospital	Menomonee Fls	100%	66
Froedtert Memorial Lutheran Hospital[2]	Milwaukee	100%	92
Howard Young Medical Center	Woodruff	100%	33
Mercy Medical Center of Oshkosh	Oshkosh	100%	38
Ministry Saint Josephs Hospital	Marshfield	100%	128
Ministry St Michaels Hosp-Stevens Pt	Stevens Point	100%	46
Sacred Heart Hospital[2]	Eau Claire	100%	70
Saint Agnes Hospital	Fond Du Lac	100%	72
Saint Clare Hospital Health Services	Baraboo	100%	27
Saint Clares Hospital of Weston	Weston	100%	37
Saint Marys Hospital Medical Center	Green Bay	100%	38
Theda Clark Medical Center	Neenah	100%	130
United Hospital System	Kenosha	100%	79
Univ of WI Hosps & Clinics Authority[2]	Madison	100%	42
Waukesha Memorial Hospital	Waukesha	100%	110
Wheaton Franciscan Saint Joseph[2]	Milwaukee	100%	81
Gundersen Lutheran Medical Center	La Crosse	99%	113
Mayo Clinic Hlth Sys-Eau Claire Hosp	Eau Claire	99%	97
Saint Elizabeth Hospital	Appleton	99%	77
Wheaton Franciscan Healthcare All Saints[2]	Racine	99%	126
Wheaton Franciscan Hlthcare St Francis	Milwaukee	99%	69
Columbia Saint Marys Hospital Ozaukee	Mequon	98%	61
Mayo Clinic Hlth Sys Franciscan Med Ctr	La Crosse	98%	47
Mercy Health System Corp	Janesville	98%	59
Meriter Hospital	Madison	98%	87
Saint Vincent Hospital[2]	Green Bay	98%	55
Bellin Memorial Hospital	Green Bay	97%	68
Beloit Memorial Hospital	Beloit	97%	35
Holy Family Memorial	Manitowoc	97%	36
Saint Marys Hospital	Madison	97%	172
Aspirus Wausau Hospital[2]	Wausau	96%	52
St Joseph's Comm Hosp of West Bend	West Bend	96%	27
Saint Nicholas Hospital	Sheboygan	95%	57

Assessed for Rehabilitation

Hospital Name	City	Rate	Cases
Aurora Lakeland Medical Center	Elkhorn	100%	26
Aurora Medical Center	Summit	100%	32
Aurora Medical Center Kenosha	Kenosha	100%	38
Aurora Saint Lukes Medical Center	Milwaukee	100%	488
Aurora Sheboygan Memorial Medical Center	Sheboygan	100%	43
Aurora West Allis Medical Center	West Allis	100%	76
Beloit Memorial Hospital	Beloit	100%	33
Columbia Saint Marys Hospital Milwaukee	Milwaukee	100%	138
Community Memorial Hospital	Menomonee Fls	100%	86
Mayo Clinic Hlth Sys-Eau Claire Hosp	Eau Claire	100%	121
Mercy Health System Corp	Janesville	100%	88
Mercy Medical Center of Oshkosh	Oshkosh	100%	46
Meriter Hospital	Madison	100%	111
Ministry Saint Josephs Hospital	Marshfield	100%	215
Saint Clare Hospital Health Services	Baraboo	100%	28
Saint Clares Hospital of Weston	Weston	100%	38
Saint Elizabeth Hospital	Appleton	100%	85
St Joseph's Comm Hosp of West Bend	West Bend	100%	27
Saint Marys Hospital Medical Center	Green Bay	100%	50
Theda Clark Medical Center	Neenah	100%	190
Wheaton Franciscan Hlthcare St Francis	Milwaukee	100%	84
Aspirus Wausau Hospital[2]	Wausau	99%	72
Aurora Baycare Medical Center	Green Bay	99%	120
Aurora Medical Center	Grafton	99%	103
Columbia Saint Marys Hospital Ozaukee	Mequon	99%	78
Froedtert Memorial Lutheran Hospital[2]	Milwaukee	99%	144
Saint Agnes Hospital	Fond Du Lac	99%	108
United Hospital System	Kenosha	99%	77
Gundersen Lutheran Medical Center	La Crosse	98%	180
Oconomowoc Memorial Hospital	Oconomowoc	98%	42
Saint Marys Hospital	Madison	98%	227
Saint Nicholas Hospital	Sheboygan	98%	54
Wheaton Franciscan Saint Joseph[2]	Milwaukee	98%	105

Aurora Medical Center Oshkosh	Oshkosh	97%	33
Bellin Memorial Hospital	Green Bay	97%	93
Howard Young Medical Center	Woodruff	97%	35
Wheaton Franciscan Healthcare All Saints[2]	Racine	97%	139
Appleton Medical Center	Appleton	96%	45
Ministry St Michaels Hosp-Stevens Pt	Stevens Point	96%	47
Sacred Heart Hospital[2]	Eau Claire	96%	108
Waukesha Memorial Hospital	Waukesha	96%	160
Saint Vincent Hospital[2]	Green Bay	95%	84
Univ of WI Hosps & Clinics Authority[2]	Madison	94%	107
Bay Area Medical Center	Marinette	91%	33
Holy Family Memorial	Manitowoc	91%	35
Mayo Clinic Hlth Sys Franciscan Med Ctr	La Crosse	91%	65

Discharged on Antithrombotic Therapy

Hospital Name	City	Rate	Cases
Appleton Medical Center	Appleton	100%	43
Aspirus Wausau Hospital[2]	Wausau	100%	63
Aurora Medical Center	Summit	100%	30
Aurora Medical Center Kenosha	Kenosha	100%	36
Aurora Medical Center Oshkosh	Oshkosh	100%	31
Aurora Saint Lukes Medical Center	Milwaukee	100%	373
Bay Area Medical Center	Marinette	100%	31
Columbia Saint Marys Hospital Ozaukee	Mequon	100%	72
Community Memorial Hospital	Menomonee Fls	100%	75
Gundersen Lutheran Medical Center	La Crosse	100%	152
Howard Young Medical Center	Woodruff	100%	35
Mayo Clinic Hlth Sys Franciscan Med Ctr	La Crosse	100%	59
Mayo Clinic Hlth Sys-Eau Claire Hosp	Eau Claire	100%	107
Ministry St Michaels Hosp-Stevens Pt	Stevens Point	100%	47
Oconomowoc Memorial Hospital	Oconomowoc	100%	41
Sacred Heart Hospital[2]	Eau Claire	100%	92
Saint Clare Hospital Health Services	Baraboo	100%	26
Saint Clares Hospital of Weston	Weston	100%	38
Saint Elizabeth Hospital	Appleton	100%	74
Saint Marys Hospital	Madison	100%	201
Theda Clark Medical Center	Neenah	100%	131
United Hospital System	Kenosha	100%	72
Univ of WI Hosps & Clinics Authority[2]	Madison	100%	70
Waukesha Memorial Hospital	Waukesha	100%	146
Wheaton Franciscan Healthcare All Saints[2]	Racine	100%	126
Aurora Baycare Medical Center	Green Bay	99%	86
Aurora Medical Center	Grafton	99%	95
Aurora West Allis Medical Center	West Allis	99%	74
Bellin Memorial Hospital	Green Bay	99%	88
Froedtert Memorial Lutheran Hospital[2]	Milwaukee	99%	119
Meriter Hospital	Madison	99%	104
Ministry Saint Josephs Hospital	Marshfield	99%	169
Saint Agnes Hospital	Fond Du Lac	99%	104
Wheaton Franciscan Hlthcare St Francis	Milwaukee	99%	77
Aurora Sheboygan Memorial Medical Center	Sheboygan	98%	41
Columbia Saint Marys Hospital Milwaukee	Milwaukee	98%	124
Mercy Medical Center of Oshkosh	Oshkosh	98%	40
Saint Nicholas Hospital	Sheboygan	98%	53
Wheaton Franciscan Saint Joseph[2]	Milwaukee	98%	91
Holy Family Memorial	Manitowoc	97%	31
Mercy Health System Corp	Janesville	97%	74
Aurora Lakeland Medical Center	Elkhorn	96%	25
Beloit Memorial Hospital	Beloit	94%	31
St Joseph's Comm Hosp of West Bend	West Bend	93%	27
Saint Marys Hospital Medical Center	Green Bay	91%	45
Saint Vincent Hospital[2]	Green Bay	87%	67

Discharged on Statin Medication

Hospital Name	City	Rate	Cases
Appleton Medical Center	Appleton	100%	30
Aurora Medical Center	Grafton	100%	71
Aurora Sheboygan Memorial Medical Center	Sheboygan	100%	28
Aurora West Allis Medical Center	West Allis	100%	55
Columbia Saint Marys Hospital Ozaukee	Mequon	100%	55
Howard Young Medical Center	Woodruff	100%	26
Ministry St Michaels Hosp-Stevens Pt	Stevens Point	100%	31
Aurora Baycare Medical Center	Green Bay	99%	67
Columbia Saint Marys Hospital Milwaukee	Milwaukee	99%	81
Froedtert Memorial Lutheran Hospital[2]	Milwaukee	99%	93
Gundersen Lutheran Medical Center	La Crosse	99%	114
Ministry Saint Josephs Hospital	Marshfield	99%	135
Saint Agnes Hospital	Fond Du Lac	99%	74
Aurora Saint Lukes Medical Center	Milwaukee	98%	274
Mayo Clinic Hlth Sys Franciscan Med Ctr	La Crosse	98%	49
Mayo Clinic Hlth Sys-Eau Claire Hosp	Eau Claire	98%	80
Meriter Hospital	Madison	98%	81
Saint Elizabeth Hospital	Appleton	98%	57
Saint Marys Hospital	Madison	98%	160
Aurora Medical Center Kenosha	Kenosha	97%	33
Theda Clark Medical Center	Neenah	97%	100
Bellin Memorial Hospital	Green Bay	96%	67
Community Memorial Hospital	Menomonee Fls	96%	55
Waukesha Memorial Hospital	Waukesha	95%	110
Wheaton Franciscan Hlthcare St Francis	Milwaukee	95%	65

NOTE: Hospital profiles are in alphabetical order by state, then city, then hospital within the city; Rankings exclude hospitals with less than 25 cases except for patient surveys which excludes hospitals with less than 100 cases; (a) 100-299 cases; (1) The number of cases/patients is too few to report; (2) Data submitted were based on a sample of cases/patients; (3) Results are based on a shorter time period than required; (4) Data suppressed by CMS for one or more quarters; (5) Results are not available for this reporting period; (6) Fewer than 100 patients completed the HCAHPS survey; (7) No cases met the criteria for this measure; (8) The lower limit of the confidence interval cannot be calculated if the number of observed infections equals zero; (9) No data are available from the state/territory for this reporting period; (10) The scores shown reflect fewer than 50 completed surveys; (11) There were discrepancies in the data collection process; (12) This measure does not apply to this hospital for this reporting period; (13) Results cannot be calculated for this reporting period; (14) The results for this state are combined with nearby states to protect confidentiality; Please refer to the User's Guide for a full explanation of data.

Hospital Name	City	Rate	Cases
Wheaton Franciscan Saint Joseph[2]	Milwaukee	95%	86
Oconomowoc Memorial Hospital	Oconomowoc	94%	31
Sacred Heart Hospital[2]	Eau Claire	94%	77
Bay Area Medical Center	Marinette	93%	27
Mercy Medical Center of Oshkosh	Oshkosh	92%	26
Saint Marys Hospital Medical Center	Green Bay	92%	37
Univ of WI Hosps & Clinics Authority[2]	Madison	92%	49
United Hospital System	Kenosha	90%	51
Wheaton Franciscan Healthcare All Saints[2]	Racine	90%	90
Aspirus Wausau Hospital[2]	Wausau	89%	54
Saint Clares Hospital of Weston	Weston	89%	28
Mercy Health System Corp	Janesville	88%	59
Saint Vincent Hospital[2]	Green Bay	85%	55
Beloit Memorial Hospital	Beloit	80%	30
Saint Nicholas Hospital	Sheboygan	73%	45
Holy Family Memorial	Manitowoc	59%	27

Venous Thromboembolism (VTE) Prophylaxis

Hospital Name	City	Rate	Cases
Aurora Baycare Medical Center	Green Bay	100%	106
Columbia Saint Marys Hospital Milwaukee	Milwaukee	100%	138
Howard Young Medical Center	Woodruff	100%	32
Mercy Medical Center of Oshkosh	Oshkosh	100%	42
Ministry St Michaels Hosp-Stevens Pt	Stevens Point	100%	48
Saint Clare Hospital Health Services	Baraboo	100%	29
Saint Clares Hospital of Weston	Weston	100%	37
Saint Marys Hospital	Madison	100%	218
Bellin Memorial Hospital	Green Bay	99%	85
Gundersen Lutheran Medical Center	La Crosse	99%	165
Theda Clark Medical Center	Neenah	99%	201
Aurora Medical Center	Grafton	98%	91
Aurora Saint Lukes Medical Center	Milwaukee	98%	498
Columbia Saint Marys Hospital Ozaukee	Mequon	98%	66
Mercy Health System Corp	Janesville	98%	81
Sacred Heart Hospital[2]	Eau Claire	98%	108
Saint Elizabeth Hospital	Appleton	98%	86
Aurora Medical Center Kenosha	Kenosha	97%	39
Aurora Sheboygan Memorial Medical Center	Sheboygan	97%	39
Meriter Hospital	Madison	97%	100
Ministry Saint Josephs Hospital	Marshfield	97%	220
Saint Agnes Hospital	Fond Du Lac	97%	88
United Hospital System	Kenosha	97%	90
Mayo Clinic Hlth Sys-Eau Claire Hosp	Eau Claire	96%	126
Oconomowoc Memorial Hospital	Oconomowoc	96%	28
St Joseph's Comm Hosp of West Bend	West Bend	96%	26
Saint Marys Hospital Medical Center	Green Bay	96%	47
Aurora West Allis Medical Center	West Allis	95%	81
Froedtert Memorial Lutheran Hospital[2]	Milwaukee	95%	144
Waukesha Memorial Hospital	Waukesha	95%	143
Wheaton Franciscan Saint Joseph[2]	Milwaukee	95%	95
Mayo Clinic Hlth Sys Franciscan Med Ctr	La Crosse	94%	52
Univ of WI Hosps & Clinics Authority[2]	Madison	94%	97
Aspirus Wausau Hospital[2]	Wausau	92%	75
Community Memorial Hospital	Menomonee Fls	92%	84
Riverview Hospital Assoc[2]	Wisc. Rapids	92%	25
Saint Vincent Hospital[2]	Green Bay	91%	86
Beloit Memorial Hospital	Beloit	89%	35
Appleton Medical Center	Appleton	88%	49
Wheaton Franciscan Hlthcare St Francis	Milwaukee	84%	79
Wheaton Franciscan Healthcare All Saints[2]	Racine	82%	141
Holy Family Memorial	Manitowoc	79%	38
Bay Area Medical Center	Marinette	77%	31
Saint Nicholas Hospital	Sheboygan	72%	64
Saint Marys Janesville Hospital	Janesville	60%	25

Written Stroke Educational Materials Given

Hospital Name	City	Rate	Cases
Aurora Sheboygan Memorial Medical Center	Sheboygan	100%	26
Bellin Memorial Hospital	Green Bay	100%	51
Columbia Saint Marys Hospital Ozaukee	Mequon	100%	35
Aurora Baycare Medical Center	Green Bay	98%	66
Theda Clark Medical Center	Neenah	98%	100
Waukesha Memorial Hospital	Waukesha	98%	89
Columbia Saint Marys Hospital Milwaukee	Milwaukee	97%	60
Community Memorial Hospital	Menomonee Fls	97%	35
Saint Agnes Hospital	Fond Du Lac	97%	72
Saint Elizabeth Hospital	Appleton	97%	36
Saint Vincent Hospital[2]	Green Bay	97%	38
Aurora Saint Lukes Medical Center	Milwaukee	96%	252
Mercy Health System Corp	Janesville	96%	48
Ministry Saint Josephs Hospital	Marshfield	95%	91
Saint Marys Hospital	Madison	95%	128
Gundersen Lutheran Medical Center	La Crosse	94%	89
Mayo Clinic Hlth Sys-Eau Claire Hosp	Eau Claire	94%	49
Mayo Clinic Hlth Sys Franciscan Med Ctr	La Crosse	92%	38
Meriter Hospital	Madison	92%	63
Sacred Heart Hospital[2]	Eau Claire	92%	53
Aurora West Allis Medical Center	West Allis	91%	46
Appleton Medical Center	Appleton	89%	27
Aurora Medical Center	Grafton	89%	55

Hospital Name	City	Rate	Cases
United Hospital System	Kenosha	80%	45
Univ of WI Hosps & Clinics Authority[2]	Madison	76%	62
Wheaton Franciscan Hlthcare St Francis	Milwaukee	75%	53
Wheaton Franciscan Saint Joseph[2]	Milwaukee	72%	47
Wheaton Franciscan Healthcare All Saints[2]	Racine	69%	77
Froedtert Memorial Lutheran Hospital[2]	Milwaukee	64%	94
Aspirus Wausau Hospital[2]	Wausau	61%	31

Surgical Care Improvement Project

Appropriate Beta Blocker Usage

Hospital Name	City	Rate	Cases
Appleton Medical Center[2]	Appleton	100%	439
Aurora Baycare Medical Center[2]	Green Bay	100%	229
Aurora Lakeland Medical Center[2]	Elkhorn	100%	39
Aurora Medical Center[2]	Summit	100%	109
Aurora Medical Center Manitowoc County[2]	Two Rivers	100%	79
Aurora Medical Center Oshkosh[2]	Oshkosh	100%	103
Aurora Memorial Hospital Burlington[2]	Burlington	100%	79
Aurora West Allis Medical Center[2]	West Allis	100%	98
Calumet Medical Center	Chilton	100%	29
Community Memorial Hospital[2]	Menomonee Fls	100%	203
Froedtert Memorial Lutheran Hospital[2]	Milwaukee	100%	273
Lakeview Medical Center[2]	Rice Lake	100%	109
Mayo Clinic Hlth Sys-Eau Claire Hosp	Eau Claire	100%	550
Mayo Clinic Health System - Red Cedar	Menomonie	100%	25
Mercy Medical Center of Oshkosh[2]	Oshkosh	100%	102
Mercy Walworth Hospital & Medical Center	Lake Geneva	100%	59
Richland Hospital	Richland Center	100%	25
River Falls Area Hospital	River Falls	100%	33
Saint Elizabeth Hospital[2]	Appleton	100%	176
St Joseph's Comm Hosp of West Bend	West Bend	100%	76
Saint Joseph's Hospital	Chippewa Falls	100%	38
Saint Marys Hospital[2]	Madison	100%	606
Shawano Medical Center	Shawano	100%	32
Theda Clark Medical Center[2]	Neenah	100%	110
Univ of WI Hosps & Clinics Authority[2]	Madison	100%	205
Westfields Hospital	New Richmond	100%	37
Wheaton Franciscan Healthcare All Saints[2]	Racine	100%	210
Wheaton Franciscan Healthcare Franklin	Franklin	100%	25
Aspirus Wausau Hospital[2]	Wausau	99%	235
Aurora Medical Center[2]	Grafton	99%	282
Aurora Medical Center Kenosha[2]	Kenosha	99%	126
Aurora Saint Lukes Medical Center	Milwaukee	99%	1295
Aurora Sheboygan Memorial Medical Center[2]	Sheboygan	99%	190
Bay Area Medical Center	Marinette	99%	89
Bellin Memorial Hospital[2]	Green Bay	99%	272
Columbia Saint Marys Hospital Milwaukee[2]	Milwaukee	99%	113
Howard Young Medical Center	Woodruff	99%	146
Madison VA Medical Center[2]	Madison	99%	116
Mercy Health System Corp	Janesville	99%	224
Meriter Hospital[2]	Madison	99%	206
Ministry Saint Josephs Hospital	Marshfield	99%	581
Ministry Saint Marys Hospital	Rhinelander	99%	115
Ministry St Michaels Hosp-Stevens Pt	Stevens Point	99%	144
The Monroe Clinic	Monroe	99%	145
Oak Leaf Surgical Hospital	Eau Claire	99%	100
Riverview Hospital Assoc[2]	Wisc. Rapids	99%	75
Saint Agnes Hospital	Fond Du Lac	99%	177
Saint Clares Hospital of Weston	Weston	99%	275
United Hospital System	Kenosha	99%	229
UW Hlth Partners Watertown Reg Med Ctr	Watertown	99%	85
Vernon Memorial Hospital	Viroqua	99%	140
Waukesha Memorial Hospital[2]	Waukesha	99%	205
Wheaton Franciscan Saint Joseph[2]	Milwaukee	99%	282
Columbia Saint Marys Hospital Ozaukee[2]	Mequon	98%	110
Gundersen Lutheran Medical Center[2]	La Crosse	98%	420
Hudson Hospital	Hudson	98%	41
Midwest Orthopedic Specialty Hospital[2]	Franklin	98%	66
Orthopaedic Hospital of Wisconsin[2]	Glendale	98%	56
Sacred Heart Hospital[2]	Eau Claire	98%	287
Saint Vincent Hospital[2]	Green Bay	98%	260
Beaver Dam Com Hospital	Beaver Dam	97%	68
Mayo Clinic Hlth Sys Franciscan Med Ctr	La Crosse	97%	274
Oconomowoc Memorial Hospital[2]	Oconomowoc	97%	59
Saint Clare Hospital Health Services	Baraboo	97%	37
Saint Marys Hospital Medical Center[2]	Green Bay	97%	92
Saint Nicholas Hospital[2]	Sheboygan	97%	90
Sauk Prairie Hospital	Prairie Du Sac	97%	157
Wheaton Franciscan Hlthcare St Francis	Milwaukee	97%	140
Aurora Medical Center Washington County[2]	Hartford	96%	48
Beloit Memorial Hospital[2]	Beloit	96%	131
Divine Savior Healthcare	Portage	96%	26
Fort Memorial Hospital[2]	Fort Atkinson	96%	69
Saint Marys Janesville Hospital	Janesville	96%	92
Milwaukee VA Medical Center[2]	Milwaukee	95%	170
Memorial Medical Center	Ashland	94%	34
Ministry Door County Medical Center	Sturgeon Bay	94%	47
Holy Family Memorial	Manitowoc	93%	147
Columbus Community Hospital	Columbus	88%	25

Appropriate VTP Within 24 Hours

Hospital Name	City	Rate	Cases
Amery Regional Medical Center[3]	Amery	100%	83
Appleton Medical Center[2]	Appleton	100%	864
Aurora Lakeland Medical Center[2]	Elkhorn	100%	133
Aurora Medical Center[2]	Grafton	100%	689
Aurora Medical Center[2]	Summit	100%	247
Aurora Medical Center Kenosha[2]	Kenosha	100%	416
Aurora Medical Center Manitowoc County[2]	Two Rivers	100%	143
Aurora Medical Center Oshkosh[2]	Oshkosh	100%	330
Aurora Medical Center Washington County[2]	Hartford	100%	188
Aurora Sheboygan Memorial Medical Center[2]	Sheboygan	100%	553
Aurora West Allis Medical Center[2]	West Allis	100%	332
Beaver Dam Com Hospital	Beaver Dam	100%	223
Berlin Memorial Hospital[2]	Berlin	100%	123
Calumet Medical Center	Chilton	100%	52
Community Memorial Hospital[2]	Menomonee Fls	100%	427
Froedtert Memorial Lutheran Hospital[2]	Milwaukee	100%	496
Hudson Hospital	Hudson	100%	108
Ladd Memorial Hospital	Osceola	100%	82
Lakeview Medical Center[2]	Rice Lake	100%	271
Langlade Hospital	Antigo	100%	48
Mayo Clinic Hlth Sys Franciscan Med Ctr	La Crosse	100%	679
Mayo Clinic Health System - Northland	Barron	100%	29
Mercy Walworth Hospital & Medical Center	Lake Geneva	100%	223
Midwest Orthopedic Specialty Hospital[2]	Franklin	100%	229
Ministry Saint Marys Hospital	Rhinelander	100%	333
The Monroe Clinic	Monroe	100%	380
Orthopaedic Hospital of Wisconsin[2]	Glendale	100%	226
Prairie Du Chien Memorial Hospital	Prairie Du Chien	100%	47
Richland Hospital	Richland Center	100%	53
River Falls Area Hospital	River Falls	100%	124
Saint Clares Hospital of Weston	Weston	100%	533
St Joseph's Comm Hosp of West Bend	West Bend	100%	277
Saint Marys Hospital Medical Center[2]	Green Bay	100%	312
Shawano Medical Center	Shawano	100%	102
Stoughton Hospital	Stoughton	100%	54
Univ of WI Hosps & Clinics Authority[2]	Madison	100%	384
Vernon Memorial Hospital	Viroqua	100%	502
Waupun Memorial Hospital	Waupun	100%	64
Wheaton Franciscan Healthcare All Saints[2]	Racine	100%	447
Wheaton Franciscan Saint Joseph[2]	Milwaukee	100%	708
Aurora Baycare Medical Center[2]	Green Bay	99%	405
Aurora Memorial Hospital Burlington[2]	Burlington	99%	228
Aurora Saint Lukes Medical Center	Milwaukee	99%	2126
Beloit Memorial Hospital[2]	Beloit	99%	313
Divine Savior Healthcare	Portage	99%	100
Gundersen Lutheran Medical Center[2]	La Crosse	99%	570
Howard Young Medical Center	Woodruff	99%	321
Madison VA Medical Center[2]	Madison	99%	162
Mayo Clinic Hlth Sys-Eau Claire Hosp	Eau Claire	99%	893
Mercy Medical Center of Oshkosh[2]	Oshkosh	99%	280
Milwaukee VA Medical Center[2]	Milwaukee	99%	265
Ministry Saint Josephs Hospital	Marshfield	99%	1235
Ministry St Michaels Hosp-Stevens Pt	Stevens Point	99%	336
Oak Leaf Surgical Hospital	Eau Claire	99%	396
Saint Agnes Hospital	Fond Du Lac	99%	467
Saint Clare Hospital Health Services	Baraboo	99%	133
Saint Elizabeth Hospital[2]	Appleton	99%	338
Saint Joseph's Hospital	Chippewa Falls	99%	97
Saint Marys Hospital[2]	Madison	99%	1226
Saint Nicholas Hospital[2]	Sheboygan	99%	247
Saint Vincent Hospital[2]	Green Bay	99%	400
Sauk Prairie Hospital	Prairie Du Sac	99%	545
United Hospital System	Kenosha	99%	563
Wheaton Franciscan Hlthcare St Francis	Milwaukee	99%	261
Holy Family Memorial	Manitowoc	98%	399
Mercy Health System Corp	Janesville	98%	539
Meriter Hospital[2]	Madison	98%	347
Reedsburg Area Medical Center	Reedsburg	98%	65
Theda Clark Medical Center[2]	Neenah	98%	386
Wheaton Franciscan Healthcare Franklin	Franklin	98%	97
Aspirus Wausau Hospital[2]	Wausau	97%	232
Bay Area Medical Center	Marinette	97%	239
Community Memorial Hospital	Oconto Falls	97%	36
Fort Memorial Hospital[2]	Fort Atkinson	97%	237
Ministry Door County Medical Center	Sturgeon Bay	97%	118
Oconomowoc Memorial Hospital[2]	Oconomowoc	97%	202
Riverview Hospital Assoc[2]	Wisc. Rapids	97%	176
Waukesha Memorial Hospital[2]	Waukesha	97%	343
Westfields Hospital	New Richmond	97%	126
Columbia Saint Marys Hospital Milwaukee[2]	Milwaukee	96%	268
Columbia Saint Marys Hospital Ozaukee[2]	Mequon	95%	259
Memorial Health Center	Medford	95%	37
Sacred Heart Hospital[2]	Eau Claire	95%	386
Saint Marys Janesville Hospital	Janesville	95%	297
UW Hlth Partners Watertown Reg Med Ctr	Watertown	95%	249
Bellin Memorial Hospital[2]	Green Bay	94%	414
Upland Hills Health	Dodgeville	89%	70
Memorial Medical Center	Ashland	85%	87

NOTE: Hospital profiles are in alphabetical order by state, then city, then hospital within the city; Rankings exclude hospitals with less than 25 cases except for patient surveys which excludes hospitals with less than 100 cases; (a) 100-299 cases; (1) The number of cases/patients is too few to report; (2) Data submitted were based on a sample of cases/patients; (3) Results are based on a shorter time period than required; (4) Data suppressed by CMS for one or more quarters; (5) Results are not available for this reporting period; (6) Fewer than 100 patients completed the HCAHPS survey; (7) No cases met the criteria for this measure; (8) The lower limit of the confidence interval cannot be calculated if the number of observed infections equals zero; (9) No data are available from the state/territory for this reporting period; (10) The scores shown reflect fewer than 50 completed surveys; (11) There were discrepancies in the data collection process; (12) This measure does not apply to this hospital for this reporting period; (13) Results cannot be calculated for this reporting period; (14) The results for this state are combined with nearby states to protect confidentiality; Please refer to the User's Guide for a full explanation of data.

Columbus Community Hospital	Columbus	83%	54
Grant Regional Health Center	Lancaster	81%	31
Mile Bluff Medical Center	Mauston	70%	40

Controlled Postoperative Blood Glucose

Hospital Name	City	Rate	Cases
Aurora Baycare Medical Center[2]	Green Bay	100%	94
Mayo Clinic Hlth Sys-Eau Claire Hosp	Eau Claire	100%	167
United Hospital System	Kenosha	99%	92
Waukesha Memorial Hospital[2]	Waukesha	99%	135
Aurora Saint Lukes Medical Center	Milwaukee	98%	892
Milwaukee VA Medical Center[2]	Milwaukee	98%	84
Ministry Saint Josephs Hospital	Marshfield	98%	273
Saint Agnes Hospital	Fond Du Lac	98%	62
Wheaton Franciscan Healthcare All Saints[2]	Racine	98%	88
Wheaton Franciscan Hlthcare St Francis	Milwaukee	98%	54
Froedtert Memorial Lutheran Hospital[2]	Milwaukee	97%	141
Madison VA Medical Center[2]	Madison	97%	37
Mercy Health System Corp	Janesville	97%	58
Saint Clares Hospital of Weston	Weston	97%	108
Saint Elizabeth Hospital[2]	Appleton	97%	157
Saint Vincent Hospital[2]	Green Bay	97%	134
Aurora Medical Center[2]	Grafton	96%	103
Community Memorial Hospital[2]	Menomonee Fls	96%	113
Gundersen Lutheran Medical Center[2]	La Crosse	96%	221
Sacred Heart Hospital[2]	Eau Claire	96%	145
Appleton Medical Center[2]	Appleton	95%	261
Wheaton Franciscan Saint Joseph[2]	Milwaukee	95%	113
Bellin Memorial Hospital[2]	Green Bay	94%	246
Columbia Saint Marys Hospital Milwaukee[2]	Milwaukee	94%	67
Aspirus Wausau Hospital[2]	Wausau	93%	109
Beloit Memorial Hospital[2]	Beloit	92%	49
Meriter Hospital[2]	Madison	92%	138
Univ of WI Hosps & Clinics Authority[2]	Madison	92%	119
Columbia Saint Marys Hospital Ozaukee[2]	Mequon	91%	76
Saint Marys Hospital[2]	Madison	91%	305

Perioperative Temperature Management

Hospital Name	City	Rate	Cases
Amery Regional Medical Center[3]	Amery	100%	94
Appleton Medical Center[2]	Appleton	100%	982
Aspirus Wausau Hospital[2]	Wausau	100%	464
Aurora Baycare Medical Center[2]	Green Bay	100%	632
Aurora Lakeland Medical Center[2]	Elkhorn	100%	147
Aurora Medical Center[2]	Grafton	100%	816
Aurora Medical Center[2]	Summit	100%	315
Aurora Medical Center Kenosha[2]	Kenosha	100%	448
Aurora Medical Center Manitowoc County[2]	Two Rivers	100%	186
Aurora Medical Center Oshkosh[2]	Oshkosh	100%	361
Aurora Medical Center Washington County[2]	Hartford	100%	212
Aurora Memorial Hospital Burlington[2]	Burlington	100%	274
Aurora Saint Lukes Medical Center	Milwaukee	100%	2777
Aurora Sheboygan Memorial Medical Center[2]	Sheboygan	100%	600
Aurora West Allis Medical Center[2]	West Allis	100%	403
Bay Area Medical Center	Marinette	100%	269
Beaver Dam Com Hospital	Beaver Dam	100%	238
Bellin Memorial Hospital[2]	Green Bay	100%	469
Berlin Memorial Hospital[2]	Berlin	100%	149
Black River Memorial Hospital	Black River Falls	100%	71
Calumet Medical Center	Chilton	100%	76
Columbia Saint Marys Hospital Milwaukee[2]	Milwaukee	100%	335
Columbia Saint Marys Hospital Ozaukee[2]	Mequon	100%	344
Columbus Community Hospital	Columbus	100%	75
Community Memorial Hospital[2]	Menomonee Fls	100%	636
Divine Savior Healthcare	Portage	100%	116
Fort Memorial Hospital[2]	Fort Atkinson	100%	266
Good Samaritan Health Center	Merrill	100%	29
Grant Regional Health Center	Lancaster	100%	32
Gundersen Lutheran Medical Center[2]	La Crosse	100%	794
Holy Family Memorial	Manitowoc	100%	444
Howard Young Medical Center	Woodruff	100%	436
Hudson Hospital	Hudson	100%	138
Ladd Memorial Hospital	Osceola	100%	92
Lakeview Medical Center[2]	Rice Lake	100%	343
Langlade Hospital	Antigo	100%	58
Mayo Clinic Hlth Sys Franciscan Med Ctr	La Crosse	100%	863
Mayo Clinic Hlth Sys-Eau Claire Hosp	Eau Claire	100%	1110
Mayo Clinic Health System - Northland	Barron	100%	35
Mayo Clinic Health System - Red Cedar	Menomonie	100%	94
Memorial Health Center	Medford	100%	44
Mercy Health System Corp	Janesville	100%	622
Mercy Medical Center of Oshkosh[2]	Oshkosh	100%	314
Mercy Walworth Hospital & Medical Center	Lake Geneva	100%	247
Meriter Hospital[2]	Madison	100%	484
Midwest Orthopedic Specialty Hospital[2]	Franklin	100%	243
Ministry Door County Medical Center	Sturgeon Bay	100%	134
Ministry Saint Josephs Hospital	Marshfield	100%	1506
Ministry Saint Marys Hospital	Rhinelander	100%	389
Ministry St Michaels Hosp-Stevens Pt	Stevens Point	100%	493
The Monroe Clinic	Monroe	100%	404
Oak Leaf Surgical Hospital	Eau Claire	100%	416
Oconomowoc Memorial Hospital[2]	Oconomowoc	100%	250
Orthopaedic Hospital of Wisconsin[2]	Glendale	100%	240
Prairie Du Chien Memorial Hospital	Prairie Du Chien	100%	56
Reedsburg Area Medical Center	Reedsburg	100%	72
Richland Hospital	Richland Center	100%	56
Ripon Medical Center[3]	Ripon	100%	46
River Falls Area Hospital	River Falls	100%	142
Sacred Heart Hospital[2]	Eau Claire	100%	510
Saint Agnes Hospital	Fond Du Lac	100%	543
Saint Clare Hospital Health Services	Baraboo	100%	139
Saint Clares Hospital of Weston	Weston	100%	641
Saint Croix Regional Medical Center	Saint Croix Falls	100%	129
Saint Elizabeth Hospital[2]	Appleton	100%	372
St Joseph's Comm Hosp of West Bend	West Bend	100%	308
Saint Joseph's Hospital	Chippewa Falls	100%	137
Saint Marys Hospital[2]	Madison	100%	1400
Saint Marys Hospital Medical Center[2]	Green Bay	100%	338
Saint Marys Janesville Hospital	Janesville	100%	351
Saint Nicholas Hospital[2]	Sheboygan	100%	307
Saint Vincent Hospital[2]	Green Bay	100%	513
Sauk Prairie Hospital	Prairie Du Sac	100%	687
Shawano Medical Center	Shawano	100%	123
Stoughton Hospital	Stoughton	100%	59
Theda Clark Medical Center[2]	Neenah	100%	463
United Hospital System	Kenosha	100%	657
Univ of WI Hosps & Clinics Authority[2]	Madison	100%	530
Upland Hills Health	Dodgeville	100%	74
UW Hlth Partners Watertown Reg Med Ctr	Watertown	100%	273
Vernon Memorial Hospital	Viroqua	100%	553
Waukesha Memorial Hospital[2]	Waukesha	100%	561
Waupun Memorial Hospital	Waupun	100%	76
Wheaton Franciscan Healthcare All Saints[2]	Racine	100%	523
Wheaton Franciscan Healthcare Franklin	Franklin	100%	110
Wheaton Franciscan Hlthcare St Francis	Milwaukee	100%	343
Wheaton Franciscan Saint Joseph[2]	Milwaukee	100%	866
Froedtert Memorial Lutheran Hospital[2]	Milwaukee	99%	651
Madison VA Medical Center[2]	Madison	99%	252
Mile Bluff Medical Center	Mauston	99%	82
Milwaukee VA Medical Center[2]	Milwaukee	99%	347
Riverview Hospital Assoc[2]	Wisc. Rapids	99%	242
Westfields Hospital	New Richmond	99%	138
Beloit Memorial Hospital[2]	Beloit	97%	343
Memorial Medical Center	Ashland	95%	96

Prophylactic Antibiotic Selection

Hospital Name	City	Rate	Cases
Amery Regional Medical Center[3]	Amery	100%	78
Aurora Lakeland Medical Center[2]	Elkhorn	100%	70
Aurora Medical Center[2]	Grafton	100%	788
Aurora Medical Center Kenosha[2]	Kenosha	100%	332
Aurora Medical Center Oshkosh[2]	Oshkosh	100%	279
Aurora Sheboygan Memorial Medical Center[2]	Sheboygan	100%	479
Aurora West Allis Medical Center[2]	West Allis	100%	261
Bay Area Medical Center	Marinette	100%	159
Beaver Dam Com Hospital	Beaver Dam	100%	193
Calumet Medical Center	Chilton	100%	59
Columbia Saint Marys Hospital Milwaukee[2]	Milwaukee	100%	241
Columbus Community Hospital	Columbus	100%	52
Community Memorial Hospital	Oconto Falls	100%	33
Divine Savior Healthcare	Portage	100%	86
Froedtert Memorial Lutheran Hospital[2]	Milwaukee	100%	417
Grant Regional Health Center	Lancaster	100%	27
Gundersen Lutheran Medical Center[2]	La Crosse	100%	628
Howard Young Medical Center	Woodruff	100%	284
Hudson Hospital	Hudson	100%	112
Madison VA Medical Center	Madison	100%	152
Mayo Clinic Hlth Sys Franciscan Med Ctr	La Crosse	100%	652
Mayo Clinic Hlth Sys-Eau Claire Hosp	Eau Claire	100%	800
Mayo Clinic Health System - Red Cedar	Menomonie	100%	71
Memorial Health Center	Medford	100%	34
Mercy Walworth Hospital & Medical Center	Lake Geneva	100%	173
Meriter Hospital[2]	Madison	100%	454
Midwest Orthopedic Specialty Hospital[2]	Franklin	100%	178
Milwaukee VA Medical Center	Milwaukee	100%	279
Oak Leaf Surgical Hospital	Eau Claire	100%	340
Orthopaedic Hospital of Wisconsin[2]	Glendale	100%	185
Prairie Du Chien Memorial Hospital	Prairie Du Chien	100%	39
Richland Hospital	Richland Center	100%	52
River Falls Area Hospital	River Falls	100%	98
Saint Clare Hospital Health Services	Baraboo	100%	124
Saint Clares Hospital of Weston	Weston	100%	570
Saint Croix Regional Medical Center	Saint Croix Falls	100%	120
Saint Elizabeth Hospital[2]	Appleton	100%	376
St Joseph's Comm Hosp of West Bend	West Bend	100%	242
Saint Marys Hospital[2]	Madison	100%	1397
Saint Marys Janesville Hospital	Janesville	100%	242
Saint Nicholas Hospital[2]	Sheboygan	100%	215
Sauk Prairie Hospital	Prairie Du Sac	100%	617
Stoughton Hospital	Stoughton	100%	38
Theda Clark Medical Center[2]	Neenah	100%	305
United Hospital System	Kenosha	100%	527
Upland Hills Health	Dodgeville	100%	28
UW Hlth Partners Watertown Reg Med Ctr	Watertown	100%	199
Vernon Memorial Hospital	Viroqua	100%	488
Wheaton Franciscan Healthcare All Saints[2]	Racine	100%	375
Wheaton Franciscan Healthcare Franklin	Franklin	100%	68
Wheaton Franciscan Saint Joseph[2]	Milwaukee	100%	615
Appleton Medical Center[2]	Appleton	99%	1019
Aspirus Wausau Hospital[2]	Wausau	99%	385
Aurora Baycare Medical Center[2]	Green Bay	99%	539
Aurora Medical Center[2]	Summit	99%	234
Aurora Medical Center Manitowoc County[2]	Two Rivers	99%	131
Aurora Medical Center Washington County[2]	Hartford	99%	172
Aurora Memorial Hospital Burlington[2]	Burlington	99%	150
Aurora Saint Lukes Medical Center	Milwaukee	99%	1862
Bellin Memorial Hospital[2]	Green Bay	99%	509
Berlin Memorial Hospital[2]	Berlin	99%	135
Columbia Saint Marys Hospital Ozaukee[2]	Mequon	99%	253
Community Memorial Hospital[2]	Menomonee Fls	99%	475
Lakeview Medical Center[2]	Rice Lake	99%	283
Memorial Medical Center	Ashland	99%	85
Mercy Health System Corp	Janesville	99%	348
Mercy Medical Center of Oshkosh[2]	Oshkosh	99%	190
Ministry Saint Josephs Hospital	Marshfield	99%	990
Ministry Saint Marys Hospital	Rhinelander	99%	308
Ministry St Michaels Hosp-Stevens Pt	Stevens Point	99%	360
The Monroe Clinic	Monroe	99%	289
Oconomowoc Memorial Hospital[2]	Oconomowoc	99%	197
Saint Agnes Hospital	Fond Du Lac	99%	383
Saint Vincent Hospital[2]	Green Bay	99%	438
Shawano Medical Center	Shawano	99%	100
Univ of WI Hosps & Clinics Authority[2]	Madison	99%	368
Waukesha Memorial Hospital[2]	Waukesha	99%	383
Wheaton Franciscan Hlthcare St Francis	Milwaukee	99%	236
Beloit Memorial Hospital[2]	Beloit	98%	285
Fort Memorial Hospital[2]	Fort Atkinson	98%	179
Reedsburg Area Medical Center	Reedsburg	98%	63
Sacred Heart Hospital[2]	Eau Claire	98%	399
Saint Marys Hospital Medical Center[2]	Green Bay	98%	212
Waupun Memorial Hospital	Waupun	98%	61
Westfields Hospital	New Richmond	98%	97
Holy Family Memorial	Manitowoc	97%	330
Ministry Door County Medical Center	Sturgeon Bay	97%	101
Riverview Hospital Assoc[2]	Wisc. Rapids	97%	185
Saint Joseph's Hospital	Chippewa Falls	97%	108
Black River Memorial Hospital	Black River Falls	91%	69
Mile Bluff Medical Center	Mauston	91%	67
Baldwin Area Medical Center	Baldwin	81%	26

Prophylactic Antibiotic Selection (Outpatient)

Hospital Name	City	Rate	Cases
Aurora Lakeland Medical Center	Elkhorn	100%	28
Aurora Memorial Hospital Burlington	Burlington	100%	139
Aurora Sheboygan Memorial Medical Center	Sheboygan	100%	325
Aurora West Allis Medical Center	West Allis	100%	457
Gundersen Lutheran Medical Center	La Crosse	100%	758
Mayo Clinic Hlth Sys-Eau Claire Hosp	Eau Claire	100%	495
Midwest Orthopedic Specialty Hospital	Franklin	100%	190
Ministry St Michaels Hosp-Stevens Pt	Stevens Point	100%	37
Oak Leaf Surgical Hospital	Eau Claire	100%	91
Orthopaedic Hospital of Wisconsin	Glendale	100%	117
River Falls Area Hospital	River Falls	100%	40
Riverview Hospital Assoc	Wisc. Rapids	100%	42
Saint Clares Hospital of Weston	Weston	100%	122
Saint Joseph's Hospital	Chippewa Falls	100%	33
Saint Marys Janesville Hospital	Janesville	100%	45
Saint Nicholas Hospital	Sheboygan	100%	78
Wheaton Franciscan Healthcare Franklin	Franklin	100%	36
Wheaton Franciscan Saint Joseph	Milwaukee	100%	627
Aspirus Wausau Hospital	Wausau	99%	486
Aurora Baycare Medical Center	Green Bay	99%	530
Berlin Memorial Hospital	Berlin	99%	77
Froedtert Memorial Lutheran Hospital	Milwaukee	99%	619
Mayo Clinic Hlth Sys Franciscan Med Ctr	La Crosse	99%	304
Mercy Medical Center of Oshkosh	Oshkosh	99%	289
Meriter Hospital	Madison	99%	329
Ministry Saint Josephs Hospital	Marshfield	99%	453
Sacred Heart Hospital	Eau Claire	99%	382
Saint Agnes Hospital	Fond Du Lac	99%	365
Saint Elizabeth Hospital	Appleton	99%	507
Saint Marys Hospital	Madison	99%	932
Sauk Prairie Hospital	Prairie Du Sac	99%	127
Theda Clark Medical Center	Neenah	99%	546
Univ of WI Hosps & Clinics Authority	Madison	99%	471
Waukesha Memorial Hospital	Waukesha	99%	435
Aurora Medical Center	Grafton	98%	250
Aurora Medical Center Manitowoc County	Two Rivers	98%	130
Beaver Dam Com Hospital	Beaver Dam	98%	86
Bellin Memorial Hospital	Green Bay	98%	627
Columbia Saint Marys Hospital Ozaukee	Mequon	98%	204
Fort Memorial Hospital	Fort Atkinson	98%	158

NOTE: Hospital profiles are in alphabetical order by state, then city, then hospital within the city; Rankings exclude hospitals with less than 25 cases except for patient surveys which excludes hospitals with less than 100 cases; (a) 100-299 cases; (1) The number of cases/patients is too few to report; (2) Data submitted were based on a sample of cases/patients; (3) Results are based on a shorter time period than required; (4) Data suppressed by CMS for one or more quarters; (5) Results are not available for this reporting period; (6) Fewer than 100 patients completed the HCAHPS survey; (7) No cases met the criteria for this measure; (8) The lower limit of the confidence interval cannot be calculated if the number of observed infections equals zero; (9) No data are available from the state/territory for this reporting period; (10) The scores shown reflect fewer than 50 completed surveys; (11) There were discrepancies in the data collection process; (12) This measure does not apply to this hospital for this reporting period; (13) Results cannot be calculated for this reporting period; (14) The results for this state are combined with nearby states to protect confidentiality; Please refer to the User's Guide for a full explanation of data.

Howard Young Medical Center	Woodruff	98%	41
Lakeview Medical Center	Rice Lake	98%	62
Mercy Health System Corp	Janesville	98%	265
Reedsburg Area Medical Center	Reedsburg	98%	64
United Hospital System	Kenosha	98%	376
Wheaton Franciscan Healthcare All Saints	Racine	98%	322
Aurora Medical Center	Summit	97%	164
Aurora Medical Center Oshkosh	Oshkosh	97%	231
Aurora Saint Lukes Medical Center	Milwaukee	97%	846
Bay Area Medical Center	Marinette	97%	76
Columbia Saint Marys Hospital Milwaukee	Milwaukee	97%	410
Community Memorial Hospital	Menomonee Fls	97%	230
Ministry Saint Marys Hospital	Rhinelander	97%	38
Oconomowoc Memorial Hospital	Oconomowoc	97%	60
Saint Vincent Hospital	Green Bay	97%	205
UW Hlth Partners Watertown Reg Med Ctr	Watertown	97%	124
Wheaton Franciscan Hlthcare St Francis	Milwaukee	97%	123
Appleton Medical Center	Appleton	96%	333
Aurora Medical Center Washington County	Hartford	96%	26
The Monroe Clinic	Monroe	96%	221
St Joseph's Comm Hosp of West Bend	West Bend	96%	97
Holy Family Memorial	Manitowoc	95%	97
Mile Bluff Medical Center	Mauston	95%	62
Aurora Medical Center Kenosha	Kenosha	93%	243
Beloit Memorial Hospital	Beloit	93%	113
Saint Clare Hospital Health Services	Baraboo	93%	43
Black River Memorial Hospital	Black River Falls	92%	25
Saint Marys Hospital Medical Center	Green Bay	91%	300
Saint Marys Hospital Superior	Superior	89%	27

Prophylactic Antibiotic Stopped

Hospital Name	City	Rate	Cases
Aurora Baycare Medical Center[2]	Green Bay	100%	529
Aurora Lakeland Medical Center[2]	Elkhorn	100%	67
Aurora Medical Center[2]	Grafton	100%	783
Aurora Medical Center Oshkosh[2]	Oshkosh	100%	272
Aurora Medical Center Washington County[2]	Hartford	100%	166
Aurora West Allis Medical Center[2]	West Allis	100%	246
Baldwin Area Medical Center	Baldwin	100%	26
Calumet Medical Center	Chilton	100%	59
Community Memorial Hospital[2]	Menomonee Fls	100%	470
Community Memorial Hospital	Oconto Falls	100%	33
Grant Regional Health Center	Lancaster	100%	25
Howard Young Medical Center	Woodruff	100%	282
Hudson Hospital	Hudson	100%	112
Mayo Clinic Hlth Sys Franciscan Med Ctr	La Crosse	100%	640
Mayo Clinic Hlth Sys-Eau Claire Hosp	Eau Claire	100%	762
Mayo Clinic Health System - Red Cedar	Menomonie	100%	70
Midwest Orthopedic Specialty Hospital[2]	Franklin	100%	178
Ministry Saint Marys Hospital	Rhinelander	100%	302
Orthopaedic Hospital of Wisconsin[2]	Glendale	100%	185
River Falls Area Hospital	River Falls	100%	98
Saint Elizabeth Hospital[2]	Appleton	100%	360
United Hospital System	Kenosha	100%	506
Wheaton Franciscan Healthcare Franklin	Franklin	100%	67
Wheaton Franciscan Saint Joseph[2]	Milwaukee	100%	602
Appleton Medical Center[2]	Appleton	99%	995
Aurora Medical Center Kenosha[2]	Kenosha	99%	318
Aurora Medical Center Manitowoc County[2]	Two Rivers	99%	130
Aurora Memorial Hospital Burlington[2]	Burlington	99%	146
Aurora Saint Lukes Medical Center	Milwaukee	99%	1800
Aurora Sheboygan Memorial Medical Center[2]	Sheboygan	99%	476
Bellin Memorial Hospital[2]	Green Bay	99%	504
Black River Memorial Hospital	Black River Falls	99%	69
Fort Memorial Hospital[2]	Fort Atkinson	99%	178
Froedtert Memorial Lutheran Hospital[2]	Milwaukee	99%	404
Gundersen Lutheran Medical Center[2]	La Crosse	99%	621
Lakeview Medical Center[2]	Rice Lake	99%	282
Madison VA Medical Center	Madison	99%	150
Meriter Hospital[2]	Madison	99%	445
Milwaukee VA Medical Center	Milwaukee	99%	277
Ministry St Michaels Hosp-Stevens Pt	Stevens Point	99%	359
The Monroe Clinic	Monroe	99%	279
Oconomowoc Memorial Hospital[2]	Oconomowoc	99%	196
Riverview Hospital Assoc[2]	Wisc. Rapids	99%	183
Saint Clare Hospital Health Services	Baraboo	99%	124
Saint Clares Hospital of Weston	Weston	99%	565
St Joseph's Comm Hosp of West Bend	West Bend	99%	229
Saint Joseph's Hospital	Chippewa Falls	99%	107
Saint Marys Hospital[2]	Madison	99%	1376
Saint Marys Hospital Medical Center[2]	Green Bay	99%	211
Saint Vincent Hospital[2]	Green Bay	99%	424
Univ of WI Hosps & Clinics Authority[2]	Madison	99%	357
Vernon Memorial Hospital	Viroqua	99%	485
Westfields Hospital	New Richmond	99%	96
Aurora Medical Center[2]	Summit	98%	231
Beaver Dam Com Hospital	Beaver Dam	98%	188
Berlin Memorial Hospital[2]	Berlin	98%	133
Columbia Saint Marys Hospital Ozaukee[2]	Mequon	98%	239
Holy Family Memorial	Manitowoc	98%	326
Ministry Saint Josephs Hospital	Marshfield	98%	965
Oak Leaf Surgical Hospital	Eau Claire	98%	339
Saint Agnes Hospital	Fond Du Lac	98%	366
Saint Nicholas Hospital[2]	Sheboygan	98%	211
Shawano Medical Center	Shawano	98%	100
UW Hlth Partners Watertown Reg Med Ctr	Watertown	98%	195
Waupun Memorial Hospital	Waupun	98%	61
Wheaton Franciscan Healthcare All Saints[2]	Racine	98%	357
Amery Regional Medical Center[3]	Amery	97%	78
Aspirus Wausau Hospital[2]	Wausau	97%	378
Columbia Saint Marys Hospital Milwaukee[2]	Milwaukee	97%	231
Mercy Health System Corp	Janesville	97%	337
Prairie Du Chien Memorial Hospital	Prairie Du Chien	97%	38
Reedsburg Area Medical Center	Reedsburg	97%	63
Saint Croix Regional Medical Center	Saint Croix Falls	97%	118
Saint Marys Janesville Hospital	Janesville	97%	236
Sauk Prairie Hospital	Prairie Du Sac	97%	616
Stoughton Hospital	Stoughton	97%	37
Waukesha Memorial Hospital[2]	Waukesha	97%	383
Wheaton Franciscan Hlthcare St Francis	Milwaukee	97%	222
Bay Area Medical Center	Marinette	96%	153
Columbus Community Hospital	Columbus	96%	52
Mercy Medical Center of Oshkosh[2]	Oshkosh	96%	190
Mercy Walworth Hospital & Medical Center	Lake Geneva	96%	170
Ministry Door County Medical Center	Sturgeon Bay	96%	95
Richland Hospital	Richland Center	96%	52
Sacred Heart Hospital[2]	Eau Claire	96%	389
Theda Clark Medical Center[2]	Neenah	96%	298
Upland Hills Health	Dodgeville	96%	27
Beloit Memorial Hospital[2]	Beloit	95%	281
Divine Savior Healthcare	Portage	94%	86
Memorial Health Center	Medford	94%	34
Mile Bluff Medical Center	Mauston	94%	66
Memorial Medical Center	Ashland	88%	84

Prophylactic Antibiotic Timing

Hospital Name	City	Rate	Cases
Appleton Medical Center[2]	Appleton	100%	1020
Aurora Baycare Medical Center[2]	Green Bay	100%	539
Aurora Lakeland Medical Center[2]	Elkhorn	100%	70
Aurora Medical Center[2]	Grafton	100%	788
Aurora Medical Center[2]	Summit	100%	234
Aurora Medical Center Washington County[2]	Hartford	100%	172
Aurora Sheboygan Memorial Medical Center[2]	Sheboygan	100%	479
Aurora West Allis Medical Center[2]	West Allis	100%	261
Beaver Dam Com Hospital	Beaver Dam	100%	193
Black River Memorial Hospital	Black River Falls	100%	69
Calumet Medical Center	Chilton	100%	59
Divine Savior Healthcare	Portage	100%	86
Ministry St Michaels Hosp-Stevens Pt	Stevens Point	100%	360
Orthopaedic Hospital of Wisconsin[2]	Glendale	100%	185
Prairie Du Chien Memorial Hospital	Prairie Du Chien	100%	39
River Falls Area Hospital	River Falls	100%	98
Saint Agnes Hospital	Fond Du Lac	100%	384
Saint Clares Hospital of Weston	Weston	100%	570
Saint Joseph's Hospital	Chippewa Falls	100%	108
Sauk Prairie Hospital	Prairie Du Sac	100%	618
Shawano Medical Center	Shawano	100%	100
Stoughton Hospital	Stoughton	100%	38
United Hospital System	Kenosha	100%	527
Wheaton Franciscan Healthcare Franklin	Franklin	100%	68
Aspirus Wausau Hospital[2]	Wausau	99%	385
Aurora Medical Center Kenosha[2]	Kenosha	99%	333
Aurora Medical Center Oshkosh[2]	Oshkosh	99%	279
Aurora Memorial Hospital Burlington[2]	Burlington	99%	150
Aurora Saint Lukes Medical Center	Milwaukee	99%	1862
Bay Area Medical Center	Marinette	99%	159
Columbia Saint Marys Hospital Milwaukee[2]	Milwaukee	99%	241
Community Memorial Hospital[2]	Menomonee Fls	99%	475
Fort Memorial Hospital[2]	Fort Atkinson	99%	179
Holy Family Memorial	Manitowoc	99%	330
Howard Young Medical Center	Woodruff	99%	285
Lakeview Medical Center[2]	Rice Lake	99%	283
Madison VA Medical Center	Madison	99%	152
Mayo Clinic Hlth Sys Franciscan Med Ctr	La Crosse	99%	652
Mayo Clinic Hlth Sys-Eau Claire Hosp	Eau Claire	99%	800
Mayo Clinic Health System - Red Cedar	Menomonie	99%	71
Mercy Medical Center of Oshkosh[2]	Oshkosh	99%	190
Mercy Walworth Hospital & Medical Center	Lake Geneva	99%	174
Midwest Orthopedic Specialty Hospital[2]	Franklin	99%	178
Milwaukee VA Medical Center	Milwaukee	99%	279
Ministry Saint Marys Hospital	Rhinelander	99%	311
The Monroe Clinic	Monroe	99%	289
Oak Leaf Surgical Hospital	Eau Claire	99%	340
Riverview Hospital Assoc[2]	Wisc. Rapids	99%	185
Sacred Heart Hospital[2]	Eau Claire	99%	399
Saint Elizabeth Hospital[2]	Appleton	99%	376
St Joseph's Comm Hosp of West Bend	West Bend	99%	242
Saint Marys Hospital[2]	Madison	99%	1399
Saint Marys Hospital Medical Center[2]	Green Bay	99%	212
Saint Nicholas Hospital[2]	Sheboygan	99%	215
Theda Clark Medical Center[2]	Neenah	99%	305
Univ of WI Hosps & Clinics Authority[2]	Madison	99%	368
UW Hlth Partners Watertown Reg Med Ctr	Watertown	99%	201
Wheaton Franciscan Healthcare All Saints[2]	Racine	99%	377
Wheaton Franciscan Hlthcare St Francis	Milwaukee	99%	236
Columbia Saint Marys Hospital Ozaukee[2]	Mequon	98%	253
Gundersen Lutheran Medical Center[2]	La Crosse	98%	632
Ministry Door County Medical Center	Sturgeon Bay	98%	101
Ministry Saint Josephs Hospital	Marshfield	98%	991
Oconomowoc Memorial Hospital[2]	Oconomowoc	98%	198
Reedsburg Area Medical Center	Reedsburg	98%	63
Saint Clare Hospital Health Services	Baraboo	98%	124
Saint Vincent Hospital[2]	Green Bay	98%	441
Waukesha Memorial Hospital[2]	Waukesha	98%	384
Waupun Memorial Hospital	Waupun	98%	61
Wheaton Franciscan Saint Joseph[2]	Milwaukee	98%	616
Bellin Memorial Hospital[2]	Green Bay	97%	509
Berlin Memorial Hospital[2]	Berlin	97%	135
Community Memorial Hospital	Oconto Falls	97%	34
Froedtert Memorial Lutheran Hospital[2]	Milwaukee	97%	420
Hudson Hospital	Hudson	97%	112
Memorial Health Center	Medford	97%	34
Mercy Health System Corp	Janesville	97%	348
Meriter Hospital[2]	Madison	97%	454
Mile Bluff Medical Center	Mauston	97%	67
Saint Croix Regional Medical Center	Saint Croix Falls	97%	120
Vernon Memorial Hospital	Viroqua	97%	489
Aurora Medical Center Manitowoc County[2]	Two Rivers	96%	132
Columbus Community Hospital	Columbus	96%	52
Grant Regional Health Center	Lancaster	96%	27
Saint Marys Janesville Hospital	Janesville	95%	242
Westfields Hospital	New Richmond	95%	97
Baldwin Area Medical Center	Baldwin	92%	26
Beloit Memorial Hospital[2]	Beloit	92%	287
Amery Regional Medical Center[3]	Amery	90%	79
Richland Hospital	Richland Center	90%	52
Memorial Medical Center	Ashland	86%	85
Upland Hills Health	Dodgeville	82%	28

Prophylactic Antibiotic Timing (Outpatient)

Hospital Name	City	Rate	Cases
Aurora West Allis Medical Center	West Allis	100%	456
Bay Area Medical Center	Marinette	100%	76
Ministry Saint Josephs Hospital	Marshfield	100%	454
Oak Leaf Surgical Hospital	Eau Claire	100%	91
Orthopaedic Hospital of Wisconsin	Glendale	100%	117
Saint Clare Hospital Health Services	Baraboo	100%	43
St Joseph's Comm Hosp of West Bend	West Bend	100%	96
Saint Vincent Hospital	Green Bay	100%	203
Aspirus Wausau Hospital	Wausau	99%	488
Aurora Medical Center	Grafton	99%	250
Aurora Medical Center	Summit	99%	164
Aurora Sheboygan Memorial Medical Center	Sheboygan	99%	326
Beaver Dam Com Hospital	Beaver Dam	99%	86
Bellin Memorial Hospital	Green Bay	99%	631
Berlin Memorial Hospital	Berlin	99%	76
Holy Family Memorial	Manitowoc	99%	98
Midwest Orthopedic Specialty Hospital	Franklin	99%	190
Saint Clares Hospital of Weston	Weston	99%	123
Saint Elizabeth Hospital	Appleton	99%	510
Sauk Prairie Hospital	Prairie Du Sac	99%	127
Theda Clark Medical Center	Neenah	99%	548
Wheaton Franciscan Hlthcare St Francis	Milwaukee	99%	123
Howard Young Medical Center	Woodruff	98%	42
Lakeview Medical Center	Rice Lake	98%	62
Mayo Clinic Hlth Sys Franciscan Med Ctr	La Crosse	98%	276
Mayo Clinic Hlth Sys-Eau Claire Hosp	Eau Claire	98%	495
Riverview Hospital Assoc	Wisc. Rapids	98%	42
Saint Agnes Hospital	Fond Du Lac	98%	367
Univ of WI Hosps & Clinics Authority	Madison	98%	303
Waukesha Memorial Hospital	Waukesha	98%	428
Wheaton Franciscan Healthcare All Saints	Racine	98%	269
Aurora Baycare Medical Center	Green Bay	97%	538
Aurora Medical Center Manitowoc County	Two Rivers	97%	133
Aurora Saint Lukes Medical Center	Milwaukee	97%	857
Froedtert Memorial Lutheran Hospital	Milwaukee	97%	517
Mercy Medical Center of Oshkosh	Oshkosh	97%	282
Meriter Hospital	Madison	97%	329
Ministry Saint Marys Hospital	Rhinelander	97%	39
Ministry St Michaels Hosp-Stevens Pt	Stevens Point	97%	37
Reedsburg Area Medical Center	Reedsburg	97%	66
Saint Joseph's Hospital	Chippewa Falls	97%	33
Saint Marys Hospital	Madison	97%	931
Wheaton Franciscan Saint Joseph	Milwaukee	97%	582
Aurora Lakeland Medical Center	Elkhorn	96%	28
Aurora Medical Center Oshkosh	Oshkosh	96%	235
Aurora Medical Center Washington County	Hartford	96%	27
Community Memorial Hospital	Menomonee Fls	96%	229
Fort Memorial Hospital	Fort Atkinson	96%	118
Gundersen Lutheran Medical Center	La Crosse	96%	721
Mercy Health System Corp	Janesville	96%	268
Sacred Heart Hospital	Eau Claire	96%	384

NOTE: Hospital profiles are in alphabetical order by state, then city, then hospital within the city; Rankings exclude hospitals with less than 25 cases except for patient surveys which excludes hospitals with less than 100 cases; (a) 100-299 cases; (1) The number of cases/patients is too few to report; (2) Data submitted were based on a sample of cases/patients; (3) Results are based on a shorter time period than required; (4) Data suppressed by CMS for one or more quarters; (5) Results are not available for this reporting period; (6) Fewer than 100 patients completed the HCAHPS survey; (7) No cases met the criteria for this measure; (8) The lower limit of the confidence interval cannot be calculated if the number of observed infections equals zero; (9) No data are available from the state/territory for this reporting period; (10) The scores shown reflect fewer than 50 completed surveys; (11) There were discrepancies in the data collection process; (12) This measure does not apply to this hospital for this reporting period; (13) Results cannot be calculated for this reporting period; (14) The results for this state are combined with nearby states to protect confidentiality; Please refer to the User's Guide for a full explanation of data.

Saint Marys Hospital Medical Center	Green Bay	96%	301
United Hospital System	Kenosha	96%	300
Appleton Medical Center	Appleton	95%	328
Aurora Medical Center Kenosha	Kenosha	95%	250
Beloit Memorial Hospital	Beloit	95%	93
Oconomowoc Memorial Hospital	Oconomowoc	95%	60
River Falls Area Hospital	River Falls	95%	40
Aurora Memorial Hospital Burlington	Burlington	94%	65
The Monroe Clinic	Monroe	94%	186
Saint Nicholas Hospital	Sheboygan	94%	80
Wheaton Franciscan Healthcare Franklin	Franklin	94%	36
Columbia Saint Marys Hospital Milwaukee	Milwaukee	92%	403
Saint Marys Janesville Hospital	Janesville	88%	50
Columbia Saint Marys Hospital Ozaukee	Mequon	86%	208
Langlade Hospital[3]	Antigo	84%	25
UW Hlth Partners Watertown Reg Med Ctr	Watertown	82%	106
Mile Bluff Medical Center	Mauston	71%	79

Urinary Catheter Removal

Hospital Name	City	Rate	Cases
Aurora Lakeland Medical Center[2]	Elkhorn	100%	89
Aurora Medical Center[2]	Grafton	100%	718
Aurora Medical Center[2]	Summit	100%	214
Aurora Sheboygan Memorial Medical Center[2]	Sheboygan	100%	531
Berlin Memorial Hospital[2]	Berlin	100%	136
Hudson Hospital	Hudson	100%	109
Lakeview Medical Center[2]	Rice Lake	100%	268
Madison VA Medical Center[2]	Madison	100%	108
Mayo Clinic Health System - Red Cedar	Menomonie	100%	56
Mercy Medical Center of Oshkosh[2]	Oshkosh	100%	234
Midwest Orthopedic Specialty Hospital[2]	Franklin	100%	107
Milwaukee VA Medical Center[2]	Milwaukee	100%	284
Ministry St Michaels Hosp-Stevens Pt	Stevens Point	100%	282
Orthopaedic Hospital of Wisconsin[2]	Glendale	100%	190
Prairie Du Chien Memorial Hospital	Prairie Du Chien	100%	38
River Falls Area Hospital	River Falls	100%	102
Saint Clare Hospital Health Services	Baraboo	100%	108
St Joseph's Comm Hosp of West Bend	West Bend	100%	250
Saint Marys Hospital Medical Center[2]	Green Bay	100%	277
Sauk Prairie Hospital	Prairie Du Sac	100%	531
Aurora Medical Center Kenosha[2]	Kenosha	99%	377
Aurora Medical Center Washington County[2]	Hartford	99%	173
Aurora Memorial Hospital Burlington[2]	Burlington	99%	195
Aurora Saint Lukes Medical Center	Milwaukee	99%	1914
Bay Area Medical Center	Marinette	99%	125
Columbia Saint Marys Hospital Ozaukee[2]	Mequon	99%	285
Froedtert Memorial Lutheran Hospital[2]	Milwaukee	99%	522
Gundersen Lutheran Medical Center[2]	La Crosse	99%	635
Holy Family Memorial	Manitowoc	99%	339
Howard Young Medical Center	Woodruff	99%	287
Mayo Clinic Hlth Sys Franciscan Med Ctr	La Crosse	99%	621
Mayo Clinic Hlth Sys-Eau Claire Hosp	Eau Claire	99%	673
Ministry Door County Medical Center	Sturgeon Bay	99%	111
Ministry Saint Marys Hospital	Rhinelander	99%	90
Oak Leaf Surgical Hospital	Eau Claire	99%	139
Sacred Heart Hospital[2]	Eau Claire	99%	337
Saint Clares Hospital of Weston	Weston	99%	393
Saint Elizabeth Hospital[2]	Appleton	99%	336
Saint Marys Hospital[2]	Madison	99%	1371
Saint Vincent Hospital[2]	Green Bay	99%	234
United Hospital System	Kenosha	99%	558
Waukesha Memorial Hospital[2]	Waukesha	99%	382
Westfields Hospital	New Richmond	99%	103
Appleton Medical Center[2]	Appleton	98%	666
Aurora Medical Center Manitowoc County[2]	Two Rivers	98%	43
Community Memorial Hospital[2]	Menomonee Fls	98%	346
Mercy Health System Corp	Janesville	98%	504
Ministry Saint Josephs Hospital	Marshfield	98%	803
The Monroe Clinic	Monroe	98%	195
Oconomowoc Memorial Hospital[2]	Oconomowoc	98%	162
Saint Joseph's Hospital	Chippewa Falls	98%	62
Waupun Memorial Hospital	Waupun	98%	61
Wheaton Franciscan Healthcare All Saints[2]	Racine	98%	216
Wheaton Franciscan Saint Joseph[2]	Milwaukee	98%	532
Mercy Walworth Hospital & Medical Center	Lake Geneva	97%	186
Meriter Hospital[2]	Madison	97%	182
Saint Agnes Hospital	Fond Du Lac	97%	346
Stoughton Hospital	Stoughton	97%	34
Univ of WI Hosps & Clinics Authority[2]	Madison	97%	262
Aurora Medical Center Oshkosh[2]	Oshkosh	96%	80
Aurora West Allis Medical Center[2]	West Allis	96%	164
Beaver Dam Com Hospital	Beaver Dam	96%	195
Bellin Memorial Hospital[2]	Green Bay	96%	315
Richland Hospital	Richland Center	96%	50
Vernon Memorial Hospital	Viroqua	96%	50
Aurora Baycare Medical Center[2]	Green Bay	95%	145
Columbia Saint Marys Hospital Milwaukee[2]	Milwaukee	95%	206
Ripon Medical Center[3]	Ripon	95%	37
Theda Clark Medical Center[2]	Neenah	95%	275
UW Hlth Partners Watertown Reg Med Ctr	Watertown	95%	120
Fort Memorial Hospital[2]	Fort Atkinson	94%	52
Saint Nicholas Hospital[2]	Sheboygan	94%	219
Upland Hills Health	Dodgeville	94%	64
Wheaton Franciscan Hlthcare St Francis	Milwaukee	94%	139
Riverview Hospital Assoc[2]	Wisc. Rapids	92%	26
Saint Marys Janesville Hospital	Janesville	92%	238
Beloit Memorial Hospital[2]	Beloit	91%	157
Columbus Community Hospital	Columbus	91%	58
Aspirus Wausau Hospital[2]	Wausau	89%	256
Divine Savior Healthcare	Portage	89%	28
Wheaton Franciscan Healthcare Franklin	Franklin	85%	41
Mile Bluff Medical Center	Mauston	78%	36

Survey of Patients' Hospital Experiences

Area Around Room 'Always' Quiet at Night

Hospital Name	City	Rate	Cases
Midwest Orthopedic Specialty Hospital	Franklin	84%	300+
Oak Leaf Surgical Hospital	Eau Claire	81%	300+
Hayward Area Memorial Hospital	Hayward	77%	(a)
Orthopaedic Hospital of Wisconsin	Glendale	76%	300+
Columbia Center	Mequon	75%	(a)
Ministry Eagle River Memorial Hospital	Eagle River	75%	(a)
Ministry Door County Medical Center	Sturgeon Bay	74%	300+
Aurora Medical Center	Summit	73%	300+
Riverview Hospital Assoc	Wisc. Rapids	73%	300+
Spooner Health System	Spooner	73%	(a)
Black River Memorial Hospital	Black River Falls	72%	(a)
Calumet Medical Center	Chilton	71%	(a)
Memorial Health Center	Medford	71%	(a)
Sauk Prairie Hospital	Prairie Du Sac	71%	300+
Waupun Memorial Hospital	Waupun	71%	(a)
River Falls Area Hospital	River Falls	70%	(a)
Saint Clare Hospital Health Services[11]	Baraboo	70%	300+
Tomah Memorial Hospital	Tomah	70%	(a)
Waukesha Memorial Hospital	Waukesha	70%	300+
Amery Regional Medical Center	Amery	69%	(a)
Grant Regional Health Center	Lancaster	69%	(a)
Ladd Memorial Hospital	Osceola	69%	(a)
The Monroe Clinic	Monroe	69%	300+
Prairie Du Chien Memorial Hospital	Prairie Du Chien	69%	300+
St Joseph's Comm Hosp of West Bend	West Bend	69%	300+
Saint Marys Janesville Hospital	Janesville	69%	300+
Southwest Health Center	Platteville	69%	(a)
Wheaton Franciscan Healthcare Franklin	Franklin	69%	300+
Oconomowoc Memorial Hospital	Oconomowoc	68%	300+
Stoughton Hospital	Stoughton	68%	(a)
Upland Hills Health	Dodgeville	68%	300+
Fort Memorial Hospital	Fort Atkinson	67%	300+
Hudson Hospital	Hudson	67%	300+
Reedsburg Area Medical Center	Reedsburg	67%	300+
Saint Joseph's Hospital	Chippewa Falls	67%	300+
Aurora Baycare Medical Center	Green Bay	66%	300+
Aurora Medical Center	Grafton	66%	300+
Bellin Memorial Hospital[11]	Green Bay	66%	300+
Lakeview Medical Center	Rice Lake	66%	300+
Mayo Clinic Health System - Red Cedar	Menomonie	66%	300+
Ministry St Michaels Hosp-Stevens Pt	Stevens Point	66%	300+
Riverside Medical Center	Waupaca	66%	(a)
Vernon Memorial Hospital	Viroqua	66%	300+
Aurora Medical Center Manitowoc County	Two Rivers	65%	300+
Saint Marys Hospital[11]	Madison	65%	300+
Aurora West Allis Medical Center	West Allis	64%	300+
Bay Area Medical Center	Marinette	64%	300+
Flambeau Hospital	Park Falls	64%	(a)
Memorial Hospital Lafayette Cty	Darlington	64%	(a)
Mercy Health System Corp	Janesville	64%	300+
Aurora Sheboygan Memorial Medical Center	Sheboygan	63%	300+
Community Memorial Hospital	Oconto Falls	63%	(a)
Memorial Medical Center	Ashland	63%	300+
Saint Marys Hospital Medical Center	Green Bay	63%	300+
Saint Vincent Hospital	Green Bay	63%	300+
Westfields Hospital	New Richmond	63%	300+
Wheaton Franciscan Saint Joseph	Milwaukee	63%	300+
Aspirus Wausau Hospital	Wausau	62%	300+
Columbia Saint Marys Hospital Ozaukee	Mequon	62%	300+
Langlade Hospital	Antigo	62%	(a)
Richland Hospital	Richland Center	62%	(a)
Saint Croix Regional Medical Center	Saint Croix Falls	62%	300+
Aurora Lakeland Medical Center	Elkhorn	61%	300+
Good Samaritan Health Center	Merrill	61%	(a)
Mayo Clinic Hlth Sys-Eau Claire Hosp	Eau Claire	61%	300+
Mayo Clinic Health System - Northland	Barron	61%	(a)
Saint Elizabeth Hospital	Appleton	61%	300+
Univ of WI Hosps & Clinics Authority	Madison	61%	300+
Columbus Community Hospital	Columbus	60%	(a)
Divine Savior Healthcare	Portage	60%	300+
Rusk County Memorial Hospital	Ladysmith	60%	(a)
UW Hlth Partners Watertown Reg Med Ctr	Watertown	60%	300+
Aurora Medical Center Kenosha	Kenosha	59%	300+
Aurora Medical Center Washington County	Hartford	59%	300+
Beaver Dam Com Hospital	Beaver Dam	59%	300+
Columbia Saint Marys Hospital Milwaukee	Milwaukee	59%	300+
Froedtert Memorial Lutheran Hospital	Milwaukee	59%	300+
Meriter Hospital	Madison	59%	300+
Sacred Heart Hospital	Eau Claire	59%	300+
Berlin Memorial Hospital	Berlin	58%	300+
Burnett Medical Center	Grantsburg	58%	(a)
Community Memorial Hospital	Menomonee Fls	58%	300+
Mercy Medical Center of Oshkosh	Oshkosh	58%	300+
Saint Agnes Hospital	Fond Du Lac	58%	300+
Saint Clares Hospital of Weston	Weston	58%	300+
Saint Nicholas Hospital	Sheboygan	58%	300+
Appleton Medical Center	Appleton	57%	300+
Aurora Medical Center Oshkosh	Oshkosh	57%	300+
Aurora Memorial Hospital Burlington	Burlington	57%	300+
New London Family Medical Center	New London	57%	(a)
Shawano Medical Center	Shawano	56%	300+
Wheaton Franciscan Healthcare All Saints	Racine	56%	300+
Aurora Saint Lukes Medical Center	Milwaukee	55%	300+
Holy Family Memorial	Manitowoc	55%	300+
Ministry Saint Marys Hospital	Rhinelander	55%	300+
Theda Clark Medical Center	Neenah	55%	300+
Beloit Memorial Hospital	Beloit	54%	300+
Mayo Clinic Hlth Sys Franciscan Med Ctr	La Crosse	54%	300+
United Hospital System	Kenosha	53%	300+
Wheaton Franciscan Hlthcare St Francis	Milwaukee	53%	300+
Howard Young Medical Center	Woodruff	52%	300+
Mile Bluff Medical Center	Mauston	51%	300+
Ripon Medical Center	Ripon	51%	(a)
Gundersen Lutheran Medical Center	La Crosse	47%	300+
Ministry Saint Josephs Hospital	Marshfield	47%	300+

Doctors 'Always' Communicated Well

Hospital Name	City	Rate	Cases
Orthopaedic Hospital of Wisconsin	Glendale	92%	300+
Grant Regional Health Center	Lancaster	91%	(a)
Black River Memorial Hospital	Black River Falls	90%	(a)
Memorial Hospital Lafayette Cty	Darlington	90%	(a)
Flambeau Hospital	Park Falls	89%	(a)
Midwest Orthopedic Specialty Hospital	Franklin	89%	300+
Sauk Prairie Hospital	Prairie Du Sac	89%	300+
Spooner Health System	Spooner	89%	(a)
Stoughton Hospital	Stoughton	89%	(a)
Vernon Memorial Hospital	Viroqua	89%	300+
Aurora Medical Center	Summit	88%	300+
Columbia Center	Mequon	88%	(a)
Upland Hills Health	Dodgeville	88%	300+
Burnett Medical Center	Grantsburg	87%	(a)
Hudson Hospital	Hudson	87%	300+
Mayo Clinic Health System - Red Cedar	Menomonie	87%	300+
Southwest Health Center	Platteville	87%	(a)
Columbus Community Hospital	Columbus	86%	(a)
Langlade Hospital	Antigo	86%	(a)
Ministry Eagle River Memorial Hospital	Eagle River	86%	(a)
River Falls Area Hospital	River Falls	86%	(a)
Hayward Area Memorial Hospital	Hayward	85%	(a)
Howard Young Medical Center	Woodruff	85%	300+
Memorial Health Center	Medford	85%	(a)
Memorial Medical Center	Ashland	85%	300+
Ministry Door County Medical Center	Sturgeon Bay	85%	300+
Oak Leaf Surgical Hospital	Eau Claire	85%	300+
Reedsburg Area Medical Center	Reedsburg	85%	300+
Saint Clare Hospital Health Services[11]	Baraboo	85%	300+
Saint Joseph's Hospital	Chippewa Falls	85%	300+
Tomah Memorial Hospital	Tomah	85%	(a)
Waupun Memorial Hospital	Waupun	85%	(a)
Aurora Lakeland Medical Center	Elkhorn	84%	300+
Aurora Medical Center	Grafton	84%	300+
Aurora Medical Center Washington County	Hartford	84%	300+
Lakeview Medical Center	Rice Lake	84%	300+
Ministry St Michaels Hosp-Stevens Pt	Stevens Point	84%	300+
Rusk County Memorial Hospital	Ladysmith	84%	(a)
Calumet Medical Center	Chilton	83%	(a)
Ladd Memorial Hospital	Osceola	83%	(a)
Mayo Clinic Hlth Sys Franciscan Med Ctr	La Crosse	83%	300+
Mayo Clinic Hlth Sys-Eau Claire Hosp	Eau Claire	83%	300+
Mercy Medical Center of Oshkosh	Oshkosh	83%	300+
Mile Bluff Medical Center	Mauston	83%	300+
Oconomowoc Memorial Hospital	Oconomowoc	83%	300+
Prairie Du Chien Memorial Hospital	Prairie Du Chien	83%	300+
Richland Hospital	Richland Center	83%	(a)
Riverside Medical Center	Waupaca	83%	(a)
Saint Marys Hospital[11]	Madison	83%	300+
Saint Marys Hospital Medical Center	Green Bay	83%	300+
Saint Marys Janesville Hospital	Janesville	83%	300+
Wheaton Franciscan Healthcare All Saints	Racine	83%	300+
Aspirus Wausau Hospital	Wausau	82%	300+
Aurora Sheboygan Memorial Medical Center	Sheboygan	82%	300+
Bay Area Medical Center	Marinette	82%	300+
Bellin Memorial Hospital[11]	Green Bay	82%	300+
Community Memorial Hospital	Oconto Falls	82%	(a)

NOTE: Hospital profiles are in alphabetical order by state, then city, then hospital within the city; Rankings exclude hospitals with less than 25 cases except for patient surveys which excludes hospitals with less than 100 cases; (a) 100-299 cases; (1) The number of cases/patients is too few to report; (2) Data submitted were based on a sample of cases/patients; (3) Results are based on a shorter time period than required; (4) Data suppressed by CMS for one or more quarters; (5) Results are not available for this reporting period; (6) Fewer than 100 patients completed the HCAHPS survey; (7) No cases met the criteria for this measure; (8) The lower limit of the confidence interval cannot be calculated if the number of observed infections equals zero; (9) No data are available from the state/territory for this reporting period; (10) The scores shown reflect fewer than 50 completed surveys; (11) There were discrepancies in the data collection process; (12) This measure does not apply to this hospital for this reporting period; (13) Results cannot be calculated for this reporting period; (14) The results for this state are combined with nearby states to protect confidentiality; Please refer to the User's Guide for a full explanation of data.

Gundersen Lutheran Medical Center	La Crosse	82%	300+
Meriter Hospital	Madison	82%	300+
Ministry Saint Marys Hospital	Rhinelander	82%	300+
Riverview Hospital Assoc	Wisc. Rapids	82%	300+
Sacred Heart Hospital	Eau Claire	82%	300+
Saint Elizabeth Hospital	Appleton	82%	300+
Saint Nicholas Hospital	Sheboygan	82%	300+
Theda Clark Medical Center	Neenah	82%	300+
Univ of WI Hosps & Clinics Authority	Madison	82%	300+
Westfields Hospital	New Richmond	82%	300+
Aurora Baycare Medical Center	Green Bay	81%	300+
Aurora Medical Center Manitowoc County	Two Rivers	81%	300+
Beaver Dam Com Hospital	Beaver Dam	81%	300+
Berlin Memorial Hospital	Berlin	81%	300+
Columbia Saint Marys Hospital Milwaukee	Milwaukee	81%	300+
Fort Memorial Hospital	Fort Atkinson	81%	300+
Mayo Clinic Health System - Northland	Barron	81%	(a)
The Monroe Clinic	Monroe	81%	300+
New London Family Medical Center	New London	81%	(a)
Saint Clares Hospital of Weston	Weston	81%	300+
St Joseph's Comm Hosp of West Bend	West Bend	81%	300+
Shawano Medical Center	Shawano	81%	300+
Wheaton Franciscan Healthcare Franklin	Franklin	81%	300+
Wheaton Franciscan Saint Joseph	Milwaukee	81%	300+
Amery Regional Medical Center	Amery	80%	(a)
Appleton Medical Center	Appleton	80%	300+
Aurora Medical Center Oshkosh	Oshkosh	80%	300+
Aurora Saint Lukes Medical Center	Milwaukee	80%	300+
Beloit Memorial Hospital	Beloit	80%	300+
Community Memorial Hospital	Menomonee Fls	80%	300+
Divine Savior Healthcare	Portage	80%	300+
Ripon Medical Center	Ripon	80%	(a)
Saint Agnes Hospital	Fond Du Lac	80%	300+
Saint Vincent Hospital	Green Bay	80%	300+
Waukesha Memorial Hospital	Waukesha	80%	300+
Aurora West Allis Medical Center	West Allis	79%	300+
Froedtert Memorial Lutheran Hospital	Milwaukee	79%	300+
Good Samaritan Health Center	Merrill	79%	(a)
Holy Family Memorial	Manitowoc	79%	300+
United Hospital System	Kenosha	79%	300+
Wheaton Franciscan Hlthcare St Francis	Milwaukee	79%	300+
Aurora Medical Center Kenosha	Kenosha	78%	300+
Columbia Saint Marys Hospital Ozaukee	Mequon	78%	300+
Mercy Health System Corp	Janesville	78%	300+
Saint Croix Regional Medical Center	Saint Croix Falls	78%	300+
Aurora Memorial Hospital Burlington	Burlington	77%	300+
UW Hlth Partners Watertown Reg Med Ctr	Watertown	76%	300+
Ministry Saint Josephs Hospital	Marshfield	74%	300+

Home Recovery Information Given

Hospital Name	City	Rate	Cases
Black River Memorial Hospital	Black River Falls	94%	(a)
Flambeau Hospital	Park Falls	94%	(a)
Orthopaedic Hospital of Wisconsin	Glendale	94%	300+
Midwest Orthopedic Specialty Hospital	Franklin	93%	300+
Oak Leaf Surgical Hospital	Eau Claire	93%	300+
Aurora Medical Center Oshkosh	Oshkosh	92%	300+
Aurora Sheboygan Memorial Medical Center	Sheboygan	92%	300+
Mayo Clinic Health System - Northland	Barron	92%	(a)
Ministry Eagle River Memorial Hospital	Eagle River	92%	(a)
River Falls Area Hospital	River Falls	92%	(a)
Sauk Prairie Hospital	Prairie Du Sac	92%	300+
Vernon Memorial Hospital	Viroqua	92%	300+
Waupun Memorial Hospital	Waupun	92%	(a)
Langlade Hospital	Antigo	91%	(a)
Memorial Health Center	Medford	91%	(a)
Stoughton Hospital	Stoughton	91%	(a)
Upland Hills Health	Dodgeville	91%	300+
Amery Regional Medical Center	Amery	90%	(a)
Aspirus Wausau Hospital	Wausau	90%	300+
Aurora Medical Center	Grafton	90%	300+
Aurora Medical Center	Summit	90%	300+
Bellin Memorial Hospital[11]	Green Bay	90%	300+
Calumet Medical Center	Chilton	90%	(a)
Columbus Community Hospital	Columbus	90%	(a)
Gundersen Lutheran Medical Center	La Crosse	90%	300+
Holy Family Memorial	Manitowoc	90%	300+
Ladd Memorial Hospital	Osceola	90%	(a)
Mayo Clinic Hlth Sys-Eau Claire Hosp	Eau Claire	90%	300+
Ministry St Michaels Hosp-Stevens Pt	Stevens Point	90%	300+
The Monroe Clinic	Monroe	90%	300+
Saint Clare Hospital Health Services[11]	Baraboo	90%	300+
Saint Clares Hospital of Weston	Weston	90%	300+
Saint Croix Regional Medical Center	Saint Croix Falls	90%	300+
Saint Marys Hospital[11]	Madison	90%	300+
Tomah Memorial Hospital	Tomah	90%	(a)
Univ of WI Hosps & Clinics Authority	Madison	90%	300+
Waukesha Memorial Hospital	Waukesha	90%	300+
Appleton Medical Center	Appleton	89%	300+
Aurora Medical Center Washington County	Hartford	89%	300+
Beaver Dam Com Hospital	Beaver Dam	89%	300+
Columbia Center	Mequon	89%	(a)
Fort Memorial Hospital	Fort Atkinson	89%	300+
Howard Young Medical Center	Woodruff	89%	300+
Lakeview Medical Center	Rice Lake	89%	300+
Mercy Medical Center of Oshkosh	Oshkosh	89%	300+
Ministry Saint Marys Hospital	Rhinelander	89%	300+
New London Family Medical Center	New London	89%	(a)
Prairie Du Chien Memorial Hospital	Prairie Du Chien	89%	300+
Saint Elizabeth Hospital	Appleton	89%	300+
Southwest Health Center	Platteville	89%	(a)
Spooner Health System	Spooner	89%	(a)
Theda Clark Medical Center	Neenah	89%	300+
Aurora Medical Center Manitowoc County	Two Rivers	88%	300+
Berlin Memorial Hospital	Berlin	88%	300+
Froedtert Memorial Lutheran Hospital	Milwaukee	88%	300+
Grant Regional Health Center	Lancaster	88%	(a)
Mayo Clinic Hlth Sys Franciscan Med Ctr	La Crosse	88%	300+
Mayo Clinic Health System - Red Cedar	Menomonie	88%	300+
Ministry Saint Josephs Hospital	Marshfield	88%	300+
Oconomowoc Memorial Hospital	Oconomowoc	88%	300+
Ripon Medical Center	Ripon	88%	(a)
Riverside Medical Center	Waupaca	88%	(a)
Riverview Hospital Assoc	Wisc. Rapids	88%	300+
Saint Joseph's Hospital	Chippewa Falls	88%	300+
Saint Marys Janesville Hospital	Janesville	88%	300+
Wheaton Franciscan Healthcare All Saints	Racine	88%	300+
Wheaton Franciscan Healthcare Franklin	Franklin	88%	300+
Wheaton Franciscan Hlthcare St Francis	Milwaukee	88%	300+
Aurora Baycare Medical Center	Green Bay	87%	300+
Aurora Lakeland Medical Center	Elkhorn	87%	300+
Beloit Memorial Hospital	Beloit	87%	300+
Burnett Medical Center	Grantsburg	87%	(a)
Community Memorial Hospital	Menomonee Fls	87%	300+
Good Samaritan Health Center	Merrill	87%	(a)
Hayward Area Memorial Hospital	Hayward	87%	(a)
Meriter Hospital	Madison	87%	300+
Ministry Door County Medical Center	Sturgeon Bay	87%	300+
Reedsburg Area Medical Center	Reedsburg	87%	300+
Richland Hospital	Richland Center	87%	(a)
Sacred Heart Hospital	Eau Claire	87%	300+
St Joseph's Comm Hosp of West Bend	West Bend	87%	300+
Saint Marys Hospital Medical Center	Green Bay	87%	300+
Saint Nicholas Hospital	Sheboygan	87%	300+
Saint Vincent Hospital	Green Bay	87%	300+
Shawano Medical Center	Shawano	87%	300+
Westfields Hospital	New Richmond	87%	300+
Aurora Memorial Hospital Burlington	Burlington	86%	300+
Aurora West Allis Medical Center	West Allis	86%	300+
Columbia Saint Marys Hospital Milwaukee	Milwaukee	86%	300+
Columbia Saint Marys Hospital Ozaukee	Mequon	86%	300+
Community Memorial Hospital	Oconto Falls	86%	(a)
Hudson Hospital	Hudson	86%	300+
Memorial Hospital Lafayette Cty	Darlington	86%	(a)
Mercy Health System Corp	Janesville	86%	300+
Mile Bluff Medical Center	Mauston	86%	300+
Rusk County Memorial Hospital	Ladysmith	86%	(a)
Saint Agnes Hospital	Fond Du Lac	86%	300+
UW Hlth Partners Watertown Reg Med Ctr	Watertown	86%	300+
Aurora Saint Lukes Medical Center	Milwaukee	85%	300+
Memorial Medical Center	Ashland	85%	300+
Wheaton Franciscan Saint Joseph	Milwaukee	85%	300+
Aurora Medical Center Kenosha	Kenosha	84%	300+
Bay Area Medical Center	Marinette	84%	300+
Divine Savior Healthcare	Portage	84%	300+
United Hospital System	Kenosha	83%	300+

Hospital Given 9 or 10 on 10 Point Scale

Hospital Name	City	Rate	Cases
Columbia Center	Mequon	94%	(a)
Orthopaedic Hospital of Wisconsin	Glendale	94%	300+
Midwest Orthopedic Specialty Hospital	Franklin	93%	300+
Oak Leaf Surgical Hospital	Eau Claire	90%	300+
Sauk Prairie Hospital	Prairie Du Sac	87%	300+
Stoughton Hospital	Stoughton	87%	(a)
River Falls Area Hospital	River Falls	85%	(a)
Upland Hills Health	Dodgeville	85%	300+
Vernon Memorial Hospital	Viroqua	84%	300+
Grant Regional Health Center	Lancaster	83%	(a)
Memorial Hospital Lafayette Cty	Darlington	83%	(a)
Ministry Door County Medical Center	Sturgeon Bay	83%	300+
Saint Marys Janesville Hospital	Janesville	83%	300+
Aurora Medical Center	Grafton	82%	300+
Aurora Medical Center	Summit	82%	300+
Black River Memorial Hospital	Black River Falls	82%	(a)
Langlade Hospital	Antigo	82%	(a)
Mayo Clinic Hlth Sys-Eau Claire Hosp	Eau Claire	82%	300+
Bellin Memorial Hospital[11]	Green Bay	81%	300+
Waukesha Memorial Hospital	Waukesha	81%	300+
Wheaton Franciscan Healthcare Franklin	Franklin	81%	300+
Froedtert Memorial Lutheran Hospital	Milwaukee	80%	300+
Hudson Hospital	Hudson	80%	300+
Memorial Health Center	Medford	80%	(a)
Saint Marys Hospital[11]	Madison	80%	300+
Ladd Memorial Hospital	Osceola	79%	(a)
Lakeview Medical Center	Rice Lake	79%	300+
Saint Clare Hospital Health Services[11]	Baraboo	79%	300+
Saint Joseph's Hospital	Chippewa Falls	79%	300+
Aspirus Wausau Hospital	Wausau	78%	300+
Calumet Medical Center	Chilton	78%	(a)
Mercy Medical Center of Oshkosh	Oshkosh	78%	300+
Meriter Hospital	Madison	78%	300+
Univ of WI Hosps & Clinics Authority	Madison	78%	300+
Waupun Memorial Hospital	Waupun	78%	(a)
Aurora Baycare Medical Center	Green Bay	77%	300+
Flambeau Hospital	Park Falls	77%	(a)
Prairie Du Chien Memorial Hospital	Prairie Du Chien	77%	300+
Richland Hospital	Richland Center	77%	(a)
Appleton Medical Center	Appleton	76%	300+
Aurora Medical Center Manitowoc County	Two Rivers	76%	300+
Columbus Community Hospital	Columbus	76%	(a)
Fort Memorial Hospital	Fort Atkinson	76%	300+
Mayo Clinic Health System - Red Cedar	Menomonie	76%	300+
The Monroe Clinic	Monroe	76%	300+
Saint Clares Hospital of Weston	Weston	76%	300+
Theda Clark Medical Center	Neenah	76%	300+
Tomah Memorial Hospital	Tomah	76%	(a)
Gundersen Lutheran Medical Center	La Crosse	75%	300+
Mayo Clinic Hlth Sys Franciscan Med Ctr	La Crosse	75%	300+
Oconomowoc Memorial Hospital	Oconomowoc	75%	300+
Reedsburg Area Medical Center	Reedsburg	75%	300+
Sacred Heart Hospital	Eau Claire	74%	300+
Saint Elizabeth Hospital	Appleton	74%	300+
Southwest Health Center	Platteville	74%	(a)
Aurora Medical Center Oshkosh	Oshkosh	73%	300+
Memorial Medical Center	Ashland	73%	300+
Spooner Health System	Spooner	73%	(a)
Aurora Sheboygan Memorial Medical Center	Sheboygan	72%	300+
Aurora West Allis Medical Center	West Allis	72%	300+
Community Memorial Hospital	Menomonee Fls	72%	300+
Good Samaritan Health Center	Merrill	72%	(a)
Ministry Eagle River Memorial Hospital	Eagle River	72%	(a)
Ministry St Michaels Hosp-Stevens Pt	Stevens Point	72%	300+
Riverview Hospital Assoc	Wisc. Rapids	72%	300+
Saint Marys Hospital Medical Center	Green Bay	72%	300+
United Hospital System	Kenosha	72%	300+
UW Hlth Partners Watertown Reg Med Ctr	Watertown	72%	300+
Aurora Saint Lukes Medical Center	Milwaukee	71%	300+
Burnett Medical Center	Grantsburg	71%	(a)
Columbia Saint Marys Hospital Ozaukee	Mequon	71%	300+
Holy Family Memorial	Manitowoc	71%	300+
Howard Young Medical Center	Woodruff	71%	300+
Saint Croix Regional Medical Center	Saint Croix Falls	71%	300+
Saint Vincent Hospital	Green Bay	71%	300+
Westfields Hospital	New Richmond	71%	300+
Wheaton Franciscan Saint Joseph	Milwaukee	71%	300+
Columbia Saint Marys Hospital Milwaukee	Milwaukee	70%	300+
Mayo Clinic Health System - Northland	Barron	70%	(a)
Mercy Health System Corp	Janesville	70%	300+
Riverside Medical Center	Waupaca	70%	(a)
St Joseph's Comm Hosp of West Bend	West Bend	70%	300+
Beaver Dam Com Hospital	Beaver Dam	69%	300+
Hayward Area Memorial Hospital	Hayward	69%	(a)
Ministry Saint Marys Hospital	Rhinelander	69%	300+
Amery Regional Medical Center	Amery	68%	(a)
Aurora Medical Center Washington County	Hartford	68%	300+
Berlin Memorial Hospital	Berlin	68%	300+
Saint Nicholas Hospital	Sheboygan	68%	300+
Wheaton Franciscan Healthcare All Saints	Racine	68%	300+
Bay Area Medical Center	Marinette	67%	300+
Beloit Memorial Hospital	Beloit	67%	300+
Ministry Saint Josephs Hospital	Marshfield	67%	300+
Saint Agnes Hospital	Fond Du Lac	67%	300+
Wheaton Franciscan Hlthcare St Francis	Milwaukee	67%	300+
Aurora Medical Center Kenosha	Kenosha	66%	300+
Community Memorial Hospital	Oconto Falls	66%	(a)
Divine Savior Healthcare	Portage	66%	300+
Mile Bluff Medical Center	Mauston	66%	300+
Aurora Lakeland Medical Center	Elkhorn	65%	300+
New London Family Medical Center	New London	62%	(a)
Ripon Medical Center	Ripon	61%	(a)
Rusk County Memorial Hospital	Ladysmith	61%	(a)
Shawano Medical Center	Shawano	60%	300+
Aurora Memorial Hospital Burlington	Burlington	58%	300+

Meds 'Always' Explained Before Given

Hospital Name	City	Rate	Cases
Oak Leaf Surgical Hospital	Eau Claire	80%	300+
Orthopaedic Hospital of Wisconsin	Glendale	79%	300+
Memorial Health Center	Medford	78%	(a)
Midwest Orthopedic Specialty Hospital	Franklin	77%	300+
Prairie Du Chien Memorial Hospital	Prairie Du Chien	77%	300+
River Falls Area Hospital	River Falls	77%	(a)

NOTE: Hospital profiles are in alphabetical order by state, then city, then hospital within the city; Rankings exclude hospitals with less than 25 cases except for patient surveys which excludes hospitals with less than 100 cases; (a) 100-299 cases; (1) The number of cases/patients is too few to report; (2) Data submitted were based on a sample of cases/patients; (3) Results are based on a shorter time period than required; (4) Data suppressed by CMS for one or more quarters; (5) Results are not available for this reporting period; (6) Fewer than 100 patients completed the HCAHPS survey; (7) No cases met the criteria for this measure; (8) The lower limit of the confidence interval cannot be calculated if the number of observed infections equals zero; (9) No data are available from the state/territory for this reporting period; (10) The scores shown reflect fewer than 50 completed surveys; (11) There were discrepancies in the data collection process; (12) This measure does not apply to this hospital for this reporting period; (13) Results cannot be calculated for this reporting period; (14) The results for this state are combined with nearby states to protect confidentiality; Please refer to the User's Guide for a full explanation of data.

Hospital Name	City	Rate	Cases
Sauk Prairie Hospital	Prairie Du Sac	77%	300+
Calumet Medical Center	Chilton	76%	(a)
Ministry Eagle River Memorial Hospital	Eagle River	76%	(a)
Spooner Health System	Spooner	76%	(a)
Aurora Medical Center	Summit	75%	300+
Stoughton Hospital	Stoughton	75%	(a)
Grant Regional Health Center	Lancaster	74%	(a)
Vernon Memorial Hospital	Viroqua	74%	300+
Black River Memorial Hospital	Black River Falls	73%	(a)
Columbia Center	Mequon	73%	(a)
Flambeau Hospital	Park Falls	73%	(a)
Memorial Hospital Lafayette Cty	Darlington	73%	(a)
Saint Marys Janesville Hospital	Janesville	73%	300+
Howard Young Medical Center	Woodruff	72%	300+
Ministry Door County Medical Center	Sturgeon Bay	72%	300+
Saint Marys Hospital[11]	Madison	72%	300+
Columbus Community Hospital	Columbus	71%	(a)
Good Samaritan Health Center	Merrill	71%	(a)
Ladd Memorial Hospital	Osceola	71%	(a)
Langlade Hospital	Antigo	71%	(a)
Ministry St Michaels Hosp-Stevens Pt	Stevens Point	71%	300+
The Monroe Clinic	Monroe	71%	300+
Riverview Hospital Assoc	Wisc. Rapids	71%	300+
Upland Hills Health	Dodgeville	71%	300+
Waupun Memorial Hospital	Waupun	71%	(a)
Divine Savior Healthcare	Portage	70%	300+
Lakeview Medical Center	Rice Lake	70%	300+
Mercy Medical Center of Oshkosh	Oshkosh	70%	300+
Reedsburg Area Medical Center	Reedsburg	70%	300+
Wheaton Franciscan Healthcare Franklin	Franklin	70%	300+
Aurora Medical Center	Grafton	69%	300+
Bellin Memorial Hospital[11]	Green Bay	69%	300+
Gundersen Lutheran Medical Center	La Crosse	69%	300+
Hudson Hospital	Hudson	69%	300+
Mayo Clinic Health System - Northland	Barron	69%	(a)
Memorial Medical Center	Ashland	69%	300+
Saint Clare Hospital Health Services[11]	Baraboo	69%	300+
Saint Elizabeth Hospital	Appleton	69%	300+
Saint Joseph's Hospital	Chippewa Falls	69%	300+
Amery Regional Medical Center	Amery	68%	(a)
Aurora Sheboygan Memorial Medical Center	Sheboygan	68%	300+
Fort Memorial Hospital	Fort Atkinson	68%	300+
Meriter Hospital	Madison	68%	300+
Ministry Saint Marys Hospital	Rhinelander	68%	300+
Tomah Memorial Hospital	Tomah	68%	(a)
UW Hlth Partners Watertown Reg Med Ctr	Watertown	68%	300+
Aurora Medical Center Manitowoc County	Two Rivers	67%	300+
Aurora Medical Center Oshkosh	Oshkosh	67%	300+
Berlin Memorial Hospital	Berlin	67%	300+
Froedtert Memorial Lutheran Hospital	Milwaukee	67%	300+
Mayo Clinic Hlth Sys Franciscan Med Ctr	La Crosse	67%	300+
Saint Clares Hospital of Weston	Weston	67%	300+
Saint Marys Hospital Medical Center	Green Bay	67%	300+
Aurora Baycare Medical Center	Green Bay	66%	300+
Bay Area Medical Center	Marinette	66%	300+
Beaver Dam Com Hospital	Beaver Dam	66%	300+
Hayward Area Memorial Hospital	Hayward	66%	(a)
Mayo Clinic Hlth Sys-Eau Claire Hosp	Eau Claire	66%	300+
Mile Bluff Medical Center	Mauston	66%	300+
Ministry Saint Josephs Hospital	Marshfield	66%	300+
Oconomowoc Memorial Hospital	Oconomowoc	66%	300+
Richland Hospital	Richland Center	66%	(a)
Riverside Medical Center	Waupaca	66%	(a)
Sacred Heart Hospital	Eau Claire	66%	300+
Saint Croix Regional Medical Center	Saint Croix Falls	66%	300+
Univ of WI Hosps & Clinics Authority	Madison	66%	300+
Waukesha Memorial Hospital	Waukesha	66%	300+
Aurora Saint Lukes Medical Center	Milwaukee	65%	300+
Mayo Clinic Health System - Red Cedar	Menomonie	65%	300+
Mercy Health System Corp	Janesville	65%	300+
Rusk County Memorial Hospital	Ladysmith	65%	(a)
St Joseph's Comm Hosp of West Bend	West Bend	65%	300+
Theda Clark Medical Center	Neenah	65%	300+
Aurora Lakeland Medical Center	Elkhorn	64%	300+
Aurora West Allis Medical Center	West Allis	64%	300+
Community Memorial Hospital	Menomonee Fls	64%	300+
Community Memorial Hospital	Oconto Falls	64%	(a)
Saint Vincent Hospital	Green Bay	64%	300+
Wheaton Franciscan Healthcare All Saints	Racine	64%	300+
Wheaton Franciscan Saint Joseph	Milwaukee	64%	300+
Appleton Medical Center	Appleton	63%	300+
Aurora Medical Center Washington County	Hartford	63%	300+
Beloit Memorial Hospital	Beloit	63%	300+
Columbia Saint Marys Hospital Ozaukee	Mequon	63%	300+
Holy Family Memorial	Manitowoc	63%	300+
Saint Nicholas Hospital	Sheboygan	63%	300+
Westfields Hospital	New Richmond	63%	300+
Wheaton Franciscan Hlthcare St Francis	Milwaukee	63%	300+
Aspirus Wausau Hospital	Wausau	62%	300+
Columbia Saint Marys Hospital Milwaukee	Milwaukee	62%	300+
Ripon Medical Center	Ripon	62%	(a)
Saint Agnes Hospital	Fond Du Lac	62%	300+
Southwest Health Center	Platteville	62%	(a)
United Hospital System	Kenosha	62%	300+
Aurora Medical Center Kenosha	Kenosha	60%	300+
Shawano Medical Center	Shawano	60%	300+
Aurora Memorial Hospital Burlington	Burlington	59%	300+
Burnett Medical Center	Grantsburg	59%	(a)
New London Family Medical Center	New London	59%	(a)

Nurses 'Always' Communicated Well

Hospital Name	City	Rate	Cases
Oak Leaf Surgical Hospital	Eau Claire	94%	300+
Orthopaedic Hospital of Wisconsin	Glendale	94%	300+
Midwest Orthopedic Specialty Hospital	Franklin	92%	300+
Stoughton Hospital	Stoughton	90%	(a)
Grant Regional Health Center	Lancaster	89%	(a)
River Falls Area Hospital	River Falls	89%	(a)
Sauk Prairie Hospital	Prairie Du Sac	89%	300+
Spooner Health System	Spooner	89%	(a)
Black River Memorial Hospital	Black River Falls	88%	(a)
Calumet Medical Center	Chilton	88%	(a)
Columbia Center	Mequon	88%	(a)
Flambeau Hospital	Park Falls	87%	(a)
Memorial Hospital Lafayette Cty	Darlington	87%	(a)
Saint Marys Hospital[11]	Madison	87%	300+
Vernon Memorial Hospital	Viroqua	87%	300+
Saint Clare Hospital Health Services[11]	Baraboo	86%	300+
Waupun Memorial Hospital	Waupun	86%	(a)
Aurora Medical Center	Grafton	85%	300+
Aurora Medical Center	Summit	85%	300+
Langlade Hospital	Antigo	85%	(a)
Ministry Door County Medical Center	Sturgeon Bay	85%	300+
The Monroe Clinic	Monroe	85%	300+
Saint Marys Janesville Hospital	Janesville	85%	300+
Upland Hills Health	Dodgeville	85%	300+
Howard Young Medical Center	Woodruff	84%	300+
Hudson Hospital	Hudson	84%	300+
Memorial Health Center	Medford	84%	(a)
Ministry Eagle River Memorial Hospital	Eagle River	84%	(a)
Prairie Du Chien Memorial Hospital	Prairie Du Chien	84%	300+
Richland Hospital	Richland Center	84%	(a)
Saint Joseph's Hospital	Chippewa Falls	84%	300+
Wheaton Franciscan Healthcare Franklin	Franklin	84%	300+
Aurora Medical Center Oshkosh	Oshkosh	83%	300+
Bellin Memorial Hospital[11]	Green Bay	83%	300+
Froedtert Memorial Lutheran Hospital	Milwaukee	83%	300+
Good Samaritan Health Center	Merrill	83%	(a)
Ministry St Michaels Hosp-Stevens Pt	Stevens Point	83%	300+
Univ of WI Hosps & Clinics Authority	Madison	83%	300+
Aurora Baycare Medical Center	Green Bay	82%	300+
Bay Area Medical Center	Marinette	82%	300+
Fort Memorial Hospital	Fort Atkinson	82%	300+
Hayward Area Memorial Hospital	Hayward	82%	(a)
Memorial Medical Center	Ashland	82%	300+
Mercy Medical Center of Oshkosh	Oshkosh	82%	300+
Oconomowoc Memorial Hospital	Oconomowoc	82%	300+
Riverview Hospital Assoc	Wisc. Rapids	82%	300+
Sacred Heart Hospital	Eau Claire	82%	300+
Saint Clares Hospital of Weston	Weston	82%	300+
Tomah Memorial Hospital	Tomah	82%	(a)
Waukesha Memorial Hospital	Waukesha	82%	300+
Aspirus Wausau Hospital	Wausau	81%	300+
Aurora Medical Center Manitowoc County	Two Rivers	81%	300+
Aurora Medical Center Washington County	Hartford	81%	300+
Aurora Sheboygan Memorial Medical Center	Sheboygan	81%	300+
Beaver Dam Com Hospital	Beaver Dam	81%	300+
Burnett Medical Center	Grantsburg	81%	(a)
Columbus Community Hospital	Columbus	81%	(a)
Ladd Memorial Hospital	Osceola	81%	(a)
Lakeview Medical Center	Rice Lake	81%	300+
Mercy Health System Corp	Janesville	81%	300+
Ministry Saint Marys Hospital	Rhinelander	81%	300+
Beloit Memorial Hospital	Beloit	80%	300+
Berlin Memorial Hospital	Berlin	80%	300+
Holy Family Memorial	Manitowoc	80%	300+
Mayo Clinic Hlth Sys Franciscan Med Ctr	La Crosse	80%	300+
Mayo Clinic Hlth Sys-Eau Claire Hosp	Eau Claire	80%	300+
Meriter Hospital	Madison	80%	300+
Reedsburg Area Medical Center	Reedsburg	80%	300+
UW Hlth Partners Watertown Reg Med Ctr	Watertown	80%	300+
Wheaton Franciscan Healthcare All Saints	Racine	80%	300+
Amery Regional Medical Center	Amery	79%	(a)
Aurora Saint Lukes Medical Center	Milwaukee	79%	300+
Community Memorial Hospital	Menomonee Fls	79%	300+
Community Memorial Hospital	Oconto Falls	79%	(a)
Divine Savior Healthcare	Portage	79%	300+
Mayo Clinic Health System - Red Cedar	Menomonie	79%	300+
Rusk County Memorial Hospital	Ladysmith	79%	(a)
Saint Croix Regional Medical Center	Saint Croix Falls	79%	300+
Saint Elizabeth Hospital	Appleton	79%	300+
Saint Marys Hospital Medical Center	Green Bay	79%	300+
Theda Clark Medical Center	Neenah	79%	300+
Wheaton Franciscan Saint Joseph	Milwaukee	79%	300+
Appleton Medical Center	Appleton	78%	300+
Aurora Lakeland Medical Center	Elkhorn	78%	300+
Aurora West Allis Medical Center	West Allis	78%	300+
Columbia Saint Marys Hospital Ozaukee	Mequon	78%	300+
Gundersen Lutheran Medical Center	La Crosse	78%	300+
Ministry Saint Josephs Hospital	Marshfield	78%	300+
Ripon Medical Center	Ripon	78%	(a)
Saint Nicholas Hospital	Sheboygan	78%	300+
Saint Vincent Hospital	Green Bay	78%	300+
Southwest Health Center	Platteville	78%	(a)
Columbia Saint Marys Hospital Milwaukee	Milwaukee	77%	300+
Mile Bluff Medical Center	Mauston	77%	300+
Saint Agnes Hospital	Fond Du Lac	77%	300+
Shawano Medical Center	Shawano	77%	300+
Westfields Hospital	New Richmond	77%	300+
United Hospital System	Kenosha	76%	300+
Wheaton Franciscan Hlthcare St Francis	Milwaukee	76%	300+
Aurora Medical Center Kenosha	Kenosha	75%	300+
Mayo Clinic Health System - Northland	Barron	75%	(a)
New London Family Medical Center	New London	75%	(a)
Riverside Medical Center	Waupaca	75%	(a)
St Joseph's Comm Hosp of West Bend	West Bend	75%	300+
Aurora Memorial Hospital Burlington	Burlington	73%	300+

Pain 'Always' Well Controlled

Hospital Name	City	Rate	Cases
Stoughton Hospital	Stoughton	83%	(a)
Midwest Orthopedic Specialty Hospital	Franklin	82%	300+
Ministry Eagle River Memorial Hospital	Eagle River	81%	(a)
Oak Leaf Surgical Hospital	Eau Claire	81%	300+
Orthopaedic Hospital of Wisconsin	Glendale	81%	300+
Vernon Memorial Hospital	Viroqua	80%	300+
Spooner Health System	Spooner	79%	(a)
Black River Memorial Hospital	Black River Falls	78%	(a)
River Falls Area Hospital	River Falls	78%	(a)
Upland Hills Health	Dodgeville	78%	300+
Ministry Door County Medical Center	Sturgeon Bay	77%	300+
Prairie Du Chien Memorial Hospital	Prairie Du Chien	77%	300+
Aurora Medical Center	Summit	76%	300+
Columbia Center	Mequon	76%	(a)
Flambeau Hospital	Park Falls	76%	(a)
Memorial Health Center	Medford	76%	(a)
Saint Marys Hospital[11]	Madison	76%	300+
Bellin Memorial Hospital[11]	Green Bay	75%	300+
Grant Regional Health Center	Lancaster	75%	(a)
Howard Young Medical Center	Woodruff	75%	300+
Langlade Hospital	Antigo	75%	(a)
Mayo Clinic Health System - Northland	Barron	75%	(a)
Ministry St Michaels Hosp-Stevens Pt	Stevens Point	75%	300+
The Monroe Clinic	Monroe	75%	300+
Sauk Prairie Hospital	Prairie Du Sac	75%	300+
Univ of WI Hosps & Clinics Authority	Madison	75%	300+
Waupun Memorial Hospital	Waupun	75%	(a)
Aurora Medical Center	Grafton	74%	300+
Saint Joseph's Hospital	Chippewa Falls	74%	300+
Saint Marys Janesville Hospital	Janesville	74%	300+
Tomah Memorial Hospital	Tomah	74%	(a)
Wheaton Franciscan Healthcare Franklin	Franklin	74%	300+
Aurora Medical Center Manitowoc County	Two Rivers	73%	300+
Aurora Medical Center Oshkosh	Oshkosh	73%	300+
Aurora Sheboygan Memorial Medical Center	Sheboygan	73%	300+
Burnett Medical Center	Grantsburg	73%	(a)
Hudson Hospital	Hudson	73%	300+
Ladd Memorial Hospital	Osceola	73%	(a)
Mercy Medical Center of Oshkosh	Oshkosh	73%	300+
Saint Marys Hospital Medical Center	Green Bay	73%	300+
Aurora Baycare Medical Center	Green Bay	72%	300+
Berlin Memorial Hospital	Berlin	72%	300+
Calumet Medical Center	Chilton	72%	(a)
Hayward Area Memorial Hospital	Hayward	72%	(a)
Riverview Hospital Assoc	Wisc. Rapids	72%	300+
Sacred Heart Hospital	Eau Claire	72%	300+
Saint Clares Hospital of Weston	Weston	72%	300+
UW Hlth Partners Watertown Reg Med Ctr	Watertown	72%	300+
Wheaton Franciscan Saint Joseph	Milwaukee	72%	300+
Aurora Lakeland Medical Center	Elkhorn	71%	300+
Aurora Medical Center Washington County	Hartford	71%	300+
Aurora Saint Lukes Medical Center	Milwaukee	71%	300+
Beaver Dam Com Hospital	Beaver Dam	71%	300+
Columbus Community Hospital	Columbus	71%	(a)
Community Memorial Hospital	Menomonee Fls	71%	300+
Froedtert Memorial Lutheran Hospital	Milwaukee	71%	300+
Mayo Clinic Hlth Sys Franciscan Med Ctr	La Crosse	71%	300+
Memorial Medical Center	Ashland	71%	300+
Mercy Health System Corp	Janesville	71%	300+
Ministry Saint Josephs Hospital	Marshfield	71%	300+
Ministry Saint Marys Hospital	Rhinelander	71%	300+
Oconomowoc Memorial Hospital	Oconomowoc	71%	300+
Richland Hospital	Richland Center	71%	(a)

NOTE: Hospital profiles are in alphabetical order by state, then city, then hospital within the city; Rankings exclude hospitals with less than 25 cases except for patient surveys which excludes hospitals with less than 100 cases; (a) 100-299 cases; (1) The number of cases/patients is too few to report; (2) Data submitted were based on a sample of cases/patients; (3) Results are based on a shorter time period than required; (4) Data suppressed by CMS for one or more quarters; (5) Results are not available for this reporting period; (6) Fewer than 100 patients completed the HCAHPS survey; (7) No cases met the criteria for this measure; (8) The lower limit of the confidence interval cannot be calculated if the number of observed infections equals zero; (9) No data are available from the state/territory for this reporting period; (10) The scores shown reflect fewer than 50 completed surveys; (11) There were discrepancies in the data collection process; (12) This measure does not apply to this hospital for this reporting period; (13) Results cannot be calculated for this reporting period; (14) The results for this state are combined with nearby states to protect confidentiality; Please refer to the User's Guide for a full explanation of data.

Hospital Name	City	Rate	Cases
Wheaton Franciscan Healthcare All Saints	Racine	71%	300+
Appleton Medical Center	Appleton	70%	300+
Aspirus Wausau Hospital	Wausau	70%	300+
Columbia Saint Marys Hospital Milwaukee	Milwaukee	70%	300+
Lakeview Medical Center	Rice Lake	70%	300+
Mayo Clinic Hlth Sys-Eau Claire Hosp	Eau Claire	70%	300+
Mayo Clinic Health System - Red Cedar	Menomonie	70%	300+
Memorial Hospital Lafayette Cty	Darlington	70%	(a)
Reedsburg Area Medical Center	Reedsburg	70%	300+
Saint Elizabeth Hospital	Appleton	70%	300+
Theda Clark Medical Center	Neenah	70%	300+
Waukesha Memorial Hospital	Waukesha	70%	300+
Aurora West Allis Medical Center	West Allis	69%	300+
Bay Area Medical Center	Marinette	69%	300+
Meriter Hospital	Madison	69%	300+
Riverside Medical Center	Waupaca	69%	(a)
Rusk County Memorial Hospital	Ladysmith	69%	(a)
Saint Clare Hospital Health Services[11]	Baraboo	69%	300+
Saint Croix Regional Medical Center	Saint Croix Falls	69%	300+
United Hospital System	Kenosha	69%	300+
Amery Regional Medical Center	Amery	68%	(a)
Beloit Memorial Hospital	Beloit	68%	300+
Fort Memorial Hospital	Fort Atkinson	68%	300+
Holy Family Memorial	Manitowoc	68%	300+
Ripon Medical Center	Ripon	68%	(a)
St Joseph's Comm Hosp of West Bend	West Bend	68%	300+
Saint Vincent Hospital	Green Bay	68%	300+
Shawano Medical Center	Shawano	68%	300+
Aurora Medical Center Kenosha	Kenosha	67%	300+
Divine Savior Healthcare	Portage	67%	300+
Gundersen Lutheran Medical Center	La Crosse	67%	300+
Saint Nicholas Hospital	Sheboygan	67%	300+
Southwest Health Center	Platteville	67%	(a)
Westfields Hospital	New Richmond	67%	300+
Wheaton Franciscan Hlthcare St Francis	Milwaukee	67%	300+
Aurora Memorial Hospital Burlington	Burlington	66%	300+
Saint Agnes Hospital	Fond Du Lac	66%	300+
Columbia Saint Marys Hospital Ozaukee	Mequon	65%	300+
Good Samaritan Health Center	Merrill	65%	(a)
Mile Bluff Medical Center	Mauston	64%	300+
New London Family Medical Center	New London	64%	(a)
Community Memorial Hospital	Oconto Falls	61%	(a)

Room and Bathroom 'Always' Clean

Hospital Name	City	Rate	Cases
Stoughton Hospital	Stoughton	94%	(a)
Ministry Door County Medical Center	Sturgeon Bay	91%	300+
River Falls Area Hospital	River Falls	91%	(a)
Rusk County Memorial Hospital	Ladysmith	91%	(a)
Oak Leaf Surgical Hospital	Eau Claire	90%	300+
Vernon Memorial Hospital	Viroqua	89%	300+
Calumet Medical Center	Chilton	88%	(a)
Midwest Orthopedic Specialty Hospital	Franklin	88%	300+
Prairie Du Chien Memorial Hospital	Prairie Du Chien	88%	300+
Spooner Health System	Spooner	88%	(a)
Aurora Medical Center Manitowoc County	Two Rivers	87%	300+
Burnett Medical Center	Grantsburg	87%	(a)
Flambeau Hospital	Park Falls	87%	(a)
Ministry Eagle River Memorial Hospital	Eagle River	87%	(a)
Richland Hospital	Richland Center	87%	(a)
Upland Hills Health	Dodgeville	87%	300+
Lakeview Medical Center	Rice Lake	86%	300+
Orthopaedic Hospital of Wisconsin	Glendale	86%	300+
Riverview Hospital Assoc	Wisc. Rapids	86%	300+
Saint Marys Janesville Hospital	Janesville	86%	300+
Memorial Hospital Lafayette Cty	Darlington	85%	(a)
Sauk Prairie Hospital	Prairie Du Sac	85%	300+
Fort Memorial Hospital	Fort Atkinson	84%	300+
Reedsburg Area Medical Center	Reedsburg	84%	300+
Southwest Health Center	Platteville	84%	(a)
Amery Regional Medical Center	Amery	83%	(a)
Columbus Community Hospital	Columbus	83%	(a)
Grant Regional Health Center	Lancaster	83%	(a)
Columbia Center	Mequon	82%	(a)
Good Samaritan Health Center	Merrill	82%	(a)
Memorial Medical Center	Ashland	82%	300+
Ministry St Michaels Hosp-Stevens Pt	Stevens Point	82%	300+
Riverside Medical Center	Waupaca	82%	(a)
Wheaton Franciscan Healthcare Franklin	Franklin	82%	300+
Aurora Medical Center	Summit	81%	300+
Aurora Medical Center Oshkosh	Oshkosh	81%	300+
Saint Clare Hospital Health Services[11]	Baraboo	81%	300+
Saint Marys Hospital[11]	Madison	81%	300+
Waukesha Memorial Hospital	Waukesha	81%	300+
Aurora Baycare Medical Center	Green Bay	80%	300+
Memorial Health Center	Medford	80%	(a)
The Monroe Clinic	Monroe	80%	300+
New London Family Medical Center	New London	80%	(a)
Oconomowoc Memorial Hospital	Oconomowoc	80%	300+
Saint Agnes Hospital	Fond Du Lac	80%	300+
Aurora Medical Center Washington County	Hartford	79%	300+
Beaver Dam Com Hospital	Beaver Dam	79%	300+
Berlin Memorial Hospital	Berlin	79%	300+
Langlade Hospital	Antigo	79%	(a)
Mayo Clinic Hlth Sys-Eau Claire Hosp	Eau Claire	79%	300+
Saint Croix Regional Medical Center	Saint Croix Falls	79%	300+
Saint Joseph's Hospital	Chippewa Falls	79%	300+
Saint Vincent Hospital	Green Bay	79%	300+
Tomah Memorial Hospital	Tomah	79%	(a)
Ladd Memorial Hospital	Osceola	78%	(a)
Saint Clares Hospital of Weston	Weston	78%	300+
St Joseph's Comm Hosp of West Bend	West Bend	78%	300+
Saint Marys Hospital Medical Center	Green Bay	78%	300+
Westfields Hospital	New Richmond	78%	300+
Aurora Medical Center	Grafton	77%	300+
Bellin Memorial Hospital[11]	Green Bay	77%	300+
Hayward Area Memorial Hospital	Hayward	77%	(a)
Holy Family Memorial	Manitowoc	77%	300+
Meriter Hospital	Madison	77%	300+
Ministry Saint Marys Hospital	Rhinelander	77%	300+
Ripon Medical Center	Ripon	77%	(a)
Sacred Heart Hospital	Eau Claire	77%	300+
UW Hlth Partners Watertown Reg Med Ctr	Watertown	77%	300+
Appleton Medical Center	Appleton	76%	300+
Bay Area Medical Center	Marinette	76%	300+
Black River Memorial Hospital	Black River Falls	76%	(a)
Howard Young Medical Center	Woodruff	76%	300+
Mayo Clinic Health System - Red Cedar	Menomonie	76%	300+
Mercy Medical Center of Oshkosh	Oshkosh	76%	300+
Theda Clark Medical Center	Neenah	76%	300+
United Hospital System	Kenosha	76%	300+
Divine Savior Healthcare	Portage	75%	300+
Mayo Clinic Health System - Northland	Barron	75%	(a)
Mercy Health System Corp	Janesville	75%	300+
Aurora Lakeland Medical Center	Elkhorn	74%	300+
Aurora Sheboygan Memorial Medical Center	Sheboygan	74%	300+
Beloit Memorial Hospital	Beloit	74%	300+
Gundersen Lutheran Medical Center	La Crosse	74%	300+
Mayo Clinic Hlth Sys Franciscan Med Ctr	La Crosse	74%	300+
Mile Bluff Medical Center	Mauston	74%	300+
Saint Elizabeth Hospital	Appleton	74%	300+
Saint Nicholas Hospital	Sheboygan	74%	300+
Univ of WI Hosps & Clinics Authority	Madison	74%	300+
Hudson Hospital	Hudson	73%	300+
Ministry Saint Josephs Hospital	Marshfield	73%	300+
Aurora Medical Center Kenosha	Kenosha	72%	300+
Aurora Memorial Hospital Burlington	Burlington	72%	300+
Aurora Saint Lukes Medical Center	Milwaukee	71%	300+
Aurora West Allis Medical Center	West Allis	71%	300+
Community Memorial Hospital	Menomonee Fls	71%	300+
Wheaton Franciscan Saint Joseph	Milwaukee	71%	300+
Aspirus Wausau Hospital	Wausau	70%	300+
Froedtert Memorial Lutheran Hospital	Milwaukee	70%	300+
Shawano Medical Center	Shawano	70%	300+
Waupun Memorial Hospital	Waupun	70%	(a)
Wheaton Franciscan Healthcare All Saints	Racine	70%	300+
Wheaton Franciscan Hlthcare St Francis	Milwaukee	70%	300+
Community Memorial Hospital	Oconto Falls	67%	(a)
Columbia Saint Marys Hospital Milwaukee	Milwaukee	66%	300+
Columbia Saint Marys Hospital Ozaukee	Mequon	66%	300+

Timely Help 'Always' Received

Hospital Name	City	Rate	Cases
Oak Leaf Surgical Hospital	Eau Claire	92%	300+
Grant Regional Health Center	Lancaster	87%	(a)
Midwest Orthopedic Specialty Hospital	Franklin	86%	300+
Vernon Memorial Hospital	Viroqua	86%	300+
Orthopaedic Hospital of Wisconsin	Glendale	85%	300+
Calumet Medical Center	Chilton	84%	(a)
Ladd Memorial Hospital	Osceola	84%	(a)
Ministry Eagle River Memorial Hospital	Eagle River	84%	(a)
Ministry Door County Medical Center	Sturgeon Bay	83%	300+
River Falls Area Hospital	River Falls	83%	(a)
Sauk Prairie Hospital	Prairie Du Sac	83%	300+
Stoughton Hospital	Stoughton	83%	(a)
Prairie Du Chien Memorial Hospital	Prairie Du Chien	82%	300+
Black River Memorial Hospital	Black River Falls	80%	(a)
Upland Hills Health	Dodgeville	80%	300+
Columbia Center	Mequon	79%	(a)
Memorial Hospital Lafayette Cty	Darlington	79%	(a)
Southwest Health Center	Platteville	79%	(a)
Saint Clare Hospital Health Services[11]	Baraboo	78%	300+
Bellin Memorial Hospital[11]	Green Bay	77%	300+
Flambeau Hospital	Park Falls	77%	(a)
Langlade Hospital	Antigo	77%	(a)
Spooner Health System	Spooner	77%	(a)
Waupun Memorial Hospital	Waupun	77%	(a)
Amery Regional Medical Center	Amery	76%	(a)
The Monroe Clinic	Monroe	76%	300+
Saint Joseph's Hospital	Chippewa Falls	76%	300+
Wheaton Franciscan Healthcare Franklin	Franklin	76%	300+
Hudson Hospital	Hudson	75%	300+
Rusk County Memorial Hospital	Ladysmith	75%	(a)
Aurora Medical Center	Grafton	74%	300+
Aurora Medical Center Oshkosh	Oshkosh	74%	300+
Community Memorial Hospital	Oconto Falls	74%	(a)
Divine Savior Healthcare	Portage	74%	300+
Good Samaritan Health Center	Merrill	74%	(a)
Hayward Area Memorial Hospital	Hayward	74%	(a)
Mayo Clinic Health System - Red Cedar	Menomonie	74%	300+
Memorial Health Center	Medford	74%	(a)
Tomah Memorial Hospital	Tomah	74%	(a)
UW Hlth Partners Watertown Reg Med Ctr	Watertown	74%	300+
Westfields Hospital	New Richmond	74%	300+
Aurora Medical Center Washington County	Hartford	73%	300+
Bay Area Medical Center	Marinette	73%	300+
Beaver Dam Com Hospital	Beaver Dam	73%	300+
Burnett Medical Center	Grantsburg	73%	(a)
Lakeview Medical Center	Rice Lake	73%	300+
Memorial Medical Center	Ashland	73%	300+
Mercy Medical Center of Oshkosh	Oshkosh	73%	300+
Saint Clares Hospital of Weston	Weston	73%	300+
Saint Croix Regional Medical Center	Saint Croix Falls	73%	300+
Saint Marys Hospital[11]	Madison	73%	300+
Saint Marys Janesville Hospital	Janesville	73%	300+
Berlin Memorial Hospital	Berlin	72%	300+
Mayo Clinic Health System - Northland	Barron	72%	(a)
Richland Hospital	Richland Center	72%	(a)
Sacred Heart Hospital	Eau Claire	72%	300+
Aurora Medical Center	Summit	71%	300+
Aurora Medical Center Manitowoc County	Two Rivers	71%	300+
Columbus Community Hospital	Columbus	71%	(a)
Howard Young Medical Center	Woodruff	71%	300+
Mile Bluff Medical Center	Mauston	71%	300+
Riverview Hospital Assoc	Wisc. Rapids	71%	300+
Aurora Baycare Medical Center	Green Bay	70%	300+
Holy Family Memorial	Manitowoc	70%	300+
Mayo Clinic Hlth Sys-Eau Claire Hosp	Eau Claire	70%	300+
Mercy Health System Corp	Janesville	70%	300+
Ripon Medical Center	Ripon	70%	(a)
Riverside Medical Center	Waupaca	70%	(a)
Saint Marys Hospital Medical Center	Green Bay	70%	300+
Univ of WI Hosps & Clinics Authority	Madison	70%	300+
Mayo Clinic Hlth Sys Franciscan Med Ctr	La Crosse	69%	300+
Ministry Saint Marys Hospital	Rhinelander	69%	300+
Ministry St Michaels Hosp-Stevens Pt	Stevens Point	69%	300+
Oconomowoc Memorial Hospital	Oconomowoc	69%	300+
Reedsburg Area Medical Center	Reedsburg	69%	300+
Theda Clark Medical Center	Neenah	69%	300+
Aurora Lakeland Medical Center	Elkhorn	68%	300+
United Hospital System	Kenosha	68%	300+
Fort Memorial Hospital	Fort Atkinson	67%	300+
Waukesha Memorial Hospital	Waukesha	67%	300+
Meriter Hospital	Madison	66%	300+
New London Family Medical Center	New London	66%	(a)
Saint Elizabeth Hospital	Appleton	66%	300+
Appleton Medical Center	Appleton	65%	300+
Aspirus Wausau Hospital	Wausau	65%	300+
Aurora Medical Center Kenosha	Kenosha	65%	300+
Froedtert Memorial Lutheran Hospital	Milwaukee	65%	300+
Shawano Medical Center	Shawano	65%	300+
Wheaton Franciscan Saint Joseph	Milwaukee	65%	300+
Beloit Memorial Hospital	Beloit	64%	300+
Community Memorial Hospital	Menomonee Fls	64%	300+
Saint Nicholas Hospital	Sheboygan	64%	300+
Wheaton Franciscan Hlthcare St Francis	Milwaukee	64%	300+
Aurora Saint Lukes Medical Center	Milwaukee	63%	300+
Aurora Sheboygan Memorial Medical Center	Sheboygan	63%	300+
Gundersen Lutheran Medical Center	La Crosse	63%	300+
Aurora West Allis Medical Center	West Allis	62%	300+
Saint Vincent Hospital	Green Bay	62%	300+
Wheaton Franciscan Healthcare All Saints	Racine	61%	300+
Saint Agnes Hospital	Fond Du Lac	60%	300+
Columbia Saint Marys Hospital Milwaukee	Milwaukee	59%	300+
Ministry Saint Josephs Hospital	Marshfield	59%	300+
St Joseph's Comm Hosp of West Bend	West Bend	57%	300+
Columbia Saint Marys Hospital Ozaukee	Mequon	56%	300+
Aurora Memorial Hospital Burlington	Burlington	52%	300+

Would Definitely Recommend Hospital

Hospital Name	City	Rate	Cases
Midwest Orthopedic Specialty Hospital	Franklin	94%	300+
Orthopaedic Hospital of Wisconsin	Glendale	94%	300+
Columbia Center	Mequon	93%	(a)
Oak Leaf Surgical Hospital	Eau Claire	91%	300+
Sauk Prairie Hospital	Prairie Du Sac	89%	300+
Upland Hills Health	Dodgeville	87%	300+
Saint Marys Janesville Hospital	Janesville	86%	300+
Stoughton Hospital	Stoughton	86%	(a)
Mayo Clinic Hlth Sys-Eau Claire Hosp	Eau Claire	85%	300+
Univ of WI Hosps & Clinics Authority	Madison	85%	300+
Bellin Memorial Hospital[11]	Green Bay	84%	300+
Hudson Hospital	Hudson	84%	300+

NOTE: Hospital profiles are in alphabetical order by state, then city, then hospital within the city; Rankings exclude hospitals with less than 25 cases except for patient surveys which excludes hospitals with less than 100 cases; (a) 100-299 cases; (1) The number of cases/patients is too few to report; (2) Data submitted were based on a sample of cases/patients; (3) Results are based on a shorter time period than required; (4) Data suppressed by CMS for one or more quarters; (5) Results are not available for this reporting period; (6) Fewer than 100 patients completed the HCAHPS survey; (7) No cases met the criteria for this measure; (8) The lower limit of the confidence interval cannot be calculated if the number of observed infections equals zero; (9) No data are available from the state/territory for this reporting period; (10) The scores shown reflect fewer than 50 completed surveys; (11) There were discrepancies in the data collection process; (12) This measure does not apply to this hospital for this reporting period; (13) Results cannot be calculated for this reporting period; (14) The results for this state are combined with nearby states to protect confidentiality; Please refer to the User's Guide for a full explanation of data.

Hospital Name	City	Rate	Cases
Ministry Door County Medical Center	Sturgeon Bay	84%	300+
Aurora Medical Center	Grafton	83%	300+
Froedtert Memorial Lutheran Hospital	Milwaukee	83%	300+
Grant Regional Health Center	Lancaster	83%	(a)
Saint Marys Hospital[11]	Madison	83%	300+
Aurora Medical Center	Summit	82%	300+
Black River Memorial Hospital	Black River Falls	82%	(a)
Vernon Memorial Hospital	Viroqua	82%	300+
Wheaton Franciscan Healthcare Franklin	Franklin	82%	300+
Ladd Memorial Hospital	Osceola	81%	(a)
Lakeview Medical Center	Rice Lake	81%	300+
River Falls Area Hospital	River Falls	81%	(a)
Waukesha Memorial Hospital	Waukesha	81%	300+
Aspirus Wausau Hospital	Wausau	80%	300+
Gundersen Lutheran Medical Center	La Crosse	80%	300+
Memorial Hospital Lafayette Cty	Darlington	80%	(a)
Theda Clark Medical Center	Neenah	80%	300+
Aurora Baycare Medical Center	Green Bay	79%	300+
Meriter Hospital	Madison	79%	300+
Appleton Medical Center	Appleton	78%	300+
Aurora Medical Center Manitowoc County	Two Rivers	78%	300+
Langlade Hospital	Antigo	78%	(a)
Mayo Clinic Hlth Sys Franciscan Med Ctr	La Crosse	78%	300+
Oconomowoc Memorial Hospital	Oconomowoc	78%	300+
Mayo Clinic Health System - Red Cedar	Menomonie	77%	300+
Mercy Medical Center of Oshkosh	Oshkosh	77%	300+
The Monroe Clinic	Monroe	77%	300+
Saint Clare Hospital Health Services[11]	Baraboo	77%	300+
Saint Clares Hospital of Weston	Weston	77%	300+
Saint Elizabeth Hospital	Appleton	77%	300+
Saint Joseph's Hospital	Chippewa Falls	77%	300+
Prairie Du Chien Memorial Hospital	Prairie Du Chien	76%	300+
Sacred Heart Hospital	Eau Claire	76%	300+
Aurora Medical Center Oshkosh	Oshkosh	75%	300+
Aurora West Allis Medical Center	West Allis	75%	300+
Columbia Saint Marys Hospital Milwaukee	Milwaukee	75%	300+
Waupun Memorial Hospital	Waupun	75%	(a)
Columbia Saint Marys Hospital Ozaukee	Mequon	74%	300+
Columbus Community Hospital	Columbus	74%	(a)
Community Memorial Hospital	Menomonee Fls	74%	300+
Fort Memorial Hospital	Fort Atkinson	74%	300+
Howard Young Medical Center	Woodruff	74%	300+
Richland Hospital	Richland Center	74%	(a)
Tomah Memorial Hospital	Tomah	74%	(a)
Aurora Saint Lukes Medical Center	Milwaukee	73%	300+
Calumet Medical Center	Chilton	73%	(a)
Holy Family Memorial	Manitowoc	73%	300+
Saint Croix Regional Medical Center	Saint Croix Falls	73%	300+
Saint Marys Hospital Medical Center	Green Bay	73%	300+
Saint Vincent Hospital	Green Bay	73%	300+
United Hospital System	Kenosha	73%	300+
Aurora Sheboygan Memorial Medical Center	Sheboygan	72%	300+
Memorial Health Center	Medford	72%	(a)
Reedsburg Area Medical Center	Reedsburg	72%	300+
Riverview Hospital Assoc	Wisc. Rapids	72%	300+
Burnett Medical Center	Grantsburg	71%	(a)
Ministry Saint Josephs Hospital	Marshfield	71%	300+
Spooner Health System	Spooner	71%	(a)
Westfields Hospital	New Richmond	71%	300+
Good Samaritan Health Center	Merrill	70%	(a)
Saint Nicholas Hospital	Sheboygan	70%	300+
Wheaton Franciscan Saint Joseph	Milwaukee	70%	300+
Aurora Medical Center Kenosha	Kenosha	69%	300+
Berlin Memorial Hospital	Berlin	69%	300+
Flambeau Hospital	Park Falls	69%	(a)
Southwest Health Center	Platteville	69%	(a)
Mayo Clinic Health System - Northland	Barron	68%	(a)
Mercy Health System Corp	Janesville	68%	300+
Ministry Eagle River Memorial Hospital	Eagle River	68%	(a)
St Joseph's Comm Hosp of West Bend	West Bend	68%	300+
Aurora Medical Center Washington County	Hartford	67%	300+
Ministry St Michaels Hosp-Stevens Pt	Stevens Point	67%	300+
Riverside Medical Center	Waupaca	67%	(a)
Wheaton Franciscan Healthcare All Saints	Racine	67%	300+
Beloit Memorial Hospital	Beloit	66%	300+
Memorial Medical Center	Ashland	66%	300+
Ministry Saint Marys Hospital	Rhinelander	66%	300+
UW Hlth Partners Watertown Reg Med Ctr	Watertown	66%	300+
Wheaton Franciscan Hlthcare St Francis	Milwaukee	66%	300+
Amery Regional Medical Center	Amery	65%	(a)
Beaver Dam Com Hospital	Beaver Dam	65%	300+
Mile Bluff Medical Center	Mauston	65%	300+
Saint Agnes Hospital	Fond Du Lac	65%	300+
Hayward Area Memorial Hospital	Hayward	64%	(a)
Aurora Lakeland Medical Center	Elkhorn	63%	300+
Community Memorial Hospital	Oconto Falls	63%	(a)
Ripon Medical Center	Ripon	63%	(a)
Bay Area Medical Center	Marinette	61%	300+
Divine Savior Healthcare	Portage	61%	300+
Shawano Medical Center	Shawano	60%	300+
Aurora Memorial Hospital Burlington	Burlington	57%	300+
New London Family Medical Center	New London	56%	(a)
Rusk County Memorial Hospital	Ladysmith	48%	(a)

Use of Medical Imaging

Cardiac Imaging Stress Test before OP Surgery

Hospital Name	City	Rate	Cases
Berlin Memorial Hospital	Berlin	0.0%	77
Saint Marys Hospital	Madison	1.1%	190
Flambeau Hospital	Park Falls	2.0%	51
Sauk Prairie Hospital	Prairie Du Sac	2.0%	51
Southwest Health Center	Platteville	2.0%	49
Vernon Memorial Hospital	Viroqua	2.1%	47
Mile Bluff Medical Center	Mauston	2.6%	194
Aurora Medical Center Oshkosh	Oshkosh	2.8%	213
Meriter Hospital	Madison	2.8%	180
Saint Clare Hospital Health Services	Baraboo	2.9%	102
Reedsburg Area Medical Center	Reedsburg	3.0%	99
Saint Croix Regional Medical Center	Saint Croix Falls	3.0%	101
Saint Elizabeth Hospital	Appleton	3.1%	225
Beaver Dam Com Hospital	Beaver Dam	3.4%	208
Amery Regional Medical Center	Amery	3.8%	53
Mayo Clinic Hlth Sys-Eau Claire Hosp	Eau Claire	3.8%	422
Saint Marys Hospital Medical Center	Green Bay	3.8%	236
Lakeview Medical Center	Rice Lake	3.9%	203
Aspirus Wausau Hospital	Wausau	4.0%	124
Columbia Saint Marys Hospital Milwaukee	Milwaukee	4.2%	523
Shawano Medical Center	Shawano	4.2%	143
Aurora Lakeland Medical Center	Elkhorn	4.3%	516
Fort Memorial Hospital	Fort Atkinson	4.3%	188
Aurora Medical Center	Summit	4.4%	251
Aurora Medical Center Washington County	Hartford	4.4%	113
Hudson Hospital	Hudson	4.4%	68
Oconomowoc Memorial Hospital	Oconomowoc	4.5%	201
UW Hlth Partners Watertown Reg Med Ctr	Watertown	4.5%	155
Wheaton Franciscan Saint Joseph	Milwaukee	4.5%	645
Aurora Memorial Hospital Burlington	Burlington	4.8%	269
Aurora Medical Center	Grafton	4.9%	205
Boscobel Area Health Care	Boscobel	4.9%	61
Mercy Medical Center of Oshkosh	Oshkosh	4.9%	182
Aurora West Allis Medical Center	West Allis	5.0%	239
Appleton Medical Center	Appleton	5.1%	651
Theda Clark Medical Center	Neenah	5.1%	136
Wheaton Franciscan Healthcare Franklin	Franklin	5.1%	99
Bellin Memorial Hospital	Green Bay	5.2%	542
Aurora Medical Center Kenosha	Kenosha	5.3%	755
Aurora Medical Center Manitowoc County	Two Rivers	5.4%	167
Columbia Saint Marys Hospital Ozaukee	Mequon	5.4%	294
The Monroe Clinic	Monroe	5.4%	386
St Joseph's Comm Hosp of West Bend	West Bend	5.5%	236
Univ of WI Hosps & Clinics Authority	Madison	5.5%	833
Aurora Saint Lukes Medical Center	Milwaukee	5.6%	1039
Beloit Memorial Hospital	Beloit	5.6%	378
Mercy Walworth Hospital & Medical Center	Lake Geneva	5.7%	70
Saint Agnes Hospital	Fond Du Lac	5.8%	463
Divine Savior Healthcare	Portage	5.9%	135
Saint Vincent Hospital	Green Bay	6.0%	302
Mercy Health System Corp	Janesville	6.1%	542
Aurora Baycare Medical Center	Green Bay	6.2%	276
Froedtert Memorial Lutheran Hospital	Milwaukee	6.2%	617
Ministry Door County Medical Center	Sturgeon Bay	6.2%	113
Ministry Saint Josephs Hospital	Marshfield	6.2%	389
Community Memorial Hospital	Menomonee Fls	6.3%	300
Memorial Hospital Lafayette Cty	Darlington	6.3%	63
Ministry Saint Marys Hospital	Rhinelander	6.4%	204
Bay Area Medical Center	Marinette	6.6%	226
Community Memorial Hospital	Oconto Falls	6.6%	61
Waukesha Memorial Hospital	Waukesha	6.8%	720
Langlade Hospital	Antigo	6.9%	131
Sacred Heart Hospital	Eau Claire	6.9%	130
Holy Family Memorial	Manitowoc	7.1%	238
Ministry St Michaels Hosp-Stevens Pt	Stevens Point	7.2%	221
Mayo Clinic Hlth Sys Franciscan Med Ctr	La Crosse	7.4%	433
Riverview Hospital Assoc	Wisc. Rapids	7.5%	147
Wheaton Franciscan Hlthcare St Francis	Milwaukee	7.6%	197
Wheaton Franciscan Healthcare All Saints	Racine	8.0%	689
Riverside Medical Center	Waupaca	8.2%	97
United Hospital System	Kenosha	9.5%	749

Combination Abdominal CT Scan

Hospital Name	City	Rate	Cases
Riverview Hospital Assoc	Wisc. Rapids	0.5%	368
Saint Marys Hospital	Madison	0.8%	382
Saint Clares Hospital of Weston	Weston	1.0%	103
Saint Marys Janesville Hospital	Janesville	1.0%	98
Community Memorial Hospital	Menomonee Fls	1.2%	412
Reedsburg Area Medical Center	Reedsburg	1.2%	163
Boscobel Area Health Care	Boscobel	1.5%	65
Gundersen Lutheran Medical Center	La Crosse	1.5%	341
Mercy Medical Center of Oshkosh	Oshkosh	1.7%	288
Shawano Medical Center	Shawano	1.8%	166
Howard Young Medical Center	Woodruff	2.0%	150
Aurora Sheboygan Memorial Medical Center	Sheboygan	2.1%	235
Calumet Medical Center	Chilton	2.1%	48
Saint Joseph's Hospital	Chippewa Falls	2.1%	281
Tomah Memorial Hospital	Tomah	2.1%	140
Hayward Area Memorial Hospital	Hayward	2.2%	178
Hudson Hospital	Hudson	2.3%	219
Prairie Du Chien Memorial Hospital	Prairie Du Chien	2.6%	153
Beaver Dam Com Hospital	Beaver Dam	2.7%	519
Berlin Memorial Hospital	Berlin	2.7%	186
Good Samaritan Health Center	Merrill	2.7%	147
Ministry Door County Medical Center	Sturgeon Bay	2.7%	365
Appleton Medical Center	Appleton	2.8%	458
Mercy Health System Corp	Janesville	2.9%	858
Saint Marys Hospital Superior	Superior	3.2%	186
Lakeview Medical Center	Rice Lake	3.3%	398
Aspirus Wausau Hospital	Wausau	3.4%	387
Saint Elizabeth Hospital	Appleton	3.5%	374
UW Hlth Partners Watertown Reg Med Ctr	Watertown	3.5%	345
Univ of WI Hosps & Clinics Authority	Madison	3.6%	2479
Southwest Health Center	Platteville	3.7%	109
Aurora West Allis Medical Center	West Allis	3.8%	744
Riverside Medical Center	Waupaca	3.8%	263
St Joseph's Comm Hosp of West Bend	West Bend	3.8%	313
River Falls Area Hospital	River Falls	3.9%	204
Bellin Memorial Hospital	Green Bay	4.0%	722
Columbia Saint Marys Hospital Milwaukee	Milwaukee	4.2%	778
Chippewa Valley Hospital	Durand	4.3%	46
Flambeau Hospital	Park Falls	4.4%	160
Ministry Saint Josephs Hospital	Marshfield	4.5%	66
United Hospital System	Kenosha	4.5%	845
Bay Area Medical Center	Marinette	4.6%	525
Saint Clare Hospital Health Services	Baraboo	4.6%	347
Aurora Memorial Hospital Burlington	Burlington	4.7%	534
Vernon Memorial Hospital	Viroqua	4.7%	127
Aurora Medical Center Kenosha	Kenosha	4.8%	691
Meriter Hospital	Madison	5.0%	484
Aurora Lakeland Medical Center	Elkhorn	5.2%	439
Langlade Hospital	Antigo	5.2%	346
Saint Marys Hospital Medical Center	Green Bay	5.3%	475
Stoughton Hospital	Stoughton	5.3%	94
Wheaton Franciscan Healthcare All Saints	Racine	5.4%	951
Ministry Saint Marys Hospital	Rhinelander	5.5%	559
Aurora Medical Center Oshkosh	Oshkosh	5.6%	340
Saint Nicholas Hospital	Sheboygan	5.6%	323
Fort Memorial Hospital	Fort Atkinson	5.8%	365
Memorial Health Center	Medford	5.8%	156
Saint Vincent Hospital	Green Bay	5.8%	589
Theda Clark Medical Center	Neenah	5.8%	397
Froedtert Memorial Lutheran Hospital	Milwaukee	6.0%	2417
Ministry St Michaels Hosp-Stevens Pt	Stevens Point	6.0%	485
New London Family Medical Center	New London	6.0%	200
Columbia Saint Marys Hospital Ozaukee	Mequon	6.1%	578
Sauk Prairie Hospital	Prairie Du Sac	6.2%	146
Oconomowoc Memorial Hospital	Oconomowoc	6.4%	376
Aurora Medical Center Manitowoc County	Two Rivers	6.5%	245
The Monroe Clinic	Monroe	6.6%	500
Amery Regional Medical Center	Amery	6.7%	149
Saint Croix Regional Medical Center	Saint Croix Falls	6.7%	282
Ministry Sacred Heart Hospital	Tomahawk	6.8%	103
Divine Savior Healthcare	Portage	6.9%	204
Aurora Medical Center	Grafton	7.1%	312
Mayo Clinic Hlth Sys-Eau Claire Hosp	Eau Claire	7.1%	917
Waukesha Memorial Hospital	Waukesha	7.1%	1224
Wheaton Franciscan Hlthcare St Francis	Milwaukee	7.2%	433
Spooner Health System	Spooner	7.5%	120
Black River Memorial Hospital	Black River Falls	7.6%	105
Memorial Hospital Lafayette Cty	Darlington	7.6%	66
Aurora Baycare Medical Center	Green Bay	7.7%	495
Mercy Walworth Hospital & Medical Center	Lake Geneva	7.9%	216
Mile Bluff Medical Center	Mauston	8.2%	255
Mayo Clinic Hlth Sys Franciscan Med Ctr	La Crosse	8.6%	755
Wheaton Franciscan Healthcare Franklin	Franklin	8.9%	302
Ministry Eagle River Memorial Hospital	Eagle River	9.1%	175
Aurora Saint Lukes Medical Center	Milwaukee	9.3%	2043
Saint Agnes Hospital	Fond Du Lac	9.3%	655
Sacred Heart Hospital	Eau Claire	9.7%	535
Wheaton Franciscan Saint Joseph	Milwaukee	9.7%	1074
Community Memorial Hospital	Oconto Falls	11.4%	132
Aurora Medical Center Washington County	Hartford	11.9%	270
Rusk County Memorial Hospital	Ladysmith	12.1%	91
Moundview Memorial Hospital & Clinics	Friendship	12.6%	87
Aurora Medical Center	Summit	15.1%	391
Holy Family Memorial	Manitowoc	15.5%	187
Beloit Memorial Hospital	Beloit	55.5%	598

Combination Brain/Sinus CT Scan

Hospital Name	City	Rate	Cases
Amery Regional Medical Center	Amery	0.0%	144
Aurora Baycare Medical Center	Green Bay	0.0%	246

NOTE: Hospital profiles are in alphabetical order by state, then city, then hospital within the city; Rankings exclude hospitals with less than 25 cases except for patient surveys which excludes hospitals with less than 100 cases; (a) 100-299 cases; (1) The number of cases/patients is too few to report; (2) Data submitted were based on a sample of cases/patients; (3) Results are based on a shorter time period than required; (4) Data suppressed by CMS for one or more quarters; (5) Results are not available for this reporting period; (6) Fewer than 100 patients completed the HCAHPS survey; (7) No cases met the criteria for this measure; (8) The lower limit of the confidence interval cannot be calculated if the number of observed infections equals zero; (9) No data are available from the state/territory for this reporting period; (10) The scores shown reflect fewer than 50 completed surveys; (11) There were discrepancies in the data collection process; (12) This measure does not apply to this hospital for this reporting period; (13) Results cannot be calculated for this reporting period; (14) The results for this state are combined with nearby states to protect confidentiality; Please refer to the User's Guide for a full explanation of data.

Chippewa Valley Hospital	Durand	0.0%	63
Community Memorial Hospital	Oconto Falls	0.0%	105
Rusk County Memorial Hospital	Ladysmith	0.0%	87
Saint Croix Regional Medical Center	Saint Croix Falls	0.0%	168
St Joseph's Comm Hosp of West Bend	West Bend	0.0%	339
Saint Joseph's Health Services	Hillsboro	0.0%	32
Oconomowoc Memorial Hospital	Oconomowoc	0.4%	227
Ministry Door County Medical Center	Sturgeon Bay	0.7%	286
Riverview Hospital Assoc	Wisc. Rapids	0.7%	304
Aspirus Wausau Hospital	Wausau	0.8%	373
Community Memorial Hospital	Menomonee Fls	0.8%	592
Wheaton Franciscan Healthcare All Saints	Racine	0.8%	1004
Sacred Heart Hospital	Eau Claire	0.9%	229
Shawano Medical Center	Shawano	0.9%	325
Divine Savior Healthcare	Portage	1.0%	206
Aurora Memorial Hospital Burlington	Burlington	1.2%	494
Lakeview Medical Center	Rice Lake	1.2%	255
Ministry Sacred Heart Hospital	Tomahawk	1.2%	167
Saint Marys Hospital	Madison	1.2%	602
Aurora Lakeland Medical Center	Elkhorn	1.3%	454
Bay Area Medical Center	Marinette	1.4%	514
Waukesha Memorial Hospital	Waukesha	1.4%	864
Univ of WI Hosps & Clinics Authority	Madison	1.6%	1025
Fort Memorial Hospital	Fort Atkinson	1.7%	353
Mayo Clinic Hlth Sys Franciscan Med Ctr	La Crosse	1.7%	418
UW Hlth Partners Watertown Reg Med Ctr	Watertown	1.7%	356
Mayo Clinic Hlth Sys-Eau Claire Hosp	Eau Claire	1.9%	702
Columbia Saint Marys Hospital Ozaukee	Mequon	2.0%	508
Mercy Health System Corp	Janesville	2.0%	547
Meriter Hospital	Madison	2.0%	605
Saint Agnes Hospital	Fond Du Lac	2.0%	659
The Monroe Clinic	Monroe	2.2%	455
Aurora Medical Center Kenosha	Kenosha	2.4%	625
Bellin Memorial Hospital	Green Bay	2.4%	584
Columbia Saint Marys Hospital Milwaukee	Milwaukee	2.4%	694
United Hospital System	Kenosha	2.4%	796
Aurora Saint Lukes Medical Center	Milwaukee	3.0%	1535
Froedtert Memorial Lutheran Hospital	Milwaukee	3.0%	1187
Wheaton Franciscan Saint Joseph	Milwaukee	3.0%	1070
Aurora West Allis Medical Center	West Allis	3.8%	702
Aurora Medical Center Manitowoc County	Two Rivers	4.3%	281
Riverside Medical Center	Waupaca	6.7%	285

Combination Chest CT Scan

Hospital Name	City	Rate	Cases
Appleton Medical Center	Appleton	0.0%	369
Aspirus Wausau Hospital	Wausau	0.0%	246
Aurora Baycare Medical Center	Green Bay	0.0%	334
Aurora Medical Center	Grafton	0.0%	203
Aurora Medical Center	Summit	0.0%	257
Aurora Medical Center Manitowoc County	Two Rivers	0.0%	181
Aurora Medical Center Washington County	Hartford	0.0%	215
Aurora Sheboygan Memorial Medical Center	Sheboygan	0.0%	155
Aurora West Allis Medical Center	West Allis	0.0%	456
Bellin Memorial Hospital	Green Bay	0.0%	671
Flambeau Hospital	Park Falls	0.0%	94
Fort Memorial Hospital	Fort Atkinson	0.0%	209
Froedtert Memorial Lutheran Hospital	Milwaukee	0.0%	2711
Good Samaritan Health Center	Merrill	0.0%	63
Hudson Hospital	Hudson	0.0%	100
Mercy Medical Center of Oshkosh	Oshkosh	0.0%	187
Ministry Eagle River Memorial Hospital	Eagle River	0.0%	91
Ministry Sacred Heart Hospital	Tomahawk	0.0%	56
Moundview Memorial Hospital & Clinics	Friendship	0.0%	57
Riverside Medical Center	Waupaca	0.0%	140
Saint Marys Hospital Medical Center	Green Bay	0.0%	291
Saint Marys Hospital Superior	Superior	0.0%	102
Saint Vincent Hospital	Green Bay	0.0%	478
Shawano Medical Center	Shawano	0.0%	89
Spooner Health System	Spooner	0.0%	99
Theda Clark Medical Center	Neenah	0.0%	174
Tomah Memorial Hospital	Tomah	0.0%	55
United Hospital System	Kenosha	0.0%	441
UW Hlth Partners Watertown Reg Med Ctr	Watertown	0.0%	252
Wheaton Franciscan Healthcare All Saints	Racine	0.0%	957
Mayo Clinic Hlth Sys-Eau Claire Hosp	Eau Claire	0.1%	766
Mayo Clinic Hlth Sys Franciscan Med Ctr	La Crosse	0.2%	547
Aurora Medical Center Oshkosh	Oshkosh	0.3%	324
Langlade Hospital	Antigo	0.3%	332
Ministry Saint Marys Hospital	Rhinelander	0.3%	346
Univ of WI Hosps & Clinics Authority	Madison	0.3%	2402
Ministry St Michaels Hosp-Stevens Pt	Stevens Point	0.4%	230
Sacred Heart Hospital	Eau Claire	0.4%	452
Saint Elizabeth Hospital	Appleton	0.4%	248
Saint Nicholas Hospital	Sheboygan	0.4%	255
Riverview Hospital Assoc	Wisc. Rapids	0.5%	215
Hayward Area Memorial Hospital	Hayward	0.7%	153
River Falls Area Hospital	River Falls	0.7%	149
Saint Joseph's Hospital	Chippewa Falls	0.7%	145
Wheaton Franciscan Healthcare Franklin	Franklin	0.7%	152
Aurora Saint Lukes Medical Center	Milwaukee	0.8%	1993

Lakeview Medical Center	Rice Lake	0.8%	394
Memorial Health Center	Medford	0.8%	120
Saint Croix Regional Medical Center	Saint Croix Falls	0.8%	129
Amery Regional Medical Center	Amery	1.1%	90
Beaver Dam Com Hospital	Beaver Dam	1.1%	354
Berlin Memorial Hospital	Berlin	1.1%	87
Divine Savior Healthcare	Portage	1.1%	186
Beloit Memorial Hospital	Beloit	1.2%	247
Howard Young Medical Center	Woodruff	1.2%	81
Reedsburg Area Medical Center	Reedsburg	1.2%	86
Aurora Medical Center Kenosha	Kenosha	1.3%	617
Black River Memorial Hospital	Black River Falls	1.3%	77
The Monroe Clinic	Monroe	1.3%	308
Aurora Memorial Hospital Burlington	Burlington	1.4%	501
Ministry Door County Medical Center	Sturgeon Bay	1.4%	219
Oconomowoc Memorial Hospital	Oconomowoc	1.4%	221
Mile Bluff Medical Center	Mauston	1.5%	259
Rusk County Memorial Hospital	Ladysmith	1.6%	61
Columbia Saint Marys Hospital Ozaukee	Mequon	1.7%	654
Bay Area Medical Center	Marinette	1.8%	223
Mercy Health System Corp	Janesville	1.8%	715
Meriter Hospital	Madison	1.8%	221
New London Family Medical Center	New London	2.0%	99
Waukesha Memorial Hospital	Waukesha	2.1%	1102
Wheaton Franciscan Hlthcare St Francis	Milwaukee	2.1%	238
Wheaton Franciscan Saint Joseph	Milwaukee	2.4%	548
Aurora Lakeland Medical Center	Elkhorn	2.9%	489
Vernon Memorial Hospital	Viroqua	2.9%	69
Saint Clare Hospital Health Services	Baraboo	3.2%	157
Saint Agnes Hospital	Fond Du Lac	3.7%	486
Columbia Saint Marys Hospital Milwaukee	Milwaukee	4.0%	746
Community Memorial Hospital	Oconto Falls	4.0%	149
Community Memorial Hospital	Menomonee Fls	4.2%	426
St Joseph's Comm Hosp of West Bend	West Bend	4.8%	189
Sauk Prairie Hospital	Prairie Du Sac	4.8%	83
Mercy Walworth Hospital & Medical Center	Lake Geneva	5.8%	121
Holy Family Memorial	Manitowoc	6.4%	171

Follow-up Mammogram/Ultrasound

A follow-up rate near zero may indicate missed cancer; a rate higher than 14% may mean there is unnecessary follow up.

Hospital Name	City	Rate	Cases
Saint Joseph's Health Services	Hillsboro	2.4%	84
River Falls Area Hospital	River Falls	3.0%	330
Saint Croix Regional Medical Center	Saint Croix Falls	3.4%	406
Ladd Memorial Hospital	Osceola	3.5%	114
Beloit Memorial Hospital	Beloit	3.7%	1162
Memorial Health Center	Medford	4.3%	325
Aurora Baycare Medical Center	Green Bay	4.8%	805
Aurora Medical Center Kenosha	Kenosha	4.8%	1005
Bellin Memorial Hospital	Green Bay	4.8%	1239
Our Lady of Victory Hospital	Stanley	5.2%	116
Hudson Hospital	Hudson	5.3%	303
Bay Area Medical Center	Marinette	5.4%	631
Saint Vincent Hospital	Green Bay	5.6%	322
United Hospital System	Kenosha	5.6%	1931
Aurora West Allis Medical Center	West Allis	5.7%	1934
Mercy Health System Corp	Janesville	5.7%	1214
Saint Marys Hospital Superior	Superior	5.7%	388
Berlin Memorial Hospital	Berlin	5.8%	360
Good Samaritan Health Center	Merrill	5.8%	292
Oconomowoc Memorial Hospital	Oconomowoc	5.9%	929
Spooner Health System	Spooner	6.0%	234
Froedtert Memorial Lutheran Hospital	Milwaukee	6.1%	3483
Ministry Saint Marys Hospital	Rhinelander	6.2%	918
Vernon Memorial Hospital	Viroqua	6.2%	291
Saint Elizabeth Hospital	Appleton	6.5%	755
Stoughton Hospital	Stoughton	6.5%	199
Prairie Du Chien Memorial Hospital	Prairie Du Chien	6.7%	240
Saint Clare Hospital Health Services	Baraboo	6.7%	285
Aurora Medical Center	Grafton	6.8%	176
Community Memorial Hospital	Oconto Falls	6.8%	147
Mile Bluff Medical Center	Mauston	6.8%	532
Boscobel Area Health Care	Boscobel	6.9%	101
Ministry Eagle River Memorial Hospital	Eagle River	6.9%	288
Mercy Medical Center of Oshkosh	Oshkosh	7.0%	727
The Monroe Clinic	Monroe	7.2%	1597
Aurora Medical Center Oshkosh	Oshkosh	7.3%	1042
UW Hlth Partners Watertown Reg Med Ctr	Watertown	7.3%	735
Aurora Memorial Hospital Burlington	Burlington	7.4%	1034
Aurora Medical Center	Summit	7.8%	670
Amery Regional Medical Center	Amery	8.0%	249
Ministry Sacred Heart Hospital	Tomahawk	8.0%	224
Univ of WI Hosps & Clinics Authority	Madison	8.1%	2288
Southwest Health Center	Platteville	8.2%	194
Community Memorial Hospital	Menomonee Fls	8.3%	193
Wheaton Franciscan Healthcare All Saints	Racine	8.4%	2642
Ministry Door County Medical Center	Sturgeon Bay	8.7%	855
Riverview Hospital Assoc	Wisc. Rapids	8.8%	478
Waukesha Memorial Hospital	Waukesha	8.8%	2682
Howard Young Medical Center	Woodruff	9.0%	67

Beaver Dam Com Hospital	Beaver Dam	9.1%	875
New London Family Medical Center	New London	9.1%	297
Wheaton Franciscan Saint Joseph	Milwaukee	9.1%	3350
Holy Family Memorial	Manitowoc	9.2%	708
Lakeview Medical Center	Rice Lake	9.2%	783
Rusk County Memorial Hospital	Ladysmith	9.2%	403
Wheaton Franciscan Healthcare Franklin	Franklin	9.2%	632
Aspirus Wausau Hospital	Wausau	9.3%	1199
Mercy Walworth Hospital & Medical Center	Lake Geneva	9.3%	268
Flambeau Hospital	Park Falls	9.4%	149
Langlade Hospital	Antigo	9.5%	462
Saint Marys Hospital Medical Center	Green Bay	9.5%	200
Fort Memorial Hospital	Fort Atkinson	9.7%	943
Calumet Medical Center	Chilton	9.8%	143
Hayward Area Memorial Hospital	Hayward	9.8%	440
Saint Agnes Hospital	Fond Du Lac	10.1%	1341
Memorial Hospital Lafayette Cty	Darlington	10.3%	97
Aurora Lakeland Medical Center	Elkhorn	10.4%	960
Ministry St Michaels Hosp-Stevens Pt	Stevens Point	10.5%	1050
Saint Joseph's Hospital	Chippewa Falls	10.5%	228
Chippewa Valley Hospital	Durand	10.6%	141
Aurora Saint Lukes Medical Center	Milwaukee	10.7%	2451
Grant Regional Health Center	Lancaster	10.8%	212
Wheaton Franciscan Hlthcare St Francis	Milwaukee	10.9%	753
Columbia Saint Marys Hospital Ozaukee	Mequon	11.1%	1536
Columbia Saint Marys Hospital Milwaukee	Milwaukee	11.2%	2658
Saint Nicholas Hospital	Sheboygan	11.3%	346
Theda Clark Medical Center	Neenah	11.9%	604
Sacred Heart Hospital	Eau Claire	12.1%	314
Moundview Memorial Hospital & Clinics	Friendship	12.6%	175
Sauk Prairie Hospital	Prairie Du Sac	12.8%	439
Divine Savior Healthcare	Portage	15.5%	601
Reedsburg Area Medical Center	Reedsburg	15.8%	292

Lumbar Spine MRI for Low Back Pain

Hospital Name	City	Rate	Cases
St Joseph's Comm Hosp of West Bend	West Bend	21.7%	92
Fort Memorial Hospital	Fort Atkinson	26.7%	75
Aurora Medical Center Kenosha	Kenosha	26.8%	149
Beaver Dam Com Hospital	Beaver Dam	26.8%	56
United Hospital System	Kenosha	27.5%	167
Wheaton Franciscan Saint Joseph	Milwaukee	29.0%	224
Ministry St Michaels Hosp-Stevens Pt	Stevens Point	29.3%	82
Community Memorial Hospital	Menomonee Fls	29.4%	68
Divine Savior Healthcare	Portage	29.6%	54
The Monroe Clinic	Monroe	30.4%	115
Froedtert Memorial Lutheran Hospital	Milwaukee	30.9%	486
Aurora Medical Center Washington County	Hartford	32.0%	50
Bellin Memorial Hospital	Green Bay	32.3%	167
Mayo Clinic Hlth Sys-Eau Claire Hosp	Eau Claire	32.8%	183
Mercy Medical Center of Oshkosh	Oshkosh	32.8%	58
Wheaton Franciscan Healthcare All Saints	Racine	33.0%	209
Aurora Saint Lukes Medical Center	Milwaukee	33.5%	248
Sauk Prairie Hospital	Prairie Du Sac	33.7%	98
Wheaton Franciscan Hlthcare St Francis	Milwaukee	33.7%	83
Mercy Walworth Hospital & Medical Center	Lake Geneva	34.0%	53
Mercy Health System Corp	Janesville	34.1%	176
Sacred Heart Hospital	Eau Claire	34.2%	79
Aurora Baycare Medical Center	Green Bay	34.3%	169
Univ of WI Hosps & Clinics Authority	Madison	34.7%	274
Amery Regional Medical Center	Amery	35.3%	51
Mayo Clinic Hlth Sys Franciscan Med Ctr	La Crosse	35.8%	162
Wheaton Franciscan Healthcare Franklin	Franklin	36.0%	114
Columbia Saint Marys Hospital Milwaukee	Milwaukee	36.2%	149
Ministry Saint Marys Hospital	Rhinelander	36.4%	77
Orthopaedic Hospital of Wisconsin	Glendale	36.4%	88
Aurora Memorial Hospital Burlington	Burlington	37.0%	108
Aurora Medical Center	Summit	37.1%	62
Lakeview Medical Center	Rice Lake	37.1%	116
UW Hlth Partners Watertown Reg Med Ctr	Watertown	37.3%	51
Saint Marys Hospital Medical Center	Green Bay	37.5%	72
Waukesha Memorial Hospital	Waukesha	37.6%	266
Oconomowoc Memorial Hospital	Oconomowoc	37.9%	95
Theda Clark Medical Center	Neenah	38.0%	50
Saint Agnes Hospital	Fond Du Lac	38.3%	128
Saint Croix Regional Medical Center	Saint Croix Falls	38.3%	47
Bay Area Medical Center	Marinette	38.4%	73
Columbia Saint Marys Hospital Ozaukee	Mequon	38.5%	78
Beloit Memorial Hospital	Beloit	39.4%	94
Saint Vincent Hospital	Green Bay	40.6%	96
Aurora Medical Center	Grafton	41.1%	56
Aurora Medical Center Manitowoc County	Two Rivers	41.4%	58
Langlade Hospital	Antigo	41.5%	82
Mile Bluff Medical Center	Mauston	41.5%	41
Aspirus Wausau Hospital	Wausau	41.7%	48
Aurora Medical Center Oshkosh	Oshkosh	42.4%	85
Holy Family Memorial	Manitowoc	43.0%	93
Aurora West Allis Medical Center	West Allis	44.2%	77
Aurora Lakeland Medical Center	Elkhorn	45.0%	80
Reedsburg Area Medical Center	Reedsburg	48.6%	70
Ministry Door County Medical Center	Sturgeon Bay	51.1%	94
Shawano Medical Center	Shawano	52.8%	36

NOTE: Hospital profiles are in alphabetical order by state, then city, then hospital within the city; Rankings exclude hospitals with less than 25 cases except for patient surveys which excludes hospitals with less than 100 cases; (a) 100-299 cases; (1) The number of cases/patients is too few to report; (2) Data submitted were based on a sample of cases/patients; (3) Results are based on a shorter time period than required; (4) Data suppressed by CMS for one or more quarters; (5) Results are not available for this reporting period; (6) Fewer than 100 patients completed the HCAHPS survey; (7) No cases met the criteria for this measure; (8) The lower limit of the confidence interval cannot be calculated if the number of observed infections equals zero; (9) No data are available from the state/territory for this reporting period; (10) The scores shown reflect fewer than 50 completed surveys; (11) There were discrepancies in the data collection process; (12) This measure does not apply to this hospital for this reporting period; (13) Results cannot be calculated for this reporting period; (14) The results for this state are combined with nearby states to protect confidentiality; Please refer to the User's Guide for a full explanation of data.

Amery Regional Medical Center

265 Griffin Street East
Amery, WI 54001
Phone: 715-268-0300
Fax: 715-268-1376
Type: Critical Access Hospitals
Emergency Services: Yes
Ownership: Voluntary non-profit - Private
Beds: 29

Key Personnel:
Hemotology Center . . . . Pat Derrington
CEO . . . . Michael Karuschak Jr
Infection Control. . . . . Nancy Magnine
Radiology. . . . . Thomas M Pelant
Chief of Medical Staff . . . . James Quenan, MD, FACS
Operating Room. . . . . James P Quenan
Quality Assurance . . . . Sandi Reed, RN, BSN, MS
Emergency Room . . . . Patrick Sura, MD

Measure	Cases	This Hosp.	State Avg.	U.S. Avg.
Blood Clot Prevention and Treatment				
Anticoagulation Overlap Therapy[5]	-	-	95%	93%
ICU Venous Thromboembolism Prophylaxis[5]	-	-	91%	92%
Incidence of Potentially Preventable VTE[5]	-	-	10%	10%
UFH with Dosages/Platelet Monitoring[5]	-	-	96%	97%
Venous Thromboembolism Prophylaxis[5]	-	-	85%	85%
Warfarin Therapy Discharge Instructions[5]	-	-	70%	75%
Chest Pain/Possible Heart Attack Care				
Aspirin Given Within 24 Hours of Arrival[3]	13	92%	98%	96%
Fibrinolytic Meds Within 30 Min. of Arrival[3,7]	-	-	52%	58%
Average Time to ECG (minutes)[3]	12	11	7	7
Average Time to Transfer (minutes)[1,3]	-	-	58	60
Children's Asthma Care				
Received Home Management Plan of Care	-	-	-	88%
Received Reliever Medication	-	-	-	100%
Received Systemic Corticosteroids	-	-	-	100%
Emergency Department				
Admittance Decision Time (minutes)[5]	-	-	65	98
Head CT Results Within 45 Min. of Arrival[5]	-	-	61%	57%
Patients Who Left ER Before Being Seen[5]	-	-	1%	2%
Time from ER Arrival to Admit. (minutes)[5]	-	-	207	274
Time from ER Arrival to Discharge (minutes)[3]	318	98	121	134
Time in ER Before Being Evaluated (minutes)[3]	325	24	19	26
Time to Pain Meds for Fractures (minutes)[5]	-	-	42	57
Heart Attack Care				
Aspirin Given at Discharge[5]	-	-	99%	99%
Fibrinolytic Meds Within 30 Min. of Arrival[5]	-	-	67%	54%
PCI Within 90 Minutes of Arrival[5]	-	-	96%	96%
Statin Prescribed at Discharge[5]	-	-	99%	98%
Heart Failure Care				
ACE Inhibitor or ARB for LVSD[1,3]	-	-	97%	97%
Discharge Instructions Given[3]	13	92%	96%	94%
Evaluation of LVS Function[3]	22	73%	99%	99%
Medicare Spending				
Medicare Spending per Patient (ratio)	-	-	0.94	0.98
Pneumonia Care				
Appropriate Initial Antibiotic Given[1,3]	-	-	96%	95%
Blood Culture Timing[3]	23	78%	98%	98%
Pregnancy and Delivery Care				
Newborn Deliveries Scheduled Early[5]	-	-	4%	6%
Preventive Care				
Immunization for Influenza[5]	-	-	90%	90%
Immunization for Pneumonia[5]	-	-	92%	92%
Stroke Care				
Anticoagulation Therapy for Atrial Fibrillation[5]	-	-	94%	95%
Antithrombotic Therapy Timing[5]	-	-	99%	98%
Assessed for Rehabilitation[5]	-	-	98%	97%
Discharged on Antithrombotic Therapy[5]	-	-	99%	99%
Discharged on Statin Medication[5]	-	-	94%	94%
Thrombolytic Therapy Timing[5]	-	-	60%	66%
Venous Thromboembolism Prophylaxis[5]	-	-	95%	94%
Written Stroke Educational Materials Given[5]	-	-	88%	88%
Surgical Care Improvement Project				
Appropriate Beta Blocker Usage[3]	22	91%	99%	98%
Appropriate VTP Within 24 Hours[3]	83	100%	99%	98%
Controlled Postoperative Blood Glucose[3,7]	-	-	96%	97%
Perioperative Temperature Management[3]	94	100%	100%	100%
Prophylactic Antibiotic Selection[3]	78	100%	99%	99%
Prophylactic Antibiotic Selection (Outpatient)[5]	-	-	98%	98%
Prophylactic Antibiotic Stopped[3]	78	97%	99%	98%
Prophylactic Antibiotic Timing[3]	79	90%	99%	99%
Prophylactic Antibiotic Timing (Outpatient)[5]	-	-	97%	98%
Urinary Catheter Removal[1,3]	-	-	98%	97%
Survey of Patients' Hospital Experiences				
Area Around Room 'Always' Quiet at Night	(a)	69%	63%	61%
Doctors 'Always' Communicated Well	(a)	80%	83%	82%
Home Recovery Information Given	(a)	90%	89%	85%
Hospital Given 9 or 10 on 10 Point Scale	(a)	68%	74%	71%
Meds 'Always' Explained Before Given	(a)	68%	68%	64%
Nurses 'Always' Communicated Well	(a)	79%	82%	79%
Pain 'Always' Well Controlled	(a)	68%	72%	71%
Room and Bathroom 'Always' Clean	(a)	83%	79%	73%
Timely Help 'Always' Received	(a)	76%	72%	68%
Would Definitely Recommend Hospital	(a)	65%	74%	71%
Use of Medical Imaging				
Cardiac Imaging Stress Test before Surgery	53	3.8%	5.4%	5.3%
Combination Abdominal CT Scan	149	6.7%	6.3%	10.5%
Combination Brain/Sinus CT Scan	144	0.0%	2.1%	2.7%
Combination Chest CT Scan	90	1.1%	1%	2.7%
Follow-up Mammogram/Ultrasound	249	8.0%	8.1%	8.8%
Lumbar Spine MRI for Low Back Pain	51	35.3%	34.9%	37.2%

Langlade Hospital

112 E Fifth St
Antigo, WI 54409
Phone: 715-623-2331
Fax: 715-623-9440
URL: www.langlادememorial.org
Type: Critical Access Hospitals
Emergency Services: Yes
Ownership: Voluntary non-profit - Church
Beds: 25

Key Personnel:
Patient Relations . . . . Sherry Bunten
Operating Room. . . . . Frank Burkett, RN
Anesthesiology. . . . . Jim Leek, MD
Infection Control. . . . . Sandy Leider
Radiology. . . . . Joseph McCausli
CEO/President. . . . . Dave Schneider
Chief of Medical Staff . . . . Jay Turnbull
Emergency Room . . . . Randy Waskin

Measure	Cases	This Hosp.	State Avg.	U.S. Avg.
Blood Clot Prevention and Treatment				
Anticoagulation Overlap Therapy[5]	-	-	95%	93%
ICU Venous Thromboembolism Prophylaxis[5]	-	-	91%	92%
Incidence of Potentially Preventable VTE[5]	-	-	10%	10%
UFH with Dosages/Platelet Monitoring[5]	-	-	96%	97%
Venous Thromboembolism Prophylaxis[5]	-	-	85%	85%
Warfarin Therapy Discharge Instructions[5]	-	-	70%	75%
Chest Pain/Possible Heart Attack Care				
Aspirin Given Within 24 Hours of Arrival	28	96%	98%	96%
Fibrinolytic Meds Within 30 Min. of Arrival[7]	-	-	52%	58%
Average Time to ECG (minutes)	26	8	7	7
Average Time to Transfer (minutes)[7]	-	-	58	60
Children's Asthma Care				
Received Home Management Plan of Care	-	-	-	88%
Received Reliever Medication	-	-	-	100%
Received Systemic Corticosteroids	-	-	-	100%
Emergency Department				
Admittance Decision Time (minutes)[5]	-	-	65	98
Head CT Results Within 45 Min. of Arrival[1,3]	-	-	61%	57%
Patients Who Left ER Before Being Seen	11,319	1%	1%	2%
Time from ER Arrival to Admit. (minutes)[5]	-	-	207	274
Time from ER Arrival to Discharge (minutes)[3]	208	126	121	134
Time in ER Before Being Evaluated (minutes)[3]	235	19	19	26
Time to Pain Meds for Fractures (minutes)[3]	20	45	42	57
Heart Attack Care				
Aspirin Given at Discharge[5]	-	-	99%	99%
Fibrinolytic Meds Within 30 Min. of Arrival[5]	-	-	67%	54%
PCI Within 90 Minutes of Arrival[5]	-	-	96%	96%
Statin Prescribed at Discharge[5]	-	-	99%	98%
Heart Failure Care				
ACE Inhibitor or ARB for LVSD[1]	-	-	97%	97%
Discharge Instructions Given	34	94%	96%	94%
Evaluation of LVS Function	44	100%	99%	99%
Medicare Spending				
Medicare Spending per Patient (ratio)	-	-	0.94	0.98
Pneumonia Care				
Appropriate Initial Antibiotic Given	51	98%	96%	95%
Blood Culture Timing	73	100%	98%	98%
Pregnancy and Delivery Care				
Newborn Deliveries Scheduled Early[5]	-	-	4%	6%
Preventive Care				
Immunization for Influenza[5]	-	-	90%	90%
Immunization for Pneumonia[5]	-	-	92%	92%
Stroke Care				
Anticoagulation Therapy for Atrial Fibrillation[5]	-	-	94%	95%
Antithrombotic Therapy Timing[5]	-	-	99%	98%
Assessed for Rehabilitation[5]	-	-	98%	97%
Discharged on Antithrombotic Therapy[5]	-	-	99%	99%
Discharged on Statin Medication[5]	-	-	94%	94%
Thrombolytic Therapy Timing[5]	-	-	60%	66%
Venous Thromboembolism Prophylaxis[5]	-	-	95%	94%
Written Stroke Educational Materials Given[5]	-	-	88%	88%
Surgical Care Improvement Project				
Appropriate Beta Blocker Usage	18	89%	99%	98%
Appropriate VTP Within 24 Hours	48	100%	99%	98%
Controlled Postoperative Blood Glucose[3,7]	-	-	96%	97%
Perioperative Temperature Management	58	100%	100%	100%
Prophylactic Antibiotic Selection	17	100%	99%	99%
Prophylactic Antibiotic Selection (Outpatient)[3]	22	95%	98%	98%
Prophylactic Antibiotic Stopped	17	94%	99%	98%
Prophylactic Antibiotic Timing	17	100%	99%	99%
Prophylactic Antibiotic Timing (Outpatient)[3]	25	84%	97%	98%
Urinary Catheter Removal	18	94%	98%	97%
Survey of Patients' Hospital Experiences				
Area Around Room 'Always' Quiet at Night	(a)	62%	63%	61%
Doctors 'Always' Communicated Well	(a)	86%	83%	82%
Home Recovery Information Given	(a)	91%	89%	85%
Hospital Given 9 or 10 on 10 Point Scale	(a)	82%	74%	71%
Meds 'Always' Explained Before Given	(a)	71%	68%	64%
Nurses 'Always' Communicated Well	(a)	85%	82%	79%
Pain 'Always' Well Controlled	(a)	75%	72%	71%
Room and Bathroom 'Always' Clean	(a)	79%	79%	73%
Timely Help 'Always' Received	(a)	77%	72%	68%
Would Definitely Recommend Hospital	(a)	78%	74%	71%
Use of Medical Imaging				
Cardiac Imaging Stress Test before Surgery	131	6.9%	5.4%	5.3%
Combination Abdominal CT Scan	346	5.2%	6.3%	10.5%
Combination Brain/Sinus CT Scan[1]	-	-	2.1%	2.7%
Combination Chest CT Scan	332	0.3%	1%	2.7%
Follow-up Mammogram/Ultrasound	462	9.5%	8.1%	8.8%
Lumbar Spine MRI for Low Back Pain	82	41.5%	34.9%	37.2%

Appleton Medical Center

1818 N Meade St
Appleton, WI 54911
Phone: 920-731-4101
Fax: 920-738-6319
URL: www.thedacare.org
Type: Acute Care Hospitals
Emergency Services: Yes
Ownership: Voluntary non-profit - Private
Beds: 160

Key Personnel:
Radiology. . . . . Timothy A Bernauer, MD
Operating Room. . . . . Sherry Cheadle
Infection Control. . . . . Steve DuBois
President . . . . Dean Gruner, MD
Pediatric Ambulatory Care . . . . . Eileen C Jekot, MD
Pediatric In-Patient Care . . . . . . Eileen C Jekot, MD
Chief of Medical Staff . . . . Greg Long, MD
Quality Assurance . . . . Sally Podoski

Measure	Cases	This Hosp.	State Avg.	U.S. Avg.
Blood Clot Prevention and Treatment				
Anticoagulation Overlap Therapy[2]	92	90%	95%	93%
ICU Venous Thromboembolism Prophylaxis[2]	77	88%	91%	92%
Incidence of Potentially Preventable VTE[1,2]	-	-	10%	10%
UFH with Dosages/Platelet Monitoring[2]	28	100%	96%	97%
Venous Thromboembolism Prophylaxis[2]	339	78%	85%	85%
Warfarin Therapy Discharge Instructions[2]	75	0%	70%	75%
Chest Pain/Possible Heart Attack Care				
Aspirin Given Within 24 Hours of Arrival[1,3]	-	-	98%	96%
Fibrinolytic Meds Within 30 Min. of Arrival[5]	-	-	52%	58%
Average Time to ECG (minutes)[1,3]	-	-	7	7

NOTE: Hospital profiles are in alphabetical order by state, then city, then hospital within the city; Rankings exclude hospitals with less than 25 cases except for patient surveys which excludes hospitals with less than 100 cases; (a) 100-299 cases; (1) The number of cases/patients is too few to report; (2) Data submitted were based on a sample of cases/patients; (3) Results are based on a shorter time period than required; (4) Data suppressed by CMS for one or more quarters; (5) Results are not available for this reporting period; (6) Fewer than 100 patients completed the HCAHPS survey; (7) No cases met the criteria for this measure; (8) The lower limit of the confidence interval cannot be calculated if the number of observed infections equals zero; (9) No data are available from the state/territory for this reporting period; (10) The scores shown reflect fewer than 50 completed surveys; (11) There were discrepancies in the data collection process; (12) This measure does not apply to this hospital for this reporting period; (13) Results cannot be calculated for this reporting period; (14) The results for this state are combined with nearby states to protect confidentiality; Please refer to the User's Guide for a full explanation of data.

Measure	Cases	This Hosp.	State Avg.	U.S. Avg.
Average Time to Transfer (minutes)[5]	-	-	58	60
Children's Asthma Care				
Received Home Management Plan of Care	-	-	-	88%
Received Reliever Medication	-	-	-	100%
Received Systemic Corticosteroids	-	-	-	100%
Emergency Department				
Admittance Decision Time (minutes)[2]	328	34	65	98
Head CT Results Within 45 Min. of Arrival	24	21%	61%	57%
Patients Who Left ER Before Being Seen	21,541	0%	1%	2%
Time from ER Arrival to Admit. (minutes)[2]	334	181	207	274
Time from ER Arrival to Discharge (minutes)	401	134	121	134
Time in ER Before Being Evaluated (minutes)	424	20	19	26
Time to Pain Meds for Fractures (minutes)	191	47	42	57
Heart Attack Care				
Aspirin Given at Discharge	273	100%	99%	99%
Fibrinolytic Meds Within 30 Min. of Arrival[1]	-	-	67%	54%
PCI Within 90 Minutes of Arrival	39	95%	96%	96%
Statin Prescribed at Discharge	275	100%	99%	98%
Heart Failure Care				
ACE Inhibitor or ARB for LVSD	55	95%	97%	97%
Discharge Instructions Given	174	97%	96%	94%
Evaluation of LVS Function	206	99%	99%	99%
Medicare Spending				
Medicare Spending per Patient (ratio)	-	0.95	0.94	0.98
Pneumonia Care				
Appropriate Initial Antibiotic Given	127	93%	96%	95%
Blood Culture Timing	147	99%	98%	98%
Pregnancy and Delivery Care				
Newborn Deliveries Scheduled Early	111	5%	4%	6%
Preventive Care				
Immunization for Influenza[2]	555	94%	90%	90%
Immunization for Pneumonia[2]	663	91%	92%	92%
Stroke Care				
Anticoagulation Therapy for Atrial Fibrillation[1]	-	-	94%	95%
Antithrombotic Therapy Timing	41	100%	99%	98%
Assessed for Rehabilitation	45	96%	98%	97%
Discharged on Antithrombotic Therapy	43	100%	99%	99%
Discharged on Statin Medication	30	100%	94%	94%
Thrombolytic Therapy Timing[1]	-	-	60%	66%
Venous Thromboembolism Prophylaxis	49	88%	95%	94%
Written Stroke Educational Materials Given	27	89%	88%	88%
Surgical Care Improvement Project				
Appropriate Beta Blocker Usage[2]	439	100%	99%	98%
Appropriate VTP Within 24 Hours[2]	864	100%	99%	98%
Controlled Postoperative Blood Glucose[2]	261	95%	96%	97%
Perioperative Temperature Management[2]	982	100%	100%	100%
Prophylactic Antibiotic Selection[2]	1,019	99%	99%	99%
Prophylactic Antibiotic Selection (Outpatient)	333	96%	98%	98%
Prophylactic Antibiotic Stopped[2]	995	99%	99%	98%
Prophylactic Antibiotic Timing[2]	1,020	100%	99%	99%
Prophylactic Antibiotic Timing (Outpatient)	328	95%	97%	98%
Urinary Catheter Removal[2]	666	98%	98%	97%
Survey of Patients' Hospital Experiences				
Area Around Room 'Always' Quiet at Night	300+	57%	63%	61%
Doctors 'Always' Communicated Well	300+	80%	83%	82%
Home Recovery Information Given	300+	89%	89%	85%
Hospital Given 9 or 10 on 10 Point Scale	300+	76%	74%	71%
Meds 'Always' Explained Before Given	300+	63%	68%	64%
Nurses 'Always' Communicated Well	300+	78%	82%	79%
Pain 'Always' Well Controlled	300+	70%	72%	71%
Room and Bathroom 'Always' Clean	300+	76%	79%	73%
Timely Help 'Always' Received	300+	65%	72%	68%
Would Definitely Recommend Hospital	300+	78%	74%	71%
Use of Medical Imaging				
Cardiac Imaging Stress Test before Surgery	651	5.1%	5.4%	5.3%
Combination Abdominal CT Scan	458	2.8%	6.3%	10.5%
Combination Brain/Sinus CT Scan[1]	-	-	2.1%	2.7%
Combination Chest CT Scan	369	0.0%	1%	2.7%
Follow-up Mammogram/Ultrasound[1]	-	-	8.1%	8.8%
Lumbar Spine MRI for Low Back Pain[1]	-	-	34.9%	37.2%

Saint Elizabeth Hospital

1506 S Oneida St
Appleton, WI 54915
URL: www.affinityhealth.org
Type: Acute Care Hospitals
Ownership: Voluntary non-profit - Private
Phone: 920-738-2000
Fax: 920-831-1324
Emergency Services: Yes
Beds: 352

Key Personnel:
Emergency Room . . . . Rosemary Dvorachek, RN
Pediatric In-Patient Care . . . . C Green, MD
Radiology. . . . . Robert Kinde, MD
Operating Room. . . . . Eileen Leinweber
CEO/President. . . . . Daniel E Neufelder
Quality Assurance . . . . Cheryl Schmidt

Measure	Cases	This Hosp.	State Avg.	U.S. Avg.
Blood Clot Prevention and Treatment				
Anticoagulation Overlap Therapy[2]	59	95%	95%	93%
ICU Venous Thromboembolism Prophylaxis[2]	70	97%	91%	92%
Incidence of Potentially Preventable VTE[1,2]	-	-	10%	10%
UFH with Dosages/Platelet Monitoring[1,2]	-	-	96%	97%
Venous Thromboembolism Prophylaxis[2]	256	97%	85%	85%
Warfarin Therapy Discharge Instructions[2]	53	96%	70%	75%
Chest Pain/Possible Heart Attack Care				
Aspirin Given Within 24 Hours of Arrival[1,3]	-	-	98%	96%
Fibrinolytic Meds Within 30 Min. of Arrival[3,7]	-	-	52%	58%
Average Time to ECG (minutes)[1,3]	-	-	7	7
Average Time to Transfer (minutes)[3,7]	-	-	58	60
Children's Asthma Care				
Received Home Management Plan of Care	-	-	-	88%
Received Reliever Medication	-	-	-	100%
Received Systemic Corticosteroids	-	-	-	100%
Emergency Department				
Admittance Decision Time (minutes)[2]	454	63	65	98
Head CT Results Within 45 Min. of Arrival[1]	-	-	61%	57%
Patients Who Left ER Before Being Seen	31,110	0%	1%	2%
Time from ER Arrival to Admit. (minutes)[2]	454	203	207	274
Time from ER Arrival to Discharge (minutes)	349	100	121	134
Time in ER Before Being Evaluated (minutes)	392	15	19	26
Time to Pain Meds for Fractures (minutes)	125	34	42	57
Heart Attack Care				
Aspirin Given at Discharge	125	100%	99%	99%
Fibrinolytic Meds Within 30 Min. of Arrival[7]	-	-	67%	54%
PCI Within 90 Minutes of Arrival	23	100%	96%	96%
Statin Prescribed at Discharge	122	100%	99%	98%
Heart Failure Care				
ACE Inhibitor or ARB for LVSD	19	100%	97%	97%
Discharge Instructions Given	122	100%	96%	94%
Evaluation of LVS Function	154	100%	99%	99%
Medicare Spending				
Medicare Spending per Patient (ratio)	-	0.93	0.94	0.98
Pneumonia Care				
Appropriate Initial Antibiotic Given	90	99%	96%	95%
Blood Culture Timing	118	99%	98%	98%
Pregnancy and Delivery Care				
Newborn Deliveries Scheduled Early	97	8%	4%	6%
Preventive Care				
Immunization for Influenza[2]	557	97%	90%	90%
Immunization for Pneumonia[2]	518	98%	92%	92%
Stroke Care				
Anticoagulation Therapy for Atrial Fibrillation	13	100%	94%	95%
Antithrombotic Therapy Timing	77	99%	99%	98%
Assessed for Rehabilitation	85	100%	98%	97%
Discharged on Antithrombotic Therapy	74	100%	99%	99%
Discharged on Statin Medication	57	98%	94%	94%
Thrombolytic Therapy Timing[1]	-	-	60%	66%
Venous Thromboembolism Prophylaxis	86	98%	95%	94%
Written Stroke Educational Materials Given	36	97%	88%	88%
Surgical Care Improvement Project				
Appropriate Beta Blocker Usage[2]	176	100%	99%	98%
Appropriate VTP Within 24 Hours[2]	338	99%	99%	98%
Controlled Postoperative Blood Glucose[2]	157	97%	96%	97%
Perioperative Temperature Management[2]	372	100%	100%	100%
Prophylactic Antibiotic Selection[2]	376	100%	99%	99%
Prophylactic Antibiotic Selection (Outpatient)	507	99%	98%	98%
Prophylactic Antibiotic Stopped[2]	360	100%	99%	98%
Prophylactic Antibiotic Timing[2]	376	99%	99%	99%
Prophylactic Antibiotic Timing (Outpatient)	510	99%	97%	98%
Urinary Catheter Removal[2]	336	99%	98%	97%
Survey of Patients' Hospital Experiences				
Area Around Room 'Always' Quiet at Night	300+	61%	63%	61%
Doctors 'Always' Communicated Well	300+	82%	83%	82%
Home Recovery Information Given	300+	89%	89%	85%
Hospital Given 9 or 10 on 10 Point Scale	300+	74%	74%	71%
Meds 'Always' Explained Before Given	300+	69%	68%	64%
Nurses 'Always' Communicated Well	300+	79%	82%	79%
Pain 'Always' Well Controlled	300+	70%	72%	71%
Room and Bathroom 'Always' Clean	300+	74%	79%	73%
Timely Help 'Always' Received	300+	66%	72%	68%
Would Definitely Recommend Hospital	300+	77%	74%	71%
Use of Medical Imaging				
Cardiac Imaging Stress Test before Surgery	225	3.1%	5.4%	5.3%
Combination Abdominal CT Scan	374	3.5%	6.3%	10.5%
Combination Brain/Sinus CT Scan[1]	-	-	2.1%	2.7%
Combination Chest CT Scan	248	0.4%	1%	2.7%
Follow-up Mammogram/Ultrasound	755	6.5%	8.1%	8.8%
Lumbar Spine MRI for Low Back Pain[1]	-	-	34.9%	37.2%

Memorial Medical Center

1615 Maple Ln
Ashland, WI 54806
URL: www.ashlandmmc.com
Type: Critical Access Hospitals
Ownership: Voluntary non-profit - Private
Phone: 715-685-5500
Fax: 715-682-4022
Emergency Services: Yes
Beds: 100

Key Personnel:
Patient Relations . . . . Dan Adams
Radiology. . . . . Fredrick E Ekberg
Infection Control. . . . . Keith Henry, MD
CEO/President. . . . . Daniel J Hymans
Chief of Medical Staff . . . . Andrew Matheus
Emergency Room . . . . Donald Patton

Measure	Cases	This Hosp.	State Avg.	U.S. Avg.
Blood Clot Prevention and Treatment				
Anticoagulation Overlap Therapy[5]	-	-	95%	93%
ICU Venous Thromboembolism Prophylaxis[5]	-	-	91%	92%
Incidence of Potentially Preventable VTE[5]	-	-	10%	10%
UFH with Dosages/Platelet Monitoring[5]	-	-	96%	97%
Venous Thromboembolism Prophylaxis[5]	-	-	85%	85%
Warfarin Therapy Discharge Instructions[5]	-	-	70%	75%
Chest Pain/Possible Heart Attack Care				
Aspirin Given Within 24 Hours of Arrival	-	-	98%	96%
Fibrinolytic Meds Within 30 Min. of Arrival	-	-	52%	58%
Average Time to ECG (minutes)	-	-	7	7
Average Time to Transfer (minutes)	-	-	58	60
Children's Asthma Care				
Received Home Management Plan of Care	-	-	-	88%
Received Reliever Medication	-	-	-	100%
Received Systemic Corticosteroids	-	-	-	100%
Emergency Department				
Admittance Decision Time (minutes)[5]	-	-	65	98
Head CT Results Within 45 Min. of Arrival	-	-	61%	57%
Patients Who Left ER Before Being Seen	-	-	1%	2%
Time from ER Arrival to Admit. (minutes)[5]	-	-	207	274
Time from ER Arrival to Discharge (minutes)	-	-	121	134
Time in ER Before Being Evaluated (minutes)	-	-	19	26
Time to Pain Meds for Fractures (minutes)	-	-	42	57
Heart Attack Care				
Aspirin Given at Discharge	16	94%	99%	99%
Fibrinolytic Meds Within 30 Min. of Arrival[7]	-	-	67%	54%
PCI Within 90 Minutes of Arrival[7]	-	-	96%	96%
Statin Prescribed at Discharge	15	60%	99%	98%
Heart Failure Care				
ACE Inhibitor or ARB for LVSD	11	91%	97%	97%
Discharge Instructions Given	31	81%	96%	94%
Evaluation of LVS Function	40	88%	99%	99%
Medicare Spending				
Medicare Spending per Patient (ratio)	-	-	0.94	0.98
Pneumonia Care				
Appropriate Initial Antibiotic Given	54	100%	96%	95%
Blood Culture Timing	66	92%	98%	98%

NOTE: Hospital profiles are in alphabetical order by state, then city, then hospital within the city; Rankings exclude hospitals with less than 25 cases except for patient surveys which excludes hospitals with less than 100 cases; (a) 100-299 cases; (1) The number of cases/patients is too few to report; (2) Data submitted were based on a sample of cases/patients; (3) Results are based on a shorter time period than required; (4) Data suppressed by CMS for one or more quarters; (5) Results are not available for this reporting period; (6) Fewer than 100 patients completed the HCAHPS survey; (7) No cases met the criteria for this measure; (8) The lower limit of the confidence interval cannot be calculated if the number of observed infections equals zero; (9) No data are available from the state/territory for this reporting period; (10) The scores shown reflect fewer than 50 completed surveys; (11) There were discrepancies in the data collection process; (12) This measure does not apply to this hospital for this reporting period; (13) Results cannot be calculated for this reporting period; (14) The results for this state are combined with nearby states to protect confidentiality; Please refer to the User's Guide for a full explanation of data.

Measure	Cases	This Hosp.	State Avg.	U.S. Avg.
Pregnancy and Delivery Care				
Newborn Deliveries Scheduled Early[5]	-	-	4%	6%
Preventive Care				
Immunization for Influenza[5]	-	-	90%	90%
Immunization for Pneumonia[5]	-	-	92%	92%
Stroke Care				
Anticoagulation Therapy for Atrial Fibrillation[5]	-	-	94%	95%
Antithrombotic Therapy Timing[5]	-	-	99%	98%
Assessed for Rehabilitation[5]	-	-	98%	97%
Discharged on Antithrombotic Therapy[5]	-	-	99%	99%
Discharged on Statin Medication[5]	-	-	94%	94%
Thrombolytic Therapy Timing[5]	-	-	60%	66%
Venous Thromboembolism Prophylaxis[5]	-	-	95%	94%
Written Stroke Educational Materials Given[5]	-	-	88%	88%
Surgical Care Improvement Project				
Appropriate Beta Blocker Usage	34	94%	99%	98%
Appropriate VTP Within 24 Hours	87	85%	99%	98%
Controlled Postoperative Blood Glucose[3,7]	-	-	96%	97%
Perioperative Temperature Management	96	95%	100%	100%
Prophylactic Antibiotic Selection	85	99%	99%	99%
Prophylactic Antibiotic Selection (Outpatient)	-	-	98%	98%
Prophylactic Antibiotic Stopped	84	88%	99%	98%
Prophylactic Antibiotic Timing	85	86%	99%	99%
Prophylactic Antibiotic Timing (Outpatient)	-	-	97%	98%
Urinary Catheter Removal	19	79%	98%	97%
Survey of Patients' Hospital Experiences				
Area Around Room 'Always' Quiet at Night	300+	63%	63%	61%
Doctors 'Always' Communicated Well	300+	85%	83%	82%
Home Recovery Information Given	300+	85%	89%	85%
Hospital Given 9 or 10 on 10 Point Scale	300+	73%	74%	71%
Meds 'Always' Explained Before Given	300+	69%	68%	64%
Nurses 'Always' Communicated Well	300+	82%	82%	79%
Pain 'Always' Well Controlled	300+	71%	72%	71%
Room and Bathroom 'Always' Clean	300+	82%	79%	73%
Timely Help 'Always' Received	300+	73%	72%	68%
Would Definitely Recommend Hospital	300+	66%	74%	71%
Use of Medical Imaging				
Cardiac Imaging Stress Test before Surgery	-	-	5.4%	5.3%
Combination Abdominal CT Scan	-	-	6.3%	10.5%
Combination Brain/Sinus CT Scan	-	-	2.1%	2.7%
Combination Chest CT Scan	-	-	1%	2.7%
Follow-up Mammogram/Ultrasound	-	-	8.1%	8.8%
Lumbar Spine MRI for Low Back Pain	-	-	34.9%	37.2%

Baldwin Area Medical Center

730 10th Ave
Baldwin, WI 54002
Phone: 715-684-3311
Fax: 715-684-4757
E-mail: baldhosp@baldwin-telecom.net
URL: www.baldwin-hospital.com
Type: Critical Access Hospitals
Emergency Services: Yes
Ownership: Voluntary non-profit - Private
Beds: 33

Key Personnel:
Radiology. . . . . Mark Doyscher
CEO/President. . . . . Alison Page
Patient Relations . . . . Jean Peavey
Emergency Room . . . . Joel Stoeckeler, MD
Quality Assurance . . . . Peggy Swedine

Measure	Cases	This Hosp.	State Avg.	U.S. Avg.
Blood Clot Prevention and Treatment				
Anticoagulation Overlap Therapy[5]	-	-	95%	93%
ICU Venous Thromboembolism Prophylaxis[5]	-	-	91%	92%
Incidence of Potentially Preventable VTE[5]	-	-	10%	10%
UFH with Dosages/Platelet Monitoring[5]	-	-	96%	97%
Venous Thromboembolism Prophylaxis[5]	-	-	85%	85%
Warfarin Therapy Discharge Instructions[5]	-	-	70%	75%
Chest Pain/Possible Heart Attack Care				
Aspirin Given Within 24 Hours of Arrival	-	-	98%	96%
Fibrinolytic Meds Within 30 Min. of Arrival	-	-	52%	58%
Average Time to ECG (minutes)	-	-	7	7
Average Time to Transfer (minutes)	-	-	58	60
Children's Asthma Care				
Received Home Management Plan of Care	-	-	-	88%
Received Reliever Medication	-	-	-	100%
Received Systemic Corticosteroids	-	-	-	100%
Emergency Department				
Admittance Decision Time (minutes)[5]	-	-	65	98
Head CT Results Within 45 Min. of Arrival	-	-	61%	57%
Patients Who Left ER Before Being Seen	-	-	1%	2%
Time from ER Arrival to Admit. (minutes)[5]	-	-	207	274
Time from ER Arrival to Discharge (minutes)	-	-	121	134
Time in ER Before Being Evaluated (minutes)	-	-	19	26
Time to Pain Meds for Fractures (minutes)	-	-	42	57
Heart Attack Care				
Aspirin Given at Discharge[5]	-	-	99%	99%
Fibrinolytic Meds Within 30 Min. of Arrival[5]	-	-	67%	54%
PCI Within 90 Minutes of Arrival[5]	-	-	96%	96%
Statin Prescribed at Discharge[5]	-	-	99%	98%
Heart Failure Care				
ACE Inhibitor or ARB for LVSD[1]	-	-	97%	97%
Discharge Instructions Given	25	88%	96%	94%
Evaluation of LVS Function	37	84%	99%	99%
Medicare Spending				
Medicare Spending per Patient (ratio)	-	-	0.94	0.98
Pneumonia Care				
Appropriate Initial Antibiotic Given	15	93%	96%	95%
Blood Culture Timing[1]	-	-	98%	98%
Pregnancy and Delivery Care				
Newborn Deliveries Scheduled Early[5]	-	-	4%	6%
Preventive Care				
Immunization for Influenza[5]	-	-	90%	90%
Immunization for Pneumonia[5]	-	-	92%	92%
Stroke Care				
Anticoagulation Therapy for Atrial Fibrillation[5]	-	-	94%	95%
Antithrombotic Therapy Timing[5]	-	-	99%	98%
Assessed for Rehabilitation[5]	-	-	98%	97%
Discharged on Antithrombotic Therapy[5]	-	-	99%	99%
Discharged on Statin Medication[5]	-	-	94%	94%
Thrombolytic Therapy Timing[5]	-	-	60%	66%
Venous Thromboembolism Prophylaxis[5]	-	-	95%	94%
Written Stroke Educational Materials Given[5]	-	-	88%	88%
Surgical Care Improvement Project				
Appropriate Beta Blocker Usage[1,3]	-	-	99%	98%
Appropriate VTP Within 24 Hours[5]	-	-	99%	98%
Controlled Postoperative Blood Glucose[3,7]	-	-	96%	97%
Perioperative Temperature Management[5]	-	-	100%	100%
Prophylactic Antibiotic Selection	26	81%	99%	99%
Prophylactic Antibiotic Selection (Outpatient)	-	-	98%	98%
Prophylactic Antibiotic Stopped	26	100%	99%	98%
Prophylactic Antibiotic Timing	26	92%	99%	99%
Prophylactic Antibiotic Timing (Outpatient)	-	-	97%	98%
Urinary Catheter Removal[5]	-	-	98%	97%
Survey of Patients' Hospital Experiences				
Area Around Room 'Always' Quiet at Night[5]	-	-	63%	61%
Doctors 'Always' Communicated Well[5]	-	-	83%	82%
Home Recovery Information Given[5]	-	-	89%	85%
Hospital Given 9 or 10 on 10 Point Scale[5]	-	-	74%	71%
Meds 'Always' Explained Before Given[5]	-	-	68%	64%
Nurses 'Always' Communicated Well[5]	-	-	82%	79%
Pain 'Always' Well Controlled[5]	-	-	72%	71%
Room and Bathroom 'Always' Clean[5]	-	-	79%	73%
Timely Help 'Always' Received[5]	-	-	72%	68%
Would Definitely Recommend Hospital[5]	-	-	74%	71%
Use of Medical Imaging				
Cardiac Imaging Stress Test before Surgery	-	-	5.4%	5.3%
Combination Abdominal CT Scan	-	-	6.3%	10.5%
Combination Brain/Sinus CT Scan	-	-	2.1%	2.7%
Combination Chest CT Scan	-	-	1%	2.7%
Follow-up Mammogram/Ultrasound	-	-	8.1%	8.8%
Lumbar Spine MRI for Low Back Pain	-	-	34.9%	37.2%

Saint Clare Hospital Health Services

707 14th St
Baraboo, WI 53913
Phone: 608-356-1400
Fax: 608-356-1367
URL: www.stclare.com
Type: Acute Care Hospitals
Emergency Services: Yes
Ownership: Voluntary non-profit - Private
Beds: 62

Key Personnel:
CEO/President. . . . . Sandra Anderson
Chief of Medical Staff . . . . Erich Herbest
Emergency Room . . . . Theresa Weiland

Measure	Cases	This Hosp.	State Avg.	U.S. Avg.
Blood Clot Prevention and Treatment				
Anticoagulation Overlap Therapy[2]	16	100%	95%	93%
ICU Venous Thromboembolism Prophylaxis[2]	40	100%	91%	92%
Incidence of Potentially Preventable VTE[2,7]	-	-	10%	10%
UFH with Dosages/Platelet Monitoring[1,2]	-	-	96%	97%
Venous Thromboembolism Prophylaxis[2]	132	98%	85%	85%
Warfarin Therapy Discharge Instructions[2]	11	100%	70%	75%
Chest Pain/Possible Heart Attack Care				
Aspirin Given Within 24 Hours of Arrival	59	100%	98%	96%
Fibrinolytic Meds Within 30 Min. of Arrival[7]	-	-	52%	58%
Average Time to ECG (minutes)	62	9	7	7
Average Time to Transfer (minutes)	20	67	58	60
Children's Asthma Care				
Received Home Management Plan of Care	-	-	-	88%
Received Reliever Medication	-	-	-	100%
Received Systemic Corticosteroids	-	-	-	100%
Emergency Department				
Admittance Decision Time (minutes)[2]	181	59	65	98
Head CT Results Within 45 Min. of Arrival[1]	-	-	61%	57%
Patients Who Left ER Before Being Seen	19,894	0%	1%	2%
Time from ER Arrival to Admit. (minutes)[2]	182	180	207	274
Time from ER Arrival to Discharge (minutes)	358	104	121	134
Time in ER Before Being Evaluated (minutes)	406	10	19	26
Time to Pain Meds for Fractures (minutes)	66	26	42	57
Heart Attack Care				
Aspirin Given at Discharge[1]	-	-	99%	99%
Fibrinolytic Meds Within 30 Min. of Arrival[7]	-	-	67%	54%
PCI Within 90 Minutes of Arrival[7]	-	-	96%	96%
Statin Prescribed at Discharge[1]	-	-	99%	98%
Heart Failure Care				
ACE Inhibitor or ARB for LVSD	15	100%	97%	97%
Discharge Instructions Given	38	100%	96%	94%
Evaluation of LVS Function	58	100%	99%	99%
Medicare Spending				
Medicare Spending per Patient (ratio)	-	0.97	0.94	0.98
Pneumonia Care				
Appropriate Initial Antibiotic Given	64	100%	96%	95%
Blood Culture Timing	96	100%	98%	98%
Pregnancy and Delivery Care				
Newborn Deliveries Scheduled Early	17	0%	4%	6%
Preventive Care				
Immunization for Influenza[2]	263	98%	90%	90%
Immunization for Pneumonia[2]	323	99%	92%	92%
Stroke Care				
Anticoagulation Therapy for Atrial Fibrillation[1]	-	-	94%	95%
Antithrombotic Therapy Timing	27	100%	99%	98%
Assessed for Rehabilitation	28	100%	98%	97%
Discharged on Antithrombotic Therapy	26	100%	99%	99%
Discharged on Statin Medication	23	100%	94%	94%
Thrombolytic Therapy Timing[7]	-	-	60%	66%
Venous Thromboembolism Prophylaxis	29	100%	95%	94%
Written Stroke Educational Materials Given	11	100%	88%	88%
Surgical Care Improvement Project				
Appropriate Beta Blocker Usage	37	97%	99%	98%
Appropriate VTP Within 24 Hours	133	99%	99%	98%
Controlled Postoperative Blood Glucose[7]	-	-	96%	97%
Perioperative Temperature Management	139	100%	100%	100%
Prophylactic Antibiotic Selection	124	100%	99%	99%
Prophylactic Antibiotic Selection (Outpatient)	43	93%	98%	98%
Prophylactic Antibiotic Stopped	124	99%	99%	98%
Prophylactic Antibiotic Timing	124	98%	99%	99%
Prophylactic Antibiotic Timing (Outpatient)	43	100%	97%	98%
Urinary Catheter Removal	108	100%	98%	97%
Survey of Patients' Hospital Experiences				
Area Around Room 'Always' Quiet at Night[11]	300+	70%	63%	61%
Doctors 'Always' Communicated Well[11]	300+	85%	83%	82%
Home Recovery Information Given[11]	300+	90%	89%	85%
Hospital Given 9 or 10 on 10 Point Scale[11]	300+	79%	74%	71%
Meds 'Always' Explained Before Given[11]	300+	69%	68%	64%

NOTE: Hospital profiles are in alphabetical order by state, then city, then hospital within the city; Rankings exclude hospitals with less than 25 cases except for patient surveys which excludes hospitals with less than 100 cases; (a) 100-299 cases; (1) The number of cases/patients is too few to report; (2) Data submitted were based on a sample of cases/patients; (3) Results are based on a shorter time period than required; (4) Data suppressed by CMS for one or more quarters; (5) Results are not available for this reporting period; (6) Fewer than 100 patients completed the HCAHPS survey; (7) No cases met the criteria for this measure; (8) The lower limit of the confidence interval cannot be calculated if the number of observed infections equals zero; (9) No data are available from the state/territory for this reporting period; (10) The scores shown reflect fewer than 50 completed surveys; (11) There were discrepancies in the data collection process; (12) This measure does not apply to this hospital for this reporting period; (13) Results cannot be calculated for this reporting period; (14) The results for this state are combined with nearby states to protect confidentiality; Please refer to the User's Guide for a full explanation of data.

Measure	Cases	This Hosp.	State Avg.	U.S. Avg.
Nurses 'Always' Communicated Well[11]	300+	86%	82%	79%
Pain 'Always' Well Controlled[11]	300+	69%	72%	71%
Room and Bathroom 'Always' Clean[11]	300+	81%	79%	73%
Timely Help 'Always' Received[11]	300+	78%	72%	68%
Would Definitely Recommend Hospital[11]	300+	77%	74%	71%
Use of Medical Imaging				
Cardiac Imaging Stress Test before Surgery	102	2.9%	5.4%	5.3%
Combination Abdominal CT Scan	347	4.6%	6.3%	10.5%
Combination Brain/Sinus CT Scan[1]		-	2.1%	2.7%
Combination Chest CT Scan	157	3.2%	1%	2.7%
Follow-up Mammogram/Ultrasound	285	6.7%	8.1%	8.8%
Lumbar Spine MRI for Low Back Pain[1]		-	34.9%	37.2%

Mayo Clinic Health System - Northland

1222 E Woodland Ave
Barron, WI 54812
URL: www.luthermidelfortnorthland.org
Phone: 715-537-3186
Fax: 715-537-9023
Type: Critical Access Hospitals
Emergency Services: Yes
Ownership: Voluntary non-profit - Other
Beds: 29

Key Personnel:
Chief of Medical Staff.......... Michael Damroth
Infection Control.............. Kim Droege
Emergency Room .... Lorna Larson, RN
Operating Room.............. Lorna Larson, RN
Quality Assurance .... Lori Springer
Anesthesiology............... Tom Thomsen

Measure	Cases	This Hosp.	State Avg.	U.S. Avg.
Blood Clot Prevention and Treatment				
Anticoagulation Overlap Therapy[5]	-	-	95%	93%
ICU Venous Thromboembolism Prophylaxis[5]	-	-	91%	92%
Incidence of Potentially Preventable VTE[5]	-	-	10%	10%
UFH with Dosages/Platelet Monitoring[5]	-	-	96%	97%
Venous Thromboembolism Prophylaxis[5]	-	-	85%	85%
Warfarin Therapy Discharge Instructions[5]	-	-	70%	75%
Chest Pain/Possible Heart Attack Care				
Aspirin Given Within 24 Hours of Arrival	-	-	98%	96%
Fibrinolytic Meds Within 30 Min. of Arrival	-	-	52%	58%
Average Time to ECG (minutes)	-	-	7	7
Average Time to Transfer (minutes)	-	-	58	60
Children's Asthma Care				
Received Home Management Plan of Care	-	-	-	88%
Received Reliever Medication	-	-	-	100%
Received Systemic Corticosteroids	-	-	-	100%
Emergency Department				
Admittance Decision Time (minutes)[5]	-	-	65	98
Head CT Results Within 45 Min. of Arrival	-	-	61%	57%
Patients Who Left ER Before Being Seen	-	-	1%	2%
Time from ER Arrival to Admit. (minutes)[5]	-	-	207	274
Time from ER Arrival to Discharge (minutes)	-	-	121	134
Time in ER Before Being Evaluated (minutes)	-	-	19	26
Time to Pain Meds for Fractures (minutes)	-	-	42	57
Heart Attack Care				
Aspirin Given at Discharge[1,3]	-	-	99%	99%
Fibrinolytic Meds Within 30 Min. of Arrival[3,7]	-	-	67%	54%
PCI Within 90 Minutes of Arrival[5]	-	-	96%	96%
Statin Prescribed at Discharge[1,3]	-	-	99%	98%
Heart Failure Care				
ACE Inhibitor or ARB for LVSD[1]	-	-	97%	97%
Discharge Instructions Given	14	100%	96%	94%
Evaluation of LVS Function	24	96%	99%	99%
Medicare Spending				
Medicare Spending per Patient (ratio)	-	-	0.94	0.98
Pneumonia Care				
Appropriate Initial Antibiotic Given	25	100%	96%	95%
Blood Culture Timing	40	100%	98%	98%
Pregnancy and Delivery Care				
Newborn Deliveries Scheduled Early[5]	-	-	4%	6%
Preventive Care				
Immunization for Influenza[5]	-	-	90%	90%
Immunization for Pneumonia[5]	-	-	92%	92%
Stroke Care				
Anticoagulation Therapy for Atrial Fibrillation[5]	-	-	94%	95%
Antithrombotic Therapy Timing[5]	-	-	99%	98%
Assessed for Rehabilitation[5]	-	-	98%	97%
Discharged on Antithrombotic Therapy[5]	-	-	99%	99%
Discharged on Statin Medication[5]	-	-	94%	94%
Thrombolytic Therapy Timing[5]	-	-	60%	66%
Venous Thromboembolism Prophylaxis[5]	-	-	95%	94%
Written Stroke Educational Materials Given[5]	-	-	88%	88%
Surgical Care Improvement Project				
Appropriate Beta Blocker Usage[1]	-	-	99%	98%
Appropriate VTP Within 24 Hours	29	100%	99%	98%
Controlled Postoperative Blood Glucose[3,7]	-	-	96%	97%
Perioperative Temperature Management	35	100%	100%	100%
Prophylactic Antibiotic Selection	19	95%	99%	99%
Prophylactic Antibiotic Selection (Outpatient)	-	-	98%	98%
Prophylactic Antibiotic Stopped	19	100%	99%	98%
Prophylactic Antibiotic Timing	19	100%	99%	99%
Prophylactic Antibiotic Timing (Outpatient)	-	-	97%	98%
Urinary Catheter Removal[1]	-	-	98%	97%
Survey of Patients' Hospital Experiences				
Area Around Room 'Always' Quiet at Night	(a)	61%	63%	61%
Doctors 'Always' Communicated Well	(a)	81%	83%	82%
Home Recovery Information Given	(a)	92%	89%	85%
Hospital Given 9 or 10 on 10 Point Scale	(a)	70%	74%	71%
Meds 'Always' Explained Before Given	(a)	69%	68%	64%
Nurses 'Always' Communicated Well	(a)	75%	82%	79%
Pain 'Always' Well Controlled	(a)	75%	72%	71%
Room and Bathroom 'Always' Clean	(a)	75%	79%	73%
Timely Help 'Always' Received	(a)	72%	72%	68%
Would Definitely Recommend Hospital	(a)	68%	74%	71%
Use of Medical Imaging				
Cardiac Imaging Stress Test before Surgery	-	-	5.4%	5.3%
Combination Abdominal CT Scan	-	-	6.3%	10.5%
Combination Brain/Sinus CT Scan	-	-	2.1%	2.7%
Combination Chest CT Scan	-	-	1%	2.7%
Follow-up Mammogram/Ultrasound	-	-	8.1%	8.8%
Lumbar Spine MRI for Low Back Pain	-	-	34.9%	37.2%

Beaver Dam Com Hospital

707 S University Ave
Beaver Dam, WI 53916
Phone: 920-887-7181
Fax: 920-887-3422
Type: Acute Care Hospitals
Emergency Services: Yes
Ownership: Voluntary non-profit - Private
Beds: 125

Key Personnel:
Chair/CEO.................. Jim Kirsh
CEO/President............... John R Landdeck
Emergency Room .... Judy MacDonald
Operating Room.............. Julie Nampel
Radiology.................... John Sweeney
Ambulatory Care .... Sandra Tiedt
Quality Assurance .... Sue Williams
Chief of Medical Staff.......... Julia S. Wright

Measure	Cases	This Hosp.	State Avg.	U.S. Avg.
Blood Clot Prevention and Treatment				
Anticoagulation Overlap Therapy[2]	17	88%	95%	93%
ICU Venous Thromboembolism Prophylaxis[2]	26	100%	91%	92%
Incidence of Potentially Preventable VTE[1,2]	-	-	10%	10%
UFH with Dosages/Platelet Monitoring[1,2]	-	-	96%	97%
Venous Thromboembolism Prophylaxis[2]	118	92%	85%	85%
Warfarin Therapy Discharge Instructions[2]	15	100%	70%	75%
Chest Pain/Possible Heart Attack Care				
Aspirin Given Within 24 Hours of Arrival	137	99%	98%	96%
Fibrinolytic Meds Within 30 Min. of Arrival[7]	-	-	52%	58%
Average Time to ECG (minutes)	138	4	7	7
Average Time to Transfer (minutes)[1]	-	-	58	60
Children's Asthma Care				
Received Home Management Plan of Care	-	-	-	88%
Received Reliever Medication	-	-	-	100%
Received Systemic Corticosteroids	-	-	-	100%
Emergency Department				
Admittance Decision Time (minutes)[2]	298	53	65	98
Head CT Results Within 45 Min. of Arrival	19	32%	61%	57%
Patients Who Left ER Before Being Seen	29,940	0%	1%	2%
Time from ER Arrival to Admit. (minutes)[2]	299	220	207	274
Time from ER Arrival to Discharge (minutes)	368	138	121	134
Time in ER Before Being Evaluated (minutes)	412	23	19	26
Time to Pain Meds for Fractures (minutes)	57	41	42	57
Heart Attack Care				
Aspirin Given at Discharge[1]	-	-	99%	99%
Fibrinolytic Meds Within 30 Min. of Arrival[7]	-	-	67%	54%
PCI Within 90 Minutes of Arrival[7]	-	-	96%	96%
Statin Prescribed at Discharge[1]	-	-	99%	98%
Heart Failure Care				
ACE Inhibitor or ARB for LVSD	12	92%	97%	97%
Discharge Instructions Given	46	89%	96%	94%
Evaluation of LVS Function	52	98%	99%	99%
Medicare Spending				
Medicare Spending per Patient (ratio)	-	0.91	0.94	0.98
Pneumonia Care				
Appropriate Initial Antibiotic Given	53	91%	96%	95%
Blood Culture Timing	77	95%	98%	98%
Pregnancy and Delivery Care				
Newborn Deliveries Scheduled Early[2]	24	0%	4%	6%
Preventive Care				
Immunization for Influenza[2]	271	89%	90%	90%
Immunization for Pneumonia[2]	325	93%	92%	92%
Stroke Care				
Anticoagulation Therapy for Atrial Fibrillation[1]	-	-	94%	95%
Antithrombotic Therapy Timing	18	94%	99%	98%
Assessed for Rehabilitation	20	95%	98%	97%
Discharged on Antithrombotic Therapy	18	100%	99%	99%
Discharged on Statin Medication	18	83%	94%	94%
Thrombolytic Therapy Timing[1]	-	-	60%	66%
Venous Thromboembolism Prophylaxis	19	95%	95%	94%
Written Stroke Educational Materials Given[1]	-	-	88%	88%
Surgical Care Improvement Project				
Appropriate Beta Blocker Usage	68	97%	99%	98%
Appropriate VTP Within 24 Hours	223	100%	99%	98%
Controlled Postoperative Blood Glucose[7]	-	-	96%	97%
Perioperative Temperature Management	238	100%	100%	100%
Prophylactic Antibiotic Selection	193	100%	99%	99%
Prophylactic Antibiotic Selection (Outpatient)	86	98%	98%	98%
Prophylactic Antibiotic Stopped	188	98%	99%	98%
Prophylactic Antibiotic Timing	193	100%	99%	99%
Prophylactic Antibiotic Timing (Outpatient)	86	99%	97%	98%
Urinary Catheter Removal	195	96%	98%	97%
Survey of Patients' Hospital Experiences				
Area Around Room 'Always' Quiet at Night	300+	59%	63%	61%
Doctors 'Always' Communicated Well	300+	81%	83%	82%
Home Recovery Information Given	300+	89%	89%	85%
Hospital Given 9 or 10 on 10 Point Scale	300+	69%	74%	71%
Meds 'Always' Explained Before Given	300+	66%	68%	64%
Nurses 'Always' Communicated Well	300+	81%	82%	79%
Pain 'Always' Well Controlled	300+	71%	72%	71%
Room and Bathroom 'Always' Clean	300+	79%	79%	73%
Timely Help 'Always' Received	300+	73%	72%	68%
Would Definitely Recommend Hospital	300+	65%	74%	71%
Use of Medical Imaging				
Cardiac Imaging Stress Test before Surgery	208	3.4%	5.4%	5.3%
Combination Abdominal CT Scan	519	2.7%	6.3%	10.5%
Combination Brain/Sinus CT Scan[1]		-	2.1%	2.7%
Combination Chest CT Scan	354	1.1%	1%	2.7%
Follow-up Mammogram/Ultrasound	875	9.1%	8.1%	8.8%
Lumbar Spine MRI for Low Back Pain	56	26.8%	34.9%	37.2%

Beloit Memorial Hospital

1969 W Hart Rd
Beloit, WI 53511
Phone: 608-364-5011
Fax: 608-364-5356
Type: Acute Care Hospitals
Emergency Services: Yes
Ownership: Voluntary non-profit - Private
Beds: 174

Key Personnel:
Radiology.................... Bilal A Ahmed
Chief of Medical Staff.......... Shamshad A Anjum
Cardiac Laboratory............ Larry Bergen
Infection Control.............. Karen Draves
Operating Room.............. Shirley Fischer
CEO/President............... Timothy McKevett

Measure	Cases	This Hosp.	State Avg.	U.S. Avg.
Blood Clot Prevention and Treatment				
Anticoagulation Overlap Therapy[2]	43	100%	95%	93%
ICU Venous Thromboembolism Prophylaxis[2]	56	95%	91%	92%

NOTE: Hospital profiles are in alphabetical order by state, then city, then hospital within the city; Rankings exclude hospitals with less than 25 cases except for patient surveys which excludes hospitals with less than 100 cases; (a) 100-299 cases; (1) The number of cases/patients is too few to report; (2) Data submitted were based on a sample of cases/patients; (3) Results are based on a shorter time period than required; (4) Data suppressed by CMS for one or more quarters; (5) Results are not available for this reporting period; (6) Fewer than 100 patients completed the HCAHPS survey; (7) No cases met the criteria for this measure; (8) The lower limit of the confidence interval cannot be calculated if the number of observed infections equals zero; (9) No data are available from the state/territory for this reporting period; (10) The scores shown reflect fewer than 50 completed surveys; (11) There were discrepancies in the data collection process; (12) This measure does not apply to this hospital for this reporting period; (13) Results cannot be calculated for this reporting period; (14) The results for this state are combined with nearby states to protect confidentiality; Please refer to the User's Guide for a full explanation of data.

Incidence of Potentially Preventable VTE[1,2]	-	-	10%	10%
UFH with Dosages/Platelet Monitoring[2]	16	94%	96%	97%
Venous Thromboembolism Prophylaxis[2]	297	87%	85%	85%
Warfarin Therapy Discharge Instructions[2]	39	79%	70%	75%
Chest Pain/Possible Heart Attack Care				
Aspirin Given Within 24 Hours of Arrival[3]	20	100%	98%	96%
Fibrinolytic Meds Within 30 Min. of Arrival[3,7]	-	-	52%	58%
Average Time to ECG (minutes)[3]	20	10	7	7
Average Time to Transfer (minutes)[1,3]	-	-	58	60
Children's Asthma Care				
Received Home Management Plan of Care	-	-	-	88%
Received Reliever Medication	-	-	-	100%
Received Systemic Corticosteroids	-	-	-	100%
Emergency Department				
Admittance Decision Time (minutes)[2]	439	56	65	98
Head CT Results Within 45 Min. of Arrival	23	87%	61%	57%
Patients Who Left ER Before Being Seen	39,846	2%	1%	2%
Time from ER Arrival to Admit. (minutes)[2]	439	226	207	274
Time from ER Arrival to Discharge (minutes)	397	127	121	134
Time in ER Before Being Evaluated (minutes)	245	39	19	26
Time to Pain Meds for Fractures (minutes)	102	72	42	57
Heart Attack Care				
Aspirin Given at Discharge	90	96%	99%	99%
Fibrinolytic Meds Within 30 Min. of Arrival[7]	-	-	67%	54%
PCI Within 90 Minutes of Arrival[1]	-	-	96%	96%
Statin Prescribed at Discharge	91	93%	99%	98%
Heart Failure Care				
ACE Inhibitor or ARB for LVSD	37	89%	97%	97%
Discharge Instructions Given	115	91%	96%	94%
Evaluation of LVS Function	147	100%	99%	99%
Medicare Spending				
Medicare Spending per Patient (ratio)	-	0.99	0.94	0.98
Pneumonia Care				
Appropriate Initial Antibiotic Given	35	94%	96%	95%
Blood Culture Timing	67	100%	98%	98%
Pregnancy and Delivery Care				
Newborn Deliveries Scheduled Early	80	2%	4%	6%
Preventive Care				
Immunization for Influenza[2]	366	96%	90%	90%
Immunization for Pneumonia[2]	458	97%	92%	92%
Stroke Care				
Anticoagulation Therapy for Atrial Fibrillation[1]	-	-	94%	95%
Antithrombotic Therapy Timing	35	97%	99%	98%
Assessed for Rehabilitation	33	100%	98%	97%
Discharged on Antithrombotic Therapy	31	94%	99%	99%
Discharged on Statin Medication	30	80%	94%	94%
Thrombolytic Therapy Timing	13	0%	60%	66%
Venous Thromboembolism Prophylaxis	35	89%	95%	94%
Written Stroke Educational Materials Given	19	42%	88%	88%
Surgical Care Improvement Project				
Appropriate Beta Blocker Usage[2]	131	96%	99%	98%
Appropriate VTP Within 24 Hours[2]	313	99%	99%	98%
Controlled Postoperative Blood Glucose[2]	49	92%	96%	97%
Perioperative Temperature Management[2]	343	97%	100%	100%
Prophylactic Antibiotic Selection[2]	285	98%	99%	99%
Prophylactic Antibiotic Selection (Outpatient)	113	93%	98%	98%
Prophylactic Antibiotic Stopped[2]	281	95%	99%	98%
Prophylactic Antibiotic Timing[2]	287	92%	99%	99%
Prophylactic Antibiotic Timing (Outpatient)	93	95%	97%	98%
Urinary Catheter Removal[2]	157	91%	98%	97%
Survey of Patients' Hospital Experiences				
Area Around Room 'Always' Quiet at Night	300+	54%	63%	61%
Doctors 'Always' Communicated Well	300+	80%	83%	82%
Home Recovery Information Given	300+	87%	89%	85%
Hospital Given 9 or 10 on 10 Point Scale	300+	67%	74%	71%
Meds 'Always' Explained Before Given	300+	63%	68%	64%
Nurses 'Always' Communicated Well	300+	80%	82%	79%
Pain 'Always' Well Controlled	300+	68%	72%	71%
Room and Bathroom 'Always' Clean	300+	74%	79%	73%
Timely Help 'Always' Received	300+	64%	72%	68%
Would Definitely Recommend Hospital	300+	66%	74%	71%
Use of Medical Imaging				
Cardiac Imaging Stress Test before Surgery	378	5.6%	5.4%	5.3%
Combination Abdominal CT Scan	598	55.5%	6.3%	10.5%
Combination Brain/Sinus CT Scan[1]	-	-	2.1%	2.7%
Combination Chest CT Scan	247	1.2%	1%	2.7%
Follow-up Mammogram/Ultrasound	1,162	3.7%	8.1%	8.8%
Lumbar Spine MRI for Low Back Pain	94	39.4%	34.9%	37.2%

Berlin Memorial Hospital

225 Memorial Drive
Berlin, WI 54923
Phone: 920-361-1313
Fax: 920-361-5318
Type: Critical Access Hospitals
Emergency Services: Yes
Ownership: Voluntary non-profit - Private
Beds: 61

Key Personnel:
Infection Control. . . . . Kathy Beier
Quality Assurance . . . . Kathy Beier
Chief of Medical Staff. . . . . Jeff Carroll, MD
CEO/President. . . . . John Feeney
Emergency Room . . . . Dan Perrault, MD
Anesthesiology. . . . . Daniel Resop, MD
Intensive Care Unit. . . . . Kelly Schmude

Measure	Cases	This Hosp.	State Avg.	U.S. Avg.
Blood Clot Prevention and Treatment				
Anticoagulation Overlap Therapy[5]	-	-	95%	93%
ICU Venous Thromboembolism Prophylaxis[5]	-	-	91%	92%
Incidence of Potentially Preventable VTE[5]	-	-	10%	10%
UFH with Dosages/Platelet Monitoring[5]	-	-	96%	97%
Venous Thromboembolism Prophylaxis[5]	-	-	85%	85%
Warfarin Therapy Discharge Instructions[5]	-	-	70%	75%
Chest Pain/Possible Heart Attack Care				
Aspirin Given Within 24 Hours of Arrival	40	100%	98%	96%
Fibrinolytic Meds Within 30 Min. of Arrival[7]	-	-	52%	58%
Average Time to ECG (minutes)	41	4	7	7
Average Time to Transfer (minutes)[7]	-	-	58	60
Children's Asthma Care				
Received Home Management Plan of Care	-	-	-	88%
Received Reliever Medication	-	-	-	100%
Received Systemic Corticosteroids	-	-	-	100%
Emergency Department				
Admittance Decision Time (minutes)[1]	-	-	65	98
Head CT Results Within 45 Min. of Arrival[5]	-	-	61%	57%
Patients Who Left ER Before Being Seen[5]	-	-	1%	2%
Time from ER Arrival to Admit. (minutes)	134	198	207	274
Time from ER Arrival to Discharge (minutes)	337	120	121	134
Time in ER Before Being Evaluated (minutes)	404	14	19	26
Time to Pain Meds for Fractures (minutes)[5]	-	-	42	57
Heart Attack Care				
Aspirin Given at Discharge[5]	-	-	99%	99%
Fibrinolytic Meds Within 30 Min. of Arrival[5]	-	-	67%	54%
PCI Within 90 Minutes of Arrival[5]	-	-	96%	96%
Statin Prescribed at Discharge[5]	-	-	99%	98%
Heart Failure Care				
ACE Inhibitor or ARB for LVSD	11	82%	97%	97%
Discharge Instructions Given	26	96%	96%	94%
Evaluation of LVS Function	39	90%	99%	99%
Medicare Spending				
Medicare Spending per Patient (ratio)	-	-	0.94	0.98
Pneumonia Care				
Appropriate Initial Antibiotic Given	26	88%	96%	95%
Blood Culture Timing	54	100%	98%	98%
Pregnancy and Delivery Care				
Newborn Deliveries Scheduled Early[5]	-	-	4%	6%
Preventive Care				
Immunization for Influenza	153	85%	90%	90%
Immunization for Pneumonia	232	88%	92%	92%
Stroke Care				
Anticoagulation Therapy for Atrial Fibrillation[1]	-	-	94%	95%
Antithrombotic Therapy Timing	16	100%	99%	98%
Assessed for Rehabilitation	15	100%	98%	97%
Discharged on Antithrombotic Therapy	13	92%	99%	99%
Discharged on Statin Medication[1]	-	-	94%	94%
Thrombolytic Therapy Timing[1]	-	-	60%	66%
Venous Thromboembolism Prophylaxis	18	72%	95%	94%
Written Stroke Educational Materials Given[1]	-	-	88%	88%
Surgical Care Improvement Project				
Appropriate Beta Blocker Usage[2]	22	100%	99%	98%
Appropriate VTP Within 24 Hours[2]	123	100%	99%	98%
Controlled Postoperative Blood Glucose[2,3]	-	-	96%	97%
Perioperative Temperature Management[2]	149	100%	100%	100%
Prophylactic Antibiotic Selection[2]	135	99%	99%	99%
Prophylactic Antibiotic Selection (Outpatient)	77	99%	98%	98%
Prophylactic Antibiotic Stopped[2]	133	98%	99%	98%
Prophylactic Antibiotic Timing[2]	135	97%	99%	99%
Prophylactic Antibiotic Timing (Outpatient)	76	99%	97%	98%
Urinary Catheter Removal[2]	136	100%	98%	97%
Survey of Patients' Hospital Experiences				
Area Around Room 'Always' Quiet at Night	300+	58%	63%	61%
Doctors 'Always' Communicated Well	300+	81%	83%	82%
Home Recovery Information Given	300+	88%	89%	85%
Hospital Given 9 or 10 on 10 Point Scale	300+	68%	74%	71%
Meds 'Always' Explained Before Given	300+	67%	68%	64%
Nurses 'Always' Communicated Well	300+	80%	82%	79%
Pain 'Always' Well Controlled	300+	72%	72%	71%
Room and Bathroom 'Always' Clean	300+	79%	79%	73%
Timely Help 'Always' Received	300+	72%	72%	68%
Would Definitely Recommend Hospital	300+	69%	74%	71%
Use of Medical Imaging				
Cardiac Imaging Stress Test before Surgery	77	0.0%	5.4%	5.3%
Combination Abdominal CT Scan	186	2.7%	6.3%	10.5%
Combination Brain/Sinus CT Scan[1]	-	-	2.1%	2.7%
Combination Chest CT Scan	87	1.1%	1%	2.7%
Follow-up Mammogram/Ultrasound	360	5.8%	8.1%	8.8%
Lumbar Spine MRI for Low Back Pain[1]	-	-	34.9%	37.2%

Black River Memorial Hospital

711 W Adams St
Black River Falls, WI 54615
Phone: 715-284-5361
Fax: 715-284-7166
URL: www.brmh.net
Type: Critical Access Hospitals
Emergency Services: Yes
Ownership: Voluntary non-profit - Private
Beds: 51

Key Personnel:
Surgery . . . . Darrin Antonelli, MD
Quality Assurance . . . . Mary Bestwait
Cardiology . . . . Ward Brown, MD
Pulmonology . . . . Kyle Dettbarn, MD
Radiology. . . . . Mary Ewing
CEO/President. . . . . Stanley J Gaynor
Emergency Room . . . . Barb Holderman, RN

Measure	Cases	This Hosp.	State Avg.	U.S. Avg.
Blood Clot Prevention and Treatment				
Anticoagulation Overlap Therapy[5]	-	-	95%	93%
ICU Venous Thromboembolism Prophylaxis[5]	-	-	91%	92%
Incidence of Potentially Preventable VTE[5]	-	-	10%	10%
UFH with Dosages/Platelet Monitoring[5]	-	-	96%	97%
Venous Thromboembolism Prophylaxis[5]	-	-	85%	85%
Warfarin Therapy Discharge Instructions[5]	-	-	70%	75%
Chest Pain/Possible Heart Attack Care				
Aspirin Given Within 24 Hours of Arrival	53	96%	98%	96%
Fibrinolytic Meds Within 30 Min. of Arrival[1]	-	-	52%	58%
Average Time to ECG (minutes)	53	8	7	7
Average Time to Transfer (minutes)[1]	-	-	58	60
Children's Asthma Care				
Received Home Management Plan of Care	-	-	-	88%
Received Reliever Medication	-	-	-	100%
Received Systemic Corticosteroids	-	-	-	100%
Emergency Department				
Admittance Decision Time (minutes)[5]	-	-	65	98
Head CT Results Within 45 Min. of Arrival[5]	-	-	61%	57%
Patients Who Left ER Before Being Seen[5]	-	-	1%	2%
Time from ER Arrival to Admit. (minutes)[5]	-	-	207	274
Time from ER Arrival to Discharge (minutes)[5]	-	-	121	134
Time in ER Before Being Evaluated (minutes)[5]	-	-	19	26
Time to Pain Meds for Fractures (minutes)[5]	-	-	42	57
Heart Attack Care				
Aspirin Given at Discharge[1,3]	-	-	99%	99%
Fibrinolytic Meds Within 30 Min. of Arrival[3,7]	-	-	67%	54%
PCI Within 90 Minutes of Arrival[5]	-	-	96%	96%
Statin Prescribed at Discharge[1,3]	-	-	99%	98%
Heart Failure Care				

NOTE: Hospital profiles are in alphabetical order by state, then city, then hospital within the city; Rankings exclude hospitals with less than 25 cases except for patient surveys which excludes hospitals with less than 100 cases; (a) 100-299 cases; (1) The number of cases/patients is too few to report; (2) Data submitted were based on a sample of cases/patients; (3) Results are based on a shorter time period than required; (4) Data suppressed by CMS for one or more quarters; (5) Results are not available for this reporting period; (6) Fewer than 100 patients completed the HCAHPS survey; (7) No cases met the criteria for this measure; (8) The lower limit of the confidence interval cannot be calculated if the number of observed infections equals zero; (9) No data are available from the state/territory for this reporting period; (10) The scores shown reflect fewer than 50 completed surveys; (11) There were discrepancies in the data collection process; (12) This measure does not apply to this hospital for this reporting period; (13) Results cannot be calculated for this reporting period; (14) The results for this state are combined with nearby states to protect confidentiality; Please refer to the User's Guide for a full explanation of data.

ACE Inhibitor or ARB for LVSD[1]	-	-	97%	97%
Discharge Instructions Given	24	100%	96%	94%
Evaluation of LVS Function	33	97%	99%	99%
Medicare Spending				
Medicare Spending per Patient (ratio)	-	-	0.94	0.98
Pneumonia Care				
Appropriate Initial Antibiotic Given	45	100%	96%	95%
Blood Culture Timing	38	92%	98%	98%
Pregnancy and Delivery Care				
Newborn Deliveries Scheduled Early[5]	-	-	4%	6%
Preventive Care				
Immunization for Influenza[5]	-	-	90%	90%
Immunization for Pneumonia[5]	-	-	92%	92%
Stroke Care				
Anticoagulation Therapy for Atrial Fibrillation[5]	-	-	94%	95%
Antithrombotic Therapy Timing[5]	-	-	99%	98%
Assessed for Rehabilitation[5]	-	-	98%	97%
Discharged on Antithrombotic Therapy[5]	-	-	99%	99%
Discharged on Statin Medication[5]	-	-	94%	94%
Thrombolytic Therapy Timing[5]	-	-	60%	66%
Venous Thromboembolism Prophylaxis[5]	-	-	95%	94%
Written Stroke Educational Materials Given[5]	-	-	88%	88%
Surgical Care Improvement Project				
Appropriate Beta Blocker Usage	19	95%	99%	98%
Appropriate VTP Within 24 Hours	12	100%	99%	98%
Controlled Postoperative Blood Glucose[3,7]	-	-	96%	97%
Perioperative Temperature Management	71	100%	100%	100%
Prophylactic Antibiotic Selection	69	91%	99%	99%
Prophylactic Antibiotic Selection (Outpatient)	25	92%	98%	98%
Prophylactic Antibiotic Stopped	69	99%	99%	98%
Prophylactic Antibiotic Timing	69	100%	99%	99%
Prophylactic Antibiotic Timing (Outpatient)	24	96%	97%	98%
Urinary Catheter Removal[1]	-	-	98%	97%
Survey of Patients' Hospital Experiences				
Area Around Room 'Always' Quiet at Night	(a)	72%	63%	61%
Doctors 'Always' Communicated Well	(a)	90%	83%	82%
Home Recovery Information Given	(a)	94%	89%	85%
Hospital Given 9 or 10 on 10 Point Scale	(a)	82%	74%	71%
Meds 'Always' Explained Before Given	(a)	73%	68%	64%
Nurses 'Always' Communicated Well	(a)	88%	82%	79%
Pain 'Always' Well Controlled	(a)	78%	72%	71%
Room and Bathroom 'Always' Clean	(a)	76%	79%	73%
Timely Help 'Always' Received	(a)	80%	72%	68%
Would Definitely Recommend Hospital	(a)	82%	74%	71%
Use of Medical Imaging				
Cardiac Imaging Stress Test before Surgery[1]	-	-	5.4%	5.3%
Combination Abdominal CT Scan	105	7.6%	6.3%	10.5%
Combination Brain/Sinus CT Scan[1]	-	-	2.1%	2.7%
Combination Chest CT Scan	77	1.3%	1%	2.7%
Follow-up Mammogram/Ultrasound[7]	-	-	8.1%	8.8%
Lumbar Spine MRI for Low Back Pain[1]	-	-	34.9%	37.2%

Mayo Clinic Health System - Chippewa Valley

1501 Thompson St
Bloomer, WI 54724
Phone: 715-568-2000
Fax: 715-568-2000
E-mail: kerg.mary@mayo.edu
Type: Critical Access Hospitals
Emergency Services: Yes
Ownership: Voluntary non-profit - Other
Beds: 37

Key Personnel:
Operating Room. . . . . Gail Anderson
Infection Control. . . . . Mel Crisp
Quality Assurance . . . . Kay Dahlka
Chief of Medical Staff. . . . . Richard Gladitsch, MD
CEO/President. . . . . John Larson, MD

Measure	Cases	This Hosp.	State Avg.	U.S. Avg.
Blood Clot Prevention and Treatment				
Anticoagulation Overlap Therapy[5]	-	-	95%	93%
ICU Venous Thromboembolism Prophylaxis[5]	-	-	91%	92%
Incidence of Potentially Preventable VTE[5]	-	-	10%	10%
UFH with Dosages/Platelet Monitoring[5]	-	-	96%	97%
Venous Thromboembolism Prophylaxis[5]	-	-	85%	85%
Warfarin Therapy Discharge Instructions[5]	-	-	70%	75%
Chest Pain/Possible Heart Attack Care				
Aspirin Given Within 24 Hours of Arrival	-	-	98%	96%
Fibrinolytic Meds Within 30 Min. of Arrival	-	-	52%	58%
Average Time to ECG (minutes)	-	-	7	7
Average Time to Transfer (minutes)	-	-	58	60
Children's Asthma Care				
Received Home Management Plan of Care	-	-	-	88%
Received Reliever Medication	-	-	-	100%
Received Systemic Corticosteroids	-	-	-	100%
Emergency Department				
Admittance Decision Time (minutes)[5]	-	-	65	98
Head CT Results Within 45 Min. of Arrival	-	-	61%	57%
Patients Who Left ER Before Being Seen	-	-	1%	2%
Time from ER Arrival to Admit. (minutes)[5]	-	-	207	274
Time from ER Arrival to Discharge (minutes)	-	-	121	134
Time in ER Before Being Evaluated (minutes)	-	-	19	26
Time to Pain Meds for Fractures (minutes)	-	-	42	57
Heart Attack Care				
Aspirin Given at Discharge[1,3]	-	-	99%	99%
Fibrinolytic Meds Within 30 Min. of Arrival[3,7]	-	-	67%	54%
PCI Within 90 Minutes of Arrival[5]	-	-	96%	96%
Statin Prescribed at Discharge[1,3]	-	-	99%	98%
Heart Failure Care				
ACE Inhibitor or ARB for LVSD[1]	-	-	97%	97%
Discharge Instructions Given[1]	-	-	96%	94%
Evaluation of LVS Function[1]	-	-	99%	99%
Medicare Spending				
Medicare Spending per Patient (ratio)	-	-	0.94	0.98
Pneumonia Care				
Appropriate Initial Antibiotic Given	16	94%	96%	95%
Blood Culture Timing	17	100%	98%	98%
Pregnancy and Delivery Care				
Newborn Deliveries Scheduled Early[5]	-	-	4%	6%
Preventive Care				
Immunization for Influenza[5]	-	-	90%	90%
Immunization for Pneumonia[5]	-	-	92%	92%
Stroke Care				
Anticoagulation Therapy for Atrial Fibrillation[5]	-	-	94%	95%
Antithrombotic Therapy Timing[5]	-	-	99%	98%
Assessed for Rehabilitation[5]	-	-	98%	97%
Discharged on Antithrombotic Therapy[5]	-	-	99%	99%
Discharged on Statin Medication[5]	-	-	94%	94%
Thrombolytic Therapy Timing[5]	-	-	60%	66%
Venous Thromboembolism Prophylaxis[5]	-	-	95%	94%
Written Stroke Educational Materials Given[5]	-	-	88%	88%
Surgical Care Improvement Project				
Appropriate Beta Blocker Usage[5]	-	-	99%	98%
Appropriate VTP Within 24 Hours[5]	-	-	99%	98%
Controlled Postoperative Blood Glucose[5]	-	-	96%	97%
Perioperative Temperature Management[5]	-	-	100%	100%
Prophylactic Antibiotic Selection[5]	-	-	99%	99%
Prophylactic Antibiotic Selection (Outpatient)	-	-	98%	98%
Prophylactic Antibiotic Stopped[5]	-	-	99%	98%
Prophylactic Antibiotic Timing[5]	-	-	99%	99%
Prophylactic Antibiotic Timing (Outpatient)	-	-	97%	98%
Urinary Catheter Removal[5]	-	-	98%	97%
Survey of Patients' Hospital Experiences				
Area Around Room 'Always' Quiet at Night[6]	<100	49%	63%	61%
Doctors 'Always' Communicated Well[6]	<100	88%	83%	82%
Home Recovery Information Given[6]	<100	86%	89%	85%
Hospital Given 9 or 10 on 10 Point Scale[6]	<100	76%	74%	71%
Meds 'Always' Explained Before Given[6]	<100	56%	68%	64%
Nurses 'Always' Communicated Well[6]	<100	85%	82%	79%
Pain 'Always' Well Controlled[6]	<100	59%	72%	71%
Room and Bathroom 'Always' Clean[6]	<100	74%	79%	73%
Timely Help 'Always' Received[6]	<100	68%	72%	68%
Would Definitely Recommend Hospital[6]	<100	71%	74%	71%
Use of Medical Imaging				
Cardiac Imaging Stress Test before Surgery	-	-	5.4%	5.3%
Combination Abdominal CT Scan	-	-	6.3%	10.5%
Combination Brain/Sinus CT Scan	-	-	2.1%	2.7%
Combination Chest CT Scan	-	-	1%	2.7%
Follow-up Mammogram/Ultrasound	-	-	8.1%	8.8%
Lumbar Spine MRI for Low Back Pain	-	-	34.9%	37.2%

Boscobel Area Health Care

205 Parker St
Boscobel, WI 53805
Phone: 608-375-4112
Fax: 608-375-5463
URL: www.boscobelhealth.com
Type: Critical Access Hospitals
Emergency Services: Yes
Ownership: Voluntary non-profit - Private
Beds: 123

Key Personnel:
CEO . . . . David Hartberg
Intensive Care Unit. . . . . Nancy Nelson
Chief of Medical Staff. . . . . Thomas Pelz
Infection Control. . . . . Sally N Rosemeyer, RN
Quality Assurance . . . . Sally N Rosemeyer, RN

Measure	Cases	This Hosp.	State Avg.	U.S. Avg.
Blood Clot Prevention and Treatment				
Anticoagulation Overlap Therapy[5]	-	-	95%	93%
ICU Venous Thromboembolism Prophylaxis[5]	-	-	91%	92%
Incidence of Potentially Preventable VTE[5]	-	-	10%	10%
UFH with Dosages/Platelet Monitoring[5]	-	-	96%	97%
Venous Thromboembolism Prophylaxis[5]	-	-	85%	85%
Warfarin Therapy Discharge Instructions[5]	-	-	70%	75%
Chest Pain/Possible Heart Attack Care				
Aspirin Given Within 24 Hours of Arrival	24	92%	98%	96%
Fibrinolytic Meds Within 30 Min. of Arrival[1,3]	-	-	52%	58%
Average Time to ECG (minutes)	26	8	7	7
Average Time to Transfer (minutes)[1,3]	-	-	58	60
Children's Asthma Care				
Received Home Management Plan of Care	-	-	-	88%
Received Reliever Medication	-	-	-	100%
Received Systemic Corticosteroids	-	-	-	100%
Emergency Department				
Admittance Decision Time (minutes)	143	55	65	98
Head CT Results Within 45 Min. of Arrival[5]	-	-	61%	57%
Patients Who Left ER Before Being Seen[5]	-	-	1%	2%
Time from ER Arrival to Admit. (minutes)	154	184	207	274
Time from ER Arrival to Discharge (minutes)[5]	-	-	121	134
Time in ER Before Being Evaluated (minutes)[5]	-	-	19	26
Time to Pain Meds for Fractures (minutes)[5]	-	-	42	57
Heart Attack Care				
Aspirin Given at Discharge[5]	-	-	99%	99%
Fibrinolytic Meds Within 30 Min. of Arrival[5]	-	-	67%	54%
PCI Within 90 Minutes of Arrival[5]	-	-	96%	96%
Statin Prescribed at Discharge[5]	-	-	99%	98%
Heart Failure Care				
ACE Inhibitor or ARB for LVSD[1]	-	-	97%	97%
Discharge Instructions Given	12	92%	96%	94%
Evaluation of LVS Function	18	72%	99%	99%
Medicare Spending				
Medicare Spending per Patient (ratio)	-	-	0.94	0.98
Pneumonia Care				
Appropriate Initial Antibiotic Given	13	100%	96%	95%
Blood Culture Timing	13	100%	98%	98%
Pregnancy and Delivery Care				
Newborn Deliveries Scheduled Early[5]	-	-	4%	6%
Preventive Care				
Immunization for Influenza[5]	-	-	90%	90%
Immunization for Pneumonia[5]	-	-	92%	92%
Stroke Care				
Anticoagulation Therapy for Atrial Fibrillation[5]	-	-	94%	95%
Antithrombotic Therapy Timing[5]	-	-	99%	98%
Assessed for Rehabilitation[5]	-	-	98%	97%
Discharged on Antithrombotic Therapy[5]	-	-	99%	99%
Discharged on Statin Medication[5]	-	-	94%	94%
Thrombolytic Therapy Timing[5]	-	-	60%	66%
Venous Thromboembolism Prophylaxis[5]	-	-	95%	94%
Written Stroke Educational Materials Given[5]	-	-	88%	88%
Surgical Care Improvement Project				
Appropriate Beta Blocker Usage[3,7]	-	-	99%	98%
Appropriate VTP Within 24 Hours[1]	-	-	99%	98%
Controlled Postoperative Blood Glucose[3,7]	-	-	96%	97%
Perioperative Temperature Management[1,3]	-	-	100%	100%
Prophylactic Antibiotic Selection[1]	-	-	99%	99%
Prophylactic Antibiotic Selection (Outpatient)[3,7]	-	-	98%	98%

NOTE: Hospital profiles are in alphabetical order by state, then city, then hospital within the city; Rankings exclude hospitals with less than 25 cases except for patient surveys which excludes hospitals with less than 100 cases; (a) 100-299 cases; (1) The number of cases/patients is too few to report; (2) Data submitted were based on a sample of cases/patients; (3) Results are based on a shorter time period than required; (4) Data suppressed by CMS for one or more quarters; (5) Results are not available for this reporting period; (6) Fewer than 100 patients completed the HCAHPS survey; (7) No cases met the criteria for this measure; (8) The lower limit of the confidence interval cannot be calculated if the number of observed infections equals zero; (9) No data are available from the state/territory for this reporting period; (10) The scores shown reflect fewer than 50 completed surveys; (11) There were discrepancies in the data collection process; (12) This measure does not apply to this hospital for this reporting period; (13) Results cannot be calculated for this reporting period; (14) The results for this state are combined with nearby states to protect confidentiality; Please refer to the User's Guide for a full explanation of data.

Measure	Cases	This Hosp.	State Avg.	U.S. Avg.
Prophylactic Antibiotic Stopped[1]	-	-	99%	98%
Prophylactic Antibiotic Timing[1]	-	-	99%	99%
Prophylactic Antibiotic Timing (Outpatient)[1,3]	-	-	97%	98%
Urinary Catheter Removal[1,3]	-	-	98%	97%
Survey of Patients' Hospital Experiences				
Area Around Room 'Always' Quiet at Night[6]	<100	74%	63%	61%
Doctors 'Always' Communicated Well[6]	<100	82%	83%	82%
Home Recovery Information Given[6]	<100	93%	89%	85%
Hospital Given 9 or 10 on 10 Point Scale[6]	<100	75%	74%	71%
Meds 'Always' Explained Before Given[6]	<100	68%	68%	64%
Nurses 'Always' Communicated Well[6]	<100	86%	82%	79%
Pain 'Always' Well Controlled[6]	<100	83%	72%	71%
Room and Bathroom 'Always' Clean[6]	<100	92%	79%	73%
Timely Help 'Always' Received[6]	<100	78%	72%	68%
Would Definitely Recommend Hospital[6]	<100	67%	74%	71%
Use of Medical Imaging				
Cardiac Imaging Stress Test before Surgery	61	4.9%	5.4%	5.3%
Combination Abdominal CT Scan	65	1.5%	6.3%	10.5%
Combination Brain/Sinus CT Scan[1]	-	-	2.1%	2.7%
Combination Chest CT Scan[1]	-	-	1%	2.7%
Follow-up Mammogram/Ultrasound	101	6.9%	8.1%	8.8%
Lumbar Spine MRI for Low Back Pain[1]	-	-	34.9%	37.2%

Aurora Memorial Hospital Burlington

252 Mchenry St Phone: 262-767-6000
Burlington, WI 53105 Fax: 262-767-6380
URL: www.aurorahealthcare.org
Type: Acute Care Hospitals Emergency Services: Yes
Ownership: Voluntary non-profit - Private Beds: 123

Key Personnel:
Quality Assurance . . . . Barb Bigler
Chief of Medical Staff. . . . . Michael Brophy, MD
Intensive Care Unit. . . . . Diane Huck
Anesthesiology. . . . . S Joshi, MD
Emergency Room . . . . John Linstroth, MD
Operating Room. . . . . Joseph Majewski
Infection Control. . . . . Gwria McPeek
President/CEO. . . . . Nick Turkal, MD

Measure	Cases	This Hosp.	State Avg.	U.S. Avg.
Blood Clot Prevention and Treatment				
Anticoagulation Overlap Therapy[2]	31	100%	95%	93%
ICU Venous Thromboembolism Prophylaxis[2]	87	100%	91%	92%
Incidence of Potentially Preventable VTE[1,2]	-	-	10%	10%
UFH with Dosages/Platelet Monitoring[1,2]	-	-	96%	97%
Venous Thromboembolism Prophylaxis[2]	193	94%	85%	85%
Warfarin Therapy Discharge Instructions[2]	30	100%	70%	75%
Chest Pain/Possible Heart Attack Care				
Aspirin Given Within 24 Hours of Arrival	34	100%	98%	96%
Fibrinolytic Meds Within 30 Min. of Arrival[1]	-	-	52%	58%
Average Time to ECG (minutes)	36	6	7	7
Average Time to Transfer (minutes)[1]	-	-	58	60
Children's Asthma Care				
Received Home Management Plan of Care	-	-	-	88%
Received Reliever Medication	-	-	-	100%
Received Systemic Corticosteroids	-	-	-	100%
Emergency Department				
Admittance Decision Time (minutes)[2]	320	78	65	98
Head CT Results Within 45 Min. of Arrival[1]	-	-	61%	57%
Patients Who Left ER Before Being Seen	14,171	1%	1%	2%
Time from ER Arrival to Admit. (minutes)[2]	356	246	207	274
Time from ER Arrival to Discharge (minutes)	346	148	121	134
Time in ER Before Being Evaluated (minutes)	332	24	19	26
Time to Pain Meds for Fractures (minutes)	62	41	42	57
Heart Attack Care				
Aspirin Given at Discharge	26	100%	99%	99%
Fibrinolytic Meds Within 30 Min. of Arrival[7]	-	-	67%	54%
PCI Within 90 Minutes of Arrival[7]	-	-	96%	96%
Statin Prescribed at Discharge	24	100%	99%	98%
Heart Failure Care				
ACE Inhibitor or ARB for LVSD	19	100%	97%	97%
Discharge Instructions Given	75	99%	96%	94%
Evaluation of LVS Function	92	100%	99%	99%
Medicare Spending				
Medicare Spending per Patient (ratio)	-	0.93	0.94	0.98
Pneumonia Care				
Appropriate Initial Antibiotic Given	80	99%	96%	95%
Blood Culture Timing	170	99%	98%	98%
Pregnancy and Delivery Care				
Newborn Deliveries Scheduled Early[2]	16	31%	4%	6%
Preventive Care				
Immunization for Influenza[2]	271	96%	90%	90%
Immunization for Pneumonia[2]	387	99%	92%	92%
Stroke Care				
Anticoagulation Therapy for Atrial Fibrillation[1]	-	-	94%	95%
Antithrombotic Therapy Timing	20	95%	99%	98%
Assessed for Rehabilitation	24	100%	98%	97%
Discharged on Antithrombotic Therapy	22	100%	99%	99%
Discharged on Statin Medication	20	100%	94%	94%
Thrombolytic Therapy Timing[7]	-	-	60%	66%
Venous Thromboembolism Prophylaxis	23	96%	95%	94%
Written Stroke Educational Materials Given	12	92%	88%	88%
Surgical Care Improvement Project				
Appropriate Beta Blocker Usage[2]	79	100%	99%	98%
Appropriate VTP Within 24 Hours[2]	228	99%	99%	98%
Controlled Postoperative Blood Glucose[2,7]	-	-	96%	97%
Perioperative Temperature Management[2]	274	100%	100%	100%
Prophylactic Antibiotic Selection[2]	150	99%	99%	99%
Prophylactic Antibiotic Selection (Outpatient)	139	100%	98%	98%
Prophylactic Antibiotic Stopped[2]	146	99%	99%	98%
Prophylactic Antibiotic Timing[2]	150	99%	99%	99%
Prophylactic Antibiotic Timing (Outpatient)	65	94%	97%	98%
Urinary Catheter Removal[2]	195	99%	98%	97%
Survey of Patients' Hospital Experiences				
Area Around Room 'Always' Quiet at Night	300+	57%	63%	61%
Doctors 'Always' Communicated Well	300+	77%	83%	82%
Home Recovery Information Given	300+	86%	89%	85%
Hospital Given 9 or 10 on 10 Point Scale	300+	58%	74%	71%
Meds 'Always' Explained Before Given	300+	59%	68%	64%
Nurses 'Always' Communicated Well	300+	73%	82%	79%
Pain 'Always' Well Controlled	300+	66%	72%	71%
Room and Bathroom 'Always' Clean	300+	72%	79%	73%
Timely Help 'Always' Received	300+	52%	72%	68%
Would Definitely Recommend Hospital	300+	57%	74%	71%
Use of Medical Imaging				
Cardiac Imaging Stress Test before Surgery	269	4.8%	5.4%	5.3%
Combination Abdominal CT Scan	534	4.7%	6.3%	10.5%
Combination Brain/Sinus CT Scan	494	1.2%	2.1%	2.7%
Combination Chest CT Scan	501	1.4%	1%	2.7%
Follow-up Mammogram/Ultrasound	1,034	7.4%	8.1%	8.8%
Lumbar Spine MRI for Low Back Pain	108	37.0%	34.9%	37.2%

Calumet Medical Center

614 Memorial Dr Phone: 920-849-2386
Chilton, WI 53014 Fax: 920-849-7510
URL: www.ministryhealth.org
Type: Critical Access Hospitals Emergency Services: Yes
Ownership: Voluntary non-profit - Private Beds: 29

Key Personnel:
CEO/President. . . . . Travis Anderson
Radiology. . . . . Corbin Asbury

Measure	Cases	This Hosp.	State Avg.	U.S. Avg.
Blood Clot Prevention and Treatment				
Anticoagulation Overlap Therapy[5]	-	-	95%	93%
ICU Venous Thromboembolism Prophylaxis[5]	-	-	91%	92%
Incidence of Potentially Preventable VTE[5]	-	-	10%	10%
UFH with Dosages/Platelet Monitoring[5]	-	-	96%	97%
Venous Thromboembolism Prophylaxis[5]	-	-	85%	85%
Warfarin Therapy Discharge Instructions[5]	-	-	70%	75%
Chest Pain/Possible Heart Attack Care				
Aspirin Given Within 24 Hours of Arrival	13	100%	98%	96%
Fibrinolytic Meds Within 30 Min. of Arrival[7]	-	-	52%	58%
Average Time to ECG (minutes)	14	6	7	7
Average Time to Transfer (minutes)[1]	-	-	58	60
Children's Asthma Care				
Received Home Management Plan of Care	-	-	-	88%
Received Reliever Medication	-	-	-	100%
Received Systemic Corticosteroids	-	-	-	100%
Emergency Department				
Admittance Decision Time (minutes)[5]	-	-	65	98
Head CT Results Within 45 Min. of Arrival[5]	-	-	61%	57%
Patients Who Left ER Before Being Seen[5]	-	-	1%	2%
Time from ER Arrival to Admit. (minutes)[5]	-	-	207	274
Time from ER Arrival to Discharge (minutes)[5]	-	-	121	134
Time in ER Before Being Evaluated (minutes)[5]	-	-	19	26
Time to Pain Meds for Fractures (minutes)[5]	-	-	42	57
Heart Attack Care				
Aspirin Given at Discharge[5]	-	-	99%	99%
Fibrinolytic Meds Within 30 Min. of Arrival[5]	-	-	67%	54%
PCI Within 90 Minutes of Arrival[5]	-	-	96%	96%
Statin Prescribed at Discharge[5]	-	-	99%	98%
Heart Failure Care				
ACE Inhibitor or ARB for LVSD[1]	-	-	97%	97%
Discharge Instructions Given	16	100%	96%	94%
Evaluation of LVS Function	22	100%	99%	99%
Medicare Spending				
Medicare Spending per Patient (ratio)	-	-	0.94	0.98
Pneumonia Care				
Appropriate Initial Antibiotic Given[1]	-	-	96%	95%
Blood Culture Timing	16	100%	98%	98%
Pregnancy and Delivery Care				
Newborn Deliveries Scheduled Early[5]	-	-	4%	6%
Preventive Care				
Immunization for Influenza[5]	-	-	90%	90%
Immunization for Pneumonia[5]	-	-	92%	92%
Stroke Care				
Anticoagulation Therapy for Atrial Fibrillation[5]	-	-	94%	95%
Antithrombotic Therapy Timing[5]	-	-	99%	98%
Assessed for Rehabilitation[5]	-	-	98%	97%
Discharged on Antithrombotic Therapy[5]	-	-	99%	99%
Discharged on Statin Medication[5]	-	-	94%	94%
Thrombolytic Therapy Timing[5]	-	-	60%	66%
Venous Thromboembolism Prophylaxis[5]	-	-	95%	94%
Written Stroke Educational Materials Given[5]	-	-	88%	88%
Surgical Care Improvement Project				
Appropriate Beta Blocker Usage	29	100%	99%	98%
Appropriate VTP Within 24 Hours	52	100%	99%	98%
Controlled Postoperative Blood Glucose[7]	-	-	96%	97%
Perioperative Temperature Management	76	100%	100%	100%
Prophylactic Antibiotic Selection	59	100%	99%	99%
Prophylactic Antibiotic Selection (Outpatient)[5]	-	-	98%	98%
Prophylactic Antibiotic Stopped	59	100%	99%	98%
Prophylactic Antibiotic Timing	59	100%	99%	99%
Prophylactic Antibiotic Timing (Outpatient)[5]	-	-	97%	98%
Urinary Catheter Removal[1]	-	-	98%	97%
Survey of Patients' Hospital Experiences				
Area Around Room 'Always' Quiet at Night	(a)	71%	63%	61%
Doctors 'Always' Communicated Well	(a)	83%	83%	82%
Home Recovery Information Given	(a)	90%	89%	85%
Hospital Given 9 or 10 on 10 Point Scale	(a)	78%	74%	71%
Meds 'Always' Explained Before Given	(a)	76%	68%	64%
Nurses 'Always' Communicated Well	(a)	88%	82%	79%
Pain 'Always' Well Controlled	(a)	72%	72%	71%
Room and Bathroom 'Always' Clean	(a)	88%	79%	73%
Timely Help 'Always' Received	(a)	84%	72%	68%
Would Definitely Recommend Hospital	(a)	73%	74%	71%
Use of Medical Imaging				
Cardiac Imaging Stress Test before Surgery[1]	-	-	5.4%	5.3%
Combination Abdominal CT Scan	48	2.1%	6.3%	10.5%
Combination Brain/Sinus CT Scan[1]	-	-	2.1%	2.7%
Combination Chest CT Scan[1]	-	-	1%	2.7%
Follow-up Mammogram/Ultrasound	143	9.8%	8.1%	8.8%
Lumbar Spine MRI for Low Back Pain[1]	-	-	34.9%	37.2%

Saint Joseph's Hospital

2661 Cty Hwy I Phone: 715-717-7200
Chippewa Falls, WI 54729 Fax: 715-726-3204
URL: www.stjoeschipfalls.com
Type: Acute Care Hospitals Emergency Services: Yes
Ownership: Voluntary non-profit - Church Beds: 193

Key Personnel:
Radiology. . . . . Mark A Augustyn

NOTE: Hospital profiles are in alphabetical order by state, then city, then hospital within the city; Rankings exclude hospitals with less than 25 cases except for patient surveys which excludes hospitals with less than 100 cases; (a) 100-299 cases; (1) The number of cases/patients is too few to report; (2) Data submitted were based on a sample of cases/patients; (3) Results are based on a shorter time period than required; (4) Data suppressed by CMS for one or more quarters; (5) Results are not available for this reporting period; (6) Fewer than 100 patients completed the HCAHPS survey; (7) No cases met the criteria for this measure; (8) The lower limit of the confidence interval cannot be calculated if the number of observed infections equals zero; (9) No data are available from the state/territory for this reporting period; (10) The scores shown reflect fewer than 50 completed surveys; (11) There were discrepancies in the data collection process; (12) This measure does not apply to this hospital for this reporting period; (13) Results cannot be calculated for this reporting period; (14) The results for this state are combined with nearby states to protect confidentiality; Please refer to the User's Guide for a full explanation of data.

Emergency Room . . . . Patrick Ayer
Chief of Medical Staff . . . . Jeffrey Brown, MD
CEO/President . . . . David Fish
Quality Assurance . . . . Raymond Myers
Infection Control . . . . Debra Neitge
Ambulatory Care . . . . Gary Wolff, RN
Operating Room . . . . Gary Wulff, RN

Measure	Cases	This Hosp.	State Avg.	U.S. Avg.
Blood Clot Prevention and Treatment				
Anticoagulation Overlap Therapy[2]	18	89%	95%	93%
ICU Venous Thromboembolism Prophylaxis[2]	21	71%	91%	92%
Incidence of Potentially Preventable VTE[1,2]	-	-	10%	10%
UFH with Dosages/Platelet Monitoring[1,2]	-	-	96%	97%
Venous Thromboembolism Prophylaxis[2]	134	87%	85%	85%
Warfarin Therapy Discharge Instructions[2]	14	71%	70%	75%
Chest Pain/Possible Heart Attack Care				
Aspirin Given Within 24 Hours of Arrival	50	100%	98%	96%
Fibrinolytic Meds Within 30 Min. of Arrival[7]	-	-	52%	58%
Average Time to ECG (minutes)	51	13	7	7
Average Time to Transfer (minutes)[1]	-	-	58	60
Children's Asthma Care				
Received Home Management Plan of Care	-	-	-	88%
Received Reliever Medication	-	-	-	100%
Received Systemic Corticosteroids	-	-	-	100%
Emergency Department				
Admittance Decision Time (minutes)[2]	192	76	65	98
Head CT Results Within 45 Min. of Arrival[1]	-	-	61%	57%
Patients Who Left ER Before Being Seen	16,829	0%	1%	2%
Time from ER Arrival to Admit. (minutes)[2]	195	214	207	274
Time from ER Arrival to Discharge (minutes)	443	137	121	134
Time in ER Before Being Evaluated (minutes)	501	18	19	26
Time to Pain Meds for Fractures (minutes)	37	48	42	57
Heart Attack Care				
Aspirin Given at Discharge[1,3]	-	-	99%	99%
Fibrinolytic Meds Within 30 Min. of Arrival[3,7]	-	-	67%	54%
PCI Within 90 Minutes of Arrival[3,7]	-	-	96%	96%
Statin Prescribed at Discharge[1,3]	-	-	99%	98%
Heart Failure Care				
ACE Inhibitor or ARB for LVSD[1]	-	-	97%	97%
Discharge Instructions Given	32	91%	96%	94%
Evaluation of LVS Function	53	100%	99%	99%
Medicare Spending				
Medicare Spending per Patient (ratio)	-	0.85	0.94	0.98
Pneumonia Care				
Appropriate Initial Antibiotic Given	30	100%	96%	95%
Blood Culture Timing	70	99%	98%	98%
Pregnancy and Delivery Care				
Newborn Deliveries Scheduled Early[2]	16	0%	4%	6%
Preventive Care				
Immunization for Influenza[2]	320	79%	90%	90%
Immunization for Pneumonia[2]	265	68%	92%	92%
Stroke Care				
Anticoagulation Therapy for Atrial Fibrillation[1,3]	-	-	94%	95%
Antithrombotic Therapy Timing[1,3]	-	-	99%	98%
Assessed for Rehabilitation[1,3]	-	-	98%	97%
Discharged on Antithrombotic Therapy[1,3]	-	-	99%	99%
Discharged on Statin Medication[1,3]	-	-	94%	94%
Thrombolytic Therapy Timing[3,7]	-	-	60%	66%
Venous Thromboembolism Prophylaxis[1,3]	-	-	95%	94%
Written Stroke Educational Materials Given[1,3]	-	-	88%	88%
Surgical Care Improvement Project				
Appropriate Beta Blocker Usage	38	100%	99%	98%
Appropriate VTP Within 24 Hours	97	99%	99%	98%
Controlled Postoperative Blood Glucose[7]	-	-	96%	97%
Perioperative Temperature Management	137	100%	100%	100%
Prophylactic Antibiotic Selection	108	97%	99%	99%
Prophylactic Antibiotic Selection (Outpatient)	33	100%	98%	98%
Prophylactic Antibiotic Stopped	107	99%	99%	98%
Prophylactic Antibiotic Timing	108	100%	99%	99%
Prophylactic Antibiotic Timing (Outpatient)	33	97%	97%	98%
Urinary Catheter Removal	62	98%	98%	97%
Survey of Patients' Hospital Experiences				
Area Around Room 'Always' Quiet at Night	300+	67%	63%	61%
Doctors 'Always' Communicated Well	300+	85%	83%	82%
Home Recovery Information Given	300+	88%	89%	85%
Hospital Given 9 or 10 on 10 Point Scale	300+	79%	74%	71%
Meds 'Always' Explained Before Given	300+	69%	68%	64%
Nurses 'Always' Communicated Well	300+	84%	82%	79%
Pain 'Always' Well Controlled	300+	74%	72%	71%
Room and Bathroom 'Always' Clean	300+	79%	79%	73%
Timely Help 'Always' Received	300+	76%	72%	68%
Would Definitely Recommend Hospital	300+	77%	74%	71%
Use of Medical Imaging				
Cardiac Imaging Stress Test before Surgery[1]	-	-	5.4%	5.3%
Combination Abdominal CT Scan	281	2.1%	6.3%	10.5%
Combination Brain/Sinus CT Scan[1]	-	-	2.1%	2.7%
Combination Chest CT Scan	145	0.7%	1%	2.7%
Follow-up Mammogram/Ultrasound	228	10.5%	8.1%	8.8%
Lumbar Spine MRI for Low Back Pain[1]	-	-	34.9%	37.2%

Columbus Community Hospital

1515 Park Ave
Columbus, WI 53925
Phone: 920-623-2200
Type: Critical Access Hospitals
Emergency Services: Yes
Ownership: Voluntary non-profit - Private

Key Personnel:
Radiology . . . . Mark F. Rich, MD
CEO/President . . . . John Russell

Measure	Cases	This Hosp.	State Avg.	U.S. Avg.
Blood Clot Prevention and Treatment				
Anticoagulation Overlap Therapy[5]	-	-	95%	93%
ICU Venous Thromboembolism Prophylaxis[5]	-	-	91%	92%
Incidence of Potentially Preventable VTE[5]	-	-	10%	10%
UFH with Dosages/Platelet Monitoring[5]	-	-	96%	97%
Venous Thromboembolism Prophylaxis[5]	-	-	85%	85%
Warfarin Therapy Discharge Instructions[5]	-	-	70%	75%
Chest Pain/Possible Heart Attack Care				
Aspirin Given Within 24 Hours of Arrival	-	-	98%	96%
Fibrinolytic Meds Within 30 Min. of Arrival	-	-	52%	58%
Average Time to ECG (minutes)	-	-	7	7
Average Time to Transfer (minutes)	-	-	58	60
Children's Asthma Care				
Received Home Management Plan of Care	-	-	-	88%
Received Reliever Medication	-	-	-	100%
Received Systemic Corticosteroids	-	-	-	100%
Emergency Department				
Admittance Decision Time (minutes)[5]	-	-	65	98
Head CT Results Within 45 Min. of Arrival	-	-	61%	57%
Patients Who Left ER Before Being Seen	-	-	1%	2%
Time from ER Arrival to Admit. (minutes)[5]	-	-	207	274
Time from ER Arrival to Discharge (minutes)	-	-	121	134
Time in ER Before Being Evaluated (minutes)	-	-	19	26
Time to Pain Meds for Fractures (minutes)	-	-	42	57
Heart Attack Care				
Aspirin Given at Discharge[5]	-	-	99%	99%
Fibrinolytic Meds Within 30 Min. of Arrival[5]	-	-	67%	54%
PCI Within 90 Minutes of Arrival[5]	-	-	96%	96%
Statin Prescribed at Discharge[5]	-	-	99%	98%
Heart Failure Care				
ACE Inhibitor or ARB for LVSD[1]	-	-	97%	97%
Discharge Instructions Given	29	93%	96%	94%
Evaluation of LVS Function	36	100%	99%	99%
Medicare Spending				
Medicare Spending per Patient (ratio)	-	-	0.94	0.98
Pneumonia Care				
Appropriate Initial Antibiotic Given	30	87%	96%	95%
Blood Culture Timing	39	95%	98%	98%
Pregnancy and Delivery Care				
Newborn Deliveries Scheduled Early[5]	-	-	4%	6%
Preventive Care				
Immunization for Influenza[5]	-	-	90%	90%
Immunization for Pneumonia[5]	-	-	92%	92%
Stroke Care				
Anticoagulation Therapy for Atrial Fibrillation[5]	-	-	94%	95%
Antithrombotic Therapy Timing[5]	-	-	99%	98%
Assessed for Rehabilitation[5]	-	-	98%	97%
Discharged on Antithrombotic Therapy[5]	-	-	99%	99%
Discharged on Statin Medication[5]	-	-	94%	94%
Thrombolytic Therapy Timing[5]	-	-	60%	66%
Venous Thromboembolism Prophylaxis[5]	-	-	95%	94%
Written Stroke Educational Materials Given[5]	-	-	88%	88%
Surgical Care Improvement Project				
Appropriate Beta Blocker Usage	25	88%	99%	98%
Appropriate VTP Within 24 Hours	54	83%	99%	98%
Controlled Postoperative Blood Glucose[7]	-	-	96%	97%
Perioperative Temperature Management	75	100%	100%	100%
Prophylactic Antibiotic Selection	52	100%	99%	99%
Prophylactic Antibiotic Selection (Outpatient)	-	-	98%	98%
Prophylactic Antibiotic Stopped	52	96%	99%	98%
Prophylactic Antibiotic Timing	52	96%	99%	99%
Prophylactic Antibiotic Timing (Outpatient)	-	-	97%	98%
Urinary Catheter Removal	58	91%	98%	97%
Survey of Patients' Hospital Experiences				
Area Around Room 'Always' Quiet at Night	(a)	60%	63%	61%
Doctors 'Always' Communicated Well	(a)	86%	83%	82%
Home Recovery Information Given	(a)	90%	89%	85%
Hospital Given 9 or 10 on 10 Point Scale	(a)	76%	74%	71%
Meds 'Always' Explained Before Given	(a)	71%	68%	64%
Nurses 'Always' Communicated Well	(a)	81%	82%	79%
Pain 'Always' Well Controlled	(a)	71%	72%	71%
Room and Bathroom 'Always' Clean	(a)	83%	79%	73%
Timely Help 'Always' Received	(a)	71%	72%	68%
Would Definitely Recommend Hospital	(a)	74%	74%	71%
Use of Medical Imaging				
Cardiac Imaging Stress Test before Surgery	-	-	5.4%	5.3%
Combination Abdominal CT Scan	-	-	6.3%	10.5%
Combination Brain/Sinus CT Scan	-	-	2.1%	2.7%
Combination Chest CT Scan	-	-	1%	2.7%
Follow-up Mammogram/Ultrasound	-	-	8.1%	8.8%
Lumbar Spine MRI for Low Back Pain	-	-	34.9%	37.2%

Cumberland Memorial Hospital

1110 7th Avenue
Cumberland, WI 54829
Phone: 715-822-2741
Fax: 715-822-2740
URL: www.cumberlandhelathcare.com
Type: Critical Access Hospitals
Emergency Services: Yes
Ownership: Voluntary non-profit - Other
Beds: 40

Key Personnel:
Chief of Medical Staff . . . . B Ankarlo, MD
CEO/President . . . . Robert J Hansen
Infection Control . . . . Toniann Knutson, RN
Anesthesiology . . . . Jeff Kuehn, CRNA
Radiology . . . . Laurie Lien
Operating Room . . . . Sarah Lunquist, RN
Emergency Room . . . . Janet Peterson, RN
Quality Assurance . . . . Nancy Ruppel

Measure	Cases	This Hosp.	State Avg.	U.S. Avg.
Blood Clot Prevention and Treatment				
Anticoagulation Overlap Therapy[5]	-	-	95%	93%
ICU Venous Thromboembolism Prophylaxis[5]	-	-	91%	92%
Incidence of Potentially Preventable VTE[5]	-	-	10%	10%
UFH with Dosages/Platelet Monitoring[5]	-	-	96%	97%
Venous Thromboembolism Prophylaxis[5]	-	-	85%	85%
Warfarin Therapy Discharge Instructions[5]	-	-	70%	75%
Chest Pain/Possible Heart Attack Care				
Aspirin Given Within 24 Hours of Arrival	-	-	98%	96%
Fibrinolytic Meds Within 30 Min. of Arrival	-	-	52%	58%
Average Time to ECG (minutes)	-	-	7	7
Average Time to Transfer (minutes)	-	-	58	60
Children's Asthma Care				
Received Home Management Plan of Care	-	-	-	88%
Received Reliever Medication	-	-	-	100%
Received Systemic Corticosteroids	-	-	-	100%
Emergency Department				
Admittance Decision Time (minutes)[3]	99	28	65	98
Head CT Results Within 45 Min. of Arrival	-	-	61%	57%
Patients Who Left ER Before Being Seen	-	-	1%	2%
Time from ER Arrival to Admit. (minutes)[3]	100	100	207	274
Time from ER Arrival to Discharge (minutes)	-	-	121	134
Time in ER Before Being Evaluated (minutes)	-	-	19	26

NOTE: Hospital profiles are in alphabetical order by state, then city, then hospital within the city; Rankings exclude hospitals with less than 25 cases except for patient surveys which excludes hospitals with less than 100 cases; (a) 100-299 cases; (1) The number of cases/patients is too few to report; (2) Data submitted were based on a sample of cases/patients; (3) Results are based on a shorter time period than required; (4) Data suppressed by CMS for one or more quarters; (5) Results are not available for this reporting period; (6) Fewer than 100 patients completed the HCAHPS survey; (7) No cases met the criteria for this measure; (8) The lower limit of the confidence interval cannot be calculated if the number of observed infections equals zero; (9) No data are available from the state/territory for this reporting period; (10) The scores shown reflect fewer than 50 completed surveys; (11) There were discrepancies in the data collection process; (12) This measure does not apply to this hospital for this reporting period; (13) Results cannot be calculated for this reporting period; (14) The results for this state are combined with nearby states to protect confidentiality; Please refer to the User's Guide for a full explanation of data.

Measure	Cases	This Hosp.	State Avg.	U.S. Avg.
Time to Pain Meds for Fractures (minutes)	-	-	42	57
Heart Attack Care				
Aspirin Given at Discharge[5]	-	-	99%	99%
Fibrinolytic Meds Within 30 Min. of Arrival[5]	-	-	67%	54%
PCI Within 90 Minutes of Arrival[5]	-	-	96%	96%
Statin Prescribed at Discharge[5]	-	-	99%	98%
Heart Failure Care				
ACE Inhibitor or ARB for LVSD[5]	-	-	97%	97%
Discharge Instructions Given[5]	-	-	96%	94%
Evaluation of LVS Function[5]	-	-	99%	99%
Medicare Spending				
Medicare Spending per Patient (ratio)	-	-	0.94	0.98
Pneumonia Care				
Appropriate Initial Antibiotic Given	25	84%	96%	95%
Blood Culture Timing[1]	-	-	98%	98%
Pregnancy and Delivery Care				
Newborn Deliveries Scheduled Early[5]	-	-	4%	6%
Preventive Care				
Immunization for Influenza[5]	-	-	90%	90%
Immunization for Pneumonia[3]	75	71%	92%	92%
Stroke Care				
Anticoagulation Therapy for Atrial Fibrillation[5]	-	-	94%	95%
Antithrombotic Therapy Timing[5]	-	-	99%	98%
Assessed for Rehabilitation[5]	-	-	98%	97%
Discharged on Antithrombotic Therapy[5]	-	-	99%	99%
Discharged on Statin Medication[5]	-	-	94%	94%
Thrombolytic Therapy Timing[5]	-	-	60%	66%
Venous Thromboembolism Prophylaxis[5]	-	-	95%	94%
Written Stroke Educational Materials Given[5]	-	-	88%	88%
Surgical Care Improvement Project				
Appropriate Beta Blocker Usage[5]	-	-	99%	98%
Appropriate VTP Within 24 Hours[5]	-	-	99%	98%
Controlled Postoperative Blood Glucose[5]	-	-	96%	97%
Perioperative Temperature Management[5]	-	-	100%	100%
Prophylactic Antibiotic Selection[5]	-	-	99%	99%
Prophylactic Antibiotic Selection (Outpatient)	-	-	98%	98%
Prophylactic Antibiotic Stopped[5]	-	-	99%	98%
Prophylactic Antibiotic Timing[5]	-	-	99%	99%
Prophylactic Antibiotic Timing (Outpatient)	-	-	97%	98%
Urinary Catheter Removal[5]	-	-	98%	97%
Survey of Patients' Hospital Experiences				
Area Around Room 'Always' Quiet at Night[5]	-	-	63%	61%
Doctors 'Always' Communicated Well[5]	-	-	83%	82%
Home Recovery Information Given[5]	-	-	89%	85%
Hospital Given 9 or 10 on 10 Point Scale[5]	-	-	74%	71%
Meds 'Always' Explained Before Given[5]	-	-	68%	64%
Nurses 'Always' Communicated Well[5]	-	-	82%	79%
Pain 'Always' Well Controlled[5]	-	-	72%	71%
Room and Bathroom 'Always' Clean[5]	-	-	79%	73%
Timely Help 'Always' Received[5]	-	-	72%	68%
Would Definitely Recommend Hospital[5]	-	-	74%	71%
Use of Medical Imaging				
Cardiac Imaging Stress Test before Surgery	-	-	5.4%	5.3%
Combination Abdominal CT Scan	-	-	6.3%	10.5%
Combination Brain/Sinus CT Scan	-	-	2.1%	2.7%
Combination Chest CT Scan	-	-	1%	2.7%
Follow-up Mammogram/Ultrasound	-	-	8.1%	8.8%
Lumbar Spine MRI for Low Back Pain	-	-	34.9%	37.2%

Memorial Hospital Lafayette Cty

800 Clay St
Darlington, WI 53530
URL: www.mhlc-mhf.org
Type: Critical Access Hospitals
Ownership: Government - Local
Phone: 608-776-4466
Fax: 608-776-5701
Emergency Services: Yes
Beds: 25

Key Personnel:
Quality Assurance . . . . Karla Blackbourn
Radiology. Dr Mark F Rich
Operating Room. . . . . Dr Scott Gibson, RN
Infection Control . . . . Pamela Gould
Chief of Medical Staff . . . . Michael Robiolio, MD

Measure	Cases	This Hosp.	State Avg.	U.S. Avg.
Blood Clot Prevention and Treatment				
Anticoagulation Overlap Therapy[1]	-	-	95%	93%
ICU Venous Thromboembolism Prophylaxis[7]	-	-	91%	92%
Incidence of Potentially Preventable VTE[7]	-	-	10%	10%
UFH with Dosages/Platelet Monitoring[7]	-	-	96%	97%
Venous Thromboembolism Prophylaxis	160	84%	85%	85%
Warfarin Therapy Discharge Instructions[7]	-	-	70%	75%
Chest Pain/Possible Heart Attack Care				
Aspirin Given Within 24 Hours of Arrival	14	100%	98%	96%
Fibrinolytic Meds Within 30 Min. of Arrival[3,7]	-	-	52%	58%
Average Time to ECG (minutes)	14	14	7	7
Average Time to Transfer (minutes)[1,3]	-	-	58	60
Children's Asthma Care				
Received Home Management Plan of Care	-	-	-	88%
Received Reliever Medication	-	-	-	100%
Received Systemic Corticosteroids	-	-	-	100%
Emergency Department				
Admittance Decision Time (minutes)	175	15	65	98
Head CT Results Within 45 Min. of Arrival[1,3]	-	-	61%	57%
Patients Who Left ER Before Being Seen[5]	-	-	1%	2%
Time from ER Arrival to Admit. (minutes)	175	152	207	274
Time from ER Arrival to Discharge (minutes)	202	98	121	134
Time in ER Before Being Evaluated (minutes)	258	18	19	26
Time to Pain Meds for Fractures (minutes)	22	34	42	57
Heart Attack Care				
Aspirin Given at Discharge[1,3]	-	-	99%	99%
Fibrinolytic Meds Within 30 Min. of Arrival[3,7]	-	-	67%	54%
PCI Within 90 Minutes of Arrival[3,7]	-	-	96%	96%
Statin Prescribed at Discharge[1,3]	-	-	99%	98%
Heart Failure Care				
ACE Inhibitor or ARB for LVSD[1]	-	-	97%	97%
Discharge Instructions Given[1]	-	-	96%	94%
Evaluation of LVS Function	14	86%	99%	99%
Medicare Spending				
Medicare Spending per Patient (ratio)	-	-	0.94	0.98
Pneumonia Care				
Appropriate Initial Antibiotic Given	13	100%	96%	95%
Blood Culture Timing[1]	-	-	98%	98%
Pregnancy and Delivery Care				
Newborn Deliveries Scheduled Early[1]	-	-	4%	6%
Preventive Care				
Immunization for Influenza	168	89%	90%	90%
Immunization for Pneumonia	237	96%	92%	92%
Stroke Care				
Anticoagulation Therapy for Atrial Fibrillation[3,7]	-	-	94%	95%
Antithrombotic Therapy Timing[1,3]	-	-	99%	98%
Assessed for Rehabilitation[1,3]	-	-	98%	97%
Discharged on Antithrombotic Therapy[1,3]	-	-	99%	99%
Discharged on Statin Medication[1,3]	-	-	94%	94%
Thrombolytic Therapy Timing[3,7]	-	-	60%	66%
Venous Thromboembolism Prophylaxis[1,3]	-	-	95%	94%
Written Stroke Educational Materials Given[3,7]	-	-	88%	88%
Surgical Care Improvement Project				
Appropriate Beta Blocker Usage[1]	-	-	99%	98%
Appropriate VTP Within 24 Hours	12	92%	99%	98%
Controlled Postoperative Blood Glucose[3,7]	-	-	96%	97%
Perioperative Temperature Management	15	100%	100%	100%
Prophylactic Antibiotic Selection	14	86%	99%	99%
Prophylactic Antibiotic Selection (Outpatient)[1,3]	-	-	98%	98%
Prophylactic Antibiotic Stopped	13	92%	99%	98%
Prophylactic Antibiotic Timing	14	100%	99%	99%
Prophylactic Antibiotic Timing (Outpatient)[1,3]	-	-	97%	98%
Urinary Catheter Removal[1]	-	-	98%	97%
Survey of Patients' Hospital Experiences				
Area Around Room 'Always' Quiet at Night	(a)	64%	63%	61%
Doctors 'Always' Communicated Well	(a)	90%	83%	82%
Home Recovery Information Given	(a)	86%	89%	85%
Hospital Given 9 or 10 on 10 Point Scale	(a)	83%	74%	71%
Meds 'Always' Explained Before Given	(a)	73%	68%	64%
Nurses 'Always' Communicated Well	(a)	87%	82%	79%
Pain 'Always' Well Controlled	(a)	70%	72%	71%
Room and Bathroom 'Always' Clean	(a)	85%	79%	73%
Timely Help 'Always' Received	(a)	79%	72%	68%
Would Definitely Recommend Hospital	(a)	80%	74%	71%
Use of Medical Imaging				
Cardiac Imaging Stress Test before Surgery	63	6.3%	5.4%	5.3%
Combination Abdominal CT Scan	66	7.6%	6.3%	10.5%
Combination Brain/Sinus CT Scan[1]	-	-	2.1%	2.7%
Combination Chest CT Scan[1]	-	-	1%	2.7%
Follow-up Mammogram/Ultrasound	97	10.3%	8.1%	8.8%
Lumbar Spine MRI for Low Back Pain[1]	-	-	34.9%	37.2%

Upland Hills Health

800 Compassion Way
Dodgeville, WI 53533
URL: www.uplandhillshealth.org
Type: Critical Access Hospitals
Ownership: Voluntary non-profit - Private
Phone: 608-930-8000
Fax: 608-930-7250
Emergency Services: Yes
Beds: 69

Key Personnel:
Radiology. . . . . Lynette Collins, MD
Pediatric Ambulatory Care . . . . . . Samy Desouky
Chief of Medical Staff . . . . Phyllis Fritsch
Emergency Room . . . . Gary Grunow
Quality Assurance . . . . Christine Harrsion
Operating Room. . . . . Dr Young Kim
Infection Control. . . . . Maria Leary
CEO/President. . . . . Lisa Schnedler

Measure	Cases	This Hosp.	State Avg.	U.S. Avg.
Blood Clot Prevention and Treatment				
Anticoagulation Overlap Therapy[5]	-	-	95%	93%
ICU Venous Thromboembolism Prophylaxis[5]	-	-	91%	92%
Incidence of Potentially Preventable VTE[5]	-	-	10%	10%
UFH with Dosages/Platelet Monitoring[5]	-	-	96%	97%
Venous Thromboembolism Prophylaxis[5]	-	-	85%	85%
Warfarin Therapy Discharge Instructions[5]	-	-	70%	75%
Chest Pain/Possible Heart Attack Care				
Aspirin Given Within 24 Hours of Arrival	-	-	98%	96%
Fibrinolytic Meds Within 30 Min. of Arrival	-	-	52%	58%
Average Time to ECG (minutes)	-	-	7	7
Average Time to Transfer (minutes)	-	-	58	60
Children's Asthma Care				
Received Home Management Plan of Care	-	-	-	88%
Received Reliever Medication	-	-	-	100%
Received Systemic Corticosteroids	-	-	-	100%
Emergency Department				
Admittance Decision Time (minutes)[5]	-	-	65	98
Head CT Results Within 45 Min. of Arrival	-	-	61%	57%
Patients Who Left ER Before Being Seen	-	-	1%	2%
Time from ER Arrival to Admit. (minutes)[5]	-	-	207	274
Time from ER Arrival to Discharge (minutes)	-	-	121	134
Time in ER Before Being Evaluated (minutes)	-	-	19	26
Time to Pain Meds for Fractures (minutes)	-	-	42	57
Heart Attack Care				
Aspirin Given at Discharge[5]	-	-	99%	99%
Fibrinolytic Meds Within 30 Min. of Arrival[5]	-	-	67%	54%
PCI Within 90 Minutes of Arrival[5]	-	-	96%	96%
Statin Prescribed at Discharge[5]	-	-	99%	98%
Heart Failure Care				
ACE Inhibitor or ARB for LVSD[1]	-	-	97%	97%
Discharge Instructions Given	11	100%	96%	94%
Evaluation of LVS Function	12	100%	99%	99%
Medicare Spending				
Medicare Spending per Patient (ratio)	-	-	0.94	0.98
Pneumonia Care				
Appropriate Initial Antibiotic Given	18	94%	96%	95%
Blood Culture Timing	22	100%	98%	98%
Pregnancy and Delivery Care				
Newborn Deliveries Scheduled Early[5]	-	-	4%	6%
Preventive Care				
Immunization for Influenza[5]	-	-	90%	90%
Immunization for Pneumonia[5]	-	-	92%	92%
Stroke Care				
Anticoagulation Therapy for Atrial Fibrillation[5]	-	-	94%	95%
Antithrombotic Therapy Timing[5]	-	-	99%	98%
Assessed for Rehabilitation[5]	-	-	98%	97%
Discharged on Antithrombotic Therapy[5]	-	-	99%	99%
Discharged on Statin Medication[5]	-	-	94%	94%
Thrombolytic Therapy Timing[5]	-	-	60%	66%

NOTE: Hospital profiles are in alphabetical order by state, then city, then hospital within the city; Rankings exclude hospitals with less than 25 cases except for patient surveys which excludes hospitals with less than 100 cases; (a) 100-299 cases; (1) The number of cases/patients is too few to report; (2) Data submitted were based on a sample of cases/patients; (3) Results are based on a shorter time period than required; (4) Data suppressed by CMS for one or more quarters; (5) Results are not available for this reporting period; (6) Fewer than 100 patients completed the HCAHPS survey; (7) No cases met the criteria for this measure; (8) The lower limit of the confidence interval cannot be calculated if the number of observed infections equals zero; (9) No data are available from the state/territory for this reporting period; (10) The scores shown reflect fewer than 50 completed surveys; (11) There were discrepancies in the data collection process; (12) This measure does not apply to this hospital for this reporting period; (13) Results cannot be calculated for this reporting period; (14) The results for this state are combined with nearby states to protect confidentiality; Please refer to the User's Guide for a full explanation of data.

Measure	Cases	This Hosp.	State Avg.	U.S. Avg.
Venous Thromboembolism Prophylaxis[5]	-	-	95%	94%
Written Stroke Educational Materials Given[5]	-	-	88%	88%
Surgical Care Improvement Project				
Appropriate Beta Blocker Usage	16	94%	99%	98%
Appropriate VTP Within 24 Hours	70	89%	99%	98%
Controlled Postoperative Blood Glucose[3,7]	-	-	96%	97%
Perioperative Temperature Management	74	100%	100%	100%
Prophylactic Antibiotic Selection	28	100%	99%	99%
Prophylactic Antibiotic Selection (Outpatient)	-	-	98%	98%
Prophylactic Antibiotic Stopped	27	96%	99%	98%
Prophylactic Antibiotic Timing	28	82%	99%	99%
Prophylactic Antibiotic Timing (Outpatient)	-	-	97%	98%
Urinary Catheter Removal	64	94%	98%	97%
Survey of Patients' Hospital Experiences				
Area Around Room 'Always' Quiet at Night	300+	68%	63%	61%
Doctors 'Always' Communicated Well	300+	88%	83%	82%
Home Recovery Information Given	300+	91%	89%	85%
Hospital Given 9 or 10 on 10 Point Scale	300+	85%	74%	71%
Meds 'Always' Explained Before Given	300+	71%	68%	64%
Nurses 'Always' Communicated Well	300+	85%	82%	79%
Pain 'Always' Well Controlled	300+	78%	72%	71%
Room and Bathroom 'Always' Clean	300+	87%	79%	73%
Timely Help 'Always' Received	300+	80%	72%	68%
Would Definitely Recommend Hospital	300+	87%	74%	71%
Use of Medical Imaging				
Cardiac Imaging Stress Test before Surgery	-	-	5.4%	5.3%
Combination Abdominal CT Scan	-	-	6.3%	10.5%
Combination Brain/Sinus CT Scan	-	-	2.1%	2.7%
Combination Chest CT Scan	-	-	1%	2.7%
Follow-up Mammogram/Ultrasound	-	-	8.1%	8.8%
Lumbar Spine MRI for Low Back Pain	-	-	34.9%	37.2%

Chippewa Valley Hospital

1220 3rd Ave W Phone: 715-672-4211
Durand, WI 54736
Type: Critical Access Hospitals Emergency Services: Yes
Ownership: Voluntary non-profit - Church

Measure	Cases	This Hosp.	State Avg.	U.S. Avg.
Blood Clot Prevention and Treatment				
Anticoagulation Overlap Therapy	-	-	95%	93%
ICU Venous Thromboembolism Prophylaxis	-	-	91%	92%
Incidence of Potentially Preventable VTE	-	-	10%	10%
UFH with Dosages/Platelet Monitoring	-	-	96%	97%
Venous Thromboembolism Prophylaxis	-	-	85%	85%
Warfarin Therapy Discharge Instructions	-	-	70%	75%
Chest Pain/Possible Heart Attack Care				
Aspirin Given Within 24 Hours of Arrival[1]	-	-	98%	96%
Fibrinolytic Meds Within 30 Min. of Arrival[3,7]	-	-	52%	58%
Average Time to ECG (minutes)[1]	-	-	7	7
Average Time to Transfer (minutes)[1,3]	-	-	58	60
Children's Asthma Care				
Received Home Management Plan of Care	-	-	-	88%
Received Reliever Medication	-	-	-	100%
Received Systemic Corticosteroids	-	-	-	100%
Emergency Department				
Admittance Decision Time (minutes)	-	-	65	98
Head CT Results Within 45 Min. of Arrival[1]	-	-	61%	57%
Patients Who Left ER Before Being Seen[5]	-	-	1%	2%
Time from ER Arrival to Admit. (minutes)	-	-	207	274
Time from ER Arrival to Discharge (minutes)	494	87	121	134
Time in ER Before Being Evaluated (minutes)	569	16	19	26
Time to Pain Meds for Fractures (minutes)	11	55	42	57
Heart Attack Care				
Aspirin Given at Discharge	-	-	99%	99%
Fibrinolytic Meds Within 30 Min. of Arrival	-	-	67%	54%
PCI Within 90 Minutes of Arrival	-	-	96%	96%
Statin Prescribed at Discharge	-	-	99%	98%
Heart Failure Care				
ACE Inhibitor or ARB for LVSD	-	-	97%	97%
Discharge Instructions Given	-	-	96%	94%
Evaluation of LVS Function	-	-	99%	99%
Medicare Spending				
Medicare Spending per Patient (ratio)	-	-	0.94	0.98
Pneumonia Care				
Appropriate Initial Antibiotic Given	-	-	96%	95%
Blood Culture Timing	-	-	98%	98%
Pregnancy and Delivery Care				
Newborn Deliveries Scheduled Early	-	-	4%	6%
Preventive Care				
Immunization for Influenza	-	-	90%	90%
Immunization for Pneumonia	-	-	92%	92%
Stroke Care				
Anticoagulation Therapy for Atrial Fibrillation	-	-	94%	95%
Antithrombotic Therapy Timing	-	-	99%	98%
Assessed for Rehabilitation	-	-	98%	97%
Discharged on Antithrombotic Therapy	-	-	99%	99%
Discharged on Statin Medication	-	-	94%	94%
Thrombolytic Therapy Timing	-	-	60%	66%
Venous Thromboembolism Prophylaxis	-	-	95%	94%
Written Stroke Educational Materials Given	-	-	88%	88%
Surgical Care Improvement Project				
Appropriate Beta Blocker Usage	-	-	99%	98%
Appropriate VTP Within 24 Hours	-	-	99%	98%
Controlled Postoperative Blood Glucose	-	-	96%	97%
Perioperative Temperature Management	-	-	100%	100%
Prophylactic Antibiotic Selection	-	-	99%	99%
Prophylactic Antibiotic Selection (Outpatient)[5]	-	-	98%	98%
Prophylactic Antibiotic Stopped	-	-	99%	98%
Prophylactic Antibiotic Timing	-	-	99%	99%
Prophylactic Antibiotic Timing (Outpatient)[5]	-	-	97%	98%
Urinary Catheter Removal	-	-	98%	97%
Survey of Patients' Hospital Experiences				
Area Around Room 'Always' Quiet at Night	-	-	63%	61%
Doctors 'Always' Communicated Well	-	-	83%	82%
Home Recovery Information Given	-	-	89%	85%
Hospital Given 9 or 10 on 10 Point Scale	-	-	74%	71%
Meds 'Always' Explained Before Given	-	-	68%	64%
Nurses 'Always' Communicated Well	-	-	82%	79%
Pain 'Always' Well Controlled	-	-	72%	71%
Room and Bathroom 'Always' Clean	-	-	79%	73%
Timely Help 'Always' Received	-	-	72%	68%
Would Definitely Recommend Hospital	-	-	74%	71%
Use of Medical Imaging				
Cardiac Imaging Stress Test before Surgery[7]	-	-	5.4%	5.3%
Combination Abdominal CT Scan	46	4.3%	6.3%	10.5%
Combination Brain/Sinus CT Scan	63	0.0%	2.1%	2.7%
Combination Chest CT Scan[1]	-	-	1%	2.7%
Follow-up Mammogram/Ultrasound	141	10.6%	8.1%	8.8%
Lumbar Spine MRI for Low Back Pain[1]	-	-	34.9%	37.2%

Ministry Eagle River Memorial Hospital

201 Hospital Rd Phone: 715-479-7411
Eagle River, WI 54521 Fax: 715-479-0395
Type: Critical Access Hospitals Emergency Services: Yes
Ownership: Voluntary non-profit - Church Beds: 29

Key Personnel:
Operating Room. . . . . Rich Foster, RN
Chief of Medical Staff. . . . . Terrance Moe, MD
Emergency Room . . . . Karen Sturdevent

Measure	Cases	This Hosp.	State Avg.	U.S. Avg.
Blood Clot Prevention and Treatment				
Anticoagulation Overlap Therapy[7]	-	-	95%	93%
ICU Venous Thromboembolism Prophylaxis[7]	-	-	91%	92%
Incidence of Potentially Preventable VTE[7]	-	-	10%	10%
UFH with Dosages/Platelet Monitoring[7]	-	-	96%	97%
Venous Thromboembolism Prophylaxis	167	100%	85%	85%
Warfarin Therapy Discharge Instructions[7]	-	-	70%	75%
Chest Pain/Possible Heart Attack Care				
Aspirin Given Within 24 Hours of Arrival	45	100%	98%	96%
Fibrinolytic Meds Within 30 Min. of Arrival[1]	-	-	52%	58%
Average Time to ECG (minutes)	47	10	7	7
Average Time to Transfer (minutes)[7]	-	-	58	60
Children's Asthma Care				
Received Home Management Plan of Care	-	-	-	88%
Received Reliever Medication	-	-	-	100%
Received Systemic Corticosteroids	-	-	-	100%
Emergency Department				
Admittance Decision Time (minutes)	299	40	65	98
Head CT Results Within 45 Min. of Arrival[1]	-	-	61%	57%
Patients Who Left ER Before Being Seen	5,067	1%	1%	2%
Time from ER Arrival to Admit. (minutes)	300	206	207	274
Time from ER Arrival to Discharge (minutes)	488	114	121	134
Time in ER Before Being Evaluated (minutes)	556	27	19	26
Time to Pain Meds for Fractures (minutes)	26	42	42	57
Heart Attack Care				
Aspirin Given at Discharge[5]	-	-	99%	99%
Fibrinolytic Meds Within 30 Min. of Arrival[5]	-	-	67%	54%
PCI Within 90 Minutes of Arrival[5]	-	-	96%	96%
Statin Prescribed at Discharge[5]	-	-	99%	98%
Heart Failure Care				
ACE Inhibitor or ARB for LVSD[1]	-	-	97%	97%
Discharge Instructions Given	17	94%	96%	94%
Evaluation of LVS Function	19	95%	99%	99%
Medicare Spending				
Medicare Spending per Patient (ratio)	-	-	0.94	0.98
Pneumonia Care				
Appropriate Initial Antibiotic Given	19	89%	96%	95%
Blood Culture Timing	20	100%	98%	98%
Pregnancy and Delivery Care				
Newborn Deliveries Scheduled Early[5]	-	-	4%	6%
Preventive Care				
Immunization for Influenza	189	100%	90%	90%
Immunization for Pneumonia	305	99%	92%	92%
Stroke Care				
Anticoagulation Therapy for Atrial Fibrillation[1]	-	-	94%	95%
Antithrombotic Therapy Timing	12	100%	99%	98%
Assessed for Rehabilitation	13	100%	98%	97%
Discharged on Antithrombotic Therapy	13	100%	99%	99%
Discharged on Statin Medication[1]	-	-	94%	94%
Thrombolytic Therapy Timing[7]	-	-	60%	66%
Venous Thromboembolism Prophylaxis	11	100%	95%	94%
Written Stroke Educational Materials Given[1]	-	-	88%	88%
Surgical Care Improvement Project				
Appropriate Beta Blocker Usage[1]	-	-	99%	98%
Appropriate VTP Within 24 Hours[1]	-	-	99%	98%
Controlled Postoperative Blood Glucose[7]	-	-	96%	97%
Perioperative Temperature Management	18	100%	100%	100%
Prophylactic Antibiotic Selection	14	100%	99%	99%
Prophylactic Antibiotic Selection (Outpatient)[1,3]	-	-	98%	98%
Prophylactic Antibiotic Stopped	14	100%	99%	98%
Prophylactic Antibiotic Timing	14	100%	99%	99%
Prophylactic Antibiotic Timing (Outpatient)[1,3]	-	-	97%	98%
Urinary Catheter Removal[7]	-	-	98%	97%
Survey of Patients' Hospital Experiences				
Area Around Room 'Always' Quiet at Night	(a)	75%	63%	61%
Doctors 'Always' Communicated Well	(a)	86%	83%	82%
Home Recovery Information Given	(a)	92%	89%	85%
Hospital Given 9 or 10 on 10 Point Scale	(a)	72%	74%	71%
Meds 'Always' Explained Before Given	(a)	76%	68%	64%
Nurses 'Always' Communicated Well	(a)	84%	82%	79%
Pain 'Always' Well Controlled	(a)	81%	72%	71%
Room and Bathroom 'Always' Clean	(a)	87%	79%	73%
Timely Help 'Always' Received	(a)	84%	72%	68%
Would Definitely Recommend Hospital	(a)	68%	74%	71%
Use of Medical Imaging				
Cardiac Imaging Stress Test before Surgery[7]	-	-	5.4%	5.3%
Combination Abdominal CT Scan	175	9.1%	6.3%	10.5%
Combination Brain/Sinus CT Scan[1]	-	-	2.1%	2.7%
Combination Chest CT Scan	91	0.0%	1%	2.7%
Follow-up Mammogram/Ultrasound	288	6.9%	8.1%	8.8%
Lumbar Spine MRI for Low Back Pain[1]	-	-	34.9%	37.2%

NOTE: Hospital profiles are in alphabetical order by state, then city, then hospital within the city; Rankings exclude hospitals with less than 25 cases except for patient surveys which excludes hospitals with less than 100 cases; (a) 100-299 cases; (1) The number of cases/patients is too few to report; (2) Data submitted were based on a sample of cases/patients; (3) Results are based on a shorter time period than required; (4) Data suppressed by CMS for one or more quarters; (5) Results are not available for this reporting period; (6) Fewer than 100 patients completed the HCAHPS survey; (7) No cases met the criteria for this measure; (8) The lower limit of the confidence interval cannot be calculated if the number of observed infections equals zero; (9) No data are available from the state/territory for this reporting period; (10) The scores shown reflect fewer than 50 completed surveys; (11) There were discrepancies in the data collection process; (12) This measure does not apply to this hospital for this reporting period; (13) Results cannot be calculated for this reporting period; (14) The results for this state are combined with nearby states to protect confidentiality; Please refer to the User's Guide for a full explanation of data.

Mayo Clinic Health System - Eau Claire Hospital

1221 Whipple St Phone: 715-838-3311
Eau Claire, WI 54703
URL: www.luthermidelfort.org
Type: Acute Care Hospitals Emergency Services: Yes
Ownership: Voluntary non-profit - Private Beds: 304

Key Personnel:
Pediatric In-Patient Care . . . . Kelly Buchheltz
Radiology. . . . . Zan Degen
Pediatric Ambulatory Care . . . . . . Melody Dodge
CEO/President. . . . . Randall Linton, MD
Chief of Medical Staff . . . . Robert Peck, MD
Infection Control. . . . . Susan Shea
Operating Room. . . . . Gary Welch
Quality Assurance . . . . Ed Wittrock

Measure	Cases	This Hosp.	State Avg.	U.S. Avg.
Blood Clot Prevention and Treatment				
Anticoagulation Overlap Therapy[2]	91	96%	95%	93%
ICU Venous Thromboembolism Prophylaxis[2]	93	95%	91%	92%
Incidence of Potentially Preventable VTE[2]	28	39%	10%	10%
UFH with Dosages/Platelet Monitoring[2]	83	100%	96%	97%
Venous Thromboembolism Prophylaxis[2]	291	96%	85%	85%
Warfarin Therapy Discharge Instructions[2]	77	64%	70%	75%
Chest Pain/Possible Heart Attack Care				
Aspirin Given Within 24 Hours of Arrival[5]	-	-	98%	96%
Fibrinolytic Meds Within 30 Min. of Arrival[5]	-	-	52%	58%
Average Time to ECG (minutes)[5]	-	-	7	7
Average Time to Transfer (minutes)[5]	-	-	58	60
Children's Asthma Care				
Received Home Management Plan of Care	-	-	-	88%
Received Reliever Medication	-	-	-	100%
Received Systemic Corticosteroids	-	-	-	100%
Emergency Department				
Admittance Decision Time (minutes)[2]	445	102	65	98
Head CT Results Within 45 Min. of Arrival[3,7]	-	-	61%	57%
Patients Who Left ER Before Being Seen	30,116	0%	1%	2%
Time from ER Arrival to Admit. (minutes)[2]	474	247	207	274
Time from ER Arrival to Discharge (minutes)	383	147	121	134
Time in ER Before Being Evaluated (minutes)	414	15	19	26
Time to Pain Meds for Fractures (minutes)	55	44	42	57
Heart Attack Care				
Aspirin Given at Discharge	218	100%	99%	99%
Fibrinolytic Meds Within 30 Min. of Arrival[7]	-	-	67%	54%
PCI Within 90 Minutes of Arrival	29	97%	96%	96%
Statin Prescribed at Discharge	217	100%	99%	98%
Heart Failure Care				
ACE Inhibitor or ARB for LVSD	50	100%	97%	97%
Discharge Instructions Given	224	98%	96%	94%
Evaluation of LVS Function	317	100%	99%	99%
Medicare Spending				
Medicare Spending per Patient (ratio)	-	0.98	0.94	0.98
Pneumonia Care				
Appropriate Initial Antibiotic Given	119	97%	96%	95%
Blood Culture Timing	178	99%	98%	98%
Pregnancy and Delivery Care				
Newborn Deliveries Scheduled Early[2]	28	0%	4%	6%
Preventive Care				
Immunization for Influenza[2]	555	89%	90%	90%
Immunization for Pneumonia[2]	702	92%	92%	92%
Stroke Care				
Anticoagulation Therapy for Atrial Fibrillation	20	95%	94%	95%
Antithrombotic Therapy Timing	97	99%	99%	98%
Assessed for Rehabilitation	121	100%	98%	97%
Discharged on Antithrombotic Therapy	107	100%	99%	99%
Discharged on Statin Medication	80	98%	94%	94%
Thrombolytic Therapy Timing[1]	-	-	60%	66%
Venous Thromboembolism Prophylaxis	126	96%	95%	94%
Written Stroke Educational Materials Given	49	94%	88%	88%
Surgical Care Improvement Project				
Appropriate Beta Blocker Usage	550	100%	99%	98%
Appropriate VTP Within 24 Hours	893	99%	99%	98%
Controlled Postoperative Blood Glucose	167	100%	96%	97%
Perioperative Temperature Management	1,110	100%	100%	100%
Prophylactic Antibiotic Selection	800	100%	99%	99%
Prophylactic Antibiotic Selection (Outpatient)	495	100%	98%	98%
Prophylactic Antibiotic Stopped	762	100%	99%	98%
Prophylactic Antibiotic Timing	800	99%	99%	99%
Prophylactic Antibiotic Timing (Outpatient)	495	98%	97%	98%
Urinary Catheter Removal	673	99%	98%	97%
Survey of Patients' Hospital Experiences				
Area Around Room 'Always' Quiet at Night	300+	61%	63%	61%
Doctors 'Always' Communicated Well	300+	83%	83%	82%
Home Recovery Information Given	300+	90%	89%	85%
Hospital Given 9 or 10 on 10 Point Scale	300+	82%	74%	71%
Meds 'Always' Explained Before Given	300+	66%	68%	64%
Nurses 'Always' Communicated Well	300+	80%	82%	79%
Pain 'Always' Well Controlled	300+	70%	72%	71%
Room and Bathroom 'Always' Clean	300+	79%	79%	73%
Timely Help 'Always' Received	300+	70%	72%	68%
Would Definitely Recommend Hospital	300+	85%	74%	71%
Use of Medical Imaging				
Cardiac Imaging Stress Test before Surgery	422	3.8%	5.4%	5.3%
Combination Abdominal CT Scan	917	7.1%	6.3%	10.5%
Combination Brain/Sinus CT Scan	702	1.9%	2.1%	2.7%
Combination Chest CT Scan	766	0.1%	1%	2.7%
Follow-up Mammogram/Ultrasound[7]	-	-	8.1%	8.8%
Lumbar Spine MRI for Low Back Pain	183	32.8%	34.9%	37.2%

Oak Leaf Surgical Hospital

3802 Oakwood Mall Dr Phone: 715-831-8130
Eau Claire, WI 54701
E-mail: info@oakleafsurgical.com
URL: www.oakleafsurgical.com
Type: Acute Care Hospitals Emergency Services: Yes
Ownership: Proprietary Beds: 13

Measure	Cases	This Hosp.	State Avg.	U.S. Avg.
Blood Clot Prevention and Treatment				
Anticoagulation Overlap Therapy[7]	-	-	95%	93%
ICU Venous Thromboembolism Prophylaxis[7]	-	-	91%	92%
Incidence of Potentially Preventable VTE[7]	-	-	10%	10%
UFH with Dosages/Platelet Monitoring[7]	-	-	96%	97%
Venous Thromboembolism Prophylaxis	19	100%	85%	85%
Warfarin Therapy Discharge Instructions[7]	-	-	70%	75%
Chest Pain/Possible Heart Attack Care				
Aspirin Given Within 24 Hours of Arrival[5]	-	-	98%	96%
Fibrinolytic Meds Within 30 Min. of Arrival[5]	-	-	52%	58%
Average Time to ECG (minutes)[5]	-	-	7	7
Average Time to Transfer (minutes)[5]	-	-	58	60
Children's Asthma Care				
Received Home Management Plan of Care	-	-	-	88%
Received Reliever Medication	-	-	-	100%
Received Systemic Corticosteroids	-	-	-	100%
Emergency Department				
Admittance Decision Time (minutes)[2,7]	-	-	65	98
Head CT Results Within 45 Min. of Arrival[5]	-	-	61%	57%
Patients Who Left ER Before Being Seen[5]	-	-	1%	2%
Time from ER Arrival to Admit. (minutes)[2,7]	-	-	207	274
Time from ER Arrival to Discharge (minutes)[5]	-	-	121	134
Time in ER Before Being Evaluated (minutes)[5]	-	-	19	26
Time to Pain Meds for Fractures (minutes)[5]	-	-	42	57
Heart Attack Care				
Aspirin Given at Discharge[5]	-	-	99%	99%
Fibrinolytic Meds Within 30 Min. of Arrival[5]	-	-	67%	54%
PCI Within 90 Minutes of Arrival[5]	-	-	96%	96%
Statin Prescribed at Discharge[5]	-	-	99%	98%
Heart Failure Care				
ACE Inhibitor or ARB for LVSD[5]	-	-	97%	97%
Discharge Instructions Given[5]	-	-	96%	94%
Evaluation of LVS Function[5]	-	-	99%	99%
Medicare Spending				
Medicare Spending per Patient (ratio)	-	0.88	0.94	0.98
Pneumonia Care				
Appropriate Initial Antibiotic Given[5]	-	-	96%	95%
Blood Culture Timing[5]	-	-	98%	98%
Pregnancy and Delivery Care				
Newborn Deliveries Scheduled Early[7]	-	-	4%	6%
Preventive Care				
Immunization for Influenza	259	96%	90%	90%
Immunization for Pneumonia[2]	255	97%	92%	92%
Stroke Care				
Anticoagulation Therapy for Atrial Fibrillation[5]	-	-	94%	95%
Antithrombotic Therapy Timing[5]	-	-	99%	98%
Assessed for Rehabilitation[5]	-	-	98%	97%
Discharged on Antithrombotic Therapy[5]	-	-	99%	99%
Discharged on Statin Medication[5]	-	-	94%	94%
Thrombolytic Therapy Timing[5]	-	-	60%	66%
Venous Thromboembolism Prophylaxis[5]	-	-	95%	94%
Written Stroke Educational Materials Given[5]	-	-	88%	88%
Surgical Care Improvement Project				
Appropriate Beta Blocker Usage	100	99%	99%	98%
Appropriate VTP Within 24 Hours	396	99%	99%	98%
Controlled Postoperative Blood Glucose[7]	-	-	96%	97%
Perioperative Temperature Management	416	100%	100%	100%
Prophylactic Antibiotic Selection	340	100%	99%	99%
Prophylactic Antibiotic Selection (Outpatient)	91	100%	98%	98%
Prophylactic Antibiotic Stopped	339	98%	99%	98%
Prophylactic Antibiotic Timing	340	99%	99%	99%
Prophylactic Antibiotic Timing (Outpatient)	91	100%	97%	98%
Urinary Catheter Removal	139	99%	98%	97%
Survey of Patients' Hospital Experiences				
Area Around Room 'Always' Quiet at Night	300+	81%	63%	61%
Doctors 'Always' Communicated Well	300+	85%	83%	82%
Home Recovery Information Given	300+	93%	89%	85%
Hospital Given 9 or 10 on 10 Point Scale	300+	90%	74%	71%
Meds 'Always' Explained Before Given	300+	80%	68%	64%
Nurses 'Always' Communicated Well	300+	94%	82%	79%
Pain 'Always' Well Controlled	300+	81%	72%	71%
Room and Bathroom 'Always' Clean	300+	90%	79%	73%
Timely Help 'Always' Received	300+	92%	72%	68%
Would Definitely Recommend Hospital	300+	91%	74%	71%
Use of Medical Imaging				
Cardiac Imaging Stress Test before Surgery[7]	-	-	5.4%	5.3%
Combination Abdominal CT Scan[7]	-	-	6.3%	10.5%
Combination Brain/Sinus CT Scan[7]	-	-	2.1%	2.7%
Combination Chest CT Scan[7]	-	-	1%	2.7%
Follow-up Mammogram/Ultrasound[7]	-	-	8.1%	8.8%
Lumbar Spine MRI for Low Back Pain[7]	-	-	34.9%	37.2%

Sacred Heart Hospital

900 W Clairemont Ave Phone: 715-717-4121
Eau Claire, WI 54701
URL: www.sacredhearteauclaire.org
Type: Acute Care Hospitals Emergency Services: Yes
Ownership: Voluntary non-profit - Church Beds: 344

Key Personnel:
Chief of Medical Staff . . . . Richard Daniels, MD
Cardiac Laboratory. . . . . Nancy DeMars
Radiology. . . . . Michael Dillon
Quality Assurance . . . . Dawn Garcia
Operating Room. . . . . Loren Lortscher
CEO/President. . . . . Julie Manas
Infection Control. . . . . Donna Moraska
Pediatric In-Patient Care . . . . Brook Steele

Measure	Cases	This Hosp.	State Avg.	U.S. Avg.
Blood Clot Prevention and Treatment				
Anticoagulation Overlap Therapy[2]	81	86%	95%	93%
ICU Venous Thromboembolism Prophylaxis[2]	84	58%	91%	92%
Incidence of Potentially Preventable VTE[2]	15	27%	10%	10%
UFH with Dosages/Platelet Monitoring[2]	51	100%	96%	97%
Venous Thromboembolism Prophylaxis[2]	298	73%	85%	85%
Warfarin Therapy Discharge Instructions[2]	65	37%	70%	75%
Chest Pain/Possible Heart Attack Care				
Aspirin Given Within 24 Hours of Arrival[1,3]	-	-	98%	96%
Fibrinolytic Meds Within 30 Min. of Arrival[5]	-	-	52%	58%
Average Time to ECG (minutes)[1,3]	-	-	7	7
Average Time to Transfer (minutes)[5]	-	-	58	60
Children's Asthma Care				
Received Home Management Plan of Care	-	-	-	88%
Received Reliever Medication	-	-	-	100%
Received Systemic Corticosteroids	-	-	-	100%
Emergency Department				

NOTE: *Hospital profiles are in alphabetical order by state, then city, then hospital within the city; Rankings exclude hospitals with less than 25 cases except for patient surveys which excludes hospitals with less than 100 cases; (a) 100-299 cases; (1) The number of cases/patients is too few to report; (2) Data submitted were based on a sample of cases/patients; (3) Results are based on a shorter time period than required; (4) Data suppressed by CMS for one or more quarters; (5) Results are not available for this reporting period; (6) Fewer than 100 patients completed the HCAHPS survey; (7) No cases met the criteria for this measure; (8) The lower limit of the confidence interval cannot be calculated if the number of observed infections equals zero; (9) No data are available from the state/territory for this reporting period; (10) The scores shown reflect fewer than 50 completed surveys; (11) There were discrepancies in the data collection process; (12) This measure does not apply to this hospital for this reporting period; (13) Results cannot be calculated for this reporting period; (14) The results for this state are combined with nearby states to protect confidentiality; Please refer to the User's Guide for a full explanation of data.*

Measure	Cases	This Hosp.	State Avg.	U.S. Avg.
Admittance Decision Time (minutes)[2]	364	74	65	98
Head CT Results Within 45 Min. of Arrival[1]	-	-	61%	57%
Patients Who Left ER Before Being Seen	19,992	1%	1%	2%
Time from ER Arrival to Admit. (minutes)[2]	365	207	207	274
Time from ER Arrival to Discharge (minutes)	370	134	121	134
Time in ER Before Being Evaluated (minutes)	397	22	19	26
Time to Pain Meds for Fractures (minutes)	89	52	42	57
Heart Attack Care				
Aspirin Given at Discharge[2]	285	100%	99%	99%
Fibrinolytic Meds Within 30 Min. of Arrival[2,7]	-	-	67%	54%
PCI Within 90 Minutes of Arrival[2]	14	100%	96%	96%
Statin Prescribed at Discharge[2]	266	98%	99%	98%
Heart Failure Care				
ACE Inhibitor or ARB for LVSD	44	82%	97%	97%
Discharge Instructions Given	119	97%	96%	94%
Evaluation of LVS Function	178	99%	99%	99%
Medicare Spending				
Medicare Spending per Patient (ratio)	-	0.96	0.94	0.98
Pneumonia Care				
Appropriate Initial Antibiotic Given[2]	115	96%	96%	95%
Blood Culture Timing[2]	144	97%	98%	98%
Pregnancy and Delivery Care				
Newborn Deliveries Scheduled Early[2]	26	4%	4%	6%
Preventive Care				
Immunization for Influenza[2]	545	98%	90%	90%
Immunization for Pneumonia[2]	667	92%	92%	92%
Stroke Care				
Anticoagulation Therapy for Atrial Fibrillation[2]	20	100%	94%	95%
Antithrombotic Therapy Timing[2]	70	100%	99%	98%
Assessed for Rehabilitation[2]	108	96%	98%	97%
Discharged on Antithrombotic Therapy[2]	92	100%	99%	99%
Discharged on Statin Medication[2]	77	94%	94%	94%
Thrombolytic Therapy Timing[1,2]	-	-	60%	66%
Venous Thromboembolism Prophylaxis[2]	108	98%	95%	94%
Written Stroke Educational Materials Given[2]	53	92%	88%	88%
Surgical Care Improvement Project				
Appropriate Beta Blocker Usage[2]	287	98%	99%	98%
Appropriate VTP Within 24 Hours[2]	386	95%	99%	98%
Controlled Postoperative Blood Glucose[2]	145	96%	96%	97%
Perioperative Temperature Management[2]	510	100%	100%	100%
Prophylactic Antibiotic Selection[2]	399	98%	99%	99%
Prophylactic Antibiotic Selection (Outpatient)	382	99%	98%	98%
Prophylactic Antibiotic Stopped[2]	389	96%	99%	98%
Prophylactic Antibiotic Timing[2]	399	99%	99%	99%
Prophylactic Antibiotic Timing (Outpatient)	384	96%	97%	98%
Urinary Catheter Removal[2]	337	99%	98%	97%
Survey of Patients' Hospital Experiences				
Area Around Room 'Always' Quiet at Night	300+	59%	63%	61%
Doctors 'Always' Communicated Well	300+	82%	83%	82%
Home Recovery Information Given	300+	87%	89%	85%
Hospital Given 9 or 10 on 10 Point Scale	300+	74%	74%	71%
Meds 'Always' Explained Before Given	300+	66%	68%	64%
Nurses 'Always' Communicated Well	300+	82%	82%	79%
Pain 'Always' Well Controlled	300+	72%	72%	71%
Room and Bathroom 'Always' Clean	300+	77%	79%	73%
Timely Help 'Always' Received	300+	72%	72%	68%
Would Definitely Recommend Hospital	300+	76%	74%	71%
Use of Medical Imaging				
Cardiac Imaging Stress Test before Surgery	130	6.9%	5.4%	5.3%
Combination Abdominal CT Scan	535	9.7%	6.3%	10.5%
Combination Brain/Sinus CT Scan	229	0.9%	2.1%	2.7%
Combination Chest CT Scan	452	0.4%	1%	2.7%
Follow-up Mammogram/Ultrasound	314	12.1%	8.1%	8.8%
Lumbar Spine MRI for Low Back Pain	79	34.2%	34.9%	37.2%

Edgerton Hospital & Health Services

11101 N Sherman Road
Edgerton, WI 53534
Phone: 608-884-3441
Fax: 608-884-1659
E-mail: mchinfo@edgertonhospital.com
URL: www.edgertonhospital.com
Type: Critical Access Hospitals
Emergency Services: Yes
Ownership: Voluntary non-profit - Private
Beds: 86

Key Personnel:

Quality Assurance . . . . Sue Alusin, POPP
Emergency Room . . . . Christine Langemo, MD
Chief of Medical Staff . . . . Dennis Litsheim, MD
Operating Room. . . . . Shelley Mcguire
Radiology. . . . . Roberta Nelson
CEO/President. . . . . Jim Pernau

Measure	Cases	This Hosp.	State Avg.	U.S. Avg.
Blood Clot Prevention and Treatment				
Anticoagulation Overlap Therapy[5]	-	-	95%	93%
ICU Venous Thromboembolism Prophylaxis[5]	-	-	91%	92%
Incidence of Potentially Preventable VTE[5]	-	-	10%	10%
UFH with Dosages/Platelet Monitoring[5]	-	-	96%	97%
Venous Thromboembolism Prophylaxis[5]	-	-	85%	85%
Warfarin Therapy Discharge Instructions[5]	-	-	70%	75%
Chest Pain/Possible Heart Attack Care				
Aspirin Given Within 24 Hours of Arrival	-	-	98%	96%
Fibrinolytic Meds Within 30 Min. of Arrival	-	-	52%	58%
Average Time to ECG (minutes)	-	-	7	7
Average Time to Transfer (minutes)	-	-	58	60
Children's Asthma Care				
Received Home Management Plan of Care	-	-	-	88%
Received Reliever Medication	-	-	-	100%
Received Systemic Corticosteroids	-	-	-	100%
Emergency Department				
Admittance Decision Time (minutes)[3]	14	34	65	98
Head CT Results Within 45 Min. of Arrival	-	-	61%	57%
Patients Who Left ER Before Being Seen	-	-	1%	2%
Time from ER Arrival to Admit. (minutes)[3]	27	213	207	274
Time from ER Arrival to Discharge (minutes)	-	-	121	134
Time in ER Before Being Evaluated (minutes)	-	-	19	26
Time to Pain Meds for Fractures (minutes)	-	-	42	57
Heart Attack Care				
Aspirin Given at Discharge[5]	-	-	99%	99%
Fibrinolytic Meds Within 30 Min. of Arrival[5]	-	-	67%	54%
PCI Within 90 Minutes of Arrival[5]	-	-	96%	96%
Statin Prescribed at Discharge[5]	-	-	99%	98%
Heart Failure Care				
ACE Inhibitor or ARB for LVSD[3,7]	-	-	97%	97%
Discharge Instructions Given[1,3]	-	-	96%	94%
Evaluation of LVS Function[1,3]	-	-	99%	99%
Medicare Spending				
Medicare Spending per Patient (ratio)	-	-	0.94	0.98
Pneumonia Care				
Appropriate Initial Antibiotic Given[1]	-	-	96%	95%
Blood Culture Timing[1]	-	-	98%	98%
Pregnancy and Delivery Care				
Newborn Deliveries Scheduled Early[5]	-	-	4%	6%
Preventive Care				
Immunization for Influenza[5]	-	-	90%	90%
Immunization for Pneumonia[5]	-	-	92%	92%
Stroke Care				
Anticoagulation Therapy for Atrial Fibrillation[5]	-	-	94%	95%
Antithrombotic Therapy Timing[5]	-	-	99%	98%
Assessed for Rehabilitation[5]	-	-	98%	97%
Discharged on Antithrombotic Therapy[5]	-	-	99%	99%
Discharged on Statin Medication[5]	-	-	94%	94%
Thrombolytic Therapy Timing[5]	-	-	60%	66%
Venous Thromboembolism Prophylaxis[5]	-	-	95%	94%
Written Stroke Educational Materials Given[5]	-	-	88%	88%
Surgical Care Improvement Project				
Appropriate Beta Blocker Usage[5]	-	-	99%	98%
Appropriate VTP Within 24 Hours[5]	-	-	99%	98%
Controlled Postoperative Blood Glucose[5]	-	-	96%	97%
Perioperative Temperature Management[5]	-	-	100%	100%
Prophylactic Antibiotic Selection[5]	-	-	99%	99%
Prophylactic Antibiotic Selection (Outpatient)	-	-	98%	98%
Prophylactic Antibiotic Stopped[5]	-	-	99%	98%
Prophylactic Antibiotic Timing[5]	-	-	99%	99%
Prophylactic Antibiotic Timing (Outpatient)	-	-	97%	98%
Urinary Catheter Removal[5]	-	-	98%	97%
Survey of Patients' Hospital Experiences				
Area Around Room 'Always' Quiet at Night[6]	<100	69%	63%	61%
Doctors 'Always' Communicated Well[6]	<100	79%	83%	82%
Home Recovery Information Given[6]	<100	97%	89%	85%
Hospital Given 9 or 10 on 10 Point Scale[6]	<100	82%	74%	71%
Meds 'Always' Explained Before Given[6]	<100	80%	68%	64%
Nurses 'Always' Communicated Well[6]	<100	86%	82%	79%
Pain 'Always' Well Controlled[6]	<100	81%	72%	71%
Room and Bathroom 'Always' Clean[6]	<100	89%	79%	73%
Timely Help 'Always' Received[6]	<100	68%	72%	68%
Would Definitely Recommend Hospital[6]	<100	81%	74%	71%
Use of Medical Imaging				
Cardiac Imaging Stress Test before Surgery	-	-	5.4%	5.3%
Combination Abdominal CT Scan	-	-	6.3%	10.5%
Combination Brain/Sinus CT Scan	-	-	2.1%	2.7%
Combination Chest CT Scan	-	-	1%	2.7%
Follow-up Mammogram/Ultrasound	-	-	8.1%	8.8%
Lumbar Spine MRI for Low Back Pain	-	-	34.9%	37.2%

Aurora Lakeland Medical Center

W3985 Cty Rd Nn
Elkhorn, WI 53121
Phone: 262-741-2000
URL: www.aurorahealthcare.org/facilities
Type: Acute Care Hospitals
Emergency Services: Yes
Ownership: Voluntary non-profit - Private
Beds: 99

Measure	Cases	This Hosp.	State Avg.	U.S. Avg.
Blood Clot Prevention and Treatment				
Anticoagulation Overlap Therapy[2]	33	97%	95%	93%
ICU Venous Thromboembolism Prophylaxis[2]	84	100%	91%	92%
Incidence of Potentially Preventable VTE[1,2]	-	-	10%	10%
UFH with Dosages/Platelet Monitoring[1,2]	-	-	96%	97%
Venous Thromboembolism Prophylaxis[2]	148	98%	85%	85%
Warfarin Therapy Discharge Instructions[2]	30	100%	70%	75%
Chest Pain/Possible Heart Attack Care				
Aspirin Given Within 24 Hours of Arrival	51	96%	98%	96%
Fibrinolytic Meds Within 30 Min. of Arrival[7]	-	-	52%	58%
Average Time to ECG (minutes)	54	3	7	7
Average Time to Transfer (minutes)	14	41	58	60
Children's Asthma Care				
Received Home Management Plan of Care	-	-	-	88%
Received Reliever Medication	-	-	-	100%
Received Systemic Corticosteroids	-	-	-	100%
Emergency Department				
Admittance Decision Time (minutes)[2]	295	83	65	98
Head CT Results Within 45 Min. of Arrival	11	91%	61%	57%
Patients Who Left ER Before Being Seen	16,126	1%	1%	2%
Time from ER Arrival to Admit. (minutes)[2]	296	218	207	274
Time from ER Arrival to Discharge (minutes)	332	120	121	134
Time in ER Before Being Evaluated (minutes)	373	20	19	26
Time to Pain Meds for Fractures (minutes)	105	40	42	57
Heart Attack Care				
Aspirin Given at Discharge[1]	-	-	99%	99%
Fibrinolytic Meds Within 30 Min. of Arrival[7]	-	-	67%	54%
PCI Within 90 Minutes of Arrival[7]	-	-	96%	96%
Statin Prescribed at Discharge[1]	-	-	99%	98%
Heart Failure Care				
ACE Inhibitor or ARB for LVSD	20	100%	97%	97%
Discharge Instructions Given	30	93%	96%	94%
Evaluation of LVS Function	44	100%	99%	99%
Medicare Spending				
Medicare Spending per Patient (ratio)	-	1.00	0.94	0.98
Pneumonia Care				
Appropriate Initial Antibiotic Given	80	99%	96%	95%
Blood Culture Timing	124	100%	98%	98%
Pregnancy and Delivery Care				
Newborn Deliveries Scheduled Early	50	10%	4%	6%
Preventive Care				
Immunization for Influenza[2]	291	98%	90%	90%
Immunization for Pneumonia[2]	338	99%	92%	92%
Stroke Care				
Anticoagulation Therapy for Atrial Fibrillation[1]	-	-	94%	95%
Antithrombotic Therapy Timing	24	100%	99%	98%
Assessed for Rehabilitation	26	100%	98%	97%
Discharged on Antithrombotic Therapy	25	96%	99%	99%
Discharged on Statin Medication	19	95%	94%	94%

NOTE: Hospital profiles are in alphabetical order by state, then city, then hospital within the city; Rankings exclude hospitals with less than 25 cases except for patient surveys which excludes hospitals with less than 100 cases; (a) 100-299 cases; (1) The number of cases/patients is too few to report; (2) Data submitted were based on a sample of cases/patients; (3) Results are based on a shorter time period than required; (4) Data suppressed by CMS for one or more quarters; (5) Results are not available for this reporting period; (6) Fewer than 100 patients completed the HCAHPS survey; (7) No cases met the criteria for this measure; (8) The lower limit of the confidence interval cannot be calculated if the number of observed infections equals zero; (9) No data are available from the state/territory for this reporting period; (10) The scores shown reflect fewer than 50 completed surveys; (11) There were discrepancies in the data collection process; (12) This measure does not apply to this hospital for this reporting period; (13) Results cannot be calculated for this reporting period; (14) The results for this state are combined with nearby states to protect confidentiality; Please refer to the User's Guide for a full explanation of data.

Measure	Cases	This Hosp.	State Avg.	U.S. Avg.
Thrombolytic Therapy Timing[7]	-	-	60%	66%
Venous Thromboembolism Prophylaxis	23	100%	95%	94%
Written Stroke Educational Materials Given	12	100%	88%	88%
Surgical Care Improvement Project				
Appropriate Beta Blocker Usage[2]	39	100%	99%	98%
Appropriate VTP Within 24 Hours[2]	133	100%	99%	98%
Controlled Postoperative Blood Glucose[2,7]	-	-	96%	97%
Perioperative Temperature Management[2]	147	100%	100%	100%
Prophylactic Antibiotic Selection[2]	70	100%	99%	99%
Prophylactic Antibiotic Selection (Outpatient)	28	100%	98%	98%
Prophylactic Antibiotic Stopped[2]	67	100%	99%	98%
Prophylactic Antibiotic Timing[2]	70	100%	99%	99%
Prophylactic Antibiotic Timing (Outpatient)	28	96%	97%	98%
Urinary Catheter Removal[2]	89	100%	98%	97%
Survey of Patients' Hospital Experiences				
Area Around Room 'Always' Quiet at Night	300+	61%	63%	61%
Doctors 'Always' Communicated Well	300+	84%	83%	82%
Home Recovery Information Given	300+	87%	89%	85%
Hospital Given 9 or 10 on 10 Point Scale	300+	65%	74%	71%
Meds 'Always' Explained Before Given	300+	64%	68%	64%
Nurses 'Always' Communicated Well	300+	78%	82%	79%
Pain 'Always' Well Controlled	300+	71%	72%	71%
Room and Bathroom 'Always' Clean	300+	74%	79%	73%
Timely Help 'Always' Received	300+	68%	72%	68%
Would Definitely Recommend Hospital	300+	63%	74%	71%
Use of Medical Imaging				
Cardiac Imaging Stress Test before Surgery	516	4.3%	5.4%	5.3%
Combination Abdominal CT Scan	439	5.2%	6.3%	10.5%
Combination Brain/Sinus CT Scan	454	1.3%	2.1%	2.7%
Combination Chest CT Scan	489	2.9%	1%	2.7%
Follow-up Mammogram/Ultrasound	960	10.4%	8.1%	8.8%
Lumbar Spine MRI for Low Back Pain	80	45.0%	34.9%	37.2%

Saint Agnes Hospital

430 E Divison St
Fond Du Lac, WI 54935
Phone: 920-929-2300
Fax: 920-926-4306
URL: www.agnesian.com
Type: Acute Care Hospitals
Emergency Services: Yes
Ownership: Voluntary non-profit - Private
Beds: 330

Key Personnel:

Quality Assurance . . . . Cathic Aschenbrenner
Operating Room. . . . . James Avery
Infection Control. . . . . Kayla Ericksen
CEO/President. . . . . Robert A Fale
Chief of Medical Staff . . . . Theodore Miller, MD
Cardiac Laboratory. . . . . Jim Mugan
Radiology. . . . . Missy Tate
Pediatric In-Patient Care . . . . Maria Zahn

Measure	Cases	This Hosp.	State Avg.	U.S. Avg.
Blood Clot Prevention and Treatment				
Anticoagulation Overlap Therapy[2]	63	100%	95%	93%
ICU Venous Thromboembolism Prophylaxis[2]	62	90%	91%	92%
Incidence of Potentially Preventable VTE[1,2]	-	-	10%	10%
UFH with Dosages/Platelet Monitoring[2]	13	100%	96%	97%
Venous Thromboembolism Prophylaxis[2]	406	89%	85%	85%
Warfarin Therapy Discharge Instructions[2]	54	89%	70%	75%
Chest Pain/Possible Heart Attack Care				
Aspirin Given Within 24 Hours of Arrival[1,3]	-	-	98%	96%
Fibrinolytic Meds Within 30 Min. of Arrival[5]	-	-	52%	58%
Average Time to ECG (minutes)[1,3]	-	-	7	7
Average Time to Transfer (minutes)[5]	-	-	58	60
Children's Asthma Care				
Received Home Management Plan of Care	-	-	-	88%
Received Reliever Medication	-	-	-	100%
Received Systemic Corticosteroids	-	-	-	100%
Emergency Department				
Admittance Decision Time (minutes)[2]	536	64	65	98
Head CT Results Within 45 Min. of Arrival	15	80%	61%	57%
Patients Who Left ER Before Being Seen	28,614	0%	1%	2%
Time from ER Arrival to Admit. (minutes)[2]	668	199	207	274
Time from ER Arrival to Discharge (minutes)	562	113	121	134
Time in ER Before Being Evaluated (minutes)	617	17	19	26
Time to Pain Meds for Fractures (minutes)	94	36	42	57
Heart Attack Care				
Aspirin Given at Discharge	229	99%	99%	99%
Fibrinolytic Meds Within 30 Min. of Arrival[7]	-	-	67%	54%
PCI Within 90 Minutes of Arrival	37	100%	96%	96%
Statin Prescribed at Discharge	219	100%	99%	98%
Heart Failure Care				
ACE Inhibitor or ARB for LVSD	43	100%	97%	97%
Discharge Instructions Given	158	92%	96%	94%
Evaluation of LVS Function	219	100%	99%	99%
Medicare Spending				
Medicare Spending per Patient (ratio)	-	0.94	0.94	0.98
Pneumonia Care				
Appropriate Initial Antibiotic Given	127	95%	96%	95%
Blood Culture Timing	251	98%	98%	98%
Pregnancy and Delivery Care				
Newborn Deliveries Scheduled Early	101	5%	4%	6%
Preventive Care				
Immunization for Influenza[2]	677	96%	90%	90%
Immunization for Pneumonia[2]	758	94%	92%	92%
Stroke Care				
Anticoagulation Therapy for Atrial Fibrillation[1]	-	-	94%	95%
Antithrombotic Therapy Timing	72	100%	99%	98%
Assessed for Rehabilitation	108	99%	98%	97%
Discharged on Antithrombotic Therapy	104	99%	99%	99%
Discharged on Statin Medication	74	99%	94%	94%
Thrombolytic Therapy Timing[1]	-	-	60%	66%
Venous Thromboembolism Prophylaxis	88	97%	95%	94%
Written Stroke Educational Materials Given	72	97%	88%	88%
Surgical Care Improvement Project				
Appropriate Beta Blocker Usage	177	99%	99%	98%
Appropriate VTP Within 24 Hours	467	99%	99%	98%
Controlled Postoperative Blood Glucose	62	98%	96%	97%
Perioperative Temperature Management	543	100%	100%	100%
Prophylactic Antibiotic Selection	383	99%	99%	99%
Prophylactic Antibiotic Selection (Outpatient)	365	99%	98%	98%
Prophylactic Antibiotic Stopped	366	98%	99%	98%
Prophylactic Antibiotic Timing	384	100%	99%	99%
Prophylactic Antibiotic Timing (Outpatient)	367	98%	97%	98%
Urinary Catheter Removal	346	97%	98%	97%
Survey of Patients' Hospital Experiences				
Area Around Room 'Always' Quiet at Night	300+	58%	63%	61%
Doctors 'Always' Communicated Well	300+	80%	83%	82%
Home Recovery Information Given	300+	86%	89%	85%
Hospital Given 9 or 10 on 10 Point Scale	300+	67%	74%	71%
Meds 'Always' Explained Before Given	300+	62%	68%	64%
Nurses 'Always' Communicated Well	300+	77%	82%	79%
Pain 'Always' Well Controlled	300+	66%	72%	71%
Room and Bathroom 'Always' Clean	300+	80%	79%	73%
Timely Help 'Always' Received	300+	60%	72%	68%
Would Definitely Recommend Hospital	300+	65%	74%	71%
Use of Medical Imaging				
Cardiac Imaging Stress Test before Surgery	463	5.8%	5.4%	5.3%
Combination Abdominal CT Scan	655	9.3%	6.3%	10.5%
Combination Brain/Sinus CT Scan	659	2.0%	2.1%	2.7%
Combination Chest CT Scan	486	3.7%	1%	2.7%
Follow-up Mammogram/Ultrasound	1,341	10.1%	8.1%	8.8%
Lumbar Spine MRI for Low Back Pain	128	38.3%	34.9%	37.2%

Fort Memorial Hospital

611 Sherman Ave E
Fort Atkinson, WI 53538
Phone: 920-568-5000
Fax: 920-568-5412
E-mail: sally.hink@famhs.org
URL: www.forthealthcare.com
Type: Acute Care Hospitals
Emergency Services: Yes
Ownership: Voluntary non-profit - Private
Beds: 110

Key Personnel:

Radiology. . . . . Edgardo Jiongco, MD
Chief of Medical Staff. . . . . Pam Kuehl, MD
Coronary Care. . . . . Linda Smith, RN
President/CEO. . . . . Michael S. Wallace
Quality Assurance . . . . Marie Wiesmann, RN
Emergency Room . . . . Harold Wilson, RN

Measure	Cases	This Hosp.	State Avg.	U.S. Avg.
Blood Clot Prevention and Treatment				
Anticoagulation Overlap Therapy[2]	26	96%	95%	93%
ICU Venous Thromboembolism Prophylaxis[2]	46	96%	91%	92%
Incidence of Potentially Preventable VTE[1,2]	-	-	10%	10%
UFH with Dosages/Platelet Monitoring[2]	11	100%	96%	97%
Venous Thromboembolism Prophylaxis[2]	130	97%	85%	85%
Warfarin Therapy Discharge Instructions[2]	23	96%	70%	75%
Chest Pain/Possible Heart Attack Care				
Aspirin Given Within 24 Hours of Arrival	91	98%	98%	96%
Fibrinolytic Meds Within 30 Min. of Arrival[7]	-	-	52%	58%
Average Time to ECG (minutes)	91	2	7	7
Average Time to Transfer (minutes)[1]	-	-	58	60
Children's Asthma Care				
Received Home Management Plan of Care	-	-	-	88%
Received Reliever Medication	-	-	-	100%
Received Systemic Corticosteroids	-	-	-	100%
Emergency Department				
Admittance Decision Time (minutes)[2]	282	64	65	98
Head CT Results Within 45 Min. of Arrival[1]	-	-	61%	57%
Patients Who Left ER Before Being Seen	16,458	0%	1%	2%
Time from ER Arrival to Admit. (minutes)[2]	295	225	207	274
Time from ER Arrival to Discharge (minutes)	360	130	121	134
Time in ER Before Being Evaluated (minutes)	306	24	19	26
Time to Pain Meds for Fractures (minutes)	41	53	42	57
Heart Attack Care				
Aspirin Given at Discharge[1]	-	-	99%	99%
Fibrinolytic Meds Within 30 Min. of Arrival[7]	-	-	67%	54%
PCI Within 90 Minutes of Arrival[7]	-	-	96%	96%
Statin Prescribed at Discharge[1]	-	-	99%	98%
Heart Failure Care				
ACE Inhibitor or ARB for LVSD[1]	-	-	97%	97%
Discharge Instructions Given	54	89%	96%	94%
Evaluation of LVS Function	72	100%	99%	99%
Medicare Spending				
Medicare Spending per Patient (ratio)	-	0.87	0.94	0.98
Pneumonia Care				
Appropriate Initial Antibiotic Given	55	93%	96%	95%
Blood Culture Timing	88	98%	98%	98%
Pregnancy and Delivery Care				
Newborn Deliveries Scheduled Early[2]	53	0%	4%	6%
Preventive Care				
Immunization for Influenza[2]	256	94%	90%	90%
Immunization for Pneumonia[2]	310	93%	92%	92%
Stroke Care				
Anticoagulation Therapy for Atrial Fibrillation[1]	-	-	94%	95%
Antithrombotic Therapy Timing	17	94%	99%	98%
Assessed for Rehabilitation	21	100%	98%	97%
Discharged on Antithrombotic Therapy	21	100%	99%	99%
Discharged on Statin Medication	20	100%	94%	94%
Thrombolytic Therapy Timing[1]	-	-	60%	66%
Venous Thromboembolism Prophylaxis	16	100%	95%	94%
Written Stroke Educational Materials Given[1]	-	-	88%	88%
Surgical Care Improvement Project				
Appropriate Beta Blocker Usage[2]	69	96%	99%	98%
Appropriate VTP Within 24 Hours[2]	237	97%	99%	98%
Controlled Postoperative Blood Glucose[2,7]	-	-	96%	97%
Perioperative Temperature Management[2]	266	100%	100%	100%
Prophylactic Antibiotic Selection[2]	179	98%	99%	99%
Prophylactic Antibiotic Selection (Outpatient)	158	98%	98%	98%
Prophylactic Antibiotic Stopped[2]	178	99%	99%	98%
Prophylactic Antibiotic Timing[2]	179	99%	99%	99%
Prophylactic Antibiotic Timing (Outpatient)	118	96%	97%	98%
Urinary Catheter Removal[2]	52	94%	98%	97%
Survey of Patients' Hospital Experiences				
Area Around Room 'Always' Quiet at Night	300+	67%	63%	61%
Doctors 'Always' Communicated Well	300+	81%	83%	82%
Home Recovery Information Given	300+	89%	89%	85%
Hospital Given 9 or 10 on 10 Point Scale	300+	76%	74%	71%
Meds 'Always' Explained Before Given	300+	68%	68%	64%
Nurses 'Always' Communicated Well	300+	82%	82%	79%
Pain 'Always' Well Controlled	300+	68%	72%	71%
Room and Bathroom 'Always' Clean	300+	84%	79%	73%
Timely Help 'Always' Received	300+	67%	72%	68%
Would Definitely Recommend Hospital	300+	74%	74%	71%

NOTE: Hospital profiles are in alphabetical order by state, then city, then hospital within the city; Rankings exclude hospitals with less than 25 cases except for patient surveys which excludes hospitals with less than 100 cases; (a) 100-299 cases; (1) The number of cases/patients is too few to report; (2) Data submitted were based on a sample of cases/patients; (3) Results are based on a shorter time period than required; (4) Data suppressed by CMS for one or more quarters; (5) Results are not available for this reporting period; (6) Fewer than 100 patients completed the HCAHPS survey; (7) No cases met the criteria for this measure; (8) The lower limit of the confidence interval cannot be calculated if the number of observed infections equals zero; (9) No data are available from the state/territory for this reporting period; (10) The scores shown reflect fewer than 50 completed surveys; (11) There were discrepancies in the data collection process; (12) This measure does not apply to this hospital for this reporting period; (13) Results cannot be calculated for this reporting period; (14) The results for this state are combined with nearby states to protect confidentiality; Please refer to the User's Guide for a full explanation of data.

Use of Medical Imaging				
Cardiac Imaging Stress Test before Surgery	188	4.3%	5.4%	5.3%
Combination Abdominal CT Scan	365	5.8%	6.3%	10.5%
Combination Brain/Sinus CT Scan	353	1.7%	2.1%	2.7%
Combination Chest CT Scan	209	0.0%	1%	2.7%
Follow-up Mammogram/Ultrasound	943	9.7%	8.1%	8.8%
Lumbar Spine MRI for Low Back Pain	75	26.7%	34.9%	37.2%

Midwest Orthopedic Specialty Hospital

10101 South 27th Saint 2nd Floor
Franklin, WI 53132
Phone: 414-817-5800
URL: www.mymosh.com
Type: Acute Care Hospitals
Emergency Services: No
Ownership: Voluntary non-profit - Private
Beds: 31

Measure	Cases	This Hosp.	State Avg.	U.S. Avg.
Blood Clot Prevention and Treatment				
Anticoagulation Overlap Therapy[1,2]	-	-	95%	93%
ICU Venous Thromboembolism Prophylaxis[2,7]	-	-	91%	92%
Incidence of Potentially Preventable VTE[2]	14	0%	10%	10%
UFH with Dosages/Platelet Monitoring[1,2]	-	-	96%	97%
Venous Thromboembolism Prophylaxis[2]	48	100%	85%	85%
Warfarin Therapy Discharge Instructions[1,2]	-	-	70%	75%
Chest Pain/Possible Heart Attack Care				
Aspirin Given Within 24 Hours of Arrival[5]	-	-	98%	96%
Fibrinolytic Meds Within 30 Min. of Arrival[5]	-	-	52%	58%
Average Time to ECG (minutes)[5]	-	-	7	7
Average Time to Transfer (minutes)[5]	-	-	58	60
Children's Asthma Care				
Received Home Management Plan of Care	-	-	-	88%
Received Reliever Medication	-	-	-	100%
Received Systemic Corticosteroids	-	-	-	100%
Emergency Department				
Admittance Decision Time (minutes)[2,7]	-	-	65	98
Head CT Results Within 45 Min. of Arrival[5]	-	-	61%	57%
Patients Who Left ER Before Being Seen[5]	-	-	1%	2%
Time from ER Arrival to Admit. (minutes)[2,7]	-	-	207	274
Time from ER Arrival to Discharge (minutes)[5]	-	-	121	134
Time in ER Before Being Evaluated (minutes)[5]	-	-	19	26
Time to Pain Meds for Fractures (minutes)[5]	-	-	42	57
Heart Attack Care				
Aspirin Given at Discharge[5]	-	-	99%	99%
Fibrinolytic Meds Within 30 Min. of Arrival[5]	-	-	67%	54%
PCI Within 90 Minutes of Arrival[5]	-	-	96%	96%
Statin Prescribed at Discharge[5]	-	-	99%	98%
Heart Failure Care				
ACE Inhibitor or ARB for LVSD[5]	-	-	97%	97%
Discharge Instructions Given[5]	-	-	96%	94%
Evaluation of LVS Function[5]	-	-	99%	99%
Medicare Spending				
Medicare Spending per Patient (ratio)	-	0.93	0.94	0.98
Pneumonia Care				
Appropriate Initial Antibiotic Given[5]	-	-	96%	95%
Blood Culture Timing[5]	-	-	98%	98%
Pregnancy and Delivery Care				
Newborn Deliveries Scheduled Early[7]	-	-	4%	6%
Preventive Care				
Immunization for Influenza[2]	320	98%	90%	90%
Immunization for Pneumonia[2]	395	84%	92%	92%
Stroke Care				
Anticoagulation Therapy for Atrial Fibrillation[5]	-	-	94%	95%
Antithrombotic Therapy Timing[5]	-	-	99%	98%
Assessed for Rehabilitation[5]	-	-	98%	97%
Discharged on Antithrombotic Therapy[5]	-	-	99%	99%
Discharged on Statin Medication[5]	-	-	94%	94%
Thrombolytic Therapy Timing[5]	-	-	60%	66%
Venous Thromboembolism Prophylaxis[5]	-	-	95%	94%
Written Stroke Educational Materials Given[5]	-	-	88%	88%
Surgical Care Improvement Project				
Appropriate Beta Blocker Usage[2]	66	98%	99%	98%
Appropriate VTP Within 24 Hours[2]	229	100%	99%	98%
Controlled Postoperative Blood Glucose[2,7]	-	-	96%	97%
Perioperative Temperature Management[2]	243	100%	100%	100%

Prophylactic Antibiotic Selection[2]	178	100%	99%	99%
Prophylactic Antibiotic Selection (Outpatient)	190	100%	98%	98%
Prophylactic Antibiotic Stopped[2]	178	100%	99%	98%
Prophylactic Antibiotic Timing[2]	178	99%	99%	99%
Prophylactic Antibiotic Timing (Outpatient)	190	99%	97%	98%
Urinary Catheter Removal[2]	107	100%	98%	97%
Survey of Patients' Hospital Experiences				
Area Around Room 'Always' Quiet at Night	300+	84%	63%	61%
Doctors 'Always' Communicated Well	300+	89%	83%	82%
Home Recovery Information Given	300+	93%	89%	85%
Hospital Given 9 or 10 on 10 Point Scale	300+	93%	74%	71%
Meds 'Always' Explained Before Given	300+	77%	68%	64%
Nurses 'Always' Communicated Well	300+	92%	82%	79%
Pain 'Always' Well Controlled	300+	82%	72%	71%
Room and Bathroom 'Always' Clean	300+	88%	79%	73%
Timely Help 'Always' Received	300+	86%	72%	68%
Would Definitely Recommend Hospital	300+	94%	74%	71%
Use of Medical Imaging				
Cardiac Imaging Stress Test before Surgery[7]	-	-	5.4%	5.3%
Combination Abdominal CT Scan[7]	-	-	6.3%	10.5%
Combination Brain/Sinus CT Scan[7]	-	-	2.1%	2.7%
Combination Chest CT Scan[7]	-	-	1%	2.7%
Follow-up Mammogram/Ultrasound[7]	-	-	8.1%	8.8%
Lumbar Spine MRI for Low Back Pain[7]	-	-	34.9%	37.2%

Wheaton Franciscan Healthcare Franklin

10101 South 27th St
Franklin, WI 53132
Phone: 414-325-4518
URL: www.mywheaton.org
Type: Acute Care Hospitals
Emergency Services: Yes
Ownership: Voluntary non-profit - Private
Key Personnel:
President . . . . Daniel Mattes

Measure	Cases	This Hosp.	State Avg.	U.S. Avg.
Blood Clot Prevention and Treatment				
Anticoagulation Overlap Therapy[2]	48	92%	95%	93%
ICU Venous Thromboembolism Prophylaxis[2]	24	100%	91%	92%
Incidence of Potentially Preventable VTE[1,2]	-	-	10%	10%
UFH with Dosages/Platelet Monitoring[2]	20	100%	96%	97%
Venous Thromboembolism Prophylaxis[2]	193	79%	85%	85%
Warfarin Therapy Discharge Instructions[2]	40	18%	70%	75%
Chest Pain/Possible Heart Attack Care				
Aspirin Given Within 24 Hours of Arrival	44	100%	98%	96%
Fibrinolytic Meds Within 30 Min. of Arrival[7]	-	-	52%	58%
Average Time to ECG (minutes)	45	7	7	7
Average Time to Transfer (minutes)[1]	-	-	58	60
Children's Asthma Care				
Received Home Management Plan of Care	-	-	-	88%
Received Reliever Medication	-	-	-	100%
Received Systemic Corticosteroids	-	-	-	100%
Emergency Department				
Admittance Decision Time (minutes)[2]	647	80	65	98
Head CT Results Within 45 Min. of Arrival[1]	-	-	61%	57%
Patients Who Left ER Before Being Seen	22,355	0%	1%	2%
Time from ER Arrival to Admit. (minutes)[2]	647	240	207	274
Time from ER Arrival to Discharge (minutes)	375	156	121	134
Time in ER Before Being Evaluated (minutes)	396	18	19	26
Time to Pain Meds for Fractures (minutes)	53	32	42	57
Heart Attack Care				
Aspirin Given at Discharge[1]	-	-	99%	99%
Fibrinolytic Meds Within 30 Min. of Arrival[7]	-	-	67%	54%
PCI Within 90 Minutes of Arrival[7]	-	-	96%	96%
Statin Prescribed at Discharge[1]	-	-	99%	98%
Heart Failure Care				
ACE Inhibitor or ARB for LVSD[1]	-	-	97%	97%
Discharge Instructions Given	36	97%	96%	94%
Evaluation of LVS Function	56	100%	99%	99%
Medicare Spending				
Medicare Spending per Patient (ratio)	-	1.00	0.94	0.98
Pneumonia Care				
Appropriate Initial Antibiotic Given	68	97%	96%	95%
Blood Culture Timing	136	99%	98%	98%
Pregnancy and Delivery Care				

Newborn Deliveries Scheduled Early[7]	-	-	4%	6%
Preventive Care				
Immunization for Influenza[2]	310	95%	90%	90%
Immunization for Pneumonia[2]	512	89%	92%	92%
Stroke Care				
Anticoagulation Therapy for Atrial Fibrillation[1]	-	-	94%	95%
Antithrombotic Therapy Timing	14	100%	99%	98%
Assessed for Rehabilitation	14	93%	98%	97%
Discharged on Antithrombotic Therapy	14	100%	99%	99%
Discharged on Statin Medication[1]	-	-	94%	94%
Thrombolytic Therapy Timing[1]	-	-	60%	66%
Venous Thromboembolism Prophylaxis	15	80%	95%	94%
Written Stroke Educational Materials Given	12	0%	88%	88%
Surgical Care Improvement Project				
Appropriate Beta Blocker Usage	25	100%	99%	98%
Appropriate VTP Within 24 Hours	97	98%	99%	98%
Controlled Postoperative Blood Glucose[7]	-	-	96%	97%
Perioperative Temperature Management	110	100%	100%	100%
Prophylactic Antibiotic Selection	68	100%	99%	99%
Prophylactic Antibiotic Selection (Outpatient)	36	100%	98%	98%
Prophylactic Antibiotic Stopped	67	100%	99%	98%
Prophylactic Antibiotic Timing	68	100%	99%	99%
Prophylactic Antibiotic Timing (Outpatient)	36	94%	97%	98%
Urinary Catheter Removal	41	85%	98%	97%
Survey of Patients' Hospital Experiences				
Area Around Room 'Always' Quiet at Night	300+	69%	63%	61%
Doctors 'Always' Communicated Well	300+	81%	83%	82%
Home Recovery Information Given	300+	88%	89%	85%
Hospital Given 9 or 10 on 10 Point Scale	300+	81%	74%	71%
Meds 'Always' Explained Before Given	300+	70%	68%	64%
Nurses 'Always' Communicated Well	300+	84%	82%	79%
Pain 'Always' Well Controlled	300+	74%	72%	71%
Room and Bathroom 'Always' Clean	300+	82%	79%	73%
Timely Help 'Always' Received	300+	76%	72%	68%
Would Definitely Recommend Hospital	300+	82%	74%	71%
Use of Medical Imaging				
Cardiac Imaging Stress Test before Surgery	99	5.1%	5.4%	5.3%
Combination Abdominal CT Scan	302	8.9%	6.3%	10.5%
Combination Brain/Sinus CT Scan[1]	-	-	2.1%	2.7%
Combination Chest CT Scan	152	0.7%	1%	2.7%
Follow-up Mammogram/Ultrasound	632	9.2%	8.1%	8.8%
Lumbar Spine MRI for Low Back Pain	114	36.0%	34.9%	37.2%

Moundview Memorial Hospital & Clinics

402 W Lake St
Friendship, WI 53934
Phone: 608-339-3331
Fax: 608-339-9385
E-mail: medwards@acmh.com
URL: www.acmh.com
Type: Critical Access Hospitals
Emergency Services: Yes
Ownership: Government - Local
Beds: 29
Key Personnel:
Emergency Room . . . . M Esmaili, MD
Chief of Medical Staff . . . . Martin Janssen, MD

Measure	Cases	This Hosp.	State Avg.	U.S. Avg.
Blood Clot Prevention and Treatment				
Anticoagulation Overlap Therapy[7]	-	-	95%	93%
ICU Venous Thromboembolism Prophylaxis[7]	-	-	91%	92%
Incidence of Potentially Preventable VTE[7]	-	-	10%	10%
UFH with Dosages/Platelet Monitoring[7]	-	-	96%	97%
Venous Thromboembolism Prophylaxis	71	51%	85%	85%
Warfarin Therapy Discharge Instructions[7]	-	-	70%	75%
Chest Pain/Possible Heart Attack Care				
Aspirin Given Within 24 Hours of Arrival	34	94%	98%	96%
Fibrinolytic Meds Within 30 Min. of Arrival[1]	-	-	52%	58%
Average Time to ECG (minutes)	34	8	7	7
Average Time to Transfer (minutes)[7]	-	-	58	60
Children's Asthma Care				
Received Home Management Plan of Care	-	-	-	88%
Received Reliever Medication	-	-	-	100%
Received Systemic Corticosteroids	-	-	-	100%
Emergency Department				
Admittance Decision Time (minutes)	81	20	65	98
Head CT Results Within 45 Min. of Arrival[1]	-	-	61%	57%

NOTE: Hospital profiles are in alphabetical order by state, then city, then hospital within the city; Rankings exclude hospitals with less than 25 cases except for patient surveys which excludes hospitals with less than 100 cases; (a) 100-299 cases; (1) The number of cases/patients is too few to report; (2) Data submitted were based on a sample of cases/patients; (3) Results are based on a shorter time period than required; (4) Data suppressed by CMS for one or more quarters; (5) Results are not available for this reporting period; (6) Fewer than 100 patients completed the HCAHPS survey; (7) No cases met the criteria for this measure; (8) The lower limit of the confidence interval cannot be calculated if the number of observed infections equals zero; (9) No data are available from the state/territory for this reporting period; (10) The scores shown reflect fewer than 50 completed surveys; (11) There were discrepancies in the data collection process; (12) This measure does not apply to this hospital for this reporting period; (13) Results cannot be calculated for this reporting period; (14) The results for this state are combined with nearby states to protect confidentiality; Please refer to the User's Guide for a full explanation of data.

Measure	Cases	This Hosp.	State Avg.	U.S. Avg.
Patients Who Left ER Before Being Seen[5]	-	-	1%	2%
Time from ER Arrival to Admit. (minutes)	96	159	207	274
Time from ER Arrival to Discharge (minutes)	550	83	121	134
Time in ER Before Being Evaluated (minutes)	496	22	19	26
Time to Pain Meds for Fractures (minutes)	11	39	42	57
Heart Attack Care				
Aspirin Given at Discharge[5]	-	-	99%	99%
Fibrinolytic Meds Within 30 Min. of Arrival[5]	-	-	67%	54%
PCI Within 90 Minutes of Arrival[5]	-	-	96%	96%
Statin Prescribed at Discharge[5]	-	-	99%	98%
Heart Failure Care				
ACE Inhibitor or ARB for LVSD[1]	-	-	97%	97%
Discharge Instructions Given[1]	-	-	96%	94%
Evaluation of LVS Function	11	91%	99%	99%
Medicare Spending				
Medicare Spending per Patient (ratio)	-	-	0.94	0.98
Pneumonia Care				
Appropriate Initial Antibiotic Given[1]	-	-	96%	95%
Blood Culture Timing[1]	-	-	98%	98%
Pregnancy and Delivery Care				
Newborn Deliveries Scheduled Early[5]	-	-	4%	6%
Preventive Care				
Immunization for Influenza	60	77%	90%	90%
Immunization for Pneumonia	92	72%	92%	92%
Stroke Care				
Anticoagulation Therapy for Atrial Fibrillation[3,7]	-	-	94%	95%
Antithrombotic Therapy Timing[1,3]	-	-	99%	98%
Assessed for Rehabilitation[1,3]	-	-	98%	97%
Discharged on Antithrombotic Therapy[1,3]	-	-	99%	99%
Discharged on Statin Medication[1,3]	-	-	94%	94%
Thrombolytic Therapy Timing[3,7]	-	-	60%	66%
Venous Thromboembolism Prophylaxis[1,3]	-	-	95%	94%
Written Stroke Educational Materials Given[1,3]	-	-	88%	88%
Surgical Care Improvement Project				
Appropriate Beta Blocker Usage[5]	-	-	99%	98%
Appropriate VTP Within 24 Hours[5]	-	-	99%	98%
Controlled Postoperative Blood Glucose[5]	-	-	96%	97%
Perioperative Temperature Management[5]	-	-	100%	100%
Prophylactic Antibiotic Selection[5]	-	-	99%	99%
Prophylactic Antibiotic Selection (Outpatient)[1,3]	-	-	98%	98%
Prophylactic Antibiotic Stopped[5]	-	-	99%	98%
Prophylactic Antibiotic Timing[5]	-	-	99%	99%
Prophylactic Antibiotic Timing (Outpatient)[1,3]	-	-	97%	98%
Urinary Catheter Removal[5]	-	-	98%	97%
Survey of Patients' Hospital Experiences				
Area Around Room 'Always' Quiet at Night[10]	<100	45%	63%	61%
Doctors 'Always' Communicated Well[10]	<100	74%	83%	82%
Home Recovery Information Given[10]	<100	82%	89%	85%
Hospital Given 9 or 10 on 10 Point Scale[10]	<100	56%	74%	71%
Meds 'Always' Explained Before Given[10]	<100	67%	68%	64%
Nurses 'Always' Communicated Well[10]	<100	84%	82%	79%
Pain 'Always' Well Controlled[10]	<100	66%	72%	71%
Room and Bathroom 'Always' Clean[10]	<100	77%	79%	73%
Timely Help 'Always' Received[10]	<100	81%	72%	68%
Would Definitely Recommend Hospital[10]	<100	47%	74%	71%
Use of Medical Imaging				
Cardiac Imaging Stress Test before Surgery[1]	-	-	5.4%	5.3%
Combination Abdominal CT Scan	87	12.6%	6.3%	10.5%
Combination Brain/Sinus CT Scan[1]	-	-	2.1%	2.7%
Combination Chest CT Scan	57	0.0%	1%	2.7%
Follow-up Mammogram/Ultrasound	175	12.6%	8.1%	8.8%
Lumbar Spine MRI for Low Back Pain[1]	-	-	34.9%	37.2%

Orthopaedic Hospital of Wisconsin

475 W River Woods Pkwy
Glendale, WI 53212
Phone: 414-961-6800
Fax: 414-961-6738
URL: www.ohow.org
Type: Acute Care Hospitals
Emergency Services: No
Ownership: Voluntary non-profit - Other
Key Personnel:
CEO/President. . . . . Susan Henckel

Measure	Cases	This Hosp.	State Avg.	U.S. Avg.
Blood Clot Prevention and Treatment				
Anticoagulation Overlap Therapy[1,2]	-	-	95%	93%
ICU Venous Thromboembolism Prophylaxis[2,7]	-	-	91%	92%
Incidence of Potentially Preventable VTE[1,2]	-	-	10%	10%
UFH with Dosages/Platelet Monitoring[2,7]	-	-	96%	97%
Venous Thromboembolism Prophylaxis[2]	35	100%	85%	85%
Warfarin Therapy Discharge Instructions[1,2]	-	-	70%	75%
Chest Pain/Possible Heart Attack Care				
Aspirin Given Within 24 Hours of Arrival[5]	-	-	98%	96%
Fibrinolytic Meds Within 30 Min. of Arrival[5]	-	-	52%	58%
Average Time to ECG (minutes)[5]	-	-	7	7
Average Time to Transfer (minutes)[5]	-	-	58	60
Children's Asthma Care				
Received Home Management Plan of Care	-	-	-	88%
Received Reliever Medication	-	-	-	100%
Received Systemic Corticosteroids	-	-	-	100%
Emergency Department				
Admittance Decision Time (minutes)[2,7]	-	-	65	98
Head CT Results Within 45 Min. of Arrival[5]	-	-	61%	57%
Patients Who Left ER Before Being Seen[5]	-	-	1%	2%
Time from ER Arrival to Admit. (minutes)[2,7]	-	-	207	274
Time from ER Arrival to Discharge (minutes)[5]	-	-	121	134
Time in ER Before Being Evaluated (minutes)[5]	-	-	19	26
Time to Pain Meds for Fractures (minutes)[5]	-	-	42	57
Heart Attack Care				
Aspirin Given at Discharge[5]	-	-	99%	99%
Fibrinolytic Meds Within 30 Min. of Arrival[5]	-	-	67%	54%
PCI Within 90 Minutes of Arrival[5]	-	-	96%	96%
Statin Prescribed at Discharge[5]	-	-	99%	98%
Heart Failure Care				
ACE Inhibitor or ARB for LVSD[5]	-	-	97%	97%
Discharge Instructions Given[5]	-	-	96%	94%
Evaluation of LVS Function[5]	-	-	99%	99%
Medicare Spending				
Medicare Spending per Patient (ratio)	-	0.86	0.94	0.98
Pneumonia Care				
Appropriate Initial Antibiotic Given[5]	-	-	96%	95%
Blood Culture Timing[5]	-	-	98%	98%
Pregnancy and Delivery Care				
Newborn Deliveries Scheduled Early[7]	-	-	4%	6%
Preventive Care				
Immunization for Influenza[2]	318	39%	90%	90%
Immunization for Pneumonia[2]	429	69%	92%	92%
Stroke Care				
Anticoagulation Therapy for Atrial Fibrillation[5]	-	-	94%	95%
Antithrombotic Therapy Timing[5]	-	-	99%	98%
Assessed for Rehabilitation[5]	-	-	98%	97%
Discharged on Antithrombotic Therapy[5]	-	-	99%	99%
Discharged on Statin Medication[5]	-	-	94%	94%
Thrombolytic Therapy Timing[5]	-	-	60%	66%
Venous Thromboembolism Prophylaxis[5]	-	-	95%	94%
Written Stroke Educational Materials Given[5]	-	-	88%	88%
Surgical Care Improvement Project				
Appropriate Beta Blocker Usage[2]	56	98%	99%	98%
Appropriate VTP Within 24 Hours[2]	226	100%	99%	98%
Controlled Postoperative Blood Glucose[2,7]	-	-	96%	97%
Perioperative Temperature Management[2]	240	100%	100%	100%
Prophylactic Antibiotic Selection[2]	185	100%	99%	99%
Prophylactic Antibiotic Selection (Outpatient)	117	100%	98%	98%
Prophylactic Antibiotic Stopped[2]	185	100%	99%	98%
Prophylactic Antibiotic Timing[2]	185	100%	99%	99%
Prophylactic Antibiotic Timing (Outpatient)	117	100%	97%	98%
Urinary Catheter Removal[2]	190	100%	98%	97%
Survey of Patients' Hospital Experiences				
Area Around Room 'Always' Quiet at Night	300+	76%	63%	61%
Doctors 'Always' Communicated Well	300+	92%	83%	82%
Home Recovery Information Given	300+	94%	89%	85%
Hospital Given 9 or 10 on 10 Point Scale	300+	94%	74%	71%
Meds 'Always' Explained Before Given	300+	79%	68%	64%
Nurses 'Always' Communicated Well	300+	94%	82%	79%
Pain 'Always' Well Controlled	300+	81%	72%	71%
Room and Bathroom 'Always' Clean	300+	86%	79%	73%
Timely Help 'Always' Received	300+	85%	72%	68%
Would Definitely Recommend Hospital	300+	94%	74%	71%
Use of Medical Imaging				
Cardiac Imaging Stress Test before Surgery[7]	-	-	5.4%	5.3%
Combination Abdominal CT Scan[7]	-	-	6.3%	10.5%
Combination Brain/Sinus CT Scan[1]	-	-	2.1%	2.7%
Combination Chest CT Scan[7]	-	-	1%	2.7%
Follow-up Mammogram/Ultrasound[7]	-	-	8.1%	8.8%
Lumbar Spine MRI for Low Back Pain	88	36.4%	34.9%	37.2%

Aurora Medical Center

975 Port Washington Road
Grafton, WI 53024
Phone: 262-329-1000
Type: Acute Care Hospitals
Emergency Services: Yes
Ownership: Voluntary non-profit - Private

Measure	Cases	This Hosp.	State Avg.	U.S. Avg.
Blood Clot Prevention and Treatment				
Anticoagulation Overlap Therapy[2]	55	91%	95%	93%
ICU Venous Thromboembolism Prophylaxis[2]	79	97%	91%	92%
Incidence of Potentially Preventable VTE[2]	18	0%	10%	10%
UFH with Dosages/Platelet Monitoring[2]	30	97%	96%	97%
Venous Thromboembolism Prophylaxis[2]	247	87%	85%	85%
Warfarin Therapy Discharge Instructions[2]	44	61%	70%	75%
Chest Pain/Possible Heart Attack Care				
Aspirin Given Within 24 Hours of Arrival[1,3]	-	-	98%	96%
Fibrinolytic Meds Within 30 Min. of Arrival[5]	-	-	52%	58%
Average Time to ECG (minutes)[1,3]	-	-	7	7
Average Time to Transfer (minutes)[5]	-	-	58	60
Children's Asthma Care				
Received Home Management Plan of Care	-	-	-	88%
Received Reliever Medication	-	-	-	100%
Received Systemic Corticosteroids	-	-	-	100%
Emergency Department				
Admittance Decision Time (minutes)[2]	464	69	65	98
Head CT Results Within 45 Min. of Arrival[3,7]	-	-	61%	57%
Patients Who Left ER Before Being Seen	11,788	0%	1%	2%
Time from ER Arrival to Admit. (minutes)[2]	471	188	207	274
Time from ER Arrival to Discharge (minutes)	347	125	121	134
Time in ER Before Being Evaluated (minutes)	369	10	19	26
Time to Pain Meds for Fractures (minutes)	91	39	42	57
Heart Attack Care				
Aspirin Given at Discharge	180	99%	99%	99%
Fibrinolytic Meds Within 30 Min. of Arrival[7]	-	-	67%	54%
PCI Within 90 Minutes of Arrival	32	94%	96%	96%
Statin Prescribed at Discharge	176	99%	99%	98%
Heart Failure Care				
ACE Inhibitor or ARB for LVSD	26	100%	97%	97%
Discharge Instructions Given	66	97%	96%	94%
Evaluation of LVS Function	103	100%	99%	99%
Medicare Spending				
Medicare Spending per Patient (ratio)	-	0.95	0.94	0.98
Pneumonia Care				
Appropriate Initial Antibiotic Given	61	98%	96%	95%
Blood Culture Timing	103	100%	98%	98%
Pregnancy and Delivery Care				
Newborn Deliveries Scheduled Early	116	4%	4%	6%
Preventive Care				
Immunization for Influenza[2]	545	96%	90%	90%
Immunization for Pneumonia[2]	699	96%	92%	92%
Stroke Care				
Anticoagulation Therapy for Atrial Fibrillation	16	100%	94%	95%
Antithrombotic Therapy Timing	78	100%	99%	98%
Assessed for Rehabilitation	103	99%	98%	97%
Discharged on Antithrombotic Therapy	95	99%	99%	99%
Discharged on Statin Medication	71	100%	94%	94%
Thrombolytic Therapy Timing[1]	-	-	60%	66%
Venous Thromboembolism Prophylaxis	91	98%	95%	94%
Written Stroke Educational Materials Given	55	89%	88%	88%
Surgical Care Improvement Project				
Appropriate Beta Blocker Usage[2]	282	99%	99%	98%
Appropriate VTP Within 24 Hours[2]	689	100%	99%	98%
Controlled Postoperative Blood Glucose[2]	103	96%	96%	97%
Perioperative Temperature Management[2]	816	100%	100%	100%

NOTE: Hospital profiles are in alphabetical order by state, then city, then hospital within the city; Rankings exclude hospitals with less than 25 cases except for patient surveys which excludes hospitals with less than 100 cases; (a) 100-299 cases; (1) The number of cases/patients is too few to report; (2) Data submitted were based on a sample of cases/patients; (3) Results are based on a shorter time period than required; (4) Data suppressed by CMS for one or more quarters; (5) Results are not available for this reporting period; (6) Fewer than 100 patients completed the HCAHPS survey; (7) No cases met the criteria for this measure; (8) The lower limit of the confidence interval cannot be calculated if the number of observed infections equals zero; (9) No data are available from the state/territory for this reporting period; (10) The scores shown reflect fewer than 50 completed surveys; (11) There were discrepancies in the data collection process; (12) This measure does not apply to this hospital for this reporting period; (13) Results cannot be calculated for this reporting period; (14) The results for this state are combined with nearby states to protect confidentiality; Please refer to the User's Guide for a full explanation of data.

Prophylactic Antibiotic Selection[2]	788	100%	99%	99%
Prophylactic Antibiotic Selection (Outpatient)	250	98%	98%	98%
Prophylactic Antibiotic Stopped[2]	783	100%	99%	98%
Prophylactic Antibiotic Timing[2]	788	100%	99%	99%
Prophylactic Antibiotic Timing (Outpatient)	250	99%	97%	98%
Urinary Catheter Removal[2]	718	100%	98%	97%
Survey of Patients' Hospital Experiences				
Area Around Room 'Always' Quiet at Night	300+	66%	63%	61%
Doctors 'Always' Communicated Well	300+	84%	83%	82%
Home Recovery Information Given	300+	90%	89%	85%
Hospital Given 9 or 10 on 10 Point Scale	300+	82%	74%	71%
Meds 'Always' Explained Before Given	300+	69%	68%	64%
Nurses 'Always' Communicated Well	300+	85%	82%	79%
Pain 'Always' Well Controlled	300+	74%	72%	71%
Room and Bathroom 'Always' Clean	300+	77%	79%	73%
Timely Help 'Always' Received	300+	74%	72%	68%
Would Definitely Recommend Hospital	300+	83%	74%	71%
Use of Medical Imaging				
Cardiac Imaging Stress Test before Surgery	205	4.9%	5.4%	5.3%
Combination Abdominal CT Scan	312	7.1%	6.3%	10.5%
Combination Brain/Sinus CT Scan[1]	-	-	2.1%	2.7%
Combination Chest CT Scan	203	0.0%	1%	2.7%
Follow-up Mammogram/Ultrasound	176	6.8%	8.1%	8.8%
Lumbar Spine MRI for Low Back Pain	56	41.1%	34.9%	37.2%

Burnett Medical Center

257 W Saint George Ave
Grantsburg, WI 54840
Phone: 715-463-5353
Fax: 715-463-2423
E-mail: info@burnettmedicalcenter.com
URL: www.burnettmedicalcenter.com
Type: Critical Access Hospitals
Emergency Services: Yes
Ownership: Voluntary non-profit - Private
Beds: 78

Key Personnel:
Cardiac Laboratory. . . . . Terry Giles
CEO/President. . . . . Gordy Lewis
Anesthesiology. . . . . Gregory Pekkala
Quality Assurance . . . . Susan Smith
Infection Control. . . . . Debra Stigar
Chief of Medical Staff. . . . . Blas_ Vitale

Measure	Cases	This Hosp.	State Avg.	U.S. Avg.
Blood Clot Prevention and Treatment				
Anticoagulation Overlap Therapy[5]	-	-	95%	93%
ICU Venous Thromboembolism Prophylaxis[5]	-	-	91%	92%
Incidence of Potentially Preventable VTE[5]	-	-	10%	10%
UFH with Dosages/Platelet Monitoring[5]	-	-	96%	97%
Venous Thromboembolism Prophylaxis[5]	-	-	85%	85%
Warfarin Therapy Discharge Instructions[5]	-	-	70%	75%
Chest Pain/Possible Heart Attack Care				
Aspirin Given Within 24 Hours of Arrival	-	-	98%	96%
Fibrinolytic Meds Within 30 Min. of Arrival	-	-	52%	58%
Average Time to ECG (minutes)	-	-	7	7
Average Time to Transfer (minutes)	-	-	58	60
Children's Asthma Care				
Received Home Management Plan of Care	-	-	-	88%
Received Reliever Medication	-	-	-	100%
Received Systemic Corticosteroids	-	-	-	100%
Emergency Department				
Admittance Decision Time (minutes)[5]	-	-	65	98
Head CT Results Within 45 Min. of Arrival	-	-	61%	57%
Patients Who Left ER Before Being Seen	-	-	1%	2%
Time from ER Arrival to Admit. (minutes)[5]	-	-	207	274
Time from ER Arrival to Discharge (minutes)	-	-	121	134
Time in ER Before Being Evaluated (minutes)	-	-	19	26
Time to Pain Meds for Fractures (minutes)	-	-	42	57
Heart Attack Care				
Aspirin Given at Discharge[5]	-	-	99%	99%
Fibrinolytic Meds Within 30 Min. of Arrival[5]	-	-	67%	54%
PCI Within 90 Minutes of Arrival[5]	-	-	96%	96%
Statin Prescribed at Discharge[5]	-	-	99%	98%
Heart Failure Care				
ACE Inhibitor or ARB for LVSD[1]	-	-	97%	97%
Discharge Instructions Given	12	100%	96%	94%
Evaluation of LVS Function	15	93%	99%	99%
Medicare Spending				
Medicare Spending per Patient (ratio)	-	-	0.94	0.98
Pneumonia Care				
Appropriate Initial Antibiotic Given	24	88%	96%	95%
Blood Culture Timing	23	96%	98%	98%
Pregnancy and Delivery Care				
Newborn Deliveries Scheduled Early[5]	-	-	4%	6%
Preventive Care				
Immunization for Influenza[5]	-	-	90%	90%
Immunization for Pneumonia[5]	-	-	92%	92%
Stroke Care				
Anticoagulation Therapy for Atrial Fibrillation[5]	-	-	94%	95%
Antithrombotic Therapy Timing[5]	-	-	99%	98%
Assessed for Rehabilitation[5]	-	-	98%	97%
Discharged on Antithrombotic Therapy[5]	-	-	99%	99%
Discharged on Statin Medication[5]	-	-	94%	94%
Thrombolytic Therapy Timing[5]	-	-	60%	66%
Venous Thromboembolism Prophylaxis[5]	-	-	95%	94%
Written Stroke Educational Materials Given[5]	-	-	88%	88%
Surgical Care Improvement Project				
Appropriate Beta Blocker Usage[1,3]	-	-	99%	98%
Appropriate VTP Within 24 Hours[5]	-	-	99%	98%
Controlled Postoperative Blood Glucose[3,7]	-	-	96%	97%
Perioperative Temperature Management	18	100%	100%	100%
Prophylactic Antibiotic Selection	17	82%	99%	99%
Prophylactic Antibiotic Selection (Outpatient)	-	-	98%	98%
Prophylactic Antibiotic Stopped	17	88%	99%	98%
Prophylactic Antibiotic Timing	17	100%	99%	99%
Prophylactic Antibiotic Timing (Outpatient)	-	-	97%	98%
Urinary Catheter Removal[7]	-	-	98%	97%
Survey of Patients' Hospital Experiences				
Area Around Room 'Always' Quiet at Night	(a)	58%	63%	61%
Doctors 'Always' Communicated Well	(a)	87%	83%	82%
Home Recovery Information Given	(a)	87%	89%	85%
Hospital Given 9 or 10 on 10 Point Scale	(a)	71%	74%	71%
Meds 'Always' Explained Before Given	(a)	59%	68%	64%
Nurses 'Always' Communicated Well	(a)	81%	82%	79%
Pain 'Always' Well Controlled	(a)	73%	72%	71%
Room and Bathroom 'Always' Clean	(a)	87%	79%	73%
Timely Help 'Always' Received	(a)	73%	72%	68%
Would Definitely Recommend Hospital	(a)	71%	74%	71%
Use of Medical Imaging				
Cardiac Imaging Stress Test before Surgery	-	-	5.4%	5.3%
Combination Abdominal CT Scan	-	-	6.3%	10.5%
Combination Brain/Sinus CT Scan	-	-	2.1%	2.7%
Combination Chest CT Scan	-	-	1%	2.7%
Follow-up Mammogram/Ultrasound	-	-	8.1%	8.8%
Lumbar Spine MRI for Low Back Pain	-	-	34.9%	37.2%

Aurora Baycare Medical Center

2845 Greenbrier Rd
Green Bay, WI 54311
Phone: 920-288-8000
URL: www.aurorabaycare.com
Type: Acute Care Hospitals
Emergency Services: Yes
Ownership: Proprietary
Beds: 167

Key Personnel:
Chief of Medical Staff. . . . . J. Richard Ludgin, MD, JD
President . . . . Daniel Meyer

Measure	Cases	This Hosp.	State Avg.	U.S. Avg.
Blood Clot Prevention and Treatment				
Anticoagulation Overlap Therapy[2]	65	97%	95%	93%
ICU Venous Thromboembolism Prophylaxis[2]	102	96%	91%	92%
Incidence of Potentially Preventable VTE[1,2]	-	-	10%	10%
UFH with Dosages/Platelet Monitoring[2]	24	96%	96%	97%
Venous Thromboembolism Prophylaxis[2]	241	90%	85%	85%
Warfarin Therapy Discharge Instructions[2]	55	49%	70%	75%
Chest Pain/Possible Heart Attack Care				
Aspirin Given Within 24 Hours of Arrival[1,3]	-	-	98%	96%
Fibrinolytic Meds Within 30 Min. of Arrival[5]	-	-	52%	58%
Average Time to ECG (minutes)[1,3]	-	-	7	7
Average Time to Transfer (minutes)[5]	-	-	58	60
Children's Asthma Care				
Received Home Management Plan of Care	-	-	-	88%
Received Reliever Medication	-	-	-	100%
Received Systemic Corticosteroids	-	-	-	100%
Emergency Department				
Admittance Decision Time (minutes)[2]	211	75	65	98
Head CT Results Within 45 Min. of Arrival[3,7]	-	-	61%	57%
Patients Who Left ER Before Being Seen	26,292	0%	1%	2%
Time from ER Arrival to Admit. (minutes)[2]	258	192	207	274
Time from ER Arrival to Discharge (minutes)	348	110	121	134
Time in ER Before Being Evaluated (minutes)	360	20	19	26
Time to Pain Meds for Fractures (minutes)	102	46	42	57
Heart Attack Care				
Aspirin Given at Discharge	152	100%	99%	99%
Fibrinolytic Meds Within 30 Min. of Arrival[7]	-	-	67%	54%
PCI Within 90 Minutes of Arrival	21	100%	96%	96%
Statin Prescribed at Discharge	148	100%	99%	98%
Heart Failure Care				
ACE Inhibitor or ARB for LVSD	19	100%	97%	97%
Discharge Instructions Given	50	98%	96%	94%
Evaluation of LVS Function	55	100%	99%	99%
Medicare Spending				
Medicare Spending per Patient (ratio)	-	0.96	0.94	0.98
Pneumonia Care				
Appropriate Initial Antibiotic Given	53	100%	96%	95%
Blood Culture Timing	72	100%	98%	98%
Pregnancy and Delivery Care				
Newborn Deliveries Scheduled Early	156	1%	4%	6%
Preventive Care				
Immunization for Influenza[2]	495	91%	90%	90%
Immunization for Pneumonia[2]	459	90%	92%	92%
Stroke Care				
Anticoagulation Therapy for Atrial Fibrillation	13	100%	94%	95%
Antithrombotic Therapy Timing	52	100%	99%	98%
Assessed for Rehabilitation	120	99%	98%	97%
Discharged on Antithrombotic Therapy	86	99%	99%	99%
Discharged on Statin Medication	67	99%	94%	94%
Thrombolytic Therapy Timing[1]	-	-	60%	66%
Venous Thromboembolism Prophylaxis	106	100%	95%	94%
Written Stroke Educational Materials Given	66	98%	88%	88%
Surgical Care Improvement Project				
Appropriate Beta Blocker Usage[2]	229	100%	99%	98%
Appropriate VTP Within 24 Hours[2]	405	99%	99%	98%
Controlled Postoperative Blood Glucose[2]	94	100%	96%	97%
Perioperative Temperature Management[2]	632	100%	100%	100%
Prophylactic Antibiotic Selection[2]	539	99%	99%	99%
Prophylactic Antibiotic Selection (Outpatient)	530	99%	98%	98%
Prophylactic Antibiotic Stopped[2]	529	100%	99%	98%
Prophylactic Antibiotic Timing[2]	539	100%	99%	99%
Prophylactic Antibiotic Timing (Outpatient)	538	97%	97%	98%
Urinary Catheter Removal[2]	145	95%	98%	97%
Survey of Patients' Hospital Experiences				
Area Around Room 'Always' Quiet at Night	300+	66%	63%	61%
Doctors 'Always' Communicated Well	300+	81%	83%	82%
Home Recovery Information Given	300+	87%	89%	85%
Hospital Given 9 or 10 on 10 Point Scale	300+	77%	74%	71%
Meds 'Always' Explained Before Given	300+	66%	68%	64%
Nurses 'Always' Communicated Well	300+	82%	82%	79%
Pain 'Always' Well Controlled	300+	72%	72%	71%
Room and Bathroom 'Always' Clean	300+	80%	79%	73%
Timely Help 'Always' Received	300+	70%	72%	68%
Would Definitely Recommend Hospital	300+	79%	74%	71%
Use of Medical Imaging				
Cardiac Imaging Stress Test before Surgery	276	6.2%	5.4%	5.3%
Combination Abdominal CT Scan	495	7.7%	6.3%	10.5%
Combination Brain/Sinus CT Scan	246	0.0%	2.1%	2.7%
Combination Chest CT Scan	334	0.0%	1%	2.7%
Follow-up Mammogram/Ultrasound	805	4.8%	8.1%	8.8%
Lumbar Spine MRI for Low Back Pain	169	34.3%	34.9%	37.2%

NOTE: Hospital profiles are in alphabetical order by state, then city, then hospital within the city; Rankings exclude hospitals with less than 25 cases except for patient surveys which excludes hospitals with less than 100 cases; (a) 100-299 cases; (1) The number of cases/patients is too few to report; (2) Data submitted were based on a sample of cases/patients; (3) Results are based on a shorter time period than required; (4) Data suppressed by CMS for one or more quarters; (5) Results are not available for this reporting period; (6) Fewer than 100 patients completed the HCAHPS survey; (7) No cases met the criteria for this measure; (8) The lower limit of the confidence interval cannot be calculated if the number of observed infections equals zero; (9) No data are available from the state/territory for this reporting period; (10) The scores shown reflect fewer than 50 completed surveys; (11) There were discrepancies in the data collection process; (12) This measure does not apply to this hospital for this reporting period; (13) Results cannot be calculated for this reporting period; (14) The results for this state are combined with nearby states to protect confidentiality; Please refer to the User's Guide for a full explanation of data.

Bellin Memorial Hospital

744 S Webster Ave
Green Bay, WI 54305
URL: www.bellin.org
Type: Acute Care Hospitals
Ownership: Voluntary non-profit - Private

Phone: 920-433-3500
Fax: 920-433-7971
Emergency Services: Yes
Beds: 167

Key Personnel:
CEO/President . . . . George F Kerwin
President . . . . Steve Maricque
CEO . . . . Gail McNutt

Measure	Cases	This Hosp.	State Avg.	U.S. Avg.
Blood Clot Prevention and Treatment				
Anticoagulation Overlap Therapy[2]	69	97%	95%	93%
ICU Venous Thromboembolism Prophylaxis[2]	131	85%	91%	92%
Incidence of Potentially Preventable VTE[2]	16	6%	10%	10%
UFH with Dosages/Platelet Monitoring[2]	33	100%	96%	97%
Venous Thromboembolism Prophylaxis[2]	232	87%	85%	85%
Warfarin Therapy Discharge Instructions[2]	53	100%	70%	75%
Chest Pain/Possible Heart Attack Care				
Aspirin Given Within 24 Hours of Arrival[1,3]	-	-	98%	96%
Fibrinolytic Meds Within 30 Min. of Arrival[5]	-	-	52%	58%
Average Time to ECG (minutes)[1,3]	-	-	7	7
Average Time to Transfer (minutes)[5]	-	-	58	60
Children's Asthma Care				
Received Home Management Plan of Care	-	-	-	88%
Received Reliever Medication	-	-	-	100%
Received Systemic Corticosteroids	-	-	-	100%
Emergency Department				
Admittance Decision Time (minutes)[2]	389	49	65	98
Head CT Results Within 45 Min. of Arrival[1]	-	-	61%	57%
Patients Who Left ER Before Being Seen	31,685	1%	1%	2%
Time from ER Arrival to Admit. (minutes)[2]	389	204	207	274
Time from ER Arrival to Discharge (minutes)	367	128	121	134
Time in ER Before Being Evaluated (minutes)	259	34	19	26
Time to Pain Meds for Fractures (minutes)	94	56	42	57
Heart Attack Care				
Aspirin Given at Discharge[2]	378	99%	99%	99%
Fibrinolytic Meds Within 30 Min. of Arrival[2,7]	-	-	67%	54%
PCI Within 90 Minutes of Arrival[2]	37	95%	96%	96%
Statin Prescribed at Discharge[2]	360	100%	99%	98%
Heart Failure Care				
ACE Inhibitor or ARB for LVSD	47	98%	97%	97%
Discharge Instructions Given	157	96%	96%	94%
Evaluation of LVS Function	195	100%	99%	99%
Medicare Spending				
Medicare Spending per Patient (ratio)	-	0.96	0.94	0.98
Pneumonia Care				
Appropriate Initial Antibiotic Given	48	85%	96%	95%
Blood Culture Timing	88	98%	98%	98%
Pregnancy and Delivery Care				
Newborn Deliveries Scheduled Early[2]	108	8%	4%	6%
Preventive Care				
Immunization for Influenza[2]	584	91%	90%	90%
Immunization for Pneumonia[2]	722	95%	92%	92%
Stroke Care				
Anticoagulation Therapy for Atrial Fibrillation	19	100%	94%	95%
Antithrombotic Therapy Timing	68	97%	99%	98%
Assessed for Rehabilitation	93	97%	98%	97%
Discharged on Antithrombotic Therapy	88	99%	99%	99%
Discharged on Statin Medication	67	96%	94%	94%
Thrombolytic Therapy Timing[1]	-	-	60%	66%
Venous Thromboembolism Prophylaxis	85	99%	95%	94%
Written Stroke Educational Materials Given	51	100%	88%	88%
Surgical Care Improvement Project				
Appropriate Beta Blocker Usage[2]	272	99%	99%	98%
Appropriate VTP Within 24 Hours[2]	414	94%	99%	98%
Controlled Postoperative Blood Glucose[2]	246	94%	96%	97%
Perioperative Temperature Management[2]	469	100%	100%	100%
Prophylactic Antibiotic Selection[2]	509	99%	99%	99%
Prophylactic Antibiotic Selection (Outpatient)	627	98%	98%	98%
Prophylactic Antibiotic Stopped[2]	504	99%	99%	98%
Prophylactic Antibiotic Timing[2]	509	97%	99%	99%
Prophylactic Antibiotic Timing (Outpatient)	631	99%	97%	98%
Urinary Catheter Removal[2]	315	96%	98%	97%
Survey of Patients' Hospital Experiences				
Area Around Room 'Always' Quiet at Night[11]	300+	66%	63%	61%
Doctors 'Always' Communicated Well[11]	300+	82%	83%	82%
Home Recovery Information Given[11]	300+	90%	89%	85%
Hospital Given 9 or 10 on 10 Point Scale[11]	300+	81%	74%	71%
Meds 'Always' Explained Before Given[11]	300+	69%	68%	64%
Nurses 'Always' Communicated Well[11]	300+	83%	82%	79%
Pain 'Always' Well Controlled[11]	300+	75%	72%	71%
Room and Bathroom 'Always' Clean[11]	300+	77%	79%	73%
Timely Help 'Always' Received[11]	300+	77%	72%	68%
Would Definitely Recommend Hospital[11]	300+	84%	74%	71%
Use of Medical Imaging				
Cardiac Imaging Stress Test before Surgery	542	5.2%	5.4%	5.3%
Combination Abdominal CT Scan	722	4.0%	6.3%	10.5%
Combination Brain/Sinus CT Scan	584	2.4%	2.1%	2.7%
Combination Chest CT Scan	671	0.0%	1%	2.7%
Follow-up Mammogram/Ultrasound	1,239	4.8%	8.1%	8.8%
Lumbar Spine MRI for Low Back Pain	167	32.3%	34.9%	37.2%

Saint Marys Hospital Medical Center

1726 Shawano Ave
Green Bay, WI 54303
E-mail: info@stmgb.org
URL: www.stmgb.org
Type: Acute Care Hospitals
Ownership: Voluntary non-profit - Other

Phone: 920-498-4200
Fax: 920-498-1861
Emergency Services: Yes
Beds: 94

Key Personnel:
Operating Room. . . . . Jane Beyer
CEO/President. . . . . James G Coller
Ambulatory Care . . . . Lawrence Connors
Cardiac Laboratory. . . . . Daniel Doran
Radiology. . . . . Henry Kenneth Feider
Emergency Room . . . . Karen Ann Stanlaw

Measure	Cases	This Hosp.	State Avg.	U.S. Avg.
Blood Clot Prevention and Treatment				
Anticoagulation Overlap Therapy[2]	37	97%	95%	93%
ICU Venous Thromboembolism Prophylaxis[2]	17	76%	91%	92%
Incidence of Potentially Preventable VTE[1,2]	-	-	10%	10%
UFH with Dosages/Platelet Monitoring[1,2]	-	-	96%	97%
Venous Thromboembolism Prophylaxis[2]	292	75%	85%	85%
Warfarin Therapy Discharge Instructions[2]	31	81%	70%	75%
Chest Pain/Possible Heart Attack Care				
Aspirin Given Within 24 Hours of Arrival[1,3]	-	-	98%	96%
Fibrinolytic Meds Within 30 Min. of Arrival[5]	-	-	52%	58%
Average Time to ECG (minutes)[1,3]	-	-	7	7
Average Time to Transfer (minutes)[5]	-	-	58	60
Children's Asthma Care				
Received Home Management Plan of Care	-	-	-	88%
Received Reliever Medication	-	-	-	100%
Received Systemic Corticosteroids	-	-	-	100%
Emergency Department				
Admittance Decision Time (minutes)[2]	421	129	65	98
Head CT Results Within 45 Min. of Arrival[1]	-	-	61%	57%
Patients Who Left ER Before Being Seen	32,670	0%	1%	2%
Time from ER Arrival to Admit. (minutes)[2]	430	182	207	274
Time from ER Arrival to Discharge (minutes)	391	115	121	134
Time in ER Before Being Evaluated (minutes)	374	18	19	26
Time to Pain Meds for Fractures (minutes)	71	54	42	57
Heart Attack Care				
Aspirin Given at Discharge	119	99%	99%	99%
Fibrinolytic Meds Within 30 Min. of Arrival[7]	-	-	67%	54%
PCI Within 90 Minutes of Arrival	18	100%	96%	96%
Statin Prescribed at Discharge	114	100%	99%	98%
Heart Failure Care				
ACE Inhibitor or ARB for LVSD	31	90%	97%	97%
Discharge Instructions Given	77	99%	96%	94%
Evaluation of LVS Function	94	100%	99%	99%
Medicare Spending				
Medicare Spending per Patient (ratio)	-	0.89	0.94	0.98
Pneumonia Care				
Appropriate Initial Antibiotic Given	77	95%	96%	95%
Blood Culture Timing	118	99%	98%	98%
Pregnancy and Delivery Care				
Newborn Deliveries Scheduled Early[2]	31	3%	4%	6%
Preventive Care				
Immunization for Influenza[2]	524	90%	90%	90%
Immunization for Pneumonia[2]	600	93%	92%	92%
Stroke Care				
Anticoagulation Therapy for Atrial Fibrillation[1]	-	-	94%	95%
Antithrombotic Therapy Timing	38	100%	99%	98%
Assessed for Rehabilitation	50	100%	98%	97%
Discharged on Antithrombotic Therapy	45	91%	99%	99%
Discharged on Statin Medication	37	92%	94%	94%
Thrombolytic Therapy Timing[1]	-	-	60%	66%
Venous Thromboembolism Prophylaxis	47	96%	95%	94%
Written Stroke Educational Materials Given	22	100%	88%	88%
Surgical Care Improvement Project				
Appropriate Beta Blocker Usage[2]	92	97%	99%	98%
Appropriate VTP Within 24 Hours[2]	312	100%	99%	98%
Controlled Postoperative Blood Glucose[2,7]	-	-	96%	97%
Perioperative Temperature Management[2]	338	100%	100%	100%
Prophylactic Antibiotic Selection[2]	212	98%	99%	99%
Prophylactic Antibiotic Selection (Outpatient)	300	91%	98%	98%
Prophylactic Antibiotic Stopped[2]	211	99%	99%	98%
Prophylactic Antibiotic Timing[2]	212	99%	99%	99%
Prophylactic Antibiotic Timing (Outpatient)	301	96%	97%	98%
Urinary Catheter Removal[2]	277	100%	98%	97%
Survey of Patients' Hospital Experiences				
Area Around Room 'Always' Quiet at Night	300+	63%	63%	61%
Doctors 'Always' Communicated Well	300+	83%	83%	82%
Home Recovery Information Given	300+	87%	89%	85%
Hospital Given 9 or 10 on 10 Point Scale	300+	72%	74%	71%
Meds 'Always' Explained Before Given	300+	67%	68%	64%
Nurses 'Always' Communicated Well	300+	79%	82%	79%
Pain 'Always' Well Controlled	300+	73%	72%	71%
Room and Bathroom 'Always' Clean	300+	78%	79%	73%
Timely Help 'Always' Received	300+	70%	72%	68%
Would Definitely Recommend Hospital	300+	73%	74%	71%
Use of Medical Imaging				
Cardiac Imaging Stress Test before Surgery	236	3.8%	5.4%	5.3%
Combination Abdominal CT Scan	475	5.3%	6.3%	10.5%
Combination Brain/Sinus CT Scan[1]	-	-	2.1%	2.7%
Combination Chest CT Scan	291	0.0%	1%	2.7%
Follow-up Mammogram/Ultrasound	200	9.5%	8.1%	8.8%
Lumbar Spine MRI for Low Back Pain	72	37.5%	34.9%	37.2%

Saint Vincent Hospital

835 S Van Buren St
Green Bay, WI 54301
URL: www.stvincenthospital.org
Type: Acute Care Hospitals
Ownership: Voluntary non-profit - Church

Phone: 920-433-0111
Fax: 920-431-3151
Emergency Services: Yes
Beds: 547

Key Personnel:
Pediatric In-Patient Care . . . . Joel Anent, MD
CEO/President. . . . . James Coller
Radiology. . . . . Henry Feider, MD
Anesthesiology. . . . . Brian Johnson, MD
Emergency Room . . . . Kenneth Johnson
Infection Control. . . . . Nancy Lorenzoni
Chief of Medical Staff. . . . . David Rentmeester, MD
Operating Room. . . . . Mary Ann Sallenbach

Measure	Cases	This Hosp.	State Avg.	U.S. Avg.
Blood Clot Prevention and Treatment				
Anticoagulation Overlap Therapy[2]	80	89%	95%	93%
ICU Venous Thromboembolism Prophylaxis[2]	46	85%	91%	92%
Incidence of Potentially Preventable VTE[2]	14	29%	10%	10%
UFH with Dosages/Platelet Monitoring[2]	27	78%	96%	97%
Venous Thromboembolism Prophylaxis[2]	306	73%	85%	85%
Warfarin Therapy Discharge Instructions[2]	68	68%	70%	75%
Chest Pain/Possible Heart Attack Care				
Aspirin Given Within 24 Hours of Arrival[1,3]	-	-	98%	96%
Fibrinolytic Meds Within 30 Min. of Arrival[5]	-	-	52%	58%
Average Time to ECG (minutes)[1,3]	-	-	7	7
Average Time to Transfer (minutes)[5]	-	-	58	60
Children's Asthma Care				
Received Home Management Plan of Care	-	-	-	88%
Received Reliever Medication	-	-	-	100%

NOTE: Hospital profiles are in alphabetical order by state, then city, then hospital within the city; Rankings exclude hospitals with less than 25 cases except for patient surveys which excludes hospitals with less than 100 cases; (a) 100-299 cases; (1) The number of cases/patients is too few to report; (2) Data submitted were based on a sample of cases/patients; (3) Results are based on a shorter time period than required; (4) Data suppressed by CMS for one or more quarters; (5) Results are not available for this reporting period; (6) Fewer than 100 patients completed the HCAHPS survey; (7) No cases met the criteria for this measure; (8) The lower limit of the confidence interval cannot be calculated if the number of observed infections equals zero; (9) No data are available from the state/territory for this reporting period; (10) The scores shown reflect fewer than 50 completed surveys; (11) There were discrepancies in the data collection process; (12) This measure does not apply to this hospital for this reporting period; (13) Results cannot be calculated for this reporting period; (14) The results for this state are combined with nearby states to protect confidentiality; Please refer to the User's Guide for a full explanation of data.

Measure	Cases	This Hosp.	State Avg.	U.S. Avg.
Received Systemic Corticosteroids	-	-	-	100%
Emergency Department				
Admittance Decision Time (minutes)[2]	364	109	65	98
Head CT Results Within 45 Min. of Arrival[1]	-	-	61%	57%
Patients Who Left ER Before Being Seen	37,289	0%	1%	2%
Time from ER Arrival to Admit. (minutes)[2]	374	180	207	274
Time from ER Arrival to Discharge (minutes)	385	120	121	134
Time in ER Before Being Evaluated (minutes)	370	19	19	26
Time to Pain Meds for Fractures (minutes)	81	45	42	57
Heart Attack Care				
Aspirin Given at Discharge	188	97%	99%	99%
Fibrinolytic Meds Within 30 Min. of Arrival[7]	-	-	67%	54%
PCI Within 90 Minutes of Arrival	24	92%	96%	96%
Statin Prescribed at Discharge	184	96%	99%	98%
Heart Failure Care				
ACE Inhibitor or ARB for LVSD	30	87%	97%	97%
Discharge Instructions Given	103	95%	96%	94%
Evaluation of LVS Function	124	98%	99%	99%
Medicare Spending				
Medicare Spending per Patient (ratio)	-	0.92	0.94	0.98
Pneumonia Care				
Appropriate Initial Antibiotic Given[2]	80	94%	96%	95%
Blood Culture Timing[2]	130	98%	98%	98%
Pregnancy and Delivery Care				
Newborn Deliveries Scheduled Early[2]	30	0%	4%	6%
Preventive Care				
Immunization for Influenza[2]	549	88%	90%	90%
Immunization for Pneumonia[2]	633	88%	92%	92%
Stroke Care				
Anticoagulation Therapy for Atrial Fibrillation[2]	13	77%	94%	95%
Antithrombotic Therapy Timing[2]	55	98%	99%	98%
Assessed for Rehabilitation[2]	84	95%	98%	97%
Discharged on Antithrombotic Therapy[2]	67	87%	99%	99%
Discharged on Statin Medication[2]	55	85%	94%	94%
Thrombolytic Therapy Timing[1,2]	-	-	60%	66%
Venous Thromboembolism Prophylaxis[2]	86	91%	95%	94%
Written Stroke Educational Materials Given[2]	38	97%	88%	88%
Surgical Care Improvement Project				
Appropriate Beta Blocker Usage[2]	260	98%	99%	98%
Appropriate VTP Within 24 Hours[2]	400	99%	99%	98%
Controlled Postoperative Blood Glucose[2]	134	97%	96%	97%
Perioperative Temperature Management[2]	513	100%	100%	100%
Prophylactic Antibiotic Selection[2]	438	99%	99%	99%
Prophylactic Antibiotic Selection (Outpatient)	205	97%	98%	98%
Prophylactic Antibiotic Stopped[2]	424	99%	99%	98%
Prophylactic Antibiotic Timing[2]	441	98%	99%	99%
Prophylactic Antibiotic Timing (Outpatient)	203	100%	97%	98%
Urinary Catheter Removal[2]	234	99%	98%	97%
Survey of Patients' Hospital Experiences				
Area Around Room 'Always' Quiet at Night	300+	63%	63%	61%
Doctors 'Always' Communicated Well	300+	80%	83%	82%
Home Recovery Information Given	300+	87%	89%	85%
Hospital Given 9 or 10 on 10 Point Scale	300+	71%	74%	71%
Meds 'Always' Explained Before Given	300+	64%	68%	64%
Nurses 'Always' Communicated Well	300+	78%	82%	79%
Pain 'Always' Well Controlled	300+	68%	72%	71%
Room and Bathroom 'Always' Clean	300+	79%	79%	73%
Timely Help 'Always' Received	300+	62%	72%	68%
Would Definitely Recommend Hospital	300+	73%	74%	71%
Use of Medical Imaging				
Cardiac Imaging Stress Test before Surgery	302	6.0%	5.4%	5.3%
Combination Abdominal CT Scan	589	5.8%	6.3%	10.5%
Combination Brain/Sinus CT Scan[1]	-	-	2.1%	2.7%
Combination Chest CT Scan	478	0.0%	1%	2.7%
Follow-up Mammogram/Ultrasound	322	5.6%	8.1%	8.8%
Lumbar Spine MRI for Low Back Pain	96	40.6%	34.9%	37.2%

Aurora Medical Center Washington County

1032 E Sumner St
Hartford, WI 53027
Phone: 262-673-2300
URL: www.aurorahealthcare.org
Type: Acute Care Hospitals
Emergency Services: Yes
Ownership: Voluntary non-profit - Private
Key Personnel:
Administrator . . . . Mark Schwartz

Measure	Cases	This Hosp.	State Avg.	U.S. Avg.
Blood Clot Prevention and Treatment				
Anticoagulation Overlap Therapy[2]	32	100%	95%	93%
ICU Venous Thromboembolism Prophylaxis[2]	33	97%	91%	92%
Incidence of Potentially Preventable VTE[1,2]	-	-	10%	10%
UFH with Dosages/Platelet Monitoring[2]	12	100%	96%	97%
Venous Thromboembolism Prophylaxis[2]	140	92%	85%	85%
Warfarin Therapy Discharge Instructions[2]	24	88%	70%	75%
Chest Pain/Possible Heart Attack Care				
Aspirin Given Within 24 Hours of Arrival	47	100%	98%	96%
Fibrinolytic Meds Within 30 Min. of Arrival[7]	-	-	52%	58%
Average Time to ECG (minutes)	48	10	7	7
Average Time to Transfer (minutes)[1]	-	-	58	60
Children's Asthma Care				
Received Home Management Plan of Care	-	-	-	88%
Received Reliever Medication	-	-	-	100%
Received Systemic Corticosteroids	-	-	-	100%
Emergency Department				
Admittance Decision Time (minutes)[2]	395	52	65	98
Head CT Results Within 45 Min. of Arrival	13	77%	61%	57%
Patients Who Left ER Before Being Seen	8,564	0%	1%	2%
Time from ER Arrival to Admit. (minutes)[2]	404	202	207	274
Time from ER Arrival to Discharge (minutes)	351	126	121	134
Time in ER Before Being Evaluated (minutes)	381	15	19	26
Time to Pain Meds for Fractures (minutes)	43	35	42	57
Heart Attack Care				
Aspirin Given at Discharge	13	100%	99%	99%
Fibrinolytic Meds Within 30 Min. of Arrival[7]	-	-	67%	54%
PCI Within 90 Minutes of Arrival[7]	-	-	96%	96%
Statin Prescribed at Discharge[1]	-	-	99%	98%
Heart Failure Care				
ACE Inhibitor or ARB for LVSD	12	100%	97%	97%
Discharge Instructions Given	59	98%	96%	94%
Evaluation of LVS Function	83	100%	99%	99%
Medicare Spending				
Medicare Spending per Patient (ratio)	-	0.98	0.94	0.98
Pneumonia Care				
Appropriate Initial Antibiotic Given	38	100%	96%	95%
Blood Culture Timing	60	97%	98%	98%
Pregnancy and Delivery Care				
Newborn Deliveries Scheduled Early[7]	-	-	4%	6%
Preventive Care				
Immunization for Influenza[2]	293	94%	90%	90%
Immunization for Pneumonia[2]	433	97%	92%	92%
Stroke Care				
Anticoagulation Therapy for Atrial Fibrillation[3,7]	-	-	94%	95%
Antithrombotic Therapy Timing[1,3]	-	-	99%	98%
Assessed for Rehabilitation[1,3]	-	-	98%	97%
Discharged on Antithrombotic Therapy[1,3]	-	-	99%	99%
Discharged on Statin Medication[3,7]	-	-	94%	94%
Thrombolytic Therapy Timing[3,7]	-	-	60%	66%
Venous Thromboembolism Prophylaxis[1,3]	-	-	95%	94%
Written Stroke Educational Materials Given[1,3]	-	-	88%	88%
Surgical Care Improvement Project				
Appropriate Beta Blocker Usage[2]	48	96%	99%	98%
Appropriate VTP Within 24 Hours[2]	188	100%	99%	98%
Controlled Postoperative Blood Glucose[2,7]	-	-	96%	97%
Perioperative Temperature Management[2]	212	100%	100%	100%
Prophylactic Antibiotic Selection[2]	172	99%	99%	99%
Prophylactic Antibiotic Selection (Outpatient)	26	96%	98%	98%
Prophylactic Antibiotic Stopped[2]	166	100%	99%	98%
Prophylactic Antibiotic Timing[2]	172	100%	99%	99%
Prophylactic Antibiotic Timing (Outpatient)	27	96%	97%	98%
Urinary Catheter Removal[2]	173	99%	98%	97%
Survey of Patients' Hospital Experiences				
Area Around Room 'Always' Quiet at Night	300+	59%	63%	61%
Doctors 'Always' Communicated Well	300+	84%	83%	82%
Home Recovery Information Given	300+	89%	89%	85%
Hospital Given 9 or 10 on 10 Point Scale	300+	68%	74%	71%
Meds 'Always' Explained Before Given	300+	63%	68%	64%
Nurses 'Always' Communicated Well	300+	81%	82%	79%
Pain 'Always' Well Controlled	300+	71%	72%	71%
Room and Bathroom 'Always' Clean	300+	79%	79%	73%
Timely Help 'Always' Received	300+	73%	72%	68%
Would Definitely Recommend Hospital	300+	67%	74%	71%
Use of Medical Imaging				
Cardiac Imaging Stress Test before Surgery	113	4.4%	5.4%	5.3%
Combination Abdominal CT Scan	270	11.9%	6.3%	10.5%
Combination Brain/Sinus CT Scan[1]	-	-	2.1%	2.7%
Combination Chest CT Scan	215	0.0%	1%	2.7%
Follow-up Mammogram/Ultrasound[7]	-	-	8.1%	8.8%
Lumbar Spine MRI for Low Back Pain	50	32.0%	34.9%	37.2%

Hayward Area Memorial Hospital

11040 N State Rd 77
Hayward, WI 54843
Phone: 715-934-4321
Fax: 715-934-4272
URL: www.hamhnh.com
Type: Critical Access Hospitals
Emergency Services: Yes
Ownership: Voluntary non-profit - Private
Beds: 25
Key Personnel:
Operating Room. . . . . Jane McPeak
CEO/President. . . . . Barbara Peickert
Chief of Medical Staff . . . . Ravinder Vir, MD

Measure	Cases	This Hosp.	State Avg.	U.S. Avg.
Blood Clot Prevention and Treatment				
Anticoagulation Overlap Therapy[1,2]	-	-	95%	93%
ICU Venous Thromboembolism Prophylaxis[2,3]	-	-	91%	92%
Incidence of Potentially Preventable VTE[2,7]	-	-	10%	10%
UFH with Dosages/Platelet Monitoring[1,2]	-	-	96%	97%
Venous Thromboembolism Prophylaxis[2]	114	38%	85%	85%
Warfarin Therapy Discharge Instructions[1,2]	-	-	70%	75%
Chest Pain/Possible Heart Attack Care				
Aspirin Given Within 24 Hours of Arrival	43	93%	98%	96%
Fibrinolytic Meds Within 30 Min. of Arrival[1]	-	-	52%	58%
Average Time to ECG (minutes)	44	18	7	7
Average Time to Transfer (minutes)[1]	-	-	58	60
Children's Asthma Care				
Received Home Management Plan of Care	-	-	-	88%
Received Reliever Medication	-	-	-	100%
Received Systemic Corticosteroids	-	-	-	100%
Emergency Department				
Admittance Decision Time (minutes)[2]	323	30	65	98
Head CT Results Within 45 Min. of Arrival[1]	-	-	61%	57%
Patients Who Left ER Before Being Seen[5]	-	-	1%	2%
Time from ER Arrival to Admit. (minutes)[2]	323	192	207	274
Time from ER Arrival to Discharge (minutes)	399	113	121	134
Time in ER Before Being Evaluated (minutes)	444	31	19	26
Time to Pain Meds for Fractures (minutes)	60	52	42	57
Heart Attack Care				
Aspirin Given at Discharge[5]	-	-	99%	99%
Fibrinolytic Meds Within 30 Min. of Arrival[5]	-	-	67%	54%
PCI Within 90 Minutes of Arrival[5]	-	-	96%	96%
Statin Prescribed at Discharge[5]	-	-	99%	98%
Heart Failure Care				
ACE Inhibitor or ARB for LVSD[1]	-	-	97%	97%
Discharge Instructions Given	24	100%	96%	94%
Evaluation of LVS Function	33	94%	99%	99%
Medicare Spending				
Medicare Spending per Patient (ratio)	-	-	0.94	0.98
Pneumonia Care				
Appropriate Initial Antibiotic Given	34	97%	96%	95%
Blood Culture Timing	45	84%	98%	98%
Pregnancy and Delivery Care				
Newborn Deliveries Scheduled Early[5]	-	-	4%	6%
Preventive Care				
Immunization for Influenza[2]	242	95%	90%	90%
Immunization for Pneumonia[2]	318	90%	92%	92%
Stroke Care				

NOTE: Hospital profiles are in alphabetical order by state, then city, then hospital within the city; Rankings exclude hospitals with less than 25 cases except for patient surveys which excludes hospitals with less than 100 cases; (a) 100-299 cases; (1) The number of cases/patients is too few to report; (2) Data submitted were based on a sample of cases/patients; (3) Results are based on a shorter time period than required; (4) Data suppressed by CMS for one or more quarters; (5) Results are not available for this reporting period; (6) Fewer than 100 patients completed the HCAHPS survey; (7) No cases met the criteria for this measure; (8) The lower limit of the confidence interval cannot be calculated if the number of observed infections equals zero; (9) No data are available from the state/territory for this reporting period; (10) The scores shown reflect fewer than 50 completed surveys; (11) There were discrepancies in the data collection process; (12) This measure does not apply to this hospital for this reporting period; (13) Results cannot be calculated for this reporting period; (14) The results for this state are combined with nearby states to protect confidentiality; Please refer to the User's Guide for a full explanation of data.

Measure	Cases	This Hosp.	State Avg.	U.S. Avg.
Anticoagulation Therapy for Atrial Fibrillation[1]	-	-	94%	95%
Antithrombotic Therapy Timing[1]	-	-	99%	98%
Assessed for Rehabilitation	11	100%	98%	97%
Discharged on Antithrombotic Therapy	11	100%	99%	99%
Discharged on Statin Medication	11	82%	94%	94%
Thrombolytic Therapy Timing[1]	-	-	60%	66%
Venous Thromboembolism Prophylaxis	12	58%	95%	94%
Written Stroke Educational Materials Given[1]	-	-	88%	88%
Surgical Care Improvement Project				
Appropriate Beta Blocker Usage[3,7]	-	-	99%	98%
Appropriate VTP Within 24 Hours[1,3]	-	-	99%	98%
Controlled Postoperative Blood Glucose[5]	-	-	96%	97%
Perioperative Temperature Management[1,3]	-	-	100%	100%
Prophylactic Antibiotic Selection[1,3]	-	-	99%	99%
Prophylactic Antibiotic Selection (Outpatient)[1,3]	-	-	98%	98%
Prophylactic Antibiotic Stopped[1,3]	-	-	99%	98%
Prophylactic Antibiotic Timing[1,3]	-	-	99%	99%
Prophylactic Antibiotic Timing (Outpatient)[1,3]	-	-	97%	98%
Urinary Catheter Removal[1,3]	-	-	98%	97%
Survey of Patients' Hospital Experiences				
Area Around Room 'Always' Quiet at Night	(a)	77%	63%	61%
Doctors 'Always' Communicated Well	(a)	85%	83%	82%
Home Recovery Information Given	(a)	87%	89%	85%
Hospital Given 9 or 10 on 10 Point Scale	(a)	69%	74%	71%
Meds 'Always' Explained Before Given	(a)	66%	68%	64%
Nurses 'Always' Communicated Well	(a)	82%	82%	79%
Pain 'Always' Well Controlled	(a)	72%	72%	71%
Room and Bathroom 'Always' Clean	(a)	77%	79%	73%
Timely Help 'Always' Received	(a)	74%	72%	68%
Would Definitely Recommend Hospital	(a)	64%	74%	71%
Use of Medical Imaging				
Cardiac Imaging Stress Test before Surgery[7]	-	-	5.4%	5.3%
Combination Abdominal CT Scan	178	2.2%	6.3%	10.5%
Combination Brain/Sinus CT Scan[1]	-	-	2.1%	2.7%
Combination Chest CT Scan	153	0.7%	1%	2.7%
Follow-up Mammogram/Ultrasound	440	9.8%	8.1%	8.8%
Lumbar Spine MRI for Low Back Pain[1]	-	-	34.9%	37.2%

Saint Joseph's Health Services

400 Water Ave
Hillsboro, WI 54634
Phone: 608-489-8000
Fax: 608-489-8181
E-mail: kcoblentz@stjhealthcare.org
URL: www.stjhealthcare.org
Type: Critical Access Hospitals
Emergency Services: Yes
Ownership: Voluntary non-profit - Private
Beds: 125

Key Personnel:
Chief of Medical Staff. . . . . Tima Brieske
CEO/President. . . . . Bill Bruce
Emergency Room . . . . Mary Charles, RN

Measure	Cases	This Hosp.	State Avg.	U.S. Avg.
Blood Clot Prevention and Treatment				
Anticoagulation Overlap Therapy[5]	-	-	95%	93%
ICU Venous Thromboembolism Prophylaxis[5]	-	-	91%	92%
Incidence of Potentially Preventable VTE[5]	-	-	10%	10%
UFH with Dosages/Platelet Monitoring[5]	-	-	96%	97%
Venous Thromboembolism Prophylaxis[5]	-	-	85%	85%
Warfarin Therapy Discharge Instructions[5]	-	-	70%	75%
Chest Pain/Possible Heart Attack Care				
Aspirin Given Within 24 Hours of Arrival	14	100%	98%	96%
Fibrinolytic Meds Within 30 Min. of Arrival[1]	-	-	52%	58%
Average Time to ECG (minutes)	15	11	7	7
Average Time to Transfer (minutes)[7]	-	-	58	60
Children's Asthma Care				
Received Home Management Plan of Care	-	-	-	88%
Received Reliever Medication	-	-	-	100%
Received Systemic Corticosteroids	-	-	-	100%
Emergency Department				
Admittance Decision Time (minutes)	122	8	65	98
Head CT Results Within 45 Min. of Arrival[1,3]	-	-	61%	57%
Patients Who Left ER Before Being Seen[5]	-	-	1%	2%
Time from ER Arrival to Admit. (minutes)	129	130	207	274
Time from ER Arrival to Discharge (minutes)	780	98	121	134
Time in ER Before Being Evaluated (minutes)	868	14	19	26
Time to Pain Meds for Fractures (minutes)[1]	-	-	42	57
Heart Attack Care				
Aspirin Given at Discharge[5]	-	-	99%	99%
Fibrinolytic Meds Within 30 Min. of Arrival[5]	-	-	67%	54%
PCI Within 90 Minutes of Arrival[5]	-	-	96%	96%
Statin Prescribed at Discharge[5]	-	-	99%	98%
Heart Failure Care				
ACE Inhibitor or ARB for LVSD[1]	-	-	97%	97%
Discharge Instructions Given	14	79%	96%	94%
Evaluation of LVS Function	19	84%	99%	99%
Medicare Spending				
Medicare Spending per Patient (ratio)	-	-	0.94	0.98
Pneumonia Care				
Appropriate Initial Antibiotic Given	19	100%	96%	95%
Blood Culture Timing	14	100%	98%	98%
Pregnancy and Delivery Care				
Newborn Deliveries Scheduled Early[5]	-	-	4%	6%
Preventive Care				
Immunization for Influenza	113	70%	90%	90%
Immunization for Pneumonia	183	83%	92%	92%
Stroke Care				
Anticoagulation Therapy for Atrial Fibrillation[5]	-	-	94%	95%
Antithrombotic Therapy Timing[5]	-	-	99%	98%
Assessed for Rehabilitation[5]	-	-	98%	97%
Discharged on Antithrombotic Therapy[5]	-	-	99%	99%
Discharged on Statin Medication[5]	-	-	94%	94%
Thrombolytic Therapy Timing[5]	-	-	60%	66%
Venous Thromboembolism Prophylaxis[5]	-	-	95%	94%
Written Stroke Educational Materials Given[5]	-	-	88%	88%
Surgical Care Improvement Project				
Appropriate Beta Blocker Usage[1]	-	-	99%	98%
Appropriate VTP Within 24 Hours	12	92%	99%	98%
Controlled Postoperative Blood Glucose[7]	-	-	96%	97%
Perioperative Temperature Management	15	100%	100%	100%
Prophylactic Antibiotic Selection	12	100%	99%	99%
Prophylactic Antibiotic Selection (Outpatient)[5]	-	-	98%	98%
Prophylactic Antibiotic Stopped	12	92%	99%	98%
Prophylactic Antibiotic Timing	12	92%	99%	99%
Prophylactic Antibiotic Timing (Outpatient)[5]	-	-	97%	98%
Urinary Catheter Removal[1]	-	-	98%	97%
Survey of Patients' Hospital Experiences				
Area Around Room 'Always' Quiet at Night[6]	<100	60%	63%	61%
Doctors 'Always' Communicated Well[6]	<100	84%	83%	82%
Home Recovery Information Given[6]	<100	91%	89%	85%
Hospital Given 9 or 10 on 10 Point Scale[6]	<100	75%	74%	71%
Meds 'Always' Explained Before Given[6]	<100	75%	68%	64%
Nurses 'Always' Communicated Well[6]	<100	86%	82%	79%
Pain 'Always' Well Controlled[6]	<100	72%	72%	71%
Room and Bathroom 'Always' Clean[6]	<100	80%	79%	73%
Timely Help 'Always' Received[6]	<100	80%	72%	68%
Would Definitely Recommend Hospital[6]	<100	68%	74%	71%
Use of Medical Imaging				
Cardiac Imaging Stress Test before Surgery[1]	-	-	5.4%	5.3%
Combination Abdominal CT Scan[1]	-	-	6.3%	10.5%
Combination Brain/Sinus CT Scan	32	0.0%	2.1%	2.7%
Combination Chest CT Scan[1]	-	-	1%	2.7%
Follow-up Mammogram/Ultrasound	84	2.4%	8.1%	8.8%
Lumbar Spine MRI for Low Back Pain[1]	-	-	34.9%	37.2%

Hudson Hospital

405 Stageline Road
Hudson, WI 54016
Phone: 715-531-6000
Fax: 715-531-6011
E-mail: codonovan@hudsonhospital.org
URL: www.hudsonhospital.org
Type: Critical Access Hospitals
Emergency Services: Yes
Ownership: Voluntary non-profit - Other
Beds: 29

Key Personnel:
Emergency Room . . . . Luke Albretch
Quality Assurance . . . . Linda Ehlers
CEO/President. . . . . Marian Furlong
Chief of Medical Staff. . . . . Gregory Young

Measure	Cases	This Hosp.	State Avg.	U.S. Avg.
Blood Clot Prevention and Treatment				
Anticoagulation Overlap Therapy[5]	-	-	95%	93%
ICU Venous Thromboembolism Prophylaxis[5]	-	-	91%	92%
Incidence of Potentially Preventable VTE[5]	-	-	10%	10%
UFH with Dosages/Platelet Monitoring[5]	-	-	96%	97%
Venous Thromboembolism Prophylaxis[5]	-	-	85%	85%
Warfarin Therapy Discharge Instructions[5]	-	-	70%	75%
Chest Pain/Possible Heart Attack Care				
Aspirin Given Within 24 Hours of Arrival	59	100%	98%	96%
Fibrinolytic Meds Within 30 Min. of Arrival[7]	-	-	52%	58%
Average Time to ECG (minutes)	60	7	7	7
Average Time to Transfer (minutes)[7]	-	-	58	60
Children's Asthma Care				
Received Home Management Plan of Care	-	-	-	88%
Received Reliever Medication	-	-	-	100%
Received Systemic Corticosteroids	-	-	-	100%
Emergency Department				
Admittance Decision Time (minutes)[5]	-	-	65	98
Head CT Results Within 45 Min. of Arrival[1]	-	-	61%	57%
Patients Who Left ER Before Being Seen	9,919	0%	1%	2%
Time from ER Arrival to Admit. (minutes)[5]	-	-	207	274
Time from ER Arrival to Discharge (minutes)	367	107	121	134
Time in ER Before Being Evaluated (minutes)	384	17	19	26
Time to Pain Meds for Fractures (minutes)	74	34	42	57
Heart Attack Care				
Aspirin Given at Discharge[5]	-	-	99%	99%
Fibrinolytic Meds Within 30 Min. of Arrival[5]	-	-	67%	54%
PCI Within 90 Minutes of Arrival[5]	-	-	96%	96%
Statin Prescribed at Discharge[5]	-	-	99%	98%
Heart Failure Care				
ACE Inhibitor or ARB for LVSD[1]	-	-	97%	97%
Discharge Instructions Given	22	100%	96%	94%
Evaluation of LVS Function	28	100%	99%	99%
Medicare Spending				
Medicare Spending per Patient (ratio)	-	-	0.94	0.98
Pneumonia Care				
Appropriate Initial Antibiotic Given	26	100%	96%	95%
Blood Culture Timing	17	100%	98%	98%
Pregnancy and Delivery Care				
Newborn Deliveries Scheduled Early[5]	-	-	4%	6%
Preventive Care				
Immunization for Influenza[5]	-	-	90%	90%
Immunization for Pneumonia[5]	-	-	92%	92%
Stroke Care				
Anticoagulation Therapy for Atrial Fibrillation[5]	-	-	94%	95%
Antithrombotic Therapy Timing[5]	-	-	99%	98%
Assessed for Rehabilitation[5]	-	-	98%	97%
Discharged on Antithrombotic Therapy[5]	-	-	99%	99%
Discharged on Statin Medication[5]	-	-	94%	94%
Thrombolytic Therapy Timing[5]	-	-	60%	66%
Venous Thromboembolism Prophylaxis[5]	-	-	95%	94%
Written Stroke Educational Materials Given[5]	-	-	88%	88%
Surgical Care Improvement Project				
Appropriate Beta Blocker Usage	41	98%	99%	98%
Appropriate VTP Within 24 Hours	108	100%	99%	98%
Controlled Postoperative Blood Glucose[7]	-	-	96%	97%
Perioperative Temperature Management	138	100%	100%	100%
Prophylactic Antibiotic Selection	112	100%	99%	99%
Prophylactic Antibiotic Selection (Outpatient)[3]	16	94%	98%	98%
Prophylactic Antibiotic Stopped	112	100%	99%	98%
Prophylactic Antibiotic Timing	112	97%	99%	99%
Prophylactic Antibiotic Timing (Outpatient)[3]	17	94%	97%	98%
Urinary Catheter Removal	109	100%	98%	97%
Survey of Patients' Hospital Experiences				
Area Around Room 'Always' Quiet at Night	300+	67%	63%	61%
Doctors 'Always' Communicated Well	300+	87%	83%	82%
Home Recovery Information Given	300+	86%	89%	85%
Hospital Given 9 or 10 on 10 Point Scale	300+	80%	74%	71%
Meds 'Always' Explained Before Given	300+	69%	68%	64%
Nurses 'Always' Communicated Well	300+	84%	82%	79%
Pain 'Always' Well Controlled	300+	73%	72%	71%
Room and Bathroom 'Always' Clean	300+	73%	79%	73%
Timely Help 'Always' Received	300+	75%	72%	68%
Would Definitely Recommend Hospital	300+	84%	74%	71%

NOTE: Hospital profiles are in alphabetical order by state, then city, then hospital within the city; Rankings exclude hospitals with less than 25 cases except for patient surveys which excludes hospitals with less than 100 cases; (a) 100-299 cases; (1) The number of cases/patients is too few to report; (2) Data submitted were based on a sample of cases/patients; (3) Results are based on a shorter time period than required; (4) Data suppressed by CMS for one or more quarters; (5) Results are not available for this reporting period; (6) Fewer than 100 patients completed the HCAHPS survey; (7) No cases met the criteria for this measure; (8) The lower limit of the confidence interval cannot be calculated if the number of observed infections equals zero; (9) No data are available from the state/territory for this reporting period; (10) The scores shown reflect fewer than 50 completed surveys; (11) There were discrepancies in the data collection process; (12) This measure does not apply to this hospital for this reporting period; (13) Results cannot be calculated for this reporting period; (14) The results for this state are combined with nearby states to protect confidentiality; Please refer to the User's Guide for a full explanation of data.

Use of Medical Imaging				
Cardiac Imaging Stress Test before Surgery	68	4.4%	5.4%	5.3%
Combination Abdominal CT Scan	219	2.3%	6.3%	10.5%
Combination Brain/Sinus CT Scan[1]	-	-	2.1%	2.7%
Combination Chest CT Scan	100	0.0%	1%	2.7%
Follow-up Mammogram/Ultrasound	303	5.3%	8.1%	8.8%
Lumbar Spine MRI for Low Back Pain[1]	-	-	34.9%	37.2%

Mercy Health System Corp

1000 Mineral Point Ave
Janesville, WI 53548
Phone: 608-756-6080
Fax: 608-756-6168
URL: www.mercyhealthsystem.org
Type: Acute Care Hospitals
Emergency Services: Yes
Ownership: Voluntary non-profit - Private
Beds: 275

Key Personnel:
CEO/President. . . . . Javon R Bea
Cardiac Laboratory. . . . . Lubin Kan
Emergency Room . . . . France Keilhauer
Operating Room. . . . . Linda Nevenschwander
Chief of Medical Staff . . . . Blaine Nowak

Measure	Cases	This Hosp.	State Avg.	U.S. Avg.
Blood Clot Prevention and Treatment				
Anticoagulation Overlap Therapy[2]	77	99%	95%	93%
ICU Venous Thromboembolism Prophylaxis[2]	57	93%	91%	92%
Incidence of Potentially Preventable VTE[1,2]	-	-	10%	10%
UFH with Dosages/Platelet Monitoring[2]	42	100%	96%	97%
Venous Thromboembolism Prophylaxis[2]	263	90%	85%	85%
Warfarin Therapy Discharge Instructions[2]	63	79%	70%	75%
Chest Pain/Possible Heart Attack Care				
Aspirin Given Within 24 Hours of Arrival[1]	-	-	98%	96%
Fibrinolytic Meds Within 30 Min. of Arrival[3,7]	-	-	52%	58%
Average Time to ECG (minutes)[1]	-	-	7	7
Average Time to Transfer (minutes)[3,7]	-	-	58	60
Children's Asthma Care				
Received Home Management Plan of Care	-	-	-	88%
Received Reliever Medication	-	-	-	100%
Received Systemic Corticosteroids	-	-	-	100%
Emergency Department				
Admittance Decision Time (minutes)[2]	580	41	65	98
Head CT Results Within 45 Min. of Arrival[1]	-	-	61%	57%
Patients Who Left ER Before Being Seen	29,768	1%	1%	2%
Time from ER Arrival to Admit. (minutes)[2]	583	163	207	274
Time from ER Arrival to Discharge (minutes)	440	103	121	134
Time in ER Before Being Evaluated (minutes)	472	8	19	26
Time to Pain Meds for Fractures (minutes)	96	36	42	57
Heart Attack Care				
Aspirin Given at Discharge	166	99%	99%	99%
Fibrinolytic Meds Within 30 Min. of Arrival[7]	-	-	67%	54%
PCI Within 90 Minutes of Arrival	37	100%	96%	96%
Statin Prescribed at Discharge	155	97%	99%	98%
Heart Failure Care				
ACE Inhibitor or ARB for LVSD	34	100%	97%	97%
Discharge Instructions Given	129	98%	96%	94%
Evaluation of LVS Function	155	97%	99%	99%
Medicare Spending				
Medicare Spending per Patient (ratio)	-	0.91	0.94	0.98
Pneumonia Care				
Appropriate Initial Antibiotic Given	82	99%	96%	95%
Blood Culture Timing	147	98%	98%	98%
Pregnancy and Delivery Care				
Newborn Deliveries Scheduled Early	107	0%	4%	6%
Preventive Care				
Immunization for Influenza[2]	620	97%	90%	90%
Immunization for Pneumonia[2]	695	97%	92%	92%
Stroke Care				
Anticoagulation Therapy for Atrial Fibrillation	12	92%	94%	95%
Antithrombotic Therapy Timing	59	98%	99%	98%
Assessed for Rehabilitation	88	100%	98%	97%
Discharged on Antithrombotic Therapy	74	97%	99%	99%
Discharged on Statin Medication	59	88%	94%	94%
Thrombolytic Therapy Timing[1]	-	-	60%	66%
Venous Thromboembolism Prophylaxis	81	98%	95%	94%
Written Stroke Educational Materials Given	48	96%	88%	88%
Surgical Care Improvement Project				
Appropriate Beta Blocker Usage	224	99%	99%	98%
Appropriate VTP Within 24 Hours	539	98%	99%	98%
Controlled Postoperative Blood Glucose	58	97%	96%	97%
Perioperative Temperature Management	622	100%	100%	100%
Prophylactic Antibiotic Selection	348	99%	99%	99%
Prophylactic Antibiotic Selection (Outpatient)	265	98%	98%	98%
Prophylactic Antibiotic Stopped	337	97%	99%	98%
Prophylactic Antibiotic Timing	348	97%	99%	99%
Prophylactic Antibiotic Timing (Outpatient)	268	96%	97%	98%
Urinary Catheter Removal	504	98%	98%	97%
Survey of Patients' Hospital Experiences				
Area Around Room 'Always' Quiet at Night	300+	64%	63%	61%
Doctors 'Always' Communicated Well	300+	78%	83%	82%
Home Recovery Information Given	300+	86%	89%	85%
Hospital Given 9 or 10 on 10 Point Scale	300+	70%	74%	71%
Meds 'Always' Explained Before Given	300+	65%	68%	64%
Nurses 'Always' Communicated Well	300+	81%	82%	79%
Pain 'Always' Well Controlled	300+	71%	72%	71%
Room and Bathroom 'Always' Clean	300+	75%	79%	73%
Timely Help 'Always' Received	300+	70%	72%	68%
Would Definitely Recommend Hospital	300+	68%	74%	71%
Use of Medical Imaging				
Cardiac Imaging Stress Test before Surgery	542	6.1%	5.4%	5.3%
Combination Abdominal CT Scan	858	2.9%	6.3%	10.5%
Combination Brain/Sinus CT Scan	547	2.0%	2.1%	2.7%
Combination Chest CT Scan	715	1.8%	1%	2.7%
Follow-up Mammogram/Ultrasound	1,214	5.7%	8.1%	8.8%
Lumbar Spine MRI for Low Back Pain	176	34.1%	34.9%	37.2%

Saint Marys Janesville Hospital

3400 East Racine Street
Janesville, WI 53546
Phone: 608-373-8000
URL: www.stmarysjanesville.com
Type: Acute Care Hospitals
Emergency Services: Yes
Ownership: Voluntary non-profit - Other

Measure	Cases	This Hosp.	State Avg.	U.S. Avg.
Blood Clot Prevention and Treatment				
Anticoagulation Overlap Therapy[2]	19	68%	95%	93%
ICU Venous Thromboembolism Prophylaxis[2]	22	82%	91%	92%
Incidence of Potentially Preventable VTE[1,2]	-	-	10%	10%
UFH with Dosages/Platelet Monitoring[1,2]	-	-	96%	97%
Venous Thromboembolism Prophylaxis[2]	228	78%	85%	85%
Warfarin Therapy Discharge Instructions[1,2]	-	-	70%	75%
Chest Pain/Possible Heart Attack Care				
Aspirin Given Within 24 Hours of Arrival	77	95%	98%	96%
Fibrinolytic Meds Within 30 Min. of Arrival[7]	-	-	52%	58%
Average Time to ECG (minutes)	78	8	7	7
Average Time to Transfer (minutes)[1]	-	-	58	60
Children's Asthma Care				
Received Home Management Plan of Care	-	-	-	88%
Received Reliever Medication	-	-	-	100%
Received Systemic Corticosteroids	-	-	-	100%
Emergency Department				
Admittance Decision Time (minutes)[2]	264	48	65	98
Head CT Results Within 45 Min. of Arrival[1]	-	-	61%	57%
Patients Who Left ER Before Being Seen	12,343	0%	1%	2%
Time from ER Arrival to Admit. (minutes)[2]	268	194	207	274
Time from ER Arrival to Discharge (minutes)	374	104	121	134
Time in ER Before Being Evaluated (minutes)	407	11	19	26
Time to Pain Meds for Fractures (minutes)	43	41	42	57
Heart Attack Care				
Aspirin Given at Discharge[1]	-	-	99%	99%
Fibrinolytic Meds Within 30 Min. of Arrival[7]	-	-	67%	54%
PCI Within 90 Minutes of Arrival[7]	-	-	96%	96%
Statin Prescribed at Discharge[1]	-	-	99%	98%
Heart Failure Care				
ACE Inhibitor or ARB for LVSD	12	92%	97%	97%
Discharge Instructions Given	49	90%	96%	94%
Evaluation of LVS Function	77	100%	99%	99%
Medicare Spending				
Medicare Spending per Patient (ratio)	-	1.01	0.94	0.98
Pneumonia Care				
Appropriate Initial Antibiotic Given	56	95%	96%	95%
Blood Culture Timing	74	97%	98%	98%
Pregnancy and Delivery Care				
Newborn Deliveries Scheduled Early	50	12%	4%	6%
Preventive Care				
Immunization for Influenza[2]	304	97%	90%	90%
Immunization for Pneumonia[2]	395	97%	92%	92%
Stroke Care				
Anticoagulation Therapy for Atrial Fibrillation[1]	-	-	94%	95%
Antithrombotic Therapy Timing	22	95%	99%	98%
Assessed for Rehabilitation	24	96%	98%	97%
Discharged on Antithrombotic Therapy	22	100%	99%	99%
Discharged on Statin Medication	21	100%	94%	94%
Thrombolytic Therapy Timing	12	0%	60%	66%
Venous Thromboembolism Prophylaxis	25	60%	95%	94%
Written Stroke Educational Materials Given	15	27%	88%	88%
Surgical Care Improvement Project				
Appropriate Beta Blocker Usage	92	96%	99%	98%
Appropriate VTP Within 24 Hours	297	95%	99%	98%
Controlled Postoperative Blood Glucose[7]	-	-	96%	97%
Perioperative Temperature Management	351	100%	100%	100%
Prophylactic Antibiotic Selection	242	100%	99%	99%
Prophylactic Antibiotic Selection (Outpatient)	45	100%	98%	98%
Prophylactic Antibiotic Stopped	236	97%	99%	98%
Prophylactic Antibiotic Timing	242	95%	99%	99%
Prophylactic Antibiotic Timing (Outpatient)	50	88%	97%	98%
Urinary Catheter Removal	238	92%	98%	97%
Survey of Patients' Hospital Experiences				
Area Around Room 'Always' Quiet at Night	300+	69%	63%	61%
Doctors 'Always' Communicated Well	300+	83%	83%	82%
Home Recovery Information Given	300+	88%	89%	85%
Hospital Given 9 or 10 on 10 Point Scale	300+	83%	74%	71%
Meds 'Always' Explained Before Given	300+	73%	68%	64%
Nurses 'Always' Communicated Well	300+	85%	82%	79%
Pain 'Always' Well Controlled	300+	74%	72%	71%
Room and Bathroom 'Always' Clean	300+	86%	79%	73%
Timely Help 'Always' Received	300+	73%	72%	68%
Would Definitely Recommend Hospital	300+	86%	74%	71%
Use of Medical Imaging				
Cardiac Imaging Stress Test before Surgery[1]	-	-	5.4%	5.3%
Combination Abdominal CT Scan	98	1.0%	6.3%	10.5%
Combination Brain/Sinus CT Scan[1]	-	-	2.1%	2.7%
Combination Chest CT Scan[1]	-	-	1%	2.7%
Follow-up Mammogram/Ultrasound[7]	-	-	8.1%	8.8%
Lumbar Spine MRI for Low Back Pain[1]	-	-	34.9%	37.2%

Aurora Medical Center Kenosha

10400 75th St
Kenosha, WI 53142
Phone: 262-948-5600
Fax: 262-942-5828
URL: www.aurorahealthcare.org
Type: Acute Care Hospitals
Emergency Services: Yes
Ownership: Voluntary non-profit - Private
Beds: 72

Key Personnel:
Chief of Medical Staff. . . . . John M Agaiby
Radiology. . . . . Martin R Crain
CEO/President. . . . . Chris Olson

Measure	Cases	This Hosp.	State Avg.	U.S. Avg.
Blood Clot Prevention and Treatment				
Anticoagulation Overlap Therapy[2]	48	90%	95%	93%
ICU Venous Thromboembolism Prophylaxis[2]	51	92%	91%	92%
Incidence of Potentially Preventable VTE[1,2]	-	-	10%	10%
UFH with Dosages/Platelet Monitoring[2]	13	100%	96%	97%
Venous Thromboembolism Prophylaxis[2]	317	91%	85%	85%
Warfarin Therapy Discharge Instructions[2]	36	56%	70%	75%
Chest Pain/Possible Heart Attack Care				
Aspirin Given Within 24 Hours of Arrival	33	91%	98%	96%
Fibrinolytic Meds Within 30 Min. of Arrival[7]	-	-	52%	58%
Average Time to ECG (minutes)	33	7	7	7
Average Time to Transfer (minutes)[1]	-	-	58	60
Children's Asthma Care				
Received Home Management Plan of Care	-	-	-	88%
Received Reliever Medication	-	-	-	100%
Received Systemic Corticosteroids	-	-	-	100%

NOTE: Hospital profiles are in alphabetical order by state, then city, then hospital within the city; Rankings exclude hospitals with less than 25 cases except for patient surveys which excludes hospitals with less than 100 cases; (a) 100-299 cases; (1) The number of cases/patients is too few to report; (2) Data submitted were based on a sample of cases/patients; (3) Results are based on a shorter time period than required; (4) Data suppressed by CMS for one or more quarters; (5) Results are not available for this reporting period; (6) Fewer than 100 patients completed the HCAHPS survey; (7) No cases met the criteria for this measure; (8) The lower limit of the confidence interval cannot be calculated if the number of observed infections equals zero; (9) No data are available from the state/territory for this reporting period; (10) The scores shown reflect fewer than 50 completed surveys; (11) There were discrepancies in the data collection process; (12) This measure does not apply to this hospital for this reporting period; (13) Results cannot be calculated for this reporting period; (14) The results for this state are combined with nearby states to protect confidentiality; Please refer to the User's Guide for a full explanation of data.

Emergency Department				
Admittance Decision Time (minutes)[2]	452	68	65	98
Head CT Results Within 45 Min. of Arrival	12	58%	61%	57%
Patients Who Left ER Before Being Seen	25,070	1%	1%	2%
Time from ER Arrival to Admit. (minutes)[2]	528	223	207	274
Time from ER Arrival to Discharge (minutes)	352	146	121	134
Time in ER Before Being Evaluated (minutes)	295	21	19	26
Time to Pain Meds for Fractures (minutes)	79	42	42	57
Heart Attack Care				
Aspirin Given at Discharge[1]	-	-	99%	99%
Fibrinolytic Meds Within 30 Min. of Arrival[7]	-	-	67%	54%
PCI Within 90 Minutes of Arrival[7]	-	-	96%	96%
Statin Prescribed at Discharge[1]	-	-	99%	98%
Heart Failure Care				
ACE Inhibitor or ARB for LVSD	33	100%	97%	97%
Discharge Instructions Given	81	88%	96%	94%
Evaluation of LVS Function	105	100%	99%	99%
Medicare Spending				
Medicare Spending per Patient (ratio)	-	1.03	0.94	0.98
Pneumonia Care				
Appropriate Initial Antibiotic Given	123	98%	96%	95%
Blood Culture Timing	168	100%	98%	98%
Pregnancy and Delivery Care				
Newborn Deliveries Scheduled Early	101	6%	4%	6%
Preventive Care				
Immunization for Influenza[2]	473	82%	90%	90%
Immunization for Pneumonia[2]	556	93%	92%	92%
Stroke Care				
Anticoagulation Therapy for Atrial Fibrillation[1]	-	-	94%	95%
Antithrombotic Therapy Timing	36	100%	99%	98%
Assessed for Rehabilitation	38	100%	98%	97%
Discharged on Antithrombotic Therapy	36	100%	99%	99%
Discharged on Statin Medication	33	97%	94%	94%
Thrombolytic Therapy Timing[1]	-	-	60%	66%
Venous Thromboembolism Prophylaxis	39	97%	95%	94%
Written Stroke Educational Materials Given	23	87%	88%	88%
Surgical Care Improvement Project				
Appropriate Beta Blocker Usage[2]	126	99%	99%	98%
Appropriate VTP Within 24 Hours[2]	416	100%	99%	98%
Controlled Postoperative Blood Glucose[2,7]	-	-	96%	97%
Perioperative Temperature Management[2]	448	100%	100%	100%
Prophylactic Antibiotic Selection[2]	332	100%	99%	99%
Prophylactic Antibiotic Selection (Outpatient)	243	93%	98%	98%
Prophylactic Antibiotic Stopped[2]	318	99%	99%	98%
Prophylactic Antibiotic Timing[2]	333	99%	99%	99%
Prophylactic Antibiotic Timing (Outpatient)	250	95%	97%	98%
Urinary Catheter Removal[2]	377	99%	98%	97%
Survey of Patients' Hospital Experiences				
Area Around Room 'Always' Quiet at Night	300+	59%	63%	61%
Doctors 'Always' Communicated Well	300+	78%	83%	82%
Home Recovery Information Given	300+	84%	89%	85%
Hospital Given 9 or 10 on 10 Point Scale	300+	66%	74%	71%
Meds 'Always' Explained Before Given	300+	60%	68%	64%
Nurses 'Always' Communicated Well	300+	75%	82%	79%
Pain 'Always' Well Controlled	300+	67%	72%	71%
Room and Bathroom 'Always' Clean	300+	72%	79%	73%
Timely Help 'Always' Received	300+	65%	72%	68%
Would Definitely Recommend Hospital	300+	69%	74%	71%
Use of Medical Imaging				
Cardiac Imaging Stress Test before Surgery	755	5.3%	5.4%	5.3%
Combination Abdominal CT Scan	691	4.8%	6.3%	10.5%
Combination Brain/Sinus CT Scan	625	2.4%	2.1%	2.7%
Combination Chest CT Scan	617	1.3%	1%	2.7%
Follow-up Mammogram/Ultrasound	1,005	4.8%	8.1%	8.8%
Lumbar Spine MRI for Low Back Pain	149	26.8%	34.9%	37.2%

United Hospital System

6308 Eighth Ave
Kenosha, WI 53143
Phone: 262-656-2011
Fax: 262-656-2124
E-mail: webmaster@uhsi.org
Type: Acute Care Hospitals
Emergency Services: Yes
Ownership: Government - Local
Beds: 315

Key Personnel:

Operating Room. . . . . Dorothy Barca, RN
Quality Assurance . . . . Mary Becker
CEO/President. . . . . Robert Cook
Infection Control. . . . . Jim Johnson

Measure	Cases	This Hosp.	State Avg.	U.S. Avg.
Blood Clot Prevention and Treatment				
Anticoagulation Overlap Therapy[2]	72	89%	95%	93%
ICU Venous Thromboembolism Prophylaxis[2]	77	96%	91%	92%
Incidence of Potentially Preventable VTE[2]	12	0%	10%	10%
UFH with Dosages/Platelet Monitoring[2]	18	94%	96%	97%
Venous Thromboembolism Prophylaxis[2]	359	98%	85%	85%
Warfarin Therapy Discharge Instructions[2]	53	98%	70%	75%
Chest Pain/Possible Heart Attack Care				
Aspirin Given Within 24 Hours of Arrival[1,3]	-	-	98%	96%
Fibrinolytic Meds Within 30 Min. of Arrival[5]	-	-	52%	58%
Average Time to ECG (minutes)[3,7]	-	-	7	7
Average Time to Transfer (minutes)[5]	-	-	58	60
Children's Asthma Care				
Received Home Management Plan of Care	-	-	-	88%
Received Reliever Medication	-	-	-	100%
Received Systemic Corticosteroids	-	-	-	100%
Emergency Department				
Admittance Decision Time (minutes)[2]	665	82	65	98
Head CT Results Within 45 Min. of Arrival	32	75%	61%	57%
Patients Who Left ER Before Being Seen	70,560	0%	1%	2%
Time from ER Arrival to Admit. (minutes)[2]	666	226	207	274
Time from ER Arrival to Discharge (minutes)	351	113	121	134
Time in ER Before Being Evaluated (minutes)	381	26	19	26
Time to Pain Meds for Fractures (minutes)	152	58	42	57
Heart Attack Care				
Aspirin Given at Discharge	120	100%	99%	99%
Fibrinolytic Meds Within 30 Min. of Arrival[7]	-	-	67%	54%
PCI Within 90 Minutes of Arrival	28	89%	96%	96%
Statin Prescribed at Discharge	109	99%	99%	98%
Heart Failure Care				
ACE Inhibitor or ARB for LVSD	106	99%	97%	97%
Discharge Instructions Given	241	92%	96%	94%
Evaluation of LVS Function	313	100%	99%	99%
Medicare Spending				
Medicare Spending per Patient (ratio)	-	1.03	0.94	0.98
Pneumonia Care				
Appropriate Initial Antibiotic Given	154	100%	96%	95%
Blood Culture Timing	308	96%	98%	98%
Pregnancy and Delivery Care				
Newborn Deliveries Scheduled Early[2]	36	0%	4%	6%
Preventive Care				
Immunization for Influenza[2]	578	99%	90%	90%
Immunization for Pneumonia[2]	721	100%	92%	92%
Stroke Care				
Anticoagulation Therapy for Atrial Fibrillation	14	79%	94%	95%
Antithrombotic Therapy Timing	79	100%	99%	98%
Assessed for Rehabilitation	77	99%	98%	97%
Discharged on Antithrombotic Therapy	72	100%	99%	99%
Discharged on Statin Medication	51	90%	94%	94%
Thrombolytic Therapy Timing[7]	-	-	60%	66%
Venous Thromboembolism Prophylaxis	90	97%	95%	94%
Written Stroke Educational Materials Given	45	80%	88%	88%
Surgical Care Improvement Project				
Appropriate Beta Blocker Usage	229	99%	99%	98%
Appropriate VTP Within 24 Hours	563	99%	99%	98%
Controlled Postoperative Blood Glucose	92	99%	96%	97%
Perioperative Temperature Management	657	100%	100%	100%
Prophylactic Antibiotic Selection	527	100%	99%	99%
Prophylactic Antibiotic Selection (Outpatient)	376	98%	98%	98%
Prophylactic Antibiotic Stopped	506	100%	99%	98%
Prophylactic Antibiotic Timing	527	100%	99%	99%
Prophylactic Antibiotic Timing (Outpatient)	300	96%	97%	98%
Urinary Catheter Removal	558	99%	98%	97%
Survey of Patients' Hospital Experiences				
Area Around Room 'Always' Quiet at Night	300+	53%	63%	61%
Doctors 'Always' Communicated Well	300+	79%	83%	82%
Home Recovery Information Given	300+	83%	89%	85%
Hospital Given 9 or 10 on 10 Point Scale	300+	72%	74%	71%
Meds 'Always' Explained Before Given	300+	62%	68%	64%
Nurses 'Always' Communicated Well	300+	76%	82%	79%
Pain 'Always' Well Controlled	300+	69%	72%	71%
Room and Bathroom 'Always' Clean	300+	76%	79%	73%
Timely Help 'Always' Received	300+	68%	72%	68%
Would Definitely Recommend Hospital	300+	73%	74%	71%
Use of Medical Imaging				
Cardiac Imaging Stress Test before Surgery	749	9.5%	5.4%	5.3%
Combination Abdominal CT Scan	845	4.5%	6.3%	10.5%
Combination Brain/Sinus CT Scan	796	2.4%	2.1%	2.7%
Combination Chest CT Scan	441	0.0%	1%	2.7%
Follow-up Mammogram/Ultrasound	1,931	5.6%	8.1%	8.8%
Lumbar Spine MRI for Low Back Pain	167	27.5%	34.9%	37.2%

Gundersen Lutheran Medical Center

1910 South Ave
La Crosse, WI 54601
Phone: 608-782-7300
Fax: 608-775-5594
E-mail: careers@gundluth.org
URL: www.gundluth.org
Type: Acute Care Hospitals
Emergency Services: Yes
Ownership: Voluntary non-profit - Private
Beds: 325

Key Personnel:

Infection Control. . . . . William Agger, MD
Hemotology Center . . . . Wayne Bottner, MD
Intensive Care Unit. . . . . Mary Lu Gerke, RN
Quality Assurance . . . . Jean Krause
Emergency Room . . . . Stephanie Schwartz
Chief of Medical Staff. . . . . Greg Thompson, MD
CEO/President. . . . . Jeffrey E Thompson, MD
Radiology. . . . . Eugene Valentini, MD

Measure	Cases	This Hosp.	State Avg.	U.S. Avg.
Blood Clot Prevention and Treatment				
Anticoagulation Overlap Therapy[2]	70	100%	95%	93%
ICU Venous Thromboembolism Prophylaxis[2]	112	94%	91%	92%
Incidence of Potentially Preventable VTE[2]	13	0%	10%	10%
UFH with Dosages/Platelet Monitoring[2]	34	88%	96%	97%
Venous Thromboembolism Prophylaxis[2]	281	97%	85%	85%
Warfarin Therapy Discharge Instructions[2]	52	67%	70%	75%
Chest Pain/Possible Heart Attack Care				
Aspirin Given Within 24 Hours of Arrival[1,3]	-	-	98%	96%
Fibrinolytic Meds Within 30 Min. of Arrival[5]	-	-	52%	58%
Average Time to ECG (minutes)[1,3]	-	-	7	7
Average Time to Transfer (minutes)[5]	-	-	58	60
Children's Asthma Care				
Received Home Management Plan of Care	-	-	-	88%
Received Reliever Medication	-	-	-	100%
Received Systemic Corticosteroids	-	-	-	100%
Emergency Department				
Admittance Decision Time (minutes)[2]	377	68	65	98
Head CT Results Within 45 Min. of Arrival[1]	-	-	61%	57%
Patients Who Left ER Before Being Seen	29,703	1%	1%	2%
Time from ER Arrival to Admit. (minutes)[2]	391	181	207	274
Time from ER Arrival to Discharge (minutes)	1,406	129	121	134
Time in ER Before Being Evaluated (minutes)	1,566	15	19	26
Time to Pain Meds for Fractures (minutes)	51	53	42	57
Heart Attack Care				
Aspirin Given at Discharge	325	99%	99%	99%
Fibrinolytic Meds Within 30 Min. of Arrival[1]	-	-	67%	54%
PCI Within 90 Minutes of Arrival	23	100%	96%	96%
Statin Prescribed at Discharge	321	100%	99%	98%
Heart Failure Care				
ACE Inhibitor or ARB for LVSD	70	97%	97%	97%
Discharge Instructions Given	198	100%	96%	94%
Evaluation of LVS Function	240	100%	99%	99%
Medicare Spending				
Medicare Spending per Patient (ratio)	-	0.89	0.94	0.98
Pneumonia Care				
Appropriate Initial Antibiotic Given	106	95%	96%	95%
Blood Culture Timing	191	99%	98%	98%
Pregnancy and Delivery Care				
Newborn Deliveries Scheduled Early	99	0%	4%	6%
Preventive Care				
Immunization for Influenza[2]	580	55%	90%	90%
Immunization for Pneumonia[2]	642	81%	92%	92%

NOTE: Hospital profiles are in alphabetical order by state, then city, then hospital within the city; Rankings exclude hospitals with less than 25 cases except for patient surveys which excludes hospitals with less than 100 cases; (a) 100-299 cases; (1) The number of cases/patients is too few to report; (2) Data submitted were based on a sample of cases/patients; (3) Results are based on a shorter time period than required; (4) Data suppressed by CMS for one or more quarters; (5) Results are not available for this reporting period; (6) Fewer than 100 patients completed the HCAHPS survey; (7) No cases met the criteria for this measure; (8) The lower limit of the confidence interval cannot be calculated if the number of observed infections equals zero; (9) No data are available from the state/territory for this reporting period; (10) The scores shown reflect fewer than 50 completed surveys; (11) There were discrepancies in the data collection process; (12) This measure does not apply to this hospital for this reporting period; (13) Results cannot be calculated for this reporting period; (14) The results for this state are combined with nearby states to protect confidentiality; Please refer to the User's Guide for a full explanation of data.

Measure	Cases	This Hosp.	State Avg.	U.S. Avg.
Stroke Care				
Anticoagulation Therapy for Atrial Fibrillation	26	92%	94%	95%
Antithrombotic Therapy Timing	113	99%	99%	98%
Assessed for Rehabilitation	180	98%	98%	97%
Discharged on Antithrombotic Therapy	152	100%	99%	99%
Discharged on Statin Medication	114	99%	94%	94%
Thrombolytic Therapy Timing	14	93%	60%	66%
Venous Thromboembolism Prophylaxis	165	99%	95%	94%
Written Stroke Educational Materials Given	89	94%	88%	88%
Surgical Care Improvement Project				
Appropriate Beta Blocker Usage[2]	420	98%	99%	98%
Appropriate VTP Within 24 Hours[2]	570	99%	99%	98%
Controlled Postoperative Blood Glucose[2]	221	96%	96%	97%
Perioperative Temperature Management[2]	794	100%	100%	100%
Prophylactic Antibiotic Selection[2]	628	100%	99%	99%
Prophylactic Antibiotic Selection (Outpatient)	758	100%	98%	98%
Prophylactic Antibiotic Stopped[2]	621	99%	99%	98%
Prophylactic Antibiotic Timing[2]	632	98%	99%	99%
Prophylactic Antibiotic Timing (Outpatient)	721	96%	97%	98%
Urinary Catheter Removal[2]	635	99%	98%	97%
Survey of Patients' Hospital Experiences				
Area Around Room 'Always' Quiet at Night	300+	47%	63%	61%
Doctors 'Always' Communicated Well	300+	82%	83%	82%
Home Recovery Information Given	300+	90%	89%	85%
Hospital Given 9 or 10 on 10 Point Scale	300+	75%	74%	71%
Meds 'Always' Explained Before Given	300+	69%	68%	64%
Nurses 'Always' Communicated Well	300+	78%	82%	79%
Pain 'Always' Well Controlled	300+	67%	72%	71%
Room and Bathroom 'Always' Clean	300+	74%	79%	73%
Timely Help 'Always' Received	300+	63%	72%	68%
Would Definitely Recommend Hospital	300+	80%	74%	71%
Use of Medical Imaging				
Cardiac Imaging Stress Test before Surgery[1]	-	-	5.4%	5.3%
Combination Abdominal CT Scan	341	1.5%	6.3%	10.5%
Combination Brain/Sinus CT Scan[1]	-	-	2.1%	2.7%
Combination Chest CT Scan[1]	-	-	1%	2.7%
Follow-up Mammogram/Ultrasound[7]	-	-	8.1%	8.8%
Lumbar Spine MRI for Low Back Pain[1]	-	-	34.9%	37.2%

Mayo Clinic Health Sys Franciscan Medical Center

700 West Avenue South
La Crosse, WI 54601
Phone: 608-785-0940
Fax: 608-791-9504
URL: www.mayohealthsytem.org
Type: Acute Care Hospitals
Emergency Services: Yes
Ownership: Voluntary non-profit - Private
Beds: 350

Key Personnel:
Operating Room. . . . . Charlotte Baier, RN
Infection Control. . . . . Ala Dababneh, MD
Intensive Care Unit. . . . . Kristof Gehrke, MD
Emergency Room . . . . Eric Grube, DO
Patient Relations . . . . Diane Holmay
CEO/President. . . . . Timothy Johnson, MD
Pediatric In-Patient Care . . . . Douglas Nelson, MD
Radiology. . . . . Martin Nelson, MD

Measure	Cases	This Hosp.	State Avg.	U.S. Avg.
Blood Clot Prevention and Treatment				
Anticoagulation Overlap Therapy[2]	42	98%	95%	93%
ICU Venous Thromboembolism Prophylaxis[2]	52	98%	91%	92%
Incidence of Potentially Preventable VTE[1,2]	-	-	10%	10%
UFH with Dosages/Platelet Monitoring[2]	34	100%	96%	97%
Venous Thromboembolism Prophylaxis[2]	235	93%	85%	85%
Warfarin Therapy Discharge Instructions[2]	34	38%	70%	75%
Chest Pain/Possible Heart Attack Care				
Aspirin Given Within 24 Hours of Arrival[1,3]	-	-	98%	96%
Fibrinolytic Meds Within 30 Min. of Arrival[5]	-	-	52%	58%
Average Time to ECG (minutes)[1,3]	-	-	7	7
Average Time to Transfer (minutes)[5]	-	-	58	60
Children's Asthma Care				
Received Home Management Plan of Care	-	-	-	88%
Received Reliever Medication	-	-	-	100%
Received Systemic Corticosteroids	-	-	-	100%
Emergency Department				
Admittance Decision Time (minutes)[2]	425	99	65	98
Head CT Results Within 45 Min. of Arrival[1,3]	-	-	61%	57%
Patients Who Left ER Before Being Seen	33,534	0%	1%	2%
Time from ER Arrival to Admit. (minutes)[2]	432	222	207	274
Time from ER Arrival to Discharge (minutes)	344	124	121	134
Time in ER Before Being Evaluated (minutes)	415	13	19	26
Time to Pain Meds for Fractures (minutes)	50	41	42	57
Heart Attack Care				
Aspirin Given at Discharge	111	99%	99%	99%
Fibrinolytic Meds Within 30 Min. of Arrival[7]	-	-	67%	54%
PCI Within 90 Minutes of Arrival	13	85%	96%	96%
Statin Prescribed at Discharge	109	99%	99%	98%
Heart Failure Care				
ACE Inhibitor or ARB for LVSD	39	100%	97%	97%
Discharge Instructions Given	98	92%	96%	94%
Evaluation of LVS Function	137	100%	99%	99%
Medicare Spending				
Medicare Spending per Patient (ratio)	-	0.90	0.94	0.98
Pneumonia Care				
Appropriate Initial Antibiotic Given	91	100%	96%	95%
Blood Culture Timing	136	96%	98%	98%
Pregnancy and Delivery Care				
Newborn Deliveries Scheduled Early	36	0%	4%	6%
Preventive Care				
Immunization for Influenza[2]	550	95%	90%	90%
Immunization for Pneumonia[2]	567	96%	92%	92%
Stroke Care				
Anticoagulation Therapy for Atrial Fibrillation	13	100%	94%	95%
Antithrombotic Therapy Timing	47	98%	99%	98%
Assessed for Rehabilitation	65	91%	98%	97%
Discharged on Antithrombotic Therapy	59	100%	99%	99%
Discharged on Statin Medication	49	98%	94%	94%
Thrombolytic Therapy Timing[1]	-	-	60%	66%
Venous Thromboembolism Prophylaxis	52	94%	95%	94%
Written Stroke Educational Materials Given	38	92%	88%	88%
Surgical Care Improvement Project				
Appropriate Beta Blocker Usage	274	97%	99%	98%
Appropriate VTP Within 24 Hours	679	100%	99%	98%
Controlled Postoperative Blood Glucose[7]	-	-	96%	97%
Perioperative Temperature Management	863	100%	100%	100%
Prophylactic Antibiotic Selection	652	100%	99%	99%
Prophylactic Antibiotic Selection (Outpatient)	304	99%	98%	98%
Prophylactic Antibiotic Stopped	640	100%	99%	98%
Prophylactic Antibiotic Timing	652	99%	99%	99%
Prophylactic Antibiotic Timing (Outpatient)	276	98%	97%	98%
Urinary Catheter Removal	621	99%	98%	97%
Survey of Patients' Hospital Experiences				
Area Around Room 'Always' Quiet at Night	300+	54%	63%	61%
Doctors 'Always' Communicated Well	300+	83%	83%	82%
Home Recovery Information Given	300+	88%	89%	85%
Hospital Given 9 or 10 on 10 Point Scale	300+	75%	74%	71%
Meds 'Always' Explained Before Given	300+	67%	68%	64%
Nurses 'Always' Communicated Well	300+	80%	82%	79%
Pain 'Always' Well Controlled	300+	71%	72%	71%
Room and Bathroom 'Always' Clean	300+	74%	79%	73%
Timely Help 'Always' Received	300+	69%	72%	68%
Would Definitely Recommend Hospital	300+	78%	74%	71%
Use of Medical Imaging				
Cardiac Imaging Stress Test before Surgery	433	7.4%	5.4%	5.3%
Combination Abdominal CT Scan	755	8.6%	6.3%	10.5%
Combination Brain/Sinus CT Scan	418	1.7%	2.1%	2.7%
Combination Chest CT Scan	547	0.2%	1%	2.7%
Follow-up Mammogram/Ultrasound[7]	-	-	8.1%	8.8%
Lumbar Spine MRI for Low Back Pain	162	35.8%	34.9%	37.2%

Rusk County Memorial Hospital

900 College Ave West
Ladysmith, WI 54848
Phone: 715-532-5561
Fax: 715-532-9809
E-mail: info@ruskhospital.org
URL: www.ruskhospital.org
Type: Critical Access Hospitals
Emergency Services: Yes
Ownership: Voluntary non-profit - Other
Beds: 25

Key Personnel:
Radiology. . . . . Mark A Augustyn
CEO . . . . Charisse Oland
Quality Assurance . . . . Lorene Reisner
Emergency Room . . . . Mary Schneider
President. . . . . Eldon Skogen
Chief of Medical Staff. . . . . Dr John Ziemer

Measure	Cases	This Hosp.	State Avg.	U.S. Avg.
Blood Clot Prevention and Treatment				
Anticoagulation Overlap Therapy[5]	-	-	95%	93%
ICU Venous Thromboembolism Prophylaxis[5]	-	-	91%	92%
Incidence of Potentially Preventable VTE[5]	-	-	10%	10%
UFH with Dosages/Platelet Monitoring[5]	-	-	96%	97%
Venous Thromboembolism Prophylaxis[5]	-	-	85%	85%
Warfarin Therapy Discharge Instructions[5]	-	-	70%	75%
Chest Pain/Possible Heart Attack Care				
Aspirin Given Within 24 Hours of Arrival[3]	24	100%	98%	96%
Fibrinolytic Meds Within 30 Min. of Arrival[1,3]	-	-	52%	58%
Average Time to ECG (minutes)[3]	24	18	7	7
Average Time to Transfer (minutes)[1,3]	-	-	58	60
Children's Asthma Care				
Received Home Management Plan of Care	-	-	-	88%
Received Reliever Medication	-	-	-	100%
Received Systemic Corticosteroids	-	-	-	100%
Emergency Department				
Admittance Decision Time (minutes)[5]	-	-	65	98
Head CT Results Within 45 Min. of Arrival[1]	-	-	61%	57%
Patients Who Left ER Before Being Seen[5]	-	-	1%	2%
Time from ER Arrival to Admit. (minutes)[5]	-	-	207	274
Time from ER Arrival to Discharge (minutes)[5]	-	-	121	134
Time in ER Before Being Evaluated (minutes)[5]	-	-	19	26
Time to Pain Meds for Fractures (minutes)	20	53	42	57
Heart Attack Care				
Aspirin Given at Discharge[1,3]	-	-	99%	99%
Fibrinolytic Meds Within 30 Min. of Arrival[3,7]	-	-	67%	54%
PCI Within 90 Minutes of Arrival[3,7]	-	-	96%	96%
Statin Prescribed at Discharge[5]	-	-	99%	98%
Heart Failure Care				
ACE Inhibitor or ARB for LVSD[1]	-	-	97%	97%
Discharge Instructions Given	17	35%	96%	94%
Evaluation of LVS Function	23	70%	99%	99%
Medicare Spending				
Medicare Spending per Patient (ratio)	-	-	0.94	0.98
Pneumonia Care				
Appropriate Initial Antibiotic Given	14	79%	96%	95%
Blood Culture Timing[1]	-	-	98%	98%
Pregnancy and Delivery Care				
Newborn Deliveries Scheduled Early[5]	-	-	4%	6%
Preventive Care				
Immunization for Influenza[5]	-	-	90%	90%
Immunization for Pneumonia[5]	-	-	92%	92%
Stroke Care				
Anticoagulation Therapy for Atrial Fibrillation[5]	-	-	94%	95%
Antithrombotic Therapy Timing[5]	-	-	99%	98%
Assessed for Rehabilitation[5]	-	-	98%	97%
Discharged on Antithrombotic Therapy[5]	-	-	99%	99%
Discharged on Statin Medication[5]	-	-	94%	94%
Thrombolytic Therapy Timing[5]	-	-	60%	66%
Venous Thromboembolism Prophylaxis[5]	-	-	95%	94%
Written Stroke Educational Materials Given[5]	-	-	88%	88%
Surgical Care Improvement Project				
Appropriate Beta Blocker Usage[1,3]	-	-	99%	98%
Appropriate VTP Within 24 Hours[1,3]	-	-	99%	98%
Controlled Postoperative Blood Glucose[3,7]	-	-	96%	97%
Perioperative Temperature Management[1,3]	-	-	100%	100%
Prophylactic Antibiotic Selection[1,3]	-	-	99%	99%
Prophylactic Antibiotic Selection (Outpatient)[1,3]	-	-	98%	98%
Prophylactic Antibiotic Stopped[1,3]	-	-	99%	98%
Prophylactic Antibiotic Timing[1,3]	-	-	99%	99%
Prophylactic Antibiotic Timing (Outpatient)[1,3]	-	-	97%	98%
Urinary Catheter Removal[1,3]	-	-	98%	97%
Survey of Patients' Hospital Experiences				
Area Around Room 'Always' Quiet at Night	(a)	60%	63%	61%
Doctors 'Always' Communicated Well	(a)	84%	83%	82%
Home Recovery Information Given	(a)	86%	89%	85%
Hospital Given 9 or 10 on 10 Point Scale	(a)	61%	74%	71%
Meds 'Always' Explained Before Given	(a)	65%	68%	64%

NOTE: Hospital profiles are in alphabetical order by state, then city, then hospital within the city; Rankings exclude hospitals with less than 25 cases except for patient surveys which excludes hospitals with less than 100 cases; (a) 100-299 cases; (1) The number of cases/patients is too few to report; (2) Data submitted were based on a sample of cases/patients; (3) Results are based on a shorter time period than required; (4) Data suppressed by CMS for one or more quarters; (5) Results are not available for this reporting period; (6) Fewer than 100 patients completed the HCAHPS survey; (7) No cases met the criteria for this measure; (8) The lower limit of the confidence interval cannot be calculated if the number of observed infections equals zero; (9) No data are available from the state/territory for this reporting period; (10) The scores shown reflect fewer than 50 completed surveys; (11) There were discrepancies in the data collection process; (12) This measure does not apply to this hospital for this reporting period; (13) Results cannot be calculated for this reporting period; (14) The results for this state are combined with nearby states to protect confidentiality; Please refer to the User's Guide for a full explanation of data.

Measure	Cases	This Hosp.	State Avg.	U.S. Avg.
Nurses 'Always' Communicated Well	(a)	79%	82%	79%
Pain 'Always' Well Controlled	(a)	69%	72%	71%
Room and Bathroom 'Always' Clean	(a)	91%	79%	73%
Timely Help 'Always' Received	(a)	75%	72%	68%
Would Definitely Recommend Hospital	(a)	48%	74%	71%
Use of Medical Imaging				
Cardiac Imaging Stress Test before Surgery[1]	-	-	5.4%	5.3%
Combination Abdominal CT Scan	91	12.1%	6.3%	10.5%
Combination Brain/Sinus CT Scan	87	0.0%	2.1%	2.7%
Combination Chest CT Scan	61	1.6%	1%	2.7%
Follow-up Mammogram/Ultrasound	403	9.2%	8.1%	8.8%
Lumbar Spine MRI for Low Back Pain[1]	-	-	34.9%	37.2%

Mercy Walworth Hospital & Medical Center

N2950 State Road 67 Phone: 262-245-0535
Lake Geneva, WI 53147
Type: Critical Access Hospitals Emergency Services: Yes
Ownership: Voluntary non-profit - Private
Key Personnel:
CEO/President. . . . . Sheridan Yerk

Measure	Cases	This Hosp.	State Avg.	U.S. Avg.
Blood Clot Prevention and Treatment				
Anticoagulation Overlap Therapy[1,2]	-	-	95%	93%
ICU Venous Thromboembolism Prophylaxis[1,2]	-	-	91%	92%
Incidence of Potentially Preventable VTE[2,7]	-	-	10%	10%
UFH with Dosages/Platelet Monitoring[2,7]	-	-	96%	97%
Venous Thromboembolism Prophylaxis[2]	90	99%	85%	85%
Warfarin Therapy Discharge Instructions[1,2]	-	-	70%	75%
Chest Pain/Possible Heart Attack Care				
Aspirin Given Within 24 Hours of Arrival	57	98%	98%	96%
Fibrinolytic Meds Within 30 Min. of Arrival[3,7]	-	-	52%	58%
Average Time to ECG (minutes)	63	7	7	7
Average Time to Transfer (minutes)[1,3]	-	-	58	60
Children's Asthma Care				
Received Home Management Plan of Care	-	-	-	88%
Received Reliever Medication	-	-	-	100%
Received Systemic Corticosteroids	-	-	-	100%
Emergency Department				
Admittance Decision Time (minutes)	626	40	65	98
Head CT Results Within 45 Min. of Arrival[1]	-	-	61%	57%
Patients Who Left ER Before Being Seen[5]	-	-	1%	2%
Time from ER Arrival to Admit. (minutes)	627	189	207	274
Time from ER Arrival to Discharge (minutes)	437	113	121	134
Time in ER Before Being Evaluated (minutes)	537	14	19	26
Time to Pain Meds for Fractures (minutes)	88	37	42	57
Heart Attack Care				
Aspirin Given at Discharge[5]	-	-	99%	99%
Fibrinolytic Meds Within 30 Min. of Arrival[5]	-	-	67%	54%
PCI Within 90 Minutes of Arrival[5]	-	-	96%	96%
Statin Prescribed at Discharge[5]	-	-	99%	98%
Heart Failure Care				
ACE Inhibitor or ARB for LVSD[1]	-	-	97%	97%
Discharge Instructions Given	18	89%	96%	94%
Evaluation of LVS Function	24	96%	99%	99%
Medicare Spending				
Medicare Spending per Patient (ratio)	-	-	0.94	0.98
Pneumonia Care				
Appropriate Initial Antibiotic Given	30	100%	96%	95%
Blood Culture Timing	43	98%	98%	98%
Pregnancy and Delivery Care				
Newborn Deliveries Scheduled Early	26	0%	4%	6%
Preventive Care				
Immunization for Influenza	564	97%	90%	90%
Immunization for Pneumonia	661	96%	92%	92%
Stroke Care				
Anticoagulation Therapy for Atrial Fibrillation[1,3]	-	-	94%	95%
Antithrombotic Therapy Timing[1,3]	-	-	99%	98%
Assessed for Rehabilitation[1,3]	-	-	98%	97%
Discharged on Antithrombotic Therapy[1,3]	-	-	99%	99%
Discharged on Statin Medication[1,3]	-	-	94%	94%
Thrombolytic Therapy Timing[3,7]	-	-	60%	66%
Venous Thromboembolism Prophylaxis[1,3]	-	-	95%	94%
Written Stroke Educational Materials Given[1,3]	-	-	88%	88%
Surgical Care Improvement Project				
Appropriate Beta Blocker Usage	59	100%	99%	98%
Appropriate VTP Within 24 Hours	223	100%	99%	98%
Controlled Postoperative Blood Glucose[7]	-	-	96%	97%
Perioperative Temperature Management	247	100%	100%	100%
Prophylactic Antibiotic Selection	173	100%	99%	99%
Prophylactic Antibiotic Selection (Outpatient)	15	100%	98%	98%
Prophylactic Antibiotic Stopped	170	96%	99%	98%
Prophylactic Antibiotic Timing	174	99%	99%	99%
Prophylactic Antibiotic Timing (Outpatient)	15	93%	97%	98%
Urinary Catheter Removal	186	97%	98%	97%
Survey of Patients' Hospital Experiences				
Area Around Room 'Always' Quiet at Night[5]	-	-	63%	61%
Doctors 'Always' Communicated Well[5]	-	-	83%	82%
Home Recovery Information Given[5]	-	-	89%	85%
Hospital Given 9 or 10 on 10 Point Scale[5]	-	-	74%	71%
Meds 'Always' Explained Before Given[5]	-	-	68%	64%
Nurses 'Always' Communicated Well[5]	-	-	82%	79%
Pain 'Always' Well Controlled[5]	-	-	72%	71%
Room and Bathroom 'Always' Clean[5]	-	-	79%	73%
Timely Help 'Always' Received[5]	-	-	72%	68%
Would Definitely Recommend Hospital[5]	-	-	74%	71%
Use of Medical Imaging				
Cardiac Imaging Stress Test before Surgery	70	5.7%	5.4%	5.3%
Combination Abdominal CT Scan	216	7.9%	6.3%	10.5%
Combination Brain/Sinus CT Scan[1]	-	-	2.1%	2.7%
Combination Chest CT Scan	121	5.8%	1%	2.7%
Follow-up Mammogram/Ultrasound	268	9.3%	8.1%	8.8%
Lumbar Spine MRI for Low Back Pain	53	34.0%	34.9%	37.2%

Grant Regional Health Center

507 S Monroe St Phone: 608-723-2143
Lancaster, WI 53813 Fax: 608-723-4464
URL: www.grantregional.com
Type: Critical Access Hospitals Emergency Services: Yes
Ownership: Voluntary non-profit - Private Beds: 29
Key Personnel:
Infection Control. . . . . Kandi Auel
Anesthesiology. . . . . David Bainbridge
CEO/President. . . . . Nicole Clapp
Patient Relations . . . . Nicole Clapp
Quality Assurance . . . . Nicole Clapp, RN
Chief of Medical Staff. . . . . Sunil Sharma, MD
Emergency Room . . . . Robert Smith, MD
Operating Room. . . . . James Yurcek

Measure	Cases	This Hosp.	State Avg.	U.S. Avg.
Blood Clot Prevention and Treatment				
Anticoagulation Overlap Therapy[5]	-	-	95%	93%
ICU Venous Thromboembolism Prophylaxis[5]	-	-	91%	92%
Incidence of Potentially Preventable VTE[5]	-	-	10%	10%
UFH with Dosages/Platelet Monitoring[5]	-	-	96%	97%
Venous Thromboembolism Prophylaxis[5]	-	-	85%	85%
Warfarin Therapy Discharge Instructions[5]	-	-	70%	75%
Chest Pain/Possible Heart Attack Care				
Aspirin Given Within 24 Hours of Arrival[5]	-	-	98%	96%
Fibrinolytic Meds Within 30 Min. of Arrival[5]	-	-	52%	58%
Average Time to ECG (minutes)[5]	-	-	7	7
Average Time to Transfer (minutes)[5]	-	-	58	60
Children's Asthma Care				
Received Home Management Plan of Care	-	-	-	88%
Received Reliever Medication	-	-	-	100%
Received Systemic Corticosteroids	-	-	-	100%
Emergency Department				
Admittance Decision Time (minutes)[5]	-	-	65	98
Head CT Results Within 45 Min. of Arrival[5]	-	-	61%	57%
Patients Who Left ER Before Being Seen	5,986	0%	1%	2%
Time from ER Arrival to Admit. (minutes)[5]	-	-	207	274
Time from ER Arrival to Discharge (minutes)[5]	-	-	121	134
Time in ER Before Being Evaluated (minutes)[5]	-	-	19	26
Time to Pain Meds for Fractures (minutes)[5]	-	-	42	57
Heart Attack Care				
Aspirin Given at Discharge[5]	-	-	99%	99%
Fibrinolytic Meds Within 30 Min. of Arrival[5]	-	-	67%	54%
PCI Within 90 Minutes of Arrival[5]	-	-	96%	96%
Statin Prescribed at Discharge[5]	-	-	99%	98%
Heart Failure Care				
ACE Inhibitor or ARB for LVSD[1]	-	-	97%	97%
Discharge Instructions Given	13	92%	96%	94%
Evaluation of LVS Function	22	86%	99%	99%
Medicare Spending				
Medicare Spending per Patient (ratio)	-	-	0.94	0.98
Pneumonia Care				
Appropriate Initial Antibiotic Given	13	100%	96%	95%
Blood Culture Timing	14	93%	98%	98%
Pregnancy and Delivery Care				
Newborn Deliveries Scheduled Early	30	17%	4%	6%
Preventive Care				
Immunization for Influenza	289	96%	90%	90%
Immunization for Pneumonia	330	95%	92%	92%
Stroke Care				
Anticoagulation Therapy for Atrial Fibrillation[1,3]	-	-	94%	95%
Antithrombotic Therapy Timing[1,3]	-	-	99%	98%
Assessed for Rehabilitation[1,3]	-	-	98%	97%
Discharged on Antithrombotic Therapy[1,3]	-	-	99%	99%
Discharged on Statin Medication[1,3]	-	-	94%	94%
Thrombolytic Therapy Timing[3,7]	-	-	60%	66%
Venous Thromboembolism Prophylaxis[1,3]	-	-	95%	94%
Written Stroke Educational Materials Given[1,3]	-	-	88%	88%
Surgical Care Improvement Project				
Appropriate Beta Blocker Usage[1]	-	-	99%	98%
Appropriate VTP Within 24 Hours	31	81%	99%	98%
Controlled Postoperative Blood Glucose[7]	-	-	96%	97%
Perioperative Temperature Management	32	100%	100%	100%
Prophylactic Antibiotic Selection	27	100%	99%	99%
Prophylactic Antibiotic Selection (Outpatient)[5]	-	-	98%	98%
Prophylactic Antibiotic Stopped	25	100%	99%	98%
Prophylactic Antibiotic Timing	27	96%	99%	99%
Prophylactic Antibiotic Timing (Outpatient)[5]	-	-	97%	98%
Urinary Catheter Removal	17	94%	98%	97%
Survey of Patients' Hospital Experiences				
Area Around Room 'Always' Quiet at Night	(a)	69%	63%	61%
Doctors 'Always' Communicated Well	(a)	91%	83%	82%
Home Recovery Information Given	(a)	88%	89%	85%
Hospital Given 9 or 10 on 10 Point Scale	(a)	83%	74%	71%
Meds 'Always' Explained Before Given	(a)	74%	68%	64%
Nurses 'Always' Communicated Well	(a)	89%	82%	79%
Pain 'Always' Well Controlled	(a)	75%	72%	71%
Room and Bathroom 'Always' Clean	(a)	83%	79%	73%
Timely Help 'Always' Received	(a)	87%	72%	68%
Would Definitely Recommend Hospital	(a)	83%	74%	71%
Use of Medical Imaging				
Cardiac Imaging Stress Test before Surgery[1]	-	-	5.4%	5.3%
Combination Abdominal CT Scan[1]	-	-	6.3%	10.5%
Combination Brain/Sinus CT Scan[1]	-	-	2.1%	2.7%
Combination Chest CT Scan[1]	-	-	1%	2.7%
Follow-up Mammogram/Ultrasound	212	10.8%	8.1%	8.8%
Lumbar Spine MRI for Low Back Pain[1]	-	-	34.9%	37.2%

Madison VA Medical Center

2500 Overlook Terrace Phone: 608-256-1901
Madison, WI 53705 Fax: 608-280-7096
URL: www.madison.va.gov
Type: Acute Care - VA Emergency Services: No
Ownership: Government Federal Beds: 87
Key Personnel:
Coronary Care . . . . Karen Anderson, RN
Chief of Medical Staff. . . . . Alan J Bridges, MD
Operating Room. . . . . Tami Essman, RN
Infection Control. . . . . Linda McKinley, RN
Radiology. . . . . James J Vesely, MD
Cardiac Laboratory. . . . . Judith Werner, RN

Measure	Cases	This Hosp.	State Avg.	U.S. Avg.
Blood Clot Prevention and Treatment				
Anticoagulation Overlap Therapy	-	-	95%	93%
ICU Venous Thromboembolism Prophylaxis	-	-	91%	92%
Incidence of Potentially Preventable VTE	-	-	10%	10%
UFH with Dosages/Platelet Monitoring	-	-	96%	97%
Venous Thromboembolism Prophylaxis	-	-	85%	85%

NOTE: Hospital profiles are in alphabetical order by state, then city, then hospital within the city; Rankings exclude hospitals with less than 25 cases except for patient surveys which excludes hospitals with less than 100 cases; (a) 100-299 cases; (1) The number of cases/patients is too few to report; (2) Data submitted were based on a sample of cases/patients; (3) Results are based on a shorter time period than required; (4) Data suppressed by CMS for one or more quarters; (5) Results are not available for this reporting period; (6) Fewer than 100 patients completed the HCAHPS survey; (7) No cases met the criteria for this measure; (8) The lower limit of the confidence interval cannot be calculated if the number of observed infections equals zero; (9) No data are available from the state/territory for this reporting period; (10) The scores shown reflect fewer than 50 completed surveys; (11) There were discrepancies in the data collection process; (12) This measure does not apply to this hospital for this reporting period; (13) Results cannot be calculated for this reporting period; (14) The results for this state are combined with nearby states to protect confidentiality; Please refer to the User's Guide for a full explanation of data.

Measure	Cases	This Hosp.	State Avg.	U.S. Avg.
Warfarin Therapy Discharge Instructions	-	-	70%	75%
Chest Pain/Possible Heart Attack Care				
Aspirin Given Within 24 Hours of Arrival	-	-	98%	96%
Fibrinolytic Meds Within 30 Min. of Arrival	-	-	52%	58%
Average Time to ECG (minutes)	-	-	7	7
Average Time to Transfer (minutes)	-	-	58	60
Children's Asthma Care				
Received Home Management Plan of Care	-	-	-	88%
Received Reliever Medication	-	-	-	100%
Received Systemic Corticosteroids	-	-	-	100%
Emergency Department				
Admittance Decision Time (minutes)	-	-	65	98
Head CT Results Within 45 Min. of Arrival	-	-	61%	57%
Patients Who Left ER Before Being Seen	-	-	1%	2%
Time from ER Arrival to Admit. (minutes)	-	-	207	274
Time from ER Arrival to Discharge (minutes)	-	-	121	134
Time in ER Before Being Evaluated (minutes)	-	-	19	26
Time to Pain Meds for Fractures (minutes)	-	-	42	57
Heart Attack Care				
Aspirin Given at Discharge	58	100%	99%	99%
Fibrinolytic Meds Within 30 Min. of Arrival[5]	-	-	67%	54%
PCI Within 90 Minutes of Arrival[1]	-	-	96%	96%
Statin Prescribed at Discharge	57	100%	99%	98%
Heart Failure Care				
ACE Inhibitor or ARB for LVSD	50	98%	97%	97%
Discharge Instructions Given	159	97%	96%	94%
Evaluation of LVS Function	182	100%	99%	99%
Medicare Spending				
Medicare Spending per Patient (ratio)	-	-	0.94	0.98
Pneumonia Care				
Appropriate Initial Antibiotic Given[1]	18	100%	96%	95%
Blood Culture Timing	67	99%	98%	98%
Pregnancy and Delivery Care				
Newborn Deliveries Scheduled Early	-	-	4%	6%
Preventive Care				
Immunization for Influenza[5]	-	-	90%	90%
Immunization for Pneumonia[5]	-	-	92%	92%
Stroke Care				
Anticoagulation Therapy for Atrial Fibrillation	-	-	94%	95%
Antithrombotic Therapy Timing	-	-	99%	98%
Assessed for Rehabilitation	-	-	98%	97%
Discharged on Antithrombotic Therapy	-	-	99%	99%
Discharged on Statin Medication	-	-	94%	94%
Thrombolytic Therapy Timing	-	-	60%	66%
Venous Thromboembolism Prophylaxis	-	-	95%	94%
Written Stroke Educational Materials Given	-	-	88%	88%
Surgical Care Improvement Project				
Appropriate Beta Blocker Usage[2]	116	99%	99%	98%
Appropriate VTP Within 24 Hours[2]	162	99%	99%	98%
Controlled Postoperative Blood Glucose[2]	37	97%	96%	97%
Perioperative Temperature Management[2]	252	99%	100%	100%
Prophylactic Antibiotic Selection	152	100%	99%	99%
Prophylactic Antibiotic Selection (Outpatient)	-	-	98%	98%
Prophylactic Antibiotic Stopped	150	99%	99%	98%
Prophylactic Antibiotic Timing	152	99%	99%	99%
Prophylactic Antibiotic Timing (Outpatient)	-	-	97%	98%
Urinary Catheter Removal[2]	108	100%	98%	97%
Survey of Patients' Hospital Experiences				
Area Around Room 'Always' Quiet at Night	-	-	63%	61%
Doctors 'Always' Communicated Well	-	-	83%	82%
Home Recovery Information Given	-	-	89%	85%
Hospital Given 9 or 10 on 10 Point Scale	-	-	74%	71%
Meds 'Always' Explained Before Given	-	-	68%	64%
Nurses 'Always' Communicated Well	-	-	82%	79%
Pain 'Always' Well Controlled	-	-	72%	71%
Room and Bathroom 'Always' Clean	-	-	79%	73%
Timely Help 'Always' Received	-	-	72%	68%
Would Definitely Recommend Hospital	-	-	74%	71%
Use of Medical Imaging				
Cardiac Imaging Stress Test before Surgery	-	-	5.4%	5.3%
Combination Abdominal CT Scan	-	-	6.3%	10.5%
Combination Brain/Sinus CT Scan	-	-	2.1%	2.7%
Combination Chest CT Scan	-	-	1%	2.7%
Follow-up Mammogram/Ultrasound	-	-	8.1%	8.8%
Lumbar Spine MRI for Low Back Pain	-	-	34.9%	37.2%

Meriter Hospital

202 S Park St
Madison, WI 53715
URL: www.meriter.com
Phone: 608-417-6000
Fax: 608-417-6568
Type: Acute Care Hospitals
Emergency Services: Yes
Ownership: Voluntary non-profit - Private
Beds: 448

Key Personnel:
Chair/CEO . . . . Virginia Graves
Chief of Medical Staff . . . . Geoffrey Priest, MD
CEO/President . . . . James L Woodward

Measure	Cases	This Hosp.	State Avg.	U.S. Avg.
Blood Clot Prevention and Treatment				
Anticoagulation Overlap Therapy[2]	96	100%	95%	93%
ICU Venous Thromboembolism Prophylaxis[2]	63	95%	91%	92%
Incidence of Potentially Preventable VTE[2]	12	0%	10%	10%
UFH with Dosages/Platelet Monitoring[2]	35	100%	96%	97%
Venous Thromboembolism Prophylaxis[2]	431	88%	85%	85%
Warfarin Therapy Discharge Instructions[2]	74	92%	70%	75%
Chest Pain/Possible Heart Attack Care				
Aspirin Given Within 24 Hours of Arrival[5]	-	-	98%	96%
Fibrinolytic Meds Within 30 Min. of Arrival[5]	-	-	52%	58%
Average Time to ECG (minutes)[5]	-	-	7	7
Average Time to Transfer (minutes)[5]	-	-	58	60
Children's Asthma Care				
Received Home Management Plan of Care	-	-	-	88%
Received Reliever Medication	-	-	-	100%
Received Systemic Corticosteroids	-	-	-	100%
Emergency Department				
Admittance Decision Time (minutes)[2]	482	62	65	98
Head CT Results Within 45 Min. of Arrival[1]	-	-	61%	57%
Patients Who Left ER Before Being Seen	44,764	0%	1%	2%
Time from ER Arrival to Admit. (minutes)[2]	482	190	207	274
Time from ER Arrival to Discharge (minutes)	1,087	105	121	134
Time in ER Before Being Evaluated (minutes)	1,149	10	19	26
Time to Pain Meds for Fractures (minutes)	89	31	42	57
Heart Attack Care				
Aspirin Given at Discharge	325	100%	99%	99%
Fibrinolytic Meds Within 30 Min. of Arrival[7]	-	-	67%	54%
PCI Within 90 Minutes of Arrival	50	94%	96%	96%
Statin Prescribed at Discharge	315	97%	99%	98%
Heart Failure Care				
ACE Inhibitor or ARB for LVSD	71	99%	97%	97%
Discharge Instructions Given	251	99%	96%	94%
Evaluation of LVS Function	307	100%	99%	99%
Medicare Spending				
Medicare Spending per Patient (ratio)	-	0.93	0.94	0.98
Pneumonia Care				
Appropriate Initial Antibiotic Given	136	95%	96%	95%
Blood Culture Timing	174	99%	98%	98%
Pregnancy and Delivery Care				
Newborn Deliveries Scheduled Early[2]	52	0%	4%	6%
Preventive Care				
Immunization for Influenza[2]	637	83%	90%	90%
Immunization for Pneumonia[2]	583	92%	92%	92%
Stroke Care				
Anticoagulation Therapy for Atrial Fibrillation	13	100%	94%	95%
Antithrombotic Therapy Timing	87	98%	99%	98%
Assessed for Rehabilitation	111	100%	98%	97%
Discharged on Antithrombotic Therapy	104	99%	99%	99%
Discharged on Statin Medication	81	98%	94%	94%
Thrombolytic Therapy Timing	23	26%	60%	66%
Venous Thromboembolism Prophylaxis	100	97%	95%	94%
Written Stroke Educational Materials Given	63	92%	88%	88%
Surgical Care Improvement Project				
Appropriate Beta Blocker Usage[2]	206	99%	99%	98%
Appropriate VTP Within 24 Hours[2]	347	98%	99%	98%
Controlled Postoperative Blood Glucose[2]	138	92%	96%	97%
Perioperative Temperature Management[2]	484	100%	100%	100%
Prophylactic Antibiotic Selection[2]	454	100%	99%	99%
Prophylactic Antibiotic Selection (Outpatient)	329	99%	98%	98%
Prophylactic Antibiotic Stopped[2]	445	99%	99%	98%
Prophylactic Antibiotic Timing[2]	454	97%	99%	99%
Prophylactic Antibiotic Timing (Outpatient)	329	97%	97%	98%
Urinary Catheter Removal[2]	182	97%	98%	97%
Survey of Patients' Hospital Experiences				
Area Around Room 'Always' Quiet at Night	300+	59%	63%	61%
Doctors 'Always' Communicated Well	300+	82%	83%	82%
Home Recovery Information Given	300+	87%	89%	85%
Hospital Given 9 or 10 on 10 Point Scale	300+	78%	74%	71%
Meds 'Always' Explained Before Given	300+	68%	68%	64%
Nurses 'Always' Communicated Well	300+	80%	82%	79%
Pain 'Always' Well Controlled	300+	69%	72%	71%
Room and Bathroom 'Always' Clean	300+	77%	79%	73%
Timely Help 'Always' Received	300+	66%	72%	68%
Would Definitely Recommend Hospital	300+	79%	74%	71%
Use of Medical Imaging				
Cardiac Imaging Stress Test before Surgery	180	2.8%	5.4%	5.3%
Combination Abdominal CT Scan	484	5.0%	6.3%	10.5%
Combination Brain/Sinus CT Scan	605	2.0%	2.1%	2.7%
Combination Chest CT Scan	221	1.8%	1%	2.7%
Follow-up Mammogram/Ultrasound[7]	-	-	8.1%	8.8%
Lumbar Spine MRI for Low Back Pain[1]	-	-	34.9%	37.2%

Saint Marys Hospital

700 South Park St
Madison, WI 53715
URL: www.stmarysmadison.com
Phone: 608-251-6100
Fax: 608-258-5711
Type: Acute Care Hospitals
Emergency Services: Yes
Ownership: Voluntary non-profit - Other
Beds: 440

Key Personnel:
Operating Room. . . . . Beverly Beine
Chief of Medical Staff . . . . Joan V Brown, MD
Pediatric In-Patient Care . . . . Diane Buss
CEO/President. . . . . Frank Byrne
Coronary Care . . . . Jody De Rosa
Quality Assurance . . . . Vicki Scheel
Emergency Room . . . . Audra Thompson
Infection Control. . . . . Chuck Zeisser

Measure	Cases	This Hosp.	State Avg.	U.S. Avg.
Blood Clot Prevention and Treatment				
Anticoagulation Overlap Therapy[2]	157	99%	95%	93%
ICU Venous Thromboembolism Prophylaxis[2]	25	96%	91%	92%
Incidence of Potentially Preventable VTE[2]	24	25%	10%	10%
UFH with Dosages/Platelet Monitoring[2]	102	100%	96%	97%
Venous Thromboembolism Prophylaxis[2]	346	87%	85%	85%
Warfarin Therapy Discharge Instructions[2]	125	90%	70%	75%
Chest Pain/Possible Heart Attack Care				
Aspirin Given Within 24 Hours of Arrival[1]	-	-	98%	96%
Fibrinolytic Meds Within 30 Min. of Arrival[3,7]	-	-	52%	58%
Average Time to ECG (minutes)[1]	-	-	7	7
Average Time to Transfer (minutes)[1,3]	-	-	58	60
Children's Asthma Care				
Received Home Management Plan of Care	-	-	-	88%
Received Reliever Medication	-	-	-	100%
Received Systemic Corticosteroids	-	-	-	100%
Emergency Department				
Admittance Decision Time (minutes)[2]	357	67	65	98
Head CT Results Within 45 Min. of Arrival	12	75%	61%	57%
Patients Who Left ER Before Being Seen	49,988	0%	1%	2%
Time from ER Arrival to Admit. (minutes)[2]	361	190	207	274
Time from ER Arrival to Discharge (minutes)	376	108	121	134
Time in ER Before Being Evaluated (minutes)	407	8	19	26
Time to Pain Meds for Fractures (minutes)	152	30	42	57
Heart Attack Care				
Aspirin Given at Discharge	488	100%	99%	99%
Fibrinolytic Meds Within 30 Min. of Arrival[7]	-	-	67%	54%
PCI Within 90 Minutes of Arrival	39	97%	96%	96%
Statin Prescribed at Discharge	487	100%	99%	98%
Heart Failure Care				
ACE Inhibitor or ARB for LVSD	113	95%	97%	97%
Discharge Instructions Given	425	96%	96%	94%
Evaluation of LVS Function	514	100%	99%	99%
Medicare Spending				

NOTE: Hospital profiles are in alphabetical order by state, then city, then hospital within the city; Rankings exclude hospitals with less than 25 cases except for patient surveys which excludes hospitals with less than 100 cases; (a) 100-299 cases; (1) The number of cases/patients is too few to report; (2) Data submitted were based on a sample of cases/patients; (3) Results are based on a shorter time period than required; (4) Data suppressed by CMS for one or more quarters; (5) Results are not available for this reporting period; (6) Fewer than 100 patients completed the HCAHPS survey; (7) No cases met the criteria for this measure; (8) The lower limit of the confidence interval cannot be calculated if the number of observed infections equals zero; (9) No data are available from the state/territory for this reporting period; (10) The scores shown reflect fewer than 50 completed surveys; (11) There were discrepancies in the data collection process; (12) This measure does not apply to this hospital for this reporting period; (13) Results cannot be calculated for this reporting period; (14) The results for this state are combined with nearby states to protect confidentiality; Please refer to the User's Guide for a full explanation of data.

Medicare Spending per Patient (ratio)	-	0.95	0.94	0.98
Pneumonia Care				
Appropriate Initial Antibiotic Given	139	99%	96%	95%
Blood Culture Timing	269	96%	98%	98%
Pregnancy and Delivery Care				
Newborn Deliveries Scheduled Early[2]	53	4%	4%	6%
Preventive Care				
Immunization for Influenza[2]	522	98%	90%	90%
Immunization for Pneumonia[2]	615	97%	92%	92%
Stroke Care				
Anticoagulation Therapy for Atrial Fibrillation	35	86%	94%	95%
Antithrombotic Therapy Timing	172	97%	99%	98%
Assessed for Rehabilitation	227	98%	98%	97%
Discharged on Antithrombotic Therapy	201	100%	99%	99%
Discharged on Statin Medication	160	98%	94%	94%
Thrombolytic Therapy Timing[1]	-	-	60%	66%
Venous Thromboembolism Prophylaxis	218	100%	95%	94%
Written Stroke Educational Materials Given	128	95%	88%	88%
Surgical Care Improvement Project				
Appropriate Beta Blocker Usage[2]	606	100%	99%	98%
Appropriate VTP Within 24 Hours[2]	1,226	99%	99%	98%
Controlled Postoperative Blood Glucose[2]	305	91%	96%	97%
Perioperative Temperature Management[2]	1,400	100%	100%	100%
Prophylactic Antibiotic Selection[2]	1,397	100%	99%	99%
Prophylactic Antibiotic Selection (Outpatient)	932	99%	98%	98%
Prophylactic Antibiotic Stopped[2]	1,376	99%	99%	98%
Prophylactic Antibiotic Timing[2]	1,399	99%	99%	99%
Prophylactic Antibiotic Timing (Outpatient)	931	97%	97%	98%
Urinary Catheter Removal[2]	1,371	99%	98%	97%
Survey of Patients' Hospital Experiences				
Area Around Room 'Always' Quiet at Night[11]	300+	65%	63%	61%
Doctors 'Always' Communicated Well[11]	300+	83%	83%	82%
Home Recovery Information Given[11]	300+	90%	89%	85%
Hospital Given 9 or 10 on 10 Point Scale[11]	300+	80%	74%	71%
Meds 'Always' Explained Before Given[11]	300+	72%	68%	64%
Nurses 'Always' Communicated Well[11]	300+	87%	82%	79%
Pain 'Always' Well Controlled[11]	300+	76%	72%	71%
Room and Bathroom 'Always' Clean[11]	300+	81%	79%	73%
Timely Help 'Always' Received[11]	300+	73%	72%	68%
Would Definitely Recommend Hospital[11]	300+	83%	74%	71%
Use of Medical Imaging				
Cardiac Imaging Stress Test before Surgery	190	1.1%	5.4%	5.3%
Combination Abdominal CT Scan	382	0.8%	6.3%	10.5%
Combination Brain/Sinus CT Scan	602	1.2%	2.1%	2.7%
Combination Chest CT Scan[1]	-	-	1%	2.7%
Follow-up Mammogram/Ultrasound[7]	-	-	8.1%	8.8%
Lumbar Spine MRI for Low Back Pain[1]	-	-	34.9%	37.2%

University of Wisconsin Hospitals & Clinics Authority

600 Highland Avenue
Madison, WI 53792
Phone: 608-263-8991
Fax: 608-263-9830
URL: www.uwhealth.org
Type: Acute Care Hospitals
Emergency Services: Yes
Ownership: Govt - Hospital Dist/Auth
Beds: 592

Key Personnel:
Emergency Room . . . . Joseph Cline, MD
Chief of Medical Staff. . . . . Christopher Green, MD
Radiology. . . . . Thomas Grist
CEO/President. . . . . Donna Katen-Bahansky
Quality Assurance . . . . Mark S Kirschbaum
Infection Control. . . . . Dennis Maki, MD
Anesthesiology. . . . . Robert Pearce, MD
Pediatric Ambulatory Care . . . . . Ellen Wald

Measure	Cases	This Hosp.	State Avg.	U.S. Avg.
Blood Clot Prevention and Treatment				
Anticoagulation Overlap Therapy[2]	161	99%	95%	93%
ICU Venous Thromboembolism Prophylaxis[2]	60	93%	91%	92%
Incidence of Potentially Preventable VTE[2]	61	3%	10%	10%
UFH with Dosages/Platelet Monitoring[2]	121	62%	96%	97%
Venous Thromboembolism Prophylaxis[2]	311	87%	85%	85%
Warfarin Therapy Discharge Instructions[2]	128	70%	70%	75%
Chest Pain/Possible Heart Attack Care				
Aspirin Given Within 24 Hours of Arrival[1,3]	-	-	98%	96%
Fibrinolytic Meds Within 30 Min. of Arrival[5]	-	-	52%	58%
Average Time to ECG (minutes)[1,3]	-	-	7	7
Average Time to Transfer (minutes)[5]	-	-	58	60
Children's Asthma Care				
Received Home Management Plan of Care	-	-	-	88%
Received Reliever Medication	-	-	-	100%
Received Systemic Corticosteroids	-	-	-	100%
Emergency Department				
Admittance Decision Time (minutes)[2]	356	74	65	98
Head CT Results Within 45 Min. of Arrival[1]	-	-	61%	57%
Patients Who Left ER Before Being Seen	46,937	0%	1%	2%
Time from ER Arrival to Admit. (minutes)[2]	366	267	207	274
Time from ER Arrival to Discharge (minutes)	340	196	121	134
Time in ER Before Being Evaluated (minutes)	380	21	19	26
Time to Pain Meds for Fractures (minutes)	108	53	42	57
Heart Attack Care				
Aspirin Given at Discharge[2]	280	100%	99%	99%
Fibrinolytic Meds Within 30 Min. of Arrival[2,7]	-	-	67%	54%
PCI Within 90 Minutes of Arrival[2]	23	96%	96%	96%
Statin Prescribed at Discharge[2]	271	99%	99%	98%
Heart Failure Care				
ACE Inhibitor or ARB for LVSD[2]	98	96%	97%	97%
Discharge Instructions Given[2]	231	99%	96%	94%
Evaluation of LVS Function[2]	269	100%	99%	99%
Medicare Spending				
Medicare Spending per Patient (ratio)	-	0.95	0.94	0.98
Pneumonia Care				
Appropriate Initial Antibiotic Given[2]	37	97%	96%	95%
Blood Culture Timing[2]	72	100%	98%	98%
Pregnancy and Delivery Care				
Newborn Deliveries Scheduled Early[2,7]	-	-	4%	6%
Preventive Care				
Immunization for Influenza[2]	583	97%	90%	90%
Immunization for Pneumonia[2]	588	97%	92%	92%
Stroke Care				
Anticoagulation Therapy for Atrial Fibrillation[2]	13	92%	94%	95%
Antithrombotic Therapy Timing[2]	42	100%	99%	98%
Assessed for Rehabilitation[2]	107	94%	98%	97%
Discharged on Antithrombotic Therapy[2]	70	100%	99%	99%
Discharged on Statin Medication[2]	49	92%	94%	94%
Thrombolytic Therapy Timing[1,2]	-	-	60%	66%
Venous Thromboembolism Prophylaxis[2]	97	94%	95%	94%
Written Stroke Educational Materials Given[2]	62	76%	88%	88%
Surgical Care Improvement Project				
Appropriate Beta Blocker Usage[2]	205	100%	99%	98%
Appropriate VTP Within 24 Hours[2]	384	100%	99%	98%
Controlled Postoperative Blood Glucose[2]	119	92%	96%	97%
Perioperative Temperature Management[2]	530	100%	100%	100%
Prophylactic Antibiotic Selection[2]	368	99%	99%	99%
Prophylactic Antibiotic Selection (Outpatient)	471	99%	98%	98%
Prophylactic Antibiotic Stopped[2]	357	99%	99%	98%
Prophylactic Antibiotic Timing[2]	368	99%	99%	99%
Prophylactic Antibiotic Timing (Outpatient)	303	98%	97%	98%
Urinary Catheter Removal[2]	262	97%	98%	97%
Survey of Patients' Hospital Experiences				
Area Around Room 'Always' Quiet at Night	300+	61%	63%	61%
Doctors 'Always' Communicated Well	300+	82%	83%	82%
Home Recovery Information Given	300+	90%	89%	85%
Hospital Given 9 or 10 on 10 Point Scale	300+	78%	74%	71%
Meds 'Always' Explained Before Given	300+	66%	68%	64%
Nurses 'Always' Communicated Well	300+	83%	82%	79%
Pain 'Always' Well Controlled	300+	75%	72%	71%
Room and Bathroom 'Always' Clean	300+	74%	79%	73%
Timely Help 'Always' Received	300+	70%	72%	68%
Would Definitely Recommend Hospital	300+	85%	74%	71%
Use of Medical Imaging				
Cardiac Imaging Stress Test before Surgery	833	5.5%	5.4%	5.3%
Combination Abdominal CT Scan	2,479	3.6%	6.3%	10.5%
Combination Brain/Sinus CT Scan	1,025	1.6%	2.1%	2.7%
Combination Chest CT Scan	2,402	0.3%	1%	2.7%
Follow-up Mammogram/Ultrasound	2,288	8.1%	8.1%	8.8%
Lumbar Spine MRI for Low Back Pain	274	34.7%	34.9%	37.2%

Holy Family Memorial

2300 Western Ave
Manitowoc, WI 54221
Phone: 920-320-2011
Fax: 920-320-8576
URL: www.hfmhealth.org
Type: Acute Care Hospitals
Emergency Services: Yes
Ownership: Voluntary non-profit - Other
Beds: 303

Key Personnel:
Emergency Room . . . . Mary Coenen
Intensive Care Unit. . . . . Mary Coenen
Chief of Medical Staff . . . . Steven Driggers, MD
Infection Control. . . . . Mike Helgesen
CEO/President. . . . . Mark P. Herzog, FACHE
Quality Assurance . . . . Betty Hove
Operating Room. . . . . Lisa Sherman
Radiology. . . . . Carrie Wasmuth

Measure	Cases	This Hosp.	State Avg.	U.S. Avg.
Blood Clot Prevention and Treatment				
Anticoagulation Overlap Therapy[2]	20	85%	95%	93%
ICU Venous Thromboembolism Prophylaxis[2]	60	72%	91%	92%
Incidence of Potentially Preventable VTE[1,2]	-	-	10%	10%
UFH with Dosages/Platelet Monitoring[1,2]	-	-	96%	97%
Venous Thromboembolism Prophylaxis[2]	188	82%	85%	85%
Warfarin Therapy Discharge Instructions[2]	15	27%	70%	75%
Chest Pain/Possible Heart Attack Care				
Aspirin Given Within 24 Hours of Arrival[1]	-	-	98%	96%
Fibrinolytic Meds Within 30 Min. of Arrival[5]	-	-	52%	58%
Average Time to ECG (minutes)[1]	-	-	7	7
Average Time to Transfer (minutes)[5]	-	-	58	60
Children's Asthma Care				
Received Home Management Plan of Care	-	-	-	88%
Received Reliever Medication	-	-	-	100%
Received Systemic Corticosteroids	-	-	-	100%
Emergency Department				
Admittance Decision Time (minutes)[2]	286	49	65	98
Head CT Results Within 45 Min. of Arrival[1,3]	-	-	61%	57%
Patients Who Left ER Before Being Seen	12,884	0%	1%	2%
Time from ER Arrival to Admit. (minutes)[2]	329	157	207	274
Time from ER Arrival to Discharge (minutes)	376	95	121	134
Time in ER Before Being Evaluated (minutes)	367	23	19	26
Time to Pain Meds for Fractures (minutes)	38	44	42	57
Heart Attack Care				
Aspirin Given at Discharge	66	100%	99%	99%
Fibrinolytic Meds Within 30 Min. of Arrival[1]	-	-	67%	54%
PCI Within 90 Minutes of Arrival	23	87%	96%	96%
Statin Prescribed at Discharge	62	98%	99%	98%
Heart Failure Care				
ACE Inhibitor or ARB for LVSD	21	100%	97%	97%
Discharge Instructions Given	81	99%	96%	94%
Evaluation of LVS Function	104	100%	99%	99%
Medicare Spending				
Medicare Spending per Patient (ratio)	-	0.94	0.94	0.98
Pneumonia Care				
Appropriate Initial Antibiotic Given	46	100%	96%	95%
Blood Culture Timing	85	100%	98%	98%
Pregnancy and Delivery Care				
Newborn Deliveries Scheduled Early	23	0%	4%	6%
Preventive Care				
Immunization for Influenza[2]	296	94%	90%	90%
Immunization for Pneumonia[2]	397	95%	92%	92%
Stroke Care				
Anticoagulation Therapy for Atrial Fibrillation[1]	-	-	94%	95%
Antithrombotic Therapy Timing	36	97%	99%	98%
Assessed for Rehabilitation	35	91%	98%	97%
Discharged on Antithrombotic Therapy	31	97%	99%	99%
Discharged on Statin Medication	27	59%	94%	94%
Thrombolytic Therapy Timing[7]	-	-	60%	66%
Venous Thromboembolism Prophylaxis	38	79%	95%	94%
Written Stroke Educational Materials Given	12	0%	88%	88%
Surgical Care Improvement Project				
Appropriate Beta Blocker Usage	147	93%	99%	98%
Appropriate VTP Within 24 Hours	399	98%	99%	98%
Controlled Postoperative Blood Glucose[7]	-	-	96%	97%
Perioperative Temperature Management	444	100%	100%	100%
Prophylactic Antibiotic Selection	330	97%	99%	99%

NOTE: Hospital profiles are in alphabetical order by state, then city, then hospital within the city; Rankings exclude hospitals with less than 25 cases except for patient surveys which excludes hospitals with less than 100 cases; (a) 100-299 cases; (1) The number of cases/patients is too few to report; (2) Data submitted were based on a sample of cases/patients; (3) Results are based on a shorter time period than required; (4) Data suppressed by CMS for one or more quarters; (5) Results are not available for this reporting period; (6) Fewer than 100 patients completed the HCAHPS survey; (7) No cases met the criteria for this measure; (8) The lower limit of the confidence interval cannot be calculated if the number of observed infections equals zero; (9) No data are available from the state/territory for this reporting period; (10) The scores shown reflect fewer than 50 completed surveys; (11) There were discrepancies in the data collection process; (12) This measure does not apply to this hospital for this reporting period; (13) Results cannot be calculated for this reporting period; (14) The results for this state are combined with nearby states to protect confidentiality; Please refer to the User's Guide for a full explanation of data.

Measure	Cases	This Hosp.	State Avg.	U.S. Avg.
Prophylactic Antibiotic Selection (Outpatient)	97	95%	98%	98%
Prophylactic Antibiotic Stopped	326	98%	99%	98%
Prophylactic Antibiotic Timing	330	99%	99%	99%
Prophylactic Antibiotic Timing (Outpatient)	98	99%	97%	98%
Urinary Catheter Removal	339	99%	98%	97%
Survey of Patients' Hospital Experiences				
Area Around Room 'Always' Quiet at Night	300+	55%	63%	61%
Doctors 'Always' Communicated Well	300+	79%	83%	82%
Home Recovery Information Given	300+	90%	89%	85%
Hospital Given 9 or 10 on 10 Point Scale	300+	71%	74%	71%
Meds 'Always' Explained Before Given	300+	63%	68%	64%
Nurses 'Always' Communicated Well	300+	80%	82%	79%
Pain 'Always' Well Controlled	300+	68%	72%	71%
Room and Bathroom 'Always' Clean	300+	77%	79%	73%
Timely Help 'Always' Received	300+	70%	72%	68%
Would Definitely Recommend Hospital	300+	73%	74%	71%
Use of Medical Imaging				
Cardiac Imaging Stress Test before Surgery	238	7.1%	5.4%	5.3%
Combination Abdominal CT Scan	187	15.5%	6.3%	10.5%
Combination Brain/Sinus CT Scan[1]	-	-	2.1%	2.7%
Combination Chest CT Scan	171	6.4%	1%	2.7%
Follow-up Mammogram/Ultrasound	708	9.2%	8.1%	8.8%
Lumbar Spine MRI for Low Back Pain	93	43.0%	34.9%	37.2%

Bay Area Medical Center

3100 Shore Dr
Marinette, WI 54143
Phone: 715-735-6621
Fax: 715-735-6241
URL: www.bamc.org
Type: Acute Care Hospitals
Emergency Services: Yes
Ownership: Voluntary non-profit - Private
Beds: 99

Key Personnel:
Radiology. . . . . David J Balison
Chair/CEO . . . . Tony Furton
CEO/President. . . . . David Olson

Measure	Cases	This Hosp.	State Avg.	U.S. Avg.
Blood Clot Prevention and Treatment				
Anticoagulation Overlap Therapy[2]	39	100%	95%	93%
ICU Venous Thromboembolism Prophylaxis[2]	55	91%	91%	92%
Incidence of Potentially Preventable VTE[1,2]	-	-	10%	10%
UFH with Dosages/Platelet Monitoring[2]	24	100%	96%	97%
Venous Thromboembolism Prophylaxis[2]	305	82%	85%	85%
Warfarin Therapy Discharge Instructions[2]	27	93%	70%	75%
Chest Pain/Possible Heart Attack Care				
Aspirin Given Within 24 Hours of Arrival	83	99%	98%	96%
Fibrinolytic Meds Within 30 Min. of Arrival[1]	-	-	52%	58%
Average Time to ECG (minutes)	84	4	7	7
Average Time to Transfer (minutes)[1]	-	-	58	60
Children's Asthma Care				
Received Home Management Plan of Care	-	-	-	88%
Received Reliever Medication	-	-	-	100%
Received Systemic Corticosteroids	-	-	-	100%
Emergency Department				
Admittance Decision Time (minutes)[2]	522	70	65	98
Head CT Results Within 45 Min. of Arrival	16	100%	61%	57%
Patients Who Left ER Before Being Seen	21,795	1%	1%	2%
Time from ER Arrival to Admit. (minutes)[2]	522	196	207	274
Time from ER Arrival to Discharge (minutes)	363	106	121	134
Time in ER Before Being Evaluated (minutes)	398	21	19	26
Time to Pain Meds for Fractures (minutes)	76	32	42	57
Heart Attack Care				
Aspirin Given at Discharge	83	98%	99%	99%
Fibrinolytic Meds Within 30 Min. of Arrival[7]	-	-	67%	54%
PCI Within 90 Minutes of Arrival[1]	-	-	96%	96%
Statin Prescribed at Discharge	85	95%	99%	98%
Heart Failure Care				
ACE Inhibitor or ARB for LVSD	36	81%	97%	97%
Discharge Instructions Given	134	93%	96%	94%
Evaluation of LVS Function	174	100%	99%	99%
Medicare Spending				
Medicare Spending per Patient (ratio)	-	0.94	0.94	0.98
Pneumonia Care				
Appropriate Initial Antibiotic Given	68	91%	96%	95%
Blood Culture Timing	101	96%	98%	98%
Pregnancy and Delivery Care				
Newborn Deliveries Scheduled Early	28	0%	4%	6%
Preventive Care				
Immunization for Influenza[2]	378	85%	90%	90%
Immunization for Pneumonia[2]	519	90%	92%	92%
Stroke Care				
Anticoagulation Therapy for Atrial Fibrillation[1]	-	-	94%	95%
Antithrombotic Therapy Timing	30	100%	99%	98%
Assessed for Rehabilitation	33	91%	98%	97%
Discharged on Antithrombotic Therapy	31	100%	99%	99%
Discharged on Statin Medication	27	93%	94%	94%
Thrombolytic Therapy Timing[1]	-	-	60%	66%
Venous Thromboembolism Prophylaxis	31	77%	95%	94%
Written Stroke Educational Materials Given	21	81%	88%	88%
Surgical Care Improvement Project				
Appropriate Beta Blocker Usage	89	99%	99%	98%
Appropriate VTP Within 24 Hours	239	97%	99%	98%
Controlled Postoperative Blood Glucose[7]	-	-	96%	97%
Perioperative Temperature Management	269	100%	100%	100%
Prophylactic Antibiotic Selection	159	100%	99%	99%
Prophylactic Antibiotic Selection (Outpatient)	76	97%	98%	98%
Prophylactic Antibiotic Stopped	153	96%	99%	98%
Prophylactic Antibiotic Timing	159	99%	99%	99%
Prophylactic Antibiotic Timing (Outpatient)	76	100%	97%	98%
Urinary Catheter Removal	125	99%	98%	97%
Survey of Patients' Hospital Experiences				
Area Around Room 'Always' Quiet at Night	300+	64%	63%	61%
Doctors 'Always' Communicated Well	300+	82%	83%	82%
Home Recovery Information Given	300+	84%	89%	85%
Hospital Given 9 or 10 on 10 Point Scale	300+	67%	74%	71%
Meds 'Always' Explained Before Given	300+	66%	68%	64%
Nurses 'Always' Communicated Well	300+	82%	82%	79%
Pain 'Always' Well Controlled	300+	69%	72%	71%
Room and Bathroom 'Always' Clean	300+	76%	79%	73%
Timely Help 'Always' Received	300+	73%	72%	68%
Would Definitely Recommend Hospital	300+	61%	74%	71%
Use of Medical Imaging				
Cardiac Imaging Stress Test before Surgery	226	6.6%	5.4%	5.3%
Combination Abdominal CT Scan	525	4.6%	6.3%	10.5%
Combination Brain/Sinus CT Scan	514	1.4%	2.1%	2.7%
Combination Chest CT Scan	223	1.8%	1%	2.7%
Follow-up Mammogram/Ultrasound	631	5.4%	8.1%	8.8%
Lumbar Spine MRI for Low Back Pain	73	38.4%	34.9%	37.2%

Ministry Saint Josephs Hospital

611 Saint Joseph Ave
Marshfield, WI 54449
Phone: 715-387-7850
Fax: 715-387-5240
E-mail: sjhweb@stjosephs-marshfield.org
URL: www.stjosephs-marshfield.org
Type: Acute Care Hospitals
Emergency Services: Yes
Ownership: Voluntary non-profit - Church
Beds: 500

Key Personnel:
Pediatric Ambulatory Care . . . . . . George J Hoehn, III, DP
Pediatric In-Patient Care . . . . George J Hoehn, III, DP
Quality Assurance . . . . Paul Nedd
CEO/President. . . . . Michael A Schmidt
Infection Control. . . . . Thomas L Sell, MD
Radiology. . . . . Tim Swan, MD
Chief of Medical Staff . . . . Fredrick Wesbrook, MD

Measure	Cases	This Hosp.	State Avg.	U.S. Avg.
Blood Clot Prevention and Treatment				
Anticoagulation Overlap Therapy[2]	154	100%	95%	93%
ICU Venous Thromboembolism Prophylaxis[2]	112	98%	91%	92%
Incidence of Potentially Preventable VTE[2]	45	0%	10%	10%
UFH with Dosages/Platelet Monitoring[2]	150	100%	96%	97%
Venous Thromboembolism Prophylaxis[2]	493	94%	85%	85%
Warfarin Therapy Discharge Instructions[2]	112	97%	70%	75%
Chest Pain/Possible Heart Attack Care				
Aspirin Given Within 24 Hours of Arrival[5]	-	-	98%	96%
Fibrinolytic Meds Within 30 Min. of Arrival[5]	-	-	52%	58%
Average Time to ECG (minutes)[5]	-	-	7	7
Average Time to Transfer (minutes)[5]	-	-	58	60
Children's Asthma Care				
Received Home Management Plan of Care	-	-	-	88%
Received Reliever Medication	-	-	-	100%
Received Systemic Corticosteroids	-	-	-	100%
Emergency Department				
Admittance Decision Time (minutes)[2]	758	65	65	98
Head CT Results Within 45 Min. of Arrival[3,7]	-	-	61%	57%
Patients Who Left ER Before Being Seen	22,095	0%	1%	2%
Time from ER Arrival to Admit. (minutes)[2]	841	182	207	274
Time from ER Arrival to Discharge (minutes)	669	115	121	134
Time in ER Before Being Evaluated (minutes)	514	26	19	26
Time to Pain Meds for Fractures (minutes)	93	44	42	57
Heart Attack Care				
Aspirin Given at Discharge	352	100%	99%	99%
Fibrinolytic Meds Within 30 Min. of Arrival[7]	-	-	67%	54%
PCI Within 90 Minutes of Arrival	31	100%	96%	96%
Statin Prescribed at Discharge	332	100%	99%	98%
Heart Failure Care				
ACE Inhibitor or ARB for LVSD	71	100%	97%	97%
Discharge Instructions Given	327	99%	96%	94%
Evaluation of LVS Function	410	100%	99%	99%
Medicare Spending				
Medicare Spending per Patient (ratio)	-	0.94	0.94	0.98
Pneumonia Care				
Appropriate Initial Antibiotic Given	82	95%	96%	95%
Blood Culture Timing	87	100%	98%	98%
Pregnancy and Delivery Care				
Newborn Deliveries Scheduled Early	77	6%	4%	6%
Preventive Care				
Immunization for Influenza[2]	1,091	97%	90%	90%
Immunization for Pneumonia[2]	1,333	97%	92%	92%
Stroke Care				
Anticoagulation Therapy for Atrial Fibrillation	42	100%	94%	95%
Antithrombotic Therapy Timing	128	100%	99%	98%
Assessed for Rehabilitation	215	100%	98%	97%
Discharged on Antithrombotic Therapy	169	99%	99%	99%
Discharged on Statin Medication	135	99%	94%	94%
Thrombolytic Therapy Timing[1]	-	-	60%	66%
Venous Thromboembolism Prophylaxis	220	97%	95%	94%
Written Stroke Educational Materials Given	91	95%	88%	88%
Surgical Care Improvement Project				
Appropriate Beta Blocker Usage	581	99%	99%	98%
Appropriate VTP Within 24 Hours	1,235	99%	99%	98%
Controlled Postoperative Blood Glucose	273	98%	96%	97%
Perioperative Temperature Management	1,506	100%	100%	100%
Prophylactic Antibiotic Selection	990	99%	99%	99%
Prophylactic Antibiotic Selection (Outpatient)	453	99%	98%	98%
Prophylactic Antibiotic Stopped	965	98%	99%	98%
Prophylactic Antibiotic Timing	991	98%	99%	99%
Prophylactic Antibiotic Timing (Outpatient)	454	100%	97%	98%
Urinary Catheter Removal	803	98%	98%	97%
Survey of Patients' Hospital Experiences				
Area Around Room 'Always' Quiet at Night	300+	47%	63%	61%
Doctors 'Always' Communicated Well	300+	74%	83%	82%
Home Recovery Information Given	300+	88%	89%	85%
Hospital Given 9 or 10 on 10 Point Scale	300+	67%	74%	71%
Meds 'Always' Explained Before Given	300+	66%	68%	64%
Nurses 'Always' Communicated Well	300+	78%	82%	79%
Pain 'Always' Well Controlled	300+	71%	72%	71%
Room and Bathroom 'Always' Clean	300+	73%	79%	73%
Timely Help 'Always' Received	300+	59%	72%	68%
Would Definitely Recommend Hospital	300+	71%	74%	71%
Use of Medical Imaging				
Cardiac Imaging Stress Test before Surgery	389	6.2%	5.4%	5.3%
Combination Abdominal CT Scan	66	4.5%	6.3%	10.5%
Combination Brain/Sinus CT Scan[1]	-	-	2.1%	2.7%
Combination Chest CT Scan[1]	-	-	1%	2.7%
Follow-up Mammogram/Ultrasound[7]	-	-	8.1%	8.8%
Lumbar Spine MRI for Low Back Pain[1]	-	-	34.9%	37.2%

NOTE: Hospital profiles are in alphabetical order by state, then city, then hospital within the city; Rankings exclude hospitals with less than 25 cases except for patient surveys which excludes hospitals with less than 100 cases; (a) 100-299 cases; (1) The number of cases/patients is too few to report; (2) Data submitted were based on a sample of cases/patients; (3) Results are based on a shorter time period than required; (4) Data suppressed by CMS for one or more quarters; (5) Results are not available for this reporting period; (6) Fewer than 100 patients completed the HCAHPS survey; (7) No cases met the criteria for this measure; (8) The lower limit of the confidence interval cannot be calculated if the number of observed infections equals zero; (9) No data are available from the state/territory for this reporting period; (10) The scores shown reflect fewer than 50 completed surveys; (11) There were discrepancies in the data collection process; (12) This measure does not apply to this hospital for this reporting period; (13) Results cannot be calculated for this reporting period; (14) The results for this state are combined with nearby states to protect confidentiality; Please refer to the User's Guide for a full explanation of data.

Mile Bluff Medical Center

1050 Division St
Mauston, WI 53948
Phone: 608-847-6161
Fax: 608-847-6017
Type: Acute Care Hospitals
Emergency Services: Yes
Ownership: Proprietary
Beds: 100
Key Personnel:
CEO/President. . . . . James M O'Keefe

Measure	Cases	This Hosp.	State Avg.	U.S. Avg.
Blood Clot Prevention and Treatment				
Anticoagulation Overlap Therapy	11	91%	95%	93%
ICU Venous Thromboembolism Prophylaxis[7]	-	-	91%	92%
Incidence of Potentially Preventable VTE[7]	-	-	10%	10%
UFH with Dosages/Platelet Monitoring[1]	-	-	96%	97%
Venous Thromboembolism Prophylaxis	523	75%	85%	85%
Warfarin Therapy Discharge Instructions[1]	-	-	70%	75%
Chest Pain/Possible Heart Attack Care				
Aspirin Given Within 24 Hours of Arrival	65	95%	98%	96%
Fibrinolytic Meds Within 30 Min. of Arrival[7]	-	-	52%	58%
Average Time to ECG (minutes)	67	8	7	7
Average Time to Transfer (minutes)[1]	-	-	58	60
Children's Asthma Care				
Received Home Management Plan of Care	-	-	-	88%
Received Reliever Medication	-	-	-	100%
Received Systemic Corticosteroids	-	-	-	100%
Emergency Department				
Admittance Decision Time (minutes)	533	106	65	98
Head CT Results Within 45 Min. of Arrival	11	18%	61%	57%
Patients Who Left ER Before Being Seen	7,523	0%	1%	2%
Time from ER Arrival to Admit. (minutes)	586	203	207	274
Time from ER Arrival to Discharge (minutes)	390	119	121	134
Time in ER Before Being Evaluated (minutes)	423	4	19	26
Time to Pain Meds for Fractures (minutes)	30	40	42	57
Heart Attack Care				
Aspirin Given at Discharge[1]	-	-	99%	99%
Fibrinolytic Meds Within 30 Min. of Arrival[7]	-	-	67%	54%
PCI Within 90 Minutes of Arrival[7]	-	-	96%	96%
Statin Prescribed at Discharge[1]	-	-	99%	98%
Heart Failure Care				
ACE Inhibitor or ARB for LVSD[1]	-	-	97%	97%
Discharge Instructions Given	26	88%	96%	94%
Evaluation of LVS Function	35	89%	99%	99%
Medicare Spending				
Medicare Spending per Patient (ratio)	-	0.84	0.94	0.98
Pneumonia Care				
Appropriate Initial Antibiotic Given	24	79%	96%	95%
Blood Culture Timing	24	96%	98%	98%
Pregnancy and Delivery Care				
Newborn Deliveries Scheduled Early	49	43%	4%	6%
Preventive Care				
Immunization for Influenza	609	95%	90%	90%
Immunization for Pneumonia	712	92%	92%	92%
Stroke Care				
Anticoagulation Therapy for Atrial Fibrillation[1]	-	-	94%	95%
Antithrombotic Therapy Timing[1]	-	-	99%	98%
Assessed for Rehabilitation[1]	-	-	98%	97%
Discharged on Antithrombotic Therapy[1]	-	-	99%	99%
Discharged on Statin Medication[1]	-	-	94%	94%
Thrombolytic Therapy Timing[1]	-	-	60%	66%
Venous Thromboembolism Prophylaxis[1]	-	-	95%	94%
Written Stroke Educational Materials Given[1]	-	-	88%	88%
Surgical Care Improvement Project				
Appropriate Beta Blocker Usage	20	70%	99%	98%
Appropriate VTP Within 24 Hours	40	70%	99%	98%
Controlled Postoperative Blood Glucose[7]	-	-	96%	97%
Perioperative Temperature Management	82	99%	100%	100%
Prophylactic Antibiotic Selection	67	91%	99%	99%
Prophylactic Antibiotic Selection (Outpatient)	62	95%	98%	98%
Prophylactic Antibiotic Stopped	66	94%	99%	98%
Prophylactic Antibiotic Timing	67	97%	99%	99%
Prophylactic Antibiotic Timing (Outpatient)	79	71%	97%	98%
Urinary Catheter Removal	36	78%	98%	97%
Survey of Patients' Hospital Experiences				
Area Around Room 'Always' Quiet at Night	300+	51%	63%	61%
Doctors 'Always' Communicated Well	300+	83%	83%	82%
Home Recovery Information Given	300+	86%	89%	85%
Hospital Given 9 or 10 on 10 Point Scale	300+	66%	74%	71%
Meds 'Always' Explained Before Given	300+	66%	68%	64%
Nurses 'Always' Communicated Well	300+	77%	82%	79%
Pain 'Always' Well Controlled	300+	64%	72%	71%
Room and Bathroom 'Always' Clean	300+	74%	79%	73%
Timely Help 'Always' Received	300+	71%	72%	68%
Would Definitely Recommend Hospital	300+	65%	74%	71%
Use of Medical Imaging				
Cardiac Imaging Stress Test before Surgery	194	2.6%	5.4%	5.3%
Combination Abdominal CT Scan	255	8.2%	6.3%	10.5%
Combination Brain/Sinus CT Scan[1]	-	-	2.1%	2.7%
Combination Chest CT Scan	259	1.5%	1%	2.7%
Follow-up Mammogram/Ultrasound	532	6.8%	8.1%	8.8%
Lumbar Spine MRI for Low Back Pain	41	41.5%	34.9%	37.2%

Memorial Health Center

135 S Gibson St
Medford, WI 54451
Phone: 715-748-8100
Fax: 715-748-8199
URL: www.memhc.com
Type: Critical Access Hospitals
Emergency Services: Yes
Ownership: Voluntary non-profit - Other
Beds: 164
Key Personnel:
Quality Assurance . . . . Carol Ahles
Operating Room. . . . . Erik Branstetter
Chairman/CEO . . . . Bruce Czech
Radiology. . . . . Steve Liegel, MD
CEO/President. . . . . Gregg Olson
Chief of Medical Staff . . . . Mark Reuter
Infection Control. . . . . Jane Schiszik

Measure	Cases	This Hosp.	State Avg.	U.S. Avg.
Blood Clot Prevention and Treatment				
Anticoagulation Overlap Therapy[5]	-	-	95%	93%
ICU Venous Thromboembolism Prophylaxis[5]	-	-	91%	92%
Incidence of Potentially Preventable VTE[5]	-	-	10%	10%
UFH with Dosages/Platelet Monitoring[5]	-	-	96%	97%
Venous Thromboembolism Prophylaxis[5]	-	-	85%	85%
Warfarin Therapy Discharge Instructions[5]	-	-	70%	75%
Chest Pain/Possible Heart Attack Care				
Aspirin Given Within 24 Hours of Arrival	37	100%	98%	96%
Fibrinolytic Meds Within 30 Min. of Arrival[7]	-	-	52%	58%
Average Time to ECG (minutes)	38	4	7	7
Average Time to Transfer (minutes)[1]	-	-	58	60
Children's Asthma Care				
Received Home Management Plan of Care	-	-	-	88%
Received Reliever Medication	-	-	-	100%
Received Systemic Corticosteroids	-	-	-	100%
Emergency Department				
Admittance Decision Time (minutes)[5]	-	-	65	98
Head CT Results Within 45 Min. of Arrival[5]	-	-	61%	57%
Patients Who Left ER Before Being Seen	7,213	0%	1%	2%
Time from ER Arrival to Admit. (minutes)[5]	-	-	207	274
Time from ER Arrival to Discharge (minutes)[5]	-	-	121	134
Time in ER Before Being Evaluated (minutes)[5]	-	-	19	26
Time to Pain Meds for Fractures (minutes)[5]	-	-	42	57
Heart Attack Care				
Aspirin Given at Discharge[5]	-	-	99%	99%
Fibrinolytic Meds Within 30 Min. of Arrival[5]	-	-	67%	54%
PCI Within 90 Minutes of Arrival[5]	-	-	96%	96%
Statin Prescribed at Discharge[5]	-	-	99%	98%
Heart Failure Care				
ACE Inhibitor or ARB for LVSD[1]	-	-	97%	97%
Discharge Instructions Given	13	100%	96%	94%
Evaluation of LVS Function	20	100%	99%	99%
Medicare Spending				
Medicare Spending per Patient (ratio)	-	-	0.94	0.98
Pneumonia Care				
Appropriate Initial Antibiotic Given	21	95%	96%	95%
Blood Culture Timing	31	100%	98%	98%
Pregnancy and Delivery Care				
Newborn Deliveries Scheduled Early[5]	-	-	4%	6%
Preventive Care				
Immunization for Influenza	232	89%	90%	90%
Immunization for Pneumonia	335	92%	92%	92%
Stroke Care				
Anticoagulation Therapy for Atrial Fibrillation[5]	-	-	94%	95%
Antithrombotic Therapy Timing[5]	-	-	99%	98%
Assessed for Rehabilitation[5]	-	-	98%	97%
Discharged on Antithrombotic Therapy[5]	-	-	99%	99%
Discharged on Statin Medication[5]	-	-	94%	94%
Thrombolytic Therapy Timing[5]	-	-	60%	66%
Venous Thromboembolism Prophylaxis[5]	-	-	95%	94%
Written Stroke Educational Materials Given[5]	-	-	88%	88%
Surgical Care Improvement Project				
Appropriate Beta Blocker Usage[1]	-	-	99%	98%
Appropriate VTP Within 24 Hours	37	95%	99%	98%
Controlled Postoperative Blood Glucose[7]	-	-	96%	97%
Perioperative Temperature Management	44	100%	100%	100%
Prophylactic Antibiotic Selection	34	100%	99%	99%
Prophylactic Antibiotic Selection (Outpatient)[1]	-	-	98%	98%
Prophylactic Antibiotic Stopped	34	94%	99%	98%
Prophylactic Antibiotic Timing	34	97%	99%	99%
Prophylactic Antibiotic Timing (Outpatient)[1]	-	-	97%	98%
Urinary Catheter Removal[1]	-	-	98%	97%
Survey of Patients' Hospital Experiences				
Area Around Room 'Always' Quiet at Night	(a)	71%	63%	61%
Doctors 'Always' Communicated Well	(a)	85%	83%	82%
Home Recovery Information Given	(a)	91%	89%	85%
Hospital Given 9 or 10 on 10 Point Scale	(a)	80%	74%	71%
Meds 'Always' Explained Before Given	(a)	78%	68%	64%
Nurses 'Always' Communicated Well	(a)	84%	82%	79%
Pain 'Always' Well Controlled	(a)	76%	72%	71%
Room and Bathroom 'Always' Clean	(a)	80%	79%	73%
Timely Help 'Always' Received	(a)	74%	72%	68%
Would Definitely Recommend Hospital	(a)	72%	74%	71%
Use of Medical Imaging				
Cardiac Imaging Stress Test before Surgery[1]	-	-	5.4%	5.3%
Combination Abdominal CT Scan	156	5.8%	6.3%	10.5%
Combination Brain/Sinus CT Scan[1]	-	-	2.1%	2.7%
Combination Chest CT Scan	120	0.8%	1%	2.7%
Follow-up Mammogram/Ultrasound	325	4.3%	8.1%	8.8%
Lumbar Spine MRI for Low Back Pain[1]	-	-	34.9%	37.2%

Community Memorial Hospital

W180 N8085 Town Hall Rd
Menomonee Falls, WI 53051
Phone: 262-251-1000
Fax: 262-253-7169
E-mail: jkohlbeck@communitymemorial.com
URL: www.communitymemorial.com
Type: Acute Care Hospitals
Emergency Services: Yes
Ownership: Voluntary non-profit - Private
Beds: 237
Key Personnel:
Operating Room. . . . . Saleem Bakhtiar
Infection Control. . . . . Margaret Bell
CEO/President. . . . . William E Bestor
Quality Assurance . . . . Georgeann Ellison
Chief of Medical Staff. . . . . Charles Holmburg, MD
Radiology. . . . . Robert Nichols
Cardiac Laboratory. . . . . Karl Raaum

Measure	Cases	This Hosp.	State Avg.	U.S. Avg.
Blood Clot Prevention and Treatment				
Anticoagulation Overlap Therapy[2]	46	87%	95%	93%
ICU Venous Thromboembolism Prophylaxis[2]	22	86%	91%	92%
Incidence of Potentially Preventable VTE[1,2]	-	-	10%	10%
UFH with Dosages/Platelet Monitoring[2]	14	100%	96%	97%
Venous Thromboembolism Prophylaxis[2]	357	80%	85%	85%
Warfarin Therapy Discharge Instructions[2]	30	73%	70%	75%
Chest Pain/Possible Heart Attack Care				
Aspirin Given Within 24 Hours of Arrival[1]	-	-	98%	96%
Fibrinolytic Meds Within 30 Min. of Arrival[3,7]	-	-	52%	58%
Average Time to ECG (minutes)[1]	-	-	7	7
Average Time to Transfer (minutes)[1,3]	-	-	58	60
Children's Asthma Care				
Received Home Management Plan of Care	-	-	-	88%
Received Reliever Medication	-	-	-	100%
Received Systemic Corticosteroids	-	-	-	100%
Emergency Department				

NOTE: Hospital profiles are in alphabetical order by state, then city, then hospital within the city; Rankings exclude hospitals with less than 25 cases except for patient surveys which excludes hospitals with less than 100 cases; (a) 100-299 cases; (1) The number of cases/patients is too few to report; (2) Data submitted were based on a sample of cases/patients; (3) Results are based on a shorter time period than required; (4) Data suppressed by CMS for one or more quarters; (5) Results are not available for this reporting period; (6) Fewer than 100 patients completed the HCAHPS survey; (7) No cases met the criteria for this measure; (8) The lower limit of the confidence interval cannot be calculated if the number of observed infections equals zero; (9) No data are available from the state/territory for this reporting period; (10) The scores shown reflect fewer than 50 completed surveys; (11) There were discrepancies in the data collection process; (12) This measure does not apply to this hospital for this reporting period; (13) Results cannot be calculated for this reporting period; (14) The results for this state are combined with nearby states to protect confidentiality; Please refer to the User's Guide for a full explanation of data.

Admittance Decision Time (minutes)[2]	589	60	65	98
Head CT Results Within 45 Min. of Arrival	17	53%	61%	57%
Patients Who Left ER Before Being Seen	20,263	0%	1%	2%
Time from ER Arrival to Admit. (minutes)[2]	592	213	207	274
Time from ER Arrival to Discharge (minutes)	371	154	121	134
Time in ER Before Being Evaluated (minutes)	421	16	19	26
Time to Pain Meds for Fractures (minutes)	103	45	42	57
Heart Attack Care				
Aspirin Given at Discharge	117	100%	99%	99%
Fibrinolytic Meds Within 30 Min. of Arrival[7]	-	-	67%	54%
PCI Within 90 Minutes of Arrival	24	96%	96%	96%
Statin Prescribed at Discharge	106	100%	99%	98%
Heart Failure Care				
ACE Inhibitor or ARB for LVSD	53	100%	97%	97%
Discharge Instructions Given	170	99%	96%	94%
Evaluation of LVS Function	226	100%	99%	99%
Medicare Spending				
Medicare Spending per Patient (ratio)	-	1.00	0.94	0.98
Pneumonia Care				
Appropriate Initial Antibiotic Given	114	97%	96%	95%
Blood Culture Timing	202	100%	98%	98%
Pregnancy and Delivery Care				
Newborn Deliveries Scheduled Early	108	6%	4%	6%
Preventive Care				
Immunization for Influenza[2]	559	85%	90%	90%
Immunization for Pneumonia[2]	760	94%	92%	92%
Stroke Care				
Anticoagulation Therapy for Atrial Fibrillation	15	100%	94%	95%
Antithrombotic Therapy Timing	66	100%	99%	98%
Assessed for Rehabilitation	86	100%	98%	97%
Discharged on Antithrombotic Therapy	75	100%	99%	99%
Discharged on Statin Medication	55	96%	94%	94%
Thrombolytic Therapy Timing[1]	-	-	60%	66%
Venous Thromboembolism Prophylaxis	84	92%	95%	94%
Written Stroke Educational Materials Given	35	97%	88%	88%
Surgical Care Improvement Project				
Appropriate Beta Blocker Usage[2]	203	100%	99%	98%
Appropriate VTP Within 24 Hours[2]	427	100%	99%	98%
Controlled Postoperative Blood Glucose[2]	113	96%	96%	97%
Perioperative Temperature Management[2]	636	100%	100%	100%
Prophylactic Antibiotic Selection[2]	475	99%	99%	99%
Prophylactic Antibiotic Selection (Outpatient)	230	97%	98%	98%
Prophylactic Antibiotic Stopped[2]	470	100%	99%	98%
Prophylactic Antibiotic Timing[2]	475	99%	99%	99%
Prophylactic Antibiotic Timing (Outpatient)	229	96%	97%	98%
Urinary Catheter Removal[2]	346	98%	98%	97%
Survey of Patients' Hospital Experiences				
Area Around Room 'Always' Quiet at Night	300+	58%	63%	61%
Doctors 'Always' Communicated Well	300+	80%	83%	82%
Home Recovery Information Given	300+	87%	89%	85%
Hospital Given 9 or 10 on 10 Point Scale	300+	72%	74%	71%
Meds 'Always' Explained Before Given	300+	64%	68%	64%
Nurses 'Always' Communicated Well	300+	79%	82%	79%
Pain 'Always' Well Controlled	300+	71%	72%	71%
Room and Bathroom 'Always' Clean	300+	71%	79%	73%
Timely Help 'Always' Received	300+	64%	72%	68%
Would Definitely Recommend Hospital	300+	74%	74%	71%
Use of Medical Imaging				
Cardiac Imaging Stress Test before Surgery	300	6.3%	5.4%	5.3%
Combination Abdominal CT Scan	412	1.2%	6.3%	10.5%
Combination Brain/Sinus CT Scan	592	0.8%	2.1%	2.7%
Combination Chest CT Scan	426	4.2%	1%	2.7%
Follow-up Mammogram/Ultrasound	193	8.3%	8.1%	8.8%
Lumbar Spine MRI for Low Back Pain	68	29.4%	34.9%	37.2%

Mayo Clinic Health System - Red Cedar

2321 Stout Rd
Menomonie, WI 54751
URL: www.mayohealthsystem.org
Type: Critical Access Hospitals
Ownership: Voluntary non-profit - Private
Phone: 715-235-5531
Fax: 715-233-7645
Emergency Services: Yes
Beds: 25

Key Personnel:
Administrator .... Steve Lindberg
CEO .... Hank Simpson
Chief of Medical Staff .... D Spendsen, MD

Measure	Cases	This Hosp.	State Avg.	U.S. Avg.
Blood Clot Prevention and Treatment				
Anticoagulation Overlap Therapy[5]	-	-	95%	93%
ICU Venous Thromboembolism Prophylaxis[5]	-	-	91%	92%
Incidence of Potentially Preventable VTE[5]	-	-	10%	10%
UFH with Dosages/Platelet Monitoring[5]	-	-	96%	97%
Venous Thromboembolism Prophylaxis[5]	-	-	85%	85%
Warfarin Therapy Discharge Instructions[5]	-	-	70%	75%
Chest Pain/Possible Heart Attack Care				
Aspirin Given Within 24 Hours of Arrival	-	-	98%	96%
Fibrinolytic Meds Within 30 Min. of Arrival	-	-	52%	58%
Average Time to ECG (minutes)	-	-	7	7
Average Time to Transfer (minutes)	-	-	58	60
Children's Asthma Care				
Received Home Management Plan of Care	-	-	-	88%
Received Reliever Medication	-	-	-	100%
Received Systemic Corticosteroids	-	-	-	100%
Emergency Department				
Admittance Decision Time (minutes)[5]	-	-	65	98
Head CT Results Within 45 Min. of Arrival	-	-	61%	57%
Patients Who Left ER Before Being Seen	-	-	1%	2%
Time from ER Arrival to Admit. (minutes)[5]	-	-	207	274
Time from ER Arrival to Discharge (minutes)	-	-	121	134
Time in ER Before Being Evaluated (minutes)	-	-	19	26
Time to Pain Meds for Fractures (minutes)	-	-	42	57
Heart Attack Care				
Aspirin Given at Discharge[1,3]	-	-	99%	99%
Fibrinolytic Meds Within 30 Min. of Arrival[3,7]	-	-	67%	54%
PCI Within 90 Minutes of Arrival[3,7]	-	-	96%	96%
Statin Prescribed at Discharge[1,3]	-	-	99%	98%
Heart Failure Care				
ACE Inhibitor or ARB for LVSD[1]	-	-	97%	97%
Discharge Instructions Given	27	96%	96%	94%
Evaluation of LVS Function	39	100%	99%	99%
Medicare Spending				
Medicare Spending per Patient (ratio)	-	-	0.94	0.98
Pneumonia Care				
Appropriate Initial Antibiotic Given	32	100%	96%	95%
Blood Culture Timing	39	95%	98%	98%
Pregnancy and Delivery Care				
Newborn Deliveries Scheduled Early[5]	-	-	4%	6%
Preventive Care				
Immunization for Influenza[5]	-	-	90%	90%
Immunization for Pneumonia[5]	-	-	92%	92%
Stroke Care				
Anticoagulation Therapy for Atrial Fibrillation[5]	-	-	94%	95%
Antithrombotic Therapy Timing[5]	-	-	99%	98%
Assessed for Rehabilitation[5]	-	-	98%	97%
Discharged on Antithrombotic Therapy[5]	-	-	99%	99%
Discharged on Statin Medication[5]	-	-	94%	94%
Thrombolytic Therapy Timing[5]	-	-	60%	66%
Venous Thromboembolism Prophylaxis[5]	-	-	95%	94%
Written Stroke Educational Materials Given[5]	-	-	88%	88%
Surgical Care Improvement Project				
Appropriate Beta Blocker Usage	25	100%	99%	98%
Appropriate VTP Within 24 Hours[3]	19	95%	99%	98%
Controlled Postoperative Blood Glucose[3,7]	-	-	96%	97%
Perioperative Temperature Management	94	100%	100%	100%
Prophylactic Antibiotic Selection	71	100%	99%	99%
Prophylactic Antibiotic Selection (Outpatient)	-	-	98%	98%
Prophylactic Antibiotic Stopped	70	100%	99%	98%
Prophylactic Antibiotic Timing	71	99%	99%	99%
Prophylactic Antibiotic Timing (Outpatient)	-	-	97%	98%
Urinary Catheter Removal	56	100%	98%	97%
Survey of Patients' Hospital Experiences				
Area Around Room 'Always' Quiet at Night	300+	66%	63%	61%
Doctors 'Always' Communicated Well	300+	87%	83%	82%
Home Recovery Information Given	300+	88%	89%	85%
Hospital Given 9 or 10 on 10 Point Scale	300+	76%	74%	71%
Meds 'Always' Explained Before Given	300+	65%	68%	64%
Nurses 'Always' Communicated Well	300+	79%	82%	79%
Pain 'Always' Well Controlled	300+	70%	72%	71%
Room and Bathroom 'Always' Clean	300+	76%	79%	73%
Timely Help 'Always' Received	300+	74%	72%	68%
Would Definitely Recommend Hospital	300+	77%	74%	71%
Use of Medical Imaging				
Cardiac Imaging Stress Test before Surgery	-	-	5.4%	5.3%
Combination Abdominal CT Scan	-	-	6.3%	10.5%
Combination Brain/Sinus CT Scan	-	-	2.1%	2.7%
Combination Chest CT Scan	-	-	1%	2.7%
Follow-up Mammogram/Ultrasound	-	-	8.1%	8.8%
Lumbar Spine MRI for Low Back Pain	-	-	34.9%	37.2%

Columbia Center

13125 N Port Washington Rd
Mequon, WI 53097
URL: www.columbiacenter.org
Type: Acute Care Hospitals
Ownership: Voluntary non-profit - Private
Phone: 262-243-7408
Emergency Services: No

Measure	Cases	This Hosp.	State Avg.	U.S. Avg.
Blood Clot Prevention and Treatment				
Anticoagulation Overlap Therapy[5]	-	-	95%	93%
ICU Venous Thromboembolism Prophylaxis[5]	-	-	91%	92%
Incidence of Potentially Preventable VTE[5]	-	-	10%	10%
UFH with Dosages/Platelet Monitoring[5]	-	-	96%	97%
Venous Thromboembolism Prophylaxis[5]	-	-	85%	85%
Warfarin Therapy Discharge Instructions[5]	-	-	70%	75%
Chest Pain/Possible Heart Attack Care				
Aspirin Given Within 24 Hours of Arrival[5]	-	-	98%	96%
Fibrinolytic Meds Within 30 Min. of Arrival[5]	-	-	52%	58%
Average Time to ECG (minutes)[5]	-	-	7	7
Average Time to Transfer (minutes)[5]	-	-	58	60
Children's Asthma Care				
Received Home Management Plan of Care	-	-	-	88%
Received Reliever Medication	-	-	-	100%
Received Systemic Corticosteroids	-	-	-	100%
Emergency Department				
Admittance Decision Time (minutes)[5]	-	-	65	98
Head CT Results Within 45 Min. of Arrival[5]	-	-	61%	57%
Patients Who Left ER Before Being Seen[5]	-	-	1%	2%
Time from ER Arrival to Admit. (minutes)[5]	-	-	207	274
Time from ER Arrival to Discharge (minutes)[5]	-	-	121	134
Time in ER Before Being Evaluated (minutes)[5]	-	-	19	26
Time to Pain Meds for Fractures (minutes)[5]	-	-	42	57
Heart Attack Care				
Aspirin Given at Discharge[5]	-	-	99%	99%
Fibrinolytic Meds Within 30 Min. of Arrival[5]	-	-	67%	54%
PCI Within 90 Minutes of Arrival[5]	-	-	96%	96%
Statin Prescribed at Discharge[5]	-	-	99%	98%
Heart Failure Care				
ACE Inhibitor or ARB for LVSD[5]	-	-	97%	97%
Discharge Instructions Given[5]	-	-	96%	94%
Evaluation of LVS Function[5]	-	-	99%	99%
Medicare Spending				
Medicare Spending per Patient (ratio)[1]	-	-	0.94	0.98
Pneumonia Care				
Appropriate Initial Antibiotic Given[5]	-	-	96%	95%
Blood Culture Timing[5]	-	-	98%	98%
Pregnancy and Delivery Care				
Newborn Deliveries Scheduled Early[5]	-	-	4%	6%
Preventive Care				
Immunization for Influenza[5]	-	-	90%	90%
Immunization for Pneumonia[5]	-	-	92%	92%
Stroke Care				
Anticoagulation Therapy for Atrial Fibrillation[5]	-	-	94%	95%
Antithrombotic Therapy Timing[5]	-	-	99%	98%
Assessed for Rehabilitation[5]	-	-	98%	97%
Discharged on Antithrombotic Therapy[5]	-	-	99%	99%
Discharged on Statin Medication[5]	-	-	94%	94%
Thrombolytic Therapy Timing[5]	-	-	60%	66%
Venous Thromboembolism Prophylaxis[5]	-	-	95%	94%
Written Stroke Educational Materials Given[5]	-	-	88%	88%

NOTE: Hospital profiles are in alphabetical order by state, then city, then hospital within the city; Rankings exclude hospitals with less than 25 cases except for patient surveys which excludes hospitals with less than 100 cases; (a) 100-299 cases; (1) The number of cases/patients is too few to report; (2) Data submitted were based on a sample of cases/patients; (3) Results are based on a shorter time period than required; (4) Data suppressed by CMS for one or more quarters; (5) Results are not available for this reporting period; (6) Fewer than 100 patients completed the HCAHPS survey; (7) No cases met the criteria for this measure; (8) The lower limit of the confidence interval cannot be calculated if the number of observed infections equals zero; (9) No data are available from the state/territory for this reporting period; (10) The scores shown reflect fewer than 50 completed surveys; (11) There were discrepancies in the data collection process; (12) This measure does not apply to this hospital for this reporting period; (13) Results cannot be calculated for this reporting period; (14) The results for this state are combined with nearby states to protect confidentiality; Please refer to the User's Guide for a full explanation of data.

Surgical Care Improvement Project				
Appropriate Beta Blocker Usage[5]	-	-	99%	98%
Appropriate VTP Within 24 Hours[5]	-	-	99%	98%
Controlled Postoperative Blood Glucose[5]	-	-	96%	97%
Perioperative Temperature Management[5]	-	-	100%	100%
Prophylactic Antibiotic Selection[5]	-	-	99%	99%
Prophylactic Antibiotic Selection (Outpatient)[5]	-	-	98%	98%
Prophylactic Antibiotic Stopped[5]	-	-	99%	98%
Prophylactic Antibiotic Timing[5]	-	-	99%	99%
Prophylactic Antibiotic Timing (Outpatient)[5]	-	-	97%	98%
Urinary Catheter Removal[5]	-	-	98%	97%
Survey of Patients' Hospital Experiences				
Area Around Room 'Always' Quiet at Night	(a)	75%	63%	61%
Doctors 'Always' Communicated Well	(a)	88%	83%	82%
Home Recovery Information Given	(a)	89%	89%	85%
Hospital Given 9 or 10 on 10 Point Scale	(a)	94%	74%	71%
Meds 'Always' Explained Before Given	(a)	73%	68%	64%
Nurses 'Always' Communicated Well	(a)	88%	82%	79%
Pain 'Always' Well Controlled	(a)	76%	72%	71%
Room and Bathroom 'Always' Clean	(a)	82%	79%	73%
Timely Help 'Always' Received	(a)	79%	72%	68%
Would Definitely Recommend Hospital	(a)	93%	74%	71%
Use of Medical Imaging				
Cardiac Imaging Stress Test before Surgery[7]	-	-	5.4%	5.3%
Combination Abdominal CT Scan[7]	-	-	6.3%	10.5%
Combination Brain/Sinus CT Scan[7]	-	-	2.1%	2.7%
Combination Chest CT Scan[7]	-	-	1%	2.7%
Follow-up Mammogram/Ultrasound[7]	-	-	8.1%	8.8%
Lumbar Spine MRI for Low Back Pain[7]	-	-	34.9%	37.2%

Columbia Saint Marys Hospital Ozaukee

13111 N Port Washington Rd Phone: 262-243-7300
Mequon, WI 53097
URL: www.columbia-stmarys.org
Type: Acute Care Hospitals Emergency Services: Yes
Ownership: Voluntary non-profit - Church
Key Personnel:
CEO/President. . . . . Travis Andersen

Measure	Cases	This Hosp.	State Avg.	U.S. Avg.
Blood Clot Prevention and Treatment				
Anticoagulation Overlap Therapy[2]	56	96%	95%	93%
ICU Venous Thromboembolism Prophylaxis[2]	65	83%	91%	92%
Incidence of Potentially Preventable VTE[1,2]	-	-	10%	10%
UFH with Dosages/Platelet Monitoring[2]	16	100%	96%	97%
Venous Thromboembolism Prophylaxis[2]	325	80%	85%	85%
Warfarin Therapy Discharge Instructions[2]	45	89%	70%	75%
Chest Pain/Possible Heart Attack Care				
Aspirin Given Within 24 Hours of Arrival[5]	-	-	98%	96%
Fibrinolytic Meds Within 30 Min. of Arrival[5]	-	-	52%	58%
Average Time to ECG (minutes)[5]	-	-	7	7
Average Time to Transfer (minutes)[5]	-	-	58	60
Children's Asthma Care				
Received Home Management Plan of Care	-	-	-	88%
Received Reliever Medication	-	-	-	100%
Received Systemic Corticosteroids	-	-	-	100%
Emergency Department				
Admittance Decision Time (minutes)[2]	648	78	65	98
Head CT Results Within 45 Min. of Arrival	13	46%	61%	57%
Patients Who Left ER Before Being Seen	17,354	0%	1%	2%
Time from ER Arrival to Admit. (minutes)[2]	657	208	207	274
Time from ER Arrival to Discharge (minutes)	368	138	121	134
Time in ER Before Being Evaluated (minutes)	406	17	19	26
Time to Pain Meds for Fractures (minutes)	78	56	42	57
Heart Attack Care				
Aspirin Given at Discharge	127	98%	99%	99%
Fibrinolytic Meds Within 30 Min. of Arrival[7]	-	-	67%	54%
PCI Within 90 Minutes of Arrival	24	92%	96%	96%
Statin Prescribed at Discharge	119	97%	99%	98%
Heart Failure Care				
ACE Inhibitor or ARB for LVSD	55	98%	97%	97%
Discharge Instructions Given	125	97%	96%	94%
Evaluation of LVS Function	173	100%	99%	99%
Medicare Spending				
Medicare Spending per Patient (ratio)	-	0.98	0.94	0.98
Pneumonia Care				
Appropriate Initial Antibiotic Given	110	94%	96%	95%
Blood Culture Timing	139	98%	98%	98%
Pregnancy and Delivery Care				
Newborn Deliveries Scheduled Early[7]	-	-	4%	6%
Preventive Care				
Immunization for Influenza[2]	429	93%	90%	90%
Immunization for Pneumonia[2]	680	93%	92%	92%
Stroke Care				
Anticoagulation Therapy for Atrial Fibrillation	20	95%	94%	95%
Antithrombotic Therapy Timing	61	98%	99%	98%
Assessed for Rehabilitation	78	99%	98%	97%
Discharged on Antithrombotic Therapy	72	100%	99%	99%
Discharged on Statin Medication	55	100%	94%	94%
Thrombolytic Therapy Timing[1]	-	-	60%	66%
Venous Thromboembolism Prophylaxis	66	98%	95%	94%
Written Stroke Educational Materials Given	35	100%	88%	88%
Surgical Care Improvement Project				
Appropriate Beta Blocker Usage[2]	110	98%	99%	98%
Appropriate VTP Within 24 Hours[2]	259	95%	99%	98%
Controlled Postoperative Blood Glucose[2]	76	91%	96%	97%
Perioperative Temperature Management[2]	344	100%	100%	100%
Prophylactic Antibiotic Selection[2]	253	99%	99%	99%
Prophylactic Antibiotic Selection (Outpatient)	204	98%	98%	98%
Prophylactic Antibiotic Stopped[2]	239	98%	99%	98%
Prophylactic Antibiotic Timing[2]	253	98%	99%	99%
Prophylactic Antibiotic Timing (Outpatient)	208	86%	97%	98%
Urinary Catheter Removal[2]	285	99%	98%	97%
Survey of Patients' Hospital Experiences				
Area Around Room 'Always' Quiet at Night	300+	62%	63%	61%
Doctors 'Always' Communicated Well	300+	78%	83%	82%
Home Recovery Information Given	300+	86%	89%	85%
Hospital Given 9 or 10 on 10 Point Scale	300+	71%	74%	71%
Meds 'Always' Explained Before Given	300+	63%	68%	64%
Nurses 'Always' Communicated Well	300+	78%	82%	79%
Pain 'Always' Well Controlled	300+	65%	72%	71%
Room and Bathroom 'Always' Clean	300+	66%	79%	73%
Timely Help 'Always' Received	300+	56%	72%	68%
Would Definitely Recommend Hospital	300+	74%	74%	71%
Use of Medical Imaging				
Cardiac Imaging Stress Test before Surgery	294	5.4%	5.4%	5.3%
Combination Abdominal CT Scan	578	6.1%	6.3%	10.5%
Combination Brain/Sinus CT Scan	508	2.0%	2.1%	2.7%
Combination Chest CT Scan	654	1.7%	1%	2.7%
Follow-up Mammogram/Ultrasound	1,536	11.1%	8.1%	8.8%
Lumbar Spine MRI for Low Back Pain	78	38.5%	34.9%	37.2%

Good Samaritan Health Center

601 S Center Ave Phone: 715-536-5511
Merrill, WI 54452 Fax: 715-539-2170
URL: www.ministryhealth.org/GSHC/home.nws
Type: Critical Access Hospitals Emergency Services: Yes
Ownership: Voluntary non-profit - Church Beds: 73
Key Personnel:
CEO/President. . . . . Michael Hammer
Infection Control. . . . . Cheryl Jahns, RN
Operating Room. . . . . Cheryl Johns
Chief of Medical Staff. . . . . Ronald Krajnik
Emergency Room . . . . Jeffrey Moore, MD
Anesthesiology. . . . . James J Schuh, MD

Measure	Cases	This Hosp.	State Avg.	U.S. Avg.
Blood Clot Prevention and Treatment				
Anticoagulation Overlap Therapy[1,2]	-	-	95%	93%
ICU Venous Thromboembolism Prophylaxis[1,2]	-	-	91%	92%
Incidence of Potentially Preventable VTE[1,2]	-	-	10%	10%
UFH with Dosages/Platelet Monitoring[2,7]	-	-	96%	97%
Venous Thromboembolism Prophylaxis[2]	91	100%	85%	85%
Warfarin Therapy Discharge Instructions[1,2]	-	-	70%	75%
Chest Pain/Possible Heart Attack Care				
Aspirin Given Within 24 Hours of Arrival	46	98%	98%	96%
Fibrinolytic Meds Within 30 Min. of Arrival[1,3]	-	-	52%	58%
Average Time to ECG (minutes)	49	7	7	7
Average Time to Transfer (minutes)[1,3]	-	-	58	60
Children's Asthma Care				
Received Home Management Plan of Care	-	-	-	88%
Received Reliever Medication	-	-	-	100%
Received Systemic Corticosteroids	-	-	-	100%
Emergency Department				
Admittance Decision Time (minutes)[2]	443	14	65	98
Head CT Results Within 45 Min. of Arrival[1,3]	-	-	61%	57%
Patients Who Left ER Before Being Seen	6,063	0%	1%	2%
Time from ER Arrival to Admit. (minutes)[2]	453	213	207	274
Time from ER Arrival to Discharge (minutes)	354	126	121	134
Time in ER Before Being Evaluated (minutes)	365	17	19	26
Time to Pain Meds for Fractures (minutes)	31	28	42	57
Heart Attack Care				
Aspirin Given at Discharge[1,3]	-	-	99%	99%
Fibrinolytic Meds Within 30 Min. of Arrival[3,7]	-	-	67%	54%
PCI Within 90 Minutes of Arrival[3,7]	-	-	96%	96%
Statin Prescribed at Discharge[1,3]	-	-	99%	98%
Heart Failure Care				
ACE Inhibitor or ARB for LVSD[1]	-	-	97%	97%
Discharge Instructions Given	18	94%	96%	94%
Evaluation of LVS Function	21	90%	99%	99%
Medicare Spending				
Medicare Spending per Patient (ratio)	-	-	0.94	0.98
Pneumonia Care				
Appropriate Initial Antibiotic Given	30	93%	96%	95%
Blood Culture Timing	47	98%	98%	98%
Pregnancy and Delivery Care				
Newborn Deliveries Scheduled Early[5]	-	-	4%	6%
Preventive Care				
Immunization for Influenza[2]	275	85%	90%	90%
Immunization for Pneumonia[2]	443	87%	92%	92%
Stroke Care				
Anticoagulation Therapy for Atrial Fibrillation[1,3]	-	-	94%	95%
Antithrombotic Therapy Timing[1,3]	-	-	99%	98%
Assessed for Rehabilitation[1,3]	-	-	98%	97%
Discharged on Antithrombotic Therapy[1,3]	-	-	99%	99%
Discharged on Statin Medication[1,3]	-	-	94%	94%
Thrombolytic Therapy Timing[3,7]	-	-	60%	66%
Venous Thromboembolism Prophylaxis[1,3]	-	-	95%	94%
Written Stroke Educational Materials Given[1,3]	-	-	88%	88%
Surgical Care Improvement Project				
Appropriate Beta Blocker Usage	12	100%	99%	98%
Appropriate VTP Within 24 Hours	14	93%	99%	98%
Controlled Postoperative Blood Glucose[7]	-	-	96%	97%
Perioperative Temperature Management	29	100%	100%	100%
Prophylactic Antibiotic Selection	18	94%	99%	99%
Prophylactic Antibiotic Selection (Outpatient)[3,7]	-	-	98%	98%
Prophylactic Antibiotic Stopped	18	100%	99%	98%
Prophylactic Antibiotic Timing	19	89%	99%	99%
Prophylactic Antibiotic Timing (Outpatient)[1,3]	-	-	97%	98%
Urinary Catheter Removal[1]	-	-	98%	97%
Survey of Patients' Hospital Experiences				
Area Around Room 'Always' Quiet at Night	(a)	61%	63%	61%
Doctors 'Always' Communicated Well	(a)	79%	83%	82%
Home Recovery Information Given	(a)	87%	89%	85%
Hospital Given 9 or 10 on 10 Point Scale	(a)	72%	74%	71%
Meds 'Always' Explained Before Given	(a)	71%	68%	64%
Nurses 'Always' Communicated Well	(a)	83%	82%	79%
Pain 'Always' Well Controlled	(a)	65%	72%	71%
Room and Bathroom 'Always' Clean	(a)	82%	79%	73%
Timely Help 'Always' Received	(a)	74%	72%	68%
Would Definitely Recommend Hospital	(a)	70%	74%	71%
Use of Medical Imaging				
Cardiac Imaging Stress Test before Surgery[1]	-	-	5.4%	5.3%
Combination Abdominal CT Scan	147	2.7%	6.3%	10.5%
Combination Brain/Sinus CT Scan[1]	-	-	2.1%	2.7%
Combination Chest CT Scan	63	0.0%	1%	2.7%
Follow-up Mammogram/Ultrasound	292	5.8%	8.1%	8.8%
Lumbar Spine MRI for Low Back Pain[1]	-	-	34.9%	37.2%

NOTE: Hospital profiles are in alphabetical order by state, then city, then hospital within the city; Rankings exclude hospitals with less than 25 cases except for patient surveys which excludes hospitals with less than 100 cases; (a) 100-299 cases; (1) The number of cases/patients is too few to report; (2) Data submitted were based on a sample of cases/patients; (3) Results are based on a shorter time period than required; (4) Data suppressed by CMS for one or more quarters; (5) Results are not available for this reporting period; (6) Fewer than 100 patients completed the HCAHPS survey; (7) No cases met the criteria for this measure; (8) The lower limit of the confidence interval cannot be calculated if the number of observed infections equals zero; (9) No data are available from the state/territory for this reporting period; (10) The scores shown reflect fewer than 50 completed surveys; (11) There were discrepancies in the data collection process; (12) This measure does not apply to this hospital for this reporting period; (13) Results cannot be calculated for this reporting period; (14) The results for this state are combined with nearby states to protect confidentiality; Please refer to the User's Guide for a full explanation of data.

Aurora Saint Lukes Medical Center

2900 W Oklahoma Ave — Phone: 414-649-6000
Milwaukee, WI 53215 — Fax: 414-649-7982
URL: www.aurorahealthcare.org
Type: Acute Care Hospitals — Emergency Services: Yes
Ownership: Voluntary non-profit - Private — Beds: 600
Key Personnel:
CEO/President. . . . . Mark Ambrosius
Infection Control. . . . . Lousie Cunningham
Emergency Room . . . . Heidi J Harkins
Operating Room. . . . . Lisa Hillyer, RN
Quality Assurance . . . . Kathy Ptak
Pediatric Ambulatory Care . . . . . . Ruth Rademacher
Pediatric In-Patient Care . . . . Ruth Rademacher
Chief of Medical Staff. . . . . Ann Tylenda

Measure	Cases	This Hosp.	State Avg.	U.S. Avg.
Blood Clot Prevention and Treatment				
Anticoagulation Overlap Therapy[2]	369	91%	95%	93%
ICU Venous Thromboembolism Prophylaxis[2]	245	93%	91%	92%
Incidence of Potentially Preventable VTE[2]	74	9%	10%	10%
UFH with Dosages/Platelet Monitoring[2]	292	100%	96%	97%
Venous Thromboembolism Prophylaxis[2]	827	77%	85%	85%
Warfarin Therapy Discharge Instructions[2]	270	67%	70%	75%
Chest Pain/Possible Heart Attack Care				
Aspirin Given Within 24 Hours of Arrival[1,3]	-	-	98%	96%
Fibrinolytic Meds Within 30 Min. of Arrival[5]	-	-	52%	58%
Average Time to ECG (minutes)[1,3]	-	-	7	7
Average Time to Transfer (minutes)[5]	-	-	58	60
Children's Asthma Care				
Received Home Management Plan of Care	-	-	-	88%
Received Reliever Medication	-	-	-	100%
Received Systemic Corticosteroids	-	-	-	100%
Emergency Department				
Admittance Decision Time (minutes)[2]	1,696	100	65	98
Head CT Results Within 45 Min. of Arrival[1,3]	-	-	61%	57%
Patients Who Left ER Before Being Seen	>100k	2%	1%	2%
Time from ER Arrival to Admit. (minutes)[2]	1,722	252	207	274
Time from ER Arrival to Discharge (minutes)	1,055	155	121	134
Time in ER Before Being Evaluated (minutes)	978	25	19	26
Time to Pain Meds for Fractures (minutes)	173	53	42	57
Heart Attack Care				
Aspirin Given at Discharge	916	100%	99%	99%
Fibrinolytic Meds Within 30 Min. of Arrival[7]	-	-	67%	54%
PCI Within 90 Minutes of Arrival	111	98%	96%	96%
Statin Prescribed at Discharge	884	100%	99%	98%
Heart Failure Care				
ACE Inhibitor or ARB for LVSD	457	100%	97%	97%
Discharge Instructions Given	1,166	98%	96%	94%
Evaluation of LVS Function	1,387	100%	99%	99%
Medicare Spending				
Medicare Spending per Patient (ratio)	-	0.99	0.94	0.98
Pneumonia Care				
Appropriate Initial Antibiotic Given	540	98%	96%	95%
Blood Culture Timing	1,046	99%	98%	98%
Pregnancy and Delivery Care				
Newborn Deliveries Scheduled Early	181	2%	4%	6%
Preventive Care				
Immunization for Influenza[2]	1,581	89%	90%	90%
Immunization for Pneumonia[2]	2,029	94%	92%	92%
Stroke Care				
Anticoagulation Therapy for Atrial Fibrillation	42	98%	94%	95%
Antithrombotic Therapy Timing	326	100%	99%	98%
Assessed for Rehabilitation	488	100%	98%	97%
Discharged on Antithrombotic Therapy	373	100%	99%	99%
Discharged on Statin Medication	274	98%	94%	94%
Thrombolytic Therapy Timing	17	76%	60%	66%
Venous Thromboembolism Prophylaxis	498	98%	95%	94%
Written Stroke Educational Materials Given	252	96%	88%	88%
Surgical Care Improvement Project				
Appropriate Beta Blocker Usage	1,295	99%	99%	98%
Appropriate VTP Within 24 Hours	2,126	99%	99%	98%
Controlled Postoperative Blood Glucose	892	98%	96%	97%
Perioperative Temperature Management	2,777	100%	100%	100%
Prophylactic Antibiotic Selection	1,862	99%	99%	99%
Prophylactic Antibiotic Selection (Outpatient)	846	97%	98%	98%
Prophylactic Antibiotic Stopped	1,800	99%	99%	98%
Prophylactic Antibiotic Timing	1,862	99%	99%	99%
Prophylactic Antibiotic Timing (Outpatient)	857	97%	97%	98%
Urinary Catheter Removal	1,914	99%	98%	97%
Survey of Patients' Hospital Experiences				
Area Around Room 'Always' Quiet at Night	300+	55%	63%	61%
Doctors 'Always' Communicated Well	300+	80%	83%	82%
Home Recovery Information Given	300+	85%	89%	85%
Hospital Given 9 or 10 on 10 Point Scale	300+	71%	74%	71%
Meds 'Always' Explained Before Given	300+	65%	68%	64%
Nurses 'Always' Communicated Well	300+	79%	82%	79%
Pain 'Always' Well Controlled	300+	71%	72%	71%
Room and Bathroom 'Always' Clean	300+	71%	79%	73%
Timely Help 'Always' Received	300+	63%	72%	68%
Would Definitely Recommend Hospital	300+	73%	74%	71%
Use of Medical Imaging				
Cardiac Imaging Stress Test before Surgery	1,039	5.6%	5.4%	5.3%
Combination Abdominal CT Scan	2,043	9.3%	6.3%	10.5%
Combination Brain/Sinus CT Scan	1,535	3.0%	2.1%	2.7%
Combination Chest CT Scan	1,993	0.8%	1%	2.7%
Follow-up Mammogram/Ultrasound	2,451	10.7%	8.1%	8.8%
Lumbar Spine MRI for Low Back Pain	248	33.5%	34.9%	37.2%

Columbia Saint Marys Hospital Milwaukee

2323 N Lake Dr — Phone: 414-291-1210
Milwaukee, WI 53211 — Fax: 414-291-1048
URL: www.columbia-stmarys.com
Type: Acute Care Hospitals — Emergency Services: Yes
Ownership: Voluntary non-profit - Church — Beds: 314
Key Personnel:
Coronary Care . . . . Andrew W Allen
CEO/President. . . . . Travis Andersen
Quality Assurance . . . . James K Beckmann, Jr
Operating Room. . . . . Jane Ryan

Measure	Cases	This Hosp.	State Avg.	U.S. Avg.
Blood Clot Prevention and Treatment				
Anticoagulation Overlap Therapy[2]	96	99%	95%	93%
ICU Venous Thromboembolism Prophylaxis[2]	139	94%	91%	92%
Incidence of Potentially Preventable VTE[2]	17	24%	10%	10%
UFH with Dosages/Platelet Monitoring[2]	38	100%	96%	97%
Venous Thromboembolism Prophylaxis[2]	234	83%	85%	85%
Warfarin Therapy Discharge Instructions[2]	84	82%	70%	75%
Chest Pain/Possible Heart Attack Care				
Aspirin Given Within 24 Hours of Arrival[5]	-	-	98%	96%
Fibrinolytic Meds Within 30 Min. of Arrival[5]	-	-	52%	58%
Average Time to ECG (minutes)[5]	-	-	7	7
Average Time to Transfer (minutes)[5]	-	-	58	60
Children's Asthma Care				
Received Home Management Plan of Care	-	-	-	88%
Received Reliever Medication	-	-	-	100%
Received Systemic Corticosteroids	-	-	-	100%
Emergency Department				
Admittance Decision Time (minutes)[2]	490	96	65	98
Head CT Results Within 45 Min. of Arrival[1]	-	-	61%	57%
Patients Who Left ER Before Being Seen	57,146	2%	1%	2%
Time from ER Arrival to Admit. (minutes)[2]	498	246	207	274
Time from ER Arrival to Discharge (minutes)	367	144	121	134
Time in ER Before Being Evaluated (minutes)	405	26	19	26
Time to Pain Meds for Fractures (minutes)	93	60	42	57
Heart Attack Care				
Aspirin Given at Discharge	136	100%	99%	99%
Fibrinolytic Meds Within 30 Min. of Arrival[7]	-	-	67%	54%
PCI Within 90 Minutes of Arrival	38	97%	96%	96%
Statin Prescribed at Discharge	138	99%	99%	98%
Heart Failure Care				
ACE Inhibitor or ARB for LVSD	100	99%	97%	97%
Discharge Instructions Given	242	97%	96%	94%
Evaluation of LVS Function	299	100%	99%	99%
Medicare Spending				
Medicare Spending per Patient (ratio)	-	0.95	0.94	0.98
Pneumonia Care				
Appropriate Initial Antibiotic Given	183	98%	96%	95%
Blood Culture Timing	267	98%	98%	98%
Pregnancy and Delivery Care				
Newborn Deliveries Scheduled Early	254	1%	4%	6%
Preventive Care				
Immunization for Influenza[2]	552	81%	90%	90%
Immunization for Pneumonia[2]	539	87%	92%	92%
Stroke Care				
Anticoagulation Therapy for Atrial Fibrillation[1]	-	-	94%	95%
Antithrombotic Therapy Timing	104	100%	99%	98%
Assessed for Rehabilitation	138	100%	98%	97%
Discharged on Antithrombotic Therapy	124	98%	99%	99%
Discharged on Statin Medication	81	99%	94%	94%
Thrombolytic Therapy Timing[1]	-	-	60%	66%
Venous Thromboembolism Prophylaxis	138	100%	95%	94%
Written Stroke Educational Materials Given	60	97%	88%	88%
Surgical Care Improvement Project				
Appropriate Beta Blocker Usage[2]	113	99%	99%	98%
Appropriate VTP Within 24 Hours[2]	268	96%	99%	98%
Controlled Postoperative Blood Glucose[2]	67	94%	96%	97%
Perioperative Temperature Management[2]	335	100%	100%	100%
Prophylactic Antibiotic Selection[2]	241	100%	99%	99%
Prophylactic Antibiotic Selection (Outpatient)	410	97%	98%	98%
Prophylactic Antibiotic Stopped[2]	231	97%	99%	98%
Prophylactic Antibiotic Timing[2]	241	99%	99%	99%
Prophylactic Antibiotic Timing (Outpatient)	403	92%	97%	98%
Urinary Catheter Removal[2]	206	95%	98%	97%
Survey of Patients' Hospital Experiences				
Area Around Room 'Always' Quiet at Night	300+	59%	63%	61%
Doctors 'Always' Communicated Well	300+	81%	83%	82%
Home Recovery Information Given	300+	86%	89%	85%
Hospital Given 9 or 10 on 10 Point Scale	300+	70%	74%	71%
Meds 'Always' Explained Before Given	300+	62%	68%	64%
Nurses 'Always' Communicated Well	300+	77%	82%	79%
Pain 'Always' Well Controlled	300+	70%	72%	71%
Room and Bathroom 'Always' Clean	300+	66%	79%	73%
Timely Help 'Always' Received	300+	59%	72%	68%
Would Definitely Recommend Hospital	300+	75%	74%	71%
Use of Medical Imaging				
Cardiac Imaging Stress Test before Surgery	523	4.2%	5.4%	5.3%
Combination Abdominal CT Scan	778	4.2%	6.3%	10.5%
Combination Brain/Sinus CT Scan	694	2.4%	2.1%	2.7%
Combination Chest CT Scan	746	4.0%	1%	2.7%
Follow-up Mammogram/Ultrasound	2,658	11.2%	8.1%	8.8%
Lumbar Spine MRI for Low Back Pain	149	36.2%	34.9%	37.2%

Froedtert Memorial Lutheran Hospital

9200 W Wisconsin Ave — Phone: 414-805-3000
Milwaukee, WI 53226 — Fax: 414-805-7790
URL: www.froedtert.com
Type: Acute Care Hospitals — Emergency Services: Yes
Ownership: Voluntary non-profit - Private — Beds: 413
Key Personnel:
Chief of Medical Staff. . . . . Lee Biblo, MD
CEO/President. . . . . Catherine Buck, MSN, RN
Infection Control. . . . . Michael Frank, MD
Coronary Care . . . . Safwan Jaradeh, MD
Pediatric Ambulatory Care . . . . . . Robert M Kliegman, MD
Pediatric In-Patient Care . . . . Robert M Kliegman, MD
Quality Assurance . . . . Mary Wolbert
Radiology. . . . . James Youker, MD

Measure	Cases	This Hosp.	State Avg.	U.S. Avg.
Blood Clot Prevention and Treatment				
Anticoagulation Overlap Therapy[2]	176	99%	95%	93%
ICU Venous Thromboembolism Prophylaxis[2]	105	96%	91%	92%
Incidence of Potentially Preventable VTE[2]	56	2%	10%	10%
UFH with Dosages/Platelet Monitoring[2]	167	100%	96%	97%
Venous Thromboembolism Prophylaxis[2]	301	92%	85%	85%
Warfarin Therapy Discharge Instructions[2]	133	69%	70%	75%
Chest Pain/Possible Heart Attack Care				
Aspirin Given Within 24 Hours of Arrival[5]	-	-	98%	96%
Fibrinolytic Meds Within 30 Min. of Arrival[5]	-	-	52%	58%
Average Time to ECG (minutes)[5]	-	-	7	7
Average Time to Transfer (minutes)[5]	-	-	58	60
Children's Asthma Care				

NOTE: Hospital profiles are in alphabetical order by state, then city, then hospital within the city; Rankings exclude hospitals with less than 25 cases except for patient surveys which excludes hospitals with less than 100 cases; (a) 100-299 cases; (1) The number of cases/patients is too few to report; (2) Data submitted were based on a sample of cases/patients; (3) Results are based on a shorter time period than required; (4) Data suppressed by CMS for one or more quarters; (5) Results are not available for this reporting period; (6) Fewer than 100 patients completed the HCAHPS survey; (7) No cases met the criteria for this measure; (8) The lower limit of the confidence interval cannot be calculated if the number of observed infections equals zero; (9) No data are available from the state/territory for this reporting period; (10) The scores shown reflect fewer than 50 completed surveys; (11) There were discrepancies in the data collection process; (12) This measure does not apply to this hospital for this reporting period; (13) Results cannot be calculated for this reporting period; (14) The results for this state are combined with nearby states to protect confidentiality; Please refer to the User's Guide for a full explanation of data.

Measure	Cases	This Hosp.	State Avg.	U.S. Avg.
Received Home Management Plan of Care	-	-	-	88%
Received Reliever Medication	-	-	-	100%
Received Systemic Corticosteroids	-	-	-	100%
Emergency Department				
Admittance Decision Time (minutes)[2]	494	44	65	98
Head CT Results Within 45 Min. of Arrival[3,7]	-	-	61%	57%
Patients Who Left ER Before Being Seen	64,923	3%	1%	2%
Time from ER Arrival to Admit. (minutes)[2]	495	238	207	274
Time from ER Arrival to Discharge (minutes)	371	184	121	134
Time in ER Before Being Evaluated (minutes)	407	17	19	26
Time to Pain Meds for Fractures (minutes)	148	42	42	57
Heart Attack Care				
Aspirin Given at Discharge	216	100%	99%	99%
Fibrinolytic Meds Within 30 Min. of Arrival[7]	-	-	67%	54%
PCI Within 90 Minutes of Arrival	40	95%	96%	96%
Statin Prescribed at Discharge	212	100%	99%	98%
Heart Failure Care				
ACE Inhibitor or ARB for LVSD[2]	112	100%	97%	97%
Discharge Instructions Given[2]	274	99%	96%	94%
Evaluation of LVS Function[2]	313	100%	99%	99%
Medicare Spending				
Medicare Spending per Patient (ratio)	-	0.95	0.94	0.98
Pneumonia Care				
Appropriate Initial Antibiotic Given[2]	72	96%	96%	95%
Blood Culture Timing[2]	170	99%	98%	98%
Pregnancy and Delivery Care				
Newborn Deliveries Scheduled Early	108	5%	4%	6%
Preventive Care				
Immunization for Influenza[2]	572	87%	90%	90%
Immunization for Pneumonia[2]	624	92%	92%	92%
Stroke Care				
Anticoagulation Therapy for Atrial Fibrillation[2]	18	94%	94%	95%
Antithrombotic Therapy Timing[2]	92	100%	99%	98%
Assessed for Rehabilitation[2]	144	99%	98%	97%
Discharged on Antithrombotic Therapy[2]	119	99%	99%	99%
Discharged on Statin Medication[2]	93	99%	94%	94%
Thrombolytic Therapy Timing[1,2]	-	-	60%	66%
Venous Thromboembolism Prophylaxis[2]	144	95%	95%	94%
Written Stroke Educational Materials Given[2]	94	64%	88%	88%
Surgical Care Improvement Project				
Appropriate Beta Blocker Usage[2]	273	100%	99%	98%
Appropriate VTP Within 24 Hours[2]	496	100%	99%	98%
Controlled Postoperative Blood Glucose[2]	141	97%	96%	97%
Perioperative Temperature Management[2]	651	99%	100%	100%
Prophylactic Antibiotic Selection[2]	417	100%	99%	99%
Prophylactic Antibiotic Selection (Outpatient)	619	99%	98%	98%
Prophylactic Antibiotic Stopped[2]	404	99%	99%	98%
Prophylactic Antibiotic Timing[2]	420	97%	99%	99%
Prophylactic Antibiotic Timing (Outpatient)	517	97%	97%	98%
Urinary Catheter Removal[2]	522	99%	98%	97%
Survey of Patients' Hospital Experiences				
Area Around Room 'Always' Quiet at Night	300+	59%	63%	61%
Doctors 'Always' Communicated Well	300+	79%	83%	82%
Home Recovery Information Given	300+	88%	89%	85%
Hospital Given 9 or 10 on 10 Point Scale	300+	80%	74%	71%
Meds 'Always' Explained Before Given	300+	67%	68%	64%
Nurses 'Always' Communicated Well	300+	83%	82%	79%
Pain 'Always' Well Controlled	300+	71%	72%	71%
Room and Bathroom 'Always' Clean	300+	70%	79%	73%
Timely Help 'Always' Received	300+	65%	72%	68%
Would Definitely Recommend Hospital	300+	83%	74%	71%
Use of Medical Imaging				
Cardiac Imaging Stress Test before Surgery	617	6.2%	5.4%	5.3%
Combination Abdominal CT Scan	2,417	6.0%	6.3%	10.5%
Combination Brain/Sinus CT Scan	1,187	3.0%	2.1%	2.7%
Combination Chest CT Scan	2,711	0.0%	1%	2.7%
Follow-up Mammogram/Ultrasound	3,483	6.1%	8.1%	8.8%
Lumbar Spine MRI for Low Back Pain	486	30.9%	34.9%	37.2%

Milwaukee VA Medical Center

5000 W. National Avenue
Milwaukee, WI 53295
Phone: 414-384-2000
URL: www.milwaukee.va.gov
Type: Acute Care - VA
Ownership: Government Federal
Emergency Services: No
Beds: 168

Measure	Cases	This Hosp.	State Avg.	U.S. Avg.
Blood Clot Prevention and Treatment				
Anticoagulation Overlap Therapy	-	-	95%	93%
ICU Venous Thromboembolism Prophylaxis	-	-	91%	92%
Incidence of Potentially Preventable VTE	-	-	10%	10%
UFH with Dosages/Platelet Monitoring	-	-	96%	97%
Venous Thromboembolism Prophylaxis	-	-	85%	85%
Warfarin Therapy Discharge Instructions	-	-	70%	75%
Chest Pain/Possible Heart Attack Care				
Aspirin Given Within 24 Hours of Arrival	-	-	98%	96%
Fibrinolytic Meds Within 30 Min. of Arrival	-	-	52%	58%
Average Time to ECG (minutes)	-	-	7	7
Average Time to Transfer (minutes)	-	-	58	60
Children's Asthma Care				
Received Home Management Plan of Care	-	-	-	88%
Received Reliever Medication	-	-	-	100%
Received Systemic Corticosteroids	-	-	-	100%
Emergency Department				
Admittance Decision Time (minutes)	-	-	65	98
Head CT Results Within 45 Min. of Arrival	-	-	61%	57%
Patients Who Left ER Before Being Seen	-	-	1%	2%
Time from ER Arrival to Admit. (minutes)	-	-	207	274
Time from ER Arrival to Discharge (minutes)	-	-	121	134
Time in ER Before Being Evaluated (minutes)	-	-	19	26
Time to Pain Meds for Fractures (minutes)	-	-	42	57
Heart Attack Care				
Aspirin Given at Discharge	65	98%	99%	99%
Fibrinolytic Meds Within 30 Min. of Arrival[5]	-	-	67%	54%
PCI Within 90 Minutes of Arrival[5]	-	-	96%	96%
Statin Prescribed at Discharge	62	100%	99%	98%
Heart Failure Care				
ACE Inhibitor or ARB for LVSD	101	97%	97%	97%
Discharge Instructions Given	257	100%	96%	94%
Evaluation of LVS Function	279	100%	99%	99%
Medicare Spending				
Medicare Spending per Patient (ratio)	-	-	0.94	0.98
Pneumonia Care				
Appropriate Initial Antibiotic Given	43	93%	96%	95%
Blood Culture Timing	70	97%	98%	98%
Pregnancy and Delivery Care				
Newborn Deliveries Scheduled Early	-	-	4%	6%
Preventive Care				
Immunization for Influenza[5]	-	-	90%	90%
Immunization for Pneumonia[5]	-	-	92%	92%
Stroke Care				
Anticoagulation Therapy for Atrial Fibrillation	-	-	94%	95%
Antithrombotic Therapy Timing	-	-	99%	98%
Assessed for Rehabilitation	-	-	98%	97%
Discharged on Antithrombotic Therapy	-	-	99%	99%
Discharged on Statin Medication	-	-	94%	94%
Thrombolytic Therapy Timing	-	-	60%	66%
Venous Thromboembolism Prophylaxis	-	-	95%	94%
Written Stroke Educational Materials Given	-	-	88%	88%
Surgical Care Improvement Project				
Appropriate Beta Blocker Usage[2]	170	95%	99%	98%
Appropriate VTP Within 24 Hours[2]	265	99%	99%	98%
Controlled Postoperative Blood Glucose[2]	84	98%	96%	97%
Perioperative Temperature Management[2]	347	99%	100%	100%
Prophylactic Antibiotic Selection	279	100%	99%	99%
Prophylactic Antibiotic Selection (Outpatient)	-	-	98%	98%
Prophylactic Antibiotic Stopped	277	99%	99%	98%
Prophylactic Antibiotic Timing	279	99%	99%	99%
Prophylactic Antibiotic Timing (Outpatient)	-	-	97%	98%
Urinary Catheter Removal[2]	284	100%	98%	97%
Survey of Patients' Hospital Experiences				
Area Around Room 'Always' Quiet at Night	-	-	63%	61%
Doctors 'Always' Communicated Well	-	-	83%	82%
Home Recovery Information Given	-	-	89%	85%
Hospital Given 9 or 10 on 10 Point Scale	-	-	74%	71%
Meds 'Always' Explained Before Given	-	-	68%	64%
Nurses 'Always' Communicated Well	-	-	82%	79%
Pain 'Always' Well Controlled	-	-	72%	71%
Room and Bathroom 'Always' Clean	-	-	79%	73%
Timely Help 'Always' Received	-	-	72%	68%
Would Definitely Recommend Hospital	-	-	74%	71%
Use of Medical Imaging				
Cardiac Imaging Stress Test before Surgery	-	-	5.4%	5.3%
Combination Abdominal CT Scan	-	-	6.3%	10.5%
Combination Brain/Sinus CT Scan	-	-	2.1%	2.7%
Combination Chest CT Scan	-	-	1%	2.7%
Follow-up Mammogram/Ultrasound	-	-	8.1%	8.8%
Lumbar Spine MRI for Low Back Pain	-	-	34.9%	37.2%

Wheaton Franciscan Healthcare Saint Francis

3237 S 16th St
Milwaukee, WI 53215
Phone: 414-647-5000
Fax: 414-647-5565
URL: www.mywheaton.org
Type: Acute Care Hospitals
Ownership: Voluntary non-profit - Private
Emergency Services: Yes
Beds: 260

Key Personnel:
Radiology. . . . . Bruce Cardone, MD
Chief of Medical Staff. . . . . Parmod Kumar, MD
Quality Assurance . . . . Joanne Mercer
Pediatric Ambulatory Care . . . . . . Chandra Shivpuri, MD
Infection Control. . . . . Pat Skonieczny, RN
Operating Room. . . . . Jean Tetlaff, RN

Measure	Cases	This Hosp.	State Avg.	U.S. Avg.
Blood Clot Prevention and Treatment				
Anticoagulation Overlap Therapy[2]	79	86%	95%	93%
ICU Venous Thromboembolism Prophylaxis[2]	71	86%	91%	92%
Incidence of Potentially Preventable VTE[2]	24	17%	10%	10%
UFH with Dosages/Platelet Monitoring[2]	56	100%	96%	97%
Venous Thromboembolism Prophylaxis[2]	300	55%	85%	85%
Warfarin Therapy Discharge Instructions[2]	47	34%	70%	75%
Chest Pain/Possible Heart Attack Care				
Aspirin Given Within 24 Hours of Arrival[1,3]	-	-	98%	96%
Fibrinolytic Meds Within 30 Min. of Arrival[5]	-	-	52%	58%
Average Time to ECG (minutes)[1,3]	-	-	7	7
Average Time to Transfer (minutes)[5]	-	-	58	60
Children's Asthma Care				
Received Home Management Plan of Care	-	-	-	88%
Received Reliever Medication	-	-	-	100%
Received Systemic Corticosteroids	-	-	-	100%
Emergency Department				
Admittance Decision Time (minutes)[2]	689	97	65	98
Head CT Results Within 45 Min. of Arrival[1]	-	-	61%	57%
Patients Who Left ER Before Being Seen	48,611	1%	1%	2%
Time from ER Arrival to Admit. (minutes)[2]	689	264	207	274
Time from ER Arrival to Discharge (minutes)	364	164	121	134
Time in ER Before Being Evaluated (minutes)	397	27	19	26
Time to Pain Meds for Fractures (minutes)	47	40	42	57
Heart Attack Care				
Aspirin Given at Discharge	118	98%	99%	99%
Fibrinolytic Meds Within 30 Min. of Arrival[7]	-	-	67%	54%
PCI Within 90 Minutes of Arrival	23	100%	96%	96%
Statin Prescribed at Discharge	124	97%	99%	98%
Heart Failure Care				
ACE Inhibitor or ARB for LVSD	64	100%	97%	97%
Discharge Instructions Given	167	98%	96%	94%
Evaluation of LVS Function	213	98%	99%	99%
Medicare Spending				
Medicare Spending per Patient (ratio)	-	0.96	0.94	0.98
Pneumonia Care				
Appropriate Initial Antibiotic Given[2]	103	98%	96%	95%
Blood Culture Timing[2]	205	99%	98%	98%
Pregnancy and Delivery Care				
Newborn Deliveries Scheduled Early[2]	92	2%	4%	6%
Preventive Care				
Immunization for Influenza[2]	613	92%	90%	90%
Immunization for Pneumonia[2]	794	91%	92%	92%

NOTE: Hospital profiles are in alphabetical order by state, then city, then hospital within the city; Rankings exclude hospitals with less than 25 cases except for patient surveys which excludes hospitals with less than 100 cases; (a) 100-299 cases; (1) The number of cases/patients is too few to report; (2) Data submitted were based on a sample of cases/patients; (3) Results are based on a shorter time period than required; (4) Data suppressed by CMS for one or more quarters; (5) Results are not available for this reporting period; (6) Fewer than 100 patients completed the HCAHPS survey; (7) No cases met the criteria for this measure; (8) The lower limit of the confidence interval cannot be calculated if the number of observed infections equals zero; (9) No data are available from the state/territory for this reporting period; (10) The scores shown reflect fewer than 50 completed surveys; (11) There were discrepancies in the data collection process; (12) This measure does not apply to this hospital for this reporting period; (13) Results cannot be calculated for this reporting period; (14) The results for this state are combined with nearby states to protect confidentiality; Please refer to the User's Guide for a full explanation of data.

Measure	Cases	This Hosp.	State Avg.	U.S. Avg.
Stroke Care				
Anticoagulation Therapy for Atrial Fibrillation	16	69%	94%	95%
Antithrombotic Therapy Timing	69	99%	99%	98%
Assessed for Rehabilitation	84	100%	98%	97%
Discharged on Antithrombotic Therapy	77	99%	99%	99%
Discharged on Statin Medication	65	95%	94%	94%
Thrombolytic Therapy Timing[1]	-	-	60%	66%
Venous Thromboembolism Prophylaxis	79	84%	95%	94%
Written Stroke Educational Materials Given	53	75%	88%	88%
Surgical Care Improvement Project				
Appropriate Beta Blocker Usage	140	97%	99%	98%
Appropriate VTP Within 24 Hours	261	99%	99%	98%
Controlled Postoperative Blood Glucose	54	98%	96%	97%
Perioperative Temperature Management	343	100%	100%	100%
Prophylactic Antibiotic Selection	236	99%	99%	99%
Prophylactic Antibiotic Selection (Outpatient)	123	97%	98%	98%
Prophylactic Antibiotic Stopped	222	97%	99%	98%
Prophylactic Antibiotic Timing	236	99%	99%	99%
Prophylactic Antibiotic Timing (Outpatient)	123	99%	97%	98%
Urinary Catheter Removal	139	94%	98%	97%
Survey of Patients' Hospital Experiences				
Area Around Room 'Always' Quiet at Night	300+	53%	63%	61%
Doctors 'Always' Communicated Well	300+	79%	83%	82%
Home Recovery Information Given	300+	88%	89%	85%
Hospital Given 9 or 10 on 10 Point Scale	300+	67%	74%	71%
Meds 'Always' Explained Before Given	300+	63%	68%	64%
Nurses 'Always' Communicated Well	300+	76%	82%	79%
Pain 'Always' Well Controlled	300+	67%	72%	71%
Room and Bathroom 'Always' Clean	300+	70%	79%	73%
Timely Help 'Always' Received	300+	64%	72%	68%
Would Definitely Recommend Hospital	300+	66%	74%	71%
Use of Medical Imaging				
Cardiac Imaging Stress Test before Surgery	197	7.6%	5.4%	5.3%
Combination Abdominal CT Scan	433	7.2%	6.3%	10.5%
Combination Brain/Sinus CT Scan[1]	-	-	2.1%	2.7%
Combination Chest CT Scan	238	2.1%	1%	2.7%
Follow-up Mammogram/Ultrasound	753	10.9%	8.1%	8.8%
Lumbar Spine MRI for Low Back Pain	83	33.7%	34.9%	37.2%

Wheaton Franciscan Saint Joseph

5000 W Chambers St
Milwaukee, WI 53210
Phone: 414-447-2000
Fax: 414-874-4394
URL: www.wfhealthcare.org
Type: Acute Care Hospitals
Emergency Services: Yes
Ownership: Voluntary non-profit - Church
Beds: 595

Key Personnel:

Cardiac Laboratory. . . . . David Kasun
Infection Control. . . . . Mary Luzinski
Operating Room. . . . . Kathy Madsen
Chief of Medical Staff. . . . . Tod Poremski, MD
CEO/President. . . . . Debra Standridge
Quality Assurance . . . . Patty Vail
Radiology. . . . . Rob Weisbecker

Measure	Cases	This Hosp.	State Avg.	U.S. Avg.
Blood Clot Prevention and Treatment				
Anticoagulation Overlap Therapy[2]	130	84%	95%	93%
ICU Venous Thromboembolism Prophylaxis[2]	73	74%	91%	92%
Incidence of Potentially Preventable VTE[2]	17	6%	10%	10%
UFH with Dosages/Platelet Monitoring[2]	69	99%	96%	97%
Venous Thromboembolism Prophylaxis[2]	334	78%	85%	85%
Warfarin Therapy Discharge Instructions[2]	90	40%	70%	75%
Chest Pain/Possible Heart Attack Care				
Aspirin Given Within 24 Hours of Arrival	21	86%	98%	96%
Fibrinolytic Meds Within 30 Min. of Arrival[5]	-	-	52%	58%
Average Time to ECG (minutes)	22	4	7	7
Average Time to Transfer (minutes)[5]	-	-	58	60
Children's Asthma Care				
Received Home Management Plan of Care	-	-	-	88%
Received Reliever Medication	-	-	-	100%
Received Systemic Corticosteroids	-	-	-	100%
Emergency Department				
Admittance Decision Time (minutes)[2]	650	86	65	98
Head CT Results Within 45 Min. of Arrival	32	84%	61%	57%
Patients Who Left ER Before Being Seen	>100k	2%	1%	2%
Time from ER Arrival to Admit. (minutes)[2]	653	243	207	274
Time from ER Arrival to Discharge (minutes)	387	112	121	134
Time in ER Before Being Evaluated (minutes)	388	20	19	26
Time to Pain Meds for Fractures (minutes)	152	35	42	57
Heart Attack Care				
Aspirin Given at Discharge	299	100%	99%	99%
Fibrinolytic Meds Within 30 Min. of Arrival[7]	-	-	67%	54%
PCI Within 90 Minutes of Arrival	77	90%	96%	96%
Statin Prescribed at Discharge	303	99%	99%	98%
Heart Failure Care				
ACE Inhibitor or ARB for LVSD[2]	135	99%	97%	97%
Discharge Instructions Given[2]	358	99%	96%	94%
Evaluation of LVS Function[2]	410	100%	99%	99%
Medicare Spending				
Medicare Spending per Patient (ratio)	-	0.94	0.94	0.98
Pneumonia Care				
Appropriate Initial Antibiotic Given[2]	129	98%	96%	95%
Blood Culture Timing[2]	227	99%	98%	98%
Pregnancy and Delivery Care				
Newborn Deliveries Scheduled Early	334	2%	4%	6%
Preventive Care				
Immunization for Influenza[2]	610	91%	90%	90%
Immunization for Pneumonia[2]	720	90%	92%	92%
Stroke Care				
Anticoagulation Therapy for Atrial Fibrillation[2]	20	85%	94%	95%
Antithrombotic Therapy Timing[2]	81	100%	99%	98%
Assessed for Rehabilitation[2]	105	98%	98%	97%
Discharged on Antithrombotic Therapy[2]	91	98%	99%	99%
Discharged on Statin Medication[2]	86	95%	94%	94%
Thrombolytic Therapy Timing[2]	18	50%	60%	66%
Venous Thromboembolism Prophylaxis[2]	95	95%	95%	94%
Written Stroke Educational Materials Given[2]	47	72%	88%	88%
Surgical Care Improvement Project				
Appropriate Beta Blocker Usage[2]	282	99%	99%	98%
Appropriate VTP Within 24 Hours[2]	708	100%	99%	98%
Controlled Postoperative Blood Glucose[2]	113	95%	96%	97%
Perioperative Temperature Management[2]	866	100%	100%	100%
Prophylactic Antibiotic Selection[2]	615	100%	99%	99%
Prophylactic Antibiotic Selection (Outpatient)	627	100%	98%	98%
Prophylactic Antibiotic Stopped[2]	602	100%	99%	98%
Prophylactic Antibiotic Timing[2]	616	98%	99%	99%
Prophylactic Antibiotic Timing (Outpatient)	582	97%	97%	98%
Urinary Catheter Removal[2]	532	98%	98%	97%
Survey of Patients' Hospital Experiences				
Area Around Room 'Always' Quiet at Night	300+	63%	63%	61%
Doctors 'Always' Communicated Well	300+	81%	83%	82%
Home Recovery Information Given	300+	85%	89%	85%
Hospital Given 9 or 10 on 10 Point Scale	300+	71%	74%	71%
Meds 'Always' Explained Before Given	300+	64%	68%	64%
Nurses 'Always' Communicated Well	300+	79%	82%	79%
Pain 'Always' Well Controlled	300+	72%	72%	71%
Room and Bathroom 'Always' Clean	300+	71%	79%	73%
Timely Help 'Always' Received	300+	65%	72%	68%
Would Definitely Recommend Hospital	300+	70%	74%	71%
Use of Medical Imaging				
Cardiac Imaging Stress Test before Surgery	645	4.5%	5.4%	5.3%
Combination Abdominal CT Scan	1,074	9.7%	6.3%	10.5%
Combination Brain/Sinus CT Scan	1,070	3.0%	2.1%	2.7%
Combination Chest CT Scan	548	2.4%	1%	2.7%
Follow-up Mammogram/Ultrasound	3,350	9.1%	8.1%	8.8%
Lumbar Spine MRI for Low Back Pain	224	29.0%	34.9%	37.2%

The Monroe Clinic

2005 5th Street
Monroe, WI 53566
Phone: 608-324-1000
Fax: 608-324-1114
E-mail: questions@monroeclinic.org
URL: www.themonroeclinic.org
Type: Acute Care Hospitals
Emergency Services: Yes
Ownership: Voluntary non-profit - Church
Beds: 221

Key Personnel:

Emergency Room . . . . Amy Fargo-Young
Chief of Medical Staff. . . . . John Frey, MD
Operating Room. . . . . Nicholas Maxwell
Quality Assurance . . . . Dorothy White
CEO/President. . . . . Julie Wilke

Measure	Cases	This Hosp.	State Avg.	U.S. Avg.
Blood Clot Prevention and Treatment				
Anticoagulation Overlap Therapy[2]	31	77%	95%	93%
ICU Venous Thromboembolism Prophylaxis[2]	149	87%	91%	92%
Incidence of Potentially Preventable VTE[1,2]	-	-	10%	10%
UFH with Dosages/Platelet Monitoring[1,2]	-	-	96%	97%
Venous Thromboembolism Prophylaxis[2]	722	91%	85%	85%
Warfarin Therapy Discharge Instructions[2]	25	88%	70%	75%
Chest Pain/Possible Heart Attack Care				
Aspirin Given Within 24 Hours of Arrival	14	93%	98%	96%
Fibrinolytic Meds Within 30 Min. of Arrival[3,7]	-	-	52%	58%
Average Time to ECG (minutes)	15	8	7	7
Average Time to Transfer (minutes)[1,3]	-	-	58	60
Children's Asthma Care				
Received Home Management Plan of Care	-	-	-	88%
Received Reliever Medication	-	-	-	100%
Received Systemic Corticosteroids	-	-	-	100%
Emergency Department				
Admittance Decision Time (minutes)[2]	1,226	56	65	98
Head CT Results Within 45 Min. of Arrival[1]	-	-	61%	57%
Patients Who Left ER Before Being Seen	20,480	0%	1%	2%
Time from ER Arrival to Admit. (minutes)[2]	1,256	214	207	274
Time from ER Arrival to Discharge (minutes)	10,422	134	121	134
Time in ER Before Being Evaluated (minutes)	11,678	18	19	26
Time to Pain Meds for Fractures (minutes)	78	50	42	57
Heart Attack Care				
Aspirin Given at Discharge	31	100%	99%	99%
Fibrinolytic Meds Within 30 Min. of Arrival[7]	-	-	67%	54%
PCI Within 90 Minutes of Arrival	14	86%	96%	96%
Statin Prescribed at Discharge	30	97%	99%	98%
Heart Failure Care				
ACE Inhibitor or ARB for LVSD	18	100%	97%	97%
Discharge Instructions Given	68	99%	96%	94%
Evaluation of LVS Function	93	100%	99%	99%
Medicare Spending				
Medicare Spending per Patient (ratio)	-	0.95	0.94	0.98
Pneumonia Care				
Appropriate Initial Antibiotic Given	87	94%	96%	95%
Blood Culture Timing	158	96%	98%	98%
Pregnancy and Delivery Care				
Newborn Deliveries Scheduled Early	38	3%	4%	6%
Preventive Care				
Immunization for Influenza[2]	1,363	74%	90%	90%
Immunization for Pneumonia[2]	1,481	83%	92%	92%
Stroke Care				
Anticoagulation Therapy for Atrial Fibrillation[1]	-	-	94%	95%
Antithrombotic Therapy Timing	18	94%	99%	98%
Assessed for Rehabilitation	21	95%	98%	97%
Discharged on Antithrombotic Therapy	20	100%	99%	99%
Discharged on Statin Medication	16	100%	94%	94%
Thrombolytic Therapy Timing[7]	-	-	60%	66%
Venous Thromboembolism Prophylaxis	22	95%	95%	94%
Written Stroke Educational Materials Given	15	73%	88%	88%
Surgical Care Improvement Project				
Appropriate Beta Blocker Usage	145	99%	99%	98%
Appropriate VTP Within 24 Hours	380	100%	99%	98%
Controlled Postoperative Blood Glucose[7]	-	-	96%	97%
Perioperative Temperature Management	404	100%	100%	100%
Prophylactic Antibiotic Selection	289	99%	99%	99%
Prophylactic Antibiotic Selection (Outpatient)	221	96%	98%	98%
Prophylactic Antibiotic Stopped	279	99%	99%	98%
Prophylactic Antibiotic Timing	289	99%	99%	99%
Prophylactic Antibiotic Timing (Outpatient)	186	94%	97%	98%
Urinary Catheter Removal	195	98%	98%	97%
Survey of Patients' Hospital Experiences				
Area Around Room 'Always' Quiet at Night	300+	69%	63%	61%
Doctors 'Always' Communicated Well	300+	81%	83%	82%
Home Recovery Information Given	300+	90%	89%	85%
Hospital Given 9 or 10 on 10 Point Scale	300+	76%	74%	71%
Meds 'Always' Explained Before Given	300+	71%	68%	64%
Nurses 'Always' Communicated Well	300+	85%	82%	79%
Pain 'Always' Well Controlled	300+	75%	72%	71%

NOTE: Hospital profiles are in alphabetical order by state, then city, then hospital within the city; Rankings exclude hospitals with less than 25 cases except for patient surveys which excludes hospitals with less than 100 cases; (a) 100-299 cases; (1) The number of cases/patients is too few to report; (2) Data submitted were based on a sample of cases/patients; (3) Results are based on a shorter time period than required; (4) Data suppressed by CMS for one or more quarters; (5) Results are not available for this reporting period; (6) Fewer than 100 patients completed the HCAHPS survey; (7) No cases met the criteria for this measure; (8) The lower limit of the confidence interval cannot be calculated if the number of observed infections equals zero; (9) No data are available from the state/territory for this reporting period; (10) The scores shown reflect fewer than 50 completed surveys; (11) There were discrepancies in the data collection process; (12) This measure does not apply to this hospital for this reporting period; (13) Results cannot be calculated for this reporting period; (14) The results for this state are combined with nearby states to protect confidentiality; Please refer to the User's Guide for a full explanation of data.

Room and Bathroom 'Always' Clean	300+	80%	79%	73%
Timely Help 'Always' Received	300+	76%	72%	68%
Would Definitely Recommend Hospital	300+	77%	74%	71%
Use of Medical Imaging				
Cardiac Imaging Stress Test before Surgery	386	5.4%	5.4%	5.3%
Combination Abdominal CT Scan	500	6.6%	6.3%	10.5%
Combination Brain/Sinus CT Scan	455	2.2%	2.1%	2.7%
Combination Chest CT Scan	308	1.3%	1%	2.7%
Follow-up Mammogram/Ultrasound	1,597	7.2%	8.1%	8.8%
Lumbar Spine MRI for Low Back Pain	115	30.4%	34.9%	37.2%

Theda Clark Medical Center

130 2nd St
Neenah, WI 54956
Phone: 920-729-3100
Fax: 920-729-3167
URL: www.thedacare.org
Type: Acute Care Hospitals
Emergency Services: Yes
Ownership: Voluntary non-profit - Private
Beds: 250

Key Personnel:
Operating Room. . . . . Sherry Cheadle
Pediatric Ambulatory Care . . . . . . Eileen Jekot, MD
Pediatric In-Patient Care . . . . Eileen Jekot, MD
Chief of Medical Staff . . . . Steven Knaus, MD
Quality Assurance . . . . Sally Podoski
Radiology. . . . . Thomas Tolly, MD
CEO/President. . . . . John Toussaint, MD

Measure	Cases	This Hosp.	State Avg.	U.S. Avg.
Blood Clot Prevention and Treatment				
Anticoagulation Overlap Therapy[2]	51	92%	95%	93%
ICU Venous Thromboembolism Prophylaxis[2]	59	95%	91%	92%
Incidence of Potentially Preventable VTE[2]	14	7%	10%	10%
UFH with Dosages/Platelet Monitoring[2]	22	100%	96%	97%
Venous Thromboembolism Prophylaxis[2]	284	92%	85%	85%
Warfarin Therapy Discharge Instructions[2]	40	0%	70%	75%
Chest Pain/Possible Heart Attack Care				
Aspirin Given Within 24 Hours of Arrival[1,3]	-	-	98%	96%
Fibrinolytic Meds Within 30 Min. of Arrival[5]	-	-	52%	58%
Average Time to ECG (minutes)[1,3]	-	-	7	7
Average Time to Transfer (minutes)[5]	-	-	58	60
Children's Asthma Care				
Received Home Management Plan of Care[1]	-	-	-	88%
Received Reliever Medication[1]	-	-	-	100%
Received Systemic Corticosteroids[1]	-	-	-	100%
Emergency Department				
Admittance Decision Time (minutes)[2]	340	50	65	98
Head CT Results Within 45 Min. of Arrival[1,3]	-	-	61%	57%
Patients Who Left ER Before Being Seen	16,381	0%	1%	2%
Time from ER Arrival to Admit. (minutes)[2]	350	169	207	274
Time from ER Arrival to Discharge (minutes)	400	113	121	134
Time in ER Before Being Evaluated (minutes)	420	18	19	26
Time to Pain Meds for Fractures (minutes)	107	42	42	57
Heart Attack Care				
Aspirin Given at Discharge	50	100%	99%	99%
Fibrinolytic Meds Within 30 Min. of Arrival[7]	-	-	67%	54%
PCI Within 90 Minutes of Arrival	19	100%	96%	96%
Statin Prescribed at Discharge	50	100%	99%	98%
Heart Failure Care				
ACE Inhibitor or ARB for LVSD	24	100%	97%	97%
Discharge Instructions Given	75	91%	96%	94%
Evaluation of LVS Function	99	99%	99%	99%
Medicare Spending				
Medicare Spending per Patient (ratio)	-	0.94	0.94	0.98
Pneumonia Care				
Appropriate Initial Antibiotic Given	47	98%	96%	95%
Blood Culture Timing	49	92%	98%	98%
Pregnancy and Delivery Care				
Newborn Deliveries Scheduled Early	108	9%	4%	6%
Preventive Care				
Immunization for Influenza[2]	520	87%	90%	90%
Immunization for Pneumonia[2]	526	83%	92%	92%
Stroke Care				
Anticoagulation Therapy for Atrial Fibrillation	21	100%	94%	95%
Antithrombotic Therapy Timing	130	100%	99%	98%
Assessed for Rehabilitation	190	100%	98%	97%
Discharged on Antithrombotic Therapy	131	100%	99%	99%
Discharged on Statin Medication	100	97%	94%	94%
Thrombolytic Therapy Timing[1]	-	-	60%	66%
Venous Thromboembolism Prophylaxis	201	99%	95%	94%
Written Stroke Educational Materials Given	100	98%	88%	88%
Surgical Care Improvement Project				
Appropriate Beta Blocker Usage[2]	110	100%	99%	98%
Appropriate VTP Within 24 Hours[2]	386	98%	99%	98%
Controlled Postoperative Blood Glucose[2,7]	-	-	96%	97%
Perioperative Temperature Management[2]	463	100%	100%	100%
Prophylactic Antibiotic Selection[2]	305	100%	99%	99%
Prophylactic Antibiotic Selection (Outpatient)	546	99%	98%	98%
Prophylactic Antibiotic Stopped[2]	298	96%	99%	98%
Prophylactic Antibiotic Timing[2]	305	99%	99%	99%
Prophylactic Antibiotic Timing (Outpatient)	548	99%	97%	98%
Urinary Catheter Removal[2]	275	95%	98%	97%
Survey of Patients' Hospital Experiences				
Area Around Room 'Always' Quiet at Night	300+	55%	63%	61%
Doctors 'Always' Communicated Well	300+	82%	83%	82%
Home Recovery Information Given	300+	89%	89%	85%
Hospital Given 9 or 10 on 10 Point Scale	300+	76%	74%	71%
Meds 'Always' Explained Before Given	300+	65%	68%	64%
Nurses 'Always' Communicated Well	300+	79%	82%	79%
Pain 'Always' Well Controlled	300+	70%	72%	71%
Room and Bathroom 'Always' Clean	300+	76%	79%	73%
Timely Help 'Always' Received	300+	69%	72%	68%
Would Definitely Recommend Hospital	300+	80%	74%	71%
Use of Medical Imaging				
Cardiac Imaging Stress Test before Surgery	136	5.1%	5.4%	5.3%
Combination Abdominal CT Scan	397	5.8%	6.3%	10.5%
Combination Brain/Sinus CT Scan[1]	-	-	2.1%	2.7%
Combination Chest CT Scan	174	0.0%	1%	2.7%
Follow-up Mammogram/Ultrasound	604	11.9%	8.1%	8.8%
Lumbar Spine MRI for Low Back Pain	50	38.0%	34.9%	37.2%

Memorial Medical Center

216 Sunset Place
Neillsville, WI 54456
Phone: 715-743-3101
Fax: 715-743-6245
Type: Critical Access Hospitals
Emergency Services: Yes
Ownership: Voluntary non-profit - Other
Beds: 28

Key Personnel:
Quality Assurance . . . . Ruth Ann Burris
Emergency Room . . . . Karen King, RN
Operating Room. . . . . Karen King
CEO . . . . Daryn J. Kumar
Chief of Medical Staff. . . . . Timothy Meyer, MD
Infection Control. . . . . Ann Rust

Measure	Cases	This Hosp.	State Avg.	U.S. Avg.
Blood Clot Prevention and Treatment				
Anticoagulation Overlap Therapy[1]	-	-	95%	93%
ICU Venous Thromboembolism Prophylaxis[7]	-	-	91%	92%
Incidence of Potentially Preventable VTE[1]	-	-	10%	10%
UFH with Dosages/Platelet Monitoring[1]	-	-	96%	97%
Venous Thromboembolism Prophylaxis	87	90%	85%	85%
Warfarin Therapy Discharge Instructions[1]	-	-	70%	75%
Chest Pain/Possible Heart Attack Care				
Aspirin Given Within 24 Hours of Arrival	48	98%	98%	96%
Fibrinolytic Meds Within 30 Min. of Arrival[7]	-	-	52%	58%
Average Time to ECG (minutes)	50	5	7	7
Average Time to Transfer (minutes)[1]	-	-	58	60
Children's Asthma Care				
Received Home Management Plan of Care	-	-	-	88%
Received Reliever Medication	-	-	-	100%
Received Systemic Corticosteroids	-	-	-	100%
Emergency Department				
Admittance Decision Time (minutes)	144	65	65	98
Head CT Results Within 45 Min. of Arrival[1,3]	-	-	61%	57%
Patients Who Left ER Before Being Seen[5]	-	-	1%	2%
Time from ER Arrival to Admit. (minutes)	165	203	207	274
Time from ER Arrival to Discharge (minutes)	199	98	121	134
Time in ER Before Being Evaluated (minutes)	230	20	19	26
Time to Pain Meds for Fractures (minutes)	18	41	42	57
Heart Attack Care				
Aspirin Given at Discharge[5]	-	-	99%	99%
Fibrinolytic Meds Within 30 Min. of Arrival[5]	-	-	67%	54%
PCI Within 90 Minutes of Arrival[5]	-	-	96%	96%
Statin Prescribed at Discharge[5]	-	-	99%	98%
Heart Failure Care				
ACE Inhibitor or ARB for LVSD[1]	-	-	97%	97%
Discharge Instructions Given	13	85%	96%	94%
Evaluation of LVS Function	17	100%	99%	99%
Medicare Spending				
Medicare Spending per Patient (ratio)	-	-	0.94	0.98
Pneumonia Care				
Appropriate Initial Antibiotic Given[1]	-	-	96%	95%
Blood Culture Timing[1]	-	-	98%	98%
Pregnancy and Delivery Care				
Newborn Deliveries Scheduled Early[5]	-	-	4%	6%
Preventive Care				
Immunization for Influenza	112	82%	90%	90%
Immunization for Pneumonia	146	87%	92%	92%
Stroke Care				
Anticoagulation Therapy for Atrial Fibrillation[3,7]	-	-	94%	95%
Antithrombotic Therapy Timing[1,3]	-	-	99%	98%
Assessed for Rehabilitation[1,3]	-	-	98%	97%
Discharged on Antithrombotic Therapy[1,3]	-	-	99%	99%
Discharged on Statin Medication[3,7]	-	-	94%	94%
Thrombolytic Therapy Timing[1,3]	-	-	60%	66%
Venous Thromboembolism Prophylaxis[1,3]	-	-	95%	94%
Written Stroke Educational Materials Given[3,7]	-	-	88%	88%
Surgical Care Improvement Project				
Appropriate Beta Blocker Usage[5]	-	-	99%	98%
Appropriate VTP Within 24 Hours[5]	-	-	99%	98%
Controlled Postoperative Blood Glucose[5]	-	-	96%	97%
Perioperative Temperature Management[5]	-	-	100%	100%
Prophylactic Antibiotic Selection[5]	-	-	99%	99%
Prophylactic Antibiotic Selection (Outpatient)[5]	-	-	98%	98%
Prophylactic Antibiotic Stopped[5]	-	-	99%	98%
Prophylactic Antibiotic Timing[5]	-	-	99%	99%
Prophylactic Antibiotic Timing (Outpatient)[5]	-	-	97%	98%
Urinary Catheter Removal[5]	-	-	98%	97%
Survey of Patients' Hospital Experiences				
Area Around Room 'Always' Quiet at Night[6]	<100	72%	63%	61%
Doctors 'Always' Communicated Well[6]	<100	85%	83%	82%
Home Recovery Information Given[6]	<100	89%	89%	85%
Hospital Given 9 or 10 on 10 Point Scale[6]	<100	71%	74%	71%
Meds 'Always' Explained Before Given[6]	<100	74%	68%	64%
Nurses 'Always' Communicated Well[6]	<100	80%	82%	79%
Pain 'Always' Well Controlled[6]	<100	69%	72%	71%
Room and Bathroom 'Always' Clean[6]	<100	88%	79%	73%
Timely Help 'Always' Received[6]	<100	76%	72%	68%
Would Definitely Recommend Hospital[6]	<100	70%	74%	71%
Use of Medical Imaging				
Cardiac Imaging Stress Test before Surgery[1]	-	-	5.4%	5.3%
Combination Abdominal CT Scan[1]	-	-	6.3%	10.5%
Combination Brain/Sinus CT Scan[1]	-	-	2.1%	2.7%
Combination Chest CT Scan[1]	-	-	1%	2.7%
Follow-up Mammogram/Ultrasound[1]	-	-	8.1%	8.8%
Lumbar Spine MRI for Low Back Pain[1]	-	-	34.9%	37.2%

New London Family Medical Center

1405 Mill St
New London, WI 54961
Phone: 920-531-2000
Fax: 920-531-2098
E-mail: dmente@ahs.fv.org
URL: www.thedacare.org
Type: Critical Access Hospitals
Emergency Services: Yes
Ownership: Voluntary non-profit - Private
Beds: 75

Key Personnel:
CEO/President. . . . . Paul Gurgel
Quality Assurance . . . . Barb Neely
Emergency Room . . . . Randy Schoenrock
Intensive Care Unit. . . . . Randy Shoenrock

Measure	Cases	This Hosp.	State Avg.	U.S. Avg.
Blood Clot Prevention and Treatment				
Anticoagulation Overlap Therapy[5]	-	-	95%	93%
ICU Venous Thromboembolism Prophylaxis[5]	-	-	91%	92%
Incidence of Potentially Preventable VTE[5]	-	-	10%	10%

NOTE: Hospital profiles are in alphabetical order by state, then city, then hospital within the city; Rankings exclude hospitals with less than 25 cases except for patient surveys which excludes hospitals with less than 100 cases; (a) 100-299 cases; (1) The number of cases/patients is too few to report; (2) Data submitted were based on a sample of cases/patients; (3) Results are based on a shorter time period than required; (4) Data suppressed by CMS for one or more quarters; (5) Results are not available for this reporting period; (6) Fewer than 100 patients completed the HCAHPS survey; (7) No cases met the criteria for this measure; (8) The lower limit of the confidence interval cannot be calculated if the number of observed infections equals zero; (9) No data are available from the state/territory for this reporting period; (10) The scores shown reflect fewer than 50 completed surveys; (11) There were discrepancies in the data collection process; (12) This measure does not apply to this hospital for this reporting period; (13) Results cannot be calculated for this reporting period; (14) The results for this state are combined with nearby states to protect confidentiality; Please refer to the User's Guide for a full explanation of data.

Measure	Cases	This Hosp.	State Avg.	U.S. Avg.
UFH with Dosages/Platelet Monitoring[5]	-	-	96%	97%
Venous Thromboembolism Prophylaxis[5]	-	-	85%	85%
Warfarin Therapy Discharge Instructions[5]	-	-	70%	75%
Chest Pain/Possible Heart Attack Care				
Aspirin Given Within 24 Hours of Arrival[5]	-	-	98%	96%
Fibrinolytic Meds Within 30 Min. of Arrival[5]	-	-	52%	58%
Average Time to ECG (minutes)[5]	-	-	7	7
Average Time to Transfer (minutes)[5]	-	-	58	60
Children's Asthma Care				
Received Home Management Plan of Care	-	-	-	88%
Received Reliever Medication	-	-	-	100%
Received Systemic Corticosteroids	-	-	-	100%
Emergency Department				
Admittance Decision Time (minutes)[5]	-	-	65	98
Head CT Results Within 45 Min. of Arrival[5]	-	-	61%	57%
Patients Who Left ER Before Being Seen	8,792	0%	1%	2%
Time from ER Arrival to Admit. (minutes)[5]	-	-	207	274
Time from ER Arrival to Discharge (minutes)[5]	-	-	121	134
Time in ER Before Being Evaluated (minutes)[5]	-	-	19	26
Time to Pain Meds for Fractures (minutes)[5]	-	-	42	57
Heart Attack Care				
Aspirin Given at Discharge[5]	-	-	99%	99%
Fibrinolytic Meds Within 30 Min. of Arrival[5]	-	-	67%	54%
PCI Within 90 Minutes of Arrival[5]	-	-	96%	96%
Statin Prescribed at Discharge[5]	-	-	99%	98%
Heart Failure Care				
ACE Inhibitor or ARB for LVSD[1]	-	-	97%	97%
Discharge Instructions Given	23	91%	96%	94%
Evaluation of LVS Function	36	86%	99%	99%
Medicare Spending				
Medicare Spending per Patient (ratio)	-	-	0.94	0.98
Pneumonia Care				
Appropriate Initial Antibiotic Given	50	98%	96%	95%
Blood Culture Timing	37	95%	98%	98%
Pregnancy and Delivery Care				
Newborn Deliveries Scheduled Early[5]	-	-	4%	6%
Preventive Care				
Immunization for Influenza[5]	-	-	90%	90%
Immunization for Pneumonia[5]	-	-	92%	92%
Stroke Care				
Anticoagulation Therapy for Atrial Fibrillation[5]	-	-	94%	95%
Antithrombotic Therapy Timing[5]	-	-	99%	98%
Assessed for Rehabilitation[5]	-	-	98%	97%
Discharged on Antithrombotic Therapy[5]	-	-	99%	99%
Discharged on Statin Medication[5]	-	-	94%	94%
Thrombolytic Therapy Timing[5]	-	-	60%	66%
Venous Thromboembolism Prophylaxis[5]	-	-	95%	94%
Written Stroke Educational Materials Given[5]	-	-	88%	88%
Surgical Care Improvement Project				
Appropriate Beta Blocker Usage[5]	-	-	99%	98%
Appropriate VTP Within 24 Hours[5]	-	-	99%	98%
Controlled Postoperative Blood Glucose[5]	-	-	96%	97%
Perioperative Temperature Management[5]	-	-	100%	100%
Prophylactic Antibiotic Selection[5]	-	-	99%	99%
Prophylactic Antibiotic Selection (Outpatient)[5]	-	-	98%	98%
Prophylactic Antibiotic Stopped[5]	-	-	99%	98%
Prophylactic Antibiotic Timing[5]	-	-	99%	99%
Prophylactic Antibiotic Timing (Outpatient)[5]	-	-	97%	98%
Urinary Catheter Removal[5]	-	-	98%	97%
Survey of Patients' Hospital Experiences				
Area Around Room 'Always' Quiet at Night	(a)	57%	63%	61%
Doctors 'Always' Communicated Well	(a)	81%	83%	82%
Home Recovery Information Given	(a)	89%	89%	85%
Hospital Given 9 or 10 on 10 Point Scale	(a)	62%	74%	71%
Meds 'Always' Explained Before Given	(a)	59%	68%	64%
Nurses 'Always' Communicated Well	(a)	75%	82%	79%
Pain 'Always' Well Controlled	(a)	64%	72%	71%
Room and Bathroom 'Always' Clean	(a)	80%	79%	73%
Timely Help 'Always' Received	(a)	66%	72%	68%
Would Definitely Recommend Hospital	(a)	56%	74%	71%
Use of Medical Imaging				
Cardiac Imaging Stress Test before Surgery[1]	-	-	5.4%	5.3%
Combination Abdominal CT Scan	200	6.0%	6.3%	10.5%
Combination Brain/Sinus CT Scan[1]	-	-	2.1%	2.7%
Combination Chest CT Scan	99	2.0%	1%	2.7%
Follow-up Mammogram/Ultrasound	297	9.1%	8.1%	8.8%
Lumbar Spine MRI for Low Back Pain[1]	-	-	34.9%	37.2%

Westfields Hospital

535 Hospital Rd
New Richmond, WI 54017
Phone: 715-246-2101
Fax: 715-243-7203
Type: Critical Access Hospitals
Emergency Services: Yes
Ownership: Voluntary non-profit - Private
Beds: 227

Key Personnel:

Radiology.................... Todd M Arsenault
Emergency Room .... David De Gear, MD
Chief of Medical Staff.......... David O DeGear, MD
Infection Control.............. Charlene Mayry, RN
Quality Assurance .... Charlene Mayry, RN
Operating Room.............. Michael Melby

Measure	Cases	This Hosp.	State Avg.	U.S. Avg.
Blood Clot Prevention and Treatment				
Anticoagulation Overlap Therapy[5]	-	-	95%	93%
ICU Venous Thromboembolism Prophylaxis[5]	-	-	91%	92%
Incidence of Potentially Preventable VTE[5]	-	-	10%	10%
UFH with Dosages/Platelet Monitoring[5]	-	-	96%	97%
Venous Thromboembolism Prophylaxis[5]	-	-	85%	85%
Warfarin Therapy Discharge Instructions[5]	-	-	70%	75%
Chest Pain/Possible Heart Attack Care				
Aspirin Given Within 24 Hours of Arrival[5]	-	-	98%	96%
Fibrinolytic Meds Within 30 Min. of Arrival[5]	-	-	52%	58%
Average Time to ECG (minutes)[5]	-	-	7	7
Average Time to Transfer (minutes)[5]	-	-	58	60
Children's Asthma Care				
Received Home Management Plan of Care	-	-	-	88%
Received Reliever Medication	-	-	-	100%
Received Systemic Corticosteroids	-	-	-	100%
Emergency Department				
Admittance Decision Time (minutes)[5]	-	-	65	98
Head CT Results Within 45 Min. of Arrival[5]	-	-	61%	57%
Patients Who Left ER Before Being Seen[5]	-	-	1%	2%
Time from ER Arrival to Admit. (minutes)[5]	-	-	207	274
Time from ER Arrival to Discharge (minutes)[5]	-	-	121	134
Time in ER Before Being Evaluated (minutes)[5]	-	-	19	26
Time to Pain Meds for Fractures (minutes)[5]	-	-	42	57
Heart Attack Care				
Aspirin Given at Discharge[5]	-	-	99%	99%
Fibrinolytic Meds Within 30 Min. of Arrival[5]	-	-	67%	54%
PCI Within 90 Minutes of Arrival[5]	-	-	96%	96%
Statin Prescribed at Discharge[5]	-	-	99%	98%
Heart Failure Care				
ACE Inhibitor or ARB for LVSD[1]	-	-	97%	97%
Discharge Instructions Given	16	75%	96%	94%
Evaluation of LVS Function	22	100%	99%	99%
Medicare Spending				
Medicare Spending per Patient (ratio)	-	-	0.94	0.98
Pneumonia Care				
Appropriate Initial Antibiotic Given	19	89%	96%	95%
Blood Culture Timing	28	93%	98%	98%
Pregnancy and Delivery Care				
Newborn Deliveries Scheduled Early[5]	-	-	4%	6%
Preventive Care				
Immunization for Influenza[5]	-	-	90%	90%
Immunization for Pneumonia[5]	-	-	92%	92%
Stroke Care				
Anticoagulation Therapy for Atrial Fibrillation[5]	-	-	94%	95%
Antithrombotic Therapy Timing[5]	-	-	99%	98%
Assessed for Rehabilitation[5]	-	-	98%	97%
Discharged on Antithrombotic Therapy[5]	-	-	99%	99%
Discharged on Statin Medication[5]	-	-	94%	94%
Thrombolytic Therapy Timing[5]	-	-	60%	66%
Venous Thromboembolism Prophylaxis[5]	-	-	95%	94%
Written Stroke Educational Materials Given[5]	-	-	88%	88%
Surgical Care Improvement Project				
Appropriate Beta Blocker Usage	37	100%	99%	98%
Appropriate VTP Within 24 Hours	126	97%	99%	98%
Controlled Postoperative Blood Glucose[3,7]	-	-	96%	97%
Perioperative Temperature Management	138	99%	100%	100%
Prophylactic Antibiotic Selection	97	98%	99%	99%
Prophylactic Antibiotic Selection (Outpatient)[5]	-	-	98%	98%
Prophylactic Antibiotic Stopped	96	99%	99%	98%
Prophylactic Antibiotic Timing	97	95%	99%	99%
Prophylactic Antibiotic Timing (Outpatient)[5]	-	-	97%	98%
Urinary Catheter Removal	103	99%	98%	97%
Survey of Patients' Hospital Experiences				
Area Around Room 'Always' Quiet at Night	300+	63%	63%	61%
Doctors 'Always' Communicated Well	300+	82%	83%	82%
Home Recovery Information Given	300+	87%	89%	85%
Hospital Given 9 or 10 on 10 Point Scale	300+	71%	74%	71%
Meds 'Always' Explained Before Given	300+	63%	68%	64%
Nurses 'Always' Communicated Well	300+	77%	82%	79%
Pain 'Always' Well Controlled	300+	67%	72%	71%
Room and Bathroom 'Always' Clean	300+	78%	79%	73%
Timely Help 'Always' Received	300+	74%	72%	68%
Would Definitely Recommend Hospital	300+	71%	74%	71%
Use of Medical Imaging				
Cardiac Imaging Stress Test before Surgery[5]	-	-	5.4%	5.3%
Combination Abdominal CT Scan[5]	-	-	6.3%	10.5%
Combination Brain/Sinus CT Scan[5]	-	-	2.1%	2.7%
Combination Chest CT Scan[5]	-	-	1%	2.7%
Follow-up Mammogram/Ultrasound[5]	-	-	8.1%	8.8%
Lumbar Spine MRI for Low Back Pain[5]	-	-	34.9%	37.2%

Oconomowoc Memorial Hospital

791 E Summit Ave
Oconomowoc, WI 53066
Phone: 262-569-9400
Fax: 262-560-4527
Type: Acute Care Hospitals
Emergency Services: Yes
Ownership: Voluntary non-profit - Other
Beds: 77

Key Personnel:

CEO/President................ Douglas Guy
Patient Relations .... Martha Klug
Chief of Medical Staff........... Brian Lipman, MD

Measure	Cases	This Hosp.	State Avg.	U.S. Avg.
Blood Clot Prevention and Treatment				
Anticoagulation Overlap Therapy[2]	22	100%	95%	93%
ICU Venous Thromboembolism Prophylaxis[2]	56	98%	91%	92%
Incidence of Potentially Preventable VTE[1,2]	-	-	10%	10%
UFH with Dosages/Platelet Monitoring[1,2]	-	-	96%	97%
Venous Thromboembolism Prophylaxis[2]	191	92%	85%	85%
Warfarin Therapy Discharge Instructions[2]	18	56%	70%	75%
Chest Pain/Possible Heart Attack Care				
Aspirin Given Within 24 Hours of Arrival[1,3]	-	-	98%	96%
Fibrinolytic Meds Within 30 Min. of Arrival[3,7]	-	-	52%	58%
Average Time to ECG (minutes)[1,3]	-	-	7	7
Average Time to Transfer (minutes)[3,7]	-	-	58	60
Children's Asthma Care				
Received Home Management Plan of Care	-	-	-	88%
Received Reliever Medication	-	-	-	100%
Received Systemic Corticosteroids	-	-	-	100%
Emergency Department				
Admittance Decision Time (minutes)[2]	358	82	65	98
Head CT Results Within 45 Min. of Arrival[1]	-	-	61%	57%
Patients Who Left ER Before Being Seen	13,387	0%	1%	2%
Time from ER Arrival to Admit. (minutes)[2]	361	216	207	274
Time from ER Arrival to Discharge (minutes)	382	122	121	134
Time in ER Before Being Evaluated (minutes)	263	15	19	26
Time to Pain Meds for Fractures (minutes)	74	34	42	57
Heart Attack Care				
Aspirin Given at Discharge	52	100%	99%	99%
Fibrinolytic Meds Within 30 Min. of Arrival[7]	-	-	67%	54%
PCI Within 90 Minutes of Arrival	16	94%	96%	96%
Statin Prescribed at Discharge	50	96%	99%	98%
Heart Failure Care				
ACE Inhibitor or ARB for LVSD	16	100%	97%	97%
Discharge Instructions Given	61	97%	96%	94%
Evaluation of LVS Function	95	100%	99%	99%
Medicare Spending				
Medicare Spending per Patient (ratio)	-	0.95	0.94	0.98
Pneumonia Care				

NOTE: Hospital profiles are in alphabetical order by state, then city, then hospital within the city; Rankings exclude hospitals with less than 25 cases except for patient surveys which excludes hospitals with less than 100 cases; (a) 100-299 cases; (1) The number of cases/patients is too few to report; (2) Data submitted were based on a sample of cases/patients; (3) Results are based on a shorter time period than required; (4) Data suppressed by CMS for one or more quarters; (5) Results are not available for this reporting period; (6) Fewer than 100 patients completed the HCAHPS survey; (7) No cases met the criteria for this measure; (8) The lower limit of the confidence interval cannot be calculated if the number of observed infections equals zero; (9) No data are available from the state/territory for this reporting period; (10) The scores shown reflect fewer than 50 completed surveys; (11) There were discrepancies in the data collection process; (12) This measure does not apply to this hospital for this reporting period; (13) Results cannot be calculated for this reporting period; (14) The results for this state are combined with nearby states to protect confidentiality; Please refer to the User's Guide for a full explanation of data.

Appropriate Initial Antibiotic Given	69	97%	96%	95%
Blood Culture Timing	97	100%	98%	98%
Pregnancy and Delivery Care				
Newborn Deliveries Scheduled Early[2]	44	0%	4%	6%
Preventive Care				
Immunization for Influenza[2]	295	95%	90%	90%
Immunization for Pneumonia[2]	360	95%	92%	92%
Stroke Care				
Anticoagulation Therapy for Atrial Fibrillation[1]	-	-	94%	95%
Antithrombotic Therapy Timing	23	100%	99%	98%
Assessed for Rehabilitation	42	98%	98%	97%
Discharged on Antithrombotic Therapy	41	100%	99%	99%
Discharged on Statin Medication	31	94%	94%	94%
Thrombolytic Therapy Timing[1]	-	-	60%	66%
Venous Thromboembolism Prophylaxis	28	96%	95%	94%
Written Stroke Educational Materials Given	20	100%	88%	88%
Surgical Care Improvement Project				
Appropriate Beta Blocker Usage[2]	59	97%	99%	98%
Appropriate VTP Within 24 Hours[2]	202	97%	99%	98%
Controlled Postoperative Blood Glucose[2,7]	-	-	96%	97%
Perioperative Temperature Management[2]	250	100%	100%	100%
Prophylactic Antibiotic Selection[2]	197	99%	99%	99%
Prophylactic Antibiotic Selection (Outpatient)	60	97%	98%	98%
Prophylactic Antibiotic Stopped[2]	196	99%	99%	98%
Prophylactic Antibiotic Timing[2]	198	98%	99%	99%
Prophylactic Antibiotic Timing (Outpatient)	60	95%	97%	98%
Urinary Catheter Removal[2]	162	98%	98%	97%
Survey of Patients' Hospital Experiences				
Area Around Room 'Always' Quiet at Night	300+	68%	63%	61%
Doctors 'Always' Communicated Well	300+	83%	83%	82%
Home Recovery Information Given	300+	88%	89%	85%
Hospital Given 9 or 10 on 10 Point Scale	300+	75%	74%	71%
Meds 'Always' Explained Before Given	300+	66%	68%	64%
Nurses 'Always' Communicated Well	300+	82%	82%	79%
Pain 'Always' Well Controlled	300+	71%	72%	71%
Room and Bathroom 'Always' Clean	300+	80%	79%	73%
Timely Help 'Always' Received	300+	69%	72%	68%
Would Definitely Recommend Hospital	300+	78%	74%	71%
Use of Medical Imaging				
Cardiac Imaging Stress Test before Surgery	201	4.5%	5.4%	5.3%
Combination Abdominal CT Scan	376	6.4%	6.3%	10.5%
Combination Brain/Sinus CT Scan	227	0.4%	2.1%	2.7%
Combination Chest CT Scan	221	1.4%	1%	2.7%
Follow-up Mammogram/Ultrasound	929	5.9%	8.1%	8.8%
Lumbar Spine MRI for Low Back Pain	95	37.9%	34.9%	37.2%

Bellin Health Oconto Hospital

820 Arbutus Ave - PO Box 357 Phone: 920-835-1100
Oconto, WI 54153
URL: www.ocontohospital.com
Type: Critical Access Hospitals Emergency Services: Yes
Ownership: Voluntary non-profit - Private

Measure	Cases	This Hosp.	State Avg.	U.S. Avg.
Blood Clot Prevention and Treatment				
Anticoagulation Overlap Therapy[5]	-	-	95%	93%
ICU Venous Thromboembolism Prophylaxis[5]	-	-	91%	92%
Incidence of Potentially Preventable VTE[5]	-	-	10%	10%
UFH with Dosages/Platelet Monitoring[5]	-	-	96%	97%
Venous Thromboembolism Prophylaxis[5]	-	-	85%	85%
Warfarin Therapy Discharge Instructions[5]	-	-	70%	75%
Chest Pain/Possible Heart Attack Care				
Aspirin Given Within 24 Hours of Arrival[3]	12	100%	98%	96%
Fibrinolytic Meds Within 30 Min. of Arrival[3,7]	-	-	52%	58%
Average Time to ECG (minutes)[3]	12	2	7	7
Average Time to Transfer (minutes)[3,7]	-	-	58	60
Children's Asthma Care				
Received Home Management Plan of Care	-	-	-	88%
Received Reliever Medication	-	-	-	100%
Received Systemic Corticosteroids	-	-	-	100%
Emergency Department				
Admittance Decision Time (minutes)[3]	53	19	65	98
Head CT Results Within 45 Min. of Arrival[5]	-	-	61%	57%
Patients Who Left ER Before Being Seen[5]	-	-	1%	2%
Time from ER Arrival to Admit. (minutes)[3]	57	153	207	274
Time from ER Arrival to Discharge (minutes)[3]	131	79	121	134
Time in ER Before Being Evaluated (minutes)[3]	30	20	19	26
Time to Pain Meds for Fractures (minutes)[1,3]	-	-	42	57
Heart Attack Care				
Aspirin Given at Discharge[5]	-	-	99%	99%
Fibrinolytic Meds Within 30 Min. of Arrival[5]	-	-	67%	54%
PCI Within 90 Minutes of Arrival[5]	-	-	96%	96%
Statin Prescribed at Discharge[5]	-	-	99%	98%
Heart Failure Care				
ACE Inhibitor or ARB for LVSD[5]	-	-	97%	97%
Discharge Instructions Given[5]	-	-	96%	94%
Evaluation of LVS Function[5]	-	-	99%	99%
Medicare Spending				
Medicare Spending per Patient (ratio)	-	-	0.94	0.98
Pneumonia Care				
Appropriate Initial Antibiotic Given[1,3]	-	-	96%	95%
Blood Culture Timing[1,3]	-	-	98%	98%
Pregnancy and Delivery Care				
Newborn Deliveries Scheduled Early[3,7]	-	-	4%	6%
Preventive Care				
Immunization for Influenza[5]	-	-	90%	90%
Immunization for Pneumonia[3]	63	90%	92%	92%
Stroke Care				
Anticoagulation Therapy for Atrial Fibrillation[5]	-	-	94%	95%
Antithrombotic Therapy Timing[5]	-	-	99%	98%
Assessed for Rehabilitation[5]	-	-	98%	97%
Discharged on Antithrombotic Therapy[5]	-	-	99%	99%
Discharged on Statin Medication[5]	-	-	94%	94%
Thrombolytic Therapy Timing[5]	-	-	60%	66%
Venous Thromboembolism Prophylaxis[5]	-	-	95%	94%
Written Stroke Educational Materials Given[5]	-	-	88%	88%
Surgical Care Improvement Project				
Appropriate Beta Blocker Usage[5]	-	-	99%	98%
Appropriate VTP Within 24 Hours[5]	-	-	99%	98%
Controlled Postoperative Blood Glucose[5]	-	-	96%	97%
Perioperative Temperature Management[5]	-	-	100%	100%
Prophylactic Antibiotic Selection[5]	-	-	99%	99%
Prophylactic Antibiotic Selection (Outpatient)[5]	-	-	98%	98%
Prophylactic Antibiotic Stopped[5]	-	-	99%	98%
Prophylactic Antibiotic Timing[5]	-	-	99%	99%
Prophylactic Antibiotic Timing (Outpatient)[5]	-	-	97%	98%
Urinary Catheter Removal[5]	-	-	98%	97%
Survey of Patients' Hospital Experiences				
Area Around Room 'Always' Quiet at Night[5]	-	-	63%	61%
Doctors 'Always' Communicated Well[5]	-	-	83%	82%
Home Recovery Information Given[5]	-	-	89%	85%
Hospital Given 9 or 10 on 10 Point Scale[5]	-	-	74%	71%
Meds 'Always' Explained Before Given[5]	-	-	68%	64%
Nurses 'Always' Communicated Well[5]	-	-	82%	79%
Pain 'Always' Well Controlled[5]	-	-	72%	71%
Room and Bathroom 'Always' Clean[5]	-	-	79%	73%
Timely Help 'Always' Received[5]	-	-	72%	68%
Would Definitely Recommend Hospital[5]	-	-	74%	71%
Use of Medical Imaging				
Cardiac Imaging Stress Test before Surgery[7]	-	-	5.4%	5.3%
Combination Abdominal CT Scan[1]	-	-	6.3%	10.5%
Combination Brain/Sinus CT Scan[1]	-	-	2.1%	2.7%
Combination Chest CT Scan[1]	-	-	1%	2.7%
Follow-up Mammogram/Ultrasound[7]	-	-	8.1%	8.8%
Lumbar Spine MRI for Low Back Pain[1]	-	-	34.9%	37.2%

Community Memorial Hospital

855 S Main St Phone: 920-846-3444
Oconto Falls, WI 54154 Fax: 920-846-4244
URL: www.cmhospital.org
Type: Critical Access Hospitals Emergency Services: Yes
Ownership: Voluntary non-profit - Private Beds: 25

Key Personnel:
Emergency Room .... Vallie Kaprelian
Chief of Medical Staff .... Genadi Maltinski, MD
Operating Room............... Kathy Micoley
Radiology..................... Arthur Stiennon
Hemotology Center .... Judy Sylema
CEO/President................. Jim VanDornick
Infection Control............... Debbie Wesolowski
Quality Assurance .... Debbie Wesolowski

Measure	Cases	This Hosp.	State Avg.	U.S. Avg.
Blood Clot Prevention and Treatment				
Anticoagulation Overlap Therapy[1]	-	-	95%	93%
ICU Venous Thromboembolism Prophylaxis	27	81%	91%	92%
Incidence of Potentially Preventable VTE[7]	-	-	10%	10%
UFH with Dosages/Platelet Monitoring[7]	-	-	96%	97%
Venous Thromboembolism Prophylaxis	12	92%	85%	85%
Warfarin Therapy Discharge Instructions[1]	-	-	70%	75%
Chest Pain/Possible Heart Attack Care				
Aspirin Given Within 24 Hours of Arrival	22	100%	98%	96%
Fibrinolytic Meds Within 30 Min. of Arrival[7]	-	-	52%	58%
Average Time to ECG (minutes)	22	14	7	7
Average Time to Transfer (minutes)[1]	-	-	58	60
Children's Asthma Care				
Received Home Management Plan of Care	-	-	-	88%
Received Reliever Medication	-	-	-	100%
Received Systemic Corticosteroids	-	-	-	100%
Emergency Department				
Admittance Decision Time (minutes)	103	60	65	98
Head CT Results Within 45 Min. of Arrival[5]	-	-	61%	57%
Patients Who Left ER Before Being Seen[5]	-	-	1%	2%
Time from ER Arrival to Admit. (minutes)	116	160	207	274
Time from ER Arrival to Discharge (minutes)[5]	-	-	121	134
Time in ER Before Being Evaluated (minutes)[5]	-	-	19	26
Time to Pain Meds for Fractures (minutes)[3]	22	39	42	57
Heart Attack Care				
Aspirin Given at Discharge[5]	-	-	99%	99%
Fibrinolytic Meds Within 30 Min. of Arrival[5]	-	-	67%	54%
PCI Within 90 Minutes of Arrival[5]	-	-	96%	96%
Statin Prescribed at Discharge[5]	-	-	99%	98%
Heart Failure Care				
ACE Inhibitor or ARB for LVSD[1]	-	-	97%	97%
Discharge Instructions Given	16	100%	96%	94%
Evaluation of LVS Function	25	96%	99%	99%
Medicare Spending				
Medicare Spending per Patient (ratio)	-	-	0.94	0.98
Pneumonia Care				
Appropriate Initial Antibiotic Given	23	87%	96%	95%
Blood Culture Timing	24	100%	98%	98%
Pregnancy and Delivery Care				
Newborn Deliveries Scheduled Early[5]	-	-	4%	6%
Preventive Care				
Immunization for Influenza	72	97%	90%	90%
Immunization for Pneumonia	114	95%	92%	92%
Stroke Care				
Anticoagulation Therapy for Atrial Fibrillation[7]	-	-	94%	95%
Antithrombotic Therapy Timing	13	100%	99%	98%
Assessed for Rehabilitation	11	100%	98%	97%
Discharged on Antithrombotic Therapy[1]	-	-	99%	99%
Discharged on Statin Medication[1]	-	-	94%	94%
Thrombolytic Therapy Timing[1]	-	-	60%	66%
Venous Thromboembolism Prophylaxis	14	43%	95%	94%
Written Stroke Educational Materials Given[1]	-	-	88%	88%
Surgical Care Improvement Project				
Appropriate Beta Blocker Usage[5]	-	-	99%	98%
Appropriate VTP Within 24 Hours	36	97%	99%	98%
Controlled Postoperative Blood Glucose[3,7]	-	-	96%	97%
Perioperative Temperature Management[5]	-	-	100%	100%
Prophylactic Antibiotic Selection	33	100%	99%	99%
Prophylactic Antibiotic Selection (Outpatient)[3]	13	100%	98%	98%
Prophylactic Antibiotic Stopped	33	100%	99%	98%
Prophylactic Antibiotic Timing	34	97%	99%	99%
Prophylactic Antibiotic Timing (Outpatient)[3]	13	100%	97%	98%
Urinary Catheter Removal[5]	-	-	98%	97%
Survey of Patients' Hospital Experiences				
Area Around Room 'Always' Quiet at Night	(a)	63%	63%	61%
Doctors 'Always' Communicated Well	(a)	82%	83%	82%
Home Recovery Information Given	(a)	86%	89%	85%
Hospital Given 9 or 10 on 10 Point Scale	(a)	66%	74%	71%

NOTE: Hospital profiles are in alphabetical order by state, then city, then hospital within the city; Rankings exclude hospitals with less than 25 cases except for patient surveys which excludes hospitals with less than 100 cases; (a) 100-299 cases; (1) The number of cases/patients is too few to report; (2) Data submitted were based on a sample of cases/patients; (3) Results are based on a shorter time period than required; (4) Data suppressed by CMS for one or more quarters; (5) Results are not available for this reporting period; (6) Fewer than 100 patients completed the HCAHPS survey; (7) No cases met the criteria for this measure; (8) The lower limit of the confidence interval cannot be calculated if the number of observed infections equals zero; (9) No data are available from the state/territory for this reporting period; (10) The scores shown reflect fewer than 50 completed surveys; (11) There were discrepancies in the data collection process; (12) This measure does not apply to this hospital for this reporting period; (13) Results cannot be calculated for this reporting period; (14) The results for this state are combined with nearby states to protect confidentiality; Please refer to the User's Guide for a full explanation of data.

Meds 'Always' Explained Before Given	(a)	64%	68%	64%
Nurses 'Always' Communicated Well	(a)	79%	82%	79%
Pain 'Always' Well Controlled	(a)	61%	72%	71%
Room and Bathroom 'Always' Clean	(a)	67%	79%	73%
Timely Help 'Always' Received	(a)	74%	72%	68%
Would Definitely Recommend Hospital	(a)	63%	74%	71%
Use of Medical Imaging				
Cardiac Imaging Stress Test before Surgery	61	6.6%	5.4%	5.3%
Combination Abdominal CT Scan	132	11.4%	6.3%	10.5%
Combination Brain/Sinus CT Scan	105	0.0%	2.1%	2.7%
Combination Chest CT Scan	149	4.0%	1%	2.7%
Follow-up Mammogram/Ultrasound	147	6.8%	8.1%	8.8%
Lumbar Spine MRI for Low Back Pain[1]	-	-	34.9%	37.2%

Ladd Memorial Hospital

2600 65th Avenue
Osceola, WI 54020
Phone: 715-294-2111
URL: www.osceolamedicalcenter.com
Type: Critical Access Hospitals
Emergency Services: Yes
Ownership: Voluntary non-profit - Private
Beds: 42

Key Personnel:

Operating Room. . . . . Warren Abell, DO
Infection Control. . . . . Pam Carlson, RN
Chief of Medical Staff. . . . . Robert Dybvig, MD
Radiology. . . . . Brad Feltz, RT, RRT
Emergency Room . . . . Kelly Johnson, RN
Hemotology Center . . . . Dody Lunde, RN
CEO/President. . . . . Jeff Meyer
Quality Assurance . . . . Dawn Olson

Measure	Cases	This Hosp.	State Avg.	U.S. Avg.
Blood Clot Prevention and Treatment				
Anticoagulation Overlap Therapy[5]	-	-	95%	93%
ICU Venous Thromboembolism Prophylaxis[5]	-	-	91%	92%
Incidence of Potentially Preventable VTE[5]	-	-	10%	10%
UFH with Dosages/Platelet Monitoring[5]	-	-	96%	97%
Venous Thromboembolism Prophylaxis[5]	-	-	85%	85%
Warfarin Therapy Discharge Instructions[5]	-	-	70%	75%
Chest Pain/Possible Heart Attack Care				
Aspirin Given Within 24 Hours of Arrival[5]	-	-	98%	96%
Fibrinolytic Meds Within 30 Min. of Arrival[5]	-	-	52%	58%
Average Time to ECG (minutes)[5]	-	-	7	7
Average Time to Transfer (minutes)[5]	-	-	58	60
Children's Asthma Care				
Received Home Management Plan of Care	-	-	-	88%
Received Reliever Medication	-	-	-	100%
Received Systemic Corticosteroids	-	-	-	100%
Emergency Department				
Admittance Decision Time (minutes)[5]	-	-	65	98
Head CT Results Within 45 Min. of Arrival[5]	-	-	61%	57%
Patients Who Left ER Before Being Seen[5]	-	-	1%	2%
Time from ER Arrival to Admit. (minutes)[5]	-	-	207	274
Time from ER Arrival to Discharge (minutes)[5]	-	-	121	134
Time in ER Before Being Evaluated (minutes)[5]	-	-	19	26
Time to Pain Meds for Fractures (minutes)[5]	-	-	42	57
Heart Attack Care				
Aspirin Given at Discharge[5]	-	-	99%	99%
Fibrinolytic Meds Within 30 Min. of Arrival[5]	-	-	67%	54%
PCI Within 90 Minutes of Arrival[5]	-	-	96%	96%
Statin Prescribed at Discharge[5]	-	-	99%	98%
Heart Failure Care				
ACE Inhibitor or ARB for LVSD[1]	-	-	97%	97%
Discharge Instructions Given[1]	-	-	96%	94%
Evaluation of LVS Function	16	69%	99%	99%
Medicare Spending				
Medicare Spending per Patient (ratio)	-	-	0.94	0.98
Pneumonia Care				
Appropriate Initial Antibiotic Given	12	100%	96%	95%
Blood Culture Timing[1]	-	-	98%	98%
Pregnancy and Delivery Care				
Newborn Deliveries Scheduled Early[5]	-	-	4%	6%
Preventive Care				
Immunization for Influenza[5]	-	-	90%	90%
Immunization for Pneumonia[5]	-	-	92%	92%
Stroke Care				
Anticoagulation Therapy for Atrial Fibrillation[5]	-	-	94%	95%
Antithrombotic Therapy Timing[5]	-	-	99%	98%
Assessed for Rehabilitation[5]	-	-	98%	97%
Discharged on Antithrombotic Therapy[5]	-	-	99%	99%
Discharged on Statin Medication[5]	-	-	94%	94%
Thrombolytic Therapy Timing[5]	-	-	60%	66%
Venous Thromboembolism Prophylaxis[5]	-	-	95%	94%
Written Stroke Educational Materials Given[5]	-	-	88%	88%
Surgical Care Improvement Project				
Appropriate Beta Blocker Usage	20	100%	99%	98%
Appropriate VTP Within 24 Hours	82	100%	99%	98%
Controlled Postoperative Blood Glucose[3,7]	-	-	96%	97%
Perioperative Temperature Management	92	100%	100%	100%
Prophylactic Antibiotic Selection[7]	-	-	99%	99%
Prophylactic Antibiotic Selection (Outpatient)[5]	-	-	98%	98%
Prophylactic Antibiotic Stopped[7]	-	-	99%	98%
Prophylactic Antibiotic Timing[7]	-	-	99%	99%
Prophylactic Antibiotic Timing (Outpatient)[5]	-	-	97%	98%
Urinary Catheter Removal[1]	-	-	98%	97%
Survey of Patients' Hospital Experiences				
Area Around Room 'Always' Quiet at Night	(a)	69%	63%	61%
Doctors 'Always' Communicated Well	(a)	83%	83%	82%
Home Recovery Information Given	(a)	90%	89%	85%
Hospital Given 9 or 10 on 10 Point Scale	(a)	79%	74%	71%
Meds 'Always' Explained Before Given	(a)	71%	68%	64%
Nurses 'Always' Communicated Well	(a)	81%	82%	79%
Pain 'Always' Well Controlled	(a)	73%	72%	71%
Room and Bathroom 'Always' Clean	(a)	78%	79%	73%
Timely Help 'Always' Received	(a)	84%	72%	68%
Would Definitely Recommend Hospital	(a)	81%	74%	71%
Use of Medical Imaging				
Cardiac Imaging Stress Test before Surgery[1]	-	-	5.4%	5.3%
Combination Abdominal CT Scan[1]	-	-	6.3%	10.5%
Combination Brain/Sinus CT Scan[1]	-	-	2.1%	2.7%
Combination Chest CT Scan[1]	-	-	1%	2.7%
Follow-up Mammogram/Ultrasound	114	3.5%	8.1%	8.8%
Lumbar Spine MRI for Low Back Pain[1]	-	-	34.9%	37.2%

Aurora Medical Center Oshkosh

855 N Westhaven Drive
Oshkosh, WI 54904
Phone: 920-456-6000
URL: www.aurorahealthcare.org
Type: Acute Care Hospitals
Emergency Services: Yes
Ownership: Voluntary non-profit - Private
Beds: 49

Key Personnel:

Chief of Medical Staff. . . . . D Erbes, MD
Emergency Room . . . . David Madenburg, DO
CEO/President. . . . . Mark A Schwartz

Measure	Cases	This Hosp.	State Avg.	U.S. Avg.
Blood Clot Prevention and Treatment				
Anticoagulation Overlap Therapy[2]	33	100%	95%	93%
ICU Venous Thromboembolism Prophylaxis[2]	73	93%	91%	92%
Incidence of Potentially Preventable VTE[1,2]	-	-	10%	10%
UFH with Dosages/Platelet Monitoring[2]	12	100%	96%	97%
Venous Thromboembolism Prophylaxis[2]	151	89%	85%	85%
Warfarin Therapy Discharge Instructions[2]	30	100%	70%	75%
Chest Pain/Possible Heart Attack Care				
Aspirin Given Within 24 Hours of Arrival[1,3]	-	-	98%	96%
Fibrinolytic Meds Within 30 Min. of Arrival[5]	-	-	52%	58%
Average Time to ECG (minutes)[1,3]	-	-	7	7
Average Time to Transfer (minutes)[5]	-	-	58	60
Children's Asthma Care				
Received Home Management Plan of Care	-	-	-	88%
Received Reliever Medication	-	-	-	100%
Received Systemic Corticosteroids	-	-	-	100%
Emergency Department				
Admittance Decision Time (minutes)[2]	183	71	65	98
Head CT Results Within 45 Min. of Arrival[1]	-	-	61%	57%
Patients Who Left ER Before Being Seen	12,778	1%	1%	2%
Time from ER Arrival to Admit. (minutes)[2]	262	210	207	274
Time from ER Arrival to Discharge (minutes)	358	96	121	134
Time in ER Before Being Evaluated (minutes)	296	20	19	26
Time to Pain Meds for Fractures (minutes)	56	40	42	57
Heart Attack Care				
Aspirin Given at Discharge	58	100%	99%	99%
Fibrinolytic Meds Within 30 Min. of Arrival[7]	-	-	67%	54%
PCI Within 90 Minutes of Arrival	19	100%	96%	96%
Statin Prescribed at Discharge	55	100%	99%	98%
Heart Failure Care				
ACE Inhibitor or ARB for LVSD	11	100%	97%	97%
Discharge Instructions Given	30	100%	96%	94%
Evaluation of LVS Function	39	100%	99%	99%
Medicare Spending				
Medicare Spending per Patient (ratio)	-	0.97	0.94	0.98
Pneumonia Care				
Appropriate Initial Antibiotic Given	39	97%	96%	95%
Blood Culture Timing	71	100%	98%	98%
Pregnancy and Delivery Care				
Newborn Deliveries Scheduled Early	45	0%	4%	6%
Preventive Care				
Immunization for Influenza[2]	286	86%	90%	90%
Immunization for Pneumonia[2]	349	92%	92%	92%
Stroke Care				
Anticoagulation Therapy for Atrial Fibrillation[1]	-	-	94%	95%
Antithrombotic Therapy Timing	24	100%	99%	98%
Assessed for Rehabilitation	33	97%	98%	97%
Discharged on Antithrombotic Therapy	31	100%	99%	99%
Discharged on Statin Medication	23	91%	94%	94%
Thrombolytic Therapy Timing[1]	-	-	60%	66%
Venous Thromboembolism Prophylaxis	23	100%	95%	94%
Written Stroke Educational Materials Given	16	88%	88%	88%
Surgical Care Improvement Project				
Appropriate Beta Blocker Usage[2]	103	100%	99%	98%
Appropriate VTP Within 24 Hours[2]	330	100%	99%	98%
Controlled Postoperative Blood Glucose[2,7]	-	-	96%	97%
Perioperative Temperature Management[2]	361	100%	100%	100%
Prophylactic Antibiotic Selection[2]	279	100%	99%	99%
Prophylactic Antibiotic Selection (Outpatient)	231	97%	98%	98%
Prophylactic Antibiotic Stopped[2]	272	100%	99%	98%
Prophylactic Antibiotic Timing[2]	279	99%	99%	99%
Prophylactic Antibiotic Timing (Outpatient)	235	96%	97%	98%
Urinary Catheter Removal[2]	80	96%	98%	97%
Survey of Patients' Hospital Experiences				
Area Around Room 'Always' Quiet at Night	300+	57%	63%	61%
Doctors 'Always' Communicated Well	300+	80%	83%	82%
Home Recovery Information Given	300+	92%	89%	85%
Hospital Given 9 or 10 on 10 Point Scale	300+	73%	74%	71%
Meds 'Always' Explained Before Given	300+	67%	68%	64%
Nurses 'Always' Communicated Well	300+	83%	82%	79%
Pain 'Always' Well Controlled	300+	73%	72%	71%
Room and Bathroom 'Always' Clean	300+	81%	79%	73%
Timely Help 'Always' Received	300+	74%	72%	68%
Would Definitely Recommend Hospital	300+	75%	74%	71%
Use of Medical Imaging				
Cardiac Imaging Stress Test before Surgery	213	2.8%	5.4%	5.3%
Combination Abdominal CT Scan	340	5.6%	6.3%	10.5%
Combination Brain/Sinus CT Scan[1]	-	-	2.1%	2.7%
Combination Chest CT Scan	324	0.3%	1%	2.7%
Follow-up Mammogram/Ultrasound	1,042	7.3%	8.1%	8.8%
Lumbar Spine MRI for Low Back Pain	85	42.4%	34.9%	37.2%

Mercy Medical Center of Oshkosh

500 S Oakwood Rd
Oshkosh, WI 54904
Phone: 920-223-2000
Fax: 920-223-0599
URL: www.ministryhealth.org
Type: Acute Care Hospitals
Emergency Services: Yes
Ownership: Voluntary non-profit - Private
Beds: 234

Key Personnel:

Chief of Medical Staff. . . . . JJ Hanusa, MD
Pediatric Ambulatory Care . . . . . . Mark Kehrberg
Pediatric In-Patient Care . . . . Mark Kehrberg
CEO/President. . . . . Kevin Nolan
Operating Room. . . . . Florette Raffi

Measure	Cases	This Hosp.	State Avg.	U.S. Avg.
Blood Clot Prevention and Treatment				
Anticoagulation Overlap Therapy[2]	31	94%	95%	93%
ICU Venous Thromboembolism Prophylaxis[2]	61	93%	91%	92%

NOTE: Hospital profiles are in alphabetical order by state, then city, then hospital within the city; Rankings exclude hospitals with less than 25 cases except for patient surveys which excludes hospitals with less than 100 cases; (a) 100-299 cases; (1) The number of cases/patients is too few to report; (2) Data submitted were based on a sample of cases/patients; (3) Results are based on a shorter time period than required; (4) Data suppressed by CMS for one or more quarters; (5) Results are not available for this reporting period; (6) Fewer than 100 patients completed the HCAHPS survey; (7) No cases met the criteria for this measure; (8) The lower limit of the confidence interval cannot be calculated if the number of observed infections equals zero; (9) No data are available from the state/territory for this reporting period; (10) The scores shown reflect fewer than 50 completed surveys; (11) There were discrepancies in the data collection process; (12) This measure does not apply to this hospital for this reporting period; (13) Results cannot be calculated for this reporting period; (14) The results for this state are combined with nearby states to protect confidentiality; Please refer to the User's Guide for a full explanation of data.

Measure	Cases	This Hosp.	State Avg.	U.S. Avg.
Incidence of Potentially Preventable VTE[1,2]	-	-	10%	10%
UFH with Dosages/Platelet Monitoring[1,2]	-	-	96%	97%
Venous Thromboembolism Prophylaxis[2]	246	95%	85%	85%
Warfarin Therapy Discharge Instructions[2]	25	100%	70%	75%
Chest Pain/Possible Heart Attack Care				
Aspirin Given Within 24 Hours of Arrival[1,3]	-	-	98%	96%
Fibrinolytic Meds Within 30 Min. of Arrival[3,7]	-	-	52%	58%
Average Time to ECG (minutes)[1,3]	-	-	7	7
Average Time to Transfer (minutes)[3,7]	-	-	58	60
Children's Asthma Care				
Received Home Management Plan of Care	-	-	-	88%
Received Reliever Medication	-	-	-	100%
Received Systemic Corticosteroids	-	-	-	100%
Emergency Department				
Admittance Decision Time (minutes)[2]	418	72	65	98
Head CT Results Within 45 Min. of Arrival[1]	-	-	61%	57%
Patients Who Left ER Before Being Seen	18,436	1%	1%	2%
Time from ER Arrival to Admit. (minutes)[2]	420	197	207	274
Time from ER Arrival to Discharge (minutes)	365	105	121	134
Time in ER Before Being Evaluated (minutes)	392	16	19	26
Time to Pain Meds for Fractures (minutes)	69	34	42	57
Heart Attack Care				
Aspirin Given at Discharge	81	100%	99%	99%
Fibrinolytic Meds Within 30 Min. of Arrival[7]	-	-	67%	54%
PCI Within 90 Minutes of Arrival	16	100%	96%	96%
Statin Prescribed at Discharge	77	100%	99%	98%
Heart Failure Care				
ACE Inhibitor or ARB for LVSD	31	100%	97%	97%
Discharge Instructions Given	95	97%	96%	94%
Evaluation of LVS Function	116	100%	99%	99%
Medicare Spending				
Medicare Spending per Patient (ratio)	-	0.90	0.94	0.98
Pneumonia Care				
Appropriate Initial Antibiotic Given	70	97%	96%	95%
Blood Culture Timing	100	100%	98%	98%
Pregnancy and Delivery Care				
Newborn Deliveries Scheduled Early	77	17%	4%	6%
Preventive Care				
Immunization for Influenza[2]	532	96%	90%	90%
Immunization for Pneumonia[2]	554	98%	92%	92%
Stroke Care				
Anticoagulation Therapy for Atrial Fibrillation[1]	-	-	94%	95%
Antithrombotic Therapy Timing	38	100%	99%	98%
Assessed for Rehabilitation	46	100%	98%	97%
Discharged on Antithrombotic Therapy	40	98%	99%	99%
Discharged on Statin Medication	26	92%	94%	94%
Thrombolytic Therapy Timing[1]	-	-	60%	66%
Venous Thromboembolism Prophylaxis	42	100%	95%	94%
Written Stroke Educational Materials Given	24	96%	88%	88%
Surgical Care Improvement Project				
Appropriate Beta Blocker Usage[2]	102	100%	99%	98%
Appropriate VTP Within 24 Hours[2]	280	99%	99%	98%
Controlled Postoperative Blood Glucose[2,7]	-	-	96%	97%
Perioperative Temperature Management[2]	314	100%	100%	100%
Prophylactic Antibiotic Selection[2]	190	99%	99%	99%
Prophylactic Antibiotic Selection (Outpatient)	289	99%	98%	98%
Prophylactic Antibiotic Stopped[2]	190	96%	99%	98%
Prophylactic Antibiotic Timing[2]	190	99%	99%	99%
Prophylactic Antibiotic Timing (Outpatient)	282	97%	97%	98%
Urinary Catheter Removal[2]	234	100%	98%	97%
Survey of Patients' Hospital Experiences				
Area Around Room 'Always' Quiet at Night	300+	58%	63%	61%
Doctors 'Always' Communicated Well	300+	83%	83%	82%
Home Recovery Information Given	300+	89%	89%	85%
Hospital Given 9 or 10 on 10 Point Scale	300+	78%	74%	71%
Meds 'Always' Explained Before Given	300+	70%	68%	64%
Nurses 'Always' Communicated Well	300+	82%	82%	79%
Pain 'Always' Well Controlled	300+	73%	72%	71%
Room and Bathroom 'Always' Clean	300+	76%	79%	73%
Timely Help 'Always' Received	300+	73%	72%	68%
Would Definitely Recommend Hospital	300+	77%	74%	71%
Use of Medical Imaging				
Cardiac Imaging Stress Test before Surgery	182	4.9%	5.4%	5.3%
Combination Abdominal CT Scan	288	1.7%	6.3%	10.5%
Combination Brain/Sinus CT Scan[1]	-	-	2.1%	2.7%
Combination Chest CT Scan	187	0.0%	1%	2.7%
Follow-up Mammogram/Ultrasound	727	7.0%	8.1%	8.8%
Lumbar Spine MRI for Low Back Pain	58	32.8%	34.9%	37.2%

Mayo Clinic Health System - Oakridge

13025 8th St
Osseo, WI 54758
Phone: 715-597-3121
Fax: 715-597-6250
URL: www.mhs.mayo.edu
Type: Critical Access Hospitals
Emergency Services: Yes
Ownership: Voluntary non-profit - Other
Beds: 68

Key Personnel:
Infection Control. . . . . Sarah Berquist
Emergency Room . . . . Margaret Lunde, RN
Patient Relations . . . . Cori Mc Reynolds
CEO/President. . . . . Mike Ryan
Chief of Medical Staff. . . . . Thomas Screneck

Measure	Cases	This Hosp.	State Avg.	U.S. Avg.
Blood Clot Prevention and Treatment				
Anticoagulation Overlap Therapy[5]	-	-	95%	93%
ICU Venous Thromboembolism Prophylaxis[5]	-	-	91%	92%
Incidence of Potentially Preventable VTE[5]	-	-	10%	10%
UFH with Dosages/Platelet Monitoring[5]	-	-	96%	97%
Venous Thromboembolism Prophylaxis[5]	-	-	85%	85%
Warfarin Therapy Discharge Instructions[5]	-	-	70%	75%
Chest Pain/Possible Heart Attack Care				
Aspirin Given Within 24 Hours of Arrival	-	-	98%	96%
Fibrinolytic Meds Within 30 Min. of Arrival	-	-	52%	58%
Average Time to ECG (minutes)	-	-	7	7
Average Time to Transfer (minutes)	-	-	58	60
Children's Asthma Care				
Received Home Management Plan of Care	-	-	-	88%
Received Reliever Medication	-	-	-	100%
Received Systemic Corticosteroids	-	-	-	100%
Emergency Department				
Admittance Decision Time (minutes)[5]	-	-	65	98
Head CT Results Within 45 Min. of Arrival	-	-	61%	57%
Patients Who Left ER Before Being Seen	-	-	1%	2%
Time from ER Arrival to Admit. (minutes)[5]	-	-	207	274
Time from ER Arrival to Discharge (minutes)	-	-	121	134
Time in ER Before Being Evaluated (minutes)	-	-	19	26
Time to Pain Meds for Fractures (minutes)	-	-	42	57
Heart Attack Care				
Aspirin Given at Discharge[5]	-	-	99%	99%
Fibrinolytic Meds Within 30 Min. of Arrival[5]	-	-	67%	54%
PCI Within 90 Minutes of Arrival[5]	-	-	96%	96%
Statin Prescribed at Discharge[5]	-	-	99%	98%
Heart Failure Care				
ACE Inhibitor or ARB for LVSD[1,3]	-	-	97%	97%
Discharge Instructions Given[1,3]	-	-	96%	94%
Evaluation of LVS Function[1,3]	-	-	99%	99%
Medicare Spending				
Medicare Spending per Patient (ratio)	-	-	0.94	0.98
Pneumonia Care				
Appropriate Initial Antibiotic Given[1]	-	-	96%	95%
Blood Culture Timing[1]	-	-	98%	98%
Pregnancy and Delivery Care				
Newborn Deliveries Scheduled Early[5]	-	-	4%	6%
Preventive Care				
Immunization for Influenza[5]	-	-	90%	90%
Immunization for Pneumonia[5]	-	-	92%	92%
Stroke Care				
Anticoagulation Therapy for Atrial Fibrillation[5]	-	-	94%	95%
Antithrombotic Therapy Timing[5]	-	-	99%	98%
Assessed for Rehabilitation[5]	-	-	98%	97%
Discharged on Antithrombotic Therapy[5]	-	-	99%	99%
Discharged on Statin Medication[5]	-	-	94%	94%
Thrombolytic Therapy Timing[5]	-	-	60%	66%
Venous Thromboembolism Prophylaxis[5]	-	-	95%	94%
Written Stroke Educational Materials Given[5]	-	-	88%	88%
Surgical Care Improvement Project				
Appropriate Beta Blocker Usage[5]	-	-	99%	98%
Appropriate VTP Within 24 Hours[5]	-	-	99%	98%
Controlled Postoperative Blood Glucose[5]	-	-	96%	97%
Perioperative Temperature Management[5]	-	-	100%	100%
Prophylactic Antibiotic Selection[5]	-	-	99%	99%
Prophylactic Antibiotic Selection (Outpatient)	-	-	98%	98%
Prophylactic Antibiotic Stopped[5]	-	-	99%	98%
Prophylactic Antibiotic Timing[5]	-	-	99%	99%
Prophylactic Antibiotic Timing (Outpatient)	-	-	97%	98%
Urinary Catheter Removal[5]	-	-	98%	97%
Survey of Patients' Hospital Experiences				
Area Around Room 'Always' Quiet at Night[10]	<100	60%	63%	61%
Doctors 'Always' Communicated Well[10]	<100	83%	83%	82%
Home Recovery Information Given[10]	<100	91%	89%	85%
Hospital Given 9 or 10 on 10 Point Scale[10]	<100	71%	74%	71%
Meds 'Always' Explained Before Given[10]	<100	69%	68%	64%
Nurses 'Always' Communicated Well[10]	<100	78%	82%	79%
Pain 'Always' Well Controlled[10]	<100	60%	72%	71%
Room and Bathroom 'Always' Clean[10]	<100	75%	79%	73%
Timely Help 'Always' Received[10]	<100	75%	72%	68%
Would Definitely Recommend Hospital[10]	<100	79%	74%	71%
Use of Medical Imaging				
Cardiac Imaging Stress Test before Surgery	-	-	5.4%	5.3%
Combination Abdominal CT Scan	-	-	6.3%	10.5%
Combination Brain/Sinus CT Scan	-	-	2.1%	2.7%
Combination Chest CT Scan	-	-	1%	2.7%
Follow-up Mammogram/Ultrasound	-	-	8.1%	8.8%
Lumbar Spine MRI for Low Back Pain	-	-	34.9%	37.2%

Flambeau Hospital

98 Sherry Ave
Park Falls, WI 54552
Phone: 715-762-7500
Fax: 715-762-7545
URL: www.ministryhealth.org
Type: Critical Access Hospitals
Emergency Services: Yes
Ownership: Voluntary non-profit - Private
Beds: 25

Key Personnel:
Emergency Room . . . . Robert C Becker, MD
Infection Control. . . . . Timothy J Lindgren, MD
Quality Assurance . . . . Robert Pflanz
Operating Room. . . . . Liz Schreiber
Chief of Medical Staff. . . . . Sue Seidl

Measure	Cases	This Hosp.	State Avg.	U.S. Avg.
Blood Clot Prevention and Treatment				
Anticoagulation Overlap Therapy[5]	-	-	95%	93%
ICU Venous Thromboembolism Prophylaxis[5]	-	-	91%	92%
Incidence of Potentially Preventable VTE[5]	-	-	10%	10%
UFH with Dosages/Platelet Monitoring[5]	-	-	96%	97%
Venous Thromboembolism Prophylaxis[5]	-	-	85%	85%
Warfarin Therapy Discharge Instructions[5]	-	-	70%	75%
Chest Pain/Possible Heart Attack Care				
Aspirin Given Within 24 Hours of Arrival	16	100%	98%	96%
Fibrinolytic Meds Within 30 Min. of Arrival[3,7]	-	-	52%	58%
Average Time to ECG (minutes)	15	5	7	7
Average Time to Transfer (minutes)[1,3]	-	-	58	60
Children's Asthma Care				
Received Home Management Plan of Care	-	-	-	88%
Received Reliever Medication	-	-	-	100%
Received Systemic Corticosteroids	-	-	-	100%
Emergency Department				
Admittance Decision Time (minutes)	459	44	65	98
Head CT Results Within 45 Min. of Arrival[1,3]	-	-	61%	57%
Patients Who Left ER Before Being Seen[5]	-	-	1%	2%
Time from ER Arrival to Admit. (minutes)	459	155	207	274
Time from ER Arrival to Discharge (minutes)	383	90	121	134
Time in ER Before Being Evaluated (minutes)	443	15	19	26
Time to Pain Meds for Fractures (minutes)[1]	-	-	42	57
Heart Attack Care				
Aspirin Given at Discharge[1]	-	-	99%	99%
Fibrinolytic Meds Within 30 Min. of Arrival[7]	-	-	67%	54%
PCI Within 90 Minutes of Arrival[7]	-	-	96%	96%
Statin Prescribed at Discharge[1]	-	-	99%	98%
Heart Failure Care				
ACE Inhibitor or ARB for LVSD[1]	-	-	97%	97%
Discharge Instructions Given	28	100%	96%	94%

NOTE: Hospital profiles are in alphabetical order by state, then city, then hospital within the city; Rankings exclude hospitals with less than 25 cases except for patient surveys which excludes hospitals with less than 100 cases; (a) 100-299 cases; (1) The number of cases/patients is too few to report; (2) Data submitted were based on a sample of cases/patients; (3) Results are based on a shorter time period than required; (4) Data suppressed by CMS for one or more quarters; (5) Results are not available for this reporting period; (6) Fewer than 100 patients completed the HCAHPS survey; (7) No cases met the criteria for this measure; (8) The lower limit of the confidence interval cannot be calculated if the number of observed infections equals zero; (9) No data are available from the state/territory for this reporting period; (10) The scores shown reflect fewer than 50 completed surveys; (11) There were discrepancies in the data collection process; (12) This measure does not apply to this hospital for this reporting period; (13) Results cannot be calculated for this reporting period; (14) The results for this state are combined with nearby states to protect confidentiality; Please refer to the User's Guide for a full explanation of data.

Evaluation of LVS Function	38	87%	99%	99%
Medicare Spending				
Medicare Spending per Patient (ratio)	-	-	0.94	0.98
Pneumonia Care				
Appropriate Initial Antibiotic Given[7]	-	-	96%	95%
Blood Culture Timing[7]	-	-	98%	98%
Pregnancy and Delivery Care				
Newborn Deliveries Scheduled Early[5]	-	-	4%	6%
Preventive Care				
Immunization for Influenza	262	99%	90%	90%
Immunization for Pneumonia	442	100%	92%	92%
Stroke Care				
Anticoagulation Therapy for Atrial Fibrillation[5]	-	-	94%	95%
Antithrombotic Therapy Timing[5]	-	-	99%	98%
Assessed for Rehabilitation[5]	-	-	98%	97%
Discharged on Antithrombotic Therapy[5]	-	-	99%	99%
Discharged on Statin Medication[5]	-	-	94%	94%
Thrombolytic Therapy Timing[5]	-	-	60%	66%
Venous Thromboembolism Prophylaxis[5]	-	-	95%	94%
Written Stroke Educational Materials Given[5]	-	-	88%	88%
Surgical Care Improvement Project				
Appropriate Beta Blocker Usage[5]	-	-	99%	98%
Appropriate VTP Within 24 Hours[5]	-	-	99%	98%
Controlled Postoperative Blood Glucose[5]	-	-	96%	97%
Perioperative Temperature Management[5]	-	-	100%	100%
Prophylactic Antibiotic Selection[5]	-	-	99%	99%
Prophylactic Antibiotic Selection (Outpatient)[5]	-	-	98%	98%
Prophylactic Antibiotic Stopped[5]	-	-	99%	98%
Prophylactic Antibiotic Timing[5]	-	-	99%	99%
Prophylactic Antibiotic Timing (Outpatient)[5]	-	-	97%	98%
Urinary Catheter Removal[5]	-	-	98%	97%
Survey of Patients' Hospital Experiences				
Area Around Room 'Always' Quiet at Night	(a)	64%	63%	61%
Doctors 'Always' Communicated Well	(a)	89%	83%	82%
Home Recovery Information Given	(a)	94%	89%	85%
Hospital Given 9 or 10 on 10 Point Scale	(a)	77%	74%	71%
Meds 'Always' Explained Before Given	(a)	73%	68%	64%
Nurses 'Always' Communicated Well	(a)	87%	82%	79%
Pain 'Always' Well Controlled	(a)	76%	72%	71%
Room and Bathroom 'Always' Clean	(a)	87%	79%	73%
Timely Help 'Always' Received	(a)	77%	72%	68%
Would Definitely Recommend Hospital	(a)	69%	74%	71%
Use of Medical Imaging				
Cardiac Imaging Stress Test before Surgery	51	2.0%	5.4%	5.3%
Combination Abdominal CT Scan	160	4.4%	6.3%	10.5%
Combination Brain/Sinus CT Scan[1]	-	-	2.1%	2.7%
Combination Chest CT Scan	94	0.0%	1%	2.7%
Follow-up Mammogram/Ultrasound	149	9.4%	8.1%	8.8%
Lumbar Spine MRI for Low Back Pain[1]	-	-	34.9%	37.2%

Southwest Health Center

1400 East Side Rd
Platteville, WI 53818
E-mail: hr@southwesthealth.org
URL: www.southwesthealth.org
Type: Critical Access Hospitals
Ownership: Voluntary non-profit - Other
Phone: 608-348-2331
Fax: 608-342-5035
Emergency Services: Yes
Beds: 119

Key Personnel:
Chief of Medical Staff .... Kevin Carr
CEO/President .... Anne Klawiter
Emergency Room .... Paul Mariskanish
Quality Assurance .... Pat Moxness
Operating Room .... Allen Rebchook
CEO .... Dan Rohrbach
Chair/CEO .... James Schneller

Measure	Cases	This Hosp.	State Avg.	U.S. Avg.
Blood Clot Prevention and Treatment				
Anticoagulation Overlap Therapy[5]	-	-	95%	93%
ICU Venous Thromboembolism Prophylaxis[5]	-	-	91%	92%
Incidence of Potentially Preventable VTE[5]	-	-	10%	10%
UFH with Dosages/Platelet Monitoring[5]	-	-	96%	97%
Venous Thromboembolism Prophylaxis[5]	-	-	85%	85%
Warfarin Therapy Discharge Instructions[5]	-	-	70%	75%
Chest Pain/Possible Heart Attack Care				
Aspirin Given Within 24 Hours of Arrival	23	100%	98%	96%
Fibrinolytic Meds Within 30 Min. of Arrival[7]	-	-	52%	58%
Average Time to ECG (minutes)	25	6	7	7
Average Time to Transfer (minutes)[1]	-	-	58	60
Children's Asthma Care				
Received Home Management Plan of Care	-	-	-	88%
Received Reliever Medication	-	-	-	100%
Received Systemic Corticosteroids	-	-	-	100%
Emergency Department				
Admittance Decision Time (minutes)[5]	-	-	65	98
Head CT Results Within 45 Min. of Arrival[5]	-	-	61%	57%
Patients Who Left ER Before Being Seen[5]	-	-	1%	2%
Time from ER Arrival to Admit. (minutes)[5]	-	-	207	274
Time from ER Arrival to Discharge (minutes)[5]	-	-	121	134
Time in ER Before Being Evaluated (minutes)[5]	-	-	19	26
Time to Pain Meds for Fractures (minutes)[5]	-	-	42	57
Heart Attack Care				
Aspirin Given at Discharge[5]	-	-	99%	99%
Fibrinolytic Meds Within 30 Min. of Arrival[5]	-	-	67%	54%
PCI Within 90 Minutes of Arrival[5]	-	-	96%	96%
Statin Prescribed at Discharge[5]	-	-	99%	98%
Heart Failure Care				
ACE Inhibitor or ARB for LVSD[1]	-	-	97%	97%
Discharge Instructions Given	25	96%	96%	94%
Evaluation of LVS Function	39	92%	99%	99%
Medicare Spending				
Medicare Spending per Patient (ratio)	-	-	0.94	0.98
Pneumonia Care				
Appropriate Initial Antibiotic Given	26	96%	96%	95%
Blood Culture Timing	31	100%	98%	98%
Pregnancy and Delivery Care				
Newborn Deliveries Scheduled Early[1]	-	-	4%	6%
Preventive Care				
Immunization for Influenza[5]	-	-	90%	90%
Immunization for Pneumonia[5]	-	-	92%	92%
Stroke Care				
Anticoagulation Therapy for Atrial Fibrillation[5]	-	-	94%	95%
Antithrombotic Therapy Timing[5]	-	-	99%	98%
Assessed for Rehabilitation[5]	-	-	98%	97%
Discharged on Antithrombotic Therapy[5]	-	-	99%	99%
Discharged on Statin Medication[5]	-	-	94%	94%
Thrombolytic Therapy Timing[5]	-	-	60%	66%
Venous Thromboembolism Prophylaxis[5]	-	-	95%	94%
Written Stroke Educational Materials Given[5]	-	-	88%	88%
Surgical Care Improvement Project				
Appropriate Beta Blocker Usage[1]	-	-	99%	98%
Appropriate VTP Within 24 Hours[1,3]	-	-	99%	98%
Controlled Postoperative Blood Glucose[3,7]	-	-	96%	97%
Perioperative Temperature Management[5]	-	-	100%	100%
Prophylactic Antibiotic Selection	15	100%	99%	99%
Prophylactic Antibiotic Selection (Outpatient)	15	87%	98%	98%
Prophylactic Antibiotic Stopped	15	100%	99%	98%
Prophylactic Antibiotic Timing	15	100%	99%	99%
Prophylactic Antibiotic Timing (Outpatient)	15	100%	97%	98%
Urinary Catheter Removal[5]	-	-	98%	97%
Survey of Patients' Hospital Experiences				
Area Around Room 'Always' Quiet at Night	(a)	69%	63%	61%
Doctors 'Always' Communicated Well	(a)	87%	83%	82%
Home Recovery Information Given	(a)	89%	89%	85%
Hospital Given 9 or 10 on 10 Point Scale	(a)	74%	74%	71%
Meds 'Always' Explained Before Given	(a)	62%	68%	64%
Nurses 'Always' Communicated Well	(a)	78%	82%	79%
Pain 'Always' Well Controlled	(a)	67%	72%	71%
Room and Bathroom 'Always' Clean	(a)	84%	79%	73%
Timely Help 'Always' Received	(a)	79%	72%	68%
Would Definitely Recommend Hospital	(a)	69%	74%	71%
Use of Medical Imaging				
Cardiac Imaging Stress Test before Surgery	49	2.0%	5.4%	5.3%
Combination Abdominal CT Scan	109	3.7%	6.3%	10.5%
Combination Brain/Sinus CT Scan[1]	-	-	2.1%	2.7%
Combination Chest CT Scan[1]	-	-	1%	2.7%
Follow-up Mammogram/Ultrasound	194	8.2%	8.1%	8.8%
Lumbar Spine MRI for Low Back Pain[1]	-	-	34.9%	37.2%

Divine Savior Healthcare

2817 New Pinery Road
Portage, WI 53901
URL: www.dshealthcare.com
Type: Acute Care Hospitals
Ownership: Voluntary non-profit - Private
Phone: 608-742-4131
Fax: 608-742-6098
Emergency Services: Yes
Beds: 162

Key Personnel:
Cardiology .... Brian Bachhuber
Intensive Care Unit .... Melissa Bradbury, RN
CEO/President .... Michael T Decker
Chief of Medical Staff .... Susan Kreckman
Quality Assurance .... Laura Lindquist, RN
Infection Control .... Wanda Lowry
Operating Room .... Allison Mitchell, RN
Emergency Room .... Jeffry Snyder, MD

Measure	Cases	This Hosp.	State Avg.	U.S. Avg.
Blood Clot Prevention and Treatment				
Anticoagulation Overlap Therapy	16	81%	95%	93%
ICU Venous Thromboembolism Prophylaxis	44	91%	91%	92%
Incidence of Potentially Preventable VTE[1]	-	-	10%	10%
UFH with Dosages/Platelet Monitoring[1]	-	-	96%	97%
Venous Thromboembolism Prophylaxis	626	57%	85%	85%
Warfarin Therapy Discharge Instructions	16	88%	70%	75%
Chest Pain/Possible Heart Attack Care				
Aspirin Given Within 24 Hours of Arrival	45	98%	98%	96%
Fibrinolytic Meds Within 30 Min. of Arrival[7]	-	-	52%	58%
Average Time to ECG (minutes)	52	7	7	7
Average Time to Transfer (minutes)	11	53	58	60
Children's Asthma Care				
Received Home Management Plan of Care	-	-	-	88%
Received Reliever Medication	-	-	-	100%
Received Systemic Corticosteroids	-	-	-	100%
Emergency Department				
Admittance Decision Time (minutes)	1,067	56	65	98
Head CT Results Within 45 Min. of Arrival[1]	-	-	61%	57%
Patients Who Left ER Before Being Seen	13,144	0%	1%	2%
Time from ER Arrival to Admit. (minutes)	1,068	221	207	274
Time from ER Arrival to Discharge (minutes)	10,990	113	121	134
Time in ER Before Being Evaluated (minutes)	11,929	24	19	26
Time to Pain Meds for Fractures (minutes)	97	38	42	57
Heart Attack Care				
Aspirin Given at Discharge[1,3]	-	-	99%	99%
Fibrinolytic Meds Within 30 Min. of Arrival[3,7]	-	-	67%	54%
PCI Within 90 Minutes of Arrival[3,7]	-	-	96%	96%
Statin Prescribed at Discharge[1,3]	-	-	99%	98%
Heart Failure Care				
ACE Inhibitor or ARB for LVSD[1]	-	-	97%	97%
Discharge Instructions Given	26	88%	96%	94%
Evaluation of LVS Function	36	92%	99%	99%
Medicare Spending				
Medicare Spending per Patient (ratio)	-	0.90	0.94	0.98
Pneumonia Care				
Appropriate Initial Antibiotic Given	58	95%	96%	95%
Blood Culture Timing	58	98%	98%	98%
Pregnancy and Delivery Care				
Newborn Deliveries Scheduled Early	24	4%	4%	6%
Preventive Care				
Immunization for Influenza	874	83%	90%	90%
Immunization for Pneumonia	989	87%	92%	92%
Stroke Care				
Anticoagulation Therapy for Atrial Fibrillation[1]	-	-	94%	95%
Antithrombotic Therapy Timing	16	100%	99%	98%
Assessed for Rehabilitation	16	100%	98%	97%
Discharged on Antithrombotic Therapy	14	100%	99%	99%
Discharged on Statin Medication	11	45%	94%	94%
Thrombolytic Therapy Timing[1]	-	-	60%	66%
Venous Thromboembolism Prophylaxis	17	59%	95%	94%
Written Stroke Educational Materials Given[1]	-	-	88%	88%
Surgical Care Improvement Project				
Appropriate Beta Blocker Usage	26	96%	99%	98%
Appropriate VTP Within 24 Hours	100	99%	99%	98%
Controlled Postoperative Blood Glucose[7]	-	-	96%	97%

NOTE: Hospital profiles are in alphabetical order by state, then city, then hospital within the city; Rankings exclude hospitals with less than 25 cases except for patient surveys which excludes hospitals with less than 100 cases; (a) 100-299 cases; (1) The number of cases/patients is too few to report; (2) Data submitted were based on a sample of cases/patients; (3) Results are based on a shorter time period than required; (4) Data suppressed by CMS for one or more quarters; (5) Results are not available for this reporting period; (6) Fewer than 100 patients completed the HCAHPS survey; (7) No cases met the criteria for this measure; (8) The lower limit of the confidence interval cannot be calculated if the number of observed infections equals zero; (9) No data are available from the state/territory for this reporting period; (10) The scores shown reflect fewer than 50 completed surveys; (11) There were discrepancies in the data collection process; (12) This measure does not apply to this hospital for this reporting period; (13) Results cannot be calculated for this reporting period; (14) The results for this state are combined with nearby states to protect confidentiality; Please refer to the User's Guide for a full explanation of data.

Measure	Cases	This Hosp.	State Avg.	U.S. Avg.
Perioperative Temperature Management	116	100%	100%	100%
Prophylactic Antibiotic Selection	86	100%	99%	99%
Prophylactic Antibiotic Selection (Outpatient)[1,3]	-	-	98%	98%
Prophylactic Antibiotic Stopped	86	94%	99%	98%
Prophylactic Antibiotic Timing	86	100%	99%	99%
Prophylactic Antibiotic Timing (Outpatient)[1,3]	-	-	97%	98%
Urinary Catheter Removal	28	89%	98%	97%
Survey of Patients' Hospital Experiences				
Area Around Room 'Always' Quiet at Night	300+	60%	63%	61%
Doctors 'Always' Communicated Well	300+	80%	83%	82%
Home Recovery Information Given	300+	84%	89%	85%
Hospital Given 9 or 10 on 10 Point Scale	300+	66%	74%	71%
Meds 'Always' Explained Before Given	300+	70%	68%	64%
Nurses 'Always' Communicated Well	300+	79%	82%	79%
Pain 'Always' Well Controlled	300+	67%	72%	71%
Room and Bathroom 'Always' Clean	300+	75%	79%	73%
Timely Help 'Always' Received	300+	74%	72%	68%
Would Definitely Recommend Hospital	300+	61%	74%	71%
Use of Medical Imaging				
Cardiac Imaging Stress Test before Surgery	135	5.9%	5.4%	5.3%
Combination Abdominal CT Scan	204	6.9%	6.3%	10.5%
Combination Brain/Sinus CT Scan	206	1.0%	2.1%	2.7%
Combination Chest CT Scan	186	1.1%	1%	2.7%
Follow-up Mammogram/Ultrasound	601	15.5%	8.1%	8.8%
Lumbar Spine MRI for Low Back Pain	54	29.6%	34.9%	37.2%

Prairie Du Chien Memorial Hospital

705 E Taylor St
Prairie Du Chien, WI 53821
Phone: 608-357-2000
Fax: 608-357-2100
Type: Critical Access Hospitals
Emergency Services: Yes
Ownership: Voluntary non-profit - Private
Beds: 43

Key Personnel:
Intensive Care Unit. . . . . Jean Bacon, RN
Chief of Medical Staff. . . . . Walter Boisrert, MD
CEO/President. . . . . Harold W Brown
Quality Assurance . . . . Jacqueline Johnsrud, RN
Emergency Room . . . . Kurt Jorgensen, MD
Operating Room. . . . . Kathy Kurt, RN
Infection Control. . . . . Ruth Mundt, RN

Measure	Cases	This Hosp.	State Avg.	U.S. Avg.
Blood Clot Prevention and Treatment				
Anticoagulation Overlap Therapy[5]	-	-	95%	93%
ICU Venous Thromboembolism Prophylaxis[5]	-	-	91%	92%
Incidence of Potentially Preventable VTE[5]	-	-	10%	10%
UFH with Dosages/Platelet Monitoring[5]	-	-	96%	97%
Venous Thromboembolism Prophylaxis[5]	-	-	85%	85%
Warfarin Therapy Discharge Instructions[5]	-	-	70%	75%
Chest Pain/Possible Heart Attack Care				
Aspirin Given Within 24 Hours of Arrival	43	98%	98%	96%
Fibrinolytic Meds Within 30 Min. of Arrival[1]	-	-	52%	58%
Average Time to ECG (minutes)	43	5	7	7
Average Time to Transfer (minutes)[1]	-	-	58	60
Children's Asthma Care				
Received Home Management Plan of Care	-	-	-	88%
Received Reliever Medication	-	-	-	100%
Received Systemic Corticosteroids	-	-	-	100%
Emergency Department				
Admittance Decision Time (minutes)	612	55	65	98
Head CT Results Within 45 Min. of Arrival[1]	-	-	61%	57%
Patients Who Left ER Before Being Seen[5]	-	-	1%	2%
Time from ER Arrival to Admit. (minutes)	614	181	207	274
Time from ER Arrival to Discharge (minutes)	418	106	121	134
Time in ER Before Being Evaluated (minutes)	525	13	19	26
Time to Pain Meds for Fractures (minutes)	33	25	42	57
Heart Attack Care				
Aspirin Given at Discharge[5]	-	-	99%	99%
Fibrinolytic Meds Within 30 Min. of Arrival[5]	-	-	67%	54%
PCI Within 90 Minutes of Arrival[5]	-	-	96%	96%
Statin Prescribed at Discharge[5]	-	-	99%	98%
Heart Failure Care				
ACE Inhibitor or ARB for LVSD[1]	-	-	97%	97%
Discharge Instructions Given	22	91%	96%	94%
Evaluation of LVS Function	31	87%	99%	99%
Medicare Spending				
Medicare Spending per Patient (ratio)	-	-	0.94	0.98
Pneumonia Care				
Appropriate Initial Antibiotic Given	23	100%	96%	95%
Blood Culture Timing	39	97%	98%	98%
Pregnancy and Delivery Care				
Newborn Deliveries Scheduled Early[5]	-	-	4%	6%
Preventive Care				
Immunization for Influenza	418	85%	90%	90%
Immunization for Pneumonia	572	95%	92%	92%
Stroke Care				
Anticoagulation Therapy for Atrial Fibrillation[5]	-	-	94%	95%
Antithrombotic Therapy Timing[5]	-	-	99%	98%
Assessed for Rehabilitation[5]	-	-	98%	97%
Discharged on Antithrombotic Therapy[5]	-	-	99%	99%
Discharged on Statin Medication[5]	-	-	94%	94%
Thrombolytic Therapy Timing[5]	-	-	60%	66%
Venous Thromboembolism Prophylaxis[5]	-	-	95%	94%
Written Stroke Educational Materials Given[5]	-	-	88%	88%
Surgical Care Improvement Project				
Appropriate Beta Blocker Usage	16	100%	99%	98%
Appropriate VTP Within 24 Hours	47	100%	99%	98%
Controlled Postoperative Blood Glucose[3,7]	-	-	96%	97%
Perioperative Temperature Management	56	100%	100%	100%
Prophylactic Antibiotic Selection	39	100%	99%	99%
Prophylactic Antibiotic Selection (Outpatient)[1,3]	-	-	98%	98%
Prophylactic Antibiotic Stopped	38	97%	99%	98%
Prophylactic Antibiotic Timing	39	100%	99%	99%
Prophylactic Antibiotic Timing (Outpatient)[3,7]	-	-	97%	98%
Urinary Catheter Removal	38	100%	98%	97%
Survey of Patients' Hospital Experiences				
Area Around Room 'Always' Quiet at Night	300+	69%	63%	61%
Doctors 'Always' Communicated Well	300+	83%	83%	82%
Home Recovery Information Given	300+	89%	89%	85%
Hospital Given 9 or 10 on 10 Point Scale	300+	77%	74%	71%
Meds 'Always' Explained Before Given	300+	77%	68%	64%
Nurses 'Always' Communicated Well	300+	84%	82%	79%
Pain 'Always' Well Controlled	300+	77%	72%	71%
Room and Bathroom 'Always' Clean	300+	88%	79%	73%
Timely Help 'Always' Received	300+	82%	72%	68%
Would Definitely Recommend Hospital	300+	76%	74%	71%
Use of Medical Imaging				
Cardiac Imaging Stress Test before Surgery[1]	-	-	5.4%	5.3%
Combination Abdominal CT Scan	153	2.6%	6.3%	10.5%
Combination Brain/Sinus CT Scan[1]	-	-	2.1%	2.7%
Combination Chest CT Scan[1]	-	-	1%	2.7%
Follow-up Mammogram/Ultrasound	240	6.7%	8.1%	8.8%
Lumbar Spine MRI for Low Back Pain[1]	-	-	34.9%	37.2%

Sauk Prairie Hospital

260 26th Street
Prairie Du Sac, WI 53578
Phone: 608-643-3311
Fax: 608-643-7151
URL: www.spmh.org
Type: Acute Care Hospitals
Emergency Services: Yes
Ownership: Voluntary non-profit - Private
Beds: 36

Key Personnel:
CEO . . . . Chad Cooper
Operating Room. . . . . John A DeGiovanni, RN
Chief of Medical Staff. . . . . Mark Heggam, MD
Emergency Room . . . . Connie Henery
Infection Control. . . . . Sandra Schlender, RN
Quality Assurance . . . . Jackie Smith
Anesthesiology. . . . . Mark Sparr

Measure	Cases	This Hosp.	State Avg.	U.S. Avg.
Blood Clot Prevention and Treatment				
Anticoagulation Overlap Therapy	11	100%	95%	93%
ICU Venous Thromboembolism Prophylaxis	48	88%	91%	92%
Incidence of Potentially Preventable VTE[7]	-	-	10%	10%
UFH with Dosages/Platelet Monitoring[7]	-	-	96%	97%
Venous Thromboembolism Prophylaxis	234	87%	85%	85%
Warfarin Therapy Discharge Instructions[1]	-	-	70%	75%
Chest Pain/Possible Heart Attack Care				
Aspirin Given Within 24 Hours of Arrival	43	98%	98%	96%
Fibrinolytic Meds Within 30 Min. of Arrival[7]	-	-	52%	58%
Average Time to ECG (minutes)	43	10	7	7
Average Time to Transfer (minutes)[1]	-	-	58	60
Children's Asthma Care				
Received Home Management Plan of Care	-	-	-	88%
Received Reliever Medication	-	-	-	100%
Received Systemic Corticosteroids	-	-	-	100%
Emergency Department				
Admittance Decision Time (minutes)[2]	147	45	65	98
Head CT Results Within 45 Min. of Arrival[1,3]	-	-	61%	57%
Patients Who Left ER Before Being Seen	6,940	1%	1%	2%
Time from ER Arrival to Admit. (minutes)[2]	151	194	207	274
Time from ER Arrival to Discharge (minutes)	396	116	121	134
Time in ER Before Being Evaluated (minutes)	443	24	19	26
Time to Pain Meds for Fractures (minutes)	69	33	42	57
Heart Attack Care				
Aspirin Given at Discharge[1]	-	-	99%	99%
Fibrinolytic Meds Within 30 Min. of Arrival[7]	-	-	67%	54%
PCI Within 90 Minutes of Arrival[7]	-	-	96%	96%
Statin Prescribed at Discharge[1]	-	-	99%	98%
Heart Failure Care				
ACE Inhibitor or ARB for LVSD[1]	-	-	97%	97%
Discharge Instructions Given[1]	-	-	96%	94%
Evaluation of LVS Function	11	100%	99%	99%
Medicare Spending				
Medicare Spending per Patient (ratio)	-	0.84	0.94	0.98
Pneumonia Care				
Appropriate Initial Antibiotic Given	23	100%	96%	95%
Blood Culture Timing	19	100%	98%	98%
Pregnancy and Delivery Care				
Newborn Deliveries Scheduled Early[2]	17	0%	4%	6%
Preventive Care				
Immunization for Influenza[2]	276	99%	90%	90%
Immunization for Pneumonia[2]	334	96%	92%	92%
Stroke Care				
Anticoagulation Therapy for Atrial Fibrillation[1]	-	-	94%	95%
Antithrombotic Therapy Timing	11	100%	99%	98%
Assessed for Rehabilitation	13	100%	98%	97%
Discharged on Antithrombotic Therapy	12	100%	99%	99%
Discharged on Statin Medication	11	91%	94%	94%
Thrombolytic Therapy Timing[7]	-	-	60%	66%
Venous Thromboembolism Prophylaxis[1]	-	-	95%	94%
Written Stroke Educational Materials Given[1]	-	-	88%	88%
Surgical Care Improvement Project				
Appropriate Beta Blocker Usage	157	97%	99%	98%
Appropriate VTP Within 24 Hours	545	99%	99%	98%
Controlled Postoperative Blood Glucose[7]	-	-	96%	97%
Perioperative Temperature Management	687	100%	100%	100%
Prophylactic Antibiotic Selection	617	100%	99%	99%
Prophylactic Antibiotic Selection (Outpatient)	127	99%	98%	98%
Prophylactic Antibiotic Stopped	616	97%	99%	98%
Prophylactic Antibiotic Timing	618	100%	99%	99%
Prophylactic Antibiotic Timing (Outpatient)	127	99%	97%	98%
Urinary Catheter Removal	531	100%	98%	97%
Survey of Patients' Hospital Experiences				
Area Around Room 'Always' Quiet at Night	300+	71%	63%	61%
Doctors 'Always' Communicated Well	300+	89%	83%	82%
Home Recovery Information Given	300+	92%	89%	85%
Hospital Given 9 or 10 on 10 Point Scale	300+	87%	74%	71%
Meds 'Always' Explained Before Given	300+	77%	68%	64%
Nurses 'Always' Communicated Well	300+	89%	82%	79%
Pain 'Always' Well Controlled	300+	75%	72%	71%
Room and Bathroom 'Always' Clean	300+	85%	79%	73%
Timely Help 'Always' Received	300+	83%	72%	68%
Would Definitely Recommend Hospital	300+	89%	74%	71%
Use of Medical Imaging				
Cardiac Imaging Stress Test before Surgery	51	2.0%	5.4%	5.3%
Combination Abdominal CT Scan	146	6.2%	6.3%	10.5%
Combination Brain/Sinus CT Scan[1]	-	-	2.1%	2.7%
Combination Chest CT Scan	83	4.8%	1%	2.7%
Follow-up Mammogram/Ultrasound	439	12.8%	8.1%	8.8%
Lumbar Spine MRI for Low Back Pain	98	33.7%	34.9%	37.2%

NOTE: Hospital profiles are in alphabetical order by state, then city, then hospital within the city; Rankings exclude hospitals with less than 25 cases except for patient surveys which excludes hospitals with less than 100 cases; (a) 100-299 cases; (1) The number of cases/patients is too few to report; (2) Data submitted were based on a sample of cases/patients; (3) Results are based on a shorter time period than required; (4) Data suppressed by CMS for one or more quarters; (5) Results are not available for this reporting period; (6) Fewer than 100 patients completed the HCAHPS survey; (7) No cases met the criteria for this measure; (8) The lower limit of the confidence interval cannot be calculated if the number of observed infections equals zero; (9) No data are available from the state/territory for this reporting period; (10) The scores shown reflect fewer than 50 completed surveys; (11) There were discrepancies in the data collection process; (12) This measure does not apply to this hospital for this reporting period; (13) Results cannot be calculated for this reporting period; (14) The results for this state are combined with nearby states to protect confidentiality; Please refer to the User's Guide for a full explanation of data.

Wheaton Franciscan Healthcare All Saints

3801 Spring St
Racine, WI 53405
Phone: 262-687-4011
Fax: 262-687-2674
URL: www.mywheaton.org
Type: Acute Care Hospitals
Emergency Services: Yes
Ownership: Voluntary non-profit - Church
Beds: 226

Key Personnel:
Quality Assurance . . . . Donna Brossard
Chief of Medical Staff. . . . . Sharee ChanceLawson, MD
Patient Relations . . . . Rose Fowler
Emergency Room . . . . Margrett Malnory
Coronary Care . . . . Carol Meils
Pediatric In-Patient Care . . . . Scott Meyer, MD
CEO/President. . . . . John D Oliverio
Operating Room. . . . . James Waltenberger, RN

Measure	Cases	This Hosp.	State Avg.	U.S. Avg.
Blood Clot Prevention and Treatment				
Anticoagulation Overlap Therapy[2]	133	92%	95%	93%
ICU Venous Thromboembolism Prophylaxis[2]	44	84%	91%	92%
Incidence of Potentially Preventable VTE[2]	25	24%	10%	10%
UFH with Dosages/Platelet Monitoring[2]	55	93%	96%	97%
Venous Thromboembolism Prophylaxis[2]	289	73%	85%	85%
Warfarin Therapy Discharge Instructions[2]	106	73%	70%	75%
Chest Pain/Possible Heart Attack Care				
Aspirin Given Within 24 Hours of Arrival[1,3]	-	-	98%	96%
Fibrinolytic Meds Within 30 Min. of Arrival[5]	-	-	52%	58%
Average Time to ECG (minutes)[1,3]	-	-	7	7
Average Time to Transfer (minutes)[5]	-	-	58	60
Children's Asthma Care				
Received Home Management Plan of Care	-	-	-	88%
Received Reliever Medication	-	-	-	100%
Received Systemic Corticosteroids	-	-	-	100%
Emergency Department				
Admittance Decision Time (minutes)[2]	536	94	65	98
Head CT Results Within 45 Min. of Arrival	15	40%	61%	57%
Patients Who Left ER Before Being Seen	59,574	1%	1%	2%
Time from ER Arrival to Admit. (minutes)[2]	540	270	207	274
Time from ER Arrival to Discharge (minutes)	379	140	121	134
Time in ER Before Being Evaluated (minutes)	380	34	19	26
Time to Pain Meds for Fractures (minutes)	178	52	42	57
Heart Attack Care				
Aspirin Given at Discharge	178	100%	99%	99%
Fibrinolytic Meds Within 30 Min. of Arrival[7]	-	-	67%	54%
PCI Within 90 Minutes of Arrival	42	100%	96%	96%
Statin Prescribed at Discharge	171	99%	99%	98%
Heart Failure Care				
ACE Inhibitor or ARB for LVSD	72	100%	97%	97%
Discharge Instructions Given	231	94%	96%	94%
Evaluation of LVS Function	291	100%	99%	99%
Medicare Spending				
Medicare Spending per Patient (ratio)	-	0.96	0.94	0.98
Pneumonia Care				
Appropriate Initial Antibiotic Given[2]	64	100%	96%	95%
Blood Culture Timing[2]	187	99%	98%	98%
Pregnancy and Delivery Care				
Newborn Deliveries Scheduled Early	157	3%	4%	6%
Preventive Care				
Immunization for Influenza[2]	518	85%	90%	90%
Immunization for Pneumonia[2]	633	86%	92%	92%
Stroke Care				
Anticoagulation Therapy for Atrial Fibrillation[2]	18	94%	94%	95%
Antithrombotic Therapy Timing[2]	126	99%	99%	98%
Assessed for Rehabilitation[2]	139	97%	98%	97%
Discharged on Antithrombotic Therapy[2]	126	100%	99%	99%
Discharged on Statin Medication[2]	90	90%	94%	94%
Thrombolytic Therapy Timing[1,2]	-	-	60%	66%
Venous Thromboembolism Prophylaxis[2]	141	82%	95%	94%
Written Stroke Educational Materials Given[2]	77	69%	88%	88%
Surgical Care Improvement Project				
Appropriate Beta Blocker Usage[2]	210	100%	99%	98%
Appropriate VTP Within 24 Hours[2]	447	100%	99%	98%
Controlled Postoperative Blood Glucose[2]	88	98%	96%	97%
Perioperative Temperature Management[2]	523	100%	100%	100%
Prophylactic Antibiotic Selection[2]	375	100%	99%	99%
Prophylactic Antibiotic Selection (Outpatient)	322	98%	98%	98%
Prophylactic Antibiotic Stopped[2]	357	98%	99%	98%
Prophylactic Antibiotic Timing[2]	377	99%	99%	99%
Prophylactic Antibiotic Timing (Outpatient)	269	98%	97%	98%
Urinary Catheter Removal[2]	216	98%	98%	97%
Survey of Patients' Hospital Experiences				
Area Around Room 'Always' Quiet at Night	300+	56%	63%	61%
Doctors 'Always' Communicated Well	300+	83%	83%	82%
Home Recovery Information Given	300+	88%	89%	85%
Hospital Given 9 or 10 on 10 Point Scale	300+	68%	74%	71%
Meds 'Always' Explained Before Given	300+	64%	68%	64%
Nurses 'Always' Communicated Well	300+	80%	82%	79%
Pain 'Always' Well Controlled	300+	71%	72%	71%
Room and Bathroom 'Always' Clean	300+	70%	79%	73%
Timely Help 'Always' Received	300+	61%	72%	68%
Would Definitely Recommend Hospital	300+	67%	74%	71%
Use of Medical Imaging				
Cardiac Imaging Stress Test before Surgery	689	8.0%	5.4%	5.3%
Combination Abdominal CT Scan	951	5.4%	6.3%	10.5%
Combination Brain/Sinus CT Scan	1,004	0.8%	2.1%	2.7%
Combination Chest CT Scan	957	0.0%	1%	2.7%
Follow-up Mammogram/Ultrasound	2,642	8.4%	8.1%	8.8%
Lumbar Spine MRI for Low Back Pain	209	33.0%	34.9%	37.2%

Reedsburg Area Medical Center

2000 N Dewey Ave
Reedsburg, WI 53959
Phone: 608-524-6487
Fax: 608-524-6566
URL: www.ramchealth.com
Type: Critical Access Hospitals
Emergency Services: Yes
Ownership: Voluntary non-profit - Private

Key Personnel:
Radiology. . . . . Douglas R Andrews
Emergency Room . . . . Janet Bolk
Infection Control. . . . . Peg Dobrovelny
Chief of Medical Staff. . . . . K M Hoffmann, MD
CEO/President. . . . . Bob Van Meeteren
Anesthesiology. . . . . Ken Olson, CRNA MS
Operating Room. . . . . Pat Peterson
Intensive Care Unit. . . . . Janet Volk

Measure	Cases	This Hosp.	State Avg.	U.S. Avg.
Blood Clot Prevention and Treatment				
Anticoagulation Overlap Therapy[5]	-	-	95%	93%
ICU Venous Thromboembolism Prophylaxis[5]	-	-	91%	92%
Incidence of Potentially Preventable VTE[5]	-	-	10%	10%
UFH with Dosages/Platelet Monitoring[5]	-	-	96%	97%
Venous Thromboembolism Prophylaxis[5]	-	-	85%	85%
Warfarin Therapy Discharge Instructions[5]	-	-	70%	75%
Chest Pain/Possible Heart Attack Care				
Aspirin Given Within 24 Hours of Arrival	71	100%	98%	96%
Fibrinolytic Meds Within 30 Min. of Arrival[1]	-	-	52%	58%
Average Time to ECG (minutes)	72	4	7	7
Average Time to Transfer (minutes)	13	61	58	60
Children's Asthma Care				
Received Home Management Plan of Care	-	-	-	88%
Received Reliever Medication	-	-	-	100%
Received Systemic Corticosteroids	-	-	-	100%
Emergency Department				
Admittance Decision Time (minutes)	556	82	65	98
Head CT Results Within 45 Min. of Arrival[1]	-	-	61%	57%
Patients Who Left ER Before Being Seen[5]	-	-	1%	2%
Time from ER Arrival to Admit. (minutes)	624	223	207	274
Time from ER Arrival to Discharge (minutes)	343	125	121	134
Time in ER Before Being Evaluated (minutes)	453	18	19	26
Time to Pain Meds for Fractures (minutes)	59	35	42	57
Heart Attack Care				
Aspirin Given at Discharge[5]	-	-	99%	99%
Fibrinolytic Meds Within 30 Min. of Arrival[5]	-	-	67%	54%
PCI Within 90 Minutes of Arrival[5]	-	-	96%	96%
Statin Prescribed at Discharge[5]	-	-	99%	98%
Heart Failure Care				
ACE Inhibitor or ARB for LVSD[1]	-	-	97%	97%
Discharge Instructions Given	28	75%	96%	94%
Evaluation of LVS Function	38	100%	99%	99%
Medicare Spending				
Medicare Spending per Patient (ratio)	-	-	0.94	0.98
Pneumonia Care				
Appropriate Initial Antibiotic Given	54	98%	96%	95%
Blood Culture Timing	60	98%	98%	98%
Pregnancy and Delivery Care				
Newborn Deliveries Scheduled Early[2]	17	0%	4%	6%
Preventive Care				
Immunization for Influenza	681	89%	90%	90%
Immunization for Pneumonia	797	91%	92%	92%
Stroke Care				
Anticoagulation Therapy for Atrial Fibrillation[5]	-	-	94%	95%
Antithrombotic Therapy Timing[5]	-	-	99%	98%
Assessed for Rehabilitation[5]	-	-	98%	97%
Discharged on Antithrombotic Therapy[5]	-	-	99%	99%
Discharged on Statin Medication[5]	-	-	94%	94%
Thrombolytic Therapy Timing[5]	-	-	60%	66%
Venous Thromboembolism Prophylaxis[5]	-	-	95%	94%
Written Stroke Educational Materials Given[5]	-	-	88%	88%
Surgical Care Improvement Project				
Appropriate Beta Blocker Usage	16	88%	99%	98%
Appropriate VTP Within 24 Hours	65	98%	99%	98%
Controlled Postoperative Blood Glucose[3,7]	-	-	96%	97%
Perioperative Temperature Management	72	100%	100%	100%
Prophylactic Antibiotic Selection	63	98%	99%	99%
Prophylactic Antibiotic Selection (Outpatient)	64	98%	98%	98%
Prophylactic Antibiotic Stopped	63	97%	99%	98%
Prophylactic Antibiotic Timing	63	98%	99%	99%
Prophylactic Antibiotic Timing (Outpatient)	66	97%	97%	98%
Urinary Catheter Removal	17	88%	98%	97%
Survey of Patients' Hospital Experiences				
Area Around Room 'Always' Quiet at Night	300+	67%	63%	61%
Doctors 'Always' Communicated Well	300+	85%	83%	82%
Home Recovery Information Given	300+	87%	89%	85%
Hospital Given 9 or 10 on 10 Point Scale	300+	75%	74%	71%
Meds 'Always' Explained Before Given	300+	70%	68%	64%
Nurses 'Always' Communicated Well	300+	80%	82%	79%
Pain 'Always' Well Controlled	300+	70%	72%	71%
Room and Bathroom 'Always' Clean	300+	84%	79%	73%
Timely Help 'Always' Received	300+	69%	72%	68%
Would Definitely Recommend Hospital	300+	72%	74%	71%
Use of Medical Imaging				
Cardiac Imaging Stress Test before Surgery	99	3.0%	5.4%	5.3%
Combination Abdominal CT Scan	163	1.2%	6.3%	10.5%
Combination Brain/Sinus CT Scan[1]	-	-	2.1%	2.7%
Combination Chest CT Scan	86	1.2%	1%	2.7%
Follow-up Mammogram/Ultrasound	292	15.8%	8.1%	8.8%
Lumbar Spine MRI for Low Back Pain	70	48.6%	34.9%	37.2%

Ministry Saint Marys Hospital

2251 North Shore Dr
Rhinelander, WI 54501
Phone: 715-361-2000
Fax: 715-361-2011
URL: www.ministryhealth.org
Type: Acute Care Hospitals
Emergency Services: Yes
Ownership: Voluntary non-profit - Private
Beds: 73

Key Personnel:
Cardiac Laboratory. . . . . Kathy Grill, RN
Pediatric In-Patient Care . . . . Rene Iannarelli
CEO/President. . . . . Kevin O'Donnell
Chief of Medical Staff. . . . . Judith Pagano, MD
Radiology. . . . . Kathi Senoraske
Operating Room. . . . . Gary Tiesling
Infection Control. . . . . Karen Wiedeman, RN
Quality Assurance . . . . Ann Zenk

Measure	Cases	This Hosp.	State Avg.	U.S. Avg.
Blood Clot Prevention and Treatment				
Anticoagulation Overlap Therapy[2]	33	100%	95%	93%
ICU Venous Thromboembolism Prophylaxis[2]	21	76%	91%	92%
Incidence of Potentially Preventable VTE[1,2]	-	-	10%	10%
UFH with Dosages/Platelet Monitoring[1,2]	-	-	96%	97%
Venous Thromboembolism Prophylaxis[2]	194	87%	85%	85%
Warfarin Therapy Discharge Instructions[2]	24	100%	70%	75%
Chest Pain/Possible Heart Attack Care				
Aspirin Given Within 24 Hours of Arrival	144	100%	98%	96%
Fibrinolytic Meds Within 30 Min. of Arrival	13	54%	52%	58%

NOTE: Hospital profiles are in alphabetical order by state, then city, then hospital within the city; Rankings exclude hospitals with less than 25 cases except for patient surveys which excludes hospitals with less than 100 cases; (a) 100-299 cases; (1) The number of cases/patients is too few to report; (2) Data submitted were based on a sample of cases/patients; (3) Results are based on a shorter time period than required; (4) Data suppressed by CMS for one or more quarters; (5) Results are not available for this reporting period; (6) Fewer than 100 patients completed the HCAHPS survey; (7) No cases met the criteria for this measure; (8) The lower limit of the confidence interval cannot be calculated if the number of observed infections equals zero; (9) No data are available from the state/territory for this reporting period; (10) The scores shown reflect fewer than 50 completed surveys; (11) There were discrepancies in the data collection process; (12) This measure does not apply to this hospital for this reporting period; (13) Results cannot be calculated for this reporting period; (14) The results for this state are combined with nearby states to protect confidentiality; Please refer to the User's Guide for a full explanation of data.

Measure	Cases	This Hosp.	State Avg.	U.S. Avg.
Average Time to ECG (minutes)	154	6	7	7
Average Time to Transfer (minutes)[7]	-	-	58	60
Children's Asthma Care				
Received Home Management Plan of Care	-	-	-	88%
Received Reliever Medication	-	-	-	100%
Received Systemic Corticosteroids	-	-	-	100%
Emergency Department				
Admittance Decision Time (minutes)[2]	171	90	65	98
Head CT Results Within 45 Min. of Arrival	16	31%	61%	57%
Patients Who Left ER Before Being Seen	19,395	0%	1%	2%
Time from ER Arrival to Admit. (minutes)[2]	318	250	207	274
Time from ER Arrival to Discharge (minutes)	749	127	121	134
Time in ER Before Being Evaluated (minutes)	611	15	19	26
Time to Pain Meds for Fractures (minutes)	47	37	42	57
Heart Attack Care				
Aspirin Given at Discharge	17	94%	99%	99%
Fibrinolytic Meds Within 30 Min. of Arrival[7]	-	-	67%	54%
PCI Within 90 Minutes of Arrival[7]	-	-	96%	96%
Statin Prescribed at Discharge	12	75%	99%	98%
Heart Failure Care				
ACE Inhibitor or ARB for LVSD	12	100%	97%	97%
Discharge Instructions Given	63	100%	96%	94%
Evaluation of LVS Function	79	100%	99%	99%
Medicare Spending				
Medicare Spending per Patient (ratio)	-	0.87	0.94	0.98
Pneumonia Care				
Appropriate Initial Antibiotic Given	62	100%	96%	95%
Blood Culture Timing	97	100%	98%	98%
Pregnancy and Delivery Care				
Newborn Deliveries Scheduled Early	48	2%	4%	6%
Preventive Care				
Immunization for Influenza[2]	278	97%	90%	90%
Immunization for Pneumonia[2]	405	96%	92%	92%
Stroke Care				
Anticoagulation Therapy for Atrial Fibrillation[7]	-	-	94%	95%
Antithrombotic Therapy Timing	17	100%	99%	98%
Assessed for Rehabilitation	17	94%	98%	97%
Discharged on Antithrombotic Therapy	17	100%	99%	99%
Discharged on Statin Medication	11	100%	94%	94%
Thrombolytic Therapy Timing[7]	-	-	60%	66%
Venous Thromboembolism Prophylaxis	17	94%	95%	94%
Written Stroke Educational Materials Given[1]	-	-	88%	88%
Surgical Care Improvement Project				
Appropriate Beta Blocker Usage	115	99%	99%	98%
Appropriate VTP Within 24 Hours	333	100%	99%	98%
Controlled Postoperative Blood Glucose[7]	-	-	96%	97%
Perioperative Temperature Management	389	100%	100%	100%
Prophylactic Antibiotic Selection	308	99%	99%	99%
Prophylactic Antibiotic Selection (Outpatient)	38	97%	98%	98%
Prophylactic Antibiotic Stopped	302	100%	99%	98%
Prophylactic Antibiotic Timing	311	99%	99%	99%
Prophylactic Antibiotic Timing (Outpatient)	39	97%	97%	98%
Urinary Catheter Removal	90	99%	98%	97%
Survey of Patients' Hospital Experiences				
Area Around Room 'Always' Quiet at Night	300+	55%	63%	61%
Doctors 'Always' Communicated Well	300+	82%	83%	82%
Home Recovery Information Given	300+	89%	89%	85%
Hospital Given 9 or 10 on 10 Point Scale	300+	69%	74%	71%
Meds 'Always' Explained Before Given	300+	68%	68%	64%
Nurses 'Always' Communicated Well	300+	81%	82%	79%
Pain 'Always' Well Controlled	300+	71%	72%	71%
Room and Bathroom 'Always' Clean	300+	77%	79%	73%
Timely Help 'Always' Received	300+	69%	72%	68%
Would Definitely Recommend Hospital	300+	66%	74%	71%
Use of Medical Imaging				
Cardiac Imaging Stress Test before Surgery	204	6.4%	5.4%	5.3%
Combination Abdominal CT Scan	559	5.5%	6.3%	10.5%
Combination Brain/Sinus CT Scan[1]	-	-	2.1%	2.7%
Combination Chest CT Scan	346	0.3%	1%	2.7%
Follow-up Mammogram/Ultrasound	918	6.2%	8.1%	8.8%
Lumbar Spine MRI for Low Back Pain	77	36.4%	34.9%	37.2%

Lakeview Medical Center

1700 West Stout Street
Rice Lake, WI 54868
URL: www.lakeviewmedical.com
Type: Acute Care Hospitals
Ownership: Voluntary non-profit - Private

Phone: 715-234-1515
Fax: 715-234-4465
Emergency Services: Yes
Beds: 75

Measure	Cases	This Hosp.	State Avg.	U.S. Avg.
Blood Clot Prevention and Treatment				
Anticoagulation Overlap Therapy[2]	33	100%	95%	93%
ICU Venous Thromboembolism Prophylaxis[2]	29	100%	91%	92%
Incidence of Potentially Preventable VTE[1,2]	-	-	10%	10%
UFH with Dosages/Platelet Monitoring[2]	19	100%	96%	97%
Venous Thromboembolism Prophylaxis[2]	114	98%	85%	85%
Warfarin Therapy Discharge Instructions[2]	27	100%	70%	75%
Chest Pain/Possible Heart Attack Care				
Aspirin Given Within 24 Hours of Arrival	96	100%	98%	96%
Fibrinolytic Meds Within 30 Min. of Arrival[1]	-	-	52%	58%
Average Time to ECG (minutes)	96	1	7	7
Average Time to Transfer (minutes)	16	70	58	60
Children's Asthma Care				
Received Home Management Plan of Care	-	-	-	88%
Received Reliever Medication	-	-	-	100%
Received Systemic Corticosteroids	-	-	-	100%
Emergency Department				
Admittance Decision Time (minutes)[2]	195	53	65	98
Head CT Results Within 45 Min. of Arrival[1]	-	-	61%	57%
Patients Who Left ER Before Being Seen	11,471	0%	1%	2%
Time from ER Arrival to Admit. (minutes)[2]	213	204	207	274
Time from ER Arrival to Discharge (minutes)	437	108	121	134
Time in ER Before Being Evaluated (minutes)	334	20	19	26
Time to Pain Meds for Fractures (minutes)	45	45	42	57
Heart Attack Care				
Aspirin Given at Discharge[7]	-	-	99%	99%
Fibrinolytic Meds Within 30 Min. of Arrival[7]	-	-	67%	54%
PCI Within 90 Minutes of Arrival[7]	-	-	96%	96%
Statin Prescribed at Discharge[7]	-	-	99%	98%
Heart Failure Care				
ACE Inhibitor or ARB for LVSD	14	100%	97%	97%
Discharge Instructions Given	34	100%	96%	94%
Evaluation of LVS Function	52	100%	99%	99%
Medicare Spending				
Medicare Spending per Patient (ratio)	-	0.86	0.94	0.98
Pneumonia Care				
Appropriate Initial Antibiotic Given	32	100%	96%	95%
Blood Culture Timing	61	100%	98%	98%
Pregnancy and Delivery Care				
Newborn Deliveries Scheduled Early	55	4%	4%	6%
Preventive Care				
Immunization for Influenza[2]	253	92%	90%	90%
Immunization for Pneumonia[2]	319	92%	92%	92%
Stroke Care				
Anticoagulation Therapy for Atrial Fibrillation[1]	-	-	94%	95%
Antithrombotic Therapy Timing	19	95%	99%	98%
Assessed for Rehabilitation	19	95%	98%	97%
Discharged on Antithrombotic Therapy	19	100%	99%	99%
Discharged on Statin Medication	13	92%	94%	94%
Thrombolytic Therapy Timing[1]	-	-	60%	66%
Venous Thromboembolism Prophylaxis	19	100%	95%	94%
Written Stroke Educational Materials Given	12	100%	88%	88%
Surgical Care Improvement Project				
Appropriate Beta Blocker Usage[2]	109	100%	99%	98%
Appropriate VTP Within 24 Hours[2]	271	100%	99%	98%
Controlled Postoperative Blood Glucose[2,7]	-	-	96%	97%
Perioperative Temperature Management[2]	343	100%	100%	100%
Prophylactic Antibiotic Selection[2]	283	99%	99%	99%
Prophylactic Antibiotic Selection (Outpatient)	62	98%	98%	98%
Prophylactic Antibiotic Stopped[2]	282	99%	99%	98%
Prophylactic Antibiotic Timing[2]	283	99%	99%	99%
Prophylactic Antibiotic Timing (Outpatient)	62	98%	97%	98%
Urinary Catheter Removal[2]	268	100%	98%	97%
Survey of Patients' Hospital Experiences				
Area Around Room 'Always' Quiet at Night	300+	66%	63%	61%
Doctors 'Always' Communicated Well	300+	84%	83%	82%
Home Recovery Information Given	300+	89%	89%	85%
Hospital Given 9 or 10 on 10 Point Scale	300+	79%	74%	71%
Meds 'Always' Explained Before Given	300+	70%	68%	64%
Nurses 'Always' Communicated Well	300+	81%	82%	79%
Pain 'Always' Well Controlled	300+	70%	72%	71%
Room and Bathroom 'Always' Clean	300+	86%	79%	73%
Timely Help 'Always' Received	300+	73%	72%	68%
Would Definitely Recommend Hospital	300+	81%	74%	71%
Use of Medical Imaging				
Cardiac Imaging Stress Test before Surgery	203	3.9%	5.4%	5.3%
Combination Abdominal CT Scan	398	3.3%	6.3%	10.5%
Combination Brain/Sinus CT Scan	255	1.2%	2.1%	2.7%
Combination Chest CT Scan	394	0.8%	1%	2.7%
Follow-up Mammogram/Ultrasound	783	9.2%	8.1%	8.8%
Lumbar Spine MRI for Low Back Pain	116	37.1%	34.9%	37.2%

Richland Hospital

333 E Second St
Richland Center, WI 53581
E-mail: hr@richlandhospital.com
URL: www.richlandhospital.com
Type: Critical Access Hospitals
Ownership: Voluntary non-profit - Private

Phone: 608-647-6321
Fax: 608-647-6235
Emergency Services: Yes
Beds: 25

Key Personnel:
Quality Assurance . . . . Carolyn Anderson
Administrator . . . . Cindy Chicker
Infection Control. . . . . Richard Lee
CEO . . . . Terri Potter

Measure	Cases	This Hosp.	State Avg.	U.S. Avg.
Blood Clot Prevention and Treatment				
Anticoagulation Overlap Therapy[5]	-	-	95%	93%
ICU Venous Thromboembolism Prophylaxis[5]	-	-	91%	92%
Incidence of Potentially Preventable VTE[5]	-	-	10%	10%
UFH with Dosages/Platelet Monitoring[5]	-	-	96%	97%
Venous Thromboembolism Prophylaxis[5]	-	-	85%	85%
Warfarin Therapy Discharge Instructions[5]	-	-	70%	75%
Chest Pain/Possible Heart Attack Care				
Aspirin Given Within 24 Hours of Arrival	-	-	98%	96%
Fibrinolytic Meds Within 30 Min. of Arrival	-	-	52%	58%
Average Time to ECG (minutes)	-	-	7	7
Average Time to Transfer (minutes)	-	-	58	60
Children's Asthma Care				
Received Home Management Plan of Care	-	-	-	88%
Received Reliever Medication	-	-	-	100%
Received Systemic Corticosteroids	-	-	-	100%
Emergency Department				
Admittance Decision Time (minutes)	560	46	65	98
Head CT Results Within 45 Min. of Arrival	-	-	61%	57%
Patients Who Left ER Before Being Seen	-	-	1%	2%
Time from ER Arrival to Admit. (minutes)	560	173	207	274
Time from ER Arrival to Discharge (minutes)	-	-	121	134
Time in ER Before Being Evaluated (minutes)	-	-	19	26
Time to Pain Meds for Fractures (minutes)	-	-	42	57
Heart Attack Care				
Aspirin Given at Discharge[5]	-	-	99%	99%
Fibrinolytic Meds Within 30 Min. of Arrival[5]	-	-	67%	54%
PCI Within 90 Minutes of Arrival[5]	-	-	96%	96%
Statin Prescribed at Discharge[5]	-	-	99%	98%
Heart Failure Care				
ACE Inhibitor or ARB for LVSD[1]	-	-	97%	97%
Discharge Instructions Given	24	100%	96%	94%
Evaluation of LVS Function	35	100%	99%	99%
Medicare Spending				
Medicare Spending per Patient (ratio)	-	-	0.94	0.98
Pneumonia Care				
Appropriate Initial Antibiotic Given	14	100%	96%	95%
Blood Culture Timing[1]	-	-	98%	98%
Pregnancy and Delivery Care				
Newborn Deliveries Scheduled Early[5]	-	-	4%	6%
Preventive Care				
Immunization for Influenza[5]	-	-	90%	90%
Immunization for Pneumonia[5]	-	-	92%	92%
Stroke Care				

NOTE: Hospital profiles are in alphabetical order by state, then city, then hospital within the city; Rankings exclude hospitals with less than 25 cases except for patient surveys which excludes hospitals with less than 100 cases; (a) 100-299 cases; (1) The number of cases/patients is too few to report; (2) Data submitted were based on a sample of cases/patients; (3) Results are based on a shorter time period than required; (4) Data suppressed by CMS for one or more quarters; (5) Results are not available for this reporting period; (6) Fewer than 100 patients completed the HCAHPS survey; (7) No cases met the criteria for this measure; (8) The lower limit of the confidence interval cannot be calculated if the number of observed infections equals zero; (9) No data are available from the state/territory for this reporting period; (10) The scores shown reflect fewer than 50 completed surveys; (11) There were discrepancies in the data collection process; (12) This measure does not apply to this hospital for this reporting period; (13) Results cannot be calculated for this reporting period; (14) The results for this state are combined with nearby states to protect confidentiality; Please refer to the User's Guide for a full explanation of data.

Measure	Cases	This Hosp.	State Avg.	U.S. Avg.
Anticoagulation Therapy for Atrial Fibrillation[5]	-	-	94%	95%
Antithrombotic Therapy Timing[5]	-	-	99%	98%
Assessed for Rehabilitation[5]	-	-	98%	97%
Discharged on Antithrombotic Therapy[5]	-	-	99%	99%
Discharged on Statin Medication[5]	-	-	94%	94%
Thrombolytic Therapy Timing[5]	-	-	60%	66%
Venous Thromboembolism Prophylaxis[5]	-	-	95%	94%
Written Stroke Educational Materials Given[5]	-	-	88%	88%
Surgical Care Improvement Project				
Appropriate Beta Blocker Usage	25	100%	99%	98%
Appropriate VTP Within 24 Hours	53	100%	99%	98%
Controlled Postoperative Blood Glucose[3,7]	-	-	96%	97%
Perioperative Temperature Management	56	100%	100%	100%
Prophylactic Antibiotic Selection	52	100%	99%	99%
Prophylactic Antibiotic Selection (Outpatient)	-	-	98%	98%
Prophylactic Antibiotic Stopped	52	96%	99%	98%
Prophylactic Antibiotic Timing	52	90%	99%	99%
Prophylactic Antibiotic Timing (Outpatient)	-	-	97%	98%
Urinary Catheter Removal	50	96%	98%	97%
Survey of Patients' Hospital Experiences				
Area Around Room 'Always' Quiet at Night	(a)	62%	63%	61%
Doctors 'Always' Communicated Well	(a)	83%	83%	82%
Home Recovery Information Given	(a)	87%	89%	85%
Hospital Given 9 or 10 on 10 Point Scale	(a)	77%	74%	71%
Meds 'Always' Explained Before Given	(a)	66%	68%	64%
Nurses 'Always' Communicated Well	(a)	84%	82%	79%
Pain 'Always' Well Controlled	(a)	71%	72%	71%
Room and Bathroom 'Always' Clean	(a)	87%	79%	73%
Timely Help 'Always' Received	(a)	72%	72%	68%
Would Definitely Recommend Hospital	(a)	74%	74%	71%
Use of Medical Imaging				
Cardiac Imaging Stress Test before Surgery	-	-	5.4%	5.3%
Combination Abdominal CT Scan	-	-	6.3%	10.5%
Combination Brain/Sinus CT Scan	-	-	2.1%	2.7%
Combination Chest CT Scan	-	-	1%	2.7%
Follow-up Mammogram/Ultrasound	-	-	8.1%	8.8%
Lumbar Spine MRI for Low Back Pain	-	-	34.9%	37.2%

Ripon Medical Center

933 Newbury St
Ripon, WI 54971
Phone: 920-748-3101
Fax: 920-748-9104
E-mail: info@riponmedicalcenter.com
URL: www.riponmedicalcenter.com
Type: Critical Access Hospitals
Emergency Services: Yes
Ownership: Voluntary non-profit - Private
Beds: 25

Key Personnel:
Chief of Medical Staff.......... Michael Combs, MD
Emergency Room............ Tami Moffat-Keenlanc
Operating Room.............. Cheryl O'Grady-Ritch
Cardiac Laboratory............ Sandy Schaffer
Quality Assurance............ Pam Schmitz
Patient Relations............. Jean Surguy
CEO/President................ Jim Tavary

Measure	Cases	This Hosp.	State Avg.	U.S. Avg.
Blood Clot Prevention and Treatment				
Anticoagulation Overlap Therapy[5]	-	-	95%	93%
ICU Venous Thromboembolism Prophylaxis[5]	-	-	91%	92%
Incidence of Potentially Preventable VTE[5]	-	-	10%	10%
UFH with Dosages/Platelet Monitoring[5]	-	-	96%	97%
Venous Thromboembolism Prophylaxis[5]	-	-	85%	85%
Warfarin Therapy Discharge Instructions[5]	-	-	70%	75%
Chest Pain/Possible Heart Attack Care				
Aspirin Given Within 24 Hours of Arrival	-	-	98%	96%
Fibrinolytic Meds Within 30 Min. of Arrival	-	-	52%	58%
Average Time to ECG (minutes)	-	-	7	7
Average Time to Transfer (minutes)	-	-	58	60
Children's Asthma Care				
Received Home Management Plan of Care	-	-	-	88%
Received Reliever Medication	-	-	-	100%
Received Systemic Corticosteroids	-	-	-	100%
Emergency Department				
Admittance Decision Time (minutes)[5]	-	-	65	98
Head CT Results Within 45 Min. of Arrival	-	-	61%	57%
Patients Who Left ER Before Being Seen	-	-	1%	2%
Time from ER Arrival to Admit. (minutes)[5]	-	-	207	274
Time from ER Arrival to Discharge (minutes)	-	-	121	134
Time in ER Before Being Evaluated (minutes)	-	-	19	26
Time to Pain Meds for Fractures (minutes)	-	-	42	57
Heart Attack Care				
Aspirin Given at Discharge[5]	-	-	99%	99%
Fibrinolytic Meds Within 30 Min. of Arrival[5]	-	-	67%	54%
PCI Within 90 Minutes of Arrival[5]	-	-	96%	96%
Statin Prescribed at Discharge[5]	-	-	99%	98%
Heart Failure Care				
ACE Inhibitor or ARB for LVSD[1]	-	-	97%	97%
Discharge Instructions Given[1]	-	-	96%	94%
Evaluation of LVS Function	13	100%	99%	99%
Medicare Spending				
Medicare Spending per Patient (ratio)	-	-	0.94	0.98
Pneumonia Care				
Appropriate Initial Antibiotic Given	18	100%	96%	95%
Blood Culture Timing	26	96%	98%	98%
Pregnancy and Delivery Care				
Newborn Deliveries Scheduled Early[5]	-	-	4%	6%
Preventive Care				
Immunization for Influenza[5]	-	-	90%	90%
Immunization for Pneumonia[5]	-	-	92%	92%
Stroke Care				
Anticoagulation Therapy for Atrial Fibrillation[5]	-	-	94%	95%
Antithrombotic Therapy Timing[5]	-	-	99%	98%
Assessed for Rehabilitation[5]	-	-	98%	97%
Discharged on Antithrombotic Therapy[5]	-	-	99%	99%
Discharged on Statin Medication[5]	-	-	94%	94%
Thrombolytic Therapy Timing[5]	-	-	60%	66%
Venous Thromboembolism Prophylaxis[5]	-	-	95%	94%
Written Stroke Educational Materials Given[5]	-	-	88%	88%
Surgical Care Improvement Project				
Appropriate Beta Blocker Usage[3]	17	100%	99%	98%
Appropriate VTP Within 24 Hours[3]	17	100%	99%	98%
Controlled Postoperative Blood Glucose[3,7]	-	-	96%	97%
Perioperative Temperature Management[3]	46	100%	100%	100%
Prophylactic Antibiotic Selection[3]	12	100%	99%	99%
Prophylactic Antibiotic Selection (Outpatient)	-	-	98%	98%
Prophylactic Antibiotic Stopped[3]	12	100%	99%	98%
Prophylactic Antibiotic Timing[3]	12	83%	99%	99%
Prophylactic Antibiotic Timing (Outpatient)	-	-	97%	98%
Urinary Catheter Removal[3]	37	95%	98%	97%
Survey of Patients' Hospital Experiences				
Area Around Room 'Always' Quiet at Night	(a)	51%	63%	61%
Doctors 'Always' Communicated Well	(a)	80%	83%	82%
Home Recovery Information Given	(a)	88%	89%	85%
Hospital Given 9 or 10 on 10 Point Scale	(a)	61%	74%	71%
Meds 'Always' Explained Before Given	(a)	62%	68%	64%
Nurses 'Always' Communicated Well	(a)	78%	82%	79%
Pain 'Always' Well Controlled	(a)	68%	72%	71%
Room and Bathroom 'Always' Clean	(a)	77%	79%	73%
Timely Help 'Always' Received	(a)	70%	72%	68%
Would Definitely Recommend Hospital	(a)	63%	74%	71%
Use of Medical Imaging				
Cardiac Imaging Stress Test before Surgery	-	-	5.4%	5.3%
Combination Abdominal CT Scan	-	-	6.3%	10.5%
Combination Brain/Sinus CT Scan	-	-	2.1%	2.7%
Combination Chest CT Scan	-	-	1%	2.7%
Follow-up Mammogram/Ultrasound	-	-	8.1%	8.8%
Lumbar Spine MRI for Low Back Pain	-	-	34.9%	37.2%

River Falls Area Hospital

1629 E Division St
River Falls, WI 54022
Phone: 715-307-6000
Fax: 715-426-4555
URL: www.allina.com
Type: Critical Access Hospitals
Emergency Services: Yes
Ownership: Voluntary non-profit - Private
Beds: 25

Key Personnel:
Infection Control.............. Lori Carlick
Operating Room.............. Matthew C Clayton, RN
CEO/President.............. David Miller
Emergency Room .... Karen Swenson, RN
Chief of Medical Staff.......... Dan Zimmerman

Measure	Cases	This Hosp.	State Avg.	U.S. Avg.
Blood Clot Prevention and Treatment				
Anticoagulation Overlap Therapy[1,2]	-	-	95%	93%
ICU Venous Thromboembolism Prophylaxis[2,7]	-	-	91%	92%
Incidence of Potentially Preventable VTE[1,2]	-	-	10%	10%
UFH with Dosages/Platelet Monitoring[1,2]	-	-	96%	97%
Venous Thromboembolism Prophylaxis[2]	133	93%	85%	85%
Warfarin Therapy Discharge Instructions[1,2]	-	-	70%	75%
Chest Pain/Possible Heart Attack Care				
Aspirin Given Within 24 Hours of Arrival	46	96%	98%	96%
Fibrinolytic Meds Within 30 Min. of Arrival[7]	-	-	52%	58%
Average Time to ECG (minutes)	48	5	7	7
Average Time to Transfer (minutes)[1]	-	-	58	60
Children's Asthma Care				
Received Home Management Plan of Care	-	-	-	88%
Received Reliever Medication	-	-	-	100%
Received Systemic Corticosteroids	-	-	-	100%
Emergency Department				
Admittance Decision Time (minutes)[2]	191	75	65	98
Head CT Results Within 45 Min. of Arrival[1,3]	-	-	61%	57%
Patients Who Left ER Before Being Seen	5,720	0%	1%	2%
Time from ER Arrival to Admit. (minutes)[2]	199	141	207	274
Time from ER Arrival to Discharge (minutes)	353	92	121	134
Time in ER Before Being Evaluated (minutes)	425	7	19	26
Time to Pain Meds for Fractures (minutes)	21	38	42	57
Heart Attack Care				
Aspirin Given at Discharge[1,3]	-	-	99%	99%
Fibrinolytic Meds Within 30 Min. of Arrival[3,7]	-	-	67%	54%
PCI Within 90 Minutes of Arrival[3,7]	-	-	96%	96%
Statin Prescribed at Discharge[1,3]	-	-	99%	98%
Heart Failure Care				
ACE Inhibitor or ARB for LVSD[1]	-	-	97%	97%
Discharge Instructions Given	12	100%	96%	94%
Evaluation of LVS Function	20	100%	99%	99%
Medicare Spending				
Medicare Spending per Patient (ratio)	-	-	0.94	0.98
Pneumonia Care				
Appropriate Initial Antibiotic Given	15	87%	96%	95%
Blood Culture Timing	13	100%	98%	98%
Pregnancy and Delivery Care				
Newborn Deliveries Scheduled Early[2]	18	6%	4%	6%
Preventive Care				
Immunization for Influenza[2]	251	95%	90%	90%
Immunization for Pneumonia[2]	292	97%	92%	92%
Stroke Care				
Anticoagulation Therapy for Atrial Fibrillation[1]	-	-	94%	95%
Antithrombotic Therapy Timing[1]	-	-	99%	98%
Assessed for Rehabilitation[1]	-	-	98%	97%
Discharged on Antithrombotic Therapy[1]	-	-	99%	99%
Discharged on Statin Medication[1]	-	-	94%	94%
Thrombolytic Therapy Timing[1]	-	-	60%	66%
Venous Thromboembolism Prophylaxis[1]	-	-	95%	94%
Written Stroke Educational Materials Given[1]	-	-	88%	88%
Surgical Care Improvement Project				
Appropriate Beta Blocker Usage	33	100%	99%	98%
Appropriate VTP Within 24 Hours	124	100%	99%	98%
Controlled Postoperative Blood Glucose[3,7]	-	-	96%	97%
Perioperative Temperature Management	142	100%	100%	100%
Prophylactic Antibiotic Selection	98	100%	99%	99%
Prophylactic Antibiotic Selection (Outpatient)	40	100%	98%	98%
Prophylactic Antibiotic Stopped	98	100%	99%	98%
Prophylactic Antibiotic Timing	98	100%	99%	99%
Prophylactic Antibiotic Timing (Outpatient)	40	95%	97%	98%
Urinary Catheter Removal	102	100%	98%	97%
Survey of Patients' Hospital Experiences				
Area Around Room 'Always' Quiet at Night	(a)	70%	63%	61%
Doctors 'Always' Communicated Well	(a)	86%	83%	82%
Home Recovery Information Given	(a)	92%	89%	85%
Hospital Given 9 or 10 on 10 Point Scale	(a)	85%	74%	71%
Meds 'Always' Explained Before Given	(a)	77%	68%	64%
Nurses 'Always' Communicated Well	(a)	89%	82%	79%
Pain 'Always' Well Controlled	(a)	78%	72%	71%

NOTE: Hospital profiles are in alphabetical order by state, then city, then hospital within the city; Rankings exclude hospitals with less than 25 cases except for patient surveys which excludes hospitals with less than 100 cases; (a) 100-299 cases; (1) The number of cases/patients is too few to report; (2) Data submitted were based on a sample of cases/patients; (3) Results are based on a shorter time period than required; (4) Data suppressed by CMS for one or more quarters; (5) Results are not available for this reporting period; (6) Fewer than 100 patients completed the HCAHPS survey; (7) No cases met the criteria for this measure; (8) The lower limit of the confidence interval cannot be calculated if the number of observed infections equals zero; (9) No data are available from the state/territory for this reporting period; (10) The scores shown reflect fewer than 50 completed surveys; (11) There were discrepancies in the data collection process; (12) This measure does not apply to this hospital for this reporting period; (13) Results cannot be calculated for this reporting period; (14) The results for this state are combined with nearby states to protect confidentiality; Please refer to the User's Guide for a full explanation of data.

Measure	Cases	This Hosp.	State Avg.	U.S. Avg.
Room and Bathroom 'Always' Clean	(a)	91%	79%	73%
Timely Help 'Always' Received	(a)	83%	72%	68%
Would Definitely Recommend Hospital	(a)	81%	74%	71%
Use of Medical Imaging				
Cardiac Imaging Stress Test before Surgery[1]	-	-	5.4%	5.3%
Combination Abdominal CT Scan	204	3.9%	6.3%	10.5%
Combination Brain/Sinus CT Scan[1]	-	-	2.1%	2.7%
Combination Chest CT Scan	149	0.7%	1%	2.7%
Follow-up Mammogram/Ultrasound	330	3.0%	8.1%	8.8%
Lumbar Spine MRI for Low Back Pain[1]	-	-	34.9%	37.2%

Saint Croix Regional Medical Center

235 State Street
Saint Croix Falls, WI 54024
URL: www.scrmc.org
Type: Critical Access Hospitals
Ownership: Voluntary non-profit - Private
Phone: 715-483-3261
Fax: 340-772-7398
Emergency Services: Yes
Beds: 25

Key Personnel:
Infection Control. . . . . Wanda Brown
Radiology. . . . . Kathy Coffman
Emergency Room . . . . Mary Erickson
Cardiac Laboratory. . . . . Deb Leal
CEO/President. . . . . Lenny Libis
Intensive Care Unit. . . . . Kari Peer
Quality Assurance . . . . Carol Thornton

Measure	Cases	This Hosp.	State Avg.	U.S. Avg.
Blood Clot Prevention and Treatment				
Anticoagulation Overlap Therapy[5]	-	-	95%	93%
ICU Venous Thromboembolism Prophylaxis[5]	-	-	91%	92%
Incidence of Potentially Preventable VTE[5]	-	-	10%	10%
UFH with Dosages/Platelet Monitoring[5]	-	-	96%	97%
Venous Thromboembolism Prophylaxis[5]	-	-	85%	85%
Warfarin Therapy Discharge Instructions[5]	-	-	70%	75%
Chest Pain/Possible Heart Attack Care				
Aspirin Given Within 24 Hours of Arrival[5]	-	-	98%	96%
Fibrinolytic Meds Within 30 Min. of Arrival[5]	-	-	52%	58%
Average Time to ECG (minutes)[5]	-	-	7	7
Average Time to Transfer (minutes)[5]	-	-	58	60
Children's Asthma Care				
Received Home Management Plan of Care	-	-	-	88%
Received Reliever Medication	-	-	-	100%
Received Systemic Corticosteroids	-	-	-	100%
Emergency Department				
Admittance Decision Time (minutes)[5]	-	-	65	98
Head CT Results Within 45 Min. of Arrival[5]	-	-	61%	57%
Patients Who Left ER Before Being Seen[5]	-	-	1%	2%
Time from ER Arrival to Admit. (minutes)[5]	-	-	207	274
Time from ER Arrival to Discharge (minutes)[5]	-	-	121	134
Time in ER Before Being Evaluated (minutes)[5]	-	-	19	26
Time to Pain Meds for Fractures (minutes)[5]	-	-	42	57
Heart Attack Care				
Aspirin Given at Discharge[5]	-	-	99%	99%
Fibrinolytic Meds Within 30 Min. of Arrival[5]	-	-	67%	54%
PCI Within 90 Minutes of Arrival[5]	-	-	96%	96%
Statin Prescribed at Discharge[5]	-	-	99%	98%
Heart Failure Care				
ACE Inhibitor or ARB for LVSD	12	92%	97%	97%
Discharge Instructions Given	35	97%	96%	94%
Evaluation of LVS Function	42	100%	99%	99%
Medicare Spending				
Medicare Spending per Patient (ratio)	-	-	0.94	0.98
Pneumonia Care				
Appropriate Initial Antibiotic Given	21	90%	96%	95%
Blood Culture Timing	31	100%	98%	98%
Pregnancy and Delivery Care				
Newborn Deliveries Scheduled Early[5]	-	-	4%	6%
Preventive Care				
Immunization for Influenza[5]	-	-	90%	90%
Immunization for Pneumonia[5]	-	-	92%	92%
Stroke Care				
Anticoagulation Therapy for Atrial Fibrillation[5]	-	-	94%	95%
Antithrombotic Therapy Timing[5]	-	-	99%	98%
Assessed for Rehabilitation[5]	-	-	98%	97%
Discharged on Antithrombotic Therapy[5]	-	-	99%	99%
Discharged on Statin Medication[5]	-	-	94%	94%
Thrombolytic Therapy Timing[5]	-	-	60%	66%
Venous Thromboembolism Prophylaxis[5]	-	-	95%	94%
Written Stroke Educational Materials Given[5]	-	-	88%	88%
Surgical Care Improvement Project				
Appropriate Beta Blocker Usage[5]	-	-	99%	98%
Appropriate VTP Within 24 Hours[5]	-	-	99%	98%
Controlled Postoperative Blood Glucose[3,7]	-	-	96%	97%
Perioperative Temperature Management	129	100%	100%	100%
Prophylactic Antibiotic Selection	120	100%	99%	99%
Prophylactic Antibiotic Selection (Outpatient)[5]	-	-	98%	98%
Prophylactic Antibiotic Stopped	118	97%	99%	98%
Prophylactic Antibiotic Timing	120	97%	99%	99%
Prophylactic Antibiotic Timing (Outpatient)[5]	-	-	97%	98%
Urinary Catheter Removal	19	74%	98%	97%
Survey of Patients' Hospital Experiences				
Area Around Room 'Always' Quiet at Night	300+	62%	63%	61%
Doctors 'Always' Communicated Well	300+	78%	83%	82%
Home Recovery Information Given	300+	90%	89%	85%
Hospital Given 9 or 10 on 10 Point Scale	300+	71%	74%	71%
Meds 'Always' Explained Before Given	300+	66%	68%	64%
Nurses 'Always' Communicated Well	300+	79%	82%	79%
Pain 'Always' Well Controlled	300+	69%	72%	71%
Room and Bathroom 'Always' Clean	300+	79%	79%	73%
Timely Help 'Always' Received	300+	73%	72%	68%
Would Definitely Recommend Hospital	300+	73%	74%	71%
Use of Medical Imaging				
Cardiac Imaging Stress Test before Surgery	101	3.0%	5.4%	5.3%
Combination Abdominal CT Scan	282	6.7%	6.3%	10.5%
Combination Brain/Sinus CT Scan	168	0.0%	2.1%	2.7%
Combination Chest CT Scan	129	0.8%	1%	2.7%
Follow-up Mammogram/Ultrasound	406	3.4%	8.1%	8.8%
Lumbar Spine MRI for Low Back Pain	47	38.3%	34.9%	37.2%

Shawano Medical Center

309 N Bartlette St
Shawano, WI 54166
E-mail: smc@shawanomed.org
URL: www.shawanomed.org
Type: Critical Access Hospitals
Ownership: Voluntary non-profit - Private
Phone: 715-526-2111
Fax: 715-526-7205
Emergency Services: Yes
Beds: 25

Key Personnel:
Patient Relations . . . . Penny Block
Intensive Care Unit. . . . . Arlene Calkins, RN
CEO/President. . . . . Dorothy Erdmann
Radiology. . . . . Paul Ho
Quality Assurance . . . . Dennis Jalter, RN
Infection Control. . . . . Kim Marquardt, RN
Operating Room. . . . . Steve Schenk, RN
Chief of Medical Staff. . . . . Amy Slagle, MD

Measure	Cases	This Hosp.	State Avg.	U.S. Avg.
Blood Clot Prevention and Treatment				
Anticoagulation Overlap Therapy[5]	-	-	95%	93%
ICU Venous Thromboembolism Prophylaxis[5]	-	-	91%	92%
Incidence of Potentially Preventable VTE[5]	-	-	10%	10%
UFH with Dosages/Platelet Monitoring[5]	-	-	96%	97%
Venous Thromboembolism Prophylaxis[5]	-	-	85%	85%
Warfarin Therapy Discharge Instructions[5]	-	-	70%	75%
Chest Pain/Possible Heart Attack Care				
Aspirin Given Within 24 Hours of Arrival[5]	-	-	98%	96%
Fibrinolytic Meds Within 30 Min. of Arrival[5]	-	-	52%	58%
Average Time to ECG (minutes)[5]	-	-	7	7
Average Time to Transfer (minutes)[5]	-	-	58	60
Children's Asthma Care				
Received Home Management Plan of Care	-	-	-	88%
Received Reliever Medication	-	-	-	100%
Received Systemic Corticosteroids	-	-	-	100%
Emergency Department				
Admittance Decision Time (minutes)[5]	-	-	65	98
Head CT Results Within 45 Min. of Arrival[5]	-	-	61%	57%
Patients Who Left ER Before Being Seen	19,401	0%	1%	2%
Time from ER Arrival to Admit. (minutes)[5]	-	-	207	274
Time from ER Arrival to Discharge (minutes)[5]	-	-	121	134
Time in ER Before Being Evaluated (minutes)[5]	-	-	19	26
Time to Pain Meds for Fractures (minutes)[5]	-	-	42	57
Heart Attack Care				
Aspirin Given at Discharge[5]	-	-	99%	99%
Fibrinolytic Meds Within 30 Min. of Arrival[5]	-	-	67%	54%
PCI Within 90 Minutes of Arrival[5]	-	-	96%	96%
Statin Prescribed at Discharge[5]	-	-	99%	98%
Heart Failure Care				
ACE Inhibitor or ARB for LVSD	16	100%	97%	97%
Discharge Instructions Given	35	97%	96%	94%
Evaluation of LVS Function	51	96%	99%	99%
Medicare Spending				
Medicare Spending per Patient (ratio)	-	-	0.94	0.98
Pneumonia Care				
Appropriate Initial Antibiotic Given	82	99%	96%	95%
Blood Culture Timing	96	99%	98%	98%
Pregnancy and Delivery Care				
Newborn Deliveries Scheduled Early[5]	-	-	4%	6%
Preventive Care				
Immunization for Influenza[5]	-	-	90%	90%
Immunization for Pneumonia[5]	-	-	92%	92%
Stroke Care				
Anticoagulation Therapy for Atrial Fibrillation[5]	-	-	94%	95%
Antithrombotic Therapy Timing[5]	-	-	99%	98%
Assessed for Rehabilitation[5]	-	-	98%	97%
Discharged on Antithrombotic Therapy[5]	-	-	99%	99%
Discharged on Statin Medication[5]	-	-	94%	94%
Thrombolytic Therapy Timing[5]	-	-	60%	66%
Venous Thromboembolism Prophylaxis[5]	-	-	95%	94%
Written Stroke Educational Materials Given[5]	-	-	88%	88%
Surgical Care Improvement Project				
Appropriate Beta Blocker Usage	32	100%	99%	98%
Appropriate VTP Within 24 Hours	102	100%	99%	98%
Controlled Postoperative Blood Glucose[7]	-	-	96%	97%
Perioperative Temperature Management	123	100%	100%	100%
Prophylactic Antibiotic Selection	100	99%	99%	99%
Prophylactic Antibiotic Selection (Outpatient)[5]	-	-	98%	98%
Prophylactic Antibiotic Stopped	100	98%	99%	98%
Prophylactic Antibiotic Timing	100	100%	99%	99%
Prophylactic Antibiotic Timing (Outpatient)[5]	-	-	97%	98%
Urinary Catheter Removal	14	100%	98%	97%
Survey of Patients' Hospital Experiences				
Area Around Room 'Always' Quiet at Night	300+	56%	63%	61%
Doctors 'Always' Communicated Well	300+	81%	83%	82%
Home Recovery Information Given	300+	87%	89%	85%
Hospital Given 9 or 10 on 10 Point Scale	300+	60%	74%	71%
Meds 'Always' Explained Before Given	300+	60%	68%	64%
Nurses 'Always' Communicated Well	300+	77%	82%	79%
Pain 'Always' Well Controlled	300+	68%	72%	71%
Room and Bathroom 'Always' Clean	300+	70%	79%	73%
Timely Help 'Always' Received	300+	65%	72%	68%
Would Definitely Recommend Hospital	300+	60%	74%	71%
Use of Medical Imaging				
Cardiac Imaging Stress Test before Surgery	143	4.2%	5.4%	5.3%
Combination Abdominal CT Scan	166	1.8%	6.3%	10.5%
Combination Brain/Sinus CT Scan	325	0.9%	2.1%	2.7%
Combination Chest CT Scan	89	0.0%	1%	2.7%
Follow-up Mammogram/Ultrasound[7]	-	-	8.1%	8.8%
Lumbar Spine MRI for Low Back Pain	36	52.8%	34.9%	37.2%

Aurora Sheboygan Memorial Medical Center

2629 N 7th St
Sheboygan, WI 53083
URL: www.aurorahealthcare.org/facilities
Type: Acute Care Hospitals
Ownership: Voluntary non-profit - Private
Phone: 920-451-5000
Fax: 920-451-5333
Emergency Services: Yes

Key Personnel:
CEO/President. . . . . Bobbe Tiegen

Measure	Cases	This Hosp.	State Avg.	U.S. Avg.
Blood Clot Prevention and Treatment				
Anticoagulation Overlap Therapy[2]	38	100%	95%	93%
ICU Venous Thromboembolism Prophylaxis[2]	30	93%	91%	92%
Incidence of Potentially Preventable VTE[1,2]	-	-	10%	10%
UFH with Dosages/Platelet Monitoring[1,2]	-	-	96%	97%

NOTE: Hospital profiles are in alphabetical order by state, then city, then hospital within the city; Rankings exclude hospitals with less than 25 cases except for patient surveys which excludes hospitals with less than 100 cases; (a) 100-299 cases; (1) The number of cases/patients is too few to report; (2) Data submitted were based on a sample of cases/patients; (3) Results are based on a shorter time period than required; (4) Data suppressed by CMS for one or more quarters; (5) Results are not available for this reporting period; (6) Fewer than 100 patients completed the HCAHPS survey; (7) No cases met the criteria for this measure; (8) The lower limit of the confidence interval cannot be calculated if the number of observed infections equals zero; (9) No data are available from the state/territory for this reporting period; (10) The scores shown reflect fewer than 50 completed surveys; (11) There were discrepancies in the data collection process; (12) This measure does not apply to this hospital for this reporting period; (13) Results cannot be calculated for this reporting period; (14) The results for this state are combined with nearby states to protect confidentiality; Please refer to the User's Guide for a full explanation of data.

Measure	Cases	This Hosp.	State Avg.	U.S. Avg.
Venous Thromboembolism Prophylaxis[2]	202	93%	85%	85%
Warfarin Therapy Discharge Instructions[2]	28	96%	70%	75%
Chest Pain/Possible Heart Attack Care				
Aspirin Given Within 24 Hours of Arrival	54	100%	98%	96%
Fibrinolytic Meds Within 30 Min. of Arrival[7]	-	-	52%	58%
Average Time to ECG (minutes)	55	7	7	7
Average Time to Transfer (minutes)	15	30	58	60
Children's Asthma Care				
Received Home Management Plan of Care	-	-	-	88%
Received Reliever Medication	-	-	-	100%
Received Systemic Corticosteroids	-	-	-	100%
Emergency Department				
Admittance Decision Time (minutes)[2]	265	60	65	98
Head CT Results Within 45 Min. of Arrival	11	55%	61%	57%
Patients Who Left ER Before Being Seen	18,591	1%	1%	2%
Time from ER Arrival to Admit. (minutes)[2]	299	192	207	274
Time from ER Arrival to Discharge (minutes)	349	109	121	134
Time in ER Before Being Evaluated (minutes)	368	21	19	26
Time to Pain Meds for Fractures (minutes)	80	37	42	57
Heart Attack Care				
Aspirin Given at Discharge	36	97%	99%	99%
Fibrinolytic Meds Within 30 Min. of Arrival[7]	-	-	67%	54%
PCI Within 90 Minutes of Arrival[1]	-	-	96%	96%
Statin Prescribed at Discharge	32	97%	99%	98%
Heart Failure Care				
ACE Inhibitor or ARB for LVSD	29	100%	97%	97%
Discharge Instructions Given	90	100%	96%	94%
Evaluation of LVS Function	114	100%	99%	99%
Medicare Spending				
Medicare Spending per Patient (ratio)	-	0.90	0.94	0.98
Pneumonia Care				
Appropriate Initial Antibiotic Given	63	98%	96%	95%
Blood Culture Timing	82	100%	98%	98%
Pregnancy and Delivery Care				
Newborn Deliveries Scheduled Early	79	6%	4%	6%
Preventive Care				
Immunization for Influenza[2]	498	97%	90%	90%
Immunization for Pneumonia[2]	487	96%	92%	92%
Stroke Care				
Anticoagulation Therapy for Atrial Fibrillation[1]	-	-	94%	95%
Antithrombotic Therapy Timing	36	100%	99%	98%
Assessed for Rehabilitation	43	100%	98%	97%
Discharged on Antithrombotic Therapy	41	98%	99%	99%
Discharged on Statin Medication	28	100%	94%	94%
Thrombolytic Therapy Timing[1]	-	-	60%	66%
Venous Thromboembolism Prophylaxis	39	97%	95%	94%
Written Stroke Educational Materials Given	26	100%	88%	88%
Surgical Care Improvement Project				
Appropriate Beta Blocker Usage[2]	190	99%	99%	98%
Appropriate VTP Within 24 Hours[2]	553	100%	99%	98%
Controlled Postoperative Blood Glucose[2,7]	-	-	96%	97%
Perioperative Temperature Management[2]	600	100%	100%	100%
Prophylactic Antibiotic Selection[2]	479	100%	99%	99%
Prophylactic Antibiotic Selection (Outpatient)	325	100%	98%	98%
Prophylactic Antibiotic Stopped[2]	476	99%	99%	98%
Prophylactic Antibiotic Timing[2]	479	100%	99%	99%
Prophylactic Antibiotic Timing (Outpatient)	326	99%	97%	98%
Urinary Catheter Removal[2]	531	100%	98%	97%
Survey of Patients' Hospital Experiences				
Area Around Room 'Always' Quiet at Night	300+	63%	63%	61%
Doctors 'Always' Communicated Well	300+	82%	83%	82%
Home Recovery Information Given	300+	92%	89%	85%
Hospital Given 9 or 10 on 10 Point Scale	300+	72%	74%	71%
Meds 'Always' Explained Before Given	300+	68%	68%	64%
Nurses 'Always' Communicated Well	300+	81%	82%	79%
Pain 'Always' Well Controlled	300+	73%	72%	71%
Room and Bathroom 'Always' Clean	300+	74%	79%	73%
Timely Help 'Always' Received	300+	63%	72%	68%
Would Definitely Recommend Hospital	300+	72%	74%	71%
Use of Medical Imaging				
Cardiac Imaging Stress Test before Surgery[1]	-	-	5.4%	5.3%
Combination Abdominal CT Scan	235	2.1%	6.3%	10.5%
Combination Brain/Sinus CT Scan[1]	-	-	2.1%	2.7%
Combination Chest CT Scan	155	0.0%	1%	2.7%
Follow-up Mammogram/Ultrasound[7]	-	-	8.1%	8.8%
Lumbar Spine MRI for Low Back Pain[1]	-	-	34.9%	37.2%

Saint Nicholas Hospital

3100 Superior Ave
Sheboygan, WI 53081
Phone: 920-459-8300
Fax: 920-451-7280
URL: www.stnicholashospital.org
Type: Acute Care Hospitals
Emergency Services: Yes
Ownership: Voluntary non-profit - Private
Beds: 185

Key Personnel:
Infection Control . . . . Sally Korff
Quality Assurance . . . . Kathie Lensen
Operating Room. . . . . Christine McCann, RN
Radiology. . . . . William Pao, MD
Pediatric Ambulatory Care . . . . . . William L Trager, MD
Pediatric In-Patient Care . . . . William L Trager, MD
Chief of Medical Staff. . . . . Philip Walker, MD

Measure	Cases	This Hosp.	State Avg.	U.S. Avg.
Blood Clot Prevention and Treatment				
Anticoagulation Overlap Therapy[2]	22	95%	95%	93%
ICU Venous Thromboembolism Prophylaxis[2]	43	67%	91%	92%
Incidence of Potentially Preventable VTE[1,2]	-	-	10%	10%
UFH with Dosages/Platelet Monitoring[2]	12	100%	96%	97%
Venous Thromboembolism Prophylaxis[2]	208	73%	85%	85%
Warfarin Therapy Discharge Instructions[2]	20	90%	70%	75%
Chest Pain/Possible Heart Attack Care				
Aspirin Given Within 24 Hours of Arrival	46	91%	98%	96%
Fibrinolytic Meds Within 30 Min. of Arrival[7]	-	-	52%	58%
Average Time to ECG (minutes)	48	10	7	7
Average Time to Transfer (minutes)[1]	-	-	58	60
Children's Asthma Care				
Received Home Management Plan of Care	-	-	-	88%
Received Reliever Medication	-	-	-	100%
Received Systemic Corticosteroids	-	-	-	100%
Emergency Department				
Admittance Decision Time (minutes)[2]	261	86	65	98
Head CT Results Within 45 Min. of Arrival[1]	-	-	61%	57%
Patients Who Left ER Before Being Seen	14,293	0%	1%	2%
Time from ER Arrival to Admit. (minutes)[2]	264	188	207	274
Time from ER Arrival to Discharge (minutes)	380	126	121	134
Time in ER Before Being Evaluated (minutes)	370	22	19	26
Time to Pain Meds for Fractures (minutes)	44	40	42	57
Heart Attack Care				
Aspirin Given at Discharge[1]	-	-	99%	99%
Fibrinolytic Meds Within 30 Min. of Arrival[7]	-	-	67%	54%
PCI Within 90 Minutes of Arrival[7]	-	-	96%	96%
Statin Prescribed at Discharge[1]	-	-	99%	98%
Heart Failure Care				
ACE Inhibitor or ARB for LVSD	16	94%	97%	97%
Discharge Instructions Given	38	92%	96%	94%
Evaluation of LVS Function	64	88%	99%	99%
Medicare Spending				
Medicare Spending per Patient (ratio)	-	0.95	0.94	0.98
Pneumonia Care				
Appropriate Initial Antibiotic Given	64	97%	96%	95%
Blood Culture Timing	85	99%	98%	98%
Pregnancy and Delivery Care				
Newborn Deliveries Scheduled Early[2]	25	0%	4%	6%
Preventive Care				
Immunization for Influenza[2]	303	84%	90%	90%
Immunization for Pneumonia[2]	397	84%	92%	92%
Stroke Care				
Anticoagulation Therapy for Atrial Fibrillation[1]	-	-	94%	95%
Antithrombotic Therapy Timing	57	95%	99%	98%
Assessed for Rehabilitation	54	98%	98%	97%
Discharged on Antithrombotic Therapy	53	98%	99%	99%
Discharged on Statin Medication	45	73%	94%	94%
Thrombolytic Therapy Timing[1]	-	-	60%	66%
Venous Thromboembolism Prophylaxis	64	72%	95%	94%
Written Stroke Educational Materials Given	24	100%	88%	88%
Surgical Care Improvement Project				
Appropriate Beta Blocker Usage[2]	90	97%	99%	98%
Appropriate VTP Within 24 Hours[2]	247	99%	99%	98%
Controlled Postoperative Blood Glucose[2,7]	-	-	96%	97%
Perioperative Temperature Management[2]	307	100%	100%	100%
Prophylactic Antibiotic Selection[2]	215	100%	99%	99%
Prophylactic Antibiotic Selection (Outpatient)	78	100%	98%	98%
Prophylactic Antibiotic Stopped[2]	211	98%	99%	98%
Prophylactic Antibiotic Timing[2]	215	99%	99%	99%
Prophylactic Antibiotic Timing (Outpatient)	80	94%	97%	98%
Urinary Catheter Removal[2]	219	94%	98%	97%
Survey of Patients' Hospital Experiences				
Area Around Room 'Always' Quiet at Night	300+	58%	63%	61%
Doctors 'Always' Communicated Well	300+	82%	83%	82%
Home Recovery Information Given	300+	87%	89%	85%
Hospital Given 9 or 10 on 10 Point Scale	300+	68%	74%	71%
Meds 'Always' Explained Before Given	300+	63%	68%	64%
Nurses 'Always' Communicated Well	300+	78%	82%	79%
Pain 'Always' Well Controlled	300+	67%	72%	71%
Room and Bathroom 'Always' Clean	300+	74%	79%	73%
Timely Help 'Always' Received	300+	64%	72%	68%
Would Definitely Recommend Hospital	300+	70%	74%	71%
Use of Medical Imaging				
Cardiac Imaging Stress Test before Surgery[1]	-	-	5.4%	5.3%
Combination Abdominal CT Scan	323	5.6%	6.3%	10.5%
Combination Brain/Sinus CT Scan[1]	-	-	2.1%	2.7%
Combination Chest CT Scan	255	0.4%	1%	2.7%
Follow-up Mammogram/Ultrasound	346	11.3%	8.1%	8.8%
Lumbar Spine MRI for Low Back Pain[1]	-	-	34.9%	37.2%

Indianhead Medical Center

113 4th Ave
Shell Lake, WI 54871
Phone: 715-468-7833
Type: Critical Access Hospitals
Emergency Services: Yes
Ownership: Proprietary

Measure	Cases	This Hosp.	State Avg.	U.S. Avg.
Blood Clot Prevention and Treatment				
Anticoagulation Overlap Therapy[5]	-	-	95%	93%
ICU Venous Thromboembolism Prophylaxis[5]	-	-	91%	92%
Incidence of Potentially Preventable VTE[5]	-	-	10%	10%
UFH with Dosages/Platelet Monitoring[5]	-	-	96%	97%
Venous Thromboembolism Prophylaxis[5]	-	-	85%	85%
Warfarin Therapy Discharge Instructions[5]	-	-	70%	75%
Chest Pain/Possible Heart Attack Care				
Aspirin Given Within 24 Hours of Arrival	-	-	98%	96%
Fibrinolytic Meds Within 30 Min. of Arrival	-	-	52%	58%
Average Time to ECG (minutes)	-	-	7	7
Average Time to Transfer (minutes)	-	-	58	60
Children's Asthma Care				
Received Home Management Plan of Care	-	-	-	88%
Received Reliever Medication	-	-	-	100%
Received Systemic Corticosteroids	-	-	-	100%
Emergency Department				
Admittance Decision Time (minutes)[5]	-	-	65	98
Head CT Results Within 45 Min. of Arrival	-	-	61%	57%
Patients Who Left ER Before Being Seen	-	-	1%	2%
Time from ER Arrival to Admit. (minutes)[5]	-	-	207	274
Time from ER Arrival to Discharge (minutes)	-	-	121	134
Time in ER Before Being Evaluated (minutes)	-	-	19	26
Time to Pain Meds for Fractures (minutes)	-	-	42	57
Heart Attack Care				
Aspirin Given at Discharge[1]	-	-	99%	99%
Fibrinolytic Meds Within 30 Min. of Arrival[7]	-	-	67%	54%
PCI Within 90 Minutes of Arrival[7]	-	-	96%	96%
Statin Prescribed at Discharge[1]	-	-	99%	98%
Heart Failure Care				
ACE Inhibitor or ARB for LVSD[1]	-	-	97%	97%
Discharge Instructions Given	12	75%	96%	94%
Evaluation of LVS Function	13	46%	99%	99%
Medicare Spending				
Medicare Spending per Patient (ratio)	-	-	0.94	0.98
Pneumonia Care				
Appropriate Initial Antibiotic Given	11	91%	96%	95%
Blood Culture Timing[1]	-	-	98%	98%

NOTE: Hospital profiles are in alphabetical order by state, then city, then hospital within the city; Rankings exclude hospitals with less than 25 cases except for patient surveys which excludes hospitals with less than 100 cases; (a) 100-299 cases; (1) The number of cases/patients is too few to report; (2) Data submitted were based on a sample of cases/patients; (3) Results are based on a shorter time period than required; (4) Data suppressed by CMS for one or more quarters; (5) Results are not available for this reporting period; (6) Fewer than 100 patients completed the HCAHPS survey; (7) No cases met the criteria for this measure; (8) The lower limit of the confidence interval cannot be calculated if the number of observed infections equals zero; (9) No data are available from the state/territory for this reporting period; (10) The scores shown reflect fewer than 50 completed surveys; (11) There were discrepancies in the data collection process; (12) This measure does not apply to this hospital for this reporting period; (13) Results cannot be calculated for this reporting period; (14) The results for this state are combined with nearby states to protect confidentiality; Please refer to the User's Guide for a full explanation of data.

Measure	Cases	This Hosp.	State Avg.	U.S. Avg.
Pregnancy and Delivery Care				
Newborn Deliveries Scheduled Early[5]	-	-	4%	6%
Preventive Care				
Immunization for Influenza[5]	-	-	90%	90%
Immunization for Pneumonia[5]	-	-	92%	92%
Stroke Care				
Anticoagulation Therapy for Atrial Fibrillation[5]	-	-	94%	95%
Antithrombotic Therapy Timing[5]	-	-	99%	98%
Assessed for Rehabilitation[5]	-	-	98%	97%
Discharged on Antithrombotic Therapy[5]	-	-	99%	99%
Discharged on Statin Medication[5]	-	-	94%	94%
Thrombolytic Therapy Timing[5]	-	-	60%	66%
Venous Thromboembolism Prophylaxis[5]	-	-	95%	94%
Written Stroke Educational Materials Given[5]	-	-	88%	88%
Surgical Care Improvement Project				
Appropriate Beta Blocker Usage[5]	-	-	99%	98%
Appropriate VTP Within 24 Hours[5]	-	-	99%	98%
Controlled Postoperative Blood Glucose[5]	-	-	96%	97%
Perioperative Temperature Management[5]	-	-	100%	100%
Prophylactic Antibiotic Selection[5]	-	-	99%	99%
Prophylactic Antibiotic Selection (Outpatient)	-	-	98%	98%
Prophylactic Antibiotic Stopped[5]	-	-	99%	98%
Prophylactic Antibiotic Timing[5]	-	-	99%	99%
Prophylactic Antibiotic Timing (Outpatient)	-	-	97%	98%
Urinary Catheter Removal[5]	-	-	98%	97%
Survey of Patients' Hospital Experiences				
Area Around Room 'Always' Quiet at Night[5]	-	-	63%	61%
Doctors 'Always' Communicated Well[5]	-	-	83%	82%
Home Recovery Information Given[5]	-	-	89%	85%
Hospital Given 9 or 10 on 10 Point Scale[5]	-	-	74%	71%
Meds 'Always' Explained Before Given[5]	-	-	68%	64%
Nurses 'Always' Communicated Well[5]	-	-	82%	79%
Pain 'Always' Well Controlled[5]	-	-	72%	71%
Room and Bathroom 'Always' Clean[5]	-	-	79%	73%
Timely Help 'Always' Received[5]	-	-	72%	68%
Would Definitely Recommend Hospital[5]	-	-	74%	71%
Use of Medical Imaging				
Cardiac Imaging Stress Test before Surgery	-	-	5.4%	5.3%
Combination Abdominal CT Scan	-	-	6.3%	10.5%
Combination Brain/Sinus CT Scan	-	-	2.1%	2.7%
Combination Chest CT Scan	-	-	1%	2.7%
Follow-up Mammogram/Ultrasound	-	-	8.1%	8.8%
Lumbar Spine MRI for Low Back Pain	-	-	34.9%	37.2%

Mayo Clinic Health Sys Franciscan Hlthcare Sparta

310 W Main St
Sparta, WI 54656
Phone: 608-269-2132
Fax: 608-269-4562
URL: www.mayohealthsystem.org/mhs/live/page.cfm
Type: Critical Access Hospitals
Emergency Services: Yes
Ownership: Voluntary non-profit - Church
Beds: 25

Key Personnel:
Patient Relations . . . . John T Brennan
Operating Room. . . . . Toni Eddy-Ballman
CEO/President. . . . . Darlene Feltes, MD
Chief of Medical Staff. . . . . J Alan Fleischmann
Surgery . . . . Christopher Huiras
Emergency Room . . . . Milton McMillen
Quality Assurance . . . . Vicki Williams

Measure	Cases	This Hosp.	State Avg.	U.S. Avg.
Blood Clot Prevention and Treatment				
Anticoagulation Overlap Therapy[1,2]	-	-	95%	93%
ICU Venous Thromboembolism Prophylaxis[2,7]	-	-	91%	92%
Incidence of Potentially Preventable VTE[2,7]	-	-	10%	10%
UFH with Dosages/Platelet Monitoring[1,2]	-	-	96%	97%
Venous Thromboembolism Prophylaxis[2]	103	92%	85%	85%
Warfarin Therapy Discharge Instructions[1,2]	-	-	70%	75%
Chest Pain/Possible Heart Attack Care				
Aspirin Given Within 24 Hours of Arrival	-	-	98%	96%
Fibrinolytic Meds Within 30 Min. of Arrival	-	-	52%	58%
Average Time to ECG (minutes)	-	-	7	7
Average Time to Transfer (minutes)	-	-	58	60
Children's Asthma Care				
Received Home Management Plan of Care	-	-	-	88%
Received Reliever Medication	-	-	-	100%
Received Systemic Corticosteroids	-	-	-	100%
Emergency Department				
Admittance Decision Time (minutes)[5]	-	-	65	98
Head CT Results Within 45 Min. of Arrival	-	-	61%	57%
Patients Who Left ER Before Being Seen	-	-	1%	2%
Time from ER Arrival to Admit. (minutes)[5]	-	-	207	274
Time from ER Arrival to Discharge (minutes)	-	-	121	134
Time in ER Before Being Evaluated (minutes)	-	-	19	26
Time to Pain Meds for Fractures (minutes)	-	-	42	57
Heart Attack Care				
Aspirin Given at Discharge[5]	-	-	99%	99%
Fibrinolytic Meds Within 30 Min. of Arrival[5]	-	-	67%	54%
PCI Within 90 Minutes of Arrival[5]	-	-	96%	96%
Statin Prescribed at Discharge[5]	-	-	99%	98%
Heart Failure Care				
ACE Inhibitor or ARB for LVSD[7]	-	-	97%	97%
Discharge Instructions Given[1]	-	-	96%	94%
Evaluation of LVS Function[1]	-	-	99%	99%
Medicare Spending				
Medicare Spending per Patient (ratio)	-	-	0.94	0.98
Pneumonia Care				
Appropriate Initial Antibiotic Given	20	100%	96%	95%
Blood Culture Timing	21	100%	98%	98%
Pregnancy and Delivery Care				
Newborn Deliveries Scheduled Early[5]	-	-	4%	6%
Preventive Care				
Immunization for Influenza[5]	-	-	90%	90%
Immunization for Pneumonia[5]	-	-	92%	92%
Stroke Care				
Anticoagulation Therapy for Atrial Fibrillation[5]	-	-	94%	95%
Antithrombotic Therapy Timing[5]	-	-	99%	98%
Assessed for Rehabilitation[5]	-	-	98%	97%
Discharged on Antithrombotic Therapy[5]	-	-	99%	99%
Discharged on Statin Medication[5]	-	-	94%	94%
Thrombolytic Therapy Timing[5]	-	-	60%	66%
Venous Thromboembolism Prophylaxis[5]	-	-	95%	94%
Written Stroke Educational Materials Given[5]	-	-	88%	88%
Surgical Care Improvement Project				
Appropriate Beta Blocker Usage[5]	-	-	99%	98%
Appropriate VTP Within 24 Hours[5]	-	-	99%	98%
Controlled Postoperative Blood Glucose[5]	-	-	96%	97%
Perioperative Temperature Management[5]	-	-	100%	100%
Prophylactic Antibiotic Selection[5]	-	-	99%	99%
Prophylactic Antibiotic Selection (Outpatient)	-	-	98%	98%
Prophylactic Antibiotic Stopped[5]	-	-	99%	98%
Prophylactic Antibiotic Timing[5]	-	-	99%	99%
Prophylactic Antibiotic Timing (Outpatient)	-	-	97%	98%
Urinary Catheter Removal[5]	-	-	98%	97%
Survey of Patients' Hospital Experiences				
Area Around Room 'Always' Quiet at Night[10]	<100	69%	63%	61%
Doctors 'Always' Communicated Well[10]	<100	92%	83%	82%
Home Recovery Information Given[10]	<100	79%	89%	85%
Hospital Given 9 or 10 on 10 Point Scale[10]	<100	64%	74%	71%
Meds 'Always' Explained Before Given[10]	<100	71%	68%	64%
Nurses 'Always' Communicated Well[10]	<100	82%	82%	79%
Pain 'Always' Well Controlled[10]	<100	71%	72%	71%
Room and Bathroom 'Always' Clean[10]	<100	56%	79%	73%
Timely Help 'Always' Received[10]	<100	89%	72%	68%
Would Definitely Recommend Hospital[10]	<100	60%	74%	71%
Use of Medical Imaging				
Cardiac Imaging Stress Test before Surgery	-	-	5.4%	5.3%
Combination Abdominal CT Scan	-	-	6.3%	10.5%
Combination Brain/Sinus CT Scan	-	-	2.1%	2.7%
Combination Chest CT Scan	-	-	1%	2.7%
Follow-up Mammogram/Ultrasound	-	-	8.1%	8.8%
Lumbar Spine MRI for Low Back Pain	-	-	34.9%	37.2%

Spooner Health System

819 Ash Street
Spooner, WI 54801
Phone: 715-635-2111
Fax: 715-635-6846
E-mail: shs@spoonerhealthsystem.com
URL: www.spoonerhealthsystem.com
Type: Critical Access Hospitals
Emergency Services: Yes
Ownership: Voluntary non-profit - Private
Beds: 130

Key Personnel:
Chief of Medical Staff. . . . . Laura Boelke, MD
Chair/CEO . . . . Sheldon Johnson
Administrator . . . . Michael Schafer
Emergency Room . . . . Linda Trent

Measure	Cases	This Hosp.	State Avg.	U.S. Avg.
Blood Clot Prevention and Treatment				
Anticoagulation Overlap Therapy[5]	-	-	95%	93%
ICU Venous Thromboembolism Prophylaxis[5]	-	-	91%	92%
Incidence of Potentially Preventable VTE[5]	-	-	10%	10%
UFH with Dosages/Platelet Monitoring[5]	-	-	96%	97%
Venous Thromboembolism Prophylaxis[5]	-	-	85%	85%
Warfarin Therapy Discharge Instructions[5]	-	-	70%	75%
Chest Pain/Possible Heart Attack Care				
Aspirin Given Within 24 Hours of Arrival	43	88%	98%	96%
Fibrinolytic Meds Within 30 Min. of Arrival[1]	-	-	52%	58%
Average Time to ECG (minutes)	46	5	7	7
Average Time to Transfer (minutes)[1]	-	-	58	60
Children's Asthma Care				
Received Home Management Plan of Care	-	-	-	88%
Received Reliever Medication	-	-	-	100%
Received Systemic Corticosteroids	-	-	-	100%
Emergency Department				
Admittance Decision Time (minutes)	242	35	65	98
Head CT Results Within 45 Min. of Arrival[5]	-	-	61%	57%
Patients Who Left ER Before Being Seen[5]	-	-	1%	2%
Time from ER Arrival to Admit. (minutes)	286	191	207	274
Time from ER Arrival to Discharge (minutes)[5]	-	-	121	134
Time in ER Before Being Evaluated (minutes)[5]	-	-	19	26
Time to Pain Meds for Fractures (minutes)[5]	-	-	42	57
Heart Attack Care				
Aspirin Given at Discharge[1]	-	-	99%	99%
Fibrinolytic Meds Within 30 Min. of Arrival[7]	-	-	67%	54%
PCI Within 90 Minutes of Arrival[3,7]	-	-	96%	96%
Statin Prescribed at Discharge[3,7]	-	-	99%	98%
Heart Failure Care				
ACE Inhibitor or ARB for LVSD[1]	-	-	97%	97%
Discharge Instructions Given	15	87%	96%	94%
Evaluation of LVS Function	23	100%	99%	99%
Medicare Spending				
Medicare Spending per Patient (ratio)	-	-	0.94	0.98
Pneumonia Care				
Appropriate Initial Antibiotic Given	33	88%	96%	95%
Blood Culture Timing	31	97%	98%	98%
Pregnancy and Delivery Care				
Newborn Deliveries Scheduled Early[5]	-	-	4%	6%
Preventive Care				
Immunization for Influenza[5]	-	-	90%	90%
Immunization for Pneumonia[5]	-	-	92%	92%
Stroke Care				
Anticoagulation Therapy for Atrial Fibrillation[5]	-	-	94%	95%
Antithrombotic Therapy Timing[5]	-	-	99%	98%
Assessed for Rehabilitation[5]	-	-	98%	97%
Discharged on Antithrombotic Therapy[5]	-	-	99%	99%
Discharged on Statin Medication[5]	-	-	94%	94%
Thrombolytic Therapy Timing[5]	-	-	60%	66%
Venous Thromboembolism Prophylaxis[5]	-	-	95%	94%
Written Stroke Educational Materials Given[5]	-	-	88%	88%
Surgical Care Improvement Project				
Appropriate Beta Blocker Usage[5]	-	-	99%	98%
Appropriate VTP Within 24 Hours[5]	-	-	99%	98%
Controlled Postoperative Blood Glucose[5]	-	-	96%	97%
Perioperative Temperature Management[5]	-	-	100%	100%
Prophylactic Antibiotic Selection[5]	-	-	99%	99%
Prophylactic Antibiotic Selection (Outpatient)[1]	-	-	98%	98%
Prophylactic Antibiotic Stopped[5]	-	-	99%	98%

NOTE: Hospital profiles are in alphabetical order by state, then city, then hospital within the city; Rankings exclude hospitals with less than 25 cases except for patient surveys which excludes hospitals with less than 100 cases; (a) 100-299 cases; (1) The number of cases/patients is too few to report; (2) Data submitted were based on a sample of cases/patients; (3) Results are based on a shorter time period than required; (4) Data suppressed by CMS for one or more quarters; (5) Results are not available for this reporting period; (6) Fewer than 100 patients completed the HCAHPS survey; (7) No cases met the criteria for this measure; (8) The lower limit of the confidence interval cannot be calculated if the number of observed infections equals zero; (9) No data are available from the state/territory for this reporting period; (10) The scores shown reflect fewer than 50 completed surveys; (11) There were discrepancies in the data collection process; (12) This measure does not apply to this hospital for this reporting period; (13) Results cannot be calculated for this reporting period; (14) The results for this state are combined with nearby states to protect confidentiality; Please refer to the User's Guide for a full explanation of data.

Measure	Cases	This Hosp.	State Avg.	U.S. Avg.
Prophylactic Antibiotic Timing[5]	-	-	99%	99%
Prophylactic Antibiotic Timing (Outpatient)[1]	-	-	97%	98%
Urinary Catheter Removal[5]	-	-	98%	97%
Survey of Patients' Hospital Experiences				
Area Around Room 'Always' Quiet at Night	(a)	73%	63%	61%
Doctors 'Always' Communicated Well	(a)	89%	83%	82%
Home Recovery Information Given	(a)	89%	89%	85%
Hospital Given 9 or 10 on 10 Point Scale	(a)	73%	74%	71%
Meds 'Always' Explained Before Given	(a)	76%	68%	64%
Nurses 'Always' Communicated Well	(a)	89%	82%	79%
Pain 'Always' Well Controlled	(a)	79%	72%	71%
Room and Bathroom 'Always' Clean	(a)	88%	79%	73%
Timely Help 'Always' Received	(a)	77%	72%	68%
Would Definitely Recommend Hospital	(a)	71%	74%	71%
Use of Medical Imaging				
Cardiac Imaging Stress Test before Surgery[1]	-	-	5.4%	5.3%
Combination Abdominal CT Scan	120	7.5%	6.3%	10.5%
Combination Brain/Sinus CT Scan[1]	-	-	2.1%	2.7%
Combination Chest CT Scan	99	0.0%	1%	2.7%
Follow-up Mammogram/Ultrasound	234	6.0%	8.1%	8.8%
Lumbar Spine MRI for Low Back Pain[1]	-	-	34.9%	37.2%

Our Lady of Victory Hospital

1120 Pine St
Stanley, WI 54768
Phone: 715-644-5571
Fax: 715-644-6221
E-mail: papiernk@olvh.org
URL: www.ministryhealth.org
Type: Critical Access Hospitals
Emergency Services: Yes
Ownership: Voluntary non-profit - Other
Beds: 25

Key Personnel:
President . . . . Cynthia Eichman
Chief of Medical Staff . . . . Sharon Hayward, MD
Quality Assurance . . . . Carol Meyer
Anesthesiology. . . . . Dwight Perkins
Emergency Room . . . . Badal Raval, MD
Operating Room. . . . . Debra Savina, RN
Infection Control. . . . . Toni Smith, RN

Measure	Cases	This Hosp.	State Avg.	U.S. Avg.
Blood Clot Prevention and Treatment				
Anticoagulation Overlap Therapy[1,3]	-	-	95%	93%
ICU Venous Thromboembolism Prophylaxis[3,7]	-	-	91%	92%
Incidence of Potentially Preventable VTE[3,7]	-	-	10%	10%
UFH with Dosages/Platelet Monitoring[3,7]	-	-	96%	97%
Venous Thromboembolism Prophylaxis[3,7]	-	-	85%	85%
Warfarin Therapy Discharge Instructions[1,3]	-	-	70%	75%
Chest Pain/Possible Heart Attack Care				
Aspirin Given Within 24 Hours of Arrival	19	95%	98%	96%
Fibrinolytic Meds Within 30 Min. of Arrival[1,3]	-	-	52%	58%
Average Time to ECG (minutes)	21	8	7	7
Average Time to Transfer (minutes)[1,3]	-	-	58	60
Children's Asthma Care				
Received Home Management Plan of Care	-	-	-	88%
Received Reliever Medication	-	-	-	100%
Received Systemic Corticosteroids	-	-	-	100%
Emergency Department				
Admittance Decision Time (minutes)[2]	278	40	65	98
Head CT Results Within 45 Min. of Arrival[1]	-	-	61%	57%
Patients Who Left ER Before Being Seen[5]	-	-	1%	2%
Time from ER Arrival to Admit. (minutes)[2]	280	190	207	274
Time from ER Arrival to Discharge (minutes)[3]	33	136	121	134
Time in ER Before Being Evaluated (minutes)[3]	38	11	19	26
Time to Pain Meds for Fractures (minutes)[1,3]	-	-	42	57
Heart Attack Care				
Aspirin Given at Discharge[1,3]	-	-	99%	99%
Fibrinolytic Meds Within 30 Minutes of Arrival[3,7]	-	-	67%	54%
PCI Within 90 Minutes of Arrival[3,7]	-	-	96%	96%
Statin Prescribed at Discharge[1,3]	-	-	99%	98%
Heart Failure Care				
ACE Inhibitor or ARB for LVSD[1]	-	-	97%	97%
Discharge Instructions Given	14	100%	96%	94%
Evaluation of LVS Function	16	100%	99%	99%
Medicare Spending				
Medicare Spending per Patient (ratio)	-	-	0.94	0.98
Pneumonia Care				
Appropriate Initial Antibiotic Given	17	71%	96%	95%
Blood Culture Timing	18	100%	98%	98%
Pregnancy and Delivery Care				
Newborn Deliveries Scheduled Early[5]	-	-	4%	6%
Preventive Care				
Immunization for Influenza	122	97%	90%	90%
Immunization for Pneumonia[2]	216	97%	92%	92%
Stroke Care				
Anticoagulation Therapy for Atrial Fibrillation[1,3]	-	-	94%	95%
Antithrombotic Therapy Timing[1,3]	-	-	99%	98%
Assessed for Rehabilitation[1,3]	-	-	98%	97%
Discharged on Antithrombotic Therapy[1,3]	-	-	99%	99%
Discharged on Statin Medication[1,3]	-	-	94%	94%
Thrombolytic Therapy Timing[3,7]	-	-	60%	66%
Venous Thromboembolism Prophylaxis[1,3]	-	-	95%	94%
Written Stroke Educational Materials Given[3,7]	-	-	88%	88%
Surgical Care Improvement Project				
Appropriate Beta Blocker Usage[5]	-	-	99%	98%
Appropriate VTP Within 24 Hours[5]	-	-	99%	98%
Controlled Postoperative Blood Glucose[5]	-	-	96%	97%
Perioperative Temperature Management[5]	-	-	100%	100%
Prophylactic Antibiotic Selection[5]	-	-	99%	99%
Prophylactic Antibiotic Selection (Outpatient)[5]	-	-	98%	98%
Prophylactic Antibiotic Stopped[5]	-	-	99%	98%
Prophylactic Antibiotic Timing[5]	-	-	99%	99%
Prophylactic Antibiotic Timing (Outpatient)[5]	-	-	97%	98%
Urinary Catheter Removal[5]	-	-	98%	97%
Survey of Patients' Hospital Experiences				
Area Around Room 'Always' Quiet at Night[6]	<100	59%	63%	61%
Doctors 'Always' Communicated Well[6]	<100	90%	83%	82%
Home Recovery Information Given[6]	<100	90%	89%	85%
Hospital Given 9 or 10 on 10 Point Scale[6]	<100	77%	74%	71%
Meds 'Always' Explained Before Given[6]	<100	70%	68%	64%
Nurses 'Always' Communicated Well[6]	<100	84%	82%	79%
Pain 'Always' Well Controlled[6]	<100	63%	72%	71%
Room and Bathroom 'Always' Clean[6]	<100	83%	79%	73%
Timely Help 'Always' Received[6]	<100	85%	72%	68%
Would Definitely Recommend Hospital[6]	<100	67%	74%	71%
Use of Medical Imaging				
Cardiac Imaging Stress Test before Surgery[1]	-	-	5.4%	5.3%
Combination Abdominal CT Scan[1]	-	-	6.3%	10.5%
Combination Brain/Sinus CT Scan[1]	-	-	2.1%	2.7%
Combination Chest CT Scan[1]	-	-	1%	2.7%
Follow-up Mammogram/Ultrasound	116	5.2%	8.1%	8.8%
Lumbar Spine MRI for Low Back Pain[1]	-	-	34.9%	37.2%

Ministry Saint Michaels Hospital of Stevens Point

900 Illinois Ave
Stevens Point, WI 54481
Phone: 715-346-5000
Fax: 715-343-3133
URL: www.saintmichaelshospital.org
Type: Acute Care Hospitals
Emergency Services: Yes
Ownership: Voluntary non-profit - Church
Beds: 129

Key Personnel:
Emergency Room . . . . Paulette Bessen
Chief of Medical Staff . . . . Mark Fenlon, MD
Quality Assurance . . . . Gloria Field
Operating Room. . . . . Steve King, RN
CEO/President. . . . . Jeffrey L Martin
Pediatric In-Patient Care . . . . Thomas McIntee, MD
Infection Control. . . . . Artie Sadlemyer
Hemotology Center . . . . Russ Shifton

Measure	Cases	This Hosp.	State Avg.	U.S. Avg.
Blood Clot Prevention and Treatment				
Anticoagulation Overlap Therapy[2]	36	100%	95%	93%
ICU Venous Thromboembolism Prophylaxis[2]	33	97%	91%	92%
Incidence of Potentially Preventable VTE[1,2]	-	-	10%	10%
UFH with Dosages/Platelet Monitoring[2]	12	100%	96%	97%
Venous Thromboembolism Prophylaxis[2]	554	98%	85%	85%
Warfarin Therapy Discharge Instructions[2]	33	91%	70%	75%
Chest Pain/Possible Heart Attack Care				
Aspirin Given Within 24 Hours of Arrival	183	99%	98%	96%
Fibrinolytic Meds Within 30 Min. of Arrival[7]	-	-	52%	58%
Average Time to ECG (minutes)	205	7	7	7
Average Time to Transfer (minutes)[1]	-	-	58	60
Children's Asthma Care				
Received Home Management Plan of Care	-	-	-	88%
Received Reliever Medication	-	-	-	100%
Received Systemic Corticosteroids	-	-	-	100%
Emergency Department				
Admittance Decision Time (minutes)[2]	504	58	65	98
Head CT Results Within 45 Min. of Arrival	11	73%	61%	57%
Patients Who Left ER Before Being Seen	19,631	0%	1%	2%
Time from ER Arrival to Admit. (minutes)[2]	504	188	207	274
Time from ER Arrival to Discharge (minutes)	1,431	128	121	134
Time in ER Before Being Evaluated (minutes)	1,597	12	19	26
Time to Pain Meds for Fractures (minutes)	59	30	42	57
Heart Attack Care				
Aspirin Given at Discharge[1]	-	-	99%	99%
Fibrinolytic Meds Within 30 Min. of Arrival[7]	-	-	67%	54%
PCI Within 90 Minutes of Arrival[7]	-	-	96%	96%
Statin Prescribed at Discharge[1]	-	-	99%	98%
Heart Failure Care				
ACE Inhibitor or ARB for LVSD	26	100%	97%	97%
Discharge Instructions Given	101	98%	96%	94%
Evaluation of LVS Function	145	100%	99%	99%
Medicare Spending				
Medicare Spending per Patient (ratio)	-	0.85	0.94	0.98
Pneumonia Care				
Appropriate Initial Antibiotic Given	48	100%	96%	95%
Blood Culture Timing	149	100%	98%	98%
Pregnancy and Delivery Care				
Newborn Deliveries Scheduled Early	41	12%	4%	6%
Preventive Care				
Immunization for Influenza[2]	468	97%	90%	90%
Immunization for Pneumonia[2]	542	97%	92%	92%
Stroke Care				
Anticoagulation Therapy for Atrial Fibrillation[1]	-	-	94%	95%
Antithrombotic Therapy Timing	46	100%	99%	98%
Assessed for Rehabilitation	47	96%	98%	97%
Discharged on Antithrombotic Therapy	47	100%	99%	99%
Discharged on Statin Medication	31	100%	94%	94%
Thrombolytic Therapy Timing[1]	-	-	60%	66%
Venous Thromboembolism Prophylaxis	48	100%	95%	94%
Written Stroke Educational Materials Given	24	96%	88%	88%
Surgical Care Improvement Project				
Appropriate Beta Blocker Usage	144	99%	99%	98%
Appropriate VTP Within 24 Hours	336	99%	99%	98%
Controlled Postoperative Blood Glucose[7]	-	-	96%	97%
Perioperative Temperature Management	493	100%	100%	100%
Prophylactic Antibiotic Selection	360	99%	99%	99%
Prophylactic Antibiotic Selection (Outpatient)	37	100%	98%	98%
Prophylactic Antibiotic Stopped	359	99%	99%	98%
Prophylactic Antibiotic Timing	360	100%	99%	99%
Prophylactic Antibiotic Timing (Outpatient)	37	97%	97%	98%
Urinary Catheter Removal	282	100%	98%	97%
Survey of Patients' Hospital Experiences				
Area Around Room 'Always' Quiet at Night	300+	66%	63%	61%
Doctors 'Always' Communicated Well	300+	84%	83%	82%
Home Recovery Information Given	300+	90%	89%	85%
Hospital Given 9 or 10 on 10 Point Scale	300+	72%	74%	71%
Meds 'Always' Explained Before Given	300+	71%	68%	64%
Nurses 'Always' Communicated Well	300+	83%	82%	79%
Pain 'Always' Well Controlled	300+	75%	72%	71%
Room and Bathroom 'Always' Clean	300+	82%	79%	73%
Timely Help 'Always' Received	300+	69%	72%	68%
Would Definitely Recommend Hospital	300+	67%	74%	71%
Use of Medical Imaging				
Cardiac Imaging Stress Test before Surgery	221	7.2%	5.4%	5.3%
Combination Abdominal CT Scan	485	6.0%	6.3%	10.5%
Combination Brain/Sinus CT Scan[1]	-	-	2.1%	2.7%
Combination Chest CT Scan	230	0.4%	1%	2.7%
Follow-up Mammogram/Ultrasound	1,050	10.5%	8.1%	8.8%
Lumbar Spine MRI for Low Back Pain	82	29.3%	34.9%	37.2%

NOTE: Hospital profiles are in alphabetical order by state, then city, then hospital within the city; Rankings exclude hospitals with less than 25 cases except for patient surveys which excludes hospitals with less than 100 cases; (a) 100-299 cases; (1) The number of cases/patients is too few to report; (2) Data submitted were based on a sample of cases/patients; (3) Results are based on a shorter time period than required; (4) Data suppressed by CMS for one or more quarters; (5) Results are not available for this reporting period; (6) Fewer than 100 patients completed the HCAHPS survey; (7) No cases met the criteria for this measure; (8) The lower limit of the confidence interval cannot be calculated if the number of observed infections equals zero; (9) No data are available from the state/territory for this reporting period; (10) The scores shown reflect fewer than 50 completed surveys; (11) There were discrepancies in the data collection process; (12) This measure does not apply to this hospital for this reporting period; (13) Results cannot be calculated for this reporting period; (14) The results for this state are combined with nearby states to protect confidentiality; Please refer to the User's Guide for a full explanation of data.

Stoughton Hospital

900 Ridge St
Stoughton, WI 53589
Phone: 608-873-6611
Fax: 608-873-2234
E-mail: info@stoughtonhospital.com
URL: www.stoughtonhospital.com
Type: Critical Access Hospitals
Emergency Services: Yes
Ownership: Voluntary non-profit - Private
Beds: 32

Key Personnel:

Operating Room. . . . . Ronald E Beresky
Chief of Medical Staff. . . . . Joyce Brehm
CEO/President. . . . . Terence J Brenny
Ambulatory Care . . . . Teresa De Nucci
Infection Control. . . . . Joyce Williams
Quality Assurance . . . . Joyce Williams

Measure	Cases	This Hosp.	State Avg.	U.S. Avg.
Blood Clot Prevention and Treatment				
Anticoagulation Overlap Therapy[2]	12	100%	95%	93%
ICU Venous Thromboembolism Prophylaxis[2]	18	100%	91%	92%
Incidence of Potentially Preventable VTE[2,7]	-	-	10%	10%
UFH with Dosages/Platelet Monitoring[1,2]	-	-	96%	97%
Venous Thromboembolism Prophylaxis[2]	92	98%	85%	85%
Warfarin Therapy Discharge Instructions[1,2]	-	-	70%	75%
Chest Pain/Possible Heart Attack Care				
Aspirin Given Within 24 Hours of Arrival[5]	-	-	98%	96%
Fibrinolytic Meds Within 30 Min. of Arrival[5]	-	-	52%	58%
Average Time to ECG (minutes)[5]	-	-	7	7
Average Time to Transfer (minutes)[5]	-	-	58	60
Children's Asthma Care				
Received Home Management Plan of Care	-	-	-	88%
Received Reliever Medication	-	-	-	100%
Received Systemic Corticosteroids	-	-	-	100%
Emergency Department				
Admittance Decision Time (minutes)[2]	335	46	65	98
Head CT Results Within 45 Min. of Arrival[5]	-	-	61%	57%
Patients Who Left ER Before Being Seen[5]	-	-	1%	2%
Time from ER Arrival to Admit. (minutes)[2]	335	183	207	274
Time from ER Arrival to Discharge (minutes)	338	129	121	134
Time in ER Before Being Evaluated (minutes)	386	9	19	26
Time to Pain Meds for Fractures (minutes)[5]	-	-	42	57
Heart Attack Care				
Aspirin Given at Discharge[5]	-	-	99%	99%
Fibrinolytic Meds Within 30 Min. of Arrival[5]	-	-	67%	54%
PCI Within 90 Minutes of Arrival[5]	-	-	96%	96%
Statin Prescribed at Discharge[5]	-	-	99%	98%
Heart Failure Care				
ACE Inhibitor or ARB for LVSD[1]	-	-	97%	97%
Discharge Instructions Given	12	83%	96%	94%
Evaluation of LVS Function	16	100%	99%	99%
Medicare Spending				
Medicare Spending per Patient (ratio)	-	-	0.94	0.98
Pneumonia Care				
Appropriate Initial Antibiotic Given	18	100%	96%	95%
Blood Culture Timing	28	100%	98%	98%
Pregnancy and Delivery Care				
Newborn Deliveries Scheduled Early[5]	-	-	4%	6%
Preventive Care				
Immunization for Influenza[2]	273	99%	90%	90%
Immunization for Pneumonia[2]	424	99%	92%	92%
Stroke Care				
Anticoagulation Therapy for Atrial Fibrillation[5]	-	-	94%	95%
Antithrombotic Therapy Timing[5]	-	-	99%	98%
Assessed for Rehabilitation[5]	-	-	98%	97%
Discharged on Antithrombotic Therapy[5]	-	-	99%	99%
Discharged on Statin Medication[5]	-	-	94%	94%
Thrombolytic Therapy Timing[5]	-	-	60%	66%
Venous Thromboembolism Prophylaxis[5]	-	-	95%	94%
Written Stroke Educational Materials Given[5]	-	-	88%	88%
Surgical Care Improvement Project				
Appropriate Beta Blocker Usage	21	100%	99%	98%
Appropriate VTP Within 24 Hours	54	100%	99%	98%
Controlled Postoperative Blood Glucose[3,7]	-	-	96%	97%
Perioperative Temperature Management	59	100%	100%	100%
Prophylactic Antibiotic Selection	38	100%	99%	99%
Prophylactic Antibiotic Selection (Outpatient)[5]	-	-	98%	98%
Prophylactic Antibiotic Stopped	37	97%	99%	98%
Prophylactic Antibiotic Timing	38	100%	99%	99%
Prophylactic Antibiotic Timing (Outpatient)[5]	-	-	97%	98%
Urinary Catheter Removal	34	97%	98%	97%
Survey of Patients' Hospital Experiences				
Area Around Room 'Always' Quiet at Night	(a)	68%	63%	61%
Doctors 'Always' Communicated Well	(a)	89%	83%	82%
Home Recovery Information Given	(a)	91%	89%	85%
Hospital Given 9 or 10 on 10 Point Scale	(a)	87%	74%	71%
Meds 'Always' Explained Before Given	(a)	75%	68%	64%
Nurses 'Always' Communicated Well	(a)	90%	82%	79%
Pain 'Always' Well Controlled	(a)	83%	72%	71%
Room and Bathroom 'Always' Clean	(a)	94%	79%	73%
Timely Help 'Always' Received	(a)	83%	72%	68%
Would Definitely Recommend Hospital	(a)	86%	74%	71%
Use of Medical Imaging				
Cardiac Imaging Stress Test before Surgery[1]	-	-	5.4%	5.3%
Combination Abdominal CT Scan	94	5.3%	6.3%	10.5%
Combination Brain/Sinus CT Scan[1]	-	-	2.1%	2.7%
Combination Chest CT Scan[1]	-	-	1%	2.7%
Follow-up Mammogram/Ultrasound	199	6.5%	8.1%	8.8%
Lumbar Spine MRI for Low Back Pain[1]	-	-	34.9%	37.2%

Ministry Door County Medical Center

323 South 18th Avenue
Sturgeon Bay, WI 54235
Phone: 920-743-5566
Fax: 920-743-8165
E-mail: dcmhinfo@dcmh.org
URL: www.doorcountymemorial.org
Type: Critical Access Hospitals
Emergency Services: Yes
Ownership: Voluntary non-profit - Church
Beds: 89

Key Personnel:

Operating Room. . . . . Jody Boes, RN
Coronary Care . . . . Sherri Christenson, RN
Quality Assurance . . . . Christa Kraus
Chief of Medical Staff. . . . . James M Lewis, MD
Infection Control. . . . . Julie Pinney, RN
CEO/President . . . . Gerald M Worrick

Measure	Cases	This Hosp.	State Avg.	U.S. Avg.
Blood Clot Prevention and Treatment				
Anticoagulation Overlap Therapy[5]	-	-	95%	93%
ICU Venous Thromboembolism Prophylaxis[5]	-	-	91%	92%
Incidence of Potentially Preventable VTE[5]	-	-	10%	10%
UFH with Dosages/Platelet Monitoring[5]	-	-	96%	97%
Venous Thromboembolism Prophylaxis[5]	-	-	85%	85%
Warfarin Therapy Discharge Instructions[5]	-	-	70%	75%
Chest Pain/Possible Heart Attack Care				
Aspirin Given Within 24 Hours of Arrival[3]	27	100%	98%	96%
Fibrinolytic Meds Within 30 Min. of Arrival[1,3]	-	-	52%	58%
Average Time to ECG (minutes)[3]	26	10	7	7
Average Time to Transfer (minutes)[1,3]	-	-	58	60
Children's Asthma Care				
Received Home Management Plan of Care	-	-	-	88%
Received Reliever Medication	-	-	-	100%
Received Systemic Corticosteroids	-	-	-	100%
Emergency Department				
Admittance Decision Time (minutes)[5]	-	-	65	98
Head CT Results Within 45 Min. of Arrival[5]	-	-	61%	57%
Patients Who Left ER Before Being Seen	9,752	1%	1%	2%
Time from ER Arrival to Admit. (minutes)[5]	-	-	207	274
Time from ER Arrival to Discharge (minutes)[5]	-	-	121	134
Time in ER Before Being Evaluated (minutes)[5]	-	-	19	26
Time to Pain Meds for Fractures (minutes)[5]	-	-	42	57
Heart Attack Care				
Aspirin Given at Discharge[1]	-	-	99%	99%
Fibrinolytic Meds Within 30 Min. of Arrival[7]	-	-	67%	54%
PCI Within 90 Minutes of Arrival[7]	-	-	96%	96%
Statin Prescribed at Discharge[1]	-	-	99%	98%
Heart Failure Care				
ACE Inhibitor or ARB for LVSD[1]	-	-	97%	97%
Discharge Instructions Given	59	95%	96%	94%
Evaluation of LVS Function	66	97%	99%	99%
Medicare Spending				
Medicare Spending per Patient (ratio)	-	-	0.94	0.98
Pneumonia Care				
Appropriate Initial Antibiotic Given	43	93%	96%	95%
Blood Culture Timing	53	100%	98%	98%
Pregnancy and Delivery Care				
Newborn Deliveries Scheduled Early[5]	-	-	4%	6%
Preventive Care				
Immunization for Influenza[2]	266	98%	90%	90%
Immunization for Pneumonia[2]	381	97%	92%	92%
Stroke Care				
Anticoagulation Therapy for Atrial Fibrillation[5]	-	-	94%	95%
Antithrombotic Therapy Timing[5]	-	-	99%	98%
Assessed for Rehabilitation[5]	-	-	98%	97%
Discharged on Antithrombotic Therapy[5]	-	-	99%	99%
Discharged on Statin Medication[5]	-	-	94%	94%
Thrombolytic Therapy Timing[5]	-	-	60%	66%
Venous Thromboembolism Prophylaxis[5]	-	-	95%	94%
Written Stroke Educational Materials Given[5]	-	-	88%	88%
Surgical Care Improvement Project				
Appropriate Beta Blocker Usage	47	94%	99%	98%
Appropriate VTP Within 24 Hours	118	97%	99%	98%
Controlled Postoperative Blood Glucose[3,7]	-	-	96%	97%
Perioperative Temperature Management	134	100%	100%	100%
Prophylactic Antibiotic Selection	101	97%	99%	99%
Prophylactic Antibiotic Selection (Outpatient)[5]	-	-	98%	98%
Prophylactic Antibiotic Stopped	95	96%	99%	98%
Prophylactic Antibiotic Timing	101	98%	99%	99%
Prophylactic Antibiotic Timing (Outpatient)[5]	-	-	97%	98%
Urinary Catheter Removal	111	99%	98%	97%
Survey of Patients' Hospital Experiences				
Area Around Room 'Always' Quiet at Night	300+	74%	63%	61%
Doctors 'Always' Communicated Well	300+	85%	83%	82%
Home Recovery Information Given	300+	87%	89%	85%
Hospital Given 9 or 10 on 10 Point Scale	300+	83%	74%	71%
Meds 'Always' Explained Before Given	300+	72%	68%	64%
Nurses 'Always' Communicated Well	300+	85%	82%	79%
Pain 'Always' Well Controlled	300+	77%	72%	71%
Room and Bathroom 'Always' Clean	300+	91%	79%	73%
Timely Help 'Always' Received	300+	83%	72%	68%
Would Definitely Recommend Hospital	300+	84%	74%	71%
Use of Medical Imaging				
Cardiac Imaging Stress Test before Surgery	113	6.2%	5.4%	5.3%
Combination Abdominal CT Scan	365	2.7%	6.3%	10.5%
Combination Brain/Sinus CT Scan	286	0.7%	2.1%	2.7%
Combination Chest CT Scan	219	1.4%	1%	2.7%
Follow-up Mammogram/Ultrasound	855	8.7%	8.1%	8.8%
Lumbar Spine MRI for Low Back Pain	94	51.1%	34.9%	37.2%

Aurora Medical Center

36500 Aurora Drive
Summit, WI 53066
Phone: 262-434-1000
URL: www.aurorahealthcare.org
Type: Acute Care Hospitals
Emergency Services: Yes
Ownership: Voluntary non-profit - Private

Key Personnel:

Emergency . . . . Mike Kefer, MD
Radiology. . . . . Ellen L Ziaja, MD

Measure	Cases	This Hosp.	State Avg.	U.S. Avg.
Blood Clot Prevention and Treatment				
Anticoagulation Overlap Therapy[2]	26	100%	95%	93%
ICU Venous Thromboembolism Prophylaxis[2]	68	97%	91%	92%
Incidence of Potentially Preventable VTE[1,2]	-	-	10%	10%
UFH with Dosages/Platelet Monitoring[1,2]	-	-	96%	97%
Venous Thromboembolism Prophylaxis[2]	151	93%	85%	85%
Warfarin Therapy Discharge Instructions[2]	23	83%	70%	75%
Chest Pain/Possible Heart Attack Care				
Aspirin Given Within 24 Hours of Arrival[1,3]	-	-	98%	96%
Fibrinolytic Meds Within 30 Min. of Arrival[3,7]	-	-	52%	58%
Average Time to ECG (minutes)[1,3]	-	-	7	7
Average Time to Transfer (minutes)[3,7]	-	-	58	60
Children's Asthma Care				
Received Home Management Plan of Care	-	-	-	88%
Received Reliever Medication	-	-	-	100%
Received Systemic Corticosteroids	-	-	-	100%
Emergency Department				

NOTE: Hospital profiles are in alphabetical order by state, then city, then hospital within the city; Rankings exclude hospitals with less than 25 cases except for patient surveys which excludes hospitals with less than 100 cases; (a) 100-299 cases; (1) The number of cases/patients is too few to report; (2) Data submitted were based on a sample of cases/patients; (3) Results are based on a shorter time period than required; (4) Data suppressed by CMS for one or more quarters; (5) Results are not available for this reporting period; (6) Fewer than 100 patients completed the HCAHPS survey; (7) No cases met the criteria for this measure; (8) The lower limit of the confidence interval cannot be calculated if the number of observed infections equals zero; (9) No data are available from the state/territory for this reporting period; (10) The scores shown reflect fewer than 50 completed surveys; (11) There were discrepancies in the data collection process; (12) This measure does not apply to this hospital for this reporting period; (13) Results cannot be calculated for this reporting period; (14) The results for this state are combined with nearby states to protect confidentiality; Please refer to the User's Guide for a full explanation of data.

Admittance Decision Time (minutes)[2]	277	70	65	98
Head CT Results Within 45 Min. of Arrival[1]	-	-	61%	57%
Patients Who Left ER Before Being Seen	11,841	0%	1%	2%
Time from ER Arrival to Admit. (minutes)[2]	287	183	207	274
Time from ER Arrival to Discharge (minutes)	356	101	121	134
Time in ER Before Being Evaluated (minutes)	384	11	19	26
Time to Pain Meds for Fractures (minutes)	75	32	42	57
Heart Attack Care				
Aspirin Given at Discharge	43	100%	99%	99%
Fibrinolytic Meds Within 30 Min. of Arrival[7]	-	-	67%	54%
PCI Within 90 Minutes of Arrival	11	100%	96%	96%
Statin Prescribed at Discharge	39	100%	99%	98%
Heart Failure Care				
ACE Inhibitor or ARB for LVSD[1]	-	-	97%	97%
Discharge Instructions Given	57	93%	96%	94%
Evaluation of LVS Function	66	100%	99%	99%
Medicare Spending				
Medicare Spending per Patient (ratio)	-	0.97	0.94	0.98
Pneumonia Care				
Appropriate Initial Antibiotic Given	37	95%	96%	95%
Blood Culture Timing	43	100%	98%	98%
Pregnancy and Delivery Care				
Newborn Deliveries Scheduled Early	32	0%	4%	6%
Preventive Care				
Immunization for Influenza[2]	306	87%	90%	90%
Immunization for Pneumonia[2]	338	91%	92%	92%
Stroke Care				
Anticoagulation Therapy for Atrial Fibrillation[1]	-	-	94%	95%
Antithrombotic Therapy Timing	18	100%	99%	98%
Assessed for Rehabilitation	32	100%	98%	97%
Discharged on Antithrombotic Therapy	30	100%	99%	99%
Discharged on Statin Medication	20	100%	94%	94%
Thrombolytic Therapy Timing[1]	-	-	60%	66%
Venous Thromboembolism Prophylaxis	24	96%	95%	94%
Written Stroke Educational Materials Given	21	95%	88%	88%
Surgical Care Improvement Project				
Appropriate Beta Blocker Usage[2]	109	100%	99%	98%
Appropriate VTP Within 24 Hours[2]	247	100%	99%	98%
Controlled Postoperative Blood Glucose[2]	24	92%	96%	97%
Perioperative Temperature Management[2]	315	100%	100%	100%
Prophylactic Antibiotic Selection[2]	234	99%	99%	99%
Prophylactic Antibiotic Selection (Outpatient)	164	97%	98%	98%
Prophylactic Antibiotic Stopped[2]	231	98%	99%	98%
Prophylactic Antibiotic Timing[2]	234	100%	99%	99%
Prophylactic Antibiotic Timing (Outpatient)	164	99%	97%	98%
Urinary Catheter Removal[2]	214	100%	98%	97%
Survey of Patients' Hospital Experiences				
Area Around Room 'Always' Quiet at Night	300+	73%	63%	61%
Doctors 'Always' Communicated Well	300+	88%	83%	82%
Home Recovery Information Given	300+	90%	89%	85%
Hospital Given 9 or 10 on 10 Point Scale	300+	82%	74%	71%
Meds 'Always' Explained Before Given	300+	75%	68%	64%
Nurses 'Always' Communicated Well	300+	85%	82%	79%
Pain 'Always' Well Controlled	300+	76%	72%	71%
Room and Bathroom 'Always' Clean	300+	81%	79%	73%
Timely Help 'Always' Received	300+	71%	72%	68%
Would Definitely Recommend Hospital	300+	82%	74%	71%
Use of Medical Imaging				
Cardiac Imaging Stress Test before Surgery	251	4.4%	5.4%	5.3%
Combination Abdominal CT Scan	391	15.1%	6.3%	10.5%
Combination Brain/Sinus CT Scan[1]	-	-	2.1%	2.7%
Combination Chest CT Scan	257	0.0%	1%	2.7%
Follow-up Mammogram/Ultrasound	670	7.8%	8.1%	8.8%
Lumbar Spine MRI for Low Back Pain	62	37.1%	34.9%	37.2%

Saint Marys Hospital Superior

3500 Tower Ave
Superior, WI 54880
Phone: 715-817-7000
Fax: 715-392-8395
URL: www.smdc.org
Type: Critical Access Hospitals
Emergency Services: Yes
Ownership: Voluntary non-profit - Private
Beds: 25

Key Personnel:

Chief of Medical Staff.......... Timothy Burke, MD
Quality Assurance .... Don Diklich
CEO/President............... Peter E Person, MD
Infection Control.............. Tim Sandor

Measure	Cases	This Hosp.	State Avg.	U.S. Avg.
Blood Clot Prevention and Treatment				
Anticoagulation Overlap Therapy[1,2]	-	-	95%	93%
ICU Venous Thromboembolism Prophylaxis[2,7]	-	-	91%	92%
Incidence of Potentially Preventable VTE[2,7]	-	-	10%	10%
UFH with Dosages/Platelet Monitoring[1,2]	-	-	96%	97%
Venous Thromboembolism Prophylaxis[2]	103	78%	85%	85%
Warfarin Therapy Discharge Instructions[1,2]	-	-	70%	75%
Chest Pain/Possible Heart Attack Care				
Aspirin Given Within 24 Hours of Arrival	27	100%	98%	96%
Fibrinolytic Meds Within 30 Min. of Arrival[7]	-	-	52%	58%
Average Time to ECG (minutes)	28	12	7	7
Average Time to Transfer (minutes)[1]	-	-	58	60
Children's Asthma Care				
Received Home Management Plan of Care	-	-	-	88%
Received Reliever Medication	-	-	-	100%
Received Systemic Corticosteroids	-	-	-	100%
Emergency Department				
Admittance Decision Time (minutes)[2]	197	36	65	98
Head CT Results Within 45 Min. of Arrival[1,3]	-	-	61%	57%
Patients Who Left ER Before Being Seen	15,211	1%	1%	2%
Time from ER Arrival to Admit. (minutes)[2]	206	186	207	274
Time from ER Arrival to Discharge (minutes)	394	102	121	134
Time in ER Before Being Evaluated (minutes)	153	21	19	26
Time to Pain Meds for Fractures (minutes)	38	35	42	57
Heart Attack Care				
Aspirin Given at Discharge[5]	-	-	99%	99%
Fibrinolytic Meds Within 30 Min. of Arrival[5]	-	-	67%	54%
PCI Within 90 Minutes of Arrival[5]	-	-	96%	96%
Statin Prescribed at Discharge[5]	-	-	99%	98%
Heart Failure Care				
ACE Inhibitor or ARB for LVSD[1]	-	-	97%	97%
Discharge Instructions Given[1]	-	-	96%	94%
Evaluation of LVS Function[1]	-	-	99%	99%
Medicare Spending				
Medicare Spending per Patient (ratio)	-	-	0.94	0.98
Pneumonia Care				
Appropriate Initial Antibiotic Given	19	95%	96%	95%
Blood Culture Timing	20	85%	98%	98%
Pregnancy and Delivery Care				
Newborn Deliveries Scheduled Early[5]	-	-	4%	6%
Preventive Care				
Immunization for Influenza[2]	137	93%	90%	90%
Immunization for Pneumonia[2]	207	100%	92%	92%
Stroke Care				
Anticoagulation Therapy for Atrial Fibrillation[5]	-	-	94%	95%
Antithrombotic Therapy Timing[5]	-	-	99%	98%
Assessed for Rehabilitation[5]	-	-	98%	97%
Discharged on Antithrombotic Therapy[5]	-	-	99%	99%
Discharged on Statin Medication[5]	-	-	94%	94%
Thrombolytic Therapy Timing[5]	-	-	60%	66%
Venous Thromboembolism Prophylaxis[5]	-	-	95%	94%
Written Stroke Educational Materials Given[5]	-	-	88%	88%
Surgical Care Improvement Project				
Appropriate Beta Blocker Usage[5]	-	-	99%	98%
Appropriate VTP Within 24 Hours[5]	-	-	99%	98%
Controlled Postoperative Blood Glucose[5]	-	-	96%	97%
Perioperative Temperature Management[5]	-	-	100%	100%
Prophylactic Antibiotic Selection[5]	-	-	99%	99%
Prophylactic Antibiotic Selection (Outpatient)	27	89%	98%	98%
Prophylactic Antibiotic Stopped[5]	-	-	99%	98%
Prophylactic Antibiotic Timing[5]	-	-	99%	99%
Prophylactic Antibiotic Timing (Outpatient)	24	96%	97%	98%
Urinary Catheter Removal[5]	-	-	98%	97%
Survey of Patients' Hospital Experiences				
Area Around Room 'Always' Quiet at Night[5]	-	-	63%	61%
Doctors 'Always' Communicated Well[5]	-	-	83%	82%
Home Recovery Information Given[5]	-	-	89%	85%
Hospital Given 9 or 10 on 10 Point Scale[5]	-	-	74%	71%
Meds 'Always' Explained Before Given[5]	-	-	68%	64%
Nurses 'Always' Communicated Well[5]	-	-	82%	79%
Pain 'Always' Well Controlled[5]	-	-	72%	71%
Room and Bathroom 'Always' Clean[5]	-	-	79%	73%
Timely Help 'Always' Received[5]	-	-	72%	68%
Would Definitely Recommend Hospital[5]	-	-	74%	71%
Use of Medical Imaging				
Cardiac Imaging Stress Test before Surgery[1]	-	-	5.4%	5.3%
Combination Abdominal CT Scan	186	3.2%	6.3%	10.5%
Combination Brain/Sinus CT Scan[1]	-	-	2.1%	2.7%
Combination Chest CT Scan	102	0.0%	1%	2.7%
Follow-up Mammogram/Ultrasound	388	5.7%	8.1%	8.8%
Lumbar Spine MRI for Low Back Pain[7]	-	-	34.9%	37.2%

Tomah Memorial Hospital

321 Butts Ave
Tomah, WI 54660
Phone: 608-372-2181
Fax: 608-374-0289
URL: www.tomahhospital.org
Type: Critical Access Hospitals
Emergency Services: Yes
Ownership: Voluntary non-profit - Private
Beds: 25

Key Personnel:

Anesthesiology............... David Demask
Quality Assurance .... Shelly Egstad
Chief of Medical Staff.......... Robb Kline, MD
Emergency Room .... Robb Kline, MD
Infection Control.............. Jan Path
Administrator .... Philip J Stuart

Measure	Cases	This Hosp.	State Avg.	U.S. Avg.
Blood Clot Prevention and Treatment				
Anticoagulation Overlap Therapy[1]	-	-	95%	93%
ICU Venous Thromboembolism Prophylaxis[7]	-	-	91%	92%
Incidence of Potentially Preventable VTE[7]	-	-	10%	10%
UFH with Dosages/Platelet Monitoring[1]	-	-	96%	97%
Venous Thromboembolism Prophylaxis	310	100%	85%	85%
Warfarin Therapy Discharge Instructions[1]	-	-	70%	75%
Chest Pain/Possible Heart Attack Care				
Aspirin Given Within 24 Hours of Arrival	54	96%	98%	96%
Fibrinolytic Meds Within 30 Min. of Arrival[1]	-	-	52%	58%
Average Time to ECG (minutes)	49	7	7	7
Average Time to Transfer (minutes)	13	106	58	60
Children's Asthma Care				
Received Home Management Plan of Care	-	-	-	88%
Received Reliever Medication	-	-	-	100%
Received Systemic Corticosteroids	-	-	-	100%
Emergency Department				
Admittance Decision Time (minutes)	490	80	65	98
Head CT Results Within 45 Min. of Arrival[1]	-	-	61%	57%
Patients Who Left ER Before Being Seen[5]	-	-	1%	2%
Time from ER Arrival to Admit. (minutes)	490	224	207	274
Time from ER Arrival to Discharge (minutes)[3]	79	114	121	134
Time in ER Before Being Evaluated (minutes)[3]	93	16	19	26
Time to Pain Meds for Fractures (minutes)[5]	-	-	42	57
Heart Attack Care				
Aspirin Given at Discharge	13	100%	99%	99%
Fibrinolytic Meds Within 30 Min. of Arrival[7]	-	-	67%	54%
PCI Within 90 Minutes of Arrival[3,7]	-	-	96%	96%
Statin Prescribed at Discharge[1]	-	-	99%	98%
Heart Failure Care				
ACE Inhibitor or ARB for LVSD[1]	-	-	97%	97%
Discharge Instructions Given	29	100%	96%	94%
Evaluation of LVS Function	33	100%	99%	99%
Medicare Spending				
Medicare Spending per Patient (ratio)	-	-	0.94	0.98
Pneumonia Care				
Appropriate Initial Antibiotic Given	50	92%	96%	95%
Blood Culture Timing	50	98%	98%	98%
Pregnancy and Delivery Care				
Newborn Deliveries Scheduled Early[5]	-	-	4%	6%
Preventive Care				
Immunization for Influenza[3]	221	100%	90%	90%
Immunization for Pneumonia[3]	321	100%	92%	92%
Stroke Care				
Anticoagulation Therapy for Atrial Fibrillation[5]	-	-	94%	95%
Antithrombotic Therapy Timing[5]	-	-	99%	98%
Assessed for Rehabilitation[5]	-	-	98%	97%

NOTE: Hospital profiles are in alphabetical order by state, then city, then hospital within the city; Rankings exclude hospitals with less than 25 cases except for patient surveys which excludes hospitals with less than 100 cases; (a) 100-299 cases; (1) The number of cases/patients is too few to report; (2) Data submitted were based on a sample of cases/patients; (3) Results are based on a shorter time period than required; (4) Data suppressed by CMS for one or more quarters; (5) Results are not available for this reporting period; (6) Fewer than 100 patients completed the HCAHPS survey; (7) No cases met the criteria for this measure; (8) The lower limit of the confidence interval cannot be calculated if the number of observed infections equals zero; (9) No data are available from the state/territory for this reporting period; (10) The scores shown reflect fewer than 50 completed surveys; (11) There were discrepancies in the data collection process; (12) This measure does not apply to this hospital for this reporting period; (13) Results cannot be calculated for this reporting period; (14) The results for this state are combined with nearby states to protect confidentiality; Please refer to the User's Guide for a full explanation of data.

Measure	Cases	This Hosp.	State Avg.	U.S. Avg.
Discharged on Antithrombotic Therapy[5]	-	-	99%	99%
Discharged on Statin Medication[5]	-	-	94%	94%
Thrombolytic Therapy Timing[5]	-	-	60%	66%
Venous Thromboembolism Prophylaxis[5]	-	-	95%	94%
Written Stroke Educational Materials Given[5]	-	-	88%	88%
Surgical Care Improvement Project				
Appropriate Beta Blocker Usage[3,7]	-	-	99%	98%
Appropriate VTP Within 24 Hours[1]	-	-	99%	98%
Controlled Postoperative Blood Glucose[3,7]	-	-	96%	97%
Perioperative Temperature Management[1]	-	-	100%	100%
Prophylactic Antibiotic Selection[1]	-	-	99%	99%
Prophylactic Antibiotic Selection (Outpatient)[1,3]	-	-	98%	98%
Prophylactic Antibiotic Stopped[1]	-	-	99%	98%
Prophylactic Antibiotic Timing[1]	-	-	99%	99%
Prophylactic Antibiotic Timing (Outpatient)[1,3]	-	-	97%	98%
Urinary Catheter Removal[1]	-	-	98%	97%
Survey of Patients' Hospital Experiences				
Area Around Room 'Always' Quiet at Night	(a)	70%	63%	61%
Doctors 'Always' Communicated Well	(a)	85%	83%	82%
Home Recovery Information Given	(a)	90%	89%	85%
Hospital Given 9 or 10 on 10 Point Scale	(a)	76%	74%	71%
Meds 'Always' Explained Before Given	(a)	68%	68%	64%
Nurses 'Always' Communicated Well	(a)	82%	82%	79%
Pain 'Always' Well Controlled	(a)	74%	72%	71%
Room and Bathroom 'Always' Clean	(a)	79%	79%	73%
Timely Help 'Always' Received	(a)	74%	72%	68%
Would Definitely Recommend Hospital	(a)	74%	74%	71%
Use of Medical Imaging				
Cardiac Imaging Stress Test before Surgery[1]	-	-	5.4%	5.3%
Combination Abdominal CT Scan	140	2.1%	6.3%	10.5%
Combination Brain/Sinus CT Scan[1]	-	-	2.1%	2.7%
Combination Chest CT Scan	55	0.0%	1%	2.7%
Follow-up Mammogram/Ultrasound[7]	-	-	8.1%	8.8%
Lumbar Spine MRI for Low Back Pain[1]	-	-	34.9%	37.2%

Tomah VA Medical Center

500 East Veterans Street
Tomah, WI 54660
Phone: 608-372-3971
URL: www.tomah.va.gov
Type: Acute Care - VA
Emergency Services: No
Ownership: Government Federal

Measure	Cases	This Hosp.	State Avg.	U.S. Avg.
Blood Clot Prevention and Treatment				
Anticoagulation Overlap Therapy	-	-	95%	93%
ICU Venous Thromboembolism Prophylaxis	-	-	91%	92%
Incidence of Potentially Preventable VTE	-	-	10%	10%
UFH with Dosages/Platelet Monitoring	-	-	96%	97%
Venous Thromboembolism Prophylaxis	-	-	85%	85%
Warfarin Therapy Discharge Instructions	-	-	70%	75%
Chest Pain/Possible Heart Attack Care				
Aspirin Given Within 24 Hours of Arrival	-	-	98%	96%
Fibrinolytic Meds Within 30 Min. of Arrival	-	-	52%	58%
Average Time to ECG (minutes)	-	-	7	7
Average Time to Transfer (minutes)	-	-	58	60
Children's Asthma Care				
Received Home Management Plan of Care	-	-	-	88%
Received Reliever Medication	-	-	-	100%
Received Systemic Corticosteroids	-	-	-	100%
Emergency Department				
Admittance Decision Time (minutes)	-	-	65	98
Head CT Results Within 45 Min. of Arrival	-	-	61%	57%
Patients Who Left ER Before Being Seen	-	-	1%	2%
Time from ER Arrival to Admit. (minutes)	-	-	207	274
Time from ER Arrival to Discharge (minutes)	-	-	121	134
Time in ER Before Being Evaluated (minutes)	-	-	19	26
Time to Pain Meds for Fractures (minutes)	-	-	42	57
Heart Attack Care				
Aspirin Given at Discharge[5]	-	-	99%	99%
Fibrinolytic Meds Within 30 Min. of Arrival[5]	-	-	67%	54%
PCI Within 90 Minutes of Arrival[5]	-	-	96%	96%
Statin Prescribed at Discharge[5]	-	-	99%	98%
Heart Failure Care				
ACE Inhibitor or ARB for LVSD[5]	-	-	97%	97%
Discharge Instructions Given[5]	-	-	96%	94%
Evaluation of LVS Function[5]	-	-	99%	99%
Medicare Spending				
Medicare Spending per Patient (ratio)	-	-	0.94	0.98
Pneumonia Care				
Appropriate Initial Antibiotic Given[5]	-	-	96%	95%
Blood Culture Timing[5]	-	-	98%	98%
Pregnancy and Delivery Care				
Newborn Deliveries Scheduled Early	-	-	4%	6%
Preventive Care				
Immunization for Influenza[2,3]	147	95%	90%	90%
Immunization for Pneumonia[2,3]	250	98%	92%	92%
Stroke Care				
Anticoagulation Therapy for Atrial Fibrillation	-	-	94%	95%
Antithrombotic Therapy Timing	-	-	99%	98%
Assessed for Rehabilitation	-	-	98%	97%
Discharged on Antithrombotic Therapy	-	-	99%	99%
Discharged on Statin Medication	-	-	94%	94%
Thrombolytic Therapy Timing	-	-	60%	66%
Venous Thromboembolism Prophylaxis	-	-	95%	94%
Written Stroke Educational Materials Given	-	-	88%	88%
Surgical Care Improvement Project				
Appropriate Beta Blocker Usage[5]	-	-	99%	98%
Appropriate VTP Within 24 Hours[5]	-	-	99%	98%
Controlled Postoperative Blood Glucose[5]	-	-	96%	97%
Perioperative Temperature Management[5]	-	-	100%	100%
Prophylactic Antibiotic Selection[5]	-	-	99%	99%
Prophylactic Antibiotic Selection (Outpatient)	-	-	98%	98%
Prophylactic Antibiotic Stopped[5]	-	-	99%	98%
Prophylactic Antibiotic Timing[5]	-	-	99%	99%
Prophylactic Antibiotic Timing (Outpatient)	-	-	97%	98%
Urinary Catheter Removal[5]	-	-	98%	97%
Survey of Patients' Hospital Experiences				
Area Around Room 'Always' Quiet at Night	-	-	63%	61%
Doctors 'Always' Communicated Well	-	-	83%	82%
Home Recovery Information Given	-	-	89%	85%
Hospital Given 9 or 10 on 10 Point Scale	-	-	74%	71%
Meds 'Always' Explained Before Given	-	-	68%	64%
Nurses 'Always' Communicated Well	-	-	82%	79%
Pain 'Always' Well Controlled	-	-	72%	71%
Room and Bathroom 'Always' Clean	-	-	79%	73%
Timely Help 'Always' Received	-	-	72%	68%
Would Definitely Recommend Hospital	-	-	74%	71%
Use of Medical Imaging				
Cardiac Imaging Stress Test before Surgery	-	-	5.4%	5.3%
Combination Abdominal CT Scan	-	-	6.3%	10.5%
Combination Brain/Sinus CT Scan	-	-	2.1%	2.7%
Combination Chest CT Scan	-	-	1%	2.7%
Follow-up Mammogram/Ultrasound	-	-	8.1%	8.8%
Lumbar Spine MRI for Low Back Pain	-	-	34.9%	37.2%

Ministry Sacred Heart Hospital

401 W Mohawk Dr Ste 100
Tomahawk, WI 54487
Phone: 715-453-7700
Fax: 715-361-2006
URL: www.ministryhealth.org
Type: Critical Access Hospitals
Emergency Services: Yes
Ownership: Voluntary non-profit - Private
Beds: 18

Key Personnel:
Chief of Medical Staff.......... Ron Cortte, MD
Emergency Room .... Paula Gebauer, RN
CEO/President.............. Monica Hilt
Infection Control............ Karen Wiedema, RN
Quality Assurance .... Karen Wiedeman

Measure	Cases	This Hosp.	State Avg.	U.S. Avg.
Blood Clot Prevention and Treatment				
Anticoagulation Overlap Therapy[1,2]	-	-	95%	93%
ICU Venous Thromboembolism Prophylaxis[1,2]	-	-	91%	92%
Incidence of Potentially Preventable VTE[2,7]	-	-	10%	10%
UFH with Dosages/Platelet Monitoring[2,7]	-	-	96%	97%
Venous Thromboembolism Prophylaxis[2]	131	98%	85%	85%
Warfarin Therapy Discharge Instructions[1,2]	-	-	70%	75%
Chest Pain/Possible Heart Attack Care				
Aspirin Given Within 24 Hours of Arrival	30	100%	98%	96%
Fibrinolytic Meds Within 30 Min. of Arrival[1,3]	-	-	52%	58%
Average Time to ECG (minutes)	33	3	7	7
Average Time to Transfer (minutes)[3,7]	-	-	58	60
Children's Asthma Care				
Received Home Management Plan of Care	-	-	-	88%
Received Reliever Medication	-	-	-	100%
Received Systemic Corticosteroids	-	-	-	100%
Emergency Department				
Admittance Decision Time (minutes)[2]	186	38	65	98
Head CT Results Within 45 Min. of Arrival[1]	-	-	61%	57%
Patients Who Left ER Before Being Seen	4,194	0%	1%	2%
Time from ER Arrival to Admit. (minutes)[2]	216	148	207	274
Time from ER Arrival to Discharge (minutes)	661	88	121	134
Time in ER Before Being Evaluated (minutes)	638	16	19	26
Time to Pain Meds for Fractures (minutes)	20	39	42	57
Heart Attack Care				
Aspirin Given at Discharge[1,3]	-	-	99%	99%
Fibrinolytic Meds Within 30 Min. of Arrival[3,7]	-	-	67%	54%
PCI Within 90 Minutes of Arrival[3,7]	-	-	96%	96%
Statin Prescribed at Discharge[1,3]	-	-	99%	98%
Heart Failure Care				
ACE Inhibitor or ARB for LVSD[1]	-	-	97%	97%
Discharge Instructions Given[1]	-	-	96%	94%
Evaluation of LVS Function	16	100%	99%	99%
Medicare Spending				
Medicare Spending per Patient (ratio)	-	-	0.94	0.98
Pneumonia Care				
Appropriate Initial Antibiotic Given	27	100%	96%	95%
Blood Culture Timing	28	100%	98%	98%
Pregnancy and Delivery Care				
Newborn Deliveries Scheduled Early[5]	-	-	4%	6%
Preventive Care				
Immunization for Influenza[2]	151	99%	90%	90%
Immunization for Pneumonia[2]	267	99%	92%	92%
Stroke Care				
Anticoagulation Therapy for Atrial Fibrillation[1]	-	-	94%	95%
Antithrombotic Therapy Timing[1]	-	-	99%	98%
Assessed for Rehabilitation[1]	-	-	98%	97%
Discharged on Antithrombotic Therapy[1]	-	-	99%	99%
Discharged on Statin Medication[1]	-	-	94%	94%
Thrombolytic Therapy Timing[7]	-	-	60%	66%
Venous Thromboembolism Prophylaxis[1]	-	-	95%	94%
Written Stroke Educational Materials Given[1]	-	-	88%	88%
Surgical Care Improvement Project				
Appropriate Beta Blocker Usage[5]	-	-	99%	98%
Appropriate VTP Within 24 Hours[5]	-	-	99%	98%
Controlled Postoperative Blood Glucose[5]	-	-	96%	97%
Perioperative Temperature Management[5]	-	-	100%	100%
Prophylactic Antibiotic Selection[5]	-	-	99%	99%
Prophylactic Antibiotic Selection (Outpatient)[5]	-	-	98%	98%
Prophylactic Antibiotic Stopped[5]	-	-	99%	98%
Prophylactic Antibiotic Timing[5]	-	-	99%	99%
Prophylactic Antibiotic Timing (Outpatient)[5]	-	-	97%	98%
Urinary Catheter Removal[5]	-	-	98%	97%
Survey of Patients' Hospital Experiences				
Area Around Room 'Always' Quiet at Night[6]	<100	66%	63%	61%
Doctors 'Always' Communicated Well[6]	<100	91%	83%	82%
Home Recovery Information Given[6]	<100	91%	89%	85%
Hospital Given 9 or 10 on 10 Point Scale[6]	<100	80%	74%	71%
Meds 'Always' Explained Before Given[6]	<100	77%	68%	64%
Nurses 'Always' Communicated Well[6]	<100	86%	82%	79%
Pain 'Always' Well Controlled[6]	<100	78%	72%	71%
Room and Bathroom 'Always' Clean[6]	<100	87%	79%	73%
Timely Help 'Always' Received[6]	<100	88%	72%	68%
Would Definitely Recommend Hospital[6]	<100	74%	74%	71%
Use of Medical Imaging				
Cardiac Imaging Stress Test before Surgery[1]	-	-	5.4%	5.3%
Combination Abdominal CT Scan	103	6.8%	6.3%	10.5%
Combination Brain/Sinus CT Scan	167	1.2%	2.1%	2.7%
Combination Chest CT Scan	56	0.0%	1%	2.7%
Follow-up Mammogram/Ultrasound	224	8.0%	8.1%	8.8%

NOTE: Hospital profiles are in alphabetical order by state, then city, then hospital within the city; Rankings exclude hospitals with less than 25 cases except for patient surveys which excludes hospitals with less than 100 cases; (a) 100-299 cases; (1) The number of cases/patients is too few to report; (2) Data submitted were based on a sample of cases/patients; (3) Results are based on a shorter time period than required; (4) Data suppressed by CMS for one or more quarters; (5) Results are not available for this reporting period; (6) Fewer than 100 patients completed the HCAHPS survey; (7) No cases met the criteria for this measure; (8) The lower limit of the confidence interval cannot be calculated if the number of observed infections equals zero; (9) No data are available from the state/territory for this reporting period; (10) The scores shown reflect fewer than 50 completed surveys; (11) There were discrepancies in the data collection process; (12) This measure does not apply to this hospital for this reporting period; (13) Results cannot be calculated for this reporting period; (14) The results for this state are combined with nearby states to protect confidentiality; Please refer to the User's Guide for a full explanation of data.

Lumbar Spine MRI for Low Back Pain[7]	-	-	34.9%	37.2%

Aurora Medical Center Manitowoc County

5000 Memorial Dr
Two Rivers, WI 54241
Phone: 920-794-5000
Fax: 920-794-5487
URL: www.aurorahealthcare.org
Type: Acute Care Hospitals
Emergency Services: Yes
Ownership: Voluntary non-profit - Private
Beds: 73

Key Personnel:
Operating Room. . . . . Per Anderas, RN
Infection Control. . . . . Vicki Grimstad
Quality Assurance . . . . Vicki Grimstad
Emergency Room . . . . James Hermann, MD
Pediatric Ambulatory Care . . . . . . Ali A Mir, MD
Pediatric In-Patient Care . . . . Ali A Mir, MD
Chief of Medical Staff. . . . . Glenn Smith, MD
Intensive Care Unit. . . . . M Swoboda, RN

Measure	Cases	This Hosp.	State Avg.	U.S. Avg.
Blood Clot Prevention and Treatment				
Anticoagulation Overlap Therapy[2]	21	95%	95%	93%
ICU Venous Thromboembolism Prophylaxis[2]	25	92%	91%	92%
Incidence of Potentially Preventable VTE[1,2]	-	-	10%	10%
UFH with Dosages/Platelet Monitoring[1,2]	-	-	96%	97%
Venous Thromboembolism Prophylaxis[2]	128	88%	85%	85%
Warfarin Therapy Discharge Instructions[2]	17	82%	70%	75%
Chest Pain/Possible Heart Attack Care				
Aspirin Given Within 24 Hours of Arrival	46	98%	98%	96%
Fibrinolytic Meds Within 30 Min. of Arrival[7]	-	-	52%	58%
Average Time to ECG (minutes)	47	10	7	7
Average Time to Transfer (minutes)[1]	-	-	58	60
Children's Asthma Care				
Received Home Management Plan of Care	-	-	-	88%
Received Reliever Medication	-	-	-	100%
Received Systemic Corticosteroids	-	-	-	100%
Emergency Department				
Admittance Decision Time (minutes)[2]	213	54	65	98
Head CT Results Within 45 Min. of Arrival	15	80%	61%	57%
Patients Who Left ER Before Being Seen	12,270	0%	1%	2%
Time from ER Arrival to Admit. (minutes)[2]	255	217	207	274
Time from ER Arrival to Discharge (minutes)	344	128	121	134
Time in ER Before Being Evaluated (minutes)	357	27	19	26
Time to Pain Meds for Fractures (minutes)	46	53	42	57
Heart Attack Care				
Aspirin Given at Discharge	11	100%	99%	99%
Fibrinolytic Meds Within 30 Min. of Arrival[7]	-	-	67%	54%
PCI Within 90 Minutes of Arrival[7]	-	-	96%	96%
Statin Prescribed at Discharge[1]	-	-	99%	98%
Heart Failure Care				
ACE Inhibitor or ARB for LVSD	12	100%	97%	97%
Discharge Instructions Given	39	92%	96%	94%
Evaluation of LVS Function	51	100%	99%	99%
Medicare Spending				
Medicare Spending per Patient (ratio)	-	0.98	0.94	0.98
Pneumonia Care				
Appropriate Initial Antibiotic Given	54	94%	96%	95%
Blood Culture Timing	53	100%	98%	98%
Pregnancy and Delivery Care				
Newborn Deliveries Scheduled Early[2]	35	0%	4%	6%
Preventive Care				
Immunization for Influenza[2]	248	98%	90%	90%
Immunization for Pneumonia[2]	296	98%	92%	92%
Stroke Care				
Anticoagulation Therapy for Atrial Fibrillation[1]	-	-	94%	95%
Antithrombotic Therapy Timing	18	100%	99%	98%
Assessed for Rehabilitation	20	100%	98%	97%
Discharged on Antithrombotic Therapy	19	100%	99%	99%
Discharged on Statin Medication	14	100%	94%	94%
Thrombolytic Therapy Timing[7]	-	-	60%	66%
Venous Thromboembolism Prophylaxis	18	100%	95%	94%
Written Stroke Educational Materials Given[1]	-	-	88%	88%
Surgical Care Improvement Project				
Appropriate Beta Blocker Usage[2]	79	100%	99%	98%
Appropriate VTP Within 24 Hours[2]	143	100%	99%	98%
Controlled Postoperative Blood Glucose[2,7]	-	-	96%	97%
Perioperative Temperature Management[2]	186	100%	100%	100%
Prophylactic Antibiotic Selection[2]	131	99%	99%	99%
Prophylactic Antibiotic Selection (Outpatient)	130	98%	98%	98%
Prophylactic Antibiotic Stopped[2]	130	99%	99%	98%
Prophylactic Antibiotic Timing[2]	132	96%	99%	99%
Prophylactic Antibiotic Timing (Outpatient)	133	97%	97%	98%
Urinary Catheter Removal[2]	43	98%	98%	97%
Survey of Patients' Hospital Experiences				
Area Around Room 'Always' Quiet at Night	300+	65%	63%	61%
Doctors 'Always' Communicated Well	300+	81%	83%	82%
Home Recovery Information Given	300+	88%	89%	85%
Hospital Given 9 or 10 on 10 Point Scale	300+	76%	74%	71%
Meds 'Always' Explained Before Given	300+	67%	68%	64%
Nurses 'Always' Communicated Well	300+	81%	82%	79%
Pain 'Always' Well Controlled	300+	73%	72%	71%
Room and Bathroom 'Always' Clean	300+	87%	79%	73%
Timely Help 'Always' Received	300+	71%	72%	68%
Would Definitely Recommend Hospital	300+	78%	74%	71%
Use of Medical Imaging				
Cardiac Imaging Stress Test before Surgery	167	5.4%	5.4%	5.3%
Combination Abdominal CT Scan	245	6.5%	6.3%	10.5%
Combination Brain/Sinus CT Scan	281	4.3%	2.1%	2.7%
Combination Chest CT Scan	181	0.0%	1%	2.7%
Follow-up Mammogram/Ultrasound[7]	-	-	8.1%	8.8%
Lumbar Spine MRI for Low Back Pain	58	41.4%	34.9%	37.2%

Vernon Memorial Hospital

507 South Main St
Viroqua, WI 54665
Phone: 608-637-2101
Fax: 608-637-2141
E-mail: jsteiner@vmh.org
URL: www.vmh.org
Type: Critical Access Hospitals
Emergency Services: Yes
Ownership: Voluntary non-profit - Private
Beds: 25

Key Personnel:
CEO . . . . Kyle Bakkum
Infection Control. . . . . Romelle Heisel
Ambulatory Care . . . . Sue Heitman
Operating Room. . . . . Sue Heitman
Chief of Medical Staff. . . . . Jeff Lawrence
Emergency Room . . . . Anthony Macasaet
Anesthesiology. . . . . Arnold Nomann
Quality Assurance . . . . Sue Sullivan

Measure	Cases	This Hosp.	State Avg.	U.S. Avg.
Blood Clot Prevention and Treatment				
Anticoagulation Overlap Therapy[1]	-	-	95%	93%
ICU Venous Thromboembolism Prophylaxis[7]	-	-	91%	92%
Incidence of Potentially Preventable VTE[1]	-	-	10%	10%
UFH with Dosages/Platelet Monitoring[7]	-	-	96%	97%
Venous Thromboembolism Prophylaxis	329	64%	85%	85%
Warfarin Therapy Discharge Instructions[1]	-	-	70%	75%
Chest Pain/Possible Heart Attack Care				
Aspirin Given Within 24 Hours of Arrival	54	100%	98%	96%
Fibrinolytic Meds Within 30 Min. of Arrival[7]	-	-	52%	58%
Average Time to ECG (minutes)	55	9	7	7
Average Time to Transfer (minutes)[1]	-	-	58	60
Children's Asthma Care				
Received Home Management Plan of Care	-	-	-	88%
Received Reliever Medication	-	-	-	100%
Received Systemic Corticosteroids	-	-	-	100%
Emergency Department				
Admittance Decision Time (minutes)[2]	344	53	65	98
Head CT Results Within 45 Min. of Arrival[5]	-	-	61%	57%
Patients Who Left ER Before Being Seen[5]	-	-	1%	2%
Time from ER Arrival to Admit. (minutes)[2]	346	187	207	274
Time from ER Arrival to Discharge (minutes)	313	113	121	134
Time in ER Before Being Evaluated (minutes)	377	23	19	26
Time to Pain Meds for Fractures (minutes)[5]	-	-	42	57
Heart Attack Care				
Aspirin Given at Discharge[1]	-	-	99%	99%
Fibrinolytic Meds Within 30 Min. of Arrival[7]	-	-	67%	54%
PCI Within 90 Minutes of Arrival[7]	-	-	96%	96%
Statin Prescribed at Discharge[1]	-	-	99%	98%
Heart Failure Care				
ACE Inhibitor or ARB for LVSD[1]	-	-	97%	97%
Discharge Instructions Given	15	93%	96%	94%
Evaluation of LVS Function	23	91%	99%	99%
Medicare Spending				
Medicare Spending per Patient (ratio)	-	-	0.94	0.98
Pneumonia Care				
Appropriate Initial Antibiotic Given	65	95%	96%	95%
Blood Culture Timing	70	99%	98%	98%
Pregnancy and Delivery Care				
Newborn Deliveries Scheduled Early[5]	-	-	4%	6%
Preventive Care				
Immunization for Influenza[2]	507	96%	90%	90%
Immunization for Pneumonia[2]	718	95%	92%	92%
Stroke Care				
Anticoagulation Therapy for Atrial Fibrillation[1]	-	-	94%	95%
Antithrombotic Therapy Timing[1]	-	-	99%	98%
Assessed for Rehabilitation[1]	-	-	98%	97%
Discharged on Antithrombotic Therapy[1]	-	-	99%	99%
Discharged on Statin Medication[1]	-	-	94%	94%
Thrombolytic Therapy Timing[1]	-	-	60%	66%
Venous Thromboembolism Prophylaxis[1]	-	-	95%	94%
Written Stroke Educational Materials Given[1]	-	-	88%	88%
Surgical Care Improvement Project				
Appropriate Beta Blocker Usage	140	99%	99%	98%
Appropriate VTP Within 24 Hours	502	100%	99%	98%
Controlled Postoperative Blood Glucose[3,7]	-	-	96%	97%
Perioperative Temperature Management	553	100%	100%	100%
Prophylactic Antibiotic Selection	488	100%	99%	99%
Prophylactic Antibiotic Selection (Outpatient)[1,3]	-	-	98%	98%
Prophylactic Antibiotic Stopped	485	99%	99%	98%
Prophylactic Antibiotic Timing	489	97%	99%	99%
Prophylactic Antibiotic Timing (Outpatient)[1,3]	-	-	97%	98%
Urinary Catheter Removal	50	96%	98%	97%
Survey of Patients' Hospital Experiences				
Area Around Room 'Always' Quiet at Night	300+	66%	63%	61%
Doctors 'Always' Communicated Well	300+	89%	83%	82%
Home Recovery Information Given	300+	92%	89%	85%
Hospital Given 9 or 10 on 10 Point Scale	300+	84%	74%	71%
Meds 'Always' Explained Before Given	300+	74%	68%	64%
Nurses 'Always' Communicated Well	300+	87%	82%	79%
Pain 'Always' Well Controlled	300+	80%	72%	71%
Room and Bathroom 'Always' Clean	300+	89%	79%	73%
Timely Help 'Always' Received	300+	86%	72%	68%
Would Definitely Recommend Hospital	300+	82%	74%	71%
Use of Medical Imaging				
Cardiac Imaging Stress Test before Surgery	47	2.1%	5.4%	5.3%
Combination Abdominal CT Scan	127	4.7%	6.3%	10.5%
Combination Brain/Sinus CT Scan[1]	-	-	2.1%	2.7%
Combination Chest CT Scan	69	2.9%	1%	2.7%
Follow-up Mammogram/Ultrasound	291	6.2%	8.1%	8.8%
Lumbar Spine MRI for Low Back Pain[1]	-	-	34.9%	37.2%

UW Health Partners Watertown Regional Medical Center

125 Hospital Dr
Watertown, WI 53098
Phone: 920-261-4210
Fax: 920-261-3940
URL: www.watertownmemorialhospital.com
Type: Acute Care Hospitals
Emergency Services: Yes
Ownership: Voluntary non-profit - Private
Beds: 95

Key Personnel:
Radiology. . . . . Jeffrey Van Beek
Infection Control. . . . . Linda Gehring
CEO/President. . . . . John Kosanovich
Chief of Medical Staff. . . . . James Milford, MD
Patient Relations . . . . Tom Peterson
Quality Assurance . . . . Tricia Price
Intensive Care Unit. . . . . Barb Quest, RN
Pediatric In-Patient Care . . . . Barb Quest, RN

Measure	Cases	This Hosp.	State Avg.	U.S. Avg.
Blood Clot Prevention and Treatment				
Anticoagulation Overlap Therapy[2]	14	93%	95%	93%
ICU Venous Thromboembolism Prophylaxis[1,2]	-	-	91%	92%
Incidence of Potentially Preventable VTE[1,2]	-	-	10%	10%
UFH with Dosages/Platelet Monitoring[1,2]	-	-	96%	97%
Venous Thromboembolism Prophylaxis[2]	113	93%	85%	85%

NOTE: Hospital profiles are in alphabetical order by state, then city, then hospital within the city; Rankings exclude hospitals with less than 25 cases except for patient surveys which excludes hospitals with less than 100 cases; (a) 100-299 cases; (1) The number of cases/patients is too few to report; (2) Data submitted were based on a sample of cases/patients; (3) Results are based on a shorter time period than required; (4) Data suppressed by CMS for one or more quarters; (5) Results are not available for this reporting period; (6) Fewer than 100 patients completed the HCAHPS survey; (7) No cases met the criteria for this measure; (8) The lower limit of the confidence interval cannot be calculated if the number of observed infections equals zero; (9) No data are available from the state/territory for this reporting period; (10) The scores shown reflect fewer than 50 completed surveys; (11) There were discrepancies in the data collection process; (12) This measure does not apply to this hospital for this reporting period; (13) Results cannot be calculated for this reporting period; (14) The results for this state are combined with nearby states to protect confidentiality; Please refer to the User's Guide for a full explanation of data.

Measure	Cases	This Hosp.	State Avg.	U.S. Avg.
Warfarin Therapy Discharge Instructions[2]	13	54%	70%	75%
Chest Pain/Possible Heart Attack Care				
Aspirin Given Within 24 Hours of Arrival	63	98%	98%	96%
Fibrinolytic Meds Within 30 Min. of Arrival[1]	-	-	52%	58%
Average Time to ECG (minutes)	64	6	7	7
Average Time to Transfer (minutes)[1]	-	-	58	60
Children's Asthma Care				
Received Home Management Plan of Care	-	-	-	88%
Received Reliever Medication	-	-	-	100%
Received Systemic Corticosteroids	-	-	-	100%
Emergency Department				
Admittance Decision Time (minutes)[2]	122	66	65	98
Head CT Results Within 45 Min. of Arrival[1]	-	-	61%	57%
Patients Who Left ER Before Being Seen	20,343	0%	1%	2%
Time from ER Arrival to Admit. (minutes)[2]	171	215	207	274
Time from ER Arrival to Discharge (minutes)	408	114	121	134
Time in ER Before Being Evaluated (minutes)	450	17	19	26
Time to Pain Meds for Fractures (minutes)	53	37	42	57
Heart Attack Care				
Aspirin Given at Discharge	11	100%	99%	99%
Fibrinolytic Meds Within 30 Min. of Arrival[7]	-	-	67%	54%
PCI Within 90 Minutes of Arrival[1]	-	-	96%	96%
Statin Prescribed at Discharge[1]	-	-	99%	98%
Heart Failure Care				
ACE Inhibitor or ARB for LVSD[1]	-	-	97%	97%
Discharge Instructions Given	18	78%	96%	94%
Evaluation of LVS Function	29	100%	99%	99%
Medicare Spending				
Medicare Spending per Patient (ratio)	-	0.96	0.94	0.98
Pneumonia Care				
Appropriate Initial Antibiotic Given	52	98%	96%	95%
Blood Culture Timing	91	99%	98%	98%
Pregnancy and Delivery Care				
Newborn Deliveries Scheduled Early[2]	40	5%	4%	6%
Preventive Care				
Immunization for Influenza[2]	255	91%	90%	90%
Immunization for Pneumonia[2]	335	95%	92%	92%
Stroke Care				
Anticoagulation Therapy for Atrial Fibrillation[1]	-	-	94%	95%
Antithrombotic Therapy Timing[1]	-	-	99%	98%
Assessed for Rehabilitation[1]	-	-	98%	97%
Discharged on Antithrombotic Therapy[1]	-	-	99%	99%
Discharged on Statin Medication[1]	-	-	94%	94%
Thrombolytic Therapy Timing[7]	-	-	60%	66%
Venous Thromboembolism Prophylaxis[1]	-	-	95%	94%
Written Stroke Educational Materials Given[1]	-	-	88%	88%
Surgical Care Improvement Project				
Appropriate Beta Blocker Usage	85	99%	99%	98%
Appropriate VTP Within 24 Hours	249	95%	99%	98%
Controlled Postoperative Blood Glucose[7]	-	-	96%	97%
Perioperative Temperature Management	273	100%	100%	100%
Prophylactic Antibiotic Selection	199	100%	99%	99%
Prophylactic Antibiotic Selection (Outpatient)	124	97%	98%	98%
Prophylactic Antibiotic Stopped	195	98%	99%	98%
Prophylactic Antibiotic Timing	201	99%	99%	99%
Prophylactic Antibiotic Timing (Outpatient)	106	82%	97%	98%
Urinary Catheter Removal	120	95%	98%	97%
Survey of Patients' Hospital Experiences				
Area Around Room 'Always' Quiet at Night	300+	60%	63%	61%
Doctors 'Always' Communicated Well	300+	76%	83%	82%
Home Recovery Information Given	300+	86%	89%	85%
Hospital Given 9 or 10 on 10 Point Scale	300+	72%	74%	71%
Meds 'Always' Explained Before Given	300+	68%	68%	64%
Nurses 'Always' Communicated Well	300+	80%	82%	79%
Pain 'Always' Well Controlled	300+	72%	72%	71%
Room and Bathroom 'Always' Clean	300+	77%	79%	73%
Timely Help 'Always' Received	300+	74%	72%	68%
Would Definitely Recommend Hospital	300+	66%	74%	71%
Use of Medical Imaging				
Cardiac Imaging Stress Test before Surgery	155	4.5%	5.4%	5.3%
Combination Abdominal CT Scan	345	3.5%	6.3%	10.5%
Combination Brain/Sinus CT Scan	356	1.7%	2.1%	2.7%
Combination Chest CT Scan	252	0.0%	1%	2.7%
Follow-up Mammogram/Ultrasound	735	7.3%	8.1%	8.8%
Lumbar Spine MRI for Low Back Pain	51	37.3%	34.9%	37.2%

Waukesha Memorial Hospital

725 American Ave
Waukesha, WI 53188
URL: www.waukeshamemorial.org
Type: Acute Care Hospitals
Ownership: Voluntary non-profit - Private
Phone: 262-928-1000
Fax: 262-928-7810
Emergency Services: Yes
Beds: 301

Key Personnel:
Cardiology . . . . Murrad Abdelkarim, MD
Radiology. . . . . Andrew Adamson, MD
Emergency Room . . . . Aaron Andersen, MD
Surgery . . . . Stephen R. Bartos, MD
Anesthesiology. . . . . Jeffrey Entress, MD
Pediatrics. . . . . Sean Faris, MD
Infection Control. . . . . David Letzer, DO
CEO/President. . . . . Ed Olson

Measure	Cases	This Hosp.	State Avg.	U.S. Avg.
Blood Clot Prevention and Treatment				
Anticoagulation Overlap Therapy[2]	124	99%	95%	93%
ICU Venous Thromboembolism Prophylaxis[2]	89	94%	91%	92%
Incidence of Potentially Preventable VTE[2]	23	4%	10%	10%
UFH with Dosages/Platelet Monitoring[2]	38	100%	96%	97%
Venous Thromboembolism Prophylaxis[2]	304	80%	85%	85%
Warfarin Therapy Discharge Instructions[2]	100	50%	70%	75%
Chest Pain/Possible Heart Attack Care				
Aspirin Given Within 24 Hours of Arrival[5]	-	-	98%	96%
Fibrinolytic Meds Within 30 Min. of Arrival[5]	-	-	52%	58%
Average Time to ECG (minutes)[5]	-	-	7	7
Average Time to Transfer (minutes)[5]	-	-	58	60
Children's Asthma Care				
Received Home Management Plan of Care	-	-	-	88%
Received Reliever Medication	-	-	-	100%
Received Systemic Corticosteroids	-	-	-	100%
Emergency Department				
Admittance Decision Time (minutes)[2]	622	79	65	98
Head CT Results Within 45 Min. of Arrival[1]	-	-	61%	57%
Patients Who Left ER Before Being Seen	39,517	1%	1%	2%
Time from ER Arrival to Admit. (minutes)[2]	625	233	207	274
Time from ER Arrival to Discharge (minutes)	372	155	121	134
Time in ER Before Being Evaluated (minutes)	339	23	19	26
Time to Pain Meds for Fractures (minutes)	191	46	42	57
Heart Attack Care				
Aspirin Given at Discharge[2]	242	100%	99%	99%
Fibrinolytic Meds Within 30 Min. of Arrival[2,7]	-	-	67%	54%
PCI Within 90 Minutes of Arrival[2]	60	100%	96%	96%
Statin Prescribed at Discharge[2]	233	98%	99%	98%
Heart Failure Care				
ACE Inhibitor or ARB for LVSD[2]	66	94%	97%	97%
Discharge Instructions Given[2]	221	97%	96%	94%
Evaluation of LVS Function[2]	291	100%	99%	99%
Medicare Spending				
Medicare Spending per Patient (ratio)	-	0.97	0.94	0.98
Pneumonia Care				
Appropriate Initial Antibiotic Given[2]	99	96%	96%	95%
Blood Culture Timing[2]	156	100%	98%	98%
Pregnancy and Delivery Care				
Newborn Deliveries Scheduled Early[2]	204	0%	4%	6%
Preventive Care				
Immunization for Influenza[2]	544	88%	90%	90%
Immunization for Pneumonia[2]	685	92%	92%	92%
Stroke Care				
Anticoagulation Therapy for Atrial Fibrillation	25	100%	94%	95%
Antithrombotic Therapy Timing	110	100%	99%	98%
Assessed for Rehabilitation	160	96%	98%	97%
Discharged on Antithrombotic Therapy	146	100%	99%	99%
Discharged on Statin Medication	110	95%	94%	94%
Thrombolytic Therapy Timing[1]	-	-	60%	66%
Venous Thromboembolism Prophylaxis	143	95%	95%	94%
Written Stroke Educational Materials Given	89	98%	88%	88%
Surgical Care Improvement Project				
Appropriate Beta Blocker Usage[2]	205	99%	99%	98%
Appropriate VTP Within 24 Hours[2]	343	97%	99%	98%
Controlled Postoperative Blood Glucose[2]	135	99%	96%	97%
Perioperative Temperature Management[2]	561	100%	100%	100%
Prophylactic Antibiotic Selection[2]	383	99%	99%	99%
Prophylactic Antibiotic Selection (Outpatient)	435	99%	98%	98%
Prophylactic Antibiotic Stopped[2]	383	97%	99%	98%
Prophylactic Antibiotic Timing[2]	384	98%	99%	99%
Prophylactic Antibiotic Timing (Outpatient)	428	98%	97%	98%
Urinary Catheter Removal[2]	382	99%	98%	97%
Survey of Patients' Hospital Experiences				
Area Around Room 'Always' Quiet at Night	300+	70%	63%	61%
Doctors 'Always' Communicated Well	300+	80%	83%	82%
Home Recovery Information Given	300+	90%	89%	85%
Hospital Given 9 or 10 on 10 Point Scale	300+	81%	74%	71%
Meds 'Always' Explained Before Given	300+	66%	68%	64%
Nurses 'Always' Communicated Well	300+	82%	82%	79%
Pain 'Always' Well Controlled	300+	70%	72%	71%
Room and Bathroom 'Always' Clean	300+	81%	79%	73%
Timely Help 'Always' Received	300+	67%	72%	68%
Would Definitely Recommend Hospital	300+	81%	74%	71%
Use of Medical Imaging				
Cardiac Imaging Stress Test before Surgery	720	6.8%	5.4%	5.3%
Combination Abdominal CT Scan	1,224	7.1%	6.3%	10.5%
Combination Brain/Sinus CT Scan	864	1.4%	2.1%	2.7%
Combination Chest CT Scan	1,102	2.1%	1%	2.7%
Follow-up Mammogram/Ultrasound	2,682	8.8%	8.1%	8.8%
Lumbar Spine MRI for Low Back Pain	266	37.6%	34.9%	37.2%

Riverside Medical Center

800 Riverside Drive
Waupaca, WI 54981
URL: www.riversidemedical.org
Type: Critical Access Hospitals
Ownership: Voluntary non-profit - Private
Phone: 715-258-1000
Fax: 715-256-2083
Emergency Services: Yes
Beds: 77

Key Personnel:
Cardiology . . . . Jacob Abraham
Radiology. . . . . Daryl Adamson
Cardiology . . . . Masud Ahmed
Cardiology . . . . Melike Arsalan
Radiology. . . . . Andru Bageac
CEO/President. . . . . Phil Kambic

Measure	Cases	This Hosp.	State Avg.	U.S. Avg.
Blood Clot Prevention and Treatment				
Anticoagulation Overlap Therapy[5]	-	-	95%	93%
ICU Venous Thromboembolism Prophylaxis[5]	-	-	91%	92%
Incidence of Potentially Preventable VTE[5]	-	-	10%	10%
UFH with Dosages/Platelet Monitoring[5]	-	-	96%	97%
Venous Thromboembolism Prophylaxis[5]	-	-	85%	85%
Warfarin Therapy Discharge Instructions[5]	-	-	70%	75%
Chest Pain/Possible Heart Attack Care				
Aspirin Given Within 24 Hours of Arrival[5]	-	-	98%	96%
Fibrinolytic Meds Within 30 Min. of Arrival[5]	-	-	52%	58%
Average Time to ECG (minutes)[5]	-	-	7	7
Average Time to Transfer (minutes)[5]	-	-	58	60
Children's Asthma Care				
Received Home Management Plan of Care	-	-	-	88%
Received Reliever Medication	-	-	-	100%
Received Systemic Corticosteroids	-	-	-	100%
Emergency Department				
Admittance Decision Time (minutes)[5]	-	-	65	98
Head CT Results Within 45 Min. of Arrival[5]	-	-	61%	57%
Patients Who Left ER Before Being Seen	12,507	0%	1%	2%
Time from ER Arrival to Admit. (minutes)[5]	-	-	207	274
Time from ER Arrival to Discharge (minutes)[5]	-	-	121	134
Time in ER Before Being Evaluated (minutes)[5]	-	-	19	26
Time to Pain Meds for Fractures (minutes)[5]	-	-	42	57
Heart Attack Care				
Aspirin Given at Discharge[5]	-	-	99%	99%
Fibrinolytic Meds Within 30 Min. of Arrival[5]	-	-	67%	54%
PCI Within 90 Minutes of Arrival[5]	-	-	96%	96%
Statin Prescribed at Discharge[5]	-	-	99%	98%
Heart Failure Care				
ACE Inhibitor or ARB for LVSD	12	83%	97%	97%
Discharge Instructions Given	28	82%	96%	94%

NOTE: Hospital profiles are in alphabetical order by state, then city, then hospital within the city; Rankings exclude hospitals with less than 25 cases except for patient surveys which excludes hospitals with less than 100 cases; (a) 100-299 cases; (1) The number of cases/patients is too few to report; (2) Data submitted were based on a sample of cases/patients; (3) Results are based on a shorter time period than required; (4) Data suppressed by CMS for one or more quarters; (5) Results are not available for this reporting period; (6) Fewer than 100 patients completed the HCAHPS survey; (7) No cases met the criteria for this measure; (8) The lower limit of the confidence interval cannot be calculated if the number of observed infections equals zero; (9) No data are available from the state/territory for this reporting period; (10) The scores shown reflect fewer than 50 completed surveys; (11) There were discrepancies in the data collection process; (12) This measure does not apply to this hospital for this reporting period; (13) Results cannot be calculated for this reporting period; (14) The results for this state are combined with nearby states to protect confidentiality; Please refer to the User's Guide for a full explanation of data.

Measure	Cases	This Hosp.	State Avg.	U.S. Avg.
Evaluation of LVS Function	42	90%	99%	99%
Medicare Spending				
Medicare Spending per Patient (ratio)	-	-	0.94	0.98
Pneumonia Care				
Appropriate Initial Antibiotic Given	34	85%	96%	95%
Blood Culture Timing	53	94%	98%	98%
Pregnancy and Delivery Care				
Newborn Deliveries Scheduled Early	17	0%	4%	6%
Preventive Care				
Immunization for Influenza[5]	-	-	90%	90%
Immunization for Pneumonia[5]	-	-	92%	92%
Stroke Care				
Anticoagulation Therapy for Atrial Fibrillation[5]	-	-	94%	95%
Antithrombotic Therapy Timing[5]	-	-	99%	98%
Assessed for Rehabilitation[5]	-	-	98%	97%
Discharged on Antithrombotic Therapy[5]	-	-	99%	99%
Discharged on Statin Medication[5]	-	-	94%	94%
Thrombolytic Therapy Timing[5]	-	-	60%	66%
Venous Thromboembolism Prophylaxis[5]	-	-	95%	94%
Written Stroke Educational Materials Given[5]	-	-	88%	88%
Surgical Care Improvement Project				
Appropriate Beta Blocker Usage[5]	-	-	99%	98%
Appropriate VTP Within 24 Hours[5]	-	-	99%	98%
Controlled Postoperative Blood Glucose[5]	-	-	96%	97%
Perioperative Temperature Management[5]	-	-	100%	100%
Prophylactic Antibiotic Selection[5]	-	-	99%	99%
Prophylactic Antibiotic Selection (Outpatient)[5]	-	-	98%	98%
Prophylactic Antibiotic Stopped[5]	-	-	99%	98%
Prophylactic Antibiotic Timing[5]	-	-	99%	99%
Prophylactic Antibiotic Timing (Outpatient)[5]	-	-	97%	98%
Urinary Catheter Removal[5]	-	-	98%	97%
Survey of Patients' Hospital Experiences				
Area Around Room 'Always' Quiet at Night	(a)	66%	63%	61%
Doctors 'Always' Communicated Well	(a)	83%	83%	82%
Home Recovery Information Given	(a)	88%	89%	85%
Hospital Given 9 or 10 on 10 Point Scale	(a)	70%	74%	71%
Meds 'Always' Explained Before Given	(a)	66%	68%	64%
Nurses 'Always' Communicated Well	(a)	75%	82%	79%
Pain 'Always' Well Controlled	(a)	69%	72%	71%
Room and Bathroom 'Always' Clean	(a)	82%	79%	73%
Timely Help 'Always' Received	(a)	70%	72%	68%
Would Definitely Recommend Hospital	(a)	67%	74%	71%
Use of Medical Imaging				
Cardiac Imaging Stress Test before Surgery	97	8.2%	5.4%	5.3%
Combination Abdominal CT Scan	263	3.8%	6.3%	10.5%
Combination Brain/Sinus CT Scan	285	6.7%	2.1%	2.7%
Combination Chest CT Scan	140	0.0%	1%	2.7%
Follow-up Mammogram/Ultrasound[7]	-	-	8.1%	8.8%
Lumbar Spine MRI for Low Back Pain[1]	-	-	34.9%	37.2%

Waupun Memorial Hospital

620 W Brown St
Waupun, WI 53963
URL: www.agnesian.com
Phone: 920-324-6530
Fax: 920-324-2085
Type: Critical Access Hospitals
Ownership: Voluntary non-profit - Church
Emergency Services: Yes
Beds: 25

Key Personnel:
Emergency Room . . . . Patricia M Demery, RN
Infection Control. . . . . Kayla Ericksen, RN

Measure	Cases	This Hosp.	State Avg.	U.S. Avg.
Blood Clot Prevention and Treatment				
Anticoagulation Overlap Therapy[5]	-	-	95%	93%
ICU Venous Thromboembolism Prophylaxis[5]	-	-	91%	92%
Incidence of Potentially Preventable VTE[5]	-	-	10%	10%
UFH with Dosages/Platelet Monitoring[5]	-	-	96%	97%
Venous Thromboembolism Prophylaxis[5]	-	-	85%	85%
Warfarin Therapy Discharge Instructions[5]	-	-	70%	75%
Chest Pain/Possible Heart Attack Care				
Aspirin Given Within 24 Hours of Arrival	-	-	98%	96%
Fibrinolytic Meds Within 30 Min. of Arrival	-	-	52%	58%
Average Time to ECG (minutes)	-	-	7	7
Average Time to Transfer (minutes)	-	-	58	60
Children's Asthma Care				
Received Home Management Plan of Care	-	-	-	88%
Received Reliever Medication	-	-	-	100%
Received Systemic Corticosteroids	-	-	-	100%
Emergency Department				
Admittance Decision Time (minutes)[5]	-	-	65	98
Head CT Results Within 45 Min. of Arrival	-	-	61%	57%
Patients Who Left ER Before Being Seen	-	-	1%	2%
Time from ER Arrival to Admit. (minutes)[5]	-	-	207	274
Time from ER Arrival to Discharge (minutes)	-	-	121	134
Time in ER Before Being Evaluated (minutes)	-	-	19	26
Time to Pain Meds for Fractures (minutes)	-	-	42	57
Heart Attack Care				
Aspirin Given at Discharge[5]	-	-	99%	99%
Fibrinolytic Meds Within 30 Min. of Arrival[5]	-	-	67%	54%
PCI Within 90 Minutes of Arrival[5]	-	-	96%	96%
Statin Prescribed at Discharge[5]	-	-	99%	98%
Heart Failure Care				
ACE Inhibitor or ARB for LVSD[1]	-	-	97%	97%
Discharge Instructions Given	20	95%	96%	94%
Evaluation of LVS Function	22	100%	99%	99%
Medicare Spending				
Medicare Spending per Patient (ratio)	-	-	0.94	0.98
Pneumonia Care				
Appropriate Initial Antibiotic Given	44	100%	96%	95%
Blood Culture Timing	53	100%	98%	98%
Pregnancy and Delivery Care				
Newborn Deliveries Scheduled Early[5]	-	-	4%	6%
Preventive Care				
Immunization for Influenza[5]	-	-	90%	90%
Immunization for Pneumonia[5]	-	-	92%	92%
Stroke Care				
Anticoagulation Therapy for Atrial Fibrillation[5]	-	-	94%	95%
Antithrombotic Therapy Timing[5]	-	-	99%	98%
Assessed for Rehabilitation[5]	-	-	98%	97%
Discharged on Antithrombotic Therapy[5]	-	-	99%	99%
Discharged on Statin Medication[5]	-	-	94%	94%
Thrombolytic Therapy Timing[5]	-	-	60%	66%
Venous Thromboembolism Prophylaxis[5]	-	-	95%	94%
Written Stroke Educational Materials Given[5]	-	-	88%	88%
Surgical Care Improvement Project				
Appropriate Beta Blocker Usage	17	100%	99%	98%
Appropriate VTP Within 24 Hours	64	100%	99%	98%
Controlled Postoperative Blood Glucose[3,7]	-	-	96%	97%
Perioperative Temperature Management	76	100%	100%	100%
Prophylactic Antibiotic Selection	61	98%	99%	99%
Prophylactic Antibiotic Selection (Outpatient)	-	-	98%	98%
Prophylactic Antibiotic Stopped	61	98%	99%	98%
Prophylactic Antibiotic Timing	61	98%	99%	99%
Prophylactic Antibiotic Timing (Outpatient)	-	-	97%	98%
Urinary Catheter Removal	61	98%	98%	97%
Survey of Patients' Hospital Experiences				
Area Around Room 'Always' Quiet at Night	(a)	71%	63%	61%
Doctors 'Always' Communicated Well	(a)	85%	83%	82%
Home Recovery Information Given	(a)	92%	89%	85%
Hospital Given 9 or 10 on 10 Point Scale	(a)	78%	74%	71%
Meds 'Always' Explained Before Given	(a)	71%	68%	64%
Nurses 'Always' Communicated Well	(a)	86%	82%	79%
Pain 'Always' Well Controlled	(a)	75%	72%	71%
Room and Bathroom 'Always' Clean	(a)	70%	79%	73%
Timely Help 'Always' Received	(a)	77%	72%	68%
Would Definitely Recommend Hospital	(a)	75%	74%	71%
Use of Medical Imaging				
Cardiac Imaging Stress Test before Surgery	-	-	5.4%	5.3%
Combination Abdominal CT Scan	-	-	6.3%	10.5%
Combination Brain/Sinus CT Scan	-	-	2.1%	2.7%
Combination Chest CT Scan	-	-	1%	2.7%
Follow-up Mammogram/Ultrasound	-	-	8.1%	8.8%
Lumbar Spine MRI for Low Back Pain	-	-	34.9%	37.2%

Aspirus Wausau Hospital

333 Pine Ridge Blvd
Wausau, WI 54401
URL: www.aspirus.org
Phone: 715-847-2121
Fax: 715-847-2017
Type: Acute Care Hospitals
Ownership: Proprietary
Emergency Services: Yes
Beds: 321

Key Personnel:
Quality Assurance . . . . Michelle Boylaneuser
Infection Control. . . . . Jeanine Bresnahan
Radiology. . . . . Kevin Drorοct
Cardiac Laboratory. . . . . Scott Gavavet
Operating Room. . . . . Anne Hanzel
Chief of Medical Staff . . . . Chuck Shabirro
CEO/President. . . . . Paul A Spaude

Measure	Cases	This Hosp.	State Avg.	U.S. Avg.
Blood Clot Prevention and Treatment				
Anticoagulation Overlap Therapy[2]	92	97%	95%	93%
ICU Venous Thromboembolism Prophylaxis[2]	82	76%	91%	92%
Incidence of Potentially Preventable VTE[2]	12	17%	10%	10%
UFH with Dosages/Platelet Monitoring[2]	58	93%	96%	97%
Venous Thromboembolism Prophylaxis[2]	279	77%	85%	85%
Warfarin Therapy Discharge Instructions[2]	77	27%	70%	75%
Chest Pain/Possible Heart Attack Care				
Aspirin Given Within 24 Hours of Arrival[5]	-	-	98%	96%
Fibrinolytic Meds Within 30 Min. of Arrival[5]	-	-	52%	58%
Average Time to ECG (minutes)[5]	-	-	7	7
Average Time to Transfer (minutes)[5]	-	-	58	60
Children's Asthma Care				
Received Home Management Plan of Care	-	-	-	88%
Received Reliever Medication	-	-	-	100%
Received Systemic Corticosteroids	-	-	-	100%
Emergency Department				
Admittance Decision Time (minutes)[2]	393	54	65	98
Head CT Results Within 45 Min. of Arrival[1]	-	-	61%	57%
Patients Who Left ER Before Being Seen	29,086	0%	1%	2%
Time from ER Arrival to Admit. (minutes)[2]	402	172	207	274
Time from ER Arrival to Discharge (minutes)	363	112	121	134
Time in ER Before Being Evaluated (minutes)	246	12	19	26
Time to Pain Meds for Fractures (minutes)	126	32	42	57
Heart Attack Care				
Aspirin Given at Discharge[2]	258	99%	99%	99%
Fibrinolytic Meds Within 30 Min. of Arrival[2,7]	-	-	67%	54%
PCI Within 90 Minutes of Arrival[2]	46	100%	96%	96%
Statin Prescribed at Discharge[2]	253	99%	99%	98%
Heart Failure Care				
ACE Inhibitor or ARB for LVSD[2]	56	96%	97%	97%
Discharge Instructions Given[2]	211	98%	96%	94%
Evaluation of LVS Function[2]	261	100%	99%	99%
Medicare Spending				
Medicare Spending per Patient (ratio)	-	0.93	0.94	0.98
Pneumonia Care				
Appropriate Initial Antibiotic Given[2]	64	98%	96%	95%
Blood Culture Timing[2]	125	95%	98%	98%
Pregnancy and Delivery Care				
Newborn Deliveries Scheduled Early	122	10%	4%	6%
Preventive Care				
Immunization for Influenza[2]	538	71%	90%	90%
Immunization for Pneumonia[2]	693	85%	92%	92%
Stroke Care				
Anticoagulation Therapy for Atrial Fibrillation[2]	12	100%	94%	95%
Antithrombotic Therapy Timing[2]	52	96%	99%	98%
Assessed for Rehabilitation[2]	72	99%	98%	97%
Discharged on Antithrombotic Therapy[2]	63	100%	99%	99%
Discharged on Statin Medication[2]	54	89%	94%	94%
Thrombolytic Therapy Timing[1,2]	-	-	60%	66%
Venous Thromboembolism Prophylaxis[2]	75	92%	95%	94%
Written Stroke Educational Materials Given[2]	31	61%	88%	88%
Surgical Care Improvement Project				
Appropriate Beta Blocker Usage[2]	235	99%	99%	98%
Appropriate VTP Within 24 Hours[2]	232	97%	99%	98%
Controlled Postoperative Blood Glucose[2]	109	93%	96%	97%
Perioperative Temperature Management[2]	464	100%	100%	100%
Prophylactic Antibiotic Selection[2]	385	99%	99%	99%
Prophylactic Antibiotic Selection (Outpatient)	486	99%	98%	98%

NOTE: Hospital profiles are in alphabetical order by state, then city, then hospital within the city; Rankings exclude hospitals with less than 25 cases except for patient surveys which excludes hospitals with less than 100 cases; (a) 100-299 cases; (1) The number of cases/patients is too few to report; (2) Data submitted were based on a sample of cases/patients; (3) Results are based on a shorter time period than required; (4) Data suppressed by CMS for one or more quarters; (5) Results are not available for this reporting period; (6) Fewer than 100 patients completed the HCAHPS survey; (7) No cases met the criteria for this measure; (8) The lower limit of the confidence interval cannot be calculated if the number of observed infections equals zero; (9) No data are available from the state/territory for this reporting period; (10) The scores shown reflect fewer than 50 completed surveys; (11) There were discrepancies in the data collection process; (12) This measure does not apply to this hospital for this reporting period; (13) Results cannot be calculated for this reporting period; (14) The results for this state are combined with nearby states to protect confidentiality; Please refer to the User's Guide for a full explanation of data.

Measure	Cases	This Hosp.	State Avg.	U.S. Avg.
Prophylactic Antibiotic Stopped[2]	378	97%	99%	98%
Prophylactic Antibiotic Timing[2]	385	99%	99%	99%
Prophylactic Antibiotic Timing (Outpatient)	488	99%	97%	98%
Urinary Catheter Removal[2]	256	89%	98%	97%
Survey of Patients' Hospital Experiences				
Area Around Room 'Always' Quiet at Night	300+	62%	63%	61%
Doctors 'Always' Communicated Well	300+	82%	83%	82%
Home Recovery Information Given	300+	90%	89%	85%
Hospital Given 9 or 10 on 10 Point Scale	300+	78%	74%	71%
Meds 'Always' Explained Before Given	300+	62%	68%	64%
Nurses 'Always' Communicated Well	300+	81%	82%	79%
Pain 'Always' Well Controlled	300+	70%	72%	71%
Room and Bathroom 'Always' Clean	300+	70%	79%	73%
Timely Help 'Always' Received	300+	65%	72%	68%
Would Definitely Recommend Hospital	300+	80%	74%	71%
Use of Medical Imaging				
Cardiac Imaging Stress Test before Surgery	124	4.0%	5.4%	5.3%
Combination Abdominal CT Scan	387	3.4%	6.3%	10.5%
Combination Brain/Sinus CT Scan	373	0.8%	2.1%	2.7%
Combination Chest CT Scan	246	0.0%	1%	2.7%
Follow-up Mammogram/Ultrasound	1,199	9.3%	8.1%	8.8%
Lumbar Spine MRI for Low Back Pain	48	41.7%	34.9%	37.2%

Aurora West Allis Medical Center

8901 W Lincoln Ave
West Allis, WI 53227
Phone: 414-328-6000
Fax: 414-328-8536
URL: www.aurorahealthcare.org
Type: Acute Care Hospitals
Emergency Services: Yes
Ownership: Voluntary non-profit - Private
Beds: 250

Key Personnel:

Intensive Care Unit. . . . . Larry Conrad
Radiology. . . . . Perry M Gould, MD
Pediatric Ambulatory Care . . . . . . Michael Gutzeit, MD
Pediatric In-Patient Care . . . . Michael Gutzeit, MD
Emergency Room . . . . Wendy Roberts, RN
Chief of Medical Staff. . . . . Jeffery Showers
President/CEO. . . . . Nick Turkal, MD
Quality Assurance . . . . Vicki Volp

Measure	Cases	This Hosp.	State Avg.	U.S. Avg.
Blood Clot Prevention and Treatment				
Anticoagulation Overlap Therapy[2]	91	91%	95%	93%
ICU Venous Thromboembolism Prophylaxis[2]	71	97%	91%	92%
Incidence of Potentially Preventable VTE[1,2]	-	-	10%	10%
UFH with Dosages/Platelet Monitoring[2]	39	100%	96%	97%
Venous Thromboembolism Prophylaxis[2]	305	86%	85%	85%
Warfarin Therapy Discharge Instructions[2]	72	68%	70%	75%
Chest Pain/Possible Heart Attack Care				
Aspirin Given Within 24 Hours of Arrival	64	100%	98%	96%
Fibrinolytic Meds Within 30 Min. of Arrival[3,7]	-	-	52%	58%
Average Time to ECG (minutes)	65	15	7	7
Average Time to Transfer (minutes)[3]	16	60	58	60
Children's Asthma Care				
Received Home Management Plan of Care	-	-	-	88%
Received Reliever Medication	-	-	-	100%
Received Systemic Corticosteroids	-	-	-	100%
Emergency Department				
Admittance Decision Time (minutes)[2]	458	91	65	98
Head CT Results Within 45 Min. of Arrival	12	92%	61%	57%
Patients Who Left ER Before Being Seen	34,374	2%	1%	2%
Time from ER Arrival to Admit. (minutes)[2]	458	252	207	274
Time from ER Arrival to Discharge (minutes)	339	152	121	134
Time in ER Before Being Evaluated (minutes)	362	25	19	26
Time to Pain Meds for Fractures (minutes)	63	58	42	57
Heart Attack Care				
Aspirin Given at Discharge	26	92%	99%	99%
Fibrinolytic Meds Within 30 Min. of Arrival[7]	-	-	67%	54%
PCI Within 90 Minutes of Arrival[7]	-	-	96%	96%
Statin Prescribed at Discharge	27	89%	99%	98%
Heart Failure Care				
ACE Inhibitor or ARB for LVSD	21	100%	97%	97%
Discharge Instructions Given	95	98%	96%	94%
Evaluation of LVS Function	135	100%	99%	99%
Medicare Spending				
Medicare Spending per Patient (ratio)	-	1.00	0.94	0.98
Pneumonia Care				
Appropriate Initial Antibiotic Given	185	100%	96%	95%
Blood Culture Timing	207	100%	98%	98%
Pregnancy and Delivery Care				
Newborn Deliveries Scheduled Early	294	2%	4%	6%
Preventive Care				
Immunization for Influenza[2]	416	97%	90%	90%
Immunization for Pneumonia[2]	455	97%	92%	92%
Stroke Care				
Anticoagulation Therapy for Atrial Fibrillation	12	92%	94%	95%
Antithrombotic Therapy Timing	78	100%	99%	98%
Assessed for Rehabilitation	76	100%	98%	97%
Discharged on Antithrombotic Therapy	74	99%	99%	99%
Discharged on Statin Medication	55	100%	94%	94%
Thrombolytic Therapy Timing[7]	-	-	60%	66%
Venous Thromboembolism Prophylaxis	81	95%	95%	94%
Written Stroke Educational Materials Given	46	91%	88%	88%
Surgical Care Improvement Project				
Appropriate Beta Blocker Usage[2]	98	100%	99%	98%
Appropriate VTP Within 24 Hours[2]	332	100%	99%	98%
Controlled Postoperative Blood Glucose[2,7]	-	-	96%	97%
Perioperative Temperature Management[2]	403	100%	100%	100%
Prophylactic Antibiotic Selection[2]	261	100%	99%	99%
Prophylactic Antibiotic Selection (Outpatient)	457	100%	98%	98%
Prophylactic Antibiotic Stopped[2]	246	100%	99%	98%
Prophylactic Antibiotic Timing[2]	261	100%	99%	99%
Prophylactic Antibiotic Timing (Outpatient)	456	100%	97%	98%
Urinary Catheter Removal[2]	164	96%	98%	97%
Survey of Patients' Hospital Experiences				
Area Around Room 'Always' Quiet at Night	300+	64%	63%	61%
Doctors 'Always' Communicated Well	300+	79%	83%	82%
Home Recovery Information Given	300+	86%	89%	85%
Hospital Given 9 or 10 on 10 Point Scale	300+	72%	74%	71%
Meds 'Always' Explained Before Given	300+	64%	68%	64%
Nurses 'Always' Communicated Well	300+	78%	82%	79%
Pain 'Always' Well Controlled	300+	69%	72%	71%
Room and Bathroom 'Always' Clean	300+	71%	79%	73%
Timely Help 'Always' Received	300+	62%	72%	68%
Would Definitely Recommend Hospital	300+	75%	74%	71%
Use of Medical Imaging				
Cardiac Imaging Stress Test before Surgery	239	5.0%	5.4%	5.3%
Combination Abdominal CT Scan	744	3.8%	6.3%	10.5%
Combination Brain/Sinus CT Scan	702	3.8%	2.1%	2.7%
Combination Chest CT Scan	456	0.0%	1%	2.7%
Follow-up Mammogram/Ultrasound	1,934	5.7%	8.1%	8.8%
Lumbar Spine MRI for Low Back Pain	77	44.2%	34.9%	37.2%

Saint Joseph's Community Hospital of West Bend

3200 Pleasant Valley Road
West Bend, WI 53095
Phone: 262-334-5533
Fax: 262-334-8484
URL: www.stjosephswb.com
Type: Acute Care Hospitals
Emergency Services: Yes
Ownership: Voluntary non-profit - Private
Beds: 80

Key Personnel:

Anesthesiology. . . . . Eric Breckenridge, DO
Quality Assurance . . . . Karen Emisse
CEO/President. . . . . Michael Laird
Radiology. . . . . Donna Lawien
Emergency Room . . . . Mary Lewis, MD
Chief of Medical Staff. . . . . G Michael Mosley, MD
Infection Control. . . . . Pat Pearson

Measure	Cases	This Hosp.	State Avg.	U.S. Avg.
Blood Clot Prevention and Treatment				
Anticoagulation Overlap Therapy[2]	57	93%	95%	93%
ICU Venous Thromboembolism Prophylaxis[2]	72	93%	91%	92%
Incidence of Potentially Preventable VTE[2]	13	0%	10%	10%
UFH with Dosages/Platelet Monitoring[2]	13	100%	96%	97%
Venous Thromboembolism Prophylaxis[2]	227	84%	85%	85%
Warfarin Therapy Discharge Instructions[2]	43	40%	70%	75%
Chest Pain/Possible Heart Attack Care				
Aspirin Given Within 24 Hours of Arrival	95	99%	98%	96%
Fibrinolytic Meds Within 30 Min. of Arrival[7]	-	-	52%	58%
Average Time to ECG (minutes)	100	9	7	7
Average Time to Transfer (minutes)	26	50	58	60
Children's Asthma Care				
Received Home Management Plan of Care	-	-	-	88%
Received Reliever Medication	-	-	-	100%
Received Systemic Corticosteroids	-	-	-	100%
Emergency Department				
Admittance Decision Time (minutes)[2]	420	64	65	98
Head CT Results Within 45 Min. of Arrival	12	75%	61%	57%
Patients Who Left ER Before Being Seen	16,689	1%	1%	2%
Time from ER Arrival to Admit. (minutes)[2]	420	212	207	274
Time from ER Arrival to Discharge (minutes)	373	134	121	134
Time in ER Before Being Evaluated (minutes)	422	19	19	26
Time to Pain Meds for Fractures (minutes)	91	46	42	57
Heart Attack Care				
Aspirin Given at Discharge[1]	-	-	99%	99%
Fibrinolytic Meds Within 30 Min. of Arrival[7]	-	-	67%	54%
PCI Within 90 Minutes of Arrival[7]	-	-	96%	96%
Statin Prescribed at Discharge[1]	-	-	99%	98%
Heart Failure Care				
ACE Inhibitor or ARB for LVSD	21	100%	97%	97%
Discharge Instructions Given	66	91%	96%	94%
Evaluation of LVS Function	85	100%	99%	99%
Medicare Spending				
Medicare Spending per Patient (ratio)	-	0.96	0.94	0.98
Pneumonia Care				
Appropriate Initial Antibiotic Given	101	99%	96%	95%
Blood Culture Timing	169	98%	98%	98%
Pregnancy and Delivery Care				
Newborn Deliveries Scheduled Early[2]	29	17%	4%	6%
Preventive Care				
Immunization for Influenza[2]	360	88%	90%	90%
Immunization for Pneumonia[2]	430	91%	92%	92%
Stroke Care				
Anticoagulation Therapy for Atrial Fibrillation[1]	-	-	94%	95%
Antithrombotic Therapy Timing	27	96%	99%	98%
Assessed for Rehabilitation	27	100%	98%	97%
Discharged on Antithrombotic Therapy	27	93%	99%	99%
Discharged on Statin Medication	21	86%	94%	94%
Thrombolytic Therapy Timing[7]	-	-	60%	66%
Venous Thromboembolism Prophylaxis	26	96%	95%	94%
Written Stroke Educational Materials Given	15	67%	88%	88%
Surgical Care Improvement Project				
Appropriate Beta Blocker Usage	76	100%	99%	98%
Appropriate VTP Within 24 Hours	277	100%	99%	98%
Controlled Postoperative Blood Glucose[7]	-	-	96%	97%
Perioperative Temperature Management	308	100%	100%	100%
Prophylactic Antibiotic Selection	242	100%	99%	99%
Prophylactic Antibiotic Selection (Outpatient)	97	96%	98%	98%
Prophylactic Antibiotic Stopped	229	99%	99%	98%
Prophylactic Antibiotic Timing	242	99%	99%	99%
Prophylactic Antibiotic Timing (Outpatient)	96	100%	97%	98%
Urinary Catheter Removal	250	100%	98%	97%
Survey of Patients' Hospital Experiences				
Area Around Room 'Always' Quiet at Night	300+	69%	63%	61%
Doctors 'Always' Communicated Well	300+	81%	83%	82%
Home Recovery Information Given	300+	87%	89%	85%
Hospital Given 9 or 10 on 10 Point Scale	300+	70%	74%	71%
Meds 'Always' Explained Before Given	300+	65%	68%	64%
Nurses 'Always' Communicated Well	300+	75%	82%	79%
Pain 'Always' Well Controlled	300+	68%	72%	71%
Room and Bathroom 'Always' Clean	300+	78%	79%	73%
Timely Help 'Always' Received	300+	57%	72%	68%
Would Definitely Recommend Hospital	300+	68%	74%	71%
Use of Medical Imaging				
Cardiac Imaging Stress Test before Surgery	236	5.5%	5.4%	5.3%
Combination Abdominal CT Scan	313	3.8%	6.3%	10.5%
Combination Brain/Sinus CT Scan	339	0.0%	2.1%	2.7%
Combination Chest CT Scan	189	4.8%	1%	2.7%
Follow-up Mammogram/Ultrasound[1]	-	-	8.1%	8.8%
Lumbar Spine MRI for Low Back Pain	92	21.7%	34.9%	37.2%

NOTE: Hospital profiles are in alphabetical order by state, then city, then hospital within the city; Rankings exclude hospitals with less than 25 cases except for patient surveys which excludes hospitals with less than 100 cases; (a) 100-299 cases; (1) The number of cases/patients is too few to report; (2) Data submitted were based on a sample of cases/patients; (3) Results are based on a shorter time period than required; (4) Data suppressed by CMS for one or more quarters; (5) Results are not available for this reporting period; (6) Fewer than 100 patients completed the HCAHPS survey; (7) No cases met the criteria for this measure; (8) The lower limit of the confidence interval cannot be calculated if the number of observed infections equals zero; (9) No data are available from the state/territory for this reporting period; (10) The scores shown reflect fewer than 50 completed surveys; (11) There were discrepancies in the data collection process; (12) This measure does not apply to this hospital for this reporting period; (13) Results cannot be calculated for this reporting period; (14) The results for this state are combined with nearby states to protect confidentiality; Please refer to the User's Guide for a full explanation of data.

Saint Clares Hospital of Weston

3400 Ministry Parkway Phone: 715-393-3000
Weston, WI 54476
E-mail: saintclare@ministryhealth.org
URL: www.ministryhealth.org
Type: Acute Care Hospitals Emergency Services: Yes
Ownership: Voluntary non-profit - Private
Key Personnel:
Chief of Medical Staff.......... Larry Hegland
Patient Relations.............. Colleen Hoerneman

Measure	Cases	This Hosp.	State Avg.	U.S. Avg.
Blood Clot Prevention and Treatment				
Anticoagulation Overlap Therapy[2]	45	100%	95%	93%
ICU Venous Thromboembolism Prophylaxis[2]	64	100%	91%	92%
Incidence of Potentially Preventable VTE[1,2]	-	-	10%	10%
UFH with Dosages/Platelet Monitoring[2]	36	100%	96%	97%
Venous Thromboembolism Prophylaxis[2]	367	100%	85%	85%
Warfarin Therapy Discharge Instructions[2]	35	100%	70%	75%
Chest Pain/Possible Heart Attack Care				
Aspirin Given Within 24 Hours of Arrival[1,3]	-	-	98%	96%
Fibrinolytic Meds Within 30 Min. of Arrival[5]	-	-	52%	58%
Average Time to ECG (minutes)[1,3]	-	-	7	7
Average Time to Transfer (minutes)[5]	-	-	58	60
Children's Asthma Care				
Received Home Management Plan of Care	-	-	-	88%
Received Reliever Medication	-	-	-	100%
Received Systemic Corticosteroids	-	-	-	100%
Emergency Department				
Admittance Decision Time (minutes)[2]	388	67	65	98
Head CT Results Within 45 Min. of Arrival[1]	-	-	61%	57%
Patients Who Left ER Before Being Seen	14,731	0%	1%	2%
Time from ER Arrival to Admit. (minutes)[2]	391	195	207	274
Time from ER Arrival to Discharge (minutes)	1,022	118	121	134
Time in ER Before Being Evaluated (minutes)	1,115	26	19	26
Time to Pain Meds for Fractures (minutes)	54	37	42	57
Heart Attack Care				
Aspirin Given at Discharge	260	100%	99%	99%
Fibrinolytic Meds Within 30 Min. of Arrival[7]	-	-	67%	54%
PCI Within 90 Minutes of Arrival	13	100%	96%	96%
Statin Prescribed at Discharge	246	100%	99%	98%
Heart Failure Care				
ACE Inhibitor or ARB for LVSD	24	100%	97%	97%
Discharge Instructions Given	134	100%	96%	94%
Evaluation of LVS Function	163	100%	99%	99%
Medicare Spending				
Medicare Spending per Patient (ratio)	-	0.90	0.94	0.98
Pneumonia Care				
Appropriate Initial Antibiotic Given	36	100%	96%	95%
Blood Culture Timing	67	100%	98%	98%
Pregnancy and Delivery Care				
Newborn Deliveries Scheduled Early[2]	81	9%	4%	6%
Preventive Care				
Immunization for Influenza[2]	515	95%	90%	90%
Immunization for Pneumonia[2]	626	95%	92%	92%
Stroke Care				
Anticoagulation Therapy for Atrial Fibrillation[1]	-	-	94%	95%
Antithrombotic Therapy Timing	37	100%	99%	98%
Assessed for Rehabilitation	38	100%	98%	97%
Discharged on Antithrombotic Therapy	38	100%	99%	99%
Discharged on Statin Medication	28	89%	94%	94%
Thrombolytic Therapy Timing[7]	-	-	60%	66%
Venous Thromboembolism Prophylaxis	37	100%	95%	94%
Written Stroke Educational Materials Given	20	100%	88%	88%
Surgical Care Improvement Project				
Appropriate Beta Blocker Usage	275	99%	99%	98%
Appropriate VTP Within 24 Hours	533	100%	99%	98%
Controlled Postoperative Blood Glucose	108	97%	96%	97%
Perioperative Temperature Management	641	100%	100%	100%
Prophylactic Antibiotic Selection	570	100%	99%	99%
Prophylactic Antibiotic Selection (Outpatient)	122	100%	98%	98%
Prophylactic Antibiotic Stopped	565	99%	99%	98%
Prophylactic Antibiotic Timing	570	100%	99%	99%
Prophylactic Antibiotic Timing (Outpatient)	123	99%	97%	98%
Urinary Catheter Removal	393	99%	98%	97%
Survey of Patients' Hospital Experiences				
Area Around Room 'Always' Quiet at Night	300+	58%	63%	61%
Doctors 'Always' Communicated Well	300+	81%	83%	82%
Home Recovery Information Given	300+	90%	89%	85%
Hospital Given 9 or 10 on 10 Point Scale	300+	76%	74%	71%
Meds 'Always' Explained Before Given	300+	67%	68%	64%
Nurses 'Always' Communicated Well	300+	82%	82%	79%
Pain 'Always' Well Controlled	300+	72%	72%	71%
Room and Bathroom 'Always' Clean	300+	78%	79%	73%
Timely Help 'Always' Received	300+	73%	72%	68%
Would Definitely Recommend Hospital	300+	77%	74%	71%
Use of Medical Imaging				
Cardiac Imaging Stress Test before Surgery[1]	-	-	5.4%	5.3%
Combination Abdominal CT Scan	103	1.0%	6.3%	10.5%
Combination Brain/Sinus CT Scan[1]	-	-	2.1%	2.7%
Combination Chest CT Scan[1]	-	-	1%	2.7%
Follow-up Mammogram/Ultrasound[7]	-	-	8.1%	8.8%
Lumbar Spine MRI for Low Back Pain[1]	-	-	34.9%	37.2%

Tri County Memorial Hospital

18601 Lincoln St Phone: 715-538-4361
Whitehall, WI 54773 Fax: 715-538-4343
Type: Critical Access Hospitals Emergency Services: Yes
Ownership: Voluntary non-profit - Private Beds: 93
Key Personnel:
CEO/President................ Ronald B Fields
Chief of Medical Staff.......... Joanne Selkurt

Measure	Cases	This Hosp.	State Avg.	U.S. Avg.
Blood Clot Prevention and Treatment				
Anticoagulation Overlap Therapy[5]	-	-	95%	93%
ICU Venous Thromboembolism Prophylaxis[5]	-	-	91%	92%
Incidence of Potentially Preventable VTE[5]	-	-	10%	10%
UFH with Dosages/Platelet Monitoring[5]	-	-	96%	97%
Venous Thromboembolism Prophylaxis[5]	-	-	85%	85%
Warfarin Therapy Discharge Instructions[5]	-	-	70%	75%
Chest Pain/Possible Heart Attack Care				
Aspirin Given Within 24 Hours of Arrival	-	-	98%	96%
Fibrinolytic Meds Within 30 Min. of Arrival	-	-	52%	58%
Average Time to ECG (minutes)	-	-	7	7
Average Time to Transfer (minutes)	-	-	58	60
Children's Asthma Care				
Received Home Management Plan of Care	-	-	-	88%
Received Reliever Medication	-	-	-	100%
Received Systemic Corticosteroids	-	-	-	100%
Emergency Department				
Admittance Decision Time (minutes)[5]	-	-	65	98
Head CT Results Within 45 Min. of Arrival	-	-	61%	57%
Patients Who Left ER Before Being Seen	-	-	1%	2%
Time from ER Arrival to Admit. (minutes)[5]	-	-	207	274
Time from ER Arrival to Discharge (minutes)	-	-	121	134
Time in ER Before Being Evaluated (minutes)	-	-	19	26
Time to Pain Meds for Fractures (minutes)	-	-	42	57
Heart Attack Care				
Aspirin Given at Discharge[5]	-	-	99%	99%
Fibrinolytic Meds Within 30 Min. of Arrival[5]	-	-	67%	54%
PCI Within 90 Minutes of Arrival[5]	-	-	96%	96%
Statin Prescribed at Discharge[5]	-	-	99%	98%
Heart Failure Care				
ACE Inhibitor or ARB for LVSD[1]	-	-	97%	97%
Discharge Instructions Given[1]	-	-	96%	94%
Evaluation of LVS Function	15	87%	99%	99%
Medicare Spending				
Medicare Spending per Patient (ratio)	-	-	0.94	0.98
Pneumonia Care				
Appropriate Initial Antibiotic Given[1]	-	-	96%	95%
Blood Culture Timing	32	94%	98%	98%
Pregnancy and Delivery Care				
Newborn Deliveries Scheduled Early[5]	-	-	4%	6%
Preventive Care				
Immunization for Influenza[5]	-	-	90%	90%
Immunization for Pneumonia[5]	-	-	92%	92%
Stroke Care				
Anticoagulation Therapy for Atrial Fibrillation[5]	-	-	94%	95%
Antithrombotic Therapy Timing[5]	-	-	99%	98%
Assessed for Rehabilitation[5]	-	-	98%	97%
Discharged on Antithrombotic Therapy[5]	-	-	99%	99%
Discharged on Statin Medication[5]	-	-	94%	94%
Thrombolytic Therapy Timing[5]	-	-	60%	66%
Venous Thromboembolism Prophylaxis[5]	-	-	95%	94%
Written Stroke Educational Materials Given[5]	-	-	88%	88%
Surgical Care Improvement Project				
Appropriate Beta Blocker Usage[5]	-	-	99%	98%
Appropriate VTP Within 24 Hours[5]	-	-	99%	98%
Controlled Postoperative Blood Glucose[5]	-	-	96%	97%
Perioperative Temperature Management[5]	-	-	100%	100%
Prophylactic Antibiotic Selection[5]	-	-	99%	99%
Prophylactic Antibiotic Selection (Outpatient)	-	-	98%	98%
Prophylactic Antibiotic Stopped[5]	-	-	99%	98%
Prophylactic Antibiotic Timing[5]	-	-	99%	99%
Prophylactic Antibiotic Timing (Outpatient)	-	-	97%	98%
Urinary Catheter Removal[5]	-	-	98%	97%
Survey of Patients' Hospital Experiences				
Area Around Room 'Always' Quiet at Night[10]	<100	65%	63%	61%
Doctors 'Always' Communicated Well[10]	<100	80%	83%	82%
Home Recovery Information Given[10]	<100	83%	89%	85%
Hospital Given 9 or 10 on 10 Point Scale[10]	<100	69%	74%	71%
Meds 'Always' Explained Before Given[10]	<100	56%	68%	64%
Nurses 'Always' Communicated Well[10]	<100	86%	82%	79%
Pain 'Always' Well Controlled[10]	<100	75%	72%	71%
Room and Bathroom 'Always' Clean[10]	<100	68%	79%	73%
Timely Help 'Always' Received[10]	<100	78%	72%	68%
Would Definitely Recommend Hospital[10]	<100	79%	74%	71%
Use of Medical Imaging				
Cardiac Imaging Stress Test before Surgery	-	-	5.4%	5.3%
Combination Abdominal CT Scan	-	-	6.3%	10.5%
Combination Brain/Sinus CT Scan	-	-	2.1%	2.7%
Combination Chest CT Scan	-	-	1%	2.7%
Follow-up Mammogram/Ultrasound	-	-	8.1%	8.8%
Lumbar Spine MRI for Low Back Pain	-	-	34.9%	37.2%

Wild Rose Com Memorial Hospital

601 Grove Ave PO Box 243 Phone: 920-622-3257
Wild Rose, WI 54984 Fax: 920-622-5593
URL: www.wildrosehospital.org
Type: Critical Access Hospitals Emergency Services: Yes
Ownership: Voluntary non-profit - Private Beds: 25
Key Personnel:
Infection Control............... Becky Brooks
CEO/President................ Donald Caves
Anesthesiology................ Dan Resop, MD
Operating Room.............. Cathy Truebl
Chief of Medical Staff.......... Chad Voskuil, MD

Measure	Cases	This Hosp.	State Avg.	U.S. Avg.
Blood Clot Prevention and Treatment				
Anticoagulation Overlap Therapy[5]	-	-	95%	93%
ICU Venous Thromboembolism Prophylaxis[5]	-	-	91%	92%
Incidence of Potentially Preventable VTE[5]	-	-	10%	10%
UFH with Dosages/Platelet Monitoring[5]	-	-	96%	97%
Venous Thromboembolism Prophylaxis[5]	-	-	85%	85%
Warfarin Therapy Discharge Instructions[5]	-	-	70%	75%
Chest Pain/Possible Heart Attack Care				
Aspirin Given Within 24 Hours of Arrival	-	-	98%	96%
Fibrinolytic Meds Within 30 Min. of Arrival	-	-	52%	58%
Average Time to ECG (minutes)	-	-	7	7
Average Time to Transfer (minutes)	-	-	58	60
Children's Asthma Care				
Received Home Management Plan of Care	-	-	-	88%
Received Reliever Medication	-	-	-	100%
Received Systemic Corticosteroids	-	-	-	100%
Emergency Department				
Admittance Decision Time (minutes)[5]	-	-	65	98
Head CT Results Within 45 Min. of Arrival	-	-	61%	57%
Patients Who Left ER Before Being Seen	-	-	1%	2%
Time from ER Arrival to Admit. (minutes)[5]	-	-	207	274
Time from ER Arrival to Discharge (minutes)	-	-	121	134

NOTE: Hospital profiles are in alphabetical order by state, then city, then hospital within the city; Rankings exclude hospitals with less than 25 cases except for patient surveys which excludes hospitals with less than 100 cases; (a) 100-299 cases; (1) The number of cases/patients is too few to report; (2) Data submitted were based on a sample of cases/patients; (3) Results are based on a shorter time period than required; (4) Data suppressed by CMS for one or more quarters; (5) Results are not available for this reporting period; (6) Fewer than 100 patients completed the HCAHPS survey; (7) No cases met the criteria for this measure; (8) The lower limit of the confidence interval cannot be calculated if the number of observed infections equals zero; (9) No data are available from the state/territory for this reporting period; (10) The scores shown reflect fewer than 50 completed surveys; (11) There were discrepancies in the data collection process; (12) This measure does not apply to this hospital for this reporting period; (13) Results cannot be calculated for this reporting period; (14) The results for this state are combined with nearby states to protect confidentiality; Please refer to the User's Guide for a full explanation of data.

Measure	Cases	This Hosp.	State Avg.	U.S. Avg.
Time in ER Before Being Evaluated (minutes)	-	-	19	26
Time to Pain Meds for Fractures (minutes)	-	-	42	57
Heart Attack Care				
Aspirin Given at Discharge[5]	-	-	99%	99%
Fibrinolytic Meds Within 30 Min. of Arrival[5]	-	-	67%	54%
PCI Within 90 Minutes of Arrival[5]	-	-	96%	96%
Statin Prescribed at Discharge[5]	-	-	99%	98%
Heart Failure Care				
ACE Inhibitor or ARB for LVSD[1]	-	-	97%	97%
Discharge Instructions Given	17	82%	96%	94%
Evaluation of LVS Function	23	87%	99%	99%
Medicare Spending				
Medicare Spending per Patient (ratio)	-	-	0.94	0.98
Pneumonia Care				
Appropriate Initial Antibiotic Given	25	88%	96%	95%
Blood Culture Timing	26	100%	98%	98%
Pregnancy and Delivery Care				
Newborn Deliveries Scheduled Early[5]	-	-	4%	6%
Preventive Care				
Immunization for Influenza[5]	-	-	90%	90%
Immunization for Pneumonia[5]	-	-	92%	92%
Stroke Care				
Anticoagulation Therapy for Atrial Fibrillation[5]	-	-	94%	95%
Antithrombotic Therapy Timing[5]	-	-	99%	98%
Assessed for Rehabilitation[5]	-	-	98%	97%
Discharged on Antithrombotic Therapy[5]	-	-	99%	99%
Discharged on Statin Medication[5]	-	-	94%	94%
Thrombolytic Therapy Timing[5]	-	-	60%	66%
Venous Thromboembolism Prophylaxis[5]	-	-	95%	94%
Written Stroke Educational Materials Given[5]	-	-	88%	88%
Surgical Care Improvement Project				
Appropriate Beta Blocker Usage[5]	-	-	99%	98%
Appropriate VTP Within 24 Hours[5]	-	-	99%	98%
Controlled Postoperative Blood Glucose[5]	-	-	96%	97%
Perioperative Temperature Management[5]	-	-	100%	100%
Prophylactic Antibiotic Selection[5]	-	-	99%	99%
Prophylactic Antibiotic Selection (Outpatient)	-	-	98%	98%
Prophylactic Antibiotic Stopped[5]	-	-	99%	98%
Prophylactic Antibiotic Timing[5]	-	-	99%	99%
Prophylactic Antibiotic Timing (Outpatient)	-	-	97%	98%
Urinary Catheter Removal[5]	-	-	98%	97%
Survey of Patients' Hospital Experiences				
Area Around Room 'Always' Quiet at Night[6]	<100	66%	63%	61%
Doctors 'Always' Communicated Well[6]	<100	78%	83%	82%
Home Recovery Information Given[6]	<100	91%	89%	85%
Hospital Given 9 or 10 on 10 Point Scale[6]	<100	58%	74%	71%
Meds 'Always' Explained Before Given[6]	<100	64%	68%	64%
Nurses 'Always' Communicated Well[6]	<100	76%	82%	79%
Pain 'Always' Well Controlled[6]	<100	69%	72%	71%
Room and Bathroom 'Always' Clean[6]	<100	67%	79%	73%
Timely Help 'Always' Received[6]	<100	60%	72%	68%
Would Definitely Recommend Hospital[6]	<100	65%	74%	71%
Use of Medical Imaging				
Cardiac Imaging Stress Test before Surgery	-	-	5.4%	5.3%
Combination Abdominal CT Scan	-	-	6.3%	10.5%
Combination Brain/Sinus CT Scan	-	-	2.1%	2.7%
Combination Chest CT Scan	-	-	1%	2.7%
Follow-up Mammogram/Ultrasound	-	-	8.1%	8.8%
Lumbar Spine MRI for Low Back Pain	-	-	34.9%	37.2%

Riverview Hospital Assoc

410 Dewey St
Wisconsin Rapids, WI 54495
Phone: 715-423-6060
Fax: 715-421-7551
URL: www.riverviewhospital.net
Type: Acute Care Hospitals
Emergency Services: Yes
Ownership: Voluntary non-profit - Private
Beds: 99

Key Personnel:

CEO/President. . . . . Celse A Berard
Emergency Room . . . . Ron R Greenburg, DO
Radiology. . . . . James V Kiernan
Chief of Medical Staff. . . . . Daniel Lucas
Quality Assurance . . . . Jim Mohr
Operating Room. . . . . Kathleen Schultz, RN

Measure	Cases	This Hosp.	State Avg.	U.S. Avg.
Blood Clot Prevention and Treatment				
Anticoagulation Overlap Therapy[2]	21	100%	95%	93%
ICU Venous Thromboembolism Prophylaxis[2]	47	96%	91%	92%
Incidence of Potentially Preventable VTE[1,2]	-	-	10%	10%
UFH with Dosages/Platelet Monitoring[1,2]	-	-	96%	97%
Venous Thromboembolism Prophylaxis[2]	146	94%	85%	85%
Warfarin Therapy Discharge Instructions[2]	17	100%	70%	75%
Chest Pain/Possible Heart Attack Care				
Aspirin Given Within 24 Hours of Arrival	124	99%	98%	96%
Fibrinolytic Meds Within 30 Min. of Arrival[1]	-	-	52%	58%
Average Time to ECG (minutes)	126	10	7	7
Average Time to Transfer (minutes)	12	72	58	60
Children's Asthma Care				
Received Home Management Plan of Care	-	-	-	88%
Received Reliever Medication	-	-	-	100%
Received Systemic Corticosteroids	-	-	-	100%
Emergency Department				
Admittance Decision Time (minutes)[2]	288	49	65	98
Head CT Results Within 45 Min. of Arrival	14	86%	61%	57%
Patients Who Left ER Before Being Seen	24,911	1%	1%	2%
Time from ER Arrival to Admit. (minutes)[2]	312	190	207	274
Time from ER Arrival to Discharge (minutes)	360	117	121	134
Time in ER Before Being Evaluated (minutes)	380	18	19	26
Time to Pain Meds for Fractures (minutes)	66	41	42	57
Heart Attack Care				
Aspirin Given at Discharge[1,2]	-	-	99%	99%
Fibrinolytic Meds Within 30 Min. of Arrival[2,7]	-	-	67%	54%
PCI Within 90 Minutes of Arrival[2,7]	-	-	96%	96%
Statin Prescribed at Discharge[1,2]	-	-	99%	98%
Heart Failure Care				
ACE Inhibitor or ARB for LVSD[2]	20	85%	97%	97%
Discharge Instructions Given[2]	54	74%	96%	94%
Evaluation of LVS Function[2]	93	96%	99%	99%
Medicare Spending				
Medicare Spending per Patient (ratio)	-	0.82	0.94	0.98
Pneumonia Care				
Appropriate Initial Antibiotic Given[2]	72	93%	96%	95%
Blood Culture Timing[2]	91	97%	98%	98%
Pregnancy and Delivery Care				
Newborn Deliveries Scheduled Early	47	4%	4%	6%
Preventive Care				
Immunization for Influenza[2]	292	88%	90%	90%
Immunization for Pneumonia[2]	329	92%	92%	92%
Stroke Care				
Anticoagulation Therapy for Atrial Fibrillation[1,2]	-	-	94%	95%
Antithrombotic Therapy Timing[2]	24	100%	99%	98%
Assessed for Rehabilitation[2]	20	90%	98%	97%
Discharged on Antithrombotic Therapy[2]	20	100%	99%	99%
Discharged on Statin Medication[2]	13	69%	94%	94%
Thrombolytic Therapy Timing[2,7]	-	-	60%	66%
Venous Thromboembolism Prophylaxis[2]	25	92%	95%	94%
Written Stroke Educational Materials Given[2]	13	92%	88%	88%
Surgical Care Improvement Project				
Appropriate Beta Blocker Usage[2]	75	99%	99%	98%
Appropriate VTP Within 24 Hours[2]	176	97%	99%	98%
Controlled Postoperative Blood Glucose[2,7]	-	-	96%	97%
Perioperative Temperature Management[2]	242	99%	100%	100%
Prophylactic Antibiotic Selection[2]	185	97%	99%	99%
Prophylactic Antibiotic Selection (Outpatient)	42	100%	98%	98%
Prophylactic Antibiotic Stopped[2]	183	99%	99%	98%
Prophylactic Antibiotic Timing[2]	185	99%	99%	99%
Prophylactic Antibiotic Timing (Outpatient)	42	98%	97%	98%
Urinary Catheter Removal[2]	26	92%	98%	97%
Survey of Patients' Hospital Experiences				
Area Around Room 'Always' Quiet at Night	300+	73%	63%	61%
Doctors 'Always' Communicated Well	300+	82%	83%	82%
Home Recovery Information Given	300+	88%	89%	85%
Hospital Given 9 or 10 on 10 Point Scale	300+	72%	74%	71%
Meds 'Always' Explained Before Given	300+	71%	68%	64%
Nurses 'Always' Communicated Well	300+	82%	82%	79%
Pain 'Always' Well Controlled	300+	72%	72%	71%
Room and Bathroom 'Always' Clean	300+	86%	79%	73%
Timely Help 'Always' Received	300+	71%	72%	68%
Would Definitely Recommend Hospital	300+	72%	74%	71%
Use of Medical Imaging				
Cardiac Imaging Stress Test before Surgery	147	7.5%	5.4%	5.3%
Combination Abdominal CT Scan	368	0.5%	6.3%	10.5%
Combination Brain/Sinus CT Scan	304	0.7%	2.1%	2.7%
Combination Chest CT Scan	215	0.5%	1%	2.7%
Follow-up Mammogram/Ultrasound	478	8.8%	8.1%	8.8%
Lumbar Spine MRI for Low Back Pain[1]	-	-	34.9%	37.2%

Howard Young Medical Center

240 Maple St
Woodruff, WI 54568
Phone: 715-356-8000
Fax: 715-356-8691
URL: www.ministryhealth.org
Type: Acute Care Hospitals
Emergency Services: Yes
Ownership: Voluntary non-profit - Church
Beds: 99

Key Personnel:

Emergency Room . . . . Rick Brodhead, MD
Infection Control. . . . . Chris Brost, RN
CEO/President. . . . . Sheila Clough
Operating Room. . . . . Kim Mears
Quality Assurance . . . . Judy Nelson
Chief of Medical Staff . . . . Michael Schaars, MD

Measure	Cases	This Hosp.	State Avg.	U.S. Avg.
Blood Clot Prevention and Treatment				
Anticoagulation Overlap Therapy[2]	21	100%	95%	93%
ICU Venous Thromboembolism Prophylaxis[1,2]	-	-	91%	92%
Incidence of Potentially Preventable VTE[1,2]	-	-	10%	10%
UFH with Dosages/Platelet Monitoring[1,2]	-	-	96%	97%
Venous Thromboembolism Prophylaxis[2]	221	99%	85%	85%
Warfarin Therapy Discharge Instructions[2]	21	100%	70%	75%
Chest Pain/Possible Heart Attack Care				
Aspirin Given Within 24 Hours of Arrival	100	100%	98%	96%
Fibrinolytic Meds Within 30 Min. of Arrival	13	77%	52%	58%
Average Time to ECG (minutes)	99	5	7	7
Average Time to Transfer (minutes)[1]	-	-	58	60
Children's Asthma Care				
Received Home Management Plan of Care	-	-	-	88%
Received Reliever Medication	-	-	-	100%
Received Systemic Corticosteroids	-	-	-	100%
Emergency Department				
Admittance Decision Time (minutes)[2]	278	66	65	98
Head CT Results Within 45 Min. of Arrival	12	50%	61%	57%
Patients Who Left ER Before Being Seen	7,686	1%	1%	2%
Time from ER Arrival to Admit. (minutes)[2]	279	220	207	274
Time from ER Arrival to Discharge (minutes)	345	134	121	134
Time in ER Before Being Evaluated (minutes)	384	27	19	26
Time to Pain Meds for Fractures (minutes)	59	43	42	57
Heart Attack Care				
Aspirin Given at Discharge[1]	-	-	99%	99%
Fibrinolytic Meds Within 30 Min. of Arrival[7]	-	-	67%	54%
PCI Within 90 Minutes of Arrival[7]	-	-	96%	96%
Statin Prescribed at Discharge[1]	-	-	99%	98%
Heart Failure Care				
ACE Inhibitor or ARB for LVSD	21	100%	97%	97%
Discharge Instructions Given	69	100%	96%	94%
Evaluation of LVS Function	90	100%	99%	99%
Medicare Spending				
Medicare Spending per Patient (ratio)	-	0.85	0.94	0.98
Pneumonia Care				
Appropriate Initial Antibiotic Given	77	95%	96%	95%
Blood Culture Timing	99	96%	98%	98%
Pregnancy and Delivery Care				
Newborn Deliveries Scheduled Early	17	0%	4%	6%
Preventive Care				
Immunization for Influenza[2]	292	97%	90%	90%
Immunization for Pneumonia[2]	392	100%	92%	92%
Stroke Care				
Anticoagulation Therapy for Atrial Fibrillation[1]	-	-	94%	95%
Antithrombotic Therapy Timing	33	100%	99%	98%
Assessed for Rehabilitation	35	97%	98%	97%
Discharged on Antithrombotic Therapy	35	100%	99%	99%
Discharged on Statin Medication	26	100%	94%	94%
Thrombolytic Therapy Timing[7]	-	-	60%	66%

NOTE: Hospital profiles are in alphabetical order by state, then city, then hospital within the city; Rankings exclude hospitals with less than 25 cases except for patient surveys which excludes hospitals with less than 100 cases; (a) 100-299 cases; (1) The number of cases/patients is too few to report; (2) Data submitted were based on a sample of cases/patients; (3) Results are based on a shorter time period than required; (4) Data suppressed by CMS for one or more quarters; (5) Results are not available for this reporting period; (6) Fewer than 100 patients completed the HCAHPS survey; (7) No cases met the criteria for this measure; (8) The lower limit of the confidence interval cannot be calculated if the number of observed infections equals zero; (9) No data are available from the state/territory for this reporting period; (10) The scores shown reflect fewer than 50 completed surveys; (11) There were discrepancies in the data collection process; (12) This measure does not apply to this hospital for this reporting period; (13) Results cannot be calculated for this reporting period; (14) The results for this state are combined with nearby states to protect confidentiality; Please refer to the User's Guide for a full explanation of data.

Venous Thromboembolism Prophylaxis	32	100%	95%	94%
Written Stroke Educational Materials Given	17	100%	88%	88%
Surgical Care Improvement Project				
Appropriate Beta Blocker Usage	146	99%	99%	98%
Appropriate VTP Within 24 Hours	321	99%	99%	98%
Controlled Postoperative Blood Glucose[7]	-	-	96%	97%
Perioperative Temperature Management	436	100%	100%	100%
Prophylactic Antibiotic Selection	284	100%	99%	99%
Prophylactic Antibiotic Selection (Outpatient)	41	98%	98%	98%
Prophylactic Antibiotic Stopped	282	100%	99%	98%
Prophylactic Antibiotic Timing	285	99%	99%	99%
Prophylactic Antibiotic Timing (Outpatient)	42	98%	97%	98%
Urinary Catheter Removal	287	99%	98%	97%
Survey of Patients' Hospital Experiences				
Area Around Room 'Always' Quiet at Night	300+	52%	63%	61%
Doctors 'Always' Communicated Well	300+	85%	83%	82%
Home Recovery Information Given	300+	89%	89%	85%
Hospital Given 9 or 10 on 10 Point Scale	300+	71%	74%	71%
Meds 'Always' Explained Before Given	300+	72%	68%	64%
Nurses 'Always' Communicated Well	300+	84%	82%	79%
Pain 'Always' Well Controlled	300+	75%	72%	71%
Room and Bathroom 'Always' Clean	300+	76%	79%	73%
Timely Help 'Always' Received	300+	71%	72%	68%
Would Definitely Recommend Hospital	300+	74%	74%	71%
Use of Medical Imaging				
Cardiac Imaging Stress Test before Surgery[1]	-	-	5.4%	5.3%
Combination Abdominal CT Scan	150	2.0%	6.3%	10.5%
Combination Brain/Sinus CT Scan[1]	-	-	2.1%	2.7%
Combination Chest CT Scan	81	1.2%	1%	2.7%
Follow-up Mammogram/Ultrasound	67	9.0%	8.1%	8.8%
Lumbar Spine MRI for Low Back Pain[1]	-	-	34.9%	37.2%

NOTE: Hospital profiles are in alphabetical order by state, then city, then hospital within the city; Rankings exclude hospitals with less than 25 cases except for patient surveys which excludes hospitals with less than 100 cases; (a) 100-299 cases; (1) The number of cases/patients is too few to report; (2) Data submitted were based on a sample of cases/patients; (3) Results are based on a shorter time period than required; (4) Data suppressed by CMS for one or more quarters; (5) Results are not available for this reporting period; (6) Fewer than 100 patients completed the HCAHPS survey; (7) No cases met the criteria for this measure; (8) The lower limit of the confidence interval cannot be calculated if the number of observed infections equals zero; (9) No data are available from the state/territory for this reporting period; (10) The scores shown reflect fewer than 50 completed surveys; (11) There were discrepancies in the data collection process; (12) This measure does not apply to this hospital for this reporting period; (13) Results cannot be calculated for this reporting period; (14) The results for this state are combined with nearby states to protect confidentiality; Please refer to the User's Guide for a full explanation of data.

Appendix A: 30-Day Death (Mortality) Rates

What Do These Mortality Categories Show?

These categories show how hospitals' risk-adjusted 30-day death (mortality) rates for heart attack, heart failure, and pneumonia compare to the rate across the U.S., after making adjustments for how sick patients were before they were admitted to the hospital and taking into account differences in death rates that might be due to chance.

This first part of this appendix shows hospitals with 30-day risk-adjusted death (mortality) rates that are lower (better) or higher (worse) than the national rate for all three categories. Hospitals are shown to be better or worse than the U.S. national rate only if the data shows with 95% certainty, that the difference between their surgical complication rates and the U.S. national rate is not due to chance.

The second part of this appendix contains state and national summaries with the following column headers:

- **Better Than U.S. National Rate.** Hospitals in the Better Than U.S. National Rate category have risk-adjusted 30-day death (mortality) rates that are lower than the U.S. National Rate, with 95% certainty that this difference is not due to chance.
- **Worse Than U.S. National Rate.** Hospitals in the Worse Than U.S. National Rate category have risk-adjusted 30-day death (mortality) rates that are higher than the U.S. National Rate, with 95% certainty that this difference is not due to chance.
- **No Different Than U.S. National Rate.** Many hospitals in the No Different Than U.S. National Rate category have risk-adjusted 30-day death (mortality) rates that are about the same as the U.S. National Rate. Other hospitals in this category have rates that are higher or lower than the U.S. National Rate, without 95% certainty that these differences are not due to chance.
- **Number of Cases Too Small.** The number of cases is too small to classify the hospital.

Why are Death Rates for Individual Hospitals Not Shown?

Comparisons based on estimated death (mortality) rates alone can be misleading. Risk-adjusted death (mortality) rates are estimated for individual hospitals based on information taken from a particular time period. If a slightly different time period had been chosen, chances are that each hospital's results would have been somewhat different.

A range ("confidence interval" or in this case an "interval estimate") around estimates show how much variation might be due to this kind of chance. In this case, researchers are 95% confident that a hospital's death (mortality) rate fell somewhere within this specified range. The smaller the range, the more precise the estimate.

When hospitals treat a very large number of patients, chance differences will not have much effect on the overall rates. The range will be small, and the estimated death (mortality) rates will be more precise. In hospitals that treat smaller numbers of patients, however, even small chance differences could have a big impact on death (mortality) rates. The 95% confidence interval, or range, will be large, and the estimated death (mortality) rates will be less precise.

Because the number of patients treated at U.S. hospitals varies widely, the precision of hospitals' estimated death (mortality) rates also varies.

Calculation of 30-Day Risk-Standardized Mortality Rates

The 30-day death (mortality) measures are estimates of deaths from any cause within 30 days of a hospital admission, for patients hospitalized with one of several primary diagnoses. Deaths can be counted in the measures regardless of whether the patient dies while still in the hospital or after discharge. Using deaths within 30 days instead of inpatient deaths show a more consistent measurement time window because length of hospital stay varies across patients and hospitals. Also, mortality over longer time periods (such as 90 days) may have less to do with the care received in the hospital and more to do with other complicating illnesses, patients' own behavior, or care provided to patients after hospital discharge. *The Comparative Guide to American Hospitals* reports on the following 30-day mortality measures:

- 30-day death rate for heart attack (acute myocardial infarction [AMI]) patients
- 30-day death rate for heart failure (HF) patients
- 30-day death rate for pneumonia patients

Which Patients are Included

The 30-day death (mortality) measures include hospitalizations for Medicare beneficiaries aged 65 or older who were enrolled in Original Medicare (traditional fee-for-service Medicare) for the entire 12 months prior to their hospital admission. The AMI, heart failure, and pneumonia (death) mortality measures also include patients aged 65 or older who were admitted to Veteran's Health Administration (VA) hospitals. Beneficiaries enrolled in Medicare managed care plans are not included.

Where the Information Comes From

The Centers for Medicare & Medicaid Services (CMS) calculates hospital-specific 30-day mortality rates using Medicare claims and eligibility information. The AMI, HF, and pneumonia mortality measures are also calculated using VA administrative data. Using administrative data makes it possible to calculate mortality rates without having to do medical chart reviews or requiring hospitals to report additional information to CMS. Research conducted during development of the AMI, HF, and pneumonia death (mortality) measures showed that statistical models based on claims data performed well in estimating hospital mortality rates compared to models that are based on information from medical chart reviews.

Risk Adjustment

To make comparison of hospital performance equitable, the 30-day (death) mortality measures adjust for patient characteristics that may make death more likely, even if the hospital provided higher quality of care. These characteristics include the patient's age, past medical history, and other diseases or conditions (comorbidities) the patient had when admitted that are known to increase the patient's risk of dying.

Significance Testing

The statistical model used to calculate 30-day (death) mortality measures also determines how precise the estimates are, and provides the upper and lower bounds of the 95% interval estimates for each hospital's risk-adjusted mortality rates. Interval estimates, which are like confidence intervals, describe the level of uncertainty around the estimated mortality rates.

Comparing Individual Hospital Rates to the U.S. National Rate

To assign hospitals to performance categories, the hospital's interval estimate is compared to the U.S. national 30-day observed (death) mortality rate. If the 95% interval estimate includes the national observed rate for that measure, the hospital's performance is in the "No Different than U.S. National Rate" category. If the entire 95% interval estimate is below the national observed rate for that measure, then the hospital is performing "Better Than U.S. National Rate." If the entire 95% interval estimate is above the national observed rate for that measure, its performance is "WorseTthan U.S. National Rate." Hospitals with fewer than 25 eligible cases are placed into a separate category that indicates that the hospital did not have enough cases to reliably tell how well the hospital is performing.

Additional Information

For more detail on how the 30-day (death) mortality rates are calculated, visit QualityNet—Mortality Measures at www.qualitynet.org.

Hospitals whose Acute Myocardial Infarction (Heart Attack) 30-Day Mortality Rate is Better (Lower) than the U.S. National Rate

Hospital	City	State	Phone	Web Site
Advocate Lutheran General Hospital	Park Ridge	Illinois	847-723-2210	www.advocatehealth.com
Alexian Brothers Medical Center	Elk Grove Village	Illinois	847-437-5500	www.alexian.org
Arkansas Heart Hospital	Little Rock	Arkansas	501-219-7000	www.arheart.com
The Aroostook Medical Center	Presque Isle	Maine	207-768-4000	www.tamc.org
Avera Heart Hospital of South Dakota	Sioux Falls	South Dakota	605-977-7000	www.avera.org/heart-hospital
Baptist Memorial Hospital	Memphis	Tennessee	901-226-5000	www.bmhcc.org
Baptist Saint Anthony's Hospital	Amarillo	Texas	806-212-2000	www.bsahs.com
Beebe Medical Center	Lewes	Delaware	302-645-3300	www.beebemed.org
Beth Israel Deaconess Medical Center	Boston	Massachusetts	617-667-7000	www.bidmc.harvard.edu
Boca Raton Regional Hospital	Boca Raton	Florida	561-362-5002	www.brrh.com
Boone Hospital Center	Columbia	Missouri	573-815-8000	www.boone.org
Catholic Medical Center	Manchester	New Hampshire	603-668-3545	www.catholicmedicalcenter.org
Cedars - Sinai Medical Center	Los Angeles	California	310-423-5000	www.cedars-sinai.edu
Centegra Health System - Woodstock Hospital	Woodstock	Illinois	815-788-5823	www.centegra.org
Centinela Hospital Medical Center	Inglewood	California	310-673-4660	www.centinelafreeman.com
Chambersburg Hospital	Chambersburg	Pennsylvania	717-267-3000	www.summithealth.org
Champlain Valley Physicians Hospital Medical Center	Plattsburgh	New York	518-561-2000	www.cvph.org
Cypress Fairbanks Medical Center	Houston	Texas	281-897-3100	www.cyfairhospital.com
Doylestown Hospital	Doylestown	Pennsylvania	215-345-2200	www.dh.org
East Orange General Hospital	East Orange	New Jersey	973-266-4401	www.evh.org
Englewood Hospital & Medical Center	Englewood	New Jersey	201-894-3000	www.englewoodhospital.com
Evangelical Community Hospital	Lewisburg	Pennsylvania	570-522-2200	www.evanhospital.com
Firsthealth Moore Regional Hospital	Pinehurst	North Carolina	910-715-1000	www.firsthealth.org
French Hospital Medical Center	San Luis Obispo	California	805-543-5353	www.frenchmedicalcenter.org
Glendale Adventist Medical Center	Glendale	California	818-409-8202	www.glendaleadventist.com
Good Samaritan Hospital	Dayton	Ohio	937-278-2612	www.goodsamdayton.org
Hackensack University Medical Center	Hackensack	New Jersey	201-996-2000	www.humed.com
Hays Medical Center	Hays	Kansas	785-623-5000	www.haysmed.com
Henry Ford Hospital	Detroit	Michigan	313-916-2600	www.henryfordhospital.com
Holy Cross Hospital	Silver Spring	Maryland	301-754-7000	www.holycrosshealth.org
Holy Name Medical Center	Teaneck	New Jersey	201-833-3000	www.holyname.org
John T Mather Memorial Hospital of Port Jefferson	Port Jefferson	New York	631-473-1320	www.matherhospital.com
Lawrence Hospital Center	Bronxville	New York	914-787-1000	www.lawrencehealth.org
Lehigh Valley Hospital	Allentown	Pennsylvania	610-402-2273	www.lvhhn.org
Lehigh Valley Hospital - Hazleton	Hazleton	Pennsylvania	570-501-4000	www.ghha.org
Loyola Gottlieb Memorial Hospital	Melrose Park	Illinois	708-450-4924	www.gottliebhospital.org
Maimonides Medical Center	Brooklyn	New York	718-283-6000	www.maimonidesmed.org
Massachusetts General Hospital	Boston	Massachusetts	617-726-2000	www.massgeneral.org
Minneapolis VA Medical Center	Minneapolis	Minnesota	612-725-2000	www1.va.gov/minneapolis
Miriam Hospital	Providence	Rhode Island	401-793-2500	www.lifespan.org/partners/tmh
Missouri Baptist Medical Center	Town & Country	Missouri	314-996-5000	www.missouribaptistmedicalcenter.org
Montefiore Medical Center	Bronx	New York	718-920-4321	www.montefiore.org
Morristown Medical Center	Morristown	New Jersey	973-971-5450	www.morristownmemorialhospital.org
Mount Sinai Medical Center	Miami Beach	Florida	305-674-2121	www.msmc.com
Munson Medical Center	Traverse City	Michigan	231-935-5000	www.munsonhealthcare.org
New York - Presbyterian Hospital	New York	New York	212-746-4189	www.nyp.org
North Shore University Hospital	Manhasset	New York	516-562-0100	www.northshorelij.com
Northwestern Memorial Hospital	Chicago	Illinois	312-926-2000	www.nmh.org
NYU Hospitals Center	New York	New York	212-263-7300	www.med.nyu.edu
Oakwood Hospital - Dearborn	Dearborn	Michigan	313-593-7125	www.oakwood.org
Olympia Medical Center	Los Angeles	California	310-657-5900	www.olympiamc.com
Overlook Medical Center	Summit	New Jersey	908-522-2000	www.atlantichealth.org
Palisades Medical Center	North Bergen	New Jersey	201-854-5000	www.palisadesmedical.org
Presence Saint Joseph Hospital - Chicago	Chicago	Illinois	773-665-3000	www.res-health.org
Presence Saint Joseph Medical Center	Joliet	Illinois	815-725-7133	www.provena.org/stjoes
Providence Hospital & Medical Centers	Southfield	Michigan	248-849-3011	www.stjohn.org/providence
Rhode Island Hospital	Providence	Rhode Island	401-444-4000	www.rhodeislandhospital.org
Sarasota Memorial Hospital	Sarasota	Florida	941-917-9000	www.smh.com
Sherman Oaks Hospital	Sherman Oaks	California	818-981-7111	www.shermanoakshospital.com
Southcoast Hospital Group	Fall River	Massachusetts	508-679-3131	www.southcoast.org/charlton
Southside Hospital	Bay Shore	New York	631-968-3000	www.northshorelij.com
Saint Francis Hospital - Roslyn	Roslyn	New York	516-562-6000	www.stfrancisheartcenter.com
Saint Joseph Mercy Hospital	Ann Arbor	Michigan	734-712-3791	www.stjoesannarbor.or
Saint Luke's Hospital Bethlehem	Bethlehem	Pennsylvania	610-954-4000	www.slhn-lehighvalley.org
Saint Luke's Hospital	Chesterfield	Missouri	314-434-1500	www.goodhealthmatters.com

Hospital	City	State	Phone	Web Site
Saint Luke's Hospital of Kansas City	Kansas City	Missouri	816-932-2000	www.saintlukeshealthsystem.org
Saint Mary's Medical Center	Huntington	West Virginia	304-526-1234	www.st-marys.org
Saint Vincent Heart Center of Indiana	Indianapolis	Indiana	317-583-5000	www.theheartcenter.com
Trinity Rock Island	Rock Island	Illinois	309-779-5000	www.trinityqc.com
University of California Davis Medical Center	Sacramento	California	916-734-2011	www.ucdmc.ucdavis.edu
Valley Hospital	Ridgewood	New Jersey	201-447-8000	www.valleyhealth.com
Wakemed - Cary Hospital	Cary	North Carolina	919-350-2550	www.wakemed.org
Waterbury Hospital	Waterbury	Connecticut	203-573-6000	www.waterburyhospital.org
William Beaumont Hospital - Troy	Troy	Michigan	248-964-8800	www.beaumonthospitals.com
Winchester Hospital	Winchester	Massachusetts	781-729-9000	www.winchesterhospital.org
Yale-New Haven Hospital	New Haven	Connecticut	203-688-4242	www.ynhh.org
Yuma Regional Medical Center	Yuma	Arizona	928-336-7275	www.yumaregional.org

Note: Table shows hospitals nationwide whose acute myocardial infarction 30-day risk-adjusted mortality rate is better (lower) than U.S. rate of 15.2%

Hospitals whose Acute Myocardial Infarction (Heart Attack) 30-Day Mortality Rate is Worse (Higher) than the U.S. National Rate

Hospital	City	State	Phone	Web Site
Altru Hospital	Grand Forks	North Dakota	701-780-5000	www.altru.org
Baptist Health Corbin	Corbin	Kentucky	606-528-1212	www.baptistregional.com
Bronson Battle Creek Hospital	Battle Creek	Michigan	269-966-8000	www.bchealth.com
Dallas Regional Medical Center	Mesquite	Texas	214-320-7000	www.dallasregionalmedicalcenter.com
Desert Springs Hospital	Las Vegas	Nevada	702-369-7600	www.desertspringshospital.net/p12.html
Hurley Medical Center	Flint	Michigan	810-257-9000	www.hurleymc.com
Kaweah Delta Medical Center	Visalia	California	559-624-2000	www.kaweahdelta.org
Lafayette General Medical Center	Lafayette	Louisiana	337-289-7991	www.lafayettegeneral.org
Lakes Region General Hospital	Laconia	New Hampshire	603-524-3211	www.lrgh.org
Laredo Medical Center	Laredo	Texas	956-796-5000	www.laredomedical.com
Mclaren Bay Region	Bay City	Michigan	989-894-3000	www.baymed.org
National Park Medical Center	Hot Springs	Arkansas	501-321-1000	www.nationalparkmedical.com
North Hills Hospital	North Richland Hills	Texas	817-255-1000	www.northhillshospital.com
Penobscot Valley Hospital	Lincoln	Maine	207-794-3321	www.pvhhealthcare.org
Robert Wood Johnson University Hospital at Rahway	Rahway	New Jersey	732-381-4200	www.rwjuhr.com/about/history.html
Schuylkill Medical Center - East Norwegian Street	Pottsville	Pennsylvania	570-621-4000	www.schuylkillhealth.com
Saint Marys Regional Medical Center	Russellville	Arkansas	479-968-2841	www.saintmarysregional.com
University Hospital SUNY Health Science Center	Syracuse	New York	315-473-4240	www.upstate.edu
Winter Haven Hospital	Winter Haven	Florida	863-293-1121	www.winterhavenhospital.com

Note: Table shows hospitals nationwide whose acute myocardial infarction 30-day risk-adjusted mortality rate is worse (higher) than U.S. rate of 15.2%

Hospitals whose Heart Failure 30-Day Mortality Rate is Better (Lower) than the U.S. National Rate

Hospital	City	State	Phone	Web Site
Abbott Northwestern Hospital	Minneapolis	Minnesota	612-863-4509	www.abbottnorthwestern.com
Advocate Trinity Hospital	Chicago	Illinois	773-967-2000	www.advocatehealth.com/trin
Alexian Brothers Medical Center	Elk Grove Village	Illinois	847-437-5500	www.alexian.org
Atlanticare Regional Medical Center	Atlantic City	New Jersey	609-441-8020	www.atlanticare.org/acmc/index.html
Aurora Saint Lukes Medical Center	Milwaukee	Wisconsin	414-649-6000	www.aurorahealthcare.org
Banner Thunderbird Medical Center	Glendale	Arizona	602-588-5555	www.bannerhealth.com
Baptist Medical Center	San Antonio	Texas	210-297-1020	www.baptisthealthsystem.org
Bay Medical Center Sacred Heart Health System	Panama City	Florida	850-769-1511	www.baymedical.org
Bayhealth - Kent General Hospital	Dover	Delaware	302-744-7001	www.bayhealth.org/about/kent.asp
Beaumont Health System	Royal Oak	Michigan	248-898-5000	www.beaumonthospitals.com
Beth Israel Deaconess Medical Center	Boston	Massachusetts	617-667-7000	www.bidmc.harvard.edu
Beverly Hospital	Montebello	California	323-726-1222	www.beverly.org
Birmingham VA Medical Center	Birmingham	Alabama	205-933-4515	www.birmingham.va.gov
Boston Medical Center Corporation	Boston	Massachusetts	617-638-8000	www.bmc.org
Brigham & Women's Hospital	Boston	Massachusetts	617-732-5500	www.brighamandwomens.org
California Hospital Medical Center Los Angeles	Los Angeles	California	213-748-2411	www.chmcla.org
Cedars - Sinai Medical Center	Los Angeles	California	310-423-5000	www.cedars-sinai.edu
Centinela Hospital Medical Center	Inglewood	California	310-673-4660	www.centinelafreeman.com
Centrastate Medical Center	Freehold	New Jersey	732-431-2000	www.centrastate.com
Champlain Valley Physicians Hospital Medical Center	Plattsburgh	New York	518-561-2000	www.cvph.org
Charleston Area Medical Center	Charleston	West Virginia	304-388-6203	www.camc.org
Clara Maass Medical Center	Belleville	New Jersey	973-450-2002	www.sbhcs.com/hospitals
Cleveland - Wade Park VA Medical Center	Cleveland	Ohio	216-791-3800	www.cleveland.va.gov
Community Hospital	Munster	Indiana	219-836-1600	www.comhs.org/community
Conemaugh Valley Memorial Hospital	Johnstown	Pennsylvania	814-534-9000	www.conemaugh.org
Desert Valley Hospital	Victorville	California	760-241-8000	www.dvmc.com
East Orange General Hospital	East Orange	New Jersey	973-266-4401	www.evh.org
Edward Hospital	Naperville	Illinois	630-527-3000	www.edward.org
Emory University Hospital Midtown	Atlanta	Georgia	404-686-4411	www.emoryhealthcare.org
Essentia Health Saint Joseph's Medical Center	Brainerd	Minnesota	218-829-2861	www.sjmcmn.org
Excela Health Frick Hospital	Mount Pleasant	Pennsylvania	724-547-1500	www.excelahealth.org
Fairview Hospital	Cleveland	Ohio	216-476-7000	www.fairviewhospital.org
Falmouth Hospital	Falmouth	Massachusetts	508-548-5300	www.capecodhealth.com
Fawcett Memorial Hospital	Port Charlotte	Florida	941-629-1181	www.fawcetthospital.com
Firsthealth Moore Regional Hospital	Pinehurst	North Carolina	910-715-1000	www.firsthealth.org
Flagler Hospital	Saint Augustine	Florida	904-819-4426	www.flaglerhospital.com
Florida Hospital Heartland Medical Center	Sebring	Florida	863-314-4466	www.fhhd.org
Forbes Regional Hospital	Monroeville	Pennsylvania	412-858-2000	www.wpahs.org
Fort Duncan Medical Center	Eagle Pass	Texas	830-773-5321	www.fortduncanmedicalcenter.com
Fountain Valley Regional Hospital & Medical Center	Fountain Valley	California	714-966-7200	www.fountainvalleyhospital.com
Franciscan Saint James Health	Olympia Fields	Illinois	708-747-4000	www.franciscanalliance.org
Franciscan Saint Margaret Health - Hammond	Hammond	Indiana	219-932-2300	www.smmhc.com
Frederick Memorial Hospital	Frederick	Maryland	240-566-3300	www.fmh.org
Genesys Regional Medical Center - Health Park	Grand Blanc	Michigan	810-606-5000	www.genesys.org
Glendale Adventist Medical Center	Glendale	California	818-409-8202	www.glendaleadventist.com
Glendale Memorial Hospital & Health Center	Glendale	California	818-502-1900	www.glendalememorialhospital.org
Good Samaritan Hospital	Los Angeles	California	213-977-2121	www.goodsam.org
Good Shepherd Medical Center	Longview	Texas	903-315-2000	www.goodshepherdhealth.org
Grand View Hospital	Sellersville	Pennsylvania	215-453-4615	www.gvh.org
Hahnemann University Hospital	Philadelphia	Pennsylvania	215-762-7000	www.hahnemannhospital.com
Harper University Hospital	Detroit	Michigan	313-745-6211	www.harperhospital.org
Henry Ford Hospital	Detroit	Michigan	313-916-2600	www.henryfordhospital.com
Henry Ford Wyandotte Hospital	Wyandotte	Michigan	734-246-6000	www.henryfordwyandotte.com
Hillcrest Hospital	Mayfield Heights	Ohio	440-312-4500	www.hillcresthospital.org
Hollywood Presbyterian Medical Center	Los Angeles	California	213-413-3000	www.qahpmc.com
Holy Name Medical Center	Teaneck	New Jersey	201-833-3000	www.holyname.org
Houston VA Medical Center	Houston	Texas	713-794-7100	www.houston.med.va.gov
Howard County General Hospital	Columbia	Maryland	410-740-7890	www.hcgh.org
Huntington Beach Hospital	Huntington Beach	California	714-843-5000	www.hbhospital.com
Huron Valley - Sinai Hospital	Commerce Township	Michigan	248-937-3370	www.hvsh.org
Ingalls Memorial Hospital	Harvey	Illinois	708-333-2300	www.ingalls.org
Inova Fairfax Hospital	Falls Church	Virginia	703-776-3332	www.inova.org
Jersey Shore University Medical Center	Neptune	New Jersey	732-776-4900	www.meridianhealth.com
Jesse Brown VA Medical Center - VA Chicago	Chicago	Illinois	312-569-8387	www.va.gov
Kingsbrook Jewish Medical Center	Brooklyn	New York	718-604-5789	www.kingsbrook.org

Hospital	City	State	Phone	Web Site
Lawrence General Hospital	Lawrence	Massachusetts	978-683-4000	www.lawrencegeneral.org
Lehigh Valley Hospital	Allentown	Pennsylvania	610-402-2273	www.lvhhn.org
Lehigh Valley Hospital - Hazleton	Hazleton	Pennsylvania	570-501-4000	www.ghha.org
Lenox Hill Hospital	New York	New York	212-439-2345	www.lenoxhillhospital.org
Libertyhealth - Jersey City Medical Center Campus	Jersey City	New Jersey	201-915-2000	www.libertyhcs.org
Long Beach Memorial Medical Center	Long Beach	California	562-933-2000	www.memorialcare.com/long_beach
Louis A Weiss Memorial Hospital	Chicago	Illinois	773-878-8700	www.weisshospital.org
Maimonides Medical Center	Brooklyn	New York	718-283-6000	www.maimonidesmed.org
Main Line Hospital Bryn Mawr Campus	Bryn Mawr	Pennsylvania	610-526-3000	www.mainlinehealth.org
Main Line Hospital Lankenau	Wynnewood	Pennsylvania	610-645-2000	www.mainlinehealth.org/lh
Marymount Hospital	Garfield Heights	Ohio	216-581-0500	www.marymount.org
Mclaren Flint	Flint	Michigan	810-342-2000	www.mclaren.org
Medical Center of Southeastern Oklahoma	Durant	Oklahoma	405-924-3080	www.mcsohealth.com
Medstar Franklin Square Medical Center	Baltimore	Maryland	443-777-7850	www.franklinsquare.org
Medstar Good Samaritan Hospital	Baltimore	Maryland	443-444-3902	www.goodsam-md.org
Medstar Washington Hospital Center	Washington	District of Columbia	202-877-7000	www.whcenter.org
Mercy Fitzgerald Hospital	Darby	Pennsylvania	215-237-4000	www.mercyhealth.org
Mercy Hospital & Medical Center	Chicago	Illinois	312-567-2000	www.mercy-chicago.org
Mercy Medical Center	Springfield	Massachusetts	413-748-9000	www.mercycares.com
Mercy Saint Vincent Medical Center	Toledo	Ohio	419-251-3232	www.mhsnr.org
The Methodist Hospital	Houston	Texas	713-790-2221	www.methodisthealth.com
Mission Hospital Regional Medical Center	Mission Viejo	California	949-364-1400	www.mission4health.com
Missouri Baptist Medical Center	Town & Country	Missouri	314-996-5000	www.missouribaptistmedicalcenter.org
Montefiore Medical Center	Bronx	New York	718-920-4321	www.montefiore.org
Morristown Medical Center	Morristown	New Jersey	973-971-5450	www.morristownmemorialhospital.org
Mount Sinai Hospital	New York	New York	212-241-7981	www.mountsinai.org
Mountainview Hospital	Las Vegas	Nevada	702-255-5065	www.mountainview-hospital.com
New York Hospital Medical Center of Queens	Flushing	New York	718-670-1231	www.nyhq.org
New York - Presbyterian Hospital	New York	New York	212-746-4189	www.nyp.org
Newark Beth Israel Medical Center	Newark	New Jersey	973-926-7850	www.sbhcs.com
Newton - Wellesley Hospital	Newton	Massachusetts	617-243-6000	www.nwh.org
North Florida Regional Medical Center	Gainesville	Florida	352-333-4100	www.nfrmc.com
North Shore Medical Center	Salem	Massachusetts	978-741-1215	www.nsmc.partners.org
Northridge Hospital Medical Center	Northridge	California	818-885-8500	www.northridgehospital.org
Northwestern Memorial Hospital	Chicago	Illinois	312-926-2000	www.nmh.org
NYU Hospitals Center	New York	New York	212-263-7300	www.med.nyu.edu
Oakwood Hospital - Dearborn	Dearborn	Michigan	313-593-7125	www.oakwood.org
Oklahoma Heart Hospital South	Oklahoma City	Oklahoma	405-628-6000	www.okheart.com/south-campus
Olympia Medical Center	Los Angeles	California	310-657-5900	www.olympiamc.com
Oroville Hospital	Oroville	California	530-533-8500	www.orovillehospital.com
Palm Beach Gardens Medical Center	Palm Beach Gardens	Florida	561-622-1411	www.pbgmc.com
Palmetto Health Richland	Columbia	South Carolina	803-296-5678	www.palmettohealth.org
Paradise Valley Hospital	National City	California	619-470-4321	www.paradisevalleyhospital.org
Penn Presbyterian Medical Center	Philadelphia	Pennsylvania	215-662-8000	www.pennhealth.com
Pennsylvania Hospital of the Univ of PA Health Sys	Philadelphia	Pennsylvania	215-829-3000	www.pennmedicine.org/pahosp
Philadelphia VA Medical Center	Philadelphia	Pennsylvania	215-823-5857	www.philadelphia.va.gov
Portland VA Medical Center	Portland	Oregon	503-220-8262	www.va.gov/portland/index.asp
Presence Saint Joseph Hospital - Chicago	Chicago	Illinois	773-665-3000	www.res-health.org
Presence Saint Joseph Medical Center	Joliet	Illinois	815-725-7133	www.provena.org/stjoes
Presence Saints Mary & Elizabeth Medical Center	Chicago	Illinois	312-770-2000	www.reshealth.org
Providence Holy Cross Medical Center	Mission Hills	California	818-365-8051	www.providence.org
Providence Hospital	Washington	District of Columbia	202-269-7000	www.provhosp.org
Providence Hospital & Medical Centers	Southfield	Michigan	248-849-3011	www.stjohn.org/providence
Providence Little Co of Mary Medical Center Torrance	Torrance	California	310-540-7676	www.lcmhs.org
Providence Tarzana Medical Center	Tarzana	California	818-881-0800	www.encino-tarzana.com
Raritan Bay Medical Center	Perth Amboy	New Jersey	732-442-3700	www.rbmc.org
Regional Medical Center of San Jose	San Jose	California	408-259-5000	www.regionalmedicalsanjose.com
Rex Hospital	Raleigh	North Carolina	919-784-3100	www.rexhealth.com
Rio Grande Regional Hospital	Mcallen	Texas	956-632-6000	www.riohealth.com
Ronald Reagan UCLA Medical Center	Los Angeles	California	310-825-6301	www.uclahealth.org
Rush Oak Park Hospital	Oak Park	Illinois	708-383-9300	www.oakparkhospital.org
Rush University Medical Center	Chicago	Illinois	312-942-5000	www.ruch.edu
Saint Agnes Hospital	Baltimore	Maryland	410-368-2101	www.stagnes.org
Saint Francis Medical Center	Lynwood	California	310-900-8900	www.stfrancis.dochs.org
Saint Michael's Medical Center	Newark	New Jersey	973-877-5350	www.cathedralhealth.org
Saint Vincent Medical Center	Los Angeles	California	213-484-7111	www.stvincent.dochs.org
Santa Monica - UCLA Medical Center & Orthopaedic Hospital	Santa Monica	California	310-319-4000	www.healthcare.ucla.edu

Hospital	City	State	Phone	Web Site
Scottsdale Healthcare - Shea Medical Center	Scottsdale	Arizona	480-323-3009	www.shc.org
Scripps Green Hospital	La Jolla	California	858-554-3600	www.scrippshealth.org
Scripps Mercy Hospital	San Diego	California	619-294-8111	www.scrippshealth.org
Shore Medical Center	Somers Point	New Jersey	609-653-3545	www.shorememorial.org
Sinai Hospital of Baltimore	Baltimore	Maryland	410-601-5131	www.sinai-balt.com
Sinai - Grace Hospital	Detroit	Michigan	313-966-3300	www.sinaigrace.org
South Pointe Hospital	Warrensville Heights	Ohio	216-491-6000	www.southpointehospital.org
South Texas Health System	Edinburg	Texas	956-632-4000	www.edinburgregional.com
Southcoast Hospital Group	Fall River	Massachusetts	508-679-3131	www.southcoast.org/charlton
Southeastern Regional Medical Center	Lumberton	North Carolina	910-671-5000	www.srmc.org
SSM Saint Marys Health Center	Richmond Heights	Missouri	314-768-8000	www.ssmhealth.com/stmarys
Saint Alexius Medical Center	Hoffman Estates	Illinois	847-843-2000	www.alexianbrothershealth.org
Saint Catherine Hospital	East Chicago	Indiana	219-392-7004	www.comhs.org/stcatherine
Saint Elizabeth's Medical Center	Brighton	Massachusetts	617-789-3000	www.semc.org
Saint Francis Hospital & Medical Center	Hartford	Connecticut	860-714-4000	www.saintfranciscare.com
Saint Francis Hospital - Roslyn	Roslyn	New York	516-562-6000	www.stfrancisheartcenter.com
Saint John Hospital & Medical Center	Detroit	Michigan	313-343-4000	www.stjohnprovidence.org
Saint Luke's Hospital	Chesterfield	Missouri	314-434-1500	www.goodhealthmatters.com
Saint Luke's Hospital of Kansas City	Kansas City	Missouri	816-932-2000	www.staintlukeshealthsystem.org
Saint Vincent's Medical Center Southside	Jacksonville	Florida	904-296-3700	www.jaxhealth.com
Thomas Jefferson University Hospital	Philadelphia	Pennsylvania	215-955-6000	www.jeffersonhospital.org
Touro Infirmary	New Orleans	Louisiana	504-897-7011	www.touro.com
Tufts Medical Center	Boston	Massachusetts	617-636-5000	www.tuftsmedicalcenter.org
University Hospital of Brooklyn - Downstate Medical Center	Brooklyn	New York	718-270-1000	www.downstate.edu
University of Maryland Charles Regional Medical Center	La Plata	Maryland	301-609-4265	www.civista.org
University of Miami Hospital	Miami	Florida	305-325-5511	www.cedarsmedicalcenter.com
UPMC Mckeesport	Mc Keesport	Pennsylvania	412-664-2000	www.selectmedicalcorp.com
UPMC Passavant	Pittsburgh	Pennsylvania	412-367-6700	www.passavant.upmc.com
UT Southwestern University Hospital	Dallas	Texas	214-879-3758	www.utsouthwestern.edu
VA Boston Healthcare System - Jamaica Plain	Jamaica Plain	Massachusetts	617-232-9500	www.vaww.visn1.med.va.gov/boston
VA Greater Los Angeles Healthcare System	West Los Angeles	California	310-478-3711	www1.va.gov
VA New York Harbor Healthcare System	New York	New York	212-686-7500	www.nyharbor.va.gov
Valley Hospital	Ridgewood	New Jersey	201-447-8000	www.valleyhealth.com
Valley Presbyterian Hospital	Van Nuys	California	818-902-3906	www.valleypres.org
Wakemed - Raleigh Campus	Raleigh	North Carolina	919-350-8000	www.wakemed.org
Washington Adventist Hospital	Takoma Park	Maryland	301-891-5651	www.adventisthealthcare.com/wah
Waukesha Memorial Hospital	Waukesha	Wisconsin	262-928-1000	www.waukeshamemorial.org
West Haven VA Medical Center	West Haven	Connecticut	203-932-5711	www.visn1.med.va.gov/vact
Wheaton Franciscan Healthcare Saint Francis	Milwaukee	Wisconsin	414-647-5000	www.mywheaton.org
White Memorial Medical Center	Los Angeles	California	323-268-5000	www.whitememorial.com
William Beaumont Hospital - Troy	Troy	Michigan	248-964-8800	www.beaumonthospitals.com
Willis Knighton Medical Center	Shreveport	Louisiana	318-212-4000	www.wkhs.com//locations/medicalcenter.aspx
Winchester Hospital	Winchester	Massachusetts	781-729-9000	www.winchesterhospital.org
Wing Memorial Hospital & Medical Center	Palmer	Massachusetts	413-283-7651	www.winghealth.org
Yale-New Haven Hospital	New Haven	Connecticut	203-688-4242	www.ynhh.org

Note: Table shows hospitals nationwide whose heart failure 30-day risk-adjusted mortality rate is better (lower) than U.S. rate of 11.7%

Hospitals whose Heart Failure 30-Day Mortality Rate is Worse (Higher) than the U.S. National Rate

Hospital	City	State	Phone	Web Site
Abbeville General Hospital	Abbeville	Louisiana	337-893-5466	www.abgen.net
Abrom Kaplan Memorial Hospital	Kaplan	Louisiana	337-643-8300	www.compasshealthcare.com/site78.php
Albany Memorial Hospital	Albany	New York	518-471-3221	www.nehealth.com
Alegent Creighton Health Immanuel Medical Center	Omaha	Nebraska	402-572-2121	www.alegent.com
Anne Arundel Medical Center	Annapolis	Maryland	443-481-1307	www.aahs.org
Appleton Medical Center	Appleton	Wisconsin	920-731-4101	www.thedacare.org
Arkansas Methodist Medical Center	Paragould	Arkansas	870-239-7000	www.arkansasmethodist.org
Baptist Health Medical Center - North Little Rock	North Little Rock	Arkansas	501-202-3000	www.baptist-health.org
Baptist Memorial Hospital/Golden Triangle	Columbus	Mississippi	662-244-1500	www.bmhcc.org/facilities/goldentriangle
Baxter Regional Medical Center	Mountain Home	Arkansas	870-508-1000	www.baxterregional.org
Blanchard Valley Hospital	Findlay	Ohio	419-423-4500	www.bvha.org
Bolivar Medical Center	Cleveland	Mississippi	662-846-2551	www.bolivarmedical.com
Brattleboro Memorial Hospital	Brattleboro	Vermont	802-257-0341	www.bmhvt.org
Bronson Methodist Hospital	Kalamazoo	Michigan	269-341-6000	www.bronsonhealth.com
Capital Region Medical Center	Jefferson City	Missouri	573-632-5000	www.crmc.org
Carilion Roanoke Memorial Hospital	Roanoke	Virginia	540-981-7000	www.carilion.com/crmh
Carolinas Medical Center/Behaviorial Health	Charlotte	North Carolina	704-355-2000	www.carolinasmedicalcenter.org
Carroll Hospital Center	Westminster	Maryland	410-848-3000	www.carrollhospitalcenter.org
Carson Tahoe Regional Medical Center	Carson City	Nevada	775-445-8000	www.carsontahoehospital.com
Cayuga Medical Center at Ithaca	Ithaca	New York	607-274-4401	www.cayugamed.org
Central Maine Medical Center	Lewiston	Maine	207-795-0111	www.cmmc.org
Central Washington Hospital	Wenatchee	Washington	509-662-1511	www.cwhs.com
Cherokee Regional Medical Center	Cherokee	Iowa	712-225-5101	www.cherokeermc.org
Chicot Memorial Medical Center	Lake Village	Arkansas	870-265-5351	www.chicotmemorial.com
Christus Hospital	Beaumont	Texas	409-892-7171	www.christushealth.org
Citizens Baptist Medical Center	Talladega	Alabama	256-761-4542	www.bhsala.com
Citrus Memorial Hospital	Inverness	Florida	352-726-1551	www.citrusmh.com
Clarion Hospital	Clarion	Pennsylvania	814-226-9500	www.clarionhospital.org
Clovis Community Medical Center	Clovis	California	559-324-4000	www.communitymedical.org
Columbia Saint Marys Hospital Ozaukee	Mequon	Wisconsin	262-243-7300	www.columbia-stmarys.org
Community Hospital North	Indianapolis	Indiana	317-621-5335	www.ecommunity.com/north
Conway Regional Medical Center	Conway	Arkansas	501-329-3831	www.conwayregional.org
Copley Memorial Hospital	Aurora	Illinois	630-978-6200	www.rushcopley.com
Coshocton County Memorial Hospital	Coshocton	Ohio	740-622-6411	www.ccmh.com
Dekalb Regional Medical Center	Fort Payne	Alabama	256-845-3150	www.baptistmedical.org
Dominican Hospital	Santa Cruz	California	831-462-7700	www.dominicanhospital.org
Edward W Sparrow Hospital	Lansing	Michigan	517-364-1000	www.sparrow.org
Emerson Hospital	W Concord	Massachusetts	978-369-1400	www.emersonhospital.org
Fletcher Allen Hospital of Vermont	Burlington	Vermont	802-847-0000	www.fletcherallen.org
Floyd Medical Center	Rome	Georgia	706-509-6900	www.floydmed.org
Geisinger Medical Center	Danville	Pennsylvania	570-271-6211	www.geisinger.org
Geneva General Hospital	Geneva	New York	315-787-4175	www.flhealth.org
GHS Greenville Memorial Medical Center	Greenville	South Carolina	864-455-7000	www.ghs.org
Good Samaritan Hospital	Lebanon	Pennsylvania	717-270-7500	www.gshleb.org
Grossmont Hospital	La Mesa	California	619-465-0711	www.sharp.com
Hendrick Medical Center	Abilene	Texas	325-670-2000	www.ehendrick.org
Highland Hospital	Rochester	New York	585-473-2200	www.urmc.rochester.edu
Hilton Head Regional Medical Center	Hilton Head Island	South Carolina	843-681-6122	www.hiltonheadmedctr.com
Hopkins County Memorial Hospital	Sulphur Springs	Texas	903-885-7671	www.hcmh.com
Hutchinson Regional Medical Center	Hutchinson	Kansas	620-665-2001	www.hutchinsonhospital.com
Iberia General Hospital & Medical Center	New Iberia	Louisiana	337-364-0441	www.iberiamedicalcenter.com
Indiana University Health La Porte Hospital	La Porte	Indiana	219-326-1234	www.laportehealth.org
Integris Grove Hospital	Grove	Oklahoma	918-786-2243	www.integris-health.com
IU Health Goshen Hospital	Goshen	Indiana	574-364-1000	www.goshenhosp.com
Jane Phillips Medical Center	Bartlesville	Oklahoma	918-333-7200	www.jpmc.org
JFK Medical Center - A M Yelencsics Comm Hospital	Edison	New Jersey	732-321-7000	www.jfkmc.org
Johnson Memorial Hospital	Franklin	Indiana	317-736-3300	www.johnsonmemorial.org
Kadlec Regional Medical Center	Richland	Washington	509-946-4611	www.kadlecmed.org
Kootenai Medical Center	Coeur D'alene	Idaho	208-625-4001	www.kootenaihealth.org
Lake Cumberland Regional Hospital	Somerset	Kentucky	606-679-7441	www.lakecumberlandhospital.com
Lake Granbury Medical Center	Granbury	Texas	817-573-2683	www.lakegranburymedicalcenter.com
Lawrence & Memorial Hospital	New London	Connecticut	860-442-0711	www.lmhospital.org
Los Alamitos Medical Center	Los Alamitos	California	562-799-3220	www.losalamitosmedctr.com
Manatee Memorial Hospital	Bradenton	Florida	941-746-5111	www.manateememorial.com
Manchester Memorial Hospital	Manchester	Connecticut	860-647-4780	www.echn.org

Hospital	City	State	Phone	Web Site
Maury Regional Hospital	Columbia	Tennessee	931-381-1111	www.maurgregional.com
Mclaren - Greater Lansing	Lansing	Michigan	517-975-6000	www.mclaren.org
Meadville Medical Center	Meadville	Pennsylvania	814-333-5000	www.mmchs.org
Medcentral Health System Mansfield Hospital	Mansfield	Ohio	419-526-8000	www.medcentral.org
Memorial Hospital of South Bend	South Bend	Indiana	574-647-1000	www.qualityoflife.org
Mercy Health System Corp	Janesville	Wisconsin	608-756-6080	www.mercyhealthsystem.org
Mercy Hospital Springfield	Springfield	Missouri	417-820-2000	www.stjohns.com
Mercy Medical Center - Redding	Redding	California	530-225-6102	www.redding.mercy.org
Mercy Medical Center - North Iowa	Mason City	Iowa	641-428-7000	www.mercynorthiowa.com
Mountain View Regional Medical Center	Las Cruces	New Mexico	575-556-7600	www.mountainviewregional.com
Nathan Littauer Hospital	Gloversville	New York	518-725-8621	www.nlh.org
Nea Baptist Memorial Hospital	Jonesboro	Arkansas	870-972-7000	www.baptistonline.com
New Hanover Regional Medical Center	Wilmington	North Carolina	910-343-7000	www.nhrmc.org
New Milford Hospital	New Milford	Connecticut	860-355-2611	www.newmilfordhospital.org
Norman Regional Health System	Norman	Oklahoma	405-321-1700	www.normanregional.com
North Mississippi Medical Center	Tupelo	Mississippi	662-377-3000	www.nmhs.net/nmmc
North Shore University Hospital	Manhasset	New York	516-562-0100	www.northshorelij.com
Northwest Community Hospital	Arlington Heights	Illinois	847-618-1000	www.nch.org
Northwest Hospital	Seattle	Washington	206-364-0500	www.nwhospital.org
O'Connor Hospital	San Jose	California	408-947-2500	www.oconnorhospital.org
Olympic Medical Center	Port Angeles	Washington	360-417-7000	www.olympicmedical.org
Our Lady of the Lake Regional Medical Center	Baton Rouge	Louisiana	225-765-6565	www.ololrmc.com
Overton Brooks VA Medical Center - Shreveport	Shreveport	Louisiana	318-424-6037	www.va.gov/sta/guide/home.asp
Pinnacle Health Hospitals	Harrisburg	Pennsylvania	717-782-5181	www.pinnaclehealth.org
Poplar Bluff Regional Medical Center	Poplar Bluff	Missouri	573-785-7721	www.poplarbluffregional.com
Porter Regional Hospital	Valparaiso	Indiana	219-983-8300	www.portermemorial.org
Providence Alaska Medical Center	Anchorage	Alaska	907-261-3675	www.providence.org
Providence Sacred Heart Medical Center	Spokane	Washington	509-474-3040	www.shmc.org
Rideout Memorial Hospital	Marysville	California	530-749-4300	www.frhg.org
Riverview Hospital Assoc	Wisconsin Rapids	Wisconsin	715-423-6060	www.riverviewhospital.net
Sacred Heart Medical Center - Riverbend	Springfield	Oregon	541-222-7300	www.peacehealth.org/sacred-heart-riverbend
Saint Anthony Medical Center	Rockford	Illinois	815-226-2000	www.osfhealth.com
Saint Francis Medical Center	Peoria	Illinois	309-655-2000	www.osfsaintfrancis.org
Salem Hospital	Salem	Oregon	503-561-5200	www.salemhospital.org
Saline Memorial Hospital	Benton	Arkansas	501-776-6000	www.salinememorial.org
San Juan Regional Medical Center	Farmington	New Mexico	505-609-2000	www.sanjuanregional.com
Sanford Usd Medical Center	Sioux Falls	South Dakota	605-333-1000	www.sanfordhealth.org
Santa Rosa Memorial Hospital	Santa Rosa	California	707-525-5300	www.stjosephhealth.org
Sarasota Memorial Hospital	Sarasota	Florida	941-917-9000	www.smh.com
Scenic Mountain Medical Center	Big Spring	Texas	432-263-1211	www.smmccares.com
Sentara Obici Hospital	Suffolk	Virginia	757-934-4000	www.sentara.com
Saint Anthony's Hospital	Saint Petersburg	Florida	727-825-1100	www.stanthonys.com
Saint Bernards Medical Center	Jonesboro	Arkansas	870-972-4100	www.sbrmc.com
Saint Francis - Downtown	Greenville	South Carolina	864-255-1000	www.stfrancishealth.org
Saint Johns Hospital	Springfield	Illinois	217-544-6464	www.st-johns.org
Saint Joseph Regional Health Center	Bryan	Texas	979-776-3912	www.st-joseph.org/sjrhc
Saint Joseph's Mercy Health Center	Hot Springs	Arkansas	501-622-1000	www.saintjosephs.com
Saint Lucie Medical Center	Port Saint Lucie	Florida	772-335-4000	www.stluciemed.com
Saint Marys Hospital Medical Center	Green Bay	Wisconsin	920-498-4200	www.stmgb.org
Saint Marys Regional Medical Center	Russellville	Arkansas	479-968-2841	www.saintmarysregional.com
Saint Nicholas Hospital	Sheboygan	Wisconsin	920-459-8300	www.stnicholashospital.org
Saint Rose Dominican Hospitals - Rose De Lima Campus	Henderson	Nevada	702-616-5000	www.dignityhealth.org/las-vegas
Starr Regional Medical Center Athens	Athens	Tennessee	423-745-1411	www.athensrmc.com
Swedish Edmonds Hospital	Edmonds	Washington	425-640-4000	www.stevenshealthcare.org
Texas Health Harris Methodist Fort Worth	Fort Worth	Texas	817-250-2100	www.texashealth.org
The Nebraska Medical Center	Omaha	Nebraska	402-552-2040	www.nebraskamed.com
Theda Clark Medical Center	Neenah	Wisconsin	920-729-3100	www.thedacare.org
Thibodaux Regional Medical Center	Thibodaux	Louisiana	985-447-5500	www.thibodaux.com
Tulare Regional Medical Center	Tulare	California	559-688-0821	www.tdhs.org
Ukiah Valley Medical Center	Ukiah	California	707-462-3111	www.uvmc.org
Union General Hospital	Blairsville	Georgia	706-745-2111	www.uniongeneralhospital.com
United Health Services Hospitals	Johnson City	New York	607-763-6000	www.vhs.ent
United Regional Health Care System	Wichita Falls	Texas	940-764-3055	www.urhcs.org
University of Missouri Health Care	Columbia	Missouri	573-882-4141	www.missouri.edu
Utah Valley Regional Medical Center	Provo	Utah	801-373-7850	www.intermountainhealthcare.org/hospitals/uvrmc
VA Southern Arizona Healthcare System	Tucson	Arizona	520-629-1821	www.va.gov/sta/guide/home.asp
Valley Hospital	Spokane	Washington	509-924-6650	www.valleyhospital.org

Hospital	City	State	Phone	Web Site
Western Missouri Medical Center	Warrensburg	Missouri	660-747-2500	www.wmmc.com
White County Medical Center	Searcy	Arkansas	501-278-3100	www.centralarkhospital.com
Wilkes-Barre General Hospital	Wilkes-Barre	Pennsylvania	570-829-8111	www.wvhcs.org
Wyoming Medical Center	Casper	Wyoming	307-577-7201	www.wyomingmedicalcenter.com

Note: Table shows hospitals nationwide whose heart failure 30-day risk-adjusted mortality rate is worse (higher) than U.S. rate of 11.7%

Hospitals whose Pneumonia 30-Day Mortality Rate is Better (Lower) than the U.S. National Rate

Hospital	City	State	Phone	Web Site
Adventist La Grange Memorial Hospital	La Grange	Illinois	708-352-1200	www.keepingyouwell.com
Ahmc Anaheim Regional Medical Center	Anaheim	California	714-774-1450	www.memorialcare.org/anaheim
Akron General Medical Center	Akron	Ohio	330-344-6000	www.akrongeneral.org
Alhambra Hospital Medical Center	Alhambra	California	626-570-1606	www.alhambrahospital.com
Arnot Ogden Medical Center	Elmira	New York	607-737-4100	www.arnothealth.org
Augusta Health	Fishersville	Virginia	540-932-4000	www.augustamed.com
Aurora Saint Lukes Medical Center	Milwaukee	Wisconsin	414-649-6000	www.aurorahealthcare.org
Aventura Hospital & Medical Center	Aventura	Florida	305-682-7000	www.aventurahospital.com
Banner Thunderbird Medical Center	Glendale	Arizona	602-588-5555	www.bannerhealth.com
Baptist Hospital of Miami	Miami	Florida	786-596-1960	www.baptisthealth.net
Barnes-Jewish Saint Peters Hospital	Saint Peters	Missouri	636-916-9000	www.bjsph.org
Bay Medical Center Sacred Heart Health System	Panama City	Florida	850-769-1511	www.baymedical.org
Baylor Regional Medical Center at Grapevine	Grapevine	Texas	817-481-1588	www.baylorhealth.com
Beaumont Health System	Grosse Pointe	Michigan	313-343-1000	www.beaumonthospitals.com
Beaumont Health System	Royal Oak	Michigan	248-898-5000	www.beaumonthospitals.com
Benefis Hospitals	Great Falls	Montana	406-455-5000	www.benefis.org
Berkshire Medical Center	Pittsfield	Massachusetts	413-447-2000	www.berkshirehealthsystems.org
Beth Israel Deaconess Medical Center	Boston	Massachusetts	617-667-7000	www.bidmc.harvard.edu
Betsy Johnson Regional Hospital	Dunn	North Carolina	910-892-7161	www.bjrh.org
Cape Cod Hospital	Hyannis	Massachusetts	508-771-1800	www.capecodhealth.org
Casey County Hospital	Liberty	Kentucky	606-787-6275	
Cedars - Sinai Medical Center	Los Angeles	California	310-423-5000	www.cedars-sinai.edu
Centinela Hospital Medical Center	Inglewood	California	310-673-4660	www.centinelafreeman.com
Centura Health - Littleton Adventist Hospital	Littleton	Colorado	303-730-5888	www.littletonhosp.org
Christ Hospital	Cincinnati	Ohio	513-585-2000	www.thechristhospital.com
Cobre Valley Regional Medical Center	Globe	Arizona	928-425-3261	www.cvchospital.com
Community Medical Center	Toms River	New Jersey	732-557-8000	www.sbhcs.com
Corning Hospital	Corning	New York	607-937-7200	www.corninghospital.org
Cox Medical Center Branson	Branson	Missouri	417-335-7000	www.skaggs.net
Delray Medical Center	Delray Beach	Florida	561-498-4440	www.delraymedicalctr.com
Desert Valley Hospital	Victorville	California	760-241-8000	www.dvmc.com
Doctors Hospital at Renaissance	Edinburg	Texas	956-362-8677	www.dhr-rgv.com
Duke University Hospital	Durham	North Carolina	919-684-8111	www.dukehealth.org
East Valley Hospital Medical Center	Glendora	California	626-335-0231	www.eastvalleyhospital.org
Edward Hospital	Naperville	Illinois	630-527-3000	www.edward.org
Eisenhower Medical Center	Rancho Mirage	California	760-340-3911	www.emc.org
Elmhurst Memorial Hospital	Elmhurst	Illinois	630-833-1400	www.emhc.org
Englewood Hospital & Medical Center	Englewood	New Jersey	201-894-3000	www.englewoodhospital.com
Evanston Hospital	Evanston	Illinois	847-432-8000	www.enh.org
Evergreen Hospital Medical Center	Kirkland	Washington	425-899-1000	www.evergreenhospital.org
Exempla Lutheran Medical Center	Wheat Ridge	Colorado	303-425-4500	www.exemlpa.org
Falmouth Hospital	Falmouth	Massachusetts	508-548-5300	www.capecodhealth.com
Firsthealth Moore Regional Hospital	Pinehurst	North Carolina	910-715-1000	www.firsthealth.org
Flagler Hospital	Saint Augustine	Florida	904-819-4426	www.flaglerhospital.com
Forbes Regional Hospital	Monroeville	Pennsylvania	412-858-2000	www.wpahs.org
Fountain Valley Regional Hospital & Medical Center	Fountain Valley	California	714-966-7200	www.fountainvalleyhospital.com
Franklin Woods Community Hospital	Johnson City	Tennessee	423-302-1120	www.msha.com
Frederick Memorial Hospital	Frederick	Maryland	240-566-3300	www.fmh.org
Frisbie Memorial Hospital	Rochester	New Hampshire	603-332-5211	www.frisbiehospital.com
Garden Grove Hospital & Medical Center	Garden Grove	California	714-537-5160	www.gardengrovehospital.com
Garfield Medical Center	Monterey Park	California	626-573-2222	www.garfieldmedicalcenter.com
Geisinger - Bloomsburg Hospital	Bloomsburg	Pennsylvania	570-387-2100	www.tbhonline.org
Genesis Healthcare System	Zanesville	Ohio	740-454-5000	www.genesishcs.org
Genesys Regional Medical Center - Health Park	Grand Blanc	Michigan	810-606-5000	www.genesys.org
Glendale Adventist Medical Center	Glendale	California	818-409-8202	www.glendaleadventist.com
Grandview Hospital & Medical Center	Dayton	Ohio	937-723-3312	www.kmcnetwork.org
Greater Baltimore Medical Center	Baltimore	Maryland	443-849-2000	www.gbmc.org
Harper University Hospital	Detroit	Michigan	313-745-6211	www.harperhospital.org
Heartland Regional Medical Center	Saint Joseph	Missouri	816-271-6000	www.heartland-health.com
Henry Ford Macomb Hospital	Clinton Township	Michigan	586-263-2300	www.stjoe-macomb.com
Hillcrest Hospital	Mayfield Heights	Ohio	440-312-4500	www.hillcresthospital.org
Hinsdale Hospital	Hinsdale	Illinois	630-856-9000	www.keepingyouwell.com
Hollywood Presbyterian Medical Center	Los Angeles	California	213-413-3000	www.qahpmc.com
Holy Name Medical Center	Teaneck	New Jersey	201-833-3000	www.holyname.org
The Hospital of Central Connecticut	New Britain	Connecticut	860-224-5011	www.thocc.org

Hospital	City	State	Phone	Web Site
Huntington Beach Hospital	Huntington Beach	California	714-843-5000	www.hbhospital.com
Huntington Memorial Hospital	Pasadena	California	626-397-5000	www.huntingtonhospital.com
Indiana University Health	Indianapolis	Indiana	317-962-5900	www.iuhealth.org
Ingalls Memorial Hospital	Harvey	Illinois	708-333-2300	www.ingalls.org
Inova Loudoun Hospital	Leesburg	Virginia	703-858-6600	www.loudounhealthcare.org
Jersey Shore University Medical Center	Neptune	New Jersey	732-776-4900	www.meridianhealth.com
Jupiter Medical Center	Jupiter	Florida	561-747-2234	www.jupitermed.com
Kane Community Hospital	Kane	Pennsylvania	814-837-8585	www.kanehosp.com
Kingsbrook Jewish Medical Center	Brooklyn	New York	718-604-5789	www.kingsbrook.org
Lehigh Valley Hospital	Allentown	Pennsylvania	610-402-2273	www.lvhhn.org
Lehigh Valley Hospital - Hazleton	Hazleton	Pennsylvania	570-501-4000	www.ghha.org
Lehigh Valley Hospital - Muhlenberg	Bethlehem	Pennsylvania	610-402-2273	www.lvhn.org
Liberty Hospital	Liberty	Missouri	816-781-7200	www.libertyhospital.org
Los Angeles Community Hospital	Los Angeles	California	323-267-0477	www.altacorp.com
Los Robles Hospital & Medical Center	Thousand Oaks	California	805-497-2727	www.losrobleshospital.com
Maimonides Medical Center	Brooklyn	New York	718-283-6000	www.maimonidesmed.org
Mary Greeley Medical Center	Ames	Iowa	515-239-2011	www.mgmc.org
Mayo Clinic Hospital	Phoenix	Arizona	480-342-2000	www.mayoclinic.org
Medical Center of Southeastern Oklahoma	Durant	Oklahoma	405-924-3080	www.mcsohealth.com
Medical City Dallas Hospital	Dallas	Texas	972-566-6222	www.medicalcityhospital.com
Medstar Franklin Square Medical Center	Baltimore	Maryland	443-777-7850	www.franklinsquare.org
Medstar Good Samaritan Hospital	Baltimore	Maryland	443-444-3902	www.goodsam-md.org
Medstar Harbor Hospital	Baltimore	Maryland	410-350-3201	www.harborhospital.org
Memorial Mission Hospital & Asheville Surgery Center	Asheville	North Carolina	828-213-1111	www.missionhospitals.org
Mercy Memorial Hospital System	Monroe	Michigan	734-240-8400	www.mercymemorial.org
The Methodist Hospital	Houston	Texas	713-790-2221	www.methodisthealth.com
Methodist Sugar Land Hospital	Sugar Land	Texas	281-274-8000	www.methodisthealth.com/sugarland
Milford Regional Medical Center	Milford	Massachusetts	508-473-1190	www.milfordregional.org
Missouri Baptist Medical Center	Town & Country	Missouri	314-996-5000	www.missouribaptistmedicalcenter.org
Monmouth Medical Center - Southern Campus	Lakewood	New Jersey	732-363-1900	www.sbhcs.com
Montefiore Medical Center	Bronx	New York	718-920-4321	www.montefiore.org
Morristown Medical Center	Morristown	New Jersey	973-971-5450	www.morristownmemorialhospital.org
Mount Auburn Hospital	Cambridge	Massachusetts	617-492-3500	www.mountauburnhospital.org
Mount Sinai Hospital	New York	New York	212-241-7981	www.mountsinai.org
Mount Sinai Medical Center	Miami Beach	Florida	305-674-2121	www.msmc.com
New York - Presbyterian Hospital	New York	New York	212-746-4189	www.nyp.org
Newton Memorial Hospital	Newton	New Jersey	973-383-2121	www.itsyourlife.com
North Shore Medical Center	Salem	Massachusetts	978-741-1215	www.nsmc.partners.org
North Shore University Hospital	Manhasset	New York	516-562-0100	www.northshorelij.com
Northern Westchester Hospital	Mount Kisco	New York	914-666-1200	www.nwhc.net
Northwestern Memorial Hospital	Chicago	Illinois	312-926-2000	www.nmh.org
Norton Community Hospital	Norton	Virginia	703-679-8865	www.nchosp.org
NYU Hospitals Center	New York	New York	212-263-7300	www.med.nyu.edu
Oakwood Hospital - Dearborn	Dearborn	Michigan	313-593-7125	www.oakwood.org
Olympia Medical Center	Los Angeles	California	310-657-5900	www.olympiamc.com
Oroville Hospital	Oroville	California	530-533-8500	www.orovillehospital.com
Our Lady of Lourdes Medical Center	Camden	New Jersey	856-757-3500	www.lourdesnet.org
Overlook Medical Center	Summit	New Jersey	908-522-2000	www.atlantichealth.org
Owensboro Health Regional Hospital	Owensboro	Kentucky	270-688-2000	www.omhs.org
Palos Community Hospital	Palos Heights	Illinois	708-923-4000	www.paloshospital.org
Paradise Valley Hospital	National City	California	619-470-4321	www.paradisevalleyhospital.org
Park Plaza Hospital	Houston	Texas	713-527-5019	www.parkplazahospital.com
Parkland Health Center	Farmington	Missouri	573-431-6005	www.bjc.org
Piedmont Hospital	Atlanta	Georgia	404-605-5000	www.piedmonthospital.org
Portland VA Medical Center	Portland	Oregon	503-220-8262	www.va.gov/portland/index.asp
Presbyterian Intercommunity Hospital	Whittier	California	526-698-0811	www.whittierpres.com
Presence Resurrection Medical Center	Chicago	Illinois	773-774-8000	www.reshealthcare.org
Presence Saint Joseph Hospital - Chicago	Chicago	Illinois	773-665-3000	www.res-health.org
Presence Saint Joseph Medical Center	Joliet	Illinois	815-725-7133	www.provena.org/stjoes
Presence Saint Marys Hospital	Kankakee	Illinois	815-937-2490	www.provenastmarys.com
Providence Hospital & Medical Centers	Southfield	Michigan	248-849-3011	www.stjohn.org/providence
Providence Little Co of Mary Medical Center Torrance	Torrance	California	310-540-7676	www.lcmhs.org
Providence Saint Joseph Medical Center	Burbank	California	818-843-5111	www.providence.org/losangeles
Providence Tarzana Medical Center	Tarzana	California	818-881-0800	www.encino-tarzana.com
Randolph Hospital	Asheboro	North Carolina	336-625-5151	www.randolphhospital.org
Raritan Bay Medical Center	Perth Amboy	New Jersey	732-442-3700	www.rbmc.org
Reading Hospital	Reading	Pennsylvania	610-988-8000	www.readinghospital.org

Hospital	City	State	Phone	Web Site
Rex Hospital	Raleigh	North Carolina	919-784-3100	www.rexhealth.com
Rhode Island Hospital	Providence	Rhode Island	401-444-4000	www.rhodeislandhospital.org
Rio Grande Regional Hospital	Mcallen	Texas	956-632-6000	www.riohealth.com
Riverside Medical Center	Kankakee	Illinois	815-933-1671	www.riversidehealthcare.org
Riverview Medical Center	Red Bank	New Jersey	732-741-2700	www.meridianhealth.com
Robert Wood Johnson University Hospital	New Brunswick	New Jersey	732-937-8900	www.rwjuh.edu
Rockingham Memorial Hospital	Harrisonburg	Virginia	540-689-1000	www.rmhonline.com
Ronald Reagan UCLA Medical Center	Los Angeles	California	310-825-6301	www.uclahealth.org
Saint Clare's Hospital	Denville	New Jersey	973-625-6000	www.saintclares.org
Saint Francis Hospital	Tulsa	Oklahoma	918-494-2200	www.saintfrancis.com
Saint Vincent Medical Center	Los Angeles	California	213-484-7111	www.stvincent.dochs.org
San Francisco VA Medical Center	San Francisco	California	415-221-4810	www.sanfrancisco.va.gov
San Gabriel Valley Medical Center	San Gabriel	California	626-289-5454	www.sangabrielvalleymedctr.org
Santa Monica - UCLA Medical Center & Orthopaedic Hospital	Santa Monica	California	310-319-4000	www.healthcare.ucla.edu
Scott & White Hospital - Round Rock	Round Rock	Texas	512-509-0100	www.sw.org
Scott & White Memorial Hospital	Temple	Texas	254-724-2111	www.sw.org
Scripps Memorial Hospital La Jolla	La Jolla	California	858-626-4123	www.scrippshealth.org
Scripps Mercy Hospital	San Diego	California	619-294-8111	www.scrippshealth.org
Sharon Regional Health System	Sharon	Pennsylvania	724-983-3800	www.sharonregional.com
Sinai Hospital of Baltimore	Baltimore	Maryland	410-601-5131	www.sinai-balt.com
South Pointe Hospital	Warrensville Heights	Ohio	216-491-6000	www.southpointehospital.org
Southampton Hospital	Southampton	New York	516-726-8200	www.southamptonhospital.org
Southcoast Hospital Group	Fall River	Massachusetts	508-679-3131	www.southcoast.org/charlton
Southwest General Health Center	Middleburg Heights	Ohio	440-816-8000	www.swgeneral.com
Spartanburg Regional Medical Center	Spartanburg	South Carolina	864-560-6000	www.srhs.com
Spring Valley Hospital Medical Center	Las Vegas	Nevada	702-853-3000	www.springvalleyhospital.com
Saint Alexius Medical Center	Hoffman Estates	Illinois	847-843-2000	www.alexianbrothershealth.org
Saint Anthony Community Hospital	Warwick	New York	845-986-2276	www.stanthonycommunityhosp.org
Saint Luke's Hospital Bethlehem	Bethlehem	Pennsylvania	610-954-4000	www.slhn-lehighvalley.org
Saint Luke's Roosevelt Hospital	New York	New York	212-523-4000	www.wehealny.org
Saint Luke's Episcopal Hospital	Houston	Texas	832-355-1000	www.sleh.com
Saint Luke's Hospital	Cedar Rapids	Iowa	319-369-7211	www.crstlukes.com
Saint Luke's Hospital	Chesterfield	Missouri	314-434-1500	www.goodhealthmatters.com
Saint Marys Hospital	Madison	Wisconsin	608-251-6100	www.stmarysmadison.com
Saint Peter's Hospital	Albany	New York	518-525-1550	www.stpetershealthcare.org
Stafford Hospital	Stafford	Virginia	540-741-9000	www.marywashingtonhealthcare.com
Swedish Covenant Hospital	Chicago	Illinois	773-878-8200	www.swedishcovenant.org
Tomball Regional Medical Center	Tomball	Texas	281-351-1623	www.tomballhospital.org
Tri Valley Health System	Cambridge	Nebraska	308-697-3329	www.trivalleyhealth.com
Tri - City Regional Medical Center	Hawaiian Gardens	California	562-860-0401	www.tri-cityrmc.org
Trumbull Memorial Hospital	Warren	Ohio	330-841-9011	www.trumhosp.org
Tufts Medical Center	Boston	Massachusetts	617-636-5000	www.tuftsmedicalcenter.org
United Regional Medical Center	Manchester	Tennessee	931-728-3586	www.urmchealthcare.com
University Medical Center of Princeton at Plainsboro	Plainsboro	New Jersey	866-460-4776	www.princetonhcs.org
University Hospitals - Elyria Medical Center	Elyria	Ohio	440-329-7500	www.emh-healthcare.org
University of California San Diego Medical Center	San Diego	California	619-543-6222	www.health.ucsd.edu
University of Maryland Shore Medical Center at Easton	Easton	Maryland	410-822-1000	www.shorehealth.org
University of Michigan Health System	Ann Arbor	Michigan	734-764-1505	www.med.umich.edu
University of Texas Health Science Center at Tyler	Tyler	Texas	903-877-7777	www.uthct.edu
UPMC Mckeesport	Mc Keesport	Pennsylvania	412-664-2000	www.selectmedicalcorp.com
VA Boston Healthcare System - Jamaica Plain	Jamaica Plain	Massachusetts	617-232-9500	www.vaww.visn1.med.va.gov/boston
VA North Florida/South Georgia Healthcare System	Gainesville	Florida	352-376-1611	www.northflorida.va.gov
VA Sierra Nevada Healthcare System	Reno	Nevada	775-328-1263	www.reno.va.gov
Valley Hospital	Ridgewood	New Jersey	201-447-8000	www.valleyhealth.com
VHS Harlingen Hospital Company	Harlingen	Texas	956-389-1100	www.vbmc.org
Virginia Mason Medical Center	Seattle	Washington	206-223-6600	www.vmmc.org
W Palm Beach VA Medical Center	West Palm Beach	Florida	561-422-8600	www.va.gov
Waukesha Memorial Hospital	Waukesha	Wisconsin	262-928-1000	www.waukeshamemorial.org
Weirton Medical Center	Weirton	West Virginia	304-797-6000	www.weirtonmedical.com
West Anaheim Medical Center	Anaheim	California	714-827-3000	www.wamc.phcs.us
West Haven VA Medical Center	West Haven	Connecticut	203-932-5711	www.visn1.med.va.gov/vact
Wheaton Franciscan Healthcare Saint Francis	Milwaukee	Wisconsin	414-647-5000	www.mywheaton.org
White Memorial Medical Center	Los Angeles	California	323-268-5000	www.whitememorial.com
William Beaumont Hospital - Troy	Troy	Michigan	248-964-8800	www.beaumonthospitals.com
Willis Knighton Medical Center	Shreveport	Louisiana	318-212-4000	www.wkhs.com//locations/medicalcenter.aspx
Yale-New Haven Hospital	New Haven	Connecticut	203-688-4242	www.ynhh.org

Note: Table shows hospitals nationwide whose pneumonia 30-day risk-adjusted mortality rate is better (lower) than U.S. rate of 11.9%

Hospitals whose Pneumonia 30-Day Mortality Rate is Worse (Higher) than the U.S. National Rate

Hospital	City	State	Phone	Web Site
Abilene Regional Medical Center	Abilene	Texas	325-428-1000	www.abileneregional.com
Acmh Hospital	Kittanning	Pennsylvania	724-543-8404	www.acmh.org
Albemarle Hospital Authority	Elizabeth City	North Carolina	252-335-0531	www.albemarlehealth.org
Antelope Valley Hospital	Lancaster	California	661-949-5000	www.avhospital.org
Aspirus Grand View Hospital	Ironwood	Michigan	906-932-2525	www.gvhs.org
Augusta VA Medical Center	Augusta	Georgia	706-823-2201	www.va.gov
Auxilio Mutuo Hospital	Hato Rey	Puerto Rico	787-758-2000	www.auxiliopr.com
Avera Sacred Heart Hospital	Yankton	South Dakota	605-668-8000	www.avera.org/sacred-heart
Bacon County Hospital	Alma	Georgia	912-632-8961	www.baconcountyhospital.com
Baptist Memorial Hospital/Golden Triangle	Columbus	Mississippi	662-244-1500	www.bmhcc.org/facilities/goldentriangle
Baptist Memorial Hospital Union City	Union City	Tennessee	731-885-2410	www.bmhcc.org
Baxter Regional Medical Center	Mountain Home	Arkansas	870-508-1000	www.baxterregional.org
Bay Area Hospital	Coos Bay	Oregon	541-269-8111	www.bayareahospital.org
Bolivar Medical Center	Cleveland	Mississippi	662-846-2551	www.bolivarmedical.com
Bon Secours Maryview Medical Center	Portsmouth	Virginia	757-398-2200	www.bonsecourshamptonroads.com
Caldwell Medical Center	Princeton	Kentucky	270-365-0300	www.caldwellhosp.org
Cameron Regional Medical Center	Cameron	Missouri	816-632-2101	www.cameronregional.org
Carilion Roanoke Memorial Hospital	Roanoke	Virginia	540-981-7000	www.carilion.com/crmh
Carondelet Saint Joseph's Hospital	Tucson	Arizona	520-873-3000	www.carondelet.org
Carson Tahoe Regional Medical Center	Carson City	Nevada	775-445-8000	www.carsontahoehospital.com
Catawba Valley Medical Center	Hickory	North Carolina	828-326-3809	www.catawbavalleymc.org
Central Carolina Hospital	Sanford	North Carolina	919-774-2100	www.centralcarolinahosp.com
Citizens Memorial Hospital	Bolivar	Missouri	417-326-6000	www.citizensmemorial.com
Cleveland Regional Medical Center	Shelby	North Carolina	704-487-3000	www.clevelandregional.org
Community Hospital East	Indianapolis	Indiana	317-355-5411	www.ecommunity.com
Conway Regional Medical Center	Conway	Arkansas	501-329-3831	www.conwayregional.org
Coshocton County Memorial Hospital	Coshocton	Ohio	740-622-6411	www.ccmh.com
Dallas County Medical Center	Fordyce	Arkansas	870-352-6300	www.dallascountymedicalcenter.com
Dekalb Regional Medical Center	Fort Payne	Alabama	256-845-3150	www.baptistmedical.org
Delano Regional Medical Center	Delano	California	661-725-4800	www.drmc.com
Desert Springs Hospital	Las Vegas	Nevada	702-369-7600	www.desertspringshospital.net/p12.html
Doctors Medical Center	Modesto	California	209-578-1211	www.dmc-modesto.com
East Georgia Regional Medical Center	Statesboro	Georgia	912-486-1500	www.egrmc.com
East Liverpool City Hospital	East Liverpool	Ohio	330-385-7200	www.elch.org
Eastern Niagara Hospital	Lockport	New York	716-514-5700	www.enhs.org
El Centro Regional Medical Center	El Centro	California	760-339-7100	www.ecrmc.org
Eliza Coffee Memorial Hospital	Florence	Alabama	256-768-8400	www.chgroup.org
Erlanger Medical Center	Chattanooga	Tennessee	423-778-7000	www.erlanger.org
Essentia Health Saint Mary's Medical Center	Duluth	Minnesota	218-786-4000	www.smdc.org
Florida Hospital Deland	Deland	Florida	386-943-4772	www.fhdeland.org
Floyd County Memorial Hospital	Charles City	Iowa	641-228-6830	www.fcmc.us.com
Franklin General Hospital	Hampton	Iowa	641-456-5000	www.franklingeneral.com
Franklin Medical Center	Winnsboro	Louisiana	318-435-9411	www.fmc-cares.com
Fremont Area Medical Center	Fremont	Nebraska	402-721-1610	www.famc.org
Frye Regional Medical Center	Hickory	North Carolina	828-322-6070	www.fryemedctr.com
Fulton County Hospital	Salem	Arkansas	870-895-2691	www.fultoncountyhospital.org
GV (Sonny) Montgomery VA Medical Center Jackson	Jackson	Mississippi	601-362-4471	www.visn16.med.va.gov
Gadsden Regional Medical Center	Gadsden	Alabama	256-494-4000	www.gadsdenregional.com
Galesburg Cottage Hospital	Galesburg	Illinois	309-345-4555	www.cottagehospital.com
Gateway Medical Center	Clarksville	Tennessee	931-502-1000	www.todaysgateway.com
GHS Laurens County Memorial Hospital	Clinton	South Carolina	864-833-9100	www.lchcs.org
Glenwood Regional Medical Center	West Monroe	Louisiana	318-329-4600	www.grmc.com
Good Samaritan Hospital	Kearney	Nebraska	308-865-7100	www.gshs.org
Good Samaritan Hospital	Lebanon	Pennsylvania	717-270-7500	www.gshleb.org
Greenview Regional Hospital	Bowling Green	Kentucky	270-793-1000	www.greenviewhospital.com
Grossmont Hospital	La Mesa	California	619-465-0711	www.sharp.com
Halifax Health Medical Center	Daytona Beach	Florida	386-254-4000	www.halifax.org
Hammond Henry Hospital	Geneseo	Illinois	309-944-6431	www.hammondhenry.com
Harrison County Hospital	Corydon	Indiana	812-738-4251	www.hchin.org
Harrison Memorial Hospital	Cynthiana	Kentucky	859-234-2300	www.harrisonmemhosp.com
Harton Regional Medical Center	Tullahoma	Tennessee	931-393-3000	www.hartonmedicalcenter.com
Helen Keller Memorial Hospital	Sheffield	Alabama	256-386-4556	www.helenkeller.com
Helena Regional Medical Center	Helena	Arkansas	870-338-5800	www.helenaregionalmedicalcenter.com
Hemet Valley Medical Center	Hemet	California	951-652-2811	www.valleyhealthsystem.com/hemmain
Highland Hospital	Rochester	New York	585-473-2200	www.urmc.rochester.edu

Hospital	City	State	Phone	Web Site
Highlands Regional Medical Center	Sebring	Florida	863-385-6101	www.highlandsregional.com
Highline Medical Center	Burien	Washington	206-244-9970	www.hchnet.org
Hospital Pavia Santurce	Fernandez Juncos	Puerto Rico	787-727-6060	www.paviahospitalsanturce.com
Howard Memorial Hospital	Nashville	Arkansas	870-845-4400	www.howardmemorial.com
Hutchinson Regional Medical Center	Hutchinson	Kansas	620-665-2001	www.hutchinsonhospital.com
Iberia General Hospital & Medical Center	New Iberia	Louisiana	337-364-0441	www.iberiamedicalcenter.com
Indiana University Health Bloomington Hospital	Bloomington	Indiana	812-353-9555	www.bloomingtonhospital.org
Indiana University Health La Porte Hospital	La Porte	Indiana	219-326-1234	www.laportehealth.org
Inspira Medical Center Vineland	Vineland	New Jersey	856-641-6610	www.sjhs.com
Integris Grove Hospital	Grove	Oklahoma	918-786-2243	www.integris-health.com
IU Health Goshen Hospital	Goshen	Indiana	574-364-1000	www.goshenhosp.com
Jackson Hospital & Clinic	Montgomery	Alabama	334-293-8000	www.jackson.org
Jackson Memorial Hospital	Miami	Florida	305-585-1111	www.jhsmiami.org
Jacksonville Medical Center	Jacksonville	Alabama	256-782-4538	www.jmchealth.com
Jane Phillips Medical Center	Bartlesville	Oklahoma	918-333-7200	www.jpmc.org
Jeff Davis Hospital	Hazlehurst	Georgia	912-375-7781	www.jeffdavishospital.org
Jennie Stuart Medical Center	Hopkinsville	Kentucky	270-887-0100	www.jsmc.org
JFK Medical Center - A M Yelencsics Comm Hospital	Edison	New Jersey	732-321-7000	www.jfkmc.org
Keokuk Area Hospital	Keokuk	Iowa	319-524-7150	www.keokukhealthsystems.org
Lafayette General Medical Center	Lafayette	Louisiana	337-289-7991	www.lafayettegeneral.org
Lake Charles Memorial Hospital	Lake Charles	Louisiana	337-494-3200	www.lcmh.com
Lake Cumberland Regional Hospital	Somerset	Kentucky	606-679-7441	www.lakecumberlandhospital.com
Lake Granbury Medical Center	Granbury	Texas	817-573-2683	www.lakegranburymedicalcenter.com
Lexington Medical Center	West Columbia	South Carolina	803-791-2000	www.lexmed.com
Lexington VA Medical Center	Lexington	Kentucky	859-233-4511	www.lexington.va.gov
Livingston Regional Hospital	Livingston	Tennessee	931-823-5611	www.livingstonregionalhospital.com
Lompoc Valley Medical Center	Lompoc	California	805-737-3300	www.lompochospital.org
Louisville VA Medical Center	Louisville	Kentucky	502-287-4000	www.va.gov/603louisville
Madera Community Hospital	Madera	California	559-675-5555	www.maderahospital.org
Mahaska Health Partnership	Oskaloosa	Iowa	641-672-3100	www.mahaskahospital.com
Margaret Mary Community Hospital	Batesville	Indiana	812-934-6624	www.mmch.org
Marion General Hospital	Columbia	Mississippi	601-736-6303	
Marshall Medical Center South	Boaz	Alabama	256-593-8310	www.mmcenters.com/mmcsouth.php
McGehee Hospital	Mcgehee	Arkansas	870-222-5600	
Medical Center Hospital	Odessa	Texas	432-640-4000	www.mchodessa.com
Memorial Medical Center	Modesto	California	209-526-4500	www.memorialmedicalcenter.org
Memorial Healthcare	Owosso	Michigan	989-723-5211	www.memorialhealthcare.org
Memorial Hospital & Manor	Bainbridge	Georgia	229-246-3500	www.mh-m.org
Memorial Hospital of Martinsville & Henry County	Martinsville	Virginia	276-666-7200	www.martinsvillehospital.com
Memorial Hospital of South Bend	South Bend	Indiana	574-647-1000	www.qualityoflife.org
Memorial Medical Center of East Texas	Lufkin	Texas	936-634-8111	www.mymemorialhealth.org
Mercy Health - West Hospital	Cincinnati	Ohio	513-215-5000	www.e-mercy.com/west-hospital.aspx
Mercy Hospital Oklahoma City	Oklahoma City	Oklahoma	405-752-3754	www.mercyok.net/mhc
Mercy Hospital Springfield	Springfield	Missouri	417-820-2000	www.stjohns.com
Mercy Medical Center	Merced	California	209-564-5000	www.mercymercedcares.org
Mercy Medical Center	Rockville Centre	New York	516-705-2525	www.mercymedicalcenter.info
Mercy Medical Center - Mount Shasta	Mount Shasta	California	530-926-6111	www.mercymtshasta.org
Mercy Memorial Health Center	Ardmore	Oklahoma	405-223-5400	www.mercyok.com/mmhc
Methodist Healthcare Memphis Hospitals	Memphis	Tennessee	901-516-8274	www.methodisthealth.org
Mid Coast Hospital	Brunswick	Maine	207-729-0181	www.midcoasthealth.com
Midtown Medical Center	Columbus	Georgia	706-571-1000	www.columbusregional.com
Milford Hospital	Milford	Connecticut	203-876-4000	www.milfordhospital.org
Mississippi Baptist Medical Center	Jackson	Mississippi	601-968-1000	www.mbmc.org
Mizell Memorial Hospital	Opp	Alabama	334-493-3541	www.mizellmh.com
Mobile Infirmary	Mobile	Alabama	251-435-4700	www.mimc.com
Morris Hospital & Healthcare Centers	Morris	Illinois	815-942-2932	www.morrishospital.org
Mount Carmel West	Columbus	Ohio	614-234-5000	www.mountcarmelhealth.com
Multicare Good Samaritan Hospital	Puyallup	Washington	253-697-2102	www.multicare.org/goodsam
Neshoba County General Hospital	Philadelphia	Mississippi	601-663-1200	www.neshobageneral.com
New London Family Medical Center	New London	Wisconsin	920-531-2000	www.thedacare.org
North Mississippi Medical Center	Tupelo	Mississippi	662-377-3000	www.nmhs.net/nmmc
North Valley Hospital	Whitefish	Montana	406-863-3550	www.nvhosp.org
Northern Louisiana Medical Center	Ruston	Louisiana	318-254-2100	www.lincolnhealth.com
Novant Health Rowan Medical Center	Salisbury	North Carolina	704-210-5000	www.rowan.org
Novant Health Thomasville Medical Center	Thomasville	North Carolina	336-472-2000	www.thomasvillemedicalcenter.org
Och Regional Medical Center	Starkville	Mississippi	662-323-4320	www.och.org
Ohio Valley General Hospital	Mckees Rocks	Pennsylvania	412-777-6161	www.ohiovalleyhospital.org

Hospital	City	State	Phone	Web Site
Olympic Medical Center	Port Angeles	Washington	360-417-7000	www.olympicmedical.org
Orange Park Medical Center	Orange Park	Florida	904-276-8500	www.opmedical.com
Paris Regional Medical Center	Paris	Texas	903-785-4521	www.parisregional.com
Passavant Area Hospital	Jacksonville	Illinois	217-245-9551	www.passavanthospital.com
Petaluma Valley Hospital	Petaluma	California	707-778-1111	www.stjosephhealth.org
Peterson Regional Medical Center	Kerrville	Texas	830-896-4200	www.petersonrmc.com
Piedmont Medical Center	Rock Hill	South Carolina	803-329-1234	www.piedmontmedicalcenter.com
Pike Community Hospital	Waverly	Ohio	740-947-2186	www.adena.org
Pinnacle Health Hospitals	Harrisburg	Pennsylvania	717-782-5181	www.pinnaclehealth.org
Pottstown Memorial Medical Center	Pottstown	Pennsylvania	610-327-7000	www.pmmctr.org
Rappahannock General Hospital	Kilmarnock	Virginia	804-435-8000	www.rgh-hospital.com
Redlands Community Hospital	Redlands	California	909-335-5500	www.redlandshospital.com
River Parishes Hospital	Laplace	Louisiana	985-652-7000	www.riverparisheshospital.com
River Valley Medical Center	Dardanelle	Arkansas	479-229-4677	
Rockcastle County Hospital	Mount Vernon	Kentucky	606-256-2195	www.rockcastlehospital.com
Rush Foundation Hospital	Meridian	Mississippi	601-483-0011	www.rushhealthsystems.org
Rush Memorial Hospital	Rushville	Indiana	765-932-7513	www.rushmemorial.com
Russell Hospital	Alexander City	Alabama	256-329-7100	www.russellmedcenter.com
Saint Joseph Mount Sterling	Mount Sterling	Kentucky	859-498-1220	www.marychiles.org
San Gorgonio Memorial Hospital	Banning	California	951-769-2101	www.sgmh.org
San Juan VA Medical Center	San Juan	Puerto Rico	800-449-8729	www.visn8.med.va.gov/caribbean
Sentara Careplex Hospital	Hampton	Virginia	757-736-1000	www.sentara.com
Sentara Leigh Hospital	Norfolk	Virginia	757-261-6601	www.sentara.com
Sentara Obici Hospital	Suffolk	Virginia	757-934-4000	www.sentara.com
Seven Rivers Regional Medical Center	Crystal River	Florida	352-795-6560	www.srrmc.com
Shands Live Oak Regional Medical Center	Live Oak	Florida	904-362-1413	www.shands.org
Sierra View District Hospital	Porterville	California	559-784-1110	www.sierra-view.com
Skyridge Medical Center	Cleveland	Tennessee	423-339-4132	www.skyridgemedcenter.com
Somerset Medical Center	Somerville	New Jersey	908-685-2200	www.somersetmedicalcenter.com
South Central Regional Medical Center	Laurel	Mississippi	601-649-4000	www.scrmc.com
South Shore Hospital	South Weymouth	Massachusetts	781-340-8000	www.southshorehospital.org
Southampton Memorial Hospital	Franklin	Virginia	757-569-6100	www.smhfranklin.com
Southern Virginia Regional Medical Center	Emporia	Virginia	434-348-4400	www.svrmc.com
Spectrum Health - Reed City Campus	Reed City	Michigan	231-832-3271	www.spectrum-health.org
Spencer Municipal Hospital	Spencer	Iowa	712-264-8300	www.spencerhospital.org
Springfield Regional Medical Center	Springfield	Ohio	937-523-1000	www.communityhospital.com
Springs Memorial Hospital	Lancaster	South Carolina	803-286-1481	www.springsmemorial.com
Saint Anthony Regional Hospital & Nursing Home	Carroll	Iowa	712-792-3581	www.stanthonyhospital.org
Saint Anthony Shawnee Hospital	Shawnee	Oklahoma	405-273-2270	www.unityhealthcenter.com
Saint Catherine Hospital	Garden City	Kansas	620-272-2561	www.stcath-hosp.org
Saint Francis Community Hospital	Federal Way	Washington	253-944-8100	www.fhshealth.org
Saint Francis Hospital	Litchfield	Illinois	217-324-2191	www.stfrancis-litchfield.org
Saint Francis Hospital	Memphis	Tennessee	901-765-1000	www.saintfrancishosp.com
Saint Francis Hospital	Columbus	Georgia	706-596-4020	www.wecareforlife.com
Saint Francis - Downtown	Greenville	South Carolina	864-255-1000	www.stfrancishealth.org
Saint Joseph Hospital	Orange	California	714-633-9111	www.sjo.org
Saint Joseph Hospital & Health Center	Kokomo	Indiana	765-456-5300	www.stvincent.org
Saint Joseph's Hospital - Savannah	Savannah	Georgia	912-819-4100	www.sjchs.org
Saint Joseph's Medical Center of Stockton	Stockton	California	209-943-2000	www.stjospehscares.org
Saint Peter's Hospital	Helena	Montana	406-442-2480	www.stpetes.org
Saint Vincent Dunn Hospital	Bedford	Indiana	812-275-3331	www.stvincent.org/St-Vincent-Dunn
Saint Vincent's East	Birmingham	Alabama	205-838-3122	www.nolandhealth.com
Starr Regional Medical Center Athens	Athens	Tennessee	423-745-1411	www.athensrmc.com
Sumner Regional Medical Center	Gallatin	Tennessee	615-452-4210	www.mysumnermedical.com
Sunbury Community Hospital	Sunbury	Pennsylvania	570-286-3333	www.schopc.org
Sunrise Hospital & Medical Center	Las Vegas	Nevada	702-731-8000	www.sunrisehospital.com
Teche Regional Medical Center	Morgan City	Louisiana	985-384-2200	www.techeregional.com
Terrebonne General Medical Center	Houma	Louisiana	985-873-4141	www.tgmc.com
Texoma Medical Center	Denison	Texas	903-416-4000	www.texomamedicalcenter.net
Thibodaux Regional Medical Center	Thibodaux	Louisiana	985-447-5500	www.thibodaux.com
Thomas Memorial Hospital	South Charleston	West Virginia	304-766-3600	www.thomaswv.org
Trinity Medical Center	Birmingham	Alabama	205-592-1000	www.bhsala.com/montclair
Trinity Rock Island	Rock Island	Illinois	309-779-5000	www.trinityqc.com
Tuality Community Hospital	Hillsboro	Oregon	503-681-1111	www.tuality.com
Twin County Regional Hospital	Galax	Virginia	276-236-8181	www.tcrh.org
Union General Hospital	Farmerville	Louisiana	318-368-9751	www.uniongen.org
United Health Services Hospitals	Johnson City	New York	607-763-6000	www.vhs.ent

Hospital	City	State	Phone	Web Site
University Mcduffie County Regional Medical Center	Thomson	Georgia	706-595-1411	www.mrmc.org
University of Missouri Health Care	Columbia	Missouri	573-882-4141	www.missouri.edu
Upson Regional Medical Center	Thomaston	Georgia	706-647-8111	www.urmc.org
Upstate New York VA Healthcare System - Western NY	Buffalo	New York	716-862-3611	www.buffalo.va.gov
Utah Valley Regional Medical Center	Provo	Utah	801-373-7850	www.intermountainhealthcare.org/hospitals/uvrmc
VA Middle Tennessee Healthcare System	Nashville	Tennessee	615-327-5332	www.tennesseevalley.va.gov
VA Salt Lake City Healthcare - George E. Wahlen VA	Salt Lake City	Utah	801-584-1211	www1.va.gov/directory/guide/facility.asp?
Vidant Edgecombe Hospital	Tarboro	North Carolina	252-641-7700	www.vidanthealth.com/edgecombe
Vista Medical Center East	Waukegan	Illinois	847-360-4000	www.vistahealth.com
Western Plains Medical Complex	Dodge City	Kansas	620-225-8400	www.westernplainsmc.com
Wilkes-Barre General Hospital	Wilkes-Barre	Pennsylvania	570-829-8111	www.wvhcs.org
Wilson Medical Center	Wilson	North Carolina	252-399-8040	www.wilmed.org/contact.asp
Wise Regional Health System	Decatur	Texas	940-627-5921	www.wiseregional.com
Woodland Heights Medical Center	Lufkin	Texas	936-634-8311	www.woodlandheights.net
Woodland Memorial Hospital	Woodland	California	530-662-3961	www.woodlandhealthcare.org
Yakima Valley Memorial Hospital	Yakima	Washington	509-575-8000	www.yakimamemorialhospital.org
Yuma Regional Medical Center	Yuma	Arizona	928-336-7275	www.yumaregional.org

Note: Table shows hospitals nationwide whose pneumonia 30-day risk-adjusted mortality rate is worse (higher) than U.S. rate of 11.9%

Hospital Mortality from Heart Attack: State and National Summary

Area	Number of Hospitals			
	Better than U.S. National Rate[1]	Worse than U.S. National Rate[2]	No Different than U.S. National Rate[3]	Number of Cases Too Small[4]
U.S. and Territories	77	19	2579	1889
Alabama	0	0	50	50
Alaska	0	0	5	15
American Samoa	0	0	0	1
Arizona	1	0	49	19
Arkansas	1	2	30	40
California	7	1	219	103
Colorado	0	0	33	35
Connecticut	2	0	28	1
Delaware	1	0	5	1
District of Columbia	0	0	6	2
Florida	3	1	157	22
Georgia	0	0	74	65
Guam	0	0	1	0
Hawaii	0	0	12	4
Idaho	0	0	10	23
Illinois	8	0	112	61
Indiana	1	0	68	49
Iowa	0	0	35	81
Kansas	1	0	29	91
Kentucky	0	1	51	43
Louisiana	0	1	49	52
Maine	1	1	30	5
Maryland	1	0	40	6
Massachusetts	4	0	54	6
Michigan	6	3	72	49
Minnesota	1	0	36	85
Mississippi	0	0	34	50
Missouri	4	0	57	54
Montana	0	0	8	39
N. Mariana Islands	0	0	0	1
Nebraska	0	0	20	56
Nevada	0	1	18	13
New Hampshire	1	1	17	6
New Jersey	8	1	54	3
New Mexico	0	0	13	26
New York	10	1	141	31
North Carolina	2	0	83	24
North Dakota	0	1	8	32
Ohio	1	0	112	47
Oklahoma	0	0	35	71
Oregon	0	0	29	31
Pennsylvania	6	1	122	33
Puerto Rico	0	0	21	24
Rhode Island	2	0	9	0
South Carolina	0	0	42	20
South Dakota	1	0	10	40
Tennessee	1	0	66	46
Texas	2	3	189	149
Utah	0	0	16	19
Vermont	0	0	10	5
Virgin Islands	0	0	1	1
Virginia	0	0	73	9
Washington	0	0	44	40
West Virginia	1	0	29	24
Wisconsin	0	0	60	62
Wyoming	0	0	3	24

Note: (1) 30-day risk-adjusted mortality rate is better (lower) than U.S. rate of 15.2%; (2) 30-day risk-adjusted mortality rate is worse (higher) than U.S. rate of 15.2%; (3) 30-day risk-adjusted mortality rate is about the same as U.S. rate of 15.2%; (4) The number of cases is too small to classify the hospital

Hospital Mortality from Heart Failure: State and National Summary

Area	Number of Hospitals			
	Better than U.S. National Rate[1]	Worse than U.S. National Rate[2]	No Different than U.S. National Rate[3]	Number of Cases Too Small[4]
U.S. and Territories	181	139	3732	725
Alabama	1	2	89	8
Alaska	0	1	9	12
American Samoa	0	0	0	1
Arizona	2	1	57	17
Arkansas	0	11	59	7
California	30	10	246	51
Colorado	0	0	55	19
Connecticut	4	3	24	1
Delaware	1	0	6	0
District of Columbia	2	0	6	0
Florida	8	5	166	8
Georgia	1	2	126	15
Guam	0	0	1	0
Hawaii	0	0	14	5
Idaho	0	1	21	15
Illinois	16	5	156	7
Indiana	3	7	108	2
Iowa	0	2	95	21
Kansas	0	1	83	49
Kentucky	0	1	92	3
Louisiana	2	6	82	19
Maine	0	1	34	2
Maryland	9	2	35	1
Massachusetts	14	1	47	2
Michigan	12	3	106	14
Minnesota	2	0	81	48
Mississippi	0	3	77	18
Missouri	4	5	96	11
Montana	0	0	26	35
N. Mariana Islands	0	0	0	1
Nebraska	0	2	48	35
Nevada	1	2	27	5
New Hampshire	0	0	25	1
New Jersey	13	1	52	0
New Mexico	0	2	30	9
New York	13	7	156	7
North Carolina	4	3	97	8
North Dakota	0	0	24	20
Ohio	6	3	144	13
Oklahoma	2	3	84	29
Oregon	1	2	49	8
Pennsylvania	16	6	136	6
Puerto Rico	0	0	28	21
Rhode Island	0	0	11	1
South Carolina	1	3	57	2
South Dakota	0	1	26	26
Tennessee	0	2	107	7
Texas	8	8	294	62
Utah	0	1	24	17
Vermont	0	2	12	1
Virgin Islands	0	0	2	0
Virginia	1	2	79	2
Washington	0	7	58	24
West Virginia	1	0	47	6
Wisconsin	3	8	101	12
Wyoming	0	1	17	11

Note: (1) 30-day risk-adjusted mortality rate is better (lower) than U.S. rate of 11.7%; (2) 30-day risk-adjusted mortality rate is worse (higher) than U.S. rate of 11.7%; (3) 30-day risk-adjusted mortality rate is about the same as U.S. rate of 11.7%; (4) The number of cases is too small to classify the hospital

Hospital Mortality from Pneumonia: State and National Summary

Area	Number of Hospitals			
	Better than U.S. National Rate[1]	Worse than U.S. National Rate[2]	No Different than U.S. National Rate[3]	Number of Cases Too Small[4]
U.S. and Territories	203	223	4014	377
Alabama	0	13	84	4
Alaska	0	0	15	7
American Samoa	0	0	1	0
Arizona	3	2	66	10
Arkansas	0	8	66	3
California	34	19	244	45
Colorado	2	0	60	13
Connecticut	4	1	27	0
Delaware	0	0	7	0
District of Columbia	0	0	8	0
Florida	9	7	167	5
Georgia	1	11	128	3
Guam	0	0	1	0
Hawaii	0	0	14	8
Idaho	0	0	33	6
Illinois	16	7	157	4
Indiana	1	10	107	2
Iowa	2	6	105	5
Kansas	0	3	116	13
Kentucky	2	9	85	0
Louisiana	1	11	86	14
Maine	0	1	35	1
Maryland	8	0	37	1
Massachusetts	10	1	51	3
Michigan	10	3	116	6
Minnesota	1	1	112	17
Mississippi	0	10	78	10
Missouri	7	4	101	5
Montana	1	2	39	20
N. Mariana Islands	0	0	1	0
Nebraska	1	2	70	13
Nevada	3	3	24	6
New Hampshire	1	0	25	0
New Jersey	15	3	48	0
New Mexico	0	0	38	4
New York	14	6	161	4
North Carolina	6	9	94	4
North Dakota	0	0	39	5
Ohio	9	6	146	4
Oklahoma	2	5	101	11
Oregon	1	2	54	3
Pennsylvania	10	7	143	5
Puerto Rico	0	3	26	21
Rhode Island	1	0	10	1
South Carolina	1	5	55	2
South Dakota	0	1	49	6
Tennessee	2	13	96	5
Texas	13	10	306	48
Utah	0	2	33	7
Vermont	0	0	15	0
Virgin Islands	0	0	2	0
Virginia	5	10	67	5
Washington	2	5	73	9
West Virginia	1	1	51	1
Wisconsin	4	1	115	5
Wyoming	0	0	26	3

Note: (1) 30-day risk-adjusted mortality rate is better (lower) than U.S. rate of 11.9%; (2) 30-day risk-adjusted mortality rate is worse (higher) than U.S. rate of 11.9%; (3) 30-day risk-adjusted mortality rate is about the same as U.S. rate of 11.9%; (4) The number of cases is too small to classify the hospital

Appendix B: 30-Day Readmission Rates

What Do These Readmission Categories Show?

"Readmission" is when patients who have had a recent stay in the hospital go back into a hospital again. The information shows how often patients are readmitted within 30 days of discharge from a previous hospital stay for heart attack, heart failure, or pneumonia. Patients may have been readmitted back to the same hospital or to a different hospital or acute care facility. They may have been readmitted for the same condition as their recent hospital stay, or for a different reason.

This first part of this appendix shows hospitals with risk-adjusted 30-day unplanned readmission rates that are lower (better) or higher (worse) than the national rate for all three categories. Hospitals are shown to be better or worse than the U.S. national rate only if the data shows with 95% certainty, that the difference between their surgical complication rates and the U.S. national rate is not due to chance.

The second part of this appendix contains state and national summaries with the following column headers:

- **Better Than U.S. National Rate.** Hospitals in the Better Than U.S. National Rate category have risk-adjusted 30-day unplanned readmission rates that are lower than the U.S. National Rate, and with 95% certainty that this difference is not due to chance.
- **Worse Than U.S. National Rate.** Hospitals in the Worse Than U.S. National Rate category have risk-adjusted 30-day unplanned readmission rates that are higher than the U.S. National Rate, and with 95% certainty that this difference is not due to chance.
- **No Different Than U.S. National Rate.** Many hospitals in the No Different Than U.S. National Rate category have risk-adjusted 30-day unplanned readmission rates that are about the same as the U.S. National Rate. Other hospitals in this category have rates that are higher or lower than the U.S. National Rate, but without 95% certainty that these differences are not due to chance.
- **Number of Cases Too Small.** The number of cases is too small to classify the hospital..

Why are Readmission Rates for Individual Hospitals Not Shown?

Comparisons based on estimated readmission rates alone can be misleading. Risk-adjusted readmission rates are estimated for individual hospitals based on information taken from a particular time period. If a slightly different time period had been chosen, chances are that each hospital's results would have been somewhat different.

A range ("confidence interval" or in this case an "interval estimate") around estimates show how much variation might be due to this kind of chance. In this case, researchers are 95% confident that a hospital's readmission rate fell somewhere within this specified range. The smaller the range, the more precise the estimate.

When hospitals treat a very large number of patients, chance differences will not have much effect on the overall rates. The range will be small, and the estimated readmission rates will be more precise. In hospitals that treat smaller numbers of patients, however, even small chance differences could have a big impact on readmission rates. The 95% confidence interval, or range, will be large, and the estimated readmission rates will be less precise.

Because the number of patients treated at U.S. hospitals varies widely, the precision of hospitals' estimated readmission rates also varies.

Calculation of 30-Day Risk-Standardized Rates of Readmission

The 30-day readmission measures are estimates of unplanned readmission for any cause to any acute care hospital within 30 days of discharge from a hospitalization. Using unplanned readmissions within 30 days instead of over longer time periods (such as 90 days) eliminate factors outside hospitals' control such as other complicating illnesses, patients' own behavior, or care provided to patients after discharge. *The Comparative Guide to American Hospitals* reports the following 30-day readmission measures:

- 30-day unplanned readmission for heart attack (AMI) patients
- 30-day unplanned readmission for heart failure (HF) patients
- 30-day unplanned readmission for pneumonia patients
- 30-day unplanned readmission for hip/knee replacement patients
- 30-day overall rate of unplanned readmission after discharge from the hospital (hospital-wide readmission). Note: This measure includes patients admitted for internal medicine, surgery/gynecology, cardiorespiratory, cardiovascular, and neurology services. It is not a composite measure.

Which Patients are Included

The 30-day unplanned readmission measures include hospitalizations for Medicare beneficiaries aged 65 or older who were enrolled in Original Medicare (traditional fee-for-service Medicare) for the entire 12 months prior to their hospital admission (and for readmissions, for 30 days after their original admission). The AMI, heart failure, and pneumonia unplanned readmission measures also include patients aged 65 or older who were admitted to Veteran's Health Administration (VA) hospitals. Beneficiaries enrolled in Medicare managed care plans are not included. The unplanned readmission measures do not include patients who died during the index admission, or who left the hospital against medical advice.

Where the Information Comes From

The Centers for Medicare & Medicaid Services (CMS) calculates hospital-specific 30-day readmission rates using Medicare claims and eligibility information. The AMI, HF, and pneumonia readmission measures are also calculated using VA administrative data. Using administrative data makes it possible to calculate readmission rates without having to do medical chart reviews or requiring hospitals to report additional information to CMS.

Risk Adjustment

To make comparison of hospital performance equitable, the 30-day unplanned readmission measures adjust for patient characteristics that may make unplanned readmission more likely, even if the hospital provided higher quality of care. These characteristics include the patient's age, past medical history, and other diseases or conditions (comorbidities) the patient had when admitted that are known to increase the patient's risk of having an unplanned readmission.

Significance Testing

The statistical model used to calculate 30-day unplanned readmission measures also determines how precise the estimates are, and provides the upper and lower bounds of the 95% interval estimates for each hospital's readmission rates. Interval estimates, which are like confidence intervals, describe the level of uncertainty around the estimated readmission rates.

Comparing Individual Hospital Rates to the U.S. National Rate

To assign hospitals to performance categories, the hospital's interval estimate is compared to the U.S. national 30-day observed unplanned readmission rate. If the 95% interval estimate includes the national observed rate for that measure, the hospital's performance is in the "No Different than U.S. National Rate" category. If the entire 95% interval estimate is below the national observed rate for that measure, then the hospital is performing "Better Than U.S. National Rate." If the entire 95% interval estimate is above the national observed rate for that measure, its performance is "Worse Than U.S. National Rate." Hospitals with fewer than 25 eligible cases are placed into a separate category that indicates that the hospital did not have enough cases to reliably tell how well the hospital is performing.

Additional information

For more detail on how the 30-day unplanned readmission rates are calculated, please visit QualityNet—Readmission Measures at www.qualitynet.org.

Hospitals whose Acute Myocardial Infarction (Heart Attack) 30-Day Readmission Rate is Better (Lower) than the U.S. National Rate

Hospital	City	State	Phone	Web Site
Asante Rogue Regional Medical Center	Medford	Oregon	541-789-7000	www.asante.org
Aspirus Wausau Hospital	Wausau	Wisconsin	715-847-2121	www.aspirus.org
Aurora Saint Lukes Medical Center	Milwaukee	Wisconsin	414-649-6000	www.aurorahealthcare.org
Baylor Heart & Vascular Hospital	Dallas	Texas	214-820-0670	www.baylorhearthospital.com
Bellin Memorial Hospital	Green Bay	Wisconsin	920-433-3500	www.bellin.org
Central Washington Hospital	Wenatchee	Washington	509-662-1511	www.cwhs.com
Frye Regional Medical Center	Hickory	North Carolina	828-322-6070	www.fryemedctr.com
GHS Greenville Memorial Medical Center	Greenville	South Carolina	864-455-7000	www.ghs.org
Lancaster General Hospital	Lancaster	Pennsylvania	717-299-5511	www.lancastergeneral.org
Lovelace Medical Center	Albuquerque	New Mexico	505-727-8000	www.lovelace.com
Maine Medical Center	Portland	Maine	207-662-0111	www.mmc.org
Mercy Health Partners - Mercy Campus	Muskegon	Michigan	231-672-3901	www.mghp.com
Munroe Regional Medical Center	Ocala	Florida	352-351-7200	www.munroeregional.com
Parkview Regional Medical Center	Fort Wayne	Indiana	260-266-1000	www.parkview.com
Providence Sacred Heart Medical Center	Spokane	Washington	509-474-3040	www.shmc.org
Saint Joseph's Hospital of Atlanta	Atlanta	Georgia	678-843-5720	www.stjosephsatlanta.org
Sanford Medical Center Fargo	Fargo	North Dakota	701-234-2000	www.meritcare.com
Sarasota Memorial Hospital	Sarasota	Florida	941-917-9000	www.smh.com
Saint Luke's Episcopal Hospital	Houston	Texas	832-355-1000	www.sleh.com
Saint Vincent Heart Center of Indiana	Indianapolis	Indiana	317-583-5000	www.theheartcenter.com
Sutter Roseville Medical Center	Roseville	California	916-781-1000	www.sutterroseville.org
University Colo Health Memorial Hospital Central	Colorado Springs	Colorado	719-365-5000	www.memorialhospital.com
Venice Regional Medical Center - Bayfront Health	Venice	Florida	941-485-7711	www.veniceregional.com

Note: Table shows hospitals nationwide whose acute myocardial infarction 30-day readmission rate is better (lower) than U.S. rate of 18.3%

Hospitals whose Acute Myocardial Infarction (Heart Attack) 30-Day Readmission Rate is Worse (Higher) than the U.S. National Rate

Hospital	City	State	Phone	Web Site
Baxter Regional Medical Center	Mountain Home	Arkansas	870-508-1000	www.baxterregional.org
Boston Medical Center Corporation	Boston	Massachusetts	617-638-8000	www.bmc.org
Carolinas Hospital System	Florence	South Carolina	843-674-2500	www.carolinashospital.com
Centra Health	Lynchburg	Virginia	434-200-4789	www.centrahealth.com
Community Medical Center	Toms River	New Jersey	732-557-8000	www.sbhcs.com
Florida Hospital	Orlando	Florida	407-303-1976	www.floridahospital.com
Good Samaritan Regional Health Center	Mount Vernon	Illinois	618-899-1469	www.smgsi.com
Hillcrest Medical Center	Tulsa	Oklahoma	918-579-1000	www.hillcrest.com
Ingalls Memorial Hospital	Harvey	Illinois	708-333-2300	www.ingalls.org
Johnson City Medical Center	Johnson City	Tennessee	423-431-6111	www.msha.com
Kaleida Health	Buffalo	New York	716-859-8620	www.kaleidahealth.org
Lewisgale Medical Center	Salem	Virginia	540-776-4000	www.lewis-gale.com
Mercy Hospital & Medical Center	Chicago	Illinois	312-567-2000	www.mercy-chicago.org
Montefiore Medical Center	Bronx	New York	718-920-4321	www.montefiore.org
Newark Beth Israel Medical Center	Newark	New Jersey	973-926-7850	www.sbhcs.com
North Shore University Hospital	Manhasset	New York	516-562-0100	www.northshorelij.com
Northside Hospital	Saint Petersburg	Florida	813-521-5000	www.northsidehospital.com
Northwest Community Hospital	Arlington Heights	Illinois	847-618-1000	www.nch.org
Olympia Medical Center	Los Angeles	California	310-657-5900	www.olympiamc.com
Presence Saint Joseph Medical Center	Joliet	Illinois	815-725-7133	www.provena.org/stjoes
Raleigh General Hospital	Beckley	West Virginia	304-256-4100	www.raleighgeneral.com
Saint Clare's Hospital	Denville	New Jersey	973-625-6000	www.saintclares.org
Saint Michael's Medical Center	Newark	New Jersey	973-877-5350	www.cathedralhealth.org
San Juan VA Medical Center	San Juan	Puerto Rico	800-449-8729	www.visn8.med.va.gov/caribbean
Saint Joseph's Regional Medical Center	Paterson	New Jersey	973-754-2010	www.sjhmc.org
Saint Vincent's Medical Center	Bridgeport	Connecticut	203-576-5551	www.stvincents.org
Tampa VA Medical Center	Tampa	Florida	813-972-2000	www.tampa.va.gov
University Hospital - Stony Brook	Stony Brook	New York	631-444-4000	www.stonybrookmedicalcenter.org
Vidant Medical Center	Greenville	North Carolina	252-847-4100	www.uhseast.com

Note: Table shows hospitals nationwide whose acute myocardial infarction 30-day readmission rate is worse (higher) than U.S. rate of 18.3%

Hospitals whose Heart Failure 30-Day Readmission Rate is Better (Lower) than the U.S. National Rate

Hospital	City	State	Phone	Web Site
Abilene Regional Medical Center	Abilene	Texas	325-428-1000	www.abileneregional.com
Alegent Creighton Health Bergan Mercy Medical Center	Omaha	Nebraska	402-398-6060	www.alegent.com
Alpena Regional Medical Center	Alpena	Michigan	989-356-7390	www.agh.org
Asante Rogue Regional Medical Center	Medford	Oregon	541-789-7000	www.asante.org
Audrain Medical Center	Mexico	Missouri	573-582-5000	www.audrainmedicalcenter.com
Aurora Sheboygan Memorial Medical Center	Sheboygan	Wisconsin	920-451-5000	www.aurorahealthcare.org/facilities
Banner Boswell Medical Center	Sun City	Arizona	623-977-7211	www.bannerhealth.com
Banner Good Samaritan Medical Center	Phoenix	Arizona	602-239-2000	www.bannerhealth.com
Baptist Memorial Hospital	Memphis	Tennessee	901-226-5000	www.bmhcc.org
Baptist Saint Anthony's Hospital	Amarillo	Texas	806-212-2000	www.bsahs.com
Bay Medical Center Sacred Heart Health System	Panama City	Florida	850-769-1511	www.baymedical.org
Baylor All Saints Medical Center at FW	Fort Worth	Texas	817-926-2544	www.baylorhealth.com/locations/allsaints
Baylor Medical Center at Garland	Garland	Texas	972-487-5000	www.baylorhealth.com
Baylor University Medical Center	Dallas	Texas	214-820-0111	www.baylorhealth.com
Bellin Memorial Hospital	Green Bay	Wisconsin	920-433-3500	www.bellin.org
Billings Clinic Hospital	Billings	Montana	406-657-4000	www.billingsclinic.com
Boca Raton Regional Hospital	Boca Raton	Florida	561-362-5002	www.brrh.com
Boone Hospital Center	Columbia	Missouri	573-815-8000	www.boone.org
Boulder Community Hospital	Boulder	Colorado	303-440-2273	www.bch.org
Bronson Methodist Hospital	Kalamazoo	Michigan	269-341-6000	www.bronsonhealth.com
Bryan Medical Center	Lincoln	Nebraska	402-481-1111	www.bryan.org
Carolinas Medical Center/Behaviorial Health	Charlotte	North Carolina	704-355-2000	www.carolinasmedicalcenter.org
Carondelet Saint Marys Hospital	Tucson	Arizona	520-872-3000	www.carondelet.org
Catawba Valley Medical Center	Hickory	North Carolina	828-326-3809	www.catawbavalleymc.org
Cedars - Sinai Medical Center	Los Angeles	California	310-423-5000	www.cedars-sinai.edu
Central Maine Medical Center	Lewiston	Maine	207-795-0111	www.cmmc.org
Central Washington Hospital	Wenatchee	Washington	509-662-1511	www.cwhs.com
Chester County Hospital	West Chester	Pennsylvania	610-431-5000	www.cchosp.com
Christus Santa Rosa Hospital	San Antonio	Texas	210-704-2011	www.christussantarosa.org
Citrus Memorial Hospital	Inverness	Florida	352-726-1551	www.citrusmh.com
Columbia Saint Marys Hospital Ozaukee	Mequon	Wisconsin	262-243-7300	www.columbia-stmarys.org
Columbus Regional Hospital	Columbus	Indiana	812-379-4441	www.crh.org
Community Hospital of the Monterey Peninsula	Monterey	California	831-624-5311	www.chomp.org
Cox Medical Center	Springfield	Missouri	417-269-6000	www.coxhealth.com
Decatur Morgan Hospital - Decatur Campus	Decatur	Alabama	256-341-2000	www.decaturgeneral.org
Dixie Regional Medical Center	Saint George	Utah	435-251-2100	www.intermountainhealthcare.org
Dominican Hospital	Santa Cruz	California	831-462-7700	www.dominicanhospital.org
East Jefferson General Hospital	Metairie	Louisiana	504-454-4000	www.eastjeffhospital.org
Eisenhower Medical Center	Rancho Mirage	California	760-340-3911	www.emc.org
Eliza Coffee Memorial Hospital	Florence	Alabama	256-768-8400	www.chgroup.org
Elmhurst Memorial Hospital	Elmhurst	Illinois	630-833-1400	www.emhc.org
Emory University Hospital	Atlanta	Georgia	404-686-8500	www.emoryhealthcare.org
Exempla Lutheran Medical Center	Wheat Ridge	Colorado	303-425-4500	www.exemlpa.org
Fargo VA Medical Center	Fargo	North Dakota	701-232-3241	www.fargo.va.gov
Fremont Area Medical Center	Fremont	Nebraska	402-721-1610	www.famc.org
Frye Regional Medical Center	Hickory	North Carolina	828-322-6070	www.fryemedctr.com
Genesis Medical Center - Davenport	Davenport	Iowa	563-421-1000	www.genesishealth.com
GHS Greenville Memorial Medical Center	Greenville	South Carolina	864-455-7000	www.ghs.org
Hartford Hospital	Hartford	Connecticut	860-545-5000	www.harthosp.org
Hutchinson Regional Medical Center	Hutchinson	Kansas	620-665-2001	www.hutchinsonhospital.com
Integris Baptist Medical Center	Oklahoma City	Oklahoma	405-951-8110	www.integris-health.com
Intermountain Medical Center	Murray	Utah	801-507-7000	www.intermountainhealthcare.org
Iowa Methodist Medical Center	Des Moines	Iowa	515-241-6212	www.iowahealth.org
John D Archbold Memorial Hospital	Thomasville	Georgia	229-228-2880	www.archbold.org
John Muir Medical Center - Concord Campus	Concord	California	925-674-2002	www.johnmuirhealth.com
John Muir Medical Center - Walnut Creek Campus	Walnut Creek	California	925-939-3000	www.jmmdhs.com
Lancaster General Hospital	Lancaster	Pennsylvania	717-299-5511	www.lancastergeneral.org
Licking Memorial Hospital	Newark	Ohio	740-348-4000	www.lmhealth.org
Lima Memorial Health System	Lima	Ohio	419-998-4731	www.limamemorial.org
Maine Medical Center	Portland	Maine	207-662-0111	www.mmc.org
Marshalltown Medical & Surgical Center	Marshalltown	Iowa	641-754-5151	www.everydaychampions.org
Mary Hitchcock Memorial Hospital	Lebanon	New Hampshire	603-650-5000	www.dhmc.org
Mayo Clinic Health System - Eau Claire Hospital	Eau Claire	Wisconsin	715-838-3311	www.luthermidelfort.org
McKay Dee Hospital	Ogden	Utah	801-387-2800	www.intermountainhealthcare.org
Mclaren Bay Region	Bay City	Michigan	989-894-3000	www.baymed.org

Hospital	City	State	Phone	Web Site
Memorial Healthcare System	Chattanooga	Tennessee	423-495-2525	www.memorial.org
Memorial Hermann Hospital System	Houston	Texas	713-448-6796	www.memorialhermann.org
Memorial Hermann Memorial City Medical Center	Houston	Texas	713-242-3000	www.mhhs.org
Memorial Hospital of South Bend	South Bend	Indiana	574-647-1000	www.qualityoflife.org
Memorial Mission Hospital & Asheville Surgery Center	Asheville	North Carolina	828-213-1111	www.missionhospitals.org
Mercy Health Partners - Mercy Campus	Muskegon	Michigan	231-672-3901	www.mghp.com
Mercy Hospital Springfield	Springfield	Missouri	417-820-2000	www.stjohns.com
Mercy Medical Center - Redding	Redding	California	530-225-6102	www.redding.mercy.org
Methodist Charlton Medical Center	Dallas	Texas	214-947-7777	www.methodisthealthsystem.org
Methodist Hospital	San Antonio	Texas	210-575-4000	www.mh.sahealth.com
The Methodist Hospital	Houston	Texas	713-790-2221	www.methodisthealth.com
Morristown Medical Center	Morristown	New Jersey	973-971-5450	www.morristownmemorialhospital.org
Morton Plant Hospital	Clearwater	Florida	727-462-7000	www.measehospitals.com
Munson Medical Center	Traverse City	Michigan	231-935-5000	www.munsonhealthcare.org
Naples Community Hospital	Naples	Florida	239-436-5000	www.nchmd.org
New Hanover Regional Medical Center	Wilmington	North Carolina	910-343-7000	www.nhrmc.org
North Shore Medical Center	Salem	Massachusetts	978-741-1215	www.nsmc.partners.org
Northeast Georgia Medical Center	Gainesville	Georgia	770-535-3553	www.nghs.com
Oklahoma Heart Hospital	Oklahoma City	Oklahoma	405-608-3200	www.okheart.com
Owensboro Health Regional Hospital	Owensboro	Kentucky	270-688-2000	www.omhs.org
Parkview Regional Medical Center	Fort Wayne	Indiana	260-266-1000	www.parkview.com
Penn Highlands Dubois	Dubois	Pennsylvania	814-371-2200	www.drmc.org
Penn Presbyterian Medical Center	Philadelphia	Pennsylvania	215-662-8000	www.pennhealth.com
Pocono Medical Center	East Stroudsburg	Pennsylvania	570-476-3348	www.poconohealthsystem.org
Portneuf Medical Center	Pocatello	Idaho	208-239-1000	www.portmed.org
Providence Saint Peter Hospital	Olympia	Washington	360-491-9480	www.providence.org/swsa
Providence Saint Vincent Medical Center	Portland	Oregon	503-216-1234	www.providence.org
Reading Hospital	Reading	Pennsylvania	610-988-8000	www.readinghospital.org
Rex Hospital	Raleigh	North Carolina	919-784-3100	www.rexhealth.com
Roper Hospital	Charleston	South Carolina	843-724-2800	www.ropersaintfrancis.com
Sacred Heart Medical Center - Riverbend	Springfield	Oregon	541-222-7300	www.peacehealth.org/sacred-heart-riverbend
Saint Vincent Hospital	Erie	Pennsylvania	814-452-5000	www.svhs.org
Santa Rosa Memorial Hospital	Santa Rosa	California	707-525-5300	www.stjosephhealth.org
Sarasota Memorial Hospital	Sarasota	Florida	941-917-9000	www.smh.com
Scripps Green Hospital	La Jolla	California	858-554-3600	www.scrippshealth.org
Sisters of Charity Providence Hospitals	Columbia	South Carolina	803-256-5300	www.providencehospitals.com
Spartanburg Regional Medical Center	Spartanburg	South Carolina	864-560-6000	www.srhs.com
Spectrum Health - Butterworth Campus	Grand Rapids	Michigan	616-391-1774	www.spectrum-health.org
Saint Charles Medical Center - Bend	Bend	Oregon	541-382-4321	www.scmc.org
Saint Francis - Downtown	Greenville	South Carolina	864-255-1000	www.stfrancishealth.org
Saint Joseph's Hospital	Saint Paul	Minnesota	651-232-7707	www.stjosephs-stpaul.org
Saint Luke's Regional Medical Center	Boise	Idaho	208-381-2222	www.slrmc.org
Saint Vincent Hospital	Santa Fe	New Mexico	505-913-5201	www.stvin.org
Sutter Roseville Medical Center	Roseville	California	916-781-1000	www.sutterroseville.org
Tallahassee Memorial Hospital	Tallahassee	Florida	850-431-1155	www.tmh.org
Tennova Healthcare	Knoxville	Tennessee	865-545-8000	www.stmaryshealth.com
The Queens Medical Center	Honolulu	Hawaii	808-538-9011	www.queens.org
Trident Medical Center	Charleston	South Carolina	843-797-8800	www.tridenthealthsystem.com
University Colo Health Memorial Hospital Central	Colorado Springs	Colorado	719-365-5000	www.memorialhospital.com
UPMC Hamot	Erie	Pennsylvania	814-877-6000	www.hamot.org
Venice Regional Medical Center - Bayfront Health	Venice	Florida	941-485-7711	www.veniceregional.com
Virginia Hospital Center	Arlington	Virginia	703-558-5000	www.virginiahospitalcenter.com
Wesley Medical Center	Wichita	Kansas	316-962-2000	www.wesleymc.com
Williamsport Regional Medical Center	Williamsport	Pennsylvania	570-321-1000	www.susquehannahealth.org
Willis Knighton Medical Center	Shreveport	Louisiana	318-212-4000	www.wkhs.com//locations/medicalcenter.aspx

Note: Table shows hospitals nationwide whose heart failure 30-day readmission rate is better (lower) than U.S. rate of 23.0%

Hospitals whose Heart Failure 30-Day Readmission Rate is Worse (Higher) than the U.S. National Rate

Hospital	City	State	Phone	Web Site
Abbeville General Hospital	Abbeville	Louisiana	337-893-5466	www.abgen.net
Advocate Trinity Hospital	Chicago	Illinois	773-967-2000	www.advocatehealth.com/trin
Banner Baywood Medical Center	Mesa	Arizona	480-321-2000	www.bannerhealth.com
Baptist Health Medical Center - North Little Rock	North Little Rock	Arkansas	501-202-3000	www.baptist-health.org
Barnes-Jewish Hospital	Saint Louis	Missouri	314-747-3000	www.barnesjewish.org
Beaumont Health System	Royal Oak	Michigan	248-898-5000	www.beaumonthospitals.com
Beckley ARH Hospital	Beckley	West Virginia	304-255-3456	www.arh.org/beckley
Beth Israel Medical Center	New York	New York	212-420-2000	www.wehealny.org
Bolivar Medical Center	Cleveland	Mississippi	662-846-2551	www.bolivarmedical.com
Brookhaven Memorial Hospital Medical Center	Patchogue	New York	631-654-7100	www.brookhavenhospitalorg
Camden Clark Medical Center	Parkersburg	West Virginia	304-424-2111	www.ccmh.org
Capital Health System - Fuld Campus	Trenton	New Jersey	609-394-6000	www.capitalhealth.org
Capital Regional Medical Center	Tallahassee	Florida	850-656-5000	www.capitalregionalmedicalcenter.com
Carepoint Health - Bayonne Hospital Center	Bayonne	New Jersey	201-858-5000	www.bayonnemedicalcenter.org
Carepoint Health - Christ Hospital	Jersey City	New Jersey	201-795-8200	www.christhospital.org
Carepoint Health - Hoboken UMC	Hoboken	New Jersey	201-418-1004	www.bonsecoursnj.com
Carolinas Hospital System	Florence	South Carolina	843-674-2500	www.carolinashospital.com
Centegra Health System - Mc Henry Hospital	Mchenry	Illinois	815-344-5000	www.centegra.org
Chicot Memorial Medical Center	Lake Village	Arkansas	870-265-5351	www.chicotmemorial.com
Cincinnati VA Medical Center	Cincinnati	Ohio	513-861-3100	www.cincinnati.va.gov
Clinch Valley Medical Center	Richlands	Virginia	276-596-6000	www.clinchvalleymedicalcenter.com
Community Medical Center	Toms River	New Jersey	732-557-8000	www.sbhcs.com
Coney Island Hospital	Brooklyn	New York	718-616-3000	www.coneyislandhospital.com
Covenant Medical Center	Saginaw	Michigan	989-583-4000	www.covenanthealthcare.com
Crozer Chester Medical Center	Upland	Pennsylvania	610-447-2000	www.crozer.org
Culpeper Regional Hospital	Culpeper	Virginia	540-829-4100	www.culpeperhospital.com
Dallas VA Medical Center - VA North Texas	Dallas	Texas	214-742-8387	www.north-texas.med.va.gov
Danville Regional Medical Center	Danville	Virginia	434-799-2100	www.danvilleregional.org
Davis Memorial Hospital	Elkins	West Virginia	304-636-3300	www.davishealthcare.org
Detroit Receiving Hospital & University Health Center	Detroit	Michigan	313-745-3104	www.drhuhc.org
Doctors Hospital of Manteca	Manteca	California	209-823-3111	www.doctorsmanteca.com
East Georgia Regional Medical Center	Statesboro	Georgia	912-486-1500	www.egrmc.com
East Orange General Hospital	East Orange	New Jersey	973-266-4401	www.evh.org
Etmc Henderson	Henderson	Texas	903-657-7541	www.hmhtx.org
Florida Hospital	Orlando	Florida	407-303-1976	www.floridahospital.com
Flushing Hospital Medical Center	Flushing	New York	718-670-5000	www.flushinghospital.org
Forrest General Hospital	Hattiesburg	Mississippi	601-288-7000	www.forrestgeneral.com
Fountain Valley Regional Hospital & Medical Center	Fountain Valley	California	714-966-7200	www.fountainvalleyhospital.com
Franciscan Saint James Health	Olympia Fields	Illinois	708-747-4000	www.franciscanalliance.org
GV (Sonny) Montgomery VA Medical Center Jackson	Jackson	Mississippi	601-362-4471	www.visn16.med.va.gov
Georgetown Memorial Hospital	Georgetown	South Carolina	843-527-7000	www.gmhsc.com
Glenwood Regional Medical Center	West Monroe	Louisiana	318-329-4600	www.grmc.com
Griffin Hospital	Derby	Connecticut	203-732-7500	www.griffinhealth.org
Harlan Appalachian Regional Healthcare Hospital	Harlan	Kentucky	606-573-8100	www.arh.org
Harmon Memorial Hospital	Hollis	Oklahoma	580-688-3363	
Hazard ARH Regional Medical Center	Hazard	Kentucky	606-439-6600	www.arh.org/hazard
Henry Ford Hospital	Detroit	Michigan	313-916-2600	www.henryfordhospital.com
Hialeah Hospital	Hialeah	Florida	305-693-6100	www.hialeahhosp.com
Highlands Regional Medical Center	Prestonsburg	Kentucky	606-886-8511	www.hrmc.org
Hines VA Medical Center	Hines	Illinois	708-202-8387	www.visn12.med.va.gov/hines
Holy Name Medical Center	Teaneck	New Jersey	201-833-3000	www.holyname.org
Holzer Medical Center	Gallipolis	Ohio	740-446-5000	www.holzer.org
Howard University Hospital	Washington	District of Columbia	202-745-6100	www.huhosp.org
Huntington VA Medical Center	Huntington	West Virginia	304-429-0241	www.huntington.med.gov
Inspira Medical Center Woodbury	Woodbury	New Jersey	856-845-0100	www.umhospital.org
Interfaith Medical Center	Brooklyn	New York	718-613-4000	www.interfaithmedical.com
Jackson Memorial Hospital	Miami	Florida	305-585-1111	www.jhsmiami.org
Jamestown Regional Medical Center	Jamestown	Tennessee	931-879-3352	www.jamestownregional.org
Jefferson Regional Medical Center	Pittsburgh	Pennsylvania	412-469-5000	www.jeffersonregional.com
Jennings American Legion Hospital	Jennings	Louisiana	337-616-7000	www.jalh.com
Jesse Brown VA Medical Center - VA Chicago	Chicago	Illinois	312-569-8387	www.va.gov
JFK Medical Center	Atlantis	Florida	561-965-7300	www.jfkmc.com
Johns Hopkins Bayview Medical Center	Baltimore	Maryland	410-550-0123	www.hopkinsbayview.org
Jordan Hospital	Plymouth	Massachusetts	508-746-2000	www.jordanhospital.org
Kennedy University Hospital - Stratford Div	Stratford	New Jersey	856-346-6000	www.kennedyhealth.org

Hospital	City	State	Phone	Web Site
King's Daughters' Medical Center	Ashland	Kentucky	606-408-4000	www.kdmc.com
Leesburg Regional Medical Center	Leesburg	Florida	352-323-5762	www.leesburgregional.org
Lewisgale Hospital Pulaski	Pulaski	Virginia	540-994-8100	www.lewisgale.com
Libertyhealth - Jersey City Medical Center Campus	Jersey City	New Jersey	201-915-2000	www.libertyhcs.org
Lutheran Medical Center	Brooklyn	New York	718-630-8000	www.lmcmc.com
Madison River Oaks Medical Center	Canton	Mississippi	601-855-5323	www.madisonriveroaks.com
Mayo Clinic Health System - Fairmont	Fairmont	Minnesota	507-238-8101	www.fairmontmedicalcenter.org
Medical Center of Southeastern Oklahoma	Durant	Oklahoma	405-924-3080	www.mcsohealth.com
Medical Center of Trinity	Trinity	Florida	727-848-1733	www.communityhospitalnpr.com
Medstar Harbor Hospital	Baltimore	Maryland	410-350-3201	www.harborhospital.org
Memorial Hospital of Rhode Island	Pawtucket	Rhode Island	401-729-2000	www.mhriweb.org
Memorial Regional Hospital	Hollywood	Florida	954-987-2000	www.memorialregional.com
Mercy Fitzgerald Hospital	Darby	Pennsylvania	215-237-4000	www.mercyhealth.org
Mercy Hospital Saint Louis	Saint Louis	Missouri	314-569-6000	www.stjohnsmercy.org
Methodist Healthcare Memphis Hospitals	Memphis	Tennessee	901-516-8274	www.methodisthealth.org
Methodist Hospitals	Gary	Indiana	219-886-4642	www.methodisthospital.org
Metrosouth Medical Center	Blue Island	Illinois	708-597-2000	www.stfrancisblueisland.com
Midwest Regional Medical Center	Midwest City	Oklahoma	405-610-8530	www.midwestregional.com
Monmouth Medical Center - Southern Campus	Lakewood	New Jersey	732-363-1900	www.sbhcs.com
Montefiore Medical Center	Bronx	New York	718-920-4321	www.montefiore.org
Montefiore New Rochelle Hospital	New Rochelle	New York	914-632-5000	www.ssmc.org
Morton Hospital	Taunton	Massachusetts	508-828-7000	www.mortonhospital.org
Multicare Auburn Medical Center	Auburn	Washington	253-833-7711	www.armcuhs.com/p1.html
Nassau University Medical Center	East Meadow	New York	516-572-0123	www.numc.edu
New York Community Hospital of Brooklyn	Brooklyn	New York	718-692-5302	www.nych.com
New York Methodist Hospital	Brooklyn	New York	718-780-3000	www.nym.org
New York - Presbyterian Hospital	New York	New York	212-746-4189	www.nyp.org
North Carolina Baptist Hospital	Winston-Salem	North Carolina	336-716-2011	www.wfubmc.edu
North Shore Medical Center	Miami	Florida	305-835-6000	www.northshoremedical.com
North Shore University Hospital	Manhasset	New York	516-562-0100	www.northshorelij.com
Northwest Hospital Center	Randallstown	Maryland	410-521-5995	www.lifebridgehealth.org
Northwest Mississippi Regional Medical Center	Clarksdale	Mississippi	662-627-3211	www.nwmsregionalmedcenter.com
Oakwood Hospital - Dearborn	Dearborn	Michigan	313-593-7125	www.oakwood.org
Ochsner Medical Center	New Orleans	Louisiana	504-842-3000	www.ochsner.org
Olympia Medical Center	Los Angeles	California	310-657-5900	www.olympiamc.com
Orange Regional Medical Center	Middletown	New York	845-343-2424	www.ormc.org
Palisades Medical Center	North Bergen	New Jersey	201-854-5000	www.palisadesmedical.org
Palm Springs General Hospital	Hialeah	Florida	305-558-2500	www.psghosp.com
Pineville Community Hospital	Pineville	Kentucky	606-337-3051	www.pinevillehospital.com
Poplar Bluff VA Medical Center	Poplar Bluff	Missouri	573-686-4151	www.poplarbluff.va.gov
Port Huron Hospital	Port Huron	Michigan	810-987-5000	www.porthuronhospital.org
Presence Saint Joseph Medical Center	Joliet	Illinois	815-725-7133	www.provena.org/stjoes
Presence United Samaritans Medical Center	Danville	Illinois	217-443-5000	www.provena.org/usmc
Prince Georges Hospital Center	Cheverly	Maryland	301-618-2000	www.princegeorgeshospital.org
Providence VA Medical Center	Providence	Rhode Island	401-457-3042	www.visn1.med.va.gov/providence
Raritan Bay Medical Center	Perth Amboy	New Jersey	732-442-3700	www.rbmc.org
Riverview Regional Medical Center	Gadsden	Alabama	256-543-5200	www.riverviewregional.com
San Antonio VA Medical Center	San Antonio	Texas	210-617-5300	www.vasthcs.med.va.gov
San Juan VA Medical Center	San Juan	Puerto Rico	800-449-8729	www.visn8.med.va.gov/caribbean
Schuylkill Medical Center - East Norwegian Street	Pottsville	Pennsylvania	570-621-4000	www.schuylkillhealth.com
Sinai - Grace Hospital	Detroit	Michigan	313-966-3300	www.sinaigrace.org
Singing River Hospital	Pascagoula	Mississippi	228-809-5000	www.srhshealth.com
Skyridge Medical Center	Cleveland	Tennessee	423-339-4132	www.skyridgemedcenter.com
Somerset Medical Center	Somerville	New Jersey	908-685-2200	www.somersetmedicalcenter.com
South Nassau Communities Hospital	Oceanside	New York	516-632-3000	www.southnassau.org
Southcoast Hospital Group	Fall River	Massachusetts	508-679-3131	www.southcoast.org/charlton
Southeastern Regional Medical Center	Lumberton	North Carolina	910-671-5000	www.srmc.org
Southern Tennessee Medical Center	Winchester	Tennessee	931-967-8295	www.southerntennessee.com
Southside Regional Medical Center	Petersburg	Virginia	804-765-5000	www.srmconline.com
SSM Depaul Health Center	Bridgeton	Missouri	314-344-6000	www.ssmdepaul.com
SSM Saint Marys Health Center	Richmond Heights	Missouri	314-768-8000	www.ssmhealth.com/stmarys
Saint Catherine of Siena Hospital	Smithtown	New York	631-862-3000	www.stcatherines.chsli.org
Saint Francis Medical Center	Monroe	Louisiana	318-966-4000	www.stfran.com
Saint John Hospital & Medical Center	Detroit	Michigan	313-343-4000	www.stjohnprovidence.org
Saint John's Episcopal Hospital at South Shore	Far Rockaway	New York	718-869-7000	www.ehs.org
Saint John's Riverside Hospital	Yonkers	New York	914-964-4444	www.riversidehealth.org
Saint Joseph's Hospital	Tampa	Florida	813-870-4398	www.stjosephstampa.org

Hospital	City	State	Phone	Web Site
Saint Joseph's Regional Medical Center	Paterson	New Jersey	973-754-2010	www.sjhmc.org
Saint Louis - John Cochran VA Medical Center	Saint Louis	Missouri	314-652-4100	www.stlouis.va.gov
Saint Luke's Hospital Bethlehem	Bethlehem	Pennsylvania	610-954-4000	www.slhn-lehighvalley.org
Saint Luke's Roosevelt Hospital	New York	New York	212-523-4000	www.wehealny.org
Saint Mary Mercy Hospital	Livonia	Michigan	734-655-4800	www.stmarymercy.org
Saint Marys Hospital	Centralia	Illinois	618-436-6519	www.stmarys-goodsamaritan.com
Swedish Covenant Hospital	Chicago	Illinois	773-878-8200	www.swedishcovenant.org
Tampa VA Medical Center	Tampa	Florida	813-972-2000	www.tampa.va.gov
Univerity of MD Balto Washington Medical Center	Glen Burnie	Maryland	410-595-1967	www.bwmc.umms.org
University Hospital of Brooklyn - Downstate Medical Center	Brooklyn	New York	718-270-1000	www.downstate.edu
University of Miami Hospital	Miami	Florida	305-325-5511	www.cedarsmedicalcenter.com
VA Middle Tennessee Healthcare System	Nashville	Tennessee	615-327-5332	www.tennesseevalley.va.gov
VA New York Harbor Healthcare System	New York	New York	212-686-7500	www.nyharbor.va.gov
VA North Florida/South Georgia Healthcare System	Gainesville	Florida	352-376-1611	www.northflorida.va.gov
Valley Hospital	Ridgewood	New Jersey	201-447-8000	www.valleyhealth.com
W Palm Beach VA Medical Center	West Palm Beach	Florida	561-422-8600	www.va.gov
Wellmont Bristol Regional Medical Center	Bristol	Tennessee	423-844-1121	www.wellmont.org
Western Maryland Regional Medical Center	Cumberland	Maryland	240-964-8001	www.wmhs.com
Westlake Regional Hospital	Columbia	Kentucky	270-384-4753	www.westlake-healthcare.org
Whitesburg ARH Hospital	Whitesburg	Kentucky	606-633-3500	www.arh.org/whitesburg
William Beaumont Hospital - Troy	Troy	Michigan	248-964-8800	www.beaumonthospitals.com
Williamson ARH Hospital	South Williamson	Kentucky	606-237-1700	www.arh.org
Wuesthoff Medical Center Rockledge	Rockledge	Florida	321-637-2603	www.wuesthoff.org
Wyckoff Heights Medical Center	Brooklyn	New York	718-963-7272	www.wyckoffhospital.org

Note: Table shows hospitals nationwide whose heart failure 30-day readmission rate is worse (higher) than U.S. rate of 23.0%

Hospitals whose Pneumonia 30-Day Readmission Rate is Better (Lower) than the U.S. National Rate

Hospital	City	State	Phone	Web Site
Bay Medical Center Sacred Heart Health System	Panama City	Florida	850-769-1511	www.baymedical.org
Boca Raton Regional Hospital	Boca Raton	Florida	561-362-5002	www.brrh.com
Bronson Methodist Hospital	Kalamazoo	Michigan	269-341-6000	www.bronsonhealth.com
Cayuga Medical Center at Ithaca	Ithaca	New York	607-274-4401	www.cayugamed.org
Citrus Memorial Hospital	Inverness	Florida	352-726-1551	www.citrusmh.com
Eisenhower Medical Center	Rancho Mirage	California	760-340-3911	www.emc.org
Evergreen Hospital Medical Center	Kirkland	Washington	425-899-1000	www.evergreenhospital.org
Florida Hospital Waterman	Tavares	Florida	352-253-3300	www.fhwat.org
Freeman Health System - Freeman West	Joplin	Missouri	417-347-1111	www.freemanhealth.com
Kalispell Regional Medical Center	Kalispell	Montana	406-752-5111	www.krmc.org
Lake Regional Health System	Osage Beach	Missouri	573-348-8000	www.lakeregional.com
Memorial Healthcare System	Chattanooga	Tennessee	423-495-2525	www.memorial.org
Memorial Hermann Hospital System	Houston	Texas	713-448-6796	www.memorialhermann.org
Memorial Hermann Memorial City Medical Center	Houston	Texas	713-242-3000	www.mhhs.org
Memorial Medical Center of West Michigan	Ludington	Michigan	231-843-2591	www.mmcwm.com
Mercy Medical Center - Redding	Redding	California	530-225-6102	www.redding.mercy.org
Owensboro Health Regional Hospital	Owensboro	Kentucky	270-688-2000	www.omhs.org
Parkview Medical Center	Pueblo	Colorado	719-584-4000	www.parkviewmc.com
Parkview Regional Medical Center	Fort Wayne	Indiana	260-266-1000	www.parkview.com
Providence Saint Vincent Medical Center	Portland	Oregon	503-216-1234	www.providence.org
Rex Hospital	Raleigh	North Carolina	919-784-3100	www.rexhealth.com
Saint Joseph Regional Medical Center	Mishawaka	Indiana	574-335-5000	www.sjmed.com
Saint Joseph's Hospital of Atlanta	Atlanta	Georgia	678-843-5720	www.stjosephsatlanta.org
Salem Regional Medical Center	Salem	Ohio	330-332-1551	www.salemhosp.com
San Antonio Community Hospital	Upland	California	714-985-2811	www.sach.org
Sarasota Memorial Hospital	Sarasota	Florida	941-917-9000	www.smh.com
South Texas Health System	Edinburg	Texas	956-632-4000	www.edinburgregional.com
Spartanburg Regional Medical Center	Spartanburg	South Carolina	864-560-6000	www.srhs.com
Saint Edward Mercy Medical Center	Fort Smith	Arkansas	479-314-6000	www.stedwardmercy.com
Saint Francis Hospital - Roslyn	Roslyn	New York	516-562-6000	www.stfrancisheartcenter.com
Saint Francis - Downtown	Greenville	South Carolina	864-255-1000	www.stfrancishealth.org
Saint Mary's Regional Medical Center	Enid	Oklahoma	580-233-6100	www.stmarysregional.com
Saint Patrick Hospital	Missoula	Montana	406-543-7271	www.saintpatrick.org
Stormont - Vail Healthcare	Topeka	Kansas	785-354-6121	www.stormontvail.org
Virtua Memorial Hospital of Burlington County	Mount Holly	New Jersey	609-914-6200	www.virtua.org
Williamsport Regional Medical Center	Williamsport	Pennsylvania	570-321-1000	www.susquehannahealth.org
Willis Knighton Medical Center	Shreveport	Louisiana	318-212-4000	www.wkhs.com//locations/medicalcenter.aspx

Note: Table shows hospitals nationwide whose pneumonia 30-day readmission rate is better (lower) than U.S. rate of 17.6%

Hospitals whose Pneumonia 30-Day Readmission Rate is Worse (Higher) than the U.S. National Rate

Hospital	City	State	Phone	Web Site
Adena Regional Medical Center	Chillicothe	Ohio	740-779-7500	www.adena.org
Advocate Lutheran General Hospital	Park Ridge	Illinois	847-723-2210	www.advocatehealth.com
Advocate South Suburban Hospital	Hazel Crest	Illinois	708-799-8000	www.advocatehealth.com
Arnot Ogden Medical Center	Elmira	New York	607-737-4100	www.arnothealth.org
Baptist Memorial Hospital Desoto	Southaven	Mississippi	662-772-4000	www.bmhcc.org/facilities/desoto
Barnes-Jewish Hospital	Saint Louis	Missouri	314-747-3000	www.barnesjewish.org
Baxter Regional Medical Center	Mountain Home	Arkansas	870-508-1000	www.baxterregional.org
Bay Area Hospital	Coos Bay	Oregon	541-269-8111	www.bayareahospital.org
Bay Pines VA Medical Center	Bay Pines	Florida	727-398-6661	www.baypines.va.gov
Bayfront Health Punta Gorda	Punta Gorda	Florida	941-639-3131	www.charlotteregional.com
Beaumont Health System	Royal Oak	Michigan	248-898-5000	www.beaumonthospitals.com
Beckley VA Medical Center	Beckley	West Virginia	304-255-2121	www.beckley.va.gov
Beth Israel Medical Center	New York	New York	212-420-2000	www.wehealny.org
Blount Memorial Hospital	Maryville	Tennessee	865-983-7211	www.blountmemorial.org
Brandon Regional Hospital	Brandon	Florida	813-681-5551	www.brandonregionalhospital.com
Bronx VA Medical Center	Bronx	New York	718-584-9000	www.med.va.gov
Bronx - Lebanon Hospital Center	Bronx	New York	212-588-7000	www.bronx-leb.org
Brookhaven Memorial Hospital Medical Center	Patchogue	New York	631-654-7100	www.brookhavenhospitalorg
Cape Fear Valley Medical Center	Fayetteville	North Carolina	910-609-4000	www.capefearvalley.com
Casey County Hospital	Liberty	Kentucky	606-787-6275	
Chambers Memorial Hospital	Danville	Arkansas	479-495-2241	www.chambershospital.com
Cleveland Clinic	Cleveland	Ohio	216-444-2200	www.clevelandclinic.org
Cleveland - Wade Park VA Medical Center	Cleveland	Ohio	216-791-3800	www.cleveland.va.gov
Columbia MO VA Medical Center	Columbia	Missouri	573-814-6000	www.columbiamo.vc.gov
Community Hospital	Munster	Indiana	219-836-1600	www.comhs.org/community
Dallas VA Medical Center - VA North Texas	Dallas	Texas	214-742-8387	www.north-texas.med.va.gov
Davis Regional Medical Center	Statesville	North Carolina	704-873-0281	www.davisregional.com
Doctors' Community Hospital	Lanham	Maryland	301-552-8085	www.dchweb.org
East Orange General Hospital	East Orange	New Jersey	973-266-4401	www.evh.org
Florida Hospital	Orlando	Florida	407-303-1976	www.floridahospital.com
Florida Hospital Tampa	Tampa	Florida	813-615-7200	www.uch.org
Forest Hills Hospital	Forest Hills	New York	718-830-4000	www.northshorelij.com
Franklin Medical Center	Winnsboro	Louisiana	318-435-9411	www.fmc-cares.com
Garden City Hospital	Garden City	Michigan	734-421-3300	www.gchosp.org
Great River Medical Center	Blytheville	Arkansas	870-838-7300	www.greatrivermc.com
Harlan Appalachian Regional Healthcare Hospital	Harlan	Kentucky	606-573-8100	www.arh.org
Hazard ARH Regional Medical Center	Hazard	Kentucky	606-439-6600	www.arh.org/hazard
Heartland Regional Medical Center	Marion	Illinois	618-998-7000	www.heartlandregional.com
Henry Ford Hospital	Detroit	Michigan	313-916-2600	www.henryfordhospital.com
Highlands Regional Medical Center	Sebring	Florida	863-385-6101	www.highlandsregional.com
Hillcrest Hospital	Mayfield Heights	Ohio	440-312-4500	www.hillcresthospital.org
Hines VA Medical Center	Hines	Illinois	708-202-8387	www.visn12.med.va.gov/hines
Holzer Medical Center	Gallipolis	Ohio	740-446-5000	www.holzer.org
Houston VA Medical Center	Houston	Texas	713-794-7100	www.houston.med.va.gov
Howard County General Hospital	Columbia	Maryland	410-740-7890	www.hcgh.org
Huntington Hospital	Huntington	New York	631-351-2000	www.hunthosp.org
Huntington VA Medical Center	Huntington	West Virginia	304-429-0241	www.huntington.med.gov
Jackson Parish Hospital	Jonesboro	Louisiana	318-259-4435	www.jacksonparishhospital.com
Jewish Hospital & Saint Mary's Healthcare	Louisville	Kentucky	502-587-4011	www.jhhs.org
Johns Hopkins Bayview Medical Center	Baltimore	Maryland	410-550-0123	www.hopkinsbayview.org
Kennedy University Hospital - Stratford Div	Stratford	New Jersey	856-346-6000	www.kennedyhealth.org
King's Daughters' Medical Center	Ashland	Kentucky	606-408-4000	www.kdmc.com
Lake City Medical Center	Lake City	Florida	386-719-9000	www.lakecitymedical.com
Lake Health	Concord	Ohio	440-953-9600	www.lakehealth.org
Lehigh Valley Hospital - Hazleton	Hazleton	Pennsylvania	570-501-4000	www.ghha.org
Lenox Hill Hospital	New York	New York	212-439-2345	www.lenoxhillhospital.org
Little Company of Mary Hospital	Evergreen Park	Illinois	708-422-6200	www.lcmh.org
Livingston Regional Hospital	Livingston	Tennessee	931-823-5611	www.livingstonregionalhospital.com
Logan Regional Medical Center	Logan	West Virginia	304-831-1350	www.loganregionalmedicalcenter.com
Marymount Hospital	Garfield Heights	Ohio	216-581-0500	www.marymount.org
Medical Center of Southeastern Oklahoma	Durant	Oklahoma	405-924-3080	www.mcsohealth.com
Medstar Good Samaritan Hospital	Baltimore	Maryland	443-444-3902	www.goodsam-md.org
Memorial Hospital	Manchester	Kentucky	606-598-5104	www.manchestermemorial.com
Mercy Memorial Health Center	Ardmore	Oklahoma	405-223-5400	www.mercyok.com/mmhc
Metrosouth Medical Center	Blue Island	Illinois	708-597-2000	www.stfrancisblueisland.com

Hospital	City	State	Phone	Web Site
Mississippi Baptist Medical Center	Jackson	Mississippi	601-968-1000	www.mbmc.org
Monroe County Medical Center	Tompkinsville	Kentucky	270-487-9231	www.mcmccares.com
Mount Sinai Hospital	New York	New York	212-241-7981	www.mountsinai.org
Muskogee VA Medical Center	Muskogee	Oklahoma	918-577-3000	www.visn16.med.va.gov/muskogee.asp
Nassau University Medical Center	East Meadow	New York	516-572-0123	www.numc.edu
New York Hospital Medical Center of Queens	Flushing	New York	718-670-1231	www.nyhq.org
New York Methodist Hospital	Brooklyn	New York	718-780-3000	www.nym.org
North Carolina Baptist Hospital	Winston-Salem	North Carolina	336-716-2011	www.wfubmc.edu
North Oaks Medical Center	Hammond	Louisiana	985-345-2700	www.northoaks.org
Northern Westchester Hospital	Mount Kisco	New York	914-666-1200	www.nwhc.net
Northwest Hospital Center	Randallstown	Maryland	410-521-5995	www.lifebridgehealth.org
Northwestern Memorial Hospital	Chicago	Illinois	312-926-2000	www.nmh.org
Oakwood Hospital - Wayne	Wayne	Michigan	734-467-4175	www.oakwood.org
Orange Regional Medical Center	Middletown	New York	845-343-2424	www.ormc.org
Oroville Hospital	Oroville	California	530-533-8500	www.orovillehospital.com
Palos Community Hospital	Palos Heights	Illinois	708-923-4000	www.paloshospital.org
Piedmont Medical Center	Rock Hill	South Carolina	803-329-1234	www.piedmontmedicalcenter.com
Pineville Community Hospital	Pineville	Kentucky	606-337-3051	www.pinevillehospital.com
Presence United Samaritans Medical Center	Danville	Illinois	217-443-5000	www.provena.org/usmc
Princeton Community Hospital	Princeton	West Virginia	304-487-7260	www.pchonline.org
Raleigh General Hospital	Beckley	West Virginia	304-256-4100	www.raleighgeneral.com
Richmond VA Medical Center	Richmond	Virginia	804-675-5000	www.med.va.gov
Robert Packer Hospital	Sayre	Pennsylvania	570-888-6666	www.guthrie.org
Russell County Medical Center	Lebanon	Virginia	276-883-8100	www.msha.com
Saint Anne's Hospital	Fall River	Massachusetts	508-674-5600	www.saintanneshospital.org
Saint Thomas Rutherford Hospital	Murfreesboro	Tennessee	615-396-4100	www.mtmc.org
San Gabriel Valley Medical Center	San Gabriel	California	626-289-5454	www.sangabrielvalleymedctr.org
San Juan VA Medical Center	San Juan	Puerto Rico	800-449-8729	www.visn8.med.va.gov/caribbean
Santa Monica - UCLA Medical Center & Orthopaedic Hospital	Santa Monica	California	310-319-4000	www.healthcare.ucla.edu
Sentara Careplex Hospital	Hampton	Virginia	757-736-1000	www.sentara.com
Silver Cross Hospital & Medical Centers	New Lenox	Illinois	815-300-1100	www.silvercross.org
Sinai Hospital of Baltimore	Baltimore	Maryland	410-601-5131	www.sinai-balt.com
Singing River Hospital	Pascagoula	Mississippi	228-809-5000	www.srhshealth.com
Springfield Regional Medical Center	Springfield	Ohio	937-523-1000	www.communityhospital.com
Saint Anthony's Medical Center	Saint Louis	Missouri	314-525-1000	www.samcstl.org
Saint Bernard Hospital	Chicago	Illinois	773-962-3900	www.stbernardhospital.com
Saint Catherine of Siena Hospital	Smithtown	New York	631-862-3000	www.stcatherines.chsli.org
Saint Francis Hospital	Poughkeepsie	New York	845-483-5000	www.sfhhc.org
Saint Joseph's Hospital Health Center	Syracuse	New York	315-448-5111	www.sjhsyr.org
Saint Luke's Roosevelt Hospital	New York	New York	212-523-4000	www.wehealny.org
Saint Rose Dominican Hospitals - Rose De Lima Campus	Henderson	Nevada	702-616-5000	www.dignityhealth.org/las-vegas
Sumner Regional Medical Center	Gallatin	Tennessee	615-452-4210	www.mysumnermedical.com
Syracuse VA Medical Center	Syracuse	New York	315-425-4400	www1.va.gov/visns/visn02
Tampa VA Medical Center	Tampa	Florida	813-972-2000	www.tampa.va.gov
Univerity of MD Balto Washington Medical Center	Glen Burnie	Maryland	410-595-1967	www.bwmc.umms.org
University Hospital - Stony Brook	Stony Brook	New York	631-444-4000	www.stonybrookmedicalcenter.org
University Hospitals - Elyria Medical Center	Elyria	Ohio	440-329-7500	www.emh-healthcare.org
University of Alabama Hospital	Birmingham	Alabama	205-934-4011	www.health.uab.edu
University of Maryland Medical Center	Baltimore	Maryland	410-328-8667	www.umm.edu
University of Maryland Charles Regional Medical Center	La Plata	Maryland	301-609-4265	www.civista.org
Upper Valley Medical Center	Troy	Ohio	937-440-7853	www.uvmc.com
Upstate New York VA Healthcare System - Western NY	Buffalo	New York	716-862-3611	www.buffalo.va.gov
VA Central Arkansas Veterans Healthcare System	Little Rock	Arkansas	501-257-1000	www.visn16.med.va.gov
VA Maryland Healthcare System - Baltimore	Baltimore	Maryland	410-605-7016	www.maryland.va.gov
VA Middle Tennessee Healthcare System	Nashville	Tennessee	615-327-5332	www.tennesseevalley.va.gov
VA Pittsburgh Healthcare System	Pittsburgh	Pennsylvania	412-688-6100	www.pittsburg.va.gov
Vassar Brothers Medical Center	Poughkeepsie	New York	845-454-8500	www.vasserbrothers.org
Wadley Regional Medical Center	Texarkana	Texas	903-798-8000	www.wadleyhealth.com
Washington Hospital	Fremont	California	510-797-1111	www.whhs.com
Wayne Memorial Hospital	Goldsboro	North Carolina	919-736-1110	www.waynehealth.org
White County Medical Center	Searcy	Arkansas	501-278-3100	www.centralarkhospital.com
White Plains Hospital Center	White Plains	New York	914-681-0600	www.wphospital.org
William Beaumont Hospital - Troy	Troy	Michigan	248-964-8800	www.beaumonthospitals.com
Wing Memorial Hospital & Medical Center	Palmer	Massachusetts	413-283-7651	www.winghealth.org
Wyckoff Heights Medical Center	Brooklyn	New York	718-963-7272	www.wyckoffhospital.org

Note: Table shows hospitals nationwide whose pneumonia 30-day readmission rate is worse (higher) than U.S. rate of 17.6%

Hospitals whose Rate of Readmission After Hip/Knee Surgery is Better (Lower) than the U.S. National Rate

Hospital	City	State	Phone	Web Site
Arkansas Surgical Hospital	No Little Rock	Arkansas	501-748-8000	www.arksurgicalhospital.com
Blake Medical Center	Bradenton	Florida	941-792-6611	www.blakemedicalcenter.com
Boca Raton Regional Hospital	Boca Raton	Florida	561-362-5002	www.brrh.com
Christus Santa Rosa Hospital	San Antonio	Texas	210-704-2011	www.christussantarosa.org
Community Memorial Hospital	Hamilton	New York	315-824-1100	www.communitymemorial.org
Eisenhower Medical Center	Rancho Mirage	California	760-340-3911	www.emc.org
Elkhart General Hospital	Elkhart	Indiana	574-294-2621	www.egh.org
Emory University Hospital	Atlanta	Georgia	404-686-8500	www.emoryhealthcare.org
Evanston Hospital	Evanston	Illinois	847-432-8000	www.enh.org
Grace Medical Center	Lubbock	Texas	806-788-4100	www.highlandcommunityhospital.com
Heart of Florida Regional Medical Center	Davenport	Florida	863-422-4971	www.heartofflorida.com
Heartland Regional Medical Center	Saint Joseph	Missouri	816-271-6000	www.heartland-health.com
Hoag Orthopedic Institute	Irvine	California	949-727-5000	www.orthopedichospital.com
Holy Cross Hospital	Fort Lauderdale	Florida	954-771-8000	www.holy-cross.com
Hospital For Special Surgery	New York	New York	212-606-1000	www.hss.edu
Inova Mount Vernon Hospital	Alexandria	Virginia	703-664-7000	www.inova.com/inovapublic.srt/imvh/index.jsp
Kalispell Regional Medical Center	Kalispell	Montana	406-752-5111	www.krmc.org
Kansas Medical Center	Andover	Kansas	316-300-4000	www.ksmedcenter.com
Kettering Medical Center	Kettering	Ohio	937-298-4331	www.khnetwork.org
Maine Medical Center	Portland	Maine	207-662-0111	www.mmc.org
Meadville Medical Center	Meadville	Pennsylvania	814-333-5000	www.mmchs.org
Memorial Healthcare System	Chattanooga	Tennessee	423-495-2525	www.memorial.org
Memorial Mission Hospital & Asheville Surgery Center	Asheville	North Carolina	828-213-1111	www.missionhospitals.org
Mercy Medical Center - Cedar Rapids	Cedar Rapids	Iowa	319-398-6011	www.mercycare.org
Mercy Medical Center - Redding	Redding	California	530-225-6102	www.redding.mercy.org
New England Baptist Hospital	Boston	Massachusetts	617-754-5800	www.nebh.caregroup.org
Ocala Regional Medical Center	Ocala	Florida	352-401-1000	www.ocalaregional.com
Oklahoma Surgical Hospital	Tulsa	Oklahoma	918-477-5000	www.oklahomasurgicalhospital.com
Orthopaedic Hospital at Parkview North	Fort Wayne	Indiana	260-672-4050	www.parkview.com
Orthopaedic Hospital of Wisconsin	Glendale	Wisconsin	414-961-6800	www.ohow.org
Poudre Valley Hospital	Fort Collins	Colorado	970-495-7000	www.pvhs.org
Presbyterian Hospital	Albuquerque	New Mexico	505-724-8386	www.phs.org
Providence Saint John's Health Center	Santa Monica	California	310-829-5511	www.stjohns.org
Reading Hospital	Reading	Pennsylvania	610-988-8000	www.readinghospital.org
Sacred Heart Medical Center - Riverbend	Springfield	Oregon	541-222-7300	www.peacehealth.org/sacred-heart-riverbend
Saint Elizabeth Regional Medical Center	Lincoln	Nebraska	402-219-7700	www.stelizabethonline.com
Saint Joseph's Hospital of Atlanta	Atlanta	Georgia	678-843-5720	www.stjosephsatlanta.org
Saint Thomas West Hospital	Nashville	Tennessee	615-222-2111	www.stthomas.org
Salinas Valley Memorial Hospital	Salinas	California	831-757-4333	www.svmh.com
Samaritan Regional Health System	Ashland	Ohio	419-289-0491	www.samho.org
Sanford Medical Center Fargo	Fargo	North Dakota	701-234-2000	www.meritcare.com
Scottsdale Healthcare - Shea Medical Center	Scottsdale	Arizona	480-323-3009	www.shc.org
Sentara Leigh Hospital	Norfolk	Virginia	757-261-6601	www.sentara.com
Saint Joseph Hospital	Orange	California	714-633-9111	www.sjo.org
Saint Joseph Mercy Oakland	Pontiac	Michigan	248-858-3000	www.stjoesoakland.org
Sutter General Hospital	Sacramento	California	916-733-8999	www.suttermedicalcenter.org
The Orthopaedic Hospital of Lutheran Health Network	Fort Wayne	Indiana	260-435-2999	www.lutheranhealth.net
United Health Services Hospitals	Johnson City	New York	607-763-6000	www.vhs.ent
VHS Harlingen Hospital Company	Harlingen	Texas	956-389-1100	www.vbmc.org
Washington Hospital	Fremont	California	510-797-1111	www.whhs.com
Wythe County Community Hospital	Wytheville	Virginia	276-228-0200	www.wcch.org

Note: Table shows hospitals nationwide whose rate of readmission after hip/knee surgery is better (lower) than U.S. rate of 5.4%

Hospitals whose Rate of Readmission After Hip/Knee Surgery is Worse (Higher) than the U.S. National Rate

Hospital	City	State	Phone	Web Site
Abington Memorial Hospital	Abington	Pennsylvania	215-481-2000	www.amh.org
Advocate Christ Hospital & Medical Center	Oak Lawn	Illinois	708-684-8000	www.advocatehealth.com
Advocate Good Samaritan Hospital	Downers Grove	Illinois	630-275-5900	www.advocatehealth.com/gsam
Bayfront Health - Saint Petersburg	Saint Petersburg	Florida	727-823-1234	www.bayfront.org
Beaufort County Memorial Hospital	Beaufort	South Carolina	843-522-5200	www.bmhsc.org
Beaumont Health System	Royal Oak	Michigan	248-898-5000	www.beaumonthospitals.com
Centrastate Medical Center	Freehold	New Jersey	732-431-2000	www.centrastate.com
Christus Saint Michael Health System	Texarkana	Texas	903-614-1000	www.christusstmichael.org
Des Peres Hospital	Saint Louis	Missouri	314-966-9100	www.despereshospital.com
Doctors' Community Hospital	Lanham	Maryland	301-552-8085	www.dchweb.org
Enloe Medical Center	Chico	California	530-332-7300	www.enloe.org
Froedtert Memorial Lutheran Hospital	Milwaukee	Wisconsin	414-805-3000	www.froedtert.com
Galesburg Cottage Hospital	Galesburg	Illinois	309-345-4555	www.cottagehospital.com
Grant Medical Center	Columbus	Ohio	614-566-9978	www.ohiohealth.com
Jackson County Memorial Hospital	Altus	Oklahoma	580-379-5000	www.jcmh.com
Leesburg Regional Medical Center	Leesburg	Florida	352-323-5762	www.leesburgregional.org
Mercy Hospital Saint Louis	Saint Louis	Missouri	314-569-6000	www.stjohnsmercy.org
Mercy Saint Anne Hospital	Toledo	Ohio	419-407-2663	www.mercyweb.org
Minden Medical Center	Minden	Louisiana	318-377-2321	www.mindenmedicalcenter.com
Northwestern Memorial Hospital	Chicago	Illinois	312-926-2000	www.nmh.org
Orlando Health	Orlando	Florida	321-841-5111	www.orlandoregionalmedicalcenter.org
Parkwest Medical Center	Knoxville	Tennessee	865-970-9800	www.yesparkwest.com
Penn Presbyterian Medical Center	Philadelphia	Pennsylvania	215-662-8000	www.pennhealth.com
Pennsylvania Hospital of the Univ of PA Health Sys	Philadelphia	Pennsylvania	215-829-3000	www.pennmedicine.org/pahosp
Peterson Regional Medical Center	Kerrville	Texas	830-896-4200	www.petersonrmc.com
Providence Hospital	Washington	District of Columbia	202-269-7000	www.provhosp.org
Reston Hospital Center	Reston	Virginia	703-689-9000	www.restonhospital.com
Saint Agnes Hospital	Baltimore	Maryland	410-368-2101	www.stagnes.org
Saline Memorial Hospital	Benton	Arkansas	501-776-6000	www.salinememorial.org
Shannon Medical Center	San Angelo	Texas	325-653-6741	www.shannonhealth.com
Sinai Hospital of Baltimore	Baltimore	Maryland	410-601-5131	www.sinai-balt.com
Southside Regional Medical Center	Petersburg	Virginia	804-765-5000	www.srmconline.com
Saint Joseph Regional Health Center	Bryan	Texas	979-776-3912	www.st-joseph.org/sjrhc
Saint Joseph's Hospital	Tampa	Florida	813-870-4398	www.stjosephstampa.org
Thomas Jefferson University Hospital	Philadelphia	Pennsylvania	215-955-6000	www.jeffersonhospital.org
Wellmont Holston Valley Medical Center	Kingsport	Tennessee	423-224-4000	www.wellmont.org
Woodland Heights Medical Center	Lufkin	Texas	936-634-8311	www.woodlandheights.net

Note: Table shows hospitals nationwide whose rate of readmission after hip/knee surgery is better (lower) than U.S. rate of 5.4%

Hospitals whose Rate of Readmission After Discharge From Hospital (Hospital-wide) is Better (Lower) than the U.S. National Rate

Hospital	City	State	Phone	Web Site
Abbott Northwestern Hospital	Minneapolis	Minnesota	612-863-4509	www.abbottnorthwestern.com
Alegent Creighton Health Bergan Mercy Medical Center	Omaha	Nebraska	402-398-6060	www.alegent.com
Alexian Brothers Medical Center	Elk Grove Village	Illinois	847-437-5500	www.alexian.org
Alpena Regional Medical Center	Alpena	Michigan	989-356-7390	www.agh.org
Alta Bates Summit Medical Center	Oakland	California	510-655-4000	www.altabates.com
American Fork Hospital	American Fork	Utah	801-855-3305	www.ihc.com/facility/facilityresults.jsp
Anderson Regional Medical Center	Meridian	Mississippi	601-553-6000	www.jarmc.org
Appleton Medical Center	Appleton	Wisconsin	920-731-4101	www.thedacare.org
Arkansas Surgical Hospital	No Little Rock	Arkansas	501-748-8000	www.arksurgicalhospital.com
Asante Rogue Regional Medical Center	Medford	Oregon	541-789-7000	www.asante.org
Aspirus Wausau Hospital	Wausau	Wisconsin	715-847-2121	www.aspirus.org
Athens Regional Medical Center	Athens	Georgia	706-475-7000	www.armc.org
Augusta Health	Fishersville	Virginia	540-932-4000	www.augustamed.com
Aurora Lakeland Medical Center	Elkhorn	Wisconsin	262-741-2000	www.aurorahealthcare.org/facilities
Aurora Medical Center Manitowoc County	Two Rivers	Wisconsin	920-794-5000	www.aurorahealthcare.org
Aurora Medical Center Washington County	Hartford	Wisconsin	262-673-2300	www.aurorahealthcare.org
Aurora Saint Lukes Medical Center	Milwaukee	Wisconsin	414-649-6000	www.aurorahealthcare.org
Aurora West Allis Medical Center	West Allis	Wisconsin	414-328-6000	www.aurorahealthcare.org
Avera Mckennan Hospital & University Health Center	Sioux Falls	South Dakota	605-322-8000	www.mckennan.org
Avera Queen of Peace	Mitchell	South Dakota	605-995-2000	www.averaqueenofpeace.org
Avera Saint Lukes	Aberdeen	South Dakota	605-622-5000	www.averastlukes.org
Banner Good Samaritan Medical Center	Phoenix	Arizona	602-239-2000	www.bannerhealth.com
Baptist Health Louisville	Louisville	Kentucky	502-897-8100	www.baptisteast.com
Baptist Medical Center	San Antonio	Texas	210-297-1020	www.baptisthealthsystem.org
Baptist Memorial Hospital	Memphis	Tennessee	901-226-5000	www.bmhcc.org
Baptist Saint Anthony's Hospital	Amarillo	Texas	806-212-2000	www.bsahs.com
Baylor All Saints Medical Center at FW	Fort Worth	Texas	817-926-2544	www.baylorhealth.com/locations/allsaints
Baylor Medical Center at Garland	Garland	Texas	972-487-5000	www.baylorhealth.com
Baylor Medical Center at Irving	Irving	Texas	972-579-8100	www.baylorhealth.com
Baylor Regional Medical Center at Grapevine	Grapevine	Texas	817-481-1588	www.baylorhealth.com
Baylor University Medical Center	Dallas	Texas	214-820-0111	www.baylorhealth.com
Baystate Medical Center	Springfield	Massachusetts	413-794-0000	www.baystatehealth.com
Bellin Memorial Hospital	Green Bay	Wisconsin	920-433-3500	www.bellin.org
Billings Clinic Hospital	Billings	Montana	406-657-4000	www.billngsclinic.com
Blanchard Valley Hospital	Findlay	Ohio	419-423-4500	www.bvha.org
Bon Secours Maryview Medical Center	Portsmouth	Virginia	757-398-2200	www.bonsecourshamptonroads.com
Boone Hospital Center	Columbia	Missouri	573-815-8000	www.boone.org
Borgess Medical Center	Kalamazoo	Michigan	269-226-7000	www.borgess.com
Boulder Community Hospital	Boulder	Colorado	303-440-2273	www.bch.org
Bronson Methodist Hospital	Kalamazoo	Michigan	269-341-6000	www.bronsonhealth.com
Bryan Medical Center	Lincoln	Nebraska	402-481-1111	www.bryan.org
Caldwell Memorial Hospital	Lenoir	North Carolina	828-757-5100	www.caldwellmemorial.org
California Pacific Medical Center - Pacific Campus Hospital	San Francisco	California	415-600-6000	www.cpmc.org
Cape Cod Hospital	Hyannis	Massachusetts	508-771-1800	www.capecodhealth.org
Carolinas Medical Center - Pineville	Charlotte	North Carolina	704-379-5000	www.carolinashealthcare.org
Carondelet Saint Marys Hospital	Tucson	Arizona	520-872-3000	www.carondelet.org
Carondelet Saint Joseph's Hospital	Tucson	Arizona	520-873-3000	www.carondelet.org
Carteret General Hospital	Morehead City	North Carolina	252-808-6000	www.ccgh.org
Catawba Valley Medical Center	Hickory	North Carolina	828-326-3809	www.catawbavalleymc.org
Central Dupage Hospital	Winfield	Illinois	630-682-1600	www.cdh.org
Central Vermont Medical Center	Barre	Vermont	802-371-4100	www.cvmc.hitchcock.org
Central Washington Hospital	Wenatchee	Washington	509-662-1511	www.cwhs.com
Centura Health - Penrose Saint Francis Health Services	Colorado Springs	Colorado	719-776-5000	www.centurahealth.com
Centura Health - Saint Mary Corwin Medical Center	Pueblo	Colorado	719-557-4000	www.stmarycorwin.org
Chandler Regional Medical Center	Chandler	Arizona	480-963-4561	www.chandlerregional.com
Charlotte Hungerford Hospital	Torrington	Connecticut	860-496-6666	www.charlottesweb.hungerford.org
Cheyenne Regional Medical Center	Cheyenne	Wyoming	307-634-2273	www.crmcwy.org
Christus Health Shreveport - Bossier	Shreveport	Louisiana	318-681-5000	www.christusschumpert.org
Citizens Medical Center	Victoria	Texas	361-572-5113	www.citizensmedicalcenter.org
Citrus Memorial Hospital	Inverness	Florida	352-726-1551	www.citrusmh.com
CMC - Blue Ridge	Morganton	North Carolina	828-580-5000	www.gracehcs.org
Comanche County Memorial Hospital	Lawton	Oklahoma	580-355-8620	www.memorialhealthsource.org
Community Hospital of the Monterey Peninsula	Monterey	California	831-624-5311	www.chomp.org
Community Memorial Hospital San Buenaventura	Ventura	California	805-652-5011	www.cmhhospital.org
The Corpus Christi Medical Center	Corpus Christi	Texas	361-761-1501	www.ccmedicalcenter.com

Hospital	City	State	Phone	Web Site
Covenant Medical Center	Lubbock	Texas	806-725-6000	www.covenanthealth.org
Deaconess Hospital	Oklahoma City	Oklahoma	405-604-6109	www.deaconessokc.com
Dixie Regional Medical Center	Saint George	Utah	435-251-2100	www.intermountainhealthcare.org
Doctors Hospital of Sarasota	Sarasota	Florida	941-342-1100	www.doctorsofsarasota.com
Dominican Hospital	Santa Cruz	California	831-462-7700	www.dominicanhospital.org
East Jefferson General Hospital	Metairie	Louisiana	504-454-4000	www.eastjeffhospital.org
Eastern Idaho Regional Medical Center	Idaho Falls	Idaho	208-529-6111	www.eirmc.org
Eisenhower Medical Center	Rancho Mirage	California	760-340-3911	www.emc.org
Englewood Community Hospital	Englewood	Florida	941-475-6571	www.englewoodcommunityhospital.com
Ephrata Community Hospital	Ephrata	Pennsylvania	717-733-0311	www.ephratahospital.org
Evergreen Hospital Medical Center	Kirkland	Washington	425-899-1000	www.evergreenhospital.org
Exempla Lutheran Medical Center	Wheat Ridge	Colorado	303-425-4500	www.exemlpa.org
Fairview Southdale Hospital	Edina	Minnesota	952-924-5000	www.fairview.org
Falmouth Hospital	Falmouth	Massachusetts	508-548-5300	www.capecodhealth.com
Flagler Hospital	Saint Augustine	Florida	904-819-4426	www.flaglerhospital.com
Flagstaff Medical Center	Flagstaff	Arizona	928-773-2009	www.nahealth.com
Franciscan Saint Elizabeth Health - Lafayette East	Lafayette	Indiana	765-502-4334	www.ste.org
Freeman Health System - Freeman West	Joplin	Missouri	417-347-1111	www.freemanhealth.com
Genesis Medical Center - Davenport	Davenport	Iowa	563-421-1000	www.genesishealth.com
GHS Greenville Memorial Medical Center	Greenville	South Carolina	864-455-7000	www.ghs.org
Grand View Hospital	Sellersville	Pennsylvania	215-453-4615	www.gvh.org
Greater Baltimore Medical Center	Baltimore	Maryland	443-849-2000	www.gbmc.org
Gundersen Lutheran Medical Center	La Crosse	Wisconsin	608-782-7300	www.gundluth.org
Gwinnett Medical Center	Lawrenceville	Georgia	678-312-1000	www.gwinnettmedicalcenter.org
Harlingen Medical Center	Harlingen	Texas	956-365-1000	www.harlingenmedicalcenter.com
Harrison Memorial Center	Bremerton	Washington	360-377-3911	www.harrisonmedical.org
Hill Country Memorial Hospital	Fredericksburg	Texas	830-997-4353	www.hcmbs.org
Hinsdale Hospital	Hinsdale	Illinois	630-856-9000	www.keepingyouwell.com
Hoag Memorial Hospital Presbyterian	Newport Beach	California	949-645-8600	www.hoaghospital.org
Hoag Orthopedic Institute	Irvine	California	949-727-5000	www.orthopedichospital.com
Hospital For Special Surgery	New York	New York	212-606-1000	www.hss.edu
Huguley Memorial Medical Center	Burleson	Texas	817-568-5317	www.huguley.org
Huntington Memorial Hospital	Pasadena	California	626-397-5000	www.huntingtonhospital.com
Hutchinson Regional Medical Center	Hutchinson	Kansas	620-665-2001	www.hutchinsonhospital.com
Indian River Medical Center	Vero Beach	Florida	772-567-4311	www.irmh.com
Indiana University Health Ball Memorial Hospital	Muncie	Indiana	765-747-3111	www.accesschs.org/baal-memorial-l
Indiana University Health North Hospital	Carmel	Indiana	317-688-2000	www.iuhealth.org/north
Integris Baptist Medical Center	Oklahoma City	Oklahoma	405-951-8110	www.integris-health.com
Intermountain Medical Center	Murray	Utah	801-507-7000	www.intermountainhealthcare.org
Iowa Lutheran Hospital	Des Moines	Iowa	515-263-5612	www.ihsdesmoines.org
Iowa Methodist Medical Center	Des Moines	Iowa	515-241-6212	www.iowahealth.org
IU Health West Hospital	Avon	Indiana	317-217-3000	www.iuhealth.org/west
Jane Phillips Medical Center	Bartlesville	Oklahoma	918-333-7200	www.jpmc.org
John Muir Medical Center - Walnut Creek Campus	Walnut Creek	California	925-939-3000	www.jmmdhs.com
Kalispell Regional Medical Center	Kalispell	Montana	406-752-5111	www.krmc.org
Kaweah Delta Medical Center	Visalia	California	559-624-2000	www.kaweahdelta.org
Kenmore Mercy Hospital	Kenmore	New York	716-447-6100	www.chsbuffalo.org
Kettering Medical Center	Kettering	Ohio	937-298-4331	www.khnetwork.org
Kootenai Medical Center	Coeur D'alene	Idaho	208-625-4001	www.kootenaihealth.org
Lakeview Memorial Hospital	Stillwater	Minnesota	651-439-5330	www.lakeview.org
Lancaster General Hospital	Lancaster	Pennsylvania	717-299-5511	www.lancastergeneral.org
Lawrence & Memorial Hospital	New London	Connecticut	860-442-0711	www.lmhospital.org
Lawrence Memorial Hospital	Lawrence	Kansas	785-505-6100	www.lmh.org
Lehigh Valley Hospital	Allentown	Pennsylvania	610-402-2273	www.lvhhn.org
Lexington Medical Center	West Columbia	South Carolina	803-791-2000	www.lexmed.com
Lovelace Medical Center	Albuquerque	New Mexico	505-727-8000	www.lovelace.com
Mainegeneral Medical Center	Augusta	Maine	207-872-1000	www.mainegeneral.org
Margaret R Pardee Memorial Hospital	Hendersonville	North Carolina	828-696-1000	www.pardeehospital.org
Marian Regional Medical Center	Santa Maria	California	805-739-3000	www.marinmedicalcenter.org
Marion General Hospital	Marion	Indiana	765-660-6000	www.mgh.net
Marquette General Hospital	Marquette	Michigan	906-228-9440	www.mgh.org
Marshalltown Medical & Surgical Center	Marshalltown	Iowa	641-754-5151	www.everydaychampions.org
Mary Lanning Healthcare	Hastings	Nebraska	402-463-4521	www.marylanning.org
Maui Memorial Medical Center	Wailuku	Hawaii	808-442-5101	www.mauimemorialmedical.org
Mayo Clinic Health System - Eau Claire Hospital	Eau Claire	Wisconsin	715-838-3311	www.luthermidelfort.org
Mayo Clinic Hospital	Phoenix	Arizona	480-342-2000	www.mayoclinic.org
McBride Clinic Orthopedic Hospital	Oklahoma City	Oklahoma	405-478-1717	www.mcbrideclinic.com

Hospital	City	State	Phone	Web Site
McKay Dee Hospital	Ogden	Utah	801-387-2800	www.intermountainhealthcare.org
Mclaren - Northern Michigan	Petoskey	Michigan	231-487-4000	www.northernhealth.org
The Medical Center of Aurora	Aurora	Colorado	303-695-2600	www.auroramed.com
Medical City Dallas Hospital	Dallas	Texas	972-566-6222	www.medicalcityhospital.com
Medwest Haywood	Clyde	North Carolina	828-456-7311	www.haymed.org
Memorial Healthcare System	Chattanooga	Tennessee	423-495-2525	www.memorial.org
Memorial Hermann Hospital System	Houston	Texas	713-448-6796	www.memorialhermann.org
Memorial Hermann Memorial City Medical Center	Houston	Texas	713-242-3000	www.mhhs.org
Memorial Hospital & Health Care Center	Jasper	Indiana	812-996-2345	www.mhhcc.org
Memorial Hospital of South Bend	South Bend	Indiana	574-647-1000	www.qualityoflife.org
Memorial Medical Center of West Michigan	Ludington	Michigan	231-843-2591	www.mmcwm.com
Memorial Mission Hospital & Asheville Surgery Center	Asheville	North Carolina	828-213-1111	www.missionhospitals.org
Mercy General Hospital	Sacramento	California	916-453-4545	www.mercygeneral.org
Mercy Health Partners - Mercy Campus	Muskegon	Michigan	231-672-3901	www.mghp.com
Mercy Hospital	Iowa City	Iowa	319-339-0300	www.mercyiowacity.org
Mercy Hospital	Portland	Maine	207-879-3000	www.mercyhospital.com
Mercy Hospital	Buffalo	New York	716-826-7000	www.chsbuffalo.org
Mercy Hospital - Grayling	Grayling	Michigan	989-348-5461	www.mercygrayling.munsonhealthcare.org
Mercy Hospital Northwest Arkansas	Rogers	Arkansas	479-338-8000	www.mercy4u.com
Mercy Hospital Springfield	Springfield	Missouri	417-820-2000	www.stjohns.com
Mercy Medical Center	Canton	Ohio	330-489-1001	www.thequalityhospital.com
Mercy Medical Center	Roseburg	Oregon	541-673-0611	www.mercyrose.org
Mercy Medical Center - Redding	Redding	California	530-225-6102	www.redding.mercy.org
Mercy Medical Center - Des Moines	Des Moines	Iowa	515-247-3121	www.mercydesmoines.org
Meriter Hospital	Madison	Wisconsin	608-417-6000	www.meriter.com
Methodist Hospital	San Antonio	Texas	210-575-4000	www.mh.sahealth.com
Methodist Stone Oak Hospital	San Antonio	Texas	210-638-2100	www.stoneoakhealth.com
Methodist Sugar Land Hospital	Sugar Land	Texas	281-274-8000	www.methodisthealth.com/sugarland
Midland Memorial Hospital	Midland	Texas	432-685-1111	www.midland-memorial.com
Mills - Peninsula Medical Center	Burlingame	California	650-696-5270	www.mills-peninsula.org
Morristown Medical Center	Morristown	New Jersey	973-971-5450	www.morristownmemorialhospital.org
Morton Plant Hospital	Clearwater	Florida	727-462-7000	www.measehospitals.com
The Moses H Cone Memorial Hospital	Greensboro	North Carolina	336-832-7000	www.mosescone.com
Mother Frances Hospital	Tyler	Texas	903-593-8441	www.tmfhs.org
Munroe Regional Medical Center	Ocala	Florida	352-351-7200	www.munroeregional.com
Munson Medical Center	Traverse City	Michigan	231-935-5000	www.munsonhealthcare.org
Naples Community Hospital	Naples	Florida	239-436-5000	www.nchmd.org
Nebraska Heart Hospital	Lincoln	Nebraska	402-328-3000	www.neheart.com
New England Baptist Hospital	Boston	Massachusetts	617-754-5800	www.nebh.caregroup.org
New Hanover Regional Medical Center	Wilmington	North Carolina	910-343-7000	www.nhrmc.org
Newton Medical Center	Newton	Kansas	316-804-6001	www.newtonmedicalcenter.com
Norman Regional Health System	Norman	Oklahoma	405-321-1700	www.normanregional.com
North Memorial Medical Center	Robbinsdale	Minnesota	763-520-5200	www.northmemorial.com
North Shore Medical Center	Salem	Massachusetts	978-741-1215	www.nsmc.partners.org
Northside Hospital	Atlanta	Georgia	404-851-8000	www.northside.com
Northwest Community Hospital	Arlington Heights	Illinois	847-618-1000	www.nch.org
Northwest Hospital	Seattle	Washington	206-364-0500	www.nwhospital.org
Northwest Texas Hospital	Amarillo	Texas	806-354-1110	www.nxtexashealthcare.com
Novant Health Huntersville Medical Center	Huntersville	North Carolina	704-316-4000	www.presbyterian.org
Oklahoma Heart Hospital	Oklahoma City	Oklahoma	405-608-3200	www.okheart.com
Oklahoma Surgical Hospital	Tulsa	Oklahoma	918-477-5000	www.oklahomasurgicalhospital.com
Olympic Medical Center	Port Angeles	Washington	360-417-7000	www.olympicmedical.org
Our Lady of the Lake Regional Medical Center	Baton Rouge	Louisiana	225-765-6565	www.ololrmc.com
Overlake Hospital Medical Center	Bellevue	Washington	425-688-5000	www.overlakehospital.org
Owensboro Health Regional Hospital	Owensboro	Kentucky	270-688-2000	www.omhs.org
Palmetto Health Baptist	Columbia	South Carolina	803-296-5678	www.palmettohealth.org
Palmetto Health Richland	Columbia	South Carolina	803-296-5678	www.palmettohealth.org
Park Nicollet Methodist Hospital	Saint Louis Park	Minnesota	952-993-5000	www.parknicollet.com/methodist
Parkview Medical Center	Pueblo	Colorado	719-584-4000	www.parkviewmc.com
Parkview Regional Medical Center	Fort Wayne	Indiana	260-266-1000	www.parkview.com
Peacehealth Saint Joseph Medical Center	Bellingham	Washington	360-734-5400	www.peacehealth.org
Peninsula Regional Medical Center	Salisbury	Maryland	410-543-7111	www.peninsula.org
Penn Highlands Dubois	Dubois	Pennsylvania	814-371-2200	www.drmc.org
Petaluma Valley Hospital	Petaluma	California	707-778-1111	www.stjosephhealth.org
Phelps County Regional Medical Center	Rolla	Missouri	573-458-8899	www.rollanet.org/~pcrmc
Piedmont Fayette Hospital	Fayetteville	Georgia	770-719-7071	www.fayettehospital.org
Piedmont Hospital	Atlanta	Georgia	404-605-5000	www.piedmonthospital.org

Hospital	City	State	Phone	Web Site
Plaza Medical Center of Fort Worth	Fort Worth	Texas	817-336-2100	www.plazamedicalcenter.com
Porter Regional Hospital	Valparaiso	Indiana	219-983-8300	www.portermemorial.org
Portneuf Medical Center	Pocatello	Idaho	208-239-1000	www.portmed.org
Presbyterian Hospital	Albuquerque	New Mexico	505-724-8386	www.phs.org
Presbyterian Hospital Matthews	Matthews	North Carolina	704-384-6500	www.presbyterian.org
Providence Alaska Medical Center	Anchorage	Alaska	907-261-3675	www.providence.org
Providence Holy Family Hospital	Spokane	Washington	509-482-2450	www.holy-family.org
Providence Hospital	Mobile	Alabama	251-633-1000	www.providencehospital.org
Providence Regional Medical Center Everett	Everett	Washington	425-261-2000	www.providence.org
Providence Sacred Heart Medical Center	Spokane	Washington	509-474-3040	www.shmc.org
Providence Saint John's Health Center	Santa Monica	California	310-829-5511	www.stjohns.org
Providence Saint Mary Medical Center	Walla Walla	Washington	509-522-5900	www.smmc.com
Providence Saint Peter Hospital	Olympia	Washington	360-491-9480	www.providence.org/swsa
Providence Saint Vincent Medical Center	Portland	Oregon	503-216-1234	www.providence.org
Rapid City Regional Hospital	Rapid City	South Dakota	605-719-1000	www.rcrh.org
Reading Hospital	Reading	Pennsylvania	610-988-8000	www.readinghospital.org
Reid Hospital & Health Care Services	Richmond	Indiana	765-983-3000	www.reidhosp.com
Rex Hospital	Raleigh	North Carolina	919-784-3100	www.rexhealth.com
Roper Hospital	Charleston	South Carolina	843-724-2800	www.ropersaintfrancis.com
Sacred Heart Medical Center - Riverbend	Springfield	Oregon	541-222-7300	www.peacehealth.org/sacred-heart-riverbend
Saddleback Memorial Medical Center	Laguna Hills	California	949-837-4500	www.memorialcare.org/saddleback
Saint Barnabas Medical Center	Livingston	New Jersey	973-322-5000	www.saintbarnabas.com
Saint Elizabeth Regional Medical Center	Lincoln	Nebraska	402-219-7700	www.stelizabethonline.com
Saint Joseph Regional Medical Center	Mishawaka	Indiana	574-335-5000	www.sjmed.com
Saint Joseph's Hospital of Atlanta	Atlanta	Georgia	678-843-5720	www.stjosephsatlanta.org
Saint Mary's Health Care	Grand Rapids	Michigan	616-685-5000	www.smhealthcare.org
Saint Thomas West Hospital	Nashville	Tennessee	615-222-2111	www.stthomas.org
Saint Vincent Hospital	Erie	Pennsylvania	814-452-5000	www.svhs.org
Salem Hospital	Salem	Oregon	503-561-5200	www.salemhospital.org
Salem Regional Medical Center	Salem	Ohio	330-332-1551	www.salemhosp.com
Salina Regional Health Center	Salina	Kansas	785-452-7000	www.srhc.com
Salinas Valley Memorial Hospital	Salinas	California	831-757-4333	www.svmh.com
Samaritan Albany General Hospital	Albany	Oregon	541-812-4000	www.samhealth.org/shs_facilities
Sampson Regional Medical Center	Clinton	North Carolina	910-592-8511	www.sampsonrmc.org
San Jacinto Methodist Hospital	Baytown	Texas	281-420-8600	www.methodisthealth.com/sanjacinto
Sanford Bemidji Medical Center	Bemidji	Minnesota	218-751-5430	www.nchs.com
Sanford Medical Center Fargo	Fargo	North Dakota	701-234-2000	www.meritcare.com
Sanford Usd Medical Center	Sioux Falls	South Dakota	605-333-1000	www.sanfordhealth.org
Santa Barbara Cottage Hospital	Santa Barbara	California	805-682-7111	www.cottagehealthsystem.org
Santa Rosa Memorial Hospital	Santa Rosa	California	707-525-5300	www.stjosephhealth.org
Sarasota Memorial Hospital	Sarasota	Florida	941-917-9000	www.smh.com
Saratoga Hospital	Saratoga Springs	New York	518-587-3222	www.saratogacare.org
Scottsdale Healthcare Osborn Medical Center	Scottsdale	Arizona	480-882-4000	www.shc.org
Scottsdale Healthcare - Shea Medical Center	Scottsdale	Arizona	480-323-3009	www.shc.org
Scottsdale Healthcare - Thompson Peak Hospital	Scottsdale	Arizona	480-324-7004	www.shc.org
Scripps Memorial Hospital - Encinitas	Encinitas	California	760-753-6501	www.scripps.org
Sentara Williamsburg Regional Medical Center	Williamsburg	Virginia	757-984-6000	www.sentara.com
Sequoia Hospital	Redwood City	California	650-367-5551	www.sequoiahospital.org
Seven Rivers Regional Medical Center	Crystal River	Florida	352-795-6560	www.srrmc.com
Sisters of Charity Providence Hospitals	Columbia	South Carolina	803-256-5300	www.providencehospitals.com
Sky Lakes Medical Center	Klamath Falls	Oregon	541-274-6150	www.skylakes.org
Sky Ridge Medical Center	Lone Tree	Colorado	720-225-1000	www.skyridgemedcenter.com
Sonoma Valley Hospital	Sonoma	California	707-935-5000	www.svh.com
Sonora Regional Medical Center	Sonora	California	209-532-3161	www.sonorahospital.org
South Lake Hospital	Clermont	Florida	352-394-4071	www.southlakehospital.com
Spartanburg Regional Medical Center	Spartanburg	South Carolina	864-560-6000	www.srhs.com
Spectrum Health - Butterworth Campus	Grand Rapids	Michigan	616-391-1774	www.spectrum-health.org
Saint Agnes Hospital	Fond Du Lac	Wisconsin	920-929-2300	www.agnesian.com
Saint Alexius Medical Center	Bismarck	North Dakota	701-530-7000	www.st.alexius.org
Saint Alphonsus Regional Medical Center	Boise	Idaho	208-367-2121	www.saintalphonsus.org
Saint Bernardine Medical Center	San Bernardino	California	909-881-4440	www.stbernardinemedicalcenter.com
Saint Charles Medical Center - Bend	Bend	Oregon	541-382-4321	www.scmc.org
Saint David's Medical Center	Austin	Texas	512-476-7111	www.stdavidsrehab.com
Saint Edward Mercy Medical Center	Fort Smith	Arkansas	479-314-6000	www.stedwardmercy.com
Saint Francis Hospital	Columbus	Georgia	706-596-4020	www.wecareforlife.com
Saint Francis Hospital - Roslyn	Roslyn	New York	516-562-6000	www.stfrancisheartcenter.com
Saint Francis Medical Center	Grand Island	Nebraska	308-384-4600	www.saintfrancisgi.org

Hospital	City	State	Phone	Web Site
Saint Francis - Downtown	Greenville	South Carolina	864-255-1000	www.stfrancishealth.org
Saint Joseph Hospital	Eureka	California	707-445-8121	www.stjosepheureka.org
Saint Joseph Hospital & Health Center	Kokomo	Indiana	765-456-5300	www.stvincent.org
Saint Joseph Medical Center	Reading	Pennsylvania	610-378-2300	www.sjmcberks.org
Saint Joseph Regional Medical Center	Lewiston	Idaho	208-743-2511	www.sjrmc.org
Saint Luke's Regional Medical Center	Boise	Idaho	208-381-2222	www.slrmc.org
Saint Luke's Hospital	Cedar Rapids	Iowa	319-369-7211	www.crstlukes.com
Saint Luke's Hospital	Duluth	Minnesota	218-249-5555	www.slhduluth.com
Saint Marks Hospital	Salt Lake City	Utah	801-268-7700	www.stmarkshospital.com
Saint Mary's Regional Medical Center	Enid	Oklahoma	580-233-6100	www.stmarysregional.com
Saint Marys Hospital	Madison	Wisconsin	608-251-6100	www.stmarysmadison.com
Saint Marys Hospital & Medical Center	Grand Junction	Colorado	970-298-1950	www.stmarygj.org
Saint Marys Regional Medical Center	Lewiston	Maine	207-777-8100	www.stmarysmaine.com
Saint Patrick Hospital	Missoula	Montana	406-543-7271	www.saintpatrick.org
Saint Peter's Hospital	Albany	New York	518-525-1550	www.stpetershealthcare.org
Saint Rose Dominican Hospitals - Siena Campus	Henderson	Nevada	702-616-5000	www.strosehospitals.org
Saint Vincent Heart Center of Indiana	Indianapolis	Indiana	317-583-5000	www.theheartcenter.com
Saint Vincent Hospital	Green Bay	Wisconsin	920-433-0111	www.stvincenthospital.org
Saint Vincent Hospital & Health Services	Indianapolis	Indiana	317-338-7000	www.indianapolis.stvincent.org
Sutter Auburn Faith Hospital	Auburn	California	530-888-4500	www.sutterauburnfaith.org
Sutter Roseville Medical Center	Roseville	California	916-781-1000	www.sutterroseville.org
Tallahassee Memorial Hospital	Tallahassee	Florida	850-431-1155	www.tmh.org
Tennova Healthcare	Knoxville	Tennessee	865-545-8000	www.stmaryshealth.com
Texas Health Harris Methodist Fort Worth	Fort Worth	Texas	817-250-2100	www.texashealth.org
Texas Health Presbyterian Hospital Plano	Plano	Texas	972-981-8000	www.presbyplano.org
Texas Health Presbyterian Hospital - WNJ	Sherman	Texas	903-870-4611	www.wnj.org
Texas Orthopedic Hospital	Houston	Texas	713-799-8600	www.texasorthopedic.com
The Queens Medical Center	Honolulu	Hawaii	808-538-9011	www.queens.org
The Toledo Hospital	Toledo	Ohio	419-291-7463	www.promedica.org
Touro Infirmary	New Orleans	Louisiana	504-897-7011	www.touro.com
United Hospital	Saint Paul	Minnesota	651-241-8802	www.allinahealth.org/ahs/united.nsf
University Colo Health Memorial Hospital Central	Colorado Springs	Colorado	719-365-5000	www.memorialhospital.com
University of Wisconsin Hospitals & Clinics Authority	Madison	Wisconsin	608-263-8991	www.uwhealth.org
UPMC Altoona	Altoona	Pennsylvania	814-889-2011	www.altoonaregional.org
UPMC Hamot	Erie	Pennsylvania	814-877-6000	www.hamot.org
Utah Valley Regional Medical Center	Provo	Utah	801-373-7850	www.intermountainhealthcare.org/hospitals/uvrmc
Venice Regional Medical Center - Bayfront Health	Venice	Florida	941-485-7711	www.veniceregional.com
VHS Harlingen Hospital Company	Harlingen	Texas	956-389-1100	www.vbmc.org
Via Christi Hospital Pittsburg	Pittsburg	Kansas	620-231-6100	www.via-christi.org
Via Christi Hospitals Wichita	Wichita	Kansas	316-268-5000	www.via-christi.org
Wakemed - Raleigh Campus	Raleigh	North Carolina	919-350-8000	www.wakemed.org
Wentworth - Douglass Hospital	Dover	New Hampshire	603-740-2580	www.wdhospital.com
Wesley Medical Center	Wichita	Kansas	316-962-2000	www.wesleymc.com
West Calcasieu Cameron Hospital	Sulphur	Louisiana	337-527-7034	www.wcch.com
West Shore Medical Center	Manistee	Michigan	231-398-1000	www.westshoremedcenter.org
Williamsport Regional Medical Center	Williamsport	Pennsylvania	570-321-1000	www.susquehannahealth.org
Willis Knighton Medical Center	Shreveport	Louisiana	318-212-4000	www.wkhs.com//locations/medicalcenter.aspx
Woodland Heights Medical Center	Lufkin	Texas	936-634-8311	www.woodlandheights.net
Wooster Community Hospital	Wooster	Ohio	330-263-8100	www.woosterhospital.org

Note: Table shows hospitals nationwide whose rate of readmission after discharge from hospital (hospital-wide) is better (lower) than U.S. rate of 16.0%

Hospitals whose Rate of Readmission After Discharge From Hospital (Hospital-wide) is Worse (Higher) than the U.S. National Rate

Hospital	City	State	Phone	Web Site
Adena Regional Medical Center	Chillicothe	Ohio	740-779-7500	www.adena.org
Advocate Christ Hospital & Medical Center	Oak Lawn	Illinois	708-684-8000	www.advocatehealth.com
Advocate Illinois Masonic Medical Center	Chicago	Illinois	773-975-1600	www.advocatehealth.com/immc
Advocate Trinity Hospital	Chicago	Illinois	773-967-2000	www.advocatehealth.com/trin
Albert Einstein Medical Center	Philadelphia	Pennsylvania	215-456-6090	www.einstein.edu
Anne Arundel Medical Center	Annapolis	Maryland	443-481-1307	www.aahs.org
Aria Health	Philadelphia	Pennsylvania	215-612-4129	www.ariahealth.com
Arkansas Methodist Medical Center	Paragould	Arkansas	870-239-7000	www.arkansasmethodist.org
Atlanticare Regional Medical Center	Atlantic City	New Jersey	609-441-8020	www.atlanticare.org/acmc/index.html
Aventura Hospital & Medical Center	Aventura	Florida	305-682-7000	www.aventurahospital.com
B R F Hospital Holdings	Shreveport	Louisiana	318-675-5000	www.lsumc.edu
Banner Desert Medical Center	Mesa	Arizona	480-412-3000	www.bannerhealth.com
Baptist Beaumont Hospital	Beaumont	Texas	409-212-5012	www.mhbh.org
Baptist Memorial Hospital Desoto	Southaven	Mississippi	662-772-4000	www.bmhcc.org/facilities/desoto
Barnes-Jewish Hospital	Saint Louis	Missouri	314-747-3000	www.barnesjewish.org
Baxter Regional Medical Center	Mountain Home	Arkansas	870-508-1000	www.baxterregional.org
Beaumont Health System	Grosse Pointe	Michigan	313-343-1000	www.beaumonthospitals.com
Beaumont Health System	Royal Oak	Michigan	248-898-5000	www.beaumonthospitals.com
Beckley ARH Hospital	Beckley	West Virginia	304-255-3456	www.arh.org/beckley
Bellevue Hospital Center	New York	New York	212-561-4132	www.nyc.gov/html/hhc/html/facilities/bellevue.shtml
Beth Israel Deaconess Hospital - Milton	Milton	Massachusetts	617-696-4600	www.miltonhosital.org
Beth Israel Deaconess Medical Center	Boston	Massachusetts	617-667-7000	www.bidmc.harvard.edu
Beth Israel Medical Center	New York	New York	212-420-2000	www.wehealny.org
Bluefield Regional Medical Center	Bluefield	West Virginia	304-327-1100	www.bluefield.org
Bolivar Medical Center	Cleveland	Mississippi	662-846-2551	www.bolivarmedical.com
Boston Medical Center Corporation	Boston	Massachusetts	617-638-8000	www.bmc.org
Botsford Hospital	Farmington Hills	Michigan	248-471-8000	www.botsfordsystem.org
Bridgeport Hospital	Bridgeport	Connecticut	203-384-3000	www.bridgeporthospital.com
Brigham & Women's Faulkner Hospital	Boston	Massachusetts	617-983-7000	www.brighamandwomensfaulkner.org
Brigham & Women's Hospital	Boston	Massachusetts	617-732-5500	www.brighamandwomens.org
Bronx - Lebanon Hospital Center	Bronx	New York	212-588-7000	www.bronx-leb.org
Brookdale Hospital Medical Center	Brooklyn	New York	718-240-5966	www.brookdalehospital.org
Brookhaven Memorial Hospital Medical Center	Patchogue	New York	631-654-7100	www.brookhavenhospitalorg
Brooklyn Hospital Center at Downtown Campus	Brooklyn	New York	718-250-8000	www.tbh.org
Byrd Regional Hospital	Leesville	Louisiana	337-239-9041	www.chs.net
California Hospital Medical Center Los Angeles	Los Angeles	California	213-748-2411	www.chmcla.org
Camden Clark Medical Center	Parkersburg	West Virginia	304-424-2111	www.ccmh.org
Capital Health System - Fuld Campus	Trenton	New Jersey	609-394-6000	www.capitalhealth.org
Capital Regional Medical Center	Tallahassee	Florida	850-656-5000	www.capitalregionalmedicalcenter.com
Carepoint Health - Christ Hospital	Jersey City	New Jersey	201-795-8200	www.christhospital.org
Carepoint Health - Hoboken UMC	Hoboken	New Jersey	201-418-1004	www.bonsecoursnj.com
Carolinas Hospital System	Florence	South Carolina	843-674-2500	www.carolinashospital.com
Casey County Hospital	Liberty	Kentucky	606-787-6275	
Catskill Regional Medical Center	Harris	New York	845-794-3300	www.crmcny.org
Chambers Memorial Hospital	Danville	Arkansas	479-495-2241	www.chambershospital.com
Chesapeake General Hospital	Chesapeake	Virginia	757-312-8121	www.chesapeakehealth.com
Clay County Hospital	Flora	Illinois	618-662-2131	www.claycountyhospital.org
Cleveland Clinic	Cleveland	Ohio	216-444-2200	www.clevelandclinic.org
Cleveland Clinic Hospital	Weston	Florida	954-689-5000	www.clevelandclinic.org
Clinch Valley Medical Center	Richlands	Virginia	276-596-6000	www.clinchvalleymedicalcenter.com
Coffee Regional Medical Center	Douglas	Georgia	229-384-1900	www.coffeeregional.org
Coliseum Medical Center	Macon	Georgia	478-765-4100	www.coliseumhealthsystem.com
Community Regional Medical Center	Fresno	California	559-459-6000	www.communitymedical.org
Conemaugh Valley Memorial Hospital	Johnstown	Pennsylvania	814-534-9000	www.conemaugh.org
Coney Island Hospital	Brooklyn	New York	718-616-3000	www.coneyislandhospital.com
Cooper University Hospital	Camden	New Jersey	856-342-2000	www.cooperhealth.org
Covenant Medical Center	Saginaw	Michigan	989-583-4000	www.covenanthealthcare.com
Crittenden Health System	Marion	Kentucky	270-965-5281	www.crittenden-health.org
Danville Regional Medical Center	Danville	Virginia	434-799-2100	www.danvilleregional.org
Davis Memorial Hospital	Elkins	West Virginia	304-636-3300	www.davishealthcare.org
Desert Valley Hospital	Victorville	California	760-241-8000	www.dvmc.com
Desoto Memorial Hospital	Arcadia	Florida	863-494-3535	www.dmh.org
Detroit Receiving Hospital & University Health Center	Detroit	Michigan	313-745-3104	www.drhuhc.org
Doctors Hospital	Columbus	Ohio	614-544-1000	www.columbusregional.com
Doctors Hospital of Manteca	Manteca	California	209-823-3111	www.doctorsmanteca.com

Hospital	City	State	Phone	Web Site
Drew Memorial Hospital	Monticello	Arkansas	870-367-2411	www.drewmemorial.org
Duke University Hospital	Durham	North Carolina	919-684-8111	www.dukehealth.org
Dyersburg Regional Medical Center	Dyersburg	Tennessee	731-285-2410	www.dyersburgregionalmc.com
East Georgia Regional Medical Center	Statesboro	Georgia	912-486-1500	www.egrmc.com
East Ohio Regional Hospital	Martins Ferry	Ohio	740-633-4151	www.eastohioregionalhospital.com
East Orange General Hospital	East Orange	New Jersey	973-266-4401	www.evh.org
Eastern Niagara Hospital	Lockport	New York	716-514-5700	www.enhs.org
Eastern State Hospital	Williamsburg	Virginia	757-253-5161	www.ehs.dmhmrsas.virginia.gov
Easton Hospital	Easton	Pennsylvania	610-250-4076	www.easton-hospital.com
Elmhurst Hospital Center	Elmhurst	New York	718-334-1141	www.nyc.gov
Emanuel Medical Center	Turlock	California	209-667-4200	www.emanuelmedicalcenter.org
Excela Health Frick Hospital	Mount Pleasant	Pennsylvania	724-547-1500	www.excelahealth.org
Fauquier Hospital	Warrenton	Virginia	540-316-5000	www.fauquierhospital.org
Fayette County Hospital	Vandalia	Illinois	618-283-1231	www.fayettecountyhospital.org
Fitzgibbon Hospital	Marshall	Missouri	660-886-7431	www.fitzgibbon.org
Florida Hospital	Orlando	Florida	407-303-1976	www.floridahospital.com
Flushing Hospital Medical Center	Flushing	New York	718-670-5000	www.flushinghospital.org
Forest Hills Hospital	Forest Hills	New York	718-830-4000	www.northshorelij.com
Franciscan Saint James Health	Olympia Fields	Illinois	708-747-4000	www.franciscanalliance.org
Franciscan Saint Margaret Health - Hammond	Hammond	Indiana	219-932-2300	www.smmhc.com
Franklin Hospital	Valley Stream	New York	516-256-6000	www.northshorelij.com
Frederick Memorial Hospital	Frederick	Maryland	240-566-3300	www.fmh.org
Garden City Hospital	Garden City	Michigan	734-421-3300	www.gchosp.org
Gateway Medical Center	Clarksville	Tennessee	931-502-1000	www.todaysgateway.com
Genesis Healthcare System	Zanesville	Ohio	740-454-5000	www.genesishcs.org
George Washington Univ Hospital	Washington	District of Columbia	202-716-4605	www.gwhospital.com
Glenwood Regional Medical Center	West Monroe	Louisiana	318-329-4600	www.grmc.com
Good Samaritan Hospital of Suffern	Suffern	New York	914-368-5000	www.goodsamhosp.org
Grant Medical Center	Columbus	Ohio	614-566-9978	www.ohiohealth.com
Great River Medical Center	Blytheville	Arkansas	870-838-7300	www.greatrivermc.com
Harlan Appalachian Regional Healthcare Hospital	Harlan	Kentucky	606-573-8100	www.arh.org
Harlem Hospital Center	New York	New York	212-491-8400	www.nyc.gov/hhc
Harper University Hospital	Detroit	Michigan	313-745-6211	www.harperhospital.org
Harris Hospital	Newport	Arkansas	870-523-8911	www.harrishospital.com
Harton Regional Medical Center	Tullahoma	Tennessee	931-393-3000	www.hartonmedicalcenter.com
Hazard ARH Regional Medical Center	Hazard	Kentucky	606-439-6600	www.arh.org/hazard
Health Alliance Hospital Broadway Campus	Kingston	New York	914-331-3131	www.kingstonregionalhealth.org
Henry Ford Hospital	Detroit	Michigan	313-916-2600	www.henryfordhospital.com
Hialeah Hospital	Hialeah	Florida	305-693-6100	www.hialeahhosp.com
Highlands Regional Medical Center	Prestonsburg	Kentucky	606-886-8511	www.hrmc.org
Hollywood Presbyterian Medical Center	Los Angeles	California	213-413-3000	www.qahpmc.com
Holy Cross Hospital	Chicago	Illinois	773-471-8000	www.holycrosshospital.org
Holzer Medical Center	Gallipolis	Ohio	740-446-5000	www.holzer.org
Hospital of Univ of Pennsylvania	Philadelphia	Pennsylvania	215-662-3227	www.upenn.edu
Howard University Hospital	Washington	District of Columbia	202-745-6100	www.huhosp.org
Hudson Valley Hospital Center	Cortlandt Manor	New York	914-734-3611	www.hvhc.org
Illinois Valley Community Hospital	Peru	Illinois	815-223-3300	www.ivch.org
Ingalls Memorial Hospital	Harvey	Illinois	708-333-2300	www.ingalls.org
Jackson Memorial Hospital	Miami	Florida	305-585-1111	www.jhsmiami.org
Jackson Parish Hospital	Jonesboro	Louisiana	318-259-4435	www.jacksonparishhospital.com
Jackson Park Hospital	Chicago	Illinois	773-947-7500	www.jacksonparkhospital.org
Jacobi Medical Center	Bronx	New York	718-918-5000	www.ci.nyc.ny.us/html/hhc
Jamaica Hospital Medical Center	Jamaica	New York	718-262-6000	www.jamaicahospital.org
Jane Todd Crawford Hospital	Greensburg	Kentucky	270-932-4211	
Jeanes Hospital	Philadelphia	Pennsylvania	215-728-2000	www.jeanes.com
Jennie Stuart Medical Center	Hopkinsville	Kentucky	270-887-0100	www.jsmc.org
Jennings American Legion Hospital	Jennings	Louisiana	337-616-7000	www.jalh.com
JFK Medical Center	Atlantis	Florida	561-965-7300	www.jfkmc.com
JFK Medical Center - A M Yelencsics Comm Hospital	Edison	New Jersey	732-321-7000	www.jfkmc.org
John H Stroger Jr Hospital	Chicago	Illinois	312-864-6000	www.cookcountygov.com
Johns Hopkins Bayview Medical Center	Baltimore	Maryland	410-550-0123	www.hopkinsbayview.org
The Johns Hopkins Hospital	Baltimore	Maryland	410-955-9540	www.jhmi.edu
Johnson City Medical Center	Johnson City	Tennessee	423-431-6111	www.msha.com
Kendall Regional Medical Center	Miami	Florida	305-223-3000	www.kendallmed.com
Kennedy University Hospital - Stratford Div	Stratford	New Jersey	856-346-6000	www.kennedyhealth.org
Kent County Memorial Hospital	Warwick	Rhode Island	401-737-7000	www.kentri.org
Kentucky River Medical Center	Jackson	Kentucky	606-666-6000	www.kentuckyrivermc.com

Hospital	City	State	Phone	Web Site
King's Daughters' Medical Center	Ashland	Kentucky	606-408-4000	www.kdmc.com
Kings County Hospital Center	Brooklyn	New York	718-245-3901	www.nyc.gov/html/hhc/html/facilities/kings.shtml
Kingsbrook Jewish Medical Center	Brooklyn	New York	718-604-5789	www.kingsbrook.org
Knox County Hospital	Barbourville	Kentucky	606-546-4175	www.knoxcohospital.com
Lahey Hospital & Medical Center - Burlington	Burlington	Massachusetts	781-744-5100	www.lahey.org
Lake Pointe Medical Center	Rowlett	Texas	972-412-2273	www.lakepointemedical.com
Lake Wales Medical Center	Lake Wales	Florida	863-676-1433	www.lakewalesmedicalcenter.com
Larkin Community Hospital	South Miami	Florida	305-284-7500	www.larkinhospital.com
Laurel Regional Medical Center	Laurel	Maryland	301-725-4300	www.laurelregionalhospital.org
Lawrence Hospital Center	Bronxville	New York	914-787-1000	www.lawrencehealth.org
Leesburg Regional Medical Center	Leesburg	Florida	352-323-5762	www.leesburgregional.org
Lenox Hill Hospital	New York	New York	212-439-2345	www.lenoxhillhospital.org
Lewisgale Hospital Pulaski	Pulaski	Virginia	540-994-8100	www.lewisgale.com
Libertyhealth - Jersey City Medical Center Campus	Jersey City	New Jersey	201-915-2000	www.libertyhcs.org
Lincoln Medical & Mental Health Center	Bronx	New York	718-579-5000	www.nyc.gov/html/hhc/lincoln
Little Company of Mary Hospital	Evergreen Park	Illinois	708-422-6200	www.lcmh.org
Long Island Jewish Medical Center	New Hyde Park	New York	718-470-7000	www.northshorelij.com
Lowell General Hospital	Lowell	Massachusetts	978-937-6000	www.lowellgeneral.org
Loyola University Medical Center	Maywood	Illinois	708-216-9000	www.lumc.edu
Lutheran Medical Center	Brooklyn	New York	718-630-8000	www.lmcmc.com
Maimonides Medical Center	Brooklyn	New York	718-283-6000	www.maimonidesmed.org
Mary Immaculate Hospital	Newport News	Virginia	757-886-6000	www.bonsecourshamptonroad.com
Medical Center of Southeastern Oklahoma	Durant	Oklahoma	405-924-3080	www.mcsohealth.com
Medical College of Georgia Hospitals & Clinics	Augusta	Georgia	706-721-6569	www.mcghealth.org
Medical College of Virginia Hospitals	Richmond	Virginia	804-828-0938	www.vcuhealth.org
Medstar Good Samaritan Hospital	Baltimore	Maryland	443-444-3902	www.goodsam-md.org
Medstar Montgomery Medical Center	Olney	Maryland	301-774-8882	www.montgomerygeneral.com
Memorial Hospital	Manchester	Kentucky	606-598-5104	www.manchestermemorial.com
Memorial Hospital	Nacogdoches	Texas	936-564-4611	www.nacmem.org
Memorial Hospital of Gardena	Gardena	California	310-532-4200	www.avantihospitals.com
Memorial Hospital of Salem County	Salem	New Jersey	856-935-1000	www.mhshealth.com
Memorial Hospital of Stilwell	Stilwell	Oklahoma	918-696-3101	www.stilwellmemorialhospital.com
Memorial Regional Hospital	Hollywood	Florida	954-987-2000	www.memorialregional.com
Mercy Fitzgerald Hospital	Darby	Pennsylvania	215-237-4000	www.mercyhealth.org
Mercy Hospital & Medical Center	Chicago	Illinois	312-567-2000	www.mercy-chicago.org
Mercy Hospital Anderson	Cincinnati	Ohio	513-624-4006	www.e-mercy.com/mercy-hospital-anderson.aspx
Mercy Hospital Fairfield	Fairfield	Ohio	513-870-7197	www.e-mercy.com/mercy-hospital-fairfield.aspx
Mercy Hospital Jefferson	Crystal City	Missouri	636-933-1000	www.jeffersonmemorial.org
Mercy Medical Center	Baltimore	Maryland	410-332-9237	www.mdmercy.com
Mercy Regional Medical Center	Ville Platte	Louisiana	337-363-5684	www.vpmc.com
Methodist Hospital	Henderson	Kentucky	270-827-7700	www.methodisthospital.net
Methodist Hospitals	Gary	Indiana	219-886-4642	www.methodisthospital.org
Metrosouth Medical Center	Blue Island	Illinois	708-597-2000	www.stfrancisblueisland.com
Middlesboro Appalachian Regional Healthcare Hospital	Middlesboro	Kentucky	606-242-1101	www.arh.org/middlesboro
Midwest Regional Medical Center	Midwest City	Oklahoma	405-610-8530	www.midwestregional.com
Milford Regional Medical Center	Milford	Massachusetts	508-473-1190	www.milfordregional.org
Miriam Hospital	Providence	Rhode Island	401-793-2500	www.lifespan.org/partners/tmh
Mission Regional Medical Center	Mission	Texas	956-323-9000	www.missionhospital.org
Monmouth Medical Center - Southern Campus	Lakewood	New Jersey	732-363-1900	www.sbhcs.com
Monroe County Medical Center	Tompkinsville	Kentucky	270-487-9231	www.mcmccares.com
Montefiore Medical Center	Bronx	New York	718-920-4321	www.montefiore.org
Montefiore New Rochelle Hospital	New Rochelle	New York	914-632-5000	www.ssmc.org
Morgan County ARH Hospital	West Liberty	Kentucky	606-743-3186	www.arh.org/morgan
Morton Hospital	Taunton	Massachusetts	508-828-7000	www.mortonhospital.org
Mountainview Hospital	Las Vegas	Nevada	702-255-5065	www.mountainview-hospital.com
Musc Medical Center	Charleston	South Carolina	843-792-2300	www.musc.edu
Nacogdoches Medical Center	Nacogdoches	Texas	936-569-9481	www.nacmedicalcenter.com
Nassau University Medical Center	East Meadow	New York	516-572-0123	www.numc.edu
Natchez Community Hospital	Natchez	Mississippi	601-445-6205	www.natchezcommunityhospital.com
Nazareth Hospital	Philadelphia	Pennsylvania	215-335-6000	www.nazarethhospital.org
New York Community Hospital of Brooklyn	Brooklyn	New York	718-692-5302	www.nych.com
New York Hospital Medical Center of Queens	Flushing	New York	718-670-1231	www.nyhq.org
New York Methodist Hospital	Brooklyn	New York	718-780-3000	www.nym.org
New York - Presbyterian Hospital	New York	New York	212-746-4189	www.nyp.org
Newark Beth Israel Medical Center	Newark	New Jersey	973-926-7850	www.sbhcs.com
North Oaks Medical Center	Hammond	Louisiana	985-345-2700	www.northoaks.org
North Shore University Hospital	Manhasset	New York	516-562-0100	www.northshorelij.com

Hospital	City	State	Phone	Web Site
Northside Hospital	Saint Petersburg	Florida	813-521-5000	www.northsidehospital.com
Northwest Hospital Center	Randallstown	Maryland	410-521-5995	www.lifebridgehealth.org
Northwest Mississippi Regional Medical Center	Clarksdale	Mississippi	662-627-3211	www.nwmsregionalmedcenter.com
Northwestern Memorial Hospital	Chicago	Illinois	312-926-2000	www.nmh.org
Norwegian - American Hospital	Chicago	Illinois	773-292-8200	www.nahospital.org
Nyack Hospital	Nyack	New York	845-348-2000	www.nyackhospital.org
NYU Hospitals Center	New York	New York	212-263-7300	www.med.nyu.edu
Oakwood Hospital - Dearborn	Dearborn	Michigan	313-593-7125	www.oakwood.org
Oakwood Hospital - Taylor	Taylor	Michigan	313-295-5253	www.oakwod.org
Oakwood Hospital - Wayne	Wayne	Michigan	734-467-4175	www.oakwood.org
Ohio State University Hospitals	Columbus	Ohio	614-293-9700	www.jamesline.com
Olympia Medical Center	Los Angeles	California	310-657-5900	www.olympiamc.com
Orange Regional Medical Center	Middletown	New York	845-343-2424	www.ormc.org
Oroville Hospital	Oroville	California	530-533-8500	www.orovillehospital.com
Osceola Regional Medical Center	Kissimmee	Florida	407-846-2266	www.osceolaregional.com
Pacifica Hospital of the Valley	Sun Valley	California	818-767-3310	www.pacificahospital.com
Palisades Medical Center	North Bergen	New Jersey	201-854-5000	www.palisadesmedical.org
Palm Springs General Hospital	Hialeah	Florida	305-558-2500	www.psghosp.com
Palmetto General Hospital	Hialeah	Florida	305-823-5000	www.palmettogeneral.com
Palms West Hospital	Loxahatchee	Florida	561-753-4245	www.palmswesthospital.com
Peacehealth Southwest Medical Center	Vancouver	Washington	360-256-2000	www.swmedicalcenter.org
Peconic Bay Medical Center	Riverhead	New York	631-548-6000	www.pbmedicalcenter.org
Pekin Memorial Hospital	Pekin	Illinois	309-347-1151	www.pekinhospital.org
Pennsylvania Hospital of the Univ of PA Health Sys	Philadelphia	Pennsylvania	215-829-3000	www.pennmedicine.org/pahosp
Perry Community Hospital	Linden	Tennessee	931-589-2121	
Pineville Community Hospital	Pineville	Kentucky	606-337-3051	www.pinevillehospital.com
Poplar Bluff Regional Medical Center	Poplar Bluff	Missouri	573-785-7721	www.poplarbluffregional.com
Pottstown Memorial Medical Center	Pottstown	Pennsylvania	610-327-7000	www.pmmctr.org
Presence Saint Francis Hospital	Evanston	Illinois	847-316-4000	www.reshealth.org
Presence Saint Joseph Hospital - Chicago	Chicago	Illinois	773-665-3000	www.res-health.org
Presence Saint Joseph Medical Center	Joliet	Illinois	815-725-7133	www.provena.org/stjoes
Presence Saints Mary & Elizabeth Medical Center	Chicago	Illinois	312-770-2000	www.reshealth.org
Presence Saint Marys Hospital	Kankakee	Illinois	815-937-2490	www.provenastmarys.com
Presence United Samaritans Medical Center	Danville	Illinois	217-443-5000	www.provena.org/usmc
Providence Hospital	Washington	District of Columbia	202-269-7000	www.provhosp.org
Providence Hospital & Medical Centers	Southfield	Michigan	248-849-3011	www.stjohn.org/providence
Queens Hospital Center	Jamaica	New York	718-883-3000	www.nyc.gov/html/hhc/qhn/home.html
Raleigh General Hospital	Beckley	West Virginia	304-256-4100	www.raleighgeneral.com
Raritan Bay Medical Center	Perth Amboy	New Jersey	732-442-3700	www.rbmc.org
Reston Hospital Center	Reston	Virginia	703-689-9000	www.restonhospital.com
Rhode Island Hospital	Providence	Rhode Island	401-444-4000	www.rhodeislandhospital.org
Richmond University Medical Center	Staten Island	New York	718-818-1234	www.rumcsi.org
Riverside Methodist Hospital	Columbus	Ohio	614-566-5000	www.ohiohealth.com
Robert Packer Hospital	Sayre	Pennsylvania	570-888-6666	www.guthrie.org
Robert Wood Johnson University Hospital	New Brunswick	New Jersey	732-937-8900	www.rwjuh.edu
Ronald Reagan UCLA Medical Center	Los Angeles	California	310-825-6301	www.uclahealth.org
Roseland Community Hospital	Chicago	Illinois	773-995-3000	www.roselandhospital.org
Roxborough Memorial Hospital	Philadelphia	Pennsylvania	215-483-9900	www.roxboroughmemorial.com
Rush University Medical Center	Chicago	Illinois	312-942-5000	www.ruch.edu
Saint Francis Hospital	Tulsa	Oklahoma	918-494-2200	www.saintfrancis.com
Saint Francis Medical Center	Peoria	Illinois	309-655-2000	www.osfsaintfrancis.org
Saint Michael's Medical Center	Newark	New Jersey	973-877-5350	www.cathedralhealth.org
Saint Peter's University Hospital	New Brunswick	New Jersey	732-745-8600	www.saintpetersuh.com
Saint Thomas Rutherford Hospital	Murfreesboro	Tennessee	615-396-4100	www.mtmc.org
Saline Memorial Hospital	Benton	Arkansas	501-776-6000	www.salinememorial.org
San Joaquin Community Hospital	Bakersfield	California	661-395-3000	www.sanjoaquinhospital.org
San Luke's Memorial Hospital	Ponce	Puerto Rico	787-844-2080	www.ssepr.com/hospital_sanlucas.html
Sandhills Regional Medical Center	Hamlet	North Carolina	910-958-2361	www.hma-corp.com
Santa Monica - UCLA Medical Center & Orthopaedic Hospital	Santa Monica	California	310-319-4000	www.healthcare.ucla.edu
Scotland Memorial Hospital	Laurinburg	North Carolina	910-291-7000	www.scotlandhealth.org
Silver Cross Hospital & Medical Centers	New Lenox	Illinois	815-300-1100	www.silvercross.org
Sinai Hospital of Baltimore	Baltimore	Maryland	410-601-5131	www.sinai-balt.com
Sinai - Grace Hospital	Detroit	Michigan	313-966-3300	www.sinaigrace.org
Singing River Hospital	Pascagoula	Mississippi	228-809-5000	www.srhshealth.com
South Nassau Communities Hospital	Oceanside	New York	516-632-3000	www.southnassau.org
South Shore Hospital	Chicago	Illinois	773-768-0810	www.southshorehospital.com
Southern Tennessee Medical Center	Winchester	Tennessee	931-967-8295	www.southerntennessee.com

Hospital	City	State	Phone	Web Site
Southern Virginia Regional Medical Center	Emporia	Virginia	434-348-4400	www.svrmc.com
Southwest Healthcare System	Murrieta	California	951-696-6000	www.ivrmc-rsmc.com
Saint Anthony's Medical Center	Saint Louis	Missouri	314-525-1000	www.samcstl.org
Saint Barnabas Hospital	Bronx	New York	212-960-9000	www.stbarnabashospital.org
Saint Bernard Hospital	Chicago	Illinois	773-962-3900	www.stbernardhospital.com
Saint Catherine of Siena Hospital	Smithtown	New York	631-862-3000	www.stcatherines.chsli.org
Saint Claire Regional Medical Center	Morehead	Kentucky	606-783-6500	www.st-claire.org
Saint Elizabeth Hospital	Belleville	Illinois	618-234-2120	www.steliz.org
Saint Elizabeth's Medical Center	Brighton	Massachusetts	617-789-3000	www.semc.org
Saint Francis Hospital	Poughkeepsie	New York	845-483-5000	www.sfhhc.org
Saint John Hospital & Medical Center	Detroit	Michigan	313-343-4000	www.stjohnprovidence.org
Saint John Macomb - Oakland Hospital - Macomb Center	Warren	Michigan	586-573-5000	www.stjohn.org
Saint John's Episcopal Hospital at South Shore	Far Rockaway	New York	718-869-7000	www.ehs.org
Saint John's Riverside Hospital	Yonkers	New York	914-964-4444	www.riversidehealth.org
Saint Joseph Health Services of RI	North Providence	Rhode Island	401-456-3000	www.fatimahospital.com
Saint Joseph Mercy Oakland	Pontiac	Michigan	248-858-3000	www.stjoesoakland.org
Saint Joseph Regional Health Center	Bryan	Texas	979-776-3912	www.st-joseph.org/sjrhc
Saint Joseph's Hospital	Philadelphia	Pennsylvania	215-787-2000	www.nphs.com
Saint Joseph's Medical Center	Yonkers	New York	914-378-7000	www.saintjosephs.org
Saint Joseph's Regional Medical Center	Paterson	New Jersey	973-754-2010	www.sjhmc.org
Saint Louis University Hospital	Saint Louis	Missouri	314-577-8000	www.slucare.edu/clinical
Saint Luke's Roosevelt Hospital	New York	New York	212-523-4000	www.wehealny.org
Saint Luke's Episcopal Hospital	Houston	Texas	832-355-1000	www.sleh.com
Saint Mary Medical Center	Hobart	Indiana	219-942-0551	www.comhs.org/stmary
Saint Mary Mercy Hospital	Livonia	Michigan	734-655-4800	www.stmarymercy.org
Saint Mary's of Michigan Medical Center	Saginaw	Michigan	989-776-8000	www.stmarysofmichigan.org
Saint Marys Hospital	Centralia	Illinois	618-436-6519	www.stmarys-goodsamaritan.com
Saint Rose Hospital	Hayward	California	510-782-6200	www.strosehospital.org
Saint Vincent Hospital	Worcester	Massachusetts	508-363-5000	www.stvincenthospital.com
Saint Vincent's Medical Center	Bridgeport	Connecticut	203-576-5551	www.stvincents.org
Saint Vincent's Medical Center	Jacksonville	Florida	904-308-7300	www.jaxhealth.com
Staten Island University Hospital	Staten Island	New York	718-226-9000	www.siuh.edu
Stephens County Hospital	Toccoa	Georgia	706-282-4250	www.stephenscountyhospital.com
Strong Memorial Hospital	Rochester	New York	585-275-2121	www.urmc.rochester.edu
Summa Health System Barberton Hospital	Barberton	Ohio	330-615-3000	www.barbhosp.com
Sumner Regional Medical Center	Gallatin	Tennessee	615-452-4210	www.mysumnermedical.com
Sunrise Hospital & Medical Center	Las Vegas	Nevada	702-731-8000	www.sunrisehospital.com
Swedish Covenant Hospital	Chicago	Illinois	773-878-8200	www.swedishcovenant.org
Temple University Hospital	Philadelphia	Pennsylvania	215-707-2000	www.tuh.templehealth.org
The University of Chicago Medical Center	Chicago	Illinois	773-702-1000	www.uchospitals.edu
Thomas Jefferson University Hospital	Philadelphia	Pennsylvania	215-955-6000	www.jeffersonhospital.org
Thorek Memorial Hospital	Chicago	Illinois	312-525-6780	www.thorek.org
Trinitas Regional Medical Center	Elizabeth	New Jersey	908-994-5000	www.trinitashospital.org
Tristar Summit Medical Center	Hermitage	Tennessee	615-316-3000	www.summitmedctr.com
Tufts Medical Center	Boston	Massachusetts	617-636-5000	www.tuftsmedicalcenter.org
Tulane Medical Center	New Orleans	Louisiana	504-988-1900	www.tuhc.com
UAMS Medical Center	Little Rock	Arkansas	501-686-5000	www.uams.edu/medcenter
UF Health Shands Hospital	Gainesville	Florida	352-265-8000	www.shands.org
Umass Memorial Medical Center	Worcester	Massachusetts	508-334-1000	www.umassmemorial.org
Union Hospital	Terre Haute	Indiana	812-238-7606	www.uhhg.org
University Health Care/University Hospitals & Clinics	Salt Lake City	Utah	801-581-2121	www.healthcare.utah.edu
University Hospital	Newark	New Jersey	973-972-5658	www.theuniversityhospital.com
University Hospital - Stony Brook	Stony Brook	New York	631-444-4000	www.stonybrookmedicalcenter.org
University Hospital of Brooklyn - Downstate Medical Center	Brooklyn	New York	718-270-1000	www.downstate.edu
University Hospitals - Elyria Medical Center	Elyria	Ohio	440-329-7500	www.emh-healthcare.org
University Hospitals Ahuja Medical Center	Beachwood	Ohio	216-767-8793	www.uhhospitals.org/ahuja
University Hospitals Case Medical Center	Cleveland	Ohio	216-844-1000	www.uhhs.com
University of Alabama Hospital	Birmingham	Alabama	205-934-4011	www.health.uab.edu
University of Arizona Medical Center	Tucson	Arizona	520-694-0111	www.azumc.com
University of Cincinnati Medical Center	Cincinnati	Ohio	513-584-1000	www.universityhospitalcincinnati.com
University of Illinois Hospital	Chicago	Illinois	312-996-3900	www.uic.edu
University of Iowa Hospital & Clinics	Iowa City	Iowa	319-356-1616	www.uihealthcare.com
University of Kentucky Hospital	Lexington	Kentucky	859-323-5000	www.uhealthcare.uky.edu
University of Louisville Hospital	Louisville	Kentucky	502-562-3000	www.uoflhealthcare.org
University of Maryland Medical Center	Baltimore	Maryland	410-328-8667	www.umm.edu
University of Maryland Medical Center Midtown Campus	Baltimore	Maryland	410-225-8996	www.marylandgeneral.org
University of Miami Hospital	Miami	Florida	305-325-5511	www.cedarsmedicalcenter.com

Hospital	City	State	Phone	Web Site
University of Michigan Health System	Ann Arbor	Michigan	734-764-1505	www.med.umich.edu
University of North Carolina Hospital	Chapel Hill	North Carolina	919-966-4131	www.unchealthcare.org
University of Texas Medical Branch Galveston	Galveston	Texas	409-772-1011	www.utmb.edu
University of Virginia Medical Center	Charlottesville	Virginia	800-251-3627	www.uvahealth.com
UPMC Presbyterian Shadyside	Pittsburgh	Pennsylvania	412-647-8788	www.upmc.edu
Valley Hospital	Ridgewood	New Jersey	201-447-8000	www.valleyhealth.com
Valley Hospital Medical Center	Las Vegas	Nevada	702-388-4000	www.valleyhealthsystem.org
Vanderbilt University Hospital	Nashville	Tennessee	615-322-3454	www.mc.vanderbilt.edu
Vassar Brothers Medical Center	Poughkeepsie	New York	845-454-8500	www.vasserbrothers.org
Vidant Medical Center	Greenville	North Carolina	252-847-4100	www.uhseast.com
Vidant Roanoke Chowan Hospital	Ahoskie	North Carolina	252-209-3000	www.uhseast.com
Washington Hospital	Fremont	California	510-797-1111	www.whhs.com
Wellmont Bristol Regional Medical Center	Bristol	Tennessee	423-844-1121	www.wellmont.org
Wellmont Holston Valley Medical Center	Kingsport	Tennessee	423-224-4000	www.wellmont.org
Wesley Medical Center	Hattiesburg	Mississippi	601-268-8000	www.wesley.com
West Chester Hospital	West Chester	Ohio	513-298-3000	www.westchesterhospital.uchealth.com
West River Regional Medical Center	Hettinger	North Dakota	701-567-4561	www.wrhs.com
West Virginia University Hospitals	Morgantown	West Virginia	304-598-4000	www.wvuh.com
Westchester General Hospital	Miami	Florida	305-263-9270	www.westchestergeneralhospital.com
Westchester Medical Center	Valhalla	New York	914-285-7017	www.wcmc.com
Western Arizona Regional Medical Center	Bullhead City	Arizona	928-763-2273	www.warmc.com
Western Maryland Regional Medical Center	Cumberland	Maryland	240-964-8001	www.wmhs.com
White County Medical Center	Searcy	Arkansas	501-278-3100	www.centralarkhospital.com
White River Medical Center	Batesville	Arkansas	870-262-1200	www.wrmc.com
William Beaumont Hospital - Troy	Troy	Michigan	248-964-8800	www.beaumonthospitals.com
Williamson ARH Hospital	South Williamson	Kentucky	606-237-1700	www.arh.org
Williamson Memorial Hospital	Williamson	West Virginia	304-235-2500	www.hmawmh.com
Winter Haven Hospital	Winter Haven	Florida	863-293-1121	www.winterhavenhospital.com
Wyckoff Heights Medical Center	Brooklyn	New York	718-963-7272	www.wyckoffhospital.org
Yale-New Haven Hospital	New Haven	Connecticut	203-688-4242	www.ynhh.org

Note: Table shows hospitals nationwide whose rate of readmission after discharge from hospital (hospital-wide) is better (lower) than U.S. rate of 16.0%

Hospital Heart Attack Readmission Rates: State and National Summary

Area	Number of Hospitals			
	Better than U.S. National Rate[1]	Worse than U.S. National Rate[2]	No Different than U.S. National Rate[3]	Number of Cases Too Small[4]
U.S. and Territories	23	29	2327	2085
Alabama	0	0	39	58
Alaska	0	0	5	14
American Samoa	0	0	0	1
Arizona	0	0	47	21
Arkansas	0	1	27	46
California	1	1	201	122
Colorado	1	0	32	33
Connecticut	0	1	27	3
Delaware	0	0	6	1
District of Columbia	0	0	6	2
Florida	3	3	144	32
Georgia	1	0	64	72
Guam	0	0	1	0
Hawaii	0	0	11	5
Idaho	0	0	9	23
Illinois	0	5	103	71
Indiana	2	0	61	54
Iowa	0	0	27	82
Kansas	0	0	27	82
Kentucky	0	0	40	55
Louisiana	0	0	44	56
Maine	1	0	21	15
Maryland	0	0	39	7
Massachusetts	0	1	52	10
Michigan	1	0	76	51
Minnesota	0	0	31	89
Mississippi	0	0	30	49
Missouri	0	0	53	59
Montana	0	0	8	35
N. Mariana Islands	0	0	1	0
Nebraska	0	0	19	53
Nevada	0	0	18	14
New Hampshire	0	0	15	10
New Jersey	0	5	55	6
New Mexico	1	0	11	26
New York	0	4	132	45
North Carolina	1	1	67	40
North Dakota	1	0	7	33
Ohio	0	0	96	61
Oklahoma	0	1	31	67
Oregon	1	0	23	36
Pennsylvania	1	0	120	41
Puerto Rico	0	1	12	32
Rhode Island	0	0	11	0
South Carolina	1	1	36	22
South Dakota	0	0	9	38
Tennessee	0	1	56	55
Texas	2	0	176	153
Utah	0	0	14	20
Vermont	0	0	8	7
Virgin Islands	0	0	1	1
Virginia	0	2	62	17
Washington	2	0	40	40
West Virginia	0	1	24	28
Wisconsin	3	0	50	68
Wyoming	0	0	2	24

Note: (1) 30-day readmission rate is better (lower) than U.S. rate of 18.3%; (2) 30-day readmission rate is worse (higher) than U.S. rate of 18.3%; (3) 30-day readmission rate is about the same as U.S. rate of 18.3%; (4) The number of cases is too small to classify the hospital

Hospital Heart Failure Readmission Rates: State and National Summary

Area	Number of Hospitals			
	Better than U.S. National Rate[1]	Worse than U.S. National Rate[2]	No Different than U.S. National Rate[3]	Number of Cases Too Small[4]
U.S. and Territories	120	159	3876	631
Alabama	2	1	92	6
Alaska	0	0	12	10
American Samoa	0	0	0	1
Arizona	3	1	60	14
Arkansas	0	3	71	3
California	10	3	280	46
Colorado	3	0	54	17
Connecticut	1	2	29	0
Delaware	0	0	7	0
District of Columbia	0	1	7	0
Florida	8	16	157	6
Georgia	3	1	129	11
Guam	0	0	1	0
Hawaii	1	0	13	5
Idaho	2	0	20	16
Illinois	1	10	168	5
Indiana	3	1	113	3
Iowa	3	0	97	18
Kansas	2	0	85	46
Kentucky	1	8	86	1
Louisiana	2	5	86	16
Maine	2	0	33	2
Maryland	0	6	40	1
Massachusetts	1	3	59	1
Michigan	6	10	108	11
Minnesota	1	1	86	43
Mississippi	0	6	77	13
Missouri	4	6	101	6
Montana	1	0	30	29
N. Mariana Islands	0	0	0	1
Nebraska	3	0	47	35
Nevada	0	0	30	5
New Hampshire	1	0	24	1
New Jersey	1	16	49	1
New Mexico	1	0	32	9
New York	0	22	156	5
North Carolina	6	2	97	8
North Dakota	1	0	24	19
Ohio	2	2	153	10
Oklahoma	2	3	87	25
Oregon	4	0	51	5
Pennsylvania	9	5	144	6
Puerto Rico	0	1	28	20
Rhode Island	0	2	9	1
South Carolina	6	2	53	2
South Dakota	0	0	29	26
Tennessee	3	6	102	4
Texas	11	3	308	52
Utah	3	0	22	17
Vermont	0	0	14	1
Virgin Islands	0	0	2	0
Virginia	1	5	76	2
Washington	2	1	64	21
West Virginia	0	5	45	4
Wisconsin	4	0	111	10
Wyoming	0	0	18	11

Note: (1) 30-day readmission rate is better (lower) than U.S. rate of 23.0%; (2) 30-day readmission rate is worse (higher) than U.S. rate of 23.0%; (3) 30-day readmission rate is about the same as U.S. rate of 23.0%; (4) The number of cases is too small to classify the hospital

Hospital Pneumonia Readmission Rates: State and National Summary

Area	Number of Hospitals			
	Better than U.S. National Rate[1]	Worse than U.S. National Rate[2]	No Different than U.S. National Rate[3]	Number of Cases Too Small[4]
U.S. and Territories	37	135	4285	376
Alabama	0	1	96	5
Alaska	0	0	15	6
American Samoa	0	0	1	0
Arizona	0	0	72	9
Arkansas	1	5	68	3
California	3	5	290	46
Colorado	1	0	62	12
Connecticut	0	1	31	0
Delaware	0	0	7	0
District of Columbia	0	0	8	0
Florida	5	8	170	5
Georgia	1	0	138	4
Guam	0	0	1	0
Hawaii	0	0	14	8
Idaho	0	0	33	7
Illinois	0	11	169	5
Indiana	2	1	115	2
Iowa	0	0	113	5
Kansas	1	0	118	13
Kentucky	1	8	87	0
Louisiana	1	3	95	13
Maine	0	0	36	1
Maryland	0	11	34	1
Massachusetts	0	2	62	1
Michigan	2	5	122	6
Minnesota	0	0	112	19
Mississippi	0	3	87	8
Missouri	2	3	107	6
Montana	2	0	40	20
N. Mariana Islands	0	0	1	0
Nebraska	0	0	77	9
Nevada	0	1	29	6
New Hampshire	0	0	26	0
New Jersey	1	2	63	2
New Mexico	0	0	39	3
New York	2	24	154	5
North Carolina	1	4	104	5
North Dakota	0	0	40	4
Ohio	1	11	149	6
Oklahoma	1	3	103	12
Oregon	1	1	55	3
Pennsylvania	1	3	157	4
Puerto Rico	0	1	26	23
Rhode Island	0	0	11	1
South Carolina	2	1	58	2
South Dakota	0	0	51	5
Tennessee	1	5	105	5
Texas	3	4	325	49
Utah	0	0	37	5
Vermont	0	0	15	0
Virgin Islands	0	0	2	0
Virginia	0	3	79	7
Washington	1	0	81	7
West Virginia	0	5	48	1
Wisconsin	0	0	120	5
Wyoming	0	0	27	2

Note: (1) 30-day readmission rate is better (lower) than U.S. rate of 17.6%; (2) 30-day readmission rate is worse (higher) than U.S. rate of 17.6%; (3) 30-day readmission rate is about the same as U.S. rate of 17.6%; (4) The number of cases is too small to classify the hospital

Hospital Readmission Rate After Hip/Knee Surgery: State and National Summary

Area	Number of Hospitals			
	Better than U.S. National Rate[1]	Worse than U.S. National Rate[2]	No Different than U.S. National Rate[3]	Number of Cases Too Small[4]
U.S. and Territories	51	38	2738	665
Alabama	0	0	52	9
Alaska	0	0	8	0
American Samoa	0	0	0	0
Arizona	1	0	48	7
Arkansas	1	1	28	7
California	8	1	199	90
Colorado	1	0	49	6
Connecticut	0	1	28	0
Delaware	0	0	5	1
District of Columbia	0	1	4	2
Florida	5	4	138	15
Georgia	2	0	77	15
Guam	0	0	0	0
Hawaii	0	0	8	6
Idaho	0	0	23	5
Illinois	1	4	110	24
Indiana	3	0	78	29
Iowa	1	0	47	17
Kansas	1	0	42	12
Kentucky	0	0	42	19
Louisiana	0	1	59	15
Maine	1	0	25	6
Maryland	0	3	40	2
Massachusetts	1	0	55	5
Michigan	1	1	96	18
Minnesota	0	0	67	16
Mississippi	0	0	29	7
Missouri	1	2	64	13
Montana	1	0	19	6
N. Mariana Islands	0	0	0	0
Nebraska	1	0	31	13
Nevada	0	0	23	2
New Hampshire	0	0	22	4
New Jersey	0	1	54	7
New Mexico	1	0	21	3
New York	3	0	119	30
North Carolina	1	0	82	6
North Dakota	1	0	7	1
Ohio	2	2	133	20
Oklahoma	1	1	45	19
Oregon	1	0	39	10
Pennsylvania	2	4	123	29
Puerto Rico	0	0	8	28
Rhode Island	0	0	9	1
South Carolina	0	1	40	13
South Dakota	0	0	17	1
Tennessee	2	2	53	19
Texas	3	5	204	51
Utah	0	0	26	6
Vermont	0	0	12	1
Virgin Islands	0	0	1	0
Virginia	3	2	55	9
Washington	0	0	53	9
West Virginia	0	0	26	6
Wisconsin	1	1	82	21
Wyoming	0	0	13	4

Note: (1) 30-day readmission rate is better (lower) than U.S. rate of 5.4%; (2) 30-day readmission rate is worse (higher) than U.S. rate of 5.4%; (3) 30-day readmission rate is about the same as U.S. rate of 5.4%; (4) The number of cases is too small to classify the hospital

Hospital Readmission Rate After Discharge From Hospital (Hospital-wide): State and National Summary

Area	Number of Hospitals			
	Better than U.S. National Rate[1]	Worse than U.S. National Rate[2]	No Different than U.S. National Rate[3]	Number of Cases Too Small[4]
U.S. and Territories	316	369	3966	158
Alabama	1	1	92	3
Alaska	1	0	20	1
American Samoa	0	0	1	0
Arizona	9	3	64	5
Arkansas	3	11	60	0
California	29	17	283	10
Colorado	9	0	63	3
Connecticut	2	4	25	0
Delaware	0	0	6	0
District of Columbia	0	3	4	0
Florida	13	23	143	2
Georgia	7	5	129	1
Guam	0	0	1	0
Hawaii	2	0	13	6
Idaho	6	0	32	2
Illinois	4	37	137	1
Indiana	14	4	104	2
Iowa	7	1	106	2
Kansas	7	0	125	6
Kentucky	2	20	72	0
Louisiana	6	8	102	9
Maine	3	0	32	1
Maryland	3	14	28	0
Massachusetts	5	13	46	0
Michigan	12	20	93	6
Minnesota	8	0	119	4
Mississippi	1	6	86	5
Missouri	4	6	100	2
Montana	3	0	50	8
N. Mariana Islands	0	0	0	1
Nebraska	6	0	79	4
Nevada	1	3	28	3
New Hampshire	1	0	25	0
New Jersey	2	21	41	0
New Mexico	2	0	38	2
New York	6	57	110	4
North Carolina	15	6	88	2
North Dakota	2	1	38	2
Ohio	6	17	141	7
Oklahoma	9	4	106	6
Oregon	8	0	48	2
Pennsylvania	11	17	134	7
Puerto Rico	0	1	47	4
Rhode Island	0	4	7	0
South Carolina	8	2	52	0
South Dakota	5	0	52	2
Tennessee	4	12	96	1
Texas	31	8	341	20
Utah	6	1	34	2
Vermont	1	0	13	0
Virgin Islands	0	0	2	0
Virginia	3	11	66	4
Washington	12	1	71	2
West Virginia	0	7	42	1
Wisconsin	15	0	107	1
Wyoming	1	0	24	2

Note: (1) 30-day readmission rate is better (lower) than U.S. rate of 16.0%; (2) 30-day readmission rate is worse (higher) than U.S. rate of 16.0%; (3) 30-day readmission rate is about the same as U.S. rate of 16.0%; (4) The number of cases is too small to classify the hospital

Appendix C: Surgical Complication Rates

What Do These Surgical Complication Measures Show?

This appendix shows how hospitals' surgical complication rates compare to the rate across the U.S. The categories are:

- A Wound That Splits Open After Surgery on the Abdomen or Pelvis
- Accidental Cuts and Tears From Medical Treatment
- Collapsed Lung Due to Medical Treatment
- Deaths Among Patients With Serious Treatable Complications After Surgery
- Rate of Complications for Hip/Knee Replacement Patients
- Serious Blood Clots After Surgery
- Serious Complications (see below for details)

This first part of this appendix shows hospitals with surgical complication rates that are lower (better) or higher (worse) than the national rate for all categories. Hospitals are shown to be better or worse than the U.S. national rate only if the data shows with 95% certainty, the difference between their surgical complication rates and the U.S. national rate is not due to chance.

The second part of this appendix contains state and national summaries with the following column headers:

- **Better Than U.S. National Rate.** Hospitals in the Better Than U.S. National Rate category have surgical complication rates that are lower than the U.S. National Rate, with 95% certainty that this difference is not due to chance.
- **Worse Than U.S. National Rate.** Hospitals in the Worse Than U.S. National Rate category have surgical complication rates that are higher than the U.S. National Rate, with 95% certainty that this difference is not due to chance.
- **No Different Than U.S. National Rate.** Many hospitals in the No Different Than U.S. National Rate category have surgical complication rates that are about the same as the U.S. National Rate. Other hospitals in this category have rates that are higher or lower than the U.S. National Rate, without 95% certainty that these differences are not due to chance.
- **Number of Cases Too Small.** The number of cases is too small to classify the hospital.

Serious Complications

Measures of serious complications are drawn from the Agency for Healthcare Research and Quality (AHRQ) Patient Safety Indicators (PSIs). The overall score for serious complications is based on how often adult patients had certain serious, but potentially preventable, complications related to medical or surgical inpatient hospital care. This composite or summary measure is based on the following measures:

- Collapsed lung that results from medical treatment (Iatrogenic pneumothorax, adult)
- Blood clots, in the lung or a large vein, after surgery (Postoperative Pulmonary Embolism or Deep Vein Thrombosis Rate)
- A wound that splits open after surgery (Postoperative wound dehiscence)
- Accidental cuts and tears (Accidental puncture or laceration)
- Pressure sores (Pressure ulcers)
- Infections from a large venous catheters (Central venous catheter-related blood stream infection rate)
- Broken hip from a fall after surgery (Postoperative hip fracture rate)
- Blood stream infection after surgery (Postoperative sepsis)

Which Patients are Included

The Serious Complications measure applies only to Medicare beneficiaries enrolled in Original Medicare (traditional fee-for-service (FFS) Medicare) who were discharged from a hospital that was paid through the inpatient prospective payment system (IPPS) after the beneficiary had an inpatient stay. Non-Medicare patients and beneficiaries enrolled in Medicare managed care plans are also excluded from the data.

Where the Information Comes From

The Centers for Medicare & Medicaid Services (CMS) calculates the indicators of patient safety data from the claims hospitals submit for Medicare beneficiaries enrolled in Original Medicare(traditional FFS Medicare). The rate for each PSI is calculated by dividing the actual number of outcomes at each hospital by the number of eligible discharges for that measure at each hospital, multiplied by 1,000. The composite value reported on Hospital Compare is the weighted averages of the component indicators. PSI data are only calculated for hospitals that are paid through the IPPS, which excludes Critical Access hospitals (CAHs), long-term care hospitals (LTCHs), Maryland waiver hospitals, cancer hospitals, children's inpatient facilities, rural health clinics, federally qualified health centers, inpatient psychiatric hospitals, inpatient rehabilitation facilities, Veterans Administration/ Department of Defense hospitals, and religious, non-medical health care institutions.

Risk Adjustment

The measures of serious complications reported are risk adjusted to account for differences in hospital patients' characteristics. In addition, the rates reported are "smoothed" to reflect the fact that measures for small hospitals are measured less accurately (i.e., are less reliable) than for larger hospitals.

Comparing Individual Hospital Rates to Benchmarks

For the composite measure, CMS assigns comparative performance categories. If the interval estimate includes and/or overlaps with the national composite value, the hospital's performance is in the "no different than U.S. national rate" category. If the entire interval estimate is below the national composite value, then the hospital is performing "better than U.S. national rate." If the entire interval estimate is above the national composite value, it is "worse than U.S. national rate."

Additional Information

For more detail on Serious Complications measures (AHRQ Patient Safety Indicators) visit the Agency for Healthcare Research and Quality (AHRQ) Patient Safety Indicator Resources Web site at www.qualityindicators.ahrq.gov.

Hospitals whose Surgical Complication Rate is Better (Lower) than the U.S. National Rate

Measure: A Wound That Splits Open After Surgery on the Abdomen or Pelvis

Hospital	City	State	Phone	Web Site
No hospitals met this criteria.				

Note: Table shows hospitals nationwide whose surgical complication rate is better (lower) than U.S. rate of 0.92%

Hospitals whose Surgical Complication Rate is Worse (Higher) than the U.S. National Rate

Measure: A Wound That Splits Open After Surgery on the Abdomen or Pelvis

Hospital	City	State	Phone	Web Site
Aurora Lakeland Medical Center	Elkhorn	Wisconsin	262-741-2000	www.aurorahealthcare.org/facilities
Banner Thunderbird Medical Center	Glendale	Arizona	602-588-5555	www.bannerhealth.com
Beaumont Health System	Royal Oak	Michigan	248-898-5000	www.beaumonthospitals.com
Bronson Methodist Hospital	Kalamazoo	Michigan	269-341-6000	www.bronsonhealth.com
Central Carolina Hospital	Sanford	North Carolina	919-774-2100	www.centralcarolinahosp.com
Cjw Medical Center	Richmond	Virginia	804-330-2001	www.hcavirginia.com
Eastern Idaho Regional Medical Center	Idaho Falls	Idaho	208-529-6111	www.eirmc.org
Erlanger Medical Center	Chattanooga	Tennessee	423-778-7000	www.erlanger.org
Exeter Hospital	Exeter	New Hampshire	603-778-7311	www.exeterhospital.com
Fairfield Medical Center	Lancaster	Ohio	740-687-8009	www.fmchealth.org
Florida Hospital Deland	Deland	Florida	386-943-4772	www.fhdeland.org
Florida Hospital Fish Memorial	Orange City	Florida	386-917-5000	www.fhfishmemorial.org
Frye Regional Medical Center	Hickory	North Carolina	828-322-6070	www.fryemedctr.com
Genesys Regional Medical Center - Health Park	Grand Blanc	Michigan	810-606-5000	www.genesys.org
Good Samaritan Hospital	San Jose	California	408-559-2011	www.goodsamsj.org
Health Alliance Hospital Broadway Campus	Kingston	New York	914-331-3131	www.kingstonregionalhealth.org
Inspira Medical Center Woodbury	Woodbury	New Jersey	856-845-0100	www.umhospital.org
Lake Cumberland Regional Hospital	Somerset	Kentucky	606-679-7441	www.lakecumberlandhospital.com
Lake Regional Health System	Osage Beach	Missouri	573-348-8000	www.lakeregional.com
Lakeland Hospital - Saint Joseph	Saint Joseph	Michigan	269-983-8300	www.lakelandhealth.org
Longmont United Hospital	Longmont	Colorado	303-651-5111	www.luhcares.org
Maine Medical Center	Portland	Maine	207-662-0111	www.mmc.org
Mayo Clinic Hospital Rochester	Rochester	Minnesota	507-255-5123	www.mayoclinic.org/saintmaryshospital
The Medical Center of Aurora	Aurora	Colorado	303-695-2600	www.auroramed.com
Medstar Washington Hospital Center	Washington	District of Columbia	202-877-7000	www.whcenter.org
Memorial Health Univ Medical Center	Savannah	Georgia	912-350-8000	www.memorialhealth.com
Mercy Saint Anne Hospital	Toledo	Ohio	419-407-2663	www.mercyweb.org
Miami Valley Hospital	Dayton	Ohio	937-208-8000	www.miamivalleyhospital.com
Mountainview Hospital	Las Vegas	Nevada	702-255-5065	www.mountainview-hospital.com
Norton Hospitals	Louisville	Kentucky	502-629-6560	www.nortonhealthcare.com
Pali Momi Medical Center	Aiea	Hawaii	808-486-6000	www.kapiolani.org
Pottstown Memorial Medical Center	Pottstown	Pennsylvania	610-327-7000	www.pmmctr.org
Robert Wood Johnson University Hospital at Rahway	Rahway	New Jersey	732-381-4200	www.rwjuhr.com/about/history.html
Southeast Georgia Health System - Brunswick Campus	Brunswick	Georgia	912-466-7000	www.sghs.org
Spring Valley Hospital Medical Center	Las Vegas	Nevada	702-853-3000	www.springvalleyhospital.com
Saint Joseph Regional Health Center	Bryan	Texas	979-776-3912	www.st-joseph.org/sjrhc
Saint Luke's Episcopal Hospital	Houston	Texas	832-355-1000	www.sleh.com
Touro Infirmary	New Orleans	Louisiana	504-897-7011	www.touro.com
University of Wisconsin Hospitals & Clinics Authority	Madison	Wisconsin	608-263-8991	www.uwhealth.org
UNM Hospital	Albuquerque	New Mexico	505-272-2111	www.hospitals.unm.edu/unmh
Wayne Memorial Hospital	Honesdale	Pennsylvania	570-253-8100	www.wmh.org

Note: Table shows hospitals nationwide whose surgical complication rate is worse (higher) than U.S. rate of 0.92%

Hospitals whose Surgical Complication Rate is Better (Lower) than the U.S. National Rate

Measure: Accidental Cuts and Tears From Medical Treatment

Hospital	City	State	Phone	Web Site
Advocate Christ Hospital & Medical Center	Oak Lawn	Illinois	708-684-8000	www.advocatehealth.com
Advocate Good Samaritan Hospital	Downers Grove	Illinois	630-275-5900	www.advocatehealth.com/gsam
Advocate Lutheran General Hospital	Park Ridge	Illinois	847-723-2210	www.advocatehealth.com
Arkansas Heart Hospital	Little Rock	Arkansas	501-219-7000	www.arheart.com
Asante Rogue Regional Medical Center	Medford	Oregon	541-789-7000	www.asante.org
Atlanticare Regional Medical Center	Atlantic City	New Jersey	609-441-8020	www.atlanticare.org/acmc/index.html
Aventura Hospital & Medical Center	Aventura	Florida	305-682-7000	www.aventurahospital.com
Baptist Beaumont Hospital	Beaumont	Texas	409-212-5012	www.mhbh.org
Baystate Medical Center	Springfield	Massachusetts	413-794-0000	www.baystatehealth.com
Bethesda Hospital East	Boynton Beach	Florida	561-737-7733	www.bethesdahealthcare.com
Cape Regional Medical Center	Cape May Ct House	New Jersey	609-463-2000	www.caperegional.com
Cedars - Sinai Medical Center	Los Angeles	California	310-423-5000	www.cedars-sinai.edu
Central Dupage Hospital	Winfield	Illinois	630-682-1600	www.cdh.org
Christiana Care Health Services	Newark	Delaware	302-733-1000	www.christianacare.org
Christus Spohn Hospital Corpus Christi	Corpus Christi	Texas	361-902-4103	www.christusspohn.org
Clear Lake Regional Medical Center	Webster	Texas	281-332-2511	www.clearlakermc.com
Community Medical Center	Toms River	New Jersey	732-557-8000	www.sbhcs.com
Delray Medical Center	Delray Beach	Florida	561-498-4440	www.delraymedicalctr.com
Duke University Hospital	Durham	North Carolina	919-684-8111	www.dukehealth.org
Englewood Hospital & Medical Center	Englewood	New Jersey	201-894-3000	www.englewoodhospital.com
Florida Hospital	Orlando	Florida	407-303-1976	www.floridahospital.com
Floyd Medical Center	Rome	Georgia	706-509-6900	www.floydmed.org
Glendale Adventist Medical Center	Glendale	California	818-409-8202	www.glendaleadventist.com
Good Samaritan Hospital Medical Center	West Islip	New York	631-376-3000	www.good-samaritan-hospital.org
Good Samaritan Medical Center	Brockton	Massachusetts	508-427-3000	www.goodsamaritanmedical.org
Indiana University Health	Indianapolis	Indiana	317-962-5900	www.iuhealth.org
Integris Baptist Medical Center	Oklahoma City	Oklahoma	405-951-8110	www.integris-health.com
Integris Southwest Medical Center	Oklahoma City	Oklahoma	405-636-7000	www.integris-health.com
Jackson - Madison County General Hospital	Jackson	Tennessee	731-541-5000	www.wth.org
Lakeland Regional Medical Center	Lakeland	Florida	863-687-1100	www.lrmc.com
Laredo Medical Center	Laredo	Texas	956-796-5000	www.laredomedical.com
Lovelace Medical Center	Albuquerque	New Mexico	505-727-8000	www.lovelace.com
Marietta Memorial Hospital	Marietta	Ohio	740-374-1400	www.mmhospital.org
Marion General Hospital	Marion	Ohio	740-383-8400	www.mariongeneral.com
Mayo Clinic	Jacksonville	Florida	904-953-2000	www.mayoclinic.org/jacksonville
Mayo Clinic Hospital	Phoenix	Arizona	480-342-2000	www.mayoclinic.org
Mayo Clinic Hospital Rochester	Rochester	Minnesota	507-255-5123	www.mayoclinic.org/saintmaryshospital
Mayo Clinic Methodist- Hospital	Rochester	Minnesota	507-266-7890	www.mayoclinic.org/methodisthospital
Mclaren Bay Region	Bay City	Michigan	989-894-3000	www.baymed.org
Memorial Healthcare System	Chattanooga	Tennessee	423-495-2525	www.memorial.org
Memorial Hermann Hospital System	Houston	Texas	713-448-6796	www.memorialhermann.org
Memorial Hermann Memorial City Medical Center	Houston	Texas	713-242-3000	www.mhhs.org
Memorial Hermann Texas Medical Center	Houston	Texas	713-704-3700	www.mhhs.org
Memorial Hospital	Belleville	Illinois	618-233-7750	www.memhosp.com
Memorial Regional Hospital	Hollywood	Florida	954-987-2000	www.memorialregional.com
Mercy Hospital Fairfield	Fairfield	Ohio	513-870-7197	www.e-mercy.com/mercy-hospital-fairfield.aspx
Methodist Hospital	San Antonio	Texas	210-575-4000	www.mh.sahealth.com
The Methodist Hospital	Houston	Texas	713-790-2221	www.methodisthealth.com
Methodist Willowbrook Hospital	Houston	Texas	281-477-1000	www.houstonmethodist.org/willowbrook-hospital
Mississippi Baptist Medical Center	Jackson	Mississippi	601-968-1000	www.mbmc.org
Munroe Regional Medical Center	Ocala	Florida	352-351-7200	www.munroeregional.com
North Florida Regional Medical Center	Gainesville	Florida	352-333-4100	www.nfrmc.com
Northwestern Memorial Hospital	Chicago	Illinois	312-926-2000	www.nmh.org
Ocala Regional Medical Center	Ocala	Florida	352-401-1000	www.ocalaregional.com
Our Lady of Lourdes Medical Center	Camden	New Jersey	856-757-3500	www.lourdesnet.org
Overlook Medical Center	Summit	New Jersey	908-522-2000	www.atlantichealth.org
Palos Community Hospital	Palos Heights	Illinois	708-923-4000	www.paloshospital.org
Presence Resurrection Medical Center	Chicago	Illinois	773-774-8000	www.reshealthcare.org
Presence Saint Joseph Medical Center	Joliet	Illinois	815-725-7133	www.provena.org/stjoes
Providence Little Co of Mary Medical Center Torrance	Torrance	California	310-540-7676	www.lcmhs.org
Providence Tarzana Medical Center	Tarzana	California	818-881-0800	www.encino-tarzana.com
Roper Hospital	Charleston	South Carolina	843-724-2800	www.ropersaintfrancis.com
Saint Thomas West Hospital	Nashville	Tennessee	615-222-2111	www.stthomas.org
Scripps Memorial Hospital La Jolla	La Jolla	California	858-626-4123	www.scrippshealth.org

Hospital	City	State	Phone	Web Site
Sentara Careplex Hospital	Hampton	Virginia	757-736-1000	www.sentara.com
Sentara Leigh Hospital	Norfolk	Virginia	757-261-6601	www.sentara.com
Sentara Norfolk General Hospital	Norfolk	Virginia	757-388-3000	www.sentara.com
Sentara Virginia Beach General Hospital	Virginia Beach	Virginia	757-395-8000	www.sentara.com
Shasta Regional Medical Center	Redding	California	530-244-5454	www.shastaregional.com
South Shore Hospital	South Weymouth	Massachusetts	781-340-8000	www.southshorehospital.org
Saint Francis Hospital	Columbus	Georgia	706-596-4020	www.wecareforlife.com
Saint Francis Hospital - Roslyn	Roslyn	New York	516-562-6000	www.stfrancisheartcenter.com
Saint John Medical Center	Tulsa	Oklahoma	918-744-3606	www.sjmc.org
Saint John's Riverside Hospital	Yonkers	New York	914-964-4444	www.riversidehealth.org
Saint Luke's Episcopal Hospital	Houston	Texas	832-355-1000	www.sleh.com
Saint Mary Medical Center	Langhorne	Pennsylvania	215-750-2003	www.stmaryhealthcare.org
Saint Mary Mercy Hospital	Livonia	Michigan	734-655-4800	www.stmarymercy.org
Saint Vincent Heart Center of Indiana	Indianapolis	Indiana	317-583-5000	www.theheartcenter.com
Staten Island University Hospital	Staten Island	New York	718-226-9000	www.siuh.edu
Sutter General Hospital	Sacramento	California	916-733-8999	www.suttermedicalcenter.org
Swedish Covenant Hospital	Chicago	Illinois	773-878-8200	www.swedishcovenant.org
Tennova Healthcare	Knoxville	Tennessee	865-545-8000	www.stmaryshealth.com
The Nebraska Medical Center	Omaha	Nebraska	402-552-2040	www.nebraskamed.com
Tuomey Healthcare System	Sumter	South Carolina	803-774-8900	www.tuomey.com
UF Health Shands Hospital	Gainesville	Florida	352-265-8000	www.shands.org
United Hospital Center	Bridgeport	West Virginia	681-342-1000	www.uhcwv.org
University of Kentucky Hospital	Lexington	Kentucky	859-323-5000	www.uhealthcare.uky.edu
University of Michigan Health System	Ann Arbor	Michigan	734-764-1505	www.med.umich.edu
Valley Hospital	Ridgewood	New Jersey	201-447-8000	www.valleyhealth.com
Vanderbilt University Hospital	Nashville	Tennessee	615-322-3454	www.mc.vanderbilt.edu
Virtua West Jersey Hospitals Berlin	Berlin	New Jersey	856-322-3200	www.virtua.org
Williamsport Regional Medical Center	Williamsport	Pennsylvania	570-321-1000	www.susquehannahealth.org
Winchester Medical Center	Winchester	Virginia	540-536-8000	www.valleyhealthlink.com
Winthrop - University Hospital	Mineola	New York	516-663-0333	www.winthrop.org

Note: Table shows hospitals nationwide whose surgical complication rate is better (lower) than U.S. rate of 1.83%

Hospitals whose Surgical Complication Rate is Worse (Higher) than the U.S. National Rate

Measure: Accidental Cuts and Tears From Medical Treatment

Hospital	City	State	Phone	Web Site
Adena Regional Medical Center	Chillicothe	Ohio	740-779-7500	www.adena.org
Adirondack Medical Center	Saranac Lake	New York	518-891-4141	www.amccares.org
Aiken Regional Medical Center	Aiken	South Carolina	803-641-5900	www.aikenregional.com
Alaska Native Medical Center	Anchorage	Alaska	907-563-2662	www.anmc.org
Appleton Medical Center	Appleton	Wisconsin	920-731-4101	www.thedacare.org
Atlanta Medical Center	Atlanta	Georgia	404-265-4000	www.atlantamedcenter.com
B R F Hospital Holdings	Shreveport	Louisiana	318-675-5000	www.lsumc.edu
Baptist Saint Anthony's Hospital	Amarillo	Texas	806-212-2000	www.bsahs.com
Barnes-Jewish Hospital	Saint Louis	Missouri	314-747-3000	www.barnesjewish.org
Baylor University Medical Center	Dallas	Texas	214-820-0111	www.baylorhealth.com
Beth Israel Deaconess Medical Center	Boston	Massachusetts	617-667-7000	www.bidmc.harvard.edu
Blessing Hospital	Quincy	Illinois	217-223-5811	www.blessinghealthsystem.org
Borgess Medical Center	Kalamazoo	Michigan	269-226-7000	www.borgess.com
Boston Medical Center Corporation	Boston	Massachusetts	617-638-8000	www.bmc.org
Bridgeport Hospital	Bridgeport	Connecticut	203-384-3000	www.bridgeporthospital.com
Carney Hospital	Boston	Massachusetts	617-506-2000	www.caritascarney.org
Caromont Regional Medical Center	Gastonia	North Carolina	704-834-4891	www.caromont.org
Catholic Medical Center	Manchester	New Hampshire	603-668-3545	www.catholicmedicalcenter.org
Centra Health	Lynchburg	Virginia	434-200-4789	www.centrahealth.com
Central Texas Medical Center	San Marcos	Texas	512-753-3690	www.ctmc.org
Centrastate Medical Center	Freehold	New Jersey	732-431-2000	www.centrastate.com
Cheshire Medical Center	Keene	New Hampshire	603-354-5400	www.cheshire-med.com
Chilton Medical Center	Pompton Plains	New Jersey	973-831-5000	www.chiltonmemorial.org
Clearview Regional Medical Center	Monroe	Georgia	770-267-1792	www.clearviewregionalmedicalcenter.com
Cleveland Clinic	Cleveland	Ohio	216-444-2200	www.clevelandclinic.org
Clovis Community Medical Center	Clovis	California	559-324-4000	www.communitymedical.org
Community Regional Medical Center	Fresno	California	559-459-6000	www.communitymedical.org
Covenant Hospital Plainview	Plainview	Texas	806-296-5531	www.covenantplainview.org
Crestwood Medical Center	Huntsville	Alabama	256-882-3100	www.crestwoodmedcenter.com
Crossgates River Oaks Hospital	Brandon	Mississippi	601-825-2811	www.rankinmedcenter.com
Crouse Hospital	Syracuse	New York	315-470-7449	www.crouse.org
Dameron Hospital	Stockton	California	209-944-5550	www.dameronhospital.org
Deaconess Hospital	Spokane	Washington	509-473-5800	www.deaconessmedicalcenter.org
Deaconess Hospital	Evansville	Indiana	812-450-5000	www.deaconess.com
Desert Regional Medical Center	Palm Springs	California	760-323-6511	www.desertmedctr.com
Eisenhower Medical Center	Rancho Mirage	California	760-340-3911	www.emc.org
El Camino Hospital	Mountain View	California	650-940-7000	www.elcaminohospital.org
Eliza Coffee Memorial Hospital	Florence	Alabama	256-768-8400	www.chgroup.org
Emory University Hospital Midtown	Atlanta	Georgia	404-686-4411	www.emoryhealthcare.org
Faith Regional Health Services	Norfolk	Nebraska	402-371-4880	www.frhs.org
Firsthealth Moore Regional Hospital	Pinehurst	North Carolina	910-715-1000	www.firsthealth.org
Geisinger Medical Center	Danville	Pennsylvania	570-271-6211	www.geisinger.org
Geisinger Wyoming Valley Medical Center	Wilkes Barre	Pennsylvania	570-826-7300	www.geisinger.org
Gila Regional Medical Center	Silver City	New Mexico	575-538-4000	www.grmc.org
Good Samaritan Hospital	San Jose	California	408-559-2011	www.goodsamsj.org
Good Samaritan Hospital	Dayton	Ohio	937-278-2612	www.goodsamdayton.org
Good Shepherd Medical Center Marshall	Marshall	Texas	903-927-6712	www.marshallregional.org
Grady Memorial Hospital	Atlanta	Georgia	404-616-4252	www.gradyhealthsystem.org
Grinnell Regional Medical Center	Grinnell	Iowa	641-236-7511	www.grmc.us
Grossmont Hospital	La Mesa	California	619-465-0711	www.sharp.com
Harborview Medical Center	Seattle	Washington	206-731-3000	www.harborview.org
Hennepin County Medical Center	Minneapolis	Minnesota	612-873-3000	www.hcmc.org
Henrico Doctors' Hospital	Richmond	Virginia	804-289-4500	www.henricodoctors.com
Heritage Valley Beaver	Beaver	Pennsylvania	412-728-7000	www.heritagevalley.org
The Indiana Heart Hospital	Indianapolis	Indiana	317-621-8063	www.hearthospital.com
Inspira Medical Center Vineland	Vineland	New Jersey	856-641-6610	www.sjhs.com
Intermountain Medical Center	Murray	Utah	801-507-7000	www.intermountainhealthcare.org
Jewish Hospital & Saint Mary's Healthcare	Louisville	Kentucky	502-587-4011	www.jhhs.org
John Dempsey Hospital	Farmington	Connecticut	860-679-1145	www.uconnhealth.orgorwww.uchc.edu
JPS Health Network	Fort Worth	Texas	817-921-3431	www.jpshealthnet.org
Jupiter Medical Center	Jupiter	Florida	561-747-2234	www.jupitermed.com
Kadlec Regional Medical Center	Richland	Washington	509-946-4611	www.kadlecmed.org
Kaiser Foundation Hospital - Fontana	Fontana	California	909-427-5500	www.kaiserpermanente.com
Kaweah Delta Medical Center	Visalia	California	559-624-2000	www.kaweahdelta.org

Hospital	City	State	Phone	Web Site
Keck Hospital of USC	Los Angeles	California	323-442-8656	www.uscuh.com
Kingman Regional Medical Center	Kingman	Arizona	928-757-2101	www.azkrmc.com
Kuakini Medical Center	Honolulu	Hawaii	808-536-2236	www.kuakini.org
LDS Hospital	Salt Lake City	Utah	801-408-1100	www.intermountainhealthcare.org
Lourdes Hospital	Paducah	Kentucky	270-444-2444	www.ehealthconnection.com
Magee Womens Hospital of UPMC Health System	Pittsburgh	Pennsylvania	412-641-4010	www.magee.edu
Maine Medical Center	Portland	Maine	207-662-0111	www.mmc.org
Manchester Memorial Hospital	Manchester	Connecticut	860-647-4780	www.echn.org
Marin General Hospital	Greenbrae	California	415-925-7900	www.maringeneral.com
Mary Hitchcock Memorial Hospital	Lebanon	New Hampshire	603-650-5000	www.dhmc.org
Mat-Su Regional Medical Center	Palmer	Alaska	907-746-8600	www.matsuregional.com
Mayo Clinic Health System - Mankato	Mankato	Minnesota	507-625-4031	www.isj-mhs.org
Mayo Clinic Health System - Eau Claire Hospital	Eau Claire	Wisconsin	715-838-3311	www.luthermidelfort.org
McKay Dee Hospital	Ogden	Utah	801-387-2800	www.intermountainhealthcare.org
Medical College of Virginia Hospitals	Richmond	Virginia	804-828-0938	www.vcuhealth.org
Medical West	Bessemer	Alabama	205-481-7000	www.uab.edu
Medstar Washington Hospital Center	Washington	District of Columbia	202-877-7000	www.whcenter.org
Memorial Medical Center	Modesto	California	209-526-4500	www.memorialmedicalcenter.org
Memorial Health Univ Medical Center	Savannah	Georgia	912-350-8000	www.memorialhealth.com
Memorial Hospital	York	Pennsylvania	717-843-8623	www.mhyork.org
Memorial Hospital & Health Care Center	Jasper	Indiana	812-996-2345	www.mhhcc.org
Memorial Hospital of Carbondale	Carbondale	Illinois	618-549-0721	www.sih.net
Memorial Medical Center	Springfield	Illinois	217-788-3000	www.memorialmedical.com
Mercy General Hospital	Sacramento	California	916-453-4545	www.mercygeneral.org
Mercy Health Hackley Campus	Muskegon	Michigan	231-726-3511	www.hackley.org
Mercy Hospital - Cadillac	Cadillac	Michigan	231-876-7200	www.mercycadillac.munsonhealthcare.org
Mercy Medical Center - Des Moines	Des Moines	Iowa	515-247-3121	www.mercydesmoines.org
Mercy Memorial Health Center	Ardmore	Oklahoma	405-223-5400	www.mercyok.com/mmhc
Methodist Hospital of Sacramento	Sacramento	California	916-423-6010	www.methodistsacramento.org
Methodist Jennie Edmundson	Council Bluffs	Iowa	712-396-6000	www.bestcare.org
Metro Health Hospital	Wyoming	Michigan	616-252-7200	www.metrohealth.net
Metrohealth System	Cleveland	Ohio	216-778-7089	www.metrohealth.org
Miami Valley Hospital	Dayton	Ohio	937-208-8000	www.miamivalleyhospital.com
Milton S Hershey Medical Center	Hershey	Pennsylvania	717-531-8521	www.hmc.psu.edu
Montrose Memorial Hospital	Montrose	Colorado	970-249-2211	www.montrosehospital.com
Morton Plant Hospital	Clearwater	Florida	727-462-7000	www.measehospitals.com
Mount Sinai Hospital	New York	New York	212-241-7981	www.mountsinai.org
Muhlenberg Community Hospital	Greenville	Kentucky	270-338-8000	www.mchky.org
Multicare Good Samaritan Hospital	Puyallup	Washington	253-697-2102	www.multicare.org/goodsam
Musc Medical Center	Charleston	South Carolina	843-792-2300	www.musc.edu
Nash General Hospital	Rocky Mount	North Carolina	252-443-8000	www.nhcs.org
New Hanover Regional Medical Center	Wilmington	North Carolina	910-343-7000	www.nhrmc.org
Newport Hospital	Newport	Rhode Island	401-846-6400	www.newporthospital.org
Northwest Medical Center	Tucson	Arizona	520-742-9000	www.northwestmedicalcenter.com
Novant Health Presbyterian Medical Center	Charlotte	North Carolina	704-384-4000	www.presbyterian.org
O U Medical Center	Oklahoma City	Oklahoma	405-271-5911	www.oumedcenter.com
OHSU Hospital & Clinics	Portland	Oregon	503-494-4036	www.ohsu.edu
Oklahoma State University Medical Center	Tulsa	Oklahoma	918-587-2561	www.tulsaregional.com
Our Lady of the Lake Regional Medical Center	Baton Rouge	Louisiana	225-765-6565	www.ololrmc.com
Overland Park Regional Medical Center	Overland Park	Kansas	913-541-5301	www.oprmc.com
Parkview Medical Center	Pueblo	Colorado	719-584-4000	www.parkviewmc.com
Peacehealth Saint Joseph Medical Center	Bellingham	Washington	360-734-5400	www.peacehealth.org
Phelps County Regional Medical Center	Rolla	Missouri	573-458-8899	www.rollanet.org/~pcrmc
Physicians Regional Medical Center - Pine Ridge	Naples	Florida	239-348-4000	www.physiciansregional.com
Pinnacle Health Hospitals	Harrisburg	Pennsylvania	717-782-5181	www.pinnaclehealth.org
Providence Holy Cross Medical Center	Mission Hills	California	818-365-8051	www.providence.org
Providence Sacred Heart Medical Center	Spokane	Washington	509-474-3040	www.shmc.org
Rhode Island Hospital	Providence	Rhode Island	401-444-4000	www.rhodeislandhospital.org
Ridgeview Medical Center	Waconia	Minnesota	952-442-2191	www.ridgeviewmedical.org
Riverview Hospital Assoc	Wisconsin Rapids	Wisconsin	715-423-6060	www.riverviewhospital.net
Ronald Reagan UCLA Medical Center	Los Angeles	California	310-825-6301	www.uclahealth.org
Rush University Medical Center	Chicago	Illinois	312-942-5000	www.ruch.edu
Russellville Hospital	Russellville	Alabama	256-332-1611	www.russellvillehospital.com
Sacred Heart Hospital	Eau Claire	Wisconsin	715-717-4121	www.sacredhearteauclaire.org
Saint Anthony Medical Center	Rockford	Illinois	815-226-2000	www.osfhealth.com
Saint Francis Medical Center	Peoria	Illinois	309-655-2000	www.osfsaintfrancis.org
Saint Joseph's Hospital of Atlanta	Atlanta	Georgia	678-843-5720	www.stjosephsatlanta.org

Hospital	City	State	Phone	Web Site
Saint Mary's Health Care	Grand Rapids	Michigan	616-685-5000	www.smhealthcare.org
Saint Mary's Regional Medical Center	Reno	Nevada	775-770-3000	www.saintmarysreno.com
Salem Hospital	Salem	Oregon	503-561-5200	www.salemhospital.org
Salina Regional Health Center	Salina	Kansas	785-452-7000	www.srhc.com
Sanford Usd Medical Center	Sioux Falls	South Dakota	605-333-1000	www.sanfordhealth.org
Santiam Memorial Hospital	Stayton	Oregon	503-769-2175	www.santiamhospital.com
Sarasota Memorial Hospital	Sarasota	Florida	941-917-9000	www.smh.com
Seton Medical Center Austin	Austin	Texas	512-324-1000	www.seton.net
Sharp Memorial Hospital	San Diego	California	858-939-3400	www.sharp.com/memorial
Sky Ridge Medical Center	Lone Tree	Colorado	720-225-1000	www.skyridgemedcenter.com
Slidell Memorial Hospital	Slidell	Louisiana	985-643-2200	www.sliddelmemorial.org
Southeast Alabama Medical Center	Dothan	Alabama	334-793-8701	www.samc.org
Southwestern Vermont Medical Center	Bennington	Vermont	802-442-6361	www.svhealthcare.org
Spectrum Health - Butterworth Campus	Grand Rapids	Michigan	616-391-1774	www.spectrum-health.org
Springhill Medical Center	Mobile	Alabama	251-344-9630	www.springhillmedicalcenter.com
Saint Elizabeth Health Center	Youngstown	Ohio	330-746-7211	www.hmhs.org
Saint Elizabeth Medical Center	Utica	New York	315-798-8100	www.stemc.org
Saint Francis Health Center	Topeka	Kansas	785-295-8000	www.stfrancistopeka.org
Saint Francis - Downtown	Greenville	South Carolina	864-255-1000	www.stfrancishealth.org
Saint Helena Hospital	Saint Helena	California	707-963-3611	www.sthelenahospital.org
Saint Joseph Medical Center	Tacoma	Washington	253-627-4101	www.fhshealth.org
Saint Joseph Mercy Hospital	Ann Arbor	Michigan	734-712-3791	www.stjoesannarbor.or
Saint Joseph's Hospital & Medical Center	Phoenix	Arizona	602-406-3000	www.stjosephs-phx.org
Saint Louis University Hospital	Saint Louis	Missouri	314-577-8000	www.slucare.edu/clinical
Saint Luke's Hospital Bethlehem	Bethlehem	Pennsylvania	610-954-4000	www.slhn-lehighvalley.org
Saint Luke's Hospital	Chesterfield	Missouri	314-434-1500	www.goodhealthmatters.com
Saint Luke's Hospital of Kansas City	Kansas City	Missouri	816-932-2000	www.staintlukeshealthsystem.org
Saint Marys Hospital	Madison	Wisconsin	608-251-6100	www.stmarysmadison.com
Stanford Hospital	Stanford	California	650-723-5708	www.stanfordhospital.com
Swedish Medical Center	Seattle	Washington	206-386-6000	www.swedish.org
Swedish Medical Center - Cherry Hill	Seattle	Washington	206-320-2000	www.swedish.org
Tacoma General Allenmore Hospital	Tacoma	Washington	253-403-1000	www.multicare.org
Tampa General Hospital	Tampa	Florida	813-844-7000	www.tgh.org
Heart Hospital Baylor Plano	Plano	Texas	469-814-3278	www.thehearthospitalbaylor.com
Theda Clark Medical Center	Neenah	Wisconsin	920-729-3100	www.thedacare.org
Thomas Hospital	Fairhope	Alabama	251-928-2375	www.thomashospital.com
Town & Country Hospital	Tampa	Florida	813-882-7159	www.townandcountryhospital.com
Trinity Hospitals	Minot	North Dakota	701-857-5000	www.trinityhealth.org
Trinity Medical Center	Birmingham	Alabama	205-592-1000	www.bhsala.com/montclair
Trinity Rock Island	Rock Island	Illinois	309-779-5000	www.trinityqc.com
Trumbull Memorial Hospital	Warren	Ohio	330-841-9011	www.trumhosp.org
Tulane Medical Center	New Orleans	Louisiana	504-988-1900	www.tuhc.com
UF Health Jacksonville	Jacksonville	Florida	904-244-0411	www.shandsjacksonville.org
UMC of Southern Nevada	Las Vegas	Nevada	702-383-2000	www.umc-cares.org
University Colo Health Memorial Hospital Central	Colorado Springs	Colorado	719-365-5000	www.memorialhospital.com
University Health Care/University Hospitals & Clinics	Salt Lake City	Utah	801-581-2121	www.healthcare.utah.edu
University Health System	San Antonio	Texas	210-358-4000	www.universityhealthsystem.com
University of California Davis Medical Center	Sacramento	California	916-734-2011	www.ucdmc.ucdavis.edu
University of Cincinnati Medical Center	Cincinnati	Ohio	513-584-1000	www.universityhospitalcincinnati.com
University of Colorado Hospital	Aurora	Colorado	720-848-0000	www.uch.edu
University of Kansas Hospital	Kansas City	Kansas	913-588-7332	www.kumc.edu
University of Miami Hospital	Miami	Florida	305-325-5511	www.cedarsmedicalcenter.com
University of Minnesota Medical Center - Fairview	Minneapolis	Minnesota	612-273-3000	www.uofmmedicalcenter.org
University of Toledo Medical Center	Toledo	Ohio	419-383-3407	www.utmc.utoledo.edu
University of Wisconsin Hospitals & Clinics Authority	Madison	Wisconsin	608-263-8991	www.uwhealth.org
UPMC Hamot	Erie	Pennsylvania	814-877-6000	www.hamot.org
UPMC Passavant	Pittsburgh	Pennsylvania	412-367-6700	www.passavant.upmc.com
UPMC Presbyterian Shadyside	Pittsburgh	Pennsylvania	412-647-8788	www.upmc.edu
UT Southwestern University Hospital	Dallas	Texas	214-879-3758	www.utsouthwestern.edu
Utah Valley Regional Medical Center	Provo	Utah	801-373-7850	www.intermountainhealthcare.org/hospitals/uvrmc
Ventura County Medical Center	Ventura	California	805-652-6075	www.vchca.org
Vidant Medical Center	Greenville	North Carolina	252-847-4100	www.uhseast.com
Virginia Mason Medical Center	Seattle	Washington	206-223-6600	www.vmmc.org
Waukesha Memorial Hospital	Waukesha	Wisconsin	262-928-1000	www.waukeshamemorial.org
Wesley Medical Center	Hattiesburg	Mississippi	601-268-8000	www.wesley.com
West Virginia University Hospitals	Morgantown	West Virginia	304-598-4000	www.wvuh.com
Wheaton Franciscan Saint Joseph	Milwaukee	Wisconsin	414-447-2000	www.wfhealthcare.org

Hospital	City	State	Phone	Web Site
Winchester Hospital	Winchester	Massachusetts	781-729-9000	www.winchesterhospital.org
Women & Infants Hospital of Rhode Island	Providence	Rhode Island	401-274-1100	www.womenandinfants.com
The Women's Hospital	Newburgh	Indiana	812-842-4200	www.deaconess.com
Yavapai Regional Medical Center	Prescott	Arizona	928-771-5676	www.yrmc.org

Note: Table shows hospitals nationwide whose surgical complication rate is worse (higher) than U.S. rate of 1.83%

Hospitals whose Surgical Complication Rate is Better (Lower) than the U.S. National Rate

Measure: Collapsed Lung Due to Medical Treatment

Hospital	City	State	Phone	Web Site
Centinela Hospital Medical Center	Inglewood	California	310-673-4660	www.centinelafreeman.com
Centra Health	Lynchburg	Virginia	434-200-4789	www.centrahealth.com
Community Medical Center	Toms River	New Jersey	732-557-8000	www.sbhcs.com
Evanston Hospital	Evanston	Illinois	847-432-8000	www.enh.org
New York - Presbyterian Hospital	New York	New York	212-746-4189	www.nyp.org
Norton Hospitals	Louisville	Kentucky	502-629-6560	www.nortonhealthcare.com
Spectrum Health - Butterworth Campus	Grand Rapids	Michigan	616-391-1774	www.spectrum-health.org
Virtua West Jersey Hospitals Berlin	Berlin	New Jersey	856-322-3200	www.virtua.org
Willis Knighton Medical Center	Shreveport	Louisiana	318-212-4000	www.wkhs.com//locations/medicalcenter.aspx

Note: Table shows hospitals nationwide whose surgical complication rate is better (lower) than U.S. rate of 0.32%

Hospitals whose Surgical Complication Rate is Worse (Higher) than the U.S. National Rate

Measure: Collapsed Lung Due to Medical Treatment

Hospital	City	State	Phone	Web Site
Abilene Regional Medical Center	Abilene	Texas	325-428-1000	www.abileneregional.com
Banner Heart Hospital	Mesa	Arizona	480-854-5050	www.bannerhealth.com
Baylor Medical Center at Garland	Garland	Texas	972-487-5000	www.baylorhealth.com
Baylor Regional Medical Center at Grapevine	Grapevine	Texas	817-481-1588	www.baylorhealth.com
Bert Fish Medical Center	New Smyrna Beach	Florida	386-424-5000	www.bertfish.com
Beth Israel Deaconess Medical Center	Boston	Massachusetts	617-667-7000	www.bidmc.harvard.edu
Bryan Medical Center	Lincoln	Nebraska	402-481-1111	www.bryan.org
Capital Region Medical Center	Jefferson City	Missouri	573-632-5000	www.crmc.org
Carolinas Medical Center - Union	Monroe	North Carolina	704-283-3100	www.carolinashealthcare.org/cmc-union
Champlain Valley Physicians Hospital Medical Center	Plattsburgh	New York	518-561-2000	www.cvph.org
Community Regional Medical Center	Fresno	California	559-459-6000	www.communitymedical.org
Des Peres Hospital	Saint Louis	Missouri	314-966-9100	www.desperes hospital.com
Feather River Hospital	Paradise	California	530-877-9361	www.frhosp.org
Florida Hospital	Orlando	Florida	407-303-1976	www.floridahospital.com
Hays Medical Center	Hays	Kansas	785-623-5000	www.haysmed.com
Inova Fairfax Hospital	Falls Church	Virginia	703-776-3332	www.inova.org
Kansas Medical Center	Andover	Kansas	316-300-4000	www.ksmedcenter.com
Largo Medical Center	Largo	Florida	727-588-5200	www.largomedical.com
Lawrence Memorial Hospital	Lawrence	Kansas	785-505-6100	www.lmh.org
Loma Linda University Medical Center	Loma Linda	California	909-558-4000	www.llumc.edu
Madera Community Hospital	Madera	California	559-675-5555	www.maderahospital.org
Maine Medical Center	Portland	Maine	207-662-0111	www.mmc.org
Massachusetts General Hospital	Boston	Massachusetts	617-726-2000	www.massgeneral.org
Mclaren - Northern Michigan	Petoskey	Michigan	231-487-4000	www.northernhealth.org
Medical West	Bessemer	Alabama	205-481-7000	www.uab.edu
Midmichigan Medical Center - Midland	Midland	Michigan	989-839-3000	www.midmichigan.org
Mills - Peninsula Medical Center	Burlingame	California	650-696-5270	www.mills-peninsula.org
Norman Regional Health System	Norman	Oklahoma	405-321-1700	www.normanregional.com
Northwest Texas Hospital	Amarillo	Texas	806-354-1110	www.nxtexashealthcare.com
NYU Hospitals Center	New York	New York	212-263-7300	www.med.nyu.edu
Orange Regional Medical Center	Middletown	New York	845-343-2424	www.ormc.org
Orlando Health	Orlando	Florida	321-841-5111	www.orlandoregionalmedicalcenter.org
Parkridge Medical Center	Chattanooga	Tennessee	423-894-4220	www.tristarhealth.com
Piedmont Hospital	Atlanta	Georgia	404-605-5000	www.piedmonthospital.org
Pikeville Medical Center	Pikeville	Kentucky	606-218-3500	www.pikevillehospital.org
Providence Health Center	Waco	Texas	254-751-4000	www.providence.net
Providence Saint Vincent Medical Center	Portland	Oregon	503-216-1234	www.providence.org
Ronald Reagan UCLA Medical Center	Los Angeles	California	310-825-6301	www.uclahealth.org
Saint Francis Medical Center	Peoria	Illinois	309-655-2000	www.osfsaintfrancis.org
Saint Joseph Hospital	Lexington	Kentucky	859-313-1000	www.sjhlex.org
Saint Joseph's Hospital of Atlanta	Atlanta	Georgia	678-843-5720	www.stjosephsatlanta.org
Sanford Medical Center Fargo	Fargo	North Dakota	701-234-2000	www.meritcare.com
Self Regional Healthcare	Greenwood	South Carolina	864-227-4111	www.selfregional.org
Sentara Norfolk General Hospital	Norfolk	Virginia	757-388-3000	www.sentara.com
Sharp Memorial Hospital	San Diego	California	858-939-3400	www.sharp.com/memorial
Silver Cross Hospital & Medical Centers	New Lenox	Illinois	815-300-1100	www.silvercross.org
SSM Depaul Health Center	Bridgeton	Missouri	314-344-6000	www.ssmdepaul.com
Saint Bernards Medical Center	Jonesboro	Arkansas	870-972-4100	www.sbrmc.com
Saint John Medical Center	Tulsa	Oklahoma	918-744-3606	www.sjmc.org
Saint John's Episcopal Hospital at South Shore	Far Rockaway	New York	718-869-7000	www.ehs.org
Saint Luke's Hospital of Kansas City	Kansas City	Missouri	816-932-2000	www.saintlukeshealthsystem.org
Saint Tammany Parish Hospital	Covington	Louisiana	985-898-4000	www.stph.org
Sturdy Memorial Hospital	Attleboro	Massachusetts	508-222-5200	www.sturdymemorial.org
Theda Clark Medical Center	Neenah	Wisconsin	920-729-3100	www.thedacare.org
UMC of Southern Nevada	Las Vegas	Nevada	702-383-2000	www.umc-cares.org
University Medical Center of El Paso	El Paso	Texas	915-521-7602	www.thomasoncares.org
University of Alabama Hospital	Birmingham	Alabama	205-934-4011	www.health.uab.edu
University of Toledo Medical Center	Toledo	Ohio	419-383-3407	www.utmc.utoledo.edu
UPMC Presbyterian Shadyside	Pittsburgh	Pennsylvania	412-647-8788	www.upmc.edu
Williamsport Regional Medical Center	Williamsport	Pennsylvania	570-321-1000	www.susquehannahealth.org

Note: Table shows hospitals nationwide whose surgical complication rate is worse (higher) than U.S. rate of 0.32%

Hospitals whose Surgical Complication Rate is Better (Lower) than the U.S. National Rate

Measure: Deaths Among Patients With Serious Treatable Complications After Surgery

Hospital	City	State	Phone	Web Site
Advocate Lutheran General Hospital	Park Ridge	Illinois	847-723-2210	www.advocatehealth.com
Alexian Brothers Medical Center	Elk Grove Village	Illinois	847-437-5500	www.alexian.org
Aurora West Allis Medical Center	West Allis	Wisconsin	414-328-6000	www.aurorahealthcare.org
Banner Thunderbird Medical Center	Glendale	Arizona	602-588-5555	www.bannerhealth.com
Baptist Saint Anthony's Hospital	Amarillo	Texas	806-212-2000	www.bsahs.com
Bayfront Health Punta Gorda	Punta Gorda	Florida	941-639-3131	www.charlotteregional.com
Delray Medical Center	Delray Beach	Florida	561-498-4440	www.delraymedicalctr.com
Emory University Hospital	Atlanta	Georgia	404-686-8500	www.emoryhealthcare.org
Evanston Hospital	Evanston	Illinois	847-432-8000	www.enh.org
Fawcett Memorial Hospital	Port Charlotte	Florida	941-629-1181	www.fawcetthospital.com
Franciscan Saint Francis Health - Indianapolis	Indianapolis	Indiana	317-865-5001	www.stfrancishospitals.org
Gwinnett Medical Center	Lawrenceville	Georgia	678-312-1000	www.gwinnettmedicalcenter.org
Hackensack University Medical Center	Hackensack	New Jersey	201-996-2000	www.humed.com
Henry Ford Wyandotte Hospital	Wyandotte	Michigan	734-246-6000	www.henryfordwyandotte.com
Hinsdale Hospital	Hinsdale	Illinois	630-856-9000	www.keepingyouwell.com
Hospital For Special Surgery	New York	New York	212-606-1000	www.hss.edu
JFK Medical Center	Atlantis	Florida	561-965-7300	www.jfkmc.com
JFK Medical Center - A M Yelencsics Comm Hospital	Edison	New Jersey	732-321-7000	www.jfkmc.org
Los Robles Hospital & Medical Center	Thousand Oaks	California	805-497-2727	www.losrobleshospital.com
Martin Medical Center	Stuart	Florida	772-287-5200	www.mmhs.com
Mayo Clinic Hospital	Phoenix	Arizona	480-342-2000	www.mayoclinic.org
Mayo Clinic Methodist- Hospital	Rochester	Minnesota	507-266-7890	www.mayoclinic.org/methodisthospital
Mclaren Flint	Flint	Michigan	810-342-2000	www.mclaren.org
Memorial Hermann Memorial City Medical Center	Houston	Texas	713-242-3000	www.mhhs.org
Missouri Baptist Medical Center	Town & Country	Missouri	314-996-5000	www.missouribaptistmedicalcenter.org
Mother Frances Hospital	Tyler	Texas	903-593-8441	www.tmfhs.org
North Colorado Medical Center	Greeley	Colorado	970-352-4121	www.bannerhealth.com
North Kansas City Hospital	North Kansas City	Missouri	816-691-2000	www.nkch.org
Northwestern Memorial Hospital	Chicago	Illinois	312-926-2000	www.nmh.org
NYU Hospitals Center	New York	New York	212-263-7300	www.med.nyu.edu
OHSU Hospital & Clinics	Portland	Oregon	503-494-4036	www.ohsu.edu
Palm Beach Gardens Medical Center	Palm Beach Gardens	Florida	561-622-1411	www.pbgmc.com
Palos Community Hospital	Palos Heights	Illinois	708-923-4000	www.paloshospital.org
Providence Hospital & Medical Centers	Southfield	Michigan	248-849-3011	www.stjohn.org/providence
Saint Alexius Medical Center	Hoffman Estates	Illinois	847-843-2000	www.alexianbrothershealth.org
Saint Alexius Medical Center	Bismarck	North Dakota	701-530-7000	www.st.alexius.org
Saint David's Medical Center	Austin	Texas	512-476-7111	www.stdavidsrehab.com
Saint Elizabeth Health Center	Youngstown	Ohio	330-746-7211	www.hmhs.org
Saint John Macomb - Oakland Hospital - Macomb Center	Warren	Michigan	586-573-5000	www.stjohn.org
Saint Joseph's Hospital & Medical Center	Phoenix	Arizona	602-406-3000	www.stjosephs-phx.org
Saint Luke's Hospital	Cedar Rapids	Iowa	319-369-7211	www.crstlukes.com
Heart Hospital Baylor Plano	Plano	Texas	469-814-3278	www.thehearthospitalbaylor.com
University of Wisconsin Hospitals & Clinics Authority	Madison	Wisconsin	608-263-8991	www.uwhealth.org

Note: Table shows hospitals nationwide whose surgical complication rate is better (lower) than U.S. rate of 110.25%

Hospitals whose Surgical Complication Rate is Worse (Higher) than the U.S. National Rate

Measure: Deaths Among Patients With Serious Treatable Complications After Surgery

Hospital	City	State	Phone	Web Site
Baptist Health Medical Center - Little Rock	Little Rock	Arkansas	501-202-2000	www.baptist-health.com
Baptist Medical Center	San Antonio	Texas	210-297-1020	www.baptisthealthsystem.org
Carolinas Hospital System	Florence	South Carolina	843-674-2500	www.carolinashospital.com
Carolinas Medical Center/Behaviorial Health	Charlotte	North Carolina	704-355-2000	www.carolinasmedicalcenter.org
Christian Hospital Northeast - Northwest	Saint Louis	Missouri	314-653-5000	www.christianhospital.org
Christiana Care Health Services	Newark	Delaware	302-733-1000	www.christianacare.org
Community Regional Medical Center	Fresno	California	559-459-6000	www.communitymedical.org
Conway Medical Center	Conway	South Carolina	843-347-8037	www.conwayhospital.com
Cooper University Hospital	Camden	New Jersey	856-342-2000	www.cooperhealth.org
Cullman Regional Medical Center	Cullman	Alabama	256-737-2000	www.crmchospital.com
Doctors Hospital	Augusta	Georgia	706-651-6008	www.doctors-hospital.net
Doctors Medical Center	Modesto	California	209-578-1211	www.dmc-modesto.com
Duke University Hospital	Durham	North Carolina	919-684-8111	www.dukehealth.org
East Texas Medical Center	Tyler	Texas	903-597-0351	www.etmc.org
Erlanger Medical Center	Chattanooga	Tennessee	423-778-7000	www.erlanger.org
Fairbanks Memorial Hospital	Fairbanks	Alaska	907-452-8181	www.bannerhealth.com
Fletcher Allen Hospital of Vermont	Burlington	Vermont	802-847-0000	www.fletcherallen.org
Florida Hospital Tampa	Tampa	Florida	813-615-7200	www.uch.org
Good Samaritan Hospital Medical Center	West Islip	New York	631-376-3000	www.good-samaritan-hospital.org
Halifax Health Medical Center	Daytona Beach	Florida	386-254-4000	www.halifax.org
Health Alliance Hospital Broadway Campus	Kingston	New York	914-331-3131	www.kingstonregionalhealth.org
Hillcrest Medical Center	Tulsa	Oklahoma	918-579-1000	www.hillcrest.com
Integris Baptist Medical Center	Oklahoma City	Oklahoma	405-951-8110	www.integris-health.com
Jewish Hospital & Saint Mary's Healthcare	Louisville	Kentucky	502-587-4011	www.jhhs.org
Kaleida Health	Buffalo	New York	716-859-8620	www.kaleidahealth.org
Lake Cumberland Regional Hospital	Somerset	Kentucky	606-679-7441	www.lakecumberlandhospital.com
Lakeland Regional Medical Center	Lakeland	Florida	863-687-1100	www.lrmc.com
Magnolia Regional Health Center	Corinth	Mississippi	662-293-7660	www.mrhc.org
Marian Regional Medical Center	Santa Maria	California	805-739-3000	www.marinmedicalcenter.org
Mary Hitchcock Memorial Hospital	Lebanon	New Hampshire	603-650-5000	www.dhmc.org
Medical Center of Central Georgia	Macon	Georgia	478-633-6805	www.mccg.org
Medical Center of Plano	Plano	Texas	972-596-6800	www.medicalcenterofplano.com
Medical College of Georgia Hospitals & Clinics	Augusta	Georgia	706-721-6569	www.mcghealth.org
Methodist Healthcare Memphis Hospitals	Memphis	Tennessee	901-516-8274	www.methodisthealth.org
Milton S Hershey Medical Center	Hershey	Pennsylvania	717-531-8521	www.hmc.psu.edu
Mobile Infirmary	Mobile	Alabama	251-435-4700	www.mimc.com
Nazareth Hospital	Philadelphia	Pennsylvania	215-335-6000	www.nazarethhospital.org
North Carolina Baptist Hospital	Winston-Salem	North Carolina	336-716-2011	www.wfubmc.edu
North Mississippi Medical Center	Tupelo	Mississippi	662-377-3000	www.nmhs.net/nmmc
Northeast Alabama Regional Medical Center	Anniston	Alabama	256-235-5121	www.rmccares.org
Oklahoma State University Medical Center	Tulsa	Oklahoma	918-587-2561	www.tulsaregional.com
Phoebe Putney Memorial Hospital	Albany	Georgia	229-312-4068	www.phoebeputney.com
Renown Regional Medical Center	Reno	Nevada	775-982-4100	www.renown.org
Riverside Methodist Hospital	Columbus	Ohio	614-566-5000	www.ohiohealth.com
Robert Wood Johnson University Hospital	New Brunswick	New Jersey	732-937-8900	www.rwjuh.edu
Robert Wood Johnson University Hospital - Hamilton	Hamilton	New Jersey	609-586-7900	www.rwjhamilton.org
Saint Francis Medical Center	Peoria	Illinois	309-655-2000	www.osfsaintfrancis.org
Sentara Norfolk General Hospital	Norfolk	Virginia	757-388-3000	www.sentara.com
Saint John Medical Center	Tulsa	Oklahoma	918-744-3606	www.sjmc.org
Saint Joseph's Hospital - Savannah	Savannah	Georgia	912-819-4100	www.sjchs.org
Saint Luke's Episcopal Hospital	Houston	Texas	832-355-1000	www.sleh.com
Saint Mary's Medical Center	Huntington	West Virginia	304-526-1234	www.st-marys.org
Saint Vincent's East	Birmingham	Alabama	205-838-3122	www.nolandhealth.com
Strong Memorial Hospital	Rochester	New York	585-275-2121	www.urmc.rochester.edu
Sunrise Hospital & Medical Center	Las Vegas	Nevada	702-731-8000	www.sunrisehospital.com
Tampa General Hospital	Tampa	Florida	813-844-7000	www.tgh.org
Trident Medical Center	Charleston	South Carolina	843-797-8800	www.tridenthealthsystem.com
UF Health Shands Hospital	Gainesville	Florida	352-265-8000	www.shands.org
Umass Memorial Medical Center	Worcester	Massachusetts	508-334-1000	www.umassmemorial.org
University Hospital	Newark	New Jersey	973-972-5658	www.theuniversityhospital.com
University Medical Center	Lubbock	Texas	806-775-8200	www.teamumc.org
University of Alabama Hospital	Birmingham	Alabama	205-934-4011	www.health.uab.edu
University of Kentucky Hospital	Lexington	Kentucky	859-323-5000	www.uhealthcare.uky.edu
University of Mississippi Medical Center	Jackson	Mississippi	601-984-4100	www.umc.edu

Hospital	City	State	Phone	Web Site
University of South Alabama Medical Center	Mobile	Alabama	251-471-7110	www.southalabama.edu/usamc
Vidant Medical Center	Greenville	North Carolina	252-847-4100	www.uhseast.com
Virtua West Jersey Hospitals Berlin	Berlin	New Jersey	856-322-3200	www.virtua.org

Note: Table shows hospitals nationwide whose surgical complication rate is worse (higher) than U.S. rate of 110.25%

Hospitals whose Surgical Complication Rate is Better (Lower) than the U.S. National Rate

Measure: Rate of Complications for Hip/Knee Replacement Patients

Hospital	City	State	Phone	Web Site
Arkansas Surgical Hospital	No Little Rock	Arkansas	501-748-8000	www.arksurgicalhospital.com
Baptist Health Louisville	Louisville	Kentucky	502-897-8100	www.baptisteast.com
Barnes-Jewish Hospital	Saint Louis	Missouri	314-747-3000	www.barnesjewish.org
Beaumont Health System	Royal Oak	Michigan	248-898-5000	www.beaumonthospitals.com
Boone Hospital Center	Columbia	Missouri	573-815-8000	www.boone.org
Bronson Methodist Hospital	Kalamazoo	Michigan	269-341-6000	www.bronsonhealth.com
Cape Cod Hospital	Hyannis	Massachusetts	508-771-1800	www.capecodhealth.org
Carilion Roanoke Memorial Hospital	Roanoke	Virginia	540-981-7000	www.carilion.com/crmh
Covenant Medical Center	Lubbock	Texas	806-725-6000	www.covenanthealth.org
Crittenton Hospital Medical Center	Rochester	Michigan	248-652-5000	www.crittenton.com
Delray Medical Center	Delray Beach	Florida	561-498-4440	www.delraymedicalctr.com
Doctors Hospital at Renaissance	Edinburg	Texas	956-362-8677	www.dhr-rgv.com
Florida Hospital Memorial Medical Center	Daytona Beach	Florida	386-676-6000	www.fhmd.com
Franciscan Saint Elizabeth Health - Lafayette East	Lafayette	Indiana	765-502-4334	www.ste.org
Heart of Florida Regional Medical Center	Davenport	Florida	863-422-4971	www.heartofflorida.com
Heartland Regional Medical Center	Saint Joseph	Missouri	816-271-6000	www.heartland-health.com
Hoag Orthopedic Institute	Irvine	California	949-727-5000	www.orthopedichospital.com
Holy Cross Hospital	Fort Lauderdale	Florida	954-771-8000	www.holy-cross.com
Hospital For Special Surgery	New York	New York	212-606-1000	www.hss.edu
Indian River Medical Center	Vero Beach	Florida	772-567-4311	www.irmh.com
Indiana Orthopaedic Hospital	Indianapolis	Indiana	317-956-1000	www.indianaorthopaedichospital.com
Jupiter Medical Center	Jupiter	Florida	561-747-2234	www.jupitermed.com
Kansas Medical Center	Andover	Kansas	316-300-4000	www.ksmedcenter.com
Kansas Surgery & Recovery Center	Wichita	Kansas	316-634-0090	www.ksrc.org
Maine Medical Center	Portland	Maine	207-662-0111	www.mmc.org
Mayo Clinic Methodist- Hospital	Rochester	Minnesota	507-266-7890	www.mayoclinic.org/methodisthospital
Mclaren - Greater Lansing	Lansing	Michigan	517-975-6000	www.mclaren.org
Memorial Healthcare System	Chattanooga	Tennessee	423-495-2525	www.memorial.org
Memorial Mission Hospital & Asheville Surgery Center	Asheville	North Carolina	828-213-1111	www.missionhospitals.org
Mississippi Baptist Medical Center	Jackson	Mississippi	601-968-1000	www.mbmc.org
Nebraska Orthopaedic Hospital	Omaha	Nebraska	402-609-1600	www.neorthohospital.com
New England Baptist Hospital	Boston	Massachusetts	617-754-5800	www.nebh.caregroup.org
North Mississippi Medical Center	Tupelo	Mississippi	662-377-3000	www.nmhs.net/nmmc
Ocala Regional Medical Center	Ocala	Florida	352-401-1000	www.ocalaregional.com
Oklahoma Surgical Hospital	Tulsa	Oklahoma	918-477-5000	www.oklahomasurgicalhospital.com
Olathe Medical Center	Olathe	Kansas	913-791-4200	www.ohsi.com
Orthopaedic Hospital at Parkview North	Fort Wayne	Indiana	260-672-4050	www.parkview.com
Plaza Medical Center of Fort Worth	Fort Worth	Texas	817-336-2100	www.plazamedicalcenter.com
Poudre Valley Hospital	Fort Collins	Colorado	970-495-7000	www.pvhs.org
Proctor Hospital	Peoria	Illinois	309-691-1000	www.proctor.org
Providence Saint John's Health Center	Santa Monica	California	310-829-5511	www.stjohns.org
Quail Creek Surgical Hospital	Amarillo	Texas	806-354-6100	www.physurg.com
Riverside Medical Center	Kankakee	Illinois	815-933-1671	www.riversidehealthcare.org
Roper Hospital	Charleston	South Carolina	843-724-2800	www.ropersaintfrancis.com
Sacred Heart Hospital	Pensacola	Florida	850-416-7000	www.sacred-heart.org
Saint Elizabeth Regional Medical Center	Lincoln	Nebraska	402-219-7700	www.stelizabethonline.com
Saint Joseph Regional Medical Center	Mishawaka	Indiana	574-335-5000	www.sjmed.com
Saint Joseph's Hospital of Atlanta	Atlanta	Georgia	678-843-5720	www.stjosephsatlanta.org
Saint Thomas Midtown Hospital	Nashville	Tennessee	615-284-5555	www.baptisthospital.com
Samaritan Regional Health System	Ashland	Ohio	419-289-0491	www.samho.org
Sanford Medical Center Bismarck	Bismarck	North Dakota	701-323-6000	www.medcenterone.com
Sentara Leigh Hospital	Norfolk	Virginia	757-261-6601	www.sentara.com
Seton Medical Center Austin	Austin	Texas	512-324-1000	www.seton.net
South Nassau Communities Hospital	Oceanside	New York	516-632-3000	www.southnassau.org
Southside Hospital	Bay Shore	New York	631-968-3000	www.northshorelij.com
Southwest General Health Center	Middleburg Heights	Ohio	440-816-8000	www.swgeneral.com
Saint Francis Hospital & Medical Center	Hartford	Connecticut	860-714-4000	www.saintfranciscare.com
Saint Helena Hospital	Saint Helena	California	707-963-3611	www.sthelenahospital.org
Saint Joseph Hospital	Orange	California	714-633-9111	www.sjo.org
Saint Joseph Mercy Oakland	Pontiac	Michigan	248-858-3000	www.stjoesoakland.org
Saint Joseph's Hospital - Savannah	Savannah	Georgia	912-819-4100	www.sjchs.org
Saint Peter's Hospital	Albany	New York	518-525-1550	www.stpetershealthcare.org
Saint Vincent's Medical Center	Jacksonville	Florida	904-308-7300	www.jaxhealth.com
Sutter General Hospital	Sacramento	California	916-733-8999	www.suttermedicalcenter.org

Hospital	City	State	Phone	Web Site
Tampa General Hospital	Tampa	Florida	813-844-7000	www.tgh.org
Texas Health Presbyterian Hospital Dallas	Dallas	Texas	214-345-6789	www.texashealth.org
Torrance Memorial Medical Center	Torrance	California	310-325-9110	www.torrancememorial.org
Valley Medical Center	Renton	Washington	425-228-3450	www.valleymed.org
VHS Harlingen Hospital Company	Harlingen	Texas	956-389-1100	www.vbmc.org
Washington Hospital	Fremont	California	510-797-1111	www.whhs.com
Western Maryland Regional Medical Center	Cumberland	Maryland	240-964-8001	www.wmhs.com
William Beaumont Hospital - Troy	Troy	Michigan	248-964-8800	www.beaumonthospitals.com
Yavapai Regional Medical Center	Prescott	Arizona	928-771-5676	www.yrmc.org

Note: Table shows hospitals nationwide whose surgical complication rate is better (lower) than U.S. rate of 3.4%

Hospitals whose Surgical Complication Rate is Worse (Higher) than the U.S. National Rate

Measure: Rate of Complications for Hip/Knee Replacement Patients

Hospital	City	State	Phone	Web Site
Alegent Health Mercy Hospital	Council Bluffs	Iowa	712-328-5000	www.alegent.com/mercy
Atrium Medical Center	Franklin	Ohio	513-420-5102	www.atriummedcenter.org
Baptist Memorial Hospital	Memphis	Tennessee	901-226-5000	www.bmhcc.org
Baptist Saint Anthony's Hospital	Amarillo	Texas	806-212-2000	www.bsahs.com
Beaumont Health System	Grosse Pointe	Michigan	313-343-1000	www.beaumonthospitals.com
Bridgeport Hospital	Bridgeport	Connecticut	203-384-3000	www.bridgeporthospital.com
Carolinas Medical Center - Northeast	Concord	North Carolina	704-783-3000	www.northeastmedical.org
Central Maine Medical Center	Lewiston	Maine	207-795-0111	www.cmmc.org
Community Memorial Hospital San Buenaventura	Ventura	California	805-652-5011	www.cmhhospital.org
D C H Regional Medical Center	Tuscaloosa	Alabama	205-759-7111	www.dchsystem.com
Decatur Morgan Hospital - Decatur Campus	Decatur	Alabama	256-341-2000	www.decaturgeneral.org
Defiance Regional Medical Center	Defiance	Ohio	419-783-6955	www.promedica.org/defiance
Doctors Medical Center	Modesto	California	209-578-1211	www.dmc-modesto.com
East Ohio Regional Hospital	Martins Ferry	Ohio	740-633-4151	www.eastohioregionalhospital.com
Floyd Medical Center	Rome	Georgia	706-509-6900	www.floydmed.org
Froedtert Memorial Lutheran Hospital	Milwaukee	Wisconsin	414-805-3000	www.froedtert.com
Gadsden Regional Medical Center	Gadsden	Alabama	256-494-4000	www.gadsdenregional.com
Genesis Medical Center - Davenport	Davenport	Iowa	563-421-1000	www.genesishealth.com
Genesys Regional Medical Center - Health Park	Grand Blanc	Michigan	810-606-5000	www.genesys.org
Grant Medical Center	Columbus	Ohio	614-566-9978	www.ohiohealth.com
Henry County Medical Center	Paris	Tennessee	731-642-1220	www.hcmc-tn.org
Houston Orthopedic & Spine Hospital	Bellaire	Texas	713-622-2262	www.foundationsurgicalhospital.com
Johnson City Medical Center	Johnson City	Tennessee	423-431-6111	www.msha.com
Lancaster General Hospital	Lancaster	Pennsylvania	717-299-5511	www.lancastergeneral.org
Louis A Weiss Memorial Hospital	Chicago	Illinois	773-878-8700	www.weisshospital.org
The Medical Center of Aurora	Aurora	Colorado	303-695-2600	www.auroramed.com
Mercy Health System Corp	Janesville	Wisconsin	608-756-6080	www.mercyhealthsystem.org
Mercy Saint Anne Hospital	Toledo	Ohio	419-407-2663	www.mercyweb.org
Mountain View Hospital	Payson	Utah	801-465-7100	www.mvhpayson.com
North Colorado Medical Center	Greeley	Colorado	970-352-4121	www.bannerhealth.com
North Kansas City Hospital	North Kansas City	Missouri	816-691-2000	www.nkch.org
Northwestern Memorial Hospital	Chicago	Illinois	312-926-2000	www.nmh.org
Novant Health Rowan Medical Center	Salisbury	North Carolina	704-210-5000	www.rowan.org
NYU Hospitals Center	New York	New York	212-263-7300	www.med.nyu.edu
Onslow Memorial Hospital	Jacksonville	North Carolina	910-577-2345	www.onslowmemorial.org
Overland Park Regional Medical Center	Overland Park	Kansas	913-541-5301	www.oprmc.com
Park Ridge Health	Hendersonville	North Carolina	828-684-8501	www.parkridgehospital.org
Pennsylvania Hospital of the Univ of PA Health Sys	Philadelphia	Pennsylvania	215-829-3000	www.pennmedicine.org/pahosp
Peterson Regional Medical Center	Kerrville	Texas	830-896-4200	www.petersonrmc.com
Pinnacle Health Hospitals	Harrisburg	Pennsylvania	717-782-5181	www.pinnaclehealth.org
Poplar Bluff Regional Medical Center	Poplar Bluff	Missouri	573-785-7721	www.poplarbluffregional.com
Reston Hospital Center	Reston	Virginia	703-689-9000	www.restonhospital.com
Riddle Memorial Hospital	Media	Pennsylvania	610-566-9400	www.riddlehospital.org
Saint Michael's Medical Center	Newark	New Jersey	973-877-5350	www.cathedralhealth.org
Shady Grove Adventist Hospital	Rockville	Maryland	240-826-6517	www.adventisthealthcare.com/sgah
Shannon Medical Center	San Angelo	Texas	325-653-6741	www.shannonhealth.com
South Central Regional Medical Center	Laurel	Mississippi	601-649-4000	www.scrmc.com
South Lake Hospital	Clermont	Florida	352-394-4071	www.southlakehospital.com
Southside Regional Medical Center	Petersburg	Virginia	804-765-5000	www.srmconline.com
Spring Valley Hospital Medical Center	Las Vegas	Nevada	702-853-3000	www.springvalleyhospital.com
Saint Alexius Medical Center	Hoffman Estates	Illinois	847-843-2000	www.alexianbrothershealth.org
Saint Anthony Hospital	Oklahoma City	Oklahoma	405-272-7000	www.saintsok.com
Saint Catherine of Siena Hospital	Smithtown	New York	631-862-3000	www.stcatherines.chsli.org
Saint Clair Memorial Hospital	Pittsburgh	Pennsylvania	412-942-6209	www.stclair.org
Saint Elizabeth Hospital	Appleton	Wisconsin	920-738-2000	www.affinityhealth.org
Saint Luke's Hospital Bethlehem	Bethlehem	Pennsylvania	610-954-4000	www.slhn-lehighvalley.org
Saint Marys Hospital	Madison	Wisconsin	608-251-6100	www.stmarysmadison.com
Saint Vincent Anderson Regional Hospital	Anderson	Indiana	765-646-8373	www.stjohnshealthsystem.org
Saint Vincent Healthcare	Billings	Montana	406-657-7000	www.svh-mt.org
Saint Vincent's Medical Center	Bridgeport	Connecticut	203-576-5551	www.stvincents.org
Sutter Auburn Faith Hospital	Auburn	California	530-888-4500	www.sutterauburnfaith.org
Sutter Solano Medical Center	Vallejo	California	707-554-5280	www.suttersolano.org
Swedish Medical Center	Englewood	Colorado	303-788-5000	www.swedishhospital.com/default.asp
Trinity Medical Center	Birmingham	Alabama	205-592-1000	www.bhsala.com/montclair

Hospital	City	State	Phone	Web Site
University of Kansas Hospital	Kansas City	Kansas	913-588-7332	www.kumc.edu
University of Toledo Medical Center	Toledo	Ohio	419-383-3407	www.utmc.utoledo.edu
Wentworth - Douglass Hospital	Dover	New Hampshire	603-740-2580	www.wdhospital.com
White River Medical Center	Batesville	Arkansas	870-262-1200	www.wrmc.com

Note: Table shows hospitals nationwide whose surgical complication rate is worse (higher) than U.S. rate of 3.4%

Hospitals whose Surgical Complication Rate is Better (Lower) than the U.S. National Rate

Measure: Serious Blood Clots After Surgery

Hospital	City	State	Phone	Web Site
Abbott Northwestern Hospital	Minneapolis	Minnesota	612-863-4509	www.abbottnorthwestern.com
Advocate Condell Medical Center	Libertyville	Illinois	847-990-5200	www.condell.org
Allegiance Health	Jackson	Michigan	517-788-4800	www.footehealth.org
Arkansas Heart Hospital	Little Rock	Arkansas	501-219-7000	www.arheart.com
Asante Rogue Regional Medical Center	Medford	Oregon	541-789-7000	www.asante.org
Aurora Saint Lukes Medical Center	Milwaukee	Wisconsin	414-649-6000	www.aurorahealthcare.org
Avera Mckennan Hospital & University Health Center	Sioux Falls	South Dakota	605-322-8000	www.mckennan.org
Avera Saint Lukes	Aberdeen	South Dakota	605-622-5000	www.averastlukes.org
Bakersfield Memorial Hospital	Bakersfield	California	661-327-1792	www.bakersfieldmemorial.org
Banner Baywood Medical Center	Mesa	Arizona	480-321-2000	www.bannerhealth.com
Banner Good Samaritan Medical Center	Phoenix	Arizona	602-239-2000	www.bannerhealth.com
Baptist Beaumont Hospital	Beaumont	Texas	409-212-5012	www.mhbh.org
Baptist Health Lexington	Lexington	Kentucky	859-260-6104	www.centralbap.com
Baptist Health Louisville	Louisville	Kentucky	502-897-8100	www.baptisteast.com
Baptist Health Medical Center - Little Rock	Little Rock	Arkansas	501-202-2000	www.baptist-health.com
Baystate Medical Center	Springfield	Massachusetts	413-794-0000	www.baystatehealth.com
Benefis Hospitals	Great Falls	Montana	406-455-5000	www.benefis.org
Berkshire Medical Center	Pittsfield	Massachusetts	413-447-2000	www.berkshirehealthsystems.org
Billings Clinic Hospital	Billings	Montana	406-657-4000	www.billingsclinic.com
Camden Clark Medical Center	Parkersburg	West Virginia	304-424-2111	www.ccmh.org
Cape Cod Hospital	Hyannis	Massachusetts	508-771-1800	www.capecodhealth.org
Carilion New River Valley Medical Center	Christiansburg	Virginia	540-731-2000	www.carilion.com
Carolinas Medical Center/Behaviorial Health	Charlotte	North Carolina	704-355-2000	www.carolinasmedicalcenter.org
Caromont Regional Medical Center	Gastonia	North Carolina	704-834-4891	www.caromont.org
Carson Tahoe Regional Medical Center	Carson City	Nevada	775-445-8000	www.carsontahoehospital.com
Centra Health	Lynchburg	Virginia	434-200-4789	www.centrahealth.com
Central Maine Medical Center	Lewiston	Maine	207-795-0111	www.cmmc.org
Charlotte Hungerford Hospital	Torrington	Connecticut	860-496-6666	www.charlottesweb.hungerford.org
Comanche County Memorial Hospital	Lawton	Oklahoma	580-355-8620	www.memorialhealthsource.org
Community Hospital North	Indianapolis	Indiana	317-621-5335	www.ecommunity.com/north
Community Medical Center	Toms River	New Jersey	732-557-8000	www.sbhcs.com
Cox Medical Center	Springfield	Missouri	417-269-6000	www.coxhealth.com
Doctors Hospital of Sarasota	Sarasota	Florida	941-342-1100	www.doctorsofsarasota.com
Duke University Hospital	Durham	North Carolina	919-684-8111	www.dukehealth.org
Eastern Idaho Regional Medical Center	Idaho Falls	Idaho	208-529-6111	www.eirmc.org
Eisenhower Medical Center	Rancho Mirage	California	760-340-3911	www.emc.org
El Camino Hospital	Mountain View	California	650-940-7000	www.elcaminohospital.org
Elkhart General Hospital	Elkhart	Indiana	574-294-2621	www.egh.org
Essentia Health - Fargo	Fargo	North Dakota	701-364-8000	www.dakotaclinic.com
Exeter Hospital	Exeter	New Hampshire	603-778-7311	www.exeterhospital.com
Flagstaff Medical Center	Flagstaff	Arizona	928-773-2009	www.nahealth.com
Fort Sanders Regional Medical Center	Knoxville	Tennessee	865-541-1101	www.fsregional.com
Franciscan Saint Elizabeth Health - Lafayette East	Lafayette	Indiana	765-502-4334	www.ste.org
Geisinger - Community Medical Center	Scranton	Pennsylvania	570-969-8240	www.cmchealthsys.org
Genesis Medical Center - Davenport	Davenport	Iowa	563-421-1000	www.genesishealth.com
Glens Falls Hospital	Glens Falls	New York	518-926-1000	www.glensfallshospital.org
Good Samaritan Regional Medical Center	Corvallis	Oregon	541-768-5111	www.samhealth.org/shs_facilities
Gundersen Lutheran Medical Center	La Crosse	Wisconsin	608-782-7300	www.gundluth.org
Harrison Memorial Center	Bremerton	Washington	360-377-3911	www.harrisonmedical.org
Hays Medical Center	Hays	Kansas	785-623-5000	www.haysmed.com
Heartland Regional Medical Center	Saint Joseph	Missouri	816-271-6000	www.heartland-health.com
Hendrick Medical Center	Abilene	Texas	325-670-2000	www.ehendrick.org
Holy Cross Hospital	Fort Lauderdale	Florida	954-771-8000	www.holy-cross.com
Indiana University Health Bloomington Hospital	Bloomington	Indiana	812-353-9555	www.bloomingtonhospital.org
Indiana University Health North Hospital	Carmel	Indiana	317-688-2000	www.iuhealth.org/north
Inova Mount Vernon Hospital	Alexandria	Virginia	703-664-7000	www.inova.com/inovapublic.srt/imvh/index.jsp
Integris Baptist Medical Center	Oklahoma City	Oklahoma	405-951-8110	www.integris-health.com
Jackson Hospital & Clinic	Montgomery	Alabama	334-293-8000	www.jackson.org
Jackson - Madison County General Hospital	Jackson	Tennessee	731-541-5000	www.wth.org
John Muir Medical Center - Concord Campus	Concord	California	925-674-2002	www.johnmuirhealth.com
John Muir Medical Center - Walnut Creek Campus	Walnut Creek	California	925-939-3000	www.jmmdhs.com
Kalispell Regional Medical Center	Kalispell	Montana	406-752-5111	www.krmc.org
Kootenai Medical Center	Coeur D'alene	Idaho	208-625-4001	www.kootenaihealth.org
Lakeland Hospital - Saint Joseph	Saint Joseph	Michigan	269-983-8300	www.lakelandhealth.org

Hospital	City	State	Phone	Web Site
Marian Regional Medical Center	Santa Maria	California	805-739-3000	www.marinmedicalcenter.org
Mary Washington Hospital	Fredericksburg	Virginia	540-741-1100	www.medicorp.org
Maury Regional Hospital	Columbia	Tennessee	931-381-1111	www.maurgregional.com
Mayo Clinic Methodist- Hospital	Rochester	Minnesota	507-266-7890	www.mayoclinic.org/methodisthospital
Mcleod Regional Medical Center - Pee Dee	Florence	South Carolina	843-777-2900	www.mcleodhealth.org
Medical Center of Central Georgia	Macon	Georgia	478-633-6805	www.mccg.org
Memorial Healthcare System	Chattanooga	Tennessee	423-495-2525	www.memorial.org
Memorial Hospital at Gulfport	Gulfport	Mississippi	228-867-4000	www.gulfportmemorial.com
Memorial Hospital of Carbondale	Carbondale	Illinois	618-549-0721	www.sih.net
Memorial Mission Hospital & Asheville Surgery Center	Asheville	North Carolina	828-213-1111	www.missionhospitals.org
Mercy Hospital	Coon Rapids	Minnesota	763-236-8205	www.allinamercy.org
Mercy Medical Center - Cedar Rapids	Cedar Rapids	Iowa	319-398-6011	www.mercycare.org
Mercy Medical Center - Redding	Redding	California	530-225-6102	www.redding.mercy.org
Mercy Medical Center - North Iowa	Mason City	Iowa	641-428-7000	www.mercynorthiowa.com
Methodist Hospital	San Antonio	Texas	210-575-4000	www.mh.sahealth.com
Methodist Medical Center of Oak Ridge	Oak Ridge	Tennessee	865-835-1000	www.mmcoakridge.com
Mother Frances Hospital	Tyler	Texas	903-593-8441	www.tmfhs.org
Munson Medical Center	Traverse City	Michigan	231-935-5000	www.munsonhealthcare.org
New England Baptist Hospital	Boston	Massachusetts	617-754-5800	www.nebh.caregroup.org
Novant Health Charlotte Orthopedic Hospital	Charlotte	North Carolina	704-316-2000	www.presbyterian.org
NW Arkansas Hospitals	Springdale	Arkansas	479-751-5711	www.northwesthealth.org
Ochsner Medical Center	New Orleans	Louisiana	504-842-3000	www.ochsner.org
Oklahoma Heart Hospital	Oklahoma City	Oklahoma	405-608-3200	www.okheart.com
Olathe Medical Center	Olathe	Kansas	913-791-4200	www.ohsi.com
Parker Adventist Hospital	Parker	Colorado	303-269-4000	www.parkerhospital.org
Parkview Medical Center	Pueblo	Colorado	719-584-4000	www.parkviewmc.com
Parkview Regional Medical Center	Fort Wayne	Indiana	260-266-1000	www.parkview.com
Parkwest Medical Center	Knoxville	Tennessee	865-970-9800	www.yesparkwest.com
Peacehealth Saint Joseph Medical Center	Bellingham	Washington	360-734-5400	www.peacehealth.org
Peconic Bay Medical Center	Riverhead	New York	631-548-6000	www.pbmedicalcenter.org
Presence Covenant Medical Center	Urbana	Illinois	217-337-2000	www.provena.org/covenant
Providence Sacred Heart Medical Center	Spokane	Washington	509-474-3040	www.shmc.org
Providence Saint John's Health Center	Santa Monica	California	310-829-5511	www.stjohns.org
Providence Saint Joseph Medical Center	Burbank	California	818-843-5111	www.providence.org/losangeles
Regional Medical Center Bayonet Point	Hudson	Florida	727-819-2929	www.mchealth.comorwww.heartoftampa.com
Riverview Medical Center	Red Bank	New Jersey	732-741-2700	www.meridianhealth.com
Sacred Heart Medical Center - Riverbend	Springfield	Oregon	541-222-7300	www.peacehealth.org/sacred-heart-riverbend
Saint Francis Medical Center	Cape Girardeau	Missouri	573-331-3000	www.sfmc.net
Saint Joseph Hospital	Lexington	Kentucky	859-313-1000	www.sjhlex.org
Saint Joseph Regional Medical Center	Mishawaka	Indiana	574-335-5000	www.sjmed.com
Saint Mary's Health Care	Grand Rapids	Michigan	616-685-5000	www.smhealthcare.org
Saint Thomas West Hospital	Nashville	Tennessee	615-222-2111	www.stthomas.org
Salinas Valley Memorial Hospital	Salinas	California	831-757-4333	www.svmh.com
San Jacinto Methodist Hospital	Baytown	Texas	281-420-8600	www.methodisthealth.com/sanjacinto
Sanford Medical Center Fargo	Fargo	North Dakota	701-234-2000	www.meritcare.com
Sanford Usd Medical Center	Sioux Falls	South Dakota	605-333-1000	www.sanfordhealth.org
Sarasota Memorial Hospital	Sarasota	Florida	941-917-9000	www.smh.com
Scott & White Memorial Hospital	Temple	Texas	254-724-2111	www.sw.org
Seton Medical Center Austin	Austin	Texas	512-324-1000	www.seton.net
Shannon Medical Center	San Angelo	Texas	325-653-6741	www.shannonhealth.com
Shasta Regional Medical Center	Redding	California	530-244-5454	www.shastaregional.com
South Georgia Medical Center	Valdosta	Georgia	229-333-1020	www.sgmc.org
Saint Charles Medical Center - Bend	Bend	Oregon	541-382-4321	www.scmc.org
Saint Cloud Hospital	Saint Cloud	Minnesota	320-251-2700	www.centracare.com
Saint David's Medical Center	Austin	Texas	512-476-7111	www.stdavidsrehab.com
Saint Elizabeth Medical Center	Lakeside Park	Kentucky	859-292-2000	www.stelizabeth.com
Saint Helena Hospital	Saint Helena	California	707-963-3611	www.sthelenahospital.org
Saint Joseph Hospital	Orange	California	714-633-9111	www.sjo.org
Saint Joseph Mercy Oakland	Pontiac	Michigan	248-858-3000	www.stjoesoakland.org
Saint Joseph's Hospital Health Center	Syracuse	New York	315-448-5111	www.sjhsyr.org
Saint Joseph's Medical Center of Stockton	Stockton	California	209-943-2000	www.stjospehscares.org
Saint Luke's Hospital	Cedar Rapids	Iowa	319-369-7211	www.crstlukes.com
Saint Mary's Regional Medical Center	Enid	Oklahoma	580-233-6100	www.stmarysregional.com
Saint Marys Hospital	Madison	Wisconsin	608-251-6100	www.stmarysmadison.com
Saint Patrick Hospital	Missoula	Montana	406-543-7271	www.saintpatrick.org
Saint Vincent Healthcare	Billings	Montana	406-657-7000	www.svh-mt.org
Saint Vincent Hospital	Santa Fe	New Mexico	505-913-5201	www.stvin.org

Hospital	City	State	Phone	Web Site
Saint Vincent Hospital & Health Services	Indianapolis	Indiana	317-338-7000	www.indianapolis.stvincent.org
Saint Vincent's Medical Center	Jacksonville	Florida	904-308-7300	www.jaxhealth.com
Sutter General Hospital	Sacramento	California	916-733-8999	www.suttermedicalcenter.org
Swedish American Hospital	Rockford	Illinois	815-968-4400	www.swedishamerican.org
Swedish Medical Center	Seattle	Washington	206-386-6000	www.swedish.org
Tallahassee Memorial Hospital	Tallahassee	Florida	850-431-1155	www.tmh.org
Texas Health Harris Methodist Hurst - Euless - Bedford	Bedford	Texas	817-848-4000	www.texashealth.org
Thibodaux Regional Medical Center	Thibodaux	Louisiana	985-447-5500	www.thibodaux.com
Trinity Rock Island	Rock Island	Illinois	309-779-5000	www.trinityqc.com
United Regional Health Care System	Wichita Falls	Texas	940-764-3055	www.urhcs.org
University Health Care/University Hospitals & Clinics	Salt Lake City	Utah	801-581-2121	www.healthcare.utah.edu
University Medical Center	Lubbock	Texas	806-775-8200	www.teamumc.org
University of Washington Medical Center	Seattle	Washington	206-598-3300	www.washington.edu/medical/uwmc
Vanderbilt University Hospital	Nashville	Tennessee	615-322-3454	www.mc.vanderbilt.edu
VHS Harlingen Hospital Company	Harlingen	Texas	956-389-1100	www.vbmc.org
Via Christi Hospitals Wichita	Wichita	Kansas	316-268-5000	www.via-christi.org
Virginia Mason Medical Center	Seattle	Washington	206-223-6600	www.vmmc.org
Wakemed - Raleigh Campus	Raleigh	North Carolina	919-350-8000	www.wakemed.org
Washington Hospital	Fremont	California	510-797-1111	www.whhs.com
Wesley Medical Center	Wichita	Kansas	316-962-2000	www.wesleymc.com
Winchester Medical Center	Winchester	Virginia	540-536-8000	www.valleyhealthlink.com
Winter Haven Hospital	Winter Haven	Florida	863-293-1121	www.winterhavenhospital.com
Wyoming Medical Center	Casper	Wyoming	307-577-7201	www.wyomingmedicalcenter.com
Yakima Valley Memorial Hospital	Yakima	Washington	509-575-8000	www.yakimamemorialhospital.org

Note: Table shows hospitals nationwide whose surgical complication rate is better (lower) than U.S. rate of 4.14%

Hospitals whose Surgical Complication Rate is Worse (Higher) than the U.S. National Rate

Measure: Serious Blood Clots After Surgery

Hospital	City	State	Phone	Web Site
Advocate Good Samaritan Hospital	Downers Grove	Illinois	630-275-5900	www.advocatehealth.com/gsam
Advocate Illinois Masonic Medical Center	Chicago	Illinois	773-975-1600	www.advocatehealth.com/immc
Advocate Lutheran General Hospital	Park Ridge	Illinois	847-723-2210	www.advocatehealth.com
Albert Einstein Medical Center	Philadelphia	Pennsylvania	215-456-6090	www.einstein.edu
Alegent Health Mercy Hospital	Council Bluffs	Iowa	712-328-5000	www.alegent.com/mercy
Alexian Brothers Medical Center	Elk Grove Village	Illinois	847-437-5500	www.alexian.org
Aultman Hospital	Canton	Ohio	330-452-9911	www.aultman.com
B R F Hospital Holdings	Shreveport	Louisiana	318-675-5000	www.lsumc.edu
Baptist Memorial Hospital Desoto	Southaven	Mississippi	662-772-4000	www.bmhcc.org/facilities/desoto
Barnes-Jewish Hospital	Saint Louis	Missouri	314-747-3000	www.barnesjewish.org
Beaumont Health System	Grosse Pointe	Michigan	313-343-1000	www.beaumonthospitals.com
Beaumont Health System	Royal Oak	Michigan	248-898-5000	www.beaumonthospitals.com
Bon Secours Saint Francis Medical Center	Midlothian	Virginia	804-594-7400	www.richmond.bonsecours.com
Bridgeport Hospital	Bridgeport	Connecticut	203-384-3000	www.bridgeporthospital.com
Brigham & Women's Hospital	Boston	Massachusetts	617-732-5500	www.brighamandwomens.org
Brookdale Hospital Medical Center	Brooklyn	New York	718-240-5966	www.brookdalehospital.org
Brookwood Medical Center	Birmingham	Alabama	205-877-1000	www.bwmc.com
Cape Coral Hospital	Cape Coral	Florida	239-574-2323	www.leememorial.org
Carilion Roanoke Memorial Hospital	Roanoke	Virginia	540-981-7000	www.carilion.com/crmh
Cedars - Sinai Medical Center	Los Angeles	California	310-423-5000	www.cedars-sinai.edu
Centennial Medical Center	Frisco	Texas	972-963-3333	www.centennialmedcenter.com
Charleston Area Medical Center	Charleston	West Virginia	304-388-6203	www.camc.org
Christian Hospital Northeast - Northwest	Saint Louis	Missouri	314-653-5000	www.christianhospital.org
Christiana Care Health Services	Newark	Delaware	302-733-1000	www.christianacare.org
Christus Saint Frances Cabrini Hospital	Alexandria	Louisiana	318-487-1122	www.cabrini.org
Christus Saint Michael Health System	Texarkana	Texas	903-614-1000	www.christusstmichael.org
Cleveland Clinic	Cleveland	Ohio	216-444-2200	www.clevelandclinic.org
Conemaugh Valley Memorial Hospital	Johnstown	Pennsylvania	814-534-9000	www.conemaugh.org
Coney Island Hospital	Brooklyn	New York	718-616-3000	www.coneyislandhospital.com
Cooper University Hospital	Camden	New Jersey	856-342-2000	www.cooperhealth.org
Crouse Hospital	Syracuse	New York	315-470-7449	www.crouse.org
D C H Regional Medical Center	Tuscaloosa	Alabama	205-759-7111	www.dchsystem.com
Danbury Hospital	Danbury	Connecticut	203-797-7000	www.danburyhospital.com
Delnor Community Hospital	Geneva	Illinois	630-208-3000	www.delnor.com
Doctors Hospital	Augusta	Georgia	706-651-6008	www.doctors-hospital.net
Doctors Hospital	Coral Gables	Florida	305-666-2111	www.baptisthealth.net
Edward Hospital	Naperville	Illinois	630-527-3000	www.edward.org
El Paso Specialty Hospital	El Paso	Texas	915-544-3636	www.elpasospecialtyhospital.com
Emory University Hospital Midtown	Atlanta	Georgia	404-686-4411	www.emoryhealthcare.org
Evanston Hospital	Evanston	Illinois	847-432-8000	www.enh.org
Flagler Hospital	Saint Augustine	Florida	904-819-4426	www.flaglerhospital.com
Florida Hospital	Orlando	Florida	407-303-1976	www.floridahospital.com
Franciscan Saint Margaret Health - Hammond	Hammond	Indiana	219-932-2300	www.smmhc.com
Geisinger Medical Center	Danville	Pennsylvania	570-271-6211	www.geisinger.org
Genesys Regional Medical Center - Health Park	Grand Blanc	Michigan	810-606-5000	www.genesys.org
Glen Cove Hospital	Glen Cove	New York	516-674-7300	www.northshorelij.com
Grady Memorial Hospital	Atlanta	Georgia	404-616-4252	www.gradyhealthsystem.org
Grand View Hospital	Sellersville	Pennsylvania	215-453-4615	www.gvh.org
Gulf Coast Medical Center Lee Memorial Health System	Fort Myers	Florida	239-768-5000	www.leememorial.org
Hackensack University Medical Center	Hackensack	New Jersey	201-996-2000	www.humed.com
Hackettstown Regional Medical Center	Hackettstown	New Jersey	908-852-5100	www.hrmcnj.org
Hahnemann University Hospital	Philadelphia	Pennsylvania	215-762-7000	www.hahnemannhospital.com
Harris Health System	Houston	Texas	713-566-6417	www.hchdonline.com
Hartford Hospital	Hartford	Connecticut	860-545-5000	www.harthosp.org
Henry Ford Hospital	Detroit	Michigan	313-916-2600	www.henryfordhospital.com
Henry Ford West Bloomfield Hospital	W Bloomfield	Michigan	248-325-1000	www.henryford.com
Henry Ford Wyandotte Hospital	Wyandotte	Michigan	734-246-6000	www.henryfordwyandotte.com
Heritage Valley Beaver	Beaver	Pennsylvania	412-728-7000	www.heritagevalley.org
Heritage Valley Sewickley	Sewickley	Pennsylvania	412-741-6600	www.heritagevalley.org
Hillcrest Hospital	Mayfield Heights	Ohio	440-312-4500	www.hillcresthospital.org
Holmes Regional Medical Center	Melbourne	Florida	321-434-7000	www.healthfirst.org
Holy Name Medical Center	Teaneck	New Jersey	201-833-3000	www.holyname.org
Hospital of Univ of Pennsylvania	Philadelphia	Pennsylvania	215-662-3227	www.upenn.edu
Huntington Memorial Hospital	Pasadena	California	626-397-5000	www.huntingtonhospital.com

Hospital	City	State	Phone	Web Site
Hurley Medical Center	Flint	Michigan	810-257-9000	www.hurleymc.com
Ingalls Memorial Hospital	Harvey	Illinois	708-333-2300	www.ingalls.org
Intermountain Medical Center	Murray	Utah	801-507-7000	www.intermountainhealthcare.org
Jackson Memorial Hospital	Miami	Florida	305-585-1111	www.jhsmiami.org
Jeanes Hospital	Philadelphia	Pennsylvania	215-728-2000	www.jeanes.com
JFK Medical Center	Atlantis	Florida	561-965-7300	www.jfkmc.com
JFK Medical Center - A M Yelencsics Comm Hospital	Edison	New Jersey	732-321-7000	www.jfkmc.org
John H Stroger Jr Hospital	Chicago	Illinois	312-864-6000	www.cookcountygov.com
JPS Health Network	Fort Worth	Texas	817-921-3431	www.jpshealthnet.org
Jupiter Medical Center	Jupiter	Florida	561-747-2234	www.jupitermed.com
Lancaster General Hospital	Lancaster	Pennsylvania	717-299-5511	www.lancastergeneral.org
Lee Memorial Hospital	Fort Myers	Florida	239-332-1111	www.leememorial.org
Legacy Emanuel Medical Center	Portland	Oregon	503-413-2200	www.legacyhealth.org
Lehigh Valley Hospital	Allentown	Pennsylvania	610-402-2273	www.lvhhn.org
Lehigh Valley Hospital - Muhlenberg	Bethlehem	Pennsylvania	610-402-2273	www.lvhn.org
Lenox Hill Hospital	New York	New York	212-439-2345	www.lenoxhillhospital.org
Little Company of Mary Hospital	Evergreen Park	Illinois	708-422-6200	www.lcmh.org
Louis A Weiss Memorial Hospital	Chicago	Illinois	773-878-8700	www.weisshospital.org
Lourdes Hospital	Paducah	Kentucky	270-444-2444	www.ehealthconnection.com
Lovelace Medical Center	Albuquerque	New Mexico	505-727-8000	www.lovelace.com
Loyola University Medical Center	Maywood	Illinois	708-216-9000	www.lumc.edu
Magee Womens Hospital of UPMC Health System	Pittsburgh	Pennsylvania	412-641-4010	www.magee.edu
Maimonides Medical Center	Brooklyn	New York	718-283-6000	www.maimonidesmed.org
Marin General Hospital	Greenbrae	California	415-925-7900	www.maringeneral.com
Mary Hitchcock Memorial Hospital	Lebanon	New Hampshire	603-650-5000	www.dhmc.org
Marymount Hospital	Garfield Heights	Ohio	216-581-0500	www.marymount.org
Mclaren Flint	Flint	Michigan	810-342-2000	www.mclaren.org
The Medical Center of Aurora	Aurora	Colorado	303-695-2600	www.auroramed.com
Medical Center of Mckinney	Mckinney	Texas	972-547-8000	www.medicalcenterofmckinney.com
Medical Center of Plano	Plano	Texas	972-596-6800	www.medicalcenterofplano.com
Medstar Georgetown University Hospital	Washington	District of Columbia	202-784-3000	www.georgetownuniversityhospital.org
Memorial Healthcare	Owosso	Michigan	989-723-5211	www.memorialhealthcare.org
Memorial Hermann Texas Medical Center	Houston	Texas	713-704-3700	www.mhhs.org
Memorial Hospital Jacksonville	Jacksonville	Florida	904-399-6111	www.memorialhospitaljax.com
Memorial Medical Center	Las Cruces	New Mexico	575-522-8641	www.mmclc.org
Menorah Medical Center	Overland Park	Kansas	913-498-6773	www.menorahmedicalcenter.com
Mercy Fitzgerald Hospital	Darby	Pennsylvania	215-237-4000	www.mercyhealth.org
Mercy Hospital Springfield	Springfield	Missouri	417-820-2000	www.stjohns.com
Mercy Saint Vincent Medical Center	Toledo	Ohio	419-251-3232	www.mhsnr.org
Miami Valley Hospital	Dayton	Ohio	937-208-8000	www.miamivalleyhospital.com
Midwest Orthopedic Specialty Hospital	Franklin	Wisconsin	414-817-5800	www.mymosh.com
Milton S Hershey Medical Center	Hershey	Pennsylvania	717-531-8521	www.hmc.psu.edu
Ministry Saint Josephs Hospital	Marshfield	Wisconsin	715-387-7850	www.stjosephs-marshfield.org
Mobile Infirmary	Mobile	Alabama	251-435-4700	www.mimc.com
Montefiore Medical Center	Bronx	New York	718-920-4321	www.montefiore.org
Morristown Medical Center	Morristown	New Jersey	973-971-5450	www.morristownmemorialhospital.org
Naples Community Hospital	Naples	Florida	239-436-5000	www.nchmd.org
Nason Hospital	Roaring Spring	Pennsylvania	814-224-2141	www.nasonhospital.com
Nathan Littauer Hospital	Gloversville	New York	518-725-8621	www.nlh.org
Newark Beth Israel Medical Center	Newark	New Jersey	973-926-7850	www.sbhcs.com
North Shore University Hospital	Manhasset	New York	516-562-0100	www.northshorelij.com
North Suburban Medical Center	Thornton	Colorado	303-451-7800	www.northsuburban.com
Northside Hospital	Atlanta	Georgia	404-851-8000	www.northside.com
Northwestern Memorial Hospital	Chicago	Illinois	312-926-2000	www.nmh.org
Novant Health Rowan Medical Center	Salisbury	North Carolina	704-210-5000	www.rowan.org
NYU Hospitals Center	New York	New York	212-263-7300	www.med.nyu.edu
O U Medical Center	Oklahoma City	Oklahoma	405-271-5911	www.oumedcenter.com
Oakwood Hospital - Southshore	Trenton	Michigan	734-671-3800	www.oakwood.org/oakwood-hospital-southshore
Och Regional Medical Center	Starkville	Mississippi	662-323-4320	www.och.org
OHSU Hospital & Clinics	Portland	Oregon	503-494-4036	www.ohsu.edu
Orlando Health	Orlando	Florida	321-841-5111	www.orlandoregionalmedicalcenter.org
Our Lady of the Lake Regional Medical Center	Baton Rouge	Louisiana	225-765-6565	www.ololrmc.com
Overlook Medical Center	Summit	New Jersey	908-522-2000	www.atlantichealth.org
Owensboro Health Regional Hospital	Owensboro	Kentucky	270-688-2000	www.omhs.org
Palmetto General Hospital	Hialeah	Florida	305-823-5000	www.palmettogeneral.com
Parkland Health & Hospital System	Dallas	Texas	214-590-8000	www.parklandhospital.com
Pennsylvania Hospital of the Univ of PA Health Sys	Philadelphia	Pennsylvania	215-829-3000	www.pennmedicine.org/pahosp
Piedmont Hospital	Atlanta	Georgia	404-605-5000	www.piedmonthospital.org

Hospital	City	State	Phone	Web Site
Pinnacle Health Hospitals	Harrisburg	Pennsylvania	717-782-5181	www.pinnaclehealth.org
Plainview Hospital	Plainview	New York	516-719-3000	www.nslij.com
Pratt Regional Medical Center	Pratt	Kansas	620-450-1160	www.prmc.org
Proctor Hospital	Peoria	Illinois	309-691-1000	www.proctor.org
Providence Hospital & Medical Centers	Southfield	Michigan	248-849-3011	www.stjohn.org/providence
Providence Memorial Hospital	El Paso	Texas	915-577-6011	www.sphn.com
Raleigh General Hospital	Beckley	West Virginia	304-256-4100	www.raleighgeneral.com
Regional Medical Center at Memphis	Memphis	Tennessee	901-545-7928	www.the-med.org
Riddle Memorial Hospital	Media	Pennsylvania	610-566-9400	www.riddlehospital.org
Robert Wood Johnson University Hospital	New Brunswick	New Jersey	732-937-8900	www.rwjuh.edu
Rose Medical Center	Denver	Colorado	303-320-2121	www.rosemed.com
Saint Barnabas Medical Center	Livingston	New Jersey	973-322-5000	www.saintbarnabas.com
Saint Peter's University Hospital	New Brunswick	New Jersey	732-745-8600	www.saintpetersuh.com
Saratoga Hospital	Saratoga Springs	New York	518-587-3222	www.saratogacare.org
Scripps Memorial Hospital La Jolla	La Jolla	California	858-626-4123	www.scrippshealth.org
Scripps Mercy Hospital	San Diego	California	619-294-8111	www.scrippshealth.org
Sentara Norfolk General Hospital	Norfolk	Virginia	757-388-3000	www.sentara.com
Sharp Memorial Hospital	San Diego	California	858-939-3400	www.sharp.com/memorial
Sierra Medical Center	El Paso	Texas	915-747-4000	www.sphn.com
Sinai - Grace Hospital	Detroit	Michigan	313-966-3300	www.sinaigrace.org
Somerset Medical Center	Somerville	New Jersey	908-685-2200	www.somersetmedicalcenter.com
South Lake Hospital	Clermont	Florida	352-394-4071	www.southlakehospital.com
Saint Alphonsus Regional Medical Center	Boise	Idaho	208-367-2121	www.saintalphonsus.org
Saint Anthonys Memorial Hospital	Effingham	Illinois	217-342-2121	www.stanthonyshospital.org
Saint Catherine of Siena Hospital	Smithtown	New York	631-862-3000	www.stcatherines.chsli.org
Saint Clare Hospital	Lakewood	Washington	253-588-1711	www.fhshealth.org
Saint Elizabeth Hospital	Belleville	Illinois	618-234-2120	www.steliz.org
Saint John's Episcopal Hospital at South Shore	Far Rockaway	New York	718-869-7000	www.ehs.org
Saint Joseph Hospital	Nashua	New Hampshire	603-882-3000	www.stjosephhospital.com
Saint Joseph Medical Center	Tacoma	Washington	253-627-4101	www.fhshealth.org
Saint Louis University Hospital	Saint Louis	Missouri	314-577-8000	www.slucare.edu/clinical
Saint Luke's Hospital Bethlehem	Bethlehem	Pennsylvania	610-954-4000	www.slhn-lehighvalley.org
Saint Luke's Roosevelt Hospital	New York	New York	212-523-4000	www.wehealny.org
Saint Luke's Warren Hospital	Phillipsburg	New Jersey	908-859-6700	www.warrenhospital.org
Saint Luke's Episcopal Hospital	Houston	Texas	832-355-1000	www.sleh.com
Saint Luke's Hospital	Chesterfield	Missouri	314-434-1500	www.goodhealthmatters.com
Saint Mary's Medical Center	West Palm Beach	Florida	561-840-6202	www.stmarysmc.com
Saint Mary's of Michigan Medical Center	Saginaw	Michigan	989-776-8000	www.stmarysofmichigan.org
Saint Vincent Hospital	Worcester	Massachusetts	508-363-5000	www.stvincenthospital.com
Staten Island University Hospital	Staten Island	New York	718-226-9000	www.siuh.edu
Summa Health Systems Hospitals	Akron	Ohio	330-375-3000	www.summahealth.org
Swedish Medical Center	Englewood	Colorado	303-788-5000	www.swedishhospital.com/default.asp
Tampa General Hospital	Tampa	Florida	813-844-7000	www.tgh.org
Temple University Hospital	Philadelphia	Pennsylvania	215-707-2000	www.tuh.templehealth.org
Carle Foundation Hospital	Urbana	Illinois	217-383-3311	www.carle.com
The University of Chicago Medical Center	Chicago	Illinois	773-702-1000	www.uchospitals.edu
Thomas Jefferson University Hospital	Philadelphia	Pennsylvania	215-955-6000	www.jeffersonhospital.org
Tri - City Medical Center	Oceanside	California	760-724-8411	www.tricitymed.org
Tucson Medical Center	Tucson	Arizona	520-327-5461	www.tmcaz.com
University Hospital	Augusta	Georgia	706-722-9011	www.universityhealth.org
University Hospital	Newark	New Jersey	973-972-5658	www.theuniversityhospital.com
University Hospital - Stony Brook	Stony Brook	New York	631-444-4000	www.stonybrookmedicalcenter.org
University Hospital SUNY Health Science Center	Syracuse	New York	315-473-4240	www.upstate.edu
University of California Davis Medical Center	Sacramento	California	916-734-2011	www.ucdmc.ucdavis.edu
University of Cincinnati Medical Center	Cincinnati	Ohio	513-584-1000	www.universityhospitalcincinnati.com
University of Illinois Hospital	Chicago	Illinois	312-996-3900	www.uic.edu
University of Miami Hospital	Miami	Florida	305-325-5511	www.cedarsmedicalcenter.com
University of Mississippi Medical Center	Jackson	Mississippi	601-984-4100	www.umc.edu
University of North Carolina Hospital	Chapel Hill	North Carolina	919-966-4131	www.unchealthcare.org
University of Tn Memorial Hospital	Knoxville	Tennessee	865-544-9000	www.utmedicalcenter.org
University of Toledo Medical Center	Toledo	Ohio	419-383-3407	www.utmc.utoledo.edu
University of Virginia Medical Center	Charlottesville	Virginia	800-251-3627	www.uvahealth.com
UPMC Presbyterian Shadyside	Pittsburgh	Pennsylvania	412-647-8788	www.upmc.edu
Valley Hospital	Ridgewood	New Jersey	201-447-8000	www.valleyhealth.com
Westchester Medical Center	Valhalla	New York	914-285-7017	www.wcmc.com
Wyckoff Heights Medical Center	Brooklyn	New York	718-963-7272	www.wyckoffhospital.org
Yale-New Haven Hospital	New Haven	Connecticut	203-688-4242	www.ynhh.org

Note: Table shows hospitals nationwide whose surgical complication rate is worse (higher) than U.S. rate of 4.14%

Hospitals whose Surgical Complication Rate is Better (Lower) than the U.S. National Rate

Measure: Serious Complications

Hospital	City	State	Phone	Web Site
Advocate Christ Hospital & Medical Center	Oak Lawn	Illinois	708-684-8000	www.advocatehealth.com
Allegiance Health	Jackson	Michigan	517-788-4800	www.footehealth.org
Anmed Health	Anderson	South Carolina	864-261-1109	www.anmed.com
Arkansas Heart Hospital	Little Rock	Arkansas	501-219-7000	www.arheart.com
Asante Rogue Regional Medical Center	Medford	Oregon	541-789-7000	www.asante.org
Atlanticare Regional Medical Center	Atlantic City	New Jersey	609-441-8020	www.atlanticare.org/acmc/index.html
Avera Mckennan Hospital & University Health Center	Sioux Falls	South Dakota	605-322-8000	www.mckennan.org
Baptist Beaumont Hospital	Beaumont	Texas	409-212-5012	www.mhbh.org
Baptist Health Lexington	Lexington	Kentucky	859-260-6104	www.centralbap.com
Baptist Health Louisville	Louisville	Kentucky	502-897-8100	www.baptisteast.com
Baystate Medical Center	Springfield	Massachusetts	413-794-0000	www.baystatehealth.com
Bethesda Hospital East	Boynton Beach	Florida	561-737-7733	www.bethesdahealthcare.com
Bethesda North	Cincinnati	Ohio	513-865-1241	www.trihealth.com
Billings Clinic Hospital	Billings	Montana	406-657-4000	www.billingsclinic.com
Carolina East Medical Center	New Bern	North Carolina	252-633-8640	www.cravenhealthcare.org
Carson Tahoe Regional Medical Center	Carson City	Nevada	775-445-8000	www.carsontahoehospital.com
Centinela Hospital Medical Center	Inglewood	California	310-673-4660	www.centinelafreeman.com
Central Dupage Hospital	Winfield	Illinois	630-682-1600	www.cdh.org
Christus Hospital	Beaumont	Texas	409-892-7171	www.christushealth.org
Christus Spohn Hospital Corpus Christi	Corpus Christi	Texas	361-902-4103	www.christusspohn.org
Community Hospital	Munster	Indiana	219-836-1600	www.comhs.org/community
Community Medical Center	Toms River	New Jersey	732-557-8000	www.sbhcs.com
Conway Regional Medical Center	Conway	Arkansas	501-329-3831	www.conwayregional.org
Cox Medical Center	Springfield	Missouri	417-269-6000	www.coxhealth.com
Delray Medical Center	Delray Beach	Florida	561-498-4440	www.delraymedicalctr.com
Duke University Hospital	Durham	North Carolina	919-684-8111	www.dukehealth.org
East Texas Medical Center	Tyler	Texas	903-597-0351	www.etmc.org
Englewood Hospital & Medical Center	Englewood	New Jersey	201-894-3000	www.englewoodhospital.com
Exeter Hospital	Exeter	New Hampshire	603-778-7311	www.exeterhospital.com
Floyd Medical Center	Rome	Georgia	706-509-6900	www.floydmed.org
Floyd Memorial Hospital & Health Services	New Albany	Indiana	812-949-5500	www.floydmedical.org
Genesis Medical Center - Davenport	Davenport	Iowa	563-421-1000	www.genesishealth.com
Glens Falls Hospital	Glens Falls	New York	518-926-1000	www.glensfallshospital.org
Heartland Regional Medical Center	Saint Joseph	Missouri	816-271-6000	www.heartland-health.com
Holy Cross Hospital	Fort Lauderdale	Florida	954-771-8000	www.holy-cross.com
Indiana University Health	Indianapolis	Indiana	317-962-5900	www.iuhealth.org
Indiana University Health Arnett Hospital	Lafayette	Indiana	765-448-8000	www.iuhealth.org/arnett
Integris Baptist Medical Center	Oklahoma City	Oklahoma	405-951-8110	www.integris-health.com
Integris Southwest Medical Center	Oklahoma City	Oklahoma	405-636-7000	www.integris-health.com
Jackson - Madison County General Hospital	Jackson	Tennessee	731-541-5000	www.wth.org
John Muir Medical Center - Concord Campus	Concord	California	925-674-2002	www.johnmuirhealth.com
Lakeland Hospital - Saint Joseph	Saint Joseph	Michigan	269-983-8300	www.lakelandhealth.org
Laredo Medical Center	Laredo	Texas	956-796-5000	www.laredomedical.com
Lehigh Valley Hospital - Hazleton	Hazleton	Pennsylvania	570-501-4000	www.ghha.org
Marietta Memorial Hospital	Marietta	Ohio	740-374-1400	www.mmhospital.org
Mary Washington Hospital	Fredericksburg	Virginia	540-741-1100	www.medicorp.org
Mayo Clinic	Jacksonville	Florida	904-953-2000	www.mayoclinic.org/jacksonville
Mayo Clinic Hospital	Phoenix	Arizona	480-342-2000	www.mayoclinic.org
Mayo Clinic Methodist- Hospital	Rochester	Minnesota	507-266-7890	www.mayoclinic.org/methodisthospital
Mclaren Bay Region	Bay City	Michigan	989-894-3000	www.baymed.org
Mcleod Regional Medical Center - Pee Dee	Florence	South Carolina	843-777-2900	www.mcleodhealth.org
Medcentral Health System Mansfield Hospital	Mansfield	Ohio	419-526-8000	www.medcentral.org
Memorial Healthcare System	Chattanooga	Tennessee	423-495-2525	www.memorial.org
Memorial Hermann Hospital System	Houston	Texas	713-448-6796	www.memorialhermann.org
Memorial Mission Hospital & Asheville Surgery Center	Asheville	North Carolina	828-213-1111	www.missionhospitals.org
Mercy Medical Center - Cedar Rapids	Cedar Rapids	Iowa	319-398-6011	www.mercycare.org
Methodist Hospital	San Antonio	Texas	210-575-4000	www.mh.sahealth.com
Methodist Medical Center of Illinois	Peoria	Illinois	309-672-5522	www.mmci.org
Methodist Willowbrook Hospital	Houston	Texas	281-477-1000	www.houstonmethodist.org/willowbrook-hospital
Metrowest Medical Center	Framingham	Massachusetts	508-383-1000	www.mwmc.com
Mississippi Baptist Medical Center	Jackson	Mississippi	601-968-1000	www.mbmc.org
Monongalia County General Hospital	Morgantown	West Virginia	304-598-1200	www.mongeneral.com
Mother Frances Hospital	Tyler	Texas	903-593-8441	www.tmfhs.org
Munroe Regional Medical Center	Ocala	Florida	352-351-7200	www.munroeregional.com

Hospital	City	State	Phone	Web Site
Munson Medical Center	Traverse City	Michigan	231-935-5000	www.munsonhealthcare.org
Nebraska Heart Hospital	Lincoln	Nebraska	402-328-3000	www.neheart.com
New York Community Hospital of Brooklyn	Brooklyn	New York	718-692-5302	www.nych.com
North Mississippi Medical Center	Tupelo	Mississippi	662-377-3000	www.nmhs.net/nmmc
Oklahoma Heart Hospital	Oklahoma City	Oklahoma	405-608-3200	www.okheart.com
Our Lady of Lourdes Medical Center	Camden	New Jersey	856-757-3500	www.lourdesnet.org
Palos Community Hospital	Palos Heights	Illinois	708-923-4000	www.paloshospital.org
Parkview Regional Medical Center	Fort Wayne	Indiana	260-266-1000	www.parkview.com
Parkwest Medical Center	Knoxville	Tennessee	865-970-9800	www.yesparkwest.com
Pomona Valley Hospital Medical Center	Pomona	California	909-865-9500	www.pvhmc.com
Presence Saint Joseph Medical Center	Joliet	Illinois	815-725-7133	www.provena.org/stjoes
Providence Little Co of Mary Medical Center Torrance	Torrance	California	310-540-7676	www.lcmhs.org
Providence Saint Joseph Medical Center	Burbank	California	818-843-5111	www.providence.org/losangeles
Redmond Regional Medical Center	Rome	Georgia	706-802-3012	www.redmondregional.com
Regional Medical Center Bayonet Point	Hudson	Florida	727-819-2929	www.mchealth.comorwww.heartoftampa.com
Roper Hospital	Charleston	South Carolina	843-724-2800	www.ropersaintfrancis.com
Saint Thomas West Hospital	Nashville	Tennessee	615-222-2111	www.stthomas.org
Sentara Careplex Hospital	Hampton	Virginia	757-736-1000	www.sentara.com
Sentara Leigh Hospital	Norfolk	Virginia	757-261-6601	www.sentara.com
Shasta Regional Medical Center	Redding	California	530-244-5454	www.shastaregional.com
Southcoast Hospital Group	Fall River	Massachusetts	508-679-3131	www.southcoast.org/charlton
Saint Elizabeth Medical Center	Lakeside Park	Kentucky	859-292-2000	www.stelizabeth.com
Saint Francis Hospital	Columbus	Georgia	706-596-4020	www.wecareforlife.com
Saint Francis Hospital - Roslyn	Roslyn	New York	516-562-6000	www.stfrancisheartcenter.com
Saint Luke's Hospital	Cedar Rapids	Iowa	319-369-7211	www.crstlukes.com
Saint Mary Medical Center	Langhorne	Pennsylvania	215-750-2003	www.stmaryhealthcare.org
Saint Mary Mercy Hospital	Livonia	Michigan	734-655-4800	www.stmarymercy.org
Saint Vincent Heart Center of Indiana	Indianapolis	Indiana	317-583-5000	www.theheartcenter.com
Saint Vincent Hospital & Health Services	Indianapolis	Indiana	317-338-7000	www.indianapolis.stvincent.org
Saint Vincent's Medical Center	Jacksonville	Florida	904-308-7300	www.jaxhealth.com
Sutter General Hospital	Sacramento	California	916-733-8999	www.suttermedicalcenter.org
Texas Health Harris Methodist Hurst - Euless - Bedford	Bedford	Texas	817-848-4000	www.texashealth.org
Thibodaux Regional Medical Center	Thibodaux	Louisiana	985-447-5500	www.thibodaux.com
Tuomey Healthcare System	Sumter	South Carolina	803-774-8900	www.tuomey.com
United Hospital Center	Bridgeport	West Virginia	681-342-1000	www.uhcwv.org
University Hospitals - Elyria Medical Center	Elyria	Ohio	440-329-7500	www.emh-healthcare.org
University of Michigan Health System	Ann Arbor	Michigan	734-764-1505	www.med.umich.edu
UPMC Altoona	Altoona	Pennsylvania	814-889-2011	www.altoonaregional.org
Vanderbilt University Hospital	Nashville	Tennessee	615-322-3454	www.mc.vanderbilt.edu
Virtua West Jersey Hospitals Berlin	Berlin	New Jersey	856-322-3200	www.virtua.org
Washington Hospital	Fremont	California	510-797-1111	www.whhs.com
Williamsport Regional Medical Center	Williamsport	Pennsylvania	570-321-1000	www.susquehannahealth.org
Willis Knighton Bossier Health Center	Bossier City	Louisiana	318-212-7000	www.wkhs.com/locations/bossier.aspx
Winchester Medical Center	Winchester	Virginia	540-536-8000	www.valleyhealthlink.com

Note: Table shows hospitals nationwide whose surgical complication rate is better (lower) than U.S. rate of 0.61%

Hospitals whose Surgical Complication Rate is Worse (Higher) than the U.S. National Rate

Measure: Serious Complications

Hospital	City	State	Phone	Web Site
Adirondack Medical Center	Saranac Lake	New York	518-891-4141	www.amccares.org
Appleton Medical Center	Appleton	Wisconsin	920-731-4101	www.thedacare.org
Aurora Medical Center Kenosha	Kenosha	Wisconsin	262-948-5600	www.aurorahealthcare.org
B R F Hospital Holdings	Shreveport	Louisiana	318-675-5000	www.lsumc.edu
Baptist Memorial Hospital Desoto	Southaven	Mississippi	662-772-4000	www.bmhcc.org/facilities/desoto
Baptist Saint Anthony's Hospital	Amarillo	Texas	806-212-2000	www.bsahs.com
Barnes-Jewish Hospital	Saint Louis	Missouri	314-747-3000	www.barnesjewish.org
Baylor University Medical Center	Dallas	Texas	214-820-0111	www.baylorhealth.com
Beaumont Health System	Royal Oak	Michigan	248-898-5000	www.beaumonthospitals.com
Beth Israel Deaconess Medical Center	Boston	Massachusetts	617-667-7000	www.bidmc.harvard.edu
Blessing Hospital	Quincy	Illinois	217-223-5811	www.blessinghealthsystem.org
Boston Medical Center Corporation	Boston	Massachusetts	617-638-8000	www.bmc.org
Bridgeport Hospital	Bridgeport	Connecticut	203-384-3000	www.bridgeporthospital.com
Brigham & Women's Hospital	Boston	Massachusetts	617-732-5500	www.brighamandwomens.org
Cape Coral Hospital	Cape Coral	Florida	239-574-2323	www.leememorial.org
Carilion Roanoke Memorial Hospital	Roanoke	Virginia	540-981-7000	www.carilion.com/crmh
Centennial Medical Center	Frisco	Texas	972-963-3333	www.centennialmedcenter.com
Central Texas Medical Center	San Marcos	Texas	512-753-3690	www.ctmc.org
Charleston Area Medical Center	Charleston	West Virginia	304-388-6203	www.camc.org
Chilton Medical Center	Pompton Plains	New Jersey	973-831-5000	www.chiltonmemorial.org
Christus Saint Frances Cabrini Hospital	Alexandria	Louisiana	318-487-1122	www.cabrini.org
Clearview Regional Medical Center	Monroe	Georgia	770-267-1792	www.clearviewregionalmedicalcenter.com
Cleveland Clinic	Cleveland	Ohio	216-444-2200	www.clevelandclinic.org
Clovis Community Medical Center	Clovis	California	559-324-4000	www.communitymedical.org
Community Regional Medical Center	Fresno	California	559-459-6000	www.communitymedical.org
Conemaugh Valley Memorial Hospital	Johnstown	Pennsylvania	814-534-9000	www.conemaugh.org
Cooper University Hospital	Camden	New Jersey	856-342-2000	www.cooperhealth.org
Crouse Hospital	Syracuse	New York	315-470-7449	www.crouse.org
Dameron Hospital	Stockton	California	209-944-5550	www.dameronhospital.org
Deaconess Hospital	Spokane	Washington	509-473-5800	www.deaconessmedicalcenter.org
Emory University Hospital Midtown	Atlanta	Georgia	404-686-4411	www.emoryhealthcare.org
Evanston Hospital	Evanston	Illinois	847-432-8000	www.enh.org
Firsthealth Moore Regional Hospital	Pinehurst	North Carolina	910-715-1000	www.firsthealth.org
Geisinger Medical Center	Danville	Pennsylvania	570-271-6211	www.geisinger.org
Geisinger Wyoming Valley Medical Center	Wilkes Barre	Pennsylvania	570-826-7300	www.geisinger.org
Genesys Regional Medical Center - Health Park	Grand Blanc	Michigan	810-606-5000	www.genesys.org
Gila Regional Medical Center	Silver City	New Mexico	575-538-4000	www.grmc.org
Good Samaritan Hospital	San Jose	California	408-559-2011	www.goodsamsj.org
Good Shepherd Medical Center Marshall	Marshall	Texas	903-927-6712	www.marshallregional.org
Grady Memorial Hospital	Atlanta	Georgia	404-616-4252	www.gradyhealthsystem.org
Grand View Hospital	Sellersville	Pennsylvania	215-453-4615	www.gvh.org
Grossmont Hospital	La Mesa	California	619-465-0711	www.sharp.com
Gulf Coast Medical Center Lee Memorial Health System	Fort Myers	Florida	239-768-5000	www.leememorial.org
Hackettstown Regional Medical Center	Hackettstown	New Jersey	908-852-5100	www.hrmcnj.org
Hahnemann University Hospital	Philadelphia	Pennsylvania	215-762-7000	www.hahnemannhospital.com
Harborview Medical Center	Seattle	Washington	206-731-3000	www.harborview.org
Hartford Hospital	Hartford	Connecticut	860-545-5000	www.harthosp.org
Hennepin County Medical Center	Minneapolis	Minnesota	612-873-3000	www.hcmc.org
Henry Ford Hospital	Detroit	Michigan	313-916-2600	www.henryfordhospital.com
Henry Ford West Bloomfield Hospital	W Bloomfield	Michigan	248-325-1000	www.henryford.com
Heritage Valley Beaver	Beaver	Pennsylvania	412-728-7000	www.heritagevalley.org
Holy Cross Hospital	Taos	New Mexico	575-758-8883	www.taoshospital.org
Hospital of Univ of Pennsylvania	Philadelphia	Pennsylvania	215-662-3227	www.upenn.edu
Huntington Memorial Hospital	Pasadena	California	626-397-5000	www.huntingtonhospital.com
Inova Fairfax Hospital	Falls Church	Virginia	703-776-3332	www.inova.org
Inspira Medical Center Vineland	Vineland	New Jersey	856-641-6610	www.sjhs.com
Intermountain Medical Center	Murray	Utah	801-507-7000	www.intermountainhealthcare.org
Jackson Memorial Hospital	Miami	Florida	305-585-1111	www.jhsmiami.org
JFK Medical Center - A M Yelencsics Comm Hospital	Edison	New Jersey	732-321-7000	www.jfkmc.org
John Dempsey Hospital	Farmington	Connecticut	860-679-1145	www.uconnhealth.orgorwww.uchc.edu
JPS Health Network	Fort Worth	Texas	817-921-3431	www.jpshealthnet.org
Kaweah Delta Medical Center	Visalia	California	559-624-2000	www.kaweahdelta.org
Keck Hospital of USC	Los Angeles	California	323-442-8656	www.uscuh.com
Lancaster General Hospital	Lancaster	Pennsylvania	717-299-5511	www.lancastergeneral.org

Hospital	City	State	Phone	Web Site
LDS Hospital	Salt Lake City	Utah	801-408-1100	www.intermountainhealthcare.org
Lee Memorial Hospital	Fort Myers	Florida	239-332-1111	www.leememorial.org
Lenox Hill Hospital	New York	New York	212-439-2345	www.lenoxhillhospital.org
Lourdes Hospital	Paducah	Kentucky	270-444-2444	www.ehealthconnection.com
Lower Keys Medical Center	Key West	Florida	305-294-5531	www.lkmc.com
Loyola University Medical Center	Maywood	Illinois	708-216-9000	www.lumc.edu
Magee Womens Hospital of UPMC Health System	Pittsburgh	Pennsylvania	412-641-4010	www.magee.edu
Maine Medical Center	Portland	Maine	207-662-0111	www.mmc.org
Marin General Hospital	Greenbrae	California	415-925-7900	www.maringeneral.com
Mary Hitchcock Memorial Hospital	Lebanon	New Hampshire	603-650-5000	www.dhmc.org
Mayo Clinic Health System - Mankato	Mankato	Minnesota	507-625-4031	www.isj-mhs.org
McKay Dee Hospital	Ogden	Utah	801-387-2800	www.intermountainhealthcare.org
The Medical Center of Aurora	Aurora	Colorado	303-695-2600	www.auroramed.com
Medical Center of Plano	Plano	Texas	972-596-6800	www.medicalcenterofplano.com
Medical College of Virginia Hospitals	Richmond	Virginia	804-828-0938	www.vcuhealth.org
Medical West	Bessemer	Alabama	205-481-7000	www.uab.edu
Medstar Georgetown University Hospital	Washington	District of Columbia	202-784-3000	www.georgetownuniversityhospital.org
Medstar Washington Hospital Center	Washington	District of Columbia	202-877-7000	www.whcenter.org
Memorial Medical Center	Modesto	California	209-526-4500	www.memorialmedicalcenter.org
Memorial Hospital Jacksonville	Jacksonville	Florida	904-399-6111	www.memorialhospitaljax.com
Memorial Medical Center	Springfield	Illinois	217-788-3000	www.memorialmedical.com
Menorah Medical Center	Overland Park	Kansas	913-498-6773	www.menorahmedicalcenter.com
Mercy Hospital - Cadillac	Cadillac	Michigan	231-876-7200	www.mercycadillac.munsonhealthcare.org
Mercy Memorial Health Center	Ardmore	Oklahoma	405-223-5400	www.mercyok.com/mmhc
Mercy Saint Vincent Medical Center	Toledo	Ohio	419-251-3232	www.mhsnr.org
Metrohealth System	Cleveland	Ohio	216-778-7089	www.metrohealth.org
Miami Valley Hospital	Dayton	Ohio	937-208-8000	www.miamivalleyhospital.com
Milton S Hershey Medical Center	Hershey	Pennsylvania	717-531-8521	www.hmc.psu.edu
Ministry Saint Josephs Hospital	Marshfield	Wisconsin	715-387-7850	www.stjosephs-marshfield.org
Montefiore Medical Center	Bronx	New York	718-920-4321	www.montefiore.org
Newark Beth Israel Medical Center	Newark	New Jersey	973-926-7850	www.sbhcs.com
North Shore University Hospital	Manhasset	New York	516-562-0100	www.northshorelij.com
North Suburban Medical Center	Thornton	Colorado	303-451-7800	www.northsuburban.com
Novant Health Presbyterian Medical Center	Charlotte	North Carolina	704-384-4000	www.presbyterian.org
NYU Hospitals Center	New York	New York	212-263-7300	www.med.nyu.edu
O U Medical Center	Oklahoma City	Oklahoma	405-271-5911	www.oumedcenter.com
OHSU Hospital & Clinics	Portland	Oregon	503-494-4036	www.ohsu.edu
Our Lady of the Lake Regional Medical Center	Baton Rouge	Louisiana	225-765-6565	www.ololrmc.com
Overland Park Regional Medical Center	Overland Park	Kansas	913-541-5301	www.oprmc.com
Parkland Health & Hospital System	Dallas	Texas	214-590-8000	www.parklandhospital.com
Parkview Medical Center	Pueblo	Colorado	719-584-4000	www.parkviewmc.com
Piedmont Hospital	Atlanta	Georgia	404-605-5000	www.piedmonthospital.org
Pinnacle Health Hospitals	Harrisburg	Pennsylvania	717-782-5181	www.pinnaclehealth.org
Plainview Hospital	Plainview	New York	516-719-3000	www.nslij.com
Providence Holy Cross Medical Center	Mission Hills	California	818-365-8051	www.providence.org
Providence Sacred Heart Medical Center	Spokane	Washington	509-474-3040	www.shmc.org
Rhode Island Hospital	Providence	Rhode Island	401-444-4000	www.rhodeislandhospital.org
Ridgeview Medical Center	Waconia	Minnesota	952-442-2191	www.ridgeviewmedical.org
Robert Wood Johnson University Hospital	New Brunswick	New Jersey	732-937-8900	www.rwjuh.edu
Ronald Reagan UCLA Medical Center	Los Angeles	California	310-825-6301	www.uclahealth.org
Rose Medical Center	Denver	Colorado	303-320-2121	www.rosemed.com
Rush University Medical Center	Chicago	Illinois	312-942-5000	www.ruch.edu
Sacred Heart Hospital	Eau Claire	Wisconsin	715-717-4121	www.sacredhearteauclaire.org
Saint Anthony Medical Center	Rockford	Illinois	815-226-2000	www.osfhealth.com
Saint Barnabas Medical Center	Livingston	New Jersey	973-322-5000	www.saintbarnabas.com
Saint Francis Medical Center	Peoria	Illinois	309-655-2000	www.osfsaintfrancis.org
Saint Mary's Health Care	Grand Rapids	Michigan	616-685-5000	www.smhealthcare.org
Santa Clara Valley Medical Center	San Jose	California	408-885-5000	www.sccgov.org
Saratoga Hospital	Saratoga Springs	New York	518-587-3222	www.saratogacare.org
Sentara Norfolk General Hospital	Norfolk	Virginia	757-388-3000	www.sentara.com
Sharp Memorial Hospital	San Diego	California	858-939-3400	www.sharp.com/memorial
Sierra Medical Center	El Paso	Texas	915-747-4000	www.sphn.com
Sinai - Grace Hospital	Detroit	Michigan	313-966-3300	www.sinaigrace.org
Somerset Medical Center	Somerville	New Jersey	908-685-2200	www.somersetmedicalcenter.com
Springhill Medical Center	Mobile	Alabama	251-344-9630	www.springhillmedicalcenter.com
Saint Alphonsus Regional Medical Center	Boise	Idaho	208-367-2121	www.saintalphonsus.org
Saint Clare Hospital	Lakewood	Washington	253-588-1711	www.fhshealth.org

Hospital	City	State	Phone	Web Site
Saint Elizabeth Health Center	Youngstown	Ohio	330-746-7211	www.hmhs.org
Saint Joseph Medical Center	Tacoma	Washington	253-627-4101	www.fhshealth.org
Saint Joseph Mercy Hospital	Ann Arbor	Michigan	734-712-3791	www.stjoesannarbor.or
Saint Joseph's Hospital & Medical Center	Phoenix	Arizona	602-406-3000	www.stjosephs-phx.org
Saint Louis University Hospital	Saint Louis	Missouri	314-577-8000	www.slucare.edu/clinical
Saint Luke's Hospital Bethlehem	Bethlehem	Pennsylvania	610-954-4000	www.slhn-lehighvalley.org
Saint Luke's Episcopal Hospital	Houston	Texas	832-355-1000	www.sleh.com
Saint Luke's Hospital	Chesterfield	Missouri	314-434-1500	www.goodhealthmatters.com
Saint Luke's Hospital of Kansas City	Kansas City	Missouri	816-932-2000	www.staintlukeshealthsystem.org
Stamford Hospital	Stamford	Connecticut	203-276-1000	www.stamhealth.org
Summa Health Systems Hospitals	Akron	Ohio	330-375-3000	www.summahealth.org
Sunrise Hospital & Medical Center	Las Vegas	Nevada	702-731-8000	www.sunrisehospital.com
Swedish Medical Center	Englewood	Colorado	303-788-5000	www.swedishhospital.com/default.asp
Swedish Medical Center - Cherry Hill	Seattle	Washington	206-320-2000	www.swedish.org
Tampa General Hospital	Tampa	Florida	813-844-7000	www.tgh.org
The University of Chicago Medical Center	Chicago	Illinois	773-702-1000	www.uchospitals.edu
Theda Clark Medical Center	Neenah	Wisconsin	920-729-3100	www.thedacare.org
Thomas Hospital	Fairhope	Alabama	251-928-2375	www.thomashospital.com
Thomas Jefferson University Hospital	Philadelphia	Pennsylvania	215-955-6000	www.jeffersonhospital.org
Trinity Hospitals	Minot	North Dakota	701-857-5000	www.trinityhealth.org
Trinity Medical Center	Birmingham	Alabama	205-592-1000	www.bhsala.com/montclair
Tucson Medical Center	Tucson	Arizona	520-327-5461	www.tmcaz.com
Tulane Medical Center	New Orleans	Louisiana	504-988-1900	www.tuhc.com
UF Health Jacksonville	Jacksonville	Florida	904-244-0411	www.shandsjacksonville.org
UMC of Southern Nevada	Las Vegas	Nevada	702-383-2000	www.umc-cares.org
University Colo Health Memorial Hospital Central	Colorado Springs	Colorado	719-365-5000	www.memorialhospital.com
University Health System	San Antonio	Texas	210-358-4000	www.universityhealthsystem.com
University Hospital - Stony Brook	Stony Brook	New York	631-444-4000	www.stonybrookmedicalcenter.org
University Hospital SUNY Health Science Center	Syracuse	New York	315-473-4240	www.upstate.edu
University Medical Center of El Paso	El Paso	Texas	915-521-7602	www.thomasoncares.org
University of Alabama Hospital	Birmingham	Alabama	205-934-4011	www.health.uab.edu
University of California Davis Medical Center	Sacramento	California	916-734-2011	www.ucdmc.ucdavis.edu
University of Cincinnati Medical Center	Cincinnati	Ohio	513-584-1000	www.universityhospitalcincinnati.com
University of Illinois Hospital	Chicago	Illinois	312-996-3900	www.uic.edu
University of Kansas Hospital	Kansas City	Kansas	913-588-7332	www.kumc.edu
University of Miami Hospital	Miami	Florida	305-325-5511	www.cedarsmedicalcenter.com
University of Mississippi Medical Center	Jackson	Mississippi	601-984-4100	www.umc.edu
University of Toledo Medical Center	Toledo	Ohio	419-383-3407	www.utmc.utoledo.edu
UPMC Hamot	Erie	Pennsylvania	814-877-6000	www.hamot.org
UPMC Passavant	Pittsburgh	Pennsylvania	412-367-6700	www.passavant.upmc.com
UPMC Presbyterian Shadyside	Pittsburgh	Pennsylvania	412-647-8788	www.upmc.edu
UT Southwestern University Hospital	Dallas	Texas	214-879-3758	www.utsouthwestern.edu
Utah Valley Regional Medical Center	Provo	Utah	801-373-7850	www.intermountainhealthcare.org/hospitals/uvrmc
Valley Hospital	Ridgewood	New Jersey	201-447-8000	www.valleyhealth.com
Vidant Medical Center	Greenville	North Carolina	252-847-4100	www.uhseast.com
Waukesha Memorial Hospital	Waukesha	Wisconsin	262-928-1000	www.waukeshamemorial.org
Wesley Medical Center	Hattiesburg	Mississippi	601-268-8000	www.wesley.com
West Virginia University Hospitals	Morgantown	West Virginia	304-598-4000	www.wvuh.com
Wheaton Franciscan Saint Joseph	Milwaukee	Wisconsin	414-447-2000	www.wfhealthcare.org
Yale-New Haven Hospital	New Haven	Connecticut	203-688-4242	www.ynhh.org

Note: Table shows hospitals nationwide whose surgical complication rate is worse (higher) than U.S. rate of 0.61%

Surgical Complication Rate: State and National Summary

Measure: A Wound That Splits Open After Surgery on the Abdomen or Pelvis

Area	Number of Hospitals			
	Better than U.S. National Rate[1]	Worse than U.S. National Rate[2]	No Different than U.S. National Rate[3]	Number of Cases Too Small[4]
U.S. and Territories	0	42	2703	391
Alabama	0	0	58	18
Alaska	0	0	8	0
American Samoa	n/a	n/a	n/a	n/a
Arizona	0	1	49	9
Arkansas	0	0	35	9
California	0	2	245	49
Colorado	0	2	37	4
Connecticut	0	0	29	0
Delaware	0	0	6	0
District of Columbia	0	1	6	0
Florida	0	2	157	3
Georgia	0	2	83	15
Guam	n/a	n/a	n/a	n/a
Hawaii	0	1	11	2
Idaho	0	1	10	1
Illinois	0	0	122	3
Indiana	0	0	72	11
Iowa	0	0	30	4
Kansas	0	0	39	11
Kentucky	0	2	51	10
Louisiana	0	1	62	17
Maine	0	1	18	1
Maryland	n/a	n/a	n/a	n/a
Massachusetts	0	0	57	1
Michigan	0	4	80	6
Minnesota	0	1	40	9
Mississippi	0	0	37	7
Missouri	0	1	61	10
Montana	0	0	11	1
N. Mariana Islands	n/a	n/a	n/a	n/a
Nebraska	0	0	19	0
Nevada	0	2	19	0
New Hampshire	0	1	12	0
New Jersey	0	2	59	3
New Mexico	0	1	22	3
New York	0	1	146	9
North Carolina	0	2	79	4
North Dakota	0	0	6	0
Ohio	0	3	117	7
Oklahoma	0	0	47	21
Oregon	0	0	32	0
Pennsylvania	0	2	128	14
Puerto Rico	n/a	n/a	n/a	n/a
Rhode Island	0	0	11	0
South Carolina	0	0	49	4
South Dakota	0	0	10	7
Tennessee	0	1	66	22
Texas	0	2	205	55
Utah	0	0	23	4
Vermont	0	0	6	0
Virgin Islands	n/a	n/a	n/a	n/a
Virginia	0	1	64	7
Washington	0	0	46	2
West Virginia	0	0	28	3
Wisconsin	0	2	58	4
Wyoming	0	0	9	2

Note: (1) Surgical complication rate is better (lower) than U.S. rate of 0.92%; (2) Surgical complication rate is worse (higher) than U.S. rate of 0.92%; (3) Surgical complication rate is about the same as U.S. rate of 0.92%; (4) The number of cases is too small to classify the hospital; n/a not available

Surgical Complication Rate: State and National Summary

Measure: Accidental Cuts and Tears From Medical Treatment

Area	Number of Hospitals			
	Better than U.S. National Rate[1]	Worse than U.S. National Rate[2]	No Different than U.S. National Rate[3]	Number of Cases Too Small[4]
U.S. and Territories	95	203	3133	42
Alabama	0	8	89	0
Alaska	0	2	7	0
American Samoa	n/a	n/a	n/a	n/a
Arizona	1	4	61	1
Arkansas	1	0	45	0
California	7	22	280	1
Colorado	0	5	40	1
Connecticut	0	4	27	1
Delaware	1	0	5	0
District of Columbia	0	1	6	0
Florida	11	8	151	1
Georgia	2	6	100	0
Guam	n/a	n/a	n/a	n/a
Hawaii	0	1	13	0
Idaho	0	0	13	1
Illinois	10	7	111	1
Indiana	2	4	83	1
Iowa	0	3	31	0
Kansas	0	4	52	0
Kentucky	1	3	61	0
Louisiana	0	4	88	6
Maine	0	1	19	0
Maryland	n/a	n/a	n/a	n/a
Massachusetts	3	4	54	0
Michigan	3	7	85	0
Minnesota	2	4	46	0
Mississippi	1	2	61	3
Missouri	0	5	71	2
Montana	0	0	13	0
N. Mariana Islands	n/a	n/a	n/a	n/a
Nebraska	1	1	21	1
Nevada	0	2	22	0
New Hampshire	0	3	10	0
New Jersey	8	3	54	1
New Mexico	1	1	31	0
New York	5	4	158	2
North Carolina	1	6	82	0
North Dakota	0	1	6	0
Ohio	3	9	126	3
Oklahoma	3	3	83	2
Oregon	1	3	29	0
Pennsylvania	2	11	140	3
Puerto Rico	n/a	n/a	n/a	n/a
Rhode Island	0	3	8	0
South Carolina	2	3	52	0
South Dakota	0	1	20	0
Tennessee	5	0	92	0
Texas	11	10	301	7
Utah	0	5	26	1
Vermont	0	1	5	0
Virgin Islands	n/a	n/a	n/a	n/a
Virginia	5	3	70	2
Washington	0	11	37	0
West Virginia	1	1	29	0
Wisconsin	0	9	57	0
Wyoming	0	0	11	0

Note: (1) Surgical complication rate is better (lower) than U.S. rate of 1.83%; (2) Surgical complication rate is worse (higher) than U.S. rate of 1.83%; (3) Surgical complication rate is about the same as U.S. rate of 1.83%; (4) The number of cases is too small to classify the hospital; n/a not available

Surgical Complication Rate: State and National Summary

Measure: Collapsed Lung Due to Medical Treatment

Area	Number of Hospitals			
	Better than U.S. National Rate[1]	Worse than U.S. National Rate[2]	No Different than U.S. National Rate[3]	Number of Cases Too Small[4]
U.S. and Territories	9	60	3366	38
Alabama	0	2	95	0
Alaska	0	0	9	0
American Samoa	n/a	n/a	n/a	n/a
Arizona	0	1	65	1
Arkansas	0	1	45	0
California	1	7	302	0
Colorado	0	0	45	1
Connecticut	0	0	31	1
Delaware	0	0	6	0
District of Columbia	0	0	7	0
Florida	0	4	166	1
Georgia	0	2	106	0
Guam	n/a	n/a	n/a	n/a
Hawaii	0	0	14	0
Idaho	0	0	13	1
Illinois	1	2	125	1
Indiana	0	0	89	1
Iowa	0	0	34	0
Kansas	0	3	52	1
Kentucky	1	2	62	0
Louisiana	1	1	92	4
Maine	0	1	19	0
Maryland	n/a	n/a	n/a	n/a
Massachusetts	0	3	58	0
Michigan	1	2	92	0
Minnesota	0	0	52	0
Mississippi	0	0	64	3
Missouri	0	4	72	2
Montana	0	0	13	0
N. Mariana Islands	n/a	n/a	n/a	n/a
Nebraska	0	1	23	0
Nevada	0	1	23	0
New Hampshire	0	0	13	0
New Jersey	2	0	63	1
New Mexico	0	0	33	0
New York	1	4	162	2
North Carolina	0	1	88	0
North Dakota	0	1	6	0
Ohio	0	1	136	4
Oklahoma	0	2	88	1
Oregon	0	1	32	0
Pennsylvania	0	2	152	2
Puerto Rico	n/a	n/a	n/a	n/a
Rhode Island	0	0	11	0
South Carolina	0	1	56	0
South Dakota	0	0	21	0
Tennessee	0	1	96	0
Texas	0	6	316	7
Utah	0	0	31	1
Vermont	0	0	6	0
Virgin Islands	n/a	n/a	n/a	n/a
Virginia	1	2	75	2
Washington	0	0	48	0
West Virginia	0	0	31	0
Wisconsin	0	1	65	0
Wyoming	0	0	11	0

Note: (1) Surgical complication rate is better (lower) than U.S. rate of 0.32%; (2) Surgical complication rate is worse (higher) than U.S. rate of 0.32%; (3) Surgical complication rate is about the same as U.S. rate of 0.32%; (4) The number of cases is too small to classify the hospital; n/a not available

Surgical Complication Rate: State and National Summary

Measure: Deaths Among Patients With Serious Treatable Complications After Surgery

Area	Number of Hospitals			
	Better than U.S. National Rate[1]	Worse than U.S. National Rate[2]	No Different than U.S. National Rate[3]	Number of Cases Too Small[4]
U.S. and Territories	43	70	1831	1058
Alabama	0	6	33	29
Alaska	0	1	4	3
American Samoa	n/a	n/a	n/a	n/a
Arizona	3	0	39	15
Arkansas	0	1	20	17
California	1	3	164	116
Colorado	1	0	27	14
Connecticut	0	0	22	7
Delaware	0	1	4	1
District of Columbia	0	0	6	1
Florida	6	5	124	26
Georgia	2	5	50	41
Guam	n/a	n/a	n/a	n/a
Hawaii	0	0	5	9
Idaho	0	0	8	4
Illinois	7	1	87	29
Indiana	1	0	54	29
Iowa	1	0	22	10
Kansas	0	0	25	23
Kentucky	0	3	31	25
Louisiana	0	0	38	28
Maine	0	0	9	11
Maryland	n/a	n/a	n/a	n/a
Massachusetts	0	1	42	15
Michigan	4	0	56	28
Minnesota	1	0	23	24
Mississippi	0	3	20	16
Missouri	2	1	44	23
Montana	0	0	9	2
N. Mariana Islands	n/a	n/a	n/a	n/a
Nebraska	0	0	17	5
Nevada	0	2	14	5
New Hampshire	0	1	10	2
New Jersey	2	5	50	7
New Mexico	0	0	10	14
New York	2	4	91	58
North Carolina	0	4	57	25
North Dakota	1	0	5	0
Ohio	1	1	84	37
Oklahoma	0	4	27	27
Oregon	1	0	17	14
Pennsylvania	0	2	80	60
Puerto Rico	n/a	n/a	n/a	n/a
Rhode Island	0	0	7	4
South Carolina	0	3	29	21
South Dakota	0	0	6	9
Tennessee	0	2	45	30
Texas	5	5	147	81
Utah	0	0	16	11
Vermont	0	1	3	2
Virgin Islands	n/a	n/a	n/a	n/a
Virginia	0	1	46	21
Washington	0	0	40	6
West Virginia	0	1	19	8
Wisconsin	2	0	39	25
Wyoming	0	0	2	9

Note: (1) Surgical complication rate is better (lower) than U.S. rate of 110.25%; (2) Surgical complication rate is worse (higher) than U.S. rate of 110.25%; (3) Surgical complication rate is about the same as U.S. rate of 110.25%; (4) The number of cases is too small to classify the hospital; n/a not available

Surgical Complication Rate: State and National Summary

Measure: Rate of Complications for Hip/Knee Replacement Patients

Area	Number of Hospitals			
	Better than U.S. National Rate[1]	Worse than U.S. National Rate[2]	No Different than U.S. National Rate[3]	Number of Cases Too Small[4]
U.S. and Territories	75	68	2655	687
Alabama	0	4	46	11
Alaska	0	0	7	1
American Samoa	0	0	0	0
Arizona	1	0	48	6
Arkansas	1	1	28	7
California	7	4	196	89
Colorado	1	3	46	6
Connecticut	1	2	26	0
Delaware	0	0	5	1
District of Columbia	0	0	5	2
Florida	11	1	134	16
Georgia	2	1	76	15
Guam	0	0	0	0
Hawaii	0	0	8	6
Idaho	0	0	23	5
Illinois	2	3	108	25
Indiana	4	1	73	32
Iowa	0	2	46	17
Kansas	3	2	37	13
Kentucky	1	0	41	19
Louisiana	0	0	59	16
Maine	1	1	24	5
Maryland	2	1	41	1
Massachusetts	2	0	54	5
Michigan	6	2	88	20
Minnesota	1	0	65	17
Mississippi	2	1	24	9
Missouri	3	2	61	14
Montana	0	1	19	6
N. Mariana Islands	0	0	0	0
Nebraska	2	0	30	13
Nevada	0	1	22	2
New Hampshire	0	1	21	4
New Jersey	0	1	53	9
New Mexico	0	0	22	2
New York	4	2	116	30
North Carolina	1	4	77	8
North Dakota	1	0	7	1
Ohio	2	6	128	21
Oklahoma	1	1	46	18
Oregon	0	0	40	10
Pennsylvania	0	6	123	27
Puerto Rico	0	0	8	27
Rhode Island	0	0	9	1
South Carolina	1	0	39	14
South Dakota	0	0	16	2
Tennessee	2	3	50	21
Texas	7	4	198	54
Utah	0	1	25	6
Vermont	0	0	12	1
Virgin Islands	0	0	1	0
Virginia	2	2	54	11
Washington	1	0	52	9
West Virginia	0	0	26	6
Wisconsin	0	4	79	22
Wyoming	0	0	13	4

Note: (1) Surgical complication rate is better (lower) than U.S. rate of 3.4%; (2) Surgical complication rate is worse (higher) than U.S. rate of 3.4%; (3) Surgical complication rate is about the same as U.S. rate of 3.4%; (4) The number of cases is too small to classify the hospital; n/a not available

Surgical Complication Rate: State and National Summary

Measure: Serious Blood Clots After Surgery

Area	Number of Hospitals			
	Better than U.S. National Rate[1]	Worse than U.S. National Rate[2]	No Different than U.S. National Rate[3]	Number of Cases Too Small[4]
U.S. and Territories	155	203	2846	114
Alabama	1	3	72	5
Alaska	0	0	8	1
American Samoa	n/a	n/a	n/a	n/a
Arizona	3	1	58	1
Arkansas	3	0	41	2
California	16	8	274	5
Colorado	2	4	38	0
Connecticut	1	5	23	0
Delaware	0	1	5	0
District of Columbia	0	1	6	0
Florida	7	18	138	2
Georgia	2	6	92	4
Guam	n/a	n/a	n/a	n/a
Hawaii	0	0	14	0
Idaho	2	1	10	1
Illinois	5	20	100	2
Indiana	8	1	79	1
Iowa	4	1	29	0
Kansas	4	2	46	3
Kentucky	4	2	57	2
Louisiana	2	3	80	7
Maine	1	0	19	0
Maryland	n/a	n/a	n/a	n/a
Massachusetts	4	2	52	2
Michigan	5	13	74	0
Minnesota	4	0	47	0
Mississippi	1	3	39	9
Missouri	3	5	62	5
Montana	5	0	7	1
N. Mariana Islands	n/a	n/a	n/a	n/a
Nebraska	0	0	23	0
Nevada	1	0	20	0
New Hampshire	1	2	10	0
New Jersey	2	15	47	1
New Mexico	1	2	23	3
New York	3	21	133	5
North Carolina	6	2	79	0
North Dakota	2	0	4	0
Ohio	0	9	122	4
Oklahoma	4	1	68	11
Oregon	4	2	26	1
Pennsylvania	1	23	127	2
Puerto Rico	n/a	n/a	n/a	n/a
Rhode Island	0	0	11	0
South Carolina	1	0	54	2
South Dakota	3	0	15	1
Tennessee	8	2	77	5
Texas	13	12	257	23
Utah	1	1	27	1
Vermont	0	0	6	0
Virgin Islands	n/a	n/a	n/a	n/a
Virginia	5	4	62	1
Washington	7	2	39	0
West Virginia	1	2	28	0
Wisconsin	3	2	61	0
Wyoming	1	0	10	0

Note: (1) Surgical complication rate is better (lower) than U.S. rate of 4.14%; (2) Surgical complication rate is worse (higher) than U.S. rate of 4.14%; (3) Surgical complication rate is about the same as U.S. rate of 4.14%; (4) The number of cases is too small to classify the hospital; n/a not available

Surgical Complication Rate: State and National Summary

Measure: Serious Complications

Area	Number of Hospitals			
	Better than U.S. National Rate[1]	Worse than U.S. National Rate[2]	No Different than U.S. National Rate[3]	Number of Cases Too Small[4]
U.S. and Territories	108	182	3184	0
Alabama	0	5	92	0
Alaska	0	0	9	0
American Samoa	n/a	n/a	n/a	n/a
Arizona	1	2	64	0
Arkansas	2	0	44	0
California	8	15	287	0
Colorado	0	6	40	0
Connecticut	0	6	26	0
Delaware	0	0	6	0
District of Columbia	0	2	5	0
Florida	7	9	155	0
Georgia	3	4	101	0
Guam	n/a	n/a	n/a	n/a
Hawaii	0	0	14	0
Idaho	0	1	13	0
Illinois	5	9	115	0
Indiana	7	0	83	0
Iowa	3	0	31	0
Kansas	0	3	53	0
Kentucky	3	1	61	0
Louisiana	2	4	92	0
Maine	0	1	19	0
Maryland	n/a	n/a	n/a	n/a
Massachusetts	3	3	55	0
Michigan	6	8	81	0
Minnesota	1	3	48	0
Mississippi	2	3	62	0
Missouri	2	4	72	0
Montana	1	0	12	0
N. Mariana Islands	n/a	n/a	n/a	n/a
Nebraska	1	0	23	0
Nevada	1	2	21	0
New Hampshire	1	1	11	0
New Jersey	5	10	51	0
New Mexico	0	2	31	0
New York	3	10	157	0
North Carolina	3	3	83	0
North Dakota	0	1	6	0
Ohio	4	8	129	0
Oklahoma	3	2	86	0
Oregon	1	1	31	0
Pennsylvania	4	16	136	0
Puerto Rico	n/a	n/a	n/a	n/a
Rhode Island	0	1	10	0
South Carolina	4	0	53	0
South Dakota	1	0	20	0
Tennessee	5	0	92	0
Texas	10	13	306	0
Utah	0	4	28	0
Vermont	0	0	6	0
Virgin Islands	n/a	n/a	n/a	n/a
Virginia	4	4	72	0
Washington	0	6	42	0
West Virginia	2	2	27	0
Wisconsin	0	7	59	0
Wyoming	0	0	11	0

Note: (1) Surgical complication rate is better (lower) than U.S. rate of 0.61%; (2) Surgical complication rate is worse (higher) than U.S. rate of 0.61%; (3) Surgical complication rate is about the same as U.S. rate of 0.61%; (4) The number of cases is too small to classify the hospital; n/a not available

Appendix D: Best Hospitals by Selected Category

What Do These Tables Show?

This appendix shows the best hospitals nationwide based on their average scores in 11 categories. The categories are:

- Blood Clot Prevention and Treatment
- Children's Asthma Care
- Emergency Department Care
- Heart Care
- Pneumonia Care
- Preventative Care
- Stroke Care
- Surgical Care
- Patient's Hospital Experiences
- Use of Medical Imaging
- Lowest Medicare Spending per Beneficiary

How Were the Hospitals Selected?

Hospitals were selected for inclusion in three ways:

- Hospitals that achieved a perfect 100% average score in all qualified measures in a given category.
- Hospitals that were in the top 5% of hospitals based on their average score in a given category.
- Hospitals whose Medicare spending ratios fell below a certain threshold.

How Were Average Scores Calculated?

The average score for any given category was calculated by averaging the scores of the individual measures that made up that category. In some instances, not all measures were included in the average score calculation. A meaure was omitted if: 1) data was not available 2) the measure did not meet the 25 case threshold for inclusion (except Patient's Hospital Experiences in which the threshold was 100 or more completed surveys). Note that the Pregnancy Care category did not have enough information available to calculate an average score.

Best Hospitals for Blood Clot Prevention and Treatment

Hospital	City	State	Phone	Web Site
Baptist Hospital of Miami	Miami	Florida	786-596-1960	www.baptisthealth.net
Berkshire Medical Center	Pittsfield	Massachusetts	413-447-2000	www.berkshirehealthsystems.org
Blanchard Valley Hospital	Findlay	Ohio	419-423-4500	www.bvha.org
Boca Raton Regional Hospital	Boca Raton	Florida	561-362-5002	www.brrh.com
Brandon Regional Hospital	Brandon	Florida	813-681-5551	www.brandonregionalhospital.com
Capital Regional Medical Center	Tallahassee	Florida	850-656-5000	www.capitalregionalmedicalcenter.com
Centerpoint Medical Center	Independence	Missouri	816-698-7000	www.centerpointmedical.com
Community Hospital of the Monterey Peninsula	Monterey	California	831-624-5311	www.chomp.org
Delray Medical Center	Delray Beach	Florida	561-498-4440	www.delraymedicalctr.com
Doctors' Community Hospital	Lanham	Maryland	301-552-8085	www.dchweb.org
Fairview Southdale Hospital	Edina	Minnesota	952-924-5000	www.fairview.org
Flushing Hospital Medical Center	Flushing	New York	718-670-5000	www.flushinghospital.org
Fort Sanders Regional Medical Center	Knoxville	Tennessee	865-541-1101	www.fsregional.com
Henrico Doctors' Hospital	Richmond	Virginia	804-289-4500	www.henricodoctors.com
Heritage Valley Beaver	Beaver	Pennsylvania	412-728-7000	www.heritagevalley.org
Heritage Valley Sewickley	Sewickley	Pennsylvania	412-741-6600	www.heritagevalley.org
John Randolph Medical Center	Hopewell	Virginia	804-541-1600	www.johnrandolphmed.com
Kaiser Foundation Hospital - Roseville	Roseville	California	916-784-4000	www.kaiserpermanente.org/roseville
Kendall Regional Medical Center	Miami	Florida	305-223-3000	www.kendallmed.com
Lewisgale Medical Center	Salem	Virginia	540-776-4000	www.lewis-gale.com
Lovelace Medical Center	Albuquerque	New Mexico	505-727-8000	www.lovelace.com
Mclaren Lapeer Region	Lapeer	Michigan	810-667-5500	www.lapeerregional.org
The Medical Center of Aurora	Aurora	Colorado	303-695-2600	www.auroramed.com
Medical Center of Plano	Plano	Texas	972-596-6800	www.medicalcenterofplano.com
Memorial Hospital Pembroke	Pembroke Pines	Florida	954-962-9650	www.memorialpembroke.com\
Memorial Hospital West	Pembroke Pines	Florida	954-436-5000	www.memorialwest.com
Memorial Regional Hospital	Hollywood	Florida	954-987-2000	www.memorialregional.com
Mercy Hospital of Folsom	Folsom	California	916-983-7400	www.mercyfolsom.org
Mercy Memorial Hospital System	Monroe	Michigan	734-240-8400	www.mercymemorial.org
Methodist Dallas Medical Center	Dallas	Texas	214-947-2879	www.mhd.com
Mountain View Regional Medical Center	Las Cruces	New Mexico	575-556-7600	www.mountainviewregional.com
Nazareth Hospital	Philadelphia	Pennsylvania	215-335-6000	www.nazarethhospital.org
North Florida Regional Medical Center	Gainesville	Florida	352-333-4100	www.nfrmc.com
Northside Hospital	Atlanta	Georgia	404-851-8000	www.northside.com
Northside Hospital Cherokee	Canton	Georgia	770-720-5298	www.northside.com/cherokee
Northside Hospital Forsyth	Cumming	Georgia	404-851-8700	www.gbhcs.org
Novant Health Forsyth Medical Center	Winston-Salem	North Carolina	336-718-5000	www.forsythmedicalcenter.org
Oak Hill Hospital	Brooksville	Florida	352-596-6632	www.oakhillhospital.com
Orange Park Medical Center	Orange Park	Florida	904-276-8500	www.opmedical.com
Overland Park Regional Medical Center	Overland Park	Kansas	913-541-5301	www.oprmc.com
Rapides Regional Medical Center	Alexandria	Louisiana	318-769-3000	www.rapidesregional.com
Regional Medical Center Bayonet Point	Hudson	Florida	727-819-2929	www.mchealth.comorwww.heartoftampa.com
Riverside Medical Center	Kankakee	Illinois	815-933-1671	www.riversidehealthcare.org
Rockdale Medical Center	Conyers	Georgia	770-918-3000	www.rockdalehospital.org
Rose Medical Center	Denver	Colorado	303-320-2121	www.rosemed.com
Saint Clares Hospital of Weston	Weston	Wisconsin	715-393-3000	www.ministryhealth.org
Saint Lucie Medical Center	Port Saint Lucie	Florida	772-335-4000	www.stluciemed.com
Saint Mary Medical Center	Hobart	Indiana	219-942-0551	www.comhs.org/stmary
Saint Mary's Medical Center	West Palm Beach	Florida	561-840-6202	www.stmarysmc.com
Saint Mary's Medical Center	Blue Springs	Missouri	816-228-5900	www.stmaryskc.com
Saint Vincent's Medical Center Southside	Jacksonville	Florida	904-296-3700	www.jaxhealth.com
Sisters of Charity Hospital	Buffalo	New York	716-862-1000	www.chsbuffalo.org
South Miami Hospital	South Miami	Florida	786-662-4000	www.baptisthealth.net
Southern Hills Hospital & Medical Center	Las Vegas	Nevada	702-880-2100	www.southernhillshospital.com
Springs Memorial Hospital	Lancaster	South Carolina	803-286-1481	www.springsmemorial.com
Summa Western Reserve Hospital	Cuyahoga Falls	Ohio	330-971-7000	www.westernreservehospital.org
Texoma Medical Center	Denison	Texas	903-416-4000	www.texomamedicalcenter.net
Trinity Medical Center	Birmingham	Alabama	205-592-1000	www.bhsala.com/montclair
Tulane Medical Center	New Orleans	Louisiana	504-988-1900	www.tuhc.com
United Hospital Center	Bridgeport	West Virginia	681-342-1000	www.uhcwv.org
University Medical Center of El Paso	El Paso	Texas	915-521-7602	www.thomasoncares.org
UPMC Horizon	Greenville	Pennsylvania	724-588-2100	www.upmc.com
UPMC Mckeesport	Mc Keesport	Pennsylvania	412-664-2000	www.selectmedicalcorp.com
Venice Regional Medical Center - Bayfront Health	Venice	Florida	941-485-7711	www.veniceregional.com
Vista Medical Center East	Waukegan	Illinois	847-360-4000	www.vistahealth.com

Hospital	City	State	Phone	Web Site
Wesley Medical Center	Wichita	Kansas	316-962-2000	www.wesleymc.com
West Georgia Medical Center	Lagrange	Georgia	706-882-1411	www.wghealth.org
West Virginia University Hospitals	Morgantown	West Virginia	304-598-4000	www.wvuh.com

Note: The hospitals shown above represent the top 5% of the 1,268 hospitals nationwide for which an average score was calculated. Average scores were calculated for hospitals with qualifying data (25 cases or more) in at least 5 of 6 measures in the Blood Clot Prevention and Treatment category.

Best Hospitals for Children's Asthma Care

Hospital	City	State	Phone	Web Site
Carroll Hospital Center	Westminster	Maryland	410-848-3000	www.carrollhospitalcenter.org
Cleveland Clinic	Cleveland	Ohio	216-444-2200	www.clevelandclinic.org
Lawnwood Regional Medical Center & Heart Institute	Fort Pierce	Florida	772-461-4000	www.lawnwoodmed.com
Memorial Regional Hospital	Hollywood	Florida	954-987-2000	www.memorialregional.com
Renown Regional Medical Center	Reno	Nevada	775-982-4100	www.renown.org

Note: The hospitals shown above represent the top 5% of the 90 hospitals nationwide for which an average score was calculated. Average scores were calculated for hospitals with qualifying data (25 cases or more) in all three measures in the Children's Asthma category.

Best Hospitals for Emergency Department Care

Hospital	City	State	Phone	Web Site
Abraham Lincoln Memorial Hospital	Lincoln	Illinois	217-732-2161	www.almh.org
Albemarle Hospital Authority	Elizabeth City	North Carolina	252-335-0531	www.albemarlehealth.org
Alliance Community Hospital	Alliance	Ohio	330-596-7527	www.achosp.org
Ashtabula County Medical Center	Ashtabula	Ohio	440-997-2262	www.acmchealth.org
Aspirus Wausau Hospital	Wausau	Wisconsin	715-847-2121	www.aspirus.org
Aurora Medical Center	Summit	Wisconsin	262-434-1000	www.aurorahealthcare.org
Avera Sacred Heart Hospital	Yankton	South Dakota	605-668-8000	www.avera.org/sacred-heart
Avera Saint Mary's Hospital	Pierre	South Dakota	605-224-3100	www.st-marys.com
Avoyelles Hospital	Marksville	Louisiana	318-253-8611	www.avoyelleshospital.com
Bates County Memorial Hospital	Butler	Missouri	660-200-7000	www.bcmhospital.com
Bear River Valley Hospital	Tremonton	Utah	435-207-4708	www.intermountainhealthcare.org
Bellevue Hospital	Bellevue	Ohio	419-483-4040	www.bellevuehospital.com
Bluffton Hospital	Bluffton	Ohio	419-358-9010	www.bvhealthsystem.org
Bourbon Community Hospital	Paris	Kentucky	859-987-3600	www.bourbonhospital.com
Brigham City Community Hospital	Brigham City	Utah	435-734-9471	www.brighamcityhospital.com
Brookings Hospital	Brookings	South Dakota	605-696-7701	www.brookingshospital.org
Cache Valley Speciality Hospital	North Logan	Utah	435-713-9700	www.cachevalleyhospital.com
Cameron Regional Medical Center	Cameron	Missouri	816-632-2101	www.cameronregional.org
Carson City Hospital	Carson City	Michigan	989-584-3131	www.carsoncityhospital.com
Cogdell Memorial Hospital	Snyder	Texas	325-574-7437	www.cogdellhospital.com
Colorado Plains Medical Center	Fort Morgan	Colorado	970-867-3391	www.coloradoplainsmedicalcenter.com
Crossroads Community Hospital	Mount Vernon	Illinois	618-244-5500	www.crossroadscommnityhospital.com
Custer Regional Hospital	Custer	South Dakota	605-673-2229	www.rcrh.org/facilities
Dauterive Hospital	New Iberia	Louisiana	337-365-7311	www.dauterivehospital.com
Daviess Community Hospital	Washington	Indiana	812-254-2760	www.dchosp.org
Decatur County Memorial Hospital	Greensburg	Indiana	812-663-4331	www.dcmh.net
Detroit Receiving Hospital & University Health Center	Detroit	Michigan	313-745-3104	www.drhuhc.org
Dupont Hospital	Fort Wayne	Indiana	260-416-3000	www.theduponthospital.com
East Cooper Medical Center	Mount Pleasant	South Carolina	843-881-0100	www.eastcoopermedctr.com
El Paso Specialty Hospital	El Paso	Texas	915-544-3636	www.elpasospecialtyhospital.com
Encino Hospital Medical Center	Encino	California	818-995-5000	www.encino-tarzana.com
Englewood Community Hospital	Englewood	Florida	941-475-6571	www.englewoodcommunityhospital.com
Evanston Regional Hospital	Evanston	Wyoming	307-789-3636	www.evanstonregionalhospital.com
Excela Health Frick Hospital	Mount Pleasant	Pennsylvania	724-547-1500	www.excelahealth.org
Fairmont General Hospital	Fairmont	West Virginia	304-367-7100	www.fghi.com
Fort Hamilton Hughes Memorial Hospital	Hamilton	Ohio	513-867-2000	www.forthamiltonhospital.com
Fremont Area Medical Center	Fremont	Nebraska	402-721-1610	www.famc.org
Genesis Medical Center - Dewitt	Dewitt	Iowa	563-659-4200	www.genesishealth.com
Good Samaritan Health Center	Merrill	Wisconsin	715-536-5511	www.ministryhealth.org/GSHC/home.nws
Good Samaritan Hospital	Kearney	Nebraska	308-865-7100	www.gshs.org
Graham Hospital Association	Canton	Illinois	309-647-5240	www.grahamhospital.org
Great Bend Regional Hospital	Great Bend	Kansas	620-792-8833	www.greatbendsurgical.com
Grove City Medical Center	Grove City	Pennsylvania	724-450-7000	www.uchpa.org
Hamilton General Hospital	Hamilton	Texas	254-386-3151	www.hamiltonhospital.org
Harrington Memorial Hospital	Southbridge	Massachusetts	508-765-9771	www.harringtonhospital.org
Harris Hospital	Newport	Arkansas	870-523-8911	www.harrishospital.com
Heber Valley Medical Center	Heber City	Utah	435-654-2500	www.intermountainhealthcare.org
Henderson County Community Hospital	Lexington	Tennessee	731-968-1801	www.hendersoncchospital.com
Hill Regional Hospital	Hillsboro	Texas	254-580-8500	www.hillregionalhospital.com
Hillside Hospital	Pulaski	Tennessee	931-363-7531	www.hillsidehospital.com
Holdenville Hospital Authority	Holdenville	Oklahoma	405-379-4200	
The Hospital at Westlake Medical Center	Austin	Texas	512-327-0000	www.westlakemedical.com
Hutchinson Health	Hutchinson	Minnesota	320-234-5000	www.hahc-hmc.com
Illinois Valley Community Hospital	Peru	Illinois	815-223-3300	www.ivch.org
Integris Blackwell Regional Hospital	Blackwell	Oklahoma	580-363-2311	www.integrisblackwell.com
Integris Health Edmond	Edmond	Oklahoma	405-657-3000	www.integrisok.com/integris-health-edmond-ok
Integris Marshall County Medical Center	Madill	Oklahoma	580-795-3384	www.integris-health.com/integris
Iroquois Memorial Hospital	Watseka	Illinois	815-432-5201	www.iroquoismemorial.com
Kansas Medical Center	Andover	Kansas	316-300-4000	www.ksmedcenter.com
Lafayette Regional Health Center	Lexington	Missouri	660-259-2203	www.lafayetteregionalhealthcenter.com
Lake Region Healthcare Corporation	Fergus Falls	Minnesota	218-736-8000	www.lrhc.org
Lakeland Community Hospital	Haleyville	Alabama	205-485-7117	www.lifepointhospitals.com
Lakeland Regional Medical Center	Lakeland	Florida	863-687-1100	www.lrmc.com
Lander Regional Hospital	Lander	Wyoming	307-332-4420	www.landerhospital.com
Lawrence Medical Center	Moulton	Alabama	256-974-2200	www.lawrencemedicalcenter.com

Hospital	City	State	Phone	Web Site
Livingston Regional Hospital	Livingston	Tennessee	931-823-5611	www.livingstonregionalhospital.com
Madison Memorial Hospital	Rexburg	Idaho	208-359-6900	www.madisonhospital.org
Maple Grove Hospital	Maple Grove	Minnesota	763-581-1000	www.maplegrove.org
Mary Greeley Medical Center	Ames	Iowa	515-239-2011	www.mgmc.org
Mary Lanning Healthcare	Hastings	Nebraska	402-463-4521	www.marylanning.org
Mayo Clinic Health System - Fairmont	Fairmont	Minnesota	507-238-8101	www.fairmontmedicalcenter.org
McBride Clinic Orthopedic Hospital	Oklahoma City	Oklahoma	405-478-1717	www.mcbrideclinic.com
McCullough - Hyde Memorial Hospital	Oxford	Ohio	513-523-2111	www.mhmh.org
McDonough District Hospital	Macomb	Illinois	309-833-4101	www.mdh.org
Mercer County Joint Township Community Hospital	Coldwater	Ohio	419-678-4843	www.mercer-health.com
Mercy Health System Corp	Janesville	Wisconsin	608-756-6080	www.mercyhealthsystem.org
Mercy Medical Center	Roseburg	Oregon	541-673-0611	www.mercyrose.org
Mercy Medical Center - Dubuque	Dubuque	Iowa	563-589-8000	www.mercydubuque.com
Mercy Regional Medical Center	Ville Platte	Louisiana	337-363-5684	www.vpmc.com
Meriter Hospital	Madison	Wisconsin	608-417-6000	www.meriter.com
Mesa View Regional Hospital	Mesquite	Nevada	702-346-8040	www.mesaviewhospital.com
Minden Medical Center	Minden	Louisiana	318-377-2321	www.mindenmedicalcenter.com
Ministry Saint Michaels Hospital of Stevens Point	Stevens Point	Wisconsin	715-346-5000	www.saintmichaelshospital.org
Moore County Hospital District	Dumas	Texas	806-935-7171	www.mchd.net
Mount Pleasant Hospital	Mount Pleasant	South Carolina	843-724-2954	www.rsfh.com
Mountain View Hospital	Payson	Utah	801-465-7100	www.mvhpayson.com
Neshoba County General Hospital	Philadelphia	Mississippi	601-663-1200	www.neshobageneral.com
Nevada Regional Medical Center	Nevada	Missouri	417-667-3355	www.nrmchealth.com
Ottawa Regional Hospital & Healthcare Center	Ottawa	Illinois	815-433-3100	www.community-hospital.org
Park City Medical Center	Park City	Utah	435-658-7000	www.intermountainhealthcare.org
Parkview Lagrange Hospital	Lagrange	Indiana	260-463-9000	www.parkview.com
Ponca City Medical Center	Ponca City	Oklahoma	580-765-3321	www.poncamedcenter.com
Portage Health	Hancock	Michigan	906-483-1000	www.portagehealth.org
Prairie Lakes Hospital	Watertown	South Dakota	605-882-7000	www.prairielakes.com
Presbyterian Saint Lukes Medical Center	Denver	Colorado	303-839-6000	www.pslmc.com
Proctor Hospital	Peoria	Illinois	309-691-1000	www.proctor.org
Providence Seaside Hospital	Seaside	Oregon	503-717-7000	www.providence.org/northcoast
Pushmataha County - Town of Antlers Hospital Authority	Antlers	Oklahoma	580-298-3341	www.pushhospital.com
Riverview Regional Medical Center	Carthage	Tennessee	615-735-9815	www.sumner.org
Rockcastle County Hospital	Mount Vernon	Kentucky	606-256-2195	www.rockcastlehospital.com
Sagewest Health Care	Riverton	Wyoming	307-856-4161	www.riverton-hospital.com
Saint Charles Parish Hospital	Luling	Louisiana	985-785-6242	www.stch.net
Saint Clare Hospital Health Services	Baraboo	Wisconsin	608-356-1400	www.stclare.com
Saint Elizabeth Grant	Williamstown	Kentucky	859-824-8240	www.stelizabeth.com
Saint Elizabeth Hospital	Appleton	Wisconsin	920-738-2000	www.affinityhealth.org
Saint James Healthcare	Butte	Montana	406-723-2500	www.stjameshealthcare.org
Saint James Hospital	Pontiac	Illinois	815-842-2828	www.osfsaintjames.org
Saint John Hospital	Leavenworth	Kansas	913-596-3930	www.providence-health.org
Saint Johns Medical Center	Jackson	Wyoming	307-733-3636	www.tetonhospital.org
Saint Margarets Hospital	Spring Valley	Illinois	815-664-1176	www.aboutsmh.org
Saint Marys Hospital	Madison	Wisconsin	608-251-6100	www.stmarysmadison.com
Saint Marys Hospital Superior	Superior	Wisconsin	715-817-7000	www.smdc.org
Saint Marys Janesville Hospital	Janesville	Wisconsin	608-373-8000	www.stmarysjanesville.com
Samaritan Albany General Hospital	Albany	Oregon	541-812-4000	www.samhealth.org/shs_facilities
Sanford Medical Center Bismarck	Bismarck	North Dakota	701-323-6000	www.medcenterone.com
Sanford Worthington Medical Center	Worthington	Minnesota	507-372-2941	www.worthingtonhospital.com
Santa Ynez Valley Cottage Hospital	Solvang	California	805-688-6431	www.cottagehealthsystem.org
Seton Smithville Regional Hospital	Smithville	Texas	512-237-3214	www.srhnet.com
Share Memorial Hospital	Alva	Oklahoma	580-327-2800	www.smcok.com
Shelby Memorial Hospital	Shelbyville	Illinois	217-774-3961	www.mysmh.org
Silverton Hospital	Silverton	Oregon	503-873-1500	www.silvertonhospital.org
Smyth County Community Hospital	Marion	Virginia	276-378-1000	www.scchosp.org
South Central Kansas Medical Center	Arkansas City	Kansas	620-442-2500	www.sckrmc.com
Spearfish Regional Hospital	Spearfish	South Dakota	605-644-4000	www.rcrh.org
Spencer Municipal Hospital	Spencer	Iowa	712-264-8300	www.spencerhospital.org
Springhill Medical Center	Springhill	Louisiana	318-539-1000	www.smccare.com
Stephens Memorial Hospital	Breckenridge	Texas	254-559-2241	www.smhtx.com
Stonewall Jackson Memorial Hospital	Weston	West Virginia	304-269-8080	www.stonewallhospital.com
Swedish Issaquah	Issaquah	Washington	425-313-4000	www.swedish.org/locations/issaquah-campus
Swedish Medical Center	Seattle	Washington	206-386-6000	www.swedish.org
Taylorville Memorial Hospital	Taylorville	Illinois	217-824-3331	www.svmh.org
Toppenish Community Hospital	Toppenish	Washington	509-865-1520	www.hma-corp.com

Hospital	City	State	Phone	Web Site
Tristar Ashland City Medical Center	Ashland City	Tennessee	615-792-3030	www.centennialashlandcity.com
UPMC Bedford Memorial	Everett	Pennsylvania	814-623-6161	www.upmc.com
UPMC Northwest	Seneca	Pennsylvania	814-676-7600	www.northwest.upmc.com
Valley West Community Hospital	Sandwich	Illinois	815-786-8484	www.snd.softfarm.com/sandhosp
Via Christi Hospital Wichita Saint Teresa	Wichita	Kansas	316-796-7800	www.via-christi.org
Walla Walla General Hospital	Walla Walla	Washington	509-525-0480	www.wwgh.com
Winn Parish Medical Center	Winnfield	Louisiana	318-648-3000	www.winnparishmedical.com
Winona Health Services	Winona	Minnesota	507-454-3650	www.winonahealth.org
Woodward Regional Hospital	Woodward	Oklahoma	580-254-8492	www.woodwardhospital.com
Yampa Valley Medical Center	Steamboat Springs	Colorado	970-879-1322	www.yvmc.org
York Hospital	York	Maine	207-363-4321	www.yorkhospital.com

Note: The hospitals shown above represent the top 5% of the 2,872 hospitals nationwide for which an average score was calculated. Average scores were calculated for hospitals with qualifying data (25 cases or more) in at least 6 of 7 measures in the Emergency Department Care category.

Best Hospitals for Heart Care

Hospital	City	State	Phone	Web Site
Advocate Good Shepherd Hospital	Barrington	Illinois	847-381-9600	www.advocatehealth.com
Advocate Illinois Masonic Medical Center	Chicago	Illinois	773-975-1600	www.advocatehealth.com/immc
Alegent Creighton Health Immanuel Medical Center	Omaha	Nebraska	402-572-2121	www.alegent.com
Arkansas Heart Hospital	Little Rock	Arkansas	501-219-7000	www.arheart.com
Baptist Hospital of Miami	Miami	Florida	786-596-1960	www.baptisthealth.net
Baylor Heart & Vascular Hospital	Dallas	Texas	214-820-0670	www.baylorhearthospital.com
Beaumont Health System	Grosse Pointe	Michigan	313-343-1000	www.beaumonthospitals.com
Blanchard Valley Hospital	Findlay	Ohio	419-423-4500	www.bvha.org
Boca Raton Regional Hospital	Boca Raton	Florida	561-362-5002	www.brrh.com
Brooklyn Hospital Center at Downtown Campus	Brooklyn	New York	718-250-8000	www.tbh.org
Broward Health North	Pompano Beach	Florida	954-786-6950	www.browardhealth.org
Calvert Memorial Hospital	Prince Frederick	Maryland	410-535-8239	www.calverthospital.com
Carepoint Health - Bayonne Hospital Center	Bayonne	New Jersey	201-858-5000	www.bayonnemedicalcenter.org
Cedars - Sinai Medical Center	Los Angeles	California	310-423-5000	www.cedars-sinai.edu
Centinela Hospital Medical Center	Inglewood	California	310-673-4660	www.centinelafreeman.com
Decatur Memorial Hospital	Decatur	Illinois	217-877-8121	www.dmhcares.org
Dekalb Regional Medical Center	Fort Payne	Alabama	256-845-3150	www.baptistmedical.org
Delray Medical Center	Delray Beach	Florida	561-498-4440	www.delraymedicalctr.com
Doctors Hospital	Augusta	Georgia	706-651-6008	www.doctors-hospital.net
Doctors Hospital	Columbus	Ohio	614-544-1000	www.columbusregional.com
Eastern Idaho Regional Medical Center	Idaho Falls	Idaho	208-529-6111	www.eirmc.org
Fairview Southdale Hospital	Edina	Minnesota	952-924-5000	www.fairview.org
Florida Hospital North Pinellas	Tarpon Springs	Florida	727-942-5000	www.hemh.com
Fort Sanders Regional Medical Center	Knoxville	Tennessee	865-541-1101	www.fsregional.com
Gateway Regional Medical Center	Granite City	Illinois	618-798-3175	www.sehs.com
Good Samaritan Hospital Medical Center	West Islip	New York	631-376-3000	www.good-samaritan-hospital.org
Good Samaritan Hospital of Suffern	Suffern	New York	914-368-5000	www.goodsamhosp.org
Hackettstown Regional Medical Center	Hackettstown	New Jersey	908-852-5100	www.hrmcnj.org
Health Central	Ocoee	Florida	407-296-1820	www.health-central.org
High Point Regional Hospital	High Point	North Carolina	336-878-6000	www.highpointregional.com
Holy Name Medical Center	Teaneck	New Jersey	201-833-3000	www.holyname.org
Homestead Hospital	Homestead	Florida	786-243-8000	www.baptisthealth.net
Hospital De La Concepcion	San German	Puerto Rico	787-892-1860	www.hospitalconcepcion.org
Hospital of Univ of Pennsylvania	Philadelphia	Pennsylvania	215-662-3227	www.upenn.edu
Hudson Valley Hospital Center	Cortlandt Manor	New York	914-734-3611	www.hvhc.org
Indiana University Health Bloomington Hospital	Bloomington	Indiana	812-353-9555	www.bloomingtonhospital.org
Ingalls Memorial Hospital	Harvey	Illinois	708-333-2300	www.ingalls.org
Jamaica Hospital Medical Center	Jamaica	New York	718-262-6000	www.jamaicahospital.org
JFK Medical Center	Atlantis	Florida	561-965-7300	www.jfkmc.com
John Dempsey Hospital	Farmington	Connecticut	860-679-1145	www.uconnhealth.orgorwww.uchc.edu
Kaiser Foundation Hospital	Honolulu	Hawaii	808-432-0000	www.kaiserpermanente.com
Kaiser Foundation Hospital - Fremont/Hayward	Hayward	California	510-784-4000	www.kaiserpermanente.org
Kaiser Foundation Hospital - Manteca	Manteca	California	209-825-3700	www.healthy.kaiserpermanente.org
Kaiser Foundation Hospital - Orange Co-Anaheim	Anaheim	California	714-644-2000	www.healthy.kaiserpermanente.org
Kaiser Foundation Hospital - Redwood City	Redwood City	California	650-299-2000	www.seiu-uhw.org/aboutuhw
Kaiser Foundation Hospital - Sacramento	Sacramento	California	916-973-5000	www.kaiserpermanente.org
Kaiser Foundation Hospital - Santa Clara	Santa Clara	California	408-236-6400	www.members.kaiserpermanente.org
Kaiser Foundation Hospital - South Bay	Harbor City	California	310-517-6441	www.kaiserpermanente.org
Kaiser Foundation Hospital - South San Francisco	South San Francisco	California	650-742-3200	www.healthy.kaiserpermanente.org
Kaiser Foundation Hospital South Sacramento	Sacramento	California	916-688-2000	www.mydoctor.kaiserpermanente.org
Kansas Medical Center	Andover	Kansas	316-300-4000	www.ksmedcenter.com
Keck Hospital of USC	Los Angeles	California	323-442-8656	www.uscuh.com
La Palma Intercommunity Hospital	La Palma	California	714-670-7400	www.lapalmaintercommunityhospital.com
Lakeview Hospital	Bountiful	Utah	801-299-2211	www.lakeviewhospital.com
Lakeview Regional Medical Center	Covington	Louisiana	985-867-4443	www.lakeviewregional.com
Laredo Medical Center	Laredo	Texas	956-796-5000	www.laredomedical.com
Las Colinas Medical Center	Irving	Texas	972-969-2000	www.lascolinas.com
Lawnwood Regional Medical Center & Heart Institute	Fort Pierce	Florida	772-461-4000	www.lawnwoodmed.com
Lawrence Memorial Hospital	Lawrence	Kansas	785-505-6100	www.lmh.org
Lewisgale Medical Center	Salem	Virginia	540-776-4000	www.lewis-gale.com
Loyola University Medical Center	Maywood	Illinois	708-216-9000	www.lumc.edu
Manatee Memorial Hospital	Bradenton	Florida	941-746-5111	www.manateememorial.com
Mary Greeley Medical Center	Ames	Iowa	515-239-2011	www.mgmc.org
Medical Center of Arlington	Arlington	Texas	817-465-3241	www.medicalcenterarlington.com
Medical Center of Trinity	Trinity	Florida	727-848-1733	www.communityhospitalnpr.com

Hospital	City	State	Phone	Web Site
Memorial Regional Hospital	Hollywood	Florida	954-987-2000	www.memorialregional.com
Mercy Fitzgerald Hospital	Darby	Pennsylvania	215-237-4000	www.mercyhealth.org
Methodist Mansfield Medical Center	Mansfield	Texas	682-622-2059	www.methodisthealthsystem.com
Methodist Sugar Land Hospital	Sugar Land	Texas	281-274-8000	www.methodisthealth.com/sugarland
Metropolitan Hospital of Miami	Miami	Florida	305-264-1000	www.pahnet.org
Mid Coast Hospital	Brunswick	Maine	207-729-0181	www.midcoasthealth.com
Newark Beth Israel Medical Center	Newark	New Jersey	973-926-7850	www.sbhcs.com
North Florida Regional Medical Center	Gainesville	Florida	352-333-4100	www.nfrmc.com
North Hills Hospital	North Richland Hills	Texas	817-255-1000	www.northhillshospital.com
North Okaloosa Medical Center	Crestview	Florida	850-689-8100	www.northokaloosa.com
North Suburban Medical Center	Thornton	Colorado	303-451-7800	www.northsuburban.com
Novant Health Forsyth Medical Center	Winston-Salem	North Carolina	336-718-5000	www.forsythmedicalcenter.org
NYU Hospitals Center	New York	New York	212-263-7300	www.med.nyu.edu
Ocala Regional Medical Center	Ocala	Florida	352-401-1000	www.ocalaregional.com
Orange Park Medical Center	Orange Park	Florida	904-276-8500	www.opmedical.com
Palms West Hospital	Loxahatchee	Florida	561-753-4245	www.palmswesthospital.com
Paradise Valley Hospital	Phoenix	Arizona	602-923-5000	www.paradisevalleyhospital.com
Paradise Valley Hospital	National City	California	619-470-4321	www.paradisevalleyhospital.org
Parma Community General Hospital	Parma	Ohio	440-743-3000	www.parmahopsital.org
Penn Presbyterian Medical Center	Philadelphia	Pennsylvania	215-662-8000	www.pennhealth.com
Phelps Memorial Hospital Assn	Sleepy Hollow	New York	914-366-3000	www.phelpshospital.org
Pikeville Medical Center	Pikeville	Kentucky	606-218-3500	www.pikevillehospital.org
Plaza Medical Center of Fort Worth	Fort Worth	Texas	817-336-2100	www.plazamedicalcenter.com
Porter Regional Hospital	Valparaiso	Indiana	219-983-8300	www.portermemorial.org
Portsmouth Regional Hospital	Portsmouth	New Hampshire	603-436-5110	www.portsmouthhospital.com
Presbyterian Community Hospital	San Juan	Puerto Rico	787-721-2160	www.presbypr.com
Providence Memorial Hospital	El Paso	Texas	915-577-6011	www.sphn.com
Riverside Community Hospital	Riverside	California	951-788-3000	www.rchc.org
Riverside Methodist Hospital	Columbus	Ohio	614-566-5000	www.ohiohealth.com
Riverview Regional Medical Center	Gadsden	Alabama	256-543-5200	www.riverviewregional.com
Roper Hospital	Charleston	South Carolina	843-724-2800	www.ropersaintfrancis.com
Rose Medical Center	Denver	Colorado	303-320-2121	www.rosemed.com
Round Rock Medical Center	Round Rock	Texas	512-341-1000	www.roundrockmedicalcenter.com
Saint Anthony Hospital	Oklahoma City	Oklahoma	405-272-7000	www.saintsok.com
Saint John's Riverside Hospital	Yonkers	New York	914-964-4444	www.riversidehealth.org
Saint Luke's Magic Valley Rmc	Twin Falls	Idaho	208-814-1000	www.stlukesonline.org/magic_valley
Saint Mary Medical Center	Hobart	Indiana	219-942-0551	www.comhs.org/stmary
Saint Mary Medical Center	Langhorne	Pennsylvania	215-750-2003	www.stmaryhealthcare.org
Saint Mary's Health Center	Jefferson City	Missouri	573-761-7000	www.stmarys-jeffcity.com
Saint Mary's Hospital - Passaic	Passaic	New Jersey	973-365-4300	www.smh-nj.com
Sanford Medical Center Bismarck	Bismarck	North Dakota	701-323-6000	www.medcenterone.com
Scripps Green Hospital	La Jolla	California	858-554-3600	www.scrippshealth.org
Scripps Memorial Hospital La Jolla	La Jolla	California	858-626-4123	www.scrippshealth.org
Sebastian River Medical Center	Sebastian	Florida	772-589-3187	www.srmcenter.com
Sentara Norfolk General Hospital	Norfolk	Virginia	757-388-3000	www.sentara.com
Shady Grove Adventist Hospital	Rockville	Maryland	240-826-6517	www.adventisthealthcare.com/sgah
Sistema Integrados De Salud Del Sur Oeste	Mayaguez	Puerto Rico	787-652-9200	
Southern Hills Hospital & Medical Center	Las Vegas	Nevada	702-880-2100	www.southernhillshospital.com
Spotsylvania Regional Medical Center	Fredericksburg	Virginia	540-498-4000	www.spotsrmc.com
SSM Depaul Health Center	Bridgeton	Missouri	314-344-6000	www.ssmdepaul.com
SSM Saint Marys Health Center	Richmond Heights	Missouri	314-768-8000	www.ssmhealth.com/stmarys
Sutter Medical Center of Santa Rosa	Santa Rosa	California	707-576-4000	www.suttersantarosa.org
University Hospital	Newark	New Jersey	973-972-5658	www.theuniversityhospital.com
University of South Alabama Medical Center	Mobile	Alabama	251-471-7110	www.southalabama.edu/usamc
Venice Regional Medical Center - Bayfront Health	Venice	Florida	941-485-7711	www.veniceregional.com
Vista Medical Center East	Waukegan	Illinois	847-360-4000	www.vistahealth.com
Walker Baptist Medical Center	Jasper	Alabama	205-387-4000	www.bhsala.com/walker
Wellmont Bristol Regional Medical Center	Bristol	Tennessee	423-844-1121	www.wellmont.org
Wesley Medical Center	Wichita	Kansas	316-962-2000	www.wesleymc.com
West Florida Hospital	Pensacola	Florida	850-494-4000	www.westfloridahospital.com
West Virginia University Hospitals	Morgantown	West Virginia	304-598-4000	www.wvuh.com
Wichita VA Medical Center	Wichita	Kansas	316-685-2221	www.wichita.va.gov

Note: The 127 hospitals shown above all achieved a perfect 100% average score. Average scores were calculated for hospitals with qualifying data (25 cases or more) in at least 5 of 11 measures in the following categories: Chest Pain/Possible Heart Attack; Heart Attack; Heart Failure. A total of 2,234 hospitals nationwide were considered.

Best Hospitals for Pneumonia Care

Hospital	City	State	Phone	Web Site
Abilene Regional Medical Center	Abilene	Texas	325-428-1000	www.abileneregional.com
Advocate Christ Hospital & Medical Center	Oak Lawn	Illinois	708-684-8000	www.advocatehealth.com
Advocate Illinois Masonic Medical Center	Chicago	Illinois	773-975-1600	www.advocatehealth.com/immc
Alaska Regional Hospital	Anchorage	Alaska	907-276-1131	www.alaskaregional.com
Alegent Creighton Health Creighton University Med	Omaha	Nebraska	402-449-4000	www.creightonhospital.com
Alegent Creighton Health Midlands Hospital	Papillion	Nebraska	402-593-3000	www.alegent.com
Allegheny General Hospital	Pittsburgh	Pennsylvania	412-359-3131	www.allhealth.edu
Asante Ashland Community Hospital	Ashland	Oregon	541-201-4001	www.ashlandhospital.org
Asante Rogue Regional Medical Center	Medford	Oregon	541-789-7000	www.asante.org
Ashtabula County Medical Center	Ashtabula	Ohio	440-997-2262	www.acmchealth.org
Aurora Baycare Medical Center	Green Bay	Wisconsin	920-288-8000	www.aurorabaycare.com
Aurora West Allis Medical Center	West Allis	Wisconsin	414-328-6000	www.aurorahealthcare.org
Aventura Hospital & Medical Center	Aventura	Florida	305-682-7000	www.aventurahospital.com
Avera Marshall Regional Medical Center	Marshall	Minnesota	507-537-9661	www.averamarshall.org
Baptist Hospital of Miami	Miami	Florida	786-596-1960	www.baptisthealth.net
Baptist Memorial Hospital Huntingdon	Huntingdon	Tennessee	731-986-4461	www.bmhcc.org
Baptist Memorial Hospital North Mississippi	Oxford	Mississippi	662-232-8100	www.baptistonline.org/facilities/oxford
Baptist Memorial Hospital Union City	Union City	Tennessee	731-885-2410	www.bmhcc.org
Beaumont Health System	Grosse Pointe	Michigan	313-343-1000	www.beaumonthospitals.com
Bellevue Medical Center	Bellevue	Nebraska	402-763-3600	www.bellevuemed.com
Berkshire Medical Center	Pittsfield	Massachusetts	413-447-2000	www.berkshirehealthsystems.org
Big Bend Regional Medical Center	Alpine	Texas	432-837-3447	www.bigbendhealthcare.com
Bolivar Medical Center	Cleveland	Mississippi	662-846-2551	www.bolivarmedical.com
Bon Secours Memorial Regional Medical Center	Mechanicsville	Virginia	804-764-6000	www.bonsecours.com
Bonner General Hospital	Sandpoint	Idaho	208-263-1441	www.bonnergeneral.org
Brigham & Women's Faulkner Hospital	Boston	Massachusetts	617-983-7000	www.brighamandwomensfaulkner.org
Broadlawns Medical Center	Des Moines	Iowa	515-282-2200	www.broadlawns.org
Brookings Hospital	Brookings	South Dakota	605-696-7701	www.brookingshospital.org
Broward Health North	Pompano Beach	Florida	954-786-6950	www.browardhealth.org
Buchanan General Hospital	Grundy	Virginia	276-935-1000	www.bgh.org
Bucyrus Community Hospital	Bucyrus	Ohio	419-562-4677	www.bchonline.org
California Pacific Medical Center - Pacific Campus Hospital	San Francisco	California	415-600-6000	www.cpmc.org
California Pacific Medical Center - Saint Luke's Campus	San Francisco	California	415-641-6562	www.stlukes.sf.org
Carepoint Health - Bayonne Hospital Center	Bayonne	New Jersey	201-858-5000	www.bayonnemedicalcenter.org
Carney Hospital	Boston	Massachusetts	617-506-2000	www.caritascarney.org
Carolinas Hospital System	Florence	South Carolina	843-674-2500	www.carolinashospital.com
Centinela Hospital Medical Center	Inglewood	California	310-673-4660	www.centinelafreeman.com
Central Peninsula General Hospital	Soldotna	Alaska	907-262-4404	www.cpgh.org
Chatuge Regional Hospital	Hiawassee	Georgia	706-896-2222	www.chatugeregionalhospital.org
Coffee Regional Medical Center	Douglas	Georgia	229-384-1900	www.coffeeregional.org
Conroe Regional Medical Center	Conroe	Texas	936-539-1111	www.conroeregional.com
Coosa Valley Medical Center	Sylacauga	Alabama	256-249-5000	www.cvhealth.net
Coral Gables Hospital	Coral Gables	Florida	305-445-8461	www.coralgableshospital.com
The Corpus Christi Medical Center	Corpus Christi	Texas	361-761-1501	www.ccmedicalcenter.com
Davis Hospital & Medical Center	Layton	Utah	801-807-1000	www.davishospital.com
Delray Medical Center	Delray Beach	Florida	561-498-4440	www.delraymedicalctr.com
Detar Hospital Navarro	Victoria	Texas	361-575-7441	www.detar.com
Detroit (John D. Dingell) VA Medical Center	Detroit	Michigan	313-576-1000	www.detroit.va.gov
Doctors Hospital	Augusta	Georgia	706-651-6008	www.doctors-hospital.net
Dominican Hospital	Santa Cruz	California	831-462-7700	www.dominicanhospital.org
Down East Community Hospital	Machias	Maine	207-255-3356	www.dech.org
Dupont Hospital	Fort Wayne	Indiana	260-416-3000	www.theduponthospital.com
East Texas Medical Center - Gilmer	Gilmer	Texas	903-841-7100	www.etmc.org
Eastern Idaho Regional Medical Center	Idaho Falls	Idaho	208-529-6111	www.eirmc.org
El Camino Hospital	Mountain View	California	650-940-7000	www.elcaminohospital.org
Encino Hospital Medical Center	Encino	California	818-995-5000	www.encino-tarzana.com
Englewood Community Hospital	Englewood	Florida	941-475-6571	www.englewoodcommunityhospital.com
Excela Health Latrobe Hospital	Latrobe	Pennsylvania	724-537-1000	www.excelahealth.org
Faith Regional Health Services	Norfolk	Nebraska	402-371-4880	www.frhs.org
Falmouth Hospital	Falmouth	Massachusetts	508-548-5300	www.capecodhealth.com
Fannin Regional Hospital	Blue Ridge	Georgia	706-632-3711	www.fanninregionalhospital.com
Fawcett Memorial Hospital	Port Charlotte	Florida	941-629-1181	www.fawcetthospital.com
Florida Hospital North Pinellas	Tarpon Springs	Florida	727-942-5000	www.hemh.com
Flowers Hospital	Dothan	Alabama	334-793-5000	www.flowershospital.com
Forest Hills Hospital	Forest Hills	New York	718-830-4000	www.northshorelij.com

Hospital	City	State	Phone	Web Site
Fostoria Community Hospital	Fostoria	Ohio	419-435-7734	www.promedica.org
Franciscan Saint Anthony Health - Michigan City	Michigan City	Indiana	219-879-8511	www.samhc.org
Franciscan Saint Elizabeth Health - Lafayette East	Lafayette	Indiana	765-502-4334	www.ste.org
Frankfort Regional Medical Center	Frankfort	Kentucky	502-875-5240	www.frankfortregional.com
Garden Grove Hospital & Medical Center	Garden Grove	California	714-537-5160	www.gardengrovehospital.com
Garden Park Medical Center	Gulfport	Mississippi	228-575-7000	www.gardenparkmedical.com
Genesis Medical Center - Davenport	Davenport	Iowa	563-421-1000	www.genesishealth.com
Georgetown Memorial Hospital	Georgetown	South Carolina	843-527-7000	www.gmhsc.com
Good Samaritan Hospital Medical Center	West Islip	New York	631-376-3000	www.good-samaritan-hospital.org
Greene Memorial Hospital	Xenia	Ohio	937-352-2000	www.ketteringhealth.org/greene
Hackensack - Umc Mountainside	Montclair	New Jersey	973-429-6000	www.mountainsidenow.org
Hackettstown Regional Medical Center	Hackettstown	New Jersey	908-852-5100	www.hrmcnj.org
Hammond Henry Hospital	Geneseo	Illinois	309-944-6431	www.hammondhenry.com
Hardin Memorial Hospital	Kenton	Ohio	419-673-0761	www.hardinmemorial.org
Harlingen Medical Center	Harlingen	Texas	956-365-1000	www.harlingenmedicalcenter.com
Heart of Lancaster Regional Medical Center	Lititz	Pennsylvania	717-625-5000	www.heartoflancaster.com
Helena Regional Medical Center	Helena	Arkansas	870-338-5800	www.helenaregionalmedicalcenter.com
Henderson County Community Hospital	Lexington	Tennessee	731-968-1801	www.hendersoncchospital.com
Holy Family Memorial	Manitowoc	Wisconsin	920-320-2011	www.hfmhealth.org
Hospital Pavia Santurce	Fernandez Juncos	Puerto Rico	787-727-6060	www.paviahospitalsanturce.com
Howard Memorial Hospital	Nashville	Arkansas	870-845-4400	www.howardmemorial.com
Huntington Beach Hospital	Huntington Beach	California	714-843-5000	www.hbhospital.com
Hutchinson Health	Hutchinson	Minnesota	320-234-5000	www.hahc-hmc.com
Ingalls Memorial Hospital	Harvey	Illinois	708-333-2300	www.ingalls.org
Intermountain Medical Center	Murray	Utah	801-507-7000	www.intermountainhealthcare.org
Jackson Hospital & Clinic	Montgomery	Alabama	334-293-8000	www.jackson.org
Jamaica Hospital Medical Center	Jamaica	New York	718-262-6000	www.jamaicahospital.org
Jay Hospital	Jay	Florida	850-675-4532	www.bhcpns.org
Jefferson Medical Center	Ranson	West Virginia	304-728-1600	www.jeffmem.com
Jennings American Legion Hospital	Jennings	Louisiana	337-616-7000	www.jalh.com
JFK Medical Center	Atlantis	Florida	561-965-7300	www.jfkmc.com
The Johns Hopkins Hospital	Baltimore	Maryland	410-955-9540	www.jhmi.edu
Kaiser Foundation Hospital - Orange Co-Anaheim	Anaheim	California	714-644-2000	www.healthy.kaiserpermanente.org
Kaiser Foundation Hospital - San Jose	San Jose	California	408-972-7000	www.mydoctor.kaiserpermanente.org
Kaiser Foundation Hospital - Santa Clara	Santa Clara	California	408-236-6400	www.members.kaiserpermanente.org
Kendall Regional Medical Center	Miami	Florida	305-223-3000	www.kendallmed.com
Kenmore Mercy Hospital	Kenmore	New York	716-447-6100	www.chsbuffalo.org
Kennewick General Hospital	Kennewick	Washington	509-586-6111	www.kennewickgeneral.com
Lake City Medical Center	Lake City	Florida	386-719-9000	www.lakecitymedical.com
Lake Forest Hospital	Lake Forest	Illinois	847-234-5600	www.lakeforesthospital.com
Lake Wales Medical Center	Lake Wales	Florida	863-676-1433	www.lakewalesmedicalcenter.com
Lakeview Medical Center	Rice Lake	Wisconsin	715-234-1515	www.lakeviewmedical.com
Lakeview Regional Medical Center	Covington	Louisiana	985-867-4443	www.lakeviewregional.com
Lancaster Regional Medical Center	Lancaster	Pennsylvania	717-291-8123	www.lancasterregional.com
Laredo Medical Center	Laredo	Texas	956-796-5000	www.laredomedical.com
Largo Medical Center	Largo	Florida	727-588-5200	www.largomedical.com
Las Colinas Medical Center	Irving	Texas	972-969-2000	www.lascolinas.com
Lawnwood Regional Medical Center & Heart Institute	Fort Pierce	Florida	772-461-4000	www.lawnwoodmed.com
Lawrence Memorial Hospital	Walnut Ridge	Arkansas	870-886-1200	www.lawrencehealth.net
Lee's Summit Medical Center	Lees Summit	Missouri	816-282-5000	www.leessummithospital.com
Lehigh Regional Medical Center	Lehigh Acres	Florida	239-369-2101	www.lehighregional.com
Lewisgale Hospital Montgomery	Blacksburg	Virginia	540-951-1111	www.mrhospital.com
Lewisgale Medical Center	Salem	Virginia	540-776-4000	www.lewis-gale.com
Libertyhealth - Jersey City Medical Center Campus	Jersey City	New Jersey	201-915-2000	www.libertyhcs.org
Little Company of Mary Hospital	Evergreen Park	Illinois	708-422-6200	www.lcmh.org
Littleton Regional Healthcare	Littleton	New Hampshire	603-444-9000	www.littletonhospital.org
Lock Haven Hospital	Lock Haven	Pennsylvania	570-893-5000	www.lockhavenhospital.com
Lucas County Health Center	Chariton	Iowa	641-774-3000	www.lchcia.com
Marin General Hospital	Greenbrae	California	415-925-7900	www.maringeneral.com
Mary Greeley Medical Center	Ames	Iowa	515-239-2011	www.mgmc.org
Maryvale Hospital	Phoenix	Arizona	623-848-5000	www.maryvalehospital.com
Mat-Su Regional Medical Center	Palmer	Alaska	907-746-8600	www.matsuregional.com
Mayo Clinic Health System - Fairmont	Fairmont	Minnesota	507-238-8101	www.fairmontmedicalcenter.org
Mayo Clinic Health System - Northland	Barron	Wisconsin	715-537-3186	www.luthermidelfortnorthland.org
McKenzie Regional Hospital	Mc Kenzie	Tennessee	731-352-5344	www.mckenzieregionalhospital.com
Mease Hospital Dunedin	Dunedin	Florida	727-733-1111	www.measehospitals.com
Medical Center of Arlington	Arlington	Texas	817-465-3241	www.medicalcenterarlington.com

Hospital	City	State	Phone	Web Site
Medical Center of Trinity	Trinity	Florida	727-848-1733	www.communityhospitalnpr.com
Medical City Dallas Hospital	Dallas	Texas	972-566-6222	www.medicalcityhospital.com
Medwest Swain	Bryson City	North Carolina	828-488-2155	www.westcarehealth.org
Memorial Healthcare System	Chattanooga	Tennessee	423-495-2525	www.memorial.org
Memorial Hospital Los Banos	Los Banos	California	209-826-0591	www.memoriallosbanos.org
Memorial Hospital Pembroke	Pembroke Pines	Florida	954-962-9650	www.memorialpembroke.com\
Memorial Hospital West	Pembroke Pines	Florida	954-436-5000	www.memorialwest.com
Memorial Regional Hospital	Hollywood	Florida	954-987-2000	www.memorialregional.com
Menorah Medical Center	Overland Park	Kansas	913-498-6773	www.menorahmedicalcenter.com
Mercy General Hospital	Sacramento	California	916-453-4545	www.mercygeneral.org
Mercy Hospital - Fort Scott	Fort Scott	Kansas	620-223-7057	www.mercy.net
Mercy Hospital of Defiance	Defiance	Ohio	419-782-8444	www.mercyweb.org/mercy_defiance.aspx
Mercy Medical Center	Springfield	Massachusetts	413-748-9000	www.mercycares.com
Mercy Regional Health Center	Manhattan	Kansas	785-776-2831	www.mercyregional.org
Methodist Medical Center of Oak Ridge	Oak Ridge	Tennessee	865-835-1000	www.mmcoakridge.com
Methodist Richardson Medical Center	Richardson	Texas	972-498-4000	www.richardsonregional.com
Metroplex Hospital	Killeen	Texas	254-526-7523	www.mplex.org
Minden Medical Center	Minden	Louisiana	318-377-2321	www.mindenmedicalcenter.com
Ministry Sacred Heart Hospital	Tomahawk	Wisconsin	715-453-7700	www.ministryhealth.org
Ministry Saint Marys Hospital	Rhinelander	Wisconsin	715-361-2000	www.ministryhealth.org
Ministry Saint Michaels Hospital of Stevens Point	Stevens Point	Wisconsin	715-346-5000	www.saintmichaelshospital.org
Moberly Regional Medical Center	Moberly	Missouri	660-263-8400	www.moberlyhospital.com
Monmouth Medical Center - Southern Campus	Lakewood	New Jersey	732-363-1900	www.sbhcs.com
Mount Pleasant Hospital	Mount Pleasant	South Carolina	843-724-2954	www.rsfh.com
Mountain Home VA Medical Center	Mountain Home	Tennessee	423-926-1171	www.mountainhome.va.gov
Mountain View Hospital	Payson	Utah	801-465-7100	www.mvhpayson.com
Mountain View Regional Medical Center	Las Cruces	New Mexico	575-556-7600	www.mountainviewregional.com
Myrtue Medical Center	Harlan	Iowa	712-755-5161	www.shelbycohealth.com
New Ulm Medical Center	New Ulm	Minnesota	507-233-1000	www.newulmmedicalcenter.com
New York Community Hospital of Brooklyn	Brooklyn	New York	718-692-5302	www.nych.com
Noble Hospital	Westfield	Massachusetts	413-568-2811	www.noblehospital.org
North Austin Medical Center	Austin	Texas	512-901-1000	www.cornerstonehealthcaregroup.com
North Florida Regional Medical Center	Gainesville	Florida	352-333-4100	www.nfrmc.com
North Shore Medical Center	Miami	Florida	305-835-6000	www.northshoremedical.com
North Suburban Medical Center	Thornton	Colorado	303-451-7800	www.northsuburban.com
Northeast Regional Medical Center	Kirksville	Missouri	660-785-1000	www.nermc.com
Northern Westchester Hospital	Mount Kisco	New York	914-666-1200	www.nwhc.net
Northside Hospital	Saint Petersburg	Florida	813-521-5000	www.northsidehospital.com
Northside Hospital	Atlanta	Georgia	404-851-8000	www.northside.com
Northside Hospital Cherokee	Canton	Georgia	770-720-5298	www.northside.com/cherokee
Norwalk Hospital Association	Norwalk	Connecticut	203-852-2000	www.norwalkhosp.org
Novant Health Forsyth Medical Center	Winston-Salem	North Carolina	336-718-5000	www.forsythmedicalcenter.org
Novant Health Franklin Medical Center	Louisburg	North Carolina	919-496-5131	www.franklinregionalmedicalctr.com
Novant Health Huntersville Medical Center	Huntersville	North Carolina	704-316-4000	www.presbyterian.org
Novant Health Thomasville Medical Center	Thomasville	North Carolina	336-472-2000	www.thomasvillemedicalcenter.org
Oak Hill Hospital	Brooksville	Florida	352-596-6632	www.oakhillhospital.com
Oaklawn Hospital	Marshall	Michigan	269-781-4271	www.oaklawnhospital.org
OHSU Hospital & Clinics	Portland	Oregon	503-494-4036	www.ohsu.edu
Oklahoma State University Medical Center	Tulsa	Oklahoma	918-587-2561	www.tulsaregional.com
Orange Park Medical Center	Orange Park	Florida	904-276-8500	www.opmedical.com
Overton Brooks VA Medical Center - Shreveport	Shreveport	Louisiana	318-424-6037	www.va.gov/sta/guide/home.asp
Palm Bay Hospital	Palm Bay	Florida	321-434-8000	www.health-first.org
Parkway Regional Hospital	Fulton	Kentucky	270-472-2522	www.parkwayregionalhospital.com
Piggott Community Hospital	Piggott	Arkansas	870-598-3881	www.piggottcommunityhospital.com
Plateau Medical Center	Oak Hill	West Virginia	304-469-8600	www.plateaumedicalcenter.com
Pleasant Valley Hospital	Point Pleasant	West Virginia	304-675-4340	www.pvalley.org
Pomerene Hospital	Millersburg	Ohio	330-674-1015	www.pomerenehospital.org
Portsmouth Regional Hospital	Portsmouth	New Hampshire	603-436-5110	www.portsmouthhospital.com
Promedica Herrick Hospital	Tecumseh	Michigan	517-424-3000	www.promedica.org/herrick
Putnam General Hospital	Eatonton	Georgia	706-485-2711	www.putnamgeneral.com
Rapides Regional Medical Center	Alexandria	Louisiana	318-769-3000	www.rapidesregional.com
Raulerson Hospital	Okeechobee	Florida	863-763-2151	www.raulersonhospital.com
Regional Hospital of Jackson	Jackson	Tennessee	731-661-2000	www.regionalhospitaljackson.com
Regional Medical Center of San Jose	San Jose	California	408-259-5000	www.regionalmedicalsanjose.com
Renown South Meadows Medical Center	Reno	Nevada	775-982-7000	www.renown.org
River Parishes Hospital	Laplace	Louisiana	985-652-7000	www.riverparisheshospital.com
Riverview Medical Center	Red Bank	New Jersey	732-741-2700	www.meridianhealth.com

Hospital	City	State	Phone	Web Site
Rockford Memorial Hospital	Rockford	Illinois	815-968-6861	www.rhsnet.org
Roper Hospital	Charleston	South Carolina	843-724-2800	www.ropersaintfrancis.com
Rose Medical Center	Denver	Colorado	303-320-2121	www.rosemed.com
Roxborough Memorial Hospital	Philadelphia	Pennsylvania	215-483-9900	www.roxboroughmemorial.com
Saint Anthony Hospital	Chicago	Illinois	773-521-1710	www.cath-health.org
Saint Anthony Shawnee Hospital	Shawnee	Oklahoma	405-273-2270	www.unityhealthcenter.com
Saint Anthony's Health Center	Alton	Illinois	618-465-2571	www.sahc.org
Saint Barnabas Medical Center	Livingston	New Jersey	973-322-5000	www.saintbarnabas.com
Saint Catherine Hospital	East Chicago	Indiana	219-392-7004	www.comhs.org/stcatherine
Saint Clare Hospital Health Services	Baraboo	Wisconsin	608-356-1400	www.stclare.com
Saint Clares Hospital of Weston	Weston	Wisconsin	715-393-3000	www.ministryhealth.org
Saint Francis Hospital	Escanaba	Michigan	906-786-3311	www.osfstfrancis.or
Saint Francis Medical Center	Trenton	New Jersey	609-599-5000	www.stfrancismedical.com
Saint James Hospital	Pontiac	Illinois	815-842-2828	www.osfsaintjames.org
Saint Joseph Hospital	Fort Wayne	Indiana	260-425-3000	www.stjoehospital.com
Saint Joseph Hospital & Health Center	Kokomo	Indiana	765-456-5300	www.stvincent.org
Saint Joseph Mercy Port Huron	Port Huron	Michigan	810-985-1510	www.mercyporthuron.com
Saint Joseph Regional Medical Center - Plymouth	Plymouth	Indiana	574-948-4000	www.sjmed.com
Saint Joseph's Hospital	Breese	Illinois	618-526-4511	www.stjoebreese.com
Saint Joseph's Mercy Health Center	Hot Springs	Arkansas	501-622-1000	www.saintjosephs.com
Saint Louise Regional Hospital	Gilroy	California	408-848-2000	www.saintlouiseregionalhospital.org
Saint Lucie Medical Center	Port Saint Lucie	Florida	772-335-4000	www.stluciemed.com
Saint Luke's Magic Valley Rmc	Twin Falls	Idaho	208-814-1000	www.stlukesonline.org/magic_valley
Saint Luke's Quakertown Hospital	Quakertown	Pennsylvania	215-538-4500	www.slhn-lehighvalley.com
Saint Margarets Hospital	Spring Valley	Illinois	815-664-1176	www.aboutsmh.org
Saint Mary Medical Center	Hobart	Indiana	219-942-0551	www.comhs.org/stmary
Saint Mary's Good Samaritan Hospital	Greensboro	Georgia	706-453-7331	www.stmarysgoodsam.org
Saint Vincent Anderson Regional Hospital	Anderson	Indiana	765-646-8373	www.stjohnshealthsystem.org
Saint Vincent's Birmingham	Birmingham	Alabama	205-939-7000	www.stv.org
Saint Vincent's East	Birmingham	Alabama	205-838-3122	www.nolandhealth.com
Saint Vincent's Medical Center Southside	Jacksonville	Florida	904-296-3700	www.jaxhealth.com
Samaritan Hospital	Moses Lake	Washington	509-765-5606	www.samaritanhealthcare.com
San Angelo Community Medical Center	San Angelo	Texas	325-949-9511	www.sacmc.com
Scripps Mercy Hospital	San Diego	California	619-294-8111	www.scrippshealth.org
Sebastian River Medical Center	Sebastian	Florida	772-589-3187	www.srmcenter.com
Seton Highland Lakes	Burnet	Texas	512-715-3000	www.seton.net
Shands Lake Shore Regional Medical Center	Lake City	Florida	386-292-8000	www.shands.org
Sharp Coronado Hospital & Healthcare Center	Coronado	California	619-435-6251	www.sharp.com/coronado
Shasta Regional Medical Center	Redding	California	530-244-5454	www.shastaregional.com
Sibley Memorial Hospital	Washington	District of Columbia	202-537-4680	www.sibley.org
Signature Healthcare Brockton Hospital	Brockton	Massachusetts	508-941-7000	www.brocktonhospital.com
Silverton Hospital	Silverton	Oregon	503-873-1500	www.silvertonhospital.org
Singing River Hospital	Pascagoula	Mississippi	228-809-5000	www.srhshealth.com
Sisters of Charity Hospital	Buffalo	New York	716-862-1000	www.chsbuffalo.org
South Miami Hospital	South Miami	Florida	786-662-4000	www.baptisthealth.net
Southern Nh Medical Center	Nashua	New Hampshire	603-577-2000	www.snhmc.org
Sparks Regional Medical Center	Fort Smith	Arkansas	501-441-4000	www.sparks.org
Spokane VA Medical Center	Spokane	Washington	509-434-7000	www.spokane.med.va.gov
Spotsylvania Regional Medical Center	Fredericksburg	Virginia	540-498-4000	www.spotsrmc.com
Stafford Hospital	Stafford	Virginia	540-741-9000	www.marywashingtonhealthcare.com
Staten Island University Hospital	Staten Island	New York	718-226-9000	www.siuh.edu
Summit Medical Center	Van Buren	Arkansas	479-471-4300	www.summitmc.net
Sutter Medical Center of Santa Rosa	Santa Rosa	California	707-576-4000	www.suttersantarosa.org
Sycamore Medical Center	Miamisburg	Ohio	937-384-8776	www.khnetwork.org/sycamore
Takoma Regional Hospital	Greeneville	Tennessee	423-639-3151	www.takoma.org
Texas Health Arlington Memorial Hospital	Arlington	Texas	817-548-6100	www.texashealth.org
Texas Health Harris Methodist Hospital Alliance	Fort Worth	Texas	682-212-2004	www.texashealth.org/alliance
Texoma Medical Center	Denison	Texas	903-416-4000	www.texomamedicalcenter.net
Thorek Memorial Hospital	Chicago	Illinois	312-525-6780	www.thorek.org
Three Rivers Medical Center	Louisa	Kentucky	606-638-9451	www.threeriversmedicalcenter.com
Togus VA Medical Center	Augusta	Maine	207-623-8411	www.maine.va.gov
Transylvania Regional Hospital	Brevard	North Carolina	828-883-5302	www.tchospital.org
Trinity Medical Center	Birmingham	Alabama	205-592-1000	www.bhsala.com/montclair
Tristar Hendersonville Medical Center	Hendersonville	Tennessee	615-338-1000	www.hendersonvillemedicalcenter.com
Tristar Southern Hills Medical Center	Nashville	Tennessee	615-781-4000	www.southernhills.com
Tristar Stonecrest Medical Center	Smyrna	Tennessee	615-768-2000	www.stonecrestmedical.com
Tucson Medical Center	Tucson	Arizona	520-327-5461	www.tmcaz.com

Hospital	City	State	Phone	Web Site
Twin Cities Hospital	Niceville	Florida	850-678-4131	www.tchealthcare.com
UH Geauga Medical Center	Chardon	Ohio	440-269-6000	www.uhgeauga.org
UHHS Memorial Hospital of Geneva	Geneva	Ohio	440-466-1141	www.uhhospitals.org/geneva
University of Maryland Medical Center	Baltimore	Maryland	410-328-8667	www.umm.edu
University of Miami Hospital	Miami	Florida	305-325-5511	www.cedarsmedicalcenter.com
UPMC Mckeesport	Mc Keesport	Pennsylvania	412-664-2000	www.selectmedicalcorp.com
VA Pittsburgh Healthcare System	Pittsburgh	Pennsylvania	412-688-6100	www.pittsburg.va.gov
Valley West Community Hospital	Sandwich	Illinois	815-786-8484	www.snd.softfarm.com/sandhosp
Venice Regional Medical Center - Bayfront Health	Venice	Florida	941-485-7711	www.veniceregional.com
Viera Hospital	Melbourne	Florida	321-434-9000	www.health-first.org
Waupun Memorial Hospital	Waupun	Wisconsin	920-324-6530	www.agnesian.com
Wayne County Hospital	Monticello	Kentucky	606-348-9343	www.waynehospital.org
Weatherford Regional Medical Center	Weatherford	Texas	817-599-1190	www.campbellhealth.com
Wesley Medical Center	Wichita	Kansas	316-962-2000	www.wesleymc.com
West Palm Hospital	West Palm Beach	Florida	561-844-6141	www.columbiahospital.com
Western Pennsylvania Hospital	Pittsburgh	Pennsylvania	412-578-5000	www.wpahs.org/wph/contact/index.html
White County Medical Center	Searcy	Arkansas	501-278-3100	www.centralarkhospital.com
Wichita VA Medical Center	Wichita	Kansas	316-685-2221	www.wichita.va.gov
Wilcox Memorial Hospital	Lihue	Hawaii	808-245-1103	www.wilcoxhealth.org
William Beaumont Hospital - Troy	Troy	Michigan	248-964-8800	www.beaumonthospitals.com
Williamsport Regional Medical Center	Williamsport	Pennsylvania	570-321-1000	www.susquehannahealth.org
Woodward Regional Hospital	Woodward	Oklahoma	580-254-8492	www.woodwardhospital.com

Note: The 288 hospitals shown above all achieved a perfect 100% average score. Average scores were calculated for hospitals with qualifying data (25 cases or more) in both measures in the Pneumonia Care category. A total of 3,347 hospitals nationwide were considered.

Best Hospitals for Preventative Care

Hospital	City	State	Phone	Web Site
Abilene Regional Medical Center	Abilene	Texas	325-428-1000	www.abileneregional.com
Adena Regional Medical Center	Chillicothe	Ohio	740-779-7500	www.adena.org
Alton Memorial Hospital	Alton	Illinois	618-463-7300	www.altonmemorialhospital.org
Arizona Spine & Joint Hospital	Mesa	Arizona	480-832-4770	www.azspineandjoint.com
Atrium Medical Center	Franklin	Ohio	513-420-5102	www.atriummedcenter.org
Avera Heart Hospital of South Dakota	Sioux Falls	South Dakota	605-977-7000	www.avera.org/heart-hospital
Bailey Medical Center	Owasso	Oklahoma	918-376-8000	www.baileymedicalcenter.com
Baptist Hospital of Miami	Miami	Florida	786-596-1960	www.baptisthealth.net
Baptist Memorial Hospital Huntingdon	Huntingdon	Tennessee	731-986-4461	www.bmhcc.org
Barstow Community Hospital	Barstow	California	760-256-1761	www.barstowhospital.com
Belton Regional Medical Center	Belton	Missouri	816-348-1236	www.beltonregionalmedicalcenter.com
Biloxi Regional Medical Center	Biloxi	Mississippi	228-436-1104	www.hmabrmc.com
Broward Health North	Pompano Beach	Florida	954-786-6950	www.browardhealth.org
Byrd Regional Hospital	Leesville	Louisiana	337-239-9041	www.chs.net
Calhoun Health Services	Calhoun City	Mississippi	662-628-6611	www.nmhs.net
Carepoint Health - Bayonne Hospital Center	Bayonne	New Jersey	201-858-5000	www.bayonnemedicalcenter.org
Carrington Health Center	Carrington	North Dakota	701-652-3141	www.carringtonhealthcenter.net
Centerpoint Medical Center	Independence	Missouri	816-698-7000	www.centerpointmedical.com
Centinela Hospital Medical Center	Inglewood	California	310-673-4660	www.centinelafreeman.com
Central Mississippi Medical Center	Jackson	Mississippi	601-376-1000	www.centralmississippimedicalcenter.com
Chesterfield General Hospital	Cheraw	South Carolina	843-537-7881	www.chesterfieldgeneral.com
Clay County Hospital	Flora	Illinois	618-662-2131	www.claycountyhospital.org
Coosa Valley Medical Center	Sylacauga	Alabama	256-249-5000	www.cvhealth.net
Coral Gables Hospital	Coral Gables	Florida	305-445-8461	www.coralgableshospital.com
The Corpus Christi Medical Center	Corpus Christi	Texas	361-761-1501	www.ccmedicalcenter.com
Cypress Pointe Hospital East	Slidell	Louisiana	504-690-8200	
Delray Medical Center	Delray Beach	Florida	561-498-4440	www.delraymedicalctr.com
Detar Hospital Navarro	Victoria	Texas	361-575-7441	www.detar.com
Dyersburg Regional Medical Center	Dyersburg	Tennessee	731-285-2410	www.dyersburgregionalmc.com
Encino Hospital Medical Center	Encino	California	818-995-5000	www.encino-tarzana.com
Fannin Regional Hospital	Blue Ridge	Georgia	706-632-3711	www.fanninregionalhospital.com
Flowers Hospital	Dothan	Alabama	334-793-5000	www.flowershospital.com
Garden Grove Hospital & Medical Center	Garden Grove	California	714-537-5160	www.gardengrovehospital.com
Garden Park Medical Center	Gulfport	Mississippi	228-575-7000	www.gardenparkmedical.com
Greenbrier Valley Medical Center	Ronceverte	West Virginia	304-647-4411	www.gvmc.com
Hedrick Medical Center	Chillicothe	Missouri	660-646-1480	www.saintlukeshealthsystem.org
Helena Regional Medical Center	Helena	Arkansas	870-338-5800	www.helenaregionalmedicalcenter.com
Henderson County Community Hospital	Lexington	Tennessee	731-968-1801	www.hendersoncchospital.com
Henry County Memorial Hospital	New Castle	Indiana	765-521-0890	www.hcmhcares.org
Heritage Medical Center	Shelbyville	Tennessee	931-685-5433	www.heritagemedicalcenter.com
Highlands Regional Medical Center	Sebring	Florida	863-385-6101	www.highlandsregional.com
Holy Name Medical Center	Teaneck	New Jersey	201-833-3000	www.holyname.org
The Hospital at Westlake Medical Center	Austin	Texas	512-327-0000	www.westlakemedical.com
Huntington Beach Hospital	Huntington Beach	California	714-843-5000	www.hbhospital.com
Indiana University Health Blackford Hospital	Hartford City	Indiana	765-348-0300	www.accesschs.org
Ingalls Memorial Hospital	Harvey	Illinois	708-333-2300	www.ingalls.org
Integris Mayes County Medical Center	Pryor	Oklahoma	918-825-1600	www.integris-health.com
Jeff Davis Hospital	Hazlehurst	Georgia	912-375-7781	www.jeffdavishospital.org
JFK Medical Center	Atlantis	Florida	561-965-7300	www.jfkmc.com
John Randolph Medical Center	Hopewell	Virginia	804-541-1600	www.johnrandolphmed.com
Kansas Medical Center	Andover	Kansas	316-300-4000	www.ksmedcenter.com
Kentucky River Medical Center	Jackson	Kentucky	606-666-6000	www.kentuckyrivermc.com
L V Stabler Memorial Hospital	Greenville	Alabama	334-382-2200	www.lvstabler.com
Lafayette Regional Health Center	Lexington	Missouri	660-259-2203	www.lafayetteregionalhealthcenter.com
Lakeview Regional Medical Center	Covington	Louisiana	985-867-4443	www.lakeviewregional.com
Laredo Medical Center	Laredo	Texas	956-796-5000	www.laredomedical.com
Lawnwood Regional Medical Center & Heart Institute	Fort Pierce	Florida	772-461-4000	www.lawnwoodmed.com
Lehigh Regional Medical Center	Lehigh Acres	Florida	239-369-2101	www.lehighregional.com
Lehigh Valley Hospital - Hazleton	Hazleton	Pennsylvania	570-501-4000	www.ghha.org
Lewisgale Medical Center	Salem	Virginia	540-776-4000	www.lewis-gale.com
Livingston Regional Hospital	Livingston	Tennessee	931-823-5611	www.livingstonregionalhospital.com
Logan Regional Medical Center	Logan	West Virginia	304-831-1350	www.loganregionalmedicalcenter.com
McNairy Regional Hospital	Selmer	Tennessee	731-645-3221	www.mcnairyregionalhospital.com
Medical Center of Plano	Plano	Texas	972-596-6800	www.medicalcenterofplano.com
Medical Center of Southeastern Oklahoma	Durant	Oklahoma	405-924-3080	www.mcsohealth.com

Hospital	City	State	Phone	Web Site
Medical Center South Arkansas	El Dorado	Arkansas	870-863-2000	www.themedcenter.net
Memorial Hospital Los Banos	Los Banos	California	209-826-0591	www.memoriallosbanos.org
Memorial Hospital Pembroke	Pembroke Pines	Florida	954-962-9650	www.memorialpembroke.com\
Memorial Hospital West	Pembroke Pines	Florida	954-436-5000	www.memorialwest.com
Menorah Medical Center	Overland Park	Kansas	913-498-6773	www.menorahmedicalcenter.com
Methodist Stone Oak Hospital	San Antonio	Texas	210-638-2100	www.stoneoakhealth.com
Mills - Peninsula Medical Center	Burlingame	California	650-696-5270	www.mills-peninsula.org
Mimbres Memorial Hospital	Deming	New Mexico	575-546-5803	www.mimbresmemorial.com
Minden Medical Center	Minden	Louisiana	318-377-2321	www.mindenmedicalcenter.com
Moberly Regional Medical Center	Moberly	Missouri	660-263-8400	www.moberlyhospital.com
Mount Desert Island Hospital	Bar Harbor	Maine	207-288-5081	www.mdihospital.com
Mountain View Hospital	Idaho Falls	Idaho	208-557-2899	www.mountainviewhospital.org
Mountain View Regional Medical Center	Las Cruces	New Mexico	575-556-7600	www.mountainviewregional.com
Newberry County Memorial Hospital	Newberry	South Carolina	803-405-7145	www.newberryhospital.org
North Carolina Specialty Hospital	Durham	North Carolina	919-956-9300	www.ncspecialty.com
Northeast Regional Medical Center	Kirksville	Missouri	660-785-1000	www.nermc.com
Northern Louisiana Medical Center	Ruston	Louisiana	318-254-2100	www.lincolnhealth.com
Northern Maine Medical Center	Fort Kent	Maine	207-834-3195	www.nmmc.org
Ocala Regional Medical Center	Ocala	Florida	352-401-1000	www.ocalaregional.com
Oconee Regional Medical Center	Milledgeville	Georgia	478-454-3550	www.oconeeregional.com
Oklahoma Heart Hospital South	Oklahoma City	Oklahoma	405-628-6000	www.okheart.com/south-campus
Oklahoma Surgical Hospital	Tulsa	Oklahoma	918-477-5000	www.oklahomasurgicalhospital.com
Orange Park Medical Center	Orange Park	Florida	904-276-8500	www.opmedical.com
Palm Springs General Hospital	Hialeah	Florida	305-558-2500	www.psghosp.com
Pampa Regional Medical Center	Pampa	Texas	806-665-3721	www.prmctx.com
Parkway Regional Hospital	Fulton	Kentucky	270-472-2522	www.parkwayregionalhospital.com
Person Memorial Hospital	Roxboro	North Carolina	336-599-2121	www.personhospital.com
Ponca City Medical Center	Ponca City	Oklahoma	580-765-3321	www.poncamedcenter.com
Rapides Regional Medical Center	Alexandria	Louisiana	318-769-3000	www.rapidesregional.com
Raulerson Hospital	Okeechobee	Florida	863-763-2151	www.raulersonhospital.com
Regional Hospital of Jackson	Jackson	Tennessee	731-661-2000	www.regionalhospitaljackson.com
Regional Medical Center Bayonet Point	Hudson	Florida	727-819-2929	www.mchealth.comorwww.heartoftampa.com
The Regional Medical Center of Acadiana	Lafayette	Louisiana	337-981-2949	www.medicalcentersw.com
Renown South Meadows Medical Center	Reno	Nevada	775-982-7000	www.renown.org
Research Medical Center	Kansas City	Missouri	816-276-4000	www.researchmedicalcenter.com
Riverview Medical Center	Red Bank	New Jersey	732-741-2700	www.meridianhealth.com
Riverview Regional Medical Center	Gadsden	Alabama	256-543-5200	www.riverviewregional.com
Rolling Plains Memorial Hospital	Sweetwater	Texas	325-235-1701	www.rpmh.net
Rush University Medical Center	Chicago	Illinois	312-942-5000	www.ruch.edu
Russellville Hospital	Russellville	Alabama	256-332-1611	www.russellvillehospital.com
Saint Elizabeth Florence	Florence	Kentucky	859-212-5220	www.stlukehospitals.com
Saint Elizabeth Ft Thomas	Fort Thomas	Kentucky	859-572-3100	www.cardinalhill.org
Saint Elizabeth Grant	Williamstown	Kentucky	859-824-8240	www.stelizabeth.com
Saint Elizabeth Medical Center	Lakeside Park	Kentucky	859-292-2000	www.stelizabeth.com
Saint James Mercy Hospital	Hornell	New York	607-324-8000	www.stjamesmercy.org
Saint Joseph Hospital & Health Center	Kokomo	Indiana	765-456-5300	www.stvincent.org
Saint Luke's Miners Memorial Hospital	Coaldale	Pennsylvania	570-645-2131	www.slhn-lehighvalley.org
Saint Mary's Health Center	Jefferson City	Missouri	573-761-7000	www.stmarys-jeffcity.com
Sebastian River Medical Center	Sebastian	Florida	772-589-3187	www.srmcenter.com
Sherman Oaks Hospital	Sherman Oaks	California	818-981-7111	www.shermanoakshospital.com
Skagit Valley Hospital	Mount Vernon	Washington	360-424-4111	www.skagitvalleyhospital.org
Sonoma Developmental Center	Eldridge	California	707-938-6393	www.dds.ca.gov/sonoma/index.cfm
South Baldwin Regional Medical Center	Foley	Alabama	251-949-3400	www.southbaldwinrmc.com
South Bay Hospital	Sun City Center	Florida	813-634-3301	www.southbayhospital.com
Southwest General Hospital	San Antonio	Texas	210-921-2000	www.swgeneralhospital.com
Stones River Hospital & Dekalb Community Hospital	Smithville	Tennessee	615-215-5000	www.dekalb-hospital.com
Stormont - Vail Healthcare	Topeka	Kansas	785-354-6121	www.stormontvail.org
Temple Community Hospital	Los Angeles	California	213-382-7252	www.templecommunityhospital.com
Terre Haute Regional Hospital	Terre Haute	Indiana	812-232-0021	www.regionalhospital.com
Texas Health Harris Methodist Hospital Azle	Azle	Texas	817-444-8700	www.hmhs.org
Tomah Memorial Hospital	Tomah	Wisconsin	608-372-2181	www.tomahhospital.org
Trinity Hospital of Augusta	Augusta	Georgia	706-481-7000	www.trinityofaugusta.com
Trinity Medical Center	Birmingham	Alabama	205-592-1000	www.bhsala.com/montclair
Twin Cities Hospital	Niceville	Florida	850-678-4131	www.tchealthcare.com
Tyrone Hospital	Tyrone	Pennsylvania	814-684-1255	www.tyronehospital.org
UPMC East	Monroeville	Pennsylvania	412-357-3000	www.upmc.com
Valley West Community Hospital	Sandwich	Illinois	815-786-8484	www.snd.softfarm.com/sandhosp

Hospital	City	State	Phone	Web Site
Vaughan Regional Medical Center Parkway Campus	Selma	Alabama	334-418-4100	www.vaughanregional.com
Vista Medical Center East	Waukegan	Illinois	847-360-4000	www.vistahealth.com
Walker Baptist Medical Center	Jasper	Alabama	205-387-4000	www.bhsala.com/walker
Weatherford Regional Medical Center	Weatherford	Texas	817-599-1190	www.campbellhealth.com
West Anaheim Medical Center	Anaheim	California	714-827-3000	www.wamc.phcs.us
West Kendall Baptist Hospital	Miami	Florida	786-467-2011	www.baptisthealth.net
West Palm Hospital	West Palm Beach	Florida	561-844-6141	www.columbiahospital.com
West Virginia University Hospitals	Morgantown	West Virginia	304-598-4000	www.wvuh.com
Western Arizona Regional Medical Center	Bullhead City	Arizona	928-763-2273	www.warmc.com
Westside Regional Medical Center	Plantation	Florida	954-473-6600	www.westsidehospital.com
Woodland Heights Medical Center	Lufkin	Texas	936-634-8311	www.woodlandheights.net
Woodward Regional Hospital	Woodward	Oklahoma	580-254-8492	www.woodwardhospital.com

Note: The 144 hospitals shown above all achieved a perfect 100% average score. Average scores were calculated for hospitals with qualifying data (25 cases or more) in both measures in the Preventative Care category. A total of 3,674 hospitals nationwide were considered.

Best Hospitals for Stroke Care

Hospital	City	State	Phone	Web Site
Baptist Hospital of Miami	Miami	Florida	786-596-1960	www.baptisthealth.net
Bellevue Medical Center	Bellevue	Nebraska	402-763-3600	www.bellevuemed.com
Blanchard Valley Hospital	Findlay	Ohio	419-423-4500	www.bvha.org
Boca Raton Regional Hospital	Boca Raton	Florida	561-362-5002	www.brrh.com
Bronx - Lebanon Hospital Center	Bronx	New York	212-588-7000	www.bronx-leb.org
Brookdale Hospital Medical Center	Brooklyn	New York	718-240-5966	www.brookdalehospital.org
Cabell Huntington Hospital	Huntington	West Virginia	304-526-2000	www.cabellhuntington.org
Capital Health Medical Center - Hopewell	Pennington	New Jersey	609-303-4000	www.capitalhealth.org
Capital Regional Medical Center	Tallahassee	Florida	850-656-5000	www.capitalregionalmedicalcenter.com
Caromont Regional Medical Center	Gastonia	North Carolina	704-834-4891	www.caromont.org
Catawba Valley Medical Center	Hickory	North Carolina	828-326-3809	www.catawbavalleymc.org
Central Carolina Hospital	Sanford	North Carolina	919-774-2100	www.centralcarolinahosp.com
Cjw Medical Center	Richmond	Virginia	804-330-2001	www.hcavirginia.com
Cleveland Clinic Hospital	Weston	Florida	954-689-5000	www.clevelandclinic.org
Cox Medical Center Branson	Branson	Missouri	417-335-7000	www.skaggs.net
Delray Medical Center	Delray Beach	Florida	561-498-4440	www.delraymedicalctr.com
Detar Hospital Navarro	Victoria	Texas	361-575-7441	www.detar.com
Doctors Hospital	Augusta	Georgia	706-651-6008	www.doctors-hospital.net
Falmouth Hospital	Falmouth	Massachusetts	508-548-5300	www.capecodhealth.com
Fawcett Memorial Hospital	Port Charlotte	Florida	941-629-1181	www.fawcetthospital.com
Forest Hills Hospital	Forest Hills	New York	718-830-4000	www.northshorelij.com
Fort Walton Beach Medical Center	Fort Walton Beach	Florida	850-862-1111	www.fwbmedicalcenter.com
Good Samaritan Hospital Medical Center	West Islip	New York	631-376-3000	www.good-samaritan-hospital.org
Grant Medical Center	Columbus	Ohio	614-566-9978	www.ohiohealth.com
Heartland Regional Medical Center	Saint Joseph	Missouri	816-271-6000	www.heartland-health.com
Holland Community Hospital	Holland	Michigan	616-392-5141	www.hoho.org
Homestead Hospital	Homestead	Florida	786-243-8000	www.baptisthealth.net
John Randolph Medical Center	Hopewell	Virginia	804-541-1600	www.johnrandolphmed.com
Kaiser Foundation Hospital - Redwood City	Redwood City	California	650-299-2000	www.seiu-uhw.org/aboutuhw
Kaiser Foundation Hospital - San Diego	San Diego	California	619-528-5000	www.members.kaiserpermanente.org
Kaiser Foundation Hospital - South Bay	Harbor City	California	310-517-6441	www.kaiserpermanente.org
Kaiser Foundation Hospital - South San Francisco	South San Francisco	California	650-742-3200	www.healthy.kaiserpermanente.org
Lake Pointe Medical Center	Rowlett	Texas	972-412-2273	www.lakepointemedical.com
Lakeview Regional Medical Center	Covington	Louisiana	985-867-4443	www.lakeviewregional.com
Lawnwood Regional Medical Center & Heart Institute	Fort Pierce	Florida	772-461-4000	www.lawnwoodmed.com
Lewisgale Medical Center	Salem	Virginia	540-776-4000	www.lewis-gale.com
Libertyhealth - Jersey City Medical Center Campus	Jersey City	New Jersey	201-915-2000	www.libertyhcs.org
Los Alamitos Medical Center	Los Alamitos	California	562-799-3220	www.losalamitosmedctr.com
Lovelace Medical Center	Albuquerque	New Mexico	505-727-8000	www.lovelace.com
Main Line Hospital Paoli	Paoli	Pennsylvania	610-648-1000	www.mainlinehealth.org
Marshall Medical Center	Placerville	California	530-622-1441	www.marshallmedical.org
Mary Immaculate Hospital	Newport News	Virginia	757-886-6000	www.bonsecourshamptonroad.com
Maui Memorial Medical Center	Wailuku	Hawaii	808-442-5101	www.mauimemorialmedical.org
Memorial Hospital Pembroke	Pembroke Pines	Florida	954-962-9650	www.memorialpembroke.com\
Memorial Hospital West	Pembroke Pines	Florida	954-436-5000	www.memorialwest.com
Mercy Hospital	Bakersfield	California	661-632-5000	www.mercybakersfield.org
Methodist Dallas Medical Center	Dallas	Texas	214-947-2879	www.mhd.com
Methodist Hospital of Southern California	Arcadia	California	626-445-4441	www.methodisthospital.org
Methodist Mansfield Medical Center	Mansfield	Texas	682-622-2059	www.methodisthealthsystem.com
Methodist Medical Center of Oak Ridge	Oak Ridge	Tennessee	865-835-1000	www.mmcoakridge.com
Methodist Richardson Medical Center	Richardson	Texas	972-498-4000	www.richardsonregional.com
Methodist Stone Oak Hospital	San Antonio	Texas	210-638-2100	www.stoneoakhealth.com
Metroplex Hospital	Killeen	Texas	254-526-7523	www.mplex.org
Mills - Peninsula Medical Center	Burlingame	California	650-696-5270	www.mills-peninsula.org
Monmouth Medical Center - Southern Campus	Lakewood	New Jersey	732-363-1900	www.sbhcs.com
Morristown Hamblen Hospital Association	Morristown	Tennessee	423-586-4231	www.mhhs1.org
Newton - Wellesley Hospital	Newton	Massachusetts	617-243-6000	www.nwh.org
North Austin Medical Center	Austin	Texas	512-901-1000	www.cornerstonehealthcaregroup.com
North Cypress Medical Center	Cypress	Texas	281-890-0203	www.ncmc-hospital.com
North Hills Hospital	North Richland Hills	Texas	817-255-1000	www.northhillshospital.com
Northside Hospital	Saint Petersburg	Florida	813-521-5000	www.northsidehospital.com
Northwest Community Hospital	Arlington Heights	Illinois	847-618-1000	www.nch.org
Novant Health Forsyth Medical Center	Winston-Salem	North Carolina	336-718-5000	www.forsythmedicalcenter.org
Novant Health Thomasville Medical Center	Thomasville	North Carolina	336-472-2000	www.thomasvillemedicalcenter.org
Oak Hill Hospital	Brooksville	Florida	352-596-6632	www.oakhillhospital.com

Hospital	City	State	Phone	Web Site
Pali Momi Medical Center	Aiea	Hawaii	808-486-6000	www.kapiolani.org
Palms of Pasadena Hospital	Saint Petersburg	Florida	727-381-1000	www.palmspasadena.com
Pikeville Medical Center	Pikeville	Kentucky	606-218-3500	www.pikevillehospital.org
Portsmouth Regional Hospital	Portsmouth	New Hampshire	603-436-5110	www.portsmouthhospital.com
Presence Saints Mary & Elizabeth Medical Center	Chicago	Illinois	312-770-2000	www.reshealth.org
Reston Hospital Center	Reston	Virginia	703-689-9000	www.restonhospital.com
Richmond University Medical Center	Staten Island	New York	718-818-1234	www.rumcsi.org
Saint Catherine of Siena Hospital	Smithtown	New York	631-862-3000	www.stcatherines.chsli.org
Saint Clair Memorial Hospital	Pittsburgh	Pennsylvania	412-942-6209	www.stclair.org
Saint Joseph Medical Center	Kansas City	Missouri	816-942-4000	www.stjosehkc.com
Saint Mary's Medical Center	San Francisco	California	415-668-1000	www.stmarysmedicalcenter.org
Salinas Valley Memorial Hospital	Salinas	California	831-757-4333	www.svmh.com
San Gabriel Valley Medical Center	San Gabriel	California	626-289-5454	www.sangabrielvalleymedctr.org
San Ramon Regional Medical Center	San Ramon	California	925-275-9200	www.sanramonmedctr.com
Scripps Memorial Hospital La Jolla	La Jolla	California	858-626-4123	www.scrippshealth.org
Sebastian River Medical Center	Sebastian	Florida	772-589-3187	www.srmcenter.com
Shasta Regional Medical Center	Redding	California	530-244-5454	www.shastaregional.com
Sherman Hospital	Elgin	Illinois	847-742-9800	www.shermanhealth.com
Sierra Nevada Memorial Hospital	Grass Valley	California	530-274-6000	www.snmh.org
South Baldwin Regional Medical Center	Foley	Alabama	251-949-3400	www.southbaldwinrmc.com
South Bay Hospital	Sun City Center	Florida	813-634-3301	www.southbayhospital.com
South Miami Hospital	South Miami	Florida	786-662-4000	www.baptisthealth.net
South Pointe Hospital	Warrensville Heights	Ohio	216-491-6000	www.southpointehospital.org
Southern Nh Medical Center	Nashua	New Hampshire	603-577-2000	www.snhmc.org
Sparks Regional Medical Center	Fort Smith	Arkansas	501-441-4000	www.sparks.org
Springs Memorial Hospital	Lancaster	South Carolina	803-286-1481	www.springsmemorial.com
Sunrise Hospital & Medical Center	Las Vegas	Nevada	702-731-8000	www.sunrisehospital.com
Sutter Auburn Faith Hospital	Auburn	California	530-888-4500	www.sutterauburnfaith.org
Temple Community Hospital	Los Angeles	California	213-382-7252	www.templecommunityhospital.com
Texas Health Harris Methodist Hurst - Euless - Bedford	Bedford	Texas	817-848-4000	www.texashealth.org
Texas Health Presbyterian Hospital Plano	Plano	Texas	972-981-8000	www.presbyplano.org
Texoma Medical Center	Denison	Texas	903-416-4000	www.texomamedicalcenter.net
Thibodaux Regional Medical Center	Thibodaux	Louisiana	985-447-5500	www.thibodaux.com
Trinity Medical Center	Birmingham	Alabama	205-592-1000	www.bhsala.com/montclair
University Hospitals Case Medical Center	Cleveland	Ohio	216-844-1000	www.uhhs.com
University of Kentucky Hospital	Lexington	Kentucky	859-323-5000	www.uhealthcare.uky.edu
UPMC East	Monroeville	Pennsylvania	412-357-3000	www.upmc.com
Vaughan Regional Medical Center Parkway Campus	Selma	Alabama	334-418-4100	www.vaughanregional.com
Vista Medical Center East	Waukegan	Illinois	847-360-4000	www.vistahealth.com
Wellmont Bristol Regional Medical Center	Bristol	Tennessee	423-844-1121	www.wellmont.org
Wesley Medical Center	Wichita	Kansas	316-962-2000	www.wesleymc.com
West Florida Hospital	Pensacola	Florida	850-494-4000	www.westfloridahospital.com
West Houston Medical Center	Houston	Texas	281-588-8080	www.westhoustonmedical.com
Wilcox Memorial Hospital	Lihue	Hawaii	808-245-1103	www.wilcoxhealth.org

Note: The hospitals shown above represent the top 5% of the 1,762 hospitals nationwide for which an average score was calculated. Average scores were calculated for hospitals with qualifying data (25 cases or more) in at least 6 of 11 measures in the Stroke Care category.

Best Hospitals for Surgical Care

Hospital	City	State	Phone	Web Site
Arizona Orthopedic & Surgical Speciality Hospital	Chandler	Arizona	480-603-9000	www.azosh.com
Avera Queen of Peace	Mitchell	South Dakota	605-995-2000	www.averaqueenofpeace.org
Baptist Health Corbin	Corbin	Kentucky	606-528-1212	www.baptistregional.com
Baptist Memorial Hospital Union City	Union City	Tennessee	731-885-2410	www.bmhcc.org
Baptist Memorial Hospital Union County	New Albany	Mississippi	662-538-7631	www.baptistonline.org
Baylor Medical Center at Uptown	Dallas	Texas	214-443-3000	www.bmcuptown.com
Baylor Regional Medical Center at Plano	Plano	Texas	469-814-2000	www.baylorhealth.com
Belton Regional Medical Center	Belton	Missouri	816-348-1236	www.beltonregionalmedicalcenter.com
Boca Raton Regional Hospital	Boca Raton	Florida	561-362-5002	www.brrh.com
Broward Health Coral Springs	Coral Springs	Florida	954-344-3000	www.coralspringsmedicalcenter.org
Broward Health Imperial Point	Fort Lauderdale	Florida	954-776-8500	www.nbhd.org
Broward Health Medical Center	Fort Lauderdale	Florida	954-355-4400	www.browardhealth.org
Carolinas Medical Center - Pineville	Charlotte	North Carolina	704-379-5000	www.carolinashealthcare.org
Caromont Regional Medical Center	Gastonia	North Carolina	704-834-4891	www.caromont.org
Dauterive Hospital	New Iberia	Louisiana	337-365-7311	www.dauterivehospital.com
Doctors Hospital	Augusta	Georgia	706-651-6008	www.doctors-hospital.net
Dupont Hospital	Fort Wayne	Indiana	260-416-3000	www.theduponthospital.com
East Alabama Medical Center	Opelika	Alabama	334-749-3411	www.eamc.org
Englewood Community Hospital	Englewood	Florida	941-475-6571	www.englewoodcommunityhospital.com
Exempla Good Samaritan Medical Center	Lafayette	Colorado	303-689-4000	www.exempla.org
Fairview Park Hospital	Dublin	Georgia	478-274-3100	www.fairviewparkhospital.com
Fannin Regional Hospital	Blue Ridge	Georgia	706-632-3711	www.fanninregionalhospital.com
Flowers Hospital	Dothan	Alabama	334-793-5000	www.flowershospital.com
Fort Walton Beach Medical Center	Fort Walton Beach	Florida	850-862-1111	www.fwbmedicalcenter.com
Garden Park Medical Center	Gulfport	Mississippi	228-575-7000	www.gardenparkmedical.com
GHS Patewood Memorial Hospital	Greenville	South Carolina	864-797-1000	www.ghs.org
Holland Community Hospital	Holland	Michigan	616-392-5141	www.hoho.org
Ingalls Memorial Hospital	Harvey	Illinois	708-333-2300	www.ingalls.org
Institute For Orthopaedic Surgery	Lima	Ohio	419-224-7586	www.ioshospital.com
Jefferson Regional Medical Center	Pine Bluff	Arkansas	870-541-7100	www.jrmc.org
JFK Medical Center	Atlantis	Florida	561-965-7300	www.jfkmc.com
Jupiter Medical Center	Jupiter	Florida	561-747-2234	www.jupitermed.com
Kansas Medical Center	Andover	Kansas	316-300-4000	www.ksmedcenter.com
Lake City Medical Center	Lake City	Florida	386-719-9000	www.lakecitymedical.com
Lawnwood Regional Medical Center & Heart Institute	Fort Pierce	Florida	772-461-4000	www.lawnwoodmed.com
Lee's Summit Medical Center	Lees Summit	Missouri	816-282-5000	www.leessummithospital.com
Lewisgale Hospital Montgomery	Blacksburg	Virginia	540-951-1111	www.mrhospital.com
Magee Womens Hospital of UPMC Health System	Pittsburgh	Pennsylvania	412-641-4010	www.magee.edu
Margaret R Pardee Memorial Hospital	Hendersonville	North Carolina	828-696-1000	www.pardeehospital.org
Marion General Hospital	Marion	Ohio	740-383-8400	www.mariongeneral.com
Mary Greeley Medical Center	Ames	Iowa	515-239-2011	www.mgmc.org
McKenzie - Willamette Medical Center	Springfield	Oregon	541-726-4400	www.mckweb.com
Medical Center Enterprise	Enterprise	Alabama	334-347-0584	www.mcehospital.com
Memorial Hospital Pembroke	Pembroke Pines	Florida	954-962-9650	www.memorialpembroke.com\
Memorial Hospital West	Pembroke Pines	Florida	954-436-5000	www.memorialwest.com
Memorial Regional Hospital	Hollywood	Florida	954-987-2000	www.memorialregional.com
Mercy Medical Center	Roseburg	Oregon	541-673-0611	www.mercyrose.org
Methodist Dallas Medical Center	Dallas	Texas	214-947-2879	www.mhd.com
Methodist Mansfield Medical Center	Mansfield	Texas	682-622-2059	www.methodisthealthsystem.com
Mountain View Regional Medical Center	Las Cruces	New Mexico	575-556-7600	www.mountainviewregional.com
Mountainview Hospital	Las Vegas	Nevada	702-255-5065	www.mountainview-hospital.com
North Carolina Specialty Hospital	Durham	North Carolina	919-956-9300	www.ncspecialty.com
North Central Surgical Center	Dallas	Texas	214-265-2810	www.northcentral-sc.com
North Florida Regional Medical Center	Gainesville	Florida	352-333-4100	www.nfrmc.com
North Mississippi Medical Center	Tupelo	Mississippi	662-377-3000	www.nmhs.net/nmmc
North Suburban Medical Center	Thornton	Colorado	303-451-7800	www.northsuburban.com
Northern Westchester Hospital	Mount Kisco	New York	914-666-1200	www.nwhc.net
Northside Hospital	Atlanta	Georgia	404-851-8000	www.northside.com
Northside Hospital Cherokee	Canton	Georgia	770-720-5298	www.northside.com/cherokee
Northside Hospital Forsyth	Cumming	Georgia	404-851-8700	www.gbhcs.org
Northwest Medical Center	Margate	Florida	954-974-0400	www.northwestmed.com
Novant Health Charlotte Orthopedic Hospital	Charlotte	North Carolina	704-316-2000	www.presbyterian.org
Novant Health Forsyth Medical Center	Winston-Salem	North Carolina	336-718-5000	www.forsythmedicalcenter.org
Novant Health Park Hospital	Winston-Salem	North Carolina	336-718-0600	www.novanthealth.org
Novant Health Rowan Medical Center	Salisbury	North Carolina	704-210-5000	www.rowan.org

Hospital	City	State	Phone	Web Site
Ocala Regional Medical Center	Ocala	Florida	352-401-1000	www.ocalaregional.com
Oklahoma Surgical Hospital	Tulsa	Oklahoma	918-477-5000	www.oklahomasurgicalhospital.com
Orange Park Medical Center	Orange Park	Florida	904-276-8500	www.opmedical.com
The Orthopaedic Hospital of Lutheran Health Network	Fort Wayne	Indiana	260-435-2999	www.lutheranhealth.net
Orthopaedic Hospital of Wisconsin	Glendale	Wisconsin	414-961-6800	www.ohow.org
Oss Orthopaedic Hospital	York	Pennsylvania	717-718-2000	www.osshealth.com
Pinnacle Health Hospitals	Harrisburg	Pennsylvania	717-782-5181	www.pinnaclehealth.org
Portsmouth Regional Hospital	Portsmouth	New Hampshire	603-436-5110	www.portsmouthhospital.com
Quail Creek Surgical Hospital	Amarillo	Texas	806-354-6100	www.physurg.com
Rapides Regional Medical Center	Alexandria	Louisiana	318-769-3000	www.rapidesregional.com
Raulerson Hospital	Okeechobee	Florida	863-763-2151	www.raulersonhospital.com
Regional Hospital of Jackson	Jackson	Tennessee	731-661-2000	www.regionalhospitaljackson.com
The Regional Medical Center of Acadiana	Lafayette	Louisiana	337-981-2949	www.medicalcentersw.com
Renown South Meadows Medical Center	Reno	Nevada	775-982-7000	www.renown.org
Reston Hospital Center	Reston	Virginia	703-689-9000	www.restonhospital.com
River Oaks Hospital	Flowood	Mississippi	601-936-2390	www.riveroakshospital.org
Rose Medical Center	Denver	Colorado	303-320-2121	www.rosemed.com
Saint Anthony's Health Center	Alton	Illinois	618-465-2571	www.sahc.org
Saint Charles Hospital	Port Jefferson	New York	631-474-6000	www.stcharles.org
Saint Elizabeth Florence	Florence	Kentucky	859-212-5220	www.stlukehospitals.com
Saint Elizabeth Medical Center	Lakeside Park	Kentucky	859-292-2000	www.stelizabeth.com
Saint Francis Regional Medical Center	Shakopee	Minnesota	952-403-3000	www.stfrancis-shakopee.com
Saint Lucie Medical Center	Port Saint Lucie	Florida	772-335-4000	www.stluciemed.com
Saint Luke's Lakeside Hospital	The Woodlands	Texas	936-266-4055	www.stlukeslakeside.com
Saint Luke's South Hospital	Overland Park	Kansas	913-317-7904	www.saintlukeshealthsystem.org
Saint Mary Medical Center	Hobart	Indiana	219-942-0551	www.comhs.org/stmary
Saint Vincent Healthcare	Billings	Montana	406-657-7000	www.svh-mt.org
Saint Vincent's Medical Center Southside	Jacksonville	Florida	904-296-3700	www.jaxhealth.com
San Angelo Community Medical Center	San Angelo	Texas	325-949-9511	www.sacmc.com
Scripps Green Hospital	La Jolla	California	858-554-3600	www.scrippshealth.org
Scripps Memorial Hospital - Encinitas	Encinitas	California	760-753-6501	www.scripps.org
Sebastian River Medical Center	Sebastian	Florida	772-589-3187	www.srmcenter.com
South Baldwin Regional Medical Center	Foley	Alabama	251-949-3400	www.southbaldwinrmc.com
South Miami Hospital	South Miami	Florida	786-662-4000	www.baptisthealth.net
South Nassau Communities Hospital	Oceanside	New York	516-632-3000	www.southnassau.org
Sparks Regional Medical Center	Fort Smith	Arkansas	501-441-4000	www.sparks.org
Springs Memorial Hospital	Lancaster	South Carolina	803-286-1481	www.springsmemorial.com
Strong Memorial Hospital	Rochester	New York	585-275-2121	www.urmc.rochester.edu
Tanner Medical Center - Carrollton	Carrollton	Georgia	770-836-9580	www.tanner.org
Texas Health Harris Methodist Hospital Southlake	Southlake	Texas	817-748-8700	www.texashealthsouthlake.com
Texas Orthopedic Hospital	Houston	Texas	713-799-8600	www.texasorthopedic.com
Trinity Medical Center	Birmingham	Alabama	205-592-1000	www.bhsala.com/montclair
Twin Cities Hospital	Niceville	Florida	850-678-4131	www.tchealthcare.com
UH Geauga Medical Center	Chardon	Ohio	440-269-6000	www.uhgeauga.org
UPMC East	Monroeville	Pennsylvania	412-357-3000	www.upmc.com
Venice Regional Medical Center - Bayfront Health	Venice	Florida	941-485-7711	www.veniceregional.com
Walker Baptist Medical Center	Jasper	Alabama	205-387-4000	www.bhsala.com/walker
West Florida Hospital	Pensacola	Florida	850-494-4000	www.westfloridahospital.com
West Georgia Medical Center	Lagrange	Georgia	706-882-1411	www.wghealth.org
West Kendall Baptist Hospital	Miami	Florida	786-467-2011	www.baptisthealth.net
West Palm Hospital	West Palm Beach	Florida	561-844-6141	www.columbiahospital.com

Note: The hospitals shown above represent the top 5% of the 2,338 hospitals nationwide for which an average score was calculated. Average scores were calculated for hospitals with qualifying data (25 cases or more) in at least 9 of 10 measures in the Surgical Care Improvment Project category.

Best Hospitals in Terms of Patient's Hospital Experiences

Hospital	City	State	Phone	Web Site
Abbeville Area Medical Center	Abbeville	South Carolina	864-366-5011	www.abbevilleareamc.com
Advanced Surgical Hospital	Washington	Pennsylvania	724-884-0710	www.ashospital.net
Animas Surgical Hospital	Durango	Colorado	970-247-3537	www.animassorgical.com
Arizona Orthopedic & Surgical Speciality Hospital	Chandler	Arizona	480-603-9000	www.azosh.com
Arkansas Heart Hospital	Little Rock	Arkansas	501-219-7000	www.arheart.com
Arkansas Surgical Hospital	No Little Rock	Arkansas	501-748-8000	www.arksurgicalhospital.com
Avera Heart Hospital of South Dakota	Sioux Falls	South Dakota	605-977-7000	www.avera.org/heart-hospital
Avera Saint Anthony's Hospital	O' Neill	Nebraska	402-336-2611	www.avera-sta.org
Baptist Emergency Hospital	San Antonio	Texas	210-402-4092	www.baptistemergencyhospital.com
Barton County Memorial Hospital	Lamar	Missouri	417-682-6081	www.bcmh.net
Baylor Heart & Vascular Hospital	Dallas	Texas	214-820-0670	www.baylorhearthospital.com
Baylor Medical Center at Frisco	Frisco	Texas	214-618-2000	www.bmcf.com
Baylor Medical Center at Trophy Club	Trophy Club	Texas	817-837-4600	www.tc-mc.com
Baylor Medical Center at Uptown	Dallas	Texas	214-443-3000	www.bmcuptown.com
Baylor Orthopedic & Spine Hospital at Arlington	Arlington	Texas	817-549-2364	www.baylorarlington.com
Baylor Surgical Hospital at Las Colinas	Irving	Texas	972-868-4000	www.ic-sh.com
Bear River Valley Hospital	Tremonton	Utah	435-207-4708	www.intermountainhealthcare.org
Bigfork Valley Hospital	Bigfork	Minnesota	218-743-3177	www.bigforkvalley.org
Black Hills Surgical Hospital	Rapid City	South Dakota	605-721-4700	www.bhsh.com
Black River Memorial Hospital	Black River Falls	Wisconsin	715-284-5361	www.brmh.net
Blue Hill Memorial Hospital	Blue Hill	Maine	207-374-2836	www.bhmh.org/default.html
Bluffton Hospital	Bluffton	Ohio	419-358-9010	www.bvhealthsystem.org
Boone County Health Center	Albion	Nebraska	402-395-2191	www.boonecohealth.org
Brodstone Memorial Hospital	Superior	Nebraska	402-879-3281	www.brodstonehospital.org
Bucks County Specialty Hospital	Bensalem	Pennsylvania	215-244-7400	www.bcshospital.com
Caldwell Memorial Hospital	Columbia	Louisiana	318-649-6111	
Central Louisiana Surgical Hospital	Alexandria	Louisiana	318-449-6400	www.clshospital.com
Chickasaw Nation Medical Center	Ada	Oklahoma	580-436-3980	www.chickasaw.net
Choctaw Nation Healthcare	Talihina	Oklahoma	918-567-7000	www.choctawnationhealth.com
Citizens Medical Center	Columbia	Louisiana	318-649-6106	www.citizensmedcenter.com
Clinton County Hospital	Albany	Kentucky	606-387-6421	www.clintoncountyhospital.com
Columbia Center	Mequon	Wisconsin	262-243-7408	www.columbiacenter.org
Community Hospital	Torrington	Wyoming	307-532-4181	www.bannerhealth.com
Community Medical Center	Falls City	Nebraska	402-245-2428	www.hhs.state.ne.us/index.htm
Community Memorial Hospital	Hicksville	Ohio	419-542-6692	www.cmhosp.com
Coordinated Health Orthopedic Hospital	Bethlehem	Pennsylvania	610-691-4300	www.coordinatedhealth.com
Cypress Pointe Surgical Hospital	Hammond	Louisiana	985-510-6200	www.cpsh.org
Dakota Plains Surgical Center	Aberdeen	South Dakota	605-225-3300	www.orthopediccenterofthedakotas.com
Doctors Hospital at Deer Creek	Leesville	Louisiana	337-392-5088	www.dhdc.md
East Texas Medical Center - Gilmer	Gilmer	Texas	903-841-7100	www.etmc.org
East Texas Medical Center Pittsburg	Pittsburg	Texas	903-856-4520	www.etmc.org
Electra Memorial Hospital	Electra	Texas	940-495-3981	www.electrahospital.com
Fairview Hospital	Great Barrington	Massachusetts	413-528-0790	www.berkshirehealthsystems.com
Fairway Medical Center	Covington	Louisiana	985-801-3010	www.fairwaymedical.com
Fayette Medical Center	Fayette	Alabama	205-932-5966	www.dchsystem.com
First Care Health Center	Park River	North Dakota	701-284-7500	www.firstcarehc.com
Floyd County Memorial Hospital	Charles City	Iowa	641-228-6830	www.fcmc.us.com
Fostoria Community Hospital	Fostoria	Ohio	419-435-7734	www.promedica.org
Foundation Surgical Hospital of San Antonio	San Antonio	Texas	210-478-5400	www.fshsanantonio.com
Fresno Surgical Hospital	Fresno	California	559-431-8000	www.fresnosurgerycenter.com
GHS Patewood Memorial Hospital	Greenville	South Carolina	864-797-1000	www.ghs.org
Glacial Ridge Hospital	Glenwood	Minnesota	320-634-2208	www.glacialridge.org
Grant Regional Health Center	Lancaster	Wisconsin	608-723-2143	www.grantregional.com
Great Falls Clinic Medical Center	Great Falls	Montana	406-216-8000	www.gfclinic.com
Green Clinic Surgical Hospital	Ruston	Louisiana	318-232-7700	www.green-clinic.com
Grundy County Memorial Hospital	Grundy Center	Iowa	319-824-5421	www.grundyhospital.com
H B Magruder Memorial Hospital	Port Clinton	Ohio	419-734-3131	www.magruderhospital.com
Heart Hospital Baylor Plano	Plano	Texas	469-814-3278	www.thehearthospitalbaylor.com
Heart Hospital of Lafayette	Lafayette	Louisiana	337-521-1000	www.hearthospitaloflafayette.com
Heritage Park Surgical Hospital	Sherman	Texas	903-813-3728	www.heritageparksurgicalhospital.com
Hill Country Memorial Hospital	Fredericksburg	Texas	830-997-4353	www.hcmbs.org
Hillsboro Area Hospital	Hillsboro	Illinois	217-532-6111	www.hillsboroareahospital.org
Hoag Orthopedic Institute	Irvine	California	949-727-5000	www.orthopedichospital.com
Houston Orthopedic & Spine Hospital	Bellaire	Texas	713-622-2262	www.foundationsurgicalhospital.com
Houston Physicians' Hospital	Webster	Texas	281-335-1700	www.houstonphysicianshospital.com

Hospital	City	State	Phone	Web Site
Indiana Orthopaedic Hospital	Indianapolis	Indiana	317-956-1000	www.indianaorthopaedichospital.com
Institute For Orthopaedic Surgery	Lima	Ohio	419-224-7586	www.ioshospital.com
Integris Health Edmond	Edmond	Oklahoma	405-657-3000	www.integrisok.com/integris-health-edmond-ok
Jefferson County Health Center	Fairfield	Iowa	641-472-4111	www.jchospital.org
Kansas City Orthopaedic Institute	Leawood	Kansas	913-319-7633	www.kcoi.com
Kentuckiana Medical Center	Clarksville	Indiana	812-280-3300	www.kentuckianamedcen.com
King's Daughters Medical Center - Brookhaven	Brookhaven	Mississippi	601-833-6011	www.kdmc.org
Lady of the Sea General Hospital	Cut Off	Louisiana	985-632-6401	www.losgh.org
Lafayette Surgical Specialty Hospital	Lafayette	Louisiana	337-769-4100	www.lafayettesurgical.com
Lakeview Memorial Hospital	Stillwater	Minnesota	651-439-5330	www.lakeview.org
Lawrence County Hospital	Monticello	Mississippi	601-587-4051	www.smrmc.com/index.php
Lincoln Surgical Hospital	Lincoln	Nebraska	402-484-9090	www.lincolnsurgery.com
Mackinac Straits Hospital & Health Center	Saint Ignace	Michigan	906-643-8585	www.mackinacstraitshealth.org
Manhattan Surgical Hospital	Manhattan	Kansas	785-776-5100	www.manhattansurgical.com
Mariners Hospital	Tavernier	Florida	305-434-3000	www.baptisthealth.net
Marion Regional Medical Center	Hamilton	Alabama	205-921-6200	www.nmhs.net
Mayo Clinic Hospital	Phoenix	Arizona	480-342-2000	www.mayoclinic.org
McBride Clinic Orthopedic Hospital	Oklahoma City	Oklahoma	405-478-1717	www.mcbrideclinic.com
Menlo Park Surgical Hospital	Menlo Park	California	650-324-8500	www.pamf.org/mpsh
Mercy Willard Hospital	Willard	Ohio	419-964-5000	www.mercyweb.org/mercy_willard.aspx
Miami County Medical Center	Paola	Kansas	913-557-4385	www.olathehealth.org
Mid - Valley Hospital	Peckville	Pennsylvania	570-383-5000	
Midwest Orthopedic Specialty Hospital	Franklin	Wisconsin	414-817-5800	www.mymosh.com
Midwest Surgical Hospital	Omaha	Nebraska	402-399-1900	www.mwsurgicalhospital.com
Millinocket Regional Hospital	Millinocket	Maine	207-723-5161	www.mrhme.org
Ministry Door County Medical Center	Sturgeon Bay	Wisconsin	920-743-5566	www.doorcountymemorial.org
Mount Carmel New Albany Surgical Hospital	New Albany	Ohio	614-775-6600	www.mountcarmelhealth.com
Mount Desert Island Hospital	Bar Harbor	Maine	207-288-5081	www.mdihospital.com
Mountain View Regional Hospital	Casper	Wyoming	307-995-8100	www.monroehospital.com
Nebraska Orthopaedic Hospital	Omaha	Nebraska	402-609-1600	www.neorthohospital.com
The Neuromedical Center Hospital	Baton Rouge	Louisiana	225-763-9900	www.theneuromedicalcenter.com
North Carolina Specialty Hospital	Durham	North Carolina	919-956-9300	www.ncspecialty.com
North Central Surgical Center	Dallas	Texas	214-265-2810	www.northcentral-sc.com
Northside Medical Center	Columbus	Georgia	706-494-2100	www.hughstonsports.com
Northwest Hills Surgical Hospital	Austin	Texas	512-346-1994	www.scasurgery.com
Northwest Specialty Hospital	Post Falls	Idaho	208-262-2300	www.northwestspecialtyhospital.com
Northwest Surgical Hospital	Oklahoma City	Oklahoma	404-848-1918	www.nwsurgicalokc.com
Oak Leaf Surgical Hospital	Eau Claire	Wisconsin	715-831-8130	www.oakleafsurgical.com
Ogallala Community Hospital	Ogallala	Nebraska	308-284-4011	www.bannerhealth.com
Oklahoma Center for Orthopaedic & Multi-Spec	Oklahoma City	Oklahoma	405-602-6500	www.ocomhospital.com
Oklahoma Heart Hospital	Oklahoma City	Oklahoma	405-608-3200	www.okheart.com
Oklahoma Heart Hospital South	Oklahoma City	Oklahoma	405-628-6000	www.okheart.com/south-campus
Oklahoma Spine Hospital	Oklahoma City	Oklahoma	405-749-2700	www.oklahomaspine.com
Oklahoma Surgical Hospital	Tulsa	Oklahoma	918-477-5000	www.oklahomasurgicalhospital.com
Orange City Area Health System	Orange City	Iowa	712-737-4984	www.ochealthsystem.org
Orthopaedic Hospital of Wisconsin	Glendale	Wisconsin	414-961-6800	www.ohow.org
OSF Holy Family Medical Center	Monmouth	Illinois	309-734-3141	www.cmchospital.com
Oss Orthopaedic Hospital	York	Pennsylvania	717-718-2000	www.osshealth.com
Ouachita Community Hospital	West Monroe	Louisiana	318-322-1339	www.ouachitahospital.com
P & S Surgical Hospital	Monroe	Louisiana	318-388-4040	www.pssurgery.com
Patients' Hospital of Redding	Redding	California	530-225-8700	www.patientshospital.com
Pella Regional Health Center	Pella	Iowa	641-628-3150	www.pellahealth.org
Pender Community Hospital	Pender	Nebraska	402-385-3083	www.pendercommunityhospital.com
Physician's Care Surgical Hospital	Royersford	Pennsylvania	610-495-4793	www.phycarehospital.com
The Physicians Centre	Bryan	Texas	979-731-3100	www.thephysicianscentre.com
Physicians Medical Center	Houma	Louisiana	985-853-1390	www.physicianshouma.com
Physicians' Medical Center	New Albany	Indiana	812-206-7660	www.pmcdev.interactivemedialab.com
Physicians' Specialty Hospital	Fayetteville	Arkansas	479-571-7002	www.pshfay.com
Quail Creek Surgical Hospital	Amarillo	Texas	806-354-6100	www.physurg.com
Richland Parish Hospital - Delhi	Delhi	Louisiana	318-878-5171	www.delhihospital.com
River Falls Area Hospital	River Falls	Wisconsin	715-307-6000	www.allina.com
Rochelle Community Hospital	Rochelle	Illinois	815-562-2181	www.rcha.net
Rockcastle County Hospital	Mount Vernon	Kentucky	606-256-2195	www.rockcastlehospital.com
Rollins Brook Community Hospital	Lampasas	Texas	512-556-3682	www.mplex.org
Sacred Heart Hospital on the Gulf	Port Saint Joe	Florida	850-229-5600	www.sacred-heart.org/gulf
Saint Joseph Memorial Hospital	Murphysboro	Illinois	618-684-3156	www.sih.net
Saint Joseph's Hospital	Breese	Illinois	618-526-4511	www.stjoebreese.com

Hospital	City	State	Phone	Web Site
Saint Luke's Lakeside Hospital	The Woodlands	Texas	936-266-4055	www.stlukeslakeside.com
Saint Luke's Wood River Medical Center	Ketchum	Idaho	208-727-8800	www.stlukesonline.org/wood_river
Saint Thomas Hospital for Spinal Surgery	Nashville	Tennessee	615-515-8200	www.hospitalforspinalsurgery.com
Salina Surgical Hospital	Salina	Kansas	785-827-0610	www.salinasurgical.com
Sanford Luverne Medical Center	Luverne	Minnesota	507-283-2321	www.sanfordluverne.org
Sauk Prairie Hospital	Prairie Du Sac	Wisconsin	608-643-3311	www.spmh.org
Sharp Coronado Hospital & Healthcare Center	Coronado	California	619-435-6251	www.sharp.com/coronado
Sioux Falls Specialty Hospital	Sioux Falls	South Dakota	605-334-6730	www.sfsurgical.com
Siouxland Surgery Center	Dakota Dunes	South Dakota	605-232-3332	www.siouxlandsurg.com
South Texas Spine & Surgical Hospital	San Antonio	Texas	210-404-0800	www.southtexassurgical.com
South Texas Surgical Hospital	Corpus Christi	Texas	361-993-2000	www.nshinc.com
Southern Surgical Hospital	Slidell	Louisiana	985-641-0600	www.sshla.com
Southwestern Regional Medical Center	Tulsa	Oklahoma	918-496-5000	www.cancercenter.com/southwestern
Specialists Hospital Shreveport	Shreveport	Louisiana	318-213-3800	www.specialistshospitalshreveport.com
Stanislaus Surgical Hospital	Modesto	California	209-572-2700	www.stanislaussurgical.com
Stewart Memorial Community Hospital	Lake City	Iowa	712-464-3171	www.stewartmemorial.org
Stoughton Hospital	Stoughton	Wisconsin	608-873-6611	www.stoughtonhospital.com
Sugar Land Surgical Hospital	Sugar Land	Texas	281-243-1000	www.sugarlandsurgicalhospital.com
Surgical Hospital at Southwoods	Youngstown	Ohio	330-758-1954	www.surgeryatsouthwoods.com
Surgical Institute of Reading	Wyomissing	Pennsylvania	717-999-9999	www.sireading.com
Surgical Specialty Center at Coordinated Health	Allentown	Pennsylvania	610-871-9110	www.coordinatedhealth.com
Surgical Specialty Center of Baton Rouge	Baton Rouge	Louisiana	225-408-5730	www.sscbr.com
Sutter Surgical Hospital - North Valley	Yuba City	California	530-749-5700	www.suttersurgicalhospitalnorthvalley.org
Texas Health Center for Diagnostics & Surgery	Plano	Texas	972-403-2700	www.ppcds.com
Texas Health Harris Methodist Hospital Southlake	Southlake	Texas	817-748-8700	www.texashealthsouthlake.com
Texas Institute for Surgery at Presbyterian Hospital	Dallas	Texas	214-647-5300	www.texasinstituteforsurgery.org
Texas Spine & Joint Hospital	Tyler	Texas	903-525-3300	www.tsjh.org
Tishomingo Health Services	Iuka	Mississippi	662-423-6051	www.nmhs.net/iuka
Tops Surgical Specialty Hospital	Houston	Texas	281-539-2900	www.tops-hospital.com
Treasure Valley Hospital	Boise	Idaho	208-373-5000	www.treasurevalleyhospital.com
Tulsa Spine & Specialty Hospital	Tulsa	Oklahoma	918-388-5701	www.tulsaspinehospital.com
United Regional Medical Center	Manchester	Tennessee	931-728-3586	www.urmchealthcare.com
University Hospitals Conneaut Medical Center	Conneaut	Ohio	440-593-1131	www.uhhospitals.org/conneaut
Upland Hills Health	Dodgeville	Wisconsin	608-930-8000	www.uplandhillshealth.org
USMD Hospital at Arlington	Arlington	Texas	817-472-3400	www.usmdhospital.com
USMD Hospital at Fort Worth	Fort Worth	Texas	817-433-9100	www.usmdfortworth.com
Vernon Memorial Hospital	Viroqua	Wisconsin	608-637-2101	www.vmh.org
Vidant Bertie Hospital	Windsor	North Carolina	252-794-6600	www.vidanthealth.com/bertie
W J Mangold Memorial Hospital	Lockney	Texas	806-652-3373	www.mangoldmemorial.org
Wellspan Surgery & Rehabilitation Hospital	York	Pennsylvania	717-812-6100	www.wellspan.org
West Kendall Baptist Hospital	Miami	Florida	786-467-2011	www.baptisthealth.net
Westlake Regional Hospital	Columbia	Kentucky	270-384-4753	www.westlake-healthcare.org
Whitman Hospital & Medical Center	Colfax	Washington	509-397-3435	www.whitmanhospital.com
Wright Memorial Hospital	Trenton	Missouri	660-359-5621	www.saintlukeshealthsystem.org
York Hospital	York	Maine	207-363-4321	www.yorkhospital.com

Note: The hospitals shown above represent the top 5% of the 3,591 hospitals nationwide for which an average score was calculated. Average scores were calculated for hospitals with qualifying data (100 completed surveys or more) in all ten measures in the Survey of Patient's Hospital Experiences category.

Best Hospitals in Terms of Use of Medical Imaging

Hospital	City	State	Phone	Web Site
Alameda Hospital	Alameda	California	510-522-3700	www.alamedahospital.org
Bartlett Regional Hospital	Juneau	Alaska	907-796-8900	www.bartletthospital.org
Caldwell Memorial Hospital	Lenoir	North Carolina	828-757-5100	www.caldwellmemorial.org
Capital Regional Medical Center	Tallahassee	Florida	850-656-5000	www.capitalregionalmedicalcenter.com
Carroll County Memorial Hospital	Carrollton	Kentucky	502-732-4321	www.ccmhosp.com
Centrastate Medical Center	Freehold	New Jersey	732-431-2000	www.centrastate.com
Chandler Regional Medical Center	Chandler	Arizona	480-963-4561	www.chandlerregional.com
Chinese Hospital	San Francisco	California	415-982-2400	www.chinesehospital-sf.org
Community Regional Medical Center	Fresno	California	559-459-6000	www.communitymedical.org
Conemaugh Valley Memorial Hospital	Johnstown	Pennsylvania	814-534-9000	www.conemaugh.org
Deaconess Hospital	Spokane	Washington	509-473-5800	www.deaconessmedicalcenter.org
Doctors Medical Center	Modesto	California	209-578-1211	www.dmc-modesto.com
Doctors Medical Center - San Pablo	San Pablo	California	510-970-5000	www.doctorsmedicalcenter.org
Dominican Hospital	Santa Cruz	California	831-462-7700	www.dominicanhospital.org
Emanuel Medical Center	Turlock	California	209-667-4200	www.emanuelmedicalcenter.org
Enloe Medical Center	Chico	California	530-332-7300	www.enloe.org
Evergreen Hospital Medical Center	Kirkland	Washington	425-899-1000	www.evergreenhospital.org
Exempla Saint Joseph Hospital	Denver	Colorado	303-837-7111	www.exempla.org
Fairview Hospital	Cleveland	Ohio	216-476-7000	www.fairviewhospital.org
Fairview Park Hospital	Dublin	Georgia	478-274-3100	www.fairviewparkhospital.com
Glens Falls Hospital	Glens Falls	New York	518-926-1000	www.glensfallshospital.org
Good Samaritan Hospital	San Jose	California	408-559-2011	www.goodsamsj.org
Halifax Health Medical Center	Daytona Beach	Florida	386-254-4000	www.halifax.org
Harrison Memorial Center	Bremerton	Washington	360-377-3911	www.harrisonmedical.org
Hartford Hospital	Hartford	Connecticut	860-545-5000	www.harthosp.org
Healthalliance Hospitals	Leominster	Massachusetts	978-466-2000	www.healthalliance.com
Heart Hospital Baylor Plano	Plano	Texas	469-814-3278	www.thehearthospitalbaylor.com
Holy Redeemer Hospital & Medical Center	Meadowbrook	Pennsylvania	215-947-3000	www.holyredeemer.com
Huntington Hospital	Huntington	New York	631-351-2000	www.hunthosp.org
Huntington Memorial Hospital	Pasadena	California	626-397-5000	www.huntingtonhospital.com
Indiana University Health White Memorial Hospital	Monticello	Indiana	574-583-7111	www.whitecmh.org
Inova Fairfax Hospital	Falls Church	Virginia	703-776-3332	www.inova.org
Jefferson Medical Center	Ranson	West Virginia	304-728-1600	www.jeffmem.com
Johnson Memorial Hospital	Stafford Springs	Connecticut	860-684-4251	www.johnsonhealthnetwork.com
Lake City Medical Center	Lake City	Florida	386-719-9000	www.lakecitymedical.com
Lake Regional Health System	Osage Beach	Missouri	573-348-8000	www.lakeregional.com
Lakewood Regional Medical Center	Lakewood	California	562-602-6751	www.lakewoodregional.com
Lasalle General Hospital	Jena	Louisiana	318-992-9200	www.lasallegeneralhospital.com
Little Falls Hospital	Little Falls	New York	315-823-5261	www.lfhny.org
Long Island Jewish Medical Center	New Hyde Park	New York	718-470-7000	www.northshorelij.com
Lourdes Medical Center of Burlington County	Willingboro	New Jersey	609-835-2900	www.lourdesnet.org/lourdes
Lovelace Medical Center	Albuquerque	New Mexico	505-727-8000	www.lovelace.com
Lowell General Hospital	Lowell	Massachusetts	978-937-6000	www.lowellgeneral.org
Mainegeneral Medical Center	Augusta	Maine	207-872-1000	www.mainegeneral.org
Maria Parham Medical Center	Henderson	North Carolina	252-438-4143	www.mphosp.org
Marin General Hospital	Greenbrae	California	415-925-7900	www.maringeneral.com
Mary Greeley Medical Center	Ames	Iowa	515-239-2011	www.mgmc.org
Mary Washington Hospital	Fredericksburg	Virginia	540-741-1100	www.medicorp.org
Maui Memorial Medical Center	Wailuku	Hawaii	808-442-5101	www.mauimemorialmedical.org
Mayo Clinic Health System - Albert Lea	Albert Lea	Minnesota	507-373-2384	www.mayoclinichealthsystem.org
McKenzie - Willamette Medical Center	Springfield	Oregon	541-726-4400	www.mckweb.com
Medstar Franklin Square Medical Center	Baltimore	Maryland	443-777-7850	www.franklinsquare.org
Medstar Southern Maryland Hospital Center	Clinton	Maryland	301-868-8000	www.medstarhealth.org
Memorial Medical Center	Modesto	California	209-526-4500	www.memorialmedicalcenter.org
Mercy General Hospital	Sacramento	California	916-453-4545	www.mercygeneral.org
Mercy Gilbert Medical Center	Gilbert	Arizona	480-728-8327	www.dignityhealth.org/mercygilbert
Mercy Hospital	Coon Rapids	Minnesota	763-236-8205	www.allinamercy.org
Mercy Medical Center - Clinton	Clinton	Iowa	563-244-5555	www.mercyclinton.com
Mercy Medical Center - Redding	Redding	California	530-225-6102	www.redding.mercy.org
Mercy San Juan Medical Center	Carmichael	California	916-537-5000	www.mercysanjuan.org
Mercy Willard Hospital	Willard	Ohio	419-964-5000	www.mercyweb.org/mercy_willard.aspx
Methodist Hospital of Sacramento	Sacramento	California	916-423-6010	www.methodistsacramento.org
Methodist Hospital of Southern California	Arcadia	California	626-445-4441	www.methodisthospital.org
Metrosouth Medical Center	Blue Island	Illinois	708-597-2000	www.stfrancisblueisland.com
Miriam Hospital	Providence	Rhode Island	401-793-2500	www.lifespan.org/partners/tmh

Hospital	City	State	Phone	Web Site
Nashoba Valley Medical Center	Ayer	Massachusetts	978-784-9000	www.nashobamed.com
Newton Memorial Hospital	Newton	New Jersey	973-383-2121	www.itsyourlife.com
North Florida Regional Medical Center	Gainesville	Florida	352-333-4100	www.nfrmc.com
Northbay Medical Center	Fairfield	California	707-646-5000	www.northbay.org
Ocala Regional Medical Center	Ocala	Florida	352-401-1000	www.ocalaregional.com
Page Memorial Hospital	Luray	Virginia	540-743-4561	www.pagememorialhospital.org
Palomar Health Downtown Campus	Escondido	California	760-739-3000	www.pph.org
Paris Regional Medical Center	Paris	Texas	903-785-4521	www.parisregional.com
Peacehealth Saint Joseph Medical Center	Bellingham	Washington	360-734-5400	www.peacehealth.org
Penobscot Bay Medical Center	Rockport	Maine	207-596-8000	www.nehealth.org
PIH Hospital - Downey	Downey	California	526-904-5000	www.drmci.org
Pomerado Hospital	Poway	California	858-485-6511	www.pph.org
Providence Sacred Heart Medical Center	Spokane	Washington	509-474-3040	www.shmc.org
Regional Medical Center of San Jose	San Jose	California	408-259-5000	www.regionalmedicalsanjose.com
Riverview Hospital Assoc	Wisconsin Rapids	Wisconsin	715-423-6060	www.riverviewhospital.net
Robert Wood Johnson University Hospital	New Brunswick	New Jersey	732-937-8900	www.rwjuh.edu
Saint Alphonsus Medical Center - Ontario	Ontario	Oregon	541-881-7000	www.holyrosary-ontario.org
Saint Alphonsus Regional Medical Center	Boise	Idaho	208-367-2121	www.saintalphonsus.org
Saint David's Medical Center	Austin	Texas	512-476-7111	www.stdavidsrehab.com
Saint Joseph Mercy Port Huron	Port Huron	Michigan	810-985-1510	www.mercyporthuron.com
Saint Joseph's Hospital Health Center	Syracuse	New York	315-448-5111	www.sjhsyr.org
Saint Mary's Hospital - Troy	Troy	New York	518-272-5000	www.setonhealth.org
Saint Marys Hospital	Waterbury	Connecticut	203-574-6000	www.stmh.org
Saint Thomas Rutherford Hospital	Murfreesboro	Tennessee	615-396-4100	www.mtmc.org
Salinas Valley Memorial Hospital	Salinas	California	831-757-4333	www.svmh.com
Santa Rosa Memorial Hospital	Santa Rosa	California	707-525-5300	www.stjosephhealth.org
Santiam Memorial Hospital	Stayton	Oregon	503-769-2175	www.santiamhospital.com
Scottsdale Healthcare - Thompson Peak Hospital	Scottsdale	Arizona	480-324-7004	www.shc.org
Scottsdale Healthcare Osborn Medical Center	Scottsdale	Arizona	480-882-4000	www.shc.org
Shady Grove Adventist Hospital	Rockville	Maryland	240-826-6517	www.adventisthealthcare.com/sgah
Sharp Chula Vista Medical Center	Chula Vista	California	619-502-5800	www.sharp.com
Southwest Regional Medical Center	Georgetown	Ohio	513-378-7800	www.browncountygeneralhospital.com
Stafford Hospital	Stafford	Virginia	540-741-9000	www.marywashingtonhealthcare.com
Sutter Delta Medical Center	Antioch	California	925-779-7200	www.sutterdelta.org
Sutter General Hospital	Sacramento	California	916-733-8999	www.suttermedicalcenter.org
Sutter Roseville Medical Center	Roseville	California	916-781-1000	www.sutterroseville.org
Swedish Edmonds Hospital	Edmonds	Washington	425-640-4000	www.stevenshealthcare.org
Tallahassee Memorial Hospital	Tallahassee	Florida	850-431-1155	www.tmh.org
Texas Health Presbyterian Hospital Dallas	Dallas	Texas	214-345-6789	www.texashealth.org
Trinity Rock Island	Rock Island	Illinois	309-779-5000	www.trinityqc.com
Union Hospital Clinton	Clinton	Indiana	765-832-1234	www.unionhospitalhealthgroup.org/wcch
University Medical Center at Brackenridge	Austin	Texas	512-324-7000	www.seton.net/locations/brackenridge
University Medical Center of Princeton at Plainsboro	Plainsboro	New Jersey	866-460-4776	www.princetonhcs.org
Valley Hospital	Spokane	Washington	509-924-6650	www.valleyhospital.org
Vidant Duplin Hospital	Kenansville	North Carolina	910-296-0941	www.dgh.org
Virtua Memorial Hospital of Burlington County	Mount Holly	New Jersey	609-914-6200	www.virtua.org
Warren Memorial Hospital	Front Royal	Virginia	703-636-0300	www.valleyhealthlink.com
Waterbury Hospital	Waterbury	Connecticut	203-573-6000	www.waterburyhospital.org
Watsonville Community Hospital	Watsonville	California	831-724-4741	www.watsonvillehospital.com
West Hills Hospital & Medical Center	West Hills	California	818-676-4100	www.westhillshospital.com
West Valley Medical Center	Caldwell	Idaho	208-459-4641	www.westvalleymedctr.com
Wooster Community Hospital	Wooster	Ohio	330-263-8100	www.woosterhospital.org

Note: The hospitals shown above represent the top 5% of the 2,308 hospitals nationwide for which an average score was calculated. Average scores were calculated for hospitals with qualifying data (25 cases or more) in at least 4 of 5 measures in the Use of Medical Imaging category. The measure, Follow-up Mammogram/Ultrasound, was not included in the average score.

Hospitals with the Lowest Medicare Spending per Beneficiary

Hospital	City	State	Phone	Web Site
Basin Healthcare Center	Odessa	Texas	432-425-9510	www.bhcodessa.com
Beaver Valley Hospital	Beaver	Utah	435-438-7102	
Bob Wilson Memorial Grant County Hospital	Ulysses	Kansas	620-356-1266	www.bwmgch.com
Brighton Hospital	Brighton	Michigan	810-227-1211	www.stjohn.org/brighton
Cherokee Indian Hospital Authority	Cherokee	North Carolina	704-497-9163	
Chinle Comprehensive Health Care Facility	Chinle	Arizona	928-674-7001	
Crownpoint Healthcare Facility	Crownpoint	New Mexico	505-786-5291	www.ihs.gov
Dhhs Usphs Indian Health Services	San Fidel	New Mexico	505-552-5300	www.ihs.gov
Eastern State Hospital	Williamsburg	Virginia	757-253-5161	www.ehs.dmhmrsas.virginia.gov
Epic Medical Center	Eufaula	Oklahoma	918-689-2535	
Fort Defiance Indian Hospital	Fort Defiance	Arizona	928-729-8000	www.home.navajo.his.gov
Gallup Indian Medical Center	Gallup	New Mexico	505-722-1000	www.ihs.gov/facilitiesservices
Guadalupe County Hospital	Santa Rosa	New Mexico	575-472-3417	
Harmon Memorial Hospital	Hollis	Oklahoma	580-688-3363	
Ira Davenport Memorial Hospital	Bath	New York	607-776-8500	www.davenportandtaylor.org
Kaiser Foundation Hospital - Antioch	Antioch	California	925-813-6500	www.kaiserpermanente.org
Kaiser Foundation Hospital - Fresno	Fresno	California	559-448-4500	www.kaiserpermanente.org
Kaiser Foundation Hospital - San Diego	San Diego	California	619-528-5000	www.members.kaiserpermanente.org
Kaiser Foundation Hospital - San Francisco	San Francisco	California	415-833-2646	www.permanente.net
Kaiser Foundation Hospital - South San Francisco	South San Francisco	California	650-742-3200	www.healthy.kaiserpermanente.org
Kaiser Foundation Hospital - Vacaville	Vacaville	California	707-624-4000	www.kaiserpermanente.org
Kaiser Sunnyside Medical Center	Clackamas	Oregon	503-571-2880	www.members.kaiserpermanente.org
Keefe Memorial Hospital	Cheyenne Wells	Colorado	719-767-5661	
Laguna Honda Hospital & Rehabilitation Center	San Francisco	California	415-759-2300	www.dph.sf.ca.us/chn/lagunahondahosp
Lewis County General Hospital	Lowville	New York	315-376-5200	www.lcgh.net
Memorial Hospital of Texas County	Guymon	Oklahoma	580-338-6515	www.mhtcguymon.org
Morton County Hospital	Elkhart	Kansas	620-697-2141	www.mchswecare.com
Mount Edgecumbe Hospital	Sitka	Alaska	907-966-2411	www.searhc.org
Newman Memorial Hospital	Shattuck	Oklahoma	580-938-2551	
P H S Indian Hospital at Belcourt - Quentin N Burdick	Belcourt	North Dakota	701-477-6111	
P H S Indian Hospital at Browning - Blackfeet	Browning	Montana	406-338-6157	www.ihs.gov
Phoenix Indian Medical Center	Phoenix	Arizona	602-263-1200	www.ihs.gov
PHS Indian Hospital at Pine Ridge	Pine Ridge	South Dakota	605-867-5131	www.ihs.gov
PHS Indian Hospital at Rosebud	Rosebud	South Dakota	605-747-2231	www.ihs.gov
Provident Hospital of Chicago	Chicago	Illinois	312-572-2000	www.providentfoundation.org
Red Lake Hospital	Redlake	Minnesota	218-679-3912	
Sacred Heart University District	Eugene	Oregon	541-686-7300	www.peacehealth.org
Sonoma Developmental Center	Eldridge	California	707-938-6393	www.dds.ca.gov/sonoma/index.cfm
South Lyon Medical Center	Yerington	Nevada	775-781-3761	
Tuba City Regional Health Care Corporation	Tuba City	Arizona	928-283-2501	www.tcrhcc.org
USPHS Lawton Indian Hospital	Lawton	Oklahoma	580-354-5000	
Valley Forge Medical Center & Hospital	Norristown	Pennsylvania	215-539-8500	www.vfmc.net
Wayne Medical Center	Waynesboro	Tennessee	931-722-5411	
Whiteriver PHS Indian Hospital	Whiteriver	Arizona	928-338-4911	
Whitfield Medical Surgical Hospital	Whitfield	Mississippi	601-351-8001	
Yalobusha General Hospital	Water Valley	Mississippi	662-473-1411	
Yukon Kuskokwim Delta Regional Hospital	Bethel	Alaska	907-543-6300	www.ykhc.org
Zuni Comprehensive Community Health Center	Zuni	New Mexico	505-782-4431	www.ihs.gov

Note: These 48 hospitals had an average ratio of 0.75 or less in the Medicare Spending per Beneficiary category. A total of 3,229 hospitals had medicare spending data available.

Appendix E: Glossary

Accreditation
An evaluative process in which a healthcare organization undergoes an examination of its policies, procedures and performance by an external private sector organization ("accrediting body") to ensure that it is meeting predetermined criteria. It usually involves both on- and off-site surveys. Also see the terms American Osteopathic Association, The Joint Commission, and Medicare-Certified Hospitals.

Acute Care—VA Medical Center
The Veterans Health Administration (VA) Medical Centers deliver inpatient hospital care and related services for surgery and short-term health conditions, as well as comprehensive primary, specialty and long-term care. The VA's medical benefits package is available to Veterans (including Reservists and National Guard) who served on active duty and meet eligibility requirements. Other groups can also be eligible. For more information, visit the U.S. Department of Veterans Affairs.

Acute care hospital
A hospital that provides inpatient medical care and other related services for surgery, acute medical conditions or injuries (usually for a short-term illness or condition).

Acute myocardial infarction (AMI)
See Heart Attack.

American Hospital Association (AHA)
The national organization that represents and serves all types of hospitals, health care networks, and their patients and communities. AHA takes part in national health policy development, legislative and regulatory debates, and legal matters. It also provides education for health care leaders and is a source of information on health care issues and trends.

American Osteopathic Association (AOA)
A member association representing approximately 52,000 osteopathic physicians (D.O.s). The AOA serves as the primary certifying body for D.O.s, and is the accrediting agency for all osteopathic medical colleges and health care facilities. The AOA writes a performance report on each hospital that it checks. You can call or write to AOA to find out a hospital's level of accreditation.

Angioplasty
In angioplasty, a catheter is used to insert a balloon that is inflated to open a blocked blood vessel. Percutaneous transluminal coronary angioplasty (PTCA) is one of several procedures used to open a blocked blood vessel, known collectively as a percutaneous coronary intervention (PCI).

Angiotensin converting enzyme (ACE) inhibitor
A drug used to treat heart attacks, heart failure, or a decreased function of the left heart. It stops production of a hormone that can narrow blood vessels, which helps reduce the pressure in the heart and lower blood pressure.

Angiotensin receptor blocker (ARB)
A drug used to treat patients with heart failure and a decreased function of the left heart. ARBs block the action of a hormone that can narrow blood vessels. This helps reduce the pressure in the heart and lower blood pressure.

Antibiotic
Drugs used to fight bacteria in the body.

ASA Physical Status Classification
Assessment by the anesthesiologist of the patient's preoperative physical condition using the American Society of Anesthesiologists' (ASA) Classification of Physical Status.

Asthma
A chronic lung condition that causes problems getting air in and out of the lungs. Children with asthma may experience wheezing, coughing, chest tightness and trouble breathing.

Atherectomy
A procedure where a blade or laser on a catheter cuts through and removes blockages in blood vessels. It is one of several procedures used to open a blocked blood vessel (known as a Percutaneous Coronary Intervention or PCI).

Beta blocker
A type of drug that is used to lower blood pressure, treat chest pain (angina) and heart failure, and to help prevent a heart attack. Beta blockers relieve the stress on the heart by slowing the heart rate and reducing the force with which the heart muscles contract to pump blood. They also help keep blood vessels from constricting in the heart, brain, and body.

Blood clot
Blood clots are clumps that occur when blood hardens from a liquid to a solid. A blood clot can partly or completely block the flow of blood in a blood vessel.

Blood culture
A blood test that shows if there are bacteria in the blood and what type of bacteria exist. It helps your doctor decide which antibiotic to use to treat a bacterial infection.

Blood thinners
Blood thinners reduce the risk of heart attack and stroke by reducing the formation of blood clots in arteries and veins. There are two main types of blood thinners-anticoagulants, such as heparin or warfarin (also called Coumadin) and antiplatelet drugs, such as aspirin.

Cardiac surgery registry
A registry collects and analyzes information on certain medical topics, conditions, or procedures for hospitals or other providers. The registry then provides the hospitals or providers with information to help them improve the care they provide. A cardiac surgery registry is one example of a registry in which hospitals or providers that perform cardiac surgery can participate.

Centers for Medicare & Medicaid Services (CMS)
The federal agency that runs the Medicare program for the elderly aged and disabled. In addition, CMS works with the states to run the Medicaid program for low-income individuals. CMS works to make sure that the people in these programs are able to get high quality health care.

Centers for Medicare & Medicaid Services (CMS) National Surgical Quality Pilot
In September of 2011, CMS engaged the American College of Surgeons (ACS) to publically report surgical outcome measures on the Hospital Compare website. Hospitals volunteering in this multispecialty surgical registry are provided with nationally validated, risk-adjusted, outcomes-based surgical quality measures. Hospitals report for one or any combination of three surgical measures—elderly surgical outcomes, colectomy outcomes, and lower-extremity bypass outcomes—collected through participation in the American College of Surgeons National Surgical Quality Improvement Program (ACS NSQIP®), a nationally validated, risk-adjusted, outcomes-based program to measure and improve the quality of surgical care in the private sector.

Certification (Medicare-certified)
State government agencies inspect health care providers, including hospitals, nursing homes, dialysis facilities and home health agencies, as well as other health care providers. These providers are certified if they pass inspection. Being certified is not the same as being accredited. Medicare or Medicaid only pays for care provided by certified or accredited providers.

Cesarean section (C-section)
A cesarean section (C-section) is the delivery of a baby through a surgical opening in the mother's lower belly area. A C-section delivery is done when it is not possible or safe for the mother to deliver the baby through the vagina.

Children's hospital
A hospital with a majority of its inpatients under the age of 18, which participates and is paid in the Medicare program as a children's hospital.

Chronic illness
An illness that persists over a long period of time.

Comorbidities
Two or more diseases that are present at the same time.

Critical access hospital (CAH)
A small facility that provides outpatient services, as well as inpatient services on a limited basis, to people in rural areas.

Computerized tomography (CT) scan
An imaging test that uses multiple x-rays to produce detailed pictures of the inside of the body (bones, organs, and other body parts).

Department of Health And Human Services (DHHS)
A federal agency that administers programs for protecting the health of all Americans, including Medicare, Medicaid, and the Children's Health Insurance Program (CHIP).

Diastolic pressure
The lowest pressure in the artery, occurring when the heart is filling with blood. In a blood pressure reading, the diastolic pressure is the second number recorded.

Elective delivery
An elective delivery is a delivery performed for a nonmedical reason. Some nonmedical reasons include wanting to schedule the birth of the baby on a specific date, living far away from the hospital, or discomfort in the last weeks of pregnancy.

Fibrinolysis, fibrinolytic drugs
Fibrinolytic drugs are "clot-busting" drugs that can help dissolve blood clots in blood vessels and improve blood flow to your heart. They are important for treating heart attacks. If you have a heart attack, your doctor may give you a fibrinolytic drug, perform a percutaneous coronary intervention (PCI), or both.

Heart attack
A heart attack, also called an acute myocardial infarction (AMI), happens when one of the heart's arteries becomes blocked and the supply of blood and oxygen to part of the heart muscle is slowed or stopped. When the heart muscle doesn't get the oxygen and nutrients it needs, the affected heart tissue may die.

Heart failure
In heart failure, the heart cannot pump enough blood through the body. The heart cannot fill with enough blood or pump with enough force, or both. Heart failure develops over time as the pumping action of the heart gets weaker. It can affect the right, the left, or both sides of the heart. Heart failure does not mean that the heart has stopped working or is about to stop working.

Hemorrhagic stroke
A hemorrhagic stroke occurs when a blood vessel in part of the brain becomes weak and bursts open, causing blood to leak into the brain. Some people have defects in the blood vessels of the brain that make this more likely.

Heparin injection
Heparin is a type of anticoagulant or "blood thinner," and is used to prevent blood clots from forming in people who have certain medical conditions or who are undergoing certain medical procedures that increase the chance that clots will form. Heparin is also used to stop the growth of clots that have already formed in the blood vessels.

Index admission
An index admission is the admission with a principal diagnosis of a specified condition that meets the inclusion and exclusion criteria for the measure.

Influenza
A serious and sometimes deadly lung infection that can spread quickly in a community. Symptoms include fever-often a high temperature of more than 102° Fahrenheit (38.9° Celsius), headache, muscle aches and pains, chills, cough and chest pain when you take a breath ("pleuritic chest pain"). Although most people recover from the illness, the Centers for Disease Control and Prevention (the CDC) estimates that in the United States more than 200,000 people are hospitalized and about 36,000 people die from the flu and its complications every year.

Influenza vaccination ("Flu Shot")
The main way to keep from getting flu is to get a yearly flu vaccination. Learn more about the flu from the Centers for Disease Control and Prevention (CDC). Hospitals should check to make sure that pneumonia patients get a flu shot during flu season to protect them from another lung infection and to help prevent the spread of influenza in the community.

Inpatient hospital services
Services you get when you're admitted to a hospital, including bed and board, nursing services, diagnostic or therapeutic services, and medical or surgical services.

International Classification of Diseases, Ninth Revision, Clinical Modification (ICD-9-CM)
The classification used to code and classify mortality data from death certificates.

Ischemic stroke
Ischemic stroke occurs when a blood vessel that supplies blood to the brain is blocked by a blood clot. Ischemic strokes may be caused by clogged arteries. Fat, cholesterol, and other substances collect on the artery walls, forming a sticky substance called plaque.

Left ventricular function assessment
A test to check how well the heart is pumping.

Long-term care hospital
Acute care hospitals that provide treatment for patients who stay, on average, more than 25 days. Most patients are transferred from an intensive or critical care unit. These hospitals provide services like comprehensive rehabilitation, respiratory therapy, head trauma treatment, and pain management.

Magnetic resonance imaging (MRI)
An imaging test that uses powerful magnets and radio waves to create pictures of the body. It does not use radiation (x-rays).

Measurement
The process of collecting data to assess performance conducted at a single point in time or repeated over time.

Medicaid
A joint federal and state program that helps with medical costs for some people with low incomes and limited resources. Medicaid programs vary from state to state, but most health care costs are covered if you qualify for both Medicare and Medicaid.

Medical imaging
Tests that create images of various parts of the body to screen for or diagnose medical conditions. Examples of medical imaging include CT Scans, MRIs, and mammograms.

Medicare Advantage Plan (Part C)
A type of Medicare health plan offered by a private company that contracts with Medicare to provide you with all your Part A and Part B benefits. Medicare Advantage Plans include Health Maintenance Organizations (HMOs), Preferred Provider Organizations (PPOs), Private Fee-for-Service Plans, Special Needs Plans, and Medicare Medical Savings Account Plans. If you're enrolled in a Medicare Advantage Plan, Medicare services are covered through the plan and aren't paid for under Original Medicare. Most Medicare Advantage Plans offer prescription drug coverage.

Medicare health plan
A plan offered by a private company that contracts with Medicare to provide Part A and Part B benefits to people with Medicare who enroll in the plan. Medicare health plans include all Medicare Advantage Plans, Medicare Cost Plans, Demonstration/Pilot Programs, and Programs of All-inclusive Care for the Elderly (PACE).

Medicare Severity-Diagnosis Related Group (MS-DRG)
The Medicare Severity - Diagnosis Related Groups (MS-DRGs) are payment groups designed for the Medicare population. Patients who have similar clinical characteristics and similar costs are assigned to an MS-DRG. The MS-DRG will be linked to a fixed payment amount based on the average cost of patients in the group. Patients can be assigned to an MS-DRG based on their diagnosis, surgical procedures, age and other information. Hospitals provide this information on their bills and Medicare uses this information to decide how much the hospitals should be paid. There may be some groups of MS-DRGs that are based on complications or comorbidities (CCs) or major complications or comorbidities (MCCs). Complications are new problems that are the result of a procedure, treatment, or illness.

Medicare-certified hospital
In order to receive any payment from either the Medicare or Medicaid programs, a hospital must meet a set of basic standards for quality of care, called "conditions of participation." Medicare-certified hospitals are reviewed periodically (every three years), either by their State Survey Agency or a CMS-approved national accreditation organization, to assure that they are continuing to provide services of acceptable quality. Accreditation is optional, but most short-term acute hospitals in the United States choose to be Medicare-certified based on accreditation by a CMS approved national accreditation organization. There are currently three CMS-approved national hospital accreditation organizations: the American Osteopathic Association/health care Facilities Accreditation Program (AOA/HFAP), Det Norske Veritas Healthcare (DNV Healthcare), and The Joint Commission (TJC).

Number of completed surveys
The "number of completed surveys" is the total number of patients who completed a survey. When at least 300 patients have completed the survey for a hospital, we can be more confident that the survey results are fully representative of patients' experiences at that hospital and are reliable for assessing the hospital's performance. However, smaller hospitals could sample all of their HCAHPS-eligible discharges but, because of their small size, still have fewer than 300 completed surveys.

Original Medicare
Original Medicare is fee-for-service coverage under which the government pays your health care providers directly for your Part A and/or Part B benefits.

Osteopathic doctor
A licensed physician who can do surgery and prescribe drugs who has training in manipulative therapy. Also called a Doctor of Osteopathy (DO).

Outpatient hospital care
Medical or surgical care you get from a hospital when your doctor hasn't written an order to admit you to the hospital as an inpatient. Outpatient hospital care may include emergency department services, observation services, outpatient surgery, lab tests, or X-rays. Your care may be considered outpatient hospital care even if you spend the night at the hospital.

Outpatient Prospective Payment System (OPPS)
Under the Outpatient Prospective Payment System (OPPS), hospitals are paid a set amount of money (called the payment rate) to provide certain outpatient services to people with Medicare.

Oxygenation assessment
Test that measures the amount of oxygen in your blood to see if you need oxygen therapy.

Patient discharge
Patients are considered "discharged" from a hospital when they are released to go home or to another health care setting, or when they die during the hospital stay.

Percutaneous coronary interventions (PCI)
The procedures called percutaneous coronary interventions (PCI), such as angioplasty and atherectomy are among those that are the most effective for opening blocked blood vessels that cause heart attacks. Doctors may perform a PCI, or give certain drugs to open the blockage, and in some cases, they may do both.

Plan of care
A written plan of care created with your physician and hospital staff. It tells what services you will get to reach and keep your best physical, mental, and social wellbeing. The hospital staff keeps your doctor up-to-date on how you are doing and updates your care plan as needed.

Pneumonia
An inflammation of the lungs caused by a viral or bacterial infection. This fills your lungs with mucus and lowers the oxygen level in your blood. Symptoms can include fever, fatigue, difficulty breathing, chills, a "wet" cough, and chest pain. For more on pneumonia, visit MedlinePlus

Pneumonia (pneumococcal) vaccination
Vaccine given to prevent pneumonia, estimated to protect against 80% of bacteria causing pneumonia.

Provider
A doctor, hospital, health care professional or health care facility.

Psychiatric hospital
A facility that provides inpatient psychiatric services for the diagnosis and treatment of mental illness on a 24-hour basis, by or under the supervision of a physician.

Quality
Quality health care is how well a doctor, hospital, health plan, or other provider of health care, keeps its patients healthy or treats them when they are sick. Good quality health care means doing the right thing at the right time, in the right way, for the right person and getting the best possible results.

Quality assurance
The process of looking at how well a medical service is provided. The process may include formally reviewing health care given to a person, or group of persons, locating the problem, correcting the problem, and then checking to see if what was done worked.

Quality Improvement Organizations (QIOs)
A group of practicing doctors and other health care experts paid by the federal government to check and improve the care given to people with Medicare.

Ratio
The amount of one thing compared to the amount of another, such as the number of combination CT scans done compared to the number of all CT scans done.

Readmissions
Patients who are admitted to the hospital for treatment of medical problems sometimes get other serious injuries, complications, or conditions, and may even die. Some patients may experience problems soon after they are discharged and need to be admitted to the hospital again. These events can often be prevented if hospitals follow best practices for treating patients.

Registry
A registry collects and analyzes information on certain medical topics, conditions, or procedures for hospitals or other providers. The registry then provides the hospitals or providers with information to help them improve the care they provide. Examples of registries in which hospitals can participate include: a multispecialty surgical registry , a nursing care registry, and a stroke care registry.

Rehabilitation hospital
A hospital that specializes in improving or restoring a patient's functional ability through therapies. Sometimes called a post-acute hospital.

Reliever medications
Relievers are medications that relax the bands of muscle surrounding the airways and are used to quickly make breathing easier.

Risk-adjusted
"Risk-adjusted" means that the measure calculations take into account how sick patients were when they went in for their initial hospital stay. When rates are risk-adjusted, it means that hospitals that usually take care of sicker patients won't have a worse rate just because their patients were sicker when they arrived at the hospital. When rates are risk-adjusted, it helps make comparisons fair and meaningful.

Risk-adjusted 30-day death (mortality) rates
The 30-day Risk-Adjusted Death (Mortality) Rates are produced using a complex statistical model, that relies on Medicare claims and enrollment information. The model predicts patient deaths for any cause within 30 days of hospital admission for heart attack or heart failure, whether the patients die while still in the hospital or after discharge. Thirty-day mortality is used because this is the time period when deaths are most likely to be related to the care patients received in the hospital. Deaths that occur outside the hospital within 30 days are included along with deaths that occur in the hospital, because some hospitals discharge patients sooner than others.

Screening mammogram
A medical procedure to check for breast cancer before you or a doctor may be able to find it manually.

Stent
A small wire tube inserted in a blood vessel by a catheter to hold open a blocked blood vessel. This is one of several procedures called a percutaneous coronary intervention (PCI) that are used to open a blocked blood vessel.

Structural measures
A structural measure reflects the environment in which providers care for patients, such as whether or not a hospital uses an electronic health record.

Survey of patients' experiences
A national, standardized survey of hospital patients about their experiences during a recent inpatient hospital stay. This is also referred to as HCAHPS (Hospital Consumer Assessment of Healthcare Providers and Systems).

Survey response rate
Tells what percentage of patients who were asked to complete the survey actually did complete it. In general, the higher this response rate percentage, the more confident we can be that the survey results for a hospital are representative of patients' experiences at that hospital and are reliable for assessing the hospital's performance.

Systemic corticosteroid
Inflammation-reducing, anti-allergic medications that affect the body as a whole.

Teaching hospital
Hospitals that train residents in approved medical, osteopathic, dental or podiatry residency programs.

The Joint Commission (JC)
An independent, not-for-profit organization that accredits and certifies a large number of health care organizations and programs in the United States. The Joint Commission's hospital accreditation program has held deeming authority since the inception of the Medicare program in 1965. The Joint Commission's mission is to continuously improve health care for the public, in collaboration with other stakeholders, by evaluating health care organizations and inspiring them to excel in providing safe and effective care of the highest quality and value.

Thrombolytic therapy
Thrombolytic therapy is the use of drugs to break up or dissolve blood clots, which are the main cause of both heart attacks and stroke.

Treatment
Something done to help with a health problem. For example, giving certain drugs and performing surgery are treatments.

Treatment options
The choices you have when there is more than one way to treat your health problem.

Venous thromboembolism (VTE)
Venous thromboembolism (VTE) is a term that includes both deep vein thrombosis and pulmonary embolism. A deep vein thrombosis (DVT) is a blood clot that forms in a vein deep in the body. A pulmonary embolism (PE) is a loose blood clot that travels to an artery in the lungs and can block blood flow.

Warfarin
A medication used to prevent blood clots from forming or growing larger in your blood and blood vessels.

Source: Medicare.gov

Regional Hospital Profile Index

2014 Title List

Visit **www.GreyHouse.com** for Product Information, Table of Contents and Sample Pages

General Reference

America's College Museums
American Environmental Leaders: From Colonial Times to the Present
An African Biographical Dictionary
An Encyclopedia of Human Rights in the United States
Constitutional Amendments
Encyclopedia of African-American Writing
Encyclopedia of the Continental Congress
Encyclopedia of Gun Control & Gun Rights
Encyclopedia of Invasions & Conquests
Encyclopedia of Prisoners of War & Internment
Encyclopedia of Religion & Law in America
Encyclopedia of Rural America
Encyclopedia of the United States Cabinet, 1789-2010
Encyclopedia of War Journalism
Encyclopedia of Warrior Peoples & Fighting Groups
From Suffrage to the Senate: America's Political Women
Nations of the World
Political Corruption in America
Speakers of the House of Representatives, 1789-2009
The Environmental Debate: A Documentary History
The Evolution Wars: A Guide to the Debates
The Religious Right: A Reference Handbook
The Value of a Dollar: 1860-2009
The Value of a Dollar: Colonial Era
This is Who We Were: A Companion to the 1940 Census
This is Who We Were: The 1920s
This is Who We Were: The 1950s
This is Who We Were: The 1960s
US Land & Natural Resource Policy
Working Americans 1770-1869 Vol. IX: Revolutionary War to the Civil War
Working Americans 1880-1999 Vol. I: The Working Class
Working Americans 1880-1999 Vol. II: The Middle Class
Working Americans 1880-1999 Vol. III: The Upper Class
Working Americans 1880-1999 Vol. IV: Their Children
Working Americans 1880-2003 Vol. V: At War
Working Americans 1880-2005 Vol. VI: Women at Work
Working Americans 1880-2006 Vol. VII: Social Movements
Working Americans 1880-2007 Vol. VIII: Immigrants
Working Americans 1880-2009 Vol. X: Sports & Recreation
Working Americans 1880-2010 Vol. XI: Inventors & Entrepreneurs
Working Americans 1880-2011 Vol. XII: Our History through Music
Working Americans 1880-2012 Vol. XIII: Education & Educators
World Cultural Leaders of the 20th & 21st Centuries

Business Information

Complete Television, Radio & Cable Industry Directory
Directory of Business Information Resources
Directory of Mail Order Catalogs
Directory of Venture Capital & Private Equity Firms
Environmental Resource Handbook
Food & Beverage Market Place
Grey House Homeland Security Directory
Grey House Performing Arts Directory
Hudson's Washington News Media Contacts Directory
New York State Directory
Sports Market Place Directory

Education Information

Charter School Movement
Comparative Guide to American Elementary & Secondary Schools
Complete Learning Disabilities Directory
Educators Resource Directory
Special Education

Health Information

Comparative Guide to American Hospitals
Complete Directory for Pediatric Disorders
Complete Directory for People with Chronic Illness
Complete Directory for People with Disabilities
Complete Mental Health Directory
Diabetes in America: A Geographic & Demographic Analysis
Directory of Health Care Group Purchasing Organizations
Directory of Hospital Personnel
HMO/PPO Directory
Medical Device Register
Older Americans Information Directory

Statistics & Demographics

America's Top-Rated Cities
America's Top-Rated Small Towns & Cities
America's Top-Rated Smaller Cities
American Tally
Ancestry & Ethnicity in America
Comparative Guide to American Hospitals
Comparative Guide to American Suburbs
Profiles of America
Profiles of... Series – State Handbooks
The Hispanic Databook
Weather America

Financial Ratings Series

TheStreet.com Ratings Guide to Bond & Money Market Mutual Funds
TheStreet.com Ratings Guide to Common Stocks
TheStreet.com Ratings Guide to Exchange-Traded Funds
TheStreet.com Ratings Guide to Stock Mutual Funds
TheStreet.com Ratings Ultimate Guided Tour of Stock Investing
Weiss Ratings Consumer Guides
Weiss Ratings Guide to Banks & Thrifts
Weiss Ratings Guide to Credit Unions
Weiss Ratings Guide to Health Insurers
Weiss Ratings Guide to Life & Annuity Insurers
Weiss Ratings Guide to Property & Casualty Insurers

Bowker's Books In Print® Titles

Books In Print®
Books In Print® Supplement
American Book Publishing Record® Annual
American Book Publishing Record® Monthly
Books Out Loud™
Bowker's Complete Video Directory™
Children's Books In Print®
El-Hi Textbooks & Serials In Print®
Forthcoming Books®
Law Books & Serials In Print™
Medical & Health Care Books In Print™
Publishers, Distributors & Wholesalers of the US™
Subject Guide to Books In Print®
Subject Guide to Children's Books In Print®

Canadian General Reference

Associations Canada
Canadian Almanac & Directory
Canadian Environmental Resource Guide
Canadian Parliamentary Guide
Financial Services Canada
Governments Canada
Health Services Canada
Libraries Canada
Major Canadian Cities
The History of Canada

 SALEM PRESS

2014 Title List

Visit **www.SalemPress.com** for Product Information, Table of Contents and Sample Pages

Literature

American Ethnic Writers
Critical Insights: Authors
Critical Insights: New Literary Collection Bundles
Critical Insights: Themes
Critical Insights: Works
Critical Survey of Drama
Critical Survey of Graphic Novels: Heroes & Super Heroes
Critical Survey of Graphic Novels: History, Theme & Technique
Critical Survey of Graphic Novels: Independents & Underground Classics
Critical Survey of Graphic Novels: Manga
Critical Survey of Long Fiction
Critical Survey of Mystery & Detective Fiction
Critical Survey of Mythology and Folklore: Heroes and Heroines
Critical Survey of Mythology and Folklore: Love, Sexuality & Desire
Critical Survey of Mythology and Folklore: World Mythology
Critical Survey of Poetry
Critical Survey of Poetry: American Poetry
Critical Survey of Poetry: British, Irish & Commonwealth Poets
Critical Survey of Poetry: European Poets
Critical Survey of Poetry: European Poets
Critical Survey of Poetry: Topical Essays
Critical Survey of Poetry: World Poets
Critical Survey of Science Fiction & Fantasy Literature
Critical Survey of Shakespeare's Sonnets
Critical Survey of Short Fiction
Critical Survey of Short Fiction: American Writers
Critical Survey of Short Fiction: British, Irish & Commonwealth Poets
Critical Survey of Short Fiction: European Writers
Critical Survey of Short Fiction: Topical Essays
Critical Survey of Short Fiction: World Writers
Cyclopedia of Literary Characters
Introduction to Literary Context: American Post-Modernist Novels
Introduction to Literary Context: American Short Fiction
Introduction to Literary Context: English Literature
Introduction to Literary Context: World Literature
Magill's Literary Annual 2014
Magill's Survey of American Literature
Magill's Survey of World Literature
Masterplots
Masterplots II: African American Literature
Masterplots II: Christian Literature
Masterplots II: Drama Series
Masterplots II: Short Story Series
Notable African American Writers
Notable American Novelists
Notable Playwrights
Short Story Writers

Science, Careers & Mathematics

Applied Science
Applied Science: Engineering & Mathematics
Applied Science: Science & Medicine
Applied Science: Technology
Biomes and Ecosystems
Careers in Chemistry
Careers in Communications & Media
Careers in Healthcare
Careers in Hospitality & Tourism
Careers in Law & Criminology
Careers in Physics
Computer Technology Inventors
Contemporary Biographies in Chemistry
Contemporary Biographies in Communications & Media
Contemporary Biographies in Healthcare
Contemporary Biographies in Hospitality & Tourism
Contemporary Biographies in Law & Criminology
Contemporary Biographies in Physics
Earth Science
Earth Science: Earth Materials & Resources
Earth Science: Earth's Surface and History
Earth Science: Physics & Chemistry of the Earth
Earth Science: Weather, Water & Atmosphere
Encyclopedia of Energy
Encyclopedia of Environmental Issues
Encyclopedia of Global Resources
Encyclopedia of Global Warming
Encyclopedia of Mathematics and Society
Encyclopedia of the Ancient World
Forensic Science
Internet Innovators
Introduction to Chemistry
Magill's Encyclopedia of Science: Animal Life
Magill's Encyclopedia of Science: Plant life
Magill's Medical Guide
Notable Natural Disasters
Solar System

Health

Addictions & Substance Abuse
Cancer
Complementary & Alternative Medicine
Genetics & Inherited Conditions
Infectious Diseases & Conditions
Magill's Medical Guide
Psychology & Mental Health
Psychology Basics

Grey House Publishing | Salem Press | H.W. Wilson
4919 Route, 22 PO Box 56, Amenia NY 12501-0056

2014 Title List

Visit **www.SalemPress.com** for Product Information, Table of Contents and Sample Pages

History and Social Science

A 2000s in America
50 States
African American History
Agriculture in History (check)
American First Ladies
American Heroes
American Indian Tribes
American Presidents
American Villains
Ancient Greece
Bill of Rights, The
Cold War, The
Defining Documents: American Revolution 1754-1805
Defining Documents: Civil War 1860-1865
Defining Documents: Emergence of Modern America, 1868-1918
Defining Documents: Exploration & Colonial America 1492-1755
Defining Documents: Manifest Destiny 1803-1860
Defining Documents: Reconstruction, 1865-1880
Defining Documents: The 1920s
Defining Documents: The 1930s
Defining Documents: World War I
Eighties in America
Encyclopedia of American Immigration
Fifties in America
Forties in America
Great Athletes
Great Events from History: 17th Century
Great Events from History: 18th Century
Great Events from History: 19th Century
Great Events from History: 20th Century, 1901-1940
Great Events from History: 20th Century, 1941-1970
Great Events from History: 20th Century, 1971-200
Great Events from History: Ancient World
Great Events from History: Middle Ages
Great Events from History: Modern Scandals
Great Events from History: Renaissance & Early Modern Era
Great Lives from History: 17th Century
Great Lives from History: 18th Century
Great Lives from History: 19th Century
Great Lives from History: 20th Century
Great Lives from History: African Americans
Great Lives from History: Ancient World
Great Lives from History: Asian & Pacific Islander Americans
Great Lives from History: Incredibly Wealthy
Great Lives from History: Inventors & Inventions
Great Lives from History: Jewish Americans
Great Lives from History: Latinos
Great Lives from History: Middle Ages
Great Lives from History: Notorious Lives
Great Lives from History: Renaissance & Early Modern Era
Great Lives from History: Scientists & Science
Historical Encyclopedia of American Business
Immigration in U.S. History
Magill's Guide to Military History
Milestone Documents in African American History
Milestone Documents in American History
Milestone Documents in World History
Milestone Documents of American Leaders
Milestone Documents of World Religions
Musicians & Composers 20th Century
Nineties in America
Seventies in America
Sixties in America
Survey of American Industry and Careers
Thirties in America
Twenties in America
U.S. Court Cases
U.S. Laws, Acts, and Treaties
U.S. Legal System
U.S. Supreme Court
United States at War
USA in Space
Weapons and Warfare
World Conflicts: Asia and the Middle East

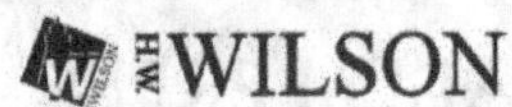

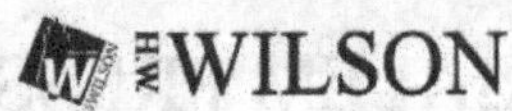

2014 Title List

Visit **www.HwWilsonInPrint.com** for Product Information, Table of Contents and Sample Pages

Current Biography
Current Biography Cumulative Index 1946-2013
Current Biography Magazine
Current Biography Yearbook-2004
Current Biography Yearbook-2005
Current Biography Yearbook-2006
Current Biography Yearbook-2007
Current Biography Yearbook-2008
Current Biography Yearbook-2009
Current Biography Yearbook-2010
Current Biography Yearbook-2011
Current Biography Yearbook-2012
Current Biography Yearbook-2013
Current Biography Yearbook-2014

Core Collections
Senior High Core Collection
Middle & Junior High School Core
Children's Core Collection
Fiction Core Collection
Public Library Core Collection: Nonfiction

Sears List
Sears List of Subject Headings
Sears: Lista de Encabezamientos de Materia

The Reference Shelf
Aging in America
Revisiting Gender
The U.S. National Debate Topic, 2014/2015
Embracing New Paradigms in education
Marijuana Reform
Representative American Speeches 2013-2014
Reality Television
The Business of Food
The Future of U.S. Economic Relations: Mexico, Cuba, and Venezuela
Sports in America
Global Climate Change
Representative American Speeches, 2012-2013
Conspiracy Theories
The Arab Spring
U.S. National Debate Topic: Transportation Infrastructure
Families: Traditional and New Structures
Faith & Science
Representative American Speeches 2011-2012
Social Networking
Dinosaurs
Space Exploration & Development
U.S. Infrastructure
Politics of the Ocean
Representative American Speeches 2010-2011
Robotics
The News and its Future
American Military Presence Overseas
Russia
Graphic Novels and Comic Books
Representative American Speeches 2009-2010

Readers' Guide
Readers Guide to Periodicals Literature
Abridged Readers' Guide to Periodical Literature
Short Story Index

Indexes
Short Story Index
Index to Legal Periodicals & Books

Facts About Series
Facts About the Presidents, Eighth Edition
Facts About China
Facts About the 20th Century
Facts About American Immigration
Facts About World's Languages

Nobel Prize Winners
Nobel Prize Winners, 2002-2013

World Authors
World Authors 2000-2005
World Authors 2006-2013

Famous First Facts
Famous First Facts, Seventh Edition
Famous First Facts About American Politics
Famous First Facts About Sports
Famous First Facts About the Environment
Famous First Facts, International Edition

American Book of Days
The American Book of Days, Fifth Edition
The International Book of Days

Junior Authors & Illustrators
Tenth Book of Junior Authors & Illustrations

Monographs
The Barnhart Dictionary of Etymology
Celebrate the World
Indexing from A to Z
Radical Change: Books for Youth in a Digital Age
The Poetry Break
Guide to the Ancient World

Wilson Chronology
Wilson Chronology of Asia and the Pacific
Wilson Chronology of Human Rights
Wilson Chronology of Ideas
Wilson Chronology of the Arts
Wilson Chronology of the World's Religions
Wilson Chronology of Women's Achievements

Book Review Digest
Book Review Digest, 2014

Grey House Publishing | Salem Press | H.W. Wilson
4919 Route, 22 PO Box 56, Amenia NY 12501-0056